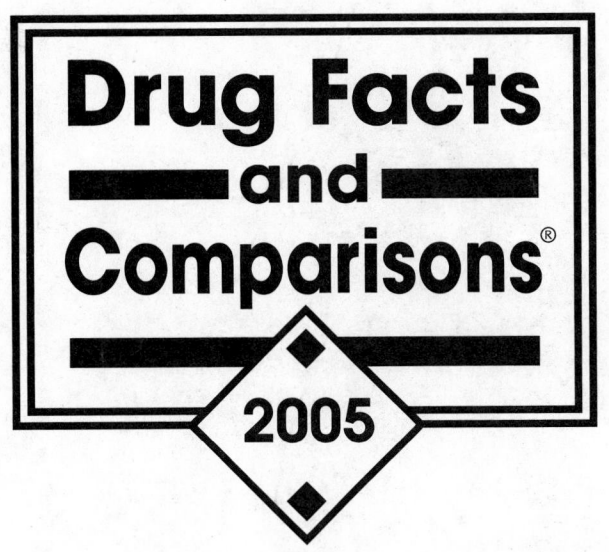

Drug Facts and Comparisons®

2005

59th edition

Drug Facts and Comparisons®

2005

59th edition

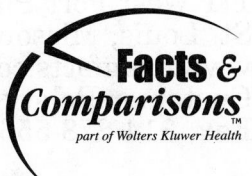

Drug Facts and Comparisons,® 2005 Edition

Manuscript indexed by Coughlin Indexing Services, Inc., Annapolis, Maryland.

ISBN 1-57439-193-3

Printed in the United States of America.

The information contained in this publication is intended to supplement the knowledge of health care professionals regarding drug information. This information is advisory only and is not intended to replace sound clinical judgment or individualized patient care in the delivery of health care services. Wolters Kluwer Health disclaims all warranties, whether expressed or implied, including any warranty as to the quality, accuracy, or suitability of this information for any particular purpose.

The information contained in *Drug Facts and Comparisons®* is available for licensing as source data. For more information on data licensing, please call 1-800-223-0554.

Facts and Comparisons®
part of Wolters Kluwer Health
111 West Port Plaza Drive, Suite 300
St. Louis, Missouri 63146-3098
www.drugfacts.com • 314-216-2100
Customer Relations 800-223-0554
Fax: 314-878-5563

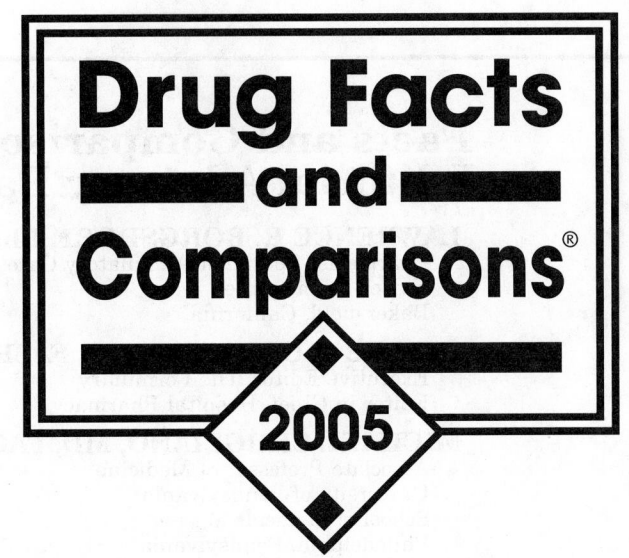

Drug Facts and Comparisons® 2005

publisher
CATHY H. REILLY

managing editor
KIRSTEN K. NOVAK

associate editors
SARAH W. LENZINI
NICHOLAS R. WEBER

assistant editors
JENNIFER A. GUIMARAES
JOHN G. HALL
KEVIN D. HARMS
JOSEPH H. HORENKAMP

senior sgml specialist
LINDA M. JONES

quality control editor
SUSAN H. SUNDERMAN

purchasing specialist
HEATHER L. GUYOTT

founding editor
ERWIN K. KASTRUP, BS PharmD, DSc†

senior managing editor
RENÉE M. WICKERSHAM

senior editor
SARA L. SCHWEAIN

senior composition specialist
JENNIFER K. WALSH

clinical director
clinical information group
RENÉE RIVARD, PharmD

clinical manager
CATHY A. MEIVES, PharmD

clinical editors
LORI A. BUSS, PharmD
KIM S. DUFNER, PharmD
PAUL JOHNSON, PharmD
NICOLE E. WILLIAMS, PharmD

† Deceased

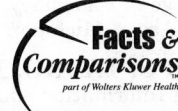

Facts & Comparisons
part of Wolters Kluwer Health

Facts and Comparisons®
Editorial Advisory Panel

LAWRENCE R. BORGSDORF, PharmD, FCSHP
Pharmacist Specialist-Ambulatory Care
Kaiser Permanente
Bakersfield, California

DENNIS J. CADA, PharmD, FASHP, FASCP
Executive Editor, The Formulary
Editor in Chief, Hospital Pharmacy

MICHAEL CIRIGLIANO, MD, FACP
Associate Professor of Medicine
University of Pennsylvania
School of Medicine
Philadelphia, Pennsylvania

TIMOTHY R. COVINGTON, PharmD, MS
Anthony and Marianne Bruno Professor of Pharmacy
Director, Managed Care Institute
School of Pharmacy, Samford University

JOYCE A. GENERALI, RPh, MS, FASHP
Director, Drug Information Center
Clinical Associate Professor
University of Kansas Medical Center
Kansas City, Kansas

DANIEL A. HUSSAR, PhD
Remington Professor of Pharmacy
Philadelphia College of Pharmacy
University of the Sciences in Philadelphia

JAMES R. SELEVAN, BSEE, MD
Founder and Member of the Board of Directors
Monarch Healthcare
Vice President of Pharmacy Relations
Syntiro Healthcare Services, Inc.

RICHARD W. SLOAN, MD, RPh
Chairman
Department of Family Practice
York Hospital, Wellspan Health
Clinical Associate Professor
Pennsylvania State University

BURGUNDA V. SWEET, PharmD
Director, Drug Information and
Investigational Drug Services
Clinical Associate Professor of Pharmacy
University of Michigan Health System and
College of Pharmacy
Ann Arbor, Michigan

DAVID S. TATRO, PharmD
Drug Information Analyst
San Carlos, California

THOMAS L. WHITSETT, MD
Professor of Medicine
Director, Vascular Medicine Program
University of Oklahoma Health Sciences Center

Contributing Review Panel

Jonathan Abrams, MD
Professor of Medicine
Cardiology Division
University of New Mexico
Albuquerque, New Mexico

Danial E. Baker, PharmD, FASHP, FASCP
Associate Dean for Clinical Programs
Professor of Pharmacotherapy
Director, Drug Information Center
Washington State University
Spokane, Washington

Jimmy D. Bartlett, OD, DOS, ScD
Professor of Optometry, School of Optometry
Professor of Pharmacology, School of Medicine
University of Alabama at Birmingham
Birmingham, Alabama

Edward S. Bennett, OD, MSEd
Associate Professor
Co-Chief, Contact Lens Service
Director of Student Services
College of Optometry
University of Missouri – St. Louis
St. Louis, Missouri

Daniel L. Brown, PharmD
Director of Early Practice Education
Wingate University
School of Pharmacy
Wingate, North Carolina

R. Keith Campbell, RPh, FAPhA, FASHP, MBA, CDE
Associate Dean/Professor of Pharmacotherapy
Washington State University
College of Pharmacy
Pullman, Washington

Melvin D. Cheitlin, MD
Emeritus Professor of Medicine
University of California, San Francisco, Cardiology Division
Former Chief, Cardiology Division
San Francisco General Hospital
San Francisco, California

Richard J. Duma, MD, PhD
Director, Department of Infectious Diseases
Infectious Disease Division
Halifax Medical Center
Daytona Beach, Florida

Kathryn M. Edwards, MD
Vice Chair for Clinical Research
Department of Pediatrics
Professor of Pediatrics
Vanderbilt University
School of Medicine
Nashville, Tennessee

Michael S. Edwards, PharmD, MBA
Assistant Director, Pharmacy Operations
The Sidney Kimmel Comprehensive Cancer Center at Johns Hopkins
Bethesda, Maryland

Mary J. Ferrill, PharmD, FASHP
Assistant Dean for Professionalization
Professor
Wingate University
School of Pharmacy
Wingate, North Carolina

Thomas A. Golper, MD
Professor of Medicine
Medical Director – Nephrology, Hypertension, and Diabetes Patient Care Center
Division of Nephrology
Vanderbilt University
Nashville, Tennessee

COL. John D. Grabenstein, RPh, PhD, FAPhA, FASHP, FRSH
Medical Service Corp.
Deputy Director for Clinical Operations
Military Vaccine Agency
U.S. Army Medical Command

Edward A. Hartshorn, PhD
Professor, Physician Assistant Studies
University of Texas Medical Branch
School of Allied Health Sciences
Galveston, Texas
Instructor
University of Texas Health Science Center
School of Nursing in Houston
Houston, Texas

Siret D. Jaanus, PhD
Professor of Pharmacology
Southern California College of Optometry
Fullerton, California

Robert E. Kates, PharmD, PhD
President
Analytical Solutions, Inc.
Sunnyvale, California

Julio R. Lopez, PharmD
Chief, Pharmacy Service
VA Northern California Health Care System
Martinez, California

Richard M. Oksas, PharmD, MPh
Family Practice Pharmacist
Natividad Medical Center
Salinas, California

J. James Rowsey, MD
St. Luke's Cataract and Laser Institute
Tarpon Springs, Florida

Mary Beth Shirk, PharmD
Specialty Practice Pharmacist,
Critical Care Medicine
Clinical Assistant Professor
The Ohio State University
  Medical Center
Columbus, Ohio

**Udho Thadani, MD, MRCP,
  FRCP(C), FACC, FAHA**
Professor Emeritus of Medicine
Cardiovascular Section
University of Oklahoma Health
  Sciences Center
Consultant Cardiologist,
  Oklahoma University
  Medical Center and
  VA Medical Center
Oklahoma City, Oklahoma

**Thom J. Zimmerman, MD,
  PhD**
Emeritus Professor and
  Chairman
Department of Ophthalmology
  and Visual Sciences
Emeritus Professor of
  Pharmacology & Toxicology
University of Louisville
School of Madicine
Global Ophthalmic Medical
  Director
Global Medical Affairs
Pharmacia Corporation
Louisville, Kentucky

Table of Contents

Foreword

Facts and Comparisons®, a part of Wolters Kluwer Health, has served the drug information needs of pharmacists and other health care professionals since its inception in 1946 by providing timely, accurate, comprehensive, unbiased, comparative information on prescription and nonprescription medications. *Drug Facts and Comparisons® (DFC)*, our flagship product, is the primary source of drug information and the reference of choice for more than 100,000 loyal subscribers because of its uncompromising editorial quality, reliability, and ease of use. *DFC* has remained unique among other drug information resources because of its organization by therapeutic use, providing single drug monographs with complete prescribing information as well as in-depth comparisons of closely related agents. Over the years, *DFC* has changed in size and scope, but the concept has never changed. That is why health care professionals continue to look to Facts and Comparisons® to keep them abreast of important information in their practice.

In addition to the annual bound edition, *DFC* is also available as the popular monthly updated loose-leaf publication and as an annual pocket-size softbound abridged version. These versions allow customers to choose the format that is best suited to their practice site and workflow.

Customers who prefer the speed and efficiency of electronic products can access *DFC* through *eFacts,* our electronic library of reference information, which is available on-line or CD ROM. In addition to *DFC*, other content sets include *Drug Interaction Facts, Med Facts* (patient drug information handouts), *Review of Natural Products, Off-Label Drug Facts, Cancer Chemotherapy, Nonprescription Drug Therapy,* and *Medi-Span Image and Imprint Database.* Information about *eFacts* can be accessed through www.drugfacts.com. Facts and Comparisons® also offers drug information for handheld personal data assistants, available for downloading at www.drugfacts.com.

Drug Facts and Comparisons® monographs are now integrated into Medi-Span's Drug Information Bridge, a pre-programmed application programming interface (API) that includes Medi-Span's drug files and clinical databases. The integration of the *DFC* referential content with Medi-Span's premier databases provides superior point-of-care solutions for our professional customers.

Facts and Comparisons® takes our mission of providing drug information to health care professionals very seriously, which is why we continue to invest in technology, improve our current publications, and stay in contact with our customers to make sure we maintain the high standards we set many years ago when Erwin Kastrup, RPh, first developed this concept. We have many people to thank for helping us achieve these goals, including our Editorial Advisory Panel, reviewers, contributors, and our excellent, dedicated employees, but more than anything we want to thank our loyal subscribers who have helped us develop and improve our drug information publications that are so widely used today.

We are dedicated to maintaining the traditions that are important to both Facts and Comparisons® and our customers, but we are also dedicated to evolving our products to meet the changing technologies and the changing needs of health care professionals. These goals only can be accomplished by responding to the comments and suggestions from our subscribers, which we encourage and appreciate. As always, let us know how we can better serve you and your drug information needs.

Cathy H. Reilly
Publisher

Preface

As the premier publisher of drug information, Facts and Comparisons® provides a broad range of print, electronic, and on-line resources to fulfill the day-to-day needs of practicing health care professionals. *Drug Facts and Comparisons® (DFC)*, our flagship publication developed in 1945 by pharmacist Erwin K. Kastrup, was initially designed to provide objective information in a format that facilitated unbiased comparisons of drug products in a timely manner. After 60 years, the basic concepts remain the same. However, the content and presentation of material in *DFC* continues to evolve to reflect the changing needs of the health care environment.

The annual bound edition is one of several formats in which *DFC* is available. The original loose-leaf version is kept up to date through monthly print updates. An electronic version, also updated monthly, is available as part of *eFacts* and can be accessed via www.drugfacts.com.

The new 58th edition of DFC incorporates 29 new drugs: abarelix (*Plenaxis*), alfuzosin HCl (*Uroxatral*), apomorphine HCl (*Apokyn*), azacitidine (*Vidaza*), bevacizumab (*Avastin*), botulism immune globulin IV (Human) (*BabyBIG*), cetuximab (*Erbitux*), cinacalcet HCl (*Sensipar*), daptomycin (*Cubicin*), efalizumab (*Raptiva*), epinastine HCl (*Elestat*), emtricitabine (*Emtriva*), fosamprenavir (*Lexiva*), flavocoxid (*Limbrel*), insulin glulisine (*Apidra*), memantine HCl (*Namenda*), miglustat (*Zavesca*), palonosetron HCl (*Aloxi*), pemetrexed (*Alimta*), rifaximin (*Xifaxan*), rosuvastatin calcium (*Crestor*), sertaconazole nitrate (*Ertaczo*), synthetic conjugated estrogens, B (*Enjuvia*), tadalafil (*Cialis*), telithromycin (*Ketek*), tinidazole (*Tindamax*), tiotropium bromide (*Spiriva*), trospium chloride (*Sanctura*), and vardenafil HCl (*Levitra*).

Significant new indications added include the following: Aldesleukin for metastatic melanoma, ciprofloxacin for bone/joint infections and complicated urinary tract infections and acute uncomplicated pyelonephritis, fluvastatin sodium for secondary prevention of coronary events, fosamprenavir for HIV infection in adults in combination with other antiretroviral agents, lamotrigine for maintenance treatment of bipolar I disorder, ophthalmic diclofenac sodium for temporary relief of pain and photophobia following corneal refractive surgery, oxcarbazepine for treatment of partial seizures in children 4 to 16 years of age, paroxetine for premenstrual dysphoric disorder, porfimer sodium for ablation of high-grade dysplasia in Barrett esophagus patients who do not undergo esophagectomy and for reduction of obstruction and palliation of symptoms in patients with completely or partially obstructive end bronchial nonsmall cell lung cancer, valacyclovir for genital herpes, valganciclovir HCl for prevention of CMV disease in kidney, heart, and kidney-pancreas transplant patients at high risk.

Sections that have undergone major revisions include the following: ACE inhibitors, childhood immunization schedule, antihypertensive treatment guidelines, antipsychotic agents, HMG-CoA reductase inhibitors, scabicides and pediculicides, and SSRIs, and a new phosphodiesterase type 5 inhibitors group monograph has been added.

As this edition goes to press, we continue to update our database daily for use in future editions and formats of *DFC*. We also continue to expand our extensive library of drug information resources to remain the full service drug information provider that our customers have come to expect. However, this can only be accomplished with feedback from the loyal health care professionals who use our information on a daily basis. Comments, criticisms, and suggestions are always welcome and encouraged. Please call or visit us at www.drugfacts.com.

Renee M. Wickersham
Senior Managing Editor

Kirsten K. Novak
Managing Editor

Introduction

Drug Facts and Comparisons® is a comprehensive drug information compendium. Organized by therapeutic drug class, the format is designed to provide a wide scope of drug information in a manner that facilitates evaluations and comparisons. A comprehensive index, a detailed table of contents for each chapter, and numerous cross references within monographs enable the reader to quickly locate needed information.

Editorial Policy

The principal editorial policy remains unchanged from the inception of *Drug Facts and Comparisons*® in 1945: Accurate, unbiased information; concise, standardized presentation; comparative, objective format; timely delivery. Review of FDA-approved product labeling, thousands of biomedical journal articles and textbooks, and policies and recommendations from many authoritative and official groups (eg, Centers for Disease Control; National Academy of Sciences; Joint National Committee on Detection, Evaluation, and Treatment of High Blood Pressure; National Heart, Lung and Blood Institute; American Thoracic Society; National Cancer Institute; FDA Office of Orphan Products Development; Food and Drug Administration) form the base of evaluation of information for *Drug Facts and Comparisons*®.

Editorial policy is guided by the distinguished Facts and Comparisons® Editorial Advisory Panel. This is an authoritative group of nationally and internationally recognized clinicians, scholars, scientists, physicians, pharmacists, and pharmacologists. In addition, many other prominent health care professionals serve on various expert panels and provide review in their specific areas of expertise for *Drug Facts and Comparisons*®. Indications and dosage recommendations are FDA-approved unless otherwise specified. Legitimate "unlabeled" uses and dosages are included when appropriate and given special emphasis. Input from an expert panel on drug interactions is also a feature.

This collection of wisdom and the world drug information literature is then molded and refined into the *Drug Facts and Comparisons*® database, monographs, and product listings. Many sources of drug information are constantly monitored so that *Drug Facts and Comparisons*® contains the most comprehensive, current drug information database available. There is not a more complete drug information compendium available presenting such clinical prescribing and drug product information.

Most of the products listed in *Drug Facts and Comparisons*® are protected by letters of patent, and their names are trademarked and registered by the firm whose name appears with the product. Identification of the product distributor is given in parentheses next to the brand name. The distributor may or may not be the actual manufacturer or fabricator of the final dosage form. When more than one company distributes a generic product, the generic product name is listed, followed by "Various, eg," in parentheses with a selected list of distributors. Listing of specific products is an indication only of market availability and is not an endorsement or recommendation. Most products listed have national or significant regional distribution.

Products that contain the same active ingredients are listed together for comparison and as an aid in product selection. However, drug product interchange is regulated by state laws; listing of products together does not imply that products are therapeutically equivalent or legally interchangeable. Caution is particularly advised when attempting to compare extended-release or delayed-release dosage forms.

How To Use *Drug Facts And Comparisons*®

Efficient use of *Drug Facts and Comparisons*® *(DFC)* requires an understanding of its organization and format.

Organization:

Information in *DFC* is organized by therapeutic use. Each of the 14 chapters is divided into groups and subgroups to facilitate comparisons of drugs and drug products with similar uses. The first page of each chapter provides a detailed outline, including page references of the information presented in that chapter.

Products most similar in content or use are listed together. This format of presenting the FACTS makes it easy to make COMPARISONS of identical, similar, or related products. Drugs with multiple uses may be listed in more than one section of the book.

Drug Monographs:

Prescribing information is presented in comprehensive drug monographs. General information on a group of closely related drugs (eg, ACE inhibitors) may be presented in a group monograph. Specific information relating to a particular drug is presented in an individual monograph under the generic name of the drug. All monographs are divided into sections identified with bold titles for ease in locating the desired information.

Indications: All indications or uses listed are FDA-approved unless specifically designated as "Unlabeled uses."

Administration and Dosage: Dosage ranges and methods of administration are presented.

Actions: This section gives a brief summary of the known pharmacologic and pharmacokinetic properties.

Contraindications: This section specifies those conditions in which the drug should NOT be used.

Warnings and Precautions: These sections list conditions in which use of the drug may be hazardous, precautions to observe, and parameters to monitor during therapy.

Drug Interactions: A brief summary of documented, clinically significant drug-drug, drug-lab test and drug-food interactions is provided.

Adverse Reactions: Reported adverse reactions are presented. Incidence data on adverse effects are included when available.

Overdosage: The clinical manifestations of toxicity and treatment of overdosage are given for most agents.

Patient Information: Essential information required by the patient for safe and effective self-administration of the medication is included.

Keeping Up:

The Keeping Up section enables the health care professional to stay up-to-date with the latest developments in drug therapy.

Orphan Drugs: Profiles the generic name and trade name of a drug, its sponsor, and the proposed use of an agent approved for marketing under the terms of the Orphan Drug Act.

Investigational Drugs: Provides brief reports on significant developments in drug therapy, including drugs currently under investigation.

Index:

The alphabetical index includes page references for all drugs by their generic name, brand name, synonyms, common abbreviations and therapeutic group names. Generic names are listed in bold type face for easy identification. A separate index of drug trade names unique to Canada is also a feature.

Product Listings:

Individual products are listed at the beginning of each monograph. The format and components of the product listings are discussed below and illustrated on the opposite page.

NOTE: Products that contain the same active ingredients are listed together for comparison and as an aid in product selection. However, drug product interchange is regulated by state laws; listing of products together does not imply that products are therapeutically equivalent or legally interchangeable. Caution is particularly advised when attempting to compare extended-release or delayed-release dosage forms.

1 Products are grouped by dosage form and strength.

2 Brand name products with the same amount of active ingredient and in the same doseform are listed in alphabetical order.

3 The name of the distributor is given in parentheses next to the product name.

4 Products available by their generic name from multiple sources are indicated as available from (Various) distributors and in selected cases, examples of generic manufacturers are listed.

5 Package sizes are given for all dosage forms and strengths of each product.

6 Product identification imprint codes are listed in parentheses.

7 Cross references to the appropriate drug monograph(s) for complete prescribing information appear at the beginning of the monograph.

8 Controlled substances are designated by their schedule (*c-ii, c-iii, c-iv,* or *c-v*).

9 Distribution status of products is indicated as *Rx* or *otc*.

10 Sugar-free liquid preparations are designated by *sf*.

11 Combination products are listed in tables to facilitate comparisons. Products most similar in formulation are listed next to each other.

12 Products with identical active ingredients are listed together.

Aminopenicillins

AMOXICILLIN

Rx	**Amoxil** (SK-Beecham)	**Tablets:** 500 mg (as trihydrate)	(Amoxil 500). Film-coated. Capsule shape. Pink. In 20s, 100s, 500s
		875 mg (as trihydrate)	(Amoxil 875). Film coated, scored. Capsule shape. Pink. In 20s, 100s, 500s.
Rx	**Amoxicillin** (Various, eg, Biocraft, Major, Rugby, Teva, URL)	**Capsules:** 250 mg (as trihydrate)	In 21s, 30s, 100s, 250s, 500s, 1000s and UD 45s and 100s.
Rx	**Amoxil** (SK-Beecham)		(Amoxil 250). Blue and pink. In 100s, 500s and UD 100s.
Rx	**Trimox** (Apothecon)		In 30s, 100s, 500s and UD 100s.
Rx	**Wymox** (Wyeth-Ayerst)		(Wyeth 559). Gray and green. In 100s and 500s.
Rx	**Amoxicillin** (Various, eg, Biocraft, Major, Teva, URL)	**Capsules:** 500 mg (as trihydrate)	In 21s, 30s, 50s, 100s, 250s, 500s and UD 45s and 100s.
Rx	**Amoxil** (SK-Beecham)		(Amoxil 500). Blue and pink. In 100s, 500s and UD 100s.
Rx	**Trimox** (Apothecon)		In 30s, 100s, 500s and UD 100s.
Rx	**Wymox** (Wyeth-Ayerst)		(Wyeth 560). Gray and green. In 50s and 500s.
Rx	**Amoxil Pediatric Drops** (SK-Beecham)	**Powder for Oral Suspension:** 50 mg/ml (as trihydrate) when reconstituted	Sucrose. Bubble gum flavor. In 15 and 30 ml.
Rx	**Trimox Pediatric Drops** (Apothecon)		Sucrose. In 15 ml.
Rx	**Amoxicillin** (Various, eg, Biocraft, Major, Teva, URL)	**Powder for Oral Suspension:** 125 mg/5 ml (as trihydrate) when reconstituted	In 80, 100, 150 and 200 ml.
Rx	**Amoxil** (SK-Beecham)		Sucrose. Strawberry flavor. In 80, 100 and 150 ml and UD 5 ml.
Rx	**Trimox** (Apothecon)		Sucrose. In 80, 100 and 150 ml.
Rx	**Wymox** (Wyeth-Ayerst)		Sucrose. In 100 and 150 ml.
Rx	**Amoxicillin** (Various, eg, Biocraft, Major, Teva, URL)	**Powder for Oral Suspension:** 250 mg/5 ml (as trihydrate) when reconstituted	In 80, 100, 150 and 200 ml.
Rx	**Amoxil** (SK-Beecham)		Sucrose. Bubble gum flavor. In 80, 100 and 150 ml and UD 5 ml.
Rx	**Trimox** (Apothecon)		Sucrose. In 80, 100 and 150 ml.
Rx	**Wymox** (Wyeth-Ayerst)		Sucrose. In 100 and 150 ml.

For complete prescribing information, refer to the Penicillins group monograph.

the advantage of more complete absorption than ampicillin, a 3-times a day regimen for most infections and less diarrhea than ampicillin.

COUGH PREPARATIONS

ANTITUSSIVE AND EXPECTORANT COMBINATIONS

Content given per tablet, 5 mL, or packet.

	Product & Distributor	Antitussive	Expectorant	Decongestant
Rx	**Levall Liquid**[1] (Athlon Pharmaceuticals[2])	20 mg carbetapentane citrate	100 mg guaifenesin	15 mg phenylephrine HCl
c-v	**Dihistine Expectorant Liquid** (Alpharma)	10 mg codeine phosphate	100 mg guaifenesin	30 mg pseudoephedrine HCl
c-v	**Guiatuss DAC Liquid**[1] (Various, eg, Alpharma, Ivax)			
c-v sf	**Halotussin DAC Syrup**[1] (Watson Laboratories)			
c-v sf	**Mytussin DAC Liquid**[1] (Morton Grove Pharmaceuticals)			
c-v	**Novagest Expectorant with Codeine Liquid**[1] (Major)			
c-iii	**Nucofed Expectorant Syrup**[1] (Monarch)			
c-iii	**Nucotuss Expectorant Syrup**[1] (Alpharma)	12.5% alcohol. In 473 mL.		
c-v	**Tussirex Syrup** (Scot-Tussin)	10 mg codeine phosphate	83.3 mg sodium citrate	4.17 mg phenylephrine HCl
c-v sf	**Tussirex Sugar Free Liquid** (Scot-Tussin)			
Rx	**Donatussin Syrup**[1] (Laser)	7.5 mg dextromethorphan HBr	100 mg guaifenesin	10 mg phenylephrine HCl
otc sf	**Tussex Cough Syrup**[1] (Alpharma)	10 mg dextromethorphan HBr	100 mg guaifenesin	5 mg phenylephrine HCl
Rx	**Tussafed Ex Syrup**[1] (Everett Laboratories)	30 mg dextromethorphan HBr	200 mg guaifenesin	10 mg phenylephrine HCl
otc	**Guiatuss CF Syrup**[1] (Alpharma)	10 mg dextromethorphan HBr	100 mg guaifenesin	30 mg pseudoephedrine HCl
otc	**Robafen CF Syrup**[1] (Major)			
otc	**Robitussin CF Syrup**[1] (Whitehall-Robins)			

Recommended Dietary Allowances (RDA) are published by the Food and Nutrition Board, National Research Council-National Academy of Sciences, as a guide for nutritional problems and to provide standards of good nutrition for different age groups. They are revised periodically.

The RDA values are *not requirements;* they are *recommended* daily intakes of certain essential nutrients. Based on available scientific knowledge, they are believed to be adequate for known nutritional needs for most *healthy* people under usual environmental stresses. The recommended allowances vary for age and sex, with extra allowances for women during pregnancy and lactation. The most commonly used RDA values (the "reference male" and "reference female") are those of adults 23 to 50 years of age. With the exception of energy (kilocalories), the RDA provide for individual requirement variations and prevent symptoms of clinical deficiency of 97% of the population.

RDA have been established for many essential nutrients; however, present knowledge of human nutritional needs of pantothenic acid and biotin is incomplete. Therefore, to ensure adequate nutrient intake, obtain the recommended allowances from as varied a selection of foods as possible. Nutritionists suggest that dietary planning include regular intake of each of the four basic food groups:

1.) Milk, cheese, dairy products – Minimum 2 servings/day.
2.) Meat, poultry, fish, beans – Minimum 2 servings/day.
3.) Vegetables, fruit – Minimum 4 servings/day.
4.) Bread, cereal (whole-grain and enriched or fortified) – Minimum 4 servings/day.

Such a balance, in sufficient quantities will provide about 1200 kcal, enough protein, and most of the vitamins and minerals required daily. A person may increase nutrient and energy intake by consuming larger quantities (or more servings/day) of the 4 basic food groups. Nutrient and energy intake may also be increased by selecting food from the fifth group, fats-sweets-alcohol, which provides mainly energy.

RDA quantities apply only to healthy people and are not intended to cover therapeutic nutritional requirements in disease or other abnormal states (ie, metabolic disorders, weight reduction, chronic disease, drug therapy). Although certain single nutrients in larger quantities may have pharmacologic actions, these are unrelated to nutritional functions. There is no convincing evidence that consuming excessive quantities of single nutrients will cure or prevent nonnutritional diseases.

The "official" listings of United States Recommended Daily Allowances (US-RDAs) should not be confused with the RDA values. US-RDA are derived from the 1968 RDA and serve as legal standards for nutritional labeling of food and dietary food and dietary supplement products controlled by the FDA. Generally, they represent the higher value of the male or female RDA and are grouped into only 3 age brackets plus 1 category for pregnant or lactating women. Prior to 1972, these allowances were erroneously listed as minimum daily requirements (MDR). A second fallacy perpetuated by US-RDA labeling of foods is the implication that a food is defective if it does not contain all the officially established nutrients in their full US-RDA quantities. No individual food is nutritionally complete, but several foods together should complement each other to provide maximal nutrient balance and to minimize naturally occurring toxic principles consumed from any individual foodstuff.

The RDA for adult males and adult females are included in each individual vitamin monograph. The table on the following page presents the listing of vitamin and mineral RDA values for all age groups as published in *Recommended Dietary Allowances*, 10th Edition, National Academy of Sciences, Washington, DC, 1989.

RECOMMENDED DIETARY ALLOWANCES OF VITAMINS AND MINERALS

RECOMMENDED DIETARY ALLOWANCES[1]

Age (years) or Condition	Weight[2] (kg)	Weight[2] (lb)	Height[2] (cm)	Height[2] (in)	Protein (g)	Vitamin A IU[3]	Vitamin D IU[4]	Vitamin E IU[5]	Vitamin K (µg)	Ascorbic acid (C) (mg)	Thiamine (B₁) (mg)	Riboflavin (B₂) (mg)	Niacin (B₃) (mg)	Pyridoxine (B₆) (mg)	Folate (µg)	Cyanocobalamin (B₁₂) (µg)	Calcium (mg)	Phosphorus (mg)	Magnesium (mg)	Iron (mg)	Zinc (mg)	Iodine (µg)	Selenium (µg)
Infants																							
0.0–0.5	6	13	60	24	13	1249	300	4	5	30	0.3	0.4	5	0.3	25	0.3	400	300	40	6	5	40	10
0.5–1	9	20	71	28	14	1249	400	6	10	35	0.4	0.5	6	0.6	35	0.5	600	500	60	10	5	50	15
Children																							
1–3	13	29	90	35	16	1332	400	9	15	40	0.7	0.8	9	1	50	0.7	800	800	80	10	10	70	20
4–6	20	44	112	44	24	1665	400	10	20	45	0.9	1.1	12	1.1	75	1	800	800	120	10	10	90	20
7–10	28	62	132	52	28	2331	400	10	30	45	1	1.2	13	1.4	100	1.4	800	800	170	10	10	120	30
Males																							
11–14	45	99	157	62	45	3330	400	15	45	50	1.3	1.5	17	1.7	150	2	1200	1200	270	12	15	150	40
15–18	66	145	176	69	59	3330	400	15	65	60	1.5	1.8	20	2	200	2	1200	1200	400	12	15	150	50
19–24	72	160	177	70	58	3330	400	15	70	60	1.5	1.7	19	2	200	2	1200	1200	350	10	15	150	70
25–50	79	174	176	70	63	3330	200	15	80	60	1.5	1.7	19	2	200	2	800	800	350	10	15	150	70
51+	77	170	173	68	63	3330	200	15	80	60	1.2	1.4	15	2	200	2	800	800	350	10	15	150	70
Females																							
11–14	46	101	157	62	46	2664	400	12	45	50	1.1	1.3	15	1.4	150	2	1200	1200	280	15	12	150	45
15–18	55	120	163	64	44	2664	400	12	55	60	1.1	1.3	15	1.5	180	2	1200	1200	300	15	12	150	50
19–24	58	128	164	65	46	2664	400	12	60	60	1.1	1.3	15	1.6	180	2	1200	1200	280	15	12	150	55
25–50	63	138	163	64	50	2664	200	12	65	60	1.1	1.3	15	1.6	180	2	800	800	280	15	12	150	55
51+	65	143	160	63	50	2664	200	12	65	60	1	1.2	13	1.6	180	2	800	800	280	10	12	150	55
Pregnant					60	2664	400	15	65	70	1.5	1.6	17	2.2	400	2.2	1200	1200	320	30	15	175	65
Lactating – 1st 6 mo.					65	4329	400	18	65	95	1.6	1.8	20	2.1	280	2.6	1200	1200	355	15	19	200	75
2nd 6 mo.					62	3996	400	16	65	90	1.6	1.7	20	2.1	260	2.6	1200	1200	340	15	16	200	75

Reproduced from: *Recommended Dietary Allowances*, 10th edition, 1989, National Academy of Sciences, National Academy Press, Washington, DC.

[1] The allowances, expressed as average daily intakes over time, are intended to provide for individual variations among most normal people as they live in the US under usual environmental stresses. Diets should be based on a variety of common foods in order to provide other nutrients for which human requirements have been less well defined.

[2] Weights and heights of Reference Adults are actual medians for the US population of the designated age, as reported by NHANES II. The median weights and heights of those < 19 years of age were taken from Hamill PV, et al. *Am J Clin Nutr.* 1979;32:607–629. The use of these figures does not imply that the height-to-weight ratios are ideal.

[3] Conversion of IU to retinol equivalents (RE): 3.33 IU = 1 mcg of retinol = 1 RE or 6 mcg. β-carotene.

[4] As cholecalciferol. 10 mcg cholecalciferol = 400 IU of vitamin D.

[5] α-Tocopherol equivalents. 1 mg d-α-tocopherol = α-TE = 1.49 IU.

VITAMIN D

phase, determine serum calcium once or twice weekly. Maintain serum calcium levels between 9 and 10 mg/dL.

Paricalcitol – During the inital phase of therapy, frequently determine serum calcium and phosphate (eg, twice weekly). Once dosage has been established, measure serum calcium and phosphate at least monthly. Measurements of serum or plasma PTH are recommended every 3 months. An intact PTH (iPTH) assay is recommended for reliable detection of biologically active PTH. During dose adjustment of paricalcitol, laboratory tests may be required more frequently.

➤*Concomitant vitamin D intake:* Evaluate vitamin D ingested in fortified foods, dietary supplements, and other concomitantly administered drugs. It may be necessary to limit dietary vitamin D and its derivatives during treatment.

➤*Hypoparathyroidism:* May need calcium, parathyroid hormone, dihydrotachysterol.

➤*Special risk:* Use caution in patients, especially in the elderly with coronary disease, renal function impairment, and arteriosclerosis.

➤*Tartrazine sensitivity:* Some of these products contain tartrazine, which may cause allergic-type reactions (including bronchial asthma) in susceptible individuals. Although the incidence of sensitivity is low, it is frequently seen in patients with aspirin hypersensitivity. Products containing tartrazine are identified in product listings.

Drug Interactions

Vitamin D Drug Interactions			
Precipitant drug	Object drug*		Description
Vitamin D	Antacids, magnesium-containing	↑	Hypermagnesemia may develop in patients on chronic renal dialysis.
Vitamin D	Digitalis glycosides	↑	Hypercalcemia in patients on digitalis may precipitate cardiac arrhythmias.
Vitamin D	Verapamil	↑	Atrial fibrillation has occurred when supplemental calcium and calciferol have induced hypercalcemia.
Cholestyramine	Vitamin D	↓	Intestinal absorption of vitamin D may be reduced.
Ketoconazole	Vitamin D	↓	Ketoconazole may inhibit both synthetic and catabolic enzymes of calcitriol. Reductions in serum endogenous calcitriol concentrations have been observed following the administration of 300 to 1200 mg/day ketoconazole for a week to healthy men.
Mineral oil	Vitamin D	↓	Absorption of vitamin D is reduced with prolonged use of mineral oil.
Phenytoin Phenobarbital	Vitamin D	↓	Endogenous synthesis of calcitriol will be inhibited. Higher doses of calcitriol may be necessary if these drugs are adminstered simultaneously.
Thiazide diuretics	Vitamin D	↑	Hypoparathyroid patients on vitamin D may develop hypercalcemia due to thiazide diuretics.

* ↑ = Object drug increased.   ↓ = Object drug decreased.

Adverse Reactions

Early – Weakness; headache; somnolence; nausea; vomiting; dry mouth; constipation; muscle pain; bone pain; metallic taste.

Late – Polyuria; polydipsia; anorexia; irritability; weight loss; nocturia; mild acidosis; hypercalciuria; anemia; reversible azotemia; generalized vascular calcification; nephrocalcinosis; conjunctivitis (calcific); pancreatitis; photophobia; rhinorrhea; pruritus; hyperthermia; decreased libido; elevated BUN; albuminuria; hypercholesterolemia; elevated AST and ALT; ectopic calcification; hypertension; cardiac arrhythmias; overt psychosis (rare).

In clinical studies on hypoparathyroidism and pseudohypoparathyroidism, hypercalcemia was noted on at least one occasion in ≈ 1 in 3 patients and hypercalciuria in ≈ 1 in 7. Elevated serum creatinine levels were observed in ≈ 1 in 6 patients (approximately one half of whom had normal levels at baseline).

Occasional mild pain on injection has been observed (*Calcijex*).

Ergocalciferol – Hypercalciuria and mental retardation have been associated with ergocalciferol.

➤*Paricalcitol:*
Lab test abnormalities – **Paricalcitol** may reduce serum total alkaline phosphatase levels.

Miscellaneous – Discontinuation of therapy caused by any adverse event occurred in 6.5% of 62 patients treated with paricalcitol and 2% of 51 patients treated with placebo for 1 to 3 months.

Nausea (13%); vomiting (13%); edema (7%); chills, fever, flu, GI bleeding, lightheadedness, pneumonia, sepsis (5%); dry mouth, feeling unwell, palpitation (3%).

Overdosage

➤*Symptoms:* Administration of vitamin D to patients in excess of their daily requirements may cause hypercalcemia, hypercalciuria, and hyperphosphatemia. Concomitant high intake of calcium and phosphate may lead to similar abnormalities. **Dihydrotachysterol** may be toxic in doses as low as 25 mg/day, and is manifested by symptoms of hypercalcemia.

Hypercalcemia leads to anorexia, nausea, weakness, headache, somnolence, vomiting, dry mouth, metallic taste, weight loss, vague aches and stiffness, constipation, diarrhea, mental retardation, tinnitus, ataxia, hypotonia, depression, amnesia, disorientation, hallucinations, syncope, coma, anemia, and mild acidosis. Impairment of renal function may cause polyuria, nocturia, hypercalciuria, polydipsia, reversible azotemia, hypertension, nephrocalcinosis, generalized vascular calcification, irreversible renal insufficiency, or proteinuria. Widespread calcification of soft tissues, including heart, blood vessels, renal tubules, skin, and lungs may occur. Bone demineralization (osteoporosis) may occur in adults; decline in average linear growth rate and increased bone mineralization may occur in infants and children (dwarfism). Effects can persist ≥ 2 months after ergocalciferol treatment, 1 month after cessation of dihydrotachysterol therapy, 2 to 4 weeks for calcifediol and 2 to 7 days for calcitriol. Death may result from cardiovascular or renal failure. Obtain serum calcium levels at least weekly after all dosage changes and subsequent dosage dosage titration. In patients receiving digitalis, obtain serial serum calcium determination, rate of urinary calcium excretion, and an assessment of ECG abnormalities due to hypercalcemia.

➤*Treatment:* Treatment of accidental overdose consists of general supportive measures. Refer to General Management of Acute Overdosage. If ingestion is discovered within a short time, emesis or gastric lavage may be beneficial. Mineral oil may promote fecal elimination.

Treatment of hypervitaminosis D with hypercalcemia consists of immediate withdrawal of vitamin D and calcium supplements, administration of a low-calcium diet, bed rest, administration of a laxative (mineral oil), attention to electrolyte imbalances, assessment of ECG abnormalities (critical in patients receiving digitalis), hemodialysis or peritoneal dialysis against a calcium-free dialysate, generous fluid intake, and urine acidification along with symptomatic and supportive treatment.

Hypercalcemic crisis with dehydration, stupor, coma, and azotemia requires more vigorous treatment. The first step is hydration; saline IV may quickly and significantly increase urinary calcium excretion. A loop diuretic (eg, furosemide) may be given with the saline infusion to further increase calcium excretion. Other measures include administration of citrates, sulfates, phosphates (do not administer with **paricalcitol**), corticosteroids, EDTA, possibly mithramycin and plicamycin. Persistent or markedly elevated serum calcium levels may be corrected by dialysis against a calcium-free dialysate. With appropriate therapy and when no permanent damage has occurred, recovery is probable.

Patient Information

Compliance with dosage instructions, diet, phosphate-binder use, and calcium supplementation is essential. Avoid use of nonprescription drugs, including magnesium-containing antacids, and natural products, unless such use has been discussed with a physician.

➤*Paricalcitol:* Instruct the patient that, to ensure effectiveness of paricalcitol therapy, it is important to adhere to a dietary regimen of calcium supplementation and phosphorus restriction. Appropriate types of phosphate-binding compounds may be needed; avoid excessive use of aluminum-containing compounds. Inform patients about the symptoms of elevated calcium.

Swallow whole; do not crush or chew.

Eating a balanced diet and periodic exposure to sunlight usually satisfies normal vitamin D requirements. Do not use vitamin supplements as a substitute for a balanced diet.

Notify physician if any of the following occurs: Weakness, lethargy, headache, anorexia, weight loss, nausea, vomiting, abdominal cramps, diarrhea, constipation, vertigo, excessive thirst, excessive urine output, dry mouth, or muscle or bone pain.

Avoid concurrent, prolonged use of mineral oil. If on chronic renal dialysis, avoid magnesium-containing antacids while taking these drugs. See Drug Interactions.

Fat Soluble Vitamins

DIHYDROTACHYSTEROL (DHT)

Dihydrotachysterol is a synthetic reduction product of tachysterol, a close isomer of vitamin D; 1 mg is approximately equivalent to 3 mg (120,000 IU) vitamin D_2.

Rx	**DHT** (Roxane)	**Tablets:** 0.125 mg	Lactose, sucrose. (54 280). White. In 50s and UD 100s.
		0.2 mg	Lactose, sucrose. (54 903). Pink. In 100s and UD 100s.
		0.4 mg	Lactose, sucrose. (54 772). White. In 50s.
		Intensol Solution: 0.2 mg/mL	20% alcohol. In 30 mL w/dropper.
Rx	**Hytakerol** (Sanofi Winthrop Pharm.)	**Capsules:** 0.125 mg	Parabens. In 50s.

For complete prescribing information, refer to the Vitamin D group monograph.

Indications

▶*Tetany:* Treatment of acute, chronic, and latent forms of postoperative tetany and idiopathic tetany.

▶*Hypoparathyroidism:* Treatment of hypoparathyroidism.

Administration and Dosage

▶*Initial dose:* 0.75 to 2.5 mg daily for several days.

▶*Maintenance dose:* 0.2 to 1.75 mg daily, as required, for normal serum calcium levels. Average dose is 0.6 mg daily. May be supplemented with 10 to 15 g oral calcium lactate or gluconate. Following thyroid operation, 0.25 mg may be given daily with 6 g calcium lactate orally, until the danger of tetany has passed.

CALCITRIOL (1α,25 dihydroxycholecalciferol; 1,25 [OH]₂D₃)

Rx	**Rocaltrol** (Roche)	**Capsules:** 0.25 mcg	Sorbitol, parabens. (Rocaltrol 0.25 Roche). Light orange. Oval. In 30s and 100s.
		0.5 mcg	Sorbitol, parabens. (Rocaltrol 0.5 Roche). Dark orange. Oblong. In 100s.
Rx	**Calcitriol** (Roxane)	**Oral solution:** 1 mcg/mL	In 15 mL with single-use graduated oral dispensers.
Rx	**Rocaltrol** (Roche)		In 15 mL bottle w/dispensers.
Rx	**Calcitriol Injection** (aaiPharma)	**Injection:** 1 mcg/mL	Sodium chloride, EDTA. In 1 mL vials.
Rx	**Calcijex** (Abbott)		In 1 mL amps.[a]
Rx	**Calcitriol Injection** (aaiPharma)	**Injection:** 2 mcg/mL	Sodium chloride, EDTA. In 1 mL vials.

[a] With 4 mg polysorbate 20, 1.5 mg sodium chloride, 10 mg sodium ascorbate, 7.6 mg dibasic sodium phosphate, anhydrous, and EDTA.

For complete prescribing information, refer to the Vitamin D group monograph.

Indications

▶*Dialysis patients (oral, IV):* Management of hypocalcemia in patients on chronic renal dialysis.

Rocaltrol also is indicated in the management of the resultant bone disease in patients undergoing chronic renal dialysis.

May significantly reduce elevated parathyroid hormone levels.

▶*Predialysis patients:* Management of secondary hyperparathyroidism and resultant metabolic bone disease in patients with moderate to severe chronic renal failure (Ccr 15 to 55 mL/min) not yet on dialysis.

▶*Hypoparathyroidism patients:* Management of hypocalcemia and its clinical manifestations in patients with postsurgical hypoparathyroidism, idiopathic hypoparathyroidism, and pseudohypoparathyroidism.

▶*Unlabeled uses:* Calcitriol, orally (initial dose of 0.25 mcg twice daily) and topically (0.1 to 0.5 mcg/g petrolatum), decreased the severity of psoriatic lesions.

Administration and Dosage

▶*Oral dosing:*

Dialysis patients – 0.25 mcg/day. If a satisfactory response is not observed, increase dosage by 0.25 mcg/day at 4- to 8-week intervals. During this titration period, obtain serum calcium levels at least twice weekly; if hypercalcemia is noted, discontinue use until normocalcemia is obtained.

Patients with normal or only slightly reduced serum calcium levels may respond to doses of 0.25 mcg every other day. Most patients undergoing hemodialysis respond to doses between 0.5 and 1 mcg/day.

Oral calcitriol may normalize plasma ionized calcium in some uremic patients, yet fail to suppress parathyroid hyperfunction. In these individuals with autonomous parathyroid hyperfunction, oral calcitriol may be useful to maintain normocalcemia but has not been shown to be adequate treatment for hyperparathyroidism.

Hypoparathyroidism – Initial dose is 0.25 mcg/day given in the morning. If a satisfactory response in the biochemical parameters and clinical manifestations of the disease are not observed, increase dose at 2- to 4-week intervals. During the dosage titration period, obtain serum calcium levels at least twice weekly, and, if hypercalcemia is noted, immediately discontinue use until normocalcemia ensues. Carefully consider lowering dietary calcium intake.

Adults and children (≥ 6 years): 0.5 to 2 mcg daily.

Children (1 to 5 years): With hypoparathyroidism, 0.25 to 0.75 mcg daily. The number of treated patients with pseudohypoparathyroidism < 6 years of age is too small to make dosage recommendations.

Predialysis patients – Initial dose is 0.25 mcg/day in adults and pediatric patients ≥ 3 years of age. Dosage may be increased if necessary to 0.5 mcg/day. Dosage is 10 to 15 ng/kg/day for pediatric patients < 3 years of age.

▶*IV dosing:* Initially, 1 mcg (0.02 mcg/kg) to 2 mcg 3 times weekly approximately every other day. Doses as small as 0.5 mcg and as large as 4 mcg 3 times weekly have been used as an initial dose.

Unsatisfactory response – The dose may be increased by 0.5 to 1 mcg at 2- to 4-week intervals. Obtain serum calcium and phosphorus levels twice weekly.

Discontinue if hypercalcemia or serum calcium times phosphate product (Ca × P) totals > 70. Reinitiate at lower dose. Doses may need to be reduced as the PTH levels decrease in response to therapy. Thus, incremental dosing must be individualized and commensurate with PTH, serum calcium, and phosphorus levels. The following table is a suggested approach in dose titration:

Suggested Approach for Calcitriol Dose Titration	
PTH Levels	IV Dose
the same or increasing	increase
decreasing by < 30%	increase
decreasing by > 30% to < 60%	maintain
decreasing by > 60%	decrease
1.5 to 3 times the ULN	maintain

▶*Storage/Stability:* Protect from light.

Fat Soluble Vitamins

ERGOCALCIFEROL (D₂)

Ergocalciferol 1 mg provides 40,000 IU of vitamin D activity.

otc	**Calciferol Drops** (Schwarz Pharma)	Liquid: 8000 IU/mL	In 60 mL.ᵃ
otc	**Drisdol Drops** (Sanofi Pharm.)		In 60 mL.ᵃ
Rx	**Drisdol** (Sanofi Pharm.)	Capsules: 50,000 IU	Tartrazine. (D92 W). In 50s.

ᵃ In propylene glycol.　　　　　　　　　　ᵇ In sesame oil.

For complete prescribing information, refer to the Vitamin D group monograph.

Indications

►*Rickets:* Treatment of refractory rickets (also known as vitamin D-resistant rickets).

►*Familial hypophosphatemia:* Treatment of familial hypophosphatemia.

►*Hypoparathyroidism:* Treatment of hypoparathyroidism.

Administration and Dosage

►*Recommended dietary allowances (RDAs):* Adults (< 25 years) 400 IU; (> 25 years) 200 IU. For a complete listing of RDAs by age, sex, and condition, refer to the RDA table. Daily dosage of 400 IU satisfies requirements for all age groups, unless there has been exposure to ultraviolet irradiation.

Individualize dosage. The range between therapeutic and toxic doses is narrow.

Blood calcium, phosphate, and BUN determinations must be made every 2 weeks or more frequently if necessary. X-ray bones monthly until the condition is corrected and stabilized. Ensure adequate calcium intake. Maintain serum calcium concentration between 9 and 10 mg/dL.

►*Vitamin D-resistant rickets:* 12,000 to 500,000 IU daily.

►*Hypoparathyroidism:* 50,000 to 200,000 IU/day plus 500 to 520 mg elemental calcium 6 times daily.

►*Familial hypophosphatemia:* 10,000 to 80,000 IU daily plus 1 to 2 g/day elemental phosphorus.

►*IM therapy:* Required in patients with GI, liver or biliary disease associated with malabsorption of vitamin D. Do not administer IV or SC.

CHOLECALCIFEROL (D₃)

Cholecalciferol 1 mg provides 40,000 IU vitamin D activity.

otc *sf*	**Delta-D** (Freeda)	Tablets: 400 IU	In 250s and 500s.
otc *sf*	**Vitamin D₃** (Freeda)	Tablets: 1000 IU₃	In 100s and 500s.

For complete prescribing information, refer the Vitamin D group monograph.

Indications

Dietary supplement; treatment of vitamin D deficiency or prophylaxis of deficiency.

Administration and Dosage

400 to 1000 IU daily.

PARICALCITOL

Rx	**Zemplar** (Abbott)	Injection: 5 mcg/mL	In 1 and 2 mL single-dose Fliptop vials.

For complete prescribing information, refer to the Vitamin D group monograph.

Indications

►*Hyperparathyroidism:* Prevention and treatment of secondary hyperparathyroidism associated with chronic renal failure.

Administration and Dosage

►*Approved by the FDA:* April 17, 1998.

The currently accepted target range for intact parathyroid hormone (iPTH) levels of CRF patients is ≤ 1.5 to 3 times the non-uremic upper limit of normal.

The recommended initial dose is 0.04 to 0.1 mcg/kg (2.8 to 7 mcg) administered as a bolus dose no more frequently than every other day at any time during dialysis. Doses as high as 0.24 mcg/kg (16.8 mcg) have been administered safely.

If a satisfactory response is not observed, the dose may be increased by 2 to 4 mcg at 2- to 4-week intervals. During any dose adjustment period, monitor serum calcium and phosphorus levels more frequently, and if an elevated calcium level or a Ca x P product > 75 is noted, immediately reduce or interrupt the drug dosage until parameters are normalized and reinitiate at a lower dose. Doses may need to be decreased as the PTH levels decrease in response to therapy. Thus, individualize incremental dosing.

The following table is a suggested approach to dose titration.

Suggested Paricalcitol Dosing Guidelines	
PTH level	Paricalcitol dose
the same or increasing	increase
decreasing by < 30%	increase
decreasing by 30% to 60%	maintain
decreasing by > 60%	decrease
1.5 to 3 times upper limit of normal	maintain

►*Storage / Stability:* Store at 25°C (77°F). Discard unused portion.

DOXERCALCIFEROL

Rx	**Hectorol** (Bone Care International)	Capsules: 2.5 mcg	BHA, ethanol. (BCI). Yellow. Oval. In 50s.

For complete prescribing information, refer to the Vitamin D group monograph.

Indications

►*Hyperparathyroidism:* Reduction of elevated intact parathyroid hormone (iPTH) levels in the management of secondary hyperparathyroidism in patients undergoing chronic renal dialysis.

Administration and Dosage

►*Approved by the FDA:* June 9, 1999.

The optimal dose of doxercalciferol must be carefully determined for each patient. The recommended initial dose is 10 mcg administered 3 times weekly at dialysis (approximately every other day). Adjust the initial dose as needed, in order to lower blood iPTH into the range of 150 to 300 pg/mL. The dose may be increased at 8-week intervals by 2.5 mcg if iPTH is not lowered by 50% and fails to reach the target range. The maximum recommended dose is 20 mcg administered 3 times a week at dialysis for a total of 60 mcg/week. Suspend drug administration if iPTH falls below 100 pg/mL, and restart 1 week later at a dose that is at least 2.5 mcg lower than the last administered dose. During titration, obtain iPTH, serum calcium, and serum phosphate levels weekly. If hypercalcemia, hyperphosphatemia, or a serum calcium times serum phosphate product (Ca × P) > 70 is noted, immediately suspend the drug until these parameters are appropriately lowered, and then restart the drug at a dose that is ≤ 2.5 mcg.

Dosing must be individualized and based on iPTH levels with monitoring of serum calcium and serum phosphate levels. The following is a suggested approach in dose titration:

Suggested Dosage for Doxercalciferol	
iPTH level	Doxercalciferol dose
Initial dosing	
> 400 pg/mL	10 mcg 3 times per week at dialysis.
Dose titration	
Decreased by < 50% and > 300 pg/mL	Increase by 2.5 mcg at 8-week intervals as necessary.
150 - 300 pg/mL	Maintain
< 100 pg/mL	Suspend for 1 week, then resume at a dose that is at least 2.5 mcg lower.

Fat Soluble Vitamins

VITAMIN E

otc	**Vitamin E** (Various, eg, Freeda)	**Tablets:** 100 IU[a]	In 100s and 250s.
		200 IU[a]	In 100s, 250s, and 500s.
		400 IU[a]	In 100s, 250s, and 500s.
		500 IU[a]	In 100s and 250s.
		800 IU[a]	In 100s.
otc	**Vitamin E with Mixed Tocopherols** (Freeda)	**Tablets:** 100 IU[b]	In 100s and 250s.
		200 IU[b]	In 100s and 250s.
		400 IU[b]	In 100s, 250s, and 500s.
otc	**Vitamin E** (Various, eg, Apothecary, Goldline, Nature's Bounty)	**Capsules:** 100 IU[b]	In 100s.
		200 IU[b]	In 100s.
		400 IU[b]	In 100s and 250s.
		1000 IU[b]	In 50s and 100s.
otc	**Mixed E 400 Softgels** (Naturally)	**Capsules:** 400 IU[b]	In 60s, 90s, and 180s.
otc *sf*	**Vita-Plus E** (Scot-Tussin)	**Capsules:** 400 IU[c]	In 50s.
otc	**d' ALPHA E 1000 Softgels** (Naturally)	**Capsules:** 1000 IU[a]	In 30s and 60s.
otc	**Mixed E 1000 Softgels** (Naturally)	**Capsules:** 1000 IU[b]	In 30s and 60s.
otc	**Aquavit-E** (Cypress)	**Drops:** 15 IU[d] per 0.3 mL	In 30 mL.
otc	**Vitamin E** (Freeda)	**Liquid:** 15 IU[b] per 30 mL	In 30, 60, and 120 mL.
otc *sf*	**Nutr-E-Sol** (Advanced Nutritional Technology)	Liquid: 798 IU[b] per 30 mL	Dye free. In 473 mL.

[a] As d-alpha tocopherol.
[b] Form of vitamin E unknown; content given in IU.
[c] As d-alpha tocopheryl acetate.
[d] As dL-alpha tocopheryl acetate.

Indications

Treatment of vitamin E deficiency.

➤*Unlabeled uses:* Vitamin E has been used in certain premature infants to reduce the toxic effects of oxygen therapy on the lung parenchyma (bronchopulmonary dysplasia) and the retina (retrolental fibroplasia). It has been investigated for the prevention of periventricular hemorrhage in premature infants.

It has also been used in cancer, skin conditions, sexual dysfunction, to reduce the incidence of nonfatal MI, to lower the incidence of coronary artery disease, aging, fibrocystic breast disease (cystic mastitis), to treat dapsone-associated hemolysis, arthritis, and tardive dyskinesia. Use of vitamin E in combination with vitamin A has been reported in the treatment of keratosis follicularis (Darier disease), pityriasis rubra pilaris, ichthyosis, and acne. Use of vitamin E (400 IU) in combination with vitamin C (1 g/day) has resulted in significant risk reduction for preeclampsia during the second half of pregnancy.

Administration and Dosage

➤*Recommended dietary allowances (RDAs):* Adult males, 15 IU; adult females, 12 IU. For a complete listing of RDAs by age, sex, and condition, refer to the RDA table.

The potencies of the several forms of vitamin E vary; therefore, dosage is usually standardized in International Units (IU), based on activity. The following table indicates the relative potency of 1 mg of the various forms of vitamin E available:

Relative Potencies of Vitamin E	
1 mg dL-alpha tocopheryl acetate = 1 IU	1 mg d-alpha tocopherol = 1.49 IU
1 mg dL-alpha tocopherol = 1.1 IU	1 mg d-alpha tocopheryl acid succinate = 1.21 IU
1 mg d-alpha tocopheryl acetate = 1.36 IU	1 mg dL-alpha tocopheryl acid succinate = 0.89 IU

➤*Storage/Stability:* Free tocopherols can be oxidized and destroyed under adverse conditions; the esters available, acetate and succinate, are very stable in light. Keep in dry, airtight container.

Actions

➤*Pharmacology:* Vitamin E is a fat-soluble vitamin with actions related to its antioxidant properties. Vitamin E protects cellular constituents from oxidation and prevents the formation of toxic oxidation products; it preserves red blood cell (RBC) wall integrity and protects RBCs against hemolysis; it stimulates a cofactor in steroid metabolism; inhibits prostaglandin production; and suppresses platelet aggregation. In combination with selenium, vitamin E protects cell membranes from oxidative damage.

There are 8 naturally occurring compounds with vitamin E activity; 4 are tocopherols and 4 are tocotrienols. Free d-alpha tocopherol is the most biologically active form of vitamin E. One IU of vitamin E activity is equivalent to 1 mg all-*rac*-α-tocopheryl acetate. Normal plasma levels of vitamin E are between 1 and 3 mg/dL in low-birth-weight infants. Infants receiving either oral or parenteral vitamin E should maintain serum vitamin levels < 3.5 mg/dL. Sources of vitamin E include vegetables, oils, seeds, corn, soy, whole wheat flour, margarine, nuts, leafy vegetables, milk, eggs, and meats.

Deficiency – Clinical deficiency of vitamin E is rare because adequate amounts are supplied in the normal diet.

Symptoms of deficiency include ataxia, muscle weakness, nystagmus, and losses in touch and pain sensations. Low tocopherol levels have been noted in the following: Premature infants; malnourished infants with macrocyticanemia; prolonged fat malabsorption (ie, cystic fibrosis, hepatic cirrhosis, sprue); malabsorption syndromes (ie, celiac disease, GI resections); patients with abetalipoproteinemia. Vitamin E deficiency in premature infants may result in hemolytic anemia, thrombocytosis, and increased platelet aggregation. Vitamin E levels < 0.5 mg/dL are suggestive of a deficiency.

Vitamin E requirements – The daily vitamin E requirement is related to the dietary intake of polyunsaturated fatty acids (PUFA), primarily linoleic acid. Vitamin E requirements may be increased in patients taking large doses of iron. Commercial infant formulas currently available provide an adequate ratio of vitamin E to PUFA; formulas for premature infants have a lower level of iron to preclude interference with vitamin E use. Thus, there is no longer a need to routinely administer vitamin E supplementation to prevent anemia.

➤*Pharmacokinetics:*

Absorption/Distribution – Vitamin E is 20% to 50% absorbed by intestinal epithelial cells in the small intestine. Bile and pancreatic juice are needed for tocopherol absorption. Absorption is increased when administered with medium-chain triglycerides. Distribution to tissues via the lymphatic system occurs as a lipoprotein complex. High concentrations of vitamin E are found in the adrenals, pituitary, testes, and thrombocytes.

Metabolism/Excretion – Vitamin E is stored unmodified in tissues (principally the liver and adipose tissue) and excreted via the feces. Excess vitamin E is converted to a lactone, esterified to glucuronic acid, and subsequently excreted in the urine.

Contraindications

Vitamin E should not be administered IV because a high mortality rate has been assoicated with 38 infant deaths.

Drug Interactions

Vitamin E Drug Interactions			
Precipitant drug	Object drug[*]		Description
Vitamin E	Anticoagulants, oral Warfarin	⬆	Vitamin E in high doses (> 4000 IU) may increase the hypoprothrombinemic effects of oral anticoagulants.
Vitamin E	Iron	⬇	Vitamin E may impair the hematologic response to iron therapy in children with iron-deficiency anemia.

[*] ⬆ = Object drug increased. ⬇ = Object drug decreased.

Adverse Reactions

Hypervitaminosis E (see Overdosage).

VITAMIN E

Overdosage

Doses < 2000 IU are not likely to cause side effects. However, large doses (> 3000 IU) have been noted to produce symptoms of hypervitaminosis E, which include nausea, weakness, intestinal cramps, headache, flatulence, diarrhea, thrombophlebitis, pulmonary embolism, severe fatigue syndrome, gynecomastia, breast tumors, increased cholesterol and triglycerides, decrease in serum thyroid hormone, and altered immunity. Doses < 2000 IU are unlikely to cause side effects. Sepsis and necrotizing enterocolitis have been reported when vitamin E levels are maintained at 5 mg/dL in low-birth-weight infants.

Patient Information

Swallow capsules whole; do not crush or chew.

VITAMIN K
PHYTONADIONE

Rx	Mephyton (Merck)	Tablets: 5 mg	Lactose. (MSD 43 Mephyton). Yellow, scored. In 100s.
Rx	AquaMEPHYTON (Merck)	Injection (aqueous colloidal solution): 2 mg per mL	In 0.5 mL amps.[a]
Rx	Phytonadione (IMS)		In 0.5 mL *Min-I-ject* prefilled syringes.

[a] With polyoxyethylated fatty acid derivative, dextrose, and benzyl alcohol.

> ### WARNING
>
> *IV use:* Severe reactions, including fatalities, have occurred during and immediately after IV injection, even with precautions to dilute the injection and to avoid rapid infusion. These severe reactions resemble hypersensitivity or anaphylaxis, including shock and cardiac or respiratory arrest. Some patients exhibit these severe reactions on receiving vitamin K for the first time. Therefore, restrict the IV route to those situations where other routes are not feasible and the serious risk involved is justified.

Indications

➤*Coagulation disorders:* Coagulation disorders caused by faulty formation of factors II, VII, IX and X when caused by vitamin K deficiency or interference with vitamin K activity.

➤*Oral:* Anticoagulant-induced prothrombin deficiency (see Warnings); hypoprothrombinemia secondary to salicylates or antibacterial therapy; hypoprothrombinemia secondary to obstructive jaundice and biliary fistulas, but only if bile salts are administered concomitantly with phytonadione.

➤*Parenteral:* Anticoagulant-induced prothrombin deficiency; hypoprothrombinemia secondary to conditions limiting absorption or synthesis of vitamin K (eg, obstructive jaundice, biliary fistula, sprue, ulcerative colitis, celiac disease, intestinal resection, cystic fibrosis of the pancreas, regional enteritis); drug-induced hypoprothrombinemias due to interference with vitamin K metabolism (eg, antibiotics, salicylates); prophylaxis and therapy of hemorrhagic disease of the newborn.

Administration and Dosage

If possible, discontinue or reduce the dosage of drugs interfering with coagulation mechanisms (eg, salicylates, antibiotics) as an alternative to phytonadione. The severity of the coagulation disorder should determine whether the immediate administration of phytonadione is required in addition to discontinuation or reduction of interfering drugs.

Inject SC or IM when possible. In older children and adults, inject IM in the upper outer quadrant of the buttocks. In infants and young children, the anterolateral aspect of the thigh or the deltoid region is preferred. When IV administration is unavoidable, inject very slowly, not exceeding 1 mg/minute.

➤*Anticoagulant-induced prothrombin deficiency in adults:* 2.5 to 10 mg or up to 25 mg (rarely, 50 mg) initially. Determine subsequent doses by PT response or clinical condition. If in 6 to 8 hours after parenteral administration (or 12 to 48 hours after oral administration) the PT has not been shortened satisfactorily, repeat dose. If shock or excessive blood loss occurs, transfusion of blood or fresh frozen plasma may be required.

➤*Hemorrhagic disease of the newborn:*

Prophylaxis – Single IM dose of 0.5 to 1 mg within 1 hour after birth. This may be repeated after 2 to 3 weeks if the mother has received anticoagulant, anticonvulsant, antituberculosal or recent antibiotic therapy during her pregnancy. Twelve to 24 hours before delivery, 1 to 5 mg may be given to the mother.

Oral doses of 2 mg are adequate for prophylaxis.

Treatment – 1 mg SC or IM. Higher doses may be necessary if the mother has been receiving oral anticoagulants. Empiric administration of vitamin K_1 should not replace proper laboratory evaluation. A prompt response (shortening of the PT in 2 to 4 hours) is usually diagnostic of hemorrhagic disease of the newborn; failure to respond indicates another diagnosis or coagulation disorder. Give blood or blood products such as fresh frozen plasma if bleeding is excessive. This therapy does not correct the underlying disorder; give phytonadione concurrently.

➤*Hypoprothrombinemia due to other causes in adults:* 2.5 to 25 mg (rarely, up to 50 mg); amount and route of administration depends on severity of condition and response obtained. Avoid oral route when clinical disorder would prevent proper absorption. Give bile salts with tablets when endogenous supply of bile to GI tract is deficient.

➤*Storage/Stability:* Protect from light at all times.

Actions

➤*Pharmacology:* Vitamin K promotes the hepatic synthesis of active prothrombin (factor II), proconvertin (factor VII), plasma thromboplastin component (factor IX) and Stuart factor (factor X). The mechanism by which vitamin K promotes formation of these clotting factors involves the hepatic post-translational carboxylation of specific glutamate residues to gamma-carboxylglutamate residues in proteins involved in coagulation, thus leading to their activation.

Phytonadione (vitamin K_1) is a lipid-soluble synthetic analog of vitamin K. Phytonadione possesses essentially the same type and degree of activity as the naturally occurring vitamin K.

➤*Pharmacokinetics:* Phytonadione is only absorbed from the GI tract via intestinal lymphatics in the presence of bile salts. Although initially concentrated in the liver, vitamin K is rapidly metabolized and very little tissue accumulation occurs. Little is known about the metabolic fate of vitamin K. Almost no free unmetabolized vitamin K appears in bile or urine.

Parenteral phytonadione is generally detectable within 1 to 2 hours. Phytonadione usually controls hemorrhage within 3 to 6 hours. A normal prothrombin level may be obtained in 12 to 14 hours. Oral phytonadione exerts its effect in 6 to 10 hours.

The US daily allowances – The US daily allowances for vitamin K have not been officially established, but have been estimated to be 10 to 20 mcg for infants, 15 to 100 mcg for children and adolescents and 70 to 140 mcg for adults. Usually, dietary vitamin K will satisfy these requirements, except during the first 5 to 8 days of the neonatal period. Naturally occurring vitamin K is found in various foods, including cabbage, cauliflower, kale, spinach, fish, liver, eggs, meats, cereal grain products, fruits and milk and dairy products.

Recommended Dietary Allowances as published by the National Academy of Sciences are as follows: Adult males, 45 to 80 mcg/day; adult females, 45 to 65 mcg/day. For a complete listing of RDA by age, sex or condition, refer to the RDA table in the Nutritionals chapter.

Contraindications

Hypersensitivity to any component of the product.

Warnings

➤*Oral anticoagulant-induced hypoprothrombinemia: Vitamin K will not counteract the anticoagulant action of heparin.*

Phytonadione promotes synthesis of prothrombin by the liver. Immediate coagulant effect should not be expected. It takes a minimum of 1 to 2 hours for a measurable improvement in the prothrombin time (PT). The prothrombin test is sensitive to the levels of factors II, VII and X. Fresh plasma or blood transfusions may be required for severe blood loss or lack of response to vitamin K.

With phytonadione use and anticoagulant therapy indicated, the patient is faced with the same clotting hazards prior to starting anticoagulant therapy. Phytonadione is not a clotting agent, but overzealous therapy may restore original thromboembolic phenomena conditions. Keep dosage as low as possible and check PT regularly.

➤*Hepatic function impairment:* Hypoprothrombinemia due to hepatocellular damage is not corrected by administration of vitamin K. Repeated large doses of vitamin K are not warranted in liver disease if the initial response is unsatisfactory (Koller test). Failure to respond to vitamin K may indicate a coagulation defect or a condition unresponsive to vitamin K. In hepatic disease, large doses may further depress liver function.

Paradoxically, giving excessive doses of vitamin K or its analogs in an attempt to correct hypoprothrombinemia associated with severe hepatitis or cirrhosis may actually result in further depression of the prothrombin concentration.

➤*Pregnancy: Category C.* Vitamin K crosses the placenta. It is not known whether vitamin K can cause fetal harm when administered to

Fat Soluble Vitamins

PHYTONADIONE

a pregnant woman or can affect reproduction capacity. Use only if clearly needed.

➤*Lactation:* Vitamin K is excreted in breast milk. Consider this if the drug must be used in a nursing mother.

➤*Children:* Safety and efficacy in children have not been established. Hemolysis, jaundice and hyperbilirubinemia in newborns, particularly in premature infants, have been reported with vitamin K. These effects may be dose-related. Therefore, do not exceed recommended dose.

Precautions

➤*Benzyl alcohol:* Benzyl alcohol contained in some products has been associated with toxicity in newborns. Specific products containing benzyl alcohol are identified in the product listings.

Drug Interactions

Vitamin K Drug Interactions			
Precipitant drug	Object drug*		Description
Vitamin K	Anticoagulants	↓	Anticoagulant effects are antagonized by vitamin K. Temporary resistance to oral anticoagulants may result. It may be necessary to increase the anticoagulant dose.

Vitamin K Drug Interactions			
Precipitant drug	Object drug*		Description
Mineral oil	Vitamin K	↓	Mineral oil may decrease GI absorption of vitamin K with concurrent oral administration.

* ↓ = Object drug decreased.

Adverse Reactions

➤*Allergic:* Anaphylactoid reactions may occur.

➤*Miscellaneous:*

Parenteral administration – Rarely, pain, swelling and tenderness at the injection site; after repeated injections, erythematous, indurated pruritic plaques have occurred. These have rarely progressed to scleroderma-like lesions that have persisted for long periods. In other cases, these lesions have resembled erythema perstans.

Transient "flushing sensations" and "peculiar" sensations of taste; rarely, dizziness, rapid and weak pulse, profuse sweating, brief hypotension, dyspnea and cyanosis.

Hyperbilirubinemia: Hyperbilirubinemia has been observed in the newborn following administration of phytonadione. This has occurred rarely and primarily with doses above those recommended (see Warnings).

Deaths have occurred after IV administration (see Warning box).

Water-Soluble Vitamins

THIAMIN (B₁)

otc	Thiamine HCl (Various, eg, Goldline, Rugby)	**Tablets**: 50 mg	In 100s and 250s.
		100 mg	In 100s, 250s, 1000s, and UD 100s.
		250 mg	In 100s, 250s.
otc	Thiamilate (Tyson)	**Tablets, enteric-coated**: 20 mg	In 100s.
Rx	Thiamine HCl (Various, eg, American Pharmaceutical Partners, ESI)	**Injection**: 100 mg/mL	≤ 9 mg benzyl alcohol. In 1 mL in 2 mL *Tubex* and 2 mL multiple-dose vials.

Indications

➤*Thiamin deficiency:* Treatment of thiamin deficiency.

➤*Parenteral:* When the oral route is not feasible (eg, severe anorexia, nausea, vomiting) or malabsorption; beriberi.

➤*Unlabeled uses:* Oral thiamin has been studied as a mosquito repellant; further verification is needed.

Administration and Dosage

➤*Recommended dietary allowances (RDAs):* Adult males, 1.2 to 1.5 mg/day; adult females, 1 to 1.1 mg/day. Thiamin is recommended at 0.5 mg/1000 Kcal intake. The need for thiamin is greater when the carbohydrate content of the diet is high. For a complete listing of RDAs by age, sex, and condition, refer to the RDA table.

➤*Thiamin deficiency:* IV doses as large as 100 mg/L to correct the deficiency as rapidly as possible. Continue parenteral doses at daily requirements only when GI disturbances prevent adequate oral absorption.

➤*Wet beriberi with myocardial failure:* Treat as an emergency cardiac condition. Administer slowly.

➤*Beriberi:* 10 to 20 mg IM 3 times/day for 2 weeks. Give an oral therapeutic multivitamin containing 5 to 10 mg thiamin daily for 1 month to achieve body tissue saturation.

Infantile beriberi – Mild infantile beriberi may respond to oral therapy. If collapse occurs, cautiously administer doses of 25 mg IV.

➤*Neuritis of pregnancy:* Patients with neuritis of pregnancy in whom vomiting is severe enough to preclude oral therapy should receive 5 to 10 mg/day IM.

➤*Wernicke-Korsakoff syndrome:* In the treatment of Wernicke-Korsakoff syndrome, administer an initial dose of 100 mg IV, followed by 50 to 100 mg/day IM until the patient is consuming a regular, balanced diet.

➤*Dextrose and patients with marginal thiamin status:* Patients with marginal thiamin status to whom dextrose is being administered should receive 100 mg in each of the first few liters of IV fluid to avoid precipitating heart failure.

➤*Incompatibility:* Vitamin B₁ is unstable in neutral or alkaline solutions; do not use in combination with alkaline solutions (eg, carbonates, citrates, barbiturates, acetates, copper ions). Solutions containing sulfites are incompatible with thiamin as are other oxidizing and reducing agents. In vitro testing of thiamin 0.1% reduced activity of erythromycin estolate, kanamycin sulfate, and streptomycin sulfate.

Actions

➤*Pharmacology:* Thiamin is a water-soluble vitamin. Sources include brewer's yeast, legumes, beef, pork, milk, liver, nuts, whole grains, enriched flour, and cereals. The primary functions of thiamin include metabolism of carbohydrates, maintenance of normal growth, transmission of nerve impulses, and acetylcholine synthesis.

Thiamin is essential for normal aerobic metabolism. Thiamin combines with adenosine triphosphate (ATP) and the enzyme thiamin diphosphokinase to form thiamin pyrophosphate, a coenzyme also known as cocarboxylase. Thiamin pyrophosphate is the active form of thiamin. It serves as a coenzyme in the carbohydrate metabolism for the decarboxylation of α keto acids (such as pyruvate) and α-ketoglutarate, as well as serving for the activity of transketolase in the pentose phosphate pathway.

Deficiency – Significant B₁ depletion can occur after 3 weeks of total thiamin dietary absence. Signs of deficiency include an increase in serum pyruvic acid. Causes of thiamin deficiency include excessive alcohol intake, long-term dialysis, decreased absorption of nutrients, excessive carbohydrate intake, excessive coffee and tea intake, anorexia, diarrhea, biliary disease, liver dysfunction, infection, hyperthyroidism, and decreased activation of thiamin pyrophosphate.

Beriberi: Beriberi is characterized by peripheral neuritis, which includes sensory disturbances in the extremities, loss of muscle strength, muscle wasting (dry beriberi), tachycardia, and an enlarged heart. Wet beriberi includes cardiovascular symptoms characterized by dyspnea on exertion, palpitations, ECG abnormalities, high-output cardiac failure, and edema. Infantile beriberi includes cardiac involvement, loss of appetite, vomiting, aphonia, and greenish stools followed by paroxysmal attacks of muscular rigidity.

Lactic acidosis: Lactic acidosis has been reported due to thiamin deficiency. A lack of thiamin pyrophosphate as a cofactor to catalyze the oxidative decarboxylation of pyruvate to acetyl coenzyme A (CoA) results in excess pyruvate. As a result, excess pyruvate is converted to lactate by lactate dehydrogenase. Release of hydrogen ions equal to the number of lactate molecules produced through hydrolysis of adenosine triphosphate during anaerobic glycolysis may result in acidosis.

Wernicke-Korsakoff syndrome: Wernicke-Korsakoff syndrome (Wernicke's disease or encephalopathy and Korsakoff's psychosis) is characterized by eye muscle paralysis, horizontal nystagmus, bilateral sixth nerve palsy, ataxia, ophthalmoplegia, and confusion. Conditions associated with development include severe thiamin deficiency, excessive alcohol consumption, prolonged IV feeding, hyperemesis gravidarum, anorexia nervosa, prolonged fasting, refeeding after starvation, and gastric plication.

➤*Pharmacokinetics:*

Absorption/Distribution – Thiamin is absorbed by a Na+ dependent active, carrier-mediated process at low concentrations in the jejunum and by passive diffusion in the jejunum and ileum at high concentrations. Maximum oral absorption is 8 to 15 mg/day. Oral absorption may be increased by administering in divided doses with food. Thiamin is mainly stored in the liver but is also found in the brain, kidney, heart, intestine, lung, spleen, and muscle. Tissue stores are saturated when intake exceeds the minimal requirement. For a complete listing of RDAs by age, sex, and condition, refer to the RDA table.

Metabolism/Excretion – Excess thiamin is excreted in the urine both as thiamin acetic acid and metabolites. Approximately 100 mcg/day of thiamin are excreted in the urine with a daily intake of 0.5 mg/1000 kcal. With normal renal function, 80% to 96% of an IV dose is excreted in the urine.

Contraindications

Hypersensitivity to thiamin.

Warnings

➤*Serious hypersensitivity/anaphylactic reactions:* Serious hypersensitivity/anaphylactic reactions can occur. Deaths have resulted from IV or IM use. An IV test dose is recommended in patients with suspected sensitivity.

➤*Wernicke's-Korsakoff syndrome:* Thiamin-deficient patients may experience a sudden onset or worsening of Wernicke's encephalopathy following glucose administration; in suspected thiamin deficiency, administer thiamin before or along with dextrose-containing fluids.

➤*Deficiency:* Simple vitamin B₁ deficiency is rare. Suspect multiple vitamin deficiencies.

➤*Pregnancy:* Category A (parenteral). (*Category C* if used in doses greater than the RDA). Studies have not shown an increased risk of fetal abnormalities if administered during pregnancy. The possibility of fetal harm appears remote; however, use during pregnancy only if clearly needed.

➤*Lactation:* It is not known whether this drug is excreted in breast milk. Use with caution in nursing women.

Adverse Reactions

Feeling of warmth; pruritus; urticaria; weakness; sweating; nausea; restlessness; tightness of the throat; angioneurotic edema; cyanosis; pulmonary edema; hemorrhage into the GI tract; cardiovascular collapse; hypersensitivity; anaphylactic shock; death.

Parenteral – Some tenderness and induration may follow IM use.

Overdosage

➤*Oral:* Hypersensitivity; anaphylactic shock. Doses of 500 mg/day for a month were administered without toxic effects.

➤*Parenteral:* Hypersensitivity; anaphylactic shock. Single parenteral doses of 100 to 500 mg have been administered without toxic effects.

Water-Soluble Vitamins

RIBOFLAVIN (B$_2$)

otc	**Riboflavin** (Various, eg, Freeda)	**Tablets**: 50 mg	In 100s and 250s.
		100 mg	In 100s and 250s.

Indications

➤*Riboflavin deficiency:* Treatment and prevention of riboflavin deficiency.

➤*Unlabeled uses:* Lactic acidosis (with hepatic steatosis) in AIDS patients taking nucleoside reverse-transcriptase inhibitors (NRTI) has been successfully treated with riboflavin 50 mg.

Administration and Dosage

➤*Recommended Dietary Allowances (RDAs):* Males, 1.4 to 1.8 mg; females, 1.2 to 1.3 mg. For a complete listing of RDAs by age, sex, or condition, refer to the RDA table.

➤*Treatment of deficiency states:* 5 to 10 mg/day.

➤*Total parenteral nutrition:*
>11 years old – 3.6 mg/day
1 to 11 years old – 1.4 mg/day.

Actions

➤*Pharmacology:* Riboflavin is a water-soluble vitamin that functions as 2 coenzymes. Flavin adenine dinucleotide (FAD) and flavin mononucleotide (FMN) catalyze many oxidation-reduction reactions including glucose oxidation, amino acid deamination, and fatty acid breakdown. Sources of riboflavin include meats, poultry, fish, dairy products, broccoli, turnips, asparagus, spinach, and enriched and fortified grains, cereals, and bakery products.

Deficiency – Early symptoms of riboflavin deficiency include sore throat and angular stomatitis. Other symptoms include achlorhydria, scrotal and vulval skin changes, normocytic anemia, corneal vascularization, cataract formation, cheilosis, glossitis, and seborrheic dermatitis. Riboflavin deficiency is marked by a decrease in the erythrocyte-glutathione-reductase enzyme activity coefficient. Causes of deficiency may include inadequate dietary intake, malabsorption syndrome, or alcohol.

➤*Pharmacokinetics:* Riboflavin is absorbed from the duodenum and is excreted with its metabolites in the urine. Small amounts of riboflavin are also excreted in the bile, feces, and sweat.

Warnings

➤*Pregnancy:* Category A. (*Category C* in doses that exceed the RDA.)

➤*Lactation:* Riboflavin is excreted in breast milk.

Precautions

➤*Deficiency:* Riboflavin deficiency seldom occurs alone and is often associated with deficiency of other vitamin deficiencies.

Overdosage

Riboflavin is not toxic in humans because of the limited absorption from the GI tract.

Patient Information

Riboflavin may cause a yellow discoloration of the urine when taken in large doses.

PANTOTHENIC ACID (B$_5$)

otc	**Calcium Pantothenate** (Various, eg, Freeda)	**Tablets**: 100 mg (equiv. to 92 mg pantothenic acid)	In 100s and 250s.
		218 mg (equiv. to 200 mg pantothenic acid)	In 100s and 250s.
		545 mg (equiv. to 500 mg pantothenic acid)	In 100s and 250s.

Indications

➤*Pantothenic acid deficiency:* Treatment of pantothenic acid deficiency.

Administration and Dosage

An approximate daily dietary intake of 4 to 7 mg/day has been recommended for adults.

➤*Total parenteral nutrition:*
> 11 years of age – 15 mg.
1 to 11 years of age – 5 mg.

Actions

➤*Pharmacology:* Pantothenic acid is a water-soluble vitamin. Pantothenic acid is a precursor of coenzyme A, which is a cofactor for a variety of enzyme-catalyzed reactions involving transfer of acetyl groups. Functions of pantothenic acid include oxidative metabolism of carbohydrates, gluconeogensis, synthesis and degradation of fatty acids, and synthesis of steroids (cholesterol), steroid hormones, sphingosine, citrate, acetoacetate, and porphyrins. Sources of pantothenic acid include meat, poultry, fish, cereals, fruits, vegetables, milk, and egg yolks.

Deficiency – Deficiency includes neuromuscular degeneration and adrenocortical insufficiency. Pantothenic acid deficiency has not been recognized in humans with a normal diet because of the ubiquitous occurrence of this vitamin in ordinary foods. Deficiency typically is seen only with severe multiple B-complex deficiencies. However, a deficiency syndrome was experimentally induced in volunteers. Symptoms included fatigue, headache, sleep disturbances, abdominal cramps, vomiting, and flatulence. Paresthesias in the extremities, muscle cramps, and impaired coordination also occurred. A total whole blood level of pantothenic acid < 100 mcg/dL is suggestive of inadequate dietary intake.

➤*Pharmacokinetics:* Pantothenic acid is absorbed from the GI tract and is distributed to all tissues. Approximately 70% of absorbed pantothenic acid is excreted in the urine.

Warnings

➤*Pregnancy:* Category A. (*Category C* in doses that exceed the RDA.) The RDA for pantothenic acid in pregnancy is 10 mg.

➤*Lactation:* Pantothenic acid is excreted in breast milk.

Overdosage

Nontoxic in humans. Diarrhea has been reported with 10 to 20 g/day of calcium pantothenate.

NIACIN (B$_3$; Nicotinic Acid)

otc[1]	**Nicotinic Acid (Niacin)** (Various, eg, Freeda, Goldline)	**Tablets**: 50 mg	In 100s and 250s.
otc[1]	**Nicotinic Acid (Niacin)** (Various, eg, Freeda, Goldline)	**Tablets**: 100 mg	In 100s and 250s.
otc[1]	**Nicotinic Acid (Niacin)** (Various, eg, Goldline)	**Tablets**: 250 mg	In 100s.
otc[1]	**Nicotinic Acid (Niacin)** (Various, eg, Freeda, Goldline)	**Tablets**: 500 mg	In 100s and 1000s.
otc[1]	**Nicotinic Acid (Niacin)** (Various, eg, Freeda)	**Tablets, timed-release**: 250 mg	In 100s and 250s.
otc[1]	**Nicotinic Acid (Niacin)** (Various, eg, Goldline)	**Tablets, timed-release**: 500 mg	In 100s and 1000s.
otc[1]	**Nicotinic Acid (Niacin)** (Various, eg, Naturally)	**Tablets, sustained-release**: 500 mg	In 100s.
otc *sf*	**Slo-Niacin** (Upsher-Smith)	**Tablets, controlled-release**: 250 mg	(250). Pink. In 100s.
		Tablets, controlled-release: 500 mg	(500). Pink. In 100s.
		Tablets, controlled-release: 750 mg	Pink. In 100s.
otc[1]	**Nicotinic Acid (Niacin)** (Various, eg, Rugby)	**Capsules, extended-release**: 250 mg	In 100s and 1000s.
otc[1]	**Nicotinic Acid (Niacin)** (Various, eg, Rugby)	**Capsules, extended-release**: 400 mg	In 100s.
otc[1]	**Nicotinic Acid (Niacin)** (Various, eg, Rugby)	**Capsules, sustained-release**: 125 mg	In 100s.
Rx	**Nicotinic Acid (Niacin)** (Various, eg, Rugby)	**Capsules, sustained-release**: 500 mg	In 100s.
Rx	**Niacor** (Upsher-Smith)		(W 901). White, scored. Biconvex. In 100s.

Water-Soluble Vitamins

NIACIN (B₃; Nicotinic Acid)

otc[1]	**Nicotinic Acid (Niacin)** (Various, eg, Goldline, Rugby)	**Capsules, timed-release** : 250 mg	In 100s.
Rx	**Nicotinic Acid (Niacin)** (Various, eg, Goldline, Rugby)	**Capsules, timed-release**: 500 mg	In 100s and 1000s.

[1] Some products may be available *Rx*, according to distributor discretion.

Refer to the Nicotinamide monograph for additional information.

Indications

➤*Niacin deficiency:* Treatment of niacin deficiency.

➤*Pellagra:* Prevention and treatment of pellagra.

➤*Hypercholesterolemia:* Adjunct to diet for the reduction of elevated total and LDL levels in patients with primary hypercholesterolemia when the response to diet and other nonpharmacologic measures alone has been inadequate.

➤*Hyperlipidemia (Types IV and V):* Adjunct therapy in adult patients at risk of pancreatitis who do not respond adequately to dietary efforts.

Administration and Dosage

➤*Recommended Dietary Allowances (RDAs):* Adult males, 15 to 20 mg; adult females, 13 to 15 mg. Niacin is recommended at 6.6 mg/1000 Kcal intake. For a complete listing of RDA by age, sex, or condition, refer to the RDA table.

The following prescribing information pertains primarily to therapeutic uses of niacin in doses exceeding basic nutritional intake (RDA levels).

➤*Oral:* To reduce flushing, begin therapy by slowly increasing the dose (100 mg 3 times a day each week).

Pellagra – Up to 500 mg/day.

Hyperlipidemia – 1 to 2 g 2 or 3 times daily. Do not exceed 6 g/day.

Sustained-release – Do not substitute sustained-release (modified-release, timed-release) nicotinic acid preparations for equivalent doses of immediate-release (crystalline) nicotinic acid.

➤*Parenteral:* Use only for vitamin deficiencies (not for treatment of hyperlipidemia) and when oral therapy is not appropriate.

➤*Pellagra:* 25 mg IV ≥ 2 times daily.

Actions

➤*Pharmacology:* Niacin, vitamin B₃, is the common name for nicotinic acid and niacinamide (nicotinamide). Nicotinic acid is present in the body as its active form, nicotinamide (niacinamide). Nicotinamide functions in the body as a component of 2 coenzymes: NAD (nicotinamide adenine dinucleotide, coenzyme I) and NADP (nicotinamide adenine dinucleotide phosphate, coenzyme II), which serve a role in oxidation-reduction reactions. Sources of niacin include niacinamide and tryptophan as well as liver, meat, fish, poultry, whole-grain and enriched breads and cereals, nuts, legumes, green vegetables, yeast, and potatoes. Approximately 60 mg of tryptophan is equivalent to 1 mg of niacin.

Deficiency – Pellagra is a state of niacin deficiency characterized by mucous membrane, GI, and CNS manifestations, a triad often referred to as dermatitis, diarrhea, and dementia. In severe cases, confusion, delusions, disorientation, and hallucinations may occur. In addition to nutritional deficiency, pellagra may also be seen in chronic alcoholism, malabsorption syndromes, patients receiving isoniazid, as part of Hartnup disease (impaired tryptophan transport), or in patients with carcinoid tumors where tryptophan is used for serotonin synthesis. Pellagra that does not respond to niacin therapy may be associated with thiamin, riboflavin, or pyridoxine deficiency. In adults, niacin deficiency is noted as a ratio of urinary 2-pyridoxine to N-methylnicotinamide < 1.

Although nicotinic acid and nicotinamide function identically as vitamins, their pharmacologic effects differ. In large doses (up to 6 g/day), nicotinic acid is effective in reducing serum lipids (LDL, HDL, triglycerides, and lipoprotein A; see Antihyperlipidemic Agents introduction). The mechanism of this action may involve decreased production of VLDL. In large doses, peripheral vasodilation is produced, predominantly in the cutaneous vessels of the face, neck, and chest. Nicotinic acid produces vasodilation and increased blood flow due to histamine release. Nicotinamide does not affect blood lipid levels or the cardiovascular system.

➤*Pharmacokinetics:* Niacin is rapidly absorbed from the GI tract; peak serum concentrations usually occur within 45 minutes. The plasma elimination half-life is ≈ 45 minutes. Major metabolites include nicotinuric acid, N-methylnicotinamide, and 2-pyridone. Approximately ⅓ of an oral dose is excreted unchanged in the urine.

Contraindications

Hepatic dysfunction; active peptic ulcer; arterial bleeding; hypersensitivity to niacin or any ingredient.

Warnings

➤*Alcohol:* Use with caution in patients who consume substantial quantities of alcohol or have a history of liver disease.

➤*Schizophrenia:* There is no evidence to support the use of nicotinic acid in the treatment of schizophrenia as part of what is referred to as "orthomolecular psychiatry."

➤*Heart disease:* People with heart disease, particularly those who have recurrent chest pain (angina) or who recently suffered a heart attack, should take niacin only under the supervision of a physician.

➤*Pregnancy: Category A. (Category C if used in doses above the RDA).* It is not known whether nicotinic acid at doses typically used for lipid disorders can cause fetal harm when administered to pregnant women. If a woman receiving nicotinic acid for primary hypercholesterolemia (Types IIa or IIb) becomes pregnant, discontinue the drug. If a woman being treated with nicotinic acid for hypertriglyceridemia (Types IV or V) conceives, assess the benefits and risks of continued drug therapy on an individual basis.

➤*Lactation:* Niacin is actively excreted in breast milk.

➤*Children:* Safety and efficacy in children have not been established in doses that exceed the RDA.

Precautions

➤*Monitoring:* Frequently monitor liver function tests and blood glucose.

Closely observe patients with gallbladder disease, a history of jaundice, glaucoma, hepatobiliary disease, liver disease, peptic ulcer, or arterial bleeding. Use caution when nicotinic acid is used in patients with unstable angina or in the acute phase of MI, particularly when such patients are also receiving vasoactive drugs such as nitrates, calcium channel blockers, or adrenergic blocking agents.

➤*Diabetes:* Observe diabetic or borderline diabetic patients closely for decreased glucose tolerance. Adjustment of diet or hypoglycemic therapy may be necessary.

➤*Gout:* Elevated uric acid levels have occurred; use caution in patients predisposed to gout.

➤*Flushing:* Flushing appears frequently with oral therapy and generally begins 20 minutes after ingestion and lasts 30 to 60 minutes. Flushing is transient and will usually subside after 3 to 6 weeks of continued therapy. The flush response can be attenuated by slowly increasing the niacin dose (100 mg 3 times daily each week), administering with food or milk, or by administering either a prostaglandin inhibitor, such as aspirin 325 mg 60 minutes prior to niacin administration, or sustained-release niacin preparations.

Drug Interactions

➤*HMG-CoA reductase inhibitors:* Coadministration of niacin and HMG-CoA reductase inhibitors (eg, lovastatin) may result in myopathy and rhabdomyolysis.

Adverse Reactions

Flushing (see Precautions), pruritus, and GI distress appear frequently with nicotinic acid oral therapy.

➤*Dermatologic:* Severe generalized flushing; sensation of warmth; acanthosis nigricans; pruritus; skin rash; dry skin; itching; tingling.

➤*GI:* Activation of peptic ulcer; nausea; vomiting; abdominal pain; diarrhea; dyspepsia.

Nicotinic acid hepatotoxicity (including cholestatic jaundice) has occurred with as little as 750 mg/day for < 3 months with either immediate- or sustained-release nicotinic acid. Crystalline (non-sustained-release) niacin may be less hepatotoxic. Cases of severe hepatic toxicity, including fulminant hepatic necrosis have occurred in patients who have substituted sustained-release (modified-release, timed-release) nicotinic acid products for immediate-release (crystalline) nicotinic acid at equivalent doses. Monitor ALT prior to treatment, every 6 to 12 weeks during the first year, and periodically thereafter (≈ 6-month intervals).

➤*Lab test abnormalities:* Decreased glucose tolerance; abnormalities of hepatic function tests; hyperuricemia; gout.

➤*Miscellaneous:* Toxic amblyopia; hypotension; transient headache; atrial fibrillation and other cardiac arrhythmias; cystoid macular edema; decreased glucose tolerance; orthostasis.

Patient Information

Cutaneous flushing and a sensation of warmth, especially in the face, may occur. Itching or tingling and headache may also occur. These effects are transient and will usually subside with continued therapy.

May cause GI upset; take with meals.

Discontinue use and consult a physician immediately if any of the following symptoms occur: Persistent flu-like symptoms (nausea, vomiting, a general "not well" feeling); loss of appetite; a decrease in urine output associated with dark-colored urine; muscle discomfort such as

Water-Soluble Vitamins

NIACIN (B$_3$; Nicotinic Acid)

tender, swollen muscles or muscle weakness; irregular heartbeat; or cloudy or blurry vision.

If dizziness (postural hypotension) occurs, avoid sudden changes in posture.

➤*Extended-release products:* Swallow whole; do not break, crush, or chew.

NIACINAMIDE (NICOTINAMIDE)

otc[1]	Niacinamide (Nicotinamide) (Various, eg, Freeda, Rugby)	**Tablets:** 100 mg	In 100s and 250s.
		500 mg	In 100s and 250s.

[1] Some products may be available *Rx*, according to distributor discretion.

For complete prescribing information, refer to the Niacin monograph.

Indications

➤*Pellagra:* Prophylaxis and treatment of pellagra.

➤*Unlabeled uses:* Treatment of several dermatologic conditions including necrobiosis lipoidica, erythema multiforme, dermatitis herpetiformis, erythema elevatum diutinum, polymorphic light eruption, erythema induratum, granuloma annulare, and psoriasis (500 mg 3 times daily).

Administration and Dosage

100 to 500 mg/day.

Actions

➤*Pharmacology:* Niacinamide is synonymous with nicotinamide, 3-pyridine carboxamide, and nicotinic acid amide. Niacinamide is the

amide of nicotinic acid (niacin, vitamin B$_3$). Nicotinamide functions as part of 2 coenzymes present in all cells, nicotinamide adenine dinucleotide (NAD) and nicotinamide adenine dinucleotide phosphate (NADP). These coenzymes participate in glycogenolysis, fatty acid metabolism, and tissue respiration. Although nicotinic acid and nicotinamide function identically as vitamins, their pharmacologic effects differ. Nicotinamide does not have the hypolipidemic or vasodilating effects characteristic of niacin (nicotinic acid). Nicotinamide has been shown to inhibit activated macrophage killing of beta cells in vitro and reduce induction of class II MHC protein on mouse beta cells.

Adverse Reactions

Liver dysfunction in high doses.

PYRIDOXINE HCl (B$_6$)

otc	Vitelle Nestrex (Fielding)	**Tablets:** 25 mg	Dextrose. In 100s.
otc	Vitamin B$_6$ (Various, eg, Freeda, Goldline, Nutro Labs)	**Tablets:** 50 mg	In 100s, 250s, and 1000s.
otc	Vitamin B$_6$ (Various, eg, Freeda, Goldline, Naturally)	**Tablets:** 100 mg	In 100s and 250s.
otc	Vitamin B$_6$ (Various, eg, Freeda)	**Tablets:** 250 mg	In 100s.
otc	Vitamin B$_6$ (Various, eg, Naturally)	**Tablets:** 500 mg	In 100s.
otc	Aminoxin (Tyson & Assoc.)	**Tablets, enteric-coated:** 20 mg[1]	In 100s.
Rx	Pyridoxine HCl (Various, eg, American Pharm. Assoc.)	**Injection:** 100 mg/mL[2]	In 1 mL vials.[3]

[1] As pyridoxal-5'-phosphate.
[2] As pyridoxine HCl.

[3] Also contains 5 mg chorobutanol anhydrous.

Indications

➤*Pyridoxine deficiency:* Treatment of pyridoxine deficiency, including drug-induced deficiency (eg, isoniazid, hydralazine, oral contraceptives).

➤*Unlabeled uses:*

Hydrazine poisoning – Although experience is limited, reversal of neurologic symptoms and CNS depression have been reported.

Premenstrual syndrome (PMS) – PMS has been treated with pyridoxine 40 to 500 mg/day, but with conflicting results.

Hyperoxaluria type I – Hyperoxaluria type I (and oxalate kidney stones) has been treated with pyridoxine in low doses (25 to 300 mg/day).

Nausea and vomiting in pregnancy – Pyridoxine may treat nausea and vomiting during pregnancy.

Carpal tunnel syndrome – 100 to 200 mg/day for ≥ 12 weeks.

Tardive dyskinesia induced by antipsychotic treatment – 100 mg/day for 4 weeks.

Administration and Dosage

➤*Recommended Dietary Allowances (RDAs):* Adult males, 1.7 to 2 mg; adult females, 1.4 to 1.6 mg. For a complete listing of RDAs by age, sex, and condition, see the RDA table.

➤*Vitamin B$_6$ dependency syndrome:* Dependence has been noted in adults administered 200 mg/day.

➤*Deficiencies due to isoniazid:* Some advocate pyridoxine prophylaxis for all isoniazid patients; others advocate prophylaxis only for those predisposed to neuropathy. Recommended prophylactic doses range from 6 to 100 mg/day, but the lower doses appear more common. Treatment of established neuropathy requires 50 to 200 mg/day.

Actions

➤*Pharmacology:* Pyridoxine, pyridoxal, or pyridoxamine (in animals) are converted to the physiologically active forms of vitamin B$_6$, pyridoxal phosphate and pyridoxamine phosphate. Pyridoxine requirements increase with increasing amounts of dietary protein.

Sources of vitamin B$_6$ include meat, liver, whole-grain breads and cereals, soybeans, vegetables, eggs, peanuts, walnuts, and corn.

Deficiency – Vitamin B$_6$ deficiency has been noted in pregnancy, uremia, liver disease, malignancies, and chronic alcoholism. Drugs that

may result in vitamin B$_6$ deficiency include the vitamin B$_6$ antagonist agents (isoniazid, cycloserine, penicillamine, hydralazine, and estrogen). Urinary excretion of 4-pyridoxic acid < 0.1 mg/24 hours is suggestive of a deficiency.

Dermatologic: Seborrheic dermatitis around the eyes, nose, and mouth; cheilosis; angular stomatitis.

Hematologic: Sideroblastic anemia. Also affects lymphocyte production and the antibody response to antigens.

Miscellaneous: Convulsions; irritability; peripheral neuropathy.

➤*Pharmacokinetics:*

Absorption/Distribution – Vitamin B$_6$ is absorbed by passive diffusion in the jejunum and to a lesser extent in the ileum.

Metabolism/Excretion – Vitamin B$_6$ is converted to pyridoxal-5-phosphate in the liver and excreted mostly as 4-pyridoxic acid in the urine.

Contraindications

Sensitivity to pyridoxine.

Warnings

➤*Pregnancy:* Category A. (*Category C* in doses that exceed the RDA.)

➤*Lactation:* Vitamin B$_6$ is excreted in breast milk and is directly proportional to maternal intake. Convulsions have been reported in infants fed a pyridoxine-deficient diet. Neonatal seizures have been noted following birth in a mother consuming pyridoxine 80 mg/day or in infants whose mothers' breast milk contained 67 mcg/day (< 20 ng/mL in a separate report). These seizures responded to pyridoxine therapy. Pyridoxine has been reported to inhibit lactation at oral doses of 600 mg/day.

➤*Children:* Safety and efficacy have not been established for use in children in doses that exceed the RDA.

Precautions

➤*Pyridoxine deficiency:* Pyridoxine deficiency alone is rare; multiple vitamin deficiencies can be expected in any inadequate diet. Some drugs may result in increased pyridoxine requirements, including the following: Cycloserine, hydralazine, isoniazid, oral contraceptives, and penicillamine.

➤*Drug abuse and dependence:* Noted in adults withdrawn from 200 mg/day.

Water-Soluble Vitamins

PYRIDOXINE HCl (B$_6$)

Drug Interactions

Pyridoxine Drug Interactions			
Precipitant drug	Object drug*		Description
Pyridoxine	Levodopa	↓	Pyridoxine reduces levodopa's effectiveness by increasing its peripheral metabolism; therefore, lower levels are available for CNS penetration.
Pyridoxine	Phenytoin	↓	Phenytoin serum levels may be decreased.

* ↓ = Object drug decreased.

Adverse Reactions

Sensory neuropathic syndromes; unstable gait; numb feet; awkwardness of hands; perioral numbness; decreased sensation to touch, temperature, and vibration; paresthesia; photoallergic reaction; ataxia.

Overdosage

Patients receiving 2 to 7 g/day (or > 0.2 g/day for > 2 months) have developed sensory neuropathy with associated ataxia and numbness of the hands and feet. When pyridoxine is discontinued, symptoms will lessen. It may take 6 months for sensation to normalize.

CYANOCOBALAMIN, ORAL (B$_{12}$)

otc	Vitamin B$_{12}$ (Various, eg, Apothecary, Goldline, Rugby)	Tablets: 100 mcg	In 100s.
otc	Vitamin B$_{12}$ (Various, eg, Goldline, Rugby)	Tablets: 500 mcg	In 100s.
		1000 mcg	In 100s.
otc	Twelve Resin-K (Key Company)	Tablets: 1000 mcg on resin.	In 60s, 250s, and 1000s.
otc	Big Shot B-12 (Naturally)	Tablets: 5000 mcg	In 30s and 60s.
otc	Big Shot B-12 (Naturally)	Tablets: 5000 mcg	In 30s and 60s.
otc	Big Shot B-12 (Naturally)	Tablets: 5000 mcg	In 30s and 60s.
otc	Vitamin B$_{12}$ (Freeda)	Lozenges: 50 mcg	Sorbitol, mannitol. In 100s.
		100 mcg	In 100s.
		250 mcg	In 100s and 250s.
		500 mcg	In 100s and 250s.

For complete prescribing information, refer to the vitamin B$_{12}$ monograph.

Indications

➤*B$_{12}$ deficiency:* Nutritional vitamin B$_{12}$ deficiency.

These products are NOT indicated for treatment of pernicious anemia.

Administration and Dosage

➤*Recommended Dietary Allowances (RDAs):* Adults, 2 mcg/day. For a complete listing of RDAs by age, sex, or condition, refer to the RDA table.

➤*Nutritional supplement:* Dosage varies. See individual product literature.

Actions

➤*Pharmacology:* Vitamin B$_{12}$ is essential to growth, cell reproduction, hematopoiesis, nucleic acid, and myelin synthesis. Sources of vitamin B$_{12}$ include liver, meat, fish, and dairy products (eg, milk and cheese). Vitamin B$_{12}$ is not present in foods of plant origin. Deficiency may result in megaloblastic anemia or pernicious anemia. Ten percent to 30% of Americans > 60 years of age experience atrophic gastritis, resulting in an inability to absorb vitamin B$_{12}$ bound to food protein.

Because of enterohepatic recycling, patients who do not absorb, or have a diet deficient in, vitamin B$_{12}$ may not see signs of deficiency for 3 to 5 years.

➤*Pharmacokinetics:* The parietal cells of the stomach secrete intrinsic factor, which regulates the amount of vitamin B$_{12}$ absorbed in the terminal ileum. Simple diffusion is responsible for absorption when > 30 mcg of vitamin B$_{12}$ is ingested. Bioavailability of oral preparations is ≈ 25%. Vitamin B$_{12}$ is primarily stored in the liver. Enterohepatic circulation plays a key role in recycling vitamin B$_{12}$ from bile and other intestinal secretions. If plasma-binding proteins are saturated, excess free vitamin B$_{12}$ will be excreted in the kidney.

Contraindications

Hypersensitivity to cyanocobalamin.

Warnings

➤*Pregnancy: Category A.* (*Category C* in doses that exceed the RDA).

➤*Lactation:* Vitamin B$_{12}$ is excreted into breast milk.

Overdosage

Vitamin B$_{12}$ is essentially nontoxic in humans. Allergic reactions and hypersensitivity have been reported.

CYANOCOBALAMIN, INTRANASAL (B$_{12}$)

Rx	Nascobal (Questcor)	Gel, intranasal: 500 mcg/0.1 mL (500 mcg/actuation)	Benzalkonium chloride. In 5 mL bottles (≈ 8 doses/bottle).

For complete prescribing information, refer to the vitamin B$_{12}$ monograph.

Indications

For maintenance of the hematologic status of patients who are in remission following IM vitamin B$_{12}$ therapy for the following conditions:
- Pernicious anemia in hematologic remission with no nervous system involvement.
- Dietary deficiency of vitamin B$_{12}$ occurring in strict vegetarians (isolated vitamin B$_{12}$ deficiency is very rare).
- Malabsorption of vitamin B$_{12}$ resulting from structural or functional damage to the stomach where intrinsic factor is secreted, or to the ileum where intrinsic factor facilitates B$_{12}$ absorption. These conditions include HIV infection, AIDS, Crohn's disease, tropical sprue, and nontropical sprue (idiopathic steatorrhea, gluten-induced enteropathy). Folate deficiency in these patients is usually more severe than vitamin B$_{12}$ deficiency.
- Inadequate secretion of intrinsic factor resulting from lesions that destroy the gastric mucosa (ingestion of corrosives, extensive neoplasia) and conditions associated with a variable degree of gastric atrophy (eg, multiple sclerosis, HIV infection, AIDS, certain endocrine disorders, iron deficiency, subtotal gastrectomy). Total gastrectomy always produces vitamin B$_{12}$ deficiency. Structural lesions leading to vitamin B$_{12}$ deficiency include regional ileitis, ileal resections, and malignancies.
- Competition for vitamin B$_{12}$ by intestinal parasites or bacteria. The fish tapeworm (*Diphyllobothrium latum*) absorbs huge quantities of vitamin B$_{12}$ and infested patients often have associated gastric atro-

phy. The blind loop syndrome may produce deficiency of vitamin B$_{12}$ or folate.
- Inadequate utilization of vitamin B$_{12}$. This may occur if antimetabolites for the vitamin are employed in the treatment of neoplasia.

Administration and Dosage

Prime prior to initial use. Repriming between doses is not necessary if the unit is upright. Administer at least 1 hour before or 1 hour after ingestion of hot foods or liquids.

➤*Vitamin B$_{12}$ malabsorption in remission following injectable vitamin B$_{12}$ therapy:* 500 mcg intranasally once weekly.

➤*Storage/Stability:* Protect from light. Keep covered in prescription vial until ready to use. Store upright at controlled room temperature (15° to 30°C; 59° to 86°F). Protect from freezing.

Actions

➤*Pharmacokinetics:* Peak concentration of B$_{12}$ after intranasal administration is 1 to 2 hours. Bioavailability is 8.9%.

Contraindications

Sensitivity to cobalt and/or vitamin B$_{12}$ or to any component of this preparation.

Warnings

➤*Optic atrophy:* Patients with early Leber's disease treated with vitamin B$_{12}$ suffered severe and swift optic atrophy.

➤*Megaloblastic anemia:* Patients with severe megaloblastic anemia intensely treated with vitamin B$_{12}$ may develop hypokalemia and sudden death. Folic acid is not a substitute for vitamin B$_{12}$, although it

CYANOCOBALAMIN, INTRANASAL (B₁₂)

may improve vitamin B_{12}-deficient megaloblastic anemia. Exclusive use of folic acid in treating vitamin B_{12}-deficient megaloblastic anemia could result in progressive and irreversible neurologic damage.

Precautions

▶*Monitoring:* Obtain hematocrit, reticulocyte count, vitamin B_{12}, folate, and iron levels prior to treatment. All parameters should be normal when beginning treatment.

Monitor vitamin B_{12} blood levels and peripheral blood counts 1 month after the start of treatment and then at 3- to 6-month intervals.

Patients with pernicious anemia have about 3 times the incidence of stomach carcinoma when compared with the general population. Perform appropriate tests.

▶*Test dose:* An intradermal test dose of parenteral vitamin B_{12} is recommended before intranasal administration to patients suspected of cyanocobalamin sensitivity.

▶*Nasal symptoms:* The effectiveness of intranasal cyanocobalamin in patients with nasal congestion, allergic rhinitis, and upper respiratory tract infections has not been determined. Defer treatment until symptoms have subsided.

Drug Interactions

Colchicine, para-aminosalicylic acid, and heavy alcohol intake for longer than 2 weeks may result in vitamin B_{12} malabsorption.

Adverse Reactions

Asthenia; headache; infection; glossitis; nausea; paresthesia; rhinitis.

▶*Lab test abnormalities:* Most antibiotics, methotrexate, or pyrimethamine invalidate folic acid and vitamin B_{12} diagnostic blood assays.

Overdosage

No overdose has been reported.

Patient Information

Administer at least 1 hour before or 1 hour after ingestion of hot foods or liquids.

Patients with pernicious anemia will require weekly vitamin B_{12} for the remainder of their lives.

Blood tests are recommended every 3 to 6 months to ensure therapy is appropriate.

AMINOBENZOATE POTASSIUM

Rx	Potaba (Glenwood)	Tablets: 500 mg	In 100s and 1000s.
Rx	Aminobenzoate Potassium (Hope Pharm)	Capsules: 500 mg	In 250s.
Rx	Potaba (Glenwood)		In 250s and 1000s.
Rx	Potaba (Glenwood)	Envules (Powder): 2 g	In 50s.

Indications

"Possibly effective" in the treatment of scleroderma, dermatomyositis, morphea, linear scleroderma, pemphigus, and Peyronie's disease.

Administration and Dosage

▶*Adults:* The average adult daily dose of aminobenzoate potassium for scleroderma, morphea, linear scleroderma, and Peyronie's disease is 12 g, usually given in 4 to 6 divided doses. Higher doses (15 to 20 g daily) are initially used in dermatomyositis. Tablets and capsules 500 mg are given at the rate of 4 tablets or capsules 6 times daily, or 6 tablets or capsules given 4 times daily usually with meals and at bedtime with a snack. Tablets must be dissolved in an adequate amount of liquid to prevent GI upset. Aminobenzoate potassium envules contain 2 g pure drug powder and constitute the individual average dose. Six envules are given for a total of 12 g aminobenzoate potassium daily.

Therapy usually requires the maintenance of adequate dosage for 2 to 3 months.

▶*Children:* 1 g daily in divided doses for each 10 lbs of body weight.

Actions

▶*Pharmacology:* Small amounts of para-aminobenzoate are present in cereal, eggs, milk, and meats. Detectable amounts are found in human blood, spinal fluid, urine, and sweat. It is suggested that aminobenzoate potassium has an antifibrosis action caused by mediation of increased oxygen uptake at the tissue level. Fibrosis is believed to occur from either too much serotonin or too little monoamine oxidase (MAO) activity over a period of time. MAO requires an adequate supply of oxygen to function properly. By increasing oxygen supply at the tissue level, aminobenzoate potassium may enhance MAO activity and prevent or cause regression of fibrosis.

Contraindications

Concurrent sulfonamide use.

Warnings

▶*Renal function impairment:* Use cautiously.

▶*Pregnancy:* Safety has not been established.

▶*Lactation:* Safety for use during lactation has not been established.

Precautions

▶*Anorexia or nausea:* If anorexia or nausea occurs, interrupt therapy until the patient is eating normally again to avoid hypoglycemia.

▶*Hypersensitivity:* If a hypersensitivity reaction occurs, discontinue the drug. Refer to Management of Acute Hypersensitivity Reactions.

Adverse Reactions

Anorexia, nausea, fever, and rash have occurred infrequently and subside with omission of the drug. Desensitization can be accomplished and treatment resumed. Hepatotoxicity also has occurred.

Overdosage

Nausea and vomiting are the most common events associated with overdose. Drug fever, dermatitis, depression of the leukocyte count, and an alleged fatal case of toxic hepatitis have been reported.

VITAMIN C (Ascorbic Acid)

Indications

▶*Scurvy:* Prevention and treatment of scurvy. Parenteral administration is desirable in an acute deficiency or when absorption of oral ascorbic acid is uncertain.

▶*Unlabeled uses:* Vitamin C in high doses has been advocated for prevention of the common cold, for treatment of asthma, atherosclerosis, wounds, schizophrenia, and cancer; however, clinical data do not justify these uses.

Vitamin C (≥ 2 g/day) may be used as a urinary acidifier either alone or in combination with methenamine therapy. Data regarding the efficacy of ascorbic acid for this purpose are conflicting. Failure to significantly lower urine pH may be attributed to inadequate dosage (< 2 g/day).

Vitamin C in doses of ≥ 150 mg have been used to control idiopathic methemoglobinemia (less effective than methylene blue).

Doses greater than the recommended RDA for vitamin C have been associated with a low incidence of senile cataract, cancer, coronary artery disease, and increase in HDL.

Risk reduction for pre-eclampsia in combination with vitamin E during the second half of pregnancy (1 g/day).

Topical – Topical vitamin C may photoprotect against UVR because of its antioxidant and anti-inflammatory properties.

Administration and Dosage

Chronic illness, infection, febrile states, hemovascular disorders, and wound healing require an increase in daily intake.

▶*Recommended Dietary Allowances (RDAs):* Adults, 60 mg. For a complete listing of RDAs by age, sex, or condition, refer to the RDA table.

▶*Nicotine use:* The RDA for smokers is 100 mg/day because of an increased utilization of vitamin C.

IM route is preferred; may administer IV or SC. Avoid rapid IV injection. IM injections may cause pain, local swelling, tenderness, and tissue necrosis.

▶*Adults:* The average protective dose is 70 to 150 mg/day. For scurvy, 300 mg to 1 g/day is recommended. However, up to 6 g/day has been administered parenterally to healthy adults without evidence of toxicity.

High-dose therapy – Taper vitamin C prior to discontinuing supplementation. Adults who abruptly stopped high-dose therapy have experienced loosened teeth and bleeding gums.

Enhanced wound healing – Doses of 300 to 500 mg/day for 7 to 10 days both preoperatively and postoperatively are adequate, although considerably larger amounts have been recommended.

Burns – Individualize dosage. For severe burns, daily doses of 1 to 2 g are recommended.

In other conditions in which the need for vitamin C is increased, 3 to 5 times the daily optimum allowance appears adequate.

Actions

▶*Pharmacology:* Vitamin C is a water-soluble vitamin with antioxidant properties. Sources of vitamin C include citrus fruits (eg, lemons,

VITAMIN C (Ascorbic Acid)

limes), strawberries, tomatoes, cabbage greens, leafy vegetables, and melons.

Physiological Roles of Vitamin C	
Catecholamine biosynthesis	Stimulates peptide synthesis and hydroxylation of proline and lysine in collagen formation
Carnitine synthesis	Epinephrine synthesis
Conversion of folic acid to folinic acid	Facilitates GI iron absorption
Tyrosine metabolism	Dopamine hydroxylation to form norepinephrine

Deficiency – Symptoms include impaired wound healing, impaired collagen synthesis, joint pain, anemia, and increased susceptibility to infections. A serum level < 0.3 mg/dL is considered to be associated with a decreased intake of vitamin C.

Scurvy: Scurvy is characterized by degenerative changes in capillaries, bone, and connective tissues manifested as perifollicular hyperkeratotic papules, dry skin, ecchymosis, muscle weakness, loose teeth caused by gum inflammation, joint pain, easy bruising, and fatigue.

➤*Pharmacokinetics:*

Absorption / Distribution – Absorption of dietary ascorbate from the distal small intestine is nearly complete. Ascorbic acid is distributed throughout water-soluble compartments of the body. The adrenal cortex, leukocytes, platelets, and the pituitary contain high ascorbic acid concentrations. Ascorbic acid body pools are > 1400 mg; ≈ 4% of this pool is used daily.

Metabolism / Excretion – Ascorbic acid is excreted in the urine.

Warnings

➤*Excessive vitamin C doses:* Diabetic patients, patients prone to recurrent renal calculi, those undergoing stool occult blood tests, and those on sodium-restricted diets or anticoagulant therapy should not take excessive doses of vitamin C over an extended period of time.

➤*Pregnancy:* Category A. (*Category C* in doses greater than the RDA.) It is not known whether ascorbic acid can cause fetal harm or can affect reproduction capacity. Give to pregnant women only if clearly needed. Do not administer ascorbic acid to pregnant women in excess of the amount needed for treatment. The fetus may adapt to high levels of vitamin C resulting in a scorbutic condition after birth when intake drops to normal levels. Clinical significance is unknown.

➤*Lactation:* Administer with caution to a nursing mother. Ascorbic acid is excreted in breast milk.

Precautions

➤*Tartrazine sensitivity:* Some of these products contain tartrazine, which may cause allergic-type reactions (including bronchial asthma) in susceptible individuals. Although the incidence of sensitivity is low, it is frequently seen in patients who also have aspirin hypersensitivity. Specific products containing tartrazine are identified in the product listings.

➤*Sulfite sensitivity:* Some of these products contain sulfites, which may cause allergic-type reactions in certain susceptible people. The overall prevalence of sulfite sensitivity in the general population is unknown and probably low. Sulfite sensitivity is seen more frequently in asthmatic than in nonasthmatic people.

Drug Interactions

➤*Drug / Lab test interactions:* Large doses (> 500 mg) of vitamin C may cause false-negative urine **glucose determinations**.

No exogenous vitamin C should be ingested for 48 to 72 hours before conducting amine-dependent stool **occult blood tests** because false-negative results may occur.

Adverse Reactions

Transient mild soreness may occur at the site of IM or SC injection. Rapid IV administration may cause temporary faintness or dizziness.

Overdosage

Nausea, vomiting, gout precipitation, rebound scurvy, increased iron absorption, impaired bacterial activity, and diarrhea (≥ 1 g). Monitor risk for developing renal calcium oxalate stones (1 to 3 g) due to excessive oxalate excretion produced by ascorbic acid metabolism.

ASCORBIC ACID

otc	**Ascorbic Acid** (Various, eg, Goldline, Nutro Labs)	**Tablets:** 250 mg	In 100s and UD 100s.
otc	**Ascorbic Acid** (Various, eg, Goldline, Naturally, Nutro Labs, Rugby[1])	**Tablets:** 500 mg	In 100s, 250s, 1000s, and UD 100s.
otc	**Cevi-Bid** (Lee)		In 100s, 500s, and UD 12s and 96s.
otc	**Ascorbic Acid** (Various, eg, Goldline, Naturally, Rugby[1])	**Tablets:** 1000 mg	In 100s and 250s.
otc	**Ascorbic Acid** (Various, eg, Naturally)	**Tablets:** 1500 mg	In 100s.
otc	**Ascorbic Acid** (Various, eg, Freeda)	**Tablets, timed-release:** 500 mg	In 100s, 250s, and 500s.
otc	**Ascorbic Acid** (Freeda)	**Tablets, timed-release:** 1000 mg	In 100s, 250s, and 500s.
otc	**Ascorbic Acid** (Various, eg, Goldine)	**Capsules:** 500 mg	In 100s.
otc	**Asco-Caps** (Key Company)		In 100s and 500s.
otc sf	**Vita-C** (Freeda)	**Crystals:** 1000 mg/¼ tsp	In 120 g and 1 lb.
otc sf	**Dull-C** (Freeda)	**Powder:** 1060 mg/¼ tsp	In 120 g and 1 lb.
otc	**Ascorbic Acid** (Humco)	**Powder:** 60 mg/¼ tsp	In 454 g.
otc	**Cecon** (Abbott)	**Solution:** 100 mg/mL	In 50 mL w/dropper.
otc	**Ascorbic Acid** (Various, eg, Rugby)	**Liquid:** 500 mg/5 mL	In 120 and 480 mL.
Rx	**Ascorbic Acid** (Various, eg, American Regent)	**Injection:** 500 mg/mL	In 50 mL vials.
Rx	**Ascor L 500** (McGuff)		0.025% EDTA. Preservative-free. In 50 mL.

[1] With or without rose hips.

For complete prescribing information, refer to the Vitamin C group monograph.

SODIUM ASCORBATE

Rx	**Cenolate** (Abbott)	**Injection:** 562.5 mg/mL (equiv. to 500 mg/mL ascorbic acid)	In 1 and 2 mL amps.[1]

[1] With 0.5% sodium hydrosulfite.

For complete prescribing information, refer to the Vitamin C group monograph.

CALCIUM ASCORBATE

otc sf	**Calcium Ascorbate** (Freeda)	**Tablets:** 500 mg	75 mg calcium. Buffered. In 100s, 250s, and 500s.
otc sf	**Calcium Ascorbate** (Freeda)	**Powder:** 814 mg/¼ tsp	100 mg calcium/¼ tsp. Buffered. In 120 g and 1 lb.

For complete prescribing information, refer to the Vitamin C group monograph.

Water-Soluble Vitamins

ASCORBIC ACID COMBINATIONS

otc	SunKist Vitamin C (Novartis)	**Tablets, chewable:** 60 mg vitamin C as sodium ascorbate and ascorbic acid	Sorbitol, sucrose, lactose. Orange flavor. In 11s.
otc *sf*	Fruit C 100 (Freeda)	**Tablets, chewable:** 100 mg vitamin C as calcium ascorbate and ascorbic acid	In 250s.
otc *sf*	Fruit C 200 (Freeda)	**Tablets, chewable:** 200 mg vitamin C as calcium ascorbate and ascorbic acid	Rose hips. In 100s and 250s.
otc	Chewable Vitamin C (Various, eg, Goldline)	**Tablets, chewable:** 250 mg vitamin C as sodium ascorbate and ascorbic acid	In 100s.
otc	SunKist Vitamin C (Novartis)		Fructose, sorbitol, sucrose, lactose. Orange flavor. In 60s.
otc	Chewable Vitamin C (Various, eg, Goldline)	**Tablets, chewable:** 500 mg vitamin C as sodium ascorbate and ascorbic acid	In 100s.
otc	SunKist Vitamin C (Novartis)		Fructose, sorbitol, sucrose, lactose. Orange flavor. In 75s.
otc	Chew-C (Key Company)		Sugar. Orange flavor. In 100s.
otc *sf*	Fruit C 500 (Freeda)	**Tablets, chewable:** 500 mg vitamin C as calcium ascorbate and ascorbic acid	Rose hips. In 100s and 250s.
otc	Vicks Vitamin C Drops (Proctor and Gamble)	**Lozenges:** 25 mg vitamin C as sodium ascorbate and ascorbic acid	Sucrose, corn syrup. Orange flavor. In 20s.

For complete prescribing information, refer to the Vitamin C group monograph.

BIOFLAVONOIDS (Vitamin P)

otc *sf*	Pan C-500 (Freeda)	**Tablets:** 100 mg hesperidin, 100 mg citrus bioflavonoids, and 500 mg vitamin C	Sodium free. In 100s, 250s, and 500s.
otc *sf*	C Factors "1000" Plus (Solgar)	**Tablets:** 1000 mg vitamin C, 25 mg rose hips, 250 mg citrus bioflavonoids complex, 50 mg rutin, 25 mg hesperidin	Sodium free. In 50s.
otc *sf*	Flavons (Freeda)	**Tablets:** 500 mg bioflavonoids[1]	In 100s and 250s.
otc	Tri-Super Flavons 1000 (Freeda)	**Tablets:** 1000 mg bioflavonoids	In 100s, 250s, and 500s.
otc	Peridin-C (Beutlich)	**Tablets:** 150 mg hesperidin complex, 50 mg hesperidin methyl cholcone (bioflavonoids), 200 mg ascorbic acid	In 100s and 500s.
otc *sf*	Span C (Freeda)	**Tablets:** 300 mg citrus bioflavonoids, 200 mg vitamin C (ascorbic acid and rose hips)[1]	In 100s, 250s, and 500s.
otc *sf*	Flavons-500 (Freeda)	**Tablets:** 500 mg citrus bioflavonoids	In 100s and 250s.
otc *sf*	Ester-C Plus 1000 mg Vitamin C (Solgar)	**Tablets:** 1000 mg vitamin C, 200 mg citrus bioflavonoid complex, 25 mg acerola, 25 mg rutin, 25 mg rose hips, 125 mg calcium	Sodium free. In 90s.
otc *sf*	Quercetin (Freeda)	**Tablets:** 50 mg quercetin (from eucalyptus)	Sodium free. In 100s and 250s.
		Tablets: 250 mg quercetin (from eucalyptus)	Sodium free. In 100s and 250s.
otc	Amino-Opti-C (Tyson)	**Tablets, sustained-release:** 1000 mg vitamin C, 250 mg lemon bioflavonoids. Rose hips powder, rutin, hesperidin[2]	In 100s.
otc *sf*	Ester-C Plus Multi-Mineral (Solgar)	**Capsules:** 425 mg vitamin C, 50 mg citrus bioflavonoid complex, 12.5 mg acerola, 12.5 mg rose hips, 5 mg rutin, 25 mg calcium, 13 mg magnesium, 12.5 mg potassium, 2.5 mg zinc	Sodium free. In 60s and 90s.
otc *sf*	Ester-C Plus 500 mg Vitamin C (Solgar)	**Capsules:** 500 mg vitamin C, 62 mg calcium, 25 mg citrus bioflavonoids, 10 mg acerola, 10 mg rose hips, 5 mg rutin	Sodium free. In 250s.

[1] Also contains calcium carbonate, calcium stearate.

[2] Also contains dicalcium phosphate, hydrogenated soybean oil.

Indications

➤*Unlabeled uses:* Bioflavonoids possess widespread activity. Some biological activities include the following: Anthelmintic, antimicrobial, antimalarial, antineoplastic, cytotoxic, mutagenic, carcinogenic, anticarcinogenic, antioxidant (free radical scavengers), inhibition of prostaglandin synthesis (anti-inflammatory), antiallergic, antiviral, antithrombotic, spasmolitic, and estrogenic. Certain flavonoids have been noted to increase lymphatic drainage and improve venous tone. Bioflavonoids are considered investigational in the treatment of HIV via HIV-1 reverse transcriptase, protease, and integrase inhibition. Unfortunately, many of these uses have not been tested in controlled clinical trials; therefore, there is little evidence that they are effective for any indication.

Administration and Dosage

There are no established recommended dietary allowances for flavonoids. However, it has been estimated that daily intake ranges from 20 mg to 1 g.

Actions

➤*Pharmacology:* Flavonoids are naturally occurring, low-molecular-weight polyphenols of plant origin, historically named "vitamin P." More than 4000 naturally occurring flavonoids have been described. Groups of flavonoids include flavones, flavonols, flavanones, and flavanols, which differ by the number and positions of hydroxyl substituents in 2 aromatic rings. Flavonoids generally occur as aglycones, glycosides, and methylated derivatives. Flavonoids are present in fruits, vegetables, nuts, seeds, grains, tea, wine, stems, and flowers. Bioflavonoid refers to extracts of citrus including lemon, orange, mandarin, or grapefruit varieties. Bioflavonoids extracted from citrus contain a variety of flavonoids. The majority of citrus flavonoids are flavanones bound as glycosides.

Flavonoid	Source
Naringin[1]	Grapefruit, pummelo
Narirutin[1]	Grapefruit
Hesperidin	Oranges, tangerines, lemons, limes
Ericotirin	Lemon, limes
Tangeretin	Tangerines, lemons, limes
Nobiletin	Tangerines, lemons, limes
Genistein	Soybeans
Quercetin	Onions, tomatoes, french beans, apples, berries, red wine

[1] Naringenin glycosides.

➤*Pharmacokinetics:*

Absorption/Distribution –

Quercetin: Quercetin peak levels are attained in < 0.7 and 2.5 hours following onion and apple ingestion, respectively. Quercetin crosses the intestinal mucosa and is tranported to the liver primarily bound to albumin.

BIOFLAVONOIDS (Vitamin P)

Metabolism / Excretion –

Quercetin: Frequent intake of quercetin-rich food resulted in elimination half-lives of 23 hours for apples and 28 hours for onion sources.

Quercetin undergoes methylation, sulphation, and glucuronidation to form various conjugates of quercetin.

Multiple dosing of grapefruit and orange juice (containing 323 mg naringenin and 44 mg hesperidin) resulted in < 25% urinary recovery.

FOLIC ACID AND DERIVATIVES
FOLIC ACID (Folacin; Pteroylglutamic Acid; Folate)

otc[1]	**Folic Acid** (Various, eg, Fibertone, Major, Rugby)	**Tablets:** 0.4 mg	In 100s.
otc[1]	**Folic Acid** (Various, eg, Fibertone, Rugby)	**Tablets:** 0.8 mg	In 100s.
Rx	**Folic Acid** (Various, eg, Genetco, Goldline, Moore, Parmed, Qualitest, Rugby)	**Tablets:** 1 mg	In 30s, 100s, 1000s and UD 100s.
Rx	**Folic Acid** (American Pharmaceutical Partners)	**Injection:** 5 mg/mL	In 10 mL vials.[2]
Rx	**Folvite** (Lederle)		In 10 mL vials.[3]

[1] Although most folic acid products carry the *Rx* legend, products which provide 0.4 mg or less (or 0.8 mg for pregnant or lactating women) may be *otc* items.

[2] With 1.5% benzyl alcohol and EDTA.
[3] With 1.5% benzyl alcohol.

Indications

➤*Megaloblastic anemia:* Treatment of megaloblastic anemias due to a deficiency of folic acid as seen in tropical or nontropical sprue, anemias of nutritional origin, pregnancy, infancy or childhood.

Administration and Dosage

Give orally, except in severe intestinal malabsorption. Although most patients with malabsorption cannot absorb food folates, they are able to absorb folic acid given orally.

Parenteral administration is not advocated but may be necessary in some individuals (eg, patients receiving parenteral or enteral alimentation). Give IM, IV or SC if disease is very severe or GI absorption is very severely impaired. Doses > 0.1 mg should not be used unless anemia due to vitamin B_{12} deficiency has been ruled out or is being adequately treated with cobalamin. Daily doses> 1 mg do not enhance the hematologic effect, and most of the excess is excreted unchanged in the urine.

➤*Usual therapeutic dosage:* Up to 1 mg daily. Resistant cases may require larger doses.

➤*Maintenance:* When clinical symptoms have subsided and the blood picture has normalized, use the dosage below. Never give < 0.1 mg/day. Keep patients under close supervision and adjust maintenance dose if relapse appears imminent. In the presence of alcoholism, hemolytic anemia, anticonvulsant therapy or chronic infection, the maintenance level may need to be increased.

Infants – 0.1 mg/day.

Children (< 4 years of age) – Up to 0.3 mg/day.

Adults and children (> 4 years of age) – 0.4 mg/day.

Pregnant and lactating women – 0.8 mg/day.

➤*Recommended dietary allowances (RDAs):* Adult males, 0.15 to 0.2 mg/day; females, 0.15 to 0.18 mg/day.

For a complete listing of RDAs by age and sex, refer to the RDA table in the Nutrients and Nutritionals chapter.

➤*Storage / Stability:* At concentrations usually used for parenteral nutrition, folate will remain stable in solution providing the pH of the solution remains above 5.

Actions

➤*Pharmacology:* Exogenous folate is required for nucleoprotein synthesis and maintenance of normal erythropoiesis. Folic acid stimulates production of red and white blood cells and platelets in certain megaloblastic anemias. Folic acid is the precursor of tetrahydrofolic acid, which is involved as a cofactor for transformylation reactions in the biosynthesis of purines and thymidylates of nucleic acids. Impairment of thymidylate synthesis in patients with folic acid deficiency is thought to account for the defective deoxyribonucleic acid (DNA) synthesis that leads to megaloblast formation and megaloblastic and macrocytic anemias.

➤*Pharmacokinetics:* Dietary folic acid is present in foods (eg, liver, dried beans, peas, lentils, oranges, whole-wheat products, vegetables such as asparagus, beets, broccoli, brussels sprouts and spinach), primarily as reduced folate polyglutamate. It must undergo hydrolysis, reduction and methylation in the GI tract before it is absorbed. Conversion to tetrahydrofolate, the active form, is B_{12}-dependent; supplies are maintained by food and enterohepatic recirculation. Oral synthetic folic acid is a monoglutamate and is completely absorbed following administration, even in the presence of malabsorption syndromes.

Folic acid appears in the plasma $\approx$ 15 to 30 minutes after an oral dose; peak levels are generally reached within 1 hour. After IV administration, the drug is rapidly cleared from the plasma. Cerebrospinal fluid levels are several times greater than serum levels of the drug. Folic acid is metabolized in the liver to 7,8–dihydrofolic acid and eventually to 5,6,7,8–tetrahydrofolic acid. Tetrahydrofolic acid derivatives are distributed to all body tissues but are stored primarily in the liver. Normal serum levels of total folate have been reported to be 5 to 15 ng/mL; nor-mal CSF levels are $\approx$ 16 to 21 ng/mL. Normal erythrocyte folate levels have been reported to range from 175 to 316 ng/mL. In general, folate serum levels < 5 ng/mL indicate folate deficiency, and levels < 2 ng/mL usually result in megaloblastic anemia.

After a single oral dose of 100 mcg of folic acid in a limited number of healthy adults, only a trace amount of the drug appeared in the urine. An oral dose of 5 mg in one study and a dose of 40 mcg/kg in another study resulted in $\approx$ 50% of the dose appearing in the urine. After a single oral dose of 15 mg, up to 90% of the dose was recovered in the urine. A majority of the metabolic products appeared in the urine after 6 hours; excretion was generally complete within 24 hours. Small amounts of orally administered folic acid have also been recovered in the feces.

Contraindications

Treatment of pernicious anemia and other megaloblastic anemias where vitamin B_{12} is deficient (not effective).

Warnings

➤*Pernicious anemia:* Folic acid in doses > 0.1 mg daily may obscure pernicious anemia in that hematologic remission can occur while neurologic manifestations remain progressive.

Except during pregnancy and lactation, folic acid should not be given in therapeutic doses > 0.4 mg daily until pernicious anemia has been ruled out. Patients with pernicious anemia receiving > 0.4 mg folic acid daily who are inadequately treated with vitamin B_{12} may show reversion of the hematologic parameters to normal, but neurologic manifestations due to vitamin B_{12} deficiency have been ruled out or are being adequately treated with cobalamin. Daily doses exceeding the Recommended Dietary Allowance should not be included in multivitamin preparations; if therapeutic amounts are necessary, folic acid should be given separately.

There is a potential danger in administering folic acid to patients with undiagnosed anemia, since folic acid may obscure the diagnosis of pernicious anemia by alleviating the hematologic manifestations of the disease while allowing the neurologic complications to progress. This may result in severe nervous system damage before the correct diagnosis is made. Adequate doses of vitamin B_{12} may prevent, halt or improve the neurologic changes caused by pernicious anemia.

➤*Benzyl alcohol:* Benzyl alcohol, contained in some of these products as a preservative, has been associated with a fatal "gasping syndrome" in premature infants.

➤*Elderly:* A recent study observed that homocysteine concentrations increase with age and low levels of folate and vitamins B_6 and B_{12}. Data suggest that high homocysteine levels may correlate with the development of occlusive vascular disease which may increase the risk of MI. Therefore, it may be prudent to consider the status of folate in persons > 65 years of age.

➤*Pregnancy: Category A.* Pregnant women are more prone to develop folate deficiency as reflected in larger dosage recommendations. Folate-deficient mothers may be more prone to complications of pregnancy and fetal abnormalities, including fetal anomalies, placental abruption, toxemia, abortions, placenta previa, low-birth-weight and premature delivery. Folic acid is usually indicated in the treatment of megaloblastic anemias of pregnancy. Folic acid requirements are markedly increased during pregnancy. The Recommended Dietary Allowance of folate during pregnancy is 0.4 mg/day.

Studies in pregnant women have not shown that folic acid increases the risk of abnormalities if administered during pregnancy. If the drug is used during pregnancy, the possibility of fetal harm appears remote. Because studies cannot rule out the possibility of harm, use folic acid during pregnancy only if clearly needed.

However, the US Public Health Service has recently recommended the use of folic acid in women of childbearing age to reduce the incidence of neural tube defects (NTDs). This is based on several studies that reported a > 50% reduced risk of NTDs in women who received 0.4 mg folic acid prior to conception and during early pregnancy. According to

Water-Soluble Vitamins

FOLIC ACID (Folacin; Pteroylglutamic Acid; Folate)

the US Public Health Service, all women of childbearing age in the US who are capable of becoming pregnant should consume 0.4 mg of folic acid per day for the purpose of reducing their risk of having a pregnancy affected with spina bifida or other NTDs. Because the effects of high intakes are not well known but include complicating the diagnosis of vitamin B_{12} deficiency, care should be taken to keep total folate consumption at < 1 mg/day, except under physician supervision. Women who have had a prior NTD-affected pregnancy are at high risk of having a subsequent affected pregnancy. When these women are planning to become pregnant, they should consult their physicians for advice.

►*Lactation:* Folic acid is excreted in breast milk; milk:plasma ratio equals ≈ 0.02.

During lactation, folic acid requirements are markedly increased; however, amounts present in human milk are adequate to fulfill infant requirements, although supplementation may be needed in low-birth-weight infants, in those who are breastfed by mothers with folic acid deficiency (50 mcg daily), or in those with infections or prolonged diarrhea. The Recommended Dietary Allowance of folate during lactation is 0.26 to 0.28 mg/day.

Drug Interactions

Folic Acid Drug Interactions			
Precipitant drug	Object drug*		Description
Aminosalicylic acid	Folic acid	↓	Decreased serum folate levels may occur during concurrent use.
Contraceptives, oral	Folic acid	↓	Oral contraceptives may impair folate metabolism and produce folate depletion, but the effect is mild and unlikely to cause anemia or megaloblastic changes.
Dihydrofolate reductase inhibitors (eg, methotrexate, trimethoprim)	Folic acid	↓	A dihydrofolate reductase deficiency caused by administration of folic acid antagonists may interfere with folic acid utilization.
Sulfasalazine	Folic acid	↓	Signs of folate deficiency have occurred.

Folic Acid Drug Interactions			
Precipitant drug	Object drug*		Description
Folic acid	Hydantoins	↓	An increase in seizure frequency and a decrease in serum concentration to subtherapeutic levels have been reported in patients receiving folic acid (particularly 5 to 30 mg/day) with phenytoin. **Phenytoin** may cause a decrease in serum folate levels, and may produce symptoms of folic acid deficiency in 27% to 91% (but clinically important megaloblastic anemia in < 1%) of patients on long-term therapy. If folic acid is required, a higher dose of phenytoin may be needed.

* ↓ = Object drug decreased.

Adverse Reactions

Folic acid is relatively nontoxic in man. Rare instances of allergic responses to folic acid preparations have occurred and have included erythema, skin rash, itching, general malaise and respiratory difficulty due to bronchospasm. One patient experienced symptoms suggesting anaphylaxis following injection of the drug.

►*CNS:* Altered sleep patterns, difficulty in concentrating, irritability, overactivity, excitement, mental depression, confusion and impaired judgement were reported in patients receiving 15 mg daily.

►*GI:* Anorexia, nausea, abdominal distention, flatulence and a bitter or bad taste have been reported in patients receiving 15 mg folic acid daily for 1 month.

►*Miscellaneous:* Allergic sensitization has been reported.

Decreased vitamin B_{12} serum levels may occur in patients receiving prolonged folic acid therapy.

Patient Information

Take only under medical supervision.

LEUCOVORIN CALCIUM (Folinic Acid; Citrovorum Factor)

Rx	Leucovorin Calcium (Various, eg, Barr, Lederle)	**Tablets:** 5 mg (as calcium)	In 30s, 100s and UD 50s.
Rx	Leucovorin Calcium (Lederle)	**Tablets:** 15 mg (as calcium)	Lactose. (LL 15 C 35). Yellowish white, scored. Oval, convex. In 12s, 24s and UD 50s.
Rx	Leucovorin Calcium (Barr)	**Tablets:** 25 mg (as calcium)	(485). Light green. In 25s.
Rx	Leucovorin Calcium (Lederle)	**Injection:** 3 mg/mL (as calcium)	In 1 mL amps.[1]
Rx	Leucovorin Calcium (American Regent)	**Injection:** 10 mg/mL (as calcium)	In 5 mg single-dose vials (25s).
Rx	Leucovorin Calcium (Lederle)	**Powder for Injection:** 50 mg/vial (as calcium)[2]	In vials.
Rx	Leucovorin Calcium (Lederle)	**Powder for Injection:** 100 mg/vial (as calcium)[2]	In vials.
Rx	Leucovorin Calcium (Mayne)	**Powder for Injection:** 350 mg/vial (as calcium)[2]	In vials.

[1] With 0.9% benzyl alcohol.
[2] Preservative free.

Indications

►*Oral and parenteral:* Leucovorin "rescue" after high-dose methotrexate therapy in osteosarcoma.

To diminish the toxicity and counteract the effects of impaired methotrexate elimination and of inadvertent overdosages of folic acid antagonists (eg, pyrimethamine, trimethoprim).

►*Parenteral:* Treatment of megaloblastic anemias due to folic acid deficiency when oral therapy is not feasible.

In combination with 5-fluorouracil to prolong survival in the palliative treatment of patients with advanced colorectal cancer.

Administration and Dosage

Oral administration of doses > 25 mg is not recommended.

►*Advanced colorectal cancer:* Either of the following two regimens are recommended:

1) Leucovorin 200 mg/m² by slow IV injection over a minimum of 3 minutes, followed by 5-FU 370 mg/m² by IV injection.

2) Leucovorin 20 mg/m² by IV injection followed by 5-FU 425 mg/m² by IV injection.

Treatment is repeated daily for 5 days. This 5 day treatment course may be repeated at 4 week (28 day) intervals for 2 courses and then repeated at 4 to 5 week (28 to 35 day) intervals provided that the patient has completely recovered from the toxic effects of the prior treatment course.

In subsequent treatment courses, adjust the dosage of 5-FU based on patient tolerance of the prior treatment course. Reduce the daily dosage of 5-FU by 20% for patients who experienced moderate hematologic or GI toxicity in the prior treatment course, and by 30% for patients who experienced severe toxicity (see Precautions). For patients who experienced no toxicity in the prior treatment course, 5-FU dosage may be increased by 10%. Leucovorin dosages are not adjusted for toxicity.

Several other doses and schedules of leucovorin/5-FU therapy have also been evaluated in patients with advanced colorectal cancer; some of these alternative regimens may also have efficacy in the treatment of this disease. However, further clinical research will be required to confirm the safety and efficacy of these alternative treatment regimens.

►*Leucovorin rescue after high-dose MTX therapy:* The recommendations for leucovorin rescue are based on an MTX dose of 12 to 15 g/m² administered by IV infusion over 4 hours (see Methotrexate monograph). Leucovorin rescue at a dose of 15 mg (≈ 10 mg/m²) every 6 hours for 10 doses starts 24 hours after the beginning of the MTX infusion. In the presence of GI toxicity, nausea or vomiting, administer leucovorin parenterally.

Determine serum creatinine and MTX levels at least once daily. Continue leucovorin administration, hydration and urinary alkalinization (pH of ≥ 7) until the MTX level is < 5 x 10⁻⁸ M (0.05 micromolar). Adjust the leucovorin dose or extend leucovorin rescue based on the following guidelines:

Guidelines for Leucovorin Rescue Dosage and Administration		
Clinical situation	Laboratory findings	Leucovorin dosage/duration
Normal MTX elimination	Serum MTX level ≈ 10 micromolar at 24 hrs after administration, 1 micromolar at 48 hrs, and < 0.2 micromolar at 72 hours	15 mg orally, IM or IV every 6 hrs for 60 hrs (10 doses starting at 24 hrs after start of MTX infusion)

LEUCOVORIN CALCIUM (Folinic Acid; Citrovorum Factor)

Guidelines for Leucovorin Rescue Dosage and Administration		
Clinical situation	Laboratory findings	Leucovorin dosage/duration
Delayed late MTX elimination	Serum MTX level remaining > 0.2 micromolar at 72 hrs and > 0.05 micromolar at 96 hrs after administration	Continue 15 mg orally, IM or IV every 6 hrs, until MTX level is < 0.05 micromolar
Delayed early MTX elimination or evidence of acute renal injury	Serum MTX level of ≥ 50 micromolar at 24 hrs, or ≥ 5 micromolar at 48 hrs after administration or a ≥ 100% increase in serum creatinine level at 24 hrs after MTX administration (eg, an increase from 0.5 mg/dL to ≥ 1 mg/dL)	150 mg IV every 3 hrs, until MTX level is < 1 micromolar; then 15 mg IV every 3 hrs until MTX level is < 0.05 micromolar

Patients who experience delayed early MTX elimination are likely to develop reversible renal failure. In addition to appropriate leucovorin therapy, these patients require continuing hydration and urinary alkalinization, and close monitoring of fluid and electrolyte status, until the serum MTX level has fallen to < 0.05 micromolar and the renal failure has resolved.

Some patients will have abnormalities in MTX elimination or renal function following administration, which are significant but less severe than the abnormalities described in the table above. These abnormalities may or may not be associated with significant clinical toxicity. If significant clinical toxicity is observed, extend leucovorin rescue for an additional 24 hours (total of 14 doses over 84 hours) in subsequent courses of therapy. Always consider the possibility that the patient is taking other medications which interact with MTX (eg, medications which may interfere with MTX elimination or binding to serum albumin) when laboratory abnormalities or clinical toxicities are observed.

➤*Impaired MTX elimination or inadvertent overdosage:* Begin leucovorin rescue as soon as possible after an inadvertent overdosage and within 24 hours of MTX administration when there is delayed excretion (see Warnings). Administer leucovorin 10 mg/m^2 IV, IM or orally every 6 hours until the serum MTX level is < 10^{-8} M. In the presence of GI toxicity, nausea or vomiting, administer leucovorin parenterally.

Determine serum creatinine and MTX levels at 24 hour intervals. If the 24 hour serum creatinine has increased 50% over baseline or if the 24 or 48 hour MTX level is > 5 x 10^{-6} M or > 9 x 10^{-7} M, respectively, increase the dose of leucovorin to 100 mg/m^2 IV every 3 hours until the MTX level is < 10^{-8} M.

Use hydration (3 L/day) and urinary alkalinization with sodium bicarbonate solution concomitantly. Adjust the bicarbonate dose to maintain the urine pH at ≥ 7.

➤*Folic acid antagonist overdosage:* Recommended dose to counteract hematologic toxicity from folic acid antagonists with less affinity for mammalian dihydrofolate reductase than MTX (eg, pyrimethamine, trimethoprim) is 5 to 15 mg/day.

➤*Megaloblastic anemia due to folic acid deficiency:* ≤ 1 mg leucovorin/day. There is no evidence that doses > 1 mg/day have greater efficacy than 1 mg doses; also, loss of folate in urine becomes roughly logarithmic as the amount given exceeds 1 mg.

➤*Storage/Stability:* Leucovorin powder for injection contains no preservative. Reconstitute with Bacteriostatic Water for Injection, USP, which contains benzyl alcohol, or with Sterile Water for Injection, USP. When reconstituted with Bacteriostatic Water for Injection, USP, the resulting solution must be used within 7 days. If the product is reconstituted with Sterile Water for Injection, USP, it must be used immediately.

Because of the benzyl alcohol contained in the 1 mL amp and in Bacteriostatic Water for Injection, USP, when doses > 10 mg/m^2 are administered, reconstitute the leucovorin amps with Sterile Water for Injection, USP, and use immediately. Because of the calcium content of the leucovorin solution, inject no more than 160 mg/min IV (16 mL of a 10 mg/mL, or 8 mL of a 20 mg/mL solution per minute). Protect from light.

Actions

➤*Pharmacology:* Leucovorin is one of several active, chemically reduced derivatives of folic acid. It is useful as an antidote to drugs which act as folic acid antagonists. Leucovorin is a mixture of the diastereoisomers of the 5-formyl derivative of tetrahydrofolic acid (THF). The biologically active compound of the mixture is the l-isomer, known as citrovorum factor or folinic acid. Leucovorin does not require reduction by the enzyme dihydrofolate reductase in order to participate in reactions utilizing folates as a source of "one-carbon" moieties. l-Leucovorin is rapidly metabolized to 1,5-methyltetrahydrofolate, which can,

in turn, be metabolized via other pathways back to 5,10-methyl-ene-tetrahydrofolate, which is converted to 5-methyltetrahydrofolate by an irreversible, enzyme-catalyzed reduction using the cofactors FADH$_2$ and NADPH.

Administration of leucovorin can counteract the therapeutic and toxic effects of folic acid antagonists such as methotrexate (MTX), which act by inhibiting dihydrofolate reductase.

In contrast, leucovorin can enhance the therapeutic and toxic effects of fluoropyrimidines used in cancer therapy, such as 5-fluorouracil (5-FU). Concurrent administration of leucovorin does not appear to alter the plasma pharmacokinetics of 5-FU. 5-FU is metabolized to fluorodeoxyuridylic acid, which binds to and inhibits the enzyme thymidylate synthase (an enzyme important in DNA repair and replication). The reduced folate, 5,10-methylenetetrahydrofolate, acts to stabilize the binding of fluorodeoxyuridylic acid to thymidylate synthase and thereby enhances the inhibition of this enzyme.

➤*Pharmacokinetics:*

Leucovorin Pharmacokinetics[1]			
Parameter	IV	IM	Oral
Total reduced folates:			
Mean peak conc. (ng/mL)	1259 (range, 897-1625)	436 (range, 240 to 725)	393 (range, 160 to 550)
Mean time to peak	10 min	52 min	2.3 hrs
Terminal half-life	6.2 hrs	6.2 hrs	5.7 hrs
5-Methyl-THF[2]			
Mean peak conc. (ng/mL)	258	226	367
Mean time to peak	1.3 hrs	2.8 hrs	2.4 hrs
5-Formyl-THF[3]			
Mean peak conc. (ng/mL)	1206	360	51
Mean time to peak	10 min	28 min	1.2 hrs

[1] Following administration of a 25 mg dose.
[2] The major metabolite to which leucovorin is primarily converted in the intestinal mucosa and which becomes the predominant circulating form of the drug.
[3] The parent compound.

The initial rise in total reduced folates is primarily due to the parent compound (5-formyl-THF). A sharp drop in parent compound follows and coincides with the appearance of the active metabolite (5-methyl-THF).

Following IV administration, the area under the plasma concentration vs time curves (AUC) for l-leucovorin, d-leucovorin and 5-methyl-THF were 28.4 ± 3.5, 956 ± 97 and 129 ± 12 mg•min/L. When a higher dose of [d,l-leucovorin] was used, similar results were obtained. The d-isomer persisted in plasma at concentrations greatly exceeding those of the l-isomer. There was no difference between IM and IV administration in the AUC for total reduced folates, 5-formyl-THF or 5-methyl-THF. The AUC of total reduced folates after oral administration was 92% of the AUC after IV administration.

Following oral administration leucovorin is rapidly absorbed and expands the serum pool of reduced folates. At a dose of 25 mg, almost 100% of the I-isomer but only 20% of the d-isomer is absorbed. Oral absorption of leucovorin is saturable at doses > 25 mg. The apparent bioavailability of leucovorin was 97% for 25 mg, 75% for 50 mg and 37% for 100 mg.

➤*Clinical trials:* In a randomized clinical study in patients with advanced metastatic colorectal cancer, three treatment regimens were compared. Leucovorin 200 mg/m^2 and 5-FU 370 mg/m^2 vs leucovorin 20 mg/m^2 and 5-FU 425 mg/m^2 vs 5-FU 500 mg/m^2. All drugs were given by slow IV infusion daily for 5 days repeated every 28 to 35 days. Response rates were 26%, 43% and 10% for the high-dose leucovorin, low-dose leucovorin and 5-FU alone groups, respectively. Respective median survival times were 12.2 months, 12 months and 7.7 months. The low-dose leucovorin regimen gave a significant improvement in weight gain of > 5%, relief of symptoms and improvement in performance status. The high-dose regimen gave a significant improvement in performance status and trended toward improvement in weight gain and in relief of symptoms.

In a second randomized clinical study, the 5-FU monotherapy was replaced by a regimen of sequentially administered MTX, 5-FU and leucovorin. Response rates with leucovorin 200 mg/m^2 and 5-FU 370 mg/m^2 vs leucovorin 20 mg/m^2 and 5-FU 425 mg/m^2 vs sequential MTX and 5-FU and leucovorin were, respectively, 33%, 31% and 4%. Respective median survival times were 402 days, 418 days and 223 days. No significant difference in weight gain of > 5% or in improvement in performance status was seen between the treatment arms.

Contraindications

Pernicious anemia and other megaloblastic anemias secondary to the lack of vitamin B$_{12}$ (see Warnings).

Warnings

➤*Anemias:* Leucovorin is improper therapy for pernicious anemia and other megaloblastic anemias secondary to the lack of vitamin B$_{12}$. A

LEUCOVORIN CALCIUM (Folinic Acid; Citrovorum Factor)

hematologic remission may occur while neurologic manifestations continue to progress.

➤*5-Fluorouracil dosage / toxicity:* Leucovorin enhances the toxicity of 5-FU. When these drugs are administered concurrently in the palliative therapy of advanced colorectal cancer, the dosage of 5-FU must be lower than usually administered. Although the toxicities observed in patients treated with the combination of leucovorin plus 5-FU are qualitatively similar to those observed in patients treated with 5-FU alone, GI toxicities (particularly stomatitis and diarrhea) are observed more commonly and may be more severe and of prolonged duration in patients treated with the combination.

In a controlled trial, toxicity, primarily GI, resulted in 7% of patients requiring hospitalization when treated with 5-FU alone or 5-FU in combination with 200 mg/m^2 leucovorin and 20% when treated with 5-FU in combination with 20 mg/m^2 leucovorin. In another trial, hospitalizations related to treatment toxicity also appeared to occur more often in patients treated with low-dose leucovorin/5-FU combination than in patients treated with the high-dose combination (11% vs 3%). Therapy with leucovorin/5-FU must not be initiated or continued in patients who have symptoms of GI toxicity of any severity, until those symptoms have completely resolved. Patients with diarrhea must be monitored with particular care until the diarrhea has resolved, as rapid clinical deterioration leading to death can occur. In an additional study utilizing higher weekly doses of 5-FU and leucovorin, elderly or debilitated patients were found to be at greater risk for severe GI toxicity.

Since leucovorin enhances the toxicity of 5-FU, administer the combination for advanced colorectal cancer under the supervision of a physician experienced in the use of antimetabolite cancer chemotherapy. Take particular care in the treatment of elderly or debilitated colorectal cancer patients, as these patients may be at increased risk of severe toxicity.

➤*Methotrexate concentrations:* Monitoring of the serum MTX concentration is essential in determining the optimal dose and duration of treatment with leucovorin. Delayed MTX excretion may be caused by a third space fluid accumulation (ie, ascites, pleural effusion), renal insufficiency or inadequate hydration. Under such circumstances, higher doses of leucovorin or prolonged administration may be indicated. Doses higher than those recommended for oral use must be given IV.

➤*Calcium content:* Because of the calcium content of the leucovorin solution, inject no more than 160 mg/min IV (16 mL of a 10 mg/mL, or 8 mL of a 20 mg/mL solution per minute).

➤*Folic acid antagonist overdosage:* In the treatment of accidental overdosages of folic acid antagonists (eg, pyrimethamine, trimethoprim), administer leucovorin as promptly as possible. As the time interval between antifolate administration (eg, MTX) and leucovorin rescue increases, leucovorin's effectiveness in counteracting toxicity decreases.

➤*Benzyl alcohol:* Because of the benzyl alcohol contained in the 1 mL amp and in certain diluents used for leucovorin injection, when doses > 10 mg/m^2 are administered, reconstitute leucovorin injection with Sterile Water for Injection, USP, and use immediately (see Administration and Dosage). Benzyl alcohol has been associated with a fatal gasping syndrome in premature infants.

➤*Pregnancy:* Category C. It is not known whether leucovorin can cause fetal harm when administered to a pregnant woman or can affect reproduction capacity. Give to a pregnant woman only if clearly needed.

➤*Lactation:* It is not known whether this drug is excreted in breast milk. Exercise caution when administering to a nursing woman.

Precautions

➤*Parenteral administration:* Parenteral administration is preferable to oral dosing if there is a possibility that the patient may vomit or not absorb the leucovorin. Leucovorin has no effect on nonhematologic toxicities of MTX such as the nephrotoxicity resulting from drug or metabolite precipitation in the kidney.

➤*Monitoring:* Obtain a CBC with differential and platelets prior to each treatment with the leucovorin/5-FU combination. During the first two courses a CBC with differential and platelets must be repeated weekly and thereafter once each cycle at the time of anticipated WBC nadir. Perform electrolyte and liver function tests prior to each treatment for the first three cycles, then prior to every other cycle. Institute dosage modifications of 5-FU as follows, based on the most severe toxicities:

5-Fluorouracil Dosage Modifications Based on Toxicities			
Diarrhea or stomatitis	WBC/mm^3 nadir	Platelets/mm^3 nadir	5-FU dose
Moderate	1000-1900	25,000-75,000	decrease 20%
Severe	< 1000	< 25,000	decrease 30%

If no toxicity occurs, the 5-FU dose may increase 10%.

Defer treatment until WBCs are 4000/mm^3 and platelets are 130,000/mm^3. If blood counts do not reach these levels within 2 weeks, discontinue treatment. Follow up patients with physical examination prior to each treatment course and with appropriate radiological examination as needed. Discontinue treatment when there is clear evidence of tumor progression.

Drug Interactions

Leucovorin Drug Interactions		
Precipitant drug	Object drug*	Description
Leucovorin	Anticonvulsants ↓	Folic acid in large amounts may counteract the antiepileptic effect of phenobarbital, phenytoin and primidone, and increase the frequency of seizures in susceptible children. Although this interaction has not been reported with leucovorin, consider the possibility when using these drugs concomitantly.
Leucovorin	5-Fluorouracil ↑	Leucovorin may enhance the toxicity of 5-FU (see Warnings).
Leucovorin	Methotrexate ↓	Small quantities of systemically administered leucovorin enter the CSF primarily as 5-methyltetrahydrofolate and remain 1 to 3 orders of magnitude lower than the usual MTX concentrations following intrathecal administration. However, high doses of leucovorin may reduce the efficacy of intrathecally administered MTX.

* ↑ = Object drug increased.   ↓ = Object drug decreased.

Adverse Reactions

Allergic sensitization, including anaphylactoid reactions and urticaria, has been reported following administration of both oral and parenteral leucovorin. No other adverse reactions have been attributed to the use of leucovorin alone.

The following table summarizes significant adverse events occurring in 316 patients treated with the leucovorin/5-FU combinations compared with 70 patients treated with 5-FU alone for advanced colorectal carcinoma.

Adverse Reactions with the Leucovorin/5-Fluorouracil Combination					
	High leucovorin[1]/ 5-FU (n=155)		Low leucovorin[2]/ 5-FU (n=161)		5-FU alone (n=70)	
Adverse reaction	Any[3] (%)	Grade 3+[4] (%)	Any[3] (%)	Grade 3+[4] (%)	Any[3] (%)	Grade 3+[4] (%)
Leukopenia	69	14	83	23	93	48
Thrombocytopenia	8	2	8	1	18	3
Infection	8	1	3	1	7	2
Nausea	74	10	80	9	60	6
Vomiting	46	8	44	9	40	7
Diarrhea	66	18	67	14	43	11
Stomatitis	75	27	84	29	59	16
Constipation	3	–	4	–	1	–
Lethargy/Malaise/ Fatigue	13	3	12	2	6	3
Alopecia	42	5	43	6	37	7
Dermatitis	21	2	25	1	13	–
Anorexia	14	1	22	4	14	–
Hospitalization for toxicity	5%		15%		7%	

[1] High leucovorin = 200 mg/m^2.
[2] Low leucovorin = 20 mg/m^2.
[3] Any = Percentage of patients reporting toxicity of any severity.
[4] Grade 3+ = Percentage of patients reporting toxicity of Grade 3 or higher.

Overdosage

Excessive amounts of leucovorin may nullify the chemotherapeutic effect of folic acid antagonists (eg, pyrimethamine, trimethoprim).

VITAMIN B$_{12}$, PARENTERAL

Indications

➤*Vitamin B$_{12}$ deficiency:* Vitamin B$_{12}$ deficiency due to malabsorption syndrome as seen in pernicious anemia; GI pathology, dysfunction or surgery; fish tapeworm infestation; malignancy of pancreas or bowel; gluten enteropathy; sprue; small bowel bacterial overgrowth; total or partial gastrectomy; accompanying folic acid deficiency.

➤*Increased vitamin B$_{12}$ requirements:* Increased vitamin B$_{12}$ requirements associated with pregnancy, thyrotoxicosis, hemolytic anemia, hemorrhage, malignancy and hepatic and renal disease.

➤*Vitamin B$_{12}$ absorption test:* (Schilling test). Cyanocobalamin (oral) is used for nutritional vitamin B$_{12}$ deficiency (see monograph).

➤*Unlabeled uses:* Hydroxocobalamin has been used to prevent and to treat cyanide toxicity associated with sodium nitroprusside. It lowers red blood cell and plasma cyanide concentrations by combining with cyanide to form cyanocobalamin, which is nontoxic and excreted in the urine.

Actions

➤*Pharmacology:* Vitamin B$_{12}$ (cyanocobalamin and hydroxocobalamin) is essential to growth, cell reproduction, hematopoiesis and nucleoprotein and myelin synthesis. Its physiologic role is associated with methylation, participating in nucleic acid and protein synthesis. Cyanocobalamin participates in red blood cell formation through activation of folic acid coenzymes. Cyanocobalamin has hematopoietic activity apparently identical to that of the anti-anemia factor in purified liver extract.Hydroxocobalamin (vitamin B$_{12a}$), an analog of cyanocobalamin in which a hydroxyl radical replaces the cyano radical, functions the same as cyanocobalamin.

The normal range of plasma B$_{12}$ is 200 to 750 pg/mL, which represents ≈ 0.1% of the total body content. The total daily loss ranges from 2 to 5 mcg. Because of its slow rate of utilization and considerable body stores, vitamin B$_{12}$ deficiency may take many months to appear.

The average diet supplies ≈ 5 to 15 mcg/day of vitamin B$_{12}$. Vitamin B$_{12}$ is bound to intrinsic factor during transit through the stomach; separation occurs in the terminal ileum in the presence of calcium, and vitamin B$_{12}$ enters the mucosal cell for absorption. It is then transported by specific B$_{12}$ binding proteins, transcobalamin I and II. Transcobalamin II is the delivery protein for vitamin B$_{12}$. In addition, ≈ 1% of the total amount ingested is absorbed by simple diffusion, but this mechanism is significant only with large doses.

For use of oral vitamin B$_{12}$ in the treatment of nutritional deficiency, see the individual monograph.

➤*Pharmacokinetics:* Absorption of vitamin B$_{12}$ depends on the presence of sufficient intrinsic factor and calcium. In general, absorption of oral B$_{12}$ is inadequate in malabsorptive states and in pernicious anemia (unless intrinsic factor is simultaneously administered).

Cyanocobalamin – Cyanocobalamin is rapidly absorbed from IM and SC injection sites; the plasma level peaks within 1 hour.Once absorbed, it is bound to plasma proteins, stored mainly in the liver and is slowly released when needed to carry out normal cellular metabolic functions. Within 48 hours after injection of 100 to 1000 mcg of vitamin B$_{12}$, 50% to 98% of the dose appears in the urine. The major portion is excreted within the first 8 hours. More rapid excretion occurs with IV administration; there is little opportunity for liver storage.

Hydroxocobalamin – Hydroxocobalamin (vitamin B$_{12a}$) is more highly protein bound and is retained in the body longer than cyanocobalamin. However, it has no advantage over cyanocobalamin. Administration of hydroxocobalamin has resulted in antibody formation to the hydroxocobalamin-transcobalamin II complex and thus cyanocobalamin may be preferred.

Contraindications

Hypersensitivity to cobalt, vitamin B$_{12}$ or any component of these products.

Warnings

➤*Inadequate response:* Parenteral administration is preferred for pernicious anemia. Avoid the IV route.

A blunted or impeded therapeutic response may be due to infection, uremia, bone marrow suppressant drugs (ie, chloramphenicol), concurrent iron or folic acid deficiency or misdiagnosis.

➤*Vitamin B$_{12}$ deficiency:* Vitamin B$_{12}$ deficiency allowed to progress for > 3 months may produce permanent degenerative lesions of the spinal cord.

➤*Optic nerve atrophy:* Patients with early Leber's disease (hereditary optic nerve atrophy) treated with cyanocobalamin suffer severe and swift optic atrophy.

➤*Hypokalemia:* Hypokalemia and sudden death may occur in severe megaloblastic anemia which is treated intensely.

➤*Benzyl alcohol:* Some of these products contain benzyl alcohol, which has been associated with a fatal "gasping syndrome" in premature infants.

➤*Pregnancy: Category C* (parenteral). Adequate and well-controlled studies have not been performed in pregnant women. However, B$_{12}$ is an essential vitamin and needs are increased during pregnancy. The National Academy of Sciences has recommended that 2.2 mcg/day should be consumed during pregnancy.

➤*Lactation:* Vitamin B$_{12}$ is excreted in breast milk in concentrations that approximate the mother's vitamin B$_{12}$blood level. Amounts of B$_{12}$ recommended by the Food and Nutrition Board, National Academy of Sciences-National Research Council (2.6 mcg daily) should be consumed during lactation.

➤*Children:* The Food and Nutrition Board, National Academy of Sciences-National Research Council recommends a daily intake of 0.3 to 0.5 mcg/day for infants < 1 year of age and 0.7 to 1.4 mcg/day for children 1 to 10 years of age.

Precautions

➤*Monitoring:* During treatment of severe megaloblastic anemia, monitor serum potassium levels closely for the first 48 hours and replace potassium if necessary. Obtain reticulocyte counts, hematocrit and vitamin B$_{12}$, iron and folic acid plasma levels prior to treatment and between the fifth and seventh days of therapy, and then frequently until the hematocrit is normal. If folate levels are low, also administer folic acid. Continue periodic hematologic evaluations throughout the patient's lifetime.

➤*Test dose:* Anaphylactic shock and death have occurred after parenteral vitamin B$_{12}$ administration. Give an intradermal test dose in patients sensitive to the cobalamins.

➤*Folate:* Doses > 10 mcg daily may produce hematologic response in patients with folate deficiency. Indiscriminate use may mask the true diagnosis of pernicious anemia.

Doses of folic acid > 0.1 mg/day may result in hematologic remission in patients with vitamin B$_{12}$ deficiency. Neurologic manifestations will not be prevented with folic acid, and if not treated with vitamin B$_{12}$, irreversible damage will result.

Single deficiency – Single deficiency (vitamin B$_{12}$ alone) is rare. Expect multiple vitamin deficiency in any dietary deficiency.

➤*Polycythemia vera:* Vitamin B$_{12}$ deficiency may suppress the signs of polycythemia vera. Treatment with vitamin B$_{12}$ may unmask this condition.

➤*Vegetarian diets:* Vegetarian diets containing no animal products (including milk products or eggs) do not supply any vitamin B$_{12}$. Vegetarians should take oral vitamin B$_{12}$ regularly.

➤*Stomach carcinoma:* Pernicious anemia patients have about 3 times the incidence of stomach carcinoma as the general population; perform appropriate tests for this condition when indicated.

➤*Immunodeficient patients:* Vitamin B$_{12}$ malabsorption may occur in patients with AIDS or HIV infection. Consider monitoring vitamin B$_{12}$ levels in these patients.

Drug Interactions

Vitamin B$_{12}$ Drug Interactions			
Precipitant drug	Object drug*		Description
Aminosalicylic acid	Vitamin B$_{12}$	↓	Biologic and therapeutic action of vitamin B$_{12}$ may be reduced. An abnormal Schilling test and symptoms of vitamin B$_{12}$ deficiency may also occur.
Chloramphenicol	Vitamin B$_{12}$	↓	The hematologic effects of vitamin B$_{12}$ may be decreased in patients with pernicious anemia.
Colchicine Alcohol	Vitamin B$_{12}$	↓	Colchicine or excessive alcohol intake (> 2 weeks) may cause malabsorption of vitamin B$_{12}$.

* ↓ = Object drug decreased.

➤*Drug/Lab test interactions:* Methotrexate, pyrimethamine and most antibiotics invalidate folic acid and vitamin B$_{12}$ diagnostic microbiological blood assays.

Adverse Reactions

The following reactions are associated with parenteral vitamin B$_{12}$:

➤*Cardiovascular:* Pulmonary edema; congestive heart failure early in treatment; peripheral vascular thrombosis.

➤*Dermatologic:* Itching; transitory exanthema.

➤*Hypersensitivity:* Anaphylactic shock and death.

➤*Miscellaneous:* Feeling of swelling of the entire body; mild transient diarrhea; polycythemia vera; pain at injection site; severe and swift optic nerve atrophy (see Warnings).

VITAMIN B$_{12}$, PARENTERAL

Patient Information

Patients with pernicious anemia will require monthly injections of vitamin B$_{12}$ for the rest of their lives. Failure to do so will result in return of the anemia and in development of incapacitating and irreversible damage to the nerves of the spinal cord.

A well balanced dietary intake is necessary; correct poor dietary habits.

Do not take folic acid instead of vitamin B$_{12}$ because folic acid may prevent anemia, but allow progression of subacute combined degeneration.

HYDROXOCOBALAMIN, CRYSTALLINE (Vitamin B$_{12}$)

Rx	Hydro-Crysti-12 (Roberts Hauck)	Injection: 1000 mcg/mL	In 30 mL.
Rx	LA-12 (Hyrex)		In 30 mL.

For complete prescribing information, refer to the Vitamin B$_{12}$ monograph.

Administration and Dosage

Administer IM only. The recommended dosage is 30 mcg/day for 5 to 10 days, followed by 100 to 200 mcg monthly. Children may be given a total of 1 to 5 mg over 2 or more weeks in doses of 100 mcg, then 30 to 50 mcg every 4 weeks for maintenance. Institute concurrent folic acid therapy at the beginning of treatment if needed.

CYANOCOBALAMIN CRYSTALLINE

otc	Vitamin B$_{12}$ (Goldline)	Tablets: 500 mcg	Pink. In 100s.
		1000 mcg	Pink. In 100s.
Rx	Vitamin B$_{12}$ (Various, eg, Goldline, Rugby)	Injection: 100 mcg per mL	In 30 mL vials.
Rx	Vitamin B$_{12}$ (Various, eg, American Regent, Geneva, Goldline, Major, Pasadena, Rugby, Schein, Warner Chilcott)	Injection: 1000 mcg per mL	In 10 and 30 mL multi-dose vials.
Rx	Crystamine (Dunhall)		In 10 and 30 mL multi-dose vials.[1]
Rx	Crysti 1000 (Roberts Hauck)		In 10 mL vials.
Rx	Cyanoject (Mayrand)		In 10 and 30 mL.[1]
Rx	Cyomin (Forest)		In 30 mL multi-dose vials.[1]
Rx	Rubesol-1000 (Central)		In 10 and 30 mL vials[1].

[1] With benzyl alcohol.

For complete prescribing information, refer to the Vitamin B$_{12}$ monograph.

Administration and Dosage

➤*Addisonian pernicious anemia:* Parenteral therapy is required for life; oral therapy is not dependable. Administer 100 mcg daily for 6 or 7 days by IM or deep SC injection. If there is clinical improvement and a reticulocyte response, give the same amount on alternate days for 7 doses, then every 3 to 4 days for another 2 to 3 weeks. By this time, hematologic values should have become normal. Follow this regimen with 100 mcg monthly for life. Administer folic acid concomitantly if needed.

➤*Other patients with vitamin B$_{12}$ deficiency:* In seriously ill patients, administer both vitamin B$_{12}$ and folic acid. It is not necessary to withhold therapy until the precise cause of B$_{12}$ deficiency is established. For hematologic signs, children may be given 10 to 50 mcg/day for 5 to 10 days followed by 100 to 250 mcg/dose every 2 to 4 weeks; for neurologic signs, 100 mcg/day for 10 to 15 days, then once or twice weekly for several months, possibly tapering to 250 to 1000 mcg monthly by 1 year.

Oral – Up to 1000 mcg/day. Oral vitamin B$_{12}$ therapy is not usually recommended for vitamin B$_{12}$ deficiency. The maximum amount of vitamin B$_{12}$ that can be absorbed from a single oral dose is 1 to 5 mcg. The percent absorbed decreases with increasing doses.

IM or SC – 30 mcg daily for 5 to 10 days followed by 100 to 200 mcg monthly. Larger doses (eg, 1000 mcg) have been recommended, even though a larger amount is lost through excretion. However, it is possible that a greater amount is retained, allowing for fewer injections.

➤*Schilling test:* The flushing dose is 1000 mcg IM.

➤*Storage/Stability:* Protect parenterals from light. Avoid freezing.

For information on parenteral calcium products, refer to Intravenous Nutritional Therapy, Minerals section.

Indications

As a dietary supplement when calcium intake may be inadequate. Conditions that may be associated with calcium deficiency include the following: Vitamin D deficiency, sprue, pregnancy and lactation, achlorhydria, chronic diarrhea, hypoparathyroidism, steatorrhea, menopause, renal failure, pancreatitis, hyperphosphatemia, and alkalosis. Some diuretics and anticonvulsants may precipitate hypocalcemia, which may validate calcium replacement therapy. Calcium salt therapy should not preclude the use of other corrective measures intended to treat the underlying cause of calcium depletion.

Oral calcium may also be used in the treatment of osteoporosis, osteomalacia, rickets, and latent tetany.

Calcium taken daily may help reduce typical premenstrual syndrome (PMS) symptoms such as bloating, cramps, fatigue, and moodiness.

➤*Calcium acetate (PhosLo):* Control of hyperphosphatemia in end-stage renal failure; does not promote aluminum absorption.

Administration and Dosage

➤*Recommended dietary allowances (RDAs):*
Men and women (19 to 24 years of age) – 1200 mg/day
Men and women (25 to 50 years of age) – 800 mg/day
Men and women (≥ 51 years of age) – 800 mg/day
➤*Dietary reference intakes (DRIs):*
Men and women (19 to 50 years of age) – 1000 mg/day
Men and women (> 51 years of age) – 1200 mg/day
Pregnant and breastfeeding women – 1000 mg/day
➤*Dietary supplement:* The usual daily dose is 500 mg to 2 g, 2 to 4 times/day.

Calcium is recommended in doses of 1500 mg/day for men > 65 years of age and for postmenopausal women not taking estrogen replacement therapy.

➤*PhosLo:* For adult dialysis patients, the initial dose is 2 tablets/capsules/gelcaps with each meal. The dosage may be increased gradually to bring the serum phosphate value < 6 mg/dL, as long as hypercalcemia does not develop. Most patients require 3 to 4 tablets with each meal.

The recommended initial dose of the half-size (333.5 mg) *PhosLo* for the adult dialysis patient is 4 capsules with each meal. The dosage may be increased gradually to bring the serum phosphate value below 6 mg/dL, as long as hypercalcemia does not develop. Most patients require 6 to 8 capsules with each meal.

➤*Florical:* 1 capsule or tablet daily.

Actions

➤*Pharmacology:* Calcium is the fifth most abundant element in the body; the major fraction is in bone. It is essential for the functional integrity of the nervous and muscular systems, for normal cardiac function, for cell permeability, and for blood coagulation. It also functions as an enzyme cofactor and affects the secretory activity of endocrine and exocrine glands.

Adequate calcium intake is particularly important during periods of bone growth in childhood and adolescence and during pregnancy and lactation. An adequate supply of calcium is necessary in adults, especially those > 40 years of age, to prevent a negative calcium balance, which may contribute to the development of osteoporosis.

Patients with advanced renal insufficiency (Ccr < 30 mL/min) exhibit phosphate retention and some degree of hyperphosphatemia. The retention of phosphate plays a pivotal role in causing secondary hyperparathyroidism associated with osteodystrophy and soft-tissue calcification. Calcium acetate, when taken with meals, combines with dietary phosphate to form insoluble calcium phosphate, which is excreted in the feces.

Elemental Calcium Content of Calcium Salts[a]		
Calcium salt	% Calcium	mEq Ca^{++}/g
Calcium glubionate	6.5	3.3
Calcium gluconate	9	4.5
Calcium lactate	13	6.5
Calcium citrate	21	10.6
Calcium acetate	25	12.6
Tricalcium phosphate	39	19.3
Calcium carbonate	40	20

[a] 1 mEq of elemental calcium = 20 mg

➤*Pharmacokinetics:*
Absorption – Calcium is absorbed from the GI tract by passive diffusion and active transport. Calcium must be in a soluble, ionized form for absorption to occur. Vitamin D is required for calcium absorption and increases the capability of the absorptive mechanisms. Calcium absorption is increased in the presence of food. Oral bioavailability in adults ranges from 25% to 35% when a 250 mg dose is given with a standardized breakfast. Absorption from milk was ≈ 29% under the same conditions. Calcium absorption varies with age, being highest during infancy (≈ 60%), decreasing to ≈ 28% in prepubertal children, and increasing again during puberty (≈ 34%). Fractional absorption remains at ≈ 25% in young adults, and increases during the last 2 trimesters of pregnancy. Calcium absorption decreases ≈ 0.21% annually in postmenopausal women and similarly in aging men.

Distribution – Calcium enters the extracellular fluid and is rapidly incorporated into skeletal tissue. Normal total serum calcium concentrations range from 9 to 10.4 mg/dL (4.5 to 5.2 mEq/L), but only ionized calcium is active. Calcium crosses the placenta and reaches higher concentrations in fetal blood than maternal blood. Calcium also is distributed in milk.

Excretion – Calcium is mainly excreted in the feces. Only small amounts are excreted in the urine. Urinary excretion of calcium may be as high as 250 to 300 mg/day in healthy adults who eat a regular diet. However, urinary excretion does not exceed 150 mg/day in patients on low calcium diets. Urinary excretion decreases with age, in the early stages of renal failure, and during pregnancy. Calcium also is excreted by the sweat glands.

Contraindications

Hypercalcemia, ventricular fibrillation.

Warnings

➤*PhosLo:* End-stage renal failure patients may develop hypercalcemia when given calcium with meals. Do not give other calcium supplements concurrently with *PhosLo*. Chronic hypercalcemia may lead to vascular and other soft tissue calcification. Monitor serum calcium levels twice weekly during the early dose adjustment period. Do not allow serum calcium times phosphate product to exceed 66.

➤*GI effects:* Calcium salts may be irritating to the GI tract when administered orally and also may cause constipation.

➤*Hypercalcemia:* Hypercalcemia may occur when large doses of calcium are administered to patients with chronic renal failure. Mild hypercalcemia may exhibit as nausea, vomiting, anorexia, or constipation, with mental changes such as stupor, delirium, coma, or confusion. By reducing calcium intake, mild hypercalcemia is usually readily controlled.

➤*Renal calculi:* Recent evidence from studies in men 40 to 75 years of age with no history of kidney stones and women 34 to 59 years of age show that high dietary intake of calcium decreases the risk of symptomatic renal calculi, while intake of supplemental calcium may increase the risk of symptomatic stones. This conflicts with the previous theory that high calcium intake contributes to the risk of renal calculi.

➤*Pregnancy: Category C (PhosLo).* It is not known whether *PhosLo* can cause fetal harm when administered to a pregnant woman or can affect reproduction capacity. Give to a pregnant woman only if clearly needed.

➤*Children:* Safety and efficacy in children have not been established (*PhosLo*).

Precautions

➤*Monitoring:* Perform frequent determinations of serum calcium concentrations. Maintain serum calcium concentrations at 9 to 10.4 mg/dL (4.5 to 5.2 mEq/L). Do not allow levels to exceed 12 mg/dL.

➤*Special risk patients:* Use calcium salts cautiously in patients with sarcoidosis, cardiac or renal disease, and in patients receiving cardiac glycosides.

➤*Calcium citrate:*
Renal function impairment – Avoid concurrent aluminum-containing antacids.

➤*Phenylketonurics:* Inform phenylketonuric patients that some of these products contain phenylalanine.

➤*Tartrazine sensitivity:* Some of these products contain tartrazine (FD&C yellow #5), which may cause allergic-type reactions (including bronchial asthma) in susceptible individuals. Although the incidence of sensitivity is low, it is frequently seen in patients who also have aspirin hypersensitivity. Specific products containing tartrazine are identified in the product listings.

Calcium

Drug Interactions

Calcium Drug Interactions			
Precipitant	Object drug*		Description
Calcium salts	Iron salts	↓	GI absorption of iron may be reduced. In order to avoid a possible interaction, separate administration times whenever possible.
Calcium carbonate	Quinolones	↓	GI absorption of quinolones may be decreased. The bioavailability of norfloxacin may be reduced; lomefloxacin and ofloxacin do not appear to be affected. Give antacids ≥ 6 hours before or 2 hours after the quinolone.
Calcium salts	Sodium polystyrene sulfonate	↓	Coadministration in patients with renal impairment may result in an unanticipated metabolic alkalosis and a reduction of the resin's binding of potassium. Separate drugs by several hours.
Calcium salts	Tetracyclines	↓	The absorption and serum levels of tetracyclines are decreased; a decreased anti-infective response may occur. Avoid simultaneous administration. Separate administration by 3 to 4 hours.

Calcium Drug Interactions			
Precipitant	Object drug*		Description
Calcium salts	Verapamil	↓	Clinical effects and toxicities of verapamil may be reversed.

* ↑ = Object drug increased.   ↓ = Object drug decreased.

Adverse Reactions

May cause constipation and headache. Mild hypercalcemia (Ca^{++} > 10.5 mg/dL) may be asymptomatic or manifest itself as anorexia, nausea, and vomiting. More severe hypercalcemia (Ca^{++} > 12 mg/dL) is associated with confusion, delirium, stupor, and coma.

Overdosage

Administration of *PhosLo* in excess of the appropriate daily dosage can cause severe hypercalcemia (see Adverse Reactions). Severe hypercalcemia can be treated by acute hemodialysis and discontinuing therapy.

Patient Information

Notify physician if any of the following occur: Anorexia, nausea, vomiting, constipation, abdominal pain, dry mouth, thirst, polyuria.

Inform phenylketonuric patients that some of these products contain phenylalanine.

Take with or following meals to enhance absorption.

Take with a large glass of water.

CALCIUM GLUCONATE

otc	**Calcium Gluconate** (Various, eg, Dixon-Shane, Freeda, Roxane, Rugby)	**Tablets:** 500 mg (45 mg elemental calcium)	In 100s.
		Tablets: 50 mg elemental calcium	In 100s and 500s.
		648 to 650 mg (58.5 to 60 mg elemental calcium)	In 1000s.
		972 to 975 mg (87.75 to 90 mg elemental calcium)	In 1000s.
otc	**Calcium Gluconate** (Freeda)	**Powder for oral suspension:** 346.7 mg elemental calcium/15 mL	In 454 g.

Complete prescribing information for these products begins in the Calcium group monograph.

CALCIUM GLUBIONATE

otc	**Calcionate** (Various, eg, Rugby, Watson)	**Syrup:** 1.8 g/5 mL	In 473 mL.
otc	**Calciquid** (Breckenridge)		In 473 mL.

Complete prescribing information for these products begins in the Calcium group monograph.

CALCIUM LACTATE

otc	**Calcium Lactate** (Various, eg, Dixon-Shane, Rugby)	**Tablets:** 648 to 650 mg (84.5 mg elemental calcium)	In 100s and 1000s.
otc	**Calcium Lactate** (Various, eg, Freeda)	**Tablets:** 100 mg elemental calcium	In 100s and 250s.
otc sf	**Cal-Lac** (Bio-Tech)	**Capsules:** 500 mg (96 mg elemental calcium)	In 100s.

Complete prescribing information for these products begins in the Calcium group monograph.

CALCIUM CITRATE

otc	**Citracal** (Mission)	**Tablets:** 200 mg elemental calcium	(CITRACAL MPC). In 100s.
otc	**Citrus Calcium** (Rugby)	**Tablets:** 200 mg as calcium citrate	Lactose free. Coated. In 100s.
otc	**Calcium Citrate** (Various, eg, Freeda, Vitaline)	**Tablets:** 250 mg elemental calcium	In 100s, 120s, 250s, 500s, 1000s.
otc	**Cal-Citrate-250** (Bio-Tech)		In 250s.
otc	**Calcium Citrate** (Various, eg, Major)	**Tablets:** 950 mg	In 100s.
otc	**Citracal Liquitab** (Mission)	**Tablets, effervescent:** 500 mg elemental calcium	Aspartame, 12 mg phenylalanine, saccharin. Orange flavor. In 30s.
otc	**Cal-Citrate-225** (Bio-Tech)	**Capsules:** 225 mg elemental calcium	In 100s and 250s.
otc	**Calcium Citrate** (Various, eg, Freeda)	**Powder for oral suspension:** 760 mg elemental calcium/5 mL	In 454 g.

Complete prescribing information for these products begins in the Calcium group monograph.

CALCIUM ACETATE

Rx	**PhosLo** (Nabi)	**Tablets:** 667 mg (169 mg elemental calcium)	Polyethylene glycol 8000. (BRA 200). White. In 200s.
		Capsules: 333.5 mg (half-size) (84.5 mg elemental calcium)	Polyethylene glycol 8000. (PhosLo 333.5 mg). White. In 400s.
		667 mg (169 mg elemental calcium)	Polyethylene glycol 8000. (PhosLo 667 mg). Blue/white. In 200s.
		Gelcaps: 667 mg (169 mg elemental calcium)	Polyethylene glycol 8000. (PhosLo 667 mg). Blue/white. In 200s.

Complete prescribing information for these products begins in the Calcium group monograph.

Calcium

TRICALCIUM PHOSPHATE (Calcium Phosphate, Tribasic)

otc sf	**Posture** (Iverness Medical)	**Tablets:** 600 mg elemental calcium	Preservative-free. In 90s.

Complete prescribing information for these products begins in the Calcium group monograph.

CALCIUM CARBONATE

otc	**Calcium Carbonate** (Various, eg, Major, Roxane, Rugby)	**Tablets:** 648 to 650 mg (260 mg elemental calcium)	In 100s and 1000s.
otc	**Calcium Carbonate** (Various, eg, Freeda)		Original and mint flavors. In 100s, 250s, and 500s.
otc	**Calcium Carbonate** (Various, eg, Roxane)	**Tablets:** 1250 mg (500 mg elemental calcium)	In 100s.
otc	**Cal-Carb Forte** (Vitaline)		Capsule shape, scored. In 100s.
otc	**Oyster Shell Calcium** (Various, eg, Major)		In 60s, 150s, 300s, and 1000s and UD 100s.
otc	**Oysco 500** (Rugby)		As oyster shell calcium. In 60s and 250s.
otc sf	**Oyst-Cal 500** (Goldline)		As oyster shell calcium. Preservative-free. Tartrazine. In 60s and 120s.
otc sf	**Os-Cal 500** (GlaxoSmithKline Consumer)		Oyster shell powder, corn syrup, parabens. In 75s.
otc	**Calcium Carbonate** (Various, eg, Major)	**Tablets:** 1500 mg (600 mg elemental calcium)	In 60s and 150s.
otc	**Calcium 600** (Rugby)		In 60s.
otc sf	**Caltrate 600** (Whitehall Robins)		Preservative-free. (CALTRATE). In 60s.
otc	**Nephro-Calci** (Watson)		(RD26). White, oval, scored. In 100s.
otc	**Tums** (GlaxoSmithKline Consumer)	**Tablets, chewable:** 500 mg (200 mg elemental calcium)	Sucrose, talc. Assorted fruit and peppermint flavors. In 75s and 150s.
otc	**Cal·Gest** (Rugby)		Dextrose. Assorted flavors. In 150s.
otc	**Calcium Antacid Extra Strength** (Various, eg, Major)	**Tablets, chewable:** 750 mg (300 mg elemental calcium)	In 96s.
otc	**Tums E-X** (GlaxoSmithKline Consumer)		Sucrose, talc. Mixed berry, assorted fruit, and sugar free orange (aspartame, < 1 mg phenylalanine, sorbitol) flavors . In 96s.
otc	**Tums Calcium for Life PMS** (GlaxoSmithKline Consumer)		Sucrose. Strawberry flavor. In 120s.
otc	**Tums Smooth Dissolve** (GlaxoSmithKline)		Sorbitol, dextrose, sucrose (2 g sugar). In peppermint and assorted fruit flavors. In 45s.
otc	**Tums Ultra** (GlaxoSmithKline Consumer)	**Tablets, chewable:** 1000 mg (400 mg elemental calcium)	Sucrose, talc. Mint flavor. In 86s.
otc	**Calcium Carbonate** (Various, eg, Major)	**Tablets, chewable:** 1250 mg (500 mg elemental calcium)	In 60s.
otc	**Cal-Carb Forte** (Vitaline)		Mint flavor. In 100s.
otc	**Calci-Chew** (Watson)		(RD05). Sugar. White. Cherry and assorted flavors. In 100s.
otc	**Os-Cal 500** (GlaxoSmithKline Consumer)		Dextrose. In 60s.
otc	**Tums Calcium for Life Bone Health** (GlaxoSmithKline Consumer)		In 90s.
otc	**Calci-Mix** (Watson)	**Capsules:** 1250 mg (500 mg elemental calcium)	In 100s.
otc	**Florical** (Mericon)	**Capsules and tablets:** 364 mg calcium carbonate (145.6 mg elemental calcium) and 8.3 mg sodium fluoride	In 100s and 500s.
otc	**Calcium Carbonate** (Various, eg, Roxane)	**Oral suspension:** 1250 mg (500 mg elemental calcium)/5 mL	In 500 mL and UD 5 mL.
otc	**Calcium Carbonate** (Various, eg, Freeda, Humco)	**Powder**	In 454 g.

Complete prescribing information for these products begins in the Calcium group monograph. For calcium carbonate antacids, see the Antacids monograph in the Gastrointestinal Agents chapter.

PHOSPHORUS REPLACEMENT PRODUCTS

Contents given per tablet or 75 mL reconstituted liquid.

	Product and distributor	Phosphorus		Potassium		Sodium		Recommended adult dose	How supplied
		mg	mEq	mg	mEq	mg	mEq		
Rx	**Uro-KP-Neutral Tablets** (Star)	250	14.25	49.4	1.27	250.5	10.9	1 or 2 tablets 4 times/day with full glass of water	Lt. peach, capsule shape. Film-coated. In 100s.
Rx	**K-Phos Neutral Tablets** (Beach)	250	14.25	45	1.1	298	13		(Beach 1125). White, capsule shape. Film-coated. In 100s and 500s.
otc sf	**Neutra-Phos Powder**[1] (Ortho-McNeil)	250	14.25	278	7.125	164	7.125	1 powder packet reconstituted in 75 mL water 4 times/day after meals and at bedtime. Provides 250 mg phosphorus per dose (1 g/day)	Fruit flavor. In 64 g bottle and UD 1.25 g packets.
otc sf	**PHOS-NaK** (Cypress)	250	unknown	280	unknown	160	unknwon	Mix 1 packet with 75 mL water or juice. Take 1 packet qid.	Fruit flavor. In 1.5 g packets (100s)
otc sf	**Neutra-Phos-K Powder**[2] (Ortho-McNeil)	250	14.25	556	14.25	0	0	1 powder packet reconstituted in 75 mL water 4 times/day after meals and at bedtime. Provides 250 mg phosphorus per dose (1 g/day)	In 71 g bottle and UD 1.45 g packets.

[1] From monobasic and dibasic sodium and potassium phosphates.

[2] From dibasic and monobasic potassium phosphates.

For information on parenteral phosphate, refer to the monograph in the IV Nutritional Therapy section.

Indications

Dietary supplements of phosphorus, particularly if the diet is restricted or needs are increased.

Neutra-Phos and *Neutra-Phos-K* are useful in the treatment of children and adults with conditions associated with excessive renal phosphate loss or inadequate GI absorption of phosphate. They are also useful as adjunct supplementation in the management of phosphate diabetes.

Administration and Dosage

➤*Recommended dietary allowances (RDAs):*

Adults (> 10 years of age) – 800 to 1200 mg.

Children (1 to 10 years of age) – 800 mg.

Infants (0.5 to 1 year of age) – 500 mg.

Infants (0 to 0.5 years of age) – 300 mg.

For a complete listing of RDAs by age, sex, and condition, refer to the RDA table.

➤*Neutra-Phos and Neutra-Phos-K powder:*

Dosage		
Age	Dose	Equivalent phosphorus dose
< 4 years of age	60 mL of oral solution 4 times/day	60 mL supplies 200 mg
Adult	75 to 600 mL (or 1 to 8 packets) taken after meals and at bedtime	75 mL (1 packet) supplies 250 mg

Powder concentrate – Patient should dissolve entire contents of 1 bottle in 3.8 L (1 gallon) of water or other desirable liquid. This solution should not be further diluted, but can be chilled to increase palatability, and can be stored for up to 60 days.

Unit-dose packets – Empty contents of 1 packet into ⅓ glassful of water (≈ 75 mL) or other liquid, such as juice, and stir well before taking.

Solubility – *Neutra-Phos* and *Neutra-Phos-K* form an oral solution by reconstitution with water or other liquids, such as juice, per label directions. The solution is neutral (pH 7.3) and isotonic active components will dissolve rapidly, while the excipients will remain in suspension.

➤*Uro-KP-Neutral:*

Adults – 1 or 2 caplets 4 times/day with a full glass of water, providing 1 g of elemental phosphorus. Dosage may be increased or decreased. Optimum daily dosage should provide 1 to 1.5 g phosphorus daily.

➤*K-Phos Neutral:* Take with a full glass of water with meals and at bedtime.

Adults – 1 or 2 tablets 4 times/day.

Children > 4 years of age – 1 tablet 4 times/day. For patients < 4 years of age, use only as directed by a physician.

➤*Storage/Stability:*

Powder – Store the powder concentrate and unit-dose packets in a dry place. When reconstituted to solution, chill if desired. Can be stored up to 60 days.

Tablets – Keep tightly closed. Store at controlled room temperature (20° to 25°C; 68° to 77°F).

Actions

➤*Pharmacology:* Phosphorus has a number of important functions in the biochemistry of the body. The bulk of the body's phosphorus is located in the bones, where it plays a key role in osteoblastic and osteoclastic activities. Enzymatically catalyzed phosphate-transfer reactions are numerous and vital in the metabolism of carbohydrate, lipid, and protein, and a proper concentration of the anion is of primary importance in assuring an orderly biochemical sequence. In addition, phosphorus plays an important role in modifying steady-state tissue concentrations of calcium. Phosphate ions are important buffers of the intracellular fluid, and also play a primary role in the renal excretion of hydrogen ion.

➤*Pharmacokinetics:*

Absorption – Approximately ⅔ of phosphate consumed by adults is absorbed from the bowel, primarily through sodium-dependent active transport, although passive diffusion does play a role mainly within the jejunum and ileum.

When reconstituted to an oral solution, phosphorus shows rapid absorption and utilization from the alimentary tract. Oral phosphate may allow serum levels to rise by as much as 1.5 mg/dL within 60 to 120 minutes after ingestion of 1000 mg phosphorus. The liquid products have an advantage over coated or uncoated tablets, as slow-dissolving tablets may cause local GI irritation or inflammation in sensitive individuals.

Metabolism – Phosphate metabolism is closely associated with calcium metabolism through vitamin D_1 parathyroid hormone, calcitonin, and the mineralization of osteoid. Reduction of plasma phosphate concentrations cause higher serum calcium levels and inhibit deposition of bone salt. An elevated plasma concentration of the phosphate anion promotes the effect of calcitonin on calcium deposition in bone.

Excretion – Over 90% of phosphate absorbed from the GI tract is excreted in the urine through filtration. The majority is then actively reabsorbed by the initial segment of the proximal tubule. A lesser amount is absorbed in the pars recta and/or loop of Henle, distal convoluted tubule, and collecting duct. Phosphate excreted into the urine represents a difference between the amount filtered and amount reabsorbed. Tubule secretion is not known to occur in the mammalian kidney. Phosphate reduces levels of urinary calcium and elevates levels of urinary pyrophosphate inhibitor. Orthophosphates have been shown to decrease the crystallization of oxalate in the urine of calculous patients.

Contraindications

Addison's disease; hyperkalemia; acidification of urine in urinary stone disease; patients with infected urolithiasis or struvite stone formation; severely impaired renal function (< 30% of normal); presence of hyperphosphatemia; hypersensitivity to active or inactive ingredients.

Warnings

➤*Pregnancy: Category C.* It is not known whether this product can cause fetal harm or affect reproduction capacity when administered to a pregnant woman. Use only when clearly needed.

➤*Lactation:* It is not known whether this drug is excreted in breast milk. Exercise caution when administering to a nursing woman.

➤*Children:* For pediatric patients < 4 years of age, use only as directed by a physician.

Precautions

➤*Monitoring:* The following determinations are important in patient monitoring (other tests may be warranted in some patients): Renal function; serum calcium; serum phosphorus; serum potassium; serum sodium. Monitor at periodic intervals during therapy.

➤*Potential GI problems:* There have been reports in the literature of small bowel lesions with some long-acting and coated potassium tablets. Orthophosphates may cause dyspepsia in patients with a history of peptic ulcer; other modes of therapy may be necessary in such patients.

➤*Sodium/Potassium restriction:* Use with caution if patient is on a sodium- or potassium-restricted diet. These products provide signifi-

PHOSPHORUS REPLACEMENT PRODUCTS

cant amounts of sodium or potassium.

►*Kidney stones:* Warn patients with kidney stones of the possibility of passing stones when phosphate therapy is started.

►*Special risk:* Use with caution when the following medical problems exist: Cardiac disease (particularly in digitalized patients); acute dehydration; renal function impairment or chronic renal disease; extensive tissue breakdown; myotonia congenita; cardiac failure; cirrhosis of the liver or severe hepatic disease; peripheral and pulmonary edema; hypernatremia; hypertension; pre-eclampsia; hypoparathyroidism; osteomalacia; acute pancreatitis; rickets (rickets may benefit from phosphate therapy; however, use caution); severe adrenal insufficiency.

Drug Interactions

Phosphate Drug Interactions			
Precipitant drug	Object drug*		Description
Androgens	Potassium and phosphate	↑	Androgens may cause retention of potassium and phosphate. Therefore, concurrent use with potassium phosphate may cause hyperkalemia or hyperphosphatemia.
Antacids	Phosphates	↓	Antacids containing magnesium, aluminum, or calcium may bind to phosphate and prevent its absorption.
Calcium Vitamin D	Phosphates	↓	The effects of phosphates may be antagonized in the treatment of hypercalcemia.
Iron supplements	Phosphate	↓	Iron-containing medications have the ability to bind phosphate and form an insoluble complex, thus preventing absorption.

Phosphate Drug Interactions			
Precipitant drug	Object drug*		Description
Phosphate	Anorexiants	↓	Acidification of urine may increase elimination and decrease therapeutic effect of anorexiants.
Phosphate	Chlorpropamide (sulfonylurea)	↑	Acidification of urine may increase bioavailability of chlorpropamide and enhance the hypoglycemic actions.
Phosphate	Methadone	↓	Acidification of the urine increases renal clearance of methadone because of increased ionization.
Phosphate	Sympatho-mimetics	↓	Acidification of urine may increase elimination and decrease therapeutic effect of sympathomimetics.

* ↑ = Object drug increased.   ↓ = Object drug decreased.

Adverse Reactions

Individuals may experience a mild laxative effect for the first few days. If this persists, reduce the daily intake until this effect subsides, or, if necessary, discontinue use.

GI upset (eg, diarrhea, nausea, stomach pain, vomiting) may occur with phosphate therapy. The following side effects have been reported less frequently: Headaches; dizziness; mental confusion; seizures; weakness or heaviness of legs; unusual tiredness or weakness; muscle cramps; numbness, tingling, pain, or weakness of hands or feet; numbness or tingling around lips; fast or irregular heartbeat; shortness of breath or troubled breathing; swelling of feet or lower legs; unusual weight gain; low urine output; unusual thirst; bone and joint pain. High serum phosphate levels may increase the incidence of extraskeletal calcification.

MAGNESIUM

otc	**Magnesium Gluconate** (Various, eg, Freeda, Rugby)	**Tablets:** ≈ 27 mg elemental magnesium	In 100s and 500s.
otc	**Magnesium** (Various, eg, Ivax)	**Tablets:** 30 mg elemental magnesium	In 100s.
otc	**Magnesium Citrate** (Various, eg, Freeda)	**Tablets:** 100 mg elemental magnesium	In 100s and 250s.
otc	**Mag-200** (Optimox)	**Tablets:** 200 mg elemental magnesium (as oxide)	300 mg PABA. In 120s.
otc sf	**Mag-Ox 400** (Blaine)	**Tablets:** 400 mg magnesium oxide (241.3 mg elemental magnesium)	(BLAINE). In 120s, 1000s, and UD 100s.
otc	**Magnesium Oxide** (Cypress)		In 120s.
otc	**Almora** (Forest)	**Tablets:** 500 mg magnesium gluconate dihydrate (27 mg elemental magnesium)	In 100s.
otc	**Mag-G** (Cypress)		In 100s.
otc	**Magonate** (Fleming)		87.5 mg Ca, 66 mg P (376 mg dibasic calcium phosphate dihydrate). In 1000s.
otc	**Magtrate** (Mission)	**Tablets:** 500 mg magnesium gluconate (29 mg elemental magnesium)	In 100s.
otc sf	**Maginex** (Geist)	**Tablets, enteric coated:** 615 magnesium-L-aspartate HCl (61 mg elemental magnesium)	In blister pack 100s, UD 100s, and robot ready 100s.
otc	**Slow-Mag** (Purdue)	**Tablets, enteric-coated:** 64 mg elemental magnesium (as chloride hexahydrate)	Calcium carbonate. In 60s.
otc	**Mag-Tab SR** (Niche)	**Tablets, sustained-release:** 84 mg elemental magnesium (as L-lactate dihydrate)	Lt. yellow, capsule shape, scored. In 60s, 100s, and 1000s.
otc sf	**Uro-Mag** (Blaine)	**Capsules:** 140 mg magnesium oxide (84.5 mg elemental magnesium)	In 100s, 1000s, and UD 100s.
otc sf	**Magonate Natal** (Fleming)	**Liquid:** 3.52 mg elemental magnesium (as gluconate)/mL	In 480 mL.
otc	**Magonate** (Fleming)	**Liquid:** 1000 mg magnesium gluconate dihydrate/5 mL (54 mg elemental magnesium/5 mL)	Sorbitol, magnesium carbonate. Melon flavor. In 473 mL.
otc	**Maginex DS** (Geist)	**Powder:** 1230 mg magnesium-L-aspartate HCl (122 mg elemental magnesium)/packet	Preservative-free. Sucrose. Lemon flavor. In 30s and robot ready 30s.

For more information on parenteral magnesium, refer to the IV Nutritional Therapy monograph in this chapter and the Anticonvulsant monograph in the CNS chapter.

Indications

As a dietary supplement.

Administration and Dosage

1 g Mg = 83.3 mEq (41.7 mmol).

►*Dietary supplement:* 40 to 400 mg/day in divided doses. Refer to product labeling.

►*Recommended dietary allowances (RDAs):*

Adult – Males, 270 to 400 mg; females, 280 to 300 mg. For a complete listing of RDAs by age, sex, and condition, refer to the RDA table.

Magnesium-containing antacids also may be used; refer to the Antacids monograph in the GI Agents chapter.

Actions

►*Pharmacology:* Magnesium is the fourth most abundant mineral in the body and the second most abundant in muscles and other organs. Only potassium levels are higher than magnesium in soft tissues (non-bone tissues). Potassium cannot be retained in soft tissues and leaks out if magnesium is deficient. An adequate amount of magnesium also is required for the absorption and utilization of calcium, favoring the deposition of calcium in bone where it belongs and preventing deposition of calcium in the soft tissues and kidneys where it does not belong. Magnesium is required in adequate amount for the normal activity of 300 enzymes, including those involved in the transfer of energy from foods to physical and mental activities. It is a very important stabilizer of polynucleic acids, substances where genetic information is stored. Unstable nucleic acids predispose to cancer.

Warnings

►*Pregnancy:* It is unknown whether magnesium supplementation will harm an unborn child or a breastfeeding child. Do not take this

MAGNESIUM

mineral without speaking to a physician if pregnant, planning a pregnancy, or breastfeeding.

Precautions

➤*Renal disease:* Do not use without physician supervision because of potential accumulation.

➤*Excessive dosage:* Excessive dosage may cause diarrhea and GI irritation.

➤*Heart disease:* Magnesium supplements may make this condition worse.

Drug Interactions

Magnesium Drug Interactions			
Precipitant drug	Object drug*		Description
Magnesium salts	Aminoquinolines (eg, chloroquine)	↓	The absorption and therapeutic effect of the aminoquinolines may be decreased.
Magnesium salts	Nitrofurantoin	↓	Adsorption of nitrofurantoin onto magnesium salts may occur, decreasing the bioavailability and possibly the anti-infective effect of nitrofurantoin.
Magnesium salts	Penicillamine	↓	The GI absorption of penicillamine may be decreased, possibly decreasing its pharmacologic effects; however, this only has been reported for magnesium-containing antacids.

Magnesium Drug Interactions			
Precipitant drug	Object drug*		Description
Magnesium salts	Tetracyclines	↓	The GI absorption and serum levels of tetracyclines may be decreased; a decreased antimicrobial response may occur.

* ↓ = Object drug decreased.

Overdosage

➤*Symptoms:* It is possible to overdose on any electrolyte if large quantities are given; magnesium is no exception. Administer magnesium cautiously, especially to patients with decreased renal function. The most common symptom of overdose is diarrhea. At serum levels between 3 to 5 mEq/L, there is a propensity for hypotension because of peripheral dilation. Severe hypotension may be seen at higher levels. Facial flushing may be seen, associated with a feeling of warmth or thirst. Nausea and vomiting may occur but are not always present. Lethargy, dysarthria, and drowsiness can appear when levels reach 5 to 7 mEq/L. Deep tendon reflexes are lost when levels reach 7 mEq/L. Shallow respirations, irregular brief periods of apnea, and, finally, prolonged apnea are expected when levels exceed 10 mEq/L. Coma occurs when serum levels are between 12 and 15 mEq/L. Finally, when levels exceed 15 to 20 mEq/L, cardiac arrest may be expected.

➤*Treatment:* Terminate exposure. Calcium administration improves many toxic symptoms. Forced diuresis intensifies the elimination of magnesium; hemodialysis is extremely effective at magnesium removal but is infrequently necessary in the absence of renal failure.

IRON-CONTAINING PRODUCTS

Indications

►*Iron deficiency:* For the prevention and treatment of iron deficiency and iron deficiency anemias.

►*Iron supplement:* As a dietary supplement for iron.

►*Unlabeled uses:* Iron supplementation may be required by most patients receiving epoetin therapy. Failure to administer iron supplements (oral or IV) during epoetin therapy can impair the hematologic response to epoetin.

Administration and Dosage

►*Iron replacement therapy in deficiency states:* Iron doses are given as elemental iron.

Premature infants – 2 to 4 mg/kg/day given in 1 to 2 divided doses. Maximum dose is 15 mg/day.

Children – 3 to 6 mg/kg/day given in 1 to 3 divided doses.

Adults – 150 to 300 mg/day given in 3 divided doses. Alternatively, 60 mg given 2 to 4 times/day may help to lessen GI effects.

The length of iron therapy depends upon the cause and severity of the iron deficiency. In general, ≈ 4 to 6 months of oral iron therapy is required to reverse uncomplicated iron deficiency anemias.

►*Recommended dietary allowances (RDAs):* Adult males (≥ 19 years old) – 10 mg; adult females (11 to 50 years old) – 15 mg, (≥ 51 years old) – 10 mg; pregnancy – 30 mg; lactation – 15 mg. For a complete listing of RDAs by age, sex or condition, refer to the RDAs section in the Nutrients and Nutritionals Chapter.

►*Iron supplementation:*

Pregnancy – 15 to 30 mg elemental iron daily (not taken with meals) should be adequate to meet the daily requirement of the last 2 trimesters.

Actions

►*Pharmacology:* Iron, an essential mineral, is a component of hemoglobin, myoglobin and a number of enzymes (eg, cytochromes, catalase, peroxidase). The total body content of iron is ≈ 50 mg/kg in men (3.5 g in the average 70 kg man), and 37 mg/kg in women. Iron is primarily stored as hemosiderin or aggregated ferritin, found in the reticuloendothelial cells of the liver, spleen and bone marrow. Approximately two-thirds of total body iron is in the circulating red blood cell mass in hemoglobin, the major factor in oxygen transport.

Iron deficiency can affect muscle metabolism, heat production and catecholamine metabolism and has been associated with behavioral or learning problems in children.

►*Pharmacokinetics:*

Absorption/Distribution – The average dietary intake of iron is 12 to 20 mg/day for males and 8 to 15 mg/day for females; however, only ≈ 10% of this iron is absorbed (1 to 2 mg/day) in individuals with adequate iron stores. Absorption is enhanced (20% to 30%) when storage iron is depleted or when erythropoiesis occurs at an increased rate.

Iron is primarily absorbed from the duodenum and upper jejunum by an active transport mechanism. The ferrous salt form is absorbed three times more readily than the ferric form. The common ferrous salts (sulfate, gluconate, fumarate) are absorbed almost on a milligram-for-milligram basis but differ in the content of elemental iron. Sustained release or enteric coated preparations reduce the amount of available iron; absorption from these doseforms is reduced because iron is transported beyond the duodenum. Dose also influences the amount of iron absorbed. The amount of iron absorbed increases progressively with larger doses; however, the percentage absorbed decreases. Food can decrease the absorption of iron by 40% to 66%; however, gastric intolerance may often necessitate administering the drug with food.

Excretion – Iron is transported via the blood and bound to transferrin. The daily loss of iron from urine, sweat and sloughing of intestinal mucosal cells amounts to ≈ 0.5 to 1 mg in healthy men. In menstruating women, ≈ 1 to 2 mg is the normal daily loss.

Elemental Iron Content of Iron Salts	
Iron salt	% Iron
Ferrous sulfate	≈ 20
Ferrous sulfate, exsiccated	≈ 30
Ferrous gluconate	≈ 12
Ferrous fumarate	≈ 33

Contraindications

Hemochromatosis; hemosiderosis; hemolytic anemias; known hypersensitivity to any ingredients.

Warnings

►*Chronic iron intake:* Individuals with normal iron balance should not take iron chronically.

►*Accidental overdose:* Accidental overdose of iron-containing products is a leading cause of fatal poisoning in children < 6 years of age.

Keep this product out of reach of children.

Precautions

►*Intolerance:* Discontinue use if symptoms of intolerance appear.

►*GI effects:* Occasional GI discomfort, such as nausea, may be minimized by taking with meals and by slowly increasing to the recommended dosage.

►*Tartrazine sensitivity:* Some of these products contain tartrazine, which may cause allergic-type reactions (including bronchial asthma) in susceptible individuals. Although the incidence of tartrazine sensitivity in the general population is low, it is frequently seen in patients who also have aspirin hypersensitivity. Specific products containing tartrazine are identified in the product listings.

►*Sulfite sensitivity:* Some of the products contain sulfites, which may cause allergic-type reactions (eg, hives, itching, wheezing, anaphylaxis) in certain susceptible persons. Although the overall prevalence of sulfite sensitivity in the general population is probably low, it is seen more frequently in asthmatics or in atopic nonasthmatic persons. Specific products containing sulfites are identified in the product listings.

Drug Interactions

Iron Salts Drug Interactions			
Precipitant drug	Object drug*		Description
Antacids	Iron salts	↓	GI absorption of iron may be reduced.
Ascorbic acid	Iron salts	↑	Ascorbic acid at doses ≥ 200 mg have been shown to enhance the absorption of iron by ≥ 30%.
Chloramphenicol	Iron salts	↑	Serum iron levels may be increased.
Cimetidine	Iron salts	↓	GI absorption of iron may be reduced.
Iron salts	Levodopa	↓	Levodopa appears to form chelates with iron salts, decreasing levodopa absorption and serum levels.
Iron salts	Levothyroxine	↓	The efficacy of levothyroxine may be decreased, resulting in hypothyroidism. Avoid concomitant administration.
Iron salts	Methyldopa	↓	Extent of methyldopa absorption may be decreased, possibly resulting in decreased efficacy.
Iron salts	Penicillamine	↓	Marked reduction in GI absorption of penicillamine may occur, possibly because of chelation.
Iron salts	Quinolones	↓	GI absorption of quinolones may be decreased because of formation of ferric ion-quinolone complex.
Iron salts	Tetracyclines	↓	Concomitant use within 2 hours may decrease absorption and serum levels of tetracyclines. Absorption of iron salts may also be decreased.
Tetracyclines	Iron salts		

* ↑ = Object drug increased.   ↓ = Object drug decreased.

►*Drug/Food interactions:* Eggs and milk inhibit iron absorption. Coffee and tea consumed with a meal or 1 hour after a meal may significantly inhibit the absorption of dietary iron; clinical significance has not been determined. Administration of calcium and iron supplements with food can reduce ferrous sulfate absorption by one-third. If combined iron and calcium supplementation is required, iron absorption is not decreased if calcium carbonate is used and the supplements are taken between meals.

Adverse Reactions

GI irritation; nausea; vomiting; constipation; diarrhea. Stools may appear darker in color.

Iron-containing liquids may temporarily stain the teeth. Dilute the liquid to reduce this possibility. When iron-containing drops are given to infants, the membrane covering the teeth may darken.

Overdosage

►*Symptoms:* The oral *lethal* dose of elemental iron is ≈ 200 to 250 mg/kg; however, considerably less has been fatal. Symptoms may present when 30 to 60 mg/kg is ingested. Acute poisoning will produce symptoms in four stages:
1.) Within 1 to 6 hours: Lethargy; nausea; vomiting; abdominal pain; tarry stools; weak-rapid pulse;, hypotension; diminished tissue perfusion; metabolic acidosis; fever; leukocytosis; hyperglycemia; dyspnea; coma.
2.) If not immediately fatal, symptoms may subside for ≈ 24 hours.
3.) Symptoms return 12 to 48 hours after ingestion and may include: Diffuse vascular congestion; pulmonary edema; shock; metabolic acidosis; convulsions; anuria; hyperthermia; death.

IRON-CONTAINING PRODUCTS

4.) If patient survives, in 2 to 6 weeks after ingestion, pyloric or antral stenosis, hepatic cirrhosis and CNS damage may be seen.

▶*Treatment:* Maintain proper airway, respiration and circulation. If the patient is a candidate for emesis, induce with syrup of ipecac; follow with gastric lavage using tepid water or 1% to 5% sodium bicarbonate to convert the ferrous sulfate to ferrous carbonate, which is poorly absorbed and less irritating. Systemic chelation therapy with deferoxamine is generally recommended for patients with serum iron levels greater than the total iron binding capacity (63 mcmol; 3.5 mg/L); IM therapy may suffice, but severe poisoning (eg, shock, coma) may require IV administration (see deferoxamine mesylate in the Antidotes section). Oral use of deferoxamine is controversial and generally discouraged. Saline cathartics may be used. Specific treatment for shock, convulsions, acidosis and renal failure may be necessary. Treatment includes usual supportive measures. Refer to General Management of Acute Overdosage.

Patient Information

Take on an empty stomach; if GI upset occurs, take after meals or with food.

Do not take within 2 hours of antacids, tetracyclines or fluoroquinolones.

Drink liquid iron preparations in water or juice and through a straw to prevent tooth stains.

Medication may cause black stools, constipation or diarrhea.

Do not crush or chew sustained release preparations.

FERROUS SULFATE
20% elemental iron.

otc	**Ferrous Sulfate** (Various, eg, Geneva, Major, Schein)	**Tablets:** 324 mg (65 mg iron)	In UD 100s.
otc	**Ferrous Sulfate** (Various, eg, Zenith-Goldline)	**Tablets:** 325 mg (65 mg iron)	In 100s.
otc	**Ferrous Sulfate** (Various, eg, Barre, Major, Rugby, Zenith-Goldline)	**Elixir:** 220 mg/5 mL (44 mg iron/5 mL)	In 473 mL.
otc	**Feosol** (SmithKline Beecham)		5% alcohol. Glucose, saccharin, sucrose. In 473 mL.
otc	**Ferrous Sulfate** (Various, eg, Barre)	**Drops:** 75 mg/0.6 mL (15 mg iron/0.6 mL)	In 50 mL.
otc	**ED-IN-SOL** (Edwards)		Alcohol, sodium benzoate, sorbitol, sucrose. In 50 mL.
otc	**Fer-In-Sol** (Mead Johnson Nutritionals)		0.2% alcohol. Sodium bisulfite, sorbitol, sugar. In 50 mL with dropper.

For complete prescribing information, refer to the Iron-Containing Products group monograph.

FERROUS SULFATE EXSICCATED
Approximately 30% elemental iron.

otc	**Feratab** (Upsher-Smith)	**Tablets:** 187 mg (60 mg iron)	In UD 100s.
otc	**Feosol** (SmithKline Beecham)	**Tablets:** 200 mg (65 mg iron)	(Fe). Glucose. In 100s.
otc	**Slow FE** (Novartis)	**Tablets, slow release:** 160 mg (50 mg iron)	Cetostearyl alcohol, lactose. (NR CIBA). In 30s, 60s and 100s.

For complete prescribing information, refer to the Iron-Containing Products group monograph.

Actions

▶*Pharmacology:* Dried ferrous sulfate is prepared by exposing well crushed crystals of ferrous sulfate to 21° to 27°C (70° to 80°F), stirring frequently and then powdering. This salt is more stable in air than the fully hydrated ferrous sulfate.

FERROUS GLUCONATE
Approximately 12% elemental iron.

otc	**Fergon** (Bayer)	**Tablets:** 240 mg (27 mg iron)	(F)Sucrose. In 100s.
otc	**Ferrous Gluconate** (Various, eg, Dixon-Shane, URL, Zenith-Goldline)	**Tablets:** 325 mg (36 mg iron)	In 100s and 1000s.

For complete prescribing information, refer to the Iron-Containing Products group monograph.

FERROUS FUMARATE
33% elemental iron.

otc	**Slow-Release Iron** (Cardinal Health)	**Tablets, extended-release:** 150 mg (50 mg iron)	Maltodextrin, mineral oil. In 30s.
otc	**Ferrous Fumarate** (Mission)	**Tablets:** 200 mg (66 mg iron)	Sugar. In 100s.
otc	**Vitron-C** (Heritage Consumer Products)		125 mg ascorbic acid. In 60s.
otc	**Hemocyte** (U.S. Pharm)	**Tablets:** 324 mg (106 mg iron)	In 100s.
otc	**Ferrous Fumarate** (Various, eg, Major)	**Tablets:** 325 mg (106 mg iron)	In 100s and 1000s.
otc	**Ferretts** (Pharmics)		Polydextrose. (P-Fe). Red, oblong, scored. Film-coated. In 60s.
otc sf	**Nephro-Fer** (R & D Labs)	**Tablets:** 350 mg (115 mg iron)	In 30s.
otc	**Feostat** (Forest)	**Tablets, chewable:** 100 mg (33 mg iron)	Chocolate flavor. In 100s and UD 100s.
otc	**Feostat** (Forest)	**Suspension:** 100 mg/5 mL (33 mg iron/5 mL)	0.2% methylparaben. Butterscotch flavor. In 240 mL.

For complete prescribing information, refer to the Iron-Containing Products group monograph.

CARBONYL IRON
Pure iron micro particles.

otc	**Feosol** (SmithKline Beecham)	**Tablets:** 50 mg iron	Lactose, sorbitol, PEG. (Fe). Capsule shape. In 60s.
otc	**Ircon** (Kenwood)	**Tablets:** 66 mg iron	In blister pack 100s.
otc	**Icar** (Hawthorn)	**Suspension:** 15 mg carbonyl iron/ 1.25 mL	Sorbitol. In 118 mL.

For complete prescribing information, refer to the Iron-Containing Products group monograph.

POLYSACCHARIDE-IRON COMPLEX

otc	**Niferex** (Ther-Rx)	**Tablets:** 50 mg iron	Lactose. In UD 100s.
otc	**Polysaccharide Iron Complex** (Various, eg, URL)	**Capsules:** 150 mg iron	In 100s.
Rx	**Ferrex 150** (Breckenridge)		(B-203). Orange/brown. In UD 100s.
otc	**Hytinic** (Hyrex)		Green and white. In 50s and 500s.
otc	**Niferex-150** (Ther-Rx)		(SP 4220). Sucrose. In UD 100s.
otc	**Nu-Iron 150** (Merz)		(NU-IRON 150 0291). In 100s.
otc sf	**Niferex** (Ther-Rx)	**Elixir:** 100 mg iron/5 mL	Sorbitol, 10% alcohol. Dye free. In 236 mL.
otc sf	**Nu-Iron** (Merz)		10% alcohol. Dye free. In 237 mL.

For complete prescribing information, refer to the Iron-Containing Products group monograph.

MODIFIED IRON PRODUCTS

otc	**Ferro-Sequels** (Self-Care)	**Tablets, timed release:** Ferrous fumarate equivalent to 50 mg iron	Docusate sodium. Lactose. In 30s and 90s.

For complete prescribing information, refer to the Iron-Containing Products group monograph.

IRON WITH VITAMIN C
Content given per capsule or tablet.

	Product and Distributor	Dose Form	Fe (mg)	Vitamin C Ascorbic Acid (mg)	Vitamin C Sodium Ascorbate (mg)	Other Content & How Supplied
otc	**Ferrex 150 Plus** (Breckenridge)	**Capsules**	150[a]	50		(B 303). Clear/yellow. In UD 100s.
otc	**Vitelle Irospan** (Fielding)	**Tablets, timed release**	65[b]	150		In 100s.
otc	**Fero-Grad-500** (Abbott)		105[c]		500	In blisterpack 30s.
otc	**Hemaspan** (Sanofi Winthrop)		110[d]	200		20 mg docusate sodium. Sugar. (Bock Hs 33). Tan. In 100s.
otc	**Vitelle Irospan** (Fielding)	**Capsules, timed release**	65[b]	150		In 60s.

[a] From polysaccharide iron and ferrous bisglycinate.
[b] From ferrous sulfate exsiccated.
[c] From ferrous sulfate.
[d] From ferrous fumarate.

For complete prescribing information, refer to the Iron-Containing Products group monograph.

Actions
➤ *Pharmacology:* ASCORBIC ACID (VITAMIN C) may enhance the absorption of iron.

IRON, PARENTERAL
IRON DEXTRAN

Rx	**InFeD** (Schein)	**Injection:** 50 mg iron/mL (as dextran)	Approximately 0.9% sodium chloride. In 2 mL single-dose vials.
Rx	**DexFerrum** (American Regent)		In 2 mL single-dose vials.

WARNING

The parenteral use of complexes of iron and carbohydrates has resulted in anaphylactic-type reactions. Deaths associated with such administration have been reported; therefore, use iron dextran injection only in those patients in whom the indications have been clearly established and laboratory investigations confirm an iron-deficient state not amenable to oral iron therapy.

Indications

➤ *Iron deficiency:* For treatment of patients with documented iron deficiency in whom oral administration is unsatisfactory or impossible.

➤ *Unlabeled uses:* Iron supplementation may be required by most patients receiving epoetin therapy. Failure to administer iron supplements (oral or IV) during epoetin therapy can impair the hematologic response to epoetin.

Administration and Dosage

➤ *Iron deficiency anemia:* Use periodic hematologic determinations as a guide. Iron storage may lag behind the appearance of normal blood morphology. Although there are significant variations in body build and weight distribution among males and females, the following table and formula represent a convenient means for estimating the total iron required. This requirement reflects the amount of iron needed to restore hemoglobin to normal or near normal levels plus an additional allowance to provide replenishment of iron stores in most individuals with moderately or severely reduced levels of hemoglobin.

Dosage – The accompanying formula and table are applicable for dosage determinations only in patients with iron deficiency anemia; they are not to be used for dosage determinations in patients requiring iron replacement for blood loss.

The total amount of iron (in mL) required to restore hemoglobin to normal levels and to replenish iron stores may be approximated from the following formula:

Dose (mL) = 0.0442 (desired Hb − observed Hb) × Weight* + (0.26 × Weight*)

*For adults and children > 15 kg (33 lbs), use the lesser of lean body weight or actual body weight in kilograms. Lean body weight is 50 kg (for males) or 45.5 kg (for females) plus 2.3 kg for each inch over 5 feet. For children 5 to 15 kg (11 to 33 lbs), use actual weight in kilograms.

Total Amount of Iron Dextran Required (to the nearest mL) for Hemoglobin and Iron Stores Replacement[a]

Lean body weight[b] kg	lb	Amount required (mL) based on observed hemoglobin 3 g/dL	4 g/dL	5 g/dL	6 g/dL	7 g/dL	8 g/dL	9 g/dL	10 g/dL
5	11	3	3	3	3	2	2	2	2
10	22	7	6	6	5	5	4	4	3
15	33	10	9	9	8	7	7	6	5
20	44	16	15	14	13	12	11	10	9
25	55	20	18	17	16	15	14	13	12
30	66	23	22	21	19	18	17	15	14
35	77	27	26	24	23	21	20	18	17
40	88	31	29	28	26	24	22	21	19
45	99	35	33	31	29	27	25	23	21
50	110	39	37	35	32	30	28	26	24
55	121	43	41	38	36	33	31	28	26
60	132	47	44	42	39	36	34	31	28
65	143	51	48	45	42	39	36	34	31
70	154	55	52	49	45	42	39	36	33
75	165	59	55	52	49	45	42	39	35
80	176	63	59	55	52	48	45	41	38
85	187	66	63	59	55	51	48	44	40
90	198	70	66	62	58	54	50	46	42
95	209	74	70	66	62	57	53	49	45
100	220	78	74	69	65	60	56	52	47
105	231	82	77	73	68	63	59	54	50
110	242	86	81	76	71	67	62	57	52

Iron

IRON DEXTRAN

Total Amount of Iron Dextran Required (to the nearest mL) for Hemoglobin and Iron Stores Replacement[a]									
Lean body weight[b]		Amount required (mL) based on observed hemoglobin							
kg	lb	3 g/dL	4 g/dL	5 g/dL	6 g/dL	7 g/dL	8 g/dL	9 g/dL	10 g/dL
115	253	90	85	80	75	70	65	59	54
120	264	94	88	83	78	73	67	62	57

[a] Table values were calculated based on a normal adult hemoglobin of 14.8 g/dL for weights > 15 kg (33 lbs) and a hemoglobin of 12 g/dL for weights ≤ 15 kg (33 lbs).

[b] For adults and children > 15 kg (33 lbs), use the lesser of lean body weight or actual body weight in kilograms. See above equation.

Administration –

IV injection: The total amount of iron dextran required for the treatment of iron deficiency anemia is determined from the preceding formula or table (see Dosage section).

• *Test dose* – Prior to administering the first therapeutic dose, give all patients an IV test dose of 0.5 mL. Administer the test dose at a gradual rate over ≥ 30 seconds (*InFeD*) or ≥ 5 minutes (*DexFerrum*). Although anaphylactic reactions known to occur following administration are usually evident within a few minutes or sooner, it is recommended that a period of ≥ 1 hour elapse before the remainder of the initial therapeutic dose is given.

Individual doses of ≤ 2 mL may be given on a daily basis until the calculated total amount required has been reached.

Give undiluted and slowly, ≤ 50 mg/min (≤ 1 mL/min).

IM injection: The total amount required for the treatment of iron deficiency anemia is determined from the preceding formula or table (see Dosage section).

• *Test dose* – Prior to administering the first therapeutic dose, give all patients an IM test dose of 0.5 mL. Administer in the same recommended test site and by the same technique as described in the last paragraph of this section. Although anaphylactic reactions known to occur following administration are usually evident within a few minutes or sooner, it is recommended that a period of ≥ 1 hour elapse before the remainder of the initial therapeutic dose is given.

If no adverse reactions are observed, the injection can be given according to the following schedule until the calculated total amount required has been reached. Each day's dose should ordinarily not exceed 0.5 mL (25 mg iron) for infants < 5 kg (11 lbs), 1 mL (50 mg iron) for children < 10 kg (22 lbs) and 2 mL (100 mg iron) for other patients.

Inject only into the muscle mass of the upper outer quadrant of the buttock (never into the arm or other exposed areas) and inject deeply with a 2 or 3 inch 19 or 20 gauge needle. If the patient is standing, have them bear their weight on the leg opposite the injection site, or if in bed, have them in a lateral position with injection site uppermost. To avoid injection or leakage into the subcutaneous tissue, a Z-track technique (displacement of the skin laterally prior to injection) is recommended.

➤*Iron replacement for blood loss:* Some individuals sustain blood losses on an intermittent or repetitive basis. Such blood losses may occur periodically in patients with hemorrhagic diatheses (eg, familial telangiectasia, hemophilia, GI bleeding) and on a repetitive basis from procedures such as renal hemodialysis. Direct iron therapy in these patients toward replacement of the equivalent amount of iron represented in the blood loss. The table and formula listed previously (under Iron deficiency anemia) are not applicable for simple iron replacement values.

Quantitative estimates of the individual's periodic blood loss and hematocrit during the bleeding episode provide a convenient method for the calculation of the required iron dose.

The following formula is based on the approximation that 1 mL of normocytic, normochromic red cells contains 1 mg elemental iron:

$$\text{Replacement iron (in mg)} = \text{Blood loss (in mL)} \times \text{hematocrit}$$

Example: Blood loss of 500 mL with 20% hematocrit

$$\text{Replacement iron} = 500 \times 0.2 = 100 \text{ mg}$$

$$\text{Iron dextran dose} = \frac{100 \text{ mg}}{50} = 2 \text{ mL}$$

➤*Incompatibility:* Do not mix iron dextran with other medications or add to parenteral nutrition solutions for IV infusion.

Actions

➤*Pharmacology:* Iron dextran, a hematinic agent, is a complex of ferric hydroxide and dextran. Circulating iron dextran is removed from the plasma by the reticuloendothelial system, which splits the complex into its components of iron and dextran. The iron is immediately bound to the available protein moieties to form hemosiderin or ferritin, the physiological forms of iron, or to a lesser extent to transferrin. This iron, which is subject to physiological control, replenishes hemoglobin

and depleted iron stores. Dextran, a polyglucose, is either metabolized or excreted.

➤*Pharmacokinetics:* The major portion of IM injections of iron dextran is absorbed within 72 hours; most of the remaining iron is absorbed over the ensuing 3 to 4 weeks. Various studies have yielded half-life values ranging from 5 hours (circulating iron dextran) to > 20 hours (total iron, both circulating and bound). These half-life values do not represent clearance of iron from the body. Iron is not easily eliminated from the body and accumulation of iron can be toxic. Negligible amounts of iron are lost via the urinary or alimentary pathways after administration of iron dextran. In vitro studies have shown that removal of iron dextran by dialysis is negligible.

Contraindications

Hypersensitivity to the product; all anemias not associated with iron deficiency; acute phase of infectious kidney disease.

Warnings

➤*Maximum dose:* 2 mL of undiluted iron dextran is the maximum recommended daily dose.

➤*Total dose infusion:* Large IV doses used with total dose infusions (TDI) have been associated with an increased incidence of adverse effects, typified by one or more of the following symptoms: Arthralgia; backache; chills; dizziness; moderate to high fever; headache; malaise; myalgia; nausea; vomiting. The onset is usually 24 to 48 hours after administration and symptoms generally subside within 3 to 4 days. These symptoms have also been reported following IM injection and generally subside within 3 to 7 days.

➤*Hypersensitivity reactions:* Have epinephrine immediately available in the event of acute hypersensitivity reactions. (Usual adult dose: 0.5 mL of a 1:1000 solution by SC or IM injection.) Refer to Management of Acute Hypersensitivity Reactions.

➤*Hepatic function impairment:* Use this preparation with extreme caution in the presence of serious impairment of liver function.

➤*Carcinogenesis:* A risk of carcinogenesis may exist for the IM injection of iron-carbohydrate complexes. Such complexes produce sarcoma when large doses are injected in rats, mice, and rabbits and possibly in hamsters.

The long latent period between the injection of a potential carcinogen and the appearance of a tumor makes it impossible to accurately measure the risk in humans. There have been, however, several reports describing tumors at the injection site in humans who previously received iron-carbohydrate complexes IM.

➤*Pregnancy: Category C.* Iron dextran is teratogenic and embryocidal in mice, rats, rabbits, dogs and monkeys when given in doses of ≈ 3 times the maximum human dose. There are no adequate and well controlled studies in pregnant women. Use during pregnancy only if the potential benefit justifies the potential risk to the fetus.

➤*Lactation:* Traces of unmetabolized iron dextran are excreted in breast milk. Exercise caution when administering to a nursing woman.

➤*Children:* Not recommended for use in infants < 4 months of age.

Precautions

➤*Monitoring:* Serum iron determinations (especially by colorimetric assays) may not be meaningful for 3 weeks; serum ferritin peaks after ≈ 7 to 9 days and slowly returns to baseline after ≈ 3 weeks; examination of the bone marrow for iron stores may not be meaningful for prolonged periods because residual iron dextran may remain in the reticuloendothelial cells.

➤*Iron overload:* Unwarranted therapy with parenteral iron will cause excess storage of iron with the consequent possibility of exogenous hemosiderosis. Such iron overload is particularly apt to occur in patients with hemoglobinopathies and other refractory anemias which might be erroneously diagnosed as iron deficiency anemia.

➤*Cardiovascular disease:* Adverse reactions of iron dextran may exacerbate cardiovascular complications in patients with preexisting cardiovascular disease.

➤*Allergies/Asthma:* Use with caution in patients with a history of significant allergies/asthma.

➤*Arthritis:* Patients with rheumatoid arthritis may have an acute exacerbation of joint pain and swelling following the administration of iron dextran.

Drug Interactions

➤*Chloramphenicol:* Serum iron levels may be increased because of decreased iron clearance and erythropoiesis due to direct bone marrow toxicity from chloramphenicol.

➤*Drug/Lab test interactions:* Large doses of iron dextran (≥ 5 mL) give a brown color to serum from a blood sample drawn 4 hours after administration; they may cause falsely elevated values of serum bilirubin and falsely decreased values of serum calcium.

Bone scans involving 99m Tc-diphosphonate have shown a dense, crescentic area of activity in the buttocks, following the contour of the iliac crest, 1 to 6 days after IM injections of iron dextran; bone scans with

IRON DEXTRAN

99m Tc-labeled bone-seeking agents have shown reduction of bony uptake, marked renal activity and excessive blood pool and soft tissue accumulation.

Adverse Reactions

Anaphylactic reactions have occurred with the use of iron dextran injection; on occasion, these reactions have been fatal (see Warning Box).

Delayed reactions include: Arthralgia; backache; chills; dizziness; fever; headache; malaise; myalgia; nausea; vomiting.

Other adverse reactions include:

➤*Cardiovascular:* Chest pain; chest tightness; shock; cardiac arrest; hypotension; hypertension; tachycardia; bradycardia; flushing; arrhythmias. Flushing and hypotension may occur from too rapid injections by the IV route.

➤*CNS:* Convulsions; seizures; syncope; headache; weakness; unresponsiveness; paresthesia; febrile episodes; chills; dizziness; disorientation; numbness; unconsciousness.

➤*Dermatologic:* Urticaria; pruritus; purpura; rash; cyanosis.

➤*GI:* Abdominal pain; nausea; vomiting; diarrhea.

➤*Hematologic/Lymphatic:* Leukocytosis; lymphadenopathy.

➤*Musculoskeletal:* Arthralgia; arthritis (may represent reactivation in patients with quiescent rheumatoid arthritis); myalgia; backache; sterile abscess; atrophy/fibrosis (IM injection site); brown skin or underlying tissue discoloration (staining); soreness or pain at or near IM injection sites; cellulitis; swelling; inflammation; local phlebitis at or near IV injection site.

➤*Respiratory:* Respiratory arrest; dyspnea; bronchospasm; wheezing.

➤*Miscellaneous:* Hematuria; febrile episodes; sweating; shivering; chills; malaise; altered taste.

SODIUM FERRIC GLUCONATE COMPLEX

Rx   **Ferrlecit** (Watson Pharma)   **Injection:** 62.5 mg/5 mL (12.5 mg/mL) elemental iron   9 mg/mL of benzyl alcohol, 20% sucrose. In 5 mL amps.

Indications

➤*Iron deficiency:* For the treatment of iron deficiency anemia in patients undergoing chronic hemodialysis who are receiving supplemental epoetin therapy.

Administration and Dosage

➤*Approved by the FDA:* February 18, 1999.

The dosage of sodium ferric gluconate complex is expressed in milligrams of elemental iron. Each 5 mL ampule contains 62.5 mg elemental iron (12.5 mg/mL).

➤*Iron deficiency:* The recommended dosage for the repletion treatment of iron deficiency in hemodialysis patients is 10 mL (125 mg elemental iron). Sodium ferric gluconate complex may be diluted in 100 mL of 0.9% sodium chloride administered by IV infusion over 1 hour. It may also be administered undiluted as a slow IV injection (at a rate of up to 12.5 mg/min). Most patients will require a minimum cumulative dose of 1 g elemental iron administered over 8 sessions at sequential dialysis treatments to achieve a favorable hemoglobin or hematocrit response. Patients may continue to require therapy with IV iron at the lowest dose necessary to maintain the target levels of hemoglobin, hematocrit, and laboratory parameters of iron storage within acceptable limits.

Sodium ferric gluconate complex has been administered at sequential dialysis sessions by infusion or by slow IV injection during the dialysis session itself.

➤*Admixture incompatibility:* Do not mix sodium ferric gluconate complex with other medications or add to parenteral nutrition solutions for IV infusion. The compatibility of sodium ferric gluconate complex with IV infusion vehicles other than 0.9% sodium chloride has not been evaluated.

➤*Storage/Stability:* Store at 20° to 25°C (68° to 77°F); excursions permitted to 15° to 30°C (59° to 86°F). Do not freeze. Use immediately after dilution in saline.

Actions

➤*Pharmacology:* Sodium ferric gluconate complex in sucrose injection is a stable macromolecular complex used to replete the total body content of iron. Iron is critical for normal hemoglobin synthesis to maintain oxygen transport. Additionally, iron is necessary for metabolism and various enzymatic processes.

The total body iron content of an adult ranges from 2 to 4 g (approximately ⅔ in hemoglobin and ⅓ in reticuloendothelial storage [bone marrow, spleen, liver] bound to intracellular ferritin). The body highly conserves iron (daily loss of 0.03%), requiring supplementation of approximately 1 mg/day to replenish losses in healthy, nonmenstruating adults. The etiology of iron deficiency in hemodialysis patients is varied and can include increased iron use (eg, from epoetin therapy) and blood loss. The administration of exogenous epoetin increases red blood cell production and iron use. The increased iron use and blood losses in the hemodialysis patient may lead to absolute or functional iron deficiency. Iron deficiency is absolute when hematologic indicators of iron stores are low. Patients with functional iron deficiency do not meet laboratory criteria for absolute iron deficiency but demonstrate an increase in hemoglobin/hematocrit or a decrease in epoetin dosage with stable hemoglobin/hematocrit when parenteral iron is administered.

➤*Pharmacokinetics:*

Absorption/Distribution – In multiple, sequential single-dose IV studies, peak drug levels (C_{max}) varied significantly by dosage and by rate of administration with the highest C_{max} observed in the regimen in which 125 mg was administered in 7 minutes (19 mg/L). The initial volume of distribution of 6 L corresponds well to calculated blood volume. The AUC for bound iron varied by dose from 17.5 mg•h/L (62.5 mg) to 35.6 mg•h/L (125 mg). Approximately 80% of drug bound iron was delivered to transferrin as a mononuclear ionic iron species within 24 hours of administration in each dosage regimen. Mean peak transferrin saturation did not exceed 100% and returned to near baseline by 40 hours after administration of each dosage regimen.

Metabolism/Excretion – The terminal elimination half-life for drug bound iron was approximately 1 hour, varying by dose but not by rate of administration. Total clearance was 3.02 to 5.35 L/h. In vitro, less than 1% of the iron species within sodium ferric gluconate complex can be dialyzed through membranes with pore sizes corresponding to 12,000 to 14,000 daltons over a period of up to 270 minutes.

Contraindications

All anemias not associated with iron deficiency; hypersensitivity to sodium ferric gluconate complex or any of its inactive components; evidence of iron overload.

Warnings

➤*Hypotension:* Hypotension associated with lightheadedness, malaise, fatigue, weakness, or severe pain in the chest, back, flanks, or groin has been associated with administration of IV iron. These hypotensive reactions are not associated with signs of hypersensitivity and have usually resolved within 1 or 2 hours. Successful treatment may consist of observation or, if the hypotension causes symptoms, volume expansion.

➤*Hypersensitivity reactions:* Serious hypersensitivity reactions have been rarely reported. One case of a life-threatening hypersensitivity reaction has been observed in a patient who received a single dose of sodium ferric gluconate complex in a postmarketing study. Three serious hypersensitivity reactions have been reported from the spontaneous reporting system (see Adverse Reactions).

➤*Mutagenesis:* Sodium ferric gluconate complex produced a clastogenic effect in an in vitro chromosomal aberration assay in Chinese hamster ovary cells.

➤*Elderly:* Clinical studies did not include sufficient numbers of subjects 65 years of age and older to determine whether they respond differently from younger subjects. Other reported clinical experience has not identified differences in responses. In general, cautiously select dose for an elderly patient, usually starting at the low end of the dosing range, reflecting the greater frequency of decreased hepatic, renal, or cardiac function and of concomitant disease or other drug therapy.

➤*Pregnancy: Category B.* There are no adequate and well-controlled studies in pregnant women. Use during pregnancy only if the potential benefit justifies the potential risk to the fetus.

➤*Lactation:* It is not known whether this drug is excreted in breast milk. Because many drugs are excreted in human milk, exercise caution when sodium ferric gluconate complex is administered to a nursing woman.

➤*Children:* Safety and efficacy have not been established. Sodium ferric gluconate complex contains benzyl alcohol; therefore, do not use in neonates.

Precautions

➤*Benzyl alcohol:* This product contains benzyl alcohol, which has been associated with a fatal "gasping syndrome" in premature infants.

➤*Iron overload:* Iron is not easily eliminated from the body and accumulation can be toxic. Unnecessary therapy with parenteral iron will cause excess storage of iron with consequent possibility of iatrogenic hemosiderosis. Iron overload is particularly apt to occur in patients with hemoglobinopathies and other refractory anemias. Do not administer sodium ferric gluconate complex to patients with iron overload.

Drug Interactions

➤*Angiotensin converting enzyme inhibitors (ACEIs):* Limited data may suggest that coadministration of an ACEI may potentiate adverse events associated with IV iron therapy.

➤*Oral iron preparations:* Coadministration of parenteral iron preparations may reduce absorption of oral iron preparations.

Iron

SODIUM FERRIC GLUCONATE COMPLEX

Adverse Reactions

➤*Hypotension:* (See Warnings). Of 226 renal dialysis patients exposed to sodium ferric gluconate complex, 3 (1.3%) patients experienced hypotensive events, which were accompanied by flushing in 2 patients. All completely reversed after 1 hour without sequelae.

Sodium ferric gluconate complex administered to patients during dialysis may cause transient hypotension. Administration may augment hypotension caused by dialysis.

Among the 126 patients evaluated in clinical studies, 1 patient experienced a transient decreased level of consciousness without hypotension. Another patient discontinued treatment prematurely because of dizziness, lightheadedness, diplopia, malaise, and weakness without hypotension that resulted in a 3- to 4-hour hospitalization for observation following drug administration. The syndrome resolved spontaneously.

➤*Hypersensitivity:* (See Warnings). In the single-dose, postmarketing safety study, 1 patient experienced a life-threatening hypersensitivity reaction (diaphoresis, nausea, vomiting, severe lower back pain, dyspnea, and wheezing for 20 minutes) following administration of sodium ferric gluconate complex. There were 9 patients (0.8%) who had an adverse reaction that precluded further sodium ferric gluconate complex administration (drug intolerance). These included 1 life-threatening reaction, 6 allergic reactions (pruritus × 2, facial flushing, chills, dyspnea/chest pain, and rash), and 2 other reactions (hypotension and nausea). Another 2 patients (0.2%) experienced allergic reactions not deemed to represent drug intolerance (nausea/malaise and nausea/dizziness) following sodium ferric gluconate complex administration.

In multiple-dose studies, hypersensitivity events associated with sodium ferric gluconate complex resulting in premature study discontinuation occurred in 3 out of a total 88 (3.4%) treated patients. The first patient withdrew after the development of pruritus and chest pain following the test dose. The second patient, in the high-dose group, experienced nausea, abdominal and flank pain, fatigue, and rash following the first dose. The third patient, in the low-dose group, experienced a "red blotchy rash" following the first dose. Of the 38 patients exposed to sodium ferric gluconate complex, none reported hypersensitivity reactions.

Many chronic renal failure patients experience cramps, pain, nausea, rash, flushing, and pruritus.

➤*Other adverse events:*

Cardiovascular – Hypotension (29%); hypertension (13%); syncope (6%); tachycardia (5%); bradycardia; vasodilation; angina pectoris; myocardial infarction; pulmonary edema.

CNS – Cramps (25%); dizziness (13%); paresthesias, fatigue (6%); agitation; somnolence.

Dermatologic – Pruritus (6%); increased sweating; rash.

GI – Nausea, vomiting, diarrhea (35%); abdominal pain (6%); anorexia; rectal disorder; dyspepsia; eructation; flatulence; GI disorder; melena.

Hematologic – Abnormal erythrocytes (11%); anemia; leukocytosis; lymphadenopathy.

Metabolic – Hyperkalemia (6%); generalized edema (5%); leg edema; peripheral edema; hypoglycemia; hypokalemia; edema; hypervolemia.

Musculoskeletal – Leg cramps (10%); myalgia; arthralgia.

Respiratory – Dyspnea (11%); coughing, upper respiratory tract infections (6%); rhinitis; pneumonia.

Special senses – Conjunctivitis; abnormal vision; ear disorder.

Miscellaneous – Injection-site reaction (33%); pain, chest pain (10%); asthenia, headache (7%); fever (5%); malaise; infection; abscess; back pain; rigors; chills; arm pain; flu-like syndrome; sepsis; carcinoma; urinary tract infection.

➤*Postmarketing:* Hypertonia; nervousness; dry mouth; hemorrhage.

Overdosage

Dosages in excess of iron needs may lead to accumulation of iron in iron storage sites and hemosiderosis. Periodic monitoring of laboratory parameters of iron storage may assist in recognition of iron accumulation. Do not administer sodium ferric gluconate complex in patients with iron overload. The sodium ferric gluconate complex is not dialyzable.

Serum iron levels greater than 300 mcg/dL may indicate iron poisoning, which is characterized by abdominal pain, diarrhea, or vomiting that progresses to pallor or cyanosis, lassitude, drowsiness, hyperventilation due to acidosis, and cardiovascular collapse.

Sodium ferric gluconate at elemental iron doses of 125, 78.8, 62.5, and 250 mg/kg caused death to mice, rats, rabbits, and dogs, respectively. The major symptoms of acute toxicity were decreased activity, staggering, ataxia, increases in the respiratory rate, tremor, and convulsions.

IRON SUCROSE

Rx	**Venofer** (American Regent Labs)	**Injection:** 20 mg elemental iron/mL	Preservative free. 300 mg/mL sucrose w/v. In 5 mL single-dose vials.

Indications

➤*Iron deficiency anemia:* For the treatment of iron deficiency anemia in patients undergoing chronic hemodialysis who are receiving supplemental erythropoietin therapy.

➤*Unlabeled uses:* Anemia in peritoneal dialysis patients; anemia in predialysis patients; bloodless surgery; autologous blood donation.

Administration and Dosage

➤*Approved by the FDA:* November 6, 2000.

The dosage of iron sucrose is expressed in terms of milligrams of elemental iron. Each 5 mL vial contains 100 mg of elemental iron (20 mg/mL).

➤*Iron deficiency anemia:* The recommended dosage of iron sucrose for the repletion treatment of iron deficiency in hemodialysis patients is 5 mL of iron sucrose (100 mg of elemental iron) delivered IV during the dialysis session. Most patients will require a minimum cumulative dose of 1000 mg of elemental iron, administered over 10 sequential dialysis sessions, to achieve a favorable hemoglobin or hematocrit response. Patients may continue to require therapy with iron sucrose or other IV iron preparations at the lowest dose necessary to maintain target levels of hemoglobin, hematocrit, and laboratory parameters of iron storage within acceptable limits.

Iron sucrose must be only administered IV (directly into the dialysis line) either by slow injection or by infusion.

➤*Slow IV injection:* In chronic renal failure patients, iron sucrose may be administered by slow IV injection into the dialysis line at a rate of 1 mL (20 mg iron) undiluted solution per minute (ie, 5 minutes/vial) not exceeding 1 vial of iron sucrose (100 mg elemental iron) per injection. Discard any unused portion.

➤*Infusion:* Iron sucrose may be also administered by infusion (into the dialysis line for hemodialysis patients). This may reduce the risk of hypotensive episodes. The content of each vial must be diluted exclusively in a maximum of 100 mL of 0.9% NaCl, immediately prior to infusion. Infuse the solution at a rate of 100 mg of iron over a period of at least 15 minutes. Discard unused diluted solution.

➤*IV incompatibility:* Do not mix iron sucrose with other medications or add to parenteral nutrition solutions for IV infusion. Inspect parenteral drug products visually for particulate matter and discoloration prior to administration, whenever the solution and container permit.

➤*Adults:* 100 mg iron administered 1 to 3 times/week to a total dose of 1000 mg in 10 doses; repeat if needed. Frequency of dosing should be no more than 3 times weekly.

➤*Storage/Stability:* Store in original carton 15° to 30°C (59° to 86°F). Do not freeze.

Actions

➤*Pharmacology:* Iron sucrose is used to replenish body iron stores in patients with iron deficiency on chronic hemodialysis and receiving erythropoietin. In these patients, iron deficiency is caused by blood loss during the dialysis procedure, increased erythropoiesis, and insufficient absorption of iron from the GI tract. Iron is essential to the synthesis of hemoglobin to maintain oxygen transport and to the function and formation of other physiologically important heme and nonheme compounds. Most hemodialysis patients require IV iron to maintain sufficient iron stores to achieve and maintain a hemoglobin of 11 to 12 g/dL.

➤*Pharmacokinetics:*

Absorption – In healthy adults treated with IV doses of iron sucrose, its iron component exhibits first order kinetics with an elimination half-life of 6 hours, total clearance of 1.2 L/hr, non-steady-state apparent volume of distribution of 10 L, and steady-state apparent volume of distribution of 7.9 L. Because iron disappearance from serum depends on the need for iron in the iron stores and iron-utilizing tissues of the body, serum clearance of iron is expected to be more rapid in iron-deficient patients treated with iron sucrose as compared with healthy individuals. The effects of age and gender on the pharmacokinetics of iron sucrose have not been studied.

Distribution – In healthy adults receiving IV doses of iron sucrose, its iron component appears to distribute mainly in blood and to some extent in extravascular fluid. A study evaluating iron sucrose containing 100 mg of iron labeled with 52Fe/59Fe in patients with iron deficiency shows that a significant amount of the administered iron distributes in the liver, spleen, and bone marrow. The bone marrow is an iron trapping compartment and not a reversible volume of distribution.

Metabolism/Excretion – Following IV administration of iron sucrose, it is dissociated into iron and sucrose by the reticuloendothelial system. The sucrose component is eliminated mainly by urinary

IRON SUCROSE

excretion. In a study evaluating a single IV dose containing 1510 mg of sucrose and 100 mg of iron in 12 healthy adults, 68.3% of the sucrose was eliminated in urine in 4 hours and 75.4% in 24 hours. Some iron also is eliminated in the urine. In this study and another study evaluating a single IV dose of iron sucrose containing 500 to 700 mg of iron in 26 anemic patients on erythropoietin therapy, ≈ 5% of the iron was eliminated in urine in 24 hours at each dose level.

Contraindications

Evidence of iron overload; known hypersensitivity to iron sucrose or any of its inactive components; anemia not caused by iron deficiency.

Warnings

➤*Hypotension:* Hypotension has been reported frequently in patients receiving IV iron. Hypotension following administration of iron sucrose may be related to rate of administration and total dose administered. Take caution to administer iron sucrose according to recommended guidelines.

➤*Hypersensitivity reactions:* Potentially fatal hypersensitivity reactions characterized by anaphylactic shock, loss of consciousness, collapse, hypotension, dyspnea, or convulsion have been reported rarely in patients receiving iron sucrose (see Adverse Reactions). Fatal immediate hypersensitivity reactions have been reported in patients receiving therapy with many iron carbohydrate complexes. Facilities for cardiopulmonary resuscitation must be available during dosing. Serious anaphylactoid reactions require appropriate resuscitation measures. Although fatal hypersensitivity reactions have not been observed in iron sucrose clinical studies, insufficient numbers of patients may have been enrolled to observe this event. Physician vigilance when administering any IV iron product is advised.

➤*Elderly:* In general, dose selection for an elderly patient should be cautious, usually starting at the low end of the dosing range, reflecting the greater frequency of decreased hepatic, renal, or cardiac function, and of concomitant disease or other drug therapy.

➤*Pregnancy: Category B.* There are no adequate and well-controlled studies in pregnant women. Use during pregnancy only if clearly needed.

➤*Lactation:* Iron sucrose is excreted in the milk of lactating rats. It is not known whether this drug is excreted in human breast milk. Because many drugs are excreted in breast milk, exercise caution when iron sucrose is administered to a nursing woman.

➤*Children:* Safety and efficacy of iron sucrose in pediatric patients have not been established.

Precautions

➤*Monitoring:* Because body iron excretion is limited and excess tissue iron can be hazardous, exercise caution to withhold iron administration in the presence of tissue iron overload. Patients receiving iron sucrose require periodic monitoring of hematologic and hematinic parameters (hemoglobin, hematocrit, serum ferritin, and transferrin saturation). Withhold iron therapy in patients with evidence of iron overload. Transferrin saturation values increase rapidly after IV administration of iron sucrose; thus, serum iron values may be reliably obtained 48 hours after IV dosing.

Drug Interactions

Drug interactions involving iron sucrose have not been studied. However, like other parenteral iron preparations, iron sucrose may be expected to reduce the absorption of concomitantly administered oral iron preparations. Do not administer concomitantly with oral iron preparations.

Adverse Reactions

Common adverse events observed in clinical trials – Adverse events, whether or not related to iron sucrose administration, reported by > 5% of treated patients are as follows: Hypotension (36%); cramps/leg cramps (23%); nausea, headache, vomiting, and diarrhea.

Adverse events, whether or not related to iron sucrose administration, reported in > 1% of treated patients are categorized below by body system.

➤*Cardiovascular:* Hypotension; chest pain; hypertension; hypervolemia.

➤*CNS:* Headache; dizziness.

➤*Dermatologic:* Pruritus; application site reaction.

➤*GI:* Nausea; vomiting; abdominal pain.

➤*Hypersensitivity:* In clinical trials, several patients experienced pruritus and 1 patient experienced a facial rash. No patients experienced generalized rashes or urticaria. No serious or life-threatening anaphylactoid reactions were observed in the trials and none of these reactions led to treatment discontinuation. From the spontaneous reporting system, 27 patients reported anaphylactoid reactions including 8 patients who experienced serious or life-threatening reactions (anaphylactic shock, loss of consciousness, collapse, hypotension, dyspnea, or convulsion) associated with iron sucrose administration in the estimated > 450,000 patients exposed to iron sucrose between 1992 and 1999.

➤*Musculoskeletal:* Cramps/leg cramps; musculoskeletal pain.

➤*Respiratory:* Dyspnea; pneumonia; cough.

➤*Miscellaneous:* Fever; pain; asthenia; unwellness; malaise; accidental injury; elevated liver enzymes.

Overdosage

Doses of iron sucrose injection in excess of iron needs may lead to accumulation of iron in storage sites leading to hemosiderosis. Periodic monitoring of iron parameters such as serum ferritin and transferrin saturation may assist in recognizing iron accumulation. Iron sucrose should not be administered to patients with iron overload and should be discontinued when serum ferritin levels equal or exceed established guidelines. Particular caution should be exercised to avoid iron overload where anemia unresponsive to treatment has been incorrectly diagnosed as iron deficiency anemia.

➤*Symptoms:* Symptoms associated with overdosage or infusing iron sucrose too rapidly included hypotension, headache, vomiting, nausea, dizziness, joint aches, paresthesia, abdominal and muscle pain, edema, and cardiovascular collapse.

➤*Treatment:* Most symptoms have been successfully treated with IV fluids, hydrocortisone, or antihistamines. Infusing the solution as recommended or at a slower rate may also alleviate symptoms.

TRACE ELEMENTS

IRON WITH VITAMINS
Content given per capsule or tablet.

	Product & Distributor	Fe mg	A IU	D IU	E IU	B1 mg	B2 mg	B3 mg	B5 mg	B6 mg	B12 mcg	C mg	FA mg	Other Content	How Supplied
Rx	**Chromagen Forte Capsules** (Ther-Rx)	151									10	60	1	Parabens	(THX 0131). In UD 100s.
Rx	**FeoGen Forte Capsules** (Rising Pharmaceuticals)[b]	151									10	60	1		(109). Brown. In UD 100s.
Rx	**Hemocyte-F Tablets** (US Pharm.)	106[a]											1		Maroon. In 100s.
Rx	**Cenogen-OB Capsules** (US Pharm.)	106[a]				10	6	30		5	15	200	1	18.2 mg Zn, Cu, Mg, Mn	In 100s.
Rx	**Nephro-Fer Rx Tablets** (R & D)	106.9[a]											1		(RD 33). Brown. Oval. Film coated. In 120s.
otc	**Ircon-FA Tablets** (Kenwood)	82[n]											0.8		In blister pack 100s.
Rx	**Chromagen FA Capsules** (Ther-Rx)	70									10	150	1	Parabens	(THX 0130). Green/Brown. In UD 100s.
Rx	**FeoGen FA Capsules** (Ther-Rx)	66									10	250	1		(116). Maroon. In UD 100s.
Rx	**Hematinic Tablets** (Cypress)	106[a]											1		In 100s.
otc	**Slow FE Slow Release Iron with Folic Acid Tablets** (Ciba)	50[d]											0.4		Lactose. In 20s.
Rx	**Nestabs CBF** (Fielding)	50	4,000	400	30	3	3	20[5]		3	8	120	1	200 mg Ca, 150 mcg I, 15 mg Zn.	(CBF). In 100s
otc	**Tolfrinic Tablets** (B.F. Ascher)	200[a]									25	100			Lactose. Dark brown. Film coated. In 100s.
Rx	**Niferex-150 Forte Capsules** (Ther-Rx)	150[f]									25		1		(SP 4330). Red, brown and white. In 100s and 1000s.
Rx	**Ferrex 150 Forte Plus Capsules** (Breckenridge)	150[m]									25	60	1		(B 398). Orange. In UD 100s.
Rx	**Fumatinic Capsules** (Laser)	66[a]									5	60			Extended release. (Laser 0181). Natural/maroon with brown, white, and off-white pellets. In 100s.
otc	**Ferralet Plus Tablets** (Mission)	46[g]									25	400	0.8		Sugar. In 60s.
otc	**Generet-500 Tablets** (Goldline)	105[h]													Timed release. In 60s.
otc	**Iberet Filmtabs** (Abbott)					6	6	30	10	5	25	150[g]			Controlled release. Film coated. In 60s.
otc	**Iron-Folic 500 Tablets** (Major)	105[d]				6	6	30	10	5	25	500[h]	0.8		(AK A101). Timed release. In 100s and 500s.
Rx	**Hematinic Plus Tablets** (Cypress)	106[a]				10	6	30	10	5	15	200	1	Cu, Mg, Mn, 18.2 mg Zn	In 100s.
otc	**Vita-Feron** (Vitaline)	150									6		0.8		In 90s.
Rx	**Nephro-Vite Rx + Fe Tablets** (R & D)	100[a]				1.5	1.7	20	10	10	6	60[i]	1	300 mcg d-biotin.	Lactose. (RD 23). Brown. Oval. Film coated. In 120s.
Rx	**Prenatal Plus w/ Betacarotene** (Rugby)	65	4000	400	11	1.8	3	20	10	10	12	120	1	Ca, Zn, Cu.	In 100s and 500s.
Rx	**Ferrex 150 Forte** (Breckenridge)	150[f]									25		1	10 mg niacinamide, 125 mg Ca, 18 mg Zn.	(B-198). Opaque maroon. In UD 100s.
Rx	**Ferrex PC Tablets** (Breckenridge)	60[e]	4000	400		3	3	2			3	50[i]	1		(B-200). Blue, oval, scored. Film coated. In UD 100s.
Rx	**Ferrex PC Forte** (Breckenridge)	60[f]	5000	400	30[i]	3	3.4			4	12	80[i]	1	250 mg Ca, 20 mg niacinamide, 0.2 mg I, 10 mg Mg, 25 mg Zn, 2 mg Cu	(B-202). White, oval, scored. Film coated. In UD 100s.

IRON WITH VITAMINS

TRACE ELEMENTS

	Product & Distributor	Fe mg	A IU	D IU	E IU	B₁ mg	B₂ mg	B₃ mg	B₅ mg	B₆ mg	B₁₂ mcg	C mg	FA mg	Other Content	How Supplied
otc	Gerivites Tablets (Rugby)	50[k]	5000	400	30[l]	1.5	1.7	20	10	2	300	60	0.4	Ca, Cl, Cr, Cu, I, K, Mg, Mn, Mo, Ni, Se, Si, P, 15 mg Zn.	In 40s.
Rx	Hemocyte Plus Tablets (US Pharm.)	106[a]				10	6	30	10	5	15	200[h]	1	Cu, Mg, Mn, 18.2 mg Zn.	In 100s.
otc sf	Parvlex Tablets (Freeda)	100[a]				20	20	20	1	10	50	50[i]	0.1	Cu, Mn.	In 100s and 250s.
otc	Prenatal H.P. (Mission)	30	4,000	400		4	2	10	1	20	2	100	0.8	50 mg Ca. Sugar.	In 100s.
Rx	Prenatal Rx (Mission)	29.5[a]	3,000	400	10[i]	4	2	20	10	20	8	240[i]	1	175 mg Ca, 2 mg Cu, 0.3 mg I, 15 mg Zn.	In 100s.
Rx	Advanced Formula Zenate Tablets (Solvay)	65[a]	3000	400	10[i]	1.5	1.6	17		2.2	2.2	70	1	Ca, I, Mg, Zn.	In UD 30s.
otc	Allbee C-800 Plus Iron Tablets (Robins)	27[a]			45[i]	15	17	100	25	25	12	800	0.4	Lactose.	Red. Film coated. Elliptical. In 60s.
otc	Theragran Stress Formula Tablets (Mead Johnson)	27[a]			30[i]	15	15	100	20	25	12	600	0.4	45 mcg biotin.	In 75s.
otc sf	StressForm "605" with Iron Tablets (NTBY)	27[j]			30[i]	15	15	100	20	5	12	605	0.4	45 mcg biotin.	In 60s.
otc	Stress Formula w/Iron Tablets (Goldline)	27[a]			30[i]	10	10	100	20	5	12	500[h]	0.4	45 mcg biotin.	In 60s.
otc	Stress Formula with Iron Tablets (NTBY)	27[k]			30[i]	10	10	100	20	5	12	500	0.4	45 mcg biotin.	In 60s.
otc	Stresstabs + Iron Tablets (Lederle)	18[a]			30[i]	10	10	100	20	5	12	500	0.4	45 mcg biotin.	(LL S2). Orange-red. Capsule shape. Film coated. In 60s.
Rx	Niferex-PN Tablets (Ther-Rx)	60[f]	4,000	400		3	3	10		2	3	50[h]	1	Ca, 18 mg Zn.	(SP 2209 131/05). Blue. Film coated. Oval. In 30s, 100s and 1000s.
Rx	Nu-Iron V Tablets (Mayrand)													Ca.	Maroon. Film coated. In 100s.
Rx	B C w/Folic Acid Plus Tablets (Geneva)	27[a]	5,000		30[i]	20	20	100	25	25	50	500	0.8	0.15 mg biotin, Cr, Cu, Mg, Mn, 22.5 mg Zn.	In 100s.
Rx	Berocca Plus Tablets (Roche)													0.15 mg biotin, Cr, Cu, Mg, Mn, 22.5 mg Zn.	(Berocca Plus/Roche). Yellow. Capsule shape. In 100s.
Rx	Formula B Plus Tablets (Major)													0.15 mg biotin, Cr, Cu, Mg, Mn, Zn.	In 100s and 500s.
otc	Mission Prenatal H.P. Tablets (Mission)	30[g]	4,000	400	30[c]	5	2	10	1	25	2	100	0.8	Ca, sugar.	In 100s.
otc	Mission Prenatal F.A. Tablets (Mission)	30[g]	4,000	400	45[i]	5	2	10	1	10	2	100	0.8	Ca, 15 mg Zn, sugar.	In 100s.
otc	Mission Prenatal Tablets (Mission)	30[g]	4,000	400	3[i]	5	2	10	1	3	2	100	0.4	Ca, sugar.	In 100s.
otc	Iromin-G Tablets (Mission)	30[g]	4,000	400	5[i]	5	2	10	1	20.6	2	100	0.8	Ca, sugar.	In 100s.
Rx sf	Vitafol Caplets (Everett)	65[a]	6,000	400	30[c]	1.1	1.8	15		2.5	5	60	1	Ca.	(EV0072). Film coated. In 100s and 1000s.
otc	Compete Tablets (Mission)	27[g]	5,000	400	45[i]	2	2.6	30		20.6	9	90	0.4	22.5 mg Zn, sugar.	In 100s.
otc sf	Freedavite Tablets (Freeda)	10[a]	5000	400	3[i]	5	3	25	5	2	2	60		Choline, inositol, potassium iodide, Ca, Cu, K, Mg, Mn, Se, 0.2 mg Zn.	In 100s and 250s.
otc	Mission Surgical Supplement Tablets (Mission)	27[g]	5000	400	45[i]	2.5	2.6	30	16.3	3.6	9	500		22.5 mg Zn, sugar.	In 100s.
otc	Therapeutic-H Tablets (Goldline)	66.7[a]	8333	133	5[i]	3.3	3.3	33.3	11.7	3.3	50	100[g]	0.33	Cu, Mg.	In 100s.
otc	Thera Hematinic Tablets (Major)													Cu, Mg.	In 250s and 1000s.
otc sf	Yelets Tablets (Freeda)	20[a]	10,000	400	10[i]	10	10	25	10	10	10	100	0.1	PABA, lysine, glutamic acid, Ca, I, Mg, Mn, Se, 4 mg Zn.	In 100s and 250s.

TRACE ELEMENTS

IRON WITH VITAMINS

	Product & Distributor	Fe mg	A IU	D IU	E IU	B_1 mg	B_2 mg	B_3 mg	B_5 mg	B_6 mg	B_{12} mcg	C mg	FA mg	Other Content	How Supplied
Rx	Zodeac-100 Tablets (Econo Med)	60[a]	8000	400	30[l]	1.7	2	20	11	4	8	120	1	300 mcg biotin, Ca, Cu, I, Mg, 15 mg Zn.	Orange. Film coated. In 100s.
otc sf	Geritol Complete Tablets (SK-Beecham)	18[k]	6000	400	30[l]	1.5	1.7	20	10	2	6	60	0.4	45 mcg biotin, Ca, Cl, Cr, Cu, I, K, Mg, Mn, Mo, Ni, P, Se, Si, Sn, V, Zn, vitamin K.	In 14s, 40s, 100s and 180s.
otc	Thera-M Tablets (Various, eg, Major)	27[k]	5000	400	30[l]	3	3.4	20	10	3	9	90	0.4	30 mcg biotin, 15 mg Zn, P, Ca, Cu, Cr, Se, Mo, K, Cl, I, Mg, Mn.	In 130s and 1000s.
otc	Multi-Vitamin Mineral w/Beta-Carotene Tablets (Mission)	27[a]	5000	400	30[l]	2.25	2.6	20	10	3	9	90	0.4	0.45 mg biotin, Ca, Cl, Cr, Cu, I, K, Mg, Mn, Mo, P, Se, 15 mg Zn, vitamin K_1.	In 130s.
otc	CertaVite Tablets (Major)	18[a]	5000	400	30[l]	1.5	1.7	20	10	2	6	60	0.4	30 mcg biotin, Ca, P, I, Mg, Cu, Mn, K, Cl, Cr, Mo, Se, Ni, Si, Sn, V, B, vitamin K_1, 15 mg Zn.	In 130s and 300s.
otc sf	ABC to Z Tablets (NTBY)													30 mcg biotin, Ca, Cl, Cr, Cu, I, K, Mg, Mn, Mo, Ni, P, Se, Si, Sn, V, Zn, vitamin K_1.	In 100s.
otc	Advanced Formula Centrum Tablets (Lederle)													30 mcg biotin, B, Ca, Cl, Cr, Cu, I, K, Mg, Mn, Mo, Ni, P, Se, Si, Sn, V, 15 mg Zn, vitamin K_1.	In 60s, 130s and 200s.
otc	Cerovite Advanced Formula Tablets (Rugby)													30 mcg biotin, Ca, Cl, Cr, Cu, I, K, Mg, Mn, Mo, Ni, P, Se, Si, Sn, V, 15 mg Zn, vitamin K_1.	In 130s.
Rx	Nephron FA (Nephro-Tech)	200[a]				1.5	1.7	20		10	6	40	1	300 mcg biotin, 75 mg docusate sodium.	(FA). In 100s.

[a] From ferrous fumarate.
[b] Rising Pharmaceuticals, 411 Sette Drive, Paramus, NJ 07652; 201-262-4200, fax 201-262-4284.
[c] As d-alpha tocopherol succinate.
[d] From ferrous sulfate.
[e] As niacinamide.
[f] From polysaccharide-iron complex.
[g] From ferrous gluconate.
[h] As sodium ascorbate.
[i] From ascorbic acid.
[j] As dl-alpha tocopheryl acetate.
[k] Form of iron content unknown.
[l] Form of vitamin E content unknown.
[m] From polysaccharide iron and ferrous bisglycinate.
[n] As carbonyl iron.

For complete prescribing information, refer to the Iron-Containing Products monograph.

Indications

Iron: Iron in combination with folic acid is used to treat iron deficiency anemia in conjunction with certain nutritional deficiencies.

B complex vitamins: B complex vitamins function as coenzymes in carbohydrate, protein or amino acid metabolism, synthesis of DNA and other molecules, maturation of red blood cells, nerve cell function or oxidation-reduction reactions.

Ascorbic acid (vitamin C): Ascorbic acid may enhance the absorption of iron.

Warnings

Pernicious anemia: Folic acid alone is improper therapy in the treatment of pernicious anemia and other megaloblastic anemias where vitamin B_{12} is deficient. Where anemia exists, establish its nature and determine underlying causes.

Folic acid, especially in doses > 0.1 mg daily, may obscure pernicious anemia, in that hematologic remission may occur while neurological manifestations remain progressive. Concomitant parenteral therapy with vitamin B_{12} may be necessary in patients with deficiency of vitamin B_{12}.

Precautions

Sulfite sensitivity: Some of these products contain sulfites that may cause allergic-type reactions (including anaphylactic symptoms and life-threatening or less severe asthmatic episodes) in certain susceptible persons. The overall prevalence of sulfite sensitivity in the general population is unknown and probably low. It is seen more frequently in asthmatic or atopic nonasthmatic persons.

TRACE ELEMENTS

IRON WITH VITAMINS, LIQUIDS
Content given per 15 mL.

	Product & Distributor	Fe mg	B1 mg	B2 mg	B3 mg	B5 mg	B6 mg	B12 mcg	C mg	FA mg	Other Content	How Supplied
Rx sf	Nu-Iron Plus Elixir (Mayrand)	300[a]						75		3	10% alcohol	Dye-free. In 237 mL.
Rx	Hemocyte-F Elixir (US Pharm)	100[a]						75		3	10% alcohol, parabens, saccharin, sorbitol	Sherry wine flavor. In 473 mL.
otc	Trophite + Iron Liquid (Menley & James)	60[b]	30					75			Saccharin, glucose, parabens	In 120 mL.
Rx	Vitafol Syrup (Everett)	90[b]			39.9		6	25.02		0.75		Raspberry-mint flavor. In 473 mL.
otc sf	Vitalize SF Liquid (Scot-Tussin)	66[b]	30				15	75			300 mg L-lysine, sorbitol, alcohol	Dye-free. In 120 mL.
otc	Geritol Tonic Liquid (SmithKline Beecham)	18[b]	2.5	2.5	50	2	0.5				25 mg methionine, 50 mg choline bitartrate, 12% alcohol	In 120 and 360 mL.

[a] From polysaccharide-iron complex.

[b] From ferric pyrophosphate.

For complete prescribing information, refer to the Iron-Containing Products group monograph.

IRON AND LIVER COMBINATIONS

For complete prescribing information refer to the Iron-Containing Products, Oral group monograph.

Indications

Iron and liver combinations are recommended for iron deficiency anemia in conjunction with certain nutritional deficiencies.

Precautions

The ingredients in these products are not sufficient, nor are they intended, for the treatment of pernicious anemia. The use of folic acid without adequate vitamin B12 therapy in patients with pernicious anemia may result in hematologic remission, but neurological progression.

▶ *Benzyl alcohol:* Some parenteral products contain benzyl alcohol, which has been associated with a fatal "gasping syndrome" in premature infants.

▶ *Liver:* Liver (concentrate, fraction or desiccated) is used as a source of vitamin B complex.

▶ *B complex vitamins:* B complex vitamins function as coenzymes in nutrient metabolism and maturation of red blood cells.

▶ *Ascorbic acid (vitamin C):* Ascorbic acid (vitamin C) may enhance the absorption of iron.

IRON AND LIVER COMBINATIONS, TABLETS
Content given per capsule or tablet.

	Product & Distributor	Fe mg	Liver	B1 mg	B2 mg	B3 mg	B5 mg	B6 mg	B12 mcg	C mg	Other Content	How Supplied
otc sf	I-L-X B12 High Potency Hematinic Caplets (Kenwood)	37.5[a]	130 mg (desiccated)	2	2	20			12	120		In 100s.

[a] From *Ferronyl* carbonyl iron.

For complete prescribing information, refer to the Iron-Containing Products group monograph.

IRON AND LIVER COMBINATIONS, LIQUIDS
Content given per 15 mL.

	Product & Distributor	Fe mg	Liver[a] mcg	B1 mg	B2 mg	B3 mg	B5 mg	B6 mg	B12 mcg	Other Content	How Supplied
otc	I-L-X B12 Elixir (Kenwood/Bradley)	102[a]	98 mg liver fraction 1	5	2	10			10	8% alcohol	In 240 mL.
otc	I-L-X Elixir (Kenwood/Bradley)	70[b]	98 mg liver concentrate 1:20	5	2	10				8% alcohol	In 240 mL.

[a] From iron ammonium citrate, brown.

[b] From ferrous gluconate.

Refer to the general discussion of these products in the Iron-Containing Products group monograph.

IRON AND LIVER COMBINATIONS, PARENTERAL

	Product & Distributor	Fe mg	Liver[a] mcg	B1 mg	B2 mg	B3 mg	B5 mg	B6 mg	B12 mcg	Other Content	How Supplied
Rx	Hytinic (Hyrex)	3[b]	1		0.75	50	1.25		15	2% procaine HCl, 2% benzyl alcohol	In 30 mL vials.

[a] B12 equivalent.

[b] From ferrous gluconate.

IRON AND LIVER COMBINATIONS, PARENTERAL

Refer to the general discussion of this product in the Iron-Containing Products group monograph.

Administration and Dosage
1 to 2 mL IM 1 to 3 times weekly.

IRON WITH VITAMIN B_{12} AND INTRINSIC FACTOR
Content given per capsule or tablet.

	Product & Distributor	Fe mg	B_{12}[a] mcg	IFC[b]	B_1 mg	B_2 mg	B_3 mg	C mg	FA mg	Other Content	How Supplied
Rx	Foltrin Capsules (Vitarine)	110[c]	15	240 mg				75	0.5		(E 5380). Maroon/red. In 100s and 1000s.
Rx	Livitrinsic-f Capsules (Goldline)										In 100s and 1000s.
Rx	Trinsicon Capsules (UCB Pharmaceuticals)										(364). Pink and red. In 60s, 500s and UD 100s.
Rx	Chromagen Capsules (Ther-Rx)	70	10 mcg B_{12}	100 mg desiccated stomach substance				150			(THX 0129). Red. In UD 100s.
Rx	FeoGen Capsules (Rising)	66	10 mcg B_{12}	100 mg desiccated stomach substance				250			(115). Maroon. IN UD 100S.

[a] B_{12} activity derived from cobalamin or liver.
[b] Intrinsic factor as concentrate or from stomach preparations.
[c] From ferrous fumarate.

Indications
These products contain Intrinsic Factor derived from stomach extract to promote the absorption of vitamin B_{12}. For treatment of anemias that respond to hematinics, including pernicious anemia and other megaloblastic anemias and also iron deficiency anemia.

MANGANESE

| otc | **Chelated Manganese** | **Tablets:** 20 mg | In 100s, 250s and 500s. |
| sf | (Freeda) | 50 mg | In 100s, 250s and 500s. |

For information on parenteral manganese, refer to the monograph in the IV Nutritional Therapy section.

Indications

As a dietary supplement.

Administration and Dosage

20 to 50 mg daily.

The need for manganese in human nutrition has been established, but no RDA has been determined. Manganese deficiency is unlikely because dietary intake usually satisfies the need; therefore, 2 to 5 mg/day via the diet is recommended.

Actions

➤*Pharmacology:* Manganese is a cofactor in many enzyme systems; it stimulates synthesis of cholesterol and fatty acids in the liver and influences mucopolysaccharide synthesis. It is concentrated in mitochondria, primarily of the pituitary gland, pancreas, liver, kidney and bone.

Zinc Supplements

For information on parenteral zinc, refer to the monograph in the IV Nutritional Therapy section.

Indications

As a dietary supplement; use to treat or prevent zinc deficiencies.

➤*Unlabeled uses:* For acrodermatitis enteropathica and delayed wound healing associated with zinc deficiency, doses of 220 mg zinc sulfate 3 times daily are used. Zinc sulfate has also been used to treat acne, rheumatoid arthritis and Wilson's disease. However, data conflict and are insufficient to recommend these uses.

In one study, zinc gluconate appeared to significantly shorten the duration of the common cold. Patients (n = 65) dissolved one tablet containing 23 mg zinc (one-half tablet for children) in the mouth every 2 hours until all symptoms were absent for 6 hours; 11% were asymptomatic within 12 hours, 22% within 24 hours. Zinc sulfate should not be used. Further study is needed.

Administration and Dosage

➤*Recommended dietary allowances (RDAs):* Adults, 12 to 15 mg. For a complete listing of RDAs by age, sex and condition, refer to the RDA table.

➤*Dietary supplement:* Average adult dose is 25 to 50 mg zinc daily. Take zinc with food to avoid gastric distress; however, some studies indicate that ingestion with some foods (eg, those that contain bran, phytates, protein, some minerals) may inhibit zinc absorption.

Actions

➤*Pharmacology:* Normal growth and tissue repair depend upon adequate zinc. Zinc acts as an integral part of several enzymes important to protein and carbohydrate metabolism.

Zinc deficiency – Zinc deficiency manifestations include: Anorexia; growth retardation; impaired taste and olfactory sensation; hypogonadism; alopecia; hepatosplenomegaly; dwarfism; rashes; cutaneous lesions; glossitis; stomatitis; blepharitis; paronychia; impaired healing.

➤*Pharmacokinetics:* Zinc salts are poorly absorbed from the GI tract; 20% to 30% of dietary zinc is absorbed. The major stores of zinc are in skeletal muscle and bone; zinc is also found in hair, nails, prostate, spermatazoa and choroid of the eye. The main excretion route is through the intestine. Only minor amounts are lost in urine ($\approx$ 2%).

Contraindications

Pregnancy (see Warnings); lactation.

Warnings

➤*Excessive intake:* Excessive intake in healthy persons may be deleterious. Eleven healthy men who ingested 150 mg zinc twice daily for 6 weeks showed significant impairment of lymphocyte and polymorphonuclear leukocyte functions and a significant decrease in high-density lipoproteins (HDL). No clinical side effects were seen during the study.

➤*Pregnancy:* Although zinc deficiency during pregnancy has been associated with adverse perinatal outcomes, other studies report no such occurrences. Therefore, since zinc deficiency is very rare, the routine use of zinc supplementation during pregnancy is not recommended. However, a dietary zinc intake of 15 mg/day is recommended.

➤*Lactation:* Breast milk concentrations of zinc decrease over time following delivery; extra dietary intake of zinc of 7 mg/day for the first 6 months of lactation and 4 mg/day during the second 6 months are recommended.

Precautions

➤*Do not exceed:* Do not exceed prescribed dosage; will cause emesis if administered in single 2 g doses.

Drug Interactions

Zinc Drug Interactions			
Precipitant drug	Object drug *		Description
Zinc salts	Fluoroquinolones	↓	The GI absorption and serum levels of some fluoroquinolones may be decreased, possibly resulting in a decreased anti-infective response.
Zinc salts	Tetracyclines	↓	The GI absorption and serum levels of tetracyclines may be decreased, possibly resulting in a decreased anti-infective response. Doxycycline does not appear to be affected.

* ↓ = Object drug decreased.

➤*Drug/Food interactions:* Bran products (including brown bread) and some foods (eg, protein, phytates, some minerals) may decrease zinc absorption.

Adverse Reactions

Nausea; vomiting.

Overdosage

➤*Symptoms:* Nausea; severe vomiting; dehydration; restlessness; sideroblastic anemia (secondary to zinc-induced copper deficiency).

➤*Treatment:* Reduce dosage or discontinue to control symptoms.

Patient Information

If GI upset occurs, take with food, but avoid foods high in calcium, phosphorus or phytate.

ZINC SULFATE (23% zinc)

otc	**Zinc 15** (Mericon)	**Tablets:** 66 mg (15 mg zinc)		In 100s.
otc	**Orazinc** (Mericon)	**Tablets:** 110 mg (25 mg zinc)		In 100s.
otc	**Zinc Sulfate** (Various, eg, Rugby)	**Tablets:** 200 mg (45 mg zinc)		In 1000s.
Rx	**Zinc Sulfate** (Various)	**Capsules:** 220 mg (50 mg zinc)		In 100s, 1000s and UD 100s.
otc	**Orazinc** (Mericon)			In 100s and 1000s.
otc	**Verazinc** (Forest)			In 100s.
otc	**Zinc-220** (Alto)			(401).Pink and blue. In 100s, 1000s and UD 100s.
Rx	**Zincate** (Paddock)			In 100s and 1000s.

Complete prescribing information for these products begins in the Zinc Supplements group monograph.

ZINC GLUCONATE (14.3% zinc)

otc	**Zinc Gluconate** (Various)	**Tablets:** 10 mg (1.4 mg zinc)	In 250s.
otc	**Zinc Gluconate** (Various, eg, Freeda)	**Tablets:** 15 mg (2 mg zinc)	In 250s.
otc	**Zinc Gluconate** (Various, eg, Major, Mission)	**Tablets:** 50 mg (7 mg zinc)	In 100s and 250s.

Complete prescribing information for these products begins in the Zinc Supplements group monograph.

ZINC ACETATE

otc	**Halls Zinc Defense** (Warner Lambert)	**Lozenges:** 5 mg	Sugar. Cherry or peppermint flavor. In 24s.

Complete prescribing information for these products begins in the Zinc Supplements group monograph.

COMPLEX ZINC CARBONATES

otc	**Zinc** (Sublingual Products)	**Liquid:** 15 mg/mL	Fructose, corn syrup solids, sorbitol, parabens. Fruit flavor. In 30 mL with dropper.

Complete prescribing information for these products begins in the Zinc Supplements group monograph.

ZINC COMBINATIONS

otc	**Zinc** (Zenith-Goldline)	**Lozenges:** 23 mg (zinc citrate/zinc gluconate)	Fructose. In 30s.

Complete prescribing information for these products begins in the Zinc Supplements group monograph.

Fluoride

Indications

▶*Prevention of dental caries:* Both neutral and acidulated phosphate fluoride effectively control dental decay. Use where water supplies are low in fluoride (< 0.7 ppm). Fluoride also controls rampant dental decay which frequently follows xerostomia-producing radiotherapy of head and neck tumors.

In communities without fluoridated water, the American Dental Association's Council on Dental Therapeutics recommends continuing fluoride supplements until the age of 13; the American Academy of Pediatrics recommends supplementation until 16 years of age.

▶*Unlabeled uses:* Sodium fluoride may be effective in treating osteoporosis. Doses (as fluoride) up to 60 mg daily or more are used in conjunction with calcium supplements, vitamin D or estrogen. However, large doses may result in a higher frequency of side effects. Some data suggest that doses < 50 mg/day are efficacious with fewer adverse reactions. No commercially available products contain high sodium fluoride doses for this use; therefore a large number of tablets would be required to obtain this dosage. Fluoride supplementation is not recommended for the prophylaxis of osteoporosis due to the potential for increased incidence of fractures (see Precautions).

Administration and Dosage

Use according to directions accompanying the product.

Fluoride Dosage	
Route/Age	Daily dose
Oral:	
Fluoride ion level in drinking water[1]	
(< 0.3 ppm):	
Birth to 6 months	None
6 months to 3 years	0.25 mg/day[2]
3 to 6 years	0.5 mg/day
6 to 16 years	1 mg/day
Fluoride content of drinking water	
(0.3 - 0.6 ppm):	
Birth to 6 months	None
6 months to 3 years	None
3 to 6 years	0.25 mg/day
6 to 16 years	0.5 mg/day
Fluoride content of drinking water (> 0.6 ppm):	
Birth to 6 months	None
6 months to 3 years	None
3 to 6 years	None
6 to 16 years	None
Topical (rinse):	
Children (6 to 12 years)	5 to 10 mL[3]
Adults and children (> 12 years)	10 mL[3]

[1] 1 ppm = 1 mg/L.
[2] 2.2 mg sodium fluoride contains 1 mg fluoride ion.
[3] Use once daily (*Point-Two,* once weekly) after thoroughly brushing teeth and rinsing mouth. Rinse around and between teeth for 1 minute, then spit out.

Actions

▶*Pharmacology:* Sodium fluoride acts systemically before tooth eruption, and topically posteruption, by increasing tooth resistance to acid dissolution, by promoting remineralization and by inhibiting the cariogenic microbial process. Acidulation provides greater topical fluoride uptake by dental enamel than neutral solutions. Phosphate protects enamel from demineralization by the acidulated formulation. Topical application of fluoride works superficially on enamel and plaque, and can reduce dental caries by 30% to 40%. Fluoride supplements may reduce the incidence of caries by up to 60%.

▶*Pharmacokinetics:* Fluoride is absorbed in the GI tract, lungs and skin. About 90% of oral fluoride is absorbed in the stomach. Absorption is related to solubility; sodium fluoride is almost completely absorbed. Calcium, iron or magnesium ions may delay absorption. Following ingestion, 50% of fluoride is deposited in bone and teeth. The major route of excretion is the kidneys; it is also excreted by sweat glands, the GI tract and in breast milk.

Contraindications

When the fluoride content of drinking water exceeds 0.7 ppm; low sodium or sodium free diets; hypersensitivity to fluoride.

Do not use 1 mg tablets in children < 3 years old or when the drinking water fluoride content is ≥ 0.3 ppm. Do not use 1 mg/5 mL rinse (as a supplement) in children < 6 years old.

Warnings

▶*Pregnancy:* Consult physician before using.
▶*Lactation:* Consult physician before using.
▶*Children:* See Contraindications.

Precautions

▶*Fractures:* Some epidemiological studies suggest that the incidence of certain types of bone fractures (crippling skeletal fluorosis) may be higher in some communities with naturally high or adjusted fluoride levels. However, other studies have not detected increased incidence of bone fractures. Crippling skeletal fluorosis is more common in parts of the world with high natural fluoride (> 10 ppm), but is extremely rare in the US.

▶*Mucositis:* Gingival tissues may be hypersensitive to some flavors or alcohol.

▶*Tartrazine sensitivity:* Some of these products contain tartrazine, which may cause allergic-type reactions (including bronchial asthma) in susceptible individuals. Although the incidence of tartrazine sensitivity in the general population is low, it is frequently seen in patients who also have aspirin hypersensitivity. Specific products containing tartrazine are identified in the product listings.

Drug Interactions

▶*Drug / Food interactions:* Incompatibility of dairy foods with systemic fluoride has occurred due to formation of calcium fluoride, which is poorly absorbed.

Adverse Reactions

▶*Dermatologic:* Eczema; atopic dermatitis; urticaria; allergic rash and other idiosyncrasies (rare).

▶*Miscellaneous:* Gastric distress; headache; weakness. Rinses and gels containing stannous fluoride may produce surface staining of the teeth; this does not occur with nonstannous fluoride topical preparations. Acidulated fluoride may dull porcelain and composite restorations.

Overdosage

▶*Chronic overdosage:* Chronic overdosage of fluorides may result in dental fluorosis (a mottling of tooth enamel) and osseous changes.

▶*Acute overdosage:*

Symptoms – In children, acute ingestion of 10 to 20 mg sodium fluoride may cause excessive salivation and GI disturbances; 500 mg may be fatal. The oral lethal dose is 70 to 140 mg/kg (5 to 10 g in adults).

GI – Salivation, nausea, abdominal pain, vomiting and diarrhea are frequent due to conversion of sodium fluoride to corrosive hydrofluoric acid in the stomach.

CNS – Because of the calcium-binding effect of fluoride, CNS irritability, paresthesias, tetany, convulsions and respiratory and cardiac failure may occur. Fluoride has a direct toxic action on muscle and nerve tissue, and it interferes with many enzyme systems.

Hypocalcemia, hypoglycemia and delayed hyperkalemia are frequent laboratory findings.

▶*Treatment:* Usual supportive measures. Refer to General Management of Acute Overdosage. Precipitate the fluoride by using gastric lavage with 0.15% calcium hydroxide. Administer IV glucose in saline for a forced diuresis; IV calcium may be indicated for tetany. Administer calcium IM (10 mL of 10% calcium gluconate, 5 mL in children) every 4 to 6 hours until recovery is complete. Maintain electrolytes, normal blood pH and adequate urine output. Removing fluoride with dialysis and hemoperfusion may also be beneficial.

Patient Information

▶*Tablets and drops:* Milk and other dairy products may decrease absorption of sodium fluoride; avoid simultaneous ingestion.

▶*Tablets:* Dissolve in the mouth, chew, swallow whole, add to drinking water or fruit juice or add to water for use in infant formulas or other food.

▶*Drops:* Take orally, undiluted, or mix with fluids or food.

▶*Rinses and gels:* Rinses and gels are most effective immediately after brushing or flossing and just prior to sleep. Expectorate any excess. Do not swallow. Do not eat, drink or rinse mouth for 30 minutes after application.

Notify dentist if tooth enamel becomes discolored.

FLUORIDE, ORAL

Rx	**EtheDent** (Ethex)	**Tablets, chewable:** 0.25 mg	In 120s.
Rx sf	**Luride Lozi-Tabs** (Colgate-Hoyt)		(COP 186). Vanilla flavor. In 120s.
Rx	**Sodium Fluoride**[a] (Various, eg, Rugby)	**Tablets, chewable:** 0.5 mg (from 1.1 mg sodium fluoride)	In 1000s.
Rx	**EtheDent** (Ethex)		In 120s and 1000s.
Rx	**Fluoritab** (Fluoritab)		Dye free. Pineapple flavor. In 1000s and 5000s.
Rx sf	**Luride Lozi-Tabs** (Colgate-Hoyt)		(COP 014). Grape and assorted fruit flavors. In 120s. Grape also in 1200s.
Rx sf	**Pharmaflur 1.1** (Pharmics)		Grape flavor. In 120s.
Rx	**Sodium Fluoride**[a] (Various, eg, Major, Rugby)	**Tablets, chewable:** 1 mg (from 2.2 mg sodium fluoride)	In 100s, 1000s and UD 1000s.
Rx	**EtheDent** (Ethex)		In 120s and 1000s.
Rx	**Karidium** (Lorvic)		White. In 180s and 1000s.
Rx sf	**Luride Lozi-Tabs** (Colgate-Hoyt)		(COP 006). Cherry and assorted fruit flavors. In 120s and 1000s. Cherry also in 5000s.
Rx sf	**Luride-SF Lozi-Tabs** (Colgate-Hoyt)		In 120s.
Rx sf	**Pharmaflur** (Pharmics)		Cherry flavor. In 1000s.
Rx sf	**Pharmaflur df** (Pharmics)		Dye free. Cherry flavor. In 120s.
Rx	**Fluoride** (Kirkman)	**Tablets:** 1 mg (from 2.2 mg sodium fluoride)	In 1000s.
Rx sf	**Flura** (Kirkman)		In 100s and 1000s.
Rx	**Sodium Fluoride** (Rugby)	**Drops:** 0.125 mg per drop (from ≈ 0.275 mg sodium fluoride)	In 30 mL.
Rx sf	**Fluoritab** (Fluoritab)	**Drops:** 0.25 mg per drop (from 0.55 mg sodium fluoride)	In 22.8 mL.
Rx sf	**Pediaflor** (Ross)	**Drops:** 0.5 mg per mL (from 1.1 mg sodium fluoride)	< 0.5% alcohol, sorbitol. Cherry flavor. In 50 mL w/dropper.
Rx sf	**Luride** (Colgate)		Peach flavor. In 50 mL.
Rx sf	**Fluoride Loz** (Kirkman)	**Lozenges:** 1 mg (from 2.2 mg sodium fluoride)	In 1000s.
Rx	**Flura-Loz** (Kirkman)		Raspberry flavor. In 100s and 1000s.
Rx sf	**Phos-Flur** (Colgate-Hoyt)	**Solution:**[b] 0.2 mg per mL (from 0.44 mg sodium fluoride)	Cherry flavor. In 250, 500 mL & gal. Cinnamon (w/saccharin), grape, wintergreen flavors. In 500 mL.

[a] May be regular or chewable.   [b] May be used as a rinse or supplement.

Complete prescribing information begins in the Fluoride group monograph.

FLUORIDE, TOPICAL

otc	**ACT** (Johnson & Johnson)	**Rinse:** 0.02% (from 0.05% sodium fluoride)	7% alcohol. In 90, 360 and 480 mL.
otc	**Fluorigard** (Colgate-Palmolive)		6% alcohol. Tartrazine. In 180, 300 & 480 mL.
otc	**Gel-Kam** (Colgate-Palmolive)	**Rinse:** 0.04% sodium fluoride	Mint, fruit and berry, bubblegum, and cinnamon flavors. In 4.3 and 7 oz.
otc sf	**MouthKote F/R** (Parnell)		Benzyl alcohol, sorbitol, menthol, EDTA. In 237 mL.
Rx	**Fluorinse** (Oral-B)	**Rinse:** 0.09% (from 0.2% sodium fluoride)	Alcohol free. Mint and cinnamon flavors. In 480 mL.
Rx	**Point-Two** (Colgate-Hoyt)		6% alcohol. Mint flavor. In 240 mL and gal.
Rx	**PreviDent Rinse** (Colgate Oral)	**Rinse:** 0.2% neutral sodium fluoride	6% alcohol. Mint flavor. In 250 mL and gal (with pump dispenser).
Rx	**Stannous Fluoride** (Cypress)	**Rinse concentrate:** 0.63% stannous fluoride	Mint flavor. In 122 g.
Rx	**Gel Kam** (Scherer)	**Gel:** 0.1% (from 0.4% stannous fluoride)	Cinnamon flavor. In 65 and 122 g and 105 g (Dental Therapy-Pak [2]).
otc	**Gel-Tin** (Young Dental)		Lime, grape, cinnamon, raspberry, mint and orange flavors. In 60 g.
otc	**Stop** (Oral-B)		Grape, cinnamon, bubblegum, piña colada and mint flavors. In 120 g.
otc	**Stannous Fluoride** (Cypress)	**Gel:** 0.4% stannous fluoride	Parabens. Mint flavor. In 122 g.

FLUORIDE, TOPICAL

Rx	**Karigel** (Lorvic)	**Gel:** 0.5% (from 1.1% sodium fluoride)	pH 5.6. Orange flavor. In 30, 130 and 250 g.
Rx	**Karigel-N** (Lorvic)		Neutral pH. In 24 and 120 g.
Rx	**Prevident** (Colgate-Hoyt)		Mint, berry, cherry and fruit sherbet flavors. In 24 and 60 g. Lime flavor in 60 g.
Rx	**Thera-Flur** (Colgate-Hoyt)	**Gel-Drops:** 0.5% (from 1.1% sodium fluoride)	pH 4.5. Lime flavor. In 24 mL.
Rx	**Thera-Flur-N** (Colgate-Hoyt)		Neutral pH. In 24 mL.
Rx	**DentaGel 1.1%** (Rising Pharmaceuticals[a])	**Gel:** 1.1% sodium fluoride	Saccharin, parabens, sorbitol. Fresh mint flavor. In 56 g.
Rx	**NeutraGard Advanced** (Pascal[b])		Wintermint flavor. In 60 g.
Rx	**Luride** (Colgate Oral)	**Gel:** 1.2% (from sodium fluoride and hydrogen fluoride)	Mint flavor. In 7 g.
Rx	**Prevident Plus** (Colgate-Hoyt)		Mint, berry, cherry and fruit sherbet flavors. In 24 and 60 g. Lime flavor in 60 g.
Rx	**Denta 5000 Plus** (Rising Pharmaceuticals[a])	**Cream:** 1.1%	Spearmint flavor. In 51 g (2s).
Rx	**EtheDent** (Ethex)		Sorbitol, saccharin. In 51 g.
Rx	**PreviDent 5000 Plus** (Colgate)		Sorbitol, saccharin. In spearmint and fruit flavors. In 51 g (1s and 2s).

[a] Rising Pharmaceuticals, 411 Sette Drive, Paramus, NJ 07652; 201-262-4200, fax 201-262-4284.

[b] Pascal Company, Inc., P.O. Box 1478, Bellevue, WA 98009–1478; 425-827-4694, 800-426-8051, fax 425-827-6893; http://www.pascaldental.com.

Complete prescribing information for these products begins in the Fluoride group monograph.

SODIUM CHLORIDE

otc	**Sustain** (Zee Medical)	**Tablets:** 220 mg sodium chloride, 18 mg calcium carbonate, 15 mg potassium chloride	In 24s.
otc	**Sodium Chloride** (Purepac)	**Tablets:** 650 mg	In 100s.
otc	**Sodium Chloride** (Various)	**Tablets:** 1 g	In 100s and 1000s.
otc	**Sodium Chloride** (Lilly)	**Tablets:** 2.25 g	In 100s and 500s.
otc	**Slo-Salt** (Mission)	**Tablets, slow release:** 600 mg	In 100s.
otc	**Slo-Salt-K** (Mission)	**Tablets, slow release:** 410 mg sodium chloride and 150 mg potassium chloride in wax matrix	In 1000s.

Indications

Prevention or treatment of extracellular volume depletion, dehydration or sodium depletion; aid in the prevention of heat prostration.

Administration and Dosage

Refer to specific product labeling for dosage guidelines.

Warnings

➤*Acclimatization:* Inappropriate salt administration in an effort to acclimatize to a hot environment can be dangerous. Balanced electrolytes and adequate hydration are essential.

➤*Salt tablets:* Salt tablets may pass through the GI tract undigested. Avoid their use in treating heat cramps since they may cause vomiting, pooling of oral fluids and potassium depletion. Use oral salt solutions instead.

➤*Pregnancy:* Seek professional advice before using these products while pregnant.

➤*Lactation:* Seek professional advice before using these products while breastfeeding.

Precautions

➤*Supplementation:* Individuals with adequate dietary sodium intake and normal renal function should not require sodium chloride supplementation. Balanced electrolyte supplements may be preferred to prevent hypokalemia.

➤*Use with caution:* Caution should be used in the presence of CHF, kidney dysfunction, peripheral or pulmonary edema or preeclampsia.

Overdosage

➤*Symptoms:* Overdosage may cause serious electrolyte disturbances. Ingestion of large amounts of sodium chloride irritates the GI mucosa and may result in nausea, vomiting, diarrhea and abdominal cramps. Edema is a sign of excess total body sodium.

Manifestations of hypernatremia may include:

Neurologic – Irritability; restlessness; weakness; obtundation progressing to convulsions and coma.

Cardiovascular – Hypertension, tachycardia, fluid accumulation.

Respiratory – Pulmonary edema; respiratory arrest.

➤*Treatment:* Treatment includes usual supportive measures. Refer to General Management of Acute Overdosage. Use appropriate measures to empty the stomach. Magnesium sulfate may be given as a cathartic. Provide an adequate airway and ventilation. Maintain vascular volume and tissue perfusion.

POTASSIUM REPLACEMENT PRODUCTS

Rx	**Potassium Chloride** (Various, eg, Abbott, Gold-line, Rugby, Warner Chil-cott)	**Tablets, controlled release:** 8 mEq (600 mg) potassium chloride in a wax matrix	In 100s and 1000s.
Rx	**Klor-Con 8** (Upsher-Smith)		(KLOR–CON 8). Blue. Film coated. In 100s, 500s and UD 100s.
Rx	**K⁺8** (Alra)	**Tablets, extended release:** 8 mEq potassium chloride	In 100s and 500s.
Rx	**K + 10** (Alra)	**Tablets, controlled release:** 10 mEq (750 mg) potassium chloride in a wax matrix	Film coated. In 100s, 500s, 1000s and UD 100s.
Rx	**Kaon Cl-10** (Savage)		Sucrose. (10). Green. Sugar coated. Capsule shape. In 1000s and Stat-Pak 100s.
Rx	**Klor-Con 10** (Upsher-Smith)		(KLOR–CON 10).Yellow. Film coated. In 100s, 500s and UD 100s.
Rx	**Klotrix** (Bristol)		(KLOTRIX BL 10 meq 770). Orange. Film coated. In 100s, 1000s and UD 100s.
Rx	**K-Tab** (Abbott)		(NM A 101)Yellow. Film coated. Oval. In 100s, 1000s, 5000s and Abbo-Pac 100s.
Rx	**Klor-Con M10** (Upsher-Smith)	**Tablets, extended-release:** 10 mEq potassium (from 750 mg potassium chloride	(KC M10). Oblong. In 90s, 100s, 1000s, and UD 100s.
Rx	**Klor-Con M15** (Upsher-Smith)	**Tablets, extended-release:** 15 mEq potassium (from 1125 mg potassium chloride	(M 15). Oblong, scored. In 100s, 1000s, and UD 100s.
Rx	**Klor-Con M20** (Upsher-Smith)	**Tablets, extended-release:** 20 mEq potassium (from 1500 mg potassium chloride	(KC M20). Oblong, scored. In 90s, 100s, 500s, 1000s, and UD 100s.
Rx	**Potassium Chloride** (Various, eg, Major, Rugby)	**Tablets, extended release:** 750 mg potassium chloride equivalent to 10 mEq potassium in a wax matrix	In 100s and 1000s.
Rx	**K-Dur 10** (Key)	**Tablets, controlled release:** 750 mg microencapsulated potassium chloride equivalent to 10 mEq potassium	(K-Dur 10). White. Oblong. In 100s and UD 100s.
Rx	**K-Dur 20** (Key)	**Tablets, controlled release:** 1500 mg microencapsulated potassium chloride equivalent to 20 mEq potassium	(20). White, scored. Oblong. In 100s, 500s, 1000s and UD 100s.
otc	**Potassium Gluconate** (Various)	**Tablets:** 500 mg potassium gluconate (83.45 mg potassium)	In 100s and 1000s.
otc	**Potassium Gluconate** (Mission)	**Tablets:** 595 mg potassium gluconate (99 mg potassium)	In 100s.
Rx	**K + Care ET** (Alra)	**Tablets, effervescent:** 20 mEq potassium (from potassium bicarbonate)	Saccharin. In 30s and 100s.
Rx sf	**Klorvess** (Sandoz)	**Tablets, effervescent:** 20 mEq potassium (from potassium chloride and bicarbonate and lysine hydrochloride)	Sodium free. Saccharin. White. In 60s and 1000s.
Rx	**K•Lyte/Cl** (Bristol)	**Tablets, effervescent:** 25 mEq potassium (from potassium Cl and bicarbonate, l-lysine monohydrochloride and citric acid)	Saccharin, docusate sodium. Fruit punch or citrus flavors. In 30s, 100s and 250s.
Rx	**K•Lyte/Cl 50** (Bristol)	**Tablets, effervescent:** 50 mEq potassium (from potassium Cl and bicarbonate, l-lysine monohydrochloride and citric acid)	Saccharin, docusate sodium. Fruit punch or citrus flavors. In 30s & 100s.
Rx	**K + Care ET** (Alra)	**Tablets, effervescent:** 25 mEq potassium (from potassium bicarbonate)	Saccharin. Orange or lime flavors. In 30s and 100s.
Rx	**Effer-K** (Nomax)	**Tablets, effervescent:** 25 mEq potassium (as bicarbonate and citrate)	Saccharin. Orange or lime flavors. In 30s, 100s & 250s.
Rx	**Effervescent Potassium** (Rugby)		Saccharin. Lime, orange or fruit punch flavors. In 30s.
Rx sf	**Klor-Con/EF** (Upsher-Smith)		Saccharin. Orange flavor. In 30s and 100s.
Rx	**K•Lyte** (Bristol)		Saccharin, docusate sodium, dextrose. Orange or lime flavor. In 30s, 100s and 250s.
Rx	**K•Lyte DS** (Bristol)	**Tablets, effervescent:** 50 mEq potassium (from potassium bicarbonate and citrate and citric acid)	Saccharin, docusate sodium, lactose. Orange or lime flavor. In 30s and 100s.
Rx	**Micro-K Extencaps** (Robins)	**Capsules, controlled release:** 600 mg potassium chloride equivalent to 8 mEq potassium. Microencapsulated particles	(Micro-K THER-RX 010). Orange. In 100s, 500s and UD 100s.
Rx	**Potassium Chloride** (Various, eg, EtheX, Gold-line, Moore, Parmed, Rugby, Warner-Chilcott)	**Capsules, controlled release:** 10 mEq (750 mg) potassium chloride. Microencapsulated particles	In 100s and 500s.
Rx	**Micro-K 10 Extencaps** (Thera-Rx)		(Micro-K 10 AHR/ 5730). Orange/white. In 100s, 500s and UD 100s.
Rx	**Potassium Chloride** (Various, eg, Barre-National, Geneva, Major, Parmed, PBI, Rugby, Schein)	**Liquid:** 20 mEq/15 mL potassium and chloride (10% KCl)	In pt and gal.
Rx sf	**Cena-K** (Century)		In pt and gal.
Rx sf	**Kay Ciel** (Forest)		4% alcohol. In 118 mL, pt and gal.
Rx sf	**Potasalan** (Lannett)		4% alcohol. Orange flavor. In pt and gal.
Rx	**Rum-K** (Fleming)	**Liquid:** 30 mEq/15 mL potassium and chloride (15% KCl)	Butter-rum flavor. In pt and gal.
Rx	**Potassium Chloride** (Various, eg, Barre-National, Major, PBI, Rugby)	**Liquid:** 40 mEq/15 mL potassium and chloride (20% KCl)	In pt and gal.
Rx sf	**Kaon-Cl 20%** (Adria)		5% alcohol, saccharin. Cherry flavor. In 480 mL.

POTASSIUM REPLACEMENT PRODUCTS

Rx	**Potassium Gluconate** (Various, eg, PBI)	**Liquid:** 20 mEq/15 mL potassium (as potassium gluconate)	In 118 mL, pt, gal and UD 5 and 15 mL (100s).
Rx sf	**Kaon** (Adria)		5% alcohol. Saccharin. Grape flavor. In 480 mL.
Rx	**Kaylixir** (Lannett)		5% alcohol. Saccharin. In pt and gal.
Rx	**Twin-K** (Boots)	**Liquid:** 20 mEq/15 mL potassium (as potassium gluconate & potassium citrate)	Sorbitol, saccharin. In 480 mL.
Rx sf	**Kolyum** (Fisons)	**Liquid:** 20 mEq potassium and 3.4 mEq chloride/15 mL (from potassium gluconate and potassium chloride)	Sorbitol, saccharin. Cherry flavor. In pt and gal.
Rx	**K + Care** (Alra)	**Powder:** 15 mEq potassium chloride per packet	Saccharin. Fruit or orange flavors. In 30s and 100s.
Rx	**Potassium Chloride** (Various, eg, Schein)	**Powder:** 20 mEq potassium chloride per packet	In 30s and 100s.
Rx sf	**Gen-K** (Goldline)		Orange/fruit flavor. In 30s.
Rx sf	**Kay Ciel** (Forest)		Saccharin. In 30s and 100s.
Rx	**K + Care** (Alta)		Saccharin. Fruit or orange flavor. In 30s and 100s.
Rx	**K-Lor** (Abbott)		Saccharin. Fruit flavor. In 30s and 100s.
Rx sf	**Klor-Con** (Upsher-Smith)		Saccharin. Fruit flavor. In 30s and 100s.
Rx	**Micro-K LS** (Robins)		Extended-release. Sucrose. In 30s and 100s.
Rx	**K + Care** (Alra)	**Powder:** 25 mEq potassium chloride per packet	Saccharin. Orange flavor. In 30s and 100s.
Rx sf	**Klor-Con/25** (Upsher-Smith)		Saccharin. Fruit flavor. In 30s, 100s and 250s.
Rx	**K-Lyte/Cl** (Mead Johnson Nutritionals)	**Powder:** 25 mEq potassium chloride per dose	Fruit punch flavor. In 225 g (30 doses).
Rx	**K-vescent Potassium Chloride** (Major)	**Powder:** 20 mEq potassium and chloride from 1.5 g potassium chloride	Saccharin. In 30 and 100 packets.

For information on parenteral potassium, refer to the IV Nutritional Therapy section.

Indications

Treatment of hypokalemia in the following conditions: With or without metabolic alkalosis; digitalis intoxication; familial periodic paralysis; diabetic acidosis; diarrhea and vomiting; surgical conditions accompanied by nitrogen loss, vomiting, suction drainage, diarrhea and increased urinary excretion of potassium; certain cases of uremia; hyperadrenalism; starvation and debilitation; corticosteroid or diuretic therapy.

Prevention of potassium depletion when dietary intake is inadequate in the following conditions: Patients receiving digitalis and diuretics for congestive heart failure; significant cardiac arrhythmias; hepatic cirrhosis with ascites; states of aldosterone excess with normal renal function; potassium-losing nephropathy; certain diarrheal states.

When hypokalemia is associated with alkalosis, use potassium chloride. When acidosis is present, use the bicarbonate, citrate, acetate or gluconate potassium salts.

▶*Unlabeled uses:* In patients with mild hypertension, the use of potassium supplements (24 to 60 mmol/day) appears to result in a long-term reduction of blood pressure.

Administration and Dosage

The usual dietary intake of potassium ranges between 40 to 150 mEq/day.

Individualize dosage. Usual range is 16 to 24 mEq/day for the prevention of hypokalemia to 40 to 100 mEq/day or more for the treatment of potassium depletion.

Potassium intoxication may result from any therapeutic dosage.

Actions

▶*Pharmacology:* Potassium, the principal intracellular cation of most body tissues, participates in a number of essential physiological processes, such as maintenance of intracellular tonicity and a proper relationship with sodium across cell membranes, cellular metabolism, transmission of nerve impulses, contraction of cardiac, skeletal and smooth muscle, acid-base balance and maintenance of normal renal function. Normal potassium serum levels range from 3.5 to 5 mEq/L. The active ion transport system maintains this gradient across the plasma membrane.

mEq/g of Various Potassium Salts	
Potassium salt	mEq/g
Potassium gluconate	4.3
Potassium citrate	9.8
Potassium bicarbonate	10
Potassium acetate	10.2
Potassium chloride	13.4

Potassium homeostasis – The potassium concentration in extracellular fluid is normally 4 to 5 mEq/L; the concentration in intracellular fluid is approximately 150 to 160 mEq/L. Plasma concentration provides a useful clinical guide to disturbances in potassium balance. By producing large differences in the ratio of intracellular to extracellular potassium, relatively small absolute changes in extracellular concentration may have important effects on neuromuscular activity.

Despite wide variations in dietary intake of potassium (eg, 40 to 120 mEq/day), plasma potassium concentration is normally stabilized within the narrow range of 4 to 5 mEq/L by virtue of close renal regulation of potassium balance. Renal potassium excretion is accomplished largely by potassium secretion in the distal portion of the nephron; essentially all filtered potassium is reabsorbed in the proximal tubule. The potassium that appears in the urine is added to the filtrate by a distal process of sodium-cation exchange. Fecal excretion of potassium is normally only a few mEq per day and does not play a significant role in potassium homeostasis.

Natural potassium sources – Foods rich in potassium include: Beef; veal; ham; chicken; turkey; fish; milk; bananas; dates; prunes; raisins; avocado; watermelon; canteloupes; apricots; molasses; beans; yams; broccoli; brussels sprouts; lentils; potatoes; spinach.

Hypokalemia – Gradual potassium depletion may occur whenever the rate of potassium loss through renal excretion or GI loss exceeds the rate of potassium intake. Potassium depletion is usually a consequence of prolonged therapy with oral diuretics, primary or secondary hyperaldosteronism, diabetic ketoacidosis, severe diarrhea (especially if associated with vomiting) or inadequate replacement during prolonged parenteral nutrition. Potassium depletion due to these causes is usually accompanied by a concomitant deficiency of chloride and is manifested by hypokalemia and metabolic alkalosis.

The use of potassium salts in patients receiving diuretics for uncomplicated essential hypertension is often unnecessary when such patients have a normal diet. However, if hypokalemia occurs, dietary supplementation with potassium-containing foods may be adequate. In more severe cases, potassium salt supplementation may be indicated.

Potassium depletion sufficient to cause 1 mEq/L drop in serum potassium requires a loss of about 100 to 200 mEq potassium from the total body store.

Symptoms: Weakness; fatigue; ileus; tetany; polydipsia; flaccid paralysis or impaired ability to concentrate urine (in advanced cases). ECG may reveal atrial and ventricular ectopy, prolongation of QT interval, ST segment depression, conduction defects, broad or flat T waves or appearance of U waves.

Contraindications

Severe renal impairment with oliguria or azotemia; untreated Addison's disease; hyperkalemia from any cause (eg, systemic acidosis, acute dehydration, extensive tissue breakdown); adynamia episodica hereditaria; acute dehydration; heat cramps; patients receiving potassium-sparing diuretics (spironolactone, triamterene or amiloride) or aldosterone-inhibiting agents.

Solid dosage forms of potassium supplements are contraindicated in any patient in whom there is cause for arrest or delay in tablet passage through the GI tract. Wax matrix potassium chloride preparations have produced esophageal ulceration in cardiac patients with esophageal

POTASSIUM REPLACEMENT PRODUCTS

compression due to an enlarged left atrium; give potassium supplementation as a liquid preparation to these patients.

Warnings

➤*Hyperkalemia:* In patients with impaired potassium excretion, potassium salts can produce hyperkalemia or cardiac arrest. This occurs most commonly in patients given IV potassium, but may also occur in patients given oral potassium. Potentially fatal hyperkalemia can develop rapidly and may be asymptomatic.

Hyperkalemia may be manifested only by an increased serum potassium concentration and characteristic ECG changes (eg, peaking of T waves, loss of P wave, depression of ST segment, prolongation of the QT interval, lengthened P-R interval, widened QRS complex). However, the following may also occur: Parasthesias; heaviness; muscle weakness and flaccid paralysis of the extremities; listlessness; mental confusion; decreased blood pressure; shock; cardiac arrhythmias; heart block.

In response to a rise in the concentration of body potassium, renal excretion of the ion is increased. With normal kidney function, it is difficult to produce potassium intoxication by oral administration. However, administer potassium supplements with caution, since the amount of deficiency and corresponding daily dose is unknown. Frequently monitor the clinical status, periodic ECG and serum potassium levels. This is particularly important in patients receiving digitalis and in patients with cardiac disease. There is a hazard in prescribing potassium in digitalis intoxication manifested by atrioventricular (AV) conduction disturbance.

➤*GI lesions:* Potassium chloride tablets have produced stenotic or ulcerative lesions of the small bowel and death. These lesions are caused by a concentration of potassium ion in the region of a rapidly dissolving tablet, which injures the bowel wall and produces obstruction, hemorrhage or perforation. The reported frequency of small bowel lesions is much less with wax matrix tablets (< 1 per 100,000 patient-years) and microencapsulated tablets than with enteric coated tablets (40 to 50 per 100,000 patient-years). Upper GI bleeding, esophageal ulceration and stricture, gastric ulceration and lower GI ulceration have occurred with wax matrix preparations. The total number of GI lesions is < 1 per 47,000 patient-years. Discontinue either type of tablet immediately and consider the possibility of bowel obstruction or perforation if severe vomiting, abdominal pain or distention or GI bleeding occurs.

Patients at greatest risk for developing potassium chloride-induced GI lesions include: The elderly, the immobile and those with scleroderma, diabetes mellitus, mitral valve replacement, cardiomegaly or esophageal stricture/compression.

Reserve slow release potassium chloride preparations for patients who cannot tolerate liquids or effervescent potassium preparations, or for patients in whom there is a problem of compliance with these preparations.

Some studies suggest the "microencapsulated" preparations are less likely to cause GI damage; however, evidence conflicts and a specific recommendation of one solid oral product over another (wax matrix or microencapsulated) cannot be made. Avoid enteric coated products.

➤*Metabolic acidosis and hyperchloremia:* In some patients (eg, those with renal tubular acidosis), potassium depletion is rarely associated with metabolic acidosis and hyperchloremia. Replace with potassium bicarbonate, citrate, acetate or gluconate.

➤*Renal function impairment:* Renal function impairment requires careful monitoring of the serum potassium concentration and appropriate dosage adjustment.

➤*Pregnancy:* Category C. It is not known whether potassium salts can cause fetal harm when administered to a pregnant woman or can affect reproduction capacity. Give to a pregnant woman only if clearly needed.

➤*Lactation:* It is not known whether this drug is excreted in breast milk. Exercise caution when administering to a nursing woman. The normal potassium content of breast milk is ≈ 13 mEq/L. As long as body potassium is not excessive, the contribution of potassium salts should have little or no effect on the level of breast milk.

➤*Children:* Safety and efficacy for use in children have not been established.

Precautions

➤*Monitoring:* When blood is drawn for analysis of plasma potassium, it is important to recognize that artificial elevations can occur after improper venipuncture technique or as a result of in vitro hemolysis of the sample.

➤*Hypokalemia:* Hypokalemia is ordinarily diagnosed by demonstrating potassium depletion in a patient and by a careful clinical history. In interpreting the serum potassium level, consider that acute alkalosis can produce hypokalemia in the absence of a deficit in total body potassium, while acute acidosis can increase the serum potassium concentration to the normal range, even in the presence of a reduced total body potassium. Treatment, particularly in the presence of cardiac disease, renal disease or acidosis, requires careful attention to acid-base balance and monitoring of serum electrolytes, ECG and clinical status of the patient.

The administration of concentrated dextrose or sodium bicarbonate may cause an intracellular potassium shift. This may cause hypokalemia which, in turn, may lead to serious cardiac arrhythmias.

Giving potassium to hypokalemic hypertensives may lower blood pressure.

➤*Tartrazine sensitivity:* Some of these products contain tartrazine, which may cause allergic-type reactions (including bronchial asthma) in susceptible individuals. Although the incidence of tartrazine sensitivity in the general population is low, it is frequently seen in patients who also have aspirin hypersensitivity. Specific products containing tartrazine are identified in the product listings.

Drug Interactions

Potassium Preparation Drug Interactions			
Precipitant drug	Object drug[*]		Description
ACE inhibitors	Potassium preparations	↑	Concurrent use may result in elevated serum potassium concentrations in certain patients.
Potassium-sparing diuretics	Potassium preparations	↑	Potassium-sparing diuretics will increase potassium retention and can produce severe hyperkalemia.
Potassium preparations	Digitalis	↑	In patients receiving digoxin, hypokalemia may result in digoxin toxicity. Therefore, use caution if discontinuing a potassium preparation in patients maintained on digoxin.

[*] ↑ = Object drug increased

In addition, potassium citrate, a urinary alkalinizer, may affect the renal excretion and pharmacologic effects of various agents (refer to the Citrate and Citric Acid Solutions monograph).

Adverse Reactions

Most common – Nausea, vomiting, diarrhea, flatulence and abdominal discomfort due to GI irritation are best managed by diluting the preparation further, by taking with meals or by dose reduction.

Rare – Skin rash.

Most severe – Hyperkalemia; GI obstruction, bleeding, ulceration or perforation.

Overdosage

For symptoms and treatment of potassium overdosage and hyperkalemia, refer to the monograph in the IV Nutritional Therapy section.

Patient Information

May cause GI upset; take after meals or with food and with a full glass of water.

Do not chew or crush tablets; swallow whole.

➤*Oral liquids, soluble powders and effervescent tablets:* Mix or dissolve completely in 3 to 8 ounces of cold water, juice or other suitable beverage and drink slowly.

Following release of potassium chloride, the expended wax matrix, which is not absorbable, can be found in the stool. This is no cause for concern.

Do not use salt substitutes concurrently, except on the advice of a physician.

Notify physician if tingling of the hands and feet, unusual tiredness or weakness, a feeling of heaviness in the legs, severe nausea, vomiting, abdominal pain or black stools (GI bleeding) occurs.

ORAL ELECTROLYTE MIXTURES

	Product	Na+	K+	Cl–	Citrate	Ca++	Mg++	Phosphate	Other Content	Calories per fl. oz.	How Supplied
		Electrolyte content									
otc	**Rehydralyte Solution** (Ross)	75[a]	20[a]	65[a]	30[a]				25 g/L dextrose	3	In 240 mL ready-to-use.
otc	**Infalyte Oral Solution** (Mead Johnson)	50[a]	25[a]	45[a]	34[a]				30 g/L rice syrup solids	4.2	Fruit flavor. In ≈ 1 L ready-to-use.
otc	**Resol Solution** (Wyeth-Ayerst)	50[a]	20[a]	50[a]	34[a]	4[a]	4[a]	5[a]	20 g/L glucose	2.5	In 240 mL ready-to-use.
otc	**Naturalyte Solution** (UBI)	45[a]	20[a]	35[a]	48[a]				25 g/L dextrose		Unflavored, fruit or bubble gum flavors. In 240 mL and 1 L.
otc	**Pedialyte Solution** (Ross)	45[a]	20[a]	35[a]	30[a]				25 g/L dextrose	3	Regular or fruit flavor. In 240 & 960 mL ready-to-use.
otc	**Pedialyte Freezer Pops** (Ross)	45[a]	20[a]	35[a]	30[a]				25 g/L dextrose, phenylalanine, aspartame	3	Grape, cherry, orange and blue raspberry flavors. In 2.1 fl oz ready-to-freeze pops (16s).
otc	**Temp Tab** (National Vitamin)	180[b]	15[b]	287[b]							Preservative- and sugar-free. In 100s.

[a] mEq/L   [b] Mg/tablet.

Indications

For maintenance of water and electrolytes following corrective parenteral therapy for severe diarrhea; for maintenance to replace mild to moderate fluid losses when food and liquid intake are discontinued; to restore fluid and minerals lost in diarrhea and vomiting in infants and children.

➤*Temp Tab:* For minimizing chronic fatigue, muscle cramps, or heat prostration because of excessive perspiration.

For use by people that are exposed to high temperatures which can cause heat fatigue.

Administration and Dosage

Individualize dosage. Follow the guidelines listed on the product labeling.

➤*Ricelyte: Children < 2 years of age:* Consult physician.

Children ≥ 2 years of age – Administer every 3 to 4 hours, up to 2 quarts per day.

➤*Resol:* Individualize dosage based on extent of weight loss and dehydration as assessed by the physician.

➤*Pedialyte/Rehydralyte:* Offer frequently in amounts tolerated. Adjust total daily intake to meet individual needs, based on thirst and response to therapy. In the following table, suggested intakes for replacement are based on fluid losses of 5% or 10% of body weight, including maintenance requirement.

Pedialyte/Rehydralyte Dosage for Infants/Young Children					
	Weight (approx.)			Rehydralyte	
Age	kg	lb	Pedialyte oz/day	Replacement for 5% dehydration (oz/day)	Replacement for 10% dehydration (oz/day)
2 wks	3.2	7	13-16	18-21	23-26
3 mos	6	13	28-32	38-42	48-52
6 mos	7.8	17	34-40	47-53	60-66
9 mos	9.2	20	38-44	53-59	68-74
1 yr	10.2	23	41-46	58-63	75-80
1.5 yr	11.4	25	45-50	64-69	83-88
2 yr	12.6	28	48-53	69-74	90-95
2.5 yr	13.6	30	51-56	74-79	97-102

Pedialyte/Rehydralyte Dosage for Infants/Young Children					
	Weight (approx.)			Rehydralyte	
Age	kg	lb	Pedialyte oz/day	Replacement for 5% dehydration (oz/day)	Replacement for 10% dehydration (oz/day)
3 yr	14.6	32	54-58	78-82	102-106
3.5 yr	16	35	56-60	83-87	110-114
4 yr	17	38	57-62	85-90	113-118

Extemporaneous oral rehydration solution[a] (Developed by the World Health Organization)				
Source	Na+/Cl–	K+	Citrate	Glucose
	NaCl or table salt	KCl or potassium salt[b]	sodium bicarbonate (baking soda)	Glucose or sucrose (cane sugar)
Weight (g)	3.5	1.5	2.5	20[c]
Household measure	0.5 tsp	0.25 tsp	0.5 tsp	2 tbsp[d]
mmol/L	90/80	20	30	111

[a] To be added to 1 L water. Follow physician's administration instructions.
[b] See potassium salt substitutes.
[c] If sucrose is used, 40 g.
[d] If sucrose is used, 4 tbsp.

➤*Temp Tab:* Take one tablet with 8 ounces of water up to 5 to 7 times/day, depending on working conditions.

Actions

➤*Pharmacology:* Used properly, mixtures with electrolytes, water and glucose prevent dehydration or achieve rehydration, and maintain strength and feeling of well being. They contain sodium, chloride, potassium and bicarbonate to replace depleted electrolytes and restore acid-base balance. Glucose facilitates sodium transport, which aids in sodium and water absorption.

Contraindications

Severe, continuing diarrhea or other critical fluid losses; intractable vomiting; prolonged shock, renal dysfunction (anuria, oliguria). These require parenteral therapy.

ELECTROLYTES

Peritonial Dialysis Solutions

PERITONEAL DIALYSIS SOLUTIONS

	Product and Distributor	Icodextrin (g/liter)	Dextrose (g/liter)	Na+	Ca++	Mg++	Cl–	Lactate	Osmolarity (mOsm/liter)	How Supplied
Rx	**Dialyte Pattern LM w/1.5% Dextrose** (Gambro)	0	15	131	3.5	0.5	94	40	345	In 1000, 2000 and 4000 mL.
Rx	**Dialyte Pattern LM w/2.5% Dextrose** (Gambro)	0	25	131.5	3.5	0.5	94	40	395	In 1000, 2000 and 4000 mL.
Rx	**Dialyte Pattern LM w/4.25% Dextrose** (Gambro)	0	42.5	131.5	3.5	0.5	94	40	485	In 1000, 2000 and 4000 mL.
Rx	**Extraneal** (Baxter)	75	0	132	3.5	0.5	96	40	282-286	In 1.5, 2, and 2.5 L *Ultrabag* and 1.5, 2, and 2.5 L *Ambu-Flex.*

Indications

Acute or chronic renal failure; acute poisoning by dialyzable toxins; intractable edema; hyperkalemia, hypercalcemia, azotemia and uremia; hepatic coma. Refer to manufacturer's package literature for specific prescribing information.

Electrolyte content given in mEq/liter.

CITRATE AND CITRIC ACID SOLUTIONS

Rx	**Cytra-3** (Cypress)	**Syrup:** 550 mg potassium citrate monohydrate, 500 mg sodium citrate dihydrate, 334 mg citric acid monohydrate per 5 mL (1 mEq potassium and 1 mEq sodium per mL and is equivalent to 2 mEq bicarbonate)	Sugar free. In 16 oz. bottles.
Rx	**Cytra-LC** (Cypress)	**Solution:** 550 mg potassium citrate monohydrate, 500 mg sodium citrate dihydrate, 334 mg citric acid monohydrate per 5 mL (1 mEq potassium and 1 mEq sodium per mL and is equivalent to 2 mEq bicarbonate)	In 16 oz. bottles.
Rx	**Cytra-K** (Cypress)	**Solution:** 1100 mg potassium citrate monohydrate and 334 mg citric acid monohydrate per 5 mL (2 mEq potassium per mL and is equivalent to 2 mEq bicarbonate)	Alcohol free. In 473 mL.
Rx	**Oracit** (Carolina Medical Products)	**Solution:** 490 mg sodium citrate and 640 mg citric acid per 5 mL (1 mEq sodium per mL and is equivalent to 1 mEq bicarbonate)	Parabens. In 500 mL and UD 15 and 30 mL.
Rx sf	**Bicitra** (Alza Corp.)	**Solution:** 500 mg sodium citrate dihydrate and 334 mg citric acid monohydrate per 5 mL (1 mEq sodium per mL and is equivalent to 1 mEq bicarbonate)	Alcohol free. In 120 and 473 mL, gal and UD 15 and 30 mL.
Rx	**Cytra-2** (Cypress)		Grape flavored. In 16 oz. bottles.
otc	**Naturalyte Oral Electrolyte Solution** (Unico)	**Solution:** 20 mEq potassium, 30 mEq citrate (20 g dextrose, 5 g fructose, 35 mEq chloride, 45 mEq sodium)/L	In unflavored, artificial fruit, bubble gum, and grape flavors. In 1 liter.

Indications

Treatment of chronic metabolic acidosis, particularly when caused by renal tubular acidosis.

Conditions where long-term maintenance of an alkaline urine is desirable, in treatment of patients with uric acid and cystine calculi of the urinary tract and in conjunction with uricosurics in gout therapy to prevent uric acid nephropathy.

Nonparticulate neutralizing buffers.

Administration and Dosage

Dilute in water before taking; follow with additional water, if desired. Monitor urinary pH with *Hydrion* paper (pH 6 to 8) or *Nitrazine* paper (pH 4.5 to 7.5).

➤*Dosage:*

Adults – 15 to 30 mL diluted with water, after meals and before bedtime.

Children – 5 to 10 mL diluted with water, after meals and before bedtime. The solution, not the crystals, is recommended for pediatric administration since dosage can be more easily regulated.

➤*Neutralizing buffer:* A single dose of 15 mL diluted with 15 mL water.

Actions

➤*Pharmacology:* Citrate and citric acid solutions are systemic and urinary alkalinizers. Preparations containing potassium citrate are preferred in patients requiring potassium or those who require sodium restriction. Conversely, sodium citrate may be administered when potassium is undesirable or contraindicated. Potassium citrate and sodium citrate are capable of buffering gastric acidity (pH > 2.5). The effects are essentially those of chlorides before absorption, and subsequently, those of bicarbonates.

➤*Pharmacokinetics:* Potassium citrate and sodium citrate are absorbed and metabolized to potassium bicarbonate and sodium bicarbonate, thus acting as systemic alkalinizers. The citric acid is metabolized to carbon dioxide and water; therefore, it has only a transient effect on systemic acid-base status. It functions as a temporary buffer component.

Oxidation is virtually complete; < 5% of the citrates are excreted in the urine unchanged.

Contraindications

Severe renal impairment with oliguria, azotemia or anuria; untreated Addison's disease; adynamia episodica hereditaria; acute dehydration; heat cramps; severe myocardial damage; hyperkalemia.

➤*Sodium citrate:* Sodium restricted patients.

Warnings

➤*Lactation:* Exercise caution when administered to a nursing woman.

Precautions

➤*Urolithiasis:* Citrate mobilizes calcium from bones and increases its renal excretion; this, along with the elevated urine pH, may predispose to urolithiasis.

➤*Hyperkalemia/Alkalosis:* Patients with low urinary output and abnormal renal mechanisms may develop hyperkalemia or alkalosis, especially in the presence of hypocalcemia.

➤*Sodium salts:* Use cautiously in patients with cardiac failure, hypertension, impaired renal function, peripheral and pulmonary edema and preeclampsia. Monitor serum electrolytes, particularly the serum bicarbonate level, in patients with renal disease.

➤*GI effects:* Dilute with water to minimize GI injury associated with the oral ingestion of concentrated potassium salts. Take after meals to avoid saline laxative effect.

Drug Interactions

Urinary Alkalinizer Drug Interactions			
Precipitant drug	Object drug *		Description
Urinary alkalinizers (eg, potassium citrate, sodium citrate)	Chlorpropamide Lithium Methenamine Methotrexate Salicylates Tetracyclines	↓	Urinary alkalinizers may increase the excretion and decrease the serum levels of these agents, possibly decreasing their pharmacologic effects.
Urinary alkalinizers (eg, potassium citrate, sodium citrate)	Anorexiants Flecainide Mecamylamine Quinidine Sympathomimetics	↑	Urinary alkalinizers may decrease the excretion and increase the serum levels of these agents, possibly increasing their pharmacologic effects.

* ↑ = Object drug increased.   ↓ = Object drug decreased.

Adverse Reactions

Hyperkalemia – Listlessness, weakness, mental confusion, tingling of extremities and other symptoms associated with high serum potassium. Hyperkalemia may exhibit the following ECG abnormalities: Disappearance of the P wave; widening or slurring of the QRS complex; changes of the ST segment; tall peaked T waves.

Overdosage

➤*Symptoms:* Overdosage with sodium salts may cause diarrhea, nausea, vomiting, hypernoia (excessive mental activity) and convulsions. Overdosage with potassium salts may cause hyperkalemia and alkalosis, especially in the presence of renal disease. Treat hyperkalemia immediately, because lethal levels can be reached in a few hours.

➤*Treatment:* For treatment of hyperkalemia, refer to the Potassium monograph in the IV Nutritional Therapy section; for treatment of sodium overdosage, refer to the Sodium Chloride monograph in the Salt Replacement Products section.

Patient Information

Dilute with water; follow with additional water, if desired.

Take after meals.

Notify physician if diarrhea, nausea, stomach pain, vomiting or convulsions occur.

SODIUM BICARBONATE

One g of sodium bicarbonate provides 11.9 mmol sodium and 11.9 mmol bicarbonate.

otc	**Sodium Bicarbonate** (Various, eg, Rugby)	**Tablets:** 325 mg	In 1000s.
		650 mg	In 1000s.
		Powder	In 120 and 300 g and 1 lb.

For information on parenteral sodium bicarbonate products, refer to the monograph in the IV Nutritional Therapy section.

Indications

A gastric, systemic and urinary alkalinizer.

Administration and Dosage

Usual dose is 325 mg to 2 g, 1 to 4 times daily. Maximum daily intake is 16 g (200 mEq) in patients < 60 years old and 8 g (100 mEq) in those older than 60 years of age.

Precautions

➤*Use cautiously:* Use caution in patients with edematous sodium-retaining states, congestive heart failure or renal impairment. Prolonged therapy may lead to systemic alkalosis.

Amino Acids

GLUTAMIC ACID

otc	**Glutamic Acid** (Various, eg, Freeda)	**Tablets:** 500 mg	In 100s and 500s.
otc	**Glutamic Acid** (J.R. Carlson)	**Powder**	In 100 g bottles.

Indications
Dietary supplement.

Administration and Dosage
500 to 1000 mg daily or as directed. Take with liquids.

L-LYSINE

otc	**L-Lysine** (Various, eg, Rugby)	**Tablets:** 312 mg	In 100s.
otc	**Enisyl** (Person & Covey)	**Tablets:** 334 mg	In 100s.
otc	**L-Lysine** (Various, eg, Goldline, Moore, Mission, Pasadena, Rugby, URL)	**Tablets:** 500 mg	In 100s.
otc	**Enisyl** (Person & Covey)		In 100s and 250s.
otc	**L-Lysine** (Approved Pharm.)	**Tablets:** 1000 mg	In 60s.
otc	**L-Lysine** (Various, eg, Miller, Tyson & Assoc.)	**Capsules:** 500 mg	In 100s and 250s.

Indications
Dietary supplement.

➤*Unlabeled uses:* Oral L-lysine has been promoted as treatment and as a prophylactic agent in herpes simplex infections; however, controlled studies do not support these claims.

Administration and Dosage
312 to 1500 mg daily.

Actions
➤*Pharmacology:* An essential amino acid which improves utilization of vegetable proteins.

METHIONINE

Rx	**Methionine** (Tyson & Assoc.)	**Capsules:** 500 mg	In 30s.

Indications
Dietary supplement.

Administration and Dosage
500 mg daily. The recommended daily allowance has not been established.

THREONINE

otc	**Threonine** (Freeda)	**Tablets:** 500 mg	In 100s and 250s.
otc	**Threonine** (Various, eg, Solgar, Tyson & Assoc.)	**Capsules:** 500 mg	In 60s.

Indications
Dietary supplement.

Administration and Dosage
500 mg daily, preferably on an empty stomach, or as directed.

AMINO ACIDS WITH VITAMINS AND MINERALS

otc	**Dequasine** (Miller)	**Tablets:** 20 mg L-lysine, 50 mg L-cysteine, 150 mg dL-methionine, 50 mg N-acetyl cysteine, 200 mg vitamin C, 40 mg Ca, 1 mg Cu, 5 mg Fe, 0.015 mg I, 20 mg K, 40 mg Mg, 5 mg Mn, 150 mcg Mo, 5 mg Zn. *Dose:* 1 tablet/day, or as recommended.	In 100s.
otc sf	**NeuroSlim** (NeuroGenesis)	**Capsules:** 500 mg dL-phenylalanine, 15 mg L-glutamine, 25 mg L-tyrosine, 10 mg L-carnitine, 10 mg L-arginine pyroglutamate, 10 mg ornithine aspartate, 0.033 mg Cr, 0.012 mg Se, 0.33 mg vitamin B$_1$, 0.5 mg B$_2$, 3.3 mg B$_3$, 0.012 mg B$_5$, 0.333 mg B$_6$, 1 mcg B$_{12}$, 5 IU E, 0.05 mg biotin, 0.066 mg FA, 1 mg Fe, 2.5 mg Zn, 35 mg Ca, 0.025 mg I, 0.33 mg Cu, 25 mg Mg. *Dose:* 2 capsules 3 times/day, 1 hour before or 2 hours after meals.	In 180s.
otc sf	**NeuRecovery-DA** (NeuroGenesis)	**Capsules:** 460 mg dL-phenylalanine, 25 mg L-glutamine, 333.3 IU vitamin A, 1.65 mg B$_1$, 0.85 mg B$_2$, 33 mg B$_3$, 15 mg B$_5$, 3 mg B$_6$, 5 mcg B$_{12}$, 0.065 mg FA, 100 mg C, 5 IU E, 0.05 mg biotin, 25 mg Ca, 0.01 mg Cr, 1.5 mg Fe, 25 mg Mg, 2.5 mg Zn. *Dose:* 2 capsules 3 times/day.	In 180s.
otc sf	**NeuRecovery-SA** (NeuroGenesis)	**Capsules:** 250 mg dL-phenylalanine, 150 mg L-tyrosine, 50 mg L-glutamine, 1.65 mg vitamin B$_1$, 2.5 mg B$_2$, 16.6 mg B$_3$, 15 mg B$_5$, 3.36 mg B$_6$, 5 mcg B$_{12}$, 0.067 mg FA, 100 mg C, 25 mg Ca, 1.5 mg Fe, 25 mg Mg, 5 mg Zn. *Dose:* ≤ 6 capsules/day.	In 180s.
otc	**A/G-Pro** (Miller)	**Tablets:** 542 mg protein hydrolysate, 50 mg L-lysine, 12.5 mg L-methionine, 0.33 mg vitamin B$_6$, 16.7 mg C, 1.66 mg iron. Cu, I, K, Mg, Mn, Zn. *Dose:* 2 tablets 3 times/day.	In 180s.
otc sf	**Jets** (Freeda)	**Tablets, chewable:** 300 mg L-lysine, 10 mg vitamin B$_1$, 5 mg B$_6$, 25 mcg B$_{12}$, 25 mg C.	In 100s.
otc sf	**Body Fortress Natural Amino** (Nature's Bounty)	**Tablets:** 1.67 g protein, 1500 mg lactalbumin hydrolysate *Dose:* 2 to 3 tablets with each meal and directly after each workout, or as directed.	Yeast and preservative free. In 150s.
otc sf	**Amina-21** (Miller)	**Capsules:** 556 mg free-form amino acids *Dose:* 1 or 2 capsules 3 times/day or as recommended.	In 100s and 300s.
otc	**PowerSleep** (Green Turtle Bay Vitamin Co.)	**Tablets:** 250 mg L-glutamine, 25 mg 5-HTP, 0.25 mg melatonin, 25 mg vitamin B$_3$, 5 mg B$_6$, 100 mg inositol, 25 mg Ca, 100 mg passion flower extract, 75 mg valerian powder *Dose:* 2 tablets 1 hour before bedtime.	In 60s.
otc sf	**PowerMate** (Green Turtle Bay Vitamin Co.)	**Tablets:** 25 mg N-acetyl-L-cysteine, 5 mg glutathione, 5000 IU vitamin A, 12.5 mg B$_3$, 250 mg C, 100 IU E, 2.5 mg Zn, 7.5 mcg Se, 5 mg gingko biloba, 100 mg green tea extract, 5 mg pine bark extract, 50 mg echinacea, 20 mg golden seal root, 2 mg coenzyme Q10 *Dose:* 2 tablets daily for 2 weeks/month.	Yeast free. In 50s.
otc	**EMF** (Wesley Pharmacal)	**Liquid:** Alanine, arginine, aspartic acid, cysteine, glutamic acid, glycine, histidine, hydroxylysine, hydroxyproline, isoleucineline, leucine, lysine, methionine, phenylalanine, proline, serine, threonine, tyrosine, valine, 15 g protein. *Dose:* 30 mL/day.	Sorbitol, saccharin. Cherry flavor. In qt.

LEVOCARNITINE (L-Carnitine)

Rx	Carnitor (Sigma-Tau)	Tablets: 330 mg	(CARNITOR ST). In 90s.
otc	L-Carnitine (Freeda Vitamins)	Tablets: 500 mg	In 50s and 100s.
otc	L-Carnitine (Various, eg, Miller Pharmacal Group, Nature's Bounty, Tyson, Watson)	Capsules: 250 mg	In 30s, 60s, and 100s.
Rx	Carnitor (Sigma-Tau)	Solution: 100 mg/mL	Sucrose, parabens. Cherry flavor. In 118 mL.
Rx	Levocarnitine (Various, eg, American Regent, Bedford)	Injection: 200 mg/mL	In single-dose vials.
Rx	Carnitor (Sigma-Tau)		Preservative-free. In single-dose vials and amps.

Indications

▶*Primary systemic carnitine deficiency:* Treatment of primary systemic carnitine deficiency.

▶*Secondary carnitine deficiency:* Acute and chronic treatment of patients with an inborn error of metabolism that results in secondary carnitine deficiency.,

▶*End-stage renal disease (ESRD):* Prevention and treatment of carnitine deficiency in patients with ESRD who are undergoing dialysis (injection only).

▶*Unlabeled uses:* Carnitine has been used to improve athletic performance and may be of use in valproate toxicity.,

Administration and Dosage

▶*Capsules:*
Nature's Bounty –
Adults: One capsule daily on an empty stomach.

Tyson – One to 3 capsules daily with meals as a dietary supplement or as directed by a physician.

▶*Injection:*
Metabolic disorders – 50 mg/kg given as a slow 2- to 3-minute bolus injection or by infusion. Often a loading dose is given in patients with severe metabolic crisis, followed by an equivalent dose over the following 24 hours. Administer every 3 or 4 hours (maximum interval every 6 hours) either by infusion or by IV injection. All subsequent daily doses are recommended to be in the range of 50 mg/kg or as therapy might require. The highest dose adminstered has been 300 mg/kg.

It is recommended that a plasma carnitine concentration be obtained prior to beginning this parenteral therapy. Weekly and monthly monitoring is recommended as well (see Precautions).

ESRD patients on hemodialysis – 10 to 20 mg/kg dry body weight as a slow 2- to 3-minute bolus injection into the venous return line after each dialysis session. Initiation of therapy may be prompted by trough (predialysis) plasma levocarnitine concentrations that are below normal (40 to 50 mcmol/L). Dose adjustments should be guided by trough (predialysis) levocarnitine concentrations and downward dose adjustments (eg, to 5 mg/kg after dialysis) may be made as early as the third or fourth week of therapy.

Compatibility/Stability – Levocarnitine injection is compatible and stable when mixed in parenteral solutions of 0.9% Sodium Chloride or Lactated Ringer's in concentrations ranging from 250 mg/500 mL (0.5 mg/mL) to 4200 mg/500 mL (8 mg/mL).

▶*Solution:*
Adults – Give 1 to 3 g/day for a 50 kg patient, administered in divided doses every 3 to 4 hours. Use higher doses with caution. Start dosage at 1 g/day, and increase slowly while assessing tolerance and response.

Infants and children – 50 to 100 mg/kg/day, administered in divided doses every 3 to 4 hours. Give higher doses with caution. Start dosage at 50 mg/kg/day, and increase slowly to a maximum of 3 g/day while assessing tolerance and therapeutic response.

Give alone or dissolve in drinks or liquid food. Space doses evenly, preferably with or after meals; consume slowly to maximize tolerance.

▶*Tablets:*
Adults – 990 mg 2 or 3 times/day, depending on clinical response.

Infants and children – 50 to 100 mg/kg/day in divided doses, with a maximum of 3 g/day. Begin with 50 mg/kg/day. Dosage depends on clinical response.

▶*Storage/Stability:*
Injection – Store reconstituted injection at room temperature (25°C; 77°F) for up to 24 hours in PVC plastic bags. Store vials and amps at controlled room temperature (25°C; 77°F) and protect from light. Discard any unused portions, as the formulation does not contain a preservative.

Solution/Tablets – Store at controlled room temperature (25°C; 77°F).

Actions

▶*Pharmacology:* L-carnitine is a naturally occurring amino acid derivative, synthesized from methionine and lysine, required in energy metabolism. It facilitates long-chain fatty acid entry into cellular mitochondria, delivering substrate and subsequent energy production. It can promote the excretion of excess organic or fatty acids in patients with defects in fatty acid metabolism or specific organic acidopathies that bioaccumulate acylCoA esters.,,

Primary carnitine deficiency – Primary systemic carnitine deficiency is characterized by low concentrations of levocarnitine in plasma, RBC, and tissues. It has not been possible to determine which symptoms are caused by carnitine deficiency and which are caused by an underlying organic acidemia, as symptoms of both abnormalities may be expected to improve with levocarnitine.

Secondary carnitine deficiency – Secondary carnitine deficiency can be a consequence of inborn errors of metabolism. L-carnitine may alleviate the metabolic abnormalities of patients with inborn errors that result in accumulation of toxic organic acids. Conditions for which this effect is demonstrated are: Glutaric aciduria II, methyl malonic aciduria, propionic acidemia, and medium chain fatty acylCoA dehydrogenase deficiency. Autointoxication occurs in these patients due to the accumulations of acylCoA compounds that disrupt intermediary metabolism. The subsequent hydrolysis of the acylCoA compound to its free acid results in acidosis that can be life-threatening. L-carnitine clears the acylCoA compound by formation of acylcarnitine, which is quickly excreted. L-carnitine deficiency is defined biochemically as abnormally low plasma levels of free carnitine < 20 mcmol/L at 1 week of age post-term and may be associated with low tissue or urine levels. Further, this condition may be associated with a ratio of plasma acylcarnitine/L-carnitine levels > 0.4 or abnormally elevated levels of acylcarnitine in the urine. In premature infants and newborns, secondary deficiency is defined as plasma L-carnitine levels below age-related normal levels.,

▶*Pharmacokinetics:*
Absorption/Distribution – L-carnitine tablets are bioequivalent to the oral solution. Following the administration of 1980 mg twice daily, the maximum plasma concentration (C_{max}) was ≈ 80 nmol/mL and the time to maximum concentration (T_{max}) occurred at 3.3 hours. Approximately 76% of free L-carnitine is eliminated in the urine. Using plasma levels uncorrected for endogenous L-carnitine, the mean distribution half-life was ≈ 0.585 hours and the mean apparent terminal elimination half-life was ≈ 17.4 hours following a single IV dose.

After correction for circulating endogenous levels in the plasma, absolute bioavailability was 15.1% from the tablets and 15.9% from the oral solution.

Total body clearance (dose/AUC including endogenous baseline levels) was a mean of 4 L/hr. L-carnitine is not bound to plasma protein or albumin.,

Metabolism/Excretion – Adult male volunteers administered a dose of L-carnitine following 15 days of a high carnitine diet and additional carnitine supplement, excreted 58% to 65% of the administered dose in 5 to 11 days in the urine and feces. Maximum concentration in serum occurred from 2 to 4.5 hours after drug administration. Major metabolites found were trimethylamine N-oxide, primarily in urine (8% to 49% of the administered dose) and [^{3}H]-g-butyrobetaine, primarily in feces (0.44% to 45% of the administered dose). Urinary excretion of carnitine was 4% to 8% of the dose. Fecal excretion of total carnitine was < 1% of total carnitine excretion.

After attainment of steady state following 4 days of L-carnitine tablets (1980 mg every 12 hours) or oral solution (2000 mg every 12 hours), urinary excretion during a single dosing interval (12 hours) was ≈ 9% of the orally administered doses (uncorrected for endogenous urinary excretion).,

Warnings

▶*Pregnancy: Category B.* There are no adequate and well-controlled studies in pregnant women. Use during pregnancy only if clearly needed.,

▶*Lactation:* Levocarnitine supplementation in nursing mothers has not been specifically studied. Any risks to the child of excess carnitine intake need to be weighed against the benefits of levocarnitine supplementation to the mother. Consideration may be given to discontinuation of nursing or of levocarnitine treatment.

Precautions

▶*Excessive doses:* Administration of high doses of the oral formulations of levocarnitine for long periods of time is not recommended in patients with severely compromised renal function or in ESRD patients on dialysis. Major metabolites formed following oral administration

LEVOCARNITINE (L-Carnitine)

(trimethylamine [TMA] and trimethylamine-N-oxide [TMAO]) will accumulate because they cannot be efficiently removed by the kidneys. This does not occur to the same extent following IV administration. TMA accumulation is not desirable because it increases the amount of nitrogenous waste to be removed in the dialysis procedure. In addition, increased levels of TMA in dialysis patients have been reported to be associated with possible neurophysiologic effects. Also, the inefficient removal of TMA may result in the development of "fishy odor" syndrome. Only the IV form of levocarnitine is indicated for use in ESRD patients on hemodialysis.

➤*Monitoring:* Monitoring should include periodic blood chemistries, vital signs, plasma carnitine concentrations, and overall clinical condition.

Adverse Reactions

➤*CNS:* Mild myasthenia has occurred in uremic patients on dL-carnitine. Seizures have been reported to occur in patients with or without pre-existing seizure activity receiving either oral or IV levocarnitine. In patients with pre-existing seizure activity, an increase in seizure frequency and severity has been reported.

➤*GI:* Transient GI complaints including nausea, vomiting, abdominal cramps, diarrhea, gastritis. Decreasing dosage may diminish or eliminate drug-related body odor or GI symptoms.,

Overdosage

There have been no reports of toxicity from levocarnitine overdosage. Levocarnitine is easily removed from plasma by dialysis. The IV LD_{50} of levocarnitine in rats is 5.4 g/kg and the oral LD_{50} of levocarnitine in mice is 19.2 g/kg. Large doses of levocarnitine may cause diarrhea.

Actions

➤*Pharmacology:* The need for lipotropics in human nutrition is not established. The lipotropic factors choline, inositol and betaine, not proven therapeutically valuable, have been used for treatment of liver disorders and disturbed fat metabolism.

Choline (trimethylethanolamine), a component of the major phospholipid, lecithin, demonstrates lipotropic action, functions as a methyl group donor and is a precursor of the neurochemical transmitter acetylcholine. Choline and lecithin (because of its choline content) have been advocated for tardive dyskinesia, Huntington's chorea, Tourette's syndrome, Friedreich's ataxia, presenile dementia, fatty liver and cirrhosis. Intestinal bacteria metabolize choline to trimethylamine, which imparts an unpleasant odor to the breath and body. Lecithin does not produce this odor. Choline also causes clinical depression in some patients.

Inositol, an isomer of glucose, is present in cell membrane phospholipids and plasma lipoproteins. No specific role in human nutrition has been established.

Linoleic and linolenic acid are polyunsaturated fatty acids that serve as precursors of important biochemical compounds, such as arachidonic acid, which gives rise to a wide variety of prostaglandins. Linoleic acid is regarded as an essential fatty acid because it cannot be synthesized in vivo and because it has a defined metabolic significance; it helps support normal growth and development and prevent essential fatty acid deficiency (EFAD). The metabolic significance of linolenic acid is unclear. Use of these precursors to alter disease states requires more research.

CHOLINE

otc	**Choline** (Various, eg, Approved Pharm, Rugby)	**Tablets:** 250 mg, 300 and 500 mg	In 100s.
		650 mg	In 90s and 100s.
otc	**Choline** (Freeda)	**Powder:** ¼ tsp equals 375 mg choline	In 16 oz.
otc	**Choline Bitartrate** (Various, eg, City Chem, Fibertone, Spectrum)	**Tablets:** 250 mg	In 100s, 250s, 500s, 1000s.
		Powder	In 120 g and 1 lb.
Rx	**Choline Chloride** (Various, eg, Baker, Biochemical, City Chem, Spectrum)	**Powder**	In 120 and 500 g and 1 and 5 lb.
otc	**Choline Dihydrogen** Citrate (Freeda)	**Tablets:** 650 mg	In 250s.
		Powder	In 120 g and 1 lb.

Refer to additional information in the Lipotropic Products monograph.

Administration and Dosage

650 mg to 2 g daily or as directed.

INOSITOL

otc	**Inositol** (Various, eg, Biochemical, Freeda, Nature's Bounty, Rugby)	**Tablets:** 250 mg	In 100s.
		500 mg	In 100s.
		650 mg	In 90s and 100s.
		Powder: ¼ tsp equals 375 mg	In 25, 60, 100, 120, 500 g & lb.
otc sf	**Inositech** (Bio-tech)	**Capsules:** 324 mg	In 100s.

Refer to additional information in the Lipotropic Products monograph.

Administration and Dosage

1 to 3 g daily in divided doses.

LIPOTROPIC COMBINATIONS

otc	**Lecithin** (Various, eg, Approved Pharm, Dixon-Shane, Goldline, Moore, Nature's Bounty, Rugby, West-Ward)	A source of choline, inositol, phosphorus, linoleic & linolenic acids	
		Capsules: 420 mg	In 60s.
		1.2 g	In 100s, 250s, 1000s.
		Tablets: 1.2 g	In 50s.
		Granules	In 210, 240, 420 g & lb.
		Liquid	In 480 mL.
otc	**PhosChol** (American Lecithin)	Phosphatidylcholine (highly purified lecithin)	
		Softgels: 565 mg	In 100s and 300s
		Softgels: 900 mg	In 100s and 300s.
		Liquid concentrate: 3000 mg/5 mL	In 240 and 480 mL.
otc	**Pertropin** (Lannett)	**Capsules:** 7 mins. linolenic acid, other essential unsaturated free fatty acids, 5 IU vitamin E	In 100s.

Refer to additional information in the Lipotropic Products monograph.

Administration and Dosage

➤*Lecithin:* One to 2 capsules daily.

➤*Pertropin:* One or 2 capsules 3 or 4 times daily.

OMEGA-3 (N-3) POLYUNSATURATED FATTY ACIDS

	Product/Distributor	mg/capsule	N-3 fat content (mg) EPA	DHA	Other Content	How Supplied
otc sf	**Promega Pearls Softgels** (Parke-Davis)	600	168	72	< 2 mg cholesterol, 1 IU vitamin E,[1] < 2% RDA of vitamins A, B$_1$, B$_2$, B$_3$, Fe and Ca	In 60s and 90s.
otc	**Cardi-Omega 3 Capsules** (Thompson Medical)	1000	180	120	< 2% RDA of vitamins A, B$_1$, B$_2$, B$_3$, C, D, Fe and Ca	Sodium free. Peppermint flavor. In 60s.
otc sf	**EPA Capsules** (Nature's Bounty)				1 IU vitamin E[1]	In 50s and 100s.
otc	**Max EPA Capsules** (Various, eg, Jones Medical, Moore, Rexall, Schein)				5 mg cholesterol, < 2% RDA of vitamins A, B$_1$, B$_2$, B$_3$, C, Ca, Fe	In 60s, 90s & 100s.
otc sf	**Promega Softgels** (Parke-Davis)	1000	280	120	< 1 mg cholesterol, 1 IU vitamin E[1] (6% RDA), vitamins A, B$_1$, B$_2$, B$_3$, Ca & Fe (< 2% RDA)	Sodium free. In 30s and 60s.
otc sf	**Sea-Omega 50 Softgels** (Rugby)	1000	300	200	1 IU vitamin E[1]	Sodium free. In 50s.
otc	**Sea-Omega 30 Softgels** (Rugby)	1200	180	140	2 IU vitamin E[1]	In 100s.
otc	**Marine Lipid Concentrate Softgels** (Vitaline)	1200	360	240	5 IU vitamin E[1]	Sodium free. In 90s.
otc	**SuperEPA 1200 Softgels** (Advanced Nutritional)	1200	360	240	5 IU vitamin E[1]	In 60s, 90s and 180s.
otc	**SuperEPA 2000 Capsules** (Advanced Nutritional)	1000	563	312	20 IU vitamin E[1]	In 30s, 60s and 90s.

[1] As d-alpha tocopherol.

Indications

Omega-3 fatty acids may be used as nondrug dietary supplements for patients at early risk of coronary artery disease primarily because of effects on platelets and lipids.

The American Heart Association recommends consumption of fish; however, it does not find justification for fish oil capsule supplementation.

➤*Unlabeled uses:* Omega-3 fatty acids have been studied as adjunctive treatment of rheumatoid arthritis (20 g/day have been used). These agents may also be of benefit in the treatment of psoriasis (10 to 15 g/day); however, data is conflicting. Omega-3 fatty acids (18 g/day) may be beneficial in preventing early restenosis after coronary angioplasty in combination with dipyridamole and aspirin in high risk male patients.

Administration and Dosage

➤*Nutritional supplement:* 1 to 2 capsules 3 times daily with meals.

Actions

➤*Pharmacology:* Cold water fish oils contain large amounts of omega-3 (N-3) polyunsaturated fatty acids, eicosapentaenoic acid (EPA) and docosahexaenoic acid (DHA). Diets high in omega-3 fatty acids may lower very low-density lipoproteins (VLDL), triglyceride and total cholesterol concentrations; increase concentrations of high-density lipoproteins (HDL); prolong bleeding times; decrease platelet aggregation; reduce plasma fibrinogen (data conflict); inhibit leukocyte function.

Studies on the effects of omega-3 fatty acids on the lipoproteins closely associated with atherosclerosis (LDL and HDL) show variable results and require further investigation.

Some studies have actually shown an increase in LDL-cholesterol levels in patients and healthy subjects receiving omega-3 fatty acids at doses currently recommended by the manufacturers (4.6 to 13.3 g/day). Although the optimal dose has not been established, significant effects of the omega-3 fatty acids may only be observed with 20 g or more per day. Some of the available products contain cholesterol and saturated fat, which may play a role in the increased LDL-cholesterol levels.

Patients on diets with high levels of fish oils have increased EPA levels and decreased arachidonic acid levels in plasma lipids and platelet membranes. Also, increased synthesis of prostaglandin I$_3$ and decreased platelet synthesis of thromboxane A$_2$ have been noted. Prostaglandin I$_3$, an antiaggregation substance, and thromboxane A$_2$, a potent stimulator of platelet aggregation and secretion, are usually in balance. It is believed EPA is utilized by vessel walls to synthesize prostaglandin I$_3$, and arachidonic acid is utilized by platelets to synthesize thromboxane A$_2$. Therefore, the higher EPA levels and lower arachidonic acid levels produced by a diet high in fish oils could cause decreased platelet aggregation. Vitamin E in the product could also contribute to decreased platelet aggregation.

Warnings

➤*Diarrhea:* Diarrhea has occurred in patients taking 4 to 6 capsules per day.

➤*Bleeding:* Increased bleeding time and inhibition of platelet aggregation have occurred. Use caution in patients receiving **anticoagulants** or **aspirin**.

➤*Diabetes mellitus:* In one study the fasting and mean glucose levels increased and insulin secretion was impaired in six patients with type 2 diabetes mellitus following 1 month of omega-3 fatty acid administration (5.4 g/day). However, increased insulin sensitivity in type 2 diabetes mellitus patients has occurred. Use with caution in type 2 diabetes mellitus patients.

➤*Pregnancy:* Until further information is available, do not use omega-3 fatty acids in these patients.

➤*Children:* Until further information is available, do not use omega-3 fatty acids in these patients.

LACTASE ENZYME

otc	**Lactrase** (Schwarz Pharma)	**Capsules:** 250 mg standardized enzyme lactase	(Kremers Urban 505). Orange/white. In 100s and blisterpack 10s and 30s.
otc	**Dairy Ease** (Blistex)	**Tablets, chewable:** 3000 FCC lactase units	Mannitol, sucrose. In 60 and 100s.

Indications

To digest lactose contained in milk for patients with lactose intolerance.

Administration and Dosage

➤*Liquid:* 5 to 15 drops per qt of milk, based on lactose conversion level desired.

➤*Tablets:* 1 to 3 tablets with the first bite of dairy food.

➤*Capsules:* 1 or 2 capsules taken with milk or dairy products. If the patient is severely intolerant to lactose, increase dosage until a satisfactory dose is achieved.

ALPHA-D-GALACTOSIDASE ENZYME

otc	**Beano** (AK Pharma)	**Liquid:** Alpha-D-galactosidase-derived from *Aspergillus niger* (≥ 175 galactose units per 5 drop dosage)	Glycerol. In 75 serving size at 5 drops per dose.
		Tablets: Alpha-galactosidase enzyme derived from *Aspergillus niger*	Cornstarch, sucrose, hydrogenated cottonseed oil, sorbitol. In 12s, 30s and 100s.

Indications

Treatment of gassiness or bloating as a result of eating a variety of grains, cereals, nuts, seeds or vegetables containing the sugars raffinose, stachyose or verbascose. This includes all or most legumes and all or most cruciferous vegetables (eg, oats, wheat, beans, peas, lentils, peanuts, soy-content foods, pistachios, broccoli, brussels sprouts, cabbage, carrots, corn, onions, squash, cauliflower).

Administration and Dosage

Use 3 to 8 drops per average serving. Approximately 5 drops on the first portion of food consumed will deal with the entire subsequent portion.

Use a higher or lower number of drops depending on the quantity of food eaten, levels of alpha-linked sugars in the food and the gas-producing propensity and tolerance of the person.

Actions

➤*Pharmacology:* Alpha-D-galactosidase enzyme hydrolyzes raffinose, verbascose and stachyose into the digestible sugars sucrose, fructose, glucose and galactose.

Precautions

➤*Galactosemics:* Galactosemics should not use without physician advice since one of the breakdown sugars is galactose.

SACROSIDASE

Rx	**Sucraid** (Orphan Medical)	**Solution:** 8500 IU/mL	In 118 mL bottles (2) with 1 mL measuring scoop.

Indications

➤*Sucrase deficiency:* Oral replacement therapy of the genetically determined sucrase deficiency, which is part of congenital sucrase-isomaltase deficiency (CSID).

Administration and Dosage

➤*Approved by the FDA:* April 9, 1998.

It is recommended that approximately half of the dosage be taken at the beginning of each meal or snack and the remainder be taken at the end of each meal or snack. Dilute with 2 to 4 ounces of water, milk or infant formula. Serve cold or at room temperature; do not warm or heat before or after addition of sacrosidase because heating is likely to decrease potency. Sacrosidase should not be reconstituted or consumed with fruit juice, since acidity may reduce the enzyme activity.

➤*Patients ≤ 15 kg (33 lbs):* 1 mL (8500 IU) – 1 full measuring scoop or 22 drops per meal or snack.

➤*Patients > 15 kg (33 lbs):* 2 mL (17,000 IU) – 2 full measuring scoops or 44 drops per meal or snack.

Dosage may be measured with the 1 mL measuring scoop (provided) or by drop count method (1 mL equals 22 drops from the sacrosidase container tip).

➤*Storage/Stability:* Store in a refrigerator at 2° to 8°C (36° to 46°F). Discard 4 weeks after first opening due to the potential for bacterial growth. Protect from heat and light.

Actions

➤*Pharmacology:* Sacrosidase is an enzyme replacement therapy for the treatment of the genetically determined sucrase deficiency, which is part of CSID. CSID is a chronic, autosomal recessive, inherited, phenotypically heterogeneous disease with highly variable enzyme activity. CSID is usually characterized by a complete or almost complete lack of endogenous sucrase activity, a very marked reduction in isomaltase activity, a moderate decrease in maltase activity and normal lactase levels. Sucrase is naturally produced in the brush border of the small intestine, primarily the distal duodenum and jejunum. Sucrase hydrolyzes the disaccharide sucrose into its component monosaccharides, glucose and fructose. Isomaltase and maltase are enzymes that break down the disaccharides isomaltose and maltose, respectively, into two molecules of glucose. Isomaltase and maltase are not components in sacrosidase.

In the absence of endogenous human sucrase, as in CSID, sucrose is not metabolized. Unhydrolyzed sucrose and starch are not absorbed from the intestine and their presence in the intestinal lumen may lead to osmotic water retention and loose stools. Unabsorbed sucrose in the colon is fermented by bacterial flora to produce increased amounts of hydrogen, methane and water. As a consequence, excessive gas, bloating, abdominal cramps, nausea and vomiting may occur. Chronic malabsorption of disaccharides may result in malnutrition. Undiagnosed or untreated CSID patients often fail to thrive and fall behind in their expected growth and development curves. Previously, the treatment of CSID has required the continual use of a strict sucrose-free diet. Approximately 4% to 10% of pediatric patients with chronic diarrhea of unknown origin have CSID. Measurement of expired breath hydrogen

under controlled conditions following a sucrose challenge (a measurement of excess hydrogen excreted in exhalation) in CSID patients has shown levels as great as 6 times that in healthy subjects. A generally accepted clinical definition of CSID is that of a condition characterized by the following: Stool pH of < 6, an increase in breath hydrogen of > 10 ppm when challenged with sucrose after fasting and a negative lactose breath test. However, because of the difficulties in diagnosing CSID, it may be warranted to conduct a short therapeutic trial (eg, 1 week) to assess response in patients suspected of having CSID.

Contraindications

Hypersensitivity to yeast, yeast products or glycerin (glycerol).

Warnings

➤*Severe wheezing:* 90 minutes after a second dose of sacrosidase necessitated admission into the ICU for a 4–year-old boy. The wheezing was probably caused by sacrosidase. He had asthma and was treated with steroids. A skin test for sacrosidase was positive.

➤*Hypersensitivity reactions:* Take care to administer initial doses of sacrosidase near a facility (within a few minutes' travel) where acute hypersensitivity reactions can be adequately treated. Alternatively, the patient may be tested for hypersensitivity to sacrosidase through skin abrasion testing. Should symptoms of hypersensitivity appear, discontinue medication and initiate symptomatic and supportive therapy. Refer to Management of Acute Hypersensitivity Reactions. Skin testing as a rechallenge has been used to verify hypersensitivity in one asthmatic child who displayed wheezing after oral sacrosidase.

➤*Pregnancy: Category C.* Sacrosidase is not expected to cause fetal harm when administered to a pregnant woman or to affect reproductive capacity. Give to a pregnant woman only if clearly needed.

➤*Lactation:* The sacrosidase enzyme is broken down in the stomach and intestines, and the component amino acids and peptides are then absorbed as nutrients.

➤*Children:* Sacrosidase has been used in patients as young as 5 months of age. Evidence from one controlled trial in primarily pediatric patients shows that sacrosidase is safe and effective for the treatment of the genetically acquired sucrase deficiency, which is part of CSID.

Precautions

➤*Starch restriction:* Although sacrosidase provides replacement therapy for the deficient sucrase, it does not provide specific replacement therapy for the deficient isomaltase. Therefore, restricting starch in the diet may still be necessary to reduce symptoms as much as possible. Evaluate the need for dietary starch restriction for patients using sacrosidase.

➤*CSID diagnosis:* The definitive test for diagnosis of CSID is the measurement of intestinal disaccharidases following small bowel biopsy. Other tests used alone may be inaccurate (eg, the breath hydrogen test [high incidence of false-negatives] or oral sucrose tolerance test [high incidence of false-positives]). Differential urinary disaccharides have been reported to show good agreement with small intestinal biopsy for diagnosis of CSID.

SACROSIDASE

It may be clinically inappropriate, difficult or inconvenient to perform a small bowel biopsy or breath hydrogen test to make a definitive diagnosis of CSID. If the diagnosis of CSID is in doubt, consider conducting a short therapeutic trial (eg, 1 week) with sacrosidase to assess response in a patient suspected of sucrase deficiency. The effects of sacrosidase have not been evaluated in patients with secondary (acquired) disaccharidase deficiencies.

▶*Diabetics:* The use of sacrosidase will enable the products of sucrose hydrolysis, glucose and fructose, to be absorbed. Carefully consider this fact in planning the diet of diabetic CSID patients using sacrosidase.

Drug Interactions

▶*Drug/Food interactions:* Sacrosidase should not be reconstituted or consumed with fruit juice, since the acidity may reduce the enzyme activity.

Adverse Reactions

Adverse experiences with sacrosidase in clinical trials were generally minor and were frequently associated with the underlying disease. In clinical studies of up to 54 months duration, a total of 52 patients received sacrosidase. The adverse experiences and respective number of patients reporting each event were as follows: Abdominal pain (4); vomiting (3); nausea, diarrhea, constipation (2); insomnia, headache, nervousness, dehydration (1). Diarrhea and abdominal pain can be a part of the clinical presentation of the genetically determined sucrase deficiency, which is part of CSID. One asthmatic child experienced a serious hypersensitivity reaction (wheezing), probably related to sacrosidase (see Warnings). The event resulted in withdrawal of the patient from the trial but resolved with no sequelae.

Overdosage

Overdosage with sacrosidase has not been reported.

Patient Information

See Patient Package Insert. Instruct patients to discard bottles of sacrosidase 4 weeks after first opening due to the potential for bacterial growth. Sacrosidase is fully soluble with water, milk and infant formula, but it is important to note that this product is sensitive to heat. Sacrosidase should not be reconstituted or consumed with fruit juice, since its acidity may reduce the enzyme activity.

LACTOBACILLUS

otc	**Bacid** (Ciba)	**Capsules:** Cultured strain ≥ 500 million viable *Lactobacillus acidophilus*	Mineral oil. In 50s and 100s.
otc	**SynBiotics-3** (NutraCea)	**Capsules:** 4.5 billion CFU *Bifidobacterium longum, Lactobacillus rhamnosus* A, *Lactobacilllus plantarum, Saccharomyces boulardii*.	Maltodextrin. In 60s and UD 200s.
otc sf	**Kala** (Freeda)	**Tablets:** 200 million units soy-based *L. acidophilus*	In 100s, 250s and 500s.
otc	**Lactinex** (Becton Dickinson)	**Granules:** Mixed culture of *L. acidophilus* and *L. bulgaricus*	In 1 g packets (12s).
		Tablets, chewable: Mixed culture of *L. acidophilus* and *L. bulgaricus*	Lactose, sucrose and mineral oil. In 50s.
otc sf	**MoreDophilus** (Freeda)	**Powder:** 4 billion units of acidophilus-carrot derivative per g	In 120 g.
otc	**Superdophilus** (Natren)	**Powder:** 2 billion *L. acidophilus* strain DDS-1 per g	In 37.5, 75 and 135 g.

Indications

Dietary supplement.

➤*Unlabeled uses:* Treatment of uncomplicated diarrhea, including that due to antibiotic therapy. The FDA has determined that these ingredients are not generally recognized as safe and effective as antidiarrheal drug products.

Treatment of acute fever blisters (cold sores).

Administration and Dosage

➤*Bacid:* 2 capsules 2 to 4 times daily. Must be refrigerated.

➤*Lactinex:*

Granules – 1 packet added to or taken with cereal, food, milk, fruit juice or water 3 or 4 times daily. Must be refrigerated.

Tablets, chewable – 4 tablets 3 or 4 times daily. May follow each dose with a small amount of milk, fruit juice or water.

➤*MoreDophilus:* 1 tsp daily with liquid. Store at room temperature.

➤*Superdophilus:* ¼ to 1 tsp 1 to 3 times daily.

Actions

➤*Pharmacology:* A viable culture of the naturally occurring metabolic products produced by *Lactobacillus acidophilus* and *L. bulgaricus*.

Contraindications

Allergy to milk or sensitivity to lactose.

Warnings

➤*Children:* Unless directed by a physician, do not use in children < 3 years old.

Precautions

➤*Fever:* Unless directed by physician, do not use for > 2 days or in the presence of high fever.

FLAVOCOXID

Rx	**Limbrel** (Primus)	**Capsule:** 250 mg	Dextrose, maltodextrin. (LIMBREL 52001). Turquoise green. In 60s.

Indications

➤*Osteoarthritis (OA):* For the clinical dietary management of OA, including associated inflammation.

Administration and Dosage

Take one 250 mg capsule every 12 hours for a total of 500 mg/day. Consume more than 500 mg/day only under direction of a physician. Do not consume food 1 hour before or after taking flavocoxid.

➤*Storage/Stability:* Store at room temperature of 15° to 30°C (59° to 86°F). Protect from light and moisture. Dispense in a light-resistant container with a child-resistant closure.

Actions

➤*Pharmacology:* Flavocoxid consists of a proprietary blend of free B-ring flavonoids and flavans from phytochemical food source materials, which are Generally Recognized as Safe.

Flavocoxid exhibits anti-inflammatory and analgesic properties in animal and human models. The mechanism of action is believed to exist because of inhibition of prostaglandin synthesis, via the inhibition of cyclo-oxygenase (COX). In addition to COX, flavocoxid has been observed to inhibit another important inflammatory pathway of arachidonic acid metabolism known as the 5-lipoxygenase (5-LO or 5-LOX) pathway. In cell-based assays, inhibition of 5-LOX has been shown to reduce the production of leukotriene-B4 (LTB4), an agent that fosters white blood cell chemotaxis and the subsequent release of reactive oxygen species and pro-inflammatory cytokines. Direct inhibition of the 5-LOX enzyme also has been observed. Reactive oxygen species (ROS) have been shown to play a key role in the degradation of cartilage in OA.

Flavocoxid also is believed to act through an antioxidant mechanism by reduction of ROS including hydroxyl radical, superoxide anion radical, and hydrogen peroxide.

Flavocoxid also has been found to reduce the pro-inflammatory cytokines interleukin-1-beta (IL-1 β) and tumor necrosis factor alpha (TNF-α) in in vitro models. This mechanism may account for the anti-inflammatory action of flavocoxid beyond that of traditional COX and 5-LOX inhibition.

Through these mechanisms, flavocoxid is beneficial for the specific dietary management of OA.

➤*Pharmacokinetics:*

Absorption – Do not consume food 1 hour before or after taking flavocoxid. Absorption under conditions of co-ingestion of flavocoxid with food is believed to be safe, but may present modest absorption limitations. This observation is based upon limited clinical experience, and testing has not been performed to confirm this observation.

Metabolism – Flavocoxid is primarily metabolized via glucuronidation and sulfation, with little hepatic metabolism involving cytochrome P450 isoenzymes (CYP). A primary ingredient constituent, baicalin, undergoes hydrolysis of the glucuronide moiety at the gut mucosal border and is absorbed as the aglycone, baicalein. Glucuronidation and sulfation of baicalein occurs intrahepatically. In vitro CYP assays using a microsomal enzyme system show CYP inhibition is nominal, ranging from 11% to 23% inhibition of selected isozymes when studied at a 10 micromolar concentration.

Contraindications

Hypersensitivity to flavocoxid or any component of flavocoxid.

Warnings

Flavocoxid has not been investigated for use in the clinical dietary management of rheumatoid arthritis, acute pain, or primary dysmenorrhea.

➤*Pregnancy:* There are no formal studies among pregnant patients; as a precaution, flavocoxid is not recommended for pregnant patients.

➤*Lactation:* There are no formal studies among lactating patients; as a precaution, flavocoxid is not recommended for lactating patients.

➤*Children:* Because there are no formal studies among patients younger than 18 years of age, as a precaution, flavocoxid is not recommended for patients younger than 18 years of age.

Precautions

➤*Corticosteroids:* Flavocoxid cannot be expected to substitute for the use of corticosteroids or to treat corticosteroid insufficiency.

➤*GI effects:* Because there are no formal studies among patients with a history of GI disorders, as a precaution, flavocoxid is not recommended for patients with a history of stomach ulcers. As with many products, GI side effects such as bleeding, ulceration, and stomach perforation can occur at any time, with or without symptoms, in patients concomitantly or previously treated with NSAIDs or COX-2 inhibitors.

Adverse Reactions

In a 90 day, well-controlled, clinical trial, the incidence of side effects for flavocoxid was comparable with placebo. Some of the adverse events reported appear to have been because of preexisting conditions.

➤*GI:* In 1 study, an isolated number of patients using flavocoxid and placebo products were found to test positive for fecal occult blood. However, the limited incidence of these adverse events was statistically the same between the flavocoxid and placebo legs of this trial. Patients experiencing these events were found to have a history of GI illness. To confirm the isolated nature of these findings, 2 fecal occult blood studies were performed, and all patients tested negative.

➤*Adverse events (at least 2% incidence):*

125 mg twice/day – Fluid accumulation in the knee; hypertension (elevation); varicose veins (increase).

250 mg twice/day – Psoriasis.

Overdosage

There are no known human cases of flavocoxid being overused. Animal studies have shown that consuming the equivalent of up to 20 times the recommended human use (500 mg/day) did not produce adverse events. However, as in most overusage situations, symptoms following an overuse of flavocoxid could vary according to the patient. If an overusage occurs, manage patients by systematic and supportive care as soon as possible following product consumption. There are no known specific antidotes for an overuse of flavocoxid.

VITAMIN A & D COMBINATIONS

	Product & Distributor	A IU	D IU	C mg	Content Given Per	Other Content and How Supplied
otc	**Vitamin A & D Tablets** (Nature's Bounty)	10,000	400		tablet	In 100s.
otc	**White Cod Liver Oil Concentrate w/ Vitamin C Tablets** (Schering-Plough)	4000	200	50	chewable tablet	Tartrazine, sugar. In 100s.
otc sf	**Tri-Vi-Sol Drops** (Mead Johnson Nutritional)	1500	400	35	1 mL	In 30 and 50 mL w/dropper.
otc	**Tri-Vitamin Infants' Drops** (Schein)					Pineapple flavor. In 50 mL w/dropper.
otc sf	**Vi-Daylin ADC Drops** (Ross)					< 0.5% alcohol, parabens. Pineapple flavor. In 50 mL.
otc	**Cod Liver Oil Capsules** (Various, eg, Apothecon, Goldline, IDE, Moore, Nature's Bounty, Rugby, Bristol-Myers Squibb)	1250	≈ 135		capsule	In 100s, 250s and 1000s.
otc	**Scott's Emulsion** (SK-Beecham)	1250	100		5 mL	Benzyl alcohol, parabens. In 187.5 and 375 mL.
otc	**Cod Liver Oil USP** (Humco)	1000	100		g	In 120 mL, pt and gal.
otc	**Cod Liver Oil Liquid USP** (Various, eg, Apothecon, Humco, Bristol-Myers Squibb)	850	85		g	In 120 and 360 mL and pt.

For additional information, refer to the Recommended Dietary Allowances monograph.

CALCIUM AND VITAMIN D

Content given per tablet or softgel.

	Product & Distributor	Ca[1] mg	D IU	P mg	Other Content and How Supplied
otc sf	**Caltrate 600 + D Tablets** (Whitehall Robins)	600	200		(C 40). (CALTRATE). In 60s.
otc sf	**Caltrate Plus Tablets** (Whitehall Robins)				7.5 mg Zn, Mg, Cu, Mn, B. (CALTRATE). In 60s.
otc sf	**Super Calcium '1200' Softgels** (Schiff)				In 60s and 120s.
otc	**Calcium Carbonate 600 mg + Vitamin D Tablets** (Major)	600	125		In 72s.
otc sf	**Calcium 600 + D Tablets** (Nature's Bounty)				In 60s.
otc sf	**Calcarb with Vitamin D** (Zenith Goldline)				In 60s.
otc sf	**Caltrate 600 + Iron/Vitamin D Tablets** (Lederle)				18 mg Fe.[2] (LL). Film coated. Capsule shape. In 60s.
otc sf	**Posture-D Tablets** (Whitehall)				Scored. Film coated. In 60s.
otc	**Calcium 600 with Vitamin D Tablets** (Mission)	600	100		In 60s.
otc sf	**Calel D Tablets** (Rhone-Poulenc Rorer)	500	200		In 75s.
otc sf	**Os-Cal 500 + D Tablets** (SK-Beecham)				Parabens. Green, oblong. In 75s and 160s.
otc sf	**Oyster Calcium 500 mg + D Tablets** (Nion)				In 120s.
otc sf	**Desert Pure Calcium** (Cal•White Mineral Co.)	500	125		Film coated. Oval. In 200s.
otc sf	**Oyster Calcium Tablets** (Nature's Bounty)	375	200		800 IU vitamin A. In 100s.
otc	**Citracal Caplets + D** (Mission)	315	200		(CITRACAL +D MISSION). In 60s.
otc	**Citracal Plus with Magnesium Tablets** (Mission)	250	125		5 mg B$_6$, B, Cu, Mg, Mn, Zn. In 150s.
otc	**Os-Cal 250 + D Tablets** (SK-Beecham)				Parabens, EDTA. (OS-CAL 250 + D). In 100s and 240s.
otc	**Oysco D Tablets** (Rugby)				In 100s, 250s and 1000s.
otc	**Oyst-Cal-D Tablets** (Goldline)				Tartrazine. Green. Film coated. In 100s, 240s and 1000s.
otc sf	**Oyster Calcium with Vitamin D Tablets** (Nion)				In 100s.
otc	**Oyster Shell Calcium with Vitamin D Tablets** (Major)				In 100s, 1000s and UD 100s.
otc	**Amino-Min-D Capsules** (Tyson)	250	100		7.5 mg Fe, 5.6 mg Zn, Mg, I, Mn, Cu, K, Cr, Se, betaine HCl, glutamic acid HCl. In 100s.
otc	**Calcet Tablets** (Mission)	152.8	100		(CALCET MPC). In 100s.
otc sf	**Bone Meal Tablets** (Nion)	236		118	In 250s.
otc sf	**Super CalciCaps Tablets** (Nion)	400	133	42	In 90s and 180s.
otc	**Dical-D Wafers** (Abbott)	232	200	180	Chewable. Sucrose, dextrose. Vanilla flavor. In 51s.
otc	**CalciCaps Tablets** (Nion)	125[3]	67	60	In 100s and 500s.
otc	**CalciCaps with Iron Tablets** (Nion)				7 mg Fe.[4] Tartrazine. In 100s and 500s.
otc	**Dical-D Tablets** (Abbott)	117[5]	133	90	In 100s.

[1] Expressed in mg elemental calcium.
[2] As ferrous fumarate.
[3] Dibasic calcium phosphate, calcium gluconate and calcium carbonate.
[4] As ferrous gluconate.
[5] Dibasic calcium phosphate hydrous as anhydrous.

For additional information, refer to the Recommended Dietary Allowances monograph.

VITAMIN COMBINATIONS, MISCELLANEOUS

Content given per capsule, tablet or mL.

	Product and Distributor	Ca[1] mg	E IU	B$_6$ mg	C mg	Other Content	How Supplied
otc sf	**Ze Caps Capsules** (Everett)		200[2]			9.6 mg Zn (as gluconate), sorbitol	In 60s.
otc sf	**Dolomite Tablets** (Nature's Bounty)	130				78 mg Mg	In 100s and 250s.
otc	**Beelith Tablets** (Beach)			20		362 mg Mg	In 100s.
otc sf	**Calcium Magnesium Zinc Tablets** (Nature's Bounty)	333				133 mg Mg, 8.3 mg Zn	In 100s.
otc sf	**KLB6 Softgels** (Nature's Bounty)			3.5		100 mg soya lecithin, 25 mg kelp, 40 mg cider vinegar	In 100s.
otc	**Ultra KLB6 Tablets** (Nature's Bounty)			16.7		400 mg lecithin, 33.3 mg kelp, 80 mg cider vinegar	In 100s.
otc sf	**Mag-Cal Tablets** (Fibertone)	416.7[3] 166.7[1]				66.7 IU D$_3$, 83.3 mg Mg, Cu, Mn, K, Zn	In 180s.
otc sf	**Bo-Cal Tablets** (Fibertone)	250				125 mg Mg, 100 IU D$_3$, B	In 120s.
otc sf	**Oesto-Mins Powder[4]** (Tyson)	250			500	250 mg Mg, 45 mg K, 100 IU vitamin D	In 200 g.
otc sf	**Mag-Cal Mega Tablets** (Freeda)	400				800 mg Mg	Kosher. In 100s and 250s.
otc sf	**Super CalciCaps M-Z Tablets** (Nion)	400				133 mg Mg, 5 mg Zn, 1667 mg vitamin A, 133 IU vitamin D, Se	In 90s.
otc	**MagneBind 200** (Nephro-Tech)	400[3] 160[1]				200 mg Mg[3]	In 150s.
otc	**MagneBind 300** (Nephro-Tech)	250[3] 101[1]				300 mg Mg[3]	In 150s.
Rx	**MagneBind 400 Rx** (Nephro-Tech)	200[3]				400 mg Mg,[3] 1 mg folic acid	In 150s.
otc	**ProSight Lutein** (Major)	22	30		60	15 mg Zn, 2 mg Cu.	In 36s.

[1] Calcium content expressed in mg elemental calcium.
[2] As dL-alpha tocopheryl acetate.
[3] Carbonate.
[4] Content given per 4.5 g.

For additional information, refer to the Recommended Dietary Allowances monograph.

VITAMIN COMBINATIONS, MISCELLANEOUS, WITH C

Content given per capsule, tablet or mL.

	Product and Distributor	A IU	E mg	B$_3$ mg	C mg	Other Content	How Supplied
otc	**Antiox** (Mayrand)	42,000[1]	100[2]		120		In 60s.
otc	**Ocuvite Extra Tablets** (Bausch & Lomb)	1000	100[2]	40	300	40 mg Zn, 3 mg B$_2$, Cu, Se, Mn, L-glutathione, 2 mg lutein	In 50s.
otc	**Pro Skin Capsules** (Marlyn)	6250[3]	100[4]		100	10 mg B$_5$, 10 mg Zn, Se	In 60s.
otc	**Protegra Softgels** (Lederle)	5000[1]	200[2]		250	7.5 mg Zn, Cu, Se, Mn	In 50s.
otc	**OcuCaps Tablets** (Akorn)	5000[1]	182[5]		400	40 mg Zn, 5 mg L-glutathione, sodium pyruvate, Cu, Se	Capsule shape. In 60s.
otc	**Ocuvite Tablets** (Bausch & Lomb)	5000[1]	30[4]		60	40 mg Zn, Cu, 40 mcg Se	In 120s.
otc	**Ocuvite Lutein Capsules** (Bausch & Lomb)		30		60	15 mg Zn, Cu, 6 mg lutein, lactose	In 36s.
otc sf	**C & E Softgels** (Nature's Bounty)		400[5]		500		In 50s.
otc sf	**Vitamin C + E Tablets** (Triage)		400[4]		500		Protein coated. Capsule shape. In 50s.
otc	**Ecee Plus Tablets** (Edwards)		165[6]		100	70 mg Mg sulfate, 80 mg Zn sulfate	In 100s.
otc	**Occuvite PreserVision Tablets** (Bausch & Lomb)	7160	100		113	17.4 mg Zn, Cu, lactose	In 120s.

[1] As beta-carotene.
[2] Form of vitamin E unknown; content given in mg.
[3] As beta, alpha and gamma carotene and lycopenes.
[4] As dL-alpha tocopheryl acetate.
[5] In IU; as mixed tocopherols complex.
[6] As d-alpha tocopheryl acid succinate.

For additional information, refer to the Recommended Dietary Allowances monograph.

NUTRITIONAL COMBINATION PRODUCTS

B VITAMIN COMBINATIONS, ORAL
Content given per capsule, tablet or 5 mL.

	Product & Distributor	B_1 mg	B_2 mg	B_3 mg	B_5 mg	B_6 mg	B_{12} mcg	FA mg	Other Content	How Supplied
otc	**B 100 Tablets** (Fibertone)	100	100	100	100	100	100	0.4	50 mcg biotin, 100 mg PABA, 100 mg choline bitartrate, 100 mg inositol	Sustained-release. In 100s.
otc sf	**B-100 Tablets** (NBTY)	100	100	100	100	100	100	0.1	100 mcg d-biotin, 100 mg base of PABA, choline, inositol and lecithin	In 50s and 100s.
otc	**Mega-B Tablets** (Arco)								100 mg PABA, 100 mg inositol, 100 mcg d-biotin, 100 mg choline bitartrate and lecithin	In 100s.
otc sf	**Super Quints-50 Tablets** (Freeda)	50	50	50	50	50	50	0.4	30 mg PABA, 50 mcg d-biotin, 50 mg inositol	Kosher. In 100s, 250s and 500s.
otc sf	**B Complex-50 Tablets** (Nion)	50	50	50	50	50	50		50 mcg biotin, 50 mg PABA, 50 mg choline bitartrate, 50 mg inositol	Sustained-release. In 100s.
otc sf	**B-50 Tablets** (NBTY)	50	50	50	50	50	50	0.1	50 mcg d-biotin, PABA, choline bitartrate, inositol	In 50s and 100s.
otc	**Iso-B Capsules** (Tyson)	25	25	75	125	50	100	0.2	2.5 mg pyridoxal 5 phosphate, 50 mg PABA, 50 mg inositol, 125 mg choline bitartrate, 100 mcg biotin	In 120s.
otc	**Neurodep-Caps Capsules** (Medical Products)	125				125	1000			In 50s.
otc	**Apatate Liquid** (Kenwood/Bradley)	15				0.5	25			Cherry flavor. In 120 and 240 mL.
otc	**Apatate Tablets** (Kenwood/Bradley)	15				0.5	25			Chewable. Cherry flavor. In 50s.
otc	**B-Complex and B-12 Tablets** (NBTY)	7	14	4.5			25		10 mg protease	In 90s.
Rx sf	**Cerefolin Tablets** (Pan American Labs)		5			50	1000		5.635 mg L-methylfolate	(PAL M5). Blue. In 90s.
otc	**Apetil Liquid** (Kenwood/Bradley)	1.7	0.3	6.7	1.67	2.5	5		14.6 mg Zn, Mg, Mn, l-lysine, sucrose, parabens, sorbitol	Alcohol free. In 237 mL.
otc	**B-Complex with B-12 Tablets** (Major)	3	2	20	0.1	1	5			In 100s.
otc sf	**B-Complex with B-12 Tablets** (Goldline)	1.5	1.7	20	10	2	6	0.4		In 100s.
otc	**Almebex Plus B$_{12}$ Liquid** (Dayton)	1	2	5		0.4	5		33 mg choline, parabens, sucrose	In 473 mL with vitamin B_{12} in separate glass container.
otc	**Gevrabon Liquid** (Lederle)	0.83	0.42	8.3	1.67	0.17	0.17		2.5 mg Fe, choline, I, Mg, Mn, 0.3 mg Zn, 18% alcohol, sucrose	In 480 mL.
otc	**Vitamin-Mineral-Supplement Liquid** (Pennex)							0.4	I, 2.5 mg Fe, Mg, 0.3 mg Zn, Mn, choline, 18% alcohol, sorbitol, methylparaben, corn syrup	Sherry wine flavor. In 473 mL.
Rx	**Senilezol Liquid** (Edwards)	0.42	0.42	1.67	0.83	0.17	0.83		3.3 mg ferric pyrophosphate, 15% alcohol, sucrose, methylparaben	In 473 mL.
otc	**Eldertonic Liquid** (Mayrand)	0.17	0.19	2.22	1.11	0.22	0.67		1.7 mg Zn, Mg, Mn, 13.5% alcohol	In 240 mL, pt and gal.
otc sf	**Brewers Yeast Tablets** (NBTY)	0.06	0.02	0.2						In 250s.
otc	**Folgard Tablets** (Upsher-Smith)					10	115	0.8		In 60s.
Rx	**Megaton Elixir** (Hyrex)		0.5	4.4	1.1	0.44	1.33	0.1	4 mg Fe, Mn, 1.7 mg Zn, 13% alcohol, parabens, sucrose	Sherry wine flavor. In 473 mL.
Rx	**PremesisRx** (Ther-Rx Corp.)					75	12	1	200 mg Ca	(Ther-Rx 019). Blue, oval. In 100s.
Rx sf	**Cardiotek Rx Tablets** (Stewart-Jackson)					50	500	2	L-arginine hydrochloride	(CAR/RX). Orange, football shape. Coated. In 30s.
Rx sf	**FOLTX** (Pan American Labs)					25	1000	2.5		Dye free. (PAL/2). Peach. In 90s.
Rx sf	**ComBgen Tablets** (Ethex)					25	500	2.2		(ETH 440). Beige, oval. In 100s.
Rx	**Folgard RX 2.2** (Upsher-Smith)					25	500	2.2		(US 016). Yellow, oval. Film-coated. In 100s.
Rx sf	**Folpace Tablets** (Alaven)					25	425	2.05	100 units E, 100 mg Mg	(AP 18). In 90s.
Rx sf	**Calafol Tablets** (Alaven)					25	425	1.6	400 mg Ca, 400 units D_3	(AP 90). In 90s.
Rx	**Folgard** (Upsher-Smith)					10	115	0.8		In 60s.

For additional information, refer to the Recommended Dietary Allowances monograph.

NUTRITIONAL COMBINATION PRODUCTS

B VITAMINS WITH VITAMIN C, ORAL
Content given per capsule, tablet or 5 mL.

	Product & Distributor	B_1 mg	B_2 mg	B_3 mg	B_5 mg	B_6 mg	B_{12} mcg	C mg	Other Content	How Supplied
otc sf	Enviro-Stress Tablets (Vitaline)	50	50	100	50	50	25	600	0.4 mg FA, 30 mg Zn, 30 IU vitamin E, Mg, Se, PABA	Slow release. In 90s and 1000s.
otc sf	T-Vites Tablets (Freeda)	25	25	150	25	25		100	30 mcg biotin, PABA, K, Mg carbonate, 2 mg Mn and 20 mg Zn gluconate	Kosher. In 100s.
otc sf	Beminal 500 Tablets (Whitehall)	25	12.5	100	20	10	5	500	Lactose	In 100s.
otc	ThexForte Tablets (Lee)	25	15	100	10	5	5	500		Capsule shape. In 75s.
otc	Vicon-C Capsules (UCB Pharma)	17.9	10	95	22	4		300	6.4 mg Mg, 15.9 mg Zn	In 60s.
otc sf	Viogen-C Capsules (Goldline)	20	10	100	20	5		300	Mg, 50 mg dried Zn sulfate, tartrazine	In 100s.
Rx	Berocca Tablets (Roche)	15	15	100	18	4	5	500	0.5 mg folic acid, sugar	(Berocca Roche). Light green. Capsule shaped. In 100s and 500s.
Rx	B-Plex Tablets (Goldline)								0.5 mg folic acid	In 100s.
Rx	Formula B Tablets (Major)									In 250s.
Rx	Strovite Tablets (Everett)								0.5 mg folic acid, lactose	In 100s.
otc	Allbee with C Tablets (Robins)	15	10.2	50	10	5		300	Saccharin, lactose	Capsule shape. In 130s.
otc	Therapeutic B Complex with C Capsules (Upsher-Smith)									Yellow/green. In UD 100s.
otc	B-Complex/Vitamin C Tablets (Geneva)									Capsule shape. Yellow. In 100s.
otc	Econo B & C Tablets (Vangard)									Capsule shape. In 100s and UD 100s.
otc	Arcobee with C Tablets (NBTY)								Tartrazine	Capsule shape. In 100s.
otc sf	B-C-Bid Tablets (Roberts)									Capsule shape. In 100s.
otc sf	Farbee with Vitamin C Tablets (Major)									Capsule shape. In 100s, 130s and 1000s.
otc sf	Gen-bee with C Tablets (Goldline)									Capsule shape. In 130s and 1000s.
otc sf	Superplex T Tablets (Major)	15	10	100	20	5	10	500		In 100s.
otc	Surbex-T Filmtabs (Abbott)									Orange. In 100s.
otc	High Potency N-Vites Tablets (Nion)									In 100s.
otc	Probec-T Tablets (Roberts)	12.2	10	100	18.4	4.1	5	600	Sucrose	In 60s.
otc	3 mg Biotin Forte Tablets (Vitaline)	10	10	40	10	25	10	200	3 mg biotin, 800 mcg FA, 30 mg Zn	In 60s and 1000s.
otc	Extra Strength 5 mg Biotin Forte Tablets (Vitaline)	10	10	40	10	25	10	100	5 mg biotin, 800 mcg FA	In 60s and 1000s.
otc	B Complex + C Tablets (Various, eg. Nion)	15	10	100	20	5	10	500		Timed release. In 100s.
otc	Surbex with C Filmtabs (Abbott)	6	6	30	10	2.5	5	250	Lactose	Film coated. In 100s.
otc	Sublingual B Total Liquid (Pharmaceutical Lab)		1.7	20	30	2	1000	60	Sorbitol	Alcohol free. In 30 mL with dropper.
Rx	Nephplex Rx Tablets (Nephro-Tech)	1.5	1.7	20	10	10	6	60	1 mg FA, 300 mcg d-biotin, 12.5 mg Zn	In 100s.
Rx	Nephro-Vite Rx Tablets (R & D)								1 mg FA, 300 mcg d-biotin	(RD 12). Yellow. Film coated. In 100s.
Rx sf	Hemovit Tablets (Dayton)								1 mg FA, 300 mcg d-biotin	Dye-free. (HT). Yellow. Film-coated. In blister 100s.
otc	Nephro-Vite Vitamin B Complex and C Supplement Tablets (R & D)								800 mcg FA, 300 mcg d-biotin	(RD 02). Yellow. Film coated. In 100s.
Rx	Nephrocaps Capsules (Fleming)	1.5	1.7	20	5	10	6	100	1 mg FA, 150 mcg biotin	(F). Black. Oval. In 100s.

NUTRITIONAL COMBINATION PRODUCTS

B VITAMINS WITH VITAMIN C, ORAL

	Product & Distributor	B1 mg	B2 mg	B3 mg	B5 mg	B6 mg	B12 mcg	C mg	Other Content	How Supplied
otc	Full Spectrum B (National Vitamin)	1.5	1.7	20	10	10	6	60	800 mcg FA, 3 mg biotin	Preservative- and sugar-free. In 100s.
otc	Dialyvite 3000 (Hillestad)	1.5	1.7	20	10	25	1000	100	3 mg FA, 300 mcg biotin, 30 units E, 70 mcg Zn.	In 90s.
Rx sf	DexFol Tablets (Rising)	1.5	1.5	20	10	50	1	60	5 mg FA, 300 mcg biotin	(R128). White. In 90s.
Rx	Diatx Tablets (Pan American)	1.5	1.5	20	10	50	1	60	5 mg FA, 300 mcg D-biotin.	Dye free. (PAL 5). Yellow. In 90s.
otc	Stress B Complex with Vitamin C Tablets (Mission)	13.8	10	50		4.1		300	15 mg Zn	Timed- release. In 60s.

For additional information, refer to the Recommended Dietary Allowances monograph.

LIPOTROPICS WITH VITAMINS
Content given per capsule or tablet.

	Product & Distributor	Choline (mg)	Inositol (mg)	Methionine (mg)	B1 mg	B2 mg	B3 mg	B5 mg	B6 mg	B12 mcg	C mg	Other Content	How Supplied
otc	Lipogen Capsules (Various, eg, Rugby)	111[1]	†	†	0.33	0.33	3.33	1.7	0.33	1.7	100	Bioflavonoids, sorbitol, lecithin	In 60s.
otc	Lipotriad Tablets (Numark)	†	†	†	1.5	1.7	20	10	2	6	60	5000 IU vitamin A (as beta carotene), 30 IU E,[2] 30 mg Zn, Cu, Se	In 60s.
otc	Lipoflavonoid Tablets (Numark)	111[1]	111	111	0.33	0.33	3.33	1.66	0.33	1.66	100	100 mg lemon bioflavonoid complex	In 100s and 500s.
otc sf	Cholinoid Capsules (Goldline)	111[1]	111	111	0.33	0.33	3.33	1.7	0.33	1.7	100	100 mg lemon bioflavonoid complex	In 100s.

* † – Amount not supplied by manufacturer.
[1] From choline bitartrate.
[2] Form of vitamin E unknown.

For additional information, refer to the Recommended Dietary Allowances monograph.

MULTIVITAMINS, CAPSULES, TABLETS, AND WAFERS
Content given per capsule, tablet, or wafer.

	Product & Distributor	A IU	D IU	E IU	B1 mg	B2 mg	B3 mg	B5 mg	B6 mg	B12 mcg	C mg	FA mg	Other Content and How Supplied
otc	Oncovite (Mission)	10,000	400	200	0.37	0.5	5	2.5	25	1.5	500	0.4	Sugar. 7.5 mg Zn. In 100s.
otc sf	Quintabs Tablets (Freeda)	10,000	400	29[1]	25	25	100	25	25	25	300	0.1	Inositol, PABA. Kosher. In 100s and 250s.
otc	Nutrox Capsules (Tyson)	10,000		150[2]	25	25	50	22			80		L-cysteine, taurine, glutathione, 15 mg zinc oxide, Se. In 90s.
otc	Optilets-500 Filmtabs (Abbott)	50,000	400	30[3]	15	10	100	20	5	12	500[4]		Film-coated. In 120s.
otc	Adavite Tablets (Hudson)	5000	400	30[1]	3	3.4	30	10	3	9	90	0.4	35 mcg biotin, 1250 IU beta carotene. In 130s.
otc	Theravee Tablets (Vangard)	5500	400	30[1]	3	3.4	30	10	3	9	120	0.4	15 mcg biotin. In 100s and UD 100s.
otc	One-A-Day Men's Vitamin Tablets (Bayer)	5000	400	45[1]	2.25	2.55	20	10	3	9	200	0.4	(One-A-Day). In 60s and 100s.
otc	Therapeutic Tablets (Goldline)	5000	400	30[3]	3	3.4	20	10	3	9	90	0.4	30 mcg d-biotin. In 100s and 130s.
otc	Therems Tablets (Rugby)	5000	400	30[3]	3	3.4	30	10	3	9	120	0.4	15 mcg biotin, 1250 IU beta carotene. In 130s and 1000s.
otc sf	One-A-Day Essential Tablets (Bayer)	5000	400	30[1]	1.5	1.7	20	10	2	6	60	0.4	In 75s and 130s.
otc	One-Tablet-Daily Tablets (Various, eg, Goldline)												In 365s and 1000s.
otc	Tab-A-Vite Tablets (Major)			30[3]									In 30s, 100s, 250s, 1000s and UD 100s.
otc	Dayalets Filmtabs (Abbott)	5000	400	30[3]	1.5	1.7	20		2	6	60	0.4	Film-coated. In 100s.
otc	Sigtab Tablets (Roberts)	5000	400	15[1]	10.3	10	100	20	6	18	333	0.4	Sucrose. In 90s and 500s.
otc	Multi-Day Tablets (NBTY)	5000	400	30[1]	1.5	1.7	20	10	2	6	60	0.4	In 100s.

NUTRITIONAL COMBINATION PRODUCTS

MULTIVITAMINS, CAPSULES, TABLETS, AND WAFERS

	Product & Distributor	A IU	D IU	E IU	B1 mg	B2 mg	B3 mg	B5 mg	B6 mg	B12 mcg	C mg	FA mg	Other Content and How Supplied
otc sf	Unicap Tablets (Upjohn)	5000	400	15[1]	1.5	1.7	20		2	6	60	0.4	Tartrazine. In 120s.
otc	Multivitamins Capsules (Solvay)	5000	400	10[3]	2.5	2.5	20	5	0.5	2	50		(0032-1204). Oval. Brown. In 100s and UD 100s.
otc sf	Oxi-Freeda Tablets (Freeda)			150[1]	20	20	40	20	20	10	100		5000 IU beta carotene, glutathione, L-cysteine, Se, 15 mg Zn. Kosher. In 100s and 250s.
otc	Sesame Street Plus Extra C Tablets (McNeil-CPC)	2750	200	10[1]	0.75	0.85	10	5	0.7	3	80	0.2	Sucrose, lactose. Chewable. Character shapes. In 50s.
otc sf	Bugs Bunny with Extra C Children's Tablets (Bayer)	2500	400	15[1]	1.05	1.2	13.5		1.05	4.5	250	0.3	Chewable. Fruit flavors. In 60s.
otc	Flintstones Plus Extra C Children's Tablets (Bayer)												Chewable. Character shapes. In 60s and 100s.
otc sf	Sunkist Multi-Vitamins + Extra C Tablets (Ciba)												5 mcg vitamin K, sorbitol, aspartame, phenylalanine. Citrus flavor. In 60s.
otc	Animal Shapes Tablets (Major)	2500	400		1.05	1.2	13.5		1.05	4.5	60	0.3	In 100s and 250s.
otc	Garfield Chewable Tablets (Menley & James)												Sucrose, lactose. Character shapes. In 60s.
otc	Bounty Bears Tablets (NBTY)												In 100s.
otc	Mediplex Plus Tablets (US Pharm)			50[3]	25	10	100	25	10	25	300	0.4	18 mg Zn, Cu, Mg, Mn. In 100s.
otc	Allbee C-800 Tablets (Robins)			45[1]	15	17	100	25	25	12	800		Lactose. (AHR). Elliptical. In 60s.
otc	Stress Formula Vitamins Capsules and Tablets (Various, eg, Goldline)			30[1]	10	10	100	20	5	12	500	0.4	**Capsules:** 45 mcg biotin. In 100s. **Tablets:** 45 mcg biotin. In 60s.
otc	Stress Formula w/Zinc Tablets (Various)			30[3]	15	10	100	20	5	12	500	0.4	45 mcg biotin, 23.9 mg Zn, Cu. In 60s.
otc	Stress Formula 600 Tablets (Vangard)			30[3]	10	10	100	20	5	12	500	0.4	45 mcg biotin. In UD 100s.
otc	Stresstabs Tablets (Lederle)			30[3]	15	10	100	20	5	12	500	0.4	45 mcg biotin. In 60s.
Rx	Cefol Filmtab Tablets (Abbott)			30[3]	15	10	100	20	5	6	750	0.5	(NJ). Green. Film coated. In 100s.

[1] Form of vitamin E unknown.
[2] As d-alpha tocopheryl acid succinate.
[3] As dL-alpha tocopheryl acetate.
[4] As d-alpha tocopheryl succinate.

For a comparison of the potencies of the various forms of vitamin E, see the vitamin E monograph.

MULTIVITAMINS, DROPS AND LIQUIDS

	Product & Distributor	Content Given Per	A IU	D IU	E IU	B1 mg	B2 mg	B3 mg	B5 mg	B6 mg	B12 mcg	C mg	Other Content	How Supplied
otc	Certagen Liquid (Goldline)	15 mL	2500	400	30[1]	1.5	1.7	20	10	2	6	60	6.6% alcohol. 300 mcg biotin, 9 mg Fe, 3 mg Zn, Cr, I, Mn, Mo	In 237 mL.
otc	Syrvite Liquid[1] (Various, eg, Major)	5 mL	2500	400	15[2]	1.05	1.2	13.5		1.05	4.5	60		In 480 mL.
otc	Daily Vitamins Liquid (Rugby)												Sugar, parabens, corn syrup, < 0.5% alcohol	In 237 and 473 mL.
otc	Vi-Daylin Multivitamin Liquid (Ross)				15[3]								≤ 0.5% alcohol, glucose, sucrose, methylparaben	Lemon/orange flavor. In 240 and 480 mL.
otc sf	LKV Infant Drops (Freeda)	0.6 mL	2500	400	5[2]	1	1	10	3	1	4	50	75 mcg biotin	In 60 mL after mixing powder and liquid.
otc	ADEKs Pediatric Drops (Scandipharm)	1 mL	1500	400	40[4]	0.5	0.6	6	3	0.6	4	45	0.1 mg vitamin K, 15 mcg biotin, 5 mg zinc, 1 mg beta carotene	In 60 mL.
otc	Poly-Vi-Sol Drops (Mead Johnson)	1 mL	1500	400	5[2]	0.5	0.6	8		0.4	2	35		In 30 and 50 mL.
otc sf	Baby Vitamin Drops (Goldline)													Alcohol free. In 50 mL.
otc sf	Poly-Vitamin Drops (Schein)				5[3]									Alcohol free. In 50 mL.
otc sf	Vi-Daylin Multivitamin Drops (Ross)	1 mL	1500	400	5[5]	0.5	0.6	8		0.4	1.5	35	< 0.5% alcohol, methylparaben, EDTA	Fruit flavor. In 50 mL.

NUTRITIONAL COMBINATION PRODUCTS

MULTIVITAMINS, DROPS AND LIQUIDS

	Product & Distributor	Content Given Per	A IU	D IU	E IU	B$_1$ mg	B$_2$ mg	B$_3$ mg	B$_5$ mg	B$_6$ mg	B$_{12}$ mcg	C mg	Other Content	How Supplied
otc	**Thera Multi-Vitamin Liquid** (Major)	5 mL	10,000	400		10	10	100	21.4	4.1	5	200	Sucrose, methylparaben	In 118 mL.
otc	**Theravite Liquid** (Barre-National)													Sugar, methylparaben	In 118 mL.

[1] May contain alcohol.
[2] Form of vitamin E unknown.
[3] As d-alpha tocopheryl acetate.
[4] As d-alpha tocopheryl polyethylene glycol-1000 succinate.
[5] As d-alpha tocopheryl acid succinate.

For a comparison of the potencies of various forms of vitamin E, see the Vitamin E monograph.

MULTIVITAMINS WITH IRON
Content given per capsule, tablet or liquid dose.

	Product & Distributor	Fe[1] mg	A IU	D IU	E IU	B$_1$ mg	B$_2$ mg	B$_3$ mg	B$_5$ mg	B$_6$ mg	B$_{12}$ mcg	C mg	FA mg	Other Content and How Supplied
otc	**CenogenUltra** (US Pharmaceutical)	106				10	6	30	10	5	15	200	1	Cu, Mn. (US CENOGEN ULTRA/140). Blue/Pink. In UD 100s.
otc	**Femiron Multi-Vitamins and Iron Tablets** (Menley & James)	20	5000	400	15²	1.5	1.7	20	10	2	6	60	0.4	In 35s, 60s and 90s.
otc	**Dayalets + Iron Filmtabs** (Abbott)	18	5000	400	30³	1.5	1.7	20		2	6	60	0.4	Film coated. In 100s.
otc sf	**One-Tablet-Daily with Iron** (Goldline)	18	5000	400	30³	1.5	1.7	20	10	2	6	60	0.4	In 100s.
otc	**Tab-A-Vite + Iron Tablets** (Major)														Tartrazine. In 100s.
otc sf	**Multi-Day Plus Iron Tablets** (NBTY)	18	5000	400	15²	1.5	1.7	20		2	6	60	0.4	In 100s.
otc	**Sesame Street Plus Iron Tablets** (McNeil-CPC)	10	2750	200	10²	0.75	0.85	10	5	0.7	3	40	0.2	Chewable. Character shapes. In 50s.
otc	**Animal Shapes + Iron Tablets** (Major)	15	2500	400	15³	1.05	1.2	13.5		1.05	4.5	60	0.3	In 100s and 250s.
otc sf	**Bounty Bears Plus Iron Tablets** (NBTY)				15²										Chewable. In 100s.
otc	**Bugs Bunny Plus Iron Tablets** (Bayer)														Chewable. In 60s.
otc	**Flintstones Plus Iron Tablets** (Bayer)														Chewable. Character shapes. In 60s and 100s.
otc	**Vi-Daylin Multivitamin + Iron Liquid** (Ross)	10	2500	400	15⁴	1.05	1.2	13.5		1.05	4.5	60		Per 5 mL. ≤ 0.5% alcohol, glucose, sucrose, parabens. Lemon/lime flavor. In 237 and 473 mL.
otc sf	**Baby Vitamin Drops with Iron** (Goldline)	10	1500	400	5²	0.5	0.6	8		0.4		35		Per 1 mL. In 50 mL.
otc	**Poly-Vi-Sol with Iron Drops** (Mead Johnson)														Per 1 mL. In 50 mL.
otc	**Polyvitamin Drops with Iron** (Various, eg. Rugby)														Per 1 mL. In 50 mL.
otc sf	**Multi-Vit Drops w/Iron** (Barre-National)														Per 1 mL. Methylparaben. In 50 mL.
otc sf	**Vi-Daylin Multivitamin + Iron Drops** (Ross)														Per 1 mL. Methylparaben, < 0.5% alcohol. Fruit flavor. In 50 mL.
Rx sf	**Diatx Fe Tablets** (Pan American)	100				1.5	1.5	20	10	50	1	60	5	300 mcg D-biotin. Dye free. (PAL 5FE). Red. In 90s.
otc sf	**Vi-Daylin ADC Vitamins + Iron Drops** (Ross)	10	1500	400								35		Per 1 mL. Methylparaben. Fruit flavor. In 50 mL.
otc	**Tri-Vi-Sol with Iron Drops** (Mead Johnson)														Per 1 mL. Fruit-like flavor. In 50 mL.
otc	**Simron Plus Capsules** (SmithKline Beecham)	10									1	3.3	50	0.1	Parabens. In 100s.

NUTRITIONAL COMBINATION PRODUCTS

MULTIVITAMINS WITH IRON

	Product & Distributor	Fe[1] mg	A IU	D IU	E IU	B₁ mg	B₂ mg	B₃ mg	B₅ mg	B₆ mg	B₁₂ mcg	C mg	FA mg	Other Content and How Supplied
Rx	NataChew (Warner Chilcott)	29[5]	1000	400	11[3]	2	3			10	12	120	1	20 mg niacinamide. Chewable. (WC 227). Tan, speckled, bisected. Wildberry flavor. In 90s.
Rx	NataFort (Warner Chilcott)	60[6]	1000	400	11	2	3			10	12	120	1	20 mg niacinamide. (NataFort). Lactose. White. Film-coated. In UDs 90s.

[1] Iron content expressed in mg elemental iron.
[2] Form of vitamin E unknown.
[3] As dL-alpha tocopheryl acetate.
[4] As d-alpha tocopheryl acid succinate.
[5] As ferrous fumarate.
[6] As carbonyl iron and ferrous sulfate.

These products contain supplemental iron; products containing therapeutic amounts of iron (>25 mg) with vitamins are listed in the blood modifiers section. For a comparison of the potencies of various forms of vitamin E, see the Vitamin E monograph.

MULTIVITAMINS WITH FLUORIDE, CAPSULES AND TABLETS

Content given per capsule or tablet.

	Product & Distributor	F[1] mg	A IU	D IU	E IU	B₁ mg	B₂ mg	B₃ mg	B₅ mg	B₆ mg	B₁₂ mcg	C mg	FA mg	Other Content and How Supplied
otc	Monocal Tablets (Mericon)	3												250 mg Ca. In 100s.
Rx	Adeflor M Tablets (Kenwood/Bradley)	1	6000	400		1.5	2.5	20	10	10	2	100		250 mg Ca, 30 mg Fe, sorbitol, sucrose. Pink. Elliptical. In 100s.
Rx	Mulvidren-F Softab Tablets (Wyeth-Ayerst)	1	4000	400		1.6	2	10	2.8	1	3	75		Saccharin. (Stuart 710). Chewable. Orange, scored. In 100s.
Rx	Poly Vitamins Fluoride Tablets[2] (Various, eg, Schein)	1	2,500	400	15[3]	1.05	1.2	13.5		1.05	4.5	60	0.3	In 100s.
Rx	Chewable Multivitamins w/Fluoride Tablets (Moore)				15[4]									Sucrose. Fruit flavor. In 100s.
Rx	Florvite Tablets (Everett)													Sucrose. Chewable. Fruit flavors. In 100s.
Rx	Poly-Vi-Flor Tablets 1.0 mg (Mead Johnson Nutritionals)													Sucrose. (MJ 474). Chewable. In 100s and 1000s.
Rx	Poly-Vi-Flor with Iron 1.0 mg Tablets (Mead Johnson Nutritionals)													Cu, 12 mg Fe, 10 mg Zn, sucrose. Chewable. In 100s and 1000s.
Rx	Polyvitamin Fluoride Tablets w/Iron (Various, eg, Rugby, Schein)													Cu, 12 mg Fe, 10 mg Zn. Chewable. In 100s.
Rx	Vi-Daylin/F Chewable Multivitamin Tablets (Ross)													Chewable. In 100s.
Rx	Vi-Daylin/F Multivitamins + Iron Chewable Tablets (Ross)													12 mg Fe, sucrose. Cherry flavor. In 100s.
Rx	Tri-Vi-Flor 1.0 mg Tablets (Mead Johnson Nutritionals)	1	2500	400								60		Sucrose. Chewable. Fruit flavor. In 100s.
Rx	Chewable Triple Vitamins with Fluoride Tablets (Major)													Dextrose, sucrose. Fruit flavor. In 100s.
Rx	Trivitamin Fluoride Tablets (Schein)													Sucrose. Chewable. Fruit flavor. In 100s.
Rx	Poly Vitamins w/Fluoride 0.5 Tablets[2] (Various, eg, Goldline, Rugby, Schein)	0.5	2500	400	15[4]	1.05	1.2	13.5		1.05	4.5	60	0.3	In 100s and 1000s.
Rx	Poly-Vi-Flor 0.5 mg Tablets (Mead Johnson Nutritionals)													Lactose, sucrose. (MJ 468). Chewable. Fruit flavor. In 100s.
Rx	Poly-Vi-Flor 0.5 mg w/Iron Tablets (Mead Johnson Nutritionals)													Cu, 12 mg Fe, 10 mg Zn, lactose, sucrose. (482 MJ). Chewable. Fruit flavor. In 100s.
Rx	Polyvitamins w/Fluoride 0.5 mg and Iron Tablets (Rugby)													Cu, 12 mg Fe, 10 mg Zn, sucrose. Chewable. Cherry flavor. In 100s.

NUTRITIONAL COMBINATION PRODUCTS

MULTIVITAMINS WITH FLUORIDE, CAPSULES AND TABLETS

	Product & Distributor	F¹ mg	A IU	D IU	E IU	B₁ mg	B₂ mg	B₃ mg	B₅ mg	B₆ mg	B₁₂ mcg	C mg	FA mg	Other Content and How Supplied
Rx	**Poly-Vi-Flor Tablets 0.25 mg** (Mead Johnson Nutritionals)	0.25	2500	400	15[4]	1.05	1.2	13.5		1.05	4.5	60	0.3	Lactose, sucrose. (MJ 487)Chewable. Fruit flavor. In 100s.
Rx	**Poly-Vi-Flor 0.25 mg Tablets w/Iron** (Mead Johnson Nutritionals)													Cu, 12 mg Fe, 10 mg Zn, lactose, sucrose. (MJ 488). Chewable. Fruit flavor. In 100s.

¹ Fluoride content expressed in mg elemental fluoride.
² May be chewable.
³ Form of vitamin E unknown.
⁴ As dL-alpha tocopheryl acetate.

For a comparison of the potencies of various forms of vitamin E, see the Vitamin E monograph.

For complete prescribing information on fluoride-containing products, refer to the Fluoride group monograph.

Indications

Used for prophylaxis of vitamin deficiencies and as an aid in the prevention of dental caries in infants and children where the fluoride content of the drinking water does not exceed 0.7 ppm.

MULTIVITAMINS WITH FLUORIDE, DROPS

	Product & Distributor	Content Given Per	F¹ mg	A IU	D IU	E IU	B₁ mg	B₂ mg	B₃ mg	B₅ mg	B₆ mg	B₁₂ mcg	C mg	Other Content and How Supplied
Rx	**Polyvitamin w/Fluoride Drops** (Various, eg, Rugby)	1 mL	0.5	1,500	400	5[2]	0.5	0.6	8		0.4	2	35	In 50 mL.
Rx	**Poly-Vi-Flor 0.5 mg Drops** (Mead Johnson Nutritionals)					5[3]								Fruit flavor. In 50 mL.
Rx	**Poly-Vi-Flor with Iron 0.5 mg Drops** (Mead Johnson Nutritionals)	1 mL	0.5	1,500	400	5[3]	0.5	0.6			0.4		35	10 mg Fe.[4] Fruit flavor. In 50 mL.
Rx	**ADC with Fluoride Drops** (Various, eg, Hi-Tech, Major)	1 mL	0.5	1,500	400								35	Methylparaben. In 50 mL.
Rx	**Tri-A-Vite F Drops** (Major)													In 50 mL.
Rx	**Tri-Vi-Flor 0.5 mg Drops** (Mead-Johnson)													Fruit flavor. In 50 mL.
Rx	**Tri-Vitamin w/Fluoride Drops** (Rugby)													In 50 mL.
Rx	**Tri Vit w/Fluoride 0.5 mg Drops** (Barre-National)													In 50 mL.
Rx sf	**Polyvitamin Fluoride Drops** (Various, eg, Goldline, Hi-Tech, Major, Rugby)	1 mL	0.25	1,500	400	5[5]	0.5	0.6	8		0.4	2	35	Alcohol free. In 50 mL.
Rx	**Poly-Vi-Flor 0.25 mg Drops** (Mead Johnson Nutritionals)					5[3]								Fruit flavor. In 50 mL.
Rx	**Florvite Drops** (Everett)					5[2]								Fruit flavor. In 50 mL.
Rx	**Multivitamin and Fluoride Drops** (Major)													In 50 mL.
Rx	**Polyvitamin Drops w/Iron and Fluoride** (Various, eg, Goldline, Hi-Tech, Rugby, Schein)	1 mL	0.25	1,500	400	5[3]	0.5	0.6	8		0.4		35	10 mg Fe.[4] In 50 mL.
Rx	**Poly-Vi-Flor with Iron 0.25 mg Drops** (Mead Johnson Nutritionals)													10 mg Fe.[4] In 50 mL.
Rx sf	**Vi-Daylin/F Multivitamin Drops** (Ross)													Methylparaben, < 0.1% alcohol. Fruit flavor. In 50 mL.
Rx sf	**Vi-Daylin/F Multivitamin + Iron Drops** (Ross)													10 mg Fe,[5] < 0.1% alcohol, methylparaben. Fruit flavor. In 50 mL.

NUTRITIONAL COMBINATION PRODUCTS

MULTIVITAMINS WITH FLUORIDE, DROPS

	Product & Distributor	Content Given Per	F[1] mg	A IU	D IU	E IU	B₁ mg	B₂ mg	B₃ mg	B₅ mg	B₆ mg	B₁₂ mcg	C mg	Other Content and How Supplied
Rx	**Tri-Vi-Flor 0.25 mg Drops** (Mead Johnson Nutritionals)	1 mL	0.25	1500	400								35	Fruit flavor. In 50 mL.
Rx sf	**Trivitamin Fluoride Drops** (Various, eg, Schein)													Alcohol free. In 50 mL.
Rx sf	**Vi-Daylin/F ADC Vitamins Drops** (Ross)													≈ 0.3% alcohol, parabens. Fruit flavor. In 50 mL.
Rx sf	**Soluvite-f Drops** (Pharmics)	0.6 mL												In 57 mL.
Rx	**Tri-Vi-Flor 0.25 mg with Iron Drops** (Mead Johnson Nutritionals)	1 mL												10 mg Fe.[4] In 50 mL.
Rx sf	**Vi-Daylin/F ADC + Iron Drops** (Ross)													10 mg Fe,[4] methylparaben. Fruit flavor. In 50 mL.
Rx	**Tri Vit w/Fluoride 0.25 mg Drops** (Barre-National)													In 50 mL.
Rx	**Apatate w/Fluoride Liquid** (Kenwood/Bradley)	5 mL	0.5				15				0.5	25		Cherry flavor. In 120 mL.

[1] Fluoride content expressed in mg elemental fluoride.
[2] As dl–alpha tocopheryl acetate.
[3] As d-alpha tocopheryl acid succinate.

[4] Iron content expressed in mg elemental iron.
[5] Form of vitamin E unknown.

For complete prescribing information on fluoride-containing products, refer to the Fluoride group monograph. For a comparison of the potencies of the various forms of vitamin E, see the vitamin E monograph.

NUTRITIONAL COMBINATION PRODUCTS

MULTIVITAMINS WITH CALCIUM AND IRON
Content given per tablet or capsule.

	Product & Distributor	Ca[a] mg	Fe[s] mg	A IU	D IU	E IU	B$_1$ mg	B$_2$ mg	B$_3$ mg	B$_5$ mg	B$_6$ mg	B$_{12}$ mcg	C mg	FA mg	Other Content	How Supplied
otc sf	**One-A-Day Women's Formula Tablets** (Bayer)	450	27	5,000	400	30[b]	1.5	1.7	20	10	2	6	60	0.4	15 mg Zn, tartrazine	In 60s and 100s.
otc sf	**K.P.N. Tablets** (Freeda)	333[c]	11	2,667	133	10[b]	2	2	10	3.3	0.83	2	33	0.27	Cu, I, K, Mg, Mn, 6.7 mg Zn, bioflavonoids	Kosher. In 100s and 250s.
Rx	**Mynatal Capsules** (ME Pharm)	300	65	5,000	400	30[d]	3	3.4	20	10	10	12	120	1	30 mcg biotin, Cr, Cu, I, Mg, Mn, Mo, 25 mg Zn	In 100s and 500s.
otc	**One-A-Day WeightSmart Tablets** (Bayer)	300	18[f]	2,500	400	30[b]	1.9	2.125	25	12.5	2.5	7.5		400[e]	Vitamin K, Mg, Zn, Se, Cu, Mn, Cr, EGCG, dextrose, glucose.	In 50s and 100s.
Rx	**Obstetrix-100** (Seyer[g])	250	100	2,700	400	30[b]	3	3.4	20		20	12	250	1	25 mg Zn, 50 mg sodium docusate	(SEYER OBX-100). Pink, oval, scored. In UD 30s.
Rx	**Prenate 90 Tablets** (Bock)	250	90	4,000	400	30[b]	3	3.4	20		20	12	120	1	DSS, Cu, I, 25 mg Zn	Dye free. Delayed-release. (Bock PN90). Film-coated. In 100s.
Rx	**Mynate 90 Plus Caplets** (ME Pharm)															Delayed-release. In 100s.
Rx	**Prenatal MR 90 Tablets** (Ethex)															Delayed-release. (Ethex 212). Oval. Film coated. In 100s.
Rx	**Par-F Tablets** (Pharmics)	250	60	5,000	400	30[b]	3	3.4	20	10	12	12	120	1	Cu, I, Mg, 15 mg Zn	In 100s.
Rx	**Mynatal FC Caplets** (ME Pharm)	250	60	5,000	400	30[b]	3	3.4	20	10	10	12	100	1	30 mcg biotin, 25 mg Zn, I, Mg, Cr, Cu, Mo, Mn	In 100s.
Rx	**Mynatal P.N. Forte Caplets** (ME Pharm)	250	60	5,000	400	30[b]	3	3.4	20		4	12	80	1	25 mg Zn, I, Mg, Cu	In 100s.
Rx	**Niferex-PN Forte Tablets** (Ther-Rx)					30[d]									Cu, I, Mg, 25 mg Zn	Dye free. (SP 2309 1 0). White. Capsule shape. Film-coated. In 100s.
Rx	**Prenatal Maternal Tablets** (Ethex)	250	60	5,000	400	30[b]	2.9	3.4	20	10	12.2	12	100	1	Cr, Cu, I, Mg, Mn, Mo, 25 mg Zn, 30 mcg biotin	In 100s.
Rx	**Marnatal-F Tablets** (Marnel)	250	60	4,000	400	30[d]	3	3.4	20	10	5	12	100	1	Mg, 25 mg Zn, Cu, I	(Marnatal-F). Lt. pink. Film-coated. In 30s and 100s.
Rx	**NovaCare Tablets** (Fielding)	250	40		240	3.5[d]	3	3.4	20	10	20	12	50	1	15 mg Zn, Cu, Mg.	(SU 01). Peach. Film-coated. In blister card 100s.
Rx	**Prenatal PC 40** (Integrity)	250	40			3.5									15 mg Zn, Cu, Mg	Polydextrose. Capsule shape. Film coated. In UD 100s.
Rx	**PreCare** (Ther-Rx Corp.)	250	40			3.5					2		50	1	6 mcg vit. D$_3$, 50 mg Mg, 15 mg Zn, 2 mg Cu, mannitol, sucrose	(THER-RX 025). Orange. Vanilla flavor. In UD 100s.
Rx	**Embrex 600 Chewable Tablets** (Andrx)	240	90	3500	400	30[h]	2	3			3	12	60	1	20 mg I, 2 mg Cu, Mg, 50 mg dioctylsulfosuccinate sodium	(CTEX P N). Blue, oval, scored. Orange flavor. In blister pack 35s and 91s.
Rx	**Advanced-RF Natal Care Tablets** (Ethex)	200	90		400	30[b]	3	3.4	20		20	12	120	1	2 mg Cu, 50 mg docusate sodium, 20 mg niacinamide, 30 mg Mg, 25 mg Zn.	Dye-free. (ETHEX/458). White, oval. In 90s.
Rx	**Ultra-NatalCare** (Ethex)	200[i]	90[i]	2,700	400	30[d]	3	3.4	20		20	12	120	1	200 mg I, 2 mg Cu, 25 mg Zn, 20 mg niacinamide, 50 mg docusate sodium.	Dye free. (PEC 123). White, oval, bisected. In UD 100s.
Rx	**Vinate GT Tablets** (Breckenridge)	200	90	2,700	400	10[b]	3	3	20	6	20	12	120	1	30 mcg biotin, 50 mg docusate sodium, 15 mg Zn, Cu, Mg.	Purple, oval. In UD 90s.
Rx	**Prenatal AD Tablets** (Cypress)	200	90	2700	400	30[d]	3	3.4	20		20	12	120	1	25 mg Zn, Cu, Mg, 5 0 mg docusate sodium.	(CYP 194). White, oval. In 90s.
Rx sf	**O-Cal f.a. Tablets** (Pharmics)	200	66	5,000	400	30[b]	3	3	20		4	12	90	1	1.1 mg F, Mg, I, Cu, 15 mg Zn	In 100s.
Rx	**Prenatal Plus** (Goldline)	200	65	4,000	400	22[b]	1.84	3	20		10	12	120	1	2 mg Cu, 25 mg Zn	In 100s.
Rx	**Prenatal Plus w/ Betacarotene Tablets** (Rugby)	200	65	4,000	400	11	1.84	3	20		10	12	120	1	25 mg Zn, Cu	In 100s and 500s.
Rx	**Prenatal Plus-Improved Tablets** (Rugby)	200	65	4,000	400	11[b]	1.5	3	20		10	12	120	1	Cu, 25 mg Zn	In 100s.
Rx	**Prenatal-1 + Iron Tablets** (Various, eg, ESI, Goldline, Qualitest, Schein)															In 100s and 500s.
Rx	**Par-Natal Plus 1 Improved Tablets** (Parmed)															In 500s.

NUTRITIONAL COMBINATION PRODUCTS

MULTIVITAMINS WITH CALCIUM AND IRON

	Product & Distributor	Ca[a] mg	Fe[s] mg	A IU	D IU	E IU	B_1 mg	B_2 mg	B_3 mg	B_5 mg	B_6 mg	B_{12} mcg	C mg	FA mg	Other Content	How Supplied
Rx	Lactocal-F Tablets (Laser)	200	65	4,000	400	30[d]	3	3.4	20		5	12	100	1	Cu, I, Mg, 15 mg Zn	(Laser 173). White. Oval. Film-coated. In 100s and 1000s.
Rx	Prenatal Z Advanced Formula (Ethex)	200	65	3,000	400	10	1.5	1.6	17		2.2	2.2	70	1	175 mcg potassium iodide, 100 mg magnesium oxide, 15 mg zinc oxide	In 100s.
Rx	NataTab Rx Tablets (Ethex)	200	29	4,000	400	30	3	3	20	7	3	8	120	1	30 mcg biotin, 15 mg Zn, Cu, I, Mg	(ETHEX 376). Yellow, oval, scored. Film-coated. In 90s.
Rx	Prenatabs RX Tablets (Cypress)														30 mcg biotin, 15 mg Zn, Cu, I, Mg	(CYP 193). White, oval. Film-coated. In 90s.
Rx	Duet Tablets (Integrity)	200	29	3,000	400	30	1.8	4	20		25	12	120	1	Cu, Zn, Mg	Sucrose. (82). Yellow, oval. In 100s.
Rx	Prenatal 19 Tablets (Cypress)	200	29	1000	400	30[d]	3	3	15	7	20	12	100	1	20 mg Zn, 25 mg docusate sodium.	(CYP196). White, oval, scored. In 100s.
Rx	Prenatal 19 Chewable Tablets (Cypress)														20 mg Zn, 25 mg docusate sodium.	(CYP 197). Orange. Orange flavor. In 100s.
Rx	Vinate Good Start Chewable Prenatal Formula Tablets (Breckenridge)														20 mg Zn.	(B 151). Off-white, mottled. In 100s.
otc	Stuart Prenatal Tablets (Integrity)	200	28	4000	400	30	1.8	1.7	20		2.6	8	120	0.8	25 mg Zn	In 100s.
Rx	StuartNatal Plus 3 Tablets (Integrity)	200	28	3000	400	22[d]	1.8	4	20		25	12	120	1	25 mg Zn, Cu, Mg	(Plus 3). Yellow, oval. In 100s.
Rx	Trinate Tablets (Cypress)														25 mg Zn, Cu, Mg.	(CYP 192). White, oval. In 100s.
Rx	Anemagen OB Capsules (Ethex)	200	28		400	30	1.6	1.8			20	12	60	1	Docusate calsium	Parabens. (ETH 052). Green. In 100s.
Rx	NatalCare Three Tablets (Ethex)	200	27	3000	400	22	1.8	4	20		25	12	120	1	25 mg Zn, Cu, Mg	(ETHEX 375). Beige, oval. In 100s.
Rx	Enfamil Natalins Rx Tablets (Mead-Johnson)	100	27	2000	200	7.5[e]	0.75	0.8	8.5	3.5	2	1.25	40	0.5	15 mcg biotin, 1.5 mg Cu, 50 mg Mg	(MJ 702). White. Oval. In 200s.
Rx	Mynatal Rx Caplets (ME Pharm)	200	60	4,000	400	15[b]	1.5	1.6	17	7	4	2.5	80	1	30 mcg biotin, 25 mg Zn, Cu, Mg	In 100s.
Rx	Prenatal Rx Tablets (Various, eg, Ethex, Goldline, Moore, Qualitest, Schein)	200	60	4,000	400	30	3	3	20				80		30 mcg biotin, Cu, Mg, 25 mg Zn	In 100s and 500s.
Rx	Natarex Prenatal Tablets (Major)	200	60	4,000	400	15[d]	1.5	1.6	17	7	4	2.5	80	1	Cu, Mg, 25 mg Zn, 30 mg biotin	In 100s.
Rx	NataTab FA (Ethex)	200	29	4,000	400	30	3	3	20		3	8	120	1	150 mcg iodine, 15 mg Zn, lactose	(ETHEX 329). Purple, oval. Film-coated. In 100s.
Rx	NataTab CFe (Ethex)	200	50	4,000	400	30	3	3	20		3	8	120	1	150 mcg iodine, 15 mg Zn, lactose	(ETHEX 328). White, oval. Film-coated. In UD 10s (100s).
Rx	Prenatal Plus Iron Tablets (Major)	200	27	4000	400	22	1.84	3			10	12	120	1	20 mg niacinamide, 2 mg Cu, and 25 mg Zn.	In 100s.
otc	Prenatal w/Folic Acid Tablets (Geneva)	200	60	4000	400	11[b]	1.5	1.7	18		2.6	4	100	0.8	25 mg Zn	Salmon. Oval. In 100s.
Rx	Nestabs FA Tablets (Fielding)	200	29	4,000	400	30[b]	3	3	20[k]		3	8	120	1	150 mcg I, 15 mg Zn	In 100s. Sugar coated.
Rx	NatalCare Plus (Ethex)	200	27	4,000	400	22	1.84	3	20		10	12	120	1	25 mg Zn, 2 mg Cu,	(Ethex/225). Pink. Film coated. In 100s.
otc	Vitelle Nestabs OTC (Fielding)	200	29	5,000	400	30[b]	3	3	20[k]		3	8	120	0.8	150 mcg I, 15 mg Zn	In 100s.
Rx	Nestabs CBF (Fielding)	200	50	4,000	400	30	3	3	20[k]		3	8	120	1	150 mcg I, 15 mg Zn	In 100s.
otc	Nutricon Tablets (Pasadena)	200	20	2,500	200	15[j]	1.5	1.5	10	5	2	5	50	0.4	Cu, I, Mg, 3.75 mg Zn, 150 mcg biotin	In 120s.
Rx	StrongStart Caplets (Savage)	200	29	1000	400	30[e]	3	3	15	7	20	12	100	1	25 mg docusate sodium, 20 mg Zn	(0343). In 30s and 100s.
Rx	StrongStart Chewable Tablets (Savage)														20 mg Zn	(0344). In 30s and 100s.
Rx	O-Cal Prenatal Tablets (Mission)	200	15	2,500	400	30[b]	1.5	1.6	17		12	12	70	1	Cu, I, Mg, 15 mg Zn	(Pharmics). White, oblong. In 100s.
otc	Centrum, Jr. + Extra Calcium Tablets (Lederle)	160	18	5,000	400	30[b]	1.5	1.7	20	10	2	6	60	0.4	Cr, Cu, I, Mg, Mn, Mo, P, 15 mg Zn, vitamin K, 45 mcg biotin, sugar	Chewable. Fruit flavor. In 60s.

NUTRITIONAL COMBINATION PRODUCTS

MULTIVITAMINS WITH CALCIUM AND IRON

	Product & Distributor	Ca[a] mg	Fe[g] mg	A IU	D IU	E IU	B₁ mg	B₂ mg	B₃ mg	B₅ mg	B₆ mg	B₁₂ mcg	C mg	FA mg	Other Content	How Supplied
otc	Calcet Plus Tablets (Mission)	152.8	18	5,000	400	30[b]	2.25	2.55	30	15	3	9	500	0.8	15 mg Zn, sugar	In 60s.
otc	My-Vitalife Capsules (ME Pharm)	130	27	6,500	400	30[b]	1.5	1.7	20	10	2	6	60	0.4	Cr, Cu, K, I, Mg, Mn, Mo, P, Se, 15 mg Zn, 30 mcg biotin	In 60s.
Rx	Vitafol-PN (Everett Laboratories)	125	65	1,700	400	30	1.6	1.8	15		2.5	5	60	1	25 mg Mg, 15 mg Zn.	Capsule shape. In UD 100s.
Rx	Multifol (Breckenridge)	125	65[f]	6000	400	30	1.1	1.8	15		2.5	5	60	1		(B126). Purple, capsule shape. In UD 100s.
Rx	Cal-Nate Tablets (Ethex)	125	27	2700	400	30[b]	3	3.4	20		20		120	1	25 mg Zn, 150 mcg iodine, 2 mg Cu, 50 mg docusate sodium.	(ETHEX/439). White, oval. In 100s.
otc	Centrum, Jr. + Extra C Tablets (Lederle)	108	18	5,000	400	30[b]	1.5	1.7	20	10	2	6	300	0.4	Cr, Cu, I, Mg, Mn, Mo, P, 15 mg Zn, vitamin K, 45 mcg biotin, sugar, lactose	Chewable. Fruit flavor. In 60s.
otc	Centrum Performance (Wyeth)	100	18	5,000	400	60	4.5	5.1	40	10	6	18	120	0.4	25 mcg vitamin K, 40 mcg biotin, chloride, 60 mg *Ginkgo biloba* leaf, 50 mg ginseng root, B, Cr, Cu, I, K, Mg, Mn, Mo, Ni, P, Se, Si, Sn, V, 15 mg Zn. Glucose, lactose, maltodextrin, sucrose	In 120s.
otc sf	Bugs Bunny Complete Tablets (Bayer)	100	18	5,000	400	30[d]	1.5	1.7	20	10	2	6	60	0.4	40 mcg biotin, Cu, I, Mg, P, aspartame, phenylalanine, 15 mg Zn	Chewable. Fruit flavor. In 60s.
Rx	Natelle-EZ (Pharmelle)	100	25	2700	400	20	3	3.5	20	8	30	12	120	1	30 mcg biotin, Cu, Mg, Se, 15 mg Zn, choline bitartrate.	(P 004). Lt. Pink, sugar-coated. Capsule shape. In 90s.
otc	4 Nails Softgel Capsules (Marlyn)	167	3	833	67	10[b]	3.3	1.7	8.3	8.3	8.3	8.3	10	33.3	8.3 mcg biotin, P, I, Mg, Cu, 3.3 mg Zn, Cr, Mn, methionine, inositol, choline bitartrate, Se, PABA, protein isolate, gelatin, lecithin, unsaturated fatty acid, predigested protein, L-cysteine, B mucopolysaccharides, silicon amino acid chelate, S	In 60s.
otc	Optimox Prenatal Tablets (Optimox)	100	5	833	67	2[k]	0.5	0.6	6.7	3.3	0.73	0.87	30	0.13	Cr, Cu, I, Mg, Mn, Se, 3.17 mg Zn	In 360s.
otc	Gynovite Plus Tablets (Optimox)	83	3	833	67	67[k]	1.7	1.7	3.3	1.7	3.3	21	30	0.07	B, betaine, biotin, Cr, Cu, hesperidin, I, inositol, Mg, Mn, PABA, pancreatin, rutin, Se, 2.5 mg Zn	In 100s.
otc	Alkavite (Vitality)	68.5	60	5000	400	30	100	3			3	12	250	1	20 mg niacin, 0.03 mg biotin, 150 mg Mg, 4 mg Zn, 0.01 mg Se.	Brown, oblong. Film-coated. In UD 100s.
otc sf	Hipotest Tablets (Marlop Pharm)	53.5	50	10,000	400	12.5[l]	25	25	50	13	15	50	150	1	Choline, betaine, PABA, rutin, bio-flavonoids, 1 mg biotin, desiccated liver, bone meal, Cu, Mg, Mn, 2.2 mg Zn, I, P, lecithin	In 100s
otc	One-A-Day Kids Scooby-Doo! Fizzy Vites Chewable Tablets (Bayer)	50	9[f]	1500	200	15	0.75	0.85	7.5	5	1	3	170	200[e]	20 mcg biotin, P, I, Mg, Zn, Cu, Na, aspartame, phenylalanine, sucrose, vegetable oil.	In 60s.
otc	Theragran-M Caplets (Mead Johnson)	40	27	5,000	400	30[d]	3	3.4	20	10	3	9	90	0.4	Cl, Cr, Cu, I, K, Mg, Mn, Mo, P, Se, 15 mg Zn, 30 mcg biotin, lactose, sucrose	(T-M). In 90s, 130s, 180s and 200s.
Rx	Mynatal PN Captabs (ME Pharm)	125	60	4,000	400		3	3	10		2	3	50	1	18 mg Zn	Blue. Film-coated. In 100s.
Rx	PreCare Prenatal Caplets (Ther-Rx)	250	40	=240	240	3.5[d]	3	3.4	20		50	12	50	1	Cu, Mg, 15 mg Zn	(Ther-Rx/118). Peach, scored. Film-coated. In UD 100s.

NUTRITIONAL COMBINATION PRODUCTS

MULTIVITAMINS WITH CALCIUM AND IRON

	Product & Distributor	Ca[a] mg	Fe[s] mg	A IU	D IU	E IU	B$_1$ mg	B$_2$ mg	B$_3$ mg	B$_5$ mg	B$_6$ mg	B$_{12}$ mcg	C mg	FA mg	Other Content	How Supplied
Rx	**PreCare Conceive Tablets** (Ther-Rx)	200	30			30[d]	3	3.4	20		50	12	60	1	2 mg Cu, 100 mg Mg, 15 mg Zn	Lactose. (Ther-Rx 014). Yellow, diamond-shape. Film-coated. In UD 100s.
Rx	**S.S.S. High Potency Vitamin Tablets** (S.S.S. Company)	100	27			50	7.5	7.5	50	10	12.5	12.5	300	200[i]	50 mg magnesium, 12 mg zinc, 1.5 mg copper, 22.5 mcg biotin.	In 20s, 40s, and 80s.

[a] Calcium and iron content expressed in mg elemental calcium and iron.
[b] Form of vitamin E unknown.
[c] As calcium carbonate and gluconate.
[d] As dL-alpha tocopheryl acetate.
[e] Content listed as mcg.
[f] As ferrous fumarate.
[g] Seyer Pharmatec, Inc., 413 St. George Street, San Juan, PR 00936; (787) 728-7044, (787) 728-7055.
[h] As dL-alpha tocopherol acetate.
[i] As calcium citrate.
[j] As carbonyl iron.
[k] As niacinamide.
[l] As d-alpha tocopheryl acid succinate.

For a comparison of the potencies of the various forms of vitamin E, see the vitamin E monograph.

NUTRITIONAL COMBINATION PRODUCTS

MULTIVITAMINS WITH MINERALS

Content given per capsule, tablet, or 5 mL.

	Product & Distributor	A IU	D IU	E IU	B₁ mg	B₂ mg	B₃ mg	B₅ mg	B₆ mg	B₁₂ mcg	C mg	FA mg	Zn[1] mg	Other Content	How Supplied
otc	Vademin-Z Capsules (Roberts/Hauck)	12,500	50	50[2]	10	5	25	10	2	25	150		2.6	Mg, Mn	In 60s.
otc sf	Total Formula-3 without Iron Tablets (Vitaline)	10,000	400	30[3]	15	15	25	25	25	25	100	0.4	30	Ca, Cr, Cu, I, K, Mg, Mn, Mo, V, B,Se, Si, vitamin K, 300 mcg biotin, hesperidin[4]	In 60s and 1000s.
Rx	Vicon Forte Capsules (Whitby)	8000		50[5]	10	5	25	10	2	10	150	1	18	Mg, Mn, lactose	(ucb 316). Orange/black. In 60s, 500s, and UD 100s.
otc sf	ICAPS Time Release Tablets (Ciba Vision)	7000		100[5]		20					200		14.25	Cu, Se	In 60s and 120s.
otc	Ondrox Tablets (LSI)	6000	300	50	0.75	0.75	10	5	1	3	125	200	7.5	50 mg Ca, 15 mcg biotin, I, Mg, Cu, P, vitamin K, K, Cr, Mn, Mo, Se, V, B, Si, citrus bioflavonoid, inositol, N-acetylcysteine, N-methionine, L-glutamine, taurine	In 60s.
otc sf	ICAPS Plus Tablets (Ciba Vision)	6000		60[5]		20					200		14.25	Cu, Se, Mn	In 60s, 120s and 180s.
Rx	Nutrifac ZX Tablets (Rising Pharmaceuticals)[6]	5000	400	50	20	20	100	25	25	50	500	1	20	Ca, Cr, Cu, Mg, Mn, Se, 200 mcg biotin	Tartrazine, mineral oil. Capsule shape. In 60s.
Rx	Glutofac-ZX Tablets (Kenwood)														Parabens, sorbitol. (GLUTOFAC-ZX). Aqua green, capsule shape. In 60s.
otc	Garfield Complete with Minerals Tablets (Menley & James)	5000	400	30[5]	1.5	1.7	20	10	2	6	60	0.4	15	Fe, Ca, Cu, P, I, Mg, 40 mcg biotin, aspartame, phenylalanine	Chewable. Character shapes. In 60s.
otc	PowerMate Tablets (Green Turtle Bay)[7]	5000		100[5]			12.5				250		2.5	Se, n-acetyl-L-cysteine	In 50s.
otc	One-A-Day Extras Antioxidant Softgel Capsules (Bayer)	5000		200[5]							250		7.5	Cu, Se, Mn, tartrazine	(One-A-Day). In 50s.
otc	Vi-Zac Capsules (Whitby)	5000		50[5]							500		18	Lactose	Orange/banded. In 60s.
otc sf	Glutofac Caplets (Kenwood/Bradley)	5000		30[5]	15	10	50	20	50		300		5	Ca, Cr, Cu, Fe, K, Mg, Mn, P, Se	In 90s.
otc	OCuSoft VMS Tablets (OCuSoft)	5000		30[5]							60			Cu, Se, 40 mg Zn	Film coated. In 60s.
Rx	Zincvit Capsules (Kenwood/Bradley)	5000	50	50[5]	10	5	25	10	2	2	300	1	9.2	Mg, Mn	(Ram/Ram). Aqua green. In 60s.
otc	Vitelle Nesentials (Fielding)	5000	400	30	3	3	25	10	2	6	120			Ca, P, Zn	In 60s.
otc	ADEKs Tablets (Scandipharm)	4000	400	150[5]	1.2	1.3	10	10	1.5	12	60	0.2	1.1	Vitamin K, 50 mcg biotin, 3 mg beta carotene, fructose	Chewable. Tan. Capsule shape. In 60s.
Rx	Eldercaps Capsules (Mayrand)	4000	400	25[5]	10	5	25	10	2		200	1	15.8	Mg, Mn, lactose	In 100s.
otc	Vicon Plus Capsules (Whitby)	4000		50[5]	10	5	25	10	2		150		18	Mg, Mn, lactose	In 60s.
otc	DermaVite (Stiefel)	3500		60		8.5			10		120	0.4	45	600 mcg biotin, 5 mg lycopene, Ca, Cr, Cu, Mn, Se, Si, sucrose	In 60s.
otc sf	Kenwood Therapeutic Liquid (Kenwood/Bradley)	3333	133	1.5[8]	2	1	20	2	0.33		50			Ca, K, Mg, Mn, P	Alcohol free. In 240 mL.
otc sf	Obtrex Tablets (Pronova)	2700	400	18	3	3.4	20		40	2	120	1	25	Se, Mg, 50 mg sodium docusate	In 60s.
otc	Flintstones Plus Calcium Tablets (Bayer)	2500	400	15[5]	1.05	1.2	13.5		1.05	4.5	60	0.3		200 mg Ca, sorbitol	Chewable. Character shapes. In 60s.
otc sf	Maximum Green Label Tablets (Vitaline)	2500	16.7	66.7[3]	16.7	8.3	31.7	66.7	16.7	16.7	200	0.13	5	Ca, Cr, I, K, Mg, Mn, Mo, Se, Si, V, 50 mcg biotin, SOD, L-lysine[4]	In 180s.
otc sf	Maximum BlueLabel Tablets (Vitaline)													Ca, Cr, Cu, I, K, Mg, Mn, Mo, Se, Si, V, 50 mcg biotin, SOD, L-lysine[4]	In 180s.
otc sf	PowerVites Tablets (Green Turtle Bay)[7]	2500	150	12.5[9]	6.3	6.3	25	25	12.5	6.3	125	0.15	2.5	B, Ca, Mg, Cu, Cr, Mn, K, Se, betaine, hesperidin, biotin[4]	In 40s, 100s and 200s.
otc sf	Vita-PMS Tablets (Bajamar)	2083	16.7	16.7[9]	4.2	4.2	4.2	4.2	50	10.4	250	0.33	4.2	Mg, Ca, Cu, Mn, K, Se, Cr, I, Fe, biotin, betaine[4]	In 100s.
otc	Po-Pon-S Tablets (Shionogi)	2000	100	5[5]	5	3	35	15	4	6	100			Ca, P	Sugar coated. In 60s and 240s.
otc	Maxovite Tablets (Tyson)	2083	16.7	16.7[9]	5	4.2	4.2	4.2	54.2	10.8	250	0.33	5	Ca, Cr, Cu, Fe, I, K, Mg, Mn, Se, 11.7 mcg biotin[4]	Sustained release. In 120s and 240s.

NUTRITIONAL COMBINATION PRODUCTS

MULTIVITAMINS WITH MINERALS

	Product & Distributor	A IU	D IU	E IU	B₁ mg	B₂ mg	B₃ mg	B₅ mg	B₆ mg	B₁₂ mcg	C mg	FA mg	Zn[1] mg	Other Content	How Supplied
otc sf	**Vita-PMS Plus Tablets** (Bajamar)	667	16.7	16.7[9]	4.2	4.2	4.2	4.2	16.7	10.4	250	0.33	4.2	Mg, Ca, Cu, Mn, K, Se, Cr, I, Fe, biotin, betaine[4]	In 100s.
otc sf	**Stress 600 w/Zinc Tablets** (Nion)			45[8]	20	10	100	25	10	25	600	0.4	5.5	Cu, 45 mcg biotin	In 60s.
otc	**Mediplex Tabules (Tablets)** (US Pharm)			60[8]	25	10	100	25	10	25	300		4	Cu, Mg, Mn	In 100s.
otc	**Bee-Zee Tablets** (Rugby)			45[8]	15	10.2	100	25	10	6	600		5.2		In 60s.
otc sf	**Z-gen Tablets** (Goldline)														In 60s.
otc	**Z-Bec Tablets** (Robins)			45[5]									22.5	Parabens	In 60s, 500s and Dis-Co pack 100s.
Rx	**Renax Caplets** (Everett)			35[9]	3	2	20	10	15	12	50	2.5	20	300 mcg biotin, Cr, Se.	*For azotemic patients with low levels of essential vitamins/minerals.* White, oblong. Film coated. In 90s.
otc sf	**Stress B-Complex Tablets** (Moore)			30[8]	15	10	100	20	5	12	500	0.4	23.9	Cu, 45 mcg biotin	In 60s.
otc sf	**Stresstabs + Zinc Tablets** (Lederle)			30[5]	10	10	100	20	5	12	500	0.4	23.9	Cu, 45 mcg biotin	(S 3). In 60s.
Rx	**Nicomide Tablets** (Sirius)											0.5		750 mg nicotinamide, 25 mg zinc oxide	In 60s.

[1] Zinc content expressed in mg elemental zinc.
[2] As dl-alpha tocopheryl succinate.
[3] As d-alpha tocopheryl succinate.
[4] Also contains bioflavonoids, choline, inositol, PABA and rutin.
[5] Form of vitamin E unknown.
[6] Rising Pharmaceuticals, Inc., 411 Sette Drive, Paramus, NJ 07652; 201-262-4200, fax 201-262-4284.
[7] The Green Turtle Bay Vitamin Co., P.O. Box 642, Summit, NJ 07902; (908) 277-2240.
[8] As dl-alpha tocopheryl acetate.
[9] As d-alpha tocopherol.

For a comparison of the potencies of various forms of vitamin E, see the Vitamin E monograph.

GERIATRIC SUPPLEMENTS WITH MULTIVITAMINS AND MINERALS
Content given per capsule, tablet or 5 mL.

	Product & Distributor	A IU	D IU	E IU	B₁ mg	B₂ mg	B₃ mg	B₅ mg	B₆ mg	B₁₂ mcg	C mg	Fe[1] mg	FA mg	Ca[1] mg	Zn mg	Other Content	How Supplied
otc sf	**Mega VM-80 Tablets** (NBTY)	10,000	1000	100[2]	80	80	80	80	80	80	250	1.2	0.4	4.5	3.58	Choline, inositol, 80 mcg biotin, PABA, bioflavonoids, betaine, hesperidin, Cu, I, K, Mg, Mn, Se	In 60s and 100s.
otc	**Vita-Plus G Softgel Capsules** (Scot-Tussin)	10,000	400	2[2]	5	2.5	40	4	1	2	75	30		75	0.5	Mg, Mn, P, K	In 100s.
otc	**One-A-Day 55 Plus Tablets** (Bayer)	6000	400	60[2]	4.5	3.4	20	20	6	25	120		0.4	220	15	30 mcg biotin, vitamin K, I, Mg, Cu, Cr, Se, Mo, Mn, K, Cl	(One-A-Day). In 50s and 80s.
otc	**Cerovite Senior Tablets** (Rugby)	6000	400	45[3]	1.5	1.7	20	10	3	25	60	9	0.2	200	15	30 mcg biotin, Cu, I, Mg, P, Cl, Cr, Mn, Mo, Ni, Se, Si, V, K, vitamin K	In 60s.
otc	**Centrum Silver Tablets** (Wyeth)	3500	400	45	1.5	1.7	20	10	3	25	60		0.4	200	15	30 mcg biotin, chloride, 250 mcg lutein, B, Cr, Cu, I, K, Mg, Mn, Mo, Ni, P, Se, Si, V, vitamin K	Sucrose, glucose. In 220s.
otc	**Certagen Senior Tablets** (Goldline)	6000	400	45[3]	1.5	1.7	20	10	3	25	60	3	0.2	80	15	30 mcg biotin, Cl, Cr, Cu, I, Mg, Mn, Mo, Ni, P, K, Se, Si, V, vitamin K	In 60s.
otc	**Gerimed Tablets** (Fielding)	5000	400	30[2]	3	3	25	2	2	6	120			370	15	P	In 60s.
Rx	**Strovite Plus Caplets** (Everett)	5000		30[3]	20	20	100	25	25	50	500	9	0.8		22.5	150 mcg biotin, Cr, Cu, Mg, Mn	(EV201). Dark red. In 100s.
otc sf	**Ultra-Freeda Tablets** (Freeda)	4166	133	66.7[2]	16.7	16.7	33	33	16.7	33	333	2	0.27	27	1.1	Choline, inositol, bioflavonoids, PABA, 100 mcg biotin, Cr, I, K, Mg, Mn, Mo, Se	In 90s, 180s and 270s.
otc sf	**Iron Free Ultra-Freeda Tablets** (Freeda)	4166	133	66.7[2]	16.7	16.7	33	33	16.7	33	333		0.27	27	1.1	Choline, inositol, bioflavonoids, PABA, 100 mcg biotin, Cr, I, K, Mg, Mn, Mo, Se	In 90s, 180s and 270s.

NUTRITIONAL COMBINATION PRODUCTS

GERIATRIC SUPPLEMENTS WITH MULTIVITAMINS AND MINERALS

	Product & Distributor	A IU	D IU	E IU	B1 mg	B2 mg	B3 mg	B5 mg	B6 mg	B12 mcg	C mg	Fe[1] mg	FA mg	Ca[1] mg	Zn mg	Other Content	How Supplied
otc	Optivite P.M.T. Tablets (Optimox)	2083	†	16.6[4]	4.2	4.2	4.2	4.2	50	10.4	250	2.5	0.03	†	4.2	Choline, Cr, Cu, I, K, Mg, Mn, Se, bioflavonoids, betaine, PABA, pancreatin, rutin, inositol, biotin	In 180s.
otc	Hep-Forte Capsules (Marlyn)	1200		10[2]	1	1	10	2	0.5	1	10		0.06		0.5	Choline, inositol, biotin, dL-methionine, desiccated liver, liver concentrate, liver fraction number 2	In 100s, 300s and 500s.
otc	Vigortol Liquid (Rugby)				0.8	0.4	8.3	1.7	0.2	0.2					0.3	Choline, I, Mg, Mn, 18% alcohol, sugar, methylparaben	Sherry wine flavor. In 473 mL.
otc	Gerivite Liquid (Goldline)											0.3				Choline, I, Mg, Mn, 18% alcohol, methylparaben, sorbitol	Rum and sherry wine flavors. In 473 mL.
otc	Viminate Liquid (Various)				2.5	1.25	25	5	0.5	0.5		7.5			1	Choline, I, Mg, Mn	In 480 mL.
otc	Geravite Elixir (Roberts-Hauck)				0.3	0.4	33.3			3.3						L-lysine, 15% alcohol, parabens, sorbitol, sucrose	Wine flavor. In 480 mL.
otc	Strovite Advance (Everett)		400	100	20	5	25	15	25	50	300		1		Zn	Carotenoids, 100 mcg biotin, alpha lipoic acid, lutein, Cr, Cu, Mg, Mn, Se, mineral oil	(EV 0208). White, oblong. In 100s.

* † – Amount not supplied by manufacturer.
[1] Calcium and iron content expressed in mg elemental calcium and iron.
[2] Form of vitamin E unknown.
[3] As dL-alpha tocopheryl acetate.
[4] As d-alpha tocopheryl acid succinate.

For a comparison of the potencies of various forms of vitamin E, see the Vitamin E monograph.

MULTIVITAMINS WITH IRON AND OTHER MINERALS

Content given per capsule, tablet or 5 mL.

	Product & Distributor	Fe[1] mg	A IU	D IU	E IU	B1 mg	B2 mg	B3 mg	B5 mg	B6 mg	B12 mcg	C mg	FA mg	Other Content	How Supplied
Rx	Prenatal-H Capsules (Cypress)	106.5												Cu, Mg, Mn, 18.2 mg Zn	(CYP187). White. In 100s.
otc	One-Tablet-Daily with Minerals (Goldline)	18	5,000	400	30[2]	1.5	1.7	20	10	2	6	60	0.4	Ca, Cl, Cr, Cu, I, K, Mg, Mn, Mo, P, Se, 30 mcg biotin, 15 mg Zn	In 100s and 1000s.
otc	Theravee-M Tablets (Vangard)	27	5,000	400	30[2]	3	3.4	30	10	3	9	120	0.4	Ca, Cl, Cr, Cu, K, I, Mg, Mn, Mo, Se, 15 mg Zn, P, 15 mcg biotin, 2,500 IU beta carotene	In 100s, 1000s and UD 100s.
otc	Therems-M Tablets (Rugby)	27	5,000[3]	400	30[2]	3	3.4	20	10	3	9	90	0.4	Ca, Cl, Cr, Cu, I, K, Mg, Mn, Mo, P, Se, 15 mg Zn, 30 mcg biotin	In 130s and 1000s.
otc	Adavite-M Tablets (Hudson)				30[3]									Ca, Cl, Cr, Cu, I, K, Mg, Mn, Mo, P, Se, 15 mg Zn, 30 mcg biotin	In 130s.
otc sf	Therapeutic-M Tablets (Goldline)				30[2]									Ca, Cl, Cr, Cu, I, K, Mg, Mn, Mo, P, Se, 15 mg Zn, 30 mcg biotin	In 1000s.
otc	Theravim-M Tablets (NBTY)				30[3]									Ca, Cl, Cr, Cu, I, K, Mg, Mn, Mo, P, Se, 15 mg Zn, 30 mcg biotin	In 130s.
Rx	Bacmin Tablets (Marnel)	27	5,000		30[2]	20	20	100	25	25	50	500	0.8	Cr, Cu, Mg, Mn, 22.5 mg Zn, 0.15 mg biotin	(EV201). Dark red. In 100s.

NUTRITIONAL COMBINATION PRODUCTS

MULTIVITAMINS WITH IRON AND OTHER MINERALS

	Product & Distributor	Fe[1] mg	A IU	D IU	E IU	B$_1$ mg	B$_2$ mg	B$_3$ mg	B$_5$ mg	B$_6$ mg	B$_{12}$ mcg	C mg	FA mg	Other Content	How Supplied
otc	Multi-Day with Calcium and Extra Iron Tablets (NBTY)	27	5,000	400	30[3]	1.5	1.7	20	10	2	6	60	0.4	Ca, 15 mg Zn, tartrazine	In 100s.
otc sf	Total Formula Tablets (Vitaline)	20	10,000	400	30[3]	15	15	25	25	25	25	100	0.4	Ca, Cr, Cu, I, K, Mg, Mn, Mo, P, Se, Si, V, vitamin K, 300 mcg biotin, 30 mg Zn, choline, bioflavonoids, hesperidin, inositol, PABA, rutin	In 90s and 100s.
otc sf	Total Formula-2 Tablets (Vitaline)													With boron. In 60s.	
otc	Optilets-M-500 Filmtabs (Abbott)	20	5,000	400	30[2]	15	10	100	20	5	12	500		Cu, I, Mg, Mn, 1.5 mg Zn	Film coated. In 120s.
otc sf	Unicap T Tablets (Upjohn)	18	5,000	400	30[3]	10	10	100	25	6	18	500	0.4	Cu, I, K, Mn, Se, 15 mg Zn, tartrazine	In 60s.
otc sf	Avail Tablets (Menley & James)	18	5,000	400	30[3]	2.25	2.55	20		3	9	90	0.4	Ca, Cr, I, Mg, Se, 22.5 mg Zn	In 60s.
otc	Myadec Tablets (Parke-Davis)	18	5,000	400	30[2]	1.7	2	20	10	3	6	60	0.4	30 mcg biotin, vitamin K, Ca, P, I, Mg, Cu, 15 mg Zn, Mn, K, Cl, Cr, Mo, Se, Ni, Si, V, B, Sn	In 130s.
otc	One-A-Day Kids Tablets (Bayer)	18	5,000	400	30	1.5	1.7	20	10	2	6	60	0.4	40 mcg biotin, Ca, Cu, P, I, Mg, 15 mg Zn	Chewable. Sorbitol, aspartame, phenylalanine. In 50s.
otc	Centrum Jr. with Iron Tablets (Lederle)	18	5,000	400	30[3]	1.5	1.7	20	10	2	6	60	0.4	Ca, Cr, Cu, I, Mg, Mn, Mo, P, 15 mg Zn, 45 mcg biotin, vitamin K	Chewable. In 60s.
otc	Cerovite Tablets (Rugby)													Ca, Cl, Cr, Cu, I, K, Mg, Mn, Mo, Ni, P, Se, Si, Sn, V, 30 mcg biotin, vitamin K, 15 mg Zn	In 130s.
otc sf	Children's SunKist Multivitamins Complete Tablets (Ciba)													Ca, 10 mg Zn, 40 mcg biotin, vitamin K, Cu, I, K, Mg, Mn, P, sorbitol, aspartame, phenylalanine, tartrazine.	Chewable. Citrus flavor. In 60s.
otc	Flintstones Complete Tablets (Bayer)													Ca, Cu, I, Mg, P, 15 mg Zn, 40 mcg biotin	Chewable. In 60s and 120s.
otc sf	Unicap M Tablets (Upjohn)													Ca, Cu, I, K, Mn, P, 15 mg Zn, tartrazine	In 120s.
otc	One-A-Day Maximum Formula Tablets (Bayer)													Ca, Cl, Cr, Cu, I, K, Mg, Mn, Mo, P, Se, 15 mg Zn, 30 mcg biotin	(One-A-Day). In 60s and 100s.
otc	Stuart Formula Tablets (J & J-Merck)	5	5,000	400	10[2]	1.5	1.7	20		1	3	50	0.1	Ca, Cu, I	In 100s.
otc	Cerovite Jr. Tablets (Rugby)	18	5,000	400	15[3]	1.5	1.7	20	10	2	6	60	0.4	Cu, I, Mg, Zn, Mn, Mo, 45 mcg biotin, Cr, sugar	In 60s.
otc	Multi-Day Plus Minerals Tablets (NBTY)	18	6,500	400	30[2]	1.5	1.7	20	10	2	6	60	0.4	Ca, Cl, Cr, Cu, I, K, Mg, Mn, Mo, P, Se, 15 mg Zn, 30 mcg biotin	In 100s.

NUTRITIONAL COMBINATION PRODUCTS

MULTIVITAMINS WITH IRON AND OTHER MINERALS

Type	Product & Distributor	Fe mg	A IU	D IU	E IU	B1 mg	B2 mg	B3 mg	B5 mg	B6 mg	B12 mcg	C mg	FA mg	Other Content	How Supplied
otc sf	Hair Booster Vitamin Tablets (NBTY)	18						35	100		6		0.4	Cu, I, Mn, 15 mg Zn, inositol, PABA, protein, choline bitartrate	In 60s.
otc sf	Quintabs-M Tablets (Freeda)	15	10,000	400	50[3]	30	30	150	30	30	30	300	0.4	Ca, Cu, Mg, Mn, Se, 30 mg Zn, PABA, K	Kosher. In 100s, 250s and 500s.
otc sf	Generix-T Tablets (Goldline)	15	10,000	400	5.5[3]	15	10	100	10	2	7.5	150		Cu, I, Mg, Mn, 1.5 mg Zn	In 100s.
otc	Multilex T & M Tablets (Rugby)	15	10,000	400	5.5[3]	15	10	100	10	2	7.5	150		Cu, I, Mg, Mn, 1.5 mg Zn	Sugar. In 100s and 1000s.
otc sf	Multilex Tabs (Rugby)	15	10,000	400	5.5[2]	10	5	30	10	1.7	3	100		Cu, I, Mg, Mn, 1.5 mg Zn	In 100s.
otc	Vitarex Tablets (Pasadena)	15	10,000	200	15[3]	15	10	100	20	5	5	250		Ca, Cu, I, K, Mg, Mn, P, 10 mg Zn	In 100s.
otc	Fosfree Tablets (Mission)	29	3,000	300		9	4	21	2	5	4	100		351 mg Ca	Sugar. In 120s.
otc	Fosfree (Mission)	14.5	1500	150		4.5	2	10.5	1	2.5	2	50		175.5 mg Ca	Sugar. In 120s.
otc sf	Monocaps Tablets (Freeda)	14	10,000	400	15[4]	15	15	41	15	15	15	125	0.1	Ca, Cu, I, K, Mg, Mn, Se, 12 mg Zn, 15 mcg biotin, L-lysine, PABA, lecithin	Kosher. In 100s, 250s and 500s.
otc	Vigomar Forte Tablets (Marlop Pharm)	12	10,000	400	15[3]	10	10	100	20	5	5	200		I, Mg, Cu, Mn, 1.5 mg Zn	In 100s.
otc	Poly-Vi-Sol w/Iron Tablets (Mead-Johnson)	12	2,500	400	15[3]	1.05	1.2	13.5		1.05	4.5	60	0.3	Cu, 8 mg Zn, sugar	Chewable. Peter Rabbit shapes. Fruit flavors. In 100s.
otc sf	Unicap Sr. Tablets (Upjohn)	10	5,000	200	15[3]	1.2	1.4	16	10	2.2	3	60	0.4	Ca, Cu, I, K, Mg, Mn, P, 15 mg Zn	In 120s.
Rx	Strovite Forte (Everett Laboratories)	10	4000[3]	400	60	20	20	100	25	25	50	500	1.0	0.15 biotin, 50 mcg Se, 50 mg MG, 15 mg Zn, 20 mcg Mo, 3 mg Cu, 0.05 mg Cr	(EV 0204). Dark green, oblong, bisect. Capsule shape. In 100s.
otc sf	Geritol Extend Caplets (SmithKline-Beecham)	10	3,333	200	15[3]	1.2	1.4	15		2	2	60	0.2	Vitamin K, Ca, I, Mg, Se, 15 mg Zn	In 40s and 100s.
otc	Advanced Formula Centrum Liquid (Lederle)	9	2,500	400	30[2]	1.5	1.7	20	10	2	6	60		300 mcg biotin, Cr, I, Mn, Mo, 3 mg Zn, 6.7% alcohol, sucrose	In 236 mL.
otc sf	Ultra Vita Time Tablets (NBTY)	6	10,000	400	13[4]	25	25	50	12.5	15	50	150	0.4	B, Ca, Cr, Cu, I, K, Mg, Mn, Mo, P, Se, 5 mg Zn, 1 mg biotin, bioflavonoids, bone meal, PABA, choline bitartrate, betaine, inositol, lecithin, desiccated liver, rutin	In 100s.
otc sf	Formula VM-2000 Tablets (Solgar)	5	12,500	200	100[3]	50	50	50	50	50	50	150	0.2	B, Ca, Cr, Cu, I, K, Mg, Mn, Mo, Se, 7.5 mg Zn, betaine, 50 mcg biotin, choline, bioflavonoids, amino acids, hesperidin, l-glutathione, PABA, rutin	In 30s, 60s, 90s and 180s.
otc	M.V.M. Capsules (Tyson & Associates)	3.6	400		60[2]	20	10	10	100	31	160	50	0.08	Ca, Cr, Cu, I, K, Mg, Mo, 6 mg Zn, 160 mcg biotin, PABA, Mn, Se, tryptophan	In 150s.

NUTRITIONAL COMBINATION PRODUCTS

MULTIVITAMINS WITH IRON AND OTHER MINERALS

	Product & Distributor	Fe[1] mg	A IU	D IU	E IU	B₁ mg	B₂ mg	B₃ mg	B₅ mg	B₆ mg	B₁₂ mcg	C mg	FA mg	Other Content	How Supplied
otc sf	**Maximum Red Label Tablets** (Vitaline)	3.3	2,500	67	66.7[3]	16.7	8.3	31.7	66.7	16.7	16.7	200	0.13	Ca, Cr, Cu, I, K, Mg, Mn, Mo, Se, Si, V, 5 mg Zn, 50 mcg biotin, choline, inositol, bioflavonoids, l-lysine, PABA	In 180s.
otc	**Androvite Tablets** (Optimox)	3	4,167	67	67[4]	8.3	8.3	8.3	16.7	16.7	20.8	167	0.06	PABA, inositol, biotin, betaine, B, Cr, Cu, I, Mg, Mn, Se, 8.3 mg Zn, pancreatin, hesperidin, rutin	In 180s.
otc sf	**ProCycle Gold Tablets** (Cyclin Pharm)	3	833.3	67	67	1.7	1.7	3.3	1.7	3.3	21	30	0.07	167 mg Ca, 2.5 mg Zn, B, Cu, Cr, I, Mg, Mn, Se, PABA, inositol, rutin, biotin, hesperidin, pancreatin, betaine	In 100s.
otc	**4 Hair Softgel Capsules** (Marlyn)	2.5	1,250		10[4]			5	25	1.5	44	25	33.3	250 mcg biotin, I, Mg, Cu, 7.5 mg Zn, choline bitartrate, inositol, Mn, methionine, PABA, B, L-cysteine, tyrosine, Si	In 60s.
otc	**S.S.S. Vitamin and Mineral Complex Liquid** (S.S.S. Company)	3	833	133[5]	10	1.7	0.57	6.7[6]	3	0.67	2	20		100 mcg biotin, 50 mcg iodine, 1 mg zinc, 0.8 mg manganese, 8 mcg chromium, 8 mcg molybdenum/5 mL	With 6.6% alcohol, sugar. In 236 mL.

[1] Iron content expressed in mg elemental iron.
[2] As dl-alpha tocopheryl acetate.
[3] Form of vitamin E unknown.

[4] As d-alpha tocopheryl acid succinate.
[5] As cholecalciferol.
[6] As niacinamide.

For a comparison of the potencies of various forms of vitamin E, see the Vitamin E monograph.

Enteral nutrition products may be administered orally, via nasogastric tube, via feeding gastrostomy or via needle-catheter jejunostomy. The defined formula diets may be monomeric or oligomeric (amino acids or short peptides and simple carbohydrates) or polymeric (more complex protein and carbohydrate sources) in composition. Modular supplements are used for individual supplementation of protein, carbohydrate or fat when formulas do not offer sufficient flexibility.

There are different criteria for evaluating and categorizing these products; no single system is ideal. Caloric density, generally in the range of 1, 1.5 or 2 Cal/mL, influences the density of other nutrients. Protein content is also a major determinant. Osmolality may be important in patients who experience diarrhea and cramping with high osmolality formulas. Consider products with low fat content in patients with significant malabsorption, hyperlipidemia or severe exocrine pancreatic insufficiency. Medium chain triglycerides are a useful energy source in patients with malabsorption, but do not provide essential fatty acids. Lactose, poorly tolerated by patients lacking lactase activity, has been eliminated from many of the nutritionally complete enteral formulas. In general, with the exception of lactose or specific allergies (eg, corn, gluten), the source of the protein or carbohydrate is not critical. Various amounts of vitamins, electrolytes and minerals are included in the formulations. Consider sodium and potassium content in patients with renal or hepatic disease. Also, consider vitamin K content in patients receiving warfarin, since the hypoprothrombinemic effect may be decreased. Although many of the products have been formulated to contain lesser amounts of vitamin K, caution is still warranted.

Some enteral preparations list the osmolality or osmolarity of the formula at standard dilution. However, when the term osmolarity is used, it cannot be determined whether the osmolarity was calculated from osmolality or if the term osmolarity is being used erroneously. Also, when samples of a specific product from the same lot or different lots were reconstituted, or if the powder was reconstituted by using the provided scoop vs reconstitution by weight, there was a wide variation in osmolality. Be aware of these potential discrepancies when utilizing osmolality information.

Cost of products is influenced by composition (oligomeric or polymeric) and form (ready-to-use or powder). In general, polymeric products cost less than oligomeric products. The form of the product indirectly affects its cost due to the amount of labor involved in preparation.

Specialized formulas are indicated for specific disease states and may be nutritionally incomplete.

Hepatic failure/encephalopathy formulas contain high concentrations of branched chain amino acids (BCAA) and low concentrations of aromatic amino acids (AAA) in an attempt to correct the abnormal plasma amino acid profiles.

Renal failure formulas contain only essential amino acids as the source of protein.

Trauma or high stress formulas contain high concentrations of BCAA, but unlike the hepatic products, are not restricted in the amounts of AAA.

Monitoring of patients receiving enteral nutritional therapy includes the following: Weight, fluid balance, serum electrolytes, glucose tolerance, liver and renal function, albumin and general condition. Watch for GI overload or obstruction and abdominal distention; check tube placement for proper position. Initiate therapy with a slow but gradual advancement in administration rate.

Several case reports and single-dose studies suggest that phenytoin administration during enteral nutritional therapy may result in decreased phenytoin concentrations; however, this has not been substantiated. Monitor phenytoin concentrations in these patients. Consider giving phenytoin 2 hours before and after the enteral feeding, or stopping the enteral therapy for 2 hours before and after phenytoin administration.

Enteral Nutritional Product Categories	
Modular Supplements	*Defined Formulas*
Protein	Milk-based formulas
Carbohydrate	Specialized formulas
Fat	Hepatic failure/encephalopathy
	Renal failure
	Trauma/stress
	Pulmonary
	Nutritionally complete,
	lactose free formulas

Content listed is based on standard dilutions. Refer to manufacturer's literature for mixing directions, other dilutions and storage conditions.

Modular Supplements

PROTEIN PRODUCTS

otc	**Gevral Protein** (Lederle)	**Powder:** Ca caseinate and sucrose. Each cup ($\approx$ 26 g) contains: 15.6 g protein, 7.05 g carbohydrate, 0.52 g fat, < 50 mg Na, $\geq$ 13 mg K and 95.3 Calories. *Dose:* 26 g in 8 oz liquid.	< 1% alcohol. In 8 oz and 5 lb.
otc	**ProMod** (Ross)	**Powder:** D-whey protein concentrate and soy lecithin. Each 26.4 g provides 20 g protein, 2.4 g fat, 2.68 g carbohydrate, 176 mg Ca, 60 mg Na, 260 mg K, 132 mg P and 112 Calories. *Dose:* Add 1 scoop (6.6 g) to liquid, food or enteral formula.	In 275 g cans.
otc	**Propac** (Sherwood)	**Powder:** Each tablespoon (4 g) contains 3 g protein (from whey protein), 0.24 g carbohydrate from lactose, 0.32 g fat, 2 mg Cl, 20 mg K, 9 mg Na, 14 mg Ca, 12 mg P, 2 mg Mg and 16 Calories. *Dose:* Add 1 tablespoon to liquid.	In 20 g packets and 350 g cans.
otc	**Essential ProPlus** (NutriSOY International, Inc.[1])	**Powder:** 16.3 g protein, 0.2 g fat, 6.4 g carbohydrates, 242.5 mg Na, 112.5 mg K, 70 mg Ca, 31.3 mg Mg, 3 mg Fe, 187.5 mg P, 0.4 mg Cu, 0.5 mg Zn, 12.9 mcg I, 0.1 mg B_1, 0.2 mg B_3, 0.1 mg folic acid/25 g. *Dose:* Add 2 tablespoons to liquid or food.	In 2 lb. containers.
otc	**Immunocal** (Immunotech Research)	**Powder:** $\approx$ 18 to 28 g whey protein/100g, $\geq$ 1.5 mg vitamin B_1/100 g. *Dose:* Mix 1 packet with liquid or food.	In 10 g packets.

[1] (888) 769-0769.

Refer to additional information in the Enteral Nutritional Therapy introduction.

GLUCOSE POLYMERS

These glucose polymers are derived from cornstarch by hydrolysis. Content given per 100 mL liquid or 100 g powder.

	Product & Distributor	CHO (g)	Calories	Sodium (mg)	Chloride (mg)	Potassium (mg)	Calcium (mg)	Phosphorus (mg)	How Supplied
otc	**Polycose Liquid** (Ross)	50	200	70	140	6	20	3	In 126 mL.
otc	**Polycose Powder** (Ross)	94	380	110	223	10	30	5	In 350 g.
otc	**Moducal Powder** (Mead Johnson Nutritional)	95[1]	380	70	150	< 10	—	—	In 368 g.[2]
otc	**Sumacal Powder** (Sherwood)	95[1]	380	100	210	< 39	< 20	< 31	In 400 g.[2]

[1] Maltodextrin. [2] Contains 0.4 g/100 g minerals (ash).

Refer to additional information in the Enteral Nutritional Therapy introduction.

Indications

Supplies calories in persons with increased caloric needs or persons unable to meet their caloric needs with usual food intake. Supplies carbohydrate calories in protein, electrolyte and fat restricted diets. Also used to increase the caloric density of traditional foods, liquid and tube feedings.

Administration and Dosage

Add to foods or beverages or mix in water. Small, frequent feedings are more desirable than large amounts given infrequently. May be used for extended periods with diets containing all other essential nutrients, or as an oral adjunct to IV administration of nutrients. Not a balanced diet; do not use as a sole source of nutrition.

CORN OIL

otc	**Lipomul** (Roberts)	**Liquid:** 10 g corn oil per 15 mL in a vehicle containing polysorbate 80, glyceride phosphates and 6.3 mg saccharin (from sodium saccharin) with 0.05% sodium benzoate, 0.05% benzoic acid, 0.07% sorbic acid, BHA and vitamin E. Each serving (45 mL) contains 270 Calories and 30 g fat.	Citrus-vanilla flavor. In 473 mL.

Refer to additional information in the Enteral Nutritional Therapy introduction.

Indications

Increasing caloric intake.

Administration and Dosage

➤*Adults:* 45 mL 2 to 4 times daily, after or between meals.

➤*Children:* 30 mL 1 to 4 times daily, after or between meals.

Precautions

Use in the presence of gallbladder disease or diabetes only on the advice of a physician.

SAFFLOWER OIL

otc	**Microlipid** (Sherwood)	**Emulsion:** 50% fat emulsion. Safflower oil, polyglycerol esters of fatty acids, soy lecithin, xanthan gum and ascorbic acid. Contains 4500 Calories and 500 g fat per L. *Osmolality* - 60 mOsm/kg water	In 120 mL.

Refer to additional information in the Enteral Nutritional Therapy introduction.

Indications

Dietary management of patients requiring caloric supplementation (ie, fatty acid deficiencies). Supplies essential fatty acids.

Administration and Dosage

➤*Oral:* May give by tablespoon. Flavor additives may improve patient acceptance.

➤*Tube feeding:* Can be added to a patient's formula depending upon the degree of caloric supplementation needed.

Shake well before using.

Precautions

Use in the presence of gallbladder disease or diabetes only on the advice of a physician.

Do not administer to patients with a severe malabsorption syndrome.

MEDIUM CHAIN TRIGLYCERIDES (MCT)

otc	**MCT** (Mead Johnson Nutritionals)	**Oil:** Lipid fraction of coconut oil consisting primarily of the triglycerides of C_8 ($\approx$ 67%) and C_{10} ($\approx$ 23%) saturated fatty acids. Contains 115 Calories/15 mL	In qt.

Refer to additional information in the Enteral Nutritional Therapy introduction.

Indications

A special dietary supplement for use in the nutritional management of patients who cannot efficiently digest and absorb conventional long chain food fats.

Administration and Dosage

15 mL, 3 to 4 times per day. Mix with fruit juices, use on salads and vegetables, incorporate into sauces or use in cooking or baking. Do not use plastic containers or utensils.

Actions

➤*Pharmacology:* Medium chain triglycerides are more rapidly hydrolyzed than conventional food fat, require less bile acid for digestion, are carried by the portal circulation and are not dependent on chylomicron formation or lymphatic transport. Does not provide essential fatty acids.

Precautions

➤*Hepatic cirrhosis:* In persons with advanced cirrhosis, large amounts of MCT may elevate blood and spinal fluid levels of medium chain fatty acids (MCFA) due to impaired hepatic clearance of MCFA which are rapidly absorbed via the portal vein. These elevated levels have caused reversible coma and precoma in subjects with advanced cirrhosis, particularly with portacaval shunts. Use with caution in persons with hepatic cirrhosis and complications such as portacaval shunts or tendency to encephalopathy.

ENTERAL NUTRITIONAL THERAPY

Defined Formula Diets

MILK-BASED FORMULAS

	Product & Distributor	Protein g	Protein Source	Carbohydrate g	Carbohydrate Source	Fat g	Fat Source	Na (mg)	K (mg)	mOsm/kg H₂O	Cal/mL	Other Content	How Supplied
otc	**Epulor** (VistaPharm)	89	milk protein, iso-leucine, leucine, lysine, methionine/cystine, phenylalanine/tyrosine, threonine, tryptophan, valine			755	soybean oil				7.1	Vit. A, B_1, B_2, B_3, B_5, B_6, B_{12}, C, D, E, K, B, Ca, Cl, Cr, Cu, Fe, I, Mg, Mn, Mo, Ni, P, Se, Si, Sn, V, Zn, biotin, folate	Lemon flavor. In 1.5 oz pouches.
otc	**NovaSource Renal** (Novartis Nutrition)	74	sodium and calcium caseinates, arginine, taurine, carnitine	200	corn syrup, fructose, hydrolyzed corn starch	100	high oleic sunflower oil, corn oil, medium chain triglycerides, soy lecithin	1000 (43.5 mEq) (complete feeding Brik Paks); 1600 (70 mEq) (closed system)	810 (20.8 mEq) (complete feeding Brik Paks); 1100 (28.2 mEq) (closed system)	700 (complete feeding Brik Paks); 960 (closed system)	2	Vit. A, B_1, B_2, B_3, B_5, B_6, B_{12}, C, D, E, K, Ca, Cl, Cu, Fe, I, Mg, Mn, P, Se, Zn, folic acid, biotin, choline	Vanilla flavor. In 237 mL Tetra Brik Paks (27s) and 1000 mL closed system containers (6s).
otc	**Meritene Powder**[1] (Sandoz Nutrition)	69.2	nonfat milk, whole milk, Ca caseinate, amino acids	119	sugar, hydrolyzed corn starch, fructose	34	soy lecithin	1077 (47 mEq)	2808 (72 mEq)	690	1.06	Vit. A, B_1, B_2, B_3, B_5, B_6, B_{12}, C, D, E, K, Ca, Cl, Cu, Fe, I, Mg, Mn, P, Zn^2	Plain (sugar free), chocolate, eggnog, vanilla and milk chocolate flavors. In 1 and 4.5 lb.
otc	**Forta Shake Powder**[3] (Ross)	9	nonfat milk	26	sucrose	< 1	unknown	115 (5 mEq)	440 (11.3 mEq)	NA	140	Vit. A, B_1, B_2, B_3, B_5, B_6, B_{12}, C, D, E, Ca, Cu, Fe, I, Mg, Mn, P, Zn^4	Vanilla, strawberry and eggnog flavors. In 470 g cans. Dutch chocolate flavor. In 530 g cans.
otc	**Ensure Pudding**[5] (Ross)	6.8	nonfat milk	34	sucrose, modified food starch	9.7	partially hydrogenated soybean oil	240	330	unknown	250	Vitamin A, D, E, K, C, folic acid, B_1, B_2, B_6, B_{12}, B_3, choline, biotin, B_5, Cl, Ca, Zn, Fe, P, Mg, I, Mn, Cu, tartrazine	Vanilla, chocolate, and butterscotch flavors. In 150 g cans.
otc	**Sustacal Pudding**[5] (Mead Johnson Nutritionals)	6.8	nonfat milk, amino acids	32	sugar, lactose, modified food starch	9.5	partially hydrogenated soy oil	120 (5.2 mEq)	320 (8.2 mEq)	NA	240	Vit. A, B_1, B_2, B_3, B_5, B_6, B_{12}, C, D, E, Ca, Cl, Cu, Fe, I, Mg, Mn, P, Zn^4, tartrazine (vanilla flavor)	Vanilla, chocolate and butterscotch flavors. In 150 g.
otc	**Nepro Liquid** (Ross)	6.6	Ca, Mg and Na caseinates	51.1	sucrose, hydrolyzed cornstarch	22.7	high-oleic safflower oil, soy oil	197	251	NA	2	Vit. A, D, E, C, B_1, B_3, B_5, B_6, B_{12}, I, biotin, FA, Na, K, Cl, Ca, P, Mg, Mn, Cu, Zn, Fe, Se^6	Lactose free. Vanilla flavor. In 240 mL ready-to-use cans.
otc	**Nutraloric Powder**[1] (Nutraloric)	91.5	Na and Ca caseinates	175	corn syrup solids, fructose	125	soybean oil, soy lecithin, mono- and diglycerides	874 (38 mEq)	3166.2 (81 mEq)	unknown	2.2	Vit. A, B_1, B_2, B_3, B_5, B_6, B_{12}, C, D, E, K, Ca, Cl, Cu, Fe, I, Mg, Mn, P, Zn^2	Chocolate, strawberry, banana nut and vanilla flavors. In 1 lb.
otc	**Immunocal**[6] (Immunotec)	37.5	milk protein isolate	0.42		0		25	30	unknown	0.15	Ca, Mg, P	In 10 g packets (30s).

1 Content given for powder mixed with whole milk.
2 Also contains folic acid, biotin and choline.
3 Content given per serving (42 g mix).
4 Also contains folic acid and biotin.
5 Content given per serving (150 g).
6 Mixed with 8 oz. of fluid per directions.

See individual product listings for specific labeled indications.

SPECIALIZED FORMULAS

Defined Formula Diets

	Product & Distributor	Protein g	Protein Source	Carbohydrate g	Carbohydrate Source	Fat g	Fat Source	Na (mg)	K (mg)	mOsm/kg H_2O	Cal/mL	Other Content	How Supplied
otc	**Amin-Aid Instant Drink Powder**[1] (McGaw)	6.6	amino acids (including phenylalanine)	124.3	maltodextrins, sucrose	15.7	partially hydrogenated soybean oil, lecithin, mono- and diglycerides	< 115 (5 mEq)	NA	700	2	Tartrazine (lemon-lime flavor)	*For acute or chronic renal failure.* Lemon-lime flavor. In 156 g packets (12s).
otc	**Boost Nutritional Pudding** (Mead Johnson Nutritionals)	7	unknown	32	unknown	9	unknown	120	320	unknown	240	Vit A, C, D, E, K, B_6, B_1, B_2, B_3, B_5, Ca, Fe, folic acid, biotin, P, I, Mg, Zn, Cu, Mn, Cr, Mo	Sugar. Vanilla, chocolate, and butterscotch flavors. In 142 g.
otc	**Boost Pudding**[2] (Mead Johnson)	10	unknown	35	unknown	7	unknown	130	400	unknown	240	Vit A, C, D, E, B_1, B_2, B_3, B_5, B_6, B_9, B_{12}, biotin, Ca, P, I, Mg, Zn, Cu, sugar, corn syrup	Vanilla, chocolate, strawberry and mocha flavors. In 237 mL.
otc	**Optimental Liquid** (Ross)	12.2	unknown	32.9	unknown	6.7	unknown	250	420	unknown	un-known	Vit A, D, E, K, C, folic acid, B_1, B_2, B_{12}, B_3, choline, biotin, B_5 chloride, Ca, P, Mg, I, Mn, Cu, Zn, Fe, Se, Cr, Mo	Sucrose, canola oil, soy oil. Vanilla and chocolate flavors. In 237 mL.
otc	**Hepatic-Aid II Instant Drink Powder**[3] (McGaw)	15	amino acids (high BCAA, low AAA)	57.3	maltodextrins, sucrose	12.3	partially hydrogenated soybean oil, lecithin, mono- and diglycerides	< 115 (5 mEq)	unknown	560	1.2	May contain tartrazine	*For chronic liver disease.* Chocolate, eggnog and custard flavors. In 93 g packets (12s).
otc	**Cyclinex-2 Powder**[4] (Ross)	15	amino acids (including carnitine, phenylalanine, tryptophan)	40	hydrolyzed corn-starch	20.7	palm oil, hydrogenated coconut oil, soy oil, mono-and diglycerides	1175 (51.1 mEq)	1830 (47 mEq)	NA	480	Vit A, B_1, B_2, B_3, B_5, B_6, B_{12}, C, D, E, K, inositol, Cl, Cu, I, Mg, Mn, P, Se, Zn, Ca, Fe^5	*For urea cycle disorder or gyrate atrophy.* Nonessential amino acid free. In 325 g.
otc	**Immun-Aid Powder**[6] (McGaw)	18.5	lactalbumin, amino acids (including carnitine, phenylalanine, taurine)	60	maltodextrins	11	medium chain triglycerides, canola oil	290 (12.6 mEq)	530 (13.6 mEq)	460	1	Vit A, B_1, B_2, B_3, B_5, B_6, B_{12}, C, D, E, K, Ca, Fe, Cl, Cu, Cr, I, Mg, Mn, Mo, P, Se, Zn^5	*For immunocompromised patients.* Custard flavor. In 123 g packets (24s).
otc	**BCAD 2 Powder**[4] (Mead Johnson Nutritionals)	24	L-glutamine, potassium aspartate, L-lysine HCl, L-tyrosine, L-proline, L-alanine, L-arginine, L-phenylalanine, L-threonine, L-serine, glycine, L-histidine, L-methionine, L-tryptophan, L-cystine, L-carnitine, taurine	57	corn syrup solids, sugar, modified corn starch	8.5	soy oil	610	1220	unknown	410	Vit A, B_1, B_2, B_3, B_5, B_6, B_{12}, C, D, E, K, inositol, Ca, Cl, Cr, Cu, Fe, I, Mg, Mn, Mo, P, Se, Zn^5	*For Maple Syrup Urine Disease or other inborn errors of branched chain amino acid metabolism.* In 1 lb cans.
otc	**Arginaid Extra Liquid** (Novartis Nutrition)	25.3	Whey protein isolate, L-arginine, L-cysteine	219.4	Sugar, hydrolyzed corn starch	0		< 295	< 93	un-known	1.05	Vitamins A, B_1, B_2, B_3, B_5, B_6, B_{12}, C, D, E, K, biotin, folic acid, Cu, Fe, I, Mn, P, Zn	For promotion of wound healing. Orange and wild berry flavors. In 8 oz Tetra Brik Paks.
otc	**Suplena Liquid** (Ross)	29.6	Ca and Na caseinates, carnitine, taurine	252.5	hydrolyzed corn starch, sucrose	95	high-oleic safflower oil, soy oil, soy lecithin	775 (34 mEq)	1104 (28.3 mEq)	un-known	2	Vit A, B_1, B_2, B_3, B_5, B_6, B_{12}, C, D, E, K, Ca, Cl, Cu, Fe, I, Mg, Mn, P, Se, Zn^5	*For renal conditions.* Vanilla flavor. In 240 mL ready-to-use cans.
otc	**Glutarex-2 Powder**[4] (Ross)	30	amino acids (including carnitine and phenylalanine)	30	hydrolyzed corn-starch	15.5	palm oil, hydrogenated coconut oil, soy oil, mono-and diglycerides	880 (38.3 mEq)	1370 (35 mEq)	NA	410	Vit A, B_1, B_2, B_3, B_5, B_6, B_{12}, C, D, E, inositol, K, Cl, Cu, I, Mg, Mn, P, Se, Zn, Ca, Fe^5	*For glutaric aciduria type I.* Lysine- and tryptophan-free. In 325 g.
otc	**Hominex-2 Powder**[4] (Ross)	30	amino acids (including carnitine, phenylalanine, tryptophan)	30	hydrolyzed corn-starch	15.5	palm oil, hydrogenated coconut oil, soy oil, mono-and diglycerides	880 (38.3 mEq)	1370 (35.1 mEq)	NA	410	Vit A, B_1, B_2, B_3, B_5, B_6, B_{12}, C, D, E, K, inositol, Cl, Cu, I, Mg, Mn, P, Se, Zn^5	*For vitamin B_6-nonresponsive homocystinuria or hypermethioninemia.* Methionine free. In 325 g.

Content per Liter

ENTERAL NUTRITIONAL THERAPY

Defined Formula Diets

SPECIALIZED FORMULAS

	Product & Distributor	Protein (g)	Protein Source	Carbohydrate (g)	Carbohydrate Source	Fat (g)	Fat Source	Na (mg)	K (mg)	mOsm/kg H₂O	Cal/mL	Other Content	How Supplied
otc	I-Valex-2 Powder[4] (Ross)	30	carnitine, phenylalanine, tryptophan, amino acids	30	hydrolyzed corn-starch	15.5	palm oil, hydrogenated coconut oil, soy oil, mono-and diglycerides	880 (38.3 mEq)	1370 (35.1 mEq)	NA	410	Vit A, B₁, B₂, B₃, B₅, B₆, B₁₂, C, D, E, K, inositol, Ca, Cl, Cu, I, Mg, Mn, P, Se, Zn⁵	*For disorder of leucine catabolism.* Leucine free. In 325 g.
otc	Ketonex-2 Powder[4] (Ross)	30	carnitine, phenylalanine, tryptophan, amino acids	30	hydrolyzed corn-starch	15.5	palm oil, hydrogenated coconut oil, soy oil, mono-and diglycerides	880 (38.3 mEq)	1370 (35.1 mEq)	NA	410	Vit A, B₁, B₂, B₃, B₅, B₆, B₁₂, C, D, E, K, inositol, Ca, Cl, Cu, I, Mg, Mn, P, Se, Zn⁵	*For maple syrup urine disease (MSUD).* Isoleucine, leucine and valine free. In 325 g.
otc	Phenex-2 Powder[2] (Ross)	30	amino acids (including carnitine, tryptophan)	30	hydrolyzed corn-starch	15.5	palm oil, hydrogenated coconut oil, soy oil, mono-and diglycerides	880 (38.3 mEq)	1370 (35.1 mEq)	NA	410	Vit A, B₁, B₂, B₃, B₅, B₆, B₁₂, C, D, E, K, inositol, Ca, Cl, Cu, I, Mg, Mn, P, Se, Zn⁵	*For phenylketonuria (PKU).* Phenylalanine free. In 325 g.
otc	Propimex-2 Powder[4] (Ross)	30	amino acids (including carnitine, phenylalanine, tryptophan)	30	hydrolyzed corn-starch	15.5	palm oil hydrogenated coconut oil, soy oil, mono-and diglycerides	880 (38.3 mEq)	1370 (35.1 mEq)	NA	410	Vit A, B₁, B₂, B₃, B₅, B₆, B₁₂, C, D, E, K, inositol, Ca, Cl, Cu, I, Mg, Mn, P, Se, Zn⁵	*For propionic or methylmalonic acidemia.* Methionine and valine free. In 325 g.
otc	Tyrex-2 Powder[4] (Ross)	30	amino acids (including carnitine, tryptophan)	30	hydrolyzed corn-starch	15.5	palm oil, hydrogenated coconut oil, soy oil	880 (38.3 mEq)	1370 (35.1 mEq)	NA	410	Vit A, B₁, B₂, B₃, B₅, B₆, B₁₂, C, D, E, K, inositol, Ca, Cl, Cu, I, Mg, Mn, P, Se, Zn⁵	*For tyrosinemia type II.* Phenylalanine and tyrosine free. In 325 g.
otc	Epulor Liquid[7] (VistaPharm)	31	unknown	4	unknown	5	unknown	7	35	NA	315	Biotin, Ca, chloride, Cr, Cu, folic acid, I, Fe, Mg, Mn, Mo, B₃, Ni, B₅, P, Se, Si, Sn, V, Vit. A, B₁, B₁₂, B₂, B₅, C, D, E, K.	Caramel flavor. In 24s.
otc	Peptamen Liquid (Nestle Clinical Nutrition)	40	enzymatically hydrolyzed whey proteins, amino acids (including carnitine, taurine)	127.2	maltodextrin, starch	39.2	MCT (fractionated coconut oil), sunflower oil, soy lecithin					Vit. A, B₁, B₂, B₃, B₅, B₆, B₁₂, C, D, E, K, Cl, Ca, P, Mg, I, Mn, Cu, Zn, Fe, Se, Cr, Mo²	*For GI impairment.* Unflavored. In ready-to-use 250 mL cans and 500 mL, 1 L, and 1.5 L UltraPak bags.
otc	Glucerna Liquid (Ross)	41	amino acids (including carnitine, taurine), Ca and Na caseinate	93	hydrolyzed corn-starch, fructose, soy fiber	55	high-oleic safflower oil, soy oil, soy lecithin	917 (40 mEq)	1542 (40 mEq)	375	1	Vit A, B₁, B₂, B₃, B₅, B₆, B₁₂, C, D, E, K, Cl, Ca, P, Mg, I, Mn, Cu, Zn, Fe, Se, Cr, Mo⁵	*For abnormal glucose tolerance.* Vanilla flavor. In 240 mL ready-to-use cans and 1 liter ready-to-hang feeding containers.
otc	Nutrament Liquid (Mead Johnson Nutritionals)	44.5	Ca and Na caseinates, skim milk, soy protein isolates (in all flavors except chocolate)	144.6	Sugar, corn syrup	27.8	canola oil, high oleic sunflower oil, corn oil, soy lecithin	695	1390	unknown	1	Vit A, B₁, B₂, B₃, B₅, B₆, B₁₂, C, D, E, K, biotin, folate, Ca, Cr, Cu, Fe, I, Mg, Mn, Mo, P, Se, Zn.	In vanilla, strawberry, chocolate, banana, coconut, and eggnog flavors. In 12 oz cans.
otc	Peptinex Liquid (Novartis Nutrition)	50	Whey protein hydrolysate, taurine, L-carnitine	160	Hydrolyzed corn starch	17	Soybean oil, medium chain triglycerides, soy lecithin	1010 (44 mEq)	1490 (38 mEq)	320	1	Vitamins A, B₁, B₂, B₃, B₅, B₆, B₁₂, C, D, E, K, biotin, choline, folic acid, Ca, Cl, Cr, Cu, Fe, I, Mg, Mn, Mo, P, Se, Zn	*For GI impaired patients.* Vanilla flavor. In 8 oz *Tetra Brik* Paks.
otc	Pulmocare Liquid[8] (Ross)	62	Ca and Na caseinate, amino acids (including carnitine, taurine)	104	hydrolyzed corn-starch, sucrose	92	corn oil, soy lecithin, canola oil, MCT (fractionated coconut oil), high-oleic safflower oil	1292 (56 mEq)	1708 (44 mEq)	475	1.5	Vit A, B₁, B₂, B₃, B₅, B₆, B₁₂, C, D, E, K, Cl, Ca, P, Mg, I, Mn, Cu, Zn, Fe, Se, Cr, Mo⁵	*For pulmonary patients.* Lactose free. Vanilla and strawberry flavors. In 240 mL ready-to-use cans and 1 liter ready-to-hang containers.
otc	NutriHeal (Nestle)	62.4	ca-K caseinate (from cow's milk), taurine	112.8	corn syrup solids, fructooligosaccharides, sugar (sucrose)	33.2	canola oil, corn oil, soy lecithin	876	1248		1	Vit A, B₁, B₂, B₃, B₅, B₆, B₁₂, C, D, E, K, beta carotene, biotin, chloride, choline, folic acid, Ca, Cr, Cu, Fe, I, Mg, Mn, Mo, P, Se, Zn.	Vanilla flavor. In 250 mL cans.

ENTERAL NUTRITIONAL THERAPY

Defined Formula Diets

SPECIALIZED FORMULAS

	Product & Distributor	Protein		Carbohydrate		Fat		Na (mg)	K (mg)	mOsm/ kg H₂O	Cal/ mL	Other Content	How Supplied
		g	Source	g	Source	g	Source						
												Content per Liter	
otc	**Jevity 1.5 Cal** (Ross)	63.4	Ca and Na caseinates, soy protein isolate, taurine, L-carnitine	214.2	corn syrup solids, corn maltodextrin, fructooligosaccharides, oat fiber, soy fiber	49.6	high oleic safflower oil, canola oil	1386	1848		1.5	Vit A, B₁, B₂, B₃, B₅, B₆, B₁₂, C, D, E, K, Cr, Ca, Cu, Fe, I, Mg, Mn, Mo, P, Se, Zn, biotin, chloride, choline, folic acid	In 237 mL cans and 1 and 1.5 L ready-to-hang containers.
otc	**Respalor Liquid** (Mead Johnson Nutritionals)	75	Ca and Na caseinate	146	corn syrup, sugar	70	MCT (fractionated coconut oil), soy lecithin, canola oil	1250 (54 mEq)	1458 (37 mEq)	580	1.5	Vit A, B₁, B₂, B₃, B₅, B₆, B₁₂, C, D, E, K, Cl, Ca, P, Mg, I, Mn, Cu, Zn, Fe, Se, Cr, Mo⁵	*For pulmonary patients.* Lactose free. Vanilla flavor. In ready-to-use 240 mL.
otc	**TraumaCal Liquid** (Mead Johnson Nutritionals)	83	Ca and Na caseinate, amino acids (including phenylalanine, tryptophan)	195	corn syrup, sugar	69	soybean oil, MCT (fractionated coconut oil), lecithin	1200 (52 mEq)	1400 (36 mEq)	490	1.5	Vit A, B₁, B₂, B₃, B₅, B₆, B₁₂, C, D, E, K, Ca, P, I, Fe, Mg, Mn, Cu, Zn, Cl⁵	*For moderately and severely stressed patients.* Lactose free. Vanilla flavor. In 237 mL ready-to-use cans.
otc	**Pro-Stat 64 Liquid**⁹ (Medical Nutrition)	500	collagen hydrolysate, amino acids (including histidine, isoleucine, leucine, lysine, methionine, phenylalanine, threonine, tryptophan, valine, alanine, arginine, aspartic acid, cystine, glutamic acid, glycine, proline, serine, tyrosine, hydroxylysine, hydroxyproline)	33	sorbitol, sucralose	0	N/A	2438	390	unknown	2.1	Cl, Mg, P, Cu	Butter pecan and cherry flavors. In 946 mL
otc	**Pro-Stat 101 Liquid**⁹ (Medical Nutrition)	500	collagen hydrolysate, amino acids (including histidine, isoleucine, leucine, lysine, methionine, phenylalanine, threonine, tryptophan, valine, alanine, arginine, aspartic acid, cystine, glutamic acid, glycine, proline, serine, tyrosine, hydroxylysine, hydroxyproline)	340	fructose, sucralose	0	N/A	2438	390	unknown	3.4	Cl, Mg, P, Cu	Butter pecan and cherry flavors. In 946 mL

¹ Content given per 156 g package.
² Content given per 237 mL.
³ Content given per ≈ 93 g packets.
⁴ Content given per 100 g.
⁵ Also contains folic acid, biotin and choline.

⁶ Content given per 123 g.
⁷ Content given per 240 mL.
⁸ Content given for vanilla flavor.
⁹ Content given per 946 mL.

See individual product listings for specific labeled indications.

ENTERAL NUTRITIONAL THERAPY

Defined Formula Diets

LACTOSE-FREE PRODUCTS

	Product & Distributor	Protein (g)	Protein Source	Carbohydrate (g)	Carbohydrate Source	Fat (g)	Fat Source	Na (mg)	K (mg)	mOsm/ kg H$_2$O	Cal/ mL	Other Content	How Supplied
otc	Nestle VHC 2.25 Liquid (Nestle Clinical Nutrition)	90	Calcium potassium caseinate, taurine, isolated soy protein	196	Corn syrup solids, sugar (sucrose)	120	Canola oil, corn oil, soy lecithin	1200	1732	950	2.25	Vit A, B$_1$, B$_2$, B$_3$, B$_5$, B$_6$, C, D, E, K, biotin, choline, FA, Na, Ca, Cr, Cu, Fe, I, Mg, Mn, Mo, P, Se, Zn	Gluten free. Vanilla flavor. In 250 mL cans.
otc	Nepro Liquid (Clintec)	69.7	Ca, Mg and Na caseinates	214.6	sucrose, hydrolyzed cornstarch	95.3	90% high-oleic safflower oil, 10% soy oil	215	1054	NA	2	Vit A, B$_1$, B$_3$, B$_5$, B$_6$, B$_{12}$, biotin, FA, Na, K, Cl, Ca, P, Mg, Mn, I, Cu, Zn, Fe, Se	Vanilla flavor. In 240 mL ready-to-use-cans.
otc	NutriFocus (Abbott)	62.16	arginine, sodium caseinates, soy and milk protein isolate	213.78	corn syrup, fiber blend, fuctooligosaccharides, sucrose	49.14	canola oil, corn oil, high oleic safflower oil, lecithin	924 (40.32 mEq)	1680 (42.84 mEq)	NA	1.5	Vit A, B$_1$, B$_2$, B$_3$, B$_5$, B$_6$, B$_{12}$, C, D, E, K, Ca, Cl, Cu, Cr, Fe, I, Mg, Mn, Mo, P, Se, Zn^1	Gluten-free. Chocolate and vanilla flavors. In 237 mL.
otc	Entrition 0.5 Liquid (Clintec)	17.5	Na and Ca caseinate	68	maltodextrin	17.5	corn oil, soy lecithin, mono- and diglycerides	350 (15.2 mEq)	600 (15.4 mEq)	120	0.5	Vit A, B$_1$, B$_2$, B$_3$, B$_5$, B$_6$, B$_{12}$, C, D, E, K, Ca, P, Mg, I, Fe, Zn, Mn, Cu, Cl^1	Unflavored. In 1 L closed system pouches.
otc	Pre-Attain Liquid (Sherwood)	20	Na caseinate	60	maltodextrin	20	corn oil, soy lecithin	340 (15 mEq)	575 (15 mEq)	150	0.5	Vit A, B$_1$, B$_2$, B$_3$, B$_5$, B$_6$, B$_{12}$, C, D, E, K, Ca, Cl, Cu, I, Fe, Mg, Mn, P, Zn^1	In 1 L pre-filled closed system containers.
otc	Citrotein Powder and Liquid^2 (Novartis)	41	egg white solids, amino acids (including phenylalanine, tryptophan)	122	sugar, hydrolyzed cornstarch	1.6	mono- and diglycerides, partially hydrogenated soybean oil	669 (29 mEq)	551 (14 mEq)	500	0.67	Vit A, B$_1$, B$_2$, B$_3$, B$_5$, B$_6$, B$_{12}$, C, D, E, Ca, P, I, Fe, Mg, Cu, Zn, Cl, Mn^1	Cholesterol and gluten free. Orange and grape flavors. In 47.1 g packets (72s) and 424 mL cans (12s).
otc	Choice dm (Mead Johnson Nutritionals)	10.6	unknown	25	unknown	12	unknown			un-known	1	Vit A, D, E, K, C, FA, B$_1$, B$_2$, B$_3$, B$_5$, B$_6$, B$_{12}$, biotin, Ca, P, I, Fe, Mg, Cu, Zn, Mn, Cl, K, Na, Se, Cr, Mo, sucrose	Vanilla flavor. In 240 mL ready-to-use cans.
otc	Vitaneed Liquid (Sherwood)	40	pureed beef, Ca and Na caseinate, dietary fiber from soy	128	maltodextrin, pureed fruits and vegetables	40	corn oil, soy lecithin	630 (27.4 mEq)	1250 (32 mEq)	300	1	Vit A, B$_1$, B$_2$, B$_3$, B$_5$, B$_6$, B$_{12}$, C, D, E, K, Ca, Cl, Cu, Fe, I, Mg, Mn, P, Zn^1	In 250 mL cans and 1 L pre-filled closed system containers.
otc	Lipisorb Powder (Mead Johnson Nutritionals)	35	Na caseinate, carnitine	117	corn syrup solids, sucrose	48	MCT, corn oil, soy lecithin	733 (32 mEq)	1250 (32 mEq)	320	1	Vit A, B$_1$, B$_2$, B$_3$, B$_5$, B$_6$, B$_{12}$, C, D, E, K, Ca, Cl, Cu, Fe, I, Mg, Mn, P, Zn^1	Vanilla flavor. In 1 lb.
otc	Introlan Half-Strength Liquid (Elan Pharma)	22.5	Na and Ca caseinate	70	maltodextrin	18	corn oil, MCT, soy lecithin	345 (15 mEq)	585 (15 mEq)	150	0.5	Vit A, B$_1$, B$_2$, B$_3$, B$_5$, B$_6$, B$_{12}$, C, D, E, K, Ca, Cl, Cu, Cr, Fe, I, Mg, Mn, Mo, P, Se, Zn^1	Gluten free. Unflavored. In 1 L closed system containers. Also available with color check.
otc	Kindercal (Mead Johnson Nutritionals)	34	Na and Ca caseinate	135	maltodextrin, sucrose	44	(oils) canola, high oleic sunflower, corn, MCT	370 (16 mEq)	1310 (34 mEq)	310	1	Vit A, B$_1$, B$_2$, B$_3$, B$_5$, B$_6$, B$_{12}$, C, D, E, K, Ca, Cr, Cu, Fe, I, Mg, Mn, Mo, P, Se, Zn, biotin, folic acid, chloride, L-carnitine, taurine	Vanilla flavor. In 240 mL cans.
otc	Profiber Liquid (Sherwood)	40	Na and Ca caseinate, dietary fiber from soy	132	hydrolyzed cornstarch	40	corn oil, soy lecithin	730 (32 mEq)	1250 (32 mEq)	300	1	Vit A, B$_1$, B$_2$, B$_3$, B$_5$, B$_6$, B$_{12}$, C, D, E, K, Ca, Cl, Cr, Cu, Fe, I, Mg, Mn, Mo, P, Se, Zn^1	In 1 L pre-filled closed system containers.
otc	Peptinex DT Liquid (Novartis Nutrition)	50	Casein hydrolysate, amino acids	164	Maltodextrin, modified corn starch	17.4	Medium chain triglycerides, soybean oil	1700 (74 mEq)	800 (21 mEq)	460	1	Vitamins A, B$_1$, B$_2$, B$_3$, B$_5$, B$_6$, B$_{12}$, C, D, E, K, biotin, choline, folic acid, Ca, Cl, Cr, Cu, Fe, I, Mg, Mn, Mo, P, Se, Zn	*For GI impaired patients.* Lactose and gluten free. In 250 mL cans and 1 and 1.5 L closed system containers.
otc	Impact Liquid (Sandoz Nutrition)	56	Na and Ca caseinate, L-arginine	130	hydrolyzed cornstarch	28	structured lipids from palm kernel oil and sunflower oil, refined menhaden oil, hydroxylated soy lecithin	1100 (48 mEq)	1300 (33 mEq)	375	1	Vit A, B$_1$, B$_2$, B$_3$, B$_5$, B$_6$, B$_{12}$, C, E, D, K, Ca, Fe, P, I, Mg, Zn, Cu, Cl, Mn, Se, Cr, Mo^1	In 250 mL ready-to-use cans.

Defined Formula Diets

LACTOSE-FREE PRODUCTS

	Product & Distributor	Protein g	Protein Source	Carbohydrate g	Carbohydrate Source	Fat g	Fat Source	Na (mg)	K (mg)	mOsm/kg H_2O	Cal/mL	Other Content	How Supplied
otc	Glucerna Weight Loss Shake (Abbott)	40.3	sodium and calcium caseinates, soy protein isolate	120.9	fructose, fructooligosaccharides, maltodextrin, soy fiber, sugar alcohols	34.1	canola oil, high oleic safflower oil, soy lecithin	868 (37.82 mEq)	1550 (39.68 mEq)	NA	0.89	Vitamin A, B_1, B_2, B_5, B_6, B_7, B_9, B_{12}, C, D_2E, K, choline, Ca, Cl, Cu, Cr, Fe, I, Mg, Mn, Mo, P, Se, Zn.	Gluten-free. Vanilla, chocolate, banana, peach, dulce de leche flavors. In 325 mL.
otc	Glucerna Select (Abbott)	50	sodium and calcium caseinates, soy protein isolate	95.7	fructose, fructooligosaccharides, maltodextrin, soy fiber, sugar alcohols	54.4	canola oil, high oleic safflower oil, soy lecithin	940 (40.9 mEq)	1810 (46.3 mEq)	470	1	Vitamin A, B_1, B_2, B_3, B_5, B_6, B_7, B_9, B_{12}, C, D, E, K, choline, Ca, Cl, Cu, Cr, Fe, I, Mg, Mn, Mo, P, Se, Zn.	Gluten-free. Vanilla flavor. In 240, 1,000, and 1,500 mL.
otc	Enlive! (Abbott)	41.2	whey protein isolate	273	maltodextrin, sucrose	0	NA	273	168	840	1.25	Vitamin A, B_1, B_2, B_3, B_5, B_6, B_{12}, C, D, E, K, biotin, choline, Ca, Cl, Cu, Cr, Fe, I, Mg, Mn, Mo, P, Se, Zn.	Gluten-free. Apple and peach flavors. In 240 mL.
otc	Nutren 1.0 Liquid (Clintec Nutrition)	40	K and Ca caseinates, taurine, carnitine	127	maltodextrin, corn syrup solids	38	MCT (fractionated coconut oil), corn oil, soy lecithin, canola oil	500 (21.7 mEq)	1252 (32 mEq)	300-390	1	Vit A, B_1, B_2, B_3, B_5, B_6, B_{12}, C, D, E, K, Ca, Cl, Cr, Cu, Fe, I, Mg, Mn, Mo, P, Se, Zn^1.	Gluten free. Unflavored and vanilla, chocolate and strawberry flavors. In 250 mL and UltraPak prefilled bags in 1 and 1.5 L.
otc	Sustacal Liquid (Mead Johnson Nutritionals)	60.4	Ca and Na caseinate, soy protein isolate	138	sugar, corn syrup	23	partially hydrogenated soy oil, soy lecithin	1000 (40 mEq)	2042 (52.4 mEq)	NA	1	Vit A, B_1, B_2, B_3, B_5, B_6, B_{12}, C, D, E, K, Ca, P, I, Fe, Mg, Cu, Zn, Mn, Cl^1.	Vanilla, chocolate, strawberry and eggnog flavors. In 240, 360 mL and qt ready-to-use cans.
otc	Vivonex T.E.N. Powder (Sandoz Nutrition)	38.2	free amino acids (phenylalanine and tryptophan)	205	unknown	2.77	linoleic acid	460 (20 mEq)	782 (20 mEq)	630	1	Vit A, B_1, B_2, B_3, B_5, B_6, B_{12}, C, D, E, K, Ca, P, I, Fe, Mg, Cu, Zn, Mn, Se, Mo, Cr, Cl^1.	In 80.4 g packets.
otc	Portagen Powder (Mead Johnson Nutritionals)	23.3	Na caseinate, amino acids (including taurine, carnitine)	77	corn syrup solids, sucrose	32	MCT (fractionated coconut oil), corn oil, soy lecithin	367 (16 mEq)	833 (21 mEq)	NA	unknown	Vit A, B_1, B_2, B_3, B_5, B_6, B_{12}, C, D, E, K, inositol, Ca, P, I, Fe, Mg, Cu, Zn, Mn, Cl^1.	In 1 lb cans.
otc	Vital High Nitrogen Powder (Ross)	41.7	essential amino acids (including phenylalanine, tryptophan), partially hydrolyzed whey, meat and soy	184.7	hydrolyzed cornstarch, sucrose	10.8	safflower oil, MCT (fractionated coconut oil, mono- and diglycerides, soy lecithin	566.7 (24.6 mEq)	1400 (36 mEq)	500	1	Vit A, B_1, B_2, B_3, B_5, B_6, B_{12}, C, D, E, K_1, Ca, P, Mg, Fe, Cu, Zn, Mn, I, Cl, folic acid, biotin, $choline^1$.	Vanilla flavor. In 79 g packets.
otc	TwoCal HN Liquid (Ross)	83	Na and Ca caseinates	214.2	hydrolyzed cornstarch, sucrose	90	MCT (fractionated coconut oil), corn oil, soy lecithin	1292 (56 mEq)	2417 (62 mEq)	unknown	2	Vit A, B_1, B_2, B_3, B_5, B_6, B_{12}, C, D, E, K, Ca, P, Mg, Fe, Cr, Cu, Se, Zn, Mn, Mo, I, Cl^1.	Vanilla flavor. In ready-to-use 240 mL cans.
otc	Criticare HN Liquid (Mead Johnson Nutritionals)	38	enzymatically hydrolyzed casein, amino acids (including phenylalanine, tryptophan)	220	maltodextrin, modified cornstarch	5.3	safflower oil, mono- and diglycerides	630 (27 mEq)	1320 (34 mEq)	650	1.06	Vit A, B_1, B_2, B_3, B_5, B_6, B_{12}, C, D, E, K, Ca, P, I, Fe, Mg, Cu, Zn, Mn, Cl^1.	Unflavored. In 240 mL ready-to-use bottles.
otc	Isocal HN Liquid (Mead Johnson Nutritionals)	44	Ca and Na caseinate, soy protein isolate, amino acids (including taurine, carnitine)	123	maltodextrin	45	soy oil, MCT (fractionated coconut oil)	930 (40 mEq)	1610 (41 mEq)	270	1.06	Vit A, B_1, B_2, B_3, B_5, B_6, B_{12}, C, D, E, K, Ca, P, I, Fe, Mg, Cu, Zn, Mn, Cl, Se, Cr, Mo^1.	Vanilla flavor. In 240 mL and qt ready-to-use cans. Unflavored In 1 L ready-to-hang bottles.
otc	Isolan Liquid (Elan)	40	caseinates	144	maltodextrin	36	MCT, corn oil	690 (30 mEq)	1170 (30 mEq)	300	1.06	Vit A, B_1, B_2, B_3, B_5, B_6, B_{12}, C, D, E, K, Ca, P, I, Fe, Mg, Cu, Zn, Mn, Cl, Se, Cr, Mo^1.	Gluten free. Unflavored. In 237 mL ready-to-use open system containers and 1 L closed system containers.

ENTERAL NUTRITIONAL THERAPY

Defined Formula Diets

LACTOSE-FREE PRODUCTS

	Product & Distributor	Protein g	Protein Source	Carbohydrate g	Carbohydrate Source	Fat g	Fat Source	Na (mg)	K (mg)	mOsm/ kg H$_2$O	Cal/ mL	Other Content	How Supplied
otc	Isotein HN Powder[3] (Sandoz Nutrition)	20	Na and Ca caseinate, lactalbumin, amino acids (including tryptophan, phenylalanine)	46.7	maltodextrin, fructose	10	MCT, hydrogenated soybean oil, mono- and diglycerides	183 (8 mEq)	317 (8.1 mEq)	300	1.19	Vit A, B$_1$, B$_2$, B$_3$, B$_5$, B$_6$, B$_{12}$, C, D, E, K, Ca, P, I, Fe, Mg, Cu, Zn, Mn, Cl, Se, Cr, Mo[1]	Gluten free. Vanilla flavor. In 87 g packets (36s).
otc	Jevity Liquid (Ross)	44	Ca and Na caseinate, soy fiber, carnitine, taurine	150.8	hydrolyzed cornstarch	35	MCT (fractionated coconut oil) canola oil, high-oleic safflower oil, soy lecithin	917 (40 mEq)	1542 (40 mEq)	300	1.06	Vit A, B$_1$, B$_2$, B$_3$, B$_5$, B$_6$, B$_{12}$, C, D, E, K, Ca, P, Mg, Fe, Mn, Cu, Zn, I, Cl, Se, Cr, Mo[1]	In 240 mL and qt ready-to-use cans and 1 L ready-to-hang bottles.
otc	Resource Liquid (Sandoz Nutrition)	37	Ca and Na caseinate, soy protein isolate, amino acids (including phenylalanine and tryptophan)	145	sugar, hydrolyzed cornstarch	37	corn oil, soy lecithin	886 (39 mEq)	1603 (41 mEq)	430	1.06	Vit A, B$_1$, B$_2$, B$_3$, B$_6$, B$_{12}$, C, D, E, K, Ca, P, I, Fe, Mg, Cu, Zn, Mn, Cl[1]	Gluten free. Vanilla, chocolate and strawberry flavors. In 240 mL ready-to-use TetraBrik paks.
otc	Osmolite Liquid (Ross)	37	Ca and Na caseinate, soy protein isolate, carnitine, taurine	143	hydrolyzed cornstarch	37	MCT (fractionated coconut oil), canola oil, high-oleic safflower oil, soy lecithin	625 (27 mEq)	1000 (26 mEq)	300	1.06	Vit A, B$_1$, B$_2$, B$_3$, B$_6$, B$_{12}$, C, D, E, K, Cl, Ca, P, Se, Mg, I, Mn, Mo, Cu, Zn, Fe[1]	Unflavored. In 240 mL and qt ready-to-use cans and 1 L ready-to-hang containers.
otc	Introlite Liquid (Ross)	22.2	Na and Ca caseinates	70.5	hydrolyzed cornstarch	18.4	MCT (fractionated coconut oil), corn oil, soy oil, soy lecithin	930 (40 mEq)	1570 (40 mEq)	200	0.53	Vit A, B$_1$, B$_2$, B$_3$, B$_6$, B$_{12}$, C, D, E, K, Cl, Ca, P, Mg, I, Mn, Cu, Zn, Fe, Se, Cr, Mo[1]	In 1 L ready-to-use ready-to-hang containers.
otc	Osmolite HN Liquid (Ross)	44	Ca and Na caseinate, soy protein isolate, carnitine, taurine	140	hydrolyzed cornstarch	35	MCT (fractionated coconut oil), high-oleic safflower oil, soy lecithin, canola oil	917 (40 mEq)	1541 (40 mEq)	300	1.06	Vit A, B$_1$, B$_2$, B$_3$, B$_6$, B$_{12}$, C, D, E, K, Cl, Ca, P, Se, Mg, I, Mn, Mo, Cu, Zn, Fe[1]	In 240 mL and qt ready-to-use cans and 1 L ready-to-hang containers.
otc	Nutrilan Liquid (Elan)	38	caseinates	143	maltodextrin	37	MCT, corn oil	632.5 (27.5 mEq)	1057 (27.1 mEq)	320	1.06	Vit A, B$_1$, B$_2$, B$_3$, B$_6$, B$_{12}$, C, D, E, K, Cl, Ca, P, Mg, I, Mn, Cu, Zn, Fe, Se, Cr, Mo[1]	Chocolate, vanilla and strawberry flavors. In ready-to-use 240 mL TetraPak open system containers.
otc	Ensure Liquid and Powder[4] (Ross)	37	Ca and Na caseinate, soy protein isolate	143	corn syrup, sucrose	37	corn oil, soy lecithin	833 (36.2 mEq)	1542 (40 mEq)	470	1.06	Vit A, B$_1$, B$_2$, B$_3$, B$_6$, B$_{12}$, C, D, E, K, Cl, Ca, Cr, P, Se, Mn, Mo, I, Mg, Cu, Zn, Fe[1]	Vanilla, chocolate, coffee, black-walnut, strawberry and eggnog flavors. In 240 mL and qt ready-to-use cans and 400 g powder.
otc	Ensure HN Liquid (Ross)	44	Ca and Na caseinate, soy protein isolate	140	corn syrup, sucrose	35	corn oil, soy lecithin	792 (34 mEq)	1042 (40 mEq)	470	1.06	Vit A, B$_1$, B$_2$, B$_3$, B$_6$, B$_{12}$, C, D, E, K, Cl, Ca, P, Mg, Fe, Mn, Cu, Zn, I[1]	Vanilla flavor. In 240 mL ready-to-use cans. Chocolate flavor. In 240 mL ready-to-use cans.
otc	Ensure High Protein Liquid (Ross)	50.4	Ca and Na caseinates, soy protein isolate	129.4	sucrose, maltodextrin	25.2	safflower oil, canola oil, soy oil	1218	2100	unknown	1	Vit A, B$_1$, B$_2$, B$_3$, B$_6$, B$_{12}$, C, D, E, K, Ca, Cl, Cr, Cu, Fe, I, Mg Mn, Mo, P, Se, Zn, folic acid	Banana, chocolate, wild berry and vanilla flavors. In 237 mL.
otc	Ultracal Liquid (Mead Johnson Nutritional)	44	Ca and Na caseinate, soy fiber, oat fiber, taurine, carnitine	123	maltodextrin	45	MCT (fractionated coconut oil), canola oil, mono- and diglycerides, soy lecithin	930 (40 mEq)	1610 (41 mEq)	310	1.06	Vit A, B$_1$, B$_2$, B$_3$, B$_6$, B$_{12}$, C, D, E, K, Ca, P, I, Fe, Mg, Cu, Zn, Mn, Cl, Se, Cr, Mo[1]	Vanilla flavor. In 240 mL and qt ready-to-use cans and 1 L ready-to-hang containers.
otc	Compleat Modified Formula Liquid (Sandoz Nutrition)	43	beef, Ca caseinate, amino acids (including phenylalanine, tryptophan)	140	maltodextrin, pureed fruits & vegetables	37	canola oil, mono- and diglycerides	1000 (43.5 mEq)	1400 (36 mEq)	300	1.07	Vit A, B$_1$, B$_2$, B$_3$, B$_5$, B$_6$, B$_{12}$, C, D, E, K, Ca, P, I, Fe, Mg, Cu, Zn, Mn, Se, Cr, Mo[1]	In ready-to-use 250 mL cans and 1000 and 1500 mL closed system containers.

ENTERAL NUTRITIONAL THERAPY

Defined Formula Diets

LACTOSE-FREE PRODUCTS

	Product & Distributor	Protein g	Protein Source	Carbohydrate g	Carbohydrate Source	Fat g	Fat Source	Na (mg)	K (mg)	mOsm/ kg H$_2$O	Cal/ mL	Other Content	How Supplied
otc	**Ensure with Fiber Liquid** (Ross)	39	Ca and Na caseinate, soy protein isolate, soy fiber	160	hydrolyzed corn-starch, sucrose	37	corn oil, soy lecithin	833 (36 mEq)	1667 (43 mEq)	480	1.1	Vit A, B_1, B_2, B_3, B_5, B_6, B_{12}, C, D, E, K, Cl, Ca, P, Mg, Fe, Mn, Cu, Zn, I, Se, Cr, Mo[1]	Vanilla and chocolate flavors. In 240 mL and qt (vanilla only) ready-to-use cans.
otc	**Fiberlan Liquid** (Elan)	50	Na and Ca caseinates	160	maltodextrin	40	MCT, corn oil, soy lecithin	920 (40 mEq)	1560 (40 mEq)	310	1.2	Vit A, B_1, B_2, B_3, B_5, B_6, B_{12}, C, D, E, K, Cl, Ca, P, Mg, Fe, Mn, Cu, Zn, I, Se, Cr, Mo[1]	Gluten free. Unflavored. In ready-to-use 237 mL open system containers and 1 L unflavored closed system containers.
otc	**Isosource Liquid** (Sandoz Nutrition)	43	Ca and Na caseinate, soy protein isolate	170	hydrolyzed corn-starch	41	MCT, canola oil, soy lecithin	1200 (52.2 mEq)	1700 (44 mEq)	360	1.2	Vit A, B_1, B_2, B_3, B_5, B_6, B_{12}, C, D, E, K, Ca, Cl, Cu, Fe, I, Mg, Mn, P, Zn, Se, Cr, Mo[1]	Fiber and gluten free. Vanilla flavor. In ready-to-use 250 mL cans, 240 mL TetraBrik packs and 1 and 1.5 L closed system containers.
otc	**Nitrolan Liquid** (Elan)	60	caseinates	160	maltodextrin	40	MCT, corn oil, soy lecithin	690 (30 mEq)	1170 (30 mEq)	310	1.24	Vit A, B_1, B_2, B_3, B_5, B_6, B_{12}, C, D, E, K, Ca, P, I, Fe, Mg, Cu, Zn, Cl, Mn, Se, Cr, Mo[1]	Gluten free. Unflavored. In ready-to-use 240 mL open system containers and 1 L closed system containers with or without color check.
otc	**Isosource HN Liquid** (Sandoz Nutrition)	53	Ca and Na caseinate, soy protein isolate, amino acids (including phenylalanine, tryptophan)	160	hydrolyzed corn-starch	41	MCT, canola oil, soy lecithin	1100 (48 mEq)	1700 (44 mEq)	330	1.2	Vit A, B_1, B_2, B_3, B_5, B_6, B_{12}, C, D, E, K, Ca, P, I, Fe, Mg, Cu, Zn, Cl, Mn, Se, Cr, Mo[1]	Vanilla flavor. In ready-to-use 250 mL cans, 240 mL TetraBrik packs and 1 and 1.5 mL closed system containers.
otc	**Comply Liquid** (Sherwood)	60	Ca and Na caseinate	180	maltodextrin, sucrose[5]	60	corn oil, soy lecithin	1100 (48 mEq)	1850 (47 mEq)	410	1.5	Vit A, B_1, B_2, B_3, B_5, B_6, B_{12}, C, D, E, K, Ca, Cl, Cu, Fe, I, Mg, Mn, P, Zn[1]	Unflavored. In 250 mL cans. Vanilla, orange and banana flavors. In 250 mL cans and 1000 mL prefilled systems.
otc	**Nutren 1.5 Liquid** (Clintec Nutrition)	60	Ca K and Na caseinate	169.2	maltodextrin	67.6	MCT (fractionated coconut oil), corn oil, canola oil, soy lecithin	752 (33 mEq)	1872 (48 mEq)	410-590	1.5	Vit A, B_1, B_2, B_3, B_5, B_6, B_{12}, C, D, E, K, Ca, Cl, Cu, Fe, I, Mg, Mn, P, Zn, Cr, Mo, Se[1]	Gluten free. Unflavored and vanilla and chocolate flavors. In 250 mL ready-to-use cans. Unflavored. In 1 L prefilled closed system containers.
otc	**Ensure Plus Liquid**[6] (Ross)	54.2	Ca and Na caseinate, soy protein isolate	197.1	corn syrup, sucrose	53	corn oil, soy lecithin	1042 (45.3 mEq)	1917 (49 mEq)	690	1.5	Vit A, B_1, B_2, B_3, B_5, B_6, B_{12}, C, D, E, K, Cl, Ca, P, Mg, Mn, I, Fe, Cu, Zn, Cr, Se, Mo[1]	Chocolate, vanilla, eggnog, strawberry and coffee flavors. In ready-to-use 240 mL and qt cans and 1 L ready-to-hang containers.
otc	**Resource Plus Liquid**[6] (Sandoz Nutrition)	55	Ca and Na caseinate, soy protein isolate	200	hydrolyzed corn-starch, sugar	53	corn oil, soy lecithin	1266 (55 mEq)	2068 (53 mEq)	600	1.5	Vit A, B_1, B_2, B_3, B_5, B_6, B_{12}, C, D, E, K, Ca, P, I, Fe, Mg, Cu, Zn, Cl, Mn[1]	Gluten free. Vanilla, chocolate and strawberry flavors. In 240 mL ready-to-use BrikPaks.
otc	**Ensure Plus HN Liquid** (Ross)	62	Ca and Na caseinate, soy protein isolate, amino acid (including carnitine, taurine)	197	hydrolyzed corn-starch, sucrose	49	corn oil, soy lecithin	1167 (51 mEq)	1792 (46 mEq)	unknown	1.5	Vit A, B_1, B_2, B_3, B_5, B_6, B_{12}, C, D, E, K, choline, Cl, Ca, P, Mg, I, Mn, Cu, Zn, Fe, Se, Cr, Mo[1]	Vanilla and chocolate flavors. In 240 mL ready-to-use cans and 1 L ready-to-hang containers.
otc	**NutriFocus** (Ross)	61.7	Na caseinate, milk protein isolate, soy protein isolate, arginine	212.3	corn syrup, sugar, fructooligosaccharides	48.8	canola oil, high oleic safflower oil, corn oil, lecithin	917	1668	unknown	1.5	Vit A, B_1, B_2, B_3, B_5, B_6, B_{12}, C, D, E, K, Ca, Cl, Cr, Cu, Fe, P, Mg, I, Mn, Zn, Fe, Se, Mo, beta carotene, biotin, choline, 417 mcg folic acid/L	20.85 g fiber/L. Lactose and gluten free. In chocolate and vanilla flavors. In 240 mL cans.
otc	**Ultralan Liquid** (Elan)	60	caseinates	202	maltodextrin	50	MCT, corn oil	1035 (45 mEq)	1755 (45 mEq)	610	1.5	Vit A, B_1, B_2, B_3, B_5, B_6, B_{12}, C, D, E, K, Ca, P, Mg, I, Mn, Cu, Zn, Fe, Se, Cr, Mo[1]	Gluten free. Unflavored. In ready-to-use 1000 mL NewPak closed system containers with and without color check.

ENTERAL NUTRITIONAL THERAPY

Defined Formula Diets

LACTOSE-FREE PRODUCTS

	Product & Distributor	Protein g	Protein Source	Carbohydrate g	Carbohydrate Source	Fat g	Fat Source	Na (mg)	K (mg)	mOsm/kg H₂O	Cal/mL	Other Content	How Supplied
otc	**Advera** (Ross)	60	soy protein hydrolysate, sodium caseinate, 127 mg/L carnitine, 212 mg/L taurine	215.8	hydrolized corn-starch, sucrose	22.8	canola oil, medium-chain triglycerides (fractionated coconut oil), refined deodorized sardine oil	1046	2827	unknown	1.3	8.9 g dietary fiber (from soy fiber), vit A, D, E, K, C, folic acid, B₁, B₂, B₃, biotin, B₅, B₆, B₁₂, Cl, Ca, Zn, Fe, P, Mg, I, Mn, Cu, Se, Cr, Mo, choline	*For dietary management in HIV infection or AIDS.* Gluten free. Chocolate flavor. In 240 mL cans.
otc	**Magnacal Liquid** (Sherwood)	70	Ca and Na caseinate	250	maltodextrin, sucrose	80	partially hydrogenated soy oil, soy lecithin, mono- and diglycerides	1000 (43.5 mEq)	1250 (32 mEq)	590	2	Vit A, B₁, B₂, B₃, B₅, B₆, B₁₂, C, D, E, K, choline, Ca, Cl, Cu, Fe, I, Mg, Mn, P, Zn	Vanilla flavor. In ready-to-use 120 and 240 mL bottles and 250 mL cans.
otc	**Isocal HCN Liquid** (Mead Johnson Nutritionals)	75	Ca and Na caseinate, amino acids (including phenylalanine, tryptophan)	200	corn syrup	102	soy oil, MCT (fractionated coconut oil), soy lecithin	800 (35 mEq)	1700 (43 mEq)	640	2	Vit A, B₁, B₂, B₃, B₅, B₆, B₁₂, C, D, E, K, Ca, P, I, Fe, Mg, Cu, Zn, Mn, Cl, Se, Cr, Mo[1]	Vanilla flavor. In 240 mL ready-to-use cans.
otc	**Nutren 2.0 Liquid** (Clintec Nutrition)	80	Ca and K caseinate, amino acids	196	maltodextrin, corn syrup solids, sucrose	106	MCT (fractionated coconut oil), corn oil, soy lecithin, canola oil	1000 (44 mEq)	2500 (64 mEq)	710	2	Vit A, B₁, B₂, B₃, B₅, B₆, B₁₂, C, D, E, K, Ca, Cl, Cu, Fe, I, Mg, Mn, P, Zn, Cr, Se, Mo[1]	Gluten free. Vanilla flavor. In 250 mL ready-to-use cans.
otc	**Forta Drink Powder**[7] (Ross)	5	whey protein concentrate	15	sucrose, pineapple juice solids	< 1	unknown	50 (2.2 mEq)	70 (1.8 mEq)	NA	85	Vit A, B₁, B₂, B₃, B₅, B₆, B₁₂, C, D, E, Ca, Cu, Fe, I, Mg, Mn, P, Zn[1]	Orange and fruit punch flavors. In 482 g cans.
otc	**Neocate One + Liquid** (SHS)	≈ 2.5	amino acids	14.6	sucrose, maltodextrin	3.5	fractionated coconut oil, canola oil, high oleic sunflower oil	20 (0.9 mEq)	93 (2.4 mEq)	835	100	Vit A, B₁, B₂, B₃, B₅, B₆, B₁₂, C, D, E, K, Ca, Cl, Cr, Cu, Fe, I, Mg, Mn, Mo, Se, Zn, FA, biotin, choline, inositol	Gluten free. Orange and pineapple flavors. In 237 mL with straw.
otc	**ReSource Just for Kids** (Novartis Nutrition)	30	sodium and calcium caseinates, whey protein concentrate, carnitine, taurine	110	hydrolyzed corn-starch, sucrose	50	high oleic sunflower oil, soybean oil, medium chain triglycerides oil	380 (17 mEq)	1300 (33 mEq)	390	1	Vit A, B₁, B₂, B₃, B₅, B₆, B₁₂, C, D, E, K, biotin, choline, folic acid, m-inositol, Ca, Cl, Cr, Cu, Fe, I, Mo, Mg, Mn, P, Se, Zn	French vanilla, chocolate, strawberry flavors. In 237 mL Tetra Brik Paks (27s).
otc	**ReSource Fruit Beverage** (Novartis Nutrition)	38	whey protein concentrates	150	sugar, hydrolyzed cornstarch	0		< 295 (< 13 mEq)	< 93 (< 2.4 mEq)	700	0.76	Vit A, B₁, B₂, B₃, B₅, B₆, B₁₂, C, D, E, K, biotin, choline, folic acid, Ca, Cl, Cu, Fe, I, Mg, Mn, P, Zn	Orange, peach, wild berry flavors. In 237 mL Tetra Brik Paks (27s).
otc	**ReSource Diabetic** (Novartis Nutrition)	63	sodium and calcium caseinates, soy protein isolates, carnitine, taurine	99	hydrolyzed cornstarch, fructose	47	high oleic sunflower oil, soybean oil	970 (42 mEq)	1100 (29 mEq)	450	1.06	Vit A, B₁, B₂, B₃, B₅, B₆, B₁₂, C, D, E, K, biotin, choline, folic acid, m-inositol, Ca, Cl, Cu, Fe, I, Mg, Mn, Mo, P, Se, Zn	French vanilla, chocolate, strawberry flavors. In 237 mL Tetra Brik Paks (27s) and 1000 and 1500 mL closed system containers (6s).
otc	**Pediasure with Fiber** (Ross)	30	sodium caseinate, low-lactose whey, carnitine, taurine	113.5	maltodextrin, sucrose, soy fiber (5 g total dietary fiber)	49.7	high-oleic safflower oil, soy oil, medium chain triglyceride oil, lecithin	380 (16.5 mEq)	1310 (33.5 mEq)	unknown	1	Vit A, B₁, B₂, B₃, B₆, B₁₂, C, D, E, K, folic acid, Ca, Fe, I, Mg, P, Se, Zn	Gluten free. Vanilla flavor. In 8 oz.

[1] Also contains folic acid, biotin and choline.
[2] Content given per orange flavor.
[3] Content given per 87 g packet.
[4] Content given per ready-to-use liquid.
[5] Unflavored does not contain sucrose.
[6] Content given per vanilla flavor.
[7] Content given per 100 mL.

See individual product listings for specific labeled indications.

INFANT FOODS

	Product & Distributor	Dilution	Protein g	Protein Source	Carbohydrate g	Carbohydrate Source	Fat g	Fat Source	Na (mg)	K (mg)	Cal	Other Content	How Supplied
otc	**Enfamil Human Milk Fortifier Powder** (Mead Johnson Nutritionals)	4 packets (3.8 g) added to breast milk	0.7	whey protein, Na caseinate	2.7	corn syrup solids, lactose	< 0.1	unknown	7 (0.3 mEq)	15.6 (0.4 mEq)	14	Vit A, B_1, B_2, B_3, B_5, B_6, B_{12}, C, D, E, K, Ca, P, Zn, Mg, Mn, Cu, Cl[1]	In 0.96 g packets (100s).
otc	**Enfamil Premature Formula Liquid** (Mead Johnson Nutritionals)	150 mL	3	nonfat milk, whey protein concentrate, amino acids	11.1	corn syrup solids, lactose	5.1	soy oil, MCT (fractionated coconut oil), mono- and diglycerides, linoleic acid	39 (1.7 mEq)	103 (2.6 mEq)	80	Vit A, B_1, B_2, B_3, B_5, B_6, B_{12}, C, D, E, K, inositol, Ca, P, Mg, Zn, Fe, Mn, Cu, I, Cl[1]	In 90 mL nursettes.
otc	**Enfamil Liquid and Powder** (Mead Johnson Nutritionals)	1 liter	15	nonfat milk, reduced minerals whey	69	lactose	37.3	soy and coconut oils, soy lecithin, mono- and diglycerides, high-oleic sunflower oil, palm olein, linoleic acid	180 (7.8 mEq)	720 (18.4 mEq)	667	Vit A, B_1, B_2, B_3, B_5, B_6, B_{12}, C, D, E, K, inositol, Ca, P, Mg, Zn, Fe, Mn, Cu, I, Cl[1]	In 390 mL concentrate, 240 mL and 1 qt ready-to-use cans 90, 180 and 240 mL nursettes and 1 and 2 lb powder.
otc	**Carnation Good-Start Liquid and Powder** (Carnation)	1 liter	16	reduced minerals whey, taurine	74.4	lactose, maltodextrin	34.5	palm olein, soy oil, coconut oil, high-oleic safflower oil	162 (7 mEq)	663 (17 mEq)	0.68	Vit A, B_1, B_2, B_3, B_5, B_6, B_{12}, C, D, E, K, inositol, Ca, Mg, P, Zn, Fe, Mn, Cu, I, Cl[1]	In 390 mL concentrated liquid, 1 qt ready-to-feed containers and 360 g powder.
otc	**PediaSure Liquid** (Ross)	1 liter	30	Na caseinate, whey protein concentrate, taurine, carnitine	108	hydrolyzed corn starch, sucrose	49	high-oleic safflower oil, soy oil, MCT (fractionated coconut oil), mono- and diglycerides, soy lecithin	375 (16.3 mEq)	1292 (33 mEq)	1000	Vit A, B_1, B_2, B_3, B_5, B_6, B_{12}, C, D, E, K, inositol, Ca, Mg, P, Zn, Fe, Mn, Cu, I, Cl, Cr, Mo, Se[1]	Gluten free. Vanilla flavor. In ready-to-use 240 mL cans.
otc	**Enfamil Next Step Liquid and Powder** (Mead Johnson Nutritionals)	1 liter	17.3	nonfat milk	74	corn syrup solids, lactose	33.3	palm olein, soy oil, coconut oil, high-oleic sunflower oil, linoleic acid	273 (11.9 mEq)	867 (22.2 mEq)	100	Vit A, B_1, B_2, B_3, B_5, B_6, B_{12}, C, D, E, K, inositol, Ca, Mg, P, Zn, Fe, Mn, Cu, I, Cl, Se[1]	In 390 mL concentrate, 1 qt ready-to-use liquid and 360 and 720 g powder.
otc	**Carnation Follow-Up Formula Liquid and Powder** (Carnation)	1 liter	17.3	nonfat milk	88	corn syrup	27.3	palm olein, coconut oil, high oleic safflower oil, soy lecithin, soy oil	260 (11.5 mEq)	900 (23 mEq)	676	Vit A, B_1, B_2, B_3, B_5, B_6, B_{12}, C, D, E, K, inositol, Ca, Mg, P, Zn, Fe, Mn, Cu, I, Cl[1]	In 390 mL concentrate, 1 qt ready-to-feed containers and 360 g powder.
otc	**Similac Human Milk Fortifier** (Ross)	4 packets (3.6 g)	1	nonfat milk, whey protein concentrate	1.8	corn syrup solids	0.36	fractionated coconut oil (medium chain triglycerides), soy lecithin	15	63	14	Vit A, B1, B2, B3, B5, B6, B12, C, D, E, K, folic acid, (folacin), biotin, Ca, Cl, Cu, Fe, Mg, Mn, P, Zn	In 0.9 g packets (50s).

[1] Also contains folic acid, biotin and choline.

Indications
See individual product listings for specific labeled indications.
Formula for bottle-fed infants; as a supplement to breast-feeding.

Precautions
In conditions where the infant is losing abnormal quantities of one or more electrolytes, it may be necessary to supply electrolytes from sources other than the formula. With premature infants weighing < 1500 g at birth, it may be necessary to supply an additional source of sodium, calcium and phosphorus during the period of very rapid growth.

INFANT FOODS WITH IRON

	Product & Distributor	Dilution	Protein g	Protein Source	Carbohydrate g	Carbohydrate Source	Fat g	Fat Source	Iron (mg)	Na (mg)	K (mg)	Cal	Other Content	How Supplied
otc	**Phenyl-Free 1** (Mead Johnson Nutritionals)	1 liter	22	casein hydrolysate, amino acids (including tryptophan, taurine, carnitine)	54.2	corn syrup solids, modified tapioca starch	16.3	corn oil	12.5	313 (14 mEq)	680 (17.4 mEq)	667	Vit A, B_1, B_2, B_3, B_5, B_6, B_{12}, C, D, E, K, inositol, Ca, P, Mg, Zn, Mn, Cu, I, Cl[1]	Low phenylalanine. In 1 lb powder.
otc	**Similac w/Iron Liquid and Powder** (Ross)	1 liter	15	nonfat milk, taurine	72.3	lactose	37	Coconut oil, corn oil, soy oil, mono- and diglycerides, soy lecithin, linoleic acid	12	180 (8 mEq)	700 (18 mEq)	676	Vit A, B_1, B_2, B_3, B_5, B_6, C, D, E, K, inositol, Ca, B_{12}, P, Mg, Zn, Mn, Cu, I, Cl[1]	In 390 mL concentrate, 240 mL and 1 qt ready-to-use cans, 120 and 240 mL nursettes and 1 lb powder.
otc	**SMA Iron Fortified Liquid and Powder** (Wyeth-Ayerst)	1 liter	15	nonfat milk, reduced minerals whey, taurine	71	lactose	35.3	oleo, coconut, safflower, sunflower and soybean oils, soy lecithin, linoleic acid	12	147 (6.4 mEq)	553 (14.2 mEq)	667	Vit A, B_1, B_2, B_3, B_5, B_6, B_{12}, C, D, E, K, Ca, P, Mg, Cl, Cu, Zn, Mn, I[1]	In 384 mL concentrate, ready-to-use 240 mL and 1 qt and 1 and 2 lb powder.

ENTERAL NUTRITIONAL THERAPY

INFANT FOODS WITH IRON

	Product & Distributor	Dilution	Protein g	Protein Source	Carbohydrate g	Carbohydrate Source	Fat g	Fat Source	Iron (mg)	Na (mg)	K (mg)	Cal	Other Content	How Supplied
otc	**Enfamil w/Iron Liquid and Powder** (Mead Johnson Nutritionals)	1 liter	15	nonfat milk, reduced minerals whey	69	lactose	37	soy and coconut oils, soy lecithin, mono- and diglycerides, palm olein, high-oleic sunflower oil, linoleic acid	12.5	180 (8 mEq)	720 (18.4 mEq)	666	Vit A, B_1, B_2, B_3, B_5, B_6, B_{12}, C, D, E, K, inositol, Ca, P, Mg, Zn, Mn, Cu, I, Cl[1]	In 390 mL concentrate, ready-to-use 240 mL and 1qt., 180 mL nursettes and 1 and 2 lb powder.
otc	**Bonamil Infant Formula w/Iron Powder or Liquid** (Wyeth-Ayerst)	150 mL	2.3	nonfat milk, taurine	10.7	lactose	5.4	soybean oil, coconut oil, soy lecithin, linoleic acid	1.8	27	93	100	Vit A, B_1, B_2, B_3, B_5, B_6, B_{12}, C, D, E, K, biotin, choline, Ca, P, Mg, Zn, Mn, Cu, I, Cl, folic acid	In 453 g powder or 946 mL ready-to-feed liquid.
otc	**EnfaCare Powder or Liquid** (Mead Johnson Nutritionals)	≈ 130 mL	2.8	nonfat milk, whey protein concentrate, taurine, L-carnitine	10.7	maltodextrin, lactose	5.3	high oleic sunflower oil, soy oil, medium chain triglycerides, coconut oil, mono- and diglycerides, soy lecithin	1.8	35	105	100	Vit A, B_1, B_2, B_3, B_5, B_6, B_{12}, C, D, E, K, 26 mcg folic acid, biotin, choline, inositol, linoleic acid, Ca, Cl, Cu, I, Mg, Mn, P, Se, Zn.	In 3 oz Nursette bottles (liquid) and 14 oz cans (powder).
otc	**Enfamil LIPIL with Iron** (Mead Johnson Nutritionals)	per 100 calories	2.1	reduced minerals whey, nonfat milk, taurine	10.9	lactose	5.3	vegetable oil (palm olein, soy, coconut, and high oleic sunflower oils), < 1% mortierella alpina oil, crypthecodinium cohnii oil, mono- and diglycerides, soy lecithin	1.8	27	108	20 cal/oz	Vit A, B_1, B_2, B_3, B_5, B_6, B_{12}, C, D, E, K, 16 mcg folic acid/100 cal, biotin, chloride, choline, inositol, linoleic acid, Ca, Cu, I, Mg, Mn, P, Se, Zn.	In 32 oz cans and 3 and 6 oz Nursette bottles (ready-to-use liquid), 13 oz cans (liquid concentrate), and 12.9 and 25.7 oz cans (powder).

[1] Also contains folic acid, biotin and choline.

See individual product listings for specific labeled indications.

SPECIALIZED INFANT FOODS

	Product & Distributor	Dilution	Protein g	Protein Source	Carbohydrate g	Carbohydrate Source	Fat g	Fat Source	Iron (mg)	Na (mg)	K (mg)	Cal	Other Content	How Supplied
otc	**RCF Liquid** (Ross)	1 liter	39.3	soy protein isolate, amino acids (including carnitine and taurine)	0.08	unknown	71	soy oil, coconut oil, mono- and diglycerides, soy lecithin	3	579 (25.2 mEq)	1429 (37 mEq)	818	Vit A, B_1, B_2, B_3, B_5, B_6, B_{12}, C, D, E, K, inositol, Ca, P, Cu, Mg, Zn, Mn, I, Cl[1]	Carbohydrate free. In 390 mL concentrate.
otc	**Nursoy Liquid and Powder** (Wyeth-Ayerst)	1 liter	21	soy protein isolate, methionine	69	sucrose	36	oleo, coconut, safflower and soybean oils, soy lecithin	11.5	200 (9 mEq)	700 (18 mEq)	667	Vit A, B_1, B_2, B_3, B_5, B_6, B_{12}, C, D, E, K, inositol, Ca, P, Cl, Mg, Mn, Cu, Zn, I[1]	In 390 mL concentrate, 1 qt ready-to-use and 1 lb powder.
otc	**Gerber Soy Formula Liquid** (Gerber)	1 liter	20	soy protein isolate, amino acids (including taurine, carnitine)	67	corn syrup solids, sugar	35.3	palm olein, soy, coconut and high oleic sunflower oils, soy lecithin, mono- and diglycerides, linoleic acid	12	313 (14 mEq)	767 (20 mEq)	667	Vit A, B_1, B_2, B_3, B_5, B_6, B_{12}, C, D, E, K, inositol, Ca, P, Cu, Mg, Zn, Mn, I, Cl[1]	In 1 qt ready-to-use.
otc	**ProSobee Liquid and Powder** (Mead Johnson Nutritionals)	1 liter	20	soy protein isolate, amino acids (including taurine, carnitine)	67	corn syrup solids	35.3	linoleic acid, coconut, corn and soy oil, palm olein, high oleic sunflower oils[2]	12.5	240 (10.5 mEq)	813 (21 mEq)	667	Vit A, B_1, B_2, B_3, B_5, B_6, B_{12}, C, D, E, K, inositol, Ca, P, Cu, Mg, Zn, Mn, I, Cl[1]	*For infants with a family history of allergies.* Sucrose, milk and lactose free. In 390 mL concentrate, 240 mL and 1 qt ready-to-use and 420 g powder.
otc	**Alimentum Liquid** (Ross)	1 liter	19	casein hydrolysate, amino acids (including tryptophan, taurine, carnitine)	69	sucrose, modified tapioca starch	36	MCT (fractionated coconut oil), safflower oil, soy oil	12	297 (13 mEq)	798 (21 mEq)	676	Vit A, B_1, B_2, B_3, B_5, B_6, B_{12}, C, D, E, K, inositol, Ca, Cl, Cu, I, Mg, Mn, P, Zn[1]	*For infants and children with severe food allergies, sensitivity to intact protein, protein maldigestion or fat malabsorption.* Corn and lactose free. In ready-to-use 240 and 360 mL.

ENTERAL NUTRITIONAL THERAPY

SPECIALIZED INFANT FOODS

	Product & Distributor	Content per Dilution											Other Content	How Supplied
		Dilution	Protein g	Protein Source	Carbohydrate g	Carbohydrate Source	Fat g	Fat Source	Iron (mg)	Na (mg)	K (mg)	Cal		
otc	**Nutramigen Liquid and Powder** (Mead Johnson Nutritionals)	1 liter	19	enzymatically hydrolyzed casein, amino acids (including tryptophan, taurine, carnitine)	89.3	corn syrup solids, modified corn-starch	26	corn oil, soy oil, linoleic acid	12.5	313 (14 mEq)	727 (19 mEq)	667	Vit A, B_1, B_2, B_3, B_5, B_6, B_{12}, C, D, E, K, inositol, Ca, P, Cu, Mg, Zn, Mn, I, Cl[1]	*For infants and children sensitive to intact proteins of milk and other foods. Lactose and sucrose free. In 1 lb powder, 390 mL concentrate and 1 qt ready-to-use.*
otc	**Pregestimil Powder** (Mead Johnson Nutritionals)	1 liter	18.7	enzymatically hydrolyzed casein, amino acids (including tryptophan, taurine, carnitine)	69	corn syrup solids, modified corn starch, dextrose	37.3	corn oil, MCT (fractionated coconut oil), high-oleic safflower oil, linoleic acid	12.5	260 (11.3 mEq)	726 (19 mEq)	667	Vit A, B_1, B_2, B_3, B_5, B_6, B_{12}, C, D, E, K, inositol, Ca, P, Cu, Mg, Zn, Mn, I, Cl[1]	*For infants with severe malabsorption disorders.* In 1 lb powder.
otc	**Isomil SF Liquid** (Ross)	1 liter	18	soy protein isolate, amino acids (including carnitine)	68.3	hydrolyzed corn-starch	37	soy oil, coconut oil, mono- and diglycerides, soy lecithin, linoleic acid	12	297 (13 mEq)	730 (19 mEq)	676	Vit A, B_1, B_2, B_3, B_5, B_6, B_{12}, C, D, E, K, inositol, Ca, P, Cu, Mg, Zn, Mn, I, Cl[1]	*For infants and children with an allergy sensitivity to cow's milk protein or intolerance to sucrose.* Sucrose and lactose free. In 390 mL concentrate.
otc	**Isomil Liquid and Powder** (Ross)	1 liter	17	soy protein isolate, amino acids (including carnitine)	70	corn syrup, sucrose, corn-starch[2]	37	corn, soy and coconut oils, mono- and diglycerides, soy lecithin	12	297 (13 mEq)	730 (18.4 mEq)	676	Vit A, B_1, B_2, B_3, B_5, B_6, B_{12}, C, D, E, K, inositol, Ca, P, Mg, Zn, Mn, Cu, I, Cl[1]	*For infants and children who are allergic or sensitive to cow's milk, lactose intolerant or deficient or are galactosemic.* Lactose free. In 390 mL concentrate, 120 mL nursing bottles, 240 mL and 1 qt ready-to-use and 420 g powder.
otc	**Similac PM 60/40 Low-Iron Liquid** (Ross)	1 liter	15.6	whey protein concentrate, Na caseinate, carnitine, taurine	68	lactose	37	coconut oil, mono- and diglycerides, soy oil, linoleic acid	1.5	160 (7 mEq)	573 (15 mEq)	100	Vit A, B_1, B_2, B_3, B_5, B_6, B_{12}, C, D, E, K, inositol, Ca, P, Cu, Mg, Zn, Mn, I, Cl	*For infants who are predisposed to hypocalcemia or those who would benefit from lowered mineral levels.* In 120 mL bottles.
otc	**Glutarex-1 Powder** (Ross)	100 g powder[3]	15	amino acids (including carnitine, phenylalanine, taurine)	47	hydrolyzed corn-starch	24	palm oil, hydrogenated coconut oil, soy oil, mono- and diglycerides, linoleic acid	9	190 (8.3 mEq)	675 (17.3 mEq)	480	Vit A, B_1, B_2, B_3, B_5, B_6, B_{12}, C, D, E, K, inositol, Ca, P, Cu, Mg, Zn, Mn, I, Cl, Se[1]	*Nutritional support of infants and toddlers with glutaric aciduria type I.* Lysine and tryptophan free. In 350 g powder.
otc	**Hominex-1 Powder** (Ross)	100 g powder[3]	15	amino acids (including phenylalanine, tryptophan, taurine, carnitine)	46.3	hydrolyzed corn-starch	24	palm oil, hydrogenated coconut oil, soy oil, mono- and diglycerides, linoleic acid	9	190 (8.3 mEq)	675 (17.3 mEq)	480	Vit A, B_1, B_2, B_3, B_5, B_6, B_{12}, C, D, E, K, inositol, Ca, P, Cu, Mg, Zn, Mn, I, Cl, Se[1]	*Nutritional support of infants and toddlers with vitamin B_6-nonresponsive homocystinuria or hypermethioninemia. Methionine free.* In 350 g powder.
otc	**I-Valex-1 Powder** (Ross)	100 g powder[3]	15	amino acids (including carnitine, phenylalanine, tryptophan, taurine)	46.3	hydrolyzed corn-starch	24	palm oil, hydrogenated coconut oil, soy oil, mono- and diglycerides, linoleic acid	9	190 (8.3 mEq)	675 (17.3 mEq)	480	Vit A, B_1, B_2, B_3, B_5, B_6, B_{12}, C, D, E, K, inositol, Ca, P, Cu, Mg, Zn, Mn, I, Cl, Se[1]	*Nutritional support of infants and toddlers with a disorder of leucine catabolism. Leucine free.* In 350 g.
otc	**Ketonex-1 Powder** (Ross)	100 g powder[3]	15	amino acids (including phenylalanine, tryptophan, carnitine, taurine)	46.3	hydrolyzed corn-starch	24	palm oil, hydrogenated coconut oil, soy oil, mono- and diglycerides, linoleic acid	9	190 (8.3 mEq)	675 (17.3 mEq)	480	Vit A, B_1, B_2, B_3, B_5, B_6, B_{12}, C, D, E, K, inositol, Ca, P, Cu, Mg, Zn, Mn, I, Cl, Se[1]	*For nutritional support of infants and toddlers with maple syrup urine disease (MSUD). Isoleucine, leucine and valine free.* In 350 g powder.
otc	**Phenex-1 Powder** (Ross)	100 g powder[3]	15	amino acids (including tryptophan, taurine, carnitine)	46.3	hydrolyzed corn-starch	24	palm oil, hydrogenated coconut oil, soy oil, mono- and diglycerides	9	190 (8.3 mEq)	675 (17.2 mEq)	480	Vit A, B_1, B_2, B_3, B_5, B_6, B_{12}, C, D, E, K, inositol, Ca, P, Cu, Mg, Zn, Mn, I, Cl, Se[1]	*Nutritional support of infants and toddlers with phenylketonuria (PKU). Phenylalanine free.* In 350 g.

ENTERAL NUTRITIONAL THERAPY

SPECIALIZED INFANT FOODS

	Product & Distributor	Dilution	Protein (g)	Protein Source	Carbohydrate (g)	Carbohydrate Source	Fat (g)	Fat Source	Iron (mg)	Na (mg)	K (mg)	Cal	Other Content	How Supplied
otc	**Propimex-1 Powder** (Ross)	100 g powder[3]	15	amino acids (including carnitine, phenylalanine, tryptophan, taurine)	46.3	hydrolyzed corn-starch	24	palm oil, hydrogenated coconut oil, soy oil, mono- and diglycerides, linoleic acid	9	190 (8.3 mEq)	675 (18 mEq)	480	Vit A, B1, B2, B3, B5, B6, B12, C, D, E, K, inositol, Ca, P, Cu, Mg, Zn, Mn, I, Cl, Se[1]	*For nutritional support of infants and toddlers with propionic or methylmalonic acidemia. Methionine- and valine-free.* In 350 g powder.
otc	**SMA Lo-Iron Infant Formula** (Wyeth Ayerst)	1 liter	15	nonfat milk, reduced minerals whey, taurine	71	lactose	353	oleo oil, coconut oil, high oleic safflower or sunflower oil, soybean oil, soy lecithin, linoleic acid	1.3	147 (6.4 mEq)	553 (14.2 mEq)	667	Vit A, B1, B2, B3, B6, C, D, E, K, inositol, Ca, P, Cu, Mg, Zn, Mn, I, Cl[1]	In 390 mL concentrate, 1 qt ready-to-use liquid and 1 lb powder.
otc	**Tyromex-1 Powder** (Ross)	100 g powder[3]	15	amino acids (including tryptophan, taurine, carnitine)	46.3	hydrolyzed corn-starch	29	palm oil, hydrogenated coconut oil, soy oil, mono- and diglycerides, linoleic acid	9	190 (8.3 mEq)	675 (17.3 mEq)	480	Vit A, B1, B2, B3, B5, B6, B12, C, D, E, K, inositol, Ca, P, Cu, Mg, Zn, Mn, I, Cl, Se[1]	*For nutritional support of infants and toddlers with tyrosinemia type I.* Phenylalanine, tyrosine and methionine free. In 350 g powder.
otc	**Lactofree Liquid and Powder** (Mead Johnson Nutritionals)	1 liter	14.7	milk protein isolate, taurine, carnitine	69.3	corn syrup solids	37	palm olein, soy, coconut and high-oleic sunflower oils, linoleic acid	12	200 (9 mEq)	733 (19 mEq)	676	Vit A, B1, B2, B3, B5, B6, B12, C, D, E, K, inositol, Ca, P, Cu, Mg, Zn, Mn, I, Cl, Se[1]	Lactose free. In 1 qt ready-to-use liquid, 390 mL concentrate and 400 g powder.
otc	**Similac Low-Iron Liquid and Powder** (Ross)	1 liter	14.3	nonfat milk, taurine	72	lactose	36	Corn, coconut and soy oils, mono- and diglycerides, soy lecithin, linoleic acid	1.5	180 (7.8 mEq)	700 (17.9 mEq)	676	Vit A, B1, B2, B3, B5, B6, B12, C, D, E, K, inositol, Ca, P, Cu, Mg, Zn, Mn, I, Cl[1]	In 390 mL concentrate, 240 mL and 1 qt ready-to-use, 120 and 240 mL nursettes and 1 lb powder.
otc	**Cyclinex-1 Powder** (Ross)	100 g powder[3]	7.5	amino acids (including phenylalanine, tryptophan, carnitine, taurine)	52	hydrolyzed corn-starch	27	palm oil, hydrogenated coconut oil, soy oil, mono- and diglycerides, linoleic acid	10	215 (9.3 mEq)	760 (19.4 mEq)	515	Vit A, B1, B2, B3, B5, B6, B12, C, D, E, K, inositol, Ca, P, Cu, Mg, Zn, Mn, I, Cl, Se[1]	*For nutritional support of infants and toddlers with a urea cycle disorder or gyrate atrophy.* Nonessential amino acid free. In 350 g.
otc	**Soyalac Liquid and Powder** (Nutricia-Loma Linda)	per 100 calories	3.1	soybean extract	10	corn syrup, sucrose	5.5	soy oil, linoleic acid	1.5	‡	‡	667	unknown	Lactose free. In 390 mL concentrate, 1 qt ready-to-use and 420 g powder.
otc	**I-Soyalac Liquid and Powder** (Nutricia-Loma Linda)	per 100 calories	3.1	soy protein isolate, amino acids	10	sucrose, tapioca dextrin, potato maltodextrin	5.5	soy oil, linoleic acid	1.9	‡	‡	100	unknown	Corn syrup solids and lactose free. In 390 mL concentrate and 1 qt ready-to-use and 420 g powder.
otc	**Isomil DF** (Ross)	per 100 calories	2.7	soybean solids, amino acids	10.1	corn syrup, sucrose	5.5	soy oil, coconut oil	1.8	44 (1.9 mEq)	108 (2.8 mEq)	676	Vit A, B1, B2, B3, B5, B6, B12, C, D, E, K, inositol, Ca, P, Cu, Mg, Zn, Mn, I, Cl, Se[1]	*For management of diarrhea in infants and toddlers.* Lactose free. In 960 mL, pre-diluted, ready-to-use cans.
otc	**Enfamil LactoFree Liquid, Liquid Concentrate, and Powder** (Mead Johnson Nutritionals)	—	2.1	‡	10.9	‡	5.3	‡	1.8	30	8 mcg	100 per serving	860 mg linoleic acid, 300 IU vit. A, 60 IU vit. D, 2 IU vit. E, 80 mcg vit. B1, 140 mcg vit. B2, 60 mcg vit. B6, 0.3 mcg vit. B12, 1000 mcg vit. B3, 16 mcg folic acid, 600 mcg vit. B5, 3 mcg biotin, 12 mg vit. C, 12 mg choline, 17 mg inositol (liquid only), 6 mg inositol (powder only), 82 mg Ca, 55 mg P, 8 mg Mg, 1 mg Zn, 15 mcg Mn, 75 mcg Xu, 15 mcg I, 2.8 mcg Se, 110 mg K, 67 mg chloride	In 397 g (powder), 384 mL (liquid concentrate, or 946 mL liquid)

ENTERAL NUTRITIONAL THERAPY

SPECIALIZED INFANT FOODS

	Product & Distributor	Dilution	Protein		Carbohydrate		Fat		Iron (mg)	Na (mg)	K (mg)	Cal	Other Content	How Supplied
			g	Source	g	Source	g	Source						
otc	**Pro-Phree Powder** (Ross)	100 g powder[3]	‡	‡	60	hydrolyzed corn-starch	31	palm oil, hydrogenated coco-nut oil, soy oil, mono- and diglycerides, linoleic acid	11.9	250 (11 mEq)	875 (22.4 mEq)	520	Vit A, B₁, B₂, B₃, B₅, B₆, B₁₂, C, D, E, K, inositol, Ca, P, Cu, Mg, Zn, Mn, I, Cl, Se,[1,4]	*For nutritional support of infants and toddlers who require extra calories, minerals, vitamins and/or protein restriction. Protein free. In 350 g powder.*

* ‡ Amount Unknown.
[1] Also contains folic acid, biotin and choline
[2] Ready-to-use contains soy lecithin and mono- and diglycerides.
[3] Content given from unreconstituted powder.
[4] Contains trace amounts of taurine and carnitine.

See individual product listings for specific labeled indications.

LACTOSE

otc	**Lactose** (Various, eg, Humco, Paddock)	**Powder**	In 1 lb.

Refer to additional information in the Enteral Nutritional Therapy introduction.

CALCIUM CASEINATE

otc	**Casec** (Mead Johnson Nutritionals)	**Powder:** Contains 88 g protein, 1.6 g calcium, 120 mg sodium, 2 g fat and 370 calories per 100 g	In 75 g.

Refer to additional information in the Enteral Nutritional Therapy introduction.

Intravenous nutritional therapy is required when normal enteral feeding is not possible or is inadequate for nutritional requirements. Specific nutritional requirements and administration mode depend on the nutritional status of the patient and the duration of parenteral therapy. To meet IV nutritional requirements, one or more of the following nutrients may be required:

Protein Substrates
  Amino Acids - General Formulations
  Amino Acids - Renal Failure Formulations
  Amino Acids - Hepatic Failure/Encephalopathy Formulations
  Amino Acids - Metabolic Stress Formulations

Energy Substrates
  Dextrose
  IV Fat Emulsion

Electrolytes

Vitamins

Trace Metals

The following general discussion reviews peripheral and central administration routes, and provides basic guidelines for use of various components of IV nutritional therapy.

►PERIPHERAL PARENTERAL NUTRITION:

Peripheral protein sparing – Amino acids with maintenance electrolytes (with or without dextrose) prevent protein catabolism, for short periods of time, in patients with adequate body fat and no clinically significant protein malnutrition. Lipolysis provides energy from oxidation of free fatty acids and ketone bodies; minimal nitrogen is lost since proteolysis does not occur. For peripheral IV infusion, 1 to 1.5 g/kg/day of amino acids achieves optimal fat mobilization and spares protein catabolism.

ProcalAmine: ProcalAmine is a unique product that provides a physiological ratio of biologically useable essential and nonessential amino acids, glycerin (glycerol) and maintenance electrolytes. Glycerin preserves body protein and participates as an active energy substrate through its phosphorylation to α-glycerophosphate.

Peripheral total parenteral nutrition (TPN) – TPN is for patients requiring parenteral nutrition when the central venous route is not indicated. Amino acids with electrolytes, combined with 5% or 10% dextrose and used with IV fat emulsions (and usually vitamins and trace metals), reduce protein catabolism in patients moderately catabolic or depleted and minimize liver glycogen depletion. Peripheral infusions may provide inadequate maintenance requirements for those with greatly increased metabolic demands or severe nutritional deficiencies requiring repletion. May add oral calories as tolerated.

►CENTRAL TOTAL PARENTERAL NUTRITION: Amino acids combined with hypertonic dextrose and IV fat emulsions infused via a central venous catheter promote protein synthesis in hypercatabolic or severely depleted patients or those requiring long-term parenteral nutrition. Appropriate electrolytes, vitamins and trace minerals are added to provide total parenteral nutrition.

►Indications: Parenteral nutrition is indicated to prevent nitrogen and weight loss or to treat negative nitrogen balance when: (1) The alimentary tract, by the oral, gastrostomy or jejunostomy route, cannot or should not be used; (2) GI absorption of protein is impaired by obstruction, inflammatory disease or its complications or antineoplastic therapy; (3) bowel rest is needed because of GI surgery or its complications such as ileus, fistulae or anastomotic leaks; (4) metabolic requirements for protein are substantially increased, as with extensive burns, infections, trauma or other hypermetabolic states; (5) morbidity and mortality may be reduced by replacing amino acids lost from tissue breakdown, thereby preserving tissue reserves, as in acute renal failure; (6) tube feeding methods alone cannot provide adequate nutrition.

After the patient's nutritional deficits, reserves and current status are assessed, set rational and precise nutritional goals. Dosage, route of administration and concomitant infusion of nonprotein calories depend on nutritional and metabolic status, anticipated duration of parenteral nutritional support and vein tolerance.

Peripheral parenteral nutrition – Administration of nutritional solutions through peripheral veins is appropriate if caloric needs are minimal, if they can be partially met by enteral alimentation, if nutritional therapy will only be required for 5 to 14 days, or if central venous access is not feasible.

Central parenteral nutrition – Amino acids, with hypertonic dextrose and IV fat emulsions infused via central venous catheter, promote protein synthesis in the hypercatabolic or severely depleted or in those requiring long-term parenteral nutrition.

Total nutrient admixtures (TNA) – A combination of amino acids, dextrose and lipids in one container has been used. Also known as multicomponent admixtures, all-in-one, 3-in-1 or triple mix, TNA offers the advantage of substituting some dextrose calories with lipids, reducing carbohydrate-related complications (eg, impaired glucose control). It also appears to be used better by the liver due to continuous lipid administration, and is less likely to interfere with immune functions. See also admixture incompatibilities/compatibilities under Administration and Dosage.

Specific disease states – Specific disease states in which TPN requires special considerations are: Renal failure, acute metabolic stress, hepatic failure/hepatic encephalopathy. See individual sections for specific discussions.

►Administration and Dosage:
Total daily dose – Total daily dose depends on daily protein requirements and on the patient's metabolic and clinical responses. The determination of nitrogen balance and accurate daily body weights, corrected for fluid balance, are probably the best means of assessing protein requirements. In addition, guide dosage by the patient's fluid intake limits, glucose and nitrogen tolerances and metabolic and clinical response.

Protein – Recommended dietary allowances of protein are approximately 0.9 g/kg for a healthy adult and 1.4 to 2.2 g/kg for healthy growing infants and children. Protein and caloric requirements in traumatized or malnourished patients may be substantially increased. Daily doses of approximately 1 to 1.5 g/kg for adults and 2 to 3 g/kg for infants are generally sufficient to promote positive nitrogen balance, although higher doses may be required in severely catabolic states. Such higher doses require frequent laboratory evaluation.

Energy requirements – To ensure proper caloric intake, estimate required calorie and energy needs using basal metabolic rate; also consider energy expenditure and disease states. The energy required for proper amino acid utilization is derived from glycogenolysis, lipolysis or infusion of dextrose or fat emulsions. After glycogen is depleted, in the absence of exogenous calories, fat becomes the major energy source. Parenteral amino acids will not be retained and utilized for anabolic purposes unless adequate nonprotein calories are provided simultaneously.

IV fat emulsion: IV fat emulsion should comprise no more than 60% of the total caloric intake, with carbohydrates and amino acids comprising the remaining 40% or more.

Electrolyte requirements – In adults, ≈ 60 to 180 mEq of potassium, 10 to 30 mEq of magnesium and 10 to 40 mM of phosphate per day appear necessary to achieve optimum metabolic response; individualize each requirement. Give sufficient quantities of the major extracellular electrolytes, sodium, calcium and chloride. (Calcium prevents hypocalcemia that may accompany phosphate administration.) Consider content of amino acid infusion when calculating daily electrolyte intake.

HepatAmine: HepatAmine contains < 3 mEq chloride/L and ≤ 10 mM/L of phosphate. Some patients, especially hypophosphatemics, may require additional phosphate.

Fluid balance – Provide sufficient water to compensate for insensible, urinary and other (eg, nasogastric suction, fistula drainage, diarrhea) fluid losses. Average daily adult fluid requirements are between 2500 and 3000 mL, but may be much higher with losses such as fistula drainage or in burn patients.

Vitamin therapy – If a patient's nutritional intake is primarily parenteral, provide vitamins (especially the water soluble vitamins). Iron is added to the solution or given IM in depot form as indicated. Folic acid and vitamin K are required additives.

Pediatric – Pediatric requirements are constrained by the greater relative fluid and caloric requirements per kg of the infant. Amino acids are best administered in a 2.5% concentration. For most pediatric patients, 2.5 g amino acids/kg/day with dextrose alone or with IV fat calories of 100 to 130 kcal/kg/day are recommended for maintenance. Start with nutritional solution of half strength at a rate of about 60 to 70 mL/kg/day. Within 24 to 48 hours, the volume and concentration of the solution can be increased until full strength pediatric solution is given at a rate of 125 to 150 mL/kg/day.

A basic central line solution for pediatric use should contain 25 g of amino acids and 200 to 250 g of glucose per 1000 mL. Such a solution given at a rate of 145 mL/kg/day provides 100 to 130 kcal/kg/day.

Give supplemental electrolytes and vitamins (including agents such as carnitine) as needed. Iron is more critical in infants because of increasing red cell mass needed for growth. Monitor serum lipids for EFAD in patients maintained on fat-free TPN.

To ensure the precise delivery of the small volumes of fluid necessary, use accurately calibrated and reliable infusion systems.

Preparation/stability of solutions – Aseptically prepare solutions under a laminar flow hood. Use promptly after mixing. Store under refrigeration for a brief period of time only (< 24 hours). Do not exceed 24 hours for administration time of a single bottle.

Admixture incompatibilities/compatibilities – Because of the potential for incompatibility in the complex formulations, keep additives to a minimum. Do not administer simultaneously with **blood** through the same infusion site because of possible pseudoagglutination. **Antibiotics, steroids** and **pressor agents** should not be added to these solutions. **Bleomycin** is incompatible with amino acids.

Vitamins, electrolytes, trace minerals, heparin and **insulin** are compatible with these solutions.

Total nutrient admixture: Total nutrient admixture (TNA; all-in-one; 3-in-1; triple mix): The combination of amino acids, dextrose and lipids (also known as total nutrient admixture) in one container is generally compatible. When utilizing this type of admixture, consider the following: (1) The order of mixing is important – add amino acids to the fat emulsion or the dextrose; (2) do not add the electrolytes directly to the fat emulsion – add them to the dextrose or amino acids first; (3) TNAs with electrolytes will eventually aggregate; (4) if not used immediately, refrigerate.

Administration sets – Replace all IV sets every 24 hours. Follow appropriate guidelines for care and maintenance of long-term indwelling catheters (eg, Broviac or Hickman).

➤*Actions:*
Pharmacology –
Amino acids: Amino acids promote the production of proteins (anabolism) needed for synthesis of structural components, reduce the rate of protein breakdown (catabolism), promote wound healing and act as buffers in the extracellular and intracellular fluids.

Dextrose: Dextrose is a source of calories; nonprotein calories are required for efficient use of amino acids. It decreases protein and nitrogen losses, promotes glycogen deposition and prevents ketosis (see individual monograph).

IV fat emulsions: IV fat emulsions provide a mixture of fatty acids to be used as a source of energy and to prevent essential fatty acid deficiency (EFAD) (see individual monograph).

Fluid/Electrolytes/Trace metals: Fluid, electrolytes, and trace metals are provided to compensate for normal sensible and insensible losses, as well as the additional losses often present in patients requiring parenteral nutrition (see individual section).

➤*Contraindications:*
Protein substrates – Hypersensitivity to any component; decreased (subcritical) circulating blood volume; inborn errors of amino acid metabolism (eg, maple syrup urine disease, isovaleric acidemia); anuria.

General amino acid formulations – Severe renal failure or liver disease; hepatic coma or encephalopathy; metabolic disorders involving impaired nitrogen utilization.

Renal failure formulations – Severe electrolyte and acid-base imbalance; hyperammonemia.

Hepatic failure/Hepatic encephalopathy formulations – Anuria.

High metabolic stress formulations – Anuria; hyperammonemia; hepatic coma; severe electrolyte or acid-base imbalance.

➤*Warnings:*
Prevention of complications – IV nutritional therapy may be associated with complications that can be prevented or minimized by careful attention to solution preparation, administration and patient monitoring. It is essential to follow a carefully prepared protocol based on current medical practices, preferably administered by an experienced team.

Amino acid metabolism – Hyperchloremic metabolic acidosis may result from amino acids provided as hydrochloride salts that release hydrochloride when utilized. To prevent or control this, supply a portion of the cations as acetate or lactate salts. Sodium and potassium phosphates are also available.

Hepatic function impairment – Hepatic function impairment may result in serum amino acid imbalances, metabolic alkalosis, prerenal azotemia, hyperammonemia, stupor and coma. Instances of asymptomatic hyperammonemia have occurred in patients without overt liver dysfunction. Amino acid products specifically formulated for patients with hepatic failure are discussed separately in this section. Give conservative doses of amino acids to patients with known or suspected hepatic dysfunction.

Hyperammonemia: Hyperammonemia occurs most often in children and adults with renal or hepatic disease and results from a diminished ability to handle a protein load. It is of special significance in infants as it can result in mental retardation. This reaction is dose-related and more likely to develop during prolonged therapy; treatment involves adjusting the dosage or decreasing amino acids.

Ketosis: Administration of amino acids without carbohydrates may result in the accumulation of ketones; correct ketonemia by administering carbohydrates.

Infection control – Parenteral nutrition is associated with a constant risk of sepsis. Careful, aseptic technique in the preparation of solutions and insertion and maintenance of central venous catheters is imperative. A 0.22 micron filter is often recommended to block particulate matter and bacteria. Presence of *Staphylococcus* or *Candida* suggests catheter sepsis. Early symptoms of infection include fever, chills, glucose intolerance and a change in the level of consciousness.

If other sources are not apparent and if fever persists, change solution, delivery system and catheter site. Culture catheter tip and draw blood cultures.

Pregnancy – *Category C.* It is not known whether IV nutritional therapy can cause fetal harm when given to a pregnant woman or can affect reproduction capacity. Use only when clearly needed and potential benefits outweigh hazards to the fetus.

Lactation – Exercise caution when administering to a nursing woman.

Children – The effect of amino acid infusions without dextrose on carbohydrate metabolism of children is not known. Use special caution in pediatric patients with acute renal failure, especially low birth weight

infants. Laboratory and clinical monitoring must be extensive and frequent.

➤*Precautions:*
Monitoring – Laboratory monitoring and clinical evaluation are necessary before and during use. Do not withdraw venous blood for blood chemistries through the same peripheral infusion site; interference with estimations of nitrogen-containing substances may occur. The following general protocol is suggested:

General Patient Monitoring During IV Nutritional Therapy
Baseline studies: CBC, platelet count, prothrombin time, weight, body length and head circumference (in infants), electrolytes, CO_2, BUN, glucose, creatinine, total protein, cholesterol, triglycerides (if on fat emulsion), uric acid, bilirubin, alkaline phosphatase, LDH, AST, albumin and other appropriate parameters.
Daily studies during stabilization (average 3 to 5 days): Urine glucose, acetone and ketones each shift, intake/output, weight, plasma and urine osmolarity, electrolytes, trace elements, CO_2, BUN, creatinine.
Routine studies after stabilization: Daily - Intake/output, weight, urine glucose and osmolarity and ketones.
Two to three times weekly: Electrolytes, BUN, blood glucose, plasma transaminases, bilirubin, blood acid-base status, ammonia, creatinine.
Weekly: CBC, prothrombin time, plasma total protein and fractions, hemoglobin, body length and head circumference (in infants), cholesterol, triglycerides, uric acid, albumin, LDH, AST, alkaline phosphatase.
Periodic: Nitrogen balance, trace elements, total lymphocyte count, iron status.

BUN – IV amino acid infusion may induce a rise in BUN, especially in GI bleeding or impaired hepatic or renal function. Perform appropriate laboratory tests periodically; discontinue if BUN exceeds normal postprandial limits and continues to rise. A modest rise in BUN normally results from increased protein intake. Azotemic patients should not receive amino acids without regard to total nitrogen intake.

Protein sparing: If daily increases in BUN (range, 10 to 15 mg/dL) for > 3 days occur, discontinue protein sparing therapy and institute a regimen with full nonprotein caloric substrates.

Cardiac effects – Avoid circulatory overload, particularly in patients with cardiac insufficiency. In patients with myocardial infarction, infusion of amino acids should always be accompanied by dextrose; in anoxia, free fatty acids cannot be used by the myocardium, and energy must be produced anaerobically from glycogen or glucose.

Hypertonic solutions – Hypertonic solutions containing dextrose should not be administered by peripheral vein infusions. Do not use hypertonic solutions in the presence of intracranial or intraspinal hemorrhage or if the patient is already dehydrated.

Glucose imbalances –
Hyperglycemia: Glucose intolerance is the most common metabolic complication; metabolic adaptation to large glucose loads requires up to 72 hours, although severely septic or hypermetabolic patients may not be able to handle the glucose load. A too rapid infusion of amino acid-carbohydrate mixtures may result in hyperglycemia, glycosuria and a hyperosmolar syndrome, characterized by mental confusion and loss of consciousness. Reducing the administration rate, decreasing the dextrose concentration or administering insulin will minimize these reactions.

Hyperglycemia may not be reflected by glycosuria in renal failure. Therefore, determine blood glucose frequently, often every 6 hours, to guide dosage of dextrose and insulin if required. Infusion of hypertonic dextrose carries a greater risk of hyperglycemia in low birth weight or septic infants.

Excess carbohydrate calories may result in fatty infiltration of the liver. Excess carbon dioxide from too much glucose can compromise weaning hypermetabolic patients from mechanical ventilation or can precipitate acute respiratory failure.

Rebound hypoglycemia: Rebound hypoglycemia may result from sudden cessation of a concentrated dextrose solution due to continued endogenous insulin production. Withdraw parenteral nutrition mixtures slowly. Administer a solution containing 5% or 10% dextrose when hypertonic dextrose infusions are abruptly discontinued.

Essential fatty acid deficiency (EFAD) – Essential fatty acid deficiency (EFAD) results from long-term fat-free IV feeding; symptoms include dry, scaly skin, eczematous rash, hair loss, poor wound healing and fatty degeneration of the liver. In adults, administer at least 500 mL fat emulsion per week to prevent EFAD (see individual monograph).

Electrolyte abnormalities – Intracellular ion deficits may arise due to two mechanisms. As protein is used for increased energy demands in a catabolic patient, intracellular ions are lost. In addition, as anabolism occurs, ions are employed in building new cells. Focus attention on supplying adequate potassium, phosphate, magnesium and calcium. Observe patients for clinical signs of paresthesias, neuromuscular weakness and changes in level of consciousness; monitor laboratory results.

The presence of impaired renal function, pulmonary disease, or cardiac insufficiency presents danger of retention of fluids.

Sodium: Use solutions containing sodium ions cautiously in patients with CHF, severe renal insufficiency, and edema with sodium retention.

Potassium: Use solutions containing potassium ions cautiously in patients with hyperkalemia or severe renal failure, and in conditions in which potassium retention is present.

Acetate: Use solutions containing acetate ions cautiously in patients with metabolic or respiratory alkalosis and in those conditions in which there is an increased level or impaired utilization of this ion, such as severe hepatic insufficiency.

Cancer chemotherapy patients – The American College of Physicians discourages the routine use of parenteral nutrition in patients undergoing cancer chemotherapy since no benefit has been determined (ie, there was no improvement in overall or short-term survival and no greater improvement in chemotherapy response).

Sulfite sensitivity – Some of these products contain sulfites which may cause allergic-type reactions including anaphylactic symptoms and life-threatening or less severe asthmatic episodes in certain susceptible persons. The overall prevalence of sulfite sensitivity in the general population is unknown and probably low. Sulfite sensitivity is seen more frequently in asthmatic or atopic persons.

➤*Drug Interactions:*

Tetracycline – Tetracycline may reduce the protein sparing effects of infused amino acids because of its antianabolic activity.

➤*Adverse Reactions:*

Catheter complications – Phlebitis and venous thrombosis may occur at the site of venipuncture or along the vein. If this occurs, discontinue use or choose another administration site. Use of large peripheral veins, inline filters and slower infusion rates may reduce the incidence of local venous irritation. Infection at the injection site and extravasation may occur.

Nausea, fever and flushing of the skin have occurred.

Metabolic complications include – Metabolic acidosis and alkalosis; hypophosphatemia; hypocalcemia; osteoporosis; glycosuria; hyperglycemia; hypo- or hypermagnesemia; osmotic diuresis; dehydration; hypervolemia; rebound hypoglycemia; hypo- or hypervitaminosis; electrolyte imbalances; hyperammonemia; elevated hepatic enzymes.

Phosphorus deficiency may lead to impaired tissue oxygenation and acute hemolytic anemia. Relative to calcium, excessive phosphorus intake can precipitate hypocalcemia with cramps, tetany and muscular hyperexcitability.

Complications known to occur from the placement of central venous catheters are pneumothorax, hemothorax, hydrothorax, artery puncture and transection, injury to the brachial plexus, malposition of the catheter, formation of arteriovenous fistula, phlebitis, thrombosis and air and catheter embolus.

Reactions reported in clinical studies as a result of infusion of the parenteral fluid were water weight gain, edema, increase in BUN and mild acidosis.

Protein Substrates

AMINO ACID INJECTION (General formulations)

For a complete discussion of the use of protein substrates as a compound of intravenous nutritional therapy, refer to the IV Nutritional Therapy general monograph.

Administration and Dosage

➤*Peripheral protein sparing:* Administer amino acids in a dose of 1 to 1.7 g/kg/day via a peripheral vein. If daily increases in BUN in the range of 10 to 15 mg/dL for > 3 days occur, discontinue and implement a regimen with full nonprotein calorie substrates.

ProcalAmine – Approximately 3 L/day will provide 90 g of amino acids, 390 nonprotein calories and recommended daily intake of principal intra- and extracellular electrolytes for the stable patient. In adults, begin with 3 L on the first day with close monitoring of the patient.

➤*Peripheral vein administration:* Mix amino acid injections with low concentrations of dextrose solutions (5% or 10%) and administer by peripheral vein with fat emulsions.

➤*Central vein administration:* Typically, 500 mL amino acid injection mixed with 500 mL concentrated dextrose injection, electrolytes and vitamins is administered over an 8 hour period.

Strongly hypertonic mixtures of amino acids and dextrose may be safely administered by continuous infusion only through a central venous catheter with the tip located in the superior vena cava. The initial rate of IV infusion should be 2 mL/min and may be increased gradually to the maximum required dose, as indicated by frequent determinations of urine and blood sugar levels. May be started with infusates containing lower concentrations of dextrose and gradually increased to estimated caloric needs as the patient's glucose tolerance increases. If the administration rate falls behind schedule, do not attempt to "catch up" to planned intake. Do not exceed 24 hours administration time for a single bottle. In addition to meeting protein needs, the administration rate is also governed by the patient's glucose tolerance, especially during the first few days of therapy.

Actions

➤*Pharmacology:* Crystalline amino acid injections are hypertonic solutions of balanced essential and nonessential l–amino acids; d–amino acids are not readily utilized by the body. Depending on the amount of caloric supplementation, these amino acids provide a substrate for protein synthesis (anabolism) or enhance conservation of existing body protein (protein sparing effect).

CRYSTALLINE AMINO ACID INFUSIONS

	Aminosyn 3.5% (Abbott)	Aminosyn II 3.5% (Abbott)	Aminosyn 5% (Abbott)	Aminosyn II 5% (Abbott)	Travasol 5.5% (Clintec)	TrophAmine 6% (McGaw)
Amino Acid Concentration	3.5%	3.5%	5%	5%	5.5%	6%
Nitrogen (g/100 mL)	0.55	0.54	0.79	0.77	0.925	0.93
Amino Acids (Essential) (mg/100 mL)						
Isoleucine	252	231	360	330	263	490
Leucine	329	350	470	500	340	840
Lysine	252	368	360	525	318	490
Methionine	140	60	200	86	318	200
Phenylalanine	154	104	220	149	340	290
Threonine	182	140	260	200	230	250
Tryptophan	56	70	80	100	99	120
Valine	280	175	400	250	252	470
Amino Acids (Nonessential) (mg/100 mL)						
Alanine	448	348	640	497	1140	320
Arginine	343	356	490	509	570	730
Histidine[a]	105	105	150	150	241	290
Proline	300	253	430	361	230	410
Serine	147	186	210	265		230
Taurine						15
Tyrosine	31	95	44	135	22	140

	Aminosyn 3.5% (Abbott)	Aminosyn II 3.5% (Abbott)	Aminosyn 5% (Abbott)	Aminosyn II 5% (Abbott)	Travasol 5.5% (Clintec)	TrophAmine 6% (McGaw)
Aminoacetic Acid (Glycine)	448	175	640	250	1140	220
Glutamic Acid		258		369		300
Aspartic Acid		245		350		190
Cysteine						< 14
Electrolytes (mEq/L)						
Sodium	7	16.3		19.3		5
Potassium			5.4			
Chloride					22	< 3
Acetate	46	25.2	86	35.9	48	56
Phosphate (mM/L)						
Osmolarity (mOsm/L)	357	308	500	438	575	525
Supplied in (mL)	1000[b]	1000[c]	500[d] 1000[d]	500[c] 1000[c]	500[e] 1000[e] 2000[e]	500[f]
Labeled Indications						
Peripheral Parenteral Nutrition	Yes	Yes	Yes	Yes	Yes	Yes
Central TPN	No	No	Yes	Yes	Yes	Yes
Protein Sparing	Yes	Yes	Yes	Yes	Yes	No

Protein Substrates

CRYSTALLINE AMINO ACID INFUSIONS

	Aminosyn 7% (Abbott)	Aminosyn-PF 7% (Abbott)	Aminosyn II 7% (Abbott)	Aminosyn 8.5% (Abbott)
Amino Acid Concentration	7%	7%	7%	8.5%
Nitrogen (g/100 mL)	1.1	1.07	1.07	1.34
Amino Acids (Essential) (mg/100 mL)				
Isoleucine	510	534	462	620
Leucine	660	831	700	810
Lysine	510	475	735	624
Methionine	280	125	120	340
Phenylalanine	310	300	209	380
Threonine	370	360	280	460
Tryptophan	120	125	140	150
Valine	560	452	350	680
Amino Acids (Nonessential) (mg/100 mL)				
Alanine	900	490	695	1100
Arginine	690	861	713	850
Histidine[a]	210	220	210	260
Proline	610	570	505	750
Serine	300	347	371	370
Taurine		50		
Tyrosine	44	44	189	44
Aminoacetic Acid (Glycine)	900	270	350	1100
Glutamic Acid		576	517	
Aspartic Acid		370	490	
Cysteine				
Electrolytes (mEq/L)				
Sodium		3.4	31.3	
Potassium	5.4			5.4
Chloride			35	
Acetate	105	32.5	50.3	90
Phosphate (mM/L)				
Osmolarity (mOsm/L)	700	586	612	850
Supplied in (mL)	500[d]	250[g] 500[g]	500[c]	500[d] 1000[d]
Labeled Indications				
Peripheral Parenteral Nutrition	Yes	Yes	Yes	Yes
Central TPN	Yes	Yes	Yes	Yes
Protein Sparing	Yes	No	Yes	Yes

	Aminosyn II 8.5% (Abbott)	Travasol 8.5% without electrolytes (Clintec)	FreAmine III 8.5% (B. Braun)
Amino Acid Concentration	8.5%	8.5%	8.5%
Nitrogen (g/100 mL)	1.3	1.43	
Amino Acids (Essential) (mg/100 mL)			
Isoleucine	561	406	590
Leucine	850	526	770
Lysine	893	492	620
Methionine	146	492	450
Phenylalanine	253	526	480
Threonine	340	356	340
Tryptophan	170	152	130
Valine	425	390	560

	Aminosyn II 8.5% (Abbott)	Travasol 8.5% without electrolytes (Clintec)	FreAmine III 8.5% (B. Braun)
Amino Acids (Nonessential) (mg/100 mL)			
Alanine	844	1760	600
Arginine	865	880	810
Histidine[a]	255	372	240
Proline	614	356	950
Serine	450		500
Taurine			
Tyrosine	230	34	
Aminoacetic Acid (Glycine)	425	1760	1190
Glutamic Acid	627		
Aspartic Acid	595		
Cysteine			< 20
Electrolytes (mEq/L)			
Sodium	33.3		10
Potassium			
Chloride		34	< 3
Acetate	61.1	73	72
Phosphate (mM/L)			10
Osmolarity (mOsm/L)	742	890	810
Supplied in (mL)	500[c] 1000[c]	500[h] 1000[h] 2000[h]	500[i] 1000[i]
Labeled Indications			
Peripheral Parenteral Nutrition	Yes	Yes	Yes
Central TPN	Yes	Yes	Yes
Protein Sparing	Yes	Yes	Yes

	TrophAmine 10% (McGaw)	Aminosyn 10% (Abbott)	Aminosyn-PF 10% (Abbott)	Aminosyn II 10% (Abbott)
Amino Acid Concentration	10%	10%	10%	10%
Nitrogen (g/100 mL)	1.55	1.57	1.52	1.53
Amino Acids (Essential) (mg/100 mL)				
Isoleucine	820	720	760	660
Leucine	1400	940	1200	1000
Lysine	820	720	677	1050
Methionine	340	400	180	172
Phenylalanine	480	440	427	298
Threonine	420	520	512	400
Tryptophan	200	160	180	200
Valine	780	800	673	500
Amino Acids (Nonessential) (mg/100 mL)				
Alanine	540	1280	698	993
Arginine	1200	980	1227	1018
Histidine[a]	480	300	312	300
Proline	680	860	812	722
Serine	380	420	495	530
Taurine	25		70	
Tyrosine	240	44	40	270
Aminoacetic Acid (Glycine)	360	1280	385	500
Glutamic Acid	500		620	738
Aspartic Acid	320		527	700
Cysteine	< 16			
Electrolytes (mEq/L)				
Sodium	5		3.4	45.3
Potassium		5.4		

Protein Substrates

CRYSTALLINE AMINO ACID INFUSIONS

	TrophAmine 10% (McGaw)	Aminosyn 10% (Abbott)	Aminosyn-PF 10% (Abbott)	Aminosyn II 10% (Abbott)
Chloride	< 3			
Acetate	97	148	46.3	71.8
Phosphate (mM/L)10				
Osmolarity (mOsm/L)	875	1000	829	873
Supplied in (mL)	500[f]	500[d] 1000[d]	1000[j]	500[c] 1000[c]
Labeled Indications				
Peripheral Parenteral Nutrition	Yes	Yes	Yes	Yes
Central TPN	Yes	Yes	Yes	Yes
Protein Sparing	No	Yes	No	Yes

	Travasol 10% (Clintec)	FreAmine III 10% (McGaw)	Novamine (Clintec)	Novamine 15% (Clintec)	Aminosyn II 15% (Abbott)
Amino Acid Concentration	10%	10%	11.4%	15%	15%
Nitrogen (g/100 mL)	1.65	1.53	1.8	2.37	2.3
Amino Acids (Essential) (mg/100 mL)					
Isoleucine	600	690	570	749	990
Leucine	730	910	790	1040	1500
Lysine	580	730	900	1180	1575
Methionine	400	530	570	749	258
Phenylalanine	560	560	790	1040	447
Threonine	420	400	570	749	600
Tryptophan	180	150	190	250	300
Valine	580	660	730	960	750
Amino Acids (Nonessential) (mg/100 mL)					
Alanine	2070	710	1650	2170	1490
Arginine	1150	950	1120	1470	1527
Histidine[a]	480	280	680	894	450
Proline	680	1120	680	894	1083
Serine	500	590	450	592	795
Taurine					
Tyrosine	40		30	39	405
Aminoacetic Acid (Glycine)	1030	1400	790	1040	750
Glutamic Acid			570	749	1107
Aspartic Acid			330	434	1050
Cysteine		< 24			
Electrolytes (mEq/L)					
Sodium		10			62.7
Potassium					
Chloride	40	< 3			
Acetate	87	≈89	114	151	107.6
Phosphate (mM/L)		10			
Osmolarity (mOsm/L)	1000	≈ 950	1057	1388	1300
Supplied in (mL)	250[l,m] 500[l,m] 1000[l,m] 2000[l]	500[i] 1000[i]	500[n] 1000[n]	500[n] 1000[n]	2000[o]
Labeled Indications					
Peripheral Parenteral Nutrition	Yes	Yes	Yes	Yes	Yes
Central TPN	Yes	Yes	Yes	Yes	Yes
Protein Sparing	Yes	Yes	Yes	No	No

[a] Histidine is considered an essential amino acid in infants and in renal failure.
[b] With 7 mEq/L sodium from the antioxidant sodium hydrosulfite.
[c] Includes 20 mg/dL sodium hydrosulfite.
[d] Includes 5.4 mEq/L potassium from the antioxidant potassium metabisulfite.
[e] With ≈ 3 mEq/L sodium bisulfite.
[f] With < 50 mg sodium metabisulfite per 100 mL.
[g] From the antioxidant sodium hydrosulfite.
[h] With 3 mEq/L sodium bisulfite.
[i] With < 0.1 g sodium bisulfite per 100 mL.
[j] With 230 mg sodium hydrosulfite per 100 mL.
[k] Potassium derived from the antioxidant potassium metabisulfite.
[l] Acetate in Viaflex container = 60 mEq/L; osmolarity is 970 mOsm/L.
[m] Sizes also come in Viaflex containers.
[n] With 30 mg sodium metabisulfite.
[o] With 60 mg sodium hydrosulfite per 100 mL.

CRYSTALLINE AMINO ACID INFUSIONS WITH ELECTROLYTES

	ProcalAmine (McGaw)	FreAmine III 3% w/Electrolytes (McGaw)	Aminosyn 3.5% M (Abbott)	Aminosyn II 3.5% M (Abbott)	3.5% Travasol w/Electrolytes (Clintec)	5.5% Travasol w/Electrolytes (Clintec)
Amino Acid Concentration	3%	3%	3.5%	3.5%	3.5%	5.5%
Nitrogen (g/100 mL)	0.46	0.46	0.55	0.54	0.591	0.925
Amino Acids (Essential) (mg/100 mL)						
Isoleucine	210	210	252	231	168	263
Leucine	270	270	329	350	217	340
Lysine	220	220	252	368	203	318
Methionine	160	160	140	60	203	318
Phenylalanine	170	170	154	104	217	340
Threonine	120	120	182	140	147	230
Tryptophan	46	46	56	70	63	99
Valine	200	200	280	175	161	252
Amino Acids (Nonessential) (mg/100 mL)						
Alanine	210	210	448	348	728	1140
Arginine	290	290	343	356	364	570
Histidine[a]	85	85	105	105	154	241
Proline	340	340	300	253	147	230
Serine	180	180	147	186		
Tyrosine			31	95	14	22
Glycine	420	420	448	175	728	1140
Glutamic Acid				258		
Aspartic Acid				245		
Cysteine	< 20	< 20				
Electrolytes (mEq/L)						
Sodium	35	35	47	36	25	70
Potassium	24	24.5	13	13	15	60
Magnesium	5	5	3	3	5	10
Chloride	41	41	40	37	25	70
Acetate	47	44	58	25	52	102
Phosphate (mM/L)	3.5	3.5	3.5	3.5	7.5	30
Osmolarity (mOsm/L)	735	≈ 405	477	425	450	850
Nonprotein Calories (g/100 mL) (glycerin)	3					
Supplied in (mL)	1000[b]	1000[c]	1000[d]	1000[e]	500[f] 1000[f]	500[f] 1000[f] 2000[f]
Labeled Indications						
Peripheral Parenteral Nutrition	Yes	Yes	Yes	Yes	Yes	Yes
Central TPN	No	No	No	No	No	Yes
Protein Sparing	Yes	Yes	Yes	Yes	Yes	Yes

Protein Substrates

CRYSTALLINE AMINO ACID INFUSIONS WITH ELECTROLYTES

	Aminosyn 7% w/Electrolytes (Abbott)	Aminosyn II 7% with Electrolytes (Abbott)	Aminosyn 8.5% w/Electrolytes (Abbott)	Aminosyn II 8.5% with Electrolytes (Abbott)	FreAmine III 8.5% w/Electrolytes (McGaw)	Travasol 8.5% w/Electrolytes (Clintec)
Amino Acid Concentration	7%	7%	8.5%	8.5%	8.5%	8.5%
Nitrogen g/100 mL	1.1	1.07	1.34	1.3	1.3	1.43
Amino Acids (Essential) (mg/100 mL)						
Isoleucine	510	462	620	561	590	406
Leucine	660	700	810	850	770	526
Lysine	510	735	624	893	620	492
Methionine	280	120	340	146	450	492
Phenylalanine	310	209	380	253	480	526
Threonine	370	280	460	340	340	356
Tryptophan	120	140	150	170	130	152
Valine	560	350	680	425	560	390
Amino Acids (Nonessential) (mg/100 mL)						
Alanine	900	695	1100	844	600	1760
Arginine	690	713	850	865	810	880
Histidine[a]	210	210	260	255	240	372
Proline	610	505	750	614	950	356
Serine	300	371	370	450	500	
Tyrosine	44	189	44	230		34
Glycine	900	350	1100	425	1190	1760
Glutamic Acid		517		627		
Aspartic Acid		490		595		
Cysteine					< 20	
Electrolytes (mEq/L)						
Sodium	70	76	70	80	60	70
Potassium	66	66	66	66	60	60
Magnesium	10	10	10	10	10	10
Chloride	96	86	98	86	60	70
Acetate	124	50	142	61	125	141
Phosphate (mM/L)	30	30	30	30	20	30
Osmolarity (mOsm/L)	1013	869	1160	999	1045	1160
Supplied in (mL)	500[g]	500[h]	500[g]	500[h]	500[i] 1000[i]	500[f] 1000[f] 2000[f]
Labeled Indications						
Peripheral Parenteral Nutrition	Yes	Yes	Yes	Yes	Yes	Yes
Central TPN	Yes	Yes	Yes	Yes	Yes	Yes
Protein Sparing	Yes	Yes	Yes	Yes	Yes	Yes

[a] Histidine is considered an essential amino acid in infants and in renal failure.
[b] With < 50 mg K+ metabisulfite and 3 mEq Ca/L.
[c] With < 0.05 g of the antioxidant potassium metabisulfite.
[d] Includes 7 mEq/L sodium from the antioxidant sodium hydrosulfite.
[e] With 20 mg sodium hydrosulfite per 100 mL.
[f] With 3 mEq/L sodium bisulfite.
[g] Includes 5.4 mEq/L potassium from the antioxidant potassium metabisulfite.
[h] Includes sodium from the antioxidant sodium hydrosulfite.
[i] With < 0.1 g sodium bisulfite per 100 mL.

CRYSTALLINE AMINO ACID INFUSIONS WITH DEXTROSE

	Travasol 2.75% in 5% Dextrose[a] (Clintec)	Travasol 2.75% in 10% Dextrose[a] (Clintec)	Travasol 2.75% in 25% Dextrose[a] (Clintec)	Aminosyn II 3.5% in 5% Dextrose[a] (Abbott)	Aminosyn II 3.5% in 25% Dextrose[a] (Abbott)
Amino Acid Concentration	2.75%	2.75%	2.75%	3.5%	3.5%
Dextrose Concentration	5%	10%	25%	5%	25%
Nitrogen (g/100 mL)	0.46	0.46	0.46	0.54	0.54
Amino Acids (Essential) (mg/100 mL)					
Isoleucine	132	132	132	231	231
Leucine	170	170	170	350	350
Lysine	159	159	159	368	368
Methionine	159	159	159	60	60
Phenylalanine	170	170	170	104	104
Threonine	115	115	115	140	140
Tryptophan	50	50	50	70	70
Valine	126	126	126	175	175
Amino Acids (Nonessential) (mg/100 mL)					
Alanine	570	570	570	348	348
Arginine	285	285	285	356	356
Histidine[b]	120	120	120	105	105
Proline	115	115	115	252	252
Serine				186	186
Tyrosine	11	11	11	94	94
Aminoacetic Acid (Glycine)	570	570	570	175	175
Glutamic Acid				258	258
Aspartic Acid				245	245
Cysteine					
Electrolytes (mEq/L)					
Sodium				18	18
Potassium					
Magnesium					
Chloride	11	11	11		
Acetate	16	16	16	25.2	25.2
Phosphate (mM/L)					
Osmolarity (mOsm/L)	530	785	1540	585	1515
Supplied in (mL)	500 mL with 500 mL dextrose	500 mL with 500 mL dextrose	500 mL with 500 mL dextrose	1000 mL with 1000 mL dextrose[c]	500 mL with 500 mL dextrose[c]
Labeled Indications					
Peripheral Parenteral Nutrition	Yes	Yes	Yes	Yes	No
Central TPN	Yes	Yes	Yes	No	Yes

	Travasol 4.25% in 5% Dextrose[a] (Clintec)	Aminosyn II 4.25% in 10% Dextrose[a] (Abbott)	Travasol 4.25% in 10% Dextrose[a] (Clintec)	Aminosyn II 4.25% in 20% Dextrose[a] (Abbott)
Amino Acid Concentration	4.25%	4.25%	4.25%	4.25%
Dextrose Concentration	5%	10%	10%	20%
Nitrogen (g/100 mL)	0.7	0.65	0.7	0.65
Amino Acids (Essential) (mg/100 mL)				
Isoleucine	203	280	203	280
Leucine	263	425	263	425
Lysine	246	446	246	446
Methionine	246	73	246	73
Phenylalanine	263	126	263	126

Protein Substrates

CRYSTALLINE AMINO ACID INFUSIONS WITH DEXTROSE

	Travasol 4.25% in 5% Dextrose[a] (Clintec)	Aminosyn II 4.25% in 10% Dextrose[a] (Abbott)	Travasol 4.25% in 10% Dextrose[a] (Clintec)	Aminosyn II 4.25% in 20% Dextrose[a] (Abbott)
Threonine	178	170	178	170
Tryptophan	76	85	76	85
Valine	195	212	195	212
Amino Acids (Nonessential) (mg/100 mL)				
Alanine	880	422	880	422
Arginine	440	432	440	432
Histidine[b]	186	128	186	128
Proline	178	307	178	307
Serine		225		225
Tyrosine	17	115	17	115
Aminoacetic Acid (Glycine)	880	212	880	212
Glutamic Acid		314		314
Aspartic Acid		298		298
Cysteine				
Electrolytes (mEq/L)				
Sodium		19		19
Potassium				
Magnesium				
Chloride	17		17	
Acetate	22	30.6	22	30.6
Phosphate (mM/L)				
Osmolarity (mOsm/L)	680	894	935	1295
Supplied in (mL)	500 mL with 500 mL dextrose	1000 mL w/1000 mL dextrose[c]	500 mL with 500 mL dextrose	1000 mL with 1000 mL dextrose[c]
Labeled Indications				
Peripheral Parenteral Nutrition	Yes	Yes	Yes	No
Central TPN	Yes	No	Yes	Yes

	Aminosyn II 4.25% in 25% Dextrose[a] (Abbott)	Travasol 4.25% in 25% Dextrose[a] (Clintec)	Aminosyn II 5% in 25% Dextrose[a] (Abbott)
Amino Acid Concentration	4.25%	4.25%	5%
Dextrose Concentration	25%	25%	25%
Nitrogen (g/100 mL)	0.65	0.65	0.77
Amino Acids (Essential) (mg/100 mL)			
Isoleucine	280	203	330
Leucine	425	263	500
Lysine	446	246	525
Methionine	73	246	86
Phenylalanine	126	263	149
Threonine	170	178	200
Tryptophan	85	76	100
Valine	212	195	250
Amino Acids (Nonessential) (mg/100 mL)			
Alanine	422	880	496
Arginine	432	440	509
Histidine[b]	128	186	150
Proline	307	178	361
Serine	225		265
Tyrosine	115	17	135
Aminoacetic Acid (Glycine)	212	880	250
Glutamic Acid	314		369
Aspartic Acid	298		350
Cysteine			
Electrolytes (mEq/L)			
Sodium	19		22.2
Potassium			
Magnesium			
Chloride		17	
Acetate	30.6	22	35.9
Phosphate (mM/L)			
Osmolarity (mOsm/L)	1536	1690	1539
Supplied in (mL)	750 and 1000 mL and 750 and 1000 mL dextrose[c]	500 mL with 500 mL dextrose[c]	500, 750 and 1000 mL and 500, 750 and 1000 mL dextrose[c]
Labeled Indications			
Peripheral Parenteral Nutrition	No	Yes	No
Central TPN	Yes	Yes	Yes

[a] Solution composition represents admixture of dual-chamber *Quick Mix* or *Nutrimix* container.
[b] Histidine is considered an essential amino acid in infants and in renal failure.
[c] With 30 mg sodium hydrosulfite per 100 mL.

CRYSTALLINE AMINO ACID INFUSIONS WITH ELECTROLYTES IN DEXTROSE

	Aminosyn II 3.5% M[a] in 5% Dextrose[b] (Abbott)	Aminosyn II 4.25% M[a] in 10% Dextrose[b] (Abbott)
Amino Acid Concentration	3.5%	4.25%
Dextrose Concentration	5%	10%
Nitrogen (g/100 mL)	0.535	0.65
Amino Acids (Essential) (mg/100 mL)		
Isoleucine	231	280
Leucine	350	425
Lysine	368	446
Methionine	60	73
Phenylalanine	104	126
Threonine	140	170
Tryptophan	70	85
Valine	175	212
Amino Acids (Nonessential) (mg/100 mL)		
Alanine	348	422
Arginine	356	432
Histidine[c]	105	128
Proline	252	307
Serine	186	225
Tyrosine	94	115
Aminoacetic Acid (Glycine)	175	212

	Aminosyn II 3.5% M[a] in 5% Dextrose[b] (Abbott)	Aminosyn II 4.25% M[a] in 10% Dextrose[b] (Abbott)
Glutamic Acid	258	314
Aspartic Acid	245	298
Cysteine		
Electrolytes (mEq/L)		
Sodium	41	43.7
Potassium	13	13
Magnesium	3	3
Chloride	36.5	36.5
Acetate	25.1	30.5
Phosphorus (mM/L)	3.5	3.5
Osmolarity (mOsm/L)	616	919
Supplied in (mL)	500 and 1000 mL and 500 and 1000 mL dextrose[d]	500 mL and 500 mL dextrose[d]
Labeled Indications		
Peripheral Parenteral Nutrition	Yes	Yes
Central TPN	No	Yes
Protein Sparing	No	No

[a] With maintenance electrolytes.
[b] Solution composition represents admixture of *Nutrimix* dual-chamber container.
[c] Histidine is considered an essential amino acid in infants and in renal failure.
[d] With 30 mg sodium hydrosulfite per 100 mL.

AMINO ACID FORMULATIONS FOR RENAL FAILURE

	Amino Acid Formulations for Renal Failure			
	Aminosyn-RF 5.2% (Abbott)	Aminess 5.2% (Clintec)	5.4% NephrAmine (McGaw)	RenAmin (Clintec)
Amino Acid Concentration	5.2%	5.2%	5.4%	6.5%
Nitrogen (g/100 mL)	0.79	0.66	0.65	1
Amino Acids (Essential) (mg/100 mL)				
Isoleucine	462	525	560	500
Leucine	726	825	880	600
Lysine	535	600	640	450
Methionine	726	825	880	500
Phenylalanine	726	825	880	490
Threonine	330	375	400	380
Tryptophan	165	188	200	160
Valine	528	600	640	820
Histidine	429	412	250	420
Amino Acids (Nonessential) (mg/100 mL)				
Cysteine			< 20	
Arginine	600			630
Alanine				560
Proline				350
Glycine				300
Serine				300
Tyrosine				40
Electrolytes (mEq/L)				
Sodium			5	
Acetate	≈ 105	50	≈ 44	60
Potassium	5.4			
Chloride			< 3	31
Osmolarity (mOsm/L)	475	416	435	600
Supplied in (mL)	300[a]	400[b]	250[c]	250[d] 500[d]

[a] With 60 mg potassium metabisulfite per 100 mL.
[b] In 500 mL bottle.
[c] With < 0.05 g sodium bisulfite per 100 mL.
[d] With ≈ 3 mEq sodium bisulfite.

For a complete discussion of the use of protein substrates for intravenous nutritional therapy, refer to the IV Nutritionals monograph.

Indications

For nutritional support of uremic patients, particularly when oral nutrition is impractical, not feasible or insufficient.

Essential amino acid injection does not replace dialysis and conventional supportive therapy in patients with renal failure. To promote urea reutilization, provide adequate calories with minimal amounts of essential amino acids and restrict the intake of nonessential nitrogen.

►*Children:* Use with caution in pediatric patients, especially low birth weight infants, due to limited clinical experience. Laboratory and clinical monitoring must be extensive and frequent. Use a low initial dose and increase slowly.

The absence of arginine in *NephrAmine* and *Aminess* may accentuate the risk of hyperammonemia in infants. *Aminosyn-RF* and *RenAmin* contain arginine.

Administration and Dosage

Provide adequate calories simultaneously. Administer essential amino acid/dextrose mixtures by continuous infusion through a central venous catheter. Use slow initial infusion rates, generally 20 to 30 mL/hour for the first 6 to 8 hours. Increase by 10 mL/hour each 24 hours, up to a maximum of 60 to 100 mL/hour.

Administration rate is governed by the patient's nitrogen, fluid and glucose tolerance. Uremic patients are frequently glucose intolerant, especially in association with peritoneal dialysis, and may require exogenous insulin to prevent hyperglycemia. To prevent rebound hypoglycemia when hypertonic dextrose infusions are abruptly discontinued, administer a 5% dextrose solution.

►*Adults:*

Aminosyn-RF – 300 to 600 mL. Mix 300 mL with 500 mL of 70% dextrose to provide a solution of 1.96% essential amino acids in 44% dextrose (calorie:nitrogen ratio = 504:1).

Aminess – 400 mL. Mix 400 mL with 500 mL of 70% dextrose to yield a solution of 2.3% essential amino acids in 39% dextrose (calorie:nitrogen ratio = 450:1).

NephrAmine – 250 to 500 mL. Mix 250 mL w/500 mL of 70% dextrose to yield solution of 1.8% essential amino acids in 47% dextrose (calorie: nitrogen ratio = 744:1).

RenAmin – 250 to 500 mL.

►*Children:* Individualize dosage. A dosage of 0.5 to 1 g/kg/day will meet the requirements of the majority of pediatric patients. Use a low initial daily dosage and increase slowly; > 1 g/kg/day is not recommended.

Actions

►*Pharmacology:* Patients with renal decompensation have different amino acid requirements than those with normal renal function. Use in uremic patients is based on the minimal requirements for each of the 8 essential amino acids. These products contain histidine, an amino acid considered essential for infant growth and for uremic patients.

In renal failure, nonspecific nitrogen-containing compounds are broken down in the intestine. The ammonia formed is absorbed and incorporated by the liver into nonessential amino acids, provided essential amino acid requirements are being met. Exogenously supplying only essential amino acids allows urea nitrogen to be recycled which can serve as a precursor for nonessential amino acid synthesis. Therefore, administration to uremic patients, particularly those who are protein deficient, results in the utilization of retained urea, and may be followed by a drop in BUN and resolution of many azotemic symptoms.

Protein Substrates

AMINO ACID FORMULATIONS FOR RENAL FAILURE

Infusion of essential amino acids and hypertonic dextrose promotes protein synthesis, improves cellular metabolic balance, decreases the rate of rise of BUN and minimizes deterioration of serum potassium, magnesium and phosphorus balance in patients with impaired renal function. This therapy may decrease morbidity associated with acute renal failure and promote earlier return of renal function. Although controversial, these formulations may have no clinically significant advantage over the general formulations containing both essential and nonessential amino acids in most uremic patients.

AMINO ACID FORMULATIONS FOR HIGH METABOLIC STRESS

For a complete discussion of the use of protein substrates as a compound of intravenous nutritional therapy, refer to the IV Nutritionals monograph.

Indications

To prevent nitrogen loss or treat negative nitrogen balance in adults if: (1) The alimentary tract, by oral, gastrostomy or jejunostomy route, cannot or should not be used, or adequate protein intake is not feasible by these routes; (2) GI protein absorption is impaired; or (3) nitrogen homeostasis is substantially impaired as with severe trauma or sepsis.

Administration and Dosage

Daily amino acid doses of ≈ 1.5 g/kg for adults with adequate calories generally satisfy protein needs and promote positive nitrogen balance. May need higher doses in severely catabolic states. Fat emulsion may help meet energy requirements.

For severely catabolic, depleted patients or those requiring long-term TPN, consider central venous nutrition. Start with infusates containing lower dextrose concentrations; gradually increase dextrose to estimated caloric needs as glucose tolerance increases. *FreAmine HBC* 750 mL and 250 mL 70% dextrose or 500 mL *Aminosyn-HBC* 7% and 500 mL concentrated dextrose, with added electrolytes, trace metals and vitamins, may be given over 8 hours. *BranchAmin* 4% must be admixed with a complete amino acid injection, with or without a concentrated caloric source.

For moderately catabolic, depleted patients in whom central venous route is not indicated, may infuse diluted *FreAmine HBC* or *Aminosyn-HBC* 7% with minimal caloric supplementation by peripheral vein; supplement, if desired, with fat emulsion.

Usual administration of 4% BCAA Injection is used as a supplement to parenteral nutrition solutions to achieve an amino acid solution that is ≈ 50% w/w BCAA. One method for achieving this ratio is the admixture of two volumes of 4% BCAA Injection at 4 g/dL concentration with one volume of an amino acid solution of 8 to 10 g/dL concentration. The supplemental amino acid mixture is given with energy substrates to provide at least 35 kcal/kg ideal body weight as nonprotein calories.

Actions

▶*Pharmacology:* These are mixtures of essential and nonessential amino acids with high concentrations of branched chain amino acids (BCAA): Isoleucine, leucine, valine.

Acute metabolic stress – Acute metabolic stress is characterized by increased urinary nitrogen excretion and hyperglycemia; glucose utilization and fat store mobilization are impaired. The primary substrates used to meet energy requirements of muscle are BCAAs.

AMINO ACID FORMULATION IN HEPATIC FAILURE/HEPATIC ENCEPHALOPATHY

Indications

For the treatment of hepatic encephalopathy in patients with cirrhosis or hepatitis. Provides nutritional support for patients with these diseases of the liver who require parenteral nutrition and are intolerant of general purpose amino acid injections, which are contraindicated in patients with hepatic coma.

Administration and Dosage

Give 80 to 120 g amino acids (12 to 18 g nitrogen)/day. Typically, 500 mL *HepatAmine* with ≈ 500 mL 50% dextrose and electrolytes and vitamins is given over 8 to 12 hours. This results in total daily fluid intake of ≈ 2 to 3 L. Patients with fluid restrictions may only tolerate 1 to 2 L. Although nitrogen requirements may be higher in severely hypercatabolic or depleted patients, provision of additional nitrogen may not be possible due to fluid intake limits, nitrogen or glucose intolerance.

Use slow initial infusion rates; gradually increase to 60 to 125 mL/hr.

▶*Peripheral vein:* Peripheral vein administration is indicated with or without parenteral carbohydrate calories for patients in whom the central venous route is not indicated and who can consume adequate calories enterally. Prepare infusates by dilution of *HepatAmine* with Sterile Water for Injection or 5% to 10% Dextrose to prepare isotonic or slightly hypertonic solutions; accompany with adequate caloric supplementation.

Actions

▶*Pharmacology:* This formulation is a mixture of essential and nonessential amino acids with high concentrations of the BCAAs, isoleucine, leucine and valine.

Hepatic failure / Hepatic encephalopathy – Etiopathology of hepatic encephalopathy is unknown and multifactorial. Rationale for BCAA therapy is based on studies in which BCAA infusions reversed abnormal plasma amino acid pattern characterized by lower BCAA levels and elevated aromatic amino acids and methionine. Normalization of these amino acids improved mental status and EEG patterns. Nitrogen balance was significantly improved and mortality reduced in these typically protein-intolerant patients who received substantial amounts of protein equivalents.

AMINO ACID FORMULATION FOR HIGH METABOLIC STRESS AND IN HEPATIC FAILURE/ HEPATIC ENCEPHALOPATHY

	STRESS FORMULATION			HEPATIC FORMULATION
	4% BranchAmin (Clintec)	FreAmine HBC 6.9% (McGaw)	Aminosyn-HBC 7% (Abbott)	HepatAmine (McGaw)
Amino Acid Concentration	4%	6.9%	7%	8%
Nitrogen (g/100 mL)	0.443	0.97	1.12	1.2
Amino Acids (Essential) (mg/100 mL)				
Isoleucine	1380	760	789	900
Leucine	1380	1370	1576	1100
Lysine		410	265	610
Methionine		250	206	100
Phenylalanine		320	228	100
Threonine		200	272	450
Tryptophan		90	88	66
Valine	1240	880	789	840
Amino Acids (Nonessential) (mg/100 mL)				
Alanine		400	660	770
Arginine		580	507	600

Protein Substrates

AMINO ACID FORMULATION FOR HIGH METABOLIC STRESS AND IN HEPATIC FAILURE/HEPATIC ENCEPHALOPATHY

	STRESS FORMULATION			HEPATIC FORMULATION
	4% BranchAmin (Clintec)	FreAmine HBC 6.9% (McGaw)	Aminosyn-HBC 7% (Abbott)	HepatAmine (McGaw)
Histidine[a]		160	154	240
Proline		630	448	800
Serine		330	221	500
Tyrosine			33	
Glycine		330	660	900
Cysteine		< 20		< 20
Electrolytes (mEq/L)				
Sodium		10	7[b]	10
Chloride		< 3		< 3
Acetate		≈ 57	72	≈ 62
Phosphate (mM/L)				10
Osmolarity (mOsm/L)	316	620	665	785
Supplied in (mL)	500	750[c,d]	500[b] 1000[b]	500[c]
Labeled Indications				
Peripheral Parenteral Nutrition	Yes[e]	Yes	Yes	Yes
Central TPN	Yes[e]	Yes	Yes	Yes

[a] Histidine is considered an essential amino acid in infants and in renal failure.
[b] With 60 mg sodium hydrosulfite.
[c] With < 100 mg sodium bisulfite/100 mL.
[d] In 1000 mL bottles.
[e] Must be admixed with a complete amino acid injection.

CYSTEINE HCl

Rx **Cysteine HCl** (Various, eg, Abbott, Gensia) **Injection:** 50 mg per mL In 10 mL additive syringe and single dose vials.

For a complete discussion of the use of protein substrates as a component of intravenous nutritional therapy, refer to the IV Nutritionals monograph.

Indications

Use only after dilution as an additive to Aminosyn to meet the IV amino acid nutritional requirements of infants receiving total parenteral nutrition.

Administration and Dosage

Use only after dilution in *Aminosyn*. Combine each 0.5 g of cysteine with 12.5 g of amino acids, such as that present in 250 mL of *Aminosyn* 5%, then dilute with 250 mL of 50% Dextrose or lesser volume as indicated. Equal volumes of *Aminosyn* 5% and 50% Dextrose produce a final solution containing *Aminosyn* 2.5% and 25% Dextrose, which is suitable for administration by central venous infusion.

➤*Storage/Stability:* Avoid excessive heat. Do not freeze. Begin administration of the final admixture within 1 hour of mixing; otherwise, immediately refrigerate the mixture and use within 24 hours.

Actions

➤*Pharmacology:* Cysteine is a sulfur-containing amino acid. It is synthesized from methionine via the trans-sulfuration pathway in the adult, but newborn infants lack the enzyme necessary to effect this conversion. Therefore, cysteine is generally considered an essential amino acid in infants.

Metabolism of cysteine produces pyruvate and inorganic sulfate as end products. Cysteine is introduced directly into the pathway of carbohydrate metabolism at the pyruvate stage with all three carbons convertible to glucose. The sulfur is primarily transformed to inorganic sulfate, which is introduced into complex polysaccharides among other structural components.

In premixed solutions of crystalline amino acids, cysteine is relatively unstable over time, eventually converting to insoluble cystine. To avoid such precipitation, cysteine is provided as an additive for use with crystalline amino acid solutions immediately prior to administration.

TROMETHAMINE

Rx **Tham** (Abbott) **Injection:** 18 g (150 mEq) per 500 mL (0.3 M) In 500 mL single dose container.[a]

[a] With acetic acid.

Indications

Prevention and correction of systemic acidosis in the following conditions: Metabolic acidosis associated with cardiac bypass surgery; correction of acidity of Acid Citrate Dextrose (ACD) blood in cardiac bypass surgery; cardiac arrest.

Administration and Dosage

Administer by slow IV infusion, by addition to pump oxygenator ACD blood or other priming fluid, or by injection into the ventricular cavity during cardiac arrest.

For peripheral vein infusion, use a large needle in the largest antecubital vein or place an indwelling catheter in a large vein of an elevated limb to minimize chemical irritation by the alkaline solution.

Avoid overtreatment (alkalosis). Measure pretreatment and subsequent blood values (eg, pH, pCO_2, pO_2, glucose, electrolytes) and urinary output to monitor dosage and progress of treatment. Limit dosage to increase blood pH to normal limits (7.35 to 7.45) and to correct acid-base derangements. Drug retention may occur, especially in patients with impaired renal function.

Dosage may be estimated from the buffer base deficit of the extracellular fluid (mEq/L) using the Siggaard-Andersen nomogram. The following formula is a general guide:

Tromethamine solution (mL of 0.3M) = body weight (kg) × base deficit (mEq/L) × 1.1†

Determine need for additional solution by serial measurements of existing base deficit.

---

† Factor of 1.1 accounts for an approximate reduction of 10% in buffering capacity due to sufficient acetic acid to lower pH of the 0.3M solution without electrolytes to ≈ 8.6.

TROMETHAMINE

➤*Acidosis during cardiac bypass surgery:* Average dose of approximately 9 mL/kg (2.7 mEq/kg or 0.32 g/kg). A total single dose of 500 mL (150 mEq or 18 g) is adequate for most adults. Larger single doses (up to 1000 mL) may be required in severe cases. Do not exceed individual doses of 500 mg/kg over a period of not less than 1 hour.

➤*Acidity of ACD priming blood:* Stored blood has a pH range from 6.22 to 6.8. Use from 0.5 to 2.5 g (15 to 77 mL) added to each 500 mL of ACD blood to correct acidity. Usually, 2 g (62 mL) added to 500 mL of ACD blood is adequate.

➤*Acidosis associated with cardiac arrest:* Administer at the same time that other standard resuscitative measures are being applied.

If the chest is open, inject 2 to 6 g (62 to 185 mL) directly into the ventricular cavity. Do not inject into the cardiac muscle. If the chest is not open, inject from 3.6 to 10.8 g (111 to 333 mL) into a large peripheral vein. Additional amounts may be required to control systemic acidosis persisting after cardiac arrest is reversed.

➤*Storage/Stability:* Highly alkaline solutions may erode glass; discard solutions of tromethamine 24 hours after reconstitution. Protect from freezing and extreme heat.

Actions

➤*Pharmacology:* Tromethamine, a highly alkaline, sodium-free organic amine, acts as a proton acceptor to prevent or correct acidosis. When administered IV as a 0.3 M solution, it combines with hydrogen ions from carbonic acid to form bicarbonate and a cationic buffer. It also acts as an osmotic diuretic, increasing urine flow, urinary pH and excretion of fixed acids, carbon dioxide and electrolytes.

➤*Pharmacokinetics:* At pH 7.4, 30% of tromethamine is not ionized and therefore is capable of reaching equilibrium in total body water. This portion may penetrate cells and may neutralize acidic ions of the intracellular fluid. The drug is rapidly eliminated by the kidneys; $\geq 75\%$ appears in urine after 8 hours and the remainder within 3 days.

Contraindications

Anuria; uremia.

Warnings

➤*Administer slowly:* Correct only the existing acidosis; avoid overdosage and alkalosis.

➤*Duration of therapy:* Because clinical experience has been limited generally to short-term use, do not administer for > 1 day except in a life-threatening situation.

➤*Respiratory depression:* Respiratory depression, although infrequent, may be more likely in patients with chronic hypoventilation or those treated with drugs which depress respiration. Large doses may depress ventilation due to increased blood pH and reduced CO_2 concentration. Adjust dosage so that blood pH does not increase above normal. If respiratory acidosis is present concomitantly with metabolic acidosis, the drug may be used with mechanical assistance to ventilation.

➤*Perivascular infiltration:* Perivascular infiltration of this highly alkaline solution may cause inflammation, vascular spasms and tissue damage (eg, necrosis, sloughing, chemical phlebitis, thrombosis). Place the needle within the largest available vein and infuse slowly (see Adverse Reactions).

➤*Hemorrhagic hepatic necrosis:* Hemorrhagic hepatic necrosis has occurred in newborns when a hypertonic solution of tromethamine was administered via the umbilical vein.

➤*Renal function impairment:* Renal function impairment demands extreme care because of potential hyperkalemia and possible decreased excretion of tromethamine. Monitor ECG and serum potassium.

➤*Pregnancy: Category C.* It is not known whether tromethamine can cause fetal harm when administered to a pregnant woman or can affect reproduction capacity. Give to a pregnant woman only if clearly needed.

➤*Children:* Severe hemorrhagic liver necrosis has occurred in neonates.

Hypoglycemia may occur when administered to premature or even full term neonates.

Precautions

➤*Monitoring:* Measure blood pH, pCO_2, bicarbonate, glucose and electrolytes before, during and after administration.

Adverse Reactions

Generally, side effects are infrequent. Transient depression of blood glucose; respiratory depression, hemorrhagic hepatic necrosis (see Warnings).

➤*Local:* Local reactions that may occur because of the solution or the technique of administration include the following: Febrile response; infection at injection site; venous thrombosis or phlebitis extending from the site of extravasation; hypervolemia.

Overdosage

➤*Symptoms:* Overdosage, in terms of total drug or too rapid administration, may cause alkalosis, overhydration, solute overload and severe prolonged hypoglycemia (several hours).

➤*Treatment:* Discontinue infusion and institute appropriate countermeasures.

Caloric Intake

DEXTROSE (d-GLUCOSE)

Rx	**D-2.5-W** (Various, eg, Abbott, Clintec)	2.5%	In 1000 mL.
Rx	**D-5-W** (Various, eg, Abbott, Clintec, IMS, McGaw)	5%	In 25, 50, 100, 150, 250, 500 and 1000 mL vials and 10 mL syringes, 25 mL fill in 150 mL, 50 mL fill in 250 mL and 100 mL fill in 250 mL vials.
Rx	**D-10-W** (Various, eg, Abbott, Clintec, Elkins-Sinn, Solopak, Winthrop)	10%	In 3 mL amps, 250, 500 and 1000 mL vials, 17 mL fill in 20 mL, 500 mL fill in 1000 mL, and 1000 mL fill in 2000 mL vials.
Rx	**D-20-W** (Various, eg, Abbott, Clintec)	20%	In 500 mL vials, 500 mL fill in 1000 mL and 1000 mL fill in 2000 mL.
Rx	**D-25-W** (Various, eg, Abbott, IMS)	25%	In 10 mL syringes.
Rx	**D-30-W** (Various, eg, Abbott, Clintec, McGaw)	30%	In 500 and 1000 mL, 500 mL fill in 1000 mL and 1000 mL fill in 2000 mL.
Rx	**D-40-W** (Various, eg, Abbott, Clintec, McGaw)	40%	In 500 and 1000 mL, 500 mL fill in 1000 mL and 1000 mL fill in 2000 mL.
Rx	**D-50-W** (Various, eg, Abbott, Astra, Clintec, IMS, McGaw, Pasadena)	50%	In 500, 1000 and 2000 mL and 50 mL amps, vials and syringes and 500 mL fill in 1000 mL and 1000 mL fill in 2000 mL.
Rx	**D-60-W** (Various, eg, Abbott, Clintec, McGaw)	60%	In 500 and 1000 mL, 500 mL fill in 1000 mL and 1000 mL fill in 2000 mL.
Rx	**D-70-W** (Various, eg, Abbott, Clintec, McGaw)	70%	In 70, 1000 and 2000 mL, 500 mL fill in 1000 mL and 1000 mL fill in 2000 mL.

Indications

➤*2.5%, 5% and 10% solutions:* Used for peripheral infusion to provide calories whenever fluid and caloric replacement are required.

➤*25% (hypertonic) solutions:* Acute symptomatic episodes of hypoglycemia in the neonate or older infant to restore depressed blood glucose levels and control symptoms.

➤*50% solution:* Used in the treatment of insulin hypoglycemia (hyperinsulinemia or insulin shock) to restore blood glucose levels.

➤*10%, 20%, 30%, 40%, 50%, 60% and 70% (hypertonic) solutions:* For infusion after admixture with other solutions such as amino acids.

➤*Unlabeled uses:* Hypertonic solutions of 25% to 50% have been used as a sclerosing agent for the treatment of varicose veins, as an irritant to produce adhesive pleuritis and to reduce cerebrospinal pressure and cerebral edema caused by delirium tremens or acute alcohol intoxication.

Administration and Dosage

Do not administer concentrated solutions SC or IM.

The concentration and dose depend on the patient's age, weight and clinical condition. Add electrolytes based on fluid and electrolyte status.

➤*Glycosuria:* The maximum rate at which dextrose can be infused without producing glycosuria is 0.5 g/kg/hour. About 95% is retained when infused at 0.8 g/kg/hour.

➤*Insulin-induced hypoglycemia:* Determine blood glucose before injecting dextrose. In emergencies, promptly administer without waiting for pretreatment test results.

Adults – 10 to 25 g. Repeated doses may be required in severe cases.

Neonates – 250 to 500 mg/kg/dose (5 to 10 mL of 25% dextrose in a 5 kg infant) to control acute symptomatic hypoglycemia.

Severe cases or older infants – Larger or repeated single doses up to 10 or 12 mL of 25% dextrose may be required. Subsequent continuous IV infusion of 10% dextrose may be needed to stabilize blood glucose levels.

➤*Admixture incompatibilities:* Additives may be incompatible. When introducing additives, use aseptic technique, mix thoroughly and do not store.

Do not administer dextrose simultaneously with blood through the same infusion set because pseudoagglutination of red cells may occur.

➤*Storage/Stability:* Do not use unless solution is clear. Discard unused portion. Protect from freezing and extreme heat.

Actions

➤*Pharmacology:* A source of calories and fluids in patients unable to obtain adequate oral intake. Parenterally injected dextrose undergoes oxidation to carbon dioxide and water, and provides 3.4 calories per gram of d–glucose monohydrate (molecular weight 198.17). A 5% solution is isotonic and is administered by IV infusion into peripheral veins. Concentrated dextrose infusions are used to provide increased caloric intake with less fluid volume; they may be irritating if given by peripheral infusions. Therefore, administer highly concentrated solutions only by central venous catheters.

Dextrose injections may induce diuresis. Dextrose is readily metabolized, may decrease body protein and nitrogen losses, promotes glycogen deposition, and decreases or prevents ketosis if sufficient doses are provided.

Caloric Content and Osmolarity of the Various Concentrations of Dextrose			
Dextrose concentration		Caloric content (Cal/L)	Osmolarity (mOsm/L)
%	g/L		
2.5	25	85	126
5	50	170	253
10	100	340	505
20	200	680	1010
25	250	850	1330
30	300	1020	1515
40	400	1360	2020
50	500	1700	2525
60	600	2040	3030
70	700	2380	3535

Contraindications

In diabetic coma while blood sugar is excessively high.

➤*Concentrated solutions:* When intracranial or intraspinal hemorrhage is present; in the presence of delirium tremens in dehydrated patients; in patients with severe hydration, anuria, hepatic coma or glucose-galactose malabsorption syndrome.

Warnings

➤*Fluid/Solute overload:* Dextrose solutions IV can cause fluid or solute overload resulting in dilution of serum electrolyte concentrations, overhydration, congested states or pulmonary edema.

➤*Hypertonic dextrose solutions:* Hypertonic dextrose solutions may cause thrombosis if infused via peripheral veins; therefore, administer via a central venous catheter.

➤*Diabetes mellitus:* Use dextrose-containing solutions with caution in patients with subclinical or overt diabetes mellitus or carbohydrate intolerance.

➤*Rapid administration:* Rapid administration of hypertonic solutions may produce significant hyperglycemia or hyperosmolar syndrome, especially in patients with chronic uremia or carbohydrate intolerance.

➤*Pregnancy: Category C.* It is not known whether dextrose can cause fetal harm when administered to a pregnant woman or can affect reproduction capacity. Use only when clearly needed. Dextrose crosses the placenta; however, insulin does not cross the placenta and the fetus is responsible for its own insulin production in response to the dextrose. Therefore, administer dextrose to a pregnant woman with caution. One report recommends an infusion rate of 3.5 to 7 g/hour since doses > 10 g/hr cause increases in fetal insulin.

➤*Lactation:* Exercise caution when administering dextrose to a nursing woman.

➤*Children:* Use with caution in infants of diabetic mothers, except as may be indicated in hypoglycemic neonates.

Precautions

➤*Monitoring:* Perform clinical evaluations and laboratory determinations to monitor fluid balance, electrolyte concentrations and acid-base balance.

➤*Hyperglycemia and glycosuria:* Hyperglycemia and glycosuria may be functions of rate of administration or metabolic insufficiency. To minimize these conditions, slow the infusion rate, monitor blood and urine glucose; if necessary, administer insulin. When concentrated dextrose infusion is abruptly withdrawn, administer 5% or 10% dextrose to avoid rebound hypoglycemia.

➤*Extravasation:* Administer so that extravasation does not occur. If thrombosis occurs during administration, stop injection and correct.

Caloric Intake

DEXTROSE (d-GLUCOSE)

➤*Hypokalemia:* Excessive administration of potassium free solutions may result in significant hypokalemia. Add potassium to dextrose solutions and administer to fasting patients with good renal function, especially those on digitalis therapy.

➤*Vitamin B complex deficiency:* Vitamin B complex deficiency may occur with dextrose administration.

Drug Interactions

➤*Corticosteroids:* Cautiously administer parenteral fluids, especially those containing sodium ions, to patients receiving corticosteroids or corticotropin.

Adverse Reactions

Febrile response; infection at the injection site; tissue necrosis; venous thrombosis or phlebitis extending from the site of injection; extravasation; hypovolemia; hypervolemia; dehydration; mental confusion or unconsciousness. These may occur because of the solution or administration technique. Use the largest available peripheral vein and a well placed small bore needle.

Hypertonic solutions – Hypertonic solutions are more likely to cause irritation; administer into larger central veins. Significant hyperglycemia, hyperosmolar syndrome and glycosuria may occur with too rapid administration of hypertonic solutions.

Overdosage

In the event of a fluid or solute overload during parenteral therapy, reevaluate the patient's condition and institute appropriate corrective treatment.

ALCOHOL (ETHANOL) IN DEXTROSE INFUSIONS

	Product/Distributor	Cal/L	mOsm/L	How Supplied
Rx	**5% Alcohol and 5% Dextrose in Water** (Various, eg, Abbott, Clintec)	450	1114	In 1000 mL.
Rx	**5% Alcohol and 5% Dextrose in Water** (McGaw)		1125	In 1000 mL.
Rx	**10% Alcohol and 5% Dextrose in Water** (McGaw)	720	1995	In 1000 mL.

For specific information on dextrose, refer to the individual monograph.

Indications

Increasing caloric intake and replenishing fluids.

➤*Unlabeled uses:*

Premature labor – Infusion of a 10% solution of ethyl alcohol IV causes a decrease in uterine activity during labor, presumably by inhibiting the release of oxytocin from the posterior pituitary, and has been used to prevent premature delivery. However, this use has largely been replaced by other therapies (eg, β-adrenergic therapy).

Administration and Dosage

Administer by slow IV infusion only; do not give SC. Individualize dosage. The average adult can metabolize approximately 10 mL/hour (200 mL of 5% solution or 100 mL of 10% solution). The usual adult dosage is 1 to 2 L and rarely exceeds 3 L of a 5% solution in a 24 hour period. Children may be given 40 mL/kg/24 hours or from 350 to 1000 mL, depending on size and clinical response.

➤*Storage/Stability:* Do not use unless solution is clear and seal is intact. Discard unused portion. Protect from freezing and extreme heat.

Actions

➤*Pharmacology:* Alcohol in dextrose solutions are an intravenous source of carbohydrate calories that restore blood glucose levels. Each mL of alcohol provides 5.6 calories; each gram of d–glucose monohydrate provides 3.4 calories. Dextrose may aid in minimizing liver glycogen depletion and exerts a protein-sparing action.

➤*Pharmacokinetics:* Ethyl alcohol is metabolized at a rate of ≈ 10 to 20 mL/hour. Sedative effects of alcohol occur if infusion rate exceeds metabolism rate. Dextrose (d-glucose) can be infused at a maximum of ≈ 0.5 to 0.85 g/kg/hour without producing significant glycosuria. Thus, the maximum rate that alcohol can be infused without producing sedative effects is well below maximum rate of dextrose utilization. Alcohol is metabolized (mostly in liver) to acetaldehyde or acetate; oxidation rate is linear with time. Starvation lowers metabolism rate and insulin increases it.

Contraindications

Epilepsy; urinary tract infection; alcoholism; diabetic coma.

Warnings

➤*Special risk patients:* Use alcohol cautiously in shock, following cranial surgery and in actual or anticipated postpartum hemorrhage.

➤*Diabetic patients:* Alcohol decreases blood sugar in these patients. In the untreated diabetic, the rate of alcohol metabolism is slowed.

➤*Vitamin deficiencies:* As a nutrient, alcohol supplies only calories; given alone it may cause or potentiate vitamin deficiencies and liver function disturbances.

➤*IV administration:* IV administration can cause fluid or solute overload resulting in dilution of serum electrolyte concentrations, overhydration, congested states or pulmonary edema.

➤*Extravasation:* Avoid extravasation during IV administration; do not give SC.

➤*Pseudoagglutination/Hemolysis:* Do not administer simultaneously with blood because of possibility of pseudoagglutination or hemolysis.

➤*Renal/Hepatic function impairment:* Use alcohol cautiously.

➤*Pregnancy: Category C.* It is not known whether alcohol can cause fetal harm when administered to a pregnant woman or can affect reproduction capacity. Use only when clearly needed. It crosses the placenta rapidly and enters fetal circulation.

Fetal Alcohol Syndrome (FAS) – Fetal alcohol syndrome (FAS), a pattern of fetal anomalies, is associated with chronic maternal alcohol consumption of 60 to 75 mL absolute alcohol (4 to 5 drinks) per day; mild FAS is associated with ingestion of as little as 30 mL per day. Features of FAS involve craniofacial, limb, growth, and CNS anomalies. Other reported problems involve cardiac and urogenital defects, liver abnormalities and hemangiomas. Behavioral problems may be long-term. Moderate drinking (> 1 ounce absolute alcohol twice/week) is associated with second trimester spontaneous abortions.

Administration of alcohol prior to delivery may cause intoxication and depression of the newborn.

➤*Lactation:* Alcohol passes freely into breast milk approximately equivalent to maternal serum levels; however, effects on the infant are generally insignificant until maternal blood levels reach 300 mg/dL. The American Academy of Pediatrics considers alcohol use in the mother compatible with breastfeeding, although adverse effects may occur.

Alcohol may cause potentiation of severe hypoprothrombic bleeding, a pseudo-Cushing syndrome and a reduction in the milk-ejecting response.

➤*Children:* Safety and efficacy are not established. See Administration and Dosage.

Precautions

➤*Monitoring:* Clinical evaluation and periodic laboratory determinations are necessary to monitor changes in electrolyte concentrations and fluid and acid-base balance.

➤*Administer slowly:* Administer slowly and observe patient for restlessness or narcosis.

➤*Gout:* Alcohol increases serum uric acid and can precipitate acute gout.

Drug Interactions

The following interactions may occur with alcohol administration. Those interactions that may only occur with long-term oral alcohol ingestion have not been included.

Alcohol Drug Interactions			
Precipitant drug	Object drug*		Description
Barbiturates Benzodiazepines Chloral hydrate Glutethimide Meprobamate Metoclopramide Phenothiazines	Alcohol	↑	Increased CNS depressant effects may occur.
Cephalosporins[a] Chlorpropamide Disulfiram Furazolidone Metronidazole Procarbazine	Alcohol	↑	A disulfiram-like reaction consisting of facial flushing, lightheadedness, weakness, sweating, tachycardia, nausea or vomiting may occur.

ALCOHOL (ETHANOL) IN DEXTROSE INFUSIONS

Alcohol Drug Interactions			
Precipitant drug	Object drug*		Description
Alcohol	Antidiabetic agents (insulin, phenformin, sulfonylureas)	↑	Because of altered glucose metabolism, the pharmacologic effects of these agents may be increased by alcohol resulting in hypoglycemia. In addition, alcohol may contribute to the lactic acidosis that is sometimes observed following phenformin administration. Both hypo- and hyperglycemia have occurred with sulfonylureas and alcohol.
Alcohol	Bromocriptine	↑	Intolerance of bromocriptine due to the severity of side effects has occurred with concurrent alcohol.
Alcohol	Salicylates	↑	Alcohol may potentiate aspirin-induced GI blood loss and bleeding time prolongation.

* ↑ = Object drug increased.
a Those agents with a methyltetrazolethiol moiety.

Adverse Reactions

Fever; injection site infection; venous thrombosis or phlebitis; extravasation; hypervolemia. These may occur because of the solution or administration technique.

Alcoholic intoxication may occur with too rapid infusion. Vertigo, flushing, disorientation (especially in elderly patients), or sedation may also occur. An alcoholic odor may be noted on the breath. Generally, these effects can be avoided by slowing the rate of infusion. Too rapid infusion of hypertonic solutions may cause local pain and, rarely, excessive vein irritation. Use the largest available peripheral vein and a well placed small bore needle.

Overdosage

In the event of alcoholic intoxication or sedation, slow the infusion or discontinue temporarily. If overhydration or solute overload occurs, reevaluate the patient and institute appropriate corrective measures.

Lipids

INTRAVENOUS FAT EMULSION

Product & Distributor	Oil (%) Safflower	Oil (%) Soybean	Fatty acid content (%) Linoleic	Oleic	Palmitic	Linolenic	Stearic	Egg yolk phospho-lipids (%)	Glycerin (%)	Calories/mL	Osmolarity (mOsm/L)	How Supplied
Intralipid[a] 10% (Clintec)		10	50	26	10	9	3.5	1.2	2.25	1.1	260	In 50, 100, 250 and 500 mL.
Intralipid 20% (Clintec)		20	50	26	10	9	3.5	1.2	2.25	2	260	In 50, 100, 250 and 500 mL.
Liposyn II[b] 10% (Abbott)	5	5	65.8	17.7	8.8	4.2	3.4	1.2	2.5	1.1	276	In 100, 200 and 500 mL.
Liposyn II[b] 20% (Abbott)	10	10	65.8	17.7	8.8	4.2	3.4	1.2	2.5	2	258	In 200 and 500 mL.
Liposyn III[b] 10% (Abbott)		10	54.5	22.4	10.5	8.3	4.2	1.2	2.5	1.1	284	In 100, 200 and 500 mL.
Liposyn III[b] 20% (Abbott)		20	54.5	22.4	10.5	8.3	4.2	1.2	2.5	2	292	In 200 and 500 mL.

[a] Store at 25°C (77°F) or below; do not freeze.
[b] Store at 30°C (86°F) or below; do not freeze.

Refer to the general discussion beginning in the IV Nutritional Therapy monograph.

> ### WARNING
>
> *Deaths in preterm infants:* Death in preterm infants after infusion of IV fat emulsions have occurred. Autopsy findings included intravascular fat accumulation in the lungs. Treatment of premature and low birth weight infants with IV fat emulsion must be based on careful benefit-risk assessment. Strict adherence to the recommended total daily dose is mandatory; hourly infusion rate should be as slow as possible and should not exceed 1 g/kg in 4 hours. Premature and small for gestational age infants have poor clearance of IV fat emulsion and increased free fatty acid plasma levels following fat emulsion infusion; therefore, administer less than the maximum recommended doses in these patients to decrease the likelihood of IV fat overload. Monitor the infant's ability to eliminate the infused fat from the circulation (such as triglycerides or plasma free fatty acid levels). The lipemia must clear between daily infusions.

Indications

Source of calories and essential fatty acids for patients requiring parenteral nutrition for extended periods of time (usually for > 5 days).

Source of essential fatty acids when a deficiency occurs.

Administration and Dosage

➤*Total parenteral nutrition:* As part of TPN, administer IV via a peripheral vein or by central venous catheter. Fat emulsion should comprise no more than 60% of the patient's total caloric intake, with carbohydrates and amino acids comprising the remaining 40% or more of caloric intake.

Adults –

10%: Initial infusion rate is 1ml/min for the first 15 to 30 minutes. If no adverse reactions occur, the infusion rate can be increased to 2 mL/min. Infuse only 500 mL the first day and increase dose the following day. Do not exceed a daily dosage of 2.5 g/kg.

20%: Initial infusion rate is 0.5 mL/min for the first 15 to 30 minutes. Infuse only 250 mL (Liposyn II;) or 500 mL *(Intralipid)* the first day and increase dose the following day. Do not exceed a daily dosage of 3 g/kg.

➤*Children:*

10% – Initial infusion rate is 0.1 mL/min for the first 10 to 15 minutes.

20% – Initial infusion rate is 0.05 mL/min for the first 10 to 15 minutes.

If no untoward reactions occur, increase rate to 1 g/kg in 4 hours. Do not exceed daily dosage of 3 g/kg.

The dosage for premature infants starts at 0.5 g fat/kg/24 hours (5 mL *Intralipid* 10%; 2.5 mL *Intralipid* 20%) and may be increased in relation to the infant's ability to eliminate fat. The maximum dosage recommended by the American Academy of Pediatrics is 3 g fat/kg/24 hours.

➤*Fatty acid deficiency:* To correct EFAD, supply 8% to 10% of the caloric intake by IV fat emulsion to provide an adequate amount of linoleic acid (4% of caloric intake as linoleate).

Fat emulsion is supplied in single dose containers; do not store partially used bottles or resterilize for later use. Do not use filters. Do not use any bottle in which there appears to be separation of the emulsion.

Fat emulsions may be simultaneously infused with amino acid-dextrose mixtures by means of a Y–connector located near the infusion site using separate flow rate controls for each solution. Keep the lipid infusion line higher than the amino acid-dextrose line. Since the lipid emulsion has a lower specific gravity, it may be taken up into the amino acid-dextrose line.

Fat emulsions may also be infused through a separate peripheral site.

➤*Total nutrient admixture (TNA):* IV fat emulsions are compatible with dextrose and amino acids, when properly mixed, for use in TPN therapy. This is also referred to as all-in-one, 3-in-1 and triple-mix. The following proper mixing sequence must be followed to minimize pH-related problems by ensuring that typically acidic dextrose injections are not mixed with lipid emulsions alone: (1) Transfer dextrose injection to the TPN admixture container; (2) transfer amino acid injection; (3) transfer the IV fat emulsion.

Amino acid injection, dextrose injection and the IV fat emulsion may be simultaneously transferred to the admixture container. Use gentle agitation to avoid localized concentration effects. Additives must not be added directly to the fat emulsion and in no case should the fat emulsion be added to the TPN container first. Shake bags gently after each addition to minimize localized concentration. If evacuated glass containers are used, add the dextrose and amino acid injections first, followed by the fat emulsion and then additives. Shake bottles gently after each addition.

Use these admixtures promptly; store under refrigeration (2° to 8°C; 36° to 46°F) for ≤ 24 hours and use completely within 24 hours after removal from refrigeration.

The prime destabilizers of emulsions are excessive acidity (low pH) and inappropriate electrolyte content. Give careful consideration to additions of divalent cations (calcium and magnesium) which cause emulsion instability. Amino acid solutions exert a buffering effect protecting the emulsion.

Inspect the admixture carefully for "breaking or oiling out" of the emulsion, which is described as the separation of the emulsion and can be visibly identified by a yellowish streaking or the accumulation of yellowish droplets in the admixed emulsion. Also examine the admixture for particulates. The admixture must be discarded if any of the above is observed.

Heparin may be added to activate lipoprotein lipase at a concentration of 1 or 2 units/mL prior to administration.

Lipid-containing fluids have a propensity to extract phthalates from phthalate-plasticized polyvinyl chloride (PVC). Although the amount is very small and no adverse clinical effects have been reported from administration of such amounts of phthalate, consider administration through a nonphthalate infusion set. Commercially available products may be accompanied by nonphthalate infusion sets.

Actions

➤*Pharmacology:* Intravenous fat emulsions are prepared from either soybean or safflower oil and provide a mixture of neutral triglycerides, predominantly unsaturated fatty acids. The major component of fatty acids are linoleic, oleic, palmitic, stearic and linolenic acids; see product listings for content. In addition, these products contain 1.2% egg yolk phospholipids as an emulsifier and glycerol to adjust tonicity. The emulsified fat particles are approximately 0.4 to 0.5 microns in diameter, similar to naturally occurring chylomicrons. IV fat emulsions are isotonic and may be given by central or peripheral venous routes.

These products are metabolized and utilized as a source of energy, causing an increase in heat production, decrease in respiratory quotient and an increase in oxygen consumption following use. The infused fat particles are cleared from the blood stream in a manner thought to be comparable to the clearing of chylomicrons.

Essential Fatty Acid Deficiency (EFAD) – Linoleic, linolenic and arachidonic acids are essential in humans. Linoleic acid, the metabolic precursor to both linolenic and arachidonic acid, cannot be synthesized in vivo. When there is a deficiency of linoleic acid, the enzyme system that converts linoleic acid to arachidonic acid (a tetraene) acts on oleic acid to synthesize eicosatrienoic acid (a triene) which lacks the physiologic functions of arachidonic acid. Biochemically, EFAD is defined as a triene to tetraene ratio > 0.4. Clinical manifestations of EFAD include scaly dermatitis, alopecia, growth retardation, poor wound healing, thrombocytopenia and fatty liver. IV fat emulsion prevents or reverses biochemical and clinical manifestations of EFAD.

INTRAVENOUS FAT EMULSION

Contraindications

Disturbance of normal fat metabolism such as pathologic hyperlipemia, lipoid nephrosis or acute pancreatitis, if accompanied by hyperlipemia. Egg yolk phospholipids are present; do not give to patients with severe egg allergies.

Warnings

➤*Special risk patients:* Exercise caution in severe liver damage, pulmonary disease, anemia, blood coagulation disorders, or when there is danger of fat embolism.

➤*Pregnancy: Category C.* It is not known whether IV fat emulsions can cause fetal harm when administered to a pregnant woman or can affect reproduction capacity. Use only when clearly needed.

Precautions

➤*Monitoring:* When IV fat emulsion is administered, monitor the patient's capacity to eliminate the infused fat from the circulation. The lipemia must clear between daily infusions. Closely monitor the hemogram, blood coagulation, liver function tests, plasma lipid profile and platelet count (especially in neonates). Discontinue use if a significant abnormality in any of these parameters is attributed to therapy.

➤*Jaundiced or premature infants:* Use with caution because free fatty acids displace bilirubin bound to albumin.

➤*Too rapid administration:* Too rapid administration can cause fluid or fat overloading. This can result in dilution of serum electrolyte concentrations, overhydration, pulmonary edema, impaired pulmonary diffusion capacity or metabolic acidosis.

Adverse Reactions

Most frequent – Sepsis due to administration equipment and thrombophlebitis due to vein irritation from concurrently administered hypertonic solutions. These adverse reactions are inseparable from the TPN procedure with or without IV fat emulsion.

Less frequent (more directly related to IV fat emulsion) –
Immediate (acute): (< 1%) – Dyspnea; cyanosis; hyperlipemia; hypercoagulability; nausea; vomiting; headache; flushing; increase in temperature; sweating; sleepiness; chest and back pain; slight pressure over the eyes; dizziness; irritation at the infusion site; thrombocytopenia in neonates (rare).

Long-term (chronic): Hepatomegaly; jaundice due to central lobular cholestasis; splenomegaly; thrombocytopenia; leukopenia; transient increases in liver function tests; overloading syndrome (focal seizures, fever, leukocytosis, splenomegaly and shock).

The deposition of brown pigmentation in the reticuloendothelial system (the so-called "IV fat pigment") has occurred. Cause and significance of this phenomenon are unknown.

Overdosage

Stop the infusion until visual inspection of the plasma, determination of triglyceride concentrations or measurement of plasma light-scattering activity by nephelometry indicates the lipid has cleared. Reevaluate the patient and institute appropriate corrective measures.

B VITAMINS, PARENTERAL
Content given per mL.

	Product & Distributor	B_1 mg	B_2 mg	B_3 mg	B_5 mg	B_6 mg	How Supplied
Rx	**B-Ject-100 Injection** (Hyrex)	100	2	100	2	2	In 30 mL vials.[a]
Rx	**Vitamin B Complex 100 Injection** (McGuff)						In 10 and 30 mL vials.[a]

[a] May contain benzyl alcohol.

B VITAMINS WITH VITAMIN C, PARENTERAL
Content given per mL.

	Product & Distributor	B_1 mg	B_2 mg	B_3 mg	B_5 mg	B_6 mg	B_{12} mcg	C mg	Other Content	How Supplied
Rx	**Key-Plex Injection** (Hyrex)	50	5	125	6	5	1000	50		In 10 mL multiple dose vials.
Rx	**Lypholized Vitamin B Complex & Vitamin C with B_{12} Injection** (McGuff)									In 10 mL vials.
Rx	**Vicam Injection** (Keene)								Benzyl alcohol	In 10 mL vials.

MULTIVITAMINS, PARENTERAL

	Product & Distributor	Content[a] given per	A IU	D IU	E IU	B_1 mg	B_2 mg	B_3 mg	B_5 mg	B_6 mg	B_{12} mcg	C mg	biotin mcg	FA mg	Other Content and How Supplied
Rx	**Berocca Parenteral Nutrition** (Roche)	1 mL	3300	200	10[b]	3	3.6	40	15	4	5	100	60	0.4	In 2 vial or ampule sets: Soln 1[c] (1 or 2 mL) and soln 2[c] (1 or 2 mL).
Rx	**M.V.I.-12 Injection** (Astra)	5 mL													In 2 vial sets: Vial 1[d] (5 mL single dose or 50 mL multiple dose) and vial 2[e] (5 mL single dose or 50 mL multiple dose).
Rx	**M.V.I.-12 Unit Vial** (Astra)	10 mL													In 10 mL two chambered vials.[d]
Rx	**M.V.I. Pediatric** (Astra)	5 mL	2300	400	7[b]	1.2	1.4	17	5	1	1	80	20	0.14	200 mcg vitamin K_1 and 375 mg mannitol. In single and multiple dose vials.[f]
Rx	**Cernevit-12** (Baxter Healthcare)	5 mL	3500	200	11.2²	3.51	4.14	46	17.25	4.53	5.5	125	60	414	In 5 mL single-dose vials.
Rx	**Infuvite Adult** (Baxter)	10 mL (after combining vials)	3300	200 IU D_3	10	6	3.6	40	15	6	5	200	60	600	150 mcg vitamin K. Polysorbate 80. In two 5 mL vials to be combined together.
Rx	**Infuvite Pediatric** (Baxter)	5 mL (after combining vials)	2300	400 IU D_3	7	1.2	1.4	17	5	1	1	80	20	140	0.2 mg vitamin K. Polysorbate 80. In two vials (4 mL and 1 mL to be combined together).
Rx	**B Complex with C and B-12 Injection** (Goldline)	1 mL				50	5	125	6	5	1,000	50			1% benzyl alcohol. In 10 mL multiple dose vials.

[a] After combining vials, if necessary.
[b] As dL-alpha tocopheryl acetate.
[c] With propylene glycol, EDTA and 1% benzyl alcohol.

[d] With propylene glycol, polysorbate 80 and polysorbate 20.
[e] With propylene glycol.
[f] With polysorbate 20 and polysorbate 80.

Minerals

CALCIUM

For information on oral calcium, refer to the Minerals, Oral section.

Indications

➤*Hypocalcemia:* For a prompt increase in plasma calcium levels (eg, neonatal tetany and tetany due to parathyroid deficiency, vitamin D deficiency, alkalosis); prevention of hypocalcemia during exchange transfusions; conditions associated with intestinal malabsorption.

➤*Calcium chloride and gluconate:* Adjunctive therapy in the treatment of insect bites or stings, such as Black Widow spider bites to relieve muscle cramping; sensitivity reactions, particularly when characterized by urticaria; depression due to overdosage of magnesium sulfate; acute symptoms of lead colic; rickets; osteomalacia.

➤*Calcium chloride:* To combat the deleterious effects of severe hyperkalemia as measured by ECG, pending correction of increased potassium in the extracellular fluid.

Cardiac resuscitation – Particularly after open heart surgery, when epinephrine fails to improve weak or ineffective myocardial contractions.

➤*Calcium gluconate:* To decrease capillary permeability in allergic conditions, nonthrombocytopenic purpura and exudative dermatoses such as dermatitis herpetiformis; for pruritus of eruptions caused by certain drugs; in hyperkalemia, calcium gluconate may aid in antagonizing the cardiac toxicity, provided the patient is not receiving digitalis therapy.

➤*Unlabeled uses:* Calcium salts have been used to treat verapamil overdose, treat acute hypotension from verapamil and prevent initial hypotension in patients requiring verapamil for whom decreases in blood pressure could be detrimental.

Administration and Dosage

Elemental Calcium Content of Calcium Salts		
Salt	% Calcium	mEq/g
Calcium chloride	27.3	13.6
Calcium gluconate	9.3	4.65

Calcium gluconate is generally preferred over calcium chloride as it is less irritating.

➤*IV:* Warm solutions to body temperature and give slowly (0.5 to 2 mL/min); stop if patient complains of discomfort. Resume when symptoms disappear. Following injection, patient should remain recumbent for a short time. Repeated injections may be needed because of the rapid calcium excretion. Inject **calcium chloride** and **gluconate** through a small needle into a large vein to minimize venous irritation.

➤*IM administration:* IM administration of **calcium gluconate** may be tolerated; however, reserve this route for emergencies when technical difficulty makes IV injection impossible. Administer **calcium gluconate** only by the IV route and **calcium chloride** by the IV or intraventricular route.

➤*Admixture incompatibilities:* Calcium salts should not generally be mixed with carbonates, phosphates, sulfates or tartrates in parenteral admixtures; they are conditionally compatible with potassium phosphates, depending on concentration. Calcium ions will chelate tetracycline.

Actions

➤*Pharmacology:* Calcium is the fifth most abundant element in the body with > 99.5% of total body stores in skeletal bone. It is essential for the functional integrity of the nervous and muscular systems, for normal cardiac contractility and the coagulation of blood. It also functions as an enzyme cofactor and affects the secretory activity of endocrine and exocrine glands. Normal levels are 8.5 to 10.5 mg/dL.

Hypocalcemia –
Symptoms: Tetany; paresthesias; laryngospasm; muscle spasms; seizures (usually grand mal); irritability; depression; psychosis; prolonged QT interval; intestinal cramps and malabsorption; respiratory arrest. Prolonged hypocalcemia may be associated with ectodermal defects including the nails, skin and teeth.

➤*Pharmacokinetics:* Approximately 80% of body calcium is excreted in the feces as insoluble salts; urinary excretion accounts for the remaining 20%.

Contraindications

Hypercalcemia; ventricular fibrillation; digitalized patients.

Warnings

➤*Extravasation:* **Calcium chloride** and **gluconate** can cause severe necrosis, sloughing and abscess formation with IM or SC administration. Take great care to avoid extravasation or accidental injection into perivascular tissues.

➤*Hypocalcemia of renal insufficiency:* **Calcium chloride** is an acidifying salt and is therefore usually undesirable for treating this condition.

➤*Pregnancy: Category C.* It is not known whether this drug can cause fetal harm when given to a pregnant woman or can affect reproduction capacity. Use only when clearly needed.

➤*Lactation:* It is not known whether **calcium gluconate** is excreted in breast milk. Exercise caution when administering to a pregnant woman.

Precautions

➤*Cardiovascular effects:* It is particularly important to prevent a high concentration of calcium from reaching the heart because of the danger of cardiac syncope.

Drug Interactions

Calcium Drug Interactions			
Precipitant	Object drug*		Description
Thiazide diuretics	Calcium salts	↑	Hypercalcemia resulting from renal tubular reabsorption, or bone release of calcium by thiazides may be amplified by exogenous calcium.
Calcium salts	Atenolol	↓	Mean peak plasma levels and bioavailability of atenolol may be decreased, possibly resulting in decreased beta blockade.
Calcium salts	Digitalis glycosides	↑	Inotropic and toxic effects are synergistic; arrhythmias may occur, especially if calcium is given IV. Avoid IV calcium in patients on digitalis glycosides; if necessary, give slowly in small amounts.
Calcium salts	Sodium polystyrene sulfonate	↓	Coadministration in patients with renal impairment may result in an unanticipated metabolic alkalosis and a reduction of the resin's binding of potassium.
Calcium salts	Verapamil	↓	Clinical effects and toxicities of verapamil may be reversed.

* ↑ = Object drug increased. ↓ = Object drug decreased.

➤*Drug/Lab test interactions:* Transient elevations of plasma 11-hydroxy-corticosteroid levels (Glenn-Nelson technique) may occur when IV calcium is administered, but levels return to control values after 1 hour. In addition, IV calcium gluconate can produce false-negative values for serum and urinary magnesium.

Adverse Reactions

IM administration – Local necrosis and abscess formation may occur with **calcium gluconate**, and severe necrosis and sloughing may occur with IM or SC administration of **calcium chloride.**

IV administration – Rapid IV administration may cause bradycardia, sense of oppression, tingling, metallic, calcium or chalky taste or "heat waves". Rapid IV **calcium gluconate** may cause vasodilation, decreased blood pressure, cardiac arrhythmias, syncope and cardiac arrest. **Calcium chloride** injections cause peripheral vasodilation and a local burning sensation; blood pressure may fall moderately.

Overdosage

➤*Symptoms:* Inadvertent systemic overloading with calcium ions can produce an acute hypercalcemic syndrome characterized by a markedly elevated plasma calcium level, weakness, lethargy, intractable nausea and vomiting, coma and sudden death.

➤*Treatment:* It may be life-saving to rapidly lower blood calcium to safe levels. It is now agreed the most effective therapy is IV sodium chloride infusion plus potent natriuretic agents, (eg, furosemide). Sodium competes with calcium for reabsorption in the distal renal tubule and furosemide potentiates this effect. Together they markedly increase renal calcium clearance and reduce hypercalcemia.

Minerals

CALCIUM GLUCONATE

1 g (10 mL) contains 93 mg (4.65 mEq) calcium.

Rx	Calcium Gluconate (Various, eg, American Regent, Astra, Elkins-Sinn, IDE, IMS, McGuff, Rugby)	Injection: 10%	In 10 mL amps and syringes, 10 and 50 mL single dose vials and 100 and 200 mL pharmacy bulk vials.[1]

[1] Not for direct infusion; dilute prior to use.

For complete prescribing information, refer to the Calcium group monograph in the Intravenous Nutritional Therapy, Electrolytes section.

Administration and Dosage

For IV use only, either directly or by infusion; SC or IM injection may cause severe necrosis and sloughing. Do not exceed a rate of 0.5 to 2 mL/minute. Calcium gluconate may also be administered by intermittent infusion at a rate not exceeding 200 mg/min, or by continuous infusion. Discontinue injection if the patient complains of discomfort. Do not use IM, as abscess formation and local necrosis may occur.

➤*Adults:* 2.3 to 9.3 mEq (5 to 20 mL) as required. Dosage range is 4.65 to 70 mEq/day.

➤*Children:* 2.3 mEq/kg/day or 56 mEq/m²/day, well diluted; give slowly in divided doses.

➤*Infants:* Not more than 0.93 mEq (2 mL).

➤*Emergency elevation of serum calcium:*

Adults – 7 to 14 mEq (15 to 30.1 mL) IV.

Children – 1 to 7 mEq (2.2 to 15 mL).

Infants – < 1 mEq (2.2 mL). Depending on patient response, these doses can be repeated every 1 to 3 days.

➤*Hypocalcemic tetany:*

Adults – 4.5 to 16 mEq of calcium (9.7 to 34.4 mL) may be given IM until therapeutic response occurs.

Children – 0.5 to 0.7 ,mEq/kg (1.1 to 1.5 mL/kg) IV 3 or 4 times daily or until tetany is controlled.

Neonates – 2.4 mEq/kg/day (5.2 mL/kg/day) in divided doses.

➤*Hyperkalemia with secondary cardiac toxicity:* Administer IV to provide 2.25 to 14 mEq (4.8 to 30.1 mL) while monitoring ECG. If necessary, repeat doses after 1 to 2 min.

➤*Magnesium intoxication:*

Adults – Initial dose is 4.5 to 9 mEq (9.7 to 19.4 mL) IV. Adjust subsequent doses to patient response. If IV use is not possible, give 2 to 5 mEq (4.3 to 10.8 mL) IM.

➤*Exchange transfusion:*

Adults – Approximately 1.35 mEq (2.9 mL) IV concurrent with each 100 mL of citrated blood.

Neonates – Administer IV at a dosage of 0.45 mEq (1 mL)/100 mL of exchanged citrated blood.

➤*Storage/Stability:* If precipitation has occurred in syringes, do not use. If precipitation is present in vials or amps dissolve by heating to 80°C (146°F) in a dry heat oven for a minimum of 1 hour. Shake vigorously; allow to cool to room temperature. Do not use if precipitate remains.

CALCIUM CHLORIDE

1 g (10 mL) contains 273 mg (13.6 mEq) calcium.

Rx	Calcium Chloride (Various, eg, Abbott, American Regent, Astra, IMS, Moore, VHA)	Injection: 10%	In 10 mL amps, vials and syringes.

For complete prescribing information, refer to the Calcium group monograph in the Intravenous Nutritional Therapy, Electrolytes section.

Administration and Dosage

➤*For IV use only.:* Injection is irritating to veins and must not be injected into tissues, since severe necrosis and sloughing may occur. Avoid extravasation. Administer slowly (not to exceed 0.5 to 1 mL/minute).

Intraventricular administration – In cardiac resuscitation, injection may be made into the ventricular cavity; do not inject into the myocardium. Intraventricular injection may be administered by personnel who are well trained in the technique and familiar with possible complications. Break off the IV needle supplied with the syringe and replace with a suitable intracardiac needle by affixing it firmly to the Luer taper provided on the syringe. After the injection has been completed, remove the needle/syringe assembly from the injection site by grasping the needle at the Luer fitting.

The intraventricular dose usually ranges from 200 to 800 mg (2 to 8 mL).

➤*Hypocalcemic disorders:*

Adults – 500 mg to 1 g at intervals of 1 to 3 days, depending on response of patient or serum calcium determinations. Repeated injections may be required.

Children – 0.2 mL/kg up to 1 to 10 mL/day.

➤*Magnesium intoxication:* Give 500 mg promptly; observe patient for signs of recovery before further doses are given.

➤*Hyperkalemic ECG disturbances of cardiac function:* Adjust dosage by constant monitoring of ECG changes during administration.

➤*Cardiac resuscitation:*

Adults – Dose ranges from 500 mg to 1 g IV or 200 to 800 mg injected into the ventricular cavity.

Children – 0.2 mL/kg.

CALCIUM PRODUCTS COMBINED, PARENTERAL

Rx	Calphosan (Glenwood)	Injection: 50 mg calcium glycerophosphate and 50 mg calcium lactate per 10 mL in sodium chloride solution (0.08 mEq Ca/mL)	In 60 mL vials.[1]

[1] With 0.25% phenol.

For complete prescribing information, refer to the Calcium group monograph in the Intravenous Nutritional Therapy, Electrolytes group monograph.

MAGNESIUM

Rx	Magnesium Chloride (Various, eg, American Regent)	Injection: 20% (1.97 mEq/mL)	In 50 mL multiple dose vials.
Rx	Magnesium Sulfate (Various, eg, Astra, Pasadena)	Injection: 10% (0.8 mEq/mL)	In 20 and 50 mL vials and 20 mL amps.
Rx	Magnesium Sulfate (Various, eg, Abbott)	Injection: 12.5% (1 mEq/mL)	In 20 mL vials.
Rx	Magnesium Sulfate (Various, eg, Abbott, American Regent, Astra, IMS, Pasadena, Smith & Nephew Solopak)	Injection: 50% (4 mEq/mL)	In 2, 5, 10, 20 and 50 mL vials, 5 and 10 mL syringes, 2 and 10 mL amps.

For information on oral magnesium, refer to the Minerals and Electrolytes, Oral section. For information on the use of magnesium sulfate as an anticonvulsant, refer to the Anticonvulsants monograph in the CNS chapter.

Indications

➤*Hypomagnesemia:* Magnesium sulfate is used as replacement therapy in magnesium deficiency especially in acute hypomagnesemia accompanied by signs of tetany similar to those observed in hypocalcemia. In such cases, the serum magnesium (Mg++) level is usually below the lower limit of normal (1.5 to 2.5 or 3 mEq/L) and the serum calcium (Ca++) level is normal (4.3 to 5.3 mEq/L) or elevated.

Total parenteral nutrition – Total parenteral nutrition patients may develop hypomagnesemia (< 1.5 mEq/L) without supplementation. Magnesium is added to correct or prevent hypomagnesemia.

➤*Preeclampsia/eclampsia/nephritis (magnesium sulfate):* Prevention and control of convulsions of severe preeclampsia and eclampsia and for control of hypertension, encephalopathy and convulsions associated with acute nephritis in children (see monograph in Anticonvulsants, Miscellaneous in the CNS chapter).

➤*Unlabeled uses:* Inhibition of premature labor (tocolytic); however, it is not a first-line agent.

In suspected acute myocardial infarction patients immediately after admission to counteract post-infarctional hypomagnesemia and subsequent arrhythmias.

Magnesium IV is effective as a bronchodilator and, therefore, may be useful in some asthmatic patients.

Since magnesium deficiency may play a role in chronic fatigue syndrome, it has been suggested that magnesium administration may be beneficial in this condition; however, there are conflicting reports and further study is needed.

Administration and Dosage

➤*IV administration:* Do not exceed 1.5 mL/min of a 10% concentration (or its equivalent), except in cases of severe eclampsia with sei-

MAGNESIUM

zures. Dilute IV infusion solutions to a concentration of ≤ 20% prior to IV administration. The most commonly used diluents are 5% Dextrose Injection and 0.9% Sodium Chloride Injection.

➤*IM administration:* Deep IM injection of the undiluted (50%) solution is appropriate for adults, but dilute to ≤ 20% concentration prior to IM injection in children.

➤*Admixture incompatibilities:* Magnesium sulfate in solution may result in a precipitate formation when mixed with solutions containing: Alcohol (in high concentrations); alkali carbonates and bicarbonates; alkali hydroxides; arsenates; barium; calcium; clindamycin phosphate; heavy metals; hydrocortisone sodium succinate; phosphates; polymyxin B sulfate; procaine HCl; salicylates; strontium; tartrates.

➤*Hyperalimentation:* Maintenance requirements are not precisely known. Maintenance dose range:

Adults – 8 to 24 mEq/day.

Infants – 2 to 10 mEq/day.

➤*Mild magnesium deficiency:*

Adults – 1 g (8.12 mEq; 2 mL of 50% solution) IM every 6 hours for 4 doses (total of 32.5 mEq/24 hours).

➤*Severe hypomagnesemia:*

IM – As much as 2 mEq/kg (0.5 mL of 50% solution) within 4 hours if necessary.

IV – 5 g (≈ 40 mEq)/L of 5% Dextrose Injection or 0.9% Sodium Chloride solution, infused over 3 hours. In treatment of deficiency states, observe caution to prevent exceeding renal excretory capacity.

➤*Seizures associated with preeclampsia/eclampsia/nephritis:* Refer to Anticonvulsants, Miscellaneous in the CNS chapter for complete dosing information.

Actions

➤*Pharmacology:* Magnesium is a cofactor in a number of enzyme systems, and is involved in neurochemical transmission and muscular excitability. As a nutritional adjunct in hyperalimentation, the precise mechanism of action is uncertain.

Magnesium deficiency – Magnesium deficiency is rare in well nourished individuals, except in malabsorption syndromes. Magnesium deficiency may occur in malabsorption syndromes, chronic alcoholism, malnutrition, intestinal bypass surgery, diuretic therapy, severe diarrhea, prolonged nasogastric suction, steatorrhea, during hemodialysis, diabetes mellitus, pancreatitis, primary aldosteronism and renal tubular damage. Early symptoms of hypomagnesemia (< 1.5 mEq/L) may develop as early as 3 to 4 days or within weeks. Predominant deficiency effects are neurological (eg, muscle irritability, clonic twitching, tremors). Hypocalcemia and hypokalemia often follow low serum levels of magnesium. While large stores of magnesium are found intracellularly and in bone in adults, they often are not mobilized sufficiently to maintain plasma levels. Parenteral magnesium therapy repairs the plasma deficit and causes deficiency signs and symptoms to cease. The normal adult body contains 20 to 30 g (2000 mEq) magnesium.

Magnesium prevents or controls convulsions by blocking neuromuscular transmission and decreasing the amount of acetylcholine liberated at the end plate by the motor nerve impulse. Magnesium is said to have a depressant effect on the CNS, but it does not adversely affect the mother, fetus or neonate when used as directed in eclampsia or preeclampsia. Normal plasma magnesium levels range from 1.5 to 2.5 mEq.

Magnesium acts peripherally to produce vasodilation. With low doses, only flushing and sweating occur; larger doses cause a lowering of blood pressure and CNS depression. The central and peripheral effects of magnesium poisoning are antagonized by IV administration of calcium.

One g of magnesium sulfate provides 8.12 mEq of magnesium.

Hypermagnesemia – As plasma magnesium rises above 4 mEq/L, the deep tendon reflexes are first decreased and then disappear as the plasma level approaches 10 mEq/L. At this level respiratory paralysis may occur. Heart block also may occur at this or lower plasma levels of magnesium. Serum magnesium concentrations in excess of 12 mEq may be fatal.

➤*Pharmacokinetics:* IM injection results in therapeutic plasma levels within 60 minutes and persists for 3 to 4 hours. IV doses provide immediate effects that last for 30 minutes. Effective anticonvulsant serum levels range from 2.5 to 7.5 mEq/L. Magnesium is excreted by the kidneys at a rate proportional to the plasma concentration and glomerular filtration.

Contraindications

➤*Magnesium sulfate:* Heart block or myocardial damage; IV magnesium to patients with preeclampsia during the 2 hours preceding delivery.

➤*Magnesium chloride:* Renal impairment; marked myocardial disease; coma.

Warnings

➤*Renal function impairment:* Because magnesium is excreted by the kidneys, use with caution. Parenteral use in the presence of renal insufficiency may lead to magnesium intoxication.

➤*Elderly:* Geriatric patients often require reduced dosage because of impaired renal function. In patients with severe impairment, dosage should not exceed 20 g in 48 hours. Monitor serum magnesium in such patients.

➤*Pregnancy: Category A.* Studies in pregnant women have not shown that magnesium sulfate injection increases the risk of fetal abnormalities if administered during all trimesters of pregnancy. If this drug is used during pregnancy, the possibility of fetal harm appears remote. However, because studies cannot rule out the possibility of harm, use during pregnancy only if clearly needed.

When administered by continuous IV infusion (especially for > 24 hours preceding delivery) to control convulsions in toxemic mothers, the newborn may show signs of magnesium toxicity, including neuromuscular or respiratory depression (see Overdosage).

➤*Lactation:* Since magnesium is distributed into milk during parenteral magnesium sulfate administration, use with caution in nursing women.

➤*Children:* Safety and efficacy in children have not been established.

Precautions

➤*Monitoring:* Maintain urine output at a level of ≥ 100 mL every 4 hours. Monitor serum magnesium levels and clinical status to avoid overdosage in preeclampsia. See Overdosage for serum level/toxicity relationships.

Clinical indications of safe dosage regimen include presence of the patellar reflex (knee jerk) and absence of respiratory depression (≈ 16 breaths or more/min). Serum magnesium levels usually sufficient to control convulsions range from 3 to 6 mg/dL (2.5 to 5 mEq/L). Strength of deep tendon reflexes begins to diminish when magnesium levels exceed 4 mEq/L. Reflexes may be absent at 10 mEq/L, where respiratory paralysis is possible. Keep an injectable calcium salt immediately available to counteract potential hazards of magnesium intoxication in eclampsia.

➤*Flushing/Sweating:* Administer with caution if flushing or sweating occurs.

➤*Hypomagnesemia:* Do not administer magnesium sulfate injection unless hypomagnesemia is confirmed.

Drug Interactions

➤*Neuromuscular blocking agents, nondepolarizing:* Neuromuscular blocking effects may be increased by concurrent magnesium sulfate. Prolonged respiratory depression with extended periods of apnea may occur.

Adverse Reactions

Adverse effects are usually the result of magnesium intoxication and include: Flushing; sweating; hypotension; stupor; depressed reflexes; flaccid paralysis; hypothermia; circulatory collapse; cardiac and CNS depression proceeding to respiratory paralysis (the most life-threatening effect).

Hypocalcemia with signs of tetany secondary to magnesium sulfate therapy for eclampsia has occurred.

Overdosage

➤*Symptoms:* Sharp drop in blood pressure and respiratory paralysis. ECG changes may include increased PR interval, increased QRS complex and prolonged QT interval. Disappearance of the patellar reflex is a useful clinical sign to detect the onset of magnesium intoxication.

Although patients usually tolerate high concentrations of magnesium in plasma, there are occasional instances when cardiac consequences may be seen in the form of complete heart block at concentrations well below 10 mEq/L.

Other signs include muscle weakness, hypotension, sedation and confusion. As plasma concentrations of magnesium begin to exceed 4 mEq/L, deep-tendon reflexes are decreased and may be absent at levels approaching 10 mEq/L.

When magnesium sulfate injection is administered parenterally in doses that are sufficient to induce hypermagnesemia, the drug has a depressant effect on the CNS and, via the peripheral neuromuscular junction, on muscle.

Approximate Correlation of Magnesium Toxicity vs Serum Level	
Serum level (mEq/L)	Effect
1.5 to 2.5	Normal serum concentration
4 to 7	"Therapeutic" level for preeclampsia/eclampsia/convulsions
7 to 10	Loss of deep tendon reflexes, hypotension, narcosis

Minerals

MAGNESIUM

Approximate Correlation of Magnesium Toxicity vs Serum Level	
Serum level (mEq/L)	Effect
12 to 15	Respiratory paralysis
> 15	Cardiac conduction affected. PR interval lengthening, QRS widening, dysrhythmias
> 25	Cardiac arrest

➤*Treatment:* Provide artificial ventilation until a calcium salt (10 to 20 mL of a 5% solution, diluted with isotonic Sodium Chloride for Injection if desired) can be injected IV to antagonize the effects of magnesium. A dose of 5 to 10 mEq calcium will usually reverse the respiratory depression and heart block. Physostigmine 0.5 to 1 mg SC may be helpful. Peritoneal dialysis or hemodialysis are also effective.

Hypermagnesemia in the newborn may require resuscitation and assisted ventilation via endotracheal intubation or intermittent positive pressure ventilation as well as IV calcium.

PHOSPHATE

Rx	**Potassium Phosphate** (Various, eg, Abbott, American Regent)	**Injection:** Provides 3 mM phosphate and 4.4 mEq potassium per mL	In 5, 10, 15, 30, and 50 mL vials.
Rx	**Sodium Phosphate** (Various, eg, Abbott, American Regent)	**Injection:** Provides 3 mM phosphate and 4 mEq sodium per mL	In 10, 15, 30 and 50 mL vials.

Indications

A source of phosphate to add to large volume IV fluids, to prevent or correct hypophosphatemia in patients with restricted oral intake.

Additive for preparing specific IV fluid formulas when needs of patient cannot be met by standard electrolyte or nutrient solutions.

Administration and Dosage

Commercial injections are mixtures of the monobasic and dibasic salt forms. To avoid confusion, prescribe and dispense in terms of millimoles (mM) of phosphorus.

For IV use only. Dilute and thoroughly mix in a larger volume of fluid. Individualize dosage. Monitor serum sodium (or potassium), inorganic phosphorus and calcium levels.

➤*Total parenteral nutrition (TPN):* Approximately 10 to 15 mM of phosphorus (equivalent to 310 to 465 mg elemental phosphorus) per liter of TPN solution is usually adequate to maintain normal serum phosphate; larger amounts may be required in hypermetabolic states. Consider the amount of sodium (or potassium) which accompanies the addition of phosphate; monitor serum electrolytes and ECG.

Infants receiving TPN – 1.5 to 2 mM/kg/day.

Actions

➤*Pharmacology:* A prominent component of all body tissues, phosphorus participates in bone deposition, regulation of calcium metabolism, buffering effects on acid-base equilibrium and various enzyme systems. In the extracellular fluid, phosphate exists as both a monovalent and a divalent form, the ratio of which is pH-dependent.

Normal serum inorganic phosphate levels –
  Adults: 3 to 4.5 mg/dL.
  Children: 4 to 7 mg/dL.

Hypophosphatemia –
  Moderate (serum level ≤ 2.5 mg/dL): Symptoms include muscle weakness, malaise, paresthesias, CNS irritability, confusion, obtundation.
  Severe (serum level < 1 mg/dL): Seizures, coma, respiratory failure, hemolytic anemia, rhabdomyolysis, tremors, platelet and leukocyte dysfunction.

➤*Pharmacokinetics:* Phosphate infused IV is excreted in the urine. Plasma phosphate is filtered by the renal glomeruli, and > 80% is actively reabsorbed by the tubules.

Contraindications

High phosphate or low calcium levels.

➤*Potassium phosphate:* Hyperkalemia.
➤*Sodium phosphate:* Hypernatremia.

Warnings

➤*Electrolyte intoxication:* To avoid phosphate, sodium or potassium intoxication, infuse solutions slowly.

➤*Hypocalcemic tetany:* Infusions of high concentrations of phosphate reduce serum calcium and produce symptoms of hypocalcemic tetany. Monitor calcium levels.

➤*Cardiac effects:* Use sodium phosphate with caution in patients with cardiac failure or who are on other edematous or sodium-retaining medications. Use potassium phosphate with caution in the presence of cardiac disease, particularly in digitalized patients. High plasma concentrations of potassium may cause death through cardiac depression or arrhythmias.

➤*Adrenal insufficiency:* Administration of phosphate products in patients with adrenal insufficiency may cause sodium or potassium phosphate intoxication.

➤*Renal function impairment:* Administration may cause sodium or potassium phosphate intoxication.

➤*Hepatic function impairment:* Use sodium phosphate with caution in patients with cirrhosis.

➤*Pregnancy: Category C.* It is not known whether sodium phosphate can cause fetal harm when administered to a pregnant woman or can affect reproduction capacity. Give phosphate to a pregnant woman only if clearly needed.

➤*Lactation:* It is not known whether this drug is excreted in breast milk. Exercise caution when administering to a nursing woman.

Precautions

➤*Monitoring:* Guide replacement therapy by the serum inorganic phosphate level and the limits imposed by the accompanying sodium or potassium ion.

Drug Interactions

For information on drug interactions involving potassium, refer to the Potassium Salts monograph.

Adverse Reactions

Phosphate intoxication results in reciprocal hypocalcemic tetany.

Overdosage

➤*Potassium phosphate:* Potassium phosphate may cause combined potassium and phosphate intoxication.

➤*Symptoms:* Paresthesias of the extremities; flaccid paralysis; listlessness; confusion; weakness and heaviness of the legs; hypotension; cardiac arrhythmias; heart block; ECG abnormalities (eg, disappearance of P waves, spreading and slurring of the QRS complex with development of a biphasic curve, cardiac arrest).

➤*Treatment:* Immediately discontinue infusions. Restore depressed serum calcium levels; reduce elevated potassium levels.

SODIUM CHLORIDE

For information on oral sodium chloride, refer to Minerals and Electrolytes, Oral section.

Indications

For parenteral restoration of sodium ion in patients with restricted oral intake. Sodium replacement is specifically indicated in patients with hyponatremia or low salt syndrome. Sodium Chloride may also be added to compatible carbohydrate solutions such as Dextrose in Water to provide electrolytes.

Sodium Chloride Injections are also indicated as pharmaceutic aids and diluents for the infusion of compatible drug additives.

➤*0.9% Sodium Chloride (Normal Saline):* Normal saline, which is isotonic, restores both water and sodium chloride losses. Other indications for parenteral 0.9% saline include: Diluting or dissolving drugs for IV, IM or SC injection; flushing of IV catheters; extracellular fluid replacement; treatment of metabolic alkalosis in the presence of fluid loss and mild sodium depletion; as a priming solution in hemodialysis procedures and to initiate and terminate blood transfusions without hemolyzing red blood cells.

➤*0.45% Sodium Chloride (Hypotonic):* Hypotonic sodium chloride is primarily a hydrating solution and may be used to assess the status of the kidneys, since more water is provided than is required for salt excretion. It may also be used in the treatment of hyperosmolar diabetes where the use of dextrose is inadvisable and there is a need for large amounts of fluid without an excess of sodium ions.

➤*3% or 5% Sodium Chloride (Hypertonic):* Hypertonic sodium chloride is used in hyponatremia and hypochloremia due to electrolyte and fluid loss replaced with sodium-free fluids; drastic dilution of body water following excessive water intake; emergency treatment of severe salt depletion.

➤*Bacteriostatic Sodium Chloride:* Only for diluting or dissolving drugs for IV, IM or SC injection. See Contraindications and Warnings.

➤*Concentrated Sodium Chloride:* As an additive in parenteral fluid therapy for use in patients who have special problems of sodium electrolyte intake or excretion. It is intended to meet the specific requirements of the patient with unusual fluid and electrolyte needs. After available clinical and laboratory information is considered and correlated, determine the appropriate number of milliequivalents of Concentrated Sodium Chloride Injection, USP and dilute for use.

Administration and Dosage

Individualize dosage. Frequent laboratory determinations and clinical evaluation are essential to monitor changes in fluid balance, blood glucose and electrolytes.

In the average adult, daily requirements of sodium and chloride are met by the infusion of 1 L of 0.9% sodium chloride (154 mEq each of sodium and chloride). Base fluid administration on calculated maintenance or replacement fluid requirements.

Do not use plastic container in series connection.

If administration is controlled by a pumping device, take care to discontinue pumping action before the container runs dry or air embolism may result.

➤*IV catheters:* Prior to and after administration of the medication, entirely flush the catheter with 0.9% Sodium Chloride for Injection. Use in accord with any warnings or precautions appropriate to the medication being administered.

➤*Calculation of sodium deficit:* To calculate the amount of sodium that must be administered to raise serum sodium to the desired level, use the following equation (TBW = total body water): Na deficit (mEq) = TBW (desired − observed plasma Na).

Base the repletion rate on the degree of urgency in the patient. Use of hypertonic saline (eg, 3% or 5%) will correct the deficit more rapidly.

➤*Concentrated Sodium Chloride:* The dosage as an additive in parenteral fluid therapy is predicated on specific requirements of the patient. The appropriate volume is then withdrawn for proper dilution. Having determined the mEq of sodium chloride to be added, divide by four to calculate the number of mL to be used. Withdraw this volume and transfer into appropriate IV solutions such as 5% Dextrose Injection. The properly diluted solution may be given IV.

➤*Admixture incompatibilities:* Some additives may be incompatible. Consult a pharmacist. When Sodium Chloride Injections are used as diluents for infusion of compatible drug additives, refer to dosage and administration information accompanying additive drugs. Check specific references for any possible incompatibility with sodium chloride.

To minimize the risk of possible incompatibilities arising from mixing this solution with other additives that may be prescribed, inspect the final infusate for cloudiness or precipitation immediately after mixing, prior to administration and periodically during administration. Do not store.

➤*Storage/Stability:* Replace IV apparatus at least once every 24 hours. Use only if solution is clear. Protect from freezing; avoid excessive heat. Store at 15° to 30°C (59° to 86°F). Brief exposure up to 40°C (104°F) does not adversely affect product.

Actions

➤*Pharmacology:* Normal osmolarity of the extracellular fluid ranges between 280 to 300 mOsm/L; it is primarily a function of sodium and its accompanying ions, chloride and bicarbonate. Sodium chloride is the principal salt involved in maintenance of plasma tonicity. One g of sodium chloride provides 17.1 mEq sodium and 17.1 mEq chloride.

Hyponatremia – Hyponatremia (< 135 mEq/L): Symptoms may include weakness, nausea, disorientation, lethargy and headache; severe cases may progress to seizures and coma.

Contraindications

Hypernatremia; fluid retention; when the administration of sodium or chloride could be clinically detrimental.

➤*3% and 5% sodium chloride solutions:* Elevated, normal or only slightly decreased plasma sodium and chloride concentrations.

➤*Bacteriostatic sodium chloride:* Newborns (see Warnings); for fluid or sodium chloride replacement.

Warnings

➤*Fluid/solute overload:* Excessive amounts of sodium chloride by any route may cause hypokalemia and acidosis. Administration of IV solutions can cause fluid or solute overload resulting in dilution of serum electrolyte concentrations, congestive heart failure (CHF), overhydration, congested states or acute pulmonary edema, especially in patients with cardiovascular disease and in patients receiving corticosteroids or corticotropin or drugs that may give rise to sodium retention. The risk of dilutional states is inversely proportional to the electrolyte concentration. The risk of solute overload causing congested states with peripheral and pulmonary edema is directly proportional to the electrolyte concentration.

Infusion of > 1 L of isotonic (0.9%) sodium chloride may supply more sodium and chloride than normally found in serum, resulting in hypernatremia; this may cause a loss of bicarbonate ions, resulting in an acidifying effect. Infusion during or immediately after surgery may result in excessive sodium retention.

➤*Hypertonic solutions:* When administered peripherally, slowly infuse through a small bore needle placed well within the lumen of a large vein to minimize venous irritation. Carefully avoid infiltration.

➤*Bacteriostatic Sodium Chloride:* Do not use in newborns. Benzyl alcohol as a preservative in Bacteriostatic Sodium Chloride Injection has been associated with toxicity in newborns. This toxicity may result from both high cumulative amounts (mg/kg) of benzyl alcohol and the limited detoxification capacity of the neonate liver. These solutions have not been reported to cause problems in older infants, children and adults. It is estimated that a 30 mL IV dose may be given to adults without toxic effects. Data are unavailable on the toxicity of other preservatives in newborns. Use preservative-free Sodium Chloride Injection for flushing intravascular catheters. Where a sodium chloride solution is required for preparing or diluting medications for use in newborns, use only preservative-free 0.9% Sodium Chloride.

➤*Concentrated Sodium Chloride Injection:* Concentrated sodium chloride injection is hypertonic and must be diluted before use. Inadvertent direct injection or absorption of concentrated Sodium Chloride Injection may give rise to sudden hypernatremia and such complications as cardiovascular shock, CNS disorders, extensive hemolysis, cortical necrosis of the kidneys and severe local tissue necrosis (if administered extravascularly). Do not use unless solution is clear.

➤*Surgical patients:* Surgical patients should seldom receive salt-containing solutions immediately following surgery unless factors producing salt depletion are present. Because of renal retention of salt during surgery, additional electrolyte given IV may result in fluid retention, edema and overloading of the circulation.

➤*Renal function impairment:* Infusions of sodium ions may result in excessive sodium retention; administer with care.

➤*Pregnancy: Category C.* It is not known whether sodium chloride can cause fetal harm when given to a pregnant woman or can affect reproduction capacity. Use only if clearly needed.

➤*Lactation:* It is not known whether sodium chloride is excreted in breast milk. Exercise caution when administering sodium chloride to a nursing woman.

➤*Children:* Safety and efficacy have not been established.

Precautions

➤*Monitoring:* Clinical evaluation and periodic laboratory determinations are necessary to monitor changes in fluid balance, electrolyte concentrations and acid-base balance during prolonged parenteral therapy or whenever the condition of the patient warrants such evaluation. Significant deviations from normal concentrations may require tailoring of the electrolyte pattern.

Extraordinary electrolyte losses (eg, during protracted nasogastric suction, vomiting, diarrhea, GI fistula drainage) may necessitate additional electrolyte supplementation. Supply additional essential electrolytes, minerals and vitamins as needed.

SODIUM CHLORIDE

➤*Hypokalemia:* Hypokalemia may result from excessive administration of potassium-free solutions.

➤*Elderly or postoperative patients:* Exercise care in administering sodium-containing solutions in renal or cardiovascular insufficiency, with or without CHF.

➤*3% and 5% sodium chloride solutions:* Infuse very slowly and use with caution to avoid pulmonary edema; observe patients constantly.

➤*Special risk:* Administer cautiously to patients with decompensated cardiovascular, cirrhotic and nephrotic disease, circulatory insufficiency, hypoproteinemia, hypervolemia, urinary tract obstruction, CHF and to patients with concurrent edema and sodium retention, those receiving corticosteroids or corticotropin and those retaining salt.

Adverse Reactions

Reactions due to solution or technique of administration – Febrile response; local tenderness; abscess; tissue necrosis or infection at injection site; venous thrombosis or phlebitis extending from injection site; extravasation; hypervolemia.

Hypernatremia – Hypernatremia may be associated with edema and exacerbation of CHF due to retention of water, resulting in expanded extracellular fluid volume.

Ion excess/deficit – Symptoms may result from an excess or deficit of one or more of the ions present in the solution; therefore, frequent monitoring of electrolyte levels is essential. If infused in large amounts, chloride ions may cause a loss of bicarbonate ions, resulting in an acidifying effect.

Postoperative salt intolerance – Symptoms include cellular dehydration, weakness, disorientation, anorexia, nausea, distention, deep respiration, oliguria, increased BUN.

Too rapid infusion – Too rapid infusion of hypertonic solutions may cause local pain and venous irritation. Adjust rate of administration according to tolerance. Use of the largest peripheral vein and a well-placed small bore needle is recommended. (See Warnings.)

If an adverse reaction occurs, discontinue the infusion, evaluate the patient, institute appropriate countermeasures and save remainder of the fluid for examination.

Overdosage

Parenteral preparations are unlikely to pose a threat of sodium chloride or fluid overload except possibly in newborn or very small infants. If these occur, reevaluate the patient and institute appropriate corrective measures.

Administration of too much sodium chloride may result in serious electrolyte disturbances with resulting retention of water, edema, loss of potassium and aggravation of an existing acidosis.

When intake of sodium chloride is excessive, excretion of crystalloids is increased in an attempt to maintain normal osmotic pressure. Thus there is increased excretion of potassium and of bicarbonate and, consequently, a tendency toward acidosis. There is also a rapid elimination of any foreign salt, such as iodide and bromide, being used for therapy.

SODIUM CHLORIDE INTRAVENOUS INFUSIONS FOR ADMIXTURES

		Sodium (mEq/L)	Chloride (mEq/L)	Osmolarity (mOsm/L)	How Supplied
Rx	**0.45% Sodium Chloride (½ Normal Saline)** (Various, eg, Abbott, Astra, Clintec, McGaw)	77	77	≈ 155	In 25, 50, 150, 250, 500 and 1000 mL.
Rx	**0.9% Sodium Chloride (Normal Saline)** (Various, eg, Abbott, Astra, Clintec, Gensia, McGaw, Rugby, Smith & Nephew SoloPak)	154	154	≈ 310	In 2, 3, 5, 10, 20, 25, 30, 50, 100, 150, 250, 500, 1000ml and 2 mL fill in 3 mL.
Rx	**3% Sodium Chloride**(Various, eg, Clintec, McGaw)	513	513	1030	In 500 mL.
Rx	**5% Sodium Chloride** (Various, eg, Abbott, Clintec, McGaw)	855	855	1710	In 500 mL.

SODIUM CHLORIDE DILUENTS

Rx	**Bacteriostatic Sodium Chloride Injection**[1] (Various, eg, American Regent, Elkins-Sinn, Rugby)	0.9% sodium chloride	In 2, 10, and 30 mL.

[1] With benzyl alcohol or parabens.

CONCENTRATED SODIUM CHLORIDE INJECTION

Rx	**Sodium Chloride Injection** (Various, eg, IMS)	14.6% sodium chloride	In 20, 40 and 200 mL.
Rx	**Sodium Chloride Injection** (Various, eg, American Regent, Gensia, IMS, Pasadena)	23.4% sodium chloride	In 30, 50, 100 and 200 mL.

Administration and Dosage

Not for direct infusion. *Must* be diluted before use.

POTASSIUM SALTS

For information on oral potassium, refer to Mineral and Electrolytes, Oral section. For information on potassium phosphate, refer to specific monograph in this section.

Indications

Prevention and treatment of moderate or severe potassium deficit when oral replacement therapy is not feasible.

➤*Potassium acetate:* Potassium acetate is useful as an additive for preparing specific IV fluid formulas when patient needs cannot be met by standard electrolyte or nutrient solutions.

Also indicated for marked loss of GI secretions by vomiting, diarrhea, GI intubation or fistulas; prolonged diuresis; prolonged parenteral use of potassium-free fluids (eg, normal saline, dextrose solutions); diabetic acidosis, especially during vigorous insulin and dextrose treatment; metabolic alkalosis; attacks of hereditary or familial periodic paralysis; hyperadrenocorticism; primary aldosteronism; overmedication with adrenocortical steroids, testosterone or corticotropin; healing phase of scalds or burns; cardiac arrhythmias, especially due to digitalis glycosides.

Administration and Dosage

mEq/g of Various Potassium Salts	
Potassium salt	mEq/g
Potassium acetate	10.2
Potassium chloride	13.4
Dibasic potassium phosphate[a]	11.5
Monobasic potassium phosphate[a]	7.3

[a] Commercial preparations of potassium phosphate injection contain a mixture of both mono- and dibasic salts (see Potassium Phosphate monograph).

➤*Do not administer undiluted potassium:* Potassium preparations must be diluted with suitable large volume parenteral solutions, mixed well and given by slow IV infusion.

Too rapid infusion of hypertonic solutions may cause local pain and, rarely, vein irritation. Adjust rate of administration according to tolerance. Use of the largest peripheral vein and a small bore needle is recommended.

The usual additive dilution of potassium chloride is 40 mEq/L of IV fluid. The maximum desirable concentration is 80 mEq/L, although extreme emergencies may dictate greater concentrations.

In critical states, potassium chloride may be administered in saline (unless saline is contraindicated) since dextrose may lower serum potassium levels by producing an intracellular shift.

Avoid "layering" of potassium by proper agitation of the prepared IV solution. Do not add potassium to an IV bottle in the hanging position.

Individualize dosage. Guide dosage and rate of infusion by ECG and serum electrolyte determinations. The following may be used as a guide:

Potassium Dosage/Rate of Infusion Guidelines			
Serum K+	Maximum infusion rate	Maximum concentration	Maximum 24 hour dose
> 2.5 mEq/L	10 mEq/hr	40 mEq/L	200 mEq
< 2 mEq/L	40 mEq/hr	80 mEq/L	400 mEq

POTASSIUM SALTS

Add electrolytes to the mixed solutions only after considering electrolytes already present and potential incompatibilities such as calcium and phosphate or sulfate.

➤*Children:* IV infusion up to 3 mEq/kg or 40 mEq/m^2/day. Adjust volume of administered fluids to body size.

Actions

➤*Pharmacology:* The principal intracellular cation, potassium is essential for maintenance of intracellular tonicity; transmission of nerve impulses; contraction of cardiac, skeletal and smooth muscle; and maintenance of normal renal function. Potassium participates in carbohydrate utilization and protein synthesis and is critical in regulating nerve conduction and muscle contraction, particularly in the heart.

Hypokalemia – Gradual potassium depletion occurs via renal excretion, through GI loss or because of inadequate intake (excretion > intake). Depletion usually results from diuretic therapy, primary or secondary hyperaldosteronism, diabetic ketoacidosis, severe diarrhea (especially if associated with vomiting) or inadequate replacement during prolonged parenteral nutrition.

Potassium depletion sufficient to cause 1 mEq/L drop in serum potassium requires a loss of about 100 to 200 mEq of potassium from the total body store.

Symptoms: Weakness; fatigue; ileus; polydipsia; flaccid paralysis or impaired ability to concentrate urine (in advanced cases).

ECG may reveal premature atrial and ventricular contractions, prolongation of QT interval, ST segment depression, broad and flat T waves or appearance of U waves. Severe cases may lead to muscular weakness, paralysis, respiratory failure.

➤*Pharmacokinetics:* Normally about 80% to 90% of potassium intake is excreted in urine with the remainder voided in stool and, to a small extent, in perspiration. Kidneys do not conserve potassium well; during fasting or in patients on a potassium-free diet, potassium loss from the body continues, resulting in potassium depletion. A deficiency of either potassium or chloride will lead to a deficit of the other.

Contraindications

Diseases where high potassium levels may be encountered; hyperkalemia; renal failure and conditions in which potassium retention is present; oliguria or azotemia; anuria; crush syndrome; severe hemolytic reactions; adrenocortical insufficiency (untreated Addison's disease); adynamica episodica hereditaria; acute dehydration; heat cramps; hyperkalemia from any cause; early postoperative oliguria except during GI drainage.

Warnings

➤*Potassium intoxication:* Do not infuse rapidly. High plasma concentrations of potassium may cause death through cardiac depression, arrhythmias or arrest. Monitor potassium replacement therapy whenever possible by continuous or serial ECG. In addition to ECG effects, local pain and phlebitis may result when a > 40 mEq/L concentration is infused.

Renal impairment or adrenal insufficiency – Renal impairments or adrenal insufficiency may cause potassium intoxication. Potassium salts can produce hyperkalemia and cardiac arrest. Potentially fatal hyperkalemia can develop rapidly and be asymptomatic. Use with great caution, if at all.

➤*Concentrated potassium:* Concentrated potassium solutions are for IV admixtures only; do not use undiluted. Direct injection may be instantaneously fatal.

Metabolic alkalosis: Potassium depletion is usually accompanied by an obligatory loss of chloride resulting in hypochloremic metabolic alkalosis. Treat the underlying cause of potassium depletion and administer IV potassium chloride.

Use solutions containing acetate ion carefully in metabolic or respiratory alkalosis, and when there is an increased level or impairment of utilization of this ion.

➤*Metabolic acidosis:* Treat associated hypokalemia with an alkalinizing potassium salt (eg, bicarbonate, citrate, gluconate, acetate).

➤*Musculoskeletal/Cardiac effects:* When serum sodium or calcium concentration is reduced, moderate elevation of serum potassium may cause toxic effects on the heart and skeletal muscle. Weakness and later paralysis of voluntary muscles, with consequent respiratory distress and dysphagia, are generally late signs, sometimes significantly preceding dangerous or fatal cardiac toxicity.

➤*Renal function impairment:* Normal kidney function permits safe potassium therapy. Although temporary elevation of serum potassium level due to renal insufficiency secondary to dehydration or shock may mask an intracellular potassium deficit, do not replenish potassium until renal function is reestablished by overcoming dehydration and shock. Discontinue potassium-containing solutions if signs of renal insufficiency develop during infusions.

➤*Pregnancy: Category C.* It is not known whether potassium salts can cause fetal harm when administered to a pregnant woman or can affect reproduction capacity. Give to a pregnant woman only if clearly needed.

➤*Lactation:* Exercise caution when administering to a nursing woman.

Precautions

➤*Monitoring:* Close medical supervision with frequent ECGs and serum potassium determinations. Plasma levels are not necessarily indicative of tissue levels.

➤*Fluid/Solute overload:* IV administration can cause fluid or solute overloading resulting in dilution of serum electrolyte concentrations, overhydration, congested states or pulmonary edema.

The risk of dilutional states is inversely proportional to the electrolyte concentration of administered parenteral solutions. The risk of solute overload causing congested states with peripheral and pulmonary edema is directly proportional to the electrolyte concentrations of such solutions.

➤*Special risk:* Use with caution in the presence of cardiac disease, particularly in digitalized patients or in the presence of renal disease, metabolic acidosis, Addison's disease, acute dehydration, prolonged or severe diarrhea, familial periodic paralysis, hypoadrenalism, hyperkalemia, hyponatremia and myotonia congenita.

Drug Interactions

Potassium Preparation Drug Interactions			
Precipitant drug	Object drug*		Description
ACE inhibitors	Potassium preparations	↑	Concurrent use may result in elevated serum potassium concentrations in certain patients.
Potassium-sparing diuretics/potassium-containing salt substitutes	Potassium preparations	↑	Potassium-sparing diuretics and potassium-containing salt substitutes will increase potassium retention and can produce severe hyperkalemia.
Potassium preparations	Digitalis	↑	In patients on digoxin, hypokalemia may result in digoxin toxicity. Use caution if discontinuing a potassium preparation in patients maintained on digoxin.

* ↑ = Object drug increased.

Adverse Reactions

Hyperkalemia – Adverse reactions involve the possibility of potassium intoxication. Signs and symptoms include: Paresthesias of extremities; flaccid paralysis; muscle or respiratory paralysis; areflexia; weakness; listlessness; mental confusion; weakness and heaviness of legs; hypotension; cardiac arrhythmias; heart block; ECG abnormalities such as disappearance of P waves, spreading and slurring of the QRS complex with development of a biphasic curve and cardiac arrest. See Overdosage.

➤*GI:* Nausea; vomiting; abdominal pain; diarrhea.

Reactions due to solution or technique of administration – Febrile response; infection at injection site; venous thrombosis; phlebitis extending from injection site; extravasation; hypervolemia; hyperkalemia; venospasm.

Overdosage

If excretory mechanisms are impaired or if potassium is administered too rapidly IV, potentially fatal hyperkalemia can result (see Contraindications and Warnings). It is important to consider the entire clinical picture and not rely solely on potassium levels since only extracellular potassium can be measured, yet intracellular potassium accounts for 98% of the total body amount.

➤*Symptoms:* Mild (> 5.5 to 6.5 mEq/L) to moderate (> 6.5 to 8 mEq/L) hyperkalemia may be asymptomatic and manifested only by increased serum potassium concentration and characteristic ECG changes. Other symptoms include muscular weakness, progressing to flaccid quadriplegia and respiratory paralysis; however, these generally do not develop unless potassium concentrations exceed 8 mEq/L. Dangerous cardiac arrhythmias often occur before onset of complete paralysis. Note that hyperkalemia produces symptoms paradoxically similar to those of hypokalemia.

ECG – Progressive increase in height and peaking of T waves; lowering of the R wave; decreased amplitude and ultimate disappearance of P waves; prolongation of PR interval and QRS complex; shortening of the QT interval; and finally, ventricular fibrillation and death.

➤*Treatment:* Terminate potassium administration. Monitor ECG. Infusion of combined dextrose and insulin in a ratio of 3 g dextrose to 1 unit regular insulin may be administered to shift potassium into cells. Administer sodium bicarbonate 50 to 100 mEq IV to reverse acidosis and also produce an intracellular shift. Give 10 to 100 mL calcium gluconate or calcium chloride 10% to reverse ECG changes. To remove potassium from the body use sodium polystyrene sulfonate resin or hemodialysis or peritoneal dialysis.

Electrolytes

POTASSIUM SALTS

In digitalized patients, too rapid lowering of serum potassium can cause digitalis toxicity (see Drug Interactions).

POTASSIUM ACETATE

Rx	**Potassium Acetate** (Various, eg, Abbott, American Regent, IMS)	**Injection:** 2 mEq/mL	In 20, 50 and 100 mL vials.
Rx	**Potassium Acetate** (Various)	**Injection:** 4 mEq/mL	In 50 mL vials.

Administration and Dosage

Must be diluted before use.

POTASSIUM CHLORIDE FOR INJECTION CONCENTRATE

Rx	**Potassium Chloride** (McGaw)	**Injection:** 2 mEq/mL	In 250 and 500 mL.
Rx	**Potassium Chloride** (Various, eg, Abbott, Baxter)	**Injection:** 10 mEq	In 5, 10, 50 and 100 mL vials and 5 mL additive syringes.
Rx	**Potassium Chloride** (Various, eg, Abbott, American Regent, Baxter)	**Injection:** 20 mEq	In 10 and 20 mL vials, 10 mL additive syringes, 10 mL amps.
Rx	**Potassium Chloride** (Various, eg, Abbott, Baxter)	**Injection:** 30 mEq	In 15, 20, 30 and 100 mL vials and 20 mL additive syringes.
Rx	**Potassium Chloride** (Various, eg, Abbott, American Regent, Baxter, McGuff)	**Injection:** 40 mEq	In 20, 30, 50 and 100 mL vials, 20 mL amps, 20 mL additive syringes.
Rx	**Potassium Chloride** (Various, eg, American Regent, McGuff)	**Injection:** 60 mEq	In 30 mL vials.
Rx	**Potassium Chloride** (Various)	**Injection:** 90 mEq	In 30 mL vials.

Administration and Dosage

Concentrate *must* be diluted before use.

SODIUM BICARBONATE

Rx	**Sodium Bicarbonate** (Abbott)	**Injection:** 4.2% (0.5 mEq/mL)	In 10 mL (5 mEq) syringes.
Rx	**Sodium Bicarbonate** (Astra)		In 2.5 and 5 mL fill in 5 and 10 mL syringes.
Rx	**Sodium Bicarbonate** (American Pharmaceutical Partners)		In 10 mL (5 mEq) *Bristoject* syringes.
Rx	**Sodium Bicarbonate** (Abbott)	**Injection:** 5% (0.6 mEq/mL)	In 500 mL[1] (297.5 mEq).
Rx	**Sodium Bicarbonate** (Baxter)		In 500 mL (297.5 mEq).
Rx	**Sodium Bicarbonate** (McGaw)		In 500 mL[1] (297.5 mEq).
Rx	**Sodium Bicarbonate** (Abbott)	**Injection:** 7.5% (0.9 mEq/mL)	In 50 mL (44.6 mEq) amps and 50 mL (44.6 mEq) syringes.
Rx	**Sodium Bicarbonate** (American Regent)		In 50 mL (44.6 mEq) vials.
Rx	**Sodium Bicarbonate** (Astra)		In 44.6 mL fill in 50 mL syringes.
Rx	**Sodium Bicarbonate** (American Pharmaceutical Partners)		In 50 mL (44.6 mEq) single-dose vials, 50 mL (44.6 mEq) *Bristoject* syringes and 200 mL (179 mEq) *MaxiVials*.
Rx	**Sodium Bicarbonate** (Abbott)	**Injection:** 8.4% (1 mEq/mL)	In 50 mL (50 mEq) fliptop vials and 10 mL (10 mEq) and 50 mL (50 mEq) syringes.
Rx	**Sodium Bicarbonate** (American Regent)		In 50 mL (50 mEq) vials.
Rx	**Sodium Bicarbonate** (Astra)		In 10 and 50 mL syringes.
Rx	**Sodium Bicarbonate** (American Pharmaceutical Partners)		In 50 mL (50 mEq) vials and 10 and 50 mEq *Bristoject* syringes.
Rx	**Neut** (Abbott)	**Neutralizing Additive Solution**[2]**:** 4% (0.48 mEq/mL)	In 5 mL (2.4 mEq) fliptop and pintop vials.[1]
Rx	**Sodium Bicarbonate** (American Pharmaceutical Partners)	**Neutralizing Additive Solution**[2]**:** 4.2% (0.5 mEq/mL)	In 5 mL fill in 6 mL vials (2.5 mEq).

[1] With EDTA.

[2] For use as a neutralizing additive solution to acidic large volume parenterals.

For information on oral sodium bicarbonate, refer to Systemic Alkalinizers.

Indications

➤*Metabolic acidosis:* In severe renal disease, uncontrolled diabetes, circulatory insufficiency due to shock, anoxia or severe dehydration, extracorporeal circulation of blood, cardiac arrest and severe primary lactic acidosis where a rapid increase in plasma total CO_2 content is crucial. Treat metabolic acidosis in addition to measures designed to control the cause of the acidosis (eg, insulin in uncomplicated diabetes, blood volume restoration in shock). Since an appreciable time interval may elapse before all ancillary effects occur, bicarbonate therapy is indicated to minimize risks inherent to acidosis itself.

At one time it was suggested to administer bicarbonate during cardiopulmonary resuscitation following cardiac arrest; however, recent evidence suggests that little benefit is provided and its use may be detrimental. For treatment of acidosis in this clinical situation, concentrate efforts on restoring ventilation and blood flow. According to the American Heart Association guidelines, use as a last resort after other standard measures have been utilized.

➤*Urinary alkalinization:* In the treatment of certain drug intoxications (eg, salicylates, lithium) and in hemolytic reactions requiring alkalinization of urine to diminish nephrotoxicity of blood pigments.

➤*Severe diarrhea:* Severe diarrhea, which is often accompanied by a significant loss of bicarbonate.

➤*Neutralizing additive solution:* To reduce the incidence of chemical phlebitis and patient discomfort due to vein irritation at or near the infusion site by raising the pH of IV acid solutions.

Administration and Dosage

Administer IV or SC following dilution to isotonicity (1.5%). For IV administration, suitable concentrations range from 1.5% (isotonic) to 8.4% (undiluted), depending on the clinical condition and requirements of the patient. Suitable dilution can be calculated from the following formula:

$$conc_1 \times volume_1 = conc_2 \times volume_2$$

Thus, 8.4% × 50 mL = 1.5% × 280 mL; or 7.5% × 50 mL = 1.5% × 250 mL; or 4.2% × 10 mL = 1.5% × 28 mL.

The diluent may be Sterile Water for Injection, Sodium Chloride Injection, 5% Dextrose or other standard electrolyte solutions. For SC administration, an isotonic solution (1.5%) of sodium bicarbonate can be prepared by diluting 1 mL (84 mg) of 8.4% solution with 4.6 mL Sterile Water for Injection. For 7.5% solution, dilute 1 mL (75 mg) with 4 mL Sterile Water for Injection. For 4.2% solution, dilute 1 mL (42 mg) with 1.8 mL Sterile Water for Injection.

Electrolytes

SODIUM BICARBONATE

►*Cardiac arrest:* Bicarbonate administration in this situation may be detrimental. See Indications. Administer according to results of arterial blood pH and $PaCO_2$ and calculation of base deficit. Flush IV lines before and after use.

Adults – A rapid IV dose of 200 to 300 mEq of bicarbonate, given as a 7.5% or 8.4% solution. Observe caution where rapid infusion of large quantities of bicarbonate is indicated. Bicarbonate solutions are hypertonic and may produce an undesirable rise in plasma sodium concentration. In cardiac arrest, however, the risks from acidosis exceed those of hypernatremia.

In emergencies, administer 300 to 500 mL of 5% sodium bicarbonate injection as rapidly as possible without overalkalinizing the patient. To avoid overalkalinizing a patient whose own body mechanisms for correcting metabolic acidosis may be maximally stimulated, only one-third to one-half of the calculated dose is administered as rapidly as indicated by the patient's cardiovascular and fluid balance status. Then, redetermine serum pH and bicarbonate concentration.

Infants (≤ 2 years of age) – 4.2% solution for IV administration at a rate not to exceed 8 mEq/kg/day to guard against the possibility of producing hypernatremia, decreasing CSF pressure and inducing intracranial hemorrhage.

Initial dose – 1 to 2 mEq/kg/min given over 1 to 2 minutes followed by 1 mEq/kg every 10 minutes of arrest. If base deficit is known, give calculated dose of $0.3 \times kg \times$ base deficit. If only 7.5% or 8.4% sodium bicarbonate is available, dilute 1:1 with 5% Dextrose in Water before administration.

►*Severe metabolic acidosis:* Administer 90 to 180 mEq/L (≈ 7.5 to 15 g) at a rate of 1 to 1.5 L during the first hour. Adjust to patient's needs for further management.

►*Less urgent forms of metabolic acidosis:* Sodium Bicarbonate Injection may be added to other IV fluids. The amount of bicarbonate to be given to older children and adults over a 4 to 8 hour period is approximately 2 to 5 mEq/kg, depending on the severity of the acidosis as judged by the lowering of total CO_2 content, blood pH and clinical condition. Initially, an infusion of 2 to 5 mEq/kg over 4 to 8 hours will produce improvement in the acid-base status of the blood.

Alternatively, estimates of the initial dose of sodium bicarbonate may be based on the following equation:

0.5 (L/kg) × body weight (kg) × desired increase in serum HCO_3^- (mEq/L) = bicarbonate dose (mEq) or 0.5 (L/kg) × body weight (kg) × base deficit (mEq/L) = bicarbonate dose (mEq).

The next step of therapy is dependent on the clinical response of the patient. If severe symptoms have abated, reduce frequency of administration and dose.

If the CO_2 plasma content is unknown, a safe average dose of sodium bicarbonate is 5 mEq (420 mg)/kg.

It is unwise to attempt full correction of a low total CO_2 content during the first 24 hours, since this may accompany an unrecognized alkalosis due to delayed readjustment of ventilation to normal. Thus, achieving total CO_2 content of about 20 mEq/L at the end of the first day will usually be associated with a normal blood pH. Further modification of the acidosis to completely normal values usually occurs in the presence of normal kidney function when and if the cause of the acidosis can be controlled. Total CO_2 brought to normal or above normal within the first day may be associated with grossly alkaline blood pH.

If administration is controlled by a pumping device, discontinue pumping action before the container runs dry or air embolism may result.

►*Neutralizing additive solution:* One vial of neutralizing additive solution added to 1 L of any of the commonly used parenteral solutions including Dextrose, Sodium Chloride, Ringer's, etc, will increase the pH to a more physiologic range (specific pH may vary slightly).

Note – Some products such as amino acid solutions and multiple electrolyte solutions containing dextrose will not be brought to near physiologic pH by the addition of sodium bicarbonate neutralizing additive solution. This is due to the relatively high buffer capacity of these fluids.

►*Admixture incompatibilities:* Avoid adding sodium bicarbonate to parenteral solutions containing **calcium**, except where compatibility is established; precipitation or haze may result. **Norepinephrine** and **dobutamine** are incompatible.

►*Storage / Stability:* Store at 15° to 30°C (59° to 86°F). Avoid excessive heat. Protect from freezing. Brief exposure up to 40°C does not adversely affect the product. Replace administration apparatus at least once every 24 hours.

Actions

►*Pharmacology:* Increases plasma bicarbonate; buffers excess hydrogen ion concentration; raises blood pH; reverses the clinical manifestations of acidosis.

One g sodium bicarbonate provides 11.9 mEq each of sodium and bicarbonate.

►*Pharmacokinetics:* Sodium bicarbonate in water dissociates to provide sodium (Na^+) and bicarbonate (HCO_3^-) ions. Sodium is the principal cation of extracellular fluid. Bicarbonate is a normal constituent of body fluids and normal plasma level ranges from 24 to 31 mEq/L. Plasma concentration is regulated by the kidney. Bicarbonate anion is considered "labile" since, at a proper concentration of hydrogen ion (H^+), it may be converted to carbonic acid (H_2CO_3), then to its volatile form, carbon dioxide (CO_2), excreted by lungs. Normally, a ratio of 1:20 (carbonic acid: bicarbonate) is present in extracellular fluid. In a healthy adult with normal kidney function, almost all the glomerular filtered bicarbonate ion is reabsorbed; < 1% is excreted in urine.

Contraindications

Losing chloride by vomiting or from continuous GI suction; receiving diuretics known to produce a hypochloremic alkalosis; metabolic and respiratory alkalosis; hypocalcemia in which alkalosis may produce tetany, hypertension, convulsions or congestive heart failure (CHF); when sodium use could be clinically detrimental.

►*Neutralizing additive solution:* Do not use as a systemic alkalinizer.

Warnings

►*Cardiac effects:*

Cardiac arrest – The risk of rapid infusion must be weighed against the potential for fatality due to acidosis.

CHF – Since sodium accompanies bicarbonate, use cautiously in patients with CHF or other edematous or sodium-retaining states.

►*Fluid / Solute overload:* IV administration can cause fluid or solute overloading resulting in dilution of serum electrolyte concentrations, overhydration, congested states or pulmonary edema. The risk of dilutional states is inversely proportional to the electrolyte concentrations of administered parenteral solutions. The risk of solute overload causing congested states with peripheral and acute pulmonary edema is directly proportional to the electrolyte concentrations of such solutions. Rapid or excessive administration of Sodium Bicarbonate Injection may produce tetany due to a decrease in ionized calcium and hypokalemia as potassium reenters the cells. Hypertonic solutions may cause vein damage. Avoid extravasation.

►*Neonates and children (< 2 years old):* Rapid injection (10 mL/min) of hypertonic sodium bicarbonate solutions may produce hypernatremia, a decrease in cerebrospinal fluid pressure and possible intracranial hemorrhage. Do not administer > 8 mEq/kg/day. A 4.2% solution is preferred for such slow administration.

►*Renal function impairment:* Administration of solutions containing sodium ions may result in sodium retention. Use with caution. Also use cautiously in oliguria or anuria.

►*Elderly:* Exercise particular care when administering sodium-containing solutions to elderly or postoperative patients with renal or cardiovascular insufficiency, with or without CHF.

►*Pregnancy: Category C.* It is not known whether sodium bicarbonate can cause fetal harm when administered to a pregnant woman. Use only if clearly needed.

►*Lactation:* It is not known whether this drug is excreted in breast milk. Exercise caution when administering to a nursing woman.

Precautions

►*Monitoring:* Adverse reactions may result from an excess or deficit of one or more of the ions in the solution; frequent monitoring of electrolyte levels is essential.

►*Avoid overdosage and alkalosis:* Avoid overdosage and alkalosis by giving repeated small doses and periodic monitoring by appropriate laboratory tests.

►*Potassium depletion:* Potassium depletion may predispose to metabolic alkalosis, and coexistent hypocalcemia may be associated with carpopedal spasm as the plasma pH rises. Minimize by treating electrolyte imbalances prior to or concomitantly with bicarbonate.

►*Chloride loss:* Patients losing chloride by vomiting or GI intubation are more susceptible to developing severe alkalosis if given alkalinizing agents.

►*Neutralizing additive solution:* Administer this solution promptly. When introducing additives, mix thoroughly and do not store. Raising pH of IV fluids with neutralizing additive solution will only reduce incidence of chemical irritation caused by infusate; it will not diminish any foreign body effects caused by needle or catheter.

Extraordinary electrolyte losses such as may occur during protracted nasogastric suction, vomiting, diarrhea or GI fistula drainage may necessitate additional electrolyte supplementation.

Electrolytes

SODIUM BICARBONATE

Drug Interactions

Sodium Bicarbonate Drug Interactions			
Precipitant drug	Object drug*		Description
Sodium bicarbonate	Chlorpropamide Lithium Methotrexate Salicylates Tetracyclines	↓	The renal clearance of these agents may be increased due to alkalinization of the urine, possibly resulting in a decreased pharmacologic effect.
Sodium bicarbonate	Anorexiants Flecainide Mecamylamine Quinidine Sympathomimetics	↑	The renal clearance of these agents may be decreased due to alkalinizaton of the urine, possibly resulting in increased pharmacologic or toxic effects.

* ↑ = Object drug increased. ↓ = Object drug decreased.

Adverse Reactions

Symptoms – Extravasation of IV hypertonic solutions of sodium bicarbonate may cause chemical cellulitis (because of their alkalinity), with tissue necrosis, ulceration or sloughing at the site of infiltration. Prompt elevation of the part, warmth and local injection of lidocaine or hyaluronidase are recommended to prevent sloughing.

Too rapid infusion of hypertonic solutions may cause local pain and venous irritation. Adjust the rate of administration according to tolerance. Use of the largest peripheral vein and a well placed small bore needle is recommended.

Too rapid or excessive administration may result in hypernatremia and alkalosis accompanied by hyperirritability or tetany. Hypernatremia may be associated with edema and exacerbation of CHF due to the retention of water, resulting in an expanded extracellular fluid volume.

Reactions that may occur because of the solution or the technique of administration include febrile response, infection at the site of injection, venous thrombosis or phlebitis extending from the injection site, extravasation and hypervolemia.

Treatment – If an adverse reaction does occur, discontinue the infusion, evaluate the patient, institute appropriate therapeutic countermeasures and save the remainder of the fluid for examination if deemed necessary.

Overdosage

➤*Symptoms:* Excessive or too rapid administration may produce alkalosis. Severe alkalosis may be accompanied by hyperirritability or tetany.

➤*Treatment:* Discontinue sodium bicarbonate. Control symptoms of alkalosis by rebreathing expired air from a paper bag or rebreathing mask or, if more severe, by parenteral injections of calcium gluconate (to control tetany and hyperexcitability). Correct severe alkalosis by IV infusion of 2.14% ammonium chloride solution, except in patients with hepatic disease, in whom ammonia use is contraindicated. Sodium chloride (0.9%) IV or potassium chloride may be indicated if there is hypokalemia.

SODIUM LACTATE

Rx	**1/6 Molar Sodium Lactate** (Various, eg, Abbott, Baxter)	**Injection:** 167 mEq/L each of sodium and lactate ions	In 500 and 1000 mL.

Complete prescribing information for these products begins in the Sodium Bicarbonate monograph.

Indications

As an alkalinizing agent for the treatment of metabolic acidosis resulting from starvation, acute infections, diabetic acidosis, diarrhea and vomiting, or renal failure.

Actions

➤*Pharmacology:* One liter of Molar sodium lactate (isotonic) administered IV is potentially equivalent in alkalinizing effect to approximately 280 mL of 5% sodium bicarbonate. One g of sodium lactate provides 8.9 mEq of sodium and of lactate.

➤*Pharmacokinetics:* Sodium lactate is metabolized to bicarbonate in the liver. The alkalinizing effects of sodium lactate result from simultaneous removal of lactate and hydrogen ions. Lactate is metabolized to glycogen and ultimately converted to carbon dioxide and water in the liver. The conversion of sodium lactate to bicarbonate requires 1 to 2 hours.

Warnings

➤*Hepatic function impairment/severe illness:* Conversion of lactate to bicarbonate may be impaired in the severely ill and in persons with hepatic disease.

➤*Severe acidosis:* Not intended nor effective for correcting severe acidotic states that require immediate restoration of plasma bicarbonate levels. Sodium lactate has no advantage over sodium bicarbonate and may be detrimental in the management of lactic acidosis.

SODIUM ACETATE

Rx	**Sodium Acetate** (Various, eg, Abbott, American Regent)	**Injection:** 2 mEq each of sodium and acetate per mL (16.4%)	In 20, 50 and 100 mL vials.
Rx	**Sodium Acetate** (Various, eg, American Regent)	**Injection:** 4 mEq each of sodium and acetate per mL (32.8%)	In 50 and 100 mL vials.

Complete prescribing information for these products begins in the Sodium Bicarbonate monograph.

Indications

Useful in acidotic states. Used as a source of sodium in large volume IV fluids to prevent or correct hyponatremia in patients with restricted intake. Useful for preparing IV fluid formulas when patient needs cannot be met by standard electrolyte or nutrient solutions.

Actions

➤*Pharmacology:* The acetate ion is metabolized to bicarbonate almost on an equimolar basis. Metabolism occurs outside the liver. One g of sodium acetate provides 7.3 mEq of sodium and of acetate.

AMMONIUM CHLORIDE

Rx	**Ammonium Chloride** (Abbott)	**Injection:** 26.75% (5 mEq/mL) To be diluted before infusion	In 20 mL (100 mEq) vials.[1]

[1] With 2 mg EDTA.

Indications

Treatment of hypochloremic states and metabolic alkalosis.

Administration and Dosage

Administer by slow IV infusion.

Dosage depends on the patient's condition and tolerance. Add the contents of one to two vials (100 to 200 mEq) to 500 or 1000 mL isotonic (0.9%) Sodium Chloride Injection. Do not exceed a concentration of 1% to 2% ammonium chloride or an administration rate of 5 mL/min in adults (≈ 3 hours for infusion of 1000 mL). Monitor dosage by repeated serum bicarbonate determinations.

➤*Storage/Stability:* Avoid excessive heat; protect from freezing. When exposed to low temperatures, concentrated solutions may crystallize. If crystals form, warm the solution to room temperature in a water bath prior to use.

Actions

➤*Pharmacology:* When loss of hydrogen and chloride ions occurs, serum bicarbonate and pH rise and serum potassium falls. The ammonium ion is converted into urea in the liver. The liberated hydrogen and chloride ions in blood and extracellular fluid result in decreased pH and corrected alkalosis. Ammonium chloride also lowers urinary pH which increases the excretion rate of basic drugs (eg, amphetamines, quinidine).

One gram of ammonium chloride provides 18.7 mEq of chloride.

Contraindications

Renal function impairment; hepatic function impairment (see Warnings); metabolic alkalosis due to vomiting of hydrochloric acid when it is accompanied by loss of sodium (excretion of sodium bicarbonate in the urine).

AMMONIUM CHLORIDE

Warnings

➤*Hepatic function impairment, severe (as occurs in uremia, cirrhosis or hepatitis):* The liver may fail to convert the ammonia to urea. This may result in marked ammonia retention with intoxication and hepatic coma.

➤*Pregnancy: Category C.* It is not known whether this drug can cause fetal harm when administered to a pregnant woman or affect reproductive capacity. Use only if clearly needed.

Precautions

➤*Ammonium toxicity:* Observe patients receiving ammonium chloride for symptoms of ammonia toxicity (eg, pallor, sweating, irregular breathing, retching, bradycardia, cardiac arrhythmias, local and general twitching, tonic convulsions, coma).

➤*Use with caution:* Use caution in primary respiratory acidosis, and high total CO_2 and buffer base.

➤*Administer slowly:* Administer slowly IV to avoid pain, toxic effects and local irritation at the venipuncture site and along the course of the vein.

Adverse Reactions

Serious metabolic acidosis (see Overdosage).

Rapid IV administration may cause pain or irritation at the injection site or along the vein.

Reactions which may occur because of solution or administration technique include: Febrile response; injection site infection; venous thrombosis or phlebitis extending from injection site; extravasation; hypervolemia (from large volume diluent).

Overdosage

➤*Symptoms:* Serious degree of metabolic acidosis; confusion; disorientation; coma.

➤*Treatment:*

Acidosis – Administer sodium bicarbonate or sodium lactate.

Trace Metals

Refer to the Trace Elements section for information on oral iodine, manganese, and zinc. Iodine is used as a thyroid agent (see monograph in Thyroid Drugs section) and as an expectorant (see monograph in Respiratory Drugs chapter).

Indications

Supplement to IV solutions given for TPN.

Administration and Dosage

Administer IV after dilution. Frequently monitor plasma levels and clinical status.

➤*Preparation:* Trace metals are usually physically compatible together, and with the electrolytes usually present in amino acid/dextrose solution used for TPN.

Actions

➤*Pharmacology:*

Chromium – Trivalent chromium is part of glucose tolerance factor, an essential activator of insulin-mediated reactions. Chromium helps maintain normal glucose metabolism and peripheral nerve function.

Serum chromium is bound to transferrin (siderophilin). Administration of chromium supplements to chromium deficient patients can result in normalization of the glucose tolerance curve from the diabetic-like curve typical of chromium deficiency. This response is viewed as a more meaningful indicator than serum chromium levels.

Copper – Copper serves as a cofactor for serum ceruloplasmin, an oxidase necessary for proper formation of the iron carrier protein, transferrin. Copper also helps maintain normal rates of red and white blood cell formation. The daily turnover of copper through ceruloplasmin is approximately 0.5 mg.

Iodine – Absorption from the GI tract is rapid and complete. Skin and lungs can also absorb iodine. On administration, iodide equilibrates in extracellular fluids and although all body cells contain iodide, it is specifically concentrated by the thyroid gland, which is estimated to contain 7 to 8 mg total iodine.

Other important organs to take up iodide are salivary glands, gastric mucosa, choroid plexus, skin, hair, mammary glands and placenta.

Iodine in saliva and gastric mucosal secretions is reabsorbed and recycled. The circulating iodine is hormonal thyroxine of which 30 to 70 mcg is protein bound and 0.5 mcg is free thyroxine.

Manganese – Manganese serves as an activator for several enzymes. During minimal intake, 20 mcg/day is retained. Manganese is bound to a specific transport protein, transmanganin, and is widely distributed, but it concentrates in mitochondria-rich tissues such as brain, kidney, pancreas and liver.

Molybdenum – Molybdenum is a constituent of the enzymes xanthine oxidase, sulfite oxidase and aldehyde oxidase. Tissue storage of molybdenum varies with the intake levels and is affected by the amount of copper and sulfate in the diet. Consistent levels are observed in liver, kidney and adrenal cortex.

Selenium – Selenium is part of glutathione peroxidase which protects cell components from oxidative damage due to peroxides produced in cellular metabolism.

Pediatric conditions, Keshan disease and Kwashiorkor have been associated with low dietary intake of selenium. The conditions are endemic to geographic areas with low selenium soil content. Dietary supplementation with selenium salts reduces the incidence of the conditions among affected children.

Zinc – Zinc serves as a cofactor for > 70 different enzymes. Zinc facilitates wound healing, helps maintain normal growth rates, normal skin hydration and the senses of taste and smell. Zinc resides in muscle, bone, skin, kidney, liver, pancreas, retina, prostate and particularly in the red and white blood cells. Zinc binds to plasma albumin, α_2-macroglobulin and some plasma amino acids including histidine, cysteine, threonine, glycine and asparagine.

At plasma levels < 20 mcg/dL, dermatitis followed by alopecia has been reported for TPN patients.

The following table summarizes deficiency symptoms, excretion routes and normal plasma levels for various trace metals. The serum level at which deficiency symptoms appear for many of these elements is not well defined.

Trace Metals: Deficiency/Excretion/Plasma Levels

Trace metal	Symptoms of deficiency	Excretion	Normal plasma levels
Copper	Leukopenia, neutropenia, anemia, decreased ceruloplasmin levels, impaired transferrin formation of secondary iron deficiency, skeletal abnormalities, defective tissue formation.	Bile (80%), intestinal wall (16%), urine (4%)	80-163 mcg/dL
Chromium	Impaired glucose tolerance, peripheral neuropathy, ataxia, confusion.	Kidneys (3-50 mcg/day), bile	1-5 mcg/L[a]
Iodine	Impaired thyroid function, goiter, cretinism.	Kidneys, bile	0.5-1.5 mcg/dL
Manganese	Nausea, vomiting, weight loss, dermatitis, changes in growth and hair color.	Bile; if obstruction present, then pancreatic juice or return to intestinal lumen. Urine (negligible)	6-12 mcg/L (whole blood)
Molybdenum	Tachycardia, tachypnea, headache, night blindness, nausea, vomiting, central scotomas, edema, lethargy, disorientation, coma, hypermethioninemia, hypouricemia, hypouricuria, low urinary excretion of inorganic sulfate and elevated urinary excretion of thiosulfate.	Primarily renal, some biliary	nd
Selenium	Muscle pain & tenderness, cardiomyopathy, Kwashiorkor, Keshan disease.	Urine, feces, lungs, skin	nd
Zinc	Diarrhea, apathy, depression, parakeratosis, hypogeusia, anorexia, dysosmia, geophagia, hypogonadism, growth retardation, anemia, hepatosplenomegaly, impaired wound healing.	90% in stools; urine, perspiration	100 ± 12 mcg/dL

[a] Not considered a meaningful index of tissue stores.

nd = No data

Contraindications

Do not give undiluted by direct injection into a peripheral vein because of the potential for infusion phlebitis, tissue irritation and potential to increase renal loss of minerals from a bolus injection.

➤*Molybdenum without copper supplement:* Copper-deficient patients. See Warnings.

Warnings

➤*Renal failure or biliary tract obstruction:* Metals may accumulate. Serial determinations of serum trace metal concentrations may be a valuable guideline.

Consider the possibility of **copper** and **manganese** retention in patients with biliary tract obstruction. Ancillary routes of manganese excretion include pancreatic secretions or reabsorption into the lumen of the duodenum, jejunum or ileum.

Adjust, reduce or omit use in renal dysfunction or GI malfunction. Consider contributions from blood transfusions. Frequently determine plasma levels.

➤*Wilson's disease:* Avoid administering **copper** supplements to patients with this genetic disorder of copper metabolism.

➤*Decreased serum levels:* Administration of **copper** in the absence of **zinc** and of zinc in the absence of copper may cause decreases in plasma levels. Perform periodic determinations of plasma zinc and copper for subsequent administrations.

➤*Copper deficiency:* **Molybdenum** promotes tissue **copper** mobilization and increases urinary copper excretion; excessive amounts produce a copper deficiency. Frequently check the metabolism of copper in patients receiving molybdenum.

➤*Multiple trace element solutions:* Multiple trace element solutions present a risk of overdosage when the need for one trace element is appreciably higher than that for the other trace elements in the formulation. Administration of trace metals as separate entities may be required.

➤*Hypersensitivity reactions:* Sensitization to **iodides** and deaths due to anaphylactic shock after use have occurred (see Adverse Reactions). Evaluate patient for hypersensitivity before initiating TPN. If patient develops a reaction, withdraw TPN immediately and institute appropriate measures. Refer to Management of Acute Hypersensitivity.

➤*Pregnancy: Category C.* It is not known whether trace metals can cause fetal harm or can affect reproductive capacity. Give to a pregnant woman only if clearly needed.

Molybdenum crosses the placenta. Presence of **selenium** in placenta and umbilical cord blood has been reported.

Precautions

➤*Replacement trace metal therapy:* Replacement trace metal therapy beyond maintenance requirements may be necessary in protracted vomiting or diarrhea, in patients with fistula drainage or nasogastric suction or in acute catabolic states.

➤*Diabetes mellitus:* In assessing the contribution of chromium supplements to maintenance of glucose homeostasis, consider that the patient may be diabetic.

➤*Iodine:* Iodine is readily absorbed through skin, lungs and mucous membranes. Give consideration to the environment, topical skin disinfection and wound treatment practices with surgical swabs and solutions containing iodine and povidone iodine. Air in the coastal areas is known to contain more iodine than inland areas.

➤*Benzyl alcohol:* Some of these products contain benzyl alcohol, which has been associated with a fatal gasping syndrome in premature infants.

Adverse Reactions

Symptoms of toxicity are unlikely to occur at recommended doses.

Hypersensitivity to **iodides** may result in angioneurotic edema, cutaneous and mucosal hemorrhages, fever, arthralgia, lymph node enlargement and eosinophilia. (See Warnings.)

Overdosage

➤*Chromium:* Nausea, vomiting, GI ulcers, renal/hepatic damage, convulsions, coma.

➤*Copper:* Prostration, behavior change, diarrhea, progressive marasmus, hypotonia, photophobia, hepatic damage and peripheral edema have occurred with a serum copper level of 286 mcg/dL. Penicillamine is an effective antidote.

➤*Iodine:* Symptoms of chronic poisoning include metallic taste, sore mouth, increased salivation, coryza, sneezing, swelling of the eyelids, severe headache, pulmonary edema, tenderness of salivary glands, acneiform skin lesions and skin eruptions. Abundant fluid and salt intake helps in elimination of iodides.

➤*Manganese:* "Manganese madness," irritability, speech disturbances, abnormal gait, headache, anorexia, apathy and impotence.

➤*Molybdenum:* Gout-like syndrome with increased blood levels of molybdenum, uric acid and xanthine oxidase.

No data on treatment of molybdenosis in humans is available. Among animals, treatment with copper, sulfate ions and tungsten enhances excretion of molybdenum. The sulfur-containing amino acids, methionine and cysteine, may afford limited protection.

➤*Selenium:* Toxicity symptoms include hair loss, weak nails, dermatitis, dental defects, GI disorders, nervousness, mental depression, metallic taste, vomiting and garlic odor of breath and sweat. Acute poisoning due to ingestion has resulted in death with histopathological changes including fulminating peripheral vascular collapse, internal vascular congestion, diffusely hemorrhagic, congested and edematous lungs and brick-red color gastric mucosa. Death was preceded by coma. No effective antidote is known.

➤*Zinc:* Single IV doses of 1 to 2 mg/kg have been given to adult leukemic patients without toxic manifestations. However, acute toxicity was reported in an adult when 10 mg zinc was infused over 1 hour on each of 4 consecutive days. Profuse sweating, decreased consciousness, blurred vision, tachycardia (140/min) and marked hypothermia (94.2°F) on the fourth day were accompanied by a serum zinc concentration of 207 mcg/dL. Symptoms abated within 3 hours.

Patients receiving an inadvertent overdose (50 to 70 mg zinc/day) developed hyperamylasemia (557 to 1850 Klein units; normal, 130 to 310).

Death resulted from 1683 mg zinc IV over 60 hours to a 72-year-old patient. Symptoms included hypotension (80/40 mm Hg), pulmonary edema, diarrhea, vomiting, jaundice and oliguria with a serum zinc level of 4184 mcg/dL.

Calcium supplements may confer a protective effect against zinc toxicity.

ZINC

Rx	**Zinc Sulfate** (Various, eg, American Regent, Loch)	**Injection:** 1 mg/mL (as sulfate [as 4.39 mg heptahydrate or 2.46 mg anhydrous])	In 10 and 30 mL vials.
Rx	**Zinca-Pak** (Smith & Nephew SoloPak)		In 10 and 30[1] mL vials.
Rx	**Zinc Sulfate** (Various, eg, Loch)	**Injection:** 5 mg/mL (as 21.95 mg sulfate)	In 5 and 10 mL vials.
Rx	**Zinca-Pak** (Smith & Nephew SoloPak)		In 5 mL vials.
Rx	**Zinc** (Various, eg, Abbott)	**Injection:** 1 mg/mL (as 2.09 mg chloride)	In 10 mL vials.

[1] With 0.9% benzyl alcohol.

Complete prescribing information begins in the Trace Metals group monograph.

Administration and Dosage

➤*Metabolically stable adults:* 2.5 to 4 mg/day. Add 2 mg/day for acute catabolic states.

➤*Stable adults with fluid loss from the small bowel:* Give an additional 12.2 mg zinc per L of TPN solution, or an additional 17.1 mg per kg of stool or ileostomy output.

➤*Full-term infants and children (≤ 5 years of age):* 100 mcg/kg/day.

➤*Premature infants (birth weight < 1500 g and up to 3 kg):* 300 mcg/kg/day.

COPPER

Rx	**Copper** (Abbott)	**Injection:** 0.4 mg/mL (as 1.07 mg cupric Cl)	In 10 mL vials.
Rx	**Cupric Sulfate** (Various, eg, American Regent, Loch)	**Injection:** 0.4 mg/mL (as 1.57 mg sulfate)	In 10 and 30 mL vials.
Rx	**Cupric Sulfate** (Various, eg, Loch)	**Injection:** 2 mg/mL (as 7.85 mg sulfate)	In 10 mL vials.

Complete prescribing information begins in the Trace Metals group monograph.

Administration and Dosage

➤*Adults:* 0.5 to 1.5 mg/day.

➤*Children:* 20 mcg/kg/day.

MANGANESE

Rx	**Manganese Chloride** (Various, eg, Abbott)	**Injection:** 0.1 mg/mL (as 0.36 mg manganese chloride)	In 10 mL vials.
Rx	**Manganese Sulfate** (Various, eg, American Regent)	**Injection:** 0.1 mg/mL (as 0.31 mg sulfate)	In 10 and 30 mL vials.

Complete prescribing information begins in the Trace Metals group monograph.

Administration and Dosage

➤*Adults:* 0.15 to 0.8 mg/day.

➤*Children:* 2 to 10 mcg/kg/day.

Trace Metals

MOLYBDENUM

Rx	**Ammonium Molybdate** (Various, eg, American Regent)	**Injection:** 25 mcg/mL (as 46 mcg/mL ammonium molybdate tetrahydrate)	In 10 mL vials.
Rx	**Molypen** (American Pharmaceutical Partners)		In 10 mL vials.

Complete prescribing information for these products begins in the Trace Metals group monograph.

➤*Deficiency state resulting from prolonged TPN support:* 163 mcg/day for 21 days reverses deficiency symptoms without toxicity.

Administration and Dosage

➤*Metabolically stable adults:* 20 to 120 mcg/day. For pediatric patients, calculate the additive dosage level by extrapolation.

CHROMIUM

Rx	**Chromium** (Various, eg, Abbott, McGuff)	**Injection:** 4 mcg/mL (as 20.5 mcg chromic chloride hexahydrate)	In 10 and 30 mL vials.
Rx	**Chromic Chloride** (Various)		In 10 and 30[1] mL vials.
Rx	**Chromium Chloride** (Various, eg, American Regent, Raway)		In 10 and 30 mL vials.
Rx	**Chroma-Pak** (Smith & Nephew SoloPak)		In 10 and 30[1] mL vials.
Rx	**Chromic Chloride** (Various)	**Injection:** 20 mcg/mL (as 102.5 mcg chromic chloride hexahydrate)	In 10 mL vials.
Rx	**Chroma-Pak** (Smith & Nephew SoloPak)		In 5 mL vials.

[1] With 0.9% benzyl alcohol.

Complete prescribing information for these products begins in the Trace Metals group monograph.

➤*Metabolically stable adults with intestinal fluid loss:* 20 mcg/day.

➤*Children:* 0.14 to 0.2 mcg/kg/day.

Administration and Dosage

➤*Adults:* 10 to 15 mcg/day.

SELENIUM

Rx	**Selenium** (Various, eg, American Regent)	**Injection:** 40 mcg/mL (as 65.4 mcg selenious acid)	In 10 mL vials.
Rx	**Sele-Pak** (Smith & Nephew SoloPak)		In 10 and 30[1] mL vials.
Rx	**Selepen** (American Pharmaceutical Partners)		In 10 and 30[1] mL vials.

[1] With 0.9% benzyl alcohol.

Complete prescribing information for these products begins in the Trace Metals group monograph.

100 mcg/day for 24 and 31 days, respectively, reverses deficiency symptoms without toxicity.

➤*Children:* 3 mcg/kg/day.

Administration and Dosage

➤*Metabolically stable adults:* 20 to 40 mcg/day.

➤*Deficiency state resulting from prolonged TPN support:*

IODINE

Rx	**Iodopen** (American Pharmaceutical Partners)	**Injection:** 100 mcg/mL (as 118 mcg sodium iodide)	In 10 mL vials.

Complete prescribing information for these products begins in the Trace Metals group monograph.

➤*Pregnant and lactating women, growing children:* 2 to 3 mcg/kg/day.

Administration and Dosage

➤*Metabolically stable adults:* 1 to 2 mcg/kg/day (normal adults, 75 to 150 mcg/day).

TRACE METAL COMBINATIONS

Content given per mL solution.

	Product and Distributor	Chromium (as chloride) mcg	Copper (as sulfate) mg	Iodine (as sodium iodine) mcg	Manganese (as sulfate) mg	Selenium (as selenious acid) mcg	Zinc (as sulfate) mg	How Supplied
Rx	**Pedtrace-4** (Fujisawa)	0.85	0.1		0.025		0.5	In 3 and 10 mL vials.
Rx	**Multiple Trace Element Neonatal** (American Regent)	0.85	0.1		0.025		1.5	In 2 mL vials.
Rx	**Neotrace-4** (Fujisawa)							In 2 mL vials.
Rx	**PedTE-PAK-4** (SoloPak)	1	0.1		0.025		1	In 3 mL vials.
Rx	**P.T.E.-4** (Fujisawa)							In 3 mL vials.
Rx	**Trace Metals Additive in 0.9% NaCl** (Abbott)	6	0.42[1]		0.37[1]		1.67[1]	In 5, 10, 50 mL vials, 5 mL syringes.
Rx	**M.T.E.-4** (Fujisawa)	4	0.4		0.1		1	In 3, 10 and 30[2] mL vials.
Rx	**MulTE-PAK-4** (SoloPak)							In 3, 10 and 30 mL vials.
Rx	**M.T.E.-4 Concentrated** (Fujisawa)	10	1		0.5		5	In 1 and 10[2] mL vials.
Rx	**PTE-5** (Fujisawa)	1	0.1		0.025	15	1	In 3 and 10 mL vials.
Rx	**M.T.E.-5** (Fujisawa)	4	0.4		0.1	20	1	In 10 mL vials.
Rx	**MulTE-PAK-5** (SoloPak)							In 3 and 10 mL vials.
Rx	**Multiple Trace Element with Selenium** (American Regent)							In 3, 10 and 30[2] mL vials.
Rx	**M.T.E.-5 Concentrated** (Fujisawa)	10	1		0.5	60	5	In 1 and 10[2] mL vials.
Rx	**Multiple Trace Element with Selenium Concentrated** (American Regent)							In 1 mL fill in 2 mL vials and 10[2] mL vials.
Rx	**Multitrace-5 Concentrate** (American Regent)							In 1 mL single-dose and 10 mL multiple-dose vials.[2]
Rx	**M.T.E.-6** (Fujisawa)	4	0.4	25	0.1	20	1	In 10 mL vials.
Rx	**M.T.E.-7**[3] (Fujisawa)							In 10 mL vials.
Rx	**M.T.E.-6 Concentrated** (Fujisawa)	10	1	75	0.5	60	5	In 1 and 10[2] mL vials.

[1] As chloride.
[2] With 0.9% benzyl alcohol.

[3] With 25 mcg molybdenum.

Complete prescribing information begins in the Trace Metals group monograph.

Therapeutic supplements to provide replacement for extraordinary losses of individual trace metals may be added.

Administration and Dosage

See manufacturers' product labeling for individual dosing information.

COMBINED ELECTROLYTE SOLUTIONS
Electrolyte content given in mEq/L.

	Product and distributor	Na⁺	K⁺	Ca⁺⁺	Mg⁺⁺	Cl⁻	Lactate	Acetate	Gluconate	Phosphate	Osmolarity (mOsm/L)	How supplied
Rx	**Normosol-M**[1] (Abbott)	40	13		3	40		16			109	In 1000 mL single-dose container.
Rx	**Ringer's Injection** (Various, eg, Abbott, Baxter, B. Braun)	≈ 147	4	≈ 4		≈ 156					≈ 310	In 500 and 1000 mL.
Rx	**Lactated Ringer's Injection** (Various, eg, Abbott, Baxter, B. Braun)	130	4	≈ 3		≈ 109	28				≈ 274	In 250, 500, and 1000 mL.
Rx	**Plasma-Lyte R**[2] (Baxter)	140	10	5	3	103	8	47			312	In 1000 mL.
Rx	**Isolyte S pH 7.4** (B. Braun)	141	5		3	98		27	23	1	295	Preservative free. In 500 and 1000 mL.
Rx	**Normosol-R**[3] (Abbott)	140	5		3	98		27	23		294	Preservative free. In 500 and 1000 mL single-dose containers.
Rx	**Normosol-R pH 7.4** (Abbott)										295	Preservative free. In 500 and 1000 mL single-dose containers.
Rx	**Plasma-Lyte 148**[2] (Baxter)										294	In 500 and 1000 mL.
Rx	**Plasma-Lyte A pH 7.4** (Baxter)										294	In 500 and 1000 mL.
Rx	**Potassium Chloride in 0.9% Sodium Chloride Injection** (Various, eg, Baxter, B. Braun)	154	20			174					≈ 350	In 1000 mL.
		154	40			194					≈ 390	In 1000 mL.

[1] pH ≈ 6.
[2] pH ≈ 5.5.
[3] pH ≈ 6.6.

Indications

For use in adults and children as a source of electrolytes and water for hydration. Additives to the solutions may help prevent certain electrolyte deficiencies in patients receiving prolonged parenteral fluid therapy (eg, magnesium) or act as alkalinizing agents.

Normosol-R and *Normosol R pH 7.4* are indicated for replacement of acute extracellular fluid volume losses in surgery, trauma, burns, or shock. Both can be used as adjunctive therapy to restore decreased circulatory volume in patients with moderate blood loss. *Normosol-R pH 7.4* also is indicated for use in starting blood (eg, as a priming solution for infusion sets) or as a diluent in packed red blood cell transfusions.

COMBINED ELECTROLYTE CONCENTRATES
Electrolyte content given in mEq/20 mL or mEq/25 mL after dilution.

	Product and distributor	Na⁺	K⁺	Ca⁺⁺	Mg⁺⁺	Cl⁻	Acetate	Gluconate	Osmolarity (mOsm/L)	How supplied
Rx	**Lypholyte**[1] (American Pharmaceutical Partners)	25	≈ 40	5	8	≈ 33	≈ 41	5	≈ 7562	In 20 and 40 mL single-dose vials, and 100 and 200 mL *Maxivials*.[2]
Rx	**Multilyte-40**[3] (American Pharmaceutical Partners)								≈ 6015	In 25 mL single-dose vials.
Rx	**Nutrilyte**[1] (American Regent)								≈ 7562	In 20 mL single-dose vials and 100 mL.[2]
Rx	**Lypholyte-II**[1] (American Pharmaceutical Partners)	35	20	4.5	5	35	29.5		≈ 6200	In 20 and 40 mL single-dose vials and 100 and 200 mL *Maxivials*[2].
Rx	**TPN Electrolytes**[1] (Abbott)	35	20	4.5	5	35	29.5		6220	In 100 mL vials.[2]
Rx	**Nutrilyte II**[1] (American Regent)	35	20	4.5	5	35	29.5		≈ 6212	In 20 mL single-dose vials and 100 mL vials.[2]
Rx	**TPN Electrolytes II**[1] (Abbott)	18	18	4.5	5	35	10.5		4320	In 20 mL single-dose and additive syringes.
Rx	**TPN Electrolytes III**[1] (Abbott)	25	40.6	5	8	33.5	40.6	5	7520	In 100 mL vials.[2]
Rx	**Hyperlyte CR**[1] (B. Braun)	25	20	5	5	30	30		5500	In 250 mL *Super-Vials*.[2]
Rx	**Multilyte-20**[3] (American Pharmaceutical Partners)	25	20	5	5	30	25		≈ 4205	In 25 mL single-dose vials.

[1] In mEq/20 mL.
[2] Pharmacy bulk packaging.
[3] In mEq/25 mL.

Indications

To facilitate amino acid utilization and maintain electrolyte balance in adults receiving parenteral nutritional solutions containing amino acids, dextrose, and other sources of calories administered by central or peripheral venous infusion. Also indicated for electrolyte replacement in adult parenteral therapy patients.

Administration and Dosage

These concentrated solutions are not for direct infusion. They are for prescription compounding of IV admixtures only. Dilute to appropriate strength with suitable IV fluid prior to administration. Recommended dosage is 20 mL (*Multilyte-40* and *Multilyte-20* is 25 mL) added to 1 L of amino acid/dextrose solution (TPN). Osmolarity is based on the concentrate.

DEXTROSE-ELECTROLYTE SOLUTIONS
Electrolyte content given in mEq/L.

	Product and distributor	Dextrose (g/L)	Calories (Cal/L)	Na⁺	K⁺	Ca⁺⁺	Mg⁺⁺	Cl⁻	Phosphate	Lactate	Acetate	Gluconate	Osmolarity (mOsm/L)	How supplied
Rx	**Dextrose 2.5% with 0.45% Sodium Chloride** (Various, eg, Abbott, Baxter, B. Braun)	25	85	77				77					280	In 500 and 1000 mL.
Rx	**Dextrose 3.3% and 0.3% Sodium Chloride** (B. Braun)	33	110	51				51					270	In 250, 500, and 1000 mL.
Rx	**Dextrose 5% with 0.2% Sodium Chloride** (Various, eg, Baxter, B. Braun)	50	170	34				34					≈ 320	In 250, 500, and 1000 mL.
Rx	**Dextrose 5% and 0.225% Sodium Chloride** (Abbott)	50	170	38.5				38.5					329	In 250, 500, and 1000 mL.
Rx	**Dextrose 5% with 0.3% Sodium Chloride** (Abbott)	50	170	51				51					355	In 250, 500, and 1000 mL.

DEXTROSE-ELECTROLYTE SOLUTIONS

	Product and distributor	Dextrose (g/L)	Calories (Cal/L)	Na⁺	K⁺	Ca⁺⁺	Mg⁺⁺	Cl⁻	Phosphate	Lactate	Acetate	Gluconate	Osmolarity (mOsm/L)	How supplied
Rx	**Dextrose 5% with 0.33% Sodium Chloride** (Various, eg, Baxter, B. Braun)	50	170	56				56					365	In 250, 500, and 1000 mL.
Rx	**Dextrose 5% with 0.45% Sodium Chloride** (Various, eg, Abbott, Baxter, B. Braun)	50	170	77				77					≈405	In 250, 500, and 1000 mL.
Rx	**Dextrose 5% with 0.9% Sodium Chloride** (Various, eg, Abbott, Baxter, B. Braun)	50	170	154				154					≈560	In 250, 500, and 1000 mL.
Rx	**Dextrose 10% with 0.2% Sodium Chloride** (Various, eg, B. Braun)	100	340	34				34					575	In 250 mL.
Rx	**Dextrose 10% with 0.225% Sodium Chloride** (Abbott)	100	340	38.5				38.5					582	In 250 and 500 mL.
Rx	**Dextrose 10% with 0.45% Sodium Chloride** (B. Braun)	100	340	77				77					660	In 1000 mL.
Rx	**Dextrose 10% and 0.9% Sodium Chloride** (Various, eg, Baxter, B. Braun)	100	340	154				154					813-815	In 500 and 1000 mL.
Rx	**Potassium Chloride in 5% Dextrose and Lactated Ringer's** (Baxter)	50	170	130	24	3		129		28			565	In 1000 mL.
		50	170	130	44	3		149		28			605	In 1000 mL.
Rx	**Potassium Chloride in 5% Dextrose** (Various, eg, Abbott, Baxter, B. Braun)	50	170		10			10					≈272	In 1000 mL.
		50	170		20			20					292-295	In 1000 mL.
		50	170		30			30					310-312	In 1000 mL.
		50	170		40			40					330-333	In 500 and 1000 mL.
Rx	**Potassium Chloride in 3.3% Dextrose and 0.3% Sodium Chloride** (B. Braun)	33	110	51	20			71					310	In 1000 mL.
Rx	**Potassium Chloride in 5% Dextrose and 0.2% Sodium Chloride** (Various, eg, Baxter, B. Braun)	50	170	34	10			44					≈340	In 1000 mL.
		50	170	34	20			54					≈360	In 250, 500, and 1000 mL.
		50	170	34	30			64					≈380	In 1000 mL.
		50	170	34	40			74					≈400	In 1000 mL.
Rx	**Potassium Chloride in 5% Dextrose and 0.33% Sodium Chloride** (Various, eg, Baxter, B. Braun)	50	170	56	20			76					405	In 500 and 1000 mL.
		50	170	56	30			86					425	In 1000 mL.
		50	170	56	40			96					446	In 1000 mL.
Rx	**Potassium Chloride in 5% Dextrose and 0.45% Sodium Chloride** (Various, eg, Baxter, B. Braun)	50	170	77	10			87					≈425	In 1000 mL.
		50	170	77	20			97					445-447	In 500 and 1000 mL.
		50	170	77	30			107					≈465	In 1000 mL.
		50	170	77	40			117					487-490	In 1000 mL.
Rx	**Potassium Chloride in 5% Dextrose and 0.9% Sodium Chloride** (Various, eg, Baxter, B. Braun)	50	170	154	20			174					≈600	In 1000 mL.
		50	170	154	40			194					≈640	In 1000 mL.
Rx	**Potassium Chloride in 10% Dextrose and 0.2% Sodium Chloride** (B. Braun)	100	340	34	20			54					615	In 250 mL.
Rx	**Dextrose 5% and Electrolyte No. 75** (Baxter)	50	180	40	35			48	15	20			402	In 250, 500, and 1000 mL.
Rx	**Isolyte M in 5% Dextrose** (B. Braun)	50	170	36	35			49	15		20		390	In 500 and 1000 mL
Rx	**Ringer's in 5% Dextrose** (Various, eg, Abbott, Baxter, B. Braun)	50	170	≈147	4	≈4.5		≈156					≈560	In 500 and 1000 mL.
Rx	**Half-Strength Lactated Ringer's in 2.5% Dextrose** (Various, eg, Abbott, Baxter, B. Braun)	25	85-89	≈65.5	2	≈1.5		≈55		14			≈264	In 250, 500, and 1000 mL.
Rx	**Lactated Ringer's in 5% Dextrose** (Various, eg, Abbott, Baxter, B. Braun)	50	170	130	4	≈3		109-112		28			525-530	In 250, 500, and 1000 mL.
Rx	**Dextrose 5% and Electrolyte No. 48** (Baxter)	50	180	25	20		3	24	3	23			348	In 250 mL.
Rx	**Isolyte H in 5% Dextrose** (B. Braun)	50	170	39	13		3	44			16		360	In 1000 mL.
Rx	**Normosol-M and 5% Dextrose** (Abbott)	50	170	40	13		3	40			16		363	In 500 and 1000 mL.
Rx	**Plasma-Lyte 56 and 5% Dextrose** (Baxter)													In 500 and 1000 mL.
Rx	**Isolyte P in 5% Dextrose** (B. Braun)	50	170	23	20		3	29	3		23		340	In 250, 500, and 1000 mL.
Rx	**Isolyte S with 5% Dextrose** (B. Braun)	50	170	140	5		3	106			27	23	550	In 1000 mL.
Rx	**Normosol-R and 5% Dextrose** (Abbott)	50	185	140	5		3	98			27	23	547	In 500 and 1000 mL.
Rx	**Plasma-Lyte 148 and 5% Dextrose** (Baxter)	50	190	140	5		3	98			27	23	547	In 500 and 1000 mL.
Rx	**Dextrose 10% and Electrolyte No. 48** (Baxter)	100	350	25	20		3	24	3	23			600	In 250 mL.[1]
Rx	**Isolyte R in 5% Dextrose** (B. Braun)	50	170	39	16	5	3	46			24		375	In 1000 mL.
Rx	**Plasma-Lyte M and 5% Dextrose** (Baxter)	50	180	40	16	5	3	40		12	12		377	In 500 and 1000 mL.
Rx	**Plasma-Lyte R and 5% Dextrose** (Baxter)	50	180	140	10	5	3	103		8	47		564	In 1000 mL.[1]

[1] With sodium bisulfite.

DEXTROSE-ELECTROLYTE SOLUTIONS

Indications

For use as a parenteral source of electrolytes, calories, or water for hydration, or as an alkalinizing agent.

INVERT SUGAR-ELECTROLYTE SOLUTIONS

Electrolyte content given in mEq/L.

	Product and distributor	Invert Sugar (g/L)	Calories (Cal/L)	Na+	K+	Mg++	Cl-	Phosphate	Lactate	Osmolarity (mOsm/L)	How supplied
Rx	**Multiple Electrolytes and 5% Travert** (Baxter)	50	196	56	25	6	56	12.5	25	449	In 1000 mL.[1]
Rx	**Multiple Electrolytes and 10% Travert** (Baxter)	100	384	56	25	6	56	12.5	25	726	In 1000 mL.[1]

[1] With sodium 5 mEq/L sodium bisulfite.

Refer to dextrose monograph for further information.

Indications

Used as a source of calories and hydration. Invert sugar is composed of equal parts of dextrose and fructose and shares the same actions and caloric value. Any supposed advantage of using invert sugar solutions would be from the fructose component.

Recombinant Human Erythropoietin

EPOETIN ALFA, RECOMBINANT (Erythropoietin; EPO)

Rx	**Epogen** (Amgen)	**Injection:** 2000 units/mL	In 1 mL single-dose vials.[1]
Rx	**Procrit** (Ortho Biotech)		In 1 mL single-dose vials.[1]
Rx	**Epogen** (Amgen)	**Injection:** 3000 units/mL	In 1 mL single-dose vials.[1]
Rx	**Procrit** (Ortho Biotech)		In 1 mL single-dose vials.[1]
Rx	**Epogen** (Amgen)	**Injection:** 4000 units/mL	In 1 mL single-dose vials.[1]
Rx	**Procrit** (Ortho Biotech)		In 1 mL single-dose vials.[1]
Rx	**Epogen** (Amgen)	**Injection:** 10,000 units/mL	In 1 mL single-dose vials[1] and 2 mL multidose vials.[2]
Rx	**Procrit** (Ortho Biotech)		In 1 mL single-dose vials[1] and 2 mL multidose vials.[2]
Rx	**Epogen** (Amgen)	**Injection:** 20,000 units/mL	In 1 mL multidose vials.[2]
Rx	**Procrit** (Ortho Biotech)		In 1 mL multidose vials.[2]
Rx	**Epogen** (Amgen)	**Injection:** 40,000 units/mL	In 1 mL single-dose vials.[1]
Rx	**Procrit** (Ortho Biotech)		In 1 mL single-dose vials.[1]

[1] Preservative free with 2.5 mg albumin (human) per mL.

[2] Preserved with 1% benzyl alcohol. With 2.5 mg albumin (human) per mL.

Indications

▶*Treatment of anemia associated with chronic renal failure (CRF):* Including adults and children 1 month of age and older on dialysis (end-stage renal disease) and adults not on dialysis, to elevate or maintain the red blood cell level (as manifested by the hematocrit or hemoglobin determinations) and to decrease the need for transfusions. Nondialysis patients with symptomatic anemia considered for therapy should have a hematocrit less than 30%. Not intended for patients who require immediate correction of severe anemia. Epoetin alfa may obviate the need for maintenance transfusions but is not a substitute for emergency transfusion.

▶*Treatment of anemia related to zidovudine therapy in HIV-infected patients:* To elevate or maintain the red blood cell level (as manifested by the hematocrit or hemoglobin determinations) and to decrease the need for transfusions. Epoetin alfa, at a dose of 100 units/kg 3 times/week, is effective in decreasing the transfusion requirement and increasing the red blood cell levels of anemic, HIV-infected patients treated with zidovudine, when the endogenous serum erythropoietin level is 500 mUnits/mL or less and when patients are receiving a dose of 4200 mg/week or less zidovudine.

▶*Treatment of anemia in cancer patients on chemotherapy:* Treatment of anemia in patients with nonmyeloid malignancies where anemia is caused by the effect of concomitantly administered chemotherapy. It is intended to decrease the need for transfusions in patients who will receive chemotherapy for a minimum of 2 months.

▶*Reduction of allogeneic blood transfusion in surgery patients:* For the treatment of anemic patients (hemoglobin 10 to 13 g/dL) scheduled to undergo elective, noncardiac, nonvascular surgery to reduce the need for allogeneic blood transfusions. Epoetin alfa is indicated for patients at high risk for perioperative transfusions with significant, anticipated blood loss. The safety of the perioperative use of epoetin alfa has been studied only in patients who are receiving anticoagulant prophylaxis.

▶*Unlabeled uses:* Use in critically ill patients to reduce the number of red blood cell transfusions; anemia of prematurity in preterm infants (25 to 100 units/kg/dose SC 3 times/week; alternatively, 200 to 300 units/kg/dose IV/SC 3 to 5 times/week for 2 to 6 weeks [total dose per week is 600 to 1400 units/kg]); anemia associated with myelodysplastic syndrome; anemia associated with chronic inflammatory disorders (eg, rheumatoid arthritis); prophylaxis of anemia associated with frequent blood donation; treatment of anemia associated with ribavirin combination therapy in hepatitis C-infected patients; treatment of anemia in cancer patients not receiving chemotherapy; once-weekly dosing regimen of cancer patients on chemotherapy: 40,000 to 60,000 units/week SC; treatment of anemia associated with CRF in children not requiring dialysis (3 months to 20 years of age: 50 to 250 units/kg SC or IV, weekly to 3 times/week); treatment of anemia related to zidovudine therapy in HIV-infected children (8 months to 17 years of age: 50 to 400 units/kg SC or IV, 2 to 3 times/week); treatment of anemia in children with cancer on chemotherapy (6 months to 18 years of age: 25 to 300 units/kg SC or IV, 3 to 7 times/week).

Administration and Dosage

▶*Approved by the FDA:* June 1, 1989.

▶*CRF patients:*

General Therapeutic Guidelines in CRF Patients for Epoetin Alfa	
Starting dose	
Adults	50 to 100 units/kg 3 times/week IV or SC
Children	50 units/kg 3 times/week IV or SC
Reduce dose when:	1) Hematocrit approaches 36% or 2) Hematocrit increases > 4 points in any 2-week period.

General Therapeutic Guidelines in CRF Patients for Epoetin Alfa	
Increase dose if:	Hematocrit does not increase by 5 to 6 points after 8 weeks of therapy and hematocrit is below suggested target range.
Maintenance dose	Individualize.
Suggested target hematocrit range	30% to 36%

Epoetin alfa may be given either as an IV or SC injection. In patients on hemodialysis, epoetin alfa usually has been administered as an IV bolus 3 times/week. While the administration is independent of the dialysis procedure, epoetin alfa may be administered into the venous line at the end of the dialysis procedure to obviate the need for additional venous access. In adult patients with CRF not on dialysis, epoetin alfa may be given either as an IV or SC injection.

Home hemodialysis patients who have been judged competent by their physicians to self-administer epoetin alfa without medical or other supervision may give themselves either an IV or SC injection. Home peritoneal dialysis patients may give themselves an SC injection.

Pretherapy evaluation – Prior to and during therapy, evaluate the patient's iron stores, including transferrin saturation and serum ferritin. Transferrin saturation should be at least 20% and ferritin should be at least 100 ng/mL. Virtually all patients will eventually require supplemental iron (see Precautions). Adequately control blood pressure prior to initiation of epoetin alfa therapy, and closely monitor and control it during therapy.

Dose adjustment – Following therapy, a period of time is required for erythroid progenitors to mature and be released into circulation resulting in an eventual increase in hematocrit. Additionally, red blood cell survival time affects hematocrit and may vary because of uremia. As a result, the time required to elicit a clinically significant change in hematocrit (increase or decrease) following any dose adjustment may be 2 to 6 weeks.

Do not adjust dose more frequently than once a month, unless clinically indicated. After any dose adjustment, determine the hematocrit twice weekly for at least 2 to 6 weeks.
- If the hematocrit is increasing and approaching 36%, reduce the dose to maintain the suggested target hematocrit range. If the reduced dose does not stop the rise in hematocrit and it exceeds 36%, temporarily withhold doses until the hematocrit begins to decrease, then reinitiate at a lower dose.
- At any time, if the hematocrit increases by more than 4 points in a 2-week period, immediately decrease the dose. After the dose reduction, monitor hematocrit twice weekly for 2 to 6 weeks; make further dose adjustments as outlined in the maintenance dose section.
- If a hematocrit increase of 5 to 6 points is not achieved after an 8-week period and iron stores are adequate (see Delayed or diminished response below), the dose may be incrementally increased. Further increases may be made at 4- to 6-week intervals until the desired response is attained.

Maintenance – Individualize dosage for each patient on dialysis.

Hemodialysis patients: Median dose of 75 units/kg 3 times/week (range, 12.5 to 525 units/kg 3 times/week) was seen in trials. Almost 10% required a dose of 25 units/kg or less and approximately 10% required more than 200 units/kg 3 times/week to maintain their hematocrit in the suggested target range.

Peritoneal dialysis patients: Median dose of 76 units/kg/week (range, 24 to 323 units/kg/week) in divided doses, 2 to 3 times/week.

Children: Median dose of 167 units/kg/week (range, 49 to 477 units/kg/week) in divided doses, 2 to 3 times/week.

Nondialysis CRF patients: Dose of 75 to 150 units/kg/week has maintained hematocrits of 36% to 38% for up to 6 months.

If the hematocrit remains below, or falls below, the suggested target range, re-evaluate iron stores. If the transferrin saturation is less than 20%, administer supplemental iron. If the transferrin saturation is

EPOETIN ALFA, RECOMBINANT (Erythropoietin; EPO)

greater than 20%, the dose of epoetin alfa may be increased. Do not make such dose increases more frequently than once a month, unless clinically indicated, as the response time of the hematocrit to a dose increase can be 2 to 6 weeks. Measure hematocrit twice weekly for 2 to 6 weeks following dose increases.

Delayed or diminished response – More than 95% of patients with CRF responded with clinically significant increases in hematocrit; virtually all patients were transfusion-independent within about 2 months of initiation of therapy.

If a patient fails to respond or maintain a response, consider other etiologies and evaluate as clinically indicated (see Delayed or diminished response).

➤*Zidovudine-treated, HIV-infected patients:* Determine endogenous serum erythropoietin level prior to transfusion. Patients taking zidovudine with erythropoietin levels more than 500 mUnits/mL are unlikely to respond.

Initial dose – For adults with serum erythropoietin levels 500 mUnits/mL or less who are receiving a dose of zidovudine 4200 mg/ week or less, the recommended starting dose is 100 units/kg as an IV or SC injection 3 times/week for 8 weeks.

Dose adjustment – If the response is not satisfactory in terms of reducing transfusion requirements or increasing hematocrit after 8 weeks of therapy, the dose can be increased by 50 to 100 units/kg 3 times/week. Evaluate response every 4 to 8 weeks thereafter and adjust the dose accordingly by 50 to 100 units/kg increments 3 times/ week. If patients have not responded satisfactorily to a 300 units/kg dose 3 times/week, it is unlikely that they will respond to higher doses.

Monitor hematocrit weekly during the dose adjustment phase of therapy.

Maintenance dose – When the desired response is attained, titrate the dose to maintain the response based on factors such as variations in zidovudine dose and the presence of intercurrent infectious or inflammatory episodes. If hematocrit exceeds 40%, stop the dose until hematocrit drops to 36%. When resuming treatment, reduce the dose by 25%, then titrate to maintain desired hematocrit.

➤*Cancer patients on chemotherapy:*

Starting dose – 150 units/kg SC 3 times weekly. In general, patients with lower baseline serum erythropoietin levels responded more vigorously to epoetin alfa. Treatment of patients with grossly elevated erythropoietin levels (eg, more than 200 mUnits/mL) is not recommended. Monitor hematocrit on a weekly basis until it is stable.

Dose adjustment – If response is not satisfactory in terms of reducing transfusion requirement or increasing hematocrit after 8 weeks of therapy, the dose may be increased up to 300 units/kg 3 times/week. If patients do not respond, it is unlikely that they will respond to higher doses. If hematocrit exceeds 40%, hold the dose until it falls to 36%. Reduce the dose by 25% when treatment is resumed and titrate to maintain desired hematocrit. If initial dose includes a very rapid hematocrit response (ie, increase of more than 4% in any 2-week period), reduce the dose.

Current guidelines – Current guidelines according to the American Society of Clinical Oncology and the American Society of Hematology recommend the use of epoetin alfa for chemotherapy-induced anemia when hemoglobin levels have decreased to 10 g/dL or less. In patients with decreasing hemoglobin levels and less severe anemia (hemoglobin levels less than 12 g/dL but have never fallen below 10 g/dL), decide to use epoetin alfa immediately or wait until levels fall below 10 g/dL based on clinical circumstances. Also, it is recommended that when the hemoglobin level has been raised to or near 12 g/dL, titrate the epoetin alfa dose to maintain that level or discontinue and restart it as the level falls to near 10 g/dL again. There is insufficient data to support raising hemoglobin levels higher than 12 g/dL.

➤*Surgery patients:* Prior to initiating treatment with epoetin alfa, obtain a hemoglobin measurement to establish that it is 10 to 13 g/dL. The recommended dose is 300 units/kg/day SC for 10 days before surgery, on the day of surgery, and for 4 days after surgery.

An alternate dose schedule is 600 units/kg SC in once-weekly doses (21, 14, and 7 days before surgery) plus a fourth dose on the day of surgery.

All patients should receive adequate iron supplementation. Initiate iron supplementation no later than the beginning of treatment with epoetin alfa and continue throughout the course of therapy.

➤*Preparation:* Do not shake. Prolonged vigorous shaking may denature the glycoprotein, rendering it biologically inactive.

Do not give in conjunction with other drug solutions. However, at time of SC administration, epoetin alfa single-dose vial may be admixed in a syringe with bacteriostatic 0.9% sodium chloride injection with benzyl alcohol 0.9% (bacteriostatic saline) at a 1:1 ratio. The benzyl alcohol acts as a local anesthetic that may ameliorate SC injection site discomfort. Multidose vials contain benzyl alcohol and admixing is not necessary.

Single-dose 1 mL vial – Contains no preservative. Use only one dose per vial; do not re-enter the vial. Discard unused portions.

Multi-dose 1 and 2 mL vial – Contains preservative. Store at 2° to 8°C (36° to 46°F) after initial entry and between doses. Discard 21 days after initial entry.

➤*Storage/Stability:* Store at 2° to 8°C (36° to 46°F). Do not freeze or shake.

Actions

➤*Pharmacology:* Erythropoietin is a glycoprotein that stimulates red blood cell production. It is produced in the kidney and stimulates the division and differentiation of erythroid progenitors in bone marrow. Epoetin alfa, a 165 amino acid glycoprotein manufactured by recombinant DNA technology, has the same biological effects as endogenous erythropoietin. It has a molecular weight of 30,400 daltons and contains the identical amino acid sequence of natural erythropoietin.

Endogenous production of erythropoietin is regulated by the level of tissue oxygenation. Hypoxia and anemia generally increase the production of erythropoietin, which in turn stimulates erythropoiesis. In healthy subjects, plasma erythropoietin levels range from 0.01 to 0.03 units/mL and increase up to 100- to 1000-fold during hypoxia or anemia. In patients with CRF, erythropoietin production is impaired; this deficiency is the primary cause of their anemia.

Epoetin alfa stimulates erythropoiesis in anemic patients on dialysis and those who do not require regular dialysis. The first evidence of a response to epoetin alfa administration is an increase in the reticulocyte count within 10 days, followed by increases in the red cell count, hemoglobin and hematocrit, usually within 2 to 6 weeks. Once the hematocrit reaches the suggested target range (30% to 36%), that level can be sustained by epoetin alfa therapy in the absence of iron deficiency and concurrent illnesses.

The rate of hematocrit increase varies among patients and depends on the dose of epoetin alfa within a therapeutic range of about 50 to 300 units/kg 3 times/week; a greater biologic response is not observed at doses exceeding 300 units/kg 3 times/week. Other factors affecting rate and extent of response include availability of iron stores, baseline hematocrit, and concurrent medical problems.

Responsiveness in HIV-infected patients is dependent on the endogenous serum erythropoietin level prior to treatment. Patients with levels of 500 mUnits/mL or less receiving zidovudine (AZT) 4200 mg/ week or less may respond; patients with endogenous levels more than 500 mUnits/mL do not appear to respond. In 4 trials, 60% to 80% of HIV-infected patients had levels of 500 mUnits/mL or less. Response is manifested by reduced transfusion requirements and increased hematocrit.

Epoetin alfa has been shown to increase hematocrit and decrease transfusion requirements after the first month of therapy (months 2 and 3) in anemic cancer patients undergoing chemotherapy.

➤*Pharmacokinetics:* Epoetin alfa IV is eliminated via first-order kinetics with a circulating half-life of about 4 to 13 hours in patients with CRF. Within the therapeutic dosage range, detectable levels of plasma erythropoietin are maintained for at least 24 hours. After SC administration of epoetin alfa to patients with CRF, peak serum levels are achieved within 5 to 24 hours after administration and decline slowly thereafter. There is no apparent difference in half-life between patients not on dialysis (serum creatinine more than 3 mg/dL) and adult patients maintained on dialysis. The half-life in healthy volunteers is about 20% shorter than in CRF patients.

➤*Clinical trials:* The rate of increase in hematocrit is dependent upon the dose of epoetin alfa administered and individual patient variation.

Hematocrit Increase Based on Epoetin Alfa Dose in Chronic Renal Failure Patients		
Starting dose (3 times weekly, IV)	Hematocrit increase	
	Hematocrit points/day	Hematocrit points/2 weeks
50 units/kg	0.11	1.5
100 units/kg	0.18	2.5
150 units/kg	0.25	3.5

Over this dosage range, about 95% of all patients responded with a clinically significant increase in hematocrit, and by the end of about 2 months of therapy, virtually all patients were transfusion-independent.

Contraindications

Uncontrolled hypertension; hypersensitivity to mammalian cell-derived products or to human albumin.

Warnings

➤*Pure red cell aplasia (PRCA):* PRCA, in association with neutralizing antibodies to native erythropoietin, has been observed in patients treated with recombinant erythropoietins. PRCA has been reported in a limited number of patients exposed to epoetin alfa. This has been reported predominantly in patients with CRF. Evaluate any patient with loss of response to epoetin alfa for the etiology of loss of effect. Discontinue epoetin alfa in any patient with evidence of PRCA and evaluate the patient for the presence of binding and neutralizing antibodies to epoetin alfa, native erythropoietin, and any other recombinant

EPOETIN ALFA, RECOMBINANT (Erythropoietin; EPO)

erythropoietin administered to the patient. Contact Amgen/Ortho Biotech Products, LP to assist in this evaluation. In patients with PRCA secondary to neutralizing antibodies to erythropoietin, do not administer epoetin alfa, and do not switch such patients to another product as anti-erythropoietin antibodies cross-react with other erythropoietins.

►*Anemia:* Not intended for CRF patients who require correction of severe anemia; epoetin alfa may obviate the need for maintenance transfusions but is not a substitute for emergency transfusion. Not indicated for treatment of anemia in HIV-infected patients or cancer patients caused by other factors such as iron or folate deficiencies, hemolysis or GI bleeding that should be managed appropriately.

Epoetin alfa is not indicated for anemic patients who are willing to donate autologous blood.

►*Thrombotic events:* During hemodialysis, patients treated with epoetin alfa may require increased anticoagulation with heparin to prevent clotting of the artificial kidney.

Clotting of the vascular access (A-V shunt) has occurred at an annualized rate of about 0.25 events per patient-year, and other thrombotic events (eg, MI, cerebrovascular accident, TIA, and pulmonary embolism) occurred at a rate of 0.04 events per patient-year in trials where the maintenance hematocrit was approximately 35% on epoetin alfa. Increased mortality was observed in a randomized placebo-controlled study in adults who did not have CRF who were undergoing coronary artery bypass surgery (7 deaths in 126 patients randomized to epoetin alfa vs no deaths among 56 patients receiving placebo). Four of these deaths occurred during the period of study drug administration and all 4 deaths were associated with thrombotic events. A causative role of epoetin alfa cannot be excluded.

In perioperative clinical trials with orthopedic surgery patients with a pretreatment hemoglobin greater than 13 g/dL treated with 300 units/kg of epoetin alfa, the possibility that epoetin alfa treatment may be associated with an increased risk of postoperative thrombotic/vascular events could not be excluded.

In 2 other orthopedic surgery studies, the overall rate (all pretreatment hemoglobin groups combined) of DVTs detected was higher in the group treated with epoetin alfa than in placebo-treated groups (11% vs 6%). This finding was attributable to the difference in DVT rates observed in the subgroup of patients with pretreatment hemoglobin levels greater than 13 g/dL. However, the incidence of DVTs was within range of that reported in the literature for orthopedic surgery patients.

In 1 study in which epoetin alfa was administered in the perioperative period to patients undergoing coronary artery bypass graft surgery, there were 7 deaths in the epoetin alfa-treated groups (N = 126) and no deaths in the placebo-treated group. The 4 deaths at the time of therapy (3%) were associated with thrombotic/vascular events. A causative role of epoetin alfa cannot be excluded.

In the orthopedic surgery study of patients with pretreatment hemoglobin of 10 to 13 g/dL, 4 (5%) of subjects in the 600 units/kg weekly dosing regimen vs no subjects in the 300 units/kg weekly dosing regimen had a thrombotic vascular event. During postmarketing, there have been rare reports of serious or unusual thromboembolic events, including migratory thrombophlebitis, microvascular thrombosis, pulmonary embolus, and thrombosis of the retinal artery and temporal and renal veins. A causal relationship to epoetin alfa has not been established.

Overall, for patients with CRF (whether on dialysis or not) in whom the target hematocrit was 32% to 40%, other thrombotic events (eg, MI, cerebrovascular accident, TIA) have occurred at an annualized rate of less than 0.04 events per patient-year of epoetin alfa. The risk of thrombotic events, including vascular access thromboses, was significantly increased in adult patients with ischemic heart disease or CHF receiving epoetin alfa therapy with the goal of reaching a normal hematocrit (42%) as compared with a target hematocrit of 30%. Closely monitor patients with pre-existing cardiovascular disease.

Because the extent of the population affected is unknown, weigh the benefits of epoetin alfa treatment against the potential for increased risks with therapy in patients at risk for thrombosis.

►*Seizures:* There have been 47 seizures in 1010 patients on dialysis treated with epoetin alfa in clinical trials, with an exposure of 986 patient-years for a rate of approximately 0.048 events per patient-year. There appeared to be a higher rate of seizures during the first 90 days of therapy (occurring in about 2.5% of patients) when compared with subsequent 90-day periods. The baseline incidence of seizures in the untreated dialysis population is difficult to determine; it appears to be in the range of 5% to 10% per patient-year. Given the potential for an increased risk of seizure during the first 90 days of therapy, closely monitor blood pressure and the presence of premonitory neurologic symptoms. Caution patients to avoid potentially hazardous activities such as driving or operating heavy machinery during this period. While the relationship between seizures and the rate of rise of the hematocrit is uncertain, it is recommended that the dose be decreased if the hematocrit increase exceeds 4 points in any 2-week period.

►*Hypertension:* Up to 80% of patients with CRF have a history of hypertension. Do not treat patients with uncontrolled hypertension; control blood pressure adequately before initiation of therapy. Although there does not appear to be any direct pressor effects of epoetin alfa, blood pressure may rise during therapy. During the early phase of treatment when the hematocrit is increasing, about 25% of patients on dialysis may require initiation of, or increases in, antihypertensive therapy. Hypertensive encephalopathy and seizures have occurred in CRF patients treated with epoetin alfa.

Take special care to closely monitor and aggressively control blood pressure in epoetin alfa-treated patients. Advise patients of the importance of compliance with antihypertensive therapy and dietary restrictions. If blood pressure is difficult to control by initiation of appropriate measures, the hematocrit may be reduced by decreasing or withholding the epoetin alfa dose. A clinically significant decrease in hematocrit may not be observed for several weeks. It is recommended that the epoetin alfa dose be decreased if the hematocrit increase exceeds 4 points in any 2-week period because of the possible association of excessive rate of rise of hematocrit with an exacerbation of hypertension.

In CRF patients on hemodialysis with clinically evident ischemic heart disease or CHF, manage the hematocrit carefully, not to exceed 36%.

Epoetin alfa has not been linked to exacerbation of hypertension, seizures, and thrombotic events in HIV-infected patients. However, withhold epoetin alfa in patients if pre-existing hypertension is uncontrolled; do not start until blood pressure is controlled.

Hypertension associated with a significant increase in hematocrit has been noted rarely in cancer patients receiving epoetin alfa. Nevertheless, monitor blood pressure carefully, particularly in patients with an underlying history of hypertension or cardiovascular disease.

For patients who respond to epoetin alfa with a rapid increase in hematocrit (eg, more than 4 points in any 2-week period), reduce the dose of epoetin alfa because of the possible association of excessive rate of rise of hematocrit with an exacerbation of hypertension.

►*Growth factor potential:* The possibility that epoetin alfa can act as a growth factor for any tumor type, particularly myeloid malignancies, cannot be excluded.

►*Hypersensitivity reactions:* Skin rashes and urticaria are rare, mild, and transient. There is no evidence of antibody development to erythropoietin, including those receiving epoetin alfa for more than 4 years. Nevertheless, if an anaphylactoid reaction occurs, immediately discontinue the drug and initiate appropriate therapy. Refer to Management of Acute Hypersensitivity Reactions.

In more than 125,000 patients treated with epoetin alfa, there have been rare reports of potentially serious allergic reactions, including urticaria with associated respiratory symptoms or circumoral edema, or urticaria alone. Most reactions occurred in situations where a causal relationship could not be established. Symptoms recurred with rechallenge in a few instances, suggesting that allergic reactivity may occasionally be associated with epoetin alfa therapy.

Two zidovudine-treated, HIV-infected patients had urticarial reactions within 48 hours of their first exposure to medication. One was treated with epoetin alfa and the other was treated with placebo. Both patients had positive immediate skin tests against their medication with a negative saline control. The basis for this apparent pre-existing hypersensitivity to components of the formulation is unknown but may be related to HIV-induced immunosuppression or prior exposure to blood products.

►*Pregnancy:* Category C. Adverse effects occurred in rats given epoetin alfa in doses 5 times the human dose. There are no adequate and well-controlled studies in pregnant women. Use in pregnancy only if the potential benefit justifies the potential risk to the fetus.

In some female patients, menses have resumed following epoetin alfa therapy; discuss the possibility of pregnancy and evaluate need for contraception.

In studies in female rats, there were decreases in body weight gain, delays in appearance of abdominal hair, delayed eye opening, delayed ossification, and decreases in the number of caudal vertebrae in the F1 fetuses of the 500 units/kg group. In female rats treated IV, there was a trend for slightly increased fetal wastage at doses of 100 and 500 units/kg.

Several case reports of intrauterine growth retardation resulting in low birth weights have been documented in pregnant patients treated with epoetin alfa. There have been reports of pre-eclampsia and worsening renal failure in pregnant women after starting epoetin alfa therapy, although it is not certain that these effects were due to the epoetin alfa therapy. There is also 1 report of abruptio placentae that resulted in fetal death at 23 weeks gestation; epoetin alfa therapy could not be excluded as a contributing factor.

►*Lactation:* It is not known whether epoetin alfa is excreted in breast milk. Exercise caution when administering to a nursing woman.

►*Children:* Safety and efficacy have not been established in patients less than 1 month of age.

Precautions

►*Monitoring:*

CRF patients – In patients with CRF not requiring dialysis, monitor blood pressure and hematocrit no less frequently than for patients maintained on dialysis. Closely monitor renal function and fluid and electrolyte balance, as an improved sense of well-being may obscure the

EPOETIN ALFA, RECOMBINANT (Erythropoietin; EPO)
need to initiate dialysis in some patients.

Determine the hematocrit twice a week until it has stabilized in the target range and the maintenance dose has been established. After any dose adjustment, determine the hematocrit twice weekly for at least 2 to 6 weeks until the hematocrit has stabilized; monitor at regular intervals.

Perform complete blood count with differential and platelet counts regularly. Modest increases have occurred in platelets and white blood cell counts, but values remained within normal ranges.

Monitor serum chemistry values (including blood urea nitrogen [BUN], uric acid, creatinine, phosphorus, and potassium) regularly. In patients on dialysis, modest increases occurred in BUN, creatinine, phosphorus, and potassium. In some patients, modest increases in serum uric acid and phosphorus were observed. The values remained within the ranges normally seen in patients with CRF.

Zidovudine-treated HIV-infected and cancer patients – Measure hematocrit once a week until it is stabilized; measure periodically thereafter.

Iron evaluation – During therapy, absolute or functional iron deficiency may develop. Functional iron deficiency, with normal ferritin levels but low transferrin saturation, is presumably caused by the inability to mobilize iron stores rapidly enough to support increased erythropoiesis. Transferrin saturation should be at least 20%, and ferritin should be at least 100 ng/mL. Prior to and during therapy, evaluate the patient's iron status, including transferrin saturation (serum iron divided by iron binding capacity) and serum ferritin. Virtually all patients will eventually require supplemental iron to increase or maintain transferrin saturation to levels that will adequately support epoetin alfa-stimulated erythropoiesis.

➤*Hematology:* The elevated bleeding time characteristic of CRF decreases toward normal after correction of anemia in epoetin alfa-treated patients. Reduction of bleeding time also occurs after correction of anemia by transfusion.

Allow sufficient time to determine a patient's responsiveness before adjusting the dose. Because of the time required for erythropoiesis and the red cell half-life, an interval of 2 to 6 weeks may occur between the time of a dose adjustment (initiation, increase, decrease, or discontinuation) and a significant change in hematocrit.

Porphyria – Exacerbation has been observed rarely in epoetin alfa-treated patients with CRF. However, epoetin alfa has not caused increased urinary excretion of porphyrin metabolites in healthy volunteers, even in the presence of a rapid erythropoietic response. Nevertheless, use with caution in patients with known porphyria.

➤*Bone marrow fibrosis:* Bone marrow fibrosis is a complication of CRF and may be related to secondary hyperparathyroidism or unknown factors. The incidence of bone marrow fibrosis was not increased in a study of adult patients on dialysis who were treated with epoetin alfa for 12 to 19 months, compared with controls.

➤*Delayed or diminished response:* If the patient fails to respond or to maintain a response to doses within the recommended range, consider and evaluate the following etiologies:

1.) Functional iron deficiency may develop with normal ferritin levels but low transferrin saturation (less than 20%), presumably caused by the inability to mobilize iron stores rapidly enough to support increased erythropoiesis. Virtually all patients will eventually require supplemental iron therapy.
2.) Underlying infectious, inflammatory, or malignant processes.
3.) Occult blood loss.
4.) Underlying hematologic diseases (eg, thalassemia, refractory anemia, other myelodysplastic disorders).
5.) Vitamin deficiencies: Folic acid or vitamin B_{12}.
6.) Hemolysis.
7.) Aluminum intoxication.
8.) Osteitis fibrosa cystica.

In the absence of another etiology, evaluate the patient for evidence of PRCA and test sera for the presence of antibodies to recombinant erythropoietins.

➤*Diet:* As the hematocrit increases and patients experience an improved sense of well-being, reinforce the importance of compliance with dietary guidelines and frequency of dialysis.

Hyperkalemia – In patients with CRF, hyperkalemia is not uncommon. In patients on dialysis, hyperkalemia has occurred at an annualized rate of about 0.11 episodes per patient-year of epoetin alfa therapy, often in association with poor compliance to medication, dietary guidelines, and frequency of dialysis.

➤*Dialysis management:* Therapy with epoetin alfa results in an increase in hematocrit and a decrease in plasma volume that could affect dialysis efficiency. This does not appear to adversely affect dialyzer function or the efficiency of high-flux hemodialysis. During hemo-

dialysis, patients treated with epoetin alfa may require increased anticoagulation with heparin to prevent clotting of the artificial kidney.

Patients who are marginally dialyzed may require adjustments in their dialysis prescription. As with all patients on dialysis, regularly monitor the serum chemistry values (including BUN, creatinine, phosphorus, and potassium) in patients treated with epoetin alfa.

➤*Benzyl alcohol:* Benzyl alcohol, which is contained in some of these products as a preservative, has been associated with an increased incidence of neurological and other complications in premature infants that are sometimes fatal.

➤*Drug abuse and dependence:* Epoetin alfa has been used by athletes to increase their performance by increasing hemoglobin ("blood doping"). Several deaths have resulted from this abuse. The hematocrit may continue to rise over several days and could result in severely high levels. Lack of proper medical supervision could result in serious adverse effects and even death.

Adverse Reactions

CRF patients – Epoetin alfa is generally well tolerated. The following adverse reactions are frequent sequelae of CRF and are not necessarily caused by epoetin alfa therapy:

Epoetin Alfa Adverse Reactions in CRF Patients (%)		
Adverse reaction	Epoetin alfa (n = 200)	Placebo (n = 135)
Hypertension	24	19
Headache	16	12
Arthralgia	11	6
Nausea	11	9
Edema	9	10
Fatigue	9	14
Diarrhea	9	6
Vomiting	8	5
Chest pain	7	9
Skin reaction (administration site)	7	12
Asthenia	7	12
Dizziness	7	13
Clotted access	7	2
Seizure	1.1	1.1
CVA/TIA	0.4	0.6
MI	0.4	1.1

Most common: Incidence (number of events per patient-year) in adult patients on dialysis (more than 567 patients): Hypertension (0.75); headache (0.4); tachycardia (0.31); nausea/vomiting (0.26); clotted vascular access (0.25); shortness of breath (0.14); hyperkalemia, diarrhea (0.11). Events that occurred within hours of administration of epoetin alfa were rare (less than 0.1%), mild and transient, and included injection site stinging in dialysis patients and flu-like symptoms (eg, arthralgias, myalgias).

Hypersensitivity: Skin rashes, urticaria (rare, mild, and transient) (see Warnings).

Children: In children with CRF on dialysis, the most common adverse events were similar to those seen with adults. Some additional adverse events seen in greater than 10% of children in either treatment group were the following: Abdominal pain; dialysis access complications, including access infections and peritonitis in those receiving peritoneal dialysis; fever; upper respiratory infection; cough; pharyngitis; and constipation. Rates were similar between the treatment groups.

Zidovudine-treated HIV-infected patients – Adverse experiences were consistent with the progression of HIV infection.

Epoetin Alfa Adverse Reactions in Zidovudine-Treated Patients (%)		
Adverse reaction	Epoetin alfa (n = 144)	Placebo (n = 153)
Pyrexia	38	29
Fatigue	25	31
Headache	19	14
Cough	18	14
Diarrhea	16	18
Rash	16	8
Nausea	15	12
Congestion, respiratory	15	10
Shortness of breath	14	13
Asthenia	11	14
Skin reaction (injection site)	10	7
Dizziness	9	10

Hypersensitivity: One zidovudine-treated HIV-infected patient had an urticarial reaction within 48 hours of the first exposure to epoetin alfa (see Warnings).

Seizures: In double-blind, placebo-controlled trials in zidovudine-treated HIV-infected patients, 10 patients have experienced seizures. These seizures appear to be related to underlying pathology such as meningitis or cerebral neoplasms, not epoetin alfa therapy.

EPOETIN ALFA, RECOMBINANT (Erythropoietin; EPO)

Surgery patients –

	Adverse Reactions in Surgery Patients Treated with Epoetin Alfa (%)				
Event	Epoetin alfa 300 units/kg (n = 112)[1]	Epoetin alfa 100 units/kg (n = 101)[1]	Placebo (n = 103)[1]	Epoetin alfa 600 units/kg (n = 73)[2]	Epoetin alfa 300 units/kg (n = 72)[2]
Pyrexia	51	50	60	47	42
Nausea	48	43	45	45	58
Constipation	43	42	43	51	53
Skin reaction (injection site)	25	19	22	26	29
Vomiting	22	12	14	21	29
Skin pain	18	18	17	5	4
Pruritus	16	16	14	14	22
Insomnia	13	16	13	21	18
Headache	13	11	9	10	19
Dizziness	12	9	12	11	21
Urinary tract infection	12	3	11	11	8
Hypertension	10	11	10	5	10
Diarrhea	10	7	12	10	6
Deep venous thrombosis[3]	10	3	5	0[4]	0[4]
Dyspepsia	9	11	6	7	8
Anxiety	7	2	11	11	4
Edema	6	11	8	11	7

[1] Study included patients undergoing orthopedic surgery treated with epoetin alfa or placebo for 15 days.
[2] Study including patients undergoing orthopedic surgery treated with epoetin alfa 600 units/kg weekly × 4 or 300 units/kg daily × 15.
[3] See Warnings.
[4] Determined by clinical symptoms.

Cancer patients on chemotherapy – Adverse reactions were consistent with the underlying disease state.

Epoetin Alfa Adverse Reactions in Cancer Patients (%)		
Adverse reaction	Epoetin alfa (n = 63)	Placebo (n = 68)
Pyrexia	29	19
Diarrhea	21	7
Nausea	17	32
Vomiting	17	15
Edema	17	1
Asthenia	13	16
Fatigue	13	15
Shortness of breath	13	9
Paresthesia	11	6

Epoetin Alfa Adverse Reactions in Cancer Patients (%)		
Adverse reaction	Epoetin alfa (n = 63)	Placebo (n = 68)
Upper respiratory infection	11	4
Dizziness	5	12
Trunk pain	3	16

Postmarketing –

Immunogenicity: Cases of antibody-induced PRCA in patients treated with recombinant human erythropoietins have been described.

Very rare occurrences of PRCA and the presence of antibodies with neutralizing activity have been reported since market introduction of epoetin alfa in the US (see Warnings). Cases have been observed in patients treated by SC and IV routes of administration. Among reported cases where the route of administration is known, PRCA has been observed more with SC administration than IV administration.

The incidence of antibody formation is highly dependent on the sensitivity and specificity of the assay. Additionally, the observed incidence of antibody positivity in an assay may be influenced by several factors, including sample handling, timing of sample collection, concomitant medications, and underlying disease. For these reasons, comparison of the incidence of antibodies to epoetin alfa with the incidence of antibodies to other products may be misleading.

Overdosage

The maximum amount that can be safely administered in single or multiple doses has not been determined. Doses up to 1500 units/kg 3 times/week for 3 to 4 weeks have been given without any direct toxic effects. Epoetin alfa can cause polycythemia if the hematocrit is not carefully monitored and the dose appropriately adjusted. If the suggested target range is exceeded, epoetin alfa may be temporarily withheld until the hematocrit returns to the target range; therapy may then be resumed using a lower dose (see Administration and Dosage). If polycythemia is of concern, phlebotomy may be indicated to decrease the hematocrit.

Patient Information

➤*Home dialysis patients:* In those situations in which the physician determines that a home dialysis patient can safely and effectively self-administer epoetin alfa, instruct the patient as to the proper dosage and administration. Refer patients to the "Information for Home Dialysis Patients" section supplied with the product.

Inform patients of the signs and symptoms of an allergic drug reaction and advise them of appropriate actions.

Thoroughly instruct the patient in the importance of proper disposal and caution against reuse of needles, syringes, or drug product. Provide a puncture-resistant container for disposal of used syringes and needles.

DARBEPOETIN ALFA

Rx	Aranesp (Amgen)	Solution for injection: 25 mcg per 0.42 mL	Preservative-free. In polysorbate or albumin solutions.[1] In single-dose, prefilled, *SingleJect* syringes.
		25 mcg per 1 mL	Preservative-free. In polysorbate or albumin solutions.[1] In 1 mL single-dose vials.
		40 mcg per 0.4 mL	Preservative-free. In polysorbate or albumin solutions.[1] In single-dose, prefilled, *SingleJect* syringes.
		40 mcg per 1 mL	Preservative-free. In polysorbate or albumin solutions.[1] In 1 mL single-dose vials.
		60 mcg per 0.3 mL	Preservative-free. In polysorbate or albumin solutions.[1] In single-dose, prefilled, *SingleJect* syringes.
		60 mcg per 1 mL	Preservative-free. In polysorbate or albumin solutions.[1] In 1 mL single-dose vials.
		100 mcg per 0.5 mL	Preservative-free. In polysorbate or albumin solutions.[1] In single-dose, prefilled, *SingleJect* syringes.
		100 mcg per 1 mL	Preservative-free. In polysorbate or albumin solutions.[1] In 1 mL single-dose vials.
		150 mcg per 0.3 mL	Preservative-free. In polysorbate or albumin solutions.[1] In single-dose, prefilled, *SingleJect* syringes.
		150 mcg per 1 mL	Preservative-free. In poly sorbate or albumin solutions.[1] In single-dose vials.
		200 mcg per 0.4 mL	Preservative-free. In polysorbate or albumin solutions.[1] In single-dose, prefilled, *SingleJect* syringes.
		200 mcg per 1 mL	Preservative-free. In polysorbate or albumin solutions.[1] In 1 mL single-dose vials.
		300 mcg per 0.6 mL	Preservative-free. In polysorbate or albumin solutions.[1] In single-dose, prefilled, *SingleJect* syringes.
		300 mcg per 1 mL	Preservative-free. In polysorbate or albumin solutions.[1] In 1 mL single-dose vials.
		500 mcg per 1 mL	Preservative-free. In polysorbate or albumin solutions.[1] In 1 mL single-dose vials and single-dose, prefilled, *SingleJect* syringes.

[1] The polysorbate solution contains 0.05 mg polysorbate 80, 2.12 mg sodium phosphate monobasic monohydrate, 0.66 mg sodium phosphate dibasic anhydrous, and 8.18 mg sodium chloride. The albumin solution contains 2.5 mg albumin (human), 2.23 mg sodium phosphate monobasic monohydrate, 0.53 mg sodium phosphate dibasic anhydrous, and 8.18 mg sodium chloride.

Indications

➤*Anemia:* For the treatment of anemia associated with chronic renal failure (CRF), including patients on and not on dialysis, and for the treatment of anemia in patients with nonmyeloid malignancies where anemia is caused by coadministered chemotherapy.

Administration and Dosage

➤*Approved by the FDA:* September 18, 2001.

DARBEPOETIN ALFA

Administer IV or SC as a single weekly injection. Start and slowly adjust the dose as described below based on hemoglobin levels. If a patient fails to respond or maintain a response, consider and evaluate other etiologies. When darbepoetin therapy is initiated or adjusted, follow the hemoglobin level weekly until stabilized, and monitor at least monthly thereafter.

For patients who respond to darbepoetin with a rapid increase in hemoglobin (eg, more than 1 g/dL in any 2-week period), the dose of darbepoetin should be reduced because of the association with excessive rate of rise of hemoglobin with adverse events.

Adjust the dose for each patient to achieve and maintain a target hemoglobin level not to exceed 12 g/dL.

►*Correction of anemia:* The recommended starting dose of darbepoetin for the correction of anemia in CRF patients is 0.45 mcg/kg body weight, administered as a single IV or SC injection once weekly. Titrate doses to not exceed a target hemoglobin concentration of 12 g/dL. For many patients, the appropriate maintenance dose will be lower than this starting dose. Predialysis patients, in particular, may require lower maintenance doses. Also, some patients have been treated successfully with SC darbepoetin administered once every 2 weeks.

►*Conversion from epoetin alfa to darbepoetin:* Estimate the starting weekly dose of darbepoetin based on the weekly epoetin alfa dose at the time of substitution. Titrate doses to maintain the target hemoglobin. Because of the longer serum half-life, administer darbepoetin less frequently than epoetin alfa. Administer once a week if patient was receiving epoetin alfa 2 to 3 times weekly. Administer darbepoetin once every 2 weeks if the patient was receiving epoetin alfa once per week. Maintain the route of administration (IV or SC).

Estimated Darbepoetin Starting Doses Based on Previous Epoetin Alfa Dose	
Previous weekly epoetin alfa dose (units/week)	Weekly starting darbepoetin dose (mcg/week)
< 2500	6.25
2500 to 4999	12.5
5000 to 10,999	25
11,000 to 17,999	40
18,000 to 33,999	60
34,000 to 89,999	100
≥ 90,000	200

►*Dose adjustment:* Allow sufficient time to determine a patient's responsiveness to a dosage of darbepoetin before adjusting the dose. Because of the time required for erythropoiesis and the red cell half-life, an interval of 2 to 6 weeks may occur between the time of a dose adjustment (eg, initiation, increase, decrease, discontinuation) and a significant change in hemoglobin.

Do not increase doses more frequently than once a month. If the hemoglobin is increasing and approaching 12 g/dL, reduce the dose by approximately 25%. If the hemoglobin continues to increase, withhold doses temporarily until the hemoglobin begins to decrease, at which point therapy should be reinitiated at a dose approximately 25% below the previous dose. If the hemoglobin increases by more than 1 g/dL in a 2-week period, decrease the dose by approximately 25%.

If the increase in hemoglobin is less than 1 g/dL over 4 weeks and iron stores are adequate, the dose of darbepoetin may be increased by approximately 25% of the previous dose. Further increases may be made at 4-week intervals until the specified hemoglobin is obtained.

►*Maintenance dose:* Adjust darbepoetin dosage to maintain a target hemoglobin not to exceed 12 g/dL. If the hemoglobin exceeds 12 g/dL, the dose may be adjusted as described above. Doses must be individualized to ensure that hemoglobin is maintained at an appropriate level for each patient.

►*Cancer patients receiving chemotherapy:* The recommended starting dose for darbepoetin alfa is 2.25 mcg/kg administered as a weekly SC injection.

The dose should be adjusted for each patient to achieve and maintain a target hemoglobin. If there is less than a 1 g/dL increase in hemoglobin after 6 weeks of therapy, increase the dose of darbepoetin alfa up to 4.5 mcg/kg. If hemoglobin increases by more than 1 g/dL in a 2-week period or if the hemoglobin exceeds 12 g/dL, reduce the dose by approximately 25%. If the hemoglobin exceeds 13 g/dL, temporarily withhold doses until the hemoglobin falls to 12 g/dL. Reinitiate therapy at a dose approximately 25% below the previous dose.

►*Preparation:* Do not shake. Vigorous shaking may denature darbepoetin, rendering it biologically inactive. Visually inspect parenteral drug products for particulate matter and discoloration prior to administration. Do not use any vials exhibiting particulate matter or discoloration. Do not dilute. Do not administer darbepoetin in conjunction with other drug solutions. Darbepoetin is packaged in single-use vials and contains no preservatives. Discard any unused portion. Do not pool unused portions.

►*Storage/Stability:* Store at 2° to 8°C (36° to 46°F). Do not freeze or shake. Protect from light.

Actions

►*Pharmacology:* Darbepoetin alfa is an erythropoiesis-stimulating protein produced in Chinese hamster ovary (CHO) cells by recombinant DNA technology. Darbepoetin stimulates erythropoiesis by the same mechanism as endogenous erythropoietin. A primary growth factor for erythroid development, erythropoietin is produced in the kidney and released into the bloodstream in response to hypoxia. In responding to hypoxia, erythropoietin interacts with progenitor stem cells to increase red cell production. Production of endogenous erythropoietin is impaired in patients with CRF, and erythropoietin deficiency is the primary cause of their anemia. Increased hemoglobin levels are not generally observed until 2 to 6 weeks after initiating treatment with darbepoetin.

►*Pharmacokinetics:* Over the therapeutic range of 0.45 to 4.5 mcg/kg, pharmacokinetic measures (C_{max}, half-life, AUC) were linear with respect to dose, and no evidence of accumulation was observed beyond an expected less than 2-fold increase in blood levels when compared with the initial dose.

Following SC administration, absorption is slow and rate-limiting and the observed half-life is 49 hours (range, 27 to 89 hours), which reflects the rate of absorption. The peak concentration occurs at 34 hours (range, 24 to 72 hours) post-SC administration in CRF patients, and bioavailability is approximately 37% (range, 30% to 50%). Peak concentrations in cancer patients are at 90 hours (range, 71 to 123 hours).

Following IV administration to adult CRF and cancer patients, darbepoetin serum concentration time profiles are biphasic, with a distribution half-life of approximately 1.4 hours and mean terminal half-life of 21 hours.

Darbepoetin has an approximately 3-fold longer terminal half-life than epoetin alfa when administered by the IV route.

►*Clinical trials:*

Exogenous erythropoietin –

CRF treatment-naive patients: In 2 open-label studies, darbepoetin or epoetin alfa were administered for the correction of anemia in CRF patients who had not been receiving prior treatment with exogenous erythropoietin. Study 1 evaluated CRF patients receiving dialysis; study 2 evaluated patients not requiring dialysis (predialysis patients). In both studies, the starting dose of darbepoetin was 0.45 mcg/kg administered once weekly. The starting dose of epoetin alfa was 50 U/kg 3 times weekly in study 1 and 50 U/kg twice weekly in study 2. Dosage adjustments were instituted to maintain hemoglobin in the study target range of 11 to 13 g/dL. (The recommended hemoglobin target is lower than the target range of these studies.) The primary efficacy endpoint was the proportion of patients who experienced at least 1 g/dL increase in hemoglobin concentration to a level of at least 11 g/dL by 20 weeks (study 1) or 24 weeks (study 2). The studies were designed to assess the safety and effectiveness of darbepoetin but not to support conclusions regarding comparisons between the 2 products.

In study 1, the hemoglobin target was achieved by 72% of the 90 patients treated with darbepoetin and 84% of the 31 patients treated with epoetin alfa. The mean increase in hemoglobin over the initial 4 weeks of darbepoetin treatment was 1.1 g/dL.

In study 2, the primary efficacy endpoint was achieved by 93% of the 129 patients treated with darbepoetin and 92% of the 37 patients treated with epoetin alfa. The mean increase in hemoglobin from baseline through the initial 4 weeks of darbepoetin treatment was 1.38 g/dL.

Conversion from other recombinant erythropoietins: Two studies were conducted in adult patients with CRF who had been receiving other recombinant erythropoietins and compared the abilities of darbepoetin and other erythropoietins to maintain hemoglobin concentrations within a study target range of 9 to 13 g/dL. (The recommended hemoglobin target is lower than the target range of these studies.) CRF patients who had been receiving stable doses of other recombinant erythropoietins were randomized to darbepoetin, or to continue with their prior erythropoietin at the previous dose and schedule. For patients randomized to darbepoetin, the initial weekly dose was determined on the basis of the previous total weekly dose of recombinant erythropoietin. Study 3 was a double-blind study in which 169 hemodialysis patients were randomized to treatment with darbepoetin and 338 patients continued on epoetin alfa. Study 4 was an open-label study in which 347 patients were randomized to treatment with darbepoetin and 175 patients were randomized to continue on epoetin alfa or epoetin beta. Of the 347 patients randomized to darbepoetin, 92% were receiving hemodialysis and 8% were receiving peritoneal dialysis.

In study 3, a median weekly dose of 0.53 mcg/kg darbepoetin was required to maintain hemoglobin in the study target range. In study 4, a median weekly dose of 0.41 mcg/kg darbepoetin was required to maintain hemoglobin in the study target range.

Cancer patients receiving chemotherapy – The safety and efficacy of darbepoetin alfa in reducing the requirement for red blood cell (RBC) transfusions in patients undergoing chemotherapy were assessed in a multinational study. This study was conducted in anemic (Hgb less than or equal to 11 g/dL) patients with advanced, small cell or non-small cell lung cancer, who received a platinum-containing chemo-

DARBEPOETIN ALFA

therapy regimen. Patients received darbepoetin alfa 2.25 mcg/kg (n = 156) or placebo (n = 158) administered as a single weekly SC injection for up to 12 weeks. The dose was escalated to 4.5 mcg/kg/week at week 6 in subjects with an inadequate response to treatment. There were 67 patients in the darbepoetin alfa arm who had their dose increased from 2.25 to 4.5 mcg/kg/week.

Efficacy was determined by a reduction in the proportion of patients who were transfused over the 12-week treatment period. With a significantly lower proportion of patients in the darbepoetin alfa arm, 26% required transfusion compared with 60% in the placebo arm. Of the 67 patients who received a dose increase, 28% had a 2 g/dL increase in hemoglobin over baseline, generally occurring between weeks 8 and 13. Of the 89 patients who did not receive a dose increase, 69% had a 2 g/dL increase in hemoglobin over baseline, generally occurring between weeks 6 and 13.

Data from these studies indicate that there is a dose response relationship with respect to hemoglobin response. The minimally effective starting dose with respect to reducing transfusion requirements was 1.5 mcg/kg/week with a plateau observed at 4.5 mcg/kg/week.

Contraindications

Uncontrolled hypertension; known hypersensitivity to the active substance or any of the excipients.

Warnings

►*Cardiovascular events:* Darbepoetin and other erythropoietic therapies may increase the risk of cardiovascular events, including death. The higher risk of cardiovascular events may be associated with higher hemoglobin or higher rates of rise of hemoglobin. The hemoglobin level should be managed to avoid exceeding a target level of 12 g/dL.

In a clinical trial of epoetin alfa treatment in hemodialysis patients with clinically evident cardiac disease, patients were randomized to a target hemoglobin of 14 ± 1 or 10 ± 1 g/dL. Higher mortality (35% vs 29%) was observed in the 634 patients randomized to a target hemoglobin of 14 g/dL than in the 631 patients assigned a target hemoglobin of 10 g/dL. The reason for the increased mortality observed in this study is unknown; however, the incidence of nonfatal MI, vascular access thrombosis, and other thrombotic events also was higher in the group randomized to a target hemoglobin of 14 g/dL.

In patients treated with darbepoetin or other recombinant erythropoietins in darbepoetin clinical trials, increases in hemoglobin greater than approximately 1 g/dL during any 2-week period were associated with increased incidence of cardiac arrest, neurologic events (including seizures and stroke), exacerbations of hypertension, CHF, vascular thrombosis/ischemia, infarction, acute MI, and fluid overload/edema. It is recommended that the dose of darbepoetin be decreased if the hemoglobin increase exceeds 1 g/dL in any 2-week period because of the association of excessive rate of rise of hemoglobin with these events.

►*Hypertension:* Do not treat patients with uncontrolled hypertension with darbepoetin; adequately control blood pressure before initiation of therapy. Blood pressure may rise during treatment of anemia with darbepoetin or epoetin alfa. In darbepoetin clinical trials, approximately 40% of patients with CRF required initiation or intensification of antihypertensive therapy during the early phase of treatment when the hemoglobin was increasing. Hypertensive encephalopathy and seizures have been observed in patients with CRF treated with darbepoetin or epoetin alfa.

Take special care to closely monitor and control blood pressure in patients treated with darbepoetin. Advise patients of the importance of compliance with antihypertensive therapy and dietary restrictions. If blood pressure is difficult to control by pharmacologic or dietary measures, reduce or withhold the dose of darbepoetin. A clinically significant decrease in hemoglobin may not be observed for several weeks.

►*Seizures:* Seizures have occurred in patients with CRF participating in clinical trials of darbepoetin and epoetin alfa. During the first several months of therapy, closely monitor blood presssure and the presence of premonitory neurologic symptoms. While the relationship between seizures and the rate of rise of hemoglobin is uncertain, it is recommended that the dose of darbepoetin be decreased if the hemoglobin increase exceeds 1 g/dL in any 2-week period.

►*Thrombotic events:* An increased incidence of thrombotic events has been observed in patients treated with erythropoietic agents. In patients with cancer who received darbepoetin alfa, pulmonary emboli, thrombophlebitis, and thrombosis occurred more frequently than in placebo controls.

►*Pure red cell aplasia:* Pure red cell aplasia (PRCA), in association with neutralizing antibodies to native erythropoietin, has been observed in patients treated with recombinant erythropoietins. This has been reported predominantly in patients with CRF. PRCA has been reported in a limited number of subjects exposed to other recombinant erythropoietin products prior to exposure to darbepoetin alfa. The contribution of darbepoetin alfa to the development of PRCA is unclear.

Darbepoetin alfa should be discontinued in any patient with evidence of PRCA and the patient evaluated for the presence of binding and neutralizing antibodies to darbepoetin alfa, native erythropoietin, and any other recombinant erythropoietin administered to the patient.

►*Albumin (human):* Darbepoetin is supplied in 2 formulations with different excipients, 1 containing polysorbate 80 and another containing albumin (human), a derivative of human blood. Based on effective donor screening and product manufacturing processes, darbepoetin formulated with albumin carries an extremely remote risk for transmission of viral diseases. A theoretical risk for transmission of Creutzfeldt-Jakob disease (CJD) also is considered extremely remote. No cases of transmission of viral disease or CJD have ever been identified for albumin.

►*Carcinogenesis:* The carcinogenic potential of darbepoetin has not been evaluated in long-term animal studies.

►*Fertility impairment:* When administered IV to male and female rats prior to and during mating, an increase in postimplantation fetal loss was seen at doses of 0.5 mcg/kg/dose or more administered 3 times/week.

►*Pregnancy:* Category C. When darbepoetin was administered IV to rats and rabbits during gestation, no evidence of a direct embryotoxic, fetotoxic, or teratogenic outcome was observed at doses up to 20 mcg/kg/day. The only adverse effect observed was a slight reduction in fetal weight, which occurred at doses causing exaggerated pharmacological effects in the dams (1 mcg/kg/day or higher).

IV injection of darbepoetin to female rats every other day from day 6 of gestation through day 23 of lactation at doses of 2.5 mcg/kg/dose and higher resulted in offspring with decreased body weights, which correlated with a low incidence of deaths, as well as delayed eye opening and delayed preputial separation.

There are no adequate and well-controlled studies in pregnant women. Use darbepoetin during pregnancy only if the potential benefit justifies the potential risk to the fetus.

►*Lactation:* It is not known whether darbepoetin is excreted in human milk. Because many drugs are excreted in human milk, exercise caution when darbepoetin is administered to a nursing woman.

►*Children:* The safety and efficacy of darbepoetin in pediatric patients have not been established.

Precautions

►*Monitoring:* After initiation of therapy, determine hemoglobin weekly until it has stabilized and the maintenance dose has been established. After a dose adjustment, determine hemoglobin weekly for at least 4 weeks until it has been determined that the hemoglobin has stabilized in response to the dose change. Then monitor hemoglobin at regular intervals.

Evaluate iron status for all patients before and during treatment, as the majority of patients will eventually require supplemental iron therapy. Supplemental iron therapy is recommended for all patients whose serum ferritin is below 100 mcg/L or whose serum transferrin saturation is below 20%.

►*Compromised erythropoietic response:* A lack of response or failure to maintain a hemoglobin response with darbepoetin doses within recommended dosing range should prompt a search for causative factors. Deficiencies of folic acid or vitamin B_{12} should be excluded or corrected. Intercurrent infections, inflammatory, or malignant processes, osteofibrosis cystica, occult blood loss, hemolysis, severe aluminum toxicity, and bone marrow fibrosis may compromise an erythropoietic response.

The safety and efficacy of darbepoetin therapy have not been established in patients with underlying hematologic diseases (eg, hemolytic anemia, sickle cell anemia, thalassemia, porphyria).

►*Patients with CRF not requiring dialysis:* Patients with CRF not yet requiring dialysis may require lower maintenance doses of darbepoetin than patients receiving dialysis. Although predialysis patients generally receive less frequent monitoring of blood pressure and laboratory parameters than dialysis patients, predialysis patients may be more responsive to the effects of darbepoetin, and require judicious monitoring of blood pressure and hemoglobin. Also closely monitor renal function and fluid and electrolyte balance.

►*Dialysis management:* Therapy with darbepoetin results in an increase in RBCs and a decrease in plasma volume, which could reduce dialysis efficiency; patients who are marginally dialyzed may require adjustments in their dialysis prescription.

►*Growth factor potential:* Darbepoetin alfa is a growth factor that primarily stimulates RBC production. The possibility that darbepoetin alfa can act as a growth factor for any tumor type, particularly myeloid malignancies, has not been evaluated. In a study of 314 subjects with advanced lung cancer, there were no statistically significant differences in time-to-progression (TTP) or overall survival (OS) observed; however, the study was not designed to detect or exclude clinically meaningful differences in either TTP or OS.

DARBEPOETIN ALFA

Adverse Reactions

Adverse Reactions Occurring in Darbepoetin-Treated Patients with CRF (%)

Adverse reaction	Patients (n = 1598)
Cardiovascular	
Hypertension	23
Hypotension	22
Cardiac arrhythmias/Cardiac arrest	10
Angina pectoris/Cardiac chest pain	8
Thrombosis vascular access	8
CHF	6
Acute MI	2
Transient ischemic attack	1
CNS	
Headache	16
Dizziness	8
Seizure	1
Stroke	1
GI	
Diarrhea	16
Vomiting	15
Nausea	14
Abdominal pain	12
Constipation	5
Musculoskeletal	
Myalgia	21
Arthralgia	11
Limb pain	10
Back pain	8
Respiratory	
Upper respiratory tract infection	14
Dyspnea	12
Cough	10
Bronchitis	6
Miscellaneous	
Infection[1]	27
Peripheral edema	11
Fatigue	9
Fever	9
Pruritus	8
Death	7
Injection site pain	7
Chest pain, unspecified	6
Fluid overload	6
Access infection	6
Influenza-like symptoms	6
Access hemorrhage	6
Asthenia	5

[1] Infection included sepsis, bacteremia, pneumonia, peritonitis, and abscess.

▶*CRF:* The most frequently reported serious adverse reactions with darbepoetin were vascular access thrombosis, CHF, sepsis, and cardiac arrhythmia. The most commonly reported adverse reactions were infection, hypertension, hypotension, myalgia, headache, and diarrhea. The most frequently reported adverse reactions resulting in clinical intervention (eg, discontinuation of darbepoetin, adjustment in dosage, the need for comedication to treat an adverse reaction symptom) were hypotension, hypertension, fever, myalgia, nausea, and chest pain.

▶*Thrombotic events:* Vascular access thrombosis in hemodialysis patients occurred in clinical trials at an annualized rate of 0.22 events per patient year of darbepoetin therapy. Rates of thrombotic events with darbepoetin therapy were similar to those observed with other recombinant erythropoietins in these trials.

▶*Cancer patients receiving chemotherapy:* The most frequently reported serious adverse events included death (10%), fever (4%), pneumonia (3%), dehydration (3%), vomiting (2%), and dyspnea (2%). The most commonly reported adverse events were fatigue, edema, nausea, vomiting, diarrhea, fever, and headache. The most frequently reported reasons for discontinuation of darbepoetin alfa were progressive disease, death, discontinuation of the chemotherapy, asthenia, dyspnea, pneumonia, and GI hemorrhage.

Adverse Events Occurring in Patients Receiving Chemotherapy (%)

Adverse reaction	Darbepoetin alfa (n = 873)	Placebo (n = 221)
Cardiovascular		
Hypertension	3.7	3.2
Thrombotic events	6.2	4.1
Pulmonary embolism	1.3	0
Thrombosis[1]	5.6	4.1
CNS		
Dizziness	14	8
Headache	12	9
Seizures/Convulsions[2]	0.6	0.5
GI		
Diarrhea	22	12
Constipation	18	17
Musculoskeletal		
Arthralgia	13	6
Myalgia	8	5
Miscellaneous		
Fatigue	33	30
Edema	21	10
Fever	19	16
Rash	7	3
Dehydration	5	3

[1] Thrombosis includes the following: Thrombophlebitis, deep thrombophlebitis, venous thrombosis, deep vein thrombosis, thromboembolism, and thrombosis.
[2] Seizures/Convusions includes the following: Convulsions, grand mal convulsions, and local convulsions.

▶*Thrombotic and cardiovascular events:* The following events were reported more frequently in darbepoetin alfa-treated patients than in placebo controls: Pulmonary embolism, thromboembolism, thrombosis, and thrombophlebitis (deep and/or superficial). Edema of any type was more frequently reported in darbepoetin alfa-treated (21%) patients than in patients who received placebo (10%).

▶*Immunogenicity:* As with all therapeutic proteins, there is a potential for immunogenicity. The incidence of antibody development in patients receiving darbepoetin has not been adequately determined. Radioimmunoprecipitation assays were performed on sera from 1534 CRF and 833 cancer patients treated with darbepoetin. High-titer antibodies were not detected in CRF patients, but assay sensitivity may be inadequate to reliably detect lower titers. Antibodies were detected by radioimmunoprecipitation in sera from 3 cancer patients; neutralizing activity, possibly related to antibodies, was detected in 1 of these 3 patients.

▶*Hypersensitivity:* There have been rare reports of potentially serious allergic reactions including skin rash and urticaria associated with darbepoetin. Symptoms have recurred with rechallenge, suggesting a causal relationship exists in some instances. If an anaphylactic reaction occurs, immediately discontinue darbepoetin and administer appropriate therapy.

Overdosage

The maximum amount of darbepoetin alfa that can be safely administered in single or multiple doses has not been determined. Doses over 3 mcg/kg/week for up to 28 weeks have been administered to CRF patients. Doses up to 8 mcg/kg/week every week and 15 mcg/kg every 3 weeks have been administered to cancer patients for up to 12 to 16 weeks. However, excessive rise and rate of rise in hemoglobin concentration have been associated with adverse events.

Patient Information

Inform patients of the possible side effects of darbepoetin and instruct them to report the side effects to the prescribing physician. Inform patients of the signs and symptoms of allergic drug reactions and advise them of appropriate actions. Counsel patients on the importance of compliance with their darbepoetin treatment, diet, and dialysis prescriptions. Stress the importance of judicious monitoring of blood pressure and hemoglobin concentration.

If it is determined that a patient can safely and effectively administer darbepoetin at home, provide appropriate instruction on the proper use of darbepoetin for the patients and their caregivers, including careful review of the "Information for Patients and Caregivers" leaflet. Caution patients and caregivers against the reuse of needles, syringes, or drug product, and thoroughly instruct the patients and caregivers in their proper disposal. A puncture-resistant container for the disposal of used syringes and needles should be made available to the patient.

Colony Stimulating Factors

FILGRASTIM (Granulocyte Colony Stimulating Factor; G-CSF)

Rx	Neupogen (Amgen)	Injection: 300 mcg/mL[1]	Preservative free. In 1 and 1.6 mL single-dose vials.
		Injection: 300 mcg/0.5 mL[2]	Preservative free. In 0.5 mL and 0.8 mL prefilled syringes.

[1] With 0.59 mg acetate, 50 mg sorbitol, 0.004% *Tween* 80 and 0.035 mg Na/mL in water for injection.

[2] With 0.295 mg acetate, 25 mg sorbitol, 0.004% *Tween* 80, and 0.0175 mg Na/mL in water for injection.

Indications

►*Cancer patients:*

Myelosuppressive chemotherapy – To decrease the incidence of infection, as manifested by febrile neutropenia, in patients with non-myeloid malignancies receiving myelosuppressive anti-cancer drugs associated with a significant incidence of severe neutropenia with fever.

Acute myeloid leukemia (AML) – To reduce the time to neutrophil recovery and the duration of fever following induction or consolidation chemotherapy treatment of adults with AML.

Bone marrow transplant (BMT) – To reduce the duration of neutropenia and neutropenia-related clinical sequelae (eg, febrile neutropenia) in patients with non-myeloid malignancies undergoing myeloablative chemotherapy followed by BMT.

Peripheral Blood Progenitor Cell (PBPC) Collection – For the mobilization of hematopoietic progenitor cells into the peripheral blood for leukapheresis collection. Mobilization allows for collection of increased progenitor cell numbers capable of engraftment compared with collection by leukapheresis without mobilization or bone marrow harvest. After myeloablative chemotherapy, the transplantation of an increased number of progenitor cells can lead to more rapid engraftment, decreasing the need for supportive care.

►*Severe chronic neutropenia (SCN):* Chronic administration to reduce the incidence and duration of sequelae of neutropenia (eg, fever, infections, oropharyngeal ulcers) in symptomatic patients with congenital, cyclic or idiopathic neutropenia.

►*Unlabeled uses:* Filgrastim may be beneficial in AIDS (0.3 to 3.6 mcg/kg/day), aplastic anemia (800 to 1200 mcg/m²/day), hairy cell leukemia, myelodysplasia (15 to 500 mcg/m²/day), drug-induced and congenital agranulocytosis, alloimmune neonatalneutropenia.

Administration and Dosage

►*Approved by the FDA:* February 1991.

►*Myelosuppressive chemotherapy:* Recommended starting dose is 5 mcg/kg/day, given as a single daily injection by SC bolus injection, by short IV infusion (15 to 30 minutes) or by continuous SC or IV infusion. Obtain CBC and platelet count before instituting therapy; monitor twice weekly during therapy. Doses may be increased in increments of 5 mcg/kg for each chemotherapy cycle according to duration and severity of the ANC nadir.

Administer no earlier than 24 hours after cytotoxic chemotherapy and not in the 24 hours before administration of chemotherapy. Give daily for up to 2 weeks until ANC has reached 10,000/mm³ following the expected chemotherapy-induced neutrophil nadir. Duration of therapy needed to attenuate chemotherapy-induced neutropenia may depend on the myelosuppressive potential of the chemotherapy regimen employed. Discontinue therapy if the ANC surpasses 10,000/mm³ after the expected chemotherapy-induced neutrophil nadir (see Precautions). In clinical trials, efficacy was observed at doses of 4 to 8 mcg/kg/day.

►*BMT:* Recommended dose following BMT is 10 mcg/kg/day given as an IV infusion of 4 or 24 hours or as a continuous 24 hour SC infusion. For patients receiving BMT, administer the first dose of filgrastim at least 24 hours after cytotoxic chemotherapy and at least 24 hours after bone marrow infusion.

During the period of neutrophil recovery, titrate the daily dose against the neutrophil response as follows:

Filgrastim Dose Based on Neutrophil Response	
Absolute neutrophil count	Filgrastim dose adjustment
When ANC > 1000/mm³ for 3 consecutive days	Reduce to 5 mcg/kg/day[1]
If ANC remains > 1000/mm³ for 3 more consecutive days	Discontinue filgrastim
If ANC decreases to < 1000/mm³	Resume at 5 mcg/kg/day

[1] If ANC decreases to < 1000/mm³ at any time during the 5 mcg/kg/day administration, increase filgrastim to 10 mcg/kg/day and follow the steps in the table.

►*PBPC collection:* 10 mcg/kg/day SC, either as a bolus or a continuous infusion. It is recommended that filgrastim be given for at least 4 days before the first leukapheresis procedure and continued until the last leukapheresis. Administration of filgrastim for 6 to 7 days with leukaphereses on days 5, 6 and 7 was found to be safe and effective.

►*SCN:*

Starting dose –
  Congenital neutropenia: 6 mcg/kg twice daily SC every day.
  Idiopathic or cyclic neutropenia: 5 mcg/kg as a single injection SC every day.

Dose adjustments – Chronic daily administration is required to maintain clinical benefit. ANC should not be used as the sole indication of efficacy. Individually adjust the dose based on the patient's clinical course as well as ANC. Reduce the dose if the ANC is persistently > 10,000/mm³.

►*Dilution of solution:* If required, filgrastim may be diluted in 5% Dextrose Solution. Filgrastim diluted to concentrations between 5 and 15 mcg/mL should be protected from adsorption to plastic materials by addition of albumin (human) to a final concentration of 2 mg/mL. When diluted in 5% Dextrose or 5% Dextrose plus albumin, filgrastim is compatible with glass bottles, PVC and polyolefin IV bags and polypropylene syringes. Dilution to a final concentration of < 5 mcg/mL is not recommended at any time. Do not dilute with saline at any time; product may precipitate.

►*Storage / Stability:* Refrigerate at 2° to 8°C (36° to 46°F). Avoid shaking. Prior to injection, filgrastim may be allowed to reach room temperature for a maximum of 24 hours. Discard any vial left at room temperature for > 24 hours. Use only one dose per vial; do not re-enter the vial. Use only one dose per prefilled syringe. Discard unused portions. Do not save unused drug for later administration. Parenteral drug products should be inspected visually for particulate matter and discoloration prior to administration whenever solution and container permit; if particulates or discoloration are observed, the container should not be used.

Actions

►*Pharmacology:* Filgrastim is a human granulocyte colony stimulating factor (G-CSF), produced by recombinant DNA technology. Filgrastim is produced by *Escherichia coli* bacteria inserted with the human G-CSF gene. G-CSF regulates the production of neutrophils within the bone marrow; endogenous G-CSF is a glycoprotein produced by monocytes, fibroblasts and endothelial cells. It has minimal direct in vivo or in vitro effects on the production of other hematopoietic cell types.

Colony stimulating factors are glycoproteins that act on hematopoietic cells by binding to specific cell surface receptors and stimulating proliferation, differentiation commitment and some end-cell functional activation. Endogenous G-CSF is a lineage-specific CSF with selectivity for neutrophil lineage. It is not species-specific and primarily affects neutrophil progenitor proliferation, differentiation and selected end-cell functional activation (including enhanced phagocytic ability, priming of the cellular metabolism associated with respiratory burst, antibody-dependent killing, and increased expression of functions associated with cell surface antigens).

►*Pharmacokinetics:* Absorption and clearance follow first-order pharmacokinetics without apparent concentration dependence. A positive linear correlation occurs between the parenteral dose and both the serum concentration and area under the concentration-time curve (AUC). Continuous IV infusion of 20 mcg/kg filgrastim over 24 hours resulted in mean and median serum concentrations of ≈ 48 and 56 ng/mL, respectively. Subcutaneous (SC) administration of 3.45 and 11.5 mcg/kg resulted in maximum serum concentrations of 4 and 49 ng/mL, respectively, within 2 to 8 hours. The volume of distribution averaged 150 mL/kg in both healthy subjects and cancer patients. The elimination half-life in both healthy subjects and cancer patients was ≈ 3.5 hours. Clearance rates were ≈ 0.5 to 0.7 mL/min/kg. Single parenteral doses or daily IV doses, over a 14-day period, resulted in comparable half-lives. The half-lives were similar for IV administration (231 minutes following doses of 34.5 mcg/kg) and for SC administration (210 minutes following doses of 3.45 mcg/kg). Continuous 24 hour IV infusions at 20 mcg/kg over an 11 to 20 day period produced steady-state serum concentrations of filgrastim with no evidence of drug accumulation over the time period investigated.

►*Clinical trials:*

Myelosuppressive chemotherapy – Filgrastim is safe and effective in accelerating the recovery of neutrophil counts across a variety of chemotherapy regimens. In a randomized, double-blind, placebo-controlled trial, patients with small-cell lung cancer received filgrastim or placebo. Filgrastim prevented infection as manifested by febrile neutropenia, decreased hospitalization and decreased IV antibiotic usage.

Bone marrow transplant (BMT) – In two separate randomized, controlled trials, patients with Hodgkin's and non-Hodgkin's lymphoma were treated with myeloablative chemotherapy and autologous bone marrow transplantation (ABMT). A statistically significant reduction in the median number of days of severe neutropenia (absolute neutrophil count [ANC] < 500/mm³) occurred in the filgrastim group vs controls. In one study, the number of days of febrile neutropenia was also reduced, as well as reductions in the number of hospitalization days and antibiotic use. Similar results were noted in myeloid and non-myeloid malignancies, breast cancer, malignant melanoma, acute lymphoblastic leukemia and germ cell tumor with ABMT.

FILGRASTIM (Granulocyte Colony Stimulating Factor; G-CSF)

Peripheral blood progenitor cells (PBPC) – Mobilization of PBPC was studied in 50 heavily pre-treated patients with non-Hodgkin's lymphoma, Hodgkin's disease, or acute lymphoblastic leukemia. Colony-forming-unit/granulocyte macrophage (CFU-GM) was used as the marker for engraftable PBPC. Both the CFU-GM and CD34+ cells reached a maximum on day 5 at > 10-fold over baseline and then remained elevated with leukapheresis.

Engraftment – In a randomized unblinded study of patients with Hodgkin's disease or non-Hodgkin's lymphoma undergoing myeloablative chemotherapy, 27 patients received filgrastim-mobilized PBPC followed by filgrastim and 31 patients received ABMT followed by filgrastim. Patients in the filgrastim-mobilized PBPC group had significantly fewer days of platelet transfusions, shorter time to a sustained platelet count, shorter time to recovery, fewer days of red blood cell transfusions and a shorter duration of post-transplant hospitalization.

Contraindications

Hypersensitivity to *E. coli*-derived proteins, filgrastim or any product components.

Warnings

➤*Hypothyroidism:* In one study, two patients with pre-existing antibodies to thyroid microsomes and to thyroglobulin and with normal thyroid function and size developed transient hypothyroidism and goiter that required thyroxine therapy.

➤*Hypersensitivity reactions:* Allergic-type reactions have occurred on initial or subsequent treatment in < 1 in 4000 patients treated with filgrastim. These have generally been characterized by systemic symptoms involving at least two body systems, most often skin (rash, urticaria, facial edema), respiratory (wheezing, dyspnea) and cardiovascular (hypotension, tachycardia). Some reactions occurred on initial exposure. Reactions tended to occur within the first 30 minutes after administration and appeared to occur more frequently in patients receiving IV filgrastim. Rapid resolution of symptoms occurred in most cases after administration of antihistamines, steroids, bronchodilators or epinephrine. Symptoms recurred in > 50% of patients who were rechallenged. Refer also to Management of Acute Hypersensitivity Reactions.

➤*Pregnancy: Category C.* There are no adequate and well-controlled studies in pregnant women. Use during pregnancy only if the potential benefit justifies the potential risk to the fetus.

➤*Lactation:* It is not known whether filgrastim is excreted in breast milk. Exercise caution if administering to a nursing woman.

➤*Children:* Serious long-term risks associated with daily filgrastim have not been identified in pediatric patients ages 4 months to 17 years with SCN.

The safety and efficacy in neonates and patients with autoimmune neutropenia of infancy have not been established.

In the cancer setting, 12 pediatric patients with neuroblastoma have received up to six cycles of cyclophosphamide, cisplatin, doxorubicin and etoposide chemo-therapy concurrently with filgrastim. In this population, filgrastim was well tolerated. There was one report of palpable splenomegaly associated with filgrastim therapy, however, the only consistently reported adverse event was musculoskeletal pain, which was no different from the experience in the adult population.

Precautions

➤*Monitoring:*

Myelosuppressive chemotherapy – Obtain complete blood count (CBC) and platelet counts prior to chemotherapy, and at regular intervals (twice per week) during therapy to avoid leukocytosis and to monitor the neutrophil count. Following cytotoxic chemotherapy, the neutrophil nadir occurred earlier during cycles when filgrastim was administered and WBC differentials demonstrated a left shift, including the appearance of promyelocytes and myeloblasts. In addition, the duration of severe neutropenia was reduced and was followed by an accelerated recovery in the neutrophil counts. Therefore, regular monitoring of WBC counts, particularly at the time of the recovery from the post-chemotherapy nadir, is recommended to avoid excessive leukocytosis. In clinical studies, therapy was discontinued when the ANC $\geq$ 10,000/mm³ after the expected chemotherapy-induced nadir.

BMT – Obtain CBC and platelet counts at a minimum of 3 times per week following marrow infusion to monitor the recovery of marrow reconstitution.

SCN – It is essential that serial complete blood cell counts with differential and platelet counts, and an evaluation of bone marrow morphology and karyotype be performed prior to initiation of therapy. The use of filgrastim prior to confirmation of SCN may impair diagnostic efforts and may thus impair or delay evaluation and treatment of an underlying condition, other than SCN, causing the neutropenia. During the initial 4 weeks of filgrastim therapy and during the 2 weeks following any dose adjustment, perform a CBC with differential and platelet count twice weekly. Once a patient is clinically stable, perform a CBC with differential and platelet count monthly.

➤*Simultaneous use with chemotherapy and radiation:* The safety and efficacy of filgrastim given simultaneously with cytotoxic chemotherapy or radiotherapy have not been established. Because of the potential sensitivity of rapidly dividing myeloid cells to cytotoxic chemotherapy, do not use filgrastim 24 hours before to 24 hours after the administration of cytotoxic chemotherapy (see Administration and Dosage).

➤*Growth factor potential:* Filgrastim is a growth factor that primarily stimulates neutrophils. However, the possibility that filgrastim can act as a growth factor for any tumor type, particularly myeloid malignancies, cannot be excluded. Therefore, exercise caution in using this drug in any malignancy with myeloid characteristics.

➤*Leukocytosis:* White blood cell counts of $\geq$ 100,000/mm³ were observed in $\approx$ 2% of patients receiving doses > 5 mcg/kg/day. There were no reports of adverse events associated with this degree of leukocytosis. To avoid potential complications of excessive leukocytosis, CBC is recommended twice per week during therapy (see Monitoring).

➤*Premature discontinuation of therapy:* A transient increase in neutrophil count is typically seen 1 to 2 days after therapy initiation. However, for a sustained therapeutic response, continue therapy until the post-setnadir ANC = 10,000/mm³. Therefore, premature discontinuation of therapy prior to recovery from the expected neutrophil nadir is generally not recommended (see Administration and Dosage).

➤*Hematologic effects:* Because of the potential of receiving higher doses of chemotherapy, the patient may be at greater risk of thrombocytopenia, anemia and non-hematologic consequences of increased chemotherapy doses. Fewer than 6% of patients had thrombocytopenia (< 50,000/mm³) during therapy, most of whom had a pre-existing history of thrombocytopenia. In most cases, thrombocytopenia was managed by dose reduction or interruption. An additional 5% of patients had platelet counts between 50,000 to 100,000/mm³. There were no associated serious hemorrhagic sequelae in these patients. Regular monitoring of the hematocrit and platelet count is recommended. Furthermore, exercise care in the use of filgrastim in conjunction with other drugs known to lower the platelet count. In septic patients, be alert to the possibility of adult respiratory distress syndrome, due to the possible influx of neutrophils at the inflammation site.

➤*Cardiac events (eg, myocardial infarctions, arrhythmias):* Such events have occurred in 11 of 375 cancer patients receiving filgrastim; the relationship to filgrastim therapy is unknown. However, closely monitor patients with pre-existing cardiac conditions.

➤*Medullary bone pain:* Occurred in 24% of patients. This bone pain was generally of mild-to-moderate severity, and could be controlled in most patients with nonnarcotic analgesics; infrequently, bone pain was severe enough to require narcotic analgesics. Bone pain occurred more frequently in patients treated with higher doses (20 to 100 mcg/kg/day) administered IV, and less frequently in patients treated with lower SC doses (3 to 10 mcg/kg/day).

➤*Cutaneous vasculitis:* There have been rare reports of cutaneous vasculitis in patients receiving filgrastim. In most cases the severity was moderate or severe. Most reports involved patients with severe chronic neutropenia receiving long-term therapy. Symptoms of vasculitis generally developed simultaneously with an increase in the ANC and abated when the ANC decreased. Many patients were able to continue therapy at a reduced dose.

Drug Interactions

Drug interactions have not been fully evaluated. Drugs that may potentiate the release of neutrophils, such as lithium, should be used with caution.

Adverse Reactions

➤*Miscellaneous:*

Myelosuppressive chemotherapy – In clinical trials, the most adverse experiences were the sequelae of the underlying malignancy or cytotoxic chemotherapy. Medullary bone pain, reported in 24% of patients, was the only consistently observed adverse reaction attributed to therapy (see Precautions).

Spontaneously reversible elevations in uric acid, lactate dehydrogenase and alkaline phosphatase occurred in 27% to 58% of patients receiving filgrastim therapy following cytotoxic chemotherapy; increases were generally mild to moderate. Transient decreases in blood pressure (< 90/60 mmHg), which did not require clinical treatment, were reported in 7 of 176 patients.

Filgrastim Adverse Reactions in Patients Receiving Myelosuppressive Chemotherapy (%)		
Adverse reactions	Filgrastim (n = 384)	Placebo (n = 257)
Nausea/Vomiting	57	64
Skeletal pain	22	11
Alopecia	18	27
Diarrhea	14	23
Neutropenic fever	13	35
Mucositis	12	20
Fever	12	11

FILGRASTIM (Granulocyte Colony Stimulating Factor; G-CSF)

Filgrastim Adverse Reactions in Patients Receiving Myelosuppressive Chemotherapy (%)		
Adverse reactions	Filgrastim (n = 384)	Placebo (n = 257)
Fatigue	11	16
Anorexia	9	11
Dyspnea	9	11
Headache	7	9
Cough	6	8
Skin rash	6	9
Chest pain	5	6
Generalized weakness	4	7
Sore throat	4	9
Stomatitis	5	10
Constipation	5	10
Pain (unspecified)	2	7

BMT – In clinical trials, the adverse reactions reported were those typically seen in patients receiving intensive chemotherapy followed by bone marrow transplantation. The most common events included stomatitis, nausea and vomiting, generally of mild-to-moderate severity and considered unrelated to filgrastim. In the randomized studies of BMT, the following occurred more frequently in patients treated with filgrastim than controls: Nausea (10%); vomiting (7%); hypertension (4%); rash (12%); peritonitis (2%); renal insufficiency, capillary leak syndrome (rare); erythema nodosum of moderate severity (1 patient).

PBPC Collection – Decreased platelet counts (97%); anemia (65%); mild to moderate musculoskeletal symptoms (44%); medullary bone pain (33%); headache (7%); increases in alkaline phosphatase (21%); increases in neutrophil counts; white blood cell > 100,000/mm³ (rare).

SCN – Mild to moderate bone pain, readily controlled with non-narcotic analgesics ($\approx$ 33%); palpable splenomegaly ($\approx$ 30%); epistaxis (15%; associated with thrombocytopenia in 2%); anemia ($\approx$ 10%, but in most cases appeared to be related to frequent diagnostic phlebotomy, chronic illness or concomitant medications); monosomy, splenomegaly (< 3%); myelodysplasia or myeloid leukemia ($\approx$ 3%); injection site reaction, rash, hepatomegaly, arthralgia, osteoporosis, increase in LDH, cutaneous vasculitis, hematuria/proteinuria, exacerbation of some pre-existing skin disorders (eg, psoriasis), alopecia (infrequent); abdominal/flank pain (infrequent); thrombocytopenia (see Precautions).

➤*Lab test abnormalities:* In clinical trials, the following laboratory results were observed. Cyclic fluctuations in the neutrophil counts were frequently observed in congenital or idiopathic neutropenia after initiation of filgrastim therapy. Platelet counts were generally at the upper limits of normal prior to therapy. With filgrastim therapy, platelet counts decreased but usually remained within normal limits. Early myeloid forms were noted in peripheral blood in most patients, including the appearance of metamyelocytes and myelocytes. Promyelocytes and myeloblasts were noted in some patients. Relative increases were occasionally noted in the number of circulating eosinophils and basophils. No consistent increases were observed with filgrastim therapy. Increases were observed in serum uric acid, lactic dehydrogenase and serum alkaline phosphatase.

Overdosage

To avoid the potential risks of excessive leukocytosis, discontinue therapy if the ANC surpasses 10,000/mm³ after the ANC nadir has occurred. Doses that increase the ANC > 10,000/mm³ may not result in any additional clinical benefit.

The maximum tolerated dose of filgrastim has not been determined. Efficacy was demonstrated at 4 to 8 mcg/kg/day in a study of non-myeloablative chemotherapy. Patients in the BMT study received up to 138 mcg/kg/day without toxic effects, although there was a flattening of the dose response curve above daily doses of > 10 mcg/kg/day. Discontinuation of therapy in patients receiving myelosuppressive chemotherapy usually results in a 50% decrease in circulating neutrophils within 1 to 2 days, with a return to pretreatment levels in 1 to 7 days.

Patient Information

If the patient can safely and effectively self administer filgrastim, instruct the patient as to the proper dosage and administration. Refer patients to the full "Information for Patients" section included with the product information; it is not a disclosure of all or possible intended effects.

PEGFILGRASTIM

Rx	Neulasta (Amgen)	Solution for Injection: 10 mg/mL	Preservative free. In dispensing pack containing single-dose syringe with needle.

Indications

➤*Myelosuppressive chemotherapy:* To decrease the incidence of infection, as manifested by febrile neutropenia, in patients with non-myeloid malignancies receiving myelosuppressive anticancer drugs associated with a clinically significant incidence of febrile neutropenia.

Administration and Dosage

➤*Approved by the FDA:* January 31, 2002.

The recommended dosage of pegfilgrastim is a single 6 mg SC injection administered once per chemotherapy cycle. Do not administer pegfilgrastim in the period between 14 days before and 24 hours after administration of cytotoxic chemotherapy.

Do not use the 6 mg fixed-dose formulation in infants, children, and smaller adolescents weighing < 45 kg.

Visually inspect pegfilgrastim for discoloration and particulate matter before administration. Do not administer pegfilgrastim if discoloration or particulates are observed.

➤*Storage / Stability:* Refrigerate pegfilgrastim at 2° to 8°C (36° to 46°F); keep syringes in their carton to protect from light until time of use. Avoid shaking. Before injection, pegfilgrastim may be allowed to reach room temperature for a maximum of 48 hours but should be protected from light. Discard pegfilgrastim left at room temperature for > 48 hours. Avoid freezing; however, if accidentally frozen, allow pegfilgrastim to thaw in the refrigerator before administration. Discard pegfilgrastim if frozen a second time.

Actions

➤*Pharmacology:* Filgrastim and pegfilgrastim are colony stimulating factors that act on hematopoietic cells by binding to specific cell surface receptors thereby stimulating proliferation, differentiation, commitment, and end cell functional activation. Studies on cellular proliferation, receptor binding, and neutrophil function demonstrate that filgrastim and pegfilgrastim have the same mechanism of action. Pegfilgrastim has reduced renal clearance and prolonged persistence in vivo as compared with filgrastim.

➤*Pharmacokinetics:* The pharmacokinetics and pharmacodynamics of pegfilgrastim were studied in 379 patients with cancer. The pharmacokinetics of pegfilgrastim were nonlinear in cancer patients and clearance decreased with increases in dose. Neutrophil receptor binding is an important component of the clearance of pegfilgrastim, and serum clearance is directly related to the number of neutrophils. For example, the concentration of pegfilgrastim declined rapidly at the onset of neutrophil recovery that followed myelosuppressive chemotherapy. In addition to numbers of neutrophils, body weight appeared to be a factor. Patients with higher body weights experienced higher systemic exposure to pegfilgrastim after receiving a dose normalized for body weight. A large variability in the pharmacokinetics of pegfilgrastim was observed in cancer patients. The half-life of pegfilgrastim ranged from 15 to 80 hours after SC injection.

➤*Clinical trials:* Pegfilgrastim was evaluated in 2 randomized, double-blind, active control studies employing 60 mg/m² doxorubicin and 75 mg/m² docetaxel administered every 21 days for up to 4 cycles for the treatment of metastatic breast cancer. Study 1 investigated the utility of a fixed dose of pegfilgrastim. Study 2 employed a weight-adjusted dose. The duration of severe neutropenia was chosen as the primary endpoint in both studies, and the efficacy of pegfilgrastim was demonstrated by establishing comparability to filgrastim-treated subjects in the mean days of severe neutropenia.

In the first study, 157 subjects were randomized to receive a single SC dose of 6 mg of pegfilgrastim on day 2 of each chemotherapy cycle or filgrastim at 5 mcg/kg/day SC beginning on day 2 of each cycle. In the second study, 310 subjects were randomized to receive a single SC injection of pegfilgrastim at 100 mcg/kg on day 2 or filgrastim at 5 mcg/kg/day SC beginning on day 2 of each cycle of chemotherapy.

The rates of febrile neutropenia in the 2 studies were comparable for pegfilgrastim and filgrastim (range, 10% to 20%).

Contraindications

Patients with known hypersensitivity to *Escherichia coli*-derived proteins, pegfilgrastim, filgrastim, or any other component of the product.

Warnings

➤*Pregnancy:* Category C. Pegfilgrastim has been shown to have adverse effects in pregnant rabbits when administered SC every other day during gestation at doses as low as 50 mcg/kg/dose ($\approx$ 4-fold higher than the recommended human dose). Pegfilgrastim doses of 200 and 250 mcg/kg/dose resulted in an increased incidence of abortions. Increased postimplantation loss caused by early resorptions was observed at doses of 200 to 1000 mcg/kg/dose and decreased numbers of live rabbit fetuses were observed at pegfilgrastim doses of 200 to 1000 mcg/kg/dose given every other day. Use pegfilgrastim in pregnancy only if the potential benefit to the mother justifies the potential risk to the fetus.

➤*Lactation:* It is not known whether pegfilgrastim is excreted in human milk. Because many drugs are excreted in human milk, exercise caution when pegfilgrastim is administered to a nursing woman.

PEGFILGRASTIM

➤*Children:* The safety and efficacy of pegfilgrastim in pediatric patients have not been established. Do not use the 6 mg fixed-dose single-use syringe formulation in infants, children, and smaller adolescents weighing < 45 kg.

Precautions

➤*Monitoring:* Obtain a CBC and platelet count before administering chemotherapy. Regular monitoring of hematocrit value and platelet count is recommended.

➤*Splenic rupture:* Rare cases of splenic rupture have been reported following the administration of the parent compound of pegfilgrastim, filgrastim, for peripheral blood progenitor cell (PBPC) mobilization in both healthy donors and patients with cancer. Some of these cases were fatal. Pegfilgrastim has not been evaluated in this setting; therefore, do not use pegfilgrastim for PBPC mobilization. Evaluate patients receiving pegfilgrastim who report left upper abdominal or shoulder tip pain for an enlarged spleen or splenic rupture.

➤*Adult respiratory distress syndrome (ARDS):* ARDS has been reported in neutropenic patients with sepsis receiving filgrastim, the parent compound of pegfilgrastim, and is postulated to be secondary to an influx of neutrophils to sites of inflammation in the lungs. Evaluate neutropenic patients receiving pegfilgrastim who develop fever, lung infiltrates, or respiratory distress for the possibility of ARDS. In the event that ARDS occurs, discontinue pegfilgrastim or withhold until resolution of ARDS and give patients appropriate medical management for this condition.

➤*Allergic reactions:* Allergic-type reactions, including anaphylaxis, skin rash, and urticaria, occurring with initial or subsequent treatment have been reported with the parent compound of pegfilgrastim, filgrastim. In some cases, symptoms have recurred with rechallenge, suggesting a causal relationship. Allergic-type reactions to pegfilgrastim have not been observed in clinical trials. If a serious allergic reaction or an anaphylactic reaction occurs, administer appropriate therapy and discontinue further use of pegfilgrastim.

➤*Sickle cell disease:* Severe sickle cell crises have been reported in patients with sickle cell disease (specifically homozygous sickle cell anemia, sickle/hemoglobin C disease, and sickle/β+ thalassemia) who received filgrastim, the parent compound of pegfilgrastim, for PBPC mobilization or following chemotherapy. One of these cases was fatal. Use pegfilgrastim with caution in patients with sickle cell disease, and only after careful consideration of the potential risks and benefits. Keep patients with sickle cell disease who receive pegfilgrastim well hydrated and monitor them for the occurrence of sickle cell crises. In the event of severe sickle cell crisis, administer supportive care and consider interventions to ameliorate the underlying event, such as therapeutic red blood cell exchange transfusion.

➤*Use with chemotherapy and/or radiation therapy:* Do not administer pegfilgrastim in the period between 14 days before and 24 hours after administration of cytotoxic chemotherapy (see Administration and Dosage) because of the potential for an increase in sensitivity of rapidly dividing myeloid cells to cytotoxic chemotherapy.

The use of pegfilgrastim has not been studied in patients receiving chemotherapy associated with delayed myelosuppression (eg, nitrosoureas, mitomycin C).

Administration of pegfilgrastim at 0, 1, and 3 days before 5-fluorouracil resulted in increased mortality in mice; administration of pegfilgrastim 24 hours after 5-fluorouracil did not adversely affect survival.

The use of pegfilgrastim has not been studied in patients receiving radiation therapy.

➤*Potential effect on malignant cells:* Pegfilgrastim is a growth factor that primarily stimulates neutrophils and neutrophil precursors; however, the G-CSF receptor through which pegfilgrastim and filgrastim act has been found on tumor cell lines, including some myeloid, T-lymphoid, lung, head and neck, and bladder tumor cell lines. The possibility that pegfilgrastim can act as a growth factor for any tumor type cannot be excluded. Use of pegfilgrastim in myeloid malignancies and myelodysplasia has not been studied.

Drug Interactions

Drugs such as lithium may potentiate the release of neutrophils; patients receiving lithium and pegfilgrastim should have more frequent monitoring of neutrophil counts.

Adverse Reactions

Most adverse experiences in clinical studies were attributed by the investigators to the underlying malignancy or cytotoxic chemotherapy and occurred at similar rates in subjects who received pegfilgrastim (n = 465) or filgrastim (n = 331). These adverse experiences occurred at rates between 72% and 15% and included the following: Nausea, fatigue, alopecia, diarrhea, vomiting, constipation, fever, anorexia, skeletal pain, headache, taste perversion, dyspepsia, myalgia, insomnia, abdominal pain, arthralgia, generalized weakness, peripheral edema, dizziness, granulocytopenia, stomatitis, mucositis, and neutropenic fever.

The most common adverse event attributed to pegfilgrastim in clinical trials was medullary bone pain, reported in 26% of subjects, which was comparable with the incidence in filgrastim-treated patients. This bone pain was generally reported to be of mild to moderate severity.

Leukocytosis (WBC counts > 100×10^9/L) was observed in < 1% of 465 subjects with nonmyeloid malignancies receiving pegfilgrastim.

The only serious event that was not deemed attributable to underlying or concurrent disease, or to concurrent therapy, was a case of hypoxia.

➤*Lab test abnormalities:* Reversible elevations in LDH, alkaline phosphatase, and uric acid, which did not require treatment intervention, were observed. The incidences of these changes, presented for pegfilgrastim relative to filgrastim, were the following: LDH (19% vs 29%), alkaline phosphatase (9% vs 16%), and uric acid (8% vs 9% [1% of reported cases for both treatment groups were classified as severe]).

➤*Miscellaneous:*
Immunogenicity – Cytopenias resulting from an antibody response to exogenous growth factors have been reported on rare occasions in patients treated with other recombinant growth factors.

Overdosage

The maximum amount of pegfilgrastim that can be administered safely in single or multiple doses has not been determined. Consider leukapheresis in the management of symptomatic individuals.

Patient Information

Inform patients of the possible side effects of pegfilgrastim, and instruct them to report side effects to the prescribing physician. Inform patients of the signs and symptoms of allergic drug reactions and advise them of appropriate actions. Counsel patients on the importance of compliance with their pegfilgrastim treatment, including regular monitoring of blood counts.

If it is determined that a patient or caregiver can safely and effectively administer pegfilgrastim at home, provide appropriate instruction on the proper use of pegfilgrastim to patients and their caregivers, including careful review of the "Information for Patients and Caregivers" insert. Caution patients and their caregivers against the reuse of needles, syringes, or drug product, and thoroughly instruct them in proper disposal techniques. Make available a puncture-resistant container for the disposal of used syringes and needles.

SARGRAMOSTIM (Granulocyte Macrophage Colony Stimulating Factor; GM-CSF)

Rx	Leukine (Berlex)	Powder for injection, lyophilized: 250 mcg	Preservative-free. In vials.[1]
		Liquid: 500 mcg/mL	1.1% benzyl alcohol. In multiple-dose vials.[1]

[1] With 40 mg mannitol, 10 mg sucrose, 1.2 mg tromethamine per mL.

Indications

➤*Myeloid reconstitution after autologous bone marrow transplantation (BMT):* In patients with non-Hodgkin's lymphoma (NHL), acute lymphoblastic leukemia (ALL), and Hodgkin's disease undergoing autologous BMT.

➤*BMT failure or engraftment delay:* For patients who have undergone allogeneic or autologous BMT in whom engraftment is delayed or has failed.

Survival benefit may be relatively greater in those patients who demonstrate ≥ 1 of the following characteristics: Autologous BMT failure or engraftment delay; no previous total body irradiation; malignancy other than leukemia; or a multiple organ failure score ≤ 2.

➤*Following induction chemotherapy in acute myelogenous leukemia (AML):* For use following induction chemotherapy in older patients with AML to shorten neutrophil recovery time and reduce the incidence of severe and life-threatening infections and infections resulting in death. Safety and efficacy have not been assessed in AML patients < 55 years of age.

➤*Mobilization and following transplantation of autologous peripheral blood progenitor cells (PBPC):* For mobilization of hematopoietic progenitor cells into peripheral blood for collection by leukapheresis. Mobilization allows collection of increased progenitor cells capable of engraftment compared with collection without mobilization. After myeloablative chemotherapy, the transplantation of an increased number of progenitor cells can lead to more rapid engraftment, which may decrease the need for supportive care. Myeloid reconstitution is also accelerated by administration following PBPC transplantation.

SARGRAMOSTIM (Granulocyte Macrophage Colony Stimulating Factor; GM-CSF)

➤*Myeloid reconstitution after allogeneic BMT:* For acceleration of myeloid recovery in patients undergoing allogeneic BMT from human lymphocyte antigen (HLA)-matched related donors. Safety and efficacy have been established in accelerating myeloid engraftment, reducing the incidence of bacteremia and other culture-positive infections and shortening the median duration of hospitalization.

➤*Unlabeled uses:* Crohn's disease, melanoma, wound healing, mucositis, stomatitis, vaccine adjuvancy.

Administration and Dosage

➤*Approved by the FDA:* March 1991.

➤*Myeloid reconstitution after autologous or allogeneic BMT:* 250 mcg/m^2/day as a 2-hour IV infusion beginning 2 to 4 hours after the bone marrow infusion and $\geq$ 24 hours after the last dose of chemotherapy or radiotherapy. If a severe adverse reaction occurs, reduce dose by 50% or temporarily discontinue the dose until the reaction abates. If blast cells appear or progression of the underlying disease occurs, discontinue treatment immediately. Interrupt or reduce dose by half if the ANC is > 20,000 cells/mm^3. Patients should not receive sargramostim until the post–marrow infusion ANC is < 500 cells/mm^3. Continue until ANC > 1500 cells/mm^3 for 3 consecutive days is attained.

To avoid potential complications of excessive leukocytosis (WBC > 50,000 cells/mm^3; ANC > 20,000 cells/mm^3), a CBC with differential is recommended twice weekly during therapy. Interrupt or reduce the dose by half if the ANC> 20,000 cells/mm^3.

➤*Neutrophil recovery following chemotherapy in AML:* 250 mcg/m^2/day IV over a 4-hour period starting approximately day 11 or 4 days following the completion of induction chemotherapy, if the day 10 bone marrow is hypoplastic with < 5% blasts. If a second cycle of induction chemotherapy is necessary, administer $\approx$ 4 days after the completion of chemotherapy if the bone marrow is hypoplastic with < 5% blasts. Continue sargramostim until ANC > 1500 cells/mm^3 for 3 consecutive days or a maximum of 42 days. Discontinue immediately if leukemic regrowth occurs. If a severe adverse reaction occurs, reduce the dose by 50% or temporarily discontinue the dose until the reaction abates.

To avoid potential complications of excessive leukocytosis (WBC > 50,000 cells/mm^3; ANC > 20,000 cells/mm^3), a CBC with differential is recommended twice weekly during therapy. Interrupt or reduce the dose by half if the ANC exceeds 20,000 cells/mm^3.

➤*Mobilization of PBPC:* 250 mcg/m^2/day IV over 24 hours or SC once daily. Continue at the same dose through the period of PBPC collection. The optimal schedule for PBPC collection has not been established. In clinical studies, PBPC collection was usually begun by day 5 and performed daily until protocol specified targets were achieved (see Clinical Trials, Mobilization of PBPC and Engraftment). If WBC > 50,000 cells/mm^3, reduce the dose by 50%. If adequate numbers of progenitor cells are not collected, consider other mobilization therapy.

➤*Post-PBPC transplantation:* 250 mcg/m^2/day IV over 24 hours or SC once daily beginning immediately following infusion of progenitor cells and continuing until an ANC > 1500 cells/mm^3 for 3 consecutive days is attained.

➤*BMT failure or engraftment delay:* 250 mcg/m^2/day for 14 days as a 2-hour IV infusion. The dose can be repeated after 7 days off therapy if engraftment has not occurred. If engraftment still has not occurred, a third course of 500 mcg/m^2/day for 14 days may be tried after another 7 days off therapy. If there is still no improvement, it is unlikely that further dose escalation will be beneficial. If a severe adverse reaction occurs, reduce the dose by 50% or temporarily discontinue the dose until the reaction abates. If blast cells appear or disease progression occurs, discontinue treatment immediately.

To avoid potential complications of excessive leukocytosis (WBC > 50,000 cells/mm^3; ANC > 20,000 cells/mm^3), a CBC with differential is recommended twice weekly during therapy. Interrupt or reduce the dose by half if the ANC> 20,000 cells/mm^3.

➤*Preparation:*

1.) Reconstitute with 1 mL Sterile Water for Injection or 1 mL Bacteriostatic Water for Injection.

2.) During reconstitution, direct the diluent at the side of the vial and gently swirl the contents to avoid foaming during dissolution. Avoid excessive or vigorous agitation; do not shake.

3.) Use sargramostim for SC injection without further dilution. Perform dilution for IV infusion in 0.9% Sodium Chloride Injection. If the final concentration is < 10 mcg/mL, add albumin (human) at a final concentration of 0.1% to the saline prior to addition of sargramostim to prevent adsorption to the components of the drug delivery system. For a final concentration of 0.1% albumin (human), add 1 mg albumin (human) per 1 mL 0.9% Sodium Chloride Injection (eg, use 1 mL 5% Albumin [Human] in 50 mL 0.9% Sodium Chloride Injection).

4.) Do not use an in-line membrane filter for IV infusion.

5.) In the absence of compatibility and stability information, do not add other medication to infusion solutions containing sargramo-

stim. Use only 0.9% Sodium Chloride Injection to prepare IV infusion solutions.

6.) Employ aseptic technique in the preparation of all sargramostim solutions. To assure correct concentration following reconstitution, take care to eliminate any air bubbles from the needle hub of the syringe used to prepare the diluent. Visually inspect parenteral drug products for particulate matter and discoloration prior to administration whenever solution and container permit. Do not use beyond the expiration date printed on the vial.

➤*Storage/Stability:* Store sargramostim liquid and reconstituted lyophilized solutions under refrigeration at 2° to 8°C (36° to 46°F). Do not freeze or shake.

Liquid sargramostim – Sargramostim liquid may be stored for up to 20 days at 2° to 8°C (36° to 46°F) once the vial has been entered. Discard any remaining solution after 20 days.

Lyophilized sargramostim – Reconstitute lyophilized sargramostim aseptically with 1 mL diluent. Do not mix together the contents of vials reconstituted with different diluents.

Sterile Water for Injection (without preservative): Lyophilized sargramostim vials contain no antibacterial preservative; therefore administer solutions prepared with Sterile Water for Injection as soon as possible, and within 6 hours following reconstitution or dilution for IV infusion. Do not re-enter or reuse the vial. Do not save any unused portion for administration > 6 hours following reconstitution.

Bacteriostatic Water for Injection (0.9% benzyl alcohol): Reconstituted solutions prepared with Bacteriostatic Water for Injection (0.9% benzyl alcohol) may be stored for up to 20 days at 2° to 8°C (36° to 46°F) prior to use. Discard reconstituted solution after 20 days. Previously reconstituted solutions mixed with freshly reconstituted solutions must be administered within 6 hours following mixing. Do not use preparations containing benzyl alcohol (including liquid sargramostim and lyophilized sargramostim reconstituted with Bacteriostatic Water for Injection) in neonates (see Precautions).

Actions

➤*Pharmacology:* Sargramostim is a recombinant human (rhu) GM-CSF produced by recombinant DNA technology in a yeast (*Saccharomyces cerevisiae*) expression system. GM-CSF is a hematopoietic growth factor that stimulates proliferation and differentiation of hematopoietic progenitor cells. Sargramostim is a glycoprotein of 127 amino acids. The amino acid sequence differs from the natural human GM-CSF by substituting leucine at position 23; the carbohydrate moiety may be different from the native protein.

GM-CSF belongs to a group of growth factors termed colony stimulating factors that support survival, clonal expansion, and differentiation of hematopoietic progenitor cells. GM-CSF induces partially committed progenitor cells to divide and differentiate in the granulocyte-macrophage pathways.

GM-CSF can activate mature granulocytes and macrophages. GM-CSF is a multilineage factor and, in addition to dose-dependent effects on the myelomonocytic lineage, can promote the proliferation of megakaryocytic and erythroid progenitors. Other factors are also required to induce complete maturation in these 2 lineages. The various cellular responses (division, maturation, activation) are induced through GM-CSF binding to specific receptors expressed on the cell surface of target cells.

The biological activity of GM-CSF is species-specific. Chemotactic, antifungal, and antiparasitic activities of granulocytes and monocytes are increased by exposure to sargramostim. Sargramostim increases the cytotoxicity of monocytes toward certain neoplastic cell lines and activates polymorphonuclear neutrophils to inhibit the growth of tumor cells.

➤*Pharmacokinetics:* Pharmacokinetic profiles have been analyzed in controlled studies of 24 healthy male volunteers. Liquid and lyophilized sargramostim, at the recommended dose of 250 mcg/m^2, have been determined to be bioequivalent based on the statistical evaluation of AUC.

When sargramostim (either liquid or lyophilized) was administered IV over 2 hours to healthy volunteers, the mean beta half-life was $\approx$ 60 minutes. Peak concentrations of GM-CSF were observed in blood samples obtained during or immediately after completion of sargramostim infusion. For sargramostim liquid, the mean maximum concentration (C_{max}) was 5 ng/mL, the mean clearance rate was $\approx$ 420 mL/min/m^2 and the mean $AUC_{0-\infty}$ was 640 ng/mL•min. Corresponding results for lyophilized sargramostim in the same subjects were mean C_{max} of 5.4 ng/mL, mean clearance rate of 431 mL/min/m^2, and mean $AUC_{0-\infty}$ of 677 ng/mL•min. GM-CSF was last detected in blood samples obtained at 3 or 6 hours.

When sargramostim (liquid or lyophilized) was administered SC to healthy volunteers, GM-CSF was detected in the serum at 15 minutes, the first sample point. The mean beta half-life was $\approx$ 162 minutes. Peak levels occurred at 1 to 3 hours postinjection, and sargramostim remained detectable for up to 6 hours after injection. The mean C_{max} was 1.5 ng/mL. For sargramostim liquid, the mean clearance was 549 mL/min/m^2 and the mean $AUC_{0-\infty}$ was 549 ng/mL•min. For lyophi-

SARGRAMOSTIM (Granulocyte Macrophage Colony Stimulating Factor; GM-CSF)

lized sargramostim, the mean clearance was 529 mL/min/m^2 and the mean AUC$_{0-\infty}$ was 501 ng/mL•min.

➤Clinical trials:

Mobilization of PBPCs and engraftment – Mobilization of PBPC and myeloid reconstitution post-transplant were compared between 4 groups of patients (n = 196) receiving sargramostim for mobilization and a historical control group that did not receive any mobilization treatment. Sequential cohorts received sargramostim. The cohorts differed by dose (125 or 250 mcg/m^2/day), route (IV over 24 hours or SC) and use of posttransplant sargramostim. Leukaphereses were initiated for all mobilization groups after the WBC reached 10,000/mm^3. PBPCs from patients treated at the 250 mcg/m^2/day dose had a significantly higher number of granulocyte-macrophage colony-forming units (CFU-GM) than those collected without mobilization. After transplantation, mobilized subjects had shorter times to myeloid engraftment and fewer days between transplantation and the last platelet transfusion compared with nonmobilized subjects.

BMT failure or engraftment delay – In 1 study, 140 patients experiencing graft failure following allogeneic or autologous BMT were evaluated in comparison with 103 historical controls; 163 had lymphoid or myeloid leukemia, 24 had NHL, 19 had Hodgkin's disease, and 37 had other diseases (eg, aplastic anemia, myelodysplasia, nonhematologic malignancy). Three categories of patients were eligible: 1) Patients displaying a delay in engraftment (ANC ≤ 100 cells/mm^3 by day 28 posttransplantation; 2) patients displaying a delay in engraftment (ANC ≤ 100 cells/mm^3 by day 21 posttransplantation) who had evidence of an active infection; and 3) patients who lost their marrow graft after a transient engraftment (manifested by an average of ANC ≥ 500 cells/mm^3 for ≥ 1 week followed by loss of engraftment with ANC < 500 cells/mm^3 for ≥ 1 week beyond day 21 posttransplantation.

One hundred day survival was improved in patients treated with sargramostim after graft failure following either autologous or allogeneic BMT. In addition, the median survival was improved by > 2-fold. Median survival of patients treated with sargramostim after autologous failure was 474 days vs 161 days for the historical patients. After allogeneic failure, median survival was 97 days vs 35 days, respectively. Improvement in survival was better in those with fewer impaired organs.

Contraindications

Excessive leukemic myeloid blasts in the bone marrow or peripheral blood (≥ 10%); known hypersensitivity to GM-CSF, yeast-derived products or any component of the product; simultaneous administration with cytotoxic chemotherapy or radiotherapy, or administration 24 hours preceding or following chemotherapy or radiotherapy.

Warnings

➤*Cardiovascular symptoms:* Occasional transient supraventricular arrhythmia has occurred during administration, particularly in patients with a previous history of cardiac arrhythmia. However, these arrhythmias have been reversible after discontinuation of sargramostim. Use with caution in patients with pre-existing cardiac disease.

➤*Respiratory symptoms:* Sequestration of granulocytes in the pulmonary circulation has occurred following sargramostim infusion, occasionally with dyspnea. Give special attention to respiratory symptoms during or immediately following infusion, especially in patients with pre-existing lung disease. In patients displaying dyspnea during administration, reduce the rate of infusion by half. Subsequent IV infusions may be administered following the standard dose schedule with careful monitoring. If respiratory symptoms worsen despite infusion rate reduction, discontinue infusion. Administer with caution in patients with hypoxia.

➤*Fluid retention:* Edema, capillary leak syndrome, and pleural or pericardial effusion have been reported in patients after sargramostim administration. In 156 patients enrolled in placebo-controlled studies using sargramostim at a dose of 250 mcg/m^2/day by 2-hour IV infusion, the reported incidences of fluid retention (sargramostim vs placebo) were as follows: Peripheral edema 11% vs 7%; pleural effusion 1% vs 0%; and pericardial effusion 4% vs 1%. Capillary leak syndrome was not observed in this limited number of studies; based on other uncontrolled studies and reports from users of marketed sargramostim, the incidence is estimated to be < 1%. In patients with pre-existing pleural and pericardial effusions, administration of sargramostim may aggravate fluid retention; however, fluid retention associated with or worsened by sargramostim has been reversible after interruption or dose reduction with or without diuretic therapy. Use with caution in pre-existing fluid retention, pulmonary infiltrates, or CHF.

➤*Hypersensitivity reactions:* Use appropriate precautions during parenteral administration of recombinant proteins in case an allergic or untoward reaction occurs. Serious allergic or anaphylactic reactions have been reported. If any serious allergic or anaphylactoid reaction occurs, immediately discontinue and initiate appropriate therapy. Refer to Management of Acute Hypersensitivity Reactions.

➤*Renal/Hepatic function impairment:* In some patients with pre-existing renal or hepatic dysfunction, sargramostim has induced elevation of serum creatinine or bilirubin and hepatic enzymes. Dose reduction or interruption has resulted in a decrease to pretreatment values. Monitoring of renal and hepatic function in patients with renal or hepatic dysfunction prior to initiation of treatment is recommended at least every other week during sargramostim administration.

➤*Pregnancy: Category C.* It is not known whether sargramostim can cause fetal harm or affect reproduction capacity when administered to a pregnant woman. Give to a pregnant woman only if clearly needed.

➤*Lactation:* It is not known whether sargramostim is excreted in breast milk. Administer sargramostim to a nursing woman only if clearly needed.

➤*Children:* Safety and efficacy have not been established; however, available data indicate that sargramostim does not exhibit any greater toxicity in children than in adults. A total of 124 pediatric subjects between the ages of 4 months and 18 years have been treated with 60 to 1000 mcg/m^2/day IV and 4 to 1500 mcg/m^2/day SC (see Precautions).

Precautions

➤*Benzyl alcohol:* Benzyl alcohol is a constituent of sargramostim liquid and Bacteriostatic Water for Injection diluent. Benzyl alcohol has been associated with a fatal "gasping syndrome" in premature infants. Do not administer liquid solutions containing benzyl alcohol (including sargramostim liquid) or lyophilized sargramostim reconstituted with Bacteriostatic Water for Injection (0.9% benzyl alcohol) to neonates.

➤*Growth factor potential:* Sargramostim is a growth factor that primarily stimulates normal myeloid precursors. However, the possibility that sargramostim can act as a growth factor for any tumor type, particularly myeloid malignancies, cannot be excluded. Exercise caution when using this drug in any malignancy with myeloid characteristics. Should disease progression be detected, discontinue therapy.

➤*First dose effects:* A syndrome with respiratory distress, hypoxia, flushing, hypotension, syncope, or tachycardia has occurred following the first administration in a particular cycle. These signs have resolved with symptomatic treatment and usually do not recur with subsequent doses in the same cycle of treatment.

➤*Increase in peripheral blood counts:* Stimulation of marrow precursors with sargramostim may result in a rapid rise in WBC count. If the ANC exceeds 20,000 cells/mm^3 or if the platelet count exceeds 500,000/mm^3, interrupt administration or reduce the dose by half. Base the decision to reduce the dose or interrupt treatment on the clinical condition of the patient. Excessive blood counts have returned to normal or baseline levels within 3 to 7 days following cessation of therapy. Perform twice-weekly monitoring of CBC with differential (including examination for the presence of blast cells) to preclude development of excessive counts.

➤*Purged bone marrow:* Sargramostim is effective in accelerating myeloid recovery in patients receiving bone marrow purged by anti-B lymphocyte monoclonal antibodies. Data obtained from uncontrolled studies suggest that if in vitro marrow purging with chemical agents causes a significant decrease in the number of responsive hematopoietic progenitors, the patient may not respond to sargramostim. When the bone marrow purging process preserves a sufficient number of progenitors (> 1.2 × 10^4/kg), a beneficial effect of sargramostim on myeloid engraftment has occurred.

➤*Previous exposure to intensive chemotherapy/radiotherapy:* In patients who have received extensive radiotherapy to hematopoietic sites for the treatment of primary disease in the abdomen or chest before autologous BMT, or have been exposed to multiple myelotoxic agents (eg, alkylating agents, anthracycline antibiotics, antimetabolites), the effect of sargramostim on myeloid reconstitution may be limited.

➤*Patients with malignancy undergoing sargramostim-mobilized PBPC collection:* When using sargramostim to mobilize PBPC, the limited in vitro data suggest that tumor cells may be released and reinfused into the patient in the leukapheresis product. The effect of reinfusion of tumor cells has not been well studied and the data are inconclusive.

➤*Concomitant use with chemotherapy and radiotherapy:* Because of potential sensitivity of rapidly dividing hematopoietic progenitor cells, do not administer within 24 hours preceding or following chemotherapy or radiotherapy (see Contraindications).

➤*Monitoring:* Sargramostim can induce variable increases in WBC or platelet counts. To avoid potential complications of excessive leukocytosis (WBC > 50,000 cells/mm^3; ANC > 20,000 cells/mm^3), perform a CBC twice weekly during therapy. Monitoring (at least biweekly) of renal and hepatic function in patients with renal or hepatic dysfunction prior to initiation of treatment is recommended. Carefully monitor body weight and hydration status during administration (see Warnings).

Drug Interactions

Use drugs that may potentiate the myeloproliferative effects of sargramostim, such as lithium and corticosteroids, with caution.

SARGRAMOSTIM (Granulocyte Macrophage Colony Stimulating Factor; GM-CSF)

Adverse Reactions

Sargramostim Adverse Reactions (%)[a]		
Adverse reaction	Sargramostim (n = 184)	Placebo (n = 180)
Cardiovascular		
Hypertension	25 to 34	32
Hemorrhage	23 to 29	30 to 43
Cardiac event	23	32
Hypotension	13	26
Tachycardia	11	9
CNS		
Neuroclinical	42	53
Headache	36	36
Neuromotor	25	26
Neuropsych	15	26
CNS disorder	11	16
Paresthesia	11	13
Insomnia	11	9
Anxiety	11	2
Neurosensory	6	11
Dermatologic		
Skin events	77	45
Rash	44 to 70	38 to 73
Alopecia	37 to 73	45 to 74
Pruritus	23	13
GI		
Nausea	58 to 90	55 to 96
Diarrhea	52 to 89	53 to 82
Vomiting	46 to 85	34 to 90
Abdominal pain	38	23
GI disorder	37	47
Stomatitis	24 to 62	29 to 63
Dyspepsia	17	20
Anorexia	13 to 54	11 to 58
Hematemesis	13	7
Dysphagia	11	7
GI hemorrhage	11 to 27	5 to 33
Constipation	8	11
Abdominal distention	4	13
GU		
GU event	50	57
Bilirubinemia	30	27
Urinary tract disorder	14	13
Hematuria	9	21
Kidney function, abnormal	8	10
Hemic/Lymphatic		
Blood dyscrasia	25	27
Thrombocytopenia	19	34
Coagulation event	19	21
Leukopenia	17	29
Petechia	6	11
Agranulocytosis	6	11
Musculoskeletal		
Bone pain	21	5
Arthralgia	11	4
Respiratory		
Pulmonary event	48	64
Pharyngitis	23	13
Lung disorder	20	23
Epistaxis	17	16
Dyspnea	15 to 28	14 to 31
Rhinitis	11	14

Sargramostim Adverse Reactions (%)[a]		
Adverse reaction	Sargramostim (n = 184)	Placebo (n = 180)
Miscellaneous		
Fever	77 to 95	74 to 96
Liver event	77	83
Mucous membrane disorder	75	78
Infection	65	68
Metabolic disorder	58	49
Malaise	57	51
Weight loss	37	28
Chills	19 to 25	20 to 26
Asthenia	17 to 66	20 to 51
Pain	17	36
Chest pain	15	9
Edema	13 to 34	11 to 35
Liver damage	13	14
Allergy	12	15
Peripheral edema	11 to 15	7 to 21
Sepsis	11	14
Eye hemorrhage	11	0
Back pain	9	18
Weight gain	8	21
Sweats	6	13
Lab test abnormalities		
Low albumin	27	36
High glucose	25 to 41	23 to 49
High BUN	23	17
High cholesterol	17	8
Increased creatinine	15	14
Hypomagnesemia	15	9
Increased ALT	13	16
Increased alkaline phosphatase	8	14
Low calcium	2	7

[a] Data pooled from separate studies, including allogeneic BMT patients, AML patients and following autologous BMT or peripheral blood progenitor transplantation.

▶*Autologous and allogeneic BMT:* In some patients with pre-existing renal or hepatic dysfunction enrolled in uncontrolled clinical trials, administration of sargramostim has induced elevation of serum creatinine or bilirubin and hepatic enzymes (see Warnings); headache (26%); pericardial effusion (25%); arthralgia (21%); myalgia (18%).

The most frequent adverse events were fever, asthenia, headache, bone pain, chills, and myalgia. These systemic events generally were mild or moderate and usually were prevented or reversed by the administration of analgesics and antipyretics such as acetaminophen. In these uncontrolled trials, other infrequent events reported were dyspnea, peripheral edema, and rash. Reports of events occurring with marketed sargramostim include arrhythmia, fainting, dizziness, eosinophilia, hypotension, injection site reactions, pain (including abdominal, back, chest and joint pain), tachycardia, thrombosis, and transient liver function abnormalities.

Overdosage

The maximum amount that can be safely administered in single or multiple doses has not been determined. Doses ≤ 100 mcg/kg/day (4000 mcg/m^2/day or 16 times the recommended dose) were administered to 4 patients for 7 to 18 days.

▶*Symptoms:* Increases in WBC ≤ 200,000 cells/mm^3 were observed. Adverse events reported were dyspnea, malaise, nausea, fever, rash, sinus tachycardia, headache, and chills. All these events were reversible after discontinuation of sargramostim.

▶*Treatment:* Discontinue therapy and carefully monitor the patient for WBC increase and respiratory symptoms.

OPRELVEKIN (Interleukin 11; IL-11)

Rx	Neumega (Genetics Institute)	**Powder for injection, lyophilized:** 5 mg	1.6 mg dibasic sodium phosphate heptahydrate, 0.55 mg monobasic sodium phosphate monohydrate. Preservative free. In single-dose vials with diluent.

Indications

➤*Thrombocytopenia, prevention:* For the prevention of severe thrombocytopenia and the reduction of the need for platelet transfusions following myelosuppressive chemotherapy in patients with non-myeloid malignancies who are at high risk of severe thrombocytopenia.

➤*Unlabeled uses:* Crohn's disease.

Administration and Dosage

➤*Approved by the FDA:* November 25, 1997.

The recommended dose in adults is 50 mcg/kg given once daily. Administer SC as a single injection in either the abdomen, thigh, or hip (or upper arm if not self-injecting). The safety and efficacy of oprelvekin has not been established in children (see Warnings).

Initiate dosing 6 to 24 hours after the completion of chemotherapy. Monitor platelet counts periodically to assess the optimal duration of therapy. Continue dosing until the post-nadir platelet count is ≥ 50,000 cells/mcL. In controlled clinical studies, doses were administered in courses of 10 to 21 days; dosing beyond 21 days per treatment course is not recommended. Discontinue treatment with oprelvekin ≥ 2 days before starting the next planned cycle of chemotherapy.

➤*Reconstitution:* Reconstitute oprelvekin aseptically with 1 mL of Sterile Water for Injection (without preservative), direct at the side of the vial and swirl the contents gently. Avoid excessive or vigorous agitation. The reconstituted solution contains 5 mg/mL of oprelvekin. Do not re-enter or reuse the single-use vial. Discard any unused portion of either reconstituted oprelvekin solution or Sterile Water for Injection.

➤*Storage/Stability:* Store lyophilized oprelvekin and diluent in a refrigerator at 2° to 8°C (36° to 46°F). Protect from light. Do not freeze. Because neither oprelvekin powder for injection, nor its accompanying diluent, Sterile Water for Injection contains a preservative; use reconstituted oprelvekin within 3 hours of reconstitution and store in the vial either at 2° to 8°C (36° to 46°F) or at room temperature ≤ 25°C (77°F). Do not freeze or shake the reconstituted solution.

Actions

➤*Pharmacology:* Interleukin eleven (IL-11) is a thrombopoietic growth factor that directly stimulates the proliferation of hematopoietic stem cells and megakaryocyte progenitor cells and induces megakaryocyte maturation, resulting in increased platelet production. IL-11 is a member of a family of human growth factors that includes human growth hormone, granulocyte colony-stimulating factor (G-CSF), and other growth factors.

Oprelvekin is produced in *Escherichia coli* by recombinant DNA methods. The protein has a molecular mass of ≈ 19,000 daltons and is non-glycosylated. The polypeptide is 177 amino acids in length and differs from the 178 amino acid length of native IL-11 only in lacking the amino-terminal proline residue. IL-11 is produced by bone marrow stromal cells and is part of the cytokine family that shares the gp130 signal transducer. Primary osteoblasts and mature osteoclasts express mRNAs for IL-11 receptor (IL-11R alpha) and gp130. Bone-forming and bone-resorbing cells are potential targets of IL-11.

The primary hematopoietic activity of oprelvekin is stimulation of megakaryocytopoiesis and thrombopoiesis. Oprelvekin has shown potent thrombopoietic activity in animal models of compromised hematopoiesis. In the models, oprelvekin improved platelet nadirs and accelerated platelet recoveries compared with controls.

Mature megakaryocytes that develop during in vivo treatment with oprelvekin are ultrastructurally normal. Platelets produced in response to oprelvekin were morphologically and functionally normal and possessed a normal lifespan.

IL-11 has nonhematopoietic activities in animals including: The regulation of intestinal epithelium growth (enhanced healing of GI lesions), the inhibition of adipogenesis, the induction of acute phase protein synthesis, inhibition of proinflammatory cytokine production by macrophages, and the stimulation of osteoclastogenesis and neurogenesis.

In a study in which oprelvekin was administered to nonmyelosuppressed cancer patients, daily SC dosing for 14 days with oprelvekin increased the platelet count in a dose-dependent manner. Platelet counts began to increase relative to baseline between 5 and 9 days after the start of dosing with oprelvekin. After cessation of treatment, platelet counts continued to increase for ≤ 7 days then returned toward baseline within 14 days.

Healthy volunteers receiving oprelvekin had a mean increase in plasma volume of > 20% and subjects receiving oprelvekin had a ≥ 10% increase in plasma volume. Red blood cell volume decreased similarly (because of repeated phlebotomy) in the oprelvekin and placebo groups. As a result, whole blood volume increased ≈ 10% and hemoglobin concentration decreased ≈ 10% in subjects receiving oprelvekin compared with placebo. Mean 24-hour sodium excretion decreased compared with placebo.

➤*Pharmacokinetics:* In a study in which a single 50 mcg/kg SC dose was administered to 18 men, the peak serum concentration (C_{max}) of 17.4 ng/mL was reached at 3.2 hours (T_{max}) following dosing. The terminal half-life was 6.9 hours. In a second study in which single 75 mcg/kg SC and IV doses were administered to 24 healthy subjects, the absolute bioavailablity of oprelvekin was > 80%.

Oprelvekin also was administered to 28 infants, children, and adolescents receiving ICE (ifosfamide, carboplatin, etoposide) chemotherapy. C_{max} and T_{max} were comparable with the adult population. The mean area under the concentration-time curve (AUC) for pediatric patients (8 months to 17 years of age) receiving 50 or 100 mcg/kg was 137 or 237 ng•hr/mL, respectively, compared with 189 ng•hr/mL in adults receiving 50 mcg/kg. Clearance of IL-11 decreases with patient age; clearance in infants and children (8 months to 11 years of age) is ≈ 1.2- to 1.6-fold higher than adults and adolescents (≥ 12 years of age).

In rats, oprelvekin was rapidly cleared from the serum and distributed to highly perfused organs. The kidney was the primary route of elimination. The amount of intact oprelvekin in the urine was low, indicating that the molecule was metabolized before excretion.

Contraindications

Hypersensitivity to oprelvekin or any component of the product.

Warnings

➤*Fluid retention:* Oprelvekin is known to cause fluid retention; use with caution in patients with clinically evident CHF, patients who may be susceptible to developing CHF, patients receiving aggressive hydration, patients with a history of heart failure who are well compensated and are receiving appropriate medical therapy, and patients with pleural or pericardial effusions.

Patients receiving oprelvekin have commonly experienced mild to moderate fluid retention, which can result in peripheral edema or dyspnea on exertion. Fluid retention also has been associated with weight gain, pulmonary edema, capillary leak syndrome, and exacerbation of pre-existing pleural effusions.

The fluid retention is reversible within several days following discontinuation of oprelvekin. During oprelvekin dosing, monitor fluid balance; appropriate medical management is advised. If a diuretic is used, carefully monitor fluid and electrolyte balance. Monitor pre-existing fluid collections, including pericardial effusions or ascites. Consider drainage if medically indicated.

Use oprelvekin with caution in patients who may develop fluid retention as a result of associated medical conditions or whose medical condition may be exacerbated by fluid retention.

Moderate decreases in hemoglobin concentration, hematocrit, and RBC (≈ 10% to 15%) without a decrease in RBC mass have occurred. These changes are predominantly caused by an increase in plasma volume (dilutional anemia) that is primarily related to renal sodium and water retention. The decrease in hemoglobin concentration typically begins within 3 to 5 days of oprelvekin initiation and is reversible over ≈ 1 week following discontinuation of oprelvekin.

Closely monitor fluid and electrolyte status in patients receiving chronic diuretic therapy. Sudden deaths have occurred in oprelvekin-treated patients receiving chronic diuretic therapy and ifosfamide who developed severe hypokalemia.

➤*Myeloablative chemotherapy:* Oprelvekin is not indicated following myeloablative chemotherapy.

➤*Renal function impairment:* Oprelvekin is eliminated primarily by the kidneys. The pharmacokinetics of oprelvekin have not been studied in mild or moderate renal impairment (creatinine clearance ≥ 15 mL/min). Fluid retention associated with oprelvekin treatment has not been studied in patients with renal impairment, but carefully monitor fluid balance in these patients.

➤*Pregnancy: Category C.* Parental toxicity has occurred when oprelvekin is given at doses of 2 to 20 times the human dose (≥ 100 mcg/kg/day) in the rat and when given in doses of 0.02 to 2 times the human dose (≥ 1 mcg/kg/day) in the rabbit. Findings in the rat consisted of transient hypoactivity and dyspnea after administration (maternal toxicity), as well as prolonged estrus cycle, increased early embryonic deaths and decreased numbers of live fetuses. In addition, low fetal body weights and a reduced number of ossified sacral and caudal vertebrae (ie, retarded fetal development) occurred in rats at 20 times the human dose. Findings in rabbits consisted of decreased (fecal/urine) eliminations (the only toxicity noted at 1 mcg/kg/day) as well as decreased food consumption, weight loss, abortion, increased embryonic and fetal deaths, and decreased numbers of live fetuses.

Adverse effects in the first generation offspring of rats given oprelvekin at maternally toxic doses ≥ 2 times the human dose (≥ 100 mcg/kg/day) during gestation and lactation included increased newborn mortality, decreased viability index on day 4 of lactation, and decreased body weights during lactation. In rats given 20 times the human dose

OPRELVEKIN (Interleukin 11; IL-11)

(1000 mcg/kg/day) during gestation and lactation, maternal toxicity and growth retardation of the first generation offspring resulted in an increased rate of fetal death of the second generation offspring.

Oprelvekin has embryocidal effects in pregnant rats and rabbits when given in doses of 0.2 to 20 times the human dose. There are no adequate and well-controlled studies in pregnant women. Use during pregnancy only if the potential benefit justifies the potential risk to the fetus.

➤*Lactation:* It is not known if oprelvekin is excreted in breast milk. Decide whether to discontinue nursing or to discontinue the drug, taking into account the importance of the drug to the mother.

➤*Children:* There are no controlled clinical trials that have established a safe and effective dose of oprelvekin in children. Therefore, the administration of oprelvekin in children, particularly those < 12 years of age, should be restricted to controlled clinical trial settings with closely monitored safety assessments. Preliminary data from a safety and pharmacokinetic trial identified papilledema in 4 of 16 children receiving doses of 100 mcg/kg/day.

Limited data from the safety and pharmacokinetic trial are available for pediatric populations receiving doses of 50 mcg/kg/day. Adequate pharmacokinetic data for doses of 50 mcg/kg/day were obtained for 7 individuals ≤ 12 years of age and 4 individuals > 12 and < 17 years of age. Children ≤ 12 years of age given doses of 50 mcg/kg/day did not achieve effective serum levels. For adolescents 13 to 16 years of age (n = 2) and young adults ≥ 17 years of age (n = 2) effective serum levels appeared to be achieved (see Pharmacokinetics).

Adverse events in this study generally were similar to those observed using oprelvekin at a dose of 50 mcg/kg in adults. However, the incidence of papilledema (14%), tachycardia (46%), and conjunctival injection (50%) were higher in the pediatric subjects than in adults. There was no evidence of a dose-response relationship for any of the oprelvekin-associated adverse events among the pediatric patients.

No studies have been performed to assess the long-term effects of oprelvekin on growth and development. In growing rodents treated with 100, 300, or 1000 mcg/kg/day for a minimum of 28 days, thickening of femoral and tibial growth plates was noted, which did not completely resolve after a 28-day nontreatment period. Primates treated for 2 to 13 weeks at doses of 10 to 1000 mcg/kg showed partially reversible joint capsule and tendon fibrosis and periosteal hyperostosis. An asymptomatic, laminated periosteal reaction in the diaphyses of the femur, tibia, and fibula has been observed in 1 patient during pediatric trials involving multiple courses of oprelvekin.

Precautions

➤*Monitoring:* During dosing with oprelvekin, monitor fluid balance; appropriate medical management is advised. If a diuretic is used, carefully monitor fluid and electrolyte balance. Obtain a complete blood count prior to chemotherapy and at regular intervals during oprelvekin therapy. Monitor platelet counts during the time of the expected nadir and until adequate recovery has occurred (postnadir counts ≥ 50,000).

➤*Timing of therapy:* Begin dosing with oprelvekin 6 to 24 hours following the completion of chemotherapy dosing. The safety and efficacy of oprelvekin given immediately prior to or concurrently with cytotoxic chemotherapy or initiated at the time of expected nadir have not been established.

➤*Duration:* The effectiveness of oprelvekin has not been evaluated in patients receiving chemotherapy regimens of > 5 days duration or regimens associated with delayed myelosuppression (eg, nitrosoureas, mitomycin-C).

➤*Cardiovascular events:* Use oprelvekin with caution in patients with a history of atrial arrhythmia and only after consideration of the potential risks in relation to anticipated benefit. In clinical trials, atrial arrhythmias (atrial fibrillation or atrial flutter) occurred in 15% of patients treated with oprelvekin at doses of 50 mcg/kg. Arrhythmias were usually brief in duration; conversion to sinus rhythm typically occurred spontaneously or after rate-control drug therapy. Approximately 50% of the patients who were rechallenged had recurrent atrial arrhythmias. Clinical sequelae, including stroke, have been reported in patients receiving oprelvekin who experienced atrial arrhythmias.

Oprelvekin has not been shown to be directly arrhythmogenic in preclinical trials. In some patients, development of atrial arrhythmias may be because of increased plama volume associated with fluid retention. A retrospective analysis of data from clinical trials suggests that advancing age and other conditions such as history of atrial fibrillation/flutter, cardiac disorder, alcohol use (moderate or more), and cardiac medication use may be associated with an increased risk of atrial arrhythmias. Ventricular arrhythmias have not been attributed to the use of oprelvekin.

➤*CNS events:* Stroke has occurred in patients who develop atrial fibrillation/flutter while receiving oprelvekin (see Cardiovascular Events).

➤*Ophthalmologic events:* Transient, mild visual blurring has been reported by patients treated with oprelvekin. Papilledema has been reported in 2% of patients in clinical trials following repeated cycles of exposure. In clinical trials, the incidence of papilledema was higher

14% in children than in adults 1%. Primates treated with 1000 mcg/kg SC once daily for 4 to 13 weeks developed papilledema, which was not associated with inflammation or any other histologic abnormality and was reversible after drug discontinuation. Use with caution in patients with pre-existing papilledema or with tumors involving the CNS because papilledema could worsen or develop during treatment.

➤*Antibody formation/allergic reactions:* A small proportion (1%) of patients developed antibodies to oprelvekin. The clinical relevance of the presence of these antibodies is unknown. No anaphylactoid or other severe adverse allergic reactions were reported following single or repeated doses of oprelvekin. Use appropriate precautions in case allergic reactions occur. Rash and rare cases of hives have been reported, but a relationship between these reactions and the development of serum antibodies has not been established.

The data reflect the percentage of patients whose test results were considered positive for antibodies to oprelvekin in an ELISA assay, and are highly dependent on the sensitivity and specificity of the assay. Additionally, the observed incidence of antibody positivity in an assay may be influenced by several factors, including sample handling, concomitant medications, and underlying disease. For these reasons, comparisons of the incidence of antibodies to oprelvekin with incidence of antibodies to other products may be misleading.

Administration of oprelvekin should be permanently discontinued in patients who experience clinically significant allergic reactions.

➤*Chronic administration:* Oprelvekin has been administered safely using the recommended dosing schedule (see Administration and Dosage) for ≤ 6 cycles following chemotherapy. The safety and efficacy of chronic administration have not been established. Continuous dosing (2 to 13 weeks) in primates produced joint capsule and tendon fibrosis and periosteal hyperostosis.

Adverse Reactions

Most adverse events were mild or moderate in severity and reversible after discontinuation of oprelvekin dosing. In general, the incidence and type of adverse events were similar between oprelvekin 50 mcg/kg and placebo groups. The following adverse events (≥ 10%) were observed at equal or greater frequency in placebo-treated patients: Asthenia; pain; chills; abdominal pain; infection; anorexia; constipation; dyspepsia; ecchymosis; myalgia; bone pain; nervousness; alopecia.

The incidence of fever, neutropenic fever, flu-like symptoms, thrombocytosis, thrombotic events, the average number of units of red blood cells transfused per patient, and the duration of neutropenia < 500 cells/mcL were similar in the oprelvekin 50 mcg/kg and the placebo groups.

Selected Oprelvekin Adverse Reactions (%)		
Adverse reaction	Oprelvekin 50 mcg/kg (n = 69)	Placebo (n = 67)
Cardiovascular		
Tachycardia	20	3
Vasodilation	19	9
Palpitations	14	3
Syncope	13	6
Atrial fibrillation/flutter	12	1
CNS		
Dizziness	38	28
Insomnia	33	27
GI		
Nausea/vomiting	77	70
Mucositis	43	37
Diarrhea	43	33
Oral moniliasis	14	1
Respiratory		
Dyspnea	48	22
Rhinitis	42	31
Cough increased	29	22
Pharyngitis	25	16
Pleural effusion	10	0
Miscellaneous		
Edema	59	15
Neutropenic fever	48	42
Headache	41	36
Fever	36	28
Rash	25	16
Conjunctival injection	19	3

The following adverse events also occurred more frequently in cancer patients receiving oprelvekin than in those receiving placebo: Amblyopia; paresthesia; dehydration; skin discoloration; exfoliative dermatitis; eye hemorrhage.

Two cancer patients treated with oprelvekin experienced sudden death, which the investigator considered possibly or probably related to oprelvekin. Both deaths occurred in patients with severe hypokalemia (< 3 mEq/L) who had received high doses of ifosfamide and were receiv-

OPRELVEKIN (Interleukin 11; IL-11)

ing daily doses of a diuretic. The relationship of these deaths to oprelvekin remains unclear.

►*Lab test abnormalities:* The most common lab abnormality was a decrease in hemoglobin concentration predominantly as a result of expansion of the plasma volume (see Warnings). The increase in plasma volume also is associated with a decrease in the serum concentration of albumin and several other proteins (eg, transferrin and gamma globulins). A parallel decrease in calcium without clinical effects has been documented. After daily SC injections, treatment with oprelvekin resulted in a 2-fold increase in plasma fibrinogen. Other acute-phase proteins also increased. These protein levels returned to normal after dosing with oprelvekin was discontinued. Von Willebrand factor concentrations increased with a normal multimer pattern in healthy subjects receiving oprelvekin.

Overdosage

Doses of oprelvekin > 100 mcg/kg have not been administered. While clinical experience is limited, doses of oprelvekin > 50 mcg/kg may be associated with an increased incidence of cardiovascular events in adult patients (see Precautions). If an overdose is administered, discontinue oprelvekin and closely observe the patient for signs of toxicity. Base reinstitution of therapy on individual patient factors (eg, evidence of toxicity, continued need for therapy).

Patient Information

In situations when oprelvekin is used outside of the hospital or office setting, instruct people who will be administering oprelvekin as to the proper dose and the method for reconstituting and administering oprelvekin. If home use is prescribed, instruct patients in the importance of proper disposal and caution against the reuse of needles, syringes, drug product, and diluent.

Inform patients of the most common adverse reactions associated with oprelvekin administration, including those symptoms related to fluid retention. Mild to moderate peripheral edema and shortness of breath on exertion can occur within the first week of treatment and may continue for the duration of administration. Advise patients who have pre-existing pleural or other effusions or a history of CHF to contact their physician if dyspnea worsens. Most patients who receive oprelvekin develop anemia. Caution patients to contact their physician if symptoms attributable to atrial arrhythmia develop. Advise female patients of childbearing potential of the possible risks of oprelvekin to the fetus.

Venous thrombi consist mainly of fibrin and red blood cells. Arterial thrombi are composed mainly of platelet aggregates. Theoretically, anticoagulant drugs should be effective for reducing risks involved with venous thrombi formation and antiplatelet drugs should be more effective for reducing risks of arterial thrombi formation.

The drugs most commonly used for their antiplatelet effects are aspirin, sulfinpyrazone, dipyridamole and ticlopidine.

Aggregation Inhibitors

CILOSTAZOL

Rx	**Pletal** (Otsuka America Pharmaceuticals)	**Tablets:** 50 mg	(PLETAL 50). White, triangular. In 60s and UD 100s.
		100 mg	(PLETAL 100). White. In 60s and UD 100s.

WARNING

Cilostazol and several of its metabolites are phosphodiesterase III inhibitors. Several drugs with this pharmacologic effect have caused decreased survival compared with placebo in patients with class III-IV CHF. Cilostazol is contraindicated in patients with CHF of any severity.

Indications

➤*Intermittent claudication:* Reduction of symptoms of intermittent claudication as indicated by an increased walking distance.

Administration and Dosage

➤*Approved by the FDA:* January 15, 1999.

➤*Intermittent claudication:* 100 mg twice daily, taken ≥ 30 minutes before or 2 hours after breakfast and dinner. Consider a dose of 50 mg twice daily during coadministration of such inhibitors of CYP3A4 as ketoconazole, itraconazole, erythromycin, and diltiazem, and during coadministration of such inhibitors of CYP2C19 as omeprazole. CYP3A4 is also inhibited by grapefruit juice. Because the magnitude and timing of this interaction have not been investigated yet, patients receiving cilostazol should avoid consuming grapefruit juice.

Patients may respond as early as 2 to 4 weeks after the initiation of therapy, but treatment for up to 12 weeks may be needed before a beneficial effect is experienced.

➤*Discontinuation of therapy:* Available data suggest that the dosage of cilostazol can be reduced or discontinued without rebound (ie, platelet hyperaggregability).

Actions

➤*Pharmacology:* Cilostazol is a quinolinone derivative that inhibits cellular phosphodiesterase and exhibits a higher specificity for phosphodiesterase III (PDE III). The mechanism of the effects of cilostazol on the symptoms of intermittent claudication is not fully understood. Cilostazol and several of its metabolites are inhibitors of cyclic AMP (cAMP) PDE III. Suppression of this isoenzyme causes increased levels of cAMP resulting in vasodilation and inhibition of platelet aggregation.

Cilostazol reversibly inhibits platelet aggregation induced by a variety of stimuli, including thrombin, ADP, collagen, arachidonic acid, epinephrine, and shear stress. Studies of circulating plasma lipids in patients taking cilostazol 100 mg twice daily for 12 weeks reported a reduction in triglycerides of 29.3 mg/dL (15%) and an increase in HDL-cholesterol of 4 mg/dL ($\approx$ 10%).

Cardiovascular effects – Cilostazol affects vascular beds and cardiovascular function. It produces nonhomogeneous dilation of vascular beds, with greater dilation in femoral beds than in vertebral, carotid, or superior mesenteric arteries. Renal arteries were not responsive to the effects of cilostazol.

In animals, cilostazol increased heart rate, myocardial contractile force, coronary blood flow, and ventricular automaticity, as would be expected for a PDE III inhibitor. Left ventricular contractility was increased at doses required to inhibit platelet aggregation. AV conduction was accelerated. In humans, heart rate increased in a dose-proportional manner by a mean of 5.1 and 7.4 beats per minute in patients treated with 50 and 100 mg twice daily, respectively. In 264 patients evaluated with Holter monitors, numerically more cilostazol-treated patients had increases in ventricular premature beats and non-sustained ventricular tachycardia events than did placebo-treated patients; the increases were not dose-related.

➤*Pharmacokinetics:*

Absorption/Distribution – Pharmacokinetics of cilostazol are approximately dose-proportional. The absolute bioavailability is not known; however, high-fat meals appear to increase absorption as indicated by an $\approx$ 90% increase in C_{max} and a 25% increase in AUC. Cilostazol and its 2 active metabolites accumulate about 2–fold with chronic administration and reach steady state within a few days.

Cilostazol is 95% to 98% protein bound, predominantly to albumin. The active metabolites, 3,4-dehydro-cilostazol (DHC) and 4'-trans-hydroxy-cilostazol (HC) are 97.4% and 66% bound, respectively. Renal impairment increased free fraction of cilostazol by 27%.

Metabolism/Excretion – Cilostazol is extensively metabolized by hepatic cytochrome P450 enzymes, primarily 3A4 and to a lesser extent 2C19. Two of the metabolites, DHC and HC, are active. DHC is 4 to 7 times as active as the parent compound and accounts for ≥ 50% of the

pharmacologic (PDE III inhibition) activity; HC is ⅕ as active as cilostazol. After oral administration, 56% of the total dose in plasma was determined to be cilostazol, 15% was DHC, and 4% was HC. There is no evidence of hepatic microenzyme induction. Cilostazol and its active metabolites have an apparent elimination half-life of 11 to 13 hours.

The primary route of excretion is urine (74%), with the remainder excreted in the feces (20%). No measurable amount of unchanged cilostazol was excreted in the urine, and < 2% of the dose was excreted as DHC. The enzyme responsible for metabolism of DHC is unknown. About 30% of the dose is excreted in the urine as HC, the remainder as other metabolites, none of which exceeded 5%.

Special populations –
   Smokers: Smoking decreased cilostazol exposure by $\approx$ 20%.
   Renal impairment: The total activity of cilostazol and its metabolites is similar in subjects with mild-to-moderate renal impairment and in healthy subjects. Severe renal impairment increases metabolite levels and alters protein binding of the parent and metabolites; however, the activity based on plasma concentrations and relative PDE III inhibiting potency showed little change. Patients on dialysis have not been studied, but it is unlikely that cilostazol can be removed efficiently by dialysis because of its high protein binding (95% to 98%).

➤*Clinical trials:* Compared with patients treated with placebo, patients treated with cilostazol 50 or 100 mg twice daily experienced statistically significant improvements in walking distances before the onset of claudication pain and the before exercise-limiting symptoms supervened (maximal walking distance). The effect of cilostazol on walking distance was seen as early as the first on-therapy observation point of 2 or 4 weeks.

Contraindications

CHF of any severity; hypersensitivity to any components of the product.

Cilostazol and several of its metabolites are inhibitors of phosphodiesterase III. Several drugs with this pharmacologic effect have caused decreased survival compared with placebo in patients with class III-IV CHF.

Warnings

➤*Cardiovascular risk:* Cilostazol is contraindicated in patients with CHF. In patients without CHF, the long-term effects of PDE III inhibitors (including cilostazol) are unknown. In the 3- to 6-month placebo-controlled trials of cilostazol, 19 deaths occurred in relatively stable (no recent MI, strokes, rest pain, or other signs of rapidly progressing disease) study patients (0.7% in the placebo group and 0.8% in the cilostazol group). There are no data on longer-term risk or risk in patients with more severe underlying heart disease.

➤*Cardiovascular lesions:* Repeated oral administration of cilostazol to dogs (≥ 30 mg/kg/day for 52 weeks, ≥ 150 mg/kg/day for 13 weeks, and 450 mg/kg/day for 2 weeks), produced cardiovascular lesions including endocardial hemorrhage, hemosiderin deposition and fibrosis in the left ventricle, hemorrhage in the right atrial wall, hemorrhage and necrosis of the smooth muscle in the wall of the coronary artery, intimal thickening of the coronary artery, and coronary arteritis and periarteritis. At the lowest dose associated with cardiovascular lesions in the 52-week study, systemic exposure (AUC) to unbound cilostazol was less than that seen in humans at the maximum recommended human dose (MRHD) of 100 mg twice daily. Similar lesions have been reported in the dog following the administration of other positive inotropic agents (including PDE III inhibitors) or vasodilating agents.

➤*Elderly:* Of the 2274 cilostazol study patients, 56% were ≥ 65 years old while 16% were ≥ 75 years old. No overall differences in safety or efficacy were observed between these subjects and younger subjects.

➤*Pregnancy: Category C.* At doses $\approx$ 5 times the MRHD, animal studies revealed decreased fetal weights, increased incidences of cardiovascular, renal, and skeletal anomalies (ventricular septal, aortic arch and subclavian artery abnormalities, renal pelvic dilation, 14th rib, and retarded ossification). When administered to rats during late pregnancy and lactation, an increased incidence of stillborn was also noted. There are no adequate and well-controlled studies in pregnant women. Use during pregnancy only if the potential benefit justifies the potential risk to the fetus.

➤*Lactation:* Transfer of cilostazol into milk has been reported in rats. Because of the potential risk to nursing infants, decide whether to discontinue nursing or to discontinue the drug.

➤*Children:* Safety and efficacy in children have not been established.

CILOSTAZOL

Drug Interactions

➤*P450 system:* Cilostazol could have pharmacokinetic interactions because of effects of other drugs on its metabolism by CYP3A4 (eg, erythromycin, ketoconazole) or CYP2C19 (eg, omeprazole). Cilostazol does not appear to inhibit CYP3A4. Strong inhibitors of CYP3A4 (eg, ketoconazole, itraconazole, fluconazole, miconazole, fluvoxamine, fluoxetine, nefazodone, sertraline) have not been studied in combination with cilostazol but would be expected to cause a greater increase in plasma levels of cilostazol and metabolites than erythromycin (see following table).

Cilostazol does not appear to cause increased blood levels of drugs metabolized by CYP3A4 (eg, lovastatin, a drug with metabolism very sensitive to CYP3A4 inhibition).

➤*Platelet function inhibitors:* Cilostazol could have pharmacodynamic interactions with other platelet function inhibitors. There is no information on the concurrent use of cilostazol and clopidogrel, a platelet aggregation inhibiting drug.

➤*Aspirin:* Short-term ($\leq$ 4 days) coadministration of aspirin with cilostazol showed a 23% to 35% increase in inhibition of ADP-induced ex vivo platelet aggregation compared with aspirin alone. No clinically significant impact on PT, aPTT, or bleeding time occurred compared with aspirin alone. There was no additive or synergistic effect on arachidonic acid-induced platelet aggregation. Effects of long-term coadministration are unknown. Of the 201 patients studied, no apparent greater incidence of hemorrhagic adverse effects were present in patients taking cilostazol and aspirin compared with equivalent doses of aspirin (75 to 325 mg/day) alone.

➤*Warfarin:* Cilostazol did not inhibit the metabolism or the pharmacologic effects of warfarin following a single dose. The effect of concomitant multiple dosing of warfarin or cilostazol on either drug is unknown.

Cilostazol Drug Interactions

Precipitant drug	Object drug*	Description
Diltiazem	Cilostazol ↑	Diltiazem (a moderate inhibitor of CYP3A4) increased cilostazol plasma concentrations by ≈ 53%. Initiate therapy at half the recommended dose.
Macrolides	Cilostazol ↑	Erythromycin (a moderately strong inhibitor of CYP3A4) increased cilostazol C_{max} by 47% and AUC by 73%; the AUC of 4'-trans-hydroxy-cilostazol was also increased by 141%. Other macrolide antibiotics would be expected to have similar effect. Initiate therapy at half the recommended dose.
Omeprazole	Cilostazol ↔	Coadministration of omeprazole did not significantly affect the metabolism of cilostazol, but the systemic exposure to 3,4-dehydro-cilostazol was increased by 69%, probably the result of omeprazole's potent inhibition of CYP2C19. Initiate therapy at half the recommended dose.

* ↑ = Object drug increased. ↔ = Undetermined clinical effect.

➤*Drug/Food interactions:* A high-fat meal increases absorption of cilostazol with an ≈ 90% increase in C_{max} and a 25% increase in AUC. Because grapefruit juice inhibits CYP3A4, avoid concurrent use with cilostazol.

Adverse Reactions

The only adverse event resulting in discontinuation of therapy in $\geq$ 3% of patients was headache, which occurred with an incidence of 1.3%, 3.5%, and 0.3% in patients treated with cilostazol 50 mg twice daily, 100 mg twice daily, or placebo, respectively. Other frequent causes of discontinuation included palpitations and diarrhea, both 1.1% for cilostazol (all doses) vs 0.1% for placebo.

Cilostazol Adverse Reactions ($\geq$ 2%)

Adverse reaction	Cilostazol 50 mg twice daily (n = 303)	Cilostazol 100 mg twice daily (n = 998)	Placebo (n = 973)
Cardiovascular			
Palpitation	5	10	1
Tachycardia	4	4	1
CNS			
Dizziness	9	10	6
Vertigo	3	1	1

Cilostazol Adverse Reactions ($\geq$ 2%)

Adverse reaction	Cilostazol 50 mg twice daily (n = 303)	Cilostazol 100 mg twice daily (n = 998)	Placebo (n = 973)
GI			
Abnormal stool	12	15	4
Diarrhea	12	19	7
Dyspepsia	6	6	4
Flatulence	2	3	2
Nausea	6	7	6
Respiratory			
Cough increased	3	4	3
Pharyngitis	7	10	7
Rhinitis	12	7	5
Miscellaneous			
Abdominal pain	4	5	3
Back pain	6	7	6
Headache	27	34	14
Infection	14	10	8
Myalgia	2	3	2
Peripheral edema	9	7	4

Other events seen with an incidence of 2% but occurring in the placebo group at least as frequently as in the 100 mg twice daily group were: Asthenia; hypertension; vomiting; leg cramps; hyperesthesia; paresthesia; dyspnea; rash; hematuria; urinary tract infection; flu syndrome; angina pectoris; arthritis; bronchitis.

Less frequent adverse events (< 2%) are listed below.

➤*Cardiovascular:* Atrial fibrillation/flutter; cerebral infarct; cerebral ischemia; CHF; heart arrest; hemorrhage; hypotension; MI; myocardial ischemia; nodal arrhythmia; postural hypotension; supraventricular tachycardia; syncope; varicose vein; vasodilation; ventricular extrasystoles/tachycardia.

➤*CNS:* Anxiety; insomnia; neuralgia.

➤*Dermatologic:* Dry skin; furunculosis; skin hypertrophy; urticaria.

➤*GI:* Anorexia; cholelithiasis; colitis; duodenal ulcer; duodenitis; esophageal hemorrhage; esophagitis; GGT increased; gastritis; gastroenteritis; gum hemorrhage; hematemesis; melena; peptic ulcer; periodontal abscess; rectal hemorrhage; stomach ulcer; tongue edema.

➤*GU:* Albuminuria; cystitis; urinary frequency; vaginal hemorrhage; vaginitis.

➤*Hematologic/Lymphatic:* Anemia; ecchymosis; iron deficiency anemia; polycythemia; purpura.

➤*Metabolic/Nutritional:* Creatinine increased; gout; hyperlipemia; hyperuricemia.

➤*Musculoskeletal:* Arthralgia; bone pain; bursitis.

➤*Respiratory:* Asthma; epistaxis; hemoptysis; pneumonia; sinusitis.

➤*Special senses:* Amblyopia; blindness; conjunctivitis; diplopia; ear pain; eye hemorrhage; retinal hemorrhage; tinnitus.

➤*Miscellaneous:* Chills; facial edema; fever; generalized edema; malaise; neck rigidity; pelvic pain; retroperitoneal hemorrhage; diabetes mellitus.

Overdosage

Information on acute overdosage with cilostazol is limited. The signs and symptoms can be anticipated to be those of excessive pharmacologic effect: Severe headache, diarrhea, hypotension, tachycardia, and possibly cardiac arrhythmias. Carefully observe the patient and give supportive treatment. Refer to General Management of Acute Overdosage. Because cilostazol is highly protein bound, it is unlikely that it can be efficiently removed by hemodialysis or peritoneal dialysis.

Patient Information

Advise patients to read the patient package insert for cilostazol carefully before starting therapy, reread it each time therapy is renewed in case the information has changed, and to take cilostazol $\geq$ 30 minutes before or 2 hours after food.

Advise patients that the beneficial effects of cilostazol on the symptoms of intermittent claudication may not be immediate. Although the patient may experience benefit in 2 to 4 weeks after initiation of therapy, treatment for up to 12 weeks may be required before a beneficial effect is experienced.

Advise patients about the uncertainty concerning cardiovascular risk in long-term use or in patients with severe underlying heart disease, as described under Warnings.

CLOPIDOGREL

Rx   **Plavix** (Sanofi-Synthelabo)   **Tablets:** 75 mg (as base)   Lactose, castor oil, mannitol. (75 1171). Pink. Film-coated. In 30s, 90s, 500s, and UD 100s.

Indications

Indicated for atherosclerotic events as follows:

➤*Recent MI or stroke, or established peripheral arterial disease:* For patients with a history of recent MI, recent stroke, or established peripheral arterial disease, clopidogrel has been shown to reduce the rate of a combined endpoint of new ischemic stroke (fatal or not), new MI (fatal or not), and other vascular death.

➤*Acute coronary syndrome:* For patients with acute coronary syndrome (unstable angina/non-Q-wave MI) including patients who are to be managed medically and those who are to be managed with percutaneous coronary intervention (with or without stent) or coronary artery bypass graft (CABG), clopidogrel has been shown to decrease the rate of a combined endpoint of cardiovascular death, MI, or stroke, as well as the rate of a combined endpoint of cardiovascular death, MI, stroke, or refractory ischemia.

Administration and Dosage

➤*Approved by the FDA:* November 18, 1997.

➤*Recent MI, recent stroke, or established peripheral arterial disease:* The recommended dose of clopidogrel is 75 mg once daily with or without food.

➤*Acute coronary syndrome:* For patients with acute coronary syndrome (unstable angina/non-Q-wave MI), initiate clopidogrel with a single 300 mg loading dose and then continue at 75 mg once daily. Initiate and continue aspirin (75 to 325 mg once daily) in combination with clopidogrel. In one study, most patients with acute coronary syndrome also received heparin acutely.

No dosage adjustment is necessary for elderly patients or patients with renal disease.

➤*Storage/Stability:* Store at 25°C (77°F); excursions permitted to 15° to 30°C (59° to 86°F).

Actions

➤*Pharmacology:* Clopidogrel is an inhibitor of ADP-induced platelet aggregation. A variety of drugs that inhibit platelet function decrease morbid events in people with established atherosclerotic cardiovascular disease as evidenced by stroke or transient ischemic attacks, MI, unstable angina, or need for vascular bypass or angioplasty. This indicates that platelets participate in the initiation or evolution of these events, and that inhibiting them can reduce the event rate.

Clopidogrel selectively inhibits the binding of adenosine diphosphate (ADP) to its platelet receptor and the subsequent ADP-mediated activation of the glycoprotein GPIIb/IIIa complex, thereby inhibiting platelet aggregation. Biotransformation of clopidogrel is necessary to produce inhibition of platelet aggregation, but an active metabolite responsible for the activity of the drug has not been isolated. Clopidogrel also inhibits platelet aggregation induced by agonists other than ADP by blocking the amplification of platelet activation by released ADP. Clopidogrel does not inhibit phosphodiesterase activity.

Clopidogrel acts by irreversibly modifying the platelet ADP receptor. Consequently, platelets exposed to clopidogrel are affected for the remainder of their lifespan.

➤*Pharmacokinetics:*

Absorption/Distribution – Clopidogrel absorption is at least 50% and is rapid after oral administration. Bioavailability is unaffected by food. Peak plasma levels (approximately 3 mg/L) of the inactive main metabolite occur approximately 1 hour after dosing. The parent compound, which also is inactive, has low and generally unquantifiable levels beyond 2 hours after dosing. An active metabolite responsible for the activity of the drug has not been isolated. The main metabolite exhibits linear kinetics in the dose range of 50 to 150 mg of clopidogrel. Both the parent compound and the main metabolite bind reversibly in vitro to plasma protein (98% and 94%, respectively); binding is non-saturable up to a concentration of 100 mg/mL.

Dose-dependent inhibition of platelet aggregation can be seen 2 hours after single oral doses of clopidogrel. Repeated doses of 75 mg/day inhibit ADP-induced platelet aggregation on the first day, reaching steady-state between days 3 and 7. At steady-state, the average inhibition level observed with a dose of 75 mg/day was between 40% and 60%. Platelet aggregation and bleeding time gradually return to baseline values after treatment is discontinued, generally in about 5 days.

Metabolism/Excretion – Clopidogrel is extensively metabolized by the liver. It undergoes rapid hydrolysis into its carboxylic acid derivative; glucuronidation also occurs. The carboxylic acid derivative represents about 85% of the circulating drug-related compounds in plasma.

The elimination half-life of the main circulating metabolite was 8 hours with approximately 50% excreted in the urine and approximately 46% in the feces 5 days after dosing. Covalent binding to platelets accounted for 2% with a half-life of 11 days.

Special populations –

Elderly: Plasma levels of the main metabolite were significantly higher in the elderly (75 years of age or older) but were not associated with differences in platelet aggregation and bleeding time. No dosage adjustment is needed.

Renal function impairment: After repeated doses of 75 mg/day, plasma levels of the main metabolite were lower in patients with severe renal impairment (Ccr from 5 to 15 mL/min) compared with subjects with moderate renal impairment (Ccr, 30 to 60 mL/min) or healthy subjects. Although inhibition of ADP-induced platelet aggregation was lower (25%) than that observed in healthy volunteers, the prolongation of bleeding time was similar to healthy volunteers receiving 75 mg/day. No dosage adjustment is needed in renally impaired patients.

Gender: In a small study comparing men and women, less inhibition of ADP-induced platelet aggregation was observed in women, but no difference in prolongation of bleeding time was evident.

➤*Clinical trials:* Efficacy of clopidogrel is derived from a randomized study comparing clopidogrel (75 mg daily) with aspirin (325 mg daily) in 19,185 patients. Patients had the following: 1) recent histories of MI (within 35 days); 2) recent histories of ischemic stroke (IS; within 6 months) with at least a week of residual neurological signs; or 3) objectively established peripheral arterial disease. Treatment averaged 1.6 years (maximum of 3 years).

The primary outcome was the time to first occurrence of new ischemic stroke (fatal or not), new MI (fatal or not), or other vascular death. Deaths not easily attributable to nonvascular causes were all classified as vascular.

Primary Outcome Events: Clopidogrel vs Aspirin (%)		
Outcome events	Clopidogrel (n = 9599)	Aspirin (n = 9586)
IS (fatal or not)	4.6	4.8
MI (fatal or not)	2.9	3.5
Other vascular death	2.4	2.4
Total	9.8	10.6

The benefit appeared to be strongest in patients who were enrolled because of peripheral vascular disease (especially those who also had a history of MI) and weaker in stroke patients. In patients who were enrolled in the trial on the sole basis of a recent MI, clopidogrel was not numerically superior to aspirin.

The overall safety profile of clopidogrel is at least as good as that of medium-dose aspirin.

Contraindications

Hypersensitivity to the drug or any component of the product; active pathological bleeding such as peptic ulcer or intracranial hemorrhage.

Warnings

➤*Thrombotic thrombocytopenic purpura (TTP):* TTP has been reported rarely following use of clopidogrel, sometimes after a short exposure (less than 2 weeks). TTP is a serious condition requiring prompt treatment. It is characterized by thrombocytopenia, microangiopathic hemolytic anemia (schistocytes [fragmented RBCs] seen on peripheral smear), neurological findings, renal dysfunction, and fever. TTP was not seen during clopidogrel's clinical trials, which included over 17,500 clopidogrel-treated patients. However, in worldwide post-marketing experience, TTP has been reported at a rate of about 4 cases per million patients exposed, or about 11 cases per million patient-years. The background rate is thought to be about 4 cases per million person-years.

➤*Hepatic function impairment:* Experience is limited in patients with severe hepatic disease, who may have bleeding diatheses. Use with caution in this population.

➤*Pregnancy: Category B.* There are no adequate and well-controlled studies in pregnant women. Use during pregnancy only if clearly needed.

➤*Lactation:* Studies in rats have shown that clopidogrel and its metabolites are excreted in milk. It is not known whether this drug is excreted in human breast milk. Because of the potential for serious adverse reactions in the nursing infant, decide whether to discontinue nursing or discontinue the drug, taking into account the importance of the drug to the mother.

➤*Children:* Safety and efficacy have not been established.

Precautions

➤*Bleeding risk:* As with other antiplatelet agents, use with caution in patients who may be at risk of increased bleeding from trauma, surgery, or other pathological conditions. If a patient is to undergo elective surgery and an antiplatelet effect is not desired, discontinue clopidogrel 5 days prior to surgery.

CLOPIDOGREL

GI bleeding – Clopidogrel prolongs the bleeding time. In the clinical trial, clopidogrel was associated with a rate of GI bleeding of 2% vs 2.7% with aspirin. Use with caution in patients who have lesions with a propensity to bleed (such as ulcers). Cautiously use drugs that might increase such lesions in patients taking clopidogrel.

Drug Interactions

At high concentrations in vitro, clopidogrel inhibits P450 2C9. Accordingly, clopidogrel may interfere with the metabolism of phenytoin, tamoxifen, tolbutamide, warfarin, torsemide, fluvastatin, and many nonsteroidal anti-inflammatory agents, but there are no data with which to predict the magnitude of these interactions. Use caution when any of these drugs is coadministered with clopidogrel.

Clopidogrel Drug Interactions			
Precipitant drug	Object drug*		Description
NSAIDs	Clopidogrel	↑	Coadministration of clopidogrel with naproxen was associated with increased occult GI blood loss. Administer NSAIDs and clopidogrel with caution.
Warfarin	Clopidogrel	↔	Clopidogrel prolongs bleeding time. The safety of coadministration with warfarin has not been established. Administer these 2 agents with caution.
Clopidogrel	Warfarin		

* ↑ = Object drug increased. ↔ = Undetermined clinical effect.

Adverse Reactions

Clopidogrel has been evaluated for safety in more than 17,500 patients, including more than 9000 patients treated for 1 year or more. The overall tolerability of clopidogrel was similar to that of aspirin, with an approximately equal incidence (13%) of patients withdrawing from treatment because of adverse reactions.

➤*CURE trial:* In this trial, clopidogrel use with aspirin was associated with an increase in bleeding compared with placebo with aspirin (see table below). There was an excess in major bleeding in patients receiving clopidogrel plus aspirin compared with placebo plus aspirin, primarily GI and at puncture sites. The incidence of intracranial hemorrhage (0.1%) and fatal bleeding (0.2%) was the same in both groups.

Incidence of Bleeding Complications in CURE Trial (%)			
Adverse reaction	Clopidogrel + aspirin[1] (n = 6259)	Placebo + aspirin[1] (n = 6303)	P-value
Major bleeding[2]	3.7[3]	2.7[4]	0.001
Life-threatening bleeding	2.2	1.8	0.13
Fatal	0.2	0.2	
5 g/dL hemoglobin drop	0.9	0.9	
Requiring surgical intervention	0.7	0.7	
Hemorrhagic strokes	0.1	0.1	
Requiring inotropes	0.5	0.5	
Requiring transfusion (≥ 4 units)	1.2	1	
Other major bleeding	1.6	1	0.005
Significantly disabling	0.4	0.3	
Intraocular bleeding with significant loss of vision	0.05	0.03	
Requiring 2 to 3 units of blood	1.3	0.9	
Minor bleeding[5]	5.1	2.4	< 0.001

[1] Other standard therapies were used as appropriate.
[2] Life threatening and other major bleeding.
[3] Major bleeding event rate for clopidogrel + aspirin was dose-dependent on aspirin: less than 100 mg = 2.6%; 100 to 200 mg = 3.5%; greater than 200 mg = 4.9%.
[4] Major bleeding event rate for placebo + aspirin was dose-dependent on aspirin: less than 100 mg = 2%; 100 to 200 mg = 2.3%; greater than 200 mg = 4%.
[5] Led to interruption of study medication.

Ninety-two percent of the patients in the CURE study received heparin/low molecular weight heparin, and the rate of bleeding in these patients was similar to the overall results.

There was no excess in major bleeds within 7 days after coronary bypass graft surgery in patients who stopped therapy more than 5 days prior to surgery (event rate 4.4% clopidogrel + aspirin and 5.3% placebo + aspirin). In patients who remained on therapy within 5 days of bypass graft surgery, the event rate was 9.6% for clopidogrel + aspirin and 6.3% for placebo + aspirin.

Adverse events occurring in 2% or more of patients on clopidogrel in the CURE controlled clinical trial are shown below regardless of relationship to clopidogrel.

Clopidogrel Adverse Reactions in CURE Trial (%)		
Adverse reaction	Clopidogrel + aspirin[1] (n = 6259)	Placebo + aspirin[1] (n = 6303)
CNS		
Headache	3.1	3.2
Dizziness	2.4	2
GI		
Abdominal pain	2.3	2.8
Dyspepsia	2	1.9
Diarrhea	2.1	2.2
Ulcers (peptic, gastric, duodenal)	0.4	0.3
Miscellaneous		
Chest pain	2.7	2.8
Rash/Skin disorders	4	3.5

[1] Other standard therapies were used as appropriate.

➤*CAPRIE:* Adverse events occurring in 2.5% or more of patients on clopidogrel in the CAPRIE controlled clinical trial are shown below regardless of relationship to clopidogrel. The median duration of therapy was 20 months, with a maximum of 3 years.

Clopidogrel Adverse Reactions in CAPRIE Trial (%)		
Adverse reaction	Clopidogrel (n = 9599)	Aspirin (n = 9586)
Cardiovascular		
Edema	4.1	4.5
Hypertension	4.3	5.1
CNS		
Headache	7.6	7.2
Dizziness	6.2	6.7
Depression	3.6	3.9
Dermatologic		
Skin/Appendage disorders	15.8	13.1
Rash	4.2	3.5
Pruritus	3.3	1.6
GI		
Abdominal pain	5.6	7.1
Dyspepsia	5.2	6.1
Diarrhea	4.5	3.4
Nausea	3.4	3.8
Hemorrhage	2	2.7
Ulcers (peptic, gastric, duodenal)	0.7	1.2
Hematologic		
Purpura	5.3	3.7
Epistaxis	2.9	2.5
Musculoskeletal		
Arthralgia	6.3	6.2
Back pain	5.8	5.3
Respiratory		
Upper respiratory tract infection	8.7	8.3
Dyspnea	4.5	4.7
Rhinitis	4.2	4.2
Bronchitis	3.7	3.7
Coughing	3.1	2.7
Miscellaneous		
Chest pain	8.3	8.3
Accidental injury	7.9	7.3
Influenza-like symptoms	7.5	7
Pain	6.4	6.3
Hypercholesterolemia	4	4.4
Urinary tract infection	3.1	3.5
Fatigue	3.3	3.4
Intracranial hemorrhage	0.4	0.5

➤*Combined adverse reactions (CURE and CAPRIE trials):* The following adverse experiences occurred in less than 1% to 2.5% of patients receiving clopidogrel in the CAPRIE or CURE trials.

Cardiovascular – Syncope, palpitation, cardiac failure, atrial fibrillation.

CNS – Hypesthesia, neuralgia, paresthesia, vertigo, anxiety, insomnia.

Dermatologic – Eczema, skin ulceration, bullous eruption, rash erythematous, rash maculopapular, urticaria.

GI – Constipation, vomiting, GI hemorrhage, gastric ulcer perforated, gastritis hemorrhagic, upper GI ulcer hemorrhagic.

CLOPIDOGREL

Overall, the incidence of GI events (eg, abdominal pain, dyspepsia, gastritis and constipation) in patients receiving clopidogrel was 27.1% compared with 29.8% in those receiving aspirin in the CAPRIE trial. In the CURE trial, the incidence of these GI events for patients receiving clopidogrel + aspirin was 11.7% compared with 12.5% for those receiving placebo + aspirin.

Hematologic – Hematoma, platelets decreased, anemia, hemarthrosis, hematuria, hemoptysis, hemorrhage intracranial, hemorrhage retroperitonial, hemorrhage of operative wound, ocular hemorrhage, pulmonary hemorrhage, purpura allergic, thrombocytopenia, aplastic anemia, anemia hypochromic, agranulocytosis, granulocytopenia, leukemia, leukopenia, neutrophils decreased.

Neutropenia / agranulocytosis: Ticlopidine, a drug chemically similar to clopidogrel, is associated with a 0.8% rate of severe neutropenia (less than 450 neutrophils/mcL). Patients in the trial were intensively monitored for neutropenia. Severe neutropenia was observed in 6 patients, 4 on clopidogrel, and 2 on aspirin. Two of the 9599 patients who received clopidogrel and none of the 9586 patients who received aspirin had neutrophil counts of 0.

One of the four clopidogrel patients was receiving cytotoxic chemotherapy, and another recovered and returned to the trial after only temporarily interrupting treatment with clopidogrel. In CURE, the numbers of patients with thrombocytopenia (19 clopidogrel + aspirin vs 24 placebo + aspirin) or neutropenia (3 vs 3) were similar.

Although the risk of myelotoxicity with clopidogrel appears to be quite low, consider this possibility when a patient receiving clopidogrel demonstrates fever or other signs of infection.

Hepatic – Hepatic enzymes increased, bilirubinemia, hepatitis infectious, fatty liver.

Respiratory – Pneumonia, sinusitis, hemothorax.

Metabolic / Nutritional – Gout, hyperuricemia, nonprotein nitrogen (NPN) increased.

Musculoskeletal – Arthritis, arthrosis.

Renal – Abnormal renal function, acute renal failure.

Special senses – Cataract, conjunctivitis.

Miscellaneous – Asthenia, fever, hernia, leg cramps, cystitis, allergic reactions, ischemic necrosis, generalized edema, menorrhagia.

➤*Postmarketing reports:* Fever, very rare cases of hypersensitivity reactions (including angioedema, bronchospasm, anaphylactoid reactions), TTP.

➤*Withdrawal rates (CURE and CAPRIE trials):*

GI – In the CAPRIE trial, the incidence of patients withdrawing from treatment because of GI adverse reactions was 3.2% for clopidogrel and 4% for aspirin. In the CURE trial, the incidence of patients withdrawing from treatment because of GI adverse reactions was 0.9% for clopidogrel + aspirin compared with 0.8% for placebo + aspirin.

Dermatologic – In the CAPRIE trial, the overall incidence of patients withdrawing from treatment because of skin and appendage disorders adverse reactions was 1.5% for clopidogrel and 0.8% for aspirin. In the CURE trial, the incidence of patients withdrawing because of skin and appendage disorders adverse reactions was 0.7% for clopidogrel + aspirin compared with 0.3% for placebo + aspirin.

Overdosage

➤*Symptoms:* No adverse events were reported after single oral administration of 600 mg in healthy volunteers. The bleeding time was prolonged by a factor of 1.7, which is similar to that typically observed with the therapeutic dose of 75 mg/day.

One case of deliberate overdosage with clopidogrel was reported in the large, controlled clinical study. A 34-year-old woman took a single 1050 mg dose. No associated adverse events occurred. No special therapy was instituted, and she recovered without sequelae.

A single oral dose of clopidogrel at 1500 or 2000 mg/kg was lethal to mice and to rats and at 3000 mg/kg to baboons. Symptoms of acute toxicity were vomiting (in baboons), prostration, difficult breathing, and GI hemorrhage in all species.

➤*Treatment:* Based on biological plausibility, platelet transfusion may be appropriate to reverse the pharmacological effects of clopidogrel if quick reversal is required.

Patient Information

Inform patients that it may take them longer to stop bleeding when they take clopidogrel and that they should report any unusual bleeding to their physician.

Patients should inform physicians and dentists that they are taking clopidogrel before any surgery is scheduled and before any new drug is taken.

TICLOPIDINE HCl

Rx	**Ticlopidine HCl** (Various, eg, Apotex Corp., Teva)	**Tablets:** 250 mg	In 30s, 60s, 100s, 500s, and 1000s.
Rx	**Ticlid** (Syntex)		(Ticlid 250). White. Oval. Film coated. In 30s, 60s, and 500s.

WARNING

Ticlopidine can cause life-threatening hematological adverse reactions, including neutropenia/agranulocytosis and thrombotic thrombocytopenic purpura (TTP).

Neutropenia / agranulocytosis: Neutropenia defined as an absolute neutrophil count (ANC) < 1200 neutrophils/mm³ occurred in 50 of 2048 (2.4%) stroke patients who received ticlopidine in clinical trials. Neutropenia is calculated as follows: ANC = WBC x % neutrophils. In 17 patients (0.8%) the neutrophil count was < 450/mm³.

Thrombotic thrombocytopenic purpura (TTP): TTP was not seen during clinical trials, but US physicians reported about 100 cases between 1992 and 1997. Based on an estimated patient exposure of 2 to 4 million, and assuming an event reporting rate of 10% (the true rate is not known), the incidence of ticlopidine-associated TTP may be as high as 1 case in every 2000 to 4000 patients exposed (see Warnings).

Monitoring clinical and hematologic status: Severe hematological adverse reactions may occur within a few days of initiating therapy. The incidence of TTP peaks after ≈ 3 to 4 weeks of therapy and neutropenia peaks at ≈ 4 to 6 weeks with both declining thereafter. Only a few cases have arisen after > 3 months of treatment. Hematological adverse reactions cannot be reliably predicted by any identified demographic or clinical characteristics. During the first 3 months of treatment, hematologically and clinically monitor patients receiving ticlopidine for evidence of neutropenia or TTP. Immediately discontinue ticlopidine if there is any evidence of neutropenia or TTP.

Indications

➤*Stroke:* To reduce the risk of thrombotic stroke (fatal or nonfatal) in patients who have experienced stroke precursors, and in patients who have had a completed thrombotic stroke.

Because ticlopidine is associated with a risk of life-threatening blood dyscrasias including TTP and neutropenia/agranulocytosis (see Warnings), reserve for patients who are intolerant or allergic to aspirin therapy or who have failed aspirin therapy.

➤*Unlabeled uses:* Ticlopidine has also been utilized in various other conditions; further study is needed:

Ticlopidine Unlabeled Uses	
Condition	Result
Intermittent claudication	Improved maximum walking and pain-free distance
Chronic arterial occlusion	Improved lower extremity ulcer healing, vascular improvement
Subarachnoid hemorrhage	Reduced incidence of neurological deficit
Uremic patients with AV shunts or fistulas	Reduced incidence of vascular occlusion
Open heart surgery	Preoperative use reduces degree of platelet count drop during extracorporeal circulation
Coronary artery bypass grafts	Decreased graft occlusion
Primary glomerulonephritis	Reduced degree of proteinuria and hematuria, improved creatinine clearance
Sickle cell disease	Reduced incidence, duration, severity of infarctive crises

Administration and Dosage

➤*Approved by the FDA:* October 1991.

➤*Recommended dose:* 250 mg twice daily taken with food.

Actions

➤*Pharmacology:* Ticlopidine is a platelet aggregation inhibitor. When taken orally, ticlopidine causes a time- and dose-dependent inhibition of both platelet aggregation and release of platelet granule constituents, as well as a prolongation of bleeding time. Ticlopidine interferes with platelet membrane function by inhibiting ADP-induced platelet-fibrinogen binding and subsequent platelet-platelet interactions. The effect on platelet function is irreversible for the life of the platelet.

In healthy volunteers > 50 years of age, substantial inhibition (> 50%) of ADP-induced platelet aggregation is detected within 4 days after administration of ticlopidine 250 mg twice daily, and maximum platelet aggregation inhibition (60% to 70%) is achieved after 8 to 11 days. Lower doses cause less and more delayed platelet aggregation inhibition, while doses > 250 mg twice daily give little additional effect on

TICLOPIDINE HCl

platelet aggregation, but an increased rate of adverse effects. After discontinuation of ticlopidine, bleeding time and other platelet function tests return to normal within 2 weeks in the majority of patients. At the recommended therapeutic dose (250 mg twice daily), ticlopidine has no known significant pharmacological actions in humans other than inhibition of platelet function and prolongation of bleeding time.

➤*Pharmacokinetics:* Ticlopidine is rapidly absorbed (> 80%), with peak plasma levels occurring ≈ 2 hours after dosing, and is extensively metabolized. Administration after meals results in a 20% increase in the area under the plasma concentration-time curve (AUC).

Ticlopidine displays non-linear pharmacokinetics and clearance decreases markedly on repeated dosing. In older volunteers, the apparent half-life after a single 250 mg dose is about 12.6 hours; with repeat dosing at 250 mg twice daily, the terminal elimination half-life rises to 4 to 5 days and steady-state levels of ticlopidine in plasma are obtained after ≈ 14 to 21 days.

Ticlopidine binds reversibly (98%) to plasma proteins, mainly to serum albumin and lipoproteins. The binding to albumin and lipoproteins is nonsaturable over a wide concentration range. Ticlopidine also binds to alpha-1 acid glycoprotein; at concentrations attained with the recommended dose, ≤ 15% in plasma is bound to this protein.

Ticlopidine is metabolized extensively by the liver; only trace amounts of intact drug are detected in the urine. Following an oral dose, 60% is recovered in the urine and 23% in the feces. Approximately, one-third of the dose excreted in the feces is intact ticlopidine, possibly excreted in the bile. Ticlopidine is a minor component in plasma (5%) after a single dose, but at steady state is the major component (15%). Approximately 40% to 50% of the metabolites circulating in plasma are covalently bound to plasma proteins, probably by acylation. Although analysis of urine and plasma indicates at least 20 metabolites, no metabolite which accounts for the activity of ticlopidine has been isolated.

Clearance decreases with age. Steady-state trough values in elderly patients (mean age, 70 years) are about twice those in younger populations.

Hepatically impaired patients – The average plasma concentration in patients with advanced cirrhosis was slightly higher than that seen in older subjects.

Renally impaired patients – Patients with mildly (creatinine clearance [Ccr] 50 to 80 mL/min) or moderately (Ccr 20 to 50 mL/min) impaired renal function were compared with healthy subjects (Ccr 80 to 150 mL/min). AUC values of ticlopidine increased by 28% and 60% in mildly and moderately impaired patients, respectively, and plasma clearance decreased by 37% and 52%, but there were no statistically significant differences in ADP-induced platelet aggregation. Bleeding times showed significant prolongation only in the moderately impaired patients.

➤*Clinical trials:*

Patients experiencing stroke precursors – In a trial comparing ticlopidine and aspirin (The Ticlopidine Aspirin Stroke Study; TASS), 3069 patients (1987 men, 1082 women) who had experienced such stroke precursors as transient ischemic attack (TIA), transient monocular blindness (amaurosis fugax), reversible ischemic neurological deficit or minor stroke were randomized to ticlopidine 250 mg twice daily or aspirin 650 mg twice daily. The study was designed to follow patients for at least 2 years and up to 5 years. Over the duration of the study, ticlopidine significantly reduced the risk of fatal and nonfatal stroke by 24% from 18.1 to 13.8 per 100 patients followed for 5 years, compared to aspirin. During the first year, when the risk of stroke is greatest, the reduction in risk of stroke (fatal and nonfatal) compared to aspirin was 48%; the reduction was similar in men and women.

Patients who had a completed atherothrombotic stroke – In a trial comparing ticlopidine with placebo (The Canadian American Ticlopidine Study; CATS) 1073 patients who had experienced a previous atherothrombotic stroke were treated with ticlopidine 250 mg twice daily or placebo for up to 3 years. Ticlopidine significantly reduced the overall risk of stroke by 24% from 24.6 to 18.6 per 100 patients followed for 3 years, compared to placebo. During the first year, the reduction in risk of fatal and nonfatal stroke over placebo was 33%.

Contraindications

Hypersensitivity to the drug; presence of hematopoietic disorders such as neutropenia and thrombocytopenia or a history of TTP; presence of a hemostatic disorder or active pathological bleeding (such as bleeding peptic ulcer or intracranial bleeding); severe liver impairment.

Warnings

➤*Neutropenia:* Neutropenia may occur suddenly. Bone-marrow examination typically shows a reduction in myeloid precursors. After withdrawal of ticlopidine, the neutrophil count usually rises to > 1200/mm^3 within 1 to 3 weeks.

➤*Thrombocytopenia:* Rarely, thrombocytopenia may occur in isolation or together with neutropenia. If clinical evaluation and repeat laboratory testing confirm the presence of thrombocytopenia (< 80,000 cells/mm^3), discontinue the drug.

➤*TTP:* Characterized by thrombocytopenia, microangiopathic hemolytic anemia (schistocytes [fragmented RBCs] seen on peripheral smear), neurological findings, renal dysfunction, and fever. The signs and symptoms can occur in any order. In particular, clinical symptoms may precede laboratory finding by hours or days. With prompt treatment (often including plasmapheresis), 70% to 80% of patients will survive with minimal or no sequelae. If possible, avoid platelet transfusions because they may accelerate thrombosis in patients with TTP on ticlopidine.

Clinically, fever might suggest neutropenia or TTP. Weakness, pallor, petechiae or purpura, dark urine (because of blood, bile pigments, or hemoglobin) or jaundice, or neurological changes might also suggest TTP. Have the patient discontinue ticlopidine and contact the physician immediately upon the occurrence of these findings.

Monitoring – Monitor patients for neutropenia, thrombocytopenia, and TTP prior to initiating ticlopidine and every 2 weeks through the third month of therapy. If therapy is stopped during this 3-month period, continue to monitor for 2 weeks after discontinuation. More frequent monitoring and monitoring after the first 3 months of therapy are necessary only in patients exhibiting clinical signs (eg, signs or symptoms suggestive of infection) or hematological laboratory signs (eg, neutrophil count < 70% of baseline count, decrease in hematocrit, or platelet count).

Laboratory monitoring includes complete blood count, especially the absolute neutrophil count (WBC x % neutrophils), platelet count, and the appearance of the peripheral smear. Thrombocytopenia induced by ticlopidine is occasionally unrelated to TTP. Further investigate for a diagnosis of TTP with the occurrence of any acute, unexplained reduction in hemoglobin or platelet count. The appearance of schistocytes on the smear is presumptive evidence of TTP. Discontinue ticlopidine if there are laboratory signs of TTP or the neutrophil count is < 1200/mm^3.

➤*Cholesterol elevation:* Ticlopidine causes increased serum cholesterol and triglycerides. Total cholesterol levels are increased 8% to 10% within 1 month of therapy and persist at that level. The ratios of lipoprotein subfractions are unchanged.

➤*Hematological effects:* Rare cases of agranulocytosis, pancytopenia, aplastic anemia, some of which have been fatal, have occurred.

➤*Anticoagulant drugs:* If a patient is switched from an anticoagulant or fibrinolytic drug to ticlopidine, discontinue the former drug prior to ticlopidine administration.

➤*Renal function impairment:* There is limited experience in patients with renal impairment. No unexpected problems have been encountered in patients having mild renal impairment, and there is no experience with dosage adjustment in patients with greater degrees of renal impairment. Nevertheless, for renally impaired patients it may be necessary to reduce ticlopidine dosage or discontinue it altogether if hemorrhagic or hematopoietic problems are encountered.

➤*Hepatic function impairment:* Because of limited experience in patients with severe hepatic disease, who may have bleeding diatheses, ticlopidine is not recommended.

➤*Elderly:* Clearance of ticlopidine is somewhat lower in elderly patients and trough levels are increased. No overall differences in safety or efficacy were observed between elderly patients and younger patients, but greater sensitivity of some older individuals cannot be ruled out.

➤*Pregnancy: Category B.* Doses of 400 mg/kg in rats, 200 mg/kg/day in mice, and 100 mg/kg in rabbits produced maternal toxicity as well as fetal toxicity. There was no evidence of a teratogenic potential of ticlopidine. There are no adequate and well controlled studies in pregnant women. Use during pregnancy only if clearly needed.

➤*Lactation:* Ticlopidine is excreted in the milk of rats. It is not known whether this drug is excreted in human breast milk. Because of the potential for serious adverse reactions in nursing infants from ticlopidine, decide whether to discontinue nursing or to discontinue the drug, taking into account the importance of the drug to the mother.

➤*Children:* Safety and efficacy in patients < 18 years of age have not been established.

Precautions

➤*Increased bleeding risk:* Use with caution in patients who may be at risk of increased bleeding from trauma, surgery, or pathological conditions. If eliminating the antiplatelet effects of ticlopidine prior to elective surgery is desired, discontinue the drug 10 to 14 days prior to surgery. Increased surgical blood loss has occurred in patients undergoing surgery during treatment with ticlopidine. In TASS and CATS clinical trials, it was recommended that patients have ticlopidine discontinued prior to elective surgery. Several hundred patients underwent surgery during the trials, and no excessive surgical bleeding was reported.

Prolonged bleeding time is normalized within 2 hours after administration of 20 mg methylprednisolone IV. Platelet transfusions may also be used to reverse the effect of ticlopidine on bleeding. If possible, avoid platelet transfusions because they may accelerate thrombosis in patients with TTP on ticlopidine.

TICLOPIDINE HCl

➤*GI bleeding:* Ticlopidine prolongs template bleeding time. Use with caution in patients who have lesions with a propensity to bleed (such as ulcers). Use drugs that might induce such lesions with caution in patients on ticlopidine.

Drug Interactions

The dose of drugs with low therapeutic ratios metabolized by hepatic microsomal enzymes may require adjustment to maintain optimal therapeutic blood levels when starting or stopping concomitant therapy with ticlopidine.

Ticlopidine Drug Interactions			
Precipitant drug	Object drug*		Description
Antacids	Ticlopidine	↓	Giving ticlopidine after antacids has resulted in an 18% decrease in ticlopidine plasma levels.
Cimetidine	Ticlopidine	↑	Chronic cimetidine administration has reduced the clearance of a single ticlopidine dose by 50%.
Ticlopidine	Aspirin	↑	Ticlopidine potentiated the effect of aspirin on collagen-induced platelet aggregation. Ticlopidine-mediated inhibition of ADP-induced platelet aggregation is not affected. Coadministration is not recommended.
Ticlopidine	Digoxin	↓	Digoxin plasma levels may decrease slightly (≈ 15%).
Ticlopidine	Phenytoin	↑	Elevated phenytoin plasma levels with associated somnolence and lethargy have been reported. Exercise caution when administering with ticlopidine. Remeasuring phenytoin levels may be useful.
Ticlopidine	Theophylline	↑	Theophylline elimination half-life was significantly increased (from 8.6 to 12.2 hr) with a comparable reduction in total plasma clearance.

* ↑ = Object drug increased.   ↓ = Object drug decreased.

➤*Drug/Food interactions:* The oral bioavailability of ticlopidine is increased by 20% when taken after a meal. Administer with food to maximize GI tolerance.

Adverse Reactions

Adverse reactions were relatively frequent, with > 50% of patients reporting at least 1. Most (30% to 40%) involved the GI tract. Most adverse effects are mild, but 21% of patients discontinued therapy because of an adverse event, principally diarrhea, rash, nausea, vomiting, GI pain, and neutropenia. Most adverse effects occur early in the course of treatment, but new adverse effects can occur after several months.

Ticlopidine Adverse Reactions vs Aspirin and Placebo (%)			
Adverse reaction	Ticlopidine (n = 2048)	Aspirin (n = 1527)	Placebo (n = 536)
Any reaction	60	53.2	34.3
Diarrhea	12.5	5.2	4.5
Nausea	7	6.2	1.7
Dyspepsia	7	9	0.9
Rash	5.1	1.5	0.6
GI pain	3.7	5.6	1.3
Neutropenia	2.4	0.8	1.1
Purpura	2.2	1.6	0
Vomiting	1.9	1.4	0.9
Flatulence	1.5	1.4	0
Pruritus	1.3	0.3	0
Dizziness	1.1	0.5	0
Anorexia	1	0.5	0
Abnormal liver function test	1	0.3	0

➤*GI:* Ticlopidine therapy has been associated with a variety of GI complaints including diarrhea and nausea. The majority of cases are mild, but about 13% of patients discontinued therapy. They usually occur within 3 months of initiation of therapy and typically are resolved within 1 to 2 weeks without discontinuation of therapy. If the effect is severe or persistent, discontinue therapy. Colitis was later diagnosed in some cases of severe or bloody diarrhea.

➤*Hematologic:* Neutropenia/thrombocytopenia, TTP (see Warning Box), agranulocytosis, eosinophilia, pancytopenia, thrombocytosis, and bone-marrow depression.

➤*Lab test abnormalities:* Elevations of alkaline phosphatase and transaminases generally occurred within 1 to 4 months of therapy initiation. The incidence of elevated alkaline phosphatase (> 2 times upper limit of normal) was 7.6% in ticlopidine patients, 6% in placebo patients, and 2.5% in aspirin patients. The incidence of elevated AST (> 2 times upper limit of normal) was 3.1% in ticlopidine patients, 4% with placebo, and 2.1% with aspirin. Occasionally patients developed minor elevations in bilirubin.

➤*Miscellaneous:* Adverse reactions occurring in the following 0.5% to 1% of patients: GI fullness; urticaria; headache; asthenia; pain; epistaxis; tinnitus.

In addition, rarer, relatively serious events have also been reported: Pancytopenia; hemolytic anemia with reticulocytosis; aplastic anemia; allergic pneumonitis; systemic lupus (positive ANA); peripheral neuropathy; vasculitis; serum sickness; arthropathy; hepatitis; cholestatic jaundice; nephrotic syndrome; myositis; hyponatremia; immune thrombocytopenia; hepatic necrosis; peptic ulcer; renal failure; sepsis; angioedema; hepatocellular jaundice; thrombocytopenic thrombotic purpura.

Hemorrhagic – Ticlopidine has been associated with a number of bleeding complications such as ecchymosis, epistaxis, hematuria, conjunctival hemorrhage, GI bleeding, posttraumatic bleeding, and perioperative bleeding. Intracerebral bleeding was rare with an incidence no greater than that seen with comparable agents (ticlopidine 0.5%, aspirin 0.6%, placebo 0.75%).

Rash – Ticlopidine has been associated with a maculopapular or urticarial rash (often with pruritus). Rash usually occurs within 3 months of initiation of therapy, with a mean onset time of 11 days. If drug is discontinued, recovery occurs within several days. Many rashes do not recur on drug rechallenge. There have been rare reports of severe rashes, including Stevens-Johnson syndrome, erythema multiforme, and exfoliative dermatitis.

Overdosage

One case of deliberate overdosage has been reported. A 38-year-old man took a single 6000 mg dose (equivalent to 24 standard 250 mg tablets). The only abnormalities reported were increased bleeding time and increased ALT. No special therapy was instituted and the patient recovered without sequelae.

Single oral doses of 1600 and 500 mg/kg were lethal to rats and mice, respectively. Symptoms of acute toxicity were GI hemorrhage, convulsions, hypothermia, dyspnea, loss of equilibrium, and abnormal gait.

Patient Information

A decrease in the number of white blood cells (neutropenia) or platelets (thrombocytopenia) can occur, especially during the first 3 months of treatment. If neutropenia is severe, it could result in an increased risk of infection. It is critically important to obtain the scheduled blood tests to detect neutropenia or thrombocytopenia. Have patients contact their physician if they experience any indication of infection such as fever, chills, or sore throat, all of which may be consequences of neutropenia. Thrombocytopenia may be part of a syndrome called TTP. Immediately report symptoms and signs of TTP, such as fever, weakness, difficulty speaking, seizures, yellowing of skin or eyes, dark or bloody urine, pallor, or petechiae (pinpoint hemorrhagic spots on the skin).

It may take longer than usual to stop bleeding when taking ticlopidine. Have patients report any unusual bleeding to their physician. Have patients tell physicians and dentists that they are taking ticlopidine before any surgery is scheduled and before any new drug is prescribed.

Promptly report side effects such as severe or persistent diarrhea, skin rashes or SC bleeding, or any signs of cholestasis, such as yellow skin or sclera, dark urine, or light colored stools.

Take ticlopidine with food or just after eating in order to minimize GI discomfort.

TREPROSTINIL SODIUM

Rx	Remodulin (United Therapeutics)	Injection: 1 mg/mL	5.3 mg sodium chloride. In 20 mL multi-use vials.
		2.5 mg/mL	5.3 mg sodium chloride. In 20 mL multi-use vials.
		5 mg/mL	5.3 mg sodium chloride. In 20 mL multi-use vials.
		10 mg/mL	4 mg sodium chloride. In 20 mL multi-use vials.

Indications

➤*Pulmonary arterial hypertension (PAH):* As a continuous SC infusion for the treatment of PAH in patients with New York Heart Association (NYHA) Class II through IV symptoms to diminish symptoms associated with exercise.

Administration and Dosage

➤*Approved by the FDA:* May 22, 2002.

Treprostinil is supplied in 20 mL vials in concentrations of 1, 2.5, 5, and 10 mg/mL. It is meant to be administered without further dilution.

During use, a single reservoir (syringe) of treprostinol can be administered up to 72 hours at 37°C (99°F). Do not use a single vial for more than 14 days after initial introduction to the vial.

➤*Initial dose:* Treprostinil is administered by continuous SC infusion. The infusion rate is initiated at 1.25 ng/kg/min. If this initial dose cannot be tolerated, reduce the infusion rate to 0.625 ng/kg/min.

➤*Dosage adjustments:* The goal of chronic dosage adjustments is to establish a dose at which PAH symptoms are improved, while minimizing excessive pharmacological effects of treprostinil (eg, headache, nausea, emesis, restlessness, anxiety, infusion site pain or reaction).

Increase the infusion rate in increments of no more than 1.25 ng/kg/min per week for the first 4 weeks and then no more than 2.5 ng/kg/min per week for the remaining duration of infusion, depending on clinical response. There is little experience with doses greater than 40 ng/kg/min. Avoid abrupt withdrawal or sudden large reductions in dosage of treprostinil as they may result in worsening of PAH symptoms.

➤*Hepatic function impairment:* In patients with mild or moderate hepatic insufficiency, decrease the initial dose to 0.625 ng/kg/min ideal body weight and increase cautiously. Treprostinil has not been studied in patients with severe hepatic insufficiency.

➤*Administration:* Treprostinil is administered by continuous SC infusion, via a self-inserted SC catheter, using an infusion pump designed for SC drug delivery. To avoid potential interruptions in drug delivery, the patient must have immediate access to a backup infusion pump and SC infusion sets. The ambulatory pump used to administer treprostinil should: (1) be small and lightweight; (2) be adjustable to approximately 0.002 mL/hr; (3) have occlusion/no delivery, low battery, programming error, and motor malfunction alarms; (4) have delivery accuracy of ± 6% or better; and (5) be positive pressure driven. The reservoir should be made of polyvinyl chloride, polypropylene, or glass.

Infusion rates are calculated using the following formula:

Infusion rate (mL/hr) = Dose (ng/kg/min) × weight (kg) × (0.00006/ treprostinil dosage strength concentration [mg/mL])

➤*Storage/Stability:* Unopened vials of treprostinil are stable until the date indicated when stored at 15° to 25°C (59° to 77°F). Store at 25°C (77°F) with excursions permitted to 15° to 30°C (59° to 86°F).

Actions

➤*Pharmacology:* The major pharmacological actions of treprostinil are direct vasodilation of pulmonary and systemic arterial vascular beds and inhibition of platelet aggregation. In animals, the vasodilatory effects reduce right and left ventricular afterload and increase cardiac output and stroke volume. Other studies have shown that treprostinil causes a dose-related negative inotropic and lusitropic effect. No major effects on cardiac conduction have been observed.

➤*Pharmacokinetics:*

Absorption – The pharmacokinetics of continuous SC treprostinil are linear over the dose range of 1.25 to 22.5 ng/kg/min (corresponding to plasma concentrations of about 0.03 to 8 mcg/L) and can be described by a 2-compartment model.

Treprostinil is relatively rapidly and completely absorbed after SC infusion, with an absolute bioavailability approximating 100%. Steady-state concentrations occurred in approximately 10 hours. Concentrations in patients treated with an average dose of 9.3 ng/kg/min were approximately 2 mcg/L.

Distribution – The volume of distribution of the drug in the central compartment is approximately 14 L/70 kg ideal body weight. Treprostinil at in vitro concentrations ranging from 330 to 10,000 mcg/L was 91% bound to human plasma protein.

Metabolism – Treprostinil is substantially metabolized by the liver, but the precise enzymes responsible are unknown. Based on the results of in vitro human hepatic cytochrome P450 studies, treprostinil does not inhibit CYP-1A2, 2C9, 2C19, 2D6, 2E1, or 3A. Whether treprostinil induces these enzymes has not been studied.

Excretion – The elimination of treprostinil is biphasic, with a terminal half-life of approximately 2 to 4 hours. Approximately 79% of an administered dose is excreted in the urine as unchanged drug (4%) and as the identified metabolite (64%). Approximately 13% of a dose is excreted in the feces. Systemic clearance is approximately 30 L/hr for a 70 kg ideal body weight person.

Special populations –

Hepatic function impairment: In patients with portopulmonary hypertension and mild (n = 4) or moderate (n = 5) hepatic insufficiency, treprostinil at an SC dose of 10 ng/kg/min for 150 minutes had a C_{max} that was increased 2- and 4-fold, respectively, and $AUC_{0-\infty}$ was increased 3- and 5-fold, respectively, compared with healthy subjects. Clearance in patients with hepatic insufficiency was reduced by up to 80%, compared with healthy adults.

Contraindications

Known hypersensitivity to treprostinil or structurally related compounds.

Warnings

➤*Renal/Hepatic function impairment:* Use caution in patients with renal or hepatic impairment.

➤*Elderly:* Clinical studies of treprostinil did not include sufficient numbers of patients 65 years of age and over to determine whether they respond differently from younger patients. In general, dose selection for an elderly patient should be cautious, reflecting the greater frequency of decreased hepatic, renal, or cardiac function, and of concomitant disease or other drug therapy.

➤*Pregnancy: Category B.* Because animal reproduction studies are not always predictive of human response, use during pregnancy only if clearly needed.

➤*Lactation:* It is not known whether treprostinil is excreted in human milk or absorbed systemically after ingestion. Because many drugs are excreted in human milk, exercise caution when treprostinil is administered to nursing women.

➤*Children:* Safety and efficacy in pediatric patients have not been established. Clinical studies of treprostinil did not include sufficient numbers of patients 16 years of age and under to determine whether they respond differently from older patients. In general, dose selections should be cautious.

Precautions

➤*Monitoring:* Treprostinil is a potent pulmonary and systemic vasodilator. Initiation of treprostinil must be performed in a setting with adequate personnel and equipment for physiological monitoring and emergency care. SC therapy with treprostinil may be used for prolonged periods. Carefully consider the patient's ability to administer treprostinil and care for an infusion system.

Drug Interactions

➤*Diuretics, antihypertensive agents, or vasodilators:* Reduction in blood pressure caused by treprostinil may be exacerbated by drugs that by themselves alter blood pressure, such as diuretics, antihypertensive agents, or vasodilators.

➤*Anticoagulants:* Because treprostinil inhibits platelet aggregation, there also is a potential for increased risk of bleeding, particularly among patients maintained on anticoagulants.

Adverse Reactions

Patients receiving treprostinil reported a wide range of adverse events, many potentially related to the underlying disease (eg, dyspnea, fatigue, chest pain, right ventricular heart failure, pallor). During clinical trials, infusion site pain and reaction were the most common adverse events among those treated with treprostinil. Infusion site reaction was defined as any local adverse event other than pain or bleeding/bruising at the infusion site and included symptoms such as erythema, induration, or rash. Infusion site reactions were sometimes severe and could lead to discontinuation of treatment.

Treprostinil Infusion Site Adverse Reactions (%)				
	Reaction		Pain	
Adverse reaction	Treprostinil	Placebo	Treprostinil	Placebo
Severe	38	1	39	2
Requiring narcotics[1]	NA[2]	NA[2]	32	1
Leading to discontinuation	3	0	7	0

[1] Based on prescriptions for narcotics, not actual use.
[2] Medications used to treat infusion site pain were not distinguished from those used to treat site reactions.

TREPROSTINIL SODIUM

Other adverse events included diarrhea, jaw pain, edema, vasodilation, and nausea.

▶*Adverse events during chronic dosing:* The following table lists adverse events that occurred at a rate of at least 3% and were more frequent in patients treated with treprostinil than with placebo in controlled trials in PAH.

Treprostinil Adverse Reactions (%)		
Adverse reaction	Treprostinil (n = 236)	Placebo (n = 233)
Infusion site pain	85	27
Infusion site reaction	83	27
Headache	27	23
Diarrhea	25	16
Nausea	22	18
Rash	14	11
Jaw pain	13	5
Vasodilation	11	5
Dizziness	9	8
Edema	9	3
Pruritus	8	6
Hypotension	4	2

Reported adverse events (at least 3%) are included except those too general to be informative, and those not plausibly attributable to the use of the drug, because they are associated with the condition being treated or are very common in the treated population.

▶*Adverse events attributable to the drug delivery system in PAH controlled trials:* There were no reports of infection related to the drug delivery system. There were 187 infusion system complications reported in 28% of patients (23% treprostinil, 33% placebo); 173 (93%) were pump related and 14 (7%) related to the infusion set. Most delivery system complications were managed easily (eg, replace syringe or battery, reprogram pump, straighten crimped infusion line). Eight of these patients (4 treprostinil, 4 placebo) reported nonserious adverse events resulting from infusion system complications. Adverse events resulting from problems with the delivery system were typically related to symptoms of excess treprostinil (eg, nausea) or return of PAH symptoms (eg, dyspnea). These events generally were resolved by correcting the delivery system pump or infusion set problem. Adverse events resulting from problems with the delivery system did not lead to clinical instability or rapid deterioration.

Overdosage

Signs and symptoms of overdose with treprostinil during clinical trials are extensions of its dose-limiting pharmacological effects and include flushing, headache, hypotension, nausea, vomiting, and diarrhea. Most events were self-limiting and resolved with reduction or withholding of treprostinil.

In controlled clinical trials, 7 patients received some level of overdose and in open-label follow-on treatment, 7 additional patients received an overdose; these occurrences resulted from accidental bolus administration of treprostinil, errors in pump programmed rate of administration, and prescription of an incorrect dose. In only 2 cases did excess delivery of treprostinil produce an event of substantial hemodynamic concern (hypotension, near-syncope).

Patient Information

Treprostinil is infused continuously through an SC catheter, via an infusion pump. Treprostinil therapy will be needed for prolonged periods, possibly years; carefully consider the patient's ability to accept, place, and care for an SC catheter and to use an infusion pump. Additionally, make patients aware that subsequent disease management may require the initiation of an IV therapy.

Indications

➤*Acute coronary syndrome:* For the treatment of acute coronary syndrome, including patients who are to be managed medically and those undergoing percutaneous coronary intervention (PCI). See individual monographs for specific indications.

Actions

➤*Pharmacology:* Tirofiban and eptifibatide are antagonists of the platelet glycoprotein (GP) IIb/IIIa receptor, the major platelet surface receptor involved in platelet aggregation. GP IIb/IIIa is found only on platelets and their progenitors. Activation of its receptor function leads to the binding of fibrinogen and von Willebrand's factor to platelets and thus, platelet aggregation. These agents reversibly prevent fibrinogen, von Willebrand's factor, and other adhesion ligands from binding to the GP IIb/IIIa receptor, thereby inhibiting platelet aggregation. They inhibit ex vivo platelet aggregation in a dose- and concentration-dependent manner. Inhibition persists over the duration of the maintenance infusion and is reversible following infusion cessation.

➤*Pharmacokinetics:*

Absorption/Distribution – The recommended regimen of a loading infusion followed by a maintenance infusion produces an early peak plasma concentration that is similar to the steady-state concentration during the infusion. Steady state is reportedly achieved within 4 to 6 hours with eptifibatide. In patients with coronary artery disease, the plasma clearance of tirofiban ranges from 152 to 267 mL/min; renal clearance accounts for 39% of plasma clearance. The steady-state volume of distribution ranges from 22 to 42 L. Unbound fraction of tirofiban in human plasma is 35%, whereas eptifibatide is 75% unbound (25% bound).

Metabolism/Excretion – The half-life is ≈ 2 hours for tirofiban and ≈ 2.5 hours for eptifibatide. Metabolism appears to be limited. Clearance of eptifibatide in patients with coronary artery disease is 55 to 58 mL/kg/hr. These agents are cleared from the plasma largely by renal excretion, ≈ 65% for tirofiban and ≈ 50% for eptifibatide.

Special populations –

Elderly: Plasma clearance of **tirofiban** is ≈ 19% to 26% lower in elderly (> 65 years of age) patients with coronary artery disease than in younger (≤ 65 years of age) patients.

Renal insufficiency: Plasma clearance of **tirofiban** is significantly decreased (> 50%) in patients with creatinine clearance < 30 mL/min, including patients requiring hemodialysis (see Administration and Dosage). Tirofiban is removed by hemodialysis.

Contraindications

Hypersensitivity to any component of the product; active internal bleeding or a history of bleeding diathesis within the previous 30 days; a history of thrombocytopenia following prior exposure to tirofiban; history of stroke within 30 days or any history of hemorrhagic stroke; major surgical procedure or severe physical trauma within the previous month; severe hypertension (systolic blood pressure > 180 mmHg [tirofiban], > 200 mmHg [eptifibatide] or diastolic blood pressure > 110 mmHg); concomitant use of another parenteral GP IIb/IIIa inhibitor, a history of intracranial hemorrhage, intracranial neoplasm, arteriovenous malformation or aneurysm, history, symptoms, or findings suggestive of aortic dissection, acute pericarditis (tirofiban). A platelet count < 100,000/mm^3, serum creatinine ≥ 2 mg/dL (for the 180 mcg/kg bolus and the 2 mcg/kg/min infusion) or ≥ 4 mg/dL (for the 135 mcg/kg bolus and the 0.5 mcg/kg/min infusion), dependency on renal dialysis (eptifibatide).

Warnings

➤*Bleeding:* Major and minor bleeding events are the most common complications encountered during therapy with tirofiban and eptifibatide. Most major bleeding occurs at the arterial access site for cardiac catheterization.

Use with caution in patients with a platelet count < 150,000/mm^3 and in patients with hemorrhagic retinopathy.

Because these agents inhibit platelet aggregation, use caution when employed with other drugs that affect hemostasis (eg, warfarin, thrombolytics, NSAIDs, dipyridamole, ticlopidine, clopidogrel). The safety of tirofiban when used in combination with thrombolytic agents has not been established. Study regimens (n = 180) of eptifibatide administered concomitantly with the approved "accelerated" regimen of alteplase did not increase the incidence of major bleeding or transfusion compared with the incidence seen when alteplase was given alone. At high study infusion rates (1.3 mcg/kg/min and 2 mcg/kg/min), eptifibatide was associated with an increase in the incidence of bleeding and transfusions compared with the incidence seen when streptokinase was given alone.

During therapy, monitor patients for potential bleeding. When bleeding cannot be controlled with pressure, discontinue infusion of the GP IIb/IIIa inhibitor and heparin.

➤*Percutaneous coronary intervention:*

Care of the femoral artery access site – Therapy with tirofiban and eptifibatide is associated with increases in bleeding rates particularly at the site of arterial access for femoral sheath placement. Take care when attempting vascular access that only the anterior wall of the

femoral artery is punctured. Prior to pulling the sheath, discontinue heparin for 3 to 4 hours and document activated clotting time (ACT) < 180 seconds or APTT < 45 seconds. Obtain proper hemostasis after removal of the sheaths using standard compressive techniques followed by close observation. While the vascular sheath is in place, maintain patients on complete bed rest with the head of the bed elevated 30° and the affected limb restrained in a straight position. Achieve sheath hemostasis ≥ 4 hours before hospital discharge.

Minimize vascular and other trauma – Minimize other arterial and venous punctures, IM injections, and the use of urinary catheters, nasotracheal intubation, and nasogastric tubes. When obtaining IV access, avoid noncompressible sites (eg, subclavian or jugular veins).

➤*Renal function impairment:* Patients with severe renal insufficiency (creatinine clearance < 30 mL/min) showed decreased plasma clearance of **tirofiban**. Reduce the dosage of tirofiban in these patients (see Administration and Dosage).

Dose adjustment is unnecessary for **eptifibatide** in mild to moderate renal impairment; no data are available for severe impairment or dialysis.

➤*Elderly:* Elderly patients receiving **tirofiban** with heparin or heparin alone had a higher incidence of bleeding complications than younger patients. The incremental risk of bleeding in patients treated with tirofiban in combination with heparin compared with heparin alone was similar regardless of age; however, the incremental risk of **eptifibatide**-associated bleeding was greater in the older patients. The overall incidence of nonbleeding adverse events was higher in older patients both for tirofiban with heparin and heparin alone. No dose adjustment is recommended.

➤*Pregnancy:* Category B. Tirofiban crosses the placenta in pregnant rats and rabbits. There are no adequate and well-controlled studies in pregnant women. Use during pregnancy only if clearly needed.

➤*Lactation:* It is not known whether GP IIb/IIIa inhibitors are excreted in breast milk. However, significant levels of tirofiban were shown to be present in rat milk. Because of the potential for adverse effects on the nursing infant, decide whether to discontinue nursing or discontinue the drug, taking into account the importance of the drug to the mother.

➤*Children:* Safety and efficacy in pediatric patients have not been established.

Precautions

➤*Monitoring:* Monitor platelet counts, hemoglobin, hematocrit, serum creatinine, and PT/APTT prior to treatment, within 6 hours following the loading infusion, and at least daily thereafter during therapy with tirofiban (or more frequently if there is evidence of significant decline). In eptifibatide patients undergoing PCI, also measure the ACT. Maintain the APTT between 50 and 70 seconds unless PCI is to be performed; during PCI, maintain the ACT between 300 and 350 seconds. If the patient experiences a platelet decrease to < 100,000/mm^3, perform additional platelet counts to exclude pseudothrombocytopenia. If thrombocytopenia is confirmed, discontinue GP IIb/IIIa inhibitors and heparin, and appropriately monitor and treat the condition.

To monitor unfractionated heparin, monitor APTT 6 hours after the start of the heparin infusion; adjust heparin to maintain APTT at ≈ 2 times control.

Drug Interactions

Glycoprotein IIb/IIIa Inhibitor Drug Interactions			
Precipitant drug	Object drug*		Description
Aspirin	GP IIb/IIIa inhibitors	↑	Concurrent use with heparin and aspirin has been associated with an increase in bleeding compared with heparin and aspirin alone. Use caution when using with other drugs that affect hemostasis (eg, warfarin) (see Warnings).
Heparin			
Levothyroxine	Tirofiban	↔	Concomitant administration increased tirofiban clearance. Clinical significance is unknown.
Omeprazole			

* ↑ = Object drug increased. ↔ = Undetermined clinical effect.

Adverse Reactions

➤*Bleeding:* The most common drug-related adverse event reported during therapy was bleeding (see Warnings).

In clinical trials, incidence of major bleeding ranged from 1.4% to 2.2% (vs 0.8% to 1.6% with heparin alone) for **tirofiban** and 4.4% to 10.8% for **eptifibatide**. Incidence of minor bleeding was 10.5% to 12% (vs 6.3% to 8% with heparin alone) for tirofiban and 10.5% to 14.2% for eptifibatide.

Intracranial bleeding in 1 study was 0.1% for **tirofiban** with heparin and 0.3% for heparin alone. The overall incidence of stroke was 0.5% to 0.7% in patients receiving **eptifibatide** and 0.7% to 0.8% in placebo patients. The incidences of retroperitoneal bleeding for tirofiban with heparin and heparin alone were 0% to 0.6% and 0.1% to 0.3%, respectively. The incidences of major GI and GU bleeding for tirofiban with heparin were 0.1% to 0.2% and 0% to 0.1%, respectively.

Female and elderly patients receiving **tirofiban** with heparin or heparin alone had a higher incidence of bleeding complications than male patients or younger patients. The incremental risk of bleeding in patients treated with tirofiban in combination with heparin over the risk in patients treated with heparin alone was comparable regardless of age or gender. No dose adjustment is recommended.

Tirofiban Non-Bleeding Adverse Reactions (> 1%)		
Adverse reaction	Tirofiban + Heparin (n = 1953)	Heparin (n = 1887)
Bradycardia	4	3
Dissection, coronary artery	5	4
Dizziness	3	2
Edema/Swelling	2	1
Pain, leg	3	2
Pain, pelvic	6	5
Reaction, vasovagal	2	1
Sweating	2	1

Other nonbleeding side effects reported at a > 1% rate with **tirofiban** administered concomitantly with heparin were nausea, fever, and headache; these side effects were reported at a similar rate in the heparin group.

TIROFIBAN HCl

Rx	**Aggrastat** (Merck)	**Injection:** 50 mcg/mL	Preservative-free. In 250[1] and 500 mL[2] single-dose *IntraVia* containers.
		Injection, concentrate: 250 mcg/mL	Preservative-free. In 25 and 50 mL vials.[3]

[1] With 2.25 g sodium chloride and 135 mg sodium citrate dihydrate.
[2] With 4.5 g sodium chloride and 270 mg sodium citrate dihydrate.

For complete prescribing information, refer to the Glycoprotein IIb/IIIa Inhibitors group monograph.

Indications

▶*Acute coronary syndrome:* In combination with heparin, for the treatment of acute coronary syndrome, including patients who are to be managed medically and those undergoing percutaneous transluminal coronary angioplasty (PTCA) or atherectomy.

Administration and Dosage

▶*Approved by the FDA:* May 14, 1998.

Tirofiban injection first must be diluted to the same strength as tirofiban injection premixed, as noted in Directions for Use below.

In clinical studies, patients received aspirin, unless it was contraindicated, and heparin. Tirofiban and heparin can be administered through the same IV catheter. In a clinical trial, tirofiban was administered in combination with heparin for 48 to 108 hours. The infusion should be continued through angiography and for 12 to 24 hours after angioplasty or atherectomy.

▶*Recommended dosage/renal function impairment:* In most patients, administer IV at an initial rate of 0.4 mcg/kg/min for 30 minutes and then continue at 0.1 mcg/kg/min. Patients with severe renal insufficiency (Ccr < 30 mL/min) should receive half the usual rate of infusion. The table below is provided as a guide to dosage adjustment by weight.

Dosage Adjustment of Tirofiban by Patient Weight				
	Most patients		Severe renal impairment	
Patient weight (kg)	30 min loading infusion rate (mL/hr)	Maintenance infusion rate (mL/hr)	30 min loading infusion rate (mL/hr)	Maintenance infusion rate (mL/hr)
30 to 37	16	4	8	2
38 to 45	20	5	10	3
46 to 54	24	6	12	3
55 to 62	28	7	14	4
63 to 70	32	8	16	4
71 to 79	36	9	18	5
80 to 87	40	10	20	5
88 to 95	44	11	22	6
96 to 104	48	12	24	6
105 to 112	52	13	26	7

The only serious nonbleeding adverse event that occurred at a rate of ≥ 1% and was more common with **eptifibatide** than placebo (7% vs 6%) was hypotension.

▶*Lab test abnormalities:* Decreases in hemoglobin (2.1%) and hematocrit (2.2%) were observed in the group receiving **tirofiban** compared with 3.1% and 2.6%, respectively, in the heparin group. Increases in the presence of urine and fecal occult blood also were observed (10.7% and 18.3%, respectively) in the group receiving tirofiban compared with 7.8% and 12.2%, respectively, in the heparin group.

Patients treated with **tirofiban** with heparin were more likely to experience decreases in platelet counts than the control group. These decreases were reversible upon discontinuation of tirofiban. The incidence of thrombocytopenia and platelet transfusions were similar between patients treated with **eptifibatide** and placebo.

Overdosage

▶*Symptoms:* In clinical trials, inadvertent overdosage with tirofiban occurred at doses ≤ 5 times and 2 times the recommended dose for bolus administration and loading infusion, respectively. Inadvertent overdosage occurred in doses ≤ 9.8 times the 0.15 mcg/kg/min maintenance infusion rate.

The most frequently reported manifestation of overdosage was bleeding, primarily minor mucocutaneous bleeding events and minor bleeding at the sites of cardiac catheterization (see Warnings).

▶*Treatment:* Treat tirofiban overdosage by assessment of the patient's clinical condition and cessation or adjustment of the drug infusion as appropriate. Tirofiban can be removed by hemodialysis.

[3] With 8 mg sodium chloride and 2.7 mg sodium citrate dihydrate.

Dosage Adjustment of Tirofiban by Patient Weight				
	Most patients		Severe renal impairment	
Patient weight (kg)	30 min loading infusion rate (mL/hr)	Maintenance infusion rate (mL/hr)	30 min loading infusion rate (mL/hr)	Maintenance infusion rate (mL/hr)
113 to 120	56	14	28	7
121 to 128	60	15	30	8
129 to 137	64	16	32	8
138 to 145	68	17	34	9
146 to 153	72	18	36	9

▶*Directions for use:* Tirofiban injection first is diluted to the same strength as tirofiban injection premixed using 1 of the following 3 methods:

1.) Withdraw and discard 100 mL from a 500 mL bag of Sterile 0.9% Sodium Chloride or 5% Dextrose in Water, and replace this volume with 100 mL of tirofiban injection (from four 25 mL vials or two 50 mL vials); or

2.) withdraw and discard 50 mL from a 250 mL bag of Sterile 0.9% Sodium Chloride or 5% Dextrose in Water, and replace this volume with 50 mL of tirofiban injection (from two 25 mL vials or one 50 mL vial); or

3.) add the contents of a 25 mL vial of tirofiban injection to a 100 mL bag of Sterile 0.9% Sodium Chloride or 5% Dextrose in Water to achieve a final concentration of 50 mcg/mL.

Mix well prior to administration.

Tirofiban injection premixed is supplied in *IntraVia* containers as 250 or 500 mL of 0.9% Sodium Chloride containing tirofiban HCl 50 mcg/mL. To open the *IntraVia* container, first tear off its foil overpouch or dust cover. The plastic may be somewhat opaque because of moisture absorption during sterilization; the opacity will diminish gradually. Do not use unless the solution is clear and the seal is intact. Do not add other drugs or remove solution directly from the bag with a syringe. Do not use plastic containers in series connections; such use can result in air embolism caused by drawing air from the first container if it is empty of solution.

▶*Admixture compatibility/incompatibility:* Tirofiban may be administered in the same IV line as heparin, dopamine, lidocaine, potassium chloride, and famotidine. Do not administer in the same IV line as diazepam.

▶*Storage/Stability:* Store at 25°C (77°F). Do not freeze. Protect from light during storage.

Glycoprotein IIb/IIIa Inhibitors

EPTIFIBATIDE

Rx	**Integrilin** (COR Therapeutics)	**Injection for solution:** 0.75 mg/mL	In 100 mL vials.
		2 mg/mL	In 10 and 100 mL vials.

For complete prescribing information, refer to the Glycoprotein IIb/IIIa Inhibitors group monograph.

Indications

➤*Acute coronary syndrome:* Treatment of patients with acute coronary syndrome (unstable angina or non-Q-wave MI), including patients who are to be medically managed and those undergoing percutaneous coronary intervention (PCI). In this setting, eptifibatide decreased the rate of a combined endpoint of death or a new MI.

➤*Treatment of patients undergoing PCI:* Treatment of patients undergoing PCI, including those undergoing intracoronary stenting. In this setting, eptifibatide decreased the rate of a combined endpoint of death, new MI, or need for urgent intervention.

Administration and Dosage

➤*Approved by the FDA:* May 18, 1998.

➤*Acute coronary syndrome:* The recommended adult dosage of eptifibatide in patients with acute coronary syndrome with a serum creatinine < 2 mg/dL is an IV bolus of 180 mcg/kg as soon as possible following diagnosis, followed by a continuous infusion of 2 mcg/kg/min until hospital discharge or initiation of coronary artery bypass graft (CABG) surgery, up to 72 hours. If a patient undergoes a PCI while receiving eptifibatide, continue the infusion up to hospital discharge or for up to 18 to 24 hours after the procedure, whichever comes first, allowing up to 96 hours of therapy. Patients weighing > 121 kg should receive a maximum bolus of 22.6 mg followed by a maximum infusion rate of 15 mg/hr.

The recommended adult dosage of eptifibatide in patients with acute coronary syndrome with serum creatinine between 2 and 4 mg/dL is an IV bolus of 180 mcg/kg as soon as possible following diagnosis, immediately followed by a continuous infusion of 1 mcg/kg/min. Patients with serum creatinine between 2 and 4 mg/dL and weighing > 121 kg should receive a maximum bolus of 22.6 mg followed by a maximum infusion rate of 7.5 mg/hr.

➤*PCI:* The recommended adult dosage of eptifibatide in patients with a serum creatinine < 2 mg/dL initiated at the time of PCI is an IV bolus of 180 mcg/kg administered immediately before the initiation of PCI followed by a continuous infusion of 2 mcg/kg/min and a second 180 mcg/kg bolus 10 minutes after the first bolus. Continue infusion until hospital discharge or for up to 18 to 24 hours, whichever comes first. A minimum of 12 hours of infusion is recommended. Patients weighing > 121 kg should receive a maximum of 22.6 mg/bolus followed by a maximum infusion rate of 15 mg/hr.

The recommended adult dose of eptifibatide in patients with a serum creatinine between 2 and 4 mg/dL initiated at the time of PCI is an IV bolus of 180 mcg/kg administered immediately before the initiation of the procedure, immediately followed by a continuous infusion of 1 mcg/kg/min and a second 180 mcg/kg bolus administered 10 minutes after the first. Patients with a serum creatinine between 2 and 4 mg/dL and weighing > 121 kg should receive a maximum of 22.6 mg/bolus followed by a maximum infusion rate of 7.5 mg/hr.

In patients undergoing CABG surgery, discontinue eptifibatide prior to surgery.

➤*Aspirin and heparin dosing:* In the clinical trials, most patients received concomitant aspirin and heparin. Doses in the clinical studies were as follows:

Acute coronary syndrome –
Aspirin:
• 160 to 325 mg by mouth initially and daily thereafter.
Heparin: Target aPTT 50 to 70 seconds during medical management.
• If weight ≥ 70 kg, 5000 U bolus followed by infusion of 1000 U/hr.
• If weight < 70 kg, 60 U/kg bolus followed by infusion of 12 U/kg/hr.

Target ACT 200 to 300 seconds during PCI

• If heparin is initiated prior to PCI, additional boluses during PCI to maintain an ACT target of 200 to 300 seconds.
• Heparin infusion after the PCI is discouraged.

PCI –
Aspirin:
• 160 to 325 mg by mouth 1 to 24 hrs prior to PCI and daily thereafter.
Heparin: Target ACT 200 to 300 seconds.
• 60 U/kg bolus initially in patients not treated with heparin within 6 hours prior to PCI.
• Additional boluses during PCI to maintain ACT within target.
• Heparin infusion after the PCI is strongly discouraged.

Stop eptifibatide infusions in patients requiring thrombolytic therapy.

➤*Directions for use:* Withdraw the bolus dose of eptifibatide from the 10 mL vial into a syringe and administer by IV push. Immediately following bolus dose administration, initiate a continuous infusion of eptifibatide. When using an IV infusion pump, administer eptifibatide undiluted directly from the 100 mL vial. Spike the 100 mL vial with a vented infusion set.

Administer eptifibatide by volume based on patient weight according to the following table:

Eptifibatide Dosing Chart by Weight					
	180 mcg/kg bolus volume	2 mcg/kg/min infusion rate		1 mcg/kg/min infusion rate	
Patient weight (kg)	from 2 mg/mL (mL)	from 2 mg/mL (mL/hr)	from 0.75 mg/mL (mL/hr)	from 2 mg/mL (mL/hr)	from 0.75 mg/mL (mL/hr)
37 to 41	3.4	2	6	1	3
42 to 46	4	2.5	7	1.3	3.5
47 to 53	4.5	3	8	1.5	4
54 to 59	5	3.5	9	1.8	4.5
60 to 65	5.6	3.8	10	1.9	5
66 to 71	6.2	4	11	2	5.5
72 to 78	6.8	4.5	12	2.3	6
79 to 84	7.3	5	13	2.5	6.5
85 to 90	7.9	5.3	14	2.7	7
91 to 96	8.5	5.6	15	2.8	7.5
97 to 103	9	6	16	3	8
104 to 109	9.5	6.4	17	3.2	8.5
110 to 115	10.2	6.8	18	3.4	9
116 to 121	10.7	7	19	3.5	9.5
> 121	11.3	7.5	20	3.7	10

➤*Admixture compatibility/incompatibility:* May administer in the same IV line as alteplase, atropine, dobutamine, heparin, lidocaine, meperidine, metoprolol, midazolam, morphine, nitroglycerin, or verapamil. Do not administer through the same IV line as furosemide.

May administer eptifibatide in the same IV line with 0.9% NaCl or 0.9% NaCl/5% dextrose. With either vehicle, the infusion may also contain up to 60 mEq/L of potassium chloride.

➤*Storage/Stability:* Refrigerate vials at 2° to 8°C (36° to 46°F). Vials may be transferred to room temperature storage (25°C [77°F]; excursions permitted between 15° and 30°C [59° and 86°F]) for a period not to exceed 2 months. Protect from light. Discard any unused portion left in the vial.

ABCIXIMAB

Rx	**ReoPro** (Lilly)	**Injection:** 2 mg/mL	In buffered solution of 0.01 M sodium phosphate, 0.15 M NaCl, and 0.001% polysorbate 80. Preservative-free. In 5 mL vials.

Indications

➤*Adjunct to percutaneous coronary intervention (PCI):* Adjunct to PCI for the prevention of acute cardiac ischemic complications in patients at high risk for abrupt closure of the treated coronary vessel.

Abciximab is intended for use with aspirin and heparin.

➤*Unlabeled uses:* For the early treatment of acute MI, abciximab has been shown to facilitate the rate and extent of thrombolysis when combined with low-dose alteplase or low-dose reteplase. Abciximab also has been shown to be safe and effective in a small study evaluating its use in the treatment of acute ischemic stroke.

Administration and Dosage

➤*Approved by the FDA:* December 22, 1994.

Abciximab is intended for use in patients undergoing PCI. The safety and efficacy of abciximab have been investigated only with concomitant administration of heparin and aspirin.

➤*Failed PCIs:* In patients with failed PCIs, stop the continuous infusion of abciximab because there is no evidence for abciximab efficacy in that setting.

➤*Serious bleeding:* In the event of serious bleeding that cannot be controlled by compression, discontinue abciximab and heparin (see Warnings).

ABCIXIMAB

►*Recommended dosage:* The recommended adult dosage is an IV bolus of 0.25 mg/kg administered 10 to 60 minutes before the start of PCI, followed by a continuous IV infusion of 0.125 mcg/kg/min (to a maximum of 10 mcg/min) for 12 hours.

Patients with unstable angina not responding to conventional medical therapy and who are planned to undergo PCI within 24 hours may be treated with an abciximab 0.25 mg/kg IV bolus followed by an 18 to 24 hour IV infusion of 10 mcg/min, concluding 1 hour after the PCI.

►*Administration instructions:*

1.) Do not use preparations of abciximab containing visibly opaque particles.

2.) Anticipate hypersensitivity reactions whenever protein solutions such as abciximab are administered. Epinephrine, dopamine, theophylline, antihistamines, and corticosteroids should be available for immediate use. If symptoms of an allergic reaction or anaphylaxis appear, stop the infusion and give appropriate treatment (see Warnings).

3.) Withdraw the necessary amount of abciximab for bolus injection into a syringe. Filter using a sterile, non-pyrogenic, low protein-binding 0.2 or 0.22 micron filter.

4.) Withdraw the necessary amount of abciximab for the continuous infusion into a syringe. Inject into an appropriate container of sterile 0.9% saline or 5% dextrose and infuse at the calculated rate via a continuous infusion pump equipped with an in-line sterile, non-pyrogenic, low protein-binding 0.2 or 0.22 micron filter or syringe filter. Discard the unused portion at the end of the infusion.

►*Admixture incompatibilities:* Administer in a separate IV line; no other medication should be added to the infusion solutions. No incompatibilities have been observed with glass bottles or polyvinyl chloride bags and administration sets.

►*Storage/Stability:* Store vials at 2° to 8°C (36° to 46°F). Do not freeze, shake, or use beyond the expiration date. Discard any unused portion left in the vial.

Actions

►*Pharmacology:* Abciximab is the Fab fragment of the chimeric human-murine monoclonal antibody 7E3. Abciximab binds to the intact glycoprotein IIb/IIIa (GPIIb/IIIa) receptor of human platelets, which is a member of the integrin family of adhesion receptors and the major platelet surface receptor involved in platelet aggregation. The drug inhibits platelet aggregation by preventing the binding of fibrinogen, von Willebrand factor, and other adhesive molecules to GPIIb/IIIa receptor sites on activated platelets. The mechanism is thought to involve steric hindrance or conformational effects to block access of large molecules to the receptor rather than interacting directly with the RGD (arginine-glycine-aspartic acid) binding site of GPIIb/IIIa.

IV administration of single bolus doses from 0.15 to 0.3 mg/kg produced rapid, dose-dependent inhibition of platelet function as measured by ex vivo platelet aggregation in response to adenosine diphosphate (ADP) or by prolongation of bleeding time. With the 2 highest doses (0.25 and 0.3 mg/kg) at 2 hours postinjection, > 80% of the GPIIb/IIIa receptors were blocked and platelet aggregation in response to 20 mcM ADP was almost abolished. The median bleeding time increased to over 30 minutes at both doses compared with a baseline value of ≈ 5 minutes.

IV administration of a single bolus dose of 0.25 mg/kg followed by a continuous 10 mcg/min infusion for periods of 12 to 96 hours produced sustained high grade GPIIb/IIIa receptor blockade (≥ 80%) and inhibition of platelet function for the duration of the infusion in most patients. Results in patients who received the 0.25 mg/kg bolus followed by a 5 mcg/min infusion for 24 hours showed a similar initial receptor blockade and inhibition of platelet aggregation, but the response was not maintained throughout the infusion period.

Low levels of GPIIb/IIIa receptor blockade are present for > 10 days following cessation of the infusion. Bleeding time returned to ≤ 12 minutes within 12 hours following the end of infusion in 75% of patients and within 24 hours in 90%. Ex vivo platelet aggregation in response to 5 mcM ADP returned to ≥ 50% of baseline within 24 hours following the end of infusion in 34% of patients and within 48 hours in 72%. In response to 20 mcM ADP, ex vivo platelet aggregation returned to ≥ 50% of baseline within 24 hours in 62% of patients and within 48 hours in 88% of patients.

►*Pharmacokinetics:* Following IV bolus administration, free plasma concentrations of abciximab decrease rapidly with an initial half-life of < 10 minutes and a second-phase half-life of ≈ 30 minutes, probably related to rapid binding to the platelet GPIIb/IIIa receptors. Platelet function generally recovers over the course of 48 hours, although abciximab remains in the circulation for ≥ 15 days in a platelet-bound state. IV administration of a 0.25 mg/kg bolus dose of abciximab followed by continuous infusion of 10 mcg/min produces almost constant free plasma concentrations throughout the infusion. At the termination of the infusion period, free plasma concentrations fall rapidly for ≈ 6 hours and then decline at a slower rate.

Contraindications

Because abciximab increases the risks of bleeding (see Warnings), it is contraindicated in the following clinical situations: Active internal bleeding; recent (within 6 weeks) GI or GU bleeding of clinical significance; history of cerebrovascular accident (CVA) within 2 years or CVA with a significant residual neurological deficit; bleeding diathesis; administration of oral anticoagulants within 7 days unless prothrombin time is ≤ 1.2 times control; thrombocytopenia (< 100,000 cells/mcL); recent (within 6 weeks) major surgery or trauma; intracranial neoplasm, arteriovenous malformation, or aneurysm; severe uncontrolled hypertension; presumed or documented history of vasculitis; use of IV dextran before PCI or intent to use it during PCI; hypersensitivity to any component of this product or to murine proteins.

Warnings

►*Bleeding:* To minimize the risk of bleeding with abciximab, it is important to use a low-dose, weight-adjusted heparin regimen, a weight-adjusted abciximab bolus and infusion, strict anticoagulation guidelines, careful vascular access site management, discontinuation of heparin after the procedure, and early femoral arterial sheath removal.

The following conditions are associated with an increased risk of bleeding in the angioplasty setting which may be additive to that of abciximab: PCI within 12 hours of the onset of symptoms for acute MI; prolonged PCI (lasting > 70 minutes); failed PCI.

Should serious bleeding occur that is not controllable with pressure, stop the infusion of abciximab and any concomitant heparin.

Bleeding sites – Therapy with abciximab requires careful attention to all potential bleeding sites (including catheter insertion, arterial and venous puncture, cutdown, needle puncture, GI, GU, and retroperitoneal sites).

Femoral artery access site: Use care when attempting vascular access so that only the anterior wall of the femoral artery is punctured, avoiding a Seldinger technique for obtaining sheath access. Avoid femoral vein sheath placement unless needed. While the vascular sheath is in place, maintain patients on complete bed rest with the head of the bed ≤ 30° and restrain the affected limb in a straight position.

Discontinuation of heparin immediately upon completion of the procedure and removal of the arterial sheath within 6 hours is strongly recommended if APTT ≤ 50 seconds or ACT ≤ 175 seconds. In all circumstances, discontinue heparin ≥ 2 hours prior to arterial sheath removal. Following sheath removal, apply pressure to the femoral artery for at least 30 minutes using either manual compression or a mechanical device for hemostasis. Apply a pressure dressing following hemostasis. Maintain the patient on bed rest for 6 to 8 hours following sheath removal or discontinuation of abciximab, or 4 hours following discontinuation of heparin, whichever is later. Remove the pressure dressing prior to ambulation.

Frequently check the sheath insertion site and distal pulses of affected leg(s) while the femoral artery sheath is in place, and for 6 hours after femoral artery sheath removal. Measure any hematoma and monitor for enlargement.

General nursing care: Arterial and venous punctures, IM injections and use of urinary catheters, nasotracheal intubation, nasogastric tubes, and automatic blood pressure cuffs should be minimized. When obtaining IV access, avoid noncompressible sites (eg, subclavian or jugular veins). Consider saline or heparin locks for blood drawing. Document and monitor vascular puncture sites. Provide gentle care when removing dressings.

►*Hypersensitivity reactions:* Administration of abciximab may result in human anti-chimeric antibody (HACA) formation that can cause allergic or hypersensitivity reactions (including anaphylaxis), thrombocytopenia, or diminished benefit upon readministration of abciximab. Patients with HACA titers may have allergic or hypersensitivity reactions when treated with other diagnostic or therapeutic monoclonal antibodies. If anaphylaxis occurs, immediately stop administration of abciximab and initiate standard appropriate resuscitative measures. Refer to Management of Acute Hypersensitivity Reactions.

►*Pregnancy:* Category C. It is not known whether abciximab can cause fetal harm when administered to a pregnant woman or can affect reproduction capacity. Give to a pregnant woman only if clearly needed.

►*Lactation:* It is not known whether this drug is excreted in breast milk or absorbed systemically after ingestion. Exercise caution when abciximab is administered to a nursing woman.

►*Children:* Safety and efficacy in children have not been established.

Precautions

►*Monitoring:* Before infusion of abciximab, measure platelet count, prothrombin time, ACT, and APTT to identify preexisting hemostatic abnormalities. During and after treatment, closely monitor platelet counts and extent of heparin anticoagulation, as assessed by activated clotting time or APTT (see Thrombocytopenia section in this monograph).

ABCIXIMAB

Based on an integrated analysis of data from all studies, the following guidelines may be used to minimize the risk for bleeding:

- When abciximab is initiated 18 to 24 hours before PCI, maintain the APTT between 60 and 85 seconds during the abciximab and heparin infusion period.
- During PCI, maintain the ACT between 200 and 300 seconds.
- If anticoagulation is continued in these patients following PCI, maintain the APTT between 55 and 75 seconds.
- Check the APTT or ACT prior to arterial sheath removal. Do not remove the sheath unless APTT ≤ 50 seconds or ACT ≤ 175 seconds.

➤*Concomitant therapy:* In clinical trials, abciximab was used concomitantly with heparin and aspirin. Because abciximab inhibits platelet aggregation, use caution when it is used with other drugs that affect hemostasis, including thrombolytics, oral anticoagulants, nonsteroidal anti-inflammatory drugs, dipyridamole, and ticlopidine.

Low molecular weight dextran and oral anticoagulants were usually given for the deployment of a coronary stent. In the 11 patients who received low molecular weight dextran with abciximab, 5 had major bleeding events and 4 had minor bleeding events.

➤*Thrombocytopenia:* Monitor platelet counts prior to treatment, 2 to 4 hours following the bolus dose of abciximab and at 24 hours or before discharge, whichever is first. If a patient experiences an acute platelet decrease (eg, decrease to < 100,000 cells/mcL or a decrease of at least 25% from pretreatment value), determine additional platelet counts. These platelet counts should be drawn in separate tubes containing EDTA, citrate, and heparin, respectively, to exclude pseudothrombocytopenia caused by in vitro anticoagulant interaction. If true thrombocytopenia is verified, immediately discontinue abciximab and appropriately monitor and treat the condition. For patients with thrombocytopenia in clinical trials, a daily platelet count was obtained until it returned to normal. If a patient's platelet count dropped to 60,000 cells/mcL, heparin and aspirin were discontinued. If a patient's platelet count dropped to < 50,000 cells/mcL, platelets were transfused.

➤*Restoration of platelet function:* In the event of serious uncontrolled bleeding or the need for emergency surgery, discontinue abciximab. If platelet function does not to return to normal, it may be restored, at least in part, with platelet transfusions.

Adverse Reactions

Abciximab Adverse Reactions Among Treated Patients in the EPIC, EPILOG, and CAPTURE Trials (%)		
Adverse reaction	Placebo (n = 2226)	Bolus + infusion (n = 3111)
Cardiovascular		
Hypotension	10.3	14.4
Bradycardia	3.5	4.5
GI		
Nausea	11.5	13.6
Vomiting	6.8	7.3
Abdominal pain	2.2	3.1
Miscellaneous		
Back pain	13.7	17.6
Chest pain	9.3	11.4
Headache	5.5	6.4
Puncture site pain	2.6	3.6
Peripheral edema	1.1	1.6

The following additional adverse events from the EPIC, EPILOG, and CAPTURE trials were reported by investigators for patients treated with a bolus plus infusion of abciximab at incidences that were < 0.5% higher than for patients in the placebo arm.

➤*Cardiovascular:* Ventricular tachycardia (1.4%); pseudoaneurysm (0.8%); palpitation (0.5%); arteriovenous fistula (0.4%); incomplete AV block (0.3%); nodal arrhythmia (0.2%); complete AV block, embolism (limb), thrombophlebitis (0.1%).

➤*CNS:* Dizziness (2.9%); anxiety (1.7%); abnormal thinking (1.3%); agitation (0.7%); hypesthesia (0.6%); confusion (0.5%); muscle contractions (0.4%); coma (0.2%); hypertonia (0.2%); diplopia (0.1%).

➤*GI:* Dyspepsia (2.1%); diarrhea (1.1%); ileus, gastroesophageal reflux (0.1%).

➤*GU:* Urinary retention (0.7%); dysuria, abnormal renal function (0.4%); frequent micturition, cystalgia, urinary incontinence, prostatitis (0.1%).

➤*Hematologic/Lymphatic:* Anemia (1.3%); leukocytosis (0.5%); petechiae (0.2%).

➤*Respiratory:* Pneumonia, rales (0.4%); pleural effusion, bronchitis, bronchospasm (0.3%); pleurisy, pulmonary embolism (0.2%); rhonchi (0.1%).

➤*Miscellaneous:* Pain (5.4%); increased sweating (1%); asthenia (0.7%); incisional pain (0.6%); pruritus (0.5%); abnormal vision, edema (0.3%); wound, abscess, cellulitis, peripheral coldness, myalgia (0.2%); injection site pain, dry mouth, pallor, diabetes mellitus, hyperkalemia, enlarged abdomen, bullous eruption, inflammation, drug toxicity (0.1%).

Bleeding – Major bleeding events were defined as either an intracranial hemorrhage or a decrease in hemoglobin > 5 g/dL. Minor bleeding events included spontaneous gross hematuria, spontaneous hematemesis, observed blood loss with a hemoglobin decrease of > 3 g/dL, or a decrease in hemoglobin of at least 4 g/dL without an identified bleeding site.

In the EPIC trial, in which a non-weight-adjusted, longer duration heparin dose regimen was used, the most common complication during abciximab therapy was bleeding during the first 36 hours. Major bleeding occurred in 10.6% of patients in the abciximab bolus plus infusion arm compared with 3.3% of patients in the placebo arm. Minor bleeding was seen in 16.8% of abciximab bolus plus infusion patients and 9.2% of placebo patients. Approximately 70% of abciximab-treated patients with major bleeding had bleeding at the arterial access site in the groin. Abciximab-treated patients also had a higher incidence of major bleeding events from GI, GU, retroperitoneal, and other sites. Bleeding rates were reduced in the CAPTURE trial and further reduced in the EPILOG and EPISTENT trials by use of modified dosing regimens and specific patient management techniques.

Abciximab treatment was not associated with excess major bleeding in patients who underwent CABG surgery. Some patients with prolonged bleeding times received platelet transfusions to correct the bleeding time prior to surgery.

Thrombocytopenia – Patients treated with abciximab were more likely to experience decreases in platelet counts and to require platelet transfusions than patients treated with placebo (see Precautions).

ANAGRELIDE HCl

Rx	**Agrylin** (Roberts)	**Capsules:** 0.5 mg	Lactose. (ROBERTS 063). Opaque, white. In 100s.
		1 mg	Lactose. (ROBERTS 064). Opaque, gray. In 100s.

Indications

►*Thrombocythemia:* For the treatment of patients with thrombocythemia, secondary to myeloproliferative disorders, to reduce the elevated platelet count and the risk of thrombosis and to ameliorate associated symptoms including thrombo-hemorrhagic events.

Administration and Dosage

►*Approved by the FDA:* March 17, 1997.

The recommended starting dose is 0.5 mg 4 times/day or 1 mg twice/day; maintain for at least 1 week, then adjust to the lowest effective dosage required to reduce and maintain platelet count below 600,000/mcL ideally to the normal range. Increase the dosage by no more than 0.5 mg/day in any 1 week. Do not exceed 10 mg/day or 2.5 mg in a single dose. Individualize the decision to treat asymptomatic young adults with essential thrombocythemia.

To monitor the effect of anagrelide and prevent the occurrence of thrombocytopenia, perform platelet counts every 2 days during the first week of treatment and at least weekly thereafter until the maintenance dosage is reached.

Typically, platelet count begins to respond within 7 to 14 days at the proper dosage. Most patients will experience an adequate response at a dose of 1.5 to 3 mg/day. Closely monitor patients with known or suspected heart disease, renal insufficiency, or hepatic dysfunction.

►*Storage/Stability:* Store at 25°C (77°F); excursions permitted to 15° to 30°C (59° to 86°F) in a light-resistant container.

Actions

►*Pharmacology:* The mechanism by which anagrelide reduces blood platelet count is under investigation. Studies support a hypothesis of dose-related reduction in platelet production resulting from a decrease in megakaryocyte hypermaturation. In blood withdrawn from healthy volunteers treated with anagrelide, a disruption was found in the postmitotic phase of megakaryocyte development and a reduction in megakaryocyte size and ploidy. At therapeutic doses, anagrelide does not produce significant changes in white cell counts or coagulation parameters and may have a small but clinically insignificant effect on red cell parameters. Platelet aggregation is inhibited in people at doses higher than those required to reduce platelet count. Anagrelide inhibits cyclic AMP phosphodiesterase and ADP- and collagen-induced platelet aggregation.

►*Pharmacokinetics:*

Absorption/Distribution – Anagrelide plasma levels peaked at 5 ng/mL at approximately 1 hour, decreased rapidly during the first 6 to 8 hours, and then declined more slowly. At fasting and at a dose of 0.5 mg, the plasma half-life is 1.3 hours and the volume of distribution is approximately 12 L/kg. Anagrelide does not accumulate in plasma after repeated administration. Bioavailability is reduced by food.

Metabolism/Excretion – Anagrelide is extensively metabolized; less than 1% is recovered unchanged in the urine. Following oral administration, more than 70% of the dose was recovered in urine. Based on limited data, there appears to be a trend towards dose linearity between doses of 0.5 and 2 mg.

Warnings

►*Cardiovascular:* Use with caution in patients with known or suspected heart disease only if the potential benefits outweigh the potential risks. Because of the positive inotropic effects and side effects of anagrelide, a pretreatment cardiovascular examination is recommended along with careful monitoring during treatment. Therapeutic doses of anagrelide may cause cardiovascular effects, including vasodilation, tachycardia, palpitations, and congestive heart failure.

►*Thrombocytopenia:* Platelet counts below 100,000/mcL occurred in 84 patients, and reduction below 50,000/mcL occurred in 44 of the 942 patients with myeloproliferative disorders while on anagrelide therapy. Thrombocytopenia promptly recovered upon discontinuation of anagrelide.

►*Renal toxicity:* Fifteen patients were found to have renal abnormalities. Eleven experienced renal failure (approximately 1%) while on anagrelide treatment; in 4 cases, the renal failure was considered to be possibly related to anagrelide treatment. The remaining 11 were found to have preexisting renal impairment. Doses ranged from 1.5 to 6 mg/day with exposure periods of 2 to 12 months. No dose adjustment was required because of renal insufficiency.

►*Renal function impairment:* It is recommended that patients with renal insufficiency (creatinine 2 mg/dL or greater) receive anagrelide when the potential benefits of therapy outweigh the potential risks. Monitor patients closely for signs of renal toxicity while receiving anagrelide.

►*Hepatic function impairment:* It is recommended that patients with evidence of hepatic dysfunction (ie, bilirubin, AST, or measures of liver function more than 1.5 times the upper limit of normal) receive anagrelide when the potential benefits of therapy outweigh the poten-

tial risks. Monitor patients closely for signs of hepatic toxicity while receiving anagrelide. Elevated liver enzymes were observed in 3 patients during anagrelide therapy.

►*Pregnancy: Category C.* A fertility and reproductive performance study performed in female rats revealed that anagrelide at oral doses of 60 mg/kg/day or more (49 times the recommended maximum human dose) disrupted implantation and exerted adverse effect on embryo/fetal survival.

Five women became pregnant while on anagrelide treatment at doses of 1 to 4 mg/day. Treatment was stopped as soon as it was realized that they were pregnant. All delivered healthy babies. There are no adequate and well-controlled studies in pregnant women. Use anagrelide during pregnancy only if the potential benefit justifies the potential risk to the fetus.

►*Lactation:* It is not known whether this drug is excreted in breast milk. Decide whether to discontinue nursing or to discontinue the drug, taking into account the importance of the drug to the mother.

►*Children:* The safety and efficacy of anagrelide in patients younger than 16 years of age have not been established. Anagrelide has been used successfully in 12 pediatric patients (age range, 6.8 to 17.4 years of age), including 8 patients with essential thrombocythemia, 2 with chronic myelogenous leukemia, 1 with polycythemia vera, and 1 with other myeloproliferative disorders. Patients were started on therapy with 0.5 mg 4 times/day to a maximum daily dose of 10 mg.

Precautions

►*Monitoring:* Anagrelide therapy requires close clinical supervision of the patient. While the platelet count is being lowered (usually during the first 2 weeks of treatment), monitor blood counts (hemoglobin, white blood cells), liver function (AST, ALT) and renal function (serum creatinine, BUN).

Blood pressure – In 9 subjects receiving a single 5 mg dose of anagrelide, standing blood pressure fell an average of 22/15 mm Hg, usually accompanied by dizziness. Only minimal changes in blood pressure were observed following a 2 mg dose.

Interruption of therapy – In general, interruption of anagrelide treatment is followed by an increase in platelet count. After sudden discontinuation of therapy, the increase in platelet count can be observed within 4 days.

►*Photosensitivity:* Photosensitization may occur; therefore, caution patients to take protective measures (ie, sunscreens, protective clothing) against exposure to ultraviolet light or sunlight until tolerance is determined.

Drug Interactions

►*Sucralfate:* A single case report suggests sucralfate may interfere with anagrelide absorption.

►*Drug/Food interactions:* When a 0.5 mg dose was taken after food, bioavailability was modestly reduced by an average of 13.8%, and plasma half-life slightly increased (to 1.8 hours), when compared with the same subjects in the fasting state. The peak plasma level was lowered by approximately 45% and delayed by 2 hours.

Adverse Reactions

While most reported adverse reactions during anagrelide therapy have been mild in intensity and have decreased in frequency with continued therapy, serious adverse events reported in patients with ET and in patients with thrombocythemias of other etiologies include the following: CHF; myocardial infarction; cardiomyopathy; cardiomegaly; complete heart block; atrial fibrillation; cerebrovascular accident; pericarditis; pericardial effusion; pleural effusion; pulmonary infiltrates; pulmonary fibrosis; pulmonary hypertension; pancreatitis; gastric/duodenal ulceration; seizure. The most common adverse events for treatment discontinuation were headache, palpitations, diarrhea, abdominal pain, and edema.

Anagrelide Adverse Reactions (≥ 5%)	
Adverse reaction	% (n = 551)
Cardiovascular	
Palpitations	26.1
Chest pain	7.8
Tachycardia	7.5
CNS	
Headache	43.5
Asthenia	23.1
Dizziness	15.4
Paresthesia	5.9
GI	
Diarrhea	25.7
Nausea	17.1
Abdominal pain	16.4

ANAGRELIDE HCl

Anagrelide Adverse Reactions (≥ 5%)	
Adverse reaction	% (n = 551)
Flatulence	10.2
Vomiting	9.7
Anorexia	7.7
Dyspepsia	5.2
Miscellaneous	
Edema	20.6
Pain	15
Dyspnea	11.9
Fever	8.9
Peripheral edema	8.5
Rash, including urticaria	8.3
Pharyngitis	6.8
Malaise	6.4
Cough	6.3
Back pain	5.9
Pruritus	5.5

Other adverse reactions (1% to less than 5%) are as follows:

➤*Cardiovascular:* Arrhythmia; hemorrhage; cardiovascular disease; angina pectoris; heart failure; postural hypotension; vasodilation; hypertension; syncope; thrombosis.

➤*CNS:* Depression; somnolence; confusion; insomnia; nervousness; amnesia; migraine.

➤*Dermatologic:* Skin disease; alopecia.

➤*GI:* Constipation; GI distress or hemorrhage; gastritis; melena; aphthous stomatitis; eructation.

➤*GU:* Dysuria; hematuria.

➤*Hematologic:* Anemia; thrombocytopenia (see Warnings); ecchymosis; lymphadenopathy.

➤*Musculoskeletal:* Arthralgia; myalgia; leg cramps.

➤*Respiratory:* Rhinitis; epistaxis; respiratory disease; sinusitis; pneumonia; bronchitis; asthma.

➤*Special senses:* Amblyopia; abnormal vision; tinnitus; visual field abnormality; diplopia.

➤*Miscellaneous:* Flu symptoms; chills; photosensitivity; elevated liver enzymes (see Warnings); dehydration.

Overdosage

➤*Symptoms:* Single oral doses of anagrelide at 2500, 1500, and 200 mg/kg in mice, rats, and monkeys, respectively, were not lethal. Symptoms of acute toxicity included decreased motor activity in mice and rats and softened stools and decreased appetite in monkeys.

There are no reports of overdosage with anagrelide. Platelet reduction from anagrelide therapy is dose related; therefore, thrombocytopenia, which can potentially cause bleeding, is expected from overdosage. Should overdosage occur, cardiac and CNS toxicity can also be expected.

➤*Treatment:* In case of overdosage, close clinical supervision of the patient is required; this especially includes monitoring of the platelet count for thrombocytopenia. Decrease dosage or stop, as appropriate, until the platelet count returns to within the normal range.

Patient Information

Anagrelide is not recommended in women who are or may become pregnant. It may cause fetal harm when administered to a pregnant woman. If this drug is used during pregnancy or if the patient becomes pregnant while taking this drug, apprise the patient of the potential harm to the fetus. Instruct women of childbearing potential that they must not be pregnant and that they should use contraception while taking anagrelide.

Advise patients that anagrelide may cause photosensitivity (sensitivity to sunlight). Advise patients to avoid prolonged exposure to the sun and other ultraviolet light. Instruct patients to use sunscreens and wear protective clothing until tolerance is determined.

DIPYRIDAMOLE

Rx	**Dipyridamole** (Various, eg, Barr, Genetco, Moore)	**Tablets**: 25 mg	In 90s, 100s, 500s, 1000s, 5000s and UD 100s,
Rx	**Persantine** (Boehringer Ingelheim)		(BI/17). Orange, sugar coated. In 100s, 1000s and UD 100s.
Rx	**Dipyridamole** (Various, eg, Barr, Genetco, Moore)	**Tablets**: 50 mg	In 100s, 500s, 1000s and UD 100s,
Rx	**Persantine** (Boehringer Ingelheim)		(BI/18). Orange, sugar coated. In 100s, 1000s and UD 100s.
Rx	**Dipyridamole** (Various, eg, Barr, Genetco, Moore)	**Tablets**: 75 mg	In 100s, 500s, 1000s and UD 100s.
Rx	**Persantine** (Boehringer Ingelheim)		(BI/19). Orange, sugar coated. In 100s, 500s and UD 100s.

Indications

➤*Thromboembolic complications:* Adjunct to coumarin anticoagulants in the prevention of postoperative thromboembolic complications of cardiac valve replacement.

➤*Unlabeled uses:* At one time, dipyridamole was indicated as a "possibly effective" long-term therapy for chronic angina pectoris. The FDA, however, has withdrawn approval for this indication.

Dipyridamole in combination with aspirin has been commonly used in the prevention of myocardial reinfarction and reduction of mortality post MI. However, combination therapy appears to be no more beneficial than the use of aspirin alone.

Administration and Dosage

➤*Adjunctive use in prophylaxis of thromboembolism after cardiac valve replacement:* The recommended dose is 75 to 100 mg, 4 times daily as an adjunct to the usual warfarin therapy. Please note that aspirin is not to be administered concomitantly with coumarin anticoagulants, which are indicated for use with dipyridamole in the prevention of thromboembolic complications (see Indications).

Actions

➤*Pharmacology:* It is believed that platelet reactivity and interaction with prosthetic cardiac valve surfaces, resulting in abnormally shortened platelet survival time, is a significant factor in thromboembolic complications occurring in connection with prosthetic heart valve replacement. Dipyridamole lengthens abnormally shortened platelet survival time in a dose-dependent manner.

Dipyridamole is a platelet adhesion inhibitor, although the mechanism of action has not been fully elucidated. The mechanism may relate to: 1) Inhibition of red blood cell uptake of adenosine, itself an inhibitor of platelet reactivity, 2) phosphodiesterase inhibition leading to increased cyclic-3', 5'-adenosine monophosphate within platelets and 3) inhibition of formation of thromboxane A_2, which is a potent stimulator of platelet activation.

Hemodynamics – In animals, intraduodenal doses of 0.5 to 4 mg/kg dipyridamole produced dose-related decreases in systemic and coronary vascular resistance leading to decreases in systemic blood pressure and increases in coronary blood flow. Onset of action in animals was about

24 minutes and effects persisted for about 3 hours.

In humans, the same qualitative hemodynamic effects have been observed. However, acute IV administration of dipyridamole may worsen regional myocardial perfusion distal to partial occlusion of coronary arteries.

➤*Pharmacokinetics:*

Metabolism – Following an oral dose of dipyridamole, the average time to peak concentration is about 75 minutes. The decline in plasma concentration fits a two-compartment model. The α half-life (the initial decline following peak concentration) is ≈ 40 minutes. The β half-life (the terminal decline in plasma concentration) is ≈ 10 hours. Dipyridamole is highly bound to plasma proteins. It is metabolized in the liver where it is conjugated as a glucuronide and excreted with the bile.

➤*Clinical trials:* In three randomized controlled clinical trials involving 854 patients who had undergone surgical placement of a prosthetic heart valve, dipyridamole with warfarin decreased the incidence of postoperative thromboembolic events by 62% to 91% compared to warfarin alone. In three additional studies involving 392 patients taking dipyridamole and coumarin-like anticoagulants, the incidence of thromboembolic events ranged from 2.3% to 6.9%. Dipyridamole does not influence prothrombin time or activity measurements when administered with warfarin.

Warnings

➤*Fertility impairment:* A significant reduction in number of corpora lutea with consequent reduction in implantations and live fetuses was observed at 155 times the maximum recommended human dose.

➤*Pregnancy:* Category B. There are no adequate and well-controlled studies in pregnant women. Use during pregnancy only if clearly needed.

➤*Lactation:* Dipyridamole is excreted in breast milk. Exercise caution when administering to a nursing woman.

➤*Children:* Safety and efficacy in children < 12 years of age have not been established.

Precautions

➤*Hypotension:* Use dipyridamole with caution in patients with hypotension because it can produce peripheral vasodilation.

DIPYRIDAMOLE

Adverse Reactions

Adverse reactions at therapeutic doses are usually minimal and transient. With long-term use, initial side effects usually disappear. The following reactions were reported in 2 heart valve replacement trials comparing dipyridamole and warfarin therapy to either warfarin alone or warfarin and placebo: Dizziness (13.6%); abdominal distress (6.1%); headache, rash (2.3%); diarrhea; vomiting; flushing; pruritus; angina pectoris, liver dysfunction (rare).

On those uncommon occasions when adverse reactions have been persistent or intolerable, they have ceased on withdrawal of the medication.

Overdosage

➤*Symptoms:* Hypotension, if it occurs, is likely to be of short duration, but a vasopressor may be used if necessary. In animals, symptoms of acute toxicity included ataxia, decreased locomotion, diarrhea, emesis, and depression.

➤*Treatment:* Since dipyridamole is highly protein bound, dialysis is not likely to be of benefit.

DIPYRIDAMOLE AND ASPIRIN

| Rx | **Aggrenox** (Boehringer Ingelheim) | **Capsules:** 200 mg extended-release dipyridamole/25 mg aspirin | Lactose, sucrose. (01A). Red/Ivory. In 60s. |

For more information, refer to the individual monographs for dipyridamole and aspirin.

Indications

➤*Stroke:* To reduce the risk of stroke in patients who have had transient ischemia of the brain or complete ischemic stroke due to thrombosis.

Administration and Dosage

➤*Approved by the FDA:* November 23, 1999.

The recommended dose of dipyridamole and aspirin combination therapy is 1 capsule given orally twice daily, 1 in the morning and 1 in the evening. Swallow whole; do not crush or chew.

Do not interchange with individual components of aspirin and dipyridamole tablets.

➤*Storage/Stability:* Store at 25°C (77°F). Protect from excessive moisture.

Actions

➤*Pharmacology:* Antithrombotic action is the result of the additive antiplatelet effects of dipyridamole and aspirin.

Dipyridamole inhibits the uptake of adenosine into platelets, endothelial cells, and erythrocytes in vitro and in vivo; the inhibition occurs in a dose-dependent manner at therapeutic concentrations (0.5 to 1.9 mcg/mL). This inhibition results in an increase in local concentrations of adenosine that acts on the platelet A_2-receptor thereby stimulating platelet adenylate cyclase and increasing platelet cyclic-3′,5′-adenosine monophosphate (cAMP) levels. Platelet aggregation is inhibited in response to various stimuli such as platelet activation factor, collagen, and adenosine diphosphate (ADP). Dipyridamole inhibits phosphodiesterase (PDE) in various tissues. While the inhibition of cAMP-PDE is weak, therapeutic levels of dipyridamole inhibit cyclic-3′,5′-guanosine monophosphate-PDE (cGMP-PDE), thereby augmenting the increase in cGMP produced by endothelium-derived relaxing factor (now identified as nitric oxide).

Aspirin inhibits platelet aggregation by irreversible inhibition of platelet cyclooxygenase and thus inhibits the generation of thromboxane A_2, a powerful inducer of platelet aggregation and vasoconstriction.

➤*Pharmacokinetics:*

Absorption –

Dipyridamole: Peak plasma levels of dipyridamole are achieved ≈ 2 hours after administration of a daily dose of 400 mg dipyridamole and aspirin combination (given as 200 mg twice daily). The peak plasma concentration at steady-state is ≈ 1.98 mcg/mL and the steady state trough concentration is ≈ 0.53 mcg/mL.

Aspirin: Peak plasma levels of aspirin are achieved ≈ 0.63 hours after administration of a 50 mg aspirin daily dose from dipyridamole and aspirin combination (given as 25 mg twice daily). The peak plasma concentration at steady-state is ≈ 319 ng/mL. Aspirin undergoes moderate hydrolysis to salicylic acid in the liver and the GI wall, with 50% to 75% of an administered dose reaching the systemic circulation as intact aspirin.

Distribution –

Dipyridamole: Dipyridamole is highly lipophilic; however, it has been shown that the drug does not cross the blood-brain barrier to any significant extent in animals. The steady-state volume of distribution of dipyridamole is ≈ 92 L. Approximately 99% of dipyridamole is bound to plasma proteins, predominantly to α1-acid glycoprotein and albumin.

Aspirin: Aspirin is poorly bound to plasma proteins and its apparent volume of distribution is low (10 L). Its metabolite, salicylic acid, is highly bound to plasma proteins, but its binding is concentration-dependent (nonlinear). At low concentrations (< 100 mcg/mL), ≈ 90% of salicylic acid is bound to albumin. Salicyclic acid is widely distributed to all tissues and fluids in the body, including the CNS, breast milk, and fetal tissues.

Metabolism/Excretion –

Dipyridamole: Dipyridamole is metabolized in the liver, primarily by conjugation with glucuronic acid, of which monoglucuronide, which has low pharmacodynamic activity, is the primary metabolite. In plasma, ≈ 80% of the total amount is present as parent compound and 20% as monoglucuronide. Most of the glucuronide metabolite (≈ 95%) is excreted via bile into the feces, with some evidence of enterohepatic circulation. Renal excretion of parent compound is negligible and urinary excretion of the glucuronide metabolite is low (≈ 5%). With IV treatment of dipyridamole, a triphasic profile is obtained: A rapid alpha phase with a half-life of ≈ 3.4 minutes, a beta phase with a half-life of ≈ 39 minutes, (which, together with the alpha phase accounts for ≈ 70% of the total area under the curve, AUC), and a prolonged elimination phase λ_Z with a half-life of ≈ 15.5 hours.

Aspirin: Aspirin is rapidly hydrolized in plasma to salicylic acid with a half-life of 20 minutes. Plasma levels of aspirin are essentially undetectable 2 to 2.5 hours after dosing, and peak salicylic acid concentra-

tion occurs 1 hour (range, 0.5 to 2 hours) after aspirin administration. Salicylic acid is primarily conjugated in the liver to form salicyluric acid, a phenolic glucuronide, an acyl glucuronide, and a number of minor metabolites. Salicylate metabolism is saturable and the total body clearance decreases at higher serum concentrations because of the limited ability of the liver to form both salicyluric acid and phenolic glucuronide. Following toxic doses (10 to 20 g), the plasma half-life may increase to > 20 hours.

The elimination of acetylsalicylic acid follows first-order kinetics with the dipyridamole and aspirin combination and has a half-life of 0.33 hours. The half-life of salicylic acid is 1.71 hours. Both values correspond well with data from the literature at a lower dose which state a resultant half-life of ≈ 2 to 3 hours. At higher doses, the elimination of salicylic acid follows zero-order kinetics (ie, the rate of elimination is constant in relation to plasma concentration) with an apparent half-life of ≥ 6 hours. Renal excretion of unchanged drug depends upon urinary pH. As urinary pH rises above 6.5, the renal clearance of free salicylate increases from < 5% to > 80%. Following therapeutic doses, ≈ 10% is excreted as salicylic acid and 75% as salicyluric acid, as the phenolic and acyl glucuronides, in urine.

Special risk –

Elderly: Plasma concentrations (determined as AUC) of dipyridamole in healthy elderly subjects > 65 years of age were ≈ 40% higher than in subjects < 55 years of age receiving treament with the dipyridamole and aspirin combination.

Hepatic function impairment: In a study conducted with an IV formulation of **dipyridamole**, patients with mild-to-severe hepatic insufficiency showed no change in plasma concentrations of dipyridamole but showed an increase in the pharmacologically inactive monoglucuronide metabolite. Dipyridamole can be dosed without restriction as long as there is no evidence of hepatic failure. Avoid **aspirin** in patients with severe hepatic insufficiency.

Renal function impairment: No changes were observed in the pharmacokinetics of **dipyridamole** or its glucuronide metabolite with creatinine clearances ranging from ≈ 15 mL/min to > 100 mL/min if data were corrected for differences in age. Avoid **aspirin** in patients with severe renal failure (glomerular filtration rate < 10 mL/min).

Contraindications

Hypersensitivity to dipyridamole, aspirin, or any of the other product components.

➤*Allergy:* Aspirin is contraindicated in patients with a known allergy to NSAIDs and in patients with asthma, rhinitis, and nasal polyps. Aspirin may cause severe urticaria, angioedema, or bronchospasms (asthma).

➤*Reye's syndrome:* Do not use in children or teenagers with viral infections with or without fever. There is a risk of Reye's syndrome with concomitant use of aspirin in certain viral illnesses.

Warnings

➤*Alcohol:* Counsel patients who consume ≥ 3 alcoholic drinks every day about the bleeding risks involved with chronic, heavy alcohol use while taking **aspirin**.

➤*Coagulation abnormalities:* Even low doses of **aspirin** can inhibit platelet function leading to an increase in bleeding time. This can adversely affect patients with inherited or acquired bleeding disorders (eg, liver disease, vitamin K deficiency).

➤*GI side effects:* GI side effects include stomach pain, heartburn, nausea, vomiting, and gross GI bleeding. Minor upper GI symptoms, such as dyspepsia, are common and can occur anytime during therapy. Watch for signs of ulceration and bleeding, even in the absence of previous GI symptoms. Inform patients about the signs and symptoms of GI side effects and what steps to take if they occur.

➤*Peptic ulcer disease:* Avoid using **aspirin**, which can cause gastric mucosal irritation and bleeding in patients with a history of active peptic ulcer disease.

➤*Renal function impairment:* Avoid aspirin in patients with severe renal failure (glomerular filtration rate < 10 mL/min).

➤*Hepatic function impairment:* Elevations of hepatic enzymes and hepatic failure have been reported in association with **dipyridamole** administration.

➤*Mutagenesis:* **Aspirin** induced chromosome aberrations in cultured human fibroblasts.

➤*Fertility impairment:*

Dipyridamole – A significant reduction in number of corpora lutea with consequent reduction in implantations and live fetuses was observed at dose of dipyridamole 1250 mg/kg/day or 7500 mg/m²/day in rats (≈ 25 times the recommended human dose on a body surface area basis).

Aspirin – Aspirin inhibits ovulation in rats.

DIPYRIDAMOLE AND ASPIRIN

➤*Pregnancy: Category B* (dipyridamole); *Category D* (aspirin).

Reproduction studies have been performed with the dipyridamole and aspirin combination in a ratio of 1:4.4 in rats and rabbits and have revealed no teratogenic evidence at doses of up to 405 mg/kg/day in rats and 135 mg/kg/day in rabbits. However, treatment with the dipyridamole and aspirin combination at 405 mg/kg/day induced abortion in rats. The doses of dipyridamole at 75 mg/kg/day represent 1.5 times the recommended human dose on a body surface area (BSA) basis. In these studies, aspirin itself was teratogenic at doses of 330 mg/kg/day (1980 mg/m²/day) in rats (eg, spina bifida, exencephaly, microphthalmia, coelosomia) and 110 mg/kg/day (1320 mg/m²/day) in rabbits (eg, congested fetuses, agenesis of skull and upper jaw, generalized edema with malformation of the head, diaphanous skin). The doses of aspirin at 330 mg/kg/day in rats and at 110 mg/kg/day in rabbits were ≈ 54 and 36 times the recommended human dose, respectively, on a BSA basis.

There are no adequate and well-controlled studies in pregnant women. Use this combination during pregnancy only if the potential benefit justifies the risk to the fetus. Because of the aspirin component, avoid the combination in the third trimester of pregnancy.

➤*Lactation:* Dipyridamole and aspirin are excreted in human breast milk in low concentrations. Exercise caution when dipyridamole and aspirin combination capsules are administered to a nursing woman.

➤*Children:* Safety and efficacy of dipyridamole and aspirin combination capsules in pediatric patients have not been studied. Because of the aspirin component, use of this product in the pediatric population is not recommended.

Precautions

Dipyridamole and aspirin combination is not interchangeable with the individual components of aspirin and dipyridamole tablets.

➤*Coronary artery disease:* Due to the vasodilatory effect of **dipyridamole**, use with caution in patients with severe coronary artery disease (eg, unstable angina, recently sustained MI). Chest pain may be aggravated in patients with underlying coronary artery disease who are receiving dipyridamole. For stroke or transient ischemic attack patients for whom **aspirin** is indicated to prevent recurrent MI or angina pectoris, the aspirin in this product may not provide adequate treatment for the cardiac indications.

➤*Hypotension:* **Dipyridamole** can produce peripheral vasodilation; use with caution in patients with hypotension.

➤*Risk of bleeding:* In 1 study, the incidence of GI bleeding was 68 patients (4.1%) in the dipyridamole and aspirin combination group, 36 patients (2.2%) in the dipyridamole group, 52 patients (3.2%) in the aspirin group, and 34 patients (2.1%) in the placebo groups. The incidence of intracranial hemorrhage was 9 patients (0.6%) in the dipyridamole and aspirin combination group, 6 patients (0.5%) in the dipyridamole group, 6 patients (0.4%) in the aspirin group, and 7 patients (0.4%) in the placebo groups.

➤*Lab test abnormalities:* **Aspirin** has been associated with elevated hepatic enzymes, blood urea nitrogen and serum creatinine, hyperkalemia, proteinuria, and prolonged bleeding time. **Dipyridamole** has been associated with elevated hepatic enzymes.

Drug Interactions

No drug-drug interaction studies were conducted with the combination of dipyridamole and aspirin. The following drug interactions are representative of the literature for each agent (dipyridamole or aspirin).

Dipyridamole and Aspirin Combination Drug Interactions			
Precipitant drug	Object drug*		Description
Dipyridamole	Adenosine	↑	Dipyridamole increases the plasma levels and cardiovascular effects of adenosine. Adjust adenosine dose as necessary.
Aspirin	ACE inhibitors	↓	Due to the indirect effect of aspirin on the renin-angiotensin conversion pathway, the hyponatremic and hypotensive effects of ACE inhibitors may be diminished by concomitant administration of aspirin.
Aspirin	Acetazolamide	↑	Concurrent use can lead to high serum concentrations of acetazolamide (and toxicity) due to competition at the renal tubule for secretion.

Dipyridamole and Aspirin Combination Drug Interactions			
Precipitant drug	Object drug*		Description
Aspirin	Anticoagulants	↑	Patients on anticoagulation therapy are at increased risk for bleeding because of effects on platelets. Aspirin can displace warfarin from protein binding sites, leading to prolongation of the prothrombin time and the bleeding time. Aspirin can also increase the anticoagulant activity of heparin, increasing bleeding risk.
Aspirin	Anticonvulsants (hydantoins, valproic acid)	↑	Increased free fraction of valproic acid, possibly leading to toxic effects of valproic acid, has occurred. The pharmacologic and toxic effects of hydantoins may be increased by coadministration of high doses of salicylates.
Aspirin	Beta blockers	↓	The hypotensive effects of beta blockers may be diminished by concomitant aspirin because of inhibition of renal prostaglandins, leading to decreased renal blood flow and salt and fluid retention.
Dipyridamole	Cholinesterase inhibitors	↓	Dipyridamole may counteract the anticholinesterase effect of cholinesterase inhibitors, thereby potentially aggravating myasthenia gravis.
Aspirin	Diuretics	↓	The effectiveness of diuretics in patients with underlying renal or cardiovascular disease may be diminished by concomitant aspirin because of inhibition of renal prostaglandins, leading to decreased renal blood flow and salt and fluid retention.
Aspirin	Methotrexate	↑	Salicylates can inhibit renal clearance of methotrexate, leading to bone marrow toxicity, especially in the elderly or renally impaired.
Aspirin	NSAIDs	↑	The concurrent use of aspirin with other NSAIDs may increase bleeding or lead to decreased renal function.
Aspirin	Oral hypoglycemics	↑	Moderate doses of aspirin may increase the effectiveness of oral hypoglycemic drugs, leading to hypoglycemia.
Aspirin	Uricosuric agents (eg, probenecid, sulfinpyrazone)	↓	Salicylates antagonize the uricosuric action of uricosuric agents.

* ↑ = Object drug increased. ↓ = Object drug decreased.

➤*Drug/Lab test interactions:* Over the course of 24 months, patients treated with dipyridamole and aspirin combination therapy showed a decline (mean change from baseline) in hemoglobin of 0.25 g/dL, hematocrit of 0.75%, and erythrocyte count of 0.13 x 10⁶/mm³.

Adverse Reactions

Dipyridamole and Aspirin Combination Therapy Adverse Events (%)				
	Individual treatment group (n = 6602)			
Adverse reaction	Dipyridamole/ Aspirin combination (n = 1650)	ER¹-DP alone (n = 1654)	ASA alone (n = 1649)	Placebo (n = 1649)
% of patients with ≥ 1 on-treatment adverse event	79.9	78.9	80.2	70.1
CNS				
Headache	39.2	38.3	33.8	32.9
Amnesia	2.4	2.4	3.5	2.1
Convulsions	1.7	0.9	1.7	1.6
Anorexia	1.2	1	0.6	0.9
Somnolence	1.2	0.8	1.1	0.5
Confusion	1.1	0.5	1.3	0.9
GI				
Abdominal pain	17.5	15.4	15.9	14.5
Dyspepsia	18.4	17.4	18.1	16.7
Nausea	16	15.4	12.7	14.1
Vomiting	8.4	7.8	6.1	7.2
Diarrhea	12.7	15.5	6.8	9.8
Melena	1.9	0.6	1.2	0.8

Antiplatelet Combination Agents

DIPYRIDAMOLE AND ASPIRIN

Dipyridamole and Aspirin Combination Therapy Adverse Events (%)				
	Individual treatment group (n = 6602)			
Adverse reaction	Dipyridamole/ Aspirin combination (n = 1650)	ER[1]-DP alone (n = 1654)	ASA alone (n = 1649)	Placebo (n = 1649)
Rectal hemorrhage	1.6	1.3	1	0.8
GI hemorrhage	1.2	0.3	0.9	0.4
Hemorrhoids	1	0.8	0.6	0.6
Hematologic				
Hemorrhage NOS[2]	3.2	1.5	2.8	1.5
Epistaxis	2.4	1	2.7	1.5
Anemia	1.6	1	1.2	0.5
Purpura	1.4	0.5	0.5	0.4
Musculoskeletal				
Arthralgia	5.5	4.5	5.5	4.6
Arthritis	2.1	1.5	1	1.2
Myalgia	1.2	1	0.7	0.7
Arthrosis	1.1	1.3	0.8	0.8
Respiratory				
Coughing	1.5	1.1	1.9	1.3
Upper respiratory tract infection	1	0.5	1	0.8
Miscellaneous				
Pain	6.4	5.3	6.2	6
Fatigue	5.8	5.6	5.9	5.5
Back pain	4.6	4.7	4.5	3.9
Accidental injury	2.5	1.5	3.1	2.2
Asthenia	1.8	1.1	1	1.1
Neoplasm NOS[2]	1.7	1	1.4	1.2
Cardiac failure	1.6	1	1.8	1.5
Malaise	1.6	1.4	1.6	1.3
Syncope	1	0.8	1	0.5

[1] Extended release.
[2] NOS = Not otherwise specified.

Discontinuation because of adverse events were 25% for dipyridamole and aspirin combination, 25% for extended-release dipyridamole, 19% for aspirin, and 21% for placebo.

Adverse reactions that occurred in < 1% or patients treated with dipyridamole and aspirin combination therapy and that were medically judged to be possibly related to either dipyridamole or aspirin are listed below.

➤*Cardiovascular:* Hypotension; tachycardia; palpitation; arrhythmia; supraventricular tachycardia.

➤*CNS:* Coma; dizziness; paresthesia; cerebral hemorrhage; intracranial hemorrhage; subarachnoid hemorrhage; agitation.

➤*Dermatologic:* Pruritus; urticaria.

➤*GI:* Gastritis; ulceration; perforation.

➤*Hematologic:* Hematoma; gingival bleeding.

➤*Hepatic:* Cholelithiasis; jaundice; abnormal hepatic function.

➤*Metabolic/Nutritional:* Hyperglycemia; thirst.

➤*Respiratory:* Hyperpnea; asthma; bronchospasm; hemoptysis; pulmonary edema.

➤*Special senses:* Tinnitus; deafness; taste loss. Patients with high frequency hearing loss may have difficulty perceiving tinnitus. In these patients, tinnitus cannot be used as a clinical indication of salicylism.

➤*Miscellaneous:* Allergic reaction; fever; flushing; uterine hemorrhage; renal insufficiency and failure; hematuria.

➤*Postmarketing reports:* The following is a list of additional adverse reactions that have been reported either in the literature or are from postmarketing spontaneous reports for either dipyridamole or aspirin.

Dermatologic – Rash; alopecia; angioedema; Stevens-Johnson syndrome.

GI – Pancreatitis; Reye's syndrome; hematemesis.

GU – Prolonged pregnancy and labor; stillbirths; lower birth weight infants; antipartum and postpartum bleeding; interstitial nephritis; papillary necrosis; proteinuria.

Hematologic – Prolongation of the prothrombin time; disseminated intravascular coagulation; coagulopathy; thrombocytopenia.

Hepatic – Hepatitis; hepatic failure.

Hypersensitivity – Acute anaphylaxis; laryngeal edema.

Lab test abnormalities – Hyperkalemia; metabolic acidosis; respiratory alkalosis; hypokalemia.

Metabolic/Nutritional – Hypoglycemia; dehydration.

Respiratory – Tachypnea; dyspnea.

Miscellaneous – Hypothermia; chest pain; angina pectoris; cerebral edema; hearing loss; rhabdomyolysis; allergic vasculitis.

Overdosage

Because of the dose ratio of dipyridamole to aspirin, overdosage of the dipyridamole and aspirin combination is likely to be dominated by signs and symptoms of dipyridamole overdose. In case of real or suspected overdose, seek medical attention or contact a Poison Control Center immediately.

➤*Symptoms:*

Dipyridamole – Based upon the known hemodynamic effects of dipyridamole, symptoms such as warm feeling, flushes, sweating, restlessness, feeling of weakness, and dizziness may occur. A drop in blood pressure and tachycardia might also be observed.

Aspirin – Salicylate toxicity may result from acute ingestion (overdose) or chronic intoxication. The early signs of salicylic overdose (salicylism), including tinnitus (ringing in the ears), occur at plasma concentrations approaching 200 mcg/mL. Plasma concentrations of aspirin > 300 mcg/mL are clearly toxic. Severe toxic effects are associated with levels > 400 mcg/mL. A single lethal dose of aspirin in adults is not known with certainty but death may be expected at 30 g.

➤*Treatment:*

Dipyridamole – Symptomatic treatment is recommended, possibly including a vasopressor drug. Consider gastic lavage. Because dipyridamole is highly protein bound, dialysis is not likely to be of benefit.

Aspirin – Treatment consists primarily of supporting vital functions, increasing salicylate elimination, and correcting the acid-base disturbance. Gastric emptying or lavage are recommended as soon as possible after ingestion, even if the patient has vomited spontaneously. After lavage or emesis, administration of activated charcoal (as a slurry) is beneficial, if < 3 hours have passed since ingestion. Do not employ charcoal absorption prior to emesis and lavage.

Severity of aspirin intoxication is determined by measuring the blood salicylate level. Closely follow acid-base status with serial blood gas and serum pH measurements. Maintain fluid and electrolyte balance.

In severe cases, hyperthermia and hypervolemia are the major immediate threats to life. Sponge children with tepid water. Administer replacement fluid IV and augment with correction of acidosis. Monitor plasma electrolytes and pH to promote alkaline diuresis of salicylate if renal function is normal. Infusion of glucose may be required to control hypoglycemia.

Hemodialysis and peritoneal dialysis can be performed to reduce the body drug content. In patients with renal insufficiency or in cases of life-threatening intoxication, dialysis is usually required. Exchange transfusion may be indicated in infants and young children.

Patient Information

Counsel patients who consume ≥ 3 alcoholic drinks every day about the bleeding risks involved with chronic, heavy alcohol use while taking **aspirin**.

Inform patients about the signs and symptoms of GI side effects and what steps to take if they occur.

Avoid using **aspirin**, which can cause gastric mucosal irritation and bleeding in patients with a history of active peptic ulcer disease.

Aspirin is contraindicated in patients with known allergy to NSAIDs and in patients with asthma, rhinitis, and nasal polyps. Aspirin may cause severe urticaria, angioedema, or bronchospams (asthma).

Do not use in children or teenagers with viral infections with or without fever. There is a risk of Reye's syndrome with concomitant use of **aspirin** in certain viral illnesses.

Blood coagulation resulting in the formation of a stable fibrin clot involves a cascade of proteolytic reactions involving the interaction of clotting factors, platelets, and tissue materials. Clotting factors (see table) exist in the blood in inactive form and must be converted to an enzymatic or activated (a) form before the next step in the clotting mechanism can be stimulated. Each factor is stimulated in turn until an insoluble fibrin clot is formed.

Two separate pathways, intrinsic and extrinsic, lead to the formation of a fibrin clot. Both pathways must function for hemostasis.

►*Intrinsic pathway:* All the protein factors necessary for coagulation are present in circulating blood. Clot formation may take several minutes and is initiated by activation of factor XII.

►*Extrinsic pathway:* Coagulation is activated by release of tissue thromboplastin, a factor not found in circulating blood. Clotting occurs in seconds because factor III bypasses the early reactions.

Refer to the complete coagulation pathway.

Anticoagulants used therapeutically include fractionated and unfractionated heparin, warfarin (a coumarin derivative), and anisindione (an indandione derivative).

Blood Clotting Factors

Factor	Synonym	Vitamin K-dependent
I	Fibrinogen	no
II	Prothrombin	yes
III	Tissue thromboplastin, tissue factor	no
IV	Calcium	no

Blood Clotting Factors

Factor	Synonym	Vitamin K-dependent
V	Labile factor, proaccelerin	no
VII	Proconvertin	yes
VIII	Antihemophilic factor, AHF	no
IX	Christmas factor, plasma thromboplastin component, PTC	yes
X	Stuart factor, Stuart-Prower factor	yes
XI	Plasma thromboplastin antecedent, PTA	no
XII	Hageman factor	no
XIII	Fibrin stabilizing factor, FSF	no
HMW-K	High molecular weight kininogen, Fitzgerald factor	no
PL	Platelets or phospholipids	no
PK	Prekallikrein, Fletcher factor	no
Protein C[1]		yes
Protein S[2]		yes

[1] Partially responsible for inhibition of the extrinsic pathway. Inactivates factors V and VIII and promotes fibrinolysis. Activity declines following warfarin administration.
[2] A cofactor to accelerate the anticoagulant activity of protein C. Decreased levels occur following warfarin administration.

COAGULATION PATHWAY

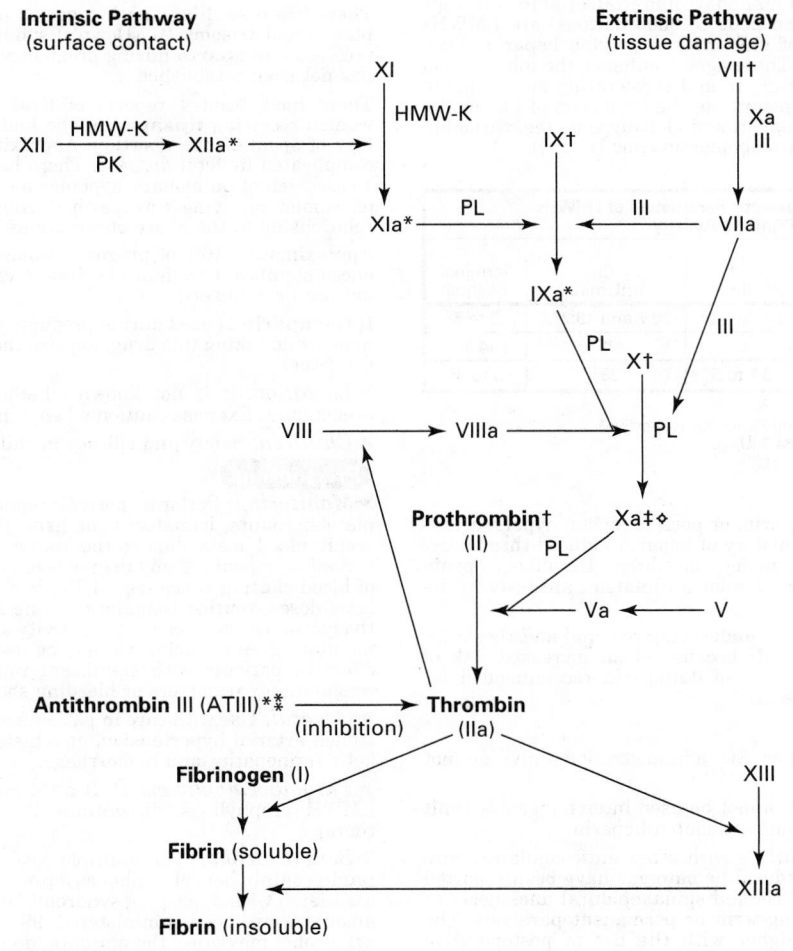

* Major site of activity for unfractionated heparin
† Site of activity for warfarin and anisindione
‡ Major site of activity for fractionated heparin
⸸ Minor site of activity for fractionated heparin
◇ Minor site of activity for unfractionated heparin

Low Molecular Weight Heparins (LMWHs)

Indications

▶*Thromboembolic/Ischemic complications:* Used for prophylaxis or treatment of thromboembolic complications following surgery or ischemic complications of unstable angina and MI. Refer to individual monographs for specific indications.

Actions

▶*Pharmacology:* **Enoxaparin** (average molecular weight distribution is ≈ 2000 to 8000 daltons), **tinzaparin** (average molecular weight ranges between 5500 to 7500 daltons), and **dalteparin** (average molecular weight ranges between 2000 to 9000 daltons) are LMWHs obtained by depolymerization of unfractionated porcine heparin. They have antithrombotic properties. These agents enhance the inhibition of Factor Xa and thrombin by binding to and accelerating antithrombin III activity. They preferentially potentiate the inhibition of Factor Xa, while only slightly affecting thrombin and clotting time (eg, thrombin time [TT] or activated partial thromboplastin time [aPTT]).

▶*Pharmacokinetics:*

Approximate Pharmacokinetic Parameters of LMWHs Based on Anti-Xa Activity					
LMWH	Bioavailability (%)	T_{max} (hrs)	Vd (L)	Cl (mL/min)	Terminal $t_{1/2}$ (hrs)
Dalteparin	≈ 87	4	2.8 to 4.2[a]	28.7 and 18.2[a,b]	3 to 5
Enoxaparin	92	3 to 5	6	15	4.5
Tinzaparin	86.7	3.7[c]	3.1 to 5	28[d]	3 to 4[c]

[a] Based on a 70 kg patient.
[b] Following 30 and 120 IU/kg doses of anti-Factor Xa, respectively.
[c] Dosing based on 4500 IU; mean dose 64.3 IU/kg.
[d] Following 4500 IU IV.

Contraindications

Hypersensitivity to LMWHs, heparin, or pork products; hypersensitivity to sulfites or benzyl alcohol, history of heparin-induced thrombocytopenia (**tinzaparin**); active major bleeding; thrombocytopenia associated with positive in vitro tests for antiplatelet antibody in the presence of a LMWH.

Do not give **dalteparin** to patients undergoing regional anesthesia for unstable angina or non-Q-wave MI because of an increased risk of bleeding associated with the dosage of dalteparin recommended for unstable angina and non-Q-wave MI.

Warnings

▶*Route of administration:* For SC administration only; do not administer IM or IV.

▶*Interchangeability:* LMWHs cannot be used interchangeably (unit for unit) with other LMWHs or unfractionated heparin.

▶*Spinal/Epidural anesthesia:* As with other anticoagulants, rare cases of neuraxial, spinal, or epidural hematomas have been reported with the concurrent use of LMWHs and spinal/epidural anesthesia or spinal puncture, resulting in long-term or permanent paralysis. The risk of these events may be higher with the use of postoperative indwelling epidural catheters or by the concomitant use of additional drugs affecting hemostasis such as NSAIDs (see Warning Box).

▶*Hemorrhage:* Use LMWHs, like other anticoagulants, with extreme caution in patients who have an increased risk of hemorrhage, such as those with severe uncontrolled hypertension, bleeding diathesis, diabetic retinopathy, bacterial endocarditis, congenital or acquired bleeding disorders (including hepatic failure and amyloidosis), active ulceration and angiodysplastic GI disease, hemorrhagic stroke or shortly after brain, spinal, or ophthalmological surgery, or in patients treated concomitantly with platelet inhibitors. As with other anticoagulants, bleeding can occur at any site during therapy with a LMWH. Search for a bleeding site if an unexpected drop in hematocrit, hemoglobin, or blood pressure occurs.

Discontinue agents that might affect hemostasis (eg, oral anticoagulants, platelet inhibitors) prior to therapy with LMWHs. Concomitant use may increase the risk of hemorrhage. Monitor patient closely if coadministration cannot be avoided (see Drug Interactions).

▶*Thrombocytopenia:* The incidence of thrombocytopenia with platelet counts between 50,000/mm^3 and 100,000/mm^3 was 1.3% in patients treated with **enoxaparin**, 1% with **tinzaparin**, and < 1% with **dalteparin**. Severe thrombocytopenia (platelet count < 50,000/mm^3) occurred in 0.13% of tinzaparin-treated patients and 0.1% of enoxaparin-treated patients.

Use extreme caution in patients with a history of heparin-induced thrombocytopenia. Closely monitor thrombocytopenia of any degree. If the platelet count falls to < 100,000/mm^3, consider discontinuing the LMWH.

▶*Priapism:* Priapism has been reported from postmarketing surveillance of **tinzaparin** as a rare occurrence. In some cases, surgical intervention was required.

▶*Renal/Hepatic function impairment:* Delayed elimination of LMWHs may occur with severe liver or kidney insufficiency. Use with caution.

▶*Elderly:* Delayed elimination of **enoxaparin** and **tinzaparin** may occur. Use with caution.

▶*Pregnancy:* Category B. There are no adequate and well-controlled studies in pregnant women. A few spontaneous postmarketing fetal deaths have been reported in **enoxaparin**-treated patients. Use during pregnancy only if clearly needed.

There has been 1 case each reported of cleft palate, optic nerve hypoplasia, and trisomy 21 (Down's) syndrome in infants of women who received **tinzaparin** during pregnancy. A cause-and-effect relationship has not been established.

There have been 4 reports of fetal death/miscarriage in pregnant women receiving **tinzaparin** who had high-risk pregnancies or a history of spontaneous abortion. Approximately 6% of pregnancies were complicated by fetal distress. There have been spontaneous reports of 1 case each of pulmonary hypoplasia or muscular hypotonia in infants of women receiving tinzaparin during pregnancy. A cause-and-effect relationship to the above observations has not been established.

Approximately 10% of pregnant women receiving **tinzaparin** experienced significant vaginal bleeding. A cause-and-effect relationship has not been established.

If **tinzaparin** is used during pregnancy, or if the patient becomes pregnant while taking this drug, apprise the patient of potential hazards to the fetus.

▶*Lactation:* It is not known whether these drugs are excreted in breast milk. Exercise caution when administering to a nursing woman.

▶*Children:* Safety and efficacy in children have not been established.

Precautions

▶*Monitoring:* Perform periodic complete blood counts, including platelet counts, hematocrit, or hemoglobin, and urinalysis; and stool occult blood tests during the course of treatment. Closely monitor thrombocytopenia of any degree (see Warnings). No special monitoring of blood clotting times (eg, aPTT) is needed. At recommended prophylaxis doses, routine coagulation tests such as PT and aPTT are relatively insensitive measures of activity and are, therefore, unsuitable for monitoring. Anti-Factor Xa may be used to monitor the anticoagulant effect in patients with significant renal impairment or if abnormal coagulation parameters or bleeding should occur.

▶*General:* Use with care in patients with a bleeding diathesis, uncontrolled arterial hypertension, or a history of recent GI ulceration, diabetic retinopathy, and hemorrhage.

▶*Thromboembolic event:* If a thromboembolic event occurs despite LMWH prophylaxis, discontinue the drug and initiate appropriate therapy.

▶*Benzyl alcohol:* The multiple-dose vials of **dalteparin** and **tinzaparin** contain benzyl alcohol as a preservative. Benzyl alcohol has been associated with a "gasping syndrome" in premature infants (when large amounts have been administered [99 to 404 mg/kg/day]). Because benzyl alcohol may cross the placenta, do not use dalteparin or tinzaparin preserved with benzyl alcohol in pregnant women.

▶*Sulfite sensitivity:* **Tinzaparin** contains metabisulfite, a sulfite that may cause allergic-type reactions including anaphylactic symptoms and life-threatening or less severe asthmatic episodes in certain susceptible people. The overall prevalence of sulfite sensitivity in the general population is unknown and probably low. Sulfite sensitivity is seen more frequently in asthmatic than in nonasthmatic people.

Low Molecular Weight Heparins (LMWHs)

Drug Interactions

➤*Anticoagulants/Platelet inhibitors:* Use LMWHs with care in patients receiving oral anticoagulants or platelet inhibitors (eg, aspirin, salicylates, NSAIDs including ketorolac tromethamine, dipyridamole, sulfinpyrazone, dextran, ticlopidine) and thrombolytics because of increased risk of bleeding. If coadministration is essential, use close clinical and laboratory monitoring of these patients.

➤*Drug/Lab test interactions:* Asymptomatic reversible increases in aspartate (AST) and alanine (ALT) aminotransferase levels have occurred in patients treated with LMWHs and heparin. Because aminotransferase determinations are important in the differential diagnosis of MI, liver disease, and pulmonary emboli, interpret elevations that might be caused by LMWHs with caution.

Adverse Reactions

LMWH Adverse Reactions (%)[a]			
Adverse reaction	Dalteparin	Enoxaparin	Tinzaparin
Hemorrhagic events			
Clinically significant bleeding[b]	0.5 to 15.9	0 to 4	0.8[e]
Hemorrhage	-	4 to 13	1.5
Injection site hematoma	0.2 to 7.1	5	≥ 1
Wound hematoma	0.1 to 3.4	-	-
Non-hemorrhagic events			
Cardiovascular			
Hypotension	-	-	≥ 1
Hypertension	-	-	≥ 1
Angina pectoris	-	-	≥ 1
Tachycardia	-	-	≥ 1
CNS			
Dizziness	-	-	≥ 1
Insomnia	-	-	≥ 1
Confusion	-	-	≥ 1
GI			
Constipation	-	-	1.3
Nausea	-	3	1.7
Vomiting	-	-	1
Abdominal pain	-	-	0.8
Diarrhea	-	-	0.6
Flatulence	-	-	≥ 1
GI disorder (NOS)	-	-	≥ 1
Dyspepsia	-	-	≥ 1
Hematologic			
Anemia	-	2 to 16	≥ 1
Hematoma	-	-	≥ 1
Thrombocythemia	-	✔	-
Thrombocytopenia	< 1	1.3	≥ 1
Hypersensitivity			
Allergic reactions[c]	✔	✔	≥ 1
Pruritus/Rash	✔	-	≥ 1
GU			
Urinary tract infection	-	-	3.7
Hematuria	-	-	≥ 1
Urinary retention	-	-	≥ 1
Dysuria	-	-	≥ 1
Respiratory			
Epistaxis	-	-	1.9
Dyspnea	-	-	1.2
Pneumonia	-	-	≥ 1
Respiratory disorder	-	-	≥ 1
Miscellaneous			
Pulmonary embolism	-	-	2.3
Back pain, pain	-	-	1.5
Fever	✔	0 to 8	1.5
Healing impaired	-	-	≥ 1
Infection	-	-	≥ 1
Edema	-	2	-
Injection site reactions[d]	1 to 3	✔	≈ 16
Peripheral edema	-	0 to 6	-
Headache	-	-	1.7
Cerebrovascular accident	-	-	-
Chest pain	-	-	2.3
Thrombophlebitis, deep	-	-	≥ 1
Thrombophlebitis, leg deep	-	-	≥ 1

[a] Data pooled from several studies and are not necessarily comparable. Percentages listed without regard to specific dosage.
[b] Defined as overt bleeding resulting in a decrease in hemoglobin ≥ 2 g/dL, transfusion of ≥ 2 units of blood, intracranial, intraocular, retroperitoneal, or intra-articular bleeding or moderate-to-severe bleeding that required discontinuation from the study or required an invasive diagnostic or therapeutic procedure.
[c] Includes maculopapular rash, vesiculobullous rash, urticaria, and bullous eruption.
[d] Includes skin necrosis, nodules, inflammation, and oozing.
[e] The 95% CI on the difference in major bleeding event rate (1.9%) was 0.33%, 3.47%.
✔ = Occurs; incidence unknown.
- = No data.

Neuraxial hematomas have occurred rarely with concurrent use of LMWHs and spinal/epidural anesthesia and postoperative indwelling catheters (see Warning Box and Warnings). Serious adverse events with enoxaparin in a clinical trial in patients with unstable angina or non-Q-wave MI include heart failure (0.95%); pneumonia (0.82%); atrial fibrillation and lung edema (0.7%).

➤*Tinzaparin:*

Cardiovascular – Angina pectoris; cardiac arrhythmia; dependent edema; MI/coronary thrombosis; thromboembolism.

Dermatologic – Bullous eruption; erythematous rash; skin necrosis.

Hematologic – Anorectal bleeding; cerebral/intracranial bleeding; epistaxis; GI hemorrhage; granulocytopenia; hemarthrosis; hematemesis; hematuria; hemorrhage (NOS); injection site bleeding; melena; purpura; retroperitoneal/intra-abdominal bleeding; thrombocytopenia; vaginal hemorrhage; wound hematoma.

Approximately 10% of pregnant women receiving **tinzaparin** experienced significant vaginal bleeding. A cause-and-effect relationship has not been established.

Miscellaneous – Congenital anomaly; fetal death; fetal distress; allergic reaction; cellulitis (local); neoplasm.

➤*Postmarketing experiences:*
   Tinzaparin: Cholestatic hepatitis; increase in hepatic enzymes; peripheral ischemia; priapism; hemoptysis; ocular hemorrhage; rectal bleeding; epidermal necrolysis; ischemic necrosis; urticaria; agranulocytosis; pancytopenia; thrombocythemia; abscess; necrosis; angioedema; neonatal hypotonia; acute febrile reaction.

There has been 1 case of spinal epidural hematoma with tinzaparin at a therapeutic dose in a patient who had not received neuraxial anesthesia or spinal puncture.

➤*Lab test abnormalities:* Asymptomatic increases in transaminase levels (AST and ALT) > 3 times the upper limit of normal of the laboratory reference range have been reported in 1.7% to 8.8% and 4.3% to 13% of patients, respectively, during treatment with LMWHs. Similar significant increases in transaminase levels have been observed in patients treated with heparin. Such elevations are fully reversible and are rarely associated with increases in bilirubin. Because transaminase determinations are important in the differential diagnosis of MI, liver disease, and pulmonary emboli, interpret elevations that might be caused by LMWHs with caution.

Overdosage

➤*Symptoms:* An excessive amount of a LMWH may lead to dose-related hemorrhagic complications.

➤*Treatment:* Effects of LMWHs may generally be stopped by the slow IV injection of protamine sulfate (1% solution) at a dose of 1 mg for every 100 anti-Xa IU of **dalteparin** and **tinzaparin** or 1 mg for every 1 mg of **enoxaparin**. A second infusion of 0.5 mg protamine per 100 anti-Xa IU of dalteparin and tinzaparin or per 1 mg of enoxaparin may be administered if the aPTT measured 2 to 4 hours after the first infusion remains prolonged. Even with these additional doses of protamine, the aPTT may remain more prolonged than would usually be found following administration of conventional heparin. In all cases, the anti-Factor Xa activity is never completely neutralized (maximum, ≈ 60% to 75%). Take particular care to avoid overdosage with protamine.

Administration of protamine sulfate can cause severe hypotensive and anaphylactoid reactions. Because fatal reactions, often resembling anaphylaxis, have been reported, give protamine only when resuscitation techniques and treatment of anaphylactic shock are readily available.

Patient Information

Contact the physician if experiencing bleeding, bruising, dizziness, lightheadedness, itching, rash, fever, swelling, or difficulty breathing.

Injections are given around the navel, upper thigh, or buttocks. Change the injection site daily.

Use proper injection technique; inject under the skin, not into muscle.

If excessive bruising occurs at the injection site, it may be lessened by an ice cube massage of the site prior to injection.

Low Molecular Weight Heparins (LMWHs)

DALTEPARIN SODIUM

Rx **Fragmin** (Pharmacia)	**Injection:** 2500 IU[1] (16 mg/0.2 mL)	Preservative free. In 0.2 mL single-dose prefilled syringes with 27-gauge × ½-inch needle.
	5000 IU[1] (32 mg/0.2 mL)	Preservative free. In 0.2 mL single-dose prefilled syringes with 27-gauge × ½-inch needle.
	7500 IU[1] (48 mg/0.3 mL)	Preservative free. In 0.3 mL single-dose prefilled syringes with 27-gauge × ½-inch needle.
	10,000 IU[1] (64mg/mL)	Preservative free. In 1 mL single-dose graduated syringes with 27-gauge × ½-inch needle.
	10,000 IU[1] (64 mg/mL)	14 mg/mL benzyl alcohol. In 9.5 mL multi-dose vials.
	25,000 IU[1] (160 mg/mL)	14 mg/mL benzyl alcohol. In 3.8 mL multi-dose vials.

[1] Anti-Factor Xa International Units.

For complete prescribing information, refer to the LMWH group monograph.

WARNING

Spinal/Epidural hematomas: When neuraxial anesthesia (spinal/epidural anesthesia) or spinal puncture is employed, patients anticoagulated or scheduled to be anticoagulated with low molecular weight heparins or heparinoids for prevention of thromboembolic complications are at risk of developing a spinal or epidural hematoma which can result in long-term or permanent paralysis.

The risk of these events is increased by the use of indwelling epidural catheters for administrations of analgesia or by the concurrent use of drugs affecting hemastasis such as nonsteroidal anti-inflammatory drugs (NSAIDs), platelet inhibitors, or other anticoagulants. The risk also appears to be increased by traumatic or repeated spinal or epidural puncture.

Frequently monitor patients for signs and symptoms of neurological impairment. If neurological compromise is noted, urgent treatment is necessary.

The physician should consider the potential benefit vs risk before neuraxial intervention in patients anticoagulated or to be anticoagulated for thromboprophylaxis.

Indications

➤*Unstable angina/Non-Q-wave MI:* For the prophylaxis of ischemic complications in unstable angina and non-Q-wave MI in patients on concurrent aspirin therapy.

➤*Deep vein thrombosis (DVT) prophylaxis:* For prophylaxis of DVT, which may lead to pulmonary embolism (PE), in patients undergoing hip replacement surgery or in patients undergoing abdominal surgery who are at risk for thromboembolic complications. Patients at risk include those who are older than 40 years of age, obese, undergoing surgery under general anesthesia lasting more than 30 minutes, or who have additional risk factors such as malignancy or a history of DVT or PE.

Administration and Dosage

➤*Approved by the FDA:* December 22, 1994.

➤*Administration:* Administer by SC injection; do not administer IM.

➤*Unstable angina/Non-Q-wave MI:* The recommended dose of dalteparin injection is 120 IU/kg of body weight (but no more than 10,000 IU) SC every 12 hours with concurrent oral aspirin (75 to 165 mg/day) therapy. Continue treatment until the patient is clinically stabilized. The usual duration of treatment is 5 to 8 days. Concurrent aspirin therapy is recommended except when contraindicated.

Volume of Dalteparin to be Administered by Patient Weight

Patient weight (lb)	< 110	110 to 131	132 to 153	154 to 175	176 to 197	≥ 198
Patient weight (kg)	< 50	50 to 59	60 to 69	70 to 79	80 to 89	≥ 90
Volume of dalteparin (mL)[a]	0.55	0.65	0.75	0.9	1	1

[a] Calculated volume based on the 9.5 mL multiple-dose vial (10,000 anti-Factor Xa IU/mL).

➤*DVT prophylaxis:*

Abdominal surgery – In patients undergoing abdominal surgery with a risk of thromboembolic complications, administer 2500 IU SC once daily, starting 1 to 2 hours prior to surgery and repeat once daily for 5 to 10 days postoperatively.

   High-risk patients: In abdominal surgery, patients at high risk for thromboembolic complications (eg, malignancy), administer 5000 IU SC the evening before surgery and repeat once daily for 5 to 10 days postoperatively. Alternatively, in patients with malignancy, administer 2500 IU SC 1 to 2 hours prior to surgery with an additional 2500 IU SC dose 12 hours later and then 5000 IU once daily for 5 to 10 days postoperatively.

Hip replacement surgery – The usual duration of administration is 5 to 10 days after surgery; up to 14 days was well tolerated in controlled clinical trials.

Dalteparin SC Dosing for Patients Undergoing Hip Replacement Surgery

Timing of first dose of dalteparin	10 o 14 hours before surgery	≤ 2 hours before surgery	4 to 8 hours after surgery[a]	Post-operative period[b]
Postoperative start	—	—	2500 IU[c]	5000 IU qd
Preoperative start — day of surgery		2500 IU	2500 IU[c]	5000 IU qd
Preoperative start — evening before surgery[d]	5000 IU		5000 IU	5000 IU qd

[a] Or later, if hemostasis has not been achieved.
[b] Up to 14 days of treatment was well tolerated in controlled clinical trials, where the usual duration of treatment was 5 to 10 days postoperatively.
[c] Allow a minimum of 6 hours between this dose and the dose to be given on postoperative day 1. Adjust the timing of the dose on postoperative day 1 accordingly.
[d] Allow ≈ 24 hours between doses.

Coagulation parameters – Dosage adjustment and routine monitoring of coagulation parameters are not required if these dosage and administration recommendations are followed.

➤*SC injection technique:* Administer by deep SC injection while patient is sitting or lying down. Dalteparin may be injected in a U-shaped area around the navel, the upper outer side of the thigh, or the upper outer quadrangle of the buttock. Vary the injection site daily. When the area around the navel or the thigh is used, use the thumb and forefinger to lift up a skin fold while giving the injection. Insert the entire length of the needle at a 45° to 90° angle.

➤*Storage/Stability:* Store at controlled room temperature, 20° to 25°C (68° to 77°F).

Low Molecular Weight Heparins (LMWHs)

ENOXAPARIN SODIUM

Rx	Lovenox (Aventis)	Injection: 30 mg/0.3 mL[1]	Preservative free. In packs of 10 amps and 10 prefilled syringes with a 27-gauge × ½-inch needle.
		40 mg/0.4 mL[1]	Preservative free. In packs of 10 prefilled syringes with a 27-gauge × ½-inch needle.
		60 mg/0.6 mL[1]	Preservative free. In packs of 10 graduated prefilled syringes with a 27-gauge × ½-inch needle.
		80 mg/0.8 mL[1]	Preservative free. In packs of 10 graduated prefilled syringes with a 27-gauge × ½-inch needle.
		100 mg/1 mL[1]	Preservative free. In packs of 10 graduated prefilled syringes with a 27-gauge × ½-inch needle.
		120 mg/0.8 mL[1]	Preservative free. In packs of 10 graduated prefilled syringes with a 27-gauge × ½-inch needle.
		150 mg/1 mL[1]	Preservative free. In packs of 10 graduated prefilled syringes with a 27-gauge × ½-inch needle.
		300 mg/3 mL[1]	15 mg/mL benzyl alcohol. In 3 mL multi-dose vials.

[1] Approximate anti-Factor Xa activity of 100 IU/1 mg enoxaparin sodium (with reference to the WHO First International Low Molecular Weight Heparin Reference Standard).

For complete prescribing information, refer to the LMWH group monograph.

WARNING

Spinal/Epidural hematomas: When neuraxial anesthesia (spinal/epidural anesthesia) or spinal puncture is employed, patients anticoagulated or scheduled to be anticoagulated with low molecular weight heparins or heparinoids for prevention of thromboembolic complications are at risk of developing a spinal or epidural hematoma which can result in long-term or permanent paralysis.

The risk of these events is increased by the use of indwelling epidural catheters for administration of analgesia or by the concomitant use of drugs affecting hemostasis such as nonsteroidal anti-inflammatory drugs (NSAIDs), platelet inhibitors, or other anticoagulants. The risk also appears to be increased by traumatic or repeated epidural or spinal puncture.

Frequently monitor patients for signs and symptoms of neurological impairment. If neurologic compromise is noted, urgent treatment is necessary.

The physician should consider the potential benefit vs risk before neuraxial intervention in patients anticoagulated or to be anticoagulated for thromboprophylaxis.

Indications

➤*Deep vein thrombosis (DVT) prophylaxis:* For prevention of DVT, which may lead to pulmonary embolism (PE) in patients undergoing hip replacement surgery (during and following hospitalization), knee replacement surgery, abdominal surgery who are at risk (ie, abdominal surgery patients at risk include those who are older than 40 years of age, obese, undergoing surgery under general anesthesia lasting more than 30 minutes, or who have additional risk factors such as malignancy or a history of DVT or PE) for thromboembolic complications, or in medical patients at risk for thromboembolic complications due to severely restricted mobility during acute illness.

➤*DVT/PE treatment:* In conjunction with warfarin sodium for inpatient treatment of acute DVT with or without PE or for outpatient treatment of acute DVT without PE.

➤*Unstable angina/Non-Q-wave MI:* For the prevention of ischemic complications of unstable angina and non-Q-wave MI when coadministered with aspirin.

Administration and Dosage

➤*Approved by the FDA:* March 29, 1993.

➤*Administration:* Administer by SC injection only; do not administer IM. Evaluate all patients for a bleeding disorder before administration of enoxaparin unless the medication is needed urgently. Since coagulation parameters are unsuitable for monitoring enoxaparin activity, routine monitoring of coagulation parameters is not required.

When using enoxaparin ampules or multi-dose vials, use a tuberculin syringe or equivalent to assure withdrawal of the appropriate volume of drug. Patients may self-inject only if their physician determines that it is appropriate and with medical follow-up as necessary.

➤*DVT prophylaxis:*

Hip or knee replacement surgery – 30 mg every 12 hours by SC injection, with the initial dose given 12 to 24 hours postoperatively provided hemostasis has been established. The usual duration of administration is 7 to 10 days; up to 14 days has been well tolerated.

For hip replacement surgery, consider a dose of 40 mg once daily SC, given initially 9 to 15 hours prior to surgery. Continue prophylaxis for 3 weeks.

Abdominal surgery – In patients at risk for thromboembolic complications, administer 40 mg once daily SC with the initial dose given 2 hours prior to surgery. The usual duration of administration is 7 to 10 days; up to 12 days has been well tolerated.

Medical patients during acute illness – In medical patients at risk for thromboembolic complications due to severely restricted mobility during acute illness, the recommended dose is 40 mg once daily SC. The usual duration of administration is 6 to 11 days; up to 14 days has been well tolerated.

➤*DVT with or without PE:*

Outpatient treatment – For patients with acute DVT without PE who can be treated at home, the recommended dose is 1 mg/kg SC every 12 hours.

Inpatient treatment – For patients with acute DVT with PE or patients with acute DVT without PE (who are not candidates for outpatient treatment), the recommended dose is 1 mg/kg SC every 12 hours or 1.5 mg/kg SC once daily (same time each day).

Outpatient and inpatient treatment – Initiate warfarin therapy when appropriate (usually within 72 hours of enoxaparin). Continue enoxaparin for a minimum of 5 days and until a therapeutic anticoagulant effect has been achieved (International Normalization Ratio [INR] 2 to 3). The average administration duration is 7 days; up to 17 days has been well tolerated.

➤*Unstable angina/Non-Q-wave MI:* In patients with unstable angina or non-Q-wave MI, the recommended dose is 1 mg/kg SC every 12 hours in conjunction with oral aspirin therapy (100 to 325 mg once daily). Treat with enoxaparin for at least 2 days and continue until clinical stabilization. The usual duration of treatment is 2 to 8 days; up to 12.5 days have been well tolerated. To minimize the risk of bleeding following vascular instrumentation during the treatment of unstable angina, adhere precisely to the intervals recommended between doses. Leave the vascular access sheath for instrumentation in place for 6 to 8 hours following a dose of enoxaparin. Give the next scheduled dose at least 6 to 8 hours after sheath removal. Observe site for signs of bleeding or hematoma formation.

➤*SC injection technique:* To avoid the loss of drug, do not expel the air bubble from the syringe before the injection. Administer by deep SC injection while patients are lying down. Alternate administration between the left and right anterolateral and left and right posterolateral abdominal wall. Introduce the whole length of the needle into a skin fold held between the thumb and forefinger; hold the skin fold throughout the injection. To minimize bruising, do not rub the injection site. Prefilled syringes and graduated prefilled syringes are available with a system that shields the needle after injection.

➤*Storage/Stability:* Store at 25°C (77°F), excursions permitted from 15° to 30°C (59° to 86°F).

TINZAPARIN SODIUM

| Rx | **Innohep** (Pharmion Corp) | Injection: 20,000 IU/mL[a] | 3.1 mg/mL sodium metabisulfite, 10 mg/mL benzyl alcohol. In 2 mL vials. |

[a] Anti-Factor Xa International Units.

For complete prescribing information, refer to the LMWH group monograph.

WARNING

Spinal/Epidural hematomas: When neuraxial anesthesia (epidural/spinal anesthesia) or spinal puncture is employed, patients anticoagulated or scheduled to be anticoagulated with low molecular weight heparins or heparinoids for prevention of thromboembolic complications are at risk of developing an epidural or spinal hematoma, which can result in long-term or permanent paralysis.

The risk of these events is increased by the use of indwelling epidural catheters for administration of analgesia or by the concomitant use of drugs affecting hemostasis such as nonsteroidal anti-inflammatory drugs (NSAIDs), platelet inhibitors, or other anticoagulants. The risk also appears to be increased by traumatic or repeated epidural or spinal puncture.

Patients should be frequently monitored for signs and symptoms of neurological impairment. If neurological compromise is noted, urgent treatment is necessary.

The physician should consider the potential benefit versus risk before neuraxial intervention in patients anticoagulated or to be anticoagulated for thromboprophylaxis.

Indications

►*Deep vein thrombosis (DVT):* Treatment of acute symptomatic DVT with or without pulmonary embolism (PE) when administered in conjunction with warfarin sodium. The safety and effectiveness of tinzaparin were established in hospitalized patients.

Administration and Dosage

►*Approved by the FDA:* July 18, 2000.

Evaluate all patients for bleeding disorders before administration of tinzaparin. Because coagulation parameters are unsuitable for monitoring tinzaparin activity, routine monitoring of coagulation parameters is not required.

►*Adults:* The recommended dose of tinzaparin for the treatment of DVT with or without PE is 175 anti-Xa IU/kg of body weight, administered SC once daily for at least 6 days and until the patient is adequately anticoagulated with warfarin (international normalizing ratio [INR] of at least 2 for 2 consecutive days). Initiate warfarin sodium therapy when appropriate (usually within 1 to 3 days of tinzaparin initiation).

As tinzaparin may theoretically affect the prothrombin time (PT)/INR, draw blood for PT/INR determination just prior to the next scheduled dose of tinzaparin for patients receiving tinzaparin and warfarin.

The following table provides tinzaparin doses for the treatment of DVT with or without PE. It is necessary to calculate the appropriate tinzaparin dose for patient weights not displayed in the table.

Use an appropriately calibrated syringe to assure withdrawal of the correct volume of drug from tinzaparin vials.

Tinzaparin Weight-Based Dosing for Treatment of DVT With or Without Symptomatic PE			
	DVT Treatment		
	175 IU/kg SC once daily 20,000 IU/mL		
Body weight (lbs)	Dose (IU)	Amount (mL)	Patient body weight (kg)
68-80	6000	0.3	31-36
81-94	7000	0.35	37-42
95-107	8000	0.4	43-48
108-118	9000	0.45	49-53
119-131	10,000	0.5	54-59
132-144	11,000	0.55	60-65
145-155	12,000	0.6	66-70
156-168	13,000	0.65	71-76
169-182	14,000	0.7	77-82
183-195	15,000	0.75	83-88
196-206	16,000	0.8	89-93
207-219	17,000	0.85	94-99
220-232	18,000	0.9	100-105
233-243	19,000	0.95	106-110
244-256	20,000	1	111-116
257-270	21,000	1.05	117-122

Use the following equation to calculate the volume (mL) of tinzaparin 175 anti-Xa IU/kg SC dose for treatment of DVT:

Patient weight (kg) $\times$ 0.00875 mL/kg = volume to be given (mL) SC.

►*Administration:* Administer tinzaparin by SC injection. Do not administer by IM or IV injection. Do not mix tinzaparin with other injections or infusions.

►*SC injection technique:* Position patients either lying down (supine) or sitting, and administer tinzaparin by deep SC injection. Alternate administration between left and right anterolateral and left and right posterolateral abdominal wall. Vary the injection site daily. Introduce the whole length of the needle into a skin fold held between the thumb and forefinger; hold the skin fold throughout the injection. To minimize bruising, do not rub the injection site after completion of the injection.

►*Storage/Stability:* Store at 25°C (77°F); excursions permitted to 15° to 30°C (59° to 86°F).

DANAPAROID SODIUM

| *Rx*   **Orgaran** (Organon) | Injection: 750 anti-Xa units/0.6 mL | Sodium sulfite. In single-dose ampules and pre-filled syringes with 25-gauge x ⅝-inch needle. In 10s. |

WARNING

When neuraxial anesthesia (epidural/spinal anesthesia) or spinal puncture is employed, patients anticoagulated or scheduled to be anticoagulated with low molecular weight heparins or heparinoids for prevention of thromboembolic complications are at risk of developing an epidural or spinal hematoma that can result in long-term or permanent paralysis.

The risk of these events is increased by the use of indwelling epidural catheters for administration of analgesia or by the concomitant use of drugs affecting hemostasis such as nonsteroidal anti-inflammatory drugs (NSAIDs), platelet inhibitors, or other anticoagulants. The risk also appears to be increased by traumatic or repeated epidural or spinal puncture.

Frequently monitor patients for signs and symptoms of neurological impairment. If neurologic compromise is noted, urgent treatment is necessary.

Consider the potential benefit vs risk before intervention in patients anticoagulated or to be an anticoagulated for thromboprophylaxis (see Warnings).

Indications

➤*Prophylaxis of postoperative deep venous thrombosis (DVT):* For the prophylaxis of postoperative DVT, which may lead to pulmonary embolism (PE), in patients undergoing elective hip replacement surgery.

➤*Unlabeled uses:* Disseminated intravascular coagulation; diabetic nephropathy; ischemic stroke or thromboembolic complications of hemorrhagic stroke; as a treatment measure for DVT; as routine anticoagulation therapy for patients requiring hemodialysis.

Danaparoid has been used clinically in the treatment of thromboembolism and to produce anticoagulation during hemodialysis, hemofiltration during cardiovascular operations and in pregnant patients at increased risk of thrombosis. It may represent a useful replacement for heparin in patients with heparin-induced thrombocytopenia, but further investigation will be necessary if the difficulties in monitoring and neutralizing its anticoagulant effects are to be overcome.

Administration and Dosage

➤*Approved by the FDA:* December 24, 1996.

➤*Usual adult dosage:* In patients undergoing hip replacement surgery, the recommended dose of danaparoid is 750 anti-Xa units twice daily administered by SC injection beginning 1 to 4 hours preoperatively, and then not sooner than 2 hours after surgery. Continue treatment throughout the period of postoperative care until the risk of DVT has diminished. The average duration of administration in clinical trials was 7 to 10 days, up to 14 days.

➤*Renal function impairment:* Carefully monitor patients with serum creatinine ≥ 2 mg/dL. In patients with renal failure undergoing hemodialysis, reduce maintenance dosages and titrate according to predialysis plasma antifactor Xa activity.

➤*Administration:* Administer SC and not by IM injection. SC injection technique: Have the patient lie down and administer by deep SC injection using a fine needle (25 to 26 gauge) to minimize tissue trauma. Alternate administration between the left and right anterolateral and left and right posterolateral abdominal wall. Introduce the whole length of the needle into a skin-fold held gently between the thumb and forefinger; hold the skin-fold throughout the injection and neither pinch nor rub afterwards.

➤*Storage/Stability:* Store ampules at a temperature of 2° to 30°C (36° to 86°F). Store syringes at a refrigerated temperature of 2° to 8°C (36° to 46°F). Protect from light.

Actions

➤*Pharmacology:* Danaparoid sodium injection is an antithrombotic agent. The average molecular weight is ≈ 5500 daltons. It is a low molecular weight sulfated glycosaminoglycans (low molecular weight heparinoid) extracted from porcine mucosa. Danaparoid prevents fibrin formation in the coagulation pathway via thrombin generation inhibition by anti-Xa and anti-IIa (thrombin) effects. The anti-Xa:anti-IIa activity ratio is > 22; inactivation of factor Xa is mediated by antithrombin-III (AT-III) while factor IIa inactivation is mediated by both AT-III and heparin cofactor II (HC II). Danaparoid has only minor effects on platelet function and platelet aggregability.

Because of its predominant anti-Xa activity, danaparoid has little effect on clotting assays (eg, prothrombin time [PT], partial thromboplastin time [PTT]). It has minimal effect on fibrinolytic activity and bleeding time.

Cross-sensitivity studies involving patients with type II heparin-induced thrombocytopenia indicate that danaparoid has a much lower in vitro cross-reactivity in platelet aggregation tests than the low molecular weight heparins.

➤*Pharmacokinetics:*

Absorption – By SC route of administration, danaparoid is ≈ 100% bioavailable, compared with the same dose administered IV. The maximum anti-Xa activity (T_{max}) occurred at ≈ 2 to 5 hours.

For single SC doses of 750, 1500, 2250, and 3250 anti-Xa units of danaparoid, the mean peak plasma anti-Xa activities were 102.4, 206.1, 283.9, and 403.4 mU/mL, respectively.

Excretion – The mean value for the terminal half-life was ≈ 24 hours and the clearance was 0.36 L/hr. Clearance was affected by body surface area in that the higher the body surface, the faster the clearance. Danaparoid is mainly eliminated via the kidneys. In patients with severely impaired renal function, the half-life of plasma anti-Xa activity may be prolonged. Monitor such patients carefully.

Special populations –

Renal function impairment: In patients with renal failure, the renal clearance of danaparoid is reduced and the beta half-life of plasma antifactor Xa activity may be prolonged. Dosage adjustments are recommended in these patients.

➤*Clinical trials:* In a US multicenter trial, danaparoid was compared with warfarin in 396 patients undergoing elective hip replacement. A significant reduction in the overall incidence of DVT was observed with danaparoid (14.6%; 29/199 patients) compared with warfarin (26.9%; 53/197 patients).

Contraindications

Severe hemorrhagic diathesis (eg, hemophilia, idiopathic thrombocytopenic purpura); active major bleeding state, including hemorrhagic stroke in the acute phase; hypersensitivity to danaparoid; Type II thrombocytopenia associated with a positive in vitro test for antiplatelet antibody in the presence of danaparoid; patients with known hypersensitivity to pork products.

Warnings

➤*IM injection:* Danaparoid is not intended for IM administration.

➤*Interchangeability:* Because a specific standard for the anti-Xa activity of danaparoid is used, the anti-Xa unit activity of danaparoid is not equivalent to that described for heparin or low molecular weight heparin. Therefore, danaparoid cannot be dosed interchangeably (unit for unit) with either heparin or low molecular weight heparins.

➤*Hemorrhage:* Hemorrhage can occur at virtually any site in patients receiving danaparoid. An unexplained fall in hematocrit or fall in blood pressure should lead to serious consideration of a hemorrhagic event. Use danaparoid, like anticoagulants, with extreme caution in disease states in which there is increased risk of hemorrhage, such as severe uncontrolled hypertension; acute bacterial endocarditis; congenital or acquired bleeding disorders; active ulcerative and angiodysplastic GI disease; nonhemorrhagic stroke; shortly after brain, spinal, or ophthalmological surgery; and postoperative indwelling epidural catheter use.

➤*Spinal or epidural hematomas:* Spinal or epidural hematomas can occur with the associated use of low molecular weight heparins or heparinoids and neuraxial (spinal/epidural) anesthesia or spinal puncture which can result in long-term or permanent paralysis. The risk of these events is higher with the use of postoperative indwelling epidural catheters or concomitant use of additional drugs affecting hemostasis such as NSAIDs (see Warning Box).

➤*Renal function impairment:* Consider the risks and benefits of danaparoid carefully before use in patients with severely impaired renal function or hemorrhagic disorders.

➤*Pregnancy: Category B.* There are no adequate and well-controlled studies in pregnant women. Use danaparoid during pregnancy only if clearly needed.

➤*Lactation:* It is not known whether danaparoid is excreted in breast milk. Exercise caution when danaparoid is administered to a nursing woman.

➤*Children:* Safety and efficacy in pediatric patients have not been established.

Precautions

➤*Monitoring:* Danaparoid only has a small effect on factor IIa (thrombin) activity; therefore, routine coagulation tests (eg, PT, activated partial thromboplastin time [aPTT], kaolin cephalin clotting time [KCCT], whole blood clotting time [WBCT], thrombin time [TT]) are unsuitable for monitoring danaparoid activity at recommended doses.

Periodic complete blood counts, including platelet count, and stool occult blood tests are recommended during the course of treatment.

➤*Thrombocytopenia:* Danaparoid shows a low cross-reactivity with antiplatelet antibodies in individuals with Type II heparin-induced

DANAPAROID SODIUM

thrombocytopenia. No cases of white-clot syndrome or cases of Type II thrombocytopenia have been reported in clinical studies for the prophylaxis of DVT in patients receiving multiple doses of danaparoid ≥ 14 days.

➤*Sulfite sensitivity:* Danaparoid contains sodium sulfite, which may cause allergic-type reactions including anaphylactic symptoms and life-threatening or less severe asthmatic episodes in certain susceptible people. The overall prevalence of sulfite sensitivity in the general population is unknown and probably low. Sulfite sensitivity is seen more frequently in asthmatic than in nonasthmatic patients.

Drug Interactions

➤*Anticoagulants:* Use with caution in patients receiving oral anticoagulants or platelet inhibitors. Monitoring of anticoagulant activity of oral anticoagulants by PT and *Thrombotest* is unreliable ≤ 5 hours after danaparoid administration.

Adverse Reactions

The following table summarizes adverse bleeding events that occurred in clinical trials that studied danaparoid injection compared with placebo, warfarin, and other agents.

Blood Loss and Transfusions: DVT and PE Prophylaxis for Orthopedic Hip Surgery (All Patients Treated)				
	Mean milliliters blood loss ± SD (n)			
Blood loss and transfusions	Danaparoid	Placebo	Warfarin	Other[1]
Intraoperative blood loss				
Males	694 ± 555 (330)	586 ± 737 (27)	689 ± 499 (141)	754 ± 661 (98)
Females	486 ± 430 (686)	416 ± 252 (66)	471 ± 306 (219)	530 ± 456 (288)
Postoperative blood loss				
Males	954 ± 879 (318)	908 ± 812 (45)	817 ± 585 (88)	1056 ± 1055 (129)
Females	700 ± 778 (639)	715 ± 520 (122)	619 ± 352 (80)	798 ± 779 (415)
Transfusions (units packed RBCs)				
Males	2.6 ± 1.8 units (258)	2.7 ± 1.4 units (35)	2.5 ± 1.4 units (87)	2.9 ± 2.1 units (82)
Females	2.6 ± 1.7 units (604)	2.8 ± 1.4 units (92)	2.1 ± 1.1 units (177)	2.8 ± 2 units (279)

[1] "Other" includes the following active reference agents: Heparin, heparin/DHE, acetylsalicylic acid, dextran, low molecular weight heparins.

Danaparoid Adverse Reactions (≥ 2%) (%)				
Adverse reaction	Danaparoid n = 645	Placebo n = 135	Warfarin n = 243	Other[1] n = 168
CNS				
Insomnia	3.1	0	13.2	0
Headache	2.6	0.7	5.3	0
Dizziness	2.3	0	5.8	0
Dermatologic				
Rash	4.8	0	7.4	1.22
Pruritus	3.9	0.7	5.8	0
GI				
Nausea	14.3	2.2	32.1	4.8
Constipation	11.3	0	28.8	1.2
Vomiting	2.9	2.2	8.2	1.8
Miscellaneous				
Fever	22.2	0.7	56.8	1.8
Injection site pain	7.6	3	0	20.2
Peripheral edema	3.3	0	7.8	2.4
Joint disorder	2.6	0	6.2	0
Urinary tract infection	2.6	0.7	2.1	3
Edema	2.6	0	5.8	1.2
Asthenia	2.3	0	4.1	0.6
Anemia	2.2	2.2	2.1	3
Urinary retention	2	0	5.8	0.6

[1] "Other" includes dextran, heparin/DHE, and aspirin.

Incidence of Adverse Reactions (≥ 2%) (%) in DVT and PE Prophylaxis Indication				
Adverse reaction	Danaparoid n = 2383	Placebo n = 276	Warfarin n = 421	Other[1] n = 1163
Injection site pain	13.7	19.2	0	13.2
Pain	8.7	0	48	1.7
Fever	7.3	0.4	35.6	1.8
Nausea	4.1	1.1	18.8	1.1
Urinary tract infection	4	1.1	6.4	5.6
Constipation	3.5	0	17.3	0.3
Rash	2.1	0	5.9	0.4
Infection	2.1	1.1	0	4

[1] "Other" includes the following active reference agents: Heparin, heparin sodium, heparin calcium, enoxaparin, dalteparin, dextran, heparin/DHE, and aspirin.

Overdosage

Single SC doses of danaparoid at 3800 anti-Xa units/kg (20.5 times the recommended human dose) and 15,200 anti-Xa units/kg (82 times the recommended human dose) were lethal to female and male rats, respectively. Symptoms of acute toxicity after IV dosing were respiratory depression, prostration, and twitching.

➤*Symptoms:* Accidental overdosage following administration of danaparoid may lead to bleeding complications.

➤*Treatment:* The effects of danaparoid on anti-Xa activity cannot be antagonized with any known agent at this time. Although protamine sulfate partially neutralizes the anti-Xa activity of danaparoid and can be safely coadministered, there is no evidence that protamine sulfate is capable of reducing severe nonsurgical bleeding during treatment with danaparoid. In the event of serious bleeding, discontinue danaparoid and administer blood or blood product transfusions as needed. Withdrawal of danaparoid may be expected to restore the coagulation balance without rebound phenomenon.

➤*Thrombosis/Embolism:* Prophylaxis and treatment of venous thrombosis and its extension; pulmonary embolism; peripheral arterial embolism; atrial fibrillation with embolization.

➤*Coagulopathies:* Diagnosis and treatment of acute and chronic consumption coagulopathies (disseminated intravascular coagulation [DIC]).

➤*Prophylaxis:* Low-dose regimen for prevention of postoperative deep venous thrombosis (DVT) and pulmonary embolism in patients undergoing major abdominothoracic surgery or who are at risk of developing thromboembolic disease.

According to the National Institutes of Health Consensus Development Conference, low-dose heparin is the treatment of choice as prophylaxis for DVT and pulmonary embolism in urology patients > 40 years of age; pregnant patients with prior thromboembolism; stroke patients; those with heart failure, acute MI or pulmonary infection; also recommended as suggested prophylaxis in high-risk surgery patients, moderate and high-risk gynecologic patients without malignancy, neurology patients with extracranial problems and patients with severe musculoskeletal trauma.

➤*Clotting prevention:* Prevention of clotting in arterial and heart surgery, blood transfusions, extracorporeal circulation, dialysis procedures and blood samples.

➤*Unlabeled uses:* Prophylaxis of left ventricular thrombi and cerebrovascular accidents post-MI.

Continuous infusion for treatment of myocardial ischemia in unstable angina refractory to conventional treatment. Heparin decreases the number of anginal attacks and silent ischemic episodes and reduces the daily duration of ischemia. Intermittent heparin is not as effective.

Prevention of cerebral thrombosis in the evolving stroke.

As an adjunct in treatment of coronary occlusion with acute MI. Although there is some controversy regarding the efficacy of heparin therapy with concurrent antiplatelet therapy (eg, aspirin) in the prevention of rethrombosis/reocclusion after primary thrombolysis with thrombolytics (eg, alteplase, anistreplase, streptokinase) during acute MI, it is recommended by the American College of Cardiology and the American Heart Association. Generally, administer heparin IV immediately after thrombolytic therapy, usually within 2 to 8 hours (depending on the thrombolytic used), and maintain the infusion for ≥ 24 hours. Begin aspirin therapy immediately as soon as the patient is admitted, and continue its administration.

Give by intermittent IV injection, continuous IV infusion or deep SC (ie, above the iliac crest of abdominal fat layer) injection. Avoid IM injection.

Continuous IV infusion is generally preferable due to the higher incidence of bleeding complications with other routes.

Adjust dosage according to coagulation test results prior to each injection. Dosage is adequate when whole blood clotting time (WBCT) is ≈ 2.5 to 3 times control value, or when aPTT is 1.5 to 2 times normal.

When given by continuous IV infusion, perform coagulation tests every 4 hours in the early stages. When administered by intermittent IV infusion, perform coagulation tests before each dose during early stages and at appropriate intervals thereafter. After deep SC injection, perform tests 4 to 6 hours after the injections.

➤*General heparin dosage guidelines:* Although dosage must be individualized, the following guidelines may be used:

Heparin Dosage Guidelines		
Method of administration	Frequency	Recommended dose[1]
Subcutaneous[2]	Initial dose	10,000 – 20,000 units[3]
	Every 8 hours	8000 – 10,000 units
	Every 12 hours	15,000 – 20,000 units
Intermittent IV	Initial dose	10,000 units[4]
	Every 4 to 6 hours	5000 – 10,000 units[4]
IV Infusion	Initial dose	In 1000 mL 0.9% sodium chloride
	Continuous	20,000 – 40,000 units/day[3]

[1] Based on a 68 kg (150 lb) patient.
[2] Use a concentrated solution.
[3] Immediately preceded by IV loading dose of 5000 units.
[4] Administer undiluted or in 50 to 100 mL 0.9% NaCl.

Heparin Dosage for DVT Treatment		
PTT (secs)	Action	Rate change
< 45	5000 units bolus	increase by 250 units/hr
45 to 54	—	increase by 150 units/hr
55 to 85	—	no change

Heparin Dosage for DVT Treatment		
PTT (secs)	Action	Rate change
86 to 110	stop infusion × 1 hr	decrease by 150 units/hr
> 110	stop infusion × 1 hr	decrease by 250 units/hr

➤*Children:* In general, the following dosage schedule may be used as a guideline:

Initial dose – 50 units/kg IV bolus.

Maintenance dose – 100 units/kg/dose IV drip every 4 hours, or 20,000 units/m^2/24 hours continuous IV infusion.

➤*Low-dose prophylaxis of postoperative thromboembolism:* Low-dose heparin prophylaxis, prior to and after surgery, will reduce the incidence of postoperative DVT in the legs and clinical pulmonary embolism. Give 5000 units SC 2 hours before surgery and 5000 units every 8 to 12 hours thereafter for 7 days or until the patient is fully ambulatory, whichever is longer. Administer by deep SC injection above the iliac crest or abdominal fat layer, arm, or thigh using a concentrated solution. Use a fine-gauge needle (25 to 26 gauge) to minimize tissue trauma. Reserve such prophylaxis for patients > 40 years of age undergoing major surgery. Exclude patients on oral anticoagulants or drugs that affect platelet function (see Drug Interactions) or in patients with bleeding disorders, brain or spinal cord injuries, spinal anesthesia, eye surgery, or potentially sanguineous operations.

If bleeding occurs during or after surgery, discontinue heparin and neutralize with protamine sulfate. If clinical evidence of thromboembolism develops despite low-dose prophylaxis, give full therapeutic doses of anticoagulants until contraindicated. Prior to heparinization, rule out bleeding disorders; perform appropriate coagulation tests just prior to surgery. Coagulation test values should be normal or only slightly elevated at these times.

➤*Surgery of the heart and blood vessels:* Give an initial dose of not less than 150 units/kg to patients undergoing total body perfusion for open heart surgery. Often, 300 units/kg is used for procedures < 60 minutes and 400 units/kg is used for procedures > 60 minutes.

➤*Extracorporeal dialysis:* Follow equipment manufacturers' operating directions.

➤*Blood transfusion:* Add 400 to 600 units per 100 mL whole blood to prevent coagulation. Add 7500 units to 100 mL 0.9% Sodium Chloride Injection (or 75,000 units/L of 0.9% Sodium Chloride Injection); from this sterile solution, add 6 to 8 mL per 100 mL whole blood. Perform leukocyte counts on heparinized blood within 2 hours of addition of heparin. Do not use heparinized blood for isoagglutinin, complement, erythrocyte fragility tests, or platelet counts.

➤*Laboratory samples:* Add 70 to 150 units per 10 to 20 mL sample of whole blood to prevent coagulation of sample (see Blood transfusion).

➤*Clearing intermittent infusion (heparin lock) sets:* To prevent clot formation in a heparin lock set, inject diluted heparin solution (Heparin Lock Flush Solution, USP; or a 10 to 100 units/mL heparin solution) via the injection hub to fill the entire set to the needle tip. Replace this solution each time the heparin lock is used. Aspirate before administering any solution via the lock to confirm patency and location of needle or catheter tip. If the administered drug is incompatible with heparin, flush the entire heparin lock set with sterile water or normal saline before and after the medication is administered; following the second flush, the dilute heparin solution may be reinstilled into the set. Consult the set manufacturer's instructions.

Because repeated injections of small doses of heparin can alter aPTT, obtain a baseline aPTT prior to insertion of a heparin lock set.

➤*Preparation of solution:* Slight discoloration does not alter potency.

When heparin is added to infusion solution for continuous IV administration, invert container ≥ 6 times to ensure adequate mixing and to prevent pooling of heparin.

➤*Converting to oral anticoagulant therapy:* Perform baseline coagulation tests to determine prothrombin activity when heparin activity is too low to affect prothrombin time (PT) or the International Normalized Ratio (INR). For immediate anticoagulant effect, give heparin in usual therapeutic doses. When results of initial prothrombin determinations are known, initiate the oral anticoagulant in the usual amount. Perform coagulation tests and prothrombin activity at appropriate intervals. To ensure continuous anticoagulation, continue full heparin therapy for several days after PT or INR has reached therapeutic range. Heparin therapy may then be discontinued. Measure PT or INR ≥ 6 hours after last IV bolus dose and 24 hours after last SC dose of heparin. If continuous IV heparin infusion is used, PT or INR can usually be measured at any time. When prothrombin activity reaches the desired therapeutic range, discontinue heparin and continue oral anticoagulants.

Actions

➤*Pharmacology:* Commercial preparations of heparin are derived from bovine lung or porcine intestinal mucosa; although chemical and biological differences exist, there are no clinical differences in the antithrombotic effects. The anticoagulant potency of heparin is standardized by bioassay and is expressed in "units" of activity. Because the number of units per milligram varies, express dosage only in "units." (Heparin sodium should contain not less than 140 heparin units/mg.)

The major rate-limiting step in the coagulation cascade is the activation of factor X, which is involved in both intrinsic and extrinsic pathways (refer to the Anticoagulant introduction). Small amounts of heparin in combination with antithrombin III (ATIII) inhibit thrombosis by inactivating factor Xa and inhibiting the conversion of prothrombin to thrombin. Once active thrombosis has developed, larger amounts of heparin in combination with heparin cofactor (HC-II) can inhibit further coagulation by inactivating thrombin and preventing the conversion of fibrinogen to fibrin. In combination with ATIII, heparin inactivates activated coagulation factors IX, X, XI, XII, plasmin, kallikrein and thrombin, inhibiting conversion of fibrinogen to fibrin. The heparin-antithrombin III complex is 100 to 1000 times more potent as an anticoagulant than antithrombin III alone. Heparin also prevents the formation of a stable fibrin clot by inhibiting the activation of factor XIII (the fibrin stabilizing factor). Other effects include the inhibition of thrombin-induced activation of factors V and VIII and variable inhibitions of platelet aggregates.

Commercial products contain both low and high molecular weight heparin fractions. Low molecular weight heparin has a greater inhibitory effect on factor Xa and less antithrombin activity than the high molecular weight fraction.

Heparin inhibits reactions that lead to clotting but does not significantly alter the concentration of the normal clotting factors of blood. Although clotting time is prolonged by full therapeutic doses, in most cases it is not measurably affected by low doses of heparin. Bleeding time is usually unaffected. The drug has no fibrinolytic activity; it will not lyse existing clots, but it can prevent extension of existing clots.

Heparin also enhances lipoprotein lipase release, (which clears plasma of circulating lipids), increases circulating free fatty acids and reduces lipoprotein levels.

➤*Pharmacokinetics:*

Absorption / Distribution – Heparin is not adsorbed from the GI tract and must be given IV or SC. An IV bolus results in immediate anticoagulant effects, the anticoagulant response to heparin at therapeutic doses is not linear but increases disproportionately both in its intensity and duration with increasing dose. Peak plasma levels of heparin are achieved 2 to 4 hours following SC use, although there are considerable individual variations. Once absorbed, heparin is distributed in plasma and is extensively and nonspecifically protein bound.

Metabolism / Excretion – Heparin is rapidly cleared from plasma with an average half-life of 30 to 180 minutes. Half-life is dose-dependent and non-linear and may be disproportionately prolonged at higher doses (30 min at 25 u/kg vs 150 minutes at 400 u/kg). Heparin is partially metabolized by liver heparinase and the reticuloendothelial system. There may be a secondary site of metabolism in the kidneys. Apparent volume of distribution is 40 to 60 mL/kg. In patients with deep venous thrombosis, plasma clearance is more rapid and half-life is shorter than in patients with pulmonary embolism. Heparin half-life may be prolonged in liver disease. Heparin is excreted in urine as unchanged drug (up to 50%), particularly after large doses. Some urinary degradation products have anticoagulant activity.

Contraindications

Hypersensitivity to heparin; severe thrombocytopenia; uncontrolled bleeding (except when it is due to DIC); any patient for whom suitable blood coagulation tests cannot be performed at the appropriate intervals (there is usually no need to monitor coagulation parameters in patients receiving low-dose heparin).

Warnings

➤*IM administration:* Avoid because of the danger of hematoma formation.

➤*Hemorrhage:* Hemorrhage can occur at virtually any site in patients receiving heparin. An unexplained fall in hematocrit, fall in blood pressure or any other unexplained symptom should lead to serious consideration of a hemorrhagic event. An overly prolonged coagulation test or bleeding can usually be controlled by withdrawing the drug. Signs and symptoms will vary according to the location and extent of bleeding and may be present as paralysis, headache, chest, abdomen, joint or other pain, shortness of breath, difficulty breathing or swallowing, unexplained swelling or unexplained shock. GI or urinary tract bleeding may indicate an underlying occult lesion. Certain hemorrhagic complications may be difficult to detect.

Adrenal hemorrhage – Adrenal hemorrhage resulting in acute adrenal insufficiency has occurred. Discontinue therapy in patients who develop signs and symptoms of acute adrenal hemorrhage or insufficiency. Initiation of therapy should not depend on laboratory confirmation of diagnosis, since any delay in an acute situation may result in death.

Ovarian (corpus luteum) hemorrhage – This type of hemorrhage has developed in a number of reproductive age women receiving anticoagulants. If unrecognized, this may be fatal.

Retroperitoneal hemorrhage – Retroperitoneal hemorrhage may occur.

Germinal matrix-intraventricular hemorrhage – Occurs fourfold higher in low-birth-weight infants receiving heparin therapy.

Use heparin with extreme caution in disease states in which there is increased danger of hemorrhage. These include:

Cardiovascular: Subacute bacterial endocarditis; severe hypertension.
CNS: During and immediately following spinal tap, spinal anesthesia or major surgery, especially of the brain, spinal cord or eye.
Hematologic: Hemophilia; some vascular purpuras; thrombocytopenia.
GI: Ulcerative lesions, diverticulitis or ulcerative colitis; continuous tube drainage of the stomach or small intestine.
Obstetric: Menstruation.
Other: Liver disease with impaired hemostasis; severe renal disease.

➤*Hyperlipidemia:* Heparin may increase free fatty acid serum levels by induction of lipoprotein lipase. The catabolism of serum lipoproteins by this enzyme produces lipid fragments rapidly processed by the liver. Patients with dysbetalipoproteinemia (type III) cannot catabolize the lipid fragments, resulting in hyperlipidemia.

➤*Benzyl alcohol:* Benzyl alcohol, which is contained in some of these products as a preservative, has been associated with a fatal "gasping syndrome" in premature infants.

➤*Resistance:* Increased resistance to the drug is frequently encountered in fever, thrombosis, thrombophlebitis, infections with thrombosing tendencies, MI, cancer and postoperative states.

➤*Thrombocytopenia:* Thrombocytopenia has occurred in patients receiving heparin with a reported incidence of up to 30%. The development of thrombocytopenia does not necessarily imply a causal relationship. Often patients have other potential causes for thrombocytopenia; they can be ill, receiving several medications or in a postoperative phase. Exclude these potential causes for thrombocytopenia before implicating heparin. The incidence of heparin-associated thrombocytopenia is higher with bovine than with porcine heparin (15.6% vs 5.8%). The severity also appears to be related to heparin dosage, with low-dose therapy resulting in fewer complications.

Early thrombocytopenia – (Type I) develops 2 to 3 days after starting heparin, tends to be mild and is due to a direct action of heparin on platelets.

Delayed thrombocytopenia – (Type II) develops 7 to 12 days after either low-dose or full-dose heparin, can have serious consequences and may reflect the presence of an immunoglobulin that induces platelet aggregation.

Mild thrombocytopenia – Mild thrombocytopenia (platelet count > 100,000/mm^3) may remain stable or reverse even if heparin is continued. However, closely monitor thrombocytopenia of any degree. If a count falls < 100,000/mm^3 or if recurrent thrombosis develops, discontinue heparin. If continued heparin therapy is essential, administration of heparin from a different organ source can be reinstituted with caution.

White clot syndrome – Patients may develop new thrombus formation in association with thrombocytopenia resulting from irreversible aggregation of platelets induced by heparin, the so-called "white clot syndrome." The process may lead to severe thromboembolic complications (eg, skin necrosis, gangrene of the extremities possibly leading to amputation, MI, pulmonary embolism, stroke, possibly death). Monitor platelet counts before and during therapy. If significant thrombocytopenia occurs, immediately terminate heparin and institute other therapeutic measures.

➤*Hypersensitivity reactions:* Give heparin to patients with documented hypersensitivity only in life-threatening situations. Before a therapeutic dose is given, a trial dose may be advisable. Have epinephrine 1:1000 immediately available. Refer to Management of Acute Hypersensitivity Reactions.

Vasospastic reactions – Vasospastic reactions may develop 6 to 10 days after starting therapy and last 4 to 6 hours. The affected limb is painful, ischemic and cyanotic. An artery to this limb may have been recently catheterized. After repeated injections, the reaction may gradually increase to generalized vasospasm with cyanosis, tachypnea, feeling of oppression and headache. Protamine sulfate has no marked effect. Itching and burning, especially on the plantar side of the feet, is possibly based on a similar allergic vasospastic reaction. Chest pain, elevated blood pressure, arthralgias or headache have also been reported in the absence of definite peripheral vasospasm.

➤*Elderly:* A higher incidence of bleeding has occurred in women > 60 years of age.

Heparin

➤*Pregnancy: Category C.* Safety for use during pregnancy has not been established. Heparin does not cross the placenta. However, its use during pregnancy has been associated with 13% to 22% unfavorable outcomes, including stillbirths and prematurity. This contrasts with a 31% incidence with coumarin derivatives. Heparin is probably the preferred anticoagulant during pregnancy, but it is not risk free. Heparin-induced osteoporosis has occurred, including collapse of vertebrae. Use with caution during pregnancy, especially during the last trimester and during the immediate postpartum period, because of the risk of maternal hemorrhage.

➤*Lactation:* Heparin is not excreted in breast milk.

➤*Children:* See Administration and Dosage. Safety and efficacy have not been determined in newborns; germinal matrix intraventricular hemorrhage occurs more often in low-birth-weight infants receiving heparin.

Use heparin lock flush solution with caution in infants with disease states in which there is an increased danger of hemorrhage. The use of the 100 unit/mL concentration is not advised because of bleeding risk, especially in low-birth-weight infants.

Precautions

➤*Monitoring:* The most common test used to monitor heparin's effect is Activated Partial Thromboplastin Time (APTT). The APTT is widely used, quick, easily done and reproducible. Other tests used include Activated Coagulation Time (ACT) and Lee White-Whole Blood Clotting Time (WBCT). The ACT is also rapid and readily available. The WBCT is time consuming and unreliable; it is used as a standard with which to compare newer tests. If the coagulation test is unduly prolonged or if hemorrhage occurs, discontinue the drug promptly (see Overdosage). Perform periodic platelet counts, hematocrit and tests for occult blood in stool during the entire course of therapy, regardless of route of administration.

➤*Hyperkalemia:* May develop, probably due to induced hypoaldosteronism. Use with caution in patients with diabetes or renal insufficiency. Monitor patient closely.

Drug Interactions

Heparin Drug Interactions			
Precipitant drug	Object drug*		Description
Cephalosporins	Heparin	↑	Several parenteral cephalosporins have caused coagulopathies; this might be additive with heparin, possibly increasing the risk of bleeding.
Nitroglycerin	Heparin	↓	The pharmacologic effects of heparin may be decreased, although information on the interaction is conflicting.
Penicillins	Heparin	↑	Parenteral penicillins can produce alterations in platelet aggregation and coagulation tests. These effects might be additive with heparin, possibly increasing the risk of bleeding.

Heparin Drug Interactions			
Precipitant drug	Object drug*		Description
Platelet inhibitors (eg, ibuprofen, indomethacin, dipyridamole, hydroxychloroquine, NSAIDs, ticlopidine phenylbutazone, aspirin, dextran)	Heparin	↑	An increased risk of bleeding is possible during concurrent administration due to interference with platelet aggregation.
Digitalis, tetracyclines, nicotine, antihistamines	Heparin	↓	May partially counteract the anticoagulant action of heparin sodium.
Streptokinase	Heparin	↓	Relative resistance to heparin anticoagulation following administration of streptokinase as a systemic thrombolytic agent may occur.

* ↑ = Object drug increased. ↓ = Object drug decreased.

➤*Drug/Lab test interactions:* Significant elevations of **aminotransferase** (AST and ALT) levels have occurred in a high percentage of patients. Cautiously interpret aminotransferase increases that might be caused by heparin.

Adverse Reactions

Hemorrhage – Hemorrhage is the chief complication (≤ 10%). See Warnings.

➤*Local: Avoid IM use.* Local irritation, erythema, mild pain, hematoma or ulceration may follow deep SC use, but are more common after IM use. Histamine-like reactions and subcutaneous and cutaneous necrosis have been observed.

➤*Hypersensitivity:*
Most common – Chills; fever; urticaria.

Rare – Asthma; rhinitis; lacrimation; headache; nausea; vomiting; shock; anaphylactoid reactions. Allergic vasospastic reactions with painful, ischemic, cyanotic limbs may develop 6 to 10 days after starting therapy and last 4 to 6 hours. Whether these are identical to thrombocytopenia-associated complications is undetermined. See Warnings.

➤*Miscellaneous:* Thrombocytopenia (see Warnings); osteoporosis (after long-term, high doses); cutaneous necrosis, suppressed aldosterone synthesis, delayed transient alopecia, priapism, rebound hyperlipidemia (after discontinuation).

Overdosage

➤*Symptoms:* Bleeding is the chief sign of heparin overdosage. Nosebleeds, hematuria or tarry stools may be the first sign of bleeding. Easy bruising or petechial formations may precede frank bleeding.

➤*Treatment:* Protamine sulfate (1% solution) will neutralize heparin (see individual monograph). Each mg of protamine neutralizes ≈ 100 USP heparin units.

HEPARIN SODIUM INJECTION, USP
A sterile solution of heparin sodium in water for injection.

Multiple Dose Vials

Rx	**Heparin Sodium** (Various, eg, Elkins-Sinn, Fujisawa, Pasadena, Solopak, Pharmacia & Upjohn)	**Injection:** 1,000 units per mL	In 1, 10 and 30 mL vials.
Rx	**Heparin Sodium** (Abbott)	**Injection:** 2,000 units per mL	In 5 and 10 mL vials.
Rx	**Heparin Sodium** (Abbott)	**Injection:** 2,500 units per mL	In 5 and 10 mL vials.
Rx	**Heparin Sodium** (Various, eg, Elkins-Sinn, Fujisawa, Pasadena,Pharmacia & Upjohn, URL)	**Injection:** 5,000 units per mL	In 1 and 10 mL vials.
Rx	**Heparin Sodium** (Various, eg, Elkins-Sinn, Lilly, Fujisawa, Pasadena, Phamacia & Upjohn)	**Injection:** 10,000 units per mL	In 0.5, 1, 4, 5 and 10 mL vials.
Rx	**Heparin Sodium** (Various, eg, Pasadena, Schein)	**Injection:** 20,000 units per mL	In 1, 2 and 5 mL vials.
Rx	**Heparin Sodium** (Various, eg, Pasadena, Schein)	**Injection:** 40,000 units per mL	In 1, 2 and 5 mL vials.

Single Dose Ampules and Vials

Rx	**Heparin Sodium** (Various, eg, Fujisawa)	**Injection:**1000 units per mL	In 1 mL vials.
Rx	**Heparin Sodium** (Various, eg, Fujisawa, Sanofi Winthrop)	**Injection:** 5000 units per mL	In 1 mL vials.
Rx	**Heparin Sodium** (Various, eg, Fujisawa, Pasadena, Pharmacia & Upjohn, Sanofi Winthrop)	**Injection:** 10,000 units per mL	In 1 mL vials.
Rx	**Heparin Sodium** (Various, eg, Fujisawa, Pasadena, Schein)	**Injection:** 20,000 units per mL	In 1 mL vials.
Rx	**Heparin Sodium** (Various, eg, Pasadena)	**Injection:** 40,000 units per mL	In 1 mL vials.

Unit-Dose

Rx	**Heparin Sodium**[1] (Elkins-Sinn)	**Injection:** 1,000 units per dose	In 1, 10 and 30 mL *Dosette* vials.[2]
Rx	**Heparin Sodium**[1] (Wyeth-Ayerst)		In 1 mL *Tubex.*[2]
Rx	**Heparin Sodium**[1] (Wyeth-Ayerst)	**Injection:** 2,500 units per dose	In 1 mL *Tubex.*[2]
Rx	**Heparin Sodium**[1] (Elkins-Sinn)	**Injection:** 5,000 units per dose	In 1 and 10 mL vial.[2]
Rx	**Heparin Sodium**[1] (Wyeth-Ayerst)		In 0.5 and 1 mL *Tubex.*[2]
Rx	**Heparin Sodium**[1] (Sanofi Winthrop)		In 1 mL fill in 2 mL *Carpuject.*[2]
Rx	**Heparin Sodium**[1] (Wyeth-Ayerst)	**Injection:** 7,500 units per dose	In 1 mL *Tubex.*[2]
Rx	**Heparin Sodium**[1] (Elkins-Sinn)	**Injection:** 10,000 units per dose	In 0.5, 1 and 4 mL vials.[2]
Rx	**Heparin Sodium**[1] (Wyeth-Ayerst)		In 1 mL *Tubex.*[2]
Rx	**Heparin Sodium**[1] (Wyeth-Ayerst)	**Injection:** 20,000 units per dose	In 1 mL *Tubex.*[2]

[1] From porcine intestinal mucosa.   [2] With benzyl alcohol.

For complete prescribing information, refer to the Heparin Group Monograph.

HEPARIN SODIUM AND SODIUM CHLORIDE

Rx	**Heparin Sodium**[1] and 0.9% Sodium Chloride (Baxter Healthcare)	**Injection:** 1000 units	In 500 mL *Viaflex.*
		2000 units	In 1000 mL *Viaflex.*
Rx	**Heparin Sodium**[1] and 0.45% Sodium Chloride (Abbott)	**Injection:** 12,500 units	In 250 mL.[2]
		25,000 units	In 250 and 500 mL.[2]

[1] From porcine intestinal mucosa.   [2] With EDTA.

For complete prescribing information, refer to the Heparin Group Monograph.

HEPARIN SODIUM LOCK FLUSH SOLUTION
Used as an IV flush to maintain patency of indwelling IV catheters in intermittent IV therapy or blood sampling; not intended for therapeutic use.

Rx	**Heparin I.V. Flush** (Medefil)	**Injection:** 1 unit per mL	In 1, 2, 2.5, 5, and 10 mL syringes.
Rx	**Heparin Lock Flush** (Various, eg, Abbott, Fujisawa)	**Injection:** 10 units per mL	In 1, 2, 5, 10, 30 and 50 mL vials; 1, 2, 2.5, 3, 5 mL disposable syringes.
Rx	**Hep-Lock**[1] (Elkins-Sinn)		In 1, 2 mL *Dosette* vials; 1, 2.5 mL *Dosette* cartridge needle units; 10, 30 mL vials.[2]
Rx	**Hep-Lock U/P**[1] (Elkins-Sinn)		Preservative free. In 1 mL *Dosette* vials.
Rx	**Hepflush-10** (American Pharmaceutical Partners)		Preservative-free. In 10 mL single-dose vials.
Rx	**Heparin Lock Flush** (Various, eg, Abbott, Fujisawa)	**Injection:** 100 units per mL	In 1, 2, 5, 10, 30 and 50 mL vials; 1 mL amps; 1, 2, 2.5, 3, 5 mL disposable syringes.
Rx	**Hep-Lock U/P**[1] (Elkins-Sinn)		Preservative free. In 1 mL *Dosette* vials.

[1] From porcine intestinal mucosa.   [2] With benzyl alcohol.

For complete prescribing information, refer to the Heparin Group Monograph.

ANTITHROMBIN III (HUMAN)

Rx	Thrombate III (Bayer)	Powder for injection, lyophilized: 500 IU	Preservative-free. In single-use vials with 10 mL Sterile Water for Injection.
		1000 IU	Preservative-free. In single-use vials with 20 mL Sterile Water for Injection.

Indications

➤*Antithrombin III deficiency:* Treatment of patients with hereditary antithrombin III deficiency in connection with surgical or obstetrical procedures or when they suffer from thromboembolism.

Administration and Dosage

Administer within 3 hours after reconstitution. Do not refrigerate after reconstitution.

Administer only by the IV route.

Once reconstituted, give alone without mixing with other agents or diluting solutions.

Product administration and handling of the needles must be done with caution. Percutaneous puncture with a needle contaminated with blood can transmit infectious viruses including HIV (AIDS) and hepatitis. Obtain immediate medical attention if injury occurs.

Place needles in sharps container after single use. Discard all equipment including any reconstituted product in accordance with biohazard procedures.

Each bottle of antithrombin III has the functional activity, in international units (IU), stated on the label of the bottle. The potency assignment has been determined with a standard calibrated against a World Health Organization antithrombin III reference preparation.

Determine dosage on an individual basis based on the pretherapy plasma AT-III level, in order to increase plasma AT-III levels to the level found in normal human plasma (100%). Dosage can be calculated from the following formula (expressed as % normal level based on functional AT-III assay):

$$\text{units required (IU)} = \frac{[\text{desired-baseline AT-III level}]}{1.4} \times \text{weight (kg)}$$

The above formula is based on an expected incremental in vivo recovery above baseline levels for antithrombin III (human) of 1.4%/IU/kg administered.

As a general recommendation, the following therapeutic program may be utilized as a starting program for treatment while modifying the program based on the actual plasma AT-III levels achieved:

1.) An initial loading dose calculated to elevate the plasma AT-III level to 120%, assuming an expected rise over the baseline plasma AT-III level of 1.4% (functional activity) per IU per kg of antithrombin III administered. Thus, if an individual has a baseline AT-III level of 57%, the initial dose would be (120 – 57)/1.4 = 45 IU/kg.

2.) Measure preinfusion and 20 minutes postinfusion (peak) plasma antithrombin III levels following the initial loading dose, the plasma antithrombin III level after 12 hours, then the level preceding the next infusion (trough level). Subsequently measure antithrombin III levels preceding and 20 minutes after each infusion until predictable peak and trough levels have been achieved, generally between 80% to 120%. Plasma levels between 80% to 120% may be maintained by administration of maintenance doses of 60% of the initial loading dose, administered every 24 hours. Adjustments in the maintenance dose or interval between doses should be made based on actual plasma AT-III levels achieved.

Monitor AT-III levels more frequently and adminster antithrombin III as necessary in situations when the half-life of antithrombin III may be shortened (following surgery, hemorrhage, or acute thrombosis, or during IV heparin administration).

When an infusion of antithrombin III is indicated for a patient with hereditary deficiency to control an acute thrombotic episode or to prevent thrombosis following surgical or obstetrical procedures, raise the antithrombin III level to normal and maintain this level for 2 to 8 days, depending on the indication for treatment, type and extensiveness of surgery, the patient's medical condition and history, and the physician's judgment. Base concomitant administration of heparin in each of these situations on the medical judgment of the physician.

➤*Reconstitution:* Reconstitute with Sterile Water for Injection and bring to room temperature prior to administration. Filter through a sterile needle as supplied in the package prior to use and administer within 3 hours following reconstitution. It may be infused over 10 to 20 minutes. It must be administered IV.

Inspect parenteral drug products visually for particulate matter and discoloration prior to administration, whenever solution and container permit.

➤*Rate of administration:* Adapt the rate of administration to the response of the individual patient, but administration of the entire dose in 10 to 20 minutes is generally well tolerated.

➤*Storage/Stability:* Store under refrigeration (2° to 8°C; 36° to 46°F). Avoid freezing as breakage of the diluent bottle might occur.

Actions

➤*Pharmacology:* Antithrombin III (AT-III), an alpha$_2$-glycoprotein of molecular weight 58,000, is normally present in human plasma at a concentration of $\approx$ 12.5 mg/dL and is the major plasma inhibitor of thrombin. Inactivation of thrombin by AT-III occurs by formation of a covalent bond resulting in an inactive 1:1 stoichiometric complex between the two, involving an interaction of the active serine of thrombin and an arginine reactive site on AT-III. AT-III is also capable of inactivating other components of the coagulation cascade including factors IXa, Xa, XIa, and XIIa, as well as plasmin.

The neutralization rate of serine proteases by AT-III proceeds slowly in the absence of heparin, but is greatly accelerated in the presence of heparin. As the therapeutic antithrombotic effect in vivo of heparin is mediated by AT-III, heparin is ineffective in the absence or near absence of AT-III.

The prevalence of the hereditary deficiency of AT-III is estimated to be 1 per 2000 to 5000 in the general population. The pattern of inheritance is autosomal-dominant. In affected individuals, spontaneous episodes of thrombosis and pulmonary embolism may be associated with AT-III levels of 40% to 60% of normal. These episodes usually appear after the age of 20, the risk increasing with age and in association with surgery, pregnancy, and delivery. The frequency of thromboembolic events in hereditary antithrombin III (AT-III) deficiency during pregnancy has been reported to be 70%, and several studies of the beneficial use of antithrombin III (Human) concentrates during pregnancy in women with hereditary deficiency have been reported. In many cases; however, no precipitating factor can be identified for venous thrombosis or pulmonary embolism. Greater than 85% of individuals with hereditary AT-III deficiency have had at least 1 thrombotic episode by the age of 50 years. In $\approx$ 60% of patients, thrombosis is recurrent. Clinical signs of pulmonary embolism occur in 40% of affected individuals. In some individuals, treatment with oral anticoagulants leads to an increase of the endogenous levels of AT-III, and treatment with oral anticoagulants may be effective in the prevention of thrombosis in such individuals.

➤*Pharmacokinetics:* The mean 50% disappearance time (the time to fall to 50% of the peak plasma level following an initial administration) was $\approx$ 22 hours, and the biologic half-life was 2.5 days based on immunologic assays and 3.8 days based on functional assays of AT-III. These values are similar to the half-life for radiolabeled antithrombin III (human) reported in the literature as 2.8 to 4.8 days.

➤*Clinical trials:* In clinical studies, none of the 13 patients with hereditary AT-III deficiency and histories of thromboembolism treated prophylactically on 16 separate occasions with antithrombin III for high thrombotic risk situations (11 surgical procedures, 5 deliveries) developed a thrombotic complication. Heparin was also admininstered in 3 of the 11 surgical procedures and in all 5 deliveries. Eight patients with hereditary AT-III deficiency were treated therapeutically with antithrombin III as well as heparin for major thrombotic or thromboembolic complications, with 7 patients recovering. Treatment reversed heparin resistance in 2 patients with hereditary AT-III deficiency being treated for thrombosis or thromboembolism.

During clinical investigation, none of 12 subjects monitored for a median of 8 months (range, 2 to 19 months) after receiving antithrombin III, became antibody-positive to HIV-1. None of 14 subjects monitored for $\geq$ 3 months demonstrated any evidence of hepatitis, either non-A, non-B hepatitis, or hepatitis B.

Warnings

➤*Viral infections:* Antithrombin III is made from human plasma. Products made from human plasma may contain infectious agents, such as viruses, that can cause disease. The risk that such products will transmit an infectious agent has been reduced by screening plasma donors for prior exposure to certain viruses, by testing for the presence of certain current virus infections, and by inactivating or removing certain viruses. Despite these measures, such products can still potentially transmit disease. There is also the possibility that unknown infectious agents may be present in such products. Individuals who receive infusions of blood or plasma products may develop signs or symptoms of some viral infections, particularly hepatitis C. All infections thought by a physician possibly to have been transmitted by this product should be reported by the physician or other health care provider to Bayer Corporation at (888) 765–3203.

Have the physician discuss the risks and benefits of this product with the patient before prescribing or administering it to a patient.

➤*Neonates:* Measure the AT-III levels in neonates of parents with hereditary AT-III deficiency immediately after birth. Fatal neonatal thromboembolism, such as aortic thrombi in children of women with hereditary antithrombin III deficiency, has been reported.

Plasma levels of AT-III are lower in neonates than adults, averaging $\approx$ 60% in normal-term infants. AT-III levels in premature infants may be much lower. Low plasma AT-III levels, especially in a premature

ANTITHROMBIN III (HUMAN)

infant, therefore, do not necessarily indicate hereditary deficiency. It is recommended that testing and treatment with antithrombin III of neonates be discussed with an expert on coagulation.

➤*Pregnancy: Category B.* Reproduction studies have been performed in rats and rabbits at doses ≤ 4 times the human dose and have revealed no evidence of impaired fertility or harm to the fetus. It is not known whether antithrombin III can cause fetal harm when administered to a pregnant women or can affect reproduction capacity. Because animal reproduction studies are not always predictive of human response, this drug should be used during pregnancy only if clearly needed.

➤*Children:* Safety and efficacy in the pediatric population have not been established.

Precautions

➤*Thrombosis:* Inform subjects with antithrombin III deficiency about the risk of thrombosis in connection with pregnancy and surgery and about the inheritance of the disease.

➤*Antithrombin* III *deficiency diagnosis:* Base the diagnosis of hereditary antithrombin III deficiency on a clear family history of venous thrombosis as well as decreased plasma antithrombin III levels and the exclusion of acquired deficiency.

Antithrombin III in plasma may be measured with amidolytic assays by using synthetic chromogenic substrates or with clotting assays or with immunoassays. The latter does not detect all congenital antithrombin III deficiencies.

➤*Lab test abnormalities:* It is recommended that AT-III plasma levels be monitored during the treatment period. Functional levels of AT-III in plasma may be measured by amidolytic assays using chromogenic substrates or by clotting assays.

Drug Interactions

➤*Heparin:* The anticoagulant effect of heparin is enhanced by concurrent treatment with antithrombin III in patients with hereditary antithrombin III deficiency. Thus, in order to avoid bleeding, reduce heparin dosage during antithrombin III treatment.

Adverse Reactions

In clinical studies adverse reactions were reported in association with 17 of the 340 infusions during the clinical studies. Included were the following: Dizziness (7); chest tightness, nausea, foul taste in mouth (3); chills, cramps (2); shortness of breath, chest pain, film over eye, lightheadedness, bowel fullness, hives, fever, oozing, hematoma formation (1). If adverse reactions are experienced, decrease the infusion rate, or if indicated, interrupt the infusion until symptoms abate.

Thrombin Inhibitor

DESIRUDIN

Rx	**Iprivask** (Aventis)	**Powder for injection, lyophilized:** 15 mg	Preservative free. In single-use vials with diluent.[1]

[1] Diluent includes 0.6 mL mannitol (3%) in water for injection.

WARNING

Spinal / Epidural hematomas: When neuraxial anesthesia (epidural/spinal anesthesia) or spinal puncture is employed, patients anticoagulated or scheduled to be anticoagulated with selective inhibitors of thrombin such as desirudin may be at risk of developing an epidural or spinal hematoma which can result in long-term or permanent paralysis.

The risk of these events may be increased by the use of indwelling spinal catheters for administration of analgesia or by the concomitant use of drugs affecting hemostasis such as non-steroidal anti-inflammatory drugs (NSAIDs), platelet inhibitors, or other anticoagulants. Likewise with such agents, the risk appears to be increased by traumatic or repeated epidural or spinal puncture.

Frequently monitor patients for signs and symptoms of neurological impairment. If neurological compromise is noted, urgent treatment is necessary.

The physician should consider the potential benefit versus risk before neuraxial intervention, in patients anticoagulated or to be anticoagulated for thromboprophylaxis.

Indications

➤*Deep vein thrombosis, prophylaxis:* Prophylaxis of deep vein thrombosis (DVT), which may lead to pulmonary embolism, in patients undergoing elective hip replacement surgery.

Administration and Dosage

➤*Approved by the FDA:* April 4, 2003.

All patients should be evaluated for bleeding disorder risk before prophylactic administration of desirudin.

➤*Initial dosage:* In patients undergoing hip replacement surgery, the recommended does of desirudin is 15 mg every 12 hours administered by SC injection with the initial dose given up to 5 to 15 minutes before surgery, but after induction of regional block anesthesia, if used (see Warnings). Up to 12 days administration (average duration, 9 to 12 days) of desirudin has been well tolerated in controlled trials.

➤*Renal function impairment:*

Desirudin Use in Renal Insufficiency		
Degree of renal insufficiency	Creatinine clearance (mL/min/1.73 m^2)	aPTT monitoring and dosing instructions
Moderate	≥ 31 to 60	Initiate therapy at 5 mg q 12 h by SC injection. Monitor aPTT and serum creatinine at least daily. If aPTT exceeds 2 times control: 1) interrupt therapy until the value returns to less than 2 times control; 2) resume therapy at a reduced dose guided by the initial degree of aPTT abnormality.
Severe	< 31	Initiate therapy at 1.7 mg q 12 h. Monitor aPTT and serum creatinine at least daily. If aPTT exceeds 2 times control: 1) interrupt therapy until the value returns to less than 2 times control; 2) consider further dose reductions guided by the initial degree of aPTT abnormality.

➤*Preparation for administration:* Reconstitution should be carried out under sterile conditions. Reconstitute each vial with 0.5 mL of provided diluent (Mannitol [3%] in water for injection). Once reconstituted, each 0.5 mL contains 15.75 mg of desirudin. Shake the vial gently until the drug is fully reconstituted. Use the reconstituted solution immediately. Discard any unused solution appropriately. Desirudin should not be mixed with other injections, solvents, or infusions. Desirudin is administered by SC injection. Do not administer by IM injection.

➤*SC injection technique:* Select a syringe with a 26- or 27-gauge needle which is approximately ½ inch in length for administration of desirudin. Withdraw the entire reconstituted solution (15.75 mg desirudin/0.5 mL) into the syringe and inject the total volume SC, which will deliver 15 mg. Patients should be sitting or lying down and desirudin injection administered by deep SC injection. Alternate administration between the left and right anterolateral and left and right posterolateral thigh or abdominal wall. Introduce the whole length of the needle into a skin fold held between the thumb and forefinger; hold the skin fold throughout the injection.

➤*Interchangeability:* Desirudin cannot be used interchangeably with other hirudins as they differ in manufacturing process and specific biological activity (ATUs). Each of these medicines has its own instructions for use.

➤*Storage / Stability:* Protect from light. Store unopened vials or ampules at 25°C (77°F); excursions permitted to 15° to 30°C (59° to 86°F). Use the reconstituted solution immediately; however, it is stable for up to 24 hours when stored at room temperature and protected from light. Discard any unused solution appropriately.

Actions

➤*Pharmacology:* Desirudin is a specific inhibitor of human thrombin. Desirudin is a selective inhibitor of free circulating and clot-bound thrombin. The anticoagulant properties of desirudin are demonstrated by its ability to prolong the clotting time of human plasma. One molecule of desirudin binds to 1 molecule of thrombin and thereby blocks the thrombogenic activity of thrombin. As a result, all thrombin-dependent coagulation assays are affected. Activated partial thromboplastin time (aPTT) is a measure of the anticoagulant activity of desirudin and increases in a dose-dependent fashion. The pharmacodynamic effect of desirudin on proteolytic activity of thrombin was assessed as an increase in aPTT. A mean aPTT prolongation of about 1.38 times baseline value (range, 0.58 to 3.41) was observed following SC twice daily injections of 15 mg desirudin. Thrombin time (TT) frequently exceeds 200 seconds even at low plasma concentrations of desirudin, which renders this test unsuitable for routine monitoring of desirudin therapy. At therapeutic serum concentrations, desirudin has no effect on other enzymes of the hemostatic system such as factors IXa, Xa, kallikrein, plasmin, tissue plasminogen activator, or activated protein C. In addition, it does not display any effect on other serine proteases, such as the digestive enzymes trypsin, chymotrypsin, or on complement activation by the classical or alternative pathways.

➤*Pharmacokinetics:*

Absorption – The absorption of desirudin is complete when administered SC at doses of 0.3 or 0.5 mg/kg. Following SC administration of single doses of 0.1 to 0.75 mg/kg, plasma concentrations of desirudin increased to a maximum level (C_{max}) between 1 and 3 hours. Both C_{max} and AUC values are dose proportional.

Distribution – Desirudin is distributed in the extracellular space with a volume of distribution at steady state of 0.25 L/kg, independent of the dose. Desirudin binds specifically and directly to thrombin, forming an extremely tight, non-covalent complex with an inhibition constant of approximately 2.6×10^{-13}. Thus, free or protein bound desirudin immediately binds circulating thrombin. The pharmacological effect of desirudin is not modified when coadministered with highly bound protein drugs (greater than 99%).

Metabolism / Excretion – Desirudin is primarily eliminated and metabolized by the kidney. Total urinary excretion of unchanged desirudin amounts to 40% to 50% of the administered dose. Metabolites lacking 1 or 2 C-terminal amino acids constitute a minor proportion of the material recovered from urine (less than 7%). There is no evidence for the presence of other metabolites. This indicates that desirudin is metabolized by stepwise degradation from the C-terminus probably catalyzed by carboxypeptidase(s) such as carboxypeptidase A, originating from the pancreas. Total clearance of desirudin is approximately 1.5 to 2.7 mL/min/kg following SC or IV administration and is independent of dose. This clearance value is close to the glomerular filtration rate. The elimination of desirudin from plasma is rapid after IV administration, with approximately 90% of the dose disappearing from the plasma within 2 hours of the injection. Plasma concentrations of desirudin then decline with a mean terminal elimination half-life of 2 to 3 hours. After SC administration, the mean terminal elimination half-life is also approximately 2 hours.

Special populations –

Renal insufficiency: In a pharmacokinetic study of renally impaired subjects, subjects with mild (Ccr between 61 and 90 mL/min/1.73 m^2), moderate (Ccr between 31 and 60 mL/min/1.73 m^2), and severe (Ccr below 31 mL/min/1.73 m^2) renal insufficiency, were administered a single IV dose of 0.5, 0.25, or 0.125 mg/kg desirudin, respectively. This resulted in mean dose-normalized AUC_{effect} increases of approximately 3-, and 9-fold for the moderate and severe renally impaired subjects, respectively. In subjects with severe renal insufficiency, terminal eliminations half-lives were prolonged up to 12 hours compared with 2 to 4 hours. Dose adjustments are recommended in certain circumstances in relation to the degree of impairment or degree of aPTT abnormality (see Warnings, Administration and Dosage).

Elderly: The mean plasma clearance of desirudin in patients at least 65 years of age is approximately 28% lower than in patients younger than 65 years of age.

➤*Clinical trials:* In the first study, desirudin 15 mg administered SC every 12 hours was compared with unfractionated heparin 5000 IU administered SC every 8 hours in 436 patients. Desirudin significantly reduced the number of total venous thromboembolism (VTE) compared with unfractionated heparin: Evaluable population: desirudin (7.5%) vs heparin (23.2%); Intent-to-Treat population: desirudin (5.8%) vs heparin (19.1%). Significantly fewer patients in the group treated with desirudin experienced proximal DVT than those patients treated with heparin: Evaluable population: desirudin (3.4%) vs heparin (16.4%); Intent-to-Treat population: desirudin (2.7%) vs heparin (13.6%).

DESIRUDIN

In a second study, desirudin 15 mg administered SC every 12 hours was compared with enoxaparin sodium 40 mg administered SC every 24 hours in 2049 patients. In both, the evaluable patient population and the intent-to-treat population, patients who received desirudin had a lower incidence of major VTE, total VTE, and proximal DVT than did patients who received enoxaparin.

Efficacy of Desirudin in Hip Replacement Surgery Patients (%)		
	Desirudin[1] 15 mg q 12 h SC	Enoxaparin[1] 40 mg qd
Evaluable hip replacement surgery patients	n = 773	n = 768
Treatment failures Major VTE[2,3] Total VTE[4] Proximal DVT	4.9 18.8 4.5	7.9 25.7 7.7
Intent-to treat hip replacement surgery patients	n = 1043	n = 1036
Treatment failures Major VTE[2] Total VTE[4] Proximal DVT	3.7 13.9 3.5	5.9 19.2 5.7

[1] Treatment was initiated ≤ 30 minutes preoperatively, but after induction of regional block anesthesia, if used.
[2] Major VTE included proximal DVT, PE, or death.
[3] Total number of patients in this evaluation: desirudin 802; enoxaparin 758.
[4] Total VTE = Venous thromboembolic events which included DVT (including proximal events), PE, or death considered to be thromboembolic in origin.

Contraindications

Known hypersensitivity to natural or recombinant hirudins and in patients with active bleeding and/or irreversible coagulation disorders.

Warnings

➤*Hemorrhagic events:* Use desirudin with caution in patients with increased risks of hemorrhage such as those with recent major surgery, organ biopsy, or puncture of a non-compressible vessel within the last month; a history of hemorrhagic stroke, intracranial or intraocular bleeding including diabetic (hemorrhagic) retinopathy, recent ischemic stroke, severe uncontrolled hypertension, bacterial endocarditis, a known hemostatic disorder (congenital or acquired [eg, hemophilia, liver disease]), or a history of GI or pulmonary bleeding within the past 3 months. Bleeding can occur at any site during therapy with desirudin. An unexplained fall in hematocrit or blood pressure should lead to a search for a bleeding site.

➤*Spinal/Epidural anesthesia:* There is a risk of neuraxial hematoma formation with the concurrent use of desirudin and spinal/epidural anesthesia, which has the potential to result in long term or permanent paralysis. The risk may be greater with the use of post-operative indwelling catheters or the concomitant use of additional drugs affecting hemostasis such as NSAIDs, platelet inhibitors, or other anticoagulants. The risk may also be increased by traumatic or repeated neuraxial puncture.

Should the physician decide to administer anticoagulation in the context of epidural/spinal anesthesia, extreme vigilance and frequent monitoring must be exercised to detect any signs and symptoms of neurological impairment such as midline back pain, sensory and motor deficits (numbness or weakness in lower limbs), or bowel and/or bladder dysfunction. If signs or symptoms of spinal hematoma are suspected, initiate urgent diagnosis and treatment including spinal cord decompression. The physician should consider the potential benefit versus risk before neuraxial intervention in patients anticoagulated or to be anticoagulated for thromboprophylaxis.

➤*Renal function impairment:* Desirudin must be used with caution in patients with renal impairment, particularly in those with moderate and severe renal impairment (Ccr less than 60 mL/min/1.73 m² body surface area). Dose reductions by factors of 3 and 9 are recommended for patients with moderate and severe renal impairment respectively. In addition, daily aPTT and serum creatinine monitoring are recommended for patients with moderate or severe renal impairment.

➤*Hepatic function impairment:* Although desirudin is not significantly metabolized by the liver, hepatic impairment or serious liver injury (eg, liver cirrhosis) may alter the anticoagulant effect of desirudin due to coagulation defects secondary to reduced generation of vitamin K-dependent coagulation factors. Use desirudin with caution in these patients.

➤*Elderly:* This drug is substantially excreted by the kidney, and the risk of adverse events because of it may be greater in patients with impaired renal function. Because elderly patients are more likely to have decreased renal function, take care in dose selection, and it may be useful to monitor renal function. Dosage adjustment in the case of moderate and severe renal impairment is necessary. Serious adverse events occurred more frequently in patients 75 years of age or older as compared with those less than 65 years of age.

➤*Pregnancy:* Category C. Teratology studies have been performed in rats at SC doses in a range of 1 to 15 mg/kg/day and in rabbits at IV doses in a range of 0.6 to 6 mg/kg/day and have revealed desirudin to be teratogenic. Observed teratogenic findings were omphalocele, asymmetric and fused sternebrae, edema, and shortened hand limbs in rats; and spina bifida, malrotated hind limb, hydrocephaly, and gastroschisis in rabbits. There are no adequate and well controlled studies in pregnant women. Desirudin should be used during pregnancy only if the potential benefit justifies the potential risk to the fetus.

➤*Lactation:* It is not known whether desirudin is excreted in human milk. Because many drugs are excreted in human milk, caution should be exercise when desirudin is administered to a breastfeeding woman.

➤*Children:* Safety and efficacy in pediatric patients have not been established.

Precautions

➤*Monitoring:* Monitor aPTT daily in patients with increased risk of bleeding and/or renal impairment. Monitor serum creatinine daily in patients with renal impairment. Peak aPTT should not exceed 2 times control. Should peak aPTT exceed this level, dose reduction is advised based on the degree of aPTT abnormality. If necessary, interrupt therapy with desirudin until aPTT falls to less than 2 times control, at which time treatment with desirudin can be resumed at a reduced dose. TT is not a suitable test for routine monitoring of desirudin therapy. Dose adjustments based on serum creatinine may be necessary (see Administration and Dosage).

Use in patients switching from oral anticoagulants to desirudin or from desirudin to oral anticoagulants – When warfarin and desirudin were coadministered, greater inhibition of hemostasis measured by aPTT, prothrombin time (PT), and international normalized ratio (INR) was observed. If a patient is switched from oral anticoagulants to desirudin therapy or from desirudin to oral anticoagulants, continue to closely monitor the anticoagulant activity with appropriate methods. Take that activity into account in the evaluation of the overall coagulation status of the patient during the switch.

➤*Antibodies/Re-exposure:* Antibodies have been reported in patients treated with hirudins. Potential for cross-sensitivity to hirudin products cannot be excluded. Irritative skin reactions were observed in 9/322 volunteers exposed to desirudin by SC injection or IV bolus or infusion in single or multiple administrations of the drug. Allergic events were reported in more than 2% of patients who were administered desirudin in Phase 3 clinical trials. Hirudin-specific IgE evaluations may not be indicative of sensitivity to desirudin as this test was not always positive in the presence of symptoms. Very rarely, anti-hirudin antibodies have been detected upon re-exposure to desirudin. Fatal anaphylactoid reactions have been reported during hirudin therapy.

Drug Interactions

Any agent which may enhance the risk of hemorrhage should be discontinued prior to initiation of desirudin therapy. These agents include medications such as Dextran 40, systemic glucocorticoids, thrombolytics, and anticoagulants.

Desirudin Drug Interactions			
Precipitant drug	Object drug*		Description
Thrombolytics (eg, alteplase, streptokinase), Glucocorticoids Dextran	Desirudin	↑	Concomitant treatment with thrombolytics may increase the risk of bleeding. Discontinue before initiations of desirudin therapy.
Anticoagulants (eg, heparin [unfractionated, and LMWH])	Desirudin	↑	During prophylaxis of venous thromboemolism, concomitant treatment is not recommended. The effects include prolongation of aPTT. As with other anticoagulants, desirudin should be used with caution.
Antiplatelets and glycoprotein IIb/IIIa antagonists (eg, salicylates, NSAIDs, ketorolac, acetylsalicylic acid, triclopidine, dipyridamole, sulfinpyrazone, clopidogrel, abciximab)	Desirudin	↑	Use with caution in conjunction with desirudin

* ↑ = Object drug increased.

Adverse Reactions

➤*Miscellaneous:*

Hemorrhagic events – The following rates of hemorrhagic events have been reported during clinical trials.

Thrombin Inhibitor

DESIRUDIN

Hemorrhage in Patients Undergoing Hip Replacement Surgery (%)			
	Desirudin 15 mg q 12 h SC (N = 1561)	Heparin 5000 IU q 8 h SC (N = 501)	Enoxaparin 40 mg qd SC (N = 1036)
Patients with any hemorrhage[1]	30	22	33
Patients with serious hemorrhage[2]	3	3	2
Patients with major hemorrhage[3]	< 1	0	< 1

[1] Includes hematomas which occurred at an incidence of 6% in the desirudin and enoxaprin treatment groups and 5% in the heparin treatment group.
[2] Bleeding complications were considered serious if perioperative transfusion requirements exceeded 5 units of whole blood or packed red cells, or if total transfusion requirements up to postoperative day 6 inclusive exceeded 7 units of whole blood or packed red cells, or total blood loss up to postoperative day 6 inclusive exceeded 3500 mL.
[3] Bleeding complications were considered major if the hemorrhage was: 1) overt and it produced a fall in hemoglobin of ≥ 2 g/dL or if it lead to a transfusion of ≥ 2 units of whole or packed cells outside the perioperative period (the time from start of surgery until ≤ 12 hours after); 2) retroperitoneal, intracranial, intraocular, intraspinal, or occurred in a major prosthetic joint.

Non-hemorrhagic events –

Adverse Events Occurring at ≥ 2% in Desirudin Treated Patients Undergoing Hip Replacement Surgery (%)			
Body System	Desirudin 15 mg q 12 h SC (N = 1561)	Heparin 5000 IU q 8 h SC (N = 501)	Enoxaparin 40 mg qd SC (N = 1036)
Injection site mass	4	6	< 1
Wound secretion	4	5	3
Anemia	3	2	4
Deep thrombophlebitis	2	8	2
Nausea	2	< 1	< 1

Related adverse events with a frequency of less than 2% and more than 0.2% (in decreasing order of frequency): Thrombosis, hypotension, leg edema, fever, decreased hemoglobin, hematuria, dizziness, epistaxis, vomiting, impaired healing, cerebrovascular disorder, leg pain, hematemesis.

Hypersensitivity – In clinical studies, allergic events were reported in less than 2% overall and in 2% of patients who were administered 15 mg desirudin.

Postmarketing – Rare reports of major hemorrhages, some of which were fatal, and anaphylactic/anaphylactoid reactions.

Overdosage

➤*Symptoms:* In case of overdose, most likely reflected in hemorrhagic complications, or suggested by excessively high aPTT values, discontinue desirudin therapy.

➤*Treatment:* No specific antidote for desirudin is available; however, the anticoagulant effect of desirudin is partially reversible using thrombin-rich plasma concentrates while aPTT levels can be reduced by the IV administration of 0.3 μg/kg DDAVP (desmopressin). The clinical effectiveness of DDAVP in treating bleeding due to desirudin overdose has not been studied. Emergency procedures should be instituted as appropriate (eg, determination of aPTT and other coagulation levels, hemoglobin, the use of blood transfusion or plasma expanders). In an open pilot, dose-ascending study to assess safety, the highest dose of desirudin (40 mg every 12 hours) caused excessive hemorrhage.

LEPIRUDIN

Rx   **Refludan** (Hoechst-Marion Roussel)   **Powder for injection:** 50 mg   Mannitol. Freeze-dried. In boxes of 10.

Indications

➤*Thrombocytopenia, heparin-induced:* For anticoagulation in patients with heparin-induced thrombocytopenia (HIT) and associated thromboembolic disease to prevent further thromboembolic complications (TECs).

➤*Unlabeled uses:* Adjunct therapy for treatment of unstable angina, acute MI without ST elevation, prevention of deep vein thrombosis, and in patients undergoing percutaneous coronary intervention.

Administration and Dosage

➤*Approved by the FDA:* March 6, 1998.

➤*Initial dosage:* Anticoagulation in adult patients with HIT and associated thromboembolic disease, 0.4 mg/kg (up to 110 kg) IV slowly (eg, over 15 to 20 seconds) as a bolus dose followed by 0.15 mg/kg (up to 110 kg/h) as a continuous IV infusion for 2 to 10 days or longer if clinically needed.

Normally the initial dosage depends on the patient's body weight; this is valid for patients up to 110 kg. In patients with a body weight exceeding 110 kg, do not increase the initial dosage beyond the 110 kg body weight dose (maximal initial bolus dose of 44 mg, maximal initial infusion dose of 16.5 mg/h).

In general, therapy with lepirudin is monitored using the activated partial thromboplastin time (aPTT) ratio (patient aPTT at a given time over an aPTT reference value, usually median of the laboratory normal range for aPTT). Determine patient baseline aPTT prior to initiation of therapy with lepirudin because lepirudin should not be started in patients presenting with a baseline aPTT ratio of 2.5 or more to avoid initial overdosing.

➤*Dose modifications:* Confirm any aPTT ratio out of the target range at once before drawing conclusions with respect to dose modifications, unless there is a clinical need to react immediately.

If the confirmed aPTT ratio is above the target range, stop the infusion for 2 hours. At restart, decrease the infusion rate by 50% (no additional IV bolus should be administered). Determine the aPTT ratio again 4 hours later.

If the confirmed aPTT ratio is below the target range, increase the infusion rate in steps of 20%. Determine the aPTT ratio again 4 hours later.

Do not exceed an infusion rate of 0.21 mg/kg/h without checking for coagulation abnormalities that might prevent an appropriate aPTT response.

➤*Renal function impairment:* As lepirudin is almost exclusively excreted in the kidneys, consider individual renal function prior to administration. In the case of renal impairment, relative overdose might occur even with the standard dosing regimen. Therefore, the bolus dose and infusion rate must be reduced in case of known or suspected renal insufficiency (Ccr less than 60 mL/min or serum creatinine above 1.5 mg/dL).

There is only limited information on the therapeutic use of lepirudin in HIT patients with significant renal impairment. The following dosage recommendations are mainly based on single-dose studies in a small number of patients with renal impairment. Therefore, these recommendations are only tentative and aPTT monitoring should be used along with monitoring of renal status.

Base dose adjustments on Ccr values, whenever available, as obtained from a reliable method (24 hour urine sampling). If Ccr is not available, base the dose adjustments on the serum creatinine.

In all patients with renal insufficiency, the bolus dose is to be reduced to 0.2 mg/kg.

The standard initial infusion rate must be reduced according to the recommendations given in the following table. Additional aPTT monitoring is highly recommended.

Reduction of Lepirudin Infusion Rate in Patients with Renal Impairment			
		Adjusted infusion rate	
Ccr (mL/min)	Serum creatinine (mg/dL)	% of standard initial infusion rate	mg/kg/h
45 to 60	1.6 to 2	50%	0.075
30 to 44	2.1 to 3	30%	0.045
15 to 29	3.1 to 6	15%	0.0225
< 15[1]	> 6[1]	avoid or stop infusion[1]	

[1] In hemodialysis patients or in case of acute renal failure (Ccr less than 15 mL/min or serum creatinine above 6 mg/dL), lepirudin infusion is to be avoided or stopped. Consider additional IV bolus doses of 0.1 mg/kg every other day only if the aPTT ratio falls below the lower therapeutic limit of 1.5.

➤*Concomitant use with thrombolytic therapy:* Clinical trials in HIT patients have provided only limited information on the combined use of lepirudin and thrombolytic agents. In the studies, the following dosage regimen of lepirudin was used in 9 HIT patients who presented with TECs at baseline and were started on lepirudin and thrombolytic therapy (alteplase, urokinase, or streptokinase).

Initial IV bolus – 0.2 mg/kg.

Continuous IV infusion – 0.1 mg/kg/h.

The number of patients receiving combined therapy was too small to identify differences in clinical outcome of patients who were started on both lepirudin and thrombolytic therapy as compared with those who were started on lepirudin alone. The combined incidences of death,

LEPIRUDIN

limb amputation, or new TEC were 22.2% and 20.7%, respectively. While there was a 47% relative increase in the overall bleeding rate in patients who were started on both lepirudin and thrombolytic therapy (55.6% vs 37.9%), there were no differences in the rates of serious bleeding events (fatal or life-threatening bleeds, bleeds that were permanently or significantly disabling, overt bleeds requiring transfusion of 2 or more units of packed red blood cells, bleeds necessitating surgical intervention, intracranial bleeds) between the groups (11.1% vs 11.2%). Although no intracranial bleeding has been observed in any of these patients, there have been reports of intracranial bleeding in the presence or absence of concomitant thrombolytic therapy (see Warnings and Adverse Reactions).

Pay special attention to the fact that thrombolytic agents may increase the aPTT ratio. Therefore, aPTT ratios with a given plasma level of lepirudin are usually higher in patients who receive concomitant thrombolysis than in those who do not.

➤*Patients scheduled to switch to oral anticoagulation:* If a patient is scheduled to receive coumarin derivatives (vitamin K antagonists) for oral anticoagulation after lepirudin therapy, the dose of lepirudin should first be gradually reduced in order to reach an aPTT ratio just above 1.5 before initiating oral anticoagulation. Initiate coumarin derivatives only when platelet counts are normalizing. The intended maintenance dose should be started with no loading dose. To avoid prothrombotic effects when initiating coumarin, continue parenteral anticoagulation for 4 to 5 days. The parenteral agent can be discontinued when the INR stabilizes within the desired target range.

➤*Preparation and dilution:* Do not mix lepirudin with other drugs except for water for injection, 0.9% sodium chloride injection, or 5% dextrose injection.

Reconstitution and further dilution are to be carried out under sterile conditions.
• For reconstitution, water for injection or 0.9% sodium chloride injection are to be used.
• For further dilution, 0.9% sodium chloride injection or 5% dextrose injection are suitable.
• For rapid, complete reconstitution, inject 1 mL of diluent into the vial and shake gently. After reconstitution, a clear, colorless solution usually is obtained in a few seconds but definitely in less than 3 minutes.
• Do not use solutions that are cloudy or contain particles.
• Use the reconstitution solution immediately. It remains stable for up to 24 hours at room temperature (eg, during infusion).
• Warm the preparation to room temperature before administration.
• Discard any unused solution appropriately.

➤*Initial IV bolus:* For IV bolus injection, use a solution with a concentration of 5 mg/mL.

Preparation of lepirudin solution with a concentration of 5 mg/mL:
• Reconstitute one vial (50 mg) with 1 mL of water for injection or 0.9% sodium chloride injection.
• The final concentration of 5 mg/mL is obtained by transferring the contents of the vial into a sterile, single-use syringe (of at least 10 mL capacity) and diluting the solution to a total volume of 10 mL using water for injection, 0.9% sodium chloride injection, or 5% dextrose injection.
• Administer the final solution according to body weight (see the following table).

IV injection of the bolus is to be carried out slowly (eg, over 15 to 20 seconds).

Standard Bolus Injection Volumes of Lepirudin According to Body Weight for a 5 mg/mL Concentration		
	Injection volume	
Body weight (kg)	Dosage 0.4 mg/kg	Dosage 0.2 mg/kg[1]
50	4 mL	2 mL
60	4.8 mL	2.4 mL
70	5.6 mL	2.8 mL
80	6.4 mL	3.2 mL
90	7.2 mL	3.6 mL
100	8 mL	4 mL
≥ 110	8.8 mL	4.4 mL

[1] Dosage recommended for all patients with renal insufficiency.

➤*IV infusion:* For continuous IV infusion, solutions with concentration of 0.2 or 0.4 mg/mL may be used.

Preparation of a lepirudin solution with a concentration of 0.2 or 0.4 mg/mL:
• Reconstitute 2 vials (each containing 50 mg) with 1 mL each using water for injection or 0.9% sodium chloride injection.
• The final concentrations of 0.2 or 0.4 mg/mL are obtained by transferring the contents of both vials into an infusion bag containing 500 or 250 mL of 0.9% sodium chloride injection or 5% dextrose injection.

The infusion rate (mL/h) is to be set according to body weight (see following table).

Standard Infusion Rates of Lepirudin According to Body Weight		
	Infusion rate at 0.15 mg/kg/h	
Body weight (kg)	500 mL infusion bag 0.2 mg/mL	250 mL infusion bag 0.4 mg/mL
50	38 mL/h	19 mL/h
60	45 mL/h	23 mL/h
70	53 mL/h	26 mL/h
80	60 mL/h	30 mL/h
90	68 mL/h	34 mL/h
100	75 mL/h	38 mL/h
≥ 110	83 mL/h	41 mL/h

➤*Storage/Stability:* Store unopened vials at 2° to 25°C (36° to 77°F). Once reconstituted, use lepirudin immediately. The reconstituted solution remains stable for up to 24 hours at room temperature (eg, during infusion). Discard any unused solution.

Actions

➤*Pharmacology:* Lepirudin (rDNA), a recombinant hirudin derived from yeast cells, is a highly specific direct inhibitor of thrombin. One antithrombin unit (ATU) is the amount of lepirudin that neutralizes one unit of World Health Organization preparation 89/588 of thrombin. The specific activity of lepirudin is approximately 16,000 ATU/mg. Its mode of action is independent of antithrombin III. Platelet factor 4 does not inhibit lepirudin. One molecule of lepirudin binds to one molecule of thrombin and thereby blocks the thrombogenic activity of thrombin. As a result, all thrombin-dependent coagulation assays are affected (eg, aPTT values increase in a dose-dependent fashion).

The pharmacodynamic effect of lepirudin on the proteolytic activity of thrombin was routinely assessed as an increase in aPTT. This was observed with increasing plasma concentrations of lepirudin, with no saturable effect up to the highest tested dose (0.5 mg/kg IV bolus). Thrombin time (TT) frequently exceeded 200 seconds even at low plasma concentrations of lepirudin, which renders this test unsuitable for routine monitoring of lepirudin therapy.

The pharmacodynamic response defined by the aPTT ratio (aPTT at a time after lepirudin administration over an aPTT reference value, usually median of the laboratory normal range for aPTT) depends on plasma drug levels, which in turn depend on the individual patient's renal function. For patients undergoing additional thrombolysis, elevated aPTT ratios were already observed at low lepirudin plasma concentrations, and further response to increasing plasma concentrations was relatively flat. In other populations, the response was steeper. At plasma concentrations of 1500 ng/mL, aPTT ratios were nearly 3 for healthy volunteers, 2.3 for patients with HIT, and 2.1 for patients with deep venous thrombosis.

➤*Pharmacokinetics:*

Absorption/Distribution – Following IV administration, distribution is essentially confined to extracellular fluids and is characterized by an initial half-life of approximately 10 minutes. Elimination follows a first-order process and is characterized by a terminal half-life of about 1.3 hours in young, healthy volunteers. As the IV dose is increased over the range of 0.1 to 0.4 mg/kg, the maximum plasma concentration and the AUC increase proportionally.

Metabolism/Excretion – Lepirudin is thought to be metabolized by release of amino acids via catabolic hydrolysis of the parent drug. Approximately 48% of the administered dose is excreted in the urine that consists of unchanged drug (35%) and other fragments of the parent drug.

The systemic clearance of lepirudin is proportional to the glomerular filtration rate or creatinine clearance. Dose adjustment, based on creatinine clearance, is recommended.

Special populations –
Women: The systemic clearance of lepirudin in women is about 25% lower than in men.
Elderly: In elderly patients, the systemic clearance of lepirudin is 20% lower than in younger patients. This may be explained by the lower creatinine clearance in elderly patients compared with younger patients.
Renal function impairment: In patients with marked renal insufficiency (creatinine clearance under 15 mL/min) and on hemodialysis, elimination half-lives are prolonged up to 2 days.

LEPIRUDIN

Systemic Clearance (Cl) and Volume of Distribution at Steady State (V_{ss}) of Lepirudin		
Patient population	Mean Cl (mL/min)	Mean Vd_{ss} (L)
Healthy young subjects (n = 18, 18 to 60 years of age)	164	12.2
Healthy elderly subjects (n = 10, 65 to 80 years of age)	139	18.7
Renally impaired patients (n = 16, Ccr < 80 mL/min)	61	18
Heparin-induced thrombocytopenia patients (n = 73)	114	32.1

Contraindications

Hypersensitivity to hirudins or to any of the components in lepirudin.

Warnings

➤*Hemorrhagic events:* As with other anticoagulants, hemorrhage can occur at any site in patients receiving lepirudin. Consider a hemorrhagic event if an unexpected fall in hemoglobin, fall in blood pressure, or any unexplained symptom occurs. While patients are being anticoagulated with lepirudin, closely monitor the anticoagulation status using an appropriate measure, such as the aPTT.

➤*Intracranial bleeding:* Intracranial bleeding following concomitant thrombolytic therapy with alteplase or streptokinase may be life-threatening. There have been reports of intracranial bleeding with lepirudin in the absence of concomitant thrombolytic therapy (see Adverse Reactions). Carefully assess the risk of lepirudin administration vs its anticipated benefit in patients with increased risk of bleeding. In particular, this includes the following conditions:
- Recent puncture of large vessels or organ biopsy
- Anomaly of vessels or organs
- Recent cerebrovascular accident, stroke, intracerebral surgery, or other neuraxial procedures
- Severe uncontrolled hypertension
- Bacterial endocarditis
- Advanced renal impairment
- Hemorrhagic diathesis
- Recent major surgery
- Recent major bleeding (eg, intracranial, GI, intraocular, or pulmonary)
- Recent active peptic ulcer

➤*Hypersensitivity reactions:* There have been reports of allergic and hypersensitivity reactions, including anaphylactic reactions. Serious anaphylactic reactions that have resulted in shock or death have been reported during initial administration or upon second or subsequent re-exposure(s).

➤*Renal function impairment:* With renal impairment, relative overdose might occur even with standard dosage regimen. In patients with marked renal insufficiency (creatinine clearance less than 15 mL/min) and on hemodialysis, elimination half-lives are prolonged up to 2 days. Reduce the bolus dose and rate of infusion in patients with known or suspected renal insufficiency (see Administration and Dosage).

➤*Pregnancy: Category B.* Lepirudin (1 mg/kg) IV crosses the placenta in pregnant rats. It is not known whether the drug crosses the placenta in humans. Following IV administration of lepirudin at 30 mg/kg/day (180 mg/m²/day, 1.2 times the recommended maximum human total daily dose) during organogenesis and perinatal-postnatal periods, pregnant rats showed an increased maternal mortality with undetermined causes. There are no adequate and well-controlled studies in pregnant women. Use during pregnancy only if clearly needed.

➤*Lactation:* It is not known whether lepirudin is excreted in breast milk. Because of the potential for serious adverse reactions in nursing infants, decide whether to discontinue nursing or to discontinue the drug, taking into account the importance of the drug to the mother.

➤*Children:* Safety and efficacy have not been established. In one study, 2 children, an 11-year-old girl and a 12-year-old boy, were treated with lepirudin. Both children presented with TECs at baseline. Lepirudin doses ranged from 0.15 to 0.22 mg/kg/h for the girl, and from 0.1 (in conjunction with urokinase) to 0.7 mg/kg/h for the boy. Treatment with lepirudin was completed after 8 and 58 days, respectively, without serious adverse events.

Precautions

➤*Monitoring:* Adjust the dosage (infusion rate) according to the aPTT ratio.

The target range for the aPTT ratio during treatment (therapeutic window) should be 1.5 to 2.5. Data from clinical trials in HIT patients suggest that with aPTT ratios higher than this target range, the risk of bleeding increases, while there is no incremental increase in clinical efficacy. Do not start in patients with a baseline aPTT ratio of 2.5 or more in order to avoid initial overdosing.

The first aPTT determination for monitoring treatment should be done 4 hours after start of the lepirudin infusion. Follow-up aPTT determinations are recommended at least once daily, as long as treatment is ongoing.

More frequent aPTT monitoring is highly recommended in patients with renal impairment or serious liver injury or with an increased risk of bleeding.

➤*Antibodies:* Formation of antihirudin antibodies was observed in about 40% of HIT patients treated with lepirudin. This may increase the anticoagulant effect of lepirudin possibly because of delayed renal elimination of active lepirudin-antihirudin complexes. Therefore, strict monitoring of aPTT is necessary also during prolonged therapy. No evidence of neutralization of lepirudin or of allergic reactions associated with positive antibody test results was found.

➤*Hepatic injury:* Serious liver injury (eg, cirrhosis) may enhance the anticoagulant effect of lepirudin caused by coagulation defects secondary to reduced generation of vitamin K-dependent coagulation factors.

➤*Re-exposure:* A total of 13 patients were re-exposed to lepirudin in two studies. One experienced a mild allergic skin reaction during the second treatment cycle. In postmarketing experience, anaphylaxis after re-exposure has been reported.

➤*Lab test abnormalities:* In general, adjust the dosage (infusion rate) according to the aPTT ratio (patient aPTT at a given time over an aPTT reference value, usually the median of the laboratory normal range for aPTT). Other thrombin-dependent coagulation assays are changed by lepirudin.

Drug Interactions

Lepirudin Drug Interactions			
Precipitant drug	Object drug*		Description
Thrombolytics (eg, alteplase, streptokinase)	Lepirudin	↑	Concomitant treatment with thrombolytics may increase the risk of bleeding complications and considerably enhance the effect of lepirudin on aPTT prolongation.
Coumarin derivatives (vitamin K antagonists)	Lepirudin	↑	Concomitant treatment with coumarin derivatives and drugs that affect platelet function may increase the risk of bleeding.

* ↑ = Object drug increased.

Adverse Reactions

➤*Miscellaneous:*

Adverse events reported in HIT patients – The following information is based on 198 patients treated with lepirudin in 2 studies. The safety profile of 113 lepirudin patients from these studies who presented with TECs at baseline was compared with 91 historical control patients. Bleeding was the most frequent adverse event observed with lepirudin.

Hemorrhagic Events[1] with Lepirudin (%)			
		Patients with TECs	
Hemorrhagic event	All patients (n = 198)	Lepirudin (n = 113)	Historical control (n = 91)
Bleeding from puncture sites and wounds	14.1	10.6	4.4
Anemia or isolated drop in hemoglobin	13.1	12.4	1.1
Other hematoma and unclassified bleeding	11.1	10.6	4.4
Hematuria	6.6	4.4	0
GI and rectal bleeding	5.1	5.3	6.6
Epistaxis	3	4.4	1.1
Hemothorax	3	0	1.1
Vaginal bleeding	1.5	1.8	0
Intracranial bleeding	0	0	2.2

[1] Patients may have suffered more than one event.

Other hemorrhagic events (eg, hemoperitoneum, hemoptysis, liver bleeding, lung bleeding, mouth bleeding, retroperitoneal bleeding) each occurred in one individual among the 198 patients treated with lepirudin.

Nonhemorrhagic Events[1] with Lepirudin (%)			
		Patients with TECs	
Adverse reaction	All patients (n = 198)	Lepirudin (n = 113)	Historical control (n = 91)
Fever	6.1	4.4	8.8
Abnormal liver function	6.1	5.3	0
Pneumonia	4	4.4	5.5

Thrombin Inhibitor

LEPIRUDIN

Nonhemorrhagic Events[1] with Lepirudin (%)			
		Patients with TECs	
Adverse reaction	All patients (n = 198)	Lepirudin (n = 113)	Historical control (n = 91)
Sepsis	4	3.5	5.5
Allergic skin reactions	3	3.5	1.1
Heart failure	3	1.8	2.2
Abnormal kidney function	2.5	1.8	4.4
Unspecified infections	2.5	1.8	1.1
Multiorgan failure	2	3.5	0
Pericardial effusion	1	0	1.1
Ventricular fibrillation	1	0	0

[1] Patients may have suffered more than one event.

Other adverse events –

Intracranial bleeding: Intracranial bleeding was the most serious adverse reaction found in populations other than HIT patients. It occurred in patients with acute MI who were started on both lepirudin and thrombolytic therapy with alteplase or streptokinase. The overall frequency of this potentially life-threatening complication among patients receiving both lepirudin and thrombolytic therapy was 0.6% (7 out of 1134 patients). Although no intracranial bleeding was observed in 1168 subjects or patients who did not receive concomitant thrombolysis, there have been postmarketing reports of intracranial bleeding with lepirudin in the absence of concomitant thrombolytic therapy.

Allergic reactions: Allergic reactions or suspected allergic reactions in populations other than HIT patients include: Airway reactions (cough, bronchospasm, stridor, dyspnea [1% to less than 10%]); unspecified allergic reactions, skin reactions (pruritus, urticaria, rash, flushes, chills [0.1% to less than 1%]); general reactions (anaphylactoid or anaphylactic [0.1% to less than 1%]); and edema (facial/tongue/larynx edema, angioedema [0.01% to less than 0.1%]).

About 53% (n = 46) of all allergic reactions or suspected allergic reactions occurred in patients who concomitantly received thrombolytic therapy (eg, streptokinase) for acute MI and/or contrast media for coronary angiography.

Postmarketing adverse events – Serious anaphylactic reactions that have resulted in shock or death have been reported (see Warnings).

Intracranial bleeding has been reported in patients treated with lepirudin with or without concomitant thrombolytic therapy. Although no intracranial bleeding was observed in clinical trials in those patients who did not receive concomitant thrombolytic therapy, there have been postmarketing reports of intracranial bleeding in patients who received lepirudin without concomitant thrombolytic therapy.

Overdosage

➤*Symptoms:* In case of overdose (eg, suggested by excessively high aPTT values) the risk of bleeding is increased.

➤*Treatment:* No specific antidote for lepirudin is available. If life-threatening bleeding occurs and excessive plasma levels of lepirudin are suspected, take the following steps:
• Immediately stop lepirudin administration.
• Determine aPTT and other coagulation levels as appropriate.
• Determine hemoglobin and prepare for blood transfusion.
• Follow the guidelines for treating patients with shock. Individual case reports and in vitro data suggest that hemofiltration or hemodialysis (using high-flux dialysis membranes with a cutoff point of 50,000 daltons [eg, AN/69]) may be useful in this situation.

ARGATROBAN

Rx **Argatroban** (GlaxoSmithKline)   **Injection:** 100 mg/mL   750 mg D-sorbitol, 1000 mg dehydrated alcohol. In 2.5 mL single-use vials.

Indications

➤*Thrombosis, prophylaxis or treatment:* An anticoagulant for prophylaxis or treatment of thrombosis in heparin-induced thrombocytopenia (HIT).

➤*Percutaneous coronary intervention (PCI):* An anticoagulant in patients with or at risk for heparin-induced thrombocytopenia undergoing PCI.

Administration and Dosage

➤*Approved by the FDA:* June 30, 2000.

Argatroban, as supplied, is a concentrated drug (100 mg/mL) that must be diluted 100-fold prior to infusion. Do not mix with other drugs prior to dilution.

➤*Preparation for IV administration:* Dilute argatroban in 0.9% sodium chloride injection, 5% dextrose injection, or lactated Ringer's injection to a final concentration of 1 mg/mL. Dilute each 2.5 mL vial 100-fold by mixing with 250 mL of diluent. Use 250 mg (2.5 mL) per 250 mL of diluent or 500 mg (5 mL) per 500 mL of diluent. The constituted solution must be mixed by repeated inversion of the diluent bag for 1 minute. Upon preparation, the solution may show slight but brief haziness because of the formation of microprecipitates that rapidly dissolve upon mixing. The pH of the IV solution prepared as recommended is 3.2 to 7.5.

➤*HIT or heparin-induced thrombocytopenia and thrombosis syndrome (HITTS):*
Initial dosage – Before giving argatroban, discontinue heparin therapy and obtain a baseline activated partial thromboplastin time (aPTT). The recommended initial dose of argatroban for adults without hepatic impairment is 2 mcg/kg/min given as a continuous infusion (see table).

Standard Infusion Rates for 2 mcg/kg/min Dose of Argatroban (1 mg/mL Final Concentration)		
Body weight (kg)	Dose (mcg/min)	Infusion rate (mL/h)
50	100	6
60	120	7
70	140	8
80	160	10
90	180	11
100	200	12
110	220	13
120	240	14
130	260	16
140	280	17

Monitoring therapy – In general, therapy with argatroban is monitored using aPTT. Tests of anticoagulant effects (including aPTT) typically attain steady-state levels within 1 to 3 hours following initiation of argatroban. Dose adjustment may be required to attain the target aPTT. Check the aPTT 2 hours after initiation of therapy to confirm the patient has attained the desired therapeutic range.

Dosage adjustment – After the initial dose of argatroban, the dose can be adjusted as clinically indicated (not to exceed 10 mcg/kg/min), until the steady-state aPTT is 1.5 to 3 times the initial baseline value (not to exceed 100 seconds). Continue argatroban therapy until platelet counts have recovered substantially (ie, more than 100×10^9/L or to pre-HIT/-HITTS baseline value).

➤*PCI in HIT/HITTS patients:*
Initial dosage – Start an infusion of argatroban at 25 mcg/kg/min and a bolus of 350 mcg/kg administered via a large bore IV line over 3 to 5 minutes. Check activated clotting time (ACT) 5 to 10 minutes after the bolus dose is completed. Proceed with the procedure if the ACT is greater than 300 seconds.

Dosage adjustment – If the ACT is less than 300 seconds, administer an additional IV bolus dose of 150 mcg/kg, increase the infusion dose to 30 mcg/kg/min, and check the ACT 5 to 10 minutes later. If the ACT is greater than 450 seconds, decrease the infusion rate to 15 mcg/kg/min, and check the ACT 5 to 10 minutes later. Once a therapeutic ACT (between 300 and 450 seconds) has been achieved, continue this infusion dose for the duration of the procedure.

Recommended Doses and Infusion Rates of Argatroban for Patients Undergoing PCI								
Body weight (kg)	For ACT 300 to 450 seconds: Initial dosage[1] 25 mcg/kg/min			If ACT < 300 seconds: Dosage adjustment[2] 30 mcg/kg/min			If ACT > 450 seconds: Dosage adjustment 15 mcg/kg/min	
	Bolus dose (mcg)	Infusion dose (mcg/min)	Infusion rate (mL/hr)	Bolus dose (mcg)	Infusion dose (mcg/min)	Infusion rate (mL/hr)	Infusion dose (mcg/min)	Infusion rate (mL/hr)
50	17500	1250	75	7500	1500	90	750	45
60	21000	1500	90	9000	1800	108	900	54
70	24500	1750	105	10500	2100	126	1050	63
80	28000	2000	120	12000	2400	144	1200	72
90	31500	2250	135	13500	2700	162	1350	81
100	35000	2500	150	15000	3000	180	1500	90
110	38500	2750	165	16500	3300	198	1650	99
120	42000	3000	180	18000	3600	216	1800	108
130	45500	3250	195	19500	3900	234	1950	117
140	49000	3500	210	21000	4200	252	2100	126

[1] Administer initial IV bolus dose of 350 mcg/kg.
[2] Administer additional IV bolus dose of 150 mcg/kg if ACT is less than 300 seconds.

In case of dissection, impending abrupt closure, thrombus formation during the procedure, or inability to achieve or maintain an ACT over

ARGATROBAN

300 seconds, additional bolus doses of 150 mcg/kg may be administered and the infusion dose increased to 40 mcg/kg/min. Check the ACT after each additional bolus or change in the rate of infusion.

Monitoring therapy – Argatroban therapy is monitored using ACT. Obtain ACTs before dosing, 5 to 10 minutes after bolus dosing and after change in infusion rate, and at the end of the PCI procedure. Draw additional ACTs about every 20 to 30 minutes during a prolonged procedure.

Continued anticoagulation after PCI – If a patient requires anticoagulation after the procedure, argatroban may be continued at a lower infusion dose. If the patient has HIT or HITTS, continue argatroban therapy until platelet counts have recovered substantially (ie, more than 100×10^9/L or to pre-HIT/-HITTS baseline value).

➤*Hepatic function impairment:* For patients with moderate hepatic impairment, an initial dose of 0.5 mcg/kg/min is recommended, based on the approximate 4-fold decrease in argatroban clearance relative to those with normal hepatic function. Monitor the aPTT closely and adjust the dosage as clinically indicated (see Warnings).

➤*Conversion to oral anticoagulant therapy:*

Initiating oral anticoagulant therapy – Recognize the potential for combined effects on International Normalized Ratio (INR) with coadministration of argatroban and warfarin. Continue to monitor argatroban using aPTT. Initiate oral anticoagulation therapy (warfarin) only after substantial recovery of platelet counts (eg, more than 100×10^9/L or to pre-HIT/-HITTS baseline value). Do not use a loading dose of warfarin. Initiate therapy using the expected daily dose of warfarin. To avoid prothrombotic effects and to ensure continuous anticoagulation when initiating warfarin, it is recommended to overlap argatroban and warfarin therapy for 4 or 5 days (see warfarin prescribing information).

Coadministration of warfarin and argatroban at doses up to 2 mcg/kg/min – Use of argatroban with warfarin results in prolongation of INR beyond that produced by warfarin alone. To avoid prothrombotic effects and to ensure continuous anticoagulation when initiating warfarin, it is recommended to continue coadministration for at least 4 or 5 days before discontinuing argatroban. The previously established relationship between INR and bleeding risk is altered. The combination of argatroban and warfarin does not cause further reduction in the vitamin K-dependent factor Xa activity than that seen with warfarin alone. The relationship between INR obtained on combined therapy and INR obtained on warfarin alone is dependent on the dose of argatroban and the thromboplastin reagent used. The INR value on warfarin alone (INR$_w$) can be calculated from the INR value on combination argatroban and warfarin therapy. Please refer to manufacturers product labeling for calculations.

Measure INR daily while argatroban and warfarin are coadministered. In general, with doses of argatroban up to 2 mcg/kg/min, argatroban can be discontinued when the INR is greater than 4 on combined therapy. After argatroban is discontinued, repeat the INR measurement in 4 to 6 hours. If the repeat INR is below the desired therapeutic range, resume the infusion of argatroban and repeat the procedure daily until the desired therapeutic range on warfarin alone is reached.

Coadministration of warfarin and argatroban at doses greater than 2 mcg/kg/min – For doses greater than 2 mcg/kg/min, the relationship of INR on warfarin alone to the INR on warfarin plus argatroban is less predictable. In this case, in order to predict the INR on warfarin alone, temporarily reduce the dose of argatroban to a dose of 2 mcg/kg/min. Repeat the INR on argatroban and warfarin 4 to 6 hours after reduction of the argatroban dose and follow the process outlined above for administering argatroban at doses up to 2 mcg/kg/min.

➤*Storage/Stability:* Argatroban is a clear, colorless to pale yellow, slightly viscous solution. Discard the vial if the solution is cloudy, or if an insoluble precipitate is noted. Store the vials in original cartons at room temperature (25°C; 77°F), with excursions permitted to 15° to 30°C (59° to 86°F). Do not freeze. Retain in the original carton to protect from light.

Solutions prepared as recommended are stable at 25°C (77°F) with excursions permitted to 15° to 30°C (59° to 86°F) in ambient indoor light for 24 hours; therefore, light-resistant measures such as foil protection for IV lines are unnecessary. Solutions are physically and chemically stable for up to 48 hours when stored at 2° to 8°C (36° to 46°F) in the dark. Do not expose prepared solutions to direct sunlight. No significant potency losses have been noted following simulated delivery of the solution through IV tubing.

Actions

➤*Pharmacology:* Argatroban is a synthetic, direct thrombin inhibitor derived from L-arginine. It reversibly binds to the thrombin active site. Argatroban does not require the cofactor antithrombin III for antithrombotic activity. It exerts its anticoagulant effects by inhibiting thrombin-catalyzed or induced reactions, including fibrin formation; activation of coagulation factors V, VIII, and XIII; protein C; and platelet aggregation.

Argatroban is highly selective for thrombin with an inhibitory constant (K_i) of 0.04 mcM. At therapeutic concentrations, argatroban has little or no effect on related serine proteases (ie, trypsin, factor Xa, plasmin, kallikrein).

Argatroban can inhibit the action of free and clot-associated thrombin. Argatroban does not interact with heparin-induced antibodies. Evaluation also did not reveal antibody formation to argatroban.

➤*Pharmacokinetics:*

Distribution – Argatroban distributes mainly in the extracellular fluid; apparent steady-state volume of distribution is 174 mL/kg (12.18 L in a 70 kg adult). Argatroban is 54% bound to human serum proteins, with binding to albumin and α_1-acid glycoprotein 20% and 34%, respectively.

Metabolism – The main route of argatroban metabolism is hydroxylation and aromatization of the 3-methyltetrahydroquinoline ring in the liver. The formation of each of the 4 known metabolites is catalyzed in vitro by the human liver microsomal cytochrome P450 enzymes CYP3A4/5. The primary metabolite (M1) exerts 3- to 5-fold weaker anticoagulant effects than argatroban. Unchanged argatroban is the major component in plasma. The plasma concentrations of M1 range between 0% and 20% of the parent drug. The other metabolites (M2 to M4) are found only in very low quantities in the urine. Data suggest that CYP3A4/5 mediated metabolism is not an important elimination pathway in vivo.

There is no interconversion of the 21-(R):21-(S) diastereoisomers. The plasma ratio of these diastereoisomers is unchanged by metabolism or hepatic impairment, remaining constant at 65:35 ($\pm$ 2%).

Excretion – Total body clearance is approximately 5.1 mL/kg/min (0.31 L/kg/h) for infusion doses up to 40 mcg/kg/min. The terminal elimination half-life of argatroban ranges between 39 and 51 minutes.

Argatroban is excreted primarily in the feces, presumably through biliary secretion. Average percent recovery of unchanged drug, relative to total dose, was 16% in urine and at least 14% in feces.

Pharmacokinetic/Pharmacodynamic relationship – When given by continuous infusion, anticoagulant effects and plasma concentrations of argatroban follow similar, predictable temporal response profiles, with low intersubject variability. Immediately upon initiation of argatroban infusion, anticoagulant effects are produced as plasma argatroban concentrations begin to rise. Steady-state levels of drug and anticoagulant effect typically are attained within 1 to 3 hours and are maintained until the infusion is discontinued or the dosage adjusted. Steady-state plasma argatroban concentrations increase proportionally with dose (for infusion doses up to 40 mcg/kg/min in healthy subjects) and are well correlated with steady-state anticoagulant effects. For infusion doses up to 40 mcg/kg/min, argatroban increases in a dose-dependent fashion in the aPTT, ACT, prothrombin time (PT) and INR, and the thrombin time (TT) in healthy volunteers and cardiac patients.

Effect on INR – Because argatroban is a direct thrombin inhibitor, coadministration of argatroban and warfarin produces a combined effect on the laboratory measurement of the INR. However, cotherapy compared with warfarin monotherapy exerts no additional effect on vitamin K dependent factor Xa activity.

The relationship between INR on cotherapy and warfarin alone is dependent on the dose of argatroban and the thromboplastin reagent used. This relationship is influenced by the International Sensitivity Index (ISI) of the thromboplastin. Thromboplastins with higher ISI values result in higher INRs on combined therapy of warfarin and argatroban.

Special populations –

Hepatic impairment: Decrease the dosage of argatroban in patients with hepatic impairment (see Administration and Dosage). Patients with hepatic impairment were not studied in PCI trials. Hepatic impairment is associated with decreased clearance and increased elimination half-life of argatroban (to 1.9 mL/kg/min and 181 minutes, respectively, for patients with a Child-Pugh score greater than 6).

Contraindications

Overt major bleeding; hypersensitivity to this product or any of its components (see Warnings).

Warnings

➤*IV Administration:* Argatroban is intended for IV administration. Discontinue all parenteral anticoagulants before administration of argatroban.

➤*Hemorrhage:* Hemorrhage can occur at any site in the body in patients receiving argatroban. Consider a hemorrhagic event if an unexplained fall in hematocrit or blood pressure, or any other unexplained symptom occurs. Use argatroban with extreme caution in disease states and other circumstances in which there is an increased danger of hemorrhage. These include severe hypertension; immediately following lumbar puncture; spinal anesthesia; major surgery, especially involving the brain, spinal cord, or eye; hematologic conditions associated with increased bleeding tendencies, such as congenital or acquired bleeding disorders, and GI lesions, such as ulcerations.

ARGATROBAN

►*Hepatic function impairment:* Exercise caution when administering argatroban to patients with hepatic disease by starting with a lower dose and carefully titrating until the desired level of anticoagulation is achieved. Also, upon cessation of argatroban infusion in the hepatically impaired patient, full reversal of anticoagulant effects may require longer than 4 hours because of decreased clearance and increased elimination half-life of argatroban (see Administration and Dosage).

Avoid use of high doses of argatroban in PCI patients with clinically significant hepatic disease or AST/ALT levels at least 3 times the upper limit of normal. Such patients were not studied in PCI trials.

►*Pregnancy:* Category B. There are no adequate and well-controlled studies in pregnant women. Use during pregnancy only if clearly needed.

►*Lactation:* Experiments in rats show that argatroban is detected in milk. It is not known whether this drug is excreted in human milk. Because many drugs are excreted in human milk and because of the potential for serious adverse reactions in nursing infants from argatroban, decide whether to discontinue nursing or to discontinue the drug, taking into account the importance of the drug to the mother.

►*Children:* The safety and efficacy of argatroban in patients below 18 years of age have not been established.

Precautions

►*Lab test abnormalities:* Anticoagulation effects associated with argatroban infusion at doses up to 40 mcg/kg/min correlate with increases in the aPTT. Although other global clot-based tests including PT, the INR, and TT are affected by argatroban, the therapeutic ranges for these tests have not been identified for argatroban therapy. Plasma argatroban concentrations also correlate well with anticoagulant effects.

In clinical trials in PCI, the ACT was used for monitoring argatroban anticoagulant activity during the procedure.

The concomitant use of argatroban and warfarin results in prolongation of the PT and INR beyond that produced by warfarin alone. Alternative approaches for monitoring concurrent argatroban and warfarin therapy are described in Administration and Dosage.

Drug Interactions

►*Heparin:* Because heparin is contraindicated in patients with HIT, the coadministration of argatroban and heparin is unlikely for this indication. However, if argatroban is initiated after cessation of heparin therapy, allow sufficient time for heparin's effect on the aPTT to decrease prior to argatroban therapy.

►*Oral anticoagulant agents:* Pharmacokinetic drug-drug interactions between argatroban and warfarin (7.5 mg single oral dose) have not been demonstrated. However, the concomitant use of argatroban and warfarin (5 to 7.5 mg initial oral dose followed by 2.5 to 6 mg/day orally for 6 to 10 days) results in prolongation of the PT and INR.

►*Other drugs affecting coagulation:* Coadministration of argatroban with antiplatelet agents, thrombolytics, and other anticoagulants may increase the risk of bleeding.

Adverse Reactions

►*HIT/HITTS patients:* The following safety information is based on 568 patients treated with argatroban. The safety profile of the patients from these studies is compared with that of 193 historical controls in which the adverse events were collected retrospectively. The adverse events reported in this section include all events regardless of relationship to treatment. Adverse events are separated into hemorrhagic and nonhemorrhagic events.

Major bleeding was defined as bleeding that was overt and associated with a hemoglobin decrease of at least 2 g/dL, that led to a transfusion of at least 2 units, or that was intracranial, retroperitoneal, or into a major prosthetic joint. Minor bleeding was overt bleeding that did not meet the criteria for major bleeding.

The following table gives an overview of the most frequently observed hemorrhagic events.

Hemorrhagic Adverse Reactions in Argatroban-Treated HIT/HITTS Patients (%)[1]		
Adverse reactions	Argatroban-treated patients (n = 568)	Control (n = 193)
Major hemorrhagic events		
Overall bleeding	5.3	6.7
GI	2.3	1.6
GU and hematuria	0.9	0.5
Decreased hemoglobin/ hematocrit	0.7	0
Multisystem hemorrhage and disseminated intravascular coagulation	0.5	1

Hemorrhagic Adverse Reactions in Argatroban-Treated HIT/HITTS Patients (%)[1]		
Adverse reactions	Argatroban-treated patients (n = 568)	Control (n = 193)
Limb and below-the-knee amputation stump	0.5	0
Intracranial hemorrhage	0[2]	0.5
Minor hemorrhagic events		
GI	14.4	18.1
GU and hematuria	11.6	0.8
Decreased hemoglobin/ hematocrit	10.4	0
Groin	5.4	3.1
Hemoptysis	2.9	0.8
Brachial	2.4	0.8

[1] Patients may have experienced more than 1 event.
[2] One patient experienced intracranial hemorrhage 4 days after discontinuation of argatroban and following therapy with urokinase and oral anticoagulation.

The following table is an overview of the most frequently observed nonhemorrhagic events.

Nonhemorrhagic Adverse Reactions in Argatroban-Treated HIT/HITTS Patients (≥ 2%)[1]		
Adverse reactions	Argatroban-treated patients (n = 568)	Control (n = 193)
Cardiovascular		
Atrial fibrillation	3	11.4
Cardiac arrest	5.8	3.1
Hypotension	7.2	2.6
Ventricular tachycardia	4.8	3.1
GI		
Abdominal pain	2.6	1.6
Diarrhea	6.2	1.6
Nausea	4.8	0.5
Vomiting	4.2	0
Respiratory		
Coughing	2.8	1.6
Dyspnea	8.1	8.8
Pneumonia	3.3	9.3
Miscellaneous		
Abnormal renal function	2.8	4.7
Cerebrovascular disorder	2.3	4.1
Fever	6.9	2.1
Infection	3.7	3.6
Pain	4.6	3.1
Sepsis	6	12.4
Urinary tract infection	4.6	5.2

[1] Patients may have experienced more than 1 event.

►*HIT/HITTS patients undergoing PCI:* The following safety information is based on 91 patients initially treated with argatroban and 21 patients subsequently re-exposed to argatroban for a total of 112 PCIs with argatroban anticoagulation. The adverse events reported in this section include all events regardless of relationship to treatment. Adverse events are separated into hemorrhagic and nonhemorrhagic events.

Major bleeding was defined as bleeding that was overt and associated with a hemoglobin decrease of at least 5 g/dL, that led to a transfusion of at least 2 units, or that was intracranial, retroperitoneal, or into a major prosthetic joint.

The rate of major bleeding events and intracranial hemorrhage in the PCI trials was 1.8% and in the placebo arm of the EPILOG (Evaluation in PTCA to Improve Long-Term Outcome with Abciximab GP IIb/IIIa blockade) study trial (placebo plus standard dose, weight-adjusted heparin) was 3.1%.

Hemorrhagic Adverse Reactions in Argatroban-Treated HIT/HITTS Patients Undergoing PCI (%)[1]	
Adverse reactions	Argatroban-treated patients (n = 112)[2]
Major hemorrhagic events	
Retroperitoneal	0.9
GI	0.9
Intracranial hemorrhage	0

ARGATROBAN

Hemorrhagic Adverse Reactions in Argatroban-Treated HIT/HITTS Patients Undergoing PCI (%)[1]	
Adverse reactions	Argatroban-treated patients (n = 112)[2]
Minor hemorrhagic events	
Groin (bleeding or hematoma)	3.6
GI (includes hematemesis)	2.6
GU (includes hematuria)	1.8
Decreased hemoglobin/hematocrit	1.8
Coronary artery bypass graft (coronary arteries)	1.8
Access site	0.9
Hemoptysis	0.9
Other	0.9

[1] Patients may have experienced more than 1 event.
[2] Ninety one patients who underwent 112 interventions.

The following table provides an overview of the most frequently observed nonhemorrhagic events (greater than 2%).

Nonhemorrhagic Adverse Reactions in Argatroban-Treated HIT/HITTS Patients Undergoing PCI (> 2%)[1]		
Adverse reactions	Argatroban procedures (n = 112)[2]	Control (n = 2226)[3]
Cardiovascular		
Bradycardia	4.5	3.5
Chest pain	15.2	9.3
Hypotension	10.7	10.3
MI	3.6	Not reported
GI		
Abdominal pain	3.6	2.2
Nausea	7.1	11.5
Vomiting	6.3	6.8
Miscellaneous		
Back pain	8	13.7
Fever	3.6	< 0.5
Headache	5.4	5.5

[1] Patients may have experienced more than 1 adverse event.
[2] Ninety one patients who underwent 112 interventions.
[3] Controls from EPIC (Evaluation of c7E3 Fab in the Prevention of Ischemic Complications), EPILOG and CAPTURE (Chimeric 7E3 Antiplatelet Therapy in Unstable angina Refractory to standard treatment) trials.

There were 22 serious adverse events in 17 PCI patients (19.6% in 112 interventions). The types of events, which are listed regardless of relationship to treatment, are shown in the following table.

Serious Adverse Reactions in HIT/HITTS Patients Undergoing PCI[1] (%)	
Adverse reaction	Argatroban procedures (n = 112)[2]
Cardiovascular	
Angina pectoris	1.8
Aortic stenosis	0.9
Arterial thrombosis	0.9
Chest pain	0.9
Coronary thrombosis	1.8
MI	3.5
Myocardial ischemia	1.8
Occlusion coronary	1.8
Vascular disorder	0.9

Serious Adverse Reactions in HIT/HITTS Patients Undergoing PCI[1] (%)	
Adverse reaction	Argatroban procedures (n = 112)[2]
GI	
GI disorder (GERD)	0.9
GI hemorrhage	0.9
Miscellaneous	
Cerebrovascular disorder	0.9
Fever	0.9
Lung edema	0.9
Retroperitoneal hemorrhage	0.9

[1] Individual events also may have been reported elsewhere (see preceding 2 tables).
[2] Ninety one patients underwent 112 procedures. Some patients may have experienced more than 1 event.

➤*Other populations:* The following safety information is based on a total of 1127 individuals who were treated with argatroban in clinical pharmacology studies (n = 211) or for other clinical indications (n = 916).

Intracranial bleeding: Intracranial bleeding only occurred in patients with acute MI who were started on argatroban and thrombolytic therapy with streptokinase. The overall frequency of this potentially life-threatening complication among patients receiving argatroban and thrombolytic therapy (streptokinase or tissue plasminogen activator) was 1% (8 out of 810 patients). Intracranial bleeding was not observed in 317 subjects or patients who did not receive concomitant thrombolysis.

Intracranial bleeding was also observed in a prospective, placebo-controlled study of argatroban in patients who had onset of acute stroke within 12 hours of study entry. Symptomatic intracranial hemorrhage was reported in 5 of 117 patients (4.3%) who received argatroban and in none of the 54 placebo patients. Asymptomatic intracranial hemorrhage occurred in 5 (4.3%) and 2 (3.7%) of the patients, respectively.

Allergic reactions: In 1127 argatroban-treated individuals, 156 allergic reactions or suspected allergic reactions were observed in clinical pharmacology studies or for other clinical indications. About 95% of these reactions occurred in patients who concomitantly received thrombolytic therapy (eg, streptokinase) for acute MI or contrast media for coronary angiography.

Allergic reactions or suspected allergic reactions include the following: Airway reactions (coughing, dyspnea [10% or more]); skin reactions (rash, bullous eruption [1% to less than 10%]); general reactions (vasodilation [1% to 10%]). The Council for International Organization of Medical Sciences III standard categories were used for classification of frequencies.

Overdosage

➤*Symptoms:* Single IV doses of argatroban at 200, 124, 150, and 200 mg/kg were lethal to mice, rats, rabbits, and dogs, respectively. The symptoms of acute toxicity were loss of righting reflex, tremors, clonic convulsions, paralysis of hind limbs, and coma.

➤*Treatment:* Excessive anticoagulation with or without bleeding may be controlled by discontinuing argatroban or by decreasing the argatroban infusion dosage (see Warnings). In clinical studies at therapeutic levels, anticoagulation parameters generally return to baseline within 2 to 4 hours after discontinuation of the drug. Reversal of anticoagulant effect may take longer in patients with hepatic impairment.

No specific antidote to argatroban is available. If life-threatening bleeding occurs and excessive plasma levels of argatroban are suspected, discontinue argatroban immediately and determine aPTT and other coagulation tests. Provide symptomatic and supportive therapy to the patient (see Warnings).

Patient Information

Inform patient the importance of reporting any signs of bleeding (eg, bruising, petechiae, hematuria) immediately to the physician.

Notify physician immediately if planning to become pregnant or are breastfeeding.

BIVALIRUDIN

Rx **Angiomax** (Medicines Company) **Powder for injection, lyophilized:** 250 mg In single-use vials.

Indications

➤*Unstable angina:* For use as an anticoagulant in patients with unstable angina undergoing percutaneous transluminal coronary angioplasty (PTCA). Bivalirudin is intended for use with aspirin and has been studied only in patients receiving concomitant aspirin.

The safety and efficacy of bivalirudin have not been established when used in conjunction with platelet inhibitors other than aspirin, such as glycoprotein IIb/IIIa inhibitors.

The safety and efficacy of bivalirudin have not been established in patients with unstable angina who are not undergoing PTCA or in patients with other acute coronary symptoms.

Administration and Dosage

➤*Approved by the FDA:* December 15, 2000.

➤*Dosage:* Recommended dosage is an IV bolus of 1 mg/kg followed by a 4-hour IV infusion at a rate of 2.5 mg/kg/h. After completion of the initial 4-hour infusion, an additional IV infusion may be initiated at a rate of 0.2 mg/kg/h for up to 20 hours, if needed. Bivalirudin is intended for use with aspirin (300 to 325 mg/day) and has been studied only in patients receiving concomitant aspirin. Initiate treatment with bivalirudin just prior to PTCA. The dose may need to be reduced, and anticoagulation status monitored, in patients with renal impairment.

➤*Administration:* Bivalirudin is intended for IV injection and infusion. To each 250 mg vial, add 5 mL of sterile water for injection. Gently swirl until all material is dissolved. Further dilute each reconstituted vial in 50 mL of 5% dextrose in water or 0.9% sodium chloride for injection to yield a final concentration of 5 mg/mL (eg, 1 vial in 50 mL, 2 vials in 100 mL, 5 vials in 250 mL). The dose to be administered is adjusted according to the patient's weight (see table below).

If the low-rate infusion is used after the initial infusion, prepare a lower concentration bag. In order to prepare this bag, reconstitute the 250 mg vial with 5 mL sterile water for injection. Gently swirl until all material is dissolved. Further dilute each reconstituted vial in 500 mL of 5% dextrose in water or 0.9% sodium chloride for injection to yield a final concentration of 0.5 mg/mL. Select the infusion rate to be administered from the right-hand column of the table below.

	Bivalirudin Dosing Table		
	Using 5 mg/mL concentration		Using 0.5 mg/mL concentration
Weight (kg)	Bolus (1 mg/kg) (mL)	Initial 4-hour infusion (2.5 mg/kg/h) (mL/h)	Subsequent low-rate infusion (0.2 mg/kg/h) (mL/h)
43 to 47	9	22.5	18
48 to 52	10	25	20
53 to 57	11	27.5	22
58 to 62	12	30	24
63 to 67	13	32.5	26
68 to 72	14	35	28
73 to 77	15	37.5	30
78 to 82	16	40	32
83 to 87	17	42.5	34
88 to 92	18	45	36
93 to 97	19	47.5	38
98 to 102	20	50	40
103 to 107	21	52.5	42
108 to 112	22	55	44
113 to 117	23	57.5	46
118 to 122	24	60	48
123 to 127	25	62.5	50
128 to 132	26	65	52
133 to 137	27	67.5	54
138 to 142	28	70	56
143 to 147	29	72.5	58
148 to 152	30	75	60

Compatabilities – No incompatibilities have been observed with glass bottles or polyvinyl chloride bags and administration sets.

Incompatabilities – Nine drugs resulted in haze formation, microparticulate formation, or gross precipitation and should not be administered in the same IV line with bivalirudin. These 9 incompatible drugs are as follows: Alteplase, amiodarone HCl, amphotericin B, chlorpromazine HCl, diazepam, prochlorperazine edisylate, reteplase, streptokinase, and vancomycin HCl.

➤*Renal function impairment:*

Bivalirudin Pharmacokinetic Parameters and Dose Adjustments in Renal Impairment			
Renal function (GFR, mL/min)	Clearance (mL/min/kg)	Half-life (minutes)	Percent reduction in infusion dose
Normal renal function (≥ 90 mL/min)	3.4	25	0
Mild renal impairment (60 to 89 mL/min)	3.4	22	0
Moderate renal impairment (30 to 59 mL/min)	2.7	34	20
Severe renal impairment (10 to 29 mL/min)	2.8	57	60
Dialysis-dependent patients (off dialysis)	1	3.5 hours	90

➤*Storage/Stability:* Store bivalirudin dosage units at 20° to 25°C (68° to 77°F). Excursions to 15° to 30°C (59° to 86°F) permitted.

Do not freeze reconstituted or diluted bivalirudin. Reconstituted material may be stored at 2° to 8°C (36° to 47°F) for up to 24 hours. Diluted bivalirudin with a concentration of between 0.5 and 5 mg/mL is stable at room temperature for up to 24 hours. Discard any unused portion of reconstituted solution remaining in the vial.

Actions

➤*Pharmacology:* Bivalirudin directly inhibits thrombin by specifically binding to the catalytic site and to the anion-binding exosite of circulating and clot-bound thrombin. Thrombin is a serine proteinase that plays a central role in the thrombotic process, acting to cleave fibrinogen into fibrin monomers and to activate factor XIII to factor XIIIa, allowing fibrin to develop a covalently cross-linked framework that stabilizes the thrombus; thrombin also activates factors V and VIII, promoting further thrombin generation, and activates platelets, stimulating aggregation and granule release. The binding of bivalirudin to thrombin is reversible as thrombin slowly cleaves the bivalirudin-Arg_3-Pro_4 bond, resulting in recovery of thrombin active site functions.

In in vitro studies, bivalirudin inhibited soluble (free) and clot-bound thrombin, was not neutralized by products of the platelet-release reaction, and prolonged the activated partial thromboplastin time (aPTT), thrombin time (TT), and prothrombin time (PT) of normal human plasma in a concentration-dependent manner. The clinical relevance of these findings is unknown.

➤*Pharmacokinetics:* Bivalirudin exhibits linear pharmacokinetics following IV administration to patients undergoing PTCA. In these patients, a mean steady-state bivalirudin concentration of about 12.3 mcg/mL is achieved following an IV bolus of 1 mg/kg and a 4-hour 2.5 mg/kg/h IV infusion. Bivalirudin is cleared from plasma by a combination of renal mechanisms and proteolytic cleavage, with a half-life in patients with normal renal function of 25 minutes. Drug elimination is related to glomular filtration rate (GFR). Total body clearance is similar for patients with normal renal function and with mild renal impairment (60 to 89 mL/min). Clearance is reduced approximately 20% in patients with moderate and severe renal impairment and reduced approximately 80% in dialysis-dependent patients. For patients with renal impairment, monitor the activated clotting time (ACT). Bivalirudin is hemodialyzable. Approximately 25% is cleared by hemodialysis.

Bivalirudin does not bind to plasma proteins (other than thrombin) or to red blood cells.

➤*Clinical trials:* Bivalirudin was evaluated in patients with unstable angina undergoing PTCA in 2 randomized, double-blind, multicenter studies with identical protocols.

The studies were designed to demonstrate the safety and efficacy of bivalirudin in patients undergoing PTCA as a treatment for unstable angina compared with a control group of similar patients receiving heparin during and up to 24 hours after initiation of PTCA. The primary protocol endpoint was a composite endpoint called procedural failure that included clinical and angiographic elements measured during hospitalization. The clinical elements were the occurrence of death, MI, or urgent revascularization, adjudicated under double-blind conditions. The angiographic elements were impending or abrupt vessel closure. The protocol-specified safety endpoint was major hemorrhage.

BIVALIRUDIN

The median duration of hospitalization was 4 days for the bivalirudin and heparin treatment groups. The rates of procedural failure were similar in the 2 groups. Study outcomes are shown in the table below.

Incidences of In-Hospital Clinical Endpoints in Randomized Clinical Trials Occurring within 7 Days (%)		
All patients	Bivalirudin (n = 2161)	Heparin (n = 2151)
Efficacy endpoints		
Procedural failure[1]	7.9	9.3
Death, MI, revascularization	6.2	7.9
Death	0.2	0.2
MI[2]	3.3	4.2
Revascularization[3]	4.2	5.6
Safety endpoint		
Major hemorrhage[4]	3.5	9.3

[1] The protocol specified primary endpoint (a composite of death or MI or clinical deterioration of cardiac origin requiring revascularization or placement of an aortic balloon pump or angiographic evidence of abrupt vessel closure).
[2] Defined as Q-wave MI; creatine kinase-MB (CK-MB) elevation 2 × ULN or greater, new ST- or T-wave abnormality, and chest pain 30 minutes or greater; or new left bundle branch block (LBBB) with chest pain 30 minutes or greater and/or elevated CK-MB enzymes; or elevated CK-MB and new ST- or T-wave abnormality without chest pain; or elevated CK-MB.
[3] Defined as any revascularization procedure, including angioplasty, coronary artery bypass graft (CABG), stenting, or placement of an intra-aortic balloon pump.
[4] Defined as the occurrence of any of the following: Intracranial bleeding, retroperitoneal bleeding, clinically overt bleeding with a decrease in hemoglobin 3 g/dL or greater or leading to a transfusion of 2 units or greater of blood.

Contraindications

Active major bleeding; hypersensitivity to bivalirudin or any of its components.

Warnings

➤*Immunogenicity / Re-exposure:* Among 494 subjects who received bivalirudin in clinical trials and were tested for antibodies, 2 subjects had treatment-emergent positive bivalirudin antibody tests. Neither subject demonstrated clinical evidence of allergic or anaphylactic reactions and repeat testing was not performed. Nine additional patients who had initial positive tests were negative on repeat testing.

➤*Elderly:* Of the total number of patients in clinical studies of bivalirudin undergoing PTCA, 41% were 65 years of age or greater, while 11% were greater than 75 years of age. A difference of 5% or greater between age groups was observed for heparin-treated but not bivalirudin-treated patients with regard to the percentage of patients with major bleeding events. There were no individual bleeding events that were observed with a difference of 5% or greater between treatment groups, although puncture site hemorrhage and catheterization site hematoma were each observed in a higher percentage of patients 65 years of age or greater than in patients less than 65 years of age. This difference between age groups was more pronounced for heparin-treated than bivalirudin-treated patients.

➤*Pregnancy: Category B.* There are no adequate and well-controlled studies in pregnant women. Bivalirudin is intended for use with aspirin (see Indications). Because of possible adverse effects on the neonate and the potential for increased maternal bleeding, particularly during the third trimester, bivalirudin and aspirin should be used together during pregnancy only if clearly needed.

➤*Lactation:* It is not known whether bivalirudin is excreted in breast milk. Because many drugs are excreted in breast milk, exercise caution when bivalirudin is administered to a nursing woman.

➤*Children:* The safety and efficacy of bivalirudin in pediatric patients have not been established.

Precautions

➤*Monitoring:* Bivalirudin is not intended for IM administration. Although most bleeding associated with the use of bivalirudin in PTCA occurs at the site of arterial puncture, hemorrhage can occur at any site. An unexplained fall in blood pressure or hematocrit, or any unexplained symptom, should lead to serious consideration of a hemorrhagic event and cessation of bivalirudin administration.

➤*Special risk:* Clinical trials have provided limited information for use of bivalirudin in patients with heparin-induced thrombocytopenia/heparin-induced thrombocytopenia-thrombosis syndrome (HIT/HITTS) undergoing PTCA. The number of HIT/HITTS patients treated is inadequate to reliably assess efficacy and safety in these patients undergoing PTCA. Bivalirudin was administered to a small number of patients with a history of HIT/HITTS or active HIT/HITTS and undergoing PTCA in an uncontrolled, open-label study and in an emergency treatment program and appeared to provide adequate anticoagulation in these patients. In in vitro studies, bivalirudin exhibited no platelet aggregation response against sera from patients with a history of HIT/HITTS.

Drug Interactions

Bivalirudin does not exhibit binding to plasma proteins (other than thrombin) or red blood cells.

Drug interaction studies have been conducted with the adenosine diphosphate (ADP) antagonist ticlopidine and the glycoprotein IIb/IIIa inhibitor abciximab and with low molecular weight heparin. Although data are limited, precluding conclusions regarding efficacy and safety in combination with these agents, the results do not suggest pharmacodynamic interactions. In patients treated with low molecular weight heparin, low molecular weight heparin was discontinued at least 8 hours prior to the procedure and administration of bivalirudin.

The safety and efficacy of bivalirudin have not been established when used in conjunction with platelet inhibitors other than aspirin, such as glycoprotein IIb/IIIa inhibitors.

In clinical trials in patients undergoing PTCA, coadministration of bivalirudin with heparin, warfarin, or thrombolytics was associated with increased risks of major bleeding events compared with patients not receiving these concomitant medications. There is no experience with coadministration of bivalirudin and plasma expanders such as dextran. Use bivalirudin with caution in patients with disease states associated with an increased risk of bleeding.

Adverse Reactions

➤*Bleeding:* In 4312 patients undergoing PTCA for treatment of unstable angina in 2 randomized, double-blind studies comparing bivalirudin to heparin, bivalirudin patients exhibited lower rates of major bleeding and lower requirements for blood transfusions. The incidence of major bleeding is presented in the following table. The incidence of major bleeding was lower in the bivalirudin group than in the heparin group.

Major Bleeding and Transfusions: All Patients[1] (%)		
	Bivalirudin (n = 2161)	Heparin (n = 2151)
Patients with major hemorrhage[2]	3.7	9.3
With ≥ 3 g/dL fall in Hgb	1.9	5.8
With ≥ 5 g/dL fall in Hgb	< 1	2.2
Retroperitoneal bleeding	< 1	< 1
Intracranial bleeding	< 1	< 1
Required transfusion	2	5.7

[1] No monitoring of ACT (or PTT) was done after a target ACT was achieved.
[2] Major hemorrhage was defined as the occurrence of any of the following: Intracranial bleeding, retroperitoneal bleeding, clinically overt bleeding with a decrease in hemoglobin 3 g/dL or greater or leading to a transfusion of 2 units of blood or greater. This table includes data from the entire hospitalization period.

➤*Other adverse events:* In 2 randomized double-blind clinical trials of bivalirudin in patients undergoing PTCA, 82% of 2161 bivalirudin-treated patients and 83% of 2151 heparin-treated patients experienced 1 or more treatment-emergent adverse event. The most frequent treatment-emergent events were back pain (42%); pain, nausea (15%); headache, hypotension (12%) in the bivalirudin-treated group. Treatment-emergent adverse events other than bleeding reported for 5% or greater of patients in either treatment group are shown in the following table.

Adverse Events Other Than Bleeding Occurring in ≥ 5% of Patients in Either Treatment Group in Randomized Clinical Trials		
	Treatment group	
Adverse reaction	Bivalirudin (n = 2161)	Heparin (n = 2151)
Cardiovascular		
Hypotension	12	17
Hypertension	6	5
Bradycardia	5	8
CNS		
Headache	12	10
Insomnia	7	6
Anxiety	6	7
Nervousness	5	4
GI		
Nausea	15	16
Vomiting	6	8
Abdominal pain	5	5
Dyspepsia	5	5
Miscellaneous		
Back pain	42	44
Pain	15	17
Injection site pain	8	13
Pelvic pain	6	8
Fever	5	5
Urinary retention	4	5

BIVALIRUDIN

Serious, nonbleeding adverse events were experienced in 2% of 2161 bivalirudin-treated patients and 2% of 2151 heparin-treated patients. The following individual serious nonbleeding adverse events were rare (greater than 0.1% to less than 1%) and similar in incidence between bivalirudin and heparin-treated patients.

Cardiovascular – Hypotension; syncope; vascular anomaly; ventricular fibrillation.

CNS – Cerebral ischemia; confusion; facial paralysis.

GU – Kidney failure; oliguria.

Miscellaneous – Lung edema; fever; infection; sepsis.

Overdosage

Discontinuation of bivalirudin leads to a gradual reduction in anticoagulant effect because of drug metabolism. There has been no experience of overdosage in human clinical trials.

➤*Treatment:* In case of overdosage, discontinue bivalirudin and closely monitor the patient for signs of bleeding. There is no known antidote for bivalirudin. Bivalirudin is hemodialyzable.

FONDAPARINUX SODIUM

Rx	**Arixtra** (Organon/Sanofi-Synthelabo)	**Injection:** 2.5 mg	In 0.5 mL single-dose prefilled syringes with needle. In 10s.

WARNING

Spinal/Epidural hematomas: When neuraxial anesthesia (epidural/spinal anesthesia) or spinal puncture is employed, patients anticoagulated or scheduled to be anticoagulated with low molecular weight heparins (LMWHs), heparinoids, or fondaparinux for prevention of thromboembolic complications are at risk of developing an epidural or spinal hematoma that can result in long-term or permanent paralysis.

The risk of these events is increased by the use of indwelling epidural catheters for administration of analgesia or by the concomitant use of drugs affecting hemostasis, such as nonsteroidal anti-inflammatory drugs (NSAIDs), platelet inhibitors, or other anticoagulants. The risk also appears to be increased by traumatic or repeated epidural or spinal puncture.

Frequently monitor patients for signs and symptoms of neurological impairment. If neurologic compromise is noted, urgent treatment is necessary.

Consider the potential benefit vs risk before neuraxial intervention in patients anticoagulated or to be anticoagulated for thromboprophylaxis (see Warnings, Precautions).

Indications

➤*Prophylaxis of deep vein thrombosis:* For the prophylaxis of deep vein thrombosis, which may lead to pulmonary embolism in patients undergoing the following:
• Hip fracture surgery;
• hip replacement surgery; or
• knee replacement surgery.

Administration and Dosage

➤*Approved by the FDA:* December 10, 2001.

➤*Administration:* Administer by SC injection. Fondaparinux must not be administered by IM injection.

➤*Dosage:* In patients undergoing hip fracture surgery, hip replacement surgery, or knee replacement surgery, the recommended dose of fondaparinux is 2.5 mg administered by SC injection once daily. After hemostasis has been established, give the initial dose 6 to 8 hours after surgery. Administration before 6 hours after surgery has been associated with an increased risk of major bleeding. The usual duration of administration is 5 to 9 days, and up to 11 days of administration has been tolerated.

➤*Admixture incompatibilities:* Do not mix fondaparinux with other injections or infusions.

➤*Storage/Stability:* Store at 25°C (77°F); excursions permitted to 15° to 30°C (59° to 86°F).

Actions

➤*Pharmacology:* The antithrombotic activity of fondaparinux is the result of antithrombin III (ATIII)-mediated selective inhibition of Factor Xa. By selectively binding to ATIII, fondaparinux potentiates (about 300 times) the innate neutralization of Factor Xa by ATIII. Neutralization of Factor Xa interrupts the blood coagulation cascade and thus inhibits thrombin formation and thrombus development.

Fondaparinux does not inactivate thrombin (activated Factor II) and has no known effect on platelet function. At the recommended dose, fondaparinux does not affect fibrinolytic activity or bleeding time.

➤*Pharmacokinetics:*

Absorption – Fondaparinux administered by SC injection is rapidly and completely absorbed (absolute bioavailability is 100%). Following a single SC dose of 2.5 mg fondaparinux in young male subjects, C_{max} of 0.34 mg/L is reached in approximately 2 hours. In patients undergoing treatment with 2.5 mg fondaparinux injection once daily, the peak steady-state plasma concentration is, on average, 0.39 to 0.5 mg/L and is reached approximately 3 hours postdose. In these patients, the minimum steady-state plasma concentration is 0.14 to 0.19 mg/L.

Distribution – In healthy adults, fondaparinux administered IV or SC distributes mainly in blood and only to a minor extent in extravascular fluid as evidenced by steady-state and non-steady-state apparent volume of distribution of 7 to 11 L. Similar fondaparinux distribution occurs in patients undergoing elective hip surgery or hip fracture surgery. In vitro, fondaparinux is highly (at least 94%) and specifically bound to ATIII and does not bind significantly to other plasma proteins (including platelet Factor 4 [PF4]) or red blood cells.

Metabolism/Excretion – In vivo metabolism of fondaparinux has not been investigated because the majority of the administered dose is eliminated unchanged in urine in individuals with normal kidney function. In healthy individuals up to 75 years of age, up to 77% of a single SC or IV fondaparinux dose is eliminated in urine as unchanged drug in 72 hours. The elimination half-life is 17 to 21 hours.

Special populations –

Renal function impairment: Fondaparinux elimination is prolonged in patients with renal impairment because the major route of elimination is urinary excretion of unchanged drug. In patients undergoing elective hip surgery or hip fracture surgery, the total clearance of fondaparinux is approximately 25% lower in patients with mild renal impairment (Ccr 50 to 80 mL/min), approximately 40% lower in patients with moderate renal impairment (Ccr 30 to 50 mL/min), and approximately 55% lower in patients with severe renal impairment (Ccr less than 30 mL/min) compared with patients with normal renal function.

Elderly: Fondaparinux elimination is prolonged in patients over 75 years of age. In studies evaluating 2.5 mg fondaparinux in hip fracture surgery or elective hip surgery, the total clearance of fondaparinux was approximately 25% lower in patients over 75 years of age as compared with patients less than 65 years of age.

Patients weighing less than 50 kg: Total clearance of fondaparinux is decreased by approximately 30% in patients weighing less than 50 kg.

➤*Clinical trials:* In 2 randomized, double-blind clinical trials in patients undergoing hip replacement surgery, 2.5 mg fondaparinux SC once daily was compared with 30 mg enoxaparin SC every 12 hours (Study 1) or to 40 mg enoxaparin SC once daily (Study 2). For both studies, both study treatments were continued for approximately 7 days. The efficacy data are provided in the following table.

Efficacy of Fondaparinux Injection in the Prophylaxis of Thromboembolic Events Following Hip Replacement Surgery				
	Study 1		Study 2	
Endpoint	Fondaparinux 2.5 mg SC once daily[1]	Enoxaparin 30 mg SC every 12 hr[2]	Fondaparinux 2.5 mg SC once daily[1]	Enoxaparin 40 mg SC once daily[3]
All treated hip replacement surgery patients	(N = 1126)	(N = 1128)	(N = 1129)	(N = 1123)
All evaluable[4] knee replacement surgery patients				
VTE[5]	48/787 6.1%[6] (4.5, 8)[7]	66/797 8.3% (6.5, 10.4)	37/908 4.1%[8] (2.9, 5.6)	85/919 9.2% (7.5, 11.3)
All DVT[9]	44/784 5.6%[10] (4.1, 7.5)	65/796 8.2% (6.4, 10.3)	36/908 4%[8] (2.8, 5.4)	83/918 9% (7.3, 11.1)
Proximal DVT	14/816 1.7%[6] (0.9, 2.9)	10/830 1.2% (0.6, 2.2)	6/922 0.7%[8] (0.2, 1.4)	23/927 2.5% (1.6, 3.7)
Symptomatic PE[11]	5/1126 0.4%[6] (0.1, 1)	1/1128 0.1% (0, 0.5)	2/1129 0.2%[6] (0, 0.6)	2/1123 0.2% (0, 0.6)

[1] Patients randomized to 2.5 mg fondaparinux received the first injection approximately 6 hours after surgery, providing that hemostasis had been achieved.
[2] Patients randomized to enoxaparin were to receive the first injection between 12 and 24 hours after surgery.
[3] Patients randomized to enoxaparin were to receive the first injection 12 hours prior to surgery except in the case of spinal anesthesia. The first postoperative enoxaparin dose was to be given between 12 and 24 hours after surgery.
[4] Evaluable patients were those who were treated and underwent the appropriate surgery (ie, elective hip replacement surgery), with an adequate efficacy assessment up to day 11.
[5] VTE = venous thromboembolism. VTE was a composite of documented DVT and/or documented symptomatic PE reported up to day 11.
[6] p value vs enoxaparin: Not significant.
[7] Number in parentheses indicates 95% confidence interval.
[8] p value vs enoxaparin in study 2: < 0.01.
[9] DVT = deep vein thrombosis.
[10] p value vs enoxaparin in study 1: < 0.05.
[11] PE = pulmonary embolism.

In a randomized, double-blind clinical trial in patients undergoing knee replacement surgery (ie, surgery requiring resection of the distal end of the femur or proximal end of the tibia) 2.5 mg fondaparinux SC once daily was compared with 30 mg enoxaparin SC every 12 hours. For both drugs, treatment was continued for approximately 7 days. The efficacy data are provided in the following table. Major bleeding was significantly greater in fondaparinux-treated patients as compared with active enoxaparin-treated patients.

FONDAPARINUX SODIUM

Efficacy of Fondaparinux Injection in the Prophylaxis of Thromboembolic Events Following Knee Replacement Surgery		
Endpoint	Fondaparinux 2.5 mg SC once daily[1]	Enoxaparin 30 mg SC every 12 hours[2]
All treated knee replacement surgery patients	(N = 517)	(N = 517)
All evaluable[3] knee replacement surgery patients		
VTE[4]	45/361 12.5%[5] (9.2, 16.3)[6]	101/363 27.8% (23.3, 32.7)
All DVT	45/361 12.5%[5] (9.2, 16.3)	98/361 27.1% (22.6, 32)
Proximal DVT	9/368 2.4%[7] (1.1, 4.6)	20/372 5.4% (3.3, 8.2)
Symptomatic PE	1/517 0.2%[7] (0, 1.1)	4/517 0.8% (0.2, 2)

[1] Patients randomized to 2.5 mg fondaparinux received the first injection approximately 6 hours after surgery, providing that hemostasis had been achieved.
[2] Patients randomized to enoxaparin received the first injection at approximately 21 hours after surgery closure, providing that hemostasis had been achieved.
[3] Evaluable patients were those who were treated and underwent the appropriate surgery (ie, knee replacement surgery), with an adequate efficacy assessment up to day 11.
[4] VTE was a composite of documented DVT and/or documented symptomatic PE reported up to day 11.
[5] p value < 0.001.
[6] Number in parentheses indicates 95% confidence interval.
[7] p value: Not significant.

Contraindications

Severe renal impairment (Ccr less than 30 mL/min); body weight less than 50 kg; active major bleeding; bacterial endocarditis; thrombocytopenia associated with a positive in vitro test for antiplatelet antibody in the presence of fondaparinux; known hypersensitivity to fondaparinux.

Warnings

➤*Injection:* Fondaparinux is not intended for IM injection.

➤*Interchangeability:* Fondaparinux cannot be used interchangeably (unit for unit) with heparin, LMWHs, or heparinoids, as they differ in manufacturing process, anti-Xa and anti-IIa activity, units, and dosage.

➤*Hemorrhage:* Fondaparinux, like other anticoagulants, should be used with extreme caution in conditions with increased risk of hemorrhage, such as congenital or acquired bleeding disorders, active ulcerative and angiodysplastic GI disease, hemorrhagic stroke, or shortly after brain, spinal, or ophthalmological surgery, or in patients treated concomitantly with platelet inhibitors.

➤*Spinal/Epidural hematomas:* Spinal or epidural hematomas, which may result in long-term or permanent paralysis, can occur with the use of anticoagulants and neuraxial (spinal/epidural) anesthesia or spinal puncture. The risk of these events may be higher with postoperative use of indwelling epidural catheters or concomitant use of other drugs affecting hemostasis, such as NSAIDs.

➤*Thrombocytopenia:* Thrombocytopenia can occur with the administration of fondaparinux. Moderate thrombocytopenia (platelet counts between 100,000/mm^3 and 50,000/mm^3) occurred at a rate of 2.9% in patients given 2.5 mg fondaparinux in clinical trials. Severe thrombocytopenia (platelet counts less than 50,000/mm^3) occurred at a rate of 0.2% in patients given 2.5 mg fondaparinux in clinical trials.

Thrombocytopenia of any degree should be monitored closely. If the platelet count falls below 100,000/mm^3, discontinue fondaparinux.

➤*Renal function impairment:* The risk of hemorrhage increases with increasing renal impairment. Occurrences of major bleeding in patients with normal renal function, mild renal impairment, moderate renal impairment, and severe renal impairment have been found to be 1.6%, 2.4%, 3.8%, and 4.8%, respectively.

Therefore, fondaparinux is contraindicated in patients with severe renal impairment (Ccr less than 30 mL/min) and should be used with caution in patients with moderate renal impairment (Ccr 30 to 50 mL/min).

Periodically assess renal function in patients receiving the drug. Immediately discontinue fondaparinux in patients who develop severe renal impairment or labile renal function while on therapy. After discontinuation of fondaparinux, its anticoagulant effects may persist for 2 to 4 days in patients with normal renal function (ie, at least 3 to 5 half-lives). The anticoagulant effects of fondaparinux may persist even longer in patients with renal impairment.

➤*Elderly:* The risk of fondaparinux-associated major bleeding increased with age: 1.8% in patients less than 65 years of age, 2.2% in those 65 to 74 years of age, and 2.7% in those 75 years of age or older. Serious adverse events increased with age for patients receiving fondaparinux. Careful attention to dosing directions and concomitant medications (especially antiplatelet medication) is advised.

Fondaparinux is substantially excreted by the kidney, and the risk of toxic reactions to fondaparinux may be greater in patients with impaired renal function. Because elderly patients are more likely to have decreased renal function, it may be useful to monitor renal function.

➤*Pregnancy:* Category B. There are no adequate and well-controlled studies in pregnant women. Because animal reproduction studies are not always predictive of human response, use during pregnancy only if clearly needed.

➤*Lactation:* Fondaparinux was found to be excreted in the milk of lactating rats. However, it is not known whether this drug is excreted in human milk. Because many drugs are excreted in human milk, exercise caution when fondaparinux is administered to a nursing mother.

➤*Children:* Safety and efficacy of fondaparinux in pediatric patients have not been established.

Precautions

➤*Monitoring:* Periodic routine CBCs (including platelet count), serum creatinine level, and stool occult blood tests are recommended during the course of treatment with fondaparinux injection.

When administered at the recommended prophylaxis dose, routine coagulation tests such as prothrombin time (PT) and activated partial thromboplastin time (aPTT) are relatively insensitive measures of fondaparinux activity and, therefore, are unsuitable for monitoring.

The anti-Factor Xa activity of fondaparinux can be measured by anti-Xa assay using the appropriate calibrator (fondaparinux). Because the international standards of heparin or LMWH are not appropriate calibrators, the activity of fondaparinux is expressed in milligrams of the fondaparinux and cannot be compared with activities of heparin or LMWHs.

If during fondaparinux therapy unexpected changes in coagulation parameters or major bleeding occurs, discontinue fondaparinux.

➤*Heparin-induced thrombocytopenia:* Use fondaparinux with caution in patients with a history of heparin-induced thrombocytopenia.

➤*Special risk:* Use fondaparinux with care in patients with a bleeding diathesis, uncontrolled arterial hypertension, or a history of recent GI ulceration, diabetic retinopathy, and hemorrhage.

Drug Interactions

Discontinue agents that may enhance the risk of hemorrhage prior to initiation of fondaparinux therapy. If coadministration is essential, close monitoring may be appropriate.

➤*Coumarin:* In an in vitro study in human liver microsomes, inhibition of CYP2A6 hydroxylation of coumarin by fondaparinux (200 mcM; ie, 350 mg/L) was 17% to 28%.

Adverse Reactions

Fondaparinux Adverse Events (≥ 2%)		
Adverse reaction	Fondaparinux 2.5 mg SC once daily (N = 3616)	Comparator: LMWH or enoxaparin[1] (N = 3956)
CNS		
Insomnia	5	5.4
Dizziness	3.6	4.2
Confusion	3.1	3.3
Headache	2	2.5
Dermatologic		
Rash	7.5	8.3
Bullous eruption	3.1	2.6
GI		
Nausea	11.3	12.2
Constipation	8.5	10.5
Vomiting	5.9	6
Diarrhea	2.5	2.6
Dyspepsia	2.4	2.6
GU		
Urinary tract infection	3.8	3.4
Urinary retention	2.9	3
Hematologic		
Anemia	19.6	16.9
Purpura	3.5	3.5
Hematoma	2.8	2.8
Postoperative hemorrhage	2.4	1.7

FONDAPARINUX SODIUM

Fondaparinux Adverse Events (≥ 2%)		
Adverse reaction	Fondaparinux 2.5 mg SC once daily (N = 3616)	Comparator: LMWH or enoxaparin[1] (N = 3956)
Miscellaneous		
Fever	13.6	15.4
Edema	8.7	8.8
Wound drainage increased	4.5	4.7
Hypokalemia	4.2	4.1
Hypotension	3.5	3.2
Pain	1.7	2.6

[1] Enoxaparin dosing regimen: 30 mg every 12 hours or 40 mg once daily.

➤*Hematologic:* During fondaparinux administration, the most common adverse reactions were bleeding complications. In knee replacement surgery, major bleeding was significantly greater in fondaparinux-treated patients than enoxaparin-treated patients.

The rates of major bleeding events reported during clinical trials with 2.5 mg fondaparinux injection are provided in the following tables.

Major Bleeding[1] Episodes Following Hip Fracture, Hip Replacement, and Knee Replacement Surgeries		
Indication	Fondaparinux 2.5 mg SC once daily	Comparator: LMWH or enoxaparin[2]
Hip fracture	2.2%	2.3%
Hip replacement	3%	2.1%
Knee replacement	2.1%[3]	0.2%

[1] Major bleeding was defined as clinically overt bleeding that was (1) fatal, (2) bleeding at critical site (eg, intracranial, retroperitoneal, intraocular, pericardial, spinal, or into adrenal gland), (3) associated with reoperation at operative site, or (4) with a bleeding index (BI) of 2 or greater. BI of 2 or greater: Overt bleeding associated only with a bleeding index of 2 or greater. (Calculated as number of whole blood or packed red blood cells transfused + [(prebleeding) − (postbleeding)] hemoglobin [g/dL] values.)
[2] Enoxaparin dosing regimen: 30 mg every 12 hours or 40 mg once daily.
[3] p value vs enoxaparin: 0.0061; 95% confidence interval: (1.1%, 3.8%) in fondaparinux group vs (0%, 1.1%) in enoxaparin group.

Bleeding Across Hip Fracture, Hip Replacement, and Knee Replacement Surgery Studies		
Indications	Fondaparinux 2.5 mg SC once daily (N = 3616) (%)	Comparator: LMWH or enoxaparin[1] (N = 3956) (%)
Major bleeding[2]	2.7	1.9
Fatal bleeding	0	< 0.1
Nonfatal bleeding at critical site	0	< 0.1

Bleeding Across Hip Fracture, Hip Replacement, and Knee Replacement Surgery Studies		
Indications	Fondaparinux 2.5 mg SC once daily (N = 3616) (%)	Comparator: LMWH or enoxaparin[1] (N = 3956) (%)
Reoperation because of bleeding	0.3	0.3
(BI) ≥ 2[3]	2.3	1.6
Minor bleeding[4]	3	2.9

[1] Enoxaparin dosing regimen: 30 mg every 12 hours or 40 mg once daily.
[2] Major bleeding was defined as clinically overt bleeding that was (1) fatal, (2) bleeding at critical site (eg, intracranial, retroperitoneal, intraocular, pericardial, spinal, or into adrenal gland), (3) associated with reoperation at operative site, or (4) with a bleeding index (BI) of 2 or greater.
[3] BI of 2 or greater: Overt bleeding associated only with a bleeding index of 2 or greater. (Calculated as number of whole blood or packed red blood cells transfused + [(prebleeding) − (postbleeding)] hemoglobin [g/dL] values.)
[4] Minor bleeding was defined as clinically overt bleeding that was not major.

Thrombocytopenia – Moderate thrombocytopenia (platelet counts between 100,000/mm^3 and 50,000/mm^3) occurred at a rate of 2.9% in patients given 2.5 mg fondaparinux in clinical trials. Severe thrombocytopenia (platelet counts less than 50,000/mm^3) occurred at a rate of 0.2% in patients given 2.5 mg fondaparinux in clinical trials (see Warnings).

➤*Lab test abnormalities:* Asymptomatic increases in AST and ALT levels greater than 3 times the upper limit of normal of the laboratory reference range have been reported in 1.7% and 2.6% of patients, respectively, during treatment with 2.5 mg fondaparinux vs 3.2% and 3.9% of patients, respectively, during treatment with 30 mg enoxaparin every 12 hours or 40 mg once daily or a LMWH comparator. Such elevations are fully reversible and are rarely associated with increases in bilirubin.

Because aminotransferase determinations are important in the differential diagnosis of MI, liver disease, and pulmonary emboli, interpret with caution elevations that might be caused by drugs like fondaparinux.

➤*Local:* Mild local irritation (eg, injection site bleeding, rash, pruritus) may occur following SC injection of fondaparinux.

Overdosage

There is no known antidote for fondaparinux. Overdose of fondaparinux may lead to hemorrhagic complications. Overdosage associated with bleeding complications should lead to treatment discontinuation and initiation of appropriate therapy.

Data obtained in patients undergoing chronic intermittent hemodialysis suggest that fondaparinux clearance can increase by 20% during hemodialysis.

WARFARIN SODIUM

Rx	**Warfarin Sodium** (Various, eg, Barr, Geneva, Taro)	**Tablets:** 1 mg	In 100s and 1000s.
Rx	**Coumadin** (Bristol-Myers Squibb)		Lactose. (COUMADIN 1). Pink, scored. In 100s, 1000s, and UD 100s.
Rx	**Jantoven** (Upsher-Smith)		Lactose, povidone. (WRF 1 832). Pink, scored. In 100s and 1000s.
Rx	**Warfarin Sodium** (Various, eg, Barr, Geneva, Taro)	2 mg	In 100s and 1000s.
Rx	**Coumadin** (Bristol-Myers Squibb)		Lactose. (COUMADIN 2). Lavender, scored. In 100s, 1000s, and UD 100s.
Rx	**Jantoven** (Upsher-Smith)		Lactose, povidone. (WRF 2 832). Lavender, scored. In 100s and 1000s.
Rx	**Warfarin Sodium** (Various, eg, Barr, Geneva, Taro)	2.5 mg	In 100s and 1000s.
Rx	**Coumadin** (Bristol-Myers Squibb)		Lactose. (COUMADIN 2½). Green, scored. In 100s, 1000s, and UD 100s.
Rx	**Jantoven** (Upsher-Smith)		Lactose, povidone. (WRF 2½ 832). Green, scored. In 100s and 1000s.
Rx	**Warfarin Sodium** (Various, eg, Barr, Geneva, Taro)	3 mg	In 100s and 1000s.
Rx	**Coumadin** (Bristol-Myers Squibb)		Lactose. (COUMADIN 3). Tan, scored. In 100s, 1000s, and UD 100s.
Rx	**Jantoven** (Upsher-Smith)		Lactose, povidone. (WRF 3 832). Tan, scored. In 100s and 1000s.
Rx	**Warfarin Sodium** (Various, eg, Barr, Geneva, Taro)	4 mg	In 100s and 1000s.
Rx	**Coumadin** (Bristol-Myers Squibb)		Lactose. (COUMADIN 4). Blue, scored. In 100s, 1000s, and UD 100s.
Rx	**Jantoven** (Upsher-Smith)		Lactose, povidone. (WRF 4 832). Blue, scored. In 100s and 1000s.
Rx	**Warfarin Sodium** (Various, eg, Barr, Geneva, Taro)	5 mg	In 100s and 1000s.
Rx	**Coumadin** (Bristol-Myers Squibb)		Lactose. (COUMADIN 5). Peach, scored. In 100s, 1000s, and UD 100s.
Rx	**Jantoven** (Upsher-Smith)		Lactose, povidone. (WRF 5 832). Peach, scored. In 100s and 1000s.
Rx	**Warfarin Sodium** (Various, eg, Barr, Geneva, Taro)	6 mg	In 100s and 1000s.
Rx	**Coumadin** (Bristol-Myers Squibb)		Lactose. (COUMADIN 6). Teal, scored. In 100s, 1000s, and UD 100s.
Rx	**Jantoven** (Upsher-Smith)		Lactose, povidone. (WRF 6 832). Teal, scored. In 100s and 1000s.
Rx	**Warfarin Sodium** (Various, eg, Barr, Geneva, Taro)	7.5 mg	In 100s and 1000s.
Rx	**Coumadin** (Bristol-Myers Squibb)		Lactose. (COUMADIN 7½). Yellow, scored. In 100s and UD 100s.
Rx	**Jantoven** (Upsher-Smith)		Lactose, povidone. (WRF 7½ 832). Yellow, scored. In 100s and 500s.
Rx	**Warfarin Sodium** (Various, eg, Barr, Geneva, Taro)	10 mg	In 100s.
Rx	**Coumadin** (Bristol-Myers Squibb)		Dye free. Lactose. (COUMADIN 10). White, scored. In 100s and UD 100s.
Rx	**Jantoven** (Upsher-Smith)		Dye free. Lactose, povidone. (WRF 10 832). White, scored. In 100s and 500s.
Rx	**Coumadin** (Bristol-Myers Squibb)	**Powder for injection, lyophilized:** 5.4 mg (2 mg/mL when reconstituted)	Mannitol. Preservative-free. In 5 mg vials.

Indications

Prophylaxis and/or treatment of venous thrombosis and its extension and pulmonary embolism.

Prophylaxis and/or treatment of the thromboembolic complications associated with atrial fibrillation and/or cardiac valve replacement.

To reduce the risk of death, recurrent MI, and thromboembolic events such as stroke or systemic embolization after MI.

➤*Unlabeled uses:* Oral anticoagulants have been used to prevent recurrent transient ischemic attack and in the treatment of antiphospholipid syndrome.

Administration and Dosage

➤*Approved by the FDA:* June 8, 1954.

➤*Initial dosage:* The dosing must be individualized according to patient's sensitivity to the drug as indicated by the prothrombin time (PT)/International Normalized Ratio (INR). Adjust dosage based on the patient's PT/INR. Use of a large loading dose may increase the incidence of hemorrhagic and other complications, does not offer more rapid protection against thrombi formation, and is not recommended.

➤*Maintenance:* Most patients are satisfactorily maintained at a dose of 2 to 10 mg/day. Gauge the individual dose and interval by the patient's prothrombin response. An INR of greater than 4 appears to provide no additional therapeutic benefit in most patients and is associated with a higher risk of bleeding.

➤*Duration of therapy:* Individualize the duration of therapy. Continue anticoagulant therapy until the danger of thrombosis and embolism has passed.

Recommendations from the American College of Chest Physicians (ACCP) for duration of anticoagulant therapy after venous thromboembolism (VTE) are included in the following table:

Duration of Anticoagulant Therapy After VTE[1]	
3 to 6 mo	First event with reversible[2] or time-limited risk factor (patient may have underlying Factor V Leiden or prothrombin 20210)
≥ 6 mo	Idiopathic VTE, first event
12 mo to lifetime	First event[3] with Cancer, until resolved Anticardiolipin antibody Antithrombin deficiency Recurrent event, idiopathic or with thrombophilia

[1] All recommendations are subject to modification by individual characteristics, including patient preference, age, comorbidity, and likelihood of recurrence.
[2] Reversible or time-limited risk factors: Surgery, trauma, immobilization, estrogen use.
[3] Proper duration of therapy is unclear in first event with homozygous Factor V Leiden, homocystinemia, deficiency of protein C or S, or multiple thrombophilias; and in recurrent events with reversible risk factors.

➤*Missed dose:* The anticoagulant effect of warfarin persists beyond 24 hours. If the patient forgets to take the prescribed dose of warfarin at the scheduled time, the dose should be taken as soon as possible on the same day. The patient should not take the missed dose by doubling the daily dose to make up for missed doses.

➤*IV route of administration:* Warfarin injection provides an alternative administration route for patients who cannot receive oral drugs. The IV dosages would be the same as those that would be used orally if the patient could take the drug by the oral route. Administer as a slow bolus injection over 1 to 2 minutes into a peripheral vein. It is not recommended for IM administration.

Reconstitution – Reconstitute the vial with 2.7 mL sterile water for injection and inspect for particulate matter and discoloration immediately prior to use. Do not use if particulate matter or discoloration is noted. After reconstitution, warfarin for injection is chemically and physically stable for 4 hours at room temperature. It does not contain any antimicrobial preservative and care must be taken to assure the sterility of the prepared solution. The vial is not recommended for multiple use; discard unused solution.

WARFARIN SODIUM

▶*Treatment during dentistry and surgery:* In patients undergoing minimal invasive procedures who must be anticoagulated prior to, during, or immediately following dental or surgical procedures, adjusting the dosage to maintain the PT/INR at the low end of the therapeutic range may safely allow for continued anticoagulation. Sufficiently limit the operative site to permit effective use of local measures for hemostasis. Under these conditions, dental and minor surgical procedures may be performed without undue risk of hemorrhage. (A severe elevation [greater than 50 seconds] in activated partial thromboplastin time [aPTT] with a PT/INR in the desired range has been identified as an indication of increased risk of postoperative hemorrhage.)

▶*Conversion from heparin therapy:* Because the anticoagulant effect of warfarin is delayed, heparin is preferred initially for rapid anticoagulation. Conversion to warfarin therapy may begin concomitantly with heparin therapy or may be delayed 3 to 6 days. To ensure continuous anticoagulation, it is advisable to continue full dose heparin therapy and that warfarin therapy be overlapped with heparin for 4 to 5 days, until warfarin therapy has produced the desired therapeutic response as determined by PT/INR. When warfarin has produced the desired PT/INR or prothrombin activity, heparin may be discontinued.

▶*Recommended INR therapeutic ranges:* Following are the recommended therapeutic ranges for oral anticoagulation therapy from the ACCP and the National Heart, Lung, and Blood Institute (NHLBI):

ACCP/NHLBI Recommended Therapeutic Range for Oral Anticoagulant Therapy		
Condition	PT ratio[1]	INR
Acute MI[2]	1.3 to 1.5	2 to 3
MI, prevent recurrent	1.4 to 1.6	2.5 to 3.5
Atrial fibrillation[2]	1.3 to 1.5	2 to 3
Mechanical prosthetic valves	1.4 to 1.6	2.5 to 3.5
Bileaflet mechanical valve in aortic position	1.3 to 1.5	2 to 3
Pulmonary embolism, treatment	1.3 to 1.5	2 to 3
Valvular heart disease[2]	1.3 to 1.5	2 to 3
Tissue heart valves[2]	1.3 to 1.5	2 to 3
Valvular heart disease[2]	1.3 to 1.5	2 to 3
Venous thrombosis		
Prophylaxis (high-risk surgery)	1.3 to 1.5	2 to 3
Treatment		2 to 3

[1] International Sensitivity Index (ISI) ratio of 2.8.
[2] To prevent systemic embolism

The INR can be calculated as INR = (observed PT ratio)^{ISI} where the ISI is the correction factor in the equation that relates the PT ratio of the local reagent to the reference preparation and is a measure of the sensitivity of a given thromboplastin to reduction of vitamin K-dependent coagulation factors; the lower the ISI, the more "sensitive" the reagent and the closer the derived INR will be to the observed PT ratio.

▶*Management of nontherapeutic INRs:* The following is a suggested approach for treatment of overanticoagulated patients:

Management of Nontherapeutic INRs			
INR	Significant bleeding	Rapid reversal	Intervention
< 5	No	No	Lower or omit a dose; resume therapy at lower dose when INR is in therapeutic range. If the INR is only minimally greater than the therapeutic range, no dose reduction may be required.
> 5 but < 9	No	No	Omit next few doses, monitor INR more frequently, resume therapy at lower dose when INR is in therapeutic range.
	Yes	No	Omit dose, give 1 to 2.5 mg vitamin K$_1$ PO.
	Yes	Yes	Give 2 to 4 mg K$_1$ PO, decrease in INR within 24 h. If INR still high, give additional dose of 1 to 2 mg K$_1$ PO.

Management of Nontherapeutic INRs			
INR	Significant bleeding	Rapid reversal	Intervention
> 9 to 20	No	No	Hold warfarin therapy, administer 3 to 5 mg K$_1$ PO; decrease in INR within 24 to 48 h; monitor INR frequently, repeat dose if necessary. Resume therapy at lower dose when INR is in therapeutic range.
> 20	Yes	Yes	Hold warfarin therapy. Give 10 mg K$_1$ slow IV infusion, may repeat dose every 12 h, supplement with plasma or prothrombin complex concentrate (PCC).
> 20 and life-threatening	Yes	Yes	Hold warfarin therapy. Give PCC supplemented with 10 mg K$_1$ slow IV. Repeat if necessary.

▶*Storage/Stability:*

Tablets – Protect from light. Store tablets in carton until contents have been used. Store at controlled room temperature (15° to 30°C; 59° to 86°F). Dispense in a tight, light-resistant container.

Injection – Protect from light. Keep vial in box until used. Store at controlled room temperature (15° to 30°C; 59° to 86°F).

After reconstitution, store at controlled room temperature (15° to 30°C; 59° to 86°F) and use within 4 hours. Do not refrigerate. Discard any unused solution.

Actions

▶*Pharmacology:* Anticoagulants act by inhibiting the synthesis of vitamin K-dependent clotting factors, which include factors II, VII, IX, and X, and the anticoagulant proteins C and S. Half-lives of these clotting factors are as follows: Factor II, 60 hours; VII, 4 to 6 hours; IX, 24 hours; X, 48 to 72 hours. The half-lives of proteins C and S are approximately 8 and 30 hours, respectively. The in vivo effect is a sequential depression of factors II, VII, IX, and X activities. Vitamin K is an essential cofactor for the post ribosomal synthesis of the vitamin K-dependent clotting factors. Warfarin is thought to interfere with clotting factor synthesis by inhibition of the regeneration of vitamin K$_1$ epoxide. Therapeutic doses of warfarin decrease the total amount of the active form of each vitamin K-dependent clotting factor made by the liver by approximately 30% to 50%.

An anticoagulant effect generally occurs within 24 hours after drug administration. However, peak anticoagulant effect may be delayed 72 to 96 hours. The duration of action of a single dose of racemic warfarin is 2 to 5 days. Anticoagulants have no direct effect on an established thrombus, nor do they reverse ischemic tissue damage. However, once a thrombus has occurred, the goal of anticoagulant treatment is to prevent further extension of the formed clot and prevent secondary thromboembolic complications that may result in serious and possibly fatal sequelae.

Warfarin is a racemic mixture of the R- and S-enantiomers. The S-enantiomer exhibits 2 to 5 times more anticoagulant activity than the R-enantiomer.

▶*Pharmacokinetics:*

Absorption – Warfarin is completely absorbed after oral administration with peak concentration generally attained within the first 4 hours.

Distribution – There are no differences in the apparent volumes of distribution after IV and oral administration of single doses of warfarin solution. Warfarin distributes into a relatively small apparent volume of distribution of about 0.14 L/kg. A distribution phase lasting 6 to 12 hours is distinguishable after rapid IV or oral administration of an aqueous solution. Approximately 99% of the drug is bound to plasma protein.

Metabolism – Warfarin is metabolized by hepatic microsomal enzymes (P450) to inactive hydroxylated metabolites and by reductases to reduced metabolites (warfarin alcohols). The warfarin alcohols have minimal anticoagulant activity. The metabolites are principally excreted into the urine and to a lesser extent into the bile.

Excretion – The terminal half-life of warfarin after a single dose is approximately 1 week; however, the effective half-life ranges from 20 to 60 hours, with a mean of about 40 hours. The half-life of R-warfarin ranges from 37 to 89 hours, while that of S-warfarin ranges from 21 to 43 hours. Up to 92% of the orally administered dose is recovered in urine. Very little warfarin is excreted unchanged in urine. Urinary excretion is in the form of metabolites.

WARFARIN SODIUM
Special populations –

Elderly: Patients 60 years of age and older appear to exhibit greater than expected PT/INR response to the anticoagulant effects of warfarin. There may be a slight decrease in the clearance of R-warfarin in the elderly as compared with the young. Therefore, as patient age increases, a lower dose of warfarin usually is required to produce a therapeutic level of anticoagulation.

Asians: Asian patients may require lower initiation and maintenance doses of warfarin.

Hepatic function impairment: Hepatic dysfunction can potentiate the response to warfarin through impaired synthesis of clotting factors and decreased metabolism of warfarin.

➤*Clinical trials:*

Atrial fibrillation (AF) – In 5 prospective, randomized, controlled clinical trials involving 3711 patients with nonrheumatic AF, warfarin significantly reduced the risk of systemic thromboembolism including stroke. The risk reduction ranged from 60% to 86%. The incidence of major bleeding in these trials ranged from 0.6% to 2.7%. These studies revealed that the effects of warfarin in reducing thromboembolic events, including stroke, were similar at moderately high INR (2 to 4.5) or low INR (1.4 to 3).

Mechanical and bioprosthetic heart valves – In a prospective, randomized, open-label, positive-controlled study in 254 patients, the thromboembolic-free interval was significantly greater in patients with mechanical prosthetic heart valves treated with warfarin alone compared with dipyridamole-aspirin ($P < 0.005$) and pentoxifylline-aspirin ($P < 0.05$) treated patients. Rates of thromboembolic events in these groups were 2.2, 8.6, and 7.9 per 100 patient years, respectively. Major bleeding rates were 2.5, 0, and 0.9 per 100 patient years, respectively.

Contraindications

Women who are pregnant or may become pregnant (see Warnings); hemorrhagic tendencies or blood dyscrasias; recent or contemplated surgery of the CNS or eye or traumatic surgery resulting in large, open surfaces; bleeding tendencies associated with active ulceration or overt bleeding of the GI, respiratory, or GU tracts, cerebrovascular hemorrhage, aneurysm (cerebral, dissecting aorta), pericarditis and pericardial effusion, or bacterial endocarditis; threatened abortion, eclampsia and preeclampsia; inadequate laboratory facilities; unsupervised patients with senility, alcoholism, or psychosis or other lack of patient cooperation; spinal puncture and other diagnostic or therapeutic procedures with potential for uncontrollable bleeding; major regional, lumbar block anesthesia; malignant hypertension; known hypersensitivity to warfarin or any other components of the product.

Warnings

➤*Hemorrhage/Necrosis:* The most serious risks associated with anticoagulant therapy with warfarin are hemorrhage in any tissue or organ and, less frequently, necrosis and/or gangrene of skin and other tissues. The risk of hemorrhage is related to the level of intensity and the duration of therapy. Bleeding that occurs during anticoagulant therapy does not always correlate with PT/INR (see Overdosage). Bleeding that occurs when the PT/INR is within the therapeutic range warrants diagnostic investigation because it may unmask a previously suspected lesion (eg, tumor, ulcer). Hemorrhage and necrosis have in some cases been reported to result in death or permanent disability. Necrosis appears to be associated with local thrombosis and usually appears within a few days of the start of therapy. In severe cases of necrosis, treatment through debridement or amputation of the affected tissue, limb, breast, or penis has been reported. Careful diagnosis is required to determine whether necrosis is caused by an underlying disease. Discontinue therapy when warfarin is suspected to be the cause of developing necrosis; heparin therapy may be considered.

➤*Special risk patients:* Exercise caution in the presence of any predisposing condition where added risk of hemorrhage, necrosis, and/or gangrene is present, as well as in the following: Severe to moderate hepatic or renal insufficiency; infectious diseases or disturbances of intestinal flora (eg, sprue, antibiotic therapy); trauma that may result in internal bleeding; surgery or trauma resulting in large exposed raw surfaces; indwelling catheters; severe to moderate hypertension; polycythemia vera; vasculitis; severe diabetes; minor and severe allergic/hypersensitivity reactions and anaphylactic reactions.

Patients with CHF may exhibit greater than expected PT/INR response to warfarin.

➤*Atheroemboli/Microemboli:* Systemic atheroemboli and cholesterol microemboli can present with a variety of signs and symptoms including purple toes syndrome, livedo reticularis, rash, gangrene, abrupt and intense pain in the leg, foot, or toes, foot ulcers, myalgia, penile gangrene, abdominal pain, flank or back pain, hematuria, renal insufficiency, hypertension, cerebral ischemia, spinal cord infarction, pancreatitis, symptoms simulating polyarteritis, or any other sequelae of vascular compromise caused by embolic occlusion. The most commonly involved visceral organs are the kidneys, followed by the pancreas, spleen, and liver. Some cases have progressed to necrosis or death. Discontinuation of warfarin therapy is recommended when such phenomena are observed.

➤*Purple toes syndrome:* Purple toes syndrome is a complication of oral anticoagulation characterized by a dark, purplish, or mottled color of the toes, usually occurring between 3 and 10 weeks, or later, after the initiation of therapy with warfarin. Major features of this syndrome include purple color of plantar surfaces and sides of the toes that blanches on moderate pressure and fades with elevation of the legs, pain and tenderness of the toes, and waxing and waning of the color over time. While the purple toes syndrome is reported to be reversible, some cases progress to gangrene or necrosis that may require debridement of the affected area or may lead to amputation.

➤*Heparin-induced thrombocytopenia:* Warfarin should be used with caution in patients with heparin-induced thrombocytopenia and deep venous thrombosis. Cases of venous limb ischemia, necrosis, and gangrene have occurred in patients with heparin-induced thrombocytopenia and deep venous thrombosis when heparin treatment was discontinued and warfarin therapy was started or continued. In some patients sequelae have included amputation of the involved area and/or death.

➤*Protein C deficiency:* Hereditary or acquired deficiencies of protein C or its cofactor, protein S, have been associated with tissue necrosis following warfarin administration. Not all patients with these conditions develop necrosis; tissue necrosis occurs in patients without these deficiencies. Concomitant anticoagulation therapy with heparin for 5 to 7 days during initiation of therapy with warfarin may minimize the incidence of tissue necrosis. Discontinue warfarin therapy when warfarin is suspected to be the cause of developing necrosis; heparin therapy may be considered for anticoagulation.

➤*Nonsteroidal anti-inflammatory drugs (NSAIDs)/aspirin:* Observe caution when warfarin is administered concomitantly with NSAIDs, including aspirin, to be certain that no change in anticoagulation dosage is required. In addition to specific drug interactions that might affect PT/INR, NSAIDs, including aspirin, can inhibit platelet aggregation and can cause GI bleeding, peptic ulceration, and/or perforation.

➤*Laboratory control:* Different thromboplastin reagents vary substantially in their sensitivity to sodium warfarin-induced effects on PT. To define the appropriate therapeutic regimen, it is important to be familiar with the sensitivity of the thromboplastin reagent used in the laboratory and its relationship to the International Reference Preparation (IRP), a sensitive thromboplastin reagent prepared from human brain.

A system of standardizing the PT in oral anticoagulant control was introduced by the World Health Organization in 1983. It is based on the determination of an INR that provides a common basis for communication of PT results and interpretations of therapeutic ranges. The INR system of reporting is based on a logarithmic relationship between the PT ratios of the test and reference preparation. The INR is the PT ratio that would be obtained if the IRP, which has an ISI of 1, was used to perform the test. Early clinical studies of oral anticoagulants, which formed the basis for recommended therapeutic ranges of 1.5 to 2.5 times control PT, used sensitive human brain thromboplastin. When using the less sensitive rabbit brain thromboplastins commonly employed in PT assays today, adjustments must be made to the targeted PT range that reflect this decrease in sensitivity.

➤*Elderly:* Patients 60 years of age and older appear to exhibit greater than expected PT/INR response to the anticoagulant effects of warfarin. Warfarin is contraindicated in any unsupervised patient with senility. Lower initiation and maintenance doses of warfarin are recommended for elderly patients.

➤*Pregnancy:* Category X. Warfarin is contraindicated in women who are or may become pregnant because the drug passes through the placental barrier and may cause fatal hemorrhage to the fetus. There have been reports of birth malformations in children born to mothers who have been treated with warfarin during pregnancy.

Embryopathy characterized by nasal hypoplasia with or without stippled epiphyses (chondrodysplasia punctata) has been reported in pregnant women exposed to warfarin during the first trimester. CNS abnormalities also have been reported, including dorsal midline dysplasia characterized by agenesis of the corpus callosum, Dandy-Walker malformation, and midline cerebellar atrophy. Ventral midline dysplasia, characterized by optic atrophy, and eye abnormalities have been observed. Mental retardation, blindness, and other CNS abnormalities have been reported in association with second and third trimester exposure. Although rare, teratogenic reports following in utero exposure to warfarin include urinary tract anomalies such as single kidney, asplenia, anencephaly, spina bifida, cranial nerve palsy, hydrocephalus, cardiac defects and congenital heart disease, polydactyly, deformities of toes, diaphragmatic hernia, corneal leukoma, cleft palate, cleft lip, schizencephaly, and microcephaly.

Spontaneous abortion and stillbirth are known to occur and a higher risk of fetal mortality is associated with the use of warfarin. Low birth weight and growth retardation also have been reported.

If the patient becomes pregnant while taking this drug, she should be apprised of the potential risks to the fetus, and the possibility of termination of the pregnancy should be discussed in light of those risks.

WARFARIN SODIUM

➤*Lactation:* Based on very limited published data, warfarin has not been detected in the breast milk of mothers treated with warfarin. The same data reports that some breast-fed infants whose mothers were treated with warfarin had prolonged prothrombin times, although not as prolonged as those of the mothers. The decision to breastfeed should be undertaken only after careful consideration of the available alternatives. Women who are breastfeeding and anticoagulated with warfarin should be very carefully monitored so that recommended PT/INR values are not exceeded. Perform coagulation tests and evaluate vitamin K status in infants at risk for bleeding tendencies before advising women taking warfarin to breastfeed. Effects in premature infants have not been evaluated.

➤*Children:* Safety and efficacy in children under 18 years of age have not been established. However, the use of warfarin in children is well-documented for the prevention and treatment of thromboembolic events. Difficulty achieving and maintaining therapeutic PT/INR ranges in the pediatric population has been reported. More frequent PT/INR determinations are recommended because of possible changing warfarin requirements.

Precautions

➤*Monitoring:*

PT – Treatment is highly individualized. Control dosage by periodic determination of PT or other suitable coagulation tests (eg, INR, APTT). Whole blood clotting and bleeding times are not effective measures. Monitor PT daily during the initiation of therapy and whenever any other drug is added to or discontinued from therapy that may alter the patient's response (see Drug Interactions). Once stabilized, monitor PT every 4 to 6 weeks.

INR – Thromboplastins vary greatly in their responsiveness to the anticoagulant effects, differing not only between manufacturers but from lot to lot as well.

Conversion from heparin therapy – As heparin may affect the PT/INR, patients receiving both heparin and warfarin should have blood for PT/INR determination drawn at least:
• 5 hours after the last IV bolus dose of heparin, or
• 4 hours after cessation of a continuous IV infusion of heparin, or
• 24 hours after the last SC heparin injection.

➤*Patient selection:* Use care in the selection of patients to ensure cooperation, especially from alcoholic, senile, or psychotic patients.

➤*Enhanced anticoagulant effects:* Endogenous factors that may be responsible for increased PT/INR response include the following: Blood dyscrasias; cancer; collagen vascular disease; CHF; diarrhea; elevated temperature; hepatic disorders (eg, infectious hepatitis, jaundice); hyperthyroidism; poor nutritional state; steatorrhea; vitamin K deficiency.

➤*Decreased anticoagulant effects:* Endogenous factors that may be responsible for decreased the PT/INR response include the following: Edema; hereditary coumarin resistance; hyperlipemia; hypothyroidism; nephrotic syndrome.

Drug Interactions

Careful monitoring and appropriate dosage adjustments usually will permit combination therapy. Critical times during therapy occur when an interacting drug is added to or discontinued from a patient stabilized on anticoagulants.

Oral Anticoagulant Drug Interactions			
Precipitant drug	Object drug*		Description
Acetaminophen Androgens Beta blockers (propranolol) Capecitabine Cephalosporins, parenteral Chenodiol Chlorpropamide Cisapride Dextran Dextrothyroxine Diazoxide Disulfiram Fibric acids Flutamide Glucagon Halothane Heparin Influenza virus vaccine Isoniazid Levamisole Methyldopa Methylphenidate NSAIDs, COX-2 selective Pentoxifylline Propoxyphen	Anticoagulants	↑	These agents may increase the anticoagulant effect. The risk of bleeding may be increased. The mechanism of the interaction is unknown or complicated.

Oral Anticoagulant Drug Interactions			
Precipitant drug	Object drug*		Description
Quinolones (eg, ciprofloxacin, levofloxacin, norfloxacin, ofloxacin) SSRIs[1] (ie, fluoxetine, fluvoxamine, paroxetine, sertraline) Streptokinase Sulfonamides Tamoxifen Thrombolytics (ie, tissue plasminogen activator [t-Pa]) Thyroid hormones Tolbutamide Tramadol Urokinase Zafirlukast Zileuton	Anticoagulants	↑	These agents may increase the anticoagulant effect. The risk of bleeding may be increased. The mechanism of the interaction is unknown or complicated.
Allopurinol Amiodarone Azole anti-fungals[2] Chloramphenicol Cimetidine HMG-CoA reductase inhibitors (ie, fluvastatin, lovastatin, simvastatin) Ifosfamide[3] Metronidazole Omeprazole Phenylbuta-zone[3] Propafenone Quinidine Quinine SMZ-TMP Sulfinpyrazone	Anticoagulants	↑	These agents may increase the anticoagulant effect of warfarin by inhibition of the anticoagulant's hepatic metabolism. The risk of bleeding may be increased.
Macrolide antibiotics	Anticoagulants	↑	These agents may increase the anticoagulant effect by reducing body clearance of warfarin. The risk of bleeding may be increased.
Loop diuretics (ie, ethacrynic acid, furose-mide) Nalidixic acid Valproate	Anticoagulants	↑	These agents may increase the anticoagulant effect of warfarin caused by displacement from binding sites. The risk of bleeding may be increased.
Amino-glycosides (oral) Tetracyclines Vitamin E	Anticoagulants	↑	These agents may increase the anticoagulant effect of warfarin through an interference with vita-min K. The risk of bleeding may be increased.
Aminosalicylic acid Diflunisal NSAIDs Penicillins, high-dose IV Salicylates Methylsalicylate ointment, topical Ticlopidine	Anticoagulants	↑	These agents may increase the anticoagulant effect of warfarin and increase the risk of bleeding caused by effects on platelet function, and, in the case of NSAIDs, GI irritant effects.
Alcohol[4] Atorvastatin Chloral hydrate Cholestyramine[5] Corticosteroids Cyclophospha-mide Methimazole Moricizine Hydantoins (eg, phenytoin) Pravastatin Prednisone Propylthiouracil Ranitidine	Anticoagulants	↑↓	Increased and decreased PT/INR responses have been reported. May increase or decrease antico-agulant effect of warfarin; mecha-nism unknown.

WARFARIN SODIUM

Oral Anticoagulant Drug Interactions

Precipitant drug	Object drug[*]		Description

Ascorbic acid, high doses
Chlordiaze-
  poxide
Clozapine
Contraceptives,
  oral[6]
Cyclosporine[7]
Estrogens
Ethchlorvynol
Griseofulvin
Haloperidol
Meprobamate
Paraldehyde
Trazodone
	Anticoagulants	↓	These agents may decrease the anticoagulant effect of warfarin. The mechanism of the interaction is unknown.

Aminoglute- thimide Barbiturates Carbamazepine Dicloxacillin[8] Glutethimide Nafcillin[8] Rifamycins Terbinafine	Anticoagulants	↓	These agents may decrease the anticoagulant effect of warfarin caused by induction of the anticoagulant's hepatic microsomal enzymes.
Spironolactone[9] Sucralfate Thiazide diuretics[9] Thiopurines[10] Vitamin K[11]	Anticoagulants	↓	These agents may decrease the anticoagulant effect of warfarin by various mechanisms (eg, possible decreased absorption or increased elimination).

[*] ↑ = Object drug increased.   ↓ = Object drug decreased.
[1] Bleeding has been reported with fluoxetine alone.
[2] Miconazole includes both intravaginal and systemic formulations.
[3] May also displace the anticoagulant from protein binding sites.
[4] Chronic consumption may increase the clearance of the anticoagulant; moderate to small doses do not alter the anticoagulant effect.
[5] Reduced anticoagulant absorption and possibly increased elimination.
[6] Rarely, increased risk of thromboembolism; this is in contrast to intended effect.
[7] Cyclosporine levels also may be decreased.
[8] Associated with warfarin resistance.
[9] Diuretic-induced hemoconcentration of clotting factors.
[10] Thiopurine-induced increase in synthesis or activation of prothrombin.
[11] Vitamin K overcomes interference of vitamin K-dependent clotting factors by anticoagulants.

➤*Herbal medicines:* Exercise caution when herbal medicines are taken concomitantly with warfarin. Specific herbals reported to affect warfarin therapy include the following:
• Bromelains, danshen, dong quai (*Angelica sinensis*), garlic, boldo, *Lycium barbarum* L., and *Ginkgo biloba* are associated most often with an increase in the effects of warfarin.
• Coenzyme Q[10] (ubidecarenone), St. John's wort, green tea, and ginseng are associated most often with a decrease in the effects of warfarin.

Some herbals may cause bleeding events when taken alone (eg, garlic, *Ginkgo biloba*) and may have anticoagulant, antiplatelet, and/or fibrinolytic properties. These effects would be expected to be additive to the anticoagulant effects of warfarin.

Some herbals that may affect coagulation are listed in the following table; however, this list should not be considered all-inclusive.

Herbals That Contain Coumarins With Potential Anticoagulant Effects

Alfalfa	Celery	Parsley
Angelica (dong quai)	Chamomile (German and Roman)	Passion flower
Aniseed		Prickly ash (Northern)
Arnica	Dandelion[3]	Quassia
Asa foetida	Fenugreek	Red clover
Bogbean[1]	Horse chestnut	Sweet clover
Boldo	Horseradish	Sweet woodruff
Buchu	Licorice[3]	Tonka beans
Capsicum[2]	Meadowsweet[1]	Wild carrot
Cassia[3]	Nettle	Wild lettuce

[1] Contains coumarins and salicylates.
[2] Contains coumarins and has fibrinolytic properties.
[3] Contains coumarins and has antiplatelet properties.

Miscellaneous Herbals With Anticoagulant Properties

Bladder wrack (*Fucus*)	Pau d'arco

Herbals That Contain Salicylate and/or Have Antiplatelet Properties

Agrimony[1]	Dandelion[3]	Meadowsweet[2]
Aloe gel	Feverfew	Onion[4]
Aspen	Garlic[4]	Policosanol
Black cohosh	German sarsaparilla	Poplar
Black haw	Ginger	Senega
Bogbean[2]	*Ginkgo biloba*	Tamarind
Cassia[3]	Ginseng (*Panax*)[4]	Willow
Clove	Licorice[3]	Wintergreen

[1] Contains salicylate and has coagulant properties.
[2] Contains coumarins and salicylates.
[3] Contains coumarins and has antiplatelet properties.
[4] Has antiplatelet and fibrinolytic properties.

Herbals With Fibrinolytic Properties

Bromelains Capsicum[1]	Garlic[2] Ginseng (*Panax*)[2]	Inositol nicotinate Onion[2]

[1] Contains coumarins and has fibrinolytic properties.
[2] Has antiplatelet and fibrinolytic properties.

Herbals with Coagulant Properties

Agrimony[1] Goldenseal	Mistletoe	Yarrow

[1] Contains salicylate and has coagulant properties.

➤*Drug/Food interactions:* Vitamin K-rich vegetables may decrease the anticoagulant effects of warfarin by interfering with absorption. Minimize consumption of vitamin K-rich foods (eg, spinach, seaweed, broccoli, turnip greens) or nutritional supplements. Mango has been shown to increase warfarin's effect.

Adverse Reactions

➤*Potential adverse events:*
Hematologic – Fatal or nonfatal hemorrhage from any organ or tissue is a consequence of the anticoagulant effect. The signs and symptoms and severity will vary according to the location and degree or extent of the bleeding. Hemorrhagic complications may present as: Paralysis; paresthesia; headache; chest, abdomen, joint, muscle, or other pain; dizziness; shortness of breath; difficult breathing or swallowing; unexplained swelling; weakness; hypotension; unexplained shock. Therefore, consider the possibility of hemorrhage in evaluating the condition of any anticoagulated patient with complaints that do not indicate an obvious diagnosis.

Dermatologic – Necrosis of skin and other tissues.

➤*Infrequent adverse events:*
Dermatologic – Rash; dermatitis, including bullous eruptions; urticaria; pruritus; alopecia.

GI – Abdominal pain, including cramping; flatulence/bloating; nausea; vomiting; diarrhea.

Hepatic – Hepatitis; cholestatic hepatic injury; jaundice; elevated liver enzymes.

Miscellaneous – Hypersensitivity/allergic reactions; systemic cholesterol microembolization; purple toes syndrome; vasculitis; edema; fever; fatigue; lethargy; malaise; asthenia; pain; headache; dizziness; taste perversion; cold intolerance; paresthesia, including feeling of cold and chills.

➤*Rare adverse events:*
Miscellaneous – Tracheal or tracheobronchial calcification (in association with long-term therapy); priapism (causal relationship not established).

Overdosage

➤*Symptoms:* Suspected or overt abnormal bleeding (eg, appearance of blood in stools or urine, hematuria, excessive menstrual bleeding, melena, petechiae, excessive bruising or persistent oozing from superficial injuries) are early manifestations of anticoagulation beyond a safe and satisfactory level.

➤*Treatment:* Excessive anticoagulation, with or without bleeding, may be controlled by discontinuing therapy and, if necessary, by administration of oral or parenteral vitamin K[1] (see individual monograph).

If minor bleeding progresses to major bleeding, give 5 to 25 mg (rarely up to 50 mg) parenteral vitamin K[1]. In emergency situations of severe hemorrhage, clotting factors can be returned to normal by administering 200 to 500 mL of fresh whole blood or fresh frozen plasma or by giving commercial Factor IX complex.

Purified Factor IX preparations should not be used because they cannot increase the levels of prothrombin, Factor VII, and Factor X, which are also depressed along with the levels of Factor IX as a result of warfarin treatment. Packed red blood cells also may be given if significant blood loss has occurred. Carefully monitor infusions of blood or plasma to avoid precipitating pulmonary edema in elderly patients or patients with heart disease.

WARFARIN SODIUM

Patient Information

Strict adherence to prescribed dosage schedule is necessary.

Do not take or discontinue any other medication, including salicylates (eg, aspirin and topical analgesics), other OTC medications, and botanical (herbal) products (eg, bromelains, coenzyme Q_{10}, danshen, dong quai, garlic, *Ginkgo biloba*, ginseng, St. John's wort) except on advice of physician or pharmacist.

Avoid alcohol consumption.

Do not take warfarin during pregnancy and do not become pregnant while taking it.

Avoid any activity or sport that may result in traumatic injury.

PT/INR tests and regular visits to physician or clinic are needed to monitor therapy.

Carry identification stating that warfarin is being taken.

If the prescribed dose of warfarin is forgotten, take the dose as soon as possible the same day, but do not take a double dose of warfarin the next day to make up for missed doses.

The amount of vitamin K in food may affect therapy with warfarin.

Avoid drastic changes in dietary habits, such as eating large amounts of green leafy vegetables.

Contact physician to report any illness, such as diarrhea, infection, or fever.

Notify physician immediately if any unusual bleeding or symptoms occur. Signs and symptoms of bleeding include the following: Pain, swelling, or discomfort; prolonged bleeding from cuts; increased menstrual flow or vaginal bleeding; nosebleeds; bleeding of gums from brushing; unusual bleeding or bruising; red or dark brown urine; red or tar black stools; headache; dizziness; weakness.

Do not change brands without consulting a physician or pharmacist.

Consult physician before undergoing dental work or elective surgery.

PROTAMINE SULFATE

Rx   **Protamine Sulfate**   **Injection:** 10 mg/mL   Preservative-free. In 5 and 25 mL vials.
      (Various, eg, American Pharmaceutical Partners [APP], Lilly)

Indications

Treatment of heparin overdosage.

Administration and Dosage

Each milligram of protamine sulfate neutralizes not less than 100 units of heparin activity derived from lung tissue or about 115 units derived from intestinal mucosa.

Because heparin disappears rapidly from circulation, the protamine dose required also decreases rapidly with time elapsed since IV heparin injection. For example, if protamine is given 30 minutes after heparin, half the usual dose may be sufficient.

Give very slowly IV over 10 minutes in doses not to exceed 50 mg. Guide dosage by blood coagulation studies.

➤*Incompatibilities:* Certain antibiotics, including several cephalosporins and penicillins.

➤*Prepared solution:* Protamine sulfate injection is for use without further dilution; if further dilution is desired, use 5% dextrose in water or normal saline.

➤*Storage/Stability:* Refrigerate at 2° to 8°C (36° to 46°F). Store at controlled room temperature 15° to 30°C (59° to 86°F); do not permit to freeze (APP only). Do not store diluted solutions; they contain no preservative.

Actions

➤*Pharmacology:* Protamines are strongly basic simple proteins of low molecular weight, rich in arginine. They occur in sperm of salmon and certain other fish species. Given alone, protamine sulfate has a weak anticoagulant effect. However, when given with heparin (strongly acidic), a stable salt forms resulting in loss of anticoagulant activity of both drugs.

➤*Pharmacokinetics:* Protamine sulfate has a rapid onset of action. Heparin is neutralized within 5 minutes after IV injection. The metabolic fate of the heparin-protamine complex is not known, but one theory is that protamine sulfate in the heparin-protamine complex may be partially metabolized or may be cleaved by fibrinolysin, thus freeing heparin.

Contraindications

Previous intolerance.

Warnings

➤*Recurrent bleeding:* Hyperheparinemia or bleeding has occurred in some patients 30 minutes to 18 hours after cardiac surgery (under cardiopulmonary bypass) in spite of complete neutralization of heparin by adequate doses of protamine at the end of the operation. Therefore, observe patients closely after cardiac surgery. Administer additional doses of protamine sulfate if indicated by coagulation studies, such as the heparin titration test with protamine and the determination of plasma thrombin time.

➤*Excessively rapid administration:* Excessively rapid administration can cause severe hypotensive and anaphylactoid reactions. Have facilities available to treat shock.

➤*Pulmonary edema:* High-protein, noncardiogenic pulmonary edema associated with the use of protamine has occurred in patients on cardiopulmonary bypass who are undergoing cardiovascular surgery. The etiologic role of protamine in the pathogenesis of this condition is uncertain, and multiple factors have been present in most cases. The condition has been reported in association with administration of certain blood products, other drugs, cardiopulmonary bypass alone and other etiologic factors. It is difficult to treat, and it can be life-threatening.

➤*Circulatory collapse:* Severe and potentially irreversible circulatory collapse associated with myocardial failure and reduced cardiac output also can occur. The mechanism(s) of this reaction and the role played by concurrent factors are unclear.

➤*Hypersensitivity reactions:* Patients with a history of allergy to fish may develop hypersensitivity reactions; although, to date, no relationship has been established between allergic reactions to protamine and fish allergy.

Previous exposure to protamine through use of protamine-containing insulins or during heparin neutralization may predispose susceptible individuals to the development of untoward reactions from the subsequent use of this drug. Reports of the presence of antiprotamine antibodies in the sera of infertile or vasectomized men suggest that some of these individuals may react to the use of protamine sulfate.

Complement activation by the heparin-protamine complexes, release of lysosomal enzymes from neutrophils, and prostaglandin and thromboxane generation have been associated with the development of anaphylactoid reactions. Fatal anaphylaxis has been reported in one patient with no prior history of allergies. Give protamine only when resuscitation techniques and treatment of anaphylactic and anaphylactoid shock are readily available. Have epinephrine 1:1000 immediately available. Refer to Management of Acute Hypersensitivity Reactions.

➤*Pregnancy: Category C.* It is not known whether the drug can cause fetal harm when administered to a pregnant woman or can affect reproduction capacity. Administer to a pregnant woman only if clearly needed.

➤*Lactation:* It is not known whether this drug is excreted in breast milk. Administer cautiously to a nursing mother.

➤*Children:* Safety and efficacy in children have not been established.

Precautions

➤*Anticoagulant effects:* Because of the anticoagulant effect, do not give more than 50 mg over 10 minutes. If additional doses are needed, do not administer more than 100 mg over a 2-hour period.

Adverse Reactions

Sudden fall in blood pressure; bradycardia; transitory flushing and feeling of warmth; dyspnea; nausea; vomiting; lassitude; back pain in conscious patients undergoing such procedures as cardiac catheterization; anaphylaxis that may result in severe respiratory distress, capillary leak and noncardiogenic pulmonary edema (see Warnings); acute pulmonary hypertension; circulatory collapse; hypersensitivity (see Warnings).

Overdosage

➤*Symptoms:* Overdose of protamine sulfate may cause bleeding. Protamine has a weak anticoagulant effect caused by an interaction with platelets and with many proteins including fibrinogen. Distinguish this effect from the rebound anticoagulation that may occur 30 minutes to 18 hours following the reversal of heparin with protamine.

Rapid administration of protamine is more likely to result in bradycardia, dyspnea, a sensation of warmth, flushing, and severe hypotension. Hypertension also has occurred.

The median lethal dose of protamine sulfate in mice is 50 mg/kg. Serum concentrations of protamine sulfate are not clinically useful. Information is not available on the amount of drug in a single dose that is associated with overdosage or is likely to be life-threatening.

➤*Treatment:* In managing overdosage, consider the possibility of multiple drug overdoses, interaction among drugs, and unusual drug kinetics.

Replace blood loss with blood transfusions or fresh frozen plasma. If the patient is hypotensive, consider fluids, epinephrine, dobutamine, or dopamine. Refer to Management of Acute Overdosage.

ALTEPLASE, RECOMBINANT

Rx	Activase	Lyophilized powder for injection[1]: 50 mg	In vials with diluent (50 mL sterile water for injection) and vacuum.
	(Genentech)	(29 million U)	
		100 mg (58 million U)	In vials with diluent (100 mL sterile water for injection) and 1 transfer device.
Rx	Cathflo Activase (Genentech)	Lyophilized powder for injection[1]: 2 mg	In vials.

[1] With L-arginine, phosphoric acid, and polysorbate 80.

Indications

➤*Acute myocardial infarction (AMI) (Activase only):* For the management of AMI in adults for the improvement of ventricular function following AMI, the reduction of the incidence of congestive heart failure, and the reduction of mortality associated with AMI. Initiate treatment as soon as possible after the onset of AMI symptoms.

➤*Acute ischemic stroke (AIS) (Activase only):* For the management of AIS in adults for improving neurological recovery and reducing the incidence of disability. Initiate treatment only within 3 hours after the onset of stroke symptoms and after exclusion of intracranial hemorrhage (ICH) by a cranial computerized tomography (CT) scan or other diagnostic imaging method sensitive for the presence of hemorrhage (see Contraindications).

➤*Pulmonary embolism (PE) (Activase only):* For the management of acute massive PE in adults for the lysis of acute PE, defined as obstruction of blood flow to a lobe or multiple segments of the lungs, and for the lysis of PE accompanied by unstable hemodynamics (eg, failure to maintain blood pressure without supportive measures).

Confirm the diagnosis by objective means such as pulmonary angiography or noninvasive procedures such as lung scanning.

➤*Restoration of function to central venous access device (Cathflo Activase only):* For the restoration of function to central venous access devices as assessed by the ability to withdraw blood.

Administration and Dosage

➤*Approved by the FDA:* February 23, 1989 (*Activase*); September 4, 2001 (*Cathflo Activase*).

For IV administration only.

➤*Restoration of function to central venous catheter (Cathflo Activase only):* Instill into dysfunctional catheter at a concentration of 1 mg/mL. For patients weighing 30 kg or more, use 2 mg in 2 mL. For patients weighing 10 kg or more to less than 30 kg, use 110% of the internal lumen volume of the catheter, not to exceed 2 mg in 2 mL. If catheter function is not restored in 120 minutes after 1 dose, a second dose may be instilled.

➤*AMI:* Administer as soon as possible after the onset of symptoms. Do not use a dose of 150 mg because it has been associated with an increase in intracranial bleeding.

Accelerated infusion – The recommended total dose is based upon patient weight, not to exceed 100 mg. For patients weighing more than 67 kg, the recommended dose administered is 100 mg as a 15 mg IV bolus, followed by 50 mg infused over the next 30 minutes, and then 35 mg infused over the next 60 minutes.

For patients weighing 67 kg or less, the recommended dose is administered as a 15 mg IV bolus, followed by 0.75 mg/kg infused over the next 30 minutes not to exceed 50 mg, and then 0.50 mg/kg over the next 60 minutes not to exceed 35 mg.

The safety and efficacy of this accelerated infusion of alteplase regimen has only been investigated with coadministration of heparin and aspirin.

3-hour infusion – The recommended dose is 100 mg administered as 60 mg (34.8 million U) in the first hour (with 6 to 10 mg administered as a bolus), 20 mg (11.6 million U) over the second hour, and 20 mg (11.6 million U) over the third hour. For smaller patients (less than 65 kg), a dose of 1.25 mg/kg administered over 3 hours, as described above, may be used.

Coadministration – Although the use of anticoagulants during and following alteplase administration has not been fully studied, heparin has been administered concomitantly for 24 hours or longer in more than 90% of patients. Aspirin and/or dipyridamole has been given either during or following heparin treatment (see Drug Interactions).

➤*AIS:* The recommended dose is 0.9 mg/kg (not to exceed 90 mg total dose) infused over 60 minutes with 10% of the total dose administered as an initial IV bolus over 1 minute. The safety and efficacy of this regimen with coadministration of heparin and aspirin during the first 24 hours after symptom onset has not been investigated. Doses greater than 0.9 mg/kg may be associated with an increased incidence of ICH. Do not use doses greater than 0.9 mg/kg (maximum 90 mg) in the management of acute ischemic stroke.

➤*PE:* The recommended dose is 100 mg administered by IV infusion over 2 hours. Institute or reinstitute heparin therapy near the end of or immediately following the alteplase infusion when the partial thromboplastin time or thrombin time returns to twice normal or less.

➤*Reconstitution:* Reconstitute only with sterile water for injection without preservatives. Do not use bacteriostatic water for injection.

The reconstituted preparation results in a colorless to pale yellow, transparent solution. Slight foaming upon reconstitution is usual; standing undisturbed for several minutes is usually sufficient to allow dissipation of any large bubbles.

50 mg vial – Do not use if vacuum is not present. Reconstitute with a large bore needle (eg, 18-gauge), directing the stream of sterile water for injection into the lyophilized cake.

100 mg vial – Use transfer device provided for reconstitution. 100 mg vials do not contain vacuum.

➤*Admixture compatibility:* May be administered as reconstituted at 1 mg/mL. As an alternative, the reconstituted solution may be further diluted immediately before administration with an equal volume of 0.9% sodium chloride injection or 5% dextrose injection to yield a concentration of 0.5 mg/mL.

➤*Admixture incompatibilities:* Do not add other medications to infusion solution.

➤*Storage/Stability:* Store lyophilized alteplase at controlled room temperature not to exceed 30°C (86°F) or under refrigeration (2° to 8°C; 36° to 46°F). During extended storage, protect from excessive exposure to light. Discard any unused solution.

The solution may be used for direct IV administration within 8 hours following reconstitution when stored between 2° and 30°C (36° and 86°F). Avoid excessive agitation during dilution; mix by gentle swirling or slow inversion. Do not use other infusion solutions.

Actions

➤*Pharmacology:* Alteplase, a tissue plasminogen activator (tPA) produced by recombinant DNA, is synthesized using the complementary DNA for natural human tissue-type plasminogen activator obtained from a human melanoma cell line. Biological potency, determined by an in vitro clot lysis assay, is expressed in International Units. The specific activity is 580,000 IU/mg.

Alteplase is an enzyme (serine protease) that has the property of fibrin-enhanced conversion of plasminogen to plasmin. It produces limited conversion of plasminogen in the absence of fibrin. When introduced into the systemic circulation at pharmacologic concentration, alteplase binds to fibrin in a thrombus and converts the entrapped plasminogen to plasmin. This initiates local fibrinolysis with limited systemic proteolysis. Following administration of 100 mg, there is a decrease (16% to 36%) in circulating fibrinogen. In a controlled trial, 8 of 73 patients (11%) receiving alteplase (1.25 mg/kg over 3 hours) experienced a decrease in fibrinogen to below 100 mg/dL.

➤*Pharmacokinetics:*

Absorption/Distribution – Because of its large molecular size, alteplase cannot easily diffuse across biological membranes and must be given parenterally, usually IV. Maximal plasma concentrations of 3 to 4 mg/L are achieved after standard administration of 90 to 100 mg doses. Steady-state concentrations for the initial infusion period were 45% higher when administered in an accelerated regimen.

Metabolism/Excretion – Alteplase is cleared rapidly from plasma at a rate of 380 to 570 mL/min, primarily by the liver. More than 50% of the drug present in plasma is cleared within 5 minutes after the infusion has been terminated, and approximately 80% is cleared within 10 minutes. Initial volume of distribution is 2.8 to 4.6 L, and it approximately doubles at steady state. Total body clearance is 34.3 to 38.4 L/h.

➤*Clinical trials:*

Accelerated infusion in AMI patients – Accelerated infusion of alteplase was studied in an international, multi-center trial (GUSTO) that randomized 41,021 patients with AMI to 4 thrombolytic regimens. Entry criteria included onset of chest pain within 6 hours of treatment and ST segment elevation of ECG. The regimens included accelerated infusion of alteplase (100 mg or less over 90 minutes) plus IV heparin (n = 10,396); streptokinase (SK) (1.5 million U over 60 minutes) plus IV heparin (n = 10,410); or SK (as above) plus SC heparin (n = 9841). A fourth regimen combined alteplase and SK. Aspirin and heparin use was directed by the GUSTO study protocol as follows: All patients were to receive 160 mg chewable aspirin administered as soon as possible, followed by 160 to 325 mg/day. IV heparin was directed to be a 5000 U IV bolus initiated as soon as possible, followed by a 1000 U/h continuous IV infusion for at least 48 hours; subsequent heparin therapy was at the discretion of the attending physician. SC heparin was directed to be 12,500 U administered 4 hours after initiation of SK therapy, followed by 12,500 U twice daily for 7 days or until discharge, whichever came first.

Subgroup analysis of patients by age, infarct location, and time from symptom onset to thrombolytic treatment showed consistently lower

ALTEPLASE, RECOMBINANT

30-day mortality for the alteplase accelerated infusion group. For patients older than 75 years of age, a predefined subgroup of 12% of patients enrolled, the incidence of stroke was 4% for the alteplase accelerated infusion group, 2.8% for SK (IV), and 3.2% for SK (SC); the incidence of combined 30-day mortality and nonfatal stroke was 20.6% for accelerated infusion of alteplase, 21.5% for SK (IV), and 22% for SK (SC).

Pulmonary emboli – In a comparative, randomized trial (n = 45), 59% of patients treated with alteplase (100 mg over 2 hours) experienced moderate or marked lysis of pulmonary emboli when assessed by pulmonary angiography 2 hours after treatment initiation. Alteplase-treated patients also experienced a significant reduction in pulmonary embolism-induced pulmonary hypertension within 2 hours of treatment. Pulmonary perfusion at 24 hours was significantly improved.

Contraindications

Hypersensitivity to alteplase or any of the components.

➤*AMI or PE (Activase only):* Active internal bleeding; history of cerebrovascular accident; recent intracranial or intraspinal surgery or trauma; intracranial neoplasm, arteriovenous malformation, or aneurysm; bleeding diathesis; severe uncontrolled hypertension.

➤*AIS (Activase only):* Evidence of ICH on pretreatment evaluation; suspicion of subarachnoid hemorrhage; recent (within 3 months) intracranial or intraspinal surgery, serious head trauma, or previous stroke; history of ICH; uncontrolled hypertension at time of treatment (eg, greater than 185 mm Hg systolic or greater than 110 mm Hg diastolic); seizure at the onset of stroke; active internal bleeding; intracranial neoplasm, arteriovenous malformation, or aneurysm; bleeding diathesis.

➤*Bleeding diathesis:* Bleeding diathesis includes, but is not limited to: Current use of oral anticoagulants (eg, warfarin sodium) with prothrombin time (PT) longer than 15 seconds; administration of heparin within 48 hours preceding stroke onset with an elevated activated partial thromboplastin time (aPTT) at presentation; platelet count below 100,000/mm^3.

Warnings

➤*Bleeding:* Bleeding is the most common complication. The bleeding associated with thrombolytic therapy can be divided into 2 broad categories:

1.) Internal bleeding involving intracranial or retroperitoneal sites or the GI, GU, or respiratory tracts.
2.) Superficial or surface bleeding, observed mainly at invaded or disturbed sites (eg, venous cutdowns, arterial punctures, sites of recent surgical intervention).

The concomitant use of heparin anticoagulation may contribute to the bleeding. Some of the hemorrhagic episodes occurred 1 or more days after alteplase effects had dissipated but while heparin therapy was continuing.

As fibrin is lysed during alteplase therapy, bleeding from recent puncture sites may occur. Therefore, thrombolytic therapy requires careful attention to all potential bleeding sites (including catheter insertion sites, arterial and venous puncture sites, cutdown sites, and needle puncture sites). Avoid IM injections and nonessential handling of the patient during treatment with alteplase. Perform venipunctures carefully and only as required. Minimize arterial and venous punctures.

Should an arterial puncture be necessary during an infusion, it is preferable to use an upper extremity vessel accessible to manual compression. Apply pressure for at least 30 minutes, apply a pressure dressing, and check the puncture site frequently for bleeding evidence. Avoid noncompressible arterial puncture (ie, avoid internal jugular and subclavian venous punctures to minimize noncompressible site bleeding).

If serious bleeding (not controllable by local pressure) occurs, immediately terminate alteplase infusion and any concomitant heparin. Protamine can be given to reverse heparin effects.

In the following conditions, the risks of alteplase therapy may be increased and should be weighed against the anticipated benefits:
- Recent major surgery (eg, coronary artery bypass graft, obstetrical delivery, organ biopsy, previous puncture of noncompressible vessels)
- Cerebrovascular disease
- Recent GI or GU bleeding
- Recent trauma
- Hypertension: Systolic BP 175 mm Hg or more or diastolic BP 110 mm Hg or more
- Likelihood of left heart thrombus (eg, mitral stenosis with atrial fibrillation)
- Acute pericarditis
- Subacute bacterial endocarditis
- Hemostatic defects including those secondary to severe hepatic or renal disease
- Significant hepatic dysfunction
- Pregnancy
- Diabetic hemorrhagic retinopathy or other hemorrhagic ophthalmic conditions
- Septic thrombophlebitis or occluded AV cannula at seriously infected site

- Advanced age (eg, older than 75 years of age)
- Patients currently receiving oral anticoagulants (eg, warfarin sodium)
- Any other condition in which bleeding constitutes a significant hazard or would be particularly difficult to manage because of its location.

➤*Cholesterol embolism:* Cholesterol embolism has been reported rarely in patients treated with all thrombolytic agents; the incidence is unknown. This serious condition, which can be lethal, is associated with invasive vascular procedures (eg, cardiac catheterization, angiography, vascular surgery) or anticoagulant therapy. Clinical features of cholesterol embolism may include livedo reticularis, "purple toe" syndrome, acute renal failure, gangrenous digits, hypertension, pancreatitis, MI, cerebral infarction, spinal cord infarction, retinal artery occlusion, bowel infarction, and rhabdomyolysis.

➤*Arrhythmias:* Coronary thrombolysis may result in arrythmias associated with reperfusion. These arrhythmias (such as sinus bradycardia, accelerated idioventricular rhythm, ventricular premature depolarizations, ventricular tachycardia) are not different from those often seen in the ordinary course of AMI and may be managed with standard antiarrhythmic measures. Have antiarrhythmic therapy for bradycardia or ventricular irritability available when alteplase infusions are administered.

➤*PE:* The treatment of PE with alteplase has not been shown to constitute treatment of underlying deep vein thrombosis. Consider the possible risk of re-embolization caused by lysis of underlying deep venous thrombi.

➤*AMI:* In AMI patients who are at low risk of death from cardiac causes (ie, no previous myocardial infarction, Killip class I) and who have high blood pressure at the time of presentation, the risk for stroke may offset the survival benefit produced by thrombolytic therapy.

➤*AIS:* The risks of alteplase therapy to treat AIS may be increased in the following conditions and should be weighed against the anticipated benefits: Severe neurological deficit (eg, NIHSS greater than 22) at presentation (increases risk of ICH) and major early infarct signs on a CT scan (eg, substantial edema, mass effect, or midline shift).

In patients without recent use of oral anticoagulants or heparin, initiate alteplase treatment prior to the availability of coagulation study results. However, discontinue infusion if either a pretreatment PT longer than 15 seconds or an elevated aPTT is identified.

In AIS, neither the incidence of ICH nor the benefits of therapy are known in patients treated with alteplase more than 3 hours after the onset of symptoms. Therefore, do not treat patients with AIS more than 3 hours after symptom onset. Because of the increased risk for misdiagnosis of AIS, special diligence is required in making this diagnosis in patients whose blood glucose values are less than 50 mg/dL or greater than 400 mg/dL.

➤*Neurological deficit:* The safety and efficacy of treatment with alteplase in patients with minor neurological deficit or with rapidly improving symptoms prior to the start of alteplase administration has not been evaluated; therefore, treatment with alteplase is not recommended.

➤*Carcinogenesis:* Cytotoxicity, as reflected by a decrease in mitotic index, was evidenced only after prolonged exposure at high concentrations.

➤*Pregnancy: Category C.* Alteplase has been shown to have an embryocidal effect because of an increased postimplantation loss rate in rabbits when administered by IV at doses approximately 100 times (3 mg/kg) the human dose. There are no adequate and well-controlled studies in pregnant women. Use during pregnancy only if the potential benefit justifies the potential risk to the fetus.

➤*Lactation:* It is not known whether alteplase is excreted in human milk. Exercise caution when administering to nursing women.

➤*Children:* Safety and efficacy of alteplase in pediatric patients have not been established (*Activase*); safety and efficacy in patients younger than 2 years of age or who weigh less than 10 kg have not been established (*Cathflo Activase*).

Precautions

➤*Monitoring:* With coadministration of heparin or aspirin, monitor for bleeding especially at arterial puncture sites. Control and monitor blood pressure frequently during and following alteplase administration to manage AIS.

Heparin has been given with and after alteplase infusions to reduce risk of rethrombosis. Either heparin or alteplase may cause bleeding complications; carefully monitor for bleeding, especially at arterial puncture sites.

➤*Infection (Cathflo Activase only):* Use with caution in the presence of suspected infection in a catheter. Use during infection may release a localized infection into the systemic circulation.

➤*Hypersensitivity:* There is no experience with readministration of alteplase. If an anaphylactoid reaction occurs, discontinue the infusion immediately and initiate appropriate therapy. Refer to Management of Acute Hypersensitivity Reactions.

ALTEPLASE, RECOMBINANT

Sustained antibody formation in patients receiving 1 dose of alteplase has not been documented, but readminister with caution. Detectable antibody levels (single point measurement) were reported in 1 patient but subsequent antibody test results were negative.

➤*Lab test abnormalities:* During therapy, if coagulation tests or measures of fibrinolytic activity are performed, the results may be unreliable unless specific precautions are taken to prevent in vitro artifacts. Alteplase present in blood in pharmacologic concentrations remains active in vitro. This can lead to degradation of fibrinogen in blood samples removed for analysis. Collection of blood samples in the presence of aprotinin (150 to 200 units/mL) can, to some extent, mitigate this phenomenon.

Drug Interactions

➤*Anticoagulants:* A potential increased risk exists when alteplase is used concomitantly with heparin and vitamin K antagonists.

➤*Drugs affecting platelet function:* Drugs that alter platelet function (ie, aspirin, dipyridamole, and abciximab) may increase the risk of bleeding if administered prior to or after alteplase therapy.

➤*Nitroglycerin:* Concomitant use decreases alteplase concentrations, therefore decreasing thrombolytic effect. Avoid use of nitroglycerin with alteplase.

Adverse Reactions

Bleeding (most frequent) – Should serious bleeding in a critical location (intracranial, GI, retroperitoneal, pericardial) occur, immediately discontinue alteplase therapy along with any concomitant therapy with heparin.

Incidence of Significant Bleeding with Alteplase for 3-Hour Infusion Regimen	
	Total dose
Site of bleeding	≤ 100 mg/3 h
GI	5%
GU	4%
Ecchymosis	1%
Retroperitoneal	< 1%
Epistaxis	< 1%
Gingival	< 1%

The incidence of ICH in AMI patients treated with alteplase is as follows:

Incidence of Intracranial Bleeding in AMI Patients with Alteplase		
Dose	Patients	%
100 mg, 3 hours	3272	0.4
≤ 100 mg, accelerated	10,396	0.7
150 mg	1779	1.3
1 to 1.4 mg/kg	237	0.4

Accelerated infusion – All strokes (1.6%); nonfatal stroke (0.9%); hemorrhagic stroke (0.7%). The incidence of all strokes, as well as that for hemorrhagic stroke, increased with increasing age.

Hypersensitivity – Allergic-type reactions (eg, anaphylactoid reaction, laryngeal edema, orolingual angioedema, rash, and urticaria) have been reported. Most reports were of patients treated for AIS and some from treatment for AMI. Many of these patients received concomitant angiotensin-converting enzyme inhibitors (ACEIs). Most cases resolved with prompt treatment.

Other adverse reactions (Activase only) –
   AMI: Arrhythmia; AV block; cardiogenic shock; heart failure; cardiac arrest; recurrent ischemia; myocardial reinfarction; myocardial rupture; electromechanical dissociation; pericardial effusion; pericarditis; mitral regurgitation; cardiac tamponade; thromboembolism; pulmonary edema; nausea and/or vomiting; hypotension; fever.
   PE: Pulmonary re-embolization; pulmonary edema; pleural effusion; thromboembolism; hypotension; fever.
   AIS: Cerebral edema; cerebral herniation; seizure; new ischemic stroke.

Other adverse reactions (Cathflo Activase only) – GI bleeding; sepsis; venous thrombosis; death; major hemorrhage; ICH; pulmonary emboli; arterial emboli; injection-site hemorrhage; upper extremity deep venous thrombosis.

RETEPLASE, RECOMBINANT

Rx	**Retavase** (Centocor)	**Powder for injection, lyophilized:** 10.4 U (18.1 mg)	Preservative-free. In kits[1] and half-kits.[2]

[1] Each kit includes a package insert, 2 single-use reteplase vials of 10.4 U (18.1 mg), 2 single-use diluent vials for reconstitution (10 mL sterile water for injection), 2 sterile 10 mL syringes, 2 sterile dispensing pins, 4 sterile needles, and 2 alcohol swabs.

[2] Each half-kit includes a package insert, 1 single-use reteplase vial 10.4 U (18.1 mg), 1 single-use diluent vial for reconstitution (10 mL sterile water for injection), and a sterile dispensing pin.

Indications

➤*Acute myocardial infarction (AMI):* For the management of AMI in adults for the improvement of ventricular function following AMI, the reduction of the incidence of congestive heart failure (CHF), and the reduction of mortality associated with AMI. Initiate treatment as soon as possible after the onset of AMI symptoms.

➤*Unlabeled uses:* For clearance of occluded venous catheters; thrombolytic treatment of acute and chronic deep venous thrombosis (DVT); treatment of massive pulmonary embolism with a double bolus; use in conjunction with heparin and percutaneous transluminal angioplasty (PTA) in the treatment of thrombosed polytetrafluoroethylene hemodialysis arteriovenous grafts (AVGs).

Administration and Dosage

➤*Approved by the FDA:* October 30, 1996.

Reteplase is for IV administration only. Reteplase is administered as a 10 + 10 U double-bolus injection. Each bolus is administered as an IV injection over 2 minutes. The second bolus is given 30 minutes after initiation of the first bolus injection. Give each bolus injection via an IV line in which no other medication is being simultaneously injected or infused. Do not add any other medications to the injection solution.

➤*Admixture incompatibility:* Do not administer heparin and reteplase simultaneously in the same IV line. If reteplase is to be injected through an IV line containing heparin, flush normal saline or 5% dextrose solution through the line prior to and following the reteplase injection.

➤*Reconstitution:* Reconstitute only with sterile water for injection (without preservatives) immediately before use. The reconstituted preparation results in a colorless solution containing 1 U/mL. Slight foaming is not unusual; allowing the vial to stand undisturbed for several minutes will usually allow dissipation of any large bubbles.

➤*Storage/Stability:* Use the solution within 4 hours after reconstitution. Store at 2° to 30°C (36° to 86°F). Keep kit sealed prior to use to protect lyophilisate from light. Store reteplase at 2° to 25°C (36° to 77°F).

Actions

➤*Pharmacology:* Reteplase is a nonglycosylated deletion mutein of tissue plasminogen activator (tPA) containing 355 of the 527 amino acids of native tPA. It is produced by recombinant DNA technology in *Escherichia coli*. It catalyzes the cleavage of endogenous plasminogen to generate plasmin. Plasmin in turn degrades the fibrin matrix of the thrombus, thereby exerting its thrombolytic action.

➤*Pharmacokinetics:* Based on the measurement of thrombolytic activity, reteplase is cleared from plasma at a rate of 250 to 450 mL/min, with an effective half-life of 13 to 16 minutes. Reteplase is cleared primarily by the liver and kidney.

➤*Clinical trials:* In 3 studies, patients were treated with aspirin (initial doses of 160 to 350 mg and subsequent doses of 75 to 350 mg) and heparin (a 5000 U IV bolus prior to administration of reteplase followed by a 1000 U/h continuous IV infusion for at least 24 hours).

Reteplase vs streptokinase – Reteplase (10 + 10 U) was compared with streptokinase (1.5 million units over 60 minutes) in a double-blind, randomized, European study. Effects upon mortality rates at 35 days were studied in 6010 patients treated within 12 hours of the symptom onset of AMI.

Incidence of Selected Outcomes				
Endpoint	Reteplase (n = 2965)	Streptokinase (n = 2971)	Reteplase-Streptokinase difference (95% CI)	P value
35-day mortality	8.9%	9.4%	−0.5	0.49[1]
6-month mortality	11%	12.1%	−1.1	0.22
Combined outcome of 35-day mortality or non-fatal stroke within 35 days	9.6%	10.2%	−0.6	0.47
Heart failure	24.8%	28.1%	−3.3	0.004
Cardiogenic shock	4.6%	5.8%	−1.2	0.03
Any stroke	1.4%	1.1%	0.3	0.34
Intracranial hemorrhage	0.8%	0.4%	0.4	0.04

[1] P value for the exploratory analysis comparing reteplase vs streptokinase.

RETEPLASE, RECOMBINANT

For mortality, stroke, and the combined outcome of mortality or stroke, the 95% confidence intervals in the table reflect the range within which the true difference in outcomes probably lies and includes the possibility of no difference. The incidences of CHF and of cardiogenic shock were significantly lower among patients treated with reteplase.

The total incidence of stroke was similar between the groups. However, more patients treated with reteplase experienced hemorrhagic strokes than patients treated with streptokinase. An exploratory analysis indicated that the incidence of intracranial hemorrhage was higher among older patients or those with elevated BP. The incidence of intracranial hemorrhage among the 698 patients treated with reteplase who were older than 70 years of age was 2.2%. Intracranial hemorrhage occurred in 2.4% patients treated with reteplase who had an initial systolic BP greater than 160 mm Hg and in 0.6% reteplase patients who had an initial systolic BP less than 160 mm Hg.

Reteplase vs alteplase – Two arteriographic studies were performed using open-label administration of the study agents and a blinded review of the arteriograms. Patients were treated within either 6 or 12 hours of the onset of symptoms. In the first study, reteplase (in doses of 10 + 10 U, 15 U, or 10 + 5 U) was compared with a 3-hour regimen of alteplase (100 mg administered over 3 hours). In the second study, reteplase (10 + 10 U) was compared with an accelerated regimen of alteplase (100 mg administered over 1.5 hours). The follow-up arteriogram was performed at a median of 8 (study 1) and 5 (study 2) days following the administration of the thrombolytics. In study 1, the best patency results were obtained with the 10 + 10 U reteplase dose. In study 2, the percentage of patients with partial or complete flow and the percentage of patients with complete flow was significantly higher with reteplase than with alteplase at 90 minutes after the initiation of therapy. In both clinical trials, the reocclusion rates were similar for reteplase and alteplase.

Contraindications

Active internal bleeding; history of cerebrovascular accident; recent intracranial or intraspinal surgery or trauma (see Warnings); intracranial neoplasm, arteriovenous malformation, or aneurysm; bleeding diathesis or severe uncontrolled hypertension because thrombolytic therapy increases the risk of bleeding.

Warnings

➤*Bleeding:* The most common complication encountered during therapy is bleeding. Bleeding sites include both internal sites (intracranial, retroperitoneal, GI, GU, respiratory) and superficial sites (venous cutdowns, arterial punctures, sites of recent surgical intervention). The concomitant use of heparin anticoagulation may contribute to bleeding. In clinical trials, some of the hemorrhage episodes occurred 1 or more days after the effects of reteplase had dissipated but while heparin therapy was continuing. Should serious bleeding (not controllable by local pressure) occur, immediately terminate concomitant anticoagulant therapy. In addition, do not give the second bolus of reteplase if serious bleeding occurs before it is administered.

The overall incidence of any bleeding event in patients treated with reteplase in clinical studies (n = 3805) was 21.1%. The severity and sites of bleeding events were comparable for reteplase and the thrombolytic agents.

Injection sites – As fibrin is lysed during reteplase therapy, bleeding from recent puncture sites may occur. Therefore, thrombolytic therapy requires careful attention to all potential bleeding sites (including catheter insertion sites, arterial and venous puncture sites, cutdown sites, and needle puncture sites). Avoid noncompressible arterial puncture and internal jugular and subclavian venous punctures to minimize bleeding from noncompressible sites. Should an arterial puncture be necessary during the administration of reteplase, it is preferable to use an upper extremity vessel accessible to manual compression. Apply pressure for at least 30 minutes, apply a pressure dressing, and check the puncture site frequently for evidence of bleeding.

IM injections: Avoid IM injections and nonessential handling of the patient during treatment. Perform venipunctures carefully and only as required.

High-risk conditions – Carefully evaluate each patient being considered for reteplase therapy and weigh the benefits against the potential risks. In the following conditions, the risks of reteplase therapy may be increased and should be weighed against the anticipated benefits:

- Recent major surgery (eg, coronary artery bypass graft, obstetrical delivery, organ biopsy)
- Previous puncture of noncompressible vessels
- Cerebrovascular disease
- Recent GI or GU bleeding
- Recent trauma
- Hypertension: Systolic BP 180 mm Hg or greater or diastolic BP 110 mm Hg or greater
- Likelihood of left heart thrombus (eg, mitral stenosis with atrial fibrillation)
- Acute pericarditis
- Subacute bacterial endocarditis

- Hemostatic defects including those secondary to severe hepatic or renal disease
- Severe hepatic or renal dysfunction
- Pregnancy
- Diabetic hemorrhagic retinopathy or other ophthalmic hemorrhaging conditions
- Septic thrombophlebitis or occluded AV cannula at a seriously infected site
- Advanced age
- Patients currently receiving oral anticoagulants (eg, warfarin sodium)
- Any other condition in which bleeding constitutes a significant hazard or would be particularly difficult to manage because of its location

➤*Cholesterol embolization:* Cholesterol embolism has been reported rarely in patients treated with thrombolytic agents; the true incidence is unknown. This serious condition, which can be lethal, is also associated with invasive vascular procedures (eg, cardiac catheterization, angiography, vascular surgery) or anticoagulant therapy. Clinical features of cholesterol embolism may include livedo reticularis, "purple toe" syndrome, acute renal failure, gangrenous digits, hypertension, pancreatitis, MI, cerebral infarction, spinal cord infarction, retinal artery occlusion, bowel infarction, and rhabdomyolysis.

➤*Arrhythmias:* Coronary thrombolysis may result in arrhythmias associated with reperfusion. These arrhythmias (eg, sinus bradycardia, accelerated idioventricular rhythm, ventricular premature depolarizations, ventricular tachycardia) are not different from those often seen in the ordinary course of AMI and should be managed with standard antiarrhythmic measures. Have antiarrhythmic therapy for bradycardia or ventricular irritability available when reteplase is administered.

➤*Pregnancy:* Category C. There are no adequate and well-controlled studies in pregnant women. The most common complication of thrombolytic therapy is bleeding; certain conditions, including pregnancy, can increase this risk. Use reteplase during pregnancy only if the potential benefit justifies the potential risk to the fetus.

➤*Lactation:* It is not known whether reteplase is excreted in human milk. Exercise caution when reteplase is administered to a nursing woman.

➤*Children:* Safety and efficacy of reteplase in pediatric patients have not been established.

Precautions

➤*Monitoring:* Heparin and aspirin have been administered concomitantly with and following the administration of reteplase in the management of AMI. Because heparin, aspirin, or reteplase may cause bleeding complications, careful monitoring for bleeding is advised, especially at arterial puncture sites.

➤*Readministration:* There is no experience with patients receiving repeat courses of therapy with reteplase. Reteplase did not induce the formation of reteplase-specific antibodies in any of the approximately 2400 patients who were tested for antibody formation. If an anaphylactoid reaction occurs, initiate appropriate therapy and do not give the second bolus of reteplase.

Drug Interactions

➤*Drugs affecting platelet function:* Drugs that alter platelet function (aspirin, dipyridamole, abciximab) may increase the risk of bleeding if administered prior to or after reteplase therapy.

➤*Anticoagulants:* A potential increased risk exists when alteplase is used concomitantly with heparin and vitamin K antagonists.

➤*Drug/Lab test interactions:* Administration of reteplase may cause decreases in plasminogen and fibrinogen. During reteplase therapy, if coagulation tests or measurements of fibrinolytic activity are performed, the results may be unreliable unless specific precautions are taken to prevent in vitro artifacts. Reteplase is an enzyme that, when present in blood in pharmacologic concentrations, remains active under in vitro conditions. This can lead to degradation of fibrinogen in blood samples removed for analysis. Collection of blood samples in the presence of PPACK (chloromethylketone) at 2 micromolar concentrations was used in clinical trials to prevent in vitro fibrinolytic artifacts.

Adverse Reactions

Bleeding – The most frequent adverse event was bleeding. The types of bleeding associated with reteplase are shown in the table below.

Reteplase Hemorrhage Rates (%)	
Bleeding site[1]	Occurrence rate
Injection site[2]	4.6 to 48.6
GI	1.8 to 9
GU	0.9 to 9.5
Anemia, site unknown	0.9 to 2.6
Intracranial hemorrhage	0.8 to 2.4

[1] See Warnings.
[2] Includes the arterial catheterization sites.

RETEPLASE, RECOMBINANT

The following adverse events are frequent sequelae of MI and may not be attributable to therapy:

➤*Cardiovascular:* Cardiogenic shock; arrhythmias (eg, sinus bradycardia, accelerated idioventricular rhythm, ventricular premature depolarizations, supraventricular tachycardia, ventricular tachycardia, ventricular fibrillation); AV block; heart failure; cardiac arrest; recurrent ischemia; reinfarction; myocardial rupture; mitral regurgitation; pericardial effusion; pericarditis; cardiac tamponade; hypotension; electromechanical dissociation.

➤*Miscellaneous:* Pulmonary edema; venous thrombosis and embolism; nausea; vomiting; fever; serious allergic or anaphylactoid reactions (rare).

TENECTEPLASE

| Rx | TNKase (Genentech) | Powder for Injection, lyophilized: 50 mg | In vials[1] with one 10 mL vial of Sterile Water for Injection and syringe. |

[1] With 0.55 g L-arginine, 0.17 g phosphoric acid, 4.3 mg polysorbate 20.

Indications

➤*Acute myocardial infarction (AMI):* For use in the reduction of mortality associated with AMI. Initiate treatment as soon as possible after the onset of AMI symptoms.

Administration and Dosage

➤*Approved by the FDA:* June 2, 2000.

Tenecteplase is for IV administration only. Do not exceed the recommended total dose of 50 mg. Base the dose upon patient weight. Initiate treatment as soon as possible after the onset of AMI symptoms.

Tenecteplase Single Bolus Dosage		
Patient weight (kg)	Tenecteplase (mg)	Volume tenecteplase[1] to be administered as a single bolus dose over 5 seconds (mL)
< 60	30	6
≥ 60 to < 70	35	7
≥ 70 to < 80	40	8
≥ 80 to < 90	45	9
≥ 90	50	10

[1] From one vial of tenecteplase reconstituted with 10 mL Sterile Water for Injection.

➤*Reconstitution:*

1.) Aseptically withdraw 10 mL of Sterile Water for Injection from the supplied diluent vial using the red hub cannula syringe filling device. Do not use Bacteriostatic Water for Injection. Do not discard shield assembly.
2.) Inject the entire contents of the syringe (10 mL) into the tenecteplase vial directing the diluent stream into the powder. Slight foaming upon reconstitution is not unusual; any large bubbles will dissipate if the product is allowed to stand undisturbed for several minutes.
3.) Gently swirl until contents are completely dissolved. Do not shake. The reconstituted preparation results in a colorless to pale yellow transparent solution containing tenecteplase at 5 mg/mL at a pH of ≈ 7.3.
4.) Determine the appropriate dose of tenecteplase (see table) and withdraw this volume (in mL) from the reconstituted vial with the syringe. Discard any unused solution.
5.) With the appropriate dose of tenecteplase in the syringe, stand the shield vertically on a flat surface (with green side down) and passively recap the red hub cannula.
6.) Remove the entire shield assembly, including the red hub cannula, by twisting counter clockwise. Note: the shield assembly also contains the clear-ended blunt plastic cannula; retain for split septum IV access.

Administer as a single IV bolus over 5 seconds. Because tenecteplase contains no antibacterial preservatives, reconstitute immediately before use.

➤*Compatibility:* Precipitation may occur when tenecteplase is administered in an IV line containing dextrose. Flush dextrose-containing lines with a saline-containing solution prior to and following single bolus administration of tenecteplase.

➤*Storage/Stability:* Store lyophilized tenecteplase at controlled room temperature not to exceed 30°C (86°F) or under refrigeration 2° to 8°C (36° to 46°F). Do not use beyond the expiration date stamped on the vial.

If the reconstituted tenecteplase is not used immediately, refrigerate the tenecteplase vial at 2° to 8°C (36° to 46°F) and use within 8 hours.

Actions

➤*Pharmacology:* Tenecteplase is a tissue plasminogen activator (tPA) produced by recombinant DNA that binds to fibrin and converts plasminogen to plasmin. In the presence of fibrin, in vitro studies demonstrate that tenecteplase conversion of plasminogen to plasmin is increased relative to its conversion in the absence of fibrin. This fibrin specificity decreases systemic activation of plasminogen and the resulting degradation of circulating fibrinogen as compared with a molecule lacking this property. Following administration of 30, 40, or 50 mg of tenecteplase, there are decreases in circulating fibrinogen (4% to 15%) and plasminogen (11% to 24%). The clinical significance of fibrin specificity on safety (eg, bleeding) or efficacy has not been established. Biological potency is determined by an in vitro clot lysis assay and is expressed in tenecteplase-specific units. The specific activity of tenecteplase has been defined as 200 units/mg.

➤*Pharmacokinetics:* In patients with AMI, tenecteplase administered as a single bolus exhibits a biphasic disposition from the plasma. Tenecteplase was cleared from the plasma with an initial half-life of 20 to 24 minutes. The terminal phase half-life of tenecteplase was 90 to 130 minutes. Liver metabolism is the major clearance mechanism for tenecteplase. In 99 of 104 patients treated with tenecteplase, mean plasma clearance ranged from 99 to 119 mL/min. The initial volume of distribution is weight-related and approximates plasma volume.

Contraindications

Tenecteplase is contraindicated in the following situations because of an increased risk of bleeding: Active internal bleeding; history of cerebrovascular accident; intracranial or intraspinal surgery or trauma within 2 months; intracranial neoplasm, arteriovenous malformation, or aneurysm; known bleeding diathesis; severe uncontrolled hypertension.

Warnings

➤*Bleeding:* The most common complication encountered during tenecteplase therapy is bleeding. The type of bleeding associated with thrombolytic therapy can be divided into 2 broad categories:
- Internal bleeding, involving intracranial and retroperitoneal sites, or the GI, GU, or respiratory tracts.
- Superficial or surface bleeding, observed mainly at vascular puncture and access sites (eg, venous cutdowns, arterial punctures) or sites of recent surgical intervention.

If serious bleeding (not controlled by local pressure) occurs, immediately discontinue any concomitant heparin or antiplatelet agents.

Heparin may contribute to the bleeding risks associated with tenecteplase.

High risk conditions – Carefully evaluate each patient being considered for therapy with tenecteplase and weigh the benefits against the potential risks. In the following conditions, weigh the increased risk of tenecteplase therapy against the anticipated benefits:
- Recent major surgery (eg, coronary artery bypass graft, obstetrical delivery, organ biopsy)
- Previous puncture of noncompressible vessels
- Cerebrovascular disease
- Recent GI or GU bleeding
- Recent trauma
- Hypertension: Systolic BP ≥ 180 mmHg or diastolic BP ≥ 110 mmHg
- High likelihood of left heart thrombus (eg, mitral stenosis with atrial fibrillation)
- Acute pericarditis
- Subacute bacterial endocarditis
- Hemostatic defects, including those secondary to severe hepatic or renal disease
- Severe hepatic dysfunction
- Pregnancy
- Diabetic hemorrhagic retinopathy or other hemorrhagic ophthalmic conditions
- Septic thrombophlebitis or occluded AV cannula at seriously infected site
- Advanced age
- Patients currently receiving oral anticoagulants (eg, warfarin sodium)
- Recent administration of GP IIb/IIIa inhibitors
- Any other condition in which bleeding constitutes a significant hazard or would be particularly difficult to manage because of its location

IM injections – Avoid IM injections and nonessential handling of the patient for the first few hours following treatment with tenecteplase. Perform and monitor venipunctures carefully.

Injection sites – Use an upper extremity vessel that is accessible to manual compression if an arterial puncture becomes necessary during the first few hours following tenecteplase therapy. Apply pressure for ≥ 30 minutes, apply a pressure dressing, and check the puncture site frequently for evidence of bleeding.

TENECTEPLASE

➤*Cholesterol embolization:* Cholesterol embolism has been reported rarely in patients treated with all types of thrombolytic agents; the true incidence is unknown. This serious condition, which can be lethal, is also associated with invasive vascular procedures (eg, cardiac catheterization, angiography, vascular surgery) or anticoagulant therapy. Clinical features of cholesterol embolism may include livedo reticularis, "purple toe" syndrome, acute renal failure, gangrenous digits, hypertension, pancreatitis, MI, cerebral infarction, spinal cord infarction, retinal artery occlusion, bowel infarction, and rhabdomyolysis.

➤*Arrhythmias:* Coronary thrombolysis may result in arrhythmias associated with reperfusion. These arrhythmias (eg, sinus bradycardia, accelerated idioventricular rhythm, ventricular premature depolarizations, ventricular tachycardia) are not different from those often seen in the ordinary course of acute MI and may be managed with standard antiarrhythmic measures. Have antiarrhythmic therapy for bradycardia or ventricular irritability available when tenecteplase is administered.

➤*Elderly:* In elderly patients, weigh the benefits of tenecteplase on mortality against the risk of increased adverse events, including bleeding.

➤*Pregnancy: Category C.* Tenecteplase has been shown to elicit maternal and embryo toxicity in rabbits given multiple IV administration. In rabbits administered 0.5, 1.5, and 5 mg/kg/day, vaginal hemorrhage resulted in maternal deaths. Subsequent embryonic deaths were secondary to maternal hemorrhage and no fetal anomalies were observed. Tenecteplase does not elicit maternal and embryo toxicity in rabbits following a single IV administration. Thus, in developmental toxicity studies conducted in rabbits, the no-observable-effect level of a single IV administration of tenecteplase on maternal or developmental toxicity was 5 mg/kg (≈ 8 to 10 times the human dose). There are no adequate and well-controlled studies in pregnant women. Use tenecteplase only if the potential benefits justify the potential risk to the fetus.

➤*Lactation:* It is not known if tenecteplase is excreted in breast milk. Because many drugs are excreted in breast milk, exercise caution when tenecteplase is administered to a nursing woman.

➤*Children:* Safety and efficacy of tenecteplase in pediatric patients have not been established.

Precautions

➤*Readministration:* Readministration of plasminogen activators, including tenecteplase, to patients who have received prior plasminogen activator therapy has not been systematically studied. Although sustained antibody formation in patients receiving 1 dose of tenecteplase has not been documented, readministration should be undertaken with caution. Administer appropriate therapy if an anaphylactic reaction occurs.

Drug Interactions

Formal interaction studies of tenecteplase with other drugs have not been performed. Patients studied in clinical trials of tenecteplase were routinely treated with heparin and aspirin. Anticoagulants (such as heparin and vitamin K antagonists) and drugs that alter platelet function (such as acetylsalicylic acid, dipyridamole, and GP IIb/IIIa inhibitors) may increase the risk of bleeding if administered prior to, during, or after tenecteplase therapy.

➤*Drug/Lab test interactions:* During tenecteplase therapy, results of coagulation tests or measures of fibrinolytic activity may be unreliable unless specific precautions are taken to prevent in vitro artifacts. Tenecteplase is an enzyme that, when present in blood in pharmacologic concentrations, remains active under in vitro conditions. This can lead to degradation of fibrinogen in blood samples removed for analysis.

Adverse Reactions

Bleeding – The most frequent adverse reaction associated with tenecteplase is bleeding. Types of major bleeding reported in ≥ 1% of the patients were hematoma (1.7%) and GI tract (1%). Types of major bleeding reported in < 1% of the patients were urinary tract, puncture site (including cardiac catheterization site), retroperitoneal, respiratory tract, and unspecified. Types of minor bleeding reported in ≥ 1% of the patients were hematoma (12.3%), urinary tract (3.7%), puncture site (including cardiac catheterization site) (3.6%), pharyngeal (3.1%), GI tract (1.9%), epistaxis (1.5%), and unspecified (1.3%).

➤*Other adverse reactions:* The following adverse reactions have been reported among patients receiving tenecteplase in clinical trials. These reactions are frequent sequelae of the underlying disease, and the effect of tenecteplase on the incidence of these events is unknown.

Cardiovascular – Cardiogenic shock; arrhythmias; atrioventricular block; heart failure; cardiac arrest; recurrent myocardial ischemia; myocardial reinfarction; myocardial rupture; cardiac tamponade; pericarditis; pericardial effusion; mitral regurgitation; thrombosis; embolism; and electromechanical dissociation.

Miscellaneous – Pulmonary edema; nausea/vomiting; hypotension; fever; serious allergic or anaphylactoid reactions (rare).

DROTRECOGIN ALFA (ACTIVATED)

| *Rx* | **Xigris** (Eli Lilly) | **Powder for infusion, lyophilized:** 5 mg | Preservative-free. Sodium chloride, sucrose. In single-use vials. |
| | | 20 mg | Preservative-free. Sodium chloride, sucrose. In single-use vials. |

Indications

▶*Sepsis:* Reduction of mortality in adult patients with severe sepsis (sepsis associated with acute organ dysfunction) who have a high risk of death.

Efficacy has not been established in adult patients with severe sepsis and lower risk of death. Safety and efficacy have not been established in pediatric patients with severe sepsis.

Administration and Dosage

▶*Approved by the FDA:* November 21, 2001.

Administer IV at an infusion rate of 24 mcg/kg/hr for a total infusion duration of 96 hours. Dose adjustment based on clinical or laboratory parameters is not recommended.

If the infusion is interrupted, restart drotrecogin alfa at the 24 mcg/kg/hr infusion rate. Dose escalation or bolus doses of drotrecogin alfa are not recommended.

In the event of clinically important bleeding, immediately stop the infusion (see Warnings).

▶*Preparation and administration instructions:*
1.) Use appropriate aseptic technique during the preparation of drotrecogin alfa for IV administration.
2.) Calculate the dose and number of drotrecogin alfa vials needed. Each vial contains 5 or 20 mg drotrecogin alfa. The vial contains an excess of drotrecogin alfa to facilitate delivery of the label amount.
3.) Prior to administration, 5 mg vials must be reconstituted with 2.5 mL Sterile Water for Injection and 20 mg vials must be reconstituted with 10 mL Sterile Water for Injection. The resulting concentration of the solution is ≈ 2 mg/mL of drotrecogin alfa. Slowly add the Sterile Water for Injection to the vial and avoid inverting or shaking the vial. Gently swirl each vial until the powder is completely dissolved.
4.) The solution of reconstituted drotrecogin alfa must be further diluted with sterile 0.9% Sodium Chloride Injection. Slowly withdraw the appropriate amount of reconstituted drotrecogin alfa solution from the vial. Add the reconstituted drotrecogin alfa into a prepared infusion bag of sterile 0.9% Sodium Chloride Injection. When adding the drotrecogin alfa into the infusion bag, direct the stream to the side of the bag to minimize the agitation of the solution. Gently invert the infusion bag to obtain a homogeneous solution. Do not transport the infusion bag between locations using mechanical delivery systems.
5.) Because drotrecogin alfa contains no antibacterial preservatives, immediately prepare the IV solution upon reconstitution of the drotrecogin alfa in the vial. If the vial of reconstituted drotrecogin alfa is not used immediately, it may be held at controlled room temperature (15° to 30°C; 59° to 86°F), but must be used within 3 hours. IV administration must be completed within 12 hours after the IV solution is prepared.
6.) Inspect parenteral drug products visually for particulate matter and discoloration prior to administration.
7.) When using an IV infusion pump to administer the drug, the solution of reconstituted drotrecogin alfa is typically diluted into an infusion bag containing sterile 0.9% Sodium Chloride Injection to a final concentration of between 100 and 200 mcg/mL.
8.) When using a syringe pump to administer the drug, the solution of reconstituted drotrecogin alfa is typically diluted with sterile 0.9% Sodium Chloride Injection to a final concentration of between 100 and 1000 mcg/mL. When administering drotrecogin alfa at low concentrations (less than ≈ 200 mcg/mL) at low flow rates (less than ≈ 5 mL/hr), the infusion set must be primed for ≈ 15 minutes at a flow rate of ≈ 5 mL/hr.
9.) Administer drotrecogin alfa via a dedicated IV line or a dedicated lumen of a multilumen central venous catheter. The only other solutions that can be administered through the same line are 0.9% Sodium Chloride Injection, Lactated Ringer's Injection, Dextrose, or Dextrose and Saline mixtures.
10.) Avoid exposing drotrecogin alfa solutions to heat and direct sunlight. No incompatibilities have been observed between drotrecogin alfa and glass infusion bottles or infusion bags and syringes made of polyvinylchloride, polyethylene, polypropylene, or polyolefin.

▶*Storage/Stability:* Refrigerate at 2° to 8°C (36° to 46°F). Do not freeze. Protect unreconstituted vials from light. Retain in carton until time of use. Do not use beyond the expiration date stamped on the vial.

Actions

▶*Pharmacology:* Activated Protein C exerts an antithrombotic effect by inhibiting Factors Va and VIIIa. In vitro data indicate that Activated Protein C has indirect profibrinolytic activity through its ability to inhibit plasminogen activator inhibitor-1 (PAI-1) and limiting generation of activated thrombin-activatable-fibrinolysis-inhibitor. Additionally, in vitro data indicate that Activated Protein C may exert an anti-inflammatory effect by inhibiting human tumor necrosis factor production by monocytes, by blocking leukocyte adhesion to selectins, and by limiting the thrombin-induced inflammatory responses within the microvascular endothelium.

▶*Pharmacokinetics:* Drotrecogin alfa and endogenous Activated Protein C are inactivated by endogenous plasma protease inhibitors. Plasma concentrations of endogenous Activated Protein C in healthy subjects and patients with severe sepsis are usually below detection limits.

In patients with severe sepsis, drotrecogin alfa infusions of 12 to 30 mcg/kg/hr rapidly produce steady-state concentrations (C_{ss}) that are proportional to infusion rates. In the Phase 3 trial, the median clearance of drotrecogin alfa was 40 L/hr (interquartile range, 27 to 52 L/hr). The median C_{ss} of 45 ng/mL (interquartile range, 35 to 62 ng/mL) was attained within 2 hours after starting infusion. In the majority of patients, plasma concentrations of drotrecogin alfa fell below the assay's quantitation limit of 10 ng/mL within 2 hours after stopping infusion. Plasma clearance of drotrecogin alfa in patients with severe sepsis is ≈ 50% higher than that in healthy subjects.

Special populations – In adult patients with severe sepsis, small differences were detected in the plasma clearance of drotrecogin alfa with regard to age, gender, hepatic dysfunction, or renal dysfunction. Dose adjustment is not required based on these factors alone or in combination.

Contraindications

Drotrecogin alfa increases the risk of bleeding and is contraindicated in patients with the following clinical situations in which bleeding could be associated with a high risk of death or significant morbidity:
• Active internal bleeding;
• recent (within 3 months) hemorrhagic stroke;
• recent (within 2 months) intracranial or intraspinal surgery or severe head trauma;
• trauma with an increased risk of life-threatening bleeding;
• presence of an epidural catheter;
• intracranial neoplasm or mass lesion or evidence of cerebral herniation.

Drotrecogin alfa is contraindicated in patients with known hypersensitivity to drotrecogin alfa (activated) or any component of the product.

Warnings

▶*Bleeding:* Bleeding is the most common serious adverse effect associated with drotrecogin alfa therapy. Carefully evaluate each patient being considered for therapy with drotrecogin alfa and weigh anticipated benefits against potential risks associated with therapy.

Certain conditions, many of which led to exclusion from the Phase 3 trial, are likely to increase the risk of bleeding with drotrecogin alfa therapy. Therefore, for patients with severe sepsis who have ≥ 1 of the following conditions, carefully consider the increased risk of bleeding when deciding to use drotrecogin alfa therapy:
• Concurrent therapeutic heparin (≥ 15 units/kg/hr);
• platelet count < 30,000 × 10⁶/L, even if the platelet count is increased after transfusions;
• prothrombin time-INR > 3;
• recent (within 6 weeks) GI bleeding;
• recent administration (within 3 days) of thrombolytic therapy;
• recent administration (within 7 days) of oral anticoagulants or glycoprotein IIb/IIIa inhibitors;
• recent adminstration (within 7 days) of aspirin > 650 mg/day or other platelet inhibitors;
• recent (within 3 months) ischemic stroke (see Contraindications);
• intracranial arteriovenous malformation or aneurysm;
• known bleeding diathesis;
• chronic severe hepatic disease; or
• any other condition in which bleeding constitutes a significant hazard or would be particularly difficult to manage because of its location.

Should clinically important bleeding occur, immediately stop the infusion of drotrecogin alfa. Carefully assess continued use of other agents affecting the coagulation system. Once adequate hemostasis has been achieved, continued use of drotrecogin alfa may be reconsidered.

Discontinue drotrecogin alfa 2 hours prior to undergoing an invasive surgical procedure or procedures with an inherent risk of bleeding. Once adequate hemostasis has been achieved, initiation of drotrecogin alfa may be reconsidered 12 hours after major invasive procedures or surgery or restarted immediately after uncomplicated less invasive procedures.

Recombinant Human Activated Protein C

DROTRECOGIN ALFA (ACTIVATED)

➤*Pregnancy: Category C.* Animal reproductive studies have not been conducted with drotrecogin alfa. It is not known whether drotrecogin alfa can cause fetal harm when administered to a pregnant woman or can affect reproduction capacity. Give drotrecogin alfa to a pregnant woman only if clearly needed.

➤*Lactation:* It is not known whether drotrecogin alfa is excreted in human milk or absorbed systemically after ingestion. Because many drugs are excreted in human milk, and because of the potential for adverse effects on the nursing infant, a decision should be made whether to discontinue nursing or discontinue the drug, taking into account the importance of the drug to the mother.

➤*Children:* The safety and efficacy of drotrecogin alfa have not been established in the age group newborn (38 weeks gestational age) to 18 years of age. The efficacy of drotrecogin alfa in adult patients with severe sepsis and high risk of death cannot be extrapolated to pediatric patients with severe sepsis.

Precautions

➤*Immunogenicity:* As with all therapeutic proteins, there is a potential for immunogenicity. The incidence of antibody development in patients receiving drotrecogin alfa has not been adequately determined, as the assay sensitivity is inadequate to reliably detect all potential antibody responses. One patient in the Phase 2 trial developed antibodies to drotrecogin alfa without clinical sequelae. One patient in the Phase 3 trial who developed antibodies to drotrecogin alfa developed superficial and deep vein thrombi during the study and died of multi-organ failure on day 36 posttreatment, but the relationship of this event to antibody is not clear.

Drotrecogin alfa has not been readministered to patients with severe sepsis.

➤*Lab test abnormalities:* Most patients with severe sepsis have a coagulopathy that is commonly associated with prolongation of the activated partial thromboplastin time (aPTT) and the prothrombin time (PT). drotrecogin alfa may variably prolong the aPTT. Therefore, the aPTT cannot be reliably used to assess the status of the coagulopathy during drotrecogin alfa infusion. Drotrecogin alfa has minimal effect on the PT and the PT can be used to monitor the status of the coagulopathy in these patients.

Drug Interactions

Drug interactions with drotrecogin alfa have not been studied in patients with severe sepsis. Use caution when drotrecogin alfa is used with other drugs that affect hemostasis (see Warnings). Approximately ⅔ of the patients in the Phase 3 study received prophylactic low dose heparin. Concomitant use of prophylactic low dose heparin did not appear to affect safety. Its effect on the efficacy of drotrecogin alfa has not been evaluated in a randomized controlled clinical trial.

➤*Drug/Lab test interactions:* Because drotrecogin alfa may affect the aPTT assay, drotrecogin alfa present in plasma samples may interfere with 1-stage coagulation assays based on the aPTT, such as factor VIII, IX, and XI assays. This interference may result in an apparent factor concentration that is lower than the true concentration. drotrecogin alfa present in plasma samples does not interfere with 1-stage factor assays based on the PT, such as factor II, V, VII, and X assays.

Adverse Reactions

➤*Hematologic:* Bleeding is the most common adverse reaction associated with drotrecogin alfa.

In the Phase 3 study, serious bleeding events were observed during the 28-day study period in 3.5% of drotrecogin alfa-treated and 2% of placebo-treated patients. The difference in serious bleeding between drotrecogin alfa and placebo occurred primarily during the infusion period and is shown in the following table. Serious bleeding events were defined as any intracranial hemorrhage, any life-threatening bleed, any bleeding event requiring the administration of ≥ 3 units of packed red blood cells/day for 2 consecutive days, or any bleeding event assessed as a serious adverse event.

Number of Patients Experiencing a Serious Bleeding Event by Site of Hemorrhage During Study Drug Infusion Period[1] in PROWESS		
	Drotrecogin alfa (n = 850)	Placebo (n = 840)
Total	20 (2.4%)	8 (1%)
Site of hemorrhage		
GI	5	4
Intra-abdominal	2	3
Intrathoracic	4	0
Retroperitoneal	3	0
Intracranial	2	0
GU	2	0
Skin/Soft tissue	1	0
Other[2]	1	1

[1] Study drug infusion period is defined as the date of initiation of study drug to the date of study drug discontinuation plus the next calendar day.
[2] Patients requiring the administration of ≥ 3 units of packed red blood cells/day for 2 consecutive days without an identified site of bleeding.

In PROWESS, 2 cases of intracranial hemorrhage (ICH) occurred during the infusion period for drotrecogin alfa-treated patients and no cases were reported in the placebo patients. The incidence of ICH during the 28-day study period was 0.2% for drotrecogin alfa-treated patients and 0.1% for placebo-treated patients. ICH has been reported in patients receiving drotrecogin alfa in nonplacebo-controlled trials with an incidence of ≈ 1% during the infusion period. The risk of ICH may be increased in patients with risk factors for bleeding such as severe coagulopathy and severe thrombocytopenia (see Warnings).

In PROWESS, 25% of the drotrecogin alfa-treated patients and 18% of the placebo-treated patients experienced ≥ 1 bleeding event during the 28-day study period. In both treatment groups, the majority of bleeding events were ecchymoses or GI tract bleeding.

➤*Miscellaneous:* Patients administered drotrecogin alfa as treatment for severe sepsis experience many events that are potential sequelae of severe sepsis and may or may not be attributable to drotrecogin alfa therapy. In clinical trials, there were no types of nonbleeding adverse events suggesting a causal association with drotrecogin alfa.

Overdosage

There is no known antidote for drotrecogin alfa. In case of overdose, immediately stop the infusion and monitor closely for hemorrhagic complications.

Thrombolytic Enzymes

Indications

➤*Streptokinase:*

Acute evolving transmural MI – Management of acute myocardial infarction (AMI) in adults, for the lysis of intracoronary thrombi, for the improvement of ventricular function and the reduction of mortality with AMI when administered by IV or the intracoronary route, as well as for reduction of infarct size and CHF associated with AMI. Earlier administration is correlated with greater clinical benefit.

Pulmonary embolism (PE) – For the lysis of objectively diagnosed (angiography or lung scan) pulmonary emboli, involving obstruction of blood flow to a lobe or multiple segments, with or without unstable hemodynamics.

Deep vein thrombosis (DVT) – For the lysis of objectively diagnosed (preferably ascending venography), acute, extensive thrombi of the deep veins such as those involving the popliteal and more proximal vessels.

Arterial thrombosis and embolism – For the lysis of acute arterial thrombi and emboli. Streptokinase is not indicated for arterial emboli originating from the left side of the heart because of the risk of new embolic phenomena such as cerebral embolism.

Occluded arteriovenous (AV) cannulae – An alternative to surgical revision for clearing totally or partially occluded AV cannulae when acceptable flow cannot be achieved.

➤*Urokinase:*

Pulmonary emboli – Indicated in adults for the lysis of acute massive pulmonary emboli, defined as obstruction of blood flow to a lobe or multiple segments.

Pulmonary emboli accompanied by unstable hemodynamics – Indicated in adults for the lysis of pulmonary emboli accompanied by unstable hemodynamics, such as failure to maintain blood pressure without supportive measures.

Confirm the diagnosis by objective means, such as pulmonary angiography or noninvasive procedures such as lung scanning.

➤*Unlabeled uses:*

Streptokinase – Appears to be an effective local thrombolytic for occluded catheters; however, its use may be limited by adverse effects. Also used to treat chronic arterial occlusions; retinal vessel thrombosis; hemolytic-uremic syndrome; renal artery thrombosis; renal cortical necrosis.

Urokinase – Used to lyse clots in AV cannulae.

Actions

➤*Pharmacology:* **Streptokinase** is a purified preparation of bacterial protein purified by group C β-hemolytic streptococci; **urokinase** is produced from human neonatal kidney cells. Both act with plasminogen to produce an "activator complex" that converts plasminogen to plasmin. Plasmin degrades fibrin clots as well as fibrinogen and other plasma proteins. IV infusion of streptokinase is followed by increased fibrinolytic activity, which decreases plasma fibrinogen levels for 24 to 36 hours. The decrease in plasma fibrinogen is associated with decreases in plasma and blood viscosity and red blood cell aggregation. The hyperfibrinolytic effect disappears within a few hours after discontinuation, but a prolonged thrombin time may persist for up to 24 hours because of the decrease in plasma levels of fibrinogen and an increase in the amount of circulating fibrin(ogen) degradation products (FDP). Depending upon the dosage and duration of infusion of streptokinase, the thrombin time will decrease to less than 2 times the normal control value within 4 hours and return to normal by 24 hours.

IV administration of streptokinase reduces blood pressure and total peripheral resistance with a corresponding reduction in cardiac afterload. Streptokinase administered by the intracoronary route results in thrombolysis, usually within 1 hour, and ensuing reperfusion results in improvement of cardiac function and reduction of mortality. Spontaneous reperfusion is known to occur. Data from 1 study show that 73% of the streptokinase-treated patients and 47% of the placebo-allocated patients reperfused during hospitalization.

Variable amounts of circulating antistreptokinase antibody are present in people as a result of recent streptococcal infections. The recommended dosage schedule obviates the need for antibody titration.

➤*Pharmacokinetics:*

Absorption/Distribution – Information regarding pharmacokinetic properties is limited. The volume of distribution of **urokinase** is 11.5 L.

Metabolism/Excretion – **Urokinase** administered by the IV infusion is rapidly cleared by the liver with an elimination half-life for biologic activity of 12.6 minutes. Small fractions of the administered dose are excreted in bile and urine. The half-life of the activator complex of streptokinase is about 23 minutes, and the complex is inactivated, in part by antistreptococcal antibodies. **Streptokinase** is cleared by sites in the liver and no metabolites have been identified.

Special populations –

Hepatic function impairment: Endogenous **urokinase**-type plasminogen activator plasma levels are elevated 2- to 4-fold in patients with moderate to severe cirrhosis. Reduced urokinase clearance in patients with hepatic impairment might be expected.

➤*Clinical trials:*

Streptokinase – In the GISSI study, the reduction in mortality was time dependent; there was a 47% reduction in mortality among patients treated within 1 hour of the onset of chest pain, a 23% reduction among patients treated within 3 hours, and a 17% reduction among patients treated between 3 and 6 hours.

In the ISIS-2 study, the reduction in mortality was also time dependent. If streptokinase and aspirin were administered within the first hour after symptom onset, the reduction in mortality was 44%. The reduction in the odds of death in patients treated within 4 hours was 53% for the combination of streptokinase and aspirin and 35% for streptokinase alone. However, the reduction was still significant when treatment was started 5 to 24 hours after symptom onset: 33% for combined therapy and 17% for streptokinase alone.

The rate of reocclusion of the infarct-related vessel has been reported to be about 15% to 20% depending on dosage, additional anticoagulant therapy, and residual stenosis. When the reinfarctions were evaluated in studies involving 8800 streptokinase-treated patients, the overall rate was 3.8% (range, 2% to 15%). In over 8500 control patients, the rate of reinfarction was 2.4%.

For DVT, the combined results of 5 randomized studies show no residual thrombotic material in 60% to 75% of streptokinase-treated patients vs 10% treated with heparin. Thrombolytic therapy also preserves venous valve function, avoiding the pathology that produces the clinical postphlebitic syndrome that occurs in 90% of the DVT patients treated with heparin.

There is a time-related decrease in effectiveness when streptokinase is used in the management of peripheral arterial thromboembolism. When administered 3 to 10 days after onset of obstruction, rates of clearance of 50% to 75% were reported.

Contraindications

➤*Streptokinase:* Active internal bleeding; recent cerebrovascular accident, intracranial or intraspinal surgery (within 2 months); intracranial neoplasm; severe uncontrolled hypertension; severe allergy to the product.

➤*Urokinase:* Active internal bleeding; recent cerebrovascular accident, intracranial or intraspinal surgery (within 2 months); recent trauma including cardiopulmonary resuscitation; intracranial neoplasm; AV malformation; aneurysm; known bleeding diatheses; severe uncontrolled arterial hypertension.

Warnings

➤*Bleeding:* The risk of serious bleeding is increased with use of thrombolytic enzymes. Fatalities caused by hemorrhage, including intracranial and retroperitoneal, have been reported in association with **urokinase**. Bleeding into the pericardium, sometimes associated with myocardial rupture, has been seen with **streptokinase** and has resulted in fatalities. Concurrent administration of urokinase with other thrombolytic agents, anticoagulants, or agents inhibiting platelet function may further increase the risk of serious bleeding.

Thrombolytic enzyme therapy requires careful attention to all potential bleeding sites (including catheter insertion sites, arterial and venous puncture sites, cutdown sites, and other needle puncture sites).

When internal bleeding occurs, it may be more difficult to manage than that which occurs with conventional anticoagulant therapy. Should potentially serious spontaneous bleeding (not controllable by direct pressure) occur, immediately terminate the infusion of the thrombolytic enzyme, and implement measures to manage the bleeding. Slowing the rate of administration will not help correct the bleeding. Serious blood loss may be managed with volume replacement, including packed red blood cells. Do not use dextran. When appropriate, consider fresh frozen plasma and/or cryoprecipitate to reverse the bleeding tendency.

Following high-dose, brief-duration IV streptokinase therapy in AMI, severe bleeding complications requiring transfusion are extremely rare (0.3% to 0.5%), and combined therapy with low-dose aspirin does not appear to increase the risk of major bleeding. The addition of aspirin to streptokinase may cause a slight increase in the risk of minor bleeding (3.1% without aspirin vs 3.9% with aspirin).

Thrombolytic enzymes will cause lysis of hemostatic fibrin deposits such as those occurring at needle puncture sites; bleeding may occur. To minimize the risk of bleeding during treatment, perform venipunctures and physical handling of the patient carefully and as infrequently as possible; avoid IM injections.

➤*High-risk patients:* Carefully evaluate each patient being considered for therapy and weigh anticipated benefits against potential risks associated with therapy.

Thrombolytic Enzymes

In the following conditions, the risks of thrombolytic enzyme therapy may be increased and should be weighed against the anticipated benefits:

- Recent (within 10 days) major surgery (eg, obstetrical delivery, organ biopsy, previous puncture of noncompressible vessels)
- Cerebrovascular disease
- Recent GI bleeding (within 10 days)
- Recent trauma (within 10 days) including cardiopulmonary resuscitation
- Hypertension (systolic BP more than 180 mm Hg and/or diastolic BP more than 110 mm Hg)
- Likelihood of left heart thrombus (eg, mitral stenosis with atrial fibrillation)
- Subacute bacterial endocarditis
- Cerebrovascular disease
- Hemostatic defects including secondary to severe hepatic or renal disease
- Pregnancy
- Age over 75 years
- Diabetic hemorrhagic retinopathy
- Septic thrombophlebitis or occluded AV cannula at a seriously infected site
- Patients currently receiving oral anticoagulants (eg, warfarin)
- Any other condition in which bleeding constitutes a significant hazard or would be particularly difficult to manage because of its location

➤*Injection sites:* If an arterial puncture is necessary, upper extremity vessels are preferable. Apply pressure for at least 30 minutes. Apply a pressure dressing and check puncture site frequently.

➤*Respiratory:* There have been reports of respiratory depression in patients receiving **streptokinase**. In some cases, it was not possible to determine whether the respiratory depression was associated with streptokinase or was a symptom of the underlying process. If respiratory depression is associated with streptokinase, the occurrence is believed to be rare.

➤*Arrhythmias:* Rapid lysis of coronary thrombi has been shown to cause reperfusion atrial or ventricular dysrhythmias requiring immediate treatment. Carefully monitor for arrhythmias during and immediately following administration of **streptokinase** for AMI. Occasionally, tachycardia and bradycardia have been observed.

➤*Hypotension:* Sometimes severe hypotension, not secondary to bleeding or anaphylaxis, may occur during or soon after IV **streptokinase** (1% to 10%). Closely monitor patients and, if symptomatic or alarming hypotension occurs, administer appropriate treatment. This may include a decrease in the IV streptokinase infusion rate. Smaller hypotensive effects are common and have not required treatment.

➤*Noncardiogenic pulmonary edema:* Noncardiogenic pulmonary edema has been reported rarely in patients treated with **streptokinase**. The risk of this appears greatest in patients who have large MIs undergoing thrombolytic therapy by the intracoronary route.

➤*Polyneuropathy:* Rarely, polyneuropathy has been temporally related to the use of **streptokinase**, with some cases described as Guillain-Barré syndrome.

➤*Anticoagulant and antiplatelets after treatment for MI:* In the treatment of AMI, aspirin has been shown to reduce the incidence of reinfarction and stroke. The addition of aspirin to **streptokinase** causes a minimal increase in the risk of minor bleeding (3.9% vs 3.1%) but does not appear to increase the incidence of major bleeding. In the treatment of AMI, aspirin, when not otherwise contraindicated, should be administered with streptokinase. The use of anticoagulants following streptokinase administration increases the risk of bleeding but has not been shown to be of unequivocal clinical benefit. Therefore, whereas the use of aspirin is recommended unless otherwise contraindicated, the use of anticoagulants should be decided by the treating physician.

➤*Anticoagulation after IV treatment for other indications:* Continuous IV infusion of heparin, without a loading dose, has been recommended following termination of **streptokinase**, infusion for treatment of PE or DVT to prevent rethrombosis. The effect of streptokinase on thrombin time (TT) and activated partial thromboplastin time (aPTT) usually will diminish within 3 to 4 hours after streptokinase therapy. Heparin therapy without a loading dose can be initiated when the TT or the aPTT is less than twice the normal control value for streptokinase and **urokinase**.

➤*Cholesterol embolism:* Cholesterol embolism has occurred rarely in patients treated with all types of thrombolytic agents; the true incidence is unknown. This serious condition, which can be lethal, is also associated with invasive vascular procedures (eg, cardiac catheterization, angiography, vascular surgery) and/or anticoagulant therapy. Clinical features of cholesterol embolism include livedo reticularis, "purple toe" syndrome, acute renal failure, gangrenous digits, hypertension, pancreatitis, MI, cerebral infarction, spinal cord infarction, retinal artery occlusion, bowel infarction, and rhabdomyolysis.

➤*PE:* If PE or recurrent PE occur during **streptokinase** therapy, complete the planned course of treatment in an attempt to lyse the embolus. While PE may occasionally occur during streptokinase treatment, the incidence is no greater than when patients are treated with heparin alone. In addition to PE, embolization to other sites during streptokinase treatment has been observed.

➤*Hypersensitivity reactions:*

Streptokinase – Anaphylactic and anaphylactoid reactions ranging in severity from minor breathing difficulty to bronchospasm, periorbital swelling, or angioneurotic edema have been observed rarely in patients treated with IV streptokinase. Fever and shivering, occurring in 1% to 4% of patients, are the most commonly reported allergic reactions with IV streptokinase in AMI. Other milder allergic effects, such as urticaria, itching, flushing, nausea, headache, and musculoskeletal pain, have been observed, as have delayed hypersensitivity reactions such as vasculitis and interstitial nephritis.

Urokinase – Hypersensitivity reactions have included the following: Anaphylaxis (with rare reports of fatal anaphylaxis), bronchospasm, orolingual edema, urticaria, fever and/or chills/rigors, hypoxia, cyanosis, dyspnea, tachycardia, hypotension, hypertension, acidosis, back pain, vomiting, nausea. Reactions generally occurred within 1 hour of beginning urokinase infusion.

Mild or moderate allergic reactions may be managed with concomitant antihistamine or corticosteroid therapy. Severe allergic reactions require immediate discontinuation of infusion with adrenergic, antihistamine, and/or corticosteroid agents administered IV as required. Refer to the Acute Management of Hypersensitivity Reactions.

➤*Pregnancy:* (*Category C* – **Streptokinase**; *Category B* – **Urokinase**). It is not known whether streptokinase can cause fetal harm when administered to a pregnant woman or can affect reproduction capacity.

Reproduction studies have been performed with urokinase in mice and rats at doses up to 1000 times the human dose and have revealed no evidence of impaired fertility or harm to the fetus. However, there are no adequate and well-controlled studies in pregnant women.

Use these drugs during pregnancy only if clearly needed.

➤*Lactation:*

Urokinase – It is not known whether urokinase is excreted in human milk. Because many drugs are excreted in human milk, exercise caution when urokinase is administered to a nursing woman.

➤*Children:*

Streptokinase – Controlled clinical studies have not been conducted in children to determine safety and efficacy in the pediatric population. The evidence of clinical benefits and risks is solely based on anecdotal reports in patients ranging in age from less than 1 month to 16 years. The largest number of patient reports have pertained to the use of streptokinase in arterial occlusions.

Urokinase – Safety and efficacy for use in children have not been established.

Precautions

➤*Monitoring:* Before therapy, determine hematocrit, platelet count, TT, aPTT, prothrombin time (PT), or fibrinogen levels.

Frequently observe clinical response and vital signs during and following **urokinase** infusion. To avoid dislodgement of possible deep vein thrombi, do not take blood pressure in the lower extremities. Results of coagulation tests and measures of fibrinolytic activity do not reliably predict efficacy or bleeding risk for patients receiving urokinase.

If heparin has been given, discontinue and start thrombolytic therapy when the TT or aPTT is less than twice the normal control value.

During the infusion, decreases in plasminogen and fibrinogen levels and an increase in the level of FDP (the latter two causing a prolongation in the clotting times of coagulation tests) generally will confirm the existence of a lytic state. Therefore, lytic therapy can be confirmed by performing the TT, aPTT, PT, or fibrinogen levels approximately 4 hours after initiation of therapy.

➤*Pancreatitis:* There have been rare cases where **streptokinase** has been administered for suspected AMI subsequently diagnosed as pancreatitis. Fatalities have occurred under these circumstances.

➤*Resistance:* Because of the increased likelihood of resistance caused by antistreptokinase antibody, **streptokinase** may not be effective if administered between 5 days and 12 months of prior streptokinase administration or streptococcal infections (ie, streptococcal pharyngitis, acute rheumatic fever or acute glomerulonephritis secondary to a streptococcal infection).

➤*Formulation with albumin (human):* The product source contains albumin, a derivative of human blood. Based on effective donor screening and product manufacturing processes, it carries an extremely remote risk for transmission of viral diseases. A theoretical risk for transmission of Creutzfeldt-Jakob disease (CJD) also is considered extremely remote. No cases of transmission of viral disease or CJD ever have been identified for albumin. All infections thought by a physician possibly to have been transmitted by these products should be reported to the appropriate manufacturer.

➤*Lab test abnormalities:* IV administration of **streptokinase** will cause marked decreases in plasminogen and fibrinogen and increases in TT, aPTT, and PT, which normalize within 12 to 24 hours. These changes may also occur in some patients with intracoronary administration of streptokinase.

Drug Interactions

►*Anticoagulants and antiplatelet agents:* Anticoagulants and agents that alter platelet function (eg, aspirin, other NSAIDs, dipyridamole, GP IIb/IIIa inhibitors) may increase the risk of serious bleeding.

►*Drug/Lab test interactions:* Transient elevations of serum transaminases have been observed when using **streptokinase**. The source of these enzyme rises and their clinical significance is not fully understood.

Adverse Reactions

►*Bleeding:*
Streptokinase: Minor bleeding can be anticipated mainly at invaded or disturbed sites. Severe and internal bleeding involving GI (including hepatic bleeding), GU, retroperitoneal, or intracerebral sites has occurred and has resulted in fatalities. In the treatment of AMI with IV streptokinase, the GISSI and ISIS-2 studies reported a rate of major bleeding (requiring transfusion) of 0.3% to 0.5%. However, rates as high as 16% have been reported in studies that required administration of anticoagulants and invasive procedures.

Urokinase: Bleeding is the most frequent adverse reaction and can be fatal. In clinical studies using a 12-hour infusion of urokinase for the treatment of PE, bleeding resulting in at least a 5% decrease in hematocrit was reported in 52 of 141 urokinase-treated patients. Significant bleeding events requiring transfusion of greater than 2 units of blood were observed during the 14-day study period in 3 of 141 urokinase-treated patients in these studies. Multiple bleeding events may have occurred in an individual patient. Most bleeding occurred at sites of external incisions and vascular puncture, with lesser frequency in GI, GU, intracranial, retroperitoneal, and IM sites.

►*Allergic:*
Streptokinase – Fever, shivering in acute MI (1% to 4%); anaphylactic and anaphylactoid reactions (rare) (eg, minor breathing difficulty, bronchospasm, periorbital swelling, angioneurotic edema); urticaria; itching; flushing; nausea; headache; musculoskeletal pain; delayed hypersensitivity reactions (eg, vasculitis and interstitial nephritis) (see Warnings); anaphylactic shock (0 to 0.1%).

Urokinase – In controlled clinical trials, allergic reaction was reported (less than 1%); anaphylaxis (rare); bronchospasm; orolingual edema; urticaria; skin rash; pruritus. Infusion reaction symptoms include hypoxia, cyanosis, dyspnea, tachycardia, hypotension, hypertension, acidosis, fever and/or chills/rigors, back pain, vomiting, and nausea.

►*Respiratory:* There have been reports of respiratory depression in patients receiving **streptokinase**. In some cases, it was not possible to determine whether the respiratory depression was associated with streptokinase or was a symptom of the underlying cause.

►*Miscellaneous:*
Streptokinase – There have been reports of back pain during infusion; cessation of pain occurred within minutes of discontinuation.

Urokinase – Regardless of causality, other adverse events in clinical studies included MI, recurrent PE, hemiplegia, stroke, decreased hematocrit, substernal pain, thrombocytopenia, and diaphoresis. Postmarketing reports included cardiac arrest, vascular embolization (cerebral and distal) including cholesterol emboli, cerebral vascular accident, pulmonary edema, reperfusion ventricular arrhythmias, and chest pain.

STREPTOKINASE

Rx	**Streptase** (Aventis Behring)	**Powder for injection, lyophilized**[1]: 250,000 IU	Preservative-free. In 6 mL vials.
		750,000 IU	Preservative-free. In 6 mL vials.
		1,500,000 IU	Preservative-free. In 6 mL vials and 50 mL infusion bottle.

[1] With 25 mg cross-linked gelatin polypeptides, 25 mg sodium l-glutamate, and 100 mg albumin (human).

For complete prescribing information, refer to the Thrombolytic Enzymes group monograph.

Indications

►*Acute evolving transmural MI:* Management of acute myocardial infarction (AMI) in adults, for the lysis of intracoronary thrombi, the improvement of ventricular function, and the reduction of mortality with AMI when administered by IV or intracoronary route, as well as for reduction of infarct size and CHF associated with MI. Earlier administration is correlated with greater clinical benefit.

►*Pulmonary embolism (PE):* For the lysis of objectively diagnosed (angiography or lung scan) pulmonary emboli involving obstruction of blood flow to a lobe or multiple segments, with or without unstable hemodynamics.

►*Deep vein thrombosis (DVT):* For the lysis of objectively diagnosed (preferably ascending venography), acute, extensive thrombi of the deep veins such as those involving the popliteal and more proximal vessels.

►*Arterial thrombosis and embolism:* For the lysis of acute arterial thrombi and emboli. Streptokinase is not indicated for arterial emboli originating from the left side of the heart because of the risk of new embolic phenomena such as cerebral embolism.

►*Occluded arteriovenous (AV) cannulae:* An alternative to surgical revision for clearing totally or partially occluded AV cannulae when acceptable flow cannot be achieved.

Administration and Dosage

►*Acute evolving transmural MI:* Administer as soon as possible after symptom onset. The greatest benefit in mortality reduction was observed when streptokinase was administered within 4 hours, but statistically significant benefit has been reported up to 24 hours.

IV infusion – Administer a total dose of 1,500,000 IU within 60 minutes.

Intracoronary infusion – Administer 20,000 IU by bolus followed by 2000 IU/min for 60 minutes for a total dose of 140,000 IU.

►*PE, DVT, arterial thrombosis, or embolism:* Institute treatment as soon as possible after thrombotic event onset, preferably within 7 days. Any delay in instituting lytic therapy to evaluate the effect of heparin therapy decreases the potential for optimal efficacy. Because human exposure to streptococci is common, antibodies to streptokinase are prevalent. Thus, a loading dose of streptokinase sufficient to neutralize these antibodies is required. A dose of 250,000 IU streptokinase infused into a peripheral vein over 30 minutes was appropriate in over 90% of patients. If the thrombin time, or any other parameter of lysis after 4 hours of therapy is not significantly different from the normal control level, discontinue streptokinase because excessive resistance is present.

Streptokinase Dosages		
Indication	Loading dose	IV infusion dosage/duration
PE	250,000 IU over 30 min	100,000 IU/h for 24 h (72 h if concurrent DVT is suspected)
DVT	250,000 IU over 30 min	100,000 IU/h for 72 h
Arterial thrombosis or embolism	250,000 IU over 30 min	100,000 IU/h for 24 to 72 h

►*AV cannulae occlusion:* Before using, try to clear the cannula by syringe technique, using heparinized saline solution. If adequate flow is not re-established, use streptokinase. Allow the effect of any pretreatment anticoagulants to diminish. Slowly instill 250,000 IU in 2 mL solution into each occluded limb of the cannula. Clamp off cannula limb(s) for 2 hours. Observe closely for adverse effects. After treatment, aspirate contents of infused cannula limb(s), flush with saline, and reconnect cannula.

►*Pediatric use:* Controlled clinical studies have not been conducted in children to determine safety and efficacy. The evidence of clinical benefits and risks is solely based on anecdotal reports in patients ranging in age from less than 1 month to 16 years. The largest number of patient reports have pertained to the use of streptokinase in arterial occlusions. For arterial occlusions, the most frequently used loading dose was 1000 IU/kg; fewer numbers of patients received 3000 IU/kg. Loading dose durations typically have ranged from 5 to 30 minutes. Continuous infusion doses were frequently 1000 IU/kg/h; fewer were at 1500 IU/kg/h. Infusions were maintained for 12 hours or less in approximately half of the published cases; a smaller proportion were between 12 and 24 hours. Reported adverse events associated with the use of streptokinase in the pediatric population are similar in nature to those associated with its use in adults. Rates of all bleeding complications have been variable and as high as 50% at catheter sites in some studies. Occasionally, bleeding has required transfusion. Careful monitoring of patient status is necessary.

►*Reconstitution (vials and infusion bottles):*
1.) Slowly add 5 mL NaCl injection or 5% dextrose injection to the streptokinase vial, directing the diluent at the side of the vacuum-packed vial rather than into the drug powder.
2.) Roll and tilt the vial gently to reconstitute. Avoid shaking (shaking may cause foaming). If necessary, total volume may be increased to a maximum of 500 mL in glass or 50 mL in plastic containers; adjust the infusion pump rate accordingly. To facilitate setting the infusion pump rate, a total volume of 45 mL, or a multiple thereof, is recommended.
3.) Withdraw the entire reconstituted contents of the vial; slowly and carefully dilute further to a total volume as recommended. Avoid shaking and agitation on dilution.

Thrombolytic Enzymes

STREPTOKINASE

4.) When diluting the 1,500,000 IU infusion bottle (50 mL), slowly add 5 mL NaCl injection or 5% dextrose injection, directing it at the side of the bottle rather than into the drug powder. Roll and tilt the bottle gently to reconstitute. Avoid shaking as it may cause foaming. Add an additional 40 mL of diluent to the bottle, avoiding shaking and agitation (total volume = 45 mL). Administer by infusion pump at the rate indicated.

5.) Inspect parenteral drug products visually for particulate matter and discoloration prior to administration (the human albumin may impart a slightly yellow color to the solution).

6.) The reconstituted solution can be filtered through a 0.8 mcm or larger pore size filter.

7.) Because streptokinase contains no preservatives, reconstitute immediately before use. The solution may be used for direct IV administration within 8 hours following reconstitution if stored at 2° to 8°C (36° to 46°F).

8.) Do not add other medication to the container.

9.) Discard unused reconstituted drug.

Streptokinase Suggested Dilutions and Infusion Rates

Indication	Infusion type	Vial size (IU)	Total solution volume	Dosage and infusion rate
AMI	Intravenous infusion	1,500,000	45 mL	Infuse 45 mL over 60 min
AMI	Intracoronary infusion	250,000	125 mL	Loading dose of 10 mL (20,000 IU); then 60 mL/h (2000 IU/min)

Streptokinase Suggested Dilutions and Infusion Rates

Indication	Infusion type	Vial size (IU)	Total solution volume	Dosage and infusion rate
PE, DVT, arterial thrombosis, embolism	IV infusion 1. Loading dose	1,500,000	90 mL	1. Infuse 30 mL/h for 30 min (250,000 IU)
	2. Maintenance dose			2. Then infuse at 6 mL/h (100,000 IU/h)
	IV infusion 1. Loading dose	1,500,000 infusion bottle	45 mL	1. 15 mL/h for 30 min (250,000 IU)
	2. Maintenance dose			2. Then infuse 3 mL/h (100,000 IU/h)

AV cannula – Slowly reconstitute contents of the 250,000 IU, vacuum-packed vial with 2 mL sodium chloride injection or 5% dextrose injection.

➤*IV incompatibilities:* Do not add other medication to streptokinase.

➤*Storage/Stability:* Store unopened vials at room temperature (15° to 30°C or 59° to 86°F). The solution may be used for direct IV administration within 8 hours following reconstitution if stored at 2° to 8°C (36° to 46°F). Discard unused reconstituted drug.

UROKINASE

Rx	**Abbokinase (Abbott)**	**Powder for injection, lyophilized:** 250,000 IU/vial	Preservative-free. With 25 mg mannitol, 250 mg albumin (human), 50 mg sodium chloride. In vials.

For complete prescribing information, refer to the Thrombolytic Enzymes group monograph.

Indications

➤*Pulmonary emboli:* Indicated in adults for the lysis of acute massive pulmonary emboli, defined as obstruction of blood flow to a lobe or multiple segments.

➤*Pulmonary emboli accompanied by unstable hemodynamics:* Indicated in adults for the lysis of pulmonary emboli accompanied by unstable hemodynamics, such as failure to maintain blood pressure without supportive measures.

Confirm the diagnosis by objective means, such as pulmonary angiography or noninvasive procedures such as lung scanning.

Administration and Dosage

For IV infusion only.

Institute urokinase treatment soon after onset of pulmonary embolism (PE). Delay in instituting therapy may decrease the potential for optimal efficacy.

➤*Reconstitution:* Do not reconstitute until immediately before use. Discard any unused portion of the reconstituted material. Reconstitute urokinase by aseptically adding 5 mL of sterile water for injection without preservatives to the vial; do not use bacteriostatic water for injection. After reconstituting, visually inspect each vial for discoloration and for the presence of particulate material. The solution should be pale and straw-colored; do not use highly colored solutions. Thin, translucent filaments occasionally occur in reconstituted urokinase vials, but do not indicate any decrease in potency of this product. To minimize formation of filaments, avoid shaking the vial during reconstitution. Roll and tilt the vial to enhance reconstitution. The solution may be terminally filtered, for example through a 0.45 micron or smaller cellulose membrane filter. Do not add other medication to this solution.

➤*Dose preparation for PE:* Prior to infusing, dilute the reconstituted urokinase with 0.9% sodium chloride injection or 5% dextrose injection. The following table may be used as an aid in the preparation of urokinase for administration.

Urokinase Dose Preparation - PE

Patient weight (lbs)	Total dose[1] of urokinase (IU)	Number of urokinase vials	Volume of urokinase after reconstitution (mL)[2]	+	Volume of diluent (mL)	=	Final volume (mL)
81-90	2,250,000	9	45		150		195
91-100	2,500,000	10	50		145		195
101-110	2,750,000	11	55		140		195
111-120	3,000,000	12	60		135		195
121-130	3,250,000	13	65		130		195
131-140	3,500,000	14	70		125		195

Urokinase Dose Preparation - PE

Patient weight (lbs)	Total dose[1] of urokinase (IU)	Number of urokinase vials	Volume of urokinase after reconstitution (mL)[2]	+	Volume of diluent (mL)	=	Final volume (mL)
141-150	3,750,000	15	75		120		195
151-160	4,000,000	16	80		115		195
161-170	4,250,000	17	85		110		195
171-180	4,500,000	18	90		105		195
181-190	4,750,000	19	95		100		195
191-200	5,000,000	20	100		95		195
201-210	5,250,000	21	105		90		195
211-220	5,500,000	22	110		85		195
221-230	5,750,000	23	115		80		195
231-240	6,000,000	24	120		75		195
241-250	6,250,000	25	125		70		195

[1] Loading dose plus dose administered during 12-hour period.
[2] After addition of 5 mL sterile water for injection per vial.

The infusion rate is a 15 mL/10 min loading dose and then 15 mL/h for 12 hours. The pump rate is 90 mL/h.

Urokinase is administered using a constant infusion pump that is capable of delivering a total volume of 195 mL. A loading dose of 2000 IU/lb (4400 IU/kg) of urokinase is given as a urokinase 0.9% sodium chloride injection or 5% dextrose injection admixture at a rate of 90 mL/h over a period of 10 minutes. This is followed by a continuous infusion of 2000 IU/lb/h (4400 IU/kg/h) of urokinase at a rate of 15 mL/h for 12 hours.

Because some urokinase admixture will remain in the tubing at the end of an infusion pump delivery cycle, perform the following flush procedure to ensure that the total dose of urokinase is administered. Administer a solution of 0.9% sodium chloride injection or 5% dextrose injection approximately equal in amount to the volume of the tubing in the infusion set via the pump to flush the urokinase admixture from the entire length of the infusion set. Set the pump to administer the flush solution at the continuous rate of 15 mL/h.

➤*Anticoagulation after terminating urokinase treatment:* After infusing urokinase, anticoagulation treatment is recommended to prevent recurrent thrombosis. Do not begin anticoagulation until the activated partial thromboplastin time has decreased to less than twice the normal control value. If heparin is used, do not administer a loading dose of heparin. Follow treatment with oral anticoagulants.

➤*Hepatic function impairment:* Endogenous urokinase-type plasminogen activator plasma levels are elevated 2- to 4-fold in patients with moderate to severe cirrhosis. Reduced urokinase clearance in patients with hepatic impairment might be expected.

➤*Storage/Stability:* Refrigerate powder at 2° to 8°C (36° to 46°F).

HYDROXYUREA

Rx	**Droxia** (Bristol-Myers Squibb Oncology)	**Capsules:** 200 mg	Lactose. (Droxia 6335). Blue-green. In 60s.
		300 mg	Lactose. (Droxia 6336). Purple. In 60s.
		400 mg	Lactose. (Droxia 6337). Reddish-orange. In 60s.

For complete prescribing and other indications information, refer to the Hydroxyurea monograph in the Antineoplastics chapter.

WARNING

Treatment of patients with hydroxyurea capsules may be complicated by severe, sometimes life-threatening, adverse effects. Administer hydroxyurea under the supervision of a physician experienced in the use of this medication for the treatment of sickle cell anemia (SCA).

Hydroxyurea is mutagenic and clastogenic, and causes cellular transformation to a tumorigenic phenotype. Hydroxyurea is thus unequivocally genotoxic and a presumed transspecies carcinogen that implies a carcinogenic risk to humans. In patients receiving long-term hydroxyurea for myeloproliferative disorders, such as polycythemia vera and thrombocythemia, secondary leukemias have been reported. It is unknown whether this leukemogenic effect is secondary to hydroxyurea or is associated with the patient's underlying disease. The physician and patient must very carefully consider the potential benefits of hydroxyurea relative to the undefined risk of developing secondary malignancies.

Indications

To reduce the frequency of painful crises and to reduce the need for blood transfusions in adults with SCA with recurrent moderate-to-severe painful crises (generally ≥ 3 crises during the preceding 12 months).

Administration and Dosage

Base dosage on patient's actual or ideal weight, whichever is less. The initial dose of hydroxyurea is 15 mg/kg/day as a single dose. The patient's blood count must be monitored every 2 weeks (see Warnings).

If blood counts are at acceptable levels, the dose may be increased by 5 mg/kg/day every 12 weeks until a maximum tolerated dose (the highest dose that does not produce toxic blood counts over 24 consecutive weeks), or 35 mg/kg/day is reached.

If blood counts are between the acceptable and toxic levels, the dose is not increased.

If blood counts are considered toxic, discontinue hydroxyurea until hematologic recovery. Treatment may then be resumed after reducing the dose by 2.5 mg/kg/day from the dose associated with hematologic toxicity. Hydroxyurea may then be titrated up or down, every 12 weeks in 2.5 mg/kg/day increments until the patient is at a stable dose that does not result in hematologic toxicity for 24 weeks. Patients who develop hematologic toxicity twice on a particular dosage should not be given that dosage again.

➤*Acceptable levels:*
• Neutrophils $\geq$ 2500 cells/mm^3,
• Platelets $\geq$ 95,000/mm^3,
• Hemoglobin > 5.3 g/dL, and
• Reticulocytes $\geq$ 95,000/mm^3 if the hemoglobin concentration < 9 g/dL.

➤*Toxic levels:*
• Neutrophils < 2000 cells/mm^3,
• Platelets < 80,000/mm^3,
• Hemoglobin < 4.5 g/dL, and
• Reticulocytes < 80,000/mm^3 if the hemoglobin concentration < 9 g/dL.

➤*Renal insufficiency:* There are no data that support specific guidance for dosage adjustment in patients with renal impairment. As renal excretion is a pathway of elimination, consider decreasing the hydroxyurea dosage in patients with renal impairment. Close monitoring of hematologic parameters is advised in these patients.

➤*Hepatic insufficiency:* There are no data that support specific guidance for dosage adjustment in patients with hepatic impairment. Close monitoring of hematologic parameters is advised in these patients.

Procedures for proper handling and disposal of cytotoxic drugs should be considered. Several guidelines on this subject have been published. There is no general agreement that all of the procedures recommended in the guidelines are necessary or appropriate.

Contraindications

Hypersensitivity to hydroxyurea or any other component of its formulation.

Warnings

➤*Pregnancy: Category D.* Hydroxyurea can cause fetal harm when administered to a pregnant woman. If this drug is used during pregnancy or if the patient becomes pregnant while taking this drug, apprise the patient of the potential harm to the fetus. Advise women of childbearing potential to avoid becoming pregnant.

Precautions

Therapy with hydroxyurea requires close supervision. Some patients treated at the recommended intial dose of 15 mg/kg/day have experienced severe or life-threatening myelosuppression, requiring interruption of treatment and dose reduction. Determine the hematologic status of the patient, as well as kidney and liver function prior to and repeatedly during treatment. Interrupt treatment if neutrophil levels fall to < 2000/mm^3; platelets fall to < 80,000/mm^3; hemoglobin declines to < 4.5 g/dL; or if reticulocytes fall below 80,000/mm^3 when the hemoglobin concentration is < 9 g/dL. Following recovery, treatment may be resumed at lower doses (see Administration and Dosage).

Adverse Reactions

The most common adverse reactions were hematologic, with neutropenia and low reticulocyte and platelet levels necessitating temporary cessation in almost all patients. Hematologic recovery usually occurred in 2 weeks.

Non-hematologic events possibly associated with treatment include hair loss, skin rash, fever, GI disturbances, weight gain, bleeding, and Parvovirus B-19 infection. Melanonychia has also been reported in patients receiving hydroxyurea for SCA.

PENTOXIFYLLINE

Rx	Pentoxifylline (Copley)	Tablets, controlled-release: 400 mg	Film-coated. In 100s, 500s, and bulk pack 5000s.
Rx	Trental (Hoechst Marion Roussel)		(Trental). Pink. Film coated. Oblong. In 100s, bulk pack 5000s and UD 100s.
Rx	Pentoxifylline Extended-Release (Purepac)	Tablets, extended-release: 400 mg	In 100s, 500s and 1000s.

Indications

➤*Intermittent claudication:* For intermittent claudication on the basis of chronic occlusive arterial disease of the limbs. Pentoxifylline improves function and symptoms but does not replace definitive therapy.

➤*Unlabeled uses:* Pentoxifylline was found superior to placebo in improving psychopathological symptoms in patients with cerebrovascular insufficiency. The drug has also been studied in diabetic angiopathies and neuropathies, transient ischemic attacks, leg ulcers, sickle cell thalassemias, strokes, high-altitude sickness, asthenozoospermia, acute and chronic hearing disorders, severe idiopathic recurrent aphthous stomatitis (400 mg three times a day for 1 month), eye circulation disorders and Raynaud's phenomenon.

Administration and Dosage

Take 400 mg 3 times daily with meals. If GI and CNS side effects occur, decrease to 400 mg twice daily. If side effects persist, discontinue the drug. While therapeutic effects may be seen within 2 to 4 weeks, continue treatment for ≥ 8 weeks.

Actions

➤*Pharmacology:* Pentoxifylline, a tri-substituted xanthine derivative, produces dose-related hemorrheologic effects, and its metabolites improve blood flow by decreasing blood viscosity and improving erythrocyte flexiblity. Leukocyte properties of hemorrheologic importance have been modified in animal and in vitro human studies. Pentoxifylline has been shown to increase leukocyte deformability and to inhibit neutrophil adhesion and activation. Tissue oxygen levels have been shown to be significantly increased by therapeutic doses of pentoxifylline in patients with peripheral arterial disease.

➤*Pharmacokinetics:*

Absorption/Distribution – After administration of the 400 mg controlled release tablet, plasma levels of the parent compound and its metabolites reach their maximum within 2 to 4 hours. Food intake shortly before dosing delays absorption of an immediate-release dosage form but does not affect total absorption. After oral administration in an aqueous solution, pentoxifylline is almost completely absorbed. Plasma levels of the parent compound and its metabolites peak within 1 hour.

Metabolism/Excretion – Pentoxifylline undergoes a first-pass effect. The major metabolites are Metabolite I and Metabolite V with plasma levels 5 and 8 times greater, respectively, than pentoxifylline. Following oral administration of aqueous solutions, the pharmacokinetics of the parent compound and Metabolite I are dose-related and not proportional (non-linear), with half-life and area under the blood level time curve (AUC) increasing with dose. The elimination kinetics of Metabolite V are not dose-dependent. Plasma half-lives of pentoxifylline and its metabolites are 0.4 to 0.8 hours and 1 to 1.6 hours, respectively. There is no evidence of accumulation or enzyme induction. The main biotransformation product is Metabolite V and excretion is primarily urinary. Essentially no parent drug is found in the urine. Less than 4% of the dose is recovered in feces.

Elderly – AUC was increased and elimination rate decreased in an older population (60 to 68 years) compared with younger individuals (22 to 30 years).

Contraindications

Patients with recent cerebral or retinal hemorrhage; intolerance to pentoxifylline or methylxanthines (eg, caffeine, theophylline, theobromine).

Warnings

➤*Hemorrhage:* Patients with risk factors complicated by hemorrhage (eg, recent surgery, peptic ulceration) should have periodic exams for bleeding including hematocrit or hemoglobin.

➤*Renal function impairment:* The clearance of pentoxifylline is reduced in patients with renal impairment, possibly resulting in toxicity. A lower dosage may be necessary in these patients.

➤*Pregnancy:* Category C. Animal studies showed no fetal malformation. Increased resorption was seen in rats of the 576 mg/kg group. No adequate studies exist in pregnant women. Use only if clearly needed.

➤*Lactation:* Pentoxifylline and its metabolites are excreted in breast milk. Because of the potential for tumorigenicity seen in rats, decide whether to discontinue nursing or discontinue the drug, taking into account the importance of the drug to the mother.

➤*Children:* Safety and efficacy for use in children are not established.

Precautions

➤*Arterial disease of the limbs:* Patients with chronic occlusive arterial disease of the limbs frequently show other manifestations of arteriosclerotic disease. There have been occasional reports of angina, hypotension and arrhythmia. Periodic systemic blood pressure monitoring is recommended, especially in patients receiving concomitant antihypertensive therapy.

Drug Interactions

Pentoxifylline Drug Interactions			
Precipitant drug	Object drug*		Description
Pentoxifylline	Warfarin	↑	Although a causal relationship has not been established, there have been reports of bleeding and prolonged prothrombin time (PT) in patients receiving pentoxifylline with or without anticoagulants or platelet aggregation inhibitors. Frequently monitor PT in patients on warfarin.
Pentoxifylline	Theophylline	↑	Concomitant administration of pentoxifylline-containing drugs leads to increased theophylline levels and theophylline toxicity in some individuals. Monitor patients closely for signs of toxicity and adjust theophylline dosage as necessary.
Pentoxifylline	Antihypertensives	↑	Small decreases in blood pressure have been observed in some patients treated with pentoxifylline; periodically monitor systemic blood pressure for patients receiving concomitant antihypertensive therapy. If indicated, reduce dosage of the antihypertensive agent.

Adverse Reactions

➤*Rare (causal relationship unknown):* Arrhythmia, tachycardia, anaphylactoid reactions, hepatitis, increased liver enzymes, jaundice, decreased serum fibrinogen, pancytopenia, aplastic anemia, leukemia, purpura, thrombocytopenia.

➤*Cardiovascular:* Angina/chest pain (0.3%); edema, hypotension, dyspnea (< 1%).

➤*GI:* Dyspepsia (2.8%); nausea (2.2%); vomiting (1.2%); belching/flatus/bloating (0.6%); anorexia, cholecystitis, constipation, dry mouth/thirst (< 1%).

➤*CNS:* Dizziness (1.9%); headache (1.2%); tremor (0.3%); anxiety, confusion, depression, seizures (< 1%).

➤*Respiratory:* Epistaxis, flu-like symptoms, laryngitis, nasal congestion (< 1%).

➤*Dermatologic:* Brittle fingernails, pruritus, rash, urticaria, angioedema (< 1%).

➤*Ophthalmic:* Blurred vision, conjunctivitis, scotomata (< 1%).

➤*Miscellaneous:* Earache, bad taste, excessive salivation, leukopenia, malaise, sore throat/swollen neck glands, weight change (< 1%).

Overdosage

➤*Symptoms:* Apparently dose-related, overdosage symptoms usually occur 4 to 5 hours after ingestion and last ≈ 12 hours. Flushing, hypotension, nervousness, tremors, convulsions, somnolence, loss of consciousness, fever and agitation have occurred. Bradycardia (30 to 40 beats/min) with first and second degree AV block occurring after 2 hours in a patient who ingested 4 to 6 g; first degree AV block persisted until 16 hours after admission.

➤*Treatment:* Treat with gastric lavage and administer activated charcoal. Monitor ECG and blood pressure. In addition to symptomatic treatment, support respiration, maintain blood pressure, treat cardiac arrhythmias and control convulsions as required.

COAGULATION FACTOR VIIa (RECOMBINANT)

Rx	**NovoSeven** (Novo Nordisk)	**Powder for injection, lyophilized:** 1.2 mg/vial (1200 mcg/vial) recombinant human coagulation Factor VIIa (rFVIIa)	In single-use vials.
		2.4 mg/vial (2400 mcg/vial) recombinant human coagulation Factor VIIa (rFVIIa)	In single-use vials.
		4.8 mg/vial (4800 mcg/vial) recombinant human coagulation Factor VIIa (rFVIIa)	In single-use vials.

Indications

▶*Bleeding episodes in hemophilia patients:* Treatment of bleeding episodes in hemophilia A or B patients with inhibitors to Factor VIII or Factor IX.

Administration and Dosage

▶*Approved by the FDA:* March 25, 1999.

▶*Dosage:* rFVIIa is intended for IV bolus administration only. Use evaluation of hemostasis to determine the effectiveness of rFVIIa and to provide a basis for modification of the treatment schedule; coagulation parameters do not necessarily correlate with or predict the effectiveness of rFVIIa.

The recommended dose of rFVIIa for hemophilia A or B patients with inhibitors is 90 mcg/kg given every 2 hours until hemostasis is achieved, or until the treatment has been judged to be inadequate. Doses between 35 and 120 mcg/kg have been used successfully in clinical trials, and both the dose and administration interval may be adjusted based on the severity of the bleeding and degree of hemostasis achieved. The minimal effective dose has not been established. For patients treated for joint or muscle bleeds, a decision on outcome was reached for a majority of patients within 8 doses although more doses were required for severe bleeds. A majority of patients who reported adverse experiences received > 12 doses.

▶*Post-hemostatic dosing:* The appropriate duration of post-hemostatic dosing has not been studied. For severe bleeds, dosing should continue at 3- to 6-hour intervals after hemostasis is achieved, to maintain the hemostatic plug. The biological and clinical effects of prolonged elevated levels of Factor VIIa have not been studied; therefore, minimize the duration of post-hemostatic dosing and appropriately monitor patients during this time period.

▶*Reconstitution:* Perform reconstitution using the following procedures:
1.) Bring rFVIIa (white, lyophilized powder) and the specified volume of Sterile Water for Injection (diluent) to room temperature, but not > 37°C (98.6°F). The specified volume of diluent corresponding to the amount of rFVIIa is as follows:

1.2 mg (1200 mcg) vial + 2.2 mL Sterile Water for Injection 4.8 mg (4800 mcg) vial + 8.5 mL Sterile Water for Injection. After reconstitution with the specified volume of diluent, each vial contains ≈ 0.6 mg/mL rFVIIa (600 mcg/mL).

2.) Remove caps from the rFVIIa vials to expose the central portion of the rubber stopper. Cleanse the rubber stoppers with an alcohol swab and allow to dry prior to use.
3.) Draw back the plunger of a sterile syringe (attached to sterile needle) and admit air into the syringe.
4.) Insert the needle of the syringe into Sterile Water for Injection vial. Inject air into the vial and withdraw the quantity required for reconstitution.
5.) Insert the syringe needle containing the diluent into the rFVIIa vial through the center of the rubber stopper, aiming the needle against the side so that the stream of liquid runs down the vial wall (the vial does not contain a vacuum). Do not inject the diluent directly on the rFVIIa powder.
6.) Gently swirl the vial until all material is dissolved. The reconstituted solution is a clear, colorless solution which may be used ≤ 3 hours after reconstitution.

▶*Administration:* Administration should take place within 3 hours after reconstitution. Discard any unused solution. Do not store reconstituted rFVIIa in syringes. It is intended for IV bolus injection only and should not be mixed with infusion solutions. Do not use if particulate matter or discoloration is observed. Perform administration using the following procedures:
1.) Draw back the plunger of a sterile syringe (attached to sterile needle) and admit air into the syringe.
2.) Insert needle into the vial of reconstituted rFVIIa. Inject air into the vial and then withdraw the appropriate amount of reconstituted rFVIIa into the syringe.
3.) Remove and discard the needle from the syringe; attach a suitable IV injection needle and administer as a slow bolus injection over 2 to 5 minutes, depending on the dose administered.
4.) Discard any unused reconstituted rFVIIa after 3 hours.

▶*Admixture incompatibility:* Do not mix rFVIIa with infusion solutions until clinical data are available to direct this use.

▶*Storage/Stability:* Prior to reconstitution, keep refrigerated (2° to 8°C/36° to 46°F). Avoid exposure to direct sunlight. Do not use past the expiration date.

After reconstitution, it may be stored either at room temperature or refrigerated for ≤ 3 hours. Do not freeze reconstituted rFVIIa or store it in syringes.

Actions

▶*Pharmacology:* Recombinant human coagulation Factor VIIa (rFVIIa) is intended for promoting hemostasis by activating the entrinsic pathway of the coagulation cascade. It is a vitamin K-dependent glycoprotein consisting of 406 amino acid residues (MW 50 K Dalton), and is structurally similar to human plasma-derived Factor VIIa. The purification process removes exogenous viruses. To eliminate the risk of human viral contamination, no human serum or other proteins are used in the production or formulation of rFVIIa. It contains trace amounts of proteins derived from the manufacturing and purification processes such as mouse IgG (maximum of 1.2 ng/mg), bovine IgG (maximum of 30 ng/mg), and protein from BHK-cells and media (maximum of 19 ng/mg).

Recombinant Factor VIIa when complexed with tissue factor can activate coagulation Factor X to Factor Xa, as well as coagulation Factor IX to Factor IXa. Factor Xa, in complex with other factors, then converts prothrombin to thrombin, which leads to the formation of a hemostatic plug by converting fibrinogen to fibrin and thereby inducing local hemostasis.

▶*Pharmacokinetics:* Single-dose pharmacokinetics of rFVIIa (17.5, 35, and 70 mcg/kg) exhibited dose-proportional kinetics in 15 subjects with hemophilia A or B. Factor VII (FVII) clotting activities were measured in plasma drawn prior to and during a 24-hour period after administration. The median apparent volume of distribution at steady state was 103 mL/kg (range, 78 to 139). Median clearance was 33 mL/kg/hr (range, 27 to 49). The median residence time was 3 hours (range, 2.4 to 3.3) and the half-life was 2.3 hours (range, 1.7 to 2.7). The median in vivo plasma recovery was 44% (30% to 71%).

Contraindications

Hypersensitivity to this product or any of its components, or to mouse, hamster, or bovine proteins.

Warnings

▶*Thrombotic events:* The extent of the risk of thrombotic adverse events after treatment is unknown, but is considered to be low. Patients with disseminated intravascular coagulation (DIC), advanced artherosclerotic disease, crush injury, or septicemia may have an increased risk of developing thrombotic events caused by circulating TF or predisposing coagulopathy (see Adverse Reactions).

Additional data on the adverse event profile in general and regarding the frequency of thrombotic events in particular is being collected through a postmarket surveillance program. The *NovoSeven* Cooperative Registry surveillance program is designed to collect data on all uses of this drug to expand the base of experience regarding its use. All prescribers can obtain information regarding contribution of patient data to this program by calling (877) 362–7355.

▶*Pregnancy:* Category C. Treatment of rats and rabbits with rFVIIa in reproduction studies has been associated with mortality at doses ≤ 6 mg/kg and 5 mg/kg. At 6 mg/kg in rats, the abortion rate was 0 out of 25 litters; in rabbits at 5 mg/kg, the abortion rate was 2 out of 25 litters. Twenty-three out of 25 female rats given 6 mg/kg gave birth successfully; however, 2 of the 23 litters died during the early period of lactation. There are no adequate and well-controlled studies in pregnant women. Use during pregnancy only if the potential benefit justifies the potential risk to the fetus.

Labor and delivery – rFVIIa was administered to a FVII-deficient patient (25 years of age, 66 kg) during a vaginal delivery (36 mcg/kg) and during a tubal ligation (90 mcg/kg). No adverse reactions were reported during labor, vaginal delivery, or the tubal ligation.

▶*Lactation:* It is not known whether rFVIIa is excreted in breast milk. Because of the potential for serious adverse reactions in nursing infants, decide whether to discontinue nursing or to discontinue the drug, taking into account the importance of the drug to the mother.

▶*Children:* Safety and efficacy were not determined to be different in various age groups, from infants to adolescents (0 to 16 years of age). Clinical trials were conducted, with dosing determined according to body weight and not according to age.

Precautions

▶*Monitoring:* Laboratory coagulation parameters may be used as an adjunct to the clinical evaluation of hemostasis in monitoring the effectiveness and treatment schedule of rFVIIa although these parameters have shown no direct correlation to achieving hemostasis. Assays of prothrombin time (PT), activated partial thromboplastin time (aPTT), and plasma FVII clotting activity (FVII:C), may give different results

COAGULATION FACTOR VIIa (RECOMBINANT)

with different reagents. Treatment has been shown to produce the following characteristics:

PT – In patients with hemophilia A/B with inhibitors, the PT shortened to an ≈ 7-second plateau at an FVII:C level of ≈ 5 U/mL. For FVII:C levels > 5 U/mL, there is no further change in PT.

aPTT – While administration of rFVIIa shortens the prolonged aPTT in hemophilia A/B patients with inhibitors, normalization usually has not been observed in doses shown to induce clinical improvement. Data indicate that clinical improvement was associated with a shortening of aPTT of 15 to 20 seconds.

FVIIa:C – FVIIa:C levels were measured 2 hours after rFVIIa administration of 35 and 90 mcg/kg following 2 days of dosing at 2-hour intervals. Average steady-state levels were 11 and 28 U/mL for the 2 dose levels, respectively.

➤*Intravascular coagulation/thrombosis:* Monitor patients receiving rFVIIa if they develop signs or symptoms of activation of the coagulation system or thrombosis. When there is laboratory confirmation of intravascular coagulation or presence of clinical thrombosis, reduce the rFVIIa dosage or stop treatment, depending on the patient's symptoms.

➤*Prolonged dosing:* Because of limited clinical studies, exercise precautions when rFVIIa is used for prolonged dosing (see Administration and Dosage).

Drug Interactions

➤*Coagulation factor concentrates:* The risk of a potential interaction between rFVIIa and coagulation factor concentrates has not been adequately evaluated in preclinical or clinical studies. Avoid simultaneous use of activated prothrombin complex concentrates or prothrombin complex concentrates.

Adverse Reactions

rFVIIa has been generally well tolerated in clinical studies in 298 patients with hemophilia A or B with inhibitors treated for 1939 bleeding episodes. The most frequent adverse events include the following: Fever (16%); hemorrhage NOS (15%); hemarthrosis (14%); fibrinogen plasma decreased (10%); hypertension (9%); allergic reaction, arthrosis, bradycardia, coagulation disorder, disseminated intravascular coagulation (DIC), edema, fibrinolysis increased, headache, hypotension, injection site reaction, pain, pneumonia, decreased prothrombin, pruritus, purpura, rash, abnormal renal function, decreased therapeutic response, vomiting (1%); thrombosis (2 patients).

Serious adverse events occurred in 14 of the 298 patients (4.7%). Six of these 14 patients died of the following conditions: Worsening of chronic renal failure, anesthesia complications during proctoscopy, renal failure complicating a retroperitoneal bleed, ruptured abscess leading to sepsis and DIC, pneumonia, and splenic hematoma and GI bleeding.

Overdosage

Two cases of accidental overdose by bolus administration have occurred in the clinical program. One hemophilia B patient (16 years of age, 68 kg) received a single dose of 352 mcg/kg and 1 hemophilia A patient (2 years of age, 14.6 kg) received doses ranging from 246 to 986 mcg/kg on 5 consecutive days. There were no reported complications in either case. Do not intentionally increase the recommended dose schedule, even in the case of lack of effect, because of the absence of information on the additional risk that may be incurred.

Patient Information

Inform patients of the benefits and risks associated with treatment. Warn patients about the early signs of hypersensitivity reactions, including hives, urticaria, tightness of the chest, wheezing, hypotension, and anaphylaxis.

ANTIHEMOPHILIC FACTOR (Factor VIII; AHF)

Rx	**Advate** (Baxter)	**Powder for Injection:** Concentrated recombinant AHF-PFM (plasma/albumin-free method). When reconstituted, contains 38 mg/mL mannitol, 10 mg/mL trehalose, 12mM histidine, 12mM Tris, 1.9 mM calcium, 0.17 mg/mL polysorbate-80, 0.1 mg/mL glutathione, and no more than 2 ng vWF/IU rAHF. Monoclonal purified and solvent-detergent treated.	108 mEq/L sodium. Preservative free. In 250, 500, 1000, and 1500 IU per single-dose vials with 5 mL of sterile water for injection, double-ended needle, filter needle, infusion set/blood collection set, and 10 mL sterile syringe.
Rx	**Alphanate** (Grifols)	**Injection, lyophilized:** Concentrate of human Factor VIII. When reconstituted, contains ≥ 5 IU FVIII:C/mg total protein, 0.3 to 0.9 g/100 mL albumin (human), ≤ 5 mmol Ca/L, ≤ 750 mcg glycine/IU FVIII:C, ≤ 1 U heparin/mL, ≤ 10 to 40 mmol histidine/L, ≤ 0.1 mg imidazole/mL, ≤ 50 to 200 mmol arginine/L, ≤ 1 mcg PEG and polysorbate 80. Solvent/detergent- and heat-treated.	≤ 0.1 mcg TNBP[1]/IU FVIII:C. In single-dose vials with diluent.[2]
Rx	**Bioclate** (Aventis)	**Powder for Injection, lyophilized:** Concentrated recombinant AHF. When reconstituted, contains 12.5 mg/mL albumin (human), 1.5 mg/mL PEG 3350, 55 mM histidine, 0.2 mg/mL Ca⁺⁺. Monoclonal purified.	180 mEq Na/L. Preservative free. In 250, 500, and 1000 IU per single-dose bottle with diluent, double-ended needle, and filter needle.
Rx	**Helixate FS** (Aventis)	**Injection, lyophilized:** Concentrate of AHF (recombinant). When reconstituted, contains 21 to 25 mg/mL glycine, ≤ 20 mcg/1000 IU imidazole, 2 to 3 mM CaCl, 32 to 40 mEq/L chloride, 18 to 23 mM histidine, < 0.6 mcg/1000 IU Cu. Solvent/detergent-treated.	27 to 36 mEq Na/L, < 5 mcg/1000 IU TNBP,[1] 28 mg sucrose. Preservative and albumin free. In 250, 500, and 1000 IU with diluent[2], double-ended needle, filter needle, and administration set.
Rx	**Hemofil M** (Baxter Healthcare)	**Injection:** A preparation of human AHF in concentrated form. When reconstituted, contains ≤ 12.5 mg/mL albumin (human), 0.07 mg/mL PEG 3350, 0.39 mg histidine, 0.1 mg glycine, and ≤ 1 ng of mouse protein. Solvent/detergent-treated. Monoclonal purified.	18 ng TNBP. In single-dose bottles with diluent,[2] double-ended needle, and filter needle.
Rx	**Hyate:C (Porcine)** (IPSEN[3])	**Powder for Injection, lyophilized:** Concentrate of AHF (VIII):C. Each vial contains 400 to 700 porcine units and 10 to 30 mmol/L citrate ions.	110 to 135 mmol/L sodium ions. Preservative free. In vials[2] with filter needle.
Rx	**Koate-DVI** (Bayer)	**Injection, lyophilized:** Concentrate of AHF (human). When reconstituted, contains ≤ 1500 mcg/mL PEG, ≤ 0.05 M glycine, ≤ 25 mcg/mL polysorbate 80, ≤ 3 mM Ca, ≤ 1 mcg/mL Al, ≤ 0.06 M histidine, ≤ 10 mg/mL albumin (human). Solvent/detergent- and heat-treated.	≤ 5 mcg/g TNBP.[1] In ≈ 250 or 500 IU Factor VIII activity and ≈ 1000 IU Factor VIII activity with diluent,[2] double-ended needle, filter needle, and administration set.
Rx	**Kogenate FS** (Bayer)	**Injection, lyophilized:** Recombinant AHF. 21 to 25 mg/mL glycine, 18 to 23 mM histidine; 2 to 3 mM CaCl, 32 to 40 mEq/L CI, ≤ 35 mcg/mL polysorbate 80, ≤ 20 mcg/1000 IU imidazole, ≤ 0.6 mcg/1000 IU Cu. Solvent/detergent-treated. Monoclonal purified.	≤ 5 mcg/1000 IU TNBP,[1] 27 to 36 mEq Na/L, 28 mg sucrose/vial. Preservative and albumin free. In 250, 500, and 1000 IU with diluent, double-ended transfer needle, filter needle, and administration set.
Rx	**Monarc-M** (American Red Cross)	**Powder for injection:** A concentrated preparation of AHF. 2 to 15 AHF IU/mg total protein, and a maximum of 12.5 mg/mL albumin (human) and 0.07 mg PEG 3350, 0.39 mg histidine, and 0.1 mg glycine/AHF IU. ≤ 0.1 ng/AHF IU mouse protein, 18 ng organic solvent (tri-n-butyl phosphate), and 50 ng detergent (octoxynol 9). Monoclonal purified.	In single-dose bottles with 10 mL Sterile Water for Injection, double-ended needle, and filter needle.

ANTIHEMOPHILIC FACTOR (Factor VIII; AHF)

Rx	**Monoclate-P** (Aventis)	**Powder for injection, lyophilized:** Concentrate of human Factor VIII: C. When reconstituted, contains ≈ 2 to 5 mM CaCl per L, ≈ 1% to 2% albumin (human), 0.8% mannitol, 1.2 mM histidine, and < 50 ng/100 IU trace murine monoclonal antibody. Heat-treated. Monoclonal purified.	≈ 300 to 450 mM/L Na ions. With diluent, double-ended needle, vented filter spike, winged infusion set, and alcohol swabs.[2]
Rx	**Recombinate** (Baxter)	**Powder for injection, lyophilized:** Concentrated recombinant AHF. When reconstituted, contains 12.5 mg/mL albumin (human), 1.5 mg/mL PEG, 55 mM histidine, 0.2 mg/mL Ca. Monoclonal purified.	180 mEq Na/L. In single-dose 250, 500, and 1000 IU bottles[2] with diluent, double-ended needle, and filter needle.
Rx	**ReFacto** (Genetics Institute)	**Powder for injection, lyophilized:** Recombinant AHF. When reconstituted, contains L-histidine, CaCl, and polysorbate 80.	NaCl, sucrose. Preservative free. In single-use vials with 250, 500, or 1000 IU/vial, with diluent, double-ended needle, filter needle for withdrawal, infusion set, and alcohol swabs.

[1] Tri-n-butyl-phosphate.
[2] Actual number of AHF units are indicated on the vials.

[3] IPSEN Inc., 27 Maple Street, Milford, MA 01757; (800) 456-7322.

Indications

➤*Classical hemophilia:* Classical hemophilia (hemophilia A) in which there is a deficiency of the plasma clotting factor, Factor VIII. Provides a means of temporarily replacing the missing clotting factor to control, correct, and/or prevent bleeding episodes. Also indicated for perioperative management of hemophilic patients.

➤*Short-term prophylaxis (ReFacto only):* For short-term routine prophylaxis to reduce the frequency of spontaneous bleeding episodes. The effect of regular routine prophylaxis on long-term morbidity and mortality is unknown.

➤*Hyate:C:* For the treatment and prevention of bleeding in congenital hemophilia A patients with antibodies (inhibitors) to human Factor VIII and also for previously nonhemophilic patients with spontaneously acquired inhibitors to human Factor VIII (acquired hemophilia). In patients with acquired hemophilia, consider porcine Factor VIII infusion as first-line therapy regardless of the initial anti-human inhibitor titer. Because of the wide individual variation in the interaction of anti-human Factor VIII antibodies with porcine Factor VIII, directly measure the patient's antibody titer against porcine Factor VIII.

Circulating antibodies (inhibitors) generally show a weaker neutralizing activity against porcine Factor VIII than against human Factor VIII. Therefore, antihemophilic factor can be used to produce a hemostatic level of Factor VIII in patients whose antibody level and kinetics preclude treatment with human Factor VIII concentrates. Determine the activity of a patient's antibody in the laboratory using porcine Factor VIII as a substrate in a modified Bethesda assay.

Administration and Dosage

Administer IV only. Use a plastic syringe; solutions may stick to the surface of glass.

Individualize dosage. The dose depends on patient weight, severity of the deficiency, severity of hemorrhage, presence of inhibitors, and the Factor VIII level desired. Clinical effect on the patient is the most important factor of therapy. When inhibitors are present, dosage requirements are extremely variable; determine by clinical response. It may be necessary to administer more AHF to obtain the desired result.

There is a linear dose-response relation with an approximate yield of 2% to 2.5% rise in Factor VIII activity for each unit of Factor VIII/kg transfused, from which an approximate factor of 0.5 IU/kg can be calculated. The following formulas provide a guide for dosage calculations:

Expected Factor VIII increase (in % of normal) =

$$\frac{\text{AHF/IU administered} \times 2}{\text{body weight (in kg)}}$$

AHF/IU required = body weight (kg) × desired Factor VIII increase (% normal) × 0.5

Physician supervision of the dosage is required. The following dosage schedule may be used as a guide.

Antihemophilic Factor Recommended Dosage Schedule		
Hemorrhage: Degree of hemorrhage	Required peak postinfusion AHF activity in the blood (as % of normal or IU/dL plasma)	Frequency of infusion
Early hemarthrosis, muscle bleed, or oral bleed	20 to 40	Begin infusion every 12 to 24 hours for 1 to 3 days until the bleeding episode as indicated by pain is resolved or healing is achieved.
More extensive hemarthrosis, muscle bleed, or hematoma	30 to 60	Repeat infusion every 12 to 24 hours for usually ≥ 3 days until pain and disability are resolved.

Antihemophilic Factor Recommended Dosage Schedule		
Life threatening bleeds such as head injury, throat bleed, severe abdominal pain	60 to 100	Repeat infusion every 8 to 24 hours until threat is resolved.
Surgery: Minor surgery, including tooth extraction	60 to 80 60 to 100 (*Advate* only)[a]	A single infusion plus oral antifibrinolytic therapy within 1 hour is sufficient in ≈ 70% of cases.
Major surgery	80 to 100 (pre- and postoperative) 80 to 120 (pre and postoperative, *Advate* only)[b]	Repeat infusion every 8 to 24 hours depending on state of healing.

[a] Give a single bolus infusion beginning within 1 hour of the operation, with optional additional dosing every 12 to 24 hours as needed to control bleeding. For dental procedures, adjunctive therapy may be considered.
[b] For bolus infusion replacement, repeat infusions every 8 to 24 hours, depending on the desired level of Factor VIII and state of wound healing.

The careful control of the substitution therapy is especially important in cases of major surgery or life-threatening hemorrhages.

Although dosage can be estimated by the calculations above, it is strongly recommended that whenever possible, appropriate laboratory tests including serial AHF assays be performed on the patient's plasma at suitable intervals to assure that adequate AHF levels have been reached and are maintained.

➤*Mild hemorrhage:* Do not repeat therapy unless further bleeding occurs. Minor episodes generally subside with a single infusion of 10 IU/kg if level ≥ 20% to 30% of normal is attained.

➤*Moderate hemorrhage and minor surgery:* These instances require plasma Factor VIII level to be raised to 30% to 50% of normal for optimum hemostasis. This usually requires an initial dose of 15 to 25 AHF/IU/kg; if further therapy is required, administer a maintenance dose of 10 to 15 AHF/IU/kg every 8 to 12 hours.

➤*Severe hemorrhage:* For life-threatening bleeding, or hemorrhage involving vital structures (CNS, retropharyngeal and retroperitoneal spaces, iliopsoas sheath), raise the Factor VIII level to 80% to 100% of normal. Administer an initial AHF dose of 40 to 50 AHF/IU/kg and a maintenance dose of 20 to 25 AHF/IU/kg every 8 to 12 hours.

➤*Major surgery:* Major surgery procedures require a dose of AHF sufficient to achieve a level of 80% to 100% of normal; give 1 hour before the procedure. Check the Factor VIII level prior to surgery to assure the level is achieved. Repeat infusions may be necessary every 6 to 12 hours initially. Maintain the Factor VIII level at a daily minimum of ≥ 30% of normal for a healing period of 10 to 14 days.

➤*Dental extraction:* Dental extraction procedures require a peak postinfusion AHF activity in the blood of 60% to 80%. A single infusion plus oral antifibrinolytic therapy within 1 hour is sufficient in ≈ 70% of cases.

➤*Prophylaxis:* Factor VIII concentrates may be administered on a regular schedule for prophylaxis of bleeding.

Incorrect diagnosis, inappropriate dosage, method of administration, and biological differences in individual patients could reduce the efficacy of these products or even result in an ill effect following its use. It is important that these products be stored properly, the directions for use be followed carefully during use, the risk of transmitting viruses be carefully weighed before a product is prescribed, and that plasma Factor VIII levels be measured in initial treatment situations or if clinical response appears inadequate.

➤*ReFacto:* For short-term routine prophylaxis to prevent or reduce the frequency of spontaneous musculoskeletal hemorrhage in patients with hemophilia A, give ≥ 2 times/week. In pediatric patients, shorter dosage intervals or higher doses may be necessary. Pharmacokinetic/pharmacodynamic modeling predicts that routine prophylactic dosing 3 times/week may be associated with a lower bleeding risk than with dosing twice weekly. No randomized comparison of different doses or frequency regimens for routine prophylaxis has been performed.

ANTIHEMOPHILIC FACTOR (Factor VIII; AHF)

►Rate of administration: Administer preparations IV at a rate of ≈ 2 mL/min. Can be given at up to 10 mL/min. Administration of the entire dose in 5 to 10 minutes is generally well tolerated. As a precaution, determine the pulse rate before and during administration of the AHF concentrate. Should a significant increase of pulse rate occur, reduce the rate of administration or discontinue.

►Storage/Stability: Store between 2° and 8°C (35° to 46°F) (except *Hyate:C*). Do not freeze. See additional storage information below. Use before the expiration date.

AHF Room Temperature Storage Recommendations	
Product	Recommendation
Advate	22° to 28°C (72° to 82°F) for ≤ 6 months[a]
Alphanate	< 30°C (80°F) for < 2 months
Bioclate	< 30°C (80°F) until expiration date
Helixate FS	< 25°C (77°F) for ≤ 2 months
Hemofil M	< 30°C (80°F) until expiration date
Koate-DVI	< 25°C (77°F) for ≤ 6 months
Kogenate	< 25°C (77°F) for ≤ 3 months
Kogenate FS	< 25°C (77°F) for ≤ 2 months
Monoclate P	< 30°C (80°F) for ≤ 6 months
Recombinate	< 30°C (80°F) until expiration date
ReFacto	< 25°C (77°F) for ≤ 3 months

[a] Should be refrigerated but may be stored at room temperature.

Advate – Refrigerate at 2° to 8°C (36° to 46°F). Avoid freezing to prevent damage to the diluent vial. Use before expiration date.

Hyate:C – Store at -15° to -20°C (5° to -4°F). Use before expiration date.

Actions

►Pharmacology: AHF is a protein found in normal plasma necessary for clot formation. Administration of AHF can temporarily correct the coagulation defect of patients with classical hemophilia (hemophilia A). Activated Factor VIII acts as a cofactor for activated Factor IX accelerating the conversion of Factor X to activated Factor X. Activated Factor X converts prothrombin into thrombin. Thrombin then converts fibrinogen into fibrin and a clot is formed. Factor VIII activity is greatly reduced in patients with hemophilia A and, therefore, replacement therapy is necessary. The biological half-life is ≈ 10 to 18 hours.

Contraindications

Hypersensitivity to mouse, hamster, or bovine protein (see Precautions), or to porcine or murine factor.

Warnings

►von Willebrand's disease: Not effective in controlling the bleeding of patients with von Willebrand's disease.

►Hepatitis and AIDS: Because antihemophilic factor is made from pooled human plasma, it may carry a risk of transmitting infectious agents (eg, viruses, and theoretically, the Creutzfeldt-Jakob disease [CJD] agent). Stringent procedures designed to reduce the risk of adventitious agent transmission have been employed in the manufacture of these products, from the screening of plasma donors and the collection and testing of plasma, through the application of viral elimination/reduction steps such as solvent detergent and heat treatment in the manufacturing process. Despite these measures, such products can still potentially transmit disease; therefore, the risk of infectious agents cannot be totally eliminated. All infections thought to by a physician possibly to have been transmitted by antihemophilic factor should be reported to the manufacturer. The physician should weigh the risks and benefits of use of the product and discuss these with the patient.

Individuals who receive infusions of blood or plasma products may develop signs or symptoms of some viral infections, particularly hepatitis C. Incubation in a solvent detergent mixture during the manufacturing process is designed to reduce the risk of transmitting viral infection. However, scientific opinion encourages hepatitis A and B vaccinations for patients with hemophilia at birth or time of diagnosis.

►Pregnancy: Category C. Safety for use during pregnancy has not been established. Use only if clearly needed.

►Children:
Bioclate, Helixate FS, Kogenate, Kogenate FS, Recombinate, ReFacto – Appropriate for use in all ages, including newborns.

Alphanate – Clinical trials in patients < 16 years of age have not been conducted. In a small, well-controlled clinical trial with patients previously treated with AHF FVII, a pediatric patient treated with *Alphanate* responded similarly to adults. No adverse events were reported.

Koate DVI – *Koate DVI* has not been studied in pediatric patients.

Advate – A total of 54 subjects 16 years of age and younger have been treated across all studies to date. Interim pharmacokinetic data for 34 subjects (per protocol analysis population) 16 years of age and younger were obtained from a combined dataset comprising subjects 10 to 16 years of age treated on the phase 2/3 pivotal study and subjects enrolled and treated on the ongoing study of pediatric previously treated subjects younger than 6 years of age. Among these, 0 were neonates (birth to younger than 1 month of age), 2 were infants (1 month to younger than 2 years of age), 15 were children (2 to 12 years of age), and 17 were adolescents (12 to 16 years of age or younger). Pharmacokinetic parameters were not significantly different for the different age categories. The mean plasma half-life was 11.21 hours (range, 8.31 to 24.7 hours). The mean AUC_{0-48h} was 1363 IU•h/dL. The mean values for C_{max} and adjusted recovery were 109 IU/dL and 2.17 IU/dL/ IU/kg, respectively.

Precautions

Identification of the clotting defect as a Factor VIII deficiency is essential before the administration of AHF FVIII:C is initiated.

►Factor VIII inhibitor: The formation of inhibitors to Factor VIII is a known complication in the management of individuals with hemophilia A. The reported prevalence of these antibodies in patients receiving plasma derived AHF is 10% to 20%. These inhibitors are invariably IgG immunoglobulins, the Factor VIII procoagulant inhibitory activity of which is expressed as Bethesda Units (BU) per mL of plasma or serum. Carefully monitor patients treated with rAHF for the development of antibodies to rAHF by appropriate clinical observations and laboratory tests. Inhibitor formation is especially common in young children with severe hemophilia during their first years of treatment, or in patients of any age who have received little previous treatment with FVIII. Nonetheless, inhibitor formation may occur at any time in the treatment of a patient with hemophilia A. Anti-inhibitor complex is available (see the Anti-Inhibitor Coagulant Complex monograph).

►Hemolysis: AHF contains naturally occurring blood group-specific antibodies (Anti-A and Anti-B isoagglutinins). When large or frequently repeated doses are needed in patients of blood group A, B, or AB, intravascular hemolysis may occur; monitor the hematocrit and Direct Coombs' test. Correct hemolytic anemia with compatible group O red blood cells or AHF from group-specific plasma.

►Monoclonal antibody-derived Factor VIII:
Formation of antibodies to mouse protein – Although no hypersensitivity reactions have been observed, they may possibly occur because of trace amounts of mouse protein.

►Laboratory tests: Ensure that adequate AHF levels have been reached and are maintained. If the AHF level fails to reach expected levels or if bleeding is not controlled after apparently adequate dosage, inhibitors may be present. The presence of inhibitors can be demonstrated and quantitated in terms of AHF units neutralized by each mL of plasma or by the total estimated plasma volume. After sufficient dosage to neutralize inhibitor, additional dosage produces predicted clinical response.

►Porcine parvovirus (PPV) (Hyate:C only): PPV is endemic in pigs throughout the world and can frequently be identified in pooled collections of porcine plasmas. The virus is highly resistant to chemical and physical methods of sterilization. The available evidence is that PPV does not cause clinical or subclinical infection in humans. The porcine plasma used in the manufacture of *Hyate:C* is screened for the presence of PPV DNA using a sensitive polymerase chain reaction test. Only plasma that is nonreactive in the test is used for the manufacture of *Hyate:C*. It is possible that extremely low levels of PPV or of other viruses, present at levels below the limit of detection of the cell screens, or small quantities of noninfective viral subunits including DNA may be present in the final product. There is no evidence that these materials are a health hazard. However, the effects, if any, of long-term exposure have not been studied systematically and are therefore unknown.

Adverse Reactions

►Cardiovascular: Mild hypotension; chest discomfort; vasodilation; angina pectoris; tachycardia.

►CNS: Headache; somnolence; lethargy; dizziness; tingling in arm, ear, and face; jittery feeling; asthenia.

►Dermatologic: Rash; facial flushing; increased perspiration; acne; pruritus.

►GI: Nausea; vomiting; taste changes; constipation; stomachache; diarrhea; anorexia; gastroenteritis; abdominal pain; dysgeusia.

►Hematologic: Forearm bleeding following venapuncture; anemia; permanent venous access catheter complications; infected hematoma; forehead bruises.

►Musculoskeletal: Myalgia; muscle weakness; joint swelling.

►Respiratory: Nose bleeds; rhinitis; dyspnea; coughing.

►Special senses: Serous otitis media; blurred vision; sore throat; eye disorder/vision abnormal.

►Miscellaneous: Fever; chills; urticaria; fatigue; depersonalization; adenopathy; pallor in an inhibitor patient with gastroenteritis; cold feet; increased amino transferase; increased bilirubin; CPK increase; cold sensation; finger pain; rigors; hot flushes; hematocrit decreased; coagulation factor VIII decreased; chest pain.

Allergic reactions – Hives, fever, urticaria, mild chills, nausea, stinging at the infusion site, tightness of the chest, hypotension, and anaphylaxis may occur.

ANTIHEMOPHILIC FACTOR (Factor VIII; AHF)

Thrombocytopenia (Hyate:C) – Acute thrombocytopenia has been reported to occur on rare occasions following infusion of *Hyate:C*. Consider monitoring of the platelet count during treatment.

Patient Information

Inform patients of the early symptoms and signs of hypersensitivity reaction, including hives, generalized urticaria, chest tightness, dyspnea, wheezing, faintness, hypotension, and anaphylaxis. Advise patients to discontinue use of the product and contact their physician or seek emergency care, depending on the severity of the reaction, if these symptoms occur.

Some viruses, such as parvovirus B19 or hepatitis A, are particularly difficult to remove or inactivate at this time. Parvovirus B19 most seriously affects seronegative pregnant women or immune-compromised individuals. The majority of parvovirus B19 and hepatitis A infections are acquired by environmental (natural) sources. Symptoms of parvovirus B19 infection include fever, drowsiness, chills, and runny nose followed $\approx$ 2 weeks later by a rash and joint pain. Evidence of hepatitis A may include several days to weeks of poor appetite, tiredness, and low-grade fever followed by nausea, vomiting, and pain in the belly. Dark urine and a yellowed complexion are also common symptoms. Encourage patients to consult their physician if such symptoms appear.

Factor VIII inhibitors are circulating antibodies that neutralize the procoagulant activity of Factor VIII. Patients with these inhibitors may not respond to treatment with AHF or the response may be much less than would otherwise be expected. Therefore, larger doses of AHF are often required. The management of bleeding in patients with inhibitors requires careful monitoring, especially if surgical procedures are indicated.

ANTI-INHIBITOR COAGULANT COMPLEX

| Rx | Autoplex T (Nabi) | Dried anti-inhibitor coagulant complex. Maximum of 2 units heparin and 2 mg polyethylene glycol/mL reconstituted material. Heat-treated. | $\approx$ 177 mEq/L Na. In vials with diluent and needles. Each bottle is labeled with the units of Factor VIII correctional activity it contains. |
| Rx | Feiba VH Immuno (Immuno-US) | Freeze-dried anti-inhibitor coagulant complex. Heparin free. Vapor-heated. | $\approx$ 8 mg/mL Na. In vials with diluent and needles. Each bottle is labeled with the units of Factor VIII inhibitor bypassing activity it contains. |

Indications

➤*Factor VIII inhibitors:* Patients with Factor VIII inhibitors who are bleeding or who are to undergo surgery.

Treat patients with anti-inhibitor coagulant complex whose present Factor VIII inhibitor levels are > 10 Bethesda Units (BU), or whose inhibitor levels are known to rise to > 10 BU following treatment with AHF (*Autoplex T*).

Patients whose present Factor VIII inhibitor levels are between 2 and 10 BU (*Autoplex T*) or 5 and 10 BU (*Feiba VH Immuno*) and whose inhibitor levels remain in this range following treatment with AHF may be treated with either AHF or anti-inhibitor coagulant complex, depending on the patient's clinical history and severity of the bleeding episode.

Patients with Factor VIII inhibitor levels of < 2 BU whose inhibitor levels are known to remain at ≤ 2 BU (*Autoplex T*) or ≤ 5 BU (*Feiba VH Immuno*) following treatment with AHF may be treated with appropriate doses of AHF.

For patients who have low levels of Factor VIII inhibitor and whose history does not include adequate laboratory indications of an anamnestic response to AHF, base the treatment of choice on clinical judgment. In patients having noncritical or minor bleeding episodes, the use of anti-inhibitor coagulant complex will maintain the inhibitor at a low level and allow the use of other coagulant therapeutic agents in subsequent major emergencies.

Feiba VH Immuno has been described in a few nonhemophiliacs with acquired inhibitors to Factors VIII, XI, and XII.

Administration and Dosage

➤*Autoplex T:* One unit of Hyland Factor VIII correctional activity is the quantity of activated prothrombin complex that, upon addition to an equal volume of Factor VIII deficient or inhibitor plasma, will correct the clotting time (ellagic acid-activated partial thromboplastin time [aPTT]) to 35 seconds (normal).

➤*Feiba VH Immuno:* One Immuno unit of activity is defined as that amount of anti-inhibitor coagulant complex that shortens the aPTT of a high titer Factor VIII inhibitor reference plasma to 50% of the blank value.

Administer by IV injection or drip only.

➤*Dosage range:*

Autoplex T – 25 to 100 Factor VIII correctional units/kg, depending upon the severity of hemorrhage. If no hemostatic improvement is observed at $\approx$ 6 hours following the initial administration, repeat the dosage. Adjust subsequent dosages and administration intervals according to the patient's clinical response.

Feiba VH Immuno – 50 to 100 Immuno Units/kg.

➤*Feiba VH Immuno:*

Joint hemorrhage – 50 U/kg at 12-hour intervals; may be increased to doses of 100 U/kg at 12-hour intervals. Continue until clear signs of clinical improvement appear (eg, pain relief, swelling reduction, joint mobilization).

Mucous membrane bleeding – 50 U/kg at 6-hour intervals under careful monitoring of visible bleeding site with repeated measurements of hematocrit. If hemorrhage does not stop, increase to 100 U/kg at 6-hour intervals; do not exceed 200 U/kg/day.

Soft tissue hemorrhage – For serious soft tissue bleeding, such as retroperitoneal bleeding, 100 U/kg at 12-hour intervals. Do not exceed 200 U/kg/day.

Other severe hemorrhages – Other severe hemorrhages, such as CNS bleeding, have been effectively treated with doses of 100 U/kg at 12-hour intervals. Anti-inhibitor coagulant complex (*Feiba VH Immuno*) may be indicated at 6-hour intervals until clear clinical improvement is achieved.

➤*Rate of administration:*

Autoplex T – Initially infuse at 2 mL/min. The rate may be gradually increased to 10 mL/min.

Feiba VH Immuno – Maximum injection or infusion rate must not exceed 2 units/kg/minute.

➤*Storage/Stability:* Refrigerate the unreconstituted complex between 2° to 8°C (35° to 46°F). Avoid freezing. Do not refrigerate after reconstitution. Complete administration within 1 hour (*Autoplex T*) to 3 hours (*Feiba VH Immuno*) after reconstitution.

Actions

➤*Pharmacology:* Control of thrombin formation is regulated by the presence of antithrombin III and other serine protease inhibitors that neutralize Factors IXa and Xa, the short biological half-lives of Factors VII and VIIa, and the presence of the circulating Factor VIII inhibitor that additionally controls overactivation of the intrinsic coagulation system.

Anti-inhibitor coagulant complex is prepared from pooled human plasma and contains variable amounts of activated and precursor clotting factors. Kinin generating system factors are also present. It is standardized by its ability to correct the clotting time of Factor VIII deficient plasma or Factor VIII deficient plasma containing inhibitors to Factor VIII.

Approximately 10% of individuals with hemophilia A have laboratory-measurable inhibitors to Factor VIII. The treatment depends upon the existing level of inhibitor, whether or not the patient responds to infusions of antihemophilic factor (AHF) with increased inhibitor levels (anamnestic rise in Factor VIII antibody), and the severity of the bleeding episode.

Contraindications

➤*Autoplex T:* Signs of fibrinolysis; disseminated intravascular coagulation (DIC).

➤*Feiba VH Immuno:* Patients with a normal coagulation mechanism.

Warnings

➤*Infectious disease transmission:* Products are prepared from large pools of human plasma. Such plasma may contain the causative agents of viral hepatitis or other viral diseases. In addition, *Feiba VH Immuno* has been subjected to a vapor heat treatment during the manufacturing process to reduce the risk of transmitting viral infections. However, no procedure is totally effective in eliminating viral infectivity.

➤*Viral infections:* Individuals who have received multiple infusions of blood or plasma products may develop signs or symptoms of certain viral infections, especially non-A, non-B hepatitis.

➤*Anamnestic responses:* Anamnestic responses with rise in Factor VIII inhibitor titer occurred in 20% of cases (*Feiba VH Immuno*).

➤*Hypersensitivity reaction:* Refer to Management of Acute Hypersensitivity Reactions.

➤*Hepatic function impairment:* Give special caution and consideration to the use of *Autoplex T* in individuals with preexisting liver disease.

➤*Pregnancy: Category C.* It is not known whether the drug can cause fetal harm when administered to a pregnant woman or can affect reproduction capacity. Use only if clearly needed.

➤*Children:* No data are available for *Feiba VH Immuno* regarding use in newborns. For *Autoplex T,* give special caution and consideration to use in newborns. A higher morbidity and mortality may be associated with hepatitis.

ANTI-INHIBITOR COAGULANT COMPLEX

Precautions

▶*Laboratory tests:* Tests used to control efficacy such as aPTT, WBCT, and TEG do not correlate with clinical improvement. Appearance of hemostatic improvement may occur without reduction of aPTT. However, expect prothrombin time to be shortened. Attempts to normalize these values by increasing the dose of anti-inhibitor coagulant complex may not be successful and are strongly discouraged because of the potential hazard of producing DIC by overdosage.

Children – Check fibrinogen levels prior to initial infusion; monitor during treatment.

▶*DIC:* If signs of DIC occur, including changes in blood pressure and pulse rate, respiratory distress, chest pain, and cough, stop the infusion and monitor the patient. Laboratory indications of DIC include prolonged thrombin time, prothrombin time, and partial thromboplastin time tests, decreased fibrinogen concentration, decreased platelet count, or the presence of fibrin split products.

▶*Identification of clotting deficiency:* Identification of clotting deficiency caused by the presence of Factor VIII inhibitors is essential before initiating administration of anti-inhibitor coagulant complex.

Feiba VH Immuno – Use only in patients with circulating inhibitors to ≥ 1 coagulation factor and do not use for the treatment of bleeding episodes resulting from coagulation factor deficiencies. Do not give to patients with significant signs of DIC or fibrinolysis. Thromboembolic events may occur, particularly following the administration of high doses or in patients with thrombotic risk factors. Monitor patients receiving > 100 units/kg for the development of DIC or symptoms of acute coronary ischemia. Give high doses only as long as absolutely necessary to stop bleeding. *Feiba VH Immuno* and antifibrinolytics have been given simultaneously without complications. However, it is recommended not to use antifibrinolytics until 12 hours after the administration of *Feiba VH Immuno.*

▶*Reconstitution/Infusion time:* If the infusion of the concentrate occurs > 1 hour following reconstitution, there may be increased prekallikrein activator (PKA) and consequent hypotension (*Autoplex T*).

▶*Nonhemophilic patients:* Nonhemophilic patients with acquired inhibitors against Factors VIII, IX, or XII may have a bleeding tendency and an increased risk of thrombosis at the same time.

Drug Interactions

▶*Epsilon-aminocaproic acid (EACA) or tranexamic acid:* The concomitant use of anti-inhibitor coagulant complex with such agents is not recommended because only limited data are available on the administration of these highly activated prothrombin complex products together with antifibrinolytic agents.

Adverse Reactions

A rapid rate of infusion may cause headache, flushing, and changes in pulse rate and blood pressure.

Laboratory and clinical signs of DIC have occasionally been observed following high doses (single infusion of > 100 U/kg and daily doses of 200 U/kg). Monitor patients on these doses carefully (see Precautions) (*Feiba VH Immuno*).

Thromboembolic events may occur, particularly after high doses and in patients with thrombotic risk factors.

MI was found to occur after high doses and prolonged administration and in the presence of risk factors predisposing to MI (*Feiba VH Immuno*).

Treat allergic reactions with antihistamines and glucocorticoids. Treat shock in the usual way.

▶*Hypersensitivity:* Fever, chills, indications of protein sensitivity, signs and symptoms of high prekallikrein activity (eg, changes in blood pressure or pulse rate); allergic reactions from mild, short-term urticarial rashes to severe anaphylactoid reactions.

FACTOR IX CONCENTRATES

Rx	**AlphaNine SD** (Grifols)	**Powder for injection:** Dried plasma fraction of Factor IX.[1] Solvent/detergent-treated. Virus-filtered.	In single-dose vials with diluent, needle, and filter.[2]
Rx	**BeneFix** (Genetics Institute)	**Powder for injection:** Nonpyrogenic lyophilized. Purified protein produced by recombinant DNA for use in Factor IX deficiency.[1]	Preservative free. In 250, 500 or 1000 IU/single-dose vial with diluent, needle, filter, infusion set, and alcohol swabs.
Rx	**Mononine** (Aventis)	**Powder for injection:** Sterile, lyophilized concentrate of Factor IX, plasma-derived.	In 250, 500, and 1000 U single-dose vials with diluent, double-ended needle, vented filter spike, winged infusion set, and alcohol swabs.[3]
Rx	**Profilnine SD** (Grifols)	**Powder for injection:** Sterile, lyophilized concentrate of Factor IX, plasma-derived. Solvent/detergent-treated.	Heparin free. Preservative free. In 250, 500, and 1000 U single-dose vials with diluent.
Rx	**Proplex T** (Baxter)	**Powder for injection:** Plasma derived concentrate of clotting Factors II, VII, IX and X.[1] Heat-treated.	In 30 mL vials with diluent and needles.[3]
Rx	**Bebulin VH** (Baxter)	**Powder for injection:** Purified freeze-dried concentrate of coagulation Factor IX, II, and X. Heat-treated.[1]	In single-dose vials with Sterile Water for Injection, double-ended needle, and filter needle.

[1] Actual number of units shown on each bottle.
[2] Contains heparin and dextrose.
[3] Contains heparin.

Indications

▶*Factor IX deficiency (hemophilia B [Christmas disease]):* To prevent or control bleeding episodes. Do not use in mild Factor IX deficiency if fresh frozen plasma is effective. (See individual package inserts for product specifications.)

▶*Factor VII deficiency (Proplex T only):* Factor IX complex has been used in hemarthroses occurring in hemophiliacs with inhibitors to Factor VIII.

The Factor VII content present in *Proplex T* has been shown to be effective in prevention or control of bleeding episodes in patients with Factor VII deficiency.

Administration and Dosage

▶*Factor IX Deficiency (hemophilia B [Christmas disease]):* For IV use only. One International Unit (IU) is defined as the activity present in 1 mL of pooled normal fresh plasma. The potency is standardized in terms of Factor IX content.

When reconstitution of Factor IX concentrate is complete, its infusion should commence within 3 hours. However, begin the infusion as promptly as is practical.

The amount of Factor IX concentrate required to restore normal hemostasis varies with circumstances and patient. Dosage depends on the degree of deficiency and desired hemostatic level of the deficient factor. Use the following formula as a guide to calculate dosage.

Units required to raise blood level percentages:

Recombinant Factor IX –

1.2 IU/kg × body weight (kg) × desired increase (% of normal)

Human-derived Factor IX –

1 IU/kg × body weight (kg) × desired increase (% of normal).

If a 70 kg (154 lb) patient needs a 25% increase in Factor IX, give
1 unit/kg × 70 kg × 25 = 1750 units.

Factor IX Dosing Guidelines in Bleeding Episodes and Surgery[1]			
Type of hemorrhage	Circulating Factor IX activity required (% or [IU/dL])	Dosing interval (hours)	Duration of therapy (days)
Minor Uncomplicated hemarthroses, superficial muscle, or soft tissue	20 to 30	12 to 24	1 to 2
Moderate Intramuscle or soft tissue with disconnection, mucous membranes, dental extractions, or hematuria	25 to 50	12 to 24	Treat until bleeding stops and healing begins; about 2 to 7 days.
Major Pharynx, retropharynx, retroperitoneum, CNS, surgery	50 to 100	12 to 24	7 to 10

[1] Adapted from: Roberts HR, Eberst ME. Current management of hemophilia B. *Hematol Oncol Clin North Am.* 1993;7:1269-1280.

FACTOR IX CONCENTRATES

As a general rule, 1 unit of human-derived Factor IX activity per kg will increase the circulating level of Factor IX by 1% of normal, and 1 IU of recombinant Factor IX per kg of body weight will increase the circulatory activity of Factor IX by 0.8 IU/dL. Determine exact dosage based on the physician's judgment of circumstances, patient condition, degree of deficiency, and the desired level of Factor IX to be achieved. If inhibitors to Factor IX appear, use sufficient additional dosage to overcome the inhibitors.

To maintain an elevated level of the deficient factor, repeat dosage as needed. Clinical studies suggest relatively high levels may be maintained by daily or twice daily doses, while the lower effective levels may require injections only once every 2 or 3 days. A single dose may stop a minor bleeding episode.

➤*Factor VII deficiency (Proplex T only):* Units required to raise blood level percentages:

0.5 unit/kg × body weight (in kg) × desired increase (% of normal).

Repeat dose every 4 to 6 hours as needed.

If a 70 kg (154 lb) patient with a Factor VII level of 0% needs to be elevated to 25%, give 0.5 unit/kg × 70 kg × 25 = 875 units.

In preparation for and following surgery, maintain levels > 25% for ≥ 1 week. Use laboratory control to assure such levels. To maintain levels > 25% for a reasonable time, calculate each dose to raise levels to 40% to 60% of normal.

➤*Factor VIII inhibitor (Proplex T only):* Employ dosage levels approximating 75 IU/kg.

Proplex T is recommended when hemarthroses occurring in hemophiliacs with inhibitors to Factor VII cannot be resolved by administration of Factor IX complex and in other types of bleeding episodes in Factor VII-inhibitor patients.

➤*Rate of administration:* This varies with the individual product; adapt to response of the patient. Infuse slowly; 2 to 3 mL/min is suggested. If headache, flushing, or changes in pulse rate or blood pressure appear, stop the infusion until symptoms subside, then resume at a slower rate.

➤*Storage/Stability:* Refrigerate between 2° to 8°C (35° to 46°F). Do not freeze diluent.

Actions

➤*Pharmacology:* Factor IX is activated by factor VII in the extrinsic coagulation pathway as well as by Factor XIa in the intrinsic coagulation pathway. Activated Factor IX, in combination with activated Factor VIII, activates Factor X. This results in the conversion of prothrombin to thrombin. Thrombin then converts fibrinogen to fibrin, and a clot can be formed.

Factor IX is the specific clotting factor deficient in patients with hemophilia B and in patients with acquired factor IX deficiencies.

The administration of Factor IX concentrate raises Factor IX plasma levels, thus minimizing the hazards of hemorrhage in patients with Factor IX deficiency.

Proplex T, Bebulin VH – Plasma levels of factors II, VII, and X may be increased following administration of these preparations.

➤*Pharmacokinetics:* The mean half-life of Factor IX administered to Factor IX-deficient patients is ≈ 22 hours (range, 11 to 36 hours). The mean increase in circulating factor IX activity after IV infusion is 0.67 to 1.15 IU/dL rise per IU/kg body weight.

Contraindications

Known hypersensitivity to mouse protein (*Mononine*) or hamster protein (*BeneFix*).

Warnings

➤*Hepatitis and AIDS:* Human-derived Factor IX products are prepared from pooled units of human plasma that may contain the causative agents of hepatitis and other viral and infectious diseases. Prescribed manufacturing procedures used at the plasma collection centers, plasma testing facilities, and the fractionation facility are designed to reduce the risk of transmitting viral infection. However, the risk of viral infectivity from these products cannot be totally eliminated.

Individuals receiving human-derived plasma product infusions may develop signs or symptoms of a viral infection, especially non-A, non-B hepatitis. Scientific opinion encourages hepatitis B and hepatitis A vaccination at birth or diagnosis for patients with hemophilia.

➤*Thromboembolic complications:* The administration of human Factor IX concentrates containing factors II, VII, IX, and X has been associated with the development of thromboembolic complications, MI, disseminated intravascular coagulation (DIC), venous thrombosis, and pulmonary embolism. Signs include change in pulse rate, blood pressure, respiratory distress, chest pain, and cough. Because of the poten-

tial risk of thromboembolic complications, exercise caution when administering these products to patients with liver disease, postoperative patients, neonates, or patients at risk for thromboembolic phenomena or DIC. In each of these situations, weigh the benefit of treatment against the risk of these complications.

If signs of DIC occur, stop the infusion promptly. To reduce the risk of enhancing intravascular coagulation, do not attempt to raise Factor IX or Factor VII levels to > 50% of normal. If it is necessary to raise the patient's Factor IX or Factor VII level higher than 50% of normal, monitor infusion to detect signs and symptoms of DIC.

➤*Nephrotic syndrome:* Nephrotic syndrome has been reported following attempted immune tolerance induction with Factor IX products in hemophilia B patients with Factor IX inhibitors and a history of severe allergic reactions to Factor IX. The safety and efficacy of using Factor IX in attempted immune tolerance induction has not been established.

➤*Hypersensitivity reactions:* Activity-neutralizing antibodies (inhibitors) have been detected in patients receiving Factor IX-containing products. Monitor patients for the development of Factor IX inhibitors. Patients with these inhibitors may be at increased risk of anaphylaxis upon subsequent challenge with Factor IX. Evaluate patients experiencing allergic reactions for the presence of inhibitor.

Allergic-type hypersensitivity reactions, including anaphylaxis, have been reported for all Factor IX products. Frequently, these events have occurred in close temporal association with the development of Factor IX inhibitors. Inform patients of the early symptoms and signs of hypersensitivity reactions, including hives, generalized urticaria, angioedema, chest tightness, dyspnea, wheezing, faintness, hypotension, tachycardia, and anaphylaxis. Advise patients to discontinue use of the product, contact physician, and seek immediate emergency care, depending on the severity of the reactions, if any of these symptoms occur.

➤*Pregnancy: Category C.* It is not known whether Factor IX can cause fetal harm when administered to a pregnant woman. Give to a pregnant woman only if clearly needed.

➤*Children:* Safety and efficacy trials in pediatric patients ≤ 6 years of age have not been conducted. Studies have been small or ongoing.

Mononine – A small trial evaluation of safety and effectiveness of *Mononine* in patients from 1 day of age to 20 years of age showed excellent hemostasis without thrombotic complications. Dosing in children is based on body weight and is based on the same adult guidelines.

Precautions

➤*Monitoring:* Monitoring the Factor IX activity using the Factor IX activity assay is advised.

Adverse Reactions

The use of high doses of Factor IX concentrates may be associated with MI, DIC, venous thrombosis, and pulmonary embolism (see Warnings).

During clinical studies conducted in previously treated patients, 60 mild adverse reactions definitely, probably, or possibly related to therapy were reported. These were nausea (16), discomfort at the IV site (13), altered taste (10), burning sensation in the jaw and skull (6), allergic rhinitis (3), lightheadedness (2), headache (2), dizziness (1), chest tightness (1), fever (1), phlebitis/cellulitis at IV site (1), drowsiness (1), dry cough/sneeze (1), rash (1), and a single hive (1). Twelve days after a dose of Factor IX, 1 hepatitis C antibody-positive patient developed a renal infarct. The relationship of the infarct to Factor IX administration is uncertain.

Postmarketing adverse events – Postmarketing adverse reactions included the following: Inadequate Factor IX recovery, inadequate therapeutic response, inhibitor development, anaphylaxis, laryngeal edema, angioedema, cyanosis, dyspnea, hypotension, thrombosis.

Rapid infusion rate – Headache, flushing, changes in blood pressure or pulse rate, transient fever, chills, tingling, urticaria, nausea, and vomiting may occur. Symptoms disappear promptly upon discontinuation. Except in the most reactive individuals, the infusion may be resumed at a slower rate.

Pyrogenic reactions – Chills and fever (particularly when large doses are used).

Profilnine SD – Adverse reactions may include the following: Urticaria, fever, chills, nausea, vomiting, headache, somnolence, lethargy, flushing, or tingling.

Patient Information

Advise patients of the early signs of hypersensitivity reactions including hives, generalized urticaria, tightness of the chest, wheezing, hypotension, anaphylaxis, dyspnea, faintness, angioedema, tachycardia, fever, nausea, rashes, and retching. Advise patients to discontinue use of the product and contact their physician if these symptoms occur.

ANTIHEMOPHILIC FACTOR/von WILLEBRAND FACTOR COMPLEX (Factor VIII/VWF; AHF/VWF)

Rx	Humate-P (Aventis Behring)	Powder for injection, lyophilized: 250 units AHF and 500 units VWF:RCo/vial[a]	In single-dose vials with 10 mL diluent, sterile transfer set for reconstitution, and a sterile filter spike for withdrawal.
		500 units AHF and 1000 units VWF:RCo/vial[a]	In single-dose vials with 20 mL diluent, sterile transfer set for reconstitution, and a sterile filter spike for withdrawal.
		1000 units AHF and 2000 units VWF:RCo/vial[a]	In single-dose vials with 30 mL diluent, sterile transfer set for reconstitution, and a sterile filter spike for withdrawal.

[a] Heat-treated. Upon reconstitution with the volume of diluent provided, each milliliter contains 20 to 40 units Factor VIII activity, 50 to 100 units von Willebrand factor:Ristocetin cofactor (VWF:RCo) activity, 15 to 33 mg of glycine, 3.5 to 9.3 mg of sodium citrate, 2 to 5.3 mg of sodium chloride, 4 to 8 mg of albumin (human), 1 to 7 mg of other proteins, and 5 to 15 mg of total proteins. Contains anti-A and anti-B blood group isoagglutinins.

Indications

►*Classical hemophilia:* In adult patients for treatment and prevention of bleeding in hemophilia A (classical hemophilia).

►*von Willebrand disease:* In adult and pediatric patients for treatment of spontaneous and trauma-induced bleeding episodes in severe von Willebrand disease, and in mild and moderate von Willebrand disease where use of desmopressin is known or suspected to be inadequate.

Controlled clinical trials to evaluate the safety and efficacy of prophylactic dosing with *Humate-P* to prevent spontaneous bleeding and to prevent excessive bleeding related to surgery have not been evaluated in von Willebrand disease patients. Adequate data are not presently available on which to evaluate or to base dosing recommendations in either of these settings.

Administration and Dosage

►*Approved by the FDA:* April 1, 1999.

Strongly consider administration of hepatitis A and hepatitis B vaccines to individuals receiving plasma derivatives. Potential risks and benefits of vaccination should be carefully weighed by the physician and discussed with the patient.

For IV administration only.

►*Hemophilia A:* As a general rule, 1 unit of Factor VIII activity per kilogram body weight will increase the circulating Factor VIII level by approximately 2 units/dL. Adequacy of treatment must be judged by the clinical effects; thus, the dosage may vary with individual cases. Although dosage must be individualized according to the needs of the patient (weight, severity of hemorrhage, presence of inhibitors), the following general dosages are recommended for adult patients

Adult Dosage Recommendations for the Treatment of Hemophilia A	
Hemorrhagic event	Dosage
Minor hemorrhage: •Early joint or muscle bleed •Severe epistaxis	Loading dose 15 units/kg to achieve FVIII:C plasma level of approximately 30% of normal; 1 infusion may be sufficient. If needed, half of the loading dose may be given once or twice daily for 1 to 2 days.
Moderate hemorrhage: •Advanced joint or muscle bleed •Neck, tongue or pharyngeal hematoma (without airway compromise) •Tooth extraction •Severe abdominal pain	Loading dose 25 units/kg to achieve FVIII:C plasma level of approximately 50% of normal, followed by 15 units/kg every 8 to 12 hours for first 1 to 2 days to maintain FVIII:C plasma level at 30% of normal, and then the same dose once or twice a day for a total of up to 7 days, or until adequate wound healing.
Life-threatening hemorrhage: •Major operations •GI bleeding •Neck, tongue, or pharyngeal hematoma with potential for airway compromise •Intracranial, intra-abdominal or intrathoracic bleeding •Fractures	Initially 40 to 50 units/kg, followed by 20 to 25 units/kg every 8 hours to maintain FVIII:C plasma level at 80% to 100% of normal for 7 days, then continue the same dose once or twice a day for another 7 days in order to maintain the FVIII:C level at 30% to 50% of normal.

Individualize dosage by clinical judgement of the potential for compromise of a vital structure, and by frequent monitoring of factor VIII activity in the patient's plasma.

►*von Willebrand disease:* The dosage should be adjusted according to the extent and location of bleeding. As a rule, 40 to 80 units VWF:RCo (corresponding to 16 to 32 units factor VIII in *Humate-P*) per kilogram body weight are given every 8 to 12 hours. Repeat doses are administered for as long as needed based on repeat monitoring of appropriate clinical and laboratory measures. Expected levels of VWF:RCo are based on an expected in vivo recovery of 1.5 units/dL rise per units/kg VWF:RCo administered. The administration of 1 units of Factor VIII per kilogram body weight can be expected to lead to a rise in circulating VWF:RCo of approximately 3.5 to 4 units/dL. The following table provides dosing guidelines for pediatric and adult patients.

Dosing Recommendations for the Treatment of von Willebrand Disease		
Classification of VWD	Hemorrhage	Dosage (units VWF:RCo/kg body weight)
Type 1 •Mild, if desmopressin is inappropriate (baseline VWF:RCo activity typically > 30%)	Major (eg, severe or refractory epistaxis, GI bleeding, CNS trauma, or traumatic hemorrhage)	Loading dose 40 to 60 units/kg, then 40 to 50 units/kg every 8 to 12 hours for 3 days to keep the nadir level of VWF:RCo > 50%; then 40 to 50 units/kg daily for a total of up to 7 days of treatment.
Type 1 •Moderate or severe (baseline VWF:RCo activity typically < 30%)	Minor (eg, epistaxis, oral bleeding, menorrhagia) Major (eg, severe or refractory epistaxis, GI bleeding, CNS trauma, hemarthrosis or traumatic hemorrhage)	40 to 50 units/kg (1 or 2 doses). Loading dose 50 to 75 units/kg, then 40 to 60 units/kg every 8 to 12 hours for 3 days to keep the nadir level of VWF:RCo > 50%; then 40 to 60 units/kg/day for a total of up to 7 days of treatment. Monitor and maintain FVIII:C levels according to the guidelines for hemophilia A therapy. See above table.
Types 2 (all variants) and 3	Minor (clinical indications above) Major (clinical indications above)	40 to 50 units/kg (1 or 2 doses). Loading dose of 60 to 80 units/kg, then 40 to 60 units/kg every 8 to 12 hours for 3 days to keep the nadir level of VWF:RCo > 50% then 40 to 60 units/kg/day for a total of up to 7 days of treatment. Monitor and maintain FVIII:C levels according to the guidelines for hemophilia A therapy. See above table.

►*Reconstitution:*
1.) Warm both diluent and *Humate-P* in unopened vials to room temperature (not above 37°C [98°F]).
2.) Pierce the double needle of the transfer set into the diluent vial. Remove the protective cap and insert the exposed (longer) needle into the upright *Humate-P* vial. The diluent will be transferred into the *Humate-P* by vacuum.
3.) Remove the diluent vial and the transfer set and discard.
4.) Gently rotate the vial. DO NOT SHAKE VIAL. Vigorous shaking will prolong the reconstitution time. Continue swirling until the powder is dissolved and the solution is ready for administration. To assure product sterility, administer within 3 hours after reconstitution.
5.) When the reconstitution procedure is precisely followed, it is not uncommon for a few small flakes or particles to remain. The filter spike provided with *Humate-P* should remove those particles and this should not influence dosage calculations.

►*Administration:* Plastic disposable syringes are recommended for administration of *Humate-P* solution. The ground glass surface of all-glass syringes tend to adhere protein solutions of this type.
1.) Attach the filter spike to a sterile disposable syringe and take the filter spike out of the package.
2.) Remove the protective cap and - without touching the tip of the filter spike - insert the disposable filter spike into the stopper of the *Humate-P* vial; inject air.
3.) Draw up the solution slowly (when using several syringes leave the filter spike in the vial). Separate the syringe from the filter spike and attach the syringe to an infusion kit or a suitable injection needle. Discard the filter spike.
4.) Slowly inject the solution (maximally 4 mL/minute) intravenously with an infusion kit or with a suitable injection needle.

►*Storage/Stability:* When stored at refrigerator temperature, 2° to 8°C (36° to 46°F), *Humate-P* is stable for the period indicated by the expiration date on its label. Within this period, *Humate-P* may be stored at room temperature not to exceed 30°C (86°F), for up to six months. Avoid freezing, which may damage the diluent container.

Actions

►*Pharmacology:* The Antihemophilic Factor/VWF complex consists of two different noncovalently bound proteins (Factor VIII and von Willebrand factor). Factor VIII is an essential cofactor in activation of Factor X leading ultimately to formation of thrombin and fibrin. The VWF

ANTIHEMOPHILIC FACTOR/von WILLEBRAND FACTOR COMPLEX (Factor VIII/VWF; AHF/VWF)

promotes platelet aggregation and platelet adhesion on damaged vascular endothelium; it also serves as a stabilizing carrier protein for the procoagulant protein Factor VIII. The activity of VWF is measured as VWF:RCo.

➤*Pharmacokinetics:* After intravenous injection of *Humate-P* in humans, there is a rapid increase of plasma Factor VIII activity (FVIII:C) followed by a rapid decrease in activity and a subsequent slower rate of decrease in activity. Studies with *Humate-P* in hemophilic patients have demonstrated a mean half-life of 12.2 hours (range, 8.4 to 17.4 hours).

The pharmacokinetics of *Humate-P* have been evaluated in 8 VWD patients (type 1, n = 1; type 2, n = 1; type 2A, n = 4; type 3, n = 2) in the non-bleeding state. The median half-life of VWF:RCo was 10.3 hours (range, 6.4 to 13.3 hours). The median in vivo recovery for VWF:RCo activity was 1.89 (units/dL)/(units/kg) (range, 1.1 to 2.74 [units/dL]/[units/kg]). In all patients, the administration of *Humate-P* resulted in a transient shortening of the bleeding time. *Humate-P* was effective in improving the VWF multimer pattern in VWD patients and in most cases this improvement was sustained through 22 to 26 hours postinfusion.

Contraindications

None known.

Warnings

➤*Thromboembolism:* Thromboembolic events have been reported in VWD patients receiving Antihemophilic Factor/von Willebrand Factor Complex replacement therapy, especially in the setting of known risk factors for thrombosis. Early reports might indicate a higher incidence in females. In addition, endogenous high levels of FVIII have also been associated with thrombosis but no causal relationship has been established. In all VWD patients in situations of high thrombotic risk receiving coagulation factor replacement therapy, caution should be exercised and antithrombotic measures should be considered (see Administration and Dosage).

➤*Transmission of infectious agents:* Antihemophilic Factor/von Willebrand Factor Complex is made from human plasma. Products made from human plasma may contain infectious agents, such as viruses, that can cause disease. The risk that such products will transmit an infectious agent has been reduced by screening plasma donors for prior exposure to certain viruses, by testing for the presence of certain current viral infections and by inactivating and/or removing certain viruses during manufacture. Despite these measures, such products can still potentially transmit disease. There is also the theoretical possibility that infectious agents not yet known or identified may be present in such products. Any infections thought by a physician possibly to have been transmitted by this product should be reported by the physician or other healthcare provider to Aventis Behring at (800) 504-5434 (in the U.S. and Canada). The physician should discuss the risks and benefits of this product with the patient.

➤*Hypersensitivity reactions:* Rare cases of allergic reaction and rise in temperature have been observed. Anaphylactic reactions can occur in rare instances. If allergic/anaphylactic reactions occur, the infusion should be discontinued and appropriate treatment given as required. In some cases, inhibitors of Factor VIII may occur. Allergic symptoms, including allergic reaction, urticaria, chest tightness, rash, pruritus, and edema, were reported in 6% of patients in a Canadian retrospective study; 2% experienced other adverse events that were considered to have a possible or probable relationship to the product. These included chills, phlebitis, vasodilation, and paresthesia. All adverse events were mild or moderate in intensity.

➤*Pregnancy:* Category C. It is not known whether *Humate-P* can cause fetal harm when administered to a pregnant woman or can affect reproduction capacity. *Humate-P* should be given to a pregnant woman only if clearly needed.

➤*Children:* Adequate and well-controlled studies with long term evaluation of joint damage have not been done in pediatric patients. Joint damage may result from suboptimal treatment of hemarthroses. For immediate control of bleeding for Hemophilia A, the general recommendations for dosing and administration for adults may be referenced (see Administration and Dosage).

The safety and effectiveness of *Humate-P* for the treatment of von Willebrand disease was demonstrated in 26 pediatric patients, including infants, children and adolescents but has not yet been evaluated in neonates. As in adults, pediatric patients should be dosed based upon weight (kg) (see Administration and Dosage).

Precautions

It is important to determine that the coagulation disorder is caused by factor VIII or VWF deficiency, since no benefit in treating other deficiencies can be expected.

➤*Isoagglutinin:* This Antihemophilic Factor/von Willebrand Factor preparation contains blood group isoagglutinins (anti-A and anti-B). When very large or frequently repeated doses are needed, as when inhibitors are present or when pre- and postsurgical care is involved, patients of blood groups A, B and AB should be monitored for signs of intravascular hemolysis and decreasing hematocrit values and be treated appropriately as required.

The replacement therapy should be monitored with the aid of coagulation tests, especially in cases of major surgery.

Adverse Reactions

Antihemophilic Factor/von Willebrand Factor (Human), Dried, Pasteurized, *Humate-P* is usually tolerated without reaction.

➤*Hypersensitivity:* See Warnings.

➤*Thromboembolism:* Reports of thromboembolic events in VWD patients with other thrombotic risk factors receiving coagulation factor replacement therapy have been obtained from spontaneous reports, published literature, and a European clinical study. Early reports might indicate a higher incidence in females. Caution should be exercised and antithrombotic measures should be considered in all VWD patients in situations of high thrombotic risk (see Warnings).

Patient Information

Some viruses, such as parvovirus B19 or hepatitis A, are particularly difficult to remove or inactivate at this time. Parvovirus B19 may most seriously affect pregnant women, or immune-compromised individuals.

Although the overwhelming number of hepatitis A and parvovirus B19 cases are community acquired, there have been reports of these infections associated with the use of some plasma-derived products. Therefore, physicians should be alert to the potential symptoms of parvovirus B19 and hepatitis A infections and inform patients under their supervision receiving plasma-derived products to report potential symptoms promptly.

Symptoms of parvovirus B19 may include low-grade fever, rash, arthralgias and transient symmetric, nondestructive arthritis. Diagnosis is often established by measuring B19 specific IgM and IgG antibodies. Symptoms of hepatitis A include low grade fever, anorexia, nausea, vomiting, fatigue and jaundice. A diagnosis may be established by determination of specific IgM antibodies.

Systemic

AMINOCAPROIC ACID

Rx	**Amicar** (Immunex)	**Tablets**: 500 mg	(LL A10). White, scored. In 100s.
Rx	**Amicar** (Immunex)	**Syrup**: 250 mg/mL	Parabens, EDTA, saccharin, sorbitol. Raspberry flavor. In 473 mL.
Rx	**Aminocaproic Acid** (VersaPharm)	**Oral solution**: 250 mg/mL	Saccharin, sorbitol, parabens. Raspberry flavor. In 237 and 473 mL.
Rx	**Aminocaproic Acid** (Various, eg, Abbott, American Regent)	**Injection**: 250 mg/mL	In 20 mL vials.
Rx	**Amicar** (Immunex)		0.9% benzyl alcohol. In 20 mL vials.

Indications

➤*Excessive bleeding:* Aminocaproic acid is useful in enhancing hemostasis when fibrinolysis contributes to bleeding. In life-threatening situations, fresh whole blood transfusions, fibrinogen infusions, and other emergency measures may be required.

➤*Unlabeled uses:* Oral or IV aminocaproic acid has been used to prevent recurrence of subarachnoid hemorrhage (SAH).

In the management of amegakaryocytic thrombocytopenia, the need for platelet transfusion may be decreased by use of aminocaproic acid.

To abort and prevent attacks of hereditary angioneurotic edema.

In patients with acute promyelocytic leukemia who develop coagulopathy associated with low levels of alpha-2-plasmin inhibitor.

To reduce postsurgical bleeding complications in patients undergoing cardiopulmonary bypass procedures.

As a bladder irrigant to control bleeding following transurethral resection of the prostate and intractable bladder hemorrhage due to radiation- or cyclophosphamide-induced cystitis.

Administration and Dosage

➤*Approved by the FDA:* 1964.

➤*Plasma levels:* An initial dose of 5 g orally or IV, followed by 1 g hourly, should achieve and sustain drug plasma levels at 0.13 mg/mL. This is the concentration apparently necessary for inhibition of fibrinolysis. Administration of more than 30 g/24 hours is not recommended.

➤*IV:* Administer by infusion, using compatible IV vehicles (eg, Sterile Water for Injection, normal saline, 5% Dextrose or Ringer's Injection). Rapid IV injection undiluted is not recommended; hypotension, bradycardia, or arrhythmias may result. For treatment of acute bleeding syndromes, give 4 to 5 g in 250 mL of diluent by infusion during the first hour, followed by continuous infusion at the rate of 1 g/hour in 50 mL of diluent. Continue for 8 hours or until bleeding is controlled.

➤*Oral:* If the patient can take oral medications, follow an identical dosage regimen.

For the treatment of acute bleeding syndromes due to elevated fibrinolytic activity, administer 5 g orally during the first hour of treatment, followed by a continuing rate of 1 g/hour. Continue this method of treatment for about 8 hours or until bleeding has been controlled.

➤*Storage/Stability:* Store between 15° and 30°C (59° and 86°F); do not freeze.

Actions

➤*Pharmacology:* Inhibits fibrinolysis via inhibition of plasminogen activator substances and, to a lesser degree, through antiplasmin activity.

➤*Pharmacokinetics:* The drug is absorbed rapidly following oral administration. Peak plasma levels occur 0.75 to 1.65 hours after an oral dose. After prolonged administration, it distributes throughout both the extravascular and intravascular compartments and readily penetrates red blood and other tissue cells.

Renal excretion is the primary route of elimination. Sixty-five percent of the dose is recovered unchanged in the urine. The terminal elimination half-life of aminocaproic acid is ≈ 2 hours.

Contraindications

Evidence of an active intravascular clotting process.

➤*Disseminated intravascular coagulation (DIC):* It is important to differentiate between hyperfibrinolysis and DIC. Criteria that may characterize primary fibrinolysis include platelet count (normal), protamine paracoagulation (negative), and euglobulin clot lysis (abnormal). Do not use aminocaproic acid in the presence of DIC without concomitant heparin.

Warnings

➤*Upper urinary tract bleeding:* Administration may cause intrarenal obstruction in the form of glomerular capillary thrombosis, or clots in the renal pelvis and ureters. Do not use in hematuria of upper urinary tract origin, unless possible benefits outweigh risks.

➤*Cardiac, hepatic, or renal disease:* Animal pathology has shown subendocardial hemorrhages and myocardial fat degeneration. Skeletal muscle weakness with necrosis of muscle fibers has been reported rarely.

Consider the possibility of cardiac muscle damage when skeletal myopathy occurs. One case of cardiac and hepatic lesions has been reported. One case of cardiac and hepatic lesions occurred following administration of 2 g aminocaproic acid every 6 hours for a total dose of

26 g. Death was due to continued cerebral vascular hemorrhage. Necrotic changes in the heart and liver were noted at autopsy.

➤*Clotting:* Inhibition of fibrinolysis by aminocaproic acid may theoretically result in clotting or thrombosis. In a few reported cases, it appears that intravascular clotting was more likely due to the patient's preexisting condition (eg, the presence of DIC), rather than to aminocaproic acid. Extravascular clots formed in vivo may not undergo spontaneous lysis as do normal clots.

➤*Benzyl alcohol:* Some of these products contain benzyl alcohol, which has been associated with a fatal "gasping syndrome" in premature infants. Benzyl alcohol is not recommended for use in newborns.

➤*Muscle weakness/Rhabdomyolysis:* Rarely, skeletal muscle weakness with necrosis of muscle fibers has been reported following prolonged administration. Clinical presentation may range from mild myalgias with weakness and fatigue to a severe proximal myopathy with rhabdomyolysis, myoglobinuria, and acute renal failure. Monitor creatine phosphokinase (CPK) levels in patients on long-term therapy; discontinue use if a rise in CPK is noted. Resolution follows discontinuation of aminocaproic acid; however, the syndrome may recur if the drug is restarted.

Guard against thrombophlebitis, a possibility with all IV therapy, by strict attention to the proper insertion of the needle and the fixing of its position.

Do not administer epsilon-aminocaproic acid with Factor IX complex concentrates or anti-inhibitor coagulant concentrates, as the risk of thrombosis may be increased.

➤*Fertility impairment:* Administration of an equivalent of the maximum human therapeutic dose impaired fertility in rats as evidenced by decreased implantations, litter sizes, and number of pups born.

➤*Pregnancy:* Category C. Safety for use during pregnancy has not been established. Use in women of childbearing potential and particularly during early pregnancy only when clearly needed and when the potential benefits outweigh the potential hazards to the fetus.

➤*Lactation:* It is not known whether this drug is excreted in human milk. Because many drugs are excreted in human milk, exercise caution when aminocaproic acid is administered to a nursing woman.

➤*Children:* Safety and efficacy have not been established.

Precautions

➤*Hyperfibrinolysis:* Aminocaproic acid inhibits both plasminogen activator substances and, to a lesser degree, plasmin activity. Do not administer without a definite diagnosis or laboratory findings indicative of hyperfibrinolysis (hyperplasminemia).

Drug Interactions

Administration of highly activated prothrombin complex products together with antifibrinolytic agents is not recommended.

Adverse Reactions

➤*Cardiovascular:* Bradycardia; hypotension; peripheral ischemia; thrombosis.

➤*CNS:* Dizziness; headache; delirium; hallucinations; confusion; intracranial hypertension; stroke; syncope.

➤*Dermatologic:* Rash; pruritus.

➤*GI:* Nausea; diarrhea; abdominal pain; vomiting.

➤*GU:* BUN increased; renal failure.

➤*Hematologic:* Agranulocytosis; coagulation disorder; leukopenia; thrombocytopenia.

➤*Local:* Injection site reactions; pain and necrosis.

➤*Musculoskeletal:* Myalgia; myositis; myopathy characterized by muscle weakness, fatigue, elevated CPK, rhabdomyolysis associated with myoglobinuria and renal failure have been reported.

➤*Respiratory:* Dyspnea; nasal congestion; pulmonary embolism.

➤*Special senses:* Tinnitus; vision decreased; watery eyes.

➤*Miscellaneous:* Edema; allergic and anaphylactoid reactions; anaphylaxis; malaise.

There have been some reports of dry ejaculation during the period of treatment. This occurred only in hemophilia patients who received the drug after undergoing dental surgical procedures. Symptoms resolved in all patients within 24 to 48 hours of completion of therapy.

There have been reports of an increased incidence of certain neurological deficits (eg, hydrocephalus, cerebral ischemia, cerebral vasospasm) associated with use of antifibrinolytic agents in the treatment of SAH.

Systemic

AMINOCAPROIC ACID

All of these events have also been described as part of the natural course of SAH, or as a consequence of diagnostic procedures such as angiography. Drug-relatedness remains unclear.

Overdosage

➤*Symptoms:* A few cases of acute overdosage with aminocaproic acid administered IV have been reported. The effects have ranged from no reaction to transient hypotension to severe acute renal failure leading to death.

➤*Treatment:* No treatment for overdosage is known, although evidence exists that aminocaproic acid is removed by hemodialysis and may be removed by peritoneal dialysis. Pharmacokinetic studies have shown that total body clearance of aminocaproic acid is markedly decreased in patients with severe renal failure.

TRANEXAMIC ACID

| *Rx* | **Cyklokapron** | **Tablets:** 500 mg | (CY). White. In 100s. |
| | (Kabi Pharmacia) | **Injection:** 100 mg/mL | In 10 mL amps. |

Indications

➤*Hemorrhage:* For short-term use (2 to 8 days) in hemophilia patients to reduce or prevent hemorrhage, and to reduce the need for replacement therapy during and following tooth extraction.

➤*Unlabeled uses:* Tranexamic acid has been used for many hemostatic purposes including prevention of bleeding after surgery or trauma (eg, tonsillectomy and adenoidectomy, prostatic surgery and cervical conization), and to prevent rebleeding of subarachnoid hemorrhage in patients. It has also been used to treat primary or IUD-induced menorrhagia, gastric and intestinal hemorrhage, recurrent epistaxis and hereditary angioneurotic edema. Tranexamic acid has been used with systemic therapy topically as a mouthwash to reduce bleeding after oral surgery in patients on anticoagulant therapy. The drug also inhibits induced hyperfibrinolysis during thrombolytic treatment with plasminogen activators.

Administration and Dosage

➤*For dental extraction in patients with hemophilia:* Immediately before surgery, substitution therapy is given with tranexamic acid, 10 mg/kg IV. After surgery, give 25 mg/kg orally 3 to 4 times daily for 2 to 8 days.

➤*Alternative:* Give 25 mg/kg orally, 3 to 4 times/day beginning 1 day prior to surgery.

➤*Parenteral:* 10 mg/kg 3 to 4 times daily for patients unable to take oral medication.

➤*Impaired renal function (moderate to severe):* The following dosages are recommended:

Tranexamic Acid Dosage		
Serum creatinine (*umol/L*)	IV Dose	Tablets
120-250 (1.36-2.83 mg/dL)	10 mg/kg bid	15 mg/kg bid
250-500 (2.83-5.66 mg/dL)	10 mg/kg/day	15 mg/kg/day
> 500 (> 5.66 mg/dL)	10 mg/kg every 48 hours or 5 mg/kg every 24 hours	15 mg/kg every 48 hours or 7.5 mg/kg every 24 hours

➤*Preparation of solution:* For IV infusion, tranexamic acid may be mixed with most solutions for infusion such as electrolyte, carbohydrate, amino acid and dextran solutions. Prepare mixture the same day solution is to be used. Heparin may be added to solution for injection. Do NOT mix with blood. This drug is a synthetic amino acid; do NOT mix with solutions containing penicillin.

Actions

➤*Pharmacology:* Tranexamic acid is a competitive inhibitor of plasminogen activation, and at much higher concentrations, a noncompetitive inhibitor of plasmin. It has actions similar to aminocaproic acid. Tranexamic acid is ≈ 10 times more potent in vitro than aminocaproic acid.

Tranexamic acid in a concentration of 1 mg/mL blood does not aggregate platelets in vitro; concentrations ≤ 10 mg/mL have no influence on platelet count, coagulation time or various coagulation factors in whole blood or citrated blood. On the other hand, tranexamic acid in concentrations of 1 and 10 mg/mL blood prolongs thrombin time.

➤*Pharmacokinetics:*

Absorption/Distribution – Absorption of tranexamic acid after oral use is ≈ 30% to 50%; bioavailability is not affected by food. The peak plasma level 3 hours after 1 g orally is 8 mg/L and after 2 g, 15 mg/L. An antifibrinolytic concentration of drug remains in different tissues for ≈ 17 hours and in serum up to 7 or 8 hours.

Tranexamic acid diffuses rapidly into joint fluid and the synovial membrane. In the joint fluid, the same concentration is obtained as in the serum. The biological half-life in the joint fluid is ≈ 3 hours.

The concentration of tranexamic acid in a number of other tissues is lower than in blood. Tranexamic acid concentration in cerebrospinal fluid is ≈ 10% that of plasma. The drug passes into the aqueous humor where the concentration is ≈ 10% of the plasma concentration.

Tranexamic acid has been detected in semen where it inhibits fibrinolytic activity but does not influence sperm migration.

The protein binding of tranexamic acid to plasminogen is ≈ 3% at therapeutic plasma levels. It does not bind to serum albumin.

Metabolism/Excretion – After an IV dose of 1 g, the plasma concentration time curve shows a triexponential decay with a half-life of ≈ 2 hours for the terminal elimination phase. The initial volume of distribution is ≈ 9 to 12 L. Urinary excretion is the main route of elimination via glomerular filtration. Overall renal clearance is equal to overall plasma clearance (110 to 116 mL/min), and > 95% of the dose is excreted unchanged in the urine. Excretion of tranexamic acid is ≈ 90% at 24 hours after IV administration of 10 mg/kg. After oral administration of 10 to 15 mg/kg, the cumulative urinary excretion at 24 and 48 hours is 39% and 41% of the ingested dose, respectively, or 78% and 82% of the absorbed material, respectively. Only a small fraction is metabolized. After oral administration, 1% of the dicarboxylic acid and 0.5% of the acetylated compound are excreted.

Contraindications

➤*Acquired defective color vision:* Prohibits measuring one endpoint of toxicity (see Warnings).

➤*Subarachnoid hemorrhage:* Cerebral edema and cerebral infarction may be caused by tranexamic acid in patients with subarachnoid hemorrhage.

Warnings

➤*Retinal changes:* No retinal changes have been reported in patients treated with tranexamic acid for weeks to months in clinical trials. However, focal areas of retinal degeneration have developed in cats, dogs, rabbits and rats following oral or IV tranexamic acid at doses between 126 and 1600 mg/kg/day (3 to 40 times the recommended human dose) from 6 days to 1 year. The incidence of such lesions has varied from 25% to 100% and was dose-related. At lower doses, some lesions are reversible.

➤*Visual abnormalities:* Often poorly characterized, visual abnormalities are the most frequently reported postmarketing adverse reaction in Sweden. For patients who are to be treated for longer than several days, perform an ophthalmological examination (including visual acuity, color vision, eyeground and visual fields) before and at regular intervals during treatment. Discontinue tranexamic acid if changes are found.

➤*Renal function impairment:* Reduce the dose in patients who have renal insufficiency because of accumulation.

➤*Carcinogenesis:* Leukemia in male mice receiving tranexamic acid up to 5 g/kg/day may have been related to treatment.

Hyperplasia of the biliary tract and cholangioma and adenocarcinoma of the intrahepatic biliary system have been reported in one strain of rats after dietary administration exceeding the maximum tolerated dose for 22 months. Subsequent similar studies in a different strain of rat have failed to show hyperplastic/neoplastic changes in the liver.

➤*Pregnancy:* Category B. There are no adequate and well controlled studies in pregnant women. However, tranexamic acid passes the placenta and appears in cord blood at concentrations approximately equal to maternal concentrations. Use only if clearly needed.

➤*Lactation:* Tranexamic acid is present in breast milk at 1% of the corresponding serum levels. Exercise caution when administering to nursing women.

➤*Children:* The drug has had limited use in children, principally in connection with tooth extraction. Limited data suggest that dosing instructions for adults can be used for children needing tranexamic acid therapy.

Adverse Reactions

➤*Miscellaneous:*

Giddiness – Has been reported occasionally.

Hypotension – Hypotension has been observed when IV injection is too rapid. Do not inject more rapidly than 1 mL/minute; this reaction has not been reported with oral use.

➤*GI:* Nausea, vomiting and diarrhea occur, but disappear when dosage is reduced.

Overdosage

There is no known case of overdosage. Symptoms may be nausea, vomiting, hypotension or orthostatic hypotension. Treatment includes the usual supportive measures. Refer to General Management of Acute Overdosage.

APROTININ

Rx	Trasylol (Bayer)	**Injection:** 10,000 KIU[1]/mL	In 100 and 200 mL vials.[2]

[1] KIU = Kallikrein Inhibitor Units.

[2] With 9 mg sodium chloride/mL.

Indications

►*Coronary artery bypass graft (CABG) patients (reduction of blood loss/need for transfusion):* For prophylactic use to reduce perioperative blood loss and the need for blood transfusion in patients undergoing cardiopulmonary bypass in the course of repeat CABG surgery.

In selected cases of primary CABG surgery where the risk of bleeding is especially high (impaired hemostasis, eg, presence of aspirin or other coagulopathy) or where transfusion is unavailable or unacceptable.

The selected use of aprotinin in primary CABG patients is based on the risk of renal dysfunction and on the risk of anaphylaxis (should a second procedure be needed).

Administration and Dosage

►*Approved by the FDA:* December 29, 1993 (1P classification).

►*Dosage regimens:*

Regimen A – 2 million KIU IV loading dose, 2 million KIU into the pump prime volume, 500,000 KIU/hr of operation as continuous IV infusion.

Regimen B – 1 million KIU IV loading dose, 1 million KIU into the pump prime volume, 250,000 KIU/hr of operation as continuous IV infusion.

Aprotinin given prophylactically in both dose regimens A and B to high-risk patients undergoing repeat CABG surgery significantly reduced the donor blood transfusion requirement relative to placebo treatment. The experience with the lower dose of aprotinin Regimen B is, however, limited. Regimen A appeared more effective than Regimen B in patients given aspirin preoperatively.

Aprotinin is supplied as a solution containing 10,000 KIU/mL, which is equal to 1.4 mg/mL. Administer all IV doses of aprotinin through a central line. Do not administer any other drug using the same line. Both regimens include a 1 mL test dose, a loading dose, a dose to be added to the priming fluid of the cardiopulmonary bypass circuit ("pump prime" dose) and a constant infusion dose. Regimen A is described in the table below:

Aprotinin Dosage: Regimen A[1]			
Test dose	Loading dose	"Pump prime" dose	Constant infusion dose
1 mL (1.4 mg or 10,000 KIU)	200 mL (280 mg or 2 million KIU)	200 mL (280 mg or 2 million KIU)	50 mL/hr (70 mg/hr or 500,000 KIU/hr)

[1] Regimen B is exactly half of Regimen A; however, both regimens include a 1 mL test dose.

Administer the 1 mL test dose IV at least 10 minutes before the loading dose. With the patient in a supine position, the loading dose is given slowly over 20 to 30 minutes, after induction of anesthesia but prior to sternotomy. When the loading dose is complete, it is followed by the constant infusion dose, which is continued until surgery is complete and the patient leaves the operating room. The "pump prime" dose is added to the priming fluid of the cardiopulmonary bypass circuit, by replacement of an aliquot of the priming fluid, prior to the institution of cardiopulmonary bypass. Total doses of > 7 million KIU have not been studied in controlled trials.

►*Renal function impairment:* In clinical trials, patients with mildly elevated pretreatment serum creatinine levels did not have a notably higher incidence of clinically significant post-treatment elevations in serum creatinine following aprotinin Regimen A compared to placebo. Changes in aprotinin pharmacokinetics with age or impaired renal function are not great enough to require any dose adjustment.

►*Admixture incompatibility:* Aprotinin is incompatible in vitro with corticosteroids, heparin, tetracyclines and nutrient solutions containing amino acids or fat emulsion. If aprotinin is to be given concomitantly with another drug, administer each drug separately through different venous lines or catheters.

►*Storage/Stability:* Protect from freezing. Store between 2° and 25°C (36° and 77°F).

Actions

►*Pharmacology:* Aprotinin is a natural protease inhibitor obtained from bovine lung with a variety of effects on the coagulation system. It inhibits plasmin and kallikrein, thus directly affecting fibrinolysis. It also inhibits the contact phase activation of coagulation which both initiates coagulation and promotes fibrinolysis. In addition to these effects on the clotting and lysis cascades in blood, aprotinin preserves the adhesive glycoproteins in the platelet membrane, making them resistant to damage from the increased plasmin levels and mechanical injury that occur during cardiopulmonary bypass (CPB). The net effect is to inhibit both fibrinolysis and turnover of coagulation factors and to decrease bleeding, although the precise mechanism of this effect is unclear.

Patients undergoing cardiac surgery with extracorporeal circulation by a heart-lung machine develop adverse changes of their blood components, blood cells and specific coagulation proteins. These changes cause a transient hemostatic defect during the intraoperative and immediate postoperative period which may result in diffuse bleeding despite correct surgical technique. At times, this blood loss is severe enough to require multiple blood transfusions and even surgical re-exploration.

►*Pharmacokinetics:*

Distribution – After IV injection, rapid distribution of aprotinin occurs into the total extracellular space, leading to a rapid initial decrease in plasma concentration. Following this distribution phase, a plasma half-life of about 150 minutes is observed. At later time points (ie, > 5 hours after dosing) there is a terminal elimination phase with a half-life of about 10 hours.

Average steady-state intraoperative plasma concentrations were 250 KIU/mL in patients (n = 20) treated during cardiac surgery by administration of the following dosage regimen: 2 million KIU IV loading dose, 2 million KIU into the pump prime volume and 500,000 KIU/hour of operation as continuous IV infusion (Regimen A). Average steady-state intraoperative plasma concentrations were 137 KIU/mL (n = 10) after administration of exactly half of Regimen A.

Metabolism/Excretion – Following a single IV dose, ≈ 25% to 40% is excreted in the urine over 48 hours. After a 30 minute infusion of 1 million KIU, ≈ 2% is excreted as unchanged drug. After a larger dose of 2 million KIU infused over 30 minutes, urinary excretion of unchanged aprotinin accounts for ≈ 9% of the dose. In animals, aprotinin is accumulated primarily in the kidney. After being filtered by the glomeruli, it is actively reabsorbed by the proximal tubules in which it is stored in phagolysosomes. Aprotinin is slowly degraded by lysosomal enzymes. The physiological renal handling is similar to that of other small proteins (eg, insulin).

►*Clinical trials:* Two placebo controlled, double-blind studies were conducted involving 236 patients undergoing repeat coronary artery bypass graft (CABG) surgery, of whom 209 were valid for efficacy analysis. The following treatments were used in the studies: Regimen A (aprotinin: 2 million KIU IV loading dose, 2 million KIU into the pump prime volume, 500,000 KIU/hour of surgery as a continuous IV infusion); Regimen B (aprotinin: 1 million KIU IV loading dose, 1 million KIU into the pump prime volume, 250,000 KIU/hour of surgery as a continuous IV infusion [exactly one-half of Regimen A]); and placebo (normal saline). Fewer patients receiving either regimen of aprotinin required any donor blood compared to placebo (pooled data): Regimen A, 30% to 42%; Regimen B, 47%; placebo, 72% to 77%. The number of units of donor blood required by patients was also reduced by both regimens (data listed by study 1 and study 2, respectively): Regimen A, 1.8 units (range, 0 to 24) and 0.4 units (range, 0 to 5); Regimen B, 2 units (range, 0 to 18); placebo, 3.5 units (range, 0 to 34) and 3.3 units (range, 0 to 20).

Study 2 also included 151 patients undergoing primary CABG surgery; 74 of the patients receiving aprotinin and 67 receiving placebo were valid for efficacy analysis. Fewer patients receiving aprotinin required any donor blood, and number of units of donor blood required was also reduced: Regimen A, 38% and 1.1 units (range, 0 to 10), respectively; placebo, 52% and 2.1 units (range, 0 to 15), respectively.

In these studies there was no diminution of benefit with age. Male and female patients received benefits from aprotinin in terms of a reduction in the average number of units of donor blood transfused. Male patients did better than females in terms of the percentage of patients who required any donor blood transfusions. However, the number of female patients studied was small.

A double-blind, randomized study compared aprotinin (n = 28) and placebo (n = 23) in primary cardiac surgery patients (mainly CABG) requiring cardiopulmonary bypass who were treated with aspirin within 48 hours of surgery. The mean total blood loss (1209.7 mL vs 2532.3 mL) and the mean number of units of packed red blood cells transfused (1.6 units vs 4.3 units) were significantly less in the aprotinin group compared to the placebo group.

In a randomized, placebo controlled study of aprotinin Regimen A vs placebo in 212 patients undergoing primary aortic or mitral valve replacement or repair, no benefit was found for aprotinin in terms of the need for transfusion or the number of units of blood required.

Contraindications

Hypersensitivity to aprotinin.

APROTININ

Warnings

►*Hypersensitivity reactions:* Patients who experience any allergic reaction to the test dose of aprotinin (see Precautions) should not receive further administration of the drug. Even after the uneventful administration of the 1 mL test dose, or without previous exposure to aprotinin, the full therapeutic dose may cause anaphylaxis. The symptoms of hypersensitivity-type reactions can range from skin eruptions, itching, dyspnea, nausea and tachycardia to fatal anaphylactic shock with circulatory failure. If hypersensitivity reactions occur during injection or infusion, stop administration immediately and initiate emergency treatment. Refer to Management of Acute Hypersensitivity Reactions. Patients with a history of allergic reactions to drugs or other agents may be at a greater risk of developing an allergic reaction.

►*Pregnancy: Category B.* There are no adequate and well controlled studies in pregnant women. Use during pregnancy only if clearly needed.

►*Children:* Safety and efficacy have not been established.

Precautions

►*Test dose:* All patients treated with aprotinin should first receive a test dose to assess the potential for allergic reactions. Administer the 1 mL test dose of aprotinin IV at least 10 minutes prior to the loading dose. Particular caution is necessary when administering aprotinin (even test doses) to patients who have received aprotinin in the past because of the risk of anaphylaxis (see Warnings). In re-exposure cases, IV administration of an antihistamine is recommended shortly before the loading dose of aprotinin.

►*Loading dose:* Give the loading dose of aprotinin IV to patients in the supine position over a 20 to 30 minute period. Rapid IV administration of aprotinin can cause a transient fall in blood pressure (see Administration and Dosage).

►*Renal failure/mortality:* An increase in both renal failure and mortality compared to age-matched historical controls has been reported in patients receiving aprotinin while undergoing deep hypothermic circulatory arrest in connection with surgery of the aortic arch. The strength of this association is uncertain because there are no data from randomized studies to confirm or refute these findings.

►*Hepatic disease:* No pharmacokinetic data from patients with pre-existing hepatic disease treated with aprotinin are available.

►*Whole blood clotting time:* Aprotinin prolongs whole blood clotting time of heparinized blood as determined by the *Hemochron* method or similar surface activation methods. In the event of prolonged extracorporeal circulation, patients may require additional heparin, even in the presence of activated clotting time (ACT) levels that appear to represent adequate anticoagulation. Therefore, in patients on cardiopulmonary bypass (CPB) who are receiving aprotinin, the standard system of monitoring heparinization during CPB, by keeping the ACT > 400 to 450 seconds, may lead to inadequate anticoagulation. In patients undergoing cardiopulmonary bypass with aprotinin therapy, employ standard loading doses of heparin. However, administer additional heparin either in a fixed-dose regimen based on patient weight and duration of CPB, or on the basis of heparin levels measured by a method, such as protamine titration, that is not affected by aprotinin.

Drug Interactions

Aprotinin Drug Interactions

Precipitant drug	Object drug*		Description
Aprotinin	Captopril	↓	In a study of nine patients with untreated hypertension, aprotinin IV infused in a dose of 2 million KIU over 2 hours blocked the acute hypotensive effect of 100 mg captopril.
Aprotinin	Fibrinolytic agents	↓	Aprotinin is known to have antifibrinolytic activity and, therefore, may inhibit the effects of fibrinolytic agents.
Aprotinin	Heparin	↑	Aprotinin, in the presence of heparin, has been found to prolong the activated clotting time. However, aprotinin should not be viewed as a heparin-sparing agent (see Precautions).

* ↑ = Object drug increased. ↓ = Object drug decreased.

Adverse Reactions

Aprotinin is generally well tolerated. The adverse events reported are frequent sequelae of open-heart surgery and are not necessarily attributable to aprotinin therapy.

Aprotinin Adverse Reactions (%)

Adverse reaction	Aprotinin (n = 364)	Placebo (n = 235)
Any event	70	70
Atrial fibrillation	25	22
Myocardial infarction	10	7
Heart failure	8	6
Atrial flutter	7	4
Ventricular tachycardia	5	4
Fever	5	3
Hypotension	4	4
Pneumonia	4	3
Respiratory disorder	4	3
Heart arrest	3	1
CHF	3	1
Supraventricular tachycardia	3	3
Kidney failure	3	1
Sepsis	3	2
Apnea	3	2
Confusion	3	2
Heart block	2	1
Shock	2	1
Asthma	2	0
Dyspnea	2	0

Other adverse reactions included: Phlebitis, kidney tubular necrosis (1.4%); convulsion, cerebral embolism (0.8%); liver damage, acute kidney failure, cerebrovascular accident, lung edema, hemolysis, allergic reaction (0.5%); pericarditis; ventricular fibrillation; pleural effusion; pneumothorax. In a pooled analysis of three placebo controlled studies, in patients undergoing cardiopulmonary bypass, there was a trend toward an increased incidence of myocardial infarction in patients given aprotinin. Furthermore, in the study of patients undergoing primary or repeat CABG (Study 2), a trend was seen toward an increased incidence of saphenous vein graft closure in patients who received aprotinin Regimen A vs placebo. No increase in mortality in the aprotinin group was observed.

►*Lab test abnormalities:* Pooled data from three placebo controlled studies showed a statistically significant increase in the incidence of postoperative renal dysfunction in the aprotinin treated group. The incidence of serum creatinine elevations ≥ 0.5 mg/dL above baseline was 23% in aprotinin (Regimen A) patients vs 12% with placebo. In patients undergoing CABG procedures only, the rates were 20% in the aprotinin group and 13% in the placebo group. Postoperative renal dysfunction was observed somewhat more frequently in association with primary cardiac valve procedures (30% for aprotinin Regimen A and 14% for Regimen B vs 8% for placebo). In the majority of instances, the renal dysfunction was not severe and was reversible.

A total of 4% of aprotinin-treated (Regimen A) patients and 1% of the placebo group had a serum creatinine increase of ≥ 2 mg/dL above the preoperative value.

Patients with baseline elevations in serum creatinine were not at increased risk of developing postoperative renal dysfunction following aprotinin treatment. In aprotinin-treated patients, there was a mean increase in creatinine of 0.16 mg/dL after the high-dose regimen (A) and a mean increase of 0.05 mg/dL after the low-dose regimen (B).

Serum glucose – In the hours after cardiopulmonary bypass surgery, the serum glucose was increased; however, the average serum glucose increase in patients treated with the high-dose regimen (61 mg/dL) was less than in the placebo-treated group (78 mg/dL).

Serum transaminases – There was a significantly greater incidence of treatment emergent abnormal liver function tests in all aprotinin-treated (Regimen A and Regimen B) patients (6%) compared with placebo-treated patients (2%). The percent of primary CABG patients developing an elevation of ALT > 1.8 times the upper limit of normal was not higher in the aprotinin-treated group compared to placebo. Among the repeat CABG patients, the percent of subjects developing an elevation of ALT of this magnitude was significantly higher in the aprotinin-treated group. This suggests an indirect effect possibly related to the risk of repeated surgery and attendant myocardial dysfunction rather than a primary drug effect. There were no differences between drug and placebo groups in the incidence of elevated ALT > 3 times the upper limit of normal.

APROTININ

Serum creatine kinase (CK) – There was a trend toward an increased incidence of elevated serum CK with increased MB fractions in aprotinin-treated patients.

Partial thromboplastin time (PTT) and activated clotting time (ACT) – Significant elevations in the PTT and ACT in aprotinin-treated patients are expected in the hours after surgery due to circulating concentrations of aprotinin, which are known to inhibit activation of the intrinsic clotting system by contact with a foreign surface, a method used in these tests (see Precautions).

➤*Hypersensitivity:* Anaphylactic reactions in patients receiving aprotinin have been reported in < 0.5% of cases. Such reactions are more likely to occur with repeated administration (see Warnings).

Reported Incidence of Anaphylaxis with Aprotinin Treatment				
	No prior aprotinin exposure		Prior aprotinin exposure	
Studies	Total	Fatal	Total	Fatal
US controlled studies	0/398	0/398	0/0	0/0
Foreign controlled studies	7/1996	1/1996	0/0	0/0
US open studies	0/299	0/299	1/6	1/6
Foreign open studies	3/1873	1/1873	1[1]	0/0
Foreign marketing	5/140,000	1/140,000	13/7000	4/7000

[1] Patient was treated a second time in violation of study protocol.

Overdosage

The maximum amount of aprotinin that can be safely administered in single or multiple doses has not been determined. Doses up to 17.5 million KIU have been administered within a 24 hour period without any apparent toxicity. There is one poorly documented case, however, of a patient who received a large, but not well determined, amount of aprotinin (in excess of 15 million KIU) in 24 hours. The patient, who had preexisting liver dysfunction, developed hepatic and renal failure postoperatively and died. The autopsy showed hepatic necrosis and extensive renal tubular and glomerular necrosis. The relationship of these findings to aprotinin therapy is unclear.

Topical

THROMBIN, TOPICAL

Rx	**Thrombin-JMI** (Jones Medical)	**Powder**	In 10,000, 20,000 and 50,000 unit vials.
Rx	**Thrombogen** (Johnson & Johnson)	**Powder**	In 5,000[3], 10,000[4] or 20,000[4] unit vials.
Rx	**Thrombostat** (Parke-Davis)	**Powder**	In 5,000[5], 10,000[6] or 20,000[6] unit vials.

[1] With 50% mannitol and 45% sodium chloride.
[2] With 50% mannitol, 45% sodium chloride and Sterile Water for Injection diluent.
[3] With Isotonic Saline diluent and transfer needle.
[4] With Isotonic Saline diluent. benzethonium chloride and transfer needle. Also in spray kit.

[5] With Isotonic Saline diluent containing 0.02 mg benzethonium chloride/mL.
[6] With Isotonic Saline diluent containing 0.02 mg benzethonium chloride/mL. Also in spray kit.

Indications

➤*Hemostasis:* As an aid in hemostasis wherever oozing blood and minor bleeding from capillaries and small venules is accessible.

In conjunction with absorbable gelatin sponges for hemostasis in various types of surgery.

Administration and Dosage

➤*Preparation of solution:* Prepare in Sterile Distilled Water or Isotonic Saline. The intended use determines the strength of the solution. For general use in plastic surgery, dental extractions, skin grafting, neurosurgery, etc, solutions containing ≈ 100 units/mL are frequently used. Where bleeding is profuse, as from cut surfaces of liver and spleen, concentrations as high as 1000 to 2000 units/mL may be required. It may often be advantageous to use thrombin in dry form on oozing surfaces.

➤*Topical use:* The recipient surface should be sponged (not wiped) free of blood before thrombin is applied. A spray may be used or the surface may be flooded using a sterile syringe and small gauge needle. The most effective hemostasis results when the thrombin mixes freely with the blood as soon as it reaches the surface. In instances where thrombin in dry form is needed, the vial is opened and the dried thrombin is then broken up into a powder. Avoid sponging of treated surfaces to ensure that the clot remains securely in place.

➤*Use in conjunction with absorbable gelatin sponge:* Immerse sponge strips in the thrombin solution. Knead the sponge strips vigorously to remove trapped air, thereby facilitating saturation of the sponge. Apply saturated sponge to bleeding area. Hold in place for 10 to 15 seconds with a pledget of cotton or a small gauze sponge.

➤*Storage / Stability:*

Thrombostat – Store at room temperature 15° to 30°C (59° to 86°F).

Thrombin JMI – Refrigerate at 2° to 8°C (36° to 46°F).

Thrombogen – Use solution immediately upon reconstitution. If necessary, refrigerate at 2° to 8°C (36° to 46°F) for up to 3 hours.

Actions

➤*Pharmacology:* Thrombin directly converts fibrinogen to fibrin, requiring no intermediate physiological agent for its action. Commercially available thrombin is derived from bovine sources. Blood fails to clot in the rare cases where the primary clotting defect is absence of fibrinogen itself. The speed with which thrombin clots blood depends on its concentration. For example, the contents of a 5000 unit vial dissolved in 5 mL of saline diluent is capable of clotting an equal volume of blood in less than a second or 1000 mL in less than a minute.

Contraindications

Sensitivity to any product components or to material of bovine origin.

Warnings

➤*Do not inject:* Thrombin must not be injected or otherwise allowed to enter large blood vessels. Extensive intravascular clotting and even death may result.

➤*Hypersensitivity reactions:* Thrombin is an antigenic substance and has caused sensitivity and allergic reactions when injected into animals. Refer to Management of Acute Hypersensitivity Reactions.

➤*Pregnancy: Category C.* It is not known whether the drug can cause fetal harm when administered to a pregnant woman or can affect reproduction capacity. Safety for use during pregnancy has not been established. Use only when clearly needed and when the potential benefits outweigh the potential hazards to the fetus.

➤*Children:* Safety and efficacy for use in children have not been established.

Adverse Reactions

Allergic reactions may be encountered in patients known to be sensitive to bovine materials.

MICROFIBRILLAR COLLAGEN HEMOSTAT

Rx	**Hemopad** (Astra)	**Fibrous absorbable collagen hemostat:** 2.5 cm x 5 cm, 5 cm x 8 cm and 8 cm x 10 cm	In 10s.
Rx	**Hemotene** (Astra)	**Fibrous absorbable collagen hemostat:** 1 g	In dispenser packs of 5.

Indications

➤*Hemostasis:* Used in surgical procedures as an adjunct to hemostasis when control of bleeding by ligature or conventional procedures is ineffective or impractical.

Administration and Dosage

This product should not be resterilized. It is not for injection or intraocular use. Moistening or wetting with saline or thrombin impairs its hemostatic efficacy. It should be used dry. Discard any unused portion.

➤*Fibrous form:* Must be applied directly to the source of bleeding. Because of its adhesiveness, it may seal over the exit site of deeper hemorrhage and conceal an underlying hematoma as in penetrating liver wounds.

Surface preparation – Compress with dry sponges immediately prior to application of the dry product, then apply pressure over the hemostat with a dry sponge; the length of time varies with the force and severity of bleeding. A minute may suffice for capillary bleeding (eg, skin graft donor sites, dermatologic curettage), but ≥ 3 to 5 minutes may be required for brisk bleeding (eg, splenic tears) or high pressure leaks in major artery suture holes.

Control of oozing from cancellous bone – Pack firmly into the spongy bone surface. After 5 to 10 minutes, tease excess away; this can usually be accomplished with blunt forceps and is facilitated by wetting with sterile 0.9% saline solution and irrigation. If breakthrough bleeding occurs in areas of thin application, apply additional hemostat. The amount required depends on the severity of bleeding.

Capillary bleeding – 1 g is usually sufficient for a 50 cm² area. Thicker coverage is required for more brisk bleeding.

Application – Adheres to wet gloves, instruments or tissue surfaces. To facilitate handling, use dry smooth forceps. Do not use gloved fingers to apply pressure.

➤*Non-woven web form:* In neurosurgical and other procedures, apply small squares to bleeding areas; then cover the sites with moist cottonoid "patties". To prevent wetting of the MCH, and to apply needed pressure, hold a suction tip against the cottonoid for one to several minutes, depending on the briskness of bleeding. After 5 to 10 minutes, remove excess MCH by teasing and irrigation.

Actions

➤*Pharmacology:* Microfibrillar collagen hemostat (MCH) is an absorbable topical hemostatic agent prepared as a dry, sterile, fibrous, water insoluble, partial hydrochloric acid salt of purified bovine corium collagen.

In contact with a bleeding surface, MCH attracts platelets that adhere to the fibrils and undergo the release phenomenon to trigger aggregation of platelets into thrombi in the interstices of the fibrous mass. The effect on platelet adhesion and aggregation is not inhibited by heparin in vitro. Platelets of patients with clinical thrombasthenia do not adhere to the hemostat in vitro. However, in clinical trials, it was effective in 50 of 68 patients receiving aspirin. It cannot control bleeding due to systemic coagulation disorders. Institute appropriate therapy to correct the underlying coagulopathy prior to use of the drug. It is tenaciously adherent to surfaces wet with blood, but excess material not involved in the hemostatic clot may be removed by teasing or irrigation, usually without restarting bleeding.

MCH stimulates a mild, chronic cellular inflammatory response. When implanted in animal tissues, it is absorbed in less than 84 days and does not predispose to stenosis at vascular anastomotic sites. These findings have not been confirmed in humans. In human studies of hemostasis in osteotomy cuts, it does not interfere with bone regeneration or healing.

Contraindications

Closure of skin incisions; it may interfere with the healing of the skin edges due to simple mechanical interposition of dry collagen.

MICROFIBRILLAR COLLAGEN HEMOSTAT

Bone surfaces to which prosthetic materials are to be attached with methylmethacrylate adhesives. By filling porosities of cancellous bone, MCH may significantly reduce the bond strength of methylmethacrylate adhesives.

Warnings

➤*Sterilization:* MCH is inactivated by autoclaving. Ethylene oxide reacts with bound hydrochloric acid to form ethylene chlorohydrin.

➤*Infection:* The presence of the hemostat does not enhance or initiate experimental staphylococcus wound infections to a greater or lesser extent than control agents. The effects on experimental wounds contaminated with a gram-negative aerobic rod and an anaerobic non-spore-forming bacteria are currently under investigation. Use in contaminated wounds may enhance infection.

➤*Pregnancy:* There are no well controlled studies in pregnant women. Safety for use during pregnancy has not been established. Use only when clearly needed and when the potential benefits outweigh the potential hazards to the fetus.

Precautions

➤*Excess material:* After several minutes, remove excess material; this is usually possible without the reinitiation of active bleeding. Failure to remove excess material may result in bowel adhesion or mechanical pressure sufficient to compromise the ureter. In otolaryngological surgery, precautions against aspiration should include removal of all excess dry material and thorough irrigation of the pharynx.

➤*Antibodies:* Contains a low level of intercalated bovine serum protein that reacts immunologically as does beef serum albumin (BSA). Increases in anti-BSA titer have been observed following treatment. About two-thirds of individuals exhibit antibody titers because of ingestion of food products of bovine origin. Intradermal skin tests have occasionally shown weak positive reactions to BSA or MCH, but these have not been correlated with IgG titers to BSA. Tests have failed to demonstrate clinically significant elicitation of antibodies of the IgE class against BSA following therapy.

➤*Blood from operative sites:* Fragments of MCH may pass through filters of blood scavenging systems. Therefore, avoid reintroduction of blood from operative sites treated with MCH.

➤*Autologous blood salvage circuits:* MCH should not be used in conjunction with autologous blood salvage circuits.

➤*Handling:* Avoid spillage on nonbleeding surfaces, particularly in abdominal or thoracic viscera.

Adverse Reactions

Most serious – Potentiation of infection (including abscess formation, hematoma, wound dehiscence and mediastinitis). Adhesion formation; allergic reaction; foreign body reaction; subgaleal seroma (single case).

The use of MCH in dental extraction sockets increases the incidence of alveolalgia. Transient laryngospasm due to aspiration of dry materials has been reported following use in tonsillectomy.

ABSORBABLE GELATIN SPONGE

Rx	**Gelfoam** (Upjohn)	**Sponges:** Size 12: 2 x 6 cm x 3 or 7 mm	In 4s and 12s (7 mm only).
		Size 50: 8 x 6.25 cm	In 4s.
		Size 100: 8 x 12.5 cm	In regular and compressed. In 6s.
		Size 200: 8 x 25 cm	In 6s.
		Packs: Size 2: 40 x 2 cm	In single jars.
		Size 6: 40 x 6 cm	In 6s.
		Dental pk: Size 4: 2 x 2 cm	In 15s.
		Prostatectomy cones: Size 13: 5″ diameter	In 6s.
		Size 18: 7″ diameter	In 6s.

Indications

➤*Hemostasis:* For use in surgical procedures as an adjunct to hemostasis when control of bleeding by ligature or conventional procedures is ineffective or impractical.

Also used in oral and dental surgery as an aid in providing hemostasis.

In open prostatic surgery, insertion into the prostatic cavity provides hemostasis.

Administration and Dosage

➤*Hemostasis:* Apply dry or saturated with NaCl injection. When bleeding is controlled, leave pieces in place. Since sponge causes little more cellular infiltration than the blood clot, the wound may be closed over it. When applied, the sponge will stay in place until it liquefies. When applied dry, compress pieces before application to bleeding surface, then hold in place with moderate pressure for 10 to 15 seconds. When used with saline solutions, immerse in solution, withdraw, squeeze to remove the air bubbles present and replace in solution where it will swell to original size. If it does not, remove and knead vigorously until all air is expelled. Leave piece wet, or blot to dampness on gauze, and apply to bleeding point. Hold in place with moderate pressure with a cotton pledget or small gauze sponge until hemostasis results.

➤*Dentistry:* When used dry, roll between fingers and lightly compress to diameter of cavity or socket. After insertion, apply light finger pressure for 1 or 2 min. When used moist, immerse in NaCl solution, then remove, squeeze thoroughly to remove air bubbles and replace in solution where it will swell to original size. Take from solution, blot on sterile gauze to remove excess fluid and place in cavity or wound.

➤*Prostatectomy cones:* These are designed for use with the Foley bag catheter.

➤*Storage/Stability:* Once package is opened, contents are subject to contamination.

Actions

➤*Pharmacology:* A sterile, pliable surgical sponge prepared from purified gelatin solution and capable of absorbing and holding many times its weight of whole blood.

When implanted into tissues, it is absorbed completely within 4 to 6 weeks without inducing excessive scar tissue formation. When applied to bleeding areas of nasal, rectal or vaginal mucosa, it completely liquefies within 2 to 5 days.

Contraindications

Closure of skin incisions (may interfere with the healing of skin edges); control of postpartum bleeding or menorrhagia.

Warnings

➤*Sterilization:* Do not resterilize by heat, since heating may change absorption time. Ethylene oxide is not recommended for resterilization; it may be trapped in the interstices of the foam and trace amounts may cause burns or irritation to tissue.

Precautions

➤*Infection:* Not recommended in the presence of infection. If signs of infection or abscess develop in the area where the sponge has been placed, reoperation may be necessary to remove the infected material and allow drainage.

➤*Compression:* Sponge may expand and impinge on nearby structures. When placing into cavities or closed tissue spaces, use minimal preliminary compression; avoid overpacking.

Adverse Reactions

Sponge may form infection and abscess (see Precautions). Giant cell granuloma in the brain has occurred at implantation site, as well as brain and spinal cord compression due to sterile fluid accumulation. Excessive fibrosis and prolonged fixation of the tendon were seen when the sponge was used at a tendon juncture.

Topical

ABSORBABLE GELATIN FILM, STERILE

Rx	Gelfilm (Upjohn)	Film: 100 mm x 125 mm	In 1s.
Rx	Gelfilm Ophthalmic (Upjohn)	Film: 25 mm x 50 mm	In 6s.

Indications

➤*Neurosurgery:* As a dural substitute; absorbable gelatin film is nonconducive to undue inflammatory reaction and absorbable at a rate slow enough to permit dural regeneration and healing of the arachnoid layer. Its use in patients undergoing craniotomies reportedly prevented the development of meningocerebral adhesions, thereby reducing the risk of postoperative sequelae.

➤*Thoracic surgery:* In the repair of pleural defects in connection with thoracotomies, thoracoplasties and extrapleural procedures, implantation has been followed by minimal tissue reaction and subsequent closure of the defect by ingrowth of regenerating pleural and fibrous tissue across the gradually resorbed implant.

➤*Ocular surgery:* In glaucoma filtration operations (ie, iridencleisis and trephination), extraocular muscle surgery and diathermy or scleral "buckling" operations for retinal detachment. There is a remarkable lack of cellular reaction to the film implanted subconjunctivally or used as a seton into the anterior chamber. Evidence shows that implants help prevent formation of adhesions between contiguous ocular structures.

Administration and Dosage

➤*Preparation:* Immerse in sterile saline solution; soak until quite pliable; cut to the desired size and shape; apply as follows:

➤*Covering dural defects:* Place over the surface of the brain. Tuck the edges of the implant beneath the dura and the wound; close the wound in the usual manner. If desired, the film can be sutured loosely to the dura. The moist film tears easily.

➤*Covering pleural defects:* Place over the defect and anchor in place by means of small interrupted sutures.

➤*As a seton in iridencleisis:* Place a small piece (≈ 4 mm x 10 mm) over the prolapsed iris pillar parallel to the limbus; Tenon's capsule and the conjunctiva are then closed with continuous absorbable sutures closely spaced to ensure tight wound closure.

➤*Diathermy or scleral "buckling" operations:* Place film over the sclera, then suture the muscle and the conjunctiva over the underlying film.

➤*Extraocular muscle surgery:* Place film over and beneath the muscle before Tenon's capsule and the conjunctiva are closed in layers.

➤*Storage / Stability:* Once the envelopes have been opened, contents are subject to contamination. To ensure sterility, use immediately after withdrawal from the envelope. Store at room temperature 15° to 30°C (59° to 86°F).

Actions

➤*Pharmacology:* A sterile, absorbable gelatin film for use in neurosurgery, thoracic and ocular surgery.

In the dry state, absorbable gelatin film has the appearance and texture of cellophane of equivalent thickness; when moistened, it assumes a rubbery consistency and can then be cut to the desired size and fitted to rounded or irregular surfaces. The rate of absorption after implantation ranges from 1 to 6 months, depending on the size of the implant and the site of implantation. Pleural and muscle implants are completely absorbed in 8 to 14 days; dural and ocular implants usually require at least 2 to 5 months for complete absorption. The absence of undue tissue reactions, with the consequent decreased likelihood of developing adhesions, has been of particular value in the case of dural and ocular implants.

Contraindications

Because the rate of absorption is likely to be increased in the presence of purulent exudation, do not implant in grossly contaminated or infected surgical wounds.

OXIDIZED CELLULOSE

Rx	Oxycel (Becton-Dickinson)	Pads: 3″ x 3″, 8 ply Pledgets: 2″ x 1″ x 1″ Strips: 18″ x 2″, 4 ply	In 10s.
Rx	Surgicel (Johnson & Johnson)	Strips: 2″ x 14″ 4″ x 8″ 2″ x 3″ ½″ x 2″	In 1s.
		Surgical Nu-knit: 1″ x 1″ 3″ x 4″ 6″ x 9″	In 1s.

Indications

➤*Hemorrhage:* Used adjunctively in surgical procedures to assist in the control of capillary, venous and small arterial hemorrhage when ligation or other conventional methods of control are impractical or ineffective. Also indicated for use in oral surgery and exodontia.

Administration and Dosage

Withdraw hemostat from the container with dry sterile forceps. Minimal amounts of an appropriate size are laid on the bleeding site or held firmly against the tissues until hemostasis is obtained.

➤*Storage / Stability:* Discard opened, unused oxidized cellulose. It cannot be resterilized.

Actions

➤*Pharmacology:* An absorbable hemostatic agent prepared from cellulose by a special process that converts it into polyanhydroglucuronic acid (cellulosic acid). Oxidation of cellulose yields an absorbable product of known acidity, soluble in alkali.

Provides hemostatic action when applied to sites of bleeding. The mechanism of action is not completely understood, but it appears to be a physical effect rather than any alteration of the normal physiologic clotting mechanism. Upon contact with blood, oxidized cellulose becomes a dark reddish-brown or almost black, tenacious, adhesive mass. It conforms and adheres readily to the bleeding surface. After 24 to 48 hours, it becomes gelatinous and can be removed, usually without causing additional bleeding. If left in situ, absorption depends on several factors, including the amount used, degree of saturation with blood and the tissue bed.

Oxidized cellulose swells upon contact with blood; the resultant pressure adds to its hemostatic action. It does not enter the normal clotting mechanism; however, within a few minutes of contact with blood, it forms an artificially produced clot in the bleeding area.

Bactericidal effects – The hemostat is bactericidal in vitro against many gram-positive and gram-negative organisms including aerobes and anaerobes: *Staphylococcus aureus, S. epidermidis, Micrococcus luteus, Streptococcus pyogenes* Groups A and B, *S. salivarius, Bacillus subtilis, Proteus vulgaris, Corynebacterium xerosis, Mycobacterium phlei, Clostridium tetani, Branhamella catarrhalis, Escherichia coli, Klebsiella aerogenes, Lactobacillus sp, Salmonella enteritidis, Shigella dysenteriae, Serratia marcescens, C. perfringens, Bacteroides fragilis, Enterococcus, Enterobacter cloacae, Pseudomonas aeruginosa, P. stutzeri* and *Proteus mirabilis*. In contrast to other hemostatic agents, it does not tend to enhance experimental infection.

Contraindications

Packing or wadding as a hemostatic agent; packing or implantation in fractures or laminectomies (it interferes with bone regeneration and can cause cyst formation); control of hemorrhage from large arteries or on nonhemorrhagic serous oozing surfaces since body fluids other than whole blood (eg, serum) do not react with oxidized cellulose to produce satisfactory hemostatic effects; do not use around the optic nerve and chiasm; as a wrap in vascular surgery because it has a stenotic effect.

Warnings

➤*Sterilization:* Do not autoclave; autoclaving causes physical breakdown.

➤*Surgery:* Not intended as a substitute for careful surgery and proper use of sutures and ligatures.

➤*Contaminated wound:* Closing oxidized cellulose in a contaminated wound without drainage may lead to complications and should be avoided.

➤*Application / Removal:* The hemostatic effect is greater when applied dry; therefore, do not moisten with water or saline. Do not impregnate with materials such as buffering or hemostatic substances. Its hemostatic effect is not enhanced by the addition of thrombin; the activity of thrombin is destroyed by the low pH of the product. If used temporarily to line the cavity of large open wounds, place so as not to overlap the skin edges.

May be left in situ when necessary, but remove it once hemostasis is achieved. It must always be removed if used in, around or in proximity to foramina in bone, areas of bony confine, the spinal cord or the optic nerve and chiasm; by swelling, it may cause nerve damage by pressure in a bony confine. Paralysis has been reported when used around the spinal cord, particularly in surgery for herniated intervertebral disc.

OXIDIZED CELLULOSE

Remove from open wounds by forceps or by irrigation with sterile water or saline solution after bleeding has stopped.

➤*Infections:* Although it is bactericidal against a wide range of pathogenic microorganisms, it is not a substitute for systemic antimicrobial agents to control or prevent postoperative infections. Do not impregnate with anti-infective agents.

Precautions

➤*Packing:* Apply by loosely packing against the bleeding surface. Avoid wadding or packing tightly, especially within the bony enclosure of the CNS and within other relatively rigid cavities where swelling may interfere with normal function or possibly cause necrosis.

➤*Use sparingly:* To control bleeding in open reduction of fractures and in cancellous bone, use sparingly. To minimize the possibility of interference with callus formation and the theoretical chance of cyst formation, remove any excess after bleeding is controlled.

➤*Urological procedures:* Use minimal amounts and exercise care to prevent plugging of the urethra, ureter or catheter.

Since absorption is prevented in chemically cauterized areas, its use should not be preceded by application of silver nitrate or any other escharotic chemicals.

➤*Otorhinolaryngologic surgery:* Exercise care so that none of the material is aspirated by the patient (eg, when controlling hemorrhage after tonsillectomy; controlling epistaxis).

Adverse Reactions

Encapsulation of fluid and foreign body reactions, with or without infection, have been reported.

Possible prolongation of drainage in cholecystectomies and difficulty passing urine per urethra after prostatectomy have been reported. There has been one report of a blocked ureter after kidney resection.

Burning has been reported when applied after nasal polyp removal and after hemorrhoidectomy. Headache, burning, stinging and sneezing in epistaxis and other rhinological procedures and stinging when applied on surface wounds (varicose ulcerations, dermabrasions and donor sites) have also been reported. These are believed to be due to the low pH of the product.

Intestinal obstruction has occurred, due to transmigration of a bolus of oxidized cellulose from gallbladder bed to terminal ileum or to adhesions in a loop of denuded intestine to which oxidized cellulose had been applied.

➤*Miscellaneous:* Necrosis of nasal mucous membrane or perforation of nasal septum due to tight packing; urethral obstruction following retropubic prostatectomy and introduction of oxidized cellulose within enucleated prostatic capsule.

Indications

Unless the condition responsible for the hypoproteinemia can be corrected, albumin in any form can provide only symptomatic relief or supportive treatment.

➤*Shock:* For shock due to burns, trauma, surgery and infections; in the treatment of injuries of such severity that shock, although not immediately present, is likely to ensue; in other similar conditions where the restoration of blood volume is urgent.

In cases in which there has been a considerable loss of red blood cells, transfusion with whole blood or red blood cells is indicated.

For the earliest emergency treatment of shock, it may be more convenient to have 25% normal serum albumin available because it is so highly concentrated. However, the concentrated solution depends (for its maximum osmotic effect) on holding additional fluids in the circulation, which are drawn from the tissues or administered separately; if patient is dehydrated, maximum effect cannot be obtained without additional fluids. Therefore, for routine hospital use, normal serum albumin 5% may be preferred, as maximum osmotic effect is obtained with no additional fluids.

Albumin 25% with appropriate crystalloids may offer therapeutic advantages in oncotic deficits or in long-standing shock where treatment has been delayed. Removal of ascitic fluid from the patient with cirrhosis may cause changes in cardiovascular function and even result in hypovolemic shock.

➤*Burns:* Albumin 5% or plasma protein 5% may be used in conjunction with adequate infusions of crystalloid to prevent hemoconcentration and to combat the water, protein and electrolyte losses which usually follow serious burns. After 24 hours, albumin 25% can be used to maintain plasma colloid osmotic pressure.

➤*Hypoproteinemia:* In clinical situations usually associated with a low concentration of plasma protein and, consequently, a reduced volume of circulating blood.

Normal serum albumin 5% or plasma protein fraction 5% may be used in hypoproteinemic patients, providing sodium restriction is not a problem. If sodium restriction is imperative, use 25% normal serum albumin.

For acute complications of chronic hypoproteinemia, use albumin 25% possibly in conjunction with a diuretic.

➤*Adult respiratory distress syndrome (ARDS):* This syndrome is characterized by deficient oxygenation caused by pulmonary interstitial edema complicating shock and postsurgical conditions. When clinical signs are those of hypoproteinemia with a fluid volume overload, albumin 25%, together with a diuretic, may play a role in therapy.

➤*Cardiopulmonary bypass:* Preoperative dilution of the blood using albumin and crystalloid is safe and well tolerated. Although the limit to which the hematocrit and plasma protein concentration can be safely lowered has not been defined, it is common to achieve a hematocrit of 20% and a plasma albumin concentration of 2.5 g/100 mL.

➤*Acute liver failure with or without coma:* Administration of albumin may serve the double purpose of supporting the colloid osmotic pressure of the plasma as well as binding excess plasma bilirubin. Albumin 25% may be considered.

➤*Sequestration of protein rich fluids:* This occurs in such conditions as acute peritonitis, pancreatitis, mediastinitis and extensive cellulitis. The magnitude of loss into the third space may require treatment of reduced volume or oncotic activity with albumin.

➤*Erythrocyte resuspension:* Albumin may be required to avoid excessive hypoproteinemia during certain types of exchange transfusion or with the use of very large volumes of previously frozen or washed red cells.

➤*Acute nephrosis:* Certain patients may not respond to cyclophosphamide or steroid therapy. A loop diuretic and albumin 25% may help control the edema and the patient may then respond to steroid treatment.

➤*Renal dialysis:* Albumin 25% may be of value in treating shock or hypotension.

➤*Hyperbilirubinemia and erythroblastosis fetalis:* Albumin can be a useful adjunct in exchange transfusions; it reduces the necessity for reexchange and increases the amount of bilirubin removed with each transfusion, lessening the risk of kernicterus.

Actions

➤*Pharmacology:* The plasma protein fractions include plasma protein fraction 5% (83% albumin with alpha and beta globulins), normal serum albumin 5% and normal serum albumin 25%.

The albumin fraction of human blood has two known functions: Maintenance of plasma colloid osmotic pressure and carrier of intermediate metabolites in the transport and exchange of tissue products. It comprises about 50% to 60% of the plasma proteins and provides approximately 70% to 80% of their colloid osmotic pressure. Thus, it is important in regulating the volume of circulating blood; its loss is critical, particularly in shock with hemorrhage or reduced plasma volume.

When plasma volume is reduced, an adequate amount of albumin quickly restores the volume in most instances. Twenty-five grams of albumin is the osmotic equivalent of approximately 2 units (500 mL) of fresh frozen plasma; or 100 mL of normal serum albumin 25% provides about as much plasma protein as does 500 mL plasma or 2 pints whole blood. Normal serum albumin 5% is osmotically equivalent to an approximately equal volume of citrated plasma. The 25% albumin solution is osmotically equivalent to 5 times the volume of citrated plasma.

Plasma protein fraction is effective in the maintenance of a normal blood volume, but it has not been proven effective to maintain oncotic pressure. When the circulating blood volume has been depleted, the hemodilution following albumin administration persists for many hours. In individuals with normal blood volume, it usually lasts only a few hours. The half-life of albumin is 15 to 20 days with a turnover of ≈ 15 g per day.

Albumin 5% increases the circulating plasma volume by approximately equal to the amount infused. Albumin 25% draws about 3.5 times its volume of additional fluid into the circulation within 15 minutes except when the patient is dehydrated. Both 5% and 25% decrease blood viscosity.

There is no evidence that normal serum albumin (human) interferes with normal coagulation mechanisms. Antibodies, especially isoagglutinins, have been removed, enabling the product to be used without regard to the patient's blood group or blood factors.

Unlike whole blood or plasma, plasma protein fractions are free of the danger of homologous serum hepatitis, because these solutions are heat treated at 60°C (140°F) for 10 hours; thus, the possibility of transmitting serum hepatitis is reduced to a minimum. No crossmatching is required and the absence of cellular elements removes the risk of sensitization with repeated infusions.

Contraindications

A history of allergic reactions to albumin; severe anemia; cardiac failure; the presence of normal or increased intravascular volume; patients on cardiopulmonary bypass.

In chronic nephrosis, infused albumin is promptly excreted by the kidneys with no relief of the chronic edema or effect on the underlying renal lesion. It is of occasional use in the rapid "priming" diuresis of nephrosis. Similarly, in hypoproteinemic states associated with chronic cirrhosis, malabsorption, protein losing enteropathies, pancreatic insufficiency and undernutrition, the infusion of albumin as a source of protein nutrition is not justified.

Warnings

➤*Pregnancy: Category C.* Safety for use has not been established. Use only when clearly needed and when the potential benefits outweigh the hazards to the fetus.

Precautions

➤*Concomitant blood administration:* When large quantities of albumin are given, supplement with or replace by whole blood to combat relative anemia.

Not a substitute for whole blood in situations where the oxygen carrying capacity of whole blood is required in addition to plasma volume expansion. Contains no recognized blood coagulating factors and should not be used for control of hemorrhage due to deficiencies or defects in the clotting mechanism.

➤*Hypotension:* Rapid infusion (> 10 mL/min) may produce hypotension. Monitor blood pressure during use and slow or discontinue infusion if hypotension occurs. Vasopressors may also help correct the hypotension.

➤*Hemorrhage:* Supplement albumin with hemodilution. When circulating blood volume has been reduced, hemodilution following the administration of albumin persists for many hours. In patients with a normal blood volume, hemodilution lasts for a much shorter period.

➤*Shock:* Monitor blood pressure frequently. Widening of the pulse pressure is correlated with an increase in stroke volume or cardiac output.

➤*Dehydration:* Patients with marked dehydration require additional fluids.

➤*Special risk patients:* Use with caution in patients with hepatic or renal failure because of the added protein load.

Certain patients (eg, those with congestive cardiac failure, renal insufficiency or with stabilized chronic anemia) are at risk of developing circulatory overload. Rapid infusion may cause vascular overload with resultant pulmonary edema. Monitor for signs of increased venous pressure.

Use caution in patients with low cardiac reserve or with no albumin deficiency. A rapid increase in plasma volume may cause circulatory embarrassment or pulmonary edema.

The quick rise in blood pressure that may follow administration of albumin after injuries or surgery necessitates observation to detect bleeding points that may have failed to bleed at the lower blood pressure; otherwise, new hemorrhage and shock may occur.

Adverse Reactions

Allergic or pyrogenic reactions – Such reactions are characterized primarily by fever and chills. Flushing, urticaria, back pain, headache, rash, nausea, vomiting, increased salivation and febrile reactions, tachycardia, hypotension, and changes in respiration, pulse and blood pressure have also been reported. If such reactions occur, discontinue the infusion and institute appropriate therapy.

➤*Cardiovascular:* Hypotension (see Precautions). In addition, rapid administration may result in vascular overload, dyspnea and pulmonary edema.

PLASMA PROTEIN FRACTION

Rx	**Plasmanate** (Bayer)	**Injection:** 5%	In 50, 250 and 500 mL vials.
Rx	**Plasma-Plex** (Centeon)		In 50, 250 and 500 mL vials with injection set.
Rx	**Protenate** (Baxter Healthcare)		In 250 and 500 mL vials.

For complete prescribing information, refer to the Plasma Protein Fractions group monograph.

Administration and Dosage

Contains 130 to 160 mEq/L sodium.

Administer by IV infusion, preferably through an area of skin at some distance from any site of infection or trauma.

➤*Hypovolemic shock:* The initial dose may be 250 or 500 mL. The rate of infusion and volume of total dose depend on the patient's condition and response. Infusion at rates exceeding 10 mL/min may result in hypotension. Monitor blood pressure during administration; slow or stop infusion if sudden hypotension occurs.

Infants and young children – Plasma protein fraction may be used in the initial therapy of shock due to dehydration or infection in infants and young children. Infuse a dose of 10 to 15 mL/lb (20 to 30 mL/kg), at a rate ≤ 10 mL per minute. Repeat, depending upon the patient's condition and response.

➤*Hypoproteinemia:* Daily doses of 1000 to 1500 mL (50 to 75 g of protein) are appropriate; larger doses may be necessary in severe hypoproteinemia with continuing loss of plasma proteins. In these and other normovolemic patients, the rate of administration should not exceed 5 to 8 mL per minute; monitor such patients for signs of hypervolemia, which include dyspnea, pulmonary edema, abnormal rise in blood and central-venous pressure.

Adjust the rate of infusion in accordance with the clinical response.

If edema is present or if large amounts of protein are continuously lost, it may be preferable to use concentrated (25%) Normal Serum Albumin because of the greater amount of protein in a given volume. However, unless the pathology responsible for the hypoproteinemia can be corrected (as by proper diet in malnutrition), plasma derivatives can provide only symptomatic relief or supportive treatment.

➤*Preparation:* Ready for use without further preparation; may be administered without regard to the recipient's blood group or type.

➤*Admixture compatibility:* The solution is compatible with the usual IV solutions of carbohydrates or electrolytes, as well as whole blood and packed red cells. However, certain solutions containing protein hydrosylates amino acid solutions or alcohol must not be infused through the same administration set, as these combinations may cause the proteins to precipitate.

➤*Storage/Stability:* Store at room temperature, not exceeding 30°C (86°F). Do not use if the solution is turbid or has been frozen, if there is a sediment in the bottle or if more than 4 hours have elapsed after the container has been entered. Contains no preservative, so the contents of each bottle should be used on one occasion only. Destroy unused portions to prevent the possibility of use of contaminated solutions.

ALBUMIN HUMAN (Normal Serum Albumin), 5%

Rx	**Albuminar-5** (Centeon)	**Injection:** 5%	In 50 and 1000 mL vials.
Rx	**Albutein 5%** (Alpha Therapeutic)		In 250 and 500 mL vials.
Rx	**Normal Serum Albumin (Human) 5% Solution** (Immuno-US)		In 50, 250 and 500 mL vials with IV set.
Rx	**Plasbumin-5** (Bayer)		In 50, 250 and 500 mL vials.

For complete prescribing information, refer to the Plasma Protein Fractions group monograph.

Administration and Dosage

Contains 130 to 160 mEq/L sodium.

Administer by IV infusion and without further dilution.

➤*Infusion rate:* Since albumin in this concentration provides additional fluid for plasma volume expansion when used in patients with normal blood volume, infusion rate should be slow enough to prevent too rapid expansion of plasma volume.

➤*Shock:* In the treatment of a patient in shock with greatly reduced blood volume, albumin 5% may be given as rapidly as necessary to improve clinical condition and restore normal blood volume. In adults, an initial dose of 500 mL of the 5% albumin solution is given as rapidly as tolerated. If response within 30 minutes is inadequate, an additional 500 mL of 5% albumin solution may be given. For pediatric use, 50 mL would be appropriate. In neonates and infants, albumin 5% may be given in large amounts. The recommended dose is 10 to 20 mL/kg. Guide therapy by the clinical response, blood pressure and assessment of relative anemia. If > 1000 mL is given, or if hemorrhage has occurred, the administration of whole blood or red blood cells may be desirable.

In patients with slightly low or normal blood volume, give at a rate of 1 to 2 mL/min. Usual administration rate for children is one-quarter to one-half the adult rate.

➤*Burns:* After a burn injury (usually beyond 24 hours), there is a correlation between the amount of albumin infused and the resultant increase in plasma colloid osmotic pressure. In severe burns, immediate therapy usually includes large volumes of crystalloid, with lesser amounts of 5% albumin solution to maintain an adequate plasma volume. After the first 24 hours, the ratio of albumin to crystalloid may be increased to establish and maintain a plasma albumin level of about 2.5 g ± 0.5 g/100 mL or a total serum protein level of about 5.2 g/100 mL. However, an optimal regimen for severe burns is not established. Duration of therapy is decided by loss of protein from burned areas and in urine. Do not consider albumin as a source of nutrition.

➤*Hypoproteinemia:* The infusion of albumin as a nutrient in the treatment of chronic hypoproteinemia is not recommended. In acute hypoproteinemia, 5% albumin may be used in replacing the protein lost in hypoproteinemic conditions. However, if edema is present or if large amounts of albumin are lost, albumin 25% is preferred because of the greater amount of protein in the concentrated solution.

➤*Preparation for administration:* Swab stopper top immediately after removing seal with suitable antiseptic prior to entering vial. Inspect visually for particulate matter and discoloration.

➤*Storage/Stability:* Store at room temperature not exceeding 30°C (86°F). Do not freeze.

Plasma Protein Fractions

ALBUMIN HUMAN (Normal Serum Albumin), 25%

Rx	**Albuminar-25** (Centeon)	Injection: 25%	In 20 mL vials.
Rx	**Albutein 25%** (Alpha Therapeutic)		In 20, 50 and 100 mL vials.
Rx	**Normal Serum Albumin (Human) 25% Solution** (Immuno-US)		In 20, 50 and 100 mL vials with IV set.
Rx	**Plasbumin-25** (Bayer)		In 20, 50 and 100 mL vials.

For complete prescribing information, refer to the Plasma Protein Fractions group monograph.

Administration and Dosage

Contains 130 to 160 mEq/L sodium. Administer by IV infusion.

➤*Preparation:* May be given undiluted or diluted in normal saline. If sodium restriction is required, administer either undiluted or diluted in a sodium free carbohydrate solution such as 5% Dextrose in Water.

➤*Hypoproteinemia with or without edema:* Unless the underlying pathology responsible for the hypoproteinemia can be corrected, IV use of albumin 25% is purely symptomatic or supportive. The usual daily dose of albumin for adults is 50 to 75 g and for children 25 g. Patients with severe hypoproteinemia who continue to lose albumin may require larger quantities. Since hypoproteinemic patients usually have approximately normal blood volumes, administration rate should not exceed 2 mL/minute, as more rapid injection may precipitate circulatory embarrassment and pulmonary edema. If slower administration is desired, 200 mL of 25% albumin may be mixed with 300 mL of 10% glucose solution and administered by continuous drip at a rate of 100 mL/hour. Although diuresis may occur soon after administration, best results are obtained if albumin is continued until the normal serum protein level is regained.

➤*Burns:* After a burn injury (usually beyond 24 hours) there is a correlation between the amount of albumin infused and the resultant increase in plasma colloid osmotic pressure. The aim should be to maintain the plasma albumin concentration in the region of 2.5 ± 0.5 g/100 mL, with a plasma oncotic pressure of 20 mmHg (equivalent to a total plasma protein concentration of 5.2 g/100 mL). This can be achieved by the IV administration of albumin 25%. The duration of therapy is decided by the loss of protein from the burned areas and in the urine. In addition, oral or parenteral feeding with amino acids should be initiated, as albumin should not be considered a source of nutrition.

Duration of treatment varies, depending upon the extent of protein loss through renal excretion, denuded areas of skin and decreased albumin synthesis. Attempts to raise albumin levels > 4 g/100 mL may result in increased rates of catabolism.

➤*Shock:* Determine initial dose by the patient's condition and response to treatment. Guide therapy by degree of venous and pulmonary congestion or hematocrit measurements.

Greatly reduced blood volume – Administer as rapidly as desired. If the initial response is inadequate, (ie, if pulse rate remains above 100/min, the blood pressure below 10 cm water, or if acrocyanosis or cold sweat is present) additional albumin may be given 15 to 30 minutes following the first dose.

Slightly low or normal blood volume – The rate of administration should be 1 mL/minute. If there is continued loss of protein, it may be desirable to give whole blood or other blood fractions.

➤*Erythrocyte resuspension:* About 25 g of albumin per liter of erythrocytes is commonly used, although the requirements in preexistent hypoproteinemia or hepatic impairment can be greater. Albumin 25% is added to the isotonic suspension of washed red cells immediately prior to transfusion.

➤*Acute nephrosis:* A loop diuretic and 100 mL albumin 25% repeated daily for 7 to 10 days may control edema and the patient may then respond to steroid treatment.

➤*Renal dialysis:* The usual volume administered is about 100 mL; avoid fluid overload. These patients cannot tolerate substantial volumes of salt solution.

➤*Hyperbilirubinemia and erythroblastosis fetalis:* The use of albumin in exchange transfusions reduces the necessity for reexchange and increases the amount of bilirubin removed with each transfusion. Administer 1 g/kg 1 to 2 hours before transfusion.

➤*Storage/Stability:* Store at room temperature not exceeding 30°C (86°F). Do not freeze.

HETASTARCH (Hydroxyethyl Starch; HES)

Rx	**Hetastarch** (Gensia Sicor Pharm)	**Injection:** 6 g/100 mL in 0.9% sodium chloride	In 500 mL IV infusion containers.

Indications

►*Shock:* Adjunct for plasma volume expansion in shock due to hemorrhage, burns, surgery, sepsis or other trauma.

►*Leukapheresis:* Adjunct to improve harvesting and increase yield of granulocytes.

Administration and Dosage

Administer by IV infusion only. Total dosage and rate of infusion depend upon the amount of blood lost and the resultant hemoconcentration.

►*Plasma volume expansion:* The usual amount is 500 to 1000 mL. Total dosage does not usually exceed 1500 mL/day (20 mL/kg). In acute hemorrhagic shock, rates approaching 20 mL/kg/hour may be used.

►*Leukapheresis:* In continuous flow centrifugation (CFC) procedures, 250 to 700 mL is typically infused at a constant fixed ratio of 1:8 to 1:13 to venous whole blood.

►*Storage/Stability:* Store at room temperature not exceeding 40°C (104°F). Do not freeze. Do not use if solution is turbid deep brown or if crystalline precipitate forms.

Actions

►*Pharmacology:* Hetastarch (HES) is a complex mixture of ethoxylated amylopectin molecules of various sizes; average molecular weight (MW) is 450,000 (range, 10,000 to > 1 million). Colloidal properties of 6% HES approximate those of human albumin. After IV infusion, plasma volume expands slightly in excess of volume infused and decreases over 24 to 36 hours. Hemodynamic status will decrease after 24 hours. Adding HES to whole blood increases the erythrocyte sedimentation rate and improves the efficiency of granulocyte collection by centrifugal means.

►*Pharmacokinetics:* Molecules < 50,000 MW are rapidly eliminated renally; ≈ 33% appear in urine in 24 hours. Larger molecules are broken down; ≈ 90% of the dose is eliminated (avg. half-life, 17 days; the remainder has a half-life of 48 days). The hydroxyethyl group remains intact and attached to glucose units when excreted.

Contraindications

Severe bleeding disorders; severe cardiac failure; renal failure with oliguria or anuria.

Warnings

►*Blood/Plasma substitute:* Not a substitute for blood or plasma, as it does not have oxygen-carrying capacity or contain plasma proteins (eg, coagulation factors).

►*Coagulation effects:* Large volumes may alter coagulation and result in transient prolongation of prothrombin time (PT), partial thromboplastin time (PTT), bleeding and clotting times, decreased hematocrit and excessive dilution of plasma proteins.

►*Leukapheresis:* Slight declines in platelet count and hemoglobin levels have been observed in donors undergoing repeated leukapheresis procedures due to the volume expanding effects of hetastarch. Hemoglobin levels usually return to normal within 24 hours. Hemodilution by hetastarch and saline may also result in 24 hour declines of total protein, albumin, calcium, and fibrinogen values.

►*Hypersensitivity reactions:* Anaphylactoid reactions (periorbital edema, urticaria, wheezing) have been reported. If these occur, discontinue the drug. If necessary, give antihistamines. See Management of Acute Hypersensitivity Reactions. Also, use caution when administering HES to a person allergic to corn.

►*Pregnancy: Category C.* Safety for use has not been established. Use only when clearly needed and when potential benefits outweigh potential hazards to the fetus.

►*Lactation:* It is not known whether hetastarch is excreted in breast milk. Exercise caution when administering to a nursing woman.

►*Children:* Safety and efficacy have not been established.

Precautions

►*Monitoring:* During leukapheresis, monitor CBC, total leukocyte and platelet counts, leukocyte differential count, hemoglobin, hematocrit, PT and PTT.

►*Special risk patients:* The possibility of circulatory overload exists. Take special care in patients with impaired renal clearance and when the risk of pulmonary edema or congestive heart failure is increased. Indirect bilirubin levels increased in two subjects receiving multiple infusions; levels returned to normal by 96 hours after infusion. Total bilirubin remained normal. Use caution in liver disease.

Adverse Reactions

Vomiting; mild temperature elevation; chills; itching; submaxillary and parotid glandular enlargement; mild influenza-like symptoms; headache; muscle pain; peripheral edema of the lower extremities; allergic reactions (see Warnings).

DEXTRAN, LOW MOLECULAR WEIGHT (Dextran 40)

Rx	**Dextran 40** (McGaw)	**Injection:** 10% dextran 40 in 0.9% sodium chloride	In 500 mL.
Rx	**Gentran 40** (Baxter)		In 500 mL.
Rx	**10% LMD** (Abbott)		In 500 mL.
Rx	**Rheomacrodex** (Medisan)		In 500 mL.
Rx	**Dextran 40** (McGaw)	**Injection:** 10% dextran 40 in 5% dextrose	In 500 mL.
Rx	**Gentran 40** (Baxter)		In 500 mL.
Rx	**10% LMD** (Abbott)		In 500 mL.
Rx	**Rheomacrodex** (Medisan)		In 500 mL.

Indications

►*Shock:* Adjunctive treatment of shock or impending shock due to hemorrhage, burns, surgery or other trauma. The solution is for emergency treatment when whole blood products are not available; it is not a substitute for whole blood or plasma proteins.

►*Priming fluid:* As a priming fluid, either as the sole primer or as an additive, in pump oxygenators during extracorporeal circulation.

►*Deep venous thrombosis (DVT)/Pulmonary embolism (PE) prophylaxis:* Prophylaxis against DVT and PE in patients undergoing procedures associated with a high incidence of thromboembolic complications, such as hip surgery.

Administration and Dosage

For IV use only.

►*Adjunctive therapy in shock:* Total dosage during the first 24 hours should not exceed 20 mL/kg. The first 10 mL/kg should be infused rapidly, with the remaining dose being administered more slowly. Monitor the central venous pressure frequently during the initial infusion. Should therapy continue beyond 24 hours, total daily dosage should not exceed 10 mL/kg, and therapy should not continue beyond 5 days.

►*Hemodiluent in extracorporeal circulation:* The dosage employed in the priming fluid will vary with the volume of pump oxygenator employed. It may be added as sole primer or as an additive. Generally, 10 to 20 mL/kg are added to the perfusion circuit. Do not exceed total dosage of 20 mL/kg; this can be limited and controlled by adding other priming fluids.

►*Prophylactic therapy of venous thrombosis and thromboembolism:* Select dosage according to the risk of thromboembolic complications (eg, type of surgery and duration of immobilization). In general, initiate treatment during surgery. Administer 500 to 1000 mL (approximately 10 mL/kg) on the day of the operation. Continue treatment at a dose of 500 mL/day for an additional 2 to 3 days. Thereafter, and according to the risk of complications, 500 mL may be administered every second or third day during the period of risk for up to 2 weeks.

►*Children:* The best guide is the body weight or surface area, and the total dosage should not exceed 20 mL/kg.

►*Storage/Stability:* Store at a constant temperature between 15° to 30°C (59° to 86°F). Protect from freezing.

Actions

►*Pharmacology:* Dextran 40 is a branched polysaccharide plasma-volume expander with an average molecular weight of 40,000 (range 10,000 to 90,000). A 2.5% solution of dextran 40 is equivalent in colloid osmotic pressure to normal plasma. Generally, plasma volume is increased onefold to twofold over the volume of dextran 40 infused. The extent and duration of volume expansion produced will depend on the preexisting blood volume, rate of infusion and rate of dextran clearance by the kidneys.

►*Pharmacokinetics:* Dextran 40 is evenly distributed in the vascular system. Its distribution according to molecular weight shifts toward higher molecular weights as the smaller molecules are excreted by the kidney. Approximately 50% administered to a normovolemic subject is excreted in the urine within 3 hours, 60% within 6 hours and 75% within 24 hours. The remaining 25% is partially hydrolyzed and

DEXTRAN, LOW MOLECULAR WEIGHT (Dextran 40)

excreted in the urine, partially excreted in the feces and partially oxidized. Unexcreted dextran molecules diffuse into the extravascular compartment and are temporarily taken up by the reticuloendothelial system. Some of these molecules are returned to the intravascular compartment via the lymphatics. Dextran is slowly degraded to glucose by the enzyme dextranase.

Adjunctive therapy in shock – Enhances blood flow, particularly in the microcirculation, by a combination of the following mechanisms: Increases blood volume, venous return and cardiac output; decreases blood viscosity and peripheral vascular resistance; reduces aggregation of erythrocytes and other cellular elements of blood by coating them and maintaining their electronegative charges.

Administration to a patient in shock usually increases blood volume, central venous pressure, cardiac output, stroke volume, arterial blood pressure, pulse pressure, capillary perfusion, venous return and urinary output; it also decreases blood viscosity, heart rate, peripheral resistance and mean transit time and prevents or reverses cellular aggregation. Hematocrit is lowered in proportion to the infusion volume.

The intense but relatively short-lived plasma expansion volume produced by dextran 40 is advantageous in the treatment of early shock because it acts rapidly to correct hypovolemia while allowing control of the plasma volume. If overexpansion occurs, the discontinuation of the infusion will result in a decline in plasma volume due to loss of dextran from the intravascular space.

Priming solution for extracorporeal circulation – Dextran 40's advantages over homologous blood and other priming fluids include: Decreased destruction of erythrocytes and platelets; reduced intravascular hemagglutination; maintenance of electronegativity of erythrocytes and platelets.

Prophylaxis against venous thrombosis, thromboembolism – The infusion of dextran 40 during and after surgical trauma reduces the incidence of DVT and PE in surgical patients subject to procedures with a high incidence of thromboembolic complications. Dextran 40 simultaneously inhibits mechanisms essential to thrombus formation such as vascular stasis and platelet adhesiveness, and alters the structure and lysability of fibrin clots.

Dextran 40 increases cardiac output, arterial, venous and microcirculatory flow and reduces mean transit time, chiefly by expanding plasma volume, by reducing blood viscosity through hemodilution and by reducing red cell aggregation.

Contraindications

Hypersensitivity to dextran; marked hemostatic defects of all types (eg, thrombocytopenia, hypofibrinogenemia), including those caused by drugs (eg, heparin, warfarin); marked cardiac decompensation; renal disease with severe oliguria or anuria.

Decreased urinary output, secondary to shock, is not a contraindication unless there is no improvement in urine output after the initial dose.

If administration of sodium or chloride could be clinically detrimental, 10% Dextran in 0.9% Sodium Chloride Injection is contraindicated.

Warnings

➤*Anaphylaxis:* Antigenicity of dextrans is directly related to their degree of branching. Because dextran 40 has a low degree of branching, it is relatively free of antigenic effect. Hypersensitivity reactions have, however, been reported (see Adverse Reactions). Infrequently, severe and fatal anaphylactoid reactions (eg, marked hypotension, cardiac and respiratory arrest) have been reported. Most of these reactions occurred early in the infusion period in patients not previously exposed to IV dextran and have appeared after administration of as little as 10 mL. Stop infusion immediately if an anaphylactoid reaction is imminent. Refer to Management of Acute Hypersensitivity Reactions. In circulatory collapse due to anaphylaxis, institute rapid volume substitution with an agent other than dextran. Dextran 1 is indicated for prophylaxis of serious anaphylactic reactions to dextran infusions.

➤*Fluid imbalance:* These products are colloid hypertonic solutions and will attract water from the extravascular space. Poorly hydrated patients will need additional fluid therapy. If given in excess, vascular overload could occur. This can be avoided by monitoring central venous pressure.

Administration of dextran IV can cause fluid or solute overloading, resulting in dilution of serum electrolyte concentrations, overhydration, congested states or pulmonary edema. The risk of dilutional states is inversely proportional to electrolyte concentrations of administered parenteral solutions.

➤*Hemorrhage:* Use with caution in patients with active hemorrhage; the increase in perfusion pressure and improved microcirculatory flow may result in additional blood loss.

Avoid administering infusions that exceed the recommended dose, as a dose-related increase in the incidence of wound hematoma, wound seroma, wound bleeding, distant bleeding (hematuria and melena) and pulmonary edema has been observed.

➤*Hematologic effects:* Use with caution in patients with thrombocytopenia. Hematocrit should not be depressed below 30% by volume. When large volumes of dextran are administered, plasma protein levels will be decreased. Do not give dextran 40 to patients with marked thrombocytopenia or hypofibrinogenemia.

In individuals with normal hemostasis, dosages of up to 15 mL/kg or > 1000 mL may prolong bleeding time and decrease coagulation due to depressed platelet function. Dosages in this range also markedly decrease factor VIII; they also decrease factors V and IX to a slightly greater degree than would be expected from hemodilution alone. Because these changes tend to be more pronounced following trauma or major surgery, observe all patients for early signs of bleeding complications.

➤*Special risk patients:* Use solutions containing sodium ions with great care, if at all, in patients with congestive heart failure, severe renal insufficiency, in clinical states in which edema exists with sodium retention (particularly in postoperative or elderly patients) and in patients receiving corticosteroids.

Use dextrose-containing solutions with caution in overt or known subclinical diabetes mellitus.

➤*Renal function impairment:* Renal excretion causes elevation of the specific gravity of the urine. In the presence of adequate urine flow, only minor elevations occur, but in patients with diminished urine flow, urine viscosity and specific gravity can be increased markedly. As osmolarity is only slightly affected by the presence of dextran molecules, assess a patient's state of hydration by determination of urine or serum osmolarity. If signs of dehydration are noted, administer additional fluids. An osmotic diuretic such as mannitol is useful in maintaining adequate urine flow.

Renal failure, sometimes irreversible, has been reported. While the pre-existing clinical condition of these patients could account for the oliguria or anuria, it is possible that dextran use may have contributed to its development. Evidence of tubular vacuolization (osmotic nephrosis) has been found following administration. The exact clinical significance is unknown.

In patients with diminished renal function, use of solutions containing sodium ions may result in sodium retention. Excessive doses may precipitate renal failure.

➤*Pregnancy: Category C.* Safety for use during pregnancy has not been established. Use only when clearly needed and when the potential benefits outweigh the potential hazards to the fetus.

➤*Lactation:* It is not known whether this drug is excreted in breast milk. Exercise caution when dextran 40 is administered to a nursing woman.

Precautions

➤*Monitoring:* Urine output should be carefully monitored. Usually, an increase in urine output occurs in oliguric patients after administration. If no increase is observed after the infusion of 500 mL, discontinue the drug until adequate diuresis develops spontaneously or can be induced by other means.

Exercise care to prevent a depression of the hematocrit below 30%.

Infusion of dextran may lead to excessive dilution of red blood cells and plasma proteins, dilution of other blood constituents (platelets, fibrinogen) or dilutional acidosis caused by dilution of the bicarbonate ion.

➤*Bleeding complications:* Observe patients for early signs of bleeding complications, particularly following surgery, major trauma or if anticoagulant drugs are being administered.

Drug Interactions

➤*Drug/Lab test interactions:* Blood sugar determinations that employ high concentrations of acid (acetic or sulfuric) may cause hydrolysis of dextran; falsely elevated glucose assays may be reported in patients receiving dextran. In other laboratory tests, the presence of dextran may result in the development of turbidity, which can interfere with bilirubin assays in which alcohol has been employed, in total protein assays employing biuret reagent and in blood sugar determinations with the ortho-toluidine method. Consider withdrawal of blood for chemical laboratory tests prior to initiating therapy.

Blood typing and crossmatching procedures employing enzyme techniques may give unreliable readings if the samples are taken after infusion. Other blood typing and crossmatching procedures are not affected. Draw blood samples for the above determinations prior to initiating infusion or, alternatively, inform the laboratory that the patient has received dextran so that suitable assay methods can be applied.

Occasional abnormal renal and hepatic function values have been reported following IV use. The specific effect on renal and hepatic function could not be determined, as most of these patients had also undergone surgery or cardiac catheterization.

Adverse Reactions

➤*Hypersensitivity:* Mild cutaneous eruptions, generalized urticaria, hypotension, nausea, vomiting, headache, dyspnea, fever, tightness of the chest, bronchospasm, wheezing and, rarely, anaphylactoid (allergic) shock (see Warnings).

➤*Miscellaneous:* Reactions which may occur because of the solution or the technique of administration include febrile response, infection at the injection site, venous thrombosis or phlebitis extending from the injection site, extravasation and hypervolemia.

DEXTRAN, LOW MOLECULAR WEIGHT (Dextran 40)

Hypernatremia may be associated with edema and exacerbation of congestive heart failure due to the retention of water, resulting in expanded extracellular fluid volume.

If solutions containing sodium chloride are infused in large volumes, chloride ions may cause a loss of bicarbonate ions, resulting in an acidifying effect.

DEXTRAN, HIGH MOLECULAR WEIGHT (Dextran 70 and 75)

Rx	Dextran 75 (Abbott)	Injection: 6% dextran 75 in 0.9% sodium chloride	In 500 mL.
Rx	Dextran 70 (McGaw)	Injection: 6% dextran 70 in 0.9% sodium chloride	In 500 mL.
Rx	Gentran 70 (Baxter)		In 500 mL.
Rx	Macrodex (Medisan)		In 500 mL.
Rx	Dextran 75 (Abbott)	Injection: 6% dextran 75 in 5% dextrose	In 500 mL.
Rx	Macrodex (Medisan)	Injection: 6% dextran 70 in 5% dextrose	In 500 mL.

Indications

➤*Shock:* Treatment of shock or impending shock due to surgery or other trauma, hemorrhage or burns. Intended for emergency treatment only when whole blood or blood products are not available; do not regard as a substitute for whole blood or plasma proteins. It should not replace other forms of therapy known to be of value in the treatment of shock.

Administration and Dosage

Administer by IV infusion only. Total dose and rate of infusion depend upon the magnitude of fluid loss and the resultant hemoconcentration. It is suggested that the total dosage not exceed 20 mL/kg during the first 24 hours.

➤*Adults:* The amount usually administered is 500 to 1000 mL, which may be given at a rate of from 20 to 40 mL/minute in an emergency.

➤*Children:* The best guide to dosage is the body weight or surface area of the patient; total dosage should not exceed 20 mL/kg.

No additives should be delivered via plasma volume expanders.

➤*Storage/Stability:* The solution has no bacteriostat; discard partially used containers. The solution must be clear. Store at a constant temperature not > 25°C (77°F).

Actions

➤*Pharmacology:* Dextrans are synthetic polysaccharides used to approximate the colloidal properties of albumin. Dextran 70 has an average molecular weight (MW) of 70,000 (range 20,000 to 200,000), and dextran 75 has an average MW of 75,000. Dextran 70 improves blood pressure, pulse rate, respiratory exchange and renal function in patients with hypovolemia or hypotensive shock. IV infusion results in an expansion of plasma volume slightly in excess of volume infused and decreases from this maximum over the next 24 hours. This plasma volume expansion improves hemodynamic status for ≥ 24 hours.

➤*Pharmacokinetics:* Dextran molecules below 50,000 molecular weight are eliminated by renal excretion, with approximately 50% appearing in the urine in 24 hours in the normovolemic patient. The remaining dextran is enzymatically degraded to glucose at a rate of about 70 to 90 mg/kg/day. This is a variable process.

Contraindications

Hypersensitivity to dextran; marked hemostatic defects of all types (thrombocytopenia, hypofibrinogenemia, etc), including those induced by drugs; marked cardiac decompensation; renal disease with severe oliguria or anuria; severe congestive heart failure, pulmonary edema and severe bleeding disorders; where use of sodium or chloride could be clinically detrimental.

Warnings

➤*Anaphylaxis:* Severe and fatal anaphylactoid reactions (eg, marked hypotension, cardiac and respiratory arrest) have occurred early in the infusion period in patients not previously exposed to IV dextran. Stop infusion immediately if an anaphylactoid reaction is imminent, provided that other means of sustaining the circulation are available. Refer to Management of Acute Hypersensitivity Reactions. In circulatory collapse due to anaphylaxis, institute rapid volume substitution with an agent other than dextran. Antihistamines may be effective in relieving some symptoms. Dextran 1 is indicated for prophylaxis of serious anaphylactic reactions associated with dextran infusions.

➤*Hematologic effects:* In individuals with normal hemostasis, dosages approximating 15 mL/kg or > 1000 mL prolong bleeding time and decrease coagulation due to depressed platelet function; use with caution in patients with thrombocytopenia. Such dosages also markedly decrease factor VIII and decrease factor V and factor IX more than would be expected from hemodilution alone. These changes tend to be more pronounced following trauma or major surgery; observe patients for early signs of bleeding complications. Transient prolongation of bleeding time may occur following doses > 1000 mL, particularly if the patient is on concomitant anticoagulation therapy. Take care to prevent depression of hematocrit below 30% by volume. When large volumes of dextran are given, plasma protein level will be decreased.

➤*Special risk patients:* Use solutions containing sodium ions with great care, if at all, in patients with congestive heart failure, pulmo-

nary edema, severe renal insufficiency, patients receiving corticosteroids or corticotropin and in clinical states in which edema exists with sodium retention. Circulatory overload may occur. Exercise special care in patients with impaired renal clearance.

Exercise care in patients with pathological abdominal conditions and in those undergoing bowel surgery.

➤*Fluid imbalance:* Fluid or solute overloading may occur, resulting in dilution of serum electrolyte concentrations, overhydration, congested states (CHF) and peripheral or pulmonary edema. The risk of dilutional states is inversely proportional to the electrolyte concentration of administered parenteral solutions.

The risk of solute overload causing congested states with peripheral and pulmonary edema is directly proportional to electrolyte concentrations of such solutions.

Monitoring central venous blood pressure is recommended to detect overexpansion of blood volume. When signs of overexpansion appear, discontinuing IV infusion allows blood volume to readjust and decline, primarily by loss of fluid to urine.

➤*Pregnancy: Category C.* Safety for use during pregnancy has not been established. There are no adequate and well controlled studies in pregnant women. Use only when clearly needed and when potential benefits outweigh potential hazards.

➤*Lactation:* It is not known whether this drug is excreted in breast milk. Exercise caution when administering to a nursing woman.

Precautions

➤*Monitoring:* Urine output should be carefully observed. An increase in urine output usually occurs in oliguric patients after the administration of dextran. If no increase is observed after the infusion of 500 mL of dextran, discontinue the drug until adequate diuresis develops spontaneously or can be provoked by other means.

➤*Bleeding complications:* Observe patients for early signs of bleeding complications, particularly following surgery or major trauma, or if anticoagulant drugs are being administered.

Drug Interactions

➤*Drug/Lab test interactions:* Blood sugar determinations that employ high concentrations of acid (acetic or sulfuric) may cause hydrolysis of dextran; falsely elevated glucose assays may be reported in patients receiving dextran. In other laboratory tests, the presence of dextran may result in the development of turbidity, which can interfere with bilirubin assays in which alcohol has been employed, in total protein assays employing biuret reagent and in blood sugar determinations with the ortho-toluidine method.

Blood typing and crossmatching procedures employing enzyme techniques may give unreliable readings if the samples are taken after infusion. If blood is drawn after the infusion, the saline-agglutination and indirect antiglobulin methods may be used for typing and crossmatching. Draw blood samples for the above determinations prior to initiating infusion or, alternatively, inform the laboratory that the patient has received dextran so that suitable assay methods can be applied.

Adverse Reactions

Infusion technique – Reactions which may occur because of the solution or the technique of administration include febrile response, infection at the injection site, venous thrombosis or phlebitis extending from the injection site, extravasation and hypervolemia. If a reaction develops, discontinue use and treat accordingly.

➤*Hypersensitivity:* Allergic reactions include urticaria, nasal congestion, wheezing, tightness of the chest, dyspnea, mild hypotension and, rarely, anaphylactoid (allergic) shock (see Warnings).

➤*Miscellaneous:* Sudden marked hypotension; nausea; vomiting; fever; joint pains.

Hypernatremia may be associated with edema and exacerbation of congestive heart failure due to water retention, resulting in expanded extracellular fluid volume.

If solutions containing sodium chloride are infused in large volumes, chloride ions may cause a loss of bicarbonate ions, resulting in an acidifying effect.

Dextran Adjunct

DEXTRAN 1

| *Rx* | **Promit** (Medisan) | **Injection:** 150 mg/mL | In 20 mL vials. |

Indications

➤*Serious anaphylactic reactions to dextran:* Prophylaxis of serious anaphylactic reactions to IV infusion of clinical dextran. Mild dextran-induced anaphylactic (allergic) reactions are not prevented by dextran 1.

Administration and Dosage

For IV use only. Do not dilute or admix with clinical dextran.

➤*Adults:* 20 mL (150 mg/mL) IV rapidly, 1 to 2 minutes before IV infusion of clinical dextran.

➤*Children:* 0.3 mL/kg in a corresponding manner.

The time interval between administration of dextran 1 and clinical dextran solutions should not exceed 15 minutes; if a longer period elapses, repeat dextran 1 dose. Repeat dextran 1 injection if 48 hours have elapsed since the last infusion of clinical dextran. Administer 1 to 2 minutes before every IV clinical dextran infusion.

May give IV through Y injection site if minimally diluted with primary solution. Do not give through an IV set used to infuse clinical dextran. May give through heparin lock.

➤*Storage/Stability:* Do not exceed 25°C (77°F). Protect from freezing.

Actions

➤*Pharmacology:* Clinical dextran is not antigenic, but its structure is similar to other antigenic polysaccharides. Some polysaccharide-reacting antibodies may crossreact with clinical dextran, forming antibody-antigen complexes that can trigger an anaphylactic reaction. This may occur in patients who have never received clinical dextran, but have enough dextran-reacting antibodies (DRA) to form large immune complexes. Dextran 1, a monovalent hapten, reacts with dextran-reactive immunoglobulin (IgG) without bridge formation and with no tendency for the formation of large immune complexes. A molar excess of monovalent hapten, given just before a clinical IV dextran solution, competitively prevents the formation of immune complexes with polyvalent clinical dextrans and impedes anaphylaxis. During the initial phase of a clinical dextran infusion, protection is affected by hapten inhibition. During the later phase and the following day, protection is exerted by dextran molecules in clinical dextran solutions because an antigen excess develops in the circulation and only small nonanaphylactogenic immune complexes can be formed. An additional injection of dextran 1 is recommended if 48 hours or more have elapsed since the previous infusion of clinical dextran.

Dextran-induced anaphylactic reactions have an incidence range of 0.002% to 0.025% per unit used (0.002% to 0.013% for dextran 40 and 0.017% to 0.025% for dextran 60/75). By means of hapten inhibition, the incidence is 15 to 20 times lower.

➤*Pharmacokinetics:* Because of its low molecular weight of 1000, dextran 1 is rapidly and completely excreted by glomerular filtration. After IV injection of a single 20 mL dose, ≈ 50% is cleared from the blood within 30 minutes. Mean urinary elimination half-life was 41 ± 11 minutes in 12 healthy individuals.

Contraindications

Do not give dextran 1 if IV use of clinical dextran solutions is contraindicated. This includes marked hemostatic defects of all types or hemorrhagic tendencies, marked cardiac decompensation and renal disease with severe oliguria or anuria.

Warnings

➤*Cardiac effects:* Severe hypotension and bradycardia have been reported.

➤*Pregnancy: Category B.* In rabbits, doses 35 to 70 times the human dose increased the incidence of fetal resorption, postimplantation fetal loss, retardation of fetal long-bone ossification and marginal fetal growth retardation. There are no adequate and well-controlled studies in pregnant women. Use only if clearly needed.

➤*Lactation:* It is not known whether dextran 1 is excreted in breast milk. Exercise caution when administering to nursing women.

Precautions

➤*Reactions:* If any reaction occurs, do not administer clinical dextran solutions.

Adverse Reactions

Cutaneous (0.016%); moderate hypotension (systolic BP > 60 mmHg; 0.014%); bradycardia (< 60 bpm) with moderate hypotension (0.013%); nausea, pallor, shivering (0.011%); bradycardia (0.004%); bradycardia with severe hypotension (systolic BP < 60 mmHg; 0.001%). Do not give subsequent infusion if adverse reactions occur.

Overdosage

The drug is rapidly cleared by renal excretion. Therefore, any overdosage should be of short duration and of minimal consequence.

HEMIN

Rx	**Panhematin** (Abbott)	**Powder for Injection:** 301 mg hematin/vial (equivalent to 7 mg hematin/mL) after reconstitution with 43 mL Sterile Water for Injection.	Preservative free. With 300 mg sorbitol. In single-dose dispensing vials.

WARNING

Hemin for injection should only be used by physicians experienced in the management of porphyrias in hospitals where the recommended clinical and laboratory diagnostic and monitoring techniques are available.

Consider hemin therapy after an appropriate period of alternate therapy (ie, 400 g glucose/day for 1 to 2 days).

Indications

➤*Porphyria:* For the amelioration of recurrent attacks of acute intermittent porphyria temporally related to the menstrual cycle in susceptible women. Manifestations such as pain, hypertension, tachycardia, abnormal mental status, and mild to progressive neurologic signs may be controlled in selected patients.

Similar findings have been reported in other patients with acute intermittent porphyria, porphyria variegata, and hereditary coproporphyria.

Administration and Dosage

For IV use only. Use a large arm vein or a central venous catheter to avoid phlebitis.

Before administering hemin for injection, consider alternate therapy (ie, 400 g glucose/day for 1 to 2 days). If improvement is unsatisfactory for the treatment of acute attacks of porphyria, administer an IV infusion containing a dose of 1 to 4 mg/kg/day of hematin over a period of 10 to 15 minutes for 3 to 14 days, based on clinical signs. In more severe cases, this dose may be repeated no earlier than every 12 hours. Give no more than 6 mg/kg in any 24-hour period.

➤*Preparation of solution:* Reconstitute by adding 43 mL of Sterile Water for Injection to the dispensing vial. Shake well for a period of 2 to 3 minutes to aid dissolution.

After reconstitution, each mL contains the equivalent of approximately 7 mg hematin (301 mg hemin/43 mL), 5 mg sodium carbonate (215 mg/43 mL), and 7 mg sorbitol (301 mg/43 mL). The drug may be administered directly from the vial.

Hemin Solution Preparation
Dosage Calculation Table
1 mg hematin equivalent = 0.14 mL
2 mg hematin equivalent = 0.28 mL
3 mg hematin equivalent = 0.42 mL
4 mg hematin equivalent = 0.56 mL

Because reconstituted hemin is not transparent, any undissolved particulate matter is difficult to see; therefore, terminal filtration through a sterile 0.45 micron or smaller filter is recommended.

➤*Admixture incompatibility:* Do not add any drug or chemical agent fluid admixture unless its effect on the chemical and physical stability has first been determined.

➤*Storage/Stability:* Because this product contains no preservative and undergoes rapid chemical decomposition in solution, do not reconstitute until immediately before use. Refrigerate lyophilized powder at 2° to 8°C (36° to 46°F) until time of use. Discard any unused portion.

Actions

➤*Pharmacology:* Hemin for injection is an enzyme inhibitor derived from processed red blood cells. It was known previously as hematin. The term hematin has been used to describe the chemical reaction product of hemin and sodium carbonate solution. Hemin is an iron-containing metalloporphyrin.

Porphyrias are rare metabolic disorders that, as a group, represent disturbances of heme synthesis and are differentiated on the basis of specific enzymatic defects. Porphyrias are characterized clinically by neurologic (psychoses, seizures, paresis) or cutaneous (photosensitivity) manifestations, and chemically by overproduction of porphyrins or their precursors. Porphyrins are byproducts of heme synthesis; heme is the iron-containing constituent of hemoglobin and respiratory pigments and is produced and required by nearly every body tissue. Heme limits the hepatic or marrow synthesis of porphyrin, which is likely due to inhibition of delta-aminolevulinic acid synthetase, the enzyme that limits the rate of porphyrin/heme biosynthetic pathway. However, the exact mechanism by which hematin produces symptomatic improvement in patients with acute episodes of the hepatic porphyrias is not known.

➤*Pharmacokinetics:* Following IV administration of hematin in nonjaundiced patients, an increase in fecal urobilinogen can be observed, which is roughly proportional to the amount of hematin administered. This suggests an enterohepatic pathway as at least 1 route of elimination. Bilirubin metabolites also are excreted in the urine following hematin injections.

➤*Clinical trials:* Hemin therapy for the acute porphyrias is not curative. After discontinuation of treatment, symptoms generally return, although remission may be prolonged. Some neurological symptoms have improved weeks to months after therapy, although little or no response was noted at the time of treatment.

Contraindications

Hypersensitivity to hemin; porphyria cutanea tarda.

Warnings

➤*Pregnancy: Category C.* Safety for use during pregnancy has not been established. Use only when clearly needed and when the potential benefits outweigh the potential hazards to the fetus.

➤*Lactation:* It is not known whether hemin for injection is excreted in breast milk. Safety for use in the nursing mother has not been established.

➤*Children:* Safety and efficacy for use in children have not been established.

Precautions

➤*Monitoring:* Drug effect will be demonstrated by a decrease in urinary concentration of 1 or more of the following compounds: ALA (delta-aminolevulinic acid); UPG (uroporphyrinogen); PBG (porphobilinogen coproporphyrin).

➤*Neuronal damage:* Clinical benefit depends on prompt administration. Attacks of porphyria may progress to irreversible neuronal damage. Hemin therapy is intended to prevent an attack from reaching the critical stage of neuronal degeneration. This agent is not effective in repairing neuronal damage.

➤*Renal effects:* Reversible renal shutdown has been observed where an excessive hematin dose (12.2 mg/kg) was administered in a single infusion. Oliguria and increased nitrogen retention occurred, although the patient remained asymptomatic. No worsening of renal function has been seen with use of recommended dosages.

➤*Diagnostic tests:* Before beginning therapy, diagnose the presence of acute porphyria using the following criteria: Presence of clinical symptoms and positive Watson-Schwartz or Hoesch test.

Drug Interactions

Hemin Drug Interactions			
Precipitant drug	Object drug*		Description
Hemin	Anticoagulants	↑	Hemin has exhibited transient, mild anticoagulant effects during clinical studies; therefore, avoid concurrent anticoagulant therapy. The extent and duration of the hypocoagulable state have not been established.
Barbiturates Estrogens Steroid metabolites	Hemin	↔	These agents increase the activity of delta-amino-levulinic acid synthetase. Because hemin therapy limits the rate of porphyria/heme biosynthesis, possibly by inhibiting the enzyme delta-aminolevulinic acid synthetase, avoid concurrent use of these agents.

* ↑ = Object drug increased. ↔ = Undetermined effect.

Adverse Reactions

Phlebitis with or without leukocytosis and with or without mild pyrexia has occurred after administration of hematin through small arm veins.

There has been 1 report of coagulopathy. This patient exhibited prolonged prothrombin time, partial thromboplastin time, thrombocytopenia, mild hypofibrinogenemia, mild elevation of fibrin split products, and a 10% fall in hematocrit.

Overdosage

Reversible renal shutdown has been observed in a case where an excessive hematin dose (12.2 mg/kg) was administered in a single infusion (see Precautions). Treatment of this case consisted of ethacrynic acid and mannitol.

WARNING

Estrogens have been reported to increase the risk of endometrial carcinoma in postmenopausal women: Studies have shown an increased risk of endometrial cancer in postmenopausal women exposed to exogenous estrogens for more than 1 year. The risk of endometrial cancer in estrogen users was 4.5 to 13.9 times greater than in nonusers and appears to depend on duration of treatment and dose. Therefore, when estrogens are used for the treatment of menopausal symptoms, use the lowest dose and discontinue medication as soon as possible. When prolonged treatment is indicated, reassess the patient at least semiannually by endometrial sampling to determine the need for continued therapy.

Close clinical surveillance of women taking estrogens is important. Adequate diagnostic measures, including endometrial sampling when indicated, should be undertaken to rule out malignancy in all cases of undiagnosed persistent or recurring abnormal vaginal bleeding.

There is no evidence that natural estrogens are more or less hazardous than synthetic estrogens at equiestrogenic doses.

Do not use estrogens during pregnancy: Estrogen therapy during pregnancy is associated with an increased risk of congenital defects in the reproductive organs of the fetus and possibly other birth defects. Studies of women who received diethylstilbestrol (DES) during pregnancy have shown that female offspring have an increased risk of vaginal adenosis, squamous cell dysplasia of the uterine cervix, and clear cell vaginal cancer later in life; male offspring have an increased risk of urogenital abnormalities and possibly testicular cancer later in life.

There is no indication for estrogen therapy during pregnancy or during the immediate postpartum period. Estrogens are ineffective for the prevention or treatment of threatened or habitual abortion. Estrogens are not indicated for the prevention of postpartum breast engorgement.

If estrogens are used during pregnancy, or if the patient becomes pregnant while taking estrogens, inform her of the potential risks to the fetus.

Cardiovascular and other risks: Do not use estrogens with or without progestins for the prevention of cardiovascular disease.

The Women's Health Initiative (WHI) reported increased risks of MI, stroke, invasive breast cancer, pulmonary emboli, and deep vein thrombosis in postmenopausal women during 5 years of treatment with conjugated equine estrogens (0.625 mg) combined with medroxyprogesterone acetate (2.5 mg) relative to placebo. Other doses of conjugated estrogens and medroxyprogesterone acetate and other combinations of estrogens and progestins were not studied in the WHI and, in the absence of comparable data, these risks should be assumed to be similar. Because of these risks, prescribe estrogens with or without progestins at the lowest effective doses and for the shortest duration consistent with treatment goals and risks for the individual woman.

The Women's Health Initiative Memory Study (WHIMS), a substudy of WHI, reported increased risk of developing probable dementia in postmenopausal women 65 years of age or older during 4 years of treatment with conjugated estrogens plus medroxyprogesterone acetate relative to placebo. It is unknown whether this finding applies to younger postmenopausal women or to women taking estrogen alone therapy.

Indications

Estrogens are most commonly used as a component of combination contraceptives or as hormone replacement therapy in postmenopausal women. Benefits in postmenopausal women include relief of moderate to severe vasomotor symptoms and decreased risk of osteoporosis. Hormone replacement therapy also may be used in vaginal and vulvar atrophy and in hypoestrogenism caused by hypogonadism, castration, or primary ovarian failure. Less commonly, select breast or prostate cancer patients with advanced disease may receive estrogens as palliative therapy. Refer to individual agents for specific indications.

➤*Unlabeled uses:* In the treatment of Turner syndrome (ovarian dysgenesis), estrogen therapy replicates the events of puberty.

Administration and Dosage

Refer to individual agents for specific administration and dosage recommendations.

➤*Moderate to severe vasomotor symptoms and/or moderate to severe symptoms of vulvar and vaginal atrophy associated with menopause:* Start at the lowest dose and discontinue as promptly as possible. Attempts to discontinue or taper medication should be made at 3- to 6-month intervals. Therapy may be given continuously with no interruption in therapy or in cyclical regimens (such as 25 days on followed by 5 days off drug) as is medically appropriate on an individualized basis.

➤*Hypoestrogenism caused by hypogonadism, castration, or primary ovarian failure:* Therapy usually is given cyclically (such as

3 weeks on and 1 week off). Adjust dose depending on severity of symptoms and patient responsiveness.

➤*Osteoporosis prevention:* Therapy may be given continuously with no interruption in therapy or in cyclical regimens (such as 25 days on followed by 5 days off drug) as is medically appropriate on an individualized basis. Discontinuation of therapy may re-establish the natural rate of bone loss.

➤*Prostate cancer (advanced androgen-dependent):* For palliation only. The effectiveness of therapy can be judged by phosphatase determinations as well as by symptomatic improvement of the patient.

➤*Breast cancer (metastatic):* For palliation only. Therapy usually is given for at least 3 months.

➤*Concomitant progestin therapy when a woman has not had a hysterectomy:* Addition of a progestin for 10 or more days of a cycle of estrogen has lowered the incidence of endometrial hyperplasia. Morphological and biochemical studies of endometrium suggest that 10 to 14 days of progestin are needed to provide maximal maturation of the endometrium and to reduce the likelihood of any hyperplastic changes. It is not established whether this will provide protection from endometrial carcinoma. There may be additional risks with the inclusion of progestin in estrogen replacement regimens, including possible increased risk of breast cancer; adverse effects on carbohydrate and lipid metabolism (lowering HDL and raising LDL); impairment of glucose tolerance; possible enhancement of mitotic activity in breast epithelial tissue, although few epidemiological data are available to address this point. Choice of progestin, regimen, and dosage may be important in minimizing risks.

Actions

➤*Pharmacology:* Estrogens occur naturally in several forms. The primary source of estrogen in normally cycling adult women is the ovarian follicle, which secretes 70 to 500 mcg of estradiol daily, depending on the phase of the menstrual cycle. This is converted primarily to estrone, which circulates in roughly equal proportion to estradiol, and to small amounts of estriol. After menopause, most endogenous estrogen is produced by conversion of androstenedione, secreted by the adrenal cortex, to estrone by peripheral tissues. Thus, estrone—especially in its sulfate ester form—is the most abundant circulating estrogen in postmenopausal women. Although circulating estrogens exist in a dynamic equilibrium of metabolic interconversions, estradiol is the principal intracellular human estrogen and is substantially more potent than estrone or estriol at the receptor.

Estrogens, important in developing and maintaining the female reproductive system and secondary sex characteristics, promote growth and development of the vagina, uterus, and fallopian tubes. With other hormones, such as pituitary hormones and progesterone, they cause enlargement of the breasts through promotion of ductal growth, stromal development, and the accretion of fat. Estrogens are intricately involved with other hormones, especially progesterone, in the processes of the ovulatory menstrual cycle and pregnancy and affect release of pituitary gonadotropins. Indirectly, they contribute to the following: Shaping of the skeleton; maintenance of tone and elasticity of urogenital structures; changes in epiphyses of long bones that allow for pubertal growth spurt and its termination; growth of axillary and pubic hair; pigmentation of nipples and genitals.

Menstruation – Decline of estrogenic activity at the end of the menstrual cycle can induce menstruation, although cessation of progesterone secretion is the most important factor in the mature ovulatory cycle. However, in the preovulatory or nonovulatory cycle, estrogen is the primary determinant of the onset of menstruation.

Menopause – After menopause, estradiol secretion from the ovaries ceases and the primary circulating estrogen is estrone. Estrone has approximately one-third the estrogenic potency of estradiol, but the estrone concentrations are about 4-fold that of estradiol after menopause.

Osteoporosis – Immobilization and prolonged bed rest produce rapid bone loss, while weight-bearing exercise has been shown to reduce bone loss and to increase bone mass. The optimal type and amount of physical activity that would prevent osteoporosis have not been established.

Estrogen reduces bone resorption and retards or halts postmenopausal bone loss. Studies have shown an approximately 60% reduction in hip and wrist fractures in women whose estrogen replacement began within a few years of menopause. Studies also suggest that estrogen reduces the rate of vertebral fractures. Even when started as late as 6 years after menopause, estrogen prevents further loss of bone mass but does not restore it to premenopausal levels.

➤*Pharmacokinetics:*

Absorption/Distribution – Estrogens used in therapy are well absorbed through the skin, mucous membranes, and GI tract. When applied for a local action, absorption is usually sufficient to cause systemic effects. When conjugated with aryl and alkyl groups for parenteral administration, the rate of absorption of oily preparations is slowed with a prolonged duration of action, such that a single IM injection of estradiol valerate or estradiol cypionate is absorbed over several weeks. Conjugated estrogens are well absorbed from the GI tract after release from the drug formulation. The tablet releases conjugated estrogens slowly over several hours. The distribution of exogenous estrogens is similar to that of endogenous estrogens. Estrogens are widely distributed in the body and are generally found in higher concentration in the sex hormone target organs. Estrogens circulate in the blood largely bound to sex hormone-binding globulin (SHBG) and albumin.

Transdermal system: In contrast to oral estradiol, the skin metabolizes estradiol via the transdermal system only to a small extent. Therefore, transdermal use produces therapeutic serum levels of estradiol with lower circulating levels of estrone and estrone conjugates and requires smaller total doses.

Metabolism / Excretion – When given orally, naturally occurring estrogens and their esters are extensively metabolized (first-pass effect) and circulate primarily as estrone sulfate, with smaller amounts of other conjugated and unconjugated estrogenic species. This results in limited oral potency. By contrast, synthetic estrogens, such as ethinyl estradiol and the nonsteroidal estrogens, are degraded very slowly in the liver and other tissues, which results in their high intrinsic potency. Estrogen drug products administered by non-oral routes are not subject to first-pass metabolism but also undergo significant hepatic uptake, metabolism, and enterohepatic recycling.

Metabolic conversion of estrogens occurs primarily in the liver (first-pass effect) but also at local target tissue sites. Complex metabolic processes result in a dynamic equilibrium of circulating conjugated and unconjugated estrogenic forms that are continually interconverted, especially between estrone and estradiol and between esterified and nonesterified forms. A certain proportion of the estrogen is excreted into the bile and then reabsorbed from the intestine. During this enterohepatic recirculation, estrogens are desulfated and resulfated and undergo degradation through conversion to less active estrogens (estriol and other estrogens), oxidation to nonestrogenic substances (catecholestrogens, which interact with catecholamine metabolism, especially in the CNS), and conjugation with glucuronic acids (which are then rapidly excreted in the urine).

➤*Clinical trials:* The WHI enrolled a total of 27,000 predominantly healthy postmenopausal women to assess the risks and benefits of either the use of 0.625 mg conjugated equine estrogens per day alone or the use of 0.625 mg conjugated equine estrogens plus 2.5 mg medroxyprogesterone acetate per day compared with placebo in the prevention of certain chronic diseases. The primary endpoint was the incidence of coronary heart disease (CHD) (nonfatal MI and CHD death), with invasive breast cancer as the primary adverse outcome studied. A global index included the earliest incidence of CHD, invasive breast cancer, stroke, pulmonary embolism (PE), endometrial cancer, colorectal cancer, hip fracture, or death from other cause.

The 0.625 mg conjugated equine estrogens per day-only substudy is continuing and results have not been reported. The 0.625 mg conjugated equine estrogens plus 2.5 mg medroxyprogesterone acetate per day study was stopped early because, according to the predefined stopping rule, the increased risk of breast cancer and cardiovascular events exceeded the specified benefits included in the global index.

For those outcomes included in the global index, absolute excess risks per 10,000 person-years in the group treated with 0.625 mg conjugated equine estrogens plus 2.5 mg medroxyprogesterone acetate per day were 7 more CHD events, 8 more strokes, 8 more PEs, and 8 more invasive breast cancers, while absolute risk reductions per 10,000 person-years were 6 fewer colorectal cancers and 5 fewer hip fractures. The absolute excess risk of events included in the global index was 19 per 10,000 person-years. There was no difference between the groups in terms of all-cause mortality (see Warning Box, Warnings, and Precautions).

Contraindications

Known or suspected breast cancer, except in appropriately selected patients being treated for metastatic disease; known or suspected estrogen-dependent neoplasia; undiagnosed abnormal genital bleeding; active deep vein thrombosis, PE, or a history of these conditions; active or recent (eg, within past year) arterial thromboembolic disease (eg, stroke, MI); active thrombophlebitis or thromboembolic disorders; history of thrombophlebitis, thrombosis or thromboembolic disorders associated with previous estrogen use (except when used in treatment of breast or prostatic malignancy); known or suspected pregnancy (see Warning Box); porphyria (estradiol vaginal tablets only); hypersensitivity to any product component.

Warnings

➤*Induction of malignant neoplasms:*

Endometrial cancer – The use of unopposed estrogens in women with intact uteri has been associated with an increased risk of endometrial cancer. The reported endometrial cancer risk among unopposed estrogen users is about 2- to 12-fold greater than in nonusers and appears dependent on duration of treatment and on estrogen dose. Most studies show no significant increased risk associated with use of estrogens for less than 1 year. The greatest risk appears associated with prolonged use, with increased risks of 15- to 24-fold for 5 to 10 years or more and this risk has been shown to persist for at least 8 to 15 years after estrogen therapy is discontinued.

Clinical surveillance of all women taking estrogen/progestin combinations is important. Adequate diagnostic measures, including endometrial sampling when indicated, should be undertaken to rule out malignancy in all cases of undiagnosed persistent or recurring abnormal vaginal bleeding. There is no evidence that the use of natural estrogens results in a different endometrial risk profile than synthetic estrogens of equivalent estrogen dose. Adding a progestin to postmenopausal estrogen therapy has been shown to reduce the risk of endometrial hyperplasia, which may be a precursor to endometrial cancer.

Breast cancer – Estrogen and estrogen/progestin therapy in postmenopausal women have been associated with an increased risk of breast cancer. In the 0.625 mg conjugated equine estrogens plus 2.5 mg medroxyprogesterone acetate per day substudy of the WHI, 26% of the women reported prior use of estrogen alone and/or estrogen/progestin combination hormone therapy. After a mean follow-up of 5.6 years during the clinical trial, the overall relative risk of invasive breast cancer was 1.24 (95% confidence interval 1.01 to 1.54), and the overall absolute risk was 41 vs 33 cases per 10,000 women-years, for estrogen plus progestin compared with placebo. among women who reported prior use of hormone therapy, the relative risk of invasive breast cancer was 1.86, and absolute risk was 46 vs 25 cases per 10,000 women-years, for estrogen plus progestin compared with placebo. Among women who reported no prior use of hormone therapy, the relative risk of invasive breast cancer was 1.09, and the absolute risk was 40 vs 36 cases per 10,000 women-years for estrogen plus progestin compared with placebo. In the WHI trial invasive breast cancers were larger and diagnosed at a more advanced stage in the estrogen plus progestin group compared with the placebo group. Metastatic disease was rare with no apparent difference between the 2 groups. Other prognostic factors such as histologic subtype, grade, and hormone receptor status did not differ between the groups.

A postmenopausal woman without a uterus who requires estrogen should receive estrogen-alone therapy and should not be exposed unnecessarily to progestins. All postmenopausal women should receive yearly breast exams by a health care provider and perform monthly breast self-examinations. In addition, mammography examinations should be scheduled based on patient age and risk factors.

Ovarian cancer – Use of estrogen-only products, in particular for 10 years or more, has been associated with an increased risk of ovarian cancer in some epidemiological studies. Other studies did not show a significant association. Data are insufficient to determine whether there is an increased risk with combined estrogen/progestin therapy in postmenopausal women.

➤*Gallbladder disease:* There is a 2-fold to 4-fold increase in risk of gallbladder disease requiring surgery in women receiving postmenopausal estrogens.

➤*Cardiovascular disorders:* Estrogen and estrogen/progestin therapy have been associated with an increased risk of cardiovascular events (eg, MI and stroke, venous thrombosis, PE [venous thromboembolism (VTE)]). Should any of these occur or be suspected, discontinue estrogens immediately.

Risk factors for cardiovascular disease (eg, hypertension, diabetes mellitus, tobacco use, hypercholesterolemia, obesity) should be managed appropriately.

CHD – In the 0.625 mg conjugated equine estrogens per day substudy of the WHI, an increase in the number of MIs and strokes has been observed compared with placebo. These observations are preliminary and the study is continuing.

In the 0.625 mg conjugated equine estrogens plus 2.5 mg medroxyprogesterone acetate per day substudy of the WHI, an increased risk of CHD events (defined as nonfatal MI and CHD death) was observed compared with placebo (37 vs 30 per 10,000 person-years). The increase in risk was observed in year 1 and persisted.

In the same substudy of the WHI, an increased risk of stroke also was observed compared with placebo (29 vs 21 per 10,000 person-years). The increase in risk was observed after the first year and persisted.

In postmenopausal women with documented heart disease (n = 2763; average age, 66.7 years) a controlled clinical trial of secondary prevention of cardiovascular disease (Heart and Estrogen/progestin Replacement Study; HERS) treatment with 0.625 mg conjugated equine estrogens plus 2.5 mg medroxyprogesterone acetate per day demonstrated no cardiovascular benefit. During an average follow-up of 4.1 years, treatment with 0.625 mg conjugated equine estrogens plus 2.5 mg medroxyprogesterone acetate per day did not reduce the overall rate of CHD events in postmenopausal women with established CHD. There were more CHD events in the 0.625 mg conjugated equine estrogens plus 2.5 mg medroxyprogesterone acetate per day-treated group than in the placebo group in year 1, but not during subsequent years.

Large doses of estrogen (5 mg conjugated estrogens per day), comparable with those used to treat cancer of the prostate and breast, have been shown in a large prospective clinical trial in men to increase the risks of nonfatal MI, PE, and thrombophlebitis.

VTE – In the 0.625 mg conjugated equine estrogens per day substudy of the WHI, an increase in VTE has been observed compared with placebo. These observations are preliminary, and the study is continuing.

In the 0.625 mg conjugated equine estrogens plus 2.5 mg medroxyprogesterone acetate per day substudy of the WHI, a 2-fold greater rate of VTE, including deep venous thrombosis and PE, was observed compared with placebo. The rate of VTE was 34 per 10,000 woman-years in the 0.625 mg conjugated equine estrogens plus 2.5 mg medroxyprogesterone acetate per day group compared with 16 per 10,000 woman-years in the placebo group. The increase in VTE risk was observed during the first year and persisted.

If feasible, discontinue estrogens at least 4 to 6 weeks before surgery of the type associated with an increased risk of thromboembolism or during periods of prolonged immobilization.

➤*Dementia:* In the WHIMS, 4,532 generally healthy postmenopausal women 65 years of age and older were studied, of whom 35% were 70 to 74 years of age and 18% were 75 years of age or older. After an average follow-up of 4 years, 40 women being treated with 0.625 mg conjugated estrogens plus 2.5 mg medroxyprogesterone acetate (1.8%, n = 2,229) and 21 women in the placebo group (0.9%, n = 2,303) received diagnoses of probable dementia. The relative risk for estrogen/progestin vs placebo was 2.05 (95% confidence interval 1.21 to 3.48), and was similar for women with and without histories of menopausal hormone use before WHIMS. The absolute risk of probable dementia for estrogen/progestin vs placebo was 45 vs 22 cases per 10,000 women-years, and the absolute excess risk for estrogen/progestin was 23 cases per 10,000 women-years. It is unknown whether these findings apply to younger postmenopausal women.

The results of the estrogen alone substudy of the WHIMS have not been reported. It is unknown whether these findings apply to estrogen alone therapy.

➤*Hepatic adenoma:* Benign hepatic adenomas appear to be associated with the use of oral contraceptives (OCs). Although benign and rare, they may rupture and may cause death through intra-abdominal hemorrhage. Such lesions have not been reported in association with other estrogen or progestogen preparations but should be considered in estrogen users having abdominal pain and tenderness, abdominal mass, or hypovolemic shock. Hepatocellular carcinoma also has been reported in women taking estrogen-containing OCs. The relationship of this malignancy to these drugs is not known.

➤*Familial hyperlipoproteinemia:* Estrogen therapy may be associated with elevations of plasma triglycerides leading to pancreatitis and other complications in patients with familial defects of lipoprotein metabolism.

➤*Hypercalcemia:* Estrogens may lead to severe hypercalcemia in patients with breast cancer and bone metastases. If this occurs, discontinue the drug and take appropriate measures to reduce the serum calcium level.

➤*Glucose tolerance:* A worsening of glucose tolerance has been observed in a significant percentage of patients on estrogen-containing OCs. Carefully observe diabetic patients receiving estrogen.

➤*Visual abnormalities:* Retinal vascular thrombosis has been reported in patients receiving estrogens. Discontinue medication pending examination if there is sudden partial or complete loss of vision or a sudden onset of proptosis, diplopia, or migraine. If examination reveals papilledema or retinal vascular lesions, discontinue estrogens.

➤*Hypothyroidism:* Estrogen administration leads to increased thyroid-binding globulin (TBG) levels. Patients with normal thyroid function can compensate for the increased TBG by making more thyroid hormone, thus maintaining free T_4 and T_3 serum concentrations in the normal range. Patients dependent on thyroid hormone replacement therapy who are also receiving estrogens may require increased doses of their thyroid replacement therapy. Monitor thyroid function in these patients in order to maintain their free thyroid hormone levels in an acceptable range.

➤*Depression:* OCs appear to be associated with an increased incidence of mental depression. Although it is not clear whether this is caused by the estrogenic or progestogenic component of the contraceptive, carefully observe patients with a history of depression.

➤*Uterine leiomyomata:* Pre-existing uterine leiomyomata may increase in size during estrogen use.

➤*Hepatic function impairment:* Exercise caution in patients with a history of cholestatic jaundice associated with past estrogen use or with pregnancy and, in the case of recurrence, discontinue medication. Estrogens may be poorly metabolized in impaired liver function; use with caution.

➤*Pregnancy: Category X.* Do not use estrogens during pregnancy. See Warning Box.

➤*Lactation:* Estrogens have been shown to decrease the quantity and quality of breast milk and detectable amounts are excreted in breast milk. Administer only when clearly needed.

➤*Children:* Estrogen therapy has been used for the induction of puberty in adolescents with some forms of pubertal delay. Safety and efficacy in pediatric patients have not otherwise been established.

Large and repeated doses of estrogen over an extended period of time have been shown to accelerate epiphyseal closure, which could result in short adult stature if treatment is initiated before the completion of physiologic puberty in normally developing children. If estrogen is administered to patients whose bone growth is not complete, periodic monitoring of bone maturation and effects on epiphyseal centers is recommended during estrogen administration.

Estrogen treatment of prepubertal girls also induces premature breast development and vaginal cornification and may induce vaginal bleeding. In boys, estrogen treatment may modify the normal pubertal process and induce gynecomastia.

Precautions

➤*Elevated blood pressure:* In a small number of case reports, substantial increases in blood pressure have been attributed to idiosyncratic reactions to estrogens. In a large, randomized, placebo-controlled clinical trial, a generalized effect of estrogen therapy on blood pressure was not seen. Monitor blood pressure at regular intervals with estrogen use.

➤*Hypercoagulability:* Some studies have shown that women taking estrogen replacement therapy have hypercoagulability, primarily related to decreased antithrombin activity. This effect appears dose- and duration-dependent and is less pronounced than that associated with oral contraceptive use. Also, postmenopausal women tend to have increased coagulation parameters at baseline compared with premenopausal women. There is some suggestion that low-dose postmenopausal mestranol may increase the risk of thromboembolism, although the majority of studies (of primarily conjugated estrogens users) report no such increase. There is insufficient information on hypercoagulability in women who have had previous thromboembolic disease. Therefore, do not use in people with active thrombophlebitis or thromboembolic disorders or in people with a history of such disorders associated with estrogen use (except in treatment of malignancy).

➤*History/Physical exam:* Before initiating estrogens, take complete medical and family history. Pretreatment and periodic history and physical exams every 12 months should include blood pressure, breasts, abdomen, pelvic organs, and a Papanicolaou smear. Generally, do not prescribe for longer than 1 year between physical examinations.

➤*Vaginal products:* Estradiol vaginal ring may not be suitable for women with narrow, short, or stenosed vaginas. Narrow vagina, vaginal stenosis, prolapse, and vaginal infections are conditions that make the vagina more susceptible to estradiol vaginal ring-caused irritation or ulceration. Women with signs or symptoms of vaginal irritation should alert their physician.

Vaginal infection is generally more common in postmenopausal women because of the lack of the normal flora of fertile women, especially lactobacillus, and the subsequent higher pH. Treat vaginal infections with appropriate antimicrobial therapy before initiation of therapy. If a vaginal infection develops during use of the estradiol vaginal ring, remove the ring and reinsert only after the infection has been appropriately treated.

Conjugated estrogens vaginal cream exposure has been reported to weaken latex condoms. Consider its potential to weaken and contribute to the failure of condoms, diaphragms, or cervical caps made of latex or rubber.

➤*Excessive estrogenic stimulation:* Certain patients may develop undesirable manifestations of excessive estrogenic stimulation (eg, abnormal or excessive uterine bleeding, mastodynia). Advise the pathologist of estrogen therapy when relevant specimens are submitted.

➤*Fluid retention:* Estrogens may cause some degree of fluid retention; conditions that might be influenced by this factor (eg, asthma, epilepsy, migraine, cardiac or renal dysfunction) require careful observation.

➤*Calcium and phosphorus metabolism:* Calcium and phosphorus metabolism is influenced by estrogens; use caution in metabolic bone diseases associated with hypercalcemia or in renal insufficiency. Use estrogens with caution in individuals with severe hypocalcemia.

➤*Endometrial hyperplasia:* Prolonged unopposed estrogen therapy may increase risk of endometrial hyperplasia.

➤*Exacerbations of other conditions:* Endometriosis may be exacerbated with administration of estrogen therapy. Estrogen therapy also may cause an exacerbation of asthma, diabetes mellitus, epilepsy, migraine, or porphyria; use with caution in patients with these conditions.

➤*Benzyl alcohol:* Benzyl alcohol, contained in some of these products as a preservative, has been associated with a fatal "gasping syndrome" in premature infants.

➤*Tartrazine sensitivity:* Some of these products contain tartrazine (FD&C yellow #5), which may cause allergic-type reactions (including bronchial asthma) in susceptible individuals. Although the incidence of sensitivity is low, it is frequently seen in patients who also have aspirin hypersensitivity. Specific products containing tartrazine are identified in the product listings.

Estrogens

Drug Interactions

Refer to the drug interaction section in the Oral Contraceptives group monograph for more information.

Estrogen Drug Interactions			
Precipitant drug	Object drug*		Description
Estrogens	Anticoagulants, oral	↓	Estrogens may theoretically reduce the effect of anticoagulants.
Estrogens	Antidepressants, tricyclic	↔	Pharmacologic effects of these agents may be altered by estrogens; the effects of this interaction may depend on the dose of the estrogen. An increased incidence of toxic reactions also may occur.
Estrogens	Corticosteroids	↑	An increase in the pharmacologic and toxicologic effects of corticosteroids may occur via inactivation of hepatic P450 enzyme.
Estrogens	Thyroid hormones	↓	In hypothyroid women, estrogens may increase serum thyroxine-binding globulin concentrations, therefore changing serum thyroxine and thyrotropin concentrations. Thyroid hormone requirements may be increased.
CYP 3A4 inducers Barbiturates Carbamazepine Rifampin St. John's wort	Estrogens	↓	Coadministration may reduce plasma concentrations of estrogens, possibly resulting in a decrease in therapeutic effects and/or changes in the uterine bleeding profile.
CYP 3A4 inhibitors Itraconazole Ketoconazole Macrolide antibiotics Ritonavir	Estrogens	↑	Coadministration may increase plasma concentrations of estrogens and may result in side effects.
Hydantoins	Estrogens	↓	Breakthrough bleeding, spotting, and pregnancy have resulted when these medications were used concurrently. A loss of seizure control also has been suggested and may be due to fluid retention.
Estrogens	Hydantoins		
Topiramate	Estrogens	↓	Topiramate may increase the metabolism of estrogens, decreasing their efficacy.

*↑ = Object drug increased. ↓ = Object drug decreased. ↔ = Undetermined clinical effect.

➤*Drug/Lab test interactions:* Certain endocrine and liver function tests may be affected by estrogen-containing OCs. Expect the following similar changes with larger doses:

Increased sulfobromophthalein retention.

Increased prothrombin time, partial thromboplastin time, platelet aggregation time, platelet count, and factors II, VII, VIII, IX, X, XII, VII-X complex, II-VII-X complex, and β-thromboglobulin; decreased antithrombin III, antifactor Xa; increased fibrinogen, plasminogen, and norepinephrine-induced platelet aggregability.

Increased thyroid binding globulin (TBG) leading to increased circulating total thyroid hormone, as measured by protein bound iodine (PBI), T_4 by column or T_4 or T_3 by radioimmunoassay. Free T_3 resin uptake is decreased, reflecting the elevated TBG; free T_4 and free T_3 concentration is unaltered.

Impaired glucose tolerance; decreased pregnanediol excretion; reduced response to metyrapone test; reduced serum folate concentration; increased serum triglyceride and phospholipid concentration.

Other binding proteins may be elevated in serum (ie, corticosteroid binding globulin [CBG], SHBG), leading to increased circulating corticosteroids and sex steroids, respectively. Free or biologically active hormone concentrations are unchanged. Other plasma proteins may be increased (angiotensinogen/renin substrate, α-1-antitrypsin, ceruloplasmin).

Increased plasma HDL and HDL-2 subfraction concentrations, reduced LDL cholesterol concentration levels, increased triglyceride levels.

➤*Drug/Food interactions:* Grapefruit juice may inhibit CYP3A4-mediated estrogen metabolism, increasing plasma concentrations of estrogens and possibly resulting in side effects.

Adverse Reactions

See Warnings regarding induction of neoplasia, adverse effects on the fetus, increased incidence of gallbladder disease, hypercalcemia, cardiovascular disease, elevated blood pressure, and adverse effects similar to those of OCs.

➤*Cardiovascular:* Venous thromboembolism; pulmonary embolism; syncope; deep and superficial venous thrombosis; thrombophlebitis; MI; stroke; increased blood pressure.

➤*CNS:* Headache; migraine; dizziness; mental depression; chorea; insomnia; anxiety; emotional lability; nervousness; mood disturbances; irritability; exacerbation of epilepsy; fatigue; sinus headache; tension headaches.

➤*Dermatologic:* Chloasma or melasma (may persist when drug is discontinued); erythema nodosum/multiforme; hemorrhagic eruption; dermatitis; skin hypertrophy; loss of scalp hair; hirsutism; pruritus; rash; pruritus ani; acne.

➤*GI:* Nausea; vomiting; abdominal cramps/pain; bloating; cholestatic jaundice; pancreatitis; diarrhea; dyspepsia; flatulence; gastritis; gastroenteritis; enlarged abdomen; hemorrhoids; increased incidence of gallbladder disease; constipation.

➤*GU:* Breakthrough bleeding; abnormal withdrawal bleeding; spotting; change in menstrual flow; dysmenorrhea; premenstrual-like syndrome; amenorrhea during and after treatment; vaginal candidiasis; change in cervical ectropion and degree of cervical secretion; cystitis-like syndrome; urinary tract infection; leukorrhea; vaginitis; vaginal discomfort/pain; vaginal hemorrhage; asymptomatic genital bacterial growth; genital moniliasis; cystitis; dysuria; genital pruritus; genital eruption; urinary incontinence; endometrial hyperplasia; increase in size of uterine leiomyomata/fibromyomata; ovarian cancer; endometrial cancer; micturition frequency; urethral disorder; vaginosis fungal; vaginal discharge.

➤*Local:* Redness/erythema and irritation at application site with the estradiol transdermal system; rash (rare).

➤*Ophthalmic:* Steepening of corneal curvature; intolerance to contact lenses; retinal vascular thrombosis.

➤*Respiratory:* Upper respiratory tract infection; sinusitis; rhinitis; bronchitis; pharyngitis; nasopharyngitis; cough; nasal congestion; pharyngolaryngeal pain.

➤*Miscellaneous:* Aggravation of porphyria; edema; changes in libido; breast pain, tenderness, enlargement, or secretion; galactorrhea; fibrocystic breast changes; breast cancer; reduced carbohydrate tolerance; pain; hypersensitivity reactions; increase or decrease in weight; back pain; arthritis; arthralgia; skeletal pain; flu-like symptoms; hot flushes; allergy; chest pain; leg edema; otitis media; toothache; tooth disorder; infection; accidental injury; asthenia; anemia; paresthesia; leg cramps; anaphylactoid/anaphylactic reactions (including urticaria and angioedema); hypocalcemia; exacerbation of asthma; increased triglycerides; neck pain; neck rigidity; candidal infection; fungal infection; herpes simplex; fluid retention.

Overdosage

Serious ill effects have not been reported following ingestion of large doses of estrogen-containing OCs by young children. Overdosage of estrogen may cause nausea and vomiting; withdrawal bleeding may occur in females.

Patient Information

Patient package insert is available with products.

Estrogens increase the chances of getting cancer of the uterus. Report any unusual vaginal bleeding right away. Vaginal bleeding after menopause may be a warning sign of cancer of the uterus.

Do not use estrogens with or without progestins to prevent heart disease, heart attacks, or strokes. Using estrogens with or without progestins may increase the chances of heart attacks, strokes, breast cancer, and blood clots.

Notify physician if any of the following occur: Pain in the calves; sharp chest pain or sudden shortness of breath; coughing blood; abnormal vaginal bleeding; missed menstrual period or suspected pregnancy; lumps in the breast; severe headache or vomiting; dizziness or fainting; vision or speech disturbance; weakness or numbness in an arm or leg; abdominal pain, swelling, or tenderness; yellowing of the skin or eyes; depression.

ESTRADIOL TOPICAL EMULSION

| Rx | Estrasorb (Novavax[1]) | **Topical emulsion:** 2.5 mg estradiol hemihydrate/g | Soybean oil, ethanol. In 1.74 g pouches.[2] |

[1] Novavax, Inc., 8320 Guilford Road, Suite C, Columbia, MD 21046; 301-854-3900; fax 301-854-3901.

[2] Each pouch contains 4.35 mg estradiol hemihydrate.

WARNING

Estrogens increase the risk of endometrial cancer: Close clinical surveillance of all women taking estrogen is important. When indicated, undertake adequate diagnostic measures, including endometrial sampling, to rule out malignancy in all cases of undiagnosed persistent or recurring abnormal vaginal bleeding. There is no evidence that the use of natural estrogens results in a different endometrial risk profile than synthetic estrogens at equivalent estrogenic doses.

Cardiovascular and other risks: Estrogens with or without progestins should not be used for the prevention of cardiovascular disease.

The Women's Health Initiative (WHI) study reported increased risks of MI, stroke, invasive breast cancer, pulmonary emboli, and deep vein thrombosis in postmenopausal women during 5 years of treatment with conjugated equine estrogens (0.625 mg) combined with medroxyprogesterone acetate (2.5 mg) relative to placebo. Other doses of conjugated estrogens and medroxyprogesterone acetate, and other combinations of estrogens and progestins were not studied in the WHI and, in the absence of comparable data, these risks should be assumed to be similar. Because of these risks, estrogens with or without progestins should be prescribed at the lowest effective doses and for the shortest duration consistent with treatment goals and risks for the individual woman.

Indications

➤*Vasomotor symptoms:* For the treatment of moderate to severe vasomotor symptoms associated with menopause.

Administration and Dosage

➤*Approved by the FDA:* October 9, 2003.

➤*Moderate to severe vasomotor symptoms:* Use the lowest effective dose and for the shortest duration consistent with treatment goals and risks for the individual women. Periodically re-evaluate patients as clinically appropriate (eg, at 3-month to 6-month intervals) to deter-

mine if treatment is still necessary. The single approved dose of estradiol topical emulsion is 3.48 g/day. The lowest effective dose for this indication has not been determined.

➤*Application:* Instructions for daily application of two 1.74 g foil-laminated pouches:

1.) Apply in a comfortable sitting position to clean, dry skin on both legs each morning. Open each pouch individually.
2.) Cut or tear the first pouch at the notches indicated near the top of the pouch.
3.) Apply the emulsion in the pouch to the top of the left thigh, being careful to push the entire contents from the bottom through the neck of the pouch.
4.) Using one or both hands, rub the emulsion into the entire left thigh and left calf for 3 minutes until thoroughly absorbed. Rub any excess material remaining on both hands on the buttocks.
5.) Cut or tear the second pouch at the notches indicated near the top of the pouch. Apply the emulsion in the pouch to the top of the right thigh, being careful to push the entire contents from the bottom through the neck of the pouch. Using one or both hands, rub the emulsion into the entire right thigh and right calf for 3 minutes until thoroughly absorbed. Rub any excess material remaining on both hands on the buttocks. Absorption was not studied on other parts of the body.
6.) Allow the application areas to dry completely before covering with clothing to avoid transfer to other individuals.
7.) On completion of application, wash both hands with soap and water to remove any residual estradiol.

➤*Concomitant progestin therapy:* When estrogen is prescribed for a postmenopausal woman with a uterus, also initiate progestin to reduce the risk of endometrial cancer. For women with a uterus, when indicated, undertake adequate diagnostic measures (eg, endometrial sampling) to rule out malignancy in cases of undiagnosed persistent or recurring abnormal vaginal bleeding.

➤*Storage/Stability:* Store at 20° to 25°C (68° to 77°F); excursions permitted to 15° to 30°C (59° to 86°F).

ESTRADIOL TRANSDERMAL SYSTEM

	Product/ Distributor	Release rate (mg/24 h)	Surface area (cm²)	Total estradiol content (mg)	How Supplied
Rx	**Menostar** (Berlex)	0.014	3.25	1	In 4s.
Rx	**Alora** (Watson)	0.025	9	0.77	In calendar packs (8 systems).
Rx	**Climara** (Berlex)		6.5	2	In 4s.
Rx	**Esclim** (Women First Healthcare)		11	5	In patient packs (8s).
Rx	**Vivelle-Dot** (Novartis)		2.5	0.39	In calendar packs (8s and 24s).
Rx	**Esclim** (Women First Healthcare)	0.0375	16.5	7.5	In patient packs (8s).
Rx	**Climara** (Berlex)		9.375	2.85	In 4s.
Rx	**Vivelle** (Novartis)		11	3.28	In calendar packs (8 and 24 systems).
Rx	**Vivelle-Dot** (Novartis)		3.75	0.585	In calendar packs (8 systems).
Rx	**Estradiol Transdermal System** (Mylan)	0.05	15.5	1.94	In 4s.
Rx	**Alora** (Watson)		18	1.5	In calendar packs (8s).
Rx	**Climara** (Berlex)		12.5	3.8	In 4s.
Rx	**Esclim** (Women First Healthcare)		22	10	In patient packs (8s).
Rx	**Estraderm** (Novartis)		10	4	In calendar packs (8 and 24 systems).
Rx	**Vivelle** (Novartis)		14.5	4.33	In calendar packs (8 and 24 systems).
Rx	**Vivelle-Dot** (Novartis)		5	0.78	In calendar packs (8 systems).
Rx	**Climara** (Berlex)	0.06 mg	15	4.55	In 4s.
Rx	**Alora** (Watson)	0.075	27	2.3	In calendar packs (8 systems).
Rx	**Climara** (Berlex)		18.75	5.7	In 4s.
Rx	**Esclim** (Women First Healthcare)		33	15	In patient pack (8s).
Rx	**Vivelle** (Novartis)		22	6.57	In calendar packs (8 and 24 systems).
Rx	**Vivelle–Dot** (Novartis)		7.5	1.17	In calendar packs (8 systems).

ESTRADIOL TRANSDERMAL SYSTEM

	Product/ Distributor	Release rate (mg/24 h)	Surface area (cm^2)	Total estradiol content (mg)	How Supplied
Rx	**Estradiol Transdermal System** (Mylan)	0.1	31	3.88	In 4s.
Rx	**Alora** (Watson)		36	3.1	In calendar packs (8 systems).
Rx	**Climara** (Berlex)		25	7.6	In 4s.
Rx	**Esclim** (Women First Healthcare)		44	20	In patient packs (8s).
Rx	**Estraderm** (Novartis)		20	8	In calendar packs (8 and 24 systems).
Rx	**Vivelle** (Novartis)		29	8.66	In calendar packs (8 and 24 systems).
Rx	**Vivelle-Dot** (Novartis)		10	1.56	In calendar packs (8 systems).

For complete prescribing information, refer to the Estrogens group monograph.

Indications

For the treatment of moderate to severe vasomotor symptoms associated with menopause (except *Menostar*); treatment of hypoestrogenism caused by hypogonadism, castration, or primary ovarian failure (except *Menostar*); vulvar and vaginal atrophy (except *Menostar*); atrophic urethritis (except *Menostar*) (*Estraderm* only); prevention of postmenopausal osteoporosis (loss of bone mass) (except *Esclim*).

Administration and Dosage

➤*Initiation of therapy:*

Treatment of menopausal symptoms – Initiate therapy with the lowest dosage necessary to control symptoms, especially in women with an intact uterus, (eg, 0.025 to 0.05 mg) applied to skin once weekly (*Climara* only) or twice weekly. Adjust dose as necessary to control symptoms. Do not make dosage increases until after the first month of therapy. Attempt to taper or discontinue the drug at 3- to 6-month intervals.

Prophylaxis to prevent postmenopausal osteoporosis – Initiate therapy with the lowest dosage necessary. Adjust dosage if necessary. Discontinuation may re-establish natural bone loss rate.

In women who are not taking oral estrogens or in women switching from another estradiol transdermal therapy, start treatment immediately. In women who are currently taking oral estrogens, start treatment 1 week after withdrawal of oral therapy or sooner if symptoms reappear in less than 1 week.

➤*Therapeutic regimen:* Therapy may be given continuously in patients who do not have an intact uterus. In patients with an intact uterus, therapy may be given on a cyclic schedule (eg, 3 weeks therapy followed by 1 week off).

Concomitant progestin therapy – When estrogen is prescribed for a postmenopausal woman with a uterus, also initiate progestin to reduce the risk of endometrial cancer. A woman without a uterus does not need progestin.

Alora, Estraderm, Esclim, Vivelle, and *Vivelle-Dot* are applied twice a week. *Climara* and *Menostar* last for 7 days and are applied once a week.

➤*Application of system:* Place adhesive side of the system on a clean, dry area of the skin on buttocks or abdomen. *Esclim* also may be placed on the femoral triangle (upper inner thigh) or upper arm. Do not apply to breasts or to a site exposed to sunlight. Rotate application site with at least a 1-week interval between applications to a particular site. The area should not be oily, damaged, or irritated. Avoid the waistline because tight clothing may rub the system off. Also avoid application to areas where sitting would dislodge the system. Apply the system immediately after opening the pouch and removing the protective liner. Press firmly in place with the palm for about 10 seconds. Make sure there is good contact, especially around the edges. In the unlikely event that a system falls off, reapply the same system (except *Climara* or *Menostar*). If necessary, apply a new system. In the event that a *Climara* or *Menostar* system falls off, apply a new system for the remainder of the 7-day dosing interval. In either case, continue the original treatment schedule.

➤*Storage/Stability:* Store at 25°C (77°F), excursions permitted to 15° to 30°C (59° to 86°F). Do not store unpouched. Apply immediately upon removal from protective pouch.

ESTRADIOL

Rx	**Estradiol** (Various, eg, Geneva, Mylan)	**Tablets:** 0.5 mg micronized estradiol	May contain lactose. In 100s.
Rx	**Estrace** (Warner Chilcott)		Lactose. (021 MJ). White, scored. In 100s.
Rx	**Gynodiol** (Fielding)		Lactose. (0768). Lavender, scored. In 30s and 100s.
Rx	**Estradiol** (Various, eg, Geneva, Mylan)	**Tablets:** 1 mg micronized estradiol	May contain lactose. In 100s and 500s.
Rx	**Estrace** (Warner Chilcott)		Lactose. (755 MJ). Lavender, scored. In 100s, 500s.
Rx	**Gynodiol** (Fielding)		Lactose. (1259). Rose, scored. In 30s and 100s.
Rx	**Gynodiol** (Fielding)	**Tablets:** 1.5 mg micronized estradiol	Lactose. (0158). Aqua, scored. In 30s and 100s.
Rx	**Estradiol** (Various, eg, Geneva, Mylan)	**Tablets:** 2 mg micronized estradiol	May contain lactose. In 100s and 500s.
Rx	**Estrace** (Warner Chilcott)		Tartrazine, lactose. (756 MJ). Turquoise, scored. In 100s and 500s.
Rx	**Gynodiol** (Fielding)		Lactose. (0748). Blue, scored. In 30s and 100s.

For complete prescribing information, refer to the Estrogens group monograph.

Indications

For the treatment of moderate to severe vasomotor symptoms associated with menopause; vulval and vaginal atrophy; hypoestrogenism caused by hypogonadism, castration, or primary ovarian failure; breast cancer (for palliation only) in appropriately selected women and men with metastatic disease; advanced androgen-dependent prostate carcinoma (for palliation only); osteoporosis prevention.

Administration and Dosage

➤*Moderate to severe vasomotor symptoms, vulval/vaginal atrophy associated with menopause:* Use the lowest dose and regimen that will control symptoms and discontinue medication as promptly as possible. Attempt to discontinue or taper medication at 3- to 6-month intervals.

Initiate treatment with 1 to 2 mg/day; adjust to control presenting symptoms. Titrate to determine the minimal effective dose for maintenance therapy. Administer cyclically (eg, 3 weeks on and 1 week off).

➤*Hypoestrogenism caused by hypogonadism, castration, or primary ovarian failure:* Treatment usually is initiated with a dose of 1 to 2 mg daily, adjusted as necessary to control presenting symptoms; determine the minimal effective dose for maintenance therapy by titration.

➤*Prostatic cancer (advanced androgen-dependent):* For palliation only. Administer 1 to 2 mg 3 times daily. Judge the effectiveness of therapy by phosphatase determinations and by symptomatic improvement of the patient.

➤*Breast cancer, metastatic:* For palliation only. The usual dose is 10 mg 3 times daily for at least 3 months.

➤*Osteoporosis prevention:* Administer cyclically (eg, 23 days on and 5 days off) 0.5 mg/day as soon as possible after menopause. Adjust dosage if necessary to control concurrent menopausal symptoms. Discontinuation may re-establish natural rate of bone loss. The mainstays of prevention and management of osteoporosis are estrogen and calcium; exercise and nutrition may be important adjuncts.

➤*Concomitant progestin therapy:* When estrogen is prescribed for a postmenopausal woman with a uterus, also initiate progestin to reduce the risk of endometrial cancer. A woman without a uterus does not need progestin.

➤*Storage/Stability:* Store at controlled room temperature 15° to 30°C (59° to 86°F). Dispense in a tight, light-resistant container.

ESTRADIOL VALERATE IN OIL

Rx	Delestrogen (Monarch)	Injection: 10 mg/mL	In 5 mL multidose vials.[1]
		20 mg/mL	In 5 mL multidose vials.[2]
		40 mg/mL	In 5 mL multidose vials.[2]

[1] In sesame oil with chlorobutanol.　　　　　　　　　　　　[2] In castor oil with benzyl benzoate and benzyl alcohol.

For complete prescribing information, refer to the Estrogens group monograph.

Indications

For the treatment of moderate to severe vasomotor symptoms associated with menopause; vulval and vaginal atrophy, hypoestrogenism caused by hypogonadism, castration, or primary ovarian failure; advanced androgen-dependent prostatic carcinoma (for palliation therapy).

Administration and Dosage

➤*Administration:* For IM injection only. Inject deeply into the upper outer quadrant of the gluteal muscle. Estradiol valerate injection may be administered with a small gauge needle. Because the 40 mg potency provides a high concentration in a small volume, observe particular care to administer the full dose.

➤*Moderate to severe vasomotor symptoms, vulval and vaginal atrophy associated with menopause:* 10 to 20 mg every 4 weeks. Choose the lowest dose and regimen that will control symptoms and discontinue medication as promptly as possible. Make attempts to discontinue or taper medication at 3- to 6-month intervals.

➤*Female hypoestrogenism caused by hypogonadism, castration, or primary ovarian failure:* 10 to 20 mg every 4 weeks.

➤*Prostatic carcinoma (advanced, androgen-dependent):* 30 mg or more every 1 or 2 weeks.

➤*Concomitant progestin therapy:* When estrogen is prescribed for a postmenopausal woman with a uterus, also initiate progestin to reduce the risk of endometrial cancer. A woman without a uterus does not need progestin.

➤*Storage/Stability:* Store at room temperature. Storage at low temperatures may result in the separation of some crystalline material that redissolves readily upon warming.

CONJUGATED ESTROGENS

Tablets contain a mixture of conjugated equine estrogens obtained exclusively from natural sources that includes sodium estrone sulfate, sodium equilin sulfate, sodium sulfate conjugates, 17α-dihydroequilin, 17α-estradiol, and 17β-dihydroequilin.

Rx	Premarin (Wyeth-Ayerst)	Tablets: 0.3 mg	Lactose, sucrose. Green, oval. In 100s and 1000s.
		0.45 mg	Lactose, sucrose. Blue, oval. In 100s and UD 100s.
		0.625 mg	Lactose, sucrose. Maroon, oval. In 1000s and UD 100s.
		0.9 mg	Lactose, sucrose. White, oval. In 100s.
		1.25 mg	Lactose, sucrose. Yellow, oval. In 100s and 1000s.
Rx	Premarin Intravenous (Wyeth-Ayerst)	Injection: 25 mg	In *Secules*[1] (vials), each with 5 mL sterile diluent.[2]

[1] With 200 mg lactose, 0.2 mg simethicone, and 12.2 mg sodium citrate.　　　　[2] With 2% benzyl alcohol.

For complete prescribing information, refer to the Estrogens group monograph.

Indications

➤*Oral:* Moderate to severe vasomotor symptoms associated with menopause; moderate to severe symptoms of vulvar and vaginal atrophy associated with menopause; prevention of postmenopausal osteoporosis (loss of bone mass); hypoestrogenism caused by hypogonadism, castration, or primary ovarian failure; breast cancer (for palliation only) in appropriately selected women and men with metastatic disease; advanced androgen-dependent prostatic carcinoma (for palliation only).

➤*Parenteral:* For the treatment of abnormal uterine bleeding caused by hormonal imbalance in the absence of organic pathology.

Administration and Dosage

➤*Concomitant progestin therapy:* When estrogen is prescribed for a postmenopausal woman with a uterus, also initiate progestin to reduce the risk of endometrial cancer. A woman without a uterus does not need progestin.

➤*Oral:* Limit the use of estrogen, alone or in combination with a progestin, to the shortest duration consistent with treatment goals and risks for the individual woman. Periodically re-evaluate patients as clinically appropriate (eg, at 3- to 6-month intervals) to determine if treatment is still necessary.

Moderate to severe vasomotor symptoms and/or moderate to severe symptoms of vulvar and vaginal atrophy associated with menopause – Start at the lowest dose. Therapy may be given continuously with no interruption, or in cyclical regimens (regimens such as 25 days on drug followed by 5 days off drug) as is medically appropriate on an individualized basis.

Female hypogonadism – 0.3 to 0.625 mg daily, administered cyclically (eg, 3 weeks on and 1 week off). Doses are adjusted depending on the severity of symptoms and responsiveness of the endometrium.

The dosage may be gradually titrated upward at 6- to 12-month intervals as needed to achieve appropriate bone age advancement and even-

tual epiphyseal closure. Chronic dosing with 0.625 mg is sufficient to induce artificial cyclic menses with sequential progestin treatment and to maintain bone mineral density after skeletal maturity is achieved.

Female castration and primary ovarian failure – 1.25 mg/day cyclically. Adjust according to severity of symptoms and patient response. For maintenance, adjust to lowest effective level.

Osteoporosis prevention – 0.625 mg/day, continuously or cyclically (such as 25 days on, 5 days off). The mainstays of prevention and management of osteoporosis are estrogen and calcium; exercise and nutrition may be important adjuncts.

Breast cancer, metastatic (for palliation) – 10 mg 3 times daily for at least 3 months.

Prostatic carcinoma (for palliation; advanced androgen-dependent) – 1.25 to 2.5 mg 3 times daily. Effectiveness can be judged by phosphatase determinations as well as by symptomatic improvement.

➤*Parenteral:* Usual dose is one 25 mg injection IV or IM. Repeat in 6 to 12 hours if necessary. Inject slowly to obviate the occurrence of flushes.

Compatibility – Infusion of conjugated estrogens with other agents is not recommended. In emergencies, however, when an infusion has already been started, make the injection into the tubing just distal to the infusion needle. Solution is compatible with normal saline, dextrose, and invert sugar solutions. It is not compatible with protein hydrolysate, ascorbic acid, or any solution with an acid pH.

➤*Storage/Stability:*

Oral – Store at room temperature (approximately 25°C). Dispense in a well-closed container.

Parenteral – Before reconstitution, refrigerate at 2° to 8°C (36° to 46°F). Use the reconstituted solution within a few hours. Refrigerated reconstituted solution is stable for 60 days. Do not use if darkening or precipitation occurs.

ESTERIFIED ESTROGENS

These products contain 75% to 85% sodium estrone sulfate and 6% to 15% sodium equilin sulfate, in such proportion that the total of these 2 components is not less than 90% of the total esterified estrogens content.

Rx	**Menest** (Monarch)	**Tablets:** 0.3 mg	Lactose. (M72). Yellow, oblong. Film-coated. In 100s.
		0.625 mg	Lactose. (M73). Orange, oblong. Film-coated. In 100s.
		1.25 mg	Lactose. (M74). Green, oblong. Film-coated. In 100s.
		2.5 mg	Lactose. (M75). Pink, oblong. Film-coated. In 50s.

For complete prescribing information, refer to the Estrogens group monograph.

Indications

For the treatment of moderate to severe vasomotor symptoms associated with menopause; atrophic vaginitis/kraurosis vulvae; female hypogonadism; female castration; primary ovarian failure; breast cancer (for palliation only) in appropriately selected women and men with metastatic disease; advanced prostate carcinoma (for palliation only).

Administration and Dosage

➤*Moderate to severe vasomotor symptoms:* 1.25 mg daily, administered cyclically (eg, 3 weeks on, 1 week off). If the patient has not menstruated within the last 2 months or more, cyclic administration is started arbitrarily. If the patient is menstruating, cyclic administration is started on day 5 of bleeding. For short-term use only; discontinue medication as promptly as possible. Re-evaluate at 3- to 6-month intervals for tapering or discontinuation of therapy.

➤*Atrophic vaginitis and kraurosis vulvae:* 0.3 to 1.25 mg or more daily, depending upon the tissue response of the individual patient. Administer cyclically. For short-term use only; discontinue medication as promptly as possible. Re-evaluate at 3- to 6-month intervals for tapering or discontinuation of therapy.

➤*Female hypogonadism:* Give cyclically. Administer 2.5 to 7.5 mg daily in divided doses for 20 days followed by a 10-day rest period. If bleeding does not occur by the end of this period, repeat the same dosage schedule. The number of courses of estrogen therapy necessary to produce bleeding varies, depending on endometrial responsiveness.

If bleeding occurs before the end of the 10-day period, begin an estrogen-progestin cyclic regimen of 2.5 to 7.5 mg daily in divided doses for 20 days. During the last 5 days of estrogen therapy, give an oral progestin. If bleeding occurs before this regimen is concluded, discontinue therapy; resume on the fifth day of bleeding.

➤*Female castration and primary ovarian failure:* Give 1.25 mg daily, cyclically. Adjust dosage up- or downward according to severity of symptoms and patient response. For maintenance, adjust dosage to lowest level that will provide effective control.

➤*Prostatic cancer (inoperable, progressing):* 1.25 to 2.5 mg 3 times a day. Judge the effectiveness of therapy by symptomatic improvement and phosphatase determinations.

➤*Breast cancer (inoperable, progressing):* 10 mg 3 times a day for at least 3 months.

➤*Concomitant progestin therapy:* When estrogen is prescribed for a postmenopausal woman with a uterus, also initiate progestin to reduce the risk of endometrial cancer. A woman without a uterus does not need progestin.

ESTROPIPATE (Piperazine Estrone Sulfate)

Estropipate is a natural substance prepared from crystalline estrone solubilized as the sulfate and stabilized with piperazine.

Rx	**Estropipate** (Various, eg, Mylan, Watson)	**Tablets:** 0.625 mg sodium estrone sulfate (equiv. to 0.75 mg estropipate)	In 30s, 100s, and 500s.
Rx	**Ogen** (Pharmacia)		Lactose. (U 3772). Yellow, scored. In 100s.
Rx	**Ortho-Est** (Women First Healthcare)		Lactose. (WFHC 101). White, diamond shape, scored. In 100s.
Rx	**Estropipate** (Various, eg, Mylan, Watson)	**Tablets:** 1.25 mg sodium estrone sulfate (equiv. to 1.5 mg estropipate)	In 30s, 100s, and 500s.
Rx	**Ogen** (Pharmacia)		Lactose. (U 3773). Peach, scored. In 100s.
Rx	**Ortho-Est** (Women First Healthcare)		Lactose. (WHFC 102). Lavender, diamond shape, scored. In 100s.
Rx	**Estropipate** (Various, eg, Watson)	**Tablets:** 2.5 mg sodium estrone sulfate (equiv. to 3 mg estropipate)	In 30s, 100s, and 500s.
Rx	**Ogen** (Pharmacia)		Lactose. (U 3774). Blue, scored. In 100s.
Rx	**Estropipate** (Various, eg, Watson)	**Tablets:** 5 mg sodium estrone sulfate (equiv. to 6 mg estropipate)	In 30s, 100s, and 500s.

For complete prescribing information, refer to the Estrogens group monograph.

Indications

For the treatment of moderate to severe vasomotor symptoms associated with menopause; vulval and vaginal atrophy; hypoestrogenism caused by hypogonadism, castration, or primary ovarian failure; osteoporosis prevention.

Administration and Dosage

➤*Moderate to severe vasomotor symptoms, vulval and vaginal atrophy associated with menopause:* Give cyclically. Choose the lowest dose and regimen that will control symptoms, and discontinue as promptly as possible. Attempt to discontinue or taper medication at 3- to 6-month intervals. Usual dosage range is 0.75 to 6 mg estropipate/day.

If a patient with vasomotor symptoms has not menstruated within the last 2 months or more, start cyclic administration arbitrarily. If the patient is menstruating, start cyclic administration on day 5 of bleeding.

➤*Female hypogonadism:* 1.5 to 9 mg estropipate/day for the first 3 weeks, followed by a rest period of 8 to 10 days. Repeat if bleeding does not occur by the end of the rest period. The number of courses of therapy necessary to produce withdrawal bleeding will vary according to the responsiveness of the endometrium. If satisfactory withdrawal bleeding does not occur, give an oral progestin in addition to estrogen during the third week of the cycle.

➤*Female castration or primary ovarian failure:* A daily dose of 1.5 to 9 mg estropipate may be given for the first 3 weeks of a theoretical cycle, followed by a rest period of 8 to 10 days. Adjust dosage upward or downward according to severity of symptoms and response of the patient. For maintenance, adjust dosage to the lowest level that will provide effective control.

➤*Osteoporosis prevention:* 0.75 mg estropipate daily for 25 days of a 31-day cycle per month. The mainstays of prevention and management of osteoporosis are estrogen and calcium; exercise and nutrition may be important adjuncts.

➤*Concomitant progestin therapy:* When estrogen is prescribed for a postmenopausal woman with a uterus, also initiate progestin to reduce the risk of endometrial cancer. A woman without a uterus does not need progestin.

➤*Storage/Stability:* Store below 30°C (86°F). Dispense in tight, light-resistant container.

SYNTHETIC CONJUGATED ESTROGENS, A

Tablets contain a blend of 9 synthetic estrogenic substances: Sodium estrone sulfate, sodium equilin sulfate, sodium 17α-dihydroequilin sulfate, sodium 17α-estradiol sulfate, sodium 17β-dihydroequilin sulfate, sodium 17α-dihydroequilenin sulfate, sodium 17β-dihydroequilenin sulfate, sodium equilenin sulfate, and sodium 17β-estradiol sulfate.

Rx	Cenestin (Duramed)	Tablets: 0.3 mg	Lactose. (dp 41). Green. Film-coated. In 30s, 100s, and 1000s.
		0.625 mg	Lactose. (dp 42). Red. Film-coated. In 30s, 100s, and 1000s.
		0.9 mg	Lactose. (dp 43). White. Film-coated. In 30s, 100s, and 1000s.
		1.25 mg	Lactose. (dp 44). Blue. Film-coated. In 30s, 100s, and 1000s.

For complete prescribing information, refer to the Estrogens group monograph.

Indications

➤*Menopause (0.625, 0.9, and 1.25 mg only):* For the treatment of moderate to severe vasomotor symptoms associated with menopause.

➤*Vulvar and vaginal atrophy (0.3 mg only):* For the treatment of vulvar and vaginal atrophy.

Administration and Dosage

➤*Menopause:* Choose the lowest dose and regimen that will control symptoms. Initial doses of 0.625 mg/day are recommended with titra-

tion up to 1.25 mg. Discontinue medication as promptly as possible. Attempt to discontinue or taper medication at 3- to 6-month intervals.

➤*Vulvar and vaginal atrophy:* 0.3 mg/day.

➤*Concomitant progestin therapy:* When estrogen is prescribed for a postmenopausal woman with a uterus, also initiate progestin to reduce the risk of endometrial cancer. A woman without a uterus does not need progestin.

➤*Storage/Stability:* Store at 25°C (77°F); excursions permitted to 15° to 30°C (59° to 86°F). Dispense in tight container and child-resistant packaging.

SYNTHETIC CONJUGATED ESTROGENS, B

Tablets contain a blend of 10 synthetic estrogenic substances: Sodium estrone sulfate, sodium equilin sulfate, sodium 17α-dihydroequilin sulfate, sodium 17α-estradiol sulfate, sodium 17β-dihydroequilin sulfate, sodium 17α-dihydroequilenin sulfate, sodium 17β-dihydroequilenin sulfate, sodium equilenin sulfate, sodium 17β-estradiol sulfate, and sodium Δ8,9-dehydroestrone sulfate.

Rx	Enjuvia (Duramed)	Tablets: 0.625 mg	EDTA, lactose. (E3). Pink, oval. Film-coated. In 100s.
		1.25 mg	EDTA, lactose. (E4). Yellow, oval. Film-coated. In 100s.

For complete prescribing information, refer to the Estrogens group monograph.

Indications

➤*Menopause:* For the treatment of moderate to severe vasomotor symptoms associated with menopause.

Administration and Dosage

➤*Approved by the FDA:* May 10, 2004.

➤*Concomitant progestin therapy:* When estrogen is prescribed for a postmenopausal woman with a uterus, initiate a progestin to reduce the risk of endometrial cancer. A woman without a uterus does not need a progestin.

➤*Menopause:* Initial dose 0.625 mg daily. Subsequent dosage adjustment may be made based upon the individual patient response. Periodically reassess dosage.

The lowest effective dose for the treatment of moderate to severe vasomotor symptoms has not been determined. Prescribe use of estrogen, alone or in combination with a progestin, with the lowest effective dose and for the shortest duration consistent with treatment goals and risks for the individual woman. Reevaluate patients periodically as clinically appropriate (eg, at 3- to 6-month intervals) to determine if treatment is still necessary (see Boxed Warnings and Warnings). For women who have a uterus, undertake adequate diagnostic measures, such as endometrial sampling, when indicated, to rule out malignancy in cases of undiagnosed persistent or recurring abnormal vaginal bleeding.

➤*Storage/Stability:* Store at controlled room temperature, 20° to 25°C (68° to 77°F); excursions are permitted to 15° to 30°C (59° to 86°F).

ESTRADIOL CYPIONATE IN OIL

Rx	Depo-Estradiol (Pharmacia)	Injection: 5 mg/mL	In 5 mL vials.[1]

[1] In cottonseed oil with 5.4 mg chlorobutanol.

For complete prescribing information, refer to the Estrogens group monograph.

Indications

For the treatment of moderate to severe vasomotor symptoms associated with menopause; hypoestrogenism caused by hypogonadism.

Administration and Dosage

For IM use only.

➤*Moderate to severe vasomotor symptoms associated with menopause:* Usual dosage range is 1 to 5 mg IM every 3 to 4 weeks. Give cyclically. For short-term use only. Choose the lowest dose that

will control symptoms, and discontinue medicine as soon as possible. Attempt to discontinue or taper medication at 3- to 6-month intervals.

➤*Female hypogonadism:* 1.5 to 2 mg IM at monthly intervals.

➤*Concomitant progestin therapy:* When estrogen is prescribed for a postmenopausal woman with a uterus, also initiate progestin to reduce the risk of endometrial cancer. A woman without a uterus does not need progestin.

➤*Storage/Stability:* Store at controlled room temperature 20° to 25°C (68° to 77°F). Warming and shaking the vial should redissolve any crystals that may have formed during storage at temperatures lower than recommended.

MISCELLANEOUS ESTROGENS, VAGINAL

Rx	Vagifem (Novo Nordisk)	Tablets, vaginal: 25 mcg estradiol (equiv. to 25.8 mcg of the hemihydrate)	Lactose. White. Film-coated. In 8s, 15s, and 18s.
Rx	Estrace Vaginal (Warner Chilcott)	Cream: 0.1 mg estradiol/g in a nonliquefying base	Stearyl alcohol, EDTA, methylparaben. In 42.5 g with calibrated applicator.
Rx	Premarin Vaginal (Wyeth-Ayerst)	Cream: 0.625 mg conjugated estrogens/g in a nonliquefying base	Benzyl and cetyl alcohols, mineral oil. In 42.5 g with or without calibrated applicator.
Rx	Ogen Vaginal (Pharmacia)	Cream: 1.5 mg estropipate/g	Cetyl alcohol, parabens, mineral oil. In 42.5 g with calibrated applicator.
Rx	Estring (Pharmacia)	Ring: 2 mg estradiol[1]	In single packs.
Rx	Femring (Galen)	Ring: 0.05 mg/day estradiol acetate[2]	In single packs.
		0.1 mg/day estradiol acetate[3]	In single packs.

[1] Releases estradiol, approximately 7.5 mcg/24 hours, in a consistent, stable manner over 90 days. Dimensions: outer diameter, 55 mm; cross-sectional diameter, 9 mm; core diameter, 2 mm.

[2] Central core contains 12.4 mg estradiol acetate that releases 0.05 mg/day for 3 months. Dimensions: outer diameter, 56 mm; cross-sectional diameter, 7.6 mm; core diameter, 2 mm.

[3] Central core contains 24.8 mg estradiol acetate that releases 0.1 mg/day for 3 months. Dimensions: outer diameter, 56 mm; cross-sectional diameter, 7.6 mm; core diameter, 2 mm.

MISCELLANEOUS ESTROGENS, VAGINAL

For complete prescribing information, refer to the Estrogens group monograph.

Indications

➤*Vulvar / Vaginal atrophy:* Treatment of urogenital symptoms associated with postmenopausal atrophy of the vagina and/or the lower urinary tract.

➤*Atrophic vaginitis (Vagifem only):* Treatment of atrophic vaginitis.

➤*Vasomotor symptoms (Femring only):* Treatment of moderate to severe vasomotor symptoms associated with menopause.

Administration and Dosage

Choose the lowest dose that will control symptoms and discontinue medication as promptly as possible. Attempt to discontinue or taper medication at 3- to 6-month intervals.

➤*Conjugated estrogens:* Administer cyclically; 3 weeks on and 1 week off. For short-term use only. Give 0.5 to 2 g/day intravaginally, depending on the severity of the condition.

➤*Estropipate:* 2 to 4 g/day intravaginally, depending on the severity of the condition.

➤*Estradiol:*

Cream – 2 to 4 g/day for 1 or 2 weeks. Gradually reduce to 50% of initial dosage for a similar period. A maintenance dose of 1 g 1 to 3 times/week may be used after restoration of the vaginal mucosa has been achieved.

Ring – Press into an oval and insert as deeply as possible into the upper ⅓ of the vaginal vault. The ring is to remain in place continu-

ously for 3 months, after which it should be removed and, if appropriate, replaced by a new ring.

If the ring is removed or falls out at any time during the 90-day treatment period, rinse the ring in lukewarm water and re-insert.

➤*Estradiol hemihydrate:* Using the supplied applicator, gently insert into the vagina as far as it can comfortably go without force.

Initial dose – 1 tablet inserted vaginally once daily for 2 weeks. Have the patient administer treatment at the same time each day.

Maintenance dose – 1 tablet inserted vaginally twice weekly.

The need to continue therapy should be assessed by the physician with the patient. Attempt to discontinue or taper medication at 3- to 6-month intervals.

➤*Concomitant progestin therapy:* When estrogen is prescribed for a postmenopausal woman with a uterus, also initiate progestin to reduce the risk of endometrial cancer. A woman without a uterus does not need progestin.

➤*Storage / Stability:* Store at controlled room temperature (15° to 30°C; 59° to 86°F). Protect from temperatures in excess of 40°C (104°F).

Patient Information

➤*Ring:* Press the ring into an oval and insert into the upper ⅓ of the vaginal vault. When the ring is in place, the patient should not feel anything. If the patient feels discomfort, the ring is probably not far enough inside; gently push the ring further into the vagina. The ring may be removed by hooking a finger through it and pulling it out.

If the ring comes out before 3 months, clean with warm water and place back into the vagina. The ring may be left in during intercourse.

MISCELLANEOUS ESTROGENS, TOPICAL

Rx	Estrogel (Unimed)	Gel: 0.06% estradiol (0.75 mg estradiol/1.25 g unit dose)	Alcohol. In 80 g tubes and 93 g pumps.

For complete prescribing information, refer to the Estrogens group monograph.

Indications

➤*Vasomotor symptoms:* For the treatment of moderate to severe vasomotor symptoms associated with menopause.

➤*Vulvar / Vaginal atrophy:* For the treatment of moderate to severe symptoms of vulvar and vaginal atrophy associated with menopause.

When prescribing solely for the treatment of symptoms of vulvar and vaginal atrophy, consider topical vaginal products.

Administration and Dosage

➤*Topical estradiol pump and tube:*

Pump – Before using the pump for the first time, it must be primed. Remove the large pump cover and fully depress the pump twice. Discard the unused gel by thoroughly rinsing down the sink or placing it in the household trash in a manner that avoids accidental exposure or ingestion by household members or pets. After priming, the pump is ready to use; 1 complete pump depression will dispense the same amount of topical estradiol gel each time.

The topical estradiol gel pump contains enough product to allow for initial priming of the pump twice and to deliver 64 daily doses. After the pump has been initially primed twice and 64 doses have been dispensed, discard the pump.

Apply topical estradiol gel at the same time each day. Apply daily dose of gel to clean, dry, unbroken skin. Apply topical estradiol gel dose after

bath, shower, or sauna. Try to leave as much time as possible between applying topical estradiol gel dose and going swimming.

Be sure skin is completely dry before applying topical estradiol gel.

To apply the dose, collect the gel into the palm of the hand by pressing the pump firmly and fully with 1 fluid motion without hesitation.

Apply the gel to one arm using the hand. Spread the gel as thinly as possible over the entire area on the inside and outside of the arm from wrist to shoulder.

Always place the cap back on the tip of the pump and the large pump cover over the top of the pump after each use.

Wash hands with soap and water after applying the gel to reduce the chance that the medicine will spread to other people.

It is not necessary to massage or rub in topical estradiol gel. Simply allow the gel to dry for up to 5 minutes before dressing.

Alcohol-based gels are flammable. Avoid fire, flame, or smoking until the gel has dried.

Never apply topical estradiol gel directly to the breast. Do not allow others to help apply the gel.

Tube – When using the topical estradiol tube, gently squeeze topical estradiol gel from the tube to fill the applicator to the halfway mark (1.25 mark). Apply the gel to one arm using the applicator. Be sure to transfer all of the gel from the applicator to the arm.

Selective Estrogen Receptor Modulator

RALOXIFENE

Rx **Evista** (Eli Lilly)	**Tablets:** 60 mg	Lactose. (LILLY 4165). White, elliptical. Film coated. In unit-of-use 30s and 100s, and 2000s.

Indications

▶*Osteoporosis, prevention and treatment:* For the treatment and prevention of osteoporosis in postmenopausal women.

Administration and Dosage

▶*Approved by the FDA:* December 9, 1997.

Postmenopausal osteoporosis may be diagnosed by history or radiographic documentation of osteoporotic fracture, bone mineral densitometry, or physical signs of vertebral crush fractures (eg, height loss, dorsal kyphosis).

The recommended dosage is 60 mg/day, which may be administered any time of day without regard to meals.

Actions

▶*Pharmacology:* Raloxifene is a selective estrogen receptor modulator (SERM) that belongs to the benzothiophene class of compounds. It reduces resorption of bone and decreases overall bone turnover as evidenced by reductions in serum and urine levels of bone turnover markers, radiocalcium kinetics studies for decreased bone resorption, and increases in bone mineral density (BMD).

Decreases in estrogen levels after oophorectomy or menopause lead to increases in bone resorption and bone loss. Bone is initially lost rapidly because the compensatory increase in bone formation is inadequate to offset resorptive losses. This imbalance between resorption and formation is related to loss of estrogen, and may also involve age-related impairment of osteoblasts or their precursors. In some women, these changes will eventually lead to decreased bone mass, osteoporosis, and increased risk for fractures, particularly of the spine, hip, and wrist. Vertebral fractures are the most common type of osteoporotic fracture in postmenopausal women.

Raloxifene's biological actions are mediated through estrogen receptor binding, resulting in activation of certain estrogenic pathways and blockade of others.

Raloxifene decreases resorption of bone and reduces biochemical markers of bone turnover to the premenopausal range. These effects on bone are manifested as reductions in the serum and urine levels of bone turnover markers, decreases in bone resorption based on radiocalcium kinetics studies, increases in BMD, and decreases in incidence of fractures. Raloxifene also has effects on lipid metabolism. Raloxifene decreases total and LDL cholesterol levels but does not increase triglyceride levels. It does not change total HDL cholesterol levels. Preclinical data demonstrate that raloxifene is an estrogen antagonist in uterine and breast tissues. Clinical trial data (through a median of 42 months) suggest that raloxifene lacks estrogen-like effects on the uterus and breast tissue.

▶*Pharmacokinetics:*

Absorption – Raloxifene is absorbed rapidly after oral administration with ≈ 60% of an oral dose absorbed. However, presystemic glucuronide conjugation is extensive, and absolute bioavailability is only 2%. Bioavailability and the time to reach average maximum plasma concentration are functions of systemic interconversion and enterohepatic cycling of raloxifene and its glucuronide metabolites. Administration with a standardized, high-fat meal increases the absorption of raloxifene (C_{max} 28% and area under the plasma concentration-time curve [AUC] 16%) but does not lead to clinically meaningful changes in systemic exposure. Raloxifene can be administered without regard to meals.

Distribution – The apparent volume of distribution is 2348 L/kg and is not dose-dependent. Raloxifene and the monoglucuronide conjugates are highly bound to plasma proteins (95%) and to albumin and α1-acid glycoprotein but not to sex steroid binding globulin.

Metabolism – Raloxifene undergoes extensive first-pass metabolism to the glucuronide conjugates: Raloxifene-4'-glucuronide, raloxifene-6-glucuronide, and raloxifene-6,4'-diglucuronide, with < 1% existing in the unconjugated form. No other metabolites have been detected, providing strong evidence that raloxifene is not metabolized by cytochrome P450 pathways. Raloxifene and its glucuronide conjugates are interconverted by reversible systemic metabolism and enterohepatic cycling, thereby prolonging its plasma elimination half-life to 27.7 hours after oral dosing.

Following IV administration, raloxifene is cleared at a rate approximating hepatic blood flow. Apparent oral clearance is 44.1 L/kg•hr. Following chronic oral dosing, clearance (Cl) ranges from 40 to 60 L/kg•hr. Increasing doses of raloxifene (ranging from 30 to 150 mg) result in slightly less than a proportional increase in AUC.

Excretion – Raloxifene is primarily excreted in the feces; < 6% of the raloxifene dose is eliminated in the urine as glucuronide conjugates and < 0.2% is excreted unchanged in urine.

Summary of Raloxifene Pharmacokinetic Parameters in Healthy Postmenopausal Women					
	C_{max}(ng/mL)/ (mg/kg)	Half-life (hr)	AUC (ng•hr/mL)/(mg/kg)	CL/F[1] (L/kg•hr)	V/F[1] (L/kg)
Single dose	0.5	27.7	27.2	44.1	2348
Multiple dose	1.36	32.5	24.2	47.4	2853

[1] F = bioavailability.

Hepatic function impairment – Raloxifene was studied, as a single dose, in Child-Pugh Class A patients with cirrhosis and total serum bilirubin ranging from 0.6 to 2 mg/dL. Plasma raloxifene concentrations were ≈ 2.5 times higher than in controls and correlated with bilirubin concentrations (see Warnings).

▶*Clinical trials:*

Effects on total body and regional BMD – In postmenopausal women, raloxifene preserves bone mass and increases BMD relative to calcium alone at 24 months. The effect on hip bone mass is similar to that for the spine.

The effects of raloxifene on BMD in postmenopausal women were examined in 3 large osteoporosis prevention trials (n = 1764). All women received calcium supplementation (400 to 600 mg/day). Women enrolled in these studies had a median age of 54 years and a median time since menopause of 5 years (< 1 up to 15 years postmenopause). Raloxifene 60 mg once daily produced increases in bone mass vs calcium supplementation alone. Compared with placebo, the increases in BMD for each of the 3 studies were statistically significant at 12 months and were maintained at 24 months. The calcium-supplemented placebo groups lost ≈ 1% of BMD over 24 months. Raloxifene also increased BMD compared with placebo in the total body by 1.3% to 2% and in Ward's Triangle (hip) by 3.1% to 4%.

Assessments of bone turnover – In a 31-week study, 33 early postmenopausal women were randomized to treatment with once-daily raloxifene 60 mg, cyclic estrogen/progestin (0.625 mg/day conjugated estrogens with 5 mg/day medroxyprogesterone acetate for the first 2 weeks of each month hormone replacement therapy [HRT]), or no treatment. Treatment with either raloxifene or HRT was associated with reduced bone resorption and a positive shift in calcium balance.

In the osteoporosis treatment and prevention trials, raloxifene therapy resulted in consistent, statistically significant suppression of bone resorption and bone formation, as reflected by changes in serum and urine markers of bone turnover. The suppression of bone turnover markers was evident by 3 months and persisted throughout the 36- and 24-month observation period.

Bone histomorphometry – In the treatment study, bone biopsies for qualitative and quantitative histomorphometry were obtained at baseline and after 2 years of treatment. In raloxifene-treated patients, there were statistically significant decreases in bone formation rate per tissue volume, consistent with a reduction in bone turnover. Normal bone quality was maintained; specifically, there was no evidence of osteomalacia, marrow fibrosis, cellular toxicity, or woven bone after 2 years of treatment. The effects of raloxifene on bone histomorphometry were determined by pre- and posttreatment biopsies in a 6-month study of postmenopausal women who received once-daily doses of raloxifene 60 mg or conjugated estrogens 0.625 mg. Ten raloxifene-treated and 8 estrogen-treated women had evaluable bone biopsies at baseline and after 6 months of therapy. Bone formation rate/bone volume and activation frequency, the primary efficacy parameters, decreased to a greater extent with conjugated estrogen treatment vs raloxifene treatment, although the differences were not statistically significant.

Effects on lipid metabolism – The effects of raloxifene on selected lipid fractions and clotting factors were evaluated in a 6-month study of 390 postmenopausal women. Raloxifene was compared with oral continuous combined estrogen/progestin (0.625 mg conjugated estrogens plus 2.5 mg medroxyprogesterone acetate, [HRT]) and placebo. Raloxifene decreased serum total and LDL cholesterol without effects on serum total HDL cholesterol or triglycerides. In addition, raloxifene significantly decreased serum fibrinogen and lipoprotein.

Raloxifene and Oral HRT Effects on Selected Lipid Fractions and Clotting Factors (Median Change from Baseline) (%)			
Endpoint	Raloxifene[1] (n = 95)	HRT (n = 96)	Placebo (n = 98)
Total cholesterol	-6.6	-4.4	0.9
LDL cholesterol	-10.9	-12.7	1
HDL cholesterol	0.7	10.6	0.9
HDL-2 cholesterol	15.4	33.3	0
HDL-3 cholesterol	-2.5	2.7	0
Fibrinogen	-12.2	-2.8	-2.1

RALOXIFENE

Raloxifene and Oral HRT Effects on Selected Lipid Fractions and Clotting Factors (Median Change from Baseline) (%)			
Endpoint	Raloxifene[1] (n = 95)	HRT (n = 96)	Placebo (n = 98)
Lipoprotein	-4.1	-16.3	3.3
Triglycerides	-4.1	20	-0.3
Plasminogen activator inhibitor-1	-2.1	-29	-9.4

[1] 60 mg once daily.

Consistent with results from the 6-month study, in the osteoporosis treatment (36 months) and prevention (24 months) studies, raloxifene statistically significantly decreased serum total and LDL cholesterol by 5% to 6% and 8% to 10%, respectively, compared with placebo. Raloxifene did not affect HDL cholesterol or triglyceride levels.

Contraindications

Women who are lactating or who are or may become pregnant (see Warnings); women with active or a history of venous thromboembolic events, including deep vein thrombosis (DVT), pulmonary embolism, and retinal vein thrombosis; hypersensitivity to raloxifene or other constituents of the drug.

Warnings

➤*Venous thromboembolic events:* An analysis of raloxifene-treated women showed an increased risk of venous thromboembolic events defined as DVT and pulmonary embolism. Other venous thromboembolic events could also occur. A less serious event, superficial thrombophlebitis, has been reported more frequently with raloxifene. The greatest risk for DVT and pulmonary embolism occurs during the first 4 months of treatment. Discontinue raloxifene ≥ 72 hours prior to and during prolonged immobilization (eg, postsurgical recovery, prolonged bed rest), and resume therapy only after the patient is fully ambulatory. Advise patients to avoid prolonged restrictions of movement during travel. Consider the risk-benefit balance in women at risk of thromboembolic disease from other reasons, such as CHF, superficial thrombophlebitis, and active malignancy.

➤*Osteoporosis risk:* No single clinical finding or test result can quantify risk of postmenopausal osteoporosis with certainty. However, clinical assessment can help to identify women at increased risk. Widely accepted risk factors include Caucasian or Asian descent, slender body build, early estrogen deficiency, smoking, alcohol consumption, low calcium diet, sedentary lifestyle, and family history of osteoporosis. Evidence of increased bone turnover from serum and urine markers and low bone mass (eg, ≥ 1 standard deviation below the mean for healthy, young adult women) as determined by densitometric techniques are also predictive. The greater the number of clinical risk factors, the greater the probability of developing postmenopausal osteoporosis.

➤*Premenopausal use:* There is no indication for premenopausal use of raloxifene. Safety of raloxifene in premenopausal women has not been established and its use is not recommended.

➤*Hepatic function impairment:* Single-dose raloxifene was studied in Child-Pugh Class A patients with cirrhosis and serum total bilirubin ranging from 0.6 to 2 mg/dL. Plasma raloxifene concentrations were ≈ 2.5 times higher than in controls and correlated with total bilirubin concentrations. Safety and efficacy have not been evaluated further in patients with severe hepatic insufficiency.

➤*Carcinogenesis:* In a 21-month carcinogenicity study in mice, there was an increased incidence of ovarian tumors in female animals given 9 to 242 mg/kg, which included benign and malignant tumors of granulosa/theca cell origin and benign tumors of epithelial cell origin. Systemic exposure (AUC) of raloxifene in this group was 0.3 to 34 times that in postmenopausal women administered a 60 mg dose. There was also an increased incidence of testicular interstitial cell tumors and prostatic adenomas and adenocarcinomas in males given 41 or 210 mg/kg (4.7 or 24 times the AUC in humans) and prostatic leiomyoblastoma in males given 210 mg/kg.

In a 2-year carcinogenicity study in rats, an increased incidence of ovarian tumors of granulosa/theca cell origin was observed in females (treated during their reproductive lives) given 279 mg/kg (≈ 400 times the AUC in humans). The clinical relevance of these tumor findings is not known.

➤*Fertility impairment:* When male and female rats were given daily doses ≥ 5 mg/kg (≥ 0.8 times the human dose) prior to and during mating, no pregnancies occurred. In female rats, at doses of 0.1 to 10 mg/kg/day (0.02 to 1.6 times the human dose), raloxifene disrupted estrous cycles and inhibited ovulation. These effects of raloxifene were reversible. In another study in rats in which raloxifene was given during the preimplantation period at doses ≥ 0.1 mg/kg (≥ 0.02 times the human dose), raloxifene delayed and disrupted embryo implantation resulting in prolonged gestation and reduced litter size. The reproductive and developmental effects observed in animals are consistent with the estrogen receptor activity of raloxifene.

➤*Pregnancy: Category X.* Do not use in women who are or may become pregnant (see Contraindications). Raloxifene may cause fetal harm when administered to a pregnant woman. In rabbit studies, abortion and a low rate of fetal heart anomalies (ventricular septal defects) occurred in rabbits at doses ≥ 0.1 mg/kg (≥ 0.04 times the human dose), and hydrocephaly was observed in fetuses at doses ≥ 10 mg/kg (≥ 4 times the human dose). In rat studies, retardation of fetal development and developmental abnormalities (eg, wavy ribs, kidney cavitation) occurred at doses ≥ 1 mg/kg (≥ 0.2 times the human dose). Treatment of rats at doses of 0.1 to 10 mg/kg (0.02 to 1.6 times the human dose) during gestation and lactation produced effects that included the following: Delayed and disrupted parturition; decreased neonatal survival and altered physical development; sex- and age-specific reductions in growth and changes in pituitary hormone content; and decreased lymphoid compartment size in offspring. At 10 mg/kg, raloxifene disrupted parturition, which resulted in maternal and progeny death and morbidity. Effects in adult offspring (4 months of age) included uterine hypoplasia and reduced fertility; however, no ovarian or vaginal pathology was observed. Warn the patient of the potential hazard to the fetus if this drug is used during pregnancy or if the patient becomes pregnant while taking this drug.

➤*Lactation:* Raloxifene should not be used by lactating women. It is not known whether raloxifene is excreted in breast milk.

➤*Children:* Do not use raloxifene in pediatric patients.

Precautions

➤*Concurrent estrogen therapy:* The concurrent use of raloxifene and systemic estrogen or hormone replacement therapy (ERT or HRT) has not been studied in prospective clinical trials; therefore, concomitant use is not recommended.

➤*Lipid metabolism:* Raloxifene lowers serum total and LDL cholesterol by 6% to 11% but does not affect serum concentrations of total HDL cholesterol or triglycerides. Take these effects into account in therapeutic decisions for patients who may require therapy for hyperlipidemia (see Clinical trials).

Limited clinical data suggest that some women with a history of marked hypertriglyceridemia (> 5.6 mmol/L or> 500 mg/dL) in response to treatment with oral estrogen or estrogen plus progestin may develop increased levels of tryglycerides when treated with raloxifene. Women with this medical history should have serum triglycerides monitored when taking raloxifene.

➤*Endometrium:* Raloxifene has not been associated with endometrial proliferation. Investigate unexplained uterine bleeding as clinically indicated.

➤*Breast abnormalities:* Raloxifene has not been associated with breast enlargement, breast pain, or an increased risk of breast cancer. Investigate any unexplained breast abnormality occurring during raloxifene therapy.

➤*Supplemental calcium:* Add supplemental calcium or vitamin D to the diet if daily intake is inadequate.

Drug Interactions

➤*Highly protein-bound drugs:* Raloxifene is > 95% bound to plasma proteins. In vitro, raloxifene did not affect the binding of warfarin, phenytoin, or tamoxifen. However, use caution when raloxifene is coadministered with other highly protein-bound drugs, such as diazepam, diazoxide, and lidocaine.

Raloxifene Drug Interactions			
Precipitant drug	Object drug*		Description
Ampicillin	Raloxifene	↓	Peak raloxifene levels and the overall extent of absorption are reduced 28% and 14%, respectively, by concurrent ampicillin. This is consistent with decreased enterohepatic cycling associated with antibiotic reduction of enteric bacteria. However, the systemic exposure and elimination rate of raloxifene were not affected. Therefore, raloxifene can be coadministered with ampicillin.
Cholestyramine	Raloxifene	↓	Raloxifene absorption and enterohepatic cycling was reduced 60%; avoid coadministration.
Raloxifene	Warfarin	↓	In single-dose studies, 10% decreases in prothrombin time (PT) have been observed. Monitor PT closely.

* ↓ = Object drug decreased.

➤*Drug/Food interactions:* Administration with a standardized, high-fat meal increases the absorption of raloxifene (C_{max} 28% and AUC 16%) but does not lead to clinically meaningful changes in systemic exposure. Raloxifene can be administered without regard to meals.

RALOXIFENE

Adverse Reactions

In the osteoporosis prevention trials, therapy was discontinued because of adverse events in 11.4% of raloxifene patients (12.2% for placebo). In the osteoporosis treatment trials, therapy was discontinued because of an adverse event in 10.9% of raloxifene patients (8.8% for placebo). Common adverse events for both sets of trials considered to be drug-related were hot flashes and leg cramps. The first occurrence of hot flashes was most commonly reported during the first 6 months of treatment.

Raloxifene Adverse Reactions (≥ 2%) (%)

Adverse reaction	Treatment		Prevention	
	Raloxifene[1] (n = 2557)	Placebo (n = 2576)	Raloxifene[1] (n = 581)	Placebo (n = 584)
Cardiovascular				
Hot flashes	9.7	6.4	24.6	18.3
Migraine	A[2]	A	2.4	2.1
Syncope	2.3	2.1	B[3]	B
Varicose vein	2.2	1.5	A	A
CNS				
Depression	A	A	6.4	6
Insomnia	A	A	5.5	4.3
Vertigo	4.1	3.7	A	A
Neuralgia	2.4	1.9	B	B
Hypesthesia	2.1	2	B	B
Dermatologic				
Rash	A	A	5.5	3.8
Sweating	2.5	2	3.1	1.7
GI				
Nausea	8.3	7.8	8.8	8.6
Diarrhea	7.2	6.9	A	A
Dyspepsia	A	A	5.9	5.8
Vomiting	4.8	4.3	3.4	3.3
Flatulence	A	A	3.1	2.4
GI disorder	A	A	3.3	2.1
Gastroenteritis	B	B	2.6	2.1
GU				
Vaginitis	A	A	4.3	3.6
Urinary tract infection	A	A	4	3.9
Cystitis	4.6	4.5	3.3	3.1
Leukorrhea	A	A	3.3	1.7
Uterine disorder[4]	3.3	2.3	A	A
Endometrial disorder	B	B	3.1	1.9
Vaginal hemorrhage	2.5	2.4	A	A
Urinary tract disorder	2.5	2.1	A	A
Metabolic/Nutritional				
Weight gain	A	A	8.8	6.8
Peripheral edema	5.2	4.4	3.3	1.9
Musculoskeletal				
Arthralgia	15.5	14	10.7	10.1
Myalgia	A	A	7.7	6.2
Leg cramps	7	3.7	5.9	1.9
Arthritis	A	A	4	3.6
Tendon disorder	3.6	3.1	A	A
Respiratory				
Sinusitis	7.9	7.5	10.3	6.5
Rhinitis	10.2	10.1	A	A
Bronchitis	9.5	8.6	A	A
Pharyngitis	5.3	5.1	7.6	7.2
Cough increased	9.3	9.2	6	5.7
Pneumonia	A	A	2.6	1.5
Laryngitis	B	B	2.2	1.4

Raloxifene Adverse Reactions (≥ 2%) (%)

Adverse reaction	Treatment		Prevention	
	Raloxifene[1] (n = 2557)	Placebo (n = 2576)	Raloxifene[1] (n = 581)	Placebo (n = 584)
Miscellaneous				
Infection	A	A	15.1	14.6
Flu syndrome	13.5	11.4	14.6	13.5
Headache	9.2	8.5	A	A
Chest pain	A	A	4	3.6
Fever	3.9	3.8	3.1	2.6
Conjunctivitis	2.2	1.7	A	A

[1] 60 mg once daily.
[2] A = placebo incidence greater than or equal to raloxifene incidence.
[3] B = < 2% incidence and more frequent with raloxifene.
[4] Actual terms most frequently referred to endometrial fluid.

Adverse Reactions: Raloxifene vs Continuous Combined or Cyclic Estrogen plus Progestin (HRT) (≥ 2%)

Adverse reaction	Raloxifene[1] (n = 317)	HRT - continuous combined[2] (n = 96)	HRT - cyclic[3] (n = 219)
Hot flashes	28.7	3.1	5.9
Infection	11	0	6.8
Abdominal pain	6.6	10.4	18.7
Vaginal bleeding	6.2	64.2	88.5
Breast pain	4.4	37.5	29.7
Chest pain	2.8	0	0.5
Flatulence	1.6	12.5	6.4

[1] 60 mg once daily.
[2] 0.625 mg conjugated estrogens plus 2.5 mg medroxyprogesterone acetate.
[3] 0.625 mg conjugated estrogens with concomitant 5 mg medroxyprogesterone acetate or 0.15 mg norgestrel on days 1 through 14 or 17 through 28.

▶*Lab test abnormalities:* The following changes in analyte concentrations are commonly observed during raloxifene therapy: Increased apolipoprotein A1; reduced serum total cholesterol, LDL cholesterol, fibrinogen, apolipoprotein B, and lipoprotein. Raloxifene modestly increases hormone-binding globulin concentrations, including sex steroid-binding globulin, thyroxine-binding globulin, and corticosteroid-binding globulin with corresponding increases in measured total hormone concentrations. There is no evidence that these changes in hormone-binding globulin concentrations affect concentrations of the corresponding free hormones.

There were small decreases in serum total calcium, inorganic phosphate, total protein, and albumin, which were generally of lesser magnitude than decreases observed during ERT/HRT. Platelet count was also decreased slightly and was not different from ERT.

Overdosage

Incidents of overdose in humans have not been reported. In an 8-week study of 63 postmenopausal women, a dose of raloxifene 600 mg/day was safely tolerated. There is no specific antidote for raloxifene.

Patient Information

For safe and effective use of raloxifene, inform patients about the following:

▶*Patient immobilization:* Discontinue raloxifene ≥ 72 hours prior to and during prolonged immobilization (eg, postsurgical recovery, prolonged bed rest), and advise patients to avoid prolonged restrictions of movement during travel because of the increased risk of venous thromboembolic events.

▶*Hot flashes or flushes:* Raloxifene is not effective in reducing hot flashes or flushes associated with estrogen deficiency. In some asymptomatic patients, hot flashes may occur upon beginning raloxifene therapy.

▶*Other preventive measures:* Instruct patients to take supplemental calcium and vitamin D if daily dietary intake is inadequate. Consider weight-bearing exercise along with the modification of certain behavioral factors, such as cigarette smoking or alcohol consumption, if these factors exist.

Instruct patients to read the patient package insert before starting therapy with raloxifene and to reread it each time the prescription is renewed.

For progestins recommended only for antineoplastic action in endometrial carcinoma, see megestrol acetate and medroxyprogesterone acetate monographs in the Antineoplastics chapter.

WARNING

Progestins have been used beginning with the first trimester of pregnancy to prevent habitual abortion or treat threatened abortion; however, there is no adequate evidence that such use is effective. There is evidence of potential harm to the fetus when given during the first 4 months of pregnancy. Therefore, the use of such drugs during the first 4 months of pregnancy is not recommended.

The cause of abortion is generally a defective ovum, which progestational agents could not be expected to influence. In addition, progestational agents have uterine relaxant properties that may cause a delay in spontaneous abortion when given to patients with fertilized defective ova.

Several reports suggest an association between intrauterine exposure to progestational drugs in the first trimester of pregnancy and genital abnormalities in male and female fetuses, and congenital anomalies, including congenital heart defects and limb-reduction defects. One study estimated that there is a 4.7-fold increased risk of limb-reduction defects in infants exposed in utero to sex hormones. The risk of hypospadias, 5 to 8 per 1000 male births in the general population, may be approximately doubled with exposure to these drugs. There are insufficient data to quantify the risk to exposed female fetuses, but because some of the more androgenic variety of these drugs induce mild virilization of the external genitalia of the female fetus, and because of the increased association of hypospadias in the male fetus, it is prudent to avoid use of these drugs during the first trimester.

If the patient is exposed to progestational drugs during the first 4 months of pregnancy or if she becomes pregnant while taking this drug, apprise her of the potential risks to the fetus.

Indications

➤*Amenorrhea:* Primary and secondary.

➤*Abnormal uterine bleeding:* Abnormal uterine bleeding caused by hormonal imbalance in the absence of organic pathology, such as fibroids or uterine cancer.

➤*Endometriosis:* Norethindrone only.

➤*AIDS wasting syndrome:* Megestrol acetate suspension only.

➤*Infertility (progesterone gel only):* Progesterone supplementation or replacement as part of an Assisted Reproductive Technology (ART) treatment for infertile women with progesterone deficiency.

➤*Unlabeled uses:* Medroxyprogesterone acetate (10 mg/day) has been used in the treatment of menopausal symptoms.

Adding progestin for ≥ 7 days of a cycle of estrogen replacement for menopause has lowered incidence of endometrial hyperplasia. Morphological and biochemical endometrium studies suggest 10 to 13 days of progestin provide maximal maturation of endometrium and eliminate any hyperplastic changes. It is not clear whether this provides protection from endometrial carcinoma. There may be additional risks with progestin in estrogen replacement regimens, including adverse effects on carbohydrate and lipid metabolism. Choice of progestin and dosage may be important in minimizing these adverse effects.

Progesterone suppositories (rectal or vaginal, 200 to 400 mg twice daily) have been used in premenstrual syndrome (PMS). Some studies report no improvements in PMS symptoms with progesterone suppositories vs placebo; however, these studies may have had methodologic flaws. One controlled trial suggested oral progesterone (100 mg in the morning, 200 mg at night for 10 days during the luteal phase) improved PMS symptoms. Further controlled studies are needed.

Progesterone has been used successfully in premature labor in late stages of pregnancy. Progesterone suppositories have been used during the luteal phase to the end of the first trimester to decrease spontaneous abortions in previous aborters and in anovulatory women receiving clomiphene citrate or human menopausal gonadotropins, and in luteal phase defects to improve fertility (see Warning Box).

Actions

➤*Pharmacology:* Progesterone, a principle of corpus luteum, is the primary endogenous progestational substance. Progestins (progesterone and derivatives) transform proliferative endometrium into secretory endometrium. Progesterone is necessary to increase endometrial receptivity for implantation of an embryo. Once an embryo is implanted, progesterone acts to maintain the pregnancy. They inhibit (at the usual dose range) or facilitate through positive feedback the secretion of pituitary gonadotropins, which in turn prevents follicular maturation and ovulation or alternatively promotes it for the "primed" follicle. They also inhibit spontaneous uterine contractions as well as other smooth muscles throughout the body. Progestins may demonstrate some anabolic or androgenic activity.

Several investigators have reported on the appetite-enhancing property of megestrol acetate and its possible use in cachexia. The precise mechanism by which megestrol produces effects in anorexia and cachexia is unknown.

➤*Pharmacokinetics:*

Absorption/Distribution –

Oral: Progestins are rapidly absorbed from the GI tract and undergo prompt hepatic degradation. Maximum concentration is acheived in 1 to 2 hours. During the first 6 hours after ingestion, half-life is ≈ 2 to 3 hours; half-life is ≈ 8 to 9 hours thereafter. Metabolites, present for several days after an oral dose, are excreted in the urine.

IM: Following IM administration, progesterone in oil is rapidly absorbed and undergoes rapid metabolism. Half-life is a few minutes. Effective concentrations of long-acting forms can be maintained for 3 to 6 months. Maximum concentration occurs in ≈ 24 hours with a half-life of ≈ 10 weeks.

Gel: Because of the gel's sustained release properties, progesterone absorption is prolonged with an absorption half-life of ≈ 25 to 50 hours, and an elimination half-life of 5 to 20 minutes. Progesterone is extensively bound to serum proteins (≈ 96% to 99%), primarily to serum albumin and corticosteroid binding globulin.

Metabolism/Excretion –

Oral/IM: The major urinary metabolite of oral progesterone is 5β-pregnan-3α, 20α-diol glucuronide. Progesterone undergoes biliary and renal elimination. Following an injection of labeled progesterone, 50% to 60% of the excretion of progesterone metabolites occurs via the kidney; ≈ 10% occurs via the bile and feces, the second major excretory pathway. Overall recovery of labeled material accounts for 70% of an administered dose, with the remainder of the dose not characterized with respect to elimination. Only a small portion of unchanged progesterone is excreted in the bile.

Gel –

Multiple Dose Pharmacokinetics of Progesterone Gel		
	Twice daily dosing for 12 days	Once daily dosing for 12 days
C_{max} (ng/ml)	14.57	15.97
C_{avg} (ng/ml)	11.6	8.99
T_{max} (hr)	3.55	5.4
AUC (ng•hr/ml)	138.72	391.98
t½ (hr)	25.91	45

Mean Single Dose Relative Bioavailability of Progesterone: Gel vs IM		
	8% gel	90 mg IM
C_{max} (ng/ml)	14.87	53.76
$C_{avg\ 0-24}$ (ng/ml)	6.98	28.98
AUC_{0-96} (ng•hr/ml)	296.78	1378.91
T_{max} (hr)	6.8	9.2
t½ (hr)	34.8	19.6

Contraindications

Hypersensitivity to progestins; thrombophlebitis, thromboembolic disorders, cerebral hemorrhage, or patients with a history of these conditions; impaired liver function or disease; carcinoma of the breast or genital organs; undiagnosed vaginal bleeding; missed abortion; as a diagnostic test for pregnancy; prophylactic use to avoid weight loss (megestrol acetate suspension).

Warnings

➤*Ophthalmologic effects:* Discontinue medication pending examination if there is a sudden partial or complete loss of vision or if there is sudden onset of proptosis, diplopia, or migraine. If papilledema or retinal vascular lesions occur, discontinue use.

➤*Thrombotic disorders:* Thrombotic disorders (eg, thrombophlebitis, cerebrovascular disorders, retinal thrombosis, pulmonary embolism) occasionally occur in patients taking progestins; be alert to the earliest manifestations of the disease. If these occur or are suspected, discontinue the drug immediately. However, this has not been shown to occur more often than that seen in a control group.

➤*HIV-infected women:* Although **megestrol** has been used extensively in women for endometrial and breast cancers, its use in HIV-infected women has been limited. All the women in the clinical trials reported breakthrough bleeding.

➤*Fertility impairment:* **Medroxyprogesterone acetate** at high doses is an antifertility drug. High doses would be expected to impair fertility until the cessation of treatment.

➤*Pregnancy:* Category D (**progesterone** injection); Category X (**norethindrone acetate**). Use is not recommended (see Warning Box). Progesterone gel is used to support embryo implantation and maintain pregnancies as part of ART treatments.

➤*Lactation:* Detectable amounts of progestins enter the milk of mothers receiving these agents. The effect on the nursing infant has not been determined.

Medroxyprogesterone does not adversely affect lactation and may increase milk production and duration of lactation if given in the puerperium.

➤*Children:* Safety and efficacy of **megestrol acetate suspension** in children have not been established.

Precautions

➤*Pretreatment physical examination:* Pretreatment physical examination should include breasts and pelvic organs, as well as Papanicolaou smear. Advise the pathologist of progestin therapy when relevant specimens are submitted. In cases of irregular vaginal bleeding, consider nonfunctional causes. Adequately diagnose all cases of vaginal bleeding.

➤*Fluid retention:* Fluid retention may occur; therefore, conditions influenced by this factor (epilepsy, migraine, asthma, cardiac or renal dysfunction) require careful observation.

➤*Depression:* Observe patients who have a history of psychic depression and discontinue the drug if depression recurs to a serious degree.

➤*Glucose tolerance:* A decrease in glucose tolerance has been observed in a small percentage of patients on estrogen-progestin combination drugs. The mechanism of this decrease is not known. For this reason, carefully observe diabetic patients receiving progestin therapy.

➤*Menopause:* The age of the patient constitutes no absolute limiting factor although treatment with progestins may mask the onset of the climacteric.

➤*Causes of weight loss:* Institute therapy with **megestrol** for weight loss only after treatable causes of weight loss are sought and addressed. These treatable causes include possible malignancies, systemic infections, GI disorders affecting absorption and endocrine, renal or psychiatric diseases.

➤*Benzyl alcohol:* Benzyl alcohol, contained in some of these products as a preservative, has been associated with a fatal "gasping syndrome" in premature infants.

Drug Interactions

Progestins Drug Interactions

Precipitant drug	Object drug*		Description
Aminoglutethimide	Medroxyprogesterone	↓	Aminoglutethimide may increase the hepatic metabolism of medroxyprogesterone, possibly decreasing its therapeutic effects.
Rifampin	Norethindrone	↓	Rifampin may reduce the plasma levels of norethindrone via hepatic microsomal enzyme induction, possibly decreasing its pharmacologic effects.

* ↓ = Object drug decreased.

➤*Drug/Lab test interactions:* Laboratory test results of hepatic function, coagulation tests (increase in prothrombin, Factors VII, VIII, IX and X), thyroid, metyrapone test and endocrine functions, may be affected by progestins.

A decrease in glucose tolerance has been observed in a small percentage of patients on estrogen-progestin combination drugs. The mechanism is obscure but appears to be related to the more androgenic progestins; observe diabetic patients who are receiving progestin therapy.

Pregnanediol – Pregnanediol determination may be altered by the use of progestins.

Adverse Reactions

For information concerning adverse reactions associated with combined estrogen-progestin therapy, refer to the Oral Contraceptives group monograph.

➤*General:*
CNS – Insomnia; somnolence; mental depression.

Dermatologic – Rash (allergic) with and without pruritus; acne; melasma or chloasma. **Progesterone** is irritating at the injection site whether the oil or aqueous vehicle is used; however, the aqueous preparation is particularly painful.

GI – Changes in weight (increase or decrease); nausea.

GU – Breakthrough bleeding; spotting; change in menstrual flow; amenorrhea; changes in cervical eversion, cervical secretions; galactorrhea.

Miscellaneous – Breast changes (tenderness); masculinization of the female fetus; edema; cholestatic jaundice; pyrexia; hirsutism.

➤*Medroxyprogesterone acetate:*
Miscellaneous – Sensitivity reactions ranging from pruritus and urticaria to generalized rash; alopecia; hirsutism.

➤*Progesterone gel:*

Progesterone Gel Adverse Reactions (%)

Adverse reaction	90 mg once daily	90 mg twice daily
CNS		
Somnolence	27	-
Headache	17	13
Nervousness	16	-
Depression	11	-
Libido decreased	10	-
Dizziness	-	5
GI		
Constipation	27	-
Nausea	22	7
Diarrhea	8	-
Vomiting	5	-
Reproductive disorders		
Breast enlargement	40	-
Breast pain	-	13
Moniliasis, genital	-	7
Vaginal discharge	-	7
Dyspareunia	6	-
Miscellaneous		
Nocturia	13	-
Arthralgia	8	-
Pruritus	-	5
Perineal pain	17	-
Cramps	-	15
Abdominal pain	12	-
Pain	-	8
Bloating	-	7

➤*Additional adverse events reported in women at a frequency < 5% include the following:*
Dermatologic – Acne; pruritus.

GI – Dyspepsia; eructation; flatulence.

GU – Dysuria; micturition frequency; UTI.

Psychiatric – Emotional lability; insomnia.

Miscellaneous – Allergy; fatigue; fever; influenza-like symptoms; water retention; asthma; back pain; leg pain; sinusitis; upper respiratory tract infection.

➤*Megestrol acetate suspension:*

Megestrol Adverse Reactions (%)[1]

Adverse reaction	Megestrol	Placebo
Diarrhea	8 to 15	8 to 15
Impotence	4 to 14	≤ 3
Rash	2 to 12	3 to 9
Flatulence	≤ 10	3 to 9
Hypertension	≤ 8	0
Asthenia	2 to 6	3 to 8
Insomnia	≤ 6	0
Nausea	≤ 5	3 to 9
Anemia	≤ 5	≤ 6
Fever	2 to 6	3
Libido decreased	≤ 5	≤ 3
Dyspepsia	≤ 4	≤ 5
Hyperglycemia	≤ 6	≤ 3
Headache	≤ 10	3 to 6
Pain	≤ 6	5 to 6
Vomiting	≤ 6	3 to 9
Pneumonia	≤ 3	3 to 6
Urinary frequency	≤ 2	≤ 5

[1] Data pooled from several studies. Percentages listed for megestrol without regard to specified dosage.

➤*Other adverse reactions reported in 1% to 3% of patients on megestrol include the following:*
Cardiovascular – Cardiomyopathy; palpitation.

CNS – Paresthesia; confusion; convulsion; depression; neuropathy; hypesthesia; abnormal thinking.

Dermatologic – Alopecia; herpes; pruritus; vesiculobullous rash; sweating; skin disorder.

GI – Constipation; dry mouth; hepatomegaly; increased salivation; oral moniliasis.

GU – Albuminuria; urinary incontinence; urinary tract infection; gynecomastia.

Respiratory – Dyspnea; cough; pharyngitis; lung disorder.

Progestins

Miscellaneous – Leukopenia; amblyopia; LDH increased; edema; peripheral edema; abdominal pain; chest pain; infection; moniliasis; sarcoma.

Patient Information

Patient package insert is available with product.

If GI upset occurs, take with food.

➤*Diabetic patients:* Glucose tolerance may be decreased; monitor urine sugar closely and report any abnormalities to physician.

Notify physician if pregnancy is suspected or if any of the following occurs: Sudden severe headache; visual disturbance; numbness in an arm or leg.

➤*Vaginal gel:* Do not use concurrently with other local intravaginal therapy. If other local intravaginal therapy is to be used concurrently, administer ≥ 6 hours before or after progesterone gel.

PROGESTERONE

Rx	**Prometrium** (Solvay)	**Capsules:** 100 mg (micronized progesterone)	Glycerin, peanut oil. (SV). Peach. In 100s.
		200 mg (micronized progesterone)	Glycerin, peanut oil. (SV2). Oval, pale yellow. In 100s.
Rx	**Progesterone In Oil** (Various, eg, APP, Watson)	**Injection:** 50 mg per mL	In sesame or peanut oil with benzyl alcohol. In 10 mL vials and 10 mL multidose vials.
Rx	**Crinone** (Serono)	**Vaginal gel:** 4% (45 mg)	Glycerin, mineral oil. In single-use, prefilled, disposable applicator delivering 1.125 g gel. In 6s.
Rx	**Prochieve** (Columbia Labs)		Glycerin, mineral oil. In single-use, prefilled, disposable applicator delivering 1.125 g gel. In 6s.
Rx	**Crinone** (Serono)	**Vaginal gel:** 8% (90 mg)	Glycerin, mineral oil. In single-use, prefilled, disposable applicator delivering 1.125 g gel. In 6s and 18s.
Rx	**Prochieve** (Columbia Labs)		Glycerin, mineral oil. In single-use, prefilled, disposable applicator delivering 1.125 g gel. In 6s and 18s.

For complete prescribing information, refer to the Progestins group monograph.

Indications

➤*Amenorrhea / Uterine bleeding (injection only):* For amenorrhea and abnormal uterine bleeding due to hormonal imbalance in the absence of organic pathology, such as submucous fibroids or uterine cancer.

➤*Assisted Reproductive Technology (ART) (gel):* The 8% gel is for progesterone supplementation or replacement as part of an ART treatment for infertile women with progesterone deficiency.

➤*Endometrial hyperplasia (capsules):* For use in the prevention of endometrial hyperplasia in nonhysterectomized postmenopausal women who are receiving conjugated estrogens tablets.

➤*Secondary amenorrhea (capsules and gel):* For use in secondary amenorrhea (capsules); the 4% gel is for the treatment of secondary amenorrhea, and the 8% gel is for women who have failed to respond to treatment with the 4% gel.

Administration and Dosage

➤*Parenteral:* For IM use. The drug is irritating at the injection site.

➤*Amenorrhea (injection only):* Administer 5 to 10 mg IM daily for 6 to 8 consecutive days. If ovarian activity has produced a proliferative endometrium, expect withdrawal bleeding 48 to 72 hours after the last injection. Spontaneous normal cycles may follow.

➤*ART (gel):* Administer 90 mg (8% gel) vaginally once daily in women who require progesterone supplementation. In women with partial or complete ovarian failure who require progesterone replacement, administer 90 mg vaginally twice daily. If pregnancy occurs, continue treatment up to 10 to 12 weeks until placental autonomy is achieved.

➤*Functional uterine bleeding (injection only):* Administer 5 to 10 mg IM daily for 6 doses. Bleeding should cease within 6 days. When estrogen also is given, begin progesterone after 2 weeks of estrogen therapy. Discontinue injections when menstrual flow begins.

➤*Prevention of endometrial hyperplasia (capsules):* Give as a single daily dose in the evening, 200 mg orally for 12 days sequentially per 28-day cycle, to postmenopausal women with a uterus who are receiving daily conjugated estrogen tablets.

➤*Secondary amenorrhea:*

Gel – Administer 45 mg (4% gel) vaginally every other day up to a total of 6 doses. For women who fail to respond, a trial of 8% gel every other day up to a total of 6 doses may be instituted. It is important to note that a dosage increase from the 4% gel can only be accomplished by using the 8% gel. Increase in the volume of gel administered does not increase the amount of progesterone absorbed.

Capsules – Give as a single daily dose of 400 mg in the evening for 10 days.

➤*Storage / Stability:* Store at 25°C (77°F); excursions permitted to 15° to 30°C (59° to 86°F).

MEDROXYPROGESTERONE ACETATE

Rx	**Medroxyprogesterone Acetate** (Various, eg, Barr, Greenstone)	**Tablets:** 2.5 mg	In 30s, 90s, 100s, 500s and 1000s.
Rx	**Provera** (Pharmacia & Upjohn)		(PROVERA 2.5). Lactose, sucrose. Orange, scored. In 30s and 100s.
Rx	**Medroxyprogesterone Acetate** (Various, eg, Barr, Greenstone)	**Tablets:** 5 mg	In 30s, 100s, 500s and 1000s.
Rx	**Provera** (Pharmacia & Upjohn)		(PROVERA 5). Lactose, sucrose. White, scored. Hexagonal. In 30s and 100s.
Rx	**Medroxyprogesterone Acetate** (Various, eg, Barr, Geneva, Greenstone)	**Tablets:** 10 mg	In 30s, 40s, 50s, 100s, 250s and 500s.
Rx	**Provera** (Pharmacia & Upjohn)		(PROVERA 10). Lactose, sucrose. White, scored. In 30s, 100s, 500s and UD 10s.

For complete prescribing information, refer to the Progestins group monograph. Parenteral medroxyprogesterone acetate is used as an antineoplastic agent; refer to the monograph in the Antineoplastics section.

Indications

➤*Endometrial hyperplasia:* To reduce the incidence of endometrial hyperplasia in nonhysterectomized postmenopausal women receiving 0.625 mg conjugated estrogens.

➤*Secondary amenorrhea / abnormal uterine bleeding:* For secondary amenorrhea and for abnormal uterine bleeding due to hormonal imbalance in the absence of organic pathology, such as fibroids or uterine cancer.

Administration and Dosage

➤*Abnormal uterine bleeding due to hormonal imbalance in the absence of organic pathology:* 5 or 10 mg daily for 5 to 10 days, beginning on the 16th or 21st day of the menstrual cycle. To produce an optimum secretory transformation of an endometrium that has been adequately primed with either endogenous or exogenous estrogen, give 10 mg daily for 10 days, beginning on the 16th day of the cycle. Withdrawal bleeding usually occurs 3 to 7 days after discontinuing therapy. Patients with recurrent episodes of abnormal uterine bleeding may benefit from planned menstrual cycling with medroxyprogesterone acetate.

➤*Endometrial hyperplasia:* 5 or 10 mg daily for 12 to 14 consecutive days per month, either beginning on the 1st day of the cycle or the 16th day of the cycle.

➤*Secondary amenorrhea:* 5 or 10 mg daily for 5 to 10 days. A dose for inducing an optimum secretory transformation of an endometrium that has been adequately primed with either endogenous or exogenous estrogen is 10 mg daily for 10 days. Start therapy any time. Withdrawal bleeding usually occurs 3 to 7 days after therapy ends.

➤*Storage / Stability:* Store at controlled room temperature, 20° to 25°C (68° to 77°F).

HYDROXYPROGESTERONE CAPROATE IN OIL

Rx	**Hydroxyprogesterone Caproate** (Various)	**Injection:** 125 mg per ml	In 10 ml vials.
Rx	**Hylutin** (Hyrex)		In 10 ml vials.[1]
Rx	**Hydroxyprogesterone Caproate** (Various, eg, Rugby, Schein)	**Injection:** 250 mg per ml	In 5 ml vials.

[1] In castor oil with benzyl benzoate and benzyl alcohol.

For complete prescribing information, refer to the Progestins group monograph.

Administration and Dosage

Hydroxyprogesterone, a long-acting progestin, has a 9 to 17 day duration of action.

For IM use.

➤*Amenorrhea (primary and secondary); dysfunctional uterine bleeding; metrorrhagia:* Usual adult dose is 375 mg.

➤*Production of secretory endometrium and desquamation:* Test for continuous endogenous estrogen production (medical D and C). Usual adult dose is 125 to 250 mg given on tenth day of cycle; repeat every 7 days until suppression is no longer desired.

NORETHINDRONE ACETATE

Rx	**Norethindrone Acetate** (Barr)	**Tablets:** 5 mg	(b 211/5). White, oval, scored. In 50s.
Rx	**Aygestin** (Barr)		Lactose. White, scored. In 50s.

For complete prescribing information, refer to the Progestins group monograph.

Indications

➤*Secondary amenorrhea, endometriosis, and abnormal uterine bleeding:* For the treatment of secondary amenorrhea, endometriosis, and abnormal uterine bleeding caused by hormonal imbalance in the absence of organic pathology, such as submucous fibroids or uterine cancer.

Administration and Dosage

Therapy must be adapted to the specific indications and therapeutic response of the individual patient. The dosage schedule assumes the interval between menses to be 28 days.

➤*Secondary amenorrhea, abnormal uterine bleeding due to hormonal imbalance in the absence of organic pathology:* Give 2.5 to 10 mg daily for 5 to 10 days during the second half of the theoretical menstrual cycle.

Withdrawal bleeding usually occurs within 3 to 7 days.

➤*Endometriosis:* Initial dose is 5 mg/day for 2 weeks; increase in increments of 2.5 mg/day every 2 weeks until 15 mg/day is reached. Therapy may be held at this level for 6 to 9 months or until breakthrough bleeding demands temporary termination.

MEGESTROL ACETATE

Rx	**Megestrol Acetate** (Various, eg, UDL)	**Tablets:** 20 mg	In 100s and UD 100s.
Rx	**Megestrol Acetate** (Various, eg, Major, UDL)	**Tablets:** 40 mg	In 100s, 500s, UD 100s, and blister package 25s.
Rx	**Megace** (Bristol-Myers Oncology)		Lactose. Lt. blue, scored. In 250s and 500s.
Rx	**Megestrol Acetate** (Various, eg, Roxane, Teva)	**Suspension:** 40 mg/mL	Alcohol, sorbitol, sucrose. In 240 mL.
Rx	**Megace** (Bristol-Myers Oncology)		≤ 0.06% alcohol, sucrose. Lemon-lime flavor. In 240 mL.

For complete prescribing information, refer to the Progestins group monograph. Megestrol is also used for advanced carcinoma of the breast or endometrium; refer to the monograph in the Antineoplastics chapter.

Indications

➤*AIDS wasting syndrome (suspension only):* Treatment of anorexia, cachexia, or an unexplained significant weight loss in patients with a diagnosis of acquired immunodeficiency syndrome (AIDS).

➤*Tumors (tablets only):* Palliative treatment of advanced carcinoma of the breast or endometrium (refer to the monograph in the Antineoplastics chapter).

Administration and Dosage

➤*AIDS wasting syndrome (suspension only):* Initial adult dose is 800 mg/day (20 mL/day). Shake the suspension well before using. In clinical trials evaluating different dose schedules, daily doses of 400 and 800 mg/day were found to be clinically effective.

➤*Storage/Stability:* Store suspension at 15° to 25°C (59° to 77°F) and dispense in a tight container. Protect from heat. Store tablets at room temperature.

ESTROGENS AND PROGESTINS COMBINED

Rx	**Prempro** (Wyeth-Ayerst)	**Tablets:** 0.3 mg conjugated estrogens/ 1.5 mg medroxyprogesterone acetate.	Cream, oval. In dial pack 28s.
		0.45 mg conjugated estrogens/1.5 mg medroxyprogesterone acetate	Gold, oval. In *EZ DIAL* 28s.
		0.625 mg conjugated estrogens/2.5 mg medroxyprogesterone acetate	Lactose, sucrose. (PREMPRO). Peach, oval. In dial pack 28s
		0.625 mg conjugated estrogens/5 mg medroxyprogesterone acetate	Lactose, sucrose. (W 0.625/5). Lt. blue, oval. In dial pack 28s.
Rx	**Premphase** (Wyeth-Ayerst)	**Tablets:** 0.625 mg conjugated estrogens; 0.625 mg conjugated estrogens/5 mg medroxyprogesterone acetate	Lactose, sucrose. (PREMARIN or PREMPHASE). **Estrogen only:** Maroon, oval. **Estrogen/Progestin:** Lt. blue, oval. In dial pack 28s (14 of each tablet).
Rx	**Femhrt** (Warner Chilcott)	**Tablets:** 5 mcg ethinyl estradiol/1 mg nor- ethindrone acetate	Lactose. (PD 144). White, D-shaped. In 90s and blister card 28s.
Rx	**Activella** (Novo Nordisk)	**Tablets:** 1 mg estradiol/0.5 mg norethin- drone acetate	Lactose. (Novo 288). White, biconvex. Film-coated. In dial pack 28s.
Rx	**Prefest** (Monarch)	**Tablets:** 1 mg estradiol; 1 mg estradiol/ 0.09 mg norgestimate	Lactose. **Estrogen only:** (1 J-C E2 O-M). Pink. **Estrogen/Progestin:** (1/90 J-C E2/N O-M). White. In blister card 30s (15 of each tablet).
Rx	**CombiPatch** (Aventis)	**Transdermal patch:** 0.05 mg estradiol/ 0.14 mg norethindrone acetate	9 cm². In 8s.
		0.05 mg estradiol/0.25 mg norethindrone acetate	16 cm². In 8s.

For complete prescribing information, refer to the Estrogens group monograph and the Progestins group monograph. Consider the information given for Oral Contraceptives (see group monograph) when using these products.

Indications

In women with an intact uterus for the treatment of moderate-to-severe vasomotor symptoms associated with menopause; treatment of vulval and vaginal atrophy (*Femhrt* excluded); osteoporosis prevention (*CombiPatch* excluded); treatment of hypoestrogenism caused by hypogonadism, castration, or primary ovarian failure (*CombiPatch* only).

Administration and Dosage

➤*Prempro:* One 0.625 mg/2.5 mg tablet once daily; can increase to 0.625 mg/5 mg once daily.

➤*Premphase:* One 0.625 mg conjugated estrogens tablet once daily on days 1 through 14 and one 0.625 mg conjugated estrogen/5 mg medroxyprogesterone tablet taken once daily on days 15 through 28.

➤*Femhrt and Activella:* One tablet/day.

➤*Ortho-Prefest:* One pink tablet/day for 3 days, followed by 1 white tablet/day for 3 days. This regimen is repeated continuously without interruption.

➤*CombiPatch:* Replace the patch system twice weekly. Advise women that monthly withdrawal bleeding often occurs.

Apply to a smooth (fold-free) clean, dry area of the skin on the lower abdomen. Do not apply to or near the breasts and avoid the waistline. The sites of application must be rotated; allow an interval of ≥ 1 week between applications to the same site.

Continuous combined regimen – Apply twice weekly during a 28-day cycle. Irregular bleeding may occur particularly in the first 6 months.

Continuous sequential regimen – It can be applied as a sequential regimen in combination with an estradiol-only transdermal delivery system.

➤*Menopause and vulval/vaginal atrophy:* Reevaluate patients at 3- to 6-month intervals to determine the need for continued treatment.

➤*Osteoporosis:* The mainstays of prevention and management of osteoporosis are estrogen and calcium; exercise and nutrition may be important adjuncts.

➤*Monitoring:* Monitor patients with an intact uterus closely for signs of endometrial cancer; evaluate recurrent or persistent abnormal vaginal bleeding appropriately to rule out malignancy.

ESTROGEN AND ANDROGEN COMBINATIONS, ORAL

Rx	**Estratest H.S.** (Solvay)	**Tablets:** 0.625 mg esterified estrogens and 1.25 mg methyltestosterone	Lactose, sucrose, parabens. (SOLVAY 1023). Lt. green, capsule shape. Sugar-coated. In 100s.
Rx	**Estratest** (Solvay)	**Tablets:** 1.25 mg esterified estrogens and 2.5 mg methyltestosterone	Lactose, sucrose, parabens. (SOLVAY 1026). Dk. green, capsule shape. Sugar-coated. In 100s and 1000s.

[a] Syntho Pharmaceuticals, Inc., 230 Sherwood Dr., Farmingdale, NY 11735; 631-755-9898.

For complete prescribing information, refer to the Estrogens and Androgens group monographs.

WARNING

Estrogens have been reported to increase the risk of endometrial carcinoma.

Close clinical surveillance of all women taking estrogens is important. In all cases of undiagnosed, persistent, or recurring abnormal vaginal bleeding, adequate diagnostic measures should be undertaken to rule out malignancy.

Do not use estrogens during pregnancy.

The use of female sex hormones, estrogens and progestogens, during early pregnancy may seriously damage the offspring.

Refer to the Warning Box in the Estrogens group monograph for more information.

Indications

➤*Moderate to severe vasomotor symptoms:* Moderate to severe vasomotor symptoms associated with menopause in patients not improved with estrogens alone.

There is no evidence that estrogens are effective for nervous symptoms or depression without associated vasomotor symptoms that may occur during menopause; do not use to treat these conditions.

Administration and Dosage

Give cyclically for short-term use only.

Use the lowest dose that will control symptoms and discontinue medication as promptly as possible.

Administer cyclically (ie, 3 weeks on and 1 week off). Make attempts to discontinue or taper medication at 3- to 6-month intervals.

➤*Usual dosage range:* One 1.25/2.5 mg tablet or one to two 0.625/1.25 mg tablets daily, as recommended by the physician.

Closely monitor treated patients with an intact uterus for signs of endometrial cancer and take appropriate diagnostic measures to rule out malignancy in the event of persistent or recurring abnormal vaginal bleeding.

➤*Storage/Stability:* Store at controlled room temperature, 15° to 30°C (59° to 86°F).

ORAL CONTRACEPTIVES

WARNING

Smoking: Cigarette smoking increases the risk of serious cardiovascular side effects from oral contraceptives (OCs). This risk increases with age and with heavy smoking ($\geq$ 15 cigarettes per day) and is quite marked in women > 35 years of age. Women who use OCs should not smoke.

Indications

➤*Contraception:* For the prevention of pregnancy.

Because of the positive association between the amount of estrogen and progestin in OCs and the risk of vascular disease and thromboembolism, minimizing exposure to these agents is in keeping with good principles of therapeutics. For any particular combination, prescribe the dosage regimen that contains the least amount of estrogen and progestin compatible with a low failure rate and needs of the individual patient. Start new patients on preparations containing $\leq$ 35 mcg estrogen.

➤*Emergency contraception (Plan B and Preven only):* For prevention of pregnancy following unprotected intercourse or a known or suspected contraceptive failure. To obtain efficacy, have the patient take the first dose as soon as possible within 72 hours of intercourse. The second dose must be taken 12 hours later.

➤*Acne vulgaris (Ortho Tri-Cyclen and Estrostep only):* For the treatment of moderate acne vulgaris in females $\geq$ 15 years of age who have no known contraindications to oral contraceptive therapy and who desire contraception, have achieved menarche, and are unresponsive to topical antiacne medications.

Administration and Dosage

➤*Acne:* The timing of dosing with *Ortho Tri-Cyclen* or *Estrostep* for acne should follow the guidelines for use of *Ortho Tri-Cyclen* or *Estrostep* as an OC. The dosage regimen for treatment of facial acne uses a 21-day active and a 7-day inert schedule. Have the patient take 1 active tablet daily for 21 days followed by 1 inert for 7 days. After 28 tablets have been taken, the patient should start a new course the next day.

➤*Emergency contraception (Plan B and Preven only):* The *Preven* emergency contraceptive kit contains a pregnancy test. This test can be used to verify an existing pregnancy resulting from intercourse that occurred earlier in the current menstrual cycle or the previous cycle. If a positive pregnancy result is obtained, advise the patient not to take the pills in the kit.

Take the initial 1 (*Plan B*) or 2 (*Preven*) pills as soon as possible but within 72 hours of unprotected intercourse. This is followed by the second dose of 1 (*Plan B*) or 2 (*Preven*) pills 12 hours later. Emergency contraception can be used at any time during the menstrual cycle. If the user vomits within 1 hour of taking either dose of the medication, she should contact her health care professional to discuss whether or not to repeat that dose or take an antinausea medication. Emergency contraceptive pills are not indicated for ongoing pregnancy protection and should not be used as a woman's routine form of contraception.

➤*Contraception:*

Progestin-only – One tablet every day at the same time. Administration is continuous, with no interruption between pill packs. Every time a pill is taken late, especially if a pill is missed, pregnancy is more likely.

Missed dose: If the patient is > 3 hours late or misses $\geq$ 1 tablet, she should take the missed pill as soon as remembered, then go back to taking progestin-only products (POPs) at the regular time, while being sure to use a backup method (eg, condom, spermicide) every time she has sexual intercourse for the next 48 hours.

Combined –

Sunday-start packaging: If the instructions recommend starting the regimen on Sunday, inform the patient to take the first tablet on the first Sunday after menstruation begins. If menstruation begins on Sunday, she should take the first tablet on that day.

21-day regimen: For day-1 start, the first day of menstrual bleeding should be counted as day 1. The cycle is to take 1 tablet per day for 21 days; no tablets are taken for 7 days. Whether bleeding has stopped or not, the patient should start a new course of the 21-day regimen. Withdrawal flow will normally occur $\approx$ 3 days after the last tablet is taken. The patient must follow the schedule whether flow occurs as expected, or whether spotting or breakthrough bleeding (BTB) occurs during the cycle.

28-day regimen: To eliminate the need to count the days between cycles, some products contain 7 inert or iron-containing tablets to permit continuous daily dosage during the entire 28-day cycle. Inform the patient to take the 7 tablets on the last 7 days of the cycle.

84-day regimen: The dosage of *Seasonale* is 1 pink (active) tablet per day for 84 consecutive days, followed by 7 days of white (inert) tablets. Withdrawal bleeding should occur during the 7 days following discontinuation of pink active tablets. During the first cycle, the patient should not place contraceptive reliance on *Seasonale* until a pink tablet

has been taken daily for 7 consecutive days; the patient should use a nonhormonal backup method of birth control (such as condoms or spermicide) during those 7 days. The patient should consider the possibility of ovulation and conception prior to initiation of medication.

The patient begins her next and all subsequent 91-day courses of tablets without interruption on the same day of the week on which she began her first course, following the same schedule. If in any cycle the patient starts tablets later than the proper day, she should protect herself against pregnancy by using a nonhormonal backup method of birth control until she has taken a pink tablet daily for 7 consecutive days.

Biphasic and triphasic OCs: Have the patient follow the instructions on the dispensers or packs; these are clearly marked, usually indicating where to start on the regimen and in what order to take the pills (usually marked with arrows), along with the appropriate week numbers. If there is any question, detailed instructions are provided in the specific package insert. As with the monophasic OCs, 1 tablet is taken each day; however, as the color of the tablet changes, the strength of the tablet also changes (ie, the estrogen/progestin ratio varies).

Missed active dose: While there is little likelihood of ovulation occurring if only 1 tablet is missed, the possibility of spotting or bleeding is increased. The possibility of ovulation occurring increases with each successive day that scheduled tablets are missed. This is particularly likely to occur if $\geq$ 2 consecutive tablets are missed. Any time $\geq$ 1 active tablets have been missed, the patient should use another method of contraception for the balance of the cycle until tablets have been taken for 7 consecutive days. If a patient forgets to take $\geq$ 1 tablet, the following is suggested:

• *One active tablet* – Have the patient take this as soon as remembered or she should take 2 tablets the next day; alternatively, the patient can take 1 tablet, discard the other missed tablet, continue as scheduled, and use another form of contraception until menses.

• *Two consecutive active tablets* – The patient should take 2 tablets as soon as remembered with the next pill at the usual time or she should take 2 tablets daily for the next 2 days, then resume the regular schedule. The patient should use an additional form of contraception for the 7 days after pills are missed, preferably for the remainder of the cycle. If 2 active pills are missed in a row in the third week and the patient is a Sunday starter, 1 pill should be taken every day until Sunday. On Sunday, the rest of the pack should be discarded and a new pack of pills started that same day. If 2 active pills are missed in a row in the third week and the patient is a day-1 starter, the rest of the pill pack should be discarded and a new pack started that same day. Menses may not occur this month but this is expected. However, if menses do not occur 2 months in a row, the health care provider or clinic should be contacted because of the possibility of pregnancy.

• *Three consecutive active tablets* – If the patient is a Sunday starter, she should keep taking 1 pill every day until Sunday. On Sunday, the rest of the pack should be discarded and a new pack of pills started that same day. If she is a day-1 starter, the rest of the pill pack should be discarded and a new pack started that same day. Menses may not occur this month, but this is expected. However, if menses do not occur 2 months in a row, the health care provider or clinic should be contacted because of the possibility of pregnancy. Pregnancy may result from sexual intercourse during the 7 days after the pills are missed. The patient should use another birth control method (eg, condoms, foam) as a backup method for those 7 days.

Switching pills – If switching from the combined pills to POPs, the patient should take the first POP the day after the last active combined pill is finished. She should not take any of the 7 inactive pills from the combined pill pack. Many women have irregular periods after switching to POPs; this is normal and to be expected. If switching from POPs to the combined pills, the patient should take the first active combined pill on the first day of menses, even if the POP pack is not finished. If switching to another brand of POPs, she should start the new brand any time. If the patient is breastfeeding, she can switch to another method of birth control at any time, except she should not switch to the combined pills until breastfeeding is stopped or until $\geq$ 6 months after delivery.

Bleeding – Bleeding that resembles menstruation occurs rarely. Persistent bleeding not controlled by this method indicates the need for reexamination of the patient; consider nonhormonal causes. If pathology has been excluded, time or a change to another formulation may solve the problem.

Missed menstrual period – If the patient has not adhered to the prescribed dosage regimen, consider possible pregnancy after the first missed period; withhold OCs until ruling out pregnancy and use a nonhormonal method of contraception. If the patient has adhered to the prescribed regimen and misses 2 consecutive periods, rule out pregnancy before continuing the contraceptive regimen.

After several months of treatment, menstrual flow may reduce to a point of virtual absence. This reduced flow may occur as a result of medication and is not indicative of pregnancy.

Postpartum administration – Postpartum administration in nonnursing mothers may begin at the first postpartum examination (4 to 6 weeks), regardless of whether spontaneous menstruation has occurred. Have the patient consider the possibility of ovulation and conception prior to initiation of medication. Also, the patient should start

Contraceptive Hormones

ORAL CONTRACEPTIVES

no earlier than 4 to 6 weeks after a midtrimester pregnancy termination. Immediate postpartum use is associated with increased risk of thromboembolism. If possible, nursing mothers should defer taking OCs until the infant is weaned (see Warnings).

If fully breastfeeding (not giving baby any food or formula), start the patient on POPs 6 weeks after delivery. If partially breastfeeding (giving baby some food or formula), the patient should start taking POPs by 3 weeks after delivery.

In the nonlactating mother, *Seasonale* may be initiated no earlier than day 28 postpartum for contraception because of the increased risk for thromboembolism. When the tablets are administered in the postpartum period, the increased risk of thromboembolic disease associated with the postpartum period must be considered. Advise the patient to use a nonhormonal backup method for the first 7 days of tablet-taking. However, if intercourse has already occurred, consider the possibility of ovulation and conception prior to initiation of medication. *Seasonale* may be initiated immediately after a first-trimester abortion; if the patient starts *Seasonale* immediately, additional contraceptive measures are not needed.

Dosage adjustments – Side effects noted during the initial cycles may be transient; if they continue, dosage adjustments may be indicated. Many side effects are related to the potency of the estrogen or progestin in the products. The following table summarizes these dose-related side effects.

Achieving Proper Hormonal Balance in an Oral Contraceptive			
Estrogen		Progestin	
Excess	Deficiency	Excess	Deficiency
Nausea, bloating Cervical mucorrhea, polyposis Melasma Hypertension Migraine headache Breast fullness or tenderness Edema	Early or mid-cycle breakthrough bleeding Increased spotting Hypomenorrhea	Increased appetite Weight gain Tiredness, fatigue Hypomenorrhea Acne, oily scalp[a] Hair loss, hirsutism[a] Depression Monilial vaginitis Breast regression	Late breakthrough bleeding Amenorrhea Hypermenorrhea

[a] Result of androgenic activity of progestins.

Pharmacological Effects of Progestins Used in Oral Contraceptives[a]			
	Progestin	Estrogen	Androgen
Desogestrel	++++	0	+++
Levonorgestrel	++++	0	++++
Norgestrel	+++	0	+++
Ethynodiol diacetate	++	+++	+
Norgestimate	++	0	++
Norethindrone acetate	++	++	++
Norethindrone	++	++	++

[a] Symbol Key: ++++ – pronounced effect; +++ – moderate effect; ++ – low effect; + – slight effect; 0 – no effect

Minimize the above effects by adjusting the estrogen/progestin balance or dosage. The following table categorizes products by their estrogenic, progestational, and androgenic activity. Because overall activity is influenced by the interaction of components, including androgenic and antiestrogenic activity, it is difficult to precisely classify products; placement in the table is only approximate. Differences between products within a group are probably not clinically significant.

Estimated Relative Oral Contraceptive Progestin/Estrogen/Androgen Activity					
	Ingredients	Brand-name examples	Progestin activity	Estrogen activity	Androgen activity
Monophasic	0.1 mg levonorgestrel/ 20 mcg EE[a]	Alesse, Aviane, Lessina, Levlite	Low	Low	Low
	0.25 mg norgestimate/35 mcg EE	Ortho-Cyclen, Sprintec		Intermediate	
	0.5 mg norethindrone/35 mcg EE	Brevicon, Modicon, Necon 0.5/35, Nortrel 0.5/35		High	
	0.4 mg norethindrone/35 mcg EE	Ovcon-35			
	0.15 mg levonorgestrel/30 mcg EE	Levlen, Levora, Nordette, Portia	Intermediate	Low	Intermediate
	0.3 mg norgestrel/30 mcg EE	Cryselle, Lo-Ovral, Low-Ogestrel			
	1 mg norethindrone/50 mcg mestranol	Necon 1/50, Norinyl 1+50, Ortho-Novum 1/50		Intermediate	
	1 mg norethindrone/35 mcg EE	Necon 1/35, Norinyl 1+35, Nortrel 1/35, Ortho-Novum 1/35		High	
	1 mg norethindrone/50 mcg EE	Ovcon-50			
	1 mg norethindrone acetate/20 mcg EE	Loestrin 21 1/20, Loestrin Fe 1/20, Microgestin Fe 1/20	High	Low	
	1.5 mg norethindrone acetate/30 mcg EE	Loestrin 21 1.5/30, Loestrin Fe 1.5/30, Microgestin Fe 1.5/30			High
	1 mg ethynodiol diacetate/35 mcg EE	Demulen 1/35, Zovia 1/35E			Low
	Desogestrel/EE 0.15 mg-20 mcg and EE 10 mcg	Kariva, Mircette			
	0.15 mg desogestrel/30 mcg EE	Apri, Desogen, Ortho-Cept	High	Intermediate	
	1 mg ethynodiol diacetate/50 mcg EE	Demulen 1/50, Zovia 1/50E			
	0.5 mg norgestrel/50 mcg EE	Ovral, Ogestrel		High	High
	3 mg drospirenone/30 mcg EE	Yasmin	No data	Intermediate[b]	None[b]
Biphasic	Norethindrone/EE 0.5-35/1-35 mg-mcg	Necon 10/11, Ortho-Novum 10/11	Intermediate	High	Low
Triphasic	Norgestimate/EE 0.18-25/0.215-25/0.25-25 mg-mcg	Ortho Tri-Cyclen Lo	Low	Low	
	Levonorgestrel/EE 0.05-30/0.075-40/0.125-30 mg-mcg	Enpresse, Tri-Levlen, Triphasil, Trivora		Intermediate	
	Norgestimate/EE 0.18-35/0.215-35/0.25-35 mg-mcg	Ortho Tri-Cyclen			
	Norethindrone/EE 0.5-35/1-35/0.5-35 mg-mcg	Tri-Norinyl		High	
	Norethindrone/EE 0.5-35/0.75-35/1-35 mg-mcg	Necon 7/7/7, Ortho-Novum 7/7/7	Intermediate		
	Norethindrone/EE 1-20/1-30/1-35 mg-mcg	Estrostep 21, Estrostep Fe	High	Low	Intermediate
	Desogestrel/EE 0.1-25/0.125-25/0.15-25 mg-mcg	Cyclessa			Low

[a] EE = ethinyl estradiol.

[b] Preclinical studies have shown that drospirenone has no androgenic, estrogenic, glucocorticoid, antiglucocorticoid, or antiandrogenic activity.

Contraceptive Hormones

ORAL CONTRACEPTIVES

Actions

➤*Pharmacology:* OCs include estrogen-progestin combinations and POPs.

Progestin-only – Progestin-only oral contraceptives prevent conception by suppressing ovulation in ≈ 50% of users, thickening the cervical mucus to inhibit sperm penetration, lowering the midcycle luteinizing hormone (LH) and follicle-stimulating hormone (FSH) peaks, slowing the movement of the ovum through the fallopian tubes, and altering the endometrium.

Combination OCs – Combination OCs inhibit ovulation by suppressing the gonadotropins, FSH, and LH. Additionally, alterations in the genital tract, including cervical mucus (which inhibits sperm penetration) and the endometrium (which reduces the likelihood of implantation), may contribute to contraceptive effectiveness.

These products differ in the type and relative potency of the components and in the relative predominance of estrogenic or progestational activity. Their ultimate effects are related to combined estrogenic, progestational, androgenic, and antiestrogenic effects.

Progestins may modify the effects of estrogens; these effects depend on the type or amount of progestin present and the ratio of progestin to estrogen. Dosage, potency, length of administration, and concomitant estrogen administration contribute to total progestational potency, making it difficult to establish equivalent doses of progestins. The total estrogenic potency of an OC is based on the combined effects of the estrogen and the estrogenic/antiestrogenic/androgenic effect of the progestin.

See the table in the Administration and Dosage section for a summary of the effects of the various progestins. Although not in the table, note that drospirenone is a spironolactone analog with antimineralocorticoid activity. Preclinical studies have shown that drospirenone has no androgenic, estrogenic, glucocorticoid, antiglucocorticoid, or antiandrogenic activity.

Contraceptive efficacy – In a study comparing the efficacy and safety of *Plan B* (1 tablet of 0.75 mg levonorgestrel taken within 72 hours of intercourse and 1 tablet taken 12 hours later) with the Yuzpe regimen (2 tablets of 0.25 mg levonorgestrel and 0.05 mg ethinyl estradiol taken within 72 hours of intercourse and 2 tablets taken 12 hours later), *Plan B* was at least as effective as the Yuzpe regimen in preventing pregnancy. After a single act of intercourse, the expected pregnancy rate of 8% (with no contraception) was reduced to ≈ 1% with *Plan B*. Thus, *Plan B* reduced the expected number of pregnancies by 89%.

If 100 women used emergency contraceptive pills (ECPs) correctly in 1 month, ≈ 2 women would become pregnant after a single act of intercourse. The use of ECPs results in a 75% reduction in the number of pregnancies expected if no ECPs were used after unprotected intercourse. Some clinical trials have shown that efficacy was greatest when ECPs were taken within 24 hours of unprotected intercourse; the efficacy decreases somewhat during each subsequent 24-hour period.

ECPs are not as effective as other forms of contraception. Efficacy in most cases depends greatly upon degree of compliance and user reliability. No other contraceptive drug or device, except levonorgestrel implant and medroxyprogesterone injection, approaches the efficacy of the combined OCs. For effectiveness rates of other contraceptive methods, refer to the following table.

Pregnancy Rates for Various Means of Contraception (%)[a]		
Method of contraception	Lowest expected[b]	Typical[c]
Oral contraceptives		3
Combined	0.1	5
Progestin-only	0.5	5
Mechanical/Chemical		
Levonorgestrel implant	0.09	0.09
Medroxyprogesterone injection	0.3	0.3
IUD		
Progesterone	1.5	2
Copper T 380A	0.8	0.6
LNg 20	0.1	0.1
Cervical cap		
Parous	26	40
Nulliparous	9	20
Condom		
Without spermicide	3	14
With spermicide[d]	1.8	4 to 6
Spermicide alone	6	26
Diaphragm (with spermicidal cream or gel)	6	20
Female condom	5	21
Periodic abstinence (ie, rhythm; all methods)	1 to 9	25

Pregnancy Rates for Various Means of Contraception (%)[a]		
Method of contraception	Lowest expected[b]	Typical[c]
Sterility		
Vasectomy	0.1	0.15
Tubal ligation	0.5	0.5
No contraception	85	85

[a] During first year of continuous use.
[b] Best guess of percentage expected to experience an accidental pregnancy among couples who initiate a method and use it consistently and correctly.
[c] A "typical" couple who initiate a method and experience an accidental pregnancy.
[d] Used as a separate product (not in condom package).

There are 3 types of combination OCs, monophasic, biphasic, and triphasic. The biphasic and triphasic OCs are intended to deliver hormones in a fashion similar to physiologic processes.

Monophasic – There is a fixed dosage of estrogen to progestin throughout the cycle.

Biphasic – The amount of estrogen remains the same for the first 21 days of the cycle. A decreased progestin:estrogen ratio in the first half of the cycle allows endometrial proliferation. An increased ratio in the second half provides adequate secretory development.

Triphasic – The estrogen amount remains the same while the progestin changes, or the dose of both estrogen and progestin change during the cycle.

Noncontraceptive health benefits – The following health benefits related to the use of combination OCs are supported by epidemiological studies that largely utilized OC formulations containing estrogen doses ≥ 35 mcg ethinyl estradiol or 50 mcg mestranol.

Effects on menses: Increased menstrual cycle regularity, decreased blood loss and decreased incidence of iron deficiency anemia, decreased incidence of dysmenorrhea.

Effects related to inhibition of ovulation: Decreased incidence of functional ovarian cysts and ectopic pregnancies.

Other effects: Decreased incidence of fibroadenomas and fibrocystic disease of the breast, acute pelvic inflammatory disease, endometrial cancer, ovarian cancer, maintenance of bone density, and decreased symptomatic endometriosis.

➤*Pharmacokinetics:*

Estrogens – Ethinyl estradiol is rapidly absorbed with peak concentrations attained within 2 hours. It undergoes considerable first-pass elimination. Mestranol is demethylated to ethinyl estradiol. Ethinyl estradiol is 97% to 98% bound to plasma albumin. Half-life varies from 6 to 20 hours. It is excreted in bile and urine as conjugates and undergoes some enterohepatic recirculation.

Progestins – Peak concentrations of norethindrone occur 0.5 to 4 hours after oral administration; it undergoes first-pass metabolism with an overall bioavailability of ≈ 65%. Levonorgestrel reaches peak concentrations between 0.5 to 2 hours, does not undergo a first-pass effect, and is completely bioavailable. Norethindrone and levonorgestrel are chiefly metabolized by reduction followed by conjugation. Desogestrel is rapidly and completely absorbed and converted into 3-keto-desogestrel, the biologically active metabolite. Relative bioavailability is ≈ 84%. Maximum concentrations of the metabolite are reached at ≈ 1.4 hours. Norgestimate is well absorbed; peak serum concentrations are observed within 2 hours followed by a rapid decline to levels generally below assay within 5 hours. However, a major metabolite, 17-deacetyl norgestimate, appears rapidly in serum with concentrations greatly exceeding that of the parent. Both norethynodrel and ethynodiol diacetate are converted to norethindrone. Peak serum concentrations of drospirenone are reached 1 to 3 hours after administration. Progestins are bound to albumin (79% to 95%) and to sex hormone binding globulin (except drospirenone). Terminal half-life of the progestins are as follows: Norethindrone, 5 to 14 hours; levonorgestrel, 11 to 45 hours; desogestrel (metabolite), 38 ± 20 hours; norgestimate (metabolite), 12 to 30 hours; drospirenone, 30 hours. Progestin-only administration results in lower steady-state serum progestin levels and a shorter elimination half-life than coadministration with estrogens.

Contraindications

Thrombophlebitis; thromboembolic disorders (eg, valvular heart disease with thrombogenic complications); history of deep-vein thrombophlebitis; cerebral vascular disease; MI; coronary artery disease; known or suspected breast carcinoma or estrogen-dependent neoplasia; carcinoma of endometrium; hepatic adenomas/carcinomas (see Warnings); undiagnosed abnormal genital bleeding; known or suspected pregnancy (see Warnings); cholestatic jaundice of pregnancy/jaundice with prior pill use; hypersensitivity to any component of the product; acute liver disease; uncontrolled hypertension; headaches with focal neurological symptoms; diabetes with vascular complications; major surgery with prolonged immobility.

➤*Yasmin:* Renal insufficiency, hepatic dysfunction, adrenal insufficiency, heavy smoking (15 or more cigarettes per day) and older than 35 years of age.

ORAL CONTRACEPTIVES

Warnings

▶*Smoking:* Cigarette smoking increases the risk of serious cardiovascular side effects from OCs. This risk increases with age and with heavy smoking (≥ 15 cigarettes per day) and is quite marked in women > 35 years of age. Women who use OCs should not smoke.

▶*Hyperkalemia: Yasmin* contains the progestin drospirenone that has antimineralocorticoid activity, including the potential for hyperkalemia in high-risk patients, comparable with 25 mg spironolactone. *Yasmin* should not be used in patients with conditions that predispose to hyperkalemia (eg, renal insufficiency, hepatic dysfunction, adrenal insufficiency). Women receiving daily, long-term treatment for chronic conditions or diseases with medications that may increase serum potassium should have their serum potassium level checked during the first treatment cycle. Drugs that may increase serum potassium include ACE inhibitors, angiotensin-II receptor antagonists, potassium-sparing diuretics, heparin, aldosterone antagonists, and NSAIDs.

▶*Risks of OC use:* The use of OCs is associated with increased risk of thromboembolism, stroke, MI, hypertension, hepatic neoplasia, and gallbladder disease, although risk of serious morbidity or mortality is very small in healthy women without underlying risk factors. Risk of morbidity/mortality increases significantly in the presence of other underlying risk factors such as hypertension, hyperlipidemias, obesity, and diabetes.

▶*Mortality:* Mortality associated with all methods of birth control is low and below that associated with childbirth, with the exception of OC use in women ≥ 35 years of age who smoke and ≥ 40 years of age who do not smoke. In 1989, the Fertility and Maternal Health Drugs Advisory Committee concluded that although cardiovascular disease risk may be increased with OC use in healthy nonsmoking women older than 40 years of age (even with the newer low-dose formulations), there also are greater potential health risks associated with pregnancy in older women and with the alternative surgical and medical procedures that may be necessary if such women do not have access to effective and acceptable means of contraception. Therefore, the committee recommended that the benefits of low-dose OC use by healthy nonsmoking women > 40 years of age may outweigh the possible risks. Of course, like all women, older women who take oral contraceptives should take an oral contraceptive that contains the least amount of estrogen and progestin that is compatible with a low failure rate and individual patient needs.

▶*Thromboembolism:* Be alert to the earliest symptoms of thromboembolic and thrombotic disorders. Should any of these occur or be suspected, discontinue the drug immediately.

In 1998, the American College of Obstetrics and Gynecology Committee on Gynecologic Practice reconfirmed that the risks of nonfatal venous thromboembolism for healthy, nonpregnant nonusers of OCs is 4 cases per 100,000 woman-years vs 10 to 15 cases per 100,000 woman-years and 20 to 30 cases per 100,000 woman-years for users of second- and third-generation OCs, respectively. The risk for pregnant women is 60 cases per 100,000 woman-years. The committee confirms that the risk of nonfatal venous thrombosis with third-generation OCs (desogestrel, gestodene, and norgestimate) is 2 to 3 times the risk of second-generation OCs. The risk of development of deep vein thrombosis was found to be 2 to 5 times higher with low-estrogen, desogestrel-containing OCs than with second-generation monophasic and triphasic preparations. The committee stated that the decision regarding the use of third-generation OCs should be left to the clinician and patient because they might have benefit in some cases (eg, patients requiring suppression of ovarian androgens or those with conditions for which they might be advantageous).

MI – MI risk associated with OC use is increased. This risk is primarily in smokers or women with other underlying risk factors for coronary artery disease such as hypertension, hypercholesterolemia, morbid obesity, and diabetes. The risk is very low in women < 30 years of age. It is estimated that the relative risk of heart attack for current OC users is 2 to 6.

Long-term use – Data suggest that the increased risk of MI persists after discontinuation of long-term OC use; the highest risk group includes women 40 to 49 years of age who used OCs for ≥ 5 years.

Smoking – Smoking in combination with OC use has been shown to contribute substantially to the incidence of MIs in women in their mid-30s or older, with smoking accounting for the majority of excess cases. Mortality rates associated with circulatory disease have been shown to increase substantially in smokers, especially in those ≥ 35 years of age who use OCs.

Cerebrovascular diseases – OCs increase the risk of cerebrovascular events (thrombotic and hemorrhagic strokes), although, in general, the risk is greatest in hypertensive women> 35 years of age who also smoke. Relative risk of thrombotic strokes ranges from 3 (normotensive users) to 14 (severe hypertensive users). Relative risk of hemorrhagic stroke for OC users is 1.2 for nonsmokers, 7.6 for smokers, 1.8 for normotensives, and 25.7 for severe hypertensives; for nonuser smokers, risk is 2.6. The attributable risk also is greater in older women.

Vascular disease – A positive association is observed between the amount of estrogen and progestin in OCs and the risk of vascular disease. A decline in serum high-density lipoproteins (HDL) has occurred with progestins and has been associated with an increased incidence of ischemic heart disease. Because estrogens increase HDL cholesterol, the net effect depends on a balance achieved between doses of estrogen and progestin and the activity of the progestin used in the contraceptives.

Age – The risk of cerebrovascular and circulatory disease in OC users is substantially increased in women ≥ 35 years of age with other risk factors (eg, smoking, uncontrolled hypertension, hypercholesterolemia [LDL 190], obesity, diabetes). Mortality rates associated with circulatory disease have been shown to increase substantially in smokers > 35 years of age and nonsmokers > 40 years of age among women who use OCs. Current clinical practice involves use of lower-estrogen dose formulations combined with careful restriction of OC use to women who do not have the various risk factors listed.

Postsurgical thromboembolism – Risk is increased 2- to 4-fold. If possible, discontinue OCs ≥ 4 weeks before and 2 weeks after surgery and during and following prolonged immobilization because OCs are associated with an increased incidence of thromboembolism.

Subarachnoid hemorrhage – Subarachnoid hemorrhage has been increased by OC use. Smoking alone increases the incidence of these accidents; smoking and OC use appear to work together to produce a combined risk greater than either alone.

Persistence of risk – An increased risk may persist for ≥ 6 years after discontinuation of OC use for cerebrovascular disease and ≥ 9 years for MI in users 40 to 49 years of age who had used OCs ≥ 5 years; this risk was not demonstrated in other age groups. This information is based on studies that used OC formulations containing ≥ 50 mcg estrogen.

NOTE – The associations between OCs and cardiovascular disease are based on epidemiological studies whose conclusions have been criticized for the following reasons: National trends of cardiovascular mortality are incompatible with these risk estimates; excess deaths may not be attributable entirely to smoking; the clinical diagnosis of thromboembolism is often unreliable.

▶*Ocular lesions:* Ocular lesions such as retinal thrombosis have been associated with the use of OCs. Discontinue medication if there is unexplained loss of vision, onset of proptosis or diplopia, papilledema, or retinal vascular lesions. Immediately undertake appropriate diagnostic therapeutic measures.

▶*Carcinoma:* Numerous epidemiological studies have been performed on the incidence of breast, endometrial, ovarian, and cervical cancer in women using OCs. While there are conflicting reports, the overall evidence in the literature suggests that use of OCs is not associated with an increase in the risk of developing breast cancer, regardless of age and parity of first use. The Cancer and Steroid Hormone study also showed no latent effect on the risk of breast cancer for at least a decade following long-term use. Some studies have shown an increased relative risk of developing breast cancer, particularly at a younger age and apparently related to duration of use. These studies have predominantly involved combined oral contraceptives; there is insufficient data to determine whether the use of POPs similarly increases the risk. Women with breast cancer should not use OCs because the role of female hormones in breast cancer has not been fully determined. Most studies have not shown such a risk; methodologies of earlier studies have been questioned. According to the CDC, there is a small subset of premenopausal-associated breast cancers, but there is no proof of cause and effect; there is no association with the postmenopausal variety.

Some studies suggest that OC use has been associated with an increase in the risk of cervical intraepithelial neoplasia in some populations of women. There is insufficient data to determine whether the use of POPs increases the risk of developing cervical intraepithelial neoplasia. There continues to be controversy about the extent to which such findings may be because of differences in sexual behavior and other factors. Other epidemiologic studies have suggested an increased risk of cervical dysplasia and carcinoma.

In spite of many studies of the relationship between OC use and breast and cervical cancers, a cause and effect relationship has not been established.

Studies have reported an increased risk of endometrial carcinoma associated with the prolonged use of estrogen in postmenopausal women. However, the risk appears to be decreased in OC users because of the progestin component. In fact, there is a protective effect; users appear about half as likely to develop ovarian and endometrial cancer as women who have never used OCs. The protective effect from endometrial cancer lasts up to 15 years after the pills are stopped.

There appears to be no increased risk of breast cancer in OC users or any subgroup of users, although the CDC states that there may be an association with a subset of young, premenopausal users. There is no increased risk of breast cancer in OC users with prior benign breast disease. Another study suggests that use prior to the first full-term pregnancy was associated with a significant relative risk of breast cancer especially when OC use began before 25 years of age.

ORAL CONTRACEPTIVES

Close clinical surveillance of all women taking OCs is essential; they should be reexamined at least once a year. In all cases of undiagnosed persistent or recurrent abnormal vaginal bleeding, rule out malignancy. Monitor women with a strong family history of breast cancer or who have breast nodules, fibrocystic disease of the breast, cervical dysplasia, or abnormal mammograms.

►*Hepatic lesions (eg, adenomas, focal nodular hyperplasia, hepatocellular carcinoma):* Benign and malignant hepatic adenomas have been associated with the use of OCs, but this is a relatively rare disease. Severe abdominal pain, shock, or death may be caused by rupture and hemorrhage of a liver tumor. Fortunately, this is quite rare; there may be some association with higher-dose mestranol preparations or duration (greater after ≥ 4 years) of OC use. While hepatic adenoma is uncommon, consider it in women presenting with abdominal pain and tenderness, abdominal mass, or shock. A few cases of hepatocellular carcinoma have been reported in women taking OCs long-term; however, an association has not been established.

►*Gallbladder disease:* Earlier studies have reported an increased risk of gallbladder surgery in OC users. More recent studies, however, have shown that the relative risk of developing gallbladder disease among OC users may be minimal. These recent findings may be related to the use of OC formulations containing lower estrogen and progestin doses.

►*Carbohydrate metabolism:* Glucose tolerance may decrease, which is directly related to estrogen dose. Progestins increase insulin secretion and create insulin resistance. These effects vary with different agents. However, OCs appear to have no effect on fasting blood glucose in nondiabetic women. Observe prediabetic and diabetic patients receiving OCs. In a recent study, OC users were less likely to develop diabetes than nonusers.

►*Lipid profile:* A small proportion of women will have persistent hypertriglyceridemia while using OCs. Changes in serum triglycerides and lipoprotein levels have been reported in OC users.

►*Elevated blood pressure:* Elevated blood pressure and hypertension may occur within a few months of beginning use. The prevalence increases with the duration of use and age. Incidence of hypertension may directly correlate with increasing dosages of progestin.

Encourage women with a history of hypertension, renal disease, or hypertension-related diseases during pregnancy to use another method of contraception. Monitor these patients if they choose to use OCs. Discontinue the OC if elevated blood pressure occurs. High blood pressure returns to normal in most women after OC discontinuation.

►*Headaches:* Onset or exacerbation of migraine or development of headache with focal neurological symptoms of a new pattern that is recurrent, persistent, or severe, requires OC discontinuation and evaluation.

►*Bleeding irregularities:* BTB and spotting are sometimes encountered in OC patients, especially during the first 3 months of use. BTB, spotting, and amenorrhea are frequent reasons for discontinuing OCs. The type and dose of progestin may be important. In BTB, consider nonhormonal causes. In undiagnosed persistent or recurrent abnormal vaginal bleeding, rule out pregnancy or malignancy. If amenorrhea occurs, rule out pregnancy. If pathology has been excluded, time or formulation change may resolve the problem. Changing to an OC with a higher estrogen content may minimize menstrual irregularity, but consider the increased risk of thromboembolic disease. Consider short-term estrogen supplements.

It was thought that women with a history of oligomenorrhea or secondary amenorrhea or young women without regular cycles may tend to remain anovulatory or become amenorrheic after discontinuation of OCs; however, this is not certain. Other factors may play a role in the development of amenorrhea after OC withdrawal, including stress, previous menstrual irregularity, psychiatric conditions, and marked weight loss. Also, the incidence may have been much higher when higher-dose products were used more regularly. Advise patients of this possibility.

Seasonale – When prescribing *Seasonale*, the convenience of fewer planned menses (4 per year instead of 13 per year) should be weighed against the inconvenience of increased intermenstrual bleeding and/or spotting. More *Seasonale* subjects, compared with subjects on the 28-day cycle regimen enrolled in a clinical trial, discontinued prematurely for unacceptable bleeding (7.7% with *Seasonale* vs 1.8% of 28-day cycle regimen).

Progestin-only products – Episodes of irregular, unpredictable spotting, and BTB within the first year are the most frequently encountered side effects and are the major reasons why women discontinue OC use.

►*Risks of use immediately preceding pregnancy:* Some extensive epidemiological studies have revealed no increased risk of birth defects in OC users prior to pregnancy.

►*Menopause:* Treatment with OCs may mask the onset of the climacteric.

►*Fertility impairment:* Fertility impairment may occur in women discontinuing OCs; however, impairment diminishes with time. In nulliparous women 25 to 29 years of age, the effect is negligible after 48 months. Among nulliparous women 30 to 34 years of age, impairment persists up to 72 months and appears more severe. For parous women, the effect is negligible and short-lived after cessation of contraception.

The limited available data indicated a rapid return of normal ovulation and fertility following discontinuation of progestin-only OCs.

►*Pregnancy: Category X.* Rule out pregnancy before initiating or continuing OCs and always consider it if withdrawal bleeding does not occur. Rule out pregnancy before continuing OCs for any patient who has missed 2 consecutive periods. If the patient has not adhered to the prescribed schedule, consider the possibility of pregnancy at the time of the first missed period and withhold further use until pregnancy has been ruled out. If pregnancy is confirmed, apprise the patient of the potential risks to the fetus. The majority of recent studies do not indicate a teratogenic effect, particularly cardiac anomalies and limb reduction defects, when OCs are taken inadvertently during early pregnancy.

The use of female sex hormones (eg, estrogens) during early pregnancy may seriously damage the offspring (see the Warning Box in the Estrogens monograph). However, there is no conclusive evidence that OC use is associated with an increase in birth defects when taken inadvertently during early pregnancy. Previously, a few studies reported that OCs might be associated with birth defects, but these findings have not been seen in more recent studies. Nevertheless, do not use during pregnancy unless clearly necessary.

Do not administer OCs to induce withdrawal bleeding as a test for pregnancy.

Do not use OCs during pregnancy to treat threatened or habitual abortion.

Ectopic pregnancy – Ectopic pregnancy, as well as intrauterine pregnancy, may occur in contraceptive failures.

The incidence of ectopic pregnancies for progestin-only OC users is 5 per 1000 women-years. Up to 10% of pregnancies reported in clinical studies of progestin-only OC users are extrauterine. Although symptoms of ectopic pregnancy should be watched for, a history of ectopic pregnancy need not be considered a contraindication for use of this contraceptive method. Health care providers should be alert to the possibility of an ectopic pregnancy in women who become pregnant or complain of lower abdominal pain while on progestin-only OCs.

►*Lactation:* Combination OCs given in the postpartum period may interfere with lactation, decreasing the quantity and quality of breast milk. Furthermore, a small amount of OC steroids is excreted in breast milk. A few adverse effects on the nursing infant have been reported, including jaundice and breast enlargement. If possible, defer use until the infant has been weaned; however, in some situations, breastfeeding is the only real alternative (see Administration and Dosage).

Small amounts of progestin pass into the breast milk resulting in steroid levels in infant plasma of 1% to 6% of maternal plasma levels.

►*Children:* Safety and efficacy has been established in women of reproductive age. Safety and efficacy are expected to be the same for postpubertal adolescents ≤ 16 years of age. Use of these products before menarche is not indicated.

Precautions

►*Monitoring:* It is good medical practice for all women to have annual history and physical examinations, including women using OCs. Physical examination may be deferred until after initiation of OCs if requested by the patient and judged appropriate by the health care provider. The physical exam should evaluate blood pressure, breasts, abdomen, and pelvic organs, including Pap smear. Perform preventative measures (ie, ensure up to date vaccinations) and screening, which should include total and HDL cholesterol within 5-year intervals. Advise the pathologist of OC therapy when relevant specimens are submitted. Do not prescribe for > 1 year without another physical exam.

►*Lipid disorders:* Closely follow women taking OCs who are being treated for hyperlipidemias. Some progestins may elevate LDL levels and decrease HDL levels (see Warnings), making hyperlipidemia control more difficult. Consider witholding the OC if the dyslipidemia does not respond (ie, LDL of 190).

HDL and total cholesterol may be increased, LDL may be increased or decreased, while LDL/HDL ratio may be decreased and triglycerides unchanged.

►*Uterine fibroids:* Pre-existing uterine leiomyomata (uterine fibroids) may increase in size. However, there is no evidence of this with low-dose OCs. In addition, data indicate that the risk of developing uterine fibroids is actually reduced with OC use.

►*Depression:* The incidence of depression in OC users ranges from < 5% to 30%. Pyridoxine deficiency may be a factor in the depression. Pyridoxine 25 to 50 mg per day has been recommended. In patients with a history of depression, discontinue if depression recurs to a serious degree. Patients becoming significantly depressed should discontinue medication to determine if the symptom is drug-related.

ORAL CONTRACEPTIVES

➤*Fluid retention:* OCs may cause fluid retention; prescribe with caution and monitor patients with conditions that might be aggravated by fluid retention (eg, convulsive disorders; migraine syndrome; asthma; cardiac, hepatic, or renal dysfunction).

➤*Hepatic function:* Patients with a history of jaundice during pregnancy have an increased risk of recurrence of jaundice; if jaundice develops, discontinue use. Steroid hormones may be poorly metabolized in patients with liver dysfunction; administer with caution.

➤*Contact lenses:* Contact lens wearers who develop changes in vision or lens tolerance should be assessed by an ophthalmologist; consider temporary or permanent cessation of wear.

➤*Serum folate levels:* Serum folate levels may be depressed by therapy. Although OCs may impair folate metabolism, the effect is mild and unlikely to cause anemia or megaloblastic changes in women who have a good dietary folate intake. Because the pregnant woman is predisposed to folate deficiency, a woman who becomes pregnant shortly after stopping therapy may have a greater chance of developing folate deficiency and its attendant complications. Folic acid supplements are recommended.

➤*Acute intermittent porphyria:* Estrogens have been reported to precipitate attacks of acute intermittent porphyria; use with caution in susceptible patients.

➤*Vomiting/Diarrhea:* Several cases of OC failure have been reported in association with vomiting or diarrhea. If significant GI disturbance occurs, a backup method of contraception for the remainder of the cycle is recommended.

➤*Sexually transmitted diseases (STDs):* Advise patients that OCs do not protect against HIV infection and other STDs.

➤*Tartrazine sensitivity:* Some of these products contain tartrazine, which may cause allergic-type reactions (including bronchial asthma) in susceptible individuals. Although the incidence of tartrazine sensitivity in the general population is low, it is frequently seen in patients who also have aspirin hypersensitivity. Specific products containing tartrazine are identified in the product listings.

Drug Interactions

Oral Contraceptive Drug Interactions

Precipitant drug	Object drug[*]		Description
Contraceptives, oral	Anticoagulants	⬌	Because OCs can increase levels of certain circulating clotting factors and reduce antithrombin III levels, therapeutic efficacy of the anticoagulants may be decreased by OCs. However, both an increased and decreased effect has occurred.
Contraceptives, oral	Antidepressants, tricyclic Beta blockers Caffeine Corticosteroids Theophyllines	↑	The hepatic metabolism of these agents may be decreased by OCs, resulting in increased therapeutic effects or toxicity.
Contraceptives, oral	Benzodiazepines	↑↓	OCs may increase the clearance of the benzodiazepines that undergo glucuronidation (eg, lorazepam, oxazepam, temazepam) because of increased metabolism. Combination OCs with alprazolam, chlordiazepoxide, diazepam, and triazolam may inhibit hepatic mixed-function oxidases leading to a decrease in benzodiazepine oxidation rate (may prolong the half-life of benzodiazepines).
Contraceptives, oral	Cyclosporine	↑	OCs may inhibit the metabolism of cyclosporine, increasing the risk of toxicity. Avoid this combination if possible. If given together, monitor cyclosporine concentrations, as well as renal and hepatic function. Adjust cyclosporine dose as indicated.
Contraceptives, oral	Lamotrigine	↓	OCs may increase lamotrigine metabolism, therefore decreasing the therapeutic effect.
Contraceptives, oral	Selegiline	↑	Coadministration may increase selegiline concentrations because of inhibition of its metabolism.

Oral Contraceptive Drug Interactions

Precipitant drug	Object drug[*]		Description
Antibiotics	Contraceptives, oral	↓	Coadministration of griseofulvin, penicillins, or tetracyclines with OCs may decrease the pharmacologic effects of the OCs, possibly because of altered steroid gut metabolism secondary to changes in the intestinal flora. Menstrual irregularities (eg, spotting, BTB) and pregnancy may occur. An alternate or additional form of birth control may be advisable during concomitant use. OCs and troleandomycin may be associated with an increased risk of intrahepatic cholestasis.
Atorvastatin	Contraceptives, oral	↑	Coadministration increased AUC values for norethindrone and ethinyl estradiol approximately 30% and 20%, respectively.
Barbiturates Carbamazepine Felbamate Griseofulvin Hydantoins[a] Modafinil Oxcarbazepine Phenytoin Protease inhibitors Rifamycins St. John's wort	Contraceptives, oral	↓	These agents may increase the hepatic metabolism of the OCs via hepatic microsomal enzyme induction, possibly resulting in decreased effectiveness of the OC; menstrual irregularities (eg, spotting, BTB) and pregnancy may occur. An alternate or additional form of birth control may be advisable during concomitant use.

[*] ↑ = Object drug increased. ↓ = Object drug decreased. ⬌ = Undetermined clinical effect.
[a] Pharmacologic effects of the hydantoins also may be altered.

➤*Drug/Lab test interactions:* Estrogen-containing OCs may cause the following alterations in serum, plasma, or blood, unless specified otherwise.

Increased – Factors I (prothrombin), VII, VIII, IX, X; fibrinogen; norepinephrine-induced platelet aggregation; thyroid-binding globulin (TBG), leading to increased total thyroid hormone (as measured by protein bound iodine, T_4 by column or radioimmunoassay); corticosteroid levels; triglycerides and phospholipids; aldosterone; amylase; gamma-glutamyltranspeptidase; iron-binding capacity; sex-hormone-binding globulins are increased and result in elevated levels of total circulating sex steroids (combination) and corticoids; transferrin; prolactin; renin activity; vitamin A.

Decreased – Antithrombin III; free T_3 resin uptake; response to metyrapone test; folate; glucose tolerance; albumin; cholinesterase; haptoglobin; tissue plasminogen activator; zinc; vitamin B_{12}; sex-hormone-binding globulin, thyroxine caused by decrease in thyroid-binding globulin (progestin-only).

Adverse Reactions

Serious – See Warnings. Arterial thromboembolism; cerebral hemorrhage; cerebral thrombosis; coronary thrombosis; gallbladder disease; hepatic adenomas or benign liver tumors; hypertension; mesenteric thrombosis MI; pulmonary embolism; thrombophlebitis and venous thrombosis with or without embolism.

➤*CNS:* Dizziness; headache; mental depression; migraine.

➤*Dermatologic:* Melasma (may persist); rash (allergic).

➤*Endocrine:* Breast tenderness, enlargement, secretion; diminution in lactation when given immediately postpartum.

➤*GI:* Abdominal cramps; bloating; cholestatic jaundice; nausea and vomiting (occurring in ≈ 10% to 30% of patients during the first cycle, less common with low doses, and the majority resolve in 3 months).

➤*GU:* Amenorrhea during and after treatment; BTB (the majority, > 80%, resolve in 3 months), spotting, change in menstrual flow; change in cervical erosion and secretions; invasive cervical cancer;temporary infertility after discontinuation; vaginal candidiasis.

➤*Ophthalmic:* Changes in corneal curvature (steepening); contact lens intolerance; neuro-ocular lesions (eg, retinal thrombosis, optic neuritis).

➤*Miscellaneous:* Edema; reduced carbohydrate tolerance; weight change (increase or decrease); prevalence of cervical chlamydia trachomatis may be increased; hirsutism (rare).

The following associations have been neither confirmed nor refuted: acne; acute hepatitis; anemia; Budd-Chiarri syndrome;cataracts; cerebrovascular disease with mitral valve prolapse; changes in appetite; changes in libido; colitis; colonic Crohn disease; cystitis-like syndrome; dizziness; EEG abnormalities; endometrial, cervical, and breast carcinoma (conflicting data; see Warnings); erythema multiforme; erythema nodosum; fatigue; gingivitis; headache; hemolytic uremic syndrome; hemorrhagic eruption; herpes gestationis; hirsutism; itching; loss of scalp hair; lupus erythematosus or lupus-like syndromes; malignant hypertension; malignant melanoma; nervousness; pancreatitis; por-

ORAL CONTRACEPTIVES

phyria; photosensitivity;pituitary tumors; premenstrual syndrome; pulmonary embolism; renal function impairment; rhinitis; sickle cell disease; vaginitis.

►*Emergency contraceptives:* The most common adverse events in the clinical trial for women receiving emergency contraceptives include the following: abdominal pain/cramps; breast tenderness; diarrhea; dizziness; fatigue; headache; menstrual irregularities; nausea; vomiting.

Overdosage

Serious ill effects have not been reported following acute overdosage of OCs in young children. Overdosage may cause nausea. Withdrawal bleeding may occur in females.

Patient Information

Patient package insert available with product.

To achieve maximum contraceptive effectiveness, inform the patient to take OCs exactly as directed at intervals not exceeding 24 hours, preferably at the same time each day, including throughout all bleeding episodes.Inform the patient to take tablets regularly with a meal or at bedtime. Efficacy depends on strict adherence to the dosage schedule. Missing a pill can cause spotting or light bleeding; the patient may be a little sick to her stomach on the days she takes the missed pill with her regularly scheduled pill. For missed doses, see Administration and Dosage.

Advise the patient to use a backup method (eg, condoms, spermicides) for the following 48 hours whenever a progestin-only OC is taken ≥ 3 hours late.

If pregnancy is terminated within the first 12 weeks, instruct the patient to start OCs immediately or within 7 days. If pregnancy is terminated after 12 weeks, instruct the patient to start OCs after 2 weeks.

OCs may cause spotting or BTB during the first few months of therapy; if bleeding occurs in > 1 cycle or lasts more than a few days, advise the patient to notify the health care provider.

Advise the patient to inform the health care provider of prolonged episodes of bleeding, amenorrhea, or severe abdominal pain.

Advise the patient to use an additional method of birth control until after the first week of administration in the initial cycle or for the entire cycle if vomiting or diarrhea occurs.

Inform patients that OCs do not protect against HIV infection and other STDs.

MONOPHASIC ORAL CONTRACEPTIVES

	Product & Distributor	Estrogen (mcg)	Progestin (mg)	How Supplied
Rx	Necon 1/50 (Watson)	50 mestranol	1 norethindrone	Lactose. (WATSON 510). Lt. blue. In 21s and 28s. With 7 white inert tablets (WATSON P) in the 28s.
Rx	Norinyl 1 + 50 (Watson)			Lactose. (Watson 265). White. In *Wallette* 28s. With 7 orange inert tablets (Watson P1).
Rx	Ortho-Novum 1/50 (Ortho-McNeil)			Lactose. (Ortho 150). Yellow. In *Dialpak* 28s. With 7 green inert tablets.
Rx	Ovcon-50 (Warner Chilcott)	50 ethinyl estradiol	1 norethindrone	Lactose. (MJ 584). Yellow. In 28s. With 7 green, capsule shape inert tablets (MJ 850).
Rx	Demulen 1/50 (Searle)		1 ethynodiol diacetate	Lactose (inert tablets). (SEARLE 71). White. In *Compack* tablet dispensers of 21s and 28s. With 7 pink inert tablets (SEARLE P) in the 28s.
Rx	Zovia 1/50E (Watson)			Lactose. (WATSON 384). Pink. In 21s and 28s. With 7 white inert tablets (WATSON P) in the 28s.
Rx	Ovral (Wyeth-Ayerst)		0.5 norgestrel	Lactose. (WYETH 56). White. In *Pilpak* 21s and 28s. With 7 pink inert tablets (WYETH 445) in the 28s.
Rx	Ogestrel 0.5/50 (Watson)			Lactose. (Watson 848). White. In 28s. With 7 peach inert tablets (Watson P1).
Rx	Necon 1/35 (Watson)	35 ethinyl estradiol	1 norethindrone	Lactose. (WATSON 508). Dk. yellow. In 21s and 28s. With 7 white inert tablets (WATSON P) in the 28s.
Rx	Norinyl 1 + 35 (Watson)			Lactose. (WATSON 259). Yellow-green. In *Wallette* 28s. With 7 orange inert tablets (WATSON P1).
Rx	Nortrel 1/35 (Barr)			Lactose. (b 949). Yellow. In 21s and 28s. With 7 white inert tablets (b 944) in the 28s.
Rx	Ortho-Novum 1/35 (Ortho-McNeil)			Lactose. (Ortho 135). Peach. In *Dialpak* and *Veridate* 28s. With 7 green inert tablets (Ortho).
Rx	Brevicon (Watson)		0.5 norethindrone	Lactose. (Watson 254). Blue. In *Wallette* 28s. With 7 orange inert tablets (Watson P1).
Rx	Modicon (Ortho-McNeil)			Lactose. (Ortho 535). White. In *Dialpak* and *Veridate* 28s. With 7 green inert tablets (Ortho).
Rx	Necon 0.5/35 (Watson)			Lactose. (WATSON 507). Lt. yellow. In 21s and 28s. With 7 white inert tablets (WATSON P) in the 28s.
Rx	Nortrel 0.5/35 (Barr)			Lactose. (b 941). Lt. yellow. In 21s and 28s. With 7 white inert tablets (b 944) in the 28s.
Rx	Ovcon-35 (Warner Chilcott)		0.4 norethindrone	Lactose. (MJ 583). Peach. In 21s and 28s. With 7 green capsule shape inert tablets (MJ 850) in the 28s.
Rx	MonoNessa (Watson)		0.25 norgestimate	(Watson 526). Blue. In 28s.
Rx	Ortho-Cyclen (Ortho-McNeil)			Lactose. (Ortho 250). Blue. In *Dialpak* and *Veridate* 28s. With 7 green inert tablets.
Rx	Sprintec (Barr)			Lactose. (b 987). Blue. In 28s. With 7 white inert tablets (b 143).
Rx	Demulen 1/35 (Searle)		1 ethynodiol diacetate	Lactose (inert tablets). (SEARLE 151). White. In *Compack* tablet dispensers of 21s and 28s. With 7 blue inert tablets (SEARLE P) in the 28s.
Rx	Zovia 1/35E (Watson)			Lactose. (WATSON 383). Lt. pink. In 21s and 28s. With 7 white inert tablets (WATSON P) in the 28s.

MONOPHASIC ORAL CONTRACEPTIVES

	Product & Distributor	Estrogen (mcg)	Progestin (mg)	How Supplied
Rx	**Yasmin** (Berlex)	30 ethinyl estradiol	3 drospirenone	Lactose. Yellow. Film-coated. In blister pack 28s. With 7 white inert film-coated tablets.
Rx	**Junel Fe 1.5/30** (Barr)		1.5 norethindrone acetate	Pink. In 28s. With 7 brown tablets (75 mg ferrous fumarate per tablet).
Rx	**Loestrin 21 1.5/30** (Duramed)			Lactose, sugar. Green. In 21s.
Rx	**Loestrin Fe 1.5/30** (Duramed)			Lactose, sugar (active tablets), sucrose (inert tablets). Green. In 28s. With 7 brown tablets (75 mg ferrous fumarate per tablet).
Rx	**Microgestin Fe 1.5/30** (Watson)			Lactose. (WATSON 631). Green. In 28s. With 7 brown tablets (75 mg ferrous fumarate per tablet; WATSON 632).
Rx	**Cryselle** (Barr)		0.3 norgestrel	White. (dp 543). In 21s and 28s. With 7 lt. green inert tablets (dp 331).
Rx	**Lo/Ovral** (Wyeth-Ayerst)			Lactose. (Wyeth 78). White. In *Pilpak* 21s and 28s. With 7 pink inert tablets (Wyeth 486) in the 28s.
Rx	**Low-Ogestrel** (Watson)			Lactose. (WATSON 847). White. In 28s. With 7 peach inert tablets (WATSON P1).
Rx	**Desogen** (Organon)		0.15 desogestrel	Lactose. (Organon T_5R). White. In 28s. With 7 green inert tablets (Organon K_2H).
Rx	**Ortho-Cept** (Ortho-McNeil)			Lactose. Orange. In *Dialpak* and *Veridate* 28s. With 7 green inert tablets.
Rx	**Apri** (Barr)			Lactose. (dp 575). Rose. In blister card 28s. With 7 white inert tablets (dp 570).
Rx	**Levlen** (Berlex)		0.15 levonor-gestrel	Lactose . (B 28). Lt. orange. In slidecase dispenser with 7 pink inert tablets.
Rx	**Levora** (Watson)			Lactose. (15/30 WATSON). White. In 28s. With 7 peach inert tablets (WATSON P1).
Rx	**Nordette** (Monarch)			Lactose. (WYETH 75). Lt. orange. In *Pilpak* 21s and 28s. With 7 pink inert tablets (WYETH 486) in the 28s.
Rx	**Portia** (Barr)			Lactose. (b 992). Pink. Film-coated. In 21s and 28s. With 7 white inert tablets (b 208) in the 28s.
Rx	**Seasonale**[a] (Duramed)			Lactose. (S 62). Pink. Film-coated. In 91s with 7 white inert tablets (S 197).
Rx	**Alesse** (Wyeth-Ayerst)	20 ethinyl estradiol	0.1 levonorgestrel	Lactose. (W 912). Pink. In 28s. With 7 lt. green inert tablets (W 650).
Rx	**Aviane** (Barr)			Lactose. (dp 016). Orange. In 28s. With 7 lt. green inert tablets (dp 519).
Rx	**Lessina** (Barr)			Lactose. (b 965). Pink. Film-coated. In 21s and 28s. With 7 white inert tablets (b 208) in the 28s.
Rx	**Levlite** (Berlex)			Lactose, sucrose. (B 22). Pink. In slidecase dispensers of 28s. With 7 white inert tablets (B 29).
Rx	**Junel Fe 1/20** (Barr)		1 norethindrone acetate	Lt. Yellow. In 28s. With 7 brown tablets (75 mg ferrous fumarate per tablet).
Rx	**Loestrin 21 1/20** (Duramed)			Lactose, sugar. White. In 21s.
Rx	**Loestrin Fe 1/20** (Duramed)			Lactose, sugar (active tablets), sucrose (inert tablets). White. In 28s. With 7 brown tablets (75 mg ferrous fumarate per tablet).
Rx	**Microgestin Fe 1/20** (Watson)			Lactose. (WATSON 630). White. In 28s. With 7 brown tablets (75 mg ferrous fumarate per tablet; WATSON 632).
Rx	**Kariva**[b] (Barr)	20 ethinyl estradiol (white tablets)/10 ethinyl estradiol (lt. blue tablets)	0.15 desogestrel (white tablets only)	Lactose. 21 white tablets (021) and 5 lt. blue tablets (022). In blister card 28s. With 2 lt. green inert tablets (331).
Rx	**Mircette**[c] (Organon)	20 ethinyl estradiol (white tablets)/10 ethinyl estradiol (yellow tablets)	0.15 desogestrel (white tablets only)	Lactose. 21 white tablets (T_4R Organon) and 5 yellow tablets (K_2S Organon). In blister card 28s. With 2 green inert tablets (K_2H Organon).
Rx	**Solia** (Prasco)	30 ethinyl estradiol	0.15 desogestrel	Lactose. 21 white tablets (T_5R Prasco). In blister card 28s. With 7 green inert tablets (K_2H Prasco).

[a] Take 1 pink (active) tablet per day for 84 consecutive days, followed by 7 days of white (inert) tablets.
[b] Take 1 white tablet daily for 21 days, followed by 1 light-green (inert) tablet daily for 2 days and 1 light-blue (active) tablet daily for 5 days.
[c] Take 1 white tablet daily for 21 days, followed by 1 green (inert) tablet daily for 2 days and 1 yellow (active) tablet daily for 5 days.

For complete prescribing information, refer to the Oral Contraceptives group monograph. The combination therapy products are listed in order of decreasing estrogen content.

BIPHASIC ORAL CONTRACEPTIVES

	Product	Phase 1	Phase 2	How Supplied
Rx	**Necon 10/11** (Watson)	0.5 mg norethindrone, 35 mcg ethinyl estradiol (10 lt. yellow tablets)	1 mg norethindrone, 35 mcg ethinyl estradiol (11 dk. yellow tablets)	Lactose. Lt. yellow = (WATSON 507). Dk. yellow = (WATSON 508). In 28s with 7 white inert tablets (WATSON P).
Rx	**Ortho-Novum 10/11** (Ortho-McNeil)	0.5 mg norethindrone, 35 mcg ethinyl estradiol (10 white tablets)	1 mg norethindrone, 35 mcg ethinyl estradiol (11 peach tablets)	Lactose. White = (Ortho 535). Peach = (Ortho 135). In *Dialpak* 28s. With 7 green inert tablets (Ortho).

For complete prescribing information, refer to the Oral Contraceptives group monograph. The combination therapy products are listed in order of decreasing estrogen content.

TRIPHASIC ORAL CONTRACEPTIVES

	Product	Phase 1	Phase 2	Phase 3	How Supplied
Rx	**Tri-Norinyl** (Watson)	0.5 mg norethindrone, 35 mcg ethinyl estradiol (7 blue tablets)	1 mg norethindrone, 35 mcg ethinyl estradiol (9 yellow-green tablets)	0.5 mg norethindrone, 35 mcg ethinyl estradiol (5 blue tablets)	Lactose. Blue = (Watson 254). Yellow-green = (Watson 259). In *Wallette* 28s. With 7 orange inert tablets (Watson P1).
Rx	**Necon 7/7/7** (Watson)	0.5 mg norethindrone, 35 mcg ethinyl estradiol (7 white tablets)	0.75 mg norethindrone, 35 mcg ethinyl estradiol (7 lt. peach tablets)	1 mg norethindrone, 35 mcg ethinyl estradiol (7 peach tablets)	In 28s. With 7 green inert tablets.
Rx	**Ortho-Novum 7/7/7** (Ortho-McNeil)				Lactose. White = (Ortho 535). Lt. peach = (Ortho 75). Peach = (Ortho 135). In *Dialpak* and *Veridate* 28s. With 7 green inert tablets (Ortho).
Rx	**Enpresse** (Barr)	0.05 mg levonorgestrel, 30 mcg ethinyl estradiol (6 pink tablets)	0.075 mg levonorgestrel, 40 mcg ethinyl estradiol (5 white tablets)	0.125 mg levonorgestrel, 30 mcg ethinyl estradiol (10 orange tablets)	Lactose. Pink = (dp 510). White = (dp 511). Orange = (dp 512). In 28s. With 7 lt. green inert tablets (dp 519).

Contraceptive Hormones

TRIPHASIC ORAL CONTRACEPTIVES

	Product	Phase 1	Phase 2	Phase 3	How Supplied
Rx	Tri-Levlen (Berlex)	0.05 mg levonorgestrel, 30 mcg ethinyl estradiol (6 brown tablets)	0.075 mg levonorgestrel, 40 mcg ethinyl estradiol (5 white tablets)	0.125 mg levonorgestrel, 30 mcg ethinyl estradiol (10 lt. yellow tablets)	Lactose. Brown = (B 95). Film-coated. White to off-white = (B 96). Film-coated. Lt. yellow = (B 97). Film-coated. In slidecase dispenser 28s. With 7 lt. green film-coated inert tablets (B 11).
Rx	Triphasil (Wyeth Labs)				Lactose. Brown = (W 641). White = (W 642). Lt. yellow = (W 643). In 21s and 28s. With 7 lt. green inert tablets (W 650) in the 28s.
Rx	Trivora (Watson)	0.05 mg levonorgestrel, 30 mcg ethinyl estradiol (6 blue tablets)	0.075 mg levonorgestrel, 40 mcg ethinyl estradiol (5 white tablets)	0.125 mg levonorgestrel, 30 mcg ethinyl estradiol (10 pink tablets)	Lactose. Blue, white, and pink tablets. In 28s. With 7 peach inert tablets (WATSON P1).
Rx	Velivet (Barr)	0.1 mg desogestrel, 25 mcg ethinyl estradiol (7 beige tablets)	0.125 mg desogestrel, 25 mcg ethinyl estradiol (7 orange tablets)	0.15 mg desogestrel, 25 mcg ethinyl estradiol (7 pink tablets)	With 7 white inert tablets. (b 334). In 28s.
Rx	Ortho Tri-Cyclen (Ortho-McNeil)	0.18 mg norgestimate, 35 mcg ethinyl estradiol (7 white tablets)	0.215 mg norgestimate, 35 mcg ethinyl estradiol (7 lt. blue tablets)	0.25 mg norgestimate, 35 mcg ethinyl estradiol (7 blue tablets)	Lactose. White = (Ortho 180). Lt. blue = (Ortho 215). Blue = (Ortho 250). In *Dialpak* and *Veridate* 28s. With 7 green inert tablets.
Rx	Tri-Previfem (Teva)				Lactose. White = (746). Lt. blue = (747). Blue = (748). In 28s. With 7 teal tablets.
Rx	TriNessa (Watson)				With 7 green inert tablets. In 28s.
Rx	Tri-Sprintec (Barr)	0.18 mg norgestimate, 35 mcg ethinyl estradiol (7 gray tablets)	0.215 mg norgestimate, 35 mcg ethinyl estradiol (7 lt. blue tablets)	0.25 mg norgestimate, 35 mcg ethinyl estradiol (7 blue tablets)	Lactose. Gray = (b 985). Lt. blue = (b 986). Blue = (b 987). White = (b 143). With 7 white inert tablets. In 28s.
Rx	Ortho Tri-Cyclen Lo (Ortho-McNeil)	0.18 mg norgestimate, 25 mcg ethinyl estradiol (7 white tablets)	0.215 mg norgestimate, 25 mcg ethinyl estradiol (7 lt. blue tablets)	0.25 mg norgestimate, 25 mcg ethinyl estradiol (7 dk. blue tablets)	Talc (green inert tablets), lactose. White = (O-M 180). Lt. blue = (O-M 215). Dk. blue = (O-M 250). In *Dialpak* and *Veridate* 28s. With 7 green inert tablets.
Rx	Estrostep 21 (Pfizer)	1 mg norethindrone acetate, 20 mcg ethinyl estradiol (5 triangular tablets)	1 mg norethindrone acetate, 30 mcg ethinyl estradiol (7 square tablets)	1 mg norethindrone acetate, 35 mcg ethinyl estradiol (9 round tablets)	Lactose. White. In 21s.
Rx	Estrostep Fe (Warner Chilcott)	1 mg norethindrone acetate, 20 mcg ethinyl estradiol (5 triangular tablets)	1 mg norethindrone acetate, 30 mcg ethinyl estradiol (7 square tablets)	1 mg norethindrone acetate, 35 mcg ethinyl estradiol (9 round tablets)	Lactose (white), sucrose (brown). White. In 28s. With 7 brown tablets (75 mg ferrous fumarate per tablet).
Rx	Cyclessa (Organon)	0.1 mg desogestrel, 25 mcg ethinyl estradiol (7 lt. yellow tablets)	0.125 mg desogestrel, 25 mcg ethinyl estradiol (7 orange tablets)	0.15 mg desogestrel, 25 mcg ethinyl estradiol (7 red tablets)	Lactose, talc. Lt. yellow = (T_0R Organon). Orange = (T_6R Organon). Red = (T_1R Organon). In 28s. With 7 green inert tablets (K_2H Organon).

For complete prescribing information, refer to the Oral Contraceptives group monograph. The combination therapy products are listed in order of decreasing estrogen content.

PROGESTIN-ONLY PRODUCTS

Rx	Camila (Barr)	**Tablets:** 0.35 mg norethindrone	Lactose. (b 715). Lt. pink. In 28s.
Rx	Errin (Barr)		Lactose. (b 344). Yellow. In 28s.
Rx	Jolivette (Watson)		Lactose. (WATSON 892). Green. In 28s.
Rx	Nor-QD (Watson)		Lactose. Yellow. In 28s.
Rx	Nora-BE (Watson)		Lactose. (Watson 629). White. In 28s.
Rx	Ortho Micronor (Ortho-McNeil)		Lactose. Green. In *Dialpak* 28s.
Rx	Ovrette (Wyeth-Ayerst)	**Tablets:** 0.075 mg norgestrel	Tartrazine, lactose. (WYETH 62). Yellow. In *Pilpak* 28s.

For complete prescribing information, refer to the Oral Contraceptives group monograph.

Administration and Dosage

Administer daily, starting on the first day of menstruation. The patient should take 1 tablet at the same time every day; administration is continuous, with no interruption between pill packs.

▶*Postpartum administration:* If patient is fully breastfeeding (not giving baby any food or formula), she may start taking progestin-only pills (POPs) 6 weeks after delivery. If she is partially breastfeeding (giving some food or formula), she should start taking POPs by 3 weeks after delivery.

▶*Switching pills:* If switching from the combined pills to POPs, the patient should take the first POP the day after the last active combined pill is finished. She should not take any of the 7 inactive pills from the combined pill pack. If switching from POPs to the combined pills, she should take the first active combined pill on the first day of menses, even if the POP pack is not finished. If switching to another brand of POPs, the patient should start the new brand any time. If the patient is breastfeeding, she can switch to another method of birth control at any time, except she cannot switch to the combined pills until breastfeeding is stopped or at least until 6 months after delivery.

▶*Missed dose:* If the patient is more than 3 hours late or misses at least 1 tablet, she should take a missed pill as soon as remembered, then go back to taking POPs at the regular time, but be sure to use a backup contraceptive method (eg, condom, spermicide) every time she has sexual intercourse for the next 48 hours.

▶*Storage/Stability:* Store at 25°C (77°F); excursions permitted to 15° to 30°C (59° to 86°F).

EMERGENCY CONTRACEPTIVES

Rx	Plan B (Duramed)	**Tablets:** 0.75 mg levonorgestrel	Lactose. (INOR). White. In blister packages of 2.
Rx	Preven (Gynétics)	**Tablets:** 0.25 mg levonorgestrel, 0.05 mg ethinyl estradiol	Lactose. (G 891). Blue. Film-coated. In blister packages of 4s.[a]

[a] Also available in a kit that contains a pregnancy test.

Indications

▶*Emergency contraception:* For prevention of pregnancy following unprotected intercourse or a known or suspected contraceptive failure. To obtain optimal efficacy, the first dose should be taken as soon as possible within 72 hours of intercourse. The second dose must be taken 12 hours later.,

Administration and Dosage

The *Preven* emergency contraceptive kit contains a pregnancy test. This test can be used to verify an existing pregnancy resulting from intercourse that occurred earlier in the current menstrual cycle or in the previous cycle. If a positive pregnancy result is obtained, advise the patient not to take the pills in the kit.

The patient should take 1 (*Plan B*) or 2 (*Preven*) tablets as soon as possible within 72 hours after unprotected intercourse. She should take the second dose of 1 (*Plan B*) or 2 (*Preven*) tablets 12 hours later. Emergency contraception can be used at any time during the menstrual cycle.

Instruct the user that if vomiting occurs within 1 hour of taking either dose of medication, to contact her health care professional to discuss whether or not to repeat that dose or take an antinausea medication.

Emergency contraceptive pills are not indicated for ongoing pregnancy protection and should not be used as a woman's routine form of contraception. Emergency contraceptives are not effective in terminating an existing pregnancy.,

▶*Storage/Stability:* Store at 25°C (77°F); excursions permitted to 15° to 30°C (59° to 86°F).,

NORELGESTROMIN/ETHINYL ESTRADIOL TRANSDERMAL SYSTEM

	Product	Release Rate	Surface Area (cm²)	Total Content	How Supplied
Rx	Ortho Evra (Ortho-McNeil)	0.15 mg norelgestromin, 0.02 mg ethinyl estradiol/ 24 h	20	6 mg norelgestromin, 0.75 mg ethinyl estradiol/patch	In cycles (3 patches) and single patches.

WARNING

Cigarette smoking increases the risk of serious cardiovascular side effects from hormonal contraceptive use. This risk increases with age and with heavy smoking (≥ 15 cigarettes per day) and is quite marked in women > 35 years of age. Strongly advise women who use hormonal contraceptives, including the norelgestromin/ethinyl estradiol transdermal patch, not to smoke.

Indications

➤*Contraception:* For prevention of pregnancy.

Administration and Dosage

➤*Approved by the FDA:* November 20, 2001.

➤*Use:* This system uses a 28-day (4-week) cycle. A new patch is applied each week for 3 weeks (21 days total). Week 4 is patch-free. Withdrawal bleeding is expected to begin during this time.

Apply every new patch on the same day of the week. This day is known as the "Patch Change Day." For example, if the first patch is applied on a Monday, apply all subsequent patches on a Monday. Wear only 1 patch at a time.

On the day after week 4 ends, a new 4-week cycle is started by applying a new patch. Under no circumstances should there be more than a 7 day patch-free interval between dosing cycles.

The patient must choose 1 option –

First day start: For first day start, the woman should apply her first patch during the first 24 hours of her menstrual period.

If therapy starts after day 1 of the menstrual cycle, a nonhormonal back-up contraceptive (eg, condoms, spermicide, diaphragm) should be used concurrently for the first 7 consecutive days of the first treatment cycle.

Sunday start: For Sunday start, the woman should apply her first patch on the first Sunday after her menstrual period starts. She must use back-up contraception for the first week of her first cycle.

If the menstrual period begins on a Sunday, the first patch should be applied on that day and no back-up contraception is needed.

➤*Application:* Apply the patch to clean, dry, intact, healthy skin on the buttock, abdomen, upper outer arm, or upper torso in a place where it will not be rubbed by tight clothing. The patch should not be placed on skin that is red, irritated, or cut, nor should it be placed on the breasts.

To prevent interference with the adhesive properties of the patch, no make-up, creams, lotions, powders, or other topical products should be applied to the skin area where the patch is or will be placed.

Patch changes may occur at any time on the change day. Apply each new patch to a new spot on the skin to help avoid irritation, although they may be kept within the same anatomic area.

➤*If a patch is partially or completely detached:*

For < 1 day (up to 24 hours) – The woman should try to reapply it to the same place or replace it with a new patch immediately. No back-up contraception is needed. The woman's "patch change day" will remain the same.

For > 1 day (≥ 24 hours) or if the woman is not sure how long the patch has been detached – The woman may not be protected from pregnancy. She should stop the current contraceptive cycle and start a new cycle immediately by applying a new patch. There is now a new "day 1" and a new "patch change day." Back-up contraception (eg, condoms, spermicide, diaphragm) must be used for the first week of the new cycle.

A patch should not be reapplied if it is no longer sticky, if it has become stuck to itself or another surface, if it has other material stuck to it, or if it has previously become loose or fallen off. If a patch cannot be reapplied, a new patch should be applied immediately. Supplemental adhesives or wraps should not be used to hold the patch in place.

➤*If the woman forgets to change her patch:*

At the start of any patch cycle (week 1/day 1) – She may not be protected from pregnancy. She should apply the first patch of the new cycle as soon as she remembers. There is now a new "patch change day" and a new "day 1." The woman must use back-up contraception (eg, condoms, spermicide, diaphragm) for the first week of the new cycle.

In the middle of the patch cycle (week 2/day 8 or week 3/day 15) –

For 1 or 2 days (up to 48 hours): She should apply a new patch immediately. The next patch should be applied on the usual "patch change day." No back-up contraception is needed.

For > 2 days (≥ 48 hours): She may not be protected from pregnancy. She should stop the current contraceptive cycle and start a new 4-week

cycle immediately by putting on a new patch. There is now a new "patch change day" and a new "day 1." The woman must use back-up contraception for 1 week.

At the end of the patch cycle (week 4/day 22) – If the woman forgets to remove her patch, she should take it off as soon as she remembers. The next cycle should be started on the usual "patch change day," which is the day after day 28. No back-up contraception is needed.

Under no circumstances should there be more than a 7-day patch-free interval between cycles. If there are > 7 patch-free days, the woman may not be protected from pregnancy and back-up contraception (eg, condoms, spermicide, diaphragm) must be used for 7 days. As with combined oral contraceptives, the risk of ovulation increases with each day beyond the recommended drug-free period. If intercourse has occurred during such an extended patch-free interval, the possibility of fertilization should be considered.

➤*Change day adjustment:* If the woman wishes to change her patch change day, she should complete her current cycle, removing the third patch on the correct day. During the patch-free week, she may select an earlier patch change day by applying a new patch on the desired day. In no case should there be > 7 consecutive patch-free days.

➤*Switching from an oral contraceptive:* Treatment with the norelgestromin/ethinyl estradiol transdermal patch should begin on the first day of withdrawal bleeding. If there is no withdrawal bleeding within 5 days of the last active (hormone-containing) tablet, pregnancy must be ruled out. If therapy starts later than the first day of withdrawal bleeding, a nonhormonal contraceptive should be used concurrently for 7 days. If > 7 days elapse after taking the last active oral contraceptive tablet, the possibility of ovulation and conception should be considered.

➤*Use after childbirth:* Women who elect not to breastfeed should start contraceptive therapy with the norelgestromin/ethinyl estradiol transdermal patch no sooner than 4 weeks after childbirth. If a woman begins using the patch postpartum and has not yet had a period, the possibility of ovulation and conception occurring prior to use of the patch should be considered, and she should be instructed to use an additional method of contraception (eg, condoms, spermicide, diaphragm) for the first 7 days.

➤*Use after abortion or miscarriage:* After an abortion or miscarriage that occurs in the first trimester, the patch may be started immediately. An additional method of contraception is not needed if the patch is started immediately. If use of the patch is not started within 5 days following a first trimester abortion, the woman should follow the instructions for a woman starting the patch for the first time. In the meantime, she should be advised to use a nonhormonal contraceptive method. Ovulation may occur within 10 days after an abortion or miscarriage.

The patch should be started no earlier than 4 weeks after a second trimester abortion or miscarriage. When the patch is used postpartum or postabortion, the increased risk of thromboembolic disease must be considered.

➤*Breakthrough bleeding or spotting:* In the event of breakthrough bleeding or spotting (bleeding that occurs on the days that the patch is worn), continue treatment. If breakthrough bleeding persists longer than a few cycles, a cause other than the patch should be considered.

In the event of no withdrawal bleeding (bleeding that should occur during the patch-free week), treatment should be resumed on the next scheduled change day. If the patch has been used correctly, the absence of withdrawal bleeding is not necessarily an indication of pregnancy. Nevertheless, the possibility of pregnancy should be considered, especially if absence of withdrawal bleeding occurs in 2 consecutive cycles. Discontinue the patch if pregnancy is confirmed.

➤*Skin irritation:* If patch use results in uncomfortable irritation, the patch may be removed and a new patch may be applied to a different location until the next change day. Only 1 patch should be worn at a time.

➤*Missed menstrual period:* If the woman has not adhered to the prescribed schedule, the possibility of pregnancy should be considered at the time of the first missed period. Discontinue hormonal contraceptive use if pregnancy is confirmed.

If the woman has adhered to the prescribed regimen and misses 1 period, she should continue using her contraceptive patches.

If the woman has adhered to the prescribed regimen and misses 2 consecutive periods, pregnancy should be ruled out. Discontinue use of the patch if pregnancy is confirmed.

➤*Storage/Stability:* Store at 25°C (77°F); excursions permitted to 15° to 30°C (59° to 86°F). Store patches in their protective pouches. Apply immediately upon removal from the protective pouch. Do not store in the refrigerator or freezer. Used patches still contain some active hormones. Each patch should be carefully folded in half so that it

NORELGESTROMIN/ETHINYL ESTRADIOL TRANSDERMAL SYSTEM

sticks to itself before throwing it away.

Actions

►*Pharmacology:* Norelgestromin is the active progestin largely responsible for the progestational activity that occurs in women following application of norelgestromin/ethinyl estradiol transdermal patch. Norelgestromin also is the primary active metabolite produced following oral administration of norgestimate.

Combination oral contraceptives act by suppression of gonadotropins. Although the primary mechanism of this action is inhibition of ovulation, other alterations include changes in the cervical mucus (which increases the difficulty of sperm entry into the uterus) and the endometrium (which reduces the likelihood of implantation).

Receptor and human sex hormone-binding globulin (SHBG) binding studies, as well as studies in animals and humans, have shown that norgestimate and norelgestromin exhibit high progestational activity with minimal intrinsic androgenicity. Transdermally administered norelgestromin, in combination with ethinyl estradiol, does not counteract the estrogen-induced increases in SHBG, resulting in lower levels of free testosterone in serum compared with baseline.

►*Pharmacokinetics:*

Absorption – Following application of the product, norelgestromin and ethinyl estradiol rapidly appear in the serum, reach a plateau by ≈ 48 hours, and are maintained at an approximate steady state throughout the wear period. C_{ss} for norelgestromin and ethinyl estradiol during 1 week of patch wear are ≈ 0.6 to 0.8 ng/mL and 40 to 50 pg/mL, respectively, and are generally consistent from all studies and application sites.

Distribution – Norelgestromin and norgestrel (a serum metabolite of norelgestromin) are highly bound (> 97%) to serum proteins. Norelgestromin is bound to albumin and not to SHBG, while norgestrel is bound primarily to SHBG, which limits its biological activity. Ethinyl estradiol is extensively bound to serum albumin.

Metabolism – Because the patch is applied transdermally, first-pass metabolism (via the GI tract or liver) of norelgestromin and ethinyl estradiol that would be expected with oral administration is avoided. Hepatic metabolism of norelgestromin occurs and metabolites include norgestrel, which is highly bound to SHBG, and various hydroxylated and conjugated metabolites. Ethinyl estradiol also is metabolized to various hydroxylated products and their glucuronide and sulfate conjugates.

Excretion – Following removal of patches, the elimination kinetics of norelgestromin and ethinyl estradiol were consistent for all studies with half-life values of ≈ 28 hours and 17 hours, respectively. The metabolites of norelgestromin and ethinyl estradiol are eliminated by renal and fecal pathways.

Special populations – The effects of age, body weight, and body surface area on the pharmacokinetics of norelgestromin and ethinyl estradiol were evaluated. For norelgestromin and ethinyl estradiol, increasing age, body weight, and body surface area each were associated with slight decreases in C_{ss} and AUC values. However, only a small fraction (10% to 25%) of the overall variability in the pharmacokinetics of norelgestromin and ethinyl estradiol following application of the norelgestromin/ethinyl estradiol transdermal patch may be associated with any or all of the above demographic parameters.

►*Clinical trials:* In 3 large clinical trials, pregnancy rates were ≈ 1 per 100 women-years of norelgestromin/ethinyl estradiol transdermal patch use. With respect to weight, 5 of the 15 pregnancies reported with norelgestromin/ethinyl estradiol transdermal patch use were among women with a baseline body weight ≥ 90 kg (198 lbs), which constituted < 3% of the study population. The greater proportion of pregnancies among women ≥ 90 kg (198 lbs) was statistically significant and suggests that the norelgestromin/ethinyl estradiol transdermal patch may be less effective in these women.

One clinical trial assessed the return of hypothalamic-pituitary-ovarian axis function posttherapy and found that FSH, LH, and estradiol mean values, though suppressed during therapy, returned to near baseline values during the 6 weeks posttherapy.

Contraindications

Thrombophlebitis; thromboembolic disorders; history of deep vein thrombophlebitis or thromboembolic disorders; cerebrovascular or coronary artery disease (current or history); valvular heart disease with complications; severe hypertension; diabetes with vascular involvement; headaches with focal neurological symptoms; major surgery with prolonged immobilization; known or suspected carcinoma of the breast or personal history of breast cancer; carcinoma of the endometrium or other known or suspected estrogen-dependent neoplasia; undiagnosed abnormal genital bleeding; cholestatic jaundice of pregnancy or jaundice with prior hormonal contraceptive use; acute or chronic hepatocellular disease with abnormal liver function; hepatic adenomas or carcinomas; known or suspected pregnancy; hypersensitivity to any component of the product.

Warnings

►*Thromboembolic disorders and other vascular problems:*

Thromboembolism – An increased risk of thromboembolic and thrombotic disease associated with the use of hormonal contraceptives is well established. Case control studies have found the relative risk of users compared with nonusers to be 3 for the first episode of superficial venous thrombosis, 4 to 11 for deep vein thrombosis or pulmonary embolism, and 1.5 to 6 for women with predisposing conditions for venous thromboembolic disease. Cohort studies have shown the relative risk to be somewhat lower, ≈ 3 for new cases and ≈ 4.5 for new cases requiring hospitalization. The risk of thromboembolic disease associated with hormonal contraceptives is not related to length of use and disappears after hormonal contraceptive use is stopped. A 2- to 4-fold increase in relative risk of postoperative thromboembolic complications has been reported with the use of hormonal contraceptives. The relative risk of venous thrombosis in women who have predisposing conditions is twice that of women without such medical conditions. If feasible, hormonal contraceptives should be discontinued ≥ 4 weeks prior to and for 2 weeks after elective surgery of a type associated with an increase in risk of thromboembolism and during and following prolonged immobilization. Since the immediate postpartum period is also associated with an increased risk of thromboembolism, hormonal contraceptives should be started no earlier than 4 weeks after delivery in women who elect not to breastfeed.

In large clinical trials (n = 3330 with 1704 women-years of exposure), 1 case of nonfatal pulmonary embolism occurred during norelgestromin/ethinyl estradiol transdermal patch use, and 1 case of postoperative nonfatal pulmonary embolism also was reported with use of the patch. It is unknown if the risk of venous thromboembolism with norelgestromin/ethinyl estradiol transdermal patch use is different than with use of combination oral contraceptives.

As with any combination hormonal contraceptives, the clinician should be alert to the earliest manifestations of thrombotic disorders (thrombophlebitis, pulmonary embolism, cerebrovascular disorders, and retinal thrombosis). Should any of these occur or be suspected, discontinue norelgestromin/ethinyl estradiol transdermal patch use immediately.

MI – An increased risk of MI has been attributed to hormonal contraceptive use. This risk is primarily in smokers or women with other underlying risk factors for coronary artery disease (eg, hypertension, hypercholesterolemia, morbid obesity, diabetes). The relative risk of heart attack for current hormonal contraceptive users has been estimated to be 2 to 6, compared with nonusers. The risk is very low under 30 years of age.

Smoking in combination with oral contraceptive use has been shown to contribute substantially to the incidence of MIs in women in their mid-30s or older, with smoking accounting for the majority of excess cases. Mortality rates associated with circulatory disease have been shown to increase substantially in smokers, especially in those ≥ 35 years of age among women who use oral contraceptives.

Hormonal contraceptives may compound the effects of well-known risk factors (eg, hypertension, diabetes, hyperlipidemias, age, obesity). In particular, some progestins are known to decrease high density lipoprotein (HDL) cholesterol and cause glucose intolerance, while estrogens may create a state of hyperinsulinism. Hormonal contraceptives have been shown to increase blood pressure among some users. Similar effects on risk factors have been associated with an increased risk of heart disease. Hormonal contraceptives, including norelgestromin/ethinyl estradiol transdermal patch, must be used with caution in women with cardiovascular disease risk factors.

Norgestimate and norelgestromin have minimal androgenic activity. There is some evidence that the risk of MI associated with hormonal contraceptives is lower when the progestin has minimal androgenic activity than when the activity is greater.

Cerebrovascular diseases – Hormonal contraceptives have been shown to increase the relative and attributable risks of cerebrovascular events (thrombotic and hemorrhagic strokes), although, in general, the risk is greatest among older (> 35 years of age), hypertensive women who also smoke. Hypertension was found to be a risk factor for users and nonusers for both types of strokes, and smoking interacted to increase the risk of stroke.

In a large study, the relative risk of thrombotic strokes has been shown to range from 3 for normotensive users to 14 for users with severe hypertension. The relative risk of hemorrhagic stroke is reported to be 1.2 for nonsmokers who used hormonal contraceptives, 2.6 for smokers who did not use hormonal contraceptives, 7.6 for smokers who used hormonal contraceptives, 1.8 for normotensive users, and 25.7 for users with severe hypertension. The attributable risk is also greater in older women.

Dose-related risk – A positive association has been observed between the amount of estrogen and progestin in hormonal contraceptives and the risk of vascular disease. A decline in serum HDL has been reported with many progestational agents. A decline in serum HDL has been associated with an increased incidence of ischemic heart disease. Because estrogens increase HDL cholesterol, the net effect of a hormonal contraceptive depends on a balance achieved between doses of

NORELGESTROMIN/ETHINYL ESTRADIOL TRANSDERMAL SYSTEM

estrogen and progestin and the activity of the progestin used in the contraceptives. The activity and amount of both hormones should be considered in the choice of a hormonal contraceptive.

Persistence of risk – There are 2 studies that have shown persistence of risk of vascular disease for ever-users of combination hormonal contraceptives. In a study in the US, the risk of developing MI after discontinuing combination hormonal contraceptives persists for ≥ 9 years for women 40 to 49 years of age who had used combination hormonal contraceptives for ≥ 5 years, but this increased risk was not demonstrated in other age groups. In another study in Great Britain, the risk of developing cerebrovascular disease persisted for ≥ 6 years after discontinuation of combination hormonal contraceptives, although excess risk was very small. However, both studies were performed with combination hormonal contraceptive formulations containing ≥ 50 mcg of estrogens.

It is unknown whether norelgestromin/ethinyl estradiol transdermal patch is distinct from other combination hormonal contraceptives with regard to the occurrence of venous and arterial thrombosis.

➤*Mortality:* With the exception of combination oral contraceptive users ≥ 35 years of age who smoke, and ≥ 40 years of age who do not smoke, mortality associated with all methods of birth control is low and below that associated with childbirth.

In 1989, the Fertility and Maternal Health Drugs Advisory Committee was asked to review the use of combination hormonal contraceptives in women ≥ 40 years of age. The Committee concluded that although cardiovascular disease risks may be increased with combination hormonal contraceptive use after 40 years of age in healthy nonsmoking women (even with the newer low-dose formulations), there are also greater potential health risks associated with pregnancy in older women and with the alternative surgical and medical procedures that may be necessary if such women do not have access to effective and acceptable means of contraception. The Committee recommended that the benefits of low-dose combination hormonal contraceptive use by healthy nonsmoking women > 40 years of age may outweigh the possible risks.

Although the data are mainly obtained with oral contraceptives, this is likely to apply to norelgestromin/ethinyl estradiol transdermal patch as well. Women of all ages who use combination hormonal contraceptives should use the lowest possible dose formulation that is effective and meets their needs.

➤*Carcinoma:* Numerous epidemiological studies give conflicting reports on the relationship between breast cancer and combination oral contraceptive (COC) use. The risk of having breast cancer diagnosed may be slightly increased among current and recent users of COCs. However, this excess risk appears to decrease over time after COC discontinuation and by 10 years after cessation the increased risk disappears. Some studies report an increased risk with duration of use while other studies do not and no consistent relationships have been found with dose or type of steroid. Some studies have found a small increase in risk for women who first use COCs before 20 years of age. Most studies show a similar pattern of risk with COC use regardless of a woman's reproductive history or her family breast cancer history.

In addition, breast cancers diagnosed in current or ever oral contraceptive users may be less clinically advanced than in never-users.

Women who currently have or have had breast cancer should not use hormonal contraceptives because breast cancer is usually a hormonally sensitive tumor.

Some studies suggest that COC use has been associated with an increase in the risk of cervical intraepithelial neoplasia in some populations of women. However, there continues to be controversy about the extent to which such findings may be because of differences in sexual behavior and other factors.

In spite of many studies of the relationship between oral contraceptive use and breast and cervical cancers, a cause-and-effect relationship has not been established. It is not known whether norelgestromin/ethinyl estradiol transdermal patch is distinct from oral contraceptives with regard to the above statements.

➤*Hepatic neoplasia:* Benign hepatic adenomas are associated with hormonal contraceptive use, although the incidence of benign tumors is rare in the US. Indirect calculations have estimated the attributable risk to be in the range of 3.3 cases/100,000 for users, a risk that increases after ≥ 4 more years of use, especially with hormonal contraceptives containing ≥ 50 mcg of estrogen. Rupture of benign, hepatic adenomas may cause death through intra-abdominal hemorrhage.

Studies from Britain and the US have shown an increased risk of developing hepatocellular carcinoma in long-term (≥ 8 years) oral contraceptive users. However, these cancers are extremely rare in the US and the attributable risk (the excess incidence) of liver cancers in oral contraceptive users approaches < 1 per million users. It is unknown whether the norelgestromin/ethinyl estradiol transdermal patch is distinct from oral contraceptives in this regard.

➤*Ocular lesions:* There have been clinical case reports of retinal thrombosis associated with the use of hormonal contraceptives. Discon-

tinue the norelgestromin/ethinyl estradiol transdermal patch if there is unexplained partial or complete loss of vision, onset of proptosis or diplopia, papilledema, or retinal vascular lesions. Undertake appropriate diagnostic and therapeutic measures immediately.

➤*Risks of use before or during early pregnancy:* Extensive epidemiological studies have revealed no increased risk of birth defects in women who have used oral contraceptives prior to pregnancy.

➤*Gallbladder disease:* Earlier studies have reported an increased lifetime relative risk of gallbladder surgery in users of hormonal contraceptives and estrogens. More recent studies, however, have shown that the relative risk of developing gallbladder disease among hormonal contraceptive users may be minimal. The recent findings of minimal risk may be related to the use of hormonal contraceptive formulations containing lower hormonal doses of estrogens and progestins.

Combination hormonal contraceptives such as norelgestromin/ethinyl estradiol transdermal patch may worsen existing gallbladder disease and may accelerate the development of this disease in previously asymptomatic women. Women with a history of combination hormonal contraceptive-related cholestasis are more likely to have the condition recur with subsequent combination hormonal contraceptive use.

➤*Carbohydrate and lipid metabolic effects:* Glucose tolerance may decrease in some users. However, in nondiabetic women, combination hormonal contraceptives appear to have no effect on fasting blood glucose. Carefully monitor prediabetic and diabetic women in particular while taking combination hormonal contraceptives such as the norelgestromin/ethinyl estradiol transdermal patch.

A small proportion of women will have persistent hypertriglyceridemia while taking hormonal contraceptives. Changes in serum triglycerides and lipoprotein levels have been reported in hormonal contraceptive users.

➤*Elevated blood pressure:* Do not start women with significant hypertension on hormonal contraception. Encourage women with a history of hypertension or hypertension-related diseases, or renal disease to use another method of contraception. If women elect to use the norelgestromin/ethinyl estradiol transdermal patch, monitor them closely and if a clinically significant elevation of blood pressure occurs, discontinue the patch. For most women, elevated blood pressure will return to normal after stopping hormonal contraceptives, and there is no difference in the occurrence of hypertension between former and never-users.

An increase in blood pressure has been reported in women taking hormonal contraceptives, and this increase is more likely in older hormonal contraceptive users and with extended duration of use. Data from the Royal College of General Practitioners and subsequent randomized trials have shown that the incidence of hypertension increases with increasing progestational activity.

➤*Headaches:* The onset or exacerbation of migraine headache or the development of headache with a new pattern that is recurrent, persistent, or severe requires discontinuation of the norelgestromin/ethinyl estradiol transdermal patch and evaluation of the cause.

➤*Bleeding irregularities and patterns:* Breakthrough bleeding and spotting are sometimes encountered in women using the norelgestromin/ethinyl estradiol transdermal patch. Consider nonhormonal causes and take adequate diagnostic measures to rule out malignancy, other pathology, or pregnancy in the event of breakthrough bleeding, as in the case of any abnormal vaginal bleeding. If pathology has been excluded, time or a change to another contraceptive product may resolve the bleeding. In the event of amenorrhea, rule out pregnancy before initiating use of the norelgestromin/ethinyl estradiol transdermal patch.

Some women may encounter amenorrhea or oligomenorrhea after discontinuation of hormonal contraceptive use, especially when such a condition was pre-existent.

In the clinical trials, most women started their withdrawal bleeding on the fourth day of the drug-free interval, and the median duration of withdrawal bleeding was 5 to 6 days. On average, 26% of women per cycle had 7 or more total days of bleeding or spotting (this includes both withdrawal flow and breakthrough bleeding or spotting).

➤*Pregnancy:* Category X. Norelgestromin was tested for its reproductive toxicity in a rabbit developmental toxicity study by the SC route of administration. Doses of 0, 1, 2, 4, and 6 mg/kg body weight, which gave systemic exposure of ≈ 25 to 125 times the human exposure with the norelgestromin/ethinyl estradiol transdermal patch, were administered daily on gestation days 7 through 19. Malformations reported were paw hyperflexion at 4 and 6 mg/kg and paw hyperextension and cleft palate at 6 mg/kg.

Ectopic pregnancy – Ectopic as well as intrauterine pregnancy may occur in contraceptive failures.

➤*Lactation:* The effects of the norelgestromin/ethinyl estradiol transdermal patch in nursing mothers have not been evaluated and are unknown. Small amounts of combination hormonal contraceptive steroids have been identified in the milk of nursing mothers and a few adverse effects on the child have been reported, including jaundice and breast enlargement. In addition, combination hormonal contraceptives

NORELGESTROMIN/ETHINYL ESTRADIOL TRANSDERMAL SYSTEM

given in the postpartum period may interfere with lactation by decreasing the quantity and quality of breast milk. Long-term follow-up of infants whose mothers used combination hormonal contraceptives while breastfeeding has shown no deleterious effects. However, advise the nursing mother not to use the norelgestromin/ethinyl estradiol transdermal patch, but to use other forms of contraception until she has completely weaned her child.

►*Children:* Safety and efficacy are expected to be the same for postpubertal adolescents < 16 years of age and for users ≥ 16 years of age. Use of this product before menarche is not indicated.

Precautions

►*Sexually transmitted diseases:* Counsel patients that this product does not protect against HIV infection (AIDS) and other sexually transmitted diseases.

►*Body weight ≥ 90 kg (198 lbs):* Results of clinical trials suggest that the norelgestromin/ethinyl estradiol transdermal patch may be less effective in women with body weight ≥ 90 kg (198 lbs) than in women with lower body weights.

►*Hepatic function:* If jaundice develops in any woman using the norelgestromin/ethinyl estradiol transdermal patch, discontinue the medication. The hormones in the patch may be poorly metabolized in women with impaired liver function.

►*Fluid retention:* Steroid hormones like those in the norelgestromin/ethinyl estradiol transdermal patch may cause some degree of fluid retention. Prescribe this product with caution, and only with careful monitoring, in patients with conditions that might be aggravated by fluid retention.

►*Emotional disorders:* Women who become significantly depressed while using combination hormonal contraceptives such as the norelgestromin/ethinyl estradiol transdermal patch should stop the medication and use another method of contraception in an attempt to determine whether the symptom is drug-related. Carefully observe women with a history of depression and discontinue the product if significant depression occurs.

►*Contact lenses:* Contact lens wearers who develop visual changes or changes in lens tolerance should be assessed by an ophthalmologist.

Drug Interactions

Most drug interactions are based on oral contraceptives.

Transdermal Contraceptive Patch Drug Interactions			
Precipitant drug	Object drug*		Description
Acetaminophen	Contraceptives, oral	↑	Ethinyl estradiol plasma levels may increase, whereas acetaminophen plasma concentrations may decrease.
Contraceptives, oral	Acetaminophen	↓	
Antibiotics	Contraceptives, oral	↓	Coadministration of griseofulvin, penicillins, or tetracyclines with OCs may decrease the pharmacologic effects of the OCs, possibly because of altered steroid gut metabolism secondary to changes in the intestinal flora. Menstrual irregularities (spotting, breakthrough bleeding) and pregnancy may occur. An alternate or additional form of birth control may be advisable during concomitant use. OCs and troleandomycin may be associated with an increased risk of intrahepatic cholestasis.
Atorvastatin	Contraceptives, oral	↑	Ethinyl estradiol AUC may increase by ≈ 20%.
Ascorbic acid	Contraceptives, oral	↑	Ethinyl estradiol plasma levels may increase.
Barbiturates Carbamazepine Felbamate Griseofulvin Hydantoins[1] Oxcarbazepine Phenylbutazone Phenytoin Primidone Rifampin Topiramate	Contraceptives, oral	↓	These agents may increase the hepatic metabolism of the OCs via hepatic microsomal enzyme induction, possibly resulting in decreased effectiveness of the OC; menstrual irregularities (spotting, breakthrough bleeding) and pregnancy may occur. An alternate or additional form of birth control may be advisable during concomitant use.
CYP3A4 inhibitors (eg, itraconazole, ketoconazole)	Contraceptives, oral	↑	Increase in plasma hormone levels may occur.
Protease inhibitors	Contraceptives, oral	↓	Increased metabolism of the OCs is suspected resulting in a loss of effectiveness of OCs. An alternate or additional form of birth control may be advisable during concomitant use.

Transdermal Contraceptive Patch Drug Interactions			
Precipitant drug	Object drug*		Description
St. John's wort	Contraceptives, oral	↓	St. John's wort may induce hepatic enzymes and p-glycoprotein transporter and may reduce the effectiveness of contraceptive steroids.
Contraceptives, oral	Anticoagulants	↔	Because OCs can increase levels of certain circulating clotting factors and reduce antithrombin III levels, therapeutic efficacy of the anticoagulants may be decreased by OCs. However, both an increased and decreased effect has occurred.
Contraceptives, oral	Antidepressants, tricyclic Beta blockers Caffeine Corticosteroids Theophyllines	↑	The hepatic metabolism of these agents may be decreased by OCs, resulting in increased therapeutic effects or toxicity.
Contraceptives, oral	Benzodiazepines	↓	OCs may increase the clearance of the benzodiazepines that undergo glucuronidation (lorazepam, oxazepam, temazepam) because of increased metabolism. Combination OCs with alprazolam, chlordiazepoxide, diazepam, and triazolam may inhibit hepatic mixed-function oxidases leading to a decrease in benzodiazepine oxidation rate (may prolong the half-life of benzodiazepines).
Contraceptives, oral	Cyclosporine Prednisolone Theophylline	↑	Increased plasma concentrations of cyclosporine, prednisolone, and theophylline have been reported with coadministration of OCs.
Contraceptives, oral	Clofibric acid Morphine Salicylic acid	↓	Increased clearance of these agents has been noted when administered with OCs.

↑ = Object drug increased. ↓ = Object drug decreased. ↔ = Undetermined clinical effect.
[1] Pharmacologic effects of the hydantoins also may be altered.

►*Drug/Lab test interactions:* Certain endocrine and liver function tests and blood components may be affected by hormonal contraceptives:

Increased – Prothrombin and factors VII, VIII, IX, and X; increased norepinephrine-induced platelet aggregability; thyroid-binding globulin (TBG) leading to increased circulating total thyroid hormone as measured by protein-bound iodine (PBI), T4 by column or by radioimmunoassay; other binding proteins may be elevated in serum; sex hormone binding globulins are increased and result in elevated levels of total circulating endogenous sex steroids and corticoids; triglycerides may be increased and levels of various other lipids and lipoproteins may be affected.

Decreased – Antithrombin III; free T3 resin uptake; glucose tolerance may be decreased; serum folate levels may be depressed by hormonal contraceptive therapy. This may be of clinical significance if a woman becomes pregnant shortly after discontinuing the norelgestromin/ethinyl estradiol transdermal patch.

Adverse Reactions

The most common adverse events reported by 9% to 22% of women using the norelgestromin/ethinyl estradiol transdermal patch in clinical trials (n = 3330) were the following, in order of decreasing incidence: Breast symptoms, headache, application site reaction, nausea, upper respiratory tract infection, menstrual cramps, and abdominal pain.

The most frequent adverse events leading to discontinuation in 1% to 2.4% of women using the norelgestromin/ethinyl estradiol transdermal patch in the trials included the following: Nausea or vomiting, application site reaction, breast symptoms, headache, emotional lability.

Listed below are adverse events that have been associated with the use of combination hormonal contraceptives. These also are likely to apply to combination transdermal hormonal contraceptives such as the norelgestromin/ethinyl estradiol transdermal patch.

►*Serious:* Thrombophlebitis and venous thrombosis with or without embolism; arterial thromboembolism; pulmonary embolism; MI; cerebral hemorrhage; cerebral thrombosis; hypertension; gallbladder disease; hepatic adenomas or benign liver tumors; mesenteric thrombosis; retinal thrombosis.

►*GI:* Cholestatic jaundice; GI symptoms (eg, abdominal cramps, bloating); nausea; vomiting.

►*GU:* Amenorrhea; breakthrough bleeding; breast changes: tenderness, enlargement, secretion; change in cervical erosion and secretion; change in menstrual flow; diminution in lactation when given immediately postpartum; spotting; temporary infertility after discontinuation of treatment; vaginal candidiasis.

►*Miscellaneous:* Change in corneal curvature (steepening); change in weight (increase or decrease); edema; intolerance to contact lenses; melasma, which may persist; mental depression; migraine; rash (allergic); reduced tolerance to carbohydrates.

NORELGESTROMIN/ETHINYL ESTRADIOL TRANS-DERMAL SYSTEM

The following adverse reactions have been reported in users of combination hormonal contraceptives and a cause-and-effect association has been neither confirmed nor refuted: Acne; Budd-Chiari syndrome; cataracts; changes in appetite; changes in libido; colitis; cystitis-like syndrome; dizziness; erythema multiforme; erythema nodosum; headache; hemolytic uremic syndrome; hemorrhagic eruption; hirsutism; impaired renal function; loss of scalp hair; nervousness; porphyria; premenstrual syndrome; vaginitis.

Overdosage

Serious ill effects have not been reported following accidental ingestion of large doses of hormonal contraceptives. Overdosage may cause nausea, vomiting, and withdrawal bleeding. Given the nature and design of the norelgestromin/ethinyl estradiol transdermal patch, it is unlikely that overdosage will occur. Serious ill effects have not been reported following acute ingestion of large doses of oral contraceptives by young children. In case of suspected overdose, remove all norelgestromin/ethinyl estradiol transdermal patches and give symptomatic treatment.

Patient Information

Counsel women that the norelgestromin/ethinyl estradiol transdermal patch does not protect against HIV infection (AIDS) and other sexually transmitted diseases.

If any of these adverse effects occur while you are using the patch, call your doctor immediately:
• Sharp chest pain, coughing of blood, sudden shortness of breath (indicating a possible clot in the lung);

• pain in the calf (indicating a possible clot in the leg);
• crushing chest pain or tightness in the chest (indicating a possible heart attack);
• audden severe headache or vomiting, dizziness or fainting, disturbances of vision or speech, weakness or numbness in an arm or leg (indicating a possible stroke);
• sudden partial or complete loss of vision (indicating a possible clot in the eye);
• breast lumps (indicating possible breast cancer or fibrocystic disease of the breast; ask your doctor or health care professional to show you how to examine your breasts);
• severe pain or tenderness in the stomach area (indicating a possibly ruptured liver tumor);
• severe problems with sleeping, weakness, lack of energy, fatigue, or change in mood (possibly indicating severe depression);
• jaundice or a yellowing of the skin or eyeballs accompanied frequently by fever, fatigue, loss of appetite, dark-colored urine, or light-colored bowel movements (indicating possible liver problems).

➤*Skin irritation:* Skin irritation, redness, or rash may occur at the site of application. If this occurs, the patch may be removed and a new patch may be applied to a new location until the next patch change day. Single replacement patches are available from pharmacies.

➤*Vaginal bleeding:* Irregular bleeding may occur during the first few months of contraceptive patch use, but also may occur after you have been using the contraceptive patch for some time. If the bleeding occurs in more than a few cycles or lasts for more than a few days, talk to your health care professional.

ETONOGESTREL/ETHINYL ESTRADIOL VAGINAL RING

	Product and Distributor	Release Rate	Total Content	How Supplied
Rx	**NuvaRing** (Organon)	0.12 mg etonogestrel, 0.015 mg ethinyl estradiol/day	11.7 mg etonogestrel 2.7 mg ethinyl estradiol/sachet	In single and 3 sachets.

WARNING

Cigarette smoking increases the risk of serious cardiovascular side effects from combination oral contraceptive use. This risk increases with age and with heavy smoking (≥ 15 cigarettes/day) and is quite marked in women > 35 years of age. Strongly advise women who use combination hormonal contraceptives, including the contraceptive vaginal ring, not to smoke.

Indications

➤*Contraception:* For the prevention of pregnancy.

Administration and Dosage

➤*Approved by the FDA:* October 3, 2001.

➤*Use:* One etonogestrel/ethinyl estradiol vaginal ring is inserted in the vagina by the woman herself. This ring is to remain in place continuously for 3 weeks. It is removed for a 1-week break, during which a withdrawal bleed usually occurs. A new ring is inserted 1 week after the last ring was removed on the same day of the week as it was inserted in the previous cycle. The withdrawal bleed usually starts on day 2 to 3 after removal of the ring and may not have finished before the next ring is inserted. In order to maintain contraceptive effectiveness, insert the new ring 1 week after the previous one was removed even if menstrual bleeding has not finished.

➤*Insertion:* The user can choose the insertion position that is most comfortable to her, for example standing with one leg up, squatting, or lying down. Compress the ring and insert it into the vagina. The exact position of the contraceptive vaginal ring inside the vagina is not critical for its function. Insert the contraceptive vaginal ring on the appropriate day and leave in place for 3 consecutive weeks.

➤*Removal:* The ring is removed 3 weeks later on the same day of the week as it was inserted and at about the same time. Remove the vaginal ring by hooking the index finger under the forward rim or by grasping the rim between the index and middle finger and pulling it out. Place the used ring in the sachet (foil pouch) and discard in a waste receptacle out of the reach of children and pets. Do not flush in the toilet.

➤*Starting the contraceptive vaginal ring:* Consider the possibility of ovulation and conception prior to the first use of the contraceptive vaginal ring.

No preceding hormonal contraceptive use in the past month – Counting the first day of menstruation as day 1, insert the contraceptive vaginal ring on or prior to day 5 of the cycle, even if the patient has not finished bleeding. During the first cycle, an additional method of contraception (eg, male condoms, spermicide) is recommended until after the first 7 days of continuous ring use.

Switching from a combination oral contraceptive – Insert the contraceptive vaginal ring anytime within 7 days after the last combined (estrogen plus progestin) oral contraceptive tablet and no later than the day that a new cycle of pills would have started. No backup method is needed.

Switching from a progestin-only method – There are several types of progestin-only methods. Insert the first contraceptive vaginal ring as follows:
• Any day of the month when switching from a progestin-only pill; do not skip any days between the last pill and the first day of contraceptive vaginal ring use;
• on the same day as contraceptive implant removal;
• on the same day as removal of a progestin-containing IUD; or
• on the day when the next contraceptive injection would be due.

In all of these cases, advise the patient to use an additional method of contraception (eg, male condoms, spermicide) for the first 7 days after insertion of the ring.

➤*Following complete first-trimester abortion:* The patient may start using the contraceptive vaginal ring within the first 5 days following a complete first trimester abortion and does not need to use an additional method of contraception. If use of the contraceptive vaginal ring is not started within 5 days following a first trimester abortion, the patient should follow the instructions for "No preceding hormonal contraceptive use in the past month." In the meantime, advise the patient to use a nonhormonal contraceptive method.

➤*Following delivery or second-trimester abortion:* Initiate the use of the contraceptive vaginal ring 4 weeks postpartum in women who elect not to breastfeed. Advise women who are breastfeeding not to use the contraceptive vaginal ring but to use other forms of contraception until the child is weaned. Initiate use of the contraceptive vaginal ring 4 weeks after a second-trimester abortion. When the contraceptive vaginal ring is used postpartum or postabortion, consider the increased risk of thromboembolic disease (see Contraindications, Warnings, and Precautions). If the patient begins using the contraceptive vaginal ring postpartum and has not yet had a period, consider the possibility of ovulation and conception occurring prior to initiation of the contraceptive vaginal ring, and instruct the patient to use an additional method of contraception (eg, male condoms, spermicide) for the first 7 days.

➤*Inadvertent removal, expulsion, or prolonged ring-free interval:* If the contraceptive vaginal ring has been out during the 3-week use period, rinse with cool to lukewarm (not hot) water and reinsert as soon as possible, at the latest within 3 hours. If the ring has been out of the vagina for > 3 hours, contraceptive effectiveness may be reduced. Use an additional method of contraception (eg, male condoms, spermicide) until the contraceptive vaginal ring has been used continuously for 7 days.

Consider the possibility of pregnancy if the ring-free interval has been extended beyond 1 week. Use an additional method of contraception (eg, male condoms, spermicide) until the contraceptive vaginal ring has been used continuously for 7 days.

➤*Prolonged use:* If the contraceptive vaginal ring has been left in place for up to 1 extra week (ie, up to 4 weeks total), remove it and insert a new ring after a 1-week ring-free interval. Rule out pregnancy if the contraceptive vaginal ring has been left in place for > 4 weeks. Use an additional method of contraception (eg, male condoms, spermi-

ETONOGESTREL/ETHINYL ESTRADIOL VAGINAL RING

cide) until the contraceptive vaginal ring has been used continuously for 7 days.

➤*In the event of a missed menstrual period:* If the patient has not adhered to the prescribed regimen (the contraceptive vaginal ring has been out of the vagina for > 3 hours or the preceding ring-free interval was extended beyond 1 week), consider the possibility of pregnancy at the time of the first missed period and discontinue the use of the contraceptive vaginal ring if pregnancy is confirmed.

Rule out pregnancy if the patient has adhered to the prescribed regimen and misses 2 consecutive periods.

Rule out pregnancy if the patient has retained 1 contraceptive vaginal ring for > 4 weeks.

➤*Storage/Stability:* Prior to dispensing to the user, store refrigerated 2° to 8°C (36° to 46°F), After dispensing to the user, the contraceptive vaginal ring can be stored for up to 4 months at 15° to 30°C (59° to 86°F). Avoid storing the contraceptive vaginal ring in direct sunlight or at temperatures above 30°C (86°F). When the contraceptive vaginal ring is dispensed to the user, place an expiration date on the label. The date should not be> 4 months from the date of dispensing or the expiration date, whichever comes first.

Actions

➤*Pharmacology:* The contraceptive vaginal ring is a nonbiodegradable, flexible, transparent, colorless to almost colorless combination contraceptive vaginal ring containing 2 active components: A progestin, etonogestrel, and an estrogen, ethinyl estradiol. When placed in the vagina, each ring releases on average 0.12 mg/day of etonogestrel and 0.015 mg/day of ethinyl estradiol over a 3-week period of use.

Combination hormonal contraceptives act by suppression of gonadotropins. Although the primary effect of this action is inhibition of ovulation, other alterations include changes in the cervical mucus (which increase the difficulty of sperm entry into the uterus) and in the endometrium (which reduce the likelihood of implantation).

Receptor binding studies, as well as studies in animals, have shown that etonogestrel, the biologically active metabolite of desogestrel, combines high progestational activity with low intrinsic androgenicity. The relevance of this latter finding in humans is unknown.

➤*Pharmacokinetics:*
Absorption – Etonogestrel released by the vaginal ring is rapidly absorbed. Bioavailability of etonogestrel after vaginal administration is ≈ 100%.

Ethinyl estradiol released by the vaginal ring is rapidly absorbed. Bioavailability of ethinyl estradiol after vaginal administration is ≈ 55.6%, which is comparable to that with oral administration of ethinyl estradiol.

Mean Serum Etonogestrel and Ethinyl Estradiol Concentrations (n = 16)			
	1 week	2 weeks	3 weeks
Etonogestrel (pg/mL)	1578	1476	1374
Ethinyl estradiol (pg/mL)	19.1	18.3	17.6

Mean Pharmacokinetic Parameters of Etonogestrel/Ethinyl Estradiol Vaginal Ring (n = 16)				
Hormone	C_{max}[1] pg/mL	T_{max}[2] hr	$t_{1/2}$[3] hr	CL[4] L/hr
Etonogestrel	1716	200.3	29.3	3.4
Ethinyl estradiol	34.7	59.3	44.7	34.8

[1] C_{max} — maximum serum concentration
[2] T_{max} — time at which maximum serum drug concentration occurs
[3] $t_{1/2}$ — elimination half-life, calculated by $0.693/K_{elim}$
[4] CL — apparent clearance

Distribution – Etonogestrel is ≈ 32% bound to sex hormone binding globulin (SHBG) and ≈ 66% bound to albumin in blood.

Ethinyl estradiol is highly but not specifically bound to serum albumin (≈ 98.5%) and induces an increase in the serum concentrations of SHBG.

Metabolism – In vitro data show that both etonogestrel and ethinyl estradiol are metabolized in liver microsomes by the cytochrome P450 3A4 isoenzyme. Ethinyl estradiol is primarily metabolized by aromatic hydroxylation, but a wide variety of hydroxylated and methylated metabolites are formed. These are present as free metabolites and as sulfate and glucuronide conjugates. The hydroxylated ethinyl estradiol metabolites have weak estrogenic activity. The biological activity of etonogestrel metabolites is unknown.

Excretion – Etonogestrel and ethinyl estradiol are primarily eliminated in urine, bile, and feces.

Contraindications

Thrombophlebitis or thromboembolic disorders; a past history of deep vein thrombophlebitis or thromboembolic disorders; cerebral vascular or coronary artery disease (current or history); valvular heart disease with complications; severe hypertension; diabetes with vascular involvement; headaches with focal neurological symptoms; major surgery with prolonged immobilization; known or suspected carcinoma of the breast or personal history of breast cancer; carcinoma of the endometrium or other known or suspected estrogen-dependent neoplasia; undiagnosed abnormal genital bleeding; cholestatic jaundice of pregnancy or jaundice with prior hormonal contraceptive use; hepatic tumors (benign or malignant); active liver disease; known or suspected pregnancy; heavy smoking (≥ 15 cigarettes/day) and > 35 years of age; hypersensitivity to any of the components of the contraceptive vaginal ring.

Warnings

➤*Thromboembolic disorders and other vascular problems:*
Thromboembolism – An increased risk of thromboembolic and thrombotic disease associated with the use of hormonal contraceptives is well-established. Case control studies have found the relative risk of users compared with nonusers to be 3 for the first episode of superficial venous thrombosis, 4 to 11 for deep vein thrombosis or pulmonary embolism, and 1.5 to 6 for women with predisposing conditions for venous thromboembolic disease. Cohort studies have shown the relative risk to be somewhat lower, ≈ 3 for new cases and ≈ 4.5 for new cases requiring hospitalization. The risk of thromboembolic disease associated with hormonal contraceptives is not related to length of use and disappears after pill use is stopped.

Several epidemiology studies indicate that third generation oral contraceptives, including those containing desogestrel (etonogestrel, the progestin in the vaginal ring, is the biologically active metabolite of desogestrel), are associated with a higher risk of venous thromboembolism than certain second generation oral contraceptives. In general, these studies indicate an ≈ 2-fold increased risk, which corresponds to an additional 1 to 2 cases of venous thromboembolism per 10,000 women-years of use. However, data from additional studies have not shown this 2-fold increase in risk. It is unknown if the vaginal ring has a different risk of venous thromboembolism than second generation oral contraceptives.

A 2- to 4-fold increase in relative risk of postoperative thromboembolic complications has been reported with the use of oral contraceptives. The relative risk of venous thrombosis in women who have predisposing conditions is twice that of women without such medical conditions. If feasible, discontinue the use of combination hormonal contraceptives, including the vaginal ring, for ≥ 4 weeks prior to and for 2 weeks after elective surgery of a type associated with an increase in risk of thromboembolism and during and following prolonged immobilization. Because the immediate postpartum period is also associated with an increased risk of thromboembolism, start combination hormonal contraceptives (eg, vaginal ring) no earlier than 4 weeks after delivery in women who elect not to breastfeed.

The clinician should be alert to the earliest manifestations of thrombotic disorders (thrombophlebitis, pulmonary embolism, cerebrovascular disorders, and retinal thrombosis). Should any of these occur or be suspected, discontinue the use of the vaginal ring immediately.

MI – An increased risk of MI has been attributed to hormonal contraceptive use. The risk is primarily in smokers or women with other underlying risk factors for coronary artery disease (eg, hypertension, hypercholesterolemia, morbid obesity, and diabetes). The relative risk of heart attack for current combination hormonal contraceptive users has been estimated to be 2 to 6. The risk is very low in women < 30 years of age.

Smoking in combination with oral contraceptive use has been shown to contribute substantially to the incidence of MI in women in their mid-30s or older with smoking accounting for the majority of excess cases. Mortality rates associated with circulatory disease have been shown to increase substantially in smokers > 35 years of age and nonsmokers > 40 years of age among women who use oral contraceptives.

Hormonal contraceptives may compound the effects of well-known risk factors (eg, hypertension, diabetes, hyperlipidemias, age, obesity). In particular, some progestogens are known to decrease high density lipoprotein (HDL) cholesterol and cause glucose intolerance, while estrogens may create a state of hyperinsulinism. Hormonal contraceptives have been shown to increase blood pressure among users. Similar effects on risk factors have been associated with an increased risk of heart disease. Use the vaginal ring with caution in women with cardiovascular disease risk factors.

Cerebrovascular diseases – Hormonal contraceptives have been shown to increase both the relative and attributable risks of cerebrovascular events (thrombotic and hemorrhagic strokes), although, in general, the risk is greatest among older (> 35 years of age), hypertensive women who also smoke. Hypertension was found to be a risk factor for both users and nonusers, for both types of strokes, while smoking interacted to increase the risk for hemorrhagic strokes.

ETONOGESTREL/ETHINYL ESTRADIOL VAGINAL RING

In a large study, the relative risk of thrombotic strokes has been shown to range from 3 for normotensive users to 14 for users with severe hypertension. The relative risk of hemorrhagic stroke is reported to be 1.2 for nonsmokers who used oral contraceptives, 2.6 for smokers who did not use oral contraceptives, 7.6 for smokers who used oral contraceptives, 1.8 for normotensive users and 25.7 for users with severe hypertension. The attributable risk is also greater in older women.

Dose-related risk – A positive association has been observed between the amount of estrogen and progestogen in hormonal contraceptives and the risk of vascular disease. A decline in serum HDL has been reported with many progestational agents. A decline in serum high-density lipoproteins has been associated with an increased incidence of ischemic heart disease. Because estrogens increase HDL cholesterol, the net effect of a hormonal contraceptive depends on a balance achieved between doses of estrogen and progestogen and the nature and absolute amount of progestogens used in the contraceptives. Consider the activity and amount of both hormones in the choice of a hormonal contraceptive.

Persistence of risk – There are 2 studies that have shown persistence of risk of vascular disease for ever-users of hormonal contraceptives. In a study in the US, the risk of developing MI after discontinuing oral contraceptives persists for ≥ 9 years for women 40 to 49 years of age who had used oral contraceptives for ≥ 5 years, but this increased risk was not demonstrated in other age groups. In another study in Great Britain, the risk of developing cerebrovascular disease persisted ≥ 6 years after discontinuation of oral contraceptives, although excess risk was very small. However, both studies were performed with oral contraceptive formulations containing ≥ 50 mcg of estrogen.

It is unknown whether the contraceptive vaginal ring is distinct from combination hormonal contraceptives with regard to the occurrence of venous or arterial thrombosis.

➤*Mortality:* With the exception of oral contraceptive users ≥ 35 years of age who smoke and ≥ 40 years of age who do not smoke, mortality associated with all methods of birth control is low and below that associated with childbirth.

In 1989, the Fertility and Maternal Health Drugs Advisory Committee was asked to review the use of combination hormonal contraceptives in women ≥ 40 years of age. The Committee concluded that although cardiovascular disease risks may be increased with oral contraceptive use after 40 years of age in healthy nonsmoking women (even with the newer low-dose formulations), there are also greater potential risks associated with pregnancy in older women and with the alternative surgical and medical procedures that may be necessary if such women do not have access to effective and acceptable means of contraception. Therefore, the Committee recommended that the benefits of low-dose oral contraceptive use by healthy nonsmoking women > 40 years of age may outweigh the possible risks. Although the data are mainly obtained with oral contraceptives, this is likely to apply to the contraceptive vaginal ring as well. Women of all ages who take hormonal contraceptives should take the lowest possible dose formulation that is effective and meets the needs of the individual patient.

➤*Carcinoma:* Numerous epidemiologic studies have been performed on the incidence of breast, endometrial, ovarian, and cervical cancer in women using combination oral contraceptives.

The risk of having breast cancer diagnosed may be slightly increased among current and recent users of combination oral contraceptives (COCs). However, this excess risk appears to decrease over time after COC discontinuation and by 10 years after cessation the increased risk disappears. Some studies report an increased risk with duration of use while other studies do not and no consistent relationships have been found with dose or type of steroid. Some studies have found a small increase in risk for women who first use COCs before 20 years of age. Most studies show a similar pattern of risk with COC use regardless of a woman's reproductive history or her family breast cancer history.

In addition, breast cancers diagnosed in current or ever oral contraceptive users may be less clinically advanced than in never-users.

Women who currently have or have had breast cancer should not use hormonal contraceptives because breast cancer is usually a hormonal sensitive tumor.

Some studies suggest that combination oral contraceptive use has been associated with an increase in the risk of cervical intraepithelial neoplasia in some populations of women. However, there continues to be controversy about the extent to which such findings may be caused by differences in sexual behavior and other factors.

In spite of many studies of the relationship between oral contraceptive use and breast and cervical cancers, a cause-and-effect relationship has not been established.

It is unknown whether the contraceptive vaginal ring is distinct from oral contraceptives with regard to the previous statements.

➤*Hepatic neoplasia:* Benign hepatic adenomas are associated with oral contraceptive use, although the incidence of benign tumors is rare in the US. Indirect calculations have estimated the attributable risk to

be in the range of 3.3 cases per 100,000 for users, a risk that increases after ≥ 4 years of use. Rupture of rare, benign, hepatic adenomas may cause death through intra-abdominal hemorrhage.

Studies from Great Britain have shown an increased risk of developing hepatocellular carcinoma in long-term (> 8 years) oral contraceptive users. However, these cancers are extremely rare in the US and the attributable risk (the excess incidence) of liver cancers in oral contraceptive users approaches < 1 per million users. It is unknown whether the contraceptive vaginal ring is distinct from oral contraceptives in this regard.

➤*Ocular lesions:* There have been clinical case reports of retinal thrombosis associated with the use of oral contraceptives. Discontinue the use of the contraceptive vaginal ring if there is unexplained partial or complete loss of vision, onset of proptosis or diplopia, papilledema, or retinal vascular lesions. Undertake appropriate diagnostic and therapeutic measures immediately.

➤*Risk of use before or during early pregnancy:* Do not use hormonal contraceptives during pregnancy. Extensive epidemiologic studies have revealed no increased risk of birth defects in women who have used oral contraceptives prior to pregnancy. Studies also do not suggest a teratogenic effect, particularly where cardiac anomalies and limb reduction defects are concerned, when oral contraceptives are taken inadvertently during early pregnancy.

➤*Gallbladder disease:* Combination hormonal contraceptives (eg, contraceptive vaginal ring) may worsen existing gallbladder disease and may accelerate the development of this disease in previously asymptomatic women. Women with a history of combination hormonal contraceptive-related cholestasis are more likely to have the condition recur with subsequent combination hormonal contraceptive use.

➤*Carbohydrate and lipid metabolic effects:* Hormonal contraceptives have been shown to cause a decrease in glucose tolerance in some users. However, in the nondiabetic woman, combination hormonal contraceptives appear to have no effect on fasting blood glucose. Carefully observe prediabetic and diabetic women while taking combination hormonal contraceptives (eg, contraceptive vaginal ring). In a clinical study involving 37 contraceptive vaginal ring-treated subjects, glucose tolerance tests showed no clinically significant changes in serum glucose levels from baseline to cycle 6.

A small proportion of women will have persistent hypertriglyceridemia while using hormonal contraceptives. Changes in serum triglycerides and lipoprotein levels have been reported in combination hormonal contraceptive users.

➤*Elevated blood pressure:* An increase in blood pressure has been reported in women taking hormonal contraceptives; this increase is more likely in older hormonal contraceptive users and with continued use. Data from the Royal College of General Practitioners and subsequent randomized trials have shown that the incidence of hypertension increases with increasing concentrations of progestogens. Encourage women with a history of hypertension or hypertension-related diseases, or renal disease to use another method of contraception. Closely monitor these women if they elect to use the contraceptive vaginal ring. Discontinue use of the contraceptive vaginal ring if significant elevation of blood pressure occurs. For most women, elevated blood pressure will return to normal after stopping hormonal contraceptives.

➤*Headache:* The onset or exacerbation of migraine or development of headache with a new pattern that is recurrent, persistent, or severe requires discontinuation of the contraceptive vaginal ring and evaluation of the cause.

➤*Bleeding irregularities and patterns:* Breakthrough bleeding and spotting are sometimes encountered in women using the contraceptive vaginal ring. If abnormal bleeding while using the contraceptive vaginal ring persists or is severe, investigate to rule out the possibility of organic pathology or pregnancy, and institute appropriate treatment when necessary. Rule out pregnancy in the event of amenorrhea.

Bleeding patterns were evaluated in 2 large clinical studies. During cycles 1 through 13, breakthrough bleeding/spotting occurred in 7.2% to 11.7% of cycles in a study of 1177 subjects and in 2.6% to 6.4% of cycles in a second study of 1145 subjects. Absence of withdrawal bleeding occurred in 2.3% to 3.8% of cycles in the first trial subjects and in 0.6% to 2.1% of cycles in the second trial subjects. Bleeding patterns for individual women over multiple cycles were not evaluated. Some women may encounter amenorrhea or oligomenorrhea after discontinuing use of the contraceptive vaginal ring, especially when a condition was preexistent.

➤*Elderly:* This medication has not been studied in women ≥ 65 years of age and is not indicated in this population.

➤*Pregnancy:* Category X. Teratology studies have been performed in rats and rabbits using the oral route of administration at doses up to 130 and 260 times, respectively, the human contraceptive vaginal ring dose (based on body surface area) and have revealed no evidence of harm to the fetus due to etonogestrel.

Ectopic pregnancy – Ectopic as well as intrauterine pregnancy may occur in contraceptive failures.

ETONOGESTREL/ETHINYL ESTRADIOL VAGINAL RING

➤*Lactation:* The effects of the contraceptive vaginal ring in nursing mothers have not been evaluated and are unknown. Small amounts of contraceptive steroids have been identified in the milk of nursing mothers and a few adverse effects on the child have been reported, including jaundice and breast enlargement. In addition, contraceptive steroids given in the postpartum period may interfere with lactation by decreasing the quantity and quality of breast milk. Long-term follow-up of children whose mothers used combination hormonal contraceptives while breastfeeding has shown no deleterious effects in infants. However, advise women who are breastfeeding not to use the contraceptive vaginal ring but to use other forms of contraception until the child is weaned.

➤*Children:* Safety and efficacy of the contraceptive vaginal ring have been established in women of reproductive age. Safety and efficacy are expected to be the same for postpubertal adolescents < 16 years of age and for users ≥ 16 years of age. Use of this product before menarche is not indicated.

Precautions

➤*Sexually transmitted diseases:* Counsel patients that this product does not protect against HIV infection (AIDS) and other sexually transmitted diseases.

➤*Lipid disorders:* Closely follow women who are being treated for hyperlipidemias if they elect to use the contraceptive vaginal ring. Some progestogens may elevate LDL levels and may render the control of hyperlipidemias more difficult.

➤*Hepatic function:* If jaundice develops in any woman using the contraceptive vaginal ring, discontinue the medication. The hormones in the contraceptive vaginal ring may be poorly metabolized in women with impaired liver function.

➤*Fluid retention:* Steroid hormones like those in the contraceptive vaginal ring may cause some degree of fluid retention. Prescribe this product with caution, and only with careful monitoring, in patients with conditions that might be aggravated by fluid retention.

➤*Emotional disorders:* Women who become significantly depressed while using combination hormonal contraceptives such as the contraceptive vaginal ring should stop the medication and use another method of contraception in an attempt to determine whether the symptom is drug-related. Carefully observe women with a history of depression and discontinue the product if significant depression occurs.

➤*Contact lenses:* Contact lens wearers who develop visual changes or changes in lens tolerance should be assessed by an ophthalmologist.

➤*Vaginal use:* The contraceptive vaginal ring may not be suitable for women with conditions that make the vagina more susceptible to vaginal irritation or ulceration. Some women are aware of the ring at random times during the 21 days of use or during intercourse. During intercourse, some sexual partners may feel the contraceptive vaginal ring in the vagina. However, clinical studies revealed that 90% of couples did not find this to be a problem.

If the contraceptive vaginal ring has been removed or expelled during the 3-week use period, it should be rinsed with cool to lukewarm (not hot) water and reinserted as soon as possible, but at the latest within 3 hours of removal or expulsion. If the contraceptive vaginal ring is lost, insert a new vaginal ring and continue the regimen without alteration. If the ring has been out of the vagina for > 3 hours, contraceptive effectiveness may be reduced and an additional method of contraception (eg, male condom, spermicide) must be used until the ring has been used continuously for 7 days. The contraceptive vaginal ring may interfere with the correct placement and position of a diaphragm. Therefore, a diaphragm is not recommended as a backup method with contraceptive vaginal ring use.

➤*Expulsion:* The contraceptive vaginal ring can be accidentally expelled, for example, when it has not been inserted properly, or while removing a tampon, moving the bowels, straining, or with severe constipation. If this occurs, rinse the vaginal ring with cool to lukewarm (not hot) water and reinsert promptly. If the contraceptive vaginal ring is lost, insert a new vaginal ring and continue the regimen without alteration. If the ring has been out of the vagina for > 3 hours, contraceptive effectiveness may be reduced and an additional method of contraception (eg, male condom, spermicide) must be used until the ring has been used continuously for 7 days. Vaginal stenosis, cervical prolapse, rectoceles, and cystoceles are conditions that under some circumstances may make expulsion more likely to occur.

Drug Interactions

Most drug interactions are based on oral contraceptives.

Contraceptive Vaginal Ring Drug Interactions			
Precipitant drug	Object drug*		Description
Acetaminophen	Contraceptives, oral	↑	Ethinyl estradiol plasma levels may increase, whereas acetaminophen plasma concentrations may decrease.
Contraceptives, oral	Acetaminophen	↓	

Contraceptive Vaginal Ring Drug Interactions			
Precipitant drug	Object drug*		Description
Antibiotics	Contraceptives, oral	↓	Coadministration of griseofulvin, penicillins, or tetracyclines with OCs may decrease the pharmacologic effects of the OCs, possibly because of altered steroid gut metabolism secondary to changes in the intestinal flora. Menstrual irregularities (spotting, breakthrough bleeding) and pregnancy may occur. An alternate or additional form of birth control may be advisable during concomitant use. OCs and troleandomycin may be associated with an increased risk of intrahepatic cholestasis.
Atorvastatin	Contraceptives, oral	↑	Ethinyl estradiol AUC may increase by ≈ 20%.
Ascorbic acid	Contraceptives, oral	↑	Ethinyl estradiol plasma levels may increase.
Barbiturates Carbamazepine Felbamate Griseofulvin Hydantoins[1] Oxcarbazepine Phenylbutazone Phenytoin Primidone Rifampin Topiramate	Contraceptives, oral	↓	These agents may increase the hepatic metabolism of the OCs via hepatic microsomal enzyme induction, possibly resulting in decreased effectiveness of the OC; menstrual irregularities (spotting, breakthrough bleeding) and pregnancy may occur. An alternate or additional form of birth control may be advisable during concomitant use.
CYP3A4 inhibitors (eg, itraconazole, ketoconazole)	Contraceptives, oral	↑	Increase in plasma hormone levels may occur.
Protease inhibitors	Contraceptives, oral	↓	Increased metabolism of the OCs is suspected, resulting in a loss of effectiveness of OCs. An alternate or additional form of birth control may be advisable during concomitant use.
St. John's wort	Contraceptives, oral	↓	St. John's wort may induce hepatic enzymes and p-glycoprotein transporter and may reduce the effectiveness of contraceptive steroids.
Miconazole	Etonogestrel/ ethinyl estradiol vaginal ring	↑	Vaginally administered oil-based miconazole capsule increased serum concentrations of etonogestrel and ethinyl estradiol by ≈ 17% and 16%, respectively.
Contraceptives, oral	Anticoagulants	↔	Therapeutic efficacy of the anticoagulants may be decreased by OCs. However, both an increased and decreased effect has occurred.
Contraceptives, oral	Antidepressants, tricyclic Beta blockers Caffeine Corticosteroids Theophyllines	↑	The hepatic metabolism of these agents may be decreased by OCs, resulting in increased therapeutic effects or toxicity.
Contraceptives, oral	Benzodiazepines	↓	OCs may increase the clearance of the benzodiazepines that undergo glucuronidation (lorazepam, oxazepam, temazepam) because of increased metabolism. Combination OCs with alprazolam, chlordiazepoxide, diazepam, and triazolam may inhibit hepatic mixed-function oxidases, leading to a decrease in benzodiazepine oxidation rate (may prolong the half-life of benzodiazepines).
Contraceptives, oral	Cyclosporine Prednisolone Theophylline	↑	Increased plasma concentrations of cyclosporine, prednisolone, and theophylline have been reported with coadministration of OCs.
Contraceptives, oral	Clofibric acid Morphine Salicylic acid	↓	Increased clearance of these agents has been noted when administered with OCs.

↑ = Object drug increased. ↓ = Object drug decreased. ↔ = Undetermined clinical effect.
[1] Pharmacologic effects of the hydantoins also may be altered.

➤*Drug/Lab test interactions:* Certain endocrine and liver function tests and blood components may be affected by hormonal contraceptives:

Increased – Prothrombin and factors VII, VIII, IX, and X; increased norepinephrine-induced platelet aggregability; thyroid binding globulin (TBG) leading to increased circulating total thyroid hormone as measured by protein-bound iodine (PBI), T4 by column or by radioimmunoassay; other binding proteins may be elevated in serum; sex hormone binding globulins are increased and result in elevated levels of total circulating endogenous sex steroids and corticoids; triglycerides may be

ETONOGESTREL/ETHINYL ESTRADIOL VAGINAL RING

increased and levels of various other lipids and lipoproteins may be affected.

Decreased – Antithrombin III; free T3 resin uptake; glucose tolerance may be decreased; serum folate levels may be depressed by hormonal contraceptive therapy. This may be of clinical significance if a woman becomes pregnant shortly after discontinuing the contraceptive vaginal ring.

Adverse Reactions

The most common adverse events reported by 5% to 14% of women using the contraceptive vaginal ring in clinical trials (n = 2501) were the following: Vaginitis, headache, upper respiratory tract infection, leukorrhea, sinusitis, weight gain, and nausea.

The most frequent system-organ class adverse events leading to discontinuation in 1% to 2.5% of women using the contraceptive vaginal ring in the trials included the following: Device-related events (foreign body sensation, coital problems, device expulsion), vaginal symptoms (discomfort/vaginitis/leukorrhea), headache, emotional lability, and weight gain.

Listed below are adverse reactions that have been associated with the use of combination hormonal contraceptives. These are also likely to apply to combination vaginal hormonal contraceptives such as the contraceptive vaginal ring.

➤*Serious:* Thrombophlebitis and venous thrombosis with or without embolism; arterial thromboembolism; pulmonary embolism; MI; cerebral hemorrhage; cerebral thrombosis; hypertension; gallbladder disease; hepatic adenomas or benign liver tumors; mesenteric thrombosis; retinal thrombosis.

➤*GI:* Cholestatic jaundice; GI symptoms (eg, abdominal cramps, bloating); nausea; vomiting.

➤*GU:* Amenorrhea; breakthrough bleeding; breast changes (tenderness, enlargement, secretion); change in cervical erosion and secretion; change in menstrual flow; diminution in lactation when given immediately postpartum; spotting; temporary infertility after discontinuation of treatment; vaginal candidiasis.

➤*Miscellaneous:* Changes in weight (increase or decrease); change in corneal curvature (steepening); edema; intolerance to contact lenses; melasma (which may persist); mental depression; migraine; rash (allergic); reduced tolerance to carbohydrates.

The following additional adverse reactions have been reported in users of combination hormonal contraceptives and a causal association has been neither confirmed nor refuted: Acne; Budd-Chiari syndrome; cataracts; changes in appetite; changes in libido; colitis; cystitis-like syndrome; dizziness; erythema multiforme; erythema nodosum; headache; hemolytic uremic syndrome; hemorrhagic eruption; hirsutism; impaired renal function; loss of scalp hair; nervousness; premenstrual syndrome; porphyria; vaginitis.

Overdosage

Overdosage of combination hormonal contraceptives may cause nausea, vomiting, vaginal bleeding, or other menstrual irregularities. Given the nature and design of the contraceptive vaginal ring, it is unlikely that overdosage will occur. If the contraceptive vaginal ring is broken, it does not release a higher dose of hormones. Serious ill effects have not been reported following acute ingestion of large doses of oral contraceptives by young children. There are no antidotes and further treatment should be symptomatic.

Patient Information

Instruct the patient regarding the proper use of the contraceptive vaginal ring.

Counsel patients that this product does not protect against HIV infection (AIDS) and other sexually transmitted diseases.

Advise patients to call their health care provider right away if they experience any of the following symptoms:
• Sharp chest pain, coughing blood, or sudden shortness of breath (possible clot in the lung);
• pain in the calf (back of lower leg; possible clot in the leg);
• crushing chest pain or heaviness in the chest (possible heart attack);
• sudden severe headache or vomiting, dizziness or fainting, problems with vision or speech, weakness or numbness in an arm or leg (possible stroke);
• sudden partial or complete loss of vision (possible clot in the eye);
• yellowing of the skin or whites of the eyes (jaundice), especially with fever, tiredness, loss of appetite, dark-colored urine, or light-colored bowel movements (possible liver problems);
• severe pain, swelling, or tenderness in the abdomen (gallbladder or liver problems);
• breast lumps (possible breast cancer or benign breast disease);
• irregular vaginal bleeding or spotting that happens in > 1 menstrual cycle or lasts for more than a few days;
• swelling (edema) of the fingers or ankles;
• difficulty in sleeping, weakness, lack of energy, fatigue, or a change in mood (possible severe depression).

INTRAUTERINE PROGESTERONE CONTRACEPTIVE SYSTEM

Rx **Progestasert** (Alza) **Intrauterine System:** T-shaped unit containing a reservoir of 38 mg progesterone with barium sulfate dispersed in medical grade silicone fluid In 6s w/ inserters.

Indications

➤*Contraception:* Intrauterine contraception in women who have had at least 1 child, are in a stable, mutually monogamous relationship, and have no history of pelvic inflammatory disease (PID).

➤*Unlabeled uses:* This system has been used in the treatment of menorrhagia.

Administration and Dosage

Insert a single system into the uterine cavity. Contraceptive effectiveness is retained for 1 year, and the system must be replaced 1 year after insertion. See manufacturer's literature for insertion and removal instructions.

Actions

➤*Pharmacology:* The *Progestasert* system, a T-shaped unit that contains a reservoir of 38 mg progesterone, is indicated for intrauterine contraception. The mechanism of action has not been demonstrated. Hypotheses include progesterone-induced inhibition of sperm capacitation or survival and alteration of the uterine milieu to prevent nidation. During use of the system, the endometrium shows progestational influence. Progesterone from the system suppresses proliferation of the endometrial tissue (an antiestrogenic effect). Following removal of the system, the endometrium rapidly returns to its normal cyclic pattern and can support pregnancy.

➤*Pharmacokinetics:* Contraceptive effectiveness is enhanced by continuous release of progesterone into the uterine cavity at an average rate of 65 mcg/day for 1 year. The mechanism is local, not systemic. The concentrations of luteinizing hormone, estradiol, and progesterone in systemic venous plasma follow regular cyclic patterns, indicative of ovulation during use of the system. For pregnancy rates for various means of contraception, refer to the Oral Contraceptives group monograph.

Contraindications

Pregnancy or suspected pregnancy; previous ectopic pregnancy; presence or history of PID; patient or partner with multiple sexual partners; sexually transmitted disease; postpartum endometritis or infected abortion; pelvic surgery; abnormalities which result in uterine distortion or uteri that measure < 6 cm or > 10 cm by sounding; uterine or cervical malignancy, including an unresolved abnormal Pap smear; genital bleeding of unknown etiology; vaginitis or cervicitis unless infection has been completely controlled and is nongonococcal and nonchlamydial; incomplete involution of the uterus following abortion or childbirth; previously inserted intrauterine device (IUD) still in place; genital actinomycosis; conditions or treatments associated with increased susceptibility to infections with microorganisms (eg, leukemia, diabetes, AIDS); IV drug abuse.

Warnings

➤*Pelvic infection:* An increased risk of PID associated with IUD use has been reported; the highest rate occurs shortly after insertion and up to 4 months thereafter. Teach patients to recognize the symptoms of PID and ectopic pregnancy. Pelvic infection may occur with an IUD in situ, and may result in tubo-ovarian abscesses or general peritonitis. If this occurs, remove the IUD and institute appropriate antibiotic treatment. PID can result in tubal damage and occlusion, threatening future fertility or predisposing to ectopic pregnancy. PID may be asymptomatic but still result in tubal damage and its sequelae.

Following diagnosis of PID, initiate antibiotic therapy promptly and remove the progesterone IUD. Guidelines for treatment are available from the CDC.

Genital actinomycosis has been associated primarily with long-term IUD use.

➤*Embedment:* Partial penetration or lodging of an IUD in the endometrium can result in difficult removal. In some cases, this can result in IUD fragmentation, necessitating surgical removal.

➤*Perforation:* Perforation, partial or total, of the uterine wall or cervix may occur. If perforation occurs, remove the device. Adhesions, foreign body reactions, peritonitis, cystic masses in the pelvis, intestinal penetrations, local inflammatory reaction with abscess formation and erosion of adjacent viscera and intestinal obstruction may result if the IUD is left in the peritoneal cavity.

➤*Mortality risks:* Refer to the Oral Contraceptives group monograph for risk of death associated with various methods of contraception.

➤*Pregnancy:* Long-term effects on the fetus are unknown.

Septic abortion – Septic abortion may be increased, associated in some instances with septicemia, septic shock, and death in patients

INTRAUTERINE PROGESTERONE CONTRACEPTIVE SYSTEM

becoming pregnant with an IUD in place, usually in the second trimester. If pregnancy occurs with a system in situ, remove it if the thread is visible or, if removal is difficult, consider termination of the pregnancy.

Continuation of pregnancy – If pregnancy is maintained and the system remains in situ, warn the patient of the increased risk of spontaneous abortion and sepsis, including death, and premature labor and delivery. Advise her to report immediately all abnormal symptoms, such as flu-like syndrome, fever, chills, abdominal cramping and pain, bleeding or vaginal discharge; generalized symptoms of septicemia may be insidious.

Congenital anomalies – Systemically administered sex steroids, including progestational agents, have been associated with an increased risk of congenital anomalies. It is not known whether there is an increased risk of such anomalies when pregnancy is continued with this system in place.

Ectopic pregnancy – The *Progestasert* system acts in the uterus to prevent uterine pregnancy, but it does not prevent either ovulation or ectopic pregnancy. Therefore, a pregnancy that occurs while a patient is using an IUD is much more likely to be ectopic. Determine whether ectopic pregnancy has occurred in patients with delayed menses or unilateral pelvic pain.

In clinical trials of the progesterone system, 1 of 3.6 pregnancies in parous women and 1 of 6.2 pregnancies in nulliparous women were ectopic. The per-year risk of ectopic pregnancy in progesterone system users is ≈ 1 ectopic pregnancy in 200 users per year. This risk is approximately the same as in noncontracepting, sexually active women.

In two clinical studies, for the first year the risk of ectopic pregnancy was approximately 6 times higher among women using progesterone systems than among women using copper systems. Over 2 years, the risk of an ectopic pregnancy with the progesterone-releasing IUD was about 10 times higher than that with copper-releasing IUDs.

Women who have previously had acute PID subsequently have an 8- to 10-fold greater than normal risk of ectopic pregnancy (see Pelvic Infection). Multiple sexual partners or a partner with multiple sexual partners, previous pelvic surgery, endometritis, endometriosis, and retrograde menstruation have also been recognized as risk factors for ectopic pregnancy.

Precautions

➤*Prior to insertion:* Prior to insertion, complete a medical and social history, and determine risk of ectopic pregnancy because of previous PID. Perform pelvic examination, Pap smear, gonorrhea and chlamydia culture and, if indicated, tests for other sexually transmitted diseases. Carefully sound the uterus prior to insertion to determine the degree of patency of the endocervical canal and the internal os, and the direction and depth of the uterine cavity. Occasionally, severe cervical stenosis may be encountered. The uterus should sound to a depth of 6 to 10 cm. Inserting the system into a uterine cavity measuring < 6.5 cm may increase the incidence of expulsion, bleeding, and pain.

To reduce the possibility of insertion in the presence of an undetermined pregnancy, insert during or shortly following menstruation.

➤*Cervicitis/Vaginitis:* Postpone use in these patients until infection has cleared and until the cervicitis has been shown not to be due to gonorrhea or chlamydia.

➤*Involution of uterus:* Do not insert postpartum or postabortion until involution of the uterus is completed. Incidence of perforation (see Warnings) and expulsion is greater if involution is not completed. Involution may be delayed in nursing mothers.

➤*Anemia:* Use cautiously in those who have anemia or history of menorrhagia or hypermenorrhea. Patients experiencing menorrhagia

or metrorrhagia following IUD insertion may be at risk of developing hypochromic microcytic anemia.

➤*Syncope/Bradycardia:* Syncope, bradycardia, or other neurovascular episodes may occur during insertion or removal, especially in patients previously disposed to these conditions or cervical stenosis.

➤*Valvular/Congenital heart disease patients:* Valvular or congenital heart disease patients are more prone to develop subacute bacterial endocarditis. The use of the IUD may represent a potential source of septic emboli.

➤*Reexamine:* Reexamine patient shortly after the first postinsertion menses, since an IUD may be expelled or displaced, but definitely within 3 months after insertion. Thereafter, perform an annual examination.

➤*Replace:* Replace the device every 12 months, since the level of contraceptive efficacy after this time decreases.

➤*Remove:* Remove the device for the following reasons: Menorrhagia/metrorrhagia-producing anemia; pelvic infection; endometritis; genital actinomycosis; intractable pelvic pain; dyspareunia; pregnancy; endometrial or cervical malignancy; uterine or cervical perforation; increase of length of the threads extending from the cervix or any other indication of partial expulsion. If retrieval threads are not visible, they may have retracted into the uterus or have been broken; therefore, consider the system displaced and remove. After menstrual period, determine that the threads still protrude from the cervix. Caution patients not to pull on the threads. If partial expulsion occurs, removal is indicated and a new system may be inserted.

➤*Bleeding and cramps:* Bleeding and cramps may occur during the first few weeks after insertion; if symptoms continue or are severe, consult health care provider.

➤*Prophylactic antibiotics:* Prophylactic antibiotics may be considered prior to IUD insertion to decrease the risk of PID; however, the utility of this treatment is still under evaluation. Regimens include doxycycline 200 mg orally 1 hour before insertion or erythromycin 500 mg orally 1 hour before and 6 hours after insertion.

Drug Interactions

➤*Anticoagulants:* Use IUDs with caution in patients receiving anticoagulants or having a coagulopathy.

Adverse Reactions

Endometritis; spontaneous abortion; septic abortion; septicemia; perforation of uterus and cervix; pelvic infection; cervical erosion; vaginitis; leukorrhea; pregnancy; ectopic pregnancy; uterine embedment; difficult removal; complete or partial expulsion; intermenstrual spotting; prolongation of menstrual flow; anemia; amenorrhea or delayed menses; pain and cramping; dysmenorrhea; backaches; dyspareunia; neurovascular episodes including bradycardia and syncope secondary to insertion; fragmentation of IUD; tubo-ovarian abscess; tubal damage; fetal damage and congenital anomalies. Perforation into the abdomen followed by peritonitis, abdominal adhesions, intestinal penetration, intestinal obstruction, local inflammatory reaction, abscess formation and erosion of adjacent viscera, and cystic masses in the pelvis have occurred. Some of these adverse reactions can lead to loss of fertility, partial or total removal of reproductive organs, hormonal imbalance, or death.

Patient Information

Patient package insert and patient instructions are available with the product. The patient must read and initial each section of the Patient Information Leaflet, and the Informed Choice Statement must be signed by the patient and by the health care provider.

Notify health care provider if any of the following occurs: Abnormal or excessive bleeding; severe cramping; abnormal or odorous vaginal discharge; fever or flu-like syndrome; pain; genital lesions or sores; missed period.

LEVONORGESTREL-RELEASING INTRAUTERINE SYSTEM

| Rx | Mirena (Berlex Labs.) | **Intrauterine system:** T-shaped unit containing a reservoir of 52 mg levonorgestrel covered by a silicone membrane | In 1s w/ inserter. |

Indications

➤*Contraception:* Intrauterine contraception ≤ 5 years. Thereafter, if continued contraception is desired, the system should be replaced.

It is recommended for women who have had at least 1 child, are in a stable, mutually monogamous relationship, have no history of pelvic inflammatory disease (PID), and have no history of ectopic pregnancy or condition that would predispose to ectopic pregnancy.

Administration and Dosage

➤*Approved by the FDA:* December 6, 2000.

Health care providers are advised to become thoroughly familiar with the insertion instructions before attempting insertion of levonorgestrel-releasing intrauterine system (LRIS).

Insert LRIS with the provided inserter into the uterine cavity within 7 days of the onset of menstruation or immediately after the first trimester abortion by carefully following the insertion instructions. It can

be replaced by a new system at any time during the menstrual cycle. The system should not remain in the uterus after 5 years. See manufacturer's literature for insertion and removal instructions.

➤*Storage/Stability:* LRIS is sterilized with ethylene oxide. Do not resterilize. For single use only. Do not use if inner package is damaged or open. Insert before the month shown on the label. Store at 25°C (77°F); with excursions permitted between 15° to 30°C (59° to 86°F).

Actions

➤*Pharmacology:* LRIS has mainly local progestogenic effects in the uterine cavity. Morphological changes of the endometrium are observed, including stromal pseudodecidualization, glandular atrophy, a leucocytic infiltration and a decrease in glandular and stromal mitoses.

Ovulation is inhibited in some women using LRIS. In a 1-year study ≈ 45% of menstrual cycles were ovulatory and in another study after 4 years, 75% of cycles were ovulatory.

LEVONORGESTREL-RELEASING INTRAUTERINE SYSTEM

The local mechanism by which continuously released levonorgestrel enhances contraceptive effectiveness of the intrauterine system (IUS) has not been conclusively demonstrated. Studies of LRIS prototypes have suggested several mechanisms that prevent pregnancy: Thickening of cervical mucus preventing passage of sperm into the uterus, inhibition of sperm capacitation or survival, and alteration of the endometrium.

➤*Pharmacokinetics:*

Absorption/Distribution – Following insertion of LRIS, the initial release of levonorgestrel into the uterine cavity is 20 mcg/day. A stable plasma level of levonorgestrel of 150 to 200 pg/ml occurs after the first few weeks following insertion of LRIS. Levonorgestrel levels after long-term use of 12, 24, and 60 months were ≈ 180 pg/ml, ≈ 192 pg/ml, and ≈ 159 pg/ml, respectively. The plasma concentrations achieved by LRIS are lower than those seen with levonorgestrel contraceptive implants and with oral contrceptives (OCs). Unlike OCs, plasma levels with LRIS do not display peaks and troughs.

The mean ± SD levonorgestrel endometrial tissue concentration in 4 women using levonorgestrel intrauterine systems releasing 30 mcg/day of levonorgestrel for 36 to 49 days was ≈ 808 ng/g wet tissue weight. The endometrial tissue concentration in 2 women who had been taking a 250 mcg levonorgestrel-containing OC for 7 days was 3.5 ng/g wet tissue weight. In contrast, fallopian tube and myometrial levonorgestrel tissue concentrations were of the same order of magnitude in the LRIS group and the OC group (between 1 and 5 ng/g of wet weight of tissue).

Levonorgestrel in serum is primarily bound to proteins (mainly sex hormone binding globulin).

Metabolism/Excretion – Levonorgestrel in serum is extensively metabolized to a large number of inactive metabolites. Metabolic clearance rates may differ among individuals by several-fold, and this may account in part for wide individual variations in levonorgestrel concentrations seen in individuals using levonorgestrel-containing contraceptive products. The elimination half-life of levonorgestrel after daily oral doses is ≈ 17 hours; both the parent drug and its metabolites are primarily excreted in the urine.

Contraindications

Pregnancy or suspicion of pregnancy; congenital or acquired uterine anomaly including fibroids if they distort the uterine cavity; acute PID or a history of PID unless there has been a subsequent intrauterine pregnancy; postpartum endometritis or infected abortion in the past 3 months; known or suspected uterine or cervical neoplasia or unresolved, abnormal Pap smear; genital bleeding of unknown etiology; untreated acute cervicitis or vaginitis, including bacterial vaginosis or other lower genital tract infections until infection is controlled; acute liver disease or liver tumor (benign or malignant); woman or her partner with multiple sexual partners; conditions associated with increased susceptibility to infections with microorganisms, including, but not limited to, leukemia, acquired immune deficiency syndrome (AIDS), and IV drug abuse; genital actinomycosis (see Warnings); a previously inserted IUD that has not been removed; hypersensitivity to any component of the product; known or suspected carcinoma of the breast; history of ectopic pregnancy or condition that would predispose to ectopic pregnancy.

Warnings

➤*Ectopic pregnancy:* In large clinical trials of LRIS, half of all pregnancies detected during the studies were ectopic. The per-year incidence of ectopic pregnancy in the clinical trials was ≈ 1 ectopic pregnancy/1000 users/year. The rate of ectopic pregnancies associated with LRIS use is not significantly different than the rate for sexually active women not using any contraception.

Clinical trials of LRIS excluded women with a history of ectopic pregnancy. It is not recommended for use in women with a history of ectopic pregnancy or conditions that increase the risk of ectopic pregnancy. Women who choose LRIS must be warned about the risks of ectopic pregnancy. They should be taught to recognize and report to their health care provider promptly any symptoms of ectopic pregnancy. Inform women that ectopic pregnancy has been associated with complications leading to loss of fertility.

➤*Intrauterine pregnancy:* In the event of an intrauterine pregnancy with LRIS, consider the following:

Septic abortion – In patients becoming pregnant with an IUD in place, septic abortion—with septicemia, septic shock, and death—may occur. If pregnancy should occur with LRIS in place, remove LRIS. Removal or manipulation of LRIS may result in pregnancy loss.

Continuation of pregnancy – If a woman becomes pregnant with LRIS in place and if LRIS cannot be removed or the woman chooses not to have it removed, she should be warned that failure to remove LRIS increases the risk of miscarriage, sepsis, premature labor, and premature delivery. She should be monitored closely and advised to report immediately any flu-like symptoms, fever, chills, cramping, pain, bleeding, vaginal discharge, or leakage of fluid.

Long-term effects and congenital anomalies – When pregnancy continues with LRIS in place, long-term effects on the offspring are unknown. Because of the intrauterine administration of levonorgestrel and local exposure to the hormone, the possibility of teratogenicity following exposure to LRIS cannot be completely excluded. Clinical experience with the outcomes of pregnancies is limited because of the small number of reported pregnancies following exposure to LRIS.

Congenital anomalies have occurred infrequently when LRIS has been in place during pregnancy. In these cases the role of LRIS in the development of the congenital anomalies is unknown. As of September 1999, 32 live births following exposure to LRIS were reported retrospectively. All but 2 of the infants were healthy at birth. One infant had pulmonary artery hypoplasia and another infant had cystic hypoplastic kidneys (a sibling of this infant had renal agenesis with no LRIS exposure).

➤*Sepsis:* As of 1999, 4 cases of Group A streptococcal sepsis (GAS) out of an estimated 1.3 million LRIS users were reported. All 4 women experienced the symptom of severe pain within hours of insertion, and this was followed by sepsis within a few days of insertion. All recovered with treatment. Since death from GAS is more likely if treatment is delayed, it is important to be aware of these rare but serious infections. Aseptic technique during LRIS insertion is essential (GAS sepsis can also occur postpartum, after minor surgery, in wounds, and is association with other IUDs).

➤*PID:* LRIS is contraindicated in the presence of known or suspected PID or in women with a history of PID unless there has been a subsequent intrauterine pregnancy. Use of IUDs has been associated with an increased risk of PID. The highest risk of PID occurs shortly after insertion (usually within the first 20 days thereafter). A decision to use LRIS must include consideration of the risks of PID.

All women who choose LRIS must be informed prior to insertion about the possibility of PID and that PID can cause tubal damage leading to ectopic pregnancy or infertility, or in infrequent cases can necessitate hysterectomy, or can cause death. Patients must be taught to recognize and report to their health care provider promptly any symptoms of PID. These symptoms include development of menstrual disorders (prolonged or heavy bleeding), unusual vaginal discharge, abdominal or pelvic pain or tenderness, dyspareunia, chills, and fever.

Women at increased risk for PID – PID is often associated with a sexually-transmitted disease, and LRIS does not protect against sexually-transmitted disease. Women who have ever had PID are at increased risk for a recurrence or reinfection.

Asymptomatic PID – PID may be asymptomatic but still result in tubal damage and its sequelae.

Treatment of PID – Following a diagnosis of PID, or suspected PID, bacteriologic specimens should be obtained and antibiotic therapy initiated promptly. Removal of LRIS after initiation of antibiotic therapy is usually appropriate. Guidelines for PID treatment are available from the Centers for Disease Control.

Actinomycosis has been associated with IUDs. Symptomatic women with IUDs should have the IUD removed and should receive antibiotics. However, the management of the asymptomatic carrier is controversial because actinomycetes can be found normally in the genital tract cultures in healthy women without IUDs. False positive findings of actinomycosis on Pap smears can be a problem. When possible, confirm the Pap smear diagnosis with cultures.

➤*Irregular bleeding and amenorrhea:* LRIS can alter the bleeding pattern. During the first 3 to 6 months of LRIS use, the number of bleeding and spotting days may be increased and bleeding patterns may be irregular. Thereafter, the number of bleeding and spotting days usually decreases but bleeding may remain irregular. If bleeding irregularities develop during prolonged treatment, appropriate diagnostic measures should be taken to rule out endometrial pathology.

Amenorrhea develops in ≈ 20% of LRIS users by 1 year. The possibility of pregnancy should be considered if menstruation does not occur within 6 weeks of the onset of previous menstruation. Once pregnancy has been excluded, repeated pregnancy tests are not necessary in amenorrheic subjects unless indicated by other signs of pregnancy or by pelvic pain.

➤*Embedment:* Partial penetration or embedment of LRIS in the myometrium may decrease contraceptive effectiveness and can result in difficult removal.

➤*Perforation:* An IUD may perforate the uterus or cervix, most often during insertion although the perforation may not be detected until some time later. If perforation occurs, the IUD must be removed and surgery may be required. Adhesions, peritonitis, intestinal perforations, intestinal obstruction, abscesses and erosion of adjacent viscera have been reported with IUDs.

It is recommended that postpartum LRIS insertion be delayed until uterine involution is complete to decrease perforation risk. There is an increased risk of perforation in women who are lactating. Inserting LRIS immediately after first trimester abortion is not known to increase the risk of perforation, but insertion after second trimester abortion should be delayed until uterine involution is complete.

LEVONORGESTREL-RELEASING INTRAUTERINE SYSTEM

➤*Ovarian cysts:* Since the contraceptive effect of LRIS is mainly caused by its local effect, ovulatory cycles with follicular rupture usually occur in women of fertile age using LRIS. Sometimes atresia of the follicle is delayed and the follicle may continue to grow. Enlarged follicles have been diagnosed in ≈ 12% of the subjects using LRIS. Most of these follicles are asymptomatic, although some may be accompanied by pelvic pain or dyspareunia. In most cases the enlarged follicles disappear spontaneously during 2 to 3 months observation. Surgical intervention is not usually required.

➤*Breast cancer:* Women who currently have or have had breast cancer should not use hormonal contraception because breast cancer is a hormone-sensitive tumor.

➤*Mortality risks:* Refer to the Oral Contaceptives group monograph for risk of death associated with various methods of contraception.

➤*Pregnancy:* Category X.

➤*Lactation:* Levonorgestrel has been identified in small quantities in the breast milk of lactating women using LRIS. In a study of 14 breastfeeding women using a LRIS prototype during lactation, mean infant serum levels of levonorgestrel were ≈ 7% of maternal serum levels. Hormonal contraceptives are not recommended as the contraceptive method of first choice during lactation.

➤*Children:* Safety and efficacy of LRIS have been established in women of reproductive age. Use of this product before menarche is not indicated.

Precautions

➤*Prior to insertion:* Obtain a complete medical and social history, including that of the partner to determine conditions that might influence the selection of an IUD for contraception (see Contraindications). Perform a physical examination including a pelvic examination, a Pap smear, and appropriate tests for any other forms of genital disease, such as gonorrhea and chlamydia, if indicated. Special attention must be given to ascertaining whether the woman is at increased risk of ectopic pregnancy or PID. LRIS is contraindicated in these women.

Carefully sound the uterus prior to LRIS insertion to determine the degree of patency of the endocervical canal and the internal os, and the direction and depth of the uterine cavity. In occasional cases, severe cervical stenosis may be encountered. Do not use excessive force to overcome this resistance.

The health care provider should determine that the patient is not pregnant. The possibility of insertion of LRIS in the presence of an existing undetermined pregnancy is reduced if insertion is performed within 7 days of the onset of a menstrual period. LRIS can be replaced by a new system at any time in the cycle. It can be inserted immediately after first trimester abortion.

Do not insert LRIS until 6 weeks postpartum or until involution of the uterus is complete in order to reduce the incidence of perforation and expulsion.

➤*Valvular / Congenital heart disease patients:* Patients with certain types of valvular or congenital heart disease and surgically constructed systemic-pulmonary shunts are at increased risk of infective endocarditis. Use of LRIS in these patients may represent a potential source of septic emboli. Patients with known congenital heart disease who may be at increased risk should be treated with appropriate antibiotics at the time of insertion and removal. Patients requiring chronic corticosteroid therapy or insulin for diabetes should be monitored with special care for infection.

➤*Coagulopathy / Anticoagulant therapy:* Use LRIS with caution in patients who have a coagulopathy or are receiving anticoagulants.

➤*Vaginitis / Cervicitis:* Use of LRIS in patients with vaginitis or cervicitis should be postponed until proper treatment has eradicated the infection and until it has been shown that the cervicitis is not caused by gonorrhea or chlamydia.

➤*Prophylactic antibiotics:* Because the presence of organisms capable of establishing PID cannot be determined by appearance, and because IUD insertion may be associated with introduction of vaginal bacteria into the uterus, strict asepsis should be observed at insertion. Consider administration of antibiotics, but the utility of this treatment is unknown.

➤*Syncope / Bradycardia:* Syncope, bradycardia, or other neurovascular episodes may occur during insertion or removal of LRIS, especially in patients with a predisposition to these conditions or cervical stenosis. If decreased pulse, perspiration, or pallor are observed, keep the patient supine until these signs have disappeared.

➤*Reexamine:* Since LRIS may be displaced, reexamine patients and evaluate shortly after the first postinsertion menses, but definitely within 3 months after insertion. Symptoms of the partial or complete expulsion of any IUD may include bleeding or pain. However, the system can be expelled from the uterine cavity without the woman noticing it. Partial expulsion may decrease the effectiveness of LRIS. As menstrual flow usually decreases after the first 3 to 6 months of LRIS use, increase of menstrual flow may be indicative of an expulsion.

If the retrieval threads are not visible, they may have retracted into the uterus or have been broken, or LRIS may have been broken, perforated the uterus, or have been expelled. Location of LRIS may be determined by sonography, x-ray, or by gentle exploration of the uterine cavity with a probe.

User complaints of pain, odorous discharge, bleeding, fever, genital lesions, or sores should be promptly responded to and prompt examination recommended (see Warnings).

➤*Replacement:* LRIS must be replaced every 5 years because contraceptive effectiveness after 5 years has not been established.

➤*Removal:* If examination during visits subsequent to insertion reveals that the length of the threads has changed from the length at time of insertion, and the system is verified as displaced, it should be removed. A new system may be inserted at that time or during the next menses if it is certain that conception has not occurred. If the threads are not visible, verify the location of the LRIS (eg, with x-ray, ultrasound, gentle probing of the uterine cavity). If the LRIS is in place with no evidence of perforation, no intervention is indicated. If expulsion has occurred, it may be replaced within 7 days of a menstrual period after pregnancy has been ruled out.

Remove LRIS for the following medical reasons: Menorrhagia or metrorrhagia producing anemia; AIDS; sexually transmitted disease; pelvic infection; endometritis; symptomatic genital actinomycosis; intractable pelvic pain; severe dyspareunia; pregnancy; endometrial or cervical malignancy; uterine or cervical perforation.

Consider removal of the system if any of the following conditions arise for the first time: Migraine, focal migraine with asymmetrical visual loss or other symptoms indicating transient cerebral ischemia; exceptionally severe headaches; jaundice; marked increase of blood pressure; severe arterial disease such as stroke or MI.

➤*Pregnancy during therapy:* In the event a pregnancy is confirmed during LRIS use, take the following steps: Determine whether pregnancy is ectopic and take appropriate measures if it is; inform patient of the risks of leaving LRIS in place or removing it during pregnancy and of the lack of data on long-term effects on the offspring of women who have had LRIS in place during conception or gestation (see Warnings); if possible, remove LRIS after the patient has been warned of the risks of removal. If removal is difficult, counsel the patient and offer pregnancy termination; if LRIS is left in place, follow the patient's course closely.

➤*Patients with diabetes:* Levonorgestrel may affect glucose tolerance, and the blood glucose concentration should be monitored in diabetic users of LRIS.

Drug Interactions

The effect of other drugs on the efficacy of LRIS has not been studied.

The effect of hormonal contraceptives may be impaired by drugs that induce liver enzymes. The influence of these drugs on the contraceptive efficacy of LRIS has not been studied.

➤*Phenytoin:* Phenytoin may decrease the efficacy of OC steroids (eg, levonorgestrel). Both hydantoin induction of progestin metabolism (CYP3A4) and sex-hormone binding globulin synthesis may reduce progestin concentrations.

Adverse Reactions

➤*Cardiovascular:* Syncope, bradycardia, hypertension (≥ 5%).

➤*CNS:* Headache, depression, nervousness (≥ 5%); migraine (< 3%).

➤*Dermatologic:* Acne, skin disorder (≥ 5%); hair loss, eczema (< 3%).

➤*GI:* Abdominal pain, nausea (≥ 5%); vomiting (< 3%).

➤*GU:* Ectopic pregnancy; septic abortion; PID; irregular or prolonged bleeding; spotting; cramping; amenorrhea; perforation; partial penetration or embedment; ovarian cysts; leukorrhea, vaginitis, dysmenorrhea, abnormal Pap smear (≥ 5%); cervicitis (< 3%).

➤*Respiratory:* Upper respiratory tract infection, sinusitis (≥ 5%).

➤*Miscellaneous:* Sepsis; back pain, breast pain, weight increase, decreased libido (≥ 5%); failed insertion, anemia, dyspareunia (< 3%).

Patient Information

Counsel patients that this product does not protect against HIV infection (AIDS) and other sexually transmitted diseases.

Prior to insertion, provide the patient with the Patient Package Insert.

Advise the patient that some bleeding, such as irregular or prolonged bleeding and spotting, or cramps may occur during the first few weeks after insertion. If her symptoms continue or are severe, she should report them to her health care provider. Instruct patient on how to check after her menstrual period to make certain that the thread still protrudes from the cervix and caution her not to pull on the thread and displace LRIS. Inform her that there is no contraceptive protection if LRIS is displaced or expelled.

About 80% of women wishing to become pregnant conceived within 12 months after removal of LRIS.

Contraceptive Hormones

MEDROXYPROGESTERONE CONTRACEPTIVE INJECTION

Rx	**Depo-Provera** (Pharmacia Corp.)	**Injection:** 150 mg/ml	In 1 ml vials.[1]

[1] With 28.9 mg PEG 3350, 2.41 mg polysorbate 80, 8.68 mg sodium chloride, 1.37 mg methylparaben and 0.15 mg propylparaben.

Medroxyprogesterone is also used for secondary amenorrhea and abnormal uterine bleeding (see the Progestins monograph) and as an antineoplastic (see monograph in Antineoplastics chapter).

Indications

►*Contraception:* Long-term injectable contraceptive in women when administered at 3-month intervals.

Administration and Dosage

Shake the vial vigorously just before use to ensure that the dose being administered represents a uniform suspension.

The recommended dose is 150 mg every 3 months administered by deep IM injection in the gluteal or deltoid muscle. To increase assurance that the patient is not pregnant at the time of the first administration, give this injection only during the first 5 days after the onset of a normal menstrual period; within 5 days postpartum if not breastfeeding; or, if breastfeeding, at 6 weeks postpartum. If the period between injections is > 14 weeks, determine that the patient is not pregnant before administering the drug.

Actions

►*Pharmacology:* Medroxyprogesterone, when administered IM at the recommended dose to women every 3 months, inhibits the secretion of gonadotropins which, in turn, prevents follicular maturation and ovulation and results in endometrial thinning. These actions produce its contraceptive effect.

►*Pharmacokinetics:* Following a single 150 mg IM dose, medroxyprogesterone concentrations increase for ≈ 3 weeks to reach peak plasma concentrations of 1 to 7 ng/ml. The levels then decrease exponentially until they become undetectable (< 100 pg/ml) between 120 to 200 days following injection. The apparent half-life following IM administration is ≈ 50 days.

Women with lower body weights conceive sooner than women with higher body weights after discontinuing medroxyprogesterone.

The effect of hepatic or renal disease on the pharmacokinetics of medroxyprogesterone is unknown.

►*Clinical trials:* In 5 clinical studies the 12-month failure rate for the group of women treated with medroxyprogesterone was 0 (no pregnancies reported) to 0.7 by Life-Table method. Pregnancy rates with contraceptive measures are typically reported for only the first year of use. The effectiveness of medroxyprogesterone is dependent on the patient returning every 3 months for re-injection.

Contraindications

Known or suspected pregnancy or as a diagnostic test for pregnancy; undiagnosed vaginal bleeding; known or suspected malignancy of breast; active thrombophlebitis, or a history of or current thromboembolic disorders, or cerebral vascular disease; liver dysfunction or disease; hypersensitivity to medroxyprogesterone or any of its other ingredients.

Warnings

►*Bleeding irregularities:* Most women using medroxyprogesterone experience disruption of menstrual bleeding patterns. Altered menstrual bleeding patterns include irregular or unpredictable bleeding or spotting, or rarely, heavy or continuous bleeding. If abnormal bleeding persists or is severe, institute appropriate investigation to rule out the possibility of organic pathology, and institute appropriate treatment when necessary.

As women continue using medroxyprogesterone, fewer experience intermenstrual bleeding and more experience amenorrhea. By month 12, amenorrhea was reported by 57% of women, and by month 24, amenorrhea was reported by 68% of women.

►*Bone mineral density changes:* Use of medroxyprogesterone may be considered among the risk factors for development of osteoporosis. The rate of bone loss is greatest in the early years of use and then subsequently approaches the normal rate of age-related fall.

►*Thromboembolic disorders:* Be alert to the earliest manifestations of thrombotic disorders (thrombophlebitis, pulmonary embolism, cerebrovascular disorders, and retinal thrombosis). If any of these occur or are suspected, do not readminister the drug.

►*Ocular disorders:* Do not readminister pending examination if there is a sudden partial or complete loss of vision or if there is a sudden onset of proptosis, diplopia, or migraine. If examination reveals papilledema or retinal vascular lesions, do not readminister.

►*Carcinogenesis:* Long-term case-controlled surveillance of users found slight or no increased overall risk of breast cancer and no overall increased risk of ovarian, liver, or cervical cancer and a prolonged, protective effect of reducing the risk of endometrial cancer in the population of users.

An increased relative risk of 2.19 of breast cancer has been associated with the use of medroxyprogesterone in women whose first exposure to the drug was within the previous 4 years and who were < 35 years of age. However, the overall relative risk for ever-users was only 1.2.

A statistically insignificant increase in relative risk estimates of invasive squamous cell cervical cancer has been associated with the use of medroxyprogesterone in women who were first exposed before 35 years of age.

►*Pregnancy: Category X.* Infants from accidental pregnancies that occur 1 to 2 months after injection of medroxyprogesterone may be at an increased risk of low birth weight, which in turn is associated with an increased risk of neonatal death. The attributable risk is low because such pregnancies are uncommon.

A significant increase in incidence of polysyndactyly and chromosomal anomalies was observed among infants of medroxyprogesterone users, the former being most pronounced in women < 30 years of age. The unrelated nature of these defects, the lack of confirmation from other studies, the distant preconceptual exposure to medroxyprogesterone, and the chance effects due to multiple statistical comparisons, make a causal association unlikely.

Children exposed to medroxyprogesterone in utero and followed to adolescence showed no evidence of any adverse effects on their health, including their physical, intellectual, sexual, or social development.

Several reports suggest an association between intrauterine exposure to progestational drugs in the first trimester of pregnancy and genital abnormalities in male and female fetuses. The risk of hypospadias (5 to 8 per 1000 male births in the general population) may be approximately doubled with exposure to these drugs. There are insufficient data to quantify the risk to exposed female fetuses, but because some of these drugs induce mild virilization of the external genitalia of the female fetus and because of the increased association of hypospadias in the male fetus, it is prudent to avoid the use of these drugs during the first trimester of pregnancy.

To ensure that medroxyprogesterone is not administered inadvertently to a pregnant woman, it is important that the first injection be given only during the first 5 days after the onset of a normal menstrual period, within 5 days postpartum if not breastfeeding and at the sixth week postpartum if breastfeeding (see Administration and Dosage).

Ectopic pregnancy – Be alert to the possibility of an ectopic pregnancy among women using medroxyprogesterone who become pregnant or complain of severe abdominal pain.

►*Lactation:* Detectable amounts of the drug have been identified in the milk of mothers receiving medroxyprogesterone. In nursing mothers treated with medroxyprogesterone, milk composition, quality, and amount are not adversely affected. Infants exposed to medroxyprogesterone via breast milk have been studied for developmental and behavioral effects through puberty; no adverse effects have been noted.

Precautions

►*Physical examination:* The pretreatment and annual history and physical examination should include special reference to breast and pelvic organs, as well as a Papanicolaou smear.

►*Fluid retention:* Because progestational drugs may cause some degree of fluid retention, conditions that might be influenced by this condition (eg, epilepsy, migraine, asthma, cardiac or renal dysfunction) require careful observation.

►*Weight changes:* There is a tendency for women to gain weight while on medroxyprogesterone therapy. From an initial average body weight of 136 lbs, women who completed 1 year of therapy gained an average of 5.4 lbs, women who completed 2 years of therapy gained an average of 8.1 lbs, women who completed 4 years gained an average of 13.8 lbs and women who completed 6 years gained an average of 16.5 lbs. Two percent of women withdrew from a large-scale clinical trial because of excessive weight gain.

►*Return of fertility:* Medroxyprogesterone has a prolonged contraceptive effect. It is expected that 68% of women who do become pregnant may conceive within 12 months, 83% may conceive within 15 months and 93% may conceive within 18 months from the last injection. The median time to conception for those who do conceive is 10 months following the last injection with a range of 4 to 31 months, and is unrelated to the duration of use.

►*CNS disorders and convulsions:* Carefully observe patients who have a history of psychic depression; do not readminister if the depression recurs.

There have been a few reported cases of convulsions. Association with drug use or preexisting conditions is not clear.

►*Carbohydrate metabolism:* A decrease in glucose tolerance has been observed in some patients. The mechanism of this decrease is

MEDROXYPROGESTERONE CONTRACEPTIVE INJECTION

obscure. For this reason, carefully observe diabetic patients during therapy.

➤*Liver function:* If jaundice develops, consider not readministering the drug.

Drug Interactions

➤*Aminoglutethimide:* Aminoglutethimide may significantly depress the serum concentrations of medroxyprogesterone. Warn users of the possibility of decreased efficacy with the use of this or any related drugs.

➤*Drug/Lab test interactions:* The following laboratory tests may be affected by medroxyprogesterone: Plasma and urinary steroid levels decreased (eg, progesterone, estradiol, pregnanediol, testosterone, cortisol); gonadotropin levels decreased; sex-hormone binding globulin concentrations decreased; protein bound iodine and butanol extractable protein bound iodine may increase; T_3 uptake values may decrease; coagulation test values for prothrombin (Factor II), and Factors VII, VIII, IX, and X may increase. Sulfobromophthalein and other liver function test values may be increased; the effects of medroxyprogesterone acetate on lipid metabolism are inconsistent. Both increases and decreases in total cholesterol, triglycerides, low-density lipoprotein (LDL) cholesterol, and high-density lipoprotein (HDL) cholesterol have been observed.

Adverse Reactions

Menstrual irregularities (bleeding or amenorrhea), weight changes, headache, nervousness, abdominal pain or discomfort, asthenia (weakness or fatigue), dizziness (> 5%); decreased libido or anorgasmia, backache, leg cramps, depression, nausea, insomnia, leukorrhea, acne, vaginitis, pelvic pain, breast pain, no hair growth or alopecia, bloating, rash, edema, hot flashes, arthralgia (1% to 5%); galactorrhea, melasma, chloasma, convulsions, changes in appetite, GI disturbances, jaundice, GU infections, vaginal cysts, dyspareunia, paresthesia, chest pain, pulmonary embolus, allergic reactions, anemia, drowsiness, syncope, dyspnea, asthma, tachycardia, fever, excessive sweating and body odor, dry skin, chills, increased thirst, hoarseness, pain at injection site, blood dyscrasia, rectal bleeding, changes in breast size, breast lumps or nipple bleeding, axillary swelling, breast cancer, prevention of lactation, sensation of pregnancy, lack of return to fertility, paralysis, facial palsy, scleroderma, osteoporosis, uterine hyperplasia, cervical cancer, varicose veins, dysmenorrhea, hirsutism, accidental pregnancy, thrombophlebitis, deep vein thrombosis (< 1%).

Patient Information

Patient labeling is included with each single dose vial. Give prospective users this labeling and inform them about the risks and benefits associated with the use of medroxyprogesterone, as compared with other forms of contraception or with no contraception at all.

Advise patients at the beginning of treatment that their menstrual cycle may be disrupted and that irregular and unpredictable bleeding or spotting results, and that this usually decreases to the point of amenorrhea as treatment continues, without other therapy being required.

MEDROXYPROGESTERONE ACETATE/ESTRADIOL CYPIONATE (MPA/E₂C)

| Rx | Lunelle (Pharmacia) | Injection: 25 mg medroxyprogesterone acetate and 5 mg estradiol cypionate per 0.5 ml | 4.28 mg NaCl. In 0.5 ml single-dose vials. |

WARNING

Cigarette smoking increases the risk of serious cardiovascular side effects from contraceptives containing estrogen. This risk increases with age and with heavy smoking (≥ 15 cigarettes/day) and is quite marked in women > 35 years of age. Women who use MPA/E₂C injection should be strongly advised not to smoke.

Indications

➤*Contraception:* For the prevention of pregnancy.

Administration and Dosage

➤*Approved by the FDA:* October 5, 2000.

The efficacy of MPA/E₂C is dependent on adherence to the recommended dosage schedule (eg, IM injections every 28 to 30 days, not to exceed 33 days). To ensure that the injection is not administered inadvertently to a pregnant woman, the first injection should be given during the first 5 days of a normal menstrual period. Administer no earlier than 4 weeks after delivery if not breastfeeding or 6 weeks after delivery if breastfeeding.

Several clinical trials of MPA/E₂C injection have reported 12-month failure rates of < 1% by Life Table analysis. Pregnancy rates for various contraceptive methods are typically reported for the first year of use. MPA/E₂C injection is effective for contraception during the first cycle of use when administered as recommended.

The recommended dose of MPA/E₂C injection is 0.5 ml administered by IM injection, into the deltoid, gluteus maximus, or anterior thigh. The aqueous suspension must be vigorously shaken just before use to ensure a uniform suspension of 25 mg MPA and 5 mg E₂C.

➤*First injection:* Within first 5 days of the onset of a normal menstrual period, or within 5 days of a complete first trimester abortion, or no earlier than 4 weeks postpartum if not breastfeeding. No earlier than 6 weeks postpartum if breastfeeding.

➤*Second and subsequent injections:* Monthly (28 to 30 days) after previous injection, not to exceed 33 days. If the patient has not adhered to the prescribed schedule (> 33 days since last injection), pregnancy should be considered and she should not receive another injection until pregnancy is ruled out. Shortening the injection interval could lead to a change in menstrual pattern. Do not use bleeding episodes to guide the injection schedule.

➤*Switching from other methods of contraception:* When switching from other contraceptive methods, MPA/E₂C injection should be given in a manner that ensures continuous contraceptive coverage based upon the mechanism of action of both methods (eg, patients switching from OCs should have their first injection of MPA/E₂C injection within 7 days after taking their last active pill).

➤*Storage/Stability:* Store at 25°C (77°F); excursions permitted to 15° to 30°C (59° to 86°F).

Actions

➤*Pharmacology:* MPA/E₂C injectable suspension when administered at the recommended dose to women every month inhibits the secretion of gonadotropins, which, in turn, prevents follicular maturation and ovulation. Although the primary mechanism of this action is inhibition of ovulation, other possible mechanisms of action include thickening and a reduction in volume of cervical mucus (which decrease sperm penetration) and thinning of the endometrium (which may reduce the likelihood of implantation).

➤*Pharmacokinetics:*

Absorption – Absorption of MPA/E₂C from the injection site is prolonged after an IM injection of medroxyprogesterone acetate (MPA) and estradiol cypionate (E₂C) injection. The time to maximum plasma concentration (T_{max}) typically occurs within 1 to 10 days postinjection for MPA and 1 to 7 days postinjection for E_2. The peak concentrations (C_{max}) generally range from 0.94 to 2.17 ng/ml for MPA and from 140 to 480 pg/ml for E_2.

Distribution – Plasma protein binding of MPA averages 86%. MPA binding occurs primarily to serum albumin; no binding of MPA occurs with sex-hormone-binding globulins (SHBG). Estrogens circulate in blood bound to albumin, SHBG, α1-glycoproteins, and transcortin. Estradiol is primarily bound to SHBG and albumin and ≈ 3% remains unbound. Unbound estrogens are known to modulate pharmacologic response.

Metabolism – MPA is extensively metabolized. Its metabolism primarily involves ring A and/or side-chain reduction, loss of the acetyl group, hydroxylation in the 2-, 6-, and 21-positions or a combination of these positions, resulting in numerous derivatives. E₂C undergoes ester hydrolysis after IM injection of MPA/E₂C, releasing the parent, active compound E_2. Exogenously delivered or endogenously derived E_2 is primarily metabolized to estrone and estriol, both of which are metabolized to their sulfate and glucuronide forms.

Excretion – Residual MPA concentrations at the end of a monthly injection of MPA/E₂C are generally < 0.5 ng/ml, consistent with its apparent elimination half-life of 15 days. Most MPA metabolites are excreted in the urine as glucuronide conjugates with only small amounts excreted as sulfates. Following the peak concentration, serum E_2 levels typically decline to 100 pg/ml by day 14 and are consistent with the apparent elimination half-life of 7 to 8 days. Estrogen metabolites are primarily excreted in the urine as glucuronides and sulfates.

Return of ovulation – Return of ovulation correlated to some extent with MPA $AUC_{0-84 \, days}$. Additionally, body weight and site of injection affected the AUC of MPA. AUC_{0-28} values are significantly higher when MPA/E₂C injection is injected into the arm compared to the anterior thigh muscle and into women with BMI ≤ 28 kg/m² compared to those with BMI > 28 kg/m². Consequently, return of ovulation may be delayed in women with BMI ≤ 28 kg/m² who receive an injection in the arm.

➤*Clinical trials:* In the clinical trials, reported 12-month pregnancy rates have been low (≤ 0.2%). Because of certain limitations of the available data (eg, loss to follow-up, lack of pregnancy testing, use of barrier contraceptive products and concomitant medications), a precise estimate of the failure rate is not possible, but is likely in the range of 0.1% to 1%.

Contraindications

Known or suspected pregnancy; thrombophlebitis or thromboembolic disorders; history of deep-vein thrombophlebitis or thromboembolic dis-

MEDROXYPROGESTERONE ACETATE/ESTRADIOL CYPIONATE (MPA/E₂C)

orders; cerebral vascular or coronary artery disease; undiagnosed abnormal genital bleeding; liver dysfunction or disease, such as history of hepatic adenoma or carcinoma; history of cholestatic jaundice of pregnancy or jaundice with prior hormonal contraceptive use including severe pruritus of pregnancy; carcinoma of the endometrium, breast, or other known or suspected estrogen-dependent neoplasia; known hypersensitivity to any of the ingredients contained in MPA/E₂C injection; heavy smoking (≥ 15 cigarettes/day) and > 35 years of age; severe hypertension; diabetes with vascular involvement; headaches with focal neurological symptoms; valvular heart disease with complications.

Warnings

➤*Risks of OC use:* The use of oral contraceptives (OC) is associated with increased risks of several serious conditions including MI, thromboembolism, stroke, hepatic neoplasia, and gallbladder disease, although the risk of serious morbidity or mortality is very small in healthy women without underlying risk factors. The risk of morbidity and mortality increases significantly in the presence of other underlying risk factors such as hypertension, hyperlipidemias, obesity, and diabetes.

➤*Thromboembolic disorders and other vascular problems:*

MI – An increased risk of MI has been attributed to OC use. This risk is primarily in smokers or women with other underlying risk factors for coronary artery disease such as hypertension, hypercholesterolemia, morbid obesity, and diabetes. The relative risk of heart attack for current OC users has been estimated to be 2% to 6%. The risk is very low in women < 30 years of age.

Smoking in combination with OC use has been shown to contribute substantially to the incidence of MI in women in their mid-30s or older with smoking accounting for the majority of excess cases. Mortality rates associated with circulatory disease have been shown to increase substantially in smokers ≥ 35 years of age and nonsmokers > 40 years of age who use OCs.

OCs may compound the effects of well-known risk factors, such as hypertension, diabetes, hyperlipidemias, age, and obesity. In particular, some progestogens are known to decrease high density lipoproteins (HDL) cholesterol and cause glucose intolerance, while estrogens may create a state of hyperinsulinism. OCs have been shown to increase blood pressure among users. Similar effects on risk factors have been associated with an increased risk of heart disease. MPA/E₂C injection must be used with caution in women with cardiovascular disease risk factors.

Thromboembolism – An increased risk of thromboembolic and thrombotic diseases associated with the use of OCs is well established. Case control studies have found the relative risk of users compared with nonusers to be 3% for the first episode of superficial venous thrombosis, 4% to 11% for deep vein thrombosis or pulmonary embolism, and 1.5% to 6% for women with predisposing conditions for venous thromboembolic disease. Cohort studies have shown the relative risk to be somewhat lower, ≈ 3% for new cases and ≈ 4.5% for new cases requiring hospitalization. The risk of thromboembolic disease caused by OCs is not related to length of use and disappears after pill use is stopped.

A 2- to 4-fold increase in relative risk of postoperative thromboembolic complications has been reported with the use of OCs. The relative risk of venous thrombosis in women who have predisposing conditions is twice that of women without such medical conditions. If feasible, OCs should be discontinued ≥ 4 weeks prior to and for 2 weeks after elective surgery of a type associated with an increase in risk of thromboembolism and during and following prolonged immobilization. Since the immediate postpartum period is also associated with an increased risk of thromboembolism, OCs, and other combined hormonal contraceptives such as MPA/E₂C injection, should be started no earlier than 4 weeks after delivery.

The clinician should be alert to the earliest manifestations of thrombotic disorders (thrombophlebitis, pulmonary embolism, cerebrovascular disorders, and retinal thrombosis). Should any of these occur or be suspected, do not readminister MPA/E₂C injection.

Cerebrovascular disease – OCs have been shown to increase the relative and attributable risks of cerebrovascular events (thrombotic and hemorrhagic strokes), although, in general, the risk is greatest among older (> 35 years of age), hypertensive women who also smoke. Hypertension was found to be a risk factor for users and nonusers, for both types of strokes, while smoking interacted to increase the risk for hemorrhagic stroke.

The relative risk of thrombotic strokes has been shown to range from 3% for normotensive users to 14% for users with severe hypertension. The relative risk of hemorrhagic stroke is reported to be 1.2% for nonsmokers who used OCs, 2.6% for smokers who did not use OCs, 7.6% for smokers who used OCs, 1.8% for normotensive users, and 25.7% for users with severe hypertension. The attributable risk is also greater in older women.

Dose-related risk of vascular disease – A positive association has been observed between the amount of estrogen and progestogen in OCs

and the risk of vascular disease. A decline in serum HDL has been reported with many progestational agents. A decline in serum HDL has been associated with an increased incidence of ischemic heart disease. Because estrogens increase HDL cholesterol, the net effect of an OC depends on a balance achieved between doses of estrogen and progestogen and the type of progestogens used in the contraceptives. The activity and amount of both hormones should be considered in the choice of a hormonal contraceptive.

Persistence of risk of vascular disease – There are 2 studies that have shown persistence of risk of vascular disease for ever-users of OCs. In a study in the US, the risk of developing MI after discontinuing OCs persists for ≥ 9 years for women 40 to 49 years of age who have used OCs for ≥ 5 years, but this increased risk was not demonstrated in other age groups. In another study in Great Britain, the risk of developing cerebrovascular disease persisted for ≥ 6 years after discontinuation of OCs, although excess risk was very small. However, both studies were performed with OC formulations containing ≥ 50 mcg of estrogen.

➤*Estimates of mortality from contraceptive use:* One study gathered data from a variety of sources that have estimated the mortality rate associated with different methods of contraception at different ages. These estimates include the combined risk of death associated with contraceptive methods plus the risk attributable to pregnancy in the event of method failure. Each method of contraception has its specific benefits and risks. The study concluded that with the exception of OC users ≥ 35 years of age who smoke and OC users ≥ 40 years of age who do not smoke, mortality associated with all methods of birth control is low and below that associated with childbirth.

The observation of a possible increase in risk of mortality with age for OC users is based on data gathered in the 1970s, but not reported until 1983. However, current clinical practice involves the use of lower estrogen-dose formulations combined with careful restriction of OC use to women who do not have the various risk factors listed.

Because of these changes in practice and because of some limited new data that suggest the risk of cardiovascular disease with the use of OCs may now be less than previously observed, the Fertility and Maternal Health Drugs Advisory Committee was asked to review the topic in 1989. The Committee concluded that although cardiovascular disease risk may be increased with OC use after age 40 in healthy nonsmoking women (even with the newer low-dose formulations), there are also greater potential health risks associated with pregnancy in older women and with the alternative surgical and medical procedures that may be necessary if such women do not have access to effective and acceptable means of contraception. Therefore, the Committee recommended that the benefits of OC use by healthy nonsmoking women > 40 years of age may outweigh the possible risks. Women of all ages who take OCs should take a product that contains the lowest amount of estrogen and progestogen that is effective.

➤*Carcinoma of the reproductive organs and breasts:* In spite of many studies of the relationship between OC use and breast and cervical cancers, a cause-and-effect relationship has not been established. No long-term studies have been conducted with MPA/E₂C injection to evaluate risk for carcinoma of the reproductive organs.

➤*Hepatic neoplasia:* Benign hepatic adenomas are associated with OC use, although the incidence of benign tumors is rare in the US. Indirect calculations have estimated the attributable risk to be in the range of 3.3 cases/100,000 cases for users, a risk that increases after ≥ 4 years of use. Rupture of benign, hepatic adenomas may cause death through intra-abdominal hemorrhage.

Studies from Britain have shown an increased risk of developing hepatocellular carcinoma in long-term (> 8 years) OC users. However, these cancers are extremely rare in the US and the attributable risk (the excess incidence) of liver cancers in OC users approaches < 1 per million users.

➤*Ocular lesions:* There have been clinical case reports of retinal thrombosis associated with the use of OCs. Discontinue MPA/E₂C injection if there is unexplained partial or complete loss of vision, onset of proptosis or diplopia, papilledema, or retinal vascular lesions. Undertake appropriate diagnostic and therapeutic measures immediately.

➤*Hormonal contraceptive use before or during pregnancy:* The use of hormonal contraceptives during pregnancy is not indicated.

The administration of combined hormonal contraceptives, such as MPA/E₂C injection, to induce withdrawal bleeding should not be used as a test for pregnancy. Do not use MPA/E₂C injection during pregnancy to treat threatened or habitual abortion. It is recommended that for any patient who has missed 2 consecutive periods, pregnancy should be considered before initiating or continuing MPA/E₂C injection. If the patient has exceeded the prescribed injection interval (> 33 days) for MPA/E₂C injection, the possibility of pregnancy should be ruled out before another injection is administered.

➤*Gallbladder disease:* In a study of 782 women taking MPA/E₂C injection for ≤ 15 cycles, cholecysitis and cholelithiasis were the only serious adverse events judged to be possibly related to the study drug. They were reported as an adverse event in 5 subjects, and 3 subjects required cholecystectomy.

MEDROXYPROGESTERONE ACETATE/ESTRADIOL CYPIONATE (MPA/E₂C)

➤*Carbohydrate and lipid metabolic effects:* Combined hormonal or progestin-only contraceptives have been shown to cause glucose intolerance in some users. However, in the nondiabetic woman, combined hormonal contraceptives appear to have no effect on fasting blood glucose. Prediabetic and diabetic patients should be carefully observed while receiving therapy with MPA/E₂C injection.

A small portion of women may have persistent hypertriglyceridemia while using OCs. Changes in serum triglycerides and lipoprotein levels have been reported in OC users.

➤*Elevated blood pressure:* An increase in blood pressure has been reported in women taking OCs and this increase is more likely in older OC users and with continued use. Data from the Royal College of General Practitioners and subsequent randomized trials have shown that the incidence of hypertension increases with increasing concentrations of progestogens. In a US clinical study, no increase in mean blood pressure was observed over 15 months use of MPA/E₂C injection.

Women with a history of hypertension or hypertension-related diseases, or renal disease should be encouraged to use another method of contraception. If women elect to use combined hormonal contraceptives such as MPA/E₂C injection, monitor closely and if significant elevation of blood pressure occurs, discontinue MPA/E₂C injection. For most women, elevated blood pressure will return to normal after stopping OCs, and there is no difference in the occurrence of hypertension among former and never-users.

➤*Headache:* The onset or exacerbation of migraine or development of headache with a new pattern that is recurrent, persistent, or severe requires evaluation of the cause before further injections of MPA/E₂C injection are given.

➤*Bleeding irregularities:* Most women using MPA/E₂C injection (58.6%) experienced alteration of menstrual bleeding patterns, including 4.1% amenorrhea, after 1 year of use. Altered bleeding patterns include frequent bleeding, irregular bleeding, prolonged bleeding, infrequent bleeding, and amenorrhea. As women continued using MPA/E₂C injection, the percent experiencing frequent or prolonged bleeding decreased, while the percent experiencing amenorrhea increased. The percent of women experiencing irregular bleeding remained fairly constant at ≈ 30% throughout the first year of use.

Regardless of the bleeding pattern, subsequent injections should be given 1 month (28 to 30 days, not to exceed 33 days) after the previous injection, unless discontinuation is medically indicated.

If abnormal bleeding associated with MPA/E₂C injection persists or is severe, appropriate investigation should be instituted to rule out the possibility of organic pathology, and appropriate treatment should be instituted when necessary. In the event of amenorrhea, pregnancy should be ruled out.

➤*Bone mineral density changes:* Use of injectable progestogen-only methods may be considered among the risk factors for development of osteoporosis. The rate of bone loss is greatest in the early years of use and then subsequently approaches the normal rate of age-related fall. Formal studies on the effect of bone mineral density changes in women receiving MPA/E₂C injection have not been conducted.

➤*Anaphylaxis and anaphylactoid reaction:* Anaphylaxis and anaphylactoid reactions have been reported with the components of MPA/E₂C injection. Allergic reactions occurring in women using MPA/E₂C injection have been mainly dermatologic, not respiratory, in nature. If an anaphylactic reaction occurs, appropriate therapy should be instituted. Serious anaphylactic reactions require emergency medical treatment.

➤*Fertility impairment:* Ovulation (signaled by a rise in serum progesterone concentrations ≥ 4.7 ng/ml) was observed 63 to 112 days after the third monthly injection of MPA/E₂C injection in 11 of 14 women participating in a pharmacodynamic study. The remaining 3 women had not ovulated by day 85 and were lost to follow-up.

In a study of 21 women who received the injection for 3 months, 52% ovulated during the first posttreatment month, and 71% during the second posttreatment month. In another study of 10 women receiving long-term administration (2 years of treatment) of MPA/E₂C injection, 60% ovulated by the third posttreatment month.

A study of 70 women who discontinued MPA/E₂C injection to become pregnant demonstrated that > 50% achieved fertility within 6 months after discontinuation, and 83% did so by 1 year.

➤*Pregnancy:* Category X.

➤*Lactation:* The effects of MPA/E₂C injection in nursing mothers have not been evaluated and are unknown. However, estrogen administration to nursing mothers has been shown to decrease the quantity and quality of breast milk. Small amounts of combined hormonal contraceptive steroids have been identified in the milk of nursing mothers and a few adverse effects on the child have been reported, including jaundice and breast enlargement. Long-term follow-up of children whose mothers used combined hormonal contraceptives while breastfeeding has shown no deleterious effects. However, women who are breastfeeding should not start taking combined hormonal contraceptives until 6 weeks postpartum.

➤*Children:* Safety and efficacy of MPA/E₂C injection have been established in women of reproductive age. Safety and efficacy are expected to be the same for postpubertal adolescents < 16 years of age and users ≥ 16 years of age. Use of this product before menarche is not indicated.

Precautions

➤*Monitoring:*

Physical examination – It is good medical practice for all women to have an annual history and physical examination, including women using combined hormonal contraceptives. The physical examination should include special reference to blood pressure, breasts, abdomen and pelvic organs, including cervical cytology, and relevant laboratory tests. In case of undiagnosed, persistent, or recurrent abnormal vaginal bleeding, appropriate measures should be conducted to rule out malignancy. Women with a strong family history of breast cancer or who have breast nodules should be monitored with particular care.

Weight change – In a study of 782 women using MPA/E₂C injection for ≤ 15 cycles, 5.7% of participants discontinued due to weight gain. Weight gain was the most common adverse event leading to discontinuation of the drug. Women gained an average of 4 pounds during the first year and an additional 2 pounds during the second year of MPA/E₂C injection use. The range of weight change during the first year of MPA/E₂C injection use was 48 pounds lost to 49 pounds gained.

Fluid retention – Progestogens and/or estrogens may cause some degree of fluid retention; therefore, use caution in treating any patient with a preexisiting medical condition that might be adversely affected by fluid retention.

Contact lenses – Contact lens wearers who develop visual changes or changes in lens tolerance should be assessed by an ophthalmologist.

Emotional disorders – Patients becoming significantly depressed while taking combined hormonal contraceptives should stop the medication and use an alternative method of contraception in an attempt to determine whether the symptoms are drug-related. Women with a history of depression should be carefully observed and consideration should be given to the discontinuation of MPA/E₂C injection if depression recurs to a serious degree.

➤*Special risk:*

Lipid disorders – Women who are being treated for hyperlipidemias should be followed closely if they use combined hormonal contraceptives. Some progestogens may elevate LDL levels and may render the control of hyperlipidemias more difficult.

Liver function – If jaundice develops in any woman receiving combined hormonal contraceptives, the medication should be discontinued. Steroid hormones may be poorly metabolized in patients with impaired liver function.

Drug Interactions

Aminoglutethimide may decrease the serum concentration of MPA. Users of MPA/E₂C injection should be informed of the possibility of decreased effectiveness with the use of this or any related drug.

MPA/E₂C Drug Interactions			
Precipitant drug	Object drug*		Description
Rifampin	Combined hormonal contraceptives	↓	Metabolism of some synthetic estrogens (eg, ethinyl estradiol) and progestins (eg, norethindrone) is increased by rifampin. A reduction in contraceptive effectiveness and an increase in menstrual irregularities have been associated with concomitant use of rifampin.
Anticonvulsants (eg, phenobarbital, phenytoin, carbamazepine)	Synthetic estrogens and progestins	↓	Anticonvulsants have been shown to increase the metabolism of some synthetic estrogens and progestins, which could result in a reduction of contraceptive effectiveness.
Antibiotics (eg, ampicillin, tetracycline, griseofulvin)	OCs	↓	Pregnancy while taking OCs have been reported when the OCs were administered with antimicrobials such as ampicillin, tetracycline, and griseofulvin. However, clinical pharmacokinetic studies have not demonstrated any consistent effects of antibiotics (other than rifampin) on plasma concentrations of synthetic steroids.
St. John's wort (*hypericum perforatum*)	Contraceptive steroids	↓	Herbal products containing St. John's wort (*hypericum perforatum*) may induce hepatic enzymes (cytochrome P450) and p-glycoprotein transporter and may reduce the effectiveness of OC steroids. This may also result in breakthrough bleeding.

MEDROXYPROGESTERONE ACETATE/ESTRADIOL CYPIONATE (MPA/E₂C)

MPA/E$_2$C Drug Interactions			
Precipitant drug	Object drug*		Description
Ascorbic acid, acetaminophen	Synthetic estrogens	↑	Ascorbic acid and acetaminophen may increase plasma concentrations of some synthetic estrogens, possibly by inhibition of conjugation.
Phenylbutazone	Synthetic estrogens	↓	A reduction in contraceptive effectiveness and an increased incidence of menstrual irregularities has been suggested with phenylbutazone.
OCs	Cyclosporine, prednisolone, theophylline	↑	Increased plasma concentrations of cyclosporine, prednisolone, and theophylline have been reported with concomitant administration of OCs. In addition, OCs may induce the conjugation of other compounds.
OCs	Temazepam, salicyclic acid, morphine, clofibric acid	↓	Decreased plasma concentrations of acetaminophen and increased clearance of temazepam, salicyclic acid, morphine, and clofibric acid have been noted when these drugs were administered with OCs.

* ↑ = Object drug increased. ↓ = Object drug decreased.

➤*Drug/Lab test interactions:* Certain endocrine and liver function tests and blood components may be affected by combined hormonal contraceptives: Increased prothrombin and factors VII, VIII, IX, and X; decreased antithrombin 3; increased norepinephrine-induced platelet aggregability; increased thyroid binding globulin (TBG) leading to increased circulating total thyroid hormone, as measured by protein-bound iodine (PBI), T4 by column or by radioimmunoassay. Free T3 resin uptake is decreased, reflecting the elevated TBG, free T4 concentration is unaltered; other binding proteins may be elevated in serum; sex-hormone-binding globulins are increased and result in elevated levels of total circulating sex steroids and corticoids; however, free or biologically active levels remain unchanged; triglycerides may be increased; glucose tolerance may be decreased; serum folate levels may be depressed by combined hormonal contraceptive therapy. This may be of clinical significance if a woman becomes pregnant shortly after discontinuing combined hormonal contraceptives.

Advise the pathologist of progestogen and estrogen therapy when relevant tissue specimens are submitted.

The following lab tests may be affected by progestins including MPA/E₂C injection: Plasma and urinary steroid levels are decreased (eg, progesterone, estradiol, pregnanediol, testosterone, cortisol); gonadotropin levels are decreased; sex-hormone-binding-globulin concentrations are decreased; sulfobromophthalein and other liver function test values may be increased.

Adverse Reactions

➤*Cardiovascular:* Arterial thromboembolism; cerebral hemorrhage; cerebral thrombosis; hypertension; MI; pulmonary embolism; thrombophlebitis; mesenteric thrombosis; retinal thrombosis.

➤*CNS:* Depression, headache (≥ 1%); dizziness; nervousness; migraine.

➤*Dermatologic:* Acne (≥ 1%); alopecia; erythema multiforme; erythema nodosum; hirsutism.

➤*GI:* Nausea (≥ 1%); colitis.

➤*GU:* Amenorrhea, dysmenorrhea, menorrhagia, metrorrhagia, breast tenderness/pain, vaginal spotting (≥ 1%); decreased libido; vaginal moniliasis; vulvovaginal disorder; breast changes, enlargement, secretion; cervical changes; temporary infertility after treatment discontinuation; diminution in lactation when given immediately postpartum; changes in libido; premenstrual syndrome; vaginitis.

➤*Hematologic:* Hemolytic uremic syndrome; porphyria; hemorrhagic eruption.

➤*Hepatic:* Hepatic adenomas or benign liver tumors; cholestatic jaundice; Budd-Chiari syndrome.

➤*Hypersensitivity:* Anaphylactic reactions; rash (allergic).

➤*Renal:* Cystitis-like syndrome; impaired renal function.

➤*Special senses:* Corneal curvature changes (eg, steepening); intolerance to contact lenses; cataracts.

➤*Miscellaneous:* Emotional lability, weight gain (≥ 1%); gallbladder disease; abdominal pain; asthenia; enlarged abdomen; weight decrease; edema; melasma that may persist; reduced carbohydrate tolerance; changes in appetite.

Overdosage

➤*Symptoms:* Overdosage of a progestin/estrogen drug combination may cause nausea and vomiting, and vaginal bleeding or other menstrual irregularities in females.

Patient Information

Give patients a copy of the patient labeling prior to administration of MPA/E₂C injection.

Advise patients that the contraceptive efficacy depends on receiving injections monthly (28 to 30 days, not to exceed 33 days). The injection schedule must be measured by the number of days, not by bleeding episodes. It is recommended that for any patient who has missed 2 consecutive menstrual periods, pregnancy should be considered before initiating or continuing MPA/E₂C injection. Thereafter, a woman who has continued amenorrhea while using MPA/E₂C injection and who has received her injections according to the recommended dosing schedule may continue to receive subsequent injections each month after the previous injection (not to exceed 33 days), unless discontinuation is medically indicated. All patients presenting for a follow-up injection of MPA/E₂C injection after day 33 should use a barrier method of contraception and should not receive another injection of MPA/E₂C injection until pregnancy has been ruled out.

Advise patients that menstrual bleeding patterns are likely be disrupted with use of MPA/E₂C injection. A few patients may experience amenorrhea. Irregular bleeding that occurs after a regular bleeding pattern has emerged should be investigated. In the presence of excessive or prolonged bleeding, other causes should be investigated and consideration should be given to alternative methods of contraception.

Counsel patients that this product does not protect against HIV infection (AIDS) and other sexually transmitted diseases.

Ovulation Stimulants

CLOMIPHENE CITRATE

Rx	**Clomiphene Citrate** (Various, eg, Lemmon)	**Tablets:** 50 mg	In 10s and 30s.
Rx	**Clomid** (Aventis Pharm.)		(Clomid 50). White, scored. In 30s.
Rx	**Milophene** (Milex)		(M50). White, scored. In 30s.
Rx	**Serophene** (Serono)		(S). White, scored. In 10s and 30s.

Indications

➤*Treatment of ovulatory failure:* Treatment of ovulatory failure in patients desiring pregnancy whose partners are fertile and potent.

➤*Unlabeled uses:* Clomiphene has been used to treat male infertility (50 to 400 mg/day for 2 to 12 months); however, this use is controversial, and further study is needed.

Administration and Dosage

Choose patients only after careful diagnostic evaluation. Ovulation and pregnancy are more attainable on 100 mg/day for 5 days. As dosage increases, however, ovarian overstimulation and other side effects may increase. A correlation may exist between dosage and multiple births.

➤*Initial therapy:* First course is 50 mg/day for 5 days. Start at any time in patients who have had no recent uterine bleeding. If progestin-induced bleeding is planned, or if spontaneous uterine bleeding occurs prior to therapy, start the regimen on or about the fifth day of the cycle. If ovulation occurs with this dosage, there is no advantage to increasing the dose in subsequent cycles of treatment. Special treatment with lower doses over a shorter duration is recommended if unusual sensitivity to pituitary gonadotropin is suspected, including patients with polycystic ovary syndrome.

➤*Second course of therapy:* Increase the dose in patients not responding to the first course. If ovulation has not occurred after the first course, administer a second course of 100 mg/day for 5 days; do not increase this dosage or duration of therapy. Start this course as early as 30 days after the previous one.

➤*Third course of therapy:* The majority of patients who are going to respond will respond to the first course of therapy; 3 courses are an adequate therapeutic trial. If ovulatory menses has not yet occurred, reevaluate diagnosis. Further treatment is not recommended in patients who do not exhibit evidence of ovulation.

➤*Pregnancy:* Before starting therapy, advise patients that multiple pregnancy is possible and poses potential hazards. Properly timed coitus is important for good results. The likelihood of conception diminishes with each succeeding course of therapy. If pregnancy has not been achieved after 3 ovulatory responses, further treatment is not recommended. Long-term cyclic therapy is not recommended.

Actions

➤*Pharmacology:* Clomiphene, an orally administered nonsteroidal agent, may induce ovulation in selected anovulatory women. Therapy appears to mediate ovulation through increased output of pituitary gonadotropins, which stimulates the maturation and endocrine activity of the ovarian follicle and the subsequent development and function of the corpus luteum. Clomiphene binds to estrogenic receptors in the cytoplasm and decreases the number of available estrogenic receptors (antiestrogen). The hypothalamus and pituitary interpret the false signal that estrogen levels are low and respond by increasing the secretion of luteinizing hormone (LH), follicle stimulating hormone (FSH), and gonadotropins. This results in ovarian stimulation.

Criteria for ovulation – Criteria for ovulation include an ovulation peak of estrogen excretion followed by a biphasic basal body temperature curve; urinary excretion of pregnanediol at postovulatory levels and endometrial histologic findings characteristic of the luteal phase.

➤*Pharmacokinetics:* Clomiphene is readily absorbed orally and is excreted principally in the feces. Excretion averaged 51% of the dose after 5 days. Drug appears in the feces 6 weeks after administration, suggesting that the remaining drug/metabolites are slowly excreted from a sequestered enterohepatic recirculation pool.

➤*Clinical trials:* In 11 studies appearing between 1964 and 1978, pregnancy occurred in 30.6% of 5413 patients with ovulatory dysfunction who received clomiphene citrate.

Contraindications

Liver disease, history of liver dysfunction or abnormal bleeding of undetermined origin; pregnancy (see Warnings); uncontrolled thyroid or adrenal dysfunction; organic intracranial lesion (eg, pituitary tumor); ovarian cysts or enlargement not due to polycystic ovarian syndrome; abnormal uterine bleeding must be evaluated prior to therapy. It is important to detect neoplastic lesions.

Warnings

➤*Criteria for therapy:* To start clomiphene therapy, the following criteria must be met: Normal liver function; normal levels of endogenous estrogen (as estimated from vaginal smears, endometrial biopsy, assay of urinary estrogen or from bleeding in response to progesterone) provide a favorable prognosis for treatment. A reduced estrogen level, although less favorable, does not preclude successful therapy.

➤*Primary pituitary/ovarian failure:* Therapy is ineffective in patients with primary pituitary or ovarian failure. Clomiphene cannot be substituted for appropriate therapy of other disturbances leading to ovulatory dysfunction (eg, thyroid or adrenal disease).

➤*Multiple pregnancy:* The incidence of multiple pregnancies was increased during those cycles in which clomiphene citrate was given. Among 2369 pregnancies, 92.1% were single and 6.9% were twins. Less than 1% of the reported deliveries resulted in triplets or more. Of these multiple pregnancies, 96% to 99% resulted in the births of live infants. Advise the patient of the frequency and potential hazards of multiple pregnancy before starting treatment.

➤*Ophthalmologic effects:* Blurring or other visual symptoms may occasionally occur; patients should use caution when driving or operating machinery, particularly in variable lighting. If visual symptoms occur, discontinue treatment and refer the patient for a complete ophthalmologic evaluation.

➤*Pregnancy:* Although no direct effect of clomiphene on the human fetus has been reported, do not administer in cases of suspected pregnancy; fetal effects have been reported in animals.

Birth defects – From 2369 delivered and reported pregnancies associated with clomiphene administration, 58 infants had birth defects. Eight of the 58 infants were born to 7 of 158 mothers who received clomiphene during the first 6 weeks after conception. Also, there were birth defects in 4 conceptions in the abortion/stillbirth category, in 14 of 357 infants from multiple pregnancies, and in 39 of 1697 infants from single pregnancies. Eight liveborn infants failed to survive.

Defects included congenital heart lesions (8 infants), Down's syndrome (5 infants), club foot (4 infants), congenital gut lesions (4 infants), and hypospadias (3 infants). Each of the following defects reportedly affected 2 infants each: Microcephaly, harelip and cleft palate, congenital hip defect, hemangioma, and undescended testes. The following also occurred: Polydactyly (both of twins), conjoined twins with teratomatous malformation, patent ductus arteriosus, amaurosis (blindness), arteriovenous fistula, inguinal hernia, umbilical hernia, syndactyly, pectus excavatum, myopathy, dermoid cyst of scalp, omphalocele, spina bifida occulta, ichthyosis, persistent lingual frenulum, and 7 infants with multiple somatic defects.

In addition to investigational studies, during the first 42 months of commercial availability of clomiphene, information was received on 7 infants with birth defects from 7 pregnancies. These reported defects were: Down's syndrome, adactyly of one hand, achondroplasia, anterior pituitary agenesis and multiple somatic lesions (3 infants).

Precautions

➤*Diagnosis prior to therapy:* A complete pelvic examination is mandatory prior to treatment; repeat before each course. Do not administer in the presence of an ovarian cyst; further enlargement may occur. The incidence of endometrial carcinoma and ovulatory disorders increases with age. Perform an endometrial biopsy before starting therapy. If abnormal bleeding is present, full diagnostic measures are mandatory.

➤*Ovarian overstimulation/enlargement:* To minimize the hazard associated with occasional abnormal ovarian enlargement, use the lowest effective dose. Some patients with polycystic ovary syndrome may have an exaggerated response to usual doses. Mid-cycle ovarian pain may be accentuated. With higher or prolonged dosage, ovarian enlargement and cyst formation may occur more frequently and the luteal phase of the cycle may be prolonged. Maximal enlargement of the ovary, whether physiologic or abnormal, does not occur until several days after discontinuation of the drug. Examine patients who complain of pelvic pain after receiving clomiphene. If ovaries are enlarged, do not give additional therapy until they return to pretreatment size; reduce the dosage or duration of the next course. Ovarian enlargement and cyst formation regress spontaneously a few days or weeks after discontinuing therapy. Unless surgical indication for laparotomy exists, manage such cystic enlargement conservatively. Rarely, massive ovarian enlargement has occurred, including a patient with polycystic ovary syndrome taking 100 mg/day for 14 days.

➤*Ophthalmic effects:* Symptoms are usually described as "blurring" spots or flashes (scintillating scotomata). They correlate with increasing total dose and disappear within a few days or weeks after discontinuation. These symptoms appear to be caused by intensification and prolongation of after-images. They often first appear or are accentuated with exposure to a more brightly lit environment. While measured visual acuity is not generally affected, one patient taking 200 mg/day developed visual blurring on day 7 of treatment, progressing to severe diminution of visual acuity by day 10. Vision returned to normal on the third day after treatment was stopped. Ophthalmologically definable scotomata and electroretinographic retinal function changes have also occurred.

CLOMIPHENE CITRATE

The following conditions have also been reported in association with clomiphene therapy; cause and effect relationship has neither been proven nor disproven: Posterior capsular cataract (all in investigational studies) (4), detachment of the posterior vitreous (1), spasm of retinal arteriole (1) and thrombosis of temporal arteries of retina (1).

➤*Hydatidiform mole:* Hydatidiform mole has been reported in 8 patients receiving clomiphene (includes 4 reported in original 2369 investigational pregnancies). A causal relationship has not been established.

Adverse Reactions

At recommended dosage, side effects are not prominent, infrequently interfere with treatment and are dose-related.

Vasomotor flushes (10.4%) – Vasomotor flushes (10.4%) resembling menopausal "hot flushes" are usually not severe and disappear promptly after treatment is discontinued.

Abdominal symptoms – Abdominal discomfort, distention, bloating (5.5%); abnormal uterine bleeding (1.25%). May resemble ovulatory (mittelschmerz) or premenstrual phenomena or discomfort caused by ovarian enlargement.

Abnormal ovarian enlargement – Abnormal ovarian enlargement (14%) is infrequent at recommended dosage (see Precautions).

➤*Miscellaneous:* Nausea, vomiting (2.2%); breast tenderness (2.1%); visual symptoms (1.5%); headache (1.3%); dizziness, lightheadedness (1%); nervousness, insomnia (0.77%); increased urination, depression, fatigue (0.7%); urticaria, allergic dermatitis (0.6%); weight gain (0.4%); reversible hair loss (0.3%); ophthalmic effects (see Precautions).

Patient Information

Notify physician if bloating, stomach or pelvic pain, blurred vision, jaundice, hot flushes, breast discomfort, headache, nausea and vomiting occur.

May cause dizziness, lightheadedness and visual disturbances; observe caution while driving or performing other tasks requiring alertness, coordination or physical dexterity.

GONADOTROPINS
FOLLITROPINS

Indications

➤*Ovulation induction:* For the induction of ovulation and pregnancy in anovulatory infertile patients in whom the cause of infertility is functional and not caused by primary ovarian failure.

Refer to individual product monographs for specific indications.

➤*Follicle stimulation:* To stimulate the development of multiple follicles in ovulatory patients undergoing Assisted Reproductive Technologies (ART), eg, in vitro fertilization.

Actions

➤*Pharmacology:* **Urofollitropin** is a preparation of highly purified follicle-stimulating hormone (FSH) extracted from the urine of postmenopausal women. **Follitropin alfa** and **follitropin beta** are human FSH preparations of recombinant DNA origin. Follitropins stimulate ovarian follicular growth in women who do not have primary ovarian failure. FSH is required for normal follicular growth, maturation and gonadal steroid production. In the female, the level of FSH is critical for the onset and duration of follicular development, and consequently for the timing and number of follicles reaching maturity. In order to affect ovulation in the absence of endogenous LH surge, human chorionic gonadotropin (hCG) must be given following the administration of urofollitropin, follitropin alfa and beta when clinical and laboratory assessment of the patient indicate that sufficient follicular maturation has occurred.

➤*Pharmacokinetics:*

Absorption/Distribution – Follitropins have absorption-rate limited pharmacokinetics; the absorption rate following IM or SC administration is slower than the elimination rate. Bioavailability ranges from ≈ 66% to 78% depending on the agent. Following a single IM or SC dose, AUCs are similar for all agents and C_{max} is similar for urofollitropin and follitropin alfa; however, the C_{max} for follitropin beta differs with respect to IM or SC administration (≈ 6.86 vs ≈ 5.41 IU/L, respectively).

Following multiple IM or SC doses, steady-state plasma levels are reached within 4 to 5 days. Peak follitropin alfa plasma levels were 6 to 12 IU/L following 150 U/day administered SC for 7 days; follitropin beta peak levels, following 75, 150 or 225 IU either SC or IM for 7 days, were ≈ 4.3 or 4.65, 8.51 or 9.46, and 13.92 or 11.3 IU/L, respectively.

Metabolism/Excretion – Total clearance of follitropin alfa following IV administration was 0.6 L/hr; data is lacking regarding clearance for the other two agents. Following multiple dosing, the terminal half-life for follitropin alfa (IM) and beta (SC) were ≈ 30 hours.

Select Pharmacokinetic Parameters of Follitropins Following SC (IM) Administration			
	Mean T_{max} (hrs)	Mean elimination t½ (hrs)[1]	Mean V_d (L)
Follitropin alfa	16 (25)	24 and 32[2]	10
Follitropin beta	(27)	(≈ 30)	8
Urofollitropin	15 (10)	-	-

[1] This value increases with body mass index.
[2] In healthy and ART patients, respectively.

Special populations –

Obesity: Body weight, measured as kg or as body mass index (BMI), was shown to influence the absorption rate and thus the AUC of follitropin alfa and beta. Increased body weight or BMI was associated with a decrease in the rate of follitropin absorption and a significantly smaller AUC. Clearance, however was essentially the same on a per kg basis.

➤*Clinical trials:*

Ovulation induction – Data from various follitropin efficacy studies for ovulation induction in oligo-anovulatory infertile women are presented below.

Follitropin Ovulation Induction: Cumulative Ovulation Rates (%)			
	Urofollitropin (n = 102)	Follitropin alfa (n = 110)	Follitropin beta (n = 105)
Cycle 1	83	64	72
Cycle 2	97	78	82
Cycle 3	100	84	85
Cumulative Pregnancy Rates (%)			
Cycle 1	14	21	14
Cycle 2	21	28	19
Cycle 3	29	35	23
Pregnancy Outcomes (%)			
	(n = 25)	(n = 39)	(n = 35)
Pregnancies not reaching term	8	20.5	31
Single birth	-	74.4	63
Multiple births	21	5.1	6

Assisted Reproductive Technologies – Data from various unrelated follitropin efficacy studies for follicular stimulation in ovulatory infertile women are depicted below. (Initial and maximal doses used in clinical studies for both urofollitropin and follitropin alfa were 225 and 450 IU.)

Follitropin–Assisted Reproductive Technologies: Follicle Stimulation Results[1]			
	Urofollitropin (n = 118)	Follitropin alfa (n = 60)	Follitropin beta (n = 585)
Oocytes recovered/patient	8.4	9.3	10.9
Mature oocytes/patient	5.9	7.8	9.1
Peak estradiol (pg/ml)[2]	1682	1576	1808
Treatment duration (days)	11.5	9.9	11
Pregnancy rate/attempt	23%	20%[3]	22.2%[4]
Pregnancy rate/transfer	27%	24%[3]	26%[4]
Pregnancy Outcomes (%)			
		(n = 12)	(n = 179)
Pregnancies not reaching term	-	20.5	28
Single birth	-	41.7	49
Multiple births	-	33.3	23

[1] All values are means.
[2] On day of hCG administration but prior to hCG dose.
[3] Pregnancy during which a fetal sac with or without heart activity was visualized by ultrasound on day 34 to 36 after hCG.
[4] A pregnancy, ≥ 12 weeks after embryo transfer, confirmed by investigator.

Contraindications

High levels of FSH indicating primary ovarian failure; uncontrolled thyroid or adrenal dysfunction; the presence of any cause of infertility other than anovulation; tumor of the ovary, breast, uterus, hypothalamus or pituitary gland; abnormal vaginal bleeding of undetermined origin; ovarian cysts or enlargement not due to polycystic ovary syndrome; hypersensitivity to the product or any of its components; pregnancy (see Warnings).

Warnings

➤*Administration:* These medications should only be used by physicians who are thoroughly familiar with infertility problems and their management. It is a potent gonadotropic substance capable of causing mild to severe adverse reactions. To minimize risks, use only at the low-

FOLLITROPINS

est effective dose. Monitor ovarian response with serum estradiol and vaginal ultrasound on a regular basis.

➤*Overstimulation of the ovary:*

Ovarian enlargement – Mild to moderate uncomplicated ovarian enlargement, which may be accompanied by abdominal distention or abdominal pain, occurs in approximately 20% of those treated with urofollitropin and hCG, and generally regresses without treatment within 2 or 3 weeks.

Ovarian Hyperstimulation Syndrome (OHSS) – The hyperstimulation syndrome is characterized by severe ovarian enlargement, abdominal pain/distention, nausea, vomiting, diarrhea, dyspnea and oliguria, and may be accompanied by ascites, pleural effusion, hypovolemia, electrolyte imbalance, hemoperitoneum and thromboembolic events. OHSS occurred in 6% of patients in trials.

If hyperstimulation occurs, stop treatment and hospitalize the patient. This syndrome develops rapidly within 24 hours to several days and generally occurs during the 7 to 10 days immediately following treatment. Hemoconcentration associated with fluid loss into the abdominal cavity has occurred and should be assessed in the following manner: 1) Fluid intake and output, 2) weight, 3) hematocrit, 4) serum and urinary electrolytes, 5) urine specific gravity, 6) BUN and creatinine and 7) abdominal girth. Perform these determinations daily or more often if the need arises. Treatment is primarily symptomatic and consists of bed rest, fluid and electrolyte replacement and analgesics. The ascitic, pleural and pericardial fluids should never be removed because of the potential danger of injury.

Hemoperitoneum from ruptured ovarian cysts is usually the result of pelvic examination. If this does occur, and if bleeding becomes such that surgery is required, design the surgical treatment to control bleeding and retain as much ovarian tissue as possible.

Intercourse should be prohibited in patients in whom significant ovarian enlargement occurs after ovulation because of the danger of hemoperitoneum resulting from ruptured ovarian cysts.

➤*Pulmonary and vascular complications:* Serious pulmonary conditions (eg, atelectasis, acute respiratory distress syndrome and exacerbation of asthma) have been reported. In addition, thromboembolic events both in association with, and separate from OHSS have been reported. Intravascular thrombosis and embolism can result in reduced blood flow to critical organs or the extremities. Sequelae of such events have included venous thrombophlebitis, pulmonary embolism, pulmonary infarction, cerebral vascular occlusion (stroke) and arterial occlusion resulting in loss of limb. In rare cases, pulmonary complications and thromboembolic events have resulted in death.

➤*Multiple births:* Reports of multiple pregnancies have been associated with these medications, including triplet and quintuplet gestations. Multiple births have occurred with **urofollitropin** (20.8%), **follitropin alfa** (12.3%) and **follotropin beta** (8%). Advise the patient of the potential risk of multiple births before starting treatment.

➤*Pregnancy: Category X.* Contraindicated in pregnancy.

➤*Lactation:* It is not known if this drug is excreted in breast milk. Exercise caution if administering to a nursing mother.

➤*Children:* Safety and efficacy in pediatric patients have not been established, although this drug is not intended for use in children.

Precautions

➤*Monitoring:* Monitor sufficient follicular maturation. This may be directly estimated by sonographic visualization of the ovaries and endometrial lining or measuring serum estradiol levels. The combination of both ultrasonography and measurement of estradiol levels is useful for monitoring the growth and development of follicles and timing hCG administration, as well as minimizing the risk of OHSS and multiple gestations.

The clinical evaluation of estrogenic activity (changes in vaginal cytology and changes in appearance and volume of cervical mucus) provides an indirect estimate of the estrogenic effect upon the target organs, and therefore it should only be used adjunctively with more direct estimates of follicular development (eg, ultrasonography and serum estradiol determinations).

The clinical confirmation of ovulation is obtained by direct and indirect indices of progesterone production. The indices most generally used are as follows: (1) a rise in basal body temperature, (2) increase in serum progesterone and (3) menstruation following the shift in basal body temperature.

When used in conjunction with indices of progesterone production, sonographic visualization of the ovaries will assist if ovulation has occurred. Sonographic evidence of ovulation may include the following: (1) fluid in the cul-de-sac, (2) follicle showing marked decrease in size and (3) collapsed follicle.

➤*Selection of patients:* Give careful attention to diagnosis in candidates for therapy. Before treatment is instituted:

1.) Perform a thorough gynecologic and endocrinologic evaluation including a hysterosalpingogram (to rule out uterine and tubal pathology) and documentation of anovulation by review of patient history, physical examination, determining serum hormonal levels as indicated and optionally performing an endometrial biopsy. Patients with tubal pathology should receive the drug only if enrolled in an in vitro fertilization program.

2.) Exclude primary ovarian failure by the determination of gonadotropin levels.

3.) Make careful examination to rule out early pregnancy.

4.) Patients in late reproductive life have a greater predilection to endometrial carcinoma and a higher incidence of anovulatory disorders. Perform a thorough diagnostic evaluation in patients who demonstrate abnormal uterine bleeding or other signs of endometrial abnormalities before starting therapy.

5.) Evaluate partner's fertility potential.

➤*Ovulation confirmation:* Treatment results in follicular growth and maturation to effect ovulation in the absence of an endogenous LH surge. HCG is given following the administration of urofollitropin and follitropin alfa and beta when clinical assessment indicates sufficient follicular maturation has occurred. This is indirectly estimated by the estrogenic effect upon the target organs. With serum or urinary estrogen determinations and ultrasonography, the estrogenic effect is an acceptable means for monitoring the growth and development of follicles, timing hCG administration and minimizing the risk of hyperstimulation. Clinically confirm ovulation, with the exception of pregnancy, by indirect indices of progesterone production. The indices most generally used are a rise in basal body temperature, increase in serum progesterone and menstruation following the shift in basal body temperature.

Other clinical parameters that may have potential use for monitoring urofollitropin therapy include changes in the vaginal cytology and appearance and volume of the cervical mucus.

Adverse Reactions

The following adverse reactions are listed in decreasing order of potential severity: Pulmonary and vascular complications (see Warnings); OHSS (see Warnings); adnexal torsion (as a complication of ovarian enlargement); mild to moderate ovarian enlargement; abdominal pain; sensitivity to urofollitropin (febrile reactions which may be accompanied by chills, musculoskeletal aches, joint pains, malaise, headache and fatigue have occurred. It is not clear whether or not these were pyrogenic responses or possible allergic reactions); ovarian cysts; GI symptoms (nausea, vomiting, diarrhea, abdominal cramps, bloating); pain, rash, swelling or irritation at the site of injection; breast tenderness; headache; dermatological symptoms (dry skin, body rash, hair loss, hives); hemoperitoneum has been reported during menotropins therapy and, therefore, may also occur during follitropin therapy.

The following adverse events have been reported in women treated with gonadotropins: Pulmonary and vascular complications (see Warnings), hemoperitoneum, adnexal torsion (as a complication of ovarian enlargement, abdominal pain), dizziness, tachycardia, dyspnea, tachypnea, febrile reactions, flu-like symptoms including fever, chills, musculoskeletal aches, joint pains, nausea, headache and malaise, ovarian cysts; gastrointestinal symptoms (nausea, vomiting, diarrhea, abdominal cramps, bloating); pain, rash, swelling, or irritation at the site of injection; breast tenderness and dermatological symptoms (dry skin, body rash, hair loss and hives).

Overdosage

Aside from possible ovarian hyperstimulation and multiple gestations (see Warnings), little is known concerning the consequences of acute overdosage.

Patient Information

Prior to therapy, inform patients of the following: Duration of treatment and monitoring required; possible adverse reactions; risk of multiple births.

Ovulation Stimulants

UROFOLLITROPIN

Rx	**Bravelle** (Ferring)	**Powder for injection, lyophilized:** 75 units FSH activity[1]	In vials[2] with 2 mL vials NaCl as diluent.

[1] Contains up to 2% luteinizing hormone (LH) activity.

[2] With 23 mg lactose monohydrate.

For complete prescribing information, refer to the Follitropins group monograph.

Indications

➤*Ovulation induction:* In conjunction with human chorionic gonadotropin (hCG) for ovulation induction in patients who previously have received pituitary suppression.

➤*Multifollicular development during ART:* In conjunction with hCG for multiple follicular development (controlled ovarian stimulation) during assisted reproductive technologies (ART) cycles in patients who have previously received pituitary suppression.

Administration and Dosage

➤*Approved by the FDA:* August 26, 1996.

➤*Infertile patients with oligo-anovulation:* The dose to stimulate development of ovarian follicles must be individualized for each patient. Use the lowest dose consistent with achieving good results based on clinical experience and reported clinical data.

The recommended initial dose for patients who have received gonadotropin-releasing hormone (GnRH) agonist or antagonist suppression is 150 units/day SC or IM for the first 5 days of treatment. Based on clinical monitoring (including serum estradiol levels and vaginal ultrasound results), adjust subsequent dosing according to individual patient response. Do not make adjustments in dose more frequently than once every 2 days and do not exceed more than 75 to 150 units/adjustment. The maximum daily dose should not exceed 450 units and, in most cases, dosing beyond 12 days is not recommended.

If patient response is appropriate, give hCG (5000 to 10,000 units) 1 day following the last dose of urofollitropin. Withhold the hCG if the serum estradiol is greater than 2000 pg/mL, if the ovaries are abnormally enlarged, or if abdominal pain occurs, and advise the patient to refrain from intercourse. These precautions may reduce the risk of Ovarian Hyperstimulation Syndrome (OHSS) and multiple gestations. Follow patients closely for at least 2 weeks after hCG administration. If there is inadequate follicle development or ovulation without subsequent pregnancy, the course of treatment may be repeated.

Encourage the couple to have intercourse daily, beginning on the day prior to the administration of hCG until ovulation becomes apparent from indices employed for the determination of progestational activity. In the light of the foregoing indices and parameters mentioned, it should become obvious that unless a physician is willing to devote considerable time to these patients and be familiar with and conduct the necessary laboratory studies, urofollitropin should not be used.

➤*ART:* The recommended initial dose of urofollitropin for patients undergoing in vitro fertilization (IVF) and donor egg patients who have received GnRH agonist or antagonist pituitary suppression is 225 units daily administered SC for the first 5 days of treatment. Based on clinical monitoring (including serum estradiol levels and vaginal ultrasound results) subsequent dosing should be adjusted according to individual patient response. Adjustments in dose should not be made more frequently than once every 2 days and should not exceed more than 75 to 150 units per adjustment. The maximum daily dose of urofollitropin given should not exceed 450 units and in most cases dosing beyond 12 days is not recommended.

Once adequate follicular development is evident, hCG (5000 to 10,000 units) should be administered to induce final follicular maturation in preparation for oocyte retrieval. The administration of hCG must be withheld in cases where the ovaries are abnormally enlarged on the last day of therapy. This should reduce the chance of developing OHSS.

➤*Reconstitution:* To prepare the solution, inject 1 mL of sterile saline for injection into the vial of urofollitropin. Do not shake, but gently swirl until the solution is clear. Generally, urofollitropin dissolves immediately. Check the liquid in the container; if it is not clear or contains particles, do not use it.

For patients requiring a single injection from multiple vials of urofollitropin, up to 6 vials can be reconstituted with 1 mL of sterile saline for injection. This can be accomplished by reconstituting a single vial as described above. Then draw the entire contents of the first vial into a syringe and inject the contents into a second vial of lyophilized urofollitropin. Gently swirl the second vial, once again checking to make sure the solution is clear and free of particles. This step can be repeated with 4 additional vials for a total of up to 6 vials of lyophilized urofollitropin into 1 mL of diluent.

Immediately administer the reconstituted urofollitropin. The recommended sites for SC injection are either side of the lower abdomen in alternating fashion. Injection into the thigh is not recommended.

➤*Storage/Stability:* Lyophilized powder may be stored in the refrigerator or at room temperature (3° to 25°C; 37° to 77°F). Protect from light. Use immediately after reconstitution. Discard unused material.

FOLLITROPIN ALFA

Rx	**Gonal-f** (Serono)	**Powder for injection, lyophilized:** 82 units FSH activity (to deliver 75 units)	30 mg sucrose. In 1 and 10 single-dose vials with sterile water for injection as diluent.
		600 units FSH activity (to deliver 450 units)	30 mg sucrose. In 1 multi-dose vial with prefilled syringe of bacteriostatic water[a] for injection as diluent and 6 syringes.
		1,200 units FSH activity (to deliver 1,050 units)	30 mg sucrose. In 1, 5, and 10 multi-dose vials with prefilled syringes of bacteriostatic water[a] for injection as diluent.
Rx	**Gonal-f RFF Pen** (Serono)	**Injection:** 415 units FSH activity (to deliver ≥ 300 units/0.05 mL)	In prefilled pens[b] with needles.
		568 units FSH activity (to deliver ≥ 450 units/0.75 mL)	
		1,026 units FSH activity (to deliver ≥ 900 units/1.5 mL)	

[a] With 0.9% benzyl alcohol.

[b] With 60 mg/mL sucrose, 3.0 mg/mL m-cresol, 1.1 mg/mL disodium hydrogen phosphate, 0.45 mg/mL sodium dihydrogen phosphate monohydrate, 0.1 mg//mL methionine, 0.1 mg/mL poloxamer 188.

For complete prescribing information, refer to the Follitropins group monograph.

Indications

➤*Ovulation induction:* For the induction of ovulation and pregnancy in oligo-anovulatory infertile patients in whom the cause of infertility is functional and not primary ovarian failure.

➤*Multifollicular development during assisted reproductive technology (ART):* To stimulate the development of multiple follicles in ovulatory patients participating in an ART program (eg, in vitro fertilization).

➤*Male infertility (except prefilled pen):* For the induction of spermatogenesis in men with primary and secondary hypogonadotropic hypogonadism in whom the cause of infertility is not primary testicular failure.

Administration and Dosage

➤*Approved by the FDA:* September 30, 1997.

For SC administration only. Individualize dosage.

➤*Ovulation induction:* The initial dose for the first cycle is 75 units/day SC. An incremental adjustment in dose of up to 37.5 units may be considered after 14 days. Further dose increases of the same magnitude can be made, if necessary, every 7 days. Do not exceed a treatment duration of 35 days unless an estradiol rise indicates imminent follicular development. To complete follicular development and effect ovulation in the absence of an endogenous luteinizing hormone surge, give 5000 units human chorionic gonadotropin (hCG) 1 day after the last dose of follitropin alfa. Withhold hCG if the serum estradiol is greater than 2000 pg/mL. If the ovaries are abnormally enlarged or abdominal pain occurs, discontinue follitropin alfa treatment, do not administer hCG, and advise the patient not to have intercourse; this may reduce the chance of developing Ovarian Hyperstimulation Syndrome (OHSS) and, should spontaneous ovulation occur, reduce the chance of multiple gestations. Conduct a follow-up visit in the luteal phase.

Individualize initial dose in subsequent cycles for each patient based on response in the preceding cycle. Doses larger than 300 units/day of follicle stimulating hormone are not routinely recommended. As in the initial cycle, 5000 units of hCG must be given 1 day after the last dose of follitropin alfa to complete follicular development and induce ovulation. Follow the above precautions to minimize the chances of developing OHSS.

FOLLITROPIN ALFA

Use the lowest dose consistent with the expectation of good results. Over the course of treatment, doses of follitropin alfa may range up to 300 units/day depending on patient response. Give until adequate follicular development is indicated by serum estradiol and vaginal ultrasonography. A response is generally evident after 5 to 7 days. Base subsequent monitoring intervals on patient response.

Encourage the couple to have intercourse daily, beginning on the day prior to hCG administration until ovulation becomes apparent. Take care to ensure insemination. In light of the indices and parameters mentioned, the drug should not be used unless a physician is willing to devote considerable time to these patients and be familiar with and conduct the necessary lab studies.

➤*Multifollicular development during ART:* Initiate in the early follicular phase (cycle day 2 or 3) at a dose of 150 units/day, until sufficient follicular development is attained. In most cases, therapy should not exceed 10 days.

In patients undergoing ART under 35 years of age, whose endogenous gonadotropin levels are suppressed, initiate follitropin alfa prefilled pens at a dose of 150 units/day. In patients undergoing ART 35 years of age and older, whose endogenous gonadotropin levels are suppressed, initiate follitropin alfa prefilled pens at a dose of 225 units/day. Continue treatment until adequate follicular development is indicated as determined by ultrasound in combination with measurement of serum estradiol levels. Consider dose adjustments after 5 days based on the patient's response; adjust subsequent dosage no more frequently than every 3 to 5 days and by no more than 75 to 150 units additionally at each adjustment. Doses greater than 450 units/day are not recommended. Once adequate follicular development is evident, administer hCG (5000 to 10,000 units) to induce final follicular maturation in preparation for oocyte retrieval. Withhold hCG in cases where the ovaries are abnormally enlarged on the last day of therapy to reduce the risk of developing OHSS.

➤*Male infertility:* The dose of follitropin alfa to induce spermatogenesis must be individualized for each patient. Give follitropin alfa in conjunction with hCG. Prior to concomitant therapy with follitropin alfa and hCG, pretreatment with hCG alone (1000 to 2250 units 2 to 3 times/week) is required. Continue treatment for a period sufficient to achieve serum testosterone levels within the normal range. Such pre-

treatment may require 3 to 6 months and the dose of hCG may need to be increased to achieve normal testosterone levels.

After normal serum testosterone levels are reached, the recommended dose of follitropin alfa is 150 units administered SC 3 times/week and the recommended dose of hCG is 1000 units (or the dose required to maintain serum testosterone levels within the normal range) 3 times/week. Use the lowest dose of follitropin alfa that induces spermatogenesis. If azoospermia persists, the dose may be increased to a maximum of 300 units 3 times/week. Follitropin alfa may need to be administered for up to 18 months to achieve adequate spermatogenesis.

➤*Reconstitution:*
Single-dose amps – Dissolve contents of 1 or more amps in 0.5 to 1 mL of sterile water for injection (concentration should not exceed 225 units/0.5 mL) and immediately give SC. Discard unused reconstituted material.

Multi-dose vials – Dissolve the contents of 1 multi-dose vial (1200 units) with the contents of 1 prefilled syringe (2 mL) containing bacteriostatic water for injection (0.9% benzyl alcohol). Resulting concentration will be 600 units/mL. Following reconstitution as directed, product will deliver approximately 1050 units FSH. Instruct patients to use the accompanying syringes calibrated in FSH units (IU FSH) for administration.

➤*Storage / Stability:*
Single-dose vials – Store vials in the refrigerator or at room temperature (2° to 25°C; 36° to 77°F). Protect from light. Use immediately after reconstitution. Discard unused material.

Multi-dose vials – Store multi-dose vials in the refrigerator or at room temperature until reconstituted (25°C; 77°F). Following reconstitution, refrigerate (2° to 8°C; 36° to 46° F) or store at room temperature (2° to 25°C; 36° to 77° F). Protect from light. Discard unused reconstituted solution after 28 days.

Prefilled pens – Store prefilled pens in the refrigerator (2° to 8°C; 36° to 46° F) until dispensed. Upon dispensing, refrigerate pen (2° to 8°C; 36° to 46° F) or store at room temperature (2° to 25°C; 36° to 77° F) for up to 1 month or until the expiration date, whichever occurs first. After the first injection, store pen in the refrigerator (2° to 8°C; 36° to 46° F) or at room temperature (2° to 25°C; 36° to 77° F) for up to 28 days. Protect from light. Do not freeze. Discard unused material after 28 days.

FOLLITROPIN BETA

Rx	Follistim (Organon)	Powder for injection, lyophilized: 75 IU FSH activity	25 mg sucrose. In vials with 5 mL Sterile Water for Injection as diluent.

For complete prescribing information, refer to the Follitropins group monograph.

Indications

➤*Follicle stimulation:* For the development of multiple follicles in ovulatory patients participating in assisted reproductive technology (ART) program, eg, in vitro fertilization.

➤*Ovulation induction:* For the induction of ovulation and pregnancy in anovulatory infertile patients in whom the cause of infertility is functional and not caused by primary ovarian failure.

Administration and Dosage

➤*Approved by the FDA:* September 29, 1997.

➤*Administration:* Administer SC or IM. The most convenient sites for SC injection are either in the abdomen around the navel where there is a lot of loose skin and layers of fatty tissue or in the upper thigh. Pinch up a large area of skin between the finger and thumb; the needle should be inserted at the base of the pinched-up skin at an angle of 45° to the skin surface. Vary the injection site with each injection.

The best site for IM injection is the upper outer quadrant of the buttock muscle. Stretching the skin helps the needle go in more easily and pushes the tissue beneath the skin out of the way. Insert the needle right up to the hilt at an angle of 90° to the skin surface. Pushing in with a quick thrust causes the least discomfort.

➤*Ovulation induction:* A variety of treatment protocols for ovulation induction exists. In studies using follitropin beta, a stepwise, gradually increasing dosing scheme was used. The starting dose was 75 IU for up to 14 days. The dose was then increased by 37.5 IU at weekly intervals until follicular growth or serum estradiol levels indicated an adequate response. The maximum individualized daily dose that has been safely used for ovulation induction patients during clinical trials is 300 IU. Treat until ultrasonic visualizations or serum estradiol determinations indicate preovulatory conditions greater than or equal to those of the normal individual followed by human chorionic gonadotropin (hCG), 5000 to 10,000 IU. If the ovaries are abnormally enlarged on the last day of therapy, withhold hCG; this reduces the risk of developing Ovarian Hyperstimulation Syndrome (OHSS).

During treatment with follitropin beta and during a 2-week posttreatment period, examine patients at least every other day for signs of excessive ovarian stimulation. Discontinue follitropin beta administration if the ovaries become abnormally enlarged or abdominal pain

occurs. Most OHSS occurs after treatment has been discontinued and reaches its maximum at about 7 to 10 days postovulation.

Encourage the couple to have intercourse daily, beginning on the day prior to the administration of hCG and until ovulation becomes apparent from the indices employed for the determination of progestational activity. Take care to ensure insemination. In the light of the foregoing indices and parameters mentioned, it should become obvious that, unless a physician is willing to devote considerable time to these patients and be familiar with and conduct these necessary laboratory studies, follitropin beta should not be used.

➤*Follicle stimulation:* A starting dose of 150 to 225 IU of follitropin beta is recommended for at least the first 4 days of treatment. The dose may be adjusted for the individual patient based upon their ovarian response. Daily maintenance dosages ranging from 75 to 300 IU for 6 to 12 days are sufficient, although longer treatment may be necessary. However, maintenance doses of 375 to 600 IU may be necessary according to individual response. The maximum daily dose used in clinical studies is 600 IU. When a sufficient number of follicles of adequate size are present, the final maturation of the follicles is induced by administering hCG at a dose of 5000 to 10,000 IU. Oocyte (egg) retrieval is performed 34 to 36 hours later. Withhold hCG in cases where the ovaries are abnormally enlarged on the last day of follitropin beta therapy; this reduces the risk of developing OHSS.

➤*Reconstitution:* Inject 1 mL Sterile Water for Injection into the follitropin beta vial. Do not shake; gently swirl until the solution is clear. Generally, follitropin beta dissolves immediately. Check the liquid in the container. Do not use if it is not clear or contains particles.

For patients requiring a single injection from multiple vials of follitropin beta, up to 4 vials can be reconstituted with 1 mL of Sterile Water for Injection. This can be accomplished by reconstituting a single vial as described above. Then draw the entire contents of the first vial into a syringe, and inject the contents into a second vial of lyophilized follitropin beta. Gently swirl the second vial, as described above, once again checking to make sure the solution is clear and free of particles. This step can be repeated with 2 additional vials for a total of up to 4 vials of lyophilized follitropin beta into 1 mL of diluent.

Immediately administer the reconstituted follitropin beta either SC or IM. Discard any unused reconstituted material.

➤*Storage / Stability:* Store powder refrigerated or at room temperature (2° to 25°C; 36° to 77°F). Protect from light. Use immediately after reconstitution. Discard unused material.

MENOTROPINS

Rx	**Pergonal** (Serono)	**Powder or pellet for injection, lyophilized:** 75 IU FSH activity, 75 IU LH activity	In amps with diluent.
Rx	**Repronex** (Ferring)		In vials with diluent.
Rx	**Pergonal** (Serono)	**Powder or pellet for injection, lyophilized:** 150 IU FSH activity, 150 IU LH activity	In amps with diluent.
Rx	**Repronex** (Ferring)		In vials with diluent.

Indications

➤*Women:* Menotropins and human chorionic gonadotropin (hCG) are given sequentially for induction of ovulation and pregnancy in the anovulatory infertile patient in whom the cause of anovulation is functional and not caused by primary ovarian failure. Also may be used to stimulate development of multiple follicles in ovulatory patients participating in an in vitro fertilization program.

➤*Men (Pergonal only):* Menotropins and concomitant hCG are given for stimulation of spermatogenesis in men with primary or secondary hypogonadotropic hypogonadism caused by a congenital factor or prepubertal hypophysectomy and in men with secondary hypogonadotropic hypogonadism caused by hypophysectomy, craniopharyngioma, cerebral aneurysm, or chromophobe adenoma.

Administration and Dosage

➤*Women:* Treatment results only in follicular growth and maturation. To effect ovulation, hCG must be given following menotropins when clinical assessment indicates sufficient follicular maturation. This is indirectly estimated by the estrogenic effect on target organs (ie, changes in the vaginal cytology, appearance and volume of cervical mucus, spinnbarkeit, ferning of cervical mucus). Only use these indices adjunctively with more direct estimates of follicular development (ie, serum estradiol, ultrasonography).

Confirmation of ovulation, with the exception of pregnancy, is obtained by indices of progesterone production, such as: 1) A rise in basal body temperature, 2) increase in serum progesterone, and 3) menstruation following the shift in basal body temperature.

Initial dosage –

Repronex: The recommended initial dose for patients who have received GnRH agonist or antagonist pituitary suppression is 150 IU SC or IM daily for the first 5 days of treatment. Based on clinical monitoring (including serum estradiol levels and vaginal ultrasound results), adjust subsequent dosing according to individual patient response. Do not make adjustments in dose more frequently than once every 2 days and do not exceed > 75 to 150 IU per adjustment. Do not exceed the maximum daily of 450 IU. Dosing beyond 12 days is not recommended.

If patient response is appropriate, give hCG 5000 to 10,000 U 1 day following the last dose of menotropins. Withhold the hCG if the serum estradiol is > 2000 pg/mL, if the ovaries are abnormally enlarged, or if abdominal pain occurs, and advise the patient to refrain from intercourse. These precautions may reduce the risk of Ovarian Hyperstimulation Syndrome (OHSS) and multiple gestation. Follow patients closely for at least 2 weeks after hCG administration. If there is inadequate follicle development or ovulation without subsequent pregnancy, the course of treatment with menotropins may be repeated.

Pergonal: Individualize dosage. Initial IM dose is 75 IU FSH/75 IU LH (1 amp) per day, for 7 to 12 days; follow by 5000 to 10,000 U hCG 1 day after the last dose of menotropins. Do not exceed 12 days of menotropins administration. Treat the patient until indices of estrogenic activity are equal to or greater than those of the normal individual. Urinary and serum estrogen determinations are useful as a guide to therapy. If the ovaries are abnormally enlarged on the last day of menotropins therapy, do not administer hCG in this course of therapy; this will reduce the chances of developing OHSS.

• *Repeat dosage* – If there is evidence of ovulation, but no pregnancy, repeat the regimen for ≥ 2 more courses before increasing the dose to 150 IU FSH/150 IU LH (2 amps) per day for 7 to 12 days. Follow by 5000 to 10,000 U hCG 1 day after the last dose of menotropins. Two amps of menotropins per day is the most effective dose. If evidence of ovulation is present, but pregnancy does not ensue, repeat the same dose for 2 more courses but larger doses are not recommended.

The couple should have intercourse daily beginning on the day prior to hCG administration until ovulation occurs; ensure insemination.

During treatment with menotropins and hCG and for 2 weeks posttreatment, examine patients at least every other day for signs of excessive ovarian stimulation. Stop treatment if the ovaries become abnormally enlarged or if abdominal pain occurs. Hyperstimulation usually occurs after treatment has been discontinued and reaches its maximum 7 to 10 days postovulation.

➤*Men (Pergonal only):* Prior to therapy with menotropins and hCG, pretreat with hCG alone (5000 U 3 times/week). Continue hCG for a sufficient period to achieve serum testosterone levels within normal range and masculinization (ie, appearance of secondary sex characteristics). Pretreatment may require 4 to 6 months. The recommended dose is 1 amp menotropins IM 3 times/week and hCG 2000 U twice a week. Continue therapy for ≥ 4 months to ensure detecting spermatozoa in ejaculate.

If the patient has not responded with increased spermatogenesis at the end of 4 months, continue treatment with 1 amp 3 times/week or increase dose to 2 amps (150 IU FSH/150 IU LH) 3 times/week, with the hCG dose unchanged.

➤*Preparation of solution:* Dissolve contents of 1 amp in 1 to 2 mL sterile saline. Administer IM immediately. Discard any unused portion.

➤*Storage/Stability:* Lyophilized powder may be refrigerated or stored at room temperature, 3° to 25°C (37° to 77°F).

Actions

➤*Pharmacology:* Menotropins is a purified preparation of gonadotropins extracted from the urine of postmenopausal women. It is biologically standardized for follicle-stimulating hormone (FSH) and luteinizing hormone (LH) activities.

Women – Produces ovarian follicular growth in women who do not have primary ovarian failure. Treatment results only in follicular growth and maturation. To effect ovulation, human chorionic gonadotropin (hCG) is given following menotropins when clinical assessment indicates sufficient follicular maturation.

Men – Menotropins administered concomitantly with hCG for ≥ 3 months induces spermatogenesis in men with primary or secondary pituitary hypofunction who have achieved adequate masculinization with prior hCG therapy.

Contraindications

➤*Women:* High gonadotropin level indicating primary ovarian failure; overt thyroid and adrenal dysfunction; any cause of infertility other than anovulation; abnormal bleeding of undetermined origin; ovarian cysts or enlargement not caused by polycystic ovary syndrome; organic intracranial lesion such as pituitary tumor; pregnancy.

➤*Men:* Normal gonadotropin levels indicating normal pituitary function; elevated gonadotropin levels indicating primary testicular failure; infertility disorders other than hypogonadotropic hypogonadism.

Warnings

➤*Physician use:* This drug should be used only by physicians thoroughly familiar with infertility problems. Menotropins can cause mild to severe adverse reactions in women.

➤*Hypersensitivity reactions:* Hypersensitivity/anaphylactic reactions associated with menotropin administration have been reported in some patients. These reactions presented as generalized urticaria, facial edema, angioneurotic edema or dyspnea suggestive of laryngeal edema.

➤*Pregnancy: Category X.* Menotropins may cause fetal harm. Birth defects occurred in 5 of 287 pregnancies. Do not use during pregnancy.

Precautions

➤*Diagnosis prior to therapy:*

Women – Perform a thorough gynecologic and endocrinologic evaluation, including a hysterosalpingogram. Document anovulation. Rule out primary ovarian failure and early pregnancy. Patients in late reproductive life have a greater predilection to endometrial carcinoma and a higher incidence of anovulatory disorders. Perform a cervical dilation and curettage before starting therapy in such patients. Evaluate the partner's fertility potential.

Men – Document lack of pituitary function. Prior to therapy, patients have low testosterone levels and low or absent gonadotropin levels. Patients with primary hypogonadotropic hypogonadism will have subnormal development of masculinization; those with secondary hypogonadotropic hypogonadism will have decreased masculinization.

➤*Overstimulation of the ovary:* To minimize the hazard of abnormal ovarian enlargement, use the lowest effective dose. Mild to moderate uncomplicated ovarian enlargement, with or without abdominal distention or abdominal pain, occurs in ≈ 20% of those treated with hCG and menotropins and generally regresses without treatment in 2 to 3 weeks. The hyperstimulation syndrome characterized by sudden ovarian enlargement and ascites, with or without pain or pleural effusion, occurs in ≈ 0.4% of patients at recommended doses. The overall incidence of this syndrome is ≈ 1.3%.

Hyperstimulation syndrome develops rapidly and generally occurs within 2 weeks following treatment; if it occurs, discontinue treatment and hospitalize patient. Hemoconcentration associated with fluid loss in the abdominal cavity has occurred; thoroughly assess by daily determination of fluid intake and output, weight, hematocrit, serum and urinary electrolytes, urine specific gravity, BUN, creatinine and abdominal girth. Treatment is primarily symptomatic and consists of bedrest, fluid and electrolyte replacement and analgesics. Never remove ascitic fluid because of the potential for injury to the ovary.

MENOTROPINS

Hemoperitoneum may occur from ruptured ovarian cysts, usually as a result of pelvic examination. If bleeding requires surgery, design the surgery to control bleeding and to retain as much ovarian tissue as possible. Prohibit intercourse when significant ovarian enlargement occurs after ovulation.

➤*Multiple births:* Pregnancies following therapy with hCG and menotropins resulted in 80% single births; 15% resulted in twins and 5% of pregnancies produced 3 or more conceptuses. Advise patient of the frequency and potential hazards of multiple pregnancy.

➤*Pulmonary/Vascular complications:* Serious pulmonary conditions (eg, atelectasis, acute respiratory distress syndrome) have been reported. In addition, thromboembolic events both in association with, and separate from, the Ovarian Hyperstimulation Syndrome have been reported following menotropin therapy. Intravascular thrombosis and embolism, which may originate in venous or arterial vessels, can result in reduced blood flow to critical organs or the extremities. Sequelae of such events have included venous thrombophlebitis, pulmonary embolism, pulmonary infarction, cerebral vascular occlusion (stroke) and arterial occlusion resulting in loss of limb. In rare cases, pulmonary complications or thromboembolic events have resulted in death.

Adverse Reactions

Women – Ovarian enlargement, ovarian cysts, adnexal torsion (as a complication of ovarian enlargement); hyperstimulation syndrome; hemoperitoneum; hypersensitivity (see Warnings); febrile reactions; fever; chills; musculoskeletal aches; joint pains; nausea; headaches; malaise; pulmonary and vascular complications (see Precautions); abdominal pain; vomiting; diarrhea; abdominal cramps; bloating; pain, rash, swelling or irritation at injection site; body rashes; dizziness; tachycardia; dyspnea; tachypnea; ectopic pregnancy.

Men – Occasional gynecomastia, breast pain, mastitis, nausea, abnormal lipoprotein fraction, abnormal AST and ALT (occasional), erythrocytosis (Hct 50%, Hgb 17.8 g%, in one patient).

CHORIONIC GONADOTROPIN

Rx	**Chorionic Gonadotropin** (Various, eg, Goldline, Rugby, Steris)	**Powder for Injection** : 5000 units per vial with 10 ml diluent (to make 500 units per ml)	In 10 ml vials.
Rx	**Chorex-5** (Hyrex)		In 10 ml vials.[2]
Rx	**Profasi** (Serono)		In 10 ml vials.[2]
Rx	**Chorionic Gonadotropin** (Various, eg, Goldline, Rugby, Steris)	**Powder for Injection:** 10,000 units per vial with 10 ml diluent (to make 1000 units per ml)	In 10 ml vials.
Rx	**Choron 10** (Forest)		In 10 ml vials.[2]
Rx	**Gonic** (Hauck)		In 10 ml vials.[2]
Rx	**Novarel** (Ferring)		In 10 ml vials.[2]
Rx	**Pregnyl** (Organon)		In 10 ml vials.[3]
Rx	**Profasi** (Serono)		In 10 ml vials.[2]
Rx	**Chorionic Gonadotropin** (Various, eg, Goldline, Steris)	**Powder for Injection** : 20,000 units per vial with 10 ml diluent (to make 2000 units per ml)	In 10 ml vials.

[1] With benzyl alcohol, < 0.2% phenol and lactose.
[2] With mannitol and 0.9% benzyl alcohol.
[3] With 0.9% benzyl alcohol.

WARNING

Human chorionic gonadotropin (hCG) has no known effect on fat mobilization, appetite, sense of hunger or body fat distribution. HCG has NOT been demonstrated to be effective adjunctive therapy in the treatment of obesity. There is no substantial evidence that it increases weight loss beyond that resulting from caloric restriction, that it causes a more attractive or "normal" distribution of fat or that it decreases the hunger and discomfort associated with calorie restricted diets.

Indications

➤*Prepubertal cryptorchidism:* Prepubertal cryptorchidism not due to anatomical obstruction. HCG is thought to induce testicular descent in situations when descent would have occurred at puberty. HCG may help predict whether orchiopexy will be needed in the future. In some cases, descent following hCG administration is permanent, but in most cases the response is temporary. Therapy is usually instituted between the ages of 4 and 9.

➤*Hypogonadism:* Selected cases of hypogonadotropic hypogonadism (hypogonadism secondary to a pituitary deficiency) in males.

➤*Ovulation induction:* Induction of ovulation in the anovulatory, infertile woman in whom the cause of anovulation is secondary and not due to primary ovarian failure, and who has been appropriately pretreated with human menotropins.

Administration and Dosage

For IM use only. There is a marked variance of opinion concerning dosage regimens. The regimen employed will depend on the indication, age and weight of the patient and the physician's preference. The following regimens have been advocated.

➤*Prepubertal cryptorchidism not caused by anatomical obstruction:*
1.) 4000 USP units, 3 times weekly for 3 weeks.
2.) 5000 USP units every second day for 4 injections.
3.) 15 injections of 500 to 1000 USP units over a period of 6 weeks.
4.) 500 USP units, 3 times weekly for 4 to 6 weeks. If this course is not successful, start another course 1 month later, giving 1000 USP units per injection.

➤*Selected cases of hypogonadotropic hypogonadism in males:*
1.) 500 to 1000 USP units 3 times a week for 3 weeks, followed by the same dose twice a week for 3 weeks.
2.) 1000 to 2000 USP units, 3 times weekly.
3.) 4000 USP units 3 times weekly for 6 to 9 months; reduce dosage to 2000 USP units 3 times weekly for an additional 3 months.

➤*Induction of ovulation and pregnancy:* In the anovulatory, infertile woman in whom the cause of anovulation is secondary and not due to primary ovarian failure, and who has been appropriately pretreated with human menotropins (see Menotropins monograph) - 5000 to 10,000 USP units 1 day following the last dose of menotropins.

The above products consist of lyophilized powder, with or without diluent, to prepare solutions for injection providing the indicated number of units of hCG. Refer to manufacturers' labeling for preparation and storage.

Actions

➤*Pharmacology:* HCG, a polypeptide hormone produced by the human placenta, is composed of an α and β subunit. The α subunit is essentially identical to the α subunits of the human pituitary gonadotropins, luteinizing hormone (LH) and follicle-stimulating hormone (FSH), as well as to the α subunit of human thyroid stimulating hormone (TSH). The β subunits of these hormones differ in amino acid sequence.

HCG's action is virtually identical to pituitary LH's, although hCG appears to have a small degree of FSH activity as well. It stimulates production of gonadal steroid hormones by stimulating interstitial cells (Leydig cells) of testis to produce androgens, and the corpus luteum of the ovary to produce progesterone. Androgen stimulation in males leads to development of secondary sex characteristics and may stimulate testicular descent when no anatomical impediment is present. The descent is usually reversible when hCG is discontinued. During the normal menstrual cycle, LH participates with FSH in development and maturation of the normal ovarian follicle, and the mid-cycle LH surge triggers ovulation; hCG can substitute for LH in this function. During a normal pregnancy, hCG secreted by the placenta maintains the corpus luteum after LH secretion decreases, supporting continued estrogen and progesterone secretion and preventing menstruation.

Contraindications

Precocious puberty; prostatic carcinoma or other androgen-dependent neoplasm; prior allergic reaction to chorionic gonadotropin; pregnancy (see Warnings).

Warnings

➤*Use for infertility:* HCG should be used in conjunction with human menopausal gonadotropins only by physicians experienced with infertility problems.

➤*Pregnancy:* Category X. HCG may cause fetal harm when administered to a pregnant woman. Combined hCG/PMS (pregnant mare's serum) therapy has been noted to induce high incidences of external congenital anomalies in the offspring of mice, in a dose-dependent manner. The potential extrapolation to humans has not been determined.

➤*Lactation:* It is not known whether this drug is excreted in breast milk. Exercise caution when hCG is administered to a nursing woman.

CHORIONIC GONADOTROPIN

➤*Children:* Safety and efficacy in children < 4 years of age have not been established.

Precautions

➤*Precocious puberty:* Induction of androgen secretion by hCG may induce phallic enlargement; testicular enlargement and redness; development of pubic hair; agressive behavior. These changes are reversible within 4 weeks of the last injection.

➤*Fluid retention:* Since androgens may cause fluid retention, use HCG with caution in patients with epilepsy, migraine, asthma, cardiac or renal disease.

Adverse Reactions

Headache; irritability; restlessness; depression; fatigue; edema; precocious puberty; gynecomastia; pain at injection site; agressive behavior; ovarian hyperstimulation syndrome; ovarian malignancy (rare); enlargement of preexisting ovarian cysts and possible rupture; arterial thromboembolism.

Ovulation induction – The principal serious adverse reactions with this indication are: Ovarian hyperstimulation (sudden ovarian enlargement); ascites with or without pain and pleural effusion; rupture of ovarian cysts with resultant hemoperitoneum; multiple births; arterial thromboembolism.

CHORIOGONADOTROPIN ALFA

Rx	**Ovidrel** (Serono)	Injection: 250 mcg/0.5 mL	28.1 mg mannitol, 505 mcg 85% O-phosphoric acid. In single-dose prefilled syringes.

Indications

➤*Final follicular maturation:* For the induction of final follicular maturation and early luteinization in infertile women who have undergone pituitary desensization and who have been appropriately pretreated with follicle stimulating hormones as part of an assisted reproductive technology (ART) program such as in vitro fertilization and embryo transfer.

➤*Ovulation induction:* For the induction of ovulation (OI) and pregnancy in anovulatory infertile patients in whom the cause of infertility is functional and not due to primary ovarian failure.

Administration and Dosage

➤*Approved by the FDA:* September 22, 2000.

Before treatment with gonadotropins is instituted, a thorough gynecologic and endocrinologic evaluation must be performed. This includes an assessment of pelvic anatomy. Patients with tubal obstruction should receive choriogonadotropin alfa only if enrolled in an in vitro fertilization program.

Exclude primary ovarian failure by the determination of gonadotropin levels.

Perform appropriate evaluation to exclude pregnancy.

Patients in later reproductive life have a greater predisposition to endometrial carcinoma as well as a higher incidence of anovulatory disorders. Always perform a thorough diagnostic evaluation in patients who demonstrate abnormal uterine bleeding or other signs of endometrial abnormalities before starting FSH and choriogonadotropin alfa therapy.

Include evaluation of the partner's fertility potential in the initial evaluation.

➤*Infertile women undergoing ART:* Administer 250 mcg choriogonadotropin alfa 1 day following the last dose of the follicle stimulating agent. Do not administer choriogonadotropin alfa until adequate follicular development is indicated by serum estradiol and vaginal ultrasonography. Withhold administration in situations in which there is an excessive ovarian response, as evidenced by clinically significant ovarian enlargement or excessive estradiol production.

➤*Infertile women undergoing OI:* Do not administer choriogonadotropin alfa until adequate follicular development is indicated by serum estradiol and vaginal ultrasonography.

Administer 250 mcg choriogonadotropin alfa 1 day following the last dose of the follicle stimulating agent.

Withhold choriogonadotropin alfa administration in situations in which there is an excessive ovarian response, as evidenced by multiple follicular development, clinically significant ovarian enlargement or excessive estradiol production.

➤*Administration:* Choriogonadotropin alfa is intended for a single SC injection to be administered following reconstition with 1 ml Sterile Water for Injection. Discard any unused reconstituted material. See package insert for further directions on self-administration by the patient.

➤*Storage/Stability:* Vials may be stored refrigerated or at room temperature (2° to 25°C; 36° to 77°F). Protect from light. Use immediately after reconstitution; discard unused material.

Actions

➤*Pharmacology:* The physicochemical, immunological, and biological activities of recombinant hCG are comparable with those of placental and human pregnancy urine-derived hCG. Choriogonadotropin alfa stimulates late follicular maturation and resumption of oocyte meiosis, and initiates rupture of the pre-ovulatory ovarian follicle. Choriogonadotropin alfa is an analog of luteinizing hormone (LH) and binds to the LH/hCG receptor of the granulosa and theca cells of the ovary to effect these changes in the absence of an endogenous LH surge. In pregnancy, hCG, secreted by the placenta, maintains the viability of the corpus luteum to provide the continued secretion of estrogen and progesterone necessary to support the first trimester of pregnancy. Choriogonadotropin alfa is administered when monitoring of the patient indicates that sufficient follicular development has occurred in response to FSH treatment for ovulation induction.

➤*Pharmacokinetics:*

Absorption – Following SC administration of 250 mcg choriogonadotropin alfa, maximum serum concentration ($\approx$ 121 IU/L) is reached after $\approx$ 12 to 24 hours. The mean absolute bioavailability of choriogonadotropin alfa following a single SC injection to healthy female volunteers is $\approx$ 40%.

Distribution – Following IV administration of 250 mcg choriogonadotropin alfa to healthy down-regulated female volunteers, the serum profile of hCG is described by a 2-compartment model with an initial half-life of $\approx$ 4.5 hours. The volume of the central compartment is $\approx$ 3 L and the steady-state volume of distribution is $\approx$ 5.9 L.

Metabolism/Excretion – Following SC administration of choriogonadotropin alfa, hCG is eliminated from the body with a mean terminal half-life of $\approx$ 29 hours. After IV administration of 250 mcg choriogonadotropin alfa to healthy down-regulated females, the mean terminal half-life is $\approx$ 26.5 hours and the total body clearance is $\approx$ 0.29 L/hr. Ten percent of the dose is excreted in the urine.

➤*Clinical trials:* The safety and efficacy of choriogonadotropin alfa have been examined in 3 well-controlled studies in women: 2 studies for ART and 1 study for OI.

ART – The safety and efficacy of 250 mcg and 500 mcg choriogonadotropin alfa administered SC vs 10,000 USP units of an approved urinary-derived hCG product administered IM were assessed in a randomized, open-label, multicenter study in infertile women undergoing in vitro fertilization and embryo transfer. The study was conducted in 20 US centers.

The primary efficacy parameter in this single-cycle study was the number of oocytes retrieved. In the study, 94 of the 297 patients were randomized to receive 250 mcg choriogonadotropin alfa. The number of oocytes retrieved was similar for the choriogonadotropin alfa and urinary-derived hCG (10,000 USP Units) treatment groups. The efficacy of 250 mcg and 500 mcg choriogonadotropin alfa were both found to be clinically and statistically equivalent to that of the approved urinary-derived hCG product and to each other.

For the 33 patients who achieved a clinical pregnancy with 250 mcg choriogonadotropin alfa, 4 pregnancies did not reach term, while 29 patients had live births (20 single births and 9 multiple births).

The safety and efficacy of 250 mcg choriogonadotropin alfa administered SC vs 5000 IU of an approved urinary-derived hCG product administered SC were assessed in a second, randomized, multicenter study in infertile women undergoing in vitro fertilization and embryo transfer. This double-blinded study was conducted in 9 centers in Europe and Israel.

The primary efficacy parameter in this single-cycle study was the number of oocytes retrieved per patient. In this study, 97 of 205 patients received 250 mcg choriogonadotropin alfa. The efficacy of 250 mcg choriogonadotropin alfa was found to be clinically and statistically equivalent to that of the approved urinary-derived hCG product.

For the 32 patients who achieved a clinical pregnancy with 250 mcg choriogonadotropin alfa, 6 pregnancies did not reach full term, while 26 had live births (18 single births and 8 multiple births).

OI – The safety and efficacy of 250 mcg choriogonadotropin alfa administered SC vs 5000 IU of an approved urinary-derived hCG product administered IM were assessed in a double-blind, randomized, multicenter study in anovulatory infertile women, which was conducted in 19 centers in Australia, Canada, Europe, and Israel.

The primary efficacy parameter in this single-cycle study was the patient ovulation rate. In this study, 99 of 242 patients received 250 mcg choriogonadotropin alfa. The efficacy of 250 mcg choriogonadotropin alfa was found to be clinically and statistically equivalent to that of the approved urinary-derived hCG product.

For the 22 patients who had a clinical pregnancy with 250 mcg choriogonadotropin alfa, 7 pregnancies did not reach full term, while 15 patients had live births (13 single births and 2 multiple births).

CHORIOGONADOTROPIN ALFA

Contraindications

Hypersensitivity to hCG preparations or one of their excipients; primary ovarian failure; uncontrolled thyroid or adrenal dysfunction; uncontrolled organic intracranial lesion such as a pituitary tumor; abnormal uterine bleeding of undetermined origin; ovarian cyst or enlargement of undetermined origin; sex hormone-dependent tumors of the reproductive tract and accessory organs; pregnancy.

Warnings

➤*Ovarian enlargement:* Mild-to-moderate uncomplicated ovarian enlargement that may be accompanied by abdominal distention and/or abdominal pain may occur in patients treated with FSH and hCG, and generally regresses without treatment within 2 or 3 weeks. Careful monitoring of ovarian response can further minimize the risk of over-stimulation.

If the ovaries are abnormally enlarged on the last day of FSH therapy, do not administer choriogonadotropin alfa in this course of therapy. This will reduce the risk of development of ovarian hyperstimulation syndrome (OHSS).

➤*OHSS:* OHSS is a medical event distinct from uncomplicated ovarian enlargement. Severe OHSS may progress rapidly (within 24 hours to several days) to become a serious medical event. It is characterized by an apparent dramatic increase in vascular permeability that can result in a rapid accumulation of fluid in the peritoneal cavity, thorax, and potentially, the pericardium. The early warning signs of development of OHSS are severe pelvic pain, nausea, vomiting, and weight gain. The following symptomatology has been seen with cases of OHSS: Abdominal pain; abdominal distension; GI symptoms, including nausea, vomiting, and diarrhea; severe ovarian enlargement; weight gain; dyspnea; and oliguria. Clinical evaluation may reveal hypovolemia, hemoconcentration, electrolyte imbalances, ascites, hemoperitoneum, pleural effusions, hydrothorax, acute pulmonary distress, and thrombo-embolic events. Transient liver function test abnormalities suggestive of hepatic dysfunction, which may be accompanied by morphologic changes on liver biopsy, have been reported in association with OHSS.

OHSS occurred in 1.7% of 236 patients treated with 250 mcg choriogonadotropin alfa during clinical trials for ART and 3% of 99 patients treated in the OI trial. OHSS occurred in 9% of 89 patients who received 500 mcg. Two patients treated with 500 mcg choriogonadotropin alfa developed severe OHSS.

OHSS may be more severe and more protracted if pregnancy occurs. OHSS develops rapidly; therefore, follow patients for at least 2 weeks after hCG administration. Most often, OHSS occurs after treatment has been discontinued and reaches its maximum at ≈ 7 to 10 days following treatment. Usually, OHSS resolves spontaneously with the onset of menses. If there is evidence that OHSS may be developing prior to hCG administration, the hCG must be withheld.

If severe OHSS occurs, stop treatment with gonadotropins and hospitalize the patient.

Consult a physician experienced in the management of this syndrome, or who is experienced in the management of fluid and electrolyte imbalances.

➤*Multiple births:* Reports of multiple births have been associated with choriogonadotropin alfa treatment. In ART, the risk of multiple births correlates to the number of embryos transferred. Multiple births occurred in 30.9% of 55 deliveries experienced by women receiving 250 mcg choriogonadotropin alfa in the ART studies. In the ovulation induction clinical trial, 13.3% of 15 live deliveries were associated with multiple births in women receiving choriogonadotropin alfa. Advise the patient of the potential risk of multiple births before starting treatment.

➤*Pulmonary and vascular complications:* Potential for the occurrence of arterial thromboembolism exists.

➤*Pregnancy:* Category X. Fetal death and impaired parturition were observed in pregnant rats given a dose of 25 mcg/day choriogonadotropin alfa equivalent to 6 times the maximum human dose of 250 mcg based on body surface area.

➤*Lactation:* It is not known whether this drug is excreted in breast milk. Because many drugs are excreted in breast milk, exercise caution if hCG is administered to a nursing woman.

Precautions

➤*Monitoring:* Gonadotropins, including choriogonadotropin alfa, should be used only by physicians who are thoroughly familiar with infertility problems and their management. Choriogonadotropin alfa is a potent gonadotropic substance capable of causing OHSS in women with or without pulmonary or vascular complications. Gonadotropin therapy requires a certain time commitment by physicians and supportive health professionals, and requires the availability of appropriate monitoring facilities. Safe and effective induction of ovulation and use of choriogonadotropin alfa in women requires monitoring of ovarian response with serum estradiol and transvaginal ultrasound on a regular basis.

In most instances, treatment of women with FSH results only in follicular recruitment and development. In the absence of an endogenous LH surge, hCG is given when monitoring of the patient indicates that sufficient follicular development has occurred. This may be estimated by ultrasound alone or in combination with measurement of serum estradiol levels. The combination of both ultrasound and serum estradiol measurement are useful for monitoring the development of follicles, for timing of the ovulatory trigger, as well as for detecting ovarian enlargement and minimizing the risk of the OHSS and multiple gestation. It is recommended that the number of growing follicles be confirmed using ultrasonography because serum estrogens do not give an indication of the size or number of follicles.

The clinical confirmation of ovulation, with the exception of pregnancy, is obtained by direct and indirect indices of progesterone production. The indices most generally used are as follows: A rise in basal body temperature, increase in serum progesterone, and menstruation following a shift in basal body temperature.

When used in conjunction with the indices of progesterone production, sonographic visualization of the ovaries will assist in determining if ovulation has occurred. Sonographic evidence of ovulation may include the following: Fluid in the cul-de-sac, ovarian stigmata, collapsed follicle, and secretory endometrium. Accurate interpretation of the indices of ovulation require a physician who is experienced in the interpretation of these tests.

➤*Lab test abnormalities:* hCG can crossreact in the radioimmunoassay of gonadotropins, especially luteinizing hormone. Each individual laboratory should establish the degree of crossreactivity with their gonadotropin assay. Physicians should make the laboratory aware of patients on hCG if gonadotropin levels are requested.

Elevations in ALT were found in 3% of 335 patients receiving 250 mcg choriogonadotropin alfa, 10% of 89 patients receiving 500 mcg choriogonadotropin alfa, and 4.8% of 328 patients receiving urinary-derived hCG. The elevations ranged up to 1.2 times the upper limit of normal. The clinical significance of these findings is not known.

Adverse Reactions

Adverse reactions in ART – Application site disorders, injection site pain/bruising, GI system disorder, abdominal pain, nausea, vomiting, post-operative pain (> 2%); injection site inflammation/reaction, flatulence, diarrhea, hiccough, ectopic pregnancy, breast pain, intermenstrual bleeding, vaginal hemorrhage, cervical lesion, leukorrhea, ovarian hyperstimulation, uterine disorders, vaginitis, vaginal discomfort, body pain, back pain, fever, dizziness, headache, hot flashes, malaise, paresthesias, rash, emotional lability, insomnia, upper respiratory tract infection, cough, dysuria, urinary tract infection, urinary incontinence, albuminuria, cardiac arrhythmia, genital moniliasis, genital herpes, leukocytosis, heart murmur, cervical carcinoma (< 2%).

Adverse reactions in OI – Application site disorders (including injection site pain/inflammation/bruising/reaction), female reproductive disorders (including ovarian cyst/hyperstimulation), GI system disorders (including abdominal pain) (> 2%); breast pain, flatulence, abdominal enlargement, pharyngitis, upper respiratory tract infection, hyperglycemia, pruritus (< 2%).

Medical events reported in pregnancies resulting from hCG therapy – Spontaneous abortion; ectopic pregnancy; premature labor; postpartum fever; congenital abnormalities.

Patient Information

Prior to hCG therapy, inform patients of the duration of treatment and monitoring of their condition that will be required. Discuss the risks of ovarian hyperstimulation syndrome and multiple births and other possible adverse reactions.

See package insert for patient self-administration directions.

NAFARELIN ACETATE

| Rx | Synarel (Syntex) | Nasal Solution: 2 mg/ml (as nafarelin base) | In 10 ml bottle with metered spray pump (delivers ≈ 200 mcg/spray).[1] |

[1] With benzalkonium chloride, glacial acetic acid and sorbitol.

Indications

➤*Endometriosis:* Endometriosis, including pain relief and reduction of endometriotic lesions. Experience has been limited to women ≥ 18 years of age treated for 6 months.

➤*Central precocious puberty:* Central precocious puberty (gonadotropin-dependent) in children of both sexes.

Administration and Dosage

➤*Approved by the FDA:* 1990.

➤*Endometriosis:* 400 mcg/day. One spray (200 mcg) into one nostril in the morning and one spray into the other nostril in the evening. Start treatment between days 2 and 4 of the menstrual cycle.

For patients with persistent regular menstruation after months of treatment, the dose may be increased to 800 mcg daily. The 800 mcg dose is given as 1 spray into each nostril in the morning (a total of 2 sprays) and again in the evening.

The recommended duration of administration is 6 months. Retreatment is not recommended since safety data are not available. If symptoms recur after a course of therapy, and further treatment with nafarelin is contemplated, assess bone density before retreatment begins to ensure that values are within normal limits.

If the use of a topical decongestant is necessary during treatment with nafarelin, the decongestant should not be used until at least 2 hours after nafarelin dosing.

At 400 mcg/day, a bottle of nafarelin provides a 30 day (about 60 sprays) supply. If the daily dose is increased, increase the supply to the patient to ensure uninterrupted treatment for the recommended duration of therapy.

➤*Central precocious puberty (CPP):* 1600 mcg/day. The dose can be increased to 1800 mcg daily if adequate suppression cannot be achieved at 1600 mcg/day.

The 1600 mcg dose is achieved by 2 sprays (400 mcg) into each nostril in the morning (4 sprays) and 2 sprays into each nostril in the evening (4 sprays), a total of 8 sprays per day. The 1800 mcg dose is achieved by 3 sprays (600 mcg) into alternating nostrils 3 times a day, a total of 9 sprays per day. The patient's head should be tilted back slightly, and 30 seconds should elapse between sprays.

If the prescribed therapy has been well tolerated by the patient, continue treatment of CPP until resumption of puberty is desired.

There appeared to be no significant effect of rhinitis on the systemic bioavailability of nafarelin; however, if the use of a nasal decongestant for rhinitis is necessary, do not use the decongestant until at least 2 hours following nafarelin.

Avoid sneezing during or immediately after dosing with nafarelin, if possible, since this may impair drug absorption.

At 1600 mcg/day, a bottle of nafarelin provides about a 7 day supply (about 56 sprays). If the daily dose is increased, increase the supply to the patient to ensure uninterrupted treatment for the duration of therapy.

➤*Storage/Stability:* Store upright at room temperature. Protect from light.

Actions

➤*Pharmacology:* Nafarelin acetate is a potent agonistic analog of gonadotropin-releasing hormone (GnRH). At the onset of administration, nafarelin stimulates the release of the pituitary gonadotropins, LH and FSH, resulting in a temporary increase of ovarian steroidogenesis. Repeated dosing abolishes the stimulatory effect on the pituitary gland. Twice daily administration leads to decreased secretion of gonadal steroids by about 4 weeks; consequently, tissues and functions that depend on gonadal steroids for their maintenance become quiescent.

When used regularly in girls and boys with CPP, nafarelin suppresses LH and sex steroid hormone levels to prepubertal levels, affects a corresponding arrest of secondary sexual development, and slows linear growth and skeletal maturation. In some cases, initial estrogen withdrawal bleeding may occur, generally within 6 weeks after initiation of therapy. Thereafter, menstruation should cease. In clinical studies the peak response of LH to GnRH stimulation was reduced from a pubertal to a prepubertal response (< 15 mIU/ml) within 1 month.

Linear growth velocity, commonly pubertal in children with CPP, is reduced in most children within the first year of treatment to values of ≤ 5 to 6 cm/year. Children with CPP are frequently taller than their chronological age peers; height for chronological age approaches normal in most children during the second or third year of treatment. Skeletal maturation rate is usually abnormal in children with CPP; in most children, bone age velocity approaches normal during the first year of treatment. This results in a narrowing of the gap between bone age and chronological age, usually by the second or third year. Mean predicted adult height increases.

➤*Pharmacokinetics:*

Absorption/Distribution – Nafarelin is rapidly absorbed into systemic circulation after intranasal administration. Maximum serum concentrations are achieved between 10 and 45 minutes. In adults, following a single dose of 200 mcg base, the observed average peak concentration is 0.6 ng/ml, whereas following a single dose of 400 mcg base, the observed average peak concentration is 1.8 ng/ml. In children, following a single dose of 400 mcg base, the observed peak concentration is 2.2 ng/ml, whereas following a single 600 mcg dose the observed peak concentration is 6.6 ng/ml. Bioavailability from a 400 mcg dose averaged 2.8%. The average serum half-life following intranasal administration is approximately 3 hours in adults and 2.5 hours in children. About 80% is bound to plasma proteins.

Metabolism/Excretion – After SC use, 44% to 55% of dose was recovered in urine and 18.5% to 44.2% in feces. About 3% of dose appears unchanged in urine. Serum half-life of metabolites is about 85.5 hours. Activity of the six identified metabolites, nafarelin metabolism by nasal mucosa, and pharmacokinetics in hepatic and renal impairment have not been determined.

➤*Clinical trials:*

Endometriosis – In controlled clinical studies, nafarelin doses of 400 and 800 mcg/day for 6 months were comparable to danazol 800 mg/day in relieving the clinical symptoms of endometriosis (pelvic pain, dysmenorrhea and dyspareunia) and in reducing the size of endometrial implants as determined by laparoscopy.

Nafarelin 400 mcg/day induced amenorrhea in ≈ 65%, 80% and 90% of the patients after 60, 90 and 120 days, respectively. Most of the rest reported only light bleeding or spotting. In post-treatment months 1, 2 and 3, normal cycles resumed in 4%, 82% and 100%, respectively, of those who did not become pregnant.

At the end of treatment, 60% of patients who received 400 mcg/day were symptom free, 32% had mild symptoms, 7% had moderate symptoms and 1% had severe symptoms. Of the 60% of patients who had complete symptom relief, 17% had moderate symptoms 6 months after treatment was discontinued, 33% had mild symptoms, 50% remained symptom free and no patient had severe symptoms.

There is no evidence that nafarelin enhances or decreases pregnancy rates.

CPP – In clinical trials, breast development was arrested or regressed in 82% of girls, and genital development was arrested or regressed in 100% of boys. Because pubic hair growth is largely controlled by adrenal androgens (unaffected by nafarelin), its development was arrested or regressed only in 54% of girls and boys.

Reversal of nafarelin's suppressive effects occurs in all children with CPP, and consists of appearance or return of menses, return of pubertal gonadotropin and gonadal sex steroid levels, or advancement of secondary sexual development. Semen analysis was normal in the two ejaculated specimens obtained thus far from boys who have been taken off therapy to resume puberty. Fertility has not been documented by pregnancies and the effect of long-term use on fertility is not known.

Contraindications

Hypersensitivity to GnRH, GnRH-agonist analogs or any excipients in the product; undiagnosed abnormal vaginal bleeding; pregnancy and lactation (see Warnings).

Warnings

➤*Establish diagnosis of CPP:* Establish diagnosis of CPP before treatment is initiated. Suspect CPP if premature development of secondary sexual characteristics occurs at or before age 8 in girls and 9 in boys, and is accompanied by significant advancement of bone age or poor adult height prediction. Confirm by pubertal gonadal sex steroid levels and pubertal LH response to stimulation by native GnRH. In females, pelvic ultrasound usually reveals enlarged uterus and ovaries, the latter often with multiple cystic formations. Brain magnetic resonance imaging or CT-scanning can detect hypothalamic or pituitary tumors, or anatomical changes associated with increased intracranial pressure. Exclude other causes of sexual precocity, such as congenital adrenal hyperplasia, testotoxicosis, testicular tumors or other autonomous feminizing or masculinizing disorders by proper clinical hormonal and diagnostic imaging examinations.

Regular monitoring is needed to assess both patient response as well as compliance. This is particularly important during the first 6 to 8 weeks of treatment to assure that suppression of pituitary-gonadal function is rapid. Begin assessment of growth velocity and bone age velocity within 3 to 6 months of treatment initiation.

Some patients may not show suppression of pituitary-gonadal axis by clinical or biochemical parameters. This may be due to lack of compliance

NAFARELIN ACETATE

with recommended treatment regimen and may be rectified by recommending that dosing be done by caregivers. If compliance problems are excluded, reconsider possible gonadotropin independent sexual precocity and conduct appropriate examinations. If compliance problems are excluded and gonadotropin-independent sexual precocity is not present, may increase dose to 1800 mcg/day as 600 mcg 3 times a day.

➤*Hypersensitivity reactions:* Reactions have occurred in 0.2% of subjects or patients. Refer to Management of Acute Hypersensitivity Reactions.

➤*Carcinogenesis:* Carcinogenicity studies of nafarelin were conducted in rats (24 months) at doses up to 100 mcg/kg/day and mice (18 months) at doses up to 500 mcg/kg/day using IM doses (up to 110 times and 560 times the maximum recommended human intranasal dose, respectively). As seen with other GnRH agonists, nafarelin induced proliferative responses (hyperplasia or neoplasia) of endocrine organs. At 24 months, there was an increase in the incidence of pituitary tumors (adenoma/carcinoma) in high-dose female rats and a dose-related increase in male rats. Pancreatic islet cell adenomas increased in both sexes, as did benign testicular and ovarian tumors in treated groups. There were dose-related increases in benign adrenal medullary tumors in treated female rats and Harderian gland tumors in male mice. Pituitary adenomas increased in high-dose female mice. No metastases of these tumors were observed. Tumorigenicity in rodents is particularly sensitive to hormonal stimulation.

➤*Fertility impairment:* In reproduction studies in male and female rats, fertility suppression fully reversed when treatment was discontinued after continuous use for up to 6 months.

➤*Pregnancy: Category X.* IM nafarelin was administered to rats throughout gestation at 0.4, 1.6 and 6.4 mcg/kg/day (about 0.5, 2 and 7 times the maximum recommended human intranasal dose). An increase in major fetal abnormalities was observed in 4/80 fetuses at the highest dose. A similar repeat study at the same doses in rats, and studies in mice and rabbits at doses up to 600 mcg/kg/day and 0.18 mcg/kg/day, respectively, failed to demonstrate an increase in fetal abnormalities. In rats and rabbits, there was a dose-related increase in fetal mortality and a decrease in fetal weight with the highest dose. The effects on rat fetal mortality are expected consequences of the alterations in hormonal levels brought about by the drug.

Safe use in pregnancy is not clinically established. Before starting treatment, exclude pregnancy. When used regularly at the recommended dose, nafarelin usually inhibits ovulation and stops menstruation. Contraception is not assured, however, particularly if patients miss successive doses. Patients should use nonhormonal methods of contraception. Advise patients that if they miss successive doses, breakthrough bleeding or ovulation may occur with the potential for conception. They should see their physician if they believe they may be pregnant. If used during pregnancy or if a patient becomes pregnant during treatment, discontinue the drug and apprise patient of potential risk to the fetus.

➤*Lactation:* It is not known whether nafarelin is excreted in breast milk. The effects on lactation or the nursing infant are not determined, do not give to nursing mothers.

➤*Children:* Nafarelin is used in children for CPP.

Precautions

➤*Menstruation:* Since menstruation should stop with effective doses of nafarelin, the patient should notify her physician if regular menstruation persists. Patients missing successive doses of nafarelin may experience breakthrough bleeding.

➤*Bone density loss:* The induced hypoestrogenic state results in a small loss in bone density over the course of treatment, some of which may not be reversible. During one 6 month treatment period, this bone loss should not be important. In patients with major risk factors for decreased bone mineral content such as chronic alcohol or tobacco use, strong family history of osteoporosis, or chronic use of drugs that can reduce bone mass such as anticonvulsants or corticosteroids, nafarelin may pose an additional risk. Weigh risks and benefits carefully before nafarelin is instituted. Repeated courses of GnRH analogs are not advisable in patients with major risk factors for loss of bone mineral content (see Adverse Reactions).

➤*Intercurrent rhinitis:* Intercurrent rhinitis patients should consult their physician for the use of a topical nasal decongestant. If the use of a topical nasal decongestant is required during treatment with nafarelin, the decongestant must be used at least 2 hours after nafarelin dosing to decrease the possibility of reducing drug absorption.

➤*Retreatment:* Retreatment for endometriosis is not recommended since safety data beyond 6 months are not available.

➤*Ovarian cysts:* As with other drugs that stimulate the release of gonadotropins or that induce ovulation in adult women with endometriosis, ovarian cysts have occurred in the first 2 months of therapy. Many, but not all, of these events occurred in women with polycystic ovarian disease. These cystic enlargements may resolve spontaneously, generally by about 4 to 6 weeks of therapy, but in some cases may

require discontinuation of drug or surgical intervention. Relevance in children is unknown.

Drug Interactions

➤*Drug/Lab test interactions:* Administration of nafarelin in therapeutic doses results in suppression of the pituitary-gonadal system. Normal function is usually restored within 4 to 8 weeks after treatment is discontinued. Therefore, diagnostic tests of pituitary gonadotropic and gonadal functions conducted during treatment and up to 4 to 8 weeks after discontinuation of nafarelin therapy may be misleading.

Adverse Reactions

CPP – In clinical trials, 2.6% of patients reported symptoms suggestive of drug sensitivity, such as shortness of breath, chest pain, urticaria, rash and pruritus. In these patients treated for an average of 41 months and as long as 80 months (6.7 years), adverse events most frequently reported consisted largely of episodes occurring during the first 6 weeks of treatment as a result of the transient stimulatory action of nafarelin upon the pituitary-gonadal axis: Acne (10%); transient breast enlargement, vaginal bleeding (8%); emotional lability (6%); transient increase in pubic hair (5%); body odor (4%); seborrhea (3%). Hot flashes, common in adult women treated for endometriosis, occurred in only 3% of treated children and were transient. Other adverse events included: Rhinitis (5%); white or brownish vaginal discharge (3%).

In one male patient with concomitant congenital adrenal hyperplasia, and who had discontinued treatment 8 months previously to resume puberty, adrenal rest tumors were found in the left testis. Relationship to nafarelin is unlikely.

Regular examination of the pituitary gland of children during long-term nafarelin therapy as well as during the post-treatment period has occasionally revealed changes in the shape and size of the pituitary gland. These changes include asymmetry and enlargement of the pituitary gland, and a pituitary microadenoma has been suspected in a few children.

➤*Endometriosis:* As would be expected with a drug that lowers serum estradiol levels, the most frequent adverse reactions were related to hypoestrogenism. In controlled studies comparing nafarelin (400 mcg/day) and danazol (600 or 800 mg/day), adverse reactions most frequently reported and thought to be drug-related are listed in the following table.

Adverse Reactions of Nafarelin Acetate vs Danazol During Treatment for Endometriosis (≈ %)		
Adverse reaction	Nafarelin (n = 203)	Danazol (n = 147)
Hypoestrogenic		
Hot flashes	90	69
Libido decrease	22	7
Vaginal dryness	19	7
Headaches	19	21
Emotional lability	15	18
Insomnia	8	4
Androgenic		
Acne	13	20
Myalgia	10	23
Breast size reduced	10	16
Edema	8	23
Seborrhea	8	17
Weight gain	8	28
Hirsutism	2	6
Libido increased	1	6
Miscellaneous		
Nasal irritation	10	3
Depression	2	5
Weight loss	1	3

Other adverse reactions (< 1%): Paresthesia; palpitations; chloasma; eye pain; maculopapular rash; urticaria; asthenia; lactation; breast engorgement; arthralgia. In formal clinical trials, immediate hypersensitivity possibly or probably related to nafarelin occurred in 3 (0.2%) of 1509 patients or healthy subjects (see Warnings).

Bone density changes: After 6 months of nafarelin, vertebral trabecular bone density and total vertebral bone mass decreased by an average 8.7% and 4.3%, respectively, compared to pretreatment. There was partial post-treatment recovery of bone density; average trabecular bone density and total bone mass were 4.9% and 3.3% less than pretreatment, respectively. Total vertebral bone mass decreased by a mean of 5.9% at the end of treatment. Mean total vertebral bone mass 6 months after post-treatment was 1.4% below pretreatment levels. There was little, if any, decrease in mineral content in compact bone of the distal radius and second metacarpal. Use for > 6 months or in the presence of other known risk factors for decreased bone mineral content may cause additional bone loss. (See Precautions.)

NAFARELIN ACETATE

Lab test abnormalities –

Plasma enzymes: AST and ALT levels were more than twice the upper limit of normal in only one patient each. There was no other clinical or laboratory evidence of abnormal liver function, and levels returned to normal in both patients after treatment was stopped.

Lipids: At enrollment, 9% of the patients in the nafarelin 400 mcg/day group and 2% of the patients in the danazol group had total cholesterol values > 250 mg/dl. These patients also had cholesterol values > 250 mg/dl at the end of treatment.

Of patients whose pretreatment cholesterol values were < 250 mg/dl, 6% on nafarelin and 18% on danazol had post-treatment values > 250 mg/dl.

Mean pretreatment values for total cholesterol from all patients were 191.8 mg/dl with nafarelin and 193.1 mg/dl with danazol. After treatment, mean total cholesterol values were 204.5 mg/dl with nafarelin and 207.7 mg/dl with danazol.

Triglycerides were increased above the upper limit of 150 mg/dl in 12% of the patients who received nafarelin and in 7% of the patients who received danazol.

At the end of treatment, no nafarelin patients had abnormally low HDL cholesterol fractions (< 30 mg/dl) vs 43% of danazol patients. No nafarelin patients had abnormally high LDL cholesterol fractions (> 190 mg/dl) vs 15% of those on danazol. There was no increase in the LDL/HDL ratio in nafarelin patients, but there was an approximate twofold increase in the LDL/HDL ratio in danazol patients.

Other changes (10% to 15%): Nafarelin was associated with elevated plasma phosphorus and eosinophil counts, and decreased serum calcium and WBC counts. Danazol was associated with an increase in hematocrit and WBC.

Overdosage

There is no clinical evidence of adverse effects following overdose of GnRH analogs. Based on animal studies, nafarelin is not absorbed after oral administration.

Patient Information

An information pamphlet for patients is included with the product.

Patients with intercurrent rhinitis should consult their physician about use of a topical nasal decongestant. Do not use until at least 2 hours after nafarelin.

Avoid sneezing during or immediately after dosing; this may impair drug absorption.

➤*Endometriosis:* Notify physician if regular menstruation persists. Breakthrough bleeding or ovulation may occur if successive doses are missed. Use a nonhormonal method of contraception during treatment.

Do not use if pregnant or breastfeeding, or if undiagnosed abnormal vaginal bleeding or allergies to any of the ingredients exist.

➤*CPP:* Reversibility of nafarelin's suppressive effects has been demonstrated by appearance or return of menses, by return of pubertal gonadotropin and gonadal sex steroid levels, or by advancement of secondary sexual development. Semen analysis was normal in two ejaculated specimens obtained thus far from boys taken off therapy to resume puberty. Fertility has not been documented by pregnancies; the effect of long-term use on fertility is not known.

Adequately counsel patients and their caregivers to ensure full compliance; irregular or incomplete daily doses may result in stimulation of the pituitary-gonadal axis.

During the first month of treatment, some signs of puberty (eg, vaginal bleeding, breast enlargement) may occur. This is the expected initial effect. Such changes should resolve soon after the first month. If it does not resolve within the first 2 months, this may be due to lack of compliance or the presence of gonadotropin-independent sexual precocity. If both possibilities are definitively excluded, the dose may be increased to 1800 mcg/day as 600 mcg 3 times/day.

HISTRELIN ACETATE

Rx	Suprelin (Roberts)	Injection: 120 mcg/0.6 ml (200 mcg/ml peptide base)	In 30 day kit of single use 0.6 ml vials.[1]
		300 mcg/0.6 ml (500 mcg/ml peptide base)	In 30 day kit of single use 0.6 ml vials.[1]
		600 mcg/0.6 ml (1000 mcg/ml peptide base)	In 30 day kit of single use 0.6 ml vials.[1]

[1] With 0.9% sodium chloride and 10% mannitol. Preservative free. With 7 syringes and needles.

Indications

For control of the biochemical and clinical manifestations of central precocious puberty. Only patients with centrally mediated precocious puberty (either idiopathic or neurogenic, and occurring before age 8 in girls or 9.5 years in boys) should receive treatment. Patients must be able to maintain compliance with a *daily* regimen of injections.

Administration and Dosage

➤*Approved by the FDA:* December 1991.

➤*Central precocious puberty:* 10 mcg/kg given as a single, daily SC injection. If prepubertal levels of sex steroids or a prepubertal gonadotropin response to GnRH testing are not achieved within the first 3 months of treatment, reevaluate the patient. Doses > 10 mcg/kg/day have not been evaluated in clinical trials. Vary injection site daily.

➤*Storage/Stability:* Histrelin contains no preservative. Vials are to be used once. Any unused solution is to be discarded. Store refrigerated at 2° to 8°C (36° to 46°F) and protect from light. Remove vial from packaging only at time of use. Allow vial to reach room temperature before injecting contents.

Actions

➤*Pharmacology:* Histrelin, a gonadotropin-releasing hormone (GnRH or LHRH) agonist, is a potent inhibitor of gonadotropin secretion when administered daily in therapeutic doses. Histrelin contains a synthetic nonapeptide agonist of the naturally occurring gonadotropin-releasing hormone. The analog possesses a greater potency than the natural sequence hormone. Following an initial stimulatory phase, chronic SC administration desensitizes responsiveness of the pituitary gonadotropin which, in turn, causes a reduction in ovarian and testicular steroidogenesis.

Although animal studies have shown that *acute* administration of histrelin results in stimulation of the reproductive system, *chronic* administration in the rat delays sexual development, inhibits estrous cyclicity and pregnancy, reduces reproductive organ weight and inhibits ovarian and testicular steroidogenesis in a reversible fashion. In the rabbit, chronic administration resulted in decreased reproductive organ weights.

In human studies, chronic administration controls the secretion of pituitary gonadotropins resulting in decreased sex steroid levels and in the regression of secondary sexual characteristics in children with precocious puberty. In girls, menses cease, serum estradiol levels are decreased to prepubertal levels, linear growth velocities decrease, skel-etal maturation is slowed and adult height predictions increase. In boys, testicular steroidogenesis is inhibited and testicular volume is reduced.

Continuous administration to patients with central precocious puberty can be monitored by standard GnRH testing and by serial determinations of sex steroid levels. The decreases in LH, FSH and sex steroid levels are evident within 3 months of therapy initiation.

Contraindications

Hypersensitivity to any components of the product; pregnancy, lactation (see Warnings).

Warnings

➤*Inadequate control:* Noncompliance with drug regimen or inadequate dosing may result in inadequate control of the pubertal process. The consequences of poor control include the return of pubertal signs such as menses, breast development and testicular growth. The long-term consequences of inadequate control of gonadal steroid secretion are unknown, but may include a further compromise of adult stature.

➤*Hypersensitivity reactions:* Serious hypersensitivity reactions (angioedema, urticaria) have been reported following histrelin administration. Clinical manifestations may include: Cardiovascular collapse; hypotension; tachycardia; loss of consciousness; angioedema; bronchospasm; dyspnea; urticaria; flushing; pruritus. If any allergic reaction occurs, discontinue therapy. Serious acute hypersensitivity reactions may require emergency medical treatment. Refer to Management of Acute Hypersensitivity Reactions.

➤*Carcinogenesis:* Carcinogenicity studies were conducted in rats for 2 years at doses of 5, 25, or 150 mcg/kg/day (up to 15 times the human dose) and in mice for 18 months at doses of 20, 200, or 2000 mcg/kg/day (up to 200 times the human dose). As seen with other GnRH agonists, histrelin was associated with an increase in tumors of hormonally responsive tissues. There was a significant increase in pituitary adenomas in rats. There was an increase in pancreatic islet cell adenomas in treated female rats and a non-dose-related increase in testicular Leydig cell tumors (highest incidence in the low-dose group). In mice, there was a significant increase in mammary gland adenocarcinomas in all treated females. In addition, there were increases in stomach papillomas in male rats given high doses, and an increase in histiocytic sarcomas in female mice at the highest dose.

➤*Fertility impairment:* Fertility studies have been conducted in rats and monkeys given SC daily doses of histrelin up to 180 mcg/kg for

HISTRELIN ACETATE

6 months and full reversibility of fertility suppression was demonstrated.

➤*Pregnancy: Category X.* Histrelin is contraindicated in women who are or may become pregnant while receiving the drug. There was increased fetal size and mortality in rats and increased fetal mortality in rabbits after histrelin administration. Other responses included dystocia, a greater incidence of unilateral hydroureter and incomplete ossification in rat fetuses. When administered to rabbits on days 6 to 18 of pregnancy at doses of 20 to 80 mcg/kg/day (2 to 8 times the human dose), histrelin produced early termination of pregnancy and increased fetal death. In rats given histrelin on days 7 to 20 of pregnancy at doses of 1 to 15 mcg/kg/day (0.1 to 1.5 times the human dose) there was an increase in fetal resorptions. The effects on fetal mortality are expected consequences of the alterations in hormonal levels brought about by the drug. If this drug is inadvertently used during pregnancy or in the rare event that a patient becomes pregnant while taking this drug, apprise the patient of the potential hazard to the fetus.

➤*Lactation:* It is not known if this drug is excreted in breast milk. Because of the potential for serious adverse reactions in nursing infants, do not give to nursing women.

➤*Children:* Safety and efficacy in children < 2 years of age have not been established.

Precautions

➤*Monitoring:* Perform an initial pelvic ultrasound to exclude other conditions before treating with histrelin. Monitor the patient carefully after 3 months and every 6 to 12 months thereafter by serial clinical evaluations, repeated height measurements, bone age determinations (yearly), and serial GnRH testing to document that gonadotropin responsiveness of the pituitary remains prepubertal while on therapy. During the initial agonistic phase of treatment, the patient may demonstrate transient increases in breast tissue, moodiness, vaginal secretions or testicular volume. After this initial agonistic phase (usually 1 to 3 weeks), control of the biochemical and physical manifestations of puberty should remain as long as chronic therapy is in effect. Discontinue treatment when the onset of puberty is desired. Following the discontinuation of treatment, document the onset of normal puberty. In addition, monitor patients to assess menstrual cyclicity, reproductive function and ultimate adult height.

➤*Physical and endocrinologic evaluation:* Before treatment is instituted, perform a thorough physical and endocrinologic evaluation which includes:

1.) Height and weight, as baseline for serial monitoring.
2.) Hand and wrist x-ray for bone age determination, to document advanced skeletal age, and as baseline for serially monitoring predicted height.
3.) Total sex steroid level (estradiol or testosterone).
4.) Adrenal steroid level, to exclude congenital adrenal hyperplasia.
5.) Beta-human chorionic gonadotropin level, to rule out a chorionic gonadotropin-secreting tumor.
6.) GnRH stimulation test, to demonstrate activation of the hypothalamic-pituitary-gonadal (HPG) axis.
7.) Pelvic/adrenal/testicular ultrasound, to rule out a steroid-secreting tumor and to document gonadal size for serial monitoring.
8.) Computerized tomography of the head, to rule out previously undiagnosed intracranial tumor.

➤*HPG axis reactivation:* Studies in rats and monkeys have indicated that all of the known biochemical and antifertility effects of histrelin are reversible. Because children who have received histrelin have not been followed long enough to ensure reactivation of the HPG axis following long-term therapy, use histrelin only when the benefits to the patient outweigh the potential risks. In addition, advise the patient or guardian that hypogonadism may result if the HPG axis fails to reactivate after the drug is discontinued.

Adverse Reactions

At least one adverse experience was reported for 139 of the 183 (76%) children in clinical studies of central precocious puberty. Three of the 183 children (2%) stopped therapy due to a hypersensitivity reaction. The following reactions have occurred in patients treated for precocious puberty (n = 183) as well as various other indications (n = 196).

➤*Cardiovascular:* Vasodilation (35%); edema (2% to 3%); palpitations, tachycardia, epistaxis, hypertension, migraine headache, pallor (1% to 3%).

➤*CNS:* Headache (22%); mood changes, nervousness, dizziness, depression, libido changes, insomnia, anxiety (1% to 10%); paresthesia, cognitive changes, syncope, somnolence, lethargy, impaired consciousness, tremor, hyperkinesia, anxiety (1% to 3%); convulsions (increased frequency), hot flashes/flushes (2%); conduct disorder (1%).

➤*Dermatologic:* Reactions at medication site such as redness, swelling and itching (12% to 45%); acne, rash (3% to 10%); sweating (1% to 10%); urticaria (4%); keratoderma, pruritus, pain, dyschromia, alopecia (1% to 3%); erythema (1%).

➤*Endocrine:* Vaginal dryness (12%); leukorrhea (2% to 6%); metrorrhagia, breast pain/edema (1% to 10%); breast discharge, decreased breast size, tenderness of female genitalia (2% to 3%); goiter, hyperlipidemia, anemia, glycosuria (1%).

➤*GI:* GI/abdominal pain, nausea, vomiting, diarrhea, flatulence, decreased appetite, dyspepsia (2% to 12%); GI cramps/distress, constipation, decreased appetite, thirst, gastritis (1% to 3%).

➤*GU:* Vaginal bleeding (usually only one episode within 1 to 3 weeks of starting therapy lasting several days) (22%); irritation/odor/pruritus/infections/pain/hypertrophy of the female genitalia, vaginitis, dysmenorrhea (1% to 10%); dyspareunia, polyuria, dysuria, urinary frequency, incontinence, hematuria, nocturia (1% to 3%).

➤*Hypersensitivity:* Acute generalized hypersensitivity reactions (angioedema, urticaria) have occurred (see Warnings).

➤*Musculoskeletal:* Arthralgia, joint stiffness, muscle cramp (3% to 10%); muscle stiffness, myalgia (2% to 3%); pain, hypotonia (1%).

➤*Respiratory:* Upper respiratory tract infection, pharyngitis, respiratory congestion, cough (1% to 10%); asthma, breathing disorder, rhinorrhea, bronchitis, sinusitis (2% to 3%); hyperventilation (1% to 3%).

➤*Special senses:* Visual disturbances (2% to 6%); ear congestion (2% to 3%); abnormal pupillary function, otalgia, hearing loss, polyopia, photophobia (1% to 3%).

➤*Miscellaneous:* Pyrexia (3% to 14%); various body pains, weight gain, fatigue, viral infection (1% to 10%); chills, malaise, purpura (1% to 3%).

Overdosage

Histrelin up to 200 mcg/kg (rats, rabbits) or 2000 mcg/kg (mice) resulted in no systemic toxicity. This represents 20 to 200 times the maximal recommended human dose of 10 mcg/kg/day.

Patient Information

Patient information is provided in each kit.

Prior to therapy, inform patients and their families of the importance of complying with the schedule of single, *daily* injections, given at approximately the same time each day. If injections are not given daily, the pubertal process may be reactivated. Histrelin contains no preservative. Inform patients that vials are to be used once and any unused solution is to be discarded. Allow medication to reach room temperature before injecting. Rotate daily injections through different body sites (upper arms, thighs, abdomen).

Make patients aware of the required monitoring of their condition and of the potential risks of therapy. Within the first month of therapy, girls being treated with histrelin may experience a light menstrual flow. This menstrual flow is common and likely is related to the lower estrogen levels brought about by treatment, and the withdrawal of estrogen support from the endometrium.

Irritation, redness or swelling at the injection sites may occur. If these reactions are severe or do not go away, notify the physician.

Advise the patients and their families to discontinue the drug and seek medical attention at the first sign of skin rash, urticaria, rapid heartbeat, difficulty in swallowing and breathing, or any swelling which may suggest angioedema (see Warnings).

GANIRELIX ACETATE

Rx **Antagon** (Organon Inc.) | **Injection:** 250 mcg/0.5 ml | In 1 ml prefilled, disposable syringes. In 1s, 5s, and 50s.

Indications

►*Infertility treatment:* For the inhibition of premature luteinizing hormone (LH) surges in women undergoing controlled ovarian hyperstimulation.

Administration and Dosage

►*Approved by the FDA:* July 29, 1999.

After initiating follicle-stimulating hormone (FSH) therapy on day 2 or 3 of the cycle, ganirelix 250 mcg may be administered SC once daily during the early-to-mid follicular phase. By taking advantage of endogenous pituitary FSH secretion, the requirement for exogenously administered FSH may be reduced. Continue treatment with ganirelix daily until the day of chorionic gonadotropin (hCG) administration. When a sufficient number of follicles of adequate size are present, as assessed by ultrasound, final maturation of follicles is induced by administering hCG. Withhold the administration of hCG in cases where the ovaries are abnormally enlarged on the last day of FSH therapy to reduce the chance of developing ovarian hyperstimulation syndrome (OHSS).

►*Directions for use:* Ganirelix is intended for SC administration only. The most convenient sites for SC injection are in the abdomen around the navel or upper thigh. Swab the injection site with a disinfectant to remove any surface bacteria. Clean ≈ 2 inches around the point where the needle will be inserted and let the disinfectant dry for ≥ 1 minute before proceeding. Pinch up a large area of skin between the finger and thumb. Vary the injection site a little with each injection. Insert the needle at the base of the pinched-up skin at an angle of 45° to 90° to the skin surface. When the needle is correctly positioned, it will be difficult to draw back on the plunger. If any blood is drawn into the syringe, the needle tip has penetrated a vein or artery. If this happens, withdraw the needle slightly and reposition the needle without removing it from the skin. Alternatively, remove the needle and use a new, sterile, prefilled syringe. Cover the injection site with a swab containing disinfectant and apply pressure; the site should stop bleeding within 1 or 2 minutes. Once the needle is correctly placed, depress the plunger slowly and steadily, so the solution is correctly injected and the skin is not damaged. Pull the syringe out quickly and apply pressure to the site with a swab containing disinfectant. Use the sterile, prefilled syringe only once and dispose of it properly.

►*Storage / Stability:* Store at 25°C (77°F). Protect from light.

Actions

►*Pharmacology:* Ganirelix is a synthetic decapeptide with high antagonistic activity against naturally occurring gonadotropin-releasing hormone (GnRH). Ganirelix is derived from native GnRH with substitutions of amino acids at positions 1, 2, 3, 6, 8, and 10.

The pulsatile release of GnRH stimulates the synthesis and secretion of LH and FSH. Ganirelix acts by competitively blocking the GnRH receptors on the pituitary gonadotroph and subsequent transduction pathway. It induces a rapid, reversible suppression of gonadotropin secretion. The suppression of pituitary LH secretion by ganirelix is more pronounced than that of FSH. An initial release of endogenous gonadotropins has not been detected with ganirelix, which is consistent with an antagonist effect. Upon discontinuation of ganirelix, pituitary LH and FSH levels are fully recovered within 48 hours.

►*Pharmacokinetics:* The pharmacokinetic parameters of single and multiple injections of ganirelix in healthy adult females are summarized in the following table. Steady-state serum concentrations are reached after 3 days of treatment. The pharmacokinetics of ganirelix are dose-proportional in the dose range of 125 to 500 mcg.

Mean Pharmacokinetic Parameters of Ganirelix	
Absorption	
Mean absolute bioavailability	91.1%[1]
C_{max}	14.8 ng/ml[1], 11.2 ng/ml[2]
T_{max}	1.1[1,2]
Distribution	
Vd	43.7 L[3], 76.5 L[2]
Protein binding	81.9%
Metabolism	
Metabolites	1 to 4 peptide and 1 to 6 peptide
Excretion	
Site	feces (75.1%)[4,5], urine (22.1%)[4,6]
Elimination t½	12.8 hr[1], 16.2 hr[2]
Clearance	2.4 L/hr[3], 3.3[2]

[1] Based on single-dose administration of 250 mcg SC.
[2] Based on multiple-dose administration of 250 mcg daily SC x 7 days.
[3] Based on single-dose administration of 250 mcg IV.
[4] Recovered over 288 hours following single-dose administration of 1 mg IV.
[5] Fecal excretion plateaus 192 hours after dosing.
[6] Urinary excretion is complete in 24 hours.

Contraindications

Hypersensitivity to ganirelix, any of its components, GnRH, or any other GnRH analog; known or suspected pregnancy (see Warnings).

Warnings

►*Latex allergy:* The packaging of this product contains natural rubber latex, which may cause allergic reactions.

►*Hypersensitivity reactions:* Caution is advised in patients with hypersensitivity to GnRH. Carefully monitor these patients after the first injection. Refer to the Management of Acute Hypersensitivity Reactions. Anaphylactic reactions or ganirelix antibody formation have not been reported in clinical trials.

►*Pregnancy: Category X.* Ganirelix is contraindicated in pregnant women. When administered from day 7 to near term to pregnant rats and rabbits at doses ≤ 10 and 30 mcg/day (≈ 0.4 to 3.2 times the human dose based on body surface area), ganirelix increased the incidence of litter resorption. There was no increase in fetal abnormalities.

The effects on fetal resorption are logical consequences of the alteration in hormonal levels brought about by the antigonadotrophic properties of this drug and could result in fetal loss in humans. Therefore, do not use this drug in pregnant women.

Ganirelix should be prescribed by physicians who are experienced in infertility treatment. Before starting treatment with ganirelix, exclude pregnancy. Safe use of ganirelix during pregnancy has not been established.

Congenital anomalies – Ongoing clinical follow-up studies of 283 newborns of women administered ganirelix were reviewed. There were 3 neonates with major congenital anomalies and 18 neonates with minor congenital anomalies. The major congenital anomalies were the following: Hydrocephalus/Meningocele, omphalocele, and Beckwith-Wiedemann syndrome. The minor congenital anomalies were the following: Nevus, skin tags, sacral sinus, hemangioma, torticollis/asymmetric skull, talipes, supernumerary digit finger, hip subluxation, torticollis/high palate, occiput/abnormal hand crease, hernia unbilicalis, hernia inguinalis, hydrocele, undescended testes, and hydronephrosis. The causal relationship between these congenital anomalies and ganirelix is unknown. Multiple factors, genetic, and others (including, but not limited to intracystoplasmatic sperm injection [ICSI], in vitro fertilization [IVF], gonadotropins, progesterone) may confound assisted reproductive technology (ART) procedures.

►*Lactation:* It is not known whether this drug is excreted in breast milk. Ganirelix should not be used by nursing women.

Drug Interactions

►*Gonadotropins:* Because ganirelix can suppress the secretion of pituitary gonadotropins, dose adjustments of exogenous gonadotropins may be necessary when used during controlled ovarian hyperstimulation.

Adverse Reactions

In clinical studies, treatment duration ranged from 1 to 14 days. The following table represents adverse events from the first day of ganirelix administration until confirmation of pregnancy by ultrasound at an incidence of ≥ 1% in ganirelix-treated subjects without regard to causality.

Ganirelix Adverse Reactions (≥ 1%)	
Adverse reaction	Ganirelix (n = 794) (%)
Abdominal pain (gynecological)	4.8
Death, fetal	3.7
Headache	3
Ovarian hyperstimulation syndrome	2.4
Vaginal bleeding	1.8
Injection site reaction	1.1
Nausea	1.1
Abdominal pain (GI)	1

►*Lab test abnormalities:* A neutrophil count ≥ 8.3 (x 10^9/L) was noted in 11.9% (≤ 16.8 x 10^9/L) of all subjects in the clinical trials. In addition, downward shifts within the ganirelix group were observed for hematocrit and total bilirubin. The clinical significance of these findings was not determined.

Patient Information

Prior to therapy with ganirelix, inform patients of the duration of treatment and monitoring procedures that will be required. Discuss the risk of possible adverse reactions (see Adverse Reactions). Do not prescribe ganirelix if the patient is pregnant.

CETRORELIX ACETATE

Rx	**Cetrotide** (ASTA Medica)	**Injection:** 0.25 mg	In trays containing 1 vial of 0.26 to 0.27 mg cetrorelix acetate, 1 ml syringe of Sterile Water for Injection, a 20-gauge needle, a 27-gauge needle, and alcohol swabs. In 1s and 7s.
		3 mg	In trays containing 1 vial of 3.12 to 3.24 mg cetrorelix acetate, a 3 ml syringe of Sterile Water for Injection, a 20-gauge needle, a 27-gauge needle, and alcohol swabs. In 1s.

Indications

➤*Infertility treatment:* For the inhibition of premature luteinizing hormone (LH) surges in women undergoing controlled ovarian stimulation.

Administration and Dosage

➤*Approved by the FDA:* August 11, 2000.

Ovarian stimulation therapy with gonadotropins (follicle stimulating hormone [FSH], human menopausal gonadotropin [hMG]) is started on cycle day 2 or 3 and may be administered SC either once daily (0.25 mg dose) or once (3 mg dose) during early-to-mid follicular phase. Adjust the dose according to individual response.

When assessment by ultrasound shows a sufficient number of follicles of adequate size, human chorionic gonadotropin (hCG) is administered to induce ovulation and final maturation of the oocytes. Do not administer hCG if the ovaries show an excessive response to the treatment with gonadotropins to reduce the chance of developing ovarian hyperstimulation syndrome (OHSS).

➤*Single-dose regimen:* 3 mg of cetrorelix acetate is administered when the serum estradiol level is indicative of an appropriate stimulation response, usually on stimulation day 7 (range, day 5 to 9). If hCG has not been administered within 4 days after injection of 3 mg cetrorelix, administer cetrorelix 0.25 mg once daily until the day of hCG administration.

➤*Multiple-dose regimen:* 0.25 mg of cetrorelix is administered on either stimulation day 5 (morning or evening) or day 6 (morning) and continued daily until the day of hCG administration

➤*Directions for use:* Cetrorelix is intended for SC administration only.
1.) Wash hands thoroughly with soap and water.
2.) Flip off the plastic cover of the vial and wipe the aluminum ring and the rubber stopper with an alcohol swab.
3.) Put the injection needle with the yellow mark (20 gauge) on the pre-filled syringe.
4.) Push the needle through the rubber stopper of the vial and slowly inject the solvent into the vial.
5.) Leaving the syringe on the vial, gently agitate the vial until the solution is clear and without residue. Avoid forming bubbles.
6.) Draw the total contents of the vial into the syringe. If necessary, invert the vial and pull back the needle as far as needed to withdraw the entire contents of the vial.
7.) Replace the needle with the yellow mark by the injection needle with the grey mark (27 gauge).
8.) Invert the syringe and push the plunger until all air bubbles have expelled.
9.) Choose an injection site at the lower abdominal wall, preferably around the navel. If you are on a multiple dose (0.25 mg) regimen, choose a different injection site each day to minimize local irritation. Use the second alcohol swab to clean the skin at the injection site. Gently pinch up the skin surrounding the site of injection.
10.) Insert the needle completely into the skin at an angle of ≈ 45°.
11.) Once you have inserted the needle completely, release your grasp of the skin.
12.) Gently pull back the plunger of the syringe to check the correct positioning of the needle. If no blood appears, inject the entire solution by slowly pushing the plunger. Thereafter, withdraw the needle and gently press the alcohol swab on the injection site. If blood appears, withdraw the needle with the syringe and gently press the alcohol swab on the injection site. Discard the syringe and the drug vial. Use a new pack and repeat the procedure.
13.) Use the syringe and needles only once. Dispose of the syringe and needles properly after use. If available, use a medical waste container for disposal.

➤*Storage/Stability:* Store 3 mg cetrorelix at 25°C (77°F). Store 0.25 mg cetrorelix under refrigeration at 2° to 8°C (36° to 46°F).

Actions

➤*Pharmacology:* Cetrorelix acetate is a synthetic decapeptide with gonadotropin-releasing hormone (GnRH) antagonistic activity. Cetrorelix acetate is an analog of native GnRH with substitutions of amino acids at positions 1, 2, 3, 6, and 10.

GnRH induces the production and release of LH and FSH from the gonadotrophic cells of the anterior pituitary. Because of a positive estradiol (E_2) feedback at midcycle, GnRH liberation is enhanced, resulting in a LH-surge. This LH-surge induces the ovulation of the dominant follicle, resumption of oocyte meiosis, and subsequently luteinization as indicated by rising progesterone levels.

Cetrorelix competes with natural GnRH for binding to membrane receptors on pituitary cells and thus controls the release of LH and FSH in a dose-dependent manner. The onset of LH suppression is ≈ 1 hour with the 3 mg dose and 2 hours with the 0.25 mg dose. This suppression is maintained by continuous treatment and there is a more pronounced effect on LH than on FSH. An initial release of endogenous gonadotropins has not been detected with cetrorelix, which is consistent with an antagonist effect.

The effects of cetrorelix on LH and FSH are reversible after discontinuation of treatment. In women, it delays the LH surge, and consequently ovulation, in a dose-dependent fashion. FSH levels are not affected at the doses used during controlled ovarian stimulation. Following a single 3 mg dose, duration of action of ≥ 4 days has been established. A dose of cetrorelix 0.25 mg every 24 hours has been shown to maintain the effect.

➤*Pharmacokinetics:*

Absorption – Cetrorelix is rapidly absorbed following SC injection, maximal plasma concentrations being achieved ≈ 1 to 2 hours after administration. The mean absolute bioavailability of cetrorelix following SC administration to healthy female subjects is 85%.

Distribution – The volume of distribution of cetrorelix following a single IV dose of 3 mg is ≈ 1 L/kg. In vitro protein binding to human plasma is 86%.

Cetrorelix concentrations in follicular fluid and plasma were similar on the day of oocyte pick-up in patients undergoing controlled ovarian stimulation. Following SC administration of cetrorelix 0.25 and 3 mg, plasma concentrations of cetrorelix were below or in the range of the lower limit of quantitation on the day of oocyte pick up and embryo transfer.

Metabolism – After SC administration of 10 mg cetrorelix to males and females, cetrorelix and small amounts of (1-9), (1-7), (1-6), and (1-4) peptides were found in bile samples over 24 hours.

In vitro studies indicate cetrorelix was stable against phase I and phase II metabolism. Cetrorelix was transformed by peptidases, and the (1-4) peptide was the predominant metabolite.

Excretion – Following SC administration of 10 mg cetrorelix to males and females, only unchanged cetrorelix was detected in urine. In 24 hours, cetrorelix and small amounts of the (1-9), (1-7), (1-6), and (1-4) peptides were found in bile samples. Two to four percent of the dose was eliminated in the urine as unchanged cetrorelix, while 5% to 10% was eliminated as cetrorelix and the 4 metabolites in bile. Therefore, only 7% to 14% of the total dose was recovered as unchanged cetrorelix and metabolites in urine and bile ≤ 24 hours. The remaining portion of the dose may not have been recovered because bile and urine were not collected for a longer period of time. The pharmacokinetic parameters of single and multiple doses of cetrorelix acetate in adult healthy female subjects are summarized in the following table.

Pharmacokinetic Parameters of Cetrorelix Following Single and Multiple (daily for 14 days) SC Administration			
	Single dose 3 mg (n = 12)	Single dose 0.25 mg (n = 12)	Multiple dose 0.25 mg (n = 12)
T_{max}[1] (hr)	1.5 (0.5 to 2)	1 (0.5 to 1.5)	1 (0.5 to 2)
$t_{1/2}$[1] (hr)	62.8 (38.2 to 108)	5 (2.4 to 48.8)	20.6 (4.1 to 179.3)
C_{max} (ng/ml)	28.5 (22.5 to 36.2)	4.97 (4.17 to 5.92)	6.42 (5.18 to 7.96)
AUC (ng•hr/ml)	536 (451 to 636)	31.4 (23.4 to 42)	44.5 (36.7 to 54.2)
CL[2] (ml/min•kg)	1.28[3]		
Vz[2] (L/kg)	1.16[3]		

[1] Median (min-max)
[2] Arithmetic mean
[3] Based on IV administration (n = 6)

Contraindications

Hypersensitivity to cetrorelix acetate, extrinsic peptide hormones, mannitol, GnRH, or any other GnRH analogs; known or suspected pregnancy and lactation (see Warnings).

Warnings

➤*Congenital anomalies:* Clinical follow-up studies of 316 newborns of women administered cetrorelix were reviewed. One infant from a set of twin neonates was found to have anencephaly at birth and died after 4 days. The other twin was healthy. Developmental findings from ongoing baby follow-ups included a child with a ventricular septal defect and another child with bilateral congenital glaucoma.

CETRORELIX ACETATE

Four pregnancies that resulted in therapeutic abortion in Phase 2 and Phase 3 controlled ovarian stimulation studies had major anomalies (diaphragmatic hernia, trisomy 21, Klinefelter syndrome, polymalformation, and trisomy 18). In 3 of these 4 cases, intracytoplasmic sperm injection (ICSI) was the fertilization method employed; in the fourth case, in vitro fertilization (IVF) was the method employed.

The minor congenital anomalies reported include the following: Supernumerary nipple, bilateral strabismus, imperforate hymen, congenital nevi, hemangiomata, and QT syndrome.

The causal relationship between the reported anomalies and cetrorelix is unknown. Multiple factors, genetic and others (including, but not limited to ICSI, IVF, gonadotropins, and progesterone) make causal attribution difficult to study.

➤*Hypersensitivity reactions:* Caution is advised in patients with hypersensitivity to GnRH. Carefully monitor these patients after the first injection. A severe anaphylactic reaction associated with cough, rash, and hypotension was observed in 1 patient after 7 months of treatment with cetrorelix (10 mg/day) in a study for an indication unrelated to infertility.

➤*Elderly:* Cetrorelix is not intended to be used in subjects ≥ 65 years of age.

➤*Pregnancy: Category X.* Cetrorelix is contraindicated in pregnant women. When administered to rats for the first 7 days of pregnancy, cetrorelix acetate did not affect the development of the implanted conceptus at doses ≤ 38 mcg/kg (≈ 1 times the recommended human therapeutic dose based on body surface area). However, a dose of 139 mcg/kg (≈ 4 times the human dose) resulted in a resorption rate and a postimplantation loss of 100%.

When administered from day 6 to near term to pregnant rats and rabbits, very early resorption and total implantation losses were seen in rats at doses from 4.6 mcg/kg (0.2 times the human dose) and in rabbits at doses from 6.8 mcg/kg (0.4 times the human dose). In animals that maintained their pregnancy, there was no increase in the incidence of fetal abnormalities.

The fetal resorption observed in animals is a logical consequence of the alteration in hormonal levels effected by the antigonadotrophic properties of cetrorelix, which could result in fetal loss in humans as well. Therefore, do not use this drug in pregnant women.

Cetrorelix should be prescribed by physicians who are experienced in fertility treatment. Before starting treatment with cetrorelix, pregnancy must be excluded.

➤*Lactation:* It is not known whether cetrorelix is excreted in human milk. Because many drugs are excreted in human milk, and because the effects of cetrorelix on lactation or the breastfed child have not been determined, do not use cetrorelix in nursing mothers.

Precautions

➤*Monitoring:* After the exclusion of preexisting conditions, enzyme elevations (ALT, AST, GGT, alkaline phosphatase) were found in 1% to 2% of patients receiving cetrorelix during controlled ovarian stimulation. The elevations ranged ≤ 3 times the upper limit of normal. The clinical significance of these findings was not determined.

During stimulation with human menopausal gonadotropin, cetrorelix had no notable effects on hormone levels aside from inhibition of LH surges.

Adverse Reactions

The safety of cetrorelix acetate for injection in 949 patients undergoing controlled ovarian stimulation (COS) in clinical studies was evaluated. Women were between 19 and 40 years of age (mean, 32 years of age). Ninety-four percent of them were Caucasian. Cetrorelix is given in doses ranging from 0.1 to 5 mg as either a single or multiple dose.

The following table shows systemic adverse events from the beginning of cetrorelix treatment until confirmation of pregnancy by ultrasound at an incidence ≥ 1% in cetrorelix-treated subjects undergoing COS.

Cetrorelix Adverse Events (≥ 1%)	
Adverse reaction	Cetrorelix (n = 949) (%)
Ovarian hyperstimulation syndrome[1]	3.5
Nausea	1.3
Headache	1.1

[1] Moderate or severe intensity, or WHO Grade II or III, respectively.

Local site reactions (eg, redness, erythema, bruising, itching, swelling, pruritus) were reported. Usually, they were of a transient nature, of mild intensity, and short duration.

Two stillbirths were reported in Phase 3 studies of cetrorelix.

Overdosage

There have been no reports of overdosage with cetrorelix 0.25 mg or 3 mg in humans. Single doses ≤ 120 mg cetrorelix have been well tolerated in patients treated for other indications without signs of overdosage.

Patient Information

Prior to therapy with cetrorelix, inform patients of the duration of treatment and monitoring procedures that will be required. Discuss the risk of possible adverse reactions.

Do not prescribe cetrorelix if a patient is pregnant.

If cetrorelix is prescribed to patients for self-administration, information for proper use is given in the patient leaflet.

ABARELIX

Rx	**Plenaxis** (Praecis[1])	**Powder for Injection:** 113 mg	Preservative-free. In kits.[2]

[1] Praecis Pharmaceuticals Incorporated, 830 Winter Street, Waltham, MA 02451-1420; (877) PRAECIS, (877) 772-3247.

[2] Kit contains a single-use 10 mL diluent vial of 0.9% sodium chloride injection, one 3 mL syringe with an 18-gauge 1½ inch needle, and one 22-gauge 1½ inch *Safety Glide* injection needle.

WARNING

Immediate-onset systemic allergic reactions, some resulting in hypotension and syncope, have occurred after administration of abarelix. These immediate-onset reactions have been reported to occur following any administration of abarelix, including after the initial dose. The cumulative risk of such a reaction increases with the duration of treatment (see Warnings). Following each injection of abarelix, observe patients for at least 30 minutes in the office and in the event of an allergic reaction, manage appropriately.

• Only physicians who have committed to the *Plenaxis* PLUS Program (*Plenaxis* User Safety Program), based on their attestation of qualifications and acceptance of prescribing responsibilities, may prescribe abarelix (see Administration and Dosage).

• Abarelix is indicated for the palliative treatment of men with advanced symptomatic prostate cancer, in whom luteinizing hormone release hormone (LHRH) agonist therapy is not appropriate and who refuse surgical castration, and have 1 or more of the following: 1) Risk of neurological compromise because of metastases, 2) ureteral or bladder outlet obstruction because of local encroachment or metastatic disease, or 3) severe bone pain from skeletal metastases persisting on narcotic analgesia.

• The effectiveness of abarelix in suppressing serum testosterone to castrate levels decreases with continued dosing in some patients. Effectiveness beyond 12 months has not been established. Treatment failure can be detected by measuring serum total testosterone concentrations just prior to administration on day 29 and every 8 weeks thereafter (see Warnings).

Indications

➤*Prostate cancer:* For the palliative treatment of men with advanced symptomatic prostate cancer in whom LHRH agonist therapy is not appropriate, who refuse surgical castration, and have 1 or more of the following: 1) Risk of neurological compromise because of metastases, 2) ureteral or bladder outlet obstruction caused by local encroachment or metastatic disease, or 3) severe bone pain from skeletal metastases persisting on narcotic analgesia.

Administration and Dosage

➤*Approved by the FDA:* November 25, 2003.

For safety reasons, abarelix is approved with marketing restrictions. Abarelix will be provided to physicians enrolled in the *Plenaxis* PLUS Program. To enroll in the abarelix prescribing program, call (866) PLENAXIS (866-753-6294) or visit http://www.plenaxisplus.com.

➤*Dose:* The recommended dose of abarelix is 100 mg IM to the buttock on days 1, 15, 29 (week 4), and every 4 weeks thereafter. Treatment failure can be detected by measuring serum testosterone concentrations just prior to abarelix administration, beginning on day 29 and every 8 weeks thereafter.

➤*Preparation for administration:* Reconstitution of 1 vial of abarelix will provide a 100 mg (50 mg/mL) dose as a single IM injection. Abarelix does not contain a preservative; administer within 1 hour following reconstitution.

1.) Prior to reconstitution, gently shake the vial of abarelix for injectable suspension. Hold the vial at a 45 degree angle and tap lightly on the table to break up any caking. Withdraw 2.2 mL of 0.9% sodium chloride injection using the enclosed 18-gauge 1½ inch needle and a 3 mL syringe. Discard the remaining diluent.

Gonadotropin-Releasing Hormone Antagonists

ABARELIX

2.) Keeping the vial upright, insert the needle all the way into the vial and inject the diluent quickly. Before withdrawing the needle, remove 2.2 mL of air. Shake immediately.

3.) Shake for approximately 15 seconds. Allow the vial to stand for approximately 2 minutes. Tap the vial to reduce foaming and swirl the vial occasionally. Again shake for approximately 15 seconds. Allow the vial to stand for approximately 2 minutes. Tap the vial to reduce foaming and swirl the vial occasionally.

4.) Do not reinject the air into the vial. Locate a second injection spot on the stopper, and then insert the 18-gauge needle. Invert the vial and draw up some of the suspension into the syringe, without removing the needle from the vial, reinject it at any remaining solids in the vial. Repeat the process until all solids are dispersed. Swirl the vial before withdrawal and withdraw the entire contents (at least 2 mL) by positioning the needle at a 45-degree angle.

5.) Pull the plunger back to recover the residual suspension in the 18-gauge 1½ inch needle. Exchange the 18-gauge 1½ inch needle with the enclosed 22-gauge 1½ inch *Safety Glide* injection needle.

6.) Insert the needle at the desired injection site and pull the plunger back to check for backflow of blood. If blood flows into the syringe, do not inject at this site. Select another injection site. Deliver the entire reconstituted suspension IM immediately. Observe the patient after injection for 30 minutes for any sign of an allergic-type response.

➤*Storage/Stability:* Store at 25°C (77°F); excursions permitted to 15° to 30°C (59° to 86°F). Abarelix does not contain a preservative; administer within 1 hour following reconstitution.

Actions

➤*Pharmacology:* Abarelix is a synthetic decapeptide with potent antagonistic activity against naturally occurring gonadotropin releasing-hormone (GnRH). Abarelix inhibits gonadotropin and related androgen production by directly and competitively blocking GnRH receptors in the pituitary. Abarelix exerts its pharmacological action by directly suppressing luteinizing hormone (LH) and follicle stimulating hormone (FSH) secretion and thereby reducing the secretion of testosterone by the testes. Because of the direct inhibition of the secretion of LH by abarelix, there is no initial increase in serum testosterone concentrations.

➤*Pharmacokinetics:*

Absorption – A single 100 mg IM dose of abarelix was given to 14 healthy male volunteers 52 to 75 years of age, with body weight of 61.6 to 110.5 kg. The pharmacokinetic information is provided below.

Abarelix Mean Pharmacokinetic Parameters					
Single dose (n = 14)	C_{max} (ng/mL)	T_{max} (days)	$AUC_{0-\infty}$ (ng·day/mL)	CL/F (L/day)	$t_{1/2}$ (days)
100 mg IM	43.4	3	500	208	13.2

Following 100 mg IM administration, abarelix is absorbed slowly with a mean peak concentration of 43.4 ng/mL observed approximately 3 days after the injection.

Distribution – The apparent volume of distribution during the terminal phase determined after IM administration of abarelix was about 4040 L, implying that abarelix probably distributes extensively within the body. Abarelix is highly bound to plasma proteins (96% to 99%).

Metabolism – In vitro hepatocyte (rat, monkey, human) studies and in vivo studies in rats and monkeys showed that the major metabolites of abarelix were formed via hydrolysis of peptide bonds. No significant oxidative or conjugated metabolites of abarelix were found either in vitro or in vivo. There is no evidence of cytochrome P450 involvement in the metabolism of abarelix.

Excretion – In humans, approximately 13% of unchanged abarelix was recovered in urine after a 15 mcg/kg IM injection; there were no detectable metabolites in urine. Renal clearance of abarelix was 14.4 L/day (or 10 mL/min) after administration of 100 mg abarelix.

Contraindications

Known hypersensitivity to any of the components in the abarelix injectable suspension.

Abarelix is not indicated in women or pediatric patients. In addition, abarelix may cause fetal harm if administered to a pregnant woman.

Warnings

➤*QT prolongation:* In a single, active-controlled clinical study comparing abarelix to LHRH agonist plus nonsteroidal antiandrogen, periodic electrocardiograms were performed. Both therapies prolonged the mean Fridericia-corrected QT interval by more than 10 msec from baseline. In approximately 20% of patients in both groups, there were either changes from baseline QTc of more than 30 msec, or end-of-treatment QTc values exceeding 450 msec. Similar results were observed in 2 other phase 3 studies with abarelix and the active-control treatments. It is unclear whether these changes were directly related to study drugs, to androgen deprivation therapy, or to other variables.

Because abarelix may prolong the QT interval, carefully consider whether the risks of abarelix outweigh the benefits in patients with baseline QTc values greater than 450 msec (eg, congenital QT prolongation) and in patients taking Class IA (eg, quinidine, procainamide) or Class III (eg, amiodarone, sotalol) antiarrhythmic medications.

➤*Decrease in effectiveness:* A decrease in overall effectiveness with increased duration of treatment as measured by failure to maintain suppression of serum testosterone below 50 ng/dL, was noted. Treatment failure can be detected by measuring serum total testosterone concentrations just prior to administration on day 29 after the initial dose and every 8 weeks thereafter. The decrease in overall effectiveness of abarelix with increased duration of treatment is greater in patients who weighed more than 102 kg (225 lbs). Strict monitoring of serum testosterone in these patients is warranted.

➤*Hypersensitivity reactions:* Immediate-onset systemic allergic reactions have occurred (see Black Box Warning). In the clinical trial of patients with advanced, symptomatic prostate cancer, 3 of 81 (3.7%) patients experienced an immediate-onset systemic allergic reaction within minutes of receiving abarelix. The allergic reactions were urticaria (day 15), urticaria and pruritus (day 29), and hypotension and syncope (day 141). Monitor patients for at least 30 minutes after each abarelix injection. In the event of an allergic reaction associated with hypotension and/or syncope, use appropriate supportive measures (eg, leg elevation, oxygen, IV fluids, antihistamines, corticosteroids, and epinephrine [alone or in combination]).

From all the prostate cancer clinical trials with abarelix (mostly in men without advanced, symptomatic disease), immediate-onset systemic allergic reactions (occurring within 30 minutes of dosing) were observed in 1.1% of patients dosed with abarelix. In 14/15 patients who experienced an allergic reaction, each developed symptoms within 8 minutes of injection. The cumulative risk of such a reaction increased with duration of treatment. The cumulative rates on days 56, 141, 365, and 676 were 0.51%, 0.8%, 1.24%, and 2.91%, respectively. Seven patients experienced hypotension or syncope as part of their allergic reaction, representing 0.5% of all patients. The cumulative rates for these types of reactions on days 56, 141, 365, and 617 after the initial dose were 0.22%, 0.32%, 0.61%, and 1.67%, respectively.

➤*Fertility impairment:* In animals, mating and fertility were significantly decreased at doses of 3 and 10 mg/kg (0.34-fold and 1.135-fold, respectively, the human therapeutic dose of 100 mg based on body surface area [BSA]), but the effects were reversible.

➤*Pregnancy:* Category X. Embryolethality occurred in pregnant rats administered a single SC dose of abarelix up to 3 mg/kg (0.228-fold the human therapeutic dose of 100 mg based on BSA). In rabbits, a dose-related increase in fetal resorptions and reduced viability was observed at doses up to 30 mg/kg (6.81-fold the human therapeutic dose of 100 mg based on BSA).

➤*Lactation:* It is not known whether abarelix is excreted in human milk. Do not use in nursing mothers.

➤*Children:* The safety and efficacy of abarelix in pediatric patients have not been studied. Abarelix is not indicated for use in pediatric patients.

Precautions

➤*Monitoring:* Monitor the response to abarelix by measuring serum total testosterone concentrations just prior to administration on day 29 and every 8 weeks thereafter. Also consider periodic measurement of serum PSA levels. Clinically meaningful transaminase elevations were observed in some patients who received abarelix or comparator drugs. Obtain serum transaminase levels before starting abarelix treatment and periodically during treatment.

➤*Decrease in bone mineral density:* Extended treatment with GnRH antagonists and LHRH agonists may result in a decrease in bone mineral density.

Adverse Reactions

Abarelix Adverse Events (≥ 10%)	
Adverse reaction	Abarelix (n = 81)
CNS	
Dizziness	12
Fatigue	10
Headache	12
Sleep disturbance[1]	44
Endocrine	
Breast enlargement[1]	30
Breast pain/nipple tenderness[1]	20
GI	
Constipation	15
Diarrhea	11
Nausea	10

ABARELIX

Abarelix Adverse Events (≥ 10%)	
Adverse reaction	Abarelix (n = 81)
GU	
Dysuria	10
Micturition frequency	10
Urinary retention	10
Urinary tract infection	10
Miscellaneous	
Back pain	17
Hot flushes[1]	79
Pain	31
Peripheral edema	15
Upper respiratory tract infection	12

[1] Pharmacological consequences of androgen deprivation.

➤*Hypersensitivity:* Immediate-onset systemic allergic reactions may occur (see Black Box Warning and Warnings).

➤*Lab test abnormalities:* Clinically meaningful increases in serum transaminases were seen in a small percentage of patients in both treatment groups in each active-controlled abarelix study. In study 1 and 2 combined, the percentage of abarelix patients reporting serum ALT greater than 2.5 times ULN or more than 200 U/L was 8.2% and 1.8%, respectively. The percentage reporting serum AST greater than 2.5 times ULN or more than 200 U/L was 3.1% and 0.8%, respectively. Similar results were reported for active comparators. Slight decreases in hemoglobin, a pharmacological consequence of castration, were observed in patients receiving abarelix and active comparator. Mean increases in serum triglycerides of approximately 10% were seen in abarelix-treated patients.

Overdosage

The maximum tolerated dose of abarelix has not been determined. The maximum dose used in clinical studies was 150 mg. There have been no reports of accidental overdose of abarelix.

Patient Information

Abarelix can cause serious or life-threatening allergic reactions that may need emergency medical treatment right away.

These serious reactions may include the following: Low blood pressure and fainting (shock); swelling of face, eyelids, tongue, or throat; asthma, wheezing, or other breathing problems such as chest tightness or shortness of breath.

Chances of getting a serious or life-threatening allergic reaction may increase with each abarelix injection.

If a serious or life-threatening allergic reaction occurs, it is usually soon after getting an abarelix injection; therefore, instruct patients to wait in the physicians's office or health care facility for 30 minutes after each abarelix injection.

Instruct patients to inform their physician right away if they feel any warmth, redness, light-headedness, swelling, or thickness in their throat; this could mean they are having a serious allergic reaction.

Inform patients to tell their physician if they or any family member have the rare heart condition known as prolongation of the QTc interval.

Abarelix can cause allergic skin reactions such as rash, hives, itching, tingling, and redness (flushing). A skin reaction may occur immediately after injection or several days later.

The most common side effects are the following: Hot flashes; problems sleeping; pain, including back pain; breast enlargement or breast pain; constipation.

Anabolic steroids are classified as a *c-iii* controlled substance under the anabolic steroids act of 1990.

An androgenic agent used in the therapy of carcinoma of the breast is listed under Antineoplastic Agents: Testolactone. (See individual monograph.)

Indications

➤*Males:* For replacement therapy in hypogonadism associated with a deficiency or absence of endogenous testosterone.

Primary hypogonadism (congenital or acquired) – Testicular failure because of cryptorchidism, bilateral torsion, orchitis, vanishing testis syndrome or orchidectomy, Klinefelter's syndrome, chemotherapy, or toxic damage from alcohol or heavy metals. These men usually have low serum testosterone levels and gonadotropins (FSH, LH) above the normal range.

Hypogonadotropic hypogonadism (congenital or acquired) – Idiopathic gonadotropin- or luteinizing hormone-releasing hormone (LHRH) deficiency or pituitary-hypothalamic injury from tumors, trauma, or radiation.

If the above conditions occur prior to puberty, androgen replacement therapy is needed for development of secondary sexual characteristics. Prolonged treatment is required to maintain sexual characteristics in these and other males who develop testosterone deficiency after puberty. However, appropriate adrenal cortical and thyroid hormone replacement therapy are still necessary and are of primary importance.

Delayed puberty – To stimulate puberty in carefully selected males with clearly delayed puberty. These patients usually have a familial pattern of delayed puberty that is not secondary to a pathological disorder; puberty is expected to occur spontaneously at a relatively late date. Brief occasional treatment with conservative doses may be justified if these patients do not respond to psychological support. Discuss the potential adverse effect on bone maturation with the patient and parents prior to androgen administration. To assess the effect of treatment on the epiphyseal centers, obtain an x-ray of the hand and wrist to determine bone age every 6 months.

➤*Females:*

Metastatic cancer – May be used secondarily in women with advancing inoperable metastatic (skeletal) mammary cancer who are 1 to 5 years postmenopausal. Primary goals of therapy include ablation of the ovaries. This treatment has been used in premenopausal women with breast cancer who have benefitted from oophorectomy and have a hormone-responsive tumor.

Androgens are not effective (lack of substantial evidence) in treating fractures or managing surgery, convalescence or functional uterine bleeding, or enhancement of athletic performance (see Warnings).

Actions

➤*Pharmacology:* Testosterone, produced by the Leydig cells of the testis, is the primary male androgen.

In many tissues, the activity of testosterone appears to depend on reduction to dihydrotestosterone, which binds to cytosol receptor proteins. The steroid-receptor complex is transported to the nucleus where it initiates transcription events and cellular changes related to androgen action.

Endogenous androgens are responsible for the normal growth and development of the male sex organs and for maintenance of secondary sex characteristics. These effects include the growth and maturation of the prostate, seminal vesicles, penis, and scrotum; the development of male hair distribution, such as facial, pubic, chest, and axillary hair; laryngeal enlargement; vocal cord thickening; alterations in body musculature and fat distribution. These drugs also cause retention of nitrogen, sodium, potassium, phosphorus, and decreased urinary excretion of calcium. Androgens have been reported to increase protein anabolism and decrease protein catabolism. Nitrogen balance is improved only when there is sufficient intake of calories and protein.

Androgens are responsible for the growth spurt of adolescence and for the termination of linear growth by fusion of the epiphyseal growth centers. In children, exogenous androgens accelerate linear growth rates but may cause a disproportionate advancement in bone maturation. Use over long periods may result in fusion of the epiphyseal growth centers and termination of the growth process. Androgens have been reported to stimulate production of red blood cells by enhancing production of the erythropoietic stimulating factor.

During administration of exogenous androgens, endogenous testosterone release is inhibited through feedback inhibition of pituitary luteinizing hormone (LH). Large doses of exogenous androgens may suppress spermatogenesis through feedback inhibition of pituitary follicle-stimulating hormone (FSH).

➤*Pharmacokinetics:*

Absorption –

Oral: Testosterone is metabolized by the gut and 44% is cleared by the liver in the first pass. Doses as high as 400 mg/day are needed to achieve clinically effective blood levels for full replacement therapy. The synthetic androgen, **methyltestosterone**, is less extensively metabolized by the liver and has a longer half-life. It is more suitable than testosterone for oral administration.

IM: Testosterone esters are less polar than free testosterone. Testosterone esters in oil injected IM are absorbed slowly from the lipid phase; thus, **testosterone cypionate** and **enanthate** can be given at intervals of 2 to 4 weeks. Suspensions of testosterone or its esters in aqueous media may cause local irritation and the rate of absorption is not always uniform.

Topical gel: In a study with the 10 g dose of topical testosterone gel (to deliver 100 mg testosterone), all patients showed an increase in serum testosterone within 30 minutes, and 8 of 9 patients had a serum testosterone concentration within the normal range by 4 hours after the initial application. Absorption of testosterone into the blood continues for the entire 24-hour dosing interval. Serum concentrations approximate the steady-state level by the end of the first 24 hours and are at steady state by the second or third day of dosing.

When the topical gel treatment is discontinued after achieving steady state, serum testosterone levels remain in the normal range for 24 to 48 hours but return to their pretreatment levels by the fifth day after the last application.

Transdermal system:

• *Testoderm* – Following placement of *Testoderm* on scrotal skin, the serum testosterone concentration rises to a maximum at 2 to 4 hours and returns toward baseline within ≈ 2 hours after system removal. Serum levels reach a plateau at 3 to 4 weeks. The testosterone levels achieved with *Testoderm* generally are within the range for normal men.

Scrotal skin is ≥ 5 times more permeable to testosterone than other skin sites. *Testoderm* and *Testoderm with Adhesive* will not produce adequate serum testosterone concentration if applied to nongenital skin.

• *Testoderm TTS* – The 3 recommended skin sites (arm, back, and upper buttocks) are interchangeable based on equivalent testosterone $AUC_{(0-27)}$ values.

• *Androderm* – Following application to nonscrotal skin, testosterone is continuously absorbed during the 24-hour dosing period. Daily application at ≈ 10 p.m. results in a serum testosterone concentration profile that mimics the normal circadian variation observed in healthy young men. Maximum concentrations occur in the early morning hours with minimum concentrations in the evening. Normal range morning serum testosterone concentrations are reached during the first day of dosing. There is no accumulation of testosterone during continuous treatment.

Distribution – Testosterone in plasma is ≈ 98% bound to a specific testosterone-estradiol-binding globulin. Generally, the amount of binding globulin will determine the percentage of free and bound testosterone; the free testosterone concentration will determine its half-life.

Metabolism / Excretion – There are considerable variations in the reported half-life of testosterone, ranging from 10 to 100 minutes. The half-life of **testosterone cypionate** IM is ≈ 8 days; for oral **fluoxymesterone**, it is ≈ 9.2 hours; **methyltestosterone** undergoes less extensive first-pass hepatic metabolism than testosterone following oral administration and has a longer half-life. Inactivation of testosterone occurs primarily in the liver. About 90% of a testosterone dose is excreted in the urine as conjugates of testosterone and its metabolites; about 6% of a dose is excreted in the feces.

Contraindications

Patients with serious cardiac, hepatic, or renal diseases; hypersensitivity to the drug or any components of the products; in men with carcinomas of the breast or known or suspected carcinoma of the prostate; women (*Testoderm*); pregnancy.

Pregnant women should avoid skin contact with *AndroGel* application sites in men. Testosterone may cause fetal harm. In the event that unwashed or unclothed skin to which *AndroGel* has been applied does come in direct contact with the skin of a pregnant woman, wash the general area of contact on the woman with soap and water as soon as possible. In vitro studies show that residual testosterone is removed from the skin surface by washing with soap and water.

Warnings

➤*Hepatic effects:* Prolonged use of high doses of androgens has been associated with the development of potentially life-threatening peliosis hepatis, hepatic neoplasms, cholestatic hepatitis, jaundice, and hepatocellular carcinoma. Long-term therapy with **testosterone enanthate**, which elevates blood levels for prolonged periods, has produced multiple hepatic adenomas. Testosterone is not known to produce these adverse effects.

Cholestatic hepatitis and jaundice occur with **fluoxymesterone** and **methyltestosterone** at relatively low doses. If cholestatic hepatitis with jaundice appears with use of any androgen, or if liver function tests become abnormal, discontinue the androgen and determine the etiology. Drug-induced jaundice is reversible when the medication is discontinued.

➤*Athletic performance:* Although the anabolic steroids are generally the agents that are abused for enhancement of athletic performance, these agents also have been used for such purposes. However, these drugs are not safe and effective for this use and have a potential risk of serious side effects.

➤*Sleep apnea:* The treatment of hypogonadal men with testosterone esters may potentiate sleep apnea in some patients, especially those with risk factors such as obesity or chronic lung diseases.

➤*Breast cancer:* In patients with breast cancer, androgen therapy may cause hypercalcemia by stimulating osteolysis. If hypercalcemia occurs, discontinue the drug.

➤*Oligospermia:* Oligospermia and reduced ejaculatory volume may occur after prolonged administration or excessive dosage.

➤*Edema:* Edema, with or without congestive heart failure, may be a serious complication in patients with preexisting cardiac, renal, or hepatic disease. In addition to discontinuation of the drug, diuretic therapy may be required.

➤*Gynecomastia:* Gynecomastia frequently develops and occasionally persists in patients being treated for hypogonadism.

➤*Bone maturation:* Use cautiously in healthy males with delayed puberty. Monitor bone maturation by assessing bone age of the wrist and hand every 6 months.

➤*Product interchange:* Do not use **testosterone cypionate** interchangeably with **testosterone propionate** because of differences in duration of action.

➤*Carcinogenesis:* Testosterone has induced cervical-uterine tumors in mice; these tumors metastasized in some cases. Injection of testosterone into some strains of female mice may increase their susceptibility to hepatoma. Testosterone is also known to increase the number of tumors and decrease the degree of differentiation of chemically-induced carcinomas of the liver in rats. There are rare reports of hepatocellular carcinoma in patients receiving long-term therapy with androgens in high doses. Drug withdrawal did not lead to tumor regression in all cases.

➤*Elderly:* Elderly males, or men in general, treated with androgens may be at an increased risk of developing prostatic hypertrophy, prostatic carcinoma, and prostatic hyperplasia.

➤*Pregnancy:* Category X. Androgens are contraindicated in women who are or who may become pregnant; androgens may cause fetal harm. Androgens cause virilization of the external genitalia of the female fetus (eg, clitoromegaly, abnormal vaginal development, fusion of genital folds to form a scrotal-like structure). The degree of masculinization is related to the amount of drug given and the age of the fetus. Masculinization is most likely to occur in the female fetus when androgens are given in the first trimester. If the patient becomes pregnant while taking these drugs, apprise her of the potential hazards to the fetus.

➤*Lactation:* It is not known whether androgens are excreted in breast milk. Decide whether to discontinue nursing or to discontinue the drug, taking into account the importance of the drug to the mother. Testosterone transdermal systems and testosterone gel are not indicated for women and must not be used in women.

➤*Children:* Use androgens cautiously in children; the drugs should only be given by specialists who are aware of the adverse effects on bone maturation.

Androgens may accelerate bone maturation without producing compensatory gain in linear growth. This adverse effect may result in compromised adult stature. The younger the child, the greater the risk of compromising final mature height.

Safety and efficacy of *Testoderm* and *Androgel* products in pediatric patients have not been established.

Benzyl alcohol – Benzyl alcohol-containing products have been associated with a fatal "gasping syndrome" in premature infants. Refer to product listings.

Precautions

➤*Monitoring:* Frequently determine urine and serum calcium levels during the course of therapy in women with disseminated breast carcinoma.

Periodically check liver function, prostate specific antigen, cholesterol, and high-density lipoprotein. To ensure proper dosing, measure serum testosterone concentrations.

Make periodic (every 6 months) x-ray examinations of bone age during treatment of prepubertal males to determine the rate of bone maturation and the effects of androgen therapy on the epiphyseal centers.

Check hemoglobin and hematocrit periodically for polycythemia in patients who are receiving high doses of androgens or who are receiving long-term administration.

➤*Virilization:* Observe women for signs of virilization (eg, deepening voice, hirsutism, acne, clitoromegaly, menstrual irregularities). Discontinue therapy at the time of evidence of mild virilism to prevent irreversible virilization. Virilization is usual following high-dose androgens. Some virilization should be tolerated during treatment for breast carcinoma.

Virilization of female partners has been reported with use of topical testosterone. Percutaneous creams leave as much as 90 mg residual testosterone on the skin. The results from one study indicated that, after removal of a *Testoderm* system, the potential for transfer of testosterone to a sexual partner was 6 mg, ¹⁄₄₅th the daily endogenous testosterone production by the female body. *Testoderm TTS* has an occlusive backing that prevents the partner from coming in contact with the active material in the system. If a *Testoderm TTS* system is inadvertently transferred to a female partner, remove it immediately and wash the contacted skin. Changes in body hair distribution or significant increases in acne of the female partner should be brought to the attention of a physician.

Patients with benign prostatic hypertrophy may develop acute urethral obstruction. Priapism or excessive sexual stimulation may develop. Oligospermia may occur after prolonged administration or excessive dosage. If any of these effects appear, stop administration. If restarted, use a lower dosage. Avoid stimulation to the point of increasing nervous, mental, and physical activities beyond the patient's cardiovascular capacity.

➤*Pellets:* Pellet implantation is much less flexible for dosage adjustment than is oral administration or IM injection of oil solutions or aqueous suspensions. Therefore, take great care when estimating the amount of testosterone needed. In the face of complications where the effects of testosterone should be discontinued, the pellets would have to be removed. In addition, there are times when the pellets may slough out. This accident is usually traceable to superficial implantation or to neglect in regard to aseptic precautions.

➤*Hypercholesterolemia:* Serum cholesterol may be altered during therapy.

➤*Tartrazine sensitivity:* Some of these products contain tartrazine, which may cause allergic-type reactions (including bronchial asthma) in susceptible individuals. Although the incidence of tartrazine sensitivity in the general population is low, it is frequently seen in patients who also have aspirin hypersensitivity. Specific products containing tartrazine are identified in the product listings.

Drug Interactions

Androgens Drug Interactions			
Precipitant drug	Object drug*		Description
Fluoxy-mesterone, Methyltestosterone	Anticoagulants	↑	The anticoagulant effect may be potentiated by 17-alkyl testosterone derivatives (eg, fluoxymesterone, methyltestosterone). Although the non-17-alkylated agent (testosterone) appears safer, ≥ 1 case report described a similar interaction. Avoid the combination with 17-alkyl derivatives if possible.
Androgens	Oxyphen-butazone	↑	Co-administration of oxyphenbutazone and androgens may result in elevated serum levels of oxyphenbutazone.
Androgens	Insulin	↓	In diabetic patients, the metabolic effects of androgens may decrease blood glucose and, therefore, insulin requirements.
Testosterone	Propranolol	↓	In a pharmacokinetic study of an injectable testosterone product, administration of testosterone cypionate led to an increased clearance of propranolol in the majority of men tested.
Testosterone	Corticosteroids, ACTH	↑	The co-administration of testosterone with ACTH or corticosteroids may enhance edema formation; thus, administer these drugs cautiously, particularly in patients with cardiac or hepatic disease.
Methyltestosterone	Cyclosporine	↑	Increased cyclosporine blood concentrations with possible toxicity (eg, nephrotoxicity) may occur. Consider monitoring serum bilirubin, serum creatinine, and cyclosporine concentrations in patients receiving cyclosporine and methyltestosterone concurrently. Adjust the doses as needed.

* ↑ = Object drug increased. ↓ = Object drug decreased.

➤*Drug/Lab test interactions:*
Thyroid function tests – Decreased levels of thyroxine-binding globulin, resulting in decreased total T_4 serum levels and increased resin uptake of T_3 and T_4. Free thyroid hormone levels remain unchanged, and there is no clinical evidence of thyroid dysfunction.

Androgens

Adverse Reactions

Female –

Most common: Amenorrhea and other menstrual irregularities; inhibition of gonadotropin secretion and virilization, including deepening voice and clitoral enlargement. The latter usually is not reversible after androgens are discontinued. When administered to a pregnant woman, androgens cause virilization of external genitalia of the female fetus.

Androgen Adverse Reactions[1] (%)

Adverse reaction	Oral	Injection	Trans-dermal	Implant	Topical (5 to 10 g dose)
Cardiovascular					
CHF	—	—	1	—	—
Hypertension	—	—	< 1	—	< 3
Tachycardia	—	—	< 1	—	—
Stroke	—	—	2	—	—
Deep vein phlebitis	—	—	1	—	—
Peripheral edema	—	—	—	—	1.4-3.1
Vasodilation	—	—	—	—	< 1
Peripheral vascular disease	—	—	< 1	—	—
CNS					
Headache	✔	✔	1-6	✔	< 4
Pain	—	—	2	—	—
Asthenia	—	—	2	—	< 3
Libido increased	✔	✔	1	✔	—
Memory loss	—	—	1	—	—
Nervousness/Anxiety	✔	✔	< 1	✔	< 3
Depression	✔	✔	< 3	✔	< 1
Dizziness/Vertigo	—	—	1-6	—	< 1
Dry mouth	—	—	< 1	—	—
Insomnia	—	—	< 1	—	—
Libido decreased	✔	✔	< 1	✔	1-3
Personality disorder	—	—	< 1	—	—
CNS stimulation	—	—	< 1	—	—
Generalized paresthesia	✔	✔	< 1	✔	< 1
Emotional lability	—	—	—	—	< 3
Amnesia	—	—	—	—	< 1
Hostility	—	—	—	—	< 1
Fatigue	—	—	< 1	—	—
Confusion	—	—	< 1	—	—
Thinking abnormalities	—	—	< 1	—	—
Dermatologic					
Application site itching	—	—	7-12	—	—
Application site erythema	—	—	3-7	—	—
Application site discomfort	—	—	4	—	—
Application site irritation	—	—	2	—	—
Pruritus	—	—	2-37	—	—
Burning sensation	—	—	3	—	—
Rash	—	—	1-2	—	—
Acne	✔	✔	1-4	✔	2.8-12.5
Alopecia	—	—	< 1	—	< 1
Male pattern baldness	✔	✔	—	✔	—
Hirsutism	✔	✔	< 1	✔	< 1
Other application site reactions	—	—	< 6	—	3.1 to 10
Injection site pain/inflammation	—	✔	—	✔	—
Burn-like blister under system	—	—	12	—	—
Seborrhea	—	✔	—	—	—
Discolored hair	—	—	—	—	< 1
Dry skin	—	—	—	—	< 1
GI					
Abdominal pain	—	—	< 1	—	—
Diarrhea	—	—	< 1	—	—
Nausea	✔	✔	< 1	✔	—
Cholestatic jaundice	✔	✔	—	✔	—
Abnormal liver function tests	✔	✔	1	✔	—
Hepatocellular neoplasms	✔	✔	—	✔	—
Peliosis hepatis	✔	✔	—	✔	—
GI bleeding	—	—	2	—	—
Increased appetite	—	—	< 1	—	—
Stomatitis	—	—	✔	—	—

Androgen Adverse Reactions[1] (%)

Adverse reaction	Oral	Injection	Trans-dermal	Implant	Topical (5 to 10 g dose)
GU					
Abnormal ejaculation	—	—	< 1	—	—
Breast pain/tenderness	—	—	1-3	—	1-3
Dysuria	—	—	< 1	—	—
UTI/Prostatitis	—	—	1-4	—	—
Impaired urination	—	—	< 1	—	< 2.8
Frequent erections	✔	✔	—	✔	—
Prolonged erection	✔	✔	—	✔	—
Oligospermia	✔	✔	—	✔	—
Scrotal cellulitis	—	—	1	—	—
BPH	—	—	1	—	—
Rectal mucosal lesion over prostate	—	—	1	—	—
Hematuria/Bladder cancer	—	—	1	—	—
Papilloma on scrotum	—	—	1	—	—
Prostate disorder	—	—	< 5	—	2.8-18.8[2]
Testes disorder	—	—	< 1	—	< 3
Penis disorder	—	—	< 1	—	< 1
Pelvic pain	—	—	< 1	—	—
Incontinence	—	—	< 1	—	—
Gynecomastia	✔	✔	1-5	✔	< 3
Hematologic					
Suppression of clotting factors	✔	✔	—	✔	—
Polycythemia	✔	✔	—	✔	—
Metabolic/Nutritional					
Hyperglycemia	—	—	< 1	—	—
Hyperlipidemia	—	—	< 1	—	—
Hyponatremia	—	—	< 1	—	—
Electrolyte imbalance	✔	✔	—	✔	—
Increased serum cholesterol	✔	✔	—	✔	—
Abnormal lab tests[3]	—	—	—	—	4.2-6.3
Musculoskeletal					
Myalgia	—	—	2	—	—
Back pain	—	—	< 1	—	—
Arthralgia	—	—	< 1	—	—
Miscellaneous					
Accidental injury	—	—	2	—	—
Flu syndrome	—	—	1	—	—
Infection	—	—	< 1	—	—
Anaphylaxis	✔	✔	—	✔	—
Accelerated growth	—	—	< 1	—	—
Bronchitis	—	—	< 1	—	—
Papillary dilation	—	—	1	—	—
Sweating	—	—	—	—	< 1

— = No data.

✔ = Reported, incidence not listed.

[1] Data pooled from separate studies and are not necessarily comparable.

[2] Including prostate enlargement, BPH, elevated PSA results, new diagnosis of prostate cancer.

[3] Including abnormal hemoglobin, hematocrit, triglycerides, serum lipids, potassium, glucose, creatinine, bilirubin, liver function tests.

Overdosage

There is one report of acute overdosage by injection of testosterone enanthate: Testosterone levels of up to 11,400 ng/dL were implicated in a cerebrovascular accident.

Patient Information

Oral tablets may cause GI upset.

Notify physician if nausea, vomiting, swelling of the ankles (edema), too frequent or persistent erections of the penis, changes in skin color, and breathing disturbances, including those associated with sleep, occur.

►*Females:* Notify physician if hoarseness, deepening of the voice, increases in facial hair, acne, or menstrual irregularities occur.

Advise male adolescent patients receiving androgens for delayed puberty to have bone development checked every 6 months.

TESTOSTERONE, LONG-ACTING

For complete prescribing information, refer to the Androgens group monograph.

Indications

➤*Replacement therapy:*

Primary hypogonadism (congenital or acquired) – Testicular failure because of cryptorchidism, bilateral torsion, orchitis, vanishing testis syndrome; or orchidectomy.

Hypogonadotropic hypogonadism (congenital or acquired) – Idiopathic gonadotropin or luteinizing hormone-releasing hormone (LHRH) deficiency, or pituitary-hypothalamic injury from tumors, trauma, or radiation. However, appropriate adrenal cortical and thyroid hormone replacement therapy are still necessary and are actually of primary importance.

If the above conditions occur prior to puberty, androgen replacement therapy will be needed during the adolescent years for development of secondary sexual characteristics. Prolonged androgen treatment will be required to maintain sexual characteristics in these and other males who develop testosterone deficiency after puberty.

Delayed puberty (testosterone enanthate only) – May be used to stimulate puberty in carefully selected males with clearly delayed puberty. These patients usually have a familial pattern of delayed puberty that is not secondary to a pathological disorder; puberty is expected to occur spontaneously at a relatively late date. Brief treatment with conservative doses may occasionally be justified in these patients if they do not repond to psychological support. Discuss the potential adverse effect on bone maturation with the patient and parents prior to androgen administration. Obtain an x-ray of the hand and wrist every 6 months to determine bone age and assess the effect of treatment on the epiphyseal centers.

➤*Metastatic mammary cancer in females (testosterone enanthate only):* May be used secondarily in women with advancing inoperable metastatic (skeletal) mammary cancer who are 1 to 5 years postmenopausal. Primary goals of therapy in these women include ablation of the ovaries. Other methods of counteracting estrogen activity are adrenalectomy, hypophysectomy, or antiestrogen therapy. This treatment also has been used in premenopausal women with breast cancer who have benefitted from oophorectomy and are considered to have a hormone-responsive tumor. Judgment concerning androgen therapy should be made by an oncologist with expertise in this field.

Administration and Dosage

For IM use only. Individualize dosage. In general, > 400 mg/month total is not required because of the prolonged action of the preparation.

Testosterone esters in oil injected IM are absorbed slowly; thus, testosterone cypionate and testosterone enanthate can be given at intervals of 2 to 4 weeks.

➤*Male hypogonadism:*

Replacement therapy (ie, for eunuchism) – 50 to 400 mg every 2 to 4 weeks.

➤*Males with delayed puberty (testosterone enanthate only):* 50 to 200 mg every 2 to 4 weeks for a limited duration (ie, 4 to 6 months).

➤*Inoperable breast cancer (testosterone enanthate only):* 200 to 400 mg every 2 to 4 weeks. Women with metastatic breast carcinoma must be followed closely because androgen therapy occasionally appears to accelerate the disease.

NOTE: Use of a wet needle or wet syringe may cause the solution to become cloudy; however, this does not affect the potency of the material.

➤*Storage / Stability:* Store at controlled room temperature, 20° to 25°C (68° to 77°F). Warming and shaking vial redissolves crystals that may have formed.

TESTOSTERONE ENANTHATE (IN OIL)

c-iii	**Delatestryl** (Savient[a])	**Injection:** 200 mg/mL	In 5 mL multidose vials and 1 mL single dose syringes with needle.[b]

[a] Savient Pharmaceuticals, Inc., 70 Wood Avenue South, Iselin, NJ, 08830; (732) 632-8800, FAX (732) 632-8844.

[b] In sesame oil with 5 mg chlorobutanol.

For complete prescribing information, refer to the Testosterone, Long-Acting monograph.

TESTOSTERONE CYPIONATE (IN OIL)

c-iii	**Depo-Testosterone** (Pharmacia)	**Injection:** 100 mg/mL	In 10 mL vials.[1]
c-iii	**Testosterone Cypionate** (Watson)	**Injection:** 200 mg/mL	Benzyl alcohol, cotton seed oil. In 10 mL multi-dose vials.
c-iii	**Depo-Testosterone** (Pharmacia)		In 1 and 10 mL vials.[2]

[1] In 736 mg cottonseed oil with 0.1 mL benzyl benzoate and 9.45 mg benzyl alcohol.

[2] In 560 mg cottonseed oil with 0.2 mL benzyl benzoate and 9.45 mg benzyl alcohol.

For complete prescribing information, refer to the Testosterone, Long-Acting monograph.

TESTOSTERONE PELLETS

c-iii	**Testopel** (Bartor Pharmacal)	**Pellets:** 75 mg	0.2 mg stearic acid, 2 mg polyvinylpyrroidone. 1 pellet/vial. In 3s, 10s, and 100s.

For complete prescribing information, refer to the Androgens group monograph.

Indications

➤*Replacement therapy:*

Primary hypogonadism (congenital or acquired) – Testicular failure caused by cryptorchidism, bilateral torsion, orchitis, vanishing testis syndrome; or orchidectomy.

Hypogonadotropic hypogonadism (congenital or acquired) – Idiopathic gonadotropin or LHRH deficiency, or pituitary-hypothalamic injury from tumors, trauma, or radiation.

If these conditions occur prior to puberty, androgen replacement therapy will be needed during the adolescent years for development of secondary sexual characteristics. Prolonged androgen treatment will be required to maintain sexual characteristics in these and other males who develop testosterone deficiency after puberty.

Delayed puberty – To stimulate puberty in carefully selected males with clearly delayed puberty. These patients usually have a familial pattern of delayed puberty that is not secondary to a pathological disorder; puberty is expected to occur spontaneously at a relatively late date. Brief treatment with conservative doses may occasionally be justified in these patients if they do not respond to psychological support. Discuss the potential adverse effect on bone maturation with the patient and parents prior to androgen administration. Obtain an x-ray of the hand and wrist every 6 months to determine bone age and assess the effect of treatment on the epiphyseal centers.

Administration and Dosage

The suggested dosage for androgens varies depending on the age and diagnosis of the individual patient. Dosage is adjusted according to the patient's response and the appearance of adverse reactions.

➤*Replacement therapy:* The dosage guideline for testosterone pellets for replacement therapy in androgen-deficient males is 150 to 450 mg SC every 3 to 6 months. Various dosage regimens have been used to induce pubertal changes in hypogonadal males; some experts have advocated lower dosages initially, gradually increasing the dose as puberty progresses, with or without a decrease to maintenance levels. Other experts emphasize that higher dosages are needed to induce pubertal changes and lower dosages can be used for maintenance after puberty. The chronological and skeletal ages must be taken into consideration, both in determining the initial dose and in adjusting the dose.

➤*Delayed puberty:* Dosages used in delayed puberty generally are in the lower range of that listed above, and for a limited time duration, for example 4 to 6 months.

➤*Determination of dose:* The number of pellets to be implanted depends upon the minimal daily requirement of testosterone propionate determined by a gradual reduction of the amount administered parenterally. The usual ratio is as follows: Implant two 75 mg pellets for each 25 mg testosterone propionate required weekly. Thus, when a patient requires injections of 75 mg/week, it is usually necessary to implant 450 mg (6 pellets). With injections of 50 mg/week, implantation of 300 mg (4 pellets) may suffice for ≈ 3 months. With lower requirements by injection, correspondingly lower amounts may be implanted. It has been found that ≈ 1/3 of the material is absorbed in the first month, 1/4 in the second month, and 1/6 in the third month. Adequate effect of the pellets ordinarily continues for 3 to 4 months, sometimes as long as 6 months.

➤*Storage / Stability:* Store in a cool place.

Androgens

TESTOSTERONE TRANSDERMAL SYSTEM

	Product/Distributor	Release rate (mg/24 hr)	Total contact surface area (cm²)	Total testosterone content (mg)	How supplied
c-iii	**Testoderm** (Alza)	4	40	10	In 30s.
c-iii	**Testoderm** (Alza)	6	60	15	In 30s.
c-iii	**Testoderm with Adhesive** (Alza)	6	60	15	In 30s.
c-iii	**Androderm** (Watson Pharma)	5	44	24.3	In 30s.
c-iii	**Androderm** (Watson Pharma)	2.5	37	12.2	In 60s.

For complete prescribing information, refer to the Androgens group monograph.

Indications

➤*Replacement therapy:*

Primary hypogonadism (congenital or acquired) – Testicular failure because of cryptorchidism, bilateral torsion, orchitis, vanishing testis syndrome, orchidectomy, Klinefelter's syndrome, chemotherapy, or toxic damage from alcohol or heavy metals. These men usually have low serum testosterone levels and gonadotropins (follicle-stimulating hormone [FSH], luteinizing hormone [LH]) above the normal range.

Hypogonadotropic hypogonadism (congenital or acquired) – Idiopathic gonadotropin or LHRH deficiency or pituitary-hypothalamic injury from tumors, trauma, or radiation. These men have low testosterone serum levels but have gonadotropins in the normal or low range.

Appropriate adrenal cortical and thyroid hormone replacement therapy may be necessary in patients with multiple pituitary or hypothalamic abnormalities.

Administration and Dosage

➤*Testoderm and Testoderm with Adhesive:* Patients should start therapy with a 6 mg/day system applied daily; if scrotal area is inadequate, use a 4 mg/day system. Place the patch on clean, dry, scrotal skin. Dry-shave scrotal hair for optimal skin contact. Do not use chemical depilatories. The system should be worn 22 to 24 hours. If the product has come off after it has been worn for > 12 hours and it cannot be reapplied, the patient may wait until the next routine application time to apply a new system.

After 3 to 4 weeks of daily system use, draw blood 2 to 4 hours after system application for determination of serum total testosterone. Because of variability in analytical values among diagnostic laboratories, perform this laboratory work and later analyses for assessing the effect of the transdermal testosterone therapy at the same laboratory.

If patients have not achieved desired results by the end of 6 to 8 weeks of use, consider another form of testosterone replacement therapy.

These systems are designed for application to scrotal skin only. Because scrotal skin is ≥ 5 times more permeable to testosterone than other skin sites, *Testoderm* or *Testoderm with Adhesive* will not produce adequate serum testosterone concentrations if applied to nonscrotal skin.

Ingestion of testosterone, or the contents of any of the *Testoderm* products will not result in clinically significant serum testosterone concentrations because of extensive first-pass metabolism. In addition, an IM injection of testosterone from any of the *Testoderm* products will not produce adequate serum testosterone levels because of its short half-life (≈ 10 minutes).

➤*Androderm:* The usual starting dose is one 5 mg system or two 2.5 mg systems applied nightly for 24 hours, providing a total dose of 5 mg/day.

Apply the adhesive side of the system to a clean, dry area of the skin on the back, abdomen, upper arms, or thighs. Avoid bony prominences or on a part of the body that may be subject to prolonged pressure during sleep or sitting (eg, the deltoid region of the upper arm, the greater trochanter of the femur and the ischial tuberosity). Application to these sites has been associated with burn-like blister reactions. Do not apply to the scrotum. Rotate the sites of application, with an interval of 7 days between applications to the same site. The area selected should not be oily, damaged, or irritated. The system does not have to be removed during sexual intercourse, nor while taking a shower or bath.

Apply the system immediately after opening the pouch and removing the protective release liner. Press the system firmly in place, making sure there is good contact with the skin, especially around the edges.

To ensure proper dosing, the morning serum testosterone concentration may be measured following system application the previous evening. If the serum concentration is outside the normal range, repeat sampling with assurance of proper system adhesion as well as appropriate application time. Confirmed serum concentrations outside the normal range may require increasing the daily dosage regimen to 7.5 mg (ie, one 5 mg and one 2.5 mg or three 2.5 mg systems), or decreasing the regimen to 2.5 mg (ie, one 2.5 mg system), maintaining nightly application. Because of variability in analytical values among diagnostic laboratories, perform this laboratory work and any later analysis for assessing the effect of therapy at the same laboratory so results can be more easily compared.

Nonvirilized patient – Dosing may be initiated with one 2.5 mg system applied nightly.

Skin irritation – Mild skin irritation may be ameliorated by treatment of the affected skin with *otc* topical hydrocortisone cream applied after system removal. Applying a small amount of 0.1% triamcinolone acetonide cream to the skin under the central drug reservoir has been shown to reduce the incidence and severity of skin irritation. The administration of 0.1% triamcinolone acetonide cream does not significantly alter transdermal absorption of testosterone from the system. Do not use ointment formulations for pretreatment as they may significantly reduce testosterone absorption.

➤*Storage/Stability:* Store at room temperature, 15° to 30°C (59° to 86°F). Do not store outside the pouch provided. Do not use damaged systems. The drug reservoir may burst from excessive pressure or heat. Discard systems in household trash in a manner that prevents accidental application or ingestion by children, pets, or others.

TESTOSTERONE GEL

c-iii	**AndroGel 1%** (Unimed Pharm.)	**Gel:** 1% testosterone	68.9% ethanol. Each packet contains 2.5 or 5 g of gel to deliver 25 or 50 mg testosterone. In 30s.
c-iii	**Testim** (Auxilium Pharm[1])		74% ethanol, glycerin. In 5 g.

[1] Auxilium Pharmaceuticals, Inc., 160 W. Germantown Pike, Suite D5, Norristown, PA 19401; 610-278-6316.

For complete prescribing information, refer to the Androgens group monograph.

Indications

➤*Replacement therapy:*

Primary hypogonadism (congenital or acquired) – For testicular failure because of cryptorchidism, bilateral torsion, orchitis, vanishing testis syndrome, orchiectomy, Klinefelter's syndrome, chemotherapy, or toxic damage from alcohol or heavy metals. These men usually have low serum testosterone levels and gonadotropins (FSH, LH) above the normal range.

Hypogonadotropic hypogonadism (congenital or acquired) – For idiopathic gonadotropin or LHRH deficiency or pituitary-hypothalamic injury from tumors, trauma, or radiation. These men have low testosterone serum levels but have gonadotropins in the normal or low range.

Administration and Dosage

The recommended starting dose of 1% testosterone gel is 5 g (to deliver 50 mg of testosterone) applied once daily (preferably in the morning) to clean, dry, intact skin of the shoulders and upper arms or abdomen. Upon opening the packet(s), squeeze the entire contents into the palm of the hand and immediately apply it to the application sites. Allow application sites to dry for a few minutes prior to dressing. Wash hands with soap and water after application. Cover the application sites with clothing after gel has dried.

Do not apply the gel to the genitals.

It is unknown for how long showering or swimming should be delayed. For optimal absorption of testosterone, it appears reasonable to wait ≥ 5 to 6 hours after application prior to showering or swimming. Nevertheless, showering or swimming after just 1 hour should have a minimal effect on the amount absorbed if done infrequently.

Measure serum testosterone levels 14 days after initiation of therapy to ensure proper dosing. If the serum testosterone concentration is below the normal range, or if the desired clinical response is not achieved, the dose may be increased from 5 to 7.5 g and from 7.5 to 10 g, as instructed by the physician.

The potential for dermal testosterone transfer following use was evaluated in vigorous skin-to-skin contact. Under study conditions, all unprotected female partners had a serum testosterone concentration > 2 times the baseline value at some time during the study. When a shirt covered the application site(s), the transfer of testosterone from the males to the female partners was completely prevented. Washing the area of contact on the other person as soon as possible with soap and water will remove residual testosterone from the skin surface.

➤*Storage/Stability:* Store at controlled room temperature (20° to 25°C (68° to 77°F).

TESTOSTERONE, BUCCAL

Rx	**Striant** (Columbia)	**Buccal system:** 30 mg testosterone	Lactose. In blister packs of 10 systems.

For complete prescribing information, refer to the Androgens group monograph.

Indications

➤*Replacement therapy:*

Primary hypogonadism (congenital or acquired) – Testicular failure caused by cryptorchidism, bilateral torsion, orchitis, vanishing testis syndrome, orchidectomy, Klinefelter syndrome, chemotherapy, or toxic damage from alcohol or heavy metals. These men usually have low serum testosterone levels and gonadotropins (FSH, LH) above the normal range.

Hypogonadotropic hypogonadism (congenital or acquired) – Idiopathic gonadotropin or LHRH deficiency, or pituitary hypothalamic injury from tumors, trauma, or radiation. These patients have low serum testosterone levels but have gonadotropins in the normal or low range.

Administration and Dosage

The recommended dosing schedule is the application of 1 buccal system (30 mg) to the gum region twice daily, morning and evening (about 12 hours apart). Testosterone buccal should be placed in a comfortable position just above the incisor tooth on either side of the mouth. With each application, testosterone should be rotated to alternate sides of the mouth.

Upon opening the packet, the rounded side surface of the buccal system should be placed against the gum and held firmly in place with a finger over the lip and against the product for 30 seconds to ensure adhesion. Testosterone buccal is designed to stay in position until removed. If the buccal system fails to properly adhere to the gum or should fall off during the 12-hour dosing interval, the old buccal system should be removed and a new one applied. If the buccal system falls out of position within 4 hours before the next dose, a new buccal system should be applied and may remain in place until the time of next regularly scheduled dosing.

Take care to avoid dislodging the buccal system and check to see if testosterone buccal is in place following toothbrushing, use of mouthwash, and consumption of food or beverages. Testosterone buccal should not be chewed or swallowed. To remove testosterone, gently slide it downwards from the gum toward the tooth to avoid scratching the gum.

➤*Storage/Stability:* Store at 20° to 25°C (68° to 77°F). Protect from heat and moisture. Damaged blister packages should not be used. Discarded testosterone buccal systems should be disposed of in household trash in a manner that prevents accidental application or ingestion by children or pets.

METHYLTESTOSTERONE

c-iii	**Methyltestosterone** (Various, eg, Global)	**Tablets:** 10 mg	In 100s.
c-iii	**Methitest** (Global)		Lactose, sugar. (7037). White, scored. In 100s.
c-iii	**Methyltestosterone** (Various, eg, Global)	**Tablets:** 25 mg	In 100s.
c-iii	**Methitest** (Global)		Lactose, sugar. (7038). Yellow, scored. In 100s and 1000s.
c-iii	**Methyltestosterone** (Various, eg, Global)	**Tablets (buccal):** 10 mg	In 100s.
c-iii	**Testred** (ICN Pharm)	**Capsules:** 10 mg	(ICN 0901). Red. In 100s.
c-iii	**Virilon** (Star)		(Virilon 10 mg). Black and clear. In 100s and 1000s.
c-iii	**Android** (ICN Pharm)		(ICN 0901). Red. In 100s.
c-iii	**Virilon IM** (Star)	**Injection:** 200 mg/mL	In 1 mL vials and 10 mL multiple dose vials.[1]

[1] In cottonseed oil with 20% benzyl benzoate and 0.9% benzyl alcohol.

For complete prescribing information, refer to the Androgens group monograph.

Indications

➤*Replacement therapy:*

Primary hypogonadism (congenital or acquired) – Testicular failure because of cryptorchidism, bilateral torsion, orchitis, vanishing testis syndrome; or orchidectomy.

Hypogonadotropic hypogonadism (congenital or acquired) – Idiopathic gonadotropin or LHRH deficiency, or pituitary-hypothalamic injury from tumors, trauma, or radiation. However, appropriate adrenal cortical and thyroid hormone replacement therapy are still necessary and are actually of primary importance.

If the above conditions occur prior to puberty, androgen replacement therapy will be needed during the adolescent years for development of secondary sexual characteristics. Prolonged androgen treatment will be required to maintain sexual characteristics in these and other males who develop testosterone deficiency after puberty.

Delayed puberty – May be used to stimulate puberty in carefully selected males with clearly delayed puberty. These patients usually have a familial pattern of delayed puberty that is not secondary to a pathological disorder; puberty is expected to occur spontaneously at a relatively late date. Brief treatment with conservative doses may occasionally be justified in these patients if they do not respond to psychological support. Discuss the potential adverse effect on bone maturation with the patient and parents prior to androgen administration. Obtain an x-ray of the hand and wrist every 6 months to determine bone age and assess the effect of treatment on the epiphyseal centers.

➤*Metastatic mammary cancer in females:* May be used secondarily in women with advancing inoperable metastatic (skeletal) mammary cancer who are 1 to 5 years postmenopausal. Primary goals of therapy in these women include ablation of the ovaries. Other methods of counteracting estrogen activity are adrenalectomy, hypophysectomy, or antiestrogen therapy. This treatment also has been used in premenopausal women with breast cancer who have benefitted from oophorectomy and are considered to have a hormone-responsive tumor. Judgment concerning androgen therapy should be made by an oncologist with expertise in this field.

Administration and Dosage

The suggested dosage for androgens varies depending on the age, sex, and diagnosis of the individual patient. Dosage is adjusted according to the patient's response and the appearance of adverse reactions.

➤*Males:*

Replacement therapy – Replacement therapy in androgen-deficient males is 10 to 50 mg of methyltestosterone daily.

Delayed puberty: Doses used in delayed puberty generally are in the lower range of that given above, and for a limited duration, for example, 4 to 6 months.

➤*Females:*

Inoperable breast cancer – 50 to 200 mg/day orally. Follow women closely because androgen therapy occasionally appears to accelerate the disease. Shorter acting androgen preparations may be preferred rather than those with prolonged activity for treating breast carcinoma, particularly during the early stages of androgen therapy.

➤*Storage/Stability:* Store at 15° to 30°C (59° to 86°F).

FLUOXYMESTERONE

c-iii	**Fluoxymesterone** (Various, eg, Major, Rosemont, United)	**Tablets**: 10 mg	In 100s.

For complete prescribing information, refer to the Androgens group monograph.

Indications

➤*Replacement therapy:*

Primary hopogonadism (congenital or acquired) – Testicular failure due to cryptorchidism, bilateral torsion, orchitis, vanishing testis syndrome, or orchidectomy.

Hypogonadotropic hypogonadism (congenital or acquired) – Idiopathic gonadotropin or LHRH deficiency, or pituitary-hypothalamic injury from tumors, trauma, or radiation.

Delayed puberty – Provided it has been definitely established as such, and is not just a familial trait.

➤*Metastatic mammary cancer in females:* For palliation of androgen-responsive recurrent mammary cancer in women who are > 1 year but < 5 years postmenopausal, or who have been proven to have a hormone-dependent tumor as shown by previous beneficial response to castration.

Administration and Dosage

Individualize dosage. Total daily oral dose may be administered in single or divided (3 or 4) doses.

➤*Males:*

Hypogonadism – 5 to 20 mg daily. It is usually preferable to begin treatment with full therapeutic doses that are later adjusted to individual requirements. Priapism is indicative of excessive dosage and is an indication for temporary withdrawal of the drug.

Delayed puberty – Carefully titrate dosage using a low dose, appropriate skeletal monitoring, and by limiting the duration of therapy to 4 to 6 months.

➤*Females:*

Inoperable breast carcinoma – 10 to 40 mg daily in divided doses. Continue for ≥ 1 month for a subjective response and 2 to 3 months for an objective response.

DANAZOL

Rx	Danazol (Various, eg, Barr)	Capsules: 50 mg	In 100s.
Rx	Danocrine (Sanofi-Synthelabo)		Orange/white. In 100s.
Rx	Danazol (Various, eg, Barr)	Capsules: 100 mg	In 100s.
Rx	Danocrine (Sanofi-Synthelabo)		(DANOCRINE 100 mg / W D04). Yellow. In 100s.
Rx	Danazol (Various, eg, Barr)	Capsules: 200 mg	In 60s, 100s, and 500s.
Rx	Danocrine (Sanofi-Synthelabo)		(DANOCRINE 200 mg / W D05). Orange. In 60s and 100s.

WARNING

Use of danazol in pregnancy is contraindicated. A sensitive test (eg, beta subunit test if available) capable of determining early pregnancy is recommended immediately prior to start of therapy. Additionally, a nonhormonal method of contraception should be used during therapy. If a patient becomes pregnant while taking danazol, discontinue administration of the drug and apprise the patient of the potential risk to the fetus.

Thromboembolism, thrombotic and thrombophlebitic events, including sagittal sinus thrombosis and life-threatening or fatal strokes have been reported.

Experience with long-term therapy with danazol is limited. Peliosis hepatis and benign hepatic adenoma have been observed with long-term use. Peliosis hepatis and hepatic adenoma may be silent until complicated by acute, potentially life-threatening intra-abdominal hemorrhage. Therefore, alert the physician to this possibility. Attempts should be made to determine the lowest dose that will provide adequate protection (see Warnings).

Danazol has been associated with several cases of benign intracranial hypertension also known as pseudotumor cerebri. Early signs and symptoms of benign intracranial hypertension include papilledema, headache, nausea and vomiting, and visual disturbances. Screen patients with these symptoms for papilledema and, if present, advise the patients to discontinue danazol immediately and refer them to a neurologist for further diagnosis and care.

Indications

➤*Endometriosis:* For the treatment of endometriosis amenable to hormonal management.

➤*Fibrocystic breast disease:* Most cases of symptomatic fibrocystic breast disease may be treated by simple measures (eg, padded bras, analgesics). Pain and tenderness may be severe enough to warrant suppression of ovarian function. Danazol is usually effective in decreasing nodularity, pain, and tenderness, but it considerably alters hormone levels. Recurrence of symptoms is very common after cessation of therapy.

➤*Hereditary angioedema:* For the prevention of attacks of angioedema (eg, cutaneous, abdominal, laryngeal) in males and females.

➤*Unlabeled uses:* Danazol has been used to treat precocious puberty, gynecomastia, and menorrhagia. It has also been studied in the treatment of idiopathic immune thrombocytopenia, lupus-associated thrombocytopenia, and autoimmune hemolytic anemia.

Administration and Dosage

➤*Endometriosis:* Begin therapy during menstruation or make sure the patient is not pregnant. In moderate-to-severe disease, or in patients infertile because of endometriosis, administer 800 mg/day in 2 divided doses to best achieve amenorrhea and rapid response to painful symptoms. Downward titration to a dose sufficient to maintain amenorrhea may be considered depending upon response. Initially, for mild cases, give 200 to 400 mg in 2 divided doses. Individualize dosage. Continue therapy uninterrupted for 3 to 6 months; may extend to 9 months. If symptoms recur after termination, treatment can be reinstituted.

➤*Fibrocystic breast disease:* Begin therapy during menstruation or make sure patient is not pregnant. Dosage ranges from 100 to 400 mg/day in 2 divided doses. A nonhormonal method of contraception is recommended when danazol is administered at this dose because ovulation may not be suppressed.

Breast pain and tenderness are usually relieved by the first month and eliminated in 2 to 3 months; elimination of nodularity requires 4 to 6 months of uninterrupted therapy. Regular or irregular menstrual patterns and amenorrhea each occur in ≈ ⅓ of patients treated with ≥ 100 mg doses. Approximately 50% of patients may have recurring symptoms within 1 year; treatment may be reinstituted.

➤*Hereditary angioedema:* Individualize dosage. Recommended starting dose is 200 mg 2 or 3 times/day. After a favorable initial response, determine continuing dosage by decreasing the dosage by ≤ 50% at intervals of ≥ 1 to 3 months if frequency of attacks prior to treatment dictates. If an attack occurs, increase dosage by ≤ 200 mg/day. During the dose-adjusting phase, monitor response closely, particularly if patient has a history of airway involvement.

➤*Storage/Stability:* Store at controlled room temperature, 15° to 30°C (59° to 86°F).

Actions

➤*Pharmacology:* A synthetic androgen derived from ethisterone, danazol suppresses the pituitary-ovarian axis by inhibiting the output of pituitary gonadotropins. It also has weak, androgenic activity. Danazol depresses the output of both follicle-stimulating hormone (FSH) and luteinizing hormone (LH). Evidence suggests direct inhibitory effect at gonadal sites and a binding of danazol to receptors of gonadal steroids at target organs. In addition, danazol has been shown to significantly decrease IgG, IgM, and IgA levels, as well as phospholipid and IgG isotope autoantibodies in patients with endometriosis and associated elevations of autoantibodies. Generally, the pituitary suppressive action is reversible. Ovulation and cyclic bleeding usually return within 60 to 90 days after therapy is discontinued.

Endometriosis – In the treatment of endometriosis, danazol alters the normal and ectopic endometrial tissue so that it becomes inactive and atrophic. Complete resolution of endometrial lesions occurs in the majority of cases. Changes in vaginal cytology and cervical mucus reflect the suppressive effect of danazol on the pituitary-ovarian axis.

Hereditary angioedema – Danazol prevents attacks of the disease characterized by episodic edema of the abdominal viscera, extremities, face, and airway that may be disabling and, if the airway is involved, fatal. In addition, danazol partially or completely corrects the primary biochemical abnormality of hereditary angioedema. It increases the levels of the deficient C1 esterase inhibitor, thereby increasing the serum levels of the C4 component of the complement system.

➤*Pharmacokinetics:* Blood levels of danazol do not increase proportionately with increases in dose. When the dose is doubled, plasma levels increase only ≈ 35% to 40%.

Contraindications

Undiagnosed abnormal genital bleeding; markedly impaired hepatic, renal, or cardiac function.

Pregnancy and lactation.

Patients with porphyria. Danazol can induce aminolevulinate acid (ALA) synthetase activity and hence porphyrin metabolism.

Warnings

➤*Thrombotic events:* Thromboembolism, thrombotic and thrombophlebitic events including sagittal sinus thrombosis and life-threatening or fatal strokes have been reported.

➤*Hepatic events:* Experience with long-term therapy with danazol is limited. Peliosis hepatis and benign hepatic adenoma have been observed with long-term use. Peliosis hepatis and hepatic adenoma may be silent until complicated by acute, potentially life-threatening intra-abdominal hemorrhage. Therefore, alert the physician to this possibility. Make attempts to determine the lowest dose that will provide adequate protection. If the drug was begun at a time of exacerbation of hereditary angioneurotic edema because of trauma, stress, or other cause, consider periodic attempts to decrease or withdraw therapy.

➤*Intracranial hypertension:* Danazol has been associated with several cases of benign intracranial hypertension (also known as pseudotumor cerebri). Early signs and symptoms of benign intracranial hypertension include papilledema, headache, nausea and vomiting, and visual disturbances. Screen patients with these symptoms for papilledema and, if present, advise the patients to discontinue danazol immediately and refer them to a neurologist for further diagnosis and care.

➤*Lipoprotein alterations:* A temporary alteration of lipoproteins in the form of decreased high density lipoproteins (HDL) and possibly increased low density lipoproteins (LDL) has been reported during danazol therapy. These alterations may be marked, and prescribers should consider the potential impact on the risk of atherosclerosis and coronary artery disease in accordance with the potential benefit of the therapy to the patient.

➤*Carcinoma of the breast:* Exclude carcinoma of the breast before initiating therapy for fibrocystic breast disease. Nodularity, pain, and tenderness because of fibrocystic disease may prevent recognition of underlying carcinoma; therefore, if any nodule persists or enlarges during treatment, rule out carcinoma.

➤*Long-term experience:* Long-term experience with danazol is limited. Long-term therapy with other steroids alkylated at the 17 position has been associated with serious toxicity (eg, cholestatic jaundice, peliosis hepatis). Similar toxicity may develop after long-term danazol. Determine the lowest dose that will provide adequate protection. If the drug was begun for exacerbation of angioneurotic edema because of trauma, stress, or another cause, consider decreasing or withdrawing therapy periodically.

DANAZOL

➤*Androgenic effects:* Androgenic effects may not be reversible even when the drug is discontinued. Watch patients closely for signs of virilization.

➤*Pregnancy: Category X.* Use of danazol in pregnancy is contraindicated. A sensitive test (eg, beta subunit test if available) capable of determining early pregnancy is recommended immediately prior to start of therapy. Additionally, a nonhormonal method of contraception should be used during therapy. If a patient becomes pregnant while taking danazol, discontinue administration of the drug and apprise the patient of the potential risk to the fetus. Exposure to danazol in utero may result in androgenic effects on the female fetus; reports of clitoral hypertrophy, labial fusion, urogenital sinus defect, vaginal atresia, and ambiguous genitalia have been received.

In rabbits, the administration of danazol on days 6 to 18 of gestation at doses of ≥ 60 mg/kg/day (2 to 4 times the human dose) resulted in inhibition of fetal development.

➤*Lactation:* Breastfeeding is contraindicated in patients taking danazol.

➤*Children:* Safety and efficacy in pediatric patients has not been established.

Precautions

➤*Monitoring:*

Fluid retention – Conditions influenced by edema (eg, epilepsy, migraine, cardiac or renal dysfunction) require careful observation.

Hepatic dysfunction – Hepatic dysfunction has been reported manifested by modest increases in serum transaminase levels; perform periodic liver function tests.

Lipoproteins – Monitor HDL and LDL periodically.

Semen – Semen should be checked for volume, viscosity, sperm count, and motility.

➤*Porphyria:* Danazol administration has been reported to cause exacerbation of the manifestations of acute intermittent porphyria.

Drug Interactions

Danazol Drug Interactions			
Precipitant drug	Object drug*		Description
Danazol	Carbamazepine	↑	Therapy with danazol may cause an increase in carbamazepine levels in patients taking both drugs.
Danazol	Cyclosporine	↑	Increased cyclosporine blood concentrations with possible toxicity (eg, nephrotoxocity) has occurred. Monitor serum bilirubin, serum creatinine, and cyclosporine concentrations in patients receiving concomitant therapy. Adjust doses of drugs as needed.
Danazol	Warfarin	↑	Prolongation of prothrombin time has been reported with concomitant use.

* ↑ = Object drug increased.

➤*Drug / Lab test interactions:* Danazol treatment may interfere with laboratory determinations of testosterone, androstenedione, and dehydroepiandrosterone.

Abnormalities in laboratory tests may occur during therapy with danazol including the following: CPK, glucose tolerance, glucagon, thyroid-binding globulin, sex hormone-binding globulin, other plasma proteins, lipids, and lipoproteins.

Adverse Reactions

Androgenic – Acne; edema; mild hirsutism; changes in the voice (eg, hoarseness, sore throat, instability, deepening of pitch); oily skin or hair; weight gain; seborrhea; hair loss; clitoral hypertrophy (rare).

➤*GU:* Menstrual disturbances including spotting; alteration of the timing of the cycle; amenorrhea. Although cyclical bleeding and ovulation usually return within 60 to 90 days after discontinuation of therapy with danazol, persistent amenorrhea has occasionally been reported. In the male, a modest reduction in spermatogenesis may occur during treatment. Abnormalities in semen volume, viscosity, sperm count, and motility may occur with long-term therapy.

Hypoestrogenic – Flushing; sweating; vaginal dryness/irritation; reduction in breast size; nervousness; emotional lability.

➤*Hepatic:* Dysfunction (elevated serum enzymes or jaundice) has been reported in patients receiving ≥ 400 mg/day. It is recommended that patients receiving danazol be monitored for hepatic dysfunction by laboratory tests and clinical observation. Serious hepatic toxicity, including cholestatic jaundice, peliosis hepatis, and hepatic adenoma has been reported.

➤*The following have been reported, but the causal relationship is not confirmed:*

CNS – Dizziness; headache; nervousness; emotional lability; fainting; weakness; Guillain-Barré syndrome; sleep disorders; fatigue; tremor; parasthesias; visual disturbances; anxiety; depression and changes in appetite; benign intracranial hypertension, convulsions (rare).

Dermatologic – Rashes (eg, maculopapular, vesicular, papular, purpuric, petechial); sun sensitivity, Stevens-Johnson syndrome (rare).

GI – Gastroenteritis; nausea; vomiting; constipation; pancreatitis (rare).

GU – Hematuria; prolonged posttherapy amenorrhea.

Hematologic – Increase in red cell and platelet count; reversible erythrocytosis, leukocytosis, or polycythemia; eosinophilia; leukopenia; thrombocytopenia.

Hypersensitivity – Urticaria, pruritus; nasal congestion (rare).

Musculoskeletal – Muscle cramps or spasms; pains; joint pain; joint lock-up; joint swelling; pain in back, neck, or extremities; carpal tunnel syndrome (rare, may be secondary to fluid retention).

Miscellaneous – Change in libido; elevated blood pressure; chills; increased insulin requirements in diabetic patients; cataracts, bleeding gums, fever, pelvic pain, nipple discharge, malignant liver tumors (after long term use) (rare).

Patient Information

Notify physician if masculinizing effects occur (eg, abnormal growth of facial or other fine body hair, deepening of the voice).

Use nonhormonal contraceptive measures during therapy. Discontinue use if pregnancy is suspected.

Androgen Hormone Inhibitor

FINASTERIDE

Rx	**Propecia** (Merck)	**Tablets:** 1 mg	Lactose. (P Propecia). Tan. Octagonal. Film-coated. In unit-of-use 30s.
Rx	**Proscar** (Merck)	**Tablets:** 5 mg	Lactose. (MSD 72 Proscar). Blue. Apple shape. Film-coated. In unit-of-use 30s and 100s and UD 100s.

Indications

►*Benign prostatic hyperplasia (BPH):* Treatment of symptomatic BPH in men with an enlarged prostate to improve symptoms, reduce acute urinary retention risk, and reduce the risk of the need for surgery including transurethral resection of the prostate (TURP) and prostatectomy.

►*Androgenetic alopecia:* Treatment of male pattern hair loss (vertex and anterior mid-scalp).

►*Unlabeled uses:* Finasteride is being investigated in combination with flutamide as adjuvant therapy following radical prostatectomy. Other potential uses include prevention of the progression of first-stage prostate cancer, treatment of acne in women, and hirsutism; however, studies are needed to assess these uses.

Administration and Dosage

►*Approved by the FDA:* June 19, 1992.

►*Benign prostatic hyperplasia:* The recommended dose is 5 mg once a day, with or without meals.

Prior to initiating therapy, appropriately evaluate to identify other conditions that might mimic BPH, such as infection, prostate cancer, stricture disease, hypotonic bladder, or other neurogenic disorders.

Although early improvement may be seen, $\geq$ 6 to 12 months of therapy may be necessary to assess whether a beneficial response has been achieved. Perform periodic follow-up evaluations to determine whether a clinical response has occurred. Most treated patients experience a rapid regression of the enlarged prostate gland; $\approx$ 50% experience an increase in urinary flow and improvement in BPH symptoms following 12 months of finasteride treatment.

►*Androgenetic alopecia:* The recommended dosage is 1 mg once a day, with or without meals. In general, daily use $\geq$ 3 months is necessary before benefit is observed. Continued use is recommended to sustain benefit. Withdrawal of treatment leads to reversal of effect within 12 months.

►*Hepatic function impairment:* Use caution in those patients with liver function abnormalities because finasteride is metabolized extensively in the liver.

Actions

►*Pharmacology:* Finasteride, a synthetic 4-azasteroid compound, is a specific inhibitor of steroid 5α-reductase, an intracellular enzyme that converts testosterone into the androgen 5α-dihydrotestosterone (DHT). It has a 100-fold selectivity for Type II 5α-reductase over the Type I isozyme and lacks affinity for the androgen receptor. The Type II 5α-reductase isozyme is primarily found in the prostate, seminal vesicles, epididymides, and hair follicles as well as the liver, and is responsible for two-thirds of circulating DHT.

Androgenetic alopecia and the development of the prostate gland is dependent on DHT. Inhibition of Type II 5α-reductase blocks the peripheral conversion of testosterone to DHT, resulting in significant decreases in serum and tissue DHT concentrations. Finasteride reduces prostatic (by $\leq$ 90%) and circulating (by $\leq$ 60% to 80%) DHT and prostate-specific antigen (PSA) levels (by 41% to 71%), and increases prostatic testosterone levels. In men with male pattern hair loss (androgenetic alopecia), the balding scalp contains miniaturized hair follicles and increased amounts of DHT; finasteride decreases scalp and serum DHT concentrations in these men.

►*Pharmacokinetics:*

Absorption/Distribution – Finasteride is well absorbed after oral administration with a bioavailability of 63% to 80%, which is unaffected by food. Maximum steady-state plasma levels of 9.2 and 37 ng/ml are reached in 1 to 2 hours after administration of 1 and 5 mg, respectively. Following IV infusion, the mean volume of distribution (Vd) is 76 L and the mean plasma clearance is 165 ml/min; mean elimination half-life is 4.8 and 6 hours following 1 and 5 mg/day dosing, respectively. Approximately 90% of circulating finasteride is bound to plasma proteins. Finasteride has been found to cross the blood-brain barrier. There is a slow accumulation phase after multiple dosing. After dosing with 5 mg/day for 17 days, plasma concentrations were 47% and 54% higher than after the first dose in men 45 to 60 years of age (n = 12) and $\geq$ 70 years of age (n = 12), respectively; mean trough concentrations were 6.2 and 8.1 ng/ml, respectively. Although steady state was not reached in this study, mean trough plasma concentration in another study in patients with BPH (mean age, 65 years) receiving 5 mg/day was 9.4 ng/ml after> 1 year of dosing. The elimination rate of finasteride is decreased in the elderly, but no dosage adjustment is necessary.

Metabolism/Excretion – Finasteride undergoes extensive hepatic metabolism through oxidative pathways to inactive compounds that are eliminated in the bile and feces; the mean urinary recovery of the parent drug within 24 hours of a dose was only 0.04%. A mean of 39% was excreted in the urine in the form of metabolites; 57% was excreted in the feces. The major compound isolated from urine was the monocarboxylic acid metabolite; virtually no unchanged drug was recovered. The t-butyl side chain monohydroxylated metabolite has been isolated from plasma. These metabolites possess $\leq$ 20% of the 5α-reductase inhibitory activity of finasteride. Approximately 90% is bound to plasma proteins. In 16 subjects receiving 5 mg/day, concentrations in semen ranged from undetectable (< 1 ng/ml) to 21 ng/ml. Based on a 5 ml ejaculate volume, the amount of finasteride in ejaculate was estimated to be 50- to 100-fold less than the dose of finasteride (5 mcg) that had no effect on circulating DHT levels in adults. In 35 men taking finasteride 1 mg daily for 6 weeks, 60% had undetectable levels. The mean finasteride level was 0.26 ng/ml and the highest level measured was 1.52 ng/ml. Estimated exposure through vaginal absorption would be up to 7.6 ng/day, 750 times lower than the no-effect dose for developmental abnormalities in Rhesus monkeys.

►*Clinical trials:*

Benign prostatic hyperplasia (BPH) – In 2 double-blind, placebo-controlled, 12-month studies in patients with BPH treated with 5 mg/day, statistically significant regression of the enlarged prostate gland was noted at the first evaluation at 3 months and was maintained through 36 months. Finasteride has also been evaluated in a separate double-blind, randomized, placebo-controlled 4-year multicenter study. A statistically significant improvement in symptoms was evident at 1 year in finasteride-treated patients vs placebo and was maintained through year 4. Data from these studies indicate an improvement in BPH-related symptoms, increased maximum urinary flow rates, and a decreasing prostate volume, suggesting that finasteride may arrest the disease process of BPH in men with an enlarged prostate.

Vertex baldness – The efficacy of finasteride was evaluated in 2 studies (n = 1553) in men with mild-to-moderate vertex baldness. Significant increases in hair count were demonstrated at 6 and 12 months in the finasteride group while significant hair loss was seen in the placebo group. At 12 months, a 107-hair difference (p < 0.001) within a 1-inch diameter circle was noted between groups. Hair count was maintained in the finasteride group for up to 24 months while the placebo group continued to show progressive hair loss. At 24 months, this resulted in a 138-hair difference between treatment groups (p < 0.001).

At 12 and 24 months, respectively, 14% and 17% of finasteride-treated men exhibited hair loss compared with 58% and 72% of men in the placebo group, while 65% and 80% of finasteride-treated men had increased hair growth compared with 37% and 47% in the placebo group. Finasteride did not appear to affect non-scalp body hair.

Anterior mid-scalp hair loss – A 12-month study (n = 326) assessed the efficacy of finasteride in men with hair loss in the anterior mid-scalp area with or without vertex balding. This study also demonstrated significant increases in hair count compared with placebo. Hair counts were obtained in the anterior mid-scalp area and did not include the area of bitemporal recession or the anterior hairline.

Contraindications

Hypersensitivity to finasteride or any component of this product; use in women or children; pregnancy or use in women who may potentially be pregnant, including handling of crushed or broken tablets (see Warnings).

Warnings

►*Hepatic function impairment:* Use caution in patients with liver function abnormalities because finasteride is metabolized extensively in the liver.

►*Carcinogenesis:* A statistically significant increase in the incidence of testicular Leydig cell adenomas and an increase in the incidence of Leydig cell hyperplasia was observed in mice at doses 228 and 23 times the human exposure, respectively.

►*Pregnancy: Category X.* In female rats, low doses of finasteride administered during pregnancy have produced abnormalities of the external genitalia in male offspring. Finasteride is contraindicated in women who are or may become pregnant. Because of the ability of 5α-reductase inhibitors to inhibit the conversion of testosterone to DHT, finasteride may cause abnormalities of the external genitalia of a male fetus of a pregnant woman who receives finasteride. No abnormalities were observed in female offspring exposed to any dose of finasteride in utero. If this drug is used during pregnancy, or if pregnancy occurs while taking this drug, apprise the woman of the potential hazard to the male fetus.

Because of the potential risk to a male fetus, a woman who is pregnant or who may become pregnant should not handle crushed or broken finasteride tablets.

►*Lactation:* Finasteride is not indicated for use in women. It is not known whether finasteride is excreted in breast milk.

FINASTERIDE

➤*Children:* Finasteride is not intended for use in pediatric patients; safety and efficacy have not been established.

Precautions

➤*Obstructive uropathy:* As not all patients with BPH demonstrate a response to finasteride, carefully monitor patients with large residual urinary volume or severely diminished urinary flow for obstructive uropathy. They may not be candidates for therapy.

➤*Prostate cancer evaluation:* Monitor patients with BPH for prostate cancer (eg, digital rectal examinations) prior to initiating therapy and periodically thereafter. A baseline PSA < 4 ng/ml does not exclude the diagnosis of prostate cancer.

Finasteride causes a decrease in serum PSA levels in patients with BPH even in the presence of prostate cancer. Consider this reduction of PSA levels when evaluating PSA laboratory data; it does not suggest a beneficial effect of finasteride on prostate cancer. In controlled clinical trials, finasteride did not appear to alter the rate of prostate cancer detection.

Carefully evaluate any sustained increases in PSA levels while on finasteride, including consideration of non-compliance to therapy.

Drug Interactions

➤*Drug/Lab test interactions:* PSA levels are decreased by ≈ 50% in patients with BPH treated with finasteride.

Adverse Reactions

Finasteride is generally well tolerated; adverse reactions usually have been mild and transient. The following reactions were reported in 12-month BPH and hair loss studies, respectively: Erectile dysfunction (3.7%, 1.3%); decreased libido (3.3%, 1.8%); decreased volume of ejaculate (2.8%, 0.8%). The annual incidence of drug-related sexual adverse experiences decreased with duration of treatment. Sexual adverse experiences resolved with continued treatment in > 60% of patients who reported them.

Post-marketing experience – Breast tenderness and enlargement; hypersensitivity reactions, including lip swelling and skin rash; and testicular pain have also been reported with finasteride.

Overdosage

Patients have received single doses up to 400 mg and multiple doses up to 80 mg/day for 3 months without adverse effects. Significant lethality was observed in male and female mice at single oral doses of 500 mg/kg and in female and male rats at single oral doses of 400 mg/kg and 1000 mg/kg, respectively.

Patient Information

Crushed or broken finasteride tablets should not be handled by a woman who is pregnant or who may become pregnant because of the potential for absorption of finasteride and the subsequent potential risk to the male fetus.

Inform patients that the volume of ejaculate may be decreased in some patients during treatment. This decrease does not appear to interfere with normal sexual function. However, impotence and decreased libido may occur.

DUTASTERIDE

| *Rx* | **Avodart** (GlaxoSmithKline) | **Capsules:** 0.5 mg | (GX CE2). Yellow, oblong. In 100s and UD 70s. |

Indications

➤*Benign prostatic hyperplasia (BPH):* For the treatment of symptomatic BPH in men with an enlarged prostate to improve symptoms, reduce the risk of acute urinary retention, and reduce the risk of the need for for BPH-related surgery.

Administration and Dosage

➤*Approved by the FDA:* October 9, 2002.

➤*Dose:* The recommended dose of dutasteride is 0.5 mg taken orally once daily. Swallow the capsules whole. Dutasteride may be administered with or without food.

➤*Storage/Stability:* Store at 25°C (77°F); excursions permitted to 15° to 30°C (59° to 86°F).

Actions

➤*Pharmacology:* Dutasteride inhibits the conversion of testosterone to 5α-dihydrotestosterone (DHT). DHT is the androgen primarily responsible for the initial development and subsequent enlargement of the prostate gland. Testosterone is converted to DHT by the enzyme 5α-reductase, which exists as 2 isoforms, type 1 and type 2. The type 2 isoenzyme is primarily active in the reproductive tissues while the type 1 isoenzyme is also responsible for testosterone conversion in the skin and liver.

Dutasteride is a competitive and specific inhibitor of type 1 and type 2 5α-reductase isoenzymes, with which it forms a stable enzyme complex. Dutasteride does not bind to the human androgen receptor.

Effect on DHT and testosterone – The maximum effect of daily doses of dutasteride on the reduction of DHT is dose dependent and is observed within 1 to 2 weeks. After 1 and 2 weeks of daily dosing with 0.5 mg dutasteride, median serum DHT concentrations were reduced by 85% and 90%, respectively. In patients with BPH treated with dutasteride 0.5 mg/day for 2 years, the median decrease in serum DHT was 94% at 1 year and 93% at 2 years. The median increase in serum testosterone was 19% at 1 and 2 years but remained within the physiologic range.

➤*Pharmacokinetics:*

Absorption – Following administration of a single 0.5 mg dose of a soft gelatin capsule, time to peak serum concentrations (T_{max}) of dutasteride occurs within 2 to 3 hours. Absolute bioavailability in 5 healthy subjects is approximately 60% (range, 40% to 94%). When the drug is administered with food, the maximum serum concentrations were reduced by 10% to 15%.

Distribution – Pharmacokinetic data following single and repeat oral doses show that dutasteride has a large volume of distribution (300 to 500 L). Dutasteride is highly bound to plasma albumin (99%) and alpha-1 acid glycoprotein (96.6%).

Metabolism/Excretion – Dutasteride is extensively metabolized in humans. While not all metabolic pathways have been identified, in vitro studies showed that dutasteride is metabolized by the CYP3A4 isoenzyme to 2 minor mono-hydroxylated metabolites. Dutasteride is not metabolized in vitro by human cytochrome P450 isozymes CYP1A2, CYP2C9, CYP2C19, and CYP2D6 at 2000 ng/mL (50-fold greater than steady-state serum concentrations). In human serum, following dosing to steady state, unchanged dutasteride, 3 major metabolites (4'-hydroxydutasteride, 1,2-dihydrodutasteride, and 6-hydroxydutasteride), and 2 minor metabolites (6,4'-dihydroxydutasteride and 15-hydroxydutasteride), as assessed by mass spectrometric response, have been detected. The absolute stereochemistry of the hydroxyl additions in the 6 and 15 positions is not known. In vitro, the 4'-hydroxydutasteride and 1,2-dihydrodutasteride metabolites are much less potent than dutasteride against both isoforms of human 5AR. The activity of 6β-hydroxydutasteride is comparable with that of dutasteride.

Dutasteride and its metabolites were excreted mainly in feces. As a percent of dose, there was approximately 5% unchanged dutasteride (approximately 1% to 15%) and 40% as dutasteride-related metabolites (approximately 2% to 90%). Only trace amounts of unchanged dutasteride were found in urine (less than 1%). Therefore, on average, the dose unaccounted for approximated 55% (range, 5% to 97%).

The terminal elimination half-life of dutasteride is approximately 5 weeks at steady state. The average steady-state serum dutasteride concentration was 40 ng/mL following 0.5 mg/day for 1 year. Following daily dosing, dutasteride serum concentrations achieve 65% of steady-state concentration after 1 month and approximately 90% after 3 months. Because of the long half-life of dutasteride, serum concentrations remain detectable (greater than 0.1 ng/mL) for up to 4 to 6 months after discontinuation of treatment.

Special populations –
Gender: Dutasteride is not indicated for use in women.
Renal function impairment: Less than 0.1% of a steady-state 0.5 mg dose of dutasteride is recovered in human urine, so no adjustment in dosage is anticipated for patients with renal impairment.
Hepatic function impairment: Because dutasteride is extensively metabolized, exposure could be higher in hepatically impaired patients.

Contraindications

In women and children; known hypersensitivity to dutasteride, other 5α-reductase inhibitors, or any component of the preparation.

Warnings

➤*Exposure of women/risk to male fetus:* Dutasteride is absorbed through the skin. Therefore, women who are pregnant or may be pregnant should not handle dutasteride capsules because of the possibility of absorption of dutasteride and the potential risk of a fetal anomaly to a male fetus. In addition, women should use caution whenever handling dutasteride capsules. If contact is made with leaking capsules, the contact area should be washed immediately with soap and water.

➤*Blood donation:* Men being treated with dutasteride should not donate blood until at least 6 months have passed following their last dose. The purpose of this deferred period is to prevent administration of dutasteride to a pregnant female transfusion recipient.

➤*CNS toxicity:* In rats and dogs, repeated oral administration of dutasteride resulted in some animals showing signs of nonspecific, reversible, centrally mediated toxicity, without associated histopathological changes at exposures 425- and 315-fold the expected clinical exposure (of parent drug), respectively.

DUTASTERIDE

➤*Hepatic function impairment:* Because dutasteride is extensively metabolized and has a half-life of approximately 5 weeks at steady state, use caution in the administration of dutasteride to patients with liver disease.

➤*Carcinogenesis:* In a 2-year carcinogenicity study in B6C3F1 mice at doses of 3, 35, 250, and 500 mg/kg/day for males and 3, 35, and 250 mg/kg/day for females, an increased incidence of benign hepatocellular adenomas was noted at 250 mg/kg/day (290-fold the expected clinical exposure to a 0.5 mg/day dose) in females only. Two of the 3 major human metabolites have been detected in mice. The exposure to these metabolites in mice is either lower than in humans or is not known.

In a 2-year carcinogenicity study in Han Wistar rats at doses of 1.5, 7.5, and 53 mg/kg/day for males and 0.8, 6.3, and 15 mg/kg/day for females, there was an increase in Leydig cell adenomas in the testes in males at 53 mg/kg/day (135-fold the expected clinical exposure). An increased incidence of Leydig cell hyperplasia was present at 7.5 mg/kg/day (52-fold the expected clinical exposure) and 53 mg/kg/day in male rats. A positive correlation between proliferative changes in the Leydig cells and an increase in circulating luteinizing hormone levels has been demonstrated with 5α-reductase inhibitors and is consistent with an effect on the hypothalamic-pituitary-testicular axis following 5α-reductase inhibition. At tumorigenic doses in rats, luteinizing hormone levels in rats were increased by 167%. In this study, the major human metabolites were tested for carcinogenicity at approximately 1 to 3 times the expected clinical exposure.

➤*Fertility impairment:* Treatment of sexually mature male rats with dutasteride at doses of 0.05, 10, 50, and 500 mg/kg/day (0.1- to 110-fold the expected clinical exposure of parent drug) for up to 31 weeks resulted in dose- and time-dependent decreases in fertility; reduced cauda epididymal (absolute) sperm counts but not sperm concentration (at 50 and 500 mg/kg/day); reduced weights of the epididymis, prostate, and seminal vesicles; and microscopic changes in the male reproductive organs. The fertility effects were reversed by week 6 of recovery at all doses, and sperm counts were normal at the end of a 14-week recovery period. The 5α-reductase-related changes consisted of cytoplasmic vacuolization of tubular epithelium in the epididymides and decreased cytoplasmic content of epithelium, consistent with decreased secretory activity in the prostate and seminal vesicles. The microscopic changes were no longer present at week 14 of recovery in the low-dose group and were partly recovered in the remaining treatment groups. Low levels of dutasteride (0.6 to 17 ng/mL) were detected in the serum of untreated female rats mated to males dosed at 10, 50, or 500 mg/kg/day for 29 to 30 weeks.

In a fertility study in female rats, oral administration of dutasteride at doses of 0.05, 2.5, 12.5, and 30 mg/kg/day resulted in reduced litter size, increased embryo resorption, and feminization of male fetuses (decreased anogenital distance) at doses of greater than or equal to 2.5 mg/kg/day (2- to 10-fold the clinical exposure of parent drug in men). Fetal body weights also were reduced at greater than or equal to 0.05 mg/kg/day in rats (less than 0.02-fold the human exposure).

➤*Pregnancy: Category X.* Dutasteride is contraindicated for use in women. It has not been studied in women because preclinical data suggest that the suppression of circulating levels of dihydrotestosterone may inhibit the development of the external genital organs in a male fetus carried by a woman exposed to dutasteride. Women who are pregnant or may be pregnant should not handle dutasteride capsules because of possible absorption of the drug.

Multiple animal studies with IV doses ranging from 400 to 2010 ng/day and oral doses ranging from 0.05 to 200 mg/kg/day showed reduction in fetal adrenal weights and fetal prostate weights, and increases in fetal ovarian and testis weights. Feminization of male fetuses and male offspring, increase in stillborn pups, reduced fetal body weight, increased incidences of skeletal variations, prolonged gestation, and a decrease in time to vaginal patency for female offspring were noted during the studies.

➤*Lactation:* It is not known whether dutasteride is excreted in human breast milk.

➤*Children:* Safety and effectiveness in the pediatric population have not been established.

Precautions

➤*Other urological diseases:* Lower urinary tract symptoms of BPH can be indicative of other urological diseases, including prostate cancer. Assess patients to rule out other urological diseases prior to treatment with dutasteride. Patients with a large residual urinary volume and/or severely diminished urinary flow may not be good candidates for 5α-reductase inhibitor therapy; carefully monitor them for obstructive uropathy.

Perform digital rectal examinations, as well as other evaluations for prostate cancer, on patients with BPH prior to initiating therapy with dutasteride and periodically thereafter.

Drug Interactions

➤*CYP450:* Based on the in vitro data, blood concentrations of dutasteride may increase in the presence of inhibitors of CYP3A4, such as ritonavir, ketoconazole, verapamil, diltiazem, cimetidine, and ciprofloxacin.

Dutasteride is not metabolized in vitro by human cytochrome P450 isozymes CYP1A2, CYP2C9, CYP2C19, and CYP2D6 at 2000 ng/mL (50-fold greater than steady-state serum concentrations). It also does not inhibit the in vitro metabolism of model substrates for the major human cytochrome P450 isoenzymes (CYP1A2, CYP2C9, CYP2C19, CYP2D6, and CYP3A4) at a concentration of 1000 ng/mL, 25 times greater than steady-state serum concentrations in humans.

➤*Drug/Lab test interactions:*

Effects on PSA – PSA levels generally decrease in patients treated with dutasteride as the prostate volume decreases. In approximately 50% of the subjects, a 20% decrease in PSA is seen within the first month of therapy. After 6 months of therapy, PSA levels stabilize to a new baseline that is approximately 50% of the pretreatment value. Results of subjects treated with dutasteride for up to 2 years indicate this 50% reduction in PSA is maintained. Therefore, establish a new baseline PSA concentration after 3 to 6 months of treatment with dutasteride.

Adverse Reactions

Dutasteride Drug-Related Adverse Events[1] over 24 Months (Pivotal Studies Pooled) (≥ 1%)				
	Adverse event onset			
Adverse events	Months 0 to 6	Months 7 to 12	Months 13 to 18	Months 19 to 24
Dutasteride (n)	(n = 2167)	(n = 1901)	(n = 1725)	(n = 1605)
Placebo (n)	(n = 2158)	(n = 1922)	(n = 1714)	(n = 1555)
Impotence				
Dutasteride	4.7	1.4	1	0.8
Placebo	1.7	1.5	0.5	0.9
Decreased libido				
Dutasteride	3	0.7	0.3	0.3
Placebo	1.4	0.6	0.2	0.1
Ejaculation disorder				
Dutasteride	1.4	0.5	0.5	0.1
Placebo	0.5	0.3	0.1	0
Gynecomastia[2]				
Dutasteride	0.5	0.8	1.1	0.6
Placebo	0.2	0.3	0.3	0.1

[1] A drug-related adverse event is one considered by the investigator to have a reasonable possibility of being caused by the study medication. In assessing causality, investigators were asked to select from 1 of 2 options: reasonably related to study medication or unrelated to study medication.

[2] Includes breast tenderness and breast enlargement.

➤*GU:*

Long-term treatment – The incidence of most drug-related sexual adverse events (impotence, decreased libido, ejaculation disorder) decreased with duration of treatment. The incidence of drug-related gynecomastia remained constant over the treatment period.

Overdosage

In volunteer studies, single doses of dutasteride up to 40 mg (80 times the therapeutic dose) for 7 days have been administered without significant safety concerns. In a clinical study, doses of 5 mg/day (10 times the therapeutic dose) were administered to 60 subjects for 6 months with no additional adverse effects to those seen at therapeutic doses of 0.5 mg.

➤*Treatment:* There is no specific antidote for dutasteride. Therefore, in cases of suspected overdosage, give symptomatic and supportive treatment as appropriate, taking the long half-life of dutasteride into consideration.

Patient Information

Instruct patients to read the Patient Information leaflet before starting therapy with dutasteride and to reread it upon prescription renewal for new information regarding the use of dutasteride.

Dutasteride capsules should not be handled by a woman who is pregnant or who may become pregnant because of the potential for absorption of dutasteride and the subsequent potential risk to a developing male fetus.

Inform patients that ejaculate volume may be decreased in some patients during treatment with dutasteride. This decrease does not appear to interfere with normal sexual function.

Men treated with dutasteride should not donate blood until at least 6 months have passed following their last dose to prevent pregnant women from receiving dutasteride through blood transfusion.

Effective February 27, 1991, these agents were switched to a *c-iii* status by the DEA because of their abuse potential.

These agents are derived from, or are closely related to, the androgen testosterone (see Androgens group monograph); they have androgenic as well as anabolic activity. Although these products possess a high-anabolic, low-androgenic activity ratio, the dissociation of anabolic from androgenic effects is incomplete and variable.

WARNING

Peliosis hepatis: Peliosis hepatis, a condition in which liver and sometimes splenic tissue is replaced with blood-filled cysts, has occurred in patients receiving androgenic anabolic steroids. These cysts are sometimes present with minimal hepatic dysfunction and have been associated with liver failure. They are often not recognized until life-threatening liver failure or intra-abdominal hemorrhage develops. Withdrawal of drug usually results in complete disappearance of lesions.

Liver cell tumors: Most often these tumors are benign and androgen-dependent, but fatal malignant tumors have occurred. Withdrawal of drug often results in regression or cessation of tumor progression. However, hepatic tumors associated with androgens or anabolic steroids are much more vascular than other hepatic tumors and may be silent until life-threatening intra-abdominal hemorrhage develops.

Blood lipid changes: Blood lipid changes associated with increased risk of atherosclerosis are seen in patients treated with androgens and anabolic steroids. These changes include decreased high-density lipoprotein and sometimes increased low-density lipoprotein. The changes may be very marked and could have a serious impact on the risk of atherosclerosis and coronary artery disease.

Indications

Refer to individual product monographs for approved indications of specific products.

➤*Anemia:* Androgens stimulate erythropoiesis and may be of value in the treatment of certain types of anemia.

➤*Hereditary angioedema:* Prophylactic use may decrease frequency and severity of attacks.

➤*Metastatic breast cancer:* For control of metastatic breast cancer in women.

Actions

➤*Pharmacology:* Anabolic steroids promote body tissue-building processes and reverse catabolic or tissue-depleting processes. Administer adequate calories and protein to achieve positive nitrogen balance. Whether this balance is of primary benefit in the utilization of protein-building dietary substances is not established.

During exogenous administration of anabolic androgens, endogenous testosterone release is inhibited through inhibition of pituitary luteinizing hormone (LH). At large doses, spermatogenesis may be suppressed through feedback inhibition of pituitary follicle-stimulating hormone (FSH).

The androgenic properties of anabolic agents may cause serious disturbances of growth and sexual development when given to young children. They suppress the gonadotropic functions of the pituitary and may exert a direct effect on testes.

Contraindications

Hypersensitivity to anabolic steroids; male patients with prostate or breast carcinoma; carcinoma of the breast in females with hypercalcemia; nephrosis; the nephrotic phase of nephritis; pregnancy (see Warnings); to enhance physical appearance or athletic performance (see Warnings).

Warnings

➤*Athletic performance:* Athletic performance is questionably modified by these agents and studies yield equivocal results. The athlete's motivation to use these steroids includes 1) increased muscle mass and strength; 2) decreased muscle recovery time allowing more frequent weight training; 3) decreased healing time after muscle injury; 4) increased aggressiveness. The increase in muscle size and weight gain is partially attributed to the increased sodium and water retention. Evidence suggests that if anabolic steroids increase lean muscle mass, the muscle tissue may be deficient in phosphate and structurally flawed. Although some athletes, previously trained in weight-lifting, who continue intensive weight-training and maintain a high-protein, high-calorie diet during steroid use may derive some benefit such as increased strength (due to reaching a chronic catabolic state), the serious health hazards associated with anabolic steroids minimize any real or perceived gain in performance. Effects of these agents may persist for up to 6 months after the last dose. Adverse effects may be serious and irreversible.

Steroid regimens – Steroid regimens used are often referred to as "stacking", "pyramiding" or "cycling". "Stacking", or "stacking the pyramid", describes the concurrent use of two or more agents at the same time, either using high doses or varying the dosage, possibly including both oral and injectable forms. This regimen is tapered upward, then downward, generally over 4 to 18 weeks, followed by a drug-free period over several months. "Pyramiding" follows the same concept but generally involves the use of a single agent. "Cycling" refers to the drug-free period which is used to aid in the preparation of an upcoming event in the hopes that the athlete will peak at the time of the contest. These regimens are used to achieve an optimal anabolic effect while minimizing side effects and detection during competition. Dosages used may be as high as 40 times the therapeutic amounts.

An abuse or addiction syndrome is now being recognized with the chronic use of these drugs. Long-term use can lead to a preoccupation with drug use, difficulty stopping despite side effects and drug craving. A type of withdrawal syndrome may be noted as well when drug levels fluctuate, with symptoms that are similar to those seen with alcohol, cocaine and narcotic withdrawal. To detect steroid use or abuse, be aware of physical, psychological and behavioral changes. Aggressive behavior is common in abusers.

In addition, athletes may ingest other drugs in an attempt to counteract short-term side effects of the steroids (eg, diuretics to minimize sodium and fluid retention).

➤*Elderly:* Geriatric patients treated with anabolic steroids may be at increased risk for the development of prostatic hypertrophy and prostatic carcinoma.

➤*Pregnancy: Category X.* Contraindicated because of possible fetal masculinization.

➤*Lactation:* It is not known whether anabolic steroids are excreted in breast milk. Because of the potential for serious adverse reactions in nursing infants, decide whether to discontinue nursing or to discontinue the drug.

➤*Children:* The adverse consequences of giving androgens to young children are not fully understood, but the possibility of causing serious disturbances does exist; weigh the possible benefits before instituting therapy in young children.

Anabolic agents may accelerate epiphyseal maturation more rapidly than linear growth in children, and the effect may continue for 6 months after the drug has been stopped. Therefore, monitor therapy by x-ray studies at 6 month intervals to avoid the risk of compromising adult height.

Safety and efficacy in children with hereditary angioedema or metastatic breast cancer (rarely found) have not been established.

Benzyl alcohol – Benzyl alcohol-containing products have been associated with a fatal "gasping syndrome" in premature infants. Refer to product listings.

Precautions

➤*Virilization:* Virilization in the female may occur. If amenorrhea or menstrual irregularities develop during treatment, discontinue the drug until etiology is determined.

➤*Leukemia:* Leukemia has been observed in patients with aplastic anemia treated with **oxymetholone**, but the role of oxymetholone is unclear.

➤*Edema:* Edema, with or without congestive heart failure, may occur. Concomitant administration of an adrenal steroid or ACTH may increase the edema. Use caution in patients with cardiac, renal or hepatic disease, epilepsy, migraine or other conditions that may be aggravated by fluid retention.

➤*Hypercalcemia:* Hypercalcemia may develop both spontaneously and as a result of hormonal therapy in women with disseminated breast carcinoma. Perform frequent urine and serum calcium level examinations. If hypercalcemia occurs, discontinue the drug.

➤*Diabetics:* Monitor carefully. Tolerance to glucose may be altered. Monitor urine or blood sugar closely.

➤*Seizure disorders:* Patients may note an increase in seizure frequency.

Drug Interactions

Anabolic Steroids Drug Interactions			
Precipitant drug	Object drug[*]		Description
Anabolic steroids	Anticoagulants	↑	The anticoagulant effect may be potentiated by 17-alkyl testosterone derivatives (eg, anabolic steroids). Avoid this combination if possible.
Anabolic steroids	Sulfonylureas	↑	The hypoglycemic action may be enhanced by methandrostenolone. Monitor blood glucose and observe patients for signs of hypoglycemia.

[*] ↑ = Object drug increased.

Anabolic Steroids

►*Drug / Lab test interactions:*

Glucose tests – Anabolic steroids have altered glucose tolerance tests. Monitor diabetics closely and adjust the insulin or oral hypoglycemic dosage accordingly.

Thyroid function tests – Decrease in protein-bound iodine (PBI), thyroxine-binding capacity, radioactive iodine uptake and an increase in T_3 uptake by resin; free thyroxine levels remain normal.

Miscellaneous – Altered metyrapone test.

Adverse Reactions

►*Endocrine:* Virilization is the most common undesirable effect. Acne occurs especially in women and prepubertal males. Anabolic steroids inhibit gonadotropin secretion.

Prepubertal males – The first signs of virilization are phallic enlargement and an increase in frequency of erections.

Postpubertal males – Acne; inhibition of testicular function with oligospermia; gynecomastia; testicular atrophy; chronic priapism; epididymitis; bladder irritability; change in libido; impotence.

Females – Hirsutism; acne; hoarseness or deepening of the voice; clitoral enlargement; change in libido; menstrual irregularities; male-pattern baldness. Voice changes, hirsutism and clitoral enlargement are usually not reversible even after prompt discontinuation. The use of estrogens with androgens will not prevent virilization in females. Masculinization of the fetus has occurred.

►*CNS:* Excitation; insomnia; habituation; depression.

►*Electrolyte disturbance:* Retention of sodium, chloride, water, potassium, phosphates and calcium; ankle swelling; decreased glucose tolerance.

►*GI:* Nausea; vomiting; diarrhea; cholestatic jaundice; hepatic necrosis; death; hepatocellular neoplasms and peliosis hepatis (long-term therapy; see Warning Box).

►*Lab test abnormalities:*

Liver function tests – BSP retention; increased AST, serum bilirubin and alkaline phosphatase.

Blood coagulation tests – May suppress clotting factors II, V, VII and X and increase prothrombin time.

►*Miscellaneous:* Increased creatinine and creatine excretion; increased serum cholesterol; premature closure of epiphyses in children; choreiform movement; increased serum cholesterol; increased serum levels of low-density lipoproteins and decreased levels of high-density lipoproteins.

Patient Information

►*Diabetic patients:* Glucose tolerance may be altered; monitor urine sugar closely and report abnormalities to physician.

►*Female patients:* Notify physician if hoarseness, deepening of the voice, male-pattern baldness, hirsutism, menstrual irregularities or acne occurs.

May cause nausea or GI upset.

Notify physician if nausea, vomiting, changes in skin color or ankle swelling occurs.

OXYMETHOLONE

c-iii	**Anadrol-50** (Syntex)	**Tablets:** 50 mg	Lactose. (Syntex 2902). White, scored. In 100s.

For complete prescribing information, refer to the Anabolic Steroids group monograph.

Indications

Anemias caused by deficient red cell production, acquired or congenital aplastic anemia, myelofibrosis and hypoplastic anemias due to the administration of myelotoxic drugs.

Administration and Dosage

►*Anemias:* 1 to 5 mg/kg/day. The usual effective dose is 1 to 2 mg/kg/day. Individualize dosage. Response is not often immediate; give for a minimum trial of 3 to 6 months. Following remission, some patients may be maintained without the drug, while others may be maintained on an established lower daily dosage. Continuous maintenance is usually necessary in patients with congenital aplastic anemia.

STANOZOLOL

c-iii	**Winstrol** (Ovation)	**Tablets:** 2 mg	Lactose. (W 53). Pink, scored. In 100s.

For complete prescribing information, refer to the Anabolic Steroids group monograph.

Indications

►*Hereditary angioedema:* Prophylactic use to decrease frequency and severity of attacks.

Administration and Dosage

Individualize dosage. Initial dosage is 2 mg 3 times a day. After a favorable response is obtained in terms of prevention of edematous attacks, decrease dosage at intervals of 1 to 3 months to a maintenance dosage of 2 mg/day. Some patients may be successfully managed on a 2 mg alternate day schedule. During dose-adjusting, closely monitor patient response, particularly if there is a history of airway involvement.

The prophylactic dose to be used prior to dental extraction, or other traumatic or stressful situations, has not been established and may be substantially larger.

Attacks of hereditary angioedema are generally infrequent in childhood, and the risks from stanozolol administration are substantially increased. Therefore, long-term prophylactic therapy is generally not recommended in children; consider the benefits and risks involved.

OXANDROLONE

c-iii	**Oxandrin** (Bio-Technology General Corp.)	**Tablets:** 2.5 mg	Lactose. (Gynex 1111). White, oval, scored. In 100s.
		10 mg	Lactose. (BTG 10). White, capsule shape. In 60s.

For complete prescribing information, refer to the Anabolic Steroids group monograph.

Indications

Adjunctive therapy to promote weight gain after weight loss following extensive surgery, chronic infections, or severe trauma, and in some patients who, without definite pathophysiologic reasons, fail to gain or to maintain normal weight; to offset the protein catabolism associated with prolonged administration of corticosteroids; for relief of the bone pain frequently accompanying osteoporosis.

►*Unlabeled uses:* Alcoholic hepatitis.

Orphan drug designation – Short stature associated with Turner syndrome; HIV wasting syndrome and HIV-associated muscle weakness.

Treatment IND – Constitutional delay of growth and puberty, which commonly is diagnosed when the height, pubertal development and bone age of an otherwise healthy adolescent are significantly below average for their chronological age.

Administration and Dosage

Individualize dosage. Use intermittent therapy.

►*Adults:* 2.5 mg 2 to 4 times daily. However, since the response of individuals to anabolic steroids varies, a daily dosage of as little as 2.5 mg or as much as 20 mg may be required to achieve the desired response. A course of therapy of 2 to 4 weeks is usually adequate. This may be repeated intermittently as indicated.

►*Children:* Total daily dosage is ≤ 0.1 mg/kg or ≤ 0.045 mg/lb. This may be repeated intermittently as indicated.

Anabolic Steroids

NANDROLONE DECANOATE

c-iii	**Nandrolone Decanoate** (Watson)	**Injection (In Oil):** 100 mg/ml	In 2 mL multiple-dose vials.[1]
c-iii	**Deca-Durabolin** (Organon)		In 2 ml vials.[1]
c-iii	**Nandrolone Decanoate** (Watson)	**Injection (In Oil):** 200 mg/ml	In 1 mL vials.[1]
c-iii	**Deca-Durabolin** (Organon)		In 1 ml vials.[1]

[1] In sesame oil with benzyl alcohol.

For complete prescribing information, refer to the Anabolic Steroids group monograph.

Indications

➤*Anemia:* Management of the anemia of renal insufficiency. This drug increases hemoglobin and red cell mass. Surgically induced anephric patients may be less responsive.

Administration and Dosage

If possible, therapy should be intermittent. Duration of therapy depends on response of the condition and appearance of adverse reactions.

Inject deeply IM, preferably into the gluteal muscle.

➤*Anemia of renal disease:*

Women – 50 to 100 mg/week.

Men – 100 to 200 mg/week.

Children (2 to 13 years of age) – Average dose is 25 to 50 mg every 3 to 4 weeks.

MIFEPRISTONE

| Rx[1] **Mifeprex** (Danco Labs) | **Tablets:** 200 mg | (MF). Light yellow, cylindrical, bi-convex. In single-dose blister packs containing 3 tablets. |

[1] Mifepristone will be supplied only to licensed physicians who sign and return a Prescriber's Agreement.

WARNING

If mifepristone results in incomplete abortion, surgical intervention may be necessary. Prescribers should determine in advance whether they will provide such care themselves or through other providers. Prescribers also should give patients clear instructions on whom to call and what to do in the event of an emergency following administration of mifepristone.

Prescribers should make sure that patients receive and have an opportunity to discuss the medication guide and patient agreement.

Indications

➤*Termination of intrauterine pregnancy:* For the medical termination of intrauterine pregnancy through 49 days of pregnancy. For purposes of this treatment, pregnancy is dated from the first day of the last menstrual period in a presumed 28-day cycle with ovulation occurring at mid-cycle. The duration of pregnancy may be determined from menstrual history and by clinical examination. Use an ultrasonographic scan if the duration of pregnancy is uncertain, or if ectopic pregnancy is suspected.

Remove any intrauterine device (IUD) before treatment with mifepristone begins.

Patients taking mifepristone must take 400 mcg of misoprostol 2 days after taking mifepristone unless a complete abortion has already been confirmed before that time.

Pregnancy termination by surgery is recommended in cases when mifepristone and misoprostol fail to cause termination of intrauterine pregnancy.

➤*Unlabeled uses:* Postcoital contraception/contragestation; intrauterine fetal death/nonviable early pregnancy; unresectable meningioma; endometriosis; Cushing's syndrome.

Administration and Dosage

Treatment with mifepristone and misoprostol for the termination of pregnancy requires 3 office visits by the patient. Mifepristone should be prescribed only by physicians who have read and understood the prescribing information. Mifepristone may be administered only in a clinic, medical office, or hospital, by or under the supervision of a physician able to assess the gestational age of an embryo and to diagnose ectopic pregnancies. Physicians must also be able to provide surgical intervention in cases of incomplete abortion or severe bleeding, or have made plans to provide such care through others, and be able to assure patient access to medical facilities equipped to provide blood transfusions and resuscitation, if necessary.

➤*Day 1:* Patients must read the medication guide and read and sign the patient agreement before mifepristone is administered.

Three 200 mg tablets (600 mg) of mifepristone are taken in a single oral dose.

➤*Day 3:* The patient returns to the health care provider 2 days after ingesting mifepristone. Unless abortion has occurred and has been confirmed by clinical examination or ultrasonographic scan, the patient takes two 200 mcg tablets (400 mcg) of misoprostol orally.

During the period immediately following the administration of misoprostol, the patient may need medication for cramps or GI symptoms. Give the patient instructions on what to do if significant discomfort, excessive bleeding or other adverse reactions occur and give a phone number to call if she has questions following the administration of misoprostol. In addition, provide the patient with the name and phone number of the physician who will be handling patient emergencies.

➤*Day-14, post-treatment examination:* Patients will return for a follow-up visit ≈ 14 days after the administration of mifepristone. The visit is very important to confirm by clinical examination or ultrasonographic scan that a complete termination of pregnancy has occurred.

According to data from US and French studies, women should expect to experience bleeding or spotting for an average of 9 to 16 days. Up to 8% of women may experience some type of bleeding for > 30 days. Persistence of heavy or moderate vaginal bleeding at this visit, however, could indicate an incomplete abortion.

Patients who have ongoing pregnancy at this visit have a risk of fetal malformation resulting from the treatment. Surgical termination is recommended to manage medical abortion treatment failures.

Adverse events, such as hospitalization, blood transfusion, ongoing pregnancy, or other major complications following the use of mifepristone and misoprostol must be reported to Danco Labs. Please provide a brief clinical and administrative synopsis of any such adverse events in writing to the following:

Medical Director
Danco Laboratories, LLC
PO Box 4816
New York, NY
10185
(877) 432-7596

For immediate consultation 24 hours a day, 7 days a week with an expert in mifepristone, call Danco Labs at (877) 432-7596.

Mifepristone will be supplied only to licensed physicians who sign and return a Prescriber's Agreement. Distribution of mifepristone will be subject to specific requirements imposed by the distributor, including procedures for storage, dosage tracking, damaged product returns, and other matters. Mifepristone is a prescription drug, although it will not be available to the public through licensed pharmacies.

➤*Storage/Stability:* Store at 25°C (77°F); excursions permitted to 15° to 30°C (59° to 86°F).

Actions

➤*Pharmacology:* The anti-progestational activity of mifepristone results from competitive interaction with progesterone at progesterone-receptor sites. Based on studies with various oral doses in several animal species (mouse, rat, rabbit, monkey), the compound inhibits the activity of endogenous or exogenous progesterone. The termination of pregnancy results.

Doses of ≥ 1 mg/kg of mifepristone antagonize the endometrial and myometrial effects of progesterone in women. During pregnancy, the compound sensitizes the myometrium to the contraction-inducing activity of prostaglandins.

Mifepristone also exhibits antiglucocorticoid and weak antiandrogenic activity. The activity of the glucocorticoid dexamethasone in rats was inhibited following doses of 10 to 25 mg/kg of mifepristone. Doses of ≥ 4.5 mg/kg in humans resulted in a compensatory elevation of adrenocorticotropic hormone (ACTH) and cortisol. Antiandrogenic activity was observed in rats following repeated administration of doses from 10 to 100 mg/kg.

➤*Pharmacokinetics:*

Absorption – Following oral administration of a single dose of 600 mg, mifepristone is rapidly absorbed, with peak plasma concentration of 1.98 mg/L occurring ≈ 90 minutes after ingestion. The absolute bioavailability of a 20 mg oral dose is 69%.

Distribution – Mifepristone is 98% bound to plasma proteins, albumin, and 1-acid glycoprotein. Binding to the latter protein is saturable, and the drug displays nonlinear kinetics with respect to plasma concentration and clearance. Following a distribution phase, elimination of mifepristone is slow at first (50% eliminated between 12 and 72 hours) and then becomes more rapid with a terminal elimination half-life of 18 hours.

Metabolism – Metabolism of mifepristone is primarily via pathways involving N-demethylation and terminal hydroxylation of the 17-propynyl chain. In vitro studies have shown that CYP450 3A4 is primarily responsible for the metabolism. The 3 major metabolites identified in humans are: 1) RU 42 633, most widely found in plasma and the N-monodemethylated metabolite; 2) RU 42 848, which results from the loss of 2 methyl groups from the 4-dimethylaminophenyl in position 11β; and 3) RU 42 698, which results from terminal hydroxylation of the 17-propynyl chain.

Excretion – By 11 days after a 600 mg dose of tritiated compound, 83% of the drug has been accounted for in the feces and 9% in the urine. Serum levels are undetectable by 11 days.

➤*Clinical trials:* Safety and efficacy data from the US clinical trials and from 2 French trials of mifepristone are reported below. The US trials provide safety data on 859 women and efficacy data on 827 women with gestation durations of ≤ 49 days (dated from the first day of the last menstrual period). In the 2 French clinical trials, safety evaluable data are available for 1800 women, while efficacy information is available for 1681 of these women. Success was defined as the complete expulsion of the products of conception without the need for surgical intervention. The overall rates of success and failure, shown by reason for failure, for the US and French studies appear in the table below.

In the US trials, 92.1% of the 827 subjects had a complete medical abortion. In 52 women (6.3%) expulsion occurred within 2 days, and resulted from the action of mifepristone (600 mg) alone, unaided by misoprostol, an analog of prostaglandin E2. All other women without an apparent expulsion took a 400 mcg dose of misoprostol 2 days after taking mifepristone. Many women (44.1%) in the US trial expelled the products of conception within 4 hours after taking misoprostol and 62.8% experienced expulsion within 24 hours after misoprostol administration. There were 65 women (7.9%) who received surgical interven-

MIFEPRISTONE

tions: 13 (1.6%) were medically indicated interventions during the study period, mostly for excessive bleeding; 5 (0.6%) interventions occurred at the patient's request; 39 women (4.7%) had incomplete abortions at the end of the study protocol; and 8 (1%) had ongoing pregnancies at the end of the study protocol.

Women who participated in the US trials reflect the racial and ethnic composition of American women. The majority of women (71.4%) were Caucasian, while 11.3% were African American, 10.9% were East Asian, and 4.7% were hispanic. A small percentage (1.7%) belonged to other racial or ethnic groups. Women aged 18 to 45 were enrolled in the trials. Nearly 66% of the women were < 30 years of age with a mean age of 27 years.

In the French trials, complete medical abortion occurred in 95.5% of the 1681 subjects, as shown in the following table. In 89 women (5.3%), complete abortion occurred within 2 days of taking mifepristone (600 mg). About 50.3% of the women in the French trials expelled the products of conception during the first 4 hours immediately following administration of misoprostol and 72.3% experienced expulsion within 24 hours after taking misoprostol. In total, 4.5% of women in the French trial ultimately received surgical intervention for excessive bleeding, incomplete abortions, or ongoing pregnancies at the end of the protocol.

Outcome Following Mifepristone and Misoprostol Treatment in US and French Trials[1] (%)		
	US trials (n = 827)	French trials (n = 1681)
Complete medical abortion	92.1	95.5
Timing of expulsion		
Before second visit	6.3	5.3
During second visit		
≤ 4 hours after misoprostol	44.1	50.3
After second visit		
> 4 hours but ≤ 24 hours after misoprostol	18.7	22
> 24 hours after misoprostol	8.2	8.6
Time of expulsion unknown	14.8	9.2
Surgical intervention	7.9	4.5
Reason for surgery		
Medically necessary interventions during study period	1.6	NA
Patient request	0.6	NA
Treatment of bleeding during study	NA	0.3
Incomplete expulsion at study end	4.7	2.9
Ongoing pregnancy at study end	1	1.3

[1] Oral mifepristone 600 mg was administered on day 1; oral misoprostol 400 mcg was given on day 3 (second visit).

Contraindications

Administration of mifepristone and misoprostol for the termination of pregnancy (the "treatment procedure") is contraindicated in patients with any of the following conditions:
- Confirmed or suspected ectopic pregnancy or undiagnosed adnexal mass (the treatment procedure will not be effective to terminate an ectopic pregnancy);
- IUD in place;
- Chronic adrenal failure;
- Concurrent long-term corticosteroid therapy;
- History of allergy to mifepristone, misoprostol, or other prostaglandin;
- Hemorrhagic disorders or concurrent anticoagulation therapy;
- Inherited porphyrias.

Because it is important to have access to appropriate medical care if an emergency develops, the treatment procedure is contraindicated if a patient does not have adequate access to medical facilities equipped to provide emergency treatment of incomplete abortion, blood transfusions, and emergency resuscitation during the period from the first visit until discharged by the administering physician.

Mifepristone should not be used by any patient who may be unable to understand the effects of the treatment procedure or to comply with its regimen. Instruct patients to review carefully the medication guide and the patient agreement provided with mifepristone and give a copy of the product label for their review. Patients should discuss their understanding of these materials with their health care providers, and retain the medication guide for later reference.

Warnings

▶*Bleeding:* Vaginal bleeding occurs in almost all patients during the treatment procedure. According to data from the US and French trials, women should expect to experience bleeding or spotting for an average of 9 to 16 days, while up to 8% of all subjects may experience some type of bleeding for ≥ 30 days. Bleeding was reported to last for 69 days in 1 patient in the French trials. In general, the duration of bleeding and spotting increased as the duration of the pregnancy increased.

In some cases, excessive bleeding may require treatment by vasoconstrictor drugs, curettage, administration of saline infusions, or blood transfusions. In the US trial, 4.8% of subjects received administration of uterotonic medications and 9 women (1%) received IV fluids. Vasoconstrictor drugs were used in 4.3% of all subjects in the French trials, and in 5.5% of women there was a decrease in hemoglobin of > 2 g/dl. Blood transfusions were administered in 1 of 859 subjects in the US trials and in 2 of 1800 subjects in the French trials. Because heavy bleeding requiring curettage occurs in ≈ 1% of patients, special care should be given to patients with hemostatic disorders, hypocoagulability, or severe anemia.

▶*Pregnancy termination confirmation:* Schedule patients for a return follow-up visit at ≈ 14 days after administration of mifepristone to confirm that the pregnancy is completely terminated and to assess the degree of bleeding. Vaginal bleeding is not evidence of the termination of pregnancy. Termination can be confirmed by clinical examination or ultrasonographic scan. Lack of bleeding following treatment, however, usually indicates failure. Medical abortion failures should be managed with surgical termination.

▶*Renal function impairment:* The effects of renal disease on the safety, efficacy, and pharmacokinetics of mifepristone have not been investigated.

▶*Hepatic function impairment:* The effects of hepatic disease on the safety, efficacy, and pharmacokinetics of mifepristone have not been investigated.

▶*Fertility impairment:* The pharmacological activity of mifepristone disrupts the estrus cycle of animals, precluding studies designed to assess effects on fertility during drug administration. Three studies have been performed in rats to determine whether there were residual effects on reproductive function after temination of the drug exposure.

In rats, administration of the lowest dose of 0.3 mg/kg/day caused severe disruption of the estrus cycles for the 3 weeks of the treatment period. Following resumption of the estrus cycle, animals were mated and no effect on reproductive performance was observed. In a neonatal exposure study in rats, the administration of a SC dose of mifepristone up to 100 mg/kg on the first day after birth had no adverse effect on future reproductive function in males or females. The onset of puberty was observed to be slightly premature in female rats neonatally exposed to mifepristone. In a separate study in rats, oviduct and ovary malformations in female rats, delayed male puberty, deficient male sexual behavior, reduced testicular size, and lowered ejaculation frequency were noted after exposure to mifepristone (1 mg every other day) as neonates.

▶*Elderly:* The effects of age on the safety, efficacy, and pharmacokinetics of mifepristone have not been investigated.

▶*Pregnancy:* Mifepristone is indicated for use in the termination of pregnancy (through 49 days of pregnancy) and has no other approved indication for use during pregnancy.

Over 620,000 women in Europe have taken mifepristone in combination with a prostaglandin to terminate pregnancy. Among these 620,000 women, ≈ 415,000 have received mifepristone together with misoprostol. As of May 2000 a total of 82 cases have been reported in which women with on-going pregnancies after using mifepristone alone or mifepristone followed by misoprostol declined to have a surgical procedure at that time. These cases are summarized in the following table.

Pregnancies Not Terminated by Surgical Abortion at the End of Mifepristone Alone or Mifepristone/Misoprostol Treatment[1]		
	Mifepristone alone (n = 42)	Mifepristone/ Misoprostol (n = 40)
Subsequently had surgical abortion	3	7
No abnormalities detected	2	7
Abnormalities detected (sirenomelia, cleft palate)	1	0
Subsequently resulted in live birth	13	13
No abnormalities detected at birth	13	13
Abnormalities detected at birth	0	0
Others/Unknown	26	20

[1] Reported cases as of May 2000.

Several reports in the literature indicate that prostaglandins, including misoprostol, may have teratogenic effects in human beings. Skull defects, cranial nerve palsies, delayed growth and psychomotor development, facial malformation, and limb defects have all been reported after first trimester exposure.

▶*Lactation:* It is not known whether mifepristone is excreted in human breast milk. Many hormones with a similar chemical structure, however, are excreted in breast milk. Because the effects of mifepristone on infants are unknown, breastfeeding women should consult with their health care provider to decide if they should discard their breast milk for a few days following administration of the medications.

▶*Children:* Safety and effectiveness in pediatric patients have not been established.

MIFEPRISTONE

Precautions

►*Monitoring:* Mifepristone is available only in single-dose packaging. Administration must be under the supervision of a qualified physician.

The use of mifepristone is assumed to require the same preventive measures as those taken prior to and during surgical abortion to prevent rhesus immunization.

There are no data on the safety and efficacy of mifepristone in women with chronic medical conditions such as cardiovascular, hypertensive, hepatic, respiratory, or renal disease; insulin-dependent diabetes mellitus; severe anemia; or heavy smoking. Treat women who are > 35 years of age and who also smoke ≥ 10 cigarettes/day with caution because such patients were generally excluded from clinical trials of mifepristone.

Although there is no clinical evidence, the effectiveness of mifepristone may be lower if misoprostol is administered > 2 days after mifepristone administration.

►*Lab test abnormalities:* Clinical examination is necessary to confirm the complete termination of pregnancy after the treatment procedure. Changes in quantitative human chorionic gonadotropin (hCG) levels will not be decisive until at least 10 days after the administration of mifepristone. A continuing pregnancy can be confirmed by ultrasonographic scan.

The existence of debris in the uterus following the treatment procedure will not necessarily require surgery for its removal.

Decreases in hemoglobin concentration, hematocrit, and red blood cell count occur in some women who bleed heavily. Hemoglobin decreases of > 2 g/dl occurred in 5.5% of subjects during the French clinical trials of mifepristone and misoprostol.

Clinically significant changes in serum enzyme (serum glutamic oxaloacetic transaminase [AST], serum glutamic pyruvic transaminase [ALT], alkaline phosphatase, gamma-glutamyltransferase [GGT]) activities were rarely reported.

Drug Interactions

Although specific drug or food interactions with mifepristone have not been studied, on the basis of this drug's metabolism by CYP 3A4, it is possible that ketoconazole, itraconazole, erythromycin, and grapefruit juice may inhibit its metabolism (increasing serum levels of mifepristone). Furthermore, rifampin, dexamethasone, St. John's wort, and certain anticonvulsants (eg, phenytoin, phenobarbital, carbamazepine) may induce mifepristone metabolism (lowering serum levels of mifepristone).

Based on in vitro inhibition information, coadministration of mifepristone may lead to an increase in serum levels of drugs that are CYP 3A4 substrates. Due to the slow elimination of mifepristone from the body, such interaction may be observed for a prolonged period after its administration. Therefore, exercise caution when mifepristone is administered with drugs that are CYP 3A4 substrates and have narrow therapeutic range, including some agents used during general anesthesia.

Adverse Reactions

The treatment procedure is designed to induce the vaginal bleeding and uterine cramping necessary to produce an abortion. Nearly all of the women who receive mifepristone and misoprostol will report adverse reactions, and many can be expected to report > 1 such reaction. About 90% of patients report adverse reactions following administration of misoprostol on day 3 of the treatment procedure. Those adverse events that occurred with a frequency > 1% in the US and French trials are shown in the following table.

Bleeding and cramping are expected consequences of the action of mifepristone as used in the treatment procedure. Following administration of mifepristone and misoprostol in the French clinical studies, 80% to 90% of women reported bleeding more heavily than they do during a heavy menstrual period. Women also typically experience abdominal pain, including uterine cramping. Other commonly reported side effects were nausea, vomiting, and diarrhea. Pelvic pain, fainting, headache, dizziness, and asthenia occurred rarely. Some adverse reactions reported during the 4 hours following administration of misoprostol were judged by women as being more severe than others: The percentage of women who considered any particular adverse event as severe ranged from 2% to 35% in the US and French trials. After the third day of the treatment procedure, the number of reports of adverse reactions declined progressively in the French trial, so that by day 14, reports were rare except for reports of bleeding and spotting.

Mifepristone and Misoprostol Adverse Events (> 1%)		
Adverse reaction	US trials	French trials
CNS		
Headache	31	2
Dizziness	12	1
Insomnia	3	NA
Anxiety	2	NA
Syncope	1	NA
Fainting	NA	2
GI		
Abdominal pain (cramping)	96	NA
Nausea	61	43
Vomiting	26	18
Diarrhea	20	12
Dyspepsia	3	NA
GU		
Uterine cramping	NA	83
Uterine hemorrhage	5	NA
Vaginitis	3	NA
Pelvic pain	NA	2
Hematologic		
Anemia	2	NA
Decrease in hemoglobin > 2 g/dl	NA	6
Miscellaneous		
Fatigue	10	NA
Back pain	9	NA
Fever	4	NA
Viral infections	4	NA
Rigors (chills/shaking)	3	NA
Asthenia	2	1
Leg pain	2	NA
Leukorrhea	2	NA
Sinusitis	2	NA
Fainting	NA	2

Overdosage

►*Symptoms:* No serious adverse reactions were reported in tolerance studies in healthy non-pregnant female and healthy male subjects in which mifepristone was administered in single doses > 3-fold that recommended for termination of pregnancy.

►*Treatment:* If a patient ingests a massive overdose, observe closely for signs of adrenal failure.

Patient Information

Fully advise patients of the treatment procedure and its effects. Give patients a copy of the medication guide and patient agreement. (Additional copies of the medication guide and patient agreement are available by contacting Danco Laboratories at [877] 432–7596.) Advise patients to review both the medication guide and the patient agreement, and give them the opportunity to discuss them and obtain answers to any questions they may have. Mifepristone should not be used by any patient who may be unable to understand the effects of the treatment procedure or to comply with its regimen. Each patient must understand the following:

• The necessity of completing the treatment schedule, including a follow-up visit ≈ 14 days after taking mifepristone;
• that vaginal bleeding and uterine cramping probably will occur;
• that prolonged or heavy vaginal bleeding is not proof of a complete expulsion;
• that if the treatment fails, there is a risk of fetal malformation;
• that medical abortion treatment failures are managed by surgical termination; and
• the steps to take in an emergency situation, including precise instructions and a telephone number that she can call if she has any problems or concerns.

Another pregnancy can occur following termination of pregnancy and before resumption of normal menses. Contraception can be initiated as soon as the termination of the pregnancy has been confirmed, or before the woman resumes sexual intercourse.

Patient information is included with each mifepristone package (see medication guide).

PROSTAGLANDINS

Dinoprostone is also used as an agent for cervical ripening. Refer to the specific monograph for complete information.

Indications

➤*For the termination of pregnancy from the following gestational weeks as calculated from the first day of the last normal menstrual period:*

Carboprost – 13 to 20 weeks.

Dinoprostone – 12 to 20 weeks.

➤*Carboprost:* Second trimester abortion characterized by failure of expulsion of the fetus during the course of treatment by another method; premature rupture of membranes in intrauterine methods with loss of drug and insufficient or absent uterine activity; requirement of a repeat intrauterine instillation of drug for expulsion of the fetus; inadvertent or spontaneous rupture of membranes in the presence of a previable fetus and absence of adequate activity for expulsion; postpartum hemorrhage due to uterine atony that has not responded to conventional management (prior treatment should include use of IV oxytocin, manipulative techniques such as uterine massage and, unless contraindicated, IM ergot preparations).

➤*Dinoprostone:* Evacuation of the uterine content in the management of missed abortion or intrauterine fetal death up to 28 weeks gestational age as calculated from the first day of the last normal menstrual period; management of nonmetastatic gestational trophoblastic disease (benign hydatidiform mole).

Actions

➤*Pharmacology:* Prostaglandins stimulate the myometrium of the gravid uterus to contract in a manner similar to that seen in the term uterus during labor. Mechanism of action has not been determined. The myometrial contractions induced are sufficient to produce uterine evacuation in the majority of cases. Postpartum, the resultant myometrial contractions provide hemostasis at the site of placentation.

These agents also stimulate the smooth muscle of the GI tract; this activity may be responsible for the vomiting or diarrhea that may occur with their use. Large doses of carboprost can elevate blood pressure, probably by contracting the vascular smooth muscle, but this has not been clinically significant with doses used for terminating pregnancy. In contrast, large doses of dinoprostone may lower blood pressure. Body temperature elevation may also occur with both drugs.

➤*Pharmacokinetics:*

Carboprost – In 2 postpartum women treated with a single IM injection of 250 mcg, the mean peak plasma concentration occurred at 15 minutes. With multiple dosing, average peak concentrations were slightly higher following each successive injection but always decreased to levels less than the preceding peak values by 2 hours after each administration.

Six metabolites have been identified. The liver appears to be the primary site for oxidation. Less than 1% of the drug is excreted unchanged in the urine. Urinary excretion of metabolites is rapid and nearly complete within 24 hours following IM administration. About 80% of the dose is excreted in the first 5 to 10 hours and an additional 5% in the next 20 hours.

Contraindications

Hypersensitivity to any of these agents; acute pelvic inflammatory disease; active cardiac, pulmonary, renal or hepatic disease.

Warnings

➤*Recommended dosages:* Use only in recommended dosages and only by medical personnel. Use in a hospital that can provide immediate intensive care and acute surgical facilities.

➤*Viable fetus:* Prostaglandins are not indicated if the fetus in utero has reached the stage of viability; they are not feticidal agents. They do not appear to directly affect the fetoplacental unit. Therefore, a previable fetus aborted by these agents could exhibit transient life signs.

➤*Pregnancy:* Category C. These drugs are embryotoxic in animals and any dose that produces increased uterine tone could put the embryo or fetus at risk. Animal studies suggest that certain prostaglandins may have teratogenic potential. Complete any failed attempts at pregnancy termination with these drugs by some other means.

Precautions

➤*Special risk patients:* Use cautiously in patients with a history of asthma, hypotension or hypertension, cardiovascular, renal or hepatic disease, anemia, jaundice, diabetes, epilepsy, or a compromised (scarred) uterus.

➤*Incomplete abortion:* Prostaglandin-induced abortion may sometimes be incomplete (incidence with **carboprost** is about 20%). In such cases, take other measures to ensure complete abortion.

➤*Chorioamnionitis:* Use **carboprost** with caution in patients with chorioamnionitis. During clinical trials, chorioamnionitis was a complication contributing to postpartum uterine atony and hemorrhage in 7% of cases, 3 of which failed to respond to carboprost. This complication

during labor may inhibit the uterine response to carboprost, similar to that reported with other oxytocic agents.

➤*Pyrexia:* Transient pyrexia due to hypothalamic thermoregulation may be seen. Temperature elevations exceeding 1.1°C (2°F) were observed in ≈ 12% of patients receiving carboprost and 50% of those receiving dinoprostone. Of those experiencing temperature elevation, ≈ 6% had a clinical diagnosis of endometritis. The remaining temperature returned to normal when therapy ended. Force fluids in patients with drug-induced fever and no clinical or bacteriological evidence of intrauterine infection. Other simple empirical measures for temperature reduction are unnecessary because of the transient or self-limiting nature of the drug-induced fever.

Differentiation of postabortion endometritis from drug-induced temperature elevations is difficult; the distinctions are summarized in the following table.

Differentiation of Endometritis vs Prostaglandin-Induced Pyrexia		
Parameter	Endometritis pyrexia	Prostaglandin-induced pyrexia
Onset	Typically, on the third day after abortion (≥ 38°C; ≥ 102°F).	Within 1 to 16 hours. after the first injection of carboprost; within 15 to 45 minutes. of dinoprostone suppository.
Duration	Untreated pyrexia and infection continue and may give rise to other pelvic infections.	Temperatures return to pretreatment levels after discontinuation of carboprost therapy (within 2 to 6 hours for dinoprostone).
Retention	Products of conception often retained in cervical os or uterine cavity.	Temperature elevation occurs whether or not tissue is retained.
Histology	Endometrium infiltrated with lymphocytes; some areas are necrotic and hemorrhagic.	Endometrial stroma may be edematous and vascular, but not inflamed.
Uterus	Remains boggy with tenderness over the fundus; pain on moving the cervix on bimanual examination.	Uterine involution normal. Uterus is not tender.
Discharge	Foul smelling lochia and leukorrhea.	Lochia normal.
Cervical culture	The culture of pathological organisms from the cervix or uterine cavity after abortion alone does not warrant the diagnosis of septic abortion in the absence of clinical evidence of sepsis. Pathogens have been cultured soon after abortion in patients with no infections. Persistent positive culture with clear clinical signs of infections are significant in the differential diagnosis.	
Blood count	Leukocytosis and differential white cell counts do not distinguish between endometritis and prostaglandin hyperthermia, because total WBCs may increase during infection and transient leukocytosis may also be drug-induced.	

➤*Cervical trauma:* Although the incidence of cervical trauma is extremely small, always carefully examine the cervix immediately postabortion.

➤*Intrauterine fetal death confirmation:* When a pregnancy diagnosed as missed abortion is electively interrupted with intravaginal **dinoprostone**, confirm intrauterine fetal death with a negative pregnancy test for chorionic gonadotropic activity (UCG test or equivalent). When a pregnancy with late fetal intrauterine death is interrupted with intravaginal dinoprostone, first confirm intrauterine fetal death.

➤*Vaginal conditions:* Use **dinoprostone** suppositories with caution in the presence of cervicitis, infected endocervical lesions or acute vaginitis.

➤*Bone effects:* High dose animal studies lasting several weeks have shown that prostaglandins of the E and F series can induce proliferation of bone. Such effects have also been noted in neonates who have received prostaglandin E$_1$ during prolonged treatment. There is no evidence that short-term use can cause similar effects.

➤*GI effects:* The pretreatment or concurrent administration of antiemetic and antidiarrheal drugs decreases the incidence of GI effects. Their use is an integral part of the management of patients undergoing abortion.

➤*Increased blood pressure:* When used for postpartum hemorrhage, 4% of patients treated with **carboprost** had a moderate increase in blood pressure. It is not certain whether this hypertension was due to a direct effect of carboprost or a return to a status of pregnancy-associated hypertension manifested by the correction of hypovolemic shock.

Drug Interactions

➤*Oxytocics:* The activity of oxytocic agents may be augmented by the prostaglandins. Concomitant use is not recommended.

Abortifacients

PROSTAGLANDINS

Adverse Reactions

Prostaglandin Adverse Reactions

Adverse reaction	Carboprost	Dinoprostone
Cardiovascular		
Arrhythmias	✓	✓
Chest pain/tightness	✓	✓
CNS		
Headache	✓	10%
Flushing	7%	✓
Anxiety/Tension	✓	✓
Hot flashes	✓	✓
Paresthesia	✓	✓
Syncope/Dizziness	✓	✓
Weakness	✓	✓
GI		
Vomiting	✓[1]	66%
Diarrhea	✓[1]	40%
Nausea	33%	33%
GU		
Endometritis	✓	✓
Uterine rupture	✓	✓
Uterine/Vaginal pain	✓	✓
Respiratory		
Coughing	✓	✓
Dyspnea/Wheezing	✓	✓
Other		
Chills/Shivering	✓	10%
Backache	✓	✓
Blurred vision	✓	✓
Breast tenderness	✓	✓

Prostaglandin Adverse Reactions

Adverse reaction	Carboprost	Dinoprostone
Diaphoresis	✓	✓
Eye pain	✓	✓
Muscle cramp/pain	✓	✓
Pyrexia/Fever	✓	✓
Rash	✓	✓
Leg cramps	✓	✓

✓ = Occurs, no incidence reported.
[1] Incidence may be decreased with pretreatment or concurrent use of antiemetics/antidiarrheals.

Other adverse reactions reported (not all clearly drug-related) include the following:

Carboprost – Hiccoughs; drowsiness; dystonia; asthma; injection site pain; tinnitus; sleep disorders; posterior cervical perforation; epigastric pain; thirst; twitching eyelids; gagging; retching; dry throat; choking sensation; thyroid storm; palpitations; vertigo; vasovagal syndrome; dry mouth; hyperventilation; respiratory distress; tachycardia; hematemesis; taste alterations; urinary tract infections; septic shock; torticollis; lethargy; endometritis from UCD; nosebleed; upper respiratory infection; retained placental fragments; shortness of breath; fullness of throat; uterine sacculation; faintness; lightheadedness; hypertension; perforated uterus; nervousness; pulmonary edema.

The most common complications when carboprost was used for abortion requiring additional treatment after hospital discharge were endometritis, retained placental fragments and excessive uterine bleeding ($\approx 2\%$).

Dinoprostone – Joint inflammation; arthralgia; myalgia; vaginitis; vulvitis; stiff neck; dehydration; tremor; hearing impairment; urine retention; pharyngitis; laryngitis; skin discoloration; vaginismus; myocardial infarction (patients with a history of cardiovascular disease); transient diastolic blood pressure decreases of > 20 mm Hg ($\approx 10\%$).

CARBOPROST TROMETHAMINE

Rx	Hemabate (Pharmacia & Upjohn)	Injection: 250 mcg carboprost and 83 mcg tromethamine per ml	9 mg sodium chloride, 9.45 mg benzyl alcohol. In 1 ml amps.[1]

[1] With 9.45% benzyl alcohol and 9 mg sodium chloride per ml.

For complete prescribing information, see the Prostaglandins group monograph.

Indications

➤*Abortion:* Indicated for aborting pregnancy between the 13th and 20th weeks of gestation as calculated from the first day of the last normal menstrual period and in the following conditions related to second trimester abortion:

1.) Failure of expulsion of the fetus during the course of treatment by another method;
2.) Premature rupture of membranes in intrauterine methods with loss of drug and insufficient or absent uterine activity;
3.) Requirement of a repeat intrauterine instillation of drug for expulsion of the fetus;
4.) Inadvertent or spontaneous rupture of membranes in the presence of a previable fetus and absence of adequate activity for expulsion.

➤*Postpartum uterine hemorrhage:* For the treatment of postpartum hemorrhage due to uterine atony that has not responded to conventional methods of managment. Prior treatment should include the use of IV administered oxytocin, manipulative techniques such as uterine massage and, unless contraindicated, IM ergot preparations.

Administration and Dosage

➤*Abortion:* For IM use only. Administer an initial dose of 250 mcg (1 ml) by deep IM injection. Give subsequent doses of 250 mcg at 1.5 to 3.5 hour intervals, depending on uterine response. The dose may be increased to 500 mcg (2 ml) if uterine contractility is inadequate after several 250 mcg (1 ml) doses.

An optional test dose – An optional test dose of 100 mcg (0.4 ml) may be administered initially.

Do not exceed a 12 mg total dose or continuous administration for > 2 days.

➤*Storage/Stability:* Refrigerate at 2° to 8°C (36° to 46°F).

DINOPROSTONE (Prostaglandin E₂)

Rx	Prostin E2 (Pharmacia & Upjohn)	Vaginal suppository: 20 mg	In foil strips of 5 individually sealed suppositories.

For complete prescribing information, refer to the Prostaglandins group monograph.

Indications

➤*Pregnancy termination:* Indicated for the termination of pregnancy from the 12th through the 20th gestational week as calculated from the first day of the last normal menstrual period.

➤*Uterine content evacuation:* Indicated for evacuation of the uterine contents in the management of missed abortion or intrauterine fetal death up to 28 weeks of gestational age as calculated from the first day of the last normal menstrual period.

➤*Nonmetastatic gestational trophoblastic disease:* Indicated in the management of nonmetastatic gestational trophoblastic disease (benign hydatidiform mole).

Administration and Dosage

Insert one suppository (20 mg) high into the vagina. The patient should remain supine for 10 minutes following insertion. Administer each subsequent suppository at 3 to 5 hour intervals until abortion occurs. Within the above recommended intervals, determine administration time by abortifacient progress, uterine contractility response, and by patient tolerance. Continuous administration for > 2 days is not advisable.

➤*Unlabeled administration and dosage:* Dinoprostone 20 mg suppositories have been used for cervical ripening by compounding into a low-dose gel formula. However, the manufacturer states that the suppository should not be used for extemporaneous preparation of any other dosage form, and that neither the suppository nor any extemporaneous formulation should be used for cervical ripening or any other indication at term pregnancy. Dinoprostone is commercially available as a vaginal insert and gel specifically for cervical ripening; only these products should be used for this purpose (see specific monograph).

➤*Storage/Stability:* Store in a freezer not above –20°C (–4°F); bring to room temperature just prior to use.

DINOPROSTONE (Prostaglandin E₂; PGE₂)

Rx	**Prepidil** (Upjohn)	**Gel:** 0.5 mg	In 3 g (2.5 ml) syringes[1] with 2 shielded catheters (10 and 20 mm tip).
Rx	**Cervidil** (Forest)	**Vaginal insert:** 10 mg	In 1s.

[1] With 240 mg colloidal silicon dioxide NF and 2760 mg triacetin, USP.

Dinoprostone is also used as an abortifacient. Refer to the Abortifacients monograph.

Indications

➤*Cervical ripening:* For initiation or continuation of cervical ripening in pregnant women at or near term with a medical or obstetrical need for labor induction.

Administration and Dosage

➤*Gel:* Use with caution in handling this product to prevent contact with skin. Wash hands thoroughly with soap and water after administration.

Preparation for use – Bring to room temperature (15° to 30°C; 59° to 86°F) just prior to administration. Do not force the warming process by using a water bath or other source of external heat (eg, microwave oven). Remove the peel-off seal from the end of the syringe, then remove the protective end cap (to serve as plunger extension) and insert the protective end cap into the plunger stopper assembly in the barrel of syringe. Choose the appropriate length shielded catheter (10 or 20 mm) and aseptically remove the sterile shielded catheter from the package. Careful vaginal examination will reveal the degree of effacement which will regulate the size of the shielded endocervical catheter to be used; use the 20 mm endocervical catheter if no effacement is present, and the 10 mm catheter if the cervix is 50% effaced. Firmly attach the catheter hub to the syringe tip as evidenced by a distinct click. Fill the catheter with sterile gel by pushing the plunger assembly to expel air from the catheter prior to administration to the patient.

Proper administration – To properly administer the product, the patient should be in a dorsal position with the cervix visualized using a speculum. Using sterile technique, introduce the gel with the catheter provided into the cervical canal just below the level of the internal os. Administer the contents of the syringe by gentle expulsion and then remove the catheter. Discard the syringe, catheter and any unused package contents after use.

Following administration, the patient should remain in the supine position for at least 15 to 30 minutes to minimize leakage from the cervical canal.

If the desired response is obtained from the starting dose of dinoprostone gel, the recommended interval before giving IV oxytocin is 6 to 12 hours. If there is no cervical/uterine response to the initial dose, repeat dosing may be given. The recommended repeat dose is 0.5 mg with a dosing interval of 6 hours. The need for additional dosing and the interval must be determined by the attending physician based on the course of clinical events. The maximum recommended cumulative dose for a 24 hour period is 1.5 mg (7.5 ml).

➤*Insert:* Dosage of dinoprostone in the insert is 10 mg, designed to be released at ≈ 0.3 mg/hr over a 12 hour period. Remove the insert upon onset of active labor or 12 hours after insertion.

One insert is placed transversely in the posterior fornix of the vagina immediately after removal from the foil package. Insertion does not require sterile conditions. Do not use the insert without its retrieval system. There is no need for previous warming of the insert. A minimal amount of a water-miscible lubricant may be used to assist in insertion of the insert; take care not to permit excess contact or coating with the lubricant and thus prevent optimal swelling and release of dinoprostone from the insert. Have patients remain supine for 2 hours following insertion; thereafter, they may be ambulatory.

➤*Storage/Stability:*

Gel – Dinoprostone gel has a shelf life of 24 months when stored under continuous refrigeration (2° to 8°C; 36° to 46°F).

Insert – Store in a freezer between −20° and −10°C (−4° and 14°F). The insert is packed in foil and is stable for a period of 3 years when stored in a freezer.

Actions

➤*Pharmacology:* Dinoprostone is the naturally occurring form of prostaglandin E₂ (PGE₂). In pregnancy, PGE₂ is secreted continuously by the fetal membranes and placenta and plays an important role in the final events leading to the initiation of labor. It is known that PGE₂ stimulates the production of PGF₂α which in turn sensitizes the myometrium to endogenous or exogenously administered oxytocin. Although PGE₂ is capable of initiating uterine contractions and may interact with oxytocin to increase uterine contractility, available evidence indicates that, in the concentrations found during the early part of labor, PGE₂ plays an important role in cervical ripening without affecting uterine contractions. This distinction serves as the basis for considering cervical ripening and induction of labor, usually by the use of oxytocin, as two separate processes.

PGE₂ plays an important role in the complex set of biochemical and structural alterations involved in cervical ripening. Cervical ripening involves a marked relaxation of the cervical smooth muscle fibers of the uterine cervix which must be transformed from a rigid structure to a softened, yielding and dilated configuration to allow passage of the fetus through the birth canal. This process involves activation of the enzyme collagenase, which is responsible for digestion of some of the structural collagen network of the cervix. This is associated with a concomitant increase in the amount of hydrophilic glycosaminoglycan and hyaluronic acid, and a decrease in dermaten sulfate. Failure of the cervix to undergo these natural physiologic changes prior to the onset of effective uterine contractions results in an unfavorable outcome for successful vaginal delivery and may result in fetal compromise. It is estimated that in ≈ 5% of pregnancies the cervix does not ripen normally. In an additional 10% to 11%, labor must be induced for medical or obstetric reasons prior to the time of cervical ripening.

Dinoprostone gel and vaginal insert provide sufficient quantities of PGE₂ to the local receptors to satisfy hormonal requirements. In the majority of patients, these local effects are manifested by changes in the consistency, dilatation and effacement of the cervix. Although some patients experience uterine hyperstimulation as a result of direct PGE₂- or PGF₂α-mediated sensitization of the myometrium to oxytocin, systemic effects of PGE₂ are rarely encountered.

Dinoprostone is also capable of stimulating smooth muscle of the GI tract. This activity may be responsible for the vomiting or diarrhea that is occasionally seen when dinoprostone is used for preinduction of cervical ripening.

Large doses can lower blood pressure, probably as a result of its effect on smooth muscle of the vascular system, and can elevate body temperature. However, with the doses used for cervical ripening these effects have not been seen.

➤*Pharmacokinetics:* When an unvalidated assay of dinoprostone gel was administered endocervically to women undergoing preinduction ripening, results from measurement of plasma levels of the metabolite 13,14-dihydro-15-keto-PGE₂ (DHK-PGE₂) showed that PGE₂ was relatively rapidly absorbed and the T_{max} was 0.5 to 0.75 hours. Plasma mean C_{max} for gel-treated subjects was 433 vs 137 pg/ml for untreated controls. In those subjects in which a clinical response was observed, mean C_{max} was 484 vs 213 pg/ml in nonresponders and 219 pg/ml in control subjects who had positive clinical progression toward normal labor. These elevated levels in gel-treated subjects appear to be largely a result of absorption of PGE₂ from the gel rather than from endogenous sources.

PGE₂ is completely metabolized. It is extensively metabolized in the lungs (≈ 95% on first pass through pulmonary circulation), and the resulting metabolites are further metabolized in the liver and kidney. The major route of elimination of the products of PGE₂ metabolism is the kidneys. Half-life is estimated to be 2.5 to 5 minutes.

Contraindications

Patients in whom oxytocic drugs are generally contraindicated or where prolonged contractions of the uterus are considered inappropriate, such as: History of cesarean section or major uterine surgery; where cephalopelvic disproportion is present; history of difficult labor or traumatic delivery; grand multiparae with ≥ 6 previous term pregnancies; non-vertex presentation; hyperactive or hypertonic uterine patterns; fetal distress where delivery is not imminent; obstetric emergencies where the benefit-to-risk ratio for fetus or mother favors surgical intervention.

Ruptured membranes.

Hypersensitivity to prostaglandins or constituents of the gel.

Placenta previa or unexplained vaginal bleeding during current pregnancy.

When vaginal delivery is not indicated such as vasa previa or active herpes genitalia.

Patients already receiving IV oxytocic drugs.

Warnings

➤*For hospital use only:* As with other potent oxytocic agents, use only with strict adherence to recommended dosages. Administer in a hospital that can provide immediate intensive care and acutesurgical facilities.

➤*Feto-pelvic relationships:* Carefully evaluate before use (see Contraindications).

➤*Special risk patients:* Exercise caution when administering to patients with asthma or history of asthma or glaucoma or raised intraocular pressure.

➤*Renal/Hepatic function impairment:* Since dinoprostone gel is extensively metabolized in the lung, liver and kidney, and the major route of elimination is the kidney, use with caution in patients with renal and hepatic dysfunction.

Agents For Cervical Ripening

DINOPROSTONE (Prostaglandin E₂; PGE₂)

➤*Pregnancy: Category C.* Prostaglandin E_2 produced an increase in skeletal anomalies in rats and rabbits. No effect would be expected clinically, when used as indicated, since dinoprostone is embryotoxic in rats and rabbits, and any dose that produces sustained increased uterine tone could put the embryo or fetus at risk (see Precautions).

Precautions

➤*Monitoring:* During use, carefully monitor uterine activity, fetal status and character of the cervix (dilation and effacement) either by auscultation or electronic fetal monitoring to detect possible evidence of undesired responses (eg, hypertonus, sustained uterine contractility, fetal distress). In cases where there is a history of hypertonic uterine contractility or tetanic uterine contractions, continuously monitor uterine activity and the state of the fetus. Consider the possibility of uterine rupture when high-tone myometrial contractions are sustained. If uterine hyperstimulation is encountered or if labor commences, or if there is any evidence of fetal distress or other maternal/fetal adverse reactions, remove the vaginal insert. Also, remove the insert prior to amniotomy.

➤*Degree of effacement:*

Gel – Use caution so as not to administer above the level of the internal os. Careful vaginal examination will reveal the degree of effacement which will regulate the size of the shielded endocervical catheter to be used. Use the 20 mm endocervical catheter if no effacement is present, and use the 10 mm catheter if the cervix is 50% effaced. Placement into the extra-amniotic space has been associated with uterine hyperstimulation.

Drug Interactions

➤*Oxytocics:* Dinoprostone gel may augment the activity of other oxytocic agents; their concomitant use is not recommended. For the sequential use of oxytocin following dinoprostone gel administration, a dosing interval of 6 to 12 hours is recommended; a dosing interval of at least 30 minutes is recommended following removal of the dinoprostone insert.

Adverse Reactions

Dinoprostone is generally well tolerated.

Gel –

Dinoprostone Gel Adverse Reactions (%)		
Adverse reaction	Dinoprostone gel (n = 884)	Control[1] (n = 847)
Maternal		
Uterine contractile abnormality	6.6	4
Any GI effect	5.7	2.6
Back pain	3.1	0
Warm feeling in vagina	1.5	0
Fever	1.4	1.2
Fetal		
Any fetal heart rate abnormality	1.7	14.5
Bradycardia	4.1	3.1
Deceleration		
Late	2.8	2.1
Variable	4.3	3.4
Unspecified	2.1	2.2

[1] Placebo gel or no treatment.

Amnionitis and intrauterine fetal sepsis have been associated with extra-amniotic intrauterine administration of PGE_2. Uterine rupture has occurred with the use of dinoprostone gel intracervically. Additional events included premature rupture of membranes, fetal depression (1 min Apgar < 7) and fetal acidosis (umbilical artery pH < 7.15).

Insert – The following adverse reactions were reported with the dinoprostone insert: Uterine hyperstimulation without fetal distress (2% to 4.7%); fetal distress without uterine hyperstimulation (2.9% to 3.8%); uterine hyperstimulation with fetal distress (2.8% to 2.9%); fever, nausea, vomiting, diarrhea, abdominal pain (< 1%).

In one study, cases of uterine hyperstimulation reversed within 2 to 13 minutes of product removal; tocolytics were required in 1 of 5 cases. Five minute Apgar scores were ≥ 7 in 98.2% of neonates whose mothers received dinoprostone inserts.

Overdosage

Overdosage may be expressed by uterine hypercontractility and uterine hypertonus. Because of the transient nature of PGE_2-induced myometrial hyperstimulation, nonsepcific, conservative management was found to be effective in the vast majority of the cases (ie, maternal position change and administration of oxygen to the mother). Beta-adrenergic drugs may be used as a treatment of hyperstimulation following the administration of PGE_2 for cervical ripening.

OXYTOCIN

| Rx | Oxytocin (Various, eg, APP) | **Injection:** 10 units/mL | In 3 and 10 mL vials. |
| Rx | Pitocin (Monarch) | | In 1 mL amps[a], 1 mL *Steri-Dose* disposable syringes, and 1 mL *Steri-Vials*.[a] |

[a] With 0.5% chlorobutanol.

WARNING

Oxytocin is indicated for the medical, rather than the elective, induction of labor. Available data and information are inadequate to define the benefit-to-risk considerations in the use of oxytocin for elective induction.

Indications

➤*Antepartum:* For the initiation or improvement of uterine contractions, when this is desirable and considered suitable for reasons of fetal or maternal concern, in order to achieve vaginal delivery. It is indicated for patients with a medical indication for the initiation of labor such as Rh problems, maternal diabetes, preeclampsia at or near term, when delivery is in the best interest of mother and fetus, or when membranes are ruptured prematurely and delivery is indicated; stimulation or reinforcement of labor, as in selected cases of uterine inertia; adjunctive therapy for the management of inevitable or incomplete abortion. In the first trimester, curettage generally is considered primary therapy. In second trimester abortion, oxytocin infusion often is successful in emptying the uterus. However, other means of therapy may be required in such cases.

➤*Postpartum:* To produce uterine contractions during the third stage of labor and to control postpartum bleeding or hemorrhage.

Administration and Dosage

The dosage of oxytocin is determined by the uterine response and, therefore, must be individualized and initiated at a very low level. The following dosage information is based upon various regimens and indications in general use.

➤*Induction or stimulation of labor:*

IV infusion (drip method) – IV infusion (drip method) is the only acceptable method of parenteral administration for the induction or stimulation of labor. Accurate control of the rate of infusion flow is essential. An infusion pump or other device and frequent monitoring of strength, frequency, and duration of contractions, resting uterine tone, and fetal heart rate are necessary for the safe administration of oxytocin for the induction or stimulation of labor.

Start an IV infusion of nonoxytocin-containing solution. Use physiologic electrolyte solution, except under unusual circumstances.

Dosage: The initial dose should be no more than 0.5 to 2 milliunits/min. Gradually increase the dose in increments of no more than 1 to 2 milliunits/min at 30- to 60-minute intervals until a contraction pattern has been established that is similar to normal labor.

Infusion rates: Infusion rates up to 6 milliunits/min give the same oxytocin levels that are found in spontaneous labor. At term, give higher infusion rates with great care; rates exceeding 9 to 10 milliunits/min rarely are required. Before term, when the sensitivity of the uterus is lower because of a lower concentration of oxytocin receptors, a higher infusion rate may be required.

Discontinue: Discontinue the oxytocin infusion immediately in the event of uterine hyperactivity or fetal distress. Administer oxygen to the mother, who preferably should be put in a lateral position. Immediately evaluate the condition of the mother and fetus; take appropriate steps. If uterine contractions become too powerful, the infusion can be stopped abruptly; oxytocic stimulation of the uterine musculature will soon wane.

➤*Control of postpartum uterine bleeding:*

IV infusion (drip method) – Add 10 to 40 units (maximum of 40 units) to 1,000 mL of a nonhydrating diluent and run at a rate necessary to control uterine atony.

IM – Administer 10 units after delivery of the placenta.

➤*Treatment of incomplete or inevitable abortion:* IV infusion of 10 units oxytocin with 500 mL physiologic saline solution or 5% dextrose in physiologic saline solution infused at a rate of 10 to 20 milliunits (20 to 40 drops) per minute. Do not exceed 30 units in a 12-hour period because of the risk of water intoxication.

➤*Reconstitution:* Add 1 mL (10 units) to 1,000 mL 0.9% aqueous sodium chloride or Ringer's lactate. The solution contains 10 milliunits/mL (0.01 units/mL). Use a constant infusion pump to accurately control the rate of infusion.

➤*Storage/Stability:*

Pitocin – Store at 2° to 8°C (36° to 46°F); may be held at 15° to 25°C (59° to 77°F) for up to 30 days. Discard after holding at 15° to 25°C (59° to 77°F).

Oxytocin – Store at controlled room temperature 15° to 30°C (59° to 86°F).

Actions

➤*Pharmacology:* Oxytocin acts on the smooth muscle of the uterus to stimulate contractions; response depends on the uterine threshold of excitability. It exerts a selective action on the smooth musculature of the uterus, particularly toward the end of pregnancy, during labor, and immediately following delivery. Oxytocin stimulates rhythmic contractions of the uterus, increases the frequency of existing contractions, and raises the tone of the uterine musculature.

➤*Pharmacokinetics:*

Absorption/Distribution – Oxytocin is distributed throughout the extracellular fluid. Small amounts of the drug probably reach the fetal circulation. Following IV administration, uterine response occurs almost immediately and subsides within 1 hour. Following IM injection, uterine response occurs within 3 to 5 minutes and persists for 2 to 3 hours.

Metabolism/Excretion – The plasma half-life is approximately 1 to 6 minutes, which is decreased in late pregnancy and lactation. Rapid removal from the plasma is accomplished mainly by the kidney and liver. Only small amounts are excreted in urine unchanged.

Contraindications

Significant cephalopelvic disproportion; unfavorable fetal positions or presentations that are undeliverable without conversion prior to delivery (eg, transverse lies); in obstetrical emergencies where the benefit-to-risk ratio for the fetus or the mother favors surgical intervention; cases of fetal distress where delivery is not imminent; prolonged use in uterine inertia or severe toxemia; hypertonic or hyperactive uterine patterns; where adequate uterine activity fails to achieve satisfactory progress; induction or augmentation of labor where vaginal delivery is contraindicated, such as invasive cervical carcinoma, active herpes genitalis, cord presentation or prolapse, total placenta previa, and vasa previa; hypersensitivity to the drug.

Warnings

➤*IV use:* When given for induction or augmentation of uterine activity, administer oxytocin only by the IV route and with adequate medical supervision in hospital. All patients receiving IV oxytocin must be under continuous observation by trained personnel who have a thorough knowledge of the drug and are qualified to identify complications.

➤*Special risk patients:* Except in unusual circumstances, do not administer oxytocin in the following conditions: fetal distress; hydramnios; partial placenta previa; prematurity; borderline cephalopelvic disproportion and any condition in which there is a predisposition for uterine rupture, such as previous major surgery on the cervix or uterus including cesarean section; overdistention of the uterus; grand multiparity; history of uterine sepsis or traumatic delivery; invasive cervical carcinoma. Weigh the potential benefits oxytocin can provide in a given case against rare but definite potential for the drug to produce hypertonicity or tetanic spasm.

➤*Maternal deaths:* Maternal deaths caused by hypertensive episodes, subarachnoid hemorrhage, or rupture of the uterus and fetal deaths caused by various causes have been associated with the use of parenteral oxytocic drugs for induction of labor or for augmentation in the first and second stages of labor.

➤*Pregnancy:* There are no known indications for use in the first and second trimester of pregnancy other than in relation to spontaneous or induced abortion. Oxytocin is not expected to present a risk of fetal abnormalities when used as indicated (see Adverse Reactions in the fetus).

➤*Lactation:* It is not known whether this drug is excreted in human milk. Because many drugs are excreted in human milk, exercise caution when administering to a nursing mother.

➤*Children:* Oxytocin is not intended for use in children.

Precautions

➤*Monitoring:* During the induction or stimulation of labor, monitor fetal heart rate, resting uterine tone, and the frequency, duration, and force of contraction. Keep in mind the possibility of increased blood and afibrinogenemia when administering the drug. Monitor for signs of water intoxication (eg, drowsiness, listlessness, confusion, headache, anuria).

Electronic fetal monitoring provides the best means for early detection of overdosage (see Overdosage). However, keep in mind that only intrauterine pressure recording can accurately measure the intrauterine pressure during contractions. A fetal scalp electrode provides a more dependable recording of the fetal heart rate than any external monitoring system.

OXYTOCIN

➤*Uterine contractions:* When properly administered, oxytocin stimulates uterine contractions comparable with those in normal labor. Overstimulation of the uterus can be hazardous to the mother and fetus. Even with proper administration and adequate supervision, hypertonic contractions can occur in patients whose uteri are hypersensitive to oxytocin. Consider this fact in exercising judgment regarding patient selection.

➤*Water intoxication:* Oxytocin has an intrinsic antidiuretic effect, acting to increase water reabsorption from the glomerular filtrate. Consider the possibility of water intoxication, particularly when oxytocin is administered by continuous infusion and the patient is receiving fluids by mouth. Severe water intoxication with convulsions and coma has occurred and is associated with a slow infusion over a 24-hour period. Maternal death caused by oxytocin-induced water intoxication has been reported.

➤*Existent labor:* When oxytocin is used for induction or reinforcement of already existent labor, carefully select patients. Consider pelvic adequacy and maternal and fetal conditions before use of the drug.

Drug Interactions

➤*Cyclopropane anesthesia:* Cyclopropane anesthesia may modify oxytocin's cardiovascular effects, producing unexpected results such as hypotension. Maternal sinus bradycardia with abnormal atrioventricular rhythms also has been noted when oxytocin was used concomitantly with cyclopropane anesthesia.

➤*Sympathomimetics:* If used concurrently with oxytocic drugs, the pressor effect of the sympathomimetics may be increased, possibly resulting in postpartum hypertension.

➤*Vasoconstrictors/caudal block anesthesia:* Severe hypertension occurred when oxytocin was given 3 to 4 hours following prophylactic administration of a vasoconstrictor in conjunction with caudal block anesthesia.

Adverse Reactions

Maternal –

Cardiovascular: Cardiac arrhythmia, hypertensive episodes, premature ventricular contractions.

GI: Nausea, vomiting.

GU: Pelvic hematoma, postpartum hemorrhage; rupture of the uterus, spasm, tetanic contraction, or uterine hypertonicity may occur from excessive dosage or hypersensitivity to the drug.

Miscellaneous: Anaphylactic reaction, fatal afibrinogenemia, subarachnoid hemorrhage; severe water intoxication with convulsions, coma, and death have been reported.

Fetal or neonate (caused by induced uterine motility) –

Cardiovascular: Bradycardia, premature ventricular contractions, and other arrhythmias.

CNS: Permanent CNS or brain damage, neonatal seizures.

Miscellaneous: Fetal death, low Apgar scores at 5 minutes, neonatal jaundice, neonatal retinal hemorrhage.

Overdosage

➤*Symptoms:* Overdosage depends essentially on uterine hyperactivity, whether or not caused by hypersensitivity to this agent. Hyperstimulation with strong (hypertonic) or prolonged (tetanic) contractions or a resting tone of at least 15 to 20 mm H_2O between contractions can lead to tumultuous labor, uterine rupture, cervical and vaginal lacerations, postpartum hemorrhage, uteroplacental hypoperfusion, and variable deceleration of fetal heart, fetal hypoxia, hypercapnia, perinatal hepatic necrosis, or death. Water intoxication with convulsions, which is caused by the inherent antidiuretic effect of oxytocin, is a serious complication that may occur if large doses (40 to 50 milliunits/min) are infused for long periods.

➤*Treatment:* To treat, discontinue drug, restrict fluid intake, initiate diuresis, administer IV hypertonic saline solution, correct electrolyte imbalance, control convulsions, and provide supportive therapy.

ERGONOVINE MALEATE

| Rx | Ergotrate (HPS Rx Enterprises) | Tablets: 0.2 mg | Mannitol. (HPS). White. In 100s, 500s, and 1000s. |

Indications

▶*Postpartum/postabortal hemorrhage:* For the prevention and treatment of postpartum and postabortal hemorrhage caused by uterine atony.

▶*Unlabeled uses:* Oxytocin challenge test.

Administration and Dosage

Immediate postpartum dose usually is 0.2 mg. Ordinarily, it is administered parenterally. To minimize late postpartum bleeding, 1 or 2 tablets may be given orally 2 to 4 times/day (every 6 to 12 hours) until the danger of uterine atony has passed (usually 48 hours). Severe cramping is evidence of effectiveness but may justify reduction in dosage. Tablets also may be administered sublingually.

▶*Storage/Stability:* Store at controlled room temperature 15° to 30°C (59° to 86°F). Dispense in a tight, light-resistant container with a child-resistant closure.

Actions

▶*Pharmacology:* When used after placental delivery, ergonovine increases the strength, duration, and frequency of uterine contractions and decreases uterine bleeding.

▶*Pharmacokinetics:* Within 6 to 15 minutes, ergonovine produces a firm tetanic contraction of the postpartum uterus that, in the course of approximately 90 minutes, gradually changes to a series of clonic contractions that persist for another 90 minutes or more.

Contraindications

Induction of labor; cases of threatened spontaneous abortion; previous allergic or idiosyncratic reactions to the drug.

Warnings

▶*Uterine effects:* All oxytocic agents are potentially dangerous. Mothers and infants have been injured, and some have died because of their injudicious use. Hyperstimulation of the uterus during labor may lead to uterine tetany and marked impairment of the uteroplacental blood flow, uterine rupture, cervical and perineal lacerations, amniotic fluid embolism, and trauma to the infant (eg, hypoxia, intracranial hemorrhage). Because of these hazards that result from overdosage, administer oxytocic agents under conditions of meticulous observation.

▶*Calcium deficiency:* Hypocalcemia may affect patient response to the drug. If the patient is not also taking digitalis, cautious administration of calcium gluconate IV may produce the desired oxytocic action.

▶*Pregnancy:*

Labor and delivery – Because of the high uterine tone produced, ergonovine is not recommended for routine use prior to the delivery of the placenta, unless the surgeon is familiar with the technique described by Davis and others and has adequate facilities and personnel at his or her disposal.

Precautions

▶*Monitoring:* Monitor blood pressure, pulse, and uterine response. Note sudden changes in vital signs or frequent periods of uterine relaxation.

▶*Duration:* Avoid prolonged use. Discontinue if symptoms of ergotism appear.

▶*Special risk patients:* Use cautiously in patients with hypertension, heart disease, venoatrial shunts, mitral-valve stenosis, obliterative vascular disease, sepsis, or hepatic or renal impairment.

▶*Vaginal bleeding:* Observe the character and amount of vaginal bleeding.

Drug Interactions

▶*Protease inhibitors:* The risk of ergot toxicity (eg, peripheral vasospasm, ischemia of the extremities) may be increased because of inhibition of hepatic metabolism. Coadministration of protease inhibitors and ergot derivatives is not recommended.

▶*Sympathomimetics:* Coadministration may result in hypertension because of additive vasoconstriction. The incidence of hypertension decreases when the sympathomimetic is not used prior to the administration of ergonovine.

Adverse Reactions

▶*Cardiovascular:* Blood pressure elevations (sometimes extreme) appear in a small percentage of patients, most frequently in association with regional anesthesia (caudal or spinal), previous administration of a vasoconstrictor, and the IV route of administration of the oxytocic. The mechanism of such hypertension is obscure because it may occur in the absence of anesthesia, vasoconstrictors, and oxytocics. These elevations are no more frequent with ergonovine than with other oxytocics. They usually subside promptly following IV administration of 15 mg chlorpromazine.

▶*GI:* Nausea and vomiting may occur, but they are uncommon.

▶*Miscellaneous:* Allergic phenomena (including shock) and ergotism have been reported.

Overdosage

▶*Symptoms:* The principal manifestations of serious overdosage are convulsions and gangrene. Symptoms of overdosage include the following: chest pain, diarrhea, dizziness, dyspnea, gangrene of the fingers and toes, hypercoagulability, loss of consciousness, numbness and coldness of the extremities, rise or fall in blood pressure, tingling, vomiting, and weak pulse.

▶*Treatment:* Treat convulsions. Control hypercoagulability by administering heparin, and maintain blood-clotting time at approximately 3 times normal. Give a vasodilator such as tolazine as an antidote; the rate of administration may be controlled by monitoring pulse rate and blood pressure. For emergency measures, delay absorption of ingested ergonovine by giving tap water, milk, or activated charcoal and then removing by gastric lavage or emesis followed by catharsis. Gangrene will require surgical amputation.

Patient Information

May cause chest pain, dizziness, headache, increased blood pressure, nausea, shortness of breath, or vomiting.

METHYLERGONOVINE MALEATE

| Rx | Methergine (Sandoz) | Injection: 0.2 mg/mL | In 1 mL ampuls. |
| | | Tablets: 0.2 mg | Lactose, FD&C Blue No.1, parabens, sucrose. (78-54 SANDOZ). Orchid, round. Coated. In 100s. |

Indications

▶*Uterine contractions/bleeding:* For routine management after delivery of the placenta; postpartum atony and hemorrhage; subinvolution. Under full obstetric supervision, it may be given in the second stage of labor following delivery of the anterior shoulder.

Administration and Dosage

▶*Orally:* 0.2 mg 3 or 4 times/day in the puerperium for a maximum of 1 week.

▶*IM:* 0.2 mg after delivery of the placenta or the anterior shoulder, or during the puerperium. Repeat as required at intervals of 2 to 4 hours.

▶*IV:* (See Warnings). Dosage same as for IM use.

▶*Storage/Stability:*

Tablets – Store below 25°C (77°F) in tight, light-resistant container.

Ampuls – Store in refrigerator 2° to 8°C (36° to 46°F). Protect from light. Administer only if solution is clear and colorless.

Actions

▶*Pharmacology:* Methylergonovine acts directly on the smooth muscle of the uterus and increases the tone, rate, and amplitude of rhythmic contractions. It induces a rapid and sustained tetanic utero-

tonic effect that shortens the third stage of labor and reduces blood loss.

▶*Pharmacokinetics:*

Absorption/Distribution – The oral bioavailability is approximately 60%, with no accumulation after repeated doses. During delivery with IM injection, bioavailability increased to 78%. Bioavailability studies have shown that oral absorption of 0.2 mg was fairly rapid, with a mean peak plasma concentration of approximately 3,243 pg/mL observed in approximately 1.12 hours. For an IM injection of 0.2 mg, the mean peak plasma concentration was approximately 5,918 pg/mL observed in approximately 0.41 hours. A delayed GI absorption of approximately 3 hours may be observed in postpartum women during oral continuous treatment. Following IV administration, methylergonovine is rapidly distributed from plasma to peripheral tissues within 2 to 3 minutes or less. The volume of distribution is approximately 56 L. The onset of action after IV administration is immediate, after IM administration 2 to 5 minutes, and after oral administration 5 to 10 minutes.

Metabolism/Excretion – Ergot alkaloids are mostly eliminated by hepatic metabolism and excretion, and the decrease in bioavailability following oral administration is probably a result of first-pass metabolism in the liver. Plasma clearance is approximately 14.4 L/h. The plasma level decline was biphasic, with a mean elimination half-life of 3.39 hours.

METHYLERGONOVINE MALEATE

Contraindications

Certain alkaloid drugs (eg, dihydroergotamine and ergotamine) are contraindicated for concomitant use with potent CYP3A4 inhibitors (eg, protease inhibitors, macrolide antibiotics, azole antifungals) because of the risk of vasospasm leading to cerebral ischemia and/or ischemia of the extremities. Although there have been no reports of such interactions with methylergonovine alone, do not use potent CYP3A4 inhibitors concomitantly with methylergonovine (see Drug Interactions).

Hypertension; toxemia; pregnancy (see Warnings); hypersensitivity.

Warnings

➤*IV use:* Do not routinely administer this drug IV because of the possibility of inducing sudden hypertensive and cerebrovascular accidents. If IV administration is considered essential as a life-saving measure, give slowly over a period of no less than 60 seconds with careful blood pressure monitoring.

➤*Pregnancy: Category C.* It is not known whether methylergonovine can cause fetal harm or affect reproductive capacity. Use is contraindicated during pregnancy because of its uterotonic effects (see Indications).

Labor and delivery – The uterotonic effect of methylergonovine is utilized after delivery to assist involution and decrease hemorrhage, shortening the third stage of labor. Use with caution during the second stage of labor. The necessity for manual removal of a retained placenta should occur only rarely with proper technique and adequate allowance of time for its spontaneous separation.

➤*Lactation:* Methylergonovine may be administered orally for a maximum of 1 week postpartum to control uterine bleeding. Recommended dosage is one 0.2 mg tablet 3 or 4 times/day. At this dosage level, a small quantity of drug appears in breast milk. Exercise caution when administering to a nursing woman.

➤*Children:* Safety and efficacy have not been established.

Precautions

➤*Special risk patients:* Exercise caution in the presence of sepsis, obliterative vascular disease, or hepatic or renal involvement.

Drug Interactions

➤*CYP3A4 inhibitors:* Do not coadminister methylergonovine with potent CYP3A4 inhibitors (see Contraindications). Examples of some of the more potent CYP3A4 inhibitors include macrolide antibiotics (eg, erythromycin, troleandomycin, clarithromycin), HIV protease or reverse transcriptase inhibitors (eg, ritonavir, indinavir, nelfinavir, delavirdine), or azole antifungals (eg, ketoconazole, itraconazole, voriconazole). Administer less potent CYP3A4 inhibitors with caution. Less potent inhibitors include saquinavir, nefazodone, fluconazole, grapefruit juice, fluoxetine, fluvoxamine, zileuton, and clotrimazole.

➤*Protease inhibitors:* The risk of ergot toxicity (peripheral vasospasm, ischemia of the extremities) may be increased because of inhibition of hepatic metabolism. Coadministration of protease inhibitors and ergot derivatives is not recommended.

➤*Sympathomimetics:* Coadministration may result in hypertension caused by additive vasoconstriction. The incidence of hypertension decreases when the sympathomimetic is not used prior to administration of methylergonovine.

Adverse Reactions

➤*Cardiovascular:* Hypertension, hypotension; acute myocardial infarction, palpitations, transient chest pains (rare).

➤*CNS:* Headache, seizure; dizziness, hallucinations (rare).

➤*GI:* Nausea, vomiting; diarrhea (rare).

➤*Miscellaneous:* Anaphylaxis, diaphoresis, dyspnea, foul taste, hematuria, leg cramps, nasal congestion, thrombophlebitis, tinnitus, water intoxication (rare).

Overdosage

➤*Symptoms:* Symptoms of acute overdose may include abdominal pain, nausea, numbness, rise in blood pressure, tingling of the extremities, and vomiting. In severe cases, these are followed by hypotension, respiratory depression, hypothermia, convulsions, and coma. Because reports of overdosage are infrequent, the lethal dose in humans has not been established. Several cases of accidental injection in newborn infants have been reported, and, in such cases, 0.2 mg represents an overdose of great magnitude. However, recovery occurred in all but one case following a period of respiratory depression, hypothermia, hypertonicity with jerking movements, and, in one case, a single convulsion.

Also, several children 1 to 3 years of age have accidentally ingested up to 10 tablets (2 mg) with no apparent ill effects. A postpartum patient took 4 tablets (0.8 mg) at one time in error and reported paresthesias and clamminess as her only symptoms.

➤*Treatment:* Treatment of acute overdosage is symptomatic and includes the usual procedures of removal of offending drug: induction of emesis, gastric lavage, catharsis, and supportive diuresis; maintenance of adequate pulmonary ventilation, especially if convulsions or coma develop; correction of hypotension with pressor drugs as needed; control of convulsions with standard anticonvulsant agents; controlling peripheral vasospasm with warmth to the extremities if needed.

Patient Information

May cause chest pain, dizziness, headache, increased blood pressure, nausea, ringing in the ears, shortness of breath, or vomiting.

Uterine Relaxant

RITODRINE HCl

Rx	**Ritodrine HCl** (Abbott)	**Injection:** 10 mg per ml	In 5 ml amps.
Rx	**Yutopar** (Astra)		In 5 ml vials and amps.[1]
Rx	**Ritodrine HCl** (Abbott)	**Injection:** 15 mg per ml	In 10 ml flip-top vials.
Rx	**Yutopar** (Astra)		In 10 ml vials[1] and syringes.[1]
Rx	**Ritodrine HCl in 5% Dextrose** (Abbott)	**Injection:** 0.3 mg per ml	In 500 ml *LifeCare* flexible containers.

[1] With 1 mg sodium metabisulfite, 4.35 mg acetic acid, 2.4 mg sodium hydroxide and 2.9 sodium chloride per ml.

Indications

➤*Preterm labor:* Management of preterm labor in suitable patients. Institute therapy as soon as the diagnosis of preterm labor is established and contraindications are ruled out in pregnancies of ≥ 20 weeks gestation.

Administration and Dosage

The optimum dose of the drug is determined by a balance of uterine response and unwanted effects. Treat recurrences of unwanted preterm labor with repeated infusion of ritodrine.

Begin as soon as possible after diagnosis. To minimize risks of hypotension, keep patient in the left lateral position during infusion and pay careful attention to hydration. *Avoid circulatory fluid overload.* Frequently monitor maternal uterine contractions, heart rate, blood pressure and fetal heart rate; individualize dosage.

Use a controlled infusion device to adjust flow rate in drops/min. An IV microdrip chamber (60 drops/ml) provides a convenient range of infusion rates.

The initial dose is 0.05 mg/min (0.17 ml/min, or 10 drops/min using a microdrip chamber at the recommended dilution), to be gradually increased by 0.05 mg/min (10 drops/min) every 10 minutes until the desired result is attained. The usual effective dosage is between 0.15 and 0.35 mg/min (30 to 70 drops/min), continued for at least 12 hours after uterine contractions cease. With the recommended dilution, the maximum volume of fluid that might be administered after 12 hours at the highest dose (0.35 mg/min) will be approximately 840 ml.

If other drugs need to be given IV, the use of "piggyback" or another site of IV administration permits continued independent control of the infusion rate of ritodrine.

➤*Preparation of solution:* 150 mg ritodrine in 500 ml fluid yields a final concentration of 0.3 mg/ml. When fluid restriction is desirable, a more concentrated solution may be prepared. For IV infusion, dilute with 5% Dextrose Solution. Use promptly after preparation.

Because of the increased probability of pulmonary edema, saline diluents (0.9% Sodium Chloride; Ringer's) and Hartmann's Solution should be reserved for cases where Dextrose Solution is undesirable (eg, diabetes mellitus).

➤*Storage/Stability:* Do not use if the solution is discolored or contains any precipitate or particulate matter. Do not use after 48 hours of preparation.

Store at room temperature, below 30°C (86°F). Protect from excessive heat.

Actions

➤*Pharmacology:* Ritodrine is a β-receptor agonist which exerts a preferential effect on β₂-adrenergic receptors such as those in the uterine smooth muscle. Stimulation of the β₂-receptors inhibits contractility of the uterine smooth muscle through the cycle of adenyl cyclase stimulation, which increases intracellular cyclic adenosine 3'-5'-monophosphate (cAMP); this leads to altering cellular calcium balance that affects smooth muscle contractility. In addition, ritodrine may directly affect the interaction between the actin and myosin of muscle through inhibition of myosin light-chain kinase.

Infusions of 0.05 to 0.3 mg/min IV decrease the intensity and frequency of uterine contractions. These effects are antagonized by β-adrenergic blocking compounds. IV administration induces an immediate dose-related elevation of heart rate (maximum mean increase 19 to 40 bpm) and widening of the pulse pressure. The average increase in systolic blood pressure is 4 mmHg, and the average decrease in diastolic pressure is 12.3 mmHg.

During IV infusion, transient elevations of blood glucose, insulin and free fatty acids have been observed. Decreased serum potassium has also been found.

➤*Pharmacokinetics:* Following a 60 minute infusion of IV ritodrine, bioavailability is 100% with peak serum levels of 32 to 52 ng/ml. Half-life of the distribution phase is 6 to 9 minutes, 1.7 to 2.6 hours for the second phase and 15 to 17 hours for the elimination phase. At 24 hours, 90% of the drug is eliminated in urine (primarily as metabolites). Protein binding is 32%. The drug crosses the placenta.

Contraindications

Before the 20th week of pregnancy and in those conditions in which continuation of pregnancy is hazardous to the mother or fetus, specifi-

cally: Antepartum hemorrhage that demands immediate delivery; eclampsia and severe preeclampsia; intrauterine fetal death; chorioamnionitis; maternal cardiac disease; pulmonary hypertension; maternal hyperthyroidism; uncontrolled maternal diabetes mellitus.

Preexisting maternal medical conditions that would be seriously affected by the pharmacologic properties of a betamimetic drug including: Hypovolemia; cardiac arrhythmias associated with tachycardia or digitalis intoxication; uncontrolled hypertension; pheochromocytoma; bronchial asthma already treated by betamimetics or steroids.

Hypersensitivity to any component of the product.

Warnings

➤*Maternal pulmonary edema:* Maternal pulmonary edema has been reported in patients treated with ritodrine, sometimes after delivery. It has occurred more often when patients were treated concomitantly with corticosteroids; however, maternal death from this condition has been reported with or without corticosteroids. Closely monitor patients and avoid fluid overload. Fluid loading IV may be aggravated by the use of betamimetics, with or without corticosteroids, and may result in circulatory overload with subsequent pulmonary edema. If pulmonary edema develops, discontinue use and manage edema by conventional means.

➤*Mild to moderate preeclampsia, hypertension or diabetes:* Do not administer to patients with these disorders unless the benefits clearly outweigh the risks.

➤*Advanced labor:* The safety and efficacy in advanced labor (cervical dilation > 4 cm or effacement > 80%) have not been established.

➤*Cardiovascular effects:* Beta-adrenergic drugs decrease cardiac output, and even in a healthy heart this added myocardial oxygen demand can sometimes lead to myocardial ischemia. Complications may include: Myocardial necrosis, which may result in death; arrhythmia, including premature atrial and ventricular contractions, ventricular tachycardia and bundle branch block; anginal pain with or without ECG changes.

Cardiovascular responses – Cardiovascular responses are common and more pronounced during IV administration; monitor these effects, including maternal pulse rate and blood pressure, fetal heart rate and maternal signs and symptoms of pulmonary edema. A persistent tachycardia (> 140 bpm) may be a sign of impending pulmonary edema. Occult cardiac disease may be unmasked with the use of ritodrine. If the patient complains of chest pain or tightness of chest, temporarily discontinue the drug and perform an ECG.

➤*Pregnancy: Category B.* here are no adequate and well controlled studies of the drug's effects in pregnant women before 20 weeks gestation; therefore, do not use this drug before the 20th week of pregnancy.

Ritodrine crosses the placenta, but studies of pregnant women from gestation week 20 have not shown increased risk of fetal abnormalities. Follow-up of children for up to 2 years has not shown harmful effects on growth or developmental or functional maturation, but the possibility cannot be excluded. Use only when clearly indicated.

Infants born before 36 weeks gestation make up < 10% of all births, but account for as many as 75% of perinatal deaths and 50% of all neurologically handicapped infants. By delaying or preventing preterm labor, the drug should cause an overall increase in neonatal survival.

Precautions

➤*Migraine headache:* Transient cerebral ischemia associated with β-sympathomimetic therapy has been reported in two patients with migraine headaches.

➤*Chorioamnionitis:* When used to manage preterm labor in a patient with premature rupture of membranes, balance benefits of delaying delivery against risk of developing chorioamnionitis.

➤*Intrauterine growth retardation (IUGR):* Among low birth weight infants, ≈ 9% may be growth retarded for gestational age. Therefore, consider IUGR in the differential diagnosis of preterm labor, especially when the gestational age is in doubt. The decision to continue or reinitiate administration will depend on an assessment of fetal maturity.

➤*Baseline ECG:* Baseline ECG should be performed to rule out occult maternal heart disease.

➤*Sulfites:* Sulfites may cause serious allergic-type reactions (eg, hives, itching, wheezing, anaphylaxis) in certain susceptible persons. Although the overall incidence of sulfite sensitivity in the general popu-

RITODRINE HCl

lation is probably low, it is seen more frequently in asthmatics or in atopic nonasthmatic persons. Specific products containing sulfites are identified in the product listings.

➤*Lab test abnormalities:* Administration of ritodrine IV elevates plasma insulin and glucose and decreases plasma potassium concentrations; monitor glucose and electrolyte levels during protracted infusions. Decrease of plasma potassium concentrations is usually transient, returning to normal within 24 hours. Pay special attention to biochemical variables when treating diabetic patients or those receiving potassium-depleting diuretics. Serial hemograms may be helpful as an index of state of hydration.

Drug Interactions

Ritodrine Drug Interactions			
Precipitant drug	Object drug*		Description
Atropine	Ritodrine	↑	Systemic hypertension may be exaggerated with parasympatholytics.
Beta blockers	Ritodrine	↓	Beta-adrenergic blockers inhibit the action of ritodrine; avoid coadministration.
Corticosteroids	Ritodrine	↑	Concomitant use may lead to pulmonary edema (see Warnings).
Diazoxide General anesthetics Magnesium sulfate Meperidine	Ritodrine	↑	Cardiovascular effects of ritodrine (especially cardiac arrhythmias or hypotension) may be potentiated by concomitant use.
Sympatho-mimetics	Ritodrine	↑	The effects of concomitant use may be additive or potentiated. A sufficient time interval should elapse prior to administration of another sympathomimetic drug.

* ↑ = Object drug increased. ↓ = Object drug decreased.

Adverse Reactions

Unwanted effects of ritodrine are usually controllable through dosage adjustment.

Dose-related alterations in maternal and fetal heart rates and in maternal blood pressure (80% to 100%). With a maximum infusion rate of 0.35 mg/min, the maximum maternal and fetal heart rates averaged, respectively, 130 bpm (range, 60 to 180) and 164 bpm (range, 130 to 200). The maximum maternal systolic blood pressures averaged an increase of 12 mmHg from pretreatment levels. The minimum maternal diastolic blood pressures averaged a decrease of 23 mmHg from pretreatment levels. In < 1% of patients, persistent maternal tachycardia or decreased diastolic blood pressure required drug withdrawal. Persistent tachycardia (> 140 bpm) may indicate impending pulmonary edema (see Warnings).

Infusion is associated with transient elevation of blood glucose and insulin, which decreases to normal after 48 to 72 hours despite continued infusion. Elevation of free fatty acids and cAMP has been reported. Expect reduced potassium levels.

Palpitations (33%); tremor, nausea, vomiting, headache, erythema (10% to 15%); nervousness, jitteriness, restlessness, emotional upset, anxiety, malaise (5% to 6%); cardiac symptoms including chest pain or tightness (rarely associated with ECG abnormalities) and arrhythmia (ventricular tachycardia), anaphylactic shock, rash, heart murmur, angina pectoris, myocardial ischemia, epigastric distress, ileus, bloating, constipation, diarrhea, dyspnea, hyperventilation, hemolytic icterus, glycosuria, lactic acidosis, sweating, chills, drowsiness, weakness (1% to 3%); impaired liver function (eg, increased transaminase levels, hepatitis; < 1%). Cases of leukopenia or agranulocytosis (in conjunction with IV infusion for > 2 to 3 weeks); leukocyte count returned to normal after cessation of therapy.

Sinus bradycardia may occur upon drug withdrawal.

➤*Miscellaneous:*

Neonatal effects – Neonatal effects infrequently reported are hypoglycemia and ileus. Hypocalcemia and hypotension have been reported in neonates whose mothers were treated with other betamimetic agents.

Overdosage

➤*Symptoms:* Excessive β-adrenergic stimulation including exaggeration of pharmacologic effects, the most prominent being tachycardia (maternal and fetal), palpitations, cardiac arrhythmia, hypotension, dyspnea, nervousness, tremor, nausea and vomiting.

➤*Treatment:* Includes usual supportive measures. Refer to General Management of Acute Overdosage. When symptoms occur as a result of IV use, discontinue the drug. Use an appropriate β-blocker as an antidote. Ritodrine is dialyzable.

Indications

➤*Osteoporosis in postmenopausal women (alendronate, risedronate):* For the treatment and prevention of osteoporosis in postmenopausal women.

➤*Osteoporosis in men (alendronate):* To increase bone mass in men with osteoporosis.

➤*Glucocorticoid-induced osteoporosis (alendronate, risedronate):* For the prevention and treatment of glucocorticoid-induced osteoporosis in men and women who are either initiating or continuing systemic glucocorticoid treatment for chronic diseases.

➤*Paget disease (osteitis deformans):* For treatment of patients with Paget disease of bone having alkaline phosphatase at least 2 times the upper limit of normal (ULN), or those who are symptomatic or at risk for future complications from their disease (**alendronate**, **risedronate**, **tiludronate**); treatment of symptomatic Paget disease (oral **etidronate**); treatment of moderate to severe Paget disease (**pamidronate**).

➤*Heterotopic ossification (oral etidronate):* Prevention and treatment of heterotopic ossification following total hip replacement or caused by spinal injury.

➤*Hypercalcemia of malignancy (HCM):* For the treatment of HCM (**zoledronic acid**); in conjunction with adequate hydration (eg, saline hydration, with or without loop diuretics) for the treatment of moderate or severe hypercalcemia associated with malignancy with or without bone metastases (**pamidronate**; patients with epidermoid or nonepidermoid tumors respond to pamidronate); when inadequately managed by dietary modification or oral hydration, concurrent therapy is recommended as soon as there is a restoration of urine output (IV **etidronate**); for HCM that persists after adequate hydration has been restored (IV **etidronate**).

➤*Breast cancer/Multiple myeloma (pamidronate):* In conjunction with standard antineoplastic therapy for the treatment of osteolytic bone metastases of breast cancer and osteolytic lesions of multiple myeloma.

➤*Multiple myeloma and bone metastases of solid tumors (zoledronic acid):* For the treatment of patients with multiple myeloma and patients with documented bone metastases from solid tumors, in conjunction with standard antineoplastic therapy. Prostate cancer should have progressed after treatment with at least 1 hormonal therapy.

➤*Unlabeled uses:*

Etidronate – Treatment and prevention of osteoporosis in postmenopausal women; prevention of corticosteroid-induced osteoporosis.

Pamidronate – Postmenopausal osteoporosis; hyperparathyroidism; prevent glucocorticoid-induced osteoporosis; reduce bone pain in patients with prostatic carcinoma; immobilization-related hypercalcemia.

Actions

➤*Pharmacology:* **Etidronate**, **tiludronate**, **pamidronate**, **risedronate**, and **alendronate** are bisphosphonates that act primarily on the bone. Their major pharmacologic action is the inhibition of normal and abnormal bone resorption. Secondarily, etidronate reduces bone formation because formation is coupled to resorption; pamidronate inhibits bone resorption apparently without inhibiting bone formation and mineralization. Alendronate shows preferential localization to sites of bone resorption, specifically under osteoclasts. The osteoclasts adhere normally to the bone surface but lack the ruffled border that is indicative of active resorption. Alendronate does not interfere with osteoclast recruitment or attachment, but it does inhibit osteoclast activity. Tiludronate disodium appears to inhibit osteoclasts through at least 2 mechanisms: Disruption of the cytoskeletal ring structure, possibly by inhibition of protein-tyrosine-phosphatase, thus leading to detachment of osteoclasts from the bone surface and the inhibition of the osteoclastic proton pump.

Reduction of abnormal bone resorption is responsible for therapeutic benefit in hypercalcemia. The exact mechanism(s) is not fully understood, but may be related to inhibition of hydroxyapatite crystal dissolution or its action on bone-resorbing cells. Pamidronate inhibits accelerated bone resorption resulting from osteoclast hyperactivity induced by various tumors in animals. The number of osteoclasts in active bone turnover sites is substantially reduced after etidronate. Etidronate also can inhibit formation and growth of hydroxyapatite crystals and their amorphous precursors at concentrations in excess of those required to inhibit crystal dissolution.

Alendronate – As a result of bone resorption inhibition, asymptomatic reductions in serum calcium and phosphate concentrations are seen after treatment with alendronate. In long-term studies, reductions from baseline in serum calcium (approximately 2%) and phosphate (approximately 4% to 6%) were seen the first month after initiation of 10 mg alendronate, but no further decreases were seen for the 5-year duration of the studies. The reduction in serum phosphate may reflect not only the positive bone mineral balance caused by alendronate but also a decrease in renal phosphate reabsorption. Alendronate decreases the rate of bone resorption directly, leading to an indirect decrease in bone formation.

In Paget disease, 40 mg alendronate once daily for 6 months produced highly significant decreases in serum alkaline phosphatase as well as in urinary markers of bone collagen degradation. As a result of the inhibition of bone resorption, alendronate induced generally mild, transient, and asymptomatic decreases in serum calcium and phosphate.

Etidronate – Etidronate does not appear to alter renal tubular reabsorption of calcium and does not affect hypercalcemia in patients with hyperparathyroidism where increased calcium reabsorption may be a factor in hypercalcemia. Hyperphosphatemia has been observed with oral etidronate, usually with doses of 10 to 20 mg/kg/day; no adverse effects have been noted, and it is not a contraindication. It is apparently caused by drug-related increased phosphate tubular reabsorption by the kidneys. Serum phosphate levels generally return to normal 2 to 4 weeks post-therapy.

In Paget disease, etidronate slows accelerated bone turnover (resorption and accretion) in pagetic lesions and to a lesser extent, in normal bone. Reduced bone turnover is often accompanied by symptomatic improvement, including reduced bone pain. Incidence of pagetic fractures may decrease, and elevated cardiac output and other vascular disorders improve.

Pamidronate – Pamidronate therapy has decreased serum phosphate levels, presumably caused by decreased release of phosphate from bone and increased renal excretion as parathyroid hormone levels (usually suppressed in HCM) return toward normal. Phosphate therapy was administered in 30% of patients; levels usually returned to normal within 7 to 10 days. Urinary calcium/creatinine and urinary hydroxyproline/creatinine ratios decrease and usually return to normal or below after treatment. The changes occur within the first week after treatment, as do decreases in serum calcium levels.

Risedronate – In pagetic patients treated with 30 mg/day risedronate for 2 months, bone turnover returned to normal in a majority of patients as evidenced by significant reductions in serum alkaline phosphatase (SAP), a marker of bone formation, and in urinary hydroxyproline/creatinine and deoxypyridinoline/creatinine, markers of bone resorption. Radiographic structural changes of bone lesions, especially improvement of a majority of lesions with an osteolytic front in weight-bearing bones, also were observed. In addition, histomorphometric data provide further support that risedronate decreases the extent of osteolysis in the appendicular and axial skeleton. Osteolytic lesions in the lower extremities improved or were unchanged in 15/16 (94%) of assessed patients; 9/16 (56%) patients showed clear improvement in osteolytic lesions. No evidence of new fractures was observed.

Tiludronate – In pagetic patients treated with 400 mg/day tiludronate for 3 months, changes in urinary hydroxyproline, a biochemical marker of bone resorption and in serum alkaline phosphatase, a marker of bone formation, indicate a reduction toward normal in the rate of bone turnover. In addition, reduced numbers of osteoclasts by histomorphometric analysis and radiological improvement of lytic lesions indicate that tiludronate can suppress the pagetic disease process.

Zoledronic acid – In vitro, zoledronic acid inhibits osteoclastic activity and induces osteoclast apoptosis. Zoledronic acid also blocks the osteoclastic resorption of mineralized bone and cartilage through its binding to bone. Zoledronic acid inhibits the increased osteoclastic activity and skeletal calcium release induced by various stimulatory factors released by tumors.

➤*Pharmacokinetics:*

Alendronate – There is no evidence that alendronate is metabolized. Relative to an IV reference dose, mean oral bioavailability in women was 0.64% for 5 to 70 mg doses after an overnight fast and 2 hours before a standardized breakfast. Oral bioavailability of the 10 mg tablet in men (0.59%) was similar to that in women given after an overnight fast and 2 hours before breakfast. In 49 postmenopausal women, bioavailability was decreased by approximately 40% when 10 mg was given either ½ or 1 hour before a standardized breakfast when compared with dosing 2 hours before eating. Bioavailability was negligible whether alendronate was given with or up to 2 hours after a standardized breakfast. Concomitant coffee or orange juice reduced bioavailability by approximately 60%. Mean steady-state volume of distribution (exclusive of bone) is at least 28 L. Protein binding in plasma is approximately 78%. After a single IV dose, approximately 50% was excreted in the urine with little or none recovered in the feces. After a single 10 mg IV dose, renal clearance was 71 mL/min; systemic clearance did not exceed 200 mL/min. Plasma levels fell by more than 95% within 6 hours after IV administration. The terminal half-life is estimated to exceed 10 years, probably reflecting alendronate release from the skeleton. Based on the above, it is estimated that after 10 years of 10 mg/day orally, the amount of alendronate released daily from the skeleton is approximately 25% of that absorbed from the GI tract.

Etidronate – Etidronate is not metabolized. The amount of drug absorbed after an oral dose is approximately 3%. In normal subjects, plasma half-life of etidronate, based on noncompartmental pharmacokinetics is 1 to 6 hours. Within 24 hours, about 50% of the absorbed dose is excreted in urine; the remainder is distributed to bone compartments from which it is slowly eliminated. Animal studies have yielded bone clearance estimates up to 165 days. In humans, the residence time on bone may vary due to such factors as specific metabolic condition and bone type. Unabsorbed drug is excreted intact in feces. Preclinical studies indicate etidronate disodium does not cross the blood-brain barrier. The mean residence time for IV etidronate in the exchangeable pool is approximately 8.7 hours. The mean volume of distribution at steady state in healthy subjects is 1370 ± 203 mL/kg while the plasma half-life is approximately 6 hours. In these same subjects, nonrenal clearance from the exchangeable pool amounts to 30% to 50% of the infused dose. This nonrenal clearance is caused by uptake by bone; subsequently, the drug is slowly eliminated through bone turnover. The half-life in bone is in excess of 90 days.

Pamidronate – Cancer patients (n = 24) who had minimal or no bony involvement were given an IV infusion of 30, 60, or 90 mg of pamidronate over 4 hours and 90 mg of pamidronate over 24 hours. The mean $\pm$ SD body retention of pamidronate was calculated to be $54\% \pm 16\%$ of the dose over 120 hours.

Pamidronate is not metabolized and is exclusively eliminated by renal excretion. After administration of 30, 60, and 90 mg of pamidronate over 4 hours, and 90 mg of pamidronate over 24 hours, an overall mean $\pm$ SD of $46\% \pm 16\%$ of the drug was excreted unchanged in the urine within 120 hours. Cumulative urinary excretion was linearly related to dose. The mean $\pm$ SD elimination half-life is 28 ± 7 hours. Mean $\pm$ SD total and renal clearances of pamidronate were 107 ± 50 mL/min and 49 ± 28 mL/min, respectively. The rate of elimination from bone has not been determined.

After IV administration in rats, approximately 50% to 60% was rapidly adsorbed by bone and slowly eliminated by the kidneys. In rats given 10 mg/kg bolus injections, approximately 30% of the compound was found in the liver shortly after administration and was then redistributed to bone or eliminated by the kidneys over 24 to 48 hours. The drug was rapidly cleared from circulation and taken up mainly by bones, liver, spleen, teeth, and tracheal cartilage. Bone uptake occurred preferentially in areas of high bone turnover. The terminal phase of elimination half-life in bone was approximately 300 days.

Risedronate – Like other bisphosphonates, no evidence supports systemic metabolism of risedronate. Absorption is relatively rapid (T_{max} approximately 1 hour) and is independent of dose. Mean oral bioavailability is 0.63%. Dosing either 0.5 hours prior to breakfast or 2 hours after dinner reduces extent of absorption by 55% as compared with the fasting state. Dosing 1 hour prior to breakfast reduces extent of absorption by 30% as compared with dosing in the fasting state.

Animal studies indicate that approximately 60% of the dose is distributed to bone with the remainder excreted in the urine. The mean steady-state volume of distribution is 6.3 L/kg; plasma protein binding is about 24%.

Approximately 50% of the absorbed dose is excreted in urine within 24 hours, and 85% of an IV dose is recovered in the urine over 28 days. Mean renal clearance is 105 mL/min and mean total clearance is 122 mL/min, with the difference primarily reflecting nonrenal clearance or clearance caused by adsorption to bone. The renal clearance is not concentration-dependent, and there is a linear relationship between renal clearance and creatinine clearance. Unabsorbed drug is eliminated unchanged in feces. Once risedronate is absorbed, the serum concentration-time profile is multiphasic with an initial half-life of about 1.5 hours and a terminal exponential half-life of 480 hours.

Tiludronate – In animals, tiludronic acid undergoes little if any metabolism. In vitro, tiludronic acid is not metabolized in human liver microsomes and hepatocytes.

Relative to IV reference dose, the mean oral bioavailability of tiludronate disodium in healthy men was 6% after an oral dose equivalent to 400 mg tiludronic acid administered after an overnight fast and 4 hours before a standard breakfast. Bioavailability is reduced by food.

After administration of a single dose equivalent to 400 mg tiludronic acid to healthy men, tiludronic acid was rapidly absorbed with peak plasma concentrations of approximately 3 mg/L occurring within 2 hours. In pagetic patients, after repeated administration of doses equivalent to 400 mg/day tiludronic acid (2 hours before or 2 hours after a meal) for durations of 12 days to 12 weeks, average plasma concentrations of tiludronic acid occurring between 1 and 2 hours after dosing ranged between 1 and 4.6 mg/L.

After oral administration of doses equivalent to 400 mg/day tiludronic acid to nonpagetic patients with osteoarthrosis, the steady state in bone was not reached after 30 days of dosing. At plasma concentrations between 1 and 10 mg/L, tiludronic acid was approximately 90% bound to human serum protein (mainly albumin).

The principal route of elimination of tiludronic acid is in the urine. After IV administration to healthy volunteers, approximately 60% of the dose was excreted in the urine as tiludronic acid within 13 days. Renal clearance is dose independent and is approximately 10 mL/min in healthy subjects. In pagetic patients treated with doses equivalent to 400 mg/day tiludronic acid for 12 days, the mean apparent plasma elimination half-life was approximately 150 hours. The elimination rate from human bone is unknown.

Special populations:

Renal insufficiency: The pharmacokinetics of **pamidronate** were studied in cancer patients (n = 19) with normal and varying degrees of renal impairment. Given the recommended dose, 90 mg infused over 4 hours, excessive accumulation of pamidronate in renally impaired patients is not anticipated if pamidronate is administered on a monthly basis.

►*Clinical trials:*
Osteoporosis –
Alendronate: Highly significant increases in bone mineral density (BMD) were seen in patients receiving 10 mg/day alendronate. Total body BMD also increased significantly, suggesting that the increases in bone mass of the spine and hip did not occur at the expense of other skeletal sites. Increases in BMD were evident as early as 3 months and continued throughout 3 years of treatment. Thus, alendronate seems to reverse the progression of osteoporosis.

One study found a 48% reduction in the proportion of patients treated with alendronate experiencing 1 or more new vertebral fractures (3.2% vs 6.2% with placebo). A reduction in the total number of new vertebral fractures (4.2% vs 11.3%) also was found In the pooled analysis, patients who received alendronate had a loss in stature that was statistically significantly less than was observed in those who received placebo (-3 mm vs -4.6 mm).

Risedronate: Risedronate 35 mg once a week (n = 485) was shown to be therapeutically equivalent to risedronate 5 mg/day (n = 480) in a 1-year, double-blind, multicenter study of postmenopausal women with osteoporosis. In the primary efficacy analysis of completers, the mean increases from baseline in lumbar spine BMD at 1 year were 4% (3.7, 4.3; 95% confidence interval [CI]) in the 5 mg/day group (n = 391) and 3.9% (3.6, 4.3; 95% CI) in the 35 mg once a week group (n = 387) and the mean difference between 5 mg/day and 35 mg/week was 0.1% (-0.42, 0.55; 95% CI). The results of the intent-to-treat analysis with the last observation carried forward were consistent with the primary efficacy analysis of completers. The 2 treatment groups also were similar with regard to BMD increases at other skeletal sites. The safety and efficacy of once-weekly 35 mg risedronate in women without osteoporosis are currently being studied, but data are not yet available.

Paget disease –
Alendronate vs etidronate: Efficacy of 40 mg alendronate once daily for 6 months was demonstrated in moderate to severe Paget disease. At 6 months, suppression of alkaline phosphatase in alendronate-treated patients was significantly greater than that with etidronate. A response occurred in approximately 85%, 30%, and 0% in alendronate-, etidronate-, and placebo-treated patients, respectively.

Pamidronate: In 1 study, 64 patients with moderate to severe Paget disease of bone received 5, 15, or 30 mg pamidronate as a single 4-hour infusion on 3 consecutive days, for total doses of 15, 45, and 90 mg. The median maximum percent decreases from baseline in serum alkaline phosphatase and urine hydroxyproline/creatinine ratios were 25%, 41%, and 57%, and 25%, 47%, and 61% for the 15, 45, and 90 mg groups, respectively. The median time to response (50% or more decrease) for serum alkaline phosphatase was approximately 1 month for the 90 mg group.

Tiludronate vs etidronate: A positive-controlled study was conducted in Europe with treatment groups of 400 mg/day tiludronate for 3 months with a 3-month treatment-free follow-up, 400 mg/day tiludronate for 6 months and 400 mg/day etidronate for 6 months. The efficacy of tiludronate was primarily assessed by SAP activity after 3 and 6 months.

Six months after the start of dosing, the decrease in SAP levels in patients who ceased dosing after a 3-month course of tiludronate was significantly greater than with 6 months of 400 mg/day etidronate, and was equivalent to levels in patients who completed a 6-month course of tiludronate.

Risedronate vs etidronate: In a double-blind, active-controlled study of patients with moderate to severe Paget disease, patients were treated with 30 mg/day risedronate for 2 months or etidronate 400 mg/day for 6 months. At day 180, 77% of risedronate-treated patients achieved normalization of serum alkaline phosphatase levels, compared with 10.5% of patients treated with etidronate. At day 540, 16 months after discontinuation of therapy, 53% of risedronate-treated patients and 14% of etidronate-treated patients with available data remained in biochemical remission.

During the first 180 days of the active-controlled study, 85% of risedronate-treated patients demonstrated a 75% or more reduction from baseline in serum alkaline phosphatase excess with 2 months of treatment compared with 20% in the etidronate-treated group with 6 months of treatment. Changes in serum alkaline phosphatase excess over time were significant following only 30 days of treatment, with a 36% reduction in serum alkaline phosphatase excess at that time compared with only a 6% reduction seen with etidronate treatment at the same time point.

Hypercalcemia of malignancy –
Etidronate: Patients with elevated calcium levels (10.1 to 17.4 mg/dL) were treated simultaneously with daily IV administration over a 3-day period and up to 3000 mL saline and 80 mg of a loop diuretic. In terms of total serum calcium changes, 88% of patients had reductions of serum calcium of 1 mg/dL or more. Total serum calcium returned to normal in 63% of patients within 7 days compared with 33% of patients treated with hydration alone. Reductions in urinary calcium excretion, which accompany reductions in excessive bone resorption, became apparent after 24 hours. This was accompanied or followed by maximum decreases in serum calcium, which were most frequently observed 72 hours after the first infusion.

When the total serum calcium values were adjusted for serum albumin levels, there was a return of normocalcemia in 24% of etidronate-treated patients and in 7% of patients treated with saline infusion. Of patients receiving etidronate, 87% vs 67% of patients on saline had albumin-adjusted serum calcium levels that returned to normal or were reduced by at least 1 mg/dL.

A second 3-day course of IV etidronate was tried in 14 patients who had a recurrence of hypercalcemia following an initial response to a 3-day infusion. All patients showed a decrease in total serum calcium of at least 1 mg/dL. Normalization of total serum calcium occurred in 11 patients.

Continuation of etidronate therapy with oral tablets may maintain clinically acceptable serum calcium levels and prolong normocalcemia.

Pamidronate: Patients who had HCM received either 30, 60, or 90 mg as a single 24-hour IV infusion if their corrected serum calcium levels were 12 mg/dL or more after 48 hours of saline hydration. The majority of patients (64%) had decreases in albumin-corrected serum calcium levels by 24 hours after initiation of treatment. Mean-corrected serum calcium levels at days 2 to 7 after treatment initiation were significantly reduced from baseline in all 3 dosage groups. As a result, by 7 days after initiation of treatment, 40%, 61%, and 100% of the patients receiving 30, 60, and 90 mg, respectively, had normal corrected serum calcium levels. Many patients (33% to 53%) in the 60 and 90 mg dosage groups continued to have normal-corrected serum calcium levels or a partial response (at least a 15% decrease of corrected serum calcium from baseline) at day 14.

Etidronate vs pamidronate: Cancer patients who had corrected serum calcium levels of 12 mg/dL or more after at least 24 hours of saline hydration were randomized to receive either 60 mg pamidronate (n = 30) as a single 24-hour IV infusion or 7.5 mg/kg etidronate (n = 35) as a 2-hour IV infusion daily for 3 days. By day 7, 70% of the patients on pamidronate and 41% on etidronate had normal corrected serum calcium levels ($P < 0.05$). When partial responders (at least a 15% decrease of serum calcium from baseline) were included, response rates were 97% for pamidronate and 65% for etidronate ($P < 0.01$). Mean corrected serum calcium for the pamidronate and etidronate groups decreased from baseline values to 10.4 and 11.2 mg/dL, respectively, on day 7. At day 14, 43% on pamidronate and 18% on etidronate still had normal corrected serum calcium levels, or maintenance of a partial response. For responders in pamidronate and etidronate groups, median duration of response was similar (7 and 5 days, respectively).

Zoledronic acid vs pamidronate: Two identical multicenter, randomized, double-blind, double-dummy studies of 4 mg zoledronic acid given as a 5-minute IV infusion or 90 mg pamidronate given as a 2-hour IV infusion were conducted in 185 patients with HCM.

To assess the effects of zoledronic acid vs those of pamidronate, the 2 multicenter HCM studies were combined in a preplanned analysis. The results of the primary analysis revealed that the proportion of patients that had normalization of corrected serum calcium by day 10 were 88% and 70% for 4 mg zoledronic acid and 90 mg pamidronate, respectively ($P = 0.002$). In these studies, no additional benefit was seen for 8 mg zoledronic acid over 4 mg zoledronic acid; however, the risk of renal toxicity of 8 mg zoledronic acid was significantly greater than that seen with 4 mg zoledronic acid.

Heterotopic ossification – **Etidronate** reduces the incidence of clinically important heterotopic bone by approximately 66% and retards the progression of immature lesions and reduces the severity by at least 50%. Follow-up data (9 months or more) suggest these benefits persist.

Contraindications

Hypersensitivity to bisphosphonates or any component of the products; hypocalcemia (**alendronate**, **risedronate**, see Precautions); abnormalities of the esophagus that delay esophageal emptying such as stricture or achalasia (**alendronate**); inability to stand or sit upright for at least 30 minutes (**alendronate**, **risedronate**); clinically overt osteomalacia (oral **etidronate**); Class Dc and higher renal impairment (serum creatinine more than 5 mg/dL; IV **etidronate** only; see Warnings).

Warnings

➤*GI irritation/disorders:* Bisphosphonates cause local irritation of the upper GI mucosa. Alert physicians to any signs or symptoms signaling a possible esophageal reaction and instruct patients to discontinue bisphosphonates and seek medical attention if they develop dysphagia, odynophagia, retrosternal pain, or new or worsening heartburn.

The risk of severe esophageal adverse experiences appears to be greater in patients who lie down after taking bisphosphonates or who fail to swallow it with a full glass (6 to 8 oz) of water, or who continue to take bisphosphonates after developing symptoms suggestive of esophageal irritation. Therefore, it is very important that the full dosing instructions are provided to and understood by the patient. In patients who cannot comply with dosing instructions because of mental disability, use bisphosphonate therapy under appropriate supervision.

Because of possible irritant effects of bisphosphonates on the upper GI mucosa and a potential for worsening of the underlying disease, use caution when bisphosphonates are given to patients with active upper GI problems (such as dysphagia, esophageal diseases, gastritis, duodenitis, or ulcers). **Etidronate** therapy has been withheld from patients with enterocolitis because diarrhea is seen in some patients, particularly at higher doses.

➤*Osteoporosis (alendronate):* Consider causes of osteoporosis other than estrogen deficiency and aging; consider glucocorticoid use.

➤*Paget disease (oral etidronate):* Response to therapy may be slow and continue for months after treatment discontinuation. Do not increase dosage prematurely. Do not initiate retreatment until after at least a 90-day drug-free interval.

➤*Asthma (zoledronic acid):* While not observed in clinical trials with zoledronic acid, administration of other bisphosphonates has been associated with bronchoconstriction in aspirin-sensitive asthmatic patients. Use zoledronic acid with caution in patients with aspirin-sensitive asthma.

➤*Renal function impairment:*

Alendronate – Although no clinical information is available, it is likely that alendronate elimination via the kidney will be reduced in impaired renal function. Therefore, somewhat greater accumulation of alendronate in bone might be expected in impaired renal function. No dosage adjustment is necessary in mild to moderate renal insufficiency (Ccr 35 to 60 mL/min). Alendronate use is not recommended in more severe renal insufficiency (Ccr less than 35 mL/min).

Etidronate (IV) – Occasional mild to moderate renal function abnormalities (elevated BUN or serum creatinine) have occurred when etidronate IV infusion was given to patients with HCM. These were reversible or remained stable without worsening after therapy completion. In some patients with preexisting renal impairment or who had received potentially nephrotoxic drugs, further renal function depression was sometimes seen. Monitor renal function.

Reduction of the etidronate dose, if used at all, may be advisable in Class Cc (Classification of Renal Function Impairment) renal function impairment (serum creatinine 2.5 to 4.9 mg/dL). Use only if the potential benefit of hypercalcemia correction will substantially exceed the potential for worsening of renal function. In patients with Class Dc and higher renal function impairment (serum creatinine greater than 5 mg/dL), withhold etidronate infusion.

Pamidronate – Bisphosphonates, including pamidronate, have been associated with renal toxicity manifested as deterioration of renal function and potential renal failure.

Because of the risk of clinically significant deterioration in renal function, which may progress to renal failure, single doses of pamidronate should not exceed 90 mg (see Administration and Dosage for appropriate infusion durations).

Pamidronate has not been tested in patients who have Class Dc renal impairment (creatinine greater than 5 mg/dL) and has been tested in few multiple myeloma patients with serum creatinine 3 mg/dL or more. For the treatment of bone metastases, the use of pamidronate in patients with severe renal impairment is not recommended. In other indications, clinical judgement should determine whether the potential benefit outweighs the potential risk in such patients.

Risedronate – Risedronate is not recommended for patients with severe renal impairment (Ccr less than 30 mL/min). No dosage adjustment is needed when Ccr is greater than 30 mL/min.

Tiludronate – Tiludronate is not recommended for patients with severe renal failure (Ccr less than 30 mL/min). The plasma elimination half-life is longer.

Zoledronic acid – Because of the risk of clinically significant deterioration in renal function, which may progress to renal failure, single doses of zoledronic acid should not exceed 4 mg and the duration of infusion should be no less than 15 minutes. Because safety and pharmacokinetic data are limited in patients with severe renal impairment, zoledronic acid treatment is not recommended in patients with bone metastases with severe renal impairment (in the clinical trials, patients with serum creatinine greater than 3 mg/dL were excluded). Consider zoledronic acid treatment in patients with HCM only after evaluating the risks and benefits of treatment (in the clinical trials, patients with serum creatinine greater than 400 mcmol/L or greater than 4.5 mg/dL were excluded).

In clinical trials, the risk for renal function deterioration (defined as an increase in serum creatinine) was significantly increased in patients who received zoledronic acid over 5 minutes compared with patients who received the same dose over 15 minutes. In addition, the risk for renal function deterioration and renal failure was significantly increased in patients who received 8 mg zoledronic acid, even when given over 15 minutes. While this risk is reduced with the 4 mg zoledronic acid dose administered over 15 minutes, deterioration in renal function can still occur. Risk factors for this deterioration include elevated baseline creatinine and multiple cycles of treatment with the bisphosphonate. Patients who receive zoledronic acid should have serum creatinine assessed prior to each treatment.

➤*Carcinogenesis:*

Alendronate – Parafollicular cell (thyroid) adenomas were increased in high-dose male rats ($P = 0.003$) at doses equivalent to 1 and 3.75 mg/kg body weight. These doses are equivalent to 0.26 and 1 times a 40 mg human daily dose based on surface area, mg/m^2.

Pamidronate – In a 104-week carcinogenicity study (daily oral pamidronate administration) in rats, there was a positive dose-response relationship for benign adrenal pheochromocytoma in males ($P < 0.00001$).

Zoledronic acid – Mice were given oral doses of zoledronic acid of 0.1, 0.5, or 2 mg/kg/day. There was an increased incidence of Harderian gland adenomas in males and females in all treatment groups (at doses of 0.002 or more times a human IV dose of 4 mg, based on a comparison of relative body surface areas).

➤*Fertility impairment:*
Pamidronate – In rats, decreased fertility occurred in first-generation offspring of parents who had received 150 mg/kg oral pamidronate; however, this occurred only when animals were mated with members of the same dose group.

Risedronate – In rats, inhibited ovulation at an oral dose of 16 mg/kg/day and decreased implantation with doses of 7 mg/kg/day or more occurred. Testicular and epididymal atrophy and inflammation were noted at 40 mg/kg/day.

Zoledronic acid – Female rats were given SC doses of 0.01, 0.03, or 0.1 mg/kg/day zoledronic acid beginning 15 days before mating and continuing through gestation. Effects observed in the high-dose group (with systemic exposure of 1.2 times the human systemic exposure following an IV dose of 4 mg, based on AUC comparison) included inhibition of ovulation and a decrease in the number of pregnant rats. Effects observed in both the mid-dose group (with systemic exposure of 0.2 times the human systemic exposure following an IV dose of 4 mg, based on AUC comparison) and high-dose group included an increase in preimplantation losses and a decrease in the number of implantations and live fetuses.

➤*Pregnancy:*
Category D. –
Pamidronate: Bolus IV studies conducted in rats and rabbits determined that pamidronate produces maternal toxicity and embryo/fetal effects when given during organogenesis at doses of 0.6 to 8.3 times the highest recommended human dose for a single IV infusion. As it has been shown that pamidronate can cross the placenta in rats and has produced marked maternal and nonterotogenic embryo/fetal effects in rats and rabbits, it should not be given to women during pregnancy.

There are no adequate and well-controlled studies in pregnant women. If the patient becomes pregnant while taking this drug, apprise the patient of the potential harm to the fetus. Advise women of childbearing potential to avoid becoming pregnant.

Zoledronic acid: There are no studies in pregnant women using zoledronic acid. If the patient becomes pregnant while taking this drug, apprise the patient of the potential harm to the fetus. Advise women of childbearing potential to avoid becoming pregnant.

Do not use zoledronic acid during pregnancy. It may cause fetal harm when administered to a pregnant woman. In reproductive studies in the pregnant rat, SC doses equivalent to 2.4 or 4.8 times the human systemic exposure (IV dose of 4 mg based on an AUC comparison) resulted in pre- and postimplantation losses, decreases in viable fetuses and fetal skeletal, visceral, and external malformations.

Category C. –
Alendronate: There are no studies in pregnant women. Use alendronate during pregnancy only if the potential benefit justifies the risk to the mother and fetus.

Reproduction studies in rats showed decreased postimplantation survival at 2 mg/kg/day and decreased body weight gain in normal pups at 1 mg/kg/day. Sites of incomplete fetal ossification were statistically significantly increased in rats beginning at 10 mg/kg/day in vertebral (cervical, thoracic, and lumbar), skull, and sternebral bones. Both total and ionized calcium decreased in pregnant rats at 15 mg/kg/day (3.9 times a 40 mg human daily dose based on surface area, mg/m²) resulting in delays and failures of delivery. Protracted parturition because of maternal hypocalcemia occurred in rats at doses as low as 0.5 mg/kg/day (0.13 times a 40 mg human daily dose based on surface area, mg/m²) when rats were treated from before mating through gestation. Maternotoxicity (late pregnancy deaths) occurred in rats treated with 15 mg/kg/day alendronate for varying periods of time; these deaths were lessened but not eliminated by treatment cessation. Calcium could not ameliorate hypocalcemia or prevent maternal and neonatal deaths caused by delay in delivery; IV calcium supplementation prevented maternal but not fetal deaths.

Oral etidronate: There are no adequate and well-controlled studies in pregnant women. Use only when clearly needed and when the potential benefits outweigh potential hazards to the fetus. Etidronate has caused skeletal abnormalities in rats when given at oral dose levels of 300 mg/kg (15 to 60 times the human dose). Other effects on the offspring (including decreased live births) occur at dosages that cause significant toxicity in the parent generation and are 25 to 200 times the human dose. The skeletal effects are thought to be the result of the pharmacological effects of the drug on bone.

IV etidronate: There are no adequate and well-controlled studies.

Risedronate: There are no adequate and well-controlled studies in pregnant women. Use during pregnancy only if the potential benefit justifies the potential risk to the fetus.

Survival of neonates was decreased in rats treated during gestation with oral doses of 16 mg/kg/day or more (approximately 5.2 times the 30 mg/day human dose based on surface area, mg/m²). Body weight was decreased in neonates from dams treated with 80 mg/kg (approximately 26 times the 30 mg/day human dose based on surface area, mg/m²). In rats treated during gestation, the number of fetuses exhibiting incomplete ossification of sternebrae or skull was statistically significantly increased at 7.1 mg/kg/day (approximately 2.3 times the 30 mg/day human dose based on surface area, mg/m²).

Tiludronate: There are no adequate and well-controlled studies in pregnant women. Use tiludronate during pregnancy only if the potential benefit justifies the potential risk to the fetus.

In rabbits at doses of 42 and 130 mg/kg/day (2 and 5 times the 400 mg/day human dose based on body surface area), there was dose-related scoliosis likely attributable to the pharmacologic properties of tiludronate. Mice receiving 375 mg/kg/day (7 times the 400 mg/day human dose based on body surface area mg/m²) showed slight maternal toxicity. Maternal toxicity also was observed in rats dosed at 375 mg/kg/day (10 times the 400 mg/day human dose).

➤*Lactation:* It is not known whether these drugs are excreted in breast milk. Exercise caution when administering **alendronate**, **etidronate, tiludronate, risedronate, pamidronate,** or **zoledronic acid** to a nursing mother. Because zoledronic acid binds to bone long-term, do not administer to a nursing woman.

➤*Children:* Safety and efficacy for use in children have not been established with most bisphosphonates (in children less than 18 years of age for **risedronate**).

Children have been treated with oral **etidronate** at doses recommended for adults to prevent heterotopic ossifications or soft tissue calcifications. A rachitic syndrome has been reported infrequently at doses of 10 mg/kg/day or more and for prolonged periods approaching or exceeding 1 year. The epiphyseal radiologic changes associated with retarded mineralization of new osteoid and cartilage, and occasional symptoms reported, have been reversible when medication is discontinued.

Precautions

➤*Monitoring:* Assess serum creatinine in patients who receive **pamidronate** prior to each treatment. Patients treated with pamidronate for bone metastases should have the dose withheld if renal function has deteriorated. Carefully monitor standard hypercalcemia-related metabolic parameters, such as serum levels of calcium, phosphate, magnesium, and potassium following pamidronate and **zoledronic acid** initiation. Asymptomatic hypophosphatemia (16%), hypomagnesemia (11%), hypokalemia (7%), and hypocalcemia (5% to 12%) have occurred. Also, closely monitor electrolytes, creatinine, CBC, differential, and hematocrit/hemoglobin. Carefully monitor patients who have pre-existing anemia, leukopenia, or thrombocytopenia in the first 2 weeks following treatment.

➤*Hypercalcemia:* Carefully monitor standard hypercalcemia-related metabolic parameters, such as serum levels of calcium, phosphate, and magnesium, as well as serum creatinine, following initiation of therapy with **zoledronic acid**. Patients with HCM must be adequately rehydrated prior to administration of zoledronic acid. Do not use loop diuretics until the patient is adequately rehydrated; use with caution in combination with zoledronic acid in order to avoid hypocalcemia. Use zoledronic acid with caution with other nephrotoxic drugs.

➤*Concomitant use with estrogen/hormone replacement therapy (alendronate):* Two clinical studies have shown that the degree of suppression of bone turnover (as assessed by mineralizing surface) was significantly greater with the combination than with either component alone. The safety and tolerability profile of the combination was consistent with those individual treatments.

➤*Nutrition:* Maintain adequate nutrition, particularly an adequate intake of calcium and vitamin D when taking oral **etidronate, risedronate,** and **alendronate**.

➤*Osteoid:* Oral **etidronate** suppresses bone turnover and may retard mineralization of osteoid laid down during the bone accretion process. These effects are dose- and time-dependent. Osteoid, which may accumulate noticeably at doses of 10 to 20 mg/kg/day, mineralizes normally post-therapy. In patients with fractures, especially of long bones, it may be advisable to delay or interrupt treatment until callus is evident.

➤*Fracture:* In Paget patients, treatment regimens of oral **etidronate** exceeding the recommended daily maximum dose of 20 mg/kg or continuous administration for periods greater than 6 months may be associated with osteomalacia and an increased risk of fracture.

Long bones predominantly affected by lytic lesions, particularly in those patients unresponsive to therapy, may be especially prone to fracture. Radiographically and biochemically monitor patients with predominantly lytic lesions to permit termination of etidronate in those patients unresponsive to treatment.

➤*Hypocalcemia:* Hypocalcemia (5% to 12%) has occurred with **pamidronate** therapy. Rare cases of symptomatic hypocalcemia (including tetany) occurred during pamidronate treatment. If hypocalcemia occurs, consider short-term calcium therapy.

Hypocalcemia must be corrected before therapy initiation with **alendronate** and **risedronate**. Also effectively treat other disturbances of mineral metabolism (eg, vitamin D deficiency). Presumably because of the effects of alendronate and risedronate on increasing bone mineral, small asymptomatic decreases in serum calcium and phosphate may occur, especially in patients with Paget disease, in whom the pretreatment rate of bone turnover may be greatly elevated and in patients receiving glucocorticoids, in whom calcium absorption may be decreased. Ensure adequate calcium and vitamin D intake to provide for these enhanced needs.

Drug Interactions

Bisphosphonate Drug Interactions

Precipitant drug	Object drug[*]		Description
Aminoglycosides	Bisphosphonates (Zoledronic acid)	↑	Caution is advised when bisphosphonates are administered with aminoglycosides, because these agents may have an additive effect to lower serum calcium levels for prolonged periods.
Aspirin	Tiludronate	↓	Aspirin may decrease the bioavailability of tiludronate by up to 50% when taken 2 hours after tiludronate.
Calcium supplements, antacids	Alendronate, Etidronate, Risedronate, Tiludronate	↓	Products containing calcium and other multivalent cations interfere with alendronate, risedronate, and etidronate absorption. The bioavailability of tiludronate is decreased by 80% by calcium when administered at the same time and 60% by some aluminum- or magnesium-containing antacids when administered 1 hour before tiludronate.
Loop diuretics	Zoledronic acid	↑	Use caution when zoledronic acid is used in combination with loop diuretics because of an increased risk of hypocalcemia.
Indomethacin	Tiludronate	↑	The bioavailability of tiludronate is increased 2- to 4-fold by indomethacin, but is not significantly altered by coadministration of diclofenac.

Bisphosphonate Drug Interactions

Precipitant drug	Object drug[*]		Description
Ranitidine	Alendronate	↑	IV ranitidine doubled alendronate bioavailability. The clinical significance is unknown.
Alendronate	Aspirin	↑	The risk of upper GI adverse effects associated with aspirin increased with alendronate doses > 10 mg/day.
Etidronate	Warfarin	↑	There have been isolated reports of patients experiencing increases in their prothrombin times when etidronate was added to warfarin therapy. Patients on warfarin should have their prothrombin time monitored.

[*] ↑ = Object drug increased.   ↓ = Object drug decreased.

►*Drug/Food interactions:* In 1 study, bioavailability of **alendronate** was decreased by 40% when 10 mg alendronate was given 0.5 or 1 hour before breakfast vs 2 hours before, and bioavailability was negligible when alendronate was given with or 2 hours after breakfast. Concomitant coffee or orange juice reduced bioavailability by 60%. Take alendronate in the morning at least 30 minutes before the first meal, beverage, or medication.

Absorption of **etidronate** may be reduced by foods. Take on an empty stomach 2 hours before a meal.

In single-dose studies, bioavailability of **tiludronate** was reduced by 90% when an oral dose equivalent to 400 mg tiludronic acid was administered with, or 2 hours after, a standard breakfast compared with the same dose administered after an overnight fast and 4 hours before a standard breakfast.

Mean oral bioavailability of **risedronate** is decreased when given with food. Take at least 30 minutes before the first food or drink of the day other than water.

Adverse Reactions

Bisphosphonate Adverse Reactions (%)[a]

Adverse reaction	Pamidronate 90 mg (n = 572)[c]	Pamidronate 60 mg over 4 hr (n = 23)	Pamidronate 60 mg over 24 hr (n = 73)	Pamidronate 90 mg over 24 hr (n = 17)	Etidronate 7.5 mg/kg x 3 days (n = 35)	Alendronate 10 mg/day[d] (n = 196)	Alendronate Fracture intervention trial[b] (n = 3236)	Tiludronate 400 mg/day (n = 75)	Tiludronate 30 mg/day x 2 months (n = 61)[e]	Risedronate 5 mg (n = 1916)	Risedronate 5 mg/day (n = 480)	Risedronate 35 mg/week (n = 485)	Zoledronic acid Hypercalcemia of malignancy 4 mg (n = 86)	Zoledronic acid Combined multiple myeloma and bone metastases of solid tumor trials 4 mg (n = 1099)
Cardiovascular														
Angina pectoris	—	—	—	—	—	—	—	—	—	2.5	—	—	—	—
Atrial fibrillation	—	—	—	6	—	—	—	—	—	—	—	—	—	—
Atrial flutter	—	—	1	—	—	—	—	—	—	—	—	—	—	—
Cardiac failure	—	—	1	—	—	—	—	—	—	—	—	—	—	—
Cardiovascular disorder	—	—	—	—	—	—	—	—	—	2.5	—	—	—	—
Chest pain	—	—	—	—	—	—	—	2.7	6.6	5	2.3	2.7	—	—
Hypertension	—	—	—	6	—	—	—	—	—	10	5.8	4.9	—	—
Hypotension	—	—	—	—	—	—	—	—	—	—	—	—	10.5	—
Syncope	—	—	—	6	—	—	—	—	—	—	0.6	2.1	—	—
Tachycardia	—	—	—	6	—	—	—	—	—	—	—	—	—	—
Vasodilation	—	—	—	—	—	—	—	—	—	—	2.3	1.4	—	—
CNS														
Agitation	—	—	—	—	—	—	—	—	—	—	—	—	12.8	—
Anxiety	14.3	—	—	—	—	—	—	—	—	4.3	0.6	2.7	14	9
Confusion	—	—	—	—	—	—	—	—	—	—	—	—	12.8	—
Convulsions	—	—	—	—	3	—	—	—	—	—	—	—	—	—
Depression	—	—	—	—	—	—	—	—	—	6.8	2.3	2.3	—	12
Dizziness	—	—	—	—	—	—	—	4	6.6	6.4	5.8	4.9	—	14
Headache	26.2	—	—	—	—	2.6	0.2	6.7	18	—	7.3	7.2	—	18
Hypertonia	—	—	—	—	—	—	—	—	—	2.2	—	—	—	—
Hypesthesia	—	—	—	—	—	—	—	—	—	—	—	—	—	10
Insomnia	22.2	—	1	—	—	—	—	—	—	4.7	—	—	15.1	14
Neuralgia	—	—	—	—	—	—	—	—	—	3.8	—	—	—	—
Paresthesia	—	—	—	—	—	—	—	4	—	2.1	—	—	—	12
Psychosis	—	4	—	—	—	—	—	—	—	—	—	—	—	—
Somnolence	—	—	1	6	—	—	—	—	—	—	—	—	—	—

Bisphosphonate Adverse Reactions (%)[a]

Adverse reaction	Pamidronate				Etidronate	Alendronate		Tiludronate	Risedronate				Zoledronic acid	
	Osteolytic bone metastases of breast cancer and osteolytic lesions of multiple myeloma (Average of 3 trials)	Hypercalcemia of malignancy study comparing these 3 dose regimens			Hypercalcemia of malignancy	Osteoporosis in postmenopausal women	Fracture intervention trial[b]	Pagetic patients	Pagetic patients	Combined osteoporosis trials	Osteoporosis study in postmenopausal women comparing these 2 doseforms		Hypercalcemia of malignancy	Combined multiple myeloma and bone metastases of solid tumor trials
	90 mg (n = 572)[c]	60 mg over 4 hr (n = 23)	60 mg over 24 hr (n = 73)	90 mg over 24 hr (n = 17)	7.5 mg/kg x 3 days (n = 35)	10 mg/day[d] (n = 196)	(n = 3236)	400 mg/day (n = 75)	30 mg/day x 2 months (n = 61)[e]	5 mg (n = 1916)	5 mg/day (n = 480)	35 mg/week (n = 485)	4 mg (n = 86)	4 mg (n = 1099)
Vertigo	—	—	—	—	—	—	—	—	—	3.3	2.1	1.6	—	—
Dermatologic														
Alopecia	—	—	—	—	—	—	—	—	—	—	—	—	—	11
Dermatitis	—	—	—	—	—	—	—	—	—	—	—	—	—	10
Pruritus	—	—	—	—	—	—	—	—	—	3	1.9	2.3	—	—
Rash	—	—	—	—	—	—	—	2.7	11.5	7.7	3.1	4.1	—	—
Skin carcinoma	—	—	—	—	—	—	—	—	—	2	—	—	—	—
Skin disorder	—	—	—	—	—	2.7	—	—	—	—	—	—	—	—
GI														
Abdominal pain	22.6	—	1	—	—	6.6	1.5	—	11.5	11.6	7.3	7.6	16.3	12
Abdominal distension	—	—	—	—	—	1	—	—	—	—	—	—	—	—
Acid regurgitation	—	—	—	—	—	2	1.1	—	—	—	—	—	—	—
Anorexia	26	4	1	12	—	—	—	—	—	—	—	—	9.3	20
Appetite decreased	—	—	—	—	—	—	—	—	—	—	—	—	—	11
Belching	—	—	—	—	—	—	—	—	3.3	—	—	—	—	—
Colitis	—	—	—	—	—	—	—	—	3.3	—	0.8	2.5	—	—
Constipation	33.2	4	—	6	3	3.1	0	—	6.6	—	12.5	12.2	26.7	28
Diarrhea	28.5	—	1	—	—	3.1	0.6	9.3	19.7	10.6	6.3	4.9	17.4	22
Dry mouth	—	—	—	—	—	—	—	—	—	—	2.5	1.4	—	—
Dyspepsia	22.6	4	—	—	—	3.6	1.1	5.3	—	—	6.9	7.6	—	—
Dysphasia	—	—	—	—	—	1	0.1	—	—	—	—	—	—	—
Esophageal ulcer	—	—	—	—	—	1.5	0.1	—	—	—	—	—	—	—
Flatulence	—	—	—	—	—	2.6	0.2	2.7	—	4.6	3.3	3.1	—	—
Gastritis	—	—	—	—	—	0.5	0.6	—	—	2.5	—	—	—	—
Gastroenteritis	—	—	—	—	—	—	—	—	—	—	3.8	3.5	—	—
GI disorder	—	—	—	—	—	—	—	—	—	2.3	1.9	2.5	—	—
GI hemorrhage	—	—	—	6	—	—	—	—	—	—	—	—	—	—
Nausea	53.5	4	—	18	6	3.6	1.1	9.3	9.8	10.9	8.5	6.2	29.1	43
Rectal disorder	—	—	—	—	—	—	—	—	—	2.2	—	—	—	—
Stomatitis	—	—	1	—	3	—	—	—	—	—	—	—	—	—
Vomiting	35.7	4	—	—	—	1	0.2	4	—	—	1.9	2.5	14	30
Weight decreased	—	—	—	—	—	—	—	—	—	—	—	—	—	13
Hemic/Lymphatic														
Anemia	42.5	—	—	6	—	—	—	—	—	2.4	—	—	22.1	29
Ecchymosis	—	—	—	—	—	—	—	—	—	4.3	—	—	—	—
Granulocytopenia	19.8	—	—	—	—	—	—	—	—	—	—	—	—	—
Leukopenia	—	4	—	—	—	—	—	—	—	—	—	—	—	—
Neutropenia	—	—	1	—	—	—	—	—	—	—	—	—	—	11
Thrombocytopenia	14	—	1	—	—	—	—	—	—	—	—	—	—	—
Lab abnormalities														
Abnormal hepatic function	—	—	—	—	3	—	—	—	—	—	—	—	—	—
Hypocalcemia	3.3	—	1	12	—	—	—	—	—	—	—	—	—	—
Hypokalemia	10.5	4	4	18	—	—	—	—	—	—	—	—	11.6	—
Hypomagnesemia	4.4	4	10	12	3	—	—	—	—	—	—	—	10.5	—
Hypophosphatemia	1.7	—	9	18	3	—	—	—	—	—	—	—	12.8	—
Serum creatinine	18.5	—	—	—	—	—	—	—	—	—	—	—	—	—
Musculoskeletal														
Arthralgia	13.6	—	—	—	—	—	—	2.7	32.8	23.7	11.5	14.2	—	18
Arthritis	—	—	—	—	—	—	—	—	—	—	4.8	4.1	—	—
Arthrosis	—	—	—	—	—	—	—	2.7	—	—	—	—	—	—
Back pain	—	—	—	—	—	8	—	—	—	26.1	9.2	8.7	—	10
Bone disorder	—	—	—	—	—	—	—	—	—	4	—	—	—	—
Bone fracture	—	—	—	—	—	—	—	—	—	—	5	6.4	—	—
Bone/skeletal pain	66.8	—	—	—	—	4.1	0.4	—	4.9	4.6	2.9	1.4	11.6	53

Bisphosphonate Adverse Reactions (%)[a]

Adverse reaction	Pamidronate — Osteolytic bone metastases of breast cancer and osteolytic lesions of multiple myeloma (Average of 3 trials) 90 mg (n = 572)[c]	Pamidronate — Hypercalcemia of malignancy study comparing these 3 dose regimens 60 mg over 4 hr (n = 23)	60 mg over 24 hr (n = 73)	90 mg over 24 hr (n = 17)	Etidronate — Hypercalcemia of malignancy 7.5 mg/kg x 3 days (n = 35)	Alendronate — Osteoporosis in postmenopausal women 10 mg/day[d] (n = 196)	Alendronate — Fracture intervention trial[b] (n = 3236)	Tiludronate — Pagetic patients 400 mg/day (n = 75)	Risedronate — Pagetic patients 30 mg/day x 2 months (n = 61)[e]	Risedronate — Combined osteoporosis trials 5 mg (n = 1916)	Risedronate — Osteoporosis study in postmenopausal women comparing these 2 doseforms 5 mg/day (n = 480)	35 mg/week (n = 485)	Zoledronic acid — Hypercalcemia of malignancy 4 mg (n = 86)	Zoledronic acid — Combined multiple myeloma and bone metastases of solid tumor trials 4 mg (n = 1099)
Bursitis	—	—	—	—	—	—	—	—	—	3	1.3	2.5	—	—
Joint disorder	—	—	—	—	—	—	—	—	—	6.8	—	—	—	—
Leg/Muscle cramps	—	—	—	—	—	—	0.2	—	3.3	3.5	—	—	—	—
Myalgia	26	—	1	—	—	—	—	—	—	6.6	4.6	6.2	—	21
Myasthenia	—	—	—	—	—	—	—	—	3.3	—	—	—	—	—
Tendon disorder	—	—	—	—	—	—	—	—	—	3	—	—	—	—
Respiratory														
Bronchitis	—	—	—	—	—	—	—	—	3.3	—	2.3	4.9	—	—
Coughing	25.7	—	—	—	—	—	—	2.7	—	—	3.1	2.5	11.6	19
Dyspnea	30.4	—	—	—	3	—	—	—	—	3.8	—	—	22.1	24
Pharyngitis	—	—	—	—	—	—	—	2.7	—	5.8	4.6	2.9	—	—
Pleural effusion	10.7	—	—	—	—	—	—	—	—	—	—	—	—	—
Pneumonia	—	—	—	—	—	—	—	—	—	3.1	0.8	2.5	—	—
Rales	—	—	—	6	—	—	—	—	—	—	—	—	—	—
Rhinitis	—	—	—	6	—	—	—	5.3	—	5.7	2.3	2.1	—	—
Sinusitis	15.6	—	—	—	—	—	—	5.3	4.9	—	4.6	4.5	—	—
URI	24.1	—	3	—	—	—	—	5.3	—	—	—	—	—	8
Special senses														
Amblyopia	—	—	—	—	—	—	—	—	3.3	—	—	—	—	—
Cataract	—	—	—	—	—	—	—	2.7	—	5.9	2.9	1.9	—	—
Conjunctivitis	—	—	—	—	—	—	—	2.7	—	3.1	—	—	—	—
Dry eye	—	—	—	—	—	—	—	—	3.3	—	—	—	—	—
Glaucoma	—	—	—	—	—	—	—	2.7	—	—	—	—	—	—
Otitis media	—	—	—	—	—	—	—	—	—	2.5	—	—	—	—
Taste perversion	—	—	—	—	3	0.5	0.1	—	—	—	—	—	—	—
Tinnitus	—	—	—	—	—	—	—	—	3.3	—	—	—	—	—
General														
Accidental injury	—	—	—	—	—	—	—	4	—	—	10.6	10.7	—	—
Asthenia	22.2	—	—	—	—	—	—	—	4.9	5.1	3.5	5.4	—	21
Edema/Peripheral edema	—	—	1	—	—	—	—	2.7	8.2	—	4.2	1.6	—	19
Fatigue	37.2	—	—	12	—	—	—	—	—	—	—	—	—	36
Fever	38.5	26	19	18	9	—	—	—	—	—	—	—	44.2	30
Fluid overload	—	—	—	—	6	—	—	—	—	—	—	—	—	—
Influenza-like symptoms	—	—	—	—	—	—	—	4	9.8	—	7.1	8.5	—	—
Infusion-site reaction	—	—	4	18	—	—	—	—	—	—	—	—	—	—
Metastases	20.5	—	—	—	—	—	—	—	—	—	—	—	11.6	—
Moniliasis	—	—	—	6	—	—	—	—	—	—	—	—	—	—
Pain	14.3	—	—	—	—	—	—	21.3	—	13.6	7.7	9.9	—	—
Miscellaneous														
Allergic reaction	—	—	—	—	—	—	—	—	—	—	1.9	2.5	—	—
Cancer progression	—	—	—	—	—	—	—	—	—	—	—	—	16.3	—
Cystitis	—	—	—	—	—	—	—	—	—	4.1	—	—	—	—
Dehydration	—	—	—	—	—	—	—	—	—	—	—	—	—	12
Hernia	—	—	—	—	—	—	—	—	—	2.9	—	—	—	—
Hyperparathyroidism	—	—	—	—	—	—	—	2.7	—	—	—	—	—	—
Hypothyroidism	—	—	—	6	—	—	—	—	—	—	—	—	—	—
Infection	—	—	—	—	—	—	—	2.7	—	29.9	19	20.6	—	—
Neck pain	—	—	—	—	—	—	—	—	—	5.3	2.7	1.2	—	—
Neoplasm	—	—	—	—	—	—	—	—	3.3	3.3	0.8	2.1	—	15
Overdose	—	—	—	—	—	—	—	—	—	—	6.9	6.8	—	—
Rigors	—	—	—	—	—	—	—	—	—	—	—	—	—	10
Tooth disorder	—	—	—	—	—	—	—	2.7	—	2.1	—	—	—	—

Bisphosphonate Adverse Reactions (%)[a]

Adverse reaction	Pamidronate — Osteolytic bone metastases of breast cancer and osteolytic lesions of multiple myeloma (Average of 3 trials) 90 mg (n = 572)[c]	Pamidronate — Hypercalcemia of malignancy study comparing these 3 dose regimens: 60 mg over 4 hr (n = 23)	60 mg over 24 hr (n = 73)	90 mg over 24 hr (n = 17)	Etidronate — Hypercalcemia of malignancy 7.5 mg/kg x 3 days (n = 35)	Alendronate — Osteoporosis in postmenopausal women 10 mg/day[d] (n = 196)	Fracture intervention trial[b] (n = 3236)	Tiludronate — Pagetic patients 400 mg/day (n = 75)	Pagetic patients 30 mg/day x 2 months (n = 61)[e]	Risedronate — Combined osteoporosis trials 5 mg (n = 1916)	Osteoporosis study in postmenopausal women comparing these 2 doseforms 5 mg/day (n = 480)	35 mg/week (n = 485)	Zoledronic acid — Hypercalcemia of malignancy 4 mg (n = 86)	Combined multiple myeloma and bone metastases of solid tumor trials 4 mg (n = 1099)
Vitamin D deficiency	—	—	—	—	—	—	—	2.7	—	—	—	—	—	—
Uremia	—	4	—	—	—	—	—	—	—	—	—	—	—	—
Urinary tract infection	18.5	—	—	—	—	—	—	—	—	10.9	2.9	5.2	14	11

— = No data.

[a] Data are pooled from separate studies and are not necessarily comparable.
[b] 5 mg/day for 2 years and 10 mg/day for either 1 or 2 additional years.
[c] Most of these adverse experiences may have been related to the underlying disease state or cancer therapy.
[d] 10 mg/day for 3 years.
[e] Considered to be possibly or probably causally related in at least 1 patient.

➤*Alendronate:*

Osteoporosis in postmenopausal women: One patient treated with 10 mg/day who had a history of peptic ulcer disease and gastrectomy and was taking concomitant aspirin developed an anastomotic ulcer with mild hemorrhage, which was considered drug-related. Aspirin and alendronate were discontinued and the patient recovered.

• *Other* – Rash, erythema (rare).

Adverse Reactions in Osteoporosis Treatment Studies in Postmenopausal Women (≥ 1%)

Adverse reaction	Alendronate 70 mg once weekly (n = 519)	Alendronate 10 mg/day (n = 370)
GI		
Abdominal distension	1	1.4
Abdominal pain	3.7	3
Acid regurgitation	1.9	2.4
Constipation	0.8	1.6
Dyspepsia	2.7	2.2
Flatulence	0.4	1.6
Gastritis	0.2	1.1
Gastric ulcer	0	1.1
Nausea	1.9	2.4
Musculoskeletal		
Muscle cramp	0.2	1.1
Musculoskeletal (bone, muscle, joint) pain	2.9	3.2

Adverse Reactions in an Osteoporosis Study in Men (≥ 2%)

Adverse reactions	Alendronate 10 mg/day (n = 146)	Placebo (n = 95)
GI		
Acid regurgitation	4.1	3.2
Flatulence	4.1	1.1
Dyspepsia	3.4	0
Abdominal pain	2.1	1.1
Nausea	2.1	0

Adverse Reactions in Osteoporosis Prevention Studies in Postmenopausal Women (≥ 1%)

Adverse reaction	2- and 3-year studies — Alendronate 5 mg/day (n = 642)	Placebo (n = 648)	1-year study — Alendronate 5 mg/day (n = 361)	Alendronate 35 mg once weekly (n = 362)
GI				
Dyspepsia	1.9	1.4	2.2	1.7
Abdominal pain	1.7	3.4	4.2	2.2
Acid regurgitation	1.4	2.5	4.2	4.7
Nausea	1.4	1.4	2.5	1.4
Diarrhea	1.1	1.7	1.1	0.6
Constipation	0.9	0.5	1.7	0.3
Abdominal distension	0.2	0.3	1.4	1.1

Adverse Reactions in Osteoporosis Prevention Studies in Postmenopausal Women (≥ 1%)

Adverse reaction	2- and 3-year studies — Alendronate 5 mg/day (n = 642)	Placebo (n = 648)	1-year study — Alendronate 5 mg/day (n = 361)	Alendronate 35 mg once weekly (n = 362)
Musculoskeletal				
Musculoskeletal (bone, muscle, or joint) pain	0.8	0.9	1.9	2.2

Adverse Reactions in 1-year Studies in Glucocorticoid-Treated Patients (≥ 1%)

Adverse reaction	Alendronate 10 mg/day (n = 157)	Alendronate 5 mg/day (n = 161)	Placebo (n = 159)
CNS			
Headache	0.6	0	1.3
GI			
Abdominal pain	3.2	1.9	0
Acid regurgitation	2.5	1.9	1.3
Constipation	1.3	0.6	0
Melena	1.3	0	0
Nausea	0.6	1.2	0.6
Diarrhea	0	0	1.3

Paget disease: In clinical studies in osteoporosis and Paget disease in patients taking 40 mg/day for 3 to 12 months, the adverse experiences were similar to those in the 10 mg/day osteoporosis study. However, there was an increased incidence of upper GI side effects in the 40 mg/day group (17.7% of the patients taking alendronate vs 10.2% placebo). One case of esophagitis and 2 cases of gastritis resulted in treatment discontinuation.

Musculoskeletal pain, which also occurs with other bisphosphonates, occurred in approximately 6% of patients treated with 40 mg/day alendronate vs approximately 1% taking placebo, rarely resulting in discontinuation. Discontinuation caused by any adverse reaction occurred in 6.4% of patients with Paget disease treated with 40 mg/day alendronate vs 2.4% of placebo-treated patients.

Lab test abnormalities – In double-blind, multicenter, controlled studies, asymptomatic, mild, and transient decreases in serum calcium and phosphate occurred in approximately 18% and 10%, respectively, of patients taking alendronate vs approximately 12% and 3% of those taking placebo. However, the incidence of decreases in serum calcium to less than 8 mg/dL (2 mM) and serum phosphate to at least 2 mg/dL (0.65 mM) were similar in both treatment groups.

Postmarketing: Hypersensitivity reactions including urticaria and rarely angioedema; esophagitis; esophageal erosions; esophageal ulcers, rarely esophageal stricture or perforation; oropharyngeal ulceration; gastric or duodenal ulcers, some severe and with complications; rash (occasionally with photosensitivity); uveitis (rare).

➤*Etidronate (oral):* The incidence of GI complaints (diarrhea, nausea) is the same at 5 mg/kg/day as for placebo (approximately 6.7%). At 10 to 20 mg/kg/day, the incidence may increase to 20% or 30%. These complaints are often alleviated by dividing the total daily dose.

Paget disease (oral): Increased or recurrent bone pain at pagetic sites or the onset of pain at previously asymptomatic sites has occurred. At 5 mg/kg/day, about 10% (vs 6.7% with placebo) report these phenomena. At higher doses, the incidence rises to about 20%. When the therapy continues, pain resolves in some patients but persists in others.

Lab test abnormalities (IV): HCM is frequently associated with abnormal elevations of serum creatinine and BUN, which improve in some patients or remain unchanged in most. However, in approximately 10% of patients, occasional mild to moderate abnormalities in renal function (increases of more than 0.5 mg/dL serum creatinine) were observed during or immediately after treatment. The possibility that etidronate IV infusion contributed to these changes cannot be excluded.

IV: Of patients who participated in the controlled hypercalcemia trials, 10 of 221 (5%) in the treatment courses reported a metallic or altered taste, or loss of taste, which usually disappeared within hours during or shortly after etidronate infusion. A few patients with Paget disease of bone have reported allergic skin rashes in association with oral etidronate.

A patient with 1 kidney and slowly rising creatinine prior to therapy received 30 mg/kg/day body weight of etidronate infusion for 18 hours (total dose 60 mg/kg). This patient reported altered taste and further gradual increase in serum creatinine from 2.1 mg/dL to 2.7 mg/dL during the week after therapy was observed.

Postmarketing:
• *Oral* – Other adverse events that have been reported and were thought to be possibly related to etidronate disodium include the following: Alopecia; arthropathies, including arthralgia and arthritis; bone fracture; esophagitis; glossitis; hypersensitivity reactions, including angioedema, follicular eruption, macular rash, maculopapular rash, pruritus, a single case of Stevens-Johnson syndrome, and urticaria; osteomalacia; neuropsychiatric events, including amnesia, confusion, depression, and hallucination; and paresthesias.

In patients receiving etidronate disodium, there have been rare reports of agranulocytosis, pancytopenia, and a report of leukopenia with recurrence on rechallenge. In addition, there have been rare reports of exacerbation of asthma. Exacerbation of existing peptic ulcer disease has been reported in a few patients. In 1 patient, perforation also occurred. In osteoporosis clinical trials, headache, gastritis, leg cramps, and arthralgia occurred at a significantly greater incidence in patients who received etidronate as compared with those who received placebo.

▶*Pamidronate:*
Hypercalcemia of malignancy: Transient mild elevation of temperature by at least 1°C was noted 24 to 48 hours after administration in 34% of patients. In trials, patients treated with pamidronate (60 or 90 mg over 24 hours) developed electrolyte abnormalities more frequently.

Drug-related local soft tissue symptoms (redness, swelling, or induration, and pain on palpation) at the site of catheter insertion were most common in patients treated with 90 mg.

Rare cases of uveitis, iritis, scleritis, and episcleritis have occurred, including 1 case of scleritis and 1 case of uveitis upon separate rechallenges.

Five of 231 patients (2%) had seizures; 2 had preexisting seizure disorders. None of the seizures were considered to be drug-related. However, a possible relationship cannot be ruled out.

Other reactions in at least 15% of patients included the following: Fluid overload; generalized/abdominal/bone pain; hypertension; anorexia; constipation; nausea; vomiting; urinary tract infection.
• *Lab test abnormalities* – Anemia; hypokalemia; hypomagnesemia; hypophosphatemia.
Paget disease: Transient mild elevation of temperature more than 1°C above pretreatment baseline was noted within 48 hours after completion of treatment in 21% of patients treated with 90 mg. Drug-related musculoskeletal pain and CNS symptoms (eg, dizziness, headache, paresthesia, increased sweating) were more common with Paget disease than with HCM treated with the same 90 mg dose.

Adverse experiences considered to be related to trial drug, which occurred in at least 5% of patients with Paget disease treated with 90 mg of pamidronate in 2 US clinical trials, were fever, nausea, back pain, and bone pain.

Other adverse reactions are as follows: Hypertension, arthrosis, bone pain, headache (10%).

Osteolytic bone metastases of breast cancer and osteolytic lesions of multiple myeloma: In multiple myeloma patients, there were 5 pamidronate-related serious and unexpected adverse experiences. Four of these were reported during the 12-month extension of the multiple myeloma trial. Three of the reports were of worsening renal function developing in patients with progressive multiple myeloma or multiple myeloma-associated amyloidosis. The fourth report was the adult respiratory distress syndrome developing in a patient recovering from pneumonia and acute gangrenous cholecystitis. One pamidronate-treated patient experienced an allergic reaction characterized by swollen and itchy eyes, runny nose, and scratchy throat within 24 hours after the sixth infusion.

In the breast cancer trials, there were 4 pamidronate-related adverse experiences, all moderate in severity, that caused a patient to discontinue participation in the trial. One was because of interstitial pneumonitis, another because of malaise and dyspnea. One pamidronate patient discontinued the trial because of asymptomatic hypocalcemia. Another pamidronate patient discontinued therapy because of severe bone pain after each infusion, which the investigator felt was trial drug-related.

Postmarketing: Rare instances of allergic manifestations have been reported, including hypotension, dyspnea, or angioedema, and very rarely, anaphylactic shock.

▶*Tiludronate:* Adverse events associated with tiludronate usually have been mild and generally have not required discontinuation of therapy. Of patients receiving 400 mg tiludronate and placebo, 1.3% and 5.4% respectively, discontinued therapy because of a clinical adverse event.

The most frequently occurring adverse events in patients who received tiludronate 400 mg/day were in the GI system: Nausea (9.3%), diarrhea (9.3%), and dyspepsia (5.3%).

Paget disease: The following reactions occurred in at least 1% of patients.

CNS – Vertigo; involuntary muscle contractions; anxiety; nervousness.

Dermatologic – Pruritus; increased sweating; Stevens-Johnson-type syndrome (rare).

GI – Dry mouth; gastritis; abdominal pain; constipation.

Miscellaneous – Asthenia; pathological fracture; bronchitis; urinary tract infection; flushing; syncope; fatigue; hypertension; anorexia; somnolence; insomnia.

▶*Risedronate:* Duodenitis and glossitis have been reported uncommonly (0.1% to 1%). There have been rare reports of abnormal liver function tests (less than 0.1%). Three patients who received risedronate 30 mg/day experienced acute iritis in 1 supportive study. All 3 patients recovered from their events. All patients were effectively treated with topical steroids.

Lab test abnormalities – Asymptomatic and small decreases were observed in serum calcium and phosphorus levels. Overall, mean decreases of 0.8% in serum calcium and of 2.7% in phosphorus were observed at 6 months in patients receiving risedronate. Throughout the phase 3 studies, serum calcium levels below 8 mg/dL were observed in 18 patients, 9 (0.5%) in each treatment arm (risedronate and placebo). Serum phosphorus levels below 2 mg/dL were observed in 14 patients, 11 (0.6%) treated with risedronate and 3 (0.2%) treated with placebo.

▶*Zoledronic acid:*
Hypercalcemia of malignancy: IV administration has been most commonly associated with fever. Occasionally, patients experience a flu-like syndrome consisting of fever, chills, bone pain or arthralgias, and myalgias. GI reactions such as nausea and vomiting have been reported following IV infusion. Local reactions at the infusion site, such as redness or swelling, were observed infrequently. In most cases, no specific treatment is required and the symptoms subside after 24 to 48 hours. Rare cases of rash, pruritus, chest pain, conjunctivitis, and hypomagnesemia have been reported.

Other adverse reactions greater than or equal to 5% but less than 10% include the following: Asthenia, chest pain, leg edema, mucositis, metastases, dysphagia, granulocytopenia, thrombocytopenia, pancytopenia, nonspecific infection, hypocalcemia, dehydration, arthralgias, headache, somnolence, pleural effusion.

Lab test abnormalities:

Grade 3 to 4 Laboratory Abnormalities in Clinical Trials for Hypercalcemia of Malignancy							
	Grade 3				Grade 4		
	Zoledronic acid 4 mg		Pamidronate 90 mg		Zoledronic acid 4 mg		Pamidronate 90 mg	
Laboratory parameter	n/N	%	n/N	%	n/N	%	n/N	%
Serum creatinine[a]	2/86	2.3	3/100	3	0/86	—	1/100	1
Hypocalcemia[b]	1/86	1.2	2/100	2	0/86	—	0/100	—
Hypophosphatemia[c]	36/70	51.4	27/81	33.3	1/70	1.4	4/81	4.9
Hypomagnesemia[d]	0/71	—	0/84	—	0/71	—	1/84	1.2

[a] Grade 3: > 3 times the ULN; Grade 4: > 6 times the ULN
[b] Grade 3: < 7 mg/dL; Grade 4: < 6 mg/dL
[c] Grade 3: < 2 mg/dL; Grade 4: < 1 mg/dL
[d] Grade 3: < 0.8 mEq/L; Grade 4: < 0.5 mEq/L

Multiple myeloma and bone metastases of solid tumors:
- *Lab test abnormalities –*

Grade 3 Laboratory Abnormalities in Clinical Trials in Patients with Bone Metastases						
Laboratory parameter	Zoledronic acid 4 mg		Pamidronate 90 mg		Placebo	
	n/N	%	n/N	%	n/N	%
Serum creatinine[a]	7/529	1.3	4/268	1.5	2/241	0.8
Hypocalcemia[b]	7/1041	0.7	4/610	0.7	0/415	—
Hypophosphatemia[c]	96/1041	9.2	40/611	6.6	13/415	3.1
Hypermagnesemia[d]	19/1039	1.8	3/609	0.5	8/415	1.9
Hypomagnesemia[e]	0/1039	—	0/609	—	1/415	0.2

[a] Grade 3: > 3 times the ULN; Grade 4: > 6 times the ULN. Serum creatinine data for all patients randomized after the 15-minute infusion amendment.
[b] Grade 3: < 7 mg/dL; Grade 4: < 6 mg/dL
[c] Grade 3: < 2 mg/dL; Grade 4: < 1 mg/dL
[d] Grade 3: > 3 mEq/L; Grade 4: > 8 mEq/L
[e] Grade 3: < 0.9 mEq/L; Grade 4: < 0.7 mEq/L

Grade 4 Laboratory Abnormalities in Clinical Trials in Patients with Bone Metastases						
Laboratory parameter	Zoledronic acid 4 mg		Pamidronate 90 mg		Placebo	
	n/N	%	n/N	%	n/N	%
Serum creatinine[a]	2/529	0.4	1/268	0.4	0/241	—
Hypocalcemia[b]	6/1041	0.6	2/610	0.3	1/415	0.2
Hypophosphatemia[c]	6/1041	0.6	0/611	—	1/415	0.2
Hypermagnesemia[d]	0/1039	—	0/609	—	2/415	0.5
Hypomagnesemia[e]	2/1039	0.2	2/609	0.3	0/415	—

[a] Grade 3: > 3 times the ULN; Grade 4: > 6 times the ULN. Serum creatinine data for all patients randomized after the 15-minute infusion amendment.
[b] Grade 3: < 7 mg/dL; Grade 4: < 6 mg/dL
[c] Grade 3: < 2 mg/dL; Grade 4: < 1 mg/dL
[d] Grade 3: > 3 mEq/L; Grade 4: > 8 mEq/L
[e] Grade 3: < 0.9 mEq/L; Grade 4: < 0.7 mEq/L

- *Renal* – In the bone metastases trials, renal deterioration was defined as an increase of 0.5 mg/dL for patients with normal baseline creatinine (less than 1.4 mg/dL) or an increase of 1 mg/dL for patients with an abnormal baseline creatinine (greater than 1.4 mg/dL). Percentage of patients with renal function deterioration who were randomized following the 15 minute 4 mg zoledronic acid infusion amendment were as follows:

  Multiple myeloma and breast cancer: Normal (9.3%), abnormal (3.8%), total (8.8%)
  Solid tumors: Normal (11%), abnormal (9.1%), total (10.9%)
  Prostate cancer: Normal (12.2%), abnormal (40%), total (15.2%)

Overdosage

➤*Alendronate:* Hypocalcemia, hypophosphatemia, and upper GI adverse events (eg, upset stomach, heartburn, esophagitis, gastritis, ulcer) may result from overdosage. Consider the administration of milk or antacids to bind alendronate. Dialysis would not be beneficial.

➤*Etidronate:*

Oral – Clinical experience with etidronate overdosage is extremely limited. Decreases in serum calcium following substantial overdosage may be expected in some patients. Signs and symptoms of hypocalcemia also may occur and some patients may develop vomiting. In 1 event, an 18-year-old female who ingested an estimated single dose of 4000 to 6000 mg (67 to 100 mg/kg) was mildly hypocalcemic (7.52 mg/dL) and experienced paresthesia of the fingers. Some patients may develop vomiting and expel the drug. Orally administered etidronate disodium may cause hematologic abnormalities in some patients. Etidronate disodium suppresses bone turnover and may retard mineralization of osteoid laid down during the bone accretion process.

Gastric lavage may remove unabsorbed drug. Standard procedures for treating hypocalcemia, including the administration of calcium IV, would be expected to restore physiologic amounts of ionized calcium and relieve signs and symptoms of hypocalcemia. Such treatment has been effective.

IV – Rapid IV administration of etidronate at doses above 27 mg/kg has produced ECG changes and bleeding problems in animals. These abnormalities are probably related to marked or rapid decreases in ionized calcium levels in blood and tissue fluids. They are thought to be caused by chelation of calcium by massive amounts of the diphosphonate. These abnormalities have been reversible in animal studies by use of ionizable calcium salts. Similar problems are not expected to occur in humans if treated with etidronate as recommended. Moreover, signs and symptoms of hypocalcemia such as paresthesias and carpopedal spasms have not been reported with either agent. The chelation effects of the diphosphonate are reversible with IV calcium gluconate.

Administration of IV etidronate at doses and possibly at rates in excess of those recommended has been associated with renal insufficiency.

➤*Pamidronate:* There have been several cases of drug maladministration of IV pamidronate in hypercalcemia patients with total doses of 225 to 300 mg given over 2.5 to 4 days. All survived but experienced hypocalcemia requiring IV or oral calcium.

One obese woman (95 kg) who was treated with pamidronate 285 mg/day for 3 days experienced high fever (39.5°C; 102°F), hypotension, and transient taste perversion noted about 6 hours after the first infusion. Fever and hypotension were rapidly corrected with steroids.

If overdosage occurs, symptomatic hypocalcemia also could result; treat such patients with short-term IV calcium.

➤*Risedronate:* Decreases in serum calcium following substantial overdose may be expected in some patients. Signs and symptoms of hypocalcemia also may occur in some of these patients.

Gastric lavage may remove unabsorbed drug. Administration of milk or antacids to chelate risedronate may be helpful. Standard procedures that are effective for treating hypocalcemia, including IV administration of calcium, would be expected to restore physiologic amounts of ionized calcium and to relieve signs and symptoms of hypocalcemia.

➤*Tiludronate:* Hypocalcemia is a potential consequence of tiludronate overdose. In 1 patient with HCM, IV administration of high doses of tiludronate (800 mg/day total dose, 6 mg/kg/day for 2 days) was associated with acute renal failure and death.

No specific information is available on the treatment of overdose with tiludronate. Dialysis would not be beneficial. Standard medical practices may be used to manage renal insufficiency or hypocalcemia if signs of these develop.

➤*Zoledronic acid:* Overdosage may cause clinically significant hypocalcemia, hypophosphatemia, and hypomagnesemia. Clinically relevant reductions in serum levels of calcium, phosphorus, and magnesium should be corrected by IV administration of calcium gluconate, potassium or sodium phosphate, and magnesium sulfate, respectively.

Patient Information

Bisphosphonates may cause GI upset (eg, nausea, diarrhea).

➤*Alendronate:* Instruct patients that the expected benefits of alendronate only may be obtained when each tablet is taken with plain water first thing in the morning and at least 30 minutes before the first food, beverage, or medication of the day. Also instruct them that waiting more than 30 minutes will improve alendronate absorption. Even dosing with orange juice or coffee markedly reduces the absorption of alendronate.

Instruct patients to take alendronate with a full glass of water (6 to 8 oz; 180 to 240 mL) and not to lie down for at least 30 minutes and until after the first food of the day following administration to facilitate delivery to the stomach and reduce the potential for esophageal irritation.

Patients should not chew or suck on the tablet because of a potential for oropharyngeal ulceration. Specifically instruct patients not to take alendronate at bedtime or before arising for the day. Inform patients that failure to follow these instructions may increase their risk of esophageal problems. Instruct patients that if they develop symptoms of esophageal disease (eg, difficulty or pain upon swallowing, retrosternal pain, new or worsening heartburn) they should stop taking alendronate and consult their physician.

Instruct patients that if they miss a dose of once-weekly alendronate they should take 1 tablet on the morning after they remember. They should not take 2 tablets on the same day but should return to taking 1 tablet once a week as originally scheduled on their chosen day.

Instruct patients to take supplemental calcium and vitamin D if dietary intake is inadequate. Consider weight-bearing exercise along with the modification of certain behavioral factors, such as excessive cigarette smoking or alcohol consumption, if these factors exist.

It is likely that calcium supplements, antacids, and some oral medications will interfere with absorption of alendronate. Therefore, patients must wait at least 30 minutes after taking alendronate before taking any other oral medications.

➤*Etidronate (oral):* Take on an empty stomach 2 hours before or after meals, including vitamin and mineral supplements or antacids, which are high in metals such as calcium, iron, magnesium, or aluminum.

➤*Risedronate:* Inform patients to pay particular attention to the dosing instructions because clinical benefits may be compromised by failure to take the drug according to instructions. Take risedronate at least 30 minutes before the first food or drink of the day other than water.

If a patient forgets to take the 5 or 35 mg risedronate tablet in the morning, inform him/her not to take it later in the day. Take only 1 risedronate 5 or 35 mg tablet the next morning and continue the usual schedule of 5 mg (1 tablet a day) or 35 mg (1 tablet on a chosen day of the week). Do not take 2 tablets on the same day.

In order to facilitate delivery to the stomach and minimize the possibility of esophageal irritation, take risedronate in an upright position, sitting or standing, with a full glass (6 to 8 oz; 180 to 240 mL) of plain water and avoid lying down for 30 minutes after taking this medication. Patients should receive supplemental calcium and vitamin D if dietary intake is inadequate (see Precautions). Calcium, magnesium or aluminum supplements, or antacids may interfere with the absorption of risedronate; take them at a different time of the day as with food. Patients should not chew or suck on tablets because of potential for oropharyngeal irritation.

Instruct patients that if they develop symptoms of esophageal disease (eg, difficulty or pain upon swallowing; retrosternal pain; severe, persistent, or worsening heartburn) they should consult their physician before continuing risedronate.

Weight-bearing exercise should be considered along with the modification of certain behavioral factors, such as excessive cigarette smoking, or alcohol consumption, if these factors exist.

Physicians should instruct their patients to read the patient information before starting therapy with 5 mg risedronate and to re-read it each time the prescription is renewed.

➤*Tiludronate:* Take tiludronate with 6 to 8 oz (180 to 240 mL) of plain water. Do not take within 2 hours of food. Maintain adequate vitamin D and calcium intake. Do not take calcium supplements, aspirin, and indomethacin within 2 hours before or after tiludronate. If needed, take aluminum- or magnesium-containing antacids at least 2 hours after tiludronate.

ALENDRONATE SODIUM

Rx	Fosamax (Merck)	Tablets: 5 mg (as base)	Lactose. (MRK 925). White. In unit-of-use 30s and 100s.
		10 mg (as base)	Lactose. (MRK 936). White, oval. In 1000s, unit-of-use 30s and 100s, *Uniblister* cards of 31, and UD 100s.
		35 mg (as base)	Lactose. (77). White, oval. In unit-of-use 4s and UD 20s.
		40 mg (as base)	Lactose. (MRK 212/Fosamax). White, triangular. In unit-of-use 30s.
		70 mg (as base)	Lactose. (31). White, oval. In unit-of-use 4s and UD 20s.
		Oral solution: 70 mg (as base)	Saccharin, parabens. Raspberry flavor. In 75 mL.

For complete prescribing information, refer to the Bisphosphonates group monograph.

Indications

➤*Glucocorticoid-induced osteoporosis:* Treatment of glucocorticoid-induced osteoporosis in men and women receiving glucocorticoids in a daily dosage equivalent to 7.5 mg or greater of prednisone and who have low bone mineral density.

➤*Osteoporosis in men:* To increase bone mass in men with osteoporosis.

➤*Osteoporosis in postmenopausal women:*

Treatment – To increase bone mass and reduce the incidence of fractures, including those of the hip and spine (vertebral compression fractures).

Prevention – Consider alendronate in postmenopausal women who are at risk of developing osteoporosis and for whom the desired clinical outcome is to maintain bone mass and reduce the risk of future fracture.

➤*Paget disease:* Treatment of Paget disease of bone in men and women who have alkaline phosphatase levels at least 2 times the ULN, who are symptomatic, or who are at risk for complications from their disease.

Administration and Dosage

➤*Approved by the FDA:* September 29, 1995.

➤*Administration:* Alendronate must be taken at least 30 minutes before the first food, beverage, or medication of the day with plain water only. Waiting less than 30 minutes or taking the drug with food, beverages (other than plain water), or other medications will lessen the effect of the drug by decreasing its absorption. To facilitate delivery to the stomach, and thus reduce the potential for esophageal irritation, advise the patient to swallow alendronate only upon arising for the day and avoid lying down for at least 30 minutes and at least until after the first food of the day. To facilitate gastric emptying, follow the oral solution with at least 2 oz (¼ cup) of water. Advise patient to take tablet with a full glass of water (6 to 8 oz; 180 to 240 mL). Do not take alendronate at bedtime or before arising for the day. Failure to follow these instructions may increase the risk of esophageal adverse reactions (see Patient Information).

Patients should receive supplemental calcium and vitamin D if dietary intake is inadequate.

➤*Glucocorticoid-induced osteoporosis:* 5 mg tablet once daily for men and women. For postmenopausal women not receiving estrogen, the recommended dose is 10 mg tablet once daily.

Patients also should receive adequate amounts of calcium and vitamin D.

➤*Osteoporosis in men:* 10 mg tablet once daily. Alternatively, one 70 mg tablet or 1 bottle of 70 mg oral solution once weekly may be considered.

➤*Osteoporosis in postmenopausal women:*

Treatment – 70 mg tablet once weekly, 10 mg tablet once daily, or 1 bottle of 70 mg oral solution once weekly.

Prevention – 35 mg tablet once weekly or 5 mg tablet once daily.

The safety of treatment and prevention of osteoporosis with alendronate has been studied for up to 7 years.

➤*Paget disease of bone:* 40 mg once a day for 6 months for men and women.

Retreatment – Relapses during the 12 months following therapy occurred in 9% of patients who responded to treatment. Specific retreatment data are not available, although responses to alendronate were similar in patients who had received prior bisphosphonate therapy and those who had not. Consider retreatment with alendronate following a 6-month post-treatment evaluation period in patients who have relapsed based on increases in serum alkaline phosphatase, which should be measured periodically. Retreatment also may be considered in those who failed to normalize their serum alkaline phosphatase.

➤*Renal function impairment:* Alendronate is not recommended for patients with severe renal insufficiency (Ccr less than 35 mL/min) because of lack of experience.

➤*Storage/Stability:*

Tablets – Store in a well-closed container at room temperature, 15° to 30°C (59° to 86°F).

Oral solution – Store at 25°C (77°F); excursions permitted to 15° to 30°C (59° to 86°F). Do not freeze.

ETIDRONATE DISODIUM (ORAL)

Rx	Didronel (Procter & Gamble Pharm.)	Tablets: 200 mg	(P & G 402). White, rectangular. In 60s.
		400 mg	(N E 406). White, scored, capsule shape. In 60s.

For complete prescribing information, refer to the Bisphosphonates group monograph.

Indications

➤*Paget disease:* For the treatment of symptomatic Paget disease of bone. Therapy usually impedes the disease process as evidenced by symptomatic relief, including decreased pain or increased mobility (experienced by 3 out of 5 patients), reductions in serum alkaline phosphatase and urinary hydroxyproline levels (30% or more in 4 out of 5 patients), histomorphometry showing reduced numbers of osteoclasts and osteoblasts and more lamellar bone formation, and bone scans showing reduced radionuclide uptake in pagetic lesions.

In addition, reductions in pagetically elevated cardiac output and skin temperature have been observed in some patients.

In many patients, the disease process will be suppressed for a period of at least 1 year following cessation of therapy. The upper limit of this period has not been determined.

The effects of etidronate treatment in patients with asymptomatic Paget disease have not been studied. However, etidronate treatment of such patients may be warranted if extensive involvement threatens irreversible neurologic damage, major joints, or major weight-bearing bones.

➤*Heterotopic ossification:* Prevention and treatment following total hip replacement or spinal cord injury. Etidronate reduces the incidence of clinically important bone by about two-thirds. Among those patients who form heterotopic bone, etidronate retards the progression of immature lesions and reduces the severity by at least 50%. Follow-up data (at least 9 months post-therapy) suggest these benefits persist.

Administration and Dosage

Administer as a single dose. However, if GI discomfort occurs, divide the dose. To maximize absorption, avoid the following within 2 hours of dosing:

1.) Food, especially items high in calcium, such as milk or milk products.

2.) Vitamins with mineral supplements or antacids high in metals (eg, calcium, iron, magnesium, aluminum).

➤*Paget disease:*

Initial treatment – 5 to 10 mg/kg/day (not to exceed 6 months) or 11 to 20 mg/kg/day (not to exceed 3 months). Reserve doses greater than 10 mg/kg/day for use when lower doses are ineffective, when there is an overriding requirement for suppression of bone turnover (especially when irreversible neurologic damage is possible) prompt reduction of elevated cardiac output is required. Doses greater than 20 mg/kg/day are not recommended.

ETIDRONATE DISODIUM (ORAL)

Retreatment – Initiate only after an etidronate-free period of at least 90 days and when there is biochemical, symptomatic, or other evidence of active disease process. Monitor patients every 3 to 6 months, although some patients may go drug-free for extended periods. Retreatment regimens are the same as for initial treatment. For most patients, the original dose will be adequate for retreatment. If not, consider increasing the dose within the recommended guidelines.

➤*Heterotopic ossification:*

Spinal cord injury – 20 mg/kg/day for 2 weeks, followed by 10 mg/kg/day for 10 weeks; total treatment period is 12 weeks. Institute therapy as soon as feasible following the injury, preferably prior to evidence of heterotopic ossification.

Total hip replacement – 20 mg/kg/day for 1 month preoperatively, then 20 mg/kg/day for 3 months postoperatively; total treatment period is 4 months.

Retreatment has not been studied.

➤*Storage/Stability:* Avoid excessive heat (over 104°F or 40°C).

ETIDRONATE DISODIUM (INTRAVENOUS)

Rx	Didronel IV (MGI Pharma)	Solution for injection: 300 mg/amp	In 6 mL amps.

For complete prescribing information, refer to the Bisphosphonates group monograph.

Indications

➤*Hypercalcemia of malignancy (HCM):* For the treatment of HCM, along with achievement and maintenance of adequate hydration, inadequately managed by dietary modification or oral hydration; treatment of HCM that persists after adequate hydration has been restored.

Patients with and without metastases and with a variety of tumors have been responsive to treatment with etidronate IV infusion.

Administration and Dosage

➤*Approved by the FDA:* April 20, 1987.

➤*Recommended dose:* 7.5 mg/kg/day infused over at least 2 hours for 3 successive days. Infusions may be continued for up to 7 days if necessary. This daily dose must be diluted in at least 250 mL of sterile normal saline.

Adequately hydrate patients throughout pamidronate treatment, but avoid overhydration, especially in those patients who have cardiac failure. Do not employ diuretic therapy prior to correction of hypovolemia.

In the treatment of HCM, it is important to initiate rehydration with saline together with "high ceiling" or loop diuretics if indicated to restore urine output. This also is intended to increase the renal excretion of calcium and initiate a reduction in serum calcium. Because increased bone resorption is usually the underlying cause of an increased flux of calcium into the vascular compartment, concurrent therapy with etidronate infusion is recommended as soon as there is a restoration of urine output. Because etidronate is excreted by the kidney, it is important to know that renal function is adequate to handle not only the increased fluid load but also the excretion of the drug itself. Etidronate infusion also is indicated for the treatment of HCM that persists after adequate hydration has been restored. Patients with and without metastases and with a variety of tumors have been responsive

to treatment with etidronate infusion. Adequate hydration of patients should be maintained, but in aged patients and in those with cardiac failure, care must be taken to avoid overhydration.

➤*Infusion time:* Administer the diluted dose IV over a period of at least 2 hours. Infusion may be added to volumes of sterile, normal saline greater than 250 mL when convenient. Single (1-day) 24-hour infusions of 25 to 30 mg/kg were administered to only a limited number of patients, and are not recommended for initial treatment. This single dose must be diluted in at least 1000 mL of sterile normal saline.

Regardless of the volume of solution in which etidronate IV infusion is diluted, slow infusion is important. Observe the minimum infusion time of 2 hours at the recommended dose or smaller doses. The usual course of treatment is 1 infusion of 7.5 mg/kg/day on each of 3 consecutive days, but some patients have been treated for up to 7 days. When patients are treated for more than 3 days, there may be an increased possibility of hypocalcemia.

➤*Retreatment:* Retreatment may be appropriate if hypercalcemia recurs. There should be at least a 7-day interval between courses of treatment. The dose and manner of retreatment is the same as that for initial treatment. Retreatment for more than 3 days has not been adequately studied. The safety and efficacy of more than 2 courses of therapy have not been studied. With renal impairment, dose reduction may be advisable.

➤*Oral etidronate:* Oral etidronate may be started on the day after the last etidronate infusion. The recommended oral dose for patients who have had hypercalcemia is 20 mg/kg/day for 30 days. If serum calcium levels remain normal or clinically acceptable, treatment may be extended. Use for more than 90 days is not adequately studied and is not recommended.

➤*Storage/Stability:* Avoid excessive heat (over 40°C; 104°F) for undiluted product.

PAMIDRONATE DISODIUM

Rx	Aredia (Novartis)	Powder for injection, lyophilized: 30 mg	470 mg mannitol. In vials.
		90 mg	375 mg mannitol. In vials.
Rx	Pamidronate Disodium (Various, eg, American Pharm Partners, Bedford, Faulding, Gensia Sicor)	Injection: 3 mg/mL	May contain mannitol. In 10 mL vials.
Rx	Pamidronate Disodium (Faulding)	Injection: 6 mg/mL	400 mg mannitol. In 10 mL vials.
Rx	Pamidronate Disodium (Various, eg, American Pharm Partners, Bedford, Faulding, Gensia Sicor)	Injection: 9 mg/mL	May contain mannitol. In 10 mL vials.

For complete prescribing information, refer to the Bisphosphonates group monograph.

Indications

➤*Hypercalcemia of malignancy (HCM):* In conjunction with adequate hydration for the treatment of moderate or severe hypercalcemia associated with malignancy, with or without bone metastases. Patients who have epidermoid or nonepidermoid tumors respond to treatment with pamidronate. The safety and efficacy of pamidronate in the treatment of hypercalcemia associated with hyperparathyroidism or non-tumor-related conditions has not been established.

➤*Paget disease:* Treatment of moderate to severe Paget disease of bone. The effectiveness of pamidronate was demonstrated primarily in patients with serum alkaline phosphatase 3 or more times the upper limit of normal. Pamidronate therapy in patients with Paget disease has been effective in reducing serum alkaline phosphatase and urinary hydroxyproline levels by 50% or more in at least 50% of patients and by 30% or more in at least 80% of patients. Pamidronate therapy has been effective in reducing these biochemical markers in patients with Paget disease who failed to respond, or no longer responded to, other treatments.

➤*Osteolytic bone metastases of breast cancer/osteolytic lesions of multiple myeloma:* In conjunction with standard antineoplastic therapy.

Administration and Dosage

➤*Approved by the FDA:* October 31, 1991.

➤*HCM:* Consider the severity and symptoms of hypercalcemia. Vigorous saline hydration alone may be sufficient for treating mild, asymptomatic hypercalcemia. Avoid overhydration in patients who have potential for cardiac failure. In hypercalcemia associated with hematologic malignancies, the use of glucocorticoid therapy may be helpful.

Moderate hypercalcemia – The recommended dose in moderate hypercalcemia (corrected serum calcium† of approximately 12 to 13.5 mg/dL) is 60 to 90 mg given as a single-dose IV infusion over 2 to 24 hours. Longer infusions (eg, more than 2 hours) may reduce the risk for renal toxicity, particularly in patients with pre-existing renal insufficiency.

Severe hypercalcemia – Recommended dose (corrected serum calcium† more than 13.5 mg/dL) is 90 mg, which must be given as a single-dose IV infusion over 2 to 24 hours. Longer infusions (eg, more than 2 hours) may reduce the risk for renal toxicity, particularly in patients with pre-existing renal insufficiency.

Retreatment – A limited number of patients have received more than 1 treatment with pamidronate for hypercalcemia. Retreatment in patients who show complete or partial response initially may be carried out if serum calcium does not return to normal or remain normal after initial treatment. Allow a minimum of 7 days to elapse before retreat-

---

† Albumin-corrected serum calcium (Cca, mg/dL) = serum calcium, mg/dL + 0.8 (4-serum albumin, g/dL).

PAMIDRONATE DISODIUM

ment to allow for full response to the initial dose. The dose and manner of retreatment are identical to that of the initial therapy.

Hydration – Initiate saline hydration promptly and attempt to restore the urine output to approximately 2 L/day throughout treatment. Mild or asymptomatic hypercalcemia may be treated with conservative measures (ie, saline hydration with or without loop diuretics). Adequately hydrate patients throughout the treatment, but avoid overhydration, especially in those patients who have cardiac failure. Do not employ diuretic therapy prior to correction of hypovolemia.

➤*Paget disease:* The recommended dose in patients with moderate to severe Paget disease of bone is 30 mg/day, given as a 4-hour infusion on 3 consecutive days for a total dose of 90 mg.

Retreatment – A limited number of patients have received more than 1 treatment in clinical trials. When clinically indicated, retreat at the dose of initial therapy.

➤*Osteolytic bone metastases of breast cancer:* The recommended dose is 90 mg administered as a 2-hour infusion every 3 to 4 weeks.

Pamidronate has been used frequently with doxorubicin, fluorouracil, cyclophosphamide, methotrexate, mitoxantrone, vinblastine, dexamethasone, prednisone, melphalan, vincristine, megesterol, and tamoxifen. It has been given less frequently with etoposide, cisplatin, cytarabine, paclitaxel, and aminoglutethimide. The optimal duration of therapy is not known; however, in 2 breast cancer studies, final analyses performed after 24 months of therapy demonstrated overall benefits.

➤*Osteolytic bone lesions of multiple myeloma:* The recommended dose is 90 mg given as a 4-hour infusion on a monthly basis. Patients with marked Bence-Jones proteinuria and dehydration should receive adequate hydration prior to pamidronate infusion.

➤*Preparation of solution:* Reconstitute by adding 10 mL sterile water for injection to each vial, resulting in a solution of 30 or 90 mg/10 mL. Allow drug to dissolve completely before withdrawing.

Method of administration – Because of the risk of clinically significant deterioration in renal function, which may progress to renal failure, single doses of of pamidronate should not exceed 90 mg (see Warnings). There must be strict adherence to the IV administration recommendations for pamidronate in order to decrease the risk of deterioration in renal function.

HCM – Administer the daily dose as an IV infusion over at least 2 to 24 hours for the 60 and 90 mg doses. Dilute in 1 L sterile 0.45% or 0.9% NaCl or 5% dextrose injection. This infusion solution is stable for up to 24 hours at room temperature.

Paget disease – Dilute the recommended daily dose of 30 mg in 500 mL sterile 0.45% or 0.9% NaCl or 5% dextrose injection and give over a 4-hour period for 3 consecutive days.

Osteolytic bone lesions of multiple myeloma – Dilute the recommended dose of 90 mg in 500 mL of sterile 0.45% or 0.9% NaCl or 5% dextrose injection and give over a 4-hour period on a monthly basis.

Osteolytic bone metastases of breast cancer – Dilute the recommended dose of 90 mg in 250 mL of sterile 0.45% or 0.9% NaCl or 5% dextrose injection and give over a 2-hour period every 3 to 4 weeks.

➤*Admixture incompatibility:* Do not mix with calcium-containing infusion solutions, such as Ringer's solution. Give in a single IV solution and line separate from all other drugs.

➤*Storage/Stability:* Do not store at or above 30°C (86°F). Pamidronate reconstituted with sterile water for injection may be stored under refrigeration at 2° to 8°C (36° to 46°F) for up to 24 hours.

TILUDRONATE DISODIUM

Rx	**Skelid** (Sanofi-Synthelabo)	**Tablets:** 240 mg (equivalent to 200 mg tiludronic acid)	Lactose. (S.W 200). White. In foil strips in cartons of 56 tablets/carton.

For complete prescribing information, refer to the Bisphosphonates group monograph.

Indications

➤*Paget disease:* Treatment of Paget disease of bone (osteitis deformans) in patients who have a level of serum alkaline phosphatase at least twice the upper limit or normal or who are symptomatic or are at risk for future complications of their disease.

Administration and Dosage

Administer a single 400 mg/day oral dose of tiludronate, taken with 6 to 8 oz (180 to 240 mL) of plain water only for a period of 3 months. Beverages other than plain water (including mineral water), food, and some medications (see Drug Interactions in the Bisphosphonates group

monograph) are likely to reduce the absorption of tiludronate. Do not take within 2 hours of food. Take calcium or mineral supplements at least 2 hours before or after tiludronate. Take aluminum- or magnesium-containing antacids at least 2 hours after taking tiludronate. Do not take within 2 hours of indomethacin.

Following therapy, allow an interval of 3 months to assess response. Specific data regarding retreatment are limited, although results from uncontrolled studies indicate favorable biochemical improvement similar to initial tiludronate treatment.

➤*Storage/Stability:* Store at 25°C (77°F); excursions permitted to 15° to 30°C (59° to 86°F). Do not remove tablets from the foil strips until they are to be used.

RISEDRONATE SODIUM

Rx	**Actonel** (Procter & Gamble)	**Tablets:** 5 mg	Lactose. (RSN 5 mg). Yellow, oval. Film-coated. In 30s and 2000s.
		30 mg	Lactose. (RSN 30 mg). White, oval. Film-coated. In 30s.
		35 mg	Lactose. (RSN 35 mg). Orange, oval. Film-coated. In dose packs of 4.

For complete prescribing information, refer to the Bisphosphonates group monograph.

Indications

➤*Postmenopausal osteoporosis:*

Treatment – In postmenopausal women with osteoporosis, risedronate increases bone mineral density (BMD) and reduces the incidence of vertebral fractures and a composite endpoint of nonvertebral osteoporosis-related fractures. Osteoporosis may be confirmed by the presence or history of osteoporotic fracture, or by the finding of low bone mass (for example, at least 2 standard deviations [SD] below the premenopausal mean).

Prevention – Consider risedronate in postmenopausal women who are at risk of developing osteoporosis and for whom the desired clinical outcome is to maintain bone mass and reduce the risk of fracture.

Factors such as a family history of osteoporosis, previous fracture, smoking, BMD (at least 1 SD below the premenopausal mean), high bone turnover, thin body frame, Caucasian or Asian race, and early menopause are associated with an increased risk of developing osteoporosis and fractures. The presence of these risk factors may be important when considering the use of risedronate for prevention of osteoporosis.

➤*Glucocorticoid-induced osteoporosis:* Prevention and treatment of glucocorticoid-induced osteoporosis in men and women initiating or continuing systemic glucocorticoid treatment (daily dosage equivalent to 7.5 mg or greater of prednisone) for chronic diseases. Give patients treated with glucocorticoids adequate amounts of calcium and vitamin D.

➤*Paget disease (osteitis deformans):* Treatment of patients with Paget disease of bone who have a level of serum alkaline phosphatase (SAP) at least 2 times the upper limit of normal, who are symptomatic, or who are at risk for future complications from their disease, to induce remission (normalization of SAP).

Administration and Dosage

➤*Approved by the FDA:* March 27, 1998.

Take at least 30 minutes before the first food or drink of the day other than water.

To facilitate delivery to the stomach, take while in an upright position with a full glass (6 to 8 oz; 180 to 240 mL) of plain water and avoid lying down for 30 minutes.

Patients should receive supplemental calcium and vitamin D if dietary intake is inadequate. Take calcium supplements and calcium-, aluminum-, and magnesium-containing medications at a different time of the day to prevent interference with risedronate absorption.

➤*Treatment/Prevention of postmenopausal osteoporosis:* 5 mg orally taken daily or one 35 mg tablet orally taken once weekly.

➤*Treatment/Prevention of glucocorticoid-induced osteoporosis:* 5 mg orally taken daily.

➤*Paget disease:* 30 mg once daily for 2 months. Retreatment may be considered (following posttreatment observation of at least 2 months) if relapse occurs or if treatment fails to normalize serum alkaline phosphatase. For retreatment, the dose and duration of therapy are the same as for initial treatment. No data are available on more than 1 course of retreatment.

➤*Renal function impairment:* Risedronate is not recommended for use in patients with severe renal impairment (Ccr less than 30 mL/min). No dosage adjustment is necessary in patients with a Ccr at least 30 mL/min or in the elderly.

➤*Storage/Stability:* Store at controlled room temperature 20° to 25°C (68° to 77°F).

ZOLEDRONIC ACID

Rx   **Zometa** (Novartis)

Powder for injection: 4.264 mg zoledronic acid monohydrate equiv. to 4 mg zoledronic acid anhydrous	220 mg mannitol, 24 mg sodium citrate. In vials.	

For complete prescribing information, refer to the Bisphosphonates group monograph.

Indications

➤*Hypercalcemia of malignancy (HCM):* For the treatment of HCM.

The safety and efficacy of zoledronic acid in the treatment of hypercalcemia associated with hyperparathyroidism or with other nontumor-related conditions has not been established.

➤*Multiple myeloma and bone metastases of solid tumors:* For treatment of patients with multiple myeloma and patients with documented bone metastases from solid tumors, in conjunction with standard antineoplastic therapy. Prostate cancer should have progressed after treatment with at least 1 hormonal therapy.

Administration and Dosage

➤*Approved by the FDA:* August 20, 2001.

➤*HCM:* Consider the severity and symptoms of tumor-induced hypercalcemia when considering use of zoledronic acid for injection. Vigorous saline hydration alone may be sufficient to treat mild, asymptomatic hypercalcemia.

Hydration – Initiate vigorous saline hydration, an integral part of hypercalcemia therapy, promptly and attempt to restore the urine output to approximately 2 L/day throughout treatment. Mild or asymptomatic hypercalcemia may be treated with conservative measures (ie, saline hydration with or without loop diuretics). Adequately hydrate patients throughout the treatment, but avoid overhydration, especially in those patients who have cardiac failure. Do not employ diuretic therapy prior to correction of hypovolemia.

Dose – The maximum recommended dose in HCM (albumin-corrected serum calcium† at least 12 mg/dL or greater [3 mmol/L]) is 4 mg. The 4 mg dose must be given as a single-dose IV infusion over no less than 15 minutes. Adequately rehydrate patients prior to administration of zoledronic acid.

Retreatment – Retreatment with 4 mg may be considered if serum calcium does not return to normal or remain normal after initial treatment. It is recommended that a minimum of 7 days elapse before retreatment to allow for a full response to the initial dose. Carefully monitor renal function in all patients receiving zoledronic acid and assess possible deterioration in renal function prior to retreatment.

➤*Multiple myeloma and metastatic bone lesions from solid tumors:* The recommended dose of zoledronic acid in patients with multiple myeloma and metastatic bone lesions from solid tumors is 4 mg infused over 15 minutes every 3 or 4 weeks. Duration of treatment in the clinical studies was 15 months for prostate cancer, 12 months for breast cancer and multiple myeloma, and 9 months for other solid tumors. Also give patients an oral calcium supplement of 500 mg and a multiple vitamin containing 400 IU vitamin D daily.

Measure serum creatinine before each zoledronic acid dose and withhold treatment for renal deterioration. In the clinical studies, renal deterioration was defined as follows:
• For patients with normal baseline creatinine, increase of 0.5 mg/dL.
• For patients with abnormal baseline creatinine, increase of 1 mg/dL.

In the clinical studies, zoledronic acid treatment was resumed only when the creatinine returned to within 10% of the baseline value.

➤*Preparation of solution:* Zoledronic acid is reconstituted by adding 5 mL of sterile water for injection to each vial. The resulting solution allows for withdrawal of 4 mg of zoledronic acid. Completely dissolve the drug before the solution is withdrawn.

The maximum recommended 4 mg dose must be further diluted in 100 mL of sterile 0.9% sodium chloride or 5% dextrose injection. The dose must be given as a single IV infusion over no less than 15 minutes.

➤*Admixture incompatibilities:* Do not mix zoledronic acid with calcium-containing infusion solutions, such as Lactated Ringer's solution, and administer it as a single IV solution in a line separate from all other drugs.

➤*Renal function deterioration:* Because of the risk of clinically significant deterioration in renal function, which may progress to renal failure, single doses of zoledronic acid should not exceed 4 mg and the duration of infusion should be no less than 15 minutes.

There must be strict adherence to the IV administration recommendations for zoledronic acid in order to decrease the risk of deterioration in renal function.

➤*Storage / Stability:* Store at 15° to 30°C (59° to 86°F).

If not used immediately after reconstitution, for microbiological integrity, refrigerate the solution at 2° to 8°C (36° to 46°F). The total time between reconstitution, dilution, storage in the refrigerator, and end of administration must not exceed 24 hours.

---

† Albumin-corrected serum calcium (Cca, mg/dL) = Ca + 0.8 (mid-range albumin-measured albumin in mg/dL)

Insulin

Indications

►*Type 1 diabetes mellitus (formerly known as insulin-dependent diabetes mellitus; IDDM):* Diabetes mellitus type 1.

►*Type 2 diabetes mellitus (formerly known as non-insulin-dependent diabetes mellitus; NIDDM):* Diabetes mellitus type 2 that cannot be properly controlled by diet, exercise, and weight reduction.

►*Hyperkalemia:* Infusion of glucose and insulin produces a shift of potassium into cells and lowers serum potassium levels.

►*Severe ketoacidosis/diabetic coma:* Insulin injection (regular insulin) may be given IV or IM for rapid effect in severe ketoacidosis or diabetic coma.

►*Highly purified (single component) and human insulins:* Local insulin allergy, immunologic insulin resistance, injection site lipodystrophy; temporary insulin use (eg, surgery, acute stress type 2 diabetes, gestational diabetes); newly diagnosed diabetics.

Administration and Dosage

The number and size of daily doses, time of administration, and diet and exercise require continuous medical supervision. Dosage adjustment may be necessary when changing types of insulin, particularly when changing from single-peak to the more purified animal or human insulins.

For insulin suspensions, ensure uniform dispersion by rolling the vial gently between hands. Avoid vigorous shaking that may result in the formation of air bubbles or foam. Regular insulin and insulin glargine should be a clear solution.

Administer maintenance doses SC. Rotate administration sites to prevent lipodystrophy. A general rule is to not administer within 1 inch of the same site for 1 month. The rate of absorption is more rapid when the injection is in the abdomen (possibly > 50% faster), followed by the upper arm, thigh, and buttocks. Therefore, it may be best to rotate sites within an area rather than rotating areas. Give regular insulin IV or IM in severe ketoacidosis or diabetic coma.

►*Dosage guidelines:* Individualize doses and monitor patients with diabetes mellitus closely; the following dosage guidelines may be considered.

Children and adults – 0.5 to 1 U/kg/day.

Insulin timing: Give insulin lispro within 15 minutes before a meal. Human regular insulin is best given 30 to 60 minutes before a meal. Give insulin glargine once daily SC at bedtime.

Insulin requirements may be altered during intercurrent conditions such as illness, emotional disturbances, or stress.

Adjust doses to achieve premeal and bedtime blood glucose levels of 80 to 140 mg/dl (children < 5 years of age, 100 to 200 mg/dl).

►*Insulin mixtures:* When mixing 2 types of insulin, always draw clear regular insulin into syringe first. Patients stabilized on mixtures should have a consistent response if the mixing is standardized. An unexpected response is most likely to occur when switching from separate injections to use of mixture or vice versa. To avoid dosage error, do not alter order of mixing insulins or change model or brand of syringe or needle. Each different type of insulin used must be of the same concentration (units/mL).

NPH/regular mixtures of insulin are now available from the manufacturer in pre-mixed formulations of 70% NPH and 30% regular. A 50/50 combination is also available. NPH/regular combinations of insulin are stable and are absorbed as if injected separately. In mixtures of regular and lente insulins, binding is detectable 5 minutes to 24 hours after mixing. If the regular/lente mixtures are not administered within the first 5 minutes after mixing, the effect of the regular insulin is diminished. The excess zinc binds with the regular and forms a lente-type insulin. Thus, it is critical that mixtures of regular with the lente insulins be mixed and injected immediately.

These mixtures remain stable for 1 month at room temperature or for 3 months refrigerated. These mixtures can also be stored in prefilled plastic or glass syringes for 1 week to possibly 14 days under refrigeration. Keep filled syringes in a vertical or oblique position with the needle pointing upward to avoid plugging problems. Prior to injection, pull back the plunger and tip the syringe back and forth, slightly agitating to remix the insulins. Check for normal appearance.

Semilente, ultralente, and lente insulins may be mixed in any ratio; they are chemically identical and differ only in size and structure of insulin particles. These mixtures are stable 1 month at room temperature or 3 months under refrigeration.

►*Insulin adsorption:* Insulin adsorption into plastic IV infusion sets has reportedly removed up to 80% of a dose, but 20% to 30% is more common. Percent adsorbed is inversely proportional to insulin concentration; it takes place within 30 to 60 minutes. Because this phenomenon cannot be accurately predicted, patient monitoring is essential.

►*Concomitant sulfonylurea therapy:* Insulin and oral sulfonylurea coadministration has been used with some success in type 2 diabetic patients who are difficult to control with diet and sulfonylurea therapy alone.

►*Storage/Stability:* Proper storage is critical. Insulin preparations being used are generally stable if stored at room temperature (and not exposed to extreme temperatures or direct sunlight) for 1 month. Always store extra bottles in the refrigerator; do not freeze.

Insulin prefilled in plastic or glass syringes is stable for 28 days under refrigeration. Insulin lispro must be mixed immediately before injection.

Actions

►*Pharmacology:* Insulin and its analogs lower blood glucose levels by stimulating peripheral glucose uptake, especially by skeletal muscle and fat, and by inhibiting hepatic glucose production. Insulin inhibits lipolysis in the adipocyte, inhibits proteolysis, and enhances protein synthesis. Insulin, secreted by the beta cells of the pancreas, is the principal hormone required for proper glucose use in normal metabolic processes. It is composed of two amino acid chains, A (acidic) and B (basic), joined together by disulfide linkages. Human insulin has minor but significant differences from animal insulin with respect to the amino acid sequence on the B-chain (see below). It is derived from a biosynthetic process with strains of *E. coli* (recombinant DNA; rDNA) or yeast (rDNA).

Insulin Amino Acids[1]							
	A-Chain Position			B-Chain Position			
Source/Types	A8	A10	A21	B28	B29	B30	B31 and B32
Beef	Ala	Val	Asn	Pro	Lys	Ala	-
Pork	Thr	Ilc	Asn	Pro	Lys	Ala	-
Human	Thr	Ilc	Asn	Pro	Lys	Thr	-
Glargine	Thr	Ilc	Gly	Pro	Lys	Thr	Arg
Aspart	Thr	Ilc	Asn	Aspartic acid	Lys	Thr	-
Lispro	Thr	Ilc	Asn	Lys	Pro	Thr	-

[1] Ala = alanine, Arg = arginine, Asn = asparagine, Gly = glycine, Ilc = isoleucine, Lys = lysine, Pro = proline, Thr = threonine, Val = valine.

Human insulin may have a more rapid onset and shorter duration of action than pork insulin in some patients. However, the bioavailability of the insulins is identical when given SC. The human insulins are slightly less antigenic than pork or beef insulins. Consider the potential for flocculation with NPH insulin. Human insulin is also the insulin of choice for patients with insulin allergy, insulin resistance, all pregnant patients with diabetes, and any patient who uses insulin intermittently.

Insulin preparations are divided into three categories according to promptness, duration, and intensity of action following SC administration: Rapid-, intermediate-, or long-acting.

Crystalline regular insulin – Crystalline regular insulin is prepared by precipitation in the presence of zinc chloride. Regular insulins available in the US are prepared at neutral pH; this improves stability. Modified forms have been developed to alter the pattern of activity.

Isophane (NPH) – A modified, crystalline protamine zinc insulin. Its effects are comparable to a mixture of 2 to 3 parts regular insulin and 1 part protamine zinc insulin.

Extended insulin zinc suspension (Ultralente) – Large crystals of insulin with high zinc content are collected and resuspended in a sodium acetate/sodium chloride solution. This relatively insoluble insulin is formed without a modifying protein.

Prompt insulin zinc suspension (Semilente) – Amorphous (noncrystalline) insulin precipitated at a high pH.

Insulin zinc suspension (Lente) – Stable mixture of 70% ultralente and 30% semilente.

Insulin Lispro – Consists of zinc-insulin lispro crystals dissolved in clear aqueous fluid. Created when the amino acids at positions 28 and 29 on the insulin B-chain are reversed.

Insulin aspart – Homologous with regular human insulin with the exception of a single substitution of the amino acid proline by aspartic acid in position B28. Produced by recombinant DNA technology utilizing *Saccharomyces cerevisiae* (baker's yeast) as the production organism.

Insulin glargine – Created when the amino acids at position 21 of human insulin are replaced by glycine and 2 arginines are added to the C terminus of the B chain.

Individual response to insulin varies and is affected by diet, exercise, concomitant drug therapy, and other factors. Characteristics of various insulins given SC are compared below:

Pharmacokinetics and Compatibility of Various Insulins					
Insulin Preparations	Half-life (hrs)	Onset (hrs)	Peak (hrs)	Duration (hrs)	Compatible mixed with
Rapid-Acting					
Insulin Injection (Regular)		0.5 to 1		8 to 12	All
Prompt Insulin Zinc Suspension (Semilente)		1 to 1.5	5 to 10	12 to 16	Lente
Lispro Insulin Solution	1	0.25	0.5 to 1.5	2 to 5	Ultralente, NPH [1]
Insulin Aspart Solution	1.5	0.25	1 to 3	3 to 5	
Intermediate-Acting					
Isophane Insulin Suspension (NPH)		1 to 1.5	4 to 12	24	Regular
Insulin Zinc Suspension (Lente)		1 to 2.5	7 to 15	24	Regular, semilente
Long-Acting					
Insulin Glargine Solution		1.1	5 [2]	24 [3]	None
Protamine Zinc Insulin Suspension (PZI)		4 to 8	14 to 24	36	Regular
Extended Insulin Zinc Suspension (Ultralente)		4 to 8	10 to 30	20 to 36	Regular, semilente

[1] See Administration and Dosage in insulin aspart monograph.
[2] No pronounced peak; small amounts of insulin glargine are slowly released resulting in a relatively constant concentration/time profile over 24 hours.
[3] Studies only conducted up to 24 hours.

Contraindications

During episodes of hypoglycemia and in patients sensitive to any ingredient of the product.

Warnings

➤*Changing insulins:* Change insulins cautiously and under medical supervision. Changes in purity, strength, brand, type, or species source may require dosage adjustment. Teach patients using insulin to self monitor blood glucose levels and keep daily records of results. Concomitant oral antidiabetic treatment may need to be adjusted.

➤*Hypersensitivity reactions:* May require discontinuation of insulin.

Local – Occasionally, redness, swelling, and itching at the injection site may develop. This reaction occurs if the injection is not properly made, if the skin is sensitive to the cleansing solution, or if the patient is allergic to insulin or insulin additives (eg, preservatives). The condition usually resolves in a few days to a few weeks. A change in the type or species source of insulin may be considered.

Systemic – Systemic reactions are less common and may present as a rash, shortness of breath, fast pulse, sweating, a drop in blood pressure, bronchospasm, shock, anaphylaxis, or angioedema and may be life-threatening.

Insulin aspart – Localized reactions and generalized myalgias have been reported with the use of cresol as an injectable excipient.

➤*Renal function impairment:* Some studies with human insulin have shown increased circulating levels of insulin in patients with renal failure. Careful glucose monitoring and dose adjustments of insulin may be necessary in patients with renal dysfunction. Insulin requirements may be reduced in patients with renal function impairment.

➤*Hepatic function impairment:* Some studies with human insulin have shown increased circulating levels of insulin in patients with hepatic failure. Careful glucose monitoring and dose adjustments of insulin may be necessary in patients with hepatic dysfunction.

➤*Fertility impairment:*

Insulin glargine – In a combined fertility and prenatal and postnatal study in male and female rats at subcutaneous doses of insulin glargine up to 0.36 mg/kg/day, which is ≈ 7 times the recommended human SC starting dose of 10 IU (0.008 mg/kg/day), based on mg/m², maternal toxicity due to dose-dependent hypoglycemia, including some deaths, was observed. Consequently, a reduction of the rearing rate occurred in the high-dose group only. Similar effects were observed with NPH human insulin.

➤*Elderly:* In elderly patients with diabetes, the initial dosing, dosing increments, and maintenance dosing should be conservative to avoid hypoglycemic reactions. Hypoglycemia may be difficult to recognize in the elderly.

➤*Pregnancy: Category B; Category C (insulin glargine, insulin aspart).* Pregnancy may make diabetes management more difficult. Human insulin does not cross the placenta, at least when given in the second trimester. Insulin is the drug of choice for diabetes control in pregnancy. Keep patients under close medical supervision. Rigid control of serum glucose and avoidance of ketoacidosis are desired throughout pregnancy. It is essential for patients with diabetes or a his-

tory of gestational diabetes to maintain good metabolic control before conception and throughout pregnancy. Insulin requirements usually fall during the first trimester and increase during the second and third trimester and rapidly decline after delivery.

Insulin glargine – Subcutaneous reproduction and teratology studies have been performed with insulin glargine and regular human insulin in rats and Himalayan rabbits. The drug was given to female rats before mating, during mating, and throughout pregnancy at doses up to 0.36 mg/kg/day, which is ≈ 7 times the recommended human SC starting dose of 10 IU (0.008 mg/kg/day), based on mg/m². In rabbits, doses of 0.072 mg/kg/day, which is ≈ 2 times the recommended human SC starting dose of 10 IU (0.008 mg/kg/day), based on mg/m², were administered during organogenesis. The effects of insulin glargine did not generally differ from those observed with regular human insulin in rats or rabbits. However, in rabbits, 5 fetuses from 2 litters of the high-dose group exhibited dilation of the cerebral ventricles. Fertility and early embryonic development appeared normal.

There are no well-controlled clinical studies of the use of insulin glargine in pregnant women. Use this drug during pregnancy only if clearly needed.

Insulin aspart – Subcutaneous reproduction and teratology studies have been performed with insulin aspart and regular human insulin in rats and rabbits. In these studies, insulin aspart was given to female rats before mating, during mating, and throughout pregnancy and to rabbits during organogenesis. The effects of insulin aspart did not differ from those observed with SC regular human insulin. Insulin aspart, like human insulin, caused pre- and post-implantation losses and visceral/skeletal abnormalities in rats at a dose of 200 U/kg/day (≈ 32 times the human SC dose of 1 U/kg/day, based on U/body surface area) and in rabbits at a dose of 10 U/kg/day (≈ 3 times the human SC dose of 1 U/kg/day, based on U/body surface area). The effects are probably secondary to maternal hypoglycemia at high doses. No significant effects were observed in rats at a dose of 50 U/kg/day and rabbits at a dose of 3 U/kg/day. These doses are ≈ 8 times the human SC dose of 1 U/kg/day for rats and equal to the human SC dose of 1 U/kg/day for rabbits, based on U/body surface area.

There are no well-controlled clinical studies of the use of insulin aspart in pregnant women. Use during pregnancy only if the potential benefit justifies the potential risk to the fetus.

➤*Lactation:* Insulin is destroyed in the GI tract when administered orally and therefore would not be expected to be absorbed intact by the breastfeeding infant. However, inadequate or excessive insulin treatment of diabetic mothers inhibits milk production. Lactating women may require adjustments in insulin dose and diet.

Insulin glargine – It is unknown whether insulin glargine is excreted in significant amounts in breast milk. Many drugs, including human insulin, are excreted in breast milk. For this reason, exercise caution when insulin glargine is administered to a nursing woman.

Insulin aspart – It is unknown whether insulin aspart is excreted in breast milk. Many drugs, including human insulin, are excreted in breast milk. For this reason, exercise caution when insulin aspart is administered to a nursing mother.

➤*Children:* Safety and efficacy in patients < 12 years of age have not been established.

Insulin glargine – Safety and effectiveness of insulin glargine have been established in children 6 to 15 years of age with type 1 diabetes.

Humalog – Humalog can be used in combination with sulfonylureas in children > 3 years of age.

Precautions

➤*Insulin resistance:* Insulin resistance occurs rarely. Insulin resistant patients require > 200 units of insulin/day for > 2 days in the absence of ketoacidosis or acute infection. Sometimes, the resistance is due to high levels of IgG antibodies to insulin. Insulin resistance may also occur in obese patients, patients with acanthosis nigricans, ketoacidosis, endocrinopathies and patients with insulin receptor defects; insulin resistance during infection may be due to a postreceptor defect. Hyperglycemia may be managed by changing insulin species source (eg, beef or mixed beef-pork to pork or human insulin). May give corticosteroids (prednisone 60 to 100 mg/day) if changing the insulin is not effective. Corticosteroids may decrease IgG production or decrease insulin binding to the antibody. Monitor closely for signs of hyperglycemia and for adverse effects of high-dose corticosteroids. Highly concentrated insulin (U-500) may also be given to insulin-resistant patients. Use caution to avoid hypoglycemia. Some Type 2 patients with insulin resistance have been treated with a combination of a sulfonylurea plus insulin (see Administration and Dosage).

➤*Hypoglycemia:* Hypoglycemia may result from excessive insulin dose or may be due to the following: Increased work or exercise without eating; food not being absorbed in the usual manner because of postponement or omission of a meal or in illness with vomiting, fever, or diarrhea; when insulin requirements decline (see Overdosage). Early warning symptoms of hypoglycemia may be different or less pronounced under certain conditions, such as long duration of diabetes, diabetic nerve disease, use of medications such as beta blockers, or

Insulin

intensified diabetes control. Such situations may result in severe hypoglycemia (and possibly loss of consciousness) prior to patients' awareness of hypoglycemia. Rapid changes in serum glucose levels may induce symptoms of hypoglycemia in people with diabetes, regardless of the glucose value.

➤*Diabetic ketoacidosis:* Diabetic ketoacidosis, a potentially life-threatening condition, requires prompt diagnosis and treatment. Hyperglucagonemia, hyperglycemia, and ketoacidosis may result. Diabetic ketoacidosis may result from stress, illness, or insulin omission or may develop slowly after a long period of insulin control. Treat with fluids, correction of acidosis and hypotension, and low-dose regular insulin IM or IV infusion.

Symptoms of Hypoglycemia vs Ketoacidosis							
Reaction	Onset	Urine glucose/ acetone	Symptoms				
			CNS	Respiration	Mouth/GI	Skin	Miscellaneous
Hypo-glycemic reaction (insulin reaction)	sudden	0/0	fatigue weakness nervous-ness confusion headache diplopia convulsions psychoses dizziness unconsci-ousness	rapid shallow	numb tingling hunger nausea	pallor moist shallow or dry	normal or non-character-istic pulse eyeballs normal
Keto-acidosis (diabetic coma)	gradual (hours or days)	+/+	drowsiness dim vision	air hunger	thirst acetone breath nausea vomiting abdominal pain loss of appetite	dry flushed	rapid pulse soft eyeballs

➤*Lipodystrophy:*

Lipoatrophy – Lipoatrophy is the breakdown of adipose tissue at the insulin injection site, causing a depression in the skin and may delay insulin absorption. It may be the result of an immune response or when less pure insulins are administered. Injection of human or purified pork insulins into the site over a 2- to 4-week period may result in SC fat accumulation.

Lipohypertrophy – Lipohypertrophy is the result of repeated insulin injection into the same site. It is the accumulation of SC fat, and it may interfere with insulin absorption from the site. This condition may be avoided by rotating the injection site.

➤*Diet:* Patients must follow a prescribed diet and exercise regularly. Determine the time, number, and amount of individual doses and distribution of food among the meals of the day. Do not change this regimen unless prescribed otherwise.

➤*Hyperthyroidism/Hypothyroidism:* Hyperthyroidism may cause an increase in the renal clearance of insulin. Therefore, patients may need more insulin to control their diabetes. Hypothyroidism may delay insulin turnover, requiring less insulin to control diabetes.

Drug Interactions

Drugs That Decrease the Hypoglycemic Effect of Insulin	
Acetazolamide	Epinephrine
AIDS antivirals	Estrogens
Albuterol	Ethacrynic acid
Asparaginase	Isoniazid
Calcitonin	Lithium carbonate
Contraceptives, oral	Morphine sulfate
Corticosteroids	Niacin
Cyclophosphamide	Nicotine
Danazol	Phenothiazines
Dextrothyroxine	Phenytoin
Diazoxide	Somatropin
Diltiazem	Terbutaline
Diuretics	Thiazide diuretics
Dobutamine	Thyroid hormones

Drugs That Increase the Hypoglycemic Effect of Insulin	
ACE inhibitors	Lithium carbonate
Alcohol	MAO inhibitors
Anabolic steroids	Mebendazole
Antidiabetic pro-ducts, oral	Pentamidine[2]
	Phenylbutazone
Beta blockers[1]	Propoxyphene
Calcium	Pyridoxine
Chloroquine	Salicylates
Clofibrate	Somatostatin analog
Clonidine	(eg, octreotide)

Drugs That Increase the Hypoglycemic Effect of Insulin	
Disopyramide	Sulfinpyrazone
Fluoxetine	Sulfonamides
Guanethidine	Tetracyclines

[1] Nonselective beta blockers may delay recovery from hypoglycemic episodes and mask their signs/symptoms. Cardioselective agents may be alternatives.
[2] May sometimes be followed by hyperglycemia.

Adverse Reactions

➤*Human insulin:* Hypoglycemia and hypokalemia are among the potential clinical adverse events associated with the use of all insulins. Other adverse events commonly associated with human insulin therapy include the following:

Miscellaneous – Allergic reactions. Sodium retention and edema may occur, particularly if previously poor metabolic control is improved by intensified insulin therapy.

Dermatologic – Injection site reaction, lipodystrophy, pruritus, rash.

Lab test abnormalities – Hypoglycemia; hypokalemia.

➤*Insulin glargine:*

Local – In clinical studies in adult patients, there was a higher incidence of treatment-emergent injection site pain in insulin glargine-treated patients (2.7%) compared with NPH insulin-treated patients (0.7%). The reports of pain at the injection site were usually mild and did not result in discontinuation of therapy. Other treatment-emergent injection site reactions occurred at similar incidences with both insulin glargine and NPH human insulin.

Ophthalmic – Retinopathy was evaluated in the clinical studies by means of retinal adverse events reported and fundus photography. The numbers of retinal adverse events reported for insulin glargine and NPH treatment groups were similar for patients with type 1 and 2 diabetes. Progression of retinopathy was investigated by fundus photography using a grading protocol derived from the Early Treatment Diabetic Retinopathy Study (ETDRS). In one clinical study involving patients with type 2 diabetes, a difference in the number of subjects with ≥ 3-step progression in ETDRS scale over a 6-month period was noted by fundus photography (7.5% in insulin glargine group vs 2.7% in NPH-treated group). The overall relevance of this isolated finding cannot be determined due to the small number of patients involved, the short follow-up period, and the fact that this finding was not observed in other clinical studies.

➤*Insulin aspart:*

Lab test abnormalities – Small, but persistent elevations in alkaline phosphatase.

Miscellaneous –

Antibody production: Insulin antibodies may develop during treatment with insulin. In large clinical trials, levels of antibodies that crossreact with human insulin and insulin aspart were higher in patients treated with insulin aspart compared with regular human insulin. The clinical significance of these antibodies is uncertain.

Overdosage

➤*Symptoms:* Hypoglycemia may result from excessive insulin dose or may be caused by the following: Increased work or exercise without eating; food not being absorbed in the usual manner because of postponement or omission of a meal or in illness with vomiting, fever, or diarrhea; when insulin requirements decline.

➤*Treatment:* Mild episodes of hypoglycemia can be treated with oral glucose or carbohydrates. Adjustments in drug dosage, meal patterns, or exercise may be needed. More severe episodes with coma, seizure, or neurologic impairment may be treated with IM/SC glucagon or concentrated IV glucose. Sustained carbohydrate intake and observation may be necessary because hypoglycemia may recur after apparent clinical recovery.

Patient Information

Use the same type and brand of syringe to avoid dosage errors. Rotate sites to prevent lipodystrophy. If using a "pen-filled" device, follow information for proper use.

Do not change the order of mixing insulins (if applicable) or change the brand, strength, type, species, or dose without your physician's knowledge.

Insulin requirements may change in patients who become ill, especially with vomiting or fever and during stress or emotional disturbances. Consult a physician.

See your dentist twice yearly; see an ophthalmologist regularly.

Patient information inserts are available; read and understand all aspects of insulin use. Patients must receive complete instructions about the nature of diabetes. Strict adherence to prescribed diet, exercise program, and personal hygiene are essential.

Periodic measurement of glycosylated hemoglobin is recommended for the monitoring of long-term glycemic control.

Insulin

Patients should wear diabetic identification (*Medic-Alert*) so appropriate treatment can be given if complications occur away from home.

Monitor blood glucose and urine for glucose and ketones as prescribed; monitor blood pressure regularly.

Patients should inform their doctor if they are pregnant or are contemplating pregnancy.

Insulin stored at room temperature will be less painful to inject compared with that stored in the refrigerator, so patients should allow refrigerated insulin to come to room temperature prior to injection.

➤*Insulin glargine:* Do not mix or dilute this type of insulin with any other insulin or solution or it will not work as intended (ie, you may lose blood sugar control).

INSULIN INJECTION (REGULAR)

otc	**Regular Iletin** II (Lilly)	**Injection:** 100 units/mL purified pork	In 10 mL vials.
otc	**Humulin R** (Lilly)	**Injection:** 100 units/mL human insulin (rDNA)	In 10 mL vials.
otc	**Novolin R** (Novo Nordisk)		In 10 mL vials.
otc	**Novolin R Prefilled** (Novo Nordisk)		In 5 × 1.5 mL prefilled syringes.
otc	**Velosulin BR** (Novo Nordisk)		In 10 mL vials.
otc	**Novolin R PenFill** (Novo Nordisk)	**Cartridges:** 100 units/mL human insulin (rDNA) (Use with *NovoPen* and *Novolin Pen*)	In 5 × 1.5 mL and 5 × 3 mL.

For complete prescribing information, refer to the Insulin group monograph.

ISOPHANE INSULIN SUSPENSION (NPH)
Insulin combined with protamine and zinc.

otc	**NPH Iletin** II (Lilly)	**Injection:** 100 units/mL purified pork	In 10 mL vials.
otc	**Humulin N** (Lilly)	**Injection:** 100 units/mL human insulin (rDNA)	In 5 × 3 mL disposable pen insulin delivery devices, and 10 mL vials.
otc	**Novolin N** (Novo Nordisk)		In 10 mL vials.
otc	**Novolin N Prefilled** (Novo Nordisk)		In 5 × 1.5 mL prefilled syringes.
otc	**Novolin N PenFill** (Novo Nordisk)	**Cartridges:** 100 units/mL human insulin (rDNA) (Use with *NovoPen* and *Novolin Pen*)	In 5 × 1.5 mL and 5 × 3 mL.

For cmplete prescribing information, refer to the Insulin group monograph.

ISOPHANE INSULIN SUSPENSION (NPH) AND INSULIN INJECTION (REGULAR)
70% isophane insulin (NPH) and 30% insulin injection (regular). Provides rapid activity (onset 30 minutes) with a duration of up to 24 hours.

otc	**Humulin 70/30** (Lilly)	**Injection:** 100 units/mL human insulin (rDNA)	In 5 × 3 mL disposable pen insulin delivery devices, and 10 mL vials.
otc	**Novolin 70/30** (Novo Nordisk)		In 10 mL vials.
otc	**Novolin 70/30 Prefilled** (Novo Nordisk)		In 5 × 1.5 mL prefilled syringes.
otc	**Novolin 70/30 PenFill** (Novo Nordisk)	**Cartridges:** 100 units/mL human insulin (rDNA) (Use with *NovoPen* and *Novolin Pen*)	In 5 × 1.5 and 5 × 3 mL.

For cmplete prescribing information, refer to the Insulin group monograph.

ISOPHANE INSULIN SUSPENSION (NPH) AND INSULIN INJECTION (REGULAR)
50% isophane insulin (NPH) and 50% insulin injection (regular). Provides rapid activity (onset 30 minutes) with a duration of up to 24 hours.

otc	**Humulin 50/50** (Lilly)	**Injection:** 100 units/mL human insulin (rDNA)	In 10 mL vials.

For cmplete prescribing information, refer to the Insulin group monograph.

INSULIN ZINC SUSPENSION (LENTE)
70% crystalline and 30% amorphous insulin suspension.

otc	**Lente Iletin** II (Lilly)	**Injection:** 100 units/mL purified pork	In 10 mL vials.
otc	**Humulin L** (Lilly)	**Injection:** 100 units/mL human insulin (rDNA)	In 10 mL vials.

For cmplete prescribing information, refer to the Insulin group monograph.

INSULIN ZINC SUSPENSION, EXTENDED (ULTRALENTE)

otc	**Humulin U** (Lilly)	**Injection:** 100 units/mL human insulin (rDNA)	In 10 mL vials.

For cmplete prescribing information, refer to the Insulin group monograph.

INSULIN ANALOG INJECTION

Rx	**Humalog** (Lilly)	**Injection:** 100 units/mL human insulin lispro (rDNA)	In 10 mL vials, 5 × 1.5 and 5 × 3 mL cartridges, and 5 × 3 mL disposable pen insulin delivery device.
Rx	**Humalog Mix75/25**[1] (Lilly)		0.28 mg protamine sulfate. In 10 mL vials and 5 × 3 mL disposable pen insulin delivery devices.
Rx	**NovoLog** (Novo Nordisk)	**Injection:** 100 units/mL human insulin aspart (rDNA)	In 3 mL *PenFill* cartridges and 10 mL vials.
Rx	**NovoLog Mix 70/30**[2] (Novo Nordisk)	**Injection:** 100 units/mL insulin aspart.	In 3 mL *Penfill* cartridges and 3 mL *FlexPen* prefilled syringes.

[1] Contains 75% insulin lispro protamine suspension and 25% insulin lispro injection (rDNA).

[2] Contains 70% insulin aspart (rDNA) protamine suspension and 30% insulin aspart (rDNA).

For complete prescribing information, refer to the Insulin group monograph.

Indications

➤*Insulin aspart:* Treatment of adults with diabetes mellitus for the control of hyperglycemia. Because insulin aspart has a more rapid onset and a shorter duration of action than human regular insulin, insulin aspart normally should be used in regimens together with an intermediate or long-acting insulin. *NovoLog* may be infused SC by external insulin pumps.

➤*Insulin lispro:* Treatment of patients with diabetes mellitus for the control of hyperglycemia. Insulin lispro has a more rapid onset and shorter duration of action than regular human insulin. Therefore, in patients with type 1 diabetes, use in regimens that include a longer-acting insulin. However, in patients with type 2 diabetes, insulin lispro may be used without a longer-acting insulin when used in combination therapy with sulfonylureas.

Children (Humalog only) — Safety and effectiveness in children less than 18 years of age have not been determined for *Humalog Mix.* Adjustment of basal insulin may be required. To improve accuracy of dosing in pediatric patients, a diluent may be used. If the diluent is added directly to the vial, the shelf life may be reduced.

Administration and Dosage

➤*Insulin aspart:* Give immediately before a meal. Individualize and determine dose based on the patient's needs. The total daily individual

INSULIN ANALOG INJECTION

insulin requirement is usually between 0.5 and 1 unit/kg/day. In a meal-related treatment regimen, 50% to 70% of this requirement may be provided by insulin aspart and the remainder provided by an intermediate-acting or long-acting insulin. Patients may require more basal insulin and more total insulin when using insulin aspart compared with regular human insulin to prevent premeal hyperglycemia. Additional basal insulin injections may be necessary.

Because of the fast onset of action of insulin aspart, administer close to a meal (start of meal within 5 to 10 minutes after injection). Regularly adjust dose according to blood glucose measurements.

Insulin pump – When used in external insulin infusion pumps, the initial programming of the pump is based on the total daily insulin dose of the previous regimen. Although there is significant interpatient variability, approximately 50% of the total dose is given as meal-related boluses and the remainder as basal infusion. Higher basal rates in external SC infusion pumps may be necessary. Infusion sets and the insulin in the infusion sets must be changed every 48 hours or sooner to assure the activity of insulin aspart and proper pump function.

Administer by SC injection in the abdominal wall, the thigh, or the upper arm, or by continuous SC infusion in the abdominal wall. Rotate injection and infusion sites within the same region. As with all insulins, the duration of action will vary according to the dose, injection site, blood flow, temperature, and level of physical activity.

▶*Insulin lispro:* Insulin lispro is intended for SC administration. Dosage regimens of insulin lispro will vary among patients and should be determined by the health care professional familiar with the patient's metabolic needs, eating habits, and other lifestyle variables. Pharmacokinetic and pharmacodynamic studies showed insulin lispro to be equipotent to human regular insulin (ie, 1 unit of insulin lispro has the same glucose-lowering capability as 1 unit of human regular insulin), but with more rapid activity and a shorter duration. *Humalog Mix75/25* has a similar glucose-lowering effect as compared with *Humulin 70/30* on a unit for unit basis. The quicker glucose-lowering effect of insulin lispro is related to the more rapid absorption rate from subcutaneous tissue. An adjustment of dose or schedule of basal insulin may be needed when a patient changes from other insulins to insulin lispro, particularly to prevent premeal hyperglycemia.

When used as a meal-time insulin, give insulin lispro within 15 minutes before or immediately after a meal. Human regular insulin is best given 30 to 60 minutes before a meal. To achieve optimal glucose control, the amount of longer-acting insulin being given may need to be adjusted when using insulin lispro.

The rate of insulin absorption and consequently the onset of activity is known to be affected by the site of injection, exercise, and other variables. Insulin lispro was absorbed at a consistently faster rate than human regular insulin in healthy male volunteers given 0.2 U/kg human regular insulin or insulin lispro at abdominal, deltoid, or femoral sites, the 3 sites often used by patients with diabetes. When not mixed in the same syringe with other insulins, insulin lispro maintains its rapid onset of action and has less variability in its onset of action among injection sites compared with human regular insulin. After abdominal administration, insulin lispro concentrations are higher than those following deltoid or thigh injections. Also, the duration of action of insulin lispro is slightly shorter following abdominal injection, compared with deltoid and femoral injections. As with all insulin preparations, the time course of action of insulin lispro may vary considerably in different individuals or within the same individual. Patients must be educated to use proper injection techniques.

Compatibility – Insulin lispro may be diluted with sterile diluent for *Humalog, Humulin N, Humulin 50/50, Humulin 70/30,* and *NPH Iletin* to a concentration of 1:10 (equivalent to U-10) or 1:2 (equivalent to U-50). Diluted insulin lispro may remain in patient use for 28 days when stored at 5°C (41°F) and for 14 days when stored at 30°C (86°F).

▶*Mixing of insulins:*

Insulin aspart – A clinical study in healthy male volunteers (n = 24) demonstrated that mixing insulin aspart with NPH human insulin immediately before injection produced some attenuation in the peak concentration of insulin aspart, but that the time to peak and the total bioavailability of insulin aspart were not significantly affected. If insulin aspart is mixed with NPH human insulin, draw insulin aspart into the syringe first. Inject immediately after mixing. Do not mix insulin aspart with crystalline zinc insulin preparations because of lack of compatability data.

The effects of mixing insulin aspart with insulins of animal source or insulin preparations produced by other manufacturers have not been studied.

Do not administer mixtures IV.

When used in external SC infusion pumps for insulin, do not mix with any other insulins or diluent.

Insulin lispro – Mixing insulin lispro with *Humulin N* or *Humulin U* does not decrease the absorption rate or the total bioavailability of insulin lispro. Given alone or mixed with *Humulin N*, insulin lispro results in a more rapid absorption and glucose-lowering effect compared with human regular insulin.

The effects of mixing insulin lispro with insulins of animal source or insulin preparations produced by other manufacturers have not been studied.

If insulin lispro is mixed with a longer-acting insulin such as *Humulin N* or *Humulin U*, insulin lispro should be drawn into the syringe first to prevent clouding of the insulin lispro by the longer-acting insulin. Injection should be made immediately after mixing. Do not give mixtures IV.

▶*Storage/Stability:*

Insulin aspart – Store between 2° and 8°C (36° and 46°F). Do not freeze. Do not use insulin aspart if it has been frozen or exposed to temperatures that exceed 37°C (98.6°F). Cartridges or vials in use may be kept at temperatures less than 30°C (86°F) for up to 28 days, but do not expose to excessive heat or sunlight. Opened vials may be refrigerated. Do not refrigerate cartridges after insertion into the *NovoPen 3*. Discard infusion sets (reservoirs, tubing, and catheters) and the *NovoLog* in the reservoir after no more than 48 hours of use or after exposure to temperatures that exceed 37°C (98.6°F).

Insulin lispro – Store in refrigerator (2° to 8°C [36° to 46°F]), but not in the freezer. If refrigeration is impossible, the vial or cartridge of insulin lispro in use can be unrefrigerated for up to 28 days, as long as it is kept as cool as possible (not greater than 30°C [86°F]) and away from direct heat and light. The *Humalog Pen* in use should not be refrigerated but should be kept as cool as possible (below 30°C [86°F]) and away from direct heat and light. Unrefrigerated insulin lispro must be used within 28 days or be discarded. Do not use insulin lispro if it has been frozen.

INSULIN GLARGINE

Rx	**Lantus** (Aventis)	**Injection:** 100 units/mL insulin glargine (rDNA)	In 10 mL vials.

For complete prescribing information, refer to the Insulin group monograph.

Indications

▶*Diabetes:* Once-daily SC administration for the treatment of adults and children with type 1 diabetes mellitus or adults with type 2 diabetes mellitus who require basal (long-acting) insulin for the control of hyperglycemia.

Insulin glargine is not the insulin of choice for the treatment of diabetic ketoacidosis. Short-acting IV insulin is the preferred treatment.

Administration and Dosage

▶*Administration:* Administer SC once daily at the same time every day. The dose may be administered at any time during the day.

Insulin glargine is not intended for IV administration. The prolonged duration of activity of insulin glargine is dependent on injection into SC tissue. IV administration of the usual SC dose could result in severe hypoglycemia.

As with all insulins, injection sites within an injection area (abdomen, thigh, or deltoid) must be rotated from one injection to the next.

In clinical studies, there was no relevant difference in insulin glargine absorption after abdominal, deltoid, or thigh SC administration. As for all insulins, the rate of absorption and, consequently, the onset and duration of action may be affected by exercise and other variables.

Insulin glargine is a recombinant human insulin analog. Its potency is approximately the same as human insulin. It exhibits a relatively constant glucose-lowering profile over 24 hours that permits once-daily dosing. The desired blood glucose levels as well as the doses and timing of antidiabetic medications must be determined individually. Blood glucose monitoring is recommended for all patients with diabetes.

▶*Children:* Insulin glargine can be safely administered to pediatric patients 6 years of age and older. Administration to pediatric patients younger than 6 years of age has not been studied. Based on the results of a study in pediatric patients, the dose recommendation for changeover to insulin glargine is the same as described for adults.

▶*Initial dosing:* In a clinical study with insulin-naïve patients with type 2 diabetes already treated with oral antidiabetic drugs, insulin glargine was started at an average dose of 10 IU once daily and subsequently adjusted according to the patient's need to a total daily dose ranging from 2 to 100 IU.

▶*Changeover to insulin glargine:* If changing from a treatment regimen with an intermediate- or long-acting insulin to a regimen with insulin glargine, the amount and timing of short-acting insulin, fast-acting insulin analog, or the dose of any oral antidiabetic drug may need to be adjusted. In clinical studies, when patients were transferred from once-daily NPH human insulin or ultralente human insulin to once-daily insulin glargine, the initial dose was usually not changed. However, when patients were transferred from twice-daily NPH to insulin glargine once daily to reduce the risk of hypoglycemia, the ini-

INSULIN GLARGINE

tial dose (IU) was usually reduced by approximately 20% (compared with total daily IU of NPH human insulin) and then adjusted based on patient response.

A program of close metabolic monitoring under medical supervision is recommended during transfer and in the initial weeks thereafter. The amount and timing of short-acting insulin or fast-acting insulin analog may need to be adjusted. This is particularly true for patients with acquired antibodies to human insulin needing high insulin doses and occurs with all insulin analogs. Dose adjustment of insulin glargine and other insulins or oral antidiabetic drugs may be required; for example, if the patient's timing of dosing, weight or lifestyle changes, or other circumstances arise that increase susceptibility to hypoglycemia or hyperglycemia.

The dose also may have to be adjusted during intercurrent illness.

➤*Preparation and handling:* Use only if clear and colorless with no visible particles.

The syringes must not contain any other medicinal product or residue.

➤*Mixing and diluting:* Insulin glargine must not be diluted or mixed with any other insulin or solution. If insulin glargine is diluted or mixed, the solution may become cloudy and the pharmacokinetic/pharmacodynamic profile (eg, onset of action, time to peak effect) of insulin glargine and/or the mixed insulin may be altered in an unpredictable manner. When insulin glargine and regular human insulin were mixed immediately before injection in dogs, a delayed onset of action and time to maximum effect for regular human insulin was observed. The total bioavailability of the mixture also was slightly decreased compared with separate injections of insulin glargine and regular human insulin. The relevance of these observations in dogs to humans is not known.

➤*Storage/Stability:* Store unopened insulin glargine vials in a refrigerator at 2° to 8°C (36° to 46°F). Do not store insulin glargine in the freezer or allow it to freeze. Discard vial if frozen.

If refrigeration is not possible, the open vial in use can be kept unrefrigerated for up to 28 days away from direct heat and light, as long as the temperature is not above 30°C (86°F). Opened vials, whether or not refrigerated, must be used within a 28-day period or they must be discarded.

INSULIN GLULISINE

Rx	**Apidra** (Aventis)	**Injection:** 100 units/mL insulin glulisine (rDNA)	In 10 mL vials.

For complete prescribing information, refer to the Insulin group monograph.

Indications

➤*Diabetes:* Treatment of adult patients with diabetes mellitus for the control of hyperglycemia.

Insulin glulisine has a more rapid onset of action and a shorter duration of action than regular human insulin. Insulin glulisine normally should be used in regimens that include a longer-acting insulin or basal insulin analog. Insulin glulisine also may be infused subcutaneously by external insulin infusion pumps.

Administration and Dosage

Insulin glulisine is a recombinant insulin analog that has been shown to be equipotent to human insulin. One unit of insulin glulisine has the same glucose-lowering effect as one unit of regular human insulin. After subcutaneous administration, it has a more rapid onset and shorter duration of action.

➤*Administration:* Give insulin glulisine within 15 minutes before a meal or within 20 minutes after starting a meal. Insulin glulisine is intended for subcutaneous administration and for use by external infusion pump.

Individualize and determine the dosage of insulin glulisine based on the physician's advice in accordance with the needs of the patient. Use in regimens that include a longer-acting insulin or basal insulin analog.

Administer by subcutaneous injection in the abdominal wall, thigh, or deltoid, or by continuous subcutaneous infusion in the abdominal wall.

As with all insulins, rotate injection sites and infusion sites within an injection area (eg, abdomen, thigh, deltoid) from one injection to the next.

As for all insulins, the rate of absorption, and consequently the onset and duration of action, may be affected by injection site, exercise, and other variables. Blood glucose monitoring is recommended for all patients with diabetes.

➤*Preparation and handling:* Only use insulin glulisine if the solution is clear and colorless with no particles visible.

➤*Mixing and diluting:* When used in a pump, do not mix insulin glulisine with other insulins or with a diluent. If glulisine is mixed with NPH human insulin, draw the glulisine into the syringe first. Make injection immediately after mixing. Do not mix glulisine with insulin preparations other than NPH.

➤*Storage/Stability:*

Unopened vial – Store unopened insulin glulisine vials in refrigerator at 2° to 8°C (36° to 46°F). Protect from light. Do not store insulin glulisine in the freezer, nor allow it to freeze. Discard vial if frozen.

Opened (in use) vial – Opened vials, whether or not refrigerated, must be used within 28 days. They must be discarded if not used within 28 days. If refrigeration is not possible, the open vial in use can be kept unrefrigerated for up to 28 days away from direct heat and light, as long as the temperature is not greater than 25°C (77°F).

Infusion sets – Discard infusion sets (eg, reservoirs, tubing, catheters) and the insulin glulisine in the reservoir after no more than 48 hours of use or after exposure to temperatures that exceed 37°C (98.6°F).

High Potency Insulin
INSULIN INJECTION CONCENTRATED

Rx	**Humulin R Regular U-500 (Concentrated)** (Lilly)	**Injection:** 500 units/mL regular human insulin (rDNA)	In 20 mL vials.[1]

[1] With 2.5 mg m-cresol and 16 mg glycerin per mL.

For complete prescribing information, refer to the Insulin group monograph.

Indications

➤*Insulin resistance:* Treatment of diabetic patients with marked insulin resistance (requirements greater than 200 units/day), because a large dose may be administered SC in a reasonable volume.

Administration and Dosage

➤*Administration:* Administer SC. Do not inject IM or IV. It is inadvisable to inject concentrated insulin IV because of possible inadvertent overdosage.

Use a tuberculin-type or insulin syringe for dosage measurement. Dosage variations are frequent in the insulin-resistant patient because the individual is unresponsive to the pharmacologic effect of the insulin. Nevertheless, encourage accuracy of measurement because of the potential danger of the preparations. Inadvertent overdose may result in irreversible insulin shock. Serious consequences may result if not used under constant medical supervision.

Concentrated insulin injection is not modified by any agent that might prolong its action. It frequently has a duration similar to repository insulin; a single dose demonstrates activity for 24 hours. This has been credited to the high concentration of the preparation.

➤*Dosage adjustments:* Closely observe every patient exhibiting insulin resistance who requires concentrated insulin for diabetic control until appropriate dosing is established. Response will vary among patients. Most patients will show a "tolerance" to insulin, so that minor dosage variations will not cause untoward symptoms of insulin shock. Some may require only 1 dose daily; others may require 2 or 3 injections per day.

Insulin resistance is frequently self-limited; after several weeks or months of high dosage, responsiveness may be regained and dosage reduced.

➤*Hypoglycemic reactions:* Hypoglycemia when using this concentrated insulin can be prolonged and severe. As with other human insulin preparations, hypoglycemic reactions may be associated with the administration of concentrated insulin. However, deep secondary hypoglycemic reactions may develop 18 to 24 hours after the original injection of concentrated insulin. Consequently, carefully observe patients and promptly initiate treatment with glucagon injections or glucose by IV injection or gavage. A few patients who have experienced hypoglycemic reactions after transfer from animal-source insulin to human insulin have reported that the early warning symptoms of hypoglycemia were less pronounced or different from those experienced with their previous insulin. Refer to Insulin group monograph.

➤*Storage/Stability:* Keep in a cold place, preferably in a refrigerator. Do not freeze. Do not use if it is not water-clear. Discoloration, turbidity, or unusual viscosity indicates deterioration or contamination.

Indications

▶*Type 2 diabetes:* As an adjunct to diet and exercise to lower the blood glucose in patients with type 2 (non-insulin-dependent) diabetes mellitus whose hyperglycemia cannot be controlled by diet and exercise alone.

▶*Unlabeled uses:* **Chlorpropamide** in doses of 200 to 500 mg/day has been used in the treatment of diabetes insipidus.

Sulfonylureas have been used as temporary adjuncts to insulin therapy in selected type 2 diabetes patients to improve diabetes control (see Administration and Dosage).

Administration and Dosage

▶*Institution of therapy:* Individualize therapy. Selection of an individual agent is influenced by the drug's potency, duration of action, metabolism, adverse reactions, patient's lack of response to other oral agents, and the patient's personal preference.

Monitor patient's blood glucose periodically to determine the minimum effective dose for the patient; to detect primary failure (ie, inadequate lowering of blood glucose at the maximum recommended dose of medication); and to detect secondary failure (ie, loss of adequate blood glucose response after an initial period of effectiveness). Glycosylated hemoglobin levels are also valuable in monitoring the patient's response to therapy.

▶*Short-term use:* Short-term administration of sulfonylureas may be sufficient during periods of transient loss of control in patients usually well controlled on diet.

▶*Transfer from other hypoglycemic agents:*
Sulfonylureas – When transferring patients from 1 oral hypoglycemic agent to another, no transitional period and no initial or priming dose is necessary. However, when transferring patients from **chlorpropamide**, exercise particular care during the first 2 weeks because the prolonged retention of chlorpropamide in the body and subsequent overlapping drug effects may provoke hypoglycemia. See specific guidelines for each agent in the individual Administration and Dosage sections.

Insulin – During insulin withdrawal period, test urine for glucose and ketones 3 times daily and report results to physician daily. For specific guidelines for each individual sulfonylurea, refer to the Administration and Dosage section for each agent.

General clinical characteristics which favor successful sulfonylureas monotherapy following insulin withdrawal include the following:
• Onset of diabetes at ≥ 35 years of age
• Obese or normal body weight
• Duration of diabetes < 10 years
• Absence of ketoacidosis
• Fasting serum glucose ≤ 200 mg/dl
• Postprandial blood glucose values < 250 mg/dl
• Insulin requirement < 40 units/day
• Absence of renal or hepatic dysfunction

▶*Elderly patients:* Elderly patients may be particularly sensitive to these agents; therefore, start with a lower initial dose before breakfast, and check blood and urine glucoseduring the first 24 hours of therapy. If control is satisfactory, continue or gradually increase dose. If there is a tendency toward hypoglycemia, reduce dose or discontinue the drug.

▶*Acute complications:* During the course of intercurrent complications (eg, ketoacidosis, severe trauma, major surgery, infections, severe diarrhea, nausea, vomiting), supportive therapy with insulin may be necessary. Continue or withdraw sulfonylurea therapy while insulin is used. Insulin is indispensable in managing acute complications; carefully instruct all diabetes patients in its use.

▶*Combination insulin therapy:* Concurrent administration of insulin and an oral sulfonylurea (generally **glipizide** or **glyburide**) has been used with some success in type 2 diabetes patients who are difficult to control with diet and sulfonylurea therapy alone. One proposed method is referred to as the BIDS system: Bedtime Insulin (usually NPH) in combination with a Daytime (morning only or morning and evening) Sulfonylurea, usually glyburide.

Actions

▶*Pharmacology:* The sulfonylurea hypoglycemic agents are sulfonamide derivatives but are devoid of antibacterial activity. These agents are divided into 2 groups: First generation (**acetohexamide, chlorpropamide, tolazamide, tolbutamide**) and second generation (**glipizide, glyburide, glimepiride**). They are used as adjuncts to diet and exercise in the treatment of type 2 diabetes, previously known as non-insulin-dependent diabetes mellitus (NIDDM). Type 2 diabetes has also been referred to as adult-onset or maturity-onset diabetes and ketosis-resistant diabetes.

Type 2 diabetes not only leads to hyperglycemia but affects several organ systems resulting in dyslipidemia, hypertension, central obesity, and accelerated atherosclerosis. This multisystem disorder, also known as the insulin resistance syndrome, contributes to high rates of morbidity and mortality that are usually manifestations of coronary artery and cerebrovascular disease. Other factors influencing premature death in these patients are the duration of diabetes, lack of glycemic control, and other cardiovascular risk factors such as smoking and physical inactivity.

Type 2 diabetes is characterized by insulin resistance, impaired insulin secretion, and overproduction of hepatic glucose. Evidence suggests that insulin resistance is the predominant factor preceding the onset of hyperglycemia. During the transition from impaired glucose tolerance to frank disease, basal hepatic glucose production rates increase, insulin resistance becomes more severe (which may be partly due to acquired conditions such as age, obesity, and an inactive lifestyle), and beta-cell function decreases affecting insulin secretory ability.

By binding to the plasma membrane of functional beta-cells in the pancreatic islets, sulfonylureas cause a decrease in potassium (K+) permeability and membrane depolarization which, in turn, leads to an increase in intracellular calcium ions and subsequent exocytosis of insulin-containing secretory granules. This process is also stimulated by glucose and other insulin-releasing fuels; however, sulfonylureas increase insulin secretion at stimulatory levels lower than that required for glucose suggesting that they enhance beta-cell response rather than change beta-cell sensitivity to glucose. The role of extrapancreatic effects of sulfonylureas in the treatment of hyperglycemia are of questionable clinical significance with the possible exception of glimepiride, which has demonstrated increased sensitivity of peripheral tissues to insulin.

Other pharmacologic activity includes: Potentiation of the effect of antidiuretic hormone (ADH); tolazamide, acetohexamide, glyburide, and glipizide may produce a mild diuresis; acetohexamide has significant uricosuric activity; chlorpropamide can cause flushing (a disulfiram-like reaction) in some patients who consume alcohol.

▶*Pharmacokinetics:* The sulfonylureas are well absorbed after oral administration. All sulfonylureas except **glipizide** can be taken with food; absorption of glipizide is delayed by food. **Tolbutamide, glyburide,** and glipizide are more effective when taken ≈ 30 minutes before a meal. **Tolazamide** is absorbed more slowly than the other sulfonylureas. They are metabolized in the liver to active and inactive metabolites and excreted primarily in the urine. The hypoglycemic effects of sulfonylureas may be prolonged in severe liver disease due to decreased metabolism.

Although the mechanisms of action and maximal hypoglycemic effects are similar, the second and first generation sulfonylureas differ. Second generation compounds possess a more nonpolar or lipophilic side chain. Therapeutically effective doses and serum concentrations of the second generation sulfonylureas are lower, due to their higher intrinsic potency. All sulfonylureas are strongly bound to plasma proteins, primarily albumin. Protein binding of the first generation sulfonylureas is ionic; that of the second generation agents is predominantly nonionic. The clinical therapeutic significance of this difference is unknown; however, because they are bound to albumin by ionic bindings, the first generation agents may be more likely to be displaced by drugs that competitively bind to proteins (eg, warfarin). Displacement of sulfonylurea agents from protein would result in greater hypoglycemic response (see Drug Interactions).

Differences exist among the sulfonylureas in the duration of hypoglycemic effects (see following table). Tolbutamide is short-acting because it is rapidly metabolized to an inactive metabolite; it may be useful in patients with kidney disease. The active metabolite of acetohexamide is 2.5 times as potent as the parent compound. Because the metabolite is excreted in the urine, the duration of action of **acetohexamide** is prolonged in renal disease. Tolazamide has 2 active metabolites which are less potent than the parent compound. The renal elimination of chlorpropamide may be sensitive to changes in urinary pH; urinary alkalinization increases its excretion in the urine. When the urine pH is < 6, urinary excretion decreases and hepatic metabolism is the primary route of elimination. The half-life of **chlorpropamide** is prolonged in renal disease.

Major Pharmacokinetic Parameters of the Sulfonylureas							
Sulfonylureas	Approximate equivalent doses (mg)	Doses/ day	Serum t½ (hrs)	Onset (hrs)	Duration (hrs)	Renal excretion (%)	Active metabolites
First generation							
Acetohexamide	500-750	1-2	≈ 6-8 (parent drug + metabolite)	1	12-24	100	Yes
Chlorpropamide	250-375	1	36	1	24-60	100	Yes
Tolazamide	250-375	1-2	7	4-6	12-24	100	Yes
Tolbutamide	1000-1500	2-3	4.5-6.5	1	6-12	100	No
Second generation							
Glipizide	10	1-2	2-4	1-3	10-24	80-85	No
Glyburide Nonmicronized	5	1-2	10	2-4	16-24	50	Yes[1]
Micronized	3	1-2	≈ 4	1	12-24	50	Yes[1]
Glimepiride	NA[2]	1	≈ 9	2-3	24	60	Yes

[1] Weakly active.
[2] Not applicable.

Contraindications

Hypersensitivity to sulfonylureas; diabetes complicated by ketoacidosis, with or without coma; sole therapy of type 1 (insulin-dependent) diabetes mellitus; diabetes when complicated by pregnancy.

Warnings

➤*Cardiovascular risk:* The administration of oral hypoglycemic drugs has been associated with increased cardiovascular mortality as compared with treatment with diet alone or diet plus insulin. Despite controversy regarding its interpretation, this warning is based on the study conducted by the University Group Diabetes Program (UGDP). This long-term prospective clinical trial involving 823 patients evaluated the effectiveness of glucose-lowering drugs in preventing or delaying vascular complications in patients with non-insulin-dependent diabetes. (*Diabetes* 1970;19]:747-830.)

Patients treated for 5 to 8 years with diet plus **tolbutamide** (1.5 g/day) had a rate of cardiovascular mortality $\approx$ 2.5 times that of patients treated with diet alone. A significant increase in total mortality was not observed. Consider this for other sulfonylureas as well.

Sulfonylurea binding to ATP-dependent K+ channels has been shown to inhibit the response to ischemia, potentially delaying the recovery of contractile function and increasing infarct size during a MI. However, prevention of channel opening during ischemia could reduce the occurrence of ventricular fibrillation during ischemia. Inform the patient of potential risks, advantages, and alternative modes of therapy.

➤*Bioavailability:* Micronized **glyburide** 3 mg tablets provide serum concentrations that are *not* bioequivalent to those from the conventional formulation (nonmicronized) 5 mg tablets. Therefore, retitrate patients when transferring patients from any hypoglycemic agent to micronized glyburide.

➤*Renal/Hepatic function impairment:* Oral hypoglycemic agents are metabolized in the liver. The drugs and most of their metabolites are excreted by the kidneys. Hepatic impairment may result in inadequate release of glucose in response to hypoglycemia. Renal impairment may cause decreased elimination of sulfonylureas leading to accumulation producing hypoglycemia. Therefore, use these agents with caution in type 2 diabetes patients with renal or hepatic impairment, and monitor renal and liver function frequently.

➤*Elderly:* In elderly, debilitated, or malnourished patients, and patients with impaired renal or hepatic function, the initial and maintenance dosing should be conservative to avoid hypoglycemic reactions.

➤*Pregnancy:* (Category C. Category B – Glynase, Micronase). Sulfonylureas (except **glyburide**) are teratogenic in animals. There are no adequate studies in pregnant women. Use only if clearly needed. In general, avoid sulfonylureas in pregnancy; they will not provide good control in patients who cannot be controlled by diet alone.

Because abnormal blood glucose levels during pregnancy may be associated with a higher incidence of congenital abnormalities, insulin is recommended to maintain blood glucose levels as close to normal as possible. However, fetal mortality and major congenital anomalies generally occur 3 to 4 times more often in offspring of diabetic mothers.

Labor and delivery – Prolonged severe hypoglycemia (4 to 10 days) has occurred in neonates born to mothers on a sulfonylurea at the time of delivery. This has been reported more frequently with agents with prolonged half-lives. If used during pregnancy, discontinue at least 2 days to 4 weeks before expected delivery date.

➤*Lactation:* **Chlorpropamide** and **tolbutamide** are excreted in breast milk. A chlorpropamide breast milk concentration of 5 mcg/ml has been detected following a 500 mg dose (normal peak blood level after 250 mg is 30 mcg/ml). It is not known if other sulfonylureas are excreted in breast milk. Because of the potential for hypoglycemia in nursing infants, decide whether to discontinue nursing or the drug.

➤*Children:* Safety and efficacy in children have not been established.

Precautions

➤*Monitoring:*

Treatment Goals for Type 2 Diabetes Mellitus		
Patient population	Average preprandial glucose (mg/dl)	HbA1c[1] (%)
ADA general recommendations[2]	80-120	< 7
Healthy, relatively young	80-120	< 8
Elderly and patients with serious medical conditions	100-140	< 9

[1] Glycosylated hemoglobin.
[2] American Diabetes Association 1999 Clinical Practice Recommendations.

Keep patients under continuous medical supervision. During the initial test period, the patient should communicate with the physician daily, and report at least weekly for the first month for physical examination and evaluation of diabetes control. After the first month, examine at monthly intervals or as indicated. Uncooperative individuals may be unsuitable for treatment with oral agents.

During the transitional period, test the urine for glucose and acetone $\geq$ 3 times daily and have the results reviewed by a physician frequently. Measurement of glycosylated hemoglobin (HbA1c) is also recommended. It is important that patients be taught to correctly and frequently self-monitor blood glucose.

Hyperglycemia is a major risk factor in the development of diabetic complications. Maintaining blood glucose levels helps prevent the progression of nephropathy, neuropathy, and retinopathy. Hyperglycemia is also associated with the risk factors of atherosclerosis.

➤*Diet and exercise:* Diet and exercise remain the primary considerations of diabetic patient management. Caloric restriction and weight loss are essential in the obese diabetic patient. These drugs are an adjunct to, not a substitute for, dietary regulation. Also, loss of blood glucose control on diet alone may be transient, thus requiring only short-term sulfonylurea therapy. Identify cardiovascular risk factors and take corrective measures where possible.

➤*Hypoglycemia:* All sulfonylureas may produce severe hypoglycemia. Proper patient selection, dosage, and instructions are important to avoid hypoglycemic episodes. Renal or hepatic insufficiency may elevate drug blood levels, and the latter may also diminish gluconeogenic capacity, both of which increase the risk of serious hypoglycemic reactions. Elderly, debilitated, or malnourished patients, and those with adrenal or pituitary insufficiency are particularly susceptible to the hypoglycemic action of glucose-lowering drugs. Hypoglycemia may be difficult to recognize in the elderly and in patients taking β-adrenergic blocking drugs. Hypoglycemia is more likely to occur when caloric intake is deficient, after severe or prolonged exercise, when alcohol is ingested, or when > 1 glucose-lowering drug is used.

Because of the long half-life of **chlorpropamide**, patients who become hypoglycemic during therapy require careful supervision of the dose and frequent feedings for at least 3 to 5 days. Hospitalization and IV glucose may be necessary.

➤*Asymptomatic patients:* Controlling blood glucose in type 2 diabetes with sulfonylureas has not been definitely established to be effective in preventing the long-term cardiovascular or neural complications of diabetes.

➤*Loss of blood glucose control:* When a patient stabilized on any diabetic regimen is exposed to stress such as fever, trauma, infection, or surgery, a loss of control may occur. At such times, it may be necessary to discontinue the drug and give insulin.

The effectiveness of any oral hypoglycemic in lowering blood glucose to a desired level decreases in many patients over time (secondary failure); this may be due to progression of the severity of the diabetes or to diminished drug responsiveness. Adequately adjust dose and assess adherence to diet before classifying a patient as a secondary failure. Primary failure occurs when the drug is ineffective in a patient when first given. Certain patients who demonstrate an inadequate response or true primary or secondary failure to 1 sulfonylurea may benefit from a transfer to another sulfonylurea.

➤*Disulfiram-like syndrome:* A sulfonylurea-induced facial flushing reaction may occur when some sulfonylureas are administered with alcohol. This syndrome is characterized by facial flushing and occasional breathlessness but without the nausea, vomiting, and hypotension seen with a true alcohol-disulfiram reaction. The facial flushing reaction occurs in $\approx$ 33% of type 2 diabetes patients taking **chlorpropamide** and alcohol. It is uncertain whether **glyburide** and **glipizide** can cause the facial flushing reaction.

➤*Syndrome of inappropriate secretion of antidiuretic hormone (SIADH):* Water retention and dilutional hyponatremia have occurred after administration of sulfonylureas to type 2 diabetes patients, especially those with CHF or hepatic cirrhosis. The drugs stimulate antidiuretic hormone (ADH) release, augmenting hypothalamic-pituitary release of ADH. The result is excessive water retention, hyponatremia, low serum osmolality, and high urine osmolality.

Glipizide, **acetohexamide**, **tolazamide**, and **glyburide** are mildly diuretic.

Drug Interactions

Sulfonylurea Drug Interactions			
Precipitant drug	Object drug*		Description
Androgens Anticoagulants Azole antifungals Chloramphenicol Clofibrate Fenfluramine Fluconazole Gemfibrozil Histamine H₂ antagonists Magnesium salts Methyldopa MAO inhibitors Probenecid Salicylates Sulfinpyrazone Sulfonamides Tricyclic antidepressants Urinary acidifiers	Sulfonylureas	↑	The hypoglycemic effect of sulfonylureas may be enhanced due to various mechanisms (eg, decreased hepatic metabolism, inhibition of renal excretion, displacement from protein-binding sites, decreased blood glucose, alteration of carbohydrate metabolism). Monitor blood glucose carefully upon initiation, cessation, or changes in therapy with any of these agents.
Beta blockers Calcium channel blockers Cholestyramine Corticosteroids Diazoxide Estrogens Hydantoins Isoniazid Nicotinic acid Oral contraceptives Phenothiazines Rifampin Sympatho-mimetics Thiazide diuretics Thyroid agents Urinary alkalinizers	Sulfonylureas	↓	The hypoglycemic effect of sulfonylureas may be decreased due to various mechanisms (eg, increased hepatic metabolism, decreased insulin release, increased renal excretion).
Charcoal	Sulfonylureas	↓	Charcoal can reduce the absorption of sulfonylureas; depending on the clinical situation, this will reduce their efficacy or toxicity.
Ciprofloxacin	Glyburide	↑	A possible interaction between glyburide and ciprofloxacin has been reported, resulting in a potentiation of the hypoglycemic action.
Ethanol	Sulfonylureas	↔	Ethanol may prolong but not augment glipizide-induced reductions in blood glucose. Chronic ethanol use may decrease the half-life of tolbutamide. Ethanol ingestion by patients taking chlorpropamide may result in a disulfiram-like reaction (see Precautions).
Chlorpropamide	Barbiturates	↑	Animal studies suggest that the action of barbiturates may be prolonged by therapy with chlorpropamide; coadminister with caution.
Glyburide	Anticoagulants	↑ ↓	Possible interactions between glyburide and coumarin derivatives have been reported that may either potentiate or weaken the effects of coumarin derivatives.
Sulfonylureas	Digitalis glycosides	↑	Concurrent administration may result in increased digitalis serum levels.

* ↑ = Object drug increased.   ↓ = Object drug decreased.   ↔ = Undetermined clinical effect.

➤*Drug/Lab test interactions:* A metabolite of **tolbutamide** in the urine may give a false-positive reaction for albumin if measured by the acidification-after-boiling test, which causes the metabolite to precipitate. There is no interference with the sulfosalicylic acid test.

➤*Drug/Food interactions:* Absorption of **glipizide** is delayed by ≈ 40 minutes when taken with food; the drug is more effective when given ≈ 30 minutes before a meal. The other sulfonylureas may be taken with food.

Adverse Reactions

Hypoglycemia – See Precautions.

➤*CNS:* Drowsiness; asthenia; nervousness; tremor; pain; insomnia; anxiety; depression; hypesthesia; chills; hypertonia; confusion; somnolence; abnormal gait; decreased libido; migraine; anorexia; arthralgia; myalgia; fatigue; weakness; paresthesia; dizziness; vertigo; malaise; headache (infrequent).

➤*Dermatologic:* Allergic skin reactions; eczema; pruritus; erythema multiforme; urticaria; morbilliform or maculopapular eruptions; lichenoid reactions; rash; sweating; exfoliative dermatitis. These may be transient and may disappear despite continued use of the drug; if skin reactions persist, discontinue the drug. Porphyria cutanea tarda; photosensitivity reactions.

➤*Endocrine:* Reactions identical to the syndrome of inappropriate secretion of antidiuretic hormone (SIADH). (See Precautions.)

➤*GI:* GI disturbances (eg, nausea, epigastric fullness, heartburn) are the most common reactions. They tend to be dose-related and may disappear when dosage is reduced. Diarrhea; taste alteration (tolbutamide); GI pain; constipation; gastralgia; dyspepsia; vomiting; hunger; proctocolitis; flatulence; cholestatic jaundice (rare, discontinue the drug if this occurs).

➤*Hematologic:* Leukopenia; thrombocytopenia (which may present as purpura); aplastic anemia; agranulocytosis; hemolytic anemia; pancytopenia; hepatic porphyria; eosinophilia.

➤*Miscellaneous:* Disulfiram-like reactions (see Precautions); tinnitus; fatigue; rhinitis; hepatic porphyria; hyponatremia; blurred vision; polyuria; trace blood in stool; thirst; edema; arrhythmia; flushing; hypertension; pharyngitis; eye pain; conjunctivitis; retinal hemorrhage; dysuria; hepatitis; dyspnea; leg cramps; syncope; vasculitis.

➤*Lab test abnormalities:* Elevated liver function tests; occasional mild-to-moderate elevations in BUN, creatinine, AST, LDH, alkaline phosphatase.

Overdosage

➤*Symptoms:* Overdosage can produce hypoglycemia. In order of general appearance, the signs and symptoms associated with hypoglycemia include: Tingling of lips and tongue; nausea; vomiting; mild epigastric pain diminished cerebral function (lethargy, yawning, confusion, agitation, nervousness); increased sympathetic activity (tachycardia, sweating, tremor, hunger) and ultimately, convulsions, stupor, coma, and death.

➤*Treatment:* Treat mild hypoglycemia without loss of consciousness or neurologic findings aggressively with oral glucose and adjustments in drug dosage or meal patterns. Continue close monitoring until the patient is stabilized. Severe hypoglycemic reactions occur infrequently, but require immediate hospitalization. If hypoglycemic coma is suspected, rapidly inject concentrated (50%) dextrose IV. Follow by a continuous infusion of more dilute (10%) dextrose at a rate that will maintain the blood glucose at a level > 100 mg/dl. Closely monitor for a minimum of 24 to 48 hours because hypoglycemia may recur after apparent clinical recovery. Because of the long half-life of **chlorpropamide**, patients who become hypoglycemic from this drug require close supervision for a minimum of 3 to 5 days.

In 1 patient with renal failure on hemodialysis, charcoal hemoperfusion shortened the half-life of chlorpropamide following an overdose. Charcoal administration also reduces the absorption of the sulfonylureas and may reduce their toxicity.

Patient Information

Patients must receive full and complete instructions about the nature of diabetes. Strict adherence to prescribed diet, an exercise program, personal hygiene, and avoidance of infection are essential. It is important to teach patients to self-monitor blood glucose.

Do not discontinue medication except on the advice of a physician.

May cause GI upset; may be taken with food. Take **glipizide** ≈ 30 minutes before a meal to increase effectiveness.

Advise patients to avoid alcohol; lack of blood sugar control may occur. Flushing has been reported with **chlorpropamide**.

Monitor urine for glucose and ketones as prescribed; monitor blood glucose as prescribed.

➤*Notify physician:* Notify physician if any of the following occurs:

Hypoglycemia – Fatigue, excessive hunger, profuse sweating, numbness of extremities.

Hyperglycemia – Excessive thirst or urination, urinary glucose, or ketones.

Other – Fever, sore throat, rash, unusual bruising or bleeding.

Sulfonylureas

CHLORPROPAMIDE

Rx	**Chlorpropamide** (Various, eg, Sidmak, UDL)	**Tablets:** 100 mg	In 100s, 500s, 1000s, and UD 100s and 600s.
Rx	**Diabinese** (Pfizer)		(393). Blue, scored. D-shaped. In 100s, 500s, and UD 100s.
Rx	**Chlorpropamide** (Various, eg, Major, Goldline, Sidmak, UDL)	**Tablets:** 250 mg	In 100s, 250s, 500s, 1000s, and UD 100s and UD 600s.
Rx	**Diabinese** (Pfizer)		(394). Blue, scored. D-shaped. In 100s, 250s, 1000s, and UD 100s.

For complete prescribing information, refer to the Sulfonylureas group monograph.

Administration and Dosage

➤*Initial dose:* 250 mg/day in the mild-to-moderately severe, middle-aged, stable type 2 diabetic patient; use 100 to 125 mg/day in older, debilitated, or malnourished patients, and patients with impaired renal/hepatic function. Take a single daily dose each morning with breakfast. In cases of GI intolerance, divide the daily dose.

➤*Maintenance therapy:* ≤ 100 to 250 mg/day. Severe diabetics may require 500 mg/day. Avoid doses > 750 mg/day.

➤*Patients on insulin:*

Transferral of Type 2 Diabetes Patients on Insulin to Chlorpropamide Monotherapy		
Insulin dose	Initial chlorpropamide dose	Insulin Withdrawal
≤ 40	250 mg/day	Not necessary; may be discontinued abruptly.
> 40	250 mg/day	Reduce insulin dose by 50%; further reduce as response is observed. Consider hospitalization during the transition period.

ACETOHEXAMIDE

Rx	**Acetohexamide** (Various, eg, Raway)	**Tablets:** 250 mg	In 100s.
Rx	**Acetohexamide** (Various)	**Tablets:** 500 mg	In 100s.

For complete prescribing information, refer to the Sulfonylureas group monograph.

Administration and Dosage

➤*Initial dose:* 250 mg to 1.5 g/day. Patients on ≤ 1 g daily can be controlled with once-daily dosage. Those receiving 1.5 g/day usually benefit from twice-daily dosage before morning and evening meals. Doses > 1.5 g/day are not recommended. Clinical reports on the efficacy of once-daily dosage of acetohexamide indicate that its effect on the blood sugar is better sustained than that of tolbutamide.

➤*Patients on other oral antidiabetic agents:* When transfer is made, the initial dose of acetohexamide should be about half the tolbutamide dose and about double the chlorpropamide dose. A transition period usually is required because of the long half-life of chlorpropa-

mide. Make subsequent dosage adjustments according to clinical response.

➤*Patients on insulin:*

Transferral of Type 2 Diabetes Patients on Insulin to Acetohexamide Monotherapy		
Insulin dose	Initial acetohexamide dose	Insulin Withdrawal
< 20	250 mg/day	Not necessary; may be discontinued abruptly.
> 20	250 mg/day	Reduce insulin dose by 25% to 30%; further reduce as response is observed. Consider hospitalization during the transition period.

TOLAZAMIDE

Rx	**Tolazamide** (Various, eg, Zenith Goldline)	**Tablets:** 100 mg	In 100s and 250s.
Rx	**Tolinase** (Pharmacia & Upjohn)		(TOLINASE 100). White, scored. In unit-of-use 100s.
Rx	**Tolazamide** (Various, eg, Mylan, Zenith Goldline)	**Tablets:** 250 mg	In 100s, 200s, 500s, and 1000s.
Rx	**Tolinase** (Pharmacia & Upjohn)		(TOLINASE 250). White, scored. In 200s, 1000s, UD 100s, and unit-of-use 100s.
Rx	**Tolazamide** (Various, eg, Mylan, Zenith Goldline)	**Tablets:** 500 mg	In 100s, 250s, and 500s.
Rx	**Tolinase** (Pharmacia & Upjohn)		(TOLINASE 500). White, scored. In unit-of-use 100s.

For complete prescribing information, refer to the Sulfonylureas group monograph.

Administration and Dosage

➤*Initial dose:* 100 to 250 mg/day for mild-to-moderately severe type 2 diabetes patients with breakfast or the first main meal. If fasting blood sugar (FBS) is < 200 mg/dl, use 100 mg/day as a single dose; if FBS is > 200 mg/dl, use 250 mg/day as a single dose. If patients are malnourished, underweight, elderly, or not eating properly, use 100 mg once a day. Adjust dose to response. If > 500 mg/day is required, give in divided doses twice daily. Doses > 1 g/day are not likely to improve control and are not recommended.

➤*Maintenance dose:* The usual maintenance dose is 100 to 1000 mg/day with the average maintenance dose being 250 to 500 mg/day. Following initiation of therapy, dosage adjustment is made in increments of 100 to 250 mg at weekly intervals based on the patient's blood glucose response.

➤*Patients on other oral antidiabetic agents:* Transfer patients from other oral antidiabetes regimens to tolazamide conservatively. When transferring patients from oral hypoglycemic agents other than chlorpropamide to tolazamide, no transition period or initial priming dose is necessary. Consider 250 mg chlorpropamide to provide approxi-

mately the same degree of blood control as 250 mg tolazamide. Observe the patient carefully for hypoglycemia during the transition period from chlorpropamide to tolazamide (1 or 2 weeks) due to the prolonged retention of chlorpropamide in the body and the possibility of a subsequent overlapping drug effect. If patient is receiving < 1 g/day tolbutamide, begin at 100 mg/day of tolazamide. If patient is receiving ≥ 1 g/day, initiate 250 mg/day tolazamide as a single dose. Consider 100 mg tolazamide to provide approximately the same degree of blood glucose control as 250 mg acetohexamide.

➤*Patients on insulin:*

Transferral of Type 2 Diabetes Patients on Insulin to Tolazamide Monotherapy		
Insulin dose	Initial tolazamide dose	Insulin Withdrawal
< 20	100 mg/day	Not necessary; may be discontinued abruptly.
20-40	250 mg/day	Not necessary; may be discontinued abruptly
> 40	250 mg/day	Reduce insulin by 50%; further reduce as response is observed. Consider hospitalization during the transition period.

TOLBUTAMIDE

Rx	**Tolbutamide** (Various, eg, Zenith Goldline, Mylan, UDL)	**Tablets:** 500 mg	In 100s and 500s.
Rx	**Orinase** (Upjohn)		Lactose. (ORINASE 500). White, scored. In 200s and unit-of-use 100s.

For complete prescribing information, refer to the Sulfonylureas group monograph.

Administration and Dosage

▶*Initial dose:* 1 to 2 g/day. Total dose may be taken in the morning, but divided doses may allow increased GI tolerance.

▶*Maintenance dose:* 0.25 to 3 g/day. A maintenance dose > 2 g/day is seldomly required. Daily doses > 3 g are not recommended.

▶*Patients on other oral antidiabetic agents:* Transfer patients from other oral antidiabetes regimens to tolbutamide conservatively. When transferring patients from oral hypoglycemic agents other than chlorpropamide to tolbutamide, no transition period and no initial or priming doses are necessary. However, when transferring patients from chlorpropamide, exercise particular care during the first 2 weeks because of the prolonged retention of chlorpropamide in the body and the possibility that subsequent overlapping drug effects might provoke hypoglycemia.

▶*Patients on insulin:*

Transferral of Type 2 Diabetes Patients on Insulin to Tolbutamide Monotherapy		
Insulin dose	Initial tolbutamide dose	Insulin withdrawal
< 20	1-2 g/day	Not necessary; may be discontinued abruptly.
20-40	1-2 g/day	Reduce insulin dose by 30% to 50%; further reduce as response is observed.
> 40	1-2 g/day	Reduce insulin dose by 20%; further reduce as response is observed. Consider hospitalization during the transition period.

Occasionally, conversion to tolbutamide in the hospital may be advisable in candidates who require > 40 units of insulin daily. During this conversion period when both insulin and tolbutamide are being used, hypoglycemia may rarely occur. During insulin withdrawal, have patients test urine for glucose and acetone ≥ 3 times daily and report results to their physician. The appearance of persistent acetonuria with glycosuria indicates that the patient is a type 1 diabetes patient who requires insulin therapy.

GLIPIZIDE

Rx	**Glipizide** (Various, eg, Endo, Mylan, UDL, Watson, Zenith Goldline)	**Tablets:** 5 mg	In 100s, 500s, 1000s, and UD 100s.
Rx	**Glucotrol** (Pfizer)		Lactose. (Pfizer 411). Dye free. White, scored. Diamond shape. In 100s, 500s, and UD 100s.
Rx	**Glipizide** (Various, eg, Endo, Mylan, UDL, Watson, Zenith Goldline)	**Tablets:** 10 mg	In 100s, 500s, 1000s, and UD 100s.
Rx	**Glucotrol** (Pfizer)		Lactose. (Pfizer 412). Dye free. White, scored. Diamond shape. In 100s, 500s, and UD 100s.
Rx	**Glipizide Extended-Release** (Andrx)	**Tablets, extended release:** 2.5 mg	(871). Blue. In 30s.
Rx	**Glucotrol XL** (Pfizer)		(Glucotrol XL 2.5). Blue, biconvex. In 30s.
Rx	**Glipizide Extended-Release** (Various, eg, Andrx, Watson)	5 mg	In 100s and 500s.
Rx	**Glucotrol XL** (Pfizer)		(Glucotrol XL 5). White, biconvex. In 100s and 500s.
Rx	**Glipizide Extended-Release** (Various, eg, Andrx, Watson)	10 mg	In 100s and 500s.
Rx	**Glucotrol XL** (Pfizer)		(GLUCOTROL XL 10). White, biconvex. In 100s and 500s.

For complete prescribing information, refer to the Sulfonylureas group monograph.

Administration and Dosage

▶*Immediate release:*

Initial dose – 5 mg/day, given ≈ 30 minutes before breakfast to achieve the greatest reduction in postprandial hyperglycemia. Geriatric patients or those with liver disease may be started on 2.5 mg/day of the immediate release formulation.

Adjust dosage in 2.5 to 5 mg increments, as determined by blood glucose response. Several days should elapse between titration steps. If response to a single dose is not satisfactory, dividing that dose may prove effective. The maximum recommended once-daily dose is 15 mg. The maximum recommended total daily dose is 40 mg.

Maintenance dose – Some patients may be controlled on a once-a-day regimen, while others show better response with divided dosing. Divide total daily doses > 15 mg and give before meals of adequate caloric content. Total daily doses > 30 mg have been safely given on a twice-daily basis to long-term patients.

▶*Extended release:*

Initial dose – 5 mg/day, given with breakfast. The recommended dose for geriatric patients is also 5 mg/day. HbA1c level measured at 3-month intervals is the preferred means of monitoring response to therapy. Measure HbA1c as extended release therapy is initiated at the 5 mg dose and repeated ≈ 3 months later. If the first test result suggests that glycemic control over the preceding 3 months was inadequate, the dose may be increased to 10 mg. Make subsequent dosage adjustments at 3-month intervals. If no improvement is seen after 3 months of therapy with a higher dose, resume the previous dose. Base decisions that use fasting blood glucose to adjust therapy on ≥ 2 similar consecutive values obtained ≥ 7 days after the previous dose adjustment.

Maintenance dose – Most patients will be controlled with 5 or 10 mg taken once daily. However, some patients may require up to the maximum recommended daily dose of 20 mg. While the glycemic control of selected patients may improve with doses that exceed 10 mg, clinical studies conducted to date have not demonstrated an additional group average reduction of HbA1c beyond what was achieved with the 10 mg dose.

Immediate vs extended release – Patients receiving immediate release glipizide may be switched safely to the extended release tablets once a day at the nearest equivalent total daily dose. Patients receiving immediate release tablets also may be titrated to the appropriate dose of the extended release tablets starting with 5 mg once daily.

Combination therapy – When used in combination with other oral blood glucose-lowering agents, add the second agent at the lowest recommended dose and observe patients carefully.

▶*Patients on other oral antidiabetic agents:* No transition period is necessary when transferring patients to the extended release tablets. Observe patients carefully (1 to 2 weeks) when being transferred from longer half-life sulfonylureas (ie, chlorpropamide) to the extended release tablets due to potential overlapping of drug effect.

▶*Patients on insulin:*

Transferral of Type 2 Diabetes Patients on Insulin to Glipizide Monotherapy		
Insulin dose	Initial glipizide dose	Insulin withdrawal
< 20	5 mg/day	Not necessary; may be discontinued abruptly.
> 20	5 mg/day	Reduce insulin dose by 50%; further reduce as response is observed. Consider hospitalization during the transition period.

Sulfonylureas

GLIMEPIRIDE

Rx	Amaryl (Hoechst-Roussel)	Tablets: 1 mg	Lactose. (AMA RYL). Pink, flat-faced, double bisect. Oblong. In 100s.
		2 mg	Lactose. (AMA RYL). Green, flat-faced, double bisect. Oblong. In 100s and UD 100s.
		4 mg	Lactose. (AMA RYL). Blue, flat-faced, double bisect. Oblong. In 100s and UD 100s.

For complete prescribing information, refer to the Sulfonylureas group monograph.

Indications

➤*Combination with insulin:* Glimepiride is also indicated for use in combination with insulin to lower blood glucose in patients whose hyperglycemia cannot be controlled by diet and exercise in conjunction with an oral hypoglycemic agent. Combined use of glimepiride and insulin may increase the potential for hypoglycemia.

Administration and Dosage

➤*Approved by the FDA:* November 30, 1995.

➤*Initial dose:* 1 to 2 mg once daily, given with breakfast or the first main meal. Patients sensitive to hypoglycemic drugs should begin at 1 mg once daily; titrate carefully.

Maximum starting dose is ≤ 2 mg.

➤*Maintenance dose:* 1 to 4 mg once daily. The maximum recommended dose is 8 mg once daily. After a dose of 2 mg is reached, increase dose at increments of ≤ 2 mg at 1- to 2-week intervals based on the patient's blood glucose response. Monitor long-term efficacy by measurement of HbA1c levels, for example, every 3 to 6 months.

➤*Combination insulin therapy:* The recommended dose is 8 mg once daily with the first main meal with low-dose insulin.

➤*Patients on other oral antidiabetic agents:* When transferring patients to glimepiride, no transition period is necessary. No exact dosage relationship exists between glimepiride and the other oral hypoglycemic agents. Observe patients carefully when being transferred from longer half-life sulfonylureas (eg, chlorpropamide) to glimepiride due to potential overlapping of drug effect.

GLYBURIDE (Glibenclamide)

Rx	Glyburide (Various, eg, Brightstone, Copley, Coventry, Geneva, Greenstone, Novopharm)	Tablets: 1.25 mg	In 50s, 100s, and 500s.
Rx	DiaBeta (Hoechst Marion Roussel)		(Hoechst Diaβ). Peach, scored. Oblong. In 50s.
Rx	Micronase (Pharmacia & Upjohn)		(MICRONASE 1.25). White, scored. In 100s.
Rx	Glyburide (Various, eg, Copley, Mova, Novopharm)	Tablets, micronized: 1.5 mg	In 100s, 500s, 1000s, and UD 100s.
Rx	Glynase PresTab (Pharmacia & Upjohn)		Lactose. (GLYNASE 1.5/PT PT). White, scored. Oval. In 100s and UD 100s.
Rx	Glyburide (Various, eg, Brightstone, Copley, Coventry, Geneva, Greenstone, Novopharm, UDL)	Tablets: 2.5 mg	In 90s, 100s, 500s, 1000s, UD 100s, and blister pack 25s, 100s, and 600s.
Rx	DiaBeta (Hoechst Marion Roussel)		(Hoechst Diaβ). Pink, scored. Oblong. In 100s and 500s.
Rx	Micronase (Pharmacia & Upjohn)		(MICRONASE 2.5). Pink, scored. In 100s, 1000s, and UD 100s.
Rx	Glyburide (Various, eg, Copley, Mova, Novopharm)	Tablets, micronized: 3 mg	In 100s, 500s, 1000s, and UD 100s.
Rx	Glynase PresTab (Pharmacia & Upjohn)		Lactose. (GLYNASE 3/PT PT). Blue, scored. Oval. In 100s, 500s, 1000s, and UD 100s.
Rx	Glyburide (Various, eg, Mova)	Tablets, micronized: 4.5 mg	In 100s, 500s, and 1000s.
Rx	Glyburide (Various, eg, Brightstone, Copley, Coventry, Geneva, Greenstone, Novopharm, UDL)	Tablets: 5 mg	In 90s, 100s, 500s, 1000s, UD 100s, and blister pack 25s, 100s, and 600s.
Rx	DiaBeta (Hoechst Marion Roussel)		(Hoechst Diaβ). Green, scored. Oblong. In 500s and 1000s.
Rx	Micronase (Pharmacia & Upjohn)		(MICRONASE 5). Blue, scored. In 100s, 500s, 1000s, and UD 100s.
Rx	Glyburide (Various, eg, Mova, Novopharm)	Tablets, micronized: 6 mg	In 100s, 500s, and 1000s.
Rx	Glynase PresTab (Pharmacia & Upjohn)		. Lactose. (GLYNASE 6/PT PT). Yellow, scored. Oval. In 100s and 500s.

For complete prescribing information, refer to the Sulfonylureas group monograph.

Indications

➤*Combination with metformin:* Glyburide may also be used concomitantly with metformin when diet and glyburide or diet and metformin alone do not result in adequate glycemic control (see Metformin monograph).

Administration and Dosage

➤*Nonmicronized:*

Initial dose – 2.5 to 5 mg daily, administered with breakfast or the first main meal. For patients who may be more sensitive to hypoglycemic drugs, start at 1.25 mg daily.

Maintenance dose – 1.25 to 20 mg daily. Give as a single dose or in divided doses. Increase in increments of ≤ 2.5 mg at weekly intervals based on the patient's blood glucose response. Daily doses > 20 mg are not recommended.

➤*Micronized:*

Initial dose – 1.5 to 3 mg/day, administered with breakfast or the first main meal. For patients who may be more sensitive to hypoglycemic drugs, start at 0.75 mg/day.

Maintenance dose – 0.75 to 12 mg/day. Give as a single dose or in divided doses; some patients, particularly those receiving > 6 mg/day, may have a more satisfactory response with twice-daily dosing. Increase in increments of ≤ 1.5 mg at weekly intervals based on the patient's blood glucose response. Daily doses > 12 mg are not recommended.

GLYBURIDE (Glibenclamide)

Concomitant metformin – Add micronized glyburide gradually to the dosing regimen of patients who have not responded to the maximum dose of metformin monotherapy after 4 weeks. (Refer to the Metformin monograph.) The desired control of blood glucose may be obtained by adjusting the dose of each drug. With concomitant therapy, the risk of hypoglycemia associated with sulfonylurea therapy continues and may be increased.

➤*Patients on other oral antidiabetic agents:* Transfer patients from other oral antidiabetic regimens to glyburide conservatively. When transferring patients from oral hypoglycemic agents other than chlorpropamide, no transition period and no initial priming dose is necessary. When transferring patients from chlorpropamide, exercise care during the first 2 weeks because the prolonged retention of chlorpropamide in the body and subsequent overlapping drug effects may provoke hypoglycemia.

➤*Patients on insulin:*

Transferral of Type 2 Diabetes Patients on Insulin to Glyburide Monotherapy		
Insulin dose	Initial glyburide dose	Insulin withdrawal
< 20	1.5-3 mg/day micronized, 2.5-5 mg/day non-micronized	Not necessary; may be discontinued abruptly.
20-40	3 mg/day micronized, 5 mg/day non-micronized	Not necessary; may be discontinued abruptly.
> 40	3 mg/day micronized, 5 mg/day non-micronized	Reduce insulin dose by 50%; further reduce as response is observed. Consider hospitalization during the transition period.

ACARBOSE

Rx	Precose (Bayer)	Tablets: 25 mg	(PRECOSE 25). White to yellow. In 100s.
		50 mg	(PRECOSE 50). White to yellow. In 100s and UD 100s.
		100 mg	(PRECOSE 100). White to yellow. In 100s and UD 100s.

Indications

➤*Type 2 diabetes mellitus:* Monotherapy as an adjunct to diet to lower blood glucose in patients with Type 2 diabetes mellitus whose hyperglycemia cannot be managed on diet alone.

Acarbose may also be used with a sulfonylurea when diet plus either acarbose or a sulfonylurea do not result in adequate glycemic control. The effect of acarbose to enhance glycemic control is additive to that of sulfonylureas, insulin, or metformin when used in combination, presumably because its mechanism of action is different.

Administration and Dosage

➤*Approved by the FDA:* September 6, 1995.

There is no fixed dosage regimen for the management of diabetes mellitus with acarbose. Dosages of acarbose must be individualized on the basis of both effectiveness and tolerance while not exceeding the maximum recommended dose of 100 mg 3 times daily. Take acarbose 3 times daily at the start (with the first bite) of each main meal. Start at a low dose, with gradual dose escalation as described below, to both reduce GI side effects and permit identification of the minimum dose required for adequate glycemic control of the patient.

During treatment initiation and dose titration (see below), use 1 hour postprandial plasma glucose to determine the therapeutic response to acarbose and identify the minimum effective dose for the patient. Thereafter, measure glycosylated hemoglobin at intervals of about 3 months. The therapeutic goal should be to decrease both postprandial plasma glucose and glycosylated hemoglobin levels to normal or near normal by using the lowest effective dose of acarbose, either as monotherapy or in combination with sulfonylureas, insulin, or metformin.

➤*Initial dosage:* The recommended starting dosage is 25 mg given orally 3 times daily at the start (with the first bite) of each main meal. However, some patients may benefit from more gradual dose titration to minimize GI side effects. This may be achieved by initiating treatment at 25 mg once per day and subsequently increasing the frequency of administration to achieve 25 mg three times daily.

➤*Maintenance dosage:* Adjust dosage at 4- to 8-week intervals based on 1 hour postprandial glucose levels and on tolerance. After the initial dosage of 25 mg 3 times daily, the dosage can be increased to 50 mg 3 times daily. Some patients may benefit from further increasing the dosage to 100 mg 3 times daily. The maintenance dose ranges from 50 to 100 mg 3 times daily. However, because patients with low body weight may be at increased risk for elevated serum transaminases, consider only patients with body weight more than 60 kg for dose titration above 50 mg 3 times daily. If no further reduction in postprandial glucose or glycosylated hemoglobin levels is observed with titration to 100 mg 3 times daily, consider lowering the dose. Once an effective and tolerated dosage has been established, it should be maintained.

➤*Maximum dosage:* The maximum recommended dosage for patients no more than 60 kg is 50 mg 3 times a day; for patients more than 60 kg, 100 mg 3 times a day.

➤*Coadministration:* Sulfonylurea agents or insulin may cause hypoglycemia. Acarbose given in combination with a sulfonylurea or insulin will cause a further lowering of blood glucose and may increase the hypoglycemic potential of the sulfonylurea. If hypoglycemia occurs, make appropriate adjustments in the dosage of these agents.

➤*Storage/Stability:* Do not store above 25°C (77°F). Protect from moisture. Keep container tightly closed.

Actions

➤*Pharmacology:* Acarbose is an oral alpha-glucosidase inhibitor for use in the management of type 2 diabetes mellitus. Acarbose is an oligosaccharide obtained from fermentation processes of the microorganism, *Actinoplanes utahensis.* Acarbose is a complex oligosaccharide that delays the digestion of ingested carbohydrates, thereby resulting in a smaller rise in blood glucose concentration following meals. As a consequence of plasma glucose reduction, acarbose reduces levels of glycosylated hemoglobin in patients with type 2 diabetes mellitus. Systemic nonenzymatic protein glycosylation, as reflected by levels of glycosylated hemoglobin, is a function of average blood glucose concentration over time.

In contrast to sulfonylureas, acarbose does not enhance insulin secretion. The antihyperglycemic action results from a competitive, reversible inhibition of pancreatic alpha-amylase and membrane-bound intestinal alpha-glucoside hydrolase enzymes. Pancreatic alpha-amylase hydrolyzes complex starches to oligosaccharides in the lumen of the small intestine while the membrane-bound intestinal alpha-glucosidases hydrolyze oligosaccharides, trisaccharides, and disaccharides to glucose and other monosaccharides in the brush border of the small

intestine. In diabetic patients, this enzyme inhibition delays glucose absorption and lowers postprandial hyperglycemia.

Because its mechanism of action is different, the effect of acarbose to enhance glycemic control is additive to that of sulfonylureas when used in combination. In addition, acarbose diminishes the insulinotropic and weight-increasing effects of sulfonylureas.

Acarbose has no inhibitory activity against lactase and consequently would not be expected to induce lactose intolerance.

➤*Pharmacokinetics:*

Absorption/Distribution – In a study of 6 healthy men, less than 2% of an oral dose was absorbed as active drug, while about 35% of total radioactivity from a ^{14}C-labeled oral dose was absorbed. An average of 51% of an oral dose was excreted in the feces as unabsorbed drug-related radioactivity within 96 hours of ingestion. Because acarbose acts locally within the GI tract, this low systemic bioavailability of parent compound is therapeutically desired. Following oral dosing of healthy volunteers with ^{14}C-labeled acarbose, peak plasma concentrations of radioactivity were attained 14 to 24 hours after dosing, while peak plasma concentrations of active drug were attained at approximately 1 hour. The delayed absorption of acarbose-related radioactivity reflects the absorption of metabolites that may be formed by either intestinal bacteria or intestinal enzymatic hydrolysis.

Metabolism – Acarbose is metabolized exclusively within the GI tract, principally by intestinal bacteria, but also by digestive enzymes. A fraction of these metabolites (approximately 34% of the dose) was absorbed and subsequently excreted in the urine. At least 13 metabolites have been identified. The major metabolites have been identified as 4-methylpyrogallol derivatives (eg, sulfate, methyl, glucuronide conjugates). One metabolite (formed by cleavage of a glucose molecule from acarbose) also has alpha-glucosidase inhibitory activity. This metabolite, together with the parent compound recovered from the urine, accounts for less than 2% of the total administered dose.

Excretion – The fraction of acarbose that is absorbed as intact drug is almost completely excreted by the kidneys. When acarbose was given IV, 89% of the dose was recovered in the urine as active drug within 48 hours. In contrast, less than 2% of an oral dose was recovered in the urine as active (eg, parent compound and active metabolite) drug. This is consistent with the low bioavailability of the parent drug. The plasma elimination half-life of acarbose activity is about 2 hours in healthy volunteers. Consequently, drug accumulation does not occur with 3 times/day dosing.

Special populations – The mean steady-state area under the curve (AUC) and maximum concentrations of acarbose were approximately 1.5 times higher in elderly compared with young volunteers; however, these differences were not statistically significant. Patients with severe renal impairment (creatinine clearance [Ccr] less than 25 mL/min/1.73 m^2) attained approximately 5 times higher peak plasma concentrations of acarbose and 6 times larger AUCs than volunteers with normal renal function.

Contraindications

Hypersensitivity to the drug; diabetic ketoacidosis or cirrhosis; inflammatory bowel disease; colonic ulceration; partial intestinal obstruction or predisposition to intestinal obstruction; chronic intestinal diseases associated with marked disorders of digestion or absorption; conditions that may deteriorate as a result of increased gas formation in the intestine.

Warnings

➤*Diet/Physical activity:* In initiating treatment for type 2 diabetes mellitus, emphasize diet as the primary form of treatment. Caloric restriction and weight loss are essential in the obese diabetic patient. Proper dietary management alone may be effective in controlling blood glucose and symptoms of hyperglycemia. Also, stress regular physical activity when appropriate. If this treatment program fails to result in adequate glycemic control, consider the use of acarbose. The use of acarbose must be viewed by both the physician and patient as a treatment in addition to diet, and not as a substitute for diet or as a convenient mechanism for avoiding dietary restraint.

➤*Renal function impairment:* Plasma concentrations of acarbose in renally impaired volunteers were proportionally increased relative to the degree of renal dysfunction. Long-term clinical trials in diabetic patients with significant renal dysfunction (serum creatinine more than 2 mg/dL) have not been conducted. Therefore, treatment of these patients with acarbose is not recommended.

➤*Carcinogenesis:* In rats, acarbose treatment resulted in a significant increase in the incidence of renal tumors (adenomas and adenocarcinomas) and benign Leydig cell tumors. Further studies were performed to separate direct carcinogenic effects of acarbose from indirect effects resulting from the carbohydrate malnutrition induced by

ACARBOSE

the large doses of acarbose employed in the studies. In these studies, the increased incidence of renal tumors found in the original studies did not occur.

➤*Pregnancy: Category B.* The safety and efficacy of acarbose in pregnant women has not been established. Use during pregnancy only if clearly needed. Because current information strongly suggests that abnormal blood glucose levels during pregnancy are associated with a higher incidence of congenital anomalies as well as increased neonatal morbidity and mortality, most experts recommend that insulin be used during pregnancy to maintain blood glucose levels as close to normal as possible.

➤*Lactation:* A small amount is excreted in the milk of lactating rats. It is not known whether this drug is excreted in human breast milk. Do not administer to a breastfeeding woman.

➤*Children:* Safety and efficacy have not been established.

Precautions

➤*Monitoring:* Monitor therapeutic response to acarbose by periodic blood glucose tests. Measurement of glycosylated hemoglobin levels is recommended for the monitoring of long-term glycemic control.

Acarbose, particularly at doses in excess of 50 mg 3 times a day, may give rise to elevations of serum transaminases (see Lab test abnormalities) and, in rare instances, hyperbilirubinemia. It is recommended that serum transaminase levels be checked every 3 months during the first year of the treatment with acarbose and periodically thereafter. If elevated transaminases are observed, a reduction in dosage or withdrawal of therapy may be indicated, particularly if the elevations persist.

➤*Hypoglycemia:* Because of its mechanism of action, acarbose alone should not cause hypoglycemia in the fasted or postprandial state. Sulfonylurea agents may cause hypoglycemia. Because acarbose given in combination with a sulfonylurea will cause a further lowering of blood glucose, it may increase the hypoglycemic potential of the sulfonylurea. Use oral glucose (dextrose), whose absorption is not inhibited by acarbose, instead of sucrose (cane sugar) in the treatment of mild-to-moderate hypoglycemia. Sucrose, in which hydrolysis to glucose and fructose is inhibited by acarbose, is unsuitable for the rapid correction of hypoglycemia. Severe hypoglycemia may require the use of either IV glucose infusion or glucagon injection. Hypoglycemia does not occur in patients receiving metformin alone under usual circumstances of use, and no increased incidence of hypoglycemia was observed in patients when acarbose was added to metformin therapy.

➤*Lab test abnormalities:*
Elevated serum transaminase levels – Long-term studies (up to 12 months, and including acarbose doses up to 300 mg 3 times daily), treatment-emergent elevations of serum transminases (AST and /or ALT) above the upper limit of normal (ULN), greater than 1.8 × ULN, and greater than 3 × ULN occurred in 14%, 6%, and 3%, respectively, of acarbose-treated patients as compared with 7%, 2%, and 1%, respectively, of placebo-treated patients. Although these differences between treatments were statistically significant, these elevations were asymptomatic, reversible, more common in females, and, in general, were not associated with other evidence of liver dysfunction. In addition, these serum transaminase elevations appeared to be dose related. Doses up to the maximum approved dose of 100 mg 3 times daily, treatment-emergent elevations of AST and/or ALT at any level of severity were similar between acarbose-treated patients and placebo-treated patients ($P \geq 0.496$).

In international postmarketing experience, 62 cases of serum transminase elevations more than 500 IU/L (29 of which were associated with jaundice) have been reported. Forty-one of these 62 cases received treatment with at least 100 mg 3 times daily and 33 of 45 patients whose reported weight was less than 60 kg. In the 59 cases where follow-up was recorded, hepatic abnormalities improved or resolved upon discontinuation of acarbose in 55. A few cases of fulminant hepatitis with fatal outcome have been reported; the relationship to acarbose is unclear.

➤*Loss of blood glucose control:* When diabetic patients are exposed to stress such as fever, trauma, infection, surgery, a temporary loss of control of blood glucose may occur. At such times, temporary insulin therapy may be necessary.

Certain drugs tend to produce hyperglycemia and may lead to loss of blood glucose control. These drugs include the thiazides and other diuretics, corticosteroids, phenothiazines, thyroid products, estrogens, oral contraceptives, phenytoin, nicotinic acid, sympathomimetics, calcium channel blocking drugs, and isoniazid. When such drugs are administered to a patient receiving acarbose, closely observe the patient for loss of blood glucose control. When such drugs are withdrawn from a patient receiving acarbose in combination with sulfonylureas or insulin, closely observe patients for any evidence of hypoglycemia.

➤*Hematocrit:* Small reductions in hematocrit occurred more often in acarbose-treated patients than in placebo-treated patients but were not associated with reductions in hemoglobin.

➤*Calcium/Vitamin B$_6$:* Low serum calcium and low plasma vitamin B$_6$ levels were associated with acarbose therapy but were thought to be either spurious or of no clinical significance.

➤*GI:* GI symptoms are the most common reaction to acarbose. In trials, the incidences of abdominal pain, diarrhea, and flatulence were 19%, 31%, and 74%, respectively, with acarbose 50 to 300 mg 3 times daily, whereas the corresponding incidences were 9%, 12%, and 29% with placebo. Abdominal pain and diarrhea tended to return to pretreatment levels over time, and the frequency and intensity of flatulence tended to abate with time. The increased GI tract symptoms in patients treated with acarbose is a manifestation of the mechanism of action of acarbose and is related to the presence of undigested carbohydrate in the lower GI tract. Rarely, these GI events may be severe and might be confused with paralytic ileus.

Drug Interactions

Acarbose Drug Interactions			
Precipitant drug	Object drug*		Description
Acarbose	Digoxin	↓	Serum digoxin concentrations may be reduced, decreasing the therapeutic effects.
Digestive enzymes (eg, amylase, pancreatin)	Acarbose	↓	Effect of acarbose may be reduced. Do not use concomitantly.
Intestinal absorbents (eg, charcoal)	Acarbose	↓	Effect of acarbose may be reduced. Do not use concomitantly.

* ↓ = Object drug decreased.

Adverse Reactions

➤*GI:* Flatulence (74%); diarrhea (31%); abdominal pain (19%) (see Precautions).

➤*Hypersensitivity:* Rarely, hypersensitive skin reactions such as rash may occur.

➤*Miscellaneous:* Edema (rare).

➤*Lab test abnormalities:* Elevated serum transaminase levels, decrease in hematocrit, low serum calcium, and low plasma vitamin B$_6$ levels have occurred (see Precautions).

Overdosage

Unlike sulfonylureas or insulin, an overdose of acarbose will not result in hypoglycemia. An overdose may result in transient increases in flatulence, diarrhea, and abdominal discomfort, which shortly subside.

Patient Information

Tell patients to take acarbose orally 3 times daily at the start (with the first bite) of main meals. It is important that patients continue to adhere to dietary instructions, a regular exercise program, and regular testing of urine and/or blood glucose.

Acarbose does not cause hypoglycemia even when administered in the fasted state. Sulfonylurea drugs and insulin, however; can lower blood sugar levels enough to cause symptoms or sometimes life-threatening hypoglycemia. Because acarbose given in combination with a sulfonylurea or insulin will cause a further lowering of blood sugar, it may increase the hypoglycemic potential of these agents. The risk of hypoglycemia, its symptoms and treatment, and conditions that predispose to its development should be well understood by the patient and family members. Because acarbose prevents the breakdown of table sugar, patients should have a readily available source of glucose (dextrose, D-glucose) to treat symptoms of low blood sugar when taking acarbose in combination with a sulfonylurea or insulin.

If side effects occur, they usually develop during the first few weeks of therapy. They are most commonly mild to moderate GI effects, such as flatulence, diarrhea or abdominal discomfort, and generally diminish in frequency and intensity with time.

Alpha-Glucosidase Inhibitors

MIGLITOL

Rx	Glyset (Pfizer)	Tablets: 25 mg	(GLYSET 25). White. In 100s.
		50 mg	(GLYSET 50). White. In 100s.
		100 mg	(GLYSET 100). White. In 100s.

Indications

➤*Type 2 diabetes mellitus:*

Monotherapy – Monotherapy adjunct to diet to improve glycemic control in patients with type 2 diabetes whose hyperglycemia cannot be managed with diet alone.

Combination therapy – In combination with a sulfonylurea when diet plus either miglitol or a sulfonylurea alone do not result in adequate glycemic control. The effect of miglitol to enhance glycemic control is additive to that of sulfonylureas when used in combination, presumably because the mechanism of action is different.

Administration and Dosage

In initiating treatment for type 2 diabetes, emphasize diet as the primary form of treatment. Caloric restriction and weight loss are essential in the obese diabetic patient. Proper dietary management alone may be effective in controlling blood glucose and symptoms of hyperglycemia. Also stress the importance of regular physical activity when appropriate. If this treatment program fails to result in adequate glycemic control, consider the use of miglitol. The use of miglitol must be viewed by the physician and patient as a treatment in addition to diet and not as a substitute for diet or as a convenient mechanism for avoiding dietary restraint.

There is no fixed dosage regimen for the management of diabetes mellitus with miglitol. Dosage of miglitol must be individualized on the basis of effectiveness and tolerance while not exceeding the maximum recommended dosage of 100 mg 3 times/day. Start miglitol at 25 mg, gradually increase dosage as described below, both to reduce GI adverse effects and to permit identification of the minimum dose required for adequate glycemic control of the patient.

During treatment initiation and dose titration, 1-hour postprandial plasma glucose may be used to determine the therapeutic response to miglitol and identify the minimum effective dose for the patient. Thereafter, measure glycosylated hemoglobin at intervals of approximately 3 months. The therapeutic goal should be to decrease both postprandial plasma glucose and glycosylate hemoglobin levels to normal or near normal by using the lowest effective dose of miglitol, either as monotherapy or in combination with a sulfonylurea.

➤*Initial dosage:* The recommended starting dosage is 25 mg, given orally 3 times/day at the start (with the first bite) of each main meal. However, some patients may benefit by starting at 25 mg once daily to minimize GI adverse effects and gradually increasing the frequency of administration to 3 times/day.

➤*Maintenance dosage:* The usual maintenance dose of miglitol is 50 mg 3 times/day although some patients may benefit from increasing the dose to 100 mg 3 times/day. In order to allow adaptation to potential adverse effects, initiate miglitol therapy at a dosage of 25 mg 3 times/day, the lowest effective dosage, and then gradually titrated upward. After 4 to 8 weeks of the 25 mg 3 times/day regimen, increase the dosage to 50 mg 3 times/day for approximately 3 months. Measure glycosylated hemoglobin at intervals of about 3 months. If, at that time, the glycosylated hemoglobin level is not satisfactory, the dosage may be further increased to 100 mg 3 times/day, the maximum recommended dosage. Pooled data from controlled studies suggest a dose-response for HbA$_{1c}$ and 1-hour postprandial plasma glucose throughout the recommended dosage range. No single study has examined the effect on glycemic control of titrating patients' doses upwards within the same study. If no further reduction in postprandial glucose or glycosylated hemoglobin levels is observed with titration to 100 mg 3 times/day, consider lowering the dose.

➤*Maximum dosage:* The maximum recommended dosage of miglitol is 100 mg 3 times/day. In 1 clinical trial, 200 mg 3 times/day gave additional improved glycemic control but increased the incidence of the GI symptoms.

➤*Combination with sulfonylureas:* Because its mechanism of action is different, the effect of miglitol to enhance glycemic control is additive to that of sulfonyureas when used in combination. In addition, miglitol diminishes the insuliotropic and weight-increasing effects of sulfonylureas. Sulfonylurea agents may cause hypoglycemia. There was no increased incidence of hypoglycemia in patients who took miglitol in combination with sulfonylurea agents compared with the incidence of hypoglycemia in patients receiving sulfonylureas alone. However, miglitol given in combination with a sulfonylurea will cause a further lowering of blood glucose and may increase the risk of hypoglycemia caused by the additive effects of the 2 agents. If hypoglycemia occurs, make appropriate adjustments in the dosage of these agents.

➤*Storage/Stability:* Store at 25°C (77°F); excursions permitted to 15° to 30°C (59° to 86°F)

Actions

➤*Pharmacology:* Miglitol is an α-glucoside inhibitor and desoxynojirimycin derivative that delays the digestion of ingested carbohydrates resulting in a smaller rise in blood glucose concentration following meals. Miglitol reduces levels of glycosylated hemoglobin in patients with type 2 (non-insulin-dependent) diabetes mellitus. Systemic nonenzymatic protein glycosylation, as reflected by levels of glycosylated hemoglobin, is a function of average blood glucose concentration over time.

In contrast to sulfonylureas, miglitol does not enhance insulin secretion. The antihyperglycemic action of miglitol results from a reversible inhibition of membrane-bound intestinal α-glucoside hydrolase enzymes. Membrane-bound intestinal α-glucosidases hydrolyze oligosaccharides and disaccharides to glucose and other monosaccharides in the brush border of the small intestine. In diabetic patients, this enzyme inhibition results in delayed glucose absorption and lowering of postprandial hyperglycemia.

Miglitol has minor inhibitory activity against lactase and, at recommended doses, would not be expected to induce lactose intolerance.

➤*Pharmacokinetics:*

Absorption – Absorption of miglitol is saturable at high doses: a dose of 25 mg is completely absorbed, whereas a dose of 100 mg is only 50% to 70% absorbed. For all doses, peak concentrations are reached in 2 to 3 hours.

Distribution – The protein binding of miglitol is negligible (less than 4%). Miglitol has a volume of distribution of 0.18 L/kg, consistent with distribution primarily into the extracellular fluid.

Metabolism – Miglitol is not metabolized. No metabolites have been detected in plasma, urine, or feces, indicating a lack of either systemic or presystemic metabolism.

Excretion – Miglitol is eliminated by renal excretion as unchanged drug. Following a 25 mg dose, more than 95% of the dose is recovered in the urine within 24 hours. At higher doses, the cumulative recovery of drug from urine is somewhat lower because of the incomplete bioavailability. The elimination half-life of miglitol from plasma is approximately 2 hours.

Renal function impairment – Because miglitol is excreted primarily by the kidneys, accumulation of miglitol is expected in patients with renal impairment. Patients with creatinine clearance less than 25 mL/min taking 25 mg 3 times/day exhibited a greater than 2-fold increase in miglitol plasma levels as compared with subjects with creatinine clearance more than 60 mL/min. Dosage adjustment to correct the increased plasma concentrations is not feasible because miglitol acts locally. Little information is available on the safety of miglitol in patients with creatinine clearance less than 25 mL/min.

Contraindications

Diabetic ketoacidosis; inflammatory bowel disease; colonic ulceration; partial intestinal obstruction; patients predisposed to intestinal obstruction; chronic intestinal diseases associated with marked disorders of digestion or absorption or with conditions that may deteriorate as a result of increased gas formation in the intestine; hypersensitivity to the drug or any of its components.

Warnings

➤*GI:* GI symptoms are the most common reactions to miglitol. The incidence of diarrhea and abdominal pain tend to diminish considerably with continued treatment (see Adverse Reactions).

➤*Renal function impairment:* Plasma concentrations of miglitol in renally impaired volunteers were proportionally increased relative to the degree of renal dysfunction. Long-term clinical trials in diabetic patients with significant renal dysfunction (serum creatinine more than 2 mg/dL) have not been conducted. Treatment of these patients with miglitol is not recommended.

➤*Pregnancy: Category B.* The highest doses tested in these studies, 450 mg/kg in the rat and 200 mg/kg in the rabbit promoted maternal and/or fetal toxicity. Fetotoxicity was indicated by a slight but significant reduction in fetal weight in the rat study and slight reduction in fetal weight, delayed ossification of the fetal skeleton, and increase in the percentage of on-viable fetuses in the rabbit study. In the peri-postnatal study in rats, the NOAEL (No Observed Adverse Effect Level) was 100 mg/kg (corresponding to approximately 4 times the exposure to humans, based on body surface area). An increase in stillborn progeny was noted at the high dose (300 mg/kg) in the rat peri-postnatal study, but not at the high dose (450 mg/kg) in the delivery segment of the rat developmental toxicity study. The safety of miglitol in pregnant women has not been established. There are no adequate and well-controlled studies in pregnant women. Use during pregnancy only if clearly needed.

MIGLITOL

►*Lactation:* Miglitol is excreted in breast milk to a very small degree. Total excretion into milk accounted for 0.02% of a 100 mg maternal dose. The estimated exposure to a nursing infant is about 0.4% of the maternal dose. Although the levels of miglitol reached in breast milk are exceedingly low, do not administer miglitol to a breastfeeding woman.

►*Children:* Safety and efficacy have not been established.

Precautions

►*Monitoring:* Monitor therapeutic response to miglitol by periodic blood glucose tests. Measurement of glycosylated hemoglobin levels is recommended for the monitoring of long-term glycemic control.

►*Hypoglycemia:* Because of its mechanism of action, miglitol, when administered alone, should not cause hypoglycemia in the fasted or postprandial state. Sulfonylurea agents may cause hypoglycemia. Because miglitol given in combination with a sulfonylurea will cause a further lowering of blood glucose, it may increase the hypoglycemic potential of the sulfonylurea, although this was not observed in clinical trials. Use oral glucose (dextrose), whose absorption is not delayed by miglitol instead of sucrose (cane sugar) in the treatment of mild-to-moderate hypoglycemia. Sucrose, whose hydrolysis to glucose and fructose is inhibited by miglitol, is unsuitable for the rapid correction of hypoglycemia. Severe hypoglycemia may require the use of either IV glucose infusion or glucagon injection.

►*Blood glucose control:* When diabetic patients are exposed to stress such as fever, trauma, infection, or surgery, a temporary loss of control of blood glucose may occur. At such times, temporary insulin therapy may be necessary.

Drug Interactions

Miglitol Drug Interactions			
Precipitant	Object drug*		Description
Miglitol	Digoxin	↓	Coadministration may reduce the average plasma concentrations of digoxin by 19% to 28%. In 1 study in diabetic patients under treatment with digoxin, plasma digoxin concentrations were not altered when coadministered with miglitol 100 mg 3 times/day × 14 days.
Miglitol	Glyburide	↓	Decreased AUC and C_{max} values for glyburide occurred when coadministered with miglitol. These differences were not statistically significant.
Miglitol	Metformin	↓	Mean AUC and C_{max} values for metformin were 12% to 13% lower when the volunteers were given miglitol as compared with placebo, but this difference was not statistically significant.
Miglitol	Propranolol	↓	Miglitol may significantly reduce the bioavailability of propranolol by 40%.

Miglitol Drug Interactions			
Precipitant	Object drug*		Description
Miglitol	Ranitidine	↓	Miglitol may significantly reduce the bioavailability of ranitidine by 60%.
Digestive enzymes (eg, amylase, pancreatin)	Miglitol	↓	Digestive enzyme preparations may reduce the effect of miglitol. Do not take concomitantly.
Intestinal adsorbents (eg, charcoal)	Miglitol	↓	Intestinal adsorbents may reduce the effect of miglitol. Do not take concomitantly.

* ↓ = Object drug decreased.

Adverse Reactions

►*Dermatologic:* Rash (4.3%, generally transient).

►*GI:* Flatulence (41.5%); diarrhea (28.7%); abdominal pain (11.7%) (see Warnings).

►*Lab test abnormalities:* Low serum iron (9.2%) usually does not persist in the majority of cases and is not associated with reductions in hemoglobin or changes in other hematologic indices.

Overdosage

Unlike sulfonylureas or insulin, an overdose of miglitol will not result in hypoglycemia. An overdose may result in transient increases in flatulence, diarrhea, and abdominal discomfort. Because of the lack of extra-intestinal effects seen with miglitol, no serious systemic reactions are expected in the event of an overdose.

Patient Information

Take orally 3 times/day at the start (with the first bite) of each main meal. It is important to continue to adhere to dietary instructions, a regular exercise program, and regular testing of urine and/or blood glucose.

Miglitol itself does not cause hypoglycemia even when administered to patients in the fasted state. Sulfonylurea drugs and insulin can lower blood sugar levels enough to cause symptoms or sometimes life-threatening hypoglycemia. Because miglitol given in combination with a sulfonylurea or insulin will cause a further lowering of blood sugar, it may increase the hypoglycemic potential of these agents. The risk of hypoglycemia, its symptoms and treatment, and conditions that predispose to its development should be well understood by patients and responsible family members. Because miglitol prevents the breakdown of table sugar, have a source of glucose (dextrose, D-glucose) available to treat the symptoms of low blood sugar when taking miglitol in combination with a sulfonylurea or insulin.

If side effects occur with miglitol, they usually develop during the first few weeks of therapy. They are most commonly mild to moderate dose-related GI effects, such as flatulence, soft stools, diarrhea, or abdominal discomfort, and they generally diminish in frequency and intensity with time. Discontinuation of drug usually results in rapid resolution of these GI symptoms.

Biguanides

METFORMIN HCl

Rx	Metformin HCl (Various, eg, Andrx, Barr, Ivax, Teva)	Tablets: 500 mg	In 100s, 500s, 1000s, 2000s, and UD 100s.
Rx	Glucophage (Bristol-Myers Squibb)		(BMS 6060 500). White to off-white. Film-coated. In 100s and 500s.
Rx	Metformin HCl (Various, eg, Andrx, Barr, Ivax, Teva)	850 mg	In 100s, 500s, 1000s, and UD 100s.
Rx	Glucophage (Bristol-Myers Squibb)		(BMS 6070 850). White to off-white. Film-coated. In 100s.
	Metformin HCl (Various, eg, Andrx, Barr, Ivax)	1000 mg	In 100s, 500s, 1000s, and UD 100s.
Rx	Glucophage (Bristol-Myers Squibb)		(BMS 6071 1000). White, oval, bisected. Film-coated. In 100s.
Rx	Metformin HCl ER (PAR)	Tablets, extended-release: 500 mg	(5053 500). White to off-white, capsule shape. In 100s.
Rx	Fortamet (Andrx)		(574). White, biconvex. Film-coated. In 60s.
Rx	Glucophage XR (Bristol-Myers Squibb)		(BMS 6063 500). White to off-white, capsule shape. In 100s and 500s.
Rx	Glucophage XR (Bristol-Myers Squibb)	Tablets, extended-release: 750 mg	(BMS 6064 750). Pale red, capsule shape. In 100s.
Rx	Fortamet (Andrx)	Tablets, extended-release: 1,000 mg	(575). White, biconvex. Film-coated. In 60s.

WARNING

Lactic acidosis: Lactic acidosis is a rare, but serious, metabolic complication that can occur because of metformin accumulation during treatment; when it occurs, it is fatal in ≈ 50% of cases. See Warnings.

Indications

▶*Type 2 diabetes:* As monotherapy, as an adjunct to diet and exercise to improve glycemic control in patients with type 2 diabetes. Metformin is indicated in patients ≥ 10 years of age and metformin extended-release (ER) tablets are indicated in patients ≥ 17 years of age.

Metformin or metformin ER may be used concomitantly with a sulfonylurea or insulin to improve glycemic control in adults ≥ 17 years of age.

Administration and Dosage

▶*Approved by the FDA:* December 29, 1994.

There is no fixed dosage regimen for the management of hyperglycemia in type 2 diabetes with metformin or any other pharmacologic agent. Dosage must be individualized on the basis of effectiveness and tolerance, while not exceeding the maximum recommended daily dose of 2550 mg in adults and 2000 mg in pediatric patients (10 to 16 years of age); the maximum recommended daily dose of metformin ER in adults is 2000 mg. Give metformin in divided doses with meals while metformin ER generally should be given once daily with the evening meal. Start at a low dose, with gradual dose escalation as described below, both to reduce GI side effects and to permit identification of the minimum dose required for adequate glycemic control of the patient.

During treatment initiation and dose titration, use fasting plasma glucose to determine therapeutic response to metformin and to identify minimum effective dose. Thereafter, measure glycosylated hemoglobin at intervals of ≈ 3 months. The therapeutic goal should be to decrease fasting plasma glucose and glycosylated hemoglobin levels to normal or near normal by using the lowest effective dose of metformin, when used as monotherapy or in combination with a sulfonylurea or insulin.

Monitoring of blood glucose and glycosylated hemoglobin also will permit detection of primary failure (ie, inadequate lowering of blood glucose at the maximum recommended dose of medication) and secondary failure (ie, loss of an adequate blood glucose-lowering response after an initial period of effectiveness).

Short-term administration may be sufficient during periods of transient loss of control in patients usually well controlled on diet alone.

Metformin ER must be swallowed whole and never crushed or chewed. Occasionally, the inactive ingredients will be eliminated in the feces as a soft, hydrated mass.

▶*Usual starting dose for adults:* In general, clinically significant responses are not seen at doses < 1500 mg/day. However, a lower recommended starting dose and gradually increased dosage is advised to minimize GI symptoms.

Metformin – The usual starting dose is 500 mg twice/day or 850 mg once/day, given with meals. Make dosage increases in increments of 500 mg/week or 850 mg every 2 weeks, up to a total of 2000 mg/day given in divided doses. Patients can be titrated from 500 mg twice/day to 850 mg twice/day after 2 weeks. For those patients requiring additional glycemic control, it may be given to a maximum daily dose of 2550 mg/day. Doses > 2000 mg may be better tolerated given 3 times/day with meals.

Metformin ER – The usual starting dose is 500 mg once/day with the evening meal. Make dosage increases in increments of 500 mg/week, up to a maximum of 2000 mg once/day with the evening meal. If glycemic control is not achieved on 2000 mg once/day, consider a trial of 1000 mg twice/day. If higher doses of metformin are required, use metformin at total daily doses up to 2550 mg administered in divided daily doses, as described above.

Conversion from metformin to metformin ER – In a randomized trial, patients currently treated with metformin were switched to metformin ER. Results of this trial suggest that patients receiving metformin treatment may be safely switched to metformin ER once daily at the same total daily dose, up to 2000 mg once/day. Following a switch from metformin to metformin ER, closely monitor glycemic control and make dosage adjustments accordingly.

▶*Pediatrics:* The usual starting dose of metformin is 500 mg twice/day, given with meals. Make dosage increases in increments of 500 mg/week up to a maximum of 2000 mg/day given in divided doses. Safety and effectiveness of metformin ER in pediatric patients have not been established.

▶*Transfer from other antidiabetic therapy:* When transferring patients from standard oral hypoglycemic agents other than chlorpropamide to metformin, generally no transition period is necessary. When transferring patients from chlorpropamide, exercise care during the first 2 weeks because of the prolonged retention of chlorpropamide leading to overlapping drug effects and possible hypoglycemia.

▶*Concomitant metformin and sulfonylurea:* If a patient has not responded to 4 weeks of the maximum dose of metformin monotherapy, consider gradual addition of an oral sulfonylurea while continuing metformin at the maximum dose, even if prior primary or secondary failure to a sulfonylurea has occurred. Clinical and pharmacokinetic drug interaction data are available only for metformin plus glyburide.

With concomitant metformin and sulfonylurea therapy, the desired control of blood glucose may be obtained by adjusting the dose of each drug. However, make attempts to identify the minimum effective dose of each drug. With concomitant metformin and sulfonylurea therapy, risk of hypoglycemia associated with sulfonylurea therapy continues and may be increased. Take appropriate precautions.

If a patient has not satisfactorily responded to 1 to 3 months of concomitant therapy with the maximum doses of metformin and an oral sulfonylurea, consider institution of insulin therapy with or without metformin.

▶*Concomitant metformin or metformin ER and insulin therapy in adults:* Continue the current insulin dose upon initiation of metformin or metformin ER therapy. Initiate metformin or metformin ER therapy at 500 mg once/day in patients on insulin therapy. For patients not responding adequately, increase the dose of metformin or metformin ER by 500 mg after ≈ 1 week and by 500 mg every week thereafter until adequate glycemic control is achieved. The maximum recommended daily dose is 2500 mg for metformin and 2000 mg for metformin ER. It is recommended that the insulin dose be decreased by 10% to 25% when fasting plasma glucose concentrations decrease to < 120 mg/dL in patients receiving concomitant insulin and metformin or metformin ER. Individualize further adjustment based on glucose-lowering response.

▶*Special patient populations:* Initial and maintenance dosing should be conservative in patients with advanced age because of the potential for decreased renal function. Base any dosage adjustment on a careful assessment of renal function. Generally, do not titrate elderly patients to the maximum dose. Do not initiate metformin and metformin ER treatment in patients ≥ 80 years of age unless measurement of Ccr demonstrates that renal function is not reduced.

METFORMIN HCl

In debilitated or malnourished patients, the dosing should also be conservative and based on a careful assessment of renal function. Do not titrate patients to the maximum dose.

Actions

➤*Pharmacology:* Metformin is an oral antihyperglycemic drug used in the management of Type 2 diabetes mellitus. It is not chemically or pharmacologically related to any other classes of oral antihyperglycemic agents. Metformin improves glucose tolerance in subjects with type 2 diabetes, lowering basal and postprandial plasma glucose. Metformin decreases hepatic glucose production, decreases intestinal absorption of glucose and improves insulin sensitivity (increases peripheral glucose uptake and utilization). Unlike sulfonylureas, metformin does not produce hypoglycemia in patients with type 2 diabetes or healthy subjects (except in special circumstances; see Precautions) and does not cause hyperinsulinemia. With metformin therapy, insulin secretion remains unchanged while fasting insulin levels and day-long plasma insulin response may actually decrease.

➤*Pharmacokinetics:*

Absorption/Distribution – The absolute bioavailability of 500 mg metformin given under fasting conditions is ≈ 50% to 60%. Studies using single oral doses of 500 and 1500 mg, and 850 to 2550 mg, indicate that there is a lack of dose proportionality with increasing doses, which is due to decreased absorption rather than an alteration in elimination. Food decreases the extent and slightly delays the absorption of metformin (see Drug Interactions).

The apparent volume of distribution following single oral doses of 850 mg averaged 654 ± 358 L. Metformin is negligibly bound to plasma proteins in contrast to sulfonylureas, which are > 90% protein bound. At usual clinical doses and dosing schedules, steady-state plasma concentrations are reached within 24 to 48 hours and are generally < 1 mcg/mL. During controlled clinical trials, maximum metformin plasma levels did not exceed 5 mcg/mL, even at maximum doses.

Following a single oral dose of metformin ER, C_{max} is achieved with a median value of 7 hours (range, 4 to 8 hours). Peak plasma levels are ≈ 20% lower compared with the same dose of metformin; however, the extent of absorption (as measured by AUC) is similar to metformin.

At steady state, the AUC and C_{max} are less than dose proportional for metformin ER within the range of 500 to 2000 mg administered once/day. Peak plasma levels are ≈ 0.6, 1.1, 1.4, and 1.8 mcg/mL for 500, 1000, 1500, and 2000 mg once/day doses, respectively. The extent of metformin absorption (as measured by AUC) from metformin ER at 2000 mg once/day dose is similar to the same total daily dose administered as metformin tablets 1000 mg twice/day. After repeated administration of metformin ER, metformin did not accumulate in plasma.

Metabolism/Excretion – Metformin is excreted unchanged in the urine and does not undergo hepatic metabolism (no metabolites have been identified in humans) nor biliary excretion. Renal clearance is ≈ 3.5 times greater than Ccr, which indicates that tubular secretion is the major route of elimination. Following oral administration, ≈ 90% of the absorbed drug is eliminated via the renal route within the first 24 hours, with a plasma elimination half-life of ≈ 6.2 hours. In blood, the elimination half-life is ≈ 17.6 hours, suggesting that the erythrocyte mass may be a compartment of distribution.

Special populations –

Renal insufficiency: In patients with decreased renal function (based on measured Ccr), the plasma and blood half-life of metformin is prolonged and the renal clearance is decreased in proportion to the decrease in Ccr.

Elderly: Limited data in healthy elderly subjects suggest that total plasma clearance of metformin is decreased, the half-life is prolonged, and C_{max} is increased, compared with healthy young subjects. From these data, it appears that the change in metformin pharmacokinetics with aging is primarily accounted for by a change in renal function. Do not initiate metformin and metformin ER treatment in patients ≥ 80 years of age unless measurement of Ccr demonstrates that renal function is not reduced.

Select Mean Metformin Pharmacokinetic Parameters Following Single or Multiple Oral Doses			
Subject groups: Metformin dose[1]	C_{max} (mcg/mL)	t_{max} (hr)	Renal clearance (mL/min)
Healthy, nondiabetic adults			
500 mg SD[2] (n = 24)	≈ 1.03	≈ 2.75	≈ 600
850 mg SD (n = 74)[3]	≈ 1.6	≈ 2.64	≈ 552
850 mg tid for 19 doses (n = 9)	≈ 2.01	≈ 1.79	≈ 642
Adults with type 2 diabetes			
850 mg SD (n = 23)	≈ 1.48	≈ 3.32	≈ 491
850 mg tid for 19 doses (n = 9)	≈ 1.9	≈ 2.01	≈ 550
Elderly,[4] healthy, nondiabetic adults			
850 mg SD (n = 12)	≈ 2.45	≈ 2.71	≈ 412
Renally impaired adults: 850 mg SD			
Mild (Ccr 61 to 90 mL/min); (n = 5)	≈ 1.86	≈ 3.2	≈ 384
Moderate (Ccr 31 to 60 mL/min); (n = 4)	≈ 4.12	≈ 3.75	≈ 108
Severe (Ccr 10 to 30 mL/min); (n = 6)	≈ 3.93	≈ 4.01	≈ 130

[1] All doses given fasting except the first 18 doses of the multiple dose studies.
[2] SD = Single dose.
[3] Combined results (average means) of 5 studies; mean age 32 years (range, 23 to 59 years of age).
[4] Elderly subjects, mean age 71 years (range, 65 to 81 years of age).

➤*Clinical trials:* A 29-week, double-blind, placebo-controlled study of metformin and glyburide, alone and in combination, was conducted in obese patients with type 2 diabetes who had failed to achieve adequate glycemic control while on maximum doses of glyburide (baseline fasting plasma glucose [FPG] of ≈ 250 mg/dL). Patients randomized to continue on glyburide experienced worsening of glycemic control, with mean increases in FPG, postprandial plasma glucose (PPG), and HbA$_{1c}$ of 14 mg/dL, 3 mg/dL, and 0.2%, respectively. In contrast, those randomized to metformin (≤ 2.5 g/day) experienced a slight improvement, with mean reductions in FPG, PPG, and HbA$_{1c}$ of 1 mg/dL, 6 mg/dL, and 0.4%, respectively. The combination of metformin and glyburide was effective in reducing FPG, PPG, and HbA$_{1c}$ levels by 63 mg/dL, 65 mg/dL, and 1.7%, respectively. Compared with results of glyburide treatment alone, the net differences with combination treatment were -77 mg/dL, -68 mg/dL, and -1.9%, respectively.

Combined Metformin/Glyburide (Combo) vs Glyburide or Metformin Monotherapy: Summary of Mean Changes from Baseline[1] in Fasting Plasma Glucose, HbA$_{1c}$, and Body Weight, at Final Visit (29-Week Study)						
	Combo (n = 213)	Glyburide (n = 209)	Metformin (n = 210)	p-Values Glyburide vs combo	p-Values metformin vs combo	Metformin vs glyburide
Fasting plasma glucose (mg/dL)						
Baseline	250.5	247.5	253.9	NS[2]	NS[2]	NS[2]
Change at final visit	−63.5	13.7	−0.9	0.001	0.001	0.025
Hemoglobin A$_{1c}$ (%)						
Baseline	8.8	8.5	8.9	NS[2]	NS[2]	0.007
Change at final visit	−1.7	0.2	−0.4	0.001	0.001	0.001
Body weight (lbs)						
Baseline	202.2	203	204	NS[2]	NS[2]	NS[2]
Change at final visit	0.9	−0.7	−8.4	0.011	0.001	0.001

[1] All patients on 20 mg/day glyburide at baseline.
[2] Not statistically significant.

In clinical studies, metformin, alone or in combination with a sulfonylurea, lowered mean fasting serum triglycerides, total cholesterol, and LDL cholesterol levels and had no adverse effects on other lipid levels.

Summary of Mean Percent Change from Baseline of Major Serum Lipid Variables at Final Visit (29-Week Studies)					
	Metformin vs placebo		Combined metformin/glyburide vs monotherapy		
	Metformin (n = 141)	Placebo (n = 145)	Metformin (n = 210)	Metformin/ Glyburide (n = 213)	Glyburide (n = 209)
Total cholesterol (mg/dL)					
Baseline	211	212.3	213.1	215.6	219.6
Mean % change at final visit	−5%	1%	−2%	−4%	1%
Total triglycerides (mg/dL)					
Baseline	236.1	203.5	242.5	215	266.1
Mean % change at final visit	−16%	1%	−3%	−8%	4%
LDL-cholesterol (mg/dL)					
Baseline	135.4	138.5	134.3	136	137.5
Mean % change at final visit	−8%	1%	−4%	−6%	3%
HDL-cholesterol (mg/dL)					
Baseline	39	40.5	37.2	39	37
Mean % change at final visit	2%	−1%	5%	3%	1%

METFORMIN HCl

Contraindications

1.) Renal disease or dysfunction (eg, as suggested by serum creatinine levels ≥ 1.5 mg/dL [males], ≥ 1.4 mg/dL [females] or abnormal Ccr), which also may result from conditions such as cardiovascular collapse (shock), acute MI, and septicemia.
2.) CHF requiring pharmacologic treatment.
3.) Temporarily discontinue metformin in patients undergoing radiologic studies involving intravascular administration of iodinated contrast materials because use of such products may result in acute alteration of renal function (see Drug Interactions).
4.) Hypersensitivity to metformin.
5.) Acute or chronic metabolic acidosis, including diabetic ketoacidosis, with or without coma. Treat diabetic ketoacidosis with insulin.

Warnings

➤*Lactic acidosis:* Lactic acidosis is a rare, but serious, metabolic complication that can occur because of metformin accumulation during treatment; when it occurs, it is fatal in ≈ 50% of cases. Lactic acidosis also may occur in association with a number of pathophysiologic conditions, including diabetes mellitus and whenever there is significant tissue hypoperfusion and hypoxemia. Lactic acidosis is characterized by elevated blood lactate levels (> 5 mmol/L), decreased blood pH, electrolyte disturbances with an increased anion gap and an increased lactate/pyruvate ratio. When metformin is implicated as the cause of lactic acidosis, metformin plasma levels > 5 mcg/mL are generally found.

The reported incidence of lactic acidosis in patients receiving metformin is very low (≈ 0.03 cases/1000 patient-years, with ≈ 0.015 fatal cases/1000 patient-years). Reported cases have occurred primarily in diabetic patients with significant renal insufficiency, including intrinsic renal disease and renal hypoperfusion, often in the setting of multiple concomitant medical/surgical problems and multiple concomitant medications. Patients with CHF requiring pharmacologic management, in particular those with unstable or acute CHF who are at risk of hypoperfusion and hypoxemia, are at increased risk of lactic acidosis. The risk of lactic acidosis increases with the degree of renal dysfunction and the patient's age. Therefore, the risk of lactic acidosis may be significantly decreased by regular monitoring of renal function in patients taking metformin and by use of the minimum effective dose. In particular, treatment of the elderly should be accompanied by careful monitoring of renal function. Do not initiate metformin treatment in patients ≥ 80 years of age unless measurement of Ccr demonstrates that renal function is not reduced, as these patients are more susceptible to developing lactic acidosis. In addition, promptly withhold metformin in the presence of any condition associated with hypoxemia, dehydration, or sepsis. Because impaired hepatic function may significantly limit the ability to clear lactate, generally avoid metformin in patients with evidence of hepatic disease. Caution patients against excessive alcohol intake (acute or chronic) because alcohol potentiates the effects of metformin on lactate metabolism. In addition, temporarily discontinue metformin prior to any intravascular radiocontrast study and for any surgical procedure.

Lactic acidosis onset is often subtle and accompanied by nonspecific symptoms such as malaise, myalgias, respiratory distress, increasing somnolence, and nonspecific abdominal distress. There may be associated hypothermia, hypotension, and resistant bradyarrhythmias with more marked acidosis. The patient and the patient's physician must be aware of the possible importance of such symptoms. Instruct the patient to notify the physician immediately if these symptoms occur. Withdraw metformin until the situation is clarified. Serum electrolytes, ketones, blood glucose and, if indicated, blood pH, lactate levels, and blood metformin levels may be useful. Once a patient is stabilized on any dose of metformin, GI symptoms, which are common during initiation of therapy, are unlikely to be drug related. Later occurrence of GI symptoms could be because of lactic acidosis or other serious disease.

Levels of fasting venous plasma lactate above the upper limit of normal but < 5 mmol/L in patients taking metformin do not necessarily indicate impending lactic acidosis and may be explainable by other mechanisms, such as poorly controlled diabetes or obesity, vigorous physical activity, or technical problems in sample handling.

Suspect lactic acidosis in any diabetic patient with metabolic acidosis lacking evidence of ketoacidosis (ketonuria and ketonemia).

Lactic acidosis is a medical emergency that must be treated in a hospital setting. In a patient with lactic acidosis who is taking metformin, discontinue the drug immediately and promptly institute general supportive measures. Because metformin is dialyzable (with a clearance of up to 170 mL/min under good hemodynamic conditions), prompt hemodialysis is recommended to correct the acidosis and remove the accumulated metformin. Such management often results in prompt reversal of symptoms and recovery.

➤*Diet/Exercise:* In initiating treatment for type 2 diabetes, emphasize diet as the primary form of treatment. Caloric restriction and weight loss are essential in the obese diabetic patient. Proper dietary management alone may be effective in controlling the blood glucose and symptoms of hyperglycemia. Loss of blood glucose control in diet-managed patients may be transient, thus requiring only short-term pharmacologic therapy. Also, stress the importance of regular physical activity and identify cardiovascular risk factors and take corrective measures where possible. If this treatment program fails to reduce symptoms or blood glucose, consider the use of metformin alone or metformin plus a sulfonylurea.

➤*Renal function impairment:* Metformin is known to be substantially excreted by the kidney, and the risk of metformin accumulation and lactic acidosis increases with the degree of impairment of renal function. Thus, patients with serum creatinine levels above the upper limit of normal for their age should not receive metformin or metformin ER. In patients with advanced age, carefully titrate metformin and metformin ER to establish the minimum dose for adequate glycemic effect, because aging is associated with reduced renal function. In elderly patients, particularly those ≥ 80 years of age, monitor renal function regularly. Generally do not titrate metformin and metformin ER to the maximum dose.

Concomitant medication(s) that affect renal function, result in significant hemodynamic change, or interfere with the disposition of metformin (ie, cationic drugs that are eliminated by renal tubular secretion; see Drug Interactions) should be used with caution.

➤*Hepatic function impairment:* Because impaired hepatic function has been associated with cases of lactic acidosis, avoid metformin in patients with clinical or laboratory evidence of hepatic disease.

➤*Elderly:* Metformin is known to be substantially excreted by the kidney and because the risk of serious adverse reactions to the drug is greater in patients with impaired renal function, only use metformin and metformin ER in patients with normal renal function (see Contraindications, Warnings, and Pharmacology). Aging is associated with reduced renal function; use with caution as age increases. Use care in dose selection and base on careful and regular monitoring of renal function. Generally, do not titrate elderly patients to the maximum dose of metformin (see Administration and Dosage).

➤*Pregnancy:* Category B. There are no adequate and well-controlled studies in pregnant women with metformin or metformin ER. Metformin was not teratogenic in rats and rabbits at ≤ 600 mg/kg/day. Balance any decision to use this drug against the benefits and risks.

Because recent information suggests that abnormal blood glucose levels during pregnancy are associated with a higher incidence of congenital abnormalities, there is a consensus among experts that insulin be used during pregnancy to maintain blood glucose levels as close to normal as possible.

➤*Lactation:* Studies in lactating rats show that metformin is excreted into milk and reaches levels comparable to those in plasma. Similar studies have not been conducted in nursing mothers, but exercise caution in such patients, and decide whether to discontinue nursing or to discontinue the drug, taking into account the importance of the drug to the mother.

➤*Children:* Safety and efficacy in children for metformin ER have not been established.

Safety and efficacy for metformin for the treatment of type 2 diabetes have been established in pediatric patients ages 10 to 16 years (studies have not been conducted in pediatric patients < 10 years). Use of metformin in this age group is supported by evidence from adequate and well-controlled studies of metformin in adults with additional data from a controlled clinical study in pediatric patients ages 10 to 16 years with type 2 diabetes, which demonstrated a similar response in glycemic control to that seen in adults. In this study, adverse effects were similar to those described in adults. A maximum daily dose of 2000 mg is recommended.

Precautions

➤*Monitoring:* Before initiation of therapy and at least annually thereafter, assess renal function and verify as normal. In patients in whom development of renal dysfunction is anticipated, assess renal function more frequently and discontinue the drug if evidence of renal impairment is present.

Evaluate a patient with diabetes previously well controlled on metformin who develops laboratory abnormalities or clinical illness (especially vague and poorly defined illness) for evidence of ketoacidosis or lactic acidosis. Tests should include serum electrolytes and ketones, blood glucose and, if indicated, blood pH, lactate, pyruvate, and metformin levels. If acidosis of either form occurs, metformin must be stopped immediately and other appropriate corrective measures initiated.

Monitor response to all diabetic therapies by periodic measurements of fasting blood glucose and glycosylated hemoglobin levels, with a goal of decreasing these levels toward the normal range. During initial dose titration, fasting glucose can be used to determine the therapeutic response. Thereafter, monitor both glucose and glycosylated hemoglobin. Measurements of glycosylated hemoglobin may be especially useful for evaluating long-term control.

Perform initial and periodic monitoring of hematologic parameters (eg, hemoglobin/hematocrit, red blood cell indices) and renal function

METFORMIN HCl

(serum creatinine) at least on an annual basis. While megaloblastic anemia has rarely been seen with metformin therapy, if this is suspected, exclude vitamin B_{12} deficiency.

➤*Hypoxic states:* Cardiovascular collapse (shock), acute CHF, acute MI, and other conditions characterized by hypoxemia have been associated with lactic acidosis and also may cause prerenal azotemia. If such events occur, discontinue metformin.

➤*Surgical procedures:* Temporarily suspend metformin for surgical procedures (unless minor and not associated with restricted intake of food and fluids). Do not restart until the patient's oral intake has resumed and renal function is normal.

➤*Vitamin B_{12} levels:* A decrease to subnormal levels of previously normal serum vitamin B_{12} levels, without clinical manifestations, was observed in ≈ 7% of patients receiving metformin in controlled clinical trials of 29 weeks duration. Such decrease, possibly because of interference with B_{12} absorption from the B_{12}-intrinsic factor complex, is, however, very rarely associated with anemia and appears to be rapidly reversible with discontinuation of metformin or vitamin B_{12} supplementation. Annual measurement of hematologic parameters is advised in patients on metformin and any apparent abnormalities should be appropriately investigated and managed.

Certain individuals with inadequate vitamin B_{12} or calcium intake or absorption appear to be predisposed to developing subnormal vitamin B_{12} levels. In these patients, routine serum vitamin B_{12} measurements at 2- to 3-year intervals may be useful.

➤*Hypoglycemia:* Hypoglycemia does not occur in patients receiving metformin alone under usual circumstances, but could occur with deficient caloric intake, strenuous exercise not compensated by caloric supplementation, or during concomitant use with other glucose-lowering agents (eg, sulfonylureas, insulin) or ethanol.

Elderly, debilitated, or malnourished patients, and those with adrenal or pituitary insufficiency or alcohol intoxication are particularly susceptible to hypoglycemic effects. Hypoglycemia may be difficult to recognize in the elderly and in those taking beta-adrenergic blocking drugs.

➤*Loss of blood glucose control :* When a patient stabilized on a diabetic regimen is exposed to stress (eg, fever, trauma, infection, surgery), a temporary loss of glycemic control may occur. At such times, it may be necessary to withhold metformin and temporarily administer insulin. Metformin may be reinstituted after the acute episode is resolved.

The effectiveness of oral antidiabetic drugs in lowering blood glucose to a targeted level decreases in many patients over a period of time. This phenomenon, which may be because of progression of the underlying disease or to diminished responsiveness to the drug, is known as secondary failure to distinguish it from primary failure in which the drug is ineffective during initial therapy. Should secondary failure occur with metformin or sulfonylurea monotherapy, combined therapy with metformin and sulfonylurea may result in a response. Should secondary failure occur with combined therapy, it may be necessary to consider therapeutic alternatives including initiation of insulin therapy.

Certain drugs tend to produce hyperglycemia and may lead to loss of glycemic control. These drugs include thiazide and other diuretics, corticosteroids, phenothiazines, thyroid products, estrogens, oral contraceptives, phenytoin, nicotinic acid, sympathomimetics, calcium channel blocking drugs, and isoniazid. When such drugs are administered to a patient receiving metformin, closely observe the patient to maintain adequate glycemic control.

Drug Interactions

Metformin Drug Interactions			
Precipitant drug	Object drug[*]		Description
Metformin	Glyburide	↓	Following coadministration of single doses, decreases in glyburide AUC and C_{max} were observed, but were highly variable. The single-dose nature of this study and the lack of correlation between glyburide blood levels and pharmacodynamic effects makes the clinical significance of this interaction uncertain.
Alcohol	Metformin	↑	Alcohol potentiates the effect of metformin on lactate metabolism. Warn patients against excessive alcohol intake, acute or chronic, while receiving metformin.
Cationic drugs (eg, amiloride, digoxin, morphine, procainamide, quinidine, quinine, ranitidine, triamterene, trimethoprim, vancomycin)	Metformin	↑	Cationic drugs that are eliminated by renal tubular secretion theoretically have the potential for interaction with metformin by competing for common renal tubular transport systems. Although such interactions remain theoretical, careful patient monitoring and dose adjustment of metformin or the interfering drug are recommended in patients who are taking cationic medications that are excreted via the proximal renal tubular secretory system.
Cimetidine	Metformin	↑	Cimetidine caused an 81% increase in peak metformin plasma concentrations, a 50% increase in AUC, and a 27% decrease in average renal clearance of metformin.
Furosemide	Metformin	↑	Furosemide increased the metformin plasma and blood C_{max} by 22% and blood AUC by 15%, without any significant change in metformin renal clearance. When administered with metformin, the C_{max} and AUC of furosemide were 31% and 12% smaller, respectively, than when administered alone, and the terminal half-life was decreased by 32%, without any significant change in furosemide renal clearance.
Metformin	Furosemide	↓	
Iodinated contrast material	Metformin	↑	Parenteral contrast studies with iodinated materials can lead to acute renal failure and have been associated with lactic acidosis in patients receiving metformin. Therefore, in patients in whom any such study is planned, withhold metformin for ≥ 48 hours prior to, and 48 hours subsequent to, the procedure and reinstitute only after renal function has been re-evaluated and found to be normal.
Nifedipine	Metformin	↑	Coadministration increased plasma metformin C_{max} and AUC by 20% and 9%, respectively, and increased the amount excreted in the urine. Nifedipine appears to enhance the absorption of metformin.

[*] ↑ = Object drug increased.   ↓ = Object drug decreased.

➤*Drug/Food interactions:* Food decreases the extent and slightly delays the absorption of a single 850 mg dose of metformin as shown by an ≈ 40% lower mean peak concentration and 25% lower AUC in plasma and a 35-minute prolongation of time to peak plasma concentration compared with the same strength administered under fasting conditions. The clinical relevance of these decreases is unknown.

Although the extent of metformin absorption (as measured by AUC) from the metformin ER tablet increases by ≈ 50% when given with food, there was no effect of food on C_{max} and T_{max}. High- and low-fat meals had the same effect on the pharmacokinetics of metformin ER.

Adverse Reactions

Metformin –

Most Common Adverse Reactions (> 5%) in a Placebo-Controlled Clinical Study of Metformin Monotherapy (%)		
Adverse reaction	Metformin monotherapy (n = 141)	Placebo (n = 145)
Diarrhea	53.2	11.7
Nausea/Vomiting	25.5	8.3
Flatulence	12.1	5.5

Most Common Adverse Reactions (> 5%) in a Placebo-Controlled Clinical Study of Metformin Monotherapy (%)		
Adverse reaction	Metformin monotherapy (n = 141)	Placebo (n = 145)
Asthenia	9.2	5.5
Ingestion	7.1	4.1
Abdominal discomfort	6.4	4.8
Headache	5.7	4.8

Diarrhea led to discontinuation of study medication in 6% of patients treated with metformin. Additionally, the following adverse reactions were reported in ≥ 1% to ≤ 5% of metformin patients and were more commonly reported with metformin than placebo: Abnormal stools, hypoglycemia, myalgia, lightheadedness, dyspnea, nail disorder, rash, sweating increased, taste disorder, chest discomfort, chills, flu syndrome, flushing, palpitation.

Metformin ER – In worldwide clinical trials, > 900 patients with type 2 diabetes have been treated with metformin ER in placebo- and active-controlled studies. In placebo-controlled trials, 781 patients were administered metformin ER and 195 patients received placebo. Adverse

METFORMIN HCl

reactions reported in > 5% of the metformin ER patients (n = 781), and that were more common in metformin ER- than placebo-treated patients (n = 195) were diarrhea (9.6%) and nausea/vomiting (6.5%).

Diarrhea led to discontinuation of study medication in 0.6% of patients treated with metformin ER. Additionally, the following adverse reactions were reported in ≥ 1% and ≤ 5% of metformin ER patients and were more commonly reported with metformin ER than placebo: Abdominal pain, constipation, abdominal distention, dyspepsia/heartburn, flatulence, dizziness, headache, upper respiratory tract infection, taste disturbance.

Overdosage

Hypoglycemia has not been seen even with ingestion of up to 85 g of metformin, although lactic acidosis has occurred in such circumstances (see Warnings). Metformin is dialyzable with a clearance of up to 170 mL/min under good hemodynamic conditions. Therefore, hemodialysis may be useful for removal of accumulated drug from patients in whom metformin overdosage is suspected.

Patient Information

Inform patients of the potential risks and advantages of metformin and of alternative modes of therapy. Also, inform them about the importance of adherence to dietary instructions, of a regular exercise program, and of regular testing of blood glucose, glycosylated hemoglobin, renal function, and hematologic parameters.

Explain the risks of lactic acidosis, its symptoms, and conditions that predispose to its development, as noted in the Warnings section. Advise patients to discontinue metformin immediately and to promptly notify their health practitioner if unexplained hyperventilation, myalgia, malaise, unusual somnolence, or other nonspecific symptoms occur. Once a patient is stabilized on metformin, GI symptoms, which are common during initiation of therapy, are unlikely to be drug related. Later occurrence of GI symptoms could be because of lactic acidosis or other serious disease.

Counsel patients against excessive alcohol intake while receiving metformin.

Inform patients that metformin ER must be swallowed whole and not crushed or chewed, and that the inactive ingredients may occasionally be eliminated in the feces as a soft mass resembling the original tablet.

REPAGLINIDE

Rx	**Prandin** (Novo Nordisk)	**Tablets:** 0.5 mg	White. In 100s, 500s, and 1000s.
		1 mg	Yellow. In 100s, 500s, and 1000s.
		2 mg	Peach. In 100s, 500s, and 1000s.

Indications

▶*Type 2 diabetes mellitus:* As an adjunct to diet and exercise to lower the blood glucose in patients with type 2 diabetes mellitus whose hyperglycemia cannot be controlled satisfactorily by diet and exercise alone.

▶*Combination therapy:* In combination with metformin or thiazolidinediones to lower blood glucose in patients whose hyperglycemia cannot be controlled by exercise, diet, and either agent alone.

Administration and Dosage

▶*Approved by the FDA:* December 23, 1997.

There is no fixed dosage regimen. Monitor the patient's blood glucose periodically to determine the minimum effective dose for the patient; to detect primary failure (ie, inadequate lowering of blood glucose at the maximum recommended dose of medication); and to detect secondary failure (ie, loss of adequate blood glucose-lowering response after an initial period of effectiveness). Glycosylated hemoglobin (HbA_{1c}) levels are of value in monitoring the patient's long-term response to therapy.

Short-term administration of repaglinide may be sufficient during periods of transient loss of control in patients usually well controlled on diet.

▶*Administration:* Repaglinide doses are usually taken within 15 minutes of the meal, but time may vary from immediately preceding the meal to as long as 30 minutes before the meal.

▶*Starting dose:* For patients not previously treated or whose HbA_{1c} is less than 8%, the starting dose is 0.5 mg with each meal. For patients previously treated with blood glucose-lowering agents and whose HbA_{1c} is 8% or more, the initial dose is 1 or 2 mg before each meal.

▶*Dose adjustment:* Determine dosing adjustments by blood glucose response, usually fasting blood glucose. Double the preprandial dose up to 4 mg with each meal until satisfactory blood glucose response is achieved. At least 1 week should elapse to assess response after each dose adjustment.

▶*Dose range:* Dose range is 0.5 to 4 mg taken with meals. Repaglinide may be dosed preprandially 2, 3, or 4 times daily in response to changes in the patient's meal pattern. Maximum recommended daily dose is 16 mg.

▶*Patient management:* Monitor long-term efficacy by measurement of HbA_{1c} levels approximately every 3 months. Failure to follow an appropriate dosage regimen may precipitate hypoglycemia or hyperglycemia. Patients who do not adhere to their prescribed dietary and drug regimen are more prone to exhibit unsatisfactory response to therapy including hypoglycemia. When hypoglycemia occurs in patients taking a combination of repaglinide and a thiazolidinedione or repaglinide and metformin, reduce the dose of repaglinide.

▶*Patients receiving other oral hypoglycemic agents:* When repaglinide is used to replace therapy with other oral hypoglycemic agents, it may be started the day after the final dose is given. Observe patients carefully for hypoglycemia because of potential overlapping of drug effects. When transferred from longer half-life sulfonylureas (eg, chlorpropamide), close monitoring may be indicated for up to 1 week or longer.

▶*Combination therapy:* If repaglinide monotherapy does not result in adequate glycemic control, metformin or a thiazolidinedione may be added. Or, if metformin or thiazolidinedione therapy does not provide adequate control, repaglinide may be added. The starting dose and dose adjustments for combination therapy are the same as repaglinide monotherapy. Carefully adjust the dose of each drug to determine the minimal dose required to achieve the desired pharmacologic effect. Failure to do so could result in an increase in the incidence of hypoglycemic episodes. Use appropriate monitoring of fasting plasma glucose (FPG) and HbA_{1c} measurements to ensure that the patient is not subjected to excessive drug exposure or increased probability of secondary drug failure.

If glucose control has not been achieved after a suitable trial of combination therapy, consider discontinuing these drugs and using insulin.

▶*Renal function impairment:* Patients with type 2 diabetes who have severe renal function impairment should initiate repaglinide with the 0.5 mg dose; subsequently, carefully titrate patients.

▶*Storage/Stability:* Do not store above 25°C (77°F). Protect from moisture; keep bottles tightly closed. Dispense in tight containers with safety closures.

Actions

▶*Pharmacology:* Repaglinide is a nonsulfonylurea hypoglycemic agent of the meglitinide class used in the management of type 2 diabetes mellitus. It lowers blood glucose levels by stimulating the release of insulin from the pancreas. This action is dependent on functioning beta cells in the pancreatic islets. Insulin release is glucose-dependent and diminishes at low glucose concentrations.

Repaglinide closes ATP-dependent potassium channels in the beta-cell membrane by binding at characterizable sites. This potassium channel blockade depolarizes the beta cell, which leads to an opening of calcium channels. The resulting increased calcium influx induces insulin secretion. The ion channel mechanism is highly tissue selective with low affinity for heart and skeletal muscle.

▶*Pharmacokinetics:*

Absorption – After oral administration, repaglinide is rapidly and completely absorbed from the GI tract. After single and multiple oral doses, peak plasma drug levels (C_{max}) occur within 1 hour (T_{max}). The mean absolute bioavailability is 56%. When given with food, the mean T_{max} was not changed, but the mean C_{max} and area under the time/plasma concentration curve (AUC) were decreased 20% and 12.4%, respectively.

Distribution – After IV dosing in healthy subjects, the volume of distribution at steady state was 31 L, and the total body clearance was 38 L/h. Protein binding and binding to human serum albumin was more than 98%.

Metabolism – Repaglinide is completely metabolized by oxidative biotransformation and direct conjugation with glucuronic acid after either an IV or oral dose. The major metabolites are an oxidized dicarboxylic acid (M2), the aromatic amine (M1), and the acyl glucuronide (M7). The cytochrome P450 enzyme system, specifically 3A4, is involved in the N-dealkylation of repaglinide to M2 and the further oxidation to M1. Metabolites do not contribute to the glucose-lowering effect.

Excretion – Repaglinide is rapidly eliminated from the blood stream with a half-life of about 1 hour. Within 96 hours after a single oral dose, about 90% was recovered in the feces and about 8% in the urine. Only 0.1% of the dose is cleared in the urine as parent compound. The major metabolite M2 accounted for 60% of the administered dose. Less than 2% of the parent drug was recovered in feces.

Special populations –
Gender: The AUC over a 0.5 to 4 mg dose range was 15% to 70% higher in females with type 2 diabetes. This difference was not reflected in the frequency of hypoglycemic episodes (male, 16%; female, 17%) or other adverse events. No change in general dosage recommendation appears indicated.

Renal function impairment: Single-dose and steady-state pharmacokinetics of repaglinide were compared between patients with type 2 diabetes and normal renal function (Ccr more than 80 mL/min), mild to moderate renal function impairment (Ccr = 40 to 80 mL/min), and severe renal function impairment (Ccr = 20 to 40 mL/min). AUC and C_{max} of repaglinide were similar in patients with normal and mild to moderately impaired renal function (mean values 56.7 ng/mL•h vs 57.2 ng/mL•h and 37.5 ng/mL vs 37.7 ng/mL, respectively). Patients with severely reduced renal function had elevated mean AUC and C_{max} values (98 ng/mL•h and 50.7 ng/mL, respectively), but this study showed only a weak correlation between repaglinide levels and creatinine clearance. Initial dose adjustment does not appear to be necessary for patients with mild to moderate renal dysfunction. However, patients with type 2 diabetes who have severe renal function impairment should initiate repaglinide with the 0.5 mg dose; subsequently, carefully titrate patients. Studies were not conducted in patients with creatinine clearances lower than 20 mL/min or patients with renal failure requiring hemodialysis.

Hepatic function impairment: In 12 healthy subjects and 12 patients with chronic liver disease (CLD), patients with moderate to severe impairment of liver function had higher and more prolonged serum concentrations of total and unbound repaglinide than healthy subjects: Healthy AUC, 91.6 ng/mL•h; C_{max}, 46.7 ng/mL; CLD AUC, 368.9 ng/mL•h; C_{max}, 105.4 ng/mL).

▶*Clinical trials:*

Repaglinide and metformin – Repaglinide was studied in combination with metformin in 83 patients not satisfactorily controlled with exercise, diet, and metformin alone. Combination therapy with repaglinide and metformin resulted in synergistic improvement in glycemic control compared with repaglinide or metformin monotherapy. HbA_{1c} was improved by 1% unit and FPG decreased by an additional 35 mg/dL.

Repaglinide and Metformin Therapy: Mean Changes from Baseline in Glycemic Parameters and Weight after 4 to 5 Months of Treatment[a]			
	Repaglinide (N = 28)	Metformin (N = 27)	Combination (N = 27)
Median final dose (mg/day)	12	1500	6 (repaglinide) 1500 (metformin)
HbA_{1c} (% units)	−0.38	−0.33	−1.41[b]
FPG (mg/dL)	8.8	−4.5	−39.2[b]
Weight (kg)	3	−0.9	2.4[c]

[a] Based on intent-to-treat analysis.
[b] $P < 0.05$ for pairwise comparisons with repaglinide and metformin.
[c] $P < 0.05$ for pairwise comparison with metformin.

REPAGLINIDE

Repaglinide and pioglitazone – A combination therapy regimen of repaglinide and pioglitazone was compared with monotherapy with either agent alone in a 24-week trial that enrolled 246 patients previously treated with sulfonylurea or metformin monotherapy (HbA_{1c} greater than 7%). Numbers of patients treated were the following: Repaglinide (N = 61), pioglitazone (N = 62), combination (N = 123). Repaglinide dosage was titrated during the first 12 weeks followed by a 12-week maintenance period. Combination therapy resulted in significantly greater improvement in glycemic control as compared with monotherapy. The changes from baseline for completers in FPG (mg/dL) and HbA_{1c} (%), respectively were as follows: −39.8 and −0.1 for repaglinide, −35.3 and −0.1 for pioglitazone, and −92.4 and −1.9 for the combination. In this study where pioglitazone dosage was kept constant, the combination therapy group showed dose-sparing effects with respect to repaglinide. The greater efficacy response of the combination group was achieved at a lower daily repaglinide dosage than in the repaglinide monotherapy group. Mean weight increases associated with combination, repaglinide, and pioglitazone therapy were 5.5, 0.3, and 2 kg, respectively.

Repaglinide and rosiglitazone – A combination therapy regimen of repaglinide and rosiglitazone was compared with monotherapy with either agent alone in a 24-week trial that enrolled 252 patients previously treated with sulfonylurea or metformin (HbA_{1c} more than 7%). Combination therapy resulted in significantly greater improvement in glycemic control as compared with a monotherapy. The glycemic effects of the combination therapy were dose-sparing with respect to total daily repaglinide dosage and total daily rosiglitazone dosage. A greater efficacy response of the combination therapy group was achieved with half the median daily dose of repaglinide and rosiglitazone, as compared with the respective monotherapy groups. Weight change associated with combination therapy was greater than that of repaglinide monotherapy.

Mean Changes from Baseline in Glycemic Parameters and Weight in a 24-week Repaglinide/Rosiglitazone Combination Study[a]

	Repaglinide (N = 63)	Rosiglitazone (N = 62)	Combination (N = 127)
Median final dose (mg/day)	12	8	6 (repaglinide) 4 (rosiglitazone)
HbA_{1c} (%)			
Baseline	9.3	9	9.1
Change by 24 weeks	−0.17	−0.56	−1.43[b]
FPG (mg/dL)			
Baseline	269	252	257
Change by 24 weeks	−54	−67	−94[b]
Change in weight (kg)	+1.3	+3.3	+4.5[c]

[a] Based on intent-to-treat analysis.
[b] $P \le 0.001$ for comparison to either monotherapy.
[c] $P < 0.001$ for comparison to repaglinide.

Contraindications

Diabetic ketoacidosis, with or without coma (treat with insulin); type 1 diabetes; hypersensitivity to the drug or its inactive ingredients.

Warnings

➤*Diet/Exercise:* In initiating treatment for patients with type 2 diabetes, emphasize diet and exercise as the primary form of treatment. Caloric restriction, weight loss, and exercise are essential in the obese diabetic patient. In addition to regular physical activity, identify cardiovascular risk factors and take corrective measures.

Use of repaglinide must be viewed as a treatment in addition to diet and not as a substitute for diet or as a convenient mechanism for avoiding dietary restraint. Furthermore, loss of blood glucose control on diet alone may be transient, thus requiring only short-term administration of repaglinide.

➤*Diabetic complications:* In patients with type 1 diabetes, the Diabetes Control and Complications Trial (DCCT) demonstrated that improved glycemic control, as reflected by HbA_{1c} and fasting glucose levels, was associated with a reduction in the diabetic complications of retinopathy, neuropathy, and nephropathy. However, controlling the blood glucose in type 2 diabetes has not been established to be effective in preventing the long-term cardiovascular and neural complications of diabetes. Nonetheless, improved glycemic control appears to be important in many patients with type 2 diabetes because it is presumed that the mechanics by which glucose causes complications is the same in both forms of diabetes.

➤*Hepatic function impairment:* Patients with impaired liver function may be exposed to higher concentrations of repaglinide and its associated metabolites than would patients with normal liver function receiving usual doses. Therefore, use repaglinide cautiously in patients with impaired liver function. Utilize longer intervals between dose adjustments to allow full assessment of response.

➤*Carcinogenesis:* In male rats, there was an increased incidence of benign adenomas of the thyroid and liver. The relevance of these findings to humans is unclear.

➤*Elderly:* There was no increase in frequency or severity of hypoglycemia in older subjects. Greater sensitivity of some older individuals to repaglinide therapy cannot be ruled out.

➤*Pregnancy: Category C.* Offspring of rat dams exposed to repaglinide at 15 times clinical exposure on a mg/m² basis during days 17 to 22 of gestation and during lactation developed nonteratogenic skeletal deformities consisting of shortening, thickening, and bending of the humerus during the postnatal period.

Safety in pregnant women has not been established. Use during pregnancy only if clearly needed. Because recent information suggests that abnormal blood glucose levels during pregnancy are associated with a higher incidence of congenital abnormalities, many experts recommend that insulin be used during pregnancy to maintain blood glucose levels as close to normal as possible.

➤*Lactation:* In rat reproduction studies, measurable levels of repaglinide were detected in the breast milk of dams and lowered blood glucose levels were observed in the pups. Cross-fostering studies indicated that skeletal changes could be induced in control pups nursed by treated dams. It is not known whether repaglinide is excreted in human breast milk. Because the potential for hypoglycemia in nursing infants may exist, decide whether to discontinue repaglinide or discontinue breastfeeding. If repaglinide is discontinued and if diet alone is inadequate for controlling blood glucose, consider insulin therapy.

➤*Children:* No studies have been performed in pediatric patients.

Precautions

➤*Monitoring:* Periodically monitor fasting blood glucose and HbA_{1c} levels with a goal of decreasing these levels towards the normal range. During dose adjustment, fasting glucose can be used to determine response. HbA_{1c} may be especially useful for evaluating long-term glycemic control. Postprandial glucose level testing may be clinically helpful in patients whose premeal blood glucose levels are satisfactory but whose overall glycemic control HbA_{1c} is inadequate.

➤*Hypoglycemia:* All oral hypoglycemic agents are capable of producing hypoglycemia. Proper patient selection, dosage, and instructions to the patients are important to avoid hypoglycemic episodes. Hepatic insufficiency may cause elevated repaglinide blood levels and may diminish gluconeogenic capacity, both of which increase the risk of serious hypoglycemia. Elderly, debilitated, or malnourished patients, and those with adrenal, pituitary, hepatic, or severe renal insufficiency are particularly susceptible to the hypoglycemic action of glucose-lowering drugs.

Hypoglycemia may be difficult to recognize in the elderly and in people taking beta-adrenergic blocking drugs. Hypoglycemia is more likely to occur when caloric intake is deficient, after severe or prolonged exercise, when alcohol is ingested, or when more than one glucose-lowering agent is used.

The frequency of hypoglycemia is greater in patients with type 2 diabetes who have not been previously treated with oral hypoglycemic agents or whose HbA_{1c} is less than 8%. Administer with meals to lessen the risk of hypoglycemia.

Patients taking repaglinide should not start taking gemfibrozil; patients taking gemfibrozil should not start taking repaglinide. Concomitant use may result in enhanced and prolonged blood glucose-lowering effects of repaglinide. Use caution in patients already on repaglinide. Monitor blood glucose levels. Repaglinide dose adjustment may be needed. Coadministration of 600 mg gemfibrozil and a single dose of 0.25 mg repaglinide (after 3 days of twice-daily 600 mg gemfibrozil) resulted in an 8.1-fold higher repaglinide AUC and prolonged repaglinide half-life from 1.3 to 3.7 h.

Gemfibrozil and itraconazole have a synergistic metabolic inhibitory effect on repaglinide. Therefore, patients taking repaglinide and gemfibrozil should not take itraconazole. Coadministration with itraconazole and a single dose of 0.25 mg repaglinide (on the third day of a regimen of 200 mg initial dose, twice-daily 100 mg itraconazole) resulted in a 1.4-fold higher repaglinide AUC. Coadministration of both gemfibrozil and itraconazole with repaglinide resulted in a 19-fold higher repaglinide AUC and prolonged repaglinide half-life to 6.1 h. Plasma repaglinide concentration at 7 h increased 28.6-fold with gemfibrozil coadministration and 70.4-fold with the gemfibrozil-itraconazole combination.

➤*Secondary failure:* It may be necessary to discontinue repaglinide and administer insulin if the patient is exposed to stress (eg, fever, trauma, infection, surgery). The effectiveness of any hypoglycemic agent in lowering blood glucose to a desired level decreases in many patients over a period of time, which may be caused by progression of the severity of diabetes or diminished responsiveness to the drug. This phenomenon is known as secondary failure, to distinguish it from primary failure in which the drug is ineffective in an individual patient when the drug is first given. Assess adequate adjustment of dose and adherence to diet before classifying a patient as a secondary failure. During maintenance programs, discontinue repaglinide if satisfactory lowering of blood glucose is no longer achieved.

REPAGLINIDE

Drug Interactions

Repaglinide Drug Interactions

Precipitant drug	Object drug*		Description
Beta blockers Chloramphenicol Coumarins MAOIs NSAIDs Probenecid Salicylates Sulfonamides	Repaglinide	↑	The action of repaglinide may be potentiated by certain drugs, including those highly protein bound. Observe for hypoglycemia and loss of glycemic control.
Calcium channel blockers Corticosteroids Estrogens Isoniazid Nicotinic acid Oral contraceptives Phenothiazines Phenytoin Sympathomimetics Thiazides and other diuretics Thyroid products	Repaglinide	↓	Certain drugs tend to produce hyperglycemia and may lead to loss of glycemic control. Observe closely.
CYP 450 inhibitors (eg, ketoconazole, macrolide antibiotics)	Repaglinide	↑	Coadministration may increase repaglinide plasma levels because of inhibition of its metabolism. Monitor blood glucose and adjust repaglinide dose as needed.
CYP 450 inducers (eg, rifampin, barbiturates, carbamazepine, clarithromycin)	Repaglinide	↓	Coadministration may decrease repaglinide plasma levels because of induction of its metabolism. Monitor blood glucose and adjust repaglinide dose as needed.
Gemfibrozil	Repaglinide	↑	Concomitant use may result in enhanced and prolonged blood glucose-lowering effects of repaglinide. Use caution in patients already on repaglinide. Monitor blood glucose levels. Repaglinide dose adjustment may be needed (see Precautions).
Gemfibrozil and Itraconazole	Repaglinide	↑	Gemfibrozil and itraconazole have a synergistic metabolic inhibitory effect on repaglinide. Therefore, patients taking repaglinide and gemfibrozil should not take itraconazole (see Precautions).
Levonorgestrel and ethinyl estradiol	Repaglinide	↑	Coadministration of a combination tablet of 0.15 mg levonorgestrel and 0.03 mg ethinyl estradiol administered once daily for 21 days with 2 mg repaglinide administered 3 times/day on days 1 to 4 and a single dose on day 5 resulted in 20% increases in repaglinide, levonorgestrel, and ethinyl estradiol C$_{max}$. Ethinyl estradiol AUC parameters were increased by 20%, while repaglinide and levonorgestrel AUC values remained unchanged.
Repaglinide	Levonorgestrel and ethinyl estradiol		
Simvastatin	Repaglinide	↑	Coadministration of 20 mg simvastatin and a single dose of 2 mg repaglinide (after 4 days of once-daily 20 mg simvastatin and 2 mg repaglinide 3 times/day) resulted in a 26% increase in repaglinide C$_{max}$.

* ↑ = Object drug increased. ↓ = Object drug decreased.

➤*Drug/Food interactions:* When given with food, mean C$_{max}$ and AUC of repaglinide were decreased 20% and 12.4%, respectively. Administer repaglinide before meals.

Adverse Reactions

Throughout 1 year in clinical trials, 13% of repaglinide patients discontinued therapy because of adverse events vs 14% of sulfonylurea patients. The most common adverse events leading to discontinuation were hyperglycemia, hypoglycemia, and related symptoms. Mild or moderate hypoglycemia occurred in 16% of repaglinide patients, 20% with glyburide, and 19% with glipizide. The adverse event profile of repaglinide was generally comparable with that for sulfonylureas.

Repaglinide Adverse Reactions (%)

Adverse reaction	Placebo study		Active study	
	Repaglinide (n = 352)	Placebo (n = 108)	Repaglinide (n = 1228)	SU[a] (n = 498)
GI				
Constipation	3	2	2	3
Diarrhea	5	2	4	6
Dyspepsia	2	2	4	2
Nausea	5	5	3	2
Vomiting	3	3	2	1
Respiratory				
Bronchitis	2	1	6	7
Rhinitis	3	3	7	8
Sinusitis	6	2	3	4
Upper respiratory tract infection	16	8	10	10
Miscellaneous				
Allergy	2	0	1	< 1
Arthralgia	6	3	3	4
Back pain	5	4	6	7
Chest pain	3	1	2	1
Headache	11	10	9	8
Hypoglycemia	31	7	16	20
Paresthesia	3	3	2	1
Tooth disorder	2	0	< 1	< 1
Urinary tract infection	2	1	3	3

[a] SU = sulfonylurea.

Cardiovascular events also occur commonly in patients with type 2 diabetes. In 1-year comparator trials, the incidence of individual events was 1% or less except for chest pain and angina (both 1.8%). The overall incidence of other cardiovascular events (hypertension, abnormal EKG, MI, arrhythmias, palpitations) was 1% or less and not different for repaglinide and the comparator drugs. The incidence of serious cardiovascular adverse events added together, including ischemia, was slightly higher for repaglinide (4%) than for sulfonylureas (3%).

Serious Repaglinide Cardiovascular Events (%)

	Repaglinide (n = 1228)	SU[a] (n = 498)
Serious CV[b] events	4	3
Cardiac ischemic events	2	2
Deaths due to CV events	0.5	0.4

[a] Glyburide and glipizide.
[b] CV = Cardiovascular.

Infrequent adverse events (less than 1%) – Less common adverse clinical or laboratory events observed in clinical trials included elevated liver enzymes, thrombocytopenia, leukopenia, and anaphylactoid reactions (1 patient).

Combination therapy with thiazolidinediones – During 24-week treatment clinical trials with repaglinide-rosiglitazone or repaglinide-pioglitazone combination therapy (a total of 250 patients in combination therapy), hypoglycemia (blood glucose less than 50 mg/dL) occurred in 7% of combination therapy patients in comparison with 7% for repaglinide monotherapy, and 2% for thiazolidinedione monotherapy.

Peripheral edema was reported in 12 of 250 repaglinide-thiazolidinedione combination therapy patients and 3 of 124 thiazolidinedione monotherapy patients, with no cases reported in these trials for repaglinide monotherapy. When corrected for dropout rates of the treatment groups, the percentage of patients having events of peripheral edema per 24 weeks of treatment were 5% for repaglinide-thiazolidinedione combination therapy, and 4% for thiazolidinedione monotherapy. There were reports in 2 of 250 patients (0.8%) treated with repaglinide-thiazolidinedione therapy of episodes of edema with CHF. Both patients had a prior history of coronary artery disease and recovered after treatment with diuretics.

Mean change in weight from baseline was + 4.9 kg for repaglinide-thiazolidinedione combination therapy. There were no patients on repaglinide-thiazolidinedione combination therapy who had elevations of liver transaminases (defined as 3 times the upper limit of normal).

➤*Postmarketing:* Although no causal relationship has been established, postmarketing experience includes reports of the following rare adverse events: alopecia, hemolytic anemia, pancreatitis, Stevens-Johnson syndrome, and severe hepatic dysfunction.

Overdosage

➤*Symptoms:* In a clinical trial, patients received increasing doses of repaglinide up to 80 mg/day for 14 days. There were few adverse effects other than those associated with the intended effect of lowering blood glucose.

REPAGLINIDE

►*Treatment:* Aggressively treat hypoglycemic symptoms without loss of consciousness or neurologic findings with oral glucose and adjustments in drug dosage and/or meal patterns. Close monitoring may continue until it is ensured that the patient is out of danger. Closely monitor patients for a minimum of 24 to 48 hours, because hypoglycemia may recur after apparent clinical recovery. There is no evidence that repaglinide is hemodialyzable. Severe hypoglycemic reactions with coma, seizure, or other neurological impairment occur infrequently but constitute medical emergencies requiring immediate hospitalization. If hypoglycemic coma is diagnosed or suspected, give the patient a rapid IV injection of concentrated (50%) glucose solution. Follow with a continuous infusion of a more dilute (10%) glucose solution at a rate that will maintain the blood glucose at a level of about 100 mg/dL.

Patient Information

Inform patients about the importance of adherence to dietary instructions, a regular exercise program, and regular testing of blood glucose and HbA_{1c}.

Explain to patients and responsible family members the risks of hypoglycemia, its symptoms and treatment, conditions that predispose to its development, and coadministration of other glucose-lowering drugs.

Instruct patients to take repaglinide before meals (2, 3, or 4 times/day). Doses are usually taken within 15 minutes of the meal, but time may vary from immediately preceding the meal to as long as 30 minutes before the meal. Instruct patients who skip a meal (or add an extra meal) to skip (or add) a dose for that meal.

NATEGLINIDE

Rx	**Starlix** (Novartis)	**Tablets:** 60 mg	Lactose. (STARLIX 60). Pink. In 100s and 500s.
		120 mg	Lactose. (STARLIX 120). Yellow, oval. In 100s and 500s.

Indications

►*Type 2 diabetes mellitus:*

Monotherapy – To lower blood glucose in patients with type 2 diabetes whose hyperglycemia cannot be adequately controlled by diet and physical exercise and who have not been chronically treated with other antidiabetic agents.

Combination therapy – In patients whose hyperglycemia is inadequately controlled with metformin or after a therapeutic response to a thiazolidinedione, nateglinide may be added to, but not substituted for, those drugs.

Do not switch patients whose hyperglycemia is not adequately controlled with glyburide or other insulin secretagogues to nateglinide; do not add nateglinide to their treatment regimen.

Administration and Dosage

►*Approved by the FDA:* December 22, 2000.

►*Monotherapy and combination with metformin or a thiazolidinedione:* The recommended starting and maintenance dose of nateglinide, alone or in combination with metformin, is 120 mg 3 times per day before meals.

The 60 mg dose of nateglinide, alone or in combination with metformin or a thiazolidinedione, may be used in patients who are near goal glycosylated hemoglobin (HbA_{1c}) when treatment is initiated.

Take 1 to 30 minutes prior to meals.

►*Storage/Stability:* Store at 25°C (77°F); excursions permitted to 15° to 30°C (59° to 86°F). Dispense in a tight container.

Actions

►*Pharmacology:* Nateglinide is an amino-acid derivative that lowers blood glucose levels by stimulating insulin secretion from the pancreas. This action is dependent upon functioning beta-cells in the pancreatic islets. Nateglinide interacts with the ATP-sensitive potassium ($K+_{ATP}$) channel on pancreatic beta-cells. The subsequent depolarization of the beta cell opens the calcium channel, producing calcium influx and insulin secretion. The extent of insulin release is glucose-dependent and diminishes at low glucose levels. Nateglinide is highly tissue selective with low affinity for heart and skeletal muscle.

Nateglinide stimulates pancreatic insulin secretion within 20 minutes of oral administration. When nateglinide is dosed 3 times/day before meals, there is a rapid rise in plasma insulin, with peak levels approximately 1 hour after dosing and a fall to baseline by 4 hours after dosing.

►*Pharmacokinetics:*

Absorption – Following oral administration immediately prior to a meal, nateglinide is rapidly absorbed with mean peak plasma drug concentrations (C_{max}) generally occurring within 1 hour (T_{max}) after dosing. When administered to patients with type 2 diabetes over the dosage range 60 to 240 mg 3 times/day for 1 week, nateglinide demonstrated linear pharmacokinetics for AUC (area under the time/plasma concentration curve) and C_{max}. T_{max} also was found to be independent of dose in this patient population. Absolute bioavailability is estimated to be approximately 73%. When given with or after meals, the extent of nateglinide absorption (AUC) remains unaffected. However, there is a delay in the rate of absorption characterized by a decrease in C_{max} and a delay in the time to peak plasma concentration T_{max}. Plasma profiles are characterized by multiple plasma concentration peaks when nateglinide is administered under fasting conditions. This effect is diminished when nateglinide is taken prior to a meal.

Distribution – Based on data following IV administration of nateglinide, the steady-state volume of distribution is estimated to be approximately 10 L in healthy subjects. Nateglinide is extensively bound (98%) to serum proteins, primarily serum albumin, and to a lesser extent α_1 acid glycoprotein. The extent of serum protein binding is independent of drug concentration over the test range of 0.1 to 10 mcg/mL.

Metabolism – Nateglinide is metabolized by the mixed-function oxidase system prior to elimination. The major routes of metabolism are hydroxylation followed by glucuronide conjugation. The major metabolites are less potent antidiabetic agents than nateglinide. The isoprene minor metabolite possesses potency similar to the parent compound nateglinide.

In vitro data demonstrate that nateglinide is predominantly metabolized by cytochrome P450 isoenzymes CYP2C9 (70%) and CYP3A4 (30%).

Excretion – Nateglinide and its metabolites are rapidly and completely eliminated following oral administration. Within 6 hours after dosing, approximately 75% of the administered ^{14}C-nateglinide was recovered in the urine. Eighty-three percent of the ^{14}C-nateglinide was excreted in the urine with an additional 10% eliminated in the feces. Approximately 16% of the ^{14}C-nateglinide was excreted in the urine as parent compound. In all studies of healthy volunteers and patients with type 2 diabetes, nateglinide plasma concentrations declined rapidly with an average elimination half-life of approximately 1.5 hours. Consistent with this short elimination half-life, there was no apparent accumulation of nateglinide upon multiple dosing of up to 240 mg 3 times/day for 7 days.

Special populations –

Renal function impairment: Patients with type 2 diabetes and renal failure on dialysis exhibited reduced overall drug exposure; however, hemodialysis patients also experienced reductions in plasma protein binding compared with the matched healthy volunteers.

Hepatic function impairment: The peak and total exposure of nateglinide in nondiabetic subjects with mild hepatic insufficiency were increased 30% compared with matched healthy subjects. Use nateglinide with caution in patients with chronic liver disease.

►*Clinical trials:* In a 24-week, double-blind, active-controlled trial, patients with type 2 diabetes who had been on a sulfonylurea for at least 3 months and who had a baseline glycosylated hemoglobin A_{1c} (HbA_{1c}) of at least 6.5% were randomized to receive 60 or 120 mg nateglinide 3 times/day before meals or 10 mg glyburide once daily. Patients randomized to nateglinide had significant increases in mean HbA_{1c} and mean fasting plasma glucose (FPG) at endpoint compared with patients randomized to glyburide.

In another randomized, double-blind, 24-week, active- and placebo-controlled study, patients with type 2 diabetes were randomized to receive 120 mg nateglinide 3 times/day before meals, 500 mg metformin 3 times/day, a combination of 120 mg nateglinide 3 times/day before meals and 500 mg metformin 3 times/day, or placebo. Fifty-seven percent of patients were previously untreated with oral antidiabetic therapy. The reductions in mean HbA_{1c} and mean FPG at endpoint with metformin monotherapy were significantly greater than the reductions in these variables with nateglinide monotherapy. Among the subset of patients naive to antidiabetic therapy, the reductions in mean HbA_{1c} and mean FBG for nateglinide monotherapy were similar to those for metformin monotherapy. Among the subset of patients previously treated with other antidiabetic agents, primarily glyburide, HbA_{1c} in the nateglinide group increased slightly from baseline, whereas HbA_{1c} was reduced in the metformin monotherapy group (see the following table).

The combination of nateglinide and metformin resulted in statistically significantly greater reductions in HbA_{1c} and FPG compared with nateglinide or metformin monotherapy. Nateglinide, alone or in combination with metformin, significantly reduced the prandial glucose elevation from premeal to 2 hours postmeal compared with placebo and metformin alone. In this study, 1 episode of severe hypoglycemia (plasma glucose up to 36 mg/dL) was reported in a patient receiving the combination of nateglinide and metformin, and 4 episodes of severe hypoglycemia were reported in a single patient in the metformin treatment arm. No patient experienced an episode of hypoglycemia that required third party assistance.

NATEGLINIDE

Endpoint Results for a 24-week Study of Nateglinide Monotherapy and Combination with Metformin				
	Placebo	Nateglinide 120 mg 3 times/day before meals	Metformin 500 mg 3 times/day	Nateglinide 120 mg before meals plus metformin[a]
HbA$_{1c}$ (%)				
All	n = 160	n = 171	n = 172	n = 162
Baseline (mean)	8.3	8.3	8.4	8.4
Change from baseline (mean)	+0.4	-0.4[b,c]	-0.8[c]	-1.5
Difference from placebo	—	-0.8[d]	-1.2[d]	-1.9[d]
Naïve	n = 98	n = 99	n = 98	n = 81
Baseline (mean)	8.2	8.1	8.3	8.2
Change from baseline (mean)	+0.3	-0.7[c]	-0.8[c]	-1.6
Difference from placebo	—	-1[d]	-1.1[d]	-1.9[d]
Non-naïve	n = 62	n = 72	n = 74	n = 81
Baseline (mean)	8.3	8.5	8.7	8.7
Change from baseline (mean)	+0.6	+0.004[b,c]	-0.8[c]	-1.4
Difference from placebo	—	-0.6[d]	-1.4[d]	-2[d]
FPG (mg/dL)				
All	n = 166	n = 173	n = 174	n = 167
Baseline (mean)	194	196.5	196	197.7
Change from baseline (mean)	+8	-13.1[b,c]	-30[c]	-44.9
Difference from placebo	—	-21.1[d]	-38[d]	-52.9[d]
Weight (kg)				
All	n = 160	n = 169	n = 169	n = 160
Baseline (mean)	85	85	86	87.4
Change from baseline (mean)	-0.4	+0.9[b,c]	-0.1	+0.2
Difference from placebo	—	+1.3[d]	+0.3	+0.6

[a] Metformin was administered 3 times/day.
[b] $P \le 0.03$ vs metformin.
[c] $P \le 0.05$ vs combination.
[d] $P \le 0.05$ vs placebo.

Contraindications

Known hypersensitivity to the drug or its inactive ingredients; type 1 diabetes; diabetic ketoacidosis (this condition should be treated with insulin).

Warnings

▶*Diet/Exercise:* In initiating treatment for patients with type 2 diabetes, emphasize diet and exercise as the primary form of treatment. Caloric restriction, weight loss, and exercise are essential in the obese diabetic patient. In addition to regular physical activity, identify cardiovascular risk factors and take corrective measures.

Use of nateglinide must be viewed as a treatment in addition to diet and not as a substitute for diet or as a convenient mechanism for avoiding dietary restraint.

▶*Hepatic function impairment:* Use nateglinide with caution in patients with chronic liver disease. Use with caution in patients with moderate to severe liver disease because such patients have not been studied.

▶*Pregnancy: Category C.* Nateglinide was not teratogenic in rats at doses up to 1000 mg/kg (approximately 60 times the human therapeutic exposure with a recommended nateglinide dose of 120 mg 3 times/day before meals). In the rabbit, embryonic development was adversely affected and the incidence of gallbladder agenesis or small gallbladder was increased at a dose of 500 mg/kg (approximately 40 times the human therapeutic exposure with a recommended nateglinide dose of 120 mg 3 times/day before meals). There are no adequate and well-controlled studies in pregnant women. Do not use nateglinide during pregnancy.

▶*Lactation:* Studies in lactating rats showed that nateglinide is excreted in the milk; the AUC$_{0-48hr}$ ratio in milk to plasma was approximately 1:4. During the peri- and postnatal period, body weights were lower in offspring of rats administered nateglinide at 1000 mg/kg (approximately 60 times the human therapeutic exposure with a recommended nateglinide dose of 120 mg 3 times/day before meals). It is not known whether nateglinide is excreted in human milk. Because many drugs are excreted in human milk, do not administer nateglinide to a nursing woman.

▶*Children:* The safety and efficacy of nateglinide in pediatric patients have not been established.

Precautions

▶*Monitoring:* Periodically assess response to therapies with glucose values and HbA$_{1c}$ levels.

▶*Hypoglycemia:* All oral blood glucose-lowering drugs that are absorbed systemically are capable of producing hypoglycemia. The frequency of hypoglycemia is related to the severity of the diabetes, the level of glycemic control, and other patient characteristics. Geriatric patients, malnourished patients, and those with adrenal or pituitary insufficiency or severe renal impairment are more susceptible to the glucose-lowering effect of these treatments. The risk of hypoglycemia

may be increased by strenuous physical exercise, ingestion of alcohol, insufficient caloric intake on an acute or chronic basis, or combinations with other oral antidiabetic agents. Hypoglycemia may be difficult to recognize in patients with autonomic neuropathy and/or those who use beta-blockers. Administer nateglinide before meals to reduce the risk of hypoglycemia. Patients who skip meals should also skip their scheduled dose of nateglinide to reduce the risk of hypoglycemia.

▶*Secondary failure:* Transient loss of glycemic control may occur with fever, infection, trauma, or surgery. Insulin therapy may be needed instead of nateglinide therapy at such times. Secondary failure, or reduced effectiveness of nateglinide over a period of time, may occur.

Drug Interactions

▶*Cytochrome P450:* In vitro metabolism studies indicate that nateglinide is predominantly metabolized by the cytochrome P450 isozyme CYP2C9 (70%) and to a lesser extent CYP3A4 (30%). Nateglinide is a potential inhibitor of the CYP2C9 isoenzyme in vivo as indicated by its ability to inhibit the in vitro metabolism of tolbutamide. Inhibition of CYP3A4 metabolic reactions was not detected in in vitro experiments.

Certain drugs, including nonsteroidal anti-inflammatory agents (NSAIDs), salicylates, monoamine oxidase inhibitors (MAOIs), and nonselective beta-adrenergic blocking agents, may potentiate the hypoglycemic action of nateglinide and other oral antidiabetic drugs.

Certain drugs including thiazides, corticosteroids, thyroid products, and sympathomimetics may reduce the hypoglycemic action of nateglinide and other oral antidiabetic drugs.

When these drugs are administered to or withdrawn from patients receiving nateglinide, closely observe the patient for changes in glycemic control.

Nateglinide Drug Interactions			
Precipitant drug	Object drug[*]		Description
Beta-adrenergic blockers, nonselective MAOIs NSAIDS Salicylates	Nateglinide	↑	These drugs may potentiate the hypoglycemic effects of nateglinide and other oral antidiabetic agents. Closely monitor blood glucose when these agents are started or stopped.
Corticosteroids Sympatho-mimetics Thiazides Thyroid products	Nateglinide	↓	These agents may reduce the hypoglycemic action of nateglinide and other oral antidiabetic agents. Closely monitor blood glucose when these agents are started or stopped.
Rifamycins (eg, rifampin)	Nateglinide	↓	Nateglinide plasma concentrations and pharmacologic effects may be decreased with coadministration. Closely monitor blood glucose levels when starting and stopping rifamycin therapy and adjust nateglinide dose as necessary.

[*] ↑ = Object drug increased. ↓ = Object drug decreased.

▶*Drug/Food interactions:* Peak plasma levels were significantly reduced when nateglinide was administered 10 minutes prior to a liquid meal.

Adverse Reactions

Hypoglycemia was relatively uncommon in all treatment arms of the clinical trials. Only 0.3% of nateglinide patients discontinued because of hypoglycemia.

Adverse Events in Nateglinide Monotherapy Trials (≥ 2%)		
Adverse reaction	Nateglinide (n = 1441)	Placebo (n = 458)
Respiratory		
Bronchitis	2.7	2.6
Coughing	2.4	2.2
Upper respiratory tract infection	10.5	8.1
Miscellaneous		
Accidental trauma	2.9	1.7
Arthropathy	3.3	2.2
Back pain	4	3.7
Diarrhea	3.2	3.1
Dizziness	3.6	2.2
Flu symptoms	3.6	2.6
Hypoglycemia	2.4	0.4

▶*Lab test abnormalities:* There were increases in mean uric acid levels for patients treated with nateglinide alone, nateglinide in combination with metformin, metformin alone, and glyburide alone. The respective differences from placebo were 0.29, 0.45, 0.28, and 0.19 mg/dL. The clinical significance of these findings is unknown.

▶*Postmarketing:* Rare cases of hypersensitivity reactions, such as rash, itching, and urticaria, have been reported.

NATEGLINIDE

Overdosage

➤*Symptoms:* In a clinical study in patients with type 2 diabetes, nateglinide was administered in increasing doses up to 720 mg/day for 7 days and there were no clinically significant adverse events reported. There have been no instances of overdose with nateglinide in clinical trials. However, an overdose may result in an exaggerated glucose-lowering effect with the development of hypoglycemic symptoms.

➤*Treatment:* Treat hypoglycemic symptoms without loss of consciousness or neurological findings with oral glucose and adjustments in dosage and/or meal patterns. Treat severe hypoglycemic reactions (coma, seizure, or other neurological symptoms) with IV glucose. As nateglinide is highly protein bound, dialysis is not an efficient means of removing it from the blood.

Patient Information

Inform patients about the importance of adherence to dietary instructions, of a regular exercise program, and of regular testing of blood glucose and HbA_{1c}.

Inform patients of the potential risks and benefits of nateglinide and of alternative modes of therapy. Explain the risks and management of hypoglycemia.

Instruct patients to take nateglinide 1 to 30 minutes before ingesting a meal, but to skip their scheduled dose if they skip the meal to reduce the risk of hypoglycemia.

Thiazolidinediones

Indications

>*Type 2 diabetes:* Monotherapy as an adjunct to diet and exercise to improve glycemic control.

In combination with metformin, insulin, or a sulfonylurea when diet, exercise, and a single agent do not result in adequate glycemic control.

Actions

>*Pharmacology:* **Rosiglitazone** and **pioglitazone**, members of the thiazolidinediones class of antidiabetic agents, improve glycemic control by improving insulin sensitivity. They depend on the presence of insulin for their mechanism of action. Studies indicate that they improve sensitivity to insulin in muscle and adipose tissue and inhibit hepatic gluconeogenesis. Thiazolidinediones are highly selective and potent agonists for the peroxisome proliferator-activated receptor-gamma (PPARγ). PPAR receptors are found in adipose tissue, skeletal muscle, and liver. Activation of PPARγ nuclear receptors regulates the transcription of insulin-responsive genes involved in the control of glucose production, transport, and utilization and participates in the regulation of fatty acid metabolism.

>*Pharmacokinetics:*

Pharmacokinetics of Thiazolidinediones		
Parameters	Pioglitazone	Rosiglitazone
Absorption		
Bioavailability	—	99%
C_{max}^a	—	1 mg[b]: 76 ng/mL 2 mg[b]: 156 ng/mL 8 mg[b]: 598 ng/mL 8 mg[c]: 432 ng/mL
T_{max}	2 hr[b] 3-4 hr[c]	1 hr
Food effect	Delays time to peak concentration; does not alter extent of absorption	28% decrease in C_{max} and delay in T_{max} (1.75 hr); no overall change in AUC
Distribution		
Volume of distribution	≈ 0.63 L/kg[a]	17.6 L
Protein binding	> 99%	≈ 99.8%
Metabolism		
Mechanism	Hydroxylation, oxidation, CYP2C8, CYP3A4, CYP1A1	N-demethylation, hydroxylation, conjugation CYP2C8, CYP2C9 (minor)
Active metabolites	MII[d], MIII[e], MIV[d]	
Excretion		
Site	Urine (15 to 30%), feces	Urine (64%), feces (23%)
Elimination half-life	Pioglitazone: 3 to 7 hr Total pioglitazone: 16 to 24 hr	3 to 4 hr
Oral clearance	5 to 7 L/hr	1 mg[b]: 3.03 L/hr 2 mg[b]: 2.89 L/hr 8 mg[b]: 2.85 L/hr 8 mg[c]: 2.97 L/hr

[a] Following single oral doses.
[b] In the fasting state.
[c] In the fed state.
[d] Hydroxy derivatives of pioglitazone.
[e] Keto derivative of pioglitazone.

Special populations –
Gender: The mean pioglitazone C_{max} and AUC values were increased 20% to 60% in females.
Hepatic function impairment:
• *Rosiglitazone* – Unbound oral clearance of rosiglitazone was significantly lower in moderate to severe liver disease patients (Child-Pugh class B/C) in comparison with healthy subjects. This resulted in an increased C_{max} by 2-fold and AUC by 3-fold, and a longer elimination half-life by 2 hours. Do not initiate rosiglitazone in patients exhibiting clinical evidence of active liver disease or increased serum transaminase levels (ALT more than 2.5 times the upper limit of normal [ULN]).
• *Pioglitazone* – Compared with healthy controls, subjects with impaired hepatic function (Child-Pugh class B/C) have approximately 45% reduction in pioglitazone and total pioglitazone mean peak concentrations but no change in the mean AUC values. Do not initiate pioglitazone if the patient exhibits clinical evidence of active liver disease or serum transaminase levels (ALT more than 2.5 times the ULN).
Obesity: Both oral clearance (CL/F) and oral steady-state volume of distribution (Vss/F) were shown to increase with increases in body weight. The range of predicted CL/F and Vss/F values varied by less than 1.7-fold and less than 2.3-fold, respectively, over the weight range observed in these analyses (50 to 150 kg).

>*Clinical trials:*
Comparative trial – In a 52-week, double-blind, glyburide-controlled trial of patients with type 2 diabetes, 195 patients were randomized to 2 mg **rosiglitazone** twice daily, 189 patients to 4 mg rosiglitazone twice daily, and 202 patients to a median titrated dose of 7.5 mg/day glyburide. Statistically significant improvement was demonstrated as a reduction in baseline in fasting blood glucose (FBG) and HbA$_{1c}$ by 40.8 mg/dL and 0.53% with 4 mg rosiglitazone twice daily, 25.4 mg/dL

and 0.27% with 2 mg rosiglitazone twice daily, and 30 mg/dL and 0.72% with glyburide. Hypoglycemia was reported in 12.1% of glyburide patients vs 0.5% (2 mg twice daily) and 1.6% (4 mg twice daily) of rosiglitazone patients. Mean weight gain was reported as 1.9 kg in glyburide patients and 1.75 kg (2 mg twice daily) and 2.95 kg (4 mg twice daily) in rosiglitazone patients.

Contraindications

Hypersensitivity to **pioglitazone** or **rosiglitazone** or any of their components.

Warnings

>*Hepatotoxicity:* Although available clinical data show no evidence of **pioglitazone**- and **rosiglitazone**-induced hepatotoxicity or ALT elevations, they are related structurally to or very similar to **troglitazone**, a thiazolidinedione no longer marketed in the United States, which was associated with idiosyncratic hepatotoxicity and cases of liver failure, liver transplants, and death during postmarketing clinical use. Do not use in patients who experienced jaundice while taking troglitazone. In preapproval clinical studies of 4598 patients treated with rosiglitazone, encompassing approximately 3600 patient-years of exposure, there was no signal of drug-induced hepatotoxicity or elevation of ALT levels. In postmarketing experience with rosiglitazone, reports of hepatitis and hepatic enzyme elevations to 3 or more times the ULN have been received. Very rarely, these reports have involved hepatic failure with and without fatal outcome, although causality has not been established. In preapproval clinical studies worldwide, over 4500 subjects were treated with pioglitazone. In US clinical studies, over 4700 patients with type 2 diabetes received pioglitazone. There was no evidence of drug-induced hepatotoxicity or elevation of ALT levels in the clinical studies. In postmarketing experience with pioglitazone, reports of hepatitis and hepatic enzyme elevations to 3 or more times the ULN have been received. Very rarely, these reports have involved hepatic failure with and without fatal outcome, although causality has not been established.

It is recommended that patients treated with pioglitazone and rosiglitazone undergo periodic monitoring of liver enzymes. Check liver enzymes prior to the initiation of therapy in all treated patients. Do not initiate therapy in patients with increased baseline liver enzyme levels (ALT more than 2.5 times the ULN). In patients with normal baseline liver enzymes following initiation of therapy, it is recommended that liver enzymes be monitored every 2 months for the first 12 months and periodically thereafter. Evaluate patients with mildly elevated liver enzymes (ALT levels less than or equal to 2.5 times the ULN) at baseline or during therapy to determine the cause of the liver enzyme elevation. Proceed with caution in the initiation of, or continuation of, therapy in patients with mild liver enzyme elevations and include appropriate close clinical follow-up, including more frequent liver enzyme monitoring, to determine if the liver enzyme elevations resolve or worsen. If, at any time, ALT levels increase to more than 3 times the ULN in patients on therapy, recheck liver enzyme levels as soon as possible. If ALT levels remain more than 3 times the ULN or if the patient is jaundiced, discontinue therapy.

If any patient develops symptoms suggesting hepatic dysfunction (eg, unexplained nausea, vomiting, abdominal pain, fatigue, anorexia, dark urine), check liver enzymes. Guide the decision by clinical judgment whether to continue the patient on therapy with pioglitazone and rosiglitazone pending laboratory evaluations. If jaundice is observed, discontinue therapy.

>*Cardiac effects:* Thiazolidinediones, alone or in combination with other antidiabetic agents, can cause fluid retention, which may exacerbate or lead to heart failure. Observe patients for signs and symptoms of heart failure. In combination with insulin, thiazolidinediones also may increase the risk of other cardiovascular adverse events. Discontinue if any deterioration in cardiac status occurs. Rosiglitazone and pioglitazone are not recommended in patients with NYHA Class 3 and 4 cardiac status.

In clinical studies, an increased incidence of edema, cardiac failure, and other cardiovascular adverse events was seen in patients on rosiglitazone and insulin combination therapy compared with insulin and placebo. Patients who experienced cardiovascular events were older on average and had a longer duration of diabetes. These cardiovascular events were noted at the 4 and 8 mg daily dose strengths. In this population, however, it was not possible to determine specific risk factors that could be used to identify all patients at risk of heart failure and other cardiovascular events on combination therapy. Three of 10 patients who developed cardiac failure on combination therapy during the double blind part of the studies had no known prior evidence of CHF, or pre-existing cardiac condition.

Monitor patients treated with combination **rosiglitazone** and insulin or combination rosiglitazone/metformin and insulin for cardiovascular adverse events. Discontinue this combination therapy in patients who do not respond as manifested by a reduction in HbA$_{1c}$ or insulin dose after 4 to 5 months of therapy or who develop any significant adverse events.

In a clinical trial involving 566 patients, 2 of 191 patients (1.1%) receiving 15 mg **pioglitazone** plus insulin and 2 of 188 patients (1.1%)

receiving 30 mg pioglitazone plus insulin developed CHF compared with none of the 187 patients on insulin therapy alone. All 4 of these patients had previous histories of cardiovascular conditions, including coronary artery disease, previous CABG procedures, and MI. In a 24-week, dose-controlled study in which pioglitazone was coadministered with insulin, 1 of 345 of patients (0.3%) on 30 mg and 3 of 345 of patients (0.9%) on 45 mg reported CHF as a serious adverse event. Analysis of data from these studies did not identify specific factors that predict increased risk of CHF in combination therapy with insulin.

In postmarketing experience with pioglitazone, cases of CHF have been reported in patients with and without previously known heart disease.

➤*Ovulation:* In premenopausal anovulatory patients, thiazolidinedione treatment may result in resumption of ovulation. These patients may be at risk for pregnancy. Recommend adequate contraception in these women.

➤*Carcinogenesis:* There was an increase in incidence of adipose hyperplasia in mice at **rosiglitazone** doses of 1.5 mg/kg/day or more (approximately 2 times human AUC at the maximum recommended human daily dose). In rats, there was a significant increase in the incidence of benign adipose tissue tumors (lipomas) at doses of 0.3 mg/kg/day or more (approximately 2 times human AUC at the maximum recommended human daily dose). These proliferative changes in both species are considered to be caused by the persistent pharmacological overstimulation of adipose tissue.

A 2-year carcinogenicity study was conducted in male and female rats at oral doses up to 63 mg/kg **pioglitazone** (approximately 14 times the maximum recommended human oral dose of 45 mg based on mg/m^2). Drug-induced tumors were not observed in any organ except for the urinary bladder. Benign and/or malignant transitional cell neoplasms were observed in male rats at 4 mg/kg/day and above (approximately equal to the maximum recommended human oral dose based on mg/m^2).

➤*Fertility impairment:* **Rosiglitazone** altered estrous cyclicity (2 mg/kg/day) and reduced fertility (40 mg/kg/day) of female rats in association with lower plasma levels of progesterone and estradiol (approximately 20 to 200 times human AUC at the maximum recommended human daily dose, respectively). In monkeys, rosiglitazone (0.6 and 4.6 mg/kg/day; approximately 3 and 15 times the human AUC at the maximum recommended human daily dose, respectively) diminished the follicular phase rise in serum estradiol with consequential reduction in the luteinizing hormone surge, lower luteal phase progesterone levels, and amenorrhea. The mechanism for these effects appears to be direct inhibition of ovarian steroidogenesis.

➤*Pregnancy:* Category C (**pioglitazone, rosiglitazone**). There are no adequate and well-controlled studies in pregnant women. Do not use pioglitazone or rosiglitazone during pregnancy unless the potential benefit justifies the potential risk to the fetus.

Treatment with rosiglitazone during mid-to-late gestation was associated with fetal death and growth retardation in rats and rabbits. Rosiglitazone caused placental pathology in rats (3 mg/kg/day). Treatment of rats during gestation through lactation reduced litter size, neonatal viability, and postnatal growth, with growth retardation reversible after puberty. For effects on the placenta, embryo/fetus, and offspring, the no-effect dose was 0.2 mg/kg/day in rats and 15 mg/kg/day in rabbits. These no-effect levels are approximately 4 times the human AUC at the maximum recommended human daily dose.

Delayed parturition and embryotoxicty (ie, increased postimplantation losses, delayed development, and reduced fetal weights) were observed in rats at oral doses of 40 mg/kg/day or more (about 10 times the maximum recommended human oral dose based on mg/m^2). No functional or behavioral toxicity was observed in the offspring of rats. In rabbits, embryotoxicity was observed at an oral dose of 160 mg/kg (about 40 times the maximum recommended human oral dose based on mg/m^2). Delayed postnatal development, attributed to decreased body weight, was observed in offspring of rats at oral doses of 10 mg/kg or more during late gestation and lactation periods (about 2 times the maximum recommended human oral dose based on mg/m^2).

Because current information strongly suggests that abnormal blood glucose levels during pregnancy are associated with a higher incidence of congenital anomalies, as well as increased neonatal morbidity and mortality, most experts recommend insulin be used during pregnancy to maintain blood glucose levels as close to normal as possible.

➤*Lactation:* It is not known whether **pioglitazone** or **rosiglitazone** are secreted in human milk. Pioglitazone and rosiglitazone are secreted in the milk of lactating rats. Do not administer to nursing women.

➤*Children:* Safety and efficacy have not been established in patients younger than 18 years of age.

Precautions

➤*Monitoring:* Perform periodic fasting blood glucose and HbA_{1c} measurements to monitor therapeutic response. Liver enzyme monitoring is recommended prior to initiation of therapy in all patients and periodically thereafter (see Warnings).

➤*Type 1 diabetes:* **Pioglitazone** and **rosiglitazone** are active only in the presence of insulin. Therefore, do not use in type 1 diabetes patients or for the treatment of diabetic ketoacidosis.

➤*Hypoglycemia:* Patients receiving **pioglitazone** and **rosiglitazone** in combination with insulin or oral hypoglycemics (eg, sulfonylureas) may be at risk for hypoglycemia; reduction in the dose of the concomitant agent may be necessary.

➤*Hematologic:* Mean decreases in hemoglobin up to 1 g/dL and hematocrit up to 3.3% were observed for **rosiglitazone** alone and in combination with other hypoglycemic agents, primarily occurring during the first 3 months or following an increase in rosiglitazone dose. White blood cell counts also decreased slightly in patients treated with rosiglitazone. **Pioglitazone** also may cause decreases in hemoglobin and hematocrit. Mean hemoglobin values declined by 2% to 4% in pioglitazone-treated patients. These changes primarily occurred within the first 4 to 12 weeks of therapy and remained relatively constant thereafter. The observed changes may be related to the increased plasma volume observed with treatment and have not been associated with any significant hematologic clinical effects.

➤*Edema:* Use **pioglitazone** and **rosiglitazone** with caution in patients with edema. In a clinical study in healthy volunteers who received rosiglitazone 8 mg once daily for 8 weeks, there was a statistically significant increase in median plasma volume compared with placebo. In controlled clinical trials of patients with type 2 diabetes, mild to moderate edema was reported in pioglitazone- and rosiglitazone-treated patients. Patients with ongoing edema are more likely to have adverse events associated with edema if started on combination therapy with insulin and rosiglitazone.

Because thiazolidinediones can cause fluid retention, which can exacerbate or lead to CHF, use with caution in patients at risk for heart failure, and monitor patients at risk for heart failure for signs and symptoms of heart failure.

➤*Weight gain:* Dose-related weight gain was seen with **rosiglitazone** and **pioglitazone** alone and in combination with other hypoglycemic agents. The mechanism of weight gain is unclear but probably involves a combination of fluid retention and fat accumulation.

In postmarketing experience, there have been rare reports of unusually rapid increases in weight and increases in excess of that generally observed in clinical trials. Assess patients who experience such increases for fluid accumulation and volume-related events (eg, excessive edema, CHF).

Drug Interactions

➤*CYP450 system:* In vitro drug metabolism studies suggest that **rosiglitazone** does not inhibit any of the major P450 enzymes at clinically relevant concentrations. In vitro data demonstrate that rosiglitazone is metabolized predominantly by CYP2C8 and, to a lesser extent, 2C9.

In vivo drug interaction studies have suggested that **pioglitazone** may be a weak inducer of CYP450 isoform 3A4 substrate. In vitro, ketoconazole appears to inhibit significantly the metabolism of pioglitazone. Pending the availability of additional data, evaluate patients receiving ketoconazole concomitantly with pioglitazone more frequently with respect to glycemic control.

Thiazolidinediones Drug Interactions,			
Precipitant drug	Object drug*		Description
Atorvastatin	Pioglitazone	↑	Concurrent use for 7 days resulted in an increase in pioglitazone and atorvastatin serum concentrations.
Pioglitazone	Atorvastatin		
Ketoconazole	Pioglitazone	↑	Coadmimistration resulted in an increase in pioglitazone AUC and C_{max}.
Pioglitazone	Midazolam	↓	Administration of pioglitazone for 15 days followed by a single 7.5 mg dose of midazolam syrup resulted in a 26% reduction in midazolam C_{max} and AUC.
Pioglitazone	Nifedipine	↑	Concurrent use of pioglitazone and extended-release nifedipine resulted in an increase in nifedipine concentrations. Clinical significance is unknown.
Pioglitazone	Oral contraceptives	↓	Coadministration of pioglitazone with an oral contraceptive (eg, ethinyl estradiol/norethindrone) for 21 days resulted in an 11% decrease in the ethinyl estradiol AUC and an 11% to 14% decrease in the C_{max}. Clinical significance is unknown. Rosiglitazone was not shown to have a clinical effect on these pharmacokinetics.

* ↑ = Object drug increased.   ↓ = Object drug decreased.

Thiazolidinediones

Adverse Reactions

Thiazolidinediones Adverse Reactions (%)[a]		
Adverse reaction	Pioglitazone (n = 606)	Rosiglitazone (n = 2526)
CNS		
Fatigue	—	3.6
Headache	9.1	5.9
GI		
Diarrhea	—	2.3
Tooth disorder	5.3	—
Metabolism		
Aggravated diabetes mellitus	5.1	—
Hyperglycemia	—	3.9
Hypoglycemia	—	0.6
Respiratory		
Pharyngitis	5.1	—
Sinusitis	6.3	3.2
Upper respiratory tract infection	13.2	9.9
Miscellaneous		
Anemia	—	1.9
Back pain	—	4
Edema	4.8	4.8
Injury	—	7.6
Myalgia	5.4	—

[a] Data are pooled from separate studies and are not necessarily comparable.

Pioglitazone – Edema was reported in 7.2% of patients treated with pioglitazone and sulfonylureas compared with 2.1% of patients on sulfonylureas alone. In combination studies with metformin, edema was reported in 6% of patients on combination therapy compared with 2.5% of patients on metformin alone.

In a 16-week, placebo-controlled, pioglitazone plus insulin trial (N = 379), 10 patients treated with pioglitazone plus insulin developed dyspnea and also, at some point during their therapy, developed either weight change or edema. Seven of these 10 patients received diuretics to treat these symptoms. This was not reported in the insulin plus placebo group. In controlled combination therapy studies with either a sulfonylurea or insulin, mild to moderate hypoglycemia, which appears to be dose-related, was reported (see Precautions).

Rosiglitazone – Overall, the types of adverse experiences reported when rosiglitazone was used in combination with metformin or a sulfonylurea were similar to those during monotherapy with rosiglitazone. Reports of anemia (7.1%) were greater in patients treated with a combination of rosiglitazone and metformin compared with rosiglitazone monotherapy or combination therapy with a sulfonylurea. Lower pretreatment hemoglobin/hematocrit levels in patients enrolled in the metformin combination clinical trials may have contributed to the higher reporting rate of anemia in these studies.

Edema was reported with higher frequency in the rosiglitazone plus insulin combination trials (insulin, 5.4%; rosiglitazone in combination with insulin, 14.7%). Reports of new onset or exacerbation of CHF occurred at rates of 1% for insulin alone, and 2% (4 mg) and 3% (8 mg) for insulin in combination with rosiglitazone. In postmarketing experience with rosiglitazone, adverse events potentially related to volume expansion (eg, CHF, pulmonary edema, pleural effusions) have been reported.

►*Lab test abnormalities:*
Hematologic – Decreases in hemoglobin, hematocrit, and white blood cell counts may be related to increased plasma volume observed with thiazolidinedione treatment. Mean decreases of up to 1 g/dL hemoglobin and up to 3.3% hematocrit occurred in **rosiglitazone**-treated patients. Mean hemoglobin values decreased by 2% to 4% in **pioglitazone**-treated patients (see Precautions).

Lipids – **Rosiglitazone** as monotherapy was associated with increases in total cholesterol, LDL, and HDL and decreases in free fatty acids. Patients treated with **pioglitazone** had mean decreases in triglycerides, mean increases in HDL cholesterol, and no consistent mean changes in LDL and total cholesterol. In placebo-controlled trials, the placebo-corrected mean changes from baseline decreased 5% to 26% for triglycerides and increased 6% to 13% for HDL in patients treated with pioglitazone.

Serum transaminase levels – In controlled trials, 0.2% of patients treated with **rosiglitazone** had reversible elevations in ALT greater than 3 times the ULN compared with 0.2% on placebo and 0.5% on active comparators. Hyperbilirubinemia was found in 0.3% of patients treated with rosiglitazone compared with 0.9% treated with placebo and 1% in patients treated with active comparators. In postmarketing experience with rosiglitazone, reports of hepatic enzyme elevations of 3 or more times the ULN and hepatitis have been received.

During clinical trials in the United States, a total of 0.3% **pioglitazone**-treated patients had ALT values 3 times or more the ULN. All patients with follow-up values had reversible elevations in ALT. In the population of patients treated with pioglitazone, mean values for bilirubin, AST, ALT, alkaline phosphatase, and GGT were decreased at the final visit compared with baseline. Fewer than 0.9% of pioglitazone-treated patients were withdrawn from clinical trials in the United States because of abnormal liver function tests.

CPK levels – During required laboratory testing in clinical trials, sporadic, transient elevations in creatine phosphokinase levels (CPK) were observed. An isolated elevation to more than 10 times the ULN (values of 2150 to 11,400 IU/L) was noted in 9 patients. Six of these patients continued to receive **pioglitazone**. Two patients completed receiving study medication at the time of the elevated value and 1 patient discontinued study medication because of the elevation. These elevations resolved without any apparent clinical sequelae. The relationship of these events to pioglitazone therapy is unknown.

Overdosage

Limited data are available with regard to overdosage in humans. In clinical studies in volunteers, **rosiglitazone** has been administered at single oral doses of up to 20 mg and was well tolerated. During controlled clinical trials, 1 case of overdose with **pioglitazone** was reported. A male patient took 120 mg/day for 4 days, then 180 mg/day for 7 days. The patient denied any clinical symptoms during this period. In the event of an overdose, initiate appropriate supportive treatment.

Patient Information

Pioglitazone and **rosiglitazone** may be taken with or without meals. If the dose is missed at the usual meal, it may be taken at the next meal. If the dose is missed on 1 day, the dose should not be doubled the following day.

Management of type 2 diabetes should include diet control. Caloric restriction, weight loss, and exercise are essential for the proper treatment of the diabetic patient because they help improve insulin sensitivity. This is important not only in the primary treatment of type 2 diabetes but in maintaining the efficacy of drug therapy.

It is important for the patient to adhere to dietary instructions and to have blood glucose and glycosylated hemoglobin tested regularly. During periods of stress, such as fever, trauma, infection, or surgery, medication requirements may change, and patients should seek the advice of their physician.

Inform patients that blood will be drawn to check their liver function prior to the start of therapy and every 2 months for the first 12 months and periodically thereafter.

When using combination therapy with insulin or an oral hypoglycemic agent, explain the risks of hypoglycemia, its symptoms, treatment, and predisposing conditions to patients and their family members.

Patients who experience an unusually rapid increase in weight or edema or who develop shortness of breath or other symptoms of heart failure while on therapy should immediately report these symptoms to their physician.

Instruct patients to immediately report any signs or symptoms of hepatic dysfunction (eg, nausea, vomiting, abdominal pain, fatigue, anorexia, dark urine, jaundice) to their physician.

Use of thiazolidinediones can cause resumption of ovulation in women. Therefore, recommend adequate contraception in premenopausal women.

Advise patients that it can take 2 weeks of rosiglitazone therapy to see a reduction in blood glucose and 2 to 3 months to see full effect.

Thiazolidinediones

ROSIGLITAZONE MALEATE

Rx	Avandia (GlaxoSmithKline)	Tablets: 2 mg	Lactose. (SB 2). Pink, pentagonal. Film-coated. In 30s, 60s, 100s, 500s, and SUP 100s.
		4 mg	Lactose. (SB 4). Orange, pentagonal. Film-coated. In 30s, 60s, 100s, 500s, and SUP 100s.
		8 mg	Lactose. (SB 8). Red-brown, pentagonal. Film-coated. In 30s, 100s, 500s, and SUP 100s.

For complete prescribing information, refer to the Thiazolidinediones group monograph.

Indications

➤*Type 2 diabetes:* Monotherapy as an adjunct to diet and exercise to improve glycemic control in patients with type 2 diabetes.

Also for use in combination with metformin, insulin, or a sulfonylurea when diet, exercise, and a single agent do not result in adequate glycemic control. For patients inadequately controlled with a maximum dose of a sulfonylurea or metformin, rosiglitazone should be added to, rather than substituted for, a sulfonylurea or metformin.

Administration and Dosage

➤*Approved by the FDA:* May 28, 1999.

Include diet control in management of type 2 diabetes. Caloric restriction, weight loss, and exercise are essential for the proper treatment of the diabetic patient because they help improve insulin sensitivity. This is important not only in the primary treatment of type 2 diabetes, but also in maintaining the efficacy of drug therapy. Prior to initiation of therapy with rosiglitazone therapy, investigate and treat secondary causes of poor glycemic control (eg, infection).

Rosiglitazone may be taken with or without food.

➤*Monotherapy:* Individualize the management of antidiabetic therapy. Rosiglitazone may be administered either at a starting dose of 4 mg once daily or divided and given in the morning and evening. For patients responding inadequately after 8 to 12 weeks of treatment, as determined by reduction in fasting plasma glucose, the dosing may be increased to 8 mg daily as indicated below. In clinical trials, the 4 mg twice daily regimen resulted in the greatest reduction in fasting blood glucose and HbA_{1c}.

➤*Combination therapy:* When rosiglitazone is added to existing therapy, the current dose of the sulfonylurea, insulin, or metformin can be continued upon initiation of rosiglitazone therapy.

Metformin – The usual starting dose of rosiglitazone in combination with metformin is 4 mg given as either a single dose once daily or in divided doses twice daily. It is unlikely that the dose of metformin will require adjustment because of hypoglycemia during combination therapy with rosiglitazone.

Insulin – For patients stabilized on insulin, continue the insulin dose upon initiation of rosiglitazone therapy. Dose rosiglitazone at 4 mg daily. Doses greater than 4 mg daily in combination with insulin are not currently indicated. It is recommended that the insulin dose be decreased 10% to 25% if the patient reports hypoglycemia or if fasting plasma glucose concentrations decrease to less than 100 mg/dL. Individualize further adjustments based on glucose-lowering response.

Sulfonylureas – When used in combination with a sulfonylurea, the recommended dose of rosiglitazone is 4 mg either as a single dose once daily or in divided doses twice daily. If patients report hypoglycemia, decrease the dose of the sulfonylurea.

Maximum recommended dose – The dose of rosiglitazone should not exceed 8 mg/day as a single dose or divided twice daily. The 8 mg/day dose has been shown to be safe and effective in clinical studies as monotherapy and in combination with metformin. Doses of rosiglitazone greater than 4 mg/day in combination with a sulfonylurea have not been studied in adequate and well-controlled clinical trials. Doses of rosiglitazone greater than 4 mg/day in combination with insulin are not currently indicated.

➤*Renal impairment:* Metformin is contraindicated in patients with renal impairment. Therefore, concomitant administration of rosiglitazone and metformin is contraindicated in these patients. However, no dosage adjustment is necessary when rosiglitazone is used as monotherapy in patients with renal impairment.

➤*Hepatic impairment:* Use with caution in patients with hepatic impairment. Do not initiate rosiglitazone therapy if the patient exhibits clinical evidence of active liver disease or increased serum transaminase levels (ALT more than 2.5 times the ULN) at start of therapy. Liver enzyme monitoring is recommended in all patients prior to initiation of therapy with rosiglitazone and periodically thereafter.

➤*Children:* The use of rosiglitazone in patients younger than 18 years of age is not recommended.

➤*Storage/Stability:* Store at 25°C (77°F); excursions 15° to 30°C (59° to 86°F). Dispense in a tight, light-resistant container.

PIOGLITAZONE HCl

Rx	Actos (Takeda Pharmaceuticals North America, Inc.)	Tablets: 15 mg	Lactose. (ACTOS 15). White to off-white. In 30s, 90s, and 500s.
		30 mg	Lactose. (ACTOS 30). White to off-white. In 30s, 90s, and 500s.
		45 mg	Lactose. (ACTOS 45). White to off-white. In 30s, 90s, and 500s.

For complete prescribing information, refer to the Thiazolidinediones group monograph.

Indications

➤*Type 2 diabetes:* Monotherapy as an adjunct to diet and exercise to improve glycemic control in patients with type 2 diabetes.

Also for use in combination with a sulfonylurea, metformin, or insulin when diet, exercise, and the single agent do not result in adequate glycemic control.

Administration and Dosage

➤*Approved by the FDA:* July 16, 1999.

Management of type 2 diabetes also should include nutritional counseling, weight reduction as needed, and exercise. These efforts are important not only in the primary treatment of type 2 diabetes, but also to maintain the efficacy of drug therapy.

Take once daily without regard to meals. It is recommended that patients be treated with pioglitazone for a period of time adequate to evaluate change in HbA_{1c} (3 months) unless glycemic control deteriorates.

➤*Monotherapy:* Initiate monotherapy in patients not adequately controlled with diet and exercise at 15 or 30 mg once daily. For patients who respond inadequately to the initial dose of pioglitazone, the dose can be increased in increments up to 45 mg once daily. Consider combination therapy for patients not responding adequately to monotherapy.

➤*Combination therapy:*

Sulfonylureas – Initiate pioglitazone in combination with a sulfonylurea at 15 or 30 mg once daily. Continue the current sulfonylurea upon initiation of pioglitazone therapy. Decrease the dose of the sulfonylurea if patient reports hypoglycemia.

Metformin – Initiate pioglitazone in combination with metformin at 15 or 30 mg once daily. Continue the current metformin dose upon initiation of pioglitazone therapy. It is unlikely that the dose of metformin will require adjustment because of hypoglycemia during combination therapy with pioglitazone.

Insulin – Initiate pioglitazone in combination with insulin at 15 or 30 mg once daily. Continue the current insulin dose upon initiation of pioglitazone therapy. Decrease the insulin dose by 10% to 25% if the patient reports hypoglycemia or if plasma glucose concentrations decrease to less than 100 mg/dL. Individualize further adjustments based on glucose-lowering response.

➤*Maximum recommended dose:* Do not exceed 45 mg once daily of pioglitazone because doses more than 45 mg once daily have not been studied in placebo-controlled clinical studies.

➤*Hepatic disease:* Do not initiate pioglitazone therapy if the patient exhibits clinical evidence of active liver disease or increased serum transaminase levels (ALT more than 2.5 times the ULN) at the start of therapy. Liver enzyme monitoring is recommended in all patients prior to initiation of therapy with pioglitazone and periodically thereafter.

➤*Children:* The use of pioglitazone in pediatric patients younger than 18 years of age is not recommended.

➤*Storage/Stability:* Store at 25°C (77°F); excursions permitted to 15° to 30°C (59° to 86°F). Keep container tightly closed, and protect from moisture and humidity.

Antidiabetic Combination Products

GLYBURIDE/METFORMIN HCl

Rx	**Glyburide/Meformin HCl** (PAR)	**Tablets:** 1.25 mg/250 mg	(6057). Pale yellow, capsule shape. Film-coated. In 100s.
Rx	**Glucovance** (Bristol-Myers Squibb)		(BMS 6072). Pale yellow, capsule shape. Film-coated. In 100s and 500s.
Rx	**Glyburide/Meformin HCl** (PAR)	**Tablets:** 2.5 mg/500 mg	(6058). Pale orange, capsule shape. Film-coated. In 100s.
Rx	**Glucovance** (Bristol-Myers Squibb)		(BMS 6073). Pale orange, capsule shape. Film-coated. In 100s and 500s.
Rx	**Glyburide/Meformin HCl** (PAR)	**Tablets:** 5 mg/500 mg	(6059). Yellow, capsule shape. Film-coated. In 100s.
Rx	**Glucovance** (Bristol-Myers Squibb)		(BMS 6074). Yellow, capsule shape. Film-coated. In 100s.

For complete prescribing information, refer to the Sulfonylureas group monograph and the Metformin HCl monograph.

WARNING

Lactic acidosis is a rare, but serious, metabolic complication that can occur because of metformin accumulation during treatment with glyburide/metformin. When it occurs, it is fatal in approximately 50% of cases. See Warnings in the Metformin MCl monograph for more information.

Indications

➤*Type 2 diabetes (initial therapy):* As initial therapy, as an adjunct to diet and exercise, to improve glycemic control in patients with type 2 diabetes whose hyperglycemia cannot be satisfactorily managed with diet and exercise alone.

➤*Type 2 diabetes (second-line therapy):* As second-line therapy when diet, exercise, and initial treatment with a sulfonylurea or metformin do not result in adequate glycemic control in patients with type 2 diabetes. For patients requiring additional therapy, a thiazolidinedione may be added to glyburide/metformin to achieve additional glycemic control.

Administration and Dosage

➤*Approved by the FDA:* July 31, 2000.

Individualize dosage on the basis of effectiveness and tolerance while not exceeding the maximum recommended daily dose of 20 mg glyburide/ 2000 mg metformin. Give with meals and initiate at a low dose, with gradual dose escalation as described below, in order to avoid hypoglycemia (largely because of glyburide), to reduce GI side effects (largely because of metformin), and to permit determination of the minimum effective dose for adequate control of blood glucose for the individual patient.

With initial treatment and during dose titration, appropriately monitor blood glucose to determine the therapeutic response to glyburide/metformin HCl and to identify the minimum effective dose for the patient. Thereafter, measure HbA_{1c} at intervals of about 3 months to assess the effectiveness of therapy.

No studies have been performed specifically examining the safety and efficacy of switching to glyburide/metformin HCl therapy in patients taking concomitant glyburide (or other sulfonylurea) plus metformin.

➤*Initial therapy:*
Starting dose – 1.25 mg/250 mg once or twice daily with meals. Increase dosage in increments of 1.25 mg/250 mg/day every 2 weeks up to the minimum effective dose necessary to achieve adequate control of blood glucose. Do not use glyburide/metformin 5 mg/500 mg as initial therapy because of an increased risk of hypoglycemia.

➤*Second-line therapy:*
Starting dose – 2.5 mg/500 mg or 5 mg/500 mg twice daily with meals. Titrate the daily dose in increments of no more than 5 mg/ 500 mg up to the minimum effective dose to achieve adequate control of blood glucose or to a maximum dose of 20 mg/2000 mg/day.

If patients previously treated with combination therapy of glyburide (or another sulfonylurea) plus metformin are switching to glyburide/metformin HCl, the starting dose should not exceed the daily dose of glyburide (or equivalent dose of another sulfonylurea) and metformin already being taken. Monitor patients closely for signs and symptoms of hypoglycemia following such a switch and titrate the dose of glyburide/metformin HCl as described above to achieve adequate control of blood glucose.

➤*Addition of thiazolidinediones to glyburide/metformin therapy:* When a thiazolidinedione is added to glyburide/metformin therapy, the current dose of glyburide/metformin can be continued and the thiazolidinedione initiated at its recommended starting dose. For patients needing additional glycemic control, the dose of the thiazolidinedione can be increased based on its recommended titration schedule. The increased glycemic control attainable with glyburide/metformin plus a thiazolidinedione may increase the potential for hypoglycemia at any time of day. In patients who develop hypoglycemia when receiving glyburide/metformin and a thiazolidinedione, consider reducing the dose of the glyburide component of glyburide/metformin. As clinically warranted, also consider adjustment of the dosages of the other components of the antidiabetic regimen.

➤*Lactic acidosis:* See Warnings in metformin HCl monograph.

➤*Specific patient populations:* Glyburide/metformin HCl is not recommended for use during pregnancy or in pediatric patients. Initial and maintenance dosing should be conservative in patients with advanced age because of the potential for decreased renal function in this population. Dosage adjustment requires a careful assessment of renal function. Do not titrate elderly, debilitated, or malnourished patients to the maximum dose to avoid the risk of hypoglycemia. Monitoring of renal function is necessary to aid in prevention of metformin-associated lactic acidosis, particular in the elderly.

➤*Storage/Stability:* Store at temperatures up to 25°C (77°F). Dispense in light-resistant containers.

GLIPIZIDE/METFORMIN HCl

Rx	**Metaglip** (Bristol-Myers Squibb)	**Tablets:** 2.5 mg/250 mg	(BMS 6081). Pink, oval. Film-coated. In 100s.
		2.5 mg/500 mg	(BMS 6077). White, oval. Film-coated. In 100s.
		5 mg/500 mg	(BMS 6078). Pink, oval. Film-coated. In 100s.

For complete prescribing information, refer to the Sulfonylureas group monograph and the Metformin HCl monograph.

WARNING

Lactic acidosis is a rare, but serious, metabolic complication that can occur due to metformin accumulation during treatment with glipizide/metformin. When it occurs, it is fatal in approximately 50% of cases. See Warnings in the Metformin HCl monograph for more information.

Indications

➤*Type 2 diabetes (initial therapy):* As initial therapy as an adjunct to diet and exercise to improve glycemic control in patients with type 2 diabetes whose hyperglycemia cannot be satisfactorily managed with diet and exercise alone.

➤*Type 2 diabetes (second-line therapy):* As second-line therapy when diet, exercise, and initial treatment with a sulfonylurea or metformin do not result in adequate glycemic control in patients with type 2 diabetes.

Administration and Dosage

➤*Approved by the FDA:* October 22, 2002.

Dosage must be individualized on the basis of effectiveness and tolerance while not exceeding the maximum recommended daily dose of 20 mg glipizide/2000 mg metformin. Give glipizide/metformin with meals and initiate at a low dose, with gradual dose escalation as described below in order to avoid hypoglycemia (largely because of glipizide), to reduce GI side effects (largely because of metformin), and to permit determination of the minimum effective dose for adequate control of blood glucose for the individual patient.

With initial treatment and during dose titration, use appropriate blood glucose monitoring to determine the therapeutic response to glipizide/ metformin and to identify the minimum effective dose for the patient. Thereafter, measure HbA_{1c} at intervals of approximately 3 months to assess the effectiveness of therapy.

No studies have been performed specifically examining the safety and efficacy of switching to glipizide/metformin therapy in patients taking concomitant glipizide (or other sulfonylurea) plus metformin.

➤*Initial therapy:* The recommended starting dose of glipizide/metformin is 2.5 mg/250 mg once a day with a meal. For patients whose fasting plasma glucose (FPG) is 280 to 320 mg/dL, consider a starting dose of 2.5 mg/500 mg twice daily. The efficacy of glipizide/metformin tablets in patients whose FPG exceeds 320 mg/dL has not been established. Increase dosage to achieve adequate glycemic control in increments of 1 tablet per day every 2 weeks up to a maximum of 10 mg/1000 mg or 10 mg/2000 mg per day given in divided doses. In clinical trials with glipizide/metformin as initial therapy, there was no experience with total daily doses greater than 10 mg/2000 mg per day.

GLIPIZIDE/METFORMIN HCl

➤*Second-line therapy:* For patients not adequately controlled on either glipizide (or another sulfonylurea) or metformin alone, the recommended starting dose is 2.5 mg/500 mg or 5 mg/500 mg twice daily with the morning and evening meals. In order to avoid hypoglycemia, the starting dose should not exceed the daily doses of glipizide or metformin already being taken. Titrate the daily dose in increments of no more than 5 mg/500 mg up to the minimum effective dose to achieve adequate control of blood glucose or to a maximum dose of 20 mg/2000 mg per day.

Patients previously treated with combination therapy of glipizide (or another sulfonylurea) plus metformin may be switched to glipizide/metformin 2.5 mg/500 mg or 5 mg/500 mg; the starting dose should not exceed the daily dose of glipizide (or equivalent dose of another sulfonylurea) and metformin already being taken. Base the decision to switch to the nearest equivalent dose or to titrate on clinical judgment.

Closely monitor patients for signs and symptoms of hypoglycemia following such a switch and titrate the dose of glipizide/metformin as described above to achieve adequate control of blood glucose.

➤*Lactic acidosis:* See Warnings in the Metformin HCl monograph.

➤*Specific patient populations:* Glipizide/metformin is not recommended for use during pregnancy or for use in pediatric patients. The initial and maintenance dosing should be conservative in patients with advanced age because of the potential for decreased renal function in this population. Any dosage adjustment requires a careful assessment of renal function. Generally, do not titrate elderly, debilitated, and malnourished patients to the maximum dose to avoid the risk of hypoglycemia. Monitoring of renal function is necessary to aid in prevention of metformin-associated lactic acidosis, particularly in the elderly.

➤*Storage / Stability:* Store at 20° to 25°C (68° to 77°F). Excursions permitted to 15° to 30°C (59° to 86°F).

ROSIGLITAZONE MALEATE/METFORMIN HCl

Rx	**Avandamet** (GlaxoSmithKline)	**Tablets:** 1 mg/500 mg	Lactose. (gsk 1/500). Yellow, oval. Film-coated. In 60s, 100s, and SUP 100s.
		2 mg/500 mg	Lactose. (gsk 2/500). Pale pink, oval. Film-coated. In 60, 100s, and SUP 100s.
		2 mg/1000 mg	Lactose. (gsk 2/1000). Yellow, oval. Film-coated. In 60 and 100s.
		4 mg/500 mg	Lactose. (gsk 4/500). Orange, oval. Film-coated. In 60s, 100s, and SUP 100s.
		4 mg/1000 mg	Lactose. (gsk 4/1000). Pink, oval. Film-coated. In 60 and100s.

For complete prescribing information, refer to the Thiazolidinedione group monograph and the Metformin HCl monograph.

> # WARNING
>
> Lactic acidosis is a rare, but serious, metabolic complication that can occur due to metformin accumulation during treatment with rosiglitazone/metformin. When it occurs, it is fatal in approximately 50% of cases. See Warnings in the Metformin HCl monograph for more information.

Indications

➤*Type 2 diabetes:* As an adjunct to diet and exercise to improve glycemic control in patients with type 2 diabetes mellitus who are already treated with combination rosiglitazone and metformin or who are not adequately controlled on metformin alone.

Administration and Dosage

➤*Approved by the FDA:* October 11, 2002.

Base the dose selection of rosiglitazone/metformin on the patient's current doses of rosiglitazone and/or metformin.

Individualize the dosage of antidiabetic therapy with rosiglitazone/metformin on the basis of effectiveness and tolerability while not exceeding the maximum recommended daily dose of 8 mg/2000 mg. Give rosiglitazone/metformin in divided doses with meals, with gradual dose escalation. This reduces GI side effects (largely because of metformin) and permits determination of the minimum effective dose for the individual patient. Give sufficient time to assess adequacy of therapeutic response. Use fasting plasma glucose (FPG) to determine the therapeutic response to rosiglitazone/metformin. After an increase in metformin dosage, dose titration is recommended if patients are not adequately controlled after 1 to 2 weeks. After an increase in rosiglitazone dosage, dose titration is recommended if patients are not adequately controlled after 8 to 12 weeks.

The safety and efficacy of rosiglitazone/metformin as initial pharmacologic therapy for patients with type 2 diabetes mellitus after a trial of caloric restriction, weight loss, and exercise has not been established.

➤*Dosage recommendations:*

Patients inadequately controlled on metformin monotherapy – The usual starting dose is 4 mg rosiglitazone (total daily dose) plus the dose of metformin already being taken (see table).

Patients inadequately controlled on rosiglitazone monotherapy – The usual starting dose is 1000 mg metformin (total daily dose) plus the dose of rosiglitazone already being taken (see table).

Rosiglitazone/Metformin Starting Dose		
	Usual *Avandamet* starting dose	
Prior therapy (total daily dose)	Tablet strength	Number of tablets
Metformin HCl[1]		
1000 mg/day	2 mg/500 mg	1 tablet bid
2000 mg/day	2 mg/1000 mg	1 tablet bid
Rosiglitazone		
4 mg/day	2 mg/500 mg	1 tablet bid
8 mg/day	4 mg/500 mg	1 tablet bid

[1] For patients on doses of metformin HCl between 1000 and 2000 mg/day, initiation of rosiglitazone/metformin requires individualization of therapy.

When switching from combination therapy of rosiglitazone plus metformin as separate tablets – The usual starting dose is the dose of rosiglitazone and metformin already being taken.

If additional glycemic control is needed – The daily dose may be increased by increments of 4 mg rosiglitazone and/or 500 mg metformin, up to the maximum recommended total daily dose of 8 mg/2000 mg.

No studies have been performed specifically examining the safety and efficacy of rosiglitazone/metformin in patients previously treated with other oral hypoglycemic agents and switched to rosiglitazone/metformin. Any change in therapy of type 2 diabetes should be undertaken with care and appropriate monitoring as changes in glycemic control can occur.

➤*Lactic acidosis:* See Warnings in the Metformin HCl monograph.

➤*Specific patient populations:* Rosiglitazone/metformin is not recommended for use in pregnancy or for use in pediatric patients. The initial and maintenance dosing should be conservative in patients with advanced age because of the potential for decreased renal function in this population. Base any dosage adjustment on a careful assessment of renal function. Generally, do not titrate elderly, debilitated, and malnourished patients to the maximum dose. Monitoring of renal function is necessary to aid in prevention of metformin-associated lactic acidosis, particularly in the elderly.

Do not initiate therapy if the patient exhibits clinical evidence of active liver disease or increased serum transaminase levels (ALT more than 2.5 times upper limit of normal at start of therapy). Liver enzyme monitoring is recommended in all patients prior to initiation of therapy with rosiglitazone/metformin and periodically thereafter.

➤*Storage / Stability:* Store at 25°C (77°F). Excursions permitted to 15° to 30°C (59° to 86°F). Dispense in a tight, light-resistant container.

GLUCAGON (rDNA Origin)

Rx	GlucaGen (Bedford)	Powder for Injection: 1 mg (1 unit)	107 mg lactose. In vials with 1 mL diluent.
Rx	Glucagon Emergency Kit (Eli Lilly)		49 mg lactose. In vials with 1 ml syringe diluent.[1]
Rx	Glucagon Diagnostic Kit (Eli Lilly)		49 mg lactose. In vials with 1 ml syringe diluent.[1]

[1] With 12 mg/ml glycerin.

Indications

➤*Hypoglycemia:* Glucagon is indicated as a treatment for severe hypoglycemia. Because patients with type 1 diabetes may have less of an increase in blood glucose levels compared with a stable type 2 diabetes patient, give supplementary carbohydrates as soon as possible, especially to a pediatric patient.

➤*Diagnostic aid:* Glucagon is indicated as a diagnostic aid in the radiologic examination of the stomach, duodenum, small bowel, and colon when diminished intestinal motility would be advantageous.

➤*Unlabeled uses:* Glucagon has been used in the treatment of propranolol overdose and in cardiovascular emergencies.

Administration and Dosage

Patient instructions are provided with the product.

Use the diluent only in preparation of glucagon for parenteral injection. Do not use glucagon at concentrations> 1 mg/ml (1 unit/ml). Use the reconstituted glucagon immediately and only if it is clear and of water-like consistency. Inspect for visual particulate matter and discoloration prior to use. Discard any unused portion.

➤*Severe hypoglycemia:* Treat severe hypoglycemia initially with IV glucose, if possible. If parenteral glucose cannot be used, prepare parenteral glucagon, and use immediately. An unconscious patient will usually awaken within 15 minutes following glucagon injection. If the response is delayed, administer an additional dose of glucagon. However, in view of the deleterious effects of cerebral hypoglycemia, seek emergency aid so that parenteral glucose can be given. After the patient responds, give supplemental carbohydrate to restore liver glycogen and to prevent secondary hypoglycemia.

Adults and children > 20 kg – 1 mg (1 unit) SC, IM, or IV.

Children < 20 kg – 0.5 mg (0.5 unit) or a dose equivalent to 20 to 30 mcg/kg.

➤*Diagnostic aid:* Administer the doses in the following chart for relaxation of the stomach, duodenum, and small bowel, depending on the time of onset of action and the duration of effect required. Because the stomach is less sensitive to the effect of glucagon, 0.5 mg IV or 2 mg IM is recommended.

Glucagon Dosing Parameters as a Diagnostic Aid			
Dose	Route	Onset (min)	Duration (min)
0.25 to 0.5 mg (0.25-0.5 unit)	IV	1	9-17
1 mg (1 unit)	IM	8-10	12-27
2 mg (2 units)[1]	IV	1	22-25
2 mg (2 units)[1]	IM	4-7	21-32

[1] 2 mg doses produce a higher incidence of nausea and vomiting.

For examination of the colon, administer 2 mg IM ≈ 10 minutes prior to initiation of the procedure.

➤*Storage/Stability:* Store at room temperature prior to reconstitution (20° to 25°C; 68° to 77°F). After reconstitution, use immediately.

Actions

➤*Pharmacology:* Glucagon, a polypeptide hormone produced by pancreatic alpha cells of the islets of Langerhans, exerts an effect on blood glucose opposite to that of insulin. Elevation in blood glucose by glucagon is due to inhibition of glycogen synthesis, enhanced formation of glucose from noncarbohydrates such as proteins and fats (gluconeogenesis), and increased hydrolysis of glycogen to glucose (glycogenolysis) in the liver. Glucagon accelerates hepatic glycogenolysis by stimulating cyclic AMP synthesis via adenylyl cyclase and enhancing phosphorylase kinase activity. Lipolysis in the adipose tissue is enhanced via adenylyl cyclase stimulation. Glucagon also increases the force of contraction in the heart and has a relaxant effect on the GI tract.

Glucagon for injection (rDNA origin) is identical to human glucagon and is synthesized in a genetically altered *Escherichia coli* strain. Parenteral administration of glucagon converts hepatic glycogen to glucose and produces relaxation of the smooth muscles of the stomach, duodenum, small bowel, and colon.

➤*Pharmacokinetics:*

Absorption/Distribution – A 1 mg dose demonstrated a mean volume of distribution of 0.25 L/kg. Maximum plasma concentrations were 7.9 ng/ml ≈ 20 minutes following SC administration and 6.9 ng/ml ≈ 13 minutes following IM dosing. Peak glucose concentrations in 25 volunteers were 136 mg/dl 30 minutes after a 1 mg SC dose and 138 mg/dl 26 minutes after a 1 mg IM dose.

Metabolism/Excretion – Glucagon is extensively degraded in the liver, kidney, and plasma. Mean clearance of a 1 mg dose was 13.5 ml/min/kg. The half-life ranged from 8 to 18 minutes.

Contraindications

Hypersensitivity to glucagon; patients with pheochromocytoma (see Warnings).

Warnings

➤*Insulinoma/Pheochromocytoma:* Administer cautiously to patients with a history of insulinoma, pheochromocytoma, or both. In patients with insulinoma, IV glucagon will produce an initial increase in blood glucose, but because of its insulin-releasing effect, it may subsequently cause hypoglycemia. Administer glucose orally, intravenously, or by gavage to a patient developing symptoms of hypoglycemia after a dose of glucagon. It also stimulates catecholamine release, causing a sudden marked increase in blood pressure in patients with pheochromocytoma. To control sudden increases in blood pressure, 5 to 10 mg of IV phentolamine mesylate may be administered.

➤*Pregnancy: Category B.* There are no adequate and well-controlled studies in pregnant women. Use during pregnancy only if clearly needed.

➤*Lactation:* It is not known whether this drug is excreted in breast milk. Exercise caution when administering to a nursing mother.

➤*Children:* The use of glucagon in pediatric patients for hypoglycemia is safe and effective. Safety and efficacy have not been established in pediatric patients for use as a diagnostic aid.

Precautions

➤*Monitoring:* Obtain blood glucose determinations in a hypoglycemic patient until the patient is asymptomatic.

➤*Hypoglycemia:* Glucagon is effective in treating hypoglycemia only if sufficient liver glycogen is present. Because glucagon is of little or no help in states of starvation, adrenal insufficiency, or chronic hypoglycemia, treat hypoglycemia in these conditions with glucose. Although glucagon may be used for emergency treatment of hypoglycemia, notify the physician when hypoglycemic reactions occur so that the insulin dose may be adjusted.

Drug Interactions

➤*Anticoagulants:* The anticoagulant effect may be enhanced by coadministration of glucagon, possibly with bleeding. The onset may be delayed. Monitor prothrombin activity and for signs of bleeding, and adjust doses accordingly.

Adverse Reactions

Nausea, vomiting (occasional; this may also occur with hypoglycemia); generalized allergic reactions including urticaria, respiratory distress, and hypotension.

Overdosage

➤*Symptoms:* Expect nausea, vomiting, gastric hypotonicity, and diarrhea without consequential toxicity if overdosage occurs. Decreased serum potassium concentration may occur, and normal limits can be obtained with potassium supplementation. IV administration has demonstrated positive inotropic and chronotropic effects. A transient increase in blood pressure and pulse rate may occur. Patients receiving beta blockers may be expected to have a greater increase in blood pressure and pulse. Increases may be transient because of glucagon's short half-life. Patients with pheochromocytoma and coronary artery disease may require therapy for increased blood pressure and pulse rate.

Because glucagon is a polypeptide, it would be rapidly destroyed by the GI tract if it were to be accidently ingested.

➤*Treatment:* In managing overdosage, consider the possibility of multiple drug overdoses, interaction among drugs, and unusual drug kinetics in the patient.

In view of the extremely short half-life of glucagon and its prompt destruction and excretion, the treatment of overdosage is symptomatic, primarily for nausea, vomiting, and possible hypokalemia.

If the patient develops a dramatic increase in blood pressure, 5 to 10 mg of phentolamine mesylate has been shown to be effective in lowering blood pressure for the short time that control would be needed.

Forced diuresis, peritoneal dialysis, hemodialysis, or charcoal hemoperfusion have not been established as beneficial for an overdose of glucagon; it is extremely unlikely that one of these procedures would ever be indicated.

Patient Information

Refer patients and family members to the patient information supplied with the product for instructions describing the method of preparing and injecting glucagon. Advise the patient and family members to become familiar with the technique of preparing glucagon before an emergency arises. Instruct patients to use 1 mg (1 unit) for adults and half the adult dose (0.5 mg [0.5 unit]) for pediatric patients weighing < 44 lbs (20 kg).

GLUCAGON (rDNA Origin)

Inform patients and family members of the following measures to prevent hypoglycemic reactions due to insulin:

- Reasonable uniformity from day to day with regard to diet, insulin, and exercise.
- Careful adjustment of the insulin program so that the type (or types) of insulin, dose, and time (or times) of administration are suited to the individual patient.
- Frequent testing of the blood or urine for glucose so that a change in insulin requirements can be foreseen.
- Routine carrying of sugar, candy, or other readily absorbable carbohydrate by the patient so that it may be taken at the first warning of an oncoming reaction.

To prevent severe hypoglycemia, inform patients and family members of the symptoms of mild hypoglycemia and how to treat it appropriately.

Inform family members to arouse the patient as quickly as possible because prolonged hypoglycemia may result in damage to the CNS. Glucagon or IV glucose should awaken the patient sufficiently so that oral carbohydrates may be taken.

Advise patients to inform their physician when hypoglycemic reactions occur so that the treatment regimen may be adjusted if necessary.

GLUCOSE

otc	**Glutose** (Paddock)	**Gel:** Liquid glucose (40% dextrose)	Dye free. In 80 g bottle and 25 g tube.
otc	**Insta-Glucose** (ICN)		Cherry flavor. In UD 30.8 g tubes.
otc	**Insulin Reaction** (Sherwood)		Lime flavor. In UD 25 g tubes.
otc	**Dex4 Glucose** (Can-Am Care)	**Tablets:** Glucose	Lemon, orange, raspberry and grape flavors. In 10s and 50s.
otc	**B-D Glucose** (Becton Dickinson)	**Tablets, chewable:** 5 g	In 36s.

Refer to parenteral dextrose (d-glucose) in Nutrients and Nutritional Agents which is also used in the treatment of acute hypoglycemia.

Indications

Management of hypoglycemia.

Administration and Dosage

Administer 10 to 20 g orally; repeat in 10 minutes if necessary. Response should occur in 10 minutes.

Glucose is not absorbed from the buccal cavity; it must be swallowed to be effective. While swallowing reflexes may be preserved in the unconscious patient, the lack of normal gag reflexes may lead to aspiration. When possible, use other methods of treating hypoglycemia in unconscious patients.

➤ *Children:* Do not give to children under 2 years of age, unless directed by a physician.

Actions

➤ *Pharmacology:* Glucose, a monosaccharide, is absorbed from the intestine after administration and then used, distributed and stored by the tissues. Direct absorption takes place, resulting in a rapid increased blood glucose concentration. Therefore, it is effective in small doses; no evidence of toxicity has been reported. Glucose provides 4 calories/gram.

Adverse Reactions

Isolated reports of nausea, which may also occur with hypoglycemia.

Cortisol, the major endogenous glucocorticoid produced in the body, is produced and secreted via the hypothalamic-anterior pituitary-adrenocortical (HPA) axis. The adrenal cortex synthesizes and secretes the steroid hormones which include mineralocorticoids (aldosterone), glucocorticoids, and to a minor extent, androgenic hormones. Aldosterone secretion is controlled mainly by potassium and the renin-angiotensin system; physiological regulation of glucocorticoid synthesis and secretion is mediated by corticotropin (ACTH), which is secreted by the anterior pituitary gland. In response to low plasma cortisol levels, ACTH is secreted; high plasma cortisol levels inhibit ACTH secretion. This relationship follows a diurnal pattern. Cholesterol and its esters are converted to pregnenolone by ACTH, which is further converted to cortisol and other intermediary products (eg, androgens). ACTH secretion is also stimulated by hypothalamic corticotropin-releasing factor, which is stimulated by serotonin, dopamine and other neurotransmitters in response to stress (emotional, physical or chemical). ACTH secretion at any given time is influenced by a negative feedback relationship from circulating glucocorticoids and the neural signals associated with stress response and the circadian pattern.

Primary adrenocortical insufficiency (Addison's disease) requires replacement therapy with physiologic doses of both mineralocorticoids and glucocorticoids. Secondary adrenocortical insufficiency due to inadequate ACTH secretion may be treated either with replacement steroid administration or with ACTH. Pharmacologic doses of exogenous glucocorticoids are used for their profound anti-inflammatory effects.

Excessive secretion of glucocorticoids (Cushing's syndrome) is due to excessive ACTH or a primary adrenal source (eg, benign adenoma, carcinoma) and is most effectively treated surgically; however, aminoglutethimide inhibits glucocorticoid synthesis and may be used to suppress excessive adrenal activity.

The agents discussed in this section are listed below:

➤*Adrenal steroid inhibitor:* Aminoglutethimide inhibits the enzymatic biosynthesis of adrenal steroids. It is useful in suppressing excessive adrenosteroid production in Cushing's syndrome.

➤*Adrenocorticotropic hormone:* Adrenocorticotropic hormone (corticotropin or ACTH), secreted by the anterior pituitary, stimulates the adrenal cortex to produce and secrete its natural steroids by activating adenyl cyclase in the cell membranes. ACTH is included in this section since the therapeutic effects of its administration are due to the activity of the liberated adrenal steroids. Adequate adrenal function is necessary for ACTH to elicit a pharmacologic response. *Cosyntropin,* a synthetic analog of ACTH, has similar corticotropic activity, but is devoid of the immunogenic properties of ACTH of porcine origin.

➤*Glucocorticoids:* Glucocorticoids cause profound and varied metabolic effects in addition to modifying the body's immune response to diverse stimuli. The naturally occurring glucocorticoids and many synthetic steroids have both glucocorticoid and mineralocorticoid activity. Other synthetic steroids have potent glucocorticoid activity without significant mineralocorticoid activity.

Glucocorticoid product listings are included in the following sections:
Oral and parenteral
Retention enemas
Respiratory inhalant
Intranasal
Ophthalmic
Topical

➤*Mineralocorticoids:* Fludrocortisone is used for partial replacement therapy in adrenocortical insufficiency and for the treatment of salt-losing adrenogenital syndrome.

Adrenal Steroid Inhibitors

AMINOGLUTETHIMIDE

| *Rx* | **Cytadren** (Ciba) | **Tablets:** 250 mg | (Ciba 24). White, scored. In 100s. |

Indications

➤*Cushing's syndrome:* For the suppression of adrenal function in selected patients with Cushing's syndrome.

➤*Unlabeled uses:* Aminoglutethimide has been used successfully in postmenopausal patients with advanced breast carcinoma and in patients with metastatic prostate carcinoma.

Aminoglutethimide was previously marketed as an anticonvulsant, but was withdrawn for that use in 1966.

Administration and Dosage

Institute treatment in a hospital until a stable dosage regimen is achieved.

Give 250 mg 4 times daily, preferably at 6 hour intervals. Follow adrenal cortical response by careful monitoring of plasma cortisol until the desired level of suppression is achieved. If cortisol suppression is inadequate, dosage may be increased in increments of 250 mg daily at intervals of 1 to 2 weeks to a total daily dose of 2 g.

Dose reduction or temporary discontinuation may be required in the event of adverse responses (ie, extreme drowsiness, severe skin rash or excessively low cortisol levels). If skin rash persists for > 5 to 8 days or becomes severe, discontinue the drug. It may be possible to reinstate therapy at a lower dosage following the disappearance of a mild or moderate rash.

Mineralocorticoid replacement therapy (ie, fludrocortisone) may be necessary. If glucocorticoid replacement therapy is needed, 20 to 30 mg hydrocortisone orally in the morning will replace endogenous secretion.

Actions

➤*Pharmacology:* Aminoglutethimide inhibits the enzymatic conversion of cholesterol to $\triangle^5$-pregnenolone, thereby reducing the synthesis of adrenal glucocorticoids, mineralocorticoids, estrogens and androgens. Aminoglutethimide blocks several other steps in steroid synthesis, including the hydroxylations required for the aromatization of androgens to estrogens. A decrease in adrenal secretion of cortisol is followed by an increased secretion of pituitary adrenocorticotropic hormone (ACTH), which will overcome the blockade of adrenocortical steroid synthesis by aminoglutethimide.

➤*Pharmacokinetics:* Aminoglutethimide is effectively absorbed orally and is minimally bound to plasma protein. Its half-life is 11 to 16 hours initially, but decreases after 1 to 2 weeks to 5 to 9 hours. Approximately 34% to 54% is excreted unchanged in the urine and 20% to 50% is excreted as the acetylated metabolite (less than one-fifth as active as the parent compound). The acetylation mechanism is genetically controlled.

➤*Clinical trials:* Morning levels of plasma cortisol in patients with adrenal carcinoma and ectopic ACTH-producing tumors were reduced on the average to about one half of the pretreatment levels, and in patients with adrenal hyperplasia to about two thirds of the pretreatment levels, during 1 to 3 months of therapy with aminoglutethimide.

Data available from the few patients with adrenal adenoma suggest similar reductions in plasma cortisol levels. Measurements of plasma cortisol showed reductions to ≥ 50% of baseline or to normal levels in one third or more of the patients studied, depending on the diagnostic groups and time of measurement.

Contraindications

Hypersensitivity to glutethimide or aminoglutethimide.

Warnings

➤*Duration of therapy:* Because aminoglutethimide does not affect the underlying disease process, it has been used primarily until more definitive therapy (ie, surgery) can be undertaken, or in cases where such therapy is not appropriate. Only a small number of patients have been treated for > 3 months. A decreased effect or escape from a favorable effect occurs more frequently in pituitary-dependent Cushing's syndrome, probably because of increasing ACTH levels in response to decreasing glucocorticoid levels.

➤*Cortical hypofunction:* May cause adrenal cortical hypofunction, especially under conditions of stress such as surgery, trauma or acute illness. Monitor patients carefully and give hydrocortisone and mineralocorticoid supplements as indicated. Do not use dexamethasone. (See Drug Interactions.)

➤*Hypotension:* Aminoglutethimide may suppress aldosterone production by the adrenal cortex and may cause orthostatic or persistent hypotension. Monitor blood pressure in all patients at appropriate intervals.

➤*Pregnancy: Category D.* Aminoglutethimide can cause fetal harm when administered to pregnant women. In about 5000 patients, two cases of pseudohermaphroditism were reported in female infants whose mothers took aminoglutethimide and concomitant anticonvulsants. Normal pregnancies have also occurred during the administration of the drug. When administered to rats at doses ½ to 3 times the maximum human dose, aminoglutethimide caused a decrease in fetal implantation, and increased fetal deaths, teratogenic effects and pseudohermaphroditism. If this drug must be used during pregnancy, or if the patient becomes pregnant while taking the drug, apprise her of the potential hazard to the fetus.

➤*Lactation:* It is not known whether this drug is excreted in breast milk. Decide whether to discontinue nursing or to discontinue the drug, taking into account the importance of the drug to the mother.

➤*Children:* Safety and efficacy have not been established.

Precautions

➤*Monitoring:* Hypothyroidism may occur. Make appropriate clinical observations and perform thyroid function studies as indicated. Supplementary thyroid hormone may be required.

Hematologic abnormalities have been reported. Elevations in AST, alkaline phosphatase and bilirubin have been reported. Perform appropriate clinical observations and regular laboratory studies before and during therapy. Determine serum electrolytes periodically.

AMINOGLUTETHIMIDE

Drug Interactions

Aminoglutethimide Drug Interactions			
Precipitant drug	Object drug*		Description
Aminoglutethimide	Anticoagulants	↓	Anticoagulant effects may be decreased.
Aminoglutethimide	Dexamethasone	↓	Possible loss of dexamethasone-induced adrenal suppression. If a corticosteroid is needed, substitute hydrocortisone.
Aminoglutethimide	Digitoxin	↓	Digitoxin clearance may be increased.
Aminoglutethimide	Medroxyprogesterone	↓	Medroxyprogesterone serum levels may be decreased.
Aminoglutethimide	Theophyllines	↓	The action of theophyllines may be reduced.

* ↓ = Object drug decreased.

Adverse Reactions

Untoward effects have been reported in ≈ 67% of patients treated for ≥ 4 weeks in Cushing's syndrome. The most frequent effects are: Drowsiness (≈ 33%), morbilliform skin rash (17%), nausea and anorexia (12.5%). These are reversible and often disappear spontaneously within 1 or 2 weeks of continued therapy.

➤*Cardiovascular:* Hypotension, occasionally orthostatic (3%); tachycardia (2.5%).

➤*CNS:* Headache and dizziness, possibly caused by decreased vascular resistance or orthostasis (5%).

➤*Dermatologic:* Rash (17%, often reversible on continued therapy); pruritus (5%). These may be allergic or hypersensitivity reactions. Urticaria has occurred rarely.

➤*Endocrine:* Adrenal insufficiency occurred during ≥ 4 weeks of therapy in 3% of patients with Cushing's syndrome. Hypothyroidism, occasionally associated with thyroid enlargement, may be detected early or confirmed by measuring the plasma levels of the thyroid hormones. Masculinization and hirsutism in females and precocious sex development in males have occasionally occurred.

➤*Hematologic:* In 4 of 27 patients with adrenal carcinoma who were treated for at least 4 weeks, there were single occurrences of neutropenia, leukopenia (patient received mitotane concomitantly) and pancytopenia. One patient with adrenal hyperplasia showed decreased hemoglobin and hematocrit during treatment. In 1214 noncushingoid patients, transient leukopenia was reported once. Coombs-negative hemolytic anemia was reported in 1 patient. In ≈ 300 patients with nonadrenal malignancy, 4% of cases showed some degree of anemia and 2 developed pancytopenia. Thrombocytopenia and agranulocytosis also have occurred.

➤*Hepatic:* Isolated abnormal liver function tests; suspected hepatotoxicity (< 0.1%); cholestatic jaundice (hypersensitivity mechanism suspected).

➤*Miscellaneous:* Vomiting, myalgia (3%). Fever, possibly related to therapy, occurred in several patients on aminoglutethimide for < 4 weeks when given with other drugs.

Overdosage

➤*Symptoms:* Overdosage has caused ataxia, somnolence, lethargy, dizziness, fatigue, coma, hyperventilation, respiratory depression, nausea and vomiting, loss of sodium and water, hyponatremia, hypochloremia, hyperkalemia, hypoglycemia, hypovolemic shock due to dehydration and hypotension. Extreme weakness has been reported with divided doses of 3 g/day. No reports of death following doses estimated as large as 7 g.

The signs and symptoms of acute overdosage with aminoglutethimide may be aggravated or modified if alcohol, hypnotics, tranquilizers, or tricyclic antidepressants have been taken at the same time.

➤*Treatment:* Gastric lavage and supportive treatment have been employed. Full consciousness following deep coma was regained ≤ 40 hours after ingestion of 3 or 4 g without lavage. No evidence of hematologic, renal or hepatic effects were subsequently found. Consider dialysis in severe intoxication. Treatment includes usual supportive measures. Refer to General Management of Acute Overdosage.

Patient Information

May produce drowsiness or dizziness; patients should observe caution while driving or performing other tasks requiring alertness, coordination, or physical dexterity.

May cause rash, fainting, weakness, or headache; notify physician if pronounced.

Nausea and loss of appetite may occur during the first 2 weeks of therapy; notify physician if these persist or become pronounced.

For complete prescribing information, refer to the Adrenocortical Steroids introduction.

Indications

➤*ACTH and cosyntropin:* For diagnostic testing of adrenocortical function and in the screening of patients presumed to have adrenocortical insufficiency. Cosyntropin is less allergenic than the exogenous ACTH preparations.

➤*ACTH:* Corticotropin has limited therapeutic value in conditions responsive to corticosteroid therapy; in such cases, corticosteroid therapy is the treatment of choice. Repository corticotropin may be used in the following disorders:

Allergic states – Control of severe or incapacitating allergic conditions intractable to adequate trials of conventional treatment: Seasonal or perennial allergic rhinitis; bronchial asthma; contact dermatitis; atopic dermatitis; serum sickness.

Collagen diseases – During an exacerbation or as maintenance therapy in selected cases of systemic lupus erythematosus; systemic dermatomyositis (polymyositis); acute rheumatic carditis.

Dermatologic diseases – Pemphigus; bullous dermatitis herpetiformis; severe erythema multiforme (Stevens-Johnson syndrome); exfoliative dermatitis; severe psoriasis; severe seborrheic dermatitis; mycosis fungoides.

Edematous state – To induce a diuresis or a remission of proteinuria in the nephrotic syndrome without uremia of the idiopathic type or that due to lupus erythematosus.

Endocrine disorders – Nonsuppurative thyroiditis; hypercalcemia associated with cancer.

GI diseases – To tide the patient over a critical period of the disease in ulcerative colitis and regional enteritis.

Hematologic disorders – Acquired (autoimmune) hemolytic anemia; secondary thrombocytopenia in adults; erythroblastopenia (RBC anemia); congenital (erythroid) hypoplastic anemia.

Neoplastic disease – For palliative management of leukemias and lymphomas in adults and acute leukemia of childhood.

Nervous system diseases – Acute exacerbations of multiple sclerosis.

Ophthalmic diseases – Severe acute and chronic allergic and inflammatory processes involving the eye and its adnexa such as the following: Allergic conjunctivitis; keratitis; herpes zoster ophthalmicus; iritis and iridocyclitis; diffuse posterior uveitis and choroiditis; optic neuritis; sympathetic ophthalmia; chorioretinitis; anterior segment inflammation; allergic corneal marginal ulcers.

Rheumatic disorders – As adjunctive therapy for short-term administration (to tide the patient over an acute episode or exacerbation) in the following: Psoriatic arthritis; rheumatoid arthritis, including juvenile rheumatoid arthritis (selected cases may require low-dose maintenance therapy); ankylosing spondylitis; acute and subacute bursitis; acute nonspecific tenosynovitis; acute gouty arthritis; post-traumatic arthritis; synovitis of osteoarthritis; epicondylitis.

Respiratory diseases – Symptomatic sarcoidosis; Loeffler's syndrome not manageable by other means; berylliosis; fulminating or disseminated pulmonary tuberculosis when used concurrently with antituberculous chemotherapy; aspiration pneumonitis.

Miscellaneous – Tuberculous meningitis with subarachnoid block or impending block when accompanied by antituberculous chemotherapy; trichinosis with neurologic or myocardial involvement.

➤*Unlabeled uses:* Treatment of infantile spasms.

Actions

➤*Pharmacology:* ACTH stimulates the adrenal cortex to secrete cortisol, corticosterone, aldosterone, and a number of weakly androgenic substances. Although ACTH does stimulate secretion of aldosterone, the rate is relatively independent. Prolonged administration of large doses of ACTH induces hyperplasia and hypertrophy of the adrenal cortex and continuous high output of cortisol, corticosterone, and weak androgens. The release of ACTH is under the influence of the nervous system via the corticotropin regulatory hormone released from the hypothalamus and by a negative corticosteroid feedback mechanism. Elevated plasma cortisol suppresses ACTH release.

Cosyntropin is a synthetic peptide corresponding to the amino acid residues 1 to 24 of human ACTH, which exhibits the full corticosteroidogenic activity of natural ACTH. A dose of 0.25 mg cosyntropin is pharmacologically equivalent to 25 units of natural ACTH. Cosyntropin is less allergenic than natural ACTH.

➤*Pharmacokinetics:* ACTH rapidly disappears from the circulation following its IV administration; in humans, the plasma half-life is about 15 minutes. The maximal effects of a trophic hormone on a target organ are achieved when optimal amounts of hormone are acting continuously. Thus, a fixed dose of ACTH will demonstrate a linear increase in adrenocortical secretion with increasing duration for the infusion.

Contraindications

➤*Repository corticotropin:* Scleroderma; osteoporosis; systemic fungal infections; ocular herpes simplex; recent surgery; history of or presence of peptic ulcer; congestive heart failure (CHF); hypertension; sensitivity to porcine proteins; IV administration. Treatment of conditions accompanied by primary adrenocortical insufficiency or adrenocortical hyperfunction.

➤*Cosyntropin:* Previous adverse reaction to drug.

Warnings

➤*Do not administer:* Do not administer until adrenal responsiveness has been verified with the route of administration (IM or SC) that will be used during treatment. A rise in urinary and plasma corticosteroid values provides direct evidence of a stimulatory effect.

➤*Chronic administration:* Chronic administration may lead to irreversible adverse effects. ACTH may suppress signs and symptoms of chronic disease without altering the natural course of the disease. Since complications with corticotropin use are dependent on the dose and duration of treatment, a risk to benefit decision must be made in each case.

➤*Prolonged use:* Prolonged use increases the risk of hypersensitivity reactions and may produce posterior subcapsular cataracts and glaucoma with possible damage to the optic nerve.

➤*Stress:* Although the action of ACTH is similar to that of exogenous adrenocortical steroids, the quantity of adrenocorticoid secreted may be variable. In patients who receive prolonged corticotropin therapy, use additional rapidly acting corticosteroids before, during, and after an unusually stressful situation.

➤*Infection:* ACTH may mask signs of infection including fungal or viral eye infections that may appear during its use. There may be decreased resistance and inability to localize infection. When infection is present, administer appropriate anti-infective therapy.

Tuberculosis – Observe patients with latent tuberculosis. During prolonged ACTH therapy, administer chemoprophylaxis.

➤*Immunosuppression:* Perform immunization procedures with caution, especially when high doses are administered, because of the possible hazards of neurological complications and lack of antibody response. While on corticotropin therapy, patients should not be vaccinated against smallpox.

➤*Blood pressure and electrolytes:* Corticotropin can elevate blood pressure, cause salt and water retention, and increase potassium and calcium excretion. Dietary salt restriction and potassium supplementation may be necessary.

➤*Hypersensitivity:* Cosyntropin exhibits slight immunologic activity, does not contain animal protein, and is less risky to use than natural ACTH. Patients known to be sensitized to natural ACTH with markedly positive skin tests will, with few exceptions, react negatively when tested intradermally with *Cortrosyn*. Most patients with a history of a previous hypersensitivity reaction to natural ACTH or a pre-existing allergic disease will tolerate cosyntropin; however, hypersensitivity reactions are possible. Refer to Management of Acute Hypersensitivity Reactions.

➤*Pregnancy: Category C.* ACTH has embryocidal effects. Use in pregnancy only when clearly needed and when potential benefits outweigh potential hazards to the fetus.

➤*Lactation:* It is not known whether this drug is excreted in breast milk. Because of the potential for serious adverse reactions in nursing infants from ACTH, decide whether to discontinue nursing or to discontinue the drug.

➤*Children:* Prolonged use of corticotropin in children will inhibit skeletal growth. If use is necessary, give intermittently and carefully observe the child.

Precautions

➤*Concomitant therapy:* Because maximal corticotropin stimulation of the adrenals may be limited during the first few days of treatment, administer other drugs when an immediate therapeutic effect is desirable.

Administer for treatment only when disease is intractable to nonsteroid treatment.

➤*Use the lowest possible dose:* Use the lowest possible dose to control the condition, and when reduction in dosage is possible, it should be gradual.

➤*Adrenocortical insufficiency:* Suppression of the pituitary adrenal axis occurs following prolonged therapy, which may be slow in returning to normal. Protect patients from the stress of trauma or surgery by the use of corticosteroids during the period of stress.

➤*Hypothyroidism and cirrhosis:* An enhanced effect of corticotropin may occur.

➤*Multiple sclerosis:* Although ACTH may speed the resolution of acute exacerbations of multiple sclerosis, it does not affect the ultimate outcome or natural course of the disease. Relatively high doses of

ACTH are necessary to demonstrate a significant effect.

➤*Acute gouty arthritis:* Limit treatment of acute gouty arthritis to a few days. Since rebound attacks may occur when corticotropin is discontinued, administer conventional concomitant therapy during corticotropin treatment and for several days after it is stopped.

➤*Mental disturbances:* Psychic symptoms may appear, or pre-existing symptoms may be enhanced. These may range from mood alteration to a psychotic state.

➤*Secondary disease:* Patients with a secondary disease may have that disease worsened. Use with caution in patients with diabetes, diverticulitis, renal insufficiency, and myasthenia gravis.

Drug Interactions

Corticotropin (ACTH) Drug Interactions			
Precipitant drug	Object drug*		Description
Corticotropin, Cosyntropin	Anticholinesterases	↓	Corticosteroids antagonize the effects of anticholinesterases in myasthenia gravis.
Corticotropin, Cosyntropin	Aspirin	↓	Corticosteroids will reduce serum salicylate levels and may decrease their effectiveness. Use aspirin cautiously in conjunction with corticotropin in hypoprothrombinemia.
Corticotropin, Cosyntropin	Diuretics	↑	Corticotropin may accentuate the electrolyte loss associated with diuretic therapy.
Barbiturates	Corticotropin, Cosyntropin	↓	Decreased pharmacologic effects of the corticosteroid may be observed. Avoid this combination if possible. Monitor closely. Increases in the corticosteroid dosage may be required.
Hydantoins (eg, phenytoin)	Corticotropin, Cosyntropin	↓	Decreased corticosteroid effects may occur. Phenytoin levels may be reduced. Monitor phenytoin levels and adjust dose of either agent if needed.
Corticotropin, Cosyntropin	Hydantoins (eg, phenytoin)		

* ↑ = Object drug increased. ↓ = Object drug decreased.

Adverse Reactions

➤*Cardiovascular:* Hypertension; CHF; necrotizing angiitis; bradycardia; tachycardia.

➤*CNS:* Convulsions; vertigo; headache; increased intracranial pressure with papilledema (pseudotumor cerebri), usually after treatment.

➤*Dermatologic:* Impaired wound healing; petechiae and ecchymoses; increased sweating; hyperpigmentation; thin fragile skin; facial erythema; acne; suppression of skin test reactions; rash.

➤*Endocrine:* Menstrual irregularities; suppression of growth in children; hirsutism; development of Cushingoid state; manifestations of latent diabetes mellitus; decreased carbohydrate tolerance; increased requirements for insulin or oral hypoglycemic agents in diabetics; secondary adrenocortical and pituitary unresponsiveness, especially during stress.

➤*GI:* Pancreatitis; ulcerative esophagitis; abdominal distention; peptic ulcer with possible perforation and hemorrhage.

➤*Hypersensitivity:* Allergic reactions may manifest as dizziness, nausea, vomiting, shock, and skin reactions. A rare hypersensitivity reaction usually associated with pre-existing allergic disease and/or a previous reaction to natural ACTH is possible. Symptoms may include slight whealing with splotchy erythema at the injection site. There have been rare reports of anaphylactic reaction.

➤*Metabolic:* Negative nitrogen balance due to protein catabolism; sodium and fluid retention; potassium and calcium loss; hypokalemic alkalosis; peripheral edema.

➤*Musculoskeletal:* Muscle weakness; steroid myopathy; loss of muscle mass; osteoporosis; vertebral compression fractures; pathologic fracture of long bones; aseptic necrosis of femoral and humeral heads.

➤*Ophthalmic:* Posterior subcapsular cataracts; increased intraocular pressure; glaucoma with possible damage to optic nerve; exophthalmos.

➤*Miscellaneous:* Abscess; prolonged use of ACTH may result in antibody production and subsequent loss of the stimulatory effect.

Overdosage

An acute overdose would present no different adverse reactions.

Patient Information

ACTH may mask signs of infection. There may be decreased resistance and inability to localize infection.

Diabetics may have increased requirements for insulin or oral hypoglycemics.

Notify physician if marked fluid retention, muscle weakness, abdominal pain, seizures, or headache occurs.

REPOSITORY CORTICOTROPIN INJECTION

Rx	H.P. Acthar Gel (Aventis)	Repository injection: 80 units/mL	In 5 mL multidose vials.[1]

[1] With 16% gelatin.

For complete prescribing information, refer to the Corticotropin group monograph.

Indications

For diagnostic testing of adrenocortical function. Corticotropin has limited therapeutic value in conditions responsive to corticosteroid therapy; in such cases, corticosteroid therapy is the treatment of choice. Repository corticotropin may be used in the following disorders:

➤*Allergic states:* Control of severe or incapacitating allergic conditions intractable to adequate trials of conventional treatment: Seasonal or perennial allergic rhinitis; bronchial asthma; contact dermatitis; atopic dermatitis; serum sickness.

➤*Collagen diseases:* During an exacerbation or as maintenance therapy in selected cases of systemic lupus erythematosus; systemic dermatomyositis (polymyositis); acute rheumatic carditis.

➤*Dermatologic diseases:* Pemphigus; bullous dermatitis herpetiformis; severe erythema multiforme (Stevens-Johnson syndrome); exfoliative dermatitis; severe psoriasis; severe seborrheic dermatitis; mycosis fungoides.

➤*Edematous state:* To induce a diuresis or a remission of proteinuria in the nephrotic syndrome without uremia of the idiopathic type or that due to lupus erythematosus.

➤*Endocrine disorders:* Nonsuppurative thyroiditis; hypercalcemia associated with cancer.

➤*GI diseases:* To tide the patient over a critical period of the disease in ulcerative colitis and regional enteritis.

➤*Hematologic disorders:* Acquired (autoimmune) hemolytic anemia; secondary thrombocytopenia in adults; erythroblastopenia (RBC anemia); congenital (erythroid) hypoplastic anemia.

➤*Neoplastic disease:* For palliative management of leukemias and lymphomas in adults and acute leukemia of childhood.

➤*Nervous system diseases:* Acute exacerbations of multiple sclerosis.

➤*Ophthalmic diseases:* Severe acute and chronic allergic and inflammatory processes involving the eye and its adnexa such as the following: Allergic conjunctivitis; keratitis; herpes zoster ophthalmicus; iritis and iridocyclitis; diffuse posterior uveitis and choroiditis; optic neuritis; sympathetic ophthalmia; chorioretinitis; anterior segment inflammation; allergic corneal marginal ulcers.

➤*Rheumatic disorders:* As adjunctive therapy for short-term administration (to tide the patient over an acute episode or exacerbation) in the following: Psoriatic arthritis; rheumatoid arthritis, including juvenile rheumatoid arthritis (selected cases may require low-dose maintenance therapy); ankylosing spondylitis; acute and subacute bursitis; acute nonspecific tenosynovitis; acute gouty arthritis; post-traumatic arthritis; synovitis of osteoarthritis; epicondylitis.

➤*Respiratory diseases:* Symptomatic sarcoidosis; Loeffler's syndrome not manageable by other means; berylliosis; fulminating or disseminated pulmonary tuberculosis when used concurrently with antituberculous chemotherapy; aspiration pneumonitis.

➤*Miscellaneous:* Tuberculous meningitis with subarachnoid block or impending block when accompanied by antituberculous chemotherapy; trichinosis with neurologic or myocardial involvement.

➤*Unlabeled uses:* Treatment of infantile spasms.

Administration and Dosage

Standard tests for verification of adrenal responsiveness to corticotropin may utilize as much as 80 units as a single injection, or 1 or more injections of a lesser dosage. Perform verification tests prior to treatment with corticotropins. The test should utilize the route(s) of administration proposed for treatment. Following verification, individualize dosage. Attempt only gradual change in dosage schedules after full drug effects have become apparent.

Chronic administration of more than 40 units/day may be associated with uncontrollable adverse effects.

When indicated, reduce dosage gradually by increasing the duration between injections or decreasing the quantity of corticotropin injected or both.

➤*Acute exacerbations of multiple sclerosis:* 80 to 120 units/day IM for 2 to 3 weeks.

➤*Usual dose:* 40 to 80 units IM or SC every 24 to 72 hours.

➤*Storage/Stability:* Refrigerate repository corticotropin injection between 2° and 8°C (36° and 46°F).

COSYNTROPIN

Rx	**Cortrosyn** (Amphastar)	**Powder for Injection, lyophilized:** 0.25 mg	In vials[1] with diluent.

[1] With 10 mg mannitol.

For complete prescribing information, refer to the Corticotropin group monograph.

Indications

For use as a diagnostic agent in the screening of patients presumed to have adrenocortical insufficiency.

➤*Unlabeled uses:* Treatment of infantile spasms.

Administration and Dosage

Administer IM or IV as a rapid screening test of adrenal function. It may also be given as an IV infusion over 4 to 8 hours to provide a greater stimulus to the adrenal glands. Doses of 0.25 to 0.75 mg have been used and a maximal response noted with the smallest dose. One suggested dose is 0.25 mg dissolved in sterile saline injected IM.

➤*Children (2 years of age or younger):* 0.125 mg will often suffice.

➤*IV infusion:* Add 0.25 mg cosyntropin to glucose or saline solutions and give at a rate of approximately 40 mcg/hour over 6 hours.

For test procedure and interpretation of results, refer to manufacturer's insert.

Glucocorticoids

For complete prescribing information, refer to the Adrenocortical Steroids introduction.

Indications

➤*Allergic states:* Control of severe or incapacitating allergic conditions intractable to conventional treatment in serum sickness and drug hypersensitivity reactions.

Parenteral therapy is indicated for urticarial transfusion reactions and acute noninfectious laryngeal edema (epinephrine is the first drug of choice).

➤*Collagen diseases:* For exacerbation or maintenance therapy in selected cases of systemic lupus erythematosus, acute rheumatic carditis or systemic dermatomyositis (polymyositis).

➤*Dermatologic diseases:* Pemphigus; bullous dermatitis herpetiformis; severe erythema multiforme (Stevens-Johnson syndrome); mycosis fungoides; severe psoriasis; angioedema or urticaria; exfoliative, severe seborrheic, contact, or atopic dermatitis.

➤*Edematous states:* To induce diuresis or remission of proteinuria in the nephrotic syndrome (without uremia) of the idiopathic type or that due to lupus erythematosus.

➤*Endocrine disorders:* Primary or secondary adrenal cortical insufficiency (hydrocortisone or cortisone is the drug of choice; synthetic analogs may be used in conjunction with mineralocorticoids; in infancy, mineralocorticoid supplementation is important); congenital adrenal hyperplasia; nonsuppurative thyroiditis; hypercalcemia associated with cancer.

Parenteral – Acute adrenal cortical insufficiency (hydrocortisone or cortisone is drug of choice); preoperatively or in serious trauma or illness with known adrenal insufficiency or when adrenal cortical reserve is doubtful; shock unresponsive to conventional therapy if adrenal cortical insufficiency exists or is suspected.

➤*GI diseases:* To tide the patient over a critical period of the disease in ulcerative colitis, regional enteritis (Crohn's disease), and intractable sprue.

➤*Hematologic disorders:* Idiopathic thrombocytopenic purpura and secondary thrombocytopenia in adults (IV only; IM use is contraindicated); acquired (autoimmune) hemolytic anemia; erythroblastopenia (RBC anemia); congenital (erythroid) hypoplastic anemia.

➤*Intra-articular or soft tissue administration:* Short-term adjunctive therapy (to tide the patient over an acute episode) in synovitis of osteoarthritis; rheumatoid arthritis; acute and subacute bursitis; acute gouty arthritis; epicondylitis; acute nonspecific tenosynovitis; post-traumatic osteoarthritis.

➤*Intralesional administration:* Keloids; localized hypertrophic, infiltrated, inflammatory lesions of lichen planus, psoriatic plaques, granuloma annulare, lichen simplex chronicus (neurodermatitis); discoid lupus erythematosus; necrobiosis lipoidica diabeticorum; alopecia areata. May be useful in cystic tumors of an aponeurosis or tendon (ganglia).

➤*Neoplastic diseases:* For palliative management of leukemias and lymphomas in adults and acute leukemia of childhood.

➤*Nervous system:* Acute exacerbations of multiple sclerosis (see Precautions).

➤*Ophthalmic:* Severe acute and chronic allergic and inflammatory processes involving the eye and its adnexa such as in the following: Allergic conjunctivitis; keratitis; allergic corneal marginal ulcers; herpes zoster ophthalmicus; iritis and iridocyclitis; chorioretinitis; diffuse posterior uveitis and choroiditis; optic neuritis; sympathetic ophthalmia and anterior segment inflammation.

➤*Respiratory diseases:* Symptomatic sarcoidosis; bronchial asthma (including status asthmaticus); Loeffler's syndrome not manageable by other means; berylliosis; fulminating or disseminated pulmonary tuberculosis when accompanied by appropriate antituberculous chemotherapy; aspiration pneumonitis; seasonal or perennial allergic rhinitis.

➤*Rheumatic disorders:* Adjunctive therapy for short-term use (acute episode or exacerbation) in the following: Ankylosing spondylitis; acute and subacute bursitis; acute nonspecific tenosynovitis; acute gouty arthritis; psoriatic arthritis; rheumatoid arthritis, including juvenile (selected cases may require low-dose maintenance therapy); post-traumatic osteoarthritis; synovitis of osteoarthritis; epicondylitis.

➤*Miscellaneous:* Tuberculous meningitis with subarachnoid block or impending block when accompanied by appropriate antituberculous chemotherapy; in trichinosis with neurologic or myocardial involvement.

➤*Dexamethasone:* Dexamethasone also is indicated for testing of adrenal cortical hyperfunction; cerebral edema associated with primary or metastatic brain tumor, craniotomy, or head injury.

➤*Triamcinolone:* Triamcinolone also is indicated for the treatment of pulmonary emphysema where bronchospasm or bronchial edema plays a significant role, and diffuse interstitial pulmonary fibrosis (Hamman-Rich syndrome); in conjunction with diuretic agents to induce a diuresis in refractory CHF and in cirrhosis of the liver with refractory ascites; and for postoperative dental inflammatory reactions.

➤*Unlabeled uses:*

Glucocorticoid Unlabeled Uses	
Use	Drug/Comment
Acute mountain sickness	Dexamethasone 4 mg q 6 h; prevention or treatment
Antiemetic	Dexamethasone most common, 16 to 20 mg
Bacterial meningitis	Dexamethasone 0.15 mg/kg q 6 h; to decrease incidence of hearing loss
Bronchopulmonary dysplasia in preterm infants	Dexamethasone 0.5 mg/kg, then taper.
COPD	Prednisone 30 to 60 mg/day for 1 to 2 weeks, then taper
Depression, diagnosis of	Dexamethasone 1 mg
Duchenne's muscular dystrophy	Prednisone 0.75 to 1.5 mg/kg/day; to improve strength and function
Graves ophthalmopathy	Prednisone 60 mg/day, taper to 20 mg/day
Hepatitis, severe alcoholic	Methylprednisolone 32 mg/day; to reduce mortality
Hirsutism	Dexamethasone 0.5 to 1 mg/day
Respiratory distress syndrome	Prevention in premature neonates (betamethasone most common); adults, methylprednisolone 30 mg/kg (controversial)
Septic shock	Methylprednisolone 30 mg/kg IV most common (very controversial)
Spinal cord injury, acute	Methylprednisolone IV within 8 hrs of injury; to improve neurologic function
Tuberculous pleurisy	Prednisolone 0.75 mg/kg/day, then taper; concurrently w/antituberculous therapy

Administration and Dosage

The maximal activity of the adrenal cortex is between 2 and 8 am, and it is minimal between 4 pm and midnight. Exogenous corticosteroids suppress adrenocortical activity the least when given at the time of maximal activity (am). Therefore, administer glucocorticoids in the morning prior to 9 am. When large doses are given, administer antacids between meals to help prevent peptic ulcers.

➤*Initiation of therapy:* The initial dosage depends on the specific disease entity being treated. Maintain or adjust the initial dosage until a satisfactory response is noted. If after a reasonable period of time there is a lack of satisfactory clinical response, discontinue the drug and transfer the patient to other appropriate therapy. It should be emphasized that dosage requirements are variable and must be individualized. For infants and children, the recommended dosage should be governed by the same considerations rather than by strict adherence to the ratio indicated by age or body weight.

➤*Maintenance therapy:* After a favorable response is observed, determine the maintenance dosage by decreasing the initial dosage in small amounts at intervals until the lowest dosage that will maintain an adequate clinical response is reached. Constant monitoring of drug dosage is required. Situations that may make dosage adjustments necessary are changes in the disease process, the patient's individual drug responsiveness, and the effect of patient exposure to stress; in this latter situation it may be necessary to increase the dosage for a period of time consistent with the patient's condition.

➤*Withdrawal of therapy:* If, after long-term therapy, the drug is to be stopped, it must be withdrawn gradually. If spontaneous remission occurs in a chronic condition, discontinue treatment gradually. Continued supervision of the patient after discontinuation of corticosteroids is essential, because there may be a sudden reappearance of severe manifestations of the disease.

➤*Alternate-day therapy:* Alternate day therapy is a dosing regimen in which twice the usual daily dose is administered every other morning. The purpose is to provide the patient requiring long-term treatment with the beneficial effects of corticosteroids while minimizing pituitary-adrenal suppression, the cushingoid state, withdrawal symptoms, and growth suppression in children. The benefits of alternate-day therapy are only achieved by using the intermediate-acting agents.

The rationale for this treatment schedule is based on 2 major premises: (a) The therapeutic effect of intermediate-acting corticosteroids persists longer than their physical presence and metabolic effects; (b) administration of the corticosteroid every other morning allows for reestablishment of a more normal hypothalamic-pituitary-adrenal (HPA) activity on the off-steroid day. Keep the following in mind when considering alternate day therapy:

1.) Benefits of alternate day therapy do not encourage indiscriminate steroid use.
2.) Alternate day therapy is primarily designed for patients in whom long-term corticosteroid therapy is anticipated.
3.) In less severe disease processes, it may be possible to initiate treatment with alternate day therapy. More severe disease states usually require daily divided high-dose therapy for initial control. Continue initial suppressive dose until satisfactory clinical response is obtained, usually 4 to 10 days in the case of many allergic and collagen diseases. Keep the period of initial suppressive dose as brief as possible, particularly when alternate day

therapy is intended. Once control is established, 2 courses are available: (a) Change to alternate day therapy, then gradually reduce the amount of corticosteroid given every other day or (b) reduce daily corticosteroid dose to the lowest effective level as rapidly as possible, then change over to an alternate day schedule. Theoretically, course (a) may be preferable.

4.) Because of the advantages of alternate day therapy, it may be desirable to try patients on this form of therapy who have been on daily corticosteroids for long periods of time (eg, patients with rheumatoid arthritis). Because these patients may already have a suppressed HPA axis, establishing them on alternate day therapy may be difficult and not always successful; however, it is recommended that such regular attempts be made. It may be helpful to triple or even quadruple the daily maintenance dose and administer this every other day rather than just doubling the daily dose if difficulty is encountered. Once the patient is controlled, attempt to reduce this dose to a minimum.

5.) Long-acting corticosteroids (eg, **dexamethasone, betamethasone**), because of their prolonged suppressive effect on adrenal activity, are not recommended for alternate day therapy.

6.) It is important to individualize therapy. Complete control of symptoms will not be possible in all patients. An explanation of the benefits of alternate day therapy will help the patient to understand and tolerate the possible flare-up in symptoms that may occur in the latter part of the off-steroid day. Other therapy to relieve symptoms may be added or increased at this time if needed.

7.) In the event of an acute flare-up of the disease process, it may be necessary to return to a full suppressive daily corticosteroid dose for control. Once control is established, alternate day therapy may be reinstituted.

➤*Intra-articular injection:* Dose depends on the joint size and varies with the severity of the condition. In chronic cases, injections may be repeated at intervals of 1 to 5 or more weeks, depending upon the degree of relief obtained from the initial injection. Injection must be made into the synovial space. Do not inject unstable joints. Repeated intra-articular injection may result in joint instability. X-ray follow-up is suggested in selected cases to detect deterioration.

Suitable sites – Suitable sites for injection are the knee, ankle, wrist, elbow, shoulder, hip, and phalangeal joints. Because difficulty is frequently encountered in entering the hip joint, avoid any large blood vessels in the area. Joints not suitable for injection are those that are anatomically inaccessible and devoid of synovial space, such as the spinal joints and the sacroiliac joints. Treatment failures frequently result from failure to enter the joint space; little or no benefit follows injection into surrounding tissue. If failures occur when injections into the synovial spaces are certain, as determined by aspiration of fluid, repeated injections are usually of no benefit. Local therapy does not alter the underlying disease process; whenever possible, employ comprehensive therapy, including physiotherapy and orthopedic correction (see Precautions).

➤*Miscellaneous (tendinitis, epicondylitis, ganglion):* In the treatment of conditions such as tendinitis or tenosynovitis, inject into the tendon sheath rather than into the substance of the tendon. When treating conditions such as epicondylitis, outline the area of greatest tenderness and infiltrate the drug into the area. For ganglia of the tendon sheaths, inject the drug directly into the cyst. In many cases, a single injection markedly decreases size of the cystic tumor and may effect disappearance. The dose varies with the condition being treated. In recurrent or chronic conditions, repeated injections may be needed.

➤*Injections for local effect in dermatologic conditions:* Avoid injection of sufficient material to cause blanching because this may be followed by a small slough. One to four injections are usually employed. Intervals between injections vary with the type of lesion being treated and duration of improvement produced by initial injection.

Actions

➤*Pharmacology:* The naturally occurring adrenocortical steroids have both anti-inflammatory (glucocorticoid) and salt-retaining (mineralocorticoid) properties. Glucocorticoids cause profound and varied metabolic effects. In addition, they modify the body's immune responses to diverse stimuli.

These compounds, including **hydrocortisone** (cortisol) and **cortisone**, are used as replacement therapy in adrenocortical deficiency states and may be used for their anti-inflammatory effects. The synthetic steroid compounds **prednisone, prednisolone,** and **fludrocortisone** also have glucocorticoid and mineralocorticoid activity. Prednisone and prednisolone are used primarily for their glucocorticoid effects.

In addition, a group of synthetic compounds with marked glucocorticoid activity are distinguished by the absence of any significant salt-retaining activity. These include **triamcinolone, dexamethasone, methylprednisolone,** and **betamethasone.** These agents are used for their potent anti-inflammatory effects.

➤*Pharmacokinetics:*

Absorption – **Hydrocortisone** and most of its congeners are readily absorbed from the GI tract; greatly altered onsets and durations are usually achieved with injections of suspensions and esters.

Distribution – **Hydrocortisone** is reversibly bound to corticosteroid-binding globulin (CBG or transcortin) and corticosteroid binding albumin (CBA). Exogenous glucocorticoids are bound to these proteins to a significantly lesser degree. In hypoproteinemic or dysproteinemic states, the total endogenous hydrocortisone levels are decreased. Conversely, with increased CBG (pregnancy, estrogen therapy), the total plasma hydrocortisone levels are elevated. These alterations are not of clinical significance because it is the unbound fraction of the hormone that is metabolically active. However, the administration of exogenous glucocorticoids to patients with altered protein-binding capacities will result in significant differences in glucocorticoid pharmacological effects.

Metabolism/Excretion – Hydrocortisone is metabolized by the liver, which is the rate-limiting step in its clearance. The metabolism and excretion of the synthetic glucocorticoids generally parallel hydrocortisone. Induction of hepatic enzymes will increase the metabolic clearance of hydrocortisone and the synthetic glucocorticoids. About 1% of its usual daily production, or about 200 mcg unchanged hormone is excreted in urine daily. Renal clearance is increased when plasma levels are increased. **Prednisone** is inactive and must be metabolized to **prednisolone**. The following table summarizes the approximate dosage equivalencies (based on glucocorticoid properties) of the various glucocorticoid preparations and several of their pharmacokinetic parameters. The half-life values refer to the intrinsic activity of each agent; insoluble salts of these drugs are used as repository injections and have sustained effects because of delayed absorption from the injection site.

Glucocorticoid Equivalencies, Potencies, and Half-Life			
Glucocorticoid	Equivalent potency dose (mg)[1]	Anti-inflammatory potency[1]	Sodium-retaining potency	Half-life plasma (min)
Short-acting				
Cortisone	25	0.8	2	30
Hydrocortisone	20	1	2	80-118
Intermediate-acting				
Prednisone	5	4	1	60
Prednisolone	5	4	1	115-212
Triamcinolone	4	5	0	200+
Methylprednisolone	4	5	0	78-188
Long-acting				
Dexamethasone	0.75	20-30	0	110-210
Betamethasone	0.6-0.75	20-30	0	300+

[1] When converting doses, use only equivalent potency column, not anti-inflammatory potency column.

Contraindications

Systemic fungal infections; hypersensitivity to the drug; IM use in idiopathic thrombocytopenic purpura; administration of live virus vaccines (eg, smallpox) in patients receiving immunosuppressive corticosteroid doses (see Warnings).

Warnings

➤*Infections:* Corticosteroids may mask signs of infection, and new infections may appear during their use. There may be decreased resistance and inability of the host defense mechanisms to prevent dissemination of the infection. If an infection occurs during therapy, it should be promptly controlled by suitable antimicrobial therapy.

Tuberculosis – Restrict use in active tuberculosis to cases of fulminating or disseminated disease in which the corticosteroid is used for disease management with appropriate chemotherapy. If corticosteroids are indicated in latent tuberculosis or tuberculin reactivity, observe closely; disease reactivation may occur. During prolonged corticosteroid use, these patients should receive chemoprophylaxis.

Fungal – Corticosteroids may exacerbate systemic fungal infections; do not use in such infections, except to control drug reactions due to amphotericin B. Concomitant use of amphotericin B and **hydrocortisone** has been followed by cardiac enlargement and CHF.

Amebiasis – Corticosteroids may activate latent amebiasis. Rule out amebiasis before giving to a patient who has been in the tropics or has unexplained diarrhea.

Cerebral malaria – A double-blind trial has shown corticosteroid use is associated with prolongation of coma and a higher incidence of pneumonia and GI bleeding.

➤*Hepatitis:* Although advocated for use in chronic active hepatitis, corticosteroids may be harmful in chronic active hepatitis positive for hepatitis B surface antigen.

➤*Ocular effects:* Prolonged use may produce posterior subcapsular cataracts, glaucoma with possible damage to the optic nerves, and may enhance the establishment of secondary ocular infections due to fungi or viruses. Use cautiously in ocular herpes simplex because of possible corneal perforation.

➤*Fluid and electrolyte balance:* Average and large doses of **hydrocortisone** or **cortisone** can cause elevation of blood pressure, salt and water retention, and increased excretion of potassium. These effects are less likely to occur with the synthetic derivatives except when used in large doses. Dietary salt restriction and potassium supplementation may be necessary. All corticosteroids increase calcium excretion.

➤*Peptic ulcer:* The relationship between peptic ulceration and glucocorticoid therapy is unclear. Patients who appear to be at risk are those being treated for nephrotic syndrome or liver disease or who are comatose postcraniotomy. Other predisposing factors include a total **prednisone** intake exceeding 1 g, a history of ulcer disease, concomitant use of known gastric irritants (as in arthritic patients), and stress. It may be desirable to use prophylactic antacids pending clarification of the relationship.

➤*Immunosuppression:* During therapy, do not use live virus vaccines (eg, smallpox). Do not immunize patients who are receiving corticosteroids, especially high doses, because of possible hazards of neurological complications and a lack of antibody response. This does not apply to patients receiving corticosteroids as replacement therapy. Corticosteroids may suppress reactions to skin tests.

➤*Adrenal suppression:* Prolonged therapy of pharmacologic doses may lead to hypothalamic-pituitary-adrenal suppression. The degree of adrenal suppression varies with the dosage, relative glucocorticoid activity, biological half-life and duration of glucocorticoid therapy within each individual. Adrenal suppression may be minimized by the use of intermediate-acting glucocorticoids (**prednisone**, **prednisolone**, **methylprednisolone**) on an alternate day schedule (see Administration and Dosage).

Following prolonged therapy, abrupt discontinuation may result in a withdrawal syndrome without evidence of adrenal insufficiency. To minimize morbidity associated with adrenal insufficiency, discontinue exogenous corticosteroid therapy gradually. During withdrawal therapy, increased supplementation may be necessary during times of stress. Symptoms of adrenal insufficiency as a result of too rapid withdrawal include the following: Nausea; fatigue; anorexia; dyspnea; hypotension; hypoglycemia; myalgia; fever; malaise; arthralgia; dizziness; desquamation of skin; fainting. Continued supervision after therapy termination is essential; severe disease manifestations may reappear suddenly.

➤*Stress:* In patients receiving or recently withdrawn from corticosteroid therapy subjected to unusual stress, increased dosage of rapidly acting corticosteroids is indicated before, during, and after stressful situations, except in patients on high-dose therapy. Relative adrenocortical insufficiency may persist for months after therapy ends; in any stress situation occurring during that period, reinstitute therapy. Because mineralocorticoid secretion may be impaired, administer salt or a mineralocorticoid concurrently.

➤*Cardiovascular:* Reports suggest an apparent association between corticosteroid use and left ventricular free wall rupture after a recent myocardial infarction. Use with great caution in these patients.

➤*Hypersensitivity reactions:* Anaphylactoid reactions have occurred rarely with corticosteroid therapy; take precautionary measures, especially in patients with a history of allergies. Refer to Management of Acute Hypersensitivity Reactions.

➤*Renal function impairment:* Edema may occur in the presence of renal disease with a fixed or decreased glomerular filtration rate. Use with caution in renal insufficiency, acute glomerulonephritis, and chronic nephritis.

➤*Elderly:* Consider the risk/benefit factors of steroid use. Consider lower doses because of body changes caused by aging (ie, diminution of muscle mass and plasma volume). Monitor blood pressure, blood glucose and electrolytes at least every 6 months.

➤*Pregnancy:* (*Category C* - **Prednisolone sodium phosphate**). Corticosteroids cross the placenta (**prednisone** has the poorest transport). In animal studies, large doses of cortisol administered early in pregnancy produced cleft palate, stillborn fetuses, and decreased fetal size. Chronic maternal ingestion during the first trimester has shown a 1% incidence of cleft palate in humans. If used in pregnancy, or in women of childbearing potential, weigh benefits against the potential hazards to the mother and fetus. Carefully observe infants born of mothers who have received substantial corticosteroid doses during pregnancy for signs of hypoadrenalism.

➤*Lactation:* Corticosteroids appear in breast milk and could suppress growth, interfere with endogenous corticosteroid production or cause other unwanted effects in the nursing infant. Advise mothers taking pharmacologic corticosteroid doses not to nurse. However, several studies suggest that amounts excreted in breast milk are negligible with **prednisone** or **prednisolone** doses ≤ 20 mg/day or **methylprednisolone** doses ≤ 8 mg/day, and large doses for short periods may not harm the infant. Alternatives to consider include waiting 3 to 4 hours after the dose before breastfeeding and using prednisolone rather than prednisone (resulting in a lower corticosteroid dose to the infant).

➤*Children:* Carefully observe growth and development of infants and children on prolonged corticosteroid therapy.

Benzyl alcohol – Some of these products contain benzyl alcohol, which has been associated with a fatal "gasping syndrome" in premature infants.

Precautions

➤*Monitoring:* Observe patients for weight increase, edema, hypertension, and excessive potassium excretion, as well as for less obvious signs of adrenocortical steroid-induced untoward effects. Monitor for a negative nitrogen balance due to protein catabolism. A liberal protein intake is essential during prolonged therapy. Evaluate blood pressure and body weight, and do routine laboratory studies, including 2-hour postprandial blood glucose and serum potassium and a chest x-ray at regular intervals during prolonged therapy. Upper GI x-rays are desirable in patients with known or suspected peptic ulcer disease or significant dyspepsia or in patients complaining of gastric distress. Observe growth and development of infants and children on prolonged therapy.

➤*Use the lowest possible dose:* Make a benefit/risk decision in each individual case as to the size of the dose, duration of treatment, and the use of daily or intermittent therapy because complications of treatment are dependent on these factors.

➤*Use with caution in:*

GI – Nonspecific ulcerative colitis if there is a probability of impending perforation, abscess or other pyogenic infection; diverticulitis; fresh intestinal anastomoses; active or latent peptic ulcer (see Warnings).

Cardiovascular – Hypertension; CHF; thromboembolitic tendencies; thrombophlebitis.

Miscellaneous – Osteoporosis; exanthema; Cushing's syndrome; antibiotic-resistant infections; convulsive disorders; metastatic carcinoma; myasthenia gravis; vaccinia; varicella; diabetes mellitus; hypothyroidism, cirrhosis (enhanced effect of corticosteroids).

➤*Steroid psychosis:* Steroid psychosis is characterized by a delirious or toxic psychosis with clouded sensorium. Other symptoms may include euphoria, insomnia, mood swings, personality changes, and severe depression. The onset of symptoms usually occurs within 15 to 30 days. Predisposing factors include doses > 40 mg **prednisone** equivalent, female predominance, and, possibly, a family history of psychiatric illness. A patient history of psychiatric problems does not correlate well with predisposition to steroid-induced psychosis. Incidence appears to correlate with dose. One study of 718 patients treated with prednisone revealed ≤ 40 mg/day = 1.3%; 41 to 80 mg/day = 4.6%; ≥ 80 mg/day = 18.4%. If the steroids cannot be discontinued, psychotropic medication is effective.

➤*Multiple sclerosis:* Although corticosteroids are effective in speeding the resolution of acute exacerbations of multiple sclerosis, they do not affect the ultimate outcome or natural history of the disease. Relatively high doses of corticosteroids are necessary to demonstrate a significant effect.

➤*Repository injections:* To minimize the likelihood and severity of atrophy, do not inject SC, avoid injection into the deltoid, and avoid repeated IM injections into the same site, if possible. Repository injections are not recommended as initial therapy in acute situations.

➤*Local injections:* Intra-articular injection may produce systemic and local effects. A marked increase in pain accompanied by local swelling, further restriction of joint motion, fever, and malaise is suggestive of septic arthritis. Appropriate examination of any joint fluid present is necessary. If a diagnosis of sepsis is confirmed, institute appropriate antimicrobial therapy. Avoid local injection into an infected site and into unstable joints.

Strongly impress patients with the importance of not overusing joints in which symptomatic benefit has been obtained as long as the inflammatory process remains active. Frequent intra-articular injection may damage joint tissues.

Avoid overdistention of the joint capsule and deposition of steroid along the needle track in intra-articular injection, as it may lead to subcutaneous atrophy. While crystals of adrenal steroids in the dermis suppress inflammatory reactions, their presence may cause disintegration of the cellular elements and physiochemical changes in the ground substance of the connective tissue.

The resultant dermal or subdermal changes may form depressions in the skin at the injection site; the degree will vary with the amount of adrenal steroid injection. Regeneration is usually complete within a few months or after all crystals of the adrenal steroid have been absorbed. In order to minimize the incidence of dermal and subdermal atrophy, exercise care not to exceed recommended doses in injections. Make multiple small injections into the area of the lesion whenever possible.

➤*Tartrazine sensitivity:* Some of these products contain tartrazine, which may cause allergic-type reactions (including bronchial asthma) in susceptible individuals. Although the incidence of tartrazine sensitivity in the general population is low, it is frequently seen in patients who also have aspirin hypersensitivity. Specific products containing tartrazine are identified in the product listings.

➤*Sulfite sensitivity:* Some of these products contain sulfites which may cause severe allergic reactions in certain susceptible individuals, particularly asthmatics. Anaphylactoid and hypersensitivity reactions have occurred. Do not use in patients allergic to sulfites. Products containing sulfites are identified in product listings.

Drug Interactions

Corticosteroid Drug Interactions			
Precipitant drug	Object drug*		Description
Aminoglutethimide	Dexamethasone	↓	Possible loss of dexamethasone-induced adrenal suppression.
Barbiturates	Corticosteroids	↓	Decreased pharmacologic effects of the corticosteroid may be observed.
Cholestyramine	Hydrocortisone	↓	The hydrocortisone AUC may be decreased.
Contraceptives, oral	Corticosteroids	↑	Corticosteroid half-life and concentration may be increased and clearance decreased.
Ephedrine	Dexamethasone	↓	A decreased half-life and increased clearance of dexamethasone may occur.
Estrogens	Corticosteroids	↑	Corticosteroid clearance may be decreased.
Hydantoins	Corticosteroids	↓	Corticosteroid clearance may be increased, resulting in reduced therapeutic effects.
Ketoconazole	Corticosteroids	↑	Corticosteroid clearance may be decreased and the AUC increased.
Macrolide antibiotics	Methylprednisolone	↑	Significant decrease in methylprednisolone clearance may require a decrease in methylprednisolone dose and the dosing interval.
Rifampin	Corticosteroids	↓	Corticosteroid clearance may be increased, resulting in decreased therapeutic effects.
Corticosteroids	Anticholinesterases	↓	Anticholinesterase effects may be antagonized in myasthenia gravis.
Corticosteroids	Anticoagulants, oral	↔	Anticoagulant dose requirements may be reduced. Conversely, corticosteroids may oppose the anticoagulant action.
Corticosteroids	Cyclosporine	↑	Although this combination is therapeutically beneficial for organ transplants, toxicity may be enhanced.
Corticosteroids	Digitalis glycosides	↑	Coadministration may enhance the possibility of digitalis toxicity associated with hypokalemia.
Corticosteroids	Isoniazid	↓	Isoniazid serum concentrations may be decreased.
Corticosteroids	Nondepolarizing muscle relaxants	↔	Corticosteroids may potentiate, counteract, or have no effect on the neuromuscular blocking action.
Corticosteroids	Potassium-depleting agents (eg, diuretics)	↑	Observe patients for hypokalemia.
Corticosteroids	Salicylates	↓	Corticosteroids will reduce serum salicylate levels and may decrease their effectiveness.
Corticosteroids	Somatrem	↓	Growth-promoting effect of somatrem may be inhibited.
Corticosteroids	Theophyllines	↔	Alterations in the pharmacologic activity of either agent may occur.
Theophyllines	Corticosteroids		

* ↑ = Object drug increased. ↓ = Object drug decreased. ↔ = Undetermined clinical effect.

➤*Drug/Lab test interactions:* Urine glucose and serum cholesterol levels may increase.

Decreased serum levels of potassium, triiodothyronine (T_3), and a minimal decrease of thyroxine (T_4) may occur. Thyroid I^{131} uptake may be decreased. False-negative results with the nitroblue-tetrazolium test for bacterial infection may occur. **Dexamethasone**, given for cerebral edema, may alter the results of a brain scan (decreased uptake of radioactive material).

Adverse Reactions

Parenteral therapy – Rare instances of blindness associated with intralesional therapy around the face and head; hyperpigmentation or hypopigmentation; SC and cutaneous atrophy; sterile abscess; Charcot-like arthropathy; burning or tingling, especially in the perineal area (after IV injection); scarring, induration, inflammation, paresthesia,

occasional irritation at the injection site or occasional brief increase in joint discomfort; transient or delayed pain or soreness; muscle twitching, ataxia, hiccoughs and nystagmus (low incidence following injection); anaphylactic reactions with or without circulatory collapse; cardiac arrest; bronchospasm; arachnoiditis after intrathecal use; foreign body granulomatous reactions involving the synovium with repeated injections.

Intra-articular: Osteonecrosis; tendon rupture; infection; skin atrophy; postinjection flare; hypersensitivity; facial flushing. Systemic reactions may also occur.

Intraspinal: Meningitis (tuberculous, bacterial, cryptococcal, aseptic, chemical); adhesive arachnoiditis; conus medullaris syndrome.

➤*Cardiovascular:* Thromboembolism or fat embolism; thrombophlebitis; necrotizing angiitis; cardiac arrhythmias or ECG changes caused by potassium deficiency; syncopal episodes; aggravation of hypertension; myocardial rupture following recent MI (see Warnings). There are reports of cardiac arrhythmias, fatal arrest, or circulatory collapse following the rapid administration of large IV doses of **methylprednisolone** (0.5 to 1 g in < 10 to 120 minutes) (see Electrolyte Disturbance).

➤*CNS:* Convulsions; increased intracranial pressure with papilledema (pseudotumor cerebri), usually after stopping treatment; vertigo; headache; neuritis/paresthesias; aggravation of pre-existing psychiatric conditions; steroid psychoses (see Precautions).

➤*Dermatologic:* Impaired wound healing; thin fragile skin; petechiae and ecchymoses; erythema; lupus erythematosus-like lesions; suppression of skin test reactions; SC fat atrophy; purpura; striae; hirsutism; acneiform eruptions; other cutaneous reactions such as allergic dermatitis; urticaria; angioneurotic edema; perineal irritation.

➤*Endocrine:* Amenorrhea, postmenopausal bleeding and other menstrual irregularities; development of cushingoid state (eg, moonface, buffalo hump, supraclavicular fat pad enlargement, central obesity); suppression of growth in children; secondary adrenocortical and pituitary unresponsiveness, particularly in times of stress (eg, trauma, surgery, illness); increased sweating; decreased carbohydrate tolerance; hyperglycemia; glycosuria; increased insulin or sulfonylurea requirements in diabetics; manifestations of latent diabetes mellitus; negative nitrogen balance caused by protein catabolism; hirsutism.

➤*Electrolyte disturbance:* Sodium and fluid retention; hypokalemia; hypokalemic alkalosis; metabolic alkalosis; hypocalcemia; CHF in susceptible patients; hypotension or shock-like reactions; hypertension (see Warnings).

➤*GI:* Pancreatitis; abdominal distension; ulcerative esophagitis; nausea; vomiting; increased appetite and weight gain; peptic ulcer with perforation and hemorrhage (see Warnings); perforation of the small and large bowel, particularly in inflammatory bowel disease.

➤*Musculoskeletal:* Muscle weakness; steroid myopathy; muscle mass loss; tendon rupture; osteoporosis; aseptic necrosis of femoral and humeral heads (1% to 37%); spontaneous fractures, including vertebral compression fractures and pathologic fracture of long bones.

➤*Ophthalmic:* Posterior subcapsular cataracts; increased IOP; glaucoma; exophthalmos.

➤*Miscellaneous:* Anaphylactoid/hypersensitivity reactions, aggravation/masking of infections (see Warnings); malaise; leukocytosis (including neonates receiving dexamethasone via maternal injection); fatigue; insomnia; increased or decreased motility and number of spermatozoa.

Overdosage

➤*Symptoms:* There are 2 categories of toxic effects from therapeutic use of glucocorticoids:

Acute adrenal insufficiency – Acute adrenal insufficiency caused by too rapid corticosteroid withdrawal after long-term use, resulting in fever, myalgia, arthralgia, malaise, anorexia, nausea, skin desquamation, orthostatic hypotension, dizziness, fainting, dyspnea, and hypoglycemia.

Cushingoid changes – Cushingoid changes from continued use of large doses resulting in moonface, central obesity, striae, hirsutism, acne, ecchymoses, hypertension, osteoporosis, myopathy, sexual dysfunction, diabetes, hyperlipidemia, peptic ulcer, increased susceptibility to infection and electrolyte and fluid imbalance. Reports of acute toxicity or death are rare.

➤*Treatment:* Recovery of normal adrenal and pituitary function may require up to 9 months. Gradually taper the steroid under the supervision of a physician. Frequent lab tests are necessary. Supplementation is required during periods of stress (eg, illness, surgery, injury). Eventually reduce to the lowest dose that will control the symptoms or discontinue the corticosteroid completely. For large, acute overdoses, treatment includes gastric lavage or emesis and usual supportive measures. Refer to General Management of Acute Overdosage.

Patient Information

May cause GI upset; take with meals or snacks. Take single daily or alternate day doses in the morning prior to 9 a.m. Take multiple doses at evenly spaced intervals throughout the day.

Glucocorticoids

Patients on chronic steroid therapy should wear or carry identification to that effect.

Notify physician if unusual weight gain, swelling of the lower extremities, muscle weakness, black tarry stools, vomiting of blood, puffing of the face, menstrual irregularities, prolonged sore throat, fever, cold, or infection occurs.

Signs of adrenal insufficiency include fatigue, anorexia, nausea, vomiting, diarrhea, weight loss, weakness, dizziness, and low blood sugar. Notify physician promptly if these symptoms occur following dosage reduction or withdrawal of therapy.

➤*High-dose or long-term therapy:* Avoid abrupt withdrawal of therapy.

BETAMETHASONE

Rx	**Celestone** (Schering)	**Syrup:** 0.6 mg/5 mL	< 1% alcohol. Sorbitol, sugar. In 118 mL.

For complete prescribing information, refer to the Glucocorticoids group monograph.

➤**Administration and Dosage**

➤*Initial dosage:* 0.6 to 7.2 mg/day; individualize.

➤*Storage/Stability:* Store between 2° and 30°C (36° and 86°F). Protect from excessive moisture.

BETAMETHASONE SODIUM PHOSPHATE

Rx	**Celestone Phosphate** (Schering)	**Injection:** 4 mg betamethasone sodium phosphate (equivalent to 3 mg betamethasone alcohol)/mL solution	In 5 mL multidose vials.[1]

[1] With EDTA, phenol, and sodium bisulfite.

For complete prescribing information, refer to the Glucocorticoids group monograph.

➤**Administration and Dosage**

➤*Initial dosage:* May vary up to 9 mg/day.

➤*Systemic:* May be given IV or IM.

➤*Local:* Intra-articular or soft tissue administration is indicated in synovitis of osteoarthritis, rheumatoid arthritis, acute and subacute

bursitis, acute gouty arthritis, epicondylitis, acute nonspecific tenosynovitis, posttraumatic osteoarthristis.

Intralesional administration is indicated for keloids; localized hypertrophic, infiltrated, inflammatory lesions of lichen planus, psoriatic plaques, granuloma annulare, and lichen simplex chronicus (neurodermatitis); discoid lupus erythematosus; necrobiosis lipoidica diabeticorum; alopecia areata.

➤*Storage/Stability:* Protect from freezing and light.

BETAMETHASONE SODIUM PHOSPHATE AND BETAMETHASONE ACETATE

Rx	**Celestone Soluspan** (Schering)	**Injection:** 3 mg betamethasone acetate and 3 mg betamethasone (as sodium phosphate)/mL suspension	In 5 mL multidose vials.[1]

[1] With EDTA and benzalkonium chloride.

For complete prescribing information, refer to the Glucocorticoids group monograph.

➤**Administration and Dosage**

Betamethasone sodium phosphate provides prompt activity, while betamethasone acetate is only slightly soluble and affords sustained activity.

➤*Systemic:* Not for IV use.

Initial dose – 0.5 to 9 mg/day IM. Dosage ranges are ⅓ to ½ the oral dose given every 12 hours. In certain acute, life-threatening situations, dosages exceeding the usual may be justified and may be in multiples of oral dosages.

➤*Bursitis, tenosynovitis, peritendinitis:* 1 mL given intrabursally.

➤*Rheumatoid arthritis and osteoarthritis:* 0.5 to 2 mL given intra-articularly.

Very large joints – 1 to 2 mL.

Large joints – 1 mL.

Medium joints – 0.5 to 1 mL.

Small joints – 0.25 to 0.5 mL.

➤*Dermatologic conditions:* 0.2 mL/cm² intradermally.

Maximum dose – 1 mL/week.

➤*Foot disorders:* The following doses are recommended at 3- to 7-day intervals:

Bursitis –
  Under heloma durum or heloma molle: 0.25 to 0.5 mL.
  Under calcaneal spur: 0.5 mL.
  Over hallux rigidus or digiti quinti varus: 0.5 mL.

Tenosynovitis, periostitis of cuboid – 0.5 mL.

Acute gouty arthritis – 0.5 to 1 mL.

➤*Storage/Stability:* Store between 2° and 25°C (36° and 77°F). Protect from light.

BUDESONIDE

Rx	**Entocort EC** (AstraZeneca)	**Capsules:** 3 mg budesonide (micronized)	Sugar spheres. (CIR 3 mg). Light gray/pink. In 100s.

For complete prescribing information, refer to the Glucocorticoids group monograph. For Respiratory Inhalant, Corticosteroids indication, refer to the monograph in the Respiratory chapter. For Respiratory Inhalant, Intranasal Steroid indication, refer to the monograph in the Respiratory chapter.

➤**Indications**

➤*Crohn's disease:* For the treatment of mild-to-moderately active Crohn's disease involving the ileum or the ascending colon.

➤**Administration and Dosage**

➤*Adults:* Take 9 mg once daily in the morning for up to 8 weeks. Swallow capsules whole; do not chew or break. Safety and efficacy of budesonide in the treatment of active Crohn's disease have not been established beyond 8 weeks. For recurring episodes of active Crohn's disease, a repeat 8-week course of budesonide can be given. Treatment

with budesonide capsules can be tapered to 6 mg/day for 2 weeks prior to complete cessation.

Patients with mild-to-moderately active Crohn's disease involving the ileum or ascending colon have been switched from oral prednisolone to budesonide with no reported episodes of adrenal insufficiency. Because prednisolone should not be stopped abruptly, tapering should begin concomitantly with initiating budesonide treatment.

Hepatic insufficiency – Consider reducing the dose of budesonide capsules in patients with hepatic insufficiency.

CYP3A4 inhibitors – If concomitant administration with a CYP3A4 inhibitor is indicated, closely monitor patients for increased signs or symptoms of hypercorticism. Consider reduction in budesonide dose.

➤*Storage/Stability:* Store at 25°C (77°F); excursions permitted to 15° to 30°C (59° to 86°F). Keep container tightly closed.

Glucocorticoids

CORTISONE

Rx	**Cortisone Acetate** (Upjohn)	**Tablets:** 5 mg	(Upjohn 15). White, scored. In 50s.
Rx	**Cortisone Acetate** (Upjohn)	**Tablets:** 10 mg	(Upjohn 23). White, scored. In 100s.
Rx	**Cortisone Acetate** (Various, eg, Bioline, Dixon-Shane, Major)	**Tablets:** 25 mg	In 100s and 500s
Rx	**Cortone Acetate** (Merck)		(MSD 219). White, scored. In 100s.

For complete prescribing information, refer to the Glucocorticoids group monograph.

Administration and Dosage

The drug is insoluble in water.

➤*Initial dosage:* 25 to 300 mg/day (oral). In less severe diseases, lower doses may suffice.

DEXAMETHASONE

Rx	**Dexamethasone** (Various, eg, Rugby)	**Tablets:** 0.25 mg	In 100s.
Rx	**Dexamethasone** (Various, eg, Bioline, Goldline, Roxane, Rugby)	**Tablets:** 0.5 mg	In 100s.
Rx	**Decadron** (MSD)		Lactose. (MSD 41). Yellow, scored. Pentagonal. In 100s and UD 100s.
Rx	**Dexameth** (Major)		In 100s.
Rx	**Dexone** (Solvay)		Lactose. (RR 3205). Yellow, scored. In 100s, UD 100s.
Rx	**Dexamethasone** (Various, eg, Bioline, Goldline, Parmed, Roxane, Rugby)	**Tablets:** 0.75 mg	In 100s and 1000s.
Rx	**Decadron** (MSD)		Lactose. (MSD 63). Bluish green, scored. Pentagonal. In 12s, 100s and UD 100s.
Rx	**Dexameth** (Major)		In 100s and Unipak 12s.
Rx	**Dexone** (Solvay)		Lactose. (RR 3210). Green, scored. In 100s, UD 100s.
Rx	**Dexamethasone** (Roxane)	**Tablets:** 1 mg	(54 489). Yellow, scored. In 100s, 1000s and UD 100s.
Rx	**Dexamethasone** (Various, eg, Bioline, Goldline, Roxane, Rugby)	**Tablets:** 1.5 mg	In 50s and 100s.
Rx	**Dexameth** (Major)		In 100s.
Rx	**Dexone** (Solvay)		Lactose. (RR 3215). Pink, scored. In 100s, UD 100s.
Rx	**Hexadrol** (Organon)		Peach, scored. In 100s.
Rx	**Dexamethasone** (Roxane)	**Tablets:** 2 mg	(54 662). White, scored. In 100s and UD 100s.
Rx	**Dexamethasone** (Various, eg, Bioline, Goldline, Rugby)	**Tablets:** 4 mg	In 50s and 100s.
Rx	**Decadron** (MSD)		Lactose. (MSD 97). White, scored. Pentagonal. In 50s & UD 100s.
Rx	**Dexameth** (Major)		In 100s.
Rx	**Dexone** (Solvay)		Lactose. (RR 3220). White, scored. In 100s, UD 100s.
Rx	**Hexadrol** (Organon)		Green, scored. In 100s.
Rx	**Dexamethasone** (Goldline)	**Tablets:** 6 mg	In 50s and 100s.
Rx	**Hexadrol** (Organon)	**Tablets:** Therapeutic Pack	Six 1.5 mg tablets (peach, scored) and eight 0.75 mg tablets (white, scored).
Rx	**Dexamethasone** (Various, eg, Bioline, Geneva, Goldline, Major, PBI, Roxane, Rugby)	**Elixir:** 0.5 mg per 5 ml	In 100, 120, 240 and 500 ml, and UD 5 and 20 ml.
Rx	**Hexadrol** (Organon)		5% alcohol. Sorbitol. Cherry flavor. In 120 ml.
Rx sf	**Dexamethasone** (Roxane)	**Oral Solution:** 0.5 mg per 5 ml	Dye free. Sorbitol. In 500 ml and UD 5 & 20 ml (100s).
Rx	**Dexamethasone Intensol** (Roxane)	**Oral Solution:** 0.5 mg per 0.5 ml	30% alcohol. In 30 ml w/dropper.

For complete prescribing information, refer to the Glucocorticoids group monograph.

Administration and Dosage

➤*Initial dosage:* 0.75 to 9 mg/day.

➤*Acute, self-limited allergic disorders or acute exacerbations of chronic allergic disorders:* In acute, self-limited allergic disorders or acute exacerbations of chronic allergic disorders, the following dosage schedule combining parenteral and oral therapy (0.75 mg tablets) is suggested: Dexamethasone sodium phosphate injection, 4 mg/ml:

First day – 1 or 2 ml IM.

Second day – 4 tablets in 2 divided doses.

Third day – 4 tablets in 2 divided doses.

Fourth day – 2 tablets in 2 divided doses.

Fifth day – 1 tablet.

Sixth day – 1 tablet.

Seventh day – No treatment.

Eighth day – Follow-up visit.

➤*Suppression tests:*

For Cushing's syndrome – Give 1 mg at 11 pm. Draw blood for plasma cortisol determination the following day at 8 am. For greater accuracy, give 0.5 mg every 6 hours for 48 hours. Collect 24 hour urine to determine 17-hydroxycorticosteroid excretion.

Test to distinguish Cushing's syndrome due to pituitary ACTH excess from Cushing's syndrome due to other causes – Give 2 mg every 6 hours for 48 hours. Collect 24 hour urine to determine 17-hydroxycorticosteroid excretion.

➤*Unlabeled uses:* The dexamethasone suppression test has been used for the detection, diagnosis and management of depression; however, pending further evaluation and research, its value is unproven.

Glucocorticoids

DEXAMETHASONE ACETATE

Rx	**Dexamethasone Acetate** (Various, eg, Bioline, Dixon-Shane, Goldline, Major, Moore, Rugby, URL)	**Injection:** 8 mg per ml (as acetate) suspension. Not for IV use.	In 5 ml vials.
Rx	**Dexasone L.A.** (Hauck)		In 5 ml vials.[1]
Rx	**Dexone LA** (Keene)		In 5 ml vials.[1]
Rx	**Cortastat LA** (Clint)		In 5 ml vials.[1]
Rx	**Dalalone D.P.** (Forest)	**Injection:** 16 mg/ml (as acetate) suspension. Not for IV or intralesional use.	In 1 and 5 ml vial.[1]

[1] With creatinine, polysorbate 80, carboxymethylcellulose, sodium bisulfite, EDTA, benzyl alcohol.

For complete prescribing information, refer to the Glucocorticoids group monograph.

Administration and Dosage

A long-acting repository preparation with prompt onset of action. Not for IV use.

➤*Systemic:* 8 to 16 mg IM, may repeat in 1 to 3 weeks.

➤*Intralesional:* 0.8 to 1.6 mg.

➤*Intra-articular and soft tissue:* 4 to 16 mg; may repeat at 1 to 3 week intervals.

DEXAMETHASONE SODIUM PHOSPHATE

Rx	**Dexamethasone Sodium Phosphate** (Various, eg, Bioline, Dixon-Shane, Elkins Sinn, Geneva Marsam, Kendall McGaw, Moore, Rugby, URL)	**Injection:** 4 mg per ml dexamethasone phosphate (as sodium phosphate) solution	In 1, 5, 10 and 30 ml vials, 1 ml disp. syringe and 1 ml fill in 2 ml vials.
Rx	**Dalalone** (Forest)		In 5 ml vials.[1]
Rx	**Decadron Phosphate** (MSD)		In 1, 5 and 25 ml vials and 2.5 ml syringes.[2]
Rx	**Dexasone** (Hauck)		In 5, 10 and 30 ml vials.[3]
Rx	**Dexone** (Keene)		In 5 and 10 ml vials.[1]
Rx	**Hexadrol Phosphate** (Organon)		In 1 and 5 ml vials and 1 ml disp. syringe.[1]
Rx	**Cortastat** (Clint)		In 5, 10 and 30 ml multiple-dose vials.[1]
Rx	**Dexamethasone Sodium Phosphate** (Various, eg, Elkins-Sinn)	**Injection:** 10 mg per ml dexamethasone phosphate (as sodium phosphate) solution	In 1 and 10 ml vials and 1 ml disp. syringe.
Rx	**Hexadrol Phosphate** (Organon)		In 10 ml (IV or IM) vials and 1 ml disp. syringe.[1]
Rx	**Hexadrol Phosphate** (Organon)	**Injection:** 20 mg per ml dexamethasone phosphate (as sodium phosphate solution)	In 5 ml vials (IV).[1]
Rx	**Decadron Phosphate** (MSD)	**Injection:** 24 mg/ml dexamethasone phosphate (as sodium phosphate) solution. For IV use only	In 5 and 10 ml vials.[4]

[1] With sodium sulfite and benzyl alcohol.
[2] With methyl and propyl parabens and sodium bisulfite.
[3] With sodium metabisulfite, EDTA and methyl and propyl parabens.
[4] With EDTA, methyl and propyl parabens and sodium bisulfite.

For complete prescribing information, refer to the Glucocorticoids group monograph.

Administration and Dosage

Has a rapid onset and short duration of action compared to less soluble preparations.

➤*Systemic:*

Initial dosage – 0.5 to 9 mg daily. Usual dose ranges are ⅓ to ½ the oral dose given every 12 hours. However, in certain acute, life-threatening situations, dosages exceeding the usual may be justified and may be in multiples of the oral dosages.

Cerebral edema – In adults, administer an initial IV dose of 10 mg, followed by 4 mg IM every 6 hours until maximum response has been noted. Response is usually noted within 12 to 24 hours. Dosage may be reduced after 2 to 4 days and gradually discontinued over 5 to 7 days.

For palliative management of patients with recurrent or inoperable brain tumors, maintenance therapy with either the injection or tablets in a dosage of 2 mg 2 or 3 times daily may be effective.

Unresponsive shock – Reported regimens range from 1 to 6 mg/kg as a single IV injection, to 40 mg initially followed by repeated IV injections every 2 to 6 hours while shock persists.

➤*Intra-articular, intralesional or soft tissue:*

Large joints – 2 to 4 mg.

Small joints – 0.8 to 1 mg.

Bursae – 2 to 3 mg.

Tendon sheaths – 0.4 to 1 mg.

Soft tissue infiltration – 2 to 6 mg.

Ganglia – 1 to 2 mg.

DEXAMETHASONE SODIUM PHOSPHATE WITH LIDOCAINE HCl

Rx	**Decadron w/Xylocaine** (MSD)	**Injection:** 4 mg dexamethasone sodium phosphate and 10 mg lidocaine HCl per ml solution	In 5 ml vials.[1]

[1] With EDTA, parabens and sodium bisulfite.

For complete prescribing information, refer to the Glucocorticoids group monograph.

Administration and Dosage

Dexamethasone sodium phosphate provides prompt activity. Lidocaine HCl is a local anesthetic with a rapid onset and a duration of 45 minutes to 1 hour (see Local Anesthetics). Steroid activity usually begins by the time the anesthesia wears off.

➤*Soft tissue injection: Acute and subacute bursitis:* 0.5 to 0.75 ml.

Acute and subacute nonspecific tenosynovitis – 0.1 to 0.25 ml.

HYDROCORTISONE (Cortisol)

Rx	**Cortef** (Upjohn)	**Tablets:** 5 mg	(Cortef 5). White, scored. In 50s.
Rx	**Hydrocortisone** (Major)	**Tablets:** 10 mg	In 100s.
Rx	**Cortef** (Upjohn)		(Cortef 10). White, scored. In 100s.
Rx	**Hydrocortone** (MSD)		(MSD 619). White, scored. Oval. In 100s.
Rx	**Hydrocortisone** (Various, eg, Major, Moore, Rugby, URL)	**Tablets:** 20 mg	In 100s.
Rx	**Cortef** (Upjohn)		(Cortef 20). White, scored. In 100s.
Rx	**Hydrocortone** (MSD)		(MSD 625). White, scored. Oval. In 100s.

For complete prescribing information, refer to the Glucocorticoids group monograph.

Administration and Dosage

Cortisol suspension is insoluble in water.

➤*Initial dosage:* 20 to 240 mg/day.

Glucocorticoids

HYDROCORTISONE ACETATE

Rx	**Hydrocortisone Acetate** (Various, eg, Dixon-Shane, Moore, Rugby, Schein, URL)	**Injection:** 25 mg per ml suspension	In 10 ml vials.
Rx	**Hydrocortone Acetate** (MSD)		In 5 ml vials.[1]
Rx	**Hydrocortisone Acetate** (Various, eg, Moore, Rugby, URL)	**Injection:** 50 mg per ml suspension	In 10 ml vials.

[1] With 4 mg polysorbate 80, 5 mg sodium carboxymethylcellulose and 9 mg benzyl alcohol per ml.

For complete prescribing information, refer to the Glucocorticoids group monograph.

Administration and Dosage

Hydrocortisone acetate has a slow onset but long duration of action when compared with more soluble preparations. Because of its insolubility, it is suitable for intra-articular, intralesional and soft tissue injection where its anti-inflammatory effects are confined mainly to the area in which it has been injected, although it is capable of producing systemic hormonal effects.

For intralesional, intra-articular or soft tissue injection only. Not for IV use.

➤*Large joints (eg, knee):* 25 mg; occasionally, 37.5 mg.

➤*Small joints (eg, interphalangeal, temporomandibular):* 10 to 25 mg.

➤*Tendon sheaths:* 5 to 12.5 mg.

➤*Soft tissue infiltration:* 25 to 50 mg; occasionally, 75 mg.

➤*Bursae:* 25 to 37.5 mg.

➤*Ganglia:* 12.5 to 25 mg.

If desired, a local anesthetic may be injected before hydrocortisone acetate or mixed in a syringe and given simultaneously.

If used prior to intra-articular injection of the steroid, inject most of the anesthetic into the soft tissues of the surrounding area and instill a small amount into the joint.

If given together, mix in the injection syringe by drawing the steroid in first, then the anesthetic. In this way, the anesthetic will not be introduced inadvertently into the vial of the steroid. The mixture must be used immediately and any unused portion discarded.

HYDROCORTISONE CYPIONATE

Rx	**Cortef** (Upjohn)	**Oral Suspension:** 10 mg per 5 ml hydrocortisone (as cypionate)	Sucrose. In 120 ml.

For complete prescribing information, refer to the Glucocorticoids group monograph.

Administration and Dosage

➤*Initial dosage:* 20 to 240 mg/day.

HYDROCORTISONE SODIUM PHOSPHATE

Rx	**Hydrocortone Phosphate** (MSD)	**Injection:** 50 mg/ml hydrocortisone (as sodium phosphate) solution	In 2 and 10 ml vials.[1]

[1] With 3.2 mg sodium bisulfite, and 1.5 mg methylparaben and 0.2 mg propylparaben.

For complete prescribing information, refer to the Glucocorticoids group monograph.

Administration and Dosage

A water soluble salt with a rapid onset but short duration of action.

Administer by IV, IM or SC injection.

➤*Initial dosage:* 15 to 240 mg/day. Usually, ⅓ to ½ the oral dose every 12 hours.

➤*Acute diseases:* Doses higher than 240 mg may be required.

HYDROCORTISONE SODIUM SUCCINATE

Rx	**A-Hydrocort** (Abbott)	**Injection:** 100 mg hydrocortisone (as sodium succinate) per vial	In 2 ml *Univials*[1] and fliptop vials.
Rx	**Solu-Cortef** (Upjohn)		In vials and 2 ml *Act-O-Vials*.[1]
Rx	**A-Hydrocort** (Abbott)	**Injection:** 250 mg hydrocortisone (as sodium succinate) per vial	In 2 ml *Univials*[1] and fliptop vials.
Rx	**Solu-Cortef** (Upjohn)		In 2 ml *Act-O-Vials*.[1]
Rx	**A-Hydrocort** (Abbott)	**Injection:** 500 mg hydrocortisone (as sodium succinate) per vial	In 4 ml *Univials*[1] and fliptop vials.
Rx	**Solu-Cortef** (Upjohn)		In 4 ml *Act-O-Vials*.[1]
Rx	**A-Hydrocort** (Abbott)	**For Injection:** 1000 mg hydrocortisone (as sodium succinate) per vial	In 8 ml *Univials*[1] and fliptop vials.
Rx	**Solu-Cortef** (Upjohn)		In 8 ml *Act-O-Vials*.[1]

[1] With benzyl alcohol.

For complete prescribing information, refer to the Glucocorticoids group monograph.

Administration and Dosage

A water soluble salt which is rapidly active.

May be administered IV or IM. The initial dose is 100 to 500 mg, and may be repeated at 2, 4 or 6 hour intervals depending on patient response and clinical condition.

METHYLPREDNISOLONE

Rx	**Methylprednisolone** (Various, eg, Geneva, Major, Moore, Parmed, Rugby)	**Tablets:** 4 mg	In 21s and 100s.
Rx	**Methylprednisolone** (Various, eg, Rugby, URL)	**Tablets:** 16 mg	In 50s.
Rx	**Medrol** (Upjohn)	**Tablets:** 2 mg[1]	(MEDROL 2). Pink, scored. Elliptical. In 100s.
		4 mg[1]	White, scored. Elliptical. In 30s, 100s, 500s, UD 100s and Dosepak 21s.
		8 mg[1]	Peach, scored. Elliptical. In 25s.
		16 mg[1]	White, scored. Elliptical. In 50s and ADT Pak 14s.
		24 mg[1]	Tartrazine. Yellow, scored. Elliptical. In 25s.
		32 mg[1]	Peach, scored. Elliptical. In 25s.

[1] With lactose and sucrose.

For complete prescribing information, refer to the Glucocorticoids group monograph.

Administration and Dosage

➤*Initial dose:* 4 to 48 mg/day; adjust until a satisfactory response is noted. Individualize dosage. Determine maintenance dose by decreasing initial dose in small decrements at appropriate intervals until reaching the lowest effective dose.

➤*Dosepak 21 therapy:* Follow manufacturer's directions.

➤*Alternate day therapy (ADT):* Twice the usual dose is administered every other morning. The patient on long-term treatment receives the beneficial effects of corticosteroids while minimizing certain undesirable effects. In less severe diseases requiring long-term therapy, treatment may be initiated with ADT.

Glucocorticoids

METHYLPREDNISOLONE ACETATE

Rx	**Methylprednisolone Acetate** (Various, eg, Rugby)	**Injection:** 20 mg per ml suspension	In 5 and 10 ml vials.
Rx	**Depo-Medrol** (Upjohn)		In 5 ml vials.[1]
Rx	**Methylprednisolone Acetate** (Various, eg, Dixon-Shane, Goldline, Moore, Rugby, URL)	**Injection:** 40 mg per ml suspension	In 5 and 10 ml vials.
Rx	**depMedalone 40** (Forest)		In 5 ml vials.[1]
Rx	**Depo-Medrol** (Upjohn)		In 1, 5 and 10 ml vials.[1]
Rx	**Depopred-40** (Hyrex)		In 5 and 10 ml vials.
Rx	**Duralone-40** (Hauck)		In 10 ml vials.[1]
Rx	**Medralone 40** (Keene)		In 5 ml vials.[1]
Rx	**Methylprednisolone Acetate** (Various, Dixon-Shane, Goldline, Moore, Rugby, URL)	**Injection:** 80 mg per ml suspension	In 5 ml vials.
Rx	**depMedalone 80** (Forest)		In 5 ml vials.[1]
Rx	**Depo-Medrol** (Upjohn)		In 1 and 5 ml vials.[1]
Rx	**Depopred-80** (Hyrex)		In 5 ml vials.
Rx	**Duralone-80** (Hauck)		In 5 ml vials.[1]
Rx	**Medralone 80** (Keene)		In 5 ml vials.[1]

[1] With polyethylene glycol and myristyl-gamma-picolinium chloride.

For complete prescribing information, refer to the Glucocorticoids group monograph.

Administration and Dosage

Because of its low solubility, methylprednisolone acetate has a sustained effect.

➤*Systemic:* Not for IV use. As a temporary substitute for oral therapy, administer the total daily dose as a single IM injection. For prolonged effect, give a single weekly dose.

Adrenogenital syndrome – A single 40 mg injection IM every 2 weeks.

Rheumatoid arthritis – Weekly IM maintenance dose varies from 40 to 120 mg.

Dermatologic lesions – 40 to 120 mg IM weekly for 1 to 4 weeks. In severe dermatitis (eg, poison ivy), relief may result within 8 to 12 hours of a single dose of 80 to 120 mg IM. In chronic contact dermatitis, repeated injections every 5 to 10 days may be necessary. In seborrheic dermatitis, a weekly dose of 80 mg IM may be adequate.

Asthma and allergic rhinitis – 80 to 120 mg IM.

➤*Intra-articular and soft tissue:*
Large joints – 20 to 80 mg.
Medium joints – 10 to 40 mg.
Small joints – 4 to 10 mg.
Ganglion, tendinitis, epicondylitis and bursitis – 4 to 30 mg.

➤*Intralesional:* 20 to 60 mg.

METHYLPREDNISOLONE SODIUM SUCCINATE

Rx	**Methylprednisolone Sodium Succinate** (Various, eg, Elkins Sinn)	**Powder for Injection:** 40 mg per vial	In 1 and 3 ml vials.
Rx	**A-Methapred** (Abbott)		In 1 ml *Univial.*[1]
Rx	**Solu-Medrol** (Upjohn)		In 1 ml *Act-O-Vial.*[1]
Rx	**Methylprednisolone Sodium Succinate** (Various, eg, Elkins Sinn)	**Powder for Injection:** 125 mg per vial	In 2 and 5 ml vials.
Rx	**A-Methapred** (Abbott)		In 2 ml *Univial.*[2]
Rx	**Solu-Medrol** (Upjohn)		In 2 ml *Act-O-Vial.*[2]
Rx	**Methylprednisolone Sodium Succinate** (Various, eg, Elkins Sinn)	**Powder for Injection:** 500 mg per vial	In 1, 4 and 20 ml vials.
Rx	**A-Methapred** (Abbott)		In 4 ml *Univial* and 500 mg ADD-Vantage vials.[3]
Rx	**Solu-Medrol** (Upjohn)		In 8 ml vials and 8 ml vials w/diluent.[3]
Rx	**Methylprednisolone Sodium Succinate** (Various, eg, Elkins Sinn)	**Powder for Injection:** 1 g per vial	In 1, 8 and 50 ml vials.
Rx	**A-Methapred** (Abbott)		In 8 ml Univial and 500 mg *ADD-Vantage* vials.[4]
Rx	**Solu-Medrol** (Upjohn)		In 1 g vials, 1 g vials w/diluent and 8 ml *Act-O-Vial.*[4]
Rx	**Solu-Medrol** (Upjohn)	**Powder for Injection:** 2 g per vial	In 2 g vials w/diluent.

[1] With sodium phosphate anhydrous (1.6 mg monobasic, 17.5 mg dibasic), 25 mg lactose and 9 mg benzyl alcohol.
[2] With sodium phosphate anhydrous (1.6 mg monobasic, 17.4 mg dibasic), ≈ 18 mg benzyl alcohol.
[3] With sodium phosphate anhydrous (6.4 mg monobasic, 69.6 mg dibasic). May contain 36 to 70.2 mg benzyl alcohol.

[4] With sodium phosphate anhydrous (12.8 mg monobasic, 139.2 mg dibasic). May contain 66.8 to 141 mg benzyl alcohol.
[5] With sodium phosphate anhydrous (25.6 mg monobasic, 278 mg dibasic), 273 mg benzyl alcohol.

For complete prescribing information, refer to the Glucocorticoids group monograph.

Administration and Dosage

Highly soluble; has rapid effect by IV or IM routes.

➤*Initial dose:* 10 to 40 mg IV, administered over 1 to several minutes.

Give subsequent doses IV or IM.

➤*Infants and children:* Not less than 0.5mg/kg/24 hours.

For high dose therapy, give 30 mg/kg IV, infused over 10 to 20 minutes. May repeat every 4 to 6 hours, not beyond 48 to 72 hours.

PREDNISOLONE

Rx	**Prednisolone** (Various, eg, Geneva, Goldline, Major, Moore, Roxane, Rugby, Schein)	**Tablets:** 5 mg	In 100s, 1000s and 5000s.
Rx	**Prelone** (Aero)	**Syrup:** 5 mg/5 ml	0.4% alcohol. EDTA, saccharin, sorbitol. Wild cherry flavor. In 120 ml.
		15 mg/5 ml	5% alcohol. Saccharin, sucrose. Cherry flavor. In 240 ml.
Rx	**Prednisolone** (Various, eg, WE Pharmaceuticals)	**Syrup:** 15 mg/5 ml	Sucrose. In 240 and 480 ml.

For complete prescribing information, refer to the Glucocorticoids group monograph.

Administration and Dosage

➤*Initial dosage:* 5 to 60 mg/day.

➤*Multiple sclerosis:* In treatment of acute exacerbations of multiple sclerosis, 200 mg daily for a week followed by 80 mg every other day for 1 month.

Glucocorticoids

PREDNISOLONE ACETATE

Rx	Prednisolone Acetate (Various, eg, Rugby, URL)	**Injection:** 25 mg per ml suspension	In 10 and 30 ml vials.
Rx	Prednisolone Acetate (Various, eg, Goldline, Moore, Rugby, URL)	**Injection:** 50 mg per ml suspension	In 10 and 30 ml vials.
Rx	Predalone 50 (Forest)		In 10 ml vials.[1]
Rx	Predcor-50 (Hauck)		In 10 ml vials.[1]

[1] With polysorbate 80, carboxymethylcellulose and benzyl alcohol.

For complete prescribing information, refer to the Glucocorticoids group monograph.

Administration and Dosage

Relatively insoluble.

➤*Systemic:* Not for IV use.

Initial dosage – 4 to 60 mg/day, IM.

➤*Intralesional, intra-articular or soft tissue injection:* 4 mg, up to 100 mg.

➤*Multiple sclerosis:* 200 mg daily for a week, followed by 80 mg every other day or 4 to 8 mg dexamethasone every other day for 1 month.

PREDNISOLONE TEBUTATE

Rx	Prednisol TBA (Pasadena)	**Injection:** 20 mg per ml suspension	In 10 ml vials.[1]

[1] With polysorbate 80, sorbitol and benzyl alcohol.

For complete prescribing information, refer to the Glucocorticoids group monograph.

Administration and Dosage

Slightly soluble with a slow onset and prolonged duration of action.

➤*Intra-articular, intralesional or soft tissue administration:*
Large joints – Large joints (eg, knee) – 20 mg; occasionally, 30 mg.

Doses > 40 mg are not recommended.

Small joints – Small joints (eg, interphalangeal, temporomandibular) - 8 to 10 mg.

Bursae – 20 to 30 mg.

Tendon sheaths – 4 to 10 mg.

Ganglia – 10 to 20 mg.

PREDNISOLONE SODIUM PHOSPHATE

Rx	Hydeltrasol (MSD)	**Injection:** 20 mg per ml prednisolone (as sodium phosphate) solution	In 2 and 5 ml vials.[1]
Rx	Key-Pred-SP (Hyrex)		In 10 ml vials.[1]
Rx sf	Pediapred (Fisons)	**Oral Liquid:** 5 mg prednisolone (as sodium phosphate) per 5 ml	Alcohol and dye free. Raspberry flavor. In 120 ml.
Rx	Orapred (Ascent Pediatrics)	**Oral solution:** 15 mg prednisolone (20.2 mg prednisolone sodium phosphate) per 5 ml	Dye free. 2% alcohol, fructose, sorbitol. Grape flavor. In 237 ml.

[1] With niacinamide, EDTA, phenol and sodium bisulfite.

For complete prescribing information, refer to the Glucocorticoids group monograph.

Administration and Dosage

Water soluble and rapid acting, but has a short duration of action.

Prednisolone sodium phosphate oral liquid produces a 20% higher peak plasma level of prednisolone which occurs approximately 15 minutes earlier than the peak seen with tablet formulations.

➤*Parenteral:* For IV or IM use.

Initial dosage – 4 to 60 mg/day.

➤*Intra-articular, intralesional or soft tissue administration:*
Large joints (eg, knee) – 10 to 20 mg.
Small joints (eg, interphalangeal, temporomandibular) – 4 to 5 mg.
Bursae – 10 to 15 mg.
Tendon sheaths – 2 to 5 mg.
Soft tissue infiltration – 10 to 30 mg.
Ganglia – 5 to 10 mg.

➤*Oral:* Initial dosage - 5 to 60 ml (5 to 60 mg base) per day.

Multiple sclerosis (acute exacerbations) – 200 mg daily for a week, followed by 80 mg every other day or 4 to 8 mg dexamethasone every other day for 1 month.

PREDNISONE

Rx	Prednisone (Various, eg, Roxane)	**Tablets:** 1 mg	In 100s, 1000s and UD 100s.
Rx	Meticorten (Schering)		Lactose. (KEM or 843). White. In 100s.
Rx	Orasone (Solvay)		Lactose. (RR 1). Pink, scored. In 100s and 1000s.
Rx	Panasol-S (Seatrace)		Pink, scored. In 100s, 1000s.
Rx	Deltasone (Upjohn)	**Tablets:** 2.5 mg	Lactose, sucrose. (Deltasone 2.5). Scored. In 100s.
Rx	Prednisone (Various, eg, Barr, Geneva, Goldline, Lannett, Major, Parmed, Rugby)	**Tablets:** 5 mg	In 100s, 500s, 1000s, 5000s and UD 100s.
Rx	Deltasone (Upjohn)		Lactose, sucrose. (Deltasone 5). Scored. In 100s, UD 100s and Dosepak 21s.
Rx	Orasone (Solvay)		Lactose. (RR 5). White, scored. In 100s and 1000s.
Rx	Prednicen-M (Central)		(131/07). Red. Film coated. In 100s, 1000s and unit pak 21s.
Rx	Sterapred (Merz)		(DAN/5052, mfg. by Danbury). (DELTASONE 5, mfg. by Upjohn). White, scored. In Uni-Pak 21s. **Sterapred 12 day.** In Uni-Pak 48s.
Rx	Prednisone (Various, eg, Barr, Geneva, Goldline, Major, Parmed, Rugby)	**Tablets:** 10 mg	In 100s, 500s, 1000s and UD 100s.
Rx	Deltasone (Upjohn)		Lactose, sucrose. (Deltasone 10). Scored. In 100s, 500s and UD 100s.
Rx	Orasone (Solvay)		Lactose. (RR 10). Blue, scored. In 100s and 1000s.
Rx	Sterapred DS (Merz)		(DAN/5442, mfg. by Danbury). (DELTASONE 10, mfg. by Upjohn). White, scored. In Uni-Pak 21s. **Sterapred DS 12 day.** In Uni-Pak 48s. **Sterapred DS 14 day.** In Uni-Pak 49s.
Rx	Prednisone (Various, eg, Barr, Bioline, Geneva, Goldline, Lannett, Major, Parmed, Rugby)	**Tablets:** 20 mg	In 100s, 500s, 1000s and UD 100s.
Rx	Deltasone (Upjohn)		Lactose, sucrose. (Deltasone 20). Scored. In 100s, 500s and UD 100s.
Rx	Orasone (Solvay)		Lactose. (RR 20). Yellow, scored. In 100s and 1000s.

Glucocorticoids

PREDNISONE

Rx	Prednisone (Various, eg, Geneva, Major, Rugby)	**Tablets:** 50 mg	In 100s and UD 100s.
Rx	Orasone (Solvay)		Lactose. (RR 50). White, scored. Film coated. In 100s.
Rx	Prednisone (Roxane)	**Oral Solution:** 5 mg per 5 ml	5% alcohol. Fructose, saccharin. Dye free. In 500 ml and UD 5 ml (40s).
Rx	Prednisone Intensol Concentrate (Roxane)	**Oral Solution:** 5 mg per ml	30% alcohol. In 30 ml.
Rx	Liquid Pred (Muro)	**Syrup:** 5 mg per 5 ml	5% alcohol. Saccharin, sorbitol and sucrose. In 120 and 240 ml.

For complete prescribing information, refer to the Glucocorticoids group monograph.

Administration and Dosage

Initial dosage varies from 5 to 60 mg/day. Prednisone is inactive and must be metabolized to prednisolone. This may be impaired in patients with liver disease.

TRIAMCINOLONE

Rx	Triamcinolone (Various, eg, Dixon-Shane, Moore, Rugby, Schein, URL)	**Tablets:** 4 mg	In 100s and 500s.
Rx	Aristocort (Fujisawa)		Lactose. (LL A4). White, scored. Oblong, flat. In 30s, 100s and *Aristo-Pak* 16s.
Rx	Kenacort (Apothecon)		Lactose. In 100s.
Rx	Aristocort (Fujisawa)	**Tablets:** 8 mg	Lactose. (LL A8). Yellow, scored. Oblong, flat. In 50s.
Rx	Kenacort (Apothecon)		Lactose, tartrazine. In 50s.
Rx	Kenacort (Apothecon)	**Syrup:** 4 mg (as diacetate) per 5 ml	Sucrose. In 120 ml.

For complete prescribing information, refer to the Glucocorticoids group monograph.

Administration and Dosage

►*Initial daily dosage in specific disorders is:*

Adrenocortical insufficiency – 4 to 12 mg, in addition to mineralocorticoid therapy.

Rheumatic and dermatological disorders and bronchial asthma – 8 to 16 mg.

Allergic states – 8 to 12 mg.

Ophthalmological diseases – 12 to 40 mg.

Respiratory diseases – 16 to 48 mg.

Hematologic disorders – 16 to 60 mg.

Tuberculous meningitis – 32 to 48 mg.

Acute rheumatic carditis – 20 to 60 mg.

Acute leukemia and lymphoma (adults) – 16 to 40 mg. It may be necessary to give as much as 100 mg/day in leukemia.
  Acute leukemia (children): 1 to 2 mg/kg.

Edematous states – 16 to 20 mg (up to 48 mg) until diuresis occurs.

Systemic lupus erythematosus – 20 to 32 mg.

TRIAMCINOLONE ACETONIDE

Rx	Tac-3 (Herbert)	**Injection:** 3 mg per ml suspension	In 5 ml vials.[1]
Rx	Kenalog-10 (Westwood-Squibb)	**Injection:** 10 mg per ml suspension	In 5 ml vials.[1]
Rx	Triamcinolone Acetonide (Various, eg, Bioline, Dixon-Shane, Geneva Marsam, Goldline)	**Injection:** 40 mg per ml suspension	In 1 and 5 ml vials.
Rx	Kenalog-40 (Westwood-Squibb)		In 1, 5 and 10 ml vials.[1]
Rx	Tac-40 (Parnell)		In 5 ml vials.
Rx	Triamonide 40 (Forest)		In 5 ml vials.[1]
Rx	Tri-Kort (Keene)		In 5 ml vials.[1]
Rx	Trilog (Hauck)		In 5 ml vials.[1]

[1] With polysorbate 80, carboxymethlcellulose and benzyl alcohol.

For complete prescribing information, refer to the Glucocorticoids group monograph.

Administration and Dosage

Relatively insoluble. Has an extended duration which may be permanent or sustained for several weeks.

►*Systemic:*
Initial IM dose – 2.5 to 60 mg/day. Not for IV use.

►*Intra-articular or intrabursal administration and for injection into tendon sheaths:*
Initial dose – 2.5 to 5 mg for smaller joints and 5 to 15 mg for larger joints. For adults, doses up to 10 mg for smaller areas and up to 40 mg for larger areas are usually sufficient.

►*Intradermal:* Use only 3 mg/ml or 10 mg/ml. Initial dose varies; limit to 1 mg per site.

Clumping results from exposure to freezing temperatures; do not use.

TRIAMCINOLONE DIACETATE

Rx	**Aristocort Intralesional** (Fujisawa)	**Injection:** 25 mg per ml suspension	In 5 ml vials.[1]
Rx	**Triamcinolone** (Various, eg, Moore, Rugby)	**Injection:** 40 mg per ml suspension	In 5 ml vials.
Rx	**Trilone** (Hauck)		In 5 ml vials.
Rx	**Amcort** (Keene)		In 5 ml vials.[1]
Rx	**Clinacort** (Clint)		In 5 ml multiple-dose vials.[1]

[1] With polysorbate 80, polyethylene glycol and benzyl alcohol.

For complete prescribing information, refer to the Glucocorticoids group monograph.

Administration and Dosage

Slightly soluble providing a prompt onset of action and a longer duration of effect.

➤*Systemic:* Not for IV use. May be administered IM for initial therapy; however, most clinicians prefer to adjust the dose orally until adequate control is attained. The average dose is 40 mg IM per week. In general, a single parenteral dose 4 to 7 times the oral daily dose controls the patient from 4 to 7 days, up to 3 to 4 weeks.

➤*Intra-articular and intrasynovial:* 5 to 40 mg.

➤*Intralesional or sublesional:* 5 to 48 mg. Do not use more than 12.5 mg per injection site. The usual average dose is 25 mg per lesion.

TRIAMCINOLONE HEXACETONIDE

Rx	**Aristospan Intralesional** (Fujisawa)	**Injection:** 5 mg per ml suspension	In 5 ml vials.[1]
Rx	**Aristospan Intra-articular** (Fujisawa)	**Injection:** 20 mg per ml suspension	In 1 and 5 ml vials.[1]

[1] With polysorbate 80, sorbitol and benzyl alcohol.

For complete prescribing information, refer to the Glucocorticoids group monograph.

Administration and Dosage

Relatively insoluble, slowly absorbed and has a prolonged action.
Not for IV use.

➤*Intra-articular:* 2 to 20 mg average.

Large joints (eg, knee, hip, shoulder) – 10 to 20 mg.

Small joints (eg, interphalangeal, metacarpophalangeal) – 2 to 6 mg.

➤*Intralesional or sublesional:* Up to 0.5 mg per square inch of affected area.

Mineralocorticoids

FLUDROCORTISONE ACETATE

| Rx | **Fludrocortisone Acetate** (Various, eg, Global) | **Tablets:** 0.1 mg | In 100s. |
| Rx | **Florinef Acetate** (Monarch) | | Lactose. (429). White, scored. In 100s. |

For complete prescribing information, refer to the Adrenocortical Steroids introduction.

Indications

Partial replacement therapy for primary and secondary adrenocortical insufficiency in Addison disease and for the treatment of salt-losing adrenogenital syndrome.

➤*Unlabeled uses:* Fludrocortisone has been used in the management of symptomatic orthostatic hypotension.

Administration and Dosage

Dosage depends on the severity of the disease and the response of the patient. Continually monitor patients for signs that indicate dosage adjustment is necessary, such as remissions or exacerbations of the disease and stress (surgery, infection, trauma).

➤*Addison disease:* The usual dose is 0.1 mg/day (range, 0.1 mg 3 times a week to 0.2 mg/day). If transient hypertension develops as a consequence of therapy, reduce the dose to 0.05 mg/day. Administration in conjunction with cortisone (10 to 37.5 mg/day in divided doses) or hydrocortisone (10 to 30 mg/day in divided doses) is preferable. In Addison disease, the combination of fludrocortisone acetate tablets with a glucocorticoid such as hydrocortisone or cortisone provides substitution therapy approximating normal adrenal activity with minimal risks of unwanted effects.

➤*Salt-losing adrenogenital syndrome:* 0.1 to 0.2 mg/day.

➤*Withdrawal:* Use the lowest possible dose of corticosteroid to control the condition being treated. Make a gradual reduction in dosage when possible. Adverse reactions to corticosteroids may be produced by too-rapid withdrawal or by continued use of large doses.

➤*Storage/Stability:* Store at room temperature; avoid excessive heat.

Actions

➤*Pharmacology:* Fludrocortisone is a synthetic, adrenocortical steroid with potent mineralocorticoid properties and high glucocorticoid activity; it is used only for its mineralocorticoid effects.

The physiological action of fludrocortisone is similar to that of hydrocortisone. However, the effects of fludrocortisone, particularly on electrolyte balance, but also on carbohydrate metabolism, are considerably heightened and prolonged. Mineralocorticoids act on the renal distal tubules to enhance the reabsorption of sodium. They increase urinary excretion of both potassium and hydrogen ions. The consequence of these 3 primary effects together with similar actions on cation transport in other tissues appears to account for the spectrum of physiological activities characteristic of mineralocorticoids.

In small oral doses, fludrocortisone produces marked sodium retention and increased urinary potassium excretion. It also causes a rise in blood pressure, apparently because of these effects on electrolyte levels. In larger doses, fludrocortisone inhibits endogenous adrenal cortical secretion, thymic activity, and pituitary corticotropin excretion, promotes the deposition of liver glycogen, and, unless protein intake is adequate, induces negative nitrogen balance.

➤*Pharmacokinetics:* Plasma half-life is approximately 3.5 hours; biological half-life ranges from 18 to 36 hours.

Contraindications

Hypersensitivity to fludrocortisone; systemic fungal infections.

Warnings

➤*Sodium retention:* Because of its marked effect on sodium retention, the use of fludrocortisone in the treatment of conditions other than those indicated is not advised.

➤*Infections:* Corticosteroids may mask some signs of infection, and new infections may appear during their use. There may be decreased resistance and inability to localize infection when corticosteroids are used. If an infection occurs during fludrocortisone acetate therapy, it should be controlled promptly by suitable antimicrobial therapy.

Tuberculosis – Restrict the use of fludrocortisone acetate tablets in patients with active tuberculosis to cases of fulminating or disseminated tuberculosis in which the corticosteroid is used for the management of the disease in conjunction with an appropriate antituberculous regimen. If corticosteroids are indicated in patients with latent tuberculosis or tuberculin reactivity, close observation is necessary because reactivation of the disease may occur. During prolonged corticosteroid therapy, these patients should receive chemoprophylaxis.

Children – Children who are on immunosuppressant drugs are more susceptible to infections than healthy children. Chicken pox and measles, for example, can have a more serious or even fatal course in children on immunosuppressant corticosteroids. In such children, or in adults who have not had these diseases, take particular care to avoid

exposure. If exposed, therapy with varicella zoster immune globulin or pooled IV immunoglobulin, as appropriate, may be indicated. If chicken pox develops, consider treatment with antiviral agents.

➤*Ocular effects:* Prolonged use of corticosteroids may produce posterior subcapsular cataracts and glaucoma with possible damage to the optic nerves and may enhance the establishment of secondary ocular infections caused by fungi or viruses.

Use corticosteroids cautiously in patients with ocular herpes simplex because of possible corneal perforation.

➤*Adrenal insufficiency:* To avoid drug-induced adrenal insufficiency, supportive dosage may be required in times of stress (eg, trauma, surgery, severe illness), both during treatment with fludrocortisone and for a year afterwards.

➤*Fluid and electrolyte balance:* Average and large doses of hydrocortisone or cortisone can cause elevation of blood pressure, retention of salt and water, and increased excretion of potassium. These effects are less likely to occur with the synthetic derivatives except when they are used in large doses. However, because fludrocortisone is a potent mineralocorticoid, carefully monitor the dosage and salt intake in order to avoid the development of hypertension, edema, or weight gain. Periodic checking of serum electrolyte levels is advisable during prolonged therapy; dietary salt restriction and potassium supplementation may be necessary. All corticosteroids increase calcium excretion.

➤*Vaccinations:* Do not vaccinate patients against smallpox while they are on corticosteroid therapy. Do not undertake other immunization procedures in patients who are on corticosteroids, especially high doses because of possible hazards of neurological complications and a lack of antibody response.

➤*Pregnancy: Category C.* Adequate animal reproduction studies have not been conducted with fludrocortisone acetate. However, many corticosteroids have been shown to be teratogenic in laboratory animals at low doses. Teratogenicity of these agents in humans has not been demonstrated. It is not known whether fludrocortisone acetate can cause fetal harm when administered to a pregnant woman or can affect reproduction capacity. Give fludrocortisone acetate to a pregnant woman only if clearly needed.

Carefully observe infants born of mothers who have received substantial doses of fludrocortisone acetate during pregnancy for signs of hypoadrenalism.

➤*Lactation:* Corticosteroids are found in the breast milk of lactating women. Exercise caution when administering these drugs to nursing women.

➤*Children:* Safety and efficacy in children have not been established. Monitor growth and development of infants and children on prolonged therapy.

Precautions

➤*Monitoring:* Regularly monitor patients for blood pressure and serum electrolyte determinations.

➤*Use with caution:*

GI – Use corticosteroids with caution in patients with nonspecific ulcerative colitis if there is a probability of impending perforation, abscess, or other pyogenic infection and in patients with diverticulitis, fresh intestinal anastomoses, or active or latent peptic ulcer.

Miscellaneous – There is an enhanced corticosteroid effect in patients with hypothyroidism and cirrhosis. Use with caution in patients with renal insufficiency, hypertension, osteoporosis, and myasthenia gravis.

➤*Psychiatric effects:* Psychic derangements may appear when corticosteroids are used. These may range from euphoria, insomnia, mood swings, personality changes, and severe depression to frank psychotic manifestations. Corticosteroids also may aggravate existing emotional instability or psychotic tendencies.

Drug Interactions

Fludrocortisone Drug Interactions			
Precipitant drug	Object drug*		Description
Anabolic steroids	Fludrocortisone	↑	Concurrent use may enhance the tendency toward edema. Use with caution, especially in patients with hepatic or cardiac disease.
Barbiturates Hydantoins Rifamycins	Fludrocortisone	↓	Fludrocortisone hepatic metabolism may be increased, resulting in decreased therapeutic effects.
Estrogens	Fludrocortisone	↑	Corticosteroid metabolism may be decreased.

FLUDROCORTISONE ACETATE

Fludrocortisone Drug Interactions			
Precipitant drug	Object drug*		Description
Fludrocortisone	Amphotericin B Potassium-depleting diuretics	↑	Coadministration may enhance hypokalemia. Check serum potassium levels at frequent intervals. Use potassium supplements if necessary.
Fludrocortisone	Anticholinesterases	↓	Although fludrocortisone is not used to treat myasthenia gravis, corticosteroids may antagonize the effects of anticholinesterases in myasthenia gravis.
Fludrocortisone	Anticoagulants, oral	↑↓	Anticoagulant dose requirements may be reduced. Conversely, corticosteroids may oppose the anticoagulant action. Monitor prothrombin time and adjust dose accordingly.
Fludrocortisone	Antidiabetic agents (oral agents and insulin)	↓	Antidiabetic effect may be decreased. Monitor for signs of hyperglycemia; adjust dose of antidiabetic agent if necessary.
Fludrocortisone	Digitalis glycosides	↑	Coadministration may enhance the possibility of arrhythmias or digitalis toxicity associated with hypokalemia. Monitor serum potassium levels and use potassium supplements if necessary.
Fludrocortisone	Nondepolarizing muscle relaxants	↓	Corticosteroids may decrease the actions of the nondepolarizing muscle relaxants.
Fludrocortisone	Salicylates	↑↓	Corticosteroids will reduce serum salicylate levels and may decrease their effectiveness. Coadministration also may increase the ulcerogenic effects of each.
Fludrocortisone	Vaccines	↑↓	Concurrent use may increase neurological complications and decrease antibody response (see Warnings).

➤*Drug/Lab test interactions:* Corticosteroids may affect the nitro-bluetetrazollum test for bacterial infection and produce false-negative results.

Adverse Reactions

Most adverse reactions are caused by fludrocortisone's mineralocorticoid activity (retention of sodium and water). When fludrocortisone is used in the small dosages recommended, the glucocorticoid side effects often seen with cortisone and its derivatives are not usually a problem; however, keep in mind the following untoward effects, particularly when fludrocortisone is used over a prolonged period of time or in conjunction with cortisone or a similar glucocorticoid.

➤*Cardiovascular:* Hypertension; CHF; cardiac enlargement.

➤*CNS:* Convulsions; increased intracranial pressure with papilledema (pseudotumor cerebri), usually after treatment; vertigo; headache; severe mental disturbances.

➤*Dermatologic:* Allergic skin rash; maculopapular rash; urticaria; impaired wound healing; thin, fragile skin; bruising; petechiae and ecchymoses; facial erythema; increased sweating; SC fat atrophy; purpura; striae; hyperpigmentation of skin and nails; hirsutism; acneiform eruptions; hives. Reactions to skin tests may be suppressed.

➤*Endocrine:* Menstrual irregularities; development of the cushingoid state; suppression of growth in children; secondary adrenocortical and pituitary unresponsiveness, particularly in times of stress (eg, trauma, surgery, illness); decreased carbohydrate tolerance; manifestations of latent diabetes mellitus; increased requirements for insulin or oral hypoglycemic agents in diabetics.

➤*GI:* Peptic ulcer with possible perforation and hemorrhage; pancreatitis; abdominal distention; ulcerative esophagitis.

➤*Metabolic:* Hyperglycemia; glycosuria; negative nitrogen balance caused by protein catabolism; potassium loss; edema; hypokalemic alkalosis.

➤*Musculoskeletal:* Muscle weakness; steroid myopathy; loss of muscle mass; osteoporosis; vertebral compression fractures; aseptic necrosis of femoral and humeral heads; pathologic fracture of long bones; spontaneous fractures.

➤*Ophthalmic:* Posterior subcapsular cataracts; increased intraocular pressure; glaucoma; exophthalmos.

➤*Miscellaneous:* Necrotizing angiitis; thrombophlebitis; aggravation or masking of infections; insomnia; syncopal episodes; anaphylactoid reactions.

Overdosage

➤*Symptoms:* Hypertension; edema; hypokalemia; excessive weight gain; increase in heart size.

➤*Treatment:* Discontinue the drug; symptoms usually subside within several days. Resume subsequent treatment with reduced doses. Muscular weakness may develop because of excessive potassium loss; treat with potassium supplements. Monitor blood pressure and serum electrolytes regularly.

Patient Information

Notify physician if dizziness, severe or continuing headaches, swelling of feet or lower legs, or unusual weight gain occurs.

Warn patients who are on immunosuppressant doses of corticosteroids to avoid exposure to chicken pox or measles and, if exposed, to obtain medical advice.

Advise the patient to use the medicine only as directed, to take a missed dose as soon as possible, unless it is almost time for the next dose, and not to double the next dose.

TERIPARATIDE (rDNA origin)

| Rx | Forteo (Eli Lilly) | Injection: 250 mcg/mL[1] | In 3 mL prefilled pen delivery device. |

[1] With 45.4 mg mannitol.

WARNING

In male and female rats, teriparatide caused an increase in the incidence of osteosarcoma (a malignant bone tumor) that was dependent on dose and treatment duration. The effect was observed at systemic exposures to teriparatide ranging from 3 to 60 times the exposure in humans given a 20 mcg dose. Because of the uncertain relevance of the rat osteosarcoma finding to humans, prescribe teriparatide only to patients for whom the potential benefits are considered to outweigh the potential risk. Do not prescribe teriparatide for patients who are at increased baseline risk for osteosarcoma (including those with Paget disease of bone or unexplained elevations of alkaline phosphatase, open epiphyses, or prior radiation therapy involving the skeleton) (see Warnings).

Indications

➤*Postmenopausal women:* For the treatment of postmenopausal women with osteoporosis who are at high risk for fracture. These include women with a history of osteoporotic fracture, who have multiple risk factors for fracture, or who have failed or are intolerant of previous osteoporosis therapy, based upon physician assessment. In postmenopausal women with osteoporosis, teriparatide increases bone mass density (BMD) and reduces the risk of vertebral and nonvertebral fractures.

➤*Men:* To increase bone mass in men with primary or hypogonadal osteoporosis who are at high risk for fracture. These include men with a history of osteoporotic fracture, who have multiple risk factors for fracture, or who have failed or are intolerant to previous osteoporosis therapy, based upon physician assessment. In men with primary or hypogonadal osteoporosis, teriparatide increases BMD. The effects of teriparatide on risk for fracture in men have not been studied.

The safety and efficacy of teriparatide have not been evaluated beyond 2 years of treatment. Consequently, use of the drug for more than 2 years is not recommended.

Administration and Dosage

➤*Approved by the FDA:* November 26, 2002.

➤*Dose:* 20 mcg once daily as an SC injection into the thigh or abdominal wall. Initially administer teriparatide under circumstances in which the patient can sit or lie down if symptoms of orthostatic hypotension occur.

➤*Storage/Stability:* Store the teriparatide pen under refrigeration at 2° to 8°C (36° to 46°F) at all times. During the use period, minimize the time out of the refrigerator; the dose may be delivered immediately following removal from the refrigerator. Recap the pen when not in use to protect the cartridge from physical damage and light. Each teriparatide pen can be used for up to 28 days after the first injection. After the 28-day use period, discard the pen even if it still contains some unused solution.

Do not freeze; do not use teriparatide if it has been frozen. Do not use if solid particles appear or if the solution is cloudy or colored.

Actions

➤*Pharmacology:* Teriparatide (rDNA origin) injection contains recombinant human parathyroid hormone (1-34), [rhPTH(1-34)], which has an identical sequence to the 34 N-terminal amino acids (the biologically active region) of the 84-amino acid human parathyroid hormone. Teriparatide is manufactured using a strain of *Escherichia coli* modified by recombinant DNA technology.

Endogenous 84-amino-acid parathyroid hormone (PTH) is the primary regulator of calcium and phosphate metabolism in bone and kidney. Physiological actions of PTH include regulation of bone metabolism, renal tubular reabsorption of calcium and phosphate, and intestinal calcium absorption. The biological actions of PTH and teriparatide are mediated through binding to specific high-affinity cell-surface receptors. Teriparatide and the 34 N-terminal amino acids of PTH bind to these receptors with the same affinity and have the same physiological actions on bone and kidney. Teriparatide is not expected to accumulate in bone or other tissues.

The skeletal effects of teriparatide depend upon the pattern of systemic exposure. Once-daily administration of teriparatide stimulates new bone formation on trabecular and cortical (periosteal and/or endosteal) bone surfaces by preferential stimulation of osteoblastic activity over osteoclastic activity. In monkey studies, teriparatide improved trabecular microarchitecture and increased bone mass and strength by stimulating new bone formation in both cancellous and cortical bone. In humans, the anabolic effects of teriparatide are manifest as an increase in skeletal mass, an increase in markers of bone formation and resorption, and an increase in bone strength. By contrast, continuous excess of endogenous PTH, as occurs in hyperparathyroidism, may be detrimental to the skeleton because bone resorption may be stimulated more than bone formation.

Pharmacodynamics – Teriparatide affects calcium and phosphorus metabolism in a pattern consistent with the known actions of endogenous PTH (eg, increases serum calcium and decreases serum phosphorus).

Serum calcium concentrations: When teriparatide 20 mcg is administered once daily, the serum calcium concentration increases transiently, beginning approximately 2 hours after dosing and reaching a maximum concentration between 4 to 6 hours (median increase, 0.4 mg/dL). The serum calcium concentration begins to decline approximately 6 hours after dosing and returns to baseline by 16 to 24 hours after each dose.

In a clinical study of postmenopausal women with osteoporosis, the median peak serum calcium concentration measured 4 to 6 hours after dosing with teriparatide 20 mcg was 2.42 mmol/L (9.68 mg/dL) at 12 months. The peak serum calcium remained below 2.76 mmol/L (11 mg/dL) in more than 99% of women at each visit. Sustained hypercalcemia was not observed.

In this study, 11.1% of women treated with teriparatide had a least 1 serum calcium value above the upper limit of normal (2.64 mmol/L [10.6 mg/dL]) compared with 1.5% of women treated with placebo. The percentage of women treated with teriparatide whose serum calcium was above the upper limit of normal on consecutive 4- to 6-hour post-dose measurements was 3% compared with 0.2% of women treated with placebo. In these women, calcium supplements and/or teriparatide doses were reduced. Teriparatide dose adjustments were made at varying intervals after the first observation of increased serum calcium (median, 21 weeks). During these intervals, there was no evidence of progressive increases in serum calcium.

In a clinical study of men with primary or hypogonadal osteoporosis, the effects on serum calcium were similar to those observed in postmenopausal women. The median peak serum calcium concentration measured 4 to 6 hours after dosing with teriparatide was 2.35 mmol/L (9.44 mg/dL) at 12 months. The peak serum calcium remained below 2.76 mmol/L (11 mg/dL) in 98% of men at each visit. Sustained hypercalcemia was not observed.

In this study, 6% of men treated with teriparatide daily had at least 1 serum calcium value above the upper limit of normal (2.64 mmol/L [10.6 mg/dL]) compared with none of the men treated with placebo. The percentage of men treated with teriparatide whose serum calcium was above the upper limit of normal on consecutive measurements was 1.3% (2 men) compared with none of the men treated with placebo. Although calcium supplements and/or teriparatide doses could have been reduced in these men, only calcium supplementation was reduced.

Urinary calcium excretion: In a clinical study of postmenopausal women with osteoporosis who received 1000 mg of supplemental calcium and at least 400 IU of vitamin D, daily teriparatide increased urinary calcium excretion. The median urinary excretion of calcium was 4.8 mmol/day (190 mg/day) at 6 months and 4.2 mmol/day (170 mg/day) at 12 months. These levels were 0.76 mmol/day (30 mg/day) and 0.3 mmol/day (12 mg/day) higher, respectively, than in women treated with placebo. The incidence of hypercalciuria (greater than 7.5 mmol Ca/day or 300 mg/day) was similar in the women treated with teriparatide or placebo.

In a clinical study of men with primary or hypogonadal osteoporosis who received 1000 mg supplemental calcium and at least 400 IU vitamin D, daily teriparatide had inconsistent effects on urinary calcium excretion. The median urinary excretion of calcium was 5.6 mmol/day (220 mg/day) at 1 month and 5.3 mmol/day (210 mg/day) at 6 months. These levels were 0.5 mmol/day (20 mg/day) higher and 0.2 mmol/day (8 mg/day) lower, respectively, than in men treated with placebo. The incidence of hypercalciuria (greater than 7.5 mmol Ca/day or 300 mg/day) was similar in the men treated with teriparatide or placebo.

Phosphorus and vitamin D: In single-dose studies, teriparatide produced transient phosphaturia and mild transient reductions in serum phosphorus concentration. In clinical trials of daily teriparatide, the median serum concentration of 1,25-dihydroxyvitamin D was increased at 12 months by 19% in women and 14% in men, compared with baseline. In the placebo group, this concentration decreased 2% in women and increased 5% in men. The median serum 25-hydroxyvitamin D concentration at 12 months was decreased 19% in women and 10% in men compared with baseline.

➤*Pharmacokinetics:*

Absorption/Distribution – Teriparatide is extensively absorbed after SC injection; the absolute bioavailability is approximately 95% based on pooled data from 20, 40, and 80 mcg doses. The rates of absorption and elimination are rapid. The peptide reaches peak serum concentrations about 30 minutes after SC injection of a 20 mcg dose and declines to nonquantifiable concentrations within 3 hours. Volume of distribution following IV injection is approximately 0.12 L/kg.

Metabolism/Excretion – Systemic clearance of teriparatide (approximately 62 L/h in women and 94 L/h in men) exceeds the rate of normal liver plasma flow, consistent with both hepatic and extrahepatic clearance. Intersubject variability in systemic clearance and volume of distribution is 25% to 50%. The half-life of teriparatide in serum is 5 minutes when administered by IV injection and approximately 1 hour

TERIPARATIDE (rDNA origin)

when administered by SC injection. The longer half-life following SC administration reflects the time required for absorption from the injection site.

No metabolism or excretion studies have been performed with teriparatide. However, the mechanisms of metabolism and elimination of PTH(1-34) and intact PTH have been extensively described in published literature. Peripheral metabolism of PTH is believed to occur by nonspecific enzymatic mechanisms in the liver followed by excretion via the kidneys.

Special populations –

Gender: Although systemic exposure to teriparatide was approximately 20% to 30% lower in men than women, the recommended dose for both genders is 20 mcg/day.

Renal function impairment: In 5 patients with severe renal insufficiency (Ccr less than 30 mL/min), the AUC and $t_{1/2}$ of teriparatide were increased by 73% and 77%, respectively. Maximum serum concentration of teriparatide was not increased. No studies have been performed in patients undergoing dialysis for chronic renal failure.

Contraindications

Hypersensitivity to teriparatide or to any of its excipients.

Warnings

➤*Osteosarcoma:* In male and female rats, teriparatide caused an increase in the incidence of osteosarcoma (a malignant bone tumor) that was dependent on dose and treatment duration (see Warning Box). The following categories of patients have increased baseline risk of osteosarcoma and, therefore, should not be treated with teriparatide:

- Paget disease of bone. Do not give teriparatide to patients with Paget disease of bone. Unexplained elevations of alkaline phosphatase may indicate Paget disease of bone.
- Pediatric populations. Teriparatide has not been studied in pediatric populations. Do not use teriparatide in pediatric patients or young adults with open epiphyses.
- Prior radiation therapy. Exclude patients with a prior history of radiation therapy involving the skeleton from treatment with teriparatide.

➤*Avoid use in:* Exclude patients with bone metastases or a history of skeletal malignancies from treatment with teriparatide.

Exclude patients with metabolic bone diseases other than osteoporosis from treatment with teriparatide.

Teriparatide has not been studied in patients with pre-existing hypercalcemia. Exclude these patients from treatment with teriparatide because of the possibility of exacerbating hypercalcemia.

➤*Carcinogenesis:* Two carcinogenicity bioassays were conducted in rats. In the first study, male and female rats were given daily SC teriparatide injections of 5, 30, or 75 mcg/kg/day for 24 months from 2 months of age. These doses resulted in systemic exposures that were respectively, 3, 20, and 60 times higher than the systemic exposure observed in humans following an SC dose of 20 mcg (based on AUC comparison). Teriparatide treatment resulted in a marked dose-related increase in the incidence of osteosarcoma, a rare malignant bone tumor, in both male and female rats. Osteosarcomas were observed at all doses and the incidence reached 40% to 50% in the high-dose groups. Teriparatide also caused a dose-related increase in osteoblastoma and osteoma in both sexes. The bone tumors in rats occurred in association with a large increase in bone mass and focal osteoblast hyperplasia.

The second 2-year study was carried out in order to determine the effect of treatment duration and animal age on the development of bone tumors. Female rats were treated for different periods between 2 and 26 months of age with SC doses of 5 and 30 mcg/kg (equivalent to 3 and 20 times the human exposure at the 20 mcg dose, based on AUC comparison). The study showed that the occurrence of osteosarcoma, osteoblastoma, and osteoma was dependent upon dose and duration of exposure. Bone tumors were observed when immature 2-month-old rats were treated with 30 mcg/kg/day for 24 months or with 5 or 30 mcg/kg/day for 6 months. Bone tumors also were observed when mature 6-month-old rats were treated with 30 mcg/kg/day for 6 or 20 months.

➤*Pregnancy:* Category C. In pregnant mice given SC doses of 225 or 1000 mcg/kg/day (greater than or equal to 60 times the human dose based on surface area [mcg/m²]) from gestation day 6 through 15, the fetuses showed an increased incidence of skeletal deviations or variations (interrupted rib, extra vertebra or rib).

Developmental effects in a perinatal/postnatal study in pregnant rats given SC doses of teriparatide from gestation day 6 through postpartum day 20 included mild growth retardation in female offspring at doses greater than or equal to 225 mcg/kg/day (greater than or equal to 120 times the human dose based on surface area [mcg/m²]), and in male offspring at 1000 mcg/kg/day (540 times the human dose based on surface area [mcg/m²]). There also was reduced motor activity in male and female offspring at 1000 mcg/kg/day. The effect of teriparatide treatment on human fetal development has not been studied. Teriparatide is not indicated for use in pregnancy.

➤*Lactation:* Because teriparatide is indicated for the treatment of osteoporosis in postmenopausal women, it should not be administered to women who are nursing their children. There have been no clinical studies to determine if teriparatide is secreted into breast milk.

➤*Children:* The safety and efficacy of teriparatide have not been established in pediatric populations. Teriparatide is not indicated for use in pediatric patients.

Precautions

➤*Urolithiasis/Pre-existing hypercalciuria:* In clinical trials, the frequency of urolithiasis was similar in patients treated with teriparatide and placebo. However, teriparatide has not been studied in patients with active urolithiasis. If active urolithiasis or pre-existing hypercalciuria are suspected, consider measurement of urinary calcium excretion. Use teriparatide with caution in patients with active or recent urolithiasis because of the potential to exacerbate this condition.

➤*Hypotension:* In short-term clinical pharmacology studies with teriparatide, transient episodes of symptomatic orthostatic hypotension were observed infrequently. Typically, an event began within 4 hours of dosing and spontaneously resolved within a few minutes to a few hours. When transient orthostatic hypotension occurred, it happened within the first several doses, it was relieved by placing the person in a reclining position; it did not preclude continued treatment.

➤*Calcium levels:* Teriparatide transiently increases serum calcium, with the maximal effect observed at approximately 4 to 6 hours postdose. By 16 hours postdose, serum calcium generally returned to or near baseline. Keep these effects in mind because serum calcium concentrations observed within 16 hours after a dose may reflect the pharmacologic effect of teriparatide. Persistent hypercalcemia was not observed in clinical trials with teriparatide. If persistent hypercalcemia is detected, discontinue treatment with teriparatide pending further evaluation of the cause of hypercalcemia.

Do not treat patients known to have an underlying hypercalcemic disorder, such as primary hyperparathyroidism, with teriparatide.

Teriparatide increases urinary calcium excretion, but the frequency of hypercalciuria in clinical trials was similar for patients treated with teriparatide and placebo.

➤*Uric acid:* Teriparatide increases serum uric acid concentrations. In clinical trials, 2.8% of teriparatide patients had serum uric acid concentrations above the upper limit of normal compared with 0.7% of placebo patients. However, the hyperuricemia did not result in an increase in gout, arthralgia, or urolithiasis.

➤*Immunogenicity:* In a large clinical trial, antibodies that cross-reacted with teriparatide were detected in 2.8% of women receiving teriparatide. Generally, antibodies were first detected following 12 months of treatment and diminished after withdrawal of therapy. There was no evidence of hypersensitivity reactions, allergic reactions, or effects on serum calcium or BMD response.

Drug Interactions

➤*Digoxin:* Sporadic case reports have suggested that hypercalcemia may predispose patients to digitalis toxicity. Because teriparatide transiently increases serum calcium, use teriparatide with caution in patients taking digitalis.

➤*Furosemide:* In a study of 9 healthy people and 17 patients with mild, moderate, or severe renal insufficiency (Ccr 13 to 72 mL/min), coadministration of IV furosemide (20 to 100 mg) with teriparatide 40 mcg resulted in small increases in the serum calcium (2%) and 24-hour urine calcium (37%) responses to teriparatide that did not appear to be clinically important.

Adverse Reactions

In the 2 Phase 3 placebo-controlled clinical trials in men and postmenopausal women, early discontinuation because of adverse events occurred in 7.1% of patients assigned to teriparatide and 5.6% of patients assigned to placebo. Reported adverse events that appeared to be increased by teriparatide treatment were dizziness and leg cramps.

Teriparatide Adverse Reactions (≥ 2%)		
Adverse reaction	Teriparatide (N = 691)	Placebo (N = 691)
Cardiovascular		
Hypertension	7.1	6.8
Syncope	2.6	1.4
Angina pectoris	2.5	1.6
CNS		
Dizziness	8	5.4
Headache	7.5	7.4
Insomnia	4.3	3.6
Depression	4.1	2.7
Vertigo	3.8	2.7
Dermatology		
Rash	4.9	4.5
Sweating	2.2	1.7
GI		
Nausea	8.5	6.7
Constipation	5.4	4.5
Dyspepsia	5.2	4.1
Diarrhea	5.1	4.6
Vomiting	3	2.3

TERIPARATIDE (rDNA origin)

Teriparatide Adverse Reactions (≥ 2%)		
Adverse reaction	Teriparatide (N = 691)	Placebo (N = 691)
GI disorder	2.3	2
Tooth disorder	2	1.3
Musculoskeletal		
Arthralgia	10.1	8.4
Leg cramps	2.6	1.3
Respiratory		
Rhinitis	9.6	8.8
Cough increased	6.4	5.5
Pharyngitis	5.5	4.8
Pneumonia	3.9	3.3
Dyspnea	3.6	2.6
Miscellaneous		
Pain	21.3	20.5
Asthenia	8.7	6.8
Neck pain	3	2.7

➤*Lab test abnormalities:* Teriparatide transiently increases serum calcium, with the maximal effect observed at approximately 4 to 6 hours postdose. Serum calcium measured at least 16 hours postdose was not different from pretreatment levels. In clinical trials, the frequency of at least 1 episode of transient hypercalcemia in the 4 to 6 hours after teriparatide administration was increased from 1.5% of women and none of the men treated with placebo to 11.1% of women and 6% of men treated with teriparatide. The percentage of patients treated with teriparatide whose transient hypercalcemia was verified on consecutive measurements was 3% of women and 1.3% of men.

Overdosage

➤*Symptoms:* Incidents of overdose in humans have not been reported in clinical trials. Teriparatide has been administered in single doses of up to 100 mcg and in repeated doses of up to 60 mcg/day for 6 weeks.

The effects of overdose that may be expected include a delayed hypercalcemic effect and risk of orthostatic hypotension. Nausea, vomiting, dizziness, and headache also may occur.

In single-dose studies in rodents using SC injection of teriparatide, no mortality was seen in rats given doses of 1000 mcg/kg (540 times the human dose based on surface area [mcg/m^2]) or in mice given 10,000 mcg/kg (2700 times the human dose based on surface area [mcg/m^2]).

➤*Treatment:* There is no specific antidote for teriparatide. The treatment of suspected overdose should include discontinuation of teriparatide, monitoring of serum calcium and phosphorus, and implementation of appropriate supportive measures, such as hydration.

Patient Information

Instruct patients to read the *Medication Guide* and pen *User Manual* before starting therapy with teriparatide and reread them each time the prescription is renewed.

Make patients aware that teriparatide caused osteosarcomas in rats and that the clinical relevance of these findings is unknown.

Initially administer teriparatide under circumstances where the patient can sit or lie down immediately if symptoms occur. Instruct patients that if they feel lightheaded or have palpitations after the injection, they should sit or lie down until the symptoms resolve. If symptoms persist or worsen, instruct patients to consult a physician before continuing treatment.

Although symptomatic hypercalcemia was not observed in clinical trials, instruct patients to contact a health care provider if they develop persistent symptoms of hypercalcemia (ie, nausea, vomiting, constipation, lethargy, muscle weakness).

Instruct patients how to properly use the delivery device (refer to *User Manual*) and dispose of needles, and advise them not to share their pens with other patients.

Inform patients regarding the roles of supplemental calcium and/or vitamin D, weight-bearing exercise, and modification of certain behavioral factors, such as cigarette smoking and/or alcohol consumption.

Thyroid Hormones

Synthetic derivatives include levothyroxine (T_4), liothyronine (T_3), and liotrix (a 4 to 1 mixture of T_4 and T_3).

WARNING

Drugs with thyroid hormone activity, alone or with other therapeutic agents, have been used for the treatment of obesity. In euthyroid patients, doses within the range of daily hormonal requirements are ineffective for weight reduction. Larger doses may produce serious or even life-threatening manifestations of toxicity, particularly when given in association with sympathomimetic amines such as those used for their anorectic effects.

Indications

►*Hypothyroidism:* As replacement or supplemental therapy in hypothyroidism of any etiology, except transient hypothyroidism during the recovery phase of subacute thyroiditis. Specific indications include the following: Cretinism, myxedema, and ordinary hypothyroidism; primary hypothyroidism resulting from functional deficiency, primary atrophy, partial or total absence of thyroid gland, or the effects of surgery, radiation, or drugs, with or without the presence of goiter; secondary (pituitary) or tertiary (hypothalamic) hypothyroidism.

►*Pituitary TSH suppressants:* In the treatment or prevention of various types of euthyroid goiters, including thyroid nodules, subacute or chronic lymphocytic thyroiditis (Hashimoto), and multinodular goiter and in the management of thyroid cancer (except liothyronine).

►*Diagnostic use (except levothyroxine):* Diagnostic use in suppression tests to differentiate suspected mild hyperthyroidism or thyroid gland autonomy.

►*Myxedema coma/precoma (injection only):* For the treatment of myxedema coma/precoma.

►*Unlabeled uses:* Thyroid hormones have been used to treat obesity; however, they are ineffective and should not be used for this condition (see Warnings).

Administration and Dosage

Individualize dosage. Determine patient response by clinical judgment in conjunction with laboratory findings.

Generally, institute thyroid therapy at relatively low doses and slowly increase in small increments until the desired response is obtained. Administer thyroid as a single daily dose, preferably before breakfast.

►*Treatment of choice:* Treatment of choice for hypothyroidism is levothyroxine (T_4) under most circumstances because of its predictable potency and prolonged half-life.

►*Thyroid cancer:* Exogenous thyroid hormone may produce regression of metastases from follicular and papillary carcinoma of the thyroid and is used as ancillary therapy of these conditions with radioactive iodine. Larger doses than those used for replacement therapy are required. Medullary thyroid carcinoma usually is unresponsive.

►*Laboratory tests:* Laboratory tests useful in the diagnosis and evaluation of thyroid function are listed in the following table, indicating the alterations noted in various thyroid disorders.

Laboratory Tests for Diagnosis and Evaluation of Thyroid Function						
↑ = Increased ↓ = Decreased N = Normal X = Contraindicated	Pregnancy	Primary hypothyroidism	Secondary hypothyroidism	Hyperthyroidism	T_3 thyrotoxicosis	Normal values
Free T_4 (unbound)	N	↓	↓	↑	N	12 to 32 pmol/L
Total T_4	↑	↓	↓	↑	N	55 to 160 nmol/L
T_3	↑	↓	↓	↑	↑	0.6 to 3.1 nmol/L
RAIU*	X	↓	-	↑	–	5% to 30%
Free thyroxine index (FT_4I)	N	↓	↓	↑	-	6.5 to 12.5[1] 1.3 to 3.9[2]
TSH*	N	↑	N/↓	↓	↓	0.4 to 4.2 mIU/L

* RAIU = radioactive iodine uptake; TSH = thyroid-stimulating hormone
[1] T_4 uptake method
[2] TT_4 × RT_3U method

►*Dosage equivalents of thyroid products:* In changing from one thyroid product to another, the following dosage equivalents may be used. However, these equivalents are only estimates; each patient still may require fine dosage adjustments.

Approximate Dosage Equivalents of Thyroid Products[1]			
Preparation	Composition ratio		Dosage equivalents
	T_4	T_3	
Thyroid desiccated	4	1	≈ 60 to 65 mg (1 grain)
Levothyroxine	1	0	≈ 50 to 60 mcg (range, 50 to 100 mcg)
Liothyronine	0	1	≈ 25 mcg (range, 15 to 37.5 mcg)
Liotrix	4	1	≈ 1 grain (12.5 mcg T_3/50 mcg T_4)

[1] References may vary in dosage equivalent recommendations.

Actions

►*Pharmacology:* Thyroid hormones include natural and synthetic derivatives. The natural product, desiccated thyroid, is derived from beef or pork. The US Pharmacopeia (USP) has standardized the total iodine content of natural preparations. Thyroid USP contains not less than 0.17% and not more than 0.23% iodine. Iodine content is only an indirect indicator of true hormonal biologic activity.

Physiological effects – The mechanisms by which thyroid hormones exert their physiologic action are not well understood. It is believed that most of their effects are exerted through control of DNA transcription and protein synthesis. These hormones enhance oxygen consumption by most tissues of the body and increase the basal metabolic rate and metabolism of carbohydrates, lipids, and proteins in the body. Thyroid hormones exert a profound influence on every organ system and are particularly important in CNS development. The physiological actions of thyroid hormones are produced predominantly by T_3, the majority of which (approximately 80%) is derived from T_4 by deiodination in peripheral tissues.

Regulation of thyroid secretion: Thyroid hormone synthesis and secretion are controlled by thyrotropin (thyroid-stimulating hormone; TSH) secreted by the anterior pituitary. TSH secretion is, in turn, controlled by a feedback mechanism effected by thyroid hormones and thyrotropin-releasing hormone (TRH), a tripeptide of hypothalamic origin. Endogenous thyroid hormone secretion is suppressed when exogenous thyroid hormones are given to euthyroid individuals in excess of the normal gland's secretion.

The normal thyroid gland contains, per gram of gland, approximately 200 mcg of T_4 and 15 mcg of T_3. The ratio of these 2 hormones in the circulation does not represent the ratio in the thyroid gland because about 80% of peripheral T_3 comes from monodeiodination of T_4. Peripheral monodeiodination of T_4 also results in the formation of reverse triiodothyronine (rT_3), which is calorigenically inactive.

Low triiodothyronine syndrome – The T_3 level is low in the fetus and newborn, in the elderly, and in cases of chronic caloric deprivation, hepatic cirrhosis, renal failure, surgical stress, and chronic illnesses.

►*Pharmacokinetics:*

Absorption – Absorption of orally administered T_4 varies from 40% to 80% of the administered dose. T_4 absorption is increased by fasting and decreased in malabsorption syndromes and by certain foods, such as soybean infant formula. Dietary fiber decreases bioavailability of T_4. Absorption also may decrease with age. In addition, many drugs and foods affect T_4 absorption. In 4 hours, T_3 is approximately 95% absorbed. The hormones in natural preparations are absorbed in a manner similar to the synthetic hormones.

Distribution – More than 99% of circulating hormones are bound to serum proteins, including thyroxine-binding globulin (TBG) and thyroxine-binding prealbumin (TBPA) and albumin (TBA), whose capacities and affinities vary for the hormones. The higher affinity of T_4 for TBG and TBPA as compared with T_3 partially explains the higher serum levels and longer half-life of T_4. Both protein-bound hormones exist in reverse equilibrium with minute amounts of free hormone, the latter accounting for the metabolic activity.

Metabolism – Approximately 80% of T_3 comes from monodeiodination of T_4. Deiodination of T_4 occurs at a number of sites, including liver, kidney, and other tissues. The conjugated hormone, in the form of glucuronide or sulfate, is found in the bile and gut where it may complete an enterohepatic circulation. Of T_4 metabolized daily, 80% to 85% is deiodinated to yield equal amounts of T_3 and reverse T_3 (rT_3). T_3 and rT_3 are further deiodinated to diiodothyronine.

Excretion – Thyroid hormones are primarily eliminated by the kidneys. A portion of the conjugated hormone reaches the colon unchanged and is eliminated in the feces. Approximately 20% of T_4 is eliminated in the stool. Urinary excretion of T_4 decreases with age.

Various Pharmacokinetic Parameters of Thyroid Hormones				
Hormone	Ratio in thyroglobulin	Biologic potency	Half-life (days)	Protein binding (%)[1]
Levothyroxine (T_4)	10 to 20	1	6 to 7[2]	99+
Liothyronine (T_3)	1	4	≤ 2.5	99+

[1] Includes TBG, TBPA, and TBA.
[2] 3 to 4 days in hyperthyroidism, 9 to 10 days in hypothyroidism.

Contraindications

In patients with diagnosed but uncorrected adrenal cortical insufficiency; untreated thyrotoxicosis; hypersensitivity to active or extraneous constituents.

Levothyroxine is contraindicated in patients with untreated subclinical (suppressed serum TSH level with normal T_3 and T_4 levels) and in patients with acute MI.

Concomitant use of *Triostat* and artificial rewarming of patients is contraindicated.

Warnings

➤*Obesity:* Obesity has been treated with thyroid hormones. In euthyroid patients, hormonal replacement doses are ineffective for weight reduction. Larger doses may produce serious or even life-threatening toxicity, particularly when given with sympathomimetic amines such as anorexiants.

➤*Infertility:* Thyroid hormone therapy is unjustified for the treatment of male or female infertility unless the condition is accompanied by hypothyroidism.

➤*Cardiovascular disease:* Use great caution when the integrity of the cardiovascular system, particularly the coronary arteries, is suspected. This includes patients with angina pectoris or the elderly, in whom there is a greater likelihood of occult cardiac disease. In these patients, initiate therapy with low doses. When, in such patients, a euthyroid state only can be reached at the expense of an aggravation of the cardiovascular disease, reduce thyroid hormone dosage.

Overtreatment with levothyroxine sodium may have adverse cardiovascular effects such as an increase in heart rate, cardiac wall thickness, and cardiac contractility and may precipitate angina or arrhythmias. During surgical procedures, closely monitor patients with coronary artery disease who are receiving levothyroxine therapy because the possibility of precipitating cardiac arrhythmias may be greater in those treated with levothyroxine. Concomitant administration of levothyroxine and sympathomimetic agents to patients with coronary artery disease may precipitate coronary insufficiency.

➤*Endocrine disorders:* Thyroid hormone therapy in patients with concomitant diabetes mellitus or insipidus or adrenal cortical insufficiency (Addison disease) exacerbates the intensity of their symptoms. Appropriate adjustments in the therapy of these concomitant endocrine diseases are required.

Autoimmune polyglandular syndrome – Occasionally, chronic autoimmune thyroiditis may occur in association with other autoimmune disorders, such as adrenal insufficiency, pernicious anemia, and insulin-dependent diabetes mellitus. Treat patients with concomitant adrenal insufficiency with replacement glucocorticoids prior to initiation of treatment. Failure to do so may precipitate an acute adrenal crisis when thyroid hormone therapy is initiated because of increased metabolic clearance of glucocorticoids by thyroid hormone. Patients with diabetes mellitus may require upward adjustments of their antidiabetic therapeutic regimens.

In patients with secondary or tertiary hypothyroidism, consider additional hypothalamic/pituitary hormone deficiencies and, if diagnosed, treat.

➤*Nontoxic diffuse goiter or nodular thyroid disease:* Exercise caution when administering levothyroxine to patients with nontoxic diffuse goiter or nodular thyroid disease in order to prevent precipitation of thyrotoxicosis. If the serum TSH is already suppressed, do not administer levothyroxine.

➤*Severe and prolonged hypothyroidism:* Severe and prolonged hypothyroidism can lead to a decreased level of adrenocortical activity commensurate with the lowered metabolic state. When thyroid replacement therapy is administered, the metabolism increases at a greater rate than adrenocortical activity, which can precipitate adrenocortical insufficiency. Therefore, in severe and prolonged hypothyroidism, supplemental adrenocortical steroids may be necessary.

➤*Morphologic hypogonadism and nephrosis:* Rule out morphologic hypogonadism and nephrosis prior to initiating therapy. If hypopituitarism is present, the adrenal deficiency must be corrected prior to starting the drug.

➤*Myxedema:* Patients with myxedema are particularly sensitive to thyroid preparations. Start dosage at a very low level and increase gradually, as acute changes may precipitate adverse cardiovascular events. Myxedema coma therapy requires simultaneous administration of glucocorticoids.

➤*Hyperthyroid effects:* In rare instances, the administration of thyroid hormone may precipitate a hyperthyroid state or may aggravate existing hyperthyroidism.

➤*Pregnancy:* Category A. Thyroid hormones cross the placental barrier to some extent, as evidenced by levels in cord blood of athyreotic fetuses being approximately one-third maternal levels. Transfer of thyroid hormone from the mother to the fetus, however, may not be adequate to prevent in utero hypothyroidism. Clinical experience does not indicate any adverse effect on the fetus when thyroid hormones are administered to a pregnant woman. Do not discontinue thyroid replacement therapy in hypothyroid women during pregnancy.

➤*Lactation:* Minimal amounts of thyroid hormones are excreted in breast milk. Thyroid is not associated with serious adverse reactions. However, exercise caution when thyroid is administered to a nursing woman.

➤*Children:* There is limited experience with liothyronine sodium injection in the pediatric population. Safety and efficacy in pediatric patients have not been established.

Congenital hypothyroidism – Pregnant women provide little or no thyroid hormone to the fetus. The incidence of congenital hypothyroidism is relatively high (1:4000) and the hypothyroid fetus would not benefit from the small amounts of hormone crossing the placenta. Routine determinations of serum T_4 and/or TSH are strongly advised in neonates in view of the deleterious effects of thyroid deficiency on growth and development.

Initiate treatment immediately upon diagnosis, and maintain for life, unless transient hypothyroidism is suspected; in this case, therapy may be interrupted for 2 to 8 weeks after 3 years of age to reassess the condition. Cessation of therapy is justified in patients who have maintained a normal TSH during those 2 to 8 weeks.

In infants, excessive doses of thyroid hormone preparations may produce craniosynostosis and may adversely affect the tempo of brain maturation and accelerate the bone age with resultant premature closure of the epiphyses and compromised adult stature.

In children, partial loss of hair may be experienced in the first few months of thyroid therapy; this usually is a transient phenomenon that results in later recovery.

Precautions

➤*Monitoring:* Treatment of patients with thyroid hormones requires the periodic assessment of thyroid status by means of appropriate laboratory tests. The TSH suppression test can be used to test the effectiveness of any thyroid preparation, keeping in mind the relative insensitivity of the infant pituitary to the negative feedback effect of thyroid hormones. Serum T_4 levels can be used to test the effectiveness of all thyroid medications except T_3. When the total serum T_4 is low but TSH is normal, a test specific to assess unbound (free) T_4 levels is warranted.

The frequency of TSH monitoring during levothyroxine dose titration depends on the clinical situation, but it is generally recommended at 6- to 8-week intervals until normalization. For patients who have recently initiated levothyroxine therapy and whose serum TSH has normalized or in patients who have had their dosage or brand of levothyroxine changed, measure the serum TSH concentration after 8 to 12 weeks. When the optimum replacement dose has been attained, clinical (physical examination) and biochemical monitoring may be performed every 6 to 12 months, depending on the clinical situation, and whenever there is a change in the patient's status.

The recommended frequency of monitoring of TSH and total or free T_4 in children is as follows: At 2 and 4 weeks after initiation of treatment; every 1 to 2 months during the first year of life; every 2 to 3 months between 1 and 3 years of age; and every 3 to 12 months thereafter until growth is completed. It is recommended that TSH and T_4 levels and a physical examination, if indicated, be performed 2 weeks after any change in levothyroxine dosage.

Specific measurements of T_4 and T_3 by competitive protein binding or radioimmunoassay are not influenced by blood levels of organic or inorganic iodine and have essentially replaced older tests (ie, PBI, BEI, T_4 by column) (see Administration and Dosage).

Persistent clinical and laboratory evidence of hypothyroidism in spite of adequate dosage replacement indicates poor patient compliance, poor absorption, excessive fecal loss, or inactivity of the preparation. Intracellular resistance to thyroid hormone is rare.

➤*Decreased bone mineral density:* In women, long-term levothyroxine therapy has been associated with increased bone resorption, thereby decreasing bone mineral density, especially in postmenopausal women on greater than replacement doses or in women who are receiving suppressive doses of levothyroxine. The increased bone resorption may be associated with increased serum levels and urinary excretion of calcium and phosphorus, elevations in bone alkaline phosphatase, and suppressed serum parathyroid hormone levels. Therefore, it is recommended that patients receiving levothyroxine be given the minimum dose necessary to achieve the desired clinical and biochemical response.

Thyroid Hormones

Drug Interactions

Thyroid Hormone Drug Interactions			
Precipitant drug	Object drug*		Description
Amiodarone Glucocorticoids (eg, dexamethasone ≥ 4 mg/day) Propylthiouracil	Thyroid hormones	↓	Concurrent use may decrease the peripheral conversion of T_4 to T_3, leading to decreased T_3 levels. However, serum T_4 levels are usually normal but occasionally may be slightly elevated.
Antacids (aluminum and magnesium hydroxides) Bile acid sequestrants (cholestyramine, colestipol) Calcium carbonate Iron salts Sodium polystyrene sulfonate Simethicone Sucralfate	Thyroid hormones	↓	Concurrent use may reduce the efficacy of the thyroid hormone because of possible binding in the GI tract, preventing absorption. Separate administration by at least 4 hours.
Beta blockers (eg, propranolol>160 mg/ day)	Thyroid hormones	↓	Concurrent use may decrease the peripheral conversion of T_4 to T_3, leading to decreased T_3 levels. However, serum T_4 levels usually are normal but occasionally may be slightly elevated.
Thyroid hormones	Beta blockers		The actions of particular beta blockers may be impaired when the hypothyroid patient is converted to the euthyroid state.
Carbamazepine Hydantoins Phenobarbital Rifamycins	Thyroid hormones	↓	Hepatic degradation of levothyroxine may increase, resulting in increased levothyroxine requirements.
Estrogens, oral contraceptives	Thyroid hormones	↓	Estrogens increase TBG and may therefore decrease the response to thyroid hormone therapy in patients with a nonfunctioning thyroid gland. An increased thyroid dose may be needed.
Furosemide (> 80 mg IV) Heparin Hydantoins NSAIDs Salicylates (> 2 g/day)	Thyroid hormones	↔	Administration of these agents with levothyroxine results in an initial transient increase in FT_4. Continued administration results in a decrease in serum T_4 and normal FT_4 and TSH; therefore, patients are clinically euthyroid.
Selective serotonin reuptake inhibitors (eg, sertraline)	Thyroid hormones	↓	Administration of sertraline in patients stabilized on levothyroxine may result in increased levothyroxine requirements.
Tricyclic antidepressants Tetracyclic antidepressants	Thyroid hormones	↑	Concurrent use of tricyclic/tetracyclic antidepressants and levothyroxine may increase the therapeutic and toxic effects of both drugs, possibly because of increased receptor sensitivity to catecholamines. Toxic effects may include increased risk of cardiac arrhythmias and CNS stimulation.
Thyroid hormones	Tricyclic antidepressants Tetracyclic antidepressants		
Thyroid hormones	Anticoagulants	↑	The anticoagulant action is increased; a decreased dose may be necessary.
Thyroid hormones	Antidiabetic agents Biguanides Meglitinides Sulfonylureas Thiazolidinediones Insulin	↓	Initiating thyroid hormones may cause increases in insulin or oral hypoglycemic requirements. Monitor closely.
Thyroid hormones	Digitalis glycosides	↓	Serum digitalis glycoside levels are reduced in hyperthyroidism or when the hypothyroid patient is converted to the euthyroid state. Therapeutic effects of digitalis glycosides may be reduced.

Thyroid Hormone Drug Interactions			
Precipitant drug	Object drug*		Description
Thyroid hormones	Growth hormones (somatrem, somatropin)	↑	Excessive use of thyroid hormones with growth hormones may accelerate epiphyseal closure. However, untreated hypothyroidism may interfere with growth response to growth hormone.
Thyroid hormones	Ketamine	↑	Concurrent use may produce marked hypertension and tachycardia. Administer with caution.
Thyroid hormones	Radiographic agents	↓	Thyroid hormones may reduce the uptake of ^{123}I, ^{131}I, ^{99m}TC.
Thyroid hormones	Sympathomimetics	↑	Concurrent use may increase the effects of either agent. Thyroid hormones may increase the risk of coronary insufficiency when sympathomimetics are given to patients with coronary artery disease. Use with caution.
Sympathomimetics	Thyroid hormones		
Thyroid hormones	Theophyllines	↑	Decreased theophylline clearance can be expected in hypothyroid patients; clearance returns to normal when euthyroid state is achieved.

* ↑ = Object drug increased ↓ = Object drug decreased ↔ = Undetermined clinical effect.

▶**Drug/Lab test interactions:** Consider changes in TBG concentration when interpreting T_4 and T_3 values. In such cases, measure the unbound (free) hormone and/or free T_4 index (FT_4I). Pregnancy, infectious hepatitis, estrogens, estrogen-containing oral contraceptives, and acute intermittent porphyria increase TBG concentrations. Decreases in TBG concentrations are observed in nephrosis, severe hypoproteinemia, severe liver disease, and acromegaly, and after androgen or corticosteroid therapy. Familial hyper- or hypothyroxine binding globulinemias have been described. The incidence of TBG deficiency approximates 1 in 9000.

Medicinal or dietary iodine interferes with all in vivo tests of radioiodine uptake, producing low uptakes that may not reflect a true decrease in hormone synthesis.

Cytokines: Interferon-α and interleukin-2 – Therapy with interferon-α has been associated with the development of antithyroid microsomal antibodies in 20% of patients and some have transient hypothyroidism, hyperthyroidism, or both. Patients who have antithyroid antibodies before treatment are at higher risk of thyroid dysfunction during treatment. Interleukin-2 has been associated with transient painless thyroiditis in 20% of patients. Interferon-β and -γ have not been reported to cause thyroid dysfunction.

Drugs That May Reduce TSH Secretion	
Dopamine/Dopamine agonists Glucocorticoids Octreotide	Use of these agents may result in a transient reduction in TSH secretion when administered at the following doses: Dopamine (≥ 1 mcg/kg/min); glucocorticoids (hydrocortisone ≥ 100 mg/day or equivalent); octreotide (> 100 mcg/day).

Drugs That May Decrease Thyroid Hormone Secretion	
Aminoglutethimide Amiodarone Iodide (including iodine-containing radiographic contrast agents) Lithium Methimazole Propylthiouracil (PTU) Sulfonamides Tolbutamide	Long-term lithium therapy can result in goiter in up to 50% of patients and in subclinical or overt hypothyroidism, each in up to 20% of patients. Oral cholecystographic agents and amiodarone slowly are excreted, producing more prolonged hypothyroidism than parenterally administered iodinated contrast agents. Long-term aminoglutethimide therapy may minimally decrease T_4 and T_3 levels and increase TSH, although all values remain within normal limits in most patients.

Drugs That May Increase Thyroid Hormone Secretion	
Amiodarone Iodide (including iodine-containing radiographic contrast agents)	Iodide and drugs that contain pharmacologic amounts of iodide may cause hyperthyroidism in euthyroid patients with Grave disease previously treated with antithyroid drugs or in euthyroid patients with thyroid autonomy (eg, multinodular goiter or hyperfunctioning thyroid adenoma). Hyperthyroidism may develop over several weeks and may persist for several months after therapy discontinuation. Amiodarone may induce hyperthyroidism by causing thyroiditis.

Drugs That May Alter Serum TBG Concentration	
Drugs that may increase serum TBG concentration	Drugs that may decrease serum TBG concentration
Estrogen-containing oral contraceptives Estrogens (oral) Heroin/Methadone 5-Fluorouracil Mitotane Tamoxifen	Androgens/Anabolic steroids Asparaginase Glucocorticoids Slow-release nicotinic acid

Drugs Associated with Thyroid Hormone and/or TSH Level Alterations by Various Mechanisms	
Chloral hydrate Diazepam Ethionamide Lovastatin Metoclopramide 6-Mercaptopurine	Nitroprusside Para-aminosalicylate sodium Perphenazine Resorcinol (excessive topical use) Thiazide diuretics

➤*Drug/Food interactions:* Consumption of certain foods may affect levothyroxine absorption, thereby necessitating adjustments in dosing. Soybean flour (infant formula), cotton seed meal, walnuts, and dietary fiber may bind and decrease the absorption of levothyroxine from the GI tract.

Adverse Reactions

Adverse reactions other than those indicating hyperthyroidism caused by therapeutic overdosage, initially or during the maintenance period, are rare. Symptoms of overdosage include the following:

➤*Cardiovascular:* Palpitations; tachycardia; arrhythmias; angina; cardiac arrest; increased pulse and blood pressure; CHF; MI.

➤*CNS:* Tremors; headache; nervousness; insomnia; hyperactivity; anxiety, irritability; emotional lability; seizures (rare).

➤*GI:* Diarrhea; vomiting; abdominal cramps.

➤*Hypersensitivity:* Allergic skin reactions (rare). Hypersensitivity reactions to inactive ingredients have occurred in patients treated with thyroid hormone products. These include the following: Urticaria, pruritus, skin rash, flushing, angioedema, various GI symptoms (eg, abdominal pain, nausea, vomiting, diarrhea), fever, arthralgia, serum sickness, and wheezing. Hypersensitivity to levothyroxine itself is not known to occur.

➤*Miscellaneous:* Weight loss; fatigue; increased appetite; menstrual irregularities; excessive sweating; heat intolerance; fever; muscle weakness; dyspnea; hair loss; flushing; decreased bone mineral density; impaired fertility; increase in liver function tests.

Pseudotumor cerebri and slipped capital femoral epiphysis have been reported in children receiving levothyroxine therapy. Overtreatment may result in craniosynostosis in infants and premature closure of the epiphyses in children with resultant compromised adult height.

Liothyronine injection only – Hypotension; phlebitis; twitching.

Overdosage

➤*Acute massive overdosage:* Large doses of antithyroid drugs (eg, methimazole, propylthiouracil) followed in 1 to 2 hours by large doses of iodine may be given to inhibit synthesis and release of thyroid hormones. Glucocorticoids may be given to inhibit the conversion of T_4 to T_3. Because T_4 is highly protein bound, very little drug will be removed by dialysis. Treatment is aimed at reducing GI absorption of the drug and counteracting central and peripheral effects, mainly those of increased sympathetic activity. Refer to General Management of Acute Overdosage. Cardiac glycosides may be indicated if CHF develops. Control fever, hypoglycemia, or fluid loss, if needed. Antiadrenergic agents, particularly propranolol (1 to 3 mg IV over 10 minutes or 80 to 160 mg orally per day), have been used to treat increased sympathetic activity.

➤*Symptoms:* Chronic excessive dosage will produce signs and symptoms of hyperthyroidism (eg, headache, irritability, nervousness, tremor, sweating, increased bowel motility, menstrual irregularities). Angina pectoris, arrhythmia, tachycardia, acute MI, or CHF may be induced or aggravated. In addition, confusion and disorientation may occur. Cerebral embolism, shock, coma, and death have been reported. Seizures have occurred in a child ingesting approximately 18 to 20 mg levothyroxine. Symptoms may not necessarily be evident or may not appear until several days after ingestion of levothyroxine sodium. Massive overdosage may result in symptoms resembling thyroid storm.

➤*Treatment:* Reduce dosage or temporarily discontinue therapy. Reinstitute treatment at a lower dosage. In healthy individuals, normal hypothalamic-pituitary-thyroid axis function is restored in 6 to 8 weeks after thyroid suppression.

Patient Information

Replacement therapy is to be taken for life, except in cases of transient hypothyroidism, usually associated with thyroiditis, and in those receiving a trial of the drug.

Take as a single daily dose, preferably at least 30 minutes before breakfast.

➤*Brand interchange:* Inform patients not to change from one brand of this drug to another without consulting their pharmacist or physician. Products manufactured by different companies may not be equally effective.

Inform patients not to discontinue medication except on the advice of a physician.

Instruct patients to notify their physician if the following symptoms occur: Rapid or irregular heartbeat, chest pain, shortness of breath, leg cramps, headache, nervousness, irritability, sleeplessness, tremors, change in appetite, weight gain or loss, vomiting, diarrhea, excessive sweating, heat intolerance, fever, changes in menstrual periods, hives or skin rash, or any other unusual medical event.

Children my experience partial hair loss in the first few months of therapy, but this is usually a transient phenomenon that results in later recovery.

Not for use as primary or adjunctive therapy in a weight-control program.

Advise patients to notify their physician if they become pregnant while taking thyroid hormones; their dose may need to be changed.

THYROID DESICCATED[1]

Rx	**Armour Thyroid** (Forest)	**Tablets:** 15 mg (¼ gr)[2]	Dextrose. (A TC). Lt. tan. In 100s.
Rx	**Armour Thyroid** (Forest)	**Tablets:** 30 mg (½ gr)[2]	Dextrose. (A TD). Lt. tan. In 100s, 1000s, 50,000s and UD 100s.
Rx	**Nature-Throid** (Western Research Laboratories)	**Tablets:** 32.4 mg (½ gr)[2]	In 100s.
Rx	**Westhroid** (Western Research Laboratories)		In 100s.
Rx	**Thyroid USP** (Various, eg, URL)	**Tablets:** 32.5 mg (½ gr)[2]	In 100s and 1000s.
Rx	**Armour Thyroid** (Forest)	**Tablets:** 60 mg (1 gr)[2]	Dextrose. (A TE). Lt. tan. In 100s, 1000s, 5000s, 50,000s, and UD 100s.
Rx	**Nature-Throid** (Western Research Laboratories)	**Tablets:** 64.8 mg (1 gr)[2]	In 100s.
Rx	**Westhroid** (Western Research Laboratories)		In 100s.
Rx	**Thyroid USP** (Various, eg, URL)	**Tablets:** 65 mg (1 gr)[2]	In 100s and 1000s.
Rx	**Armour Thyroid** (Forest)	**Tablets:** 90 mg (1½ gr)[2]	Dextrose. (A TJ). Lt. tan. In 100s.
Rx	**Armour Thyroid** (Forest)	**Tablets:** 120 mg (2 gr)[2]	Dextrose. (A TF). Lt. tan. In 100s, 1000s, 50,000s, and UD 100s.
Rx	**Nature-Throid** (Western Research Laboratories)	**Tablets:** 129.6 mg (2 gr)[2]	In 100s.
Rx	**Westhroid** (Western Research Laboratories)		In 100s.
Rx	**Thyroid USP** (Various, eg, URL)	**Tablets:** 130 mg (2 gr)[2]	In 100s and 1000s.
Rx	**Armour Thyroid** (Forest)	**Tablets:** 180 mg (3 gr)[2]	Dextrose. (A TG). Lt. tan, scored. In 100s and 1000s.
Rx	**Nature-Throid** (Western Research Laboratories)	**Tablets:** 194.4 mg (3 gr)[2]	In 100s.
Rx	**Westhroid** (Western Research Laboratories)		In 100s.
Rx	**Thyroid USP** (Various, eg, URL)	**Tablets:** 195 mg (3 gr)[2]	In 100s and 1000s.
Rx	**Armour Thyroid** (Forest)	**Tablets:** 240 mg (4 gr)[2]	Dextrose. (A TH). Lt. tan. In 100s.
Rx	**Armour Thyroid** (Forest)	**Tablets:** 300 mg (5 gr)[2]	Dextrose. (A TI). Lt. tan, scored. In 100s.

Thyroid Hormones

THYROID DESICCATED[1]

Rx	Bio-Throad (Bio-Tech)	Capsules: 7.5 mg (⅛ gr)[2]	In 100s and 1000s.
		15 mg (¼ gr)[2]	In 100s and 1000s.
		30 mg (½ gr)[2]	In 100s and 1000s.
		60 mg (1 gr)[2]	In 100s and 1000s.
		90 mg (1½ gr)[2]	In 100s and 1000s.
		120 mg (2 gr)[2]	In 100s and 1000s.
		150 mg (2½ gr)[2]	In 100s and 1000s.
		180 mg (3 gr)[2]	In 100s and 1000s.
		240 mg (4 gr)[2]	In 100s and 1000s.

[1] Porcine derived.

[2] The amounts given in grains are according to the respective manufacturers. The exact equivalent is: 1 gr = 64.8 mg.

For complete prescribing information, refer to the Thyroid Drugs group monograph.

WARNING

Drugs with thyroid hormone activity, alone or with other therapeutic agents, have been used for the treatment of obesity. In euthyroid patients, doses within the range of daily hormonal requirements are ineffective for weight reduction. Larger doses may produce serious or even life-threatening manifestations of toxicity, particularly when given in association with sympathomimetic amines such as those used for their anorectic effects.

Indications

►*Hypothyroidism:* As replacement or supplemental therapy in patients with hypothyroidism of any etiology, except transient hypothyroidism during the recovery phase of subacute thyroiditis. This category includes cretinism, myxedema, and ordinary hypothyroidism in patients of any age (children, adults, the elderly), or state (including pregnancy); primary hypothyroidism resulting from functional deficiency, primary atrophy, partial or total absence of thyroid gland, or the effects of surgery, radiation, or drugs, with or without the presence of goiter; and secondary (pituitary) or tertiary (hypothalamic) hypothyroidism.

►*Pituitary thyroid stimulating hormone (TSH) suppression:* As pituitary TSH suppressants in the treatment or prevention of various types of euthyroid goiters, including thyroid nodules, subacute or chronic lymphocytic thyroiditis (Hashimoto), and multinodular goiter and in the management of thyroid cancer.

►*Diagnostic agent:* As diagnostic agents in suppression tests to differentiate suspected mild hyperthyroidism or thyroid gland autonomy.

Administration and Dosage

Thyroid USP is composed of desiccated animal porcine thyroid glands. liothyronine (T_3) is approximately 4 times as potent as levothyroxine (T_4) on a microgram for microgram basis. They provide 38 mcg T_4 and 9 mcg T_3 per grain of thyroid.

The dosage of thyroid hormones is determined by the indication and must in every case be individualized according to patient response and laboratory findings.

►*Hypothyroidism:*
Initial dosage – Institute therapy using low doses, with increments that depend on cardiovascular status. Usual starting dose is 30 mg, with increments of 15 mg every 2 to 3 weeks. Use 15 mg/day in patients with long-standing myxedema, particularly if cardiovascular impairment is suspected. Reduce dosage if angina occurs.

Maintenance dosage – Most patients require 60 to 120 mg/day; failure to respond to 180 mg doses suggests lack of compliance or malabsorption. Adequate therapy usually results in normal TSH and T_4 levels after 2 to 3 weeks of therapy.

Dosage readjustment: Readjust dosage within the first 4 weeks of therapy after proper clinical and laboratory evaluations.

►*Thyroid cancer:* Larger amounts of thyroid hormone than those used for replacement therapy are required.

►*Diagnostic agent:* For adults, the usual suppressive dose of T_4 is 1.56 mcg/kg of body weight per day given for 7 to 10 days. These doses usually yield normal serum T_4 and T_3 levels and lack of response to TSH.

►*Children:* Follow recommendations in the following table. In infants with congenital hypothyroidism, institute therapy with full doses as soon as diagnosis is made.

Recommended Pediatric Dosage for Congenital Hypothyroidism		
Age	Dose per day (mg)	Daily dose per kg (mg)
0 to 6 mo	7.5 to 30	2.4 to 6
6 to 12 mo	30 to 45	3.6 to 4.8
1 to 5 y	45 to 60	3 to 3.6
6 to 12 y	60 to 90	2.4 to 3
> 12 y	> 90	1.2 to 1.8

►*Special populations:* Initiate therapy in low doses (15 to 30 mg) in patients with angina pectoris or the elderly, in whom there is a greater likelihood of occult cardiac disease.

►*Storage/Stability:* Store at controlled room temperature 15° to 30°C (59° to 86°F) in capped bottles or unbroken plastic strip packing. Dispense in tight, light-resistant containers.

LEVOTHYROXINE SODIUM (T_4; L-thyroxine)

Rx	Levothyroxine Sodium (Various, eg, Mylan)	Tablets: 0.025 mg	In 100s.
Rx	Levothroid (Forest)		(25). Orange, caplet shape. In 100s and 1000s.
Rx	Levoxyl (Jones Pharma)		(25). Orange, oval. In 100s and 1000s.
Rx	Synthroid (Abbott)		Sugar, lactose. (SYNTHROID 25). Orange, scored. In 100s and 1000s.
Rx	Thyro-Tabs (Lloyd[1])		(25). Orange, capsule shape. In 100s and 1000s.
Rx	Levothyroxine Sodium (Various, eg, Mylan)	Tablets 0.05 mg	In 100s.
Rx	Levothroid (Forest)		(50). White, caplet shape. In 100s and 1000s.
Rx	Levoxyl (Jones Pharma)		(50). White, oval. In 100s and 1000s.
Rx	Synthroid (Abbott)		Sugar, lactose. (SYNTHROID 50). White, scored. In 100s, 1000s, and UD 100s.
Rx	Thyro-Tabs (Lloyd[1])		(50). White, capsule shape. In 100s and 1000s.
Rx	Levothyroxine Sodium (Various, eg, Mylan)	Tablets: 0.075 mg	In 100s.
Rx	Levothroid (Forest)		(75) Violet, caplet shape. In 100s and 1000s.
Rx	Levoxyl (Jones Pharma)		(75). Purple, oval. In 100s and 1000s.
Rx	Synthroid (Abbott)		Sugar, lactose. (SYNTHROID 75). Violet, scored. In 100s, 1000s, and UD 100s.
Rx	Thyro-Tabs (Lloyd[1])		(75). Violet, capsule shape. In 100s and 1000s.

LEVOTHYROXINE SODIUM (T$_4$; L-thyroxine)

Rx	**Levothyroxine Sodium** (Various, eg, Mylan)	**Tablets:** 0.088 mg	In 100s.
Rx	**Levothroid** (Forest)		(88). Mint green, caplet shape. In 100s and 1000s.
Rx	**Levoxyl** (Jones Pharma)		(88). Olive, oval. In 100s, 1000s, and UD 100s.
Rx	**Synthroid** (Abbott)		Sugar, lactose. (SYNTHROID 88). Olive, scored. In 100s and 1000s.
Rx	**Thyro-Tabs** (Lloyd[1])		(88). Rose, capsule shape. In 100s and 1000s.
Rx	**Unithroid** (Lannett)		Lactose. (JSP 561). Olive, scored. In 100s.
Rx	**Levothyroxine Sodium** (Various, eg, Mylan)	**Tablets:** 0.1 mg	In 100s.
Rx	**Levothroid** (Forest)		(100). Yellow, caplet shape. In 100s and 1000s.
Rx	**Levoxyl** (Jones Pharma)		(100). Yellow, oval. In 100s and 1000s.
Rx	**Synthroid** (Abbott)		Sugar, lactose. (SYNTHROID 100). Yellow, scored. In 100s, 1000s, and UD 100s.
Rx	**Thyro-Tabs** (Lloyd[1])		(100). Yellow, capsule shape. In 100s and 1000s.
Rx	**Levothyroxine Sodium** (Various, eg, Mylan)	**Tablets:** 0.112 mg	In 100s.
Rx	**Levothroid** (Forest)		(112). Rose, caplet shape. In 100s and 1000s.
Rx	**Levoxyl** (Jones Pharma)		(112). Rose, oval. In 100s, 1000s, and UD 100s.
Rx	**Synthroid** (Abbott)		Sugar, lactose. (SYNTHROID 112). Rose, scored. In 100s and 1000s..
Rx	**Thyro-Tabs** (Lloyd[1])		(112). Mint green, capsule shape. In 100s and 1000s.
Rx	**Unithroid** (Lannett)		Lactose. (JSP 562). Rose, scored. In 100s.
Rx	**Levothyroxine Sodium** (Various, eg, Mylan)	**Tablets:** 0.125 mg	In 100s.
Rx	**Levothroid** (Forest)		(125). Brown, caplet shape. In 100s and 1000s.
Rx	**Levoxyl** (Jones Pharma)		(125). Brown, oval. In 100s and 1000s.
Rx	**Synthroid** (Abbott)		Sugar, lactose. (SYNTHROID 125). Brown, scored. In 100s, 1000s, and UD 100s.
Rx	**Thyro-Tabs** (Lloyd[1])		(125). Brown, capsule shape. In 100s and 1000s.
Rx	**Levoxyl** (Jones Pharma)	**Tablets:** 0.137 mg	(137). Dk blue, oval. In 100s, 1000s, and UD 100s.
Rx	**Synthroid** (Abbott)		Sugar, lactose. (SYNTHROID 137). Turquoise, scored. In 100s and 1000s.
Rx	**Levothyroxine Sodium** (Various, eg, Mylan)	**Tablets:** 0.15 mg	In 100s.
Rx	**Levothroid** (Forest)		(150). Blue, caplet shape. In 100s and 1000s.
Rx	**Levoxyl** (Jones Pharma)		(150). Blue, oval. In 100s and 1000s.
Rx	**Synthroid** (Abbott)		Sugar, lactose. (SYNTHROID 150). Blue, scored. In 100s, 1000s, and UD 100s.
Rx	**Thyro-Tabs** (Lloyd[1])		(150). Blue, capsule shape. In 100s and 1000s.
Rx	**Unithroid** (Lannett)		Lactose. (JSP 520). Blue, scored. In 100s.
Rx	**Levothyroxine Sodium** (Various, eg, Mylan)	**Tablets:** 0.175 mg	In 100s.
Rx	**Levothroid** (Forest)		(175). Lilac, caplet shape. In 100s and 1000s.
Rx	**Levoxyl** (Jones Pharma)		(175). Turquoise, oval. In 100s, 1000s, and UD 100s.
Rx	**Synthroid** (Abbott)		Sugar, lactose. (SYNTHROID 175). Lilac, scored. In 100s and 1000s.
Rx	**Thyro-Tabs** (Lloyd[1])		(175). Lilac, capsule shape. In 100s and 1000s.
Rx	**Levothyroxine Sodium** (Various, eg, Mylan)	**Tablets:** 0.2 mg	In 100s.
Rx	**Levothroid** (Forest)		(200). Pink, caplet shape. In 100s and 1000s.
Rx	**Levoxyl** (Jones Pharma)		(200). Pink, oval. In 100s and 1000s.
Rx	**Synthroid** (Abbott)		Sugar, lactose. (SYNTHROID 200). Pink, scored. In 100s, 1000s, and UD 100s.
Rx	**Thyro-Tabs** (Lloyd[1])		(200). Pink, capsule shape. In 100s and 1000s.
Rx	**Levothyroxine Sodium** (Various, eg, Mylan)	**Tablets:** 0.3 mg	In 100s.
Rx	**Levothroid** (Forest)		(300). Green, caplet shape. In 100s and 1000s.
Rx	**Levoxyl** (Jones Pharma)		(300). Green, oval. In 100s, 1000s, and UD 100s.
Rx	**Synthroid** (Abbott)		Sugar, lactose. (SYNTHROID 300). Green, scored. In 100s and 1000s.
Rx	**Thyro-Tabs** (Lloyd[1])		(300). Green, capsule shape. In 100s and 1000s.
Rx	**Unithroid** (Lannett)		Lactose. (JSP 523). Green. In 100s.
Rx	**Levothyroxine Sodium** (Various, eg, Bedford, McGuff)	**Powder for injection, lyophilized:** 200 mcg	In 10 mL vials.
Rx	**Synthroid** (Abbott)		In 10 mL vials.[2]
Rx	**Levothyroxine Sodium** (Various, eg, Bedford, McGuff)	**Powder for injection, lyophilized:** 500 mcg	In 10 mL vials.
Rx	**Synthroid** (Abbott)		In 10 mL vials.[3]

[1] Lloyd, Inc., PO Box 130, Shenandoah, IA 51601; (800) 831-0004.
[2] With 10 mg mannitol and 0.7 mg tribasic sodium phosphate, anhydrous, per vial.
[3] With 1.75 mg tribasic sodium phosphate, anhydrous, per vial.

For complete prescribing information, refer to the Thyroid Hormones group monograph.

Thyroid Hormones

LEVOTHYROXINE SODIUM (T₄; L-thyroxine)

WARNING

Thyroid hormones, alone or with other therapeutic agents, should not be used for the treatment of obesity or for weight loss. In euthyroid patients, doses within the range of daily hormonal requirements are ineffective for weight reduction. Larger doses may produce serious or even life-threatening manifestations of toxicity, particularly when given in association with sympathomimetic amines such as those used for their anorectic effects.

Indications

➤*Hypothyroidism:* As replacement or supplemental therapy in congenital or acquired hypothyroidism of any etiology, except transient hypothyroidism during the recovery phase of subacute thyroiditis. Specific indications include the following: Primary (thyroidal), secondary (pituitary), and tertiary (hypothalamic) hypothyroidism and subclinical hypothyroidism. Primary hypothyroidism may result from functional deficiency, primary atrophy, partial or total congenital absence of the thyroid gland, or from the effects of surgery, radiation, or drugs, with or without the presence of goiter.

The injection can be used IV when rapid repletion is required and IV or IM when the oral route is precluded.

➤*Pituitary thyroid stimulating hormone (TSH) suppression:* For the treatment or prevention of various types of euthyroid goiters, including thyroid nodules, subacute or chronic lymphocytic thyroiditis (Hashimoto), and multinodular goiter and as an adjunct to surgery and radioiodine therapy in the management of thyrotropin-dependent well-differentiated thyroid cancer.

Administration and Dosage

Optimal dosage is determined by patient's clinical response and laboratory findings. Take levothyroxine in the morning on an empty stomach, at least 30 minutes before any food is eaten. Take levothyroxine at least 4 hours apart from drugs that are known to interfere with its absorption.

➤*Dosage equivalence:* Approximately 50 to 60 mcg (range, 50 to 100 mcg) of levothyroxine equals approximately 60 to 65 mg (1 grain) of thyroid dessicated.

➤*Bioavailability:* Bioequivalence problems have been documented in the past for levothyroxine products marketed by different manufacturers. Brand interchange is not recommended unless comparative bioavailability data, which provide evidence of therapeutic equivalence, are available. If patients are switched from one product to another, reassess measures of thyroid function and retitrate the levothyroxine dose as necessary.

➤*Hypothyroidism in adults and children in whom growth and puberty are complete:* Therapy may begin at full replacement doses in otherwise healthy individuals younger than 50 years of age and in those older than 50 years of age who have been recently treated for hyperthyroidism or who have been hypothyroid for only a short time (eg, a few months). The average full replacement dose of levothyroxine is approximately 1.7 mcg/kg/day (eg, 100 to 125 mcg/day for a 70 kg adult). Older patients may require less than 1 mcg/kg/day. Levothyroxine sodium doses greater than than 200 mcg/day are seldom required. An inadequate response to daily doses of 300 mcg/day or more is rare and may indicate poor compliance, malabsorption, and/or drug interactions.

For most patients older than 50 years of age or for patients younger than 50 years of age with underlying cardiac disease, an initial starting dose of 25 to 50 mcg/day of levothyroxine is recommended, with gradual increments in dose at 6- to 8-week intervals, as needed. The recommended starting dose of levothyroxine sodium in elderly patients with cardiac disease is 12.5 to 25 mcg/day, with gradual dose increments at 4- to 6-week intervals.

Dosage adjustment – The levothyroxine dose generally is adjusted in 12.5 to 25 mcg increments until the patient with primary hypothyroidism is clinically euthyroid and the serum TSH has normalized.

➤*Severe hypothyroidism:* In patients with severe hypothyroidism, the recommended initial levothyroxine dose is 12.5 to 25 mcg/day with increases of 25 mcg/day every 2 to 4 weeks, accompanied by clinical and laboratory assessment, until the TSH level is normalized.

IV or IM – IV or IM injection can be substituted for the oral dosage form when oral ingestion is precluded for long periods of time. The initial parenteral dosage should be approximately one-half of the previously established oral dosage. A daily maintenance dose of 50 to 100 mcg parenterally should suffice to maintain the euthyroid state once established. Close observation of the patient, with individual adjustment of the dosage as needed, is recommended.

➤*Subclinical hypothyroidism:* If this condition is treated, a lower levothyroxine dose (eg, 1 mcg/kg/day) than that used for full replacement may be adequate to normalize the serum TSH level. Patients who are not treated should be monitored yearly for changes in clinical status and thyroid laboratory parameters.

➤*Myxedema coma:* Myxedema coma is a life-threatening emergency characterized by poor circulation and hypometabolism and may result in unpredictable absorption of levothyroxine from the GI tract. Therefore, oral thyroid hormone drug products are not recommended to treat this condition; administer thyroid hormone products formulated for IV. Sudden administration of large doses is not without cardiovascular risks; therefore, do not undertake IV therapy without weighing alternative risks. Clinical judgment may dictate smaller doses.

In myxedema coma or stupor, without concomitant severe heart disease, 200 to 500 mcg of levothyroxine for injection may be administered IV as a solution containing 100 mcg/mL. Do not add to other IV fluids. Although the patient may show evidence of increased responsivity within 6 to 8 hours, full therapeutic effect may not be evident until the following day. An additional 100 to 300 mcg or more may be given on the second day if evidence of significant and progressive improvements has not occurred. Levothyroxine for injection produces a predictable increase in the reservoir level of hormone with a 7-day half-life. This usually precludes the need for multiple injections but maintain continued daily administration of lesser amounts parenterally until the patient is fully capable of accepting a daily oral dose.

➤*TSH suppression in well-differentiated thyroid cancer and thyroid nodules:* The target level for TSH suppression in these conditions has not been established in controlled studies. In addition, the efficacy of TSH suppression for benign nodular disease is controversial. Therefore, individualize the dose of levothyroxine used for TSH suppression based on the specific disease and the patient being treated.

In the treatment of well-differentiated (papillary and follicular) thyroid cancer, levothyroxine is used as an adjunct to surgery and radioiodine therapy. Generally, TSH is suppressed to less than 0.1 mU/L, and this usually requires a levothyroxine dose of greater than 2 mcg/kg/day. However, in patients with high-risk tumors, the target level for TSH suppression may be less than 0.01 mU/L.

In the treatment of benign nodules and nontoxic multinodular goiter, TSH generally is suppressed to a higher target (eg, 0.1 to 0.5 or 1 mU/L) than that used for the treatment of thyroid cancer. Levothyroxine is contraindicated if the serum TSH already is suppressed because of the risk of precipitating overt thyrotoxicosis.

➤*Special populations:* Exercise caution when administering levothyroxine to patients with underlying cardiovascular disease, to the elderly, and to those with concomitant adrenal insufficiency.

➤*Children:* Follow the recommendations in the following table. In infants with congenital or acquired hypothyroidism, institute therapy with full doses as soon as diagnosis is made.

Levothyroxine tablets may be given to infants and children who cannot swallow intact tablets. Crush the proper dose tablet and suspend in a small amount (5 to 10 mL) of water. The suspension can be given by spoon or dropper. Do not store the suspension for any period of time. Do not use foods that decrease absorption of levothyroxine, such as soybean infant formula, for administering levothyroxine sodium tablets.

Infants and children – Levothyroxine therapy usually is initiated at full replacement doses, with the recommended dose per body weight decreasing with age (see table). However, in children with chronic or severe hypothyroidism, an initial 25 mcg/day dose of levothyroxine is recommended with increments of 25 mcg every 2 to 4 weeks until the desired effect is achieved.

Hyperactivity in an older child can be minimized if the starting dose is one-fourth of the recommended full replacement dose and the dose is then increased on a weekly basis by an amount equal to one-fourth of the full-recommended replacement dose until the full recommended replacement dose is reached.

Newborns – The recommended starting dose is 10 to 15 mcg/kg/day. Consider a lower starting dose (eg, 25 mcg/day) in infants at risk for cardiac failure; the dose should be increased in 4 to 6 weeks as needed based on clinical and laboratory response to treatment. In infants with very low (less than 5 mcg/dL) or undetectable serum T₄ concentrations, the recommended initial starting dose is 50 mcg/day of levothyroxine.

| Recommended Pediatric Dosage for Congenital Hypothyroidism ||
Age	Daily dose per kg (mcg)[1]
0 to 3 mo	10 to 15
3 to 6 mo	8 to 10
6 to 12 mo	6 to 8
1 to 5 y	5 to 6
6 to 12 y	4 to 5
> 12 y (growth/puberty incomplete)	2 to 3
> 12 y (growth/puberty complete)	1.7

[1] The dose should be adjusted based on clinical response and laboratory parameters.

➤*Preparation of injectable solution:* Reconstitute by adding 5 mL 0.9% sodium chloride injection (final volume approximately 5 mL). Shake the vial to ensure complete mixing. Use immediately after reconstitution. Do not add to other IV fluids. Discard any unused portion.

➤*Storage/Stability:* Store at 25° (77°F); excursions permitted to 15° to 30°C (59° to 86°F). Protect from light and moisture.

LIOTHYRONINE SODIUM (T$_3$)

Rx	**Cytomel** (Monarch)	**Tablets:** 5 mcg	Sucrose. (JMI D14). White. In 100s.
		25 mcg	Sucrose. (JMI D16). White, scored. In 100s.
		50 mcg	Sucrose. (JMI D17). White, scored. In 100s.
Rx	**Triostat** (Monarch)	**Injection:** 10 mcg/mL	In 1 mL vials.[1]

[1] With 6.8% alcohol, 2.19 mg ammonia (as ammonium hydroxide) per mL.

For complete prescribing information, refer to the Thyroid Hormones group monograph.

WARNING

Drugs with thyroid hormone activity, alone or with other therapeutic agents, have been used for the treatment of obesity. In euthyroid patients, doses within the range of daily hormonal requirements are ineffective for weight reduction. Larger doses may produce serious or even life-threatening manifestations of toxicity, particularly when given in association with sympathomimetic amines such as those used for their anorectic effects.

Indications

➤*Oral:*

Hypothyroidism – As replacement or supplemental therapy in patients with hypothyroidism of any etiology, except transient hypothyroidism during the recovery phase of subacute thyroiditis. This category includes cretinism, myxedema, and ordinary hypothyroidism in patients of any age (children, adults, the elderly), or state (including pregnancy); primary hypothyroidism resulting from functional deficiency, primary atrophy, partial or total absence of thyroid gland, or the effects of surgery, radiation, or drugs, with or without the presence of goiter; and secondary (pituitary), or tertiary (hypothalamic) hypothyroidism.

Pituitary thyroid stimulating hormone (TSH) suppressant – As pituitary TSH suppressants in the treatment or prevention of various types of euthyroid goiters, including thyroid nodules, subacute or chronic lymphocytic thyroiditis (Hashimoto), and multinodular goiter.

Diagnostic agent – As diagnostic agents in suppression tests to differentiate suspected mild hyperthyroidism or thyroid gland autonomy.

➤*IV:*

Myxedema coma/precoma – For the treatment of myxedema coma/precoma.

Administration and Dosage

Liothyronine sodium is a synthetic form of the natural thyroid hormone T$_3$. It has a short duration of activity that permits quick dosage adjustment and facilitates control of overdosage. It can be used in patients allergic to desiccated thyroid or thyroid extract derived from pork or beef.

➤*Dosage equivalents:* Approximately 25 mcg (range, 15 to 37.5 mcg) equals approximately 60 to 65 mg (1 grain) of desiccated thyroid.

Administer cautiously to patients in whom there is a strong suspicion of thyroid gland autonomy; exogenous hormone effects will be additive to the endogenous source.

➤*Oral:*

Mild hypothyroidism – Starting dose is 25 mcg/day. Daily dosage may then be increased by up to 25 mcg every 1 or 2 weeks. Usual maintenance dose is 25 to 75 mcg/day.

Congenital hypothyroidism – Starting dose is 5 mcg/day, with a 5 mcg increment every 3 to 4 days until the desired response is achieved. Infants a few months of age may require only 20 mcg/day for maintenance. At 1 year of age, 50 mcg/day may be required. Above 3 years of age, full adult dosage may be necessary.

Simple (nontoxic) goiter – Starting dose is 5 mcg/day. Dosage may be increased by 5 or 10 mcg/day every 1 to 2 weeks. When 25 mcg/day is reached, dosage may be increased every 1 to 2 weeks by 12.5 or 25 mcg. Usual maintenance dosage is 75 mcg/day.

Thyroid suppression therapy – 75 to 100 mcg/day for 7 days; radioactive iodine uptake is determined before and after administration of the hormone. A 50% or greater suppression of uptake indicates a normal thyroid-pituitary axis and thus rules out thyroid gland autonomy.

Myxedema – Starting dose is 5 mcg/day. This may be increased by 5 to 10 mcg/day every 1 to 2 weeks until a satisfactory therapeutic response is attained. When 25 mcg/day is reached, dosage may be increased by 5 to 25 mcg every 1 or 2 weeks. Usual maintenance dose is 50 to 100 mcg/day.

➤*IV:*

Myxedema coma/precoma – Myxedema coma, usually precipitated in the hypothyroid patient of long standing by intercurrent illness or drugs such as sedatives and anesthetics, is a medical emergency. Direct therapy at the correction of electrolyte disturbances, possible infection, or other intercurrent illness in addition to IV liothyronine administration. Simultaneous glucocorticosteroids are required.

Liothyronine injection is for IV use only; do not give IM or SC. Prompt administration of an adequate dose is important in determining clinical outcome. Base initial and subsequent doses on continuous monitoring of patient's clinical status and response. Give doses at least 4 hours, and not more than 12 hours, apart. Giving at least 65 mcg/day initially is associated with lower mortality. There is limited clinical experience with exceeding 100 mcg/day.

An initial IV dose ranging from 25 to 50 mcg is recommended in the emergency treatment of myxedema coma/precoma in adults. In patients with known or suspected cardiovascular disease, an initial dose of 10 to 20 mcg is suggested. However, base doses on continuous monitoring of the condition and response to therapy. Exercise caution in adjusting the dose because of potentially large changes to precipitate adverse cardiovascular events.

A single dose of liothyronine administered IV produces a detectable metabolic response in as little as 2 to 4 hours and a maximum therapeutic response within 2 days.

Concomitant use of *Triostat* and artificial rewarming of patients is contraindicated. It has been reported that the administration of liothyronine sodium will restore a normal body temperature in 24 to 48 hours if heat loss is prevented by keeping the patient covered with blankets in a warm room.

Switching to oral therapy: Resume oral therapy as soon as the clinical situation has been stabilized and the patient is able to take oral medication. When switching to tablets, discontinue injection, initiate oral therapy at a low dosage, and increase gradually according to response. If oral levothyroxine is used, keep in mind that there is a delay of several days in the onset of action; discontinue IV therapy gradually.

➤*Special populations:* Use with great caution in patients with angina pectoris, the elderly (in whom there is a greater likelihood of occult cardiac disease), or children. There is limited experience with liothyronine injection in the pediatric population; safety and efficacy have not been established. Initiate therapy at low doses with due consideration for its relatively rapid onset of action. Start oral therapy with 5 mcg/day; increase only by 5 mcg increments at 2-week intervals.

In patients with known or suspected cardiovascular disease, the extremely rapid onset of action of liothyronine injection may warrant initiating therapy at a dose of 10 to 20 mcg.

➤*Exchange therapy:* When switching a patient to liothyronine from thyroid levothyroxine or thyroglobulin, discontinue the other medication, initiate liothyronine at a low dosage, and increase gradually according to the patient's response. When selecting a starting dosage, keep in mind that liothyronine has a rapid onset of action and that residual effects of the other thyroid preparation may persist for the first several weeks of therapy.

➤*Storage/Stability:*

Tablets – Store between 15° and 30°C (59° to 86°F).

Injection – Store between 2° and 8°C (36° to 46°F).

Thyroid Hormones

LIOTRIX

	Product and distributor	Tablet strength (grain)	Content (mcg)[1]		Thyroid equivalent (mg)	How supplied
			T$_3$	T$_4$		
Rx	**Thyrolar** (Forest)	¼	3.1	12.5	15	Lactose. (YC). Violet/White. Two-layered. In 100s.
		½	6.25	25	30	Lactose. (YD). Peach/White. Two-layered. In 100s.
		1	12.5	50	60	Lactose. (YE). Pink/White. Two-layered. In 100s.
		2	25	100	120	Lactose. (YF). Green/White. Two-layered. In 100s.
		3	37.5	150	180	Lactose. (YH). Yellow/White. Two-layered. In 100s.

[1] Liothyronine sodium (T$_3$) is approximately 4 times as potent as levothyroxine (T$_4$) on a microgram-for-microgram basis.

For complete prescribing information, refer to the Thyroid Hormones group monograph.

WARNING

Drugs with thyroid hormone activity, alone or with other therapeutic agents have been used for the treatment of obesity. In euthyroid patients, doses within the range of daily hormonal requirements are ineffective for weight reduction. Larger doses may produce serious or even life-threatening manifestations of toxicity, particularly when given in association with sympathomimetic amines such as those used for their anorectic effects.

Indications

►*Hypothyroidism:* As replacement or supplemental therapy in patients with hypothyroidism of any etiology, except transient hypothyroidism during the recovery phase of subacute thyroiditis. This category includes cretinism, myxedema, and ordinary hypothyroidism in patients of any age (children, adults, the elderly), or state (including pregnancy); primary hypothyroidism resulting from functional deficiency, primary atrophy, partial or total absence of thyroid gland, or the effects of surgery, radiation, or drugs, with or without the presence of goiter; and secondary (pituitary) or tertiary (hypothalamic) hypothyroidism.

►*Pituitary thyroid stimulating hormone (TSH) suppression:* As pituitary TSH suppressants in the treatment or prevention of various types of euthyroid goiters, including thyroid nodules, subacute or chronic lymphocytic thyroiditis (Hashimoto), and multinodular goiter and in the management of thyroid cancer.

►*Diagnostic agent:* As diagnostic agents in suppression tests to differentiate suspected mild hyperthyroidism or thyroid gland autonomy.

Administration and Dosage

►*Dosage equivalents:* Each 60 mg liotrix tablet will usually replace approximately 60 to 65 mg (1 grain) of desiccated thyroid.

Optimal dosage is determined by patient's clinical response and laboratory findings.

►*Hypothyroidism:*

Initial dosage – Institute therapy using low doses, with increments that depend on cardiovascular status. Usual starting dose is 1 tablet of *Thyrolar ½* with increments of 1 tablet of *Thyrolar ¼* every 2 to 3 weeks. A lower starting dose, 1 tablet/day *Thyrolar ¼* is recommended in patients with long-standing myxedema, particularly if cardiovascular impairment is suspected, in which case extreme caution is recommended. Reduce dosage if angina occurs.

Maintenance dosage – Most patients require 1 tablet *Thyrolar 1* to 1 tablet *Thyrolar 2* per day; failure to respond to 1 tablet *Thyrolar 3* suggests lack of compliance or malabsorption. Maintenance dosages of 1 tablet *Thyrolar 1* to 1 tablet of *Thyrolar 2* per day usually result in normal serum levothyroxine and triiodothyronine levels. Adequate therapy usually results in normal TSH and T$_4$ levels after 2 to 3 weeks of therapy.

Dosage readjustment: Readjust dosage within the first 4 weeks of therapy after proper clinical and laboratory evaluations including serum levels of T$_4$ bound and free, and TSH.

►*Thyroid cancer:* Larger amounts of thyroid hormone than those used for replacement therapy are required. Medullary carcinoma of the thyroid usually is unresponsive to this therapy.

►*Diagnostic agent:* For adults, the usual suppressive dose of T$_4$ is 1.56 mcg/kg of body weight per day given for 7 to 10 days. These doses usually yield normal serum T$_4$ and T$_3$ levels and lack of response to TSH.

►*Children:* Follow recommendations in the following table. In infants with congenital hypothyroidism, institute therapy with full doses as soon as diagnosis is made.

Recommended Pediatric Dosage for Congenital Hypothyroidism			
	Dose per day in mcg		
Age	T$_3$/T$_4$	to	T$_3$/T$_4$
0 to 6 mo	3.1/12.5	to	6.25/25
6 to 12 mo	6.25/25	to	9.35/37.5
1 to 5 y	9.35/37.5	to	12.5/50
6 to 12 y	12.5/50	to	18.75/75
Over 12 y			> 18.75/75

►*Special populations:* In patients with angina pectoris or the elderly, in whom there is a greater likelihood of occult cardiac disease, initiate therapy with low doses (1 tablet of *Thyrolar ¼* or *Thyrolar ½*).

►*Storage/Stability:* Store at cold temperature between 2° to 8°C (36° to 46°F) in a tight, light-resistant container.

IODINE PRODUCTS

Rx	**Strong Iodine Solution (Lugol's Solution)** (Various, eg, Lannett)	**Solution:** 5% iodine and 10% potassium iodide	In 120 ml, pt and gal.

Indications

Used adjunctively with an antithyroid drug in hyperthyroid patients in preparation for thyroidectomy and to treat thyrotoxic crisis or neonatal thyrotoxicosis.

Thyroid blocking in a radiation emergency.

For use of potassium iodide as an expectorant and for other respiratory tract conditions, see the Iodine Products monograph in the Expectorant section of the Respiratories chapter.

➤*Unlabeled uses:* Potassium iodide (60 mg 3 times daily) has been used effectively in a limited number of patients for Sweet's syndrome (acute febrile neutrophilic dermatosis) in combination with a potent topical steroid, as an alternative to systemic corticosteroids.

Also effective for the treatment of lymphocutaneous sporotrichosis (a dimorphic fungus that typically infects the skin and lymphatic system).

Administration and Dosage

➤*Recommended dietary allowances (RDAs):* The RDA for iodine is 150 mcg for adults.

To prepare hyperthyroid patients for thyroidectomy, administer 2 to 6 drops strong iodine solution 3 times daily for 10 days prior to surgery.

➤*For thyroid blocking in a radiation emergency:* Use only as directed by state or local public health authorities in the event of a radiation emergency. Take for 10 days unless directed otherwise by state or local public health authorities.

Adults and children (> 1 year) – One tablet (130 mg) daily (crush tablets for small children).

Infants (< 1 year) – ½ crushed tablet (65 mg) daily.

Actions

➤*Pharmacology:* An adequate intake of iodine is necessary for normal thyroid function and the synthesis of thyroid hormones.

Elemental iodine (from the diet or as medication) is reduced in the GI tract and enters the circulation in the form of iodide, which is actively transported and concentrated by the thyroid gland. Hormone synthesis requires the oxidation of iodide and iodination of tyrosyl residues in thyroglobulin to form iodotyrosine precursors. These precursors undergo a "coupling reaction" to yield the active thyroid hormones T_3 and T_4. High concentrations of iodide greatly influence iodine metabolism by the thyroid gland. Large doses of iodides can inhibit T_4 and T_3 synthesis and rapidly inhibit proteolysis of colloid and the release of T_4 and T_3 into the bloodstream.

The effects of iodides are evident within 24 hours; maximum effects are attained after 10 to 15 days of continuous therapy. If administered chronically, therapeutic effects may persist for up to 6 weeks after the crisis has abated.

Contraindications

Hypersensitivity to iodides.

Warnings

➤*Pregnancy: Category D* (potassium iodide). Iodides readily cross the placenta and may cause hypothyroidism and goiter in the fetus or newborn when used long-term or close to term; short-term use (eg, 10 days) may not carry this risk. Administer to pregnant women only if clearly needed.

➤*Lactation:* Iodide is excreted in breast milk; however, the significance to the infant is not known. According to the American Academy of Pediatrics, these agents are not contraindicated in breastfeeding.

Drug Interactions

➤*Lithium carbonate:* Lithium carbonate and iodide preparations may have synergistic hypothyroid activity; concomitant use may result in hypothyroidism.

Adverse Reactions

Possible side effects of potassium iodide include: Skin rashes; swelling of the salivary glands; "iodism" (metallic taste, burning mouth and throat, sore teeth and gums, symptoms of a head cold and sometimes stomach upset and diarrhea); allergic reactions (ie, fever and joint pains, swelling of parts of the face and body and, at times, severe shortness of breath requiring immediate medical attention). Overactivity or underactivity of the thyroid gland or enlargement of the thyroid gland (goiter) may occur rarely.

Overdosage

➤*Acute poisoning:*

Symptoms – Iodine is corrosive, and toxic symptoms are mainly the result of local GI tract irritation. Gastroenteritis, abdominal pain and diarrhea (sometimes bloody) may be seen. Fatalities may occur from circulatory collapse due to shock, corrosive gastritis or asphyxiation from swelling of the glottis or larynx.

Treatment – Gastric lavage with a soluble starch solution (15 g cornstarch or flour in 500 ml water) is recommended for removing iodine from the stomach. A 1% oral solution of sodium thiosulfate is a specific antidote, as it will reduce iodine to iodide. Milk may help relieve gastric irritation. Correct fluid and electrolyte imbalance, and treat shock if necessary.

➤*Chronic poisoning:* Discontinue use of iodine or iodides. High sodium chloride intake will speed recovery. For iodism characterized by skin or mucous membrane reactions, give cortisone or equivalent corticosteroid 25 to 100 mg every 6 hours orally until symptoms abate.

Patient Information

➤*Strong iodine solution:* Dilute with water or fruit juice to improve taste.

Discontinue use and notify physician if fever, skin rash, metallic taste, swelling of the throat, burning of the mouth and throat, sore gums and teeth, head cold symptoms, severe GI distress or enlargement of the thyroid gland (goiter) occurs.

Antithyroid Agents

Indications

►*Hyperthyroidism:* Long-term therapy may lead to disease remission. Also used to ameliorate hyperthyroidism in preparation for subtotal thyroidectomy or radioactive iodine therapy.

Propylthiouracil (PTU) is also used when thyroidectomy is contraindicated or not advisable.

►*Unlabeled uses:* PTU (300 mg/day) may be useful in reducing the mortality due to alcoholic liver disease by reducing the hepatic hypermetabolic state induced by alcohol.

Administration and Dosage

In one study, the rate of remission and time to relapse of Grave's disease was significantly increased when antithyroid therapy was given for a prolonged duration (18 months) vs short-term (6 month) treatment. However, the monitoring of thyroid-stimulating antibody values may be a useful guide for shortening the duration of treatment in some patients.

One small study reported that single and divided daily doses of methimazole were equally effective in hyperthyroid patients. Traditionally administered in divided doses, it was suggested that a single daily dose would be effective since methimazole is present in the thyroid for 20 hours and is active for 40 hours despite a serum half-life of 6 to 13 hours. Further study is needed.

Actions

►*Pharmacology:* PTU and methimazole inhibit the synthesis of thyroid hormones and, thus, are effective in the treatment of hyperthyroidism. They do not inactivate existing thyroxine (T_4) and triiodothyronine (T_3) which are stored in the thyroid or which circulate in the blood, nor do they interfere with the effectiveness of exogenous thyroid hormones. PTU partially inhibits the peripheral conversion of T_4 to T_3.

Both drugs are concentrated in the thyroid gland. Pharmacokinetic data are summarized in the following table:

Various Pharmacokinetic Parameters of Antithyroid Agents						
Antithyroid agent	Bioavailability (%)	Protein binding (%)	Transplacental passage	Breast milk levels (M:P)[1]	Half-life(hrs)	Excreted in urine (%)
Propylthiouracil	80-95	75-80	Low	Low (0.1)	1-2	< 35
Methimazole	80-95	0	High	High (1)	6-13	< 10

[1] Approximate milk:plasma ratio.

Contraindications

Hypersensitivity to antithyroid drugs; nursing mothers (see Warnings).

Warnings

►*Agranulocytosis:* Agranulocytosis is potentially the most serious side effect of therapy. Instruct patients to report any symptoms of agranulocytosis, such as hay fever, sore throat, skin eruptions, fever, headache or general malaise. In such cases, white blood cell and differential counts should be made to determine whether agranulocytosis has developed. Exercise particular care with patients receiving additional drugs known to cause agranulocytosis. Leukopenia, thrombocytopenia and aplastic anemia (pancytopenia) may also occur. Discontinue the drug in the presence of agranulocytosis, aplastic anemia, hepatitis, fever or exfoliative dermatitis. Monitor the patient's bone marrow function.

One report recommends routine monitoring of the WBC count for at least the first 3 months of therapy, thereby potentially detecting agranulocytosis prior to becoming evident by infection.

►*Carcinogenesis:* Laboratory animals treated with PTU for > 1 year have demonstrated thyroid hyperplasia and carcinoma formation. Such animal findings are seen with continuous suppression of thyroid function by sufficient doses of a variety of antithyroid agents, as well as in dietary iodine deficiency, subtotal thyroidectomy, and implantation of autonomous thyrotropic hormone-secreting pituitary tumors. Pituitary adenomas have also been described.

►*Pregnancy: Category D.* These agents, used judiciously, are effective drugs in hyperthyroidism complicated by pregnancy. Because they readily cross the placenta and can induce goiter and even cretinism in the developing fetus, it is important that a sufficient, but not excessive, dose be given. In many pregnant women, the thyroid dysfunction diminishes as the pregnancy proceeds, thus making a reduction of dose possible. In some instances, these products can be withdrawn 2 or 3 weeks before delivery. PTU can cause fetal harm when administered to a pregnant woman. Approximately 10% will develop neonatal goiter. However, if an antithyroid agent is needed, PTU is preferred because it is less likely than methimazole to cross the placenta and induce fetal/neonatal complications (eg, aplasia cutis).

►*Lactation:* Postpartum patients receiving antithyroid preparations should not nurse their babies. However, if necessary, the preferred drug is PTU.

►*Children:* In several case reports, PTU hepatotoxicity has occurred in pediatric patients. Discontinue the drug immediately if signs and symptoms of hepatic dysfunction develop.

Precautions

►*Monitoring:* Monitor thyroid function tests periodically during therapy. Once clinical evidence of hyperthyroidism has resolved, the finding of an elevated serum TSH indicates that a lower maintenance dose of PTU should be used.

►*Hemorrhagic effects:* Because PTU may cause hypoprothrombinemia and bleeding, monitor prothrombin time during therapy, especially before surgical procedures.

Drug Interactions

►*Anticoagulants:* The activity of oral anticoagulants may be potentiated by the anti-vitamin K activity attributed to PTU.

Adverse Reactions

Adverse reactions probably occur in < 1% of patients.

Agranulocytosis is the most serious effect.

►*CNS:* Paresthesias; neuritis; headache; vertigo; drowsiness; neuropathies; CNS stimulation; depression.

►*Dermatologic:* Skin rash; urticaria; pruritus; erythema nodosum; skin pigmentation; exfoliative dermatitis; lupus-like syndrome, including splenomegaly, hepatitis, periarteritis and hypoprothrombinemia and bleeding.

►*GI:* Nausea and vomiting; epigastric distress; loss of taste; sialadenophathy.

►*Hematologic:* Inhibition of myelopoiesis (agranulocytosis, granulocytopenia and thrombocytopenia); aplastic anemia; hypoprothrombinemia; periarteritis. About 10% of patients with untreated hyperthyroidism have leukopenia (WBC count < 4000 per mm^3), often with relative granulocytopenia.

►*Hepatic:* Jaundice (which may persist for several weeks after discontinuance); hepatitis.

►*Renal:* Nephritis.

►*Miscellaneous:* Abnormal hair loss; arthralgia; myalgia; edema; lymphadenopathy; drug fever; interstitial pneumonitis insulin autoimmune syndrome (may result in hypoglycemic coma).

Overdosage

►*Symptoms:* Nausea; vomiting; epigastric distress; headache; fever; arthralgia; pruritus; edema; pancytopenia. Agranulocytosis is the most serious effect. Rarely, exfoliative dermatitis, hepatitis, neuropathies or CNS stimulation or depression may occur.

►*Treatment:* Protect the patient's airway and support ventilation and perfusion. Meticulously monitor and maintain, within acceptable limits, the patient's vital signs, blood gases, serum electrolytes, etc. Monitor the patient's bone marrow function. Refer to General Management of Acute Overdosage.

Forced diuresis, peritoneal dialysis, hemodialysis or charcoal hemoperfusion have not been established as beneficial for an overdose of propylthiouracil.

Patient Information

Take at regular intervals around the clock (usually every 8 hours), unless directed otherwise by physician.

Notify physician if fever, sore throat, unusual bleeding or bruising, headache, rash, yellowing of the skin or vomiting occurs.

PROPYLTHIOURACIL (PTU)

Rx	Propylthiouracil (Various, eg, Dixon-Shane, Rugby)	**Tablets:** 50 mg	In 100s and 1000s.

For complete prescribing information, refer to the Antithyroid Agents group monograph.

Administration and Dosage

Usually administered in 3 equal doses at ≈ 8 hour intervals.

►*Adults:*

Initial – 300 mg/day. In patients with severe hyperthyroidism, very large goiters, or both, the initial dosage is usually 400 mg/day; an occasional patient will require 600 to 900 mg/day initially.

Maintenance – Usually, 100 to 150 mg daily.

►*Children:*

6 to 10 years – Initial dose is 50 to 150 mg/day.

≥ 10 years – Initial dose is 150 to 300 mg/day.

PROPYLTHIOURACIL (PTU)

Maintenance – Determined by patient response.

Another suggested dosage for children is as follows:

➤*Initial:* 5 to 7 mg/kg/day or 150 to 200 mg/m²/day in divided doses every 8 hours.

➤*Maintenance:* ⅓ to ⅔ the initial dose beginning when the patient is euthyroid.

METHIMAZOLE

Rx	Methimazole (Par Pharm)	Tablets: 5 mg	Lactose. (EM/5). White to off-white. In 100s.
Rx	Tapazole (Lilly)		(Lilly J94). White, scored. In 100s.
Rx	Methimazole (Par Pharm)	10 mg	Lactose. (EM/10). White to off-white. In 100s.
Rx	Tapazole (Lilly)		(Lilly J95). White, scored. In 100s.

For complete prescribing information, refer to the Antithyroid Agents group monograph.

Administration and Dosage

Usually administered in 3 equal doses at ≈ 8 hour intervals.

➤*Adults:*

Initial – 15 mg daily for mild hyperthyroidism, 30 to 40 mg/day for moderately severe hyperthyroidism and 60 mg/day for severe hyperthyroidism.

Maintenance – 5 to 15 mg/day.

➤*Children:*

Initial – 0.4 mg/kg daily.

Maintenance – Approximately one-half the initial dose.

Another suggested dosage for children is as follows:

➤*Initial:* 0.5 to 0.7 mg/kg/day or 15 to 20 mg/m²/day in 3 divided doses.

➤*Maintenance:* ⅓ to ⅔ of initial dose beginning when the patient is euthyroid.

➤*Maximum:* 30 mg/24 hours.

SODIUM IODIDE I 131

Rx	Iodotope (Squibb Diagnostics)	Capsules: Radioactivity range is 8, 15, 30, 50 or 100 mCi per capsule at time of calibration	Blue/buff. In 5s, 10s,15s and 20s.
		Oral Solution:¹ Radioactivity concentration of 7.05 mCi per ml at time of calibration	In vials containing approximately 7, 14, 28, 70 or 106 mCi at time of calibration.
Rx	Sodium Iodide I 131 Therapeutic (Mallinckrodt)	Capsules: Radioactivity range is 0.75 to 100 mCi per capsule.	
		Oral Solution: Radioactivity range is 3.5 to 150 mCi per vial.	

¹ With 1 mg EDTA per ml.

Indications

Treatment of hyperthyroidism and selected cases of thyroid carcinoma. Palliative effects may be seen in patients with papillary or follicular carcinoma of the thyroid. Thyrotropin may effect stimulation of radio-iodide uptake. (Radioiodide will not be taken up by giant cell and spindle cell carcinoma of the thyroid or by amyloid solid carcinomas.)

Administration and Dosage

Measure the dose by a radioactivity calibration system just prior to administration. Consult product literature for specific calibration and dosimetry information.

➤*Hyperthyroidism:* The total amount needed to achieve a clinical remission without destruction of the entire thyroid varies widely; the usual dose range is 4 to 10 millicuries (mCi). Toxic nodular goiter and other special situations will require larger doses.

➤*Thyroid carcinoma:* Individualize dosage. The usual dose for ablation of normal thyroid tissue is 50 mCi, with subsequent therapeutic doses usually 100 to 150 mCi.

➤*Preparation of oral solution:* To prepare stock solution, dilute oral solution with Purified Water, USP containing 0.2% sodium thiosulfate as a reducing agent. Acidic diluents may cause a pH drop below 7.5 and may stimulate volatilization of iodine 131-hydriodic acid.

Actions

➤*Pharmacokinetics:* Sodium iodide I 131 is readily absorbed from the GI tract. Following absorption, the iodide is primarily distributed within the extracellular fluid of the body. It is trapped and rapidly converted to protein-bound iodine by the thyroid; it is concentrated, but not protein-bound, by the stomach and salivary glands. It is promptly excreted by the kidneys. About 90% of the local irradiation is caused by beta radiation and 10% by gamma radiation.

Iodine 131 decays by beta and gamma emissions with a physical half-life of 8.04 days. Following oral administration, about 40% of the activity has an effective half-life of 0.34 days and 60% has an effective half-life of 7.61 days. Consult product literature for specific calibration and dosimetry information.

Contraindications

Preexisting vomiting and diarrhea; pregnancy (see Warnings).

Warnings

➤*Patients < 30 years old:* Sodium iodide I 131 is not usually used for the treatment of hyperthyroidism in patients < 30 years old unless circumstances preclude other treatment.

➤*Pregnancy: Category X.* Sodium iodide I 131 can cause fetal harm when administered to a pregnant woman. Permanent damage to the fetal thyroid can occur. The drug is contraindicated in women who are or may become pregnant. If it is used during pregnancy, or if the patient becomes pregnant while taking this drug, inform her of the potential hazard to the fetus.

➤*Lactation:* Since iodine is excreted in breast milk, substitute with formula feedings.

Precautions

➤*Antithyroid therapy:* Antithyroid therapy of a severely hyperthyroid patient is usually discontinued for 3 to 4 days before administration of radioiodide.

Drug Interactions

➤*Stable iodine (any form), thyroid, antithyroid agents:* The uptake of iodine 131 will be affected by recent intake of these agents. Question the patient regarding previous medication and procedures involving radiographic contrast media.

Adverse Reactions

The immediate adverse reactions following treatment of hyperthyroidism are usually mild, but following the larger doses used in thyroid carcinoma, may be much more severe.

➤*Hematologic:* Depression of the hematopoietic system (large doses); bone marrow depression; acute leukemia; anemia; blood dyscrasias; leukopenia; thrombocytopenia.

➤*Miscellaneous:* Radiation sickness (some degree of nausea and vomiting); chest pain; tachycardia; itching skin; rash; hives; increase in clinical symptoms; acute thyroid crises; severe sialoadenitis; chromosomal abnormalities; death.

Tenderness and swelling of neck, pain on swallowing, sore throat and cough may occur around the third day after treatment and are usually amenable to analgesics.

Temporary thinning of the hair may occur 2 to 3 months after treatment.

Allergic type reactions have been reported infrequently following the administration of iodine-containing radiopharmaceuticals.

Overdosage

In the treatment of hyperthyroidism, overdosage may result in hypothyroidism, the onset of which may be delayed. Appropriate replacement therapy is recommended if hypothyroidism occurs.

Indications

➤*Growth failure associated with chronic renal insufficiency:* Treatment of children who have growth failure associated with chronic renal insufficiency up to the time of renal transplantation. Use in conjunction with optimal management of chronic renal insufficiency.

➤*Growth failure (except Serostim):* Long-term treatment of children who have growth failure caused by a lack of adequate endogenous growth hormone secretion.

➤*Turner Syndrome (Nutropin and Nutropin AQ only):* Long-term treatment of short stature associated with Turner Syndrome.

➤*Cachexia (Serostim only):* Treatment of AIDS wasting or cachexia.

➤*Somatropin deficiency syndrome (Humatrope only):* Replacement of endogenous somatropin in adults with somatropin deficiency syndrome who meet the following criteria: 1) Biochemical diagnosis of somatropin deficiency syndrome, by means of a negative response to a standard growth hormone stimulation test [maximum peak < 5 ng/ml when measured by RIA (polyclonal antibody) or < 2.5 ng/ml when measured by IRMA (monoclonal antibody)]; and 2) *Adult onset:* Patients who have somatropin deficiency syndrome, either alone or with multiple hormone deficiencies (hypopituitarism), as a result of pituitary disease, hypothalamic disease, surgery, radiation therapy; or *childhood onset:* Patients who were growth hormone-deficient during childhood who have somatropin deficiency syndrome confirmed as an adult before replacement therapy with somatropin is started.

➤*Unlabeled:* Short children due to Intrauterine Growth Retardation (IUGR), 0.5 to 5.1 U/m^2 for ≤ 18 months.

Actions

➤*Pharmacology:* **Somatrem** and **somatropin** are purified polypeptide hormones of recombinant DNA origin. Somatrem contains the identical sequence of 191 amino acids constituting pituitary-derived human growth hormone plus an additional amino acid, methionine. Somatropin's amino acid sequence is identical to that of a human growth hormone of pituitary origin.

Linear growth – The primary action is the stimulation of linear growth. This effect is demonstrated in patients lacking adequate endogenous growth hormone production. **Somatrem** and **somatropin** are therapeutically equivalent to endogenous growth hormone. Short-term clinical studies in normal adults show equivalent pharmacokinetics. Treatment of growth hormone deficient children results in an increase in growth rate and insulin-like growth factor/somatomedin-C (IGF-I) levels similar to that seen with human growth hormone (pituitary origin).

Skeletal growth – These agents stimulate skeletal growth in pediatric patients with growth hormone deficiency. The measurable increase in body length after administration of **somatropin** or human growth hormone results from its effect on the epiphyseal growth plates of long bones. Concentrations of IGF-I, which may play a role in skeletal growth, are low in the serum of growth hormone deficient children but increase during treatment. Elevations in mean serum alkaline phosphatase concentrations are seen.

Cell growth – The number of skeletal muscle cells is markedly decreased in short-stature children lacking endogenous growth hormone compared with healthy children. Treatment with growth hormone increases the number and size of muscle cells.

Organ growth – Growth hormone influences internal organ size and increases red cell mass.

Protein metabolism – Linear growth is facilitated in part by increased cellular protein synthesis. Nitrogen retention, as demonstrated by a decline in urinary nitrogen excretion and blood urea nitrogen (BUN), follows the initiation of growth hormone therapy. Treatment with **somatrem** or **somatropin** results in a similar decline in BUN.

Carbohydrate metabolism – Children with hypopituitarism sometimes experience fasting hypoglycemia that is improved by **somatropin** therapy. Large doses of growth hormone may impair glucose tolerance. Administration of growth hormone to normal adults results in increased serum insulin levels. Although the precise mechanism by which these drugs induce insulin resistance is not known, it is attributed to a decrease in insulin sensitivity. An increase in serum glucose levels is observed during somatropin treatment.

Lipid metabolism – Administration of growth hormone results in reduction in body fat stores, lipid mobilization and increased plasma fatty acids. Mean cholesterol levels decreased in patients treated with somatropin.

Mineral metabolism – Retention of sodium, potassium and phosphorus induced by growth hormone administration is thought to be caused by cell growth. Serum levels of inorganic phosphate increase in patients with growth hormone deficiency after somatropin or somatrem therapy because of metabolic activity associated with bone growth as well as increased tubular reabsorption of phosphate by the kidney. Serum calcium is not significantly altered. Although calcium excretion in the urine is increased, there is a simultaneous increase in calcium absorption from the intestine.

Connective tissue metabolism – Growth hormone stimulates the synthesis of chondroitin sulfate and collagen as well as the urinary excretion of hydroxyproline.

➤*Pharmacokinetics: Absorption* – Following SC administration of 0.1 mg/kg **somatropin** in healthy men, a mean peak concentration (C_{max}) of 56.1 ng/ml occurred at a mean time of 7.5 hrs. The extent of absorption was 626 ng•hr/ml and closely compares with that of **somatrem** (590 ng•hr/ml). The absolute bioavailability of somatropin is 75% and 63% after SC and IM administration, respectively.

Distribution – The volume of distribution of **somatropin** after IV injection is about 0.07 L/kg. The mean terminal half-life after IV administration of rhGH is 19.5 minutes.The AUC of somatropin is similar regardless of injection site. In healthy and growth hormone-deficient adults and children, the IM and SC pharmacokinetic profiles of somatropin are similar regardless of type of growth hormone or dosing regimen used.

Metabolism – Growth hormone localizes to highly perfused organs, most notably liver and kidney. In the kidney, growth hormone is filtered by the glomerulus, reabsorbed in the proximal tubule and is broken down within renal cells into amino acids that return to the circulation. A small number of dose-ranging studies suggest that clearance and AUC of **somatropin** is proportional to dose in the therapeutic dose range. The mean half-life of IV somatropin is 0.36 hours, whereas SC and IM administered somatropin have mean half-lives of 3.8 and 4.9 hours, respectively.

Excretion – In healthy volunteers, mean clearance is 0.14 L/hr/kg. Clearance of rhGH after IV administration in healthy adults and children is reported to be in the range of 116 to 1/4 ml/hr/kg. Consistent with the role of the liver and kidney as major elimination organs for exogenously administered human growth hormone, there is a reduction in growth hormone clearance in patients with severe liver or kidney dysfunction.

Contraindications

Subjects with closed epiphyses; sensitivity to benzyl alcohol (diluent supplied with some products is Bacteriostatic Water for Injection, benzyl alcohol preserved); evidence of tumor activity or active neoplasia (intracranial lesions must be inactive and antitumor therapy completed prior to instituting therapy; discontinue if there is evidence of tumor activity, recurrent tumor growth or neoplasia); sensitivity to m-cresol or glycerin (diluent supplied with *Humatrope*; see Administration and Dosage).

Warnings

➤*Weight loss:* Reevaluate treatment for AIDS wasting or cachexia in patients who continue to lose weight in the first 2 weeks of treatment.

➤*HIV:* Recombinant human growth hormone (rhGH) has been shown to potentiate HIV replication in vitro at concentrations ranging from 50 to 250 ng/ml. There was no increase in virus production when the antiretroviral agents, zidovudine, didanosine or lamivudine were added to the culture medium. Additional in vitro studies have shown that rhGH does not interfere with the antiviral activity of zalcitabine or stavudine. In controlled clinical trials, no significant growth hormone-associated increase in viral burden was observed. However, the protocol required all participants to be on concomitant nucleoside analogue therapy for the duration of the study. In view of the potential for acceleration of virus replication, it is recommended that HIV+ patients be maintained on nucleoside analogue therapy for the duration of serostim therapy.

➤*Increased tissue turgor:* Swelling (particularly in the hands and feet) and musculoskeletal discomfort (pain, swelling or stiffness) may occur during treatment with **serostim** but may resolve spontaneously with analgesic therapy or after reducing the frequency of dosing.

➤*Carpal tunnel syndrome:* Carpal tunnel syndrome may occur during treatment with **serostim**. If the symptoms of carpal tunnel syndrome do not resolve by decreasing the weekly number of doses of serostim, it is recommended that treatment be discontinued.

➤*Benzyl alcohol:* The diluents supplied with some products contain benzyl alcohol as a preservative. Benzyl alcohol has been associated with a fatal "gasping syndrome" in premature infants.

➤*Pregnancy:* Category B (**serostim** only). *Category C.* Give to a pregnant woman only if clearly needed.

➤*Lactation:* It is not known whether **somatropin** is excreted in breast milk. Exercise caution when administering to a nursing mother.

➤*Children:* Available literature data suggest that rhGH clearances are similar in adults and children.

Precautions

➤*Monitoring: Thyroid* – Serum levels of inorganic phosphorus, alkaline phosphatase and parathyroid hormone (PTH) may increase with somatropin therapy. Changes in thyroid hormone laboratory measurements may develop during treatment in children who lack adequate endogenous growth hormone secretion. Untreated hypothyroidism prevents optimal response to therapy. Therefore, periodically test thyroid function and treat with thyroid hormone when indicated.

➤*Diabetes:* Insulin resistance may be induced by growth hormone. Closely monitor patients with diabetes or glucose intolerance during somatropin therapy.

➤*Intracranial lesion:* Frequently monitor patients with growth hormone deficiency secondary to an intracranial lesion for progression or recurrence of the underlying disease process. In pediatric patients, clinical literature has demonstrated no relationship between **somatropin** replacement therapy and CNS tumor recurrence. In adults, it is unknown whether there is any relationship between somatropin replacement therapy and CNS tumor recurrence.

➤*Skin lesion:* Carefully monitor patients for any malignant transformation of skin lesions.

➤*Slipped capital epiphysis:* Periodically examine patients with growth failure secondary to chronic renal insufficiency for evidence of renal osteodystrophy progression. Slipped capital femoral epiphysis or avascular necrosis of the femoral head may be seen in children with advanced renal osteodystrophy, and it is uncertain whether these problems are affected by growth hormone therapy. Obtain x-rays of the hip prior to initiating therapy. Physicians and parents should be alert to the development of a limp or complaints of hip or knee pain in patients treated with growth hormone. Slipped capital femoral epiphysis may occur more frequently in patients with endocrine disorders or in patients undergoing rapid growth.

➤*Gynecomastia:* Gynecomastia occurs in about 70% of boys during puberty, but prepubertal gynecomastia is rare. When gynecomastia does occur before puberty, there is usually evidence of endogenous or exogenous estrogenic stimulation.

➤*Intracranial hypertension (IH):* IH with papilledema, visual changes, headache, nausea, or vomiting has been reported in a small number of patients treated with growth hormone products. Symptoms usually occurred within the first 8 weeks of the initiation of therapy. In all cases, IH-associated signs and symptoms resolved after termination of therapy or a reduction of the growth hormone dose. Funduscopic examination of patients is recommended at the initiation and periodically during the course of growth hormone therapy.

➤*Renal transplant:* No studies have been performed of **somatropin** (Nutropin) therapy in children who have received renal transplants. Treatment of patients with functioning renal allografts is not indicated.

➤*Antibody production:* As with all protein pharmaceuticals, a small percentage of patients may develop antibodies to the protein. Growth hormone antibody binding capacities < 2 mg/L have not been associated with growth attenuation. In some cases when binding capacity exceeds 2 mg/L, growth attenuation has been observed. In general, growth hormone antibodies are not neutralizing and do not interfere with the growth response. In addition to an evaluation of compliance with the prescribed treatment program and thyroid status, test for antibodies to human growth hormone in any patient who fails to respond to therapy.

Drug Interactions

➤*Glucocorticoid therapy:* Glucocorticoid therapy may inhibit growth-promoting effect. Carefully adjust the glucocorticoid replacement dose in patients with coexisting ACTH deficiency to avoid an inhibitory effect on growth.

➤*Drug/Lab test interactions:* Changes in thyroid hormone laboratory measurements may develop during **somatropin** treatment in children who lack adequate endogenous growth hormone secretion (see Precautions).

Adverse Reactions

Leukemia has occurred in a small number of children receiving **somatropin** or somatrem; however, the relationship is uncertain.

Immunologic –
  Somatrem: Approximately 30% to 40% of patients developed persistent antibodies. One of 84 subjects treated for 6 to 36 months developed antibodies associated with high binding capacities and failed to respond. In patients who had been previously treated with pituitary-derived growth hormone, 1 of 22 subjects developed persistent antibodies (see Precautions).
  Somatropin: Approximately 2% of patients developed antibodies. Of the 232 patients receiving somatropin for ≥ 6 months, 4.7% had serum binding of radiolabeled growth hormone in excess of twice the binding observed in control sera. In comparison, 74.5% of 106 patients treated for ≥ 6 months with somatrem in a similar trial had serum binding of radiolabeled growth hormone of at least twice that of the binding observed in control sera (see Precautions).

➤*Miscellaneous:*
  Nutropin AQ – Mild and transient peripheral edema (infrequent); carpal tunnel syndrome, increased growth of preexisting nevi, gynecomastia, pancreatitis (rare).

Somatropin –
  Adults: Headache; localized muscle pain; weakness; mild hyperglycemia; glucosuria; mild, transient edema early in treatment (2.5%).
  Pediatrics: Injection site pain (infrequent).

Overdosage

Acute overdosage could lead initially to hypoglycemia and subsequently to hyperglycemia. Long-term overdosage could result in signs and symptoms of gigantism or acromegaly consistent with the known effects of excess human growth hormone.

Patient Information

Inform patients being treated with growth hormone or their parents of the potential benefits and risks associated with treatment.

If home use is desired, give instructions on appropriate use, including a review of the contents of the patient information insert. Thoroughly instruct patients or parents in the importance of proper disposal and caution against any reuse of needles and syringes.

SOMATREM

Rx	Protropin (Genentech)	Powder for injection, lyophilized: 5 mg (≈ 15 IU) per vial[1]	In cartons of 2 vials and 10 mL multidose vial of diluent.[2]
		10 mg (≈ 30 IU) per vial[3]	In cartons of 2 vials and two 10 mL multidose vials of diluent.[2]

[1] With 40 mg mannitol.
[2] Bacteriostatic Water for Injection with 0.9% benzyl alcohol.

[3] With 80 mg mannitol.

For complete prescribing information, refer to the Growth Hormone group monograph.

Indications

➤*Treatment of growth failure:* For the long-term treatment of children who have growth failure caused by a lack of adequate endogenous growth hormone secretion. Exclude other etiologies of short stature.

Administration and Dosage

➤*Approved by the FDA:* October 1985.

Individualize dosage. A weekly dosage of up to 0.3 mg/kg (≈ 0.9 IU/kg) of body weight administered by daily IM or SC injection is recommended. Do not exceed a weekly dosage of 0.3 mg/kg (≈ 0.9 IU/kg) of body weight because of the potential risk of known effects of excess human growth hormone. Discontinue therapy if final height is achieved or epiphyseal fusion occurs. Evaluate patients who fail to respond adequately while on therapy to determine the cause of unresponsiveness.

➤*Preparation of solution:* Reconstitute each 5 or 10 mg vial with 1 to 5 mL or 1 to 10 mL, respectively, of Bacteriostatic Water for Injection (benzyl alcohol preserved) only; aim the stream of diluent against the glass wall of the vial. Do not shake. Gently swirl until contents are completely dissolved. Do not inject if solution is cloudy immediately after reconstitution or refrigeration. Use a small enough syringe that the prescribed dose can be drawn from the vial with reasonable accuracy.

Newborns – Benzyl alcohol as a preservative has been associated with toxicity (see Warnings). When administering to newborns, reconstitute with Sterile Water for Injection. Use only 1 dose per vial; discard the unused portion. The pH after reconstitution is ≈ 7.8.

➤*Storage/Stability:* Store at 2° to 8°C (36° to 46°F). Use reconstituted vials in 14 days. Avoid freezing.

SOMATROPIN

Rx	**Genotropin Miniquick** (Pharmacia)	Powder for injection, lyophilized: 0.2 mg/vial	Preservative free. In single-use syringe with 2-chamber cartridge. In 7s.[1]
		0.4 mg/vial	
		0.6 mg/vial	
		0.8 mg/vial	
		1 mg/vial	
		1.2 mg/vial	
		1.4 mg/vial	
		1.6 mg/vial	
		1.8 mg vial	
		2 mg/vial	
Rx	**Genotropin** (Pharmacia)	**Powder for injection, lyophilized:** 1.5 mg (≈ 4.5 IU)/vial	Preservative free. In 1.5 mg Intra-Mix 2-chamber cartridge with pressure-release needle. In 5s.
Rx	**Norditropin** (Novo Nordisk)	**Powder for injection, lyophilized:** 4 mg (≈ 12 IU)/vial	In vials[2] with diluent.[3]
Rx	**Serostim** (Serono)		Sucrose. In single-use vials with diluent.
Rx	**Nutropin** (Genentech)	**Powder for injection, lyophilized:** 5 mg (≈ 15 IU)/vial	In cartons of 2 vials[4] with a 10 mL multiple-dose vial of diluent.[5]
Rx	**Humatrope** (Eli Lilly)		In vials[6] with 5 mL diluent.[7]
Rx	**Serostim** (Serono)		Sucrose. In single-use vials with diluent.
Rx	**Saizen** (Serono)		Sucrose. In vials with diluent.[5]
Rx	**Tev-Tropin** (Gate)		30 mg mannitol. In vials with 5 mL diluent (bacteriostatic 0.9% sodium chloride for injection).
Rx	**Genotropin** (Pharmacia)	**Powder for injection, lyophilized:** 5.8 mg (≈ 17.4 IU)/vial	In 5.8 mg Intra-Mix 2-chamber cartridge with pressure-release needle and 2-chamber cartridge. In 1s and 5s.[8]
Rx	**Serostim** (Serono)	**Powder for injection, lyophilized:** 6 mg (≈ 18 IU)/vial	Sucrose. In single-use vials with diluent.
Rx	**Humatrope** (Eli Lilly)	**Powder for injection, lyophilized:** 6 mg (18 IU)/cartridge	In cartridge with prefilled syringe of diluent.[9]
Rx	**Norditropin** (Novo Nordisk)	**Powder for injection, lyophilized:** 8 mg (≈ 24 IU)/vial	In vials[2] with diluent.[3]
Rx	**Nutropin** (Genentech)	**Powder for injection, lyophilized:** 10 mg (≈ 30 IU)/vial	In cartons of 2 vials[10] with two 10 mL multiple-dose vials of diluent.[5]
Rx	**Humatrope** (Eli Lilly)	**Powder for injection, lyophilized:** 12 mg (36 IU)/cartridge	In cartridge with prefilled syringe of diluent.[11]
Rx	**Genotropin** (Pharmacia)	**Powder for injection, lyophilized:** 13.8 mg (≈ 41.4 IU)/vial	In Intra-Mix 2-chamber cartridge of 1s and 5s.[12]
Rx	**Nutropin Depot** (Genentech)	**Powder for injection:** 13.5 mg	Preservative free. In single-use vials with 1.5 mL diluent, and three 21-gauge, ½-inch needles.
		Powder for injection: 18 mg	Preservative free. In single-use vials with 1.5 mL diluent, and three 21-gauge, ½-inch needles.
		Powder for injection: 22.5 mg	Preservative free. In single-use vials with 1.5 mL diluent, and three 21-gauge, ½-inch needles.
Rx	**Humatrope** (Eli Lilly)	**Powder for injection, lyophilized:** 24 mg (72 IU)/cartridge	In cartridge with prefilled syringe of diluent.[13]
Rx	**Nutropin AQ** (Genentech)	**Injection:** 10 mg (≈ 30 IU)/vial	In 2 mL multiple-dose vials (6s).[14]
Rx	**Norditropin** (Novo Nordisk)	**Injection:** 5 mg/1.5 mL	In cartridges.[15]
		Injection: 10 mg/1.5 mL	In cartridges.[15]
		Injection: 15 mg/1.5 mL	In cartridges.[16]

[1] With 0.23 mg glycine, 13.74 mg mannitol.
[2] With 44 mg mannitol and 8.8 mg glycine.
[3] With Water for Injection with 1.5% benzyl alcohol.
[4] With 45 mg mannitol and 1.7 mg glycine.
[5] With Bacteriostatic Water for Injection with 0.9% benzyl alcohol.
[6] With 25 mg mannitol and 5 mg glycine.
[7] With Water for Injection with 0.3% Metacresol and 1.7% glycerin.
[8] With 46.8 mg mannitol.
[9] With 18 mg mannitol, 6 mg glycine, Water for Injection with 0.3% Metacresol.

[10] With 90 mg mannitol and 3.4 mg glycine.
[11] With 36 mg mannitol, 12 mg glycine, Water for Injection with 0.3% Metacresol.
[12] With 46 mg mannitol.
[13] With 72 mg mannitol, 24 mg glycine, Water for Injection with 0.3% Metacresol.
[14] With 17.4 mg sodium chloride, 5 mg phenol, 4 mg polysorbate 20, and 10 mM sodium citrate.
[15] With 4.5 mg phenol and 60 mg mannitol.
[16] With 4.5 mg phenol and 58 mg mannitol.

For complete prescribing information, refer to the Growth Hormone group monograph.

Indications

►*Growth failure (except Serostim):* Long-term treatment of children who have growth failure caused by an inadequate secretion of endogenous growth hormone (GH).

►*Growth failure (Genotropin only):* Long-term treatment of children who have growth failure caused by Prader-Willi syndrome (PWS). Confirm diagnosis by appropriate genetic testing.

►*Growth hormone deficiency (GHD) in adults (Genotropin, Nutropin, Nutropin AQ, and Humatrope only):* Long-term replacement therapy in adults with GHD of either childhood- or adult-onset etiology. Confirm GHD by an appropriate growth hormone stimulation test.

►*Growth failure associated with chronic renal insufficiency (Nutropin AQ and Nutropin only):* Treatment of growth failure associated with chronic renal insufficiency up to the time of renal transplantation.

►*Short stature associated with Turner syndrome (Nutropin, Nutropin AQ, and Humatrope only):* Long-term treatment of short stature associated with Turner syndrome.

►*AIDS wasting or cachexia (Serostim only):* Treatment of AIDS wasting or cachexia.

Administration and Dosage

Individualize dosage. Do not continue therapy if final height is achieved or epiphyseal fusion occurs. Evaluate patients who fail to respond adequately while on somatropin therapy to determine the cause of unresponsiveness.

SOMATROPIN

►Reconstitution technique (except Genotropin and Nutropin Depot): To reconstitute somatropin, inject the diluent into the vial, aiming the liquid against the glass vial wall. Swirl the vial with a gentle rotary motion until contents are dissolved completely. The solution should be clear immediately after reconstitution. Do not administer if the reconstituted product is cloudy immediately after reconstitution or refrigeration.

►Genotropin: The weekly dose should be divided into 6 to 7 SC injections. Administer in the thigh, buttocks, or abdomen; rotate the site of SC injections daily to help prevent lipoatrophy.

Pediatric GHD – 0.16 to 0.24 mg/kg body weight/week is recommended.

Pediatric PWS – 0.24 mg/kg body weight/week is recommended.

Adult GHD – Recommended starting dose is not more than 0.04 mg/kg/week. Dose may be increased at 4- to 8-week intervals according to individual patient requirements to a maximum of 0.08 mg/kg/week, depending on tolerance of treatment.

Reconstitution – Supplied as a powder, filled in a 2-chamber cartridge with the active ingredient in the front chamber and the diluent in the rear chamber. A reconstitution device is used to mix the diluent and the lyophilized powder. Follow the directions for reconstitution provided with each device. Do not shake.
   Storage/Stability: Before reconstitution, refrigerate at 2° to 8°C (36° to 46°F). Do not freeze. Protect from light. The 1.5 mg cartridge reconstituted with diluent may be refrigerated for ≤ 24 hours because it contains no preservative. Use once and discard any remaining solution.

The 5.8 and 13.8 mg cartridges are reconstituted with a diluent containing a preservative. After reconstitution, they may be stored under refrigeration for up to 21 days.

Refrigerate the *Genotropin Miniquick* prior to dispensing, but it may be stored ≤ 25°C (77°F) for up to 3 months after dispensing. The diluent has no preservative. After reconstitution, it may be stored under refrigeration for up to 24 hours before use. Use only once and then discard.

►Humatrope:
Pediatric patients – The recommended weekly dosage is 0.18 mg/kg (0.54 IU/kg) of body weight. The maximal replacement weekly dosage is 0.3 mg/kg (0.9 IU/kg) of body weight. Divide into equal doses given either on 3 alternate days, 6 times a week, or daily. Administer by SC or IM injection. Individualize dosage and administration schedule.
   Turner syndrome – A weekly dosage of up to 0.375 mg/kg (1.125 IU/kg) of body weight administered by SC injection is recommended. Divide into equal doses given either daily or on 3 alternate days.

Adult patients – The recommended dosage at the start of therapy is ≤ 0.006 mg/kg/day (0.018 IU/kg/day) given as a daily SC injection. The dose may be increased according to individual patient requirements to a maximum of 0.0125 mg/kg/day (0.0375 IU/kg/day).

Reconstitution – Reconstitute each 5 mg vial with 1.5 to 5 mL of diluent supplied.

Reconstitute each cartridge using the diluent syringe and the diluent connector that accompany the cartridge; do not reconstitute with the diluent for *Humatrope* provided with *Humatrope* vials.
   Storage/Stability: Before reconstitution, vials, cartridges, and diluent are stable when refrigerated at 2° to 8°C (36° to 46°F). Vials of somatropin are stable for ≤ 14 days after reconstitution with diluent for *Humatrope* or Bacteriostatic Water for Injection when stored in a refrigerator at 2° to 8°C (36° to 46°F). After reconstitution with Sterile Water, use only 1 dose/*Humatrope* vial and discard the unused portion. If the solution is not used immediately, it must be refrigerated at 2° to 8°C (36° to 46°F) and used within 24 hours. After reconstitution, cartridges of *Humatrope* are stable for up to 28 days when reconstituted with diluent for *Humatrope* and stored in a refrigerator at 2° to 8°C (36° to 46°F). Avoid freezing.

►Nutropin/Nutropin AQ:
Pediatric GHD – A weekly dosage of up to 0.3 mg/kg of body weight divided into daily SC injections is recommended.

Adult GHD – The recommended dosage at the start of therapy is ≤ 0.006 mg/kg given as a daily SC injection. The dose may be increased according to individual patient requirements to a maximum of 0.025 mg/kg daily in patients < 35 years of age and to a maximum of 0.0125 mg/kg daily in patients > 35 years of age.

To minimize the occurrence of adverse events in older or overweight patients, lower doses may be necessary. During therapy, decrease dosage if required by the occurrence of side effects or excessive IGF-I levels.

Chronic renal insufficiency (CRI) – A weekly dosage of up to 0.35 mg/kg of body weight divided into daily SC injections is recommended. Therapy may be continued up to the time of renal transplantation.

In order to optimize therapy for patients who require dialysis, the following guidelines for an injection schedule are recommended: 1) Hemodialysis patients should receive their injection at night just prior to going to sleep or at least 3 to 4 hours after hemodialysis to prevent hematoma formation caused by the heparin; 2) Chronic Cycling Peritoneal Dialysis (CCPD) patients should receive their injection in the morning after they have completed dialysis; 3) Chronic Ambulatory Peritoneal Dialysis (CAPD) patients should receive their injection in the evening at the time of the overnight exchange.

Turner syndrome – A weekly dosage of ≤ 0.375 mg/kg of body weight divided into equal doses 3 to 7 times/week by SC injection is recommended.

Reconstitution (Nutropin) – Reconstitute each 5 mg vial with 1 to 5 mL or each 10 mg vial with 1 to 10 mL of Bacteriostatic Water for Injection (benzyl alcohol preserved) only.
   Newborns: Benzyl alcohol has been associated with toxicity (see Warnings). When administering to newborns, reconstitute with Sterile Water for Injection. Use only one dose per vial; discard the unused portion. The pH after reconstitution with Bacteriostatic Water for Injection is ≈ 7.4.
   Storage/Stability (Nutropin): Before reconstitution, vials and diluent are stable when refrigerated at 2° to 8°C (36° to 46°F). Avoid freezing.

Reconstituted vials are stable for up to 14 days stored in a refrigerator at 2° to 8°C (36° to 46°F). Avoid freezing.

Nutropin AQ – Vial contents are stable for 28 days after initial use when stored at 2° to 8°C (36° to 46°F). Avoid freezing the vial.

►Nutropin Depot:
Once-monthly injection – Administer 1.5 mg/kg body weight SC on the same day of each month. Subjects > 15 kg will require > 1 injection per dose.

Twice-monthly injections – Administer 0.75 mg/kg body weight SC twice each month on the same days of each month (eg, days 1 and 15 of each month). Subjects > 30 kg will require > 1 injection per dose.

The following table indicates the required number of injections per dose.

Number of *Nutropin Depot* Injections Per Dose		
Patient weight (kg)	0.75 mg/kg twice monthly	1.5 mg/kg once monthly
≤ 15	1	1
> 15 to 30	1	2
> 30 to 45	2	3
> 45 to 60	2	*
> 60	3	*

* Twice monthly dosing recommended.

Reconstitution – Use only with diluent provided in the kit and administer with the supplied needles.

Using the following table, determine the volume of diluent needed to suspend. Withdraw the diluent into a 3 mL syringe using the needle supplied in the kit. Use only the diluent supplied in the kit for reconstitution and discard any remaining diluent.

Nutropin Depot Reconstitution Diluent Volume Needed	
Vial size (mg somatropin)	Volume of diluent to be added (mL)
13.5	0.8
18	1
22.5	1.2

Note: Since the suspension is viscous and prevents complete withdrawal of the entire vial contents, the vials are overfilled to ensure delivery of the labeled amount of somatropin. Using these diluent volumes for final suspension results in a final concentration of 19 mg/mL somatropin in each vial size.

Inject the diluent into the vial against the vial wall. Swirl the vial vigorously for up to 2 minutes to disperse the powder in the diluent. Mixing is complete when the suspension appears uniform, thick, and milky, and all the powder is fully dispersed. Do not store the vial after reconstitution or the suspension may settle.

Withdraw the required dose. Use only 1 vial for each injection. Replace the needle with a new needle from the kit and administer the dose immediately to avoid settling of the suspension in the syringe. Deliver the dose from the syringe at a continuous rate over not more than 5 seconds. Discard unused vial contents as the product contains no preservative. An extra needle has been provided in the kit.
   Storage/Stability – Before reconstitution, store vials and diluent at 2° to 8°C (36° to 46°F). Avoid freezing.

After suspension, all injections must be given immediately. Do not allow suspension to settle prior to withdrawal of the dose. Do not store or use suspended solution to suspend another vial.

►Serostim: Administered SC daily at bedtime according to the following dosage recommendations:

Serostim Dosage Recommendations	
Patient weight	Dose[1]
> 55 kg	6 mg SC daily
45 to 55 kg	5 mg SC daily
35 to 45 kg	4 mg SC daily

[1] Based on an approximate daily dosage of 0.1 mg/kg.

SOMATROPIN

In patients who weigh < 35 kg, administer at a dose of 0.1 mg/kg SC daily at bedtime.

Dose reductions for side effects related to treatment, which are unresponsive to symptomatic treatment, may be affected by reducing the total daily dose or the number of doses given per week.

Reconstitution – Reconstitute each vial with 1 mL Sterile Water for Injection.

  Storage/Stability: Before reconstitution, store powder and diluent at room temperature, 15° to 30°C (59° to 86°F). Use within 24 hours after reconstitution with diluent. Refrigerate the reconstituted solution at 2° to 8°C (36° to 46°F).

➤*Saizen:* Administer 0.06 mg/kg (≈ 0.18 IU/kg) SC or IM 3 times weekly.

Reconstitution – Reconstitute with 1 to 3 mL of Bacteriostatic Water for Injection (benzyl alcohol preserved).

  Storage/Stability: Before reconstitution, store at room temperature, 15° to 30°C (59° to 86°F). Reconstituted solutions are stable for up to 14 days under refrigeration. Avoid freezing.

➤*Norditropin:* The recommended dosage is 0.024 to 0.034 mg/kg body weight SC 6 to 7 times/week. Give the injections in the thighs and vary the injection site on the thigh on a rotating basis.

Cartridges must be administered using the corresponding color-coded *NordiPen* injection pen (pen sold separately). The 5 mg/1.5 mL cartridge uses the orange pen, the 10 mg/1.5 mL cartridge uses the blue pen, and the 15 mg/1.5 mL cartridge uses the green pen.

Reconstitution – Reconstitute each 4 or 8 mg vial with the 2 mL diluent.

  Storage/Stability: Before and after reconstitution, refrigerate at 2° to 8°C (36° to 46°F). Do not freeze. Avoid direct light. Use reconstituted vials within 14 days after dissolution.

Actions

➤*Pharmacology:* Posterior pituitary secretions include oxytocin and vasopressin, polypeptides containing 8 amino acids. Oxytocin is formed primarily in the paraventricular nuclei and vasopressin in the supraoptic nuclei of the hypothalamus. They are then transported in combination with a carrier protein, neurophysin, to accumulate in nerve endings in the posterior pituitary gland. Under appropriate stimuli, they are released from nerve endings and absorbed into adjacent capillaries.

Vasopressin – Vasopressin exhibits its most marked activity on the renal tubular epithelium, where it promotes water resorption of (antidiuretic hormone effect) and smooth muscle contraction throughout the vascular bed (vasopressor effects). Vasoconstriction is marked in portal and splanchnic vessels, somewhat less in peripheral, coronary, cerebral, and pulmonary vessels and slight in intrahepatic vessels. Vasopressin, and to a lesser extent, oxytocin, enhances GI motility and tone.

Neurogenic or central diabetes insipidus is a disorder of water metabolism that results from a partial or complete deficiency in the production and secretion of vasopressin from the neurohypophysis. Nephrogenic or peripheral diabetes insipidus results from an insensitivity of the renal tubules to the action of antidiuretic hormone. Vasopressin and its synthetic analogs are the principal treatment of neurogenic diabetes insipidus, but are ineffective in treating the nephrogenic variant.

Vasopressin is a purified form of the posterior pituitary, having only pressor and antidiuretic hormone (ADH) activity. Vasopressin may be obtained from natural sources or by chemical synthesis. The synthetic derivative, desmopressin, acts principally as ADH, possessing little pressor activity, and is relatively free of oxytocic activity.

Posterior Pituitary Hormone Products

Agent	Indications	Route	Concentration
Vasopressin Derivatives			
Vasopressin	Diabetes insipidus Post-op abdominal distention	Parenteral	20 u/mL
Desmopressin	Diabetes insipidus	Nasal Parenteral	0.1 mg/mL 4 mcg/mL
	Nocturnal enuresis Renal capacity testing	Nasal	0.1 mg/mL
	Hemophilia A von Willebrand's disease (Type I)	Nasal Parenteral	1.5 mg/mL 4 mcg/mL

Posterior Pituitary Hormone Products

Agent	Indications	Route	Concentration
Oxytocics[1]			
Oxytocin	Initiate/augment labor 2nd trimester abortion Postpartum hemorrhage	Parenteral	10 u/mL
Ergonovine	Postpartum/postabortal hemorrhage Migraine headache	Oral Parenteral	0.2 mg 0.2 mg/mL
Methyl-ergonovine	Postpartum/postabortal hemorrhage	Oral Parenteral	0.2 mg 0.2 mg/mL

[1] Other agents with oxytocic effects on the uterus used to induce abortion are discussed under Abortifacients.

➤*Pharmacokinetics:*

Oxytocin – Oxytocin exerts its most marked activity in inducing uterine muscle contraction and inducing contraction of the lacteal glands, which results in milk ejection in lactating women. Uterine motility is controlled by a variety of biochemical and regulatory processes including cAMP, calcium, prostaglandins, and oxytocin. The mechanism of oxytocin-facilitated smooth muscle contraction is poorly understood. The sensitivity of the uterus to oxytocin increases gradually during gestation, then increases sharply before parturition.

Naturally derived oxytocin, no longer commercially available, has been replaced by synthetic oxytocin. Oxytocin is most frequently used to induce or improve uterine contractions in labor. Ergot derivatives (ergonovine and methylergonovine) are also used for oxytocic effects on uterine muscle. These agents are most appropriately used to prevent postpartum uterine atony and hemorrhage.

VASOPRESSIN (8-Arginine-Vasopressin)

Rx	**Vasopressin** (Various, eg, American Pharmaceutical Partners, American Regent)	**Injection:** 20 pressor units/mL	With 0.5% chlorobutanol. In 0.5, 1, and 10 mL vials.
Rx	**Pitressin** (Monarch)		With 0.5% chlorobutanol. In 1 mL amps and vials.

Refer to the general discussion of these products in the Posterior Pituitary Hormones group monograph.

Indications

➤*Diabetes insipidus:* Treatment of diabetes insipidus.

➤*Abdominal distention:* Prevention and treatment of postoperative abdominal distention.

➤*Abdominal roentgenography:* To dispel interfering gas shadows in abdominal roentgenography.

➤*Unlabeled uses:* Vasopressin has been used to control acute variceal hemorrhage, treat refractory septic shock (low-dose vasopressin), and treat ventricular fibrillation/pulseless ventricular tachycardia cardiac arrest.

Administration and Dosage

May be given IM or SC.

➤*Usual dose:* 5 to 10 units usually elicit full physiologic response. Give IM at 3- or 4-hour intervals as needed. Reduce dosage proportionately for children.

➤*Diabetes insipidus:*

Intranasal – The injection solution may be administered intranasally on cotton pledgets, by nasal spray or dropper. Individualize dosage.

Parenteral – 5 to 10 units 2 or 3 times daily as needed.

➤*Abdominal distention:* To prevent or relieve postoperative distention, give 5 units initially; increase to 10 units at subsequent injections, if necessary. Give IM at 3- or 4-hour intervals. Reduce dosage proportionately for children. These recommendations also apply to distention complicating pneumonia or other acute toxemias.

➤*Abdominal roentgenography:* Administer 2 injections of 10 units each. Give 2 hours and ½ hour, respectively, before films are exposed. An enema may be given prior to first dose.

Actions

➤*Pharmacology:* Exogenous vasopressin exerts all the same mechanisms as endogenous vasopressin, also known as antidiuretic hormone. The antidiuretic action of vasopressin is attributed to increasing reabsorption of water by the renal tubules. Vasopressin can cause contraction of smooth muscle of the GI tract and of all parts of the vascular bed, especially the capillaries, small arterioles, and venules with less effect on the smooth musculature of the large veins. The direct effect on the contractile elements is neither antagonized by adrenergic blocking agents nor prevented by vascular denervation.

➤*Pharmacokinetics:* Following IM or SC injection, the duration of antidiuretic activity for vasopressin is 2 to 8 hours. Most is metabolized and rapidly destroyed in liver and kidneys. Vasopressin has a plasma half-life of ≈ 10 to 20 minutes. After 4 hours, ≈ 5% of an SC dose is excreted unchanged in urine.

Contraindications

Anaphylaxis or hypersensitivity to vasopressin or its components.

Warnings

➤*Vascular disease:* Use with extreme caution in patients with vascular disease (especially coronary artery disease) since even small doses may precipitate anginal pain; with larger doses, consider the possibility of MI.

➤*Water intoxication:* Vasopressin may produce water intoxication. Early signs of drowsiness, listlessness, and headaches precede terminal coma and convulsions.

➤*Vasoconstriction/Necrosis:* Severe vasoconstriction and local tissue necrosis may result if vasopressin extravasates during IV infusion.

➤*Chronic nephritis:* Chronic nephritis with nitrogen retention contraindicates use until reasonable nitrogen blood levels have been attained.

➤*Hypersensitivity reactions:* Local or systemic allergic reactions may occur in hypersensitive individuals (see Adverse Reactions). Anaphylaxis (cardiac arrest or shock) has been observed shortly after injection. Refer to Management of Acute Hypersensitivity Reactions.

➤*Pregnancy: Category C.* It is not known whether vasopressin causes fetal harm when administered to a pregnant woman or affects reproductive capacity. Administer to a pregnant woman only if clearly needed. Doses sufficient for an antidiuretic effect are not likely to produce tonic uterine contractions that could be harmful to the fetus or threaten the continuation of the pregnancy.

➤*Lactation:* Exercise caution when administering to a nursing woman.

VASOPRESSIN (8-Arginine-Vasopressin)

Precautions

▶*Monitoring:* Electrocardiograms and fluid and electrolyte status determinations are recommended at intervals during therapy.

▶*Special risk patients:* Use vasopressin cautiously in the presence of epilepsy, migraine, asthma, heart failure, or any state in which a rapid increase in extracellular water may result in further compromise.

Drug Interactions

Vasopressin Drug Interactions			
Precipitant drug	Object drug*		Description
Carbamazepine Chlorpropamide Clofibrate Urea Fludrocortisone Tricyclic antidepressants	Vasopressin	↑	Concomitant administration may potentiate the antidiuretic effect of vasopressin.
Demeclocycline Norepinephrine Lithium Heparin Alcohol	Vasopressin	↓	Concomitant administration may decrease the antidiuretic effect of vasopressin.
Ganglionic blocking agents	Vasopressin	↑	Ganglionic blocking agents may produce a marked increase in sensitivity to the pressor effects of vasopressin.

* ↑ = Object drug increased. ↓ = Object drug decreased.

Adverse Reactions

▶*Cardiovascular:* Cardiac arrest, circumoral pallor, arrhythmias, decreased cardiac output, angina, myocardial ischemia, peripheral vasoconstriction, gangrene.

▶*CNS:* Tremor, vertigo, "pounding" in head.

▶*Dermatologic:* Sweating, urticaria, cutaneous gangrene.

▶*GI:* Abdominal cramps, nausea, vomiting, passage of gas.

▶*Miscellaneous:* Anaphylaxis (cardiac arrest or shock), bronchial constriction.

Overdosage

Treat water intoxication with water restriction and temporary withdrawal of vasopressin until polyuria occurs. Severe water intoxication may require osmotic diuresis with mannitol, hypertonic dextrose, or urea alone or with furosemide.

Patient Information

Side effects such as skin blanching, abdominal cramps, and nausea may be reduced by taking 1 or 2 glasses of water with the dose. These side effects are usually not serious and will probably disappear within a few minutes.

DESMOPRESSIN ACETATE (1-Deamino-8-D-Arginine Vasopressin)

Rx	**DDAVP** (Aventis)	**Tablets:** 0.1 mg	Lactose. (DDAVP 0.1 rPr). White. In 100s.
		0.2 mg	Lactose. (DDAVP 0.2 rPr). White. In 100s.
Rx	**Desmopressin Acetate** (Bausch & Lomb)	**Nasal solution:** 0.1 mg/mL (10 mcg/spray)	0.5% chlorobutanol. In 5 mL nasal pump dispenser.
Rx	**DDAVP** (Aventis)	**Nasal solution:** 0.1 mg/mL (0.1 mg equals ≈ 400 IU arginine vasopressin)	**Nasal spray pump:**[1] 7.5 mg NaCl/mL. In 5 mL bottle with spray pump (50 doses of 10 mcg).
			Rhinal tube delivery system:[2] 9 mg NaCl/mL. In 2.5 mL vials with 2 applicator tubes.
Rx	**Stimate** (Centeon)	**Nasal solution:** 1.5 mg/mL	9 mg NaCl/mL. In 2.5 mL bottle[2] (25 doses of 150 mcg each).
Rx	**Minirin** (Ferring)	**Nasal spray:** 0.5 mg/mL	In 5 mL[2] (50 doses of 10 mcg).
Rx	**Desmopressin Acetate** (Various, eg, Ferring)	**Injection:** 4 mcg/mL	1 mL single-dose amps and 10 mL multidose vials.
Rx	**DDAVP** (Aventis)		9 mg NaCl/mL. In 1 mL amps and 10 mL multidose vials.[2]

[1] With 1.7 mg citric acid monohydrate, 3 mg disodium phosphate dihydrate, 0.2 mg benzalkonium chloride solution (50%) per mL.

[2] With 5 mg chlorobutanol per mL.

Refer to the general discussion of these products in the Posterior Pituitary Hormones introduction.

Indications

▶*DDAVP:*

Primary nocturnal enuresis (intranasal only) – May be used alone or adjunctive to behavioral conditioning or other nonpharmacological intervention. It is effective in some cases that are refractory to conventional therapies.

Central cranial diabetes insipidus (intranasal, oral, and parenteral) – Antidiuretic hormone (ADH) replacement therapy in the management of central cranial (neurogenic) diabetes insipidus and for temporary polyuria and polydipsia following head trauma or surgery in the pituitary region. Ineffective for the treatment of nephrogenic diabetes insipidus.

Hemophilia A (intranasal and parenteral) – Hemophilia A (intranasal and parenteral) with Factor VIII levels > 5%. Desmopressin will often maintain hemostasis in patients with hemophilia A during surgery and postoperatively when administered 30 minutes prior to procedure. The drug also will stop bleeding in hemophilia A patients with episodes of spontaneous or trauma-induced injuries such as hemarthroses, IM hematomas, or mucosal bleeding.

von Willebrand's disease (Type I) (intranasal and parenteral) – Mild-to-moderate classic von Willebrand's disease (Type I) with Factor VIII levels > 5%. Hemostasis in these patients can often be maintained during surgery and postoperatively when the drug is administered 30 minutes prior to the procedure. Episodes of spontaneous or trauma-induced injuries such as hemarthroses, IM hematomas, or mucosal bleeding can usually be stopped.

▶*Stimate:*

Hemophilia A – Hemophilia A with Factor VIII coagulant activity levels > 5%. Desmopressin will also stop bleeding in patients with hemophilia A with episodes of spontaneous or trauma-induced injuries such as hemarthroses, IM hematomas, or mucosal bleeding.

von Willebrand's disease (Type I) – Mild-to-moderate classic von Willebrand's disease (Type I) with Factor VIII levels > 5%. Desmopressin also will stop bleeding in mild-to-moderate von Willebrand's

disease patients with episodes of spontaneous or trauma-induced injuries such as hemarthroses, IM hematomas, mucosal bleeding, or menorrhagia.

▶*Unlabeled uses:*

Intranasal – Treatment of chronic autonomic failure (eg, nocturnal polyuria, overnight weight loss, morning postural hypotension).

Administration and Dosage

▶*Primary nocturnal enuresis:* Individualize dosage.

Initial dose (≥ 6 years of age) – 20 mcg (0.2 mL) intranasally at bedtime. Adjustment ≤ 40 mcg is suggested if the patient does not respond. Some patients may respond to 10 mcg and adjustment to that lower dose may be done if the patient has shown a response to 20 mcg. It is recommended that 50% of the dose be administered per nostril. Adequately controlled studies have not been conducted beyond 4 to 8 weeks.

▶*Central cranial diabetes insipidus:*

Intranasal – The nasal tube delivery system is supplied with a flexible calibrated plastic tube (rhinyle). Draw solution into the rhinyle. Insert one end of tube into nostril; blow on the other end to deposit solution deep into nasal cavity. The nasal spray pump also may be used.

   Adults: 0.1 to 0.4 mL daily, either as a single dose or divided into 2 or 3 doses. Most adults require 0.2 mL daily in 2 divided doses. Adjust morning and evening doses separately for an adequate diurnal rhythm of water turnover.

   Children (3 months to 12 years of age): 0.05 to 0.3 mL daily, either as a single dose or in 2 divided doses.

Parenteral – Administer SC or by direct IV injection.

   Adults: 0.5 to 1 mL daily in 2 divided doses, adjusted separately for an adequate diurnal rhythm of water turnover. For patients switching from intranasal to IV, the comparable IV antidiuretic dose is ≈ 1/10 the intranasal dose. Estimate response by adequate sleep duration and adequate but not excessive water turnover.

Oral – The dosage must be determined for each individual patient and adjusted according to the diurnal pattern of response. Estimate response by adequate duration of sleep and adequate, not excessive, water turnover. Begin therapy 12 hours after the last intranasal dose

DESMOPRESSIN ACETATE (1-Deamino-8-D-Arginine Vasopressin)

for patients previously on intranasal therapy. Observe patients closely during the initial dose titration period and measure appropriate safety parameters to assure adequate response. Monitor patient at regular intervals during therapy to assure adequate antidiuretic response. Implement modifications in dosage regimen as necessary to assure adequate water turnover.

Adults: Begin with 0.05 mg 2 times a day and adjust individually to their optimum therapeutic dose. Separately adjust each dose for an adequate diurnal rhythm of water turnover. Increase or decrease total daily dosage (range, 0.1 to 1.2 mg divided 2 or 3 times a day) as needed to obtain adequate antidiuresis.

Children: Begin dosing with 0.05 mg. Careful fluid intake restrictions in children is required to prevent hyponatremia and water intoxication.

➤*Hemophilia A and von Willebrand's disease (Type I):*

Parenteral – Administer 0.3 mcg/kg diluted in sterile physiologic saline; infuse IV slowly over 15 to 30 minutes. In adults and children weighing> 10 kg, use 50 mL diluent; in children weighing ≤ 10 kg, use 10 mL. Monitor blood pressure and pulse during infusion. If used preoperatively, administer 30 minutes prior to the procedure.

Determine the necessity for repeat dose or use of any blood products for hemostasis by laboratory response and patient's clinical condition. Consider the tendency toward tachyphylaxis with repeating dose more than every 48 hours.

Intranasal – Administer by nasal insufflation, 1 spray/nostril, to provide a total dose of 300 mcg. In patients weighing < 50 kg, 150 mcg administered as a single spray provided the expected effect on Factor VIII coagulant activity, Factor VIII ristocetin cofactor activity, and skin bleeding time. If used preoperatively, administer 2 hours prior to the scheduled procedure.

Determine the necessity for repeat administration or use of any blood products for hemostasis by laboratory response as well as the clinical condition of the patient. Consider the tendency toward tachyphylaxis (lessening of response) with repeated administration given more frequently than every 48 hours.

The nasal spray pump only delivers doses of 10 mcg (*DDAVP*) or 150 mcg (*Stimate*). If doses other than these are required, consider nasal tube delivery or injection.

The *Stimate* spray pump must be primed prior to the first use. To prime pump, press down 4 times. Discard the bottle after 25 doses since the amount delivered thereafter per spray may be substantially < 150 mcg of drug.

➤*Storage / Stability:*

Intranasal – Refrigerate nasal solution at 2° to 8°C (36° to 46°F). Nasal solution will maintain stability for ≤ 3 weeks when stored at room temperature (22°C; 72°F).

Injection – Refrigerate at 2° to 8°C (36° to 46°F).

Actions

➤*Pharmacology:* A synthetic analog of arginine vasopressin, the naturally occurring human ADH provides a prompt onset of action with a long duration. The antidiuretic action is more specific and more prolonged than that of the natural hormone or lypressin. The plasma half-life of lypressin is 17 to 35 minutes. Urine volume is reduced, and urine osmolality is increased.

The change in structure of arginine vasopressin to desmopressin acetate results in less vasopressor activity and decreased action on visceral smooth muscle relative to enhanced antidiuretic activity. Consequently, clinically effective antidiuretic doses are usually below the threshold for effects on vascular or visceral smooth muscle.

Desmopressin produces a dose-related increase in Factor VIII levels. The increase is rapid, becoming evident in ≤ 30 minutes and peaking in 90 to 120 minutes. The Factor VIII-related antigen and ristocetin cofactor activity are also increased to a smaller degree.

➤*Pharmacokinetics:*

Injection – Biphasic half-lives of desmopressin acetate are 7.8 and 75.5 minutes for the fast and slow phases, respectively, compared with 2.5 and 14.5 minutes for lysine vasopressin. When administered by injection, desmopressin has an antidiuretic effect ≈ 10 times that of an equivalent dose administered intranasally.

Intranasal – The half-life of the nasal spray is between 3.3 and 3.5 hours, over the range of intranasal doses, 150 to 450 mcg. Plasma concentrations of the nasal spray are maximal at ≈ 40 to 45 minutes after dosing. The bioavailability of the nasal spray when administered by the intranasal route as a 1.5 mg/mL solution is between 3.3% and 4.1%. Plasminogen activator activity increases rapidly after IV infusion, but clinically significant fibrinolysis has not occurred.

Oral – The bioavailability of the tablets is ≈ 5% and 0.15% compared with intranasal and IV desmopressin, respectively. The time to reach maximum plasma levels ranges from 0.9 to 1.5 hours following oral or intranasal administration, respectively. Following administration of tablets, the onset of antidiuretic effect occurs at ≈ 1 hour, and it reaches a maximum at ≈ 4 to 7 hours based on the measurement of increased urine osmolality. The plasma half-life of desmopressin follows a monoexponential time course with $t_{1/2}$ values of 1.5 to 2.5 hours, which is independent of dose. Increasing oral doses produces dose-dependent increases in the plasma levels of desmopressin tablets.

➤*Clinical trials:* In one study, the tablets and intranasal formulation were compared during an 8-hour dosing interval at steady-state. The doses administered to 36 hydrated (water-loaded) healthy male adult volunteers every 8 hours were 0.1, 0.2, and 0.4 mg orally and 0.01 mg intranasally by rhinal tube.

With respect to the mean values of total urine volume decrease and maximum urine osmolality increase from baseline, the 0.4 and 0.2 mg oral dose produced between 95% to 110% and 84% to 99% of pharmacodynamic activity, respectively, when compared with the 0.01 mg intranasal dose.

While both the 0.2 mg and 0.4 mg oral doses are considered pharmacodynamically similar to the 0.01 mg intranasal dose, the pharmacodynamic data on an intersubject basis was highly variable; therefore, individual dosing is recommended.

In another study in diabetes insipidus patients, the tablet and intranasal formulations were compared over a 12-hour period. Ten fluid-controlled patients < 18 years of age were administered tablet doses of 0.2 and 0.4 mg and intranasal doses of 10 and 20 mcg.

All 4 dose formulations have a similar pronounced pharmacodynamic effect on urine volume and urine osmolality. At 2 hours after study drug administration, mean urine volume was 4 mL/min and urine osmolality was > 500 mOsm/kg. Mean plasma osmolality remained relatively constant over the time course recorded (0 to 12 hours).

Contraindications

Hypersensitivity to desmopressin acetate or its components.

Intranasal delivery may be inappropriate where there is an impaired level of consciousness.

Warnings

➤*Hemophilia A:* Not indicated for treatment of hemophilia A with Factor VIII levels ≤ 5%, for the treatment of hemophilia B, or in patients who have Factor VIII antibodies. Some patients with Factor VIII levels between 2% to 5% may be treatable.

➤*von Willebrand's disease:* Patients who are least likely to respond are those with severe homozygous von Willebrand's disease with Factor VIII coagulant activity, Factor VIII antigen, and von Willebrand's factor (ristocetin cofactor) activities < 1%. Other patients may respond in a variable fashion, depending on the type of molecular defect.

Not indicated – Not indicated for the treatment of severe classic von Willebrand's disease (Type I) and when an abnormal molecular form of Factor VIII antigen is evident.

Do not use for Type IIB von Willebrand's disease; may induce platelet aggregation.

➤*Test dose:* Before the initial therapeutic administration of the nasal spray, the physician should establish that the patient shows an appropriate change in the coagulation profile following a test dose of intranasal administration.

➤*Water intoxication:* Caution very young and elderly patients to ingest only enough fluid to satisfy thirst to decrease the potential occurrence of water intoxication and hyponatremia. Pay particular attention to the possibility of the rare occurrence of an extreme decrease in plasma osmolality that may result in seizures, leading to coma.

➤*Hypersensitivity reactions:* Rare severe allergic reactions have been reported with desmopressin. Anaphylaxis has been reported with IV administration but not with intranasal or oral (tablets).

➤*Pregnancy:* Category B. Several publications of desmopressin acetate's use in the management of diabetes insipidus during pregnancy are available. However, there are no adequate and well-controlled studies in pregnant women. Safety and efficacy for use during pregnancy have not been established. Use only when clearly needed and when the potential benefits outweigh potential hazards to the fetus. Published reports stress that, as opposed to preparations containing the natural hormones, desmopressin in antidiuretic doses has no uterotonic action, but the physician will have to weigh possible therapeutic advantages against possible danger in each case.

➤*Lactation:* Safety for use in nursing women has not been established. Patients receiving desmopressin for diabetes insipidus have been reported to breastfeed without apparent problems in the infant. A single study in postpartum women showed little, if any, change in breast milk following a 10 mcg intranasal dose. However, there have been no controlled studies in nursing mothers. Exercise caution when administering desmopressin to a nursing woman.

➤*Children:* Infants and children require careful fluid intake restriction to prevent possible hyponatremia and water intoxication.

Intranasal desmopressin has been used in children with diabetes insipidus, and the tablets have been used safely in children (≥ 4 years of age) with diabetes insipidus for periods ≤ 44 months. If desmopressin is used in the very young, adjust the dose individually, with attention to the danger of an extreme decrease in plasma osmolality leading to hyponatremia with possible convulsions. Initiate doses at 0.05 mL (intranasal) or 0.05 mg (oral).

DESMOPRESSIN ACETATE (1-Deamino-8-D-Arginine Vasopressin)

Pediatric Use of Desmopressin Acetate	
Indication/Doseform	Safety and efficacy not proven in children less than age:
Central cranial diabetes insipidus Intranasal Oral Parenteral	Adjust dosage (*DDAVP*) 4 years 12 years
Hemophilia A Intranasal Oral Parenteral	11 months (*Stimate*) Not indicated. 3 months
Primary nocturnal enuresis Intranasal Oral Parenteral	6 years (*DDAVP*) Not indicated. Not indicated.
von Willebrand's disease Intranasal Oral Parenteral	11 months (*Stimate*) Not indicated. 3 months

Precautions

➤*Monitoring:*

Diabetes insipidus – Monitor urine volume/osmolality and plasma osmolality.

Hemophilia A – Determine Factor VIII coagulant activity before injecting desmopressin for hemostasis; if the activity is < 5% of normal, do not rely on desmopressin. Other tests to assess patient status include levels of Factor VIII coagulant, Factor VIII antigen and ristocetin cofactor, and activated partial thromboplastin time.

von Willebrand's disease – Assess levels of Factor VIII coagulant, Factor VIII antigen, and ristocetin cofactor. Skin bleeding time also may be helpful.

➤*Cardiovascular effects:* High intranasal dosage has infrequently produced a slight elevation of blood pressure that disappeared with dosage reduction. This effect has not been observed with single oral doses ≤ 0.6 mg. Use with caution in coronary artery insufficiency or hypertensive cardiovascular disease. Desmopressin injection has infrequently produced changes in blood pressure causing either a slight elevation in blood pressure or a transient fall in blood pressure and a compensatory increase in heart rate. Use the drug with caution in patients with coronary artery insufficiency or hypertensive cardiovascular disease.

➤*Nasal mucosa changes:* Nasal mucosa changes (eg, scarring, edema, discharge, blockage, congestion, severe atrophic rhinitis), cranial surgery (eg, transphenoidal hypophysectomy), and nasal packing compromise intranasal delivery; consider administering IV.

➤*Thrombotic events:* There have been rare reports of thrombotic events (eg, thrombosis, acute cerebrovascular thrombosis, acute myocardial infarction) following desmopressin injection in patients predisposed to thrombus formation. No causality has been determined; however, use the drug with caution in these patients.

➤*Decreased response:* There are reports of an occasional change in response to intranasal desmopressin with time, usually > 6 months. Some patients may show a decreased responsiveness, others a shortened duration of effect. There is no evidence that this effect is because of the development of binding antibodies, but it may be because of a local inactivation of the peptide. No lessening of effect has been seen in the 46 patients who were treated with desmopressin tablets for 12 to 44 months and no serum antibodies to desmopressin were detected.

➤*Fluid/Electrolyte imbalance:* Use with caution in patients with conditions associated with fluid and electrolyte imbalance, such as cystic fibrosis, because these patients are prone to hyponatremia.

Drug Interactions

Desmopressin Drug Interactions			
Precipitant drug	Object drug*		Description
Desmopressin	Pressor agents	↑	Although desmopressin pressor activity is very low, use large intranasal doses or parenteral doses as large as 0.3 mcg/kg cautiously with other pressor agents.
Carbamazepine	Desmopressin	↑	Carbamazepine, which potentiates ADH, may potentiate the effects of desmopressin.
Chlorpropamide	Desmopressin	↑	Chlorpropamide, which potentiates ADH, may potentiate the effects of desmopressin.

* ↑ = Object drug increased.

Adverse Reactions

Intranasal (DDAVP) – Adverse reactions that disappear with dosage reduction include: abdominal pain (mild); facial flushing; headache (transient); nasal congestion; nausea; rhinitis. Other adverse reactions include: Asthenia; chills; conjunctivitis; cough; dizziness; epistaxis; eye edema; GI disorder; lacrimation disorder; nosebleed; nostril pain; sore throat; upper respiratory infections.

Intranasal (Stimate) – Adverse reactions include: Agitation; balanitis; chest pain; chills; dizziness; dyspepsia; edema; insomnia; itchy or light sensitive eyes; pain; palpitations; somnolence; tachycardia; vomiting; warm feeling.

Parenteral – Adverse reactions that disappear with dosage reduction include: Abdominal pain (mild); facial flushing; headache (transient); nausea; vulval pain. Other adverse reactions include: Anaphylaxis (rare); blood pressure changes; burning pain; edema; erythema (local).

Oral – In long-term clinical studies in which patients with diabetes insipidus were followed for periods ≤ 12 to 44 months of tablet therapy, transient increases in AST ≤ 1.5 times the upper limit of normal occurred. Elevated AST returned to the normal range despite continued use of tablets.

Overdosage

➤*Symptoms:* Abdominal pain, dyspnea, facial flushing, fluid retention, headache and mucous membrane irritation may occur.

➤*Treatment:* Reduce the dosage, decrease the frequency of use or withdraw the drug according to the severity of the condition. There is no known specific antidote.

Patient Information

Patient instructions provided with intranasal product; review administration with patient.

If bleeding is not controlled, contact the physician.

Notify physician if headache, shortness of breath, heartburn, nausea, abdominal cramps or vulval pain occurs.

➤*Intranasal:* Inform patients that the bottle accurately delivers 25 or 50 doses. Discard any solution remaining after 25 or 50 doses because the amount delivered thereafter may be substantially less than prescribed. Do not attempt to transfer remaining solution to another bottle.

OCTREOTIDE ACETATE

Rx	**Sandostatin** (Novartis)	**Injection:** 0.05 mg/ml	In 1 ml amps.
		0.1 mg/ml	In 1 ml amps.
		0.2 mg/ml	In 5 ml multi-dose vials.
		0.5 mg/ml	In 1 ml amps.
		1 mg/ml	In 5 ml multi-dose vials.
Rx	**Sandostatin LAR Depot** (Novartis)	**Injection:** 10 mg/5 ml	Carboxymethylcellulose sodium. In kits w/ 2 ml diluent, 1½" 20-gauge needles and instruction booklet.
		20 mg/5 ml	
		30 mg/5 ml	

Indications

➤*Sandostatin:*

Acromegaly – To reduce blood levels of growth hormone and IGF-I in acromegaly patients who have had inadequate response to or cannot be treated with surgical resection, pituitary irradiation and bromocriptine at maximally tolerated doses. The goal is to achieve normalization of growth hormone and IGF-I levels.

Carcinoid tumors – Symptomatic treatment of patients with metastatic carcinoid tumors where it suppresses or inhibits associated severe diarrhea and flushing episodes.

Vasoactive intestinal peptide tumors (VIPomas) – Treatment of the profuse watery diarrhea associated with VIP-secreting tumors.

➤*Sandostatin LAR Depot:*

Acromegaly – For long-term maintenance therapy in acromegalic patients for whom medical treatment is appropriate and who have been shown to respond to and can tolerate octreotide acetate injection. The goal of treatment in acromegaly is to reduce GH and IGF-I levels to normal. *Sandostatin LAR Depot* can be used in patients who have had an inadequate response to surgery or in those for whom surgical resection is not an option. It may also be used in patients who have received radiation and have had an inadequate therapeutic response.

Carcinoid tumors – For long-term treatment of the severe diarrhea and flushing episodes associated with metastatic carcinoid tumors in patients in whom initial treatment with *Sandostatin* injection has been shown to be effective and tolerated.

VIPomas – For long-term treatment of the profuse watery diarrhea associated with VIP-secreting tumors in patients in whom initial treatment with *Sandostatin* injection has been shown to be effective and tolerated.

➤*Unlabeled uses:* Octreotide is effective in treating the following conditions:

GI fistula – To reduce output from GI fistulas. Dosage ranges from 50 to 200 mcg every 8 hours.

Variceal bleeding – Dosage ranges from 25 to 50 mcg/hr via continuous IV infusion. Duration is from 18 hours to 5 days.

Diarrheal states – Since octreotide prolongs intestinal transit time, it is beneficial in relieving diarrhea associated with a variety of conditions including: AIDS-related diarrhea (100 to 500 mcg SC 3 times daily); idiopathic secretory diarrhea; short bowel (ileostomy) syndrome (IV infusion of 25 mcg/hr or SC 50 mcg twice daily); diabetes; pancreatic cholera syndrome; diarrhea due to chemotherapy/radiation therapy in cancer patients (50 to 100 mcg SC 3 times daily for 1 to 3 days).

Pancreatic fistula – To reduce output from pancreatic fistulas. Dosages range from 50 to 200 mcg every 8 hours.

Irritable bowel syndrome – 100 mcg single dose to 125 mcg SC twice daily.

Dumping syndrome – 50 to 150 mcg/day.

Other uses for which octreotide may be beneficial include: Enteric fistula; pancreatitis; pancreatic surgery; glucagonoma; insulinoma; gastrinoma (Zollinger-Ellison syndrome); intestinal obstruction; local radiotherapy; chronic pain management; antineoplastic therapy; decrease insulin requirements in diabetes mellitus; thyrotropin- and TSH-secreting tumors.

Administration and Dosage

➤*Sandostatin administration:* Octreotide may be administered SC or IV. SC injection is the usual route of administration for control of symptoms. Pain with SC use may be reduced by using the smallest volume that will deliver the desired dose. Avoid multiple injections at the same site within short periods of time. Rotate sites in a systematic manner. The initial dosage is usually 50 mcg administered 2 or 3 times daily. Upward dose titration is usually required.

Although not an approved method of administration, continuous subcutaneous infusion (CSI) has been used to administer octreotide. Advantages to CSI include patient convenience, increased compliance, decreased injection site pain, minimization of GI side effects and continuous octreotide serum levels.

➤*Sandostatin LAR Depot administration:* Do not administer IV or SC. Administer immediately after mixing. Administer intragluteally at 4–week intervals. Avoid deltoid injections because of significant discomfort at the injection site.

➤*Acromegaly:*

Sandostatin – Dosage may be initiated at 50 mcg 3 times daily. This low dose may permit adaptation to adverse GI effects for patients who will require higher doses. IGF-I levels every 2 weeks can be used to guide titration. Alternatively, multiple growth hormone levels at 0 to 8 hours after octreotide administration permit more rapid titration of dose. The goal is to achieve growth hormone levels < 5 ng/ml or IGF-I levels < 1.9 U/ml in males and < 2.2 U/ml in females. The dose most commonly found to be effective is 100 mcg 3 times daily, but some require up to 500 mcg 3 times daily for maximum efficacy. Doses > 300 mcg/day seldom result in additional benefit. If an increase in dose fails to provide additional benefit, reduce the dose. Reevaluate IGF-I or growth hormone levels at 6 month intervals.

Withdraw octreotide yearly for ≈ 4 weeks from patients who have received irradiation to assess disease activity. If growth hormone or IGF-I levels increase and signs and symptoms recur, therapy may be resumed.

Sandostatin LAR Depot – Patients currently receiving *Sandostatin* injection can be switched directly to *Sandostatin LAR Depot* in a dose of 20 mg given IM intragluterally at 4 week intervals for 3 months. Avoid detoid injections because of significant discomfort at injection site. Alternate gluteal injection sites to avoid irritation.

At the end of 3 months *Sandostatin LAR Depot* dosage may be continued at the same level or increased or decreased based on the following regimen:

GH ≤ 2.5 ng/ml, IGF-I normal and clinical symptoms controlled, maintain *Sandostatin LAR Depot* dosage at 20 mg every 4 weeks.

GH > 2.5 ng/ml, IGF-I elevated, or clinical symptoms uncontrolled, increase *Sandostatin LAR Depot* dosage to 30 mg every 4 weeks.

GH ≤ 1 ng/ml, IGF-I normal and clinical symptoms controlled, reduce *Sandostatin LAR Depot* dosage to 10 mg every 4 weeks.

Patients whose GH, IGF-I, and symptoms are not adequately controlled at a dose of 30 mg may have the dose increased to 40 mg every 4 weeks. Doses> 40 mg are not recommended.

Administration of *Sandostatin LAR Depot* at intervals > 4 weeks is not recommended because there is no adequate information on whether such patients could be satisfactorily controlled.

In patients who have received pituitary irradiation, *Sandostatin LAR Depot* should be withdrawn yearly for ≈ 8 weeks to assess disease activity. If GH or IGF-I levels increase and signs and symptoms recur, *Sandostatin LAR Depot* therapy may be resumed.

➤*Carcinoid tumors:* The suggested daily dosage of octreotide during the first 2 weeks of therapy ranges from 100 to 600 mcg/day in 2 to 4 divided doses (mean daily dosage is 300 mcg). In the clinical studies, the median daily maintenance dosage was approximately 450 mcg, but clinical biochemical benefits were obtained in some patients with as little as 50 mcg, while others required doses up to 1500 mcg/day. However, experience with doses > 750 mcg per day is limited.

➤*VIPomas:* Daily dosages of 200 to 300 mcg in 2 to 4 divided doses are recommended during the initial 2 weeks of therapy (range, 150 to 750 mcg) to control symptoms of the disease. On an individual basis, dosage may be adjusted to achieve a therapeutic response, but usually doses > 450 mcg/day are not required.

➤*Sandostatin LAR Depot:* Patients not currently receiving octreotide acetate should begin therapy with *Sandostatin* injection given SC. The suggested daily dosage for carcinoid tumors during the first 2 weeks of therapy ranges from 100 to 600 mcg/day in 2 to 4 divided doses. Some patients may require ≤ 1500 mcg/day. The suggested daily dosage for VIPomas is 200 to 300 mcg in 2 to 4 divided doses; dosage may be adjusted on an individual basis to control symptoms but usually doses > 450 mcg/day are not required.

Continue *Sandostatin* injection for ≥ 2 weeks. Thereafter, patients who are considered "responders" to octreotide acetate and who tolerate the drug may be switched to *Sandostatin LAR Depot* in the dosage regimen described below.

Patients currently receiving *Sandostatin* can be switched to *Sandostatin LAR Depot* in a dosage of 20 mg given IM intragluteally at 4–week intervals for 2 months. Avoid deltoid injections because of significant discomfort at the injection site. Because of the need for serum octreotide to reach therapeutically effective levels following initial injection of *Sandostatin LAR Depot*, carcinoid tumor and VIPoma patients should continue to receive *Sandostatin* SC for at least 2 weeks

OCTREOTIDE ACETATE

in the same dosage used before the switch. Failure to continue SC injections for this period may result in exacerbation of symptoms.

After 2 months of a 20 mg dosage of *Sandostatin LAR Depot*, dosage may be increased to 30 mg every 4 weeks if symptoms are not adequately controlled. Patients who achieve good control on a 20 mg dose may have the dose lowered to 10 mg for a trial period. If symptoms recur, increase dosage to 20 mg every 4 weeks. However, many patients can be satisfactorily maintained at a 10 mg dosage every 4 weeks. A dose of 10 mg is not recommended as a starting dose.

Doses > 30 mg are not recommended because there is no information on their usefulness.

Despite good overall control of symptoms, patients with carcinoid tumors and VIPomas often experience periodic exacerbation of symptoms. During these periods they may be given *Sandostatin* SC for a few days at the dosage they were receiving prior to switching to *Sandostatin LAR Depot*. When symptoms are again controlled, the *Sandostatin* SC can be discontinued.

Administration of *Sandostatin LAR Depot* at intervals > 4 weeks are not recommended because there is no adequate information on whether such patients could be adequately controlled.

➤*Admixture incompatibility:* Although octreotide appears to be physically compatible in total parenteral nutrition (TPN) solutions for 48 hours at room temperature and for 7 days under refrigeration, it is not compatible in TPN solutions because of the formation of a glycosyl octreotide conjugate which may decrease its efficacy.

➤*Admixture compatibility:* Octreotide is stable in sterile isotonic saline solutions or sterile solutions of dextrose 5% in water for 24 hours. It may be diluted in volumes of 50 to 200 ml and infused IV over 15 to 30 min or administered by IV push over 3 min. In emergency situations (eg, carcinoid crisis) it may be given by rapid bolus.

➤*Storage/Stability:* For prolonged storage, store octreotide amps and multi-dose vials in the refrigerator at 2° to 8°C (36° to 46°F) and protect from light. At room temperature (20° to 30°C; 70° to 86°F), octreotide is stable for 14 days if protected from light. In one study, octreotide was stable in polypropylene syringes for up to 29 days at 3°C (37°F; protected from light) and for up to 22 days at 23°C (73°F; exposed to light). Following refrigeration, the solution can be allowed to come to room temperature prior to administration. Do not warm artificially. After initial use, discard multi-dose vials within 14 days. Open amps just prior to administration and discard the unused portion. Do not use if particulates or discoloration are observed.

Actions

➤*Pharmacology:* Octreotide acetate is a long-acting octapeptide with pharmacologic actions similar to those of the natural hormone somatostatin. It is an even more potent inhibitor of growth hormone, glucagon and insulin than somatostatin. Like somatostatin, it also suppresses LH response to GnRH, decreases splanchnic blood flow and inhibits release of serotonin, gastrin, vasoactive intestinal peptide, secretin, motilin and pancreatic polypeptide. Octreotide substantially reduces growth hormone or IGF-I (somatomedin C) levels in patients with acromegaly. Single doses inhibit gallbladder contractility and decrease bile secretion in healthy volunteers. In clinical trials, the incidence of gallstone or biliary sludge formation was markedly increased. Octreotide also suppresses secretion of thyroid stimulating hormone.

In patients with acromegaly, octreotide reduces growth hormone to within normal ranges in 50% of patients and reduces IGF-I to within normal ranges in 50% to 60% of patients. Since the effects of pituitary irradiation may not become maximal for several years, adjunctive therapy with octreotide to reduce blood levels of growth hormone and IGF-I offers potential benefit before the effects of irradiation are manifested. Improvement in clinical signs and symptoms or reduction in tumor size or rate of growth were not shown in clinical trials.

In patients with vasoactive intestinal peptide tumors, improvement has been noted in the overall condition of these otherwise therapeutically unresponsive patients. Therapy with octreotide results in improvement in electrolyte abnormalities (eg, hypokalemia), often enabling reduction of fluid and electrolyte support. Data are insufficient to determine whether the drug decreases size, rate of growth or development of metastases in patients with these tumors. Octreotide acetate was used in patients ranging in age from 1 month to 83 years without any drug limiting toxicity.

➤*Pharmacokinetics:*

Absorption/Distribution – After SC injection, octreotide is absorbed rapidly and completely from the injection site. Peak concentrations of 5.5 ng/ml (100 mcg dose) were reached 0.4 hours after dosing. IV and SC doses are bioequivalent. Peak concentrations and area under the curve values were dose-proportional both after SC or IV single doses of up to 400 mcg and with multiple doses of 200 mcg 3 times daily (600 mcg/day). Clearance was reduced by about 66% suggesting nonlinear kinetics of the drug at daily doses of 600 mcg/day as compared to 150 mcg/day.

The distribution of octreotide from plasma was rapid (alpha half-life = 0.2 hr), the volume of distribution (Vd) was estimated to be 13.6 L and total body clearance was 10 L/hr. In blood, the distribution into the erythrocytes was found to be negligible and about 65% was bound in

the plasma in a concentration-independent manner. Binding was mainly to lipoprotein and, to a lesser extent, to albumin.

Metabolism/Excretion – The elimination of octreotide from plasma had an apparent half-life of 1.7 hours compared with 1 to 3 minutes with the natural hormone. The duration of action is variable but extends up to 12 hours depending upon the type of tumor. About 32% of the dose is excreted unchanged in the urine. In elderly patients, dose adjustments may be necessary due to a significant increase in the half-life (46%) and a significant decrease in the clearance (26%) of octreotide.

In patients with acromegaly, the pharmacokinetics differ somewhat from those in healthy volunteers. A mean peak concentration of 2.8 ng/ml (100 mcg dose) was reached in 0.7 hours after SC dosing. The Vd_{ss} was estimated to be 21.6 ± 8.5 L and the total body clearance was increased to 18 L/hr. The mean percent of bound drug was 41.2%. Disposition and elimination half-lives were similar to healthy subjects.

In patients with severe renal failure requiring dialysis, clearance was reduced to about half that found in healthy subjects (from approximately 10 to 4.5 L/hr). The effect of hepatic diseases on the disposition of octreotide is unknown.

Contraindications

Sensitivity to this drug or any of its components.

Warnings

➤*Biliary tract effects:* Single doses have inhibited gallbladder contractility and decreased bile secretion in healthy volunteers. In clinical trials (primarily patients with acromegaly or psoriasis), the incidence of biliary tract abnormalities was 52% (27% gallstones, 22% sludge without stones, 3% biliary duct dilatation). Incidence of stones or sludge in patients who received the drug for ≥ 12 months was 48%. Among patients treated for ≤ 1 month, < 2% developed gallstones. The incidence of gallstones did not appear related to age, sex or dose. The majority of patients developing gallbladder abnormalities had GI symptoms which were not specific to gallbladder disease. A few patients developed acute cholecystitis, ascending cholangitis, biliary obstruction, cholestatic hepatitis or pancreatitis during therapy or following its withdrawal. One patient developed ascending cholangitis and died.

➤*Renal function impairment:* In patients with severe renal failure requiring dialysis, octreotide half-life may be increased, necessitating adjustment of maintenance dose.

➤*Elderly:* Dose adjustments may be necessary due to a significant increase in the half-life (46%) and a significant decrease in the clearance (26%) of octreotide.

➤*Pregnancy:* Category B. There are no adequate and well controlled studies in pregnant women. Use during pregnancy only if clearly needed.

➤*Lactation:* It is not known whether this drug is excreted in breast milk. Exercise caution when octreotide is administered to a nursing woman.

➤*Children:* The youngest patient to receive the drug was 1 month old. Doses of 1 to 10 mcg/kg were well tolerated in young patients. A single case of an infant (nesidioblastosis) was complicated by a seizure thought to be independent of octreotide.

Precautions

➤*Monitoring:* Laboratory tests that may be helpful as biochemical markers in determining and following patient response depend on the specific tumor. Based on diagnosis, measurement of the following substances may be useful in monitoring the progress of therapy:

Acromegaly – Growth hormone, IGF-I. Responsiveness to octreotide may be evaluated by determining growth hormone levels at 1 to 4 hour intervals for 8 to 12 hours post dose; alternatively, a single measurement of IGF-I level may be made 2 weeks after drug initiation or dosage change.

Carcinoid – 5-HIAA (urinary 5-hydroxyindole acetic acid), plasma serotonin, plasma Substance P.

VIPoma – VIP (plasma vasoactive intestinal peptide).

Perform baseline and periodic total or free T_4 measurements during chronic use.

➤*Hypo- or hyperglycemia:* Hypo- or hyperglycemia that may occur during therapy is usually mild, but may result in overt diabetes mellitus or necessitate dose changes in insulin or other hypoglycemic agents. Hypo- and hyperglycemia occurred in 3% and 15% of acromegalic patients, respectively. Severe hyperglycemia, subsequent pneumonia and death following initiation of octreotide was reported in one patient with no history of hyperglycemia.

➤*Hypothyroidism:* In acromegalic patients, 12% developed biochemical hypothyroidism, only 6% developed goiter and 4% required initiation of thyroid replacement therapy while receiving octreotide. Baseline and periodic assessment of thyroid function (TSH, total or free T_4) is recommended during chronic therapy.

➤*Cardiac effects:* In acromegalics, bradycardia (< 50 bpm) developed in 21%; conduction abnormalities and arrhythmias each occurred in 9% of patients during therapy. Other ECG changes observed included QT prolongation, axis shifts, early repolarization, low voltage, R/S transi-

OCTREOTIDE ACETATE

tion and early wave progression. These ECG changes are not uncommon in acromegalic patients. Dose adjustments in drugs such as beta blockers that have bradycardia effects may be necessary. In one acromegalic patient with severe CHF, initiation of octreotide resulted in worsening of CHF with improvement when the drug was discontinued. Confirmation of a drug effect was obtained with a positive rechallenge.

➤*Pancreatitis:* Several cases of pancreatitis occurred in patients receiving octreotide.

➤*Dietary fat:* Dietary fat absorption may be altered in some patients. Perform periodic quantitative 72-hour fecal fat and serum carotene determinations to aid in the assessment of possible drug-induced aggravation of fat malabsorption.

Drug Interactions

➤*Cyclosporine:* A single case of a transplant rejection episode (renal/whole pancreas) in a patient immunosuppressed with cyclosporine was reported. Octreotide used to reduce exocrine secretion and close a fistula in this patient resulted in decreases in blood levels of cyclosporine and may have contributed to the rejection episode.

➤*Drug/Food interactions:* Octreotide may alter the absorption of dietary fats in some patients. In addition, depressed vitamin B_{12} levels and abnormal Schilling's tests have been observed in some patients receiving octreotide; monitoring of vitamin B_{12} levels is recommended during chronic therapy.

Adverse Reactions

➤*Cardiovascular:* Sinus bradycardia (21% in acromegalics; see Precautions); conduction abnormalities, arrhythmias (9%; see Precautions); chest pain, shortness of breath, thrombophlebitis, ischemia, hypertensive reaction, CHF, hypertension, palpitations, orthostatic BP decrease, tachycardia (< 1%).

➤*CNS:* Headache (6%); dizziness, fatigue, weakness (1% to 4%); depression, anxiety, libido decrease, syncope, tremor, seizure, vertigo, Bell's palsy, paranoia, pituitary apoplexy, increased intraocular pressure (< 1%).

➤*Dermatologic:* Injection site pain (7.5%); flushing, edema, pruritus, hair loss (1% to 4%); rash, cellulitis, petechiae, urticaria (< 1%).

➤*Endocrine:* Hyperglycemia, hypoglycemia (15% and 3%, respectively, in acromegalics; 1.5% in others); biochemical hypothyroidism (12% in acromegalics; isolated cases in others; see Precautions).

Galactorrhea, hypoadrenalism, diabetes insipidus, gynecomastia, amenorrhea, polymenorrhea, vaginitis (< 1%).

➤*GI:* Diarrhea, loose stools, nausea, abdominal discomfort (30% to 58% acromegalics, 5% to 10% other disorders); frequency was not dose-related, but diarrhea and abdominal discomfort generally resolved more quickly in patients treated with 300 mcg/day than with 750 mcg/day. Vomiting, flatulence, abnormal stools, abdominal distention, constipation (< 10%); hepatitis, jaundice, increase in liver enzymes, GI bleeding, hemorrhoids and appendicitis (< 1%).

➤*GU:* Pollakiuria, urinary tract infection (1% to 4%); nephrolithiasis, hematuria (< 1%).

➤*Hematologic:* Injection site hematoma, bruise (1% to 4%); anemia, iron deficiency, epistaxis (< 1%).

➤*Respiratory:* Cold symptoms (1% to 4%); pneumonia, pulmonary nodule, status asthmaticus (< 1%).

➤*Musculoskeletal:* Backache, joint pain (1% to 4%); arthritis, joint effusion, muscle pain, Raynaud's phenomenon (< 1%).

➤*Miscellaneous:* Gallbladder abnormalities, especially stones or biliary sludge (frequent with chronic therapy; see Warnings); flu symptoms, fat malabsorption (see Drug Interactions), blurred vision (1% to 4%); otitis, allergic reaction, increased CK, visual disturbance (< 1%); anaphylactoid reactions, including anaphylactic shock (several patients).

Evaluation of 20 patients treated for at least 6 months has failed to demonstrate titers of antibodies exceeding background levels. However, antibody titers to octreotide were subsequently reported in three patients and resulted in prolonged duration of drug action in two patients.

Overdosage

IV bolus doses of 1 mg (healthy volunteers) or 30 mg IV over 20 minutes and 120 mg IV over 8 hours (research patients) have not resulted in serious ill effects.

Patient Information

Give careful instruction in sterile SC injection technique to patients and other persons who may administer octreotide.

PEGVISOMANT

Rx	Somavert (Pharmacia)	Powder for injection, lyophilized: 10 mg (as protein)/vial	In single-dose, sterile glass vial.[1]
		15 mg (as protein)/vial	In single-dose, sterile glass vial.[1]
		20 mg (as protein)/vial	In single-dose, sterile glass vial.[1]

[1] With sterile water for injection and 36 mg mannitol.

Indications

➤*Acromegaly:* For the treatment of acromegaly in patients who have had an inadequate response to surgery and/or radiation therapy and/or other medical therapies, or for whom these therapies are not appropriate. The goal of treatment is to normalize serum insulin-like growth factor-I (IGF-I) levels.

Administration and Dosage

➤*Approved by the FDA:* March 25, 2003.

Administer a loading dose of 40 mg of pegvisomant SC under physician supervision. Instruct patient to begin daily SC injections of 10 mg of pegvisomant. Measure serum IGF-I concentrations every 4 to 6 weeks, at which time the dosage of pegvisomant should be adjusted in 5-mg increments if IGF-I levels are still elevated (or 5 mg decrements if IGF-I levels have decreased below the normal range). While the goals of therapy are to achieve and then maintain serum IGF-I concentrations within the age-adjusted normal range and to alleviate the signs and symptoms of acromegaly, base titration of dosing on IGF-I levels. It is unknown whether patients who remain symptomatic while achieving normalized IGF-I levels would benefit from increased dosing with pegvisomant.

The maximum daily maintenance dose should not exceed 30 mg.

➤*Reconstitution/Administration:* Pegvisomant is supplied as a lyophilized powder. Reconstitute each vial of pegvisomant with 1 mL of the diluent provided in the package (sterile water for injection). To prepare the solution, withdraw 1 mL of sterile water for injection and inject it into the vial of pegvisomant, aiming the stream of liquid against the glass wall. Hold the vial between the palms of both hands and gently roll it to dissolve the powder. Do not shake the vial, as this may cause denaturation of pegvisomant. Discard the diluent vial containing the remaining water for injection. After reconstitution, each vial of pegvisomant contains 10, 15, or 20 mg of pegvisomant protein in 1 mL of solution. Visually inspect parenteral drug products for particulate matter and discoloration prior to administration. The solution should be clear after reconstitution. If the solution is cloudy, do not inject it. Administer only 1 dose from each vial. Administer pegvisomant within 6 hours after reconstitution.

➤*Storage/Stability:* Prior to reconstitution, store pegvisomant in a refrigerator at 2° to 8°C (36° to 46°F). Protect from freezing.

After reconstitution, administer pegvisomant within 6 hours. Administer only 1 dose from each vial.

Actions

➤*Pharmacology:* Pegvisomant is a protein of recombinant DNA origin containing 191 amino acid residues to which several polyethylene glycol (PEG) polymers are covalently bound (predominantly 4 to 6 PEG/protein molecule). It selectively binds to growth hormone (GH) receptors on cell surfaces, where it blocks the binding of endogenous GH, and thus interferes with GH signal transduction. Inhibition of GH action results in decreased serum concentrations of IGF-I, as well as other GH-responsive serum proteins, including IGF binding protein-3 (IGFBP-3) and the acid-labile subunit (ALS).

➤*Pharmacokinetics:*

Absorption – Following SC administration, peak serum concentrations are not generally attained until 33 to 77 hours after administration. The mean extent of absorption of a 20 mg SC dose was 57%, relative to a 10 mg IV dose.

Distribution – The mean apparent volume of distribution is 7 L (12% coefficient of variation), suggesting that pegvisomant does not distribute extensively into tissues. After a single SC administration, exposure (C_{max}, AUC) to pegvisomant increases disproportionately with increasing dose. Mean ± SEM serum concentrations after 12 weeks of therapy with daily doses of 10, 15, and 20 mg were approximately 6600, 16,000, and 27,000 ng/mL, respectively.

Metabolism/Excretion – The pegvisomant molecule contains covalently bound PEG polymers in order to reduce the clearance rate. Clearance of pegvisomant following multiple doses is lower than seen following a single dose. The mean total body systemic clearance following multiple doses is estimated to range between 36 to 28 mL/h for SC doses ranging from 10 to 20 mg/day, respectively. Clearance of pegvisomant was found to increase with body weight. Pegvisomant is eliminated from serum with a mean half-life of approximately 6 days following either single or multiple doses. Less than 1% of administered drug is recovered in the urine over 96 hours. The elimination route of pegvisomant has not been studied in humans.

Contraindications

History of hypersensitivity to any of its components. The stopper on the vial of pegvisomant contains latex.

Warnings

➤*Elderly:* Clinical studies of pegvisomant did not include sufficient numbers of subjects 65 years of age and older to determine whether they respond differently from younger subjects. In general, dose selection for an elderly patient should be cautious, usually starting at the low end of the dosing range, reflecting the greater frequency of decreased hepatic, renal, or cardiac function, and of concomitant disease or other drug therapy.

➤*Pregnancy: Category B.* At the 10 mg/kg/day dose (10 times the maximum human therapeutic dose based on body surface area), a reproducible, slight increase in postimplantation loss was observed in both studies. There are no adequate and well-controlled studies in pregnant women. Because animal reproduction studies are not always predictive of human responses, use pegvisomant during pregnancy only if clearly needed.

➤*Lactation:* It is not known whether pegvisomant is excreted in human milk. Because may drugs are excreted in milk, exercise caution when pegvisomant is administered to a nursing woman.

➤*Children:* The safety and efficacy of pegvisomant in pediatric patients have not been established.

Precautions

➤*Monitoring:* Evaluate treatment with pegvisomant by monitoring serum IGF-I concentrations 4 to 6 weeks after therapy is initiated or any dose adjustments are made and at least every 6 months after IGF-I levels have normalized. The goals of treatment should be to maintain a patient's serum IGF-I concentration within the age-adjusted normal range and to control the signs and symptoms of acromegaly.

➤*Tumor growth:* Tumors that secrete GH may expand and cause serious complications. Therefore, carefully monitor all patients with these tumors, including those who are receiving pegvisomant, with periodic imaging scans of the sella turcica. During clinical studies of pegvisomant, 2 patients manifested progressive tumor growth. Both patients had, at baseline, large globular tumors impinging on the optic chiasm, which had been relatively resistant to previous anti-acromegalic therapies. Overall, mean tumor size was unchanged during the course of treatment with pegvisomant in the clinical studies.

➤*Glucose metabolism:* GH opposes the effects of insulin on carbohydrate metabolism by decreasing insulin sensitivity; thus, glucose tolerance may increase in some patients treated with pegvisomant. Although none of the acromegalic patients with diabetes mellitus who were treated with pegvisomant during the clinical studies had clinically relevant hypoglycemia, carefully monitor these patients and reduce doses of antidiabetic drugs as necessary.

➤*GH deficiency:* A state of functional GH deficiency may result from administration of pegvisomant, despite the presence of elevated serum GH levels. Therefore, during treatment with pegvisomant, carefully observe patients for the clinical signs and symptoms of a GH-deficient state, and monitor and maintain serum IGF-I concentrations within the age-adjusted normal range (by adjustment of the dose of pegvisomant).

➤*Liver tests (LTs):* Elevations of srum concentrations of ALT and AST greater than 10 times the upper limit of normal (ULN) were reported in 2 patients (0.8%) exposed to pegvisomant during premarketing clinical studies. One patient was rechallenged with pegvisomant, and the recurrence of elevated transaminase levels suggested a probable causal relationship between administration of the drug and the elevation in liver enzymes. A liver biopsy performed on the second patient was consistent with chronic hepatitis of unknown etiology. In both patients, the transaminase elevations normalized after discontinuation of the drug.

During the premarketing clinical studies, the incidence of elevations in ALT greater than 3 times but less than or equal to 10 times the ULN in patients treated with pegvisomant and placebo were 1.2% and 2.1%, respectively.

Obtain baseline serum ALT, AST, total bilirubin (TBIL), and alkaline phosphatase (ALP) levels prior to initiating therapy with pegvisomant.

Initiation of Treatment with Pegvisomant Based on Results of Liver Tests	
Baseline LT levels	Recommendations
Normal	May treat with pegvisomant. Monitor LTs at monthly intervals during the first 6 months of treatment, quarterly for the next 6 months, and then biannually for the next year.
Elevated, but ≤ 3 × ULN	May treat with pegvisomant; however, monitor LTs monthly for ≥ 1 year after initiation of therapy and then biannually for the next year.

PEGVISOMANT

Initiation of Treatment with Pegvisomant Based on Results of Liver Tests	
Baseline LT levels	Recommendations
> 3 × ULN	Do not treat with pegvisomant until a comprehensive work-up establishes the cause of the patient's liver dysfunction. Determine if cholelithiasis or choledocholithiases is present, particularly in patients with a history of prior therapy with somatostatin analogs. Based on the work-up, consider initiation of therapy with pegvisomant. If the decision is to treat, very closely monitor LTs and clinical symptoms.

Continuation of Treatment with Pegvisomant Based on Results of Liver Tests	
LT levels and clinical signs/symptoms	Recommendations
≥ 3 but < 5 × ULN (without signs/symptoms of hepatitis or other liver injury, or increase in serum TBIL)	May continue therapy with pegvisomant. However, monitor LTs weekly to determine if further increases occur. In addition, perform a comprehensive hepatic workup to discern if an alternative cause of liver dysfunction is present.
≥ 5 × ULN, or transaminase elevations ≥ 3 × ULN associated with any increase in serum TBIL (with or without signs/symptoms of hepatitis or other liver injury)	Discontinue pegvisomant immediately. Perform a comprehensive hepatic workup, including serial LTs, to determine if and when serum levels return to normal. If LTs normalize (regardless of whether an alternative cause of the liver dysfunction is discovered), consider cautious reinitiation of therapy with pegvisomant, with frequent LT monitoring.
Signs or symptoms suggestive of hepatitis or other liver injury (eg, jaundice, bilirubinuria, fatigue, nausea, vomiting, right upper quadrant pain, ascites, unexplained edema, easy bruisability)	Immediately perform a comprehensive hepatic workup. If liver injury is confirmed, discontinue the drug.

➤*Lab test abnormalities:* Pegvisomant interferes with the measurement of serum GH concentrations by commercially available GH assays. Furthermore, even when accurately determined, GH levels usually increase during therapy with pegvisomant. Therefore, do not adjust treatment with pegvisomant based on serum GH concentrations.

Drug Interactions

➤*Insulin and/or oral hypoglycemic agents:* Acromegalic patients with diabetes mellitus being treated with insulin and/or oral hypoglycemic agents may require dose reductions of these therapeutic agents after the initiation of therapy with pegvisomant.

➤*Opioids:* In clinical studies, patients on opioids often needed higher serum pegvisomant concentrations to achieve appropriate IGF-I suppression compared with patients not receiving opioids. The mechanism of this interaction is not known.

➤*Drug/Lab test interactions:* Pegvisomant has significant structural similarity to GH, which causes it to cross-react in commercially available GH assays. Because serum concentrations of pegvisomant at therapeutically effective doses are generally 100 to 1000 times higher than endogenous serum GH levels seen in patients with acromegaly, commercially available GH assays will overestimate true GH levels. Therefore, do not monitor or adjust treatment with pegvisomant based on serum GH concentrations reported from these assays. Instead, only base monitoring and dose adjustments on serum IGF-I levels.

Adverse Reactions

Elevations of serum concentrations of ALT and AST greater than 10 times the ULN were reported in 2 subjects (0.8%) exposed to pegvisomant in pre-approval clinical studies.

Nine acromegalic patients (9.6%) withdrew from premarketing clinical studies because of adverse events, including 2 patients with marked transaminase elevations, one patient with lipohypertrophy at the injection sites, and one patient with substantial weight gain. The majority of reported adverse events were of mild to moderate intensity and limited duration. Most adverse events did not appear to be dose dependent. The table below shows the incidence of treatment-emergent adverse events that were reported in at least 2 patients treated with pegvisomant and at frequencies greater than placebo during the 12-week, placebo-controlled study.

Number of Patients with Acromegaly Reporting Adverse Events in a 12-week Placebo-Controlled Study with Pegvisomant (%)[1]				
	Pegvisomant			Placebo (n = 32)
Adverse Reaction	10 mg/day (n = 26)	15 mg/day (n = 26)	20 mg/day (n = 28)	
GI				
Diarrhea	4	0	14	3
Nausea	0	8	14	3
Miscellaneous				
Infection[2]	23	0	0	6
Abnormal LFTs	12	4	4	3
Accidental injury	8	4	0	3
Back pain	8	0	4	3
Dizziness	8	4	4	6
Injection site reaction	8	4	11	0
Pain	8	4	14	6
Peripheral edma	8	0	4	0
Sinusitis	8	0	4	3
Chest pain	4	8	0	0
Flu syndrome	4	12	7	0
Hypertension	0	8	0	0
Paresthesia	0	0	7	6

[1] Table includes only those events that were reported in at least 2 patients and at a higher incidence in patients treated with pegvisomant than in patients treated with placebo.
[2] The 6 events coded as "infection" in the group treated with 10 mg pegvisomant were reported as cold symptoms (3), upper respiratory infection (1), blister (1), and ear infection (1). The 2 events in the placebo group were reported as cold symptoms (1) and chest infection (1).

In premarketing clinical studies, approximately 17% of the patients developed low titer, nonneutralizing anti-GH antibodies. Although the presence of these antibodies did not appear to impact the efficacy of pegvisomant, the long-term clinical significance of these antibodies is not known. No assay for anti-pegvisomant antibodies is commercially available for patients receiving pegvisomant.

Overdosage

➤*Symptoms:* In 1 reported incident of acute overdose with pegvisomant during premarkting clinical studies, a patient self-administered 80 mg/day for 7 days. The patient experienced a slight increase in fatigue, had no other complaints, and demonstrated no significant clinical laboratory abnormalities.

➤*Treatment:* In cases of overdose, discontinue administration of pegvisomant and do not resume until IGF-I levels return to within or above the normal range.

Patient Information

Carefully instruct patients and any other people who may administer pegvisomant by a health care professional on how to properly reconstitute and inject the product. Inform patients about the need for serial monitoring of LTs, and to immediately discontinue therapy and contact their physician if they become jaundiced. In addition, patients should be made aware that serial IGF-I levels will need to be obtained to allow their physician to properly adjust the dose of pegvisomant.

LARONIDASE

Rx	Aldurazyme (BioMarin)	Injection: 2.9 mg laronidase per 5 mL	Preservative-free. In 5 mL single-use vials.[1]

[1] Contains 0.1% albumin (human) after dilution. Also contains 43.9 mg sodium chloride, 63.5 mg sodium phosphate monbasic monohydrate, 10.7 mg sodium phosphate dibasic heptahydrate.

Indications

➤*Mucopolysaccharidosis I (MPS I):* For patients with Hurler and Hurler-Scheie forms of MPS I and for patients with the Scheie form who have moderate to severe symptoms. The risks and benefits of treating mildly affected patients with the Scheie form have not been established.

Laronidase has been shown to improve pulmonary function and walking capacity.

Administration and Dosage

➤*Approved by the FDA:* April 30, 2003.

➤*Dosage:* The recommended dosage regimen of laronidase is 0.58 mg/kg administered once weekly as an IV infusion.

➤*Pretreatment:* Pretreatment with antipyretics and/or antihistamines is recommended 60 minutes prior to the start of infusion.

➤*Administration:* The total volume of the infusion is determined by the patient's body weight and should be delivered over approximately 3 to 4 hours. Patients with a body weight of 20 kg or less should receive a total volume of 100 mL. Patients with a body weight greater than 20 kg should receive a total volume of 250 mL. The initial infusion rate of 10 mcg/kg/hr may be incrementally increased every 15 minutes during the first hour, as tolerated, until a maximum infusion rate of 200 mcg/kg/hr is reached. The maximum rate is then maintained for the remainder of the infusion (2 to 3 hours). See tables below.

Administration of Laronidase for Patients Weighing 20 kg or Less	
Total volume of laronidase infusion = 100 mL	
2 mL/hr × 15 min (10 mcg/kg/hr)	Obtain vital signs; if stable then increase the rate to...
4 mL/hr × 15 min (20 mcg/kg/hr)	Obtain vital signs; if stable then increase the rate to...
8 mL/hr × 15 min (50 mcg/kg/hr)	Obtain vital signs; if stable then increase the rate to...
16 mL/hr × 15 min (100 mcg/kg/hr)	Obtain vital signs; if stable then increase the rate to...
32 mL/hr × approximately 3 hours (200 mcg/kg/hr)	For the remainder of the infusion.

Administration of Laronidase for Patients Weighing Greater than 20 kg	
Total volume of laronidase infusion = 250 mL	
5 mL/hr × 15 min (10 mcg/kg/hr)	Obtain vital signs; if stable then increase the rate to...
10 mL/hr × 15 min (20 mcg/kg/hr)	Obtain vital signs; if stable then increase the rate to...
20 mL/hr × 15 min (50 mcg/kg/hr)	Obtain vital signs; if stable then increase the rate to...
40 mL/hr × 15 min (100 mcg/kg/hr)	Obtain vital signs; if stable then increase the rate to...
80 mL/hr × approximately 3 hours (200 mcg/kg/hr)	For the remainder of the infusion.

➤*Dilution:* Dilute the concentrated infusion solution with 0.1% albumin (human) in 0.9% sodium chloride injection (see table below). Prepare laronidase using PVC containers and administer with a PVC infusion set equipped with an in-line, low protein binding 0.2 micrometer filter.

Amount of Albumin to be Added to Laronidase Infusion		
Total volume of laronidase infusion (mL)	Volume of albumin (human) 5% to be added (mL)	Volume of albumin (human) 25% to be added (mL)
100	2	0.4
250	5	1

➤*Compatibility:* Do not mix laronidase with other medicinal products in the same infusion.

➤*Storage/Stability:* Refrigerate at 2° to 8°C (36° to 46°F). Do not freeze or shake. Do not use laronidase after the expiration date on the vial. This product contains no preservatives; dispose of any unused product.

Use the dilution solution immediately. If immediate use is not possible, refrigerate the diluted solution at 2 to 8°C (36° to 46°F). The in-use storage should not be longer than 36 hours from the time of preparation to completion of administration. Room temperature storage of diluted solution is not recommended.

Actions

➤*Pharmacology:* Laronidase is a polymorphic variant of the human enzyme, α-L-iduronidase that is produced by recombinant DNA technology in a Chinese hamster ovary cell line. Mucopolysaccharide storage disorders are caused by the deficiency of specific lysosomal enzymes required for the catabolism of glycosaminoglycans (GAG). Mucopolysaccharidosis I (MPS I) is characterized by the deficiency of α-L-iduronidase, a lysosomal hydrolase that catalyses the hydrolysis of terminal α-L-iduronic acid residues of dermatan sulfate and heparan sulfate. Reduced or absent α-L-iduronidase activity results in the accumulation of the GAG substrates, dermatan sulfate, and heparan sulfate throughout the body and leads to widespread cellular, tissue, and organ dysfunction.

The rationale of laronidase therapy in MPS I is to provide exogenous enzyme for uptake into lysosomes and increase the catabolism of GAG. Laronidase uptake by cells into lysosomes is most likely mediated by the mannose-6-phosphate-terminated oligosaccharide chains of laronidase binding to specific mannose-6-phosphate receptors.

Most patients who received once-weekly infusions of laronidase developed antibodies to laronidase by week 12. Laronidase has a specific activity of approximately 172 U/mg.

➤*Pharmacokinetics:*

Absorption/Distribution – The pharmacokinetics of laronidase were evaluated in 12 patients with MPS I who received 0.58 mg/kg of laronidase as a 4-hour infusion. After the 1st, 12th, and 26th weekly infusions, the mean maximum plasma concentrations (C_{max}) ranged from 1.2 to 1.7 mcg/mL for the 3 time points. The mean area under the plasma concentration-time curve (AUC_∞) ranged from 4.5 to 6.9 mcg•h/mL. The mean volume of distribution (V_z) ranged from 0.24 to 0.6 L/kg.

Metabolism/Excretion – Mean plasma clearance (CL) ranged from 1.7 to 2.7 mL/min/kg, and the mean elimination half-life ($t_{1/2}$) ranged from 1.5 to 3.6 hours. Between weeks 1 and 12, increases in plasma clearance of laronidase were observed in some patients that appeared to be proportional to the antibody titer. At week 26, plasma clearance of laronidase was comparable to that at week 1 in spite of the continued and, in some cases, increased titers of antibodies.

Warnings

➤*Hypersensitivity reactions:* Patients treated with laronidase may develop infusion-related hypersensitivity reactions (see Adverse Reactions). In the clinical studies, 1 patient developed an anaphylactic reaction approximately 3 hours after the initiation of the infusion. The reaction consisted of urticaria and airway obstruction. Resuscitation required an emergency tracheostomy. This patient's pre-existing MPS I related upper airway obstruction may have contributed to the severity of this reaction.

Some infusion-related reactions may be ameliorated by slowing the rate of infusion or treatment with additional antipyretics and/or antihistamines. If severe hypersensitivity or anaphylactic reactions occur, immediately discontinue the infusion of laronidase and initiate appropriate treatment. Exercise caution if epinephrine is being considered for use in patients with MPS I due to the increased prevalance of coronary artery disease in these patients.

Consider the risks and benefits of re-administering laronidase following a severe hypersensitivity or anaphylactic reaction. Exercise extreme care, with appropriate resuscitation measures available, if the decision is made to re-administer the product.

➤*Pregnancy: Category B.* Reproduction studies have been performed in male and female rats at doses up to 6.2 times the human dose and have revealed no evidence of impaired fertility or harm to the fetus caused by laronidase. However, there are no adequate and well-controlled studies in pregnant women. Use laronidase during pregnancy only if clearly needed.

➤*Lactation:* It is not known whether the drug is excreted in human milk. Because many drugs are excreted in human milk, exercise caution when laronidase is administered to a nursing woman.

➤*Children:* Safety and efficacy in patients under 5 years of age have not been established.

Precautions

➤*Pretreatment:* Patients should receive antipyretics and/or antihistamines prior to infusion. If an infusion reaction occurs, regardless of pretreatment, decreasing the infusion rate, temporarily stopping the infusion, and/or administration of additional antipyretics and/or antihistamines may ameliorate the symptoms.

➤*Immunogenicity:* Fifty of 55 patients (91%) treated with laronidase were positive for antibodies to laronidase. The clinical significance of antibodies to laronidase is not known, including the potential for product neutralization.

LARONIDASE

Four patients in the controlled study who experienced severe infusion-related reactions were tested for laronidase specific IgE antibodies and complement activation. One of the 4 patients had an anaphylactic reaction consisting of urticaria and airway obstruction and tested positive for both laronidase specific IgE binding antibodies and complement activation.

Adverse Reactions

The most serious adverse reaction reported with laronidase was an anaphylactic reaction consisting of urticaria and airway obstruction, which occurred in 1 patient. Pre-existing upper airway obstruction may have contributed to the severity of the reaction.

The most common adverse reactions associated with laronidase treatment in the clinical studies were upper respiratory tract infection, rash, and injection site reaction (see table below).

The most common adverse reactions requiring intervention were infusion-related reactions, particularly flushing. Most infusion-related reactions requiring intervention were ameliorated with slowing the infusion rate, temporarily stopping the infusion, and/or administering additional antipyretics and/or antihistamines.

Adverse Reactions and Selected Laboratory Abnormalities in the Placebo-Controlled Study (%)		
Adverse reaction	Laronidase (N = 22)	Placebo (N = 23)
Abscess	9	0
Bilirubinemia	9	0
Chest pain	9	0
Corneal opacity	9	0
Dependent edema	9	0
Facial edema	9	0
Hyperreflexia	14	0
Hypotension	9	0

Adverse Reactions and Selected Laboratory Abnormalities in the Placebo-Controlled Study (%)		
Adverse reaction	Laronidase (N = 22)	Placebo (N = 23)
Injection site pain	9	0
Injection site reaction	18	9
Paresthesia	14	4
Rash	36	22
Thrombocytopenia	9	0
Upper respiratory tract infection	32	17
Vein disorder	14	4

➤*Infusion-related reactions:* Infusion-related reactions were reported in 7 of 22 patients treated with laronidase. Infusion-related reactions were not significantly different between the laronidase treatment group and the placebo group, who received infusions of diluent and all components of laronidase except the laronidase enzyme. The most common infusion-related reactions included flushing, fever, headache, and rash. Flushing occurred in 5 patients (23%) receiving laronidase; the other reactions were less frequent. All were mild to moderate in severity. The frequency of infusion-related reactions decreased with continued use during the open-label extended use period. There was 1 case of anaphylaxis during the open-label extension period (see Warnings). Less common infusion-related reactions include cough, bronchospasm, dyspnea, urticaria, angioedema, and pruritus.

Patient Information

Inform patients that a registry for MPS I patients has been established in order to better understand the variability and progression of MPS I disease, and to continue to monitor and evaluate treatments. Encourage patients to participate and advise them that their participation may involve long-term follow-up. Information regarding the registry program may be found at http://www.MPSIregistry.com or by calling (800) 745-4447.

AGALSIDASE BETA

Rx   **Fabrazyme** (Genzyme)

	Powder for injection, lyophilized: 5.5 mg (5 mg/mL when reconstituted)	Preservative free. In 5 mL single-use vials.[a]
	37 mg (5 mg/mL when reconstituted)	Preservative free. In 20 mL single-use vials.[b]

[a] Contains 33 mg mannitol, 3 mg sodium phosphate monobasic monohydrate, 8.8 mg sodium phosphate dibasic heptahydrate per vial.

[b] Contains 222 mg mannitol, 20.4 mg sodium phosphate monobasic monohydrate, 59.2 mg sodium phosphate dibasic heptahydrate per vial.

Indications

➤*Fabry disease:* For use in patients with Fabry disease. Agalsidase beta reduces globotriaosylceramide (GL-3) deposition in capillary endothelium of the kidney and certain other cell types.

Administration and Dosage

➤*Approved by the FDA:* April 24, 2003.

The recommended dosage of agalsidase beta is 1 mg/kg infused every 2 weeks as an IV infusion.

The initial IV infusion rate should be no more than 0.25 mg/min (15 mg/hr). The infusion rate may be slowed in the event of infusion-associated reactions. After patient tolerance to the infusion is well established, the infusion rate may be increased in increments of 0.05 to 0.08 mg/min (increments of 3 to 5 mg/hr) each subsequent infusion. Thirty-one of 58 (53%) patients have received infusions at rates of 33 mg/hr or more.

➤*Pretreatment:* Patients should receive antipyretics prior to infusion.

➤*Reconstitution:* Select a combination of 35 and 5 mg vials so that the total number of milligrams is greater than or equal to the patient's number of kilograms of body weight.

Avoid shaking or agitation of this product. Do not use filter needles during the preparation of the infusion. Allow agalsidase beta vials and diluent to reach room temperature prior to reconstitution (approximately 30 minutes). Reconstitute each 37 mg vial of agalsidase by slowly injecting 7.2 mL of sterile water for injection down the inside wall of the vial. Roll and tilt each vial gently. Total extractable amount per vial is 35 mg/7 mL.

Reconstitute each 5 mg vial of agalsidase by slowly injecting 1.1 mL of sterile water or injection down the inside wall of each vial. Roll and tilt each vial gently. Total extractable amount per vial is 5 mg/mL.

➤*Dilution:* Further dilute the reconstituted solution with 0.9% sodium chloride injection to a final total volume of 500 mL. Prior to adding the volume of reconstituted agalsidase beta required for the patient dose, remove an equal volume of 0.9% sodium chloride for injection from the 500 mL infusion bag. Discard any vial with unused reconstituted solution. Gently invert infusion bag to mix the solution, avoiding vigorous shaking and agitation.

➤*Administration:* Patient dose (in milligrams) divided by 5 mg/mL is equal to the number of milliliters of reconstituted agalsidase required for patient dose.

The diluted solution may be filtered through an in-line, low protein-binding, 0.2 micron filter during administration.

Do not infuse agalsidase beta in the same IV line with other products.

➤*Storage / Stability:* Vials are for single use only. Refrigerate between 2° to 8°C (36° to 46°F). Do not use agalsidase beta after the expiration date on the vial. Use reconstituted and diluted solutions of agalsidase beta immediately. This product contains no preservatives. If immediate use is not possible, the reconstituted and diluted solution may be stored up to 24 hours at 2° to 8°C (36° to 46°F). Discard any unused product.

Actions

➤*Pharmacology:* Agalsidase beta is recombinant human alpha-galactosidase A enzyme with the same amino acid sequence as the native enzyme. Agalsidase beta is produced by recombinant DNA technology in a Chinese hamster ovary mammalian cell expression system. Agalsidase beta is intended to provide an exogenous source of α-galactosidase A in Fabry disease patients. Alpha-galactosidase A catalyzes the hydrolysis of GL-3 and other α-galactyl-terminated neutral glycosphingolipids, such as galabiosylceramide and blood group B substances to ceramide dihexoside and galactose. The specific activity of agalsidase beta is approximately 70 U/mg.

Fabry disease is an X-linked genetic disorder of glycosphingolipid metabolism. Deficiency of the lysosomal enzyme α-galactosidase A leads to progressive accumulation of glycosphingolipids, predominantly GL-3, in many body tissues occurring over a period of years or decades. Clinical manifestations of Fabry disease include renal failure, cardiomyopathy, and cerebrovascular accidents. Accumulation of GL-3 in renal endothelial cells may play a role in renal failure.

➤*Pharmacokinetics:*

Absorption / Distribution – Plasma profiles of agalsidase beta were studied at 0.3, 1, and 3 mg/kg in 15 patients with Fabry disease. AUC and clearance did not increase proportionally with increasing doses, demonstrating that the enzyme follows nonlinear pharmacokinetics.

In 11 patients with Fabry disease given 1 mg/kg agalsidase beta every 14 days for a total of 11 infusions, the pharmacokinetic responses following repeated dosing fell into 3 categories. In some patients, pharma-cokinetic responses were maintained with repeated dosing, whereas in other patients, pharmacokinetic values decreased at infusion 7 relative to baseline and returned to baseline values by infusion 11. In the remaining patients, AUC declined and failed to return to baseline by infusion 11. In these patients, the average AUC was 25% of its initial level. Some patients with elevated titers of antibody to agalsidase were among those with decreased AUC. The development of antibodies to agalsidase did not influence half-life, but reduced apparent C_{max} and AUC. The long-term consequence of antibody development of the pharmacokinetics of agalsidase has not been established.

Metabolism / Excretion – Terminal half-life was dose independent, with a range of 45 to 102 minutes.

Warnings

➤*Infusion reactions:* Infusion reactions occurred in many patients treated with agalsidase beta (see Adverse Reactions). Some of the reactions were severe. Infusion reactions included fever, rigors, chest tightness, hypertension, hypotension, pruritus, myalgia, dyspnea, urticaria, abdominal pain, and headache. All patients were pretreated with acetaminophen and an antihistamine. Infusion reactions occurred in some patients after receiving antipyretics, antihistamines, and oral steroids.

Give patients antipyretics prior to infusion. If an infusion reaction occurs, regardless of pretreatment, decreasing the infusion rate, temporarily stopping the infusion, and/or administration of additional antipyretics, antihistamines, and/or steroids may ameliorate the symptoms. Because of the potential for severe infusion reactions, appropriate medical support measures should be readily available when agalsidase beta is administered.

➤*Women:* Fabry disease is an X-linked genetic disorder. However, some heterozygous women will develop signs and symptoms of Fabry disease due to the variability of the X chromosome inactivation within cells. Generally, the rates of progression of organ impairment are slower than in male Fabry disease patients and severity of signs and symptoms is variable.

➤*Pregnancy: Category B.* Reproduction studies have been performed in rats at doses up to 30 times the human dose and have revealed no evidence of impaired fertility or negative effects on embryo fetal development due to agalsidase beta. However, there are no adequate and well-controlled studies in pregnant women. Use this drug during pregnancy only if clearly needed. Encourage women of childbearing potential to enroll in the Fabry patient registry (see Patient Information).

➤*Lactation:* It is not known whether agalsidase beta is excreted in human milk. Because many drugs are excreted in human milk, exercise caution when agalsidase beta is administered to a nursing woman. Encourage nursing mothers to enroll in the Fabry patient registry (see Patient Information).

➤*Children:* The safety and efficacy of agalsidase beta in children have not been established.

Precautions

➤*Cardiac function:* Patients with advanced Fabry disease may have compromised cardiac function, which may predispose them to a higher risk of severe complications from infusion reactions (see Warnings). Closely monitor patients with compromised cardiac function if the decision is made to administer agalsidase beta.

➤*Immunogenicity:* Most patients develop IgG antibodies to agalsidase beta. Some patients developed IgE or skin test reactivity specific to agalsidase beta. Physicians should consider testing for IgE in patients who experienced suspected allergic reactions and consider the risks and benefits of continued treatment in patients with anti-agalsidase beta IgE.

There are no marketed tests for antibodies against agalsidase beta. If testing is warranted, contact your local Genzyme representative or Genzyme Corporation at (800) 745-4447.

Sixty-three of 71 (89%) patients in the clinical studies treated with agalsidase beta have developed antibodies to agalsidase beta. Most patients who develop antibodies do so within the first 3 months of exposure. Antibodies to agalsidase beta were purified from 15 patients with high antibody titers (at least 12,800) and studied for inhibition of in vitro enzyme activity. Under the conditions of this assay, most of these 15 patients had inhibition of in vitro enzyme activity ranging between 14% to 74% at 1 or more timepoints during the study. No general pattern was seen in individual patient reactivity over time. The clinical significance of binding and/or inhibitory antibodies to agalsidase beta is not known. In patients followed in the open-label study, reduction of GL-3 in plasma and GL-3 inclusions in superficial skin capillaries was maintained after antibody formation.

AGALSIDASE BETA

Adverse Reactions

The most serious and most common adverse reactions reported with agalsidase beta are infusion reactions. Serious and/or frequently occurring infusion reactions consisted of 1 or more of the following: Tachycardia, hypertension, throat tightness, chest pain/tightness, dyspnea, fever, chills/rigors, abdominal pain, pruritus, urticaria, nausea, vomiting, lip or ear edema, and rash (see Warnings). Infusion reactions declined in frequency with continued use of agalsidase beta. However, serious infusion reactions may occur after extended durations of agalsidase beta treatment.

Other reported serious adverse events included stroke, pain, ataxia, bradycardia, cardiac arrhythmia, cardiac arrest, decreased cardiac output, vertigo, hypoacousia, and nephrotic syndrome. These adverse events also occur as manifestations of Fabry disease; an alteration in frequency or severity cannot be determined from the small numbers of patients studied.

The data described below reflect exposure of 29 patients to 1 mg/kg agalsidase beta every 2 weeks for 5 months in a placebo-controlled study. All 58 patients continued into an open-label extension study of agalsidase beta treatment for up to 30 additional months. An additional 28 patients received open-label treatment. All patients were treated with antipyretics and antihistamines prior to the infusions.

Agalsidase Beta Adverse Reactions (%)		
Adverse Reaction	Agalsidase beta (N = 29)	Placebo (N = 29)
Cardiovascular		
Edema (dependent)	21	3
Hypotension	14	7
Hypertension	10	0
Cardiomegaly	10	3
CNS		
Headache	45	38
Anxiety	28	17
Dizziness	14	7
Depression	10	3

Agalsidase Beta Adverse Reactions (%)		
Adverse Reaction	Agalsidase beta (N = 29)	Placebo (N = 29)
GI		
Nausea	28	14
Dyspepsia	10	3
Musculoskeletal		
Skeletal pain	21	0
Arthrosis	10	0
Respiratory		
Rhinitis	38	24
Pharyngitis	28	7
Bronchitis	10	3
Bronchospasm	7	0
Laryngitis	7	0
Sinusitis	7	0
Miscellaneous		
Rigors	52	14
Fever	48	17
Pain	21	10
Chest pain	17	10
Temperature change sensation	17	3
Pallor	14	3
Paresthesia	14	7
Testicular pain	7	0

Overdosage

There have been no reports of overdose with agalsidase beta. In clinical trials, patients received doses up to 3 mg/kg body weight.

Patient Information

Inform patients that a registry has been established in order to better understand the variability and progression of Fabry disease in the population as a whole and in women, and to monitor and evaluate long-term treatment effects of agalsidase beta. The registry will also monitor the effect of agalsidase beta on pregnant women and their offspring, and determine if agalsidase is excreted in breast milk. Encourage patients to participate and advise them that their participation is voluntary and may involve long-term follow-up. For more information visit http://www.fabryregistry.com or call (800) 745-4447.

MIGLUSTAT

| Rx | **Zavesca** (Actelion) | **Capsules:** 100 mg | Sodium starch glucollate. (OGT 918, 100). White, opaque. Gelatin. In 90s and blister card 18s. |

Indications

➤*Gaucher disease:* For the treatment of adult patients with mild to moderate type 1 Gaucher disease for whom enzyme replacement therapy is not a therapeutic option (eg, because of constraints such as allergy, hypersensitivity, or poor venous access).

The efficacy and safety of miglustat has not been evaluated in patients with severe type 1 Gaucher disease, defined as a hemoglobin concentration below 9 g/dL, a platelet count below 50×10^9/L, or active bone disease.

Administration and Dosage

➤*Approved by the FDA:* July 31, 2003.

The recommended dose for the treatment of adult patients with type 1 Gaucher disease is one 100 mg capsule administered orally 3 times/day at regular intervals. May be taken with or without food.

It may be necessary to reduce the dose to one 100 mg capsule once or twice/day in some patients for adverse effects such as diarrhea or tremor.

➤*Renal insufficiency:* In patients with mild renal impairment (adjusted creatinine clearance [Ccr] 50 to 70 mL/min/1.73 m^2), start miglustat at a dose of 100 mg twice daily. In patients with moderate renal impairment (adjusted Ccr of 30 to 50 mL/min/1.73 m^2), start at a dose of 100 mg/day. Use of miglustat in patients with severe renal impairment (Ccr of less than 30 mL/min/1.73 m^2) is not recommended.

➤*Storage/Stability:* Store at 20° to 25°C (68° to 77°F). Brief exposure to 15° to 30°C (59° to 86°F) permitted.

Actions

➤*Pharmacology:* Miglustat is an N-alkylated imino sugar, a synthetic analogue of D-glucose, and functions as a competitive and reversible inhibitor of the enzyme glucosylceramide synthase, the initial enzyme in a series of reactions that result in the synthesis of most glycosphingolipids. The goal of treatment with miglustat is to reduce the rate of glycosphingolipid biosynthesis so that the amount of glycosphingolipid substrate is reduced to a level that allows the residual activity of the deficient glucocerebrosidase enzyme to be more effective (substrate reduction therapy).

Type 1 Gaucher disease is caused by a functional deficiency of glucocerebrosidase, the enzyme that mediates the degradation of the glycosphingolipid glucosylceramide. The failure to degrade glucosylceramide results in the lysosomal storage of this material within tissue macrophages, leading to widespread pathology. Macrophages containing stored glucosylceramide are typically found in the liver, spleen, and bone marrow and occasionally in the lung, kidney, and intestine. Secondary hematologic consequences include severe anemia and thrombocytopenia in addition to the characteristic progressive hepatosplenomegaly. Skeletal complications include osteonecrosis and osteopenia with secondary pathological fractures.

➤*Pharmacokinetics:*

Absorption – The time to maximize observed plasma concentration of miglustat (T_{max}) ranged from 2 to 2.5 hours in Gaucher patients. Plasma concentrations show a biexponential decline, characterized by a short distribution phase and a longer elimination phase. The effective half-life of miglustat is approximately 6 to 7 hours, which predicts that steady state will be achieved by 1.5 to 2 days following the start of 3 times daily dosing.

Coadministration of miglustat with food results in a decrease in the rate of absorption and C_{max} was decreased by 36% and T_{max} delayed 2 hours. The mean oral bioavailability is about 97% relative to an oral solution administered under fasting conditions.

Distribution – Miglustat does not bind to plasma proteins. Mean apparent volume of distribution of miglustat is 83 to 105 L in Gaucher patients, indicating that miglustat distributes into extravascular tissues.

Excretion – The major route of excretion is renal. Miglustat is excreted unchanged in the urine. Renal impairment has a significant effect on the pharmacokinetics of miglustat, resulting in increased systemic exposure of miglustat in such patients.

Special populations –

Renal function impairment: Patients with Fabry disease and impaired renal function indicate that clearance of miglustat decreases with decreasing renal function. The data suggest an approximate decrease in clearance of 40% and 60%, respectively, in mild and moderate renal impairment, justifying the need to decrease the dosing of miglustat in such patients dependent upon Ccr levels. Data in severe renal impairment are limited to 2 patients with Ccr in the range 18 to 29 mL/min and cannot be extrapolated below this range. These data suggest a decrease in clearance by at least 70% in patients with severe renal impairment. Treatment with miglustat in patients with severe renal impairment is, therefore, not recommended (see Dosage and Administration).

➤*Clinical trials:* In a study, 36 adult patients with type 1 Gaucher disease who had been receiving enzyme replacement therapy with cerezyme for a minimum of 2 years prior to study entry were randomized to 1 of 3 treatment groups, as follows: Miglustat 100 mg 3 times/day alone; cerezyme (patient's usual dose) alone; miglustat 100 mg 3 times/day plus cerezyme (usual dose). Patients were treated for 6 months.

At month 6, the results showed a significant decrease in mean percent change in liver volume in the combination treatment group compared to the cerezyme alone group. There were no significant differences between the groups for mean absolute changes in liver and spleen volume and hemoglobin concentration. However, there was a significant difference between the miglustat alone and cerezyme alone groups in platelet counts at month 6, with the miglustat alone group having a mean absolute decrease in platelet count of 21.6×10^9/L and the cerezyme alone group having a mean absolute increase in platelet count of 10.1×10^9/L.

Twenty-nine patients were enrolled in a 6-month extension study. There were significant decreases in platelet counts from month 6 to month 12 in the 2 groups originally randomized to treatment with cerezyme and to combination therapy, and a continued decrease in platelet counts in the group originally randomized to miglustat alone. In adult type 1 Gaucher disease patients who had been treated with enzyme replacement therapy for at least 2 years, switching to miglustat as monotherapy was associated with decreases in platelet counts after discontinuation of enzyme replacement therapy. Platelet counts also declined after discontinuation of enzyme replacement therapy in patients treated with combination therapy.

Contraindications

Hypersensitivity to the active substance or any of the excipients; in women who are or may become pregnant.

Warnings

➤*Peripheral neuropathy:* Cases of peripheral neuropathy have been reported in patients treated with miglustat. Advise all patients undergoing miglustat treatment to undergo baseline and repeat neurological evaluations at approximately 6-month intervals. Carefully reassess the risk/benefit of miglustat therapy in patients who develop symptoms such as numbness and tingling. Cessation of treatment may be considered.

➤*Renal function impairment:* Miglustat is known to be substantially excreted by the kidney, and the risk of adverse reactions to this drug may be greater in patients with impaired renal function. Clearance decreased by 40% to 60% in patients with mild to moderate renal impairment, and up to 70% in patients with severe renal impairment. Dose reductions are recommended for those patients with mild to moderate renal impairment, the reduction being dependent upon the level of their Ccr adjustment. For those patients with severe renal impairment, treatment with miglustat is not recommended. Because elderly patients are more likely to have decreased renal function, exercise caution in dose selection and monitor renal function.

➤*Fertility impairment:* Male rats, given 20 mg/kg/day miglustat by oral gavage 14 days prior to mating, had decreased spermatogenesis with altered sperm morphology and motility and decreased fertility. Decreased spermatogenesis was reversible following 6 weeks of drug withdrawal. A higher dose of 60 mg/kg/day resulted in seminiferous tubule and testicular atrophy/degeneration.

Female rats were given oral gavage doses of 20, 60, 180 mg/kg/day beginning 14 days before mating and continuing through gestation. Effects observed at 20 mg/kg/day included decreased corpora lutea, increased postimplantation loss, and decreased live births.

➤*Elderly:* Make dose selection for an elderly patient with caution, usually starting at the low end of the dosing range, reflecting the greater frequency of decreased hepatic, renal, and cardiac function and of concomitant disease or other drug therapy.

➤*Pregnancy: Category X.* There are no adequate and well-controlled studies of miglustat in pregnant women. Miglustat should not be used during pregnancy.

Miglustat is contraindicated in women who are or may become pregnant. If this drug is administered to a woman with reproductive potential, apprise the patient of the potential hazard to the fetus. Male patients should maintain reliable contraceptive methods while taking miglustat and for 3 months after stopping the drug.

Miglustat may cause fetal harm when administered to a pregnant woman. In female rats given miglustat by oral gavage at doses of 20, 60, 180 mg/kg/day beginning 14 days before mating and continuing through gestation day 17, decreased live births including complete litter loss and decreased fetal weight were observed in the mid- and high-dose groups. In pregnant rats given miglustat by oral gavage at doses of 20, 60, 180 mg/kg/day from gestation day 6 through lactation, dystocia and delayed parturition were observed in the mid- and high-dose groups. In addition, decreased live births and pup body weights were observed at more than 20 mg/kg/day.

MIGLUSTAT

In pregnant rabbits given miglustat by oral gavage at doses of 15, 30, 45 mg/kg/day during gestation days 6 through 18, maternal death and decreased body weight gain were observed at 15 mg/kg/day.

►*Lactation:* It is not known whether miglustat is excreted in human milk. Because many drugs are excreted in human milk and because of the potential for serious adverse reactions in nursing infants from miglustat, the drug should not be used in nursing mothers unless the potential benefit justifies the potential risk to the infant. A decision should be made whether to discontinue nursing or discontinue the drug, taking into account the importance of the drug to the lactating mother.

Studies in pregnant rats exposed to miglustat during gestation through lactation are associated with dystocia and delayed parturition at systemic exposure 2 times the human therapeutic systemic exposure.

►*Children:* The safety and efficacy of miglustat have not been evaluated in patients younger than 18 years of age. Treatment with miglustat is associated with diarrhea and weight loss in approximately 85% and up to 65%, respectively, of adult patients. The effects of miglustat on growth and development in children have not been evaluated.

Precautions

►*Monitoring:* Advise all patients undergoing miglustat treatment to undergo baseline and repeat neurological evaluations at approximately 6-month intervals.

►*Tremor:* Approximately 30% of patients have reported tremors or exacerbation of existing tremors on treatment. These tremors were described as an exaggerated physiological tremor of the hands. Tremor usually began in the first month of therapy and in many cases resolved between 1 to 3 months during treatment. Dose reduction may usually ameliorate the tremor within days, but discontinuation with treatment may sometimes be required.

►*Diarrhea and weight loss:* Diarrhea and weight loss were common in clinical studies of patients treated with miglustat, approximately 85% and up to 65%, respectively. Diarrhea appears to be the result of the disaccharidase inhibitory activity of miglustat, with a resultant osmotic diarrhea. It is unclear if weight loss results from the diarrhea and associated GI complaints, a decrease in food intake, or a combination of these or other factors. The incidence of diarrhea was noted to decrease over time with continued miglustat treatment and was noted to result in an increase in the use of antidiarrheal medications, most commonly loperamide. The incidence of weight loss was most evident in the first 12 months of treatment.

Adverse Reactions

Adverse Reactions in ≥ 5% of Patients in Two Trials of Miglustat (%)		
Adverse reaction	Study 1 (starting dose 100 mg 3 times/day) (N = 28)	Study 2 (50 mg 3 times/day) (N = 18)
CNS		
Headache	21	22
Tremor	11	11
Paresthesia	7	0
Cramps (legs)	4	11
Dizziness	0	11
Migraine	0	6
GI		
Diarrhea	89	89
Flatulence	29	44
Abdominal pain	18	50
Nausea	14	22
Anorexia	7	0
Dyspepsia	7	0
Vomiting	4	11
Bloating	0	6
Epigastric pain (not food-related)	0	6
Miscellaneous		
Weight decrease	39	67
Thrombocytopenia	7	6

Adverse Reactions in ≥ 5% of Patients in Two Trials of Miglustat (%)		
Adverse reaction	Study 1 (starting dose 100 mg 3 times/day) (N = 28)	Study 2 (50 mg 3 times/day) (N = 18)
Visual disturbance	0	17
Cramps	0	11
Menstrual disorder	0	6

Adverse Reactions in ≥ 5% of Patients in Controlled Study (%)			
Adverse reaction	Miglustat alone (N = 12)	Cerezyme alone (N = 12)	Miglustat plus cerezyme (N = 12)
CNS			
Tremor	17	0	33
Dizziness	8	0	25
Cramps (legs)	8	0	0
Gait unsteady	8	0	0
Memory loss	8	0	0
Numbness localized	0	0	8
Shaking	0	0	8
Appetite absent	0	0	8
Jitteriness	0	0	8
GI			
Diarrhea	100	0	83
Abdominal pain	67	0	58
Flatulence	50	0	42
Constipation	8	0	25
Abdominal distension	8	0	8
Nausea	8	0	8
Dry mouth	8	0	0
Abdominal distension (gaseous)	8	0	0
Special Senses			
Eye abnormality	0	0	8
Visual disturbance	0	0	8
Miscellaneous			
Weight decrease	67	0	42
Generalized weakness	17	0	8
Back pain	8	0	0
Heaviness in limbs	8	0	0
Pain	0	8	8
Chills	0	0	8
Influenza-like symptoms	0	0	8
Pain (legs)	0	0	8
Menstrual irregularity	0	0	8

Overdosage

Miglustat has been administered at doses of up to 3000 mg/day (approximately 10 times the recommended starting dose administered to Gaucher patients) for up to 6 months in human immunodeficiency virus (HIV)-positive patients. Adverse events observed in the HIV studies included granulocytopenia, dizziness, and paresthesia. Leukopenia and neutropenia also have been observed in a similar group of patients receiving 800 mg/day or above.

Patient Information

Advise patients that diarrhea, GI complaints, and weight loss are common side effects of therapy, and to adhere to dietary instructions. Also advise patients to promptly report any numbness, pain, or burning in the hands and feet, and the development of tremor or worsening in an existing tremor.

Instruct patients to avoid high carbohydrate content foods during treatment with miglustat if they present with diarrhea.

Advise male patients to maintain reliable contraceptive methods while taking miglustat. Before seeking to conceive, advise male patients to cease miglustat and maintain reliable contraceptive methods for 3 months thereafter.

IMIGLUCERASE

Rx **Cerezyme** (Genzyme)	**Powder for injection, lyophilized:** Preservative free. In vials. [1] 212 units (equiv. to a withdrawal dose of 200 units imiglucerase).

[1] Contains 155 mg mannitol and 70 mg sodium citrate (52 mg trisodium citrate, 18 mg disodium hydrogen citrate) per vial.

Indications

➤*Gaucher's disease:* Long-term enzyme replacement therapy for patients with a confirmed diagnosis of Type 1 Gaucher's disease that results in one or more of the following conditions: Anemia; thrombocytopenia; bone disease; hepatomegaly; splenomegaly.

Administration and Dosage

➤*Approved by the FDA:* March 23, 1994 (1P Classification).

Administered by IV infusion over 1 to 2 hours. Individualize dosage.

➤*Initial dosage:* Initial dosage may be as little as 2.5 U/kg 3 times a week up to as much as 60 U/kg administered as frequently as once a week or as infrequently as every 4 weeks; 60 U/kg every 2 weeks is the dosage for which the most data are available. Disease severity may dictate that treatment be initiated at a relatively high dose or relatively frequent administration.

➤*Maintenance:* After patient response is well established, a reduction in dosage may be attempted for maintenance therapy. Progressive reductions can be made at intervals of 3 to 6 months while carefully monitoring response parameters.

➤*Preparation of solution:* On the day of use, after the correct amount of imiglucerase to be administered to the patient has been determined, the appropriate number of vials are each reconstituted with 5.1 ml of Sterile Water for Injection, USP, to give a reconstituted volume of 5.3 ml (40 U/ml). A 5 ml volume is then withdrawn from each vial and pooled with 0.9% Sodium Chloride Injection, USP, to a final volume of 100 to 200 ml. Alternatively the appropriate dose of imiglucerase may be administered such that a rate of no greater than 1 U/ kg/ min is infused. Relatively low toxicity, combined with the extended time course of response, allows small dosage adjustments to be made occasionally to avoid discarding partially used bottles. Thus, the dosage administered in individual infusions may be slightly increased or decreased to fully utilize each vial as long as the monthly administered dosage remains substantially unaltered.

➤*Storage / Stability:* Store at 2° to 8°C (36° to 46°F). Any vials exhibiting particulate matter or discoloration should not be used. DO NOT USE imiglucerase after the expiration date on the vial. Since imiglucerase does not contain any preservative, after reconstitution, properly dilute vials and do not store for subsequent use. When diluted to 50 ml, imiglucerase is stable for up to 24 hours when stored at 2° to 8°C (36° to 46°F).

Actions

➤*Pharmacology:* Imiglucerase is an analogue of the human enzyme β-glucocerebrosidase, a lysosomal glycoprotein enzyme which catalyzes the hydrolysis of the glycolipid glucocerebroside to glucose and ceramide. Imiglucerase is produced by recombinant DNA technology using mammalian cell culture (Chinese hamster ovary). Purified imiglucerase is a monomeric glycoprotein of 497 amino acids. It differs from placental glucocerebrosidase by one amino acid at position 495 where histidine is substituted for arginine. The modified structures on imiglucerase are somewhat different from those on placental glucocerebrosidase. These mannose-terminated oligosaccharide chains of imiglucerase are specifically recognized by endocytic carbohydrate receptors on macrophages, the cells that accumulate lipid in Gaucher's disease.

Gaucher's disease is characterized by a deficiency of β-glucocerebrosidase activity, resulting in accumulation of glucocerebrosidase in tissue macrophages which become engorged and are typically found in the liver, spleen and bone marrow and occasionally in lung, kidney and intestine. Secondary hematologic sequelae include severe anemia and thrombocytopenia in addition to the characteristic progressive hepatosplenomegaly, skeletal complications, including osteonecrosis and osteopenia, with secondary pathological fractures. Imiglucerase improved anemia and thrombocytopenia, reduced spleen and liver size, and decreased cachexia to a degree similar to that observed with alglucerase.

➤*Pharmacokinetics:* During 1 hour IV infusions of four doses (7.5, 15, 30 and 60 U/kg) of imiglucerase, steady-state enzymatic activity was achieved by 30 minutes. Following infusion, plasma enzymatic activity declined rapidly with half-life ranging from 3.6 to 10.4 minutes. Plasma clearance ranged from 9.8 to 20.3 ml/min/kg. The volume of distribution corrected for weight ranged from 0.09 to 0.15 L/kg. These variables do not appear to be influenced by dose or duration of infusion. However, only one or two patients were studied at each dose level and infusion rate. The pharmacokinetics of imiglucerase do not appear to be different from placental-derived alglucerase. In patients who developed IgG antibody to imiglucerase, an apparent effect on serum enzyme levels resulted in diminished volume of distribution and clearance and increased elimination half-life compared to patients without antibody (see Warnings).

Contraindications

Hypersensitivity (carefully re-evaluate treatment if there is significant clinical evidence of hypersensitivity to the product).

Warnings

➤*Antibodies:* During the clinical trials (duration, 9 months), 4 of 25 patients (16%) treated with imiglucerase developed IgG antibodies reactive with imiglucerase. During the same clinical trial, 6 of 15 patients (40%) treated with placental-derived alglucerase developed IgG antibodies to alglucerase, and one of these patients had clinical allergic signs and symptoms resulting in withdrawal from the study. Of those patients treated with imiglucerase, only one patient developed a transient rash. No patients treated with imiglucerase, either initially or after changing over from alglucerase, have exhibited serious symptoms of immediate hypersensitivity, although a risk for such reactions may be present. Approach treatment with caution in patients who have exhibited symptoms of hypersensitivity to the product.

➤*Pregnancy: Category C.* It is not known whether imiglucerase can cause fetal harm when administered to a pregnant women, or can affect reproductive capacity. Do not administer during pregnancy except when the indication and need are clear and the potential benefit is judged to substantially justify the risk.

➤*Lactation:* It is not known whether this drug is excreted in breast milk. Exercise caution when imiglucerase is administered to a nursing woman.

Adverse Reactions

During clinical trials with imiglucerase involving 25 patients with Gaucher's disease, the following adverse events were noted: Headache (n = 3); nausea, abdominal discomfort, dizziness, pruritus, rash, mild decrease in blood pressure, decrease in urinary frequency (n = 1). None of these events were judged to be serious or to warrant medical intervention or interruption of therapy. All proved transient and did not recur frequently. Symptoms suggestive of allergic hypersensitivity have been noted in a number of patients treated with alglucerase (see Warnings).

Overdosage

Effects of dosages exceeding 120 U/kg per 4 weeks have not been studied and therefore dosages > 120 U/kg are not recommended.

CALCITONIN-SALMON

Rx	Miacalcin (Novartis)	Injection: 200 IU/ml	With phenol. In 2 ml vials.
Rx	Miacalcin (Novartis)	Nasal spray: 200 IU/activation (0.09 ml/dose)	8.5 mg sodium chloride. In 2 ml metered dose glass bottle with pump.

Indications

➤*Postmenopausal osteoporosis (injection and nasal):* Prevention of progressive loss of bone mass. Use nasal formulation only in patients who cannot take estrogen.

➤*Paget's disease of bone (injection only):* For patients with moderate to severe Paget's disease characterized by polyostotic involvement with elevated serum alkaline phosphatase and urinary hydroxyproline excretion.

➤*Hypercalcemia (injection only):* In early treatment of hypercalcemic emergencies, along with other appropriate agents, use when a rapid decrease in serum calcium is required, until more specific treatment can be accomplished. It may also be added to existing therapeutic regimens for hypercalcemia.

Administration and Dosage

➤*Skin testing:* Prepare a dilution at 10 IU/ml by withdrawing 0.05 ml of the 200 IU/ml solution in a tuberculin syringe and filling it to 1 ml with sodium chloride injection. Mix well, discard 0.9 ml and inject intracutaneously 0.1 ml ($\approx$ 1 IU) on the inner aspect of the forearm. Observe the injection site 15 minutes after injection. The appearance of more than mild erythema or wheal constitutes a positive response.

➤*Postmenopausal osteoporosis:*
Injection – 100 IU/day SC or IM.

Nasal – 200 IU intranasally every day, alternating nostrils daily. Before the first dose, it is necessary to activate the pump (see Patient Information).

Patients should also receive supplemental calcium carbonate 1.5 g daily and an adequate vitamin D intake (400 units daily). An adequate diet is also essential.

➤*Paget's disease (injection only):* Starting dose is 100 IU/day SC (preferred for outpatient self-administration) or IM. Monitor by periodic measurement of serum alkaline phosphatase and 24 hour urinary hydroxyproline and evaluation of symptoms. Normalization of biochemical abnormalities and decreased bone pain is usually seen in the first few months. Improvement of neurologic lesions requires > 1 year.

Doses of 50 IU/day or every other day are usually sufficient to maintain biochemical and clinical improvement. Maintain the higher dose in any patient with serious deformity or neurological involvement.

In any patient with a good response initially who later relapses (clinically or biochemically), investigate for antibody formation (see Warnings).

➤*Hypercalcemia (injection only):* Starting dose is 4 IU/kg every 12 hours, SC or IM. If response is not satisfactory after 1 or 2 days, increase to 8 IU/kg every 12 hours. If the response remains unsatisfactory after 2 more days, the dose may be further increased to a maximum of 8 IU/kg every 6 hours. If the volume to be injected exceeds 2 ml, IM injection is preferable and multiple sites of injection should be used.

➤*Storage/Stability:*
Injection – Refrigerate between 2° to 6°C (36° to 43°F).

Nasal – Store unopened bottle in the refrigerator between 2° and 8°C. Once the pump has been activated, store at room temperature.

Actions

➤*Pharmacology:* Calcitonins are polypeptide hormones secreted by parafollicular cells of the thyroid in mammals. Calcitonin has a role in the regulation of calcium and bone metabolism and it has direct renal effects and actions on the GI tract. Calcitonin appears essentially identical to mammalian calcitonins, but its potency per mg and duration of action are greater. Single injections of calcitonin transiently inhibit bone resorption. With prolonged use, there is a persistent, smaller decrease in the rate of bone resorption associated with decreased resorptive activity and number of osteoclasts. Osteocytic resorption may also be decreased. Endogenous calcitonin, with parathyroid hormone (PTH), regulates blood calcium. High blood calcium levels increase secretion of calcitonin, which inhibits bone resorption. In healthy adults, administration of exogenous calcitonin only slightly decreases serum calcium.

Paget's disease of bone (osteitis deformans) – Paget's disease of bone (osteitis deformans) is characterized by abnormal and accelerated bone formation and resorption in one or more bones. Active Paget's disease involving a large bone mass may increase the urinary hydroxyproline excretion (reflecting breakdown of collagen-containing bone matrix) and serum alkaline phosphatase (reflecting increased bone formation). Calcitonin, presumably by blocking bone resorption, improves the biochemical abnormalities (> 30% reduction). It decreases the rate of bone turnover with a resultant fall in the serum alkaline phosphatase and urinary hydroxyproline excretion in $\approx$ 66% of patients. These biochemical changes appear to correspond to more normal bone as evidenced by: 1) Radiologic regression of Pagetic lesions; 2) improvement of impaired auditory nerves (infrequent) and other neurologic func-

tions; 3) decreases in abnormally elevated cardiac output. Improvements occur rarely and spontaneously; they cannot be predicted. Some patients with Paget's disease who have good initial biochemical or symptomatic responses later relapse. Explanations are incomplete.

Hypercalcemia – Calcitonin-salmon lowers elevated serum calcium in patients with carcinoma, multiple myeloma or primary hyperparathyroidism (lesser response). Patients with higher serum calcium tend to show a greater reduction. The decrease in calcium occurs about 2 hours after injection and lasts for 6 to 8 hours. Given every 12 hours, the drug lowered calcium for 5 to 8 days. Average reduction of 8 hour postinjection serum calcium was about 9%.

Postmenopausal osteoporosis – Calcitonin, given by the intranasal route, increases spinal bone mass in postmenopausal women with established osteoporosis but not in early postmenopausal women.

Kidney – Calcitonin increases the excretion of filtered phosphate, calcium and sodium by decreasing tubular reabsorption. In some patients, the inhibition of bone resorption is of such magnitude that the consequent reduction of filtered calcium load more than compensates for the decrease in tubular reabsorption of calcium. This decreases rather than increases urinary calcium. Transient increases in sodium and water excretion may occur after the initial injection, but these changes usually return to pretreatment levels with continued therapy.

GI – Short-term administration results in marked transient decreases in the volume and acidity of gastric juice and in the volume of trypsin and amylase content of pancreatic juice. Whether this continues during chronic therapy is not known.

➤*Pharmacokinetics:* Animal studies suggest that calcitonin is rapidly converted to smaller inactive fragments, primarily in the kidneys, but also in the blood and peripheral tissues. A small amount of unchanged hormone and its inactive metabolites are excreted in the urine. Peak plasma concentration time for the injection is 16 to 25 minutes. Peak plasma concentration time for the nasal spray is 31 to 39 minutes; the calculated half-life is 43 minutes.

Contraindications

Clinical allergy to synthetic calcitonin-salmon.

Warnings

➤*Antibody formation:* Circulating antibodies to calcitonin occur after 2 to 18 months of treatment in about half the treated Paget's disease patients, but calcitonin treatment remained effective in many of these cases. Occasionally, patients with high antibody titers usually will have suffered a biochemical relapse of Paget's disease and are unresponsive to the acute hypocalcemic effects of calcitonin.

➤*Osteogenic sarcoma:* Osteogenic sarcoma is known to increase in Paget's disease. Pagetic lesions may appear by x-ray to progress markedly, possibly with some loss of definition of periosteal margins. Evaluate such lesions to differentiate them from osteogenic sarcoma.

➤*Asymptomatic Paget's disease:* There is no evidence that prophylactic use is beneficial in asymptomatic patients. Consider treatment in cases in which there is extensive involvement of the skull or spinal cord with the possibility of irreversible neurologic damage. Base treatment on demonstrated effect on Pagetic bone.

➤*Elderly:* No unusual adverse events or increased incidence of common adverse events have been noted in patients > 65 years of age receiving the nasal formulation.

➤*Pregnancy: Category C.* Calcitonin has decreased fetal birth weights in rabbits when given in doses 14 to 56 times the recommended human dose. Because calcitonin does not cross the placenta, this may be due to metabolic effects of calcitonin on the pregnant animal. There are no studies in pregnant women. Use these agents only if the potential benefits outweigh the hazards to the fetus.

➤*Lactation:* Calcitonin inhibits lactation in animals. It is not known whether it is excreted in breast milk. Safety for use during nursing has not been established.

➤*Children:* Disorders of bone in children (juvenile Paget's disease) have been reported rarely. No adequate data support usage in children.

Precautions

➤*Allergy:* The possibility of a systemic allergic reaction exists. Refer to Management of Acute Hypersensitivity Reactions. Consider skin testing prior to treatment, particularly for patients with suspected sensitivity. (See Administration and Dosage).

➤*Hypocalcemic tetany:* Hypocalcemic tetany could occur with calcitonin, although no cases have been reported. Have parenteral calcium available during the first several doses.

Periodically examine urine sediment of patients on chronic therapy. Coarse granular casts and renal tubular epithelial cell casts were reported in young adult volunteers at bed rest who were given calcitonin to study the effect on immobilization osteoporosis. The urine sediment became normal after calcitonin was stopped.

CALCITONIN-SALMON

➤*Nasal examination:* Perform a nasal examination prior to the start of treatment and at any time nasal complaints occur.

Adverse Reactions

Calcitonin Adverse Reactions (Nasal Spray)		
Adverse reaction	Nasal spray (n = 341)	Placebo (n = 131)
Rhinitis	12%	6.9%
Nasal symptoms (eg, irritation, redness, sores)	10%	16%
Back pain	5%	2.3%
Arthralgia	3.8%	5.3%
Epistaxis	3.5%	4.6%
Headache	3.2%	4.6%

➤*Cardiovascular:* Hypertension, angina pectoris (rare); tachycardia; palpitation; bundle branch block; myocardial infarction.

➤*CNS:* Dizziness, paresthesia, depression (rare); insomnia; anxiety; vertigo; migraine; neuralgia; agitation.

➤*Dermatologic:* Inflammatory reactions at the injection site (10%); flushing of face or hands (2% to 5%); pruritus of ear lobes; edema of feet; skin rash; skin ulceration; eczema; alopecia; increased sweating.

➤*Endocrine:* Goiter; hyperthyroidism.

➤*GI:* Nausea with or without vomiting (10%) is most evident when treatment is initiated and tends to decrease with continued use; anorexia; epigastric discomfort; salty taste; flatulence; increased appetite; gastritis; dry mouth; diarrhea, abdominal pain, dyspepsia, constipation (rare).

➤*GU:* Cystitis (rare); pyelonephritis; hematuria; renal calculus.

➤*Hematologic/Lymphatic:* Lymphadenopathy, infection (rare); anemia.

➤*Metabolic:* Mild tetanic symptoms, asymptomatic mild hypercalcemia (rare); cholelithiasis; thirst; hepatitis; weight increase (< 1%).

➤*Musculoskeletal:* Arthrosis, myalgia (rare); arthritis; polymyalgia rheumatica; stiffness.

➤*Ophthalmic:* Abnormal lacrimation, conjunctivitis (rare); blurred vision; vitreous floater.

➤*Respiratory:* Sinusitis, upper respiratory tract infection, bronchospasm (rare); pharyngitis; bronchitis; pneumonia; coughing; dyspnea; taste perversion; parosmia.

➤*Miscellaneous:* Nocturia; feverish sensation; eye pain; tinnitus; hearing loss; earache; cerebrovascular accident; thrombophlebitis; flu-like symptoms, fatigue (rare) (< 1%).

Overdosage

A dose of 1000 IU SC may produce nausea and vomiting as the only adverse effects. Doses of 32 units/kg/day for 1 or 2 days demonstrate no other adverse effects.

Patient Information

➤*Nasal:* Patients should notify their physician if they develop significant nasal irritation.

To activate the pump, hold the bottle upright and depress the two white side arms toward the bottle six times until a faint spray is emitted. The pump is activated once this first faint spray has been emitted. At this point, firmly place the nozzle into the nostril with the head in the upright position, and depress the pump toward the bottle. It is not necessary to reactivate the pump before each daily dose.

CINACALCET HCl

Rx	Sensipar (Amgen)	Tablets: 30 mg (as base)	(AMGEN 30). Light-green, oval. Film-coated. In 30s.
		60 mg (as base)	(AMGEN 60). Light-green, oval. Film-coated. In 30s.
		90 mg (as base)	(AMGEN 90). Light-green, oval. Film-coated. In 30s.

Indications

➤*Parathyroid carcinoma:* For the treatment of hypercalcemia in patients with parathyroid carcinoma.

➤*Secondary hyperparathyroidism (HPT):* For the treatment of secondary HPT in patients with chronic kidney disease (CKD) on dialysis.

Administration and Dosage

➤*Approved by the FDA:* March 8, 2004.

Take cinacalcet tablets whole; do not divide. Take with food or shortly after a meal. Individualize dosage.

➤*Parathyroid carcinoma:* The recommended starting oral dose of cinacalcet is 30 mg twice daily. Titrate the dosage every 2 to 4 weeks through sequential doses of 30 mg twice daily, 60 mg twice daily, 90 mg twice daily, and 90 mg 3 or 4 times/day as necessary to normalize serum calcium levels.

➤*Secondary HPT:* The recommended starting oral dose of cinacalcet is 30 mg once daily. Measure serum calcium and serum phosphorus within 1 week and measure intact parathyroid hormone (iPTH) 1 to 4 weeks after initiation or dose adjustment of cinacalcet. Titrate cinacalcet no more frequently than every 2 to 4 weeks through sequential doses of 60, 90, 120, and 180 mg once daily to target iPTH consistent with the National Kidney Foundation-Kidney Disease Outcomes Quality Initiative (NKF-K/DOQI) recommendation for CKD patients on dialysis of 150 to 300 pg/mL.

Cinacalcet can be used alone or in combination with vitamin D sterols and/or phosphate binders.

During dose titration, frequently monitor serum calcium levels. If levels decrease below the normal range, take appropriate steps to increase serum calcium levels, such as providing supplemental calcium, initiating or increasing the dose of calcium-based phosphate binder or vitamin D sterols, or temporarily withholding cinacalcet treatment (see Precautions).

If iPTH levels decrease below the NKF-K/DOQI recommended target range (150 to 300 pg/mL) in patients treated with cinacalcet, reduce the dose of cinacalcet and/or vitamin D sterols or discontinue therapy (see Precautions).

➤*Concomitant therapy:* If a patient initiates or discontinues therapy with a strong CYP3A4 inhibitor (eg, ketoconazole, erythromycin, itraconazole), dose adjustment of cinacalcet may be required. Closely monitor parathyroid hormone (PTH) and serum calcium concentrations.

➤*Storage/Stability:* Store at 25°C (77°F); excursions permitted to 15° to 30°C (59° to 86°F).

Actions

➤*Pharmacology:* Cinacalcet is a calcimimetic agent that increases the sensitivity of the calcium-sensing receptor to activation by extracellular calcium. Secondary HPT in patients with CKD is a progressive disease, associated with increases in PTH levels and derangements in calcium and phosphorus metabolism. Increased PTH stimulates osteoclastic activity, resulting in cortical bone resorption and marrow fibrosis. The goals of treatment of secondary HPT are to lower levels of PTH, calcium, and phosphorus in the blood in order to prevent progressive bone disease and the systemic consequences of disordered mineral metabolism. In CKD patients on dialysis with uncontrolled secondary HPT, reductions in PTH are associated with a favorable impact on bone-specific alkaline phosphatase, bone turnover, and bone fibrosis.

The calcium-sensing receptor on the surface of the chief cell of the parathyroid gland is the principal regulator of PTH secretion. Cinacalcet directly lowers PTH levels by increasing the sensitivity of the calcium-sensing receptor to extracellular calcium. The reduction in PTH is associated with a concomitant decrease in serum calcium levels.

➤*Pharmacokinetics:*

Absorption/Distribution – After oral administration of cinacalcet, C_{max} is achieved in approximately 2 to 6 hours. A food-effect study in healthy volunteers indicated that the C_{max} and $AUC_{(0-\infty)}$ were increased 82% and 68%, respectively, when cinacalcet was administered with a high-fat meal compared with fasting. C_{max} and $AUC_{(0-\infty)}$ of cinacalcet were increased 65% and 50%, respectively, when cinacalcet was administered with a low-fat meal compared with fasting.

Steady-state drug levels are achieved within 7 days. The mean accumulation ratio is approximately 2 with once-daily oral administration. The median accumulation ratio is approximately 2 to 5 with twice-daily oral administration. The AUC and C_{max} of cinacalcet increase proportionally over the dose range of 30 to 180 mg once daily. The pharmacokinetic profile of cinacalcet does not change over time with once-daily dosing of 30 to 180 mg. The volume of distribution is high (approximately 1000 L), indicating extensive distribution. Cinacalcet is approximately 93% to 97% bound to plasma proteins. The ratio of blood

cinacalcet concentration to plasma cinacalcet concentration is 0.8 at a blood cinacalcet concentration of 10 ng/mL.

Metabolism – Cinacalcet is metabolized by multiple enzymes, primarily CYP3A4, CYP2D6, and CYP1A2. After administration of a 75 mg radiolabeled dose to healthy volunteers, cinacalcet was rapidly and extensively metabolized via the following: 1) oxidative N-dealkylation to hydrocinnamic acid and hydroxy-hydrocinnamic acid, which are further metabolized via β-oxidation and glycine conjugation; the oxidative N-dealkylation process also generates metabolites that contain the naphthalene ring; and 2) oxidation of the naphthalene ring on the parent drug to form dihydrodiols, which are further conjugated with glucuronic acid. The plasma concentrations of the major circulating metabolites, including the cinnamic acid derivatives and glucuronidated dihydrodiols, markedly exceed parent drug concentrations. The hydrocinnamic acid metabolite was shown to be inactive at concentrations up to 10 mcM in a cell-based assay measuring calcium-receptor activation. The glucuronide conjugates formed after cinacalcet oxidation were shown to have a potency approximately 0.003 times that of cinacalcet in a cell-based assay measuring a calcimimetic response.

Excretion – After absorption, cinacalcet concentrations decline in a biphasic fashion with a terminal half-life of 30 to 40 hours. Renal excretion of metabolites was the primary route of elimination of radioactivity. Approximately 80% of the dose was recovered in the urine and 15% in the feces.

Special populations –

Hepatic function impairment: In patients with moderate and severe hepatic impairment (as indicated by the Child-Pugh method), cinacalcet (50 mg single dose) exposures as defined by the $AUC_{(0-\infty)}$ were 2.4 and 4.2 times higher, respectively, than that in normal patients. The mean half-life of cinacalcet is prolonged by 33% and 70% in patients with moderate and severe hepatic impairment, respectively. Protein binding of cinacalcet is not affected by impaired hepatic function (see Warnings).

Pharmacodynamics – Reduction in iPTH levels correlated with cinacalcet concentrations in CKD patients. The nadir in iPTH level occurs approximately 2 to 6 hours postdose, corresponding with the C_{max} of cinacalcet. After steady state is reached, serum calcium concentrations remain constant over the dosing interval in CKD patients.

Contraindications

Hypersensitivity to any component of this product.

Warnings

➤*Seizures:* In 3 clinical studies of CKD patients on dialysis, 5% of the patients in the cinacalcet and placebo groups reported a history of seizure disorder at baseline. During the trials, seizures (primarily generalized or tonic-clonic) were observed in 1.4% of cinacalcet-treated patients and 0.4% of placebo-treated patients. Five of the 9 cinacalcet-treated patients had a history of seizure disorder and 2 were receiving antiseizure medication at the time of their seizure. Both placebo-treated patients had a history of seizure disorder and were receiving antiseizure medication at the time of their seizure. While the basis for the reported difference in seizure rate is not clear, the threshold for seizures is lowered by significant reductions in serum calcium levels. Therefore, closely monitor serum calcium levels in patients receiving cinacalcet, particularly in patients with a history of a seizure disorder.

➤*Hepatic function impairment:* Cinacalcet exposure as assessed by $AUC_{(0-\infty)}$ in patients with moderate and severe hepatic impairment (as indicated by the Child-Pugh method) were 2.4 and 4.2 times higher, respectively, than that in normal patients. In patients with moderate and severe hepatic impairment, closely monitor PTH and serum calcium throughout treatment with cinacalcet.

➤*Pregnancy: Category C.* In animal studies, no teratogenicity was observed, but decreased fetal body weights were seen in some studies. This was in conjunction with maternal toxicity (decreased food consumption and body weight gain). In rats, higher doses of 15 and 25 mg/kg/day (exposures 2 to 3 times a human oral dose of 180 mg/day based on AUC comparisons) were accompanied by maternal signs of hypocalcemia (periparturient mortality and early postnatal pup loss), and reductions in postnatal maternal and pup body-weight gain. Cinacalcet has been shown to cross the placental barrier in rabbits.

There are no adequate and well-controlled studies in pregnant women. Use during pregnancy only if the potential benefit justifies the potential risk to the fetus.

➤*Lactation:* Studies in rats have shown that cinacalcet is excreted in the milk with a high milk-to-plasma ratio. It is not known whether this drug is excreted in human milk. Considering these data in rats and because many drugs are excreted in human milk and there is potential for clinically significant adverse reactions in infants, decide whether to discontinue nursing or to discontinue the drug, taking into account the importance of the drug to the lactating woman.

CINACALCET HCl

►*Children:* The safety and efficacy of cinacalcet in children have not been established.

Precautions

►*Monitoring:* In patients with CKD on dialysis with secondary HPT, measure serum calcium and serum phosphorus within 1 week and measure iPTH 1 to 4 weeks after initiation or dose adjustment of cinacalcet. Once the maintenance dose has been established, measure serum calcium and serum phosphorus approximately monthly, and PTH every 1 to 3 months (see Administration and Dosage). All iPTH measurements during cinacalcet trials were obtained using the Nichols intact immunoradiometric assay (IRMA).

In patients with end-stage renal disease, testosterone levels are often below the normal range. In a placebo-controlled trial in patients with CKD on dialysis, there were reductions in total and free testosterone in male patients following 6 months of treatment with cinacalcet. Levels of total testosterone decreased by a median of 15.8% in the cinacalcet-treated patients and by 0.6% in the placebo-treated patients. Levels of free testosterone decreased by a median of 31.3% in the cinacalcet-treated patients and by 16.3% in the placebo-treated patients. The clinical significance of these reductions in serum testosterone is unknown.

In patients with parathyroid carcinoma, measure serum calcium within 1 week after initiation of dose adjustment or cinacalcet. Once maintenance dose levels have been established, measure serum calcium every 2 months (see Administration and Dosage).

►*Hypocalcemia:* Cinacalcet lowers serum calcium; therefore, closely monitor patients for the occurrence of hypocalcemia. Potential manifestations of hypocalcemia include cramping, convulsions, myalgias, paresthesias, and tetany. Do not initiate cinacalcet treatment if serum calcium is less than the lower limit of the normal range (8.4 mg/dL). Measure serum calcium within 1 week after initiation or cinacalcet dose adjustment. Once the maintenance dose has been established, measure serum calcium approximately monthly.

If serum calcium falls below 8.4 mg/dL but remains above 7.5 mg/dL, or if symptoms of hypocalcemia occur, calcium-containing phosphate binders and/or vitamin D sterols can be used to raise serum calcium. If serum calcium falls below 7.5 mg/dL, or if symptoms of hypocalcemia persist and the dose of vitamin D cannot be increased, withhold administration of cinacalcet until serum calcium levels reach 8 mg/dL and/or symptoms of hypocalcemia have resolved. Re-initiate treatment using the next lowest dose of cinacalcet (see Administration and Dosage).

In the 26-week studies of patients with CKD on dialysis, 66% of patients receiving cinacalcet compared with 25% of patients receiving placebo developed at least 1 serum calcium value less than 8.4 mg/dL. Less than 1% of patients in each group permanently discontinued the study drug because of hypocalcemia.

In CKD patients with secondary HPT not on dialysis, the long-term safety and efficacy of cinacalcet have not been established. Exploratory investigation indicates that CKD patients not on dialysis have an increased risk for hypocalcemia compared with CKD patients on dialysis, which may be because of lower baseline calcium levels. In a small, short-term study in which the median dose of cinacalcet was 30 mg at the completion of the study, 74% of cinacalcet-treated patients experienced at least 1 serum calcium value less than 8.4 mg/dL.

►*Adynamic bone disease:* Adynamic bone disease may develop if iPTH levels are suppressed below 100 pg/mL when assessed using the standard Nichols IRMA. One clinical study evaluated bone histomorphometry in patients treated with cinacalcet for 1 year. Three patients with mild HPT bone disease at the beginning of the study developed adynamic bone disease during treatment with cinacalcet. Two of these patients had iPTH levels below 100 pg/mL at multiple time points during the study. In the three 6-month, phase 3 studies conducted in CKD patients on dialysis, 11% of patients treated with cinacalcet had mean iPTH values below 100 pg/mL during the efficacy-assessment phase. If iPTH levels decrease below the NKF-K/DOQI recommended target range (150 to 300 pg/mL) in patients treated with cinacalcet, reduce the dose of cinacalcet and/or vitamin D sterols or discontinue therapy.

Drug Interactions

►*CYP 450 system:* Cinacalcet is metabolized by multiple cytochrome P450 enzymes, primarily CYP3A4, CYP2D6, and CYP1A2. Cinacalcet is a strong in vitro inhibitor of CYP2D6. Therefore, dose adjustments may be required of concomitant medications that are predominantly metabolized by CYP2D6 and have a narrow therapeutic index (eg, flecainide, vinblastine, thioridazine, most tricyclic antidepressants). Administration with amitriptyline increased amitriptyline and nortriptyline (active metabolite) exposure by approximately 20% in CYP2D6 extensive metabolizers.

Cinacalcet is metabolized in part by CYP3A4. Coadministration with ketoconazole, a strong inhibitor of CYP3A4, increased cinacalcet exposure by 2.3 fold. Dose adjustments of cinacalcet may be required; closely monitor PTH and calcium concentrations if patient initiates or discontinues therapy with a strong CYP3A4 inhibitor (eg, ketoconazole, erythromycin, itraconazole).

►*Drug/Food interactions:* A food-effect study in healthy volunteers indicated that the C_{max} and $AUC_{(0-\infty)}$ were increased 82% and 68%, respectively, when cinacalcet was administered with a high-fat meal compared with fasting. C_{max} and $AUC_{(0-\infty)}$ of cinacalcet were increased 65% and 50%, respectively, when cinacalcet was administered with a low-fat meal compared with fasting.

Adverse Reactions

►*Secondary HPT:*

Cinacalcet Adverse Reactions in Patients with CKD on Dialysis (≥ 5%)		
Adverse reaction[a]	Cinacalcet (n = 656)	Placebo (n = 470)
GI		
Anorexia	6	4
Diarrhea	21	20
Nausea	31	19
Vomiting	27	15
Miscellaneous		
Access infection	5	4
Asthenia	7	4
Dizziness	10	8
Hypertension	7	5
Myalgia	15	14
Pain chest, noncardiac	6	4

[a] Included are events that were reported at a greater incidence in the cinacalcet group than in the placebo group.

►*Parathyroid carcinoma:* The most frequent adverse events in this patient group were nausea and vomiting.

Overdosage

Doses titrated up to 300 mg once daily have been safely administered to patients on dialysis. Overdosage of cinacalcet may lead to hypocalcemia. In the event of overdosage, monitor patients for signs and symptoms of hypocalcemia, and take appropriate measures to correct serum calcium levels. Because cinacalcet is highly protein bound, hemodialysis is not an effective treatment for overdosage of cinacalcet.

Patient Information

Instruct patients to take cinacalcet with food or shortly after a meal. Take tablets whole; do not divide.

Instruct patients to immediately report the following symptoms to their health care provider: Cramping, convulsions, myalgias, paresthesias, and tetany.

GALLIUM NITRATE

Rx	**Ganite** (Genta[a])	**Injection:** 25 mg/mL	Preservative free. In 20 mL single-dose vials.

[a] Genta Incorporated, Berkeley Heights, NJ 07922; (888) TO-GENTA.

WARNING

Concurrent use of gallium nitrate with other potentially nephrotoxic drugs (eg, aminoglycosides, amphotericin B) may increase the risk for developing severe renal insufficiency in patients with cancer-related hypercalcemia. If use of a potentially nephrotoxic drug is indicated during therapy, discontinue gallium nitrate and continue hydration for several days after administering the potentially nephrotoxic drug. Closely monitor serum creatinine and urine output during and after this period. Discontinue gallium nitrate therapy if the serum creatinine level exceeds 2.5 mg/dL.

Indications

➤*Cancer-related hypercalcemia:* For the treatment of cancer-related hypercalcemia (clearly symptomatic) unresponsive to adequate hydration.

In general, patients with a serum calcium (corrected for albumin) less than 12 mg/dL would not be expected to be symptomatic. Mild or asymptomatic hypercalcemia may be treated with conservative measures (eg, saline hydration, with or without diuretics). In the treatment of cancer-related hypercalcemia, it is important first to establish adequate hydration, preferably with IV saline, in order to increase the renal excretion of calcium and correct dehydration caused by hypercalcemia.

Administration and Dosage

➤*Approved by the FDA:* January 1991.

➤*Usual dose:* 200 mg/m²/day for 5 consecutive days. In patients with mild hypercalcemia and few symptoms, a lower dosage of 100 mg/m²/day for 5 days may be considered. If serum calcium levels are lowered into the normal range in fewer than 5 days, treatment may be discontinued early. The daily dose must be given as an IV infusion over 24 hours.

Dilute the daily dose, preferably in 1 L 0.9% sodium chloride injection or 5% dextrose injection, for administration as an IV infusion over 24 hours. Maintain adequate hydration throughout the treatment period, with careful attention to avoid overhydration in patients with compromised cardiovascular status. Controlled studies have not been undertaken to evaluate the safety and efficacy of retreatment with gallium nitrate.

➤*Storage/Stability:* When gallium nitrate is added to either 0.9% sodium chloride injection or 5% dextrose injection, it is stable for 48 hours at room temperature (15° to 30°C; 59° to 86°F) and for 7 days if stored under refrigeration (2° to 8°C; 36° to 46°F). Contains no preservative; discard unused portion. Store vials at 20° to 25°C (68° to 77°F).

Actions

➤*Pharmacology:* Gallium nitrate is a hydrated nitrate salt of the group IIIa element, gallium. Gallium exerts a hypocalcemic effect by inhibiting calcium resorption from bone, possibly by reducing increased bone turnover. The precise mechanism has not been determined. No cytotoxic effects were observed with bone cells in animals.

Cancer-related hypercalcemia – Cancer-related hypercalcemia is a common problem in hospitalized patients with malignancy. It may affect 10% to 20% of patients with cancer. Different types of malignancies seem to vary in their propensity to cause hypercalcemia. A higher incidence of hypercalcemia has been observed in patients with nonsmall cell lung cancer, breast cancer, multiple myeloma, kidney cancer, and cancer of the head and neck. Hypercalcemia of malignancy seems to result from an imbalance between the net resorption of bone and urinary excretion of calcium. Hypercalcemia may produce signs and symptoms including: Anorexia, lethargy, fatigue, nausea, vomiting, constipation, dehydration, renal insufficiency, impaired mental status, coma, and cardiac arrest. A rapid rise in serum calcium may cause more severe symptoms for a given level of hypercalcemia.

➤*Pharmacokinetics:* Gallium nitrate was infused at a daily dose of 200 mg/m² for 5 (n = 2) or 7 (n = 10) consecutive days to 12 cancer patients. Apparent steady state generally is achieved in 24 to 48 hours. The range of average steady-state plasma levels of gallium observed among 7 patients was between 1134 and 2399 ng/mL. The average plasma clearance following daily infusion of 200 mg/m² for 5 or 7 days was 0.15 L/h/kg (range, 0.12 to 0.2 L/h/kg). In 1 patient who received daily infusion doses of 100, 150, and 200 mg/m², the apparent steady-state gallium levels did not increase proportionally with a dose increase. Gallium nitrate is not metabolized either by the liver or kidneys and appears to be significantly excreted via the kidney.

➤*Clinical trials:* A randomized, double-blind clinical study comparing gallium nitrate with calcitonin was conducted in patients with a serum calcium concentration (corrected for albumin) of 12 mg/dL or more following 2 days of hydration. Gallium nitrate was given as a continuous 200 mg/m²/day IV infusion for 5 days and 8 IU/kg calcitonin IM was given every 6 hours for 5 days. Elevated serum calcium (corrected

for albumin) was normalized in 75% (18 of 24) of the patients receiving gallium nitrate and in 27% (7 of 26) of the patients receiving calcitonin. The time course of effect on serum calcium (corrected for albumin) is summarized in the following table:

Change in Serum Calcium by Gallium Nitrate vs Calcitonin		
	Mean change in serum calcium (mg/dL)[a]	
Time period[b] (hours)	Gallium nitrate	Calcitonin
24	-0.4	-1.6[c]
48	-0.9	-1.4
72	-1.5	-1.1
96	-2.9[c]	-1.1
120	-3.3[c]	-1.3

[a] Serum calcium change from baseline (corrected for albumin).
[b] Time after initiation of therapy.
[c] Comparison between treatment groups (P < 0.01).

The median duration of normocalcemia/hypocalcemia was 7.5 days for patients treated with gallium nitrate and 1 day for patients treated with calcitonin. A total of 92% of patients treated with gallium nitrate had a decrease in serum calcium (corrected for albumin) of 2 mg/dL or more vs 54% of patients treated with calcitonin (P = 0.004).

Contraindications

Severe renal impairment (serum creatinine greater than 2.5 mg/dL).

Warnings

➤*Anemia:* The use of very high doses (up to 1400 mg/m²) in treating patients with advanced cancer has been associated with anemia, and several patients have received red blood cell transfusions. Because of the serious nature of the underlying illness, it is uncertain that the anemia was caused by gallium nitrate.

➤*Renal function impairment:* Hypercalcemia in cancer patients is commonly associated with impaired renal function (elevated BUN and/or serum creatinine). It is strongly recommended that serum creatinine be monitored during therapy. It is important that such patients be adequately hydrated with oral and/or IV fluids (preferably saline) and that a satisfactory urine output (2 L/day is recommended) be established before beginning therapy. Maintain adequate hydration throughout the treatment period, and avoid overhydration in patients with compromised cardiovascular status. Do not use diuretic therapy prior to correction of hypovolemia. Discontinue gallium nitrate therapy if the serum creatinine level exceeds 2.5 mg/dL.

The use of gallium nitrate in patients with marked renal insufficiency (serum creatinine greater than 2.5 mg/dL) has not been systematically examined. If therapy is undertaken in patients with moderately impaired renal function (serum creatinine 2 to 2.5 mg/dL), frequently monitor patient's renal status. Discontinue treatment if the serum creatinine level exceeds 2.5 mg/dL.

➤*Pregnancy:* Category C. It is not known whether gallium nitrate can cause fetal harm when administered to a pregnant woman or can affect reproductive capacity. Administer to a pregnant woman only if clearly needed. Animal reproduction studies have not been conducted with gallium nitrate.

➤*Lactation:* It is not known whether gallium nitrate is excreted in breast milk. Because of the potential for serious adverse reactions in nursing infants, decide whether to discontinue nursing or discontinue the drug, taking into account the importance of the drug to the mother.

➤*Children:* The safety and efficacy of gallium nitrate have not been established.

Precautions

➤*Monitoring:* Closely monitor renal function (serum creatinine and BUN) and serum calcium during gallium nitrate therapy. In addition to baseline assessment, the suggested frequency of calcium and phosphorus determinations is daily and twice weekly, respectively. Discontinue gallium nitrate if serum creatinine is greater than 2.5 mg/dL.

Changes in total serum calcium (especially during rehydration) may not accurately reflect changes in the concentration of free-ionized calcium. Measurement of the serum albumin concentration and correction of the total serum calcium concentration may help assess the severity of hypercalcemia in the absence of a direct measurement of free-ionized calcium.

➤*Asymptomatic or mild to moderate hypocalcemia:* Asymptomatic or mild to moderate hypocalcemia (6.5 to 8 mg/dL, corrected for serum albumin) occurred in approximately 38% of patients in the controlled clinical trial. One patient exhibited a positive Chvostek's sign. If hypocalcemia occurs, stop gallium nitrate therapy; short-term calcium therapy may be necessary.

➤*Visual and auditory disturbances:* A small proportion (less than 1%) of patients treated with multiple high doses of gallium nitrate combined with other investigational anticancer drugs, have developed acute optic neuritis. While these patients were critically ill and had

GALLIUM NITRATE

received multiple drugs, a reaction to high-dose gallium nitrate is possible. Most patients had a full recovery; however, at least 1 case of permanent blindness has occurred. One patient with cancer-related hypercalcemia developed a hearing loss following gallium nitrate administration. Because of the patient's underlying condition and concurrent therapies, the relationship of this event to gallium nitrate administration is unclear. Tinnitus and partial loss of auditory acuity have occurred rarely (less than 1%) in patients who received high-dose gallium nitrate as anticancer treatment.

➤*Transient hypophosphatemia:* Transient hypophosphatemia of mild to moderate degree may occur in up to 79% of hypercalcemic patients following treatment. In a controlled clinical trial, 33% of patients had at least 1 serum phosphorus measurement between 1.5 to 2.4 mg/dL, while 46% of patients had at least 1 serum phosphorus value of less than 1.5 mg/dL. Patients who develop hypophosphatemia may require oral phosphorus therapy.

➤*Decreased serum bicarbonate:* Decreased serum bicarbonate, possibly secondary to mild respiratory alkalosis, occurred in 40% to 50% of cancer patients treated with gallium nitrate. The cause was unclear. This effect has been asymptomatic and has not required specific treatment.

➤*Hypotension:* A decrease in mean systolic and diastolic blood pressure was observed several days after treatment with gallium nitrate in a controlled clinical trial. The decrease in blood pressure was asymptomatic and did not require specific treatment.

Drug Interactions

➤*Nephrotoxic drugs (eg, aminoglycosides, amphotericin B):* Combined use of gallium nitrate with other potentially nephrotoxic drugs may increase the risk of developing renal insufficiency in patients with cancer-related hypercalcemia (see Warning Box).

➤*Cyclophosphamide:* A symptom complex of dyspnea (associated with interstitial pneumonitis in some instances), mouth soreness, and asthenia has been reported in a small number of multiple myeloma patients receiving low dose (40 mg) gallium nitrate SC in addition to oral cyclophosphamide and prednisone. The serious nature of the underlying condition of these patients precludes a precise understanding of the relationship of these events to either gallium nitrate treatment alone or with cyclophosphamide.

Adverse Reactions

➤*Cardiovascular:* Lower extremity edema, tachycardia (causal relationship unknown); hypotension (see Precautions).

➤*CNS:* Confusion, dreams and hallucinations, lethargy, paresthesia (causal relationship unknown). A single case of encephalopathy followed rapidly by coma and death has been reported after treatment in a cancer chemotherapy trial with 300 mg/m^2 gallium nitrate/day for 7 days.

➤*GI:* Constipation, diarrhea, nausea and/or vomiting (causal relationship unknown).

➤*Hematologic:* Anemia (see Warnings); leukopenia (causal relationship unknown).

➤*Metabolic:* Decreased serum bicarbonate (see Precautions), hypocalcemia, transient hypophosphatemia.

➤*Renal:* Rise in BUN and creatinine (approximately 12.5%; see Warnings). Two patients receiving gallium nitrate developed acute renal failure, but the relationship of these events to the drug was unclear.

➤*Respiratory:* Dyspnea, pleural effusion, pulmonary infiltrates, rales and rhonchi (causal relationship unknown).

➤*Special senses:* Decreased hearing, visual impairment (see Precautions).

➤*Miscellaneous:* Fever, hypothermia, skin rash (causal relationship unknown).

Overdosage

➤*Symptoms:* Rapid IV infusion of gallium nitrate or use of doses higher than recommended (200 mg/m^2) may cause nausea and vomiting and a substantially increased risk of renal insufficiency.

➤*Treatment:* Discontinue further drug administration and monitor serum calcium. Administer vigorous IV hydration, with or without diuretics, for 2 to 3 days. During this time, carefully monitor renal function and urinary output for balanced fluid intake and output.

Patient Information

Advise patients to tell their health care provider if any of the following occur:

➤*Severe:* Abnormal dreams, chills, difficulty breathing, fast heartbeat, hallucinations.

➤*Common:* Changes in vision or hearing, mouth sores, weakness, .

➤*Other:* Abnormal skin sensations, confusion, constipation, diarrhea, dry rattling of the throat, fever, lack of energy, low body temperature, nausea, rales, rash, swelling of the ankles and feet, vomiting.

SODIUM PHENYLBUTYRATE

Rx	**Buphenyl** (Ucyclyd Pharma)	**Tablets:** 500 mg	(UCY 500). Off-white, oval. In 250s and 500s.
		Powder: 3.2 g (3 g sodium phenylbutyrate) per tsp	In 500 and 950 ml bottles. Measurers provided.
		9.1 g (8.6 g sodium phenylbutyrate) per tbsp	In 500 and 950 ml bottles. Measurers provided.

Indications

➤*Cycle disorders:* Sodium phenylbutyrate is indicated as adjunctive therapy in the chronic management of patients with urea cycle disorders involving deficiencies of carbamoyl phosphate synthetase (CPS), ornithine transcarbamoylase (OTC) or argininosuccinic acid synthetase (AAS). It is indicated in all patients with neonatal-onset deficiency (complete enzymatic deficiency, presenting within the first 28 days of life). It is also indicated in patients with late-onset disease (partial enzymatic deficiency, presenting after the first month of life) who have a history of hyperammonemic encephalopathy. It is important that the diagnosis be made early and treatment initiated immediately to improve survival. Any episode of acute hyperammonemia should be treated as a life-threatening emergency.

Administration and Dosage

➤*Tablets:* For oral use only. It is indicated for children weighing > 20 kg or adults.

Usual dose – 450 to 600 mg/kg/day in patients weighing < 20 kg, or 9.9 to 13 g/m²/day in larger patients. Take in equally divided amounts with each meal (eg, three times daily). The safety and efficacy of doses > 20 g/day (40 tablets) has not been established.

➤*Powder:* For oral use via mouth, gastrostomy or nasogastric tube only. Mix with food (solid or liquid). Avoid acidic beverages. Each level teaspoon dispenses 3.2 g of powder and 3 g of sodium phenylbutyrate. Each level tablespoon dispenses 9.1 g of powder and 8.6 g of sodium phenylbutyrate. Shake lightly before use.

Usual dose – 450 to 600 mg/kg/day in patients weighing < 20 kg, or 9.9 to 13 g/m²/day in larger patients. Take in equally divided amounts with each meal or feeding, four to six times daily. The safety and efficacy of doses> 20 g/day has not been established.

➤*Storage/Stability:* Store at room temperature, 15° to 30°C (59° to 86°F). After opening, keep bottle tightly closed.

Actions

➤*Pharmacology:* Sodium phenylbutyrate is a pro-drug and is rapidly metabolized to phenylacetate. Phenylacetate is a metabolically-active compound that conjugates with glutamine via acetylation to form phenylacetylglutamine. Phenylacetylglutamine is excreted then by the kidneys. On a molar basis, it is comparable to urea (each containing two moles of nitrogen). Therefore, phenylacetylglutamine provides an alternate vehicle for waste nitrogen excretion.

➤*Pharmacokinetics:*

Absorption – Peak plasma levels of phenylbutyrate occur within 1 hour after a single dose of 5 g sodium phenylbutyrate powder with a C_{max} of 195 mcg/ml and for the tablets, a C_{max} of 218 mcg/ml under fasting conditions. The effect of food on phenylbutyrate's absorption is unknown.

Excretion – A majority of the administered compound (≈ 80% to 100%) is excreted by the kidneys within 24 hours as the conjugation product, phenylacetylglutamine. For each gram of sodium phenylbutyrate administered, it is estimated that between 0.12 to 0.15 g of phenylacetylglutamine nitrogen is produced.

Hepatic function impairment: In patients who did not have urea cycle disorders, but had impaired hepatic function, the metabolism and excretion of sodium phenylbutyrate were not affected.

Pharmacokinetic studies have not been conducted in the primary patient population (neonates, infants and children), but pharmacokinetic data were obtained from normal adult subjects.

Following oral administration of 5 g, measurable plasma levels of phenylbutyrate and phenylacetate were detected 15 and 30 min after dosing, respectively, and phenylacetylglutamine was detected shortly thereafter. The pharmacokinetic parameters for phenylbutyrate for C_{max} (mcg/ml), T_{max} (hours) and elimination half-life were 195, 1 and 0.76 hours, respectively, and for phenylacetate 45.3, 3.55 and 1.29 hours, respectively. The major sites for metabolism are the liver and kidney.

In patients with urea cycle disorders, sodium phenylbutyrate decreases elevated plasma ammonia and glutamine levels. It increases waste nitrogen excretion in the form of phenylacetylglutamine.

The pharmacokinetic parameters, AUC and C_{max} for both plasma phenylbutyrate and phenylacetate were about 30% to 50% greater in females than in males.

Contraindications

Management of acute hyperammonemia, which is a medical emergency.

Warnings

➤*Fluid retention:* Use with great care, if at all, in patients with CHF or severe renal insufficiency, and in clinical states in which there is sodium retention with edema.

➤*Pre-existing neurologic impairment:* Reversal of pre-existing neurologic impairment is not likely to occur with treatment, and neurologic deterioration may continue.

➤*Acute hyperammonemic encephalopathy:* Acute hyperammonemic encephalopathy recurred in the majority of patients.

➤*Long-term:* Sodium phenylbutyrate may be required life-long unless orthotopic liver transplantation is elected.

➤*Renal/Hepatic function impairment:* Sodium phenylbutyrate is metabolized in the liver and kidney, and phenylacetylglutamine is primarily excreted by the kidney. Use caution when administering the drug to patients with hepatic or renal insufficiency.

➤*Pregnancy: Category C.* It is not known whether sodium phenylbutyrate can cause fetal harm when administered to a pregnant woman or can affect reproduction capacity. Give sodium phenylbutyrate to a pregnant woman only if clearly needed.

➤*Lactation:* It is not known whether this drug is excreted in breast milk. Because many drugs are excreted in breast milk, exercise caution when administering sodium phenylbutyrate to a nursing woman.

➤*Children:* The use of tablets for neonates, infants and children ≤ 20 kg is not recommended (see Administration and Dosage).

Precautions

➤*Monitoring:* Maintain plasma levels of ammonia, arginine, branched-chain amino acids and serum proteins within normal limits, and maintain plasma glutamine at levels < 1000 mcmol/L. Periodically monitor serum drug levels of phenylbutyrate and its metabolites, phenylacetate and phenylacetylglutamine.

Drug Interactions

Sodium Phenylbutyrate Drug Interactions			
Precipitant drug	Object drug*		Description
Corticosteroids	Sodium phenyl-butyrate	↓	Corticosteroids may cause the breakdown of body protein and increase plasma ammonia levels.
Haloperidol/Valproate	Sodium phenyl-butyrate	↓	Haloperidol/Valproate may cause hyperammonemia.
Probenecid	Sodium phenyl-butyrate	↑	Probenecid is known to inhibit the renal transport of many organic compounds, including hippuric acid, and may affect renal excretion of the conjugation product of sodium phenylbutyrate, as well as its metabolite.

* ↑ = Object drug increased.　↓ = Object drug decreased.

Adverse Reactions

Amenorrhea/menstrual dysfunction (23%); decreased appetite (4%); body odor (probably caused by the metabolite phenylacetate), bad taste or taste aversion (3%).

Other adverse events reported in ≤ 2% of patients:

➤*Cardiovascular:* Arrhythmia; edema (one patient).

➤*CNS:* Depression; neurotoxicity (somnolence, fatigue and lightheadedness; less frequently, headache, dysgeusia, hypoacusis, disorientation, impaired memory and exacerbation of a pre-existing neuropathy). These adverse events were mainly mild in severity. The acute onset and reversibility when the phenylacetate infusion was discontinued suggest a drug effect.

➤*GI:* Abdominal pain; gastritis; nausea; vomiting; constipation; rectal bleeding; peptic ulcer disease; pancreatitis (one patient).

➤*Hematologic:* Aplastic anemia; ecchymosis (one patient).

➤*Miscellaneous:* Headache; syncope; weight gain; renal tubular acidosis; rash.

➤*Lab test abnormalities:*

Metabolic – Acidosis (14%); alkalosis, hyperchloremia (7%); hypophosphatemia (6%); hyperuricemia, hyperphosphatemia (2%); hypernatremia, hypokalemia (1%).

Nutritional – Hypoalbuminemia (11%); decreased total protein (3%).

Hepatic – Increased alkaline phosphatase (6%); increased liver transaminases (4%); hyperbilirubinemia (1%).

Hematologic – Anemia (9%); leukopenia, leukocytosis (4%); thrombocytopenia (3%); thrombocytosis (1%).

Overdosage

No adverse experiences have been reported involving overdoses of sodium phenylbutyrate in patients with urea cycle disorders.

➤*Treatment:* In the event of an overdose, discontinue the drug and institute supportive measures. Hemodialysis or peritoneal dialysis may be beneficial.

BETAINE ANHYDROUS

| *Rx* | **Cystadane** (Orphan Medical) | **Powder:** 1 g/1.7 ml | White, granular. In 180 g bottles. |

Indications

➤*Homocystinuria:* Betaine is indicated for the treatment of homocystinuria to decrease elevated homocysteine blood levels. Included within the category of homocystinuria are deficiencies or defects in: 1) Cystathionine beta-synthase (CBS); 2) 5,10–methylenetetrahydrofolate reductase (MTHFR); and 3) cobalamin cofactor metabolism (cbl).

Betaine has been administered concomitantly with vitamin B_6 (pyridoxine), vitamin B_{12} (cyanocobalamin) and folate.

Administration and Dosage

The usual dosage used in adult and pediatric patients is 6 g/day administered orally in divided doses of 3 g twice daily. Dosages of up to 20 g/day have been necessary to control homocysteine levels in some patients. In pediatric patients < 3 years of age, dosage may be started at 100 mg/kg/day and then increased weekly by 100 mg/kg increments. Dosage in all patients can be gradually increased until plasma homocysteine is undetectable or present only in small amounts.

Measure prescribed amount with the measuring scoop provided (one level 1.7 ml scoop is equal to 1 g of betaine anhydrous powder) and then dissolve in 120 to 180 ml (4 to 6 oz) of water for immediate ingestion.

➤*Storage/Stability:* Store at room temperature, 15° to 30°C (59° to 86°F).

Actions

➤*Pharmacology:* Betaine acts as a methyl group donor in the remethylation of homocysteine to methionine in patients with homocystinuria. As a result, toxic blood levels of homocysteine are reduced in these patients, usually 20% to 80% or less of pre-treatment levels.

Elevated homocysteine blood levels are associated with clinical problems such as cardiovascular thrombosis, osteoporosis, skeletal abnormalities and optic lens dislocation. Plasma levels of homocysteine were decreased in nearly all patients treated with betaine. In observational studies without concurrent controls, clinical improvement was reported by physicians in ≈ ¾ of patients taking betaine. Many of these patients were also taking other therapies such as vitamin B_6 (pyridoxine), vitamin B_{12} (cyanocobalamin) and folate with variable biochemical responses. In most cases, adding betaine resulted in a further reduction in homocysteine.

Betaine lowers plasma homocysteine levels in the three types of homocystinuria: Cystathionine beta-synthase (CBS) deficiency; 5,10–methylenetetrahydrofolate reductase (MTHFR) deficiency; and cobalamin cofactor metabolism (cbl) defect.

Betaine has also increased low plasma methionine and S-adenosylmethionine (SAM) levels in patients with MTHFR deficiency and cbl defect.

In CBS-deficient patients, large increases in methionine levels have been observed. However, the increased methionine levels do not appear to have been associated with adverse clinical consequences.

Betaine occurs naturally in the body. It is a metabolite of choline and is present in small amounts in foods (eg, beets, spinach, cereals and seafood).

➤*Pharmacokinetics:* The onset of action is within several days and a steady state in response to dosage is achieved within several weeks. Patients have taken betaine for many years without evidence of tolerance.

Warnings

➤*Pregnancy: Category C.* It is not known whether betaine can cause fetal harm when administered to a pregnant woman or can affect reproductive capacity. Give to a pregnant woman only if clearly needed.

➤*Lactation:* It is not known whether betaine is excreted in breast milk. Its metabolic precursor, choline, occurs at high levels in breast milk. Exercise caution when administering to a nursing woman.

➤*Children:* The majority of case studies of homocystinuria patients treated wih betaine have been pediatric patients. The disorder, in its most severe form, can be manifested within the first months or years of life by lethargy, failure to thrive, developmental delays, seizures or optic lens displacement. Patients have been treated successfully without adverse effects within the first months or years of life with dosages ≥ 6 g/day with resultant biochemical and clinical improvement. However, dosage titration may be preferable in pediatric patients (see Dosage and Administration).

Adverse Reactions

Betaine Anhydrous Adverse Reactions	
Adverse reaction	n = 111
Nausea	2
GI distress	2
Diarrhea	1
Aspirated the powder	1
Caused odor	1
Questionable psychological changes	1
Unspecified problem	1

Overdosage

In an acute toxicology study in rats, death frequently occurred at doses ≥ 10,000 mg/kg.

Patient Information

Shake bottle lightly before removing cap.

Measure with the scoop provided.

One level scoop (1.7 ml) is equivalent to 1 g of betaine anhydrous powder. Measure the number of scoops your physician has prescribed.

Mix with 120 to 180 ml (4 to 6 oz) of water until completely dissolved, then drink immediately.

Always replace the cap tightly after using. Protect from moisture. Do not use if powder does not completely dissolve or gives a colored solution.

CYSTEAMINE BITARTRATE

Rx	Cystagon (Mylan)	Capsules: 50 mg (as cysteamine bitartrate)	(Cysta 50 Mylan). White. In 100s and 500s.
		150 mg (as cysteamine bitartrate)	(Cystagon 150 Mylan). White. In 100s and 500s.

Indications

➤*Nephropathic cystinosis:* Management in children and adults.

Administration and Dosage

➤*Approved by the FDA:* August 15, 1994.

➤*Initial dose:* For the management of nephropathic cystinosis, initiate therapy promptly once the diagnosis is confirmed (ie, increased white cell cystine). Start new patients on ¼ to ⅙ of the maintenance dose of cysteamine. The dose should then be raised gradually over 4 to 6 weeks to avoid intolerance.

➤*Maintenance:* The recommended cysteamine maintenance dose for children up to age 12 years is 1.3 g/m²/day of the free base, given in 4 divided doses. Intact cysteamine capsules should not be administered to children under the age of ≈ 6 years due to the risk of aspiration. Cysteamine capsules may be administered to children under the age of ≈ 6 years by sprinkling the capsule contents over food. Patients > 12 years of age and > 110 lbs should receive 2 g/day, in 4 divided doses.

When cysteamine is well tolerated, the goal of therapy is to keep leukocyte cystine levels < 1 nmol/½ cystine/mg protein 5 to 6 hours following administration of cysteamine. Patients with poorer tolerability still receive significant benefit if white cell cystine levels are < 2 nmol/½ cystine/mg protein. The cysteamine dose can be increased to a maximum of 1.95 g/m²/day to achieve this level. The dose of 1.95 g/m²/day has been associated with an increased rate of withdrawal from treatment due to intolerance and an increased incidence of adverse events.

Cystinotic patients taking cysteamine HCl or phosphocysteamine solutions may be transferred to equimolar doses of cysteamine bitartrate capsules.

The recommended maintenance dose of 1.3 g/m²/day can be approximated by administering cysteamine according to the following table, which takes surface area as well as weight into consideration.

Cysteamine Maintenance Dose	
Weight (lbs)	Cysteamine free base every 6 hours (mg)
0-10	100
11-20	150
21-30	200
31-40	250
41-50	300
51-70	350
71-90	400
91-110	450
> 110	500

Patients > 12 years of age and > 110 lbs should receive 2 g/day given in 4 divided doses as a starting maintenance dose. This dose should be reached after 4 to 6 weeks of incremental dosage increases as stated above. The dose should be raised if the leukocyte cystine level remains > 2 nmol/½ cystine/mg/protein.

Obtain leukocyte cystine measurements, taken 5 to 6 hours after dose administration, for new patients after the maintenance dose is achieved. Patients being transferred from cysteamine HCl or phosphocysteamine solutions to capsules should have their white cell cystine levels measured in 2 weeks, and thereafter every 3 months to assess optimal dosage as described above.

If cysteamine is poorly tolerated initially due to GI tract symptoms or transient skin rashes, temporarily stop therapy, then reinstitute at a lower dose and gradually increase to the proper dose.

Actions

➤*Pharmacology:* Cysteamine is a cystine depleting agent that lowers the cystine content of cells in patients with cystinosis, an inherited defect of lysosomal transport. Cysteamine is an aminothiol that participates within lysosomes in a thiol-disulfide interchange reaction converting cystine into cysteine and cysteine-cysteamine mixed disulfide, both of which can exit the lysosome in patients with cystinosis.

Cystinosis is an autosomal recessive inborn error of metabolism in which the transport of cystine out of lysosomes is abnormal; in the nephropathic form, accumulation of cystine and formation of crystals damage various organs, especially the kidney, leading to renal tubular Fanconi syndrome and progressive glomerular failure, with end-stage renal failure by the end of the first decade of life. In four studies of cystinosis patients, renal death (need for transplant or dialysis) occurred at a median age of < 10 years. Patients with cystinosis also experience growth failure, rickets and photophobia due to cystine deposits in the cornea. With time, most organs are damaged, including the retina, muscles and CNS. There are approximately 200 pre-transplant cystinosis patients in the US with nephropathic cystinosis.

Healthy individuals and persons heterozygous for cystinosis have white cell cystine levels of < 0.2 and usually < 1 nmol/½cystine/mg protein, respectively. Individuals with nephropathic cystinosis have elevations of white cell cystine > 2 nmol/½ cystine/mg protein. White cell cystine is monitored in these patients to determine adequacy of dosing. In the Long Term Study (see Clinical trials) entry white cell cystine levels were 3.73 nmol/½ cystine/mg protein (range, 0.13 to 19.80) and were maintained close to 1 nmol/½ cystine/mg protein with a cysteamine dose range of 1.3 to 1.95 g/m²/day. There are approximately 200 pre-transplant cystinosis patients in the US with nephropathic cystinosis.

➤*Clinical trials:* The National Collaborative Cysteamine Study (NCCS) treated 94 children with nephropathic cystinosis with increasing doses of cysteamine HCl (mean dose, 54 mg/kg/day) to attain white cell cystine levels of < 2 nmol/½ cystine/mg protein 5 to 6 hours post-dose, and compared their outcome with a historical control group (n = 17). The principal measures of effectiveness were serum creatinine, calculated creatinine clearance (Ccr) and growth (height).

The average median white cell cystine level attained during treatment was 1.7 ± 0.2 nmol/½ cystine/mg protein. Twelve of the 94 cysteamine-treated patients required early dialysis or renal transplant. Median follow-up of cysteamine patients was > 32 months and 20% were followed > 5 years. Among cysteamine patients, glomerular function was maintained over time despite the longer period of treatment and follow-up. Placebo treated patients, in contrast, experienced a gradual rise in serum creatinine. Patients on treatment maintained growth (did not show increasing growth failure compared to healthy individuals) although growth velocity did not increase enough to allow patients to catch up to age norms. Calculated Ccr was evaluated for two groups, one with poor and one with good white cell cystine depletion. The final mean Ccr of the good depletion group was 20.8 ml/min/1.73 m² greater than the mean for the poor depletion group.

The Long Term Study, initiated in 1988, utilized both cysteamine HCl and phosphocysteamine in 46 patients who completed the NCCS (averaging 6.5 years of treatment) and 93 new patients. Patients had cystinosis diagnosed by elevated white cell cystine (mean, 3.63 nmol/½ cystine/mg protein). New patients and 46 continuing patients were required to have serum creatinine < 3 and 4 mg/dl, respectively. Patients were randomized to doses of 1.3 or 1.95 g/m²/day. Doses could be increased if white cell cystine levels were ≈ 2 nmol/½ cystine/mg protein and lowered due to intolerance.

White cell cystine levels averaged 1.72 ± 1.65 and 1.86 ± 0.92 nmol/½ cystine/mg protein in the 1.3 and 1.95 g/m²/day groups, respectively. In new patients, serum creatinine was essentially unchanged over the period of follow-up (≈ 50% followed for 24 months) and phosphocysteamine and cysteamine HCl had similar effects. The long-term follow-up group (almost 80% were followed at least 2 years) had essentially no change in renal function. Both groups maintained height (although they did not catch up from baseline). There was no apparent difference between the two doses.

Contraindications

Hypersensitivity to cysteamine or penicillamine.

Warnings

➤*Rash:* If a skin rash develops, withhold cysteamine until the rash clears. Cysteamine may be restarted at a lower dose under close supervision, then slowly titrated to the therapeutic dose. If a severe skin rash develops such as erythema multiforme bullosa or toxic epidermal necrolysis, cysteamine should not be readministered.

➤*CNS symptoms:* CNS symptoms such as seizures, lethargy, somnolence, depression and encephalopathy have been associated with cysteamine. If CNS symptoms develop, carefully evaluate the patient and adjust the dose as necessary. Neurological complications have been described in some cystinotic patients not on cysteamine treatment. This may be a manifestation of the primary disorder. Patients should not engage in hazardous activities until the effects of cysteamine on mental performance are known.

➤*Fertility impairment:* At an oral dose of 375 mg/kg/day (1.7 times the recommended human dose), cysteamine reduced the fertility of rats and offspring survival.

➤*Pregnancy: Category C.* It is not known whether cysteamine can cause fetal harm when administered to a pregnant woman. Use only when clearly needed and when the potential benefits outweigh the potential hazards to the fetus.

➤*Lactation:* It is not known whether cysteamine is excreted in breast milk. Because of the manifested potential of cysteamine for developmental toxicity in suckling rat pups when it was administered to their lactating mothers at an oral dose of 375 mg/kg/day, decide whether to discontinue nursing or to discontinue the drug, taking into account the importance of the drug to the mother.

➤*Children:* The safety and efficacy of cysteamine for cystinotic children have been established. Initiate therapy as soon as the diagnosis of nephropathic cystinosis has been confirmed.

CYSTEAMINE BITARTRATE

Precautions

➤*Monitoring:* Cysteamine has occasionally been associated with reversible leukopenia and abnormal liver function studies. Therefore, monitor blood counts and liver function studies.

Leukocyte cystine measurements are useful to determine adequate dosage and compliance. When measured 5 to 6 hours after cysteamine administration, the goal should be a level < 1 nmol/½; cystine/mg protein. In some patients with poorer tolerability for cysteamine, patients may still receive benefit with a white cell cystine level of < 2 nmol/½; cystine/mg protein. Measurements should be done every 3 months, more frequently when patients are transferred from cysteamine HCl or phosphocysteamine solutions to cysteamine bitartrate.

➤*GI symptoms:* GI symptoms, including nausea, vomiting, anorexia and abdominal pain (sometimes severe), have been associated with cysteamine. If these develop, therapy may have to be interrupted and the dose adjusted. A dose of 1.95 g/m²/day (≈ 80 to 90 mg/kg/day) was associated with an increased number of withdrawals from treatment due to intolerance and an increased incidence of adverse events.

➤*Concurrent therapy:* Cysteamine can be administered with electrolyte and mineral replacements necessary for management of the Fanconi syndrome as well as vitamin D and thyroid hormone.

Adverse Reactions

In three clinical trials, cysteamine or phosphocysteamine have been administered to 246 children with cystinosis. Causality of side effects is sometimes difficult to determine because adverse effects may result from the underlying disease.

Adverse reactions or intolerance leading to cessation of treatment occurred in 8% of patients in the US studies. Withdrawals due to intolerance, vomiting associated with medication, anorexia, lethargy and fever appeared dose-related, occurring more frequently in those patients receiving 1.95 vs 1.3 g/m²/day.

The most frequent adverse reactions seen involve the GI (see Precautions) and central nervous systems (see Warnings). These are especially prominent at the initiation of therapy. Temporarily suspending treatment, then gradual reintroduction may be effective in improving tolerance. The most common events (> 5%) were vomiting (35%), anorexia (31%), fever (22%), diarrhea (16%), lethargy (11%) and rash (7%).

Other adverse reactions are as follows:

➤*CNS:* Somnolence; encephalopathy; headache; seizures; ataxia; confusion; tremor; hyperkinesia; decreased hearing; dizziness; jitteriness.

➤*GI:* Nausea; bad breath; abdominal pain; dyspepsia; constipation; gastroenteritis; duodenitis; duodenal ulceration.

➤*Psychiatric:* Nervousness; abnormal thinking; depression; emotional lability; hallucinations; nightmares.

➤*Miscellaneous:* Abnormal liver function; anemia; leukopenia; dehydration; hypertension; urticaria.

Overdosage

➤*Symptoms:* A single oral dose of 660 mg/kg was lethal to rats. Symptoms of acute toxicity were reduction of motor activity and generalized hemorrhage in the GI tract and kidneys. One case of massive human overdosage has been reported. The patient immediately vomited the drug and did not develop any symptoms.

➤*Treatment:* Should overdose occur, appropriately support the respiratory and cardiovascular systems. No specific antidote is known. Refer to General Management of Acute Overdosage. Hemodialysis may be considered since cysteamine is poorly bound to plasma proteins.

SODIUM BENZOATE AND SODIUM PHENYLACETATE

| Rx | Ucephan (Ucyclyd Pharma) | Solution: 10 g sodium benzoate and 10 g sodium phenylacetate per 100 ml | In 100 ml multiple unit bottles. |

Indications

➤*Hyperammonemia:* Adjunctive therapy for the prevention and treatment of hyperammonemia in the chronic management of patients with UCE involving partial or complete deficiencies of carbamylphosphate synthetase, ornithine transcarbamylase or argininosuccinate synthetase.

Administration and Dosage

➤*Approved by the FDA:* December 23, 1987.

For oral use only. Must be diluted before use.

The usual total daily dose for adjunctive therapy of UCE patients is 2.5 ml/kg/day (250 mg sodium benzoate and 250 mg sodium phenylacetate) in 3 to 6 equally divided doses. Total daily dose should not exceed 100 ml (10 g each of sodium benzoate and sodium phenylacetate).

Dilute each dose in 4 to 8 ounces of infant formula or milk and administer with meals. If other beverages are used, particularly acidic beverages, precipitation of the drug may occur depending on pH and the final concentration. Inspect mixture for compatibility before administration.

Because this is a concentrated solution, exercise care in calculating the dose to avoid the possibility of overdosage.

Not intended as sole therapy for UCE patients. Combine as adjunctive therapy with dietary management (low-protein diet) and amino acid supplementation for optimal results.

Because sodium phenylacetate has a lingering odor, exercise care in mixing and administering the drug to minimize contact with skin and clothing.

➤*Storage/Stability:* Store at room temperature. Avoid excessive heat.

Actions

➤*Pharmacology:* Sodium benzoate and sodium phenylacetate are metabolically active compounds that decrease elevated blood ammonia concentrations in patients with inborn errors of ureagenesis. The mechanisms for this action are conjugation reactions involving acylation of amino acids, which result in decreased ammonia formation. Benzoate and phenylacetate activate conjugation pathways that substitute for or supplement the defective ureagenic pathway in patients with urea cycle enzymopathies (UCE), preventing the accumulation of ammonia.

The therapeutic regimens of sodium benzoate and sodium phenylacetate, which also included dietary manipulation and amino acid supplementation, were effective in long-term management of UCE patients. Survival rate in patients with complete enzyme deficiencies was ≈ 80% with this combined regimen in what was previously an almost universally fatal disease within the first year of life. The survival rate for each complete enzyme deficiency studied was: Carbamylphosphate synthetase, 75%; ornithine transcarbamylase (males), 59%; argininosuccinate synthetase, 96%. Survival in heterozygous females with partial ornithine transcarbamylase deficiency was 95%; for patients with other partial deficiencies, 86%. Early diagnosis and treatment are important in minimizing developmental disabilities. Reversal of preexisting neurologic impairment is not likely to occur with treatment, and neurologic deterioration may continue in some patients.

➤*Pharmacokinetics:* Studies have not been conducted in the primary patient population (neonates, infants and children). Preliminary pharmacokinetic data were obtained from only three healthy adult subjects and the overall disposition of sodium benzoate, sodium phenylacetate and their metabolites has not been fully characterized. Peak blood levels of benzoate or phenylacetate occur within 1 hour after a single oral dose of sodium benzoate or sodium phenylacetate. A majority of the administered compound (≈ 80% to 100%) was excreted by the kidneys within 24 hours as the respective conjugation product, hippurate or phenylacetylglutamine. The major sites for metabolism of benzoate and phenylacetate are the liver and kidneys.

Warnings

➤*Sodium:* Because of the sodium content of this product, consider the possibility of hypernatremia. Use with great care, if at all, in patients with CHF, severe renal insufficiency and in clinical states in which there is sodium retention with edema. In patients with diminished renal function, administration of solutions containing sodium ions may result in sodium retention.

➤*Benzyl alcohol:* Some of these products contain benzyl alcohol, which has been associated with fatal "gasping syndrome" in premature infants.

➤*Hypersensitivity reactions:* Do not administer to patients with known hypersensitivities to sodium benzoate or sodium phenylacetate. No such cases of hypersensitivities have been reported.

➤*Pregnancy: Category C.* Safety for use during pregnancy has not been established. Use only when clearly needed and when the potential benefits outweigh the hazards to the fetus.

➤*Lactation:* It is not known whether this drug is excreted in breast milk. Use caution when administering to a nursing woman.

Precautions

➤*Adjunctive therapy:* Not intended as sole therapy for UCE patients. Combine as adjunctive therapy with dietary management (low-protein diet) and amino acid supplementation for optimal results.

➤*Hyperbilirubinemia:* Use with caution in neonates with hyperbilirubinemia, as in vitro experiments suggest that benzoate competes for bilirubin binding sites on albumin.

➤*Neonatal hyperammonemic coma:* The benefits of treating neonatal hyperammonemic coma with this drug have not been established. The treatment of choice in neonatal hyperammonemic coma is hemodialysis. Peritoneal dialysis may be helpful if hemodialysis is not available.

Drug Interactions

Sodium Benzoate/Phenylacetate Drug Interactions			
Precipitant drug	Object drug*		Description
Penicillin	Sodium benzoate/phenylacetate	↓	Penicillin may compete with conjugated products of sodium benzoate and sodium phenylacetate for active secretion by renal tubules.
Probenecid	Sodium benzoate/phenylacetate	↓	Probenecid inhibits the renal transport of many organic compounds, including amino hippuric acid and may affect renal excretion of the conjugation products of sodium benzoate and sodium phenylacetate.
Valproic acid	Sodium benzoate/phenylacetate	↓	Valproic acid may induce hyperammonemia. Therefore, administration of valproic acid to UCE patients may exacerbate their condition and be antagonistic to the efficacy of sodium benzoate/phenylacetate.

* ↓ = Object drug decreased.

Adverse Reactions

Nausea and vomiting.

Side effects associated with salicylates such as exacerbation of peptic ulcers, mild hyperventilation and mild respiratory alkalosis may occur because of structural similarities between benzoate and salicylates.

If an adverse reaction does occur, discontinue administration, evaluate the patient and institute appropriate therapeutic countermeasures.

Overdosage

Four overdoses of sodium phenylacetate or sodium benzoate in UCE patients have been reported, two cases following the use of an IV infusion. Two patients became irritable and vomited after receiving threefold overdoses of oral sodium benzoate. Both patients recovered without treatment within 24 hours after the drug was discontinued.

➤*Treatment:* Discontinue the drug and institute supportive measures for metabolic acidosis and circulatory collapse. Hemodialysis or peritoneal dialysis may be beneficial.

BROMOCRIPTINE MESYLATE

Rx	**Parlodel**	**Tablets:** 2.5 mg (as mesylate)	Lactose. (Parlodel 2½). White, scored. In 30s and 100s.
	(Sandoz)	**Capsules:** 5 mg (as mesylate)	Lactose. (Parlodel 5 mg). Caramel and white. In 30s and 100s.

Bromocriptine is also used for Parkinson's disease; refer to the monograph in the Antiparkinson Agents section for further information.

Indications

➤*Hyperprolactinemia-associated dysfunctions:* Amenorrhea with or without galactorrhea, infertility or hypogonadism. Indicated in patients with prolactin-secreting adenomas, which may be the basic underlying endocrinopathy contributing to above clinical presentations. Reduction in tumor size has been demonstrated in both male and female patients with macroadenomas. In cases where adenectomy is elected, bromocriptine therapy may be used to reduce tumor mass prior to surgery.

➤*Acromegaly:* Bromocriptine, alone or as adjunctive therapy with pituitary irradiation or surgery, reduces serum growth hormone by ≥ 50% in ≈ 50% of patients treated, although not usually to normal levels.

➤*Parkinson's disease:* See monograph in the Antiparkinson Agents section.

➤*Unlabeled uses:* Bromocriptine has been used to treat hyperprolactinemia associated with pituitary adenomas; it has caused elevated prolactin levels to normalize, causing shrinkage of macroprolactinomas. Maintenance doses of 0.625 to 10 mg/day have been used for 6 to 52 months.

Neuroleptic malignant syndrome.

Cocaine addiction.

Cyclical mastalgia.

Bromocroptine was previously indicated for prevention of physiological lactation (secretion, congestion, engorgement) occurring after parturition when the mother does not breastfeed, or after stillbirth or abortion. However, this indication has been withdrawn by the manufacturer; it should no longer be used for this condition.

Administration and Dosage

➤*Hyperprolactinemic indications:*

Initial – 0.5 to 2.5 mg daily with meals; 2.5 mg may be added as tolerated every 3 to 7 days or until optimal therapeutic response is achieved. Therapeutic dosage usually is 5 to 7.5 mg (range, 2.5 to 15 mg/day).

➤*Acromegaly:* Virtually all patients receiving therapeutic benefit show reductions in circulating levels of growth hormone. Periodically assess growth hormone levels. If no significant reduction in hormone levels has occurred after a brief trial, consider dosage adjustment or discontinue the drug.

Initial – 1.25 to 2.5 mg for 3 days (with food) on retiring. Add an additional 1.25 to 2.5 mg as tolerated every 3 to 7 days until the patient obtains optimal therapeutic benefit. Evaluate patients monthly and adjust the dosage based on reductions of growth hormone. The usual optimal therapeutic dosage range varies from 20 to 30 mg/day. Maximal dosage should not exceed 100 mg/day.

Withdraw patients treated with pituitary irradiation from bromocriptine therapy on a yearly basis to assess both the clinical effects of radiation on the disease process as well as the effects of bromocriptine. Usually, a 4 to 8 week withdrawal period is adequate. Recurrence of symptoms or growth hormone increases indicate the disease process is still active. Consider further courses of bromocriptine.

Actions

➤*Pharmacology:* Bromocriptine mesylate is a semisynthetic ergot alkaloid derivative which inhibits prolactin secretion with no effect on other pituitary hormones, except in acromegaly, where it lowers elevated blood levels of growth hormone.

It is a dopamine receptor agonist that activates postsynaptic dopamine receptors. The dopaminergic neurons in the tuberoinfundibular process modulate the secretion of prolactin from the anterior pituitary by secreting a prolactin inhibitory factor (thought to be dopamine) in the corpus striatum; the dopaminergic neurons are involved in the control of motor function. Bromocriptine significantly reduces plasma levels of prolactin in patients with physiologically elevated prolactin and in patients with hyperprolactinemia.

Amenorrhea / galactorrhea / female infertility – In about 75% of cases of galactorrhea and amenorrhea, bromocriptine suppresses the galactorrhea and reinitiates normal ovulatory menstrual cycles, usually in 6 to 8 weeks. However, some patients respond within a few days. Others may take up to 8 months. Menses are usually reinitiated prior to complete suppression of galactorrhea.

Galactorrhea may take longer to control, depending on the degree of stimulation of mammary tissue prior to therapy. A ≥ 75% reduction in secretion usually occurs after 8 to 12 weeks. Some patients fail to respond, even after 12 months.

Acromegaly – Bromocriptine produces a prompt and sustained reduction in circulating levels of serum growth hormone. Since the effects of external pituitary radiation may not become maximal for several years, adjunctive therapy with bromocriptine offers potential benefit before the effects of irradiation are manifested (see Precautions).

➤*Pharmacokinetics:*

Absorption / Distribution – Twenty-eight percent of an oral dose is absorbed from the GI tract. Blood levels following a 2.5 mg dose range from 2 to 3 ng equivalents/ml. Plasma levels range from 4 to 6 ng equivalents/ml. The drug undergoes first-pass metabolism and only 6% of the absorbed dose reaches the systemic circulation unchanged. Plasma half-life is 6 to 8 hours. Bromocriptine is 90% to 96% bound to serum albumin.

Metabolism / Excretion – Bromocriptine is completely metabolized prior to excretion; 84.6% of the dose is excreted in the feces. Only 2.5% to 5.5% is excreted in the urine. The major route of excretion of absorbed drug is via the bile.

Contraindications

Sensitivity to ergot alkaloids; severe ischemic heart disease or peripheral vascular disease; withdraw in patients being treated for hyperprolactinemia when pregnancy is diagnosed (see Warnings).

Warnings

➤*Pituitary tumors:* Since hyperprolactinemia with amenorrhea/galactorrhea and infertility has been found in patients with pituitary tumors, perform evaluation of pituitary before treatment.

➤*Symptomatic hypotension:* In postpartum studies, hypotension (decrease in supine systolic and diastolic pressures of > 20 and 10 mm Hg, respectively) was observed in almost 30% of patients. On occasion, the drop in supine systolic pressure was as great as 50 to 59 mm Hg. However, since bromocriptine causes hypotension and, rarely, hypertension, do not initiate therapy until the vital signs are stabilized and no sooner than 4 hours after delivery.

Give particular attention to patients with preeclampsia and to those who have received within the preceding 24 hours other ergot alkaloids or drugs which can alter blood pressure. Monitor blood pressure, particularly during the first few weeks of therapy. Exercise care when bromocriptine is administered concomitantly with other medications known to lower blood pressure.

➤*Rhinorrhea:* A few cases of cerebrospinal fluid rhinorrhea occurred in patients receiving bromocriptine for treatment of large prolactinomas. This has occurred rarely, usually only in patients who have received previous transsphenoidal surgery, pituitary radiation, or both, and who were receiving bromocriptine for tumor recurrence. It may also occur in previously untreated patients whose tumor extends into the sphenoid sinus.

➤*Pregnancy: Category B.* Since pregnancy is often the therapeutic objective in many hyperprolactinemic patients presenting with amenorrhea/galactorrhea and infertility, assess pituitary to detect the presence of a prolactin secreting adenoma. Advise patients not seeking pregnancy, or those harboring large adenomas, to use contraceptive measures other than oral contraceptives during treatment. Since pregnancy may occur prior to reinitiation of menses, perform a pregnancy test at least every 4 weeks during the amenorrheic period and once menses are reinitiated, every time a patient misses a menstrual period. Discontinuation of bromocriptine treatment in patients with known macroadenomas has been associated with rapid regrowth of tumor and increase in serum prolactin in most cases.

Safe use of bromocriptine has not been demonstrated in pregnancy and use in pregnancy is contraindicated. If pregnancy occurs, discontinue treatment immediately and carefully observe these patients throughout pregnancy for signs and symptoms which may develop if a previously undetected prolactin-secreting tumor enlarges.

Prolactin-secreting adenomas may expand and compression of optic or other cranial nerves may occur and emergency pituitary surgery may be necessary. In most cases, compression resolves following delivery. Reinitiation of bromocriptine has produced improvement in visual fields of patients in whom nerve compression has occurred during pregnancy. The relative efficacy of bromocriptine vs surgery in preserving visual fields is not known. Evaluate patients with rapidly progressive visual field loss to decide on the most appropriate therapy.

Of 1276 reported pregnancies in women who took bromocriptine during early pregnancy, there were 1109 live born infants and 4 stillborn infants.

The total incidence of malformations (3.3%) and spontaneous abortions (11%) does not exceed that of the population at large. There were three hydatidiform moles, two in the same patient.

➤*Lactation:* Since bromocriptine prevents lactation, do not administer to mothers who will breastfeed.

➤*Children:* Safety and efficacy in children < 15 years of age have not been established.

BROMOCRIPTINE MESYLATE

Precautions

➤*Acromegaly:* Cold sensitive digital vasospasm has occurred in some acromegalic patients treated with bromocriptine. The response can be reversed by reducing the dosage and may be prevented by keeping the fingers warm. Cases of severe GI bleeding from peptic ulcers have been reported, some fatal. Although there is no evidence that bromocriptine increases the incidence of peptic ulcers in acromegalic patients, thoroughly investigate symptoms suggestive of peptic ulcer and treat appropriately.

Possible tumor expansion during therapy has occurred. The natural history of growth hormone secreting tumors is unknown; monitor patients. If evidence of tumor expansion develops, discontinue treatment and consider alternative procedures.

➤*Pulmonary effects:* Long-term treatment (6 to 36 months) in doses of 20 to 100 mg/day is associated with pulmonary infiltrates, pleural effusion and pleural thickening. When treatment was terminated, the changes slowly reverted toward normal.

Drug Interactions

Bromocriptine Drug Interactions			
Precipitant drug	Object drug*		Description
Erythromycin	Bromocriptine	↑	Bromocriptine levels may be increased, possibly increasing pharmacologic and toxic effects.
Phenothiazines	Bromocriptine	↓	Efficacy of bromocriptine, when used for prolactin-secreting tumors, may be inhibited.
Sympatho-mimetics Isometheptene Phenylpropa-nolamine	Bromocriptine	↑	In several case reports, bromocriptine side effects were exacerbated during concurrent use of these agents, including ventricular tachycardia and cardiac dysfunction.

* ↑ = Object drug increased.　　↓ = Object drug decreased.

Adverse Reactions

➤*Hyperprolactinemic indications:* The incidence of adverse effects is high (69%), but they are generally mild to moderate. Therapy was discontinued in approximately 5% of patients. Adverse reactions include: Nausea (49%); headache (19%); dizziness (17%); fatigue (7%); lightheadedness, vomiting (5%); abdominal cramps (4%); nasal congestion, constipation, diarrhea, drowsiness (3%); psychosis; hypotension; cerebrospinal fluid rhinorrhea (see Warnings). Occurrence of these effects may be lessened by temporarily reducing dosage to ½ tablet 2 to 3 times daily.

➤*Acromegaly:*

Cardiovascular – Postural/orthostatic hypotension (6%); arrhythmias, ventricular tachycardia (< 1%).

CNS – Digital vasospasm, drowsiness/tiredness (3%); dizziness, headache, syncope, Raynaud's syndrome (< 2%); faintness, lightheadedness, decreased sleep requirement, visual hallucinations, lassitude, vertigo, paresthesia, delusional psychosis (< 1%).

GI – Nausea (18%); constipation (14%); anorexia; dry mouth, indigestion/dyspepsia (4%); vomiting (2%); GI bleeding (< 2%).

Respiratory – Nasal stuffiness (4%); shortness of breath (< 1%).

Miscellaneous – Sluggishness, paranoia, insomnia, heavy headedness, reduced tolerance to cold, tingling of ears, facial pallor, muscle cramps, hair loss, alcohol potentiation (< 1%).

➤*Lab test abnormalities:* Elevations in BUN, AST, ALT, GGPT, CPK, alkaline phosphatase and uric acid are usually transient and not clinically significant.

Patient Information

Take with meals or food.

Dizziness or fainting may occur, particularly following the first dose; take the first dose while lying down. Avoid sudden changes in posture, such as rising from a sitting position. Observe caution while driving or performing other tasks requiring alertness, coordination or physical dexterity.

Advise patients receiving bromocriptine for hyperprolactinemic states associated with macroadenoma or those who have had previous transsphenoidal surgery to report any persistent watery nasal discharge to a physician. Advise patients receiving bromocriptine for treatment of a macroadenoma that discontinuation of drug may be associated with rapid regrowth of the tumor and recurrence of original symptoms.

Use contraceptive measures (other than oral contraceptives) during treatment.

CABERGOLINE

Rx   **Dostinex** (Pharmacia & Upjohn)   **Tablets:** 0.5 mg   (PU 700). White, scored. Capsule shaped. In bottles of 8.

Indications

➤*Hyperprolactinemia:* The treatment of hyperprolactinemic disorders, either idiopathic or because of pituitary adenomas.

➤*Unlabeled uses:* Cabergoline has caused tumor shrinkage in patients with microprolactinoma or macroprolactinoma, but more studies are needed; Parkinson's disease (7.5 mg/day); normalize androgen levels and improve menstrual cyclicity in polycystic ovary syndrome (0.5 mg/week).

Administration and Dosage

➤*Approved by the FDA:* December 23, 1996.

The recommended dosage of cabergoline for initiation of therapy is 0.25 mg twice a week. Dosage may be increased by 0.25 mg twice weekly to ≤ 1 mg twice a week according to the patient's serum prolactin level.

Dosage increases should not occur more rapidly than every 4 weeks. If the patient does not respond adequately and no additional benefit is observed with higher doses, use the lowest dose that achieved maximal response and consider other therapeutic approaches.

After a normal serum prolactin level has been maintained for 6 months, cabergoline may be discontinued. Periodically monitor the serum prolactin level to determine if or when treatment with cabergoline should be reinstituted. The durability of efficacy beyond 24 months of therapy with cabergoline has not been established.

Actions

➤*Pharmacology:* The secretion of prolactin by the anterior pituitary is mainly under hypothalmic inhibitory control, likely exerted through release of dopamine by tuberoinfundibular neurons. Cabergoline is a synthetic ergot derivative long-acting dopamine receptor agonist with a high affinity for D_2 receptors. Cabergoline inhibits basal and metoclopramide-induced prolactin secretion. Receptor-binding studies indicate that cabergoline has low affinity for dopamine D_1, alpha$_1$- and alpha$_2$-adrenergic and 5-HT$_1$- and 5-HT$_2$-serotonin receptors.

Pharmacodynamics – Dose response with inhibition of plasma prolactin, onset of maximal effect and duration of effect has been documented following single cabergoline doses to healthy volunteers (0.05 to 1.5 mg) and hyperprolactinemic patients (0.3 to 1 mg). Prolactin inhibition was evident at doses > 0.2 mg, while doses ≥ 0.5 mg caused maximal suppression in most subjects. Higher doses produce prolactin suppression in a greater proportion of subjects and with an earlier onset and longer duration of action. In 12 healthy volunteers, 0.5, 1 and 1.5 mg doses resulted in complete prolactin inhibition, with a maximum effect within 3 hours in 92% to 100% of subjects after the 1 and 1.5 mg doses compared with 50% of subjects after the 0.5 mg dose.

In hyperprolactinemic patients, the maximal prolactin decrease after a 0.6 mg single dose of cabergoline was comparable with 2.5 mg bromocriptine; however, the duration of effect was markedly longer (14 days vs 24 hours). The time to maximal effect was shorter for bromocriptine than cabergoline (6 hours vs 48 hours).

In 72 healthy volunteers, single or multiple doses (≤ 2 mg) of cabergoline resulted in selective inhibition of prolactin with no apparent effect on other anterior pituitary hormones (GH, FSH, LH, ACTH and TSH) or cortisol.

➤*Pharmacokinetics:*

Absorption – Following single oral doses of 0.5 mg to 1.5 mg given to 12 healthy adult volunteers, mean peak plasma levels of 30 to 70 picograms of cabergoline were observed within 2 to 3 hours. The absolute bioavailability of cabergoline is unknown. A significant fraction of the administered dose undergoes a first-pass effect. Absorption is not affected by food.

Distribution – Cabergoline is moderately bound (40% to 42%) to human plasma proteins in a concentration-independent manner. Concomitant dosing of highly protein-bound drugs is unlikely to affect its disposition. Over the 0.5 to 7 mg dose range, cabergoline plasma levels appeared to be dose-proportional in 12 healthy adult volunteers and nine adult parkinsonian patients. A repeat-dose study in 12 healthy volunteers suggests that steady-state levels following a once-weekly dosing schedule are expected to be 2– to 3–fold higher than after a single dose.

Metabolism – Cabergoline is extensively metabolized, predominantly via hydrolysis of the acylurea bond or the urea moiety. Cytochrome P450 mediated metabolism appears to be minimal. Hydrolysis of the acylurea or urea moiety abolishes the prolactin-lowering effect of cabergoline, and major metabolites identified thus far do not contribute to the therapeutic effect. Cytochrome P450-mediated metabolism appears to be minimal.

Excretion – After oral dosing of radioactive cabergoline to five healthy volunteers, ≈ 22% and 60% of the dose was excreted within 20 days in the urine and feces, respectively. Less than 4% of the dose was excreted unchanged in the urine. Nonrenal and renal clearances for cabergoline

are ≈ 3.2 L/min and 0.08 L/min, respectively. Urinary excretion in hyperprolactinemic patients was similar. The elimination half-life is estimated to be 63 to 69 hours. The prolonged prolactin-lowering effect of cabergoline may be related to its slow elimination and long half-life.

Special populations –

Renal function impairment: The pharmacokinetics of cabergoline were not altered in 12 patients with moderate to severe renal insufficiency as assessed by creatinine clearance.

Cabergoline Pharmacokinetic Parameters in Patients with Renal Insufficiency					
Type of Patients	C$_{max}$ (pg/ml)	T$_{max}$* (hr)	AUC$_{(0-168\ hr)}$ (pg-hr/ml)	CL$_R$ (ml/min)	Ae* $_{(0-168\ hr)}$ (mcg)
Healthy	59.1	2.5	2861	76.7	11.9
Renal insufficiency (moderate)	86.7	1.5	3778	38.9	12.6
Renal insufficiency (severe)	55.7	2.5	2834	34.2	4.4

* Total urinary excretion of unchanged drug.

Hepatic function impairment: In 12 patients with mild to moderate hepatic dysfunction, no effect on mean cabergoline C$_{max}$ or area under the plasma concentration curve (AUC) was observed. However, patients with severe insufficiency show a substantial increase in the mean cabergoline C$_{max}$ and AUC, which necessitates caution.

➤*Clinical trials:* In the 8–week, double-blind period of the comparative trial with bromocriptine (cabergoline n = 223; bromocriptine n = 236), prolactin was normalized in 77% of the patients treated with cabergoline at 0.5 mg twice weekly compared with 59% of those treated with bromocriptine at 2.5 mg twice daily. Restoration of menses occurred in 77% of the women treated with cabergoline, compared with 70% of those treated with bromocriptine. Among patients with galactorrhea, this symptom disappeared in 73% of those treated with cabergoline compared with 56% of those treated with bromocriptine.

Contraindications

Uncontrolled hypertension or known hypersensitivity to ergot derivatives.

Warnings

➤*Hepatic function impairment:* Because cabergoline is extensively metabolized by the liver, use caution and careful monitoring when administering cabergoline to patients with hepatic function impairment.

➤*Carcinogenesis:* There was a slight increase in the incidence of cervical and uterine leiomyomas and uterine leiomyosarcomas in mice. In rats, there was a slight increase in malignant tumors of the cervix and uterus and interstitial cell adenomas.

➤*Fertility impairment:* In female rats, a dose of 0.003 mg/kg/day for 2 weeks prior to mating and throughout the mating period inhibited conception.

➤*Pregnancy: Category B.* There were 24 out of 204 miscarriages and three abortions induced because of major malformations. Two of the 148 single live-born infants had significant malformations: one megaureter, one scaphocephaly. Follow-up of babies indicates normal physical and mental development. Use this drug during pregnancy only if clearly needed.

Pregnancy-induced hypertension – Do not use dopamine agonists in patients with pregnancy-induced hypertension, for example, preeclampsia and eclampsia, unless the potential benefit is judged to outweigh the possible risk.

➤*Lactation:* It is not known whether this drug is excreted in breast milk. Decide whether to discontinue nursing or to discontinue the drug, taking into account the importance of the drug to the mother. Use of cabergoline for the inhibition or suppression of physiologic lactation is not recommended.

The prolactin-lowering action of cabergoline suggests that it will interfere with lactation. Because of this interference with lactation, do not give to women postpartum who are breastfeeding or who are planning to breastfeed.

Postpartum lactation inhibition or suppression – Cabergoline is not indicated for the inhibition or suppression of physiologic lactation. Use of bromocriptine, another dopamine agonist for this purpose, has been associated with cases of hypertension, stroke and seizures.

➤*Children:* Safety and effectiveness of cabergoline in pediatric patients have not been established.

Precautions

➤*Monitoring:* Monitor prolactin levels monthly until prolactin levels are normalized (< 20 mcg/L in women and < 15 mcg/L in men).

➤*Orthostatic hypotension:* Initial doses > 1 mg may produce orthostatic hypotension. Exercise caution when administering cabergoline with other medications known to lower blood pressure.

CABERGOLINE

Drug Interactions

Cabergoline Drug Interactions

Precipitant drug	Object drug*		Description
Cabergoline	Antihypertensives	↑	Additive hypotensive effects may occur when cabergoline is administered with other hypotensive medications. In addition, antihypertensive dosage adjustments may be necessary if antihypertensive medications are administered concurrently with cabergoline.
Dopamine (D₂) antagonists (eg, phenothiazines, butyrophenones, thioxanthenes or metoclopramide)	Cabergoline	↓	Dopamine (D₂) antagonists may reduce the therapeutic effects of cabergoline. Do not administer with cabergoline.

* ↑ = Object drug increased. ↓ = Object drug decreased.

Adverse Reactions

Cabergoline Adverse Reactions Compared with Bromocriptine (%)

Adverse Reaction	Cabergoline	Bromocriptine
Cardiovascular		
Postural hypotension	4	6
Hypotension	+	6
Palpitations	+	-
CNS		
Headache	26	27
Dizziness	17	18
Somnolence	5	-
Vertigo	4	4
Paresthesia	2	3
Depression	3	-
Nervousness	2	-
Anxiety	+	-
Insomnia	+	-
GI		
Nausea	29	48
Constipation	7	9
Abdominal pain	5	8
Dyspepsia	5	7
Vomiting	4	7
Dry mouth	2	1

Cabergoline Adverse Reactions Compared with Bromocriptine (%)

Adverse Reaction	Cabergoline	Bromocriptine
Diarrhea	2	3
Flatulence	2	1
Throat irritation	1	-
Toothache	1	-
Anorexia	+	4
Weight loss/gain	+	-
GU		
Breast pain	1	-
Dysmenorrhea	1	-
Increased libido	+	-
Miscellaneous		
Nasal stuffiness	+	4
Abnormal vision	1	-
Acne	+	-
Epistaxis	+	-
Pruritus	+	-
Asthenia	6	6
Fatigue	5	8
Syncope	1	1
Influenza-like symptoms	1	-
Malaise	1	-
Periorbital edema	1	1
Peripheral edema	1	4
Hot flashes	1	-

+ Occurs, but percentage is unknown.

Compared with bromocriptine, cabergoline was discontinued because of an adverse event in 4 of 221 patients (2%), while bromocriptine was discontinued in 14 of 231 patients (6%). The most common reasons for discontinuation from cabergoline were headache, nausea and vomiting; the most common reasons for discontinuation from bromocriptine were nausea, vomiting, headache, and dizziness or vertigo.

Overdosage

Overdosage might be expected to produce nasal congestion, syncope or hallucinations. Take measures to support blood pressure if necessary.

Patient Information

Notify physician if pregnancy occurs or is suspected, or if patient intends to become pregnant during therapy. Perform a pregnancy test if there is any suspicion of pregnancy and discuss discontinuation of treatment.

Inform patients that dizziness or lightheadedness may occur if they stand up too fast. If this occurs, have them get up slowly and avoid sudden changes in posture.

In addition to the agents in this section, sulindac and indomethacin (see Nonsteroidal Anti-inflammatory Agents monograph) are indicated for the treatment of gout. See also probenecid and sulfinpyrazone in the Uricosurics section.

Uricosurics

PROBENECID

Rx   **Probenecid** (Various, eg, Geneva, Moore, Parmed, Purepac, Schein, URL)   **Tablets:** 0.5 g   In 100s and 1000s.

Indications

➤*Treatment of hyperuricemia:* Treatment of hyperuricemia associated with gout and gouty arthritis.

➤*Prolongation of plasma levels of antibiotics:* Adjuvant to therapy with penicillins or cephalosporins, for elevation and prolongation of plasma levels of the antibiotic.

Administration and Dosage

➤*Gout:* Do not start therapy until an acute gouty attack has subsided. However, if an acute attack is precipitated during therapy, probenecid may be continued. Give full therapeutic doses of colchicine or other appropriate therapy to control the acute attack.

Adults – 0.25 g twice daily for 1 week, followed by 0.5 g twice daily thereafter. Gastric intolerance may indicate overdosage and may be reduced by decreasing dosage.

Renal function impairment – Some degree of renal impairment may be present in patients with gout. A daily dosage of 1 g may be adequate. However, if necessary, the daily dosage may be increased by 0.5 g increments every 4 weeks within tolerance (usually ≤ 2 g/day) if symptoms of gouty arthritis are not controlled or the 24-hour urate excretion is not ≤ 700 mg. Probenecid may not be effective in chronic renal insufficiency, particularly when the glomerular filtration rate is ≤ 30 ml/min.

Urinary alkalinization – Urates tend to crystallize out of an acid urine; therefore, a liberal fluid intake is recommended, as well as sufficient sodium bicarbonate (3 to 7.5 g/day) or potassium citrate (7.5 g/day) to maintain an alkaline urine; continue alkalization until the serum uric acid level returns to normal limits and tophaceous deposits disappear. Thereafter, urinary alkalization and the restriction of purine-producing foods may be relaxed.

Maintenance therapy – Continue the dosage that maintains normal serum uric acid levels. When there have been no acute attacks for ≥ 6 months and serum uric acid levels have remained within normal limits, decrease the daily dosage by 0.5 g every 6 months. Do not reduce the maintenance dosage to the point where serum uric acid levels increase.

➤*Penicillin or cephalosporin therapy:* The phenolsulfonphthalein excretion test (PSP) may be used to determine the effectiveness of probenecid in retarding penicillin excretion and maintaining therapeutic levels. The renal clearance of PSP is reduced to ⅕ the normal rate when dosage of probenecid is adequate.

Adults – 2 g/day in divided doses. Reduce dosage in older patients in whom renal impairment may be present. Not recommended in conjunction with penicillin or a cephalosporin in the presence of known renal impairment.

Children (2 to 14 yrs) – Initial dose 25 mg/kg or 0.7 g/m² body surface. Maintenance dose 40 mg/kg/day or 1.2 g/m² body surface divided into 4 doses. For children weighing > 50 kg (110 lbs), use the adult dosage. Do not use in children < 2 years of age.

Gonorrhea (uncomplicated) – Give probenecid as a single 1 g dose immediately before or with 4.8 million units penicillin G procaine, aqueous, divided into at least two doses.

Neurosyphilis – Aqueous procaine penicillin G, 2.4 million units/day IM plus probenecid 500 mg orally 4 times daily, both for 10 to 14 days.†

Pelvic inflammatory disease (PID) – Cefoxitin 2 g IM plus probenecid, 1 g orally in a single dose concurrently.†

Actions

➤*Pharmacology:* A uricosuric and renal tubular blocking agent, probenecid inhibits the tubular reabsorption of urate, thus increasing the urinary excretion of uric acid and decreasing serum uric acid levels. Effective uricosuria reduces the miscible urate pool, retards urate deposition and promotes reabsorption of urate deposits.

Probenecid is most useful in gouty arthritis patients with reduced urinary excretion of uric acid (< 800 mg/day) on an unrestricted diet. Allopurinol is more appropriate for patients with excessive uric acid synthesis as indicated by > 800 mg uric acid through urinary excretion daily on a purine-free diet.

Probenecid also inhibits the tubular secretion of most penicillins and cephalosporins and usually increases plasma levels by any route the antibiotic is given. A 2- to 4-fold plasma elevation has been demonstrated.

➤*Pharmacokinetics:* Probenecid is well absorbed after oral administration and produces peak plasma concentrations in 2 to 4 hours. It is highly protein bound (85% to 95%) to plasma albumin. The half-life is dose-dependent and varies from < 5 to > 8 hours. Probenecid is hydroxylated to active metabolites and is excreted in the urine primarily in metabolite form.

Contraindications

Hypersensitivity to probenecid; children < 2 years of age; blood dyscrasias or uric acid kidney stones. Do not start therapy until an acute gouty attack has subsided.

Warnings

➤*Exacerbation of gout:* Exacerbation of gout following therapy with probenecid may occur; in such cases, colchicine or other appropriate therapy is advisable.

➤*Salicylates:* Use of salicylates is contraindicated in patients on probenecid therapy. Salicylates antagonize probenecid's uricosuric action.

➤*Sulfa drug allergy:* Probenecid is a sulfonamide; patients with a history of allergy to sulfa drugs may react to probenecid. Use with caution.

➤*Hypersensitivity reactions:* Rarely, severe allergic reactions and anaphylaxis have occurred. Most of these occur within several hours after readministration following prior use of the drug. The appearance of hypersensitivity reactions requires therapy cessation. Refer to Management of Acute Hypersensitivity Reactions.

➤*Renal function impairment:* Dosage requirements may be increased in renal impairment. Probenecid may not be effective in chronic renal insufficiency, particularly when the glomerular filtration rate is ≤ 30 ml/minute. Probenecid is not recommended in conjunction with a penicillin in the presence of known renal impairment

➤*Pregnancy: Category B.* Probenecid crosses the placenta and appears in cord blood. It has been used during pregnancy without producing adverse effects in the fetus or in the infant. Use only when clearly needed and when potential benefits outweigh potential hazards to the fetus.

➤*Children:* Do not use in children < 2 years of age.

Precautions

➤*Alkalinization of urine:* Hematuria, renal colic, costovertebral pain and formation of urate stones associated with use in gouty patients may be prevented by alkalization of urine and liberal fluid intake; monitor acid-base balance. See Administration and Dosage.

➤*Peptic ulcer history:* Use with caution.

Drug Interactions

	Probenecid Drug Interactions			
Precipitant drug	Object drug*		Description	
Probenecid	Acyclovir	↑	Decreased acyclovir renal clearance and increased bioavailability following IV use may occur.	
Probenecid	Allopurinol	↑	A beneficial interaction; coadministration may increase the uric acid lowering effect.	
Probenecid	Barbiturates	↑	The anesthesia produced by thiopental may be extended or achieved at lower doses.	
Probenecid	Benzodiazepines	↑	A more rapid onset or more prolonged benzodiazepine effect may occur.	
Probenecid	Clofibrate	↑	Accumulation of clofibric acid (active metabolite of clofibrate) may occur, leading to higher steady-state serum concentrations.	
Probenecid	Dapsone	↑	Possible accumulation of dapsone and its metabolites.	

† CDC 1993 Sexually Transmitted Diseases Treatment Guidelines. *Morbidity and Mortality Weekly Report* 1993 Sept 24;42 (No. RR-14).

PROBENECID

Probenecid Drug Interactions			
Precipitant drug	Object drug*		Description
Probenecid	Dyphylline	↑	Increased half-life and decreased clearance of dyphylline may occur. This may be beneficial in extending the dyphylline dosing interval.
Probenecid	Methotrexate	↑	Methotrexate's plasma levels, therapeutic effects and toxicity may be enhanced.
Probenecid	NSAIDs	↑	NSAID plasma levels may be increased; toxicity may be enhanced.
Probenecid	Pantothenic acid	↑	Renal transport of pantothenic acid may be inhibited; plasma levels may increase.
Probenecid	Penicillamine	↑	Pharmacologic effects of penicillamine may be attenuated.
Probenecid	Rifampin	↑	Renal transport of rifampin may be inhibited; plasma levels may increase.
Probenecid	Sulfonamides	↑	Renal transport of sulfonamides may be inhibited; plasma levels may increase.
Probenecid	Sulfonylureas	↑	Half-life of sulfonylureas may be increased.
Probenecid	Zidovudine	↑	Increased zidovudine bioavailability may occur; cutaneous eruptions accompanied by systemic symptoms including malaise, myalgia or fever have occurred.
Salicylates	Probenecid	↓	Coadministration may inhibit the uricosuric action of either drug alone.

* ↑ = Object drug increased. ↓ = Object drug decreased.

➤*Drug/Lab test interactions:* A reducing substance may appear in the urine during therapy. Although this disappears with discontinuation, a false diagnosis of glycosuria may be made. Confirm suspected glycosuria by using a test specific for glucose.

A falsely high determination of theophylline has occurred in vitro using the Schack and Waxler technique when therapeutic concentrations of theophylline and probenecid were added to human plasma.

Probenecid may inhibit the renal excretion of: Phenolsulfonphthalein (PSP), 17–ketosteroids and sulfobromophthalein (BSP).

Adverse Reactions

Headache; anorexia; nausea; vomiting; urinary frequency; hypersensitivity reactions (including anaphylaxis, dermatitis, pruritus and fever; see Warnings); sore gums; flushing; dizziness; anemia; hemolytic anemia (possibly related to G-6-PD deficiency); nephrotic syndrome; hepatic necrosis; aplastic anemia; exacerbation of gout; uric acid stones with or without hematuria; renal colic or costovertebral pain.

Patient Information

Avoid taking aspirin or other salicylates that antagonize the effects of probenecid.

May cause GI upset; may be taken with food or antacids. If nausea, vomiting or loss of appetite persists, notify physician.

Drink plenty of water, at least 6 to 8 full (8 oz) glasses daily, to prevent development of kidney stones.

SULFINPYRAZONE

Rx	**Sulfinpyrazone** (Various, eg, Barr, Goldline, Rugby)	**Tablets:** 100 mg	In 100s and 500s.
Rx	**Anturane** (Novartis)		White, scored. In 100s.
Rx	**Sulfinpyrazone** (Various, eg, Barr, Goldline, Rugby, Zenith)	**Capsules:** 200 mg	In 100s, 500s and 1000s.
Rx	**Anturane** (Novartis)		Green. In 100s.

Indications

➤*Gouty arthritis:* Treatment of chronic and intermittent gouty arthritis.

➤*Unlabeled uses:* Sulfinpyrazone may decrease the incidence of sudden cardiac death when given to patients 1 to 6 months post-myocardial infarction 300 mg 4 times daily; Sulfinpyrazone may decrease the frequency of systemic embolism in patients with rheumatic mitral stenosis.

A placebo controlled study of 186 patients with rheumatic mitral stenosis suggested that sulfinpyrazone may decrease the frequency of systemic embolism.

Administration and Dosage

➤*Initial:* 200 to 400 mg daily in two divided doses, with meals or milk, gradually increasing when necessary to full maintenance dosage in 1 week.

➤*Maintenance:* 400 mg daily in two divided doses; may increase to 800 mg daily or reduce to as low as 200 mg daily after the blood urate level has been controlled. Continue treatment without interruption even in the presence of acute exacerbations, which can be concomitantly treated with phenylbutazone or colchicine. Patients previously controlled with other uricosuric therapy may be transferred to sulfinpyrazone at full maintenance dosage.

Actions

➤*Pharmacology:* Sulfinpyrazone, a pyrazolidine derivative, is a potent uricosuric agent that inhibits renal tubular reabsorption of uric acid, thereby reducing elevated blood uric acid levels and causing a slow depletion of urate deposits from around joints and in other tissues. It also exhibits antithrombotic and platelet inhibitory effects but lacks anti-inflammatory and analgesic properties of its congener, phenylbutazone. It reduces renal tubular secretion of organic anions (eg, antibiotics, sulfonamides) and displaces other anions bound extensively to plasma proteins (eg, tolbutamide, warfarin, phenytoin). Sulfinpyrazone is not intended for relief of an acute attack of gout.

Sulfinpyrazone competitively inhibits platelet prostaglandin synthesis, which prevents platelet aggregation.

➤*Pharmacokinetics:* Sulfinpyrazone is well absorbed after oral administration; 98% to 99% is bound to plasma proteins. The plasma half-life is ≈ 4 hours after IV administration. Approximately 50% of the orally administered dose appears in the urine after 24 hours: 90% as unchanged drug and 10% as it's active metabolite, N^1-p-hydroxyphenol.

Contraindications

Active peptic ulcer or symptoms of GI inflammation or ulceration; hypersensitivity to phenylbutazone or other pyrazoles; blood dyscrasias.

Warnings

➤*Secondary hyperuricemia:* Do not use sulfinpyrazone to control hyperuricemia secondary to the treatment of malignant disease.

➤*Renal function impairment:* Periodically assess renal function. Renal failure has occurred, but a cause and effect relationship has not always been clearly established.

➤*Pregnancy:* Use only when clearly needed and when the potential benefits outweigh the potential hazards to the fetus.

Precautions

➤*Monitoring:* Keep patients under close medical supervision; perform periodic blood counts.

➤*Healed peptic ulcer:* Administer with care.

➤*Alkalinization of urine:* Because it is a potent uricosuric, sulfinpyrazone may precipitate acute gouty arthritis, urolithiasis and renal colic, especially in initial stages of therapy. Adequate fluid intake and alkalinization of the urine are recommended.

SULFINPYRAZONE

Drug Interactions

	Sulfinpyrazone Drug Interactions		
Precipitant drug	Object drug[*]		Description
Sulfinpyrazone	Acetaminophen	↔	Risk of acetaminophen hepatotoxicity may be increased. Also, therapeutic effects of acetaminophen may be reduced.
Sulfinpyrazone	Anticoagulants, oral	↑	The anticoagulant activity of warfarin will likely be enhanced; hemorrhage could occur.
Sulfinpyrazone	Theophylline	↓	Plasma theophylline clearance may be increased, thus lowering plasma levels.
Sulfinpyrazone	Tolbutamide	↑	Decreased clearance and increased half-life of tolbutamide may occur; hypoglycemia may result. Glyburide was not affected in one study.
Sulfinpyrazone	Verapamil	↓	Increased clearance and decreased bioavailability of verapamil may occur.
Niacin	Sulfinpyrazone	↓	Sulfinpyrazone's uricosuric effect may be reduced.
Salicylates	Sulfinpyrazone	↓	Sulfinpyrazone's uricosuric effect may be suppressed.

[*] ↑ = Object drug increased.   ↓ = Object drug decreased.   ↔ = Undetermined clinical effect.

Adverse Reactions

Most frequent – Upper GI disturbances. Administer with food, milk or antacids; despite this precaution, the drug may aggravate or reactivate peptic ulcer.

Less frequent – Rash (in most instances did not necessitate discontinuing therapy); rare blood dyscrasias (eg, anemia, leukopenia, agranulocytosis, thrombocytopenia, aplastic anemia); bronchoconstriction in patients with aspirin-induced asthma.

Overdosage

➤*Symptoms:* Nausea; vomiting; diarrhea; epigastric pain; ataxia; labored respiration; convulsions; coma. Possible symptoms seen after overdosage with other pyrazolidine derivatives: Anemia; jaundice; ulceration.

➤*Treatment:* No specific antidote. Treatment includes usual supportive measures. Refer to General Management of Acute Overdosage.

Patient Information

May cause GI upset; take with food, milk or antacids.

Avoid aspirin and other products containing salicylates that may antagonize the action of sulfinpyrazone.

Drink at least 10 to 12 glasses (8 ounces each) of fluid daily.

Treatment should continue without interruption even during acute exacerbations.

ALLOPURINOL

Rx	**Allopurinol** (Various, eg, Boots, Geneva, Major, Mylan, Parmed, Vangard)	**Tablets**: 100 mg	In 100s, 500s, 1000s and UD 100s.
Rx	**Zyloprim** (Faro Pharmaceuticals, Inc.)		Lactose. (Zyloprim 100). White, scored. In 100s.
Rx	**Allopurinol** (Various, eg, Boots, Geneva, Major, Mylan, Parmed, Vangard)	**Tablets**: 300 mg	In 100s, 500s, 1000s and UD 100s.
Rx	**Zyloprim** (Faro Pharmaceuticals, Inc.)		Lactose. (Zyloprim 300). Peach, scored. In 100s and 500s.

For information on allopurinol injection, please refer to the Purine Analogs and Related Agents in the Antineoplastics chapter.

Indications

➤*Gout:* Management of signs and symptoms of primary or secondary gout (acute attacks, tophi, joint destruction, uric acid lithiasis or nephropathy).

➤*Malignancies:* Management of patients with leukemia, lymphoma and malignancies receiving therapy that causes elevations of serum and urinary uric acid. Discontinue allopurinol when the potential for overproduction of uric acid is no longer present.

➤*Calcium oxalate calculi:* Management of patients with recurrent calcium oxalate calculi whose daily uric acid excretion exceeds 800 mg/day (males) or 750 mg/day (females). Carefully assess therapy initially and periodically to determine that treatment is beneficial and that the benefits outweigh the risks.

➤*Unlabeled uses:* Allopurinol mouthwash (20 mg in 3% methylcellulose; 1 mg/ml) has been used successfully to prevent fluorouracil-induced stomatitis; 600 mg/day ameliorated the granulocyte suppressant effect of fluorouracil.

Recent studies suggest a role for allopurinol in the prevention of ischemic reperfusion tissue damage; to reduce the incidence of perioperative mortality and postoperative arrhythmias in coronary artery bypass surgery patients (300 mg 12 hours and 1 hour before surgery); to reduce relapse rates of *H. pylori*-induced duodenal ulcers and treatment of hematemesis from NSAID-induced erosive gastritis (50 mg four times daily); to alleviate pain related to acute pancreatitis (50 mg 4 times/day, rectally); to ex vivo preservation and function of organs for liver and kidney transplantation by supplementing preservation solutions with allopurinol; and to reduce rejection episodes in adult cadaver renal transplant recipients by adding low-dose allopurinol 25 mg on alternate days to a triple immunosuppressive regimen of azathioprine/cyclosporine/prednisolone. Allopurinol 20 mg/kg for 15 days has been used successfully against *Leishmania* in the treatment of American cutaneous leishmaniasis and against *Trypanosoma cruzi*; for Chagas' disease (600 to 900 mg/day for 60 days); and as an alternative for patients with epileptic seizures refractory to standard therapy (150 mg/day for children < 20 kg, otherwise 300 mg/day).

Administration and Dosage

➤*Control of gout and hyperuricemia:* The average dose is 200 to 300 mg/day for mild gout and 400 to 600 mg/day for moderately severe tophaceous gout. Divide doses that are > 300 mg. The minimum effective dose is 100 to 200 mg daily; the maximum recommended dose is 800 mg/day.

Children (6 to 10 years of age) – In secondary hyperuricemia associated with malignancy, give 300 mg daily; those < 6 years old are generally given 150 mg/day. Evaluate response after ≈ 48 hours of therapy and adjust dosage if necessary.

Another suggested dose is 1 mg/kg/day divided every 6 hours, to a maximum of 600 mg/day. After 48 hours of treatment, titrate dose according to serum uric acid levels.

➤*Prevention of uric acid nephropathy during vigorous therapy of neoplastic disease:* 600 to 800 mg daily for 2 to 3 days with a high fluid intake. Similar considerations govern dosage regulation for maintenance purposes in secondary hyperuricemia.

➤*To reduce the possibility of flare-up of acute gouty attacks:* Start with 100 mg daily and increase at weekly intervals by 100 mg (without exceeding the maximum recommended dosage) until a serum uric acid level of ≤ 6 mg/dl is attained.

➤*Serum uric acid levels:* Normal serum urate levels are usually achieved in 1 to 3 weeks. The upper limit of normal is ≈ 7 mg/dl for men and postmenopausal women and 6 mg/dl for premenopausal women. Do not rely on a single reading because estimation of uric acid may be difficult. By selecting the appropriate dose and using uricosuric agents in certain patients, it is possible to reduce the serum uric acid level to normal and, if desired, to hold it as low as 2 to 3 mg/dl indefinitely.

➤*Renal function impairment:* Accumulation of allopurinol and its metabolites can occur in renal failure; consequently, reduce the dose. With a creatinine clearance (Ccr) of 10 to 20 ml/min, 200 mg/day is suitable. When the Ccr is < 10 ml/min, do not exceed 100 mg/day. With extreme renal impairment (Ccr < 3 ml/min) the interval between doses may also need to be increased. The correct dosage is best determined by using the serum uric acid level as an index.

Suggested Allopurinol doses	
Ccr (ml/min)	Dose
60	200 mg/day
40	150 mg/day
20	100 mg/day
10	100 mg on alternate days
< 10	100 mg 3 times/week

➤*Concomitant therapy:* In patients treated with colchicine or anti-inflammatory agents, continue therapy while adjusting the allopurinol dosage until a normal serum uric acid level and freedom from acute attacks have been maintained for several months.

➤*Replacement therapy:* In transferring a patient from a uricosuric agent to allopurinol, gradually reduce the dose of the uricosuric agent over several weeks and gradually increase the dose of allopurinol until a normal serum uric acid level is maintained.

➤*Recurrent calcium oxalate stones:* For hyperuricosuric patients, 200 to 300 mg/day in single or divided doses. Adjust dose up or down depending upon the resultant control of the hyperuricosuria based upon subsequent 24-hour urinary urate determinations. Patients may also benefit from dietary changes such as reduction of animal protein, sodium, refined sugars, oxalate-rich foods and excessive calcium intake as well as increase in oral fluids and dietary fiber.

➤*Storage/Stability:* Store at 15° to 25°C (59° to 77°F) in a dry place.

Actions

➤*Pharmacology:* Allopurinol inhibits xanthine oxidase, the enzyme responsible for the conversion of hypoxanthine and xanthine to uric acid. Allopurinol is metabolized to oxipurinol (alloxanthine), which is also an inhibitor of xanthine oxidase. Allopurinol acts on purine catabolism, reducing the production of uric acid, without disrupting the biosynthesis of vital purines.

Reutilization of both hypoxanthine and xanthine for nucleotide and nucleic acid synthesis is markedly enhanced when their oxidation is inhibited by allopurinol. However, this does not disrupt normal nucleic acid anabolism because feedback inhibition is an integral part of purine biosynthesis. The serum concentration of hypoxanthine plus xanthine in patients receiving allopurinol for hyperuricemia usually ranges from 0.3 to 0.4 mg/dl compared with a normal level of ≈ 0.15 mg/dl. A maximum of 0.9 mg/dl of these oxypurines has been reported when the serum urate was lowered to < 2 mg/dl by high doses of allopurinol. These values are far below the saturation levels, at which point their precipitation would occur (> 7 mg/dl).

Administration generally results in a fall in both serum and urinary uric acid within 2 to 3 days. The magnitude of this decrease is dose-dependent. One week or more of treatment may be required before the full effects of the drug are manifested; likewise, uric acid may return to pretreatment levels slowly following cessation of therapy. This reflects primarily the accumulation and slow clearance of oxipurinol. In some patients, a dramatic fall in urinary uric acid excretion may not occur, particularly in those with severe tophaceous gout. This may be caused by the mobilization of urate from tissue deposits as the serum uric acid level begins to fall.

➤*Pharmacokinetics:* Allopurinol is ≈ 90% absorbed from the GI tract. Peak plasma levels occur at 1.5 hours and 4.5 hours for allopurinol and oxipurinol, respectively. After a single 300 mg dose, maximum plasma levels of ≈ 3 mcg/ml of allopurinol and 6.5 mcg/ml of oxipurinol are produced.

Allopurinol has a plasma half-life of ≈1 to 2 hours. However, oxipurinol has a plasma half-life of ≈ 15 hours. Therefore, effective xanthine oxidase inhibition is maintained for 24 hours with single daily doses. Allopurinol is cleared essentially by glomerular filtration; oxipurinol is reabsorbed in the kidney tubules in a manner similar to the reabsorption of uric acid. Approximately 20% is excreted in the feces.

The clearance of oxipurinol is increased by uricosuric drugs, and as a consequence, the addition of a uricosuric may reduce the degree of xanthine oxidase inhibition by oxipurinol and increase the urinary uric acid excretion. Some patients may benefit from combined therapy and may achieve minimum serum uric acid levels, provided the total urinary uric acid load does not exceed the competence of the patient's renal function.

Contraindications

Do not restart patients who have developed a severe reaction to the drug.

ALLOPURINOL

Warnings

➤*Asymptomatic hyperuricemia:* This drug is not innocuous. Do not use to treat asymptomatic hyperuricemia.

Skin rash, usually maculopapular, sometimes scaly or exfoliative, is most common. Incidence of skin rash may be increased in renal disorders. Skin reactions can be severe and sometimes fatal; therefore, discontinue therapy at the first sign of rash. The most severe reactions also include: Fever; chills; arthralgias; cholestatic jaundice; eosinophilia; mild leukocytosis; leukopenia.

➤*Hepatotoxicity:* A few cases of reversible clinical hepatotoxicity have occurred; in some patients, asymptomatic rises in serum alkaline phosphatase or serum transaminase levels have been observed. If anorexia, weight loss, or pruritus develop in patients taking allopurinol, evaluation of liver function should be part of their diagnostic workup. Perform periodic liver function tests during early stages of therapy, particularly in patients with pre-existing liver disease.

➤*Hypersensitivity reactions:* Discontinue at first appearance of skin rash or other signs of allergic reactions. In some instances, rash may be followed by more severe hypersensitivity reactions such as exfoliative, urticarial or purpuric lesions, or Stevens-Johnson syndrome (erythema multiforme exudativum), generalized vasculitis, irreversible hepatotoxicity, and, rarely, death. Refer to Management of Acute Hypersensitivity Reactions.

➤*Renal function impairment:* Some patients with pre-existing renal disease or poor urate clearance have increased BUN during allopurinol administration. Although the mechanism has not been established, patients with impaired renal function require less drug and careful observation during the early stages of treatment; reduce dosage or discontinue therapy if increased abnormalities in renal function appear and persist.

In patients with severely impaired renal function or decreased urate clearance, the plasma half-life of oxipurinol is greatly prolonged (see Administration and Dosage).

Renal failure in association with allopurinol has been observed among patients with hyperuricemia secondary to neoplastic diseases. Concurrent conditions such as multiple myeloma and congestive myocardial disease were present. Renal failure is also frequently associated with gouty nephropathy and rarely with allopurinol-associated hypersensitivity reactions. Albuminuria has occurred among patients who developed clinical gout following chronic glomerulonephritis and chronic pyelonephritis.

➤*Pregnancy: Category C.* There are no adequate and well-controlled studies in pregnant women. Use only when clearly needed.

➤*Lactation:* Allopurinol and oxipurinol have been found in breast milk. Exercise caution when administering to a nursing woman.

➤*Children:* Allopurinol is rarely indicated for use in children, with the exception of those with hyperuricemia secondary to malignancy or in certain rare inborn errors of purine metabolism.

Precautions

➤*Monitoring:* Periodically determine liver and kidney function especially during the first few months of therapy. Perform BUN, serum creatinine, or creatinine clearance and reassess the patient's dosage.

➤*Acute attacks of gout:* Acute attacks of gout have increased during the early stages of allopurinol administration, even when normal or subnormal serum uric acid levels have been attained; in general, give maintenance doses of colchicine prophylactically when allopurinol is begun. The attacks usually become shorter and less severe after several months of therapy. A possible explanation for these episodes may be the mobilization of urates from tissue deposits, which causes fluctuations in the serum uric acid level. Even with adequate therapy, it may require several months to deplete the uric acid pool sufficiently to control acute episodes.

➤*Fluid intake:* Fluid intake sufficient to yield a daily urinary output of ≥ 2 L and the maintenance of a neutral or slightly alkaline urine are desirable to avoid the theoretic possibility of formation of xanthine calculi under the influence of allopurinol therapy and to help prevent renal precipitation of urates in patients receiving concomitant uricosurics.

➤*Drowsiness:* Drowsiness has occurred occasionally. Patients should observe caution while driving or performing other tasks requiring alertness, coordination, or physical dexterity.

➤*Bone marrow depression:* Bone marrow depression has occurred in patients receiving allopurinol, most of whom received concomitant drugs with the potential for causing this reaction. This has occurred as early as 6 weeks to 6 years after the initiation of therapy. Rarely, a patient may develop varying degrees of bone marrow depression, affecting one or more cell lines, while receiving allopurinol alone.

Drug Interactions

Allopurinol Drug Interactions			
Precipitant drug	Object drug*		Description
Allopurinol	Ampicillin	↑	The rate of ampicillin-induced skin rash appears much higher with allopurinol coadministration than with either drug alone.
Allopurinol	Anticoagulants, oral	↑	Data are conflicting. The anticoagulant action of some agents may be enhanced, but probably not that of warfarin.
Allopurinol	Cyclophosphamide	↑	Myelosuppressive effects of cyclophosphamide may be enhanced, possibly increasing the risk of bleeding or infection.
Allopurinol	Theophyllines	↑	Theophylline clearance may be decreased with large allopurinol doses (600 mg/day) leading to increased plasma theophylline levels and possible toxicity.
Allopurinol	Thiopurines	↑	Clinically significant increases in pharmacologic and toxic effects of oral thiopurines have occurred.
ACE Inhibitors	Allopurinol	↑	There is possibly a higher risk of hypersensitivity reaction when these agents are coadministered than when each drug is administered alone.
Aluminum salts	Allopurinol	↓	Pharmacologic effects of allopurinol may be decreased.
Thiazide diuretics	Allopurinol	↑	Coadministration may increase the incidence of hypersensitivity reactions to allopurinol.
Uricosuric agents	Allopurinol	↓	Uricosuric agents that increase the excretion of urate are also likely to increase the excretion of oxipurinol and thus lower the degree of inhibition of xanthine oxidase.

* ↑ = Object drug increased. ↓ = Object drug decreased.

Adverse Reactions

➤*CNS:* Headache; peripheral neuropathy; neuritis; paresthesia; somnolence.

➤*Dermatologic:* Skin rash (see Warnings); vesicular bullous dermatitis; eczematoid dermatitis; pruritus; urticaria; onycholysis; lichen planus; Stevens-Johnson syndrome (erythema multiforme exudativum); purpura; toxic epidermal necrolysis (Lyell's syndrome).

➤*GI:* Nausea; vomiting; diarrhea; intermittent abdominal pain; gastritis; dyspepsia.

➤*Hematologic:* Leukopenia; leukocytosis; eosinophilia; thrombocytopenia.

➤*Hepatic:* Increased alkaline phosphatase, AST, and ALT; hepatomegaly; cholestatic jaundice; granulomatous hepatitis; hepatic necrosis.

➤*Miscellaneous:* Arthralgia; acute attacks of gout; ecchymosis; fever; myopathy; epistaxis; taste loss or perversion; renal failure; uremia; alopecia; hypersensitivity vasculitis; necrotizing angitis.

➤*The following have occurred in < 1% of patients; causal relationship is unknown:*

Cardiovascular – Pericarditis; peripheral vascular disease; thrombophlebitis; bradycardia; vasodilation.

CNS – Optic neuritis; confusion; dizziness; vertigo; foot drop; depression; amnesia; tinnitis; asthenia; insomnia; malaise.

Dermatologic – Furunculosis; facial edema; sweating; skin edema.

Endocrine – Infertility, gynecomastia (male); hypercalcemia.

GI – Hemorrhagic pancreatitis; GI bleeding; stomatitis; salivary gland swelling; hyperlipidemia; tongue edema; anorexia.

GU – Nephritis; impotence; primary hematuria; albuminuria.

Hematologic – Eosinophilic fibrohistiocytic lesion of bone marrow; prothrombin decrease; reticulocytosis; lymphadenopathy; lymphocytosis; hemolytic and aplastic anemia; agranulocytosis; pancytopenia; anemia.

Ophthalmic – Macular retinitis; iritis; conjunctivitis; amblyopia; cataracts.

Respiratory – Bronchospasm; asthma; pharyngitis; rhinitis.

Miscellaneous – Myalgia; decrease in libido.

ALLOPURINOL

Overdosage

Both allopurinol and oxipurinol are dialyzable; however, the usefulness of hemodialysis or peritoneal dialysis in the management of allopurinol overdose is unknown.

Patient Information

Allopurinol is better tolerated if taken with food or milk. A fluid intake sufficient to yield a daily urinary output of ≥ 2 L and the maintenance of a neutral or, preferably, slightly alkaline urine are desirable. Drink ≥ 10 to 12 (8 oz) glasses of fluids per day.

May produce drowsiness; observe caution while driving or performing other tasks requiring alertness, coordination, or physical dexterity.

Notify physician if skin rash, painful urination, blood in the urine, irritation of the eyes, or swelling of the lips and mouth occurs.

Remind patients to continue drug therapy prescribed for gouty attacks because optimal benefit may be delayed for 2 to 6 weeks.

Urinary acidification with large doses of vitamin C may increase the possibility of kidney stone formation.

COLCHICINE

Rx	Colchicine (Abbott)	Tablets: 0.6 mg (1/100 gr)	Lactose. Yellow. In 100s
Rx	Colchicine (Various, eg, Allscripts, Integrity, Major, Qualitest, URL, Watson, West-ward)		In 30s, 60s, 100s, and 1000s.
Rx	Colchicine (Bedford)	Injection: 0.5 mg/mL	In 2 mL vials.

Indications

➤*Gout:* Colchicine is specifically indicated for treatment and relief of pain in attacks of acute gouty arthritis. Recommended for regular prophylactic use between attacks and is often effective in aborting an attack when taken at the first sign of articular discomfort.

➤*Colchicine IV:* Colchicine IV is used when rapid response is desired or GI side effects interfere with oral use. Occasionally, it is effective when the oral preparation is not. After the acute attack has subsided, the patient usually can be given oral colchicine.

➤*Unlabeled uses:* Familial Mediterranean fever (1 to 2 mg/day); for chronic prophylactic therapy to reduce the frequency and severity of painful serositis attacks or as an intermittent short-term therapy to abort an acute attack.

Hepatic cirrhosis (1 mg 5 days weekly).

Primary biliary cirrhosis (0.6 mg twice daily).

Treatment of Behçet's disease (0.5 to 1.5 mg/day).

Scleroderma (1 mg/day).

Sweet's syndrome (0.5 mg 1 to 3 times daily).

Colchicine also has been used in the treatment of amyloidosis, sarcoid arthritis, acute inflammatory calcific tendonitis, arthritis associated with erythema nodosum, leukemia, adenocarcinoma of the GI tract, mycosis fungoides, and topically to treat intraurethral condyloma acuminata in men.

Administration and Dosage

➤*Oral:*

Acute gouty arthritis – The usual dose to relieve or abort an attack is 1.2 mg (two 0.6 mg tablets). This dose may be followed by 1 tablet every hour or 2 every 2 hours until pain is relieved or until diarrhea ensues. Each patient should learn the dose needed and should keep the drug at hand for use at the first sign of an attack. After the initial dose, it is sometimes sufficient to take 0.6 mg every 2 or 3 hours. Stop the drug if there is GI discomfort or diarrhea.

The total amount of colchicine needed to control pain and inflammation during an acute attack is usually 4 to 8 mg. Articular pain and swelling typically abate within 12 hours and usually are gone in 24 to 48 hours. Wait 3 days before initiating a second course to minimize the possibility of cumulative toxicity.

If adrenocorticotropic hormone (ACTH) is used to treat a gouty arthritis attack, give at least 1 mg/day colchicine, and continue for a few days after ACTH is withdrawn.

Prophylaxis during intercritical periods – To reduce the frequency and severity of paroxysms, administer continuously. If patients have fewer than 1 attack/year, the usual dose is 0.6 mg/day for 3 or 4 days a week; if more than 1 attack/year, the usual dose is 0.6 mg/day. Severe cases may require 1.2 to 1.8 mg/day.

Prophylaxis in patients undergoing surgery – In patients with gout, an attack may be precipitated by even a minor surgical procedure. Administer 0.6 mg 3 times/day for 3 days before and 3 days after surgery.

➤*Parenteral:* For IV use only. Severe local irritation occurs if given SC or IM. If leakage into surrounding tissue or outside the vein should occur, considerable irritation and possible tissue damage may follow. There is no specific antidote. Local application of heat or cold and the use of analgesics may provide relief.

Administer over 2 to 5 minutes. Do not dilute with 5% Dextrose in Water. If a decrease in concentration of colchicine is required, use 0.9% Sodium Chloride Injection, which does not contain a bacteriostatic agent. Do not use turbid solutions.

Treatment of acute gouty arthritis – Average initial dose is 2 mg. This may be followed by 0.5 mg every 6 hours until a satisfactory response is achieved. Do not exceed a total dosage of 4 mg for a 24-hour period. Cumulative doses of colchicine above 4 mg have resulted in irreversible multiple organ failure and death. Do not exceed a total dosage

of 4 mg for one course of treatment. Some clinicians recommend a single IV dose of 3 mg, while others recommend not more than 1 mg IV for the initial dose, followed by 0.5 mg once or twice daily, if needed.

If pain recurs, it may be necessary to give 1 to 2 mg/day for several days; however, no more colchicine should be given *by any route* for at least 7 days after a full course of IV therapy (4 mg). Many patients can be transferred to oral colchicine at a dosage similar to that being given IV.

Prophylaxis or maintenance of recurrent or chronic gouty arthritis – 0.5 to 1 mg once or twice daily. Oral colchicine is preferable, usually in conjunction with a uricosuric agent. If an acute attack of gout occurs while the patient is taking colchicine as maintenance therapy, institute an alternative drug in preference to increasing the dose of colchicine.

➤*Storage/Stability:* Store tablets below 30° C (86°F) in a tight, light-resistant container. Store injection at controlled room temperature (15° to 30°C; 59° to 86°F).

Actions

➤*Pharmacology:* The exact mechanism of action of colchicine in gout is unknown. It involves reduction of lactic acid production by leukocytes that results in a decreased deposition of uric acid and reduction of phagocytosis with inflammatory response abatement.

Colchicine apparently exerts its effect by reducing the inflammatory response to the deposited crystals and also by diminishing phagocytosis. Colchicine directly diminishes lactic acid production by leukocytes and diminishes phagocytosis and thereby interrupting the cycle of urate crystal deposition and inflammatory response that sustains the acute attack. The oxidation of glucose in phagocytizing as well as in nonphagocytizing leukocytes in vitro is suppressed by colchicine.

Although it relieves pain in acute attacks, colchicine is not an analgesic. It is not a uricosuric and will not prevent the progression of gout to chronic gouty arthritis. Its prophylactic, suppressive effect helps reduce the incidence of acute attacks and relieves the patient's occasional residual pain and mild discomfort.

Colchicine can produce a temporary leukopenia, followed by leukocytosis.

➤*Pharmacokinetics:*

Absorption – Colchicine is rapidly absorbed after oral administration.

Distribution – Large amounts of the drug and metabolites enter the intestinal tract in bile and intestinal secretions. Colchicine does not appear to be tightly bound to serum protein; hence, the drug rapidly leaves the blood stream. High concentrations are found in the kidney, liver, and spleen.

Metabolism/Excretion – Colchicine is partially metabolized in the liver. The plasma half-life is about 20 minutes; colchicine has a half-life of about 60 hours in leukocytes. Excretion occurs primarily by biliary and renal routes.

Contraindications

Hypersensitivity to colchicine; serious GI, renal, hepatic, or cardiac disorders; blood dyscrasias. Do not give colchicine in the presence of combined renal and hepatic disease.

Warnings

➤*Renal/Hepatic function impairment:* Increased colchicine toxicity may occur. Do not give colchicine in the presence of combined renal and hepatic disease.

➤*Fertility impairment:* Colchicine arrests cell division in animals and plants. It has adversely affected spermatogenesis in humans and in some animal species.

➤*Elderly:* Administer colchicine with great caution to elderly and debilitated patients, especially those with renal, hepatic, GI, or heart disease.

➤*Pregnancy: Category C* (oral). *Category D* (parenteral). Colchicine can cause fetal harm when administered to a pregnant woman. Use

COLCHICINE

only when clearly needed and when the potential benefits outweigh the potential hazards to the fetus.

➤*Lactation:* It is not known whether this drug is excreted in breast milk. Exercise caution when administering colchicine to a nursing woman.

➤*Children:* Safety and efficacy for use in children have not been established.

Precautions

➤*Monitoring:* Perform periodic blood counts in patients receiving long-term therapy.

➤*GI effects:* If nausea, vomiting, or diarrhea occur, discontinue the drug. Vomiting, diarrhea, abdominal pain, and nausea may occur, especially when maximum doses are necessary for a therapeutic effect. Diarrhea may be severe. GI symptoms may occur with IV therapy, usually large doses. To avoid more serious toxicity, discontinue use when these symptoms appear, regardless of whether joint pain has been relieved.

➤*Thrombophlebitis:* Thrombophlebitis rarely occurs at the site of injection.

➤*Myopathy and neuropathy:* Colchicine myoneuropathy commonly causes weakness in patients on standard therapy who have elevated plasma levels because of altered renal function. It is often unrecognized and misdiagnosed as polymyositis or uremic neuropathy. Proximal weakness and elevated serum creatine kinase generally are present and resolve in 3 to 4 weeks following drug withdrawal. Myopathy may occur in patients on usual maintenance doses, especially in the presence of renal impairment.

➤*Malabsorption of vitamin B_{12}:* Colchicine induces reversible malabsorption of vitamin B_{12}, apparently by altering the function of ileal mucosa.

Drug Interactions

➤*Cyclosporine:* Severe adverse clinical symptoms including GI, hepatic, renal, and neuromuscular toxicity may occur during coadministration.

➤*Drug/Lab test interactions:* Decreased thrombocyte values may be obtained. Colchicine may cause false-positive results when testing urine for RBC or hemoglobin.

Adverse Reactions

Adverse reactions in decreasing order of severity are bone marrow depression with aplastic anemia, with agranulocytosis or thrombocyto-

penia (long-term therapy). Peripheral neuritis, purpura, myopathy (see Precautions), loss of hair, and reversible azoospermia also have occurred. Hypersensitivity (infrequent), dermatoses, vomiting, diarrhea, abdominal pain, and nausea also have occurred. Diarrhea may be severe.

➤*Lab test abnormalities:* Elevated alkaline phosphatase and AST.

Overdosage

➤*Symptoms:* The onset of toxic effects usually is delayed for several hours or more after the ingestion of an acute overdose. The lethal dose is estimated to be 65 mg; however, deaths have occurred with as little as 7 mg. Cumulative IV doses of greater than 4 mg have resulted in irreversible multiple organ failure and death.

The first symptoms to appear are nausea, vomiting, abdominal pain, and diarrhea. Fluid extravasation may lead to shock. Myocardial injury may be accompanied by ST-segment elevation, decreased contractility, and profound shock. Muscle weakness or paralysis may occur and progress to respiratory failure. Hepatocellular damage, renal failure, and lung parenchymal infiltrates may occur and, by the fifth day after overdose, leukopenia, thrombocytopenia, and coagulopathy also may occur. If the patient survives, alopecia and stomatitis may occur. There is no clear separation of nontoxic, toxic, and lethal doses. Diarrhea may be bloody because of hemorrhagic gastroenteritis. Burning sensations in throat, stomach, and skin may be prominent symptoms. Extensive vascular damage may result in shock. Hematuria and oliguria may indicate kidney damage. Muscular weakness may be marked, and an ascending paralysis of the CNS may develop. The patient usually remains conscious; however, delirium and convulsions may occur. Death may result from respiratory arrest.

➤*Treatment:* Use supportive measures such as ventilation support, vital signs, blood gases, and perfusion. Instigate gastric lavage and measures to prevent shock. Consider activated charcoal instead of or in addition to gastric emptying. Symptomatic and supportive treatment may include atropine and morphine for abdominal pain and artificial respiration with oxygen to combat respiratory distress. No specific antidote is known. Refer to General Management of Acute Overdosage.

Patient Information

Notify physician if skin rash, sore throat, fever, unusual bleeding, bruising, tiredness, weakness, numbness, or tingling occurs.

Discontinue medication as soon as gout pain is relieved or at the first sign of nausea, vomiting, stomach pain, or diarrhea. If symptoms persist, notify the physician.

PROBENECID AND COLCHICINE

Rx	Probenecid and Colchicine (Various, eg, Ivax, Schein)	Tablets: 500 mg probenecid, 0.5 mg colchicine	In 100s and 1000s.

For complete prescribing information see the individual probenecid and colchicine monographs.

Indications

For the treatment of chronic gouty arthritis when complicated by frequent, recurrent acute attacks of gout

Administration and Dosage

Do not start therapy with probenecid and colchicine until an acute gouty attack has subsided. However, if an acute attack is precipitated

during therapy, probenecid and colchicine may be continued without changing the dosage and additional colchicine or other appropriate therapy given to control the acute attack.

The recommended adult dosage is 1 tablet/day for 1 week followed by 1 tablet twice/day

EMERGENCY KITS

Rx   **Cyanide Antidote Package** (Various, eg, Taylor)
       Sodium nitrite, 300 mg in 10 mL (2 amps)
       Sodium thiosulfate, 12.5 g in 50 mL (2 vials)
       Amyl nitrite inhalant, 5 minim/0.3 mL (12 amps)
       Also disposable syringes, stomach tube, tourniquet, and instructions.

Indications

➤*Cyanide poisoning:* For treatment of cyanide poisoning.

Administration and Dosage

Personnel should acquire some skill in the proper method of administering the contents of this package prior to an emergency. Cyanide poisoning is rapidly fatal. The patient seldom survives many hours. The prevention of death demands a quick diagnosis and the prompt use of specific antidotes. No valuable time should be lost. Even though the diagnosis is doubtful, institute the recommended therapy immediately. For best results, the physician should be acquainted beforehand with the following steps:

1.) Instruct an assistant how to break an ampule of amyl nitrite, one at a time, in a handkerchief and hold it in front of the patient's mouth for 15 seconds, followed by a rest for 15 seconds. Then reapply until sodium nitrite can be administered. This interrupted schedule is important because continuous use of amyl nitrite may prevent adequate oxygenation.

2.) Discontinue administration of amyl nitrite and inject IV 300 mg (10 mL of a 3% solution) of sodium nitrite at the rate of 2.5 to 5 mL/min. The recommended dose of sodium nitrite for children is 6 to 8 mL/m^2 (approximately 0.2 mL/kg body weight), but is not to exceed 10 mL.

3.) Immediately thereafter, inject 12.5 g (50 mL of a 25% solution) of sodium thiosulfate for adults. The dosage for children is 7 g/m^2 of body surface area, but dosage should not exceed 12.5 g. The same needle and vein may be used.

4.) If the poison was taken by mouth, perform gastric lavage as soon as possible, but this should not delay the treatments outlined above. Lavage may be done concurrently by a third person–a physician or a nurse if one is available. One should take quick action without waiting for positive diagnostic tests.

Watch the patient closely for at least 24 to 48 hours. If signs of poisoning reappear, repeat the injection of both sodium nitrite and sodium thiosulfate, but each in 50% of the original dose. Even if the patient seems perfectly well, the medication may be given for prophylactic purposes 2 hours after the first injections.

If respiration has ceased but the pulse is palpable, apply artificial respiration at once. The purpose is not to revive, per se, but to keep the heart beating. Lay the gauze sponge or handkerchief containing the amyl nitrite over the patient's nose, for it may hasten the resumption of respiratory movements. When signs of breathing appear, promptly inject the above solutions.

Warnings

➤*Methemoglobinemia:* Both sodium nitrite and amyl nitrite in excessive doses induce dangerous methemoglobinemia and can cause death. The amounts found in a single cyanide antidote package are not excessive for an adult. Calculate the doses for children on a surface area or on a weight basis with the dosage adjusted so that excessive methemoglobin is not formed.

Various Detoxification Agents and Their Uses	
Drug (trade name)	Toxic/Overdosed substance
Dimercaprol (*BAL In Oil*)	Arsenic, gold, mercury, lead
Deferoxamine mesylate (*Desferal*)	Iron
Dexrazoxane (*Zinecard*)	Doxorubicin-induced cardio-myopathy
Digoxin immune fab (*Digibind, Digifab*)	Digoxin, digitoxin
Edetate calcium disodium (*Calcium Disodium Versenate*)	Lead
Flumazenil (*Romazicon*)	Benzodiazepines
Fomepizole (*Antizol*)	Ethylene glycol, methanol
Mesna (*Mesnex*)	Ifosfamide-induced hemorrhagic cystitis
Methylene blue (Various)	Nitrites
Narcotic antagonists Naloxone (*Narcan*) Nalmefene (*Revex*) Naltrexone (*ReVia*)	Opioids
Physostigmine salicylate (*Antilirium*)	Anticholinergics (including tricyclic antidepressants)
Pralidoxime Cl (*Protopam Cl*)	Organophosphates Anticholinesterases
Sodium thiosulfate (Various)	Cyanide
Succimer (*Chemet*)	Lead
Trientene (*Syprine*)	Copper
Other agents used additionally as antidotes:	
Acetylcysteine (*Mucomyst, Mucosil*)	Acetaminophen
Amyl nitrite, Na Nitrite, Na Thiosulfate (*Cyanide antidote kit*)	Cyanide

Various Detoxification Agents and Their Uses	
Drug (trade name)	Toxic/Overdosed substance
Anticholinesterases Pyridostigmine Br (*Mestinon, Regonol*) Neostigmine Br (*Prostigmin*) Edrophonium Cl (*Tensilon*)	Nondepolarizing muscle relaxants
Atropine (Various)	Cholinergic agents: Organo-phosphates, carbamates, pilo-carpine, physostigmine, or choline esters.
Glucagon	Insulin-induced hypoglycemia, beta blockers
Hydroxocobalamin (Various)	Cyanide poisoning
Leucovorin calcium (*Wellcovorin*)	Folic acid antagonists (eg, methotrexate)
Protamine sulfate (Various)	Heparin
Pyridoxine	Isoniazid
Vitamin K$_1$ (Various)	Oral anticoagulants
Nonspecific therapy of overdoses include the following:	
Activated charcoal (Various)	Nonspecific, supportive therapies of overdoses. See also General Management of Acute Overdosage.
Cathartics	
Osmotic diuretics	
Polyethylene glycol electrolyte solution (*GoLYTELY*)	
Syrup of ipecac (Various)	
Urinary acidifiers	
Urinary alkalinizers	

TRIENTINE HCl

| Rx | **Syprine** (Merck) | **Capsules:** 250 mg | (SYPRINE/MSD 661). Light brown. In 100s. |

Indications

➤*Wilson disease:* Treatment of patients with Wilson disease who are intolerant of penicillamine.

Administration and Dosage

➤*Approved by the FDA:* November 8, 1985.

Take on an empty stomach at least 1 hour before or 2 hours after meals and at least 1 hour apart from any other drug, food, or milk. Swallow the capsules whole and do not open or chew.

➤*Adults:* Initially, 750 to 1250 mg/day in divided doses 2, 3, or 4 times/day. May increase to a maximum of 2000 mg/day.

➤*Children 12 years of age and under:* Initially, 500 to 750 mg/day in divided doses 2, 3, or 4 times/day. May increase to a maximum of 1500 mg/day.

Increase the daily dose only when the clinical response is not adequate or the concentration of free serum copper is persistently above 20 mcg/dL. Determine optimal long-term maintenance dosage at 6- to 12-month intervals.

➤*Storage/Stability:* Store at 2° to 8°C (36° to 46°F) in a tightly closed container.

Actions

➤*Pharmacology:* Wilson disease (hepatolenticular degeneration) is an inherited metabolic defect resulting in excess copper accumulation, possibly because the liver lacks the mechanism to excrete free copper into the bile. Hepatocytes store excess copper, but when their capacity is exceeded, copper is released into the blood and is taken up into extrahepatic sites. Treat this condition with a low copper diet and chelating agents that bind copper to facilitate its excretion from the body. Trientine is a chelating compound for removal of excess copper from the body.

➤*Clinical trials:* Renal clearance studies were carried out with penicillamine and trientine on separate occasions in selected patients treated with penicillamine for at least 1 year. Six hour excretion rates of copper were determined off treatment and after a single dose of 500 mg penicillamine or 1.2 g trientine. Results demonstrated that trientine is effective as a cupriuretic agent in patients with Wilson disease, although on a molar basis, the drug appears to be less potent or less effective than penicillamine.

Contraindications

Hypersensitivity to trientine.

Warnings

➤*Not indicated for the following:* Not indicated for cystinuria; rheumatoid arthritis; biliary cirrhosis.

➤*Patient supervision:* Patients should remain under regular medical supervision throughout the period of drug administration.

➤*Iron deficiency anemia:* Closely monitor patients (especially women) for evidence of iron deficiency anemia.

➤*Elderly:* In general, dose selection should be cautious, usually starting at the low end of the dosing range, reflecting the greater frequency of decreased hepatic, renal, or cardiac function, and of concomitant disease or other drug therapy.

➤*Pregnancy: Category C.* Trientine was teratogenic in rats at doses similar to the human dose. The frequencies of resorptions and fetal abnormalities, including hemorrhage and edema, increased while fetal copper levels decreased. There are no adequate and well-controlled studies in pregnant women. Use during pregnancy only when the potential benefits outweigh the potential hazards to the fetus.

➤*Lactation:* It is not known whether this drug is excreted in breast milk. Exercise caution when administering to a nursing woman.

➤*Children:* Safety and efficacy for use in children have not been established. Trientine has been used clinically in children as young as 6 years of age with no reported adverse effects.

Precautions

➤*Monitoring:* The most reliable index for monitoring treatment is the determination of free copper in the serum, which equals the difference between quantitatively determined total copper and ceruloplasmin-copper. Adequately treated patients will usually have less than 10 mcg free copper/dL of serum.

Therapy may be monitored with a 24-hour urinary copper analysis periodically (ie, every 6 to 12 months). Urine must be collected in copper-free glassware. Because a low copper diet should keep copper absorption down to less than 1 mg/day, the patient probably will be in the desired state of negative copper balance if 0.5 to 1 mg of copper is present in a 24-hour collection of urine.

➤*Hypersensitivity:* There are no reports of hypersensitivity in patients given trientine for Wilson disease. However, there have been reports of asthma, bronchitis, and dermatitis occurring after prolonged environmental exposure in workers who use trientine as a hardener of epoxy resins. Observe patients closely for signs of possible hypersensitivity. Refer to Management of Hypersensitivity Reactions.

Drug Interactions

➤*Mineral supplements:* In general, do not give mineral supplements; they may block the absorption of trientine. However, iron deficiency may develop, especially in children and menstruating or pregnant women, or as a result of the low copper diet recommended for Wilson disease. If necessary, iron may be given in short courses, but because iron and trientine each inhibit absorption of the other, allow 2 hours to elapse between administration of trientine and iron.

➤*Drug/Food interactions:* It is important that trientene be taken on an empty stomach at least 1 hour before or 2 hours after meals and at least 1 hour apart from any other drug, food, or milk. This permits maximum absorption; also, coadministration may inactivate trientine by metal binding in the GI tract.

Adverse Reactions

Iron deficiency, systemic lupus erythematosus, dystonia, muscular spasm, and myasthenia gravis have occurred in patients with Wilson disease who were being treated with trientine.

Trientine is not indicated for treatment of biliary cirrhosis, but in 1 study of 4 patients treated with trientine for primary biliary cirrhosis, the following adverse reactions were reported: Heartburn; epigastric pain and tenderness; thickening, fissuring, and flaking of the skin; hypochromic microcytic anemia; acute gastritis; aphthoid ulcers; abdominal pain; melena; anorexia; malaise; cramps; muscle pain; weakness; rhabdomyolysis. A causal relationship to drug therapy could not be rejected or established.

Overdosage

There is a report of an adult woman who ingested 30 g trientine without apparent ill effects.

Patient Information

Take on an empty stomach at least 1 hour before or 2 hours after meals and at least 1 hour apart from any other drug, food, or milk.

Swallow capsules whole with water. Do not open or chew.

Because of the potential for contact dermatitis, promptly wash any site of exposure to the capsule contents with water.

Take temperature nightly for the first month of treatment, and report any symptoms such as fever or skin eruption.

SUCCIMER (DMSA)

| Rx | **Chemet** (Ovation) | **Capsules:** 100 mg | Sucrose. (Chemet 100). White. In 100s. |

Indications

➤*Lead poisoning:* Treatment of lead poisoning in children with blood lead levels above 45 mcg/dL. Not indicated for prophylaxis of lead poisoning in a lead-containing environment; always accompany succimer use with identification and removal of the source of lead exposure.

➤*Unlabeled uses:* Succimer may be beneficial in the treatment of other heavy metal poisonings (eg, mercury, arsenic); further study is needed.

Administration and Dosage

➤*Approved by the FDA:* February 1991.

Start dosage at 10 mg/kg or 350 mg/m^2 every 8 hours for 5 days; initiation of therapy at higher doses is not recommended (see table). Reduce frequency of administration to 10 mg/kg or 350 mg/m^2 every 12 hours (two-thirds of initial daily dosage) for an additional 2 weeks of therapy.

A course of treatment lasts 19 days. Repeated courses may be necessary if indicated by weekly monitoring of blood lead concentration. A minimum of 2 weeks between courses is recommended unless blood lead levels indicate the need for more prompt treatment.

Succimer Pediatric Dosing Chart			
Weight		Dose (mg)[1]	Number of capsules[1]
lbs	kg		
18-35	8-15	100	1
36-55	16-23	200	2
56-75	24-34	300	3
76-100	35-44	400	4
> 100	> 45	500	5

[1] To be administered every 8 hours for 5 days, followed by dosing every 12 hours for 14 days.

SUCCIMER (DMSA)

In young children who cannot swallow capsules, succimer can be administered by separating the capsule and sprinkling the medicated beads on a small amount of soft food or putting them in a spoon and following with a fruit drink.

Identification of the lead source in the child's environment and its abatement are critical to successful therapy. Chelation therapy is not a substitute for preventing further exposure to lead and should not be used to permit continued exposure to lead.

Patients who have received calcium EDTA with or without dimercaprol may use succimer for subsequent treatment after an interval of 4 weeks. Data on the concomitant use of succimer with calcium EDTA with or without dimercaprol are not available, and such use is not recommended.

Adequately hydrate all patients undergoing treatment.

➤*Storage/Stability:* Store between 15° and 25°C (59° and 77°F) and avoid excessive heat.

Actions

➤*Pharmacology:* Succimer is an orally active, heavy metal chelating agent; it forms water soluble chelates and, consequently, increases the urinary excretion of lead.

➤*Pharmacokinetics:* In a study in healthy adult volunteers, after a single dose of 16, 32, or 48 mg/kg, absorption was rapid but variable, with peak blood levels between 1 and 2 hours. Approximately 49% of the dose was excreted: 39% in the feces, 9% in the urine, and 1% as carbon dioxide from the lungs. Because fecal excretion probably represented nonabsorbed drug, most of the absorbed drug was excreted by the kidneys. The apparent elimination half-life was about 2 days.

In other studies of healthy adult volunteers receiving a single oral dose of 10 mg/kg, succimer was rapidly and extensively metabolized. Approximately 25% of the dose was excreted in the urine with the peak blood level and urinary excretion occurring between 2 and 4 hours. Of the total amount of drug eliminated in the urine, approximately 90% was eliminated in altered form as mixed succimer-cysteine disulfides; the remaining 10% was eliminated unchanged.

➤*Clinical trials:*

Effect on essential minerals – Succimer had no significant effect on the urinary elimination of iron, calcium, or magnesium. Zinc excretion doubled during treatment. The effect of succimer on the excretion of essential minerals was small compared with that of calcium EDTA, which can induce more than a 10–fold increase in urinary excretion of zinc and doubling of copper and iron excretion.

Succimer vs EDTA: A study was performed in 15 children 2 to 7 years of age with blood lead levels of 30 to 49 mcg/dL and positive calcium EDTA lead mobilization tests. Each group of 5 patients received 350, 233, or 116 mg/m² succimer every 8 hours for 5 days. These doses corresponded to 10, 6.7, and 3.3 mg/kg. Six control patients received 1000 mg/m²/day calcium EDTA IV for 5 days. Following therapy, the mean blood lead levels decreased 78%, 63%, and 42%, respectively, in the 3 groups treated with succimer. The response of the 350 mg/m² every 8 hours (10 mg/kg every 8 hours) group was significantly better than that of the other succimer-treated groups as well as that of the control group, whose mean blood lead level fell 48%. No adverse reactions or changes in essential mineral excretion were reported in the succimer-treated groups. In the calcium EDTA-treated group, the cumulative amount of urinary lead excreted was slightly but significantly greater than in the succimer group. After calcium EDTA, the urinary excretion of copper, zinc, iron, and calcium were significantly increased.

As with other chelators, adults and children experienced a rebound in blood lead levels after discontinuing succimer. In these studies, after treatment with 350 mg/m² (10 mg/kg) every 8 hours for 5 days, the mean lead level rebounded and plateaued at 60% to 85% of pretreatment levels 2 weeks after therapy. The rebound plateau was somewhat higher with lower doses of succimer and with IV calcium EDTA.

Contraindications

History of allergy to the drug.

Warnings

➤*Lead exposure:* Not a substitute for effective abatement of lead exposure.

➤*Neutropenia:* Mild to moderate neutropenia has been observed in some patients receiving succimer. While a causal relationship to succimer has not been definitely established, neutropenia has been reported with other drugs in the same chemical class. Obtain a complete blood count with white blood cell differential and direct platelet counts prior to and weekly during treatment with succimer. Withhold or discontinue therapy if the absolute neutrophil count (ANC) is below 1200/mcL and follow the patient closely to document recovery of the ANC to above 1500/mcL or to the patient's baseline neutrophil count. There is limited experience with re-exposure in patients who have developed neutropenia. Therefore, rechallenge such patients only if the benefit of succimer therapy clearly outweighs the potential risk of another episode of neutropenia and then only with careful patient monitoring.

Infection – Instruct patients treated with succimer to report promptly any signs of infection. If infection is suspected, immediately conduct the above laboratory tests.

➤*Pregnancy: Category C.* Succimer is teratogenic and fetotoxic in pregnant mice when given SC in a dose range of 410 to 1640 mg/kg/day during the period of organogenesis. There are no adequate and well-controlled studies in pregnant women. Use during pregnancy only if the potential benefit justifies the potential risk to the fetus.

➤*Lactation:* It is not known whether this drug is excreted in breast milk. Discourage mothers requiring therapy from nursing their infants.

➤*Children:* Safety and efficacy in children under 12 months of age have not been established.

Precautions

➤*Rebound blood lead levels:* Elevated blood lead levels and associated symptoms may return rapidly after discontinuation of succimer because of redistribution of lead from bone stores to soft tissues and blood. After therapy, monitor patients for rebound of blood lead levels by measuring the levels at least once weekly until stable. However, use the severity of lead intoxication (as measured by initial blood lead level and rate and degree of rebound of blood lead) as a guide for more frequent blood lead monitoring.

➤*Renal function:* Adequately hydrate all patients undergoing treatment. Exercise caution in using succimer therapy in patients with compromised renal function. Limited data suggest that succimer is dialyzable but that the lead chelates are not.

➤*Hepatic function:* Transient mild elevations of serum transaminases have been observed in 6% to 10% of patients during the course of therapy. Monitor serum transaminases before the start of therapy and at least weekly during therapy. Closely monitor patients with a history of liver disease. No data are available regarding the metabolism of succimer in patients with liver disease.

➤*Repeated courses:* Clinical experience is limited. The safety of uninterrupted dosing longer than 3 weeks has not been established and is not recommended.

➤*Allergic reactions:* The possibility of allergic or other mucocutaneous reactions must be borne in mind upon readministration (and during initial courses). Monitor patients requiring repeated courses during each treatment course. One patient experienced recurrent mucocutaneous vesicular eruptions of increasing severity affecting oral mucosa, external urethral meatus, and perianal area on third, fourth, and fifth courses. The reaction resolved between courses and upon discontinuation of therapy.

Drug Interactions

➤*Chelation therapy (eg, EDTA):* Coadministration of succimer with other chelation therapy is not recommended.

➤*Drug/Lab test interactions:* Succimer may interfere with serum and urinary laboratory tests. In vitro, succimer caused false-positive results for ketones in urine using nitroprusside reagents such as *Ketostix* and falsely decreased measurements of serum uric acid and CPK.

Adverse Reactions

The most common events attributable to succimer (ie, GI symptoms or increases in serum transaminases) have been observed in about 10% of patients (see Precautions). Rashes, some necessitating discontinuation of therapy, have been reported in about 4% of patients. If rash occurs, consider other causes (eg, measles) before ascribing the reaction to succimer. Rechallenge with succimer may be considered if lead levels are high enough to warrant retreatment. One allergic mucocutaneous reaction has been reported upon repeated administration of the drug (see Precautions). Mild to moderate neutropenia has occurred in some patients receiving succimer (see Warnings). The following table presents adverse events reported with the administration of succimer for the treatment of lead and other heavy metal intoxication.

Succimer Adverse Reactions (%)[1]		
Body system/adverse reaction	Children (n = 191)	Adults (n = 134)
GI: Nausea; vomiting; diarrhea; appetite loss; hemorrhoidal symptoms; loose stools; metallic taste in mouth	12	20.9
Body as a whole: Back, stomach, head, rib, flank pain; abdominal cramps; chills; fever; flu-like symptoms; heavy head/tired; head cold; headache; moniliasis	5.2	15.7
Metabolic: Elevated AST, ALT, alkaline phosphatase, serum cholesterol	4.2	10.4
CNS: Drowsiness; dizziness; sensorimotor neuropathy; sleepiness; paresthesia	1	12.7

Chelating Agents

SUCCIMER (DMSA)

Succimer Adverse Reactions (%)[1]		
Body system/adverse reaction	Children (n = 191)	Adults (n = 134)
Dermatologic: Papular rash; herpetic rash; rash; mucocutaneous eruptions; pruritus	2.6	11.2
Special senses: Cloudy film in eye; ears plugged; otitis media; watery eyes	1	3.7
Respiratory: Sore throat; rhinorrhea; nasal congestion; cough	3.7	0.7
GU: Decreased urination; voiding difficulty; proteinuria increased	0	3.7
Other: Arrhythmia	0	1.8
Mild to moderate neutropenia; increased platelet count; intermittent eosinophilia	0.5	1.5
Kneecap pain; leg pains	0	3

[1] Incidence regardless of attribution or dosage.

Overdosage

Doses of 2300 to 2400 mg/kg in the rat and mouse produced ataxia, convulsions, labored respiration, and frequently death. Induction of vomiting or gastric lavage followed by administration of an activated charcoal slurry and appropriate supportive therapy are recommended. Refer to General Management of Acute Overdosage.

Limited data indicate that succimer is dialyzable.

Patient Information

Instruct patients to maintain adequate fluid intake. If rash occurs, patients should consult their physician.

In young children unable to swallow capsules, the contents of the capsule can be administered in a small amount of food (see Administration and Dosage).

Instruct patients to promptly report any indication of infection, which may be a sign of neutropenia (see Warnings).

DIMERCAPROL

Rx **BAL In Oil** (Taylor) **Injection:** 10% (100 mg/mL) In peanut oil with 20% benzyl benzoate. In 3 mL amps.

Indications

➤*Poisoning:* Treatment of arsenic, gold, and mercury poisoning; acute lead poisoning when used with calcium EDTA; acute mercury poisoning if therapy is begun within 1 or 2 hours following ingestion. Not very effective for chronic mercury poisoning.

Administration and Dosage

Give by deep IM injection only. Begin therapy as early as possible along with other supportive measures.

➤*Mild arsenic or gold poisoning:* 2.5 mg/kg 4 times/day for 2 days, then 2 times on the third day, and once daily thereafter for 10 days.

➤*Severe arsenic or gold poisoning:* 3 mg/kg every 4 hours for 2 days, then 4 times on the third day, then twice daily thereafter for 10 days.

➤*Mercury poisoning:* 5 mg/kg initially, then 2.5 mg/kg 1 to 2 times/day for 10 days.

➤*Acute lead encephalopathy:* 4 mg/kg alone in the first dose and thereafter at 4-hour intervals in combination with calcium EDTA administered at a separate site. For less severe poisoning, the dose can be reduced to 3 mg/kg after the first dose. Maintain treatment for 2 to 7 days, depending on clinical response.

➤*Storage/Stability:* Store at 15° to 25°C (59° to 77°F).

Actions

➤*Pharmacology:* Dimercaprol promotes excretion of arsenic, gold, and mercury by chelation. The dimercaprol sulfhydryl groups form complexes with metals, thus preventing or reversing the metallic binding of sulfhydryl-containing enzymes.

➤*Pharmacokinetics:* After IM use, peak concentrations occur in 30 to 60 minutes. It has a short half-life; excretion is complete within 4 hours of a single dose.

Contraindications

Dimercaprol is contraindicated in most instances of hepatic insufficiency with the exception of postarsenical jaundice. Discontinue the drug or use only with extreme caution if acute renal insufficiency develops during therapy.

Iron, cadmium, or selenium poisoning; the resulting dimercaprol-metal complexes are more toxic than the metal alone, especially to the kidneys.

Warnings

➤*Other metal poisonings:* Dimercaprol is of questionable value in metal poisonings other than those listed in Indications (eg, antimony, bismuth).

➤*Renal/Hepatic function impairment:* Do not use in hepatic insufficiency unless caused by arsenic poisoning. Discontinue or use only with extreme caution if acute renal insufficiency develops during therapy.

➤*Pregnancy: Category C.* It is not known whether dimercaprol can cause fetal harm when administered to a pregnant woman or can affect reproduction capacity. Give dimercaprol to a pregnant woman only if clearly needed.

➤*Lactation:* It is not known if dimercaprol is excreted in breast milk. Use caution when administering to a nursing woman.

Precautions

➤*Urinary alkalinization:* Urinary alkalinization is recommended because the dimercaprol-metal complex breaks down easily in an acid medium. Alkaline urine protects the kidney during therapy.

➤*G-6-PD deficiency:* Use with caution in these patients; hemolysis may occur.

Drug Interactions

➤*Iron:* Do not administer to patients taking dimercaprol.

Adverse Reactions

A consistent response to dimercaprol is a rise in blood pressure accompanied by tachycardia, roughly proportional to the dose. Larger than recommended doses may cause other transitory signs and symptoms in order of frequency as follows: Nausea; vomiting; headache; burning sensation in the lips, mouth, and throat; feeling of constriction or pain in the throat, chest, or hands; conjunctivitis, lacrimation, blepharal spasm, rhinorrhea, salivation; tingling of the hands; burning sensation in the penis; sweating of the forehead, hands, and other areas; abdominal pain; occasional appearance of painful sterile abscesses. These may be accompanied by anxiety, weakness, and unrest, and may be relieved by an antihistamine.

Local pain at the site of injection may occur. A reaction apparently peculiar to children is fever, which may persist during therapy. It occurs in approximately 30% of children. A transient reduction of the percentage of polymorphonuclear leukocytes also may be observed.

Overdosage

Dosage exceeding 5 mg/kg will usually be followed by vomiting, convulsions, and stupor beginning within 30 minutes and subsiding within 6 hours following injection.

DEFEROXAMINE MESYLATE

| *Rx* | **Desferal** (Novartis) | **Powder for Injection, lyophilized:** 500 mg | In vials. |
| | | 2 g | In vials. |

Indications

➤*Acute iron intoxication:* An adjunct to standard treatment measures.

➤*Chronic iron overload:* Deferoxamine can promote iron excretion in patients with secondary iron overload from multiple transfusions (as may occur in the treatment of some chronic anemias, including thalassemia). Long-term therapy with deferoxamine slows hepatic iron accumulation; retards or eliminates hepatic fibrosis progression.

➤*Unlabeled uses:* In patients with chronic renal failure, deferoxamine has been used in the treatment of aluminum overload, commonly related to the use of aluminum-contaminated dialysate or ingestion of aluminum-containing phosphorous binding drugs.

Deferoxamine also has been used as a diagnostic test for iron storage disease in patients with normal renal function.

Administration and Dosage

➤*Acute iron intoxication:*

IM – Preferred route; use for all patients not in shock. Initially, 1 g then 500 mg every 4 hours for 2 doses. Subsequently, give 500 mg every 4 to 12 hours based on clinical response. Do not exceed 6 g/day.

IV – Use only in cardiovascular collapse and give by slow infusion. The rate of infusion should not exceed 15 mg/kg/h for the first 1 g administered. Subsequent IV dosing, if needed, must be at a slower rate, not to exceed 125 mg/h.

The reconstituted solution is added to physiologic saline, glucose in water, or lactated Ringer's solution.

Administer an initial dose of 1 g at a rate not to exceed 15 mg/kg/h. This may be followed by 500 mg over 4 hours for 2 doses. Depending on the clinical response, subsequent doses of 500 mg may be administered over 4 to 12 hours. The total amount administered should not exceed 6 g/day.

As soon as possible, stop IV and give IM.

➤*Chronic iron overload:* Individualize dosage.

IM – 500 mg to 1 g/day. Give 2 g IV with, but separate from, each unit of blood. The rate of IV infusion must not exceed 15 mg/kg/h. The total daily dose should not exceed 1 g in the absence of a transfusion, or 6 g even if transfused 3 or more units of blood or packed red blood cells.

SC – 1 to 2 g/day (20 to 40 mg/kg/day) over 8 to 24 hours with continuous mini-infusion pump. Individualize infusion duration. In some patients, iron excretion will be as much after a short infusion (8 to 12 hours) as if the same dose is given over 24 hours.

➤*Children:* Maximum dose is 6 g/24 h.

➤*Preparation:* Deferoxamine is preferably dissolved by adding 5 mL sterile water for injection to each 500 mg vial or 20 mL sterile water for injection to each 2 g vial. The reconstituted deferoxamine solution is isotonic, clear, and colorless to slightly yellowish at the recommended concentration of 10%.

In clinical situations requiring a smaller volume of solution (eg, IM injection), deferoxamine may be dissolved by adding 2 mL sterile water for injection to each 500 mg vial or 8 mL sterile water for injection to each 2 g vial. This concentration may produce a stronger yellow colored solution. Completely dissolve the drug before the solution is withdrawn.

Deferoxamine reconstituted with sterile water for injection is for single use only.

➤*Storage/Stability:* Do not store above 25°C (77°F).

Use the product immediately after reconstitution (commencement of treatment within 3 hours) for microbiological safety. When reconstitution is carried out under validated aseptic conditions (in a sterile laminar flow hood using aseptic technique), the product may be stored at room temperature for a maximum period of 24 hours before use. Do not refrigerate reconstituted solution. Reconstituting desferoxamine in solvents or under conditions other than indicated may result in precipitation. Do not use turbid solutions.

Actions

➤*Pharmacology:* Deferoxamine chelates iron by forming a stable complex that prevents the iron from entering into further chemical reactions. It readily chelates iron from ferritin and hemosiderin but not readily from transferrin; it does not combine with the iron from cytochromes and hemoglobin. One hundred parts by weight can bind approximately 8.5 parts of ferric iron. Does not demonstrably increase electrolyte/trace metal excretion.

➤*Pharmacokinetics:* Deferoxamine is metabolized principally by plasma enzymes, but the pathways have not yet been defined. Iron chelate is excreted renally, giving urine a reddish color. Some is excreted in feces via bile. Elimination half-life is about 6 hours.

Contraindications

Severe renal disease or anuria.

Warnings

➤*Primary hemochromatosis:* Deferoxamine is not indicated for the treatment of primary hemochromatosis because phlebotomy is the method of choice of removing excess iron in this disorder.

➤*Ocular and auditory disturbances:* Ocular and auditory disturbances have been reported when deferoxamine was administered over prolonged periods of time, at high doses, or in patients with low ferritin levels. The ocular disturbances observed have been blurring of vision; cataracts after prolonged administration in chronic iron overload; decreased visual acuity including visual loss, visual defects, scotoma; impaired peripheral, color, and night vision; optic neuritis, cataracts, corneal opacities, and retinal pigmentary abnormalities. The auditory abnormalities reported have been tinnitus and hearing loss including high frequency sensorineural hearing loss. In most cases, ocular and auditory disturbances were reversible upon immediate cessation of treatment.

Visual acuity tests, slit-lamp examinations, funduscopy, and audiometry are recommended periodically in patients treated for prolonged periods of time. Toxicity is more likely to be reversed if symptoms or test abnormalities are detected early.

➤*Acute respiratory distress syndrome:* Acute respiratory distress syndrome, also reported in children, has been described following treatment with excessively high IV doses in patients with acute iron intoxication or thalassemia.

➤*Mutagenesis:* Cytoxicity may occur because deferoxamine has been shown to inhibit DNA synthesis in vitro.

➤*Pregnancy:* Category C. Delayed ossification in mice and skeletal anomalies in rabbits were observed after deferoxamine was administered in daily doses up to 4.5 times the maximum daily human dose. No adverse effects were observed in similar studies in rats. There are no adequate and well-controlled studies in pregnant women. Use deferoxamine during pregnancy only if the potential benefit justifies the potential risk to the fetus.

➤*Lactation:* It is not known whether this drug is excreted in human milk. Exercise caution when deferoxamine is administered to a nursing woman.

➤*Children:* Safety and effectiveness in pediatric patients under 3 years of age have not been established. Iron mobilization by deferoxamine is relatively poor in patients under 3 years of age with relatively little iron overload. Ordinarily, do not give the drug to such patients unless significant iron mobilization (eg, 1 mg or more of iron/day) can be demonstrated.

High doses of deferoxamine and concomitant low ferritin levels also have been associated with growth retardation. After reduction of deferoxamine dose, growth velocity may partially resume to pretreatment rates.

Monitor pediatric patients receiving deferoxamine for body weight and growth every 3 months.

Precautions

➤*Infections:* Iron overload increases susceptibility of patients to *Yersinia enterocolitica* and *Yersinia pseudotuberculosis* infections. In some rare cases, treatment of deferoxamine has enhanced this susceptibility, resulting in generalized infections by providing this bacteria with a siderophore otherwise missing. In such cases, discontinue deferoxamine treatment until the infection is resolved.

In patients receiving deferoxamine, rare cases of mucormycosis, some with a fatal outcome, have been reported. If any of the suspected signs or symptoms occur, discontinue deferoxamine, carry out mycological tests, and institute appropriate treatment immediately.

➤*Aluminum overload:* In patients with aluminum-related encephalopathy, high doses of deferoxamine may exacerbate neurological dysfunction (seizures), probably owing to an acute increase in circulating aluminum. Deferoxamine may precipitate the onset of dialysis dementia. Treatment with deferoxamine in the presence of aluminum overload may result in decreased serum calcium and aggravation of hyperparathyroidism.

➤*Rapid infusion:* Flushing of the skin, urticaria, hypotension, and shock have occurred in a few patients with rapid IV injection. Therefore, give deferoxamine IM or by slow SC or IV infusion.

➤*Vitamin C use:* Patients with iron overload usually become vitamin C deficient, probably because iron oxidizes the vitamin. As an adjuvant to iron chelation therapy, vitamin C in doses up to 200 mg for adults may be given in divided doses, starting after an initial month of regular treatment with deferoxamine. Vitamin C increases availability of iron for chelation. In general, 50 mg/day suffices for children under 10 years

DEFEROXAMINE MESYLATE

of age and 100 mg/day for older children. Larger doses of vitamin C fail to produce any additional increase in excretion of iron complex.

In patients with severe chronic iron overload, impairment of cardiac function has been reported following concomitant treatment with deferoxamine and high doses of vitamin C (more than 500 mg/day in adults). The cardiac dysfunction was reversible when vitamin C was discontinued. Take the following precautions when vitamin C and deferoxamine are to be used concomitantly: a) do not give vitamin C supplements to patients with cardiac failure; b) start supplemental vitamin C only after an initial month of regular treatment with deferoxamine; c) give vitamin C only if the patient is receiving deferoxamine regularly, ideally soon after setting up the infusion pump; d) do not exceed the daily vitamin C dose of 200 mg in adults, given in divided doses; e) clinical monitoring of cardiac function is advisable during such combined therapy.

Drug Interactions

Deferoxamine Drug Interactions			
Precipitant drug	Object drug*		Description
Deferoxamine	Gallium-67	↓	Imaging results may be distorted because of the rapid urinary excretion of deferoxamine-bound gallium-67. Discontinue deferoxamine 48 hours prior to scintigraphy.
Deferoxamine	Prochlorperazine	↑	Concurrent use may lead to temporary impairment of consciousness.

* ↑ = Object drug increased. ↓ = Object drug decreased.

Adverse Reactions

The following adverse reactions have been observed, but there are not enough data to support an estimate of their frequency.

➤*Cardiovascular:* Hypotension, shock, tachycardia.

➤*CNS:* Neurological disturbances including dizziness, peripheral sensory, motor, or mixed neuropathy, paresthesias; exacerbation or precipitation of aluminum-related dialysis encephalopathy (see Precautions).

➤*GI:* Abdominal discomfort, diarrhea, nausea, vomiting.

➤*GU:* Dysuria, impaired renal function (see Contraindications); reddish urine (see Pharmacokinetics).

➤*Hematologic:* Blood dyscrasia (ie, cases of thrombocytopenia and/or leukopenia have been reported. A causal relationship has not been clearly established).

➤*Hypersensitivity:* Anaphylactic reaction with or without shock, angioedema, generalized rash, urticaria.

➤*Local:* Burning, crusting, erythema, eschar, induration, infiltration, local edema, localized irritation, pain, pruritus, swelling, vesicles, wheal formation. Injection site reactions may be associated with systemic allergic reactions.

➤*Musculoskeletal:* Leg cramps have occurred. Growth retardation and bone changes (eg, metaphyseal dysplasia) are common in chelated patients given doses above 60 mg/kg, especially those who begin iron chelation in the first 3 years of life. If doses are kept to 40 mg/kg or below, the risk may be reduced (see Warnings).

➤*Respiratory:* Acute respiratory distress syndrome (with dyspnea, cyanosis, and/or interstitial infiltrates) (see Warnings).

➤*Special senses:* High-frequency sensorineural hearing loss and/or tinnitus are uncommon if dosage guidelines are not exceeded and if dose is reduced when ferritin levels decline. Visual disturbances are rare if dosage guidelines are not exceeded. These may include decreased acuity, blurred vision, loss of vision, dyschromatopsia, night blindness, visual field defects, scotoma, retinopathy (pigmentary degeneration), optic neuritis, and cataracts (see Warnings).

➤*Miscellaneous:* Local injection site reactions may be accompanied by systemic reactions (eg, arthralgia, fever, headache, myalgia, nausea, vomiting, abdominal pain, asthma). Generalized rash has occurred very rarely.

Rare infections with *Yersinia* and mucormycosis have been reported in association with deferoxamine use (see Precautions).

Overdosage

➤*Symptoms:* Inadvertent administration of an overdose or inadvertent IV bolus administration/rapid IV infusion may be associated with hypotension, tachycardia, and GI disturbances; acute but transient loss of vision, aphasia, agitation, headache, nausea, pallor, CNS depression including coma, bradycardia, and acute renal failure have been reported.

➤*Treatment:* There is no specific antidote. Discontinue deferoxamine and undertake appropriate symptomatic measures. Deferoxamine is readily dialyzable.

Patient Information

Patients experiencing dizziness or other nervous system disturbances or impairment of vision or hearing should refrain from driving or operating potentially hazardous machines.

Inform patients that occasionally their urine may show a reddish discoloration.

EDETATE CALCIUM DISODIUM (Calcium EDTA)

Rx	Calcium Disodium Versenate (3M Pharm.)	Injection: 200 mg/mL	In 5 mL amps.

WARNING

Calcium EDTA is capable of producing toxic effects that can be fatal. Lead encephalopathy is relatively rare in adults, but occurs more often in pediatric patients in whom it may be incipient and thus overlooked. The mortality rate in pediatric patients has been high. Patients with lead encephalopathy and cerebral edema may experience a lethal increase in intracranial pressure following IV infusion; the IM route is preferred for these patients. In cases where the IV route is necessary, avoid rapid infusion. Follow the dosage schedule and at no time exceed the recommended daily dose.

Indications

➤*Lead poisoning:* Acute and chronic lead poisoning and lead encephalopathy.

Administration and Dosage

Calcium EDTA is equally effective whether administered IV or IM. The IM injection is very painful; therefore, the IV route of administration may be preferred. In patients at risk for lead encephalopathy, rapid IV infusion may increase intracranial pressure and worsen the encephalopathy.

➤*Lead poisoning:* If possible, remove the patient from the source of lead.

Blood lead level 20 to 70 mcg/dL – The recommended dose for asymptomatic adults and pediatric patients whose blood lead level is less than 70 mcg/dL but more than 20 mcg/dL (WHO recommended upper allowable level) is 1000 mg/m²/day whether given IV or IM. Therapy is continued over a period of 5 days. Therapy is then interrupted for 2 to 4 days to allow redistribution of the lead and to prevent severe depletion of zinc and other essential metals. Two courses of treatment are usually employed; however, it depends on the severity of the lead toxicity and the patient's tolerance of the drug.

Blood lead level more than 70 mcg/dL – In those with a lead level more than 70 mcg/dL or clinical symptoms consistent with lead poisoning, it is recommended that calcium EDTA be used in conjunction with dimercaprol. Therapy is initiated with an IM dose of dimercaprol,

another IM dose of dimercaprol 4 hours later, followed immediately by IV calcium EDTA as a single dose infused over several hours or as a continuous infusion.

➤*Lead encephalopathy:* Lead encephalopathy is relatively rare in adults, but is common in children and has a high mortality rate. Combination therapy of dimercaprol and calcium EDTA is usually required. IM administration of calcium EDTA may be necessary to avoid fluid overload and increased intracranial pressure.

➤*Lead nephropathy:* The following dosing regimen has been suggested. These regimens may be repeated at 1-month intervals.

Calcium EDTA Dosage Regimen for Adults with Lead Nephropathy	
Serum creatinine (mg/dL)	Calcium EDTA dose
2 to 3	500 mg/m² every 24 h for 5 days
3 to 4	500 mg/m² every 48 h for 3 doses
>4	500 mg/m² once weekly

➤*IV administration:* Add the total daily dose of calcium EDTA (1000 mg/m²/day) to 250 to 500 mL of 5% dextrose or 0.9% sodium chloride injection. Infuse the total daily dose over 4 to 24 hours.

Incompatibilities – Calcium EDTA injection is incompatible with 10% dextrose, 10% invert sugar in 0.9% sodium chloride, lactated Ringer's, Ringer's, 1/6 molar sodium lactate injections, and with injectable amphotericin B and hydralazine HCl.

➤*IM administration:* Divide the total daily dosage (1000 mg/m²/day) into equal doses spaced 8 to 12 hours apart. Add lidocaine or procaine to the calcium EDTA injection to minimize pain at the injection site. The final lidocaine or procaine concentration of 5 mg/mL (0.5%) can be obtained as follows: 0.25 mL of 10% lidocaine solution/5 mL (entire content of ampule) concentrated calcium EDTA; 1 mL of 1% lidocaine or procaine solution/mL of concentrated calcium EDTA. When used alone, regardless of method of administration, do not give calcium EDTA at doses larger than those recommended.

➤*Diagnostic test:* Several methods have been described for lead mobilization tests using calcium EDTA to assess body stores. These procedures have advantages and disadvantages that should be

EDETATE CALCIUM DISODIUM (Calcium EDTA)

reviewed in current references. Do not perform calcium EDTA mobilization tests in symptomatic patients and in patients with blood lead levels above 55 mcg/dL for whom appropriate therapy is indicated.

➤*Storage/Stability:* Store at controlled room temperature (15° to 30°C; 59° to 86°F).

Actions

➤*Pharmacology:* Calcium EDTA forms chelates with divalent and trivalent metals. A stable chelate will form with any metal that has the ability to displace calcium from the molecule, a feature shared by lead, zinc, cadmium, manganese, iron, and mercury.

The primary source of lead chelated by calcium EDTA is from bone; subsequently, soft tissue lead is redistributed to bone when chelation is stopped. There is also some reduction in kidney lead levels following chelation therapy.

➤*Pharmacokinetics:* Calcium EDTA is poorly absorbed from the GI tract. The half-life of the injection is 20 to 60 minutes. About 50% is excreted in the urine in 1 hour; over 95% is excreted in 24 hours. Calcium EDTA is distributed primarily in the extracellular fluid with only about 5% of the plasma concentration found in spinal fluid. Almost none of the compound is metabolized.

Contraindications

Anuria; active renal disease; hepatitis.

Warnings

➤*Do not exceed recommended dosage:* EDTA can produce toxic and potentially fatal effects. In lead encephalopathy, avoid rapid infusion; the IM route is preferred (see Black Box warning).

➤*Renal effects:* Treatment-induced nephrotoxicity is dose-dependent and may be reduced by assuring adequate diuresis before therapy begins. Urine flow must be monitored throughout therapy. Therapy must be stopped if anuria or severe oliguria develop. The proximal tubule hydropic degeneration usually recovers upon cessation of therapy. Calcium EDTA must be used in reduced doses in patients with pre-existing mild renal disease. Monitor patients for cardiac rhythm irregularities and other ECG changes during IV therapy.

➤*Hepatic effects:* Mild increases in ALT and AST are common but return to normal within 48 hours after discontinuing therapy.

➤*Renal function impairment:* Calcium EDTA must be used in reduced doses in patients with pre-existing mild renal disease.

➤*Pregnancy: Category B.* A reproduction study performed in rats at doses up to about 25 to 40 times the human dose revealed evidence of fetal malformations caused by calcium EDTA, which were prevented by simultaneous supplementation of dietary zinc. However, there are no adequate and well-controlled studies in pregnant women. Use during pregnancy only if clearly needed.

➤*Lactation:* It is not known whether this drug is excreted in human milk. Exercise caution when edetate calcium disodium is administered to a nursing woman.

➤*Children:* Because lead poisoning occurs in pediatric populations and adults but is frequently more severe in pediatric patients, calcium EDTA is used in patients of all ages. In cases where the IV route is necessary, avoid rapid infusion. Urine flow must be monitored throughout therapy; calcium EDTA therapy must be stopped if anuria or severe oliguria develops (see Precautions). Do not exceed the recommended daily dosage at any time.

Precautions

➤*Monitoring:* Check urinalysis and urine sediment, renal and hepatic function and serum electrolyte levels before each course of therapy and then monitor daily during therapy in severe cases; in less serious cases monitor after the second and fifth day of therapy. Therapy must be discontinued at the first sign of renal toxicity. The presence of large renal epithelial cells or increasing number of red blood cells in urinary sediment or greater proteinuria call for immediate stopping of calcium EDTA administration. Interrupt infusion for 1 hour before obtaining a blood lead level to avoid a falsely elevated value. Alkaline phosphatase values are frequently depressed (possibly because of decreased serum

zinc levels), but return to normal within 48 hours after cessation of therapy. Elevated erythrocyte protoporphyrin levels (greater than 35 mcg/dL of whole blood) indicate the need to perform a venous blood lead determination. If the whole blood lead concentration is between 25 and 55 mcg/dL, a mobilization test can be considered. An elevation of urinary coproporphyrin (adults: more than 250 mcg/day; pediatric patients under 80 lbs: more than 75 mcg/day) and elevation of urinary delta aminolevulinic acid (ALA) (adults: more than 4 mg/day; pediatric patients: more than 3 mg/m^2/day) are associated with blood lead levels of more than 40 mcg/dL. Urinary coproporphyrin may be falsely negative in terminal patients and in severely iron-depleted pediatric patients who are not regenerating heme. In growing pediatric patients, long-bone x-rays showing lead lines and abdominal x-rays showing radiopaque material in the abdomen may be of help in estimating the level of exposure to lead.

➤*Hydration:* Avoid excess fluids in patients with lead encephalopathy and increased intracranial pressure. In such cases, mix with procaine to give a final concentration of 0.5% procaine and administer IM.

Acutely ill individuals may be dehydrated from vomiting. Because EDTA is excreted almost exclusively in the urine, it is very important to establish urine flow with IV infusion before administering the first dose. Once urine flow is established, restrict further IV fluid to basal water and electrolyte requirements. Stop EDTA when urine flow ceases.

Drug Interactions

➤*Insulin zinc:* Calcium EDTA interferes with the action of zinc insulin preparations by chelating the zinc.

➤*Steroids:* Steroids enhance the renal toxicity of calcium EDTA in animals.

Adverse Reactions

➤*Cardiovascular:* Hypotension; cardiac rhythm irregularities.

➤*CNS:* Tremors; headache; numbness; tingling.

➤*GI:* Cheilosis; nausea; vomiting; anorexia; excessive thirst.

➤*GU:* Glycosuria; proteinuria; microscopic hematuria and large epithelial cells in urinary sediment.

➤*Hematologic:* Transient bone marrow depression; anemia.

➤*Hypersensitivity:* Histamine-like reactions (eg, sneezing, nasal congestion, lacrimation); rash.

➤*Metabolic:* Zinc deficiency; hypercalcemia.

➤*Renal:* Acute necrosis of proximal tubules that may result in fatal nephrosis (see Warnings); infrequent changes in distal tubules and glomeruli.

➤*Lab test abnormalities:* Mild increases in AST and ALT are common (see Warnings).

➤*Miscellaneous:* Pain at IM injection site (see Administration and Dosage); fever; chills; malaise; fatigue; myalgia; arthralgia.

Overdosage

➤*Symptoms:* Inadvertent administration of 5 times the recommended dose, infused IV over a 24-hour period, to an asymptomatic 16-month-old patient with a blood lead content of 56 mcg/dL did not cause any ill effects. Calcium EDTA can aggravate the symptoms of severe lead poisoning; therefore, most toxic effects (eg, cerebral edema, renal tubular necrosis) appear to be associated with lead poisoning. Because of cerebral edema, a therapeutic dose may be lethal to an adult or a pediatric patient with lead encephalopathy. Higher dosage of calcium EDTA may produce a more severe zinc deficiency.

➤*Treatment:* Treat cerebral edema with repeated doses of mannitol. Steroids enhance the renal toxicity of calcium EDTA in animals and, therefore, are no longer recommended. Zinc levels must be monitored. Good urinary output must be maintained because diuresis will enhance drug elimination. It is not known if calcium EDTA is dialyzable.

Patient Information

Instruct patients to immediately inform their physician if urine output stops for 12 hours.

SODIUM THIOSULFATE

Rx	Sodium Thiosulfate (American Regent)	Injection: 10% (100 mg/mL) (as pentahydrate)	Preservative-free. In 10 mL single-dose vials.
		25% (250 mg/mL) (as pentahydrate)	Preservative-free. In 50 mL single-dose vials.

Indications

➤*Cyanide poisoning:* May be used alone or as adjunctive therapy with sodium nitrite or amyl nitrite in cyanide toxicity.

➤*Unlabeled uses:* Sodium thiosulfate has been used as an antidote for cisplatin-induced nephrotoxicity. It also has been shown to be beneficial for extravasation of significant amounts of cisplatin.

Administration and Dosage

Death from cyanide poisoning occurs rapidly; avoid delays in administering sodium thiosulfate.

Sodium thiosulfate injection is meant for slow IV use only.

➤*Cyanide poisoning:*

Adults – 12.5 g IV over approximately 10 minutes, whether used alone or in combination with other cyanide antidotes.

Children – 7 g/m^2; maximum dose 12.5 g.

Monitoring – Closely monitor patients for 24 to 48 hours for symptoms to reappear. If symptoms recur, repeat administration at one-half the original dose.

➤*Storage / Stability:* Store at controlled room temperature (15° to 30°C; 59° to 86°F).

Actions

➤*Pharmacology:* The primary mechanism of cyanide detoxification involves conversion of cyanide to the relatively nontoxic thiocyanate ion. This reaction involves the enzyme rhodanese (thiosulfate cyanide sulfurtransferase) found in many body tissues, but with major activity in the liver. The body has the capability to detoxify cyanide; however, the rhodanese enzyme system responds slowly to large amounts of cyanide. The rhodanese enzyme reaction can be accelerated by supplying an exogenous source of sulfur, accomplished by administering sodium thiosulfate.

➤*Pharmacokinetics:* Following IV injection, sodium thiosulfate is distributed throughout the extracellular fluid and excreted unchanged in the urine. The biological half-life is 0.65 hours.

Warnings

➤*Pregnancy: Category C.* Safety for use during pregnancy has not been established. Use only when clearly needed and when the potential benefits outweigh the potential hazards to the fetus.

Precautions

➤*Hypovolemia:* Sodium thiosulfate is essentially nontoxic. However, studies conducted in dogs, with a constant infusion of sodium thiosulfate, showed hypovolemia that was considered to be due to an osmotic diuretic effect of sodium thiosulfate.

SODIUM NITRITE

Rx	Sodium Nitrite (Hope)	Injection: 30 mg/mL	In 10 mL vials.

Indications

➤*Cyanide poisoning:* As adjunctive therapy with sodium thiosulfate injection and amyl nitrite inhalants for the treatment of cyanide poisoning.

➤*Unlabeled uses:* Hydrogen sulfide poisoning.

Administration and Dosage

Death from cyanide poisoning occurs rapidly; avoid delays in administration.

1.) Break an ampule of amyl nitrite, one at a time, in a handkerchief and hold it in front of the patient's mouth for 15 seconds followed by a rest for 15 seconds. Then reapply until sodium nitrite can be administered. This interrupted schedule is important because continuous use of amyl nitrite may prevent adequate oxygenation.

2.) Discontinue administration of amyl nitrite. Inject 300 mg (10 mL of a 3% solution) sodium nitrite IV at the rate of 2.5 to 5 mL/minute for adults; inject 6 to 8 mL/m^2 (approximately 0.2 mL/kg of body weight), not to exceed 10 mL for children.

3.) Immediately thereafter, inject 12.5 g (50 mL of a 25% solution) sodium thiosulfate for adults; inject 7 g/m^2 of body surface area, not to exceed 12.5 g for children. The same needle and vein may be used.

Watch the patient closely for at least 24 to 48 hours. If signs of poisoning reappear, repeat injections of sodium nitrite and sodium thiosulfate, but each in one half of the original dose. Even if the patient seems well, the medication may be given for prophylactic purposes 2 hours after the first injections.

If respiration has ceased but the pulse is palpable, immediately apply artificial respiration. Lay the gauze sponge or handkerchief containing the amyl nitrite over the patient's nose, because it may hasten the resumption of respiration movements. When signs of breathing appear, promptly inject the above solutions.

➤*Storage / Stability:* Store at controlled room temperature 15° to 30°C (59° to 86°F).

Actions

➤*Pharmacology:* Sodium nitrite reacts with hemoglobin to form methemoglobin. Methemoglobin removes cyanide ions from various tissues and couples with them to become cyanmethemoglobin, which has relatively low toxicity.

The combination of sodium nitrite and sodium thiosulfate is effective therapy against cyanide and hydrocyanic acid poisoning. The 2 substances injected IV, one after the other (nitrite followed by thiosulfate), are capable of detoxifying approximately 20 lethal doses of sodium cyanide in dogs and are effective even after respiration has stopped. As long as the heart is still beating, the chances of recovery by utilizing this method are good.

There is not only a summation but also a definite potentiation of action when the nitrite and the thiosulfate are administered together.

Precautions

➤*Hypotension:* Nitrites produce significant vasodilation, and rapid administration may result in hypotension. Hypotension may be avoided or lessened by slow administration (eg, IV push over at least 5 minutes) or by diluting the dose in 50 to 100 mL of 5% dextrose in water or normal saline and beginning infusion as a slow drip then increasing to the most rapid rate tolerated. Frequently monitor blood pressure during treatment with sodium nitrite.

➤*Methemoglobinemia:* Both sodium nitrite and amyl nitrite in excessive doses induce dangerous methemoglobinemia and can cause death. The recommended dosage is not excessive for an adult. Calculate the doses for children on a surface area or weight basis, with the dosage adjusted so that excessive methemoglobin does not form. Monitor methemoglobin levels, especially when multiple doses of sodium nitrite are required. Avoid levels greater than 30% to 40%. If signs of excessive methemoglobinemia develop (ie, blue skin and mucous membranes, vomiting, shock, coma), 1% methylene blue solution IV may be useful. Note: Methylene blue use in a cyanide-intoxicated patient results in increased cyanide release and, thus, clinical deterioration. In addition, consider oxygen inhalation and transfusion of whole fresh blood.

Adverse Reactions

Dizziness, flushing, headache, hypotension, methemoglobinemia, nausea, syncope, tachycardia, and vomiting may occur.

NALMEFENE HCl

Rx	**Revex** (Ohmeda)	**Injection:** 100 mcg/mL nalmefene base	Blue label.[1] In 1 mL amps.
		1 mg/mL nalmefene base	Green label.[2] In 2 mL amps.

[1] The blue labeled product is for postoperative use.

[2] The green labeled product is for management of overdose.

Indications

➤*Reversal of opioid effects:* Complete or partial reversal of opioid drug effects, including respiratory depression, induced by either natural or synthetic opioids.

➤*Opioid overdose:* Management of known or suspected opioid overdose.

Administration and Dosage

➤*Approved by the FDA:* April 17, 1995 (1S classification).

➤*Important information - Dosage strengths:* Nalmefene is supplied in 2 concentrations that are packaged in ampules of different appearance: An amp with a blue label containing 1 mL at a concentration suitable for postoperative use (100 mcg/mL) and an amp with a green label containing 2 mL suitable for the management of overdose (1 mg/mL, 10 times as concentrated, 20 times as much drug). Take proper steps to prevent use of the incorrect dosage strength.

➤*Administration:* Titrate nalmefene to reverse the undesired effects of opioids. Once adequate reversal has been established, additional administration is not required and may actually be harmful because of unwanted reversal of analgesia or precipitated withdrawal.

➤*Duration of action:* The duration of action of nalmefene is as long as that of most opioid analgesics. However, the apparent duration of action will vary, depending on the half-life and plasma concentration of the narcotic being reversed, the presence or absence of other drugs affecting the brain or muscles of respiration, and the dose of nalmefene administered. Partially reversing doses of nalmefene (1 mcg/kg) lose their effect as the drug is redistributed through the body, and the effects of these low doses may not last more than 30 to 60 minutes in the presence of persistent opioid effects. Fully reversing doses (1 mg/70 kg) last many hours, but may complicate the management of patients who are in pain, at high cardiovascular risk, or who are physically dependent on opioids.

The recommended doses represent a compromise between a desirable controlled reversal and the need for prompt response and adequate duration of action. Using higher dosages or shorter intervals between incremental doses is likely to increase the incidence and severity of symptoms related to acute withdrawal such as nausea, vomiting, elevated blood pressure, and anxiety.

➤*Patients tolerant to or physically dependent on opioids:* Nalmefene may cause acute withdrawal symptoms in individuals who have some degree of tolerance to and dependence on opioids. Closely observe these patients for symptoms of withdrawal following administration of the initial and subsequent injections of nalmefene. Administer subsequent doses with intervals of at least 2 to 5 minutes between doses to allow the full effect of each incremental dose of nalmefene to be reached.

➤*Reversal of postoperative opioid depression:* Use the 100 mcg/mL dosage strength (blue label); refer to the following table for initial doses. The goal of treatment with nalmefene in the postoperative setting is to achieve reversal of excessive opioid effects without inducing a complete reversal and acute pain. This is best accomplished with an initial dose of 0.25 mcg/kg followed by 0.25 mcg/kg incremental doses at 2- to 5-minute intervals, stopping as soon as the desired degree of opioid reversal is obtained. A cumulative total dose > 1 mcg/kg does not provide additional therapeutic effect.

Nalmefene Dosage for Reversal of Postoperative Opioid Depression	
Body weight (kg)	Amount of nalmefene 100 mcg/mL solution (mL)
50	0.125
60	0.15
70	0.175
80	0.2
90	0.225
100	0.25

➤*Cardiovascular risk patients:* In cases where the patient is known to be at increased cardiovascular risk, it may be desirable to dilute nalmefene 1:1 with saline or sterile water and use smaller initial and incremental doses of 0.1 mcg/kg.

➤*Management of known/suspected opioid overdose:* Use 1 mg/mL dosage strength (green label). The recommended initial dose of nalmefene for nonopioid dependent patients is 0.5 mg/70 kg. If needed, this may be followed by a second dose of 1 mg/70 kg, 2 to 5 minutes later. If a total dose of 1.5 mg/70 kg has been administered without clinical response, additional nalmefene is unlikely to have an effect. Do not give patients more nalmefene than is required to restore the respiratory rate to normal, thus minimizing the likelihood of cardiovascular stress and precipitated withdrawal syndrome.

If there is a reasonable suspicion of opioid dependency, initially administer a challenge dose of 0.1 mg/70 kg. If there is no evidence of withdrawal in 2 minutes, follow the recommended dosing. Nalmefene had no effect in cases where opioids were not responsible for sedation and hypoventilation. Therefore, only treat patients with nalmefene when the likelihood of an opioid overdose is high based on a history of opioid overdose or the clinical presentation of respiratory depression with concurrent pupillary constriction.

➤*Repeated dosing:* Nalmefene is the longest acting of the currently available parenteral opioid antagonists. If recurrence of respiratory depression does occur, titrate the dose again to clinical effect using incremental doses to avoid overreversal.

➤*Hepatic and renal disease:* Hepatic disease and renal failure substantially reduce the clearance of nalmefene (see Warnings). For single episodes of opioid antagonism, adjustment of nalmefene dosage is not required. However, in patients with renal failure, slowly administer the incremental doses (over 60 seconds) to minimize the hypertension and dizziness reported following the abrupt administration of nalmefene to such patients.

➤*Loss of IV access:* Should IV access be lost or not readily obtainable, a single dose of nalmefene should be effective within 5 to 15 minutes after 1 mg IM or SC doses (see Pharmacokinetics).

Actions

➤*Pharmacology:* Nalmefene, an opioid antagonist, is a 6-methylene analog of naltrexone. Nalmefene prevents or reverses the effects of opioids, including respiratory depression, sedation, and hypotension. It has a longer duration of action than naloxone at fully reversing doses. Nalmefene has no opioid agonist activity; it does not produce respiratory depression, psychotomimetic effects, or pupillary constriction, and no pharmacological activity was observed when it was administered in the absence of opioid agonists. Nalmefene can produce acute withdrawal symptoms in individuals who are opioid-dependent.

➤*Pharmacokinetics:*

Absorption – Nalmefene was completely bioavailable following IM or SC administration in 12 male volunteers relative to IV use (relative bioavailabilities were 101.5% and 99.7%, respectively). Nalmefene will be administered primarily as an IV bolus; however, it can be given IM or SC if venous access cannot be established. While the time to maximum plasma concentration was 2.3 hours following IM and 1.5 hours following SC administrations, therapeutic plasma concentrations are likely to be reached within 5 to 15 minutes after a 1 mg dose in an emergency. Because of the variability in the speed of absorption for IM and SC dosing and the inability to titrate to effect, take great care if repeated doses must be given by these routes.

Distribution – Following a 1 mg parenteral dose, nalmefene was rapidly distributed. A 1 mg dose blocked > 80% of brain opioid receptors within 5 minutes after administration. The apparent volumes of distribution centrally and at steady state are 3.9 and 8.6 L/kg, respectively. Over a concentration range of 0.1 to 2 mcg/ml, 45% is bound to plasma proteins. In vitro, nalmefene distributed 67% into red blood cells and 39% into plasma.

Metabolism – Nalmefene is metabolized by the liver, primarily by glucuronide conjugation, and excreted in the urine; < 5% is excreted in the urine unchanged, and 17% is excreted in the feces. It also is metabolized to trace amounts of an N-dealkylated metabolite. Nalmefene glucuronide is inactive; the N-dealkylated metabolite has minimal activity. Nalmefene may undergo enterohepatic recycling.

Excretion – After IV administration of 1 mg to healthy males (19 to 32 years of age), plasma concentrations declined biexponentially with a redistribution and a terminal elimination half-life of 41 ± 34 minutes and 10.8 ± 5.2 hours, respectively. The systemic clearance of nalmefene is 0.8 L/hr/kg and the renal clearance is 0.08 L/hr/kg.

Nalmefene Pharmacokinetic Parameters in Adult Males (1 mg IV dose)		
Parameter	Young (n = 18)	Elderly (n = 11)
Age (years)	19-32	62-80
C_p at 5 min (ng/ml)	3.7	5.8
Vd_{ss} (L/kg)	8.6	8.6
V_c (L/kg)	3.9	2.8
AUC_{0-inf} (ng•hr/ml)	16.6	17.3
Terminal $t_{1/2}$ (hr)	10.8	9.4
Cl_{plasma} (L/hr/kg)	0.8	0.8

NALMEFENE HCl

➤*Clinical trials:*

Reversal of postoperative opioid depression – In five controlled trials, patients received nalmefene following morphine or fentanyl intraoperatively. Five minutes after administration, initial single doses of 0.1, 0.25, 0.5 or 1 mcg/kg had effectively reversed respiratory depression in a dose-dependent manner. Twenty minutes after initial administration, respiratory depression had been effectively reversed in most patients receiving cumulative doses within the recommended range (0.1 to 1 mcg/kg). Total doses > 1 mcg/kg did not increase the therapeutic response. The postoperative administration of nalmefene at the recommended doses did not prevent the analgesic response to subsequently administered opioids.

Reversal of the effect of intrathecally administered opioids – IV nalmefene doses of 0.5 and 1 mcg/kg were administered to 47 patients given intrathecal morphine. One to two doses reversed respiratory depression in most patients. The administration of nalmefene at the recommended doses did not prevent the analgesic response to subsequently administered opioids.

Management of known or suspected opioid overdose – Nalmefene doses of 0.5 to 2 mg were studied in four trials of patients who were presumed to have taken an opioid overdose. Doses of 0.5 to 1 mg effectively reversed respiratory depression within 2 to 5 minutes in most patients subsequently confirmed to have opioid overdose. A total dose > 1.5 mg did not increase the therapeutic response.

Contraindications

Hypersensitivity to the product.

Warnings

➤*Emergency use:* Nalmefene, like all drugs in this class, is not the primary treatment for ventilatory failure. In most emergency settings, treatment with nalmefene should follow, not precede, the establishment of a patent airway, ventilatory assistance, administration of oxygen and establishment of circulatory access.

➤*Respiratory depression:* Accidental overdose with long acting opioids (eg, methadone, levomethadyl) may result in prolonged respiratory depression. Respiratory depression in both the postoperative and overdose setting may be complex and involve the effects of anesthetic agents, neuromuscular blockers and other drugs. While nalmefene has a longer duration of action than naloxone in fully reversing doses, be aware that a recurrence of respiratory depression is possible, even after an apparently adequate initial response to nalmefene treatment. Observe patients until there is no reasonable risk of recurrent respiratory depression.

➤*Renal function impairment:* There was a statistically significant 27% decrease in plasma clearance of nalmefene in the end-stage renal disease (ESRD) population during interdialysis (0.57 L/hr/kg) and a 25% decreased plasma clearance in the ESRD population during intradialysis (0.59 L/hr/kg) compared to controls (0.79 L/hr/kg). The elimination half-life was prolonged in ESRD patients from 10.2 (controls) to 26.1 hr.

➤*Hepatic function impairment:* Subjects with hepatic disease had a 28.3% decrease in plasma clearance of nalmefene compared to controls (0.56 vs 0.78 L/hr/kg, respectively). Elimination half-life increased from 10.2 to 11.9 hours in the hepatically impaired. No dosage adjustment is recommended since nalmefene will be administered as an acute course of therapy.

➤*Elderly:* Dose proportionality was observed in nalmefene AUC following 0.5 to 2 mg IV administration to elderly male subjects. Following a 1 mg IV dose, there were no significant differences between young and elderly adult male subjects with respect to plasma clearance, steady-state volume of distribution or half-life. There was an apparent age-related decrease in the central volume of distribution that resulted in a greater initial nalmefene concentration in the elderly group. While initial plasma concentrations were transiently higher in the elderly, it would not be anticipated that this population would require dosing adjustment.

➤*Pregnancy: Category B.* There are no adequate and well controlled studies in pregnant women. Use this drug during pregnancy only if clearly needed.

➤*Lactation:* Nalmefene and its metabolites were secreted into rat milk, reaching concentrations approximately three times those in plasma at 1 hour and decreasing to about half the corresponding plasma concentrations by 24 hours following bolus administration. Exercise caution when nalmefene is administered to a nursing woman.

➤*Children:* Safety and efficacy have not been established. Only use nalmefene in the resuscitation of the newborn when the expected benefits outweigh the risks.

Precautions

➤*Cardiovascular risks:* Pulmonary edema, cardiovascular instability, hypotension, hypertension, ventricular tachycardia and ventricular fibrillation have been reported in connection with opioid reversal in both postoperative and emergency department settings. In many cases, these effects appear to be the result of abrupt reversal of opioid effects. Although nalmefene has been used safely in patients with preexisting cardiac disease, use all drugs of this class with caution in patients at high cardiovascular risk or who have received potentially cardiotoxic drugs.

➤*Risk of precipitated withdrawal:* Nalmefene is known to produce acute withdrawal symptoms and, therefore, should be used with extreme caution in patients with known physical dependence on opioids or following surgery involving high uses of opioids. Imprudent use or excessive doses of opioid antagonists in the postoperative setting has been associated with hypertension, tachycardia and excessive mortality in patients at high risk for cardiovascular complications.

➤*Incomplete reversal of buprenorphine:* In animals, nalmefene doses up to 10 mg/kg (437 times the maximum recommended human dose) produced incomplete reversal of buprenorphine-induced analgesia. This appears to be a consequence of a high affinity and slow displacement of buprenorphine from the opioid receptors. Hence, nalmefene may not completely reverse buprenorphine-induced respiratory depression.

Drug Interactions

➤*Flumazenil:* Both flumazenil and nalmefene can induce seizures in animals. Coadministration of these agents produced fewer seizures than expected in a study in rodents, based on the expected effects of each drug alone. Based on these data, an adverse interaction from the coadministration of the two drugs is not expected, but remain aware of the potential risk of seizures from agents in these classes.

Adverse Reactions

Nalmefene is well tolerated and shows no serious toxicity during experimental administration to healthy individuals, even when given at 15 times the highest recommended dose. In a small number of subjects, at doses exceeding the recommended dose, nalmefene produced symptoms suggestive of reversal of endogenous opioids, such as those that have been reported for other narcotic antagonist drugs. These symptoms (eg, nausea, chills, myalgia, dysphoria, abdominal cramps, joint pain) were usually transient and occurred at very low frequency.

Symptoms of precipitated opioid withdrawal at the recommended clinical doses were seen in both postoperative and overdose patients who were later found to have had histories of covert opioid use. Symptoms of precipitated withdrawal similar to those seen with other opioid antagonists, were transient following the lower doses used in the postoperative setting and more prolonged following the administration of the larger doses used in the treatment of overdose.

Tachycardia and nausea following the use of nalmefene in the postoperative setting were reported at the same frequencies as for naloxone at equivalent doses. The risk of both of these adverse events was low at doses giving partial reversal and increased with increases in dose. Thus, total doses > 1 mcg/kg in the postoperative setting and 1.5 mg/70 kg in the treatment of overdose are not recommended.

Nalmefene Adverse Reactions (> 1%)			
Adverse reaction	Nalmefene (n = 1127)	Naloxone (n = 369)	Placebo (n = 77)
Nausea	18%	18%	4%
Vomiting	9%	7%	6%
Tachycardia	5%	8%	-
Hypertension	5%	7%	-
Postoperative pain	4%	4%	N/A
Fever	3%	4%	-
Dizziness	3%	4%	1%
Headache	1%	1%	4%
Chills	1%	1%	-
Hypotension	1%	1%	-
Vasodilation	1%	1%	-

Other adverse reactions include the following:

➤*Cardiovascular:* Bradycardia, arrhythmia (< 1%).

➤*CNS:* Somnolence, depression, agitation, nervousness, tremor, confusion, withdrawal syndrome, myoclonus (< 1%).

➤*GI:* Diarrhea, dry mouth (< 1%).

➤*Lab test abnormalities:* Transient increases in CPK (0.5%; these increases were believed to be related to surgery and not believed to be related to the administration of nalmefene); increases in AST (0.3% with either nalmefene or naloxone).

➤*Miscellaneous:* Pharyngitis, pruritus, urinary retention (< 1%).

Overdosage

IV doses of up to 24 mg administered to healthy volunteers in the absence of opioid agonists produced no serious adverse reactions, severe signs or symptoms or clinically significant laboratory abnormalities. As with all opioid antagonists, use in patients physically dependent on opioids can result in precipitated withdrawal reactions that may result in symptoms that require medical attention. Treatment of such cases should be symptomatic and supportive. Refer to General Management of Acute Overdosage. Administration of large amounts of opioids to patients receiving opioid antagonists in an attempt to overcome a full blockade has resulted in adverse respiratory and circulatory reactions.

Antidotes

NALOXONE HCl

Rx	**Naloxone HCl** (Various, eg, Abbott, Elkins-Sinn, SoloPak)	**Injection:** 0.4 mg/ml	In 1 ml amps, 1 ml syringes and 1, 2 and 10 ml vials.
Rx	**Narcan** (DuPont Pharm.)		In 1 ml amps and 10 ml vials.[1]
Rx	**Narcan** (DuPont Pharm.)	**Injection:** 1 mg/ml	In 2 ml amps and 10 ml vials.[1]
Rx	**Naloxone HCl** (Various, eg, Abbott)	**Neonatal injection:** 0.02 mg/ml	In 2 ml vials.

[1] Available with or without parabens.

Indications

➤*Reversal of opioid effects:* For the complete or partial reversal of narcotic depression, including respiratory depression, induced by opioid including natural and synthetic narcotics, propoxyphene, methadone, nalbuphine, butorphanol and pentazocine.

➤*Opioid overdose:* For the diagnosis of suspected acute opioid overdosage.

➤*Unlabeled uses:* Naloxone has been used to improve circulation in refractory shock. Naloxone has also been used for the reversal of alcoholic coma, dementia of the Alzheimer type and schizophrenia.

Administration and Dosage

Give IV, IM or SC. The most rapid onset of action is achieved with IV use, which is recommended in emergency situations. Duration of action of some narcotics may exceed that of naloxone. Keep patients under continued surveillance and give repeat doses as necessary.

➤*Adults:*

Narcotic overdose (known or suspected) – Initial dose is 0.4 to 2 mg IV; may repeat IV at 2 to 3 minute intervals. If no response is observed after 10 mg has been administered, question the diagnosis of narcotic-induced or partial narcotic-induced toxicity. IM or SC administration may be necessary if the IV route is not available.

Postoperative narcotic depression (partial reversal) – Small doses are usually sufficient. Titrate dose according to the patient's response. Excessive dosage may result in significant reversal of analgesia and increase in blood pressure. Similarly, too rapid reversal may induce nausea, vomiting, sweating or circulatory stress.

Initial dose: Inject in increments of 0.1 to 0.2 mg IV at 2 to 3 minute intervals to the desired degree of reversal (ie, adequate ventilation and alertness without significant pain or discomfort).

Repeat dose: Repeat doses may be required within 1 or 2 hr intervals depending on the amount, type (ie, short- or long-acting) and time interval since last administration. Supplemental IM doses have produced a longer lasting effect.

➤*Children:*

Narcotic overdose (known or suspected) – Initial dose is 0.01 mg/kg IV; give a subsequent dose of 0.1 mg/kg if needed. If an IV route is not available, may be given IM or SC in divided doses. If necessary, dilute with Sterile Water for Injection.

Postoperative narcotic depression – Follow the recommendations and cautions under adult administration guidelines. For initial reversal of respiratory depression, inject in increments of 0.005 to 0.01 mg IV at 2 to 3 minute intervals to desired degree of reversal.

➤*Neonates:*

Narcotic-induced depression – Initial dose is 0.01 mg/kg IV, IM or SC; may be repeated in accordance with adult administration guidelines.

➤*Intravenous infusion:* Dilute in normal saline or 5% dextrose solutions. The addition of 2 mg in 500 ml of either solution provides a concentration of 0.004 mg/ml. Titrate the administration rate in accordance with the patient's response.

Incompatibilities – Do not mix naloxone with preparations containing bisulfite, metabisulfite, long-chain or high molecular weight anions, or any solution having an alkaline pH. Do not add any drug or chemical agent unless its effect on the chemical and physical stability of the solution has first been established.

➤*Storage/Stability:* Use mixtures within 24 hrs. After 24 hrs, discard unused solution.

Actions

➤*Pharmacology:* The narcotic antagonist naloxone is clinically useful in the reversal of narcotic-induced respiratory depression. Naloxone, a pure narcotic antagonist, will precipitate abstinence syndrome in the presence of narcotic addiction. Because it is devoid of undesirable agonist properties, naloxone is preferred for reversal of narcotic-induced respiratory depression. Naloxone prevents or reverses opioid effects including respiratory depression, sedation and hypotension; it can reverse psychotomimetic and dysphoric effects of agonist-antagonists (eg, pentazocine).

Mechanism – The mechanism of action is not fully understood; evidence suggests that it antagonizes the opioid effects by competing for the same receptor sites. Naloxone is an essentially pure narcotic antagonist, ie, it does not possess "agonistic" or morphine-like properties.

Effects – Naloxone does not produce respiratory depression, psychotomimetic effects or pupillary constriction. In the absence of narcotics or agonistic effects of other narcotic antagonists, naloxone exhibits essentially no pharmacologic activity.

➤*Pharmacokinetics:*

Distribution – After parenteral use, naloxone is rapidly distributed in the body. Onset of action of IV naloxone is generally apparent within 2 min; it is only slightly less rapid when give SC or IM. Duration of action depends upon dose and route. IM use produces a more prolonged effect than IV use. The requirement for repeat doses will also depend upon amount, type and route of the narcotic being antagonized.

Metabolism – Naloxone is metabolized in the liver, primarily by glucuronide conjugation. It is excreted in the urine. The serum of half-life in adults ranged from 30 to 81 minutes (mean 64 ± 12 minutes); in neonates, 3.1 ± 0.5 hours.

Contraindications

Hypersensitivity to these agents.

Warnings

➤*Drug dependence:* Administer cautiously to persons who are known or suspected to be physically dependent on opioids, including newborns of mothers with narcotic dependence. Reversal of narcotic effect will precipitate acute abstinence syndrome.

➤*Repeat administration:* The patient who has satisfactorily responded should be kept under continued surveillance. Administer repeated doses as necessary, because the duration of action of some narcotics may exceed that of the narcotic antagonist.

➤*Respiratory depression:* Not effective against respiratory depression due to nonopioid drugs. Reversal of buprenorphine-induced respiratory depression may be incomplete; if an incomplete response occurs, mechanically assist respiration.

➤*Pregnancy: Category B.* No adequate and well controlled studies in pregnant women. Use during pregnancy only when clearly needed.

➤*Lactation:* It is not known whether the drug is excreted in breast milk. Use caution when administering to a nursing woman.

Precautions

➤*Other supportive therapy:* Maintain a free airway and provide artificial respiration, cardiac massage and vasopressor agents; employ when necessary to counteract acute narcotic overdosage.

➤*Cardiovascular effects:* Several instances of hypotension, hypertension, pulmonary edema, ventricular tachycardia and fibrillation have been reported in postoperative patients, most of whom had preexisting cardiovascular disorders or had received other drugs that may have similar adverse cardiovascular effects. A direct cause and effect relationship is not established; use caution in patients with pre-existing cardiac disease or who have received potentially cardiotoxic drugs.

Adverse Reactions

Abrupt reversal of narcotic depression may result in nausea, vomiting, sweating, tachycardia, increased blood pressure and tremulousness.

In postoperative patients, excessive dosage may result in excitement and significant reversal of analgesia, hypotension, hypertension, pulmonary edema and ventricular tachycardia and fibrillation. Seizures have been reported infrequently.

Antidotes

NALTREXONE HCl

Rx	**Naltrexone HCl** (Various, Amide)	**Tablets:** 50 mg	In 30s, 100s, and 500s.
Rx	**ReVia** (Bristol-Myers Squibb Primary Care)	**Tablets:** 50 mg	Sugar. (DuPont NTR). Scored. In 50s.

Indications

➤*Narcotic addiction:* Blockade of the effects of exogenously administered opioids.

➤*Alcoholism:* Treatment of alcohol dependence.

➤*Unlabeled uses:* Naltrexone has been used in eating disorders and in the treatment of postconcussional syndrome unresponsive to other treatments. To increase patient compliance, an SC implant is being studied.

Administration and Dosage

If there is any question of occult opioid dependence, perform a naloxone challenge test. Do not attempt treatment until naloxone challenge is negative.

➤*Alcoholism:* A dose of 50 mg once daily is recommended for most patients.

The placebo controlled studies that demonstrated the efficacy of naltrexone as an adjunctive treatment of alcoholism used a dose regimen of 50 mg once daily for up to 12 weeks. Of patients taking naltrexone for alcoholism, 5% to 15% will complain of non-specific side effects, chiefly GI upset. An initial 25 mg dose, splitting the daily dose and adjusting the time of dosing have met with limited success. No dose or pattern of dosing has been shown to be more effective than any other in reducing these complaints for all patients.

Consider naltrexone as only one of many factors determining the success of treatment of alcoholism. Factors associated with a good outcome in the clinical trials with naltrexone were the type, intensity and duration of treatment; appropriate management of comorbid conditions; use of community-based support groups; and good medication compliance. To achieve the best possible treatment outcome, implement appropriate compliance-enhancing techniques for all components of the treatment program, especially medication compliance.

➤*Narcotic dependence:* Initiate treatment using the following guidelines:

1.) Do not attempt treatment until the patient has remained opioid-free for 7 to 10 days. Verify by analyzing urine for opioids. The patient should not be manifesting withdrawal signs or reporting withdrawal symptoms.
2.) Administer a naloxone challenge test (see below). If signs of opioid withdrawal are still observed following challenge, do not treat with naltrexone. The naloxone challenge can be repeated in 24 hours.
3.) Initiate treatment carefully, slowly increasing the dose. Administer 25 mg initially; observe patient for 1 hour. If no withdrawal signs occur, give the rest of the daily dose.

➤*Naloxone challenge test:* Do not perform in a patient showing clinical signs of opioid withdrawal or in a patient whose urine contains opioids. Administer the challenge test either IV or SC.

IV challenge – Draw 2 ampuls of naloxone, 2 ml (0.8 mg) into a syringe. Inject 0.5 ml (0.2 mg); while the needle is still in the patient's vein, observe for 30 seconds for withdrawal signs or symptoms. If there is no evidence of withdrawal, inject the remaining 1.5 ml (0.6 mg) and observe for an additional 20 minutes for signs and symptoms of withdrawal.

SC challenge – Administer 2 ml (0.8 mg) SC, and observe the patient for signs and symptoms of withdrawal for 45 minutes.

Monitor – Monitor the patient's vital signs and watch for signs and symptoms of opioid withdrawal. Question the patient carefully. The signs and symptoms of opioid withdrawal include, but are not limited to, the following: Stuffiness or runny nose, tearing, yawning, sweating, tremor, vomiting or piloerection, feeling of temperature change, joint or bone and muscle pain, abdominal cramps, skin crawling.

Interpretation of the challenge – The elicitation of the enumerated signs or symptoms indicates a potential risk for the subject, and naltrexone should not be administered. If there are no signs or symptoms of withdrawal, naltrexone may be administered. If there is any doubt in the observer's mind that the patient is not opioid-free, or is in continuing withdrawal, readminister naloxone as follows:

Confirmatory rechallenge – Inject 4 ml (1.6 mg) of naloxone IV and observe the patient again for signs and symptoms of withdrawal. If none are present, naltrexone may be given. If signs and symptoms of withdrawal are present, delay naltrexone until repeated naloxone challenge indicates the patient is no longer at risk.

➤*Maintenance treatment:* Once patient has started naltrexone, 50 mg every 24 hours will produce adequate clinical blockade of the actions of parenterally administered opioids (ie, this dose will block the effects of a 25 mg IV heroin challenge). Flexible dosing may be used. Thus, patients may receive 50 mg every weekday with a 100 mg dose on Saturday, 100 mg every other day, or 150 mg every third day. While

the degree of opioid blockade may be somewhat reduced by using higher doses at longer dosing intervals, improved patient compliance may result from dosing every 48 to 72 hours. Several studies have employed the following dosing regimen with success: 100 mg Monday, 100 mg Wednesday and 150 mg Friday.

Actions

➤*Pharmacology:* Naltrexone, a pure opioid antagonist, markedly attenuates or completely reversibly blocks the subjective effects of IV opioids. When coadministered with morphine on a chronic basis, it blocks the physical dependence to morphine, heroin and other opioids. Naltrexone is a synthetic congener of oxymorphone with no opioid agonist properties, and it is related to naloxone. It has few other, if any, intrinsic actions. However, it does produce some pupillary constriction. Administration is not associated with the development of tolerance or dependence. In subjects physically dependent on opioids, naltrexone will precipitate withdrawal symptomatology.

Naltrexone 50 mg will block the pharmacologic effects of 25 mg IV heroin for as long as 24 hours. Data suggest that doubling the dose of naltrexone provides blockade for 48 hours and tripling the dose provides blockade for about 72 hours.

Naltrexone blocks the effects of opioids by competitive binding at opioid receptors. This makes the blockade potentially surmountable, but administration of very high doses of opiates has resulted in excessive symptoms of histamine release in subjects.

The mechanism of action in alcoholism is not understood; however, involvement of the endogenous opioid system is suggested. Naltrexone competitively binds to opioid receptors and may block the effects of endogenous opioids. Opioid antagonists reduce alcohol consumption by animals, and naltrexone reduces alcohol consumption. Naltrexone is not aversive therapy and does not cause a disulfiram-like reaction either as a result of opiate use or ethanol ingestion.

➤*Pharmacokinetics:*

Absorption – Although well absorbed orally, naltrexone is subject to significant first pass metabolism with oral bioavailability estimates ranging from 5% to 40%. Following oral administration, naltrexone undergoes rapid and nearly complete absorption with ≈ 96% of the dose absorbed from the GI tract. Peak plasma levels of both naltrexone and 6–β-naltrexol occur within 1 hour of dosing.

Distribution – The volume of distribution for naltrexone after IV administration is estimated to be 1350 L. In vitro, naltrexone is 21% bound to plasma proteins.

Metabolism/Excretion – The major metabolite of naltrexone is 6–β-naltrexol. The activity of naltrexone is believed to be due to both parent and the 6–β-naltrexol metabolite. Two other minor metabolites are 2–hydroxy-3–methoxy-6–β-naltrexol and 2–hydroxy-3–methyl-naltrexone. Naltrexone and its metabolites are also conjugated to form additional metabolic products. The mean elimination half-life values for naltrexone and 6–β-naltrexol are 4 and 13 hours, respectively. The systemic clearance (after IV administration) of naltrexone is ≈ 3.5 L/min, which exceeds liver blood flow (≈ 1.2 L/min). This suggests both that naltrexone is a highly extracted drug (> 98% metabolized) and that extra-hepatic sites of drug metabolism exist.

The renal clearance for naltrexone ranges from 30 to 127 ml/min and suggests that renal elimination is primarily by glomerular filtration. In comparison, the renal clearance for 6–β-naltrexol ranges from 230 to 369 ml/min, suggesting an additional renal tubular secretory mechanism. Both parent drug and metabolites are excreted primarily by the kidney (53% to 79% of the dose), however, urinary excretion of unchanged naltrexone accounts for < 2% of an oral dose and fecal excretion is a minor elimination pathway. The urinary excretion of unchanged and conjugated 6–β-naltrexone accounts for 43% of an oral dose. Naltrexone and its metabolites may undergo enterohepatic recycling.

➤*Clinical trials:*

Alcoholism – In one study, 104 alcohol-dependent patients were randomized to receive either naltrexone 50 mg once daily or placebo. Naltrexone proved superior to placebo in measures of drinking including abstention rates (51% vs 23%), number of drinking days and relapse (31% vs 60%). In a second study with 82 alcohol-dependent patients, the group of patients receiving naltrexone had lower relapse rates (21% vs 41%), less alcohol craving and fewer drinking days compared with patients who received placebo, but these results depended on the specific analysis used.

In the clinical studies, treatment with naltrexone supported abstinence, prevented relapse and decreased alcohol consumption. In an uncontrolled study, the patterns of abstinence and relapse were similar to those observed in the controlled studies. Naltrexone was not uniformly helpful to all patients and the expected effect of the drug is a modest improvement in the outcome of conventional treatment.

NALTREXONE HCl

Treatment of narcotic addiction – Naltrexone produces complete blockade of the euphoric effects of opioids in both volunteer and addict populations. When administered by means that enforce compliance, it will produce an effective opioid blockade, but has not been shown to affect the use of cocaine or other non-opioid drugs of abuse.

The drug is reported to be of greatest use in good prognosis narcotic addicts who take the drug as part of a comprehensive occupational rehabilitative program, behavioral contract or other compliance-enhancing protocol. Unlike methadone or levomethadyl, naltrexone does not reinforce medication compliance and is expected to have a therapeutic effect only when given under external conditions that support continued use of the medication.

Contraindications

Patients receiving opioid analgesics; opioid-dependent patients; patients in acute opioid withdrawal; failed naloxone challenge; positive urine screen for opioids; history of sensitivity to naltrexone (it is not known if there is any cross-sensitivity with naloxone or other phenanthrene-containing opioids); acute hepatitis or liver failure.

Warnings

➤*Hepatotoxicity:* Naltrexone has the capacity to cause hepatocellular injury when given in excessive doses. It is contraindicated in acute hepatitis or liver failure, and its use in patients with active liver disease must be carefully considered in light of its hepatotoxic effects.

The margin of separation between the apparently safe dose of naltrexone and the dose causing hepatic injury appears to be only fivefold or less. Naltrexone does not appear to be a hepatotoxin at the recommended doses.

Warn patients of the risk of hepatic injury and advise them to stop naltrexone and seek medical attention if they experience symptoms of acute hepatitis.

Evidence of its hepatotoxic potential is derived primarily from a placebo controlled study in which naltrexone was administered to obese subjects at a dose approximately fivefold that recommended (300 mg/day). Five of 26 naltrexone recipients developed elevations of serum transaminases 3 to 19 times their baseline values after 3 to 8 weeks of treatment. The patients involved were generally clinically asymptomatic and the transaminase levels of all patients on whom follow-up was obtained returned to (or toward) baseline values in a matter of weeks. The lack of any transaminase elevations of similar magnitude in any of the 24 placebo patients indicates that naltrexone is a direct hepatotoxin.

This is also supported by evidence from other placebo controlled studies in which exposure to naltrexone at doses above the amount recommended for the treatment of alcoholism or opiate blockade (50 mg/day) consistently produced more numerous and more significant elevations of serum transaminases than did placebo. Transaminase elevations in 3 of 9 patients with Alzheimer's disease who received naltrexone (at doses up to 300 mg/day) for 5 to 8 weeks in an open clinical trial have been reported.

Although no cases of hepatic failure have ever been reported, consider this as a possible risk of treatment.

➤*Abstinence precipitation/syndrome:* Unintended precipitation of abstinence or exacerbation of a preexisting subclinical abstinence syndrome may occur; therefore, patients should remain opioid-free for a minimum of 7 to 10 days before starting naltrexone. The absence of opioid in urine is not sufficient proof that a patient is opioid-free. Perform a naloxone challenge to exclude the possibility of precipitating a withdrawal reaction (see Administration and Dosage).

➤*Severe opioid withdrawal syndromes:* Severe opioid withdrawal syndromes precipitated by accidental naltrexone ingestion have occurred in opioid-dependent individuals. Withdrawal symptoms usually appear within 5 minutes of ingestion and may last up to 48 hours. Mental status changes, including confusion, somnolence and visual hallucinations have occurred. Significant fluid losses from vomiting and diarrhea have required IV fluids.

➤*Surmountable blockade:* While naltrexone is a potent antagonist with a prolonged pharmacologic effect (24 to 72 hours), the blockade produced by naltrexone is surmountable. This poses a potential risk to individuals who attempt to overcome the blockade by self-administering large amounts of opioids. Any attempt by a patient to overcome the antagonism by taking opioids is very dangerous and may lead to fatal overdose. Also, lesser amounts of exogenous opioids are dangerous if they are taken in a manner (ie, relatively long after the last dose of naltrexone) and in an amount that persists in the body longer than effective concentrations of naltrexone and its metabolites.

When reversal of blockade is required – In an emergency situation in patients receiving full blocking doses of naltrexone, a suggested plan of management is regional analgesia, conscious sedation with a benzodiazepine, use of non-opioid analgesics or general anesthesia.

In a situation requiring opioid analgesia, the amount of opioid required may be greater than usual and resulting respiratory depression may be deeper and more prolonged. A rapid-acting analgesic which minimizes respiratory depression is preferred. Individualize dosage; monitor closely.

Additionally, nonreceptor-mediated actions may occur (eg, facial swelling, itching, generalized erythema presumably due to histamine release).

➤*Use with narcotics:* Patients taking naltrexone may not benefit from opioid-containing medicines, such as cough and cold preparations, antidiarrheal preparations and opioid analgesics. Use a nonopioid-containing alternative, if available.

In a 2 year carcinogenicity study in rats, there were small increases in the numbers of mesotheliomas in males and tumors of vascular origin in both sexes. The number of tumors were within the range seen in historical control groups, except for the vascular tumors in females, where the 4% incidence exceeded the historical maximum of 2%.

Naltrexone (100 mg/kg, ≈ 140 times the human therapeutic dose) caused a significant increase in pseudo-pregnancy in the rat. A decrease in the pregnancy rate of mated female rats also occurred.

➤*Pregnancy: Category C.* Naltrexone is embryocidal in rats and rabbits when given in doses ≈ 140 times the human therapeutic dose. There are no adequate and well controlled studies in pregnant women. Use naltrexone in pregnancy only when the potential benefit justifies the risk to the fetus.

➤*Lactation:* It is not known if naltrexone is excreted in breast milk. Exercise caution when naltrexone is administered to a nursing mother.

➤*Children:* Safety for use in children < 18 years of age has not been established.

Precautions

➤*Monitoring:* A high index of suspicion for drug-related hepatic injury is critical if the occurrence of liver damage induced by naltrexone is to be detected at the earliest possible time. Evaluations, using appropriate batteries of tests to detect liver injury, are recommended at a frequency appropriate to the clinical situation and the dose of naltrexone.

➤*Suicide:* The risk of suicide is increased in patients with substance abuse with or without concomitant depression. This risk is not abated by treatment with naltrexone.

Drug Interactions

Naltrexone Drug Interactions			
Precipitant drug	Object drug*		Description
Naltrexone	Opioid-containing products	↓	Patients taking naltrexone may not benefit from opioid-containing products such as cough/cold and antidiarrheal preparations and opioid analgesics (see Warnings).
Naltrexone	Thioridazine	↑	Lethargy and somnolence have occurred with concurrent use.

* ↑ = Object drug increased. ↓ = Object drug decreased.

Adverse Reactions

Alcoholism – Nausea (10%); headache (7%); dizziness, nervousness, fatigue (4%); insomnia, vomiting (3%); anxiety, somnolence (2%). Depression (5% to 7%), suicidal ideation (2%) and attempted suicide (< 1%) have been reported in individuals on naltrexone, placebo and in concurrent control groups undergoing treatment for alcoholism. Although no causal relationship with naltrexone is suspected, be aware that treatment with naltrexone does not reduce the risk of suicide in these patients (see Precautions).

A small fraction of patients may experience an opioid withdrawal-like symptom complex of tearfulness, mild nausea, abdominal cramps, restlessness, bone/joint pain, myalgia and nasal symptoms. This may represent the unmasking of occult opioid use, or it may represent symptoms attributable to naltrexone.

➤*Narcotic addiction:*

Cardiovascular – Phlebitis, edema, increased blood pressure, nonspecific ECG changes, palpitations, tachycardia (< 1%).

CNS – Difficulty sleeping, anxiety, nervousness, headache, low energy (> 10%); irritability, increased energy, dizziness (< 10%); depression, paranoia, fatigue, drowsiness, disorientation, restlessness, confusion, hallucinations, nightmares, bad dreams (< 1%).

Dermatologic – Skin rash (< 10%); itching, oily skin, pruritus, acne, athlete's foot, cold sores, alopecia (< 1%).

GI – Abdominal cramps/pain, nausea, vomiting (> 10%); loss of appetite, diarrhea, constipation (< 10%); excess gas, hemorrhoids, ulcer, dry mouth (< 1%); hepatotoxicity (see Warnings).

GU – Delayed ejaculation, decreased potency (< 10%); increased frequency/ discomfort during urination, increased or decreased sexual interest (< 1%).

Musculoskeletal – Joint/muscle pain (> 10%); painful shoulders/legs/knees, tremors, twitching (< 1%).

NALTREXONE HCl

Respiratory – Nasal congestion, rhinorrhea, sneezing, sore throat, excess mucus or phlegm, sinus trouble, heavy breathing, hoarseness, cough, shortness of breath (< 1%).

Special senses – Blurred vision, burning/light-sensitive/swollen/aching/strained eyes, "clogged" or aching ears, tinnitus (< 1%).

Miscellaneous – Chills, increased thirst (< 10%); increased appetite, weight loss/gain, yawning, nose bleeds, fever, inguinal pain, swollen glands, "side" pains, head "pounding", cold feet, hot spells (< 1%). Idiopathic thrombocytopenic purpura was reported in one patient but cleared without sequelae after discontinuation of naltrexone and corticosteroid treatment.

Lab test abnormalities – Liver test abnormalities, lymphocytosis.

Overdosage

➤*Symptoms:* In one study, subjects who received 800 mg/day for up to 1 week showed no evidence of toxicity. In acute toxicity studies in animals, death was due to clonic-tonic convulsions or respiratory failure.

➤*Treatment:* Treat symptomatically (see also General Management of Acute Overdosage).

Patient Information

Patients should wear identification indicating naltrexone use.

If patients attempt self-administration of heroin or any other opiate in small doses, they will perceive no effect. However, self-administration of large doses of heroin or other narcotics can overcome the blockade and may cause coma, serious injury or death.

Naltrexone is well tolerated in the recommended doses, but may cause liver injury when taken in excess or in people who develop liver disease from other causes. If patients develop abdominal pain lasting more than a few days, white bowel movements, dark urine or yellowing of eyes, they should stop taking naltrexone immediately and see their physician as soon as possible.

FLUMAZENIL

| *Rx* | **Romazicon** (Hoffman-La Roche) | **Injection:** 0.1 mg/ml | With parabens and EDTA. In 5 and 10 ml vials. |

Indications

➤*Reversal of benzodiazepine sedation:* For the complete or partial reversal of the sedative effects of benzodiazepines in cases where general anesthesia has been induced or maintained with benzodiazepines, where sedation has been produced with benzodiazepines for diagnostic and therapeutic procedures, and for the management of benzodiazepine overdose.

Administration and Dosage

➤*Approved by the FDA:* December 1991.

For IV use only. To minimize the likelihood of pain at the injection site, administer flumazenil through a freely running IV infusion into a large vein (see Precautions).

➤*Individualization of dosage:* The serious adverse effects of flumazenil are related to the reversal of benzodiazepine effects. Using more than the minimally effective dose of flumazenil is tolerated by most patients but may complicate the management of patients who are physically dependent on benzodiazepines or patients who are depending on benzodiazepines for therapeutic effect (such as suppression of seizures in cyclic antidepressant overdose).

In high-risk patients, it is important to administer the smallest amount of flumazenil that is effective. The 1 minute wait between individual doses in the dose-titration recommended for general clinical populations may be too short for high-risk patients because it takes 6 to 10 minutes for any single dose of flumazenil to reach full effects. Slow the rate of administration of flumazenil administered to high-risk patients.

➤*Reversal of conscious sedation or in general anesthesia:* For the reversal of the sedative effects of benzodiazepines administered for conscious sedation or general anesthesia, the recommended initial dose is 0.2 mg (2 ml) administered IV over 15 seconds. If the desired level of consciousness is not obtained after waiting an additional 45 seconds, a further dose of 0.2 mg (2 ml) can be injected and repeated at 60 second intervals where necessary (up to a maximum of 4 additional times) to a maximum total dose of 1 mg (10 ml). Individualize the dose based on the patient's response, with most patients responding to doses of 0.6 to 1 mg.

The major risk will be resedation because the duration of effect of a long-acting (or large dose of a short-acting) benzodiazepine may exceed that of flumazenil. In the event of resedation, repeated doses may be administered at 20 minute intervals as needed. For repeat treatment, administer ≤ 1 mg (given as 0.2 mg/min) at any one time, and give ≤ 3 mg in any 1 hour.

It is recommended that flumazenil be administered as the series of small injections described (not as a single bolus injection) to allow the practitioner to control the reversal of sedation to the approximate endpoint desired and to minimize the possibility of adverse effects.

➤*Suspected benzodiazepine overdose:* For initial management of a known or suspected benzodiazepine overdose, the recommended initial dose is 0.2 mg (2 ml) administered IV over 30 seconds. If the desired level of consciousness is not obtained after waiting 30 seconds, a further dose of 0.3 mg (3 ml) can be administered over another 30 seconds. Further doses of 0.5 mg (5 ml) can be administered over 30 seconds at 1 minute intervals up to a cumulative dose of 3 mg.

The risk of confusion, agitation, emotional lability and perceptual distortion with the doses recommended in patients with benzodiazepine overdose (3 to 5 mg administered as 0.5 mg/min) may be greater than that expected with lower doses and slower administration. The recommended doses represent a compromise between a desirable slow awakening and the need for prompt response and a persistent effect in the overdose situation. If circumstances permit, the physician may elect to use the 0.2 mg/min titration rate to slowly awaken the patient over 5 to 10 minutes, which may help to reduce signs and symptoms on emergence.

Do not rush the administration of flumazenil. Patients should have a secure airway and IV access before administration of the drug and be awakened gradually (see Precautions).

Most patients with benzodiazepine overdose will respond to a cumulative dose of 1 to 3 mg, and doses > 3 mg do not reliably produce additional effects. On rare occasions, patients with a partial response at 3 mg may require additional titration up to a total dose of 5 mg (administered slowly in the same manner).

If a patient has not responded 5 minutes after receiving a cumulative dose of 5 mg, the major cause of sedation is likely not to be due to benzodiazepines, and additional flumazenil is likely to have no effect.

In the event of resedation, repeated doses may be given at 20 minute intervals if needed. For repeat treatment, give ≤ 1 mg (given as 0.5 mg/min) at any one time and give ≤ 3 mg in any 1 hour.

➤*Admixture compatibility:* Flumazenil is compatible with 5% Dextrose in Water, Lactated Ringer's and normal saline solutions. If flumazenil is drawn into a syringe or mixed with any of these solutions, it should be discarded after 24 hours. For optimum sterility, flumazenil should remain in the vial until just before use.

Flumazenil 20 mcg/ml, in 5% Dextrose Injection, was physically compatible and chemically stable for 24 hours at 23°C (73°F) with aminophylline 2 mg/ml, dobutamine 2 mg/ml, cimetidine 2.4 mg/ml, famotidine 0.08 mg/ml, ranitidine 0.3 mg/ml, heparin sodium 50 units/ml, lidocaine HCl 4 mg/ml or procainamide HCl 4 mg/ml. Flumazenil 20 mcg/ml, in 5% Dextrose Injection, was physically compatible and chemically stable for 12 hours at 23°C (73°F) with dopamine HCl 3.2 mg/ml.

Actions

➤*Pharmacology:* Flumazenil is a benzodiazepine receptor antagonist available for IV administration. Flumazenil, an imidazobenzodiazepine derivative, antagonizes the actions of benzodiazepines on the CNS and competitively inhibits the activity at the benzodiazepine recognition site on the GABA/benzodiazepine receptor complex. It is a weak partial agonist in some animal models, but has little or no agonist activity in man. The drug does not antagonize the CNS effects of drugs affecting the GABA-ergic neurons by means other than the benzodiazepine receptor (including ethanol, barbiturates or general anesthetics) and does not reverse the effects of opioids.

Flumazenil antagonizes sedation, impairment of recall, psychomotor impairment and ventilatory depression produced by benzodiazepines in healthy volunteers. The duration and degree of reversal of benzodiazepine effects are related to the dose and plasma concentrations of flumazenil. Generally, doses of ≈ 0.1 to 0.2 mg (corresponding to peak plasma levels of 3 to 6 ng/ml) produce partial antagonism, whereas higher doses of 0.4 to 1 mg (peak plasma levels of 12 to 28 ng/ml) usually produce complete antagonism in patients who have received the usual sedating doses of benzodiazepines. The onset of reversal is usually evident within 1 to 2 minutes after the injection is completed. Within 3 minutes, 80% response will be reached, with the peak effect occurring at 6 to 10 minutes. The duration and degree of reversal are related to the plasma concentration of the sedating benzodiazepine as well as the dose of flumazenil given.

➤*Pharmacokinetics:* After IV administration, plasma concentrations of flumazenil follow a 2 compartment open pharmacokinetic model with an initial distribution half-life of 7 to 15 minutes and a terminal half-life of 41 to 79 minutes. Peak concentrations are proportional to dose, with an apparent initial volume of distribution (Vd) of 0.5 L/kg. After redistribution the apparent Vd ranges from 0.77 to 1.6 L/kg. Protein binding is ≈ 50%.

FLUMAZENIL

Flumazenil is a highly extracted drug. Clearance of flumazenil occurs primarily by hepatic metabolism and is dependent on hepatic blood flow. In healthy volunteers, total clearance ranges from 0.7 to 1.3 L/hr/kg, with < 1% of the administered dose eliminated unchanged in the urine. The major metabolites of flumazenil identified in urine are in the de-ethylated free acid and its glucuronide conjugate. In preclinical studies there was no evidence of pharmacologic activity exhibited by the de-ethylated free acid. Elimination of drug is essentially complete within 72 hours, with 90% to 95% appearing in urine and 5% to 10% in the feces.

Pharmacokinetic Parameters of Flumazenil Following a 5 min 1 mg Infusion	
Parameter	Mean (Range)
Maximum concentration	24 ng/ml (38%, 11-43)
AUC	15 ng • hr/ml (22%, 10-22)
Volume of distribution	1 L/kg (24%, 0.8-1.6)
Clearance	1 L/hr/kg (20%, 0.7-1.4)
Half-life	54 min (21%, 41-79)

The pharmacokinetics of flumazenil are not significantly affected by gender, age, renal failure (creatinine clearance < 10 ml/min) or hemodialysis beginning 1 hour after drug administration. Mean total clearance is decreased to 40% to 60% of normal in patients with moderate liver dysfunction and to 25% of normal in patients with severe liver dysfunction compared with age-matched healthy subjects. This results in a prolongation of the half-life from 0.8 hours in healthy subjects to 1.3 hours in patients with moderate hepatic impairment and 2.4 hours in severely impaired patients.

➤*Clinical trials:* Flumazenil has been administered to reverse the effects of benzodiazepines in conscious sedation, general anesthesia and the management of suspected benzodiazepine overdose.

Conscious sedation – In 4 trials in 970 patients who received an average of 30 mg diazepam or 10 mg midazolam for sedation (with or without a narcotic) flumazenil was effective in reversing the sedating and psychomotor effects of the benzodiazepine; however, amnesia was less completely and less consistently reversed. Of patients receiving flumazenil, 78% responded by becoming completely alert. Of those patients, ≈ 50% responded to doses of 0.4 to 0.6 mg, while the other half responded to doses of 0.8 to 1 mg. Reversal of sedation was not associated with any increase in the frequency of inadequate analgesia or increase in narcotic demand in these studies. While most patients remained alert throughout the 3 hour post-procedure observation period, resedation occurred in 3% to 9% of the patients, and was most common in patients who had received high doses of benzodiazepines (see Precautions).

General anesthesia – In 4 trials, 644 patients received midazolam as an induction or maintenance agent in both balanced and inhalational anesthesia. Flumazenil was effective in reversing sedation and restoring psychomotor function, but did not completely restore memory as tested by picture recall. Flumazenil was not as effective in reversal of sedation in patients who had received multiple anesthetics in addition to benzodiazepines. Of patients sedated with midazolam, 81% responded to flumazenil by becoming completely alert or just slightly drowsy. Of these patients, 36% responded to doses of 0.4 to 0.6 mg, while 64% responded to doses of 0.8 to 1 mg.

Resedation in patients who responded to flumazenil occurred in 10% to 15% and was more common with larger doses of midazolam (> 20 mg), long procedures (> 60 minutes) and use of neuromuscular blocking agents (see Precautions).

Management of suspected benzodiazepine overdose – In 2 trials, 497 patients were presumed to have taken an overdose of a benzodiazepine, either alone or in combination with a variety of other agents. In these trials, 299 patients were proven to have taken a benzodiazepine as part of the overdose, and 80% of the 148 who received flumazenil responded by an improvement in level of consciousness. Of the patients who responded to flumazenil, 75% responded to a total dose of 1 to 3 mg. Reversal of sedation was associated with an increased frequency of symptoms of CNS excitation. Of the patients treated with flumazenil, 1% to 3% were treated for agitation or anxiety.

Contraindications

Hypersensitivity to flumazenil or to benzodiazepines; benzodiazepine use for control of a potentially life-threatening condition (eg, control of intracranial pressure or status epilepticus); signs of serious cyclic antidepressant overdose (see Warnings).

Warnings

➤*Seizures:* The use of flumazenil has been associated with the occurrence of seizures. These are most frequent in patients who have been on benzodiazepines for long-term sedation or in overdose cases where patients are showing signs of serious cyclic antidepressant overdose. Individualize the dosage of flumazenil and be prepared to manage seizures.

➤*Seizure risk:* The reversal of benzodiazepine effects may be associated with the onset of seizures in certain high-risk populations. Possible risk factors for seizures include: Concurrent major sedative-hypnotic drug withdrawal; recent therapy with repeated doses of parenteral benzodiazepines; myoclonic jerking or seizure activity prior to flumazenil administration in overdose cases; concurrent cyclic antidepressant poisoning.

Flumazenil is not recommended in cases of serious cyclic antidepressant poisoning, as manifested by motor abnormalities (twitching, rigidity, focal seizure), dysrhythmia (wide QRS, ventricular dysrhythmia, heart block), anticholinergic signs (mydriasis, dry mucosa, hypoperistalsis) and cardiovascular collapse at presentation. In such cases, withhold flumazenil and allow the patient to remain sedated (with ventilatory and circulatory support as needed) until the signs of antidepressant toxicity have subsided. Treatment with flumazenil has no known benefit to the seriously ill mixed-overdose patient other than reversing sedation and should not be used in cases where seizures (from any cause) are likely.

Most convulsions associated with flumazenil administration require treatment and have been successfully managed with benzodiazepines, phenytoin or barbiturates. Because of the presence of flumazenil, higher than usual doses of benzodiazepines may be required.

➤*Hypoventilation:* Monitor patients who have received flumazenil for the reversal of benzodiazepine effects (after conscious sedation or general anesthesia) for resedation, respiratory depression or other residual benzodiazepine effects for an appropriate period (up to 120 minutes) based on the dose and duration of effect of the benzodiazepine employed, because flumazenil has not been established as an effective treatment for hypoventilation due to benzodiazepine administration. The availability of flumazenil does not diminish the need for prompt detection of hypoventilation and the ability to effectively intervene by establishing an airway and assisting ventilation.

Flumazenil may not fully reverse postoperative airway problems or ventilatory insufficiency induced by benzodiazepines. In addition, even if flumazenil is initially effective, such problems may recur because the effects of flumazenil wear off before the effects of many benzodiazepines. Always monitor overdose cases for resedation until the patients are stable and resedation is unlikely.

➤*Hepatic function impairment:* The clearance of flumazenil is reduced to 40% to 60% of normal in patients with mild to moderate hepatic disease and to 25% of normal in patients with severe hepatic dysfunction (see Pharmacokinetics). While the dose of flumazenil used for initial reversal of benzodiazepine effects is not affected, reduce the size and frequency of repeat doses of the drug in liver disease.

➤*Elderly:* The pharmacokinetics of flumazenil have been studied in the elderly and are not significantly different from younger patients. Several studies in patients > 65 years of age and one study in patients > 80 years of age suggest that while the doses of benzodiazepines used to induce sedation should be reduced, ordinary doses of flumazenil may be used for reversal.

➤*Pregnancy: Category C.* In rabbits, embryocidal effects (as evidenced by increased pre- and post-implantation losses) were observed at 50 mg/kg (200 times the human exposure from a maximum recommended IV dose of 5 mg). In rats at oral dosages of 5, 25 and 125 mg/kg/day, pup survival was decreased during the lactating period, pup liver weight at weaning was increased for the high-dose group (125 mg/kg/day) and incisor eruption and ear opening in the offspring were delayed; the delay in ear opening was associated with a delay in the appearance of the auditory startle response. There are no adequate and well controlled studies in pregnant women. Use during pregnancy only if potential benefits justify potential risks to the fetus.

Labor and delivery – The use of flumazenil to reverse the effects of benzodiazepines used during labor and delivery is not recommended because the effects of the drug in the newborn are unknown.

➤*Lactation:* Exercise caution when deciding to administer flumazenil to a nursing woman because it is not known whether flumazenil is excreted in breast milk.

➤*Children:* Flumazenil is not recommended for use in children (either for reversal of sedation, management of overdose or resuscitation of the newborn); no clinical studies have been performed to determine the risks, benefits and dosage to be used.

Precautions

➤*Monitoring:* Flumazenil may be expected to improve the alertness of patients recovering from a procedure involving sedation or anesthesia with benzodiazepines, but should not be substituted for an adequate period of post-procedure monitoring. The availability of flumazenil does not reduce the risks associated with the use of large doses of benzodiazepine for sedation. Monitor patients for resedation, respiratory depression (see Warnings) or other persistent or recurrent agonist effects for an adequate period of time after administration of flumazenil.

➤*Return of sedation:* Resedation is least likely in cases where flumazenil is administered to reverse a low dose of a short-acting benzodiazepine (< 10 mg midazolam). It is most likely in cases where a large single or cumulative dose of a benzodiazepine has been given in the course of a long procedure along with neuromuscular blocking agents and multiple anesthetic agents.

FLUMAZENIL

Profound resedation was observed in 1% to 3% of patients in the clinical studies. In clinical situations where resedation must be prevented, physicians may wish to repeat the initial dose (up to 1 mg given at 0.2 mg/min) at 30 minutes and possibly again at 60 minutes. This dosage schedule, although not studied in clinical trials, was effective in preventing resedation in healthy volunteers.

➤*Intensive Care Unit (ICU):* Use with caution in the ICU because of the increased risk of unrecognized benzodiazepine dependence in such settings. Flumazenil may produce convulsions in patients physically dependent on benzodiazepines (see Administration and Dosage and Warnings).

The use of flumazenil to diagnose benzodiazepine-induced sedation in the ICU is not recommended due to the risk of adverse events as described above. In addition, the prognostic significance of a patient's failure to respond to flumazenil in cases confounded by metabolic disorder, traumatic injury, drugs other than benzodiazepines or any other reasons not associated with benzodiazepine receptor occupancy is not known.

➤*Overdose situations:* Flumazenil is intended as an adjunct to, not a substitute for, proper management of airway, assisted breathing, circulatory access and support, internal decontamination by lavage and charcoal, and adequate clinical evaluation. Institute necessary measures to secure airway, ventilation and IV access prior to administering flumazenil. Upon arousal patients may try to withdraw endotracheal tubes or IV lines as the result of confusion and agitation following awakening.

➤*Head injury:* Use with caution in patients with head injury as flumazenil may be capable of precipitating convulsions or altering cerebral blood flow in patients receiving benzodiazepines.

➤*Neuromuscular blocking agents:* Do not use flumazenil until the effects of neuromuscular blockade have been fully reversed.

➤*Psychiatric patients:* Flumazenil may provoke panic attacks in patients with a history of panic disorder.

➤*Drug- and alcohol-dependent patients:* Use with caution in patients with alcoholism and other drug dependencies due to the increased frequency of benzodiazepine tolerance and dependence observed in these patient populations. Flumazenil is not recommended either as a treatment for benzodiazepine dependence or for the management of protracted benzodiazepine abstinence syndromes, as such use has not been studied.

The administration of flumazenil can precipitate benzodiazepine withdrawal in humans. This has been seen in healthy volunteers treated with therapeutic doses of oral lorazepam for up to 2 weeks who exhibited effects such as hot flushes, agitation and tremor when treated with cumulative doses of up to 3 mg flumazenil.

Similar adverse experiences suggestive of flumazenil precipitation of benzodiazepine withdrawal have occurred in some patients in clinical trials. Such patients had a short-lived syndrome characterized by dizziness, mild confusion, emotional lability, agitation (with signs and symptoms of anxiety) and mild sensory distortions. This response was dose-related, most common at doses > 1 mg, rarely required treatment other than reassurance and was usually short-lived. When required (5 to 10 cases), these patients were successfully treated with usual doses of a barbiturate, a benzodiazepine or other sedative drug.

Assume that flumazenil administration may trigger dose-dependent withdrawal syndromes in patients with established physical dependence on benzodiazepines and may complicate the management of withdrawal syndromes for alcohol, barbiturates and cross-tolerant sedatives.

➤*Tolerance to benzodiazepines:* Flumazenil may cause benzodiazepine withdrawal symptoms in individuals who have been taking benzodiazepines long enough to have some degree of tolerance. Patients who had been taking benzodiazepines prior to entry into the flumazenil trials who were given flumazenil in doses > 1 mg experienced withdrawal-like events 2 to 5 times more frequently than patients who received < 1 mg.

In patients who may have tolerance to benzodiazepines, as indicated by clinical history or by the need for larger than usual doses of benzodiazepines, slower titration rates of 0.1 mg/min and lower total doses may help reduce the frequency of emergent confusion and agitation. In such cases, take special care to monitor the patients for resedation because of the lower doses of flumazenil used.

➤*Pain on injection:* To minimize the likelihood of pain or inflammation at the injection site, administer flumazenil through a freely flowing IV infusion into a large vein. Local irritation may occur following extravasation into perivascular tissues.

➤*Respiratory disease:* Appropriate ventilatory support is the primary treatment of patients with serious lung disease who experience serious respiratory depression due to benzodiazepines rather than the administration of flumazenil. Flumazenil is capable of partially reversing benzodiazepine-induced alterations in ventilatory drive in healthy volunteers, but is not clinically effective.

➤*Ambulatory patients:* Effects may wear off before a long-acting benzodiazepine is completely cleared from the body. In general, if a patient shows no signs of sedation within 2 hours after a 1 mg dose, serious resedation at a later time is unlikely. Provide an adequate observation period for any patient in whom either long-acting benzodiazepines (eg, diazepam) or large doses of short-acting benzodiazepines (eg, > 10 mg midazolam) have been used (see Administration and Dosage).

Because of the increased risk of adverse reactions in patients who have been taking benzodiazepines on a regular basis, it is particularly important to carefully query about benzodiazepine, alcohol and sedative use as part of the history prior to any procedure in which the use of flumazenil is planned (see Drug and Alcohol Dependent Patients).

➤*Drug abuse and dependence:* Flumazenil acts as a benzodiazepine antagonist, blocks benzodiazepine effects in animals and man, antagonizes benzodiazepine reinforcement in animals, produces dysphoria in healthy subjects and has had no reported abuse in foreign marketing. It has a benzodiazepine-like structure, but does not act as a benzodiazepine agonist in man and is not a controlled substance.

Drug Interactions

➤*Mixed drug overdosage:* Particular caution is necessary when using flumazenil in cases of mixed drug overdosage; toxic effects (eg, convulsions, cardiac dysrhythmias) of other drugs taken in overdose (especially cyclic antidepressants) may emerge with reversal of the benzodiazepine effect by flumazenil (see Warnings).

➤*Benzodiazepine:* Benzodiazepine pharmacokinetics are unaltered in the presence of flumazenil.

➤*Drug/Food interactions:* Ingestion of food during an IV infusion of flumazenil results in a 50% increase in flumazenil clearance, most likely due to the increased hepatic blood flow that accompanies a meal.

Adverse Reactions

Serious adverse reactions – Deaths have occurred in patients who received flumazenil in a variety of clinical settings. The majority of deaths occurred in patients with serious underlying disease or in patients who had ingested large amounts of non-benzodiazepine drugs (usually cyclic antidepressants) as part of an overdose.

Serious adverse events have occurred in all clinical settings, and convulsions are the most common serious adverse event reported. Flumazenil administration has been associated with the onset of convulsions in patients who are relying on benzodiazepine effects to control seizures, are physically dependent on benzodiazepines or who have ingested large doses of other drugs (see Warnings).

Two of the 446 patients who received flumazenil in controlled clinical trials for the management of a benzodiazepine overdose had cardiac dysrhythmias (1 ventricular tachycardia, 1 junctional tachycardia).

➤*Cardiovascular:* Cutaneous vasodilation (sweating, flushing, hot flushes) (1% to 3%); arrhythmia (atrial, nodal, ventricular extrasystoles), bradycardia, tachycardia, hypertension, chest pain (< 1%).

➤*CNS:* Dizziness (vertigo, ataxia) (10%); agitation (anxiety, nervousness), dry mouth, tremors, palpitations, insomnia, dyspnea, hyperventilation (3% to 9%); emotional lability (abnormal crying, depersonalization, euphoria, increased tears, depression, dysphoria, paranoia) (1% to 3%); confusion (difficulty concentrating, delirium), convulsions (see Warnings), somnolence (stupor), speech disorder (dysphonia, thick tongue) (< 1%).

➤*GI:* Nausea, vomiting (11%); hiccups (< 1%).

➤*Special senses:* Abnormal vision (visual field defect, diplopia), blurred vision (3% to 9%); paresthesia (sensation abnormal, hypoesthesia) (1% to 3%); abnormal hearing (transient hearing impairment, hyperacusis, tinnitus) (< 1%).

➤*Miscellaneous:* Headache, injection site pain, increased sweating (3% to 9%); injection site reaction (thrombophlebitis, skin abnormality, rash), fatigue (asthenia, malaise) (1% to 3%); rigors, shivering (< 1%).

Overdosage

Large IV doses of flumazenil, when administered to healthy volunteers in the absence of a benzodiazepine agonist, produced no serious adverse reactions. In clinical studies, most adverse reactions to flumazenil were an extension of the pharmacologic effects of the drug in reversing benzodiazepine effects.

Reversal with an excessively high dose of flumazenil may produce anxiety, agitation, increased muscle tone, hyperesthesia and possibly convulsions. Convulsions have been treated with barbiturates, benzodiazepines and phenytoin, generally with prompt resolution of the seizures (see Warnings).

Patient Information

Flumazenil does not consistently reverse amnesia. Patients cannot be expected to remember information told to them in the post-procedure period; reinforce instructions given to patients in writing or give to a responsible family member. Discuss with patients, both before surgery and at discharge, that although they may feel alert at the time of discharge, the effects of the benzodiazepine may recur. Instruct the

FLUMAZENIL

patient, preferably in writing, that their memory and judgment may be impaired and specifically advise patients:

1.) Not to engage in any activities requiring complete alertness, and not to operate hazardous machinery or a motor vehicle until at least 18 to 24 hours after discharge, and it is certain no residual sedative effects of the benzodiazepine remain.

2.) Not to take any alcohol or non-prescription drugs for 18 to 24 hours after flumazenil administration or if the effects of the benzodiazepine persist.

PHYSOSTIGMINE SALICYLATE

| Rx | Antilirium (Forest) | Injection: 1 mg/ml | With 2% benzyl alcohol and 0.1% sodium bisulfite. In 2 ml ampules. |

Indications

➤*Anticholinergic toxicity:* To reverse toxic CNS effects caused by anticholinergic drugs (including tricyclic antidepressants).

➤*Unlabeled uses:* Physostigmine has been used to treat delirium tremens and Alzheimer's disease. It may also antagonize diazepam's CNS-depressant effects.

Administration and Dosage

➤*Postanesthesia:* 0.5 to 1 mg IM or IV. Administer IV slowly, ≤ 1 mg/min. Repeat at 10 to 30 minute intervals if desired response is not obtained.

➤*Anticholinergic toxicity:* 2 mg IM or IV. Administer IV slowly, ≤ 1 mg/min. Repeat if life-threatening signs such as arrhythmia, convulsions or coma occur.

➤*Pediatric:* Recommended dosage is 0.02 mg/kg IM or by slow IV injection, ≤ 0.5 mg/min. If necessary, repeat at 5 to 10 minute intervals until a therapeutic effect or a maximum dose of 2 mg is attained.

Actions

➤*Pharmacology:* The action of acetylcholine is transient because of hydrolysis by acetylcholinesterase. Physostigmine, a reversible anticholinesterase drug, increases the concentration of acetylcholine at the sites of cholinergic transmission and prolongs and exaggerates the effect of acetylcholine.

Physostigmine reverses these central and peripheral anticholinergic effects –

Central toxic effects: Anxiety, delirium, disorientation, hallucinations, hyperactivity and seizures. Severe poisoning due to anticholinergics may produce coma, medullary paralysis and death.

Peripheral toxic effects: Tachycardia, hyperpyrexia, mydriasis, vasodilation, urinary retention, decreased GI motility, decreased secretion in salivary and sweat glands, loss of secretions in the pharynx, bronchi and nasal passages.

➤*Pharmacokinetics:* Physostigmine, a tertiary amine, is readily absorbed and freely crosses the blood-brain barrier following IM or IV administration. Peak effects are seen within minutes and persist for 45 to 60 minutes following IV administration if the patient has not suffered anoxia or other trauma. Physostigmine is rapidly hydrolyzed by cholinesterase. Plasma half-life is ≈ 1 to 2 hours. Renal impairment does NOT require dosage alteration.

Contraindications

Asthma; gangrene; diabetes; cardiovascular disease; GI or GU tract obstruction; any vagotonic state; patients receiving choline esters or depolarizing neuromuscular blocking agents (decamethonium, succinylcholine).

Warnings

➤*Discontinue drug:* Discontinue the drug if symptoms of excessive salivation or emesis, frequent urination or diarrhea occur. If excessive sweating or nausea occurs, reduce dosage.

➤*Administration rate:* Rapid administration can cause bradycardia, hypersalivation leading to respiratory difficulties and seizures (see Administration and Dosage).

➤*Hypersensitivity reactions:* Because of the possibility of hypersensitivity, atropine sulfate should be available as an antagonist and antidote for physostigmine.

➤*Pregnancy: Category C.* Transient muscular weakness has been noted in neonates whose mothers were treated with other cholinesterase inhibitors for myasthenia gravis. Use only if clearly needed and potential benefits outweigh hazards to the fetus.

➤*Lactation:* Safety for use has not been established.

➤*Children:* Reserve for life-threatening situations only.

Precautions

➤*Benzyl alcohol:* Benzyl alcohol, contained in this product as a preservative, has been associated with a fatal "gasping syndrome" in premature infants.

➤*Sulfite sensitivity:* This product contains sulfites which may cause allergic-type reactions (including anaphylactic symptoms and life-threatening or less severe asthmatic episodes) in certain susceptible people. The overall prevalence of sulfite sensitivity in the general population is unknown and probably low. It is seen more frequently in asthmatic or atopic nonasthmatic people.

Adverse Reactions

Nausea, vomiting, salivation; bradycardia and convulsions (see Warnings).

Overdosage

Can cause cholinergic crisis. Atropine sulfate is an appropriate antidote.

FOMEPIZOLE (4-Methylpyrazole; 4-MP)

| Rx | Antizol (Orphan Medical) | Injection, concentrate: 1 g/mL | Preservative-free. In 1.5 mL vials. |

Indications

➤*Ethylene glycol or methanol poisoning:* As an antidote for ethylene glycol (antifreeze) and methanol poisoning or for use in suspected ethylene glycol or methanol ingestion, either alone or in combination with hemodialysis.

Administration and Dosage

➤*Treatment guidelines:* If ethylene glycol or methanol poisoning is left untreated, the natural progression of the poisoning leads to accumulation of toxic metabolites, including glycolic and oxalic acids (ethylene glycol intoxication) and formic acid (methanol intoxication). These metabolites can induce metabolic acidosis, nausea/vomiting, seizures, stupor, coma, calcium oxaluria, acute tubular necrosis, blindness, and death. The diagnosis of these poisonings may be difficult because ethylene glycol or methanol concentrations diminish in the blood as they are metabolized to their respective metabolites. Hence, frequently monitor both ethylene glycol and methanol concentrations and acid-base balance, as determined by serum electrolyte (anion gap) or arterial blood gas analysis, and use to guide treatment.

Treatment consists of blocking the formation of toxic metabolites using inhibitors of alcohol dehydrogenase, such as fomepizole, and correction of metabolic abnormalities. In patients with high ethylene glycol or methanol concentrations (≥ 50 mg/dL), significant metabolic acidosis or renal failure, consider hemodialysis to remove ethylene glycol or methanol and the respective toxic metabolites of these alcohols.

Treatment with fomepizole may be discontinued when ethylene glycol or methanol concentrations are undetectable or have been reduced to < 20 mg/dL, and the patient is asymptomatic with normal pH.

➤*Treatment:* Begin fomepizole treatment immediately upon suspicion of ethylene glycol or methanol ingestion based on patient history or anion gap metabolic acidosis, increased osmolar gap, visual disturbances, oxalate crystals in the urine or a documented serum ethylene glycol or methanol concentration of > 20 mg/dL.

Administer a loading dose of 15 mg/kg, followed by doses of 10 mg/kg every 12 hours for 4 doses, then 15 mg/kg every 12 hours thereafter until ethylene glycol or methanol concentrations are undetectable or have been reduced to < 20 mg/dL, and the patient is asymptomatic with normal pH. Administer all doses as a slow IV infusion over 30 minutes.

➤*Hemodialysis:* Consider hemodialysis in addition to fomepizole in the case of renal failure, significant or worsening metabolic acidosis, or a measured ethylene glycol or methanol concentration of ≥ 50 mg/dL. Dialyze patients to correct metabolic abnormalities and to lower the ethylene glycol concentrations to < 50 mg/dL.

Fomepizole is dialyzable; increase the frequency of dosing to every 4 hours during hemodialysis.

Fomepizole Dosing in Patients Requiring Hemodialysis	
Parameters	Dosing Schedule
At beginning of hemodialysis	
< 6 hours since last dose	Do not administer dose.
≥ 6 hours since last dose	Administer next scheduled dose.
During hemodialysis	Every 4 hours.
At end of hemodialysis	
< 1 hour since last dose	Do not administer dose.
1 to 3 hours since last dose	Administer ½ of next scheduled dose.
> 3 hours since last dose	Administer next scheduled dose.
Maintenance dosing off hemodialysis	Administer next scheduled dose 12 hours from last dose.

FOMEPIZOLE (4-Methylpyrazole; 4-MP)

➤*Preparation:* Using sterile technique, draw the appropriate dose of fomepizole from the vial with a syringe and inject into at least 100 mL of sterile 0.9% Sodium Chloride Injection or Dextrose 5% Injection. Mix well. Infuse the entire contents of the resulting solution over 30 minutes. Fomepizole, like all parenteral products, should be inspected visually for particulate matter prior to administration. Fomepizole solidifies at temperatures < 25°C (77°F). If the fomepizole solution has become solid in the vial, liquefy by running the vial under warm water or by holding in the hand. Solidification does not affect the efficacy, safety, or stability of fomepizole.

➤*Storage / Stability:* Store at controlled room temperature, 20° to 25°C (68° to 77°F). Fomepizole diluted in 0.9% Sodium Chloride Injection or Dextrose 5% Injection remains stable and sterile for ≥ 24 hours when stored refrigerated or at room temperature. Fomepizole does not contain a preservative. Therefore, maintain sterile conditions and after dilution, do not use after 24 hours. Solutions showing haziness, particulate matter, precipitate, discoloration, or leakage should not be used.

Actions

➤*Pharmacology:* Fomepizole is a competitive inhibitor of alcohol dehydrogenase that catalyzes the oxidation of ethanol to acetaldehyde. Alcohol dehydrogenase also catalyzes the initial steps in the metabolism of ethylene glycol and methanol to their toxic metabolites.

Ethylene glycol is metabolized to glycoaldehyde, which undergoes subsequent sequential oxidations to yield glycolate, glyoxylate, and oxalate. Glycolate and oxalate are the metabolic by-products primarily responsible for the metabolic acidosis and renal damage seen in ethylene glycol toxicosis. The lethal dose of ethylene glycol is ≈ 1.4 mL/kg.

Methanol, the main component of windshield wiper fluid, is slowly metabolized via alcohol dehydrogenase to formaldehyde with subsequent oxidation via formaldehyde dehydrogenase to yield formic acid. Formic acid is primarily responsible for the metabolic acidosis and visual disturbances (eg, decreased visual acuity and potential blindness) associated with methanol poisoning. A lethal dose of methanol in humans is approximately 1 to 2 mL/kg.

➤*Pharmacokinetics:*

Absorption / Distribution – After IV infusion, fomepizole rapidly distributes to total body water. The volume of distribution is between 0.6 and 1.02 L/kg. The plasma half-life varies with the dose, even in patients with normal renal function, and has not been calculated. The concentration of fomepizole at which alcohol dehydrogenase is inhibited by 50% in vitro is ≈ 0.1 mcmol/L. Fomepizole concentrations in the range of 100 to 300 mcmol/L (8.6 to 24.6 mg/L) have been targeted to ensure adequate plasma concentrations for the effective inhibition of alcohol dehydrogenase.

In healthy volunteers, oral doses of fomepizole (10 to 20 mg/kg) significantly reduced the rate of elimination of moderate doses of ethanol, which is also metabolized through the action of alcohol dehydrogenase (see Drug Interactions.)

Metabolism / Excretion – Only 1% to 3.5% of the administered dose of fomepizole (7 to 20 mg/kg oral and IV) was excreted unchanged in the urine, indicating that metabolism is the major route of elimination. In humans, the primary metabolite of fomepizole is 4-carboxypyrazole (≈ 80% to 85% of administered dose), which is excreted in the urine. With multiple doses, fomepizole rapidly induces its own metabolism via the P450 system, producing a significant increase in the elimination rate after ≈ 30 to 40 hours. After enzyme induction, elimination follows first-order kinetics. Saturable elimination occurs at therapeutic blood concentrations (100 to 300 mcmol/L, 8.2 to 24.6 mg/L).

Special populations – Fomepizole injection has not been studied sufficiently to determine whether the pharmacokinetics differ for a geriatric population.

➤*Clinical trials:* In 2 prospective US clinical trials without a concomitant control group, 14 of 16 patients in the ethylene glycol trial and 7 of 11 patients in the methanol trial underwent hemodialysis because of severe intoxication. All patients received fomepizole shortly after admission. The results of these 2 studies provided evidence that fomepizole blocks ethylene glycol and methanol metabolism mediated by alcohol dehydrogenase in the clinical setting. In both studies, plasma concentrations of toxic metabolites of ethylene glycol and methanol failed to rise in the initial phases of treatment, the relationship to fomepizole therapy was confounded by hemodialysis and significant blood ethanol concentrations in many of the patients. However, in the postdialysis period(s), when ethanol concentrations were insignificant and ethylene glycol or methanol were > 20 mg/dL, the administration of fomepizole alone blocked any rise in glycolate or formate concentrations, respectively.

In a separate French trial, 5 patients presented with ethylene glycol concentrations ranging from 46.5 to 345 mg/dL, insignificant ethanol blood concentrations and normal renal function. These patients were treated with fomepizole alone without hemodialysis, and none developed signs of renal injury.

Contraindications

Documented serious hypersensitivity reaction to fomepizole or other pyrazoles.

Warnings

➤*Fertility impairment:* In rats, fomepizole (110 mg/kg) administered orally for 40 to 42 days resulted in decreased testicular mass (≈ 8% reduction). This dose is ≈ 0.6 times the human maximum daily exposure. Reduction was similar for rats treated with either ethanol or fomepizole alone. When fomepizole was given in combination with ethanol, the decrease in testicular mass was significantly greater (≈ 30% reduction) compared with those rats treated exclusively with fomepizole or ethanol.

➤*Elderly:* Safety and effectiveness in geriatric patients have not been established.

➤*Pregnancy: Category C.* It is not known whether fomepizole can cause fetal harm when administered to pregnant women or can affect reproduction capacity. Give to pregnant women only if clearly needed.

➤*Lactation:* It is not known whether this drug is excreted in breast milk. Exercise caution when fomepizole is administered to a breastfeeding woman.

➤*Children:* Safety and efficacy have not been established.

Precautions

➤*Monitoring:* In addition to specific antidote treatment with fomepizole, patients intoxicated with ethylene glycol or methanol must be managed for metabolic acidosis, acute renal failure (ethylene glycol), adult respiratory distress syndrome, visual disturbances (methanol), and hypocalcemia. Fluid therapy and sodium bicarbonate administration are potential supportive therapies. In addition, potassium and calcium supplementation and oxygen administration are usually necessary. Hemodialysis is necessary in the anuric patient or in patients with severe metabolic acidosis or azotemia (see Administration and Dosage). Assess treatment success by frequent measurements of blood gases, pH, electrolytes, BUN, creatinine, and urinalysis, in addition to other laboratory tests as indicated by individual patient conditions. At frequent intervals throughout the treatment, patients poisoned with ethylene glycol should be monitored for ethylene glycol concentrations in serum and urine, and the presence of urinary oxalate crystals. Similarly, monitor serum methanol concentrations in patients poisoned with methanol.

Because acidosis and electrolyte imbalances can affect the cardiovascular system, perform electrocardiography. In the comatose patient, electroencephalography may also be required. In addition, monitor hepatic enzymes and WBC counts during treatment, as transient increases in serum transaminase concentrations and eosinophilia have been noted with repeated fomepizole dosing.

➤*Administration:* Do not give fomepizole undiluted or by bolus injection. Venous irritation and phlebosclerosis occurred in 2 of 6 healthy volunteers given bolus injections (over 5 minutes) of fomepizole at a concentration of 25 mg/mL.

➤*Allergic reactions:* Minor allergic reactions (mild rash, eosinophilia) have been reported in a few patients receiving fomepizole (see Adverse Reactions). Therefore, monitor patients for signs of allergic reactions.

Drug Interactions

➤*Ethanol:* Oral doses of fomepizole (10 to 20 mg/kg), via alcohol dehydrogenase inhibition, significantly reduced the rate of elimination of ethanol (by ≈ 40%) given to healthy volunteers in moderate doses. Similarly, ethanol decreased the rate of elimination of fomepizole (by ≈ 50%) by the same mechanism.

Reciprocal interactions may occur with concomitant use of fomepizole and drugs that increase or inhibit the cytochrome P450 system (eg, phenytoin, carbamazepine, cimetidine, ketoconazole), although this has not been studied.

Adverse Reactions

The most frequent adverse events reported as drug-related or unknown relationship to study drug in the 78 patients and 63 healthy volunteers who received fomepizole were headache (14%), nausea (11%), dizziness, increased drowsiness, and bad taste/metallic taste (6% each). Other adverse events reported in approximately ≤ 3% of those receiving fomepizole are listed below:

➤*Cardiovascular:* Sinus bradycardia/bradycardia; tachycardia; phlebitis; shock; hypotension; phlebosclerosis.

➤*CNS:* Seizure; vertigo; lightheadedness; nystagmus; agitation; facial flush; anxiety; feeling of drunkenness; strange feeling; decreased environmental awareness.

➤*GI:* Vomiting; diarrhea; dyspepsia; decreased appetite; transient transaminitis; heartburn.

➤*Hematologic / Lymphatic:* Lymphangitis; eosinophilia/hypereosinophilia; disseminated intravascular coagulation; anemia.

FOMEPIZOLE (4-Methylpyrazole; 4-MP)

➤*Respiratory:* Hiccups; pharyngitis.

➤*Special senses:* Abnormal smell; speech/visual disturbances; roar in ear; transient blurred vision.

➤*Miscellaneous:* Abdominal pain; fever; multiorgan system failure; pain during fomepizole injection; inflammation at injection site; anuria; lumbalgia/backache; hangover; rash; application site reaction.

Overdosage

Nausea, dizziness, and vertigo occurred in healthy volunteers receiving 50 and 100 mg/kg doses of fomepizole (at plasma concentrations of 290 to 520 mcmol/L, 23.8 to 42.6 mg/L). These doses are 3 to 6 times the recommended dose. This dose-dependent CNS effect was short-lived in most subjects and lasted up to 30 hours in 1 subject. Fomepizole is dialyzable, and hemodialysis may be useful in treating cases of overdosage.

PRALIDOXIME CHLORIDE (2-PAM)

Rx	Protopam Chloride (Wyeth-Ayerst)	Powder for injection[1]: 1 g	In 20 mL single-use vials.

[1] Porous cake.

Indications

➤*Organophosphate poisoning:* Antidote in poisoning caused by organophosphate pesticides and chemicals with anticholinesterase activity (eg, azodrin, diazinon, dichlorvos (DDVP) with chlordane, disulfoton, EPN, isoflurophate, malathion, *Metasystox* I and fenthion, methyldemeton, methylparathion, mevinphos, parathion, parathion and mevinphos, phosphamidon, sarin, *Systox*, TEPP).

➤*Anticholinesterase drug overdosage:* Control of overdosage by anticholinesterase drugs used to treat myasthenia gravis.

The principal indications for the use of pralidoxime are muscle weakness and respiratory depression. In severe poisoning, respiratory depression may be caused by muscle weakness.

Administration and Dosage

Inspect for particulate matter and discoloration prior to administration whenever solution and container permit. Discard unused solution after a dose has been withdrawn.

➤*Organophosphate poisoning:* Treatment is most effective if administered immediately after poisoning. Generally, little is accomplished if the drug is given more than 36 hours after termination of exposure. However, when the poison has been ingested, exposure may continue for some time because of slow absorption from the lower bowel, and fatal relapses have been reported after initial improvement. Continued administration for several days may be useful in such patients. Close supervision of the patient is indicated for at least 48 to 72 hours.

Severe poisoning (coma, cyanosis, respiratory depression) requires intensive management. This includes the removal of secretions, airway management, correction of acidosis and hypoxemia, and artificial ventilation. Give atropine as soon as possible after hypoxemia is improved. Do not give atropine in the presence of significant hypoxia because of the risk of atropine-induced ventricular fibrillation. In adults, atropine 2 to 4 mg IV may be given. Repeat every 5 to 10 minutes until full atropinization (secretions are inhibited) or signs of atropine toxicity appear (eg, delirium, hyperthermia, muscle twitching). Maintain atropinization for at least 48 hours and until any depressed blood cholinesterase activity is reversed. After the effects of atropine become apparent, pralidoxime may be administered.

Adults – Inject an initial dose of 1 to 2 g of pralidoxime, preferably as an infusion in 100 mL of saline over a 15- to 30-minute period. If this is not practical or if pulmonary edema is present, give slowly by IV injection as a 5% solution in water over not less than 5 minutes. After about 1 hour, give a second dose of 1 to 2 g if muscle weakness is not relieved. Give additional doses cautiously if muscle weakness persists. Too-rapid administration may result in temporary worsening of cholinergic manifestations. Do not exceed an injection rate of 200 mg/min. If IV use is not feasible, give IM or SC.

In severe cases, especially after ingestion of the poison, monitor the effect of therapy by ECG because of possible heart block caused by the anticholinesterase. Where the poison has been ingested, consider the likelihood of continuing absorption from the lower bowel; additional doses of pralidoxime may be needed every 3 to 8 hours. In effect, the patient should be titrated with pralidoxime as long as signs of poisoning recur. As in all cases of organophosphate poisoning, take care to keep the patient under observation for at least 24 hours. If convulsions interfere with respiration, they may be controlled by the slow IV injection of diazepam, up to 20 mg in adults.

Children – 25 to 50 mg/kg/dose; however, safety and efficacy in children have not been established.

➤*Anticholinesterase drug overdosage:* As an antagonist to such anticholinesterases as neostigmine, pyridostigmine, and ambenonium used in the treatment of myasthenia gravis may be given pralidoxime 1 to 2 g IV followed by increments of 250 mg every 5 minutes.

➤*Storage/Stability:* Store at controlled room temperature 20° to 25°C (68° to 77°F).

Actions

➤*Pharmacology:* Pralidoxime reactivates cholinesterase (mainly outside the CNS) that has been inactivated by phosphorylation caused by an organophosphate pesticide or related compound. Destruction of accumulated acetylcholine can then proceed, allowing neuromuscular junctions to function normally. Pralidoxime also slows the process of "aging" of phosphorylated cholinesterase to a nonreactive form and detoxifies certain organophosphates by direct chemical reaction. The drug's most critical effect is relieving respiratory muscle paralysis. Because pralidoxime is less effective in relieving depression of the respiratory center, concomitant atropine is always required to block the effect of accumulated acetylcholine at this site. Pralidoxime relieves muscarinic signs and symptoms (ie, salivation, bronchospasm), but this is relatively unimportant because atropine is adequate for this purpose.

➤*Pharmacokinetics:* Pralidoxime is distributed throughout the extracellular water; it is not bound to plasma protein. The drug is rapidly excreted in the urine partly unchanged and partly as a metabolite produced by the liver. Consequently, pralidoxime is relatively short acting and repeated doses may be needed, especially when there is any evidence of continuing absorption of the poison. The minimum therapeutic concentration of pralidoxime in plasma is 4 mcg/mL; this level is reached in about 16 minutes after a single injection of 600 mg pralidoxime. The apparent half-life of pralidoxime is 74 to 77 minutes.

Contraindications

Morphine, theophylline, aminophylline, and succinylcholine. Known hypersensitivity to the drug and other situations in which the risk of its use clearly outweighs possible benefit.

Warnings

➤*Drugs to avoid in organophosphate poisoning:* Morphine, theophylline, aminophylline, and succinylcholine are contraindicated. Tranquilizers of the reserpine or phenothiazine type are to be avoided in patients with organophosphate poisoning.

➤*Phosphorus, inorganic phosphates, or organophosphate poisoning:* Pralidoxime is not effective in the treatment of poisoning caused by phosphorus, inorganic phosphates, or organophosphates not having anticholinesterase activity.

➤*Carbamate pesticides:* Pralidoxime is not indicated as an antidote for intoxication by pesticides of the carbamate class because it may increase the toxicity of carbaryl.

➤*Dermal exposure:* If dermal exposure has occurred, remove clothing and thoroughly wash hair and skin with alcohol or sodium bicarbonate as soon as possible.

➤*Convulsions:* Diazepam may be given cautiously if convulsions are not controlled by atropine.

➤*Renal function impairment:* A decrease in renal function will result in increased drug blood levels; reduce dosage in the presence of renal insufficiency.

➤*Pregnancy: Category C.* It is not known whether pralidoxime can cause fetal harm when administered to a pregnant woman or can affect reproduction capacity. Give to a pregnant woman only if clearly needed.

➤*Lactation:* It is not known whether this drug is excreted in breast milk. Exercise caution when pralidoxime is administered to a nursing woman.

➤*Children:* Safety and efficacy in children have not been established.

Precautions

➤*Monitoring:* Institute treatment of organophosphate poisoning without waiting for laboratory test results. Red blood cell, plasma cholinesterase, and urinary paranitrophenol measurements (for parathion exposure) may help confirm diagnosis and follow the course of the illness. A reduction in red blood cell cholinesterase concentration to below 50% of normal has been seen only with organophosphate ester poisoning.

➤*Injection rate:* Administer pralidoxime IV slowly and preferably by infusion because side effects, such as tachycardia, laryngospasm, and muscle rigidity, have been attributed in a few cases to a too-rapid injection rate (see Administration and Dosage).

➤*Myasthenia gravis:* Use with caution in treating organophosphate overdosage in cases of myasthenia gravis, because it may precipitate a myasthenic crisis.

Drug Interactions

➤*Atropine:* When atropine and pralidoxime are used together, atropinization (eg, flushing, mydriasis, tachycardia, dryness of the mouth and nose) may occur earlier than expected when atropine is used alone.

PRALIDOXIME CHLORIDE (2-PAM)

This is especially true if the total dose of atropine has been large and the administration of pralidoxime has been delayed.

➤*Barbiturates:* Barbiturates are potentiated by the anticholinesterases; therefore, use with caution in the treatment of convulsions.

➤*Reserpine or phenothiazine-type tranquilizers:* Avoid tranquilizers of the reserpine or phenothiazine type.

Adverse Reactions

Mild to moderate pain at the injection site 40 to 60 minutes after IM injection; AST and ALT elevations, which return to normal in about 2 weeks; transient elevations in CPK; dizziness; blurred vision; diplopia and impaired accommodation; headache; drowsiness; nausea; tachycardia; increased systolic and diastolic blood pressure; hyperventilation; muscular weakness.

Excitement and manic behavior immediately following recovery of consciousness have been reported. However, similar behavior has occurred in cases of organophosphate poisoning that were not treated with pralidoxime.

Overdosage

➤*Symptoms:* The following symptoms were observed in healthy subjects only: Dizziness, headache, blurred vision, diplopia, impaired accommodation, nausea, slight tachycardia. In therapy, it has been difficult to differentiate side effects caused by the drug from those caused by the effects of the poison.

➤*Treatment:* Administer artificial respiration and other supportive therapy as needed.

DIGOXIN IMMUNE FAB (Ovine)

Rx	**Digibind** (GlaxoSmithKline)	**Powder for injection, lyophilized:** 38 mg/vial. Each vial will bind ≈ 0.5 mg digoxin.	28 mg sodium chloride. Preservative free. In vials.
Rx	**DigiFab** (Savage)	**Powder for injection, lyophilized:** 40 mg/vial. Each vial will bind ≈ 0.5 mg digoxin.	2 mg sodium acetate. Preservative free. In vials.

Indications

For the treatment of life-threatening or potentially life-threatening digoxin toxicity or overdose. *Digibind* also has been successfully used to treat life-threatening digitoxin (not available in the United States) overdose. Digoxin immune Fab is not indicated for milder cases of digitalis toxicity.

Clinical conditions requiring administration include the following:

- Known suicidal or accidental consumption of more than 10 mg of digoxin in previously healthy adults or 4 mg (or more than 0.1 mg/kg [*DigiFab*]) in previously healthy children, or ingestion causing steady-state serum concentrations greater than 10 ng/mL;
- chronic ingestions causing steady-state serum digoxin concentrations exceeding 6 ng/mL in adults or 4 ng/mL in children (*DigiFab*); and
- manifestations of life-threatening toxicity caused by digoxin overdose, including severe ventricular arrhythmias (eg, ventricular tachycardia or fibrillation), progressive bradycardia, and second or third degree heart block not responsive to atropine, serum potassium levels exceeding 5 mEq/L (*Digibind*) or 5.5 mEq/L in adults or 6 mEq/L in children (*DigiFab*) with rapidly progressive signs and symptoms of digoxin toxicity.

Administration and Dosage

The dosage of digoxin immune Fab varies according to the amount of digoxin or digitoxin to be neutralized.

Administer IV slowly as an IV infusion over at least 30 minutes. If infusion rate-related reactions occur, stop the infusion and restart at a slower rate. If cardiac arrest is imminent, digoxin can be given as a bolus injection. With bolus injection, an increased incidence of infusion-related reactions may be expected.

It is recommended for *Digibind* to be infused through a 0.22 micron membrane filter to ensure no undissolved particulate matter is administered.

➤*Dosage for acute ingestion of unknown amount:* Twenty vials (760 mg of *Digibind* or 800 mg of *DigiFab*) are adequate to treat most life-threatening ingestions in both adults and children. In small children, it is important to monitor for volume overload. In general, a large dose of digoxin immune Fab has a faster onset of effect, but may enhance the possibility of a febrile reaction. The physician may consider administering 10 vials, observing the patient's response, and following with an additional 10 vials if clinically indicated. Failure of the patient to respond to digoxin immune Fab should alert the physician to the possibility that the clinical problem may not be caused by digitalis toxicity.

➤*Dosage for toxicity during chronic therapy:* In adults, 6 vials (228 mg [*Digibind*] or 240 mg [*DigiFab*]) are usually adequate to reverse most cases of toxicity. This dose can be used in patients who are in acute distress or for whom a serum digoxin or digitoxin concentration is not available. In infants and small children (20 kg or less), a single vial usually should suffice.

➤*Dose determination:* Erroneous calculations may result from inaccurate estimates of the amount of digitalis ingested or absorbed or from nonsteady-state serum digitalis concentrations. Inaccurate serum digitalis concentration measurements are a possible source of error.

Dosage calculations are based on a steady-state volume of distribution of approximately 5 L/kg for digoxin (0.5 L/kg for digitoxin) to convert serum digitalis concentration to the amount of digitalis in the body. Many patients may require higher doses for complete neutralization. Ordinarily, round the doses up to the next whole vial.

If toxicity has not adequately reversed after several hours or appears to recur, readministration of *Digibind* at a dose guided by clinical judgment may be required. If a patient is in need of readministration of *DigiFab* because of recurrent toxicity, or to a new toxic episode that occurs soon after the first episode, measurement of free (unbound) serum digitalis concentrations should be considered because Fab may still be present in the body.

➤*Dosage calculation:* If in any case the dose estimated based on ingested amount differs substantially from that calculated based on the serum digoxin or digitoxin concentration, it may be preferable to use the higher dose estimate.

Acute ingestion of known amount – Each vial will bind approximately 0.5 mg of digoxin (or digitoxin).

$$\text{Dose (in \# of vials)} = \frac{\text{Total digitalis body load (mg)}}{0.5 \text{ mg of digitalis bound/vial}}$$

For toxicity from an acute ingestion, total body load in milligrams will be approximately equal to the amount ingested in milligrams for digoxin capsules or digitoxin, or the amount ingested in milligrams multiplied by 0.8 (to account for incomplete absorption) for digoxin tablets.

Approximate Dose for Reversal of a Single Large Digoxin Overdose	
Number of digoxin tablets or capsules ingested[1]	Number of vials
25	10
50	20
75	30
100	40
150	60
200	80

[1] 0.25 mg tablets (80% bioavailability); 0.2 mg *Lanoxicaps* capsules (100% bioavailability).

Calculations based on steady-state serum digoxin concentrations –

Adults: To estimate number of vials for adult patients for whom a steady-state serum digoxin concentration is known, use the following formula:

$$\text{Dose (in \# of vials)} = \frac{(\text{Serum digoxin concentration in ng/mL}) (\text{weight in kg})}{100}$$

Estimates of Fab Fragments (in Number of Vials) From Serum Digoxin Concentration in Adults							
Weight (kg)	Serum digoxin concentration (ng/mL)[1]						
	1	2	4	8	12	16	20
40	0.5 v	1 v	2 v	3 v	5 v	7 v	8 v
60	0.5 v	1 v	3 v	5 v	7 v	10 v	12 v
70	1 v	2 v	3 v	6 v	9 v	11 v	14 v
80	1 v	2 v	3 v	7 v	10 v	13 v	16 v
100	1 v	2 v	4 v	8 v	12 v	16 v	20 v

[1] v = vial

Children:

- *Digibind* – Because infants and small children can have much smaller dosage requirements, reconstitute the 38 mg vial as directed and administer with a tuberculin syringe. For very small doses, dilute the reconstituted vial with 34 mL sterile isotonic saline to achieve 1 mg/mL concentration.

$$\text{Dose (in mg)} = \frac{(\text{Dose [in \# of vials]})}{(38 \text{ mg/vial})}$$

Antidotes

DIGOXIN IMMUNE FAB (Ovine)

Dose Estimates of *Digibind* from Serum Digoxin Concentration in Infants/Small Children							
Weight (kg)	Serum digoxin concentration (ng/mL)						
	1	2	4	8	12	16	20
1	0.4 mg[1]	1 mg[1]	1.5 mg[1]	3 mg[1]	5 mg	6 mg	8 mg
3	1 mg[1]	2 mg[1]	5 mg	9 mg	14 mg	18 mg	23 mg
5	2 mg[1]	4 mg	8 mg	15 mg	23 mg	30 mg	38 mg
10	4 mg	8 mg	15 mg	30 mg	46 mg	61 mg	76 mg
20	8 mg	15 mg	30 mg	61 mg	91 mg	122 mg	152 mg

[1] Dilution of reconstituted vial to 1 mg/mL may be desirable.

• *DigiFab* – Because infants and small children can have much smaller dosage requirements, it is recommended that the 40 mg vial be reconstituted as directed and administered with a tuberculin syringe. For very small doses, a reconstituted vial can be diluted with 36 mL of sterile isotonic saline to achieve a 1 mg/mL concentration.

$$\text{Dose (in mg)} = \frac{\text{(Dose [in \# of vials])}}{\text{(40 mg/vial)}}$$

Dose Estimates of *DigiFab* from Serum Digoxin Concentration in Infants/Small Children							
Weight (kg)	Serum digoxin concentration (ng/mL)						
	1	2	4	8	12	16	20
1	0.4 mg[1]	1 mg[1]	1.5 mg[1]	3 mg[1]	5 mg	6.5 mg	8 mg
3	1 mg[1]	2.5 mg[1]	5 mg	10 mg	14 mg	19 mg	24 mg
5	2 mg[1]	4 mg	8 mg	16 mg	24 mg	32 mg	40 mg
10	4 mg	8 mg	16 mg	32 mg	48 mg	64 mg	80 mg
20	8 mg	16 mg	32 mg	64 mg	96 mg	128 mg	160 mg

[1] Dilution of reconstituted vial to 1 mg/mL may be desirable.

➤*Calculations based on steady-state digitoxin concentrations:* The dosage of digoxin immune Fab for digitoxin toxicity can be approximated using the following formula:

$$\text{Dose (in \# of vials)} = \frac{\text{(Serum digitoxin concentration in ng/mL) (weight in kg)}}{1000}$$

➤*Reconstitution:* Dissolve the contents in each vial with 4 mL of Sterile Water for Injection. Mix gently to give a protein concentration of 9.5 mg/mL (*Digibind*) or 10 mg/mL (*DigiFab*). Use reconstituted product promptly. If it is not used immediately, store at 2° to 8°C (36° to 46°F) for up to 4 hours. The reconstituted product may be diluted with sterile isotonic saline to a convenient volume.

➤*Storage/Stability:* Refrigerate at 2° to 8°C (36° to 46°F) for up to 4 hours after reconstitution.

Digibind – Unreconstituted vials can be stored at up to 30°C (86°F) for a total of 30 days.

DigiFab – Do not freeze.

Actions

➤*Pharmacology:* Digoxin immune Fab (ovine) is antigen binding fragments (Fab) derived from specific antidigoxin antibodies produced in sheep. Production involves conjugation of digoxin as a hapten to human albumin. Sheep are immunized with this material to produce antibodies specific for the digoxin molecule. The antibody is papain digested, and digoxin-specific Fab fragments are isolated and purified.

Improvement in signs and symptoms of digitalis intoxication ordinarily begins in 30 minutes or less. Digoxin immune Fab binds molecules of digoxin, making them unavailable for binding at their site of action. The Fab fragment-digoxin complex accumulates in the blood and is excreted by the kidneys. The net effect is to shift the equilibrium away from binding of digoxin to its receptors in the body, thereby reversing its effects.

➤*Pharmacokinetics:* The pharmacokinetic profiles of Fab are similar for both products. The similar volumes of distribution (0.3 L/kg and 0.4 L/kg for *DigiFab* and *Digibind*, respectively) indicate considerable penetration from the circulation into the extracellular space and are consistent with previous reports of ovine Fab distribution, as are the elimination half-life values (15 and 23 hours for *DigiFab* and *Digibind*, respectively). The elimination half-life of 15 to 20 hours in patients with normal renal function appears to be increased up to 10-fold in patients with renal impairment, although volume of distribution remains unaffected.

Contraindications

None known.

Warnings

➤*Allergy to papain or derivatives:* Patients with allergies to papain, chymopapain, other papaya extracts, or the pineapple enzyme bromelain may also be at risk for an allergic reaction to digoxin immune Fab. In addition, it has been noted in the literature that some dust mite allergens and some latex allergens share antigenic structures with papain and patients with these allergies may be allergic to papain. Do not administer digoxin immune Fab to patients with a known history of hypersensitivity to papaya or papain unless the benefits outweigh the risks and appropriate management for anaphylactic reactions is readily available.

➤*Skin testing:*

Digibind – Skin testing for allergy was performed during the clinical investigation of this agent. Only 1 patient developed erythema at the site of skin testing. The patient had no adverse reaction to systemic treatment. Allergy testing is not routinely required before treatment of life-threatening digitalis toxicity because it can delay urgently needed therapy.

Skin testing may be appropriate for high-risk individuals, especially patients with known allergies or those previously treated with digoxin immune Fab. The intradermal skin test can be performed by: 1) Diluting 0.1 mL of reconstituted drug (9.5 mg/mL) in 9.9 mL sterile isotonic saline; 2) injecting 0.1 mL of the 1:100 dilution (9.5 mcg) intradermally and observing for an urticarial wheal surrounded by a zone of erythema. Read the test at 20 minutes.

The scratch test procedure is performed by placing 1 drop of a 1:100 dilution on the skin and making a ¼-inch scratch through the drop with a needle. The area is inspected at 20 minutes for an urticarial wheal surrounded by erythema.

If skin testing causes a systemic reaction, apply a tourniquet above the site of testing and treat anaphylaxis. Avoid further administration of the drug unless its use is absolutely essential; in this case, pretreat the patient with corticosteroids and diphenhydramine and make preparations for treating anaphylaxis.

DigiFab – Skin testing has not proved useful in predicting allergic response to *Digibind*. Because of this and because it may delay urgently needed therapy, skin testing was not performed during the clinical studies of *DigiFab* and is not suggested prior to dosing with this product.

➤*Hypersensitivity reactions:* Allergic reactions have occurred rarely, but consider the possibility of anaphylactic, hypersensitivity, or febrile reactions. If an anaphylactoid reaction occurs, discontinue the drug infusion and initiate appropriate therapy. The need for epinephrine should be balanced against its potential risk in the setting of digitalis toxicity. Refer to Management of Acute Hypersensitivity Reactions.

Patients with known allergies or allergies to sheep protein would be particularly at risk, as would individuals who have previously received antibodies or Fab fragments raised in sheep. Patients with a history of allergy, especially to antibiotics, appear to be at particular risk.

➤*Renal function impairment:* The elimination half-life in renal failure has not been clearly defined. Patients with renal dysfunction have been successfully treated with digoxin immune Fab. There is no evidence to suggest any difference between these patients and patients with normal renal function, but excretion of the Fab fragment-digoxin complex from the body is probably delayed. In patients who are functionally anephric, anticipate failure to clear the Fab fragment-digoxin complex from the blood by glomerular filtration and renal excretion. Whether this would lead to reintoxication by release of newly unbound digoxin into the blood is uncertain. Monitor such patients for a prolonged period for possible recurrence of digitalis toxicity. Monitoring of free (unbound) digoxin concentrations after the administration may be appropriate in order to establish recrudescent toxicity in renal failure patients.

➤*Elderly:* Because elderly patients are more likely to have decreased renal function, it may be useful to monitor renal function and to observe for possible recurrence of toxicity.

➤*Pregnancy: Category C.* It is not known whether this agent can cause fetal harm or affect reproduction capacity. Use only if clearly needed.

➤*Lactation:* It is not known whether this drug is excreted in breast milk. Exercise caution when administering to a nursing mother.

➤*Children:* This agent has been used successfully in infants with no apparent adverse sequelae. Use of this drug in infants should be based on careful consideration of the benefits of the drug balanced against the potential risk involved.

Precautions

➤*Monitoring:* Digoxin immune Fab will interfere with digitalis immunoassay measurements. The standard serum digoxin concentration measurement can be clinically misleading until the Fab fragment is eliminated from the body. Obtain digoxin serum concentrations before digoxin immune Fab or drug administration. These measurements may be difficult to interpret if drawn soon after the last digitalis dose, because at least 6 to 8 hours are required for equilibration of digoxin between serum and tissue. Closely monitor the patient, including temperature, blood pressure, ECG, and potassium concentration during and after drug administration. The total serum digoxin concentration may rise precipitously following administration, but this will be almost entirely bound to the Fab fragment.

Potassium – Severe digitalis intoxication can cause life-threatening elevation in serum potassium concentration by shifting potassium from

DIGOXIN IMMUNE FAB (Ovine)

inside to outside the cell. This can lead to increased renal excretion of potassium. These patients may have hyperkalemia with a total body deficit of potassium. When the effect of digitalis is reversed, potassium shifts back inside the cell with a resulting decline in serum potassium concentration. Hypokalemia may develop rapidly. Monitor serum potassium concentration repeatedly, especially over the first several hours after the drug is given, and cautiously give potassium supplementation when necessary.

➤*Standard intoxication management:* Standard therapy for digitalis intoxication includes withdrawal of the drug, correction of electrolyte disturbances (especially hyperkalemia), acid-base imbalances, hypoxia, and treatment of cardiac arrhythmias. Massive digitalis intoxication can cause hyperkalemia; administration of potassium supplements in the setting of digitalis intoxication may be hazardous.

➤*Digoxin withdrawal:* In a few instances, the condition of those with low cardiac output states and CHF could have been exacerbated by withdrawal of the inotropic effects of digitalis. Patients with atrial fibrillation may develop a rapid ventricular response from withdrawal of the effects of digitalis on the AV node.

Patients with intrinsically poor cardiac function may deteriorate from withdrawal of digoxin. Additional support can be provided by use of IV inotropes (eg, dopamine or dobutamine) or vasodilators. With catechol-amines, take care not to aggravate digitalis toxic rhythm disturbances. Do not use other types of digitalis glycosides. Redigitalization should be postponed if possible until the Fab fragments have been eliminated from the body; this may require several days. Patients with impaired renal function may require a week or longer.

➤*Immunogenicity:* Prior treatment with digoxin-specific ovine immune Fab carries a theoretical risk of sensitization to ovine serum protein and possible diminution of the efficacy of the drug due to the presence of human antibodies against ovine Fab. Human antibodies to ovine Fab have been reported in some patients receiving *Digibind*; however, to date, there have been no clinical reports of human antiovine immunoglobulin antibodies causing a reduction in binding of ovine digoxin immune Fab or neutralization response to ovine digoxin immune Fab.

Adverse Reactions

Exacerbation of low cardiac output and CHF; hypokalemia; allergic reactions (rarely); rapid ventricular response in patients with atrial fibrillation caused by digoxin withdrawal (see Precautions).

Patient Information

Advise patients to contact their physician immediately if they experience any signs and symptoms of delayed allergic reactions or serum sickness (eg, rash, pruritus, urticaria) after hospital discharge.

ACETYLCYSTEINE (N-Acetylcysteine)

Rx	**Acetylcysteine** (Various, eg, Abbott, American Regent, Mayne)	**Oral solution:** 10%	EDTA. In 4, 10, and 30 mL vials.
Rx	**Mucomyst** (Sandoz)		
Rx	**Acetylcysteine** (Various, eg, Abbott, American Regent, Mayne)	**Oral solution:** 20%	EDTA. In 4, 10, and 30 mL vials.
Rx	**Mucomyst** (Sandoz)		
Rx	**Acetadote** (Cumberland)	**Injection:** 20% (200 mg/mL)	Preservative-free. 0.5 mg/mL EDTA. In 30 mL single-dose vials.

Indications

➤*Acetaminophen overdose:* To prevent or lessen hepatic injury after ingestion of a potentially hepatotoxic quantity of acetaminophen.

It is essential to initiate treatment as soon as possible after the overdose and, in any case, within 24 hours of ingestion.

➤*Mucolytic (oral solution only):* As adjuvant therapy for abdominal, viscid, or inspissated mucus secretions (refer to Acetylcysteine in the Mucolytics section of the Respiratory chapter).

➤*Unlabeled uses:* Although there is conflicting data, some studies support the use of acetylcysteine for the prevention of radiocontrast-induced nephropathy. The oral solution has been administered IV in certain cases. Please contact the Poison Control Center at (800) 222-1222 for further information.

Administration and Dosage

On admission for suspected acetaminophen overdose, draw a serum blood sample at least 4 hours after ingestion to determine the acetaminophen level; this will serve as a basis for determining the need for treatment with acetylcysteine. If the patient presents after 4 hours postingestion, immediately determine the serum acetaminophen sample.

Administer acetylcysteine within 8 hours after acetaminophen ingestion for maximum protection against hepatic injury for patients whose serum acetaminophen levels fall above the "possible" toxicity line on the Rumack-Matthew nomogram. If the time of ingestion is unknown or the serum acetaminophen level is not available, cannot be interpreted, or is not available within the 8-hour time interval from acetaminophen ingestion, immediately administer acetylcysteine if 24 hours or less have elapsed from the reported time of ingestion of an overdose of acetaminophen, regardless of the quantity reported to have been ingested. Do not await results of assays for acetaminophen level before initiating acetylcysteine treatment. Use lavage, ipecac, or activated charcoal as indicated.

The critical ingestion-treatment interval for maximum protection against severe hepatic injury is between 0 and 8 hours. Efficacy diminishes progressively after 8 hours, and treatment initiation between 15 and 24 hours postingestion of acetaminophen yields limited efficacy. However, it does not appear to worsen the condition of patients; therefore, do not withhold treatment because the reported time of ingestion may not be correct.

➤*IV:* IV administration requires dilution with 5% dextrose. See the table below for dosing guidelines for the 3 total IV infusions.

IV Acetylcysteine Dosing Guidelines			
Dose type	Dose	IV infusion rate	Dilution
Loading dose	150 mg/kg	Over 15 minutes	150 mg/kg in 200 mL of 5% dextrose
Maintenance dose 1	50 mg/kg	Over 4 hours	50 mg/kg in 500 mL of 5% dextrose
Maintenance dose 2	100 mg/kg	Over 16 hours	100 mg/kg in 1000 mL of 5% dextrose

Incompatibilities – IV acetylcysteine is not compatible with rubber and metals, particularly iron, copper, and nickel. Drug stability and safety of acetylcysteine when mixed with other drugs have not been established.

➤*Oral:* Oral administration requires dilution of 10% or 20% solution with diet cola or other diet soft drinks to a final concentration of 5%. If administered via gastric tube or Miller-Abbott tube, water may be used as the diluent. Freshly prepare the dilutions and use within 1 hour. Remaining undiluted solutions in opened vials can be stored in the refrigerator for up to 96 hours. Regardless of the quantity of acetaminophen reported to have been ingested, immediately administer oral acetylcysteine if 24 hours or less have elapsed from the reported time of ingestion of an acetaminophen overdose.

Oral Acetylcysteine Dosing Guidelines				
Dose type	Dose	Frequency	Dilution	Final concentration
Loading dose	140 mg/kg	Once	Dilute with diet cola or other diet soft drinks	5%
Maintenance doses	70 mg/kg	4 hours after loading dose and at 4-hour intervals thereafter for 17 total doses	Dilute with diet cola or other diet soft drinks	5%

If the patient vomits any oral dose within 1 hour of administration, repeat that dose. If the patient is persistently unable to retain the orally administered acetylcysteine, it may be administered by duodenal intubation.

ACETYLCYSTEINE (N-Acetylcysteine)

►*Acetaminophen assays:* The acute ingestion of acetaminophen in quantities of 150 mg/kg or greater may result in hepatic toxicity. However, the reported history of the drug quantity ingested as an overdose often is inaccurate and is not a reliable guide to therapy of the overdose. Therefore, plasma or serum acetaminophen concentrations, determined as early as possible but no sooner than 4 hours following an acute overdose, are essential in assessing the potential risk of hepatoxicity. Acetaminophen levels drawn less than 4 hours postingestion may be misleading. If an assay for acetaminophen cannot be obtained, it is necessary to assume that the overdose is potentially toxic.

►*Interpretation of acetaminophen assays:* Refer to the nomogram at the end of this section to determine if plasma concentration is in the potentially toxic range.

Interpretation of Nomogram		
Predetoxification plasma levels	Hepatic toxicity incidence	Indication
Value falls above the solid black line (probable line)	Probable	Continue with maintenance doses
Value falls above the broken line (possible line)	Possible	Continue with maintenance doses
Value falls below the broken line (possible line)	Unlikely	May discontinue acetylcysteine treatment

►*Storage / Stability:*

IV – Store unopened vials at controlled room temperature (20° to 25°C; 68° to 77°F). The reconstituted solution is stable for 24 hours at controlled room temperature. Single-dose vials are preservative-free; discard any unused portion. Do not use if vial was opened previously.

Oral – Store unopened vials at controlled room temperature, 15° to 30°C (59° to 86°F). Use diluted solutions within 1 hour. If only a portion of a vial is used, refrigerate the remaining undiluted portion and use within 96 hours.

Antidotes

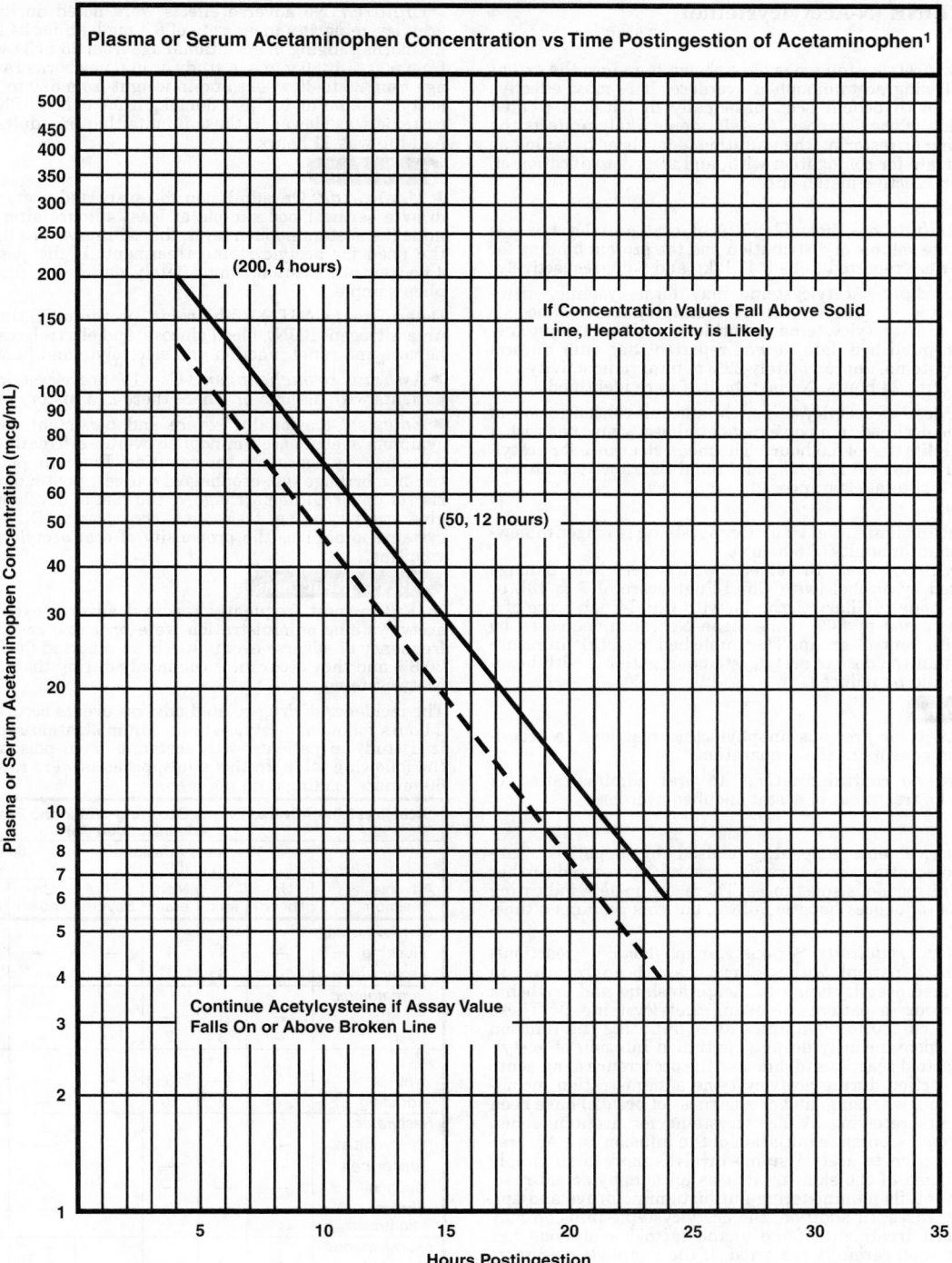

Plasma or Serum Acetaminophen Concentration vs Time Postingestion of Acetaminophen[1]

- (200, 4 hours)
- If Concentration Values Fall Above Solid Line, Hepatotoxicity is Likely
- (50, 12 hours)
- Continue Acetylcysteine if Assay Value Falls On or Above Broken Line

Plasma or Serum Acetaminophen Concentration (mcg/mL)

Hours Postingestion

[1] Adapted from Rumack and Matthews. *Pediatrics*. 1975;55:871-876.

ACETYLCYSTEINE (N-Acetylcysteine)

Actions

▶*Pharmacology:* Acetylcysteine has been shown to reduce the extent of liver injury following acetaminophen overdose. It is most effective when given early, with benefit seen principally in patients treated within 8 to 10 hours of the overdose. Acetylcysteine likely protects the liver by maintaining or restoring the glutathione levels or by acting as an alternate substrate for conjugation with, and thus detoxification of, the acetaminophen reactive metabolite.

▶*Pharmacokinetics:*

Absorption / Distribution – Bioavailability of oral acetylcysteine is low. The steady-state volume of distribution and the protein binding for IV acetylcysteine were reported to be 0.47 L/kg and 83%, respectively.

Metabolism / Excretion – Acetylcysteine may form cysteine, disulfides, and conjugates in vivo (eg, N, N'-diacetylcysteine, N-acetyl-cysteine-cysteine, N-acetylcysteine-glutathione, N-acetylcysteine-protein). Based on published data, it was reported that after an oral dose of ^{35}S-acetylcysteine, approximately 22% of total radioactivity was excreted in urine after 24 hours. No metabolites were identified.

After a single IV dose of acetylcysteine, the plasma concentration of total acetylcysteine declined in a polyexponential decay manner with a mean terminal half life ($t_{1/2}$) of 5.6 hours. The mean clearance for acetylcysteine was reported to be 0.11 L/h/kg and renal clearance constituted approximately 30% of total clearance.

Special populations –
Children: The mean elimination $t_{1/2}$ of acetylcysteine is longer in newborns (11 hours) than in adults (5.6 hours).
Hepatic function impairment: In subjects with severe liver damage (ie, cirrhosis caused by alcohol [with Child-Pugh score of 7 to 13]) or primary and/or secondary biliary cirrhosis (with Child-Pugh score of 5 to 7), mean $t_{1/2}$ increased by 80% while mean clearance decreased by 30% compared with control group. The published medical literature does not indicate that the dose of acetylcysteine in patients with hepatic impairment should be reduced.

Contraindications

▶*IV:* Hypersensitivity or previous anaphylactoid reactions to acetylcysteine or any components in the preparation.

▶*Oral:* There are no contraindications to oral administration of acetylcysteine in the treatment of acetaminophen overdose.

Warnings

▶*Encephalopathy:* If encephalopathy caused by hepatic failure becomes evident, discontinue acetylcysteine treatment to avoid further administration of nitrogenous substances. There are no data indicating that acetylcysteine influences hepatic failure, but this remains a theoretical possibility.

▶*Hypersensitivity reactions:* Serious anaphylactoid reactions, including death in a patient with asthma, have been reported in patients administered acetylcysteine IV. Acute flushing and erythema of the skin may occur in patients receiving acetylcysteine IV. These reactions usually occur 30 to 60 minutes after initiating the infusion and often resolve spontaneously despite continued infusion of acetylcysteine. Anaphylactoid reactions (defined as the occurrence of an acute hypersensitivity reaction during acetylcysteine administration including rash, hypotension, wheezing, and/or shortness of breath) have been observed in patients receiving IV acetylcysteine for acetaminophen overdose and occurred soon after initiation of the infusion (see Adverse Reactions). If a reaction to acetylcysteine involves more than simply flushing and erythema of the skin, treat it as an anaphylactoid reaction. This usually entails administering antihistaminic drugs and epinephrine in severe cases. In addition, the acetylcysteine infusion may be interrupted until treatment of the anaphylactoid symptoms has been initiated and then carefully restarted. If the anaphylactoid reaction returns upon reinitiation of treatment or increases in severity, discontinue IV acetylcysteine and consider alternative patient management. For additional information, contact a Poison Control Center at (800) 222-1222.

▶*Mutagenesis:* Acetylcysteine was positive in the in vitro mouse lymphoma cell (L5178Y/TK±) forward mutation test.

▶*Pregnancy: Category B.* In 4 pregnant women with acetaminophen toxicity, oral or IV acetylcysteine was administered at the time of delivery. Acetylcysteine crossed the placenta and was measurable in newborn circulation and cord blood of 3 viable infants following delivery and in cardiac blood of a fourth infant at autopsy (22 weeks gestational age who died 3 hours after birth). No adverse sequelae developed in the 3 viable infants. All mothers recovered and none of the infants had evidence of acetaminophen poisoning. There are no adequate and well-controlled studies in pregnant women. Use during pregnancy only if clearly needed.

▶*Lactation:* It is not known whether this drug is excreted in human milk. Because many drugs are excreted in human milk, exercise caution when administering acetylcysteine to a nursing woman.

▶*Children:* No adverse effects were noted during IV infusion with acetylcysteine at a mean rate of 8.4 mg/kg/h for 24 hours to 10 preterm newborns ranging in gestational age from 25 to 31 weeks and in weight from 500 to 1380 g in one study or in 6 newborns ranging in gestational age from 26 to 30 weeks and in weight from 520 to 1335 g infused with acetylcysteine at 0.1 to 1.3 mg/kg/h for 6 days. Elimination of acetylcysteine was slower in these infants than in adults; mean elimination half life was 11 hours.

Precautions

▶*Monitoring:* On admission for suspected acetaminophen overdose, draw a serum blood sample at least 4 hours after ingestion to determine the acetaminophen level; this will serve as a basis for determining the need for acetylcysteine treatment. If the patient presents after 4 hours postingestion, immediately determine the serum acetaminophen sample.

Determine the AST, ALT, bilirubin, prothrombin time, creatinine, blood urea nitrogen (BUN), blood glucose, and electrolytes in order to monitor hepatic and renal function and electrolyte and fluid balance.

▶*Asthma / Bronchospasm:* Use IV acetylcysteine with caution in patients with asthma or where there is a history of bronchospasm.

▶*Emesis:* Occasionally, severe and persistent vomiting occurs as a symptom of acute acetaminophen overdose. Treatment with oral acetylcysteine may aggravate the vomiting. Evaluate patients at risk of gastric hemorrhage (eg, esophageal varices, peptic ulcers) concerning the risk of upper GI hemorrhage vs the risk of developing hepatic toxicity; give acetylcysteine treatment accordingly. Dilution of the acetylcysteine minimizes the propensity of oral acetylcysteine to aggravate vomiting.

Adverse Reactions

▶*IV:* The most frequently reported adverse events attributed to IV acetylcysteine administration were pruritus, rash, and urticaria. The frequency of adverse events has been reported to be between 0.2% and 20.8% and they occur most commonly during the initial loading dose of acetylcysteine.

The incidence of drug-related adverse events occurring within the first 2 hours following acetylcysteine administration reported in a randomized study in patients with acetaminophen poisoning is presented in the following table. In this study, patients were randomized to a 15- or 60-minute loading dose regimen.

Acetylcysteine Adverse Events Occurring Within the First 2 Hours Following Administration (%)							
Adverse reaction	15-minute infusion (n = 109)				60-minute infusion (n = 71)		
	Unknown	Mild	Moderate	Severe	Unknown	Mild	Moderate	Severe
Cardiovascular								
Flushing	—	1	1	—	—	3	1	—
Tachycardia	—	4	1	—	—	3	—	—
Dermatologic								
Pruritus	—	1	—	—	—	3	—	—
Rash	—	3	2	—	—	4	—	—
GI								
Nausea	1	—	6	—	—	1	1	—
Vomiting	—	2	10	—	—	3	6	—
Respiratory								
Pharyngitis	—	—	1	—	—	—	—	—
Rhinorrhea	—	1	—	—	—	—	—	—
Rhonchi	—	—	—	—	—	1	—	—
Throat tightness	—	—	—	—	—	1	—	—
Miscellaneous								
Anaphylactoid reaction	2	6	10	1	—	6	7	1
Chest tightness	—	1	—	—	—	—	—	—
Ear pain	—	—	1	—	—	—	—	—
Feeling hot	—	—	—	—	—	1	—	—

▶*Oral:* Oral administration of acetylcysteine, especially in the large doses needed to treat acetaminophen overdose, may result in nausea, vomiting, and other GI symptoms. Rash with or without mild fever has been observed rarely.

Overdosage

Single IV doses of acetylcysteine at 1000 mg/kg in mice, 2445 mg/kg in rats, 1500 mg/kg in guinea pigs, 1200 mg/kg in rabbits, and 500 mg/kg in dogs were lethal. Symptoms of acute toxicity were ataxia, convulsions, cyanosis, hypoactivity, labored respiration, and loss of righting reflex.

IPECAC SYRUP

otc	**Ipecac** (Various, eg, Roxane)	Syrup	1.5% to 1.75% alcohol. In 15 and 30 ml.
Rx	**Ipecac** (Various, eg, Paddock)	Syrup	2% alcohol. In 15 and 30 ml.

Indications

➤*Overdose/Poisoning:* Treatment of drug overdose and in certain poisonings.

Administration and Dosage

Ipecac syrup may not work on an empty stomach. Have patient sit upright with head forward before administering dose.

➤*Children (< 1 yr):* 5 to 10 ml, then ½ to 1 glass water. Should *probably* give only with medical supervision. There is controversy over giving to children < 1 year, although it appears to be safe and effective.

➤*Children (> 1 year to 12 years):* 15 ml followed by 1 to 2 glasses of water.

➤*Adults:* 15 to 30 ml followed by 3 to 4 glasses of water.

➤*Repeat dosage:* Repeat dosage (15 ml) once, in persons older than one year, if vomiting does not occur within 20 to 30 min. If vomiting does not occur within 30 to 45 min after the second dose, perform gastric lavage.

Actions

➤*Pharmacology:* Ipecac produces vomiting by a local irritant effect on GI mucosa and a central medullary effect (stimulation of chemoreceptor trigger zone). The central effect is caused by emetine and cephaeline, the two alkaloids. An adequate dose causes vomiting within 30 min in > 90% of patients (average time is < 20 min).

Contraindications

Semiconscious or unconscious patients. Do not use if strychnine, corrosives such as alkalies and strong acids, or petroleum distillates have been ingested.

Warnings

➤*Syrup/Fluid extract:* Do not confuse ipecac syrup with ipecac fluid extract, which is 14 times stronger and has caused some deaths.

➤*Call an emergency room:* Call an emergency room, poison control center or physician before using; if vomiting does not occur within 30 to 45 minutes after the second dose, perform gastric lavage.

➤*Ipecac syrup abuse:* Ipecac syrup abuse may occur in bulimic and anorexic patients. It has been implicated as the causative factor of severe cardiomyopathies, and even death, in several persons with eating disorders who used it regularly to induce vomiting.

➤*Pregnancy: Category C.* It is not known whether the drug can cause harm when administered to a pregnant woman. Minimal systemic absorption is expected when used as directed (see Administration and Dosage).

➤*Lactation:* It is not known whether ipecac alkaloids are excreted in breast milk. Exercise caution if ipecac syrup is used for treatment of a nursing woman.

Precautions

➤*Absorption:* Ipecac syrup can be cardiotoxic if not vomited and allowed to be absorbed. Absorption of emetine may occur and cause heart conduction disturbances, atrial fibrillation or fatal myocarditis.

Drug Interactions

Activated charcoal will adsorb ipecac syrup. If both are to be used, give the activated charcoal only after vomiting has been produced by the ipecac syrup.

Adverse Reactions

Reactions are generally not significant if the dose is not exceeded. Diarrhea (25% in children < 3 years); drowsiness (20% in children < 3 years); coughing or choking in association with emesis (< 4%); mild CNS depression; GI upset (may last several hours after emesis).

Overdosage

➤*Symptoms:* Ipecac is cardiotoxic if absorbed and may cause cardiac conduction disturbances, bradycardia, atrial fibrillation, hypotension or fatal myocarditis.

➤*Treatment:* Activated charcoal may be given to adsorb ipecac syrup; perform gastric lavage. Support cardiovascular system by symptomatic treatment.

Patient Information

Always consult a physician or poison control center in cases of accidental ingestion.

Give with adequate amounts of water; do not use milk or carbonated beverages. Do not exceed recommended dosage.

CHARCOAL, ACTIVATED

otc	**Activated Charcoal** (Various)	**Powder**	In 15, 30, 40, 120 and 240 g and UD 30 g.
otc	**Activated Charcoal** (Various)	**Liquid:** 208 mg/ml	12.5 g with propylene glycol. In 60 ml bottle. 25 g with propylene glycol. In 120 ml bottle.
otc	**Actidose-Aqua** (Paddock)		25 g in 120 ml suspension. 50 g in 240 ml suspension.
otc	**Actidose with Sorbitol** (Paddock)		25 g in 120 ml suspension with sorbitol. 50 g in 240 ml suspension with sorbitol.
otc	**Liqui-Char** (Jones Medical)		12.5 g in 60 ml bottle, 15 g in 75 ml bottle, 25 g in 120 ml squeeze container, 30 g in 120 ml squeeze container, 50 g in 240 ml squeeze container.
otc	**CharcoAid** (Requa)	**Suspension:** 15 g	Sorbitol. In 120 ml.
		30 g	Sorbitol. In 150 ml.
otc	**CharcoAid 2000** (Requa)	**Liquid:** 15 g	With and without sorbitol. In 120 ml.
		50 g	With and without sorbitol. In 240 ml.
		Granules: 15 g	In 120 ml.

Indications

➤*Poisoning:* For use as an emergency treatment in poisoning by most drugs and chemicals.

Administration and Dosage

Administer to conscious persons only.

➤*Acute intoxication:*

Adult initial dose – 25 to 100 g (or 1 g/kg or approximately 10 times the amount of poison ingested) as a suspension (4 to 8 ounces water). For maximum effect, administer activated charcoal solution within 30 minutes after ingestion of poison.

➤*GI dialysis:* Multiple administration may be used in severe poisonings to prevent desorption from the charcoal; also promoted to increase GI clearance and rate of elimination of drugs that undergo an enteral recirculation pattern.

➤*Storage/Stability:* Activated charcoal adsorbs gases from the air; therefore, store in closed containers.

Actions

➤*Pharmacology:* Activated charcoal is a carbon residue derived from organic material by exposing it to an oxidizing gas compound of steam, oxygen and acids at high temperatures resulting in the production of increased surface area through the creation of external and internal pores. Activation (to make a fine network of pores) of the charcoal surface increases adsorptive properties. The maximum amount of drug adsorbed by such charcoal is approximately 100 to 1000 mg/g charcoal. Activated charcoal is insoluble in water.

Sorbitol – Sorbitol may be added to some activated charcoal products because it improves the taste, and it does not have a gritty oral residue. Sorbitol also reduces intestinal transit time from 25 hours to ≈ 1 hour.

Activated charcoal adsorbs toxic substances by forming an effective barrier between any remaining particulate material and the GI mucosa, thus inhibiting GI adsorption. The adsorptive properties of the activated charcoal in a liquid base are slightly decreased during its shelf life but are still capable of adsorbing at least 99% of the substances tested.

Contraindications

Ineffective for poisoning or overdosage of mineral acids and alkalies.

Although not necessarily contraindicated, activated charcoal is not particularly effective in poisonings of ethanol, methanol and iron salts.

Warnings

➤*Emesis:* Induce emesis before giving activated charcoal. After ipecac-induced vomiting, the patient may be intolerant of activated charcoal for 1 to 2 hours.

Antidotes

CHARCOAL, ACTIVATED

➤*Gastric lavage:* Activated charcoal can be administered in the early stages of gastric lavage. Use activated charcoal without sorbitol. The gastric lavage returns will be black.

➤*Children:* Not recommended in children < 1 year of age.

Drug Interactions

➤*Syrup of ipecac:* Do not administer concomitantly. Activated charcoal will adsorb and inactivate this agent.

The effectiveness of other medication may be decreased when used concurrently because of adsorption by the activated charcoal.

➤*Drug/Food interactions:* Do not mix charcoal with milk, ice cream or sherbet since it will decrease the adsorptive capacity of the activated charcoal.

Adverse Reactions

➤*GI:* Rapid ingestion of high doses may cause vomiting. Constipation or diarrhea may occur. Stools will be black.

Sorbitol – Sorbitol may cause loose stools, vomiting and dehydration.

➤*Respiratory:* Aspiration of activated charcoal has been reported to produce airway obstruction and a limited number of fatalities have occurred. Bronchiolitis obliterans resulting in death has developed several weeks after the aspiration of activated charcoal.

Overdosage

Bowel obstruction.

METHYLENE BLUE

| Rx | Urolene Blue (Star) | **Tablets:** 65 mg | In 100s and 1000s. |
| Rx | Methylene Blue (Various, eg, Pasadena) | **Injection:** 10 mg/ml | In 1 and 10 ml amps. |

Indications

➤*Oral:*

Cyanide poisoning – For treatment of idiopathic and drug-induced methemoglobinemia and as an antidote for cyanide poisoning.

Urinary tract calculi – May be useful in the management of patients with oxalate urinary tract calculi.

➤*Genitourinary antiseptic:* A mild GU antiseptic and stimulant for mucous surfaces.

➤*Unlabeled uses:*

Glutaricaciduria – Methylene blue may be of benefit in neonatal glutaricaciduria type II unresponsive to riboflavin.

Administration and Dosage

➤*Oral:* Take 65 to 130 mg, 3 times daily after meals with a full glass of water.

➤*Parenteral:* 1 to 2 mg/kg (0.1 to 0.2 ml/kg) (see Precautions).

➤*Storage/Stability:*

Tablets – Store in a dry place at room temperature (15° to 30°C; 59° to 86°F).

Injection – Store below 40°C (104°F), preferably between 15° and 30°C (59° and 86°F).

Actions

➤*Pharmacology:* This compound has an oxidation-reduction action and a tissue staining property. In high concentrations, methylene blue converts the ferrous iron of reduced hemoglobin in the ferric form; as a result, methemoglobin is produced. This action is the basis for the antidotal action of methylene blue in cyanide poisoning. In contrast, low concentrations of methylene blue are capable of hastening the conversion of methemoglobin to hemoglobin.

Methylene blue is a dye that is a weak germicide and is used as a mild GU antiseptic. It is primarily bacteriostatic.

Contraindications

Renal insufficiency; patients allergic to methylene blue; intraspinal injection.

Warnings

➤*Aniline-induced methemoglobulinemia:* Methylene blue should be used with caution in the treatment of aniline-induced methemoglobulinemia because it may precipitate Heinz body formation and hemolytic anemia.

➤*Alkaline urine:* Restrict drugs or foods which produce an alkaline urine.

➤*Pregnancy: Category C.* Safety for use in pregnancy has not been established. Use only if the potential benefits outweigh the risks.

Precautions

➤*G-6-PD deficiency:* Methylene blue may induce hemolysis in glucose-6–phosphate dehydrogenase (G-6–PD) deficient patients.

➤*Anemia:* Continued administration may cause a marked anemia due to accelerated destruction of erythrocytes. Therefore, perform frequent hemoglobin checks.

➤*Cyanosis and cardiovascular abnormalities:* Cyanosis and cardiovascular abnormalities have accompanied treatment in humans.

➤*Additional methemoglobin:* Inject IV slowly over a period of several minutes to prevent local high concentrations of the compound from producing additional methemoglobin.

➤*Photosensitivity:* Photosensitization (photoallergy or phototoxicity) may occur; therefore, caution patients to take protective measures against exposure to ultraviolet or sunlight (eg, sunscreens, protective clothing) until tolerance is determined.

Adverse Reactions

Oral – Turns the urine and sometimes the stool blue-green. May cause bladder irritation and, in some cases, nausea, vomiting and diarrhea. Large doses may cause fever.

Overdosage

➤*Oral:* Symptoms include vomiting, headache and diarrhea.

Patient Information

Take after meals with a glass of water.

May discolor the urine or stool blue-green.

Cardiac Glycosides

DIGOXIN

Rx	Lanoxicaps (Cardinal Health)	Capsules: 0.05 mg	Parabens, sorbitol. (A2C). Red. In 100s.
		0.1 mg	Parabens, sorbitol. (B2C). Yellow. In 100s.
		0.2 mg	Parabens, sorbitol. (C2C). Green. In 100s.
Rx	Digoxin (Various, eg, Qualitest)	Tablets: 0.125 mg	In 1000s.
Rx	Lanoxin (GlaxoWellcome)		Lactose. (Lanoxin Y3B). Yellow, scored. In 30s, 100s, 1000s, 5000s and UD 100s.
Rx	Digitek (Bertek Pharm)		Lactose. (B 145). Yellow, round, scored. In 100s, 1000s, and 5000s.
Rx	Digoxin (Various, eg, Qualitest)	Tablets: 0.25 mg	In 1000s.
Rx	Lanoxin (GlaxoWellcome)		Lactose. (Lanoxin X3A). White. In 30s, 100s, 1000s, 5000s and UD 100s.
Rx	Digitek (Bertek Pharm)		Lactose. (B 146). White, scored. In 100s, 1000s, and 5000s.
Rx	Digoxin[1] (Various, eg, Roxane)	Elixir, pediatric: 0.05 mg/mL	In 60 mL and UD 2.5 and 5 mL.
Rx	Lanoxin (GlaxoWellcome)		10% alcohol, 0.1% methylparaben. Lime flavor. In 60 mL with calibrated dropper.
Rx	Digoxin (Elkins-Sinn)	Injection: 0.25 mg/mL	In 2 mL amps.[2]
Rx	Digoxin (Various, Abbott, Wyeth-Ayerst)		In 1 and 2 mL *Tubex* or *Carpuject*.[3]
Rx	Lanoxin (GlaxoWellcome)		In 2 mL amps.[3]
Rx	Digoxin Injection, Pediatric (Abbott)	Injection, pediatric: 0.1 mg/mL	In 1 mL amps.[3]
Rx	Lanoxin (GlaxoWellcome)		In 1 mL amps.[3]

[1] May contain 10% alcohol.
[2] With 0.1 mL alcohol and 0.4 mL propylene glycol per mL.
[3] With 40% propylene glycol and 10% alcohol.

Indications

➤*Heart failure:* For the treatment of mild-to-moderate heart failure. Digoxin increases left ventricular ejection fraction and improves heart failure symptoms as evidenced by exercise capacity and heart failure-related hospitalizations and emergency care, while having no effect on mortality. Where possible, use digoxin with a diuretic and an angiotensin-converting enzyme inhibitor, but an optimal order for starting these 3 drugs cannot be specified.

➤*Atrial fibrillation:* For the control of ventricular response rate in patients with chronic atrial fibrillation.

Administration and Dosage

Recommended dosages of digoxin may require considerable modification because of individual sensitivity of the patient to the drug, the presence of associated conditions, or the use of concurrent medications. In selecting a dose of digoxin, the following factors must be considered:

1.) The body weight of the patient. Calculate doses based upon lean (ie, ideal) body weight.
2.) The patient's renal function, preferably evaluated on the basis of estimated creatinine clearance.
3.) The patient's age. Infants and children require different doses of digoxin than adults. Also advanced age may be indicative of diminished renal function even in patients with normal serum creatinine concentration (ie, < 1.5 mg/dL).
4.) Concomitant disease states, concurrent medications, or other factors likely to alter the pharmacokinetic or pharmacodynamic profile of digoxin (see Precautions).

Adult and pediatric dosage guidelines provided are based upon average patient response and substantial individual variation can be expected. Accordingly, base ultimate dosage selection upon clinical assessment of the patient.

➤*Serum digoxin concentrations:* About 66% of adults considered adequately digitalized (without evidence of toxicity) have serum digoxin concentrations ranging from 0.8 to 2 ng/mL. However, digoxin may produce clinical benefits even at serum concentrations below this range. About 66% of adult patients with clinical toxicity have serum digoxin concentrations > 2 ng/mL. However, because 33% of patients with clinical toxicity have concentrations < 2 ng/mL, values < 2 ng/mL do not rule out the possibility that a certain sign or symptom is related to digoxin therapy. Rarely, there are patients who are unable to tolerate digoxin at serum concentrations < 0.8 ng/mL. Consequently, interpret the serum concentration of digoxin in the overall clinical context, and do not use an isolated measurement as the basis for increasing or decreasing the dose of the drug.

To allow adequate time for equilibration of digoxin between serum and tissue, perform sampling of serum concentrations just before the next scheduled dose of the drug. If this is not possible, perform sampling ≥ 6 to 8 hours after the last dose, regardless of the route of administration or the formulation used. On a once-daily dosing schedule, the concentration of digoxin will be 10% to 25% lower when sampled at 24 vs 8 hours, depending upon the patient's renal function. On a twice-daily dosing schedule, there will be only minor differences in serum digoxin concentrations whether sampling is done at 8 or 12 hours after a dose.

If a discrepancy exists between the reported serum concentration and the observed clinical response, consider the following possibilities:

1.) Analytical problems in the assay procedure.
2.) Inappropriate serum sampling time.
3.) Administration of a digitalis glycoside other than digoxin.
4.) Conditions (described in Warnings and Precautions) causing an alteration in the sensitivity of the patient to digoxin.
5.) Serum digoxin concentration may decrease acutely during periods of exercise without any associated change in clinical efficacy because of increased binding of digoxin to skeletal muscle.

➤*Heart failure:*

Adults – Digitalization may be accomplished by either of 2 general approaches that vary in dosage and frequency of administration but reach the same endpoint in terms of total amount of digoxin accumulated in the body.

1.) If rapid digitalization is considered medically appropriate, it may be achieved by administering a loading dose based upon projected peak digoxin body stores. Calculate maintenance dose as a percentage of the loading dose.
2.) Obtain more gradual digitalization beginning an appropriate maintenance dose, thus allowing digoxin body stores to accumulate slowly. Steady-state serum digoxin concentration will be achieved in ≈ 5 half-lives of the drug for the individual patient. Depending upon the patient's renal function, this will take between 1 and 3 weeks.

➤*Atrial fibrillation:* Peak digoxin body stores larger than the 8 to 12 mcg/kg required for most patients with heart failure and normal sinus rhythm have been used for control of ventricular rate in patients with atrial fibrillation. Titrate doses of digoxin used for the treatment of chronic atrial fibrillation to the minimum dose that achieves the desired ventricular rate control without causing undesirable side effects. Data are not available to establish the appropriate resting or exercise target rates that should be achieved.

➤*Renal function impairment:* In children with renal disease, digoxin must be carefully titrated based upon clinical response.

➤*Rapid digitalization with a loading dose:* Peak digoxin body stores of 8 to 12 mcg/kg should provide therapeutic effect with minimum risk of toxicity in most patients with heart failure and normal sinus rhythm. Because of altered digoxin distribution and elimination, projected peak body stores for patients with renal insufficiency should be conservative (ie, 6 to 10 mcg/kg; see Precautions).

Administer the loading dose in several portions, with roughly half the total given as the first dose. Additional fractions of this planned total dose may be given at 6- to 8-hour intervals, with careful assessment of clinical response before each additional dose.

If the patient's clinical reponse necessitates a change from the calculated loading dose of digoxin, then base calculation of the maintenance dose upon the amount actually given.

Digoxin injection is frequently used to achieve rapid digitalization, with conversion to digoxin tablets or capsules for maintenance therapy. If patients are switched from IV to oral digoxin formulations, make allowances for differences in bioavailability when calculating maintenance dosages (see Pharmacology).

DIGOXIN

Tablets – A single initial dose of 500 to 750 mcg (0.5 to 0.75 mg) of digoxin tablets usually produces a detectable effect in 0.5 to 2 hours that becomes maximal in 2 to 6 hours. Additional doses of 125 to 375 mcg (0.125 to 0.375 mg) may be given cautiously at 6- to 8-hour intervals until clinical evidence of an adequate effect is noted. The usual amount of digoxin tablets that a 70 kg patient requires to achieve 8 to 12 mcg/kg peak body stores is 750 to 1250 mcg (0.75 to 1.25 mg).

Capsules – A single initial dose of 400 to 600 mcg (0.4 to 0.6 mg) digoxin capsules usually produces a detectable effect in 0.5 to 2 hours that becomes maximal in 2 to 6 hours. Additional doses of 100 to 300 mcg (0.1 to 0.3 mg) may be given cautiously at 6- to 8-hour intervals until clinical evidence of an adequate effect is noted. The usual amount of the capsules that a 70 kg patient requires to achieve 8 to 12 mcg/kg peak body stores is 600 to 1000 mcg (0.6 to 1 mg).

Injection – A single initial IV dose of 400 to 600 mcg (0.4 to 0.6 mg) of injection usually produces a detectable effect in 5 to 30 minutes that becomes maximal in 1 to 4 hours. Additional doses of 100 to 300 mcg (0.1 to 0.3 mg) may be given cautiously at 6- to 8-hour intervals until clinical evidence of an adequate effect is noted. The usual amount of injection that a 70 kg patient requires to achieve 8 to 12 mcg/kg peak body stores is 600 to 1000 mcg (0.6 to 1 mg).

➤*Dosage adjustment when changing preparations:* The difference in bioavailability between digoxin injection or capsules and pediatric elixir or tablets must be considered when changing patients from 1 dosage form to another.

The absolute bioavailability of the capsule formulation is greater than that of the standard tablets and near that of the IV dosage form. As a result, the doses recommended for the capsules are the same as those for injection. Adjustments in dosage will seldom be necessary when converting a patient from the IV formulation to capsules.

Doses of 100 mcg (0.1 mg) and 200 mcg (0.2 mg) of digoxin capsules are approximately equivalent to 125 mcg (0.125 mg) and 250 mcg (0.25 mg) doses of tablets and pediatric elixir, respectively.

➤*Maintenance dosing:* The doses of digoxin used in controlled trials in patients with heart failure have ranged from 125 to 500 mcg (0.125 to 0.5 mg) once daily. In these studies, the digoxin dose has been generally titrated according to the patient's age, lean body weight, and renal function. Therapy is generally initiated at a dose of 250 mcg (0.25 mg) once daily in patients < 70 years of age with good renal function, at a dose of 125 mcg (0.125 mg) once daily in patients > 70 years of age or with impaired renal function, and at a dose of 62.5 mcg (0.0625 mg) in patients with marked renal impairment. Doses may be increased every 2 weeks according to clinical response.

In a subset of ≈ 1800 patients enrolled in a trial (wherein dosing was based on an algorithm similar to that in the table below) the mean (± SD) serum digoxin concentrations at 1 month and 12 months were ≈ 1.01 ng/mL and ≈ 0.97 ng/mL, respectively.

Base the maintenance dose upon the percentage of the peak body stores lost each day through elimination. The following formula has had wide clinical use:

$$\text{Maintenance dose} = \text{Peak Body Stores (ie, Loading Dose)} \times \frac{\% \text{ Daily Loss}}{100} \text{ (ie, } 14 = \text{Ccr}/5)$$

Ccr is creatinine clearance, corrected to 70 kg body weight or 1.73 m^2 body surface area.

➤*Tablets:*

Maintenance dosing –

Usual Digoxin Tablet Daily Maintenance Dose Requirements (mcg) for Estimated Peak Body Stores of 10 mcg/kg							
Corrected Ccr (mL/min/70 kg)[1]	Lean Body Weight (kg/lbs)						Number of days before steady-state achieved[2]
	50/110	60/132	70/154	80/176	90/198	100/220	
0	62.5	125	125	125	187.5	187.5	22
10	125	125	125	187.5	187.5	187.5	19
20	125	125	187.5	187.5	187.5	250	16
30	125	187.5	187.5	187.5	250	250	14
40	125	187.5	187.5	250	250	250	13
50	187.5	187.5	250	250	250	250	12
60	187.5	187.5	250	250	250	375	11
70	187.5	250	250	250	250	375	10
80	187.5	250	250	250	375	375	9
90	187.5	250	250	250	375	500	8
100	250	250	250	375	375	500	7

[1] Ccr is creatinine clearance, corrected to 70 kg body weight or 1.73 m^2 body surface area. For adults, if only serum creatinine concentrations (Scr) are available, a Ccr (corrected to 70 kg body weight) may be estimated in men as (140 − Age)/Scr. For women, multiply this result by 0.85. Note: This equation cannot be used for estimating Ccr in infants or children.

[2] If no loading dose is administered.

Example – Based on the table above, give a patient in heart failure with an estimated lean body weight of 70 kg and a Ccr of 60 mL/min a dose of 250 mcg (0.25 mg) daily of digoxin tablets, usually taken after the morning meal. If no loading dose is administered, anticipate steady-state serum concentrations in this patient at ≈ 11 days.

Infants and children – In general, divided daily dosing is recommended for infants and young children < 10 years of age. In the newborn period, renal clearance of digoxin is diminished and observe suitable dosage adjustments. This is especially pronounced in the premature infant. Beyond the immediate newborn period, children generally require proportionally larger doses than adults on the basis of body weight or body surface area. Children > 10 years of age require adult dosages in proportion to their body weight. Some researchers have suggested that infants and young children tolerate slightly higher serum concentrations than do adults.

Daily maintenance doses for each age group are given in the table below and should provide therapeutic effects with minimum risk of toxicity in most patients with heart failure and normal sinus rhythm. These recommendations assume the presence of normal renal function:

Daily Digoxin Maintenance Doses in Children with Normal Renal Function	
Age	Daily maintenance dose (mcg/kg)
2 to 5 years	10 to 15
5 to 10 years	7 to 10
> 10 years	3 to 5

➤*Capsules:* Because of the more complete absorption of digoxin from soft capsules, recommended oral doses are only 80% of those for tablets and elixir. Because the significance of the higher peak serum concentrations associated with once daily capsules is not established, divided daily dosing is presently recommended for the following:

1.) Infants and children < 10 years of age.
2.) Patients requiring a daily dose of ≥ 300 mcg (0.3 mg).
3.) Patients with a history of digitalis toxicity.
4.) Patients considered likely to become toxic.
5.) Patients in whom compliance is not a problem.

Cardiac Glycosides

DIGOXIN

Corrected Ccr (mL/min/70 kg)[1]	Usual Digoxin Solution-Filled Capsule Daily Maintenance Dose Requirements (mcg) for Estimated Peak Body Stores of 10 mcg/kg						Number of days before steady-state achieved[2]
	Lean Body Weight (kg/lbs)						
	50/110	60/132	70/154	80/176	90/198	100/220	
0	50	100	100	100	150	150	22
10	100	100	100	150	150	150	19
20	100	100	150	150	150	200	16
30	100	150	150	150	200	200	14
40	100	150	150	200	200	250	13
50	150	150	200	200	250	250	12
60	150	150	200	200	250	300	11
70	150	200	200	250	250	300	10
80	150	200	200	250	300	300	9
90	150	200	250	250	300	350	8
100	200	200	250	300	300	350	7

[1] Ccr is creatinine clearance, corrected to 70 kg body weight or 1.73 m^2 body surface area. For adults, if only serum creatinine concentrations (Scr) are available, a Ccr (corrected to 70 kg body weight) may be estimated in men as $(140 - Age)/Scr$. For women, multiply this result by 0.85. Note: This equation cannot be used for estimating Ccr in infants or children.
[2] If no loading dose is administered.

Example – Based on the above table, give a patient in heart failure with an estimated lean body weight of 70 kg and a Ccr of 60 mL/min, a dose of 200 mcg (0.2 mg) daily of digoxin capsules, usually taken as a divided dose of one 100 mcg (0.1 mg) capsule after the morning and evening meals. If no loading dose is administered, anticipate steady-state serum concentrations in this patient at ≈ 11 days.

Infants and children – Individualize dosage. Divided daily dosing is recommended for infants and young children < 10 years of age. In these patients, where dosage adjustment is frequent and outside the fixed dosages available, digoxin capsules may not be the formulation of choice. In the newborn period, renal clearance of digoxin is diminished; observe suitable dosage adjustment. This is especially pronounced in the premature infant. Beyond the immediate newborn period, children generally require proportionally larger doses than adults on the basis of body weight or body surface area. Children > 10 years of age require adult dosages in proportion to body weight. Some researchers have suggested that infants and young children tolerate slightly higher serum concentrations than do adults.

Maintenance dosage – Daily maintenance doses for each age group are given below and should provide therapeutic effects with minimum risk of toxicity in most patients with heart failure and normal sinus rhythm. These recommendations assume the presence of normal renal function.

Usual Digitalizing and Maintenance Dosages for Digoxin Capsules in Children with Normal Renal Function Based on Lean Body Weight		
Age	Digitalizing[1] dose (mcg/kg)	Daily maintenance dose[2] (mcg/kg)
2 to 5 years	25 to 35	25% to 35% of the oral or IV digitalizing dose[3]
5 to 10 years	15 to 30	
> 10 years	8 to 12	

[1] IV digitalizing doses are the same as digitalizing doses of digoxin capsules.
[2] Divided daily dosing is recommended for children < 10 years of age.
[3] Projected or actual digitalizing dose providing desired clinical response.

➤*Pediatric elixir:*
Usual digitalizing and maintenance dosing –

Usual Digitalizing and Maintenance Dosages for Pediatric Elixir in Children with Normal Renal Function Based on Lean Body Weight		
Age	Oral digitalizing[1] dose (mcg/kg)	Daily maintenance dose[2] (mcg/kg)
Premature	20 to 30	20% to 30% of oral digitalizing dose[3]
Full-term	25 to 35	25% to 35% of oral digitalizing dose[3]
1 to 24 months	35 to 60	
2 to 5 years	30 to 40	
5 to 10 years	20 to 35	
> 10 years	10 to 15	

[1] IV digitalizing doses are 80% of oral digitalizing doses.
[2] Divided daily dosing is recommended for children < 10 years of age.
[3] Projected or actual digitalizing dose providing clinical response.

Gradual digitalization with a maintenance dose – More gradual digitalization can also be accomplished by beginning an appropriate maintenance dose. The range of percentages provided in the above table can be used in calculating this dose for patients with normal renal function.

➤*Injection:* Slow infusion of injection is preferable to bolus administration. Rapid infusion of digitalis glycosides has been shown to cause systemic and coronary arteriolar constriction, which may be clinically undesirable. Caution is thus advised and injection should probably be administered over a period of ≥ 5 minutes. Mixing injection with other drugs in the same container or simultaneous administration in the same intravenous line is not recommended.

Parenteral administration of digoxin should be used only when the need for rapid digitalization is urgent or when the drug cannot be taken orally. IM injection can lead to severe pain at the injection site, thus IV administration is preferred. If the drug must be administered by the IM route, it should be injected deep into the muscle followed by massage. No more than 500 mcg (2 mL) should be injected into a single site.

If tuberculin syringes are used to measure very small doses, one must be aware of the problem of inadvertent overadministration of digoxin. The syringe should not be flushed with the parenteral solution after its contents are expelled into an indwelling vascular catheter.

Admixture compatibility – Digoxin injection can be administered undiluted or diluted with a ≥ 4-fold volume of Sterile Water for Injection, 0.9% Sodium Chloride Injection, or 5% Dextrose Injection. The use of < 4-fold volume of diluent could lead to precipitation of the digoxin. Immediate use of the diluted product is recommended.

DIGOXIN
Maintenance Dose –

Usual Daily Maintenance Dose Requirements (mcg) of Digoxin Injection for Estimated Peak Body Stores of 10 mcg/kg[1]							
	Lean body weight (kg/lb)						
Corrected Ccr (mL/min/70 kg)[2]	50/110	60/132	70/154	80/176	90/198	100/220	Number of Days before steady-state achieved[3]
0	75	75	100	100	125	150	22
10	75	100	100	125	150	150	19
20	100	100	125	150	150	175	16
30	10	125	150	150	175	200	14
40	100	125	150	175	200	225	13
50	125	150	175	200	225	250	12
60	125	150	175	200	225	250	11
70	150	175	200	225	250	275	10
80	150	175	200	250	275	300	9
90	150	200	225	250	300	325	8
100	175	200	250	275	300	350	7

[1] Daily maintenance doses have been rounded to the nearest 25 mcg increment.

[2] Ccr is creatinine clearance, corrected to 70 kg body weight or 1.73 m² body surface area. For adults, if only serum creatinine concentrations (Scr) are available, a Ccr (corrected to 70 kg body weight) may be estimated in men as (140 – Age)/Scr. For women, this result should be multiplied by 0.85. Note: This equation cannot be used for estimating creatinine clearance in infants or children.

[3] If no loading dose is administered.

Example: Based on the above table, give a patient in heart failure with an estimated lean body weight of 70 kg and a Ccr of 60 mL/min a dose of 175 mcg (0.175 mg) daily of digoxin injection. If no loading dose is administered, anticipate steady-state serum concentrations in this patient at ≈ 11 days.

➤*Pediatric injection:*
Digitalizing and maintenance dosages –

Usual Digitalizing and Maintenance Dosages for Digoxin Pediatric Injection in Children with Normal Renal Function Based on Lean Body Weight		
Age	IV digitalizing[1] dose (mcg/kg)	Daily IV maintenance dose[2] (mcg/kg)
Premature	15 to 25	20% to 30% of the IV digitalizing dose[3]
Full-term	20 to 30	25% to 35% of the IV digitalizing dose[3]
1 to 24 months	30 to 50	
2 to 5 years	25 to 35	
5 to 10 years	15 to 30	
≥ 10 years	8 to 12	

[1] IV digitalizing doses are 80% of oral digitalizing doses.

[2] Divided daily dosing is recommended for children < 10 years of age.

[3] Projected or actual digitalizing dose providing clinical response.

Gradual digitalization with a maintenance dose – More gradual digitalization can also be accomplished by beginning an appropriate maintenance dose. The range of percentages provided in the table above can be used in calculating this dose for patients with normal renal function.

Actions

➤*Pharmacology:* Digoxin is a cardiac (or digitalis) glycoside derived from the plant *Digitalis lanata*. These drugs have common specific effects on the myocardium. The term "digitalis" is used to designate the whole group of glycosides. The glycosides are composed of the following 2 portions: A sugar and a cardenolide. Digoxin inhibits sodium-potassium ATPase, an enzyme that regulates the quantity of sodium and potassium inside cells. Inhibition of the enzyme leads to an increase in the intracellular concentration of sodium and thus, (by stimulation of sodium-calcium exchange) an increase in the intracellular concentration of calcium. The beneficial effects of digoxin result from direct actions on cardiac muscle, as well as indirect actions on the cardiovascular system mediated by effects on the autonomic nervous system. The autonomic effects include the following: A vagomimetic action, which is responsible for the effects of digoxin on the sinoatrial and atrioventricular (AV) nodes; and baroreceptor sensitization, which results in increased afferent inhibitory activity and reduced activity of the sympathetic nervous system and renin-angiotensin system for any given increment in mean arterial pressure. The pharmacologic consequences of these direct and indirect effects are the following: An increase in the force and velocity of myocardial systolic contraction (positive inotropic action); a decrease in the degree of activation of the sympathetic nervous system and renin-angiotensin system (neurohormonal deactivating effect); and slowing of the heart rate and decreased conduction velocity through the AV node (vagomimetic effect). The effects of digoxin in heart failure are mediated by its positive inotropic and neurohormonal deactivating effects, whereas the effects of the drug in atrial arrhythmias are related to its vagomimetic actions. In high doses, digoxin increases sympathetic outflow from the CNS. This increase in sympathetic activity may be an important factor in digitalis toxicity.

Hemodynamic effects – Digoxin produces hemodynamic improvement in patients with heart failure. Short- and long-term therapy with the drug increases cardiac output and lowers pulmonary artery pressure, pulmonary capillary wedge pressure, and systemic vascular resistance. These hemodynamic effects are accompanied by an increase in the left ventricular ejection fraction and a decrease in end-systolic and endodiastolic dimensions.

➤*Pharmacokinetics:*

Absorption – Following oral administration, peak serum concentrations of digoxin occur at 1 to 3 hours. Absorption of digoxin from the tablets has been demonstrated to be 60% to 80% complete compared with an identical IV dose of digoxin (absolute bioavailability) or capsules (relative bioavailability). When the tablets are taken after meals, the rate of absorption is slowed; however, the amount absorbed from an oral dose may be reduced. Comparisons of the systemic availability and equivalent doses for oral preparations of digoxin are shown in the table below:

Comparisons of the Systemic Availability and Equivalent Doses for Oral Preparations of Digoxin					
Product	Absolute bioavailability (%)	Equivalent doses (mcg)[1] among dosage forms			
Tablets	60 to 80	62.5	125	250	500
Pediatric elixir	70 to 85	62.5	125	250	500
Capsules	90 to 100	50	100	200	400
Injection/IV	100	50	100	200	400

[1] For example, 125 mcg tablets equivalent to 125 mcg pediatric elixir equivalent to 100 mcg capsules equivalent to 100 mcg injection/IV.

In some patients, orally-administered digoxin is converted to inactive reduction products (eg, dihydrodigoxin) by colonic bacteria in the gut. Data suggest that 1 in 10 patients treated with digoxin tablets will degrade ≥ 40% of the ingested dose. As a result, certain antibiotics may increase the absorption of digoxin in such patients. Although inactivation of these bacteria by antibiotics is rapid, the serum digoxin concentration will rise at a rate consistent with the elimination half-life of digoxin. The magnitude of rise in serum digoxin concentration relates to the extent of bacterial inactivation, and may be as much as 2-fold in some cases.

Distribution – Following drug administration, a 6- to 8-hour tissue distribution phase is observed. This is followed by a much more gradual decline in the serum concentration of the drug, which is dependent on the elimination of digoxin from the body. The peak height and slope of the early portion (absorption/distribution phases) of the serum concentration-time curve are dependent upon the route of administration and the absorption characteristics of the formulation. Clinical evidence indicates that the early high serum concentrations do not reflect the concentration of digoxin at its site of action, but that with chronic use, the steady-state postdistribution serum concentrations are in equilibrium with tissue concentrations and correlate with pharmacologic effects. In individual patients, these postdistribution serum concentrations may be useful in evaluating therapeutic and toxic effects.

Digoxin is concentrated in tissues and therefore has a large apparent volume of distribution. Digoxin crosses the blood-brain barrier and the placenta. At delivery, the serum digoxin concentration in the newborn is similar to the serum concentration in the mother. Approximately 25% of digoxin in the plasma is bound to protein. Serum digoxin concentrations are not significantly altered by large changes in fat tissue weight, so that its distribution space correlates best with lean (ie, ideal) body weight, not total body weight.

Metabolism – Only a small percentage (16%) of a dose of digoxin is metabolized. The end metabolites, which include 3 β-digoxigenin, 3-keto-digoxigenin, and their glucuronide and sulfate conjugates, are polar in nature and are postulated to be formed via hydrolysis, oxida-

DIGOXIN

tion, and conjugation. The metabolism of digoxin is not dependent upon the cytochrome P450 system, and digoxin is not known to induce or inhibit the cytochrome P450 system.

Excretion – Elimination of digoxin follows first-order kinetics (ie, the quantity of digoxin eliminated at any time is proportional to the total body content). Following IV administration to healthy volunteers, 50% to 70% of a digoxin dose is excreted unchanged in the urine. Renal excretion of digoxin is proportional to glomerular filtration rate and is largely independent of urine flow. In healthy volunteers with normal renal function, digoxin has a half-life of 1.5 to 2 days. The half-life in anuric patients is prolonged to 3.5 to 5 days. Digoxin is not effectively removed from the body by dialysis, exchange transfusion, or during cardiopulmonary bypass because most of the drug is bound to tissue and does not circulate in the blood.

Special populations –
Renal function impairment: The clearance of digoxin can be primarily correlated with renal function as indicated by Ccr. See Administration and Dosage for the table that provides the usual daily maintenance dose requirements of digoxin tablets based on Ccr (per 70 kg).

Contraindications

Ventricular fibrillation; hypersensitivity to digoxin or other digitalis preparations.

Warnings

➤*Sinus node disease and AV block:* Because digoxin slows sinoatrial and AV conduction, the drug commonly prolongs the PR interval. The drug may cause severe sinus bradycardia or sinoatrial block in patients with pre-existing sinus node disease and may cause advanced or complete heart block in patient with pre-existing incomplete AV block. In such patients, consider inserting a pacemaker before treatment with digoxin.

➤*Accessory AV pathway (Wolf-Parkinson-White syndrome):* After IV digoxin therapy, some patients with paroxysmal atrial fibrillation or flutter and a coexisting accessory AV pathway have developed increased antegrade conduction across the accessory pathway bypassing the AV node, leading to a very rapid ventricular response or ventricular fibrillation. Unless conduction down the accessory pathway has been blocked (either pharmacologically or by surgery), do not use digoxin in such patients. The treatment of paroxysmal supraventricular tachycardia in such patients is usually direct-current cardioversion.

➤*Use in patients with preserved left ventricular systolic function:* Patients with certain disorders involving heart failure associated with preserved left ventricular ejection fraction may be particularly susceptible to toxicity of the drug. Such disorders include restrictive cardiomyopathy, constructive pericarditis, amyloid heart disease, and acute cor pulmonale. Patients with idiopathic hypertrophic subaortic stenosis may have worsening of the outflow obstruction because of the inotropic effects of digoxin.

➤*Renal function impairment:* Digoxin is primarily excreted by the kidneys; therefore, patients with impaired renal function require smaller than usual maintenance doses of digoxin (see Administration and Dosage). Because of the prolonged elimination half-life, a longer period of time is required to achieve an initial or new steady-state serum concentration in patients with renal impairment than in patients with normal renal function. If appropriate care is not taken to reduce the dose of digoxin, such patients are at high risk for toxicity, and toxic effects will last longer in such patients than in patients with normal renal function.

➤*Hepatic function impairment:* Impaired hepatic function does not appear to significantly alter transformation or effects of digoxin.

➤*Elderly:* The majority of clinical experience gained with digoxin has been in the elderly population. This experience has not identified differences in response or adverse effects between the elderly and younger patients. However, this drug is known to be substantially excreted by the kidney, and the risk of toxic reactions to this drug may be greater in patients with impaired renal function. Because elderly patients are more likely to have decreased renal function, exercise care in dose selection based on renal function; monitor renal function.

➤*Pregnancy: Category C.* It is not known whether digoxin can cause fetal harm when administered to a pregnant woman or can affect reproductive capacity. Administer digoxin to a pregnant woman only if clearly needed and only if the benefit to the mother outweighs the risk to the fetus.

➤*Lactation:* Studies have shown that digoxin concentrations in the mother's serum and milk are similar. However, the estimated exposure of a nursing infant to digoxin via breastfeeding will be far below the usual infant maintenance dose. Therefore, this amount should have no pharmacologic effect upon the infant. Nevertheless, exercise caution when digoxin is administered to a nursing woman.

➤*Children:* Newborn infants display considerable variability in their tolerance to digoxin. Premature and immature infants are particularly sensitive to the effects of digoxin, and the dosage of the drug must not only be reduced but must be individualized according to their degree of maturity. Digitalis glycosides can cause poisoning in children due to accidental ingestion.

Precautions

➤*Electrolyte disorders:* In patients with hypokalemia or hypomagnesemia, toxicity may occur despite serum digoxin concentrations < 2 ng/mL, because potassium or magnesium depletion sensitizes the myocardium to digoxin. Therefore, it is desirable to maintain normal serum potassium and magnesium concentrations in patients being treated with digoxin. Deficiencies of these electrolytes may result from malnutrition, diarrhea, or prolonged vomiting, as well as the use of the following drugs or procedures: Diuretics, amphotericin B, corticosteroids, antacids, dialysis, mechanical suction of GI secretions.

Hypercalcemia from any cause predisposes the patient to digitalis toxicity. Calcium, particularly when administered rapidly by the IV route, may produce serious arrhythmias in digitalized patients. On the other hand, hypocalcemia can nullify the effects of digoxin in humans; thus, digoxin may be ineffective until serum calcium is restored to normal. These interactions are related to the fact that digoxin affects contractility and excitability of the heart in a manner similar to that of calcium.

➤*Thyroid disorders and hypermetabolic states:* Hypothyroidism may reduce the requirements for digoxin. Heart failure or atrial arrhythmias resulting from hypermetabolic or hyperdynamic states (eg, hyperthyroidism, hypoxia, arteriovenous shunt) are best treated by addressing the underlying condition. Atrial arrhythmias associated with hypermetabolic states are particularly resistant to digoxin treatment. Care must be taken to avoid toxicity if digoxin is used.

➤*Acute MI:* Use digoxin with caution in patients with acute MI. The use of inotropic drugs in some patients in this setting may result in undesirable increases in myocardial oxygen demand and ischemia.

➤*Electrical cardioversion:* It may be desirable to reduce the dose of digoxin for 1 to 2 days prior to electrical cardioversion of atrial fibrillation to avoid the induction of ventricular arrhythmias, but physicians must consider the consequences of increasing the ventricular response if digoxin is withdrawn. If digitalis toxicity is suspected, delay elective cardioversion. If it is not prudent to delay cardioversion, select the lowest possible energy level to avoid provoking ventricular arrhythmias.

➤*Lab test abnormalities:* Periodically assess serum electrolytes and renal function (serum creatinine concentrations); the frequency of assessments will depend on the clinical setting.

Drug Interactions

Because of the considerable variability of these interactions, individualize the dosage of digoxin when patients receive these medications concurrently. Furthermore, exercise caution when combining digoxin with any drug that may cause a significant deterioration in renal function, because a decline in glomerular filitration or tubular secretion may impair the excretion of digoxin.

➤*Increased digoxin serum levels:* The following agents may increase digoxin serum levels via various mechanisms (eg, altered GI flora, increased absorption, decreased clearance), possibly increasing its therapeutic and toxic effects:

Drugs That May Increase Digitalis Serum Levels	
Amiodarone	Macrolides
Benzodiazepines	(clarithromycin, erythromycin)
(alprazolam, diazepam)	Propafenone
Bepridil	Propantheline
Cyclosporine	Quinidine
Diphenoxylate	Quinine
Indomethacin	Spironolactone
Itraconazole	Tetracyclines
	Verapamil

➤*Decreased digitalis serum levels:* The following agents may decrease digitalis serum levels, possibly decreasing therapeutic effects:

Drugs That May Decrease Digitalis Serum Levels	
Aminoglycosides, oral	Colestipol
Antacids	Kaolin/pectin
(aluminum and magnesium containing)	Metoclopramide[1]
Antineoplastics, combination	Neomycin
(bleomycin, carmustine, cyclophosphamide,	Penicillamine
cytarabine, doxorubicin, methotrexate,	Rifampin
procarbazine, vincristine)[1]	St. John's wort
Charcoal, activated	Sulfasalazine
Cholestyramine[1]	

[1] The absorption of the gelatin capsule and elixir formulations of digoxin may not be affected to as great an extent.

DIGOXIN

Digoxin Drug Interactions			
Precipitant drug	Object drug*		Description
Beta blockers (eg, carvedilol)	Digoxin	↑	Although beta blockers and digoxin may be useful in combination to control atrial fibrillation, their additive effects on AV node conduction may result in advanced or complete heart block.
Calcium	Digoxin	↑	Calcium administered rapidly by the IV route may produce serious arrhythmias in digitalized patients.
Calcium channel blockers (eg, verapamil)	Digoxin	↑	Although calcium channel blockers and digoxin may be useful in combination to control atrial fibrillation, their additive effects on AV node conduction may result in advanced or complete heart block.
Succinylcholine	Digoxin	↑	Succinylcholine may cause a sudden extrusion of potassium from muscle cells, thereby causing arrhythmias in digitalized patients.
Sympathomimetics	Digoxin	↑	Concomitant use of digoxin and sympathomimetics increases the risk of cardiac arrhythmias.
Thiazide Diuretics, loop diuretics	Digoxin	↑	Diuretic-induced electrolyte disturbances may predispose to digitalis-induced arrhythmias. Measure plasma levels of potassium and magnesium and supplement low levels. Prevent further losses with dietary sodium restriction or potassium-sparing diuretics.
Thyroid hormones	Digoxin	↓	Thyroid administration to a digitalized, hypothyroid patient may increase the dose requirement of digoxin

* ↑ = Object drug increased. ↓ = Object drug decreased.

➤*Drug/Lab test interactions:* The use of therapeutic doses of digoxin may cause prolongation of the PR interval and depression of the ST segment on the electrocardiogram. Digoxin may produce false positive ST-T changes on the electrocardiogram during exercise testing. These electophysiologic effects reflect an expected effect of the drug and are not indicative of toxicity.

➤*Drug/Food interactions:* When digoxin tablets are taken after meals, the rate of absorption is slowed but total amount absorbed is usually unchanged. However, when taken with meals high in bran fiber, the amount absorbed may be reduced.

Adverse Reactions

Digoxin adverse reactions are dose-dependent and occur at doses higher than those needed to achieve a therapeutic effect. Hence, adverse reactions are less common when digoxin is used within the recommended dose range or therapeutic serum concentration range and when there is careful attention to concurrent medications and conditions.

Because some patients may be particularly susceptible to side effects with digoxin, always select the dosage of the drug carefully and adjust as the clinical condition of the patient warrants. In the past, when high doses of digoxin were used and little attention was paid to clinical status or concurrent medications, adverse reactions to digoxin were more frequent and severe. Cardiac adverse reactions accounted for ≈ ½, GI disturbances for ≈ ¼, and CNS and other toxicity for ≈ ¼ of these adverse reactions. However, available evidence suggests that the incidence and severity of digoxin toxicity has decreased substantially in recent years.

The following table summarizes the incidence of those adverse experiences for patients treated with digoxin tablets or placebo from 2 randomized, double-blind, placebo-controlled withdrawal trials. Patients in these trials were also receiving diuretics with or without angiotensin-converting enzyme inhibitors. These patients had been stable on digoxin and were randomized to digoxin or placebo. The results reflect the experience in patients following dosage titration with the use of serum digoxin concentrations and careful follow-up.

Digoxin Adverse Experiences		
Adverse event	Digoxin (n = 123)	Placebo (n = 125)
Cardiovascular		
Palpitation	1	4
Ventricular extrasystole	1	1
Tachycardia	2	1
Heart arrest	1	1

Digoxin Adverse Experiences		
Adverse event	Digoxin (n = 123)	Placebo (n = 125)
CNS		
Headache	4	4
Dizziness	6	5
Mental disturbances	5	1
GI		
Anorexia	1	4
Nausea	4	2
Vomiting	2	1
Diarrhea	4	1
Abdominal pain	0	6
Miscellaneous		
Rash	2	1
Death	4	3

➤*Cardiovascular:* Therapeutic doses of digoxin may cause heart block in patients with pre-existing sinoatrial or AV conduction disorders; avoid heart block by adjusting the dose of digoxin. Prophylactic use of a cardiac pacemaker may be considered if the risk of heart block is considered unacceptable. High doses of digoxin may produce a variety of rhythm disturbances, such as first-degree, second-degree (Wenkebach), or third-degree heart block (including asystole); atrial tachycardia with block; AV dissociation; accelerated junctional (nodal) rhythm; unifocal or multiform ventricular premature contractions (especially bigeminy or trigeminy); ventricular tachycardia; and ventricular fibrillation. Digoxin produces PR prolongation and ST segment depression that should not by themselves be considered digoxin toxicity. Cardiac toxicity can also occur at therapeutic doses in patients who have conditions that may alter their sensitivity to digoxin.

➤*CNS:* Visual disturbanes (blurred or yellow vision); headache; weakness; dizziness; apathy; confusion; mental disturbances (eg, anxiety, depression, delirium, hallucination).

➤*GI:* Anorexia; nausea; vomiting; diarrhea. Rarely, the use of digoxin has been associated with abdominal pain; intestinal ischemia; hemorrhagic necrosis of the intestines.

➤*Miscellaneous:* Gynecomastia has been occasionally observed following the prolonged use of digoxin. Thrombocytopenia and maculopapular rash and other skin reactions (rare).

Infants and children – The side effects of digoxin in infants and children differ from those seen in adults in several respects. Although digoxin may produce anorexia, nausea, vomiting, diarrhea, and CNS disturbances in young patients, these are rarely the initial symptoms of overdosage. Rather, the earliest and most frequent manifestation of excessive dosing with digoxin in infants and children is the appearance of cardiac arrhythmias, including sinus bradycardia. In children, the use of digoxin may produce any arrhythmia. The most common are conduction disturbances or supraventricular tachyarrhythmias, such as atrial tachycardia (with or without block) and junctional (nodal) tachycardia. Ventricular arrhythmias are less common. Sinus bradycardia may be a sign of impending digoxin intoxication, especially in infants, even in the absence of first-degree heart block. Assume any arrhythmia or alteration in cardiac conduction that develops in a child taking digoxin to be caused by digoxin until further evaluation proves otherwise.

Overdosage

➤*Symptoms:* Manifestations of life-threatening toxicity include ventricular tachycardia or ventricular fibrillation, or progressive bradyarrhythmias, or heart block. The administration of > 10 mg of digoxin in a previously healthy adult, > 4 mg in a previously healthy child, or a steady-state serum concentration> 10 ng/mL often results in cardiac arrest.

➤*Treatment:* Temporarily discontinue digoxin until the adverse reaction resolves. Correct factors that may contribute to the adverse reaction (eg, electrolyte disturbances, concurrent medications). Once the adverse reaction has resolved, therapy with digoxin may be reinstituted, following a careful reassessment of dose. Withdrawal of digoxin may be all that is required to treat the adverse reaction. However, when the primary manifestation of digoxin overdosage is a cardiac arrhythmia, additional therapy may be needed.

If the rhythm disturbance is a symptomatic bradyarrhythmia or heart block, consideration should be given to the reversal of toxicity with digoxin immune fab (ovine) (see below), the use of atropine, or the insertion of a temporary cardiac pacemaker. However, asymptomatic bradycardia or heart block related to digoxin may require only temporary withdrawal of the drug and cardiac monitoring of the patient.

If the rhythm disturbance is a ventricular arrhythmia, consider the correction of electrolyte disorders, particularly if hypokalemia (see below) or hypomagnesemia is present. Digoxin immune fab is a specific antidote for digoxin and may be used to reverse potentially life-threatening ventricular arrhythmias because digoxin overdosage.

DIGOXIN

Potassium administration – Maintain the serum potassium concentration between 4 and 5.5 mmol/L. Potassium is usually administered orally, but when correction of the arrhythmia is urgent and the serum potassium concentration is low, potassium may be administered cautiously by the IV route. Monitor the electrocardiogram for any evidence of potassium toxicity (eg, peaking of T waves) and to observe the effect on the arrhythmia. Potassium salts may be dangerous in patients who manifest bradycardia or heart block due to digoxin (unless primarily related to supraventricular tachycardia) and in the setting of massive digitalis overdosage.

Use digoxin immune fab to reverse the toxic effects of ingestion of a massive overdose. The decision to administer digoxin immune fab to a patient who has ingested a massive dose of digoxin but who has not yet manifested life-threatening toxicity should depend on the likelihood that life-threatening toxicity will occur (see above).

Patients with massive digitalis ingestion should receive large doses of activated charcoal to prevent absorption and bind digoxin in the gut during enteroenteric recirculation. Emesis or gastric lavage may be indicated especially if ingestion has occurred within 30 minutes of the patient's presentation at the hospital. Do not induce emesis in patients who are obtunded. If a patient presents > 2 hours after ingestion or already has toxic manifestations, it may be unsafe to induce vomiting or attempt passage of a gastric tube because such maneuvers may induce an acute vagal episode that can worsen digitalis-related arrhythmias.

Severe digitalis intoxication can cause a massive shift of potassium from inside to outside the cell, leading to life-threatening hyperkalemia. Avoid the administration of potassium supplements in the setting of massive intoxication. Hyperkalemia caused by massive digitalis toxicity is best treated with digoxin immune fab; initial treatment with glucose and insulin may also be required if hyperkalemia itself is acutely life-threatening.

INAMRINONE LACTATE

Rx	Inamrinone Lactate (Abbott Hospital)	Injection: 5 mg/mL (as lactate)	In 20 mL amps.[1]

[1] With 0.25 mg/mL sodium metabisulfite.

Indications

➤*Congestive heart failure (CHF):* For the short-term management of CHF. Use only in patients who can be closely monitored and who have not responded adequately to digitalis, diuretics or vasodilators. Duration of therapy depends on patient responsiveness.

Administration and Dosage

➤*Approved by the FDA:* July 1984.

Administer as supplied or dilute in 0.5% or 0.9% saline solution to a concentration of 1 to 3 mg/mL. Use diluted solutions within 24 hours.

➤*Initial therapy:* 0.75 mg/kg IV bolus slowly over 2 to 3 minutes.

➤*Maintenance infusion:* 5 to 10 mcg/kg/min.

An additional bolus of 0.75 mg/kg may be given 30 minutes after initiating therapy.

Do not exceed a total daily dose (including loading doses) of 10 mg/kg. A limited number of patients studied at higher doses support a dosage regimen of up to 18 mg/kg/day for shortened durations of therapy.

Adjust rate of administration and duration of therapy according to patient response.

Above dosing regimen creates a plasma concentration of ≈ 3 mcg/mL.

➤*Admixture incompatibilities:*

Dextrose solution – A chemical interaction occurs slowly over a 24-hour period when inamrinone is mixed directly with dextrose-containing solutions. Therefore, do not dilute with dextrose-containing solutions prior to injection. Inamrinone may be injected into a running dextrose infusion through a Y-connector or directly into the tubing where preferable.

Furosemide – When furosemide is injected into an IV line of inamrinone infusion, a precipitate immediately forms. Do not administer furosemide in IV lines containing inamrinone.

➤*Storage/Stability:* Protect ampules from light. Store at room temperature.

Actions

➤*Pharmacology:* Inamrinone is a positive inotropic agent with vasodilator activity, different in structure and mode of action from either digitalis glycosides or catecholamines. Its mechanism has not been fully elucidated.

Inamrinone is not a beta-adrenergic agonist. It inhibits myocardial cyclic adenosine monophosphate (cAMP) phosphodiesterase activity and increases cellular levels of cAMP. It does not inhibit sodium-potassium ATPase activity.

Inamrinone reduces afterload and preload by its direct relaxant effect on vascular smooth muscle. In patients with depressed myocardial function, inamrinone produces a prompt increase in cardiac output due to its inotropic and vasodilator actions.

Improvement in left ventricular function and relief of congestive heart failure (CHF) in patients with ischemic heart disease have been observed without inducing symptoms or electrocardiographic signs of myocardial ischemia.

Inamrinone produces hemodynamic and symptomatic benefits to patients not satisfactorily controlled by conventional therapy with diuretics and cardiac glycosides.

➤*Pharmacokinetics:*

Distribution – Inamrinone has a volume of distribution of 1.2 L/kg and a distribution half-life of ≈ 4.6 minutes. It is 10% to 49% protein bound. In CHF patients, after a loading bolus dose, steady-state plasma levels of ≈ 2.4 mcg/mL are maintained by an infusion of 5 to 10 mcg/kg/min. With associated compromised renal and hepatic perfusion, plasma levels may rise.

Metabolism/Excretion – Inamrinone is metabolized by conjugative pathways. Mean elimination half-life is ≈ 3.6 hours. In patients with CHF, the mean elimination half-life is ≈ 5.8 hours (range, 3 to 15 hours).

The primary route of excretion is via the urine as both inamrinone and metabolites. Approximately 63% of an oral dose is excreted in the urine over 96 hours. Approximately 18% is excreted in the feces in 72 hours. In a 24-hour IV inamrinone study, 10% to 40% was excreted unchanged in the urine.

Onset/Duration/Effect – Dose-related maximum increases in cardiac output occur; the peak effect occurs within 10 minutes at all doses. The duration of effect depends upon the dose, lasting ≈ 30 minutes at 0.75 mg/kg and ≈ 2 hours at 3 mg/kg. Increases in cardiac index show a linear relationship to plasma concentration.

Pulmonary capillary wedge pressure (PCWP) and total peripheral resistance show dose-related decreases. At doses up to 3 mg/kg, dose-related decreases in dia-stolic pressure (up to 13%) have been observed.

Mean arterial pressure decreases (9.7%) at a dose of 3 mg/kg. Heart rate is generally unchanged.

Children – Infants and children have a larger volume of distribution and a decreased elimination half-life.

Contraindications

Hypersensitivity to inamrinone or bisulfites.

Warnings

➤*Atrial flutter/fibrillation:* Inamrinone's inotropic effects are additive to those of digitalis. In cases of atrial flutter/fibrillation, inamrinone may increase ventricular response rate because of its slight enhancement of atrioventricular (AV) conduction. In these cases, prior treatment with digitalis is recommended.

➤*Hepatotoxicity:* If acute marked alterations in liver enzymes occur together with clinical symptoms, discontinue inamrinone. If less than marked enzyme alterations occur without clinical symptoms, continue inamrinone, reduce dosage or discontinue the drug based on benefit-to-risk considerations.

➤*Hypersensitivity reactions:* Hypersensitivity occurred in patients treated for ≈ 2 weeks with oral inamrinone (see Adverse Reactions). Consider hypersensitivity reactions in any patient maintained for a prolonged period on inamrinone. Refer to Management of Acute Hypersensitivity Reactions.

➤*Carcinogenesis:* Dystocia occurred in rats receiving 100 mg/kg/day, resulting in increased numbers of stillbirths, decreased litter size and poor pup survival.

➤*Pregnancy: Category C.* Animal studies (15 to 50 mg/kg) are conflicting. There are no adequate and well controlled studies in pregnant women. Use during pregnancy only if the potential benefit justifies the potential risk to the fetus.

➤*Lactation:* It is not known whether inamrinone is secreted in breast milk. Exercise caution when administering to nursing women.

➤*Children:* Safety and efficacy in children have not been established. In preterm infants, short-term use of inamrinone (5 mcg/kg/min) was effective in the management of CHF (see Pharmacokinetics).

Precautions

➤*Aortic or pulmonic valvular disease:* Do not use inamrinone in patients with severe aortic or pulmonic valvular disease in lieu of surgical relief of the obstruction. It may aggravate outflow tract obstruction in hypertrophic subaortic stenosis.

➤*Arrhythmias:* Supraventricular and ventricular arrhythmias have been observed in the very high-risk population treated. While inamrinone per se is not arrhythmogenic, the potential for arrhythmia present in CHF itself may be increased by any drug or drug combination.

➤*Thrombocytopenia:* Thrombocytopenia is more common in patients receiving prolonged therapy. In patients whose platelet counts were not allowed to remain depressed, no bleeding occurred.

Platelet reduction is dose-dependent and appears to be due to a decreased platelet survival time. Bone marrow examinations were normal. There is no evidence of immune response or a platelet-activating factor.

➤*Management of adverse reactions:*

Platelet count reductions – Asymptomatic platelet count reduction (to < 150,000/mm^3) may be reversed within 1 week of a decrease in drug dosage. Further, with no change in drug dosage, the count may stabilize at lower than pre-drug levels without any clinical sequelae. Pre-drug platelet counts and frequent platelet counts during therapy are recommended. If a platelet count < 150,000/mm^3 occurs, consider the following:

• Maintain total daily dose unchanged.
• Decrease total daily dose.
• Discontinue if risk exceeds the potential benefit.

➤*Acute myocardial infarction:* No clinical trials have been carried out in patients in the acute phase of postmyocardial infarction. Therefore, inamrinone is not recommended in these cases.

➤*Fluid balance:* Patients who have received vigorous diuretic therapy may have insufficient cardiac filling pressure to respond adequately to inamrinone; cautious liberalization of fluid and electrolyte intake may be indicated.

➤*Monitoring:*

Fluids and electrolytes – Monitor fluid and electrolyte changes and renal function during inamrinone therapy; improvement in cardiac output with resultant diuresis may necessitate a reduction in the dose of diuretic. Potassium loss due to excessive diuresis may predispose digitalized patients to arrhythmias. Therefore, correct hypokalemia by potassium supplementation in advance of or during inamrinone use.

Blood pressure and heart rate: Monitor blood pressure and heart rate and slow or stop the infusion rate in patients showing excessive decreases in blood pressure.

INAMRINONE LACTATE

Central venous pressure (CVP): Monitoring CVP may be valuable in assessing hypotension and fluid balance management. Also, measure urine output and body weight.

➤*Sulfite sensitivity:* This product contains sodium metabisulfite, a sulfite that may cause allergic-type reactions (including anaphylactic symptoms and life-threatening or less severe asthmatic episodes) in certain susceptible people. The overall prevalence of sulfite sensitivity in the general population is unknown and probably low. Sulfite sensitivity is seen more frequently in asthmatic people.

Adverse Reactions

➤*Cardiovascular:* Arrhythmia (3%); hypotension (1.3%).

➤*GI:* Nausea (1.7%); vomiting (0.9%); abdominal pain, anorexia (0.4%); hepatotoxicity (see Warnings). Should severe or debilitating GI effects occur, reduce dosage or discontinue the drug based on the usual benefit-to-risk considerations.

➤*Hypersensitivity:* Pericarditis, pleuritis and ascites (fatal in 1 case), myositis with interstitial shadowing on chest x–ray and elevated sedimentation rate (1 case) and vasculitis with nodular pulmonary densities, hypoxemia and jaundice with oral inamrinone (see Warnings).

➤*Miscellaneous:* Thrombocytopenia (< 100,000/mm^3) (2.4%); fever (0.9%); chest pain (0.2%); burning at the injection site (0.2%).

Overdosage

A death has occurred with a massive accidental overdose, although the causal relationship is uncertain. Exercise diligence during product preparation and administration.

Inamrinone's vasodilator effect may produce hypotension. If this occurs, reduce or discontinue administration. Institute general measures for circulatory support. Refer to Management of Acute Overdosage.

MILRINONE LACTATE

Rx	Milrinone Lactate (Bedford)	Injection: 1 mg/mL	47 mg/mL dextrose. In 10, 20, and 50 mL single-dose vials.
Rx	Primacor (Sanofi Winthrop)		47 mg anhydrous dextrose. In 10 and 20 mL single-dose vials.
Rx	Primacor (Sanofi Winthrop)	Injection, premixed: 200 mcg/mL in 5% Dextrose Injection[1]	In 100 mL.

[1] With 0.282 mg/mL lactic acid.

Indications

➤*Congestive heart failure (CHF):* Short-term IV therapy. The majority of experience has been in patients receiving digoxin and diuretics.

Administration and Dosage

➤*Approved by the FDA:* December 1987.

Administer with a loading dose followed by a continuous infusion (maintenance dose) according to the following guidelines. Adjust the infusion rate according to hemodynamic and clinical response. Most patients show an improvement in hemodynamic status as evidenced by increases in cardiac output and reductions in pulmonary capillary wedge pressure.

Milrinone Dosing		
Loading dose 50 mcg/kg: Administer slowly over 10 minutes		
Maintenance dose[1]		
	Infusion rate	Total daily dose (24 hours)
Minimum	0.375 mcg/kg/min	0.59 mg/kg
Standard	0.5 mcg/kg/min	0.77 mg/kg
Maximum	0.75 mcg/kg/min	1.13 mg/kg

[1] Administer as a continuous IV infusion.

Milrinone Rates of Infusion (mL/kg/hr)[1]			
Maintenance dose	Concentration		
Milrinone (mcg/kg/min)	100 mcg/mL[2]	150 mcg/mL[3]	200 mcg/mL[4]
0.375	0.22	0.15	0.11
0.4	0.24	0.16	0.12
0.5	0.3	0.2	0.15
0.6	0.36	0.24	0.18
0.7	0.42	0.28	0.21
0.75	0.45	0.3	0.22

[1] In order to calculate flow rate (mL/hr), multiply infusion delivery rate times patient weight (in kg).
[2] Prepare by adding 180 mL diluent per 20 mg vial (20 mL).
[3] Prepare by adding 113 mL diluent per 20 mg vial (20 mL).
[4] Prepare by adding 80 mL diluent per 20 mg vial (20 mL).

➤*Dilution:* Dilute with 0.45% or 0.9% Sodium Chloride Injection or 5% Dextrose Injection only.

➤*Renal function impairment:* Presence of renal impairment significantly increases the terminal elimination half-life of milrinone. Reductions in infusion rate may be necessary. For patients with clinical evidence of renal impairment, use the following table.

Milrinone Infusion Rate in Impaired Renal Function	
Creatinine clearance (mL/min/1.73 m^2)	Infusion rate (mcg/kg/min)
50	0.43
40	0.38
30	0.33
20	0.28
10	0.23
5	0.2

Dosage may be titrated to the maximum hemodynamic effect and should not exceed 1.13 mg/kg/day. Duration of therapy should depend on patient responsiveness.

➤*Admixture incompatibility:* There is an immediate chemical interaction which is evidenced by the formation of a precipitate when furosemide is injected into an IV line of an infusion of milrinone.

➤*Storage/Stability:* Store at room temperature 15° to 30°C (59° to 86°F).

Actions

➤*Pharmacology:* Milrinone is a member of a new class of bipyridine inotropic/vasodilator agents with phosphodiesterase inhibitor activity. It is a positive inotrope and vasodilator, with little chronotropic activity, different in structure and mode of action from either the digitalis glycosides or catecholamines.

At relevant inotropic and vasorelaxant concentrations, milrinone is a selective inhibitor of peak III cAMP phosphodiesterase isozyme in cardiac and vascular muscle. This inhibitory action is consistent with cAMP-mediated increases in intracellular ionized calcium and contractile force in cardiac muscle, as well as with cAMP-dependent contractile protein phosphorylation and relaxation in vascular muscle. Additional experimental evidence indicates that milrinone is not a beta-adrenergic agonist nor does it inhibit sodium-potassium adenosine triphosphatase activity as do the digitalis glycosides.

In patients with CHF milrinone produces dose-related and plasma drug concentration-related increases in the maximum rate of increase of left ventricular pressure. Milrinone has a direct inotropic effect and direct arterial vasodilator activity. Both the inotropic and vasodilatory effects occur over the therapeutic range of plasma concentrations of 100 to 300 ng/mL. In addition to increasing myocardial contractility, milrinone improves diastolic function as evidenced by improvements in left ventricular diastolic relaxation.

In patients with depressed myocardial function, milrinone produced a prompt increase in cardiac output and decreases in pulmonary capillary wedge pressure and vascular resistance, without a significant increase in heart rate or myocardial oxygen consumption. These hemodynamic improvements were dose and plasma concentration related. Hemodynamic improvement during IV therapy was accompanied by clinical symptomatic improvement. The great majority of patients experience improvements in hemodynamic function within 5 to 15 minutes of the initiation of therapy.

In CHF patients, milrinone (administered as a loading injection followed by a maintenance infusion) produced significant mean initial increases in cardiac index, significant decreases in pulmonary capillary wedge pressure and significant decreases in systemic vascular resistance. The heart rate was generally unchanged. Mean arterial pressure fell by up to 5% at the two lower dose regimens, but by 17% at the highest dose. Patients evaluated for 48 hours maintained improvements in hemodynamic function, with no evidence of diminished response (tachyphylaxis). A smaller number of patients have received infusions for periods up to 72 hours without evidence of tachyphylaxis.

The duration of therapy should depend on patient responsiveness. Patients have been maintained on infusions for up to 5 days.

Milrinone has a favorable inotropic effect in fully digitalized patients without causing signs of glycoside toxicity. Theoretically, in cases of atrial flutter/fibrillation, it is possible that milrinone may increase ventricular response rate because of its slight enhancement of AV node conduction. In these cases, consider digitalis prior to the institution of therapy.

MILRINONE LACTATE

Improvement in left ventricular function in patients with ischemic heart disease has occurred. The improvement has occurred without inducing symptoms or ECG signs of myocardial ischemia.

➤*Pharmacokinetics:* Steady-state plasma concentrations after ≈ 6 to 12 hours of unchanging maintenance infusion of 0.5 mcg/kg/min are ≈ 200 ng/mL. Near maximum favorable effects on cardiac output and pulmonary capillary wedge pressure are seen at plasma concentrations in the 150 to 250 ng/mL range. Following IV injections of 12.5 to 125 mcg/kg to CHF patients, milrinone had a volume of distribution of 0.38 L/kg, a mean terminal elimination half-life of 2.3 hours and a clearance of 0.13 L/kg/hr. Following IV infusions of 0.2 to 0.7 mcg/kg/min to CHF patients, the drug had a volume of distribution of about 0.45 L/kg, a mean terminal elimination half-life of 2.4 hours and a clearance of 0.14 L/kg/hr. These pharmacokinetic parameters were not dose-dependent, and the area under the plasma concentration vs time curve following injections was significantly dose-dependent. Milrinone is ≈ 70% bound to plasma protein.

The primary route of excretion is via the urine. The major urinary excretions of orally administered milrinone are milrinone (83%) and its 0-glucuronide metabolite (12%). Elimination in healthy subjects via the urine is rapid, with ≈ 60% recovered within the first 2 hours following dosing and ≈ 90% recovered within the first 8 hours following dosing. The mean renal clearance is ≈ 0.3 L/min, indicative of active secretion.

➤*Clinical trials:*

Oral – In a single, multicenter, double-blind trial of the chronic administration of oral milrinone, patients with New York Heart Association (NYHA) class III and IV heart failure and left ventricular ejection fraction of < 35% were randomized to placebo (n = 527) or oral milrinone (40 mg daily, n = 561) and followed for a median of 6 months. Statistically, the oral milrinone treatment group significantly increased all-cause mortality and cardiovascular mortality. This finding in patients on oral milrinone was not apparent during the initial period of chronic treatment (15 days) in either the overall patient population or in the NYHA class IV subgroup.

IV – The acute administration of IV milrinone has been evaluated in clinical trials in > 1600 patients with chronic heart failure, heart failure associated with cardiac surgery and heart failure associated with myocardial infarction. The total number of deaths, either on therapy or shortly thereafter (24 hours) was 15 (< 9%), few of which were thought to be drug-related.

Contraindications

Hypersensitivity to the drug.

Warnings

➤*Life-threatening arrhythmias:* Life-threatening arrhythmias were infrequent and, when present, these have been associated with certain underlying factors such as preexisting arrhythmias, metabolic abnormalities (eg, hypokalemia), abnormal digoxin levels and catheter insertion. Supraventricular arrhythmias occurred in 3.8% of the patients; the incidence of both supraventricular and ventricular arrhythmias has not been related to the dose or plasma milrinone concentration.

➤*Elderly:* There are no special dosage recommendations for the elderly patient. Patients in all age groups demonstrated clinically and statistically significant responses. No age-related effects on the incidence of adverse reactions have been observed. Controlled pharmacokinetic studies have not disclosed any age-related effects on the distribution and elimination of milrinone.

➤*Pregnancy: Category C.* An increased resorption rate was apparent at both 8 and 12 mg/kg/day doses of IV milrinone in pregnant rabbits. There are no adequate and well controlled studies in pregnant women. Use during pregnancy only if the potential benefit justifies the potential risk to the fetus.

➤*Lactation:* It is not known whether milrinone is excreted in breast milk. Exercise caution when milrinone is administered to nursing women.

➤*Children:* Safety and efficacy have not been established.

Precautions

➤*Monitoring:*

Electrolytes – Carefully monitor fluid and electrolyte changes and renal function during therapy. Improvement in cardiac output with resultant diuresis may necessitate a reduction in the dose of diuretic. Potassium loss due to excessive diuresis may predispose digitalized patients to arrhythmias. Therefore, correct hypokalemia by potassium supplementation in advance of or during use of milrinone.

Blood pressure and heart rate – During therapy monitor blood pressure and heart rate, and slow or stop the rate of infusion in patients showing excessive decreases in blood pressure. If prior vigorous diuretic therapy is suspected to have caused significant decreases in cardiac filling pressure, cautiously administer milrinone with monitoring of blood pressure, heart rate and clinical symptomatology.

➤*Cardiovascular effects:*

Obstructive aortic or pulmonic valvular disease – Do not use with severe obstructive aortic or pulmonic valvular disease in lieu of surgical relief of the obstruction. Like other inotropic agents, it may aggravate outflow tract obstruction in hypertrophic subaortic stenosis.

Supraventricular and ventricular arrhythmias – Both have occurred in the high-risk population treated. In some patients, IV and oral milrinone have increased ventricular ectopy, including nonsustained ventricular tachycardia. The potential for arrhythmia, present in CHF itself, may be increased by many drugs or combinations of drugs. Closely monitor patients receiving milrinone during infusion.

Atrial flutter/fibrillation – Milrinone produces a slight shortening of AV node conduction time, indicating a potential for an increased ventricular response rate in patients with atrial flutter/fibrillation which is not controlled with digitalis therapy.

Adverse Reactions

➤*Cardiovascular:* Ventricular arrhythmias (12.1%), including ventricular ectopic activity (8.5%); hypotension (2.9%); nonsustained ventricular tachycardia (2.8%); angina/chest pain (1.2%); sustained ventricular tachycardia (1%); ventricular fibrillation (0.2%).

➤*Miscellaneous:* Headaches, usually mild to moderate in severity (2.9%); hypokalemia (0.6%); tremors, thrombocytopenia (0.4%); bronchospasm (rare).

Overdosage

Doses of milrinone may produce hypotension because of the vasodilator effects. If this occurs, reduce or temporarily discontinue administration of milrinone until the patient's condition stabilizes. No specific antidote is known, but use general measures for circulatory support. Refer to General Management of Acute Overdosage.

Optimal therapy of cardiac arrhythmias requires documentation, accurate diagnosis and modification of precipitating causes, and if indicated, proper selection and use of antiarrhythmic drugs. Comprehensive information on individual agents is presented in the following monographs.

These drugs are classified according to their effects on the action potential of cardiac cells and their presumed mechanism of action. Although drugs within the same group are similar, that does not imply that another agent within the group would not be more effective or safer in an individual patient.

➤Group I: Local anesthetics or membrane-stabilizing agents that depress phase 0.

IA (quinidine, procainamide, disopyramide) – Depress phase 0 and prolong the action potential duration.

IB (tocainide, lidocaine, phenytoin, mexiletine) – Depress phase 0 slightly and may shorten the action potential duration. Although arrhythmia is not a labeled indication for phenytoin, it is commonly used in treatment of digitalis-induced arrhythmias.

IC (flecainide, propafenone) – Marked depression of phase 0. Slight effect on repolarization. Profound slowing of conduction.

Moricizine – A Group I agent that shares some of the characteristics of the Group IA, B and C agents.

➤Group II (propranolol, esmolol, acebutolol): Depress phase 4 depolarization.

➤Group III (bretylium, amiodarone, sotalol): Produce a prolongation of phase 3 (repolarization).

➤Group IV (verapamil): Depresses phase 4 depolarization and lengthen phases 1 and 2 of repolarization.

➤Digitalis glycosides (digoxin): Causes a decrease in maximal diastolic potential and action potential duration and increases the slope of phase 4 depolarization.

➤Adenosine: Adenosine slows conduction time through the AV node and can interrupt the reentry pathways through the AV node.

➤Serum drug levels: Some antiarrhythmic drugs (eg, quinidine) can produce toxic effects that can be easily confused with the symptoms for which the drug has been prescribed. Drug serum levels are important in evaluating toxic or subtherapeutic dosage regimens of most antiarrhythmic drugs. They also aid in monitoring active metabolites (eg, procainamide/NAPA), suspected drug interactions and subtherapeutic response due to drug failure, noncompliance, altered clearance or altered absorption.

➤Proarrhythmic effects: Antiarrhythmic agents may cause new or worsened arrhythmias. Such proarrhythmic effects range from an increase in frequency of PVCs to the development of more severe ventricular tachycardia, ventricular fibrillation or torsade de pointes (ie, tachycardia that is more sustained or more rapid), which may lead to death. It is often not possible to distinguish a proarrhythmic effect from the patient's underlying rhythm disorder. It is therefore essential that each patient be evaluated electrocardiographically and clinically prior to and during therapy to determine whether the response to the drug supports continued treatment.

➤Cardiac Arrhythmia Suppression Trial: In the National Heart, Lung and Blood Institute's Cardiac Arrhythmia Suppression Trial (CAST), a long-term, multicenter, randomized, double-blind study in patients with asymptomatic non-life-threatening ventricular ectopy who had had a myocardial infarction (MI) > 6 days but < 2 years previously, and who demonstrated mild to moderate left ventricular dysfunction, an excessive mortality or non-fatal cardiac arrest rate was seen in patients treated with encainide or flecainide (56/730) compared with that seen in patients assigned to carefully matched placebo treated groups (22/725). This led to discontinuation of those two arms of the trial. In this study, the average duration of treatment with flecainide was 10 months.

The moricizine and placebo arms of the trial were continued in CAST II. In this randomized, double-blind trial, patients with asymptomatic non-life-threatening arrhythmias who had had an MI within 4 to 90 days and left ventricular ejection fraction ≤ 0.4 prior to enrollment were evaluated. The average duration of moricizine treatment was 18 months. The study was discontinued because there was no possibility of demonstrating a benefit toward improved survival with moricizine and because of an evolving adverse trend after long-term treatment.

The applicability of these results to other populations (eg, those without recent MI) and to other antiarrhythmic drugs is uncertain, but at present it is prudent (1) to consider any IC agent (especially one documented to provoke new serious arrhythmias) to have a similar risk and (2) to consider the risks of Class IC agents, coupled with the lack of any evidence of improved survival, generally unacceptable in patients without life-threatening ventricular arrhythmias, even if the patients are experiencing unpleasant, but not life-threatening symptoms or signs.

➤Pharmacokinetics: The information in the pharmacokinetics table with clinical data and observation can be a valuable tool. However, the information must be used rationally and the data obtained properly (ie, obtaining and analyzing serum level data) to be effective. See individual monographs for more detailed explanations.

Antiarrhythmic Electrophysiology/Electrocardiogram Effects

Group	Drug	Automaticity: SA node	Automaticity: Ectopic pacemaker	Conduction velocity: Atrium	Conduction velocity: AV node	Conduction velocity: His-Purkinje	Refractory period: Atrium	Refractory period: AV node	Refractory period: His-Purkinje	Refractory period: Ventricle	Refractory period: Accessory pathways[2]	ECG: Heart rate	ECG: PR interval	ECG: QRS complex	ECG: QTc interval	ECG: JT interval
I	Moricizine[3]	0	↓	0	↓	↓	±	0	0	0-↑	↑	0-↑	↑	↑	0	↓
	Quinidine	±	↓	↓	±	↓	↑↑	0-↑[4]	↑↑	↑	↑	±	±	↑	↑	↑
	Procainamide	±	↓	↓	±	↓	↑	0-↑[4]	↑↑	↑	↑↑	±	±	↑	↑	↑
	Disopyramide	±	↓	↓	±	↓	↑↑	0-↑[4]	↑↑	↑	↑	±	±	↑	↑	↑
	Lidocaine	0	↓	—	0	0	±	±	±	↑-↓	0	0	0	0	0-↓	0
	Phenytoin	↓-0	↓	—	0	0	±	±	±	—	0	0	0-↓	0	↓	0
	Tocainide	0-↓	↓	0	0	0	↓	↓	±	↓	↑	0	0	0	0-↓	0
	Mexiletine	↓	↓	0	0	0	±	↑	↑	↑	-	0	0	0	0	0
	Flecainide	↓	↓	↓↓	↓	↓↓	0	0	↑	↑	↑↑	0	↑[5]	↑↑[5]	0-↑[5]	
	Propafenone	0	↓	0	↓	↓	0	↑	↑	↑	↑	0	↑[5]	↑↑[5]	0-↑[5]	
II	Propranolol	↓	↓	±	↓	0-↓	±	↑	0	0	0-↑	↓	0-↑	0	0-↓	↓
	Esmolol	↓	↓	±	0-	±	↑	0	0	0-↑	↓	0-↑	0	0-↓	0	
	Acebutolol	↓	↓	±	↓	0	±	↑	0	0	0-↑	↓	0-↑	0	0-↓	↓
III	Bretylium	↑	↑	0	0	0-↑	0	↓-↑[6]	↑	0-↑	±	0	0	0	0	↑
	Amiodarone	↓	↓	↓	↓	↓	↑	↑	↑	↑	↑	↓	↑	↑	↑↑	↑↑
	Sotalol[7]	↓	↓	0	↓	0	↑↑	↑	↑↑	↑↑	↑	↓	↑	0	↑↑	↑↑
IV	Verapamil	↓	↓	0	↓	0	0	↑	0	0	0	↓	↑	0	0	0
—	Digoxin	0-↓	↑	±	↓	0-↓	±	↑	0	↓	↓-↑	↓	↑	0	↓	↓
—	Adenosine	↓	↓	0	↓	0	0	↑	0	0	0	↑	↑	0	0	↓

[1] These values assume therapeutic levels.
[2] Accessory pathways occur in Wolff-Parkinson-White syndrome (preexcitation phenomena) and possibly other abnormal conditions.
[3] Does not belong to any of the 3 subclasses (A, B or C), but does have some properties of each.
[4] Retrograde AV node RP↑; antegrade RP not affected.
[5] Dose-related increases.
[6] Due to a complex balance of direct and indirect autonomic effects.
[7] Has both Group II (beta blocking) and III properties; Class III effects are seen at doses > 160 mg.

Antiarrhythmic Pharmacokinetics

Group	Antiarrhythmic Drug	Onset (hrs) (oral)[1]	Duration (hrs)	Half-life (hrs)	Protein binding (%)	Excreted unchanged (%)	Therapeutic serum level (mcg/mL)	Toxic serum levels (mcg/mL)
I A	Moricizine	2	10-24	1.5-3.5[2]	95	< 1	Not applicable	—
	Quinidine	0.5	6-8	6-7	80-90	10-50	2-6	> 8
	Procainamide	0.5	3+	2.5-4.7	14-23	40-70	4-8	> 16
	Disopyramide	0.5	6-7	4-10	20-60[3]	40-60	2-8	> 9
I B	Lidocaine	—	0.25[4]	1-2	40-80	< 3	1.5-6	> 7
	Phenytoin	0.5-1	24+	22-36[5]	87-93	< 5	10-20	> 20
	Tocainide	—	—	11-15	10-20	28-55	4-10	> 10
	Mexiletine	—	—	10-12	50-60	10	0.5-2	> 2
I C	Flecainide	—	—	12-27	40	30	0.2-1	> 1
	Propafenone	—	—	2-10[8]	97	< 1	0.06-1	—
II	Propranolol	0.5	3-5	2-3	90-95	< 1	0.05-0.1	—
	Esmolol	< 5 min	very short	0.15	55	< 2	—	—
	Acebutolol		24-30	3-4	26	15-20	—	—
III	Bretylium	—	6-8	5-10	0-8	> 80	0.5-1.5	—
	Amiodarone	1-3 wks[9]	weeks to months	26-107 days	96	negligible	0.5-2.5	> 2.5
	Sotalol			12	0	100	—	—
IV	Verapamil	0.5	6	3-7	90	3-4	0.08-0.3	—
—	Digoxin	0.5-2	24+	30-40	20-25	60	0.5-2 ng/mL	> 2.5 ng/mL
—	Adenosine	(34 sec IV)	1-2 min	< 10 sec	—	0 (enters body pool)	Not applicable	—

[1] Within 1 to 5 minutes with IV use.
[2] Half-life may be reduced in patients after multiple dosing.
[3] Protein binding is concentration-dependent.
[4] Very short after discontinuation of IV infusion.
[5] Half-life increases with increasing dosage.
[6] Half-life 10 to 32 hours in < 10% of patients (slow metabolizers).
[7] Onset of action may occur in 2 to 3 days.

MORICIZINE HCl

Rx	Ethmozine (Shire)	**Tablets:** 200 mg	Lactose. Lt. green. Film coated. Oval, convex. In 100s and UD 100s.
		250 mg	Lactose. Lt. orange. Film coated. Oval, convex. In 100s and UD 100s.
		300 mg	Lactose. Lt. blue. Film coated. Oval, convex. In 100s and UD 100s.

Refer to the general introductory discussion concerning Antiarrhythmic Agents.

WARNING

Mortality: Moricizine was 1 of 3 antiarrhythmic drugs included in the National Heart Lung and Blood Institute's Cardiac Arrhythmia Suppression Trial (CAST I), a long-term, multicenter, randomized, double-blind study in patients with asymptomatic non-life-threatening ventricular arrhythmias who had a MI more than 6 days, but less than 2 years, previously. An excessive mortality or nonfatal cardiac arrest rate was seen in patients treated with both of the Class IC agents included in the trial, which led to discontinuation of those 2 arms of the trial. Average duration of treatment was 10 months.

The moricizine and placebo arms of the trial were continued in the NHLBI-sponsored CAST II. In this randomized, double-blind trial, patients with asymptomatic non-life-threatening arrhythmias who had an MI within 4 to 90 days and left ventricular ejection fraction 0.4 or less prior to enrollment were evaluated. The average duration of treatment with moricizine in this study was 18 months. The study was discontinued because there was no possibility of demonstrating a benefit toward improved survival with moricizine and because of an evolving adverse trend after long-term treatment, although there was no statistical significance vs placebo.

The applicability of the CAST results to other populations (eg, those without recent MI) is uncertain. Considering the known proarrhythmic properties of moricizine and the lack of evidence of improved survival for any antiarrhythmic drug in patients without life-threatening arrhythmias, it is prudent to reserve the use of moricizine for patients with life-threatening ventricular arrhythmias.

Indications

Treatment of documented ventricular arrhythmias, such as sustained ventricular tachycardia, that are life-threatening. Because of the proarrhythmic effects of moricizine, reserve its use for patients in whom the benefits of treatment outweigh the risks.

Initiate treatment in the hospital.

Administration and Dosage

▶*Approved by the FDA:* June 26, 1990.

Individualize dosage. Clinical, cardiac rhythm monitoring, ECG intervals, exercise testing, and/or programmed electrical stimulation testing may be used to guide antiarrhythmic response and dosage adjustment. In general, the patients will be at high risk; hospitalize for the initiation of therapy.

▶*Usual adult dosage:* Between 600 and 900 mg/day, given every 8 hours in three equally divided doses. Within this range, the dosage can be adjusted as tolerated, in increments of 150 mg/day at 3-day intervals, until the desired effect is obtained. Patients with life-threatening arrhythmias who exhibit a beneficial response as judged by objective criteria (eg, Holter monitoring, programmed electrical stimulation, exercise testing) can be maintained on chronic moricizine therapy. As the antiarrhythmic effect of moricizine persists for longer than 12 hours, some patients whose arrhythmias are well controlled on an every 8-hour regimen may be given the same total daily dose in an every 12-hour regimen to increase convenience and help assure compliance. When higher doses are used, patients may experience more dizziness and nausea on the every 12-hour regimen.

▶*Hepatic or renal function impairment:* Start at 600 mg/day or less and monitor closely, including measurement of ECG intervals, before dosage adjustment.

▶*Transfer from another antiarrhythmic:* Recommendations for transferring patients from another antiarrhythmic to moricizine can be given based on theoretical considerations. Withdraw previous antiarrhythmic therapy for 1 to 2 plasma half-lives before starting moricizine at the recommended dosages. In patients in whom withdrawal of a previous antiarrhythmic is likely to produce life-threatening arrhythmias, hospitalize.

Transferring to Moricizine from Another Antiarrhythmic	
Agent transferred from	Start moricizine
Quinidine, disopyramide	6 to 12 hours after last dose
Procainamide	3 to 6 hours after last dose
Mexiletine, propafenone or tocainide	8 to 12 hours after last dose
Flecainide	12 to 24 hours after last dose

Actions

▶*Pharmacology:* Moricizine is a Class I antiarrhythmic agent with potent local anesthetic activity and myocardial membrane stabilizing effects. It shares some of the characteristics of the IA, B and C agents. Moricizine reduces the fast inward current carried by sodium ions. In isolated dog Purkinje fibers, moricizine shortens Phase 2 and 3 repolarization, resulting in a decreased action potential duration and effective refractory period. A dose-related decrease in the maximum rate of

MORICIZINE HCl

Phase 0 depolarization (V_{max}) occurs without effect on maximum diastolic potential or action potential amplitude. The sinus node and atrial tissue of the dog are not affected.

Although moricizine is chemically related to the neuroleptic phenothiazines, it has not demonstrated central or peripheral dopaminergic activity in animals. Moreover, in patients on chronic moricizine, serum prolactin levels did not increase.

Hemodynamic effects – In patients with impaired left ventricular function, moricizine has minimal effects on measurements of cardiac performance such as cardiac index, stroke volume index, pulmonary capillary wedge pressure, systemic or pulmonary vascular resistance or ejection fraction, either at rest or during exercise. Moricizine is associated with a small, but consistent increase in resting blood pressure and heart rate. In patients with ventricular arrhythmias, exercise tolerance is unaffected. In patients with a history of congestive heart failure (CHF) or angina pectoris, exercise duration and rate-pressure product at maximal exercise are unchanged during moricizine administration. Nonetheless, in some cases, worsened heart failure in patients with severe underlying heart disease has been attributed to moricizine.

The antiarrhythmic and electrophysiologic effects of moricizine are not related in time course or intensity to plasma moricizine concentrations or to the concentrations of any identified metabolite, all of which have short (2 to 3 hours) half-lives. Following single doses of moricizine, there is a prompt prolongation of the PR interval, which becomes normal within 2 hours, consistent with the rapid fall of plasma moricizine. JT interval shortening, however, peaks approximately 6 hours and persists for at least 10 hours. Although an effect on ventricular premature depolarizations (VPD) rates is seen within 2 hours after dosing, the full effect is seen after 10 to 14 hours and persists in full, when therapy is terminated, for longer than 10 hours, after which the effect decays slowly, and is still substantial at 24 hours. This suggests either an unidentified metabolite with an active, long half-life, or a structural or functional "deep compartment" with slow entry from, and release to, the plasma. The following description of parent compound pharmacokinetics is therefore of uncertain relevance to clinical actions.

Electrophysiology – In patients with ventricular tachycardia, moricizine 750 and 900 mg/day prolongs AV conduction. Both AV nodal conduction time (AH interval) and His-Purkinje conduction time (HV interval) are prolonged by 10% to 13% and 21% to 26%, respectively. The PR interval is prolonged by 16% to 20% and the QRS by 7% to 18%. Prolongations of 2% to 5% in the corrected QT interval result from widening of the QRS interval, but there is shortening of the JT interval, indicating an absence of significant effect on ventricular repolarization.

Intra-atrial conduction or atrial effective refractory periods are not consistently affected. In patients without sinus node dysfunction, moricizine has minimal effects on sinus cycle length and sinus node recovery time. These effects may be significant in patients with sinus node dysfunction (see Precautions).

➤*Pharmacokinetics:*

Absorption / Distribution – Following oral administration, moricizine undergoes significant first-pass metabolism resulting in an absolute bioavailability of approximately 38%. Peak plasma concentrations are usually reached within 0.5 to 2 hours. Administration 30 minutes after a meal delays the rate of absorption, resulting in lower peak plasma concentrations, but the extent of absorption is not altered. Plasma levels are proportional to dose over the recommended therapeutic dose range. The apparent volume of distribution after oral administration is very large (300 L or more) and is not significantly related to body weight. Moricizine is approximately 95% bound to plasma proteins, independent of plasma concentration.

Metabolism / Excretion – Moricizine undergoes extensive biotransformation; less than 1% is excreted unchanged in the urine. There are at least 26 metabolites, but no single metabolite has been found to represent as much as 1% of the administered dose, and as stated previously, antiarrhythmic response has relatively slow onset and offset. Two metabolites are pharmacologically active in at least one animal model: Moricizine sulfoxide and phenothiazine-2-carbamic acid ethyl ester sulfoxide. Each of these metabolites represents a small percentage of the administered dose (less than 0.6%), is present in lower plasma concentrations than the parent drug, and has a plasma elimination half-life of approximately 3 hours.

Moricizine induces its own metabolism. Average plasma concentrations in patients decrease with multiple dosing. This decrease in plasma levels of parent drug does not appear to affect clinical outcome for patients on chronic therapy. The plasma half-life is 1.5 to 3.5 hours (most values about 2 hours) following single or multiple oral doses in patients with ventricular ectopy. Approximately 56% is excreted in the feces and 39% is excreted in the urine. Some enterohepatic recycling occurs.

➤*Clinical trials:* Moricizine at daily doses of 600 to 900 mg produced a dose-related reduction in the occurrence of frequent VPD and reduced the incidence of nonsustained and sustained ventricular tachycardia (VT). In controlled clinical trials, moricizine had antiarrhythmic activity similar to that of disopyramide, propranolol and quinidine. In programmed electrical stimulation studies (PES), moricizine prevented the induction of sustained ventricular tachycardia in approximately 25% of patients. Activity of moricizine is maintained during long-term use.

Moricizine is effective in treating ventricular arrhythmias in patients with and without organic heart disease. It may be effective in patients in whom other antiarrhythmics are ineffective, not tolerated or contraindicated.

Arrhythmia exacerbation or "rebound" is not noted following discontinuation of therapy.

Contraindications

Preexisting second- or third-degree AV block; right bundle branch block when associated with left hemiblock (bifascicular block) unless a pacemaker is present; cardiogenic shock; hypersensitivity to the drug.

Warnings

➤*Mortality:* Moricizine was one of three antiarrhythmic drugs included in the National Heart Lung and Blood Institute's Cardiac Arrhythmia Suppression Trial (CAST I), a long-term, multicenter, randomized, double-blind study in patients with asymptomatic non-life-threatening ventricular arrhythmias who had a MI more than 6 days, but less than 2 years, previously. An excessive mortality or nonfatal cardiac arrest rate was seen in patients treated with both of the Class IC agents included in the trial, which led to discontinuation of those 2 arms of the trial. Average duration of treatment was 10 months.

The moricizine and placebo arms of the trial were continued in the NHLBI-sponsored CAST II. In this randomized, double-blind trial, patients with asymptomatic non-life-threatening arrhythmias who had an MI within 4 to 90 days and left ventricular ejection fraction 0.4 or less prior to enrollment were evaluated. The average duration of treatment with moricizine in this study was 18 months. The study was discontinued because there was no possibility of demonstrating a benefit toward improved survival with moricizine and because of an evolving adverse trend after long-term treatment, although there was no statistical significance vs placebo.

The applicability of the CAST results to other populations (eg, those without recent MI) is uncertain. Considering the known proarrhythmic properties of moricizine and the lack of evidence of improved survival for any antiarrhythmic drug in patients without life-threatening arrhythmias, it is prudent to reserve the use of moricizine for patients with life-threatening ventricular arrhythmias.

➤*Survival:* Antiarrhythmic drugs have not been proven to favorably affect survival or incidence of sudden death.

➤*Proarrhythmic effects:* Like other antiarrhythmic drugs, moricizine can provoke new rhythm disturbances or make existing arrhythmias worse. These proarrhythmic effects can range from an increase in the frequency of VPDs to the development of new or more severe ventricular tachycardia (eg, tachycardia that is more sustained or more resistant to conversion to sinus rhythm, with potentially fatal consequences). It is often not possible to distinguish a proarrhythmic effect from the patient's underlying rhythm disorder; therefore, consider the occurrence rates that follow approximations. Note also that drug-induced arrhythmias can generally be identified only when they occur early after starting the drug and when the rhythm can be identified, usually because the patient is being monitored. It is clear from the CAST study that some antiarrhythmic drugs can cause increased sudden death mortality, presumably due to new arrhythmias or asystole that do not appear early after treatment but that represent a sustained increased risk.

Domestic pre-marketing trials included 1072 patients given moricizine; 397 had baseline lethal arrhythmias (sustained VT or VF and non-sustained VT with hemodynamic symptoms) and 576 had potentially lethal arrhythmias (increased VPDs or NSVT in patients with known structural heart disease, active ischemia, CHF or an LVEF less than 40% and/or CI less than 2 L/min/m^2). In this population, there were 40 (3.7%) identified pro-arrhythmic events, 26 (2.5%) of which were serious, either fatal (6), new hemodynamically significant sustained VT or VF (4), new sustained VT that was not hemodynamically significant (11) or sustained VT that became syncopal/presyncopal when it had not been before (5). Proarrhythmic effects described as incessant ventricular tachycardia were observe in the postmarketing PES study and in postmarketing adverse event reports.

In general, serious proarrhythmic effects were equally common in patients with more and less severe arrhythmias, 2.5% in the patients with baseline lethal arrhythmias vs 2.8% in patients with potentially lethal arrhythmias, although the patients with serious effects were more likely to have a history of sustained VT (38% vs 23%). In the postmarketing comparative PES study, patients treated with 250 to 300 mg moricizine TID had a proarrhythmic rate of 14%.

Five of the six fatal proarrhythmic events were in patients with baseline lethal arrhythmias; four had prior cardiac arrests. Rates and severity of proarrhythmic events were similar in patients given 600 to 900 mg/day and those given higher doses. Patients with proarrhythmic events were more likely than the overall population to have coronary artery disease (85% vs 67%), history of acute MI (75% vs 53%), CHF (60% vs 43%) and cardiomegaly (55% vs 33%). All of the six proarrhythmic deaths were in patients with coronary artery disease; 5 of 6 each had documented acute MI, CHF and cardiomegaly.

MORICIZINE HCl

In two recent studies, moricizine (400 to 1000 mg/day) was ineffective in patients with refractory sustained ventricular arrhythmias (failed therapy with other class I agents) and carried a considerable risk for life threatening proarrhythmia. In one study, seven of 26 patients (27%) developed proarrhythmia during moricizine loading, and in the other study four of 21 patients (19%) had a probable proarrhythmic response.

➤*Electrolyte disturbances:* Hypokalemia, hyperkalemia or hypomagnesemia may alter the effects of Class I antiarrhythmic drugs. Correct electrolyte imbalances before administration of moricizine.

➤*Sick sinus syndrome:* Use with extreme caution in patients with sick sinus syndrome since it may cause sinus bradycardia, sinus pause or sinus arrest.

➤*Renal function impairment:* Plasma levels of intact moricizine are unchanged in hemodialysis patients, but a significant portion (39%) is metabolized and excreted in the urine. Although no identified active metabolite is known to increase in people with renal failure, metabolites of unrecognized importance could be affected. Administer cautiously. Start patients with significant renal dysfunction on lower doses and monitor for excessive pharmacologic effects, including ECG intervals, before dosage adjustment (see Administration and Dosage).

➤*Hepatic function impairment:* Patients with significant liver dysfunction have reduced plasma clearance and an increased half-life of moricizine. The precise relationship of moricizine levels to effect is not clear. Treat hepatic disease patients with lower doses. Closely monitor for excessive pharmacological effects, including ECG intervals, before dosage adjustment. Administer with particular care to patients with severe liver disease, if at all (see Administration and Dosage).

➤*Carcinogenesis:* In a 24-month mouse study in which moricizine was administered to provide up to 320 mg/kg/day, ovarian tubular adenomas and granulosa cell tumors were limited to moricizine-treated animals.

In a 24-month study in which moricizine was administered to rats at doses of 25, 50 and 100 mg/kg/day, Zymbal's Gland Carcinoma was observed in one mid-dose and two high-dose males. The rats also showed a dose-related increase in hepatocellular cholangioma in both sexes, along with fatty metamorphosis, possibly due to disruption of hepatic choline utilization for phospholipid biosynthesis.

➤*Pregnancy: Category B.* In a study in which rats were dosed with moricizine prior to and during mating, and throughout gestation and lactation, dose levels 3.4 and 6.7 times the maximum recommended human daily dose produced a dose-related decrease in pup and maternal weight gain, possibly related to a larger litter size. In a study in which dosing was begun on day 15 of gestation, moricizine, at a level 6.7 times the maximum recommended human daily dose, produced a retardation in maternal weight gain but no effect on pup growth. There are no adequate and well-controlled studies in pregnant women. Use during pregnancy only if clearly needed.

➤*Lactation:* Moricizine is excreted in the milk of animals and is present in human breast milk. Because of the potential for serious adverse reactions in nursing infants, decide whether to discontinue nursing or to discontinue the drug, taking into account the importance of the drug to the mother.

➤*Children:* Safety and efficacy in children younger than 18 years of age have not been established.

Precautions

➤*ECG changes/Conduction abnormalities:* Moricizine slows AV nodal and intraventricular conduction, producing dose-related increases in PR and QRS intervals. In clinical trials, the average increase in PR interval was 12% and QRS interval was 14%. Although the QTc interval is increased, this is due to QRS prolongation; the JT interval is shortened, indicating absence of significant slowing of ventricular repolarization. The degree of lengthening of PR and QRS intervals does not predict efficacy.

In controlled clinical trials and in open studies, the overall incidence of delayed ventricular conduction, including new bundle branch block pattern, was approximately 9.4%. In patients without baseline conduction abnormalities, the frequency of second-degree AV block was 0.2% and third-degree AV block did not occur. In patients with baseline conduction abnormalities, the frequencies of second-degree AV block and third-degree AV block were 0.9% and 1.4%, respectively.

Therapy was discontinued in 1.6% of patients due to ECG changes (0.6% due to sinus pause or asystole, 0.2% to AV block, 0.2% to junctional rhythm, 0.4% to intraventricular conduction delay and 0.2% to wide QRS and/or PR interval).

In patients with preexisting conduction abnormalities, initiate therapy cautiously. If second- or third-degree AV block occurs, discontinue therapy unless a ventricular pacemaker is in place. When changing the dose or adding concomitant medications which may also affect cardiac conduction, monitor ECG.

➤*Congestive heart failure:* Most patients with CHF have tolerated recommended daily doses without unusual toxicity or change in effect. Pharmacokinetic differences between patients with and without CHF were not apparent (see Hepatic function impairment). In some cases,

worsened heart failure has been attributed to moricizine. Carefully watch patients with preexisting heart failure when initiating therapy.

➤*Effects on pacemaker threshold:* Since the effect of moricizine on the sensing and pacing thresholds of artificial pacemakers has not been sufficiently studied, monitor pacing parameters if moricizine is used.

➤*Drug fever:* Three patients developed rechallenge-confirmed drug fever, with one patient experiencing an elevation above 39.5° to 40.6°C (103° to 105°F) with rigors. Fevers occurred at about 2 weeks in two cases, and after 21 weeks in the third. Fevers resolved within 48 hours after discontinuation of moricizine.

Drug Interactions

Moricizine Drug Interactions			
Precipitant Drug	Object Drug*		Comments
Cimetidine	Moricizine	↑	1.4-fold increase in moricizine plasma levels; 49% decrease in clearance. Initiate moricizine at low doses (not > 600 mg/day).
Digoxin	Moricizine	↑	Additive prolongation of the PR interval, but not with a significant increase in the rate of second- or third-degree AV block. Little change in serum digoxin levels or pharmacokinetics.
Diltiazem	Moricizine	↑	Diltiazem may elevate moricizine concentrations, while moricizine may reduce diltiazem concentrations. Monitor closely.
Moricizine	Diltiazem	↓	
Propranolol	Moricizine	↑	Small additive increase in PR interval; no changes in overall ECG intervals.
Moricizine	Theophylline	↓	Theophylline clearance increased 44% to 66% and plasma half-life decreased 19% to 33% (conventional and sustained-release theophylline).

*   ↑ = Object drug increased   ↓ = Object drug decreased

➤*Drug/Food interactions:* Administration of moricizine 30 minutes after a meal delays the rate of absorption, resulting in lower peak plasma concentrations, but the extent of absorption is not altered.

Adverse Reactions

The most serious adverse reaction reported is proarrhythmia (see Warnings). This occurred in 3.7% of 1072 patients with ventricular arrhythmias who received a wide range of doses under a variety of circumstances. In addition, in controlled clinical trials and in open studies, adverse reactions led to discontinuation of moricizine in 7% of 1105 patients with ventricular and supraventricular arrhythmias, including: Nausea (3.2%); ECG abnormalities (1.6%; principally conduction defects, sinus pause, junctional rhythm or AV block); CHF (1%); dizziness, anxiety, drug fever (see Precautions), urinary retention, blurred vision, GI upset, rash, laboratory abnormalities (0.3% to 0.4%).

Elderly – Adverse reactions were generally similar in patients > 65 years old (n = 375) and < 65 years of age (n = 697), although discontinuation of therapy for reasons other than proarrhythmia were more common in older patients (13.9% vs 7.7%). Overall mortality was greater in older patients (9.3% vs 3.9%), but those were not deaths attributed to treatment; older patients had more serious underlying heart disease.

➤*Cardiovascular:* Palpitations (5.8%); sustained ventricular tachycardia, cardiac chest pain, CHF, cardiac death (2% to < 5%); hypotension, hypertension, syncope, supraventricular arrhythmias (including atrial fibrillations/flutter), cardiac arrest, bradycardia, pulmonary embolism, MI, vasodilation, cerebrovascular events, thrombophlebitis (< 2%).

➤*CNS:* Dizziness (15.1%); headache (8%); fatigue (5.9%); hypesthesias, asthenia, nervousness, paresthesias, sleep disorders (2% to < 5%); tremor, anxiety, depression, euphoria, confusion, somnolence, agitation, seizure, coma, abnormal gait, hallucinations, nystagmus, diplopia, speech disorder, akathisia, memory loss, ataxia, abnormal coordination, dyskinesia, vertigo, tinnitus (< 2%).

Dizziness appears to be related to the size of each dose. In a comparison of 900 mg/day given at 450 mg twice daily or 300 mg 3 times daily, > 20% of patients experienced dizziness on the twice daily regimen vs 12% on the 3 times daily regimen.

➤*GI:* Nausea (9.6%); abdominal pain, dyspepsia, vomiting, diarrhea (2% to < 5%); anorexia, bitter taste, dysphagia, flatulence, ileus (< 2%).

➤*GU:* Urinary retention or frequency, dysuria, urinary incontinence, kidney pain, impotence, decreased libido (< 2%).

➤*Respiratory:* Dyspnea (5.7%); hyperventilation, apnea, asthma, pharyngitis, cough, sinusitis (< 2%).

➤*Miscellaneous:* Sweating, musculoskeletal pain, dry mouth, blurred vision (2% to < 5%); drug fever, hypothermia, temperature intolerance, eye pain, rash, pruritus, dry skin, urticaria, swelling of the lips and tongue, periorbital edema (< 2%).

Two patients developed thrombocytopenia that may have been drug-related. Clinically significant elevations in liver function tests (biliru-

MORICIZINE HCl

bin, serum transaminases) and jaundice consistent with hepatitis occurred rarely. Although a cause-and-effect relationship has not been established, caution is advised in patients who develop unexplained signs of hepatic dysfunction; consider discontinuing therapy.

Overdosage

➤*Symptoms:* Emesis; lethargy; coma; syncope; hypotension; conduction disturbances; exacerbation of CHF; MI; sinus arrest; arrhythmias (including junctional bradycardia, ventricular tachycardia, ventricular fibrillation and asystole); respiratory failure. Deaths have occurred after accidental or intentional overdoses of 2250 and 10,000 mg, respectively. Accidental introduction of moricizine into the lungs of monkeys resulted in rapid arrhythmic death.

➤*Treatment:* Treatment should be supportive. Hospitalize patients and monitor for cardiac, respiratory and CNS changes. Provide advanced life support systems, including an intracardiac pacing catheter where necessary. Treat acute overdosage with appropriate gastric evacuation, and with special care to avoid aspiration. Refer to General Management of Acute Overdosage.

Patient Information

Take exactly as prescribed. Dosage changes must be supervised by the physician.

Contact the physician immediately if chest pain or discomfort, pounding in the chest (palpitations), irregular heartbeat or fever occur.

Hospitalization is required when starting on this medication.

IBUTILIDE FUMARATE

| *Rx* | **Corvert** (Pharmacia & Upjohn) | **Solution:** 0.1 mg/mL | In 10 mL vials. |

Refer to the general introductory discussion concerning Antiarrhythmic Agents.

WARNING

Life-threatening arrhythmias - appropriate treatment environment: Ibutilide can cause potentially fatal arrhythmias, particularly sustained polymorphic ventricular tachycardia, usually in association with QT prolongation (torsades de pointes), but sometimes without documented QT prolongation. In clinical studies, these arrhythmias, which require cardioversion, occurred in 1.7% or treated patients during, or within a number of hours of, use of ibutilide. These arrhythmias can be reversed if treated promptly (see Warnings). It is essential that ibutilide be administered in a setting of continuous ECG monitoring and by personnel trained in identification and treatment of acute ventricular arrthymias, particularly polymorphic ventricular tachycardia.

NOTE: Patients with a trial fibrillation of > 2 to 3 days' duration must be adequately anticoagulated, generally for at least 2 weeks.

Choice of patients: Patients with chronic atrial fibrillation have a strong tendency to revert after conversion to sinus rhythm, and treatments to maintain sinus rhythm carry risks. Therefore, carefully select patients to be treated with ibutilide, such that the expected benefits of maintaining sinus rhythm outweigh the immediate risks of ibutilide, and the risks of maintenance therapy, and are likely to offer an advantage compared with alternative management.

Indications

➤*Atrial fibrillation/flutter:* For the rapid conversion of atrial fibrillation or atrial flutter of recent onset to sinus rhythm. Patients with atrial arrhythmias of longer duration are less likely to respond to ibutilide. The effectiveness of ibutilide has not been determined in patients with arrhythmias of > 90 days in duration.

Administration and Dosage

➤*Approved by the FDA:* March 1996.

The recommended dose based on controlled trials is outlined in the table below. Stop ibutilide infusion as soon as the presenting arrhythmia is terminated or in the event of sustained or nonsustained ventricular tachycardia, or marked prolongation of QT or QTc.

Recommended Dose of Ibutilide Injection		
Patient weight	Initial infusion (over 10 minutes)	Second Infusion
≥ 60 kg (132 lb)	One vial (1 mg)	If the arrhythmia does not terminate within 10 minutes after the end of the initial infusion, a second 10-minute infusion of equal strength may be administered 10 minutes after completion of the first infusion.
< 60 kg (132 lb)	0.1 mL/kg (0.01 mg/kg)	

In a trial comparing ibutilide and sotalol, 2 mg ibutilide administered as a single infusion to patients weighing > 60 kg was also effective in terminating atrial fibrillation or atrial flutter.

Observe patients with continuous ECG monitoring for at least 4 hours following infusion or until QTc has returned to baseline. Longer monitoring is required if any arrhythmic activity is noted. Skilled personnel and proper equipment, such as a cardioverter/difibrillator and medication for treatment of sustained ventribular tachycardia, including polymorphic ventricular tachycardia, must be available during administration of ibutilide and subsequent monitoring of the patient.

➤*Dilution:* Ibutilide may be administered undiluted or diluted in 50 mL diluent. Ibutilide may be added to 0.9% Sodium Chloride Injection or 5% Dextrose Injection before infusion. The contents of one 10 mL vial (0.1 mg/mL) may be added to a 50 mL infusion bag to form an admixture of ≈ 0.017 mg/mL.

➤*Admixture compatibility:* The following diluents are compatible with ibutilide (0.1 mg/mL): 5% Dextrose Injection and 0.9% Sodium Chloride Injection. The following IV solution containers are compatible

with admixtures of ibutilide (0.1 mg/mL): Polyvinyl choride plastic bags; polyolefin bags.

➤*Storage/Stability:* Admixtures of the product, with approved diluents, are chemically and physically stable for 24 hours at room temperature (15° to 30°C; 59° to 86°F) and for 48 hours at refrigerated temperatures (2°to 8°C; 36° to 46°F).

Actions

➤*Pharmacology:* Ibutilide is an antiarrhythmic drug with predominantly class III (cardiac action potential prolongation) properties according to the Vaughan Williams Classification. Ibutilide prolongs action potential duration in isolated adult cardiac myocytes and increases both atrial and ventricular refractoriness in vivo (ie, class III electrophysiologic effects). Voltage clamp studies indicate that ibutilide, at nanomolar concentrations, delays repolarization by activation of a slow, inward current (predominantly sodium), rather than by blocking outward potassium currents, which is the mechanism by which most other class III antiarrhythmics act. These effects lead to prolongation of atrial and ventricular action potential duration and refractoriness, the predominant electrophysiologic properties of ibutilide in humans that are thought to be the basis for its antiarrhythmic effect.

Electrophysiology – Ibutilide produces mild slowing of the sinus rate and AV conduction. Ibutilide produces no clinically significant effect on QRS duration at IV doses up to 0.03 mg/kg administered over a 10-minute period. Although there is no established relationship between plasma concentration and antiarrhythmic effect, ibutilide produces dose-related prolongation of the QT interval, which is thought to be associated with its antiarrhythmic activity. (See Warnings for relationship between QTc prolongation and torsades de pointes-type arrhythmias.) In a study in healthy volunteers, IV infusions of ibutilide resulted in prolongation of the QT interval that was directly correlated with ibutilide plasma concentration during and after 10-minute and 8-hour infusions. A steep ibutilide concentration/response (QT prolongation) relationship was shown. The maximum effect was a function of both the dose and the infusion rate.

Hemodynamics – A study of hemodynamic function in patients with ejection fractions both above and below 35% showed no clinically significant effects on cardiac output, mean pulmonary arterial pressure or pulmonary capillary wedge pressure at doses up to 0.03 mg/kg.

➤*Pharmacokinetics:*

Absorption/Distribution – After IV infusion, ibutilide plasma concentrations rapidly decrease in a multiexponential fashion. The pharmacokinetics of ibutilide are highly variable among subjects. Ibutilide has a high systemic plasma clearance that approximates liver blood flow (≈ 29 mL/min/kg), a large steady-state volume of distribution (≈ 11 L/kg) in healthy volunteers and minimal (≈ 40%) protein binding. The drug is cleared rapidly and highly distributed in patients being treated for atrial flutter or atrial fibrillation. The elimination half-life averages about 6 hours (range, 2 to 12 hours). The pharmacokinetics are linear with respect to the dose over the dose range of 0.01 to 0.10 mg/kg. The enantiomers of ibutilide have pharmacokinetic properties similar to each other and to ibutilide.

Metabolism/Excretion – In healthy male volunteers, ≈ 82% of a 0.01 mg/kg dose was excreted in the urine (≈ 7% of the dose as unchanged ibutilide) and the remainder (≈ 19%) was recovered in the feces. Eight metabolites of ibutilide were detected in the urine. These metabolites are thought to be formed primarily by ω-oxidation followed by sequential β-oxidation of the heptyl side chain of ibutilide. Of the eight metabolites, only the ω-hydroxy metabolite possesses class III electrophysiologic properties similar to that of ibutilide in an *in vitro* isolated rabbit myocardium model. The plasma concentrations of this active metabolite, however, are < 10% that of ibutilide.

➤*Clinical trials:* Treatment with IV ibutilide for acute termination of recent onset atrial flutter/fibrillation was evaluated in 466 patients participating in two trials. In one trial, single 10-minute infusions of 0.005 to 0.025 mg/kg were tested in parallel groups. In the second trial, up to two infusions of ibutilide were evaluated: the first 1 mg, the second given 10 minutes after completion of the first infusion, either 0.5 or 1 mg. In a third study, 319 patients with atrial fibrillation or atrial flutter were randomized to receive single, 10-minute IV infusions of either sotalol (1.5 mg/kg) or ibutilide (1 or 2 mg). Among patients with atrial

IBUTILIDE FUMARATE

flutter, 53% receiving 1 mg ibutilide and 70% receiving 2 mg ibutilide converted, compared with 18% of those receiving sotalol. In patients with atrial fibrillation, 22% and 43% receiving 1 and 2 mg ibutilide, respectively, converted compared with 10% of patients receiving sotalol.

Conversion of atrial flutter/fibrillation (70% of those who converted) usually occurred within 30 minutes of the start of infusion and was dose related. The latest conversion seen was at 90 minutes after the start of the infusion. Most converted patients remained in normal sinus rhythm for 24 hours.

Overall responses in these patients, defined as termination of arrhythmias for any length of time during or within 1 hour following completed infusion of randomized dose, were in the range of 45% to 50% at doses above 0.0125 mg/kg (vs 2% for placebo). Twenty-four hour responses were similar. For these atrial arrhythmias, ibutilide was more effective in patients with flutter than fibrillation (> 50% vs < 40%).

The number of patients who remained in the converted rhythm at the end of 24 hours were slightly less than those patients who converted intially, but the difference between conversion rates for ibutilide compared with placebo was still statistically significant. In long-term follow-up, ≈ 40% of all patients remained recurrence free, usually with chronic prophylactic treatment, 400 to 500 days after acute treatment, regardless of the method of conversion.

Patients with more recent onset of arrhythmia had a higher rate of conversion. Response rates were 42% and 50% for patients with onset of atrial fibrillation/flutter for < 30 days in the two efficacy studies compared with 16% and 31% in those with more chronic arrhythmias.

Contraindications

Hypersensitivity to ibutilide or any of the other product components.

Warnings

➤*Proarrhythmia:* Like other antiarrhythmic agents, ibutilide can induce or worsen ventricular arrhythmias in some patients. This may have potentially fatal consequences. Torsades de pointes, a polymorphic ventricular tachycardia that develops in the setting of a prolonged QT interval, may occur because of the effect ibutilide has on cardiac repolarization, but ibutilide can also cause polymorphic VT in the absence of excessive prolongation of the QT interval. In general, with drugs that prolong the QT interval, the risk of torsades de pointes is thought to increase progressively as the QT interval is prolonged and may be worsened with bradycardia, a varying heart rate and hypokalemia.

In clinical trials conducted in patients with atrial fibrillation and atrial flutter, those with QTc intervals > 440 msec were not usually allowed to participate, and serum potassium had to be above 4 mEq/L. Although change in QTc was dose dependent for ibutilide, there was no clear relationship between risk of serious proarrhythmia and dose, possibly due to the small number of events. In clinical trials of IV ibutilide, patients with a history of CHF or low left ventricular ejection fraction appeared to have a higher incidence of sustained polymorphic ventricular tachycardia (VT) than those without such underlying conditions; for sustained polymorphic VT, the rate was 6.2% in patients with a history of CHF and 0.8% without it. There was also a suggestion that women had a higher risk of proarrhythmia, but the sex difference was not observed in all studies and was most prominent for nonsustained VT. The incidence of sustained ventricular arrhythmias was similar in male (1.8%) and female (1.5%) patients, possibly due to the small number of events. Ibutilide is not recommended in patients who have demonstrated polymorphic VT (eg, torsades de pointes).

During clinical trials, 1.7% of patients with atrial flutter or atrial fibrillation treated with ibutilide developed sustained polymorphic VT requiring cardioversion. In these clinical trials, many initial episodes of polymorphic VT occurred after the infusion of ibutilide was stopped, but generally not more than 40 minutes after the start of the first infusion. There were, however, instances of recurrent polymorphic VT that occurred about 3 hours after the initial infusion. In two cases, the VT degenerated into ventricular fibrillation, requiring immediate defibrillation. Other cases were managed with cardiac pacing and magnesium sulfate infusions. Nonsustained polymorphic VT ocurred in 2.7% of patients, and nonsustained monomorphic VTs occurred in 4.9% of the patients (see Adverse Reactions).

Proarrhythmic events must be anticipated. Skilled personnel and proper equipment, including cardiac monitoring equipment, intracardiac pacing facilities, a cardioverter/defibrillator and medication for treatment of sustained VT, including polymorphic VT, must be available during and after administration of ibutilide. Before treatment, correct hypokalemia and hypomagnesemia to reduce the potential for proarrhythmia. Observe patients with continuous ECG monitoring for at least 4 hours following infusion or until QTc has returned to baseline. Longer monitoring is required if any arrhythmic activity is noted. Management of polymorphic VT includes discontinuation of ibutilide, correction of electrolyte abnormalities, especially potassium and magnesium, and overdrive cardiac pacing, electrical cardioversion or defibrillation. Pharmacologic therapies include magnesium sulfate infusions. Generally avoid treatment with antiarrhythmics.

➤*Renal/Hepatic function impairment:* It is unlikely that dosing adjustments would be necessary in patients with compromised renal or hepatic function based on the following considerations: (1) Ibutilide is indicated for rapid IV therapy (duration ≤ 30 min) and is dosed to a known, well-defined pharmacologic action (termination of arrhythmia) or to a maximum of two 10–minute infusions; (2) < 10% of the dose is excreted unchanged in the urine; and (3) drug distribution appears to be one of the primary mechanisms responsible for termination of the pharmacologic effect. Nonetheless, monitor patients with abnormal liver function by telemetry for more than the 4-hour periods generally recommended. In 285 patients with atrial fibrillation or atrial flutter who were treated with ibutilide, the clearance of ibutilide was independent of renal function, as assessed by creatinine clearance (range, 21 to 140 mL/min).

➤*Elderly:* The mean age of patients in clinical trials was 65. No age-related differences were observed in pharmacokinetic, efficacy or safety parameters for patients < 65 compared with patients ≥ 65 years of age.

➤*Pregnancy: Category C.* Ibutilide administered orally was teratogenic (adactyly, cleft pallate, scoliosis) and embryocidal in reproduction studies in rats. Do not administer to a pregnant woman unless clinical benefit outweighs potential risk to the fetus.

➤*Lactation:* The excretion of ibutilide into breast milk has not been studied; accordingly, discourage breastfeeding during therapy.

➤*Children:* Clinical trials in patients with atrial fibrillation and atrial flutter did not include anyone under the age of 18. Safety and efficacy of ibutilide in children have not been established.

Precautions

➤*Heart block:* Of the nine (1.5%) ibutilide-treated patients with reports of reversible heart block, five had first-degree, three had second-degree and one had complete heart block.

Drug Interactions

No specific pharmacokinetic or other formal drug interaction studies were conducted.

➤*Concomitant antiarrhythmics:* Class Ia antiarrhythmic drugs (Vaughan Williams Classification), such as disopyramide, quinidine and procainamide, and other class III drugs, such as amiodarone and sotalol, should not be given concomitantly with ibutilide or within 4 hours postinfusion because of their potential to prolong refractoriness. In the clinical trials, class I or other class III antiarrhythmic agents were withheld for at least 5 half-lives prior to ibutilide infusion and for 4 hours after dosing, but thereafter were allowed at the physician's discretion.

➤*Other drugs that prolong the QT interval:* The potential for proarrhythmia may increase with the administration of ibutilide to patients who are being treated with drugs that prolong the QT interval, such as phenothiazines, tricyclic and tetracyclic antidepressants and certain antihistamine drugs (H_1 receptor antagonists).

➤*Digoxin:* Supraventricular arrhythmias may mask the cardiotoxicity associated with excessive digoxin levels. Therefore, it is advisable to be particularly cautious in patients whose plasma digoxin levels are above or suspected to be above the usual therapeutic range.

Adverse Reactions

Ibutilide was generally well tolerated in clinical trials. Of the 586 patients with atrial fibrillation or atrial flutter who received ibutilide in phase II/III studies, 149 (25%) reported medical events related to the cardiovascular system, including sustained polymorphic VT (1.7%) and nonsustained polymorphic VT (2.7%).

Other clinically important adverse events include the following: Nonsustained monomorphic ventricular extrasystoles (5.1%); nonsustained monomorphic VT (4.9%); headache (3.6%); tachycardia/sinus tachycardia/supraventricular tachycardia, nonsustained polymorphic VT (2.7%); hypotension/postural hypotension (2%); bundle branch block (1.9%); sustained polymorphic VT (1.7%); AV block (1.5%); bradycardia/sinus bradycardia, QT segment prolonged, hypertension (1.2%); nausea (> 1%); palpitation (1%); supraventricular extrsystoles (0.9%); nodal arrhythmia (0.7%); congestive heart failure (0.5%); syncope, renal failure (0.3%); idioventricular rhythm, sustained monomorphic VT (0.2%).

Overdosage

Acute overdose in animals results in CNS toxicity, notably, CNS depression, rapid gasping breathing and convulsions. In clinical trials, four patients were unintentionally overdosed. The largest dose was 3.4 mg administered over 15 minutes. One patient (0.025 mg/kg) developed increased ventricular ectopy and monomorphic ventricular tachycardia, another patient (0.032 mg/kg) developed third-degree AV block and nonsustained polymorphic VT and two patients (0.038 and 0.02 mg/kg) had no medical event reports. Based on known pharmacology, the clinical effects of an overdosage with ibutilide could exaggerate the expected prolongation of repolarization seen at usual clinical doses. Treat medical events (eg, proarrhythmia, AV block) that occur after the overdosage with measures appropriate for that condition.

Quinidine

Refer to the general introductory discussion concerning Antiarrhythmic Agents.

Indications

➤*Oral:* Premature atrial, AV junctional and ventricular contractions; paroxysmal atrial (supraventricular) tachycardia; paroxysmal AV junctional rhythm; atrial flutter; paroxysmal and chronic atrial fibrillation; established atrial fibrillation when therapy is appropriate; paroxysmal ventricular tachycardia not associated with complete heart block; maintenance therapy after electrical conversion of atrial fibrillation or flutter.

➤*Parenteral:* When oral therapy is not feasible or when rapid therapeutic effect is required.

Quinidine gluconate – Life-threatening *Plasmodium falciparum* malaria: Unless impossible, start therapy in an intensive care setting with continuous ECG monitoring, frequent blood pressure monitoring and periodic monitoring of parasitemia.

Administration and Dosage

➤*Test dose:* Administer a single 200 mg tablet of quinidine sulfate or 200 mg IM quinidine gluconate to determine whether the patient has an idiosyncratic reaction. Continuously monitor ECG when quinidine is used in large doses.

Adjust the dosage to maintain the plasma concentration between 2 to 6 mcg/mL.

➤*Oral:*

Premature atrial and ventricular contractions – 200 to 300 mg 3 or 4 times daily.

Paroxysmal supraventricular tachycardias – 400 to 600 mg every 2 or 3 hours until the paroxysm is terminated.

Atrial flutter – Administer quinidine after digitalization. Individualize dosage.

Conversion of atrial fibrillation – 200 mg every 2 or 3 hours for 5 to 8 doses, with subsequent daily increases until sinus rhythm is restored or toxic effects occur. Do not exceed a total daily dose of 3 to 4 g in any regimen. Prior to quinidine administration, control the ventricular rate and CHF (if present) with digoxin.

Maintenance therapy – 200 to 300 mg 3 or 4 times daily. Other patients may require larger doses or more frequent administration than the usually recommended schedule. However, institute such an increased dosage only after careful evaluation of the patient, including ECG and quinidine serum level monitoring.

Sustained release forms – 300 to 600 mg every 8 or 12 hours. Since the rate of absorption from the various sustained release formulations may be markedly different, and since the anhydrous quinidine content is different, do not consider them interchangeable.

➤*Parenteral:* The patient must be under close clinical, ECG and blood pressure monitoring, especially during IV administration to detect any change in rate or rhythm. If the patient's condition is not critical, give quinidine gluconate IM. On the other hand, extreme palpitation, dyspnea, vomiting, and a shocklike state in patients with ventricular tachycardia are signs that IV administration may be required as a lifesaving measure when D-C cardioversion is not available.

IM – In the treatment of acute tachycardia, the initial dose is 600 mg quinidine gluconate. Subsequently, 400 mg quinidine gluconate can be repeated as often as every 2 hours. Determine successive doses by the effect of the preceding dose.

IV – In about 50% of patients who respond successfully to quinidine, the arrhythmia can be terminated by ≤ 330 mg quinidine gluconate (or its equivalent in other salts); as much as 500 to 750 mg may be required. Inject slowly. Dilute 10 mL (800 mg) of quinidine gluconate injection to 50 mL with 5% Dextrose Injection, USP. Inject the diluted solution slowly at a rate of 1 mL/min for maximum safety.

Quinidine gluconate – P. falciparum malaria – Two regimens have been empirically shown to be effective, with or without concomitant exchange transfusions. As soon as practical, institute standard oral antiplasmodial therapy.

1.) *Loading,* 15 mg/kg in 250 mL normal saline infused over 4 hours followed by: *Maintenance,* beginning 24 hours after the beginning of the loading dose, 7.5 mg/kg infused over 4 hours, every 8 hours for 7 days or until oral therapy can be instituted.

2.) *Loading,* 10 mg/kg in 250 mL normal saline infused over 1 to 2 hours, followed immediately by: *Maintenance,* 0.02 mg/kg/min for up to 72 hours or until parasitemia decreases to < 1% or oral therapy can be instituted.

➤*Children:*

The following doses have been suggested –

Oral (quinidine sulfate): 30 mg/kg/24 hours or 900 mg/m^2/24 hours in 5 divided doses.

IV (quinidine gluconate): 2 to 10 mg/kg/dose every 3 to 6 hours as needed; however, this route is not recommended.

Actions

➤*Pharmacology:* Quinidine, a class IA antiarrhythmic, depresses myocardial excitability, conduction velocity and contractility. Therapeutically, it prolongs the effective refractory period and increases conduction time, thereby preventing the reentry phenomenon. In addition, quinidine exerts an indirect anticholinergic effect; it decreases vagal tone and may facilitate conduction in the atrioventricular junction.

➤*Pharmacokinetics:*

Absorption / Distribution – There are differences in the anhydrous quinidine alkaloid content among the various salts. See table below:

Anhydrous Quinidine Alkaloid Content in Various Salts		
Quinidine salts	Quinidine content		Time to peak plasma levels (hours)
	Active drug	Absorbed	
Quinidine Gluconate	62%	70%	3-5
Quinidine Sulfate	83%	73%	1 to 3[1]

[1] 3 to 5 hours for sustained release form.

Quinidine is rapidly absorbed from the GI tract. Maximum effects of quinidine gluconate occur 30 to 90 minutes after IM administration; onset is more rapid after IV administration. Activity persists for ≥ 6 to 8 hours. The average therapeutic serum levels are reported to be 2 to 7 mcg/mL. Toxic reactions may occur at levels from 5 to ≥ 8 mcg/mL. Quinidine is 80% to 90% bound to plasma proteins; the unbound fraction may be significantly increased in patients with hepatic insufficiency. Accumulation occurs in most tissues, except the brain.

Metabolism / Excretion – From 60% to 80% of a dose is metabolized via the liver into several metabolites; the primary metabolites are 3-hydroxyquinidine and 2-oxoquinidinone. Whether or not these or other metabolites have antiarrhythmic activity is unclear and controversial. Quinidine is excreted unchanged (10% to 50%) in the urine within 24 hours. The elimination half-life ranges from 4 to 10 hours in healthy patients, with a mean of 6 to 7 hours. Urinary acidification facilitates quinidine elimination, and alkalinization retards it. In patients with cirrhosis, the elimination half-life may be prolonged and the volume of distribution increased. In congestive heart failure (CHF), total clearance and volume of distribution are decreased. In the elderly, the elimination half-life may be increased. The influence of renal dysfunction on the disposition of quinidine is controversial; volume of distribution and renal clearance may be reduced.

Contraindications

Hypersensitivity or idiosyncrasy to quinidine or other cinchona derivatives manifested by thrombocytopenia, skin eruption or febrile reactions; myasthenia gravis; history of thrombocytopenic purpura associated with quinidine administration; digitalis intoxication manifested by arrhythmias or AV conduction disorders; complete heart block; left bundle branch block or other severe intraventricular conduction defects exhibiting marked QRS widening or bizarre complexes; complete AV block with an AV nodal or idioventricular pacemaker; aberrant ectopic impulses and abnormal rhythms due to escape mechanisms; history of drug-induced torsades de pointes; history of long QT syndrome.

Warnings

➤*Hepatotoxicity:* Occurrences of hepatotoxicity (including granulomatous hepatitis) have been reported due to quinidine hypersensitivity. Unexplained fever or elevation of hepatic enzymes, particularly in the early stages of therapy, warrants consideration. Monitor liver function during the first 4 to 8 weeks of therapy. Discontinuing quinidine usually results in toxicity resolution.

➤*Atrial flutter or fibrillation:* Reversion to sinus rhythm may be preceded by a progressive reduction in degree of AV block to a 1:1 ratio, which results in an extremely rapid ventricular rate. Prior to use in atrial flutter, pretreat with a digitalis preparation.

Although quinidine reduces recurrences of atrial fibrillation after cardioversion, it may be associated with an increase in mortality.

➤*Cardiotoxicity:* Cardiotoxicity (eg, increased PR and QT intervals, 50% widening of QRS complex, ventricular tachyarrhythmias, frequent ventricular ectopic beats or tachycardia) dictates immediate discontinuation of quinidine; closely monitor the ECG. Some specialists recommend quinidine therapy be initiated only in hospitalized patients with ECG monitoring. However, this is generally reserved for patients receiving large doses or who are at high risk.

In susceptible individuals (ie, marginally compensated cardiovascular disease), quinidine may produce clinically important depression of cardiac function such as hypotension, bradycardia or heartblock.

Large oral doses may reduce the arterial pressure by means of peripheral vasodilation. Serious hypotension is more likely with parenteral use.

Use quinidine with extreme caution in incomplete AV block, since complete block and asystole may result. The drug may cause unpredictable dysrhythmias in digitalized patients; use with caution in the presence of digitalis intoxication. Use cautiously in patients with partial bundle branch block, severe CHF and hypotensive states due to the depressant effects of quinidine on myocardial contractility and arterial pressure; usefulness of quinidine is limited unless these conditions are due to or aggravated by the arrhythmia. Consider the potential disadvantages and benefits.

➤*Parenteral therapy:* The dangers of parenteral use of quinidine are increased in the presence of AV block or absence of atrial activity. Administration is more hazardous in patients with extensive myocardial damage. Use of quinidine in digitalis-induced cardiac arrhythmia is extremely dangerous because the cardiac glycoside may already have caused serious impairment of intracardiac conduction system. Too rapid IV administration of as little as 200 mg may precipitate a fall of 40 to 50 mmHg in arterial pressure. Inject slowly (see Administration and Dosage).

➤*Syncope:* Syncope occasionally occurs in patients on long-term quinidine therapy, usually resulting from ventricular tachycardia or fibrillation. It is manifested by sudden loss of consciousness and by polymorphic ventricular tachycardia. This syndrome does not appear to be related to dose or plasma levels but occurs more often with prolonged QT intervals. Syncopal episodes frequently terminate spontaneously or respond to treatment, but are sometimes fatal. Torsades de pointes is often the cause.

➤*Renal, hepatic or cardiac insufficiency:* Use with caution in renal (especially renal tubular acidosis), cardiac or hepatic insufficiency because of potential toxicity.

➤*Hypersensitivity reactions:* Asthma, muscle weakness and infection with fever prior to quinidine administration may mask hypersensitivity reactions to the drug.

Test dose – Administer a single 200 mg tablet of quinidine sulfate or 200 mg IM quinidine gluconate prior to the initiation of treatment to determine whether the patient has an idiosyncrasy to quinidine.

During the first weeks of therapy, although rare, consider hypersensitivity to quinidine including anaphylactoid reactions (eg, angioedema, purpura, acute asthmatic episode, vascular collapse). Refer to Management of Acute Hypersensitivity Reactions.

➤*Pregnancy: Category C.* Quinidine crosses the placenta and achieves fetal serum levels similar to maternal levels. Neonatal thrombocytopenia has occurred after maternal use. Safety for use during pregnancy is not established. Use only when clearly needed and when potential benefits outweigh potential hazards to fetus.

Oxytocic properties – Oxytocic properties are reported with quinidine, as with quinine; clinical significance is not known.

➤*Lactation:* Safety for use in the nursing mother has not been established. Quinidine is excreted into breast milk with a milk:serum ratio of ≈ 0.71. Use caution when quinidine is administered to a nursing woman. The American Academy of Pediatrics considers quinidine to be compatible with breastfeeding.

➤*Children:* Safety and efficacy have not been established.

Precautions

➤*Monitoring:* Perform periodic blood counts and liver and kidney function tests. Discontinue use if blood dyscrasias or signs of hepatic or renal disorders occur. Initiate therapy in the hospital and continuously monitor ECG and check quinidine levels. This is generally done when large doses are used or the patient is at increased risk. Frequently measure arterial blood pressure during IV use; discontinue if blood pressure falls significantly.

➤*Vagolytic effects:* Because quinidine has vagolytic activity on the atrium and AV node, administration of cholinergic drugs or use of any other procedure to enhance vagal activity may fail to terminate paroxysmal supraventricular tachycardia.

➤*Potassium balance:* The effect of quinidine is enhanced by potassium and reduced if hypokalemia is present. The risk of drug-induced torsades de pointes is increased by concomitant hypokalemia.

➤*Malaria (P. falciparum):* Dosing schedules known to be effective have been associated with hypotension, increased QRS and corrected QT intervals and cinchonism. Closely monitor ECG and blood pressure.

Drug Interactions

Quinidine Drug Interactions			
Precipitant drug	Object drug*		Description
Amiodarone	Quinidine	↑	Increased quinidine levels may occur with possible production of potentially fatal cardiac dysrhythmias.
Antacids	Quinidine	↑	Certain antacids may increase serum quinidine levels, which may result in toxicity.
Barbiturates	Quinidine	↓	Quinidine serum levels and elimination half-life may be decreased.

Quinidine Drug Interactions			
Precipitant drug	Object drug*		Description
Cholinergic drugs	Quinidine	↓	Since quinidine antagonizes the effect of vagal excitation upon the atrium and AV node, concurrent cholinergic agents may result in failure to terminate paroxysmal supraventricular tachycardia.
Cimetidine	Quinidine	↑	Quinidine serum levels may be increased.
Hydantoins	Quinidine	↓	A decrease in the therapeutic effect of quinidine may occur.
Nifedipine	Quinidine	↓	Serum levels and actions of quinidine may be lower than predicted by the dosage.
Rifampin	Quinidine	↓	Increased metabolism of quinidine which may be associated with a reduction in its therapeutic effects.
Sucralfate	Quinidine	↓	Serum quinidine levels may be reduced, decreasing the therapeutic effects.
Urinary alkalinizers	Quinidine	↑	Urinary elimination of quinidine is reduced. Serum quinidine levels may be increased accompanied by increased pharmacologic effects.
Verapamil	Quinidine	↑	Quinidine clearance may be reduced and its half-life prolonged, resulting in hypotension, bradycardia, ventricular tachycardia, AV block and pulmonary edema.
Quinidine	Anticholinergics	↑	Quinidine exhibits a distinct anticholinergic activity in the myocardial tissues. Concurrent use may cause an additive vagolytic effect.
Quinidine	Anticoagulants	↑	Anticoagulation may be potentiated; hemorrhage could occur.
Quinidine	Beta blockers	↑	Effects of metoprolol or propranolol may be increased in "extensive metabolizers."
Quinidine	Cardiac glycosides (digitoxin, digoxin)	↑	Plasma levels of the cardiac glycosides are markedly increased. Pharmacologic effects are increased and toxicity may occur.
Quinidine	Disopyramide	↑	Increased disopyramide levels or decreased quinidine levels may occur.
Disopyramide	Quinidine	↓	
Quinidine	Nondepolarizing neuromuscular blockers	↑	Nondepolarizing neuromuscular blocker effects may be enhanced.
Quinidine	Procainamide	↑	Pharmacologic effects of procainamide may be increased; elevated procainamide and NAPA (major metabolite) plasma levels with toxicity may occur.
Quinidine	Propafenone	↑	Serum propafenone levels may be increased in rapid extensive metabolizers of the drug (≈ 90% of patients), increasing the pharmacologic effects.
Quinidine	Succinylcholine	↑	The neuromuscular blockade produced by succinylcholine may be prolonged.
Quinidine	Tricyclic antidepressants	↑	The clearance of the tricyclic antidepressants may be reduced, possibly resulting in increased pharmacologic effects.

* ↑ = Object drug increased.   ↓ = Object drug decreased.

➤*Drug/Lab test interactions:* Triamterene and quinidine have similar fluorescence spectra; thus, triamterene will interfere with the fluorescent measurement of quinidine serum levels.

Adverse Reactions

➤*Cardiovascular:* Widening of QRS complex; cardiac asystole; ventricular ectopy; idioventricular rhythms (including ventricular tachycardia and fibrillation and torsades de pointes in some instances); paradoxical tachycardia; arterial embolism; hypotension; ventricular extrasystoles occurring at the rate of one or more every 6 normal beats; prolonged QT interval; complete AV block; ventricular flutter.

Stop use if any of these occur: Increase of > 25% in duration of QRS complex; disappearance of P waves; restoration of sinus rhythm; decrease in heart rate to 120 bpm in the ECG.

➤*CNS:* Headache; fever; vertigo; apprehension; excitement; confusion; delirium; syncope; dementia; ataxia; depression.

➤*Dermatologic:* Rash; urticaria; cutaneous flushing with intense pruritus; photosensitivity; eczema; exfoliative eruptions; psoriasis; abnormalities of pigmentation.

➤*GI:* The most common reactions seen with quinidine include the following: Nausea; vomiting; abdominal pain; diarrhea; anorexia. These may be preceded by fever.

Rarely, oral quinidine has been associated with esophageal disorders, primarily esophagitis.

➤*Hematologic:* Acute hemolytic anemia; hypoprothrombinemia; thrombocytopenic purpura; agranulocytosis; drug-induced hypoprothrombinemic hemorrhage in patients on chronic anticoagulant therapy (see Drug Interactions); thrombocytopenia; leukocytosis; shift to left in WBC differential; neutropenia.

➤*Hypersensitivity:* Angioedema; acute asthma; vascular collapse; respiratory arrest; hepatic dysfunction, including granulomatous hepatitis; hepatic toxicity; purpura; vasculitis (see Warnings).

➤*Musculoskeletal:* Arthralgia; myalgia.

➤*Ophthalmic:* Mydriasis; blurred vision; disturbed color perception; reduced vision field; photophobia; diplopia; night blindness; scotomata; optic neuritis.

➤*Special senses:* Disturbed hearing (tinnitus, decreased auditory acuity).

➤*Miscellaneous:* Increase in serum skeletal muscle creatine phosphokinase.

Cinchonism – Ringing in the ears; hearing loss; headache; nausea; dizziness; vertigo; lightheadedness; disturbed vision. These may appear after a single dose.

Renal / Hepatic – Lupus nephritis; hepatic toxicity, including granulomatous hepatitis; hepatitis.

Lupus erythematosus – Lupus erythematosus has occurred. Symptoms include hepatosplenomegaly/lymphadenopathy and a positive antinuclear antibody test. Symptoms resolve after drug withdrawal.

Overdosage

Severe quinidine intoxication may be associated with depressed mental function, even in hemodynamically stable patients. The patient progresses from lethargy to coma, including respiratory arrest; recurrent generalized motor seizures may occur. The onset of CNS manifestations may be substantially delayed beyond the onset of cardiovascular toxicity; conversely, recovery from coma is often delayed.

➤*Symptoms:*

Cardiovascular – Tachyarrhythmias (sinus tachycardia, ventricular tachycardia, ventricular fibrillation, torsades de pointes); depressed automaticity and conduction (QRS and QTc prolongation, bundle branch block, sinus bradycardia, sinoatrial block, sinus arrest, AV block, ST depression, T inversion); hypotension (depressed contractility and cardiac output, vasodilation); syncope; heart failure.

CNS – Lethargy; confusion; coma; respiratory depression or arrest; seizures; headache; paresthesia; vertigo.

GI – Vomiting; abdominal pain; diarrhea; nausea.

Miscellaneous – Cinchonism; hypokalemia; visual/auditory disturbances; tinnitus; acidosis.

➤*Treatment:* If ingestion of quinidine is recent, gastric lavage, emesis or administration of activated charcoal may reduce absorption. Management of overdosage includes the following: Symptomatic treatment; ECG, blood gases, serum electrolytes and blood pressure monitoring; cardiac pacing, if indicated; acidification of the urine. Avoid alkalinization of the urine. Mechanical ventilation and other supportive measures may be required.

IV infusion of ⅙ molar sodium lactate reportedly reduces the cardiotoxic effects of quinidine. Because marked CNS depression may occur even in the presence of convulsions, do not give CNS depressants. Hypotension may be treated, if necessary, with metaraminol or norepinephrine after adequate fluid volume replacement. Tachydysrhythmias should respond to phenytoin or lidocaine. Hemodialysis has been effective in overdosage but is rarely warranted.

Patient Information

Do not discontinue therapy unless instructed by physician.

May cause GI upset; take with food.

Notify the physician if ringing in the ears, visual disturbances, dizziness, headache, nausea, skin rash, or breathing difficulty occurs.

Do not crush or chew sustained-release tablets.

QUINIDINE SULFATE
Contains 83% anhydrous quinidine alkaloid.

Rx	**Quinidine Sulfate** (Various, eg, Danbury, Eon)	**Tablets:** 200 mg	In 100s and 1000s.
Rx	**Quinidine Sulfate** (Various, eg, Danbury, Eon)	**Tablets:** 300 mg	In 100s and 1000s.
Rx	**Quinidine Sulfate** (Various, eg, Teva)	**Tablets, sustained-release:** 300 mg	In 100s and 250s.

For complete prescribing information, refer to the Quinidine group monograph.

QUINIDINE GLUCONATE
Conains 62% anhydrous quinidine alkaloid.

Rx	**Quinidine Gluconate** (Various, eg, Geneva)	**Tablets, sustained-release:** 324 mg	In 100s, 250s, and 500s.
Rx	**Quinidine Gluconate** (Lilly)	**Injection:** 80 mg/mL (50 mg/mL quinidine)	In 10 mL multi-dose vials.[1]

[1] With 0.005% EDTA and 0.25% phenol.

For complete prescribing information, refer to the Quinidine group monograph.

PROCAINAMIDE HCl

Rx	**Procainamide HCl**[1] (Various, eg, Teva)	**Tablets, extended-release:** 250 mg	In 100s and 500s.
Rx	**Procainamide HCl**[1] (Various, eg, Teva)	**Tablets, extended-release:** 500 mg	In 100s and 500s.
Rx	**Procainamide HCl**[1] (Various, eg, Teva)	**Tablets, extended-release:** 750 mg	In 100s and 500s.
Rx	**Procanbid**[2] (Monarch)	**Tablets, extended-release:** 500 mg	(PROCANBID 500). White, elliptical. Film-coated. In 60s and UD 100s.
Rx	**Procainamide HCl**[1] (Various, eg, Teva)	**Tablets, extended-release:** 1000 mg	In 100s.
Rx	**Procanbid**[2] (Monarch)		(PROCANBID 1000). Gray, elliptical. Film-coated. In UD 100s.
Rx	**Procainamide HCl** (Various, eg, Ivax)	**Capsules:** 250 mg	May contain parabens. In 100s, 250s, and 1000s.
Rx	**Procainamide HCl** (Various, eg, Ivax)	**Capsules:** 375 mg	May contain parabens. In 100s, 250s, and 1000s.
Rx	**Procainamide HCl** (Various, eg, Ivax)	**Capsules:** 500 mg	May contain parabens. In 100s, 250s, and 1000s.
Rx	**Procainamide HCl** (Various, eg, Abbott)	**Injection:** 500 mg/mL	May contain methylparaben and sodium metabisulfite. In 2 mL vials.

[1] These extended-release tablets are dosed at 6-hour intervals.

[2] These extended-release tablets are dosed at 12-hour intervals.

Refer to the general introductory discussion concerning Antiarrhythmic Agent.

WARNING

The prolonged administration of procainamide often leads to the development of a positive antinuclear antibody (ANA) test, with or without symptoms of a lupus erythematosus-like syndrome. If a positive ANA titer develops, assess the benefit/risk ratio related to continued procainamide therapy.

Mortality: In the National Heart, Lung and Blood Institute's Cardiac Arrhythmia Suppression Trial (CAST), a long-term, multicentered, randomized, double-blind study in patients with asymptomatic non-life-threatening ventricular arrhythmias who had an MI more than 6 days but less than 2 years previously, an excessive mortality or nonfatal cardiac arrest rate was seen in patients treated with encainide or flecainide (7.7%) compared with that seen in patients assigned to matched placebo-treated groups (3%). The average duration of treatment with encainide or flecainide in this study was 10 months.

The applicability of these results to other populations (eg, those without recent MIs) is uncertain. Considering the known proarrhythmic properties of procainamide and the lack of evidence of improved survival for any antiarrhythmic drug in patients without life-threatening arrhythmias, the use of procainamide and other antiarrhythmic agents should be reserved for patients with life-threatening ventricular arrhythmias.

Blood dyscrasias: Agranulocytosis, bone marrow depression, neutropenia, hypoplastic anemia, and thrombocytopenia in patients receiving procainamide have been reported at a rate of approximately 0.5%. Most of these patients received procainamide within the recommended dosage range. Fatalities have occurred (with approximately 20% to 25% mortality in reported cases of agranulocytosis). Because most of these events have been noted during the first 12 weeks of therapy, it is recommended that complete blood counts (CBC), including white cell, differential, and platelet counts be performed at weekly intervals for the first 3 months of therapy, and periodically thereafter. Perform CBC promptly if the patient develops any signs of infection (eg, fever, chills, sore throat, stomatitis), bruising, or bleeding. If any of these hematologic disorders are identified, discontinue therapy. Blood counts usually return to normal within 1 month of discontinuation. Use caution in patients with pre-existing marrow failure or cytopenia of any type (see Adverse Reactions).

Indications

Treatment of documented ventricular arrhythmias, such as sustained ventricular tachycardia, that are judged to be life-threatening. Because of the proarrhythmic effects, use with lesser arrhythmias is generally not recommended.

Because procainamide has the potential to produce serious hematologic disorders (0.5%), particularly leukopenia or agranulocytosis (sometimes fatal), reserve its use for patients in whom the benefits of treatment clearly outweigh the risks (see Warnings).

Avoid treatment of patients with asymptomatic ventricular premature depolarizations.

➤*Unlabeled uses:*

Atrial fibrillation/flutter – Procainamide has been used to convert atrial fibrillation/flutter to sinus rhythm.

Use in children – The following doses of procainamide have been suggested:

Oral: 15 to 50 mg/kg/day divided every 3 to 6 hours. Maximum dose is 4 g/day.

IM: 20 to 30 mg/kg/day.

IV: Loading dose is 3 to 6 mg/kg infused over 5 minutes, not to exceed 100 mg/dose. Maintenance dose is 20 to 80 mcg/kg/min as continuous IV infusion; usual maximum is 2 g/day.

For the treatment of hemodynamically stable ventricular tachycardia in children, procainamide (loading dose of 15 mg/kg IV infused over 30 to 60 minutes) may be considered as an alternative agent to amiodarone.

Administration and Dosage

➤*Approved by the FDA:* June 1950.

➤*Oral:* Oral dosage forms are preferable for less urgent arrhythmias and for long-term maintenance after initial parenteral therapy. Individualize dosage based on clinical assessment of the degree of underlying myocardial disease, the patient's age and renal function.

As a general guide, for younger adult patients with normal renal function, an initial total daily oral dose of up to 50 mg/kg may be used, given in divided doses every 3 hours (or with *Procanbid*, in 2 divided doses every 12 hours), to maintain therapeutic blood levels. For older patients, especially those older than 50 years of age, or for patients with renal, hepatic, or cardiac insufficiency, lesser amounts or longer intervals may produce adequate blood levels and decrease the probability of occurrence of dose-related adverse reactions. Administer the initial total daily dose of the immediate-release form in divided doses at 3-, 4-, or 6-hour intervals and adjust according to patient response.

Guidelines to Provide up to 50 mg/kg/day Procainamide[1]					
Weight		Immediate-release		Dose every 6 hours (extended release)	Dose every 12 hours (*Procanbid* extended-release tablets only)
lb	kg	Dose every 3 hours	Dose every 6 hours		
88-110	40-50	250 mg	500 mg	500 mg	1 g
132-154	60-70	375 mg	750 mg	750 mg	1.5 g
176-198	80-90	500 mg	1 g	1 g	2 g
> 220	> 100	625 mg	1.25 g	1.25 g	2.5 g

[1] Initial dosage schedule guide only, to be adjusted for each patient individually, based on age, cardiorenal function, blood level (if available), and clinical response.

➤*Extended-release:* For patients who have been receiving another formulation of procainamide, the dose of the other formulation can function as a general guide, but retitration with extended-release procainamide is recommended. Swallow extended-release procainamide tablets whole and do not break or chew.

➤*Parenteral:* Useful for arrhythmias that require immediate suppression and for maintenance of arrhythmia control. IV therapy allows most rapid control of serious arrhythmias, including those following MI; use in circumstances where close observation and monitoring of the patient are possible, such as in hospital or emergency facilities. IM administration is less apt to produce temporary high plasma levels, but therapeutic plasma levels are not obtained as rapidly as with IV administration.

IM – Administration may be used as an alternative to the oral route for patients with less threatening arrhythmias but who are nauseated or vomiting, ordered to receive nothing by mouth preoperatively, or may have malabsorptive problems. An initial daily dose of 50 mg/kg may be estimated. Divide this amount into fractional doses of ⅛ to ¼ to be injected IM every 3 to 6 hours until oral therapy is possible. If more than 3 injections are given, assess patient factors such as age and renal function, clinical response and, if available, blood levels of procainamide and n-acetylprocainamide (NAPA) in adjusting further doses for that individual. For treatment of arrhythmias associated with anesthesia or surgery, the suggested dose is 100 to 500 mg by IM injection.

IV – Cautiously administer the IV injection to avoid a possible hypotensive response. Initial arrhythmia control, under blood pressure and ECG monitoring, may usually be accomplished safely within 30 minutes by either of the 2 methods that follow:

1.) Slowly direct injection into a vein or into tubing of an established infusion line at a rate not to exceed 50 mg/min. It is advisable to dilute the 500 mg/mL concentrations prior to IV injection to facilitate control of dosage rate. Doses of 100 mg may be administered every 5 minutes at this rate until the arrhythmia is suppressed or

PROCAINAMIDE HCl

until 500 mg has been administered, after which it is advisable to wait at least 10 minutes to allow for more distribution into tissues before resuming.

2.) Alternatively, a loading infusion containing 20 mg/mL (1 g diluted to 50 mL with 5% dextrose injection) may be administered at a constant rate of 1 mL/min for 25 to 30 minutes to deliver 500 to 600 mg. Some effects may be seen after infusion of the first 100 or 200 mg; it is unusual to require more than 600 mg to achieve satisfactory antiarrhythmic effects.

The maximum advisable dosage to be given either by repeated bolus injections or such loading infusion is 1 g.

To maintain therapeutic levels, a more dilute IV infusion at a concentration of 2 mg/mL is convenient (1 g in 500 mL 5% dextrose injection), and may be administered at 1 to 3 mL/min. If daily total fluid intake must be limited, a 4 mg/mL concentration (1 g in 250 mL of 5% dextrose injection) administered at 0.5 to 1.5 mL/min will deliver an equivalent 2 to 6 mg/min. Assess the amount needed in a given patient to maintain the therapeutic level principally from the clinical response. This will depend on the patient's weight and age, renal elimination, hepatic acetylation rate, and cardiac status, but adjust for each patient based on close observation. A maintenance infusion rate of 50 mcg/kg/min to a person with a normal renal procainamide elimination half-life of 3 hours should produce a plasma level of about 6.5 mcg/mL.

Dilutions and Rates for IV Infusions of Procainamide

Infusion	Final concentration	Infusion volume[1]	Procainamide to be added	Infusion rate
Initial loading infusion	20 mg/mL	50 mL	1000 mg	1 mL/min (for up to 25 to 30 min)
Maintenance infusion[2]	2 mg/mL or	500 mL	1000 mg	1 to 3 mL/min
	4 mg/mL	250 mL	1000 mg	0.5 to 1.5 mL/min

[1] All infusions should be made up to final volume with 5% dextrose injection.
[2] The maintenance infusion rates are calculated to deliver 2 to 6 mg/min depending on body weight, renal elimination rate, and steady-state plasma level needed to maintain control of the arrhythmia. The 4 mg/mL maintenance concentration may be preferred if total infused volume must be limited.

Because the principal route for elimination of procainamide and NAPA is renal excretion, reduced excretion will prolong the half-life of elimination and lower the dose rate needed to maintain therapeutic levels. Advancing age reduces the renal excretion of procainamide and NAPA independently of reductions in Ccr; compared with normal young adults, there is an approximately 25% reduction at 50 years of age and a 50% reduction at 75 years of age.

Terminate IV therapy if persistent conduction disturbances or hypotension develop. As soon as the patient's basic cardiac rhythm appears to be stabilized, oral antiarrhythmic maintenance therapy is preferable (if indicated and possible). A period of about 3 to 4 hours (one half-life for renal elimination, ordinarily) should elapse after the last IV dose before administering the first dose of oral procainamide.

➤*Storage / Stability:* Store capsules at 15° to 30°C (59° to 86°F); store extended-release tablets at 20° to 25°C (68° to 77°F). Dispense in well-closed, tight containers. Store injection at controlled room temperature (15° to 30°C; 59° to 86°F); do not freeze.

Actions

➤*Pharmacology:* Procainamide, a class IA antiarrhythmic, increases the effective refractory period of the atria, and to a lesser extent, the bundle of His-Purkinje system and ventricles of the heart. It reduces impulse conduction velocity in the atria, His-Purkinje fibers, and ventricular muscle, but has variable effects on the atrioventricular (AV) node, a direct slowing action and a weaker vagolytic effect that may speed AV conduction slightly.

Myocardial excitability is reduced in the atria, Purkinje fibers, papillary muscles, and ventricles by an increase in the threshold for excitation, combined with inhibition of ectopic pacemaker activity by retardation of the slow phase of diastolic depolarization, thus decreasing automaticity especially in ectopic sites. Contractility of the undamaged heart is usually not affected by therapeutic concentrations, although slight reduction of cardiac output may occur, and may be significant in the presence of myocardial damage. Therapeutic levels of procainamide may exert vagolytic effects and produce slight acceleration of heart rate, while high or toxic concentrations may prolong AV conduction time or induce AV block, or even cause abnormal automaticity and spontaneous firing by unknown mechanisms.

Electrophysiology – The ECG may reflect the above effects by showing slight sinus tachycardia (because of the anticholinergic action) and widened QRS complexes and, less regularly, prolonged QT and PR intervals (because of longer systole and slower conduction), as well as some decrease in QRS and T-wave amplitude. These direct effects on electrical activity, conduction, responsiveness, excitability, and automaticity are characteristic of a group IA antiarrhythmic agent, the prototype for which is quinidine; procainamide effects are very similar. However, procainamide has weaker vagal blocking action than does quinidine, does not induce alpha-adrenergic blockade, and is less depressing to cardiac contractility.

➤*Pharmacokinetics:*

Absorption / Distribution – Oral procainamide is resistant to digestive hydrolysis, and the drug is well absorbed from the entire small intestinal surface, but individual patients vary in their completeness of absorption. The absolute bioavailability from immediate-release procainamide capsules is approximately 85% in patients and healthy subjects. Following oral administration, plasma levels peak at about 45 to 120 minutes. Following IM injection, absorption into the bloodstream is rapid; plasma levels peak in 15 to 60 minutes, considerably faster than oral administration. IV use can produce therapeutic plasma levels within minutes after an infusion is started. About 15% to 20% is reversibly bound to plasma proteins, and considerable amounts are more slowly and reversibly bound to tissues of the heart, liver, lung, and kidney. The apparent volume of distribution eventually reaches about 2 L/kg with a half-life of approximately 5 minutes. While procainamide crosses the blood-brain barrier in the dog, it did not concentrate in the brain at levels higher than in plasma. Plasma esterases are far less active in hydrolysis of procainamide than of procaine. After administration of procainamide extended-release tablets with a high-fat meal, the extent of procainamide absorption was increased by about 20%.

Metabolism / Excretion – A significant fraction of the circulating procainamide may be metabolized in hepatocytes to NAPA, ranging from 16% to 21% of an administered dose in "slow acetylators" to 24% to 33% in "fast acetylators." Because NAPA also has significant antiarrhythmic activity and somewhat slower renal clearance than procainamide, both hepatic acetylation rate capability and renal function, as well as age, have significant effects on the effective biologic half-life of therapeutic action of administered procainamide and the NAPA derivative. The elimination half-life of procainamide is 3 to 4 hours in patients with normal renal function, but reduced creatinine clearance (Ccr) and advancing age each prolong the elimination half-life. Based upon the approximate half-life of 3 hours for procainamide, pharmacokinetic steady state would be reached within 1 day. Trace amounts may be excreted in the urine as free and conjugated p-aminobenzoic acid, 30% to 60% as unchanged procainamide, and 6% to 52% as the NAPA derivative. Both procainamide and NAPA are eliminated by active tubular secretion as well as by glomerular filtration. After IV administration of procainamide, the renal clearance of procainamide ranged from 400 to 600 mL/min. Active renal secretion ranged from 300 to 500 mL/min, and is therefore, the major elimination pathway for procainamide. Action of procainamide on the CNS is not prominent, but high plasma concentrations may cause tremors.

While therapeutic plasma levels for procainamide have been reported to be 3 to 10 mcg/mL, certain patients such as those with sustained ventricular tachycardia may need higher levels for adequate control. This may justify the increased risk of toxicity (see Overdosage). Where programmed ventricular stimulation has been used to evaluate efficacy of procainamide in preventing recurrent ventricular tachyarrhythmias, higher plasma levels (mean, 13.6 mcg/mL) were found necessary for adequate control. Plasma levels of NAPA that produce arrhythmia suppression range from 10 to 20 mcg/mL. Toxicity may occur with levels more than 30 mcg/mL, although there appears to be overlap between the therapeutic and toxic ranges.

Contraindications

Complete heart block; idiosyncratic hypersensitivity; lupus erythematosus; torsades de pointes (see Warnings).

Warnings

➤*Blood dyscrasias:* Agranulocytosis, bone marrow depression, neutropenia, hypoplastic anemia, and thrombocytopenia in patients receiving procainamide have been reported at a rate of about 0.5%. Most of these patients received procainamide within the recommended dosage range. Fatalities have occurred (with about 20% to 25% mortality in reported cases of agranulocytosis). Because most of these events have been noted during the first 12 weeks of therapy, it is recommended that CBC, including white cell, differential, and platelet counts be performed at weekly intervals for the first 3 months of therapy, and periodically thereafter. Perform CBC promptly if the patient develops any signs of infection (eg, fever, chills, sore throat, stomatitis), bruising, or bleeding. If any of these hematologic disorders are identified, discontinue therapy. Blood counts usually return to normal within 1 month of discontinuation. Use caution in patients with pre-existing marrow failure or cytopenia of any type (see Adverse Reactions).

➤*Mortality:* In the CAST study, a long-term, multicentered, randomized, double-blind study in patients with asymptomatic non-life-threatening ventricular arrhythmias who had had MIs more than 6 days but less than 2 years previously, an excessive mortality or nonfatal cardiac arrest rate (7.7%) was seen in patients treated with encainide or flecainide compared with that seen in patients assigned to matched placebo-treated groups (3%). The average duration of treatment with encainide or flecainide in this study was 10 months.

The applicability of these results to other populations (eg, those without recent MIs) is uncertain. Considering the known proarrhythmic properties of procainamide and the lack of evidence of improved survival for any antiarrhythmic drug in patients without life-threatening arrhythmias, reserve the use of procainamide and other antiarrhythmic agents for patients with life-threatening ventricular arrhythmias.

PROCAINAMIDE HCl

➤*Survival:* Antiarrhythmic drugs have not been shown to enhance survival in patients with ventricular arrhythmias.

➤*Complete heart block:* Do not administer to patients with complete heart block because of its effects in suppressing nodal or ventricular pacemakers and the hazard of asystole. It may be difficult to recognize complete heart block in patients with ventricular tachycardia, but if significant slowing of ventricular rate occurs during treatment without evidence of AV conduction appearing, stop procainamide. In cases of second-degree AV block or various types of hemiblock, avoid or discontinue procainamide because of the possibility of increased severity of block, unless ventricular rate is controlled by an electrical pacemaker.

➤*Torsades de pointes:* In the unusual ventricular arrhythmia called torsades de pointes, characterized by alternation of one or more ventricular premature beats in directions of the QRS complexes on ECG in persons with prolonged QT and often enhanced U waves, group IA antiarrhythmic drugs are contraindicated. Administration of procainamide in such cases may aggravate this special type of ventricular extrasystole or tachycardia instead of suppressing it.

➤*Lupus erythematosus:* An established diagnosis of systemic lupus erythematosus is a contraindication to procainamide therapy because aggravation of symptoms is highly likely. If the lupus erythematosus-like syndrome develops in a patient with recurrent life-threatening arrhythmias not controlled by other agents, corticosteroid suppressive therapy may be used concomitantly with procainamide. Because the procainamide-induced lupoid syndrome rarely includes the dangerous pathologic renal changes, therapy may not necessarily have to be stopped unless the symptoms of serositis and the possibility of further lupoid effects are of greater risk than the benefit of procainamide in controlling arrhythmias. Patients with rapid acetylation capability are less likely to develop the lupoid syndrome after prolonged procainamide therapy (see Black Box Warning).

➤*Digitalis intoxication:* Exercise caution in the use of procainamide in arrhythmias associated with digitalis intoxication. Procainamide can suppress digitalis-induced arrhythmias; however, if there is concomitant marked disturbance of AV conduction, additional depression of conduction and ventricular asystole or fibrillation may result. Therefore, consider use of procainamide only if discontinuation of digitalis, and therapy with potassium, lidocaine, or phenytoin, are ineffective.

➤*First-degree heart block:* Exercise caution if the patient exhibits or develops first-degree heart block while taking procainamide; dosage reduction is advised in such cases. If the block persists despite dosage reduction, continuation of procainamide must be evaluated on the basis of current benefit vs risk of increased heart block.

➤*Predigitalization for atrial flutter or fibrillation:* Cardiovert or digitalize patients with atrial flutter or fibrillation prior to procainamide administration to avoid enhancement of AV conduction that may result in ventricular rate acceleration beyond tolerable limits. Adequate digitalization reduces but does not eliminate the possibility of sudden increase in ventricular rate as the atrial rate is slowed by procainamide in these arrhythmias.

➤*Congestive heart failure (CHF):* Use with caution in patients with CHF and in those with acute ischemic heart disease or cardiomyopathy because even slight depression of myocardial contractility may further reduce cardiac output of the damaged heart.

➤*Concurrent antiarrhythmic agents:* Concurrent use of procainamide with other group IA antiarrhythmic agents (eg, quinidine, disopyramide) may produce enhanced prolongation of conduction or depression of contractility and hypotension, especially in patients with cardiac decompensation. Reserve such use for patients with serious arrhythmias unresponsive to a single drug; use only if close observation is possible (see Drug Interactions).

➤*Myasthenia gravis:* Patients may show worsening of symptoms from procainamide because of its procaine-like effect on diminishing acetylcholine release at skeletal muscle motor nerve endings. Procainamide administration may be hazardous without optimal adjustment of anticholinesterase medications and other precautions. Immediately after initiation of therapy, closely observe patients for muscular weakness if myasthenia gravis is a possibility.

➤*Hypersensitivity reactions:* In patients sensitive to procaine or other ester-type local anesthetics, cross-sensitivity to procainamide is unlikely; however, consider the possibility. Do not use procainamide if it produces acute allergic dermatitis, asthma, or anaphylactic symptoms.

➤*Renal function impairment:* Renal insufficiency may lead to accumulation of high plasma levels from conventional doses of procainamide, with effects similar to those of overdosage (see Overdosage), unless dosage is adjusted for the individual patient.

➤*Pregnancy: Category C.* Procainamide crosses the placenta. It is not known whether procainamide can cause fetal harm when administered to a pregnant woman or can affect reproduction capacity. However, use during pregnancy has not been associated with congenital anomalies or other adverse effects to the fetus. Give to a pregnant woman only if clearly needed.

➤*Lactation:* Both procainamide and NAPA are excreted in breast milk and absorbed by the nursing infant. Because of the potential for serious adverse reactions in nursing infants, decide whether to discontinue nursing or the drug, taking into account the importance of the drug to the mother.

➤*Children:* Safety and efficacy have not been established. However, see Indications.

Precautions

➤*Monitoring:* Based upon the approximate half-life of 3 hours for procainamide, pharmacokinetic steady state would be reached within 1 day. After achieving and maintaining therapeutic plasma concentrations and satisfactory ECG and clinical responses, continue frequent periodic monitoring of vital signs and ECG. If evidence of QRS widening of more than 25% or marked prolongation of the QT interval occurs, concern for overdosage is appropriate; reduction in dosage is advisable if a 50% increase occurs. Elevated serum creatinine or urea nitrogen, reduced Ccr or history of renal insufficiency, and use in older patients (over 50 years of age), provide grounds to anticipate that less than the usual dosage may suffice, because the urinary elimination of procainamide and NAPA may be reduced, leading to gradual accumulation beyond normally predicted amounts. If facilities are available for measurement of plasma procainamide and NAPA levels or acetylation capability, individual dose adjustment for optimal therapeutic levels may be easier; however, close observation of clinical effectiveness is the most important criterion.

In the longer term, periodic CBCs are useful to detect possible idiosyncratic hematologic effects of procainamide on neutrophil, platelet, or red cell homeostasis; agranulocytosis may occur occasionally in patients on long-term therapy. A rising titer of serum ANA may precede clinical symptoms of the lupoid syndrome. Laboratory tests, such as CBCs, ECG, and serum creatinine or urea nitrogen may be indicated, depending on the clinical situation; periodic rechecking of the CBC and ANA may be helpful in early detection of untoward reactions.

➤*Embolization:* In conversion of atrial fibrillation to normal sinus rhythm by any means, dislodgement of mural thrombi may lead to embolization.

➤*Sulfite sensitivity:* Some of these products contain sulfites that may cause allergic-type reactions, including anaphylactic symptoms and life-threatening or less severe asthmatic episodes in certain susceptible persons. The overall prevalence of sulfite sensitivity in the general population is unknown and probably low. It is seen more frequently in asthmatic or atopic nonasthmatic persons.

Drug Interactions

Procainamide Drug Interactions			
Precipitant drug	Object drug*		Description
Amiodarone	Procainamide	↑	Amiodarone may increase procainamide serum concentrations. Monitor procainamide concentrations closely.
Anticholinergics	Procainamide	↑	Coadministration may produce additive antivagal effects on AV conduction. This effect is not as well documented for procainamide as for quinidine.
Antiarrhythmics	Procainamide	↑	Additive effects on the heart may occur with concurrent use of procainamide and other antiarrhythmics (eg, lidocaine, quinidine, disopyramide). Dosage reduction may be necessary (see Warnings). Quinidine also may increase procainamide and NAPA concentrations.
Cimetidine Ranitidine	Procainamide	↑	Cimetidine may increase procainamide serum concentrations because of decreased renal clearance. Avoid this combination, if possible. If cimetidine is necessary, then monitor procainamide concentrations closely and adjust the dose as needed. Large (> 300 mg/day) doses of ranitidine also may have this effect.
Ethanol	Procainamide	↔	The actions of procainamide could be altered, but because the main metabolite (NAPA) is also an antiarrhythmic, specific effects are unclear.
Propranolol	Procainamide	↑	One study showed that propranolol increased procainamide serum concentrations by decreasing the plasma clearance. Another study showed no changes in procainamide clearance.

PROCAINAMIDE HCl

Procainamide Drug Interactions			
Precipitant drug	Object drug*		Description
Quinolones	Procainamide	↑	The risk of life-threatening cardiac arrhythmias, including torsades de pointes, may be increased when procainamide is given with sparfloxacin, gatifloxacin, or moxifloxacin. Sparfloxacin is contraindicated with class IA antiarrhythmics. Also, ofloxacin may increase procainamide concentrations. Monitor concentrations and adjust dose as indicated.
Thioridazine Ziprasidone	Procainamide	↑	Concurrent use may result in synergistic or additive prolongation of the QT$_c$ interval and increase the risk for life-threatening cardiac arrhythmias, including torsades de pointes.
Trimethoprim	Procainamide	↑	Elevated procainamide and NAPA serum levels may occur, possibly resulting in increased pharmacologic effects. Monitor serum concentrations.
Procainamide	Neuromuscular blockers (eg, succinylcholine)	↑	Procainamide may potentiate the neuromuscular blockade produced by agents such as succinylcholine. A reduced dose of the neuromuscular blocker may be required.

* ↑ = Object drug increased. ↔ = Undetermined clinical effect.

➤*Drug/Lab test interactions:* Suprapharmacologic concentrations of lidocaine and meprobamate may inhibit fluorescence of procainamide and NAPA. Propranolol shows a native fluorescence close to the procainamide/NAPA peak wavelengths; therefore, tests that depend on fluorescence measurement may be affected.

Adverse Reactions

➤*Cardiovascular:* Hypotension following oral administration is rare. Hypotension and serious disturbances of cardiorhythm, such as ventricular asystole or fibrillation, are more common after IV use. Second-degree heart block has occurred in 2 of almost 500 patients taking procainamide orally.

➤*CNS:* Dizziness; giddiness; weakness; mental depression; psychosis with hallucinations.

➤*Dermatologic:* Angioneurotic edema; urticaria; pruritus; flushing; maculopapular rash.

➤*GI:* Anorexia, nausea, vomiting, abdominal pain, bitter taste, diarrhea (3% to 4%; oral).

➤*Hematologic:* Neutropenia; thrombocytopenia; hemolytic anemia (rare). Agranulocytosis has occurred after repeated use of procainamide; deaths have occurred (see Warnings).

➤*Hepatic:* Elevations of transaminase with and without elevations of alkaline phosphatase and bilirubin have been reported. Some patients have had clinical symptoms (eg, malaise, right upper quadrant pain). Deaths from liver failure have been reported.

➤*Miscellaneous:*
Lupus erythematosus – A lupus erythematosus-like syndrome (eg, arthralgia, pleural or abdominal pain, and sometimes arthritis, pleural effusion, pericarditis, fever, chills, myalgia, and possibly related hematologic or skin lesions) is fairly common after prolonged administration, perhaps more often in patients who are slow acetylators (see Warnings). While some studies have reported the syndrome in less than 1 in 500, others have reported it in up to 30% of patients on long-term oral therapy. If discontinuation does not reverse the lupoid symptoms, corticosteroid treatment may be effective.

Overdosage

➤*Symptoms:* Progressive widening of the QRS complex, prolonged QT and PR intervals, lowering of the R and T waves, and increasing AV block may be seen with doses that are excessive for a given patient. Increased ventricular extrasystoles or ventricular tachycardia or fibrillation may occur. After IV administration, but seldom after oral therapy, transient high plasma levels may induce hypotension, affecting systolic more than diastolic pressures, especially in hypertensive patients. Such high levels also may produce CNS depression, tremor, and respiratory depression.

Plasma levels above 10 mcg/mL are increasingly associated with toxic findings that are seen occasionally in the 10 to 12 mcg/mL range, more often in the 12 to 15 mcg/mL range, and commonly in patients with plasma levels above 15 mcg/mL. Overdosage symptoms may result following a single oral 2 g dose, while 3 g may be dangerous, especially if the patient is a slow acetylator and has decreased renal function or underlying organic heart disease.

➤*Treatment:* Treatment includes general supportive measures, close observation, monitoring of vital signs, and possibly IV pressor agents and mechanical cardiorespiratory support. Refer to General Management of Acute Overdosage. If available, procainamide and NAPA plasma levels may be helpful in assessing the potential degree of toxicity and response to therapy. Both procainamide and NAPA are removed from the circulation by hemodialysis but not peritoneal dialysis. No specific antidote for procainamide is known.

Patient Information

Close cooperation in adhering to the prescribed dosage schedule is of great importance in safely controlling the cardiac arrhythmia. More medication is not necessarily better and may be dangerous; skipping doses or increasing intervals between doses to suit personal convenience may lead to loss of control of the heart problem, and "making up" missed doses by doubling up later may be hazardous.

The patient should disclose any history of drug sensitivity, especially to procaine, other local anesthetic agents or aspirin, and report any history of kidney disease, CHF, myasthenia gravis, liver disease, or lupus erythematosus.

The patient should report promptly any symptoms of arthralgia, myalgia, fever, chills, skin rash, easy bruising, sore throat, or sore mouth, infections, dark urine or icterus, wheezing, muscular weakness, chest or abdominal pain, palpitations, nausea, vomiting, anorexia, diarrhea, hallucinations, dizziness, or depression.

Advise patient not to break or chew the extended-release tablet formulation as this would interfere with designed dissolution characteristics. The tablet matrix may be seen in the stool because it does not disintegrate following release of procainamide.

DISOPYRAMIDE

Rx	Disopyramide Phosphate (Various, eg, Geneva, Tava)	Capsules: 100 mg (as phosphate)	In 100s and 500s.
Rx	Norpace (Pharmacia)		Lactose. (SEARLE 2752 NORPACE 100 MG). White/Orange. In 100s and 1000s.
Rx	Disopyramide Phosphate (Various, eg, Geneva, Teva)	Capsules: 150 mg (as phosphate)	In 100s and 500s.
Rx	Norpace (Pharmacia)		Lactose. (SEARLE 2762 NORPACE 150 MG). Brown/Orange. In 100s and 1000s.
Rx	Norpace CR (Pharmacia)	Capsules, extended-release: 100 mg (as phosphate)	Sucrose. (SEARLE 2732 NORPACE CR 100 mg). White/Lt. green. In 100s, 500s, and UD 100s.
Rx	Disopyramide Phosphate (Various, eg, Ethex, Geneva)	Capsules, extended-release: 150 mg (as phosphate)	In 100s.
Rx	Norpace CR (Pharmacia)		Sucrose. (SEARLE 2742 NORPACE CR 150 mg). Brown/Lt. green. In 100s, 500s, and UD 100s.

Refer to the general introductory discussion concerning Antiarrhythmic Agents.

WARNING

In the National Heart, Lung, and Blood Institute's Cardiac Arrhythmia Suppression Trial (CAST), a long-term, multi-center, randomized, double-blind study in patients with asymptomatic non-life-threatening ventricular arrhythmias who had an MI more than 6 days but less than 2 years previously, an excessive mortality or nonfatal cardiac arrest rate (7.7%) was seen in patients treated with encainide or flecainide compared with that seen in patients assigned to carefully matched placebo-treated groups (3%). The average duration of treatment with encainide or flecainide in this study was 10 months.

The applicability of the CAST results to other populations (eg, those without recent MI) is uncertain. Considering the known proarrhythmic properties of disopyramide and the lack of evidence of improved survival for any antiarrhythmic drug in patients without life-threatening arrhythmias, the use of disopyramide as well as other antiarrhythmic agents should be reserved for patients with life-threatening ventricular arrhythmias.

Indications

Treatment of documented ventricular arrhythmias (eg, sustained ventricular tachycardia) considered to be life-threatening.

➤Unlabeled uses: Disopyramide may be beneficial in the treatment of paroxysmal supraventricular tachycardia.

Administration and Dosage

➤Approved by the FDA: 1977.

Individualize dosage. Initiate treatment in the hospital. Do not break or chew extended-release capsules.

➤Adults: 400 to 800 mg/day given in divided doses. The recommended dosage for most adults is 600 mg/day given in divided doses. For patients < 50 kg (110 pounds), give 400 mg/day. Divide the total daily dose and administer every 6 hours in the immediate-release form or every 12 hours in the controlled-release form.

In the event of increased anticholinergic side effects, plasma levels of disopyramide should be monitored and the dose of the drug adjusted accordingly. A reduction of the dose by one third, from the recommended 600 mg/day to 400 mg/day, would be reasonable, without changing the dosing interval.

➤Children: Divide daily dosage and administer equal doses every 6 hours or at intervals according to patient needs. Closely monitor plasma levels and therapeutic response. Hospitalize patients during initial treatment and start dose titration at the lower end of the ranges provided below:

Suggested Total Daily Disopyramide Dosage in Children[1]	
Age (years)	Disopyramide (mg/kg/day)
< 1	10 to 30
1 to 4	10 to 20
4 to 12	10 to 15
12 to 18	6 to 15

[1] Prepare a 1 to 10 mg/mL suspension by adding contents of the immediate-release capsule to cherry syrup, NF. The resulting suspension, when refrigerated, is stable for 1 month; shake thoroughly before measuring dose. Dispense in an amber glass bottle. Do not use the controlled-release form to prepare the solution.

➤Initial loading dose: For rapid control of ventricular arrhythmia, give an initial loading dose of 300 mg immediate-release (200 mg for patients < 50 kg [110 lb]). Therapeutic effects are attained in 30 minutes to 3 hours. If there is no response or no evidence of toxicity within 6 hours of the loading dose, 200 mg every 6 hours may be administered instead of the usual 150 mg. If there is no response within 48 hours, discontinue the drug or carefully monitor subsequent immediate-release doses of 250 or 300 mg every 6 hours.

Do not use the controlled-release form initially if rapid plasma levels are desired.

➤Severe refractory ventricular tachycardia: A limited number of patients have tolerated up to 1600 mg/day (400 mg every 6 hours),

resulting in plasma levels up to 9 mcg/mL. Hospitalize patients for close evaluation and continuous monitoring.

➤Cardiomyopathy or possible cardiac decompensation: Do not administer a loading dose, and limit the initial dosage to 100 mg immediate-release every 6 to 8 hours. Make subsequent dosage adjustments gradually.

➤Renal/Hepatic function failure: For patients with moderate renal insufficiency (Ccr > 40 mL/min) or hepatic insufficiency, the recommended dosage is 400 mg/day given in divided doses (either 100 mg every 6 hours for immediate release or 200 mg every 12 hours for controlled release).

In severe renal insufficiency (Ccr ≤ 40 mL/min), the recommended dosage is 100 mg of immediate-release form given at intervals shown in the table below, with or without an initial loading dose of 150 mg.

Disopyramide (Immediate-release) Dosage in Renal Impairment			
Creatinine clearance (mL/min)	Loading dose (mg)	Dose (mg)	Dosage interval (hours)
30-40	150	100	8
15-30	150	100	12
< 15	150	100	24

➤Transfer to disopyramide: Based on theoretical considerations, use the regular maintenance schedule, without a loading dose, 6 to 12 hours after the last dose of quinidine or 3 to 6 hours after the last dose of procainamide. Where withdrawal of quinidine or procainamide is likely to produce life-threatening arrhythmias, consider hospitalization.

When transferring from immediate to controlled release, start maintenance schedule of controlled release 6 hours after the last dose of immediate release.

Actions

➤Pharmacology:

Mechanism of action – Disopyramide is a class IA antiarrhythmic agent pharmacologically similar to, but chemically unrelated to, procainamide and quinidine. It decreases the rate of diastolic depolarization (phase 4), decreases the upstroke velocity (phase 0), increases the action potential duration of normal cardiac cells, and prolongs the refractory period (phases 2 and 3). It also decreases the disparity in refractoriness between infarcted and adjacent normally perfused myocardium and does not affect alpha- or beta-adrenergic receptors.

Anticholinergic activity – In vitro anticholinergic activity is approximately 0.06% that of atropine; the usual dose of 150 mg every 6 hours or 300 mg controlled release every 12 hours compares with approximately 0.4 to 0.6 mg of atropine.

Hemodynamic effects – At recommended oral doses, disopyramide rarely produces significant alterations of blood pressure in patients without congestive heart failure (see Warnings). With IV disopyramide (dosage form not available in US), either increases in systolic/diastolic or decreases in systolic blood pressure have occurred depending on the infusion rate and the patient population. IV disopyramide may cause cardiac depression with an approximate mean 10% reduction of cardiac output, which is more pronounced in patients with cardiac dysfunction.

Electrophysiology – Disopyramide shortens sinus node recovery time and lengthens atrial and ventricular refractoriness. The effects on AV nodal conduction and refractoriness and sinus node function vary because of a depressant effect that is counteracted by a vagolytic action. The principal metabolite, mono-N-dealkyldisopyramide (MND), exhibits little antiarrhythmic activity, but is 20 to 30 times more anticholinergic than the parent drug. Little effect has been shown on the AV nodal and His-Purkinje conduction times or on QRS duration, but conduction in accessory pathways is prolonged.

➤Pharmacokinetics:

Absorption/Distribution – Following oral administration of immediate-release disopyramide, the drug is rapidly and almost completely (≈ 90%) absorbed. Peak plasma levels usually occur within 2 hours. Therapeutic plasma levels of disopyramide are 2 to 4 mcg/mL. Protein binding is concentration-dependent and varies from 50% to 65%; it is difficult to predict the concentration of the free drug when total drug is measured. After the oral administration of 200 mg disopyramide to 10 cardiac patients with borderline to moderate heart failure, the time to

DISOPYRAMIDE

peak serum concentration of 2.3 ± 1.5 hours was increased, and the mean peak serum concentration of 4.8 ± 1.6 mcg/mL was higher than in healthy volunteers.

Metabolism/Excretion – About 50% is excreted in the urine as the unchanged drug and 30% as metabolites (20% MND). The plasma concentration of MND is approximately one tenth that of disopyramide. The mean plasma half-life is 6.7 hours (range, 4 to 10 hours).

Immediate-release vs controlled-release – In a crossover study in healthy subjects, the bioavailability of the controlled-release form was similar to that from the immediate-release capsules. With a single 300 mg oral dose, peak disopyramide plasma concentrations of 3.23 ± 0.75 mcg/mL at 2.5 ± 2.3 hours were obtained with two 150 mg immediate-release capsules and 2.22 ± 0.47 mcg/mL at 4.9 ± 1.4 hours with two 150 mg controlled-release capsules. The elimination half-life was 8.31 ± 1.83 hours with the immediate-release capsules and 11.65 ± 4.72 hours with controlled-release capsules. The amount of disopyramide and MND excreted in the urine in 48 hours was 128 and 48 mg, respectively, with the immediate-release capsules and 112 and 33 mg, respectively, with controlled-release capsules.

Following multiple doses, steady-state plasma levels of between 2 and 4 mcg/mL were attained following either 150 mg every 6 hours with immediate-release capsules or 300 mg every 12 hours with controlled-release capsules.

Special populations –

Renal function impairment: A preliminary report of 3 patients on long-term hemodialysis revealed a 45% to 72% reduction in disopyramide half-life during dialysis. In contrast, another study in patients on chronic hemodialysis demonstrated little difference in disopyramide half-life with or without dialysis (16.8 vs 16.1 hours). Resin and charcoal hemoperfusion were effective in rapidly decreasing disopyramide plasma levels in acute overdosage (see Overdosage).

In impaired renal function (creatinine clearance [Ccr] < 40 mL/min), half-life values ranged from 8 to 18 hours. Therefore, decrease the dose in renal failure to avoid drug accumulation (see Administration and Dosage). Altering urinary pH does not affect plasma half-life.

Contraindications

Cardiogenic shock; preexisting second- or third-degree AV block (if no pacemaker is present); congenital QT prolongation; hypersensitivity to disopyramide.

Warnings

➤*Mortality:* In the National Heart, Lung, and Blood Institute's Cardiac Arrhythmia Suppression Trial (CAST), a long-term, multi-center, randomized, double-blind study in patients with asymptomatic non-life-threatening ventricular arrhythmias who had had an MI more than 6 days but less than 2 years previously, an excessive mortality or nonfatal cardiac arrest rate (7.7%) was seen in patients treated with encainide or flecainide compared with that seen in patients assigned to carefully matched placebo-treated groups (3%). The average duration of treatment with encainide or flecainide in this study was 10 months.

The applicability of the CAST results to other populations (eg, those without recent MI) is uncertain. Considering the known proarrhythmic properties of disopyramide and the lack of evidence of improved survival for any antiarrhythmic drug in patients without life-threatening arrhythmias, the use of disopyramide as well as other antiarrhythmic agents should be reserved for patients with life-threatening ventricular arrhythmias.

➤*Proarrhythmic effects:* Because of the proarrhythmic effects, use with lesser arrhythmias is generally not recommended.

➤*Asymptomatic ventricular premature contractions:* Avoid treatment of patients with this condition.

➤*Survival:* Antiarrhythmic drugs have not been shown to enhance survival in patients with ventricular arrhythmias.

➤*Negative inotropic properties:*

Heart failure/hypotension – May cause or aggravate CHF or produce severe hypotension, especially in patients with primary cardiomyopathy or inadequately compensated CHF. Do not use in patients with uncompensated or marginally compensated CHF or hypotension unless secondary to cardiac arrhythmia. Treat patients with a history of heart failure with careful attention to the maintenance of cardiac function, including optimal digitalization. If hypotension occurs or CHF worsens, discontinue use; restart at a lower dosage after adequate cardiac compensation has been established.

Do not give a loading dose to patients with myocarditis or other cardiomyopathy; closely monitor initial dosage and subsequent adjustments.

QRS widening – Although unusual, QRS widening (more than 25%) may occur; discontinue use in such cases.

QT$_c$ prolongation – QT$_c$ prolongation and worsening of the arrhythmia, including ventricular tachycardia and fibrillation, may occur. Patients who have QT prolongation in response to quinidine may be at particular risk. As with other Type IA antiarrhythmics, disopyramide has been associated with torsade de pointes. If QT prolongation > 25% is observed and if ectopy continues, monitor closely and consider discontinuing the drug.

➤*Atrial tachyarrhythmias:* Digitalize patients with atrial flutter or fibrillation prior to administration to ensure that enhancement of AV conduction does not increase ventricular rate beyond acceptable limits.

➤*Conduction abnormalities:* Use caution in patients with sick sinus syndrome, Wolff-Parkinson-White (WPW), syndrome or bundle branch block.

➤*Heart block:* If first degree heart block develops, reduce dosage. If the block persists, drug continuation must depend upon the benefit compared to the risk of higher degrees of heart block. Development of second- or third-degree AV block or unifascicular, bifascicular, or trifascicular block requires discontinuation of therapy, unless ventricular rate is controlled by a ventricular pacemaker.

➤*Concomitant antiarrhythmic therapy:* Reserve concomitant use of disopyramide with other class IA or class IC antiarrhythmics or propranolol for life-threatening arrhythmias unresponsive to a single agent. Such use may produce serious negative inotropic effects or may excessively prolong conduction, particularly in patients with cardiac decompensation.

➤*Hypoglycemia:* Reported in rare instances. Monitor blood glucose levels in patients with CHF, chronic malnutrition, hepatic or renal disease, and in those taking drugs which could compromise normal glucoregulatory mechanisms in the absence of food (eg, beta-adrenoceptor blockers, alcohol).

➤*Anticholinergic activity:* Do not use in patients with urinary retention, glaucoma, or myasthenia gravis unless adequate overriding measures are taken. Urinary retention may occur in either sex, but males with benign prostatic hypertrophy are at particular risk. In patients with a family history of glaucoma, measure intraocular pressure before initiating therapy. Use with special care in patients with myasthenia gravis, because disopyramide could precipitate a myasthenic crisis.

➤*Renal function impairment:* Reduce dosage in impaired renal function. Carefully monitor ECG for prolongation of PR interval, evidence of QRS widening or other signs of overdosage (see Overdosage). The controlled-release form is not recommended for patients with severe renal insufficiency (Ccr ≤ 40 mL/min).

➤*Hepatic function impairment:* Hepatic function impairment increases plasma half-life; therefore, reduce dosage in such patients. Carefully monitor the ECG. Patients with cardiac dysfunction have a higher potential for hepatic impairment.

➤*Pregnancy: Category C.* Disopyramide was associated with decreased numbers of implantation sites and decreased growth and survival of pups when administered to pregnant rats at 250 mg/kg/day (≥ 20 times the usual daily human dose), a level at which weight gain and food consumption of dams were also reduced. Increased resorption rates were reported in rabbits at 60 mg/kg/day (≥ 5 times the usual daily human dose). At a maternal concentration of 2.3 mg/L disopyramide, the fetal cord concentration is 0.9 mg/L. Well-controlled studies have not been performed in pregnant women and experience is limited. Use only when clearly needed and when the potential benefits outweigh the potential hazards to the fetus. Disopyramide has been found in human fetal blood. Disopyramide may stimulate contractions of the pregnant uterus.

➤*Lactation:* Disopyramide has been detected in breast milk at a concentration not exceeding that in maternal plasma. Therefore, decide whether to discontinue nursing or to discontinue the drug taking into account the importance of the drug to the mother.

➤*Children:* Safety and efficacy have not been established.

Precautions

➤*Potassium imbalance:* Disopyramide may be ineffective in *hypo*kalemia and its toxic effects may be enhanced in *hyper*kalemia. Correct any potassium deficit before instituting therapy.

Drug Interactions

➤*CYP 450 system:* In vitro metabolic studies indicate that disopyramide is metabolized by CYP3A4; inhibitors of this system (eg, erythromycin, clarithromycin) may elevate plasma levels of disopyramide.

Disopyramide Drug Interactions			
Precipitant drug	Object drug*		Description
Antiarrhythmics	Disopyramide	↑	Other antiarrhythmics (eg, procainamide, lidocaine) have been used with disopyramide; however, widening of the QRS complex or QT prolongation may occur.
Beta blockers	Disopyramide	↔	This interaction is difficult to predict. Disopyramide clearance may be decreased; other adverse effects (eg, sinus bradycardia, hypotension) may occur. Others report no occurrence of synergistic or additive negative inotropic effects.

DISOPYRAMIDE

Disopyramide Drug Interactions			
Precipitant drug	Object drug*		Description
Cisapride	Disopyramide	↑	The risk of life-threatening cardiac arrhythmias, including torsades de pointes, may be increased due to possibly additive prolongation of the QT interval.
Disopyramide	Cisapride		
Clarithromycin Erythromycin	Disopyramide	↑	Increased disopyramide plasma levels may occur. Arrhythmias and increased QTc intervals have occurred.
Fluoroquino-lones	Disopyramide	↑	The risk of life-threatening cardiac arrhythmias, including torsades de pointes, may be increased. Sparfloxacin is contraindicated and gatifloxacin, levofloxacin, and moxifloxacin should be avoided in patients receiving disopyramide.
Hydantoins	Disopyramide	↓	Disopyramide serum levels, half-life and bioavailability may be decreased; anticholinergic effects may be enhanced. Effects may persist for several days after hydantoin withdrawal.
Quinidine	Disopyramide	↑	Concurrent use may result in increased disopyramide serum levels and decreased quinidine levels. This may result in diso-pyramide toxicity or decreased response to quinidine.
Disopyramide	Quinidine	↓	
Rifampin	Disopyramide	↓	Disopyramide serum levels may be decreased.
Thioridazine Ziprasidone	Disopyramide	↑	The risk of life-threatening cardiac arrhythmias, including torsades de pointes, may be increased. Coadministration is contraindicated.
Verapamil	Disopyramide	↔	Until data on this interaction are available, it is recommended that disopyramide not be adminis-tered within 48 hours before or 24 hours after verapamil.
Disopyramide	Anticoagulants	↓	Decreased prothrombin time after disopyramide discontinuation may occur. However, this may be due to a hemodynamic effect and not an interaction.
Disopyramide	Digoxin	↑	Although serum digoxin levels may be increased, a clinically sig-nificant interaction appears unlikely. A beneficial interaction has also been suggested.

* ↑ = Object drug increased. ↓ = Object drug decreased. ↔ = Undetermined clinical effect.

Adverse Reactions

The most serious adverse reactions are hypotension and CHF. The most common reactions are anticholinergic and dose-dependent. These may be transitory, but may be persistent or severe. Urinary retention is the most serious anticholinergic effect.

➤*Cardiovascular:* Hypotension with or without CHF, increased CHF, edema, weight gain, cardiac conduction disturbances, shortness of breath, syncope, chest pain (1% to 3%); AV block (< 1%). There have been reports of severe myocardial depression (with hypotension and an increase in venous pressure) and unexplained severe epigastric pain following standard oral doses.

➤*CNS:* Dizziness, fatigue, headache (3% to 9%); nervousness (1% to 3%); depression, insomnia (< 1%); acute psychosis (rare, prompt rever-sal when therapy discontinued).

➤*Dermatologic:* Generalized rash, dermatoses, itching (1% to 3%).

➤*GI:* Dry mouth (32%); nausea, pain, bloating, gas (3% to 9%); anorexia, diarrhea, vomiting (1% to 3%); elevated liver enzymes (< 1%); reversible cholestatic jaundice.

➤*GU:* Urinary hesitancy (14%); constipation (11%); urinary retention, frequency and urgency (3% to 9%); impotence (1% to 3%); dysuria, elevated creatinine (< 1%).

➤*Hematologic:* Decreased hemoglobin, hematocrit (< 1%); thrombocy-topenia, reversible agranulocytosis (rare).

➤*Musculoskeletal:* Muscle weakness, malaise, aches/pain (3% to 9%);

➤*Special senses:* Blurred vision, dry nose, eyes and throat (3% to 9%).

➤*Miscellaneous:* Hypokalemia, elevated cholesterol and triglycerides (1% to 3%); numbness, tingling, elevated BUN (< 1%); hypoglycemia; fever and respiratory difficulty; gynecomastia (rare); anaphylactoid reactions; lupus erythematosus symptoms (most cases occurred in patients who had been switched to disopyramide from procainamide after developing symptoms).

Overdosage

➤*Symptoms:* Overdose may be followed by apnea, loss of conscious-ness, cardiac arrhythmias, loss of spontaneous respiration and death. Toxic plasma levels produce excessive widening of the QRS complex and QT interval, worsening of CHF, hypotension, varying conduction disturbances, bradycardia, and finally, asystole. Anticholinergic effects may also be observed.

➤*Treatment:* Prompt, vigorous treatment is necessary even in the absence of symptoms. Such treatment may be lifesaving and may include gastric lavage followed by activated charcoal by mouth or stom-ach tube.

Administration of isoproterenol, dopamine, cardiac glycosides, diuret-ics, intra-aortic balloon counterpulsation, mechanical ventilation, hemodialysis or charcoal hemoperfusion may be used. Monitor ECG.

If progressive AV block develops, implement endocardial pacing. In case of impaired renal function, measures to increase the GFR may reduce the toxicity. Altering urinary pH does not affect plasma half-life or the amount of disopyramide excreted in the urine.

Anticholinergic effects can be reversed with neostigmine.

Refer also to General Management of Acute Overdosage.

Patient Information

May cause dry mouth, difficult urination, dizziness, breathing difficulty, constipation or blurred vision. Notify physician if symptoms persist, but do not discontinue unless instructed to do so by physician.

Do not break or chew extended-release capsules.

LIDOCAINE HCl

Rx	**LidoPen Auto-Injector** (Survival Technology)	**Injection:** (for IM adminis-tration) 300 mg/3 mL	Automatic injection device.[1]
Rx	**Lidocaine HCl for Cardiac Arrhythmias** (Abbott)	**Injection:** (for direct IV administration) 1% (10 mg/mL)	In 5 mL amps, 20, 30 and 50 mL vials and 5 mL *Abboject* syringes.
Rx	**Lidocaine HCl for Cardiac Arrhythmias** (Various, eg, Abbott)	**Injection:** (for direct IV administration) 2% (20 mg/mL)	In 5, 10, 20, 30 and 50 mL vials and 5 mL syringes.
Rx	**Xylocaine HCl IV for Cardiac Arrhythmias** (Astra)		In 5 mL amps.
Rx	**Lidocaine HCl for Cardiac Arrhythmias** (Various, eg, Abbott)	**Injection:** (for IV admix-tures) 4% (40 mg/mL)	In 5 mL amps and 25 and 50 mL vials.
Rx	**Lidocaine HCl for Cardiac Arrhythmias** (Abbott)	**Injection:** (for IV admix-tures) 10% (100 mg/mL)	In 10 mL additive vials.
Rx	**Lidocaine HCl for Cardiac Arrhythmias** (Abbott)	**Injection:** (for IV admix-tures) 20% (200 mg/mL)	In 5 and 10 mL syringes and 10 mL vials.
Rx	**Lidocaine HCl in 5% Dextrose** (Various, eg, Baxter, McGaw)	**Injection:** (for IV infusion) 0.2% (2 mg/mL)	In 500 and 1000 mL.
		0.4% (4 mg/mL)	In 250 and 500 mL.
		0.8% (8 mg/mL)	In 250 and 500 mL.

[1] With EDTA and methylparaben.

Refer to the general introductory discussion concerning Antiarrhythmic Agents.

Indications

➤*IV:* Acute management of ventricular arrhythmias occurring during cardiac manipulation, such as cardiac surgery or in relation to acute myocardial infarction (MI).

LIDOCAINE HCl

➤*IM:* Single doses are justified in the following exceptional circumstances: When ECG equipment is not available to verify the diagnosis but the potential benefits outweigh the possible risks; when facilities for IV administration are not readily available; by the patient in the prehospital phase of suspected acute MI, directed by qualified medical personnel viewing the transmitted ECG.

➤*Unlabeled uses:* In pediatric patients with cardiac arrest, < 10% develop ventricular fibrillation, and others develop ventricular tachycardia; the hemodynamically compromised child may develop ventricular couplets or frequent premature ventricular beats. In these cases, lidocaine 1 mg/kg should be administered by the IV, intraosseous or endotracheal route. A second 1 mg/kg dose may be given in 10 to 15 minutes. Start a lidocaine infusion if the second dose is required; a third bolus may be needed in 10 to 15 minutes to maintain therapeutic levels.

Administration and Dosage

➤*Approved by the FDA:* November 1948.

➤*IM:* 300 mg. The deltoid muscle is preferred. Avoid intravascular injection. Use only the 10% solution for IM injection.

The *LidoPen Auto-Injector* unit is for self-administration into the deltoid muscle or anterolateral aspect of thigh. Patient instructions are provided with the product.

Replacement therapy – As soon as possible, change patient to IV lidocaine or to an oral antiarrhythmic preparation for maintenance therapy. However, if necessary, an additional IM injection may be administered after 60 to 90 minutes.

➤*IV:* Use only lidocaine injection without preservatives, clearly labeled for IV use. Monitor ECG constantly to avoid potential overdosage and toxicity.

IV bolus – Used to establish rapid therapeutic blood levels. Continuous IV infusion is necessary to maintain antiarrhythmic effects. The usual dose is 50 to 100 mg, given 25 to 50 mg/minute. If the initial injection does not produce the desired clinical response, give a second bolus dose after 5 minutes. Give no more than 200 to 300 mg/hour.

Loading (bolus) doses – Reduce in patients with CHF or reduced cardiac output and in the elderly. However, some investigators recommend the usual loading dose be administered and only the maintenance dosage be reduced.

IV continuous infusion – Used to maintain therapeutic plasma levels following loading doses in patients in whom arrhythmias tend to recur and who cannot receive oral antiarrhythmic drugs. Administer at a rate of 1 to 4 mg/min (20 to 50 mcg/kg/min). Reduce maintenance doses in patients with heart failure or liver disease, or who are also receiving other drugs known to decrease clearance of lidocaine or decrease liver blood flow (see Drug Interactions) and in patients > 70 years of age. Reassess the rate of infusion as soon as the cardiac rhythm stabilizes or at the earliest signs of toxicity. Change patients to oral antiarrhythmic agents for maintenance therapy as soon as possible. It is rarely necessary to continue IV infusions for prolonged periods. Use a precision volume control IV set for continuous IV infusion.

Children – The American Heart Association's Standards and Guidelines recommend a bolus dose of 1 mg/kg, followed by an infusion of 30 mcg/kg/min. The following dosage has also been suggested:
  Loading dose: 1 mg/kg/dose given IV or intratracheally every 5 to 10 min to desired effect, maximum total dose 5 mg/kg.
  Maintenance: 20 to 50 mcg/kg/min.

Preparation of infusion – Add 1 or 2 g lidocaine to 1 L of 5% Dextrose in Water to prepare a 0.1% to 0.2% solution; each mL will contain ≈ 1 to 2 mg lidocaine. Therefore, 1 to 4 mL/min (of a 1 mg/mL solution) will provide 1 to 4 mg lidocaine/minute. If fluid restriction is desirable, prepare a more concentrated solution.

➤*Storage/Stability:* Stable for 24 hours after dilution in 5% Dextrose in Water.

Actions

➤*Pharmacology:* Therapeutic concentrations of lidocaine attenuate phase 4 diastolic depolarization, decrease automaticity and cause a decrease or no change in excitability and membrane responsiveness. Action potential duration and effective refractory period (ERP) of Purkinje fibers and ventricular muscle are decreased, while the ratio of ERP to action potential duration is increased. The AV node ERP may increase, decrease or remain unchanged; atrial ERP is unchanged. Lidocaine raises ventricular fibrillation threshold. Lidocaine has little or no effect on autonomic tone.

Clinical electrophysiological studies have demonstrated no change in sinus node recovery time or sinoatrial conduction time. AV nodal conduction time is unchanged or shortened, and His-Purkinje conduction time is unchanged. Lidocaine increases the electrical stimulation threshold of the ventricle during diastole. In therapeutic doses, lidocaine produces no change in myocardial contractility, systolic arterial blood pressure or absolute refractory period.

➤*Pharmacokinetics:*

Absorption/Distribution – Lidocaine is ineffective orally; 60% to 70% of an oral dose is metabolized by the liver before reaching the systemic circulation. It is most commonly administered IV with an immediate onset (within minutes) and brief duration (10 to 20 minutes) of action following a bolus dose. Continuous IV infusion of lidocaine (1 to 4 mg/min) is necessary to maintain antiarrhythmic effects. Following IM administration, therapeutic serum levels are achieved in 5 to 15 minutes and may persist for up to 2 hours. Higher and more rapid serum levels are achieved by injection into the deltoid muscle, which is preferred over the gluteus or vastus lateralis. Therapeutic serum levels are 1.5 to 6 mcg/mL; serum levels > 6 to 10 mcg/mL are usually toxic. Lidocaine is about 50% protein bound (concentration dependent).

Metabolism/Excretion – Extensive biotransformation in the liver (≈ 90%) results in at least two active metabolites, monoethylglycinexylidide (MEGX) and glycinexylidide (GX). These metabolites exhibit both antiarrhythmic and convulsant properties. The hepatic extraction ratio is between 62% and 81%. Lidocaine exhibits a biphasic half-life. The distribution phase (half-life ≈ 10 minutes) accounts for the short duration of action following IV bolus administration. The elimination half-life is 1.5 to 2 hours; half-life may be ≥ 3 hours following infusions of > 24 hours. Because of the rapid rate at which lidocaine is metabolized, any condition that alters liver function, including changes in liver blood flow, which could result from severe congestive heart failure (CHF) or shock, may alter lidocaine kinetics. Less than 10% of the parent drug is excreted unchanged in the urine. Renal elimination plays an important role in the elimination of the metabolites. Accumulation of GX in patients with severely impaired renal function on prolonged infusions may contribute to lidocaine toxicity.

Contraindications

Hypersensitivity to amide local anesthetics; Stokes-Adams syndrome; Wolff-Parkinson-White syndrome; severe degrees of sinoatrial, atrioventricular (AV) or intraventricular block in the absence of an artificial pacemaker.

Warnings

➤*Survival:* Prophylactic single dose lidocaine administered in a monitored environment does not appear to affect mortality in the earliest phase of acute MI, and may harm some patients who are later shown not to have suffered an acute MI.

➤*Constant ECG monitoring:* Essential for proper administration. Have emergency resuscitative equipment and drugs immediately available to manage adverse reactions involving the cardiovascular, respiratory or central nervous systems.

➤*IV use:* Signs of excessive depression of cardiac conductivity, such as sinus node dysfunction, prolongation of PR interval, widening of the QRS complex, and the appearance or aggravation of arrhythmias, should be followed by dosage reduction and, if necessary, prompt cessation of IV infusion.

➤*IM use:* May increase creatine phosphokinase (CPK) levels. Use of the enzyme determination without isoenzyme separation, as a diagnostic test for acute MI, may be compromised.

➤*Cardiac effects:* Use with caution and in lower doses in patients with CHF, reduced cardiac output, digitalis toxicity accompanied by AV block and in the elderly.

In sinus bradycardia or incomplete heart block, lidocaine administration for the elimination of ventricular ectopy without prior acceleration in heart rate (eg, by atropine, isoproterenol or electric pacing) may promote more frequent and serious ventricular arrhythmias or complete heart block (see Contraindications). Use with caution in patients with hypovolemia and shock, and all forms of heart block.

Acceleration of ventricular rate – This may occur when administered to patients with atrial flutter or fibrillation.

➤*Hypersensitivity reactions:* Reactions may occur (see Adverse Reactions). Refer to Management of Acute Hypersensitivity Reactions.

➤*Renal/Hepatic function impairment:* Lidocaine is metabolized mainly in the liver and excreted by the kidney. Use caution with repeated or prolonged use in liver or renal disease; possible toxic accumulation of lidocaine or its metabolites may occur.

➤*Pregnancy: Category B.* Lidocaine readily crosses the placental barrier. However, there are no adequate and well controlled studies in pregnant women; therefore use during pregnancy only when clearly needed.

➤*Lactation:* In a single case report, lidocaine was excreted into breast milk at concentrations 40% of serum levels. At this level, an infant might ingest up to 1.5 mg, a very small amount that would not be expected to lead to significant accumulation. However, exercise caution when administering to a nursing woman.

➤*Children:* Safety and efficacy have not been established; reduce dosage. The IM auto-injector device is not recommended in children < 50 kg (110 lbs).

Precautions

➤*Malignant hyperthermia:* Amide local anesthetic administration has been associated with acute onset of fulminant hypermetabolism of skeletal muscle known as malignant hyperthermic crisis. Recognition of early unexplained signs of tachycardia, tachypnea, labile blood pressure and metabolic acidosis may precede temperature elevation. Successful outcome depends on early diagnosis, prompt discontinuance of the trig-

LIDOCAINE HCl

gering agent and institution of treatment, including oxygen, supportive measures and IV dantrolene sodium (see individual monograph).

The safety of amide local anesthetics in patients with genetic predisposition of malignant hyperthermia has not been fully assessed; use lidocaine with caution in such patients. In hospitals where triggering agents for malignant hyperthermia are administered, a standard protocol for management should be available.

Drug Interactions

Lidocaine Drug Interactions

Precipitant drug	Object drug[*]		Description
Beta blockers	Lidocaine	↑	Increased lidocaine levels may occur, possibly resulting in toxicity.
Cimetidine	Lidocaine	↑	Decreased lidocaine clearance with possible toxicity. Ranitidine, and perhaps other H$_2$ antagonists, do not appear to interact.
Procainamide	Lidocaine	↑	Additive cardiodepressant action may occur with potential for conduction abnormalities.
Tocainide	Lidocaine	↑	Since these agents are pharmacologically similar, concomitant use may cause an increased incidence of adverse reactions.
Lidocaine	Succinylcholine	↑	Prolongation of neuromuscular blockade may occur.

[*] ↑ = Object drug increased

Adverse Reactions

➤*Cardiovascular:* Hypotension; bradycardia; cardiovascular collapse, which may lead to cardiac arrest.

➤*CNS:* Lightheadedness; nervousness; drowsiness; dizziness; apprehension; confusion; mood changes; "doom anxiety;" hallucinations; euphoria; tinnitus; blurred or double vision; sensation of heat, cold or numbness; twitching; tremors; convulsions; unconsciousness.

➤*Hypersensitivity:* Infrequent allergic reactions may occur, characterized by cutaneous lesions, urticaria, edema or anaphylactoid reactions. Skin testing has doubtful value. See Warnings.

➤*Local:* Occasional soreness at the IM injection site; febrile response; infection at the injection site; venous thrombosis or phlebitis extending from the site of injection;

➤*Miscellaneous:* Extravasation, respiratory depression and arrest, vomiting.

Overdosage

➤*Symptoms:* Lidocaine blood concentrations may correlate with CNS toxicity (see Adverse Reactions). Mild CNS symptoms (drowsiness, dizziness, transient paresthesias) quickly resolve. General guidelines are provided in the table below:

Lidocaine Plasma[1] Concentrations and Effects

Concentration (mcg/mL)	Toxicity[2]
< 1.5	Idiosyncratic
1.5 to 4	Mild CNS and cardiovascular effects
4 to 6	Mild CNS effects common; cardiovascular in those with concomitant disease
6 to 8	Significant risk of CNS and cardiovascular depression
> 8	Seizures, obtundation, hypotension, respiratory depression, decreased cardiac output, coma

[1] Whole blood concentrations may be 10% to 30% lower.
[2] Patients with significant conduction system abnormalities or marginal hemodynamic status may develop apparent toxicity even at very low lidocaine concentrations. Metabolites also can contribute to toxicity even with modest lidocaine plasma concentrations.

➤*Treatment:* In the case of severe reaction, discontinue the drug. Institute emergency resuscitative procedures and supportive treatment. For severe convulsions, use small increments of diazepam or an ultra-short-acting barbiturate (thiopental or thiamylal); if those are not available, use a short-acting barbiturate (pentobarbital or secobarbital). If the patient is under anesthesia, succinylcholine may be given IV. Assure a patent airway and adequate ventilation. If circulatory depression occurs, administer vasopressors and, if necessary, institute CPR.

FLECAINIDE ACETATE

Rx	**Flecainide** (Various, eg, Mylan, Par)	**Tablets:** 50 mg	In 100s.	
Rx	**Tambocor** (3M Pharm.)		(TR 50 3M). White. In 100s and UD 100s.	
Rx	**Flecainide** (Various, eg, Mylan, Par)	**Tablets:** 100 mg	In 100s.	
Rx	**Tambocor** (3M Pharm.)		(TR 100 3M). White, scored. In 100s and UD 100s.	
Rx	**Flecainide** (Various, eg, Mylan, Par)	**Tablets:** 150 mg	In 100s.	
Rx	**Tambocor** (3M Pharm.)		(TR 150 3M). White, scored. Oval. In 100s.	

Refer to the general introductory discussion concerning Antiarrhythmic Agents.

WARNING

Mortality: Flecainide was included in the National Heart Lung and Blood Institute's Cardiac Arrhythmia Suppression Trial (CAST), a long-term, multicenter, randomized, double-blind study in patients with asymptomatic non-life-threatening ventricular arrhythmias who had an MI more than 6 days but less than 2 years previously. An excessive mortality or non-fatal cardiac arrest rate was seen in patients treated with flecainide compared with that seen in patients assigned to a carefully matched placebo-treated group. This rate was 5.1% for flecainide and 2.3% for the matched placebo. The average duration of treatment with flecainide in this study was 10 months.

The applicability of the CAST results to other populations (eg, those without recent MI) is uncertain, but at present, it is prudent to consider the risks of Class IC agents (including flecainide), coupled with the lack of any evidence of improved survival, generally unacceptable in patients without life-threatening ventricular arrhythmias, even if the patients are experiencing unpleasant, but not life-threatening, symptoms or signs.

Ventricular pro-arrhythmic effects in patients with atrial fibrillation/flutter: A review of the world literature revealed reports of 568 patients treated with oral flecainide for paroxysmal atrial fibrillation/flutter (PAF). Ventricular tachycardia was experienced in 0.4% of these patients. Of 19 patients in the literature with chronic atrial fibrillation (CAF), 10.5% experienced ventricular tachycardia (VT) or ventricular fibrillation (VF). Flecainide is not recommended for use in patients with CAF. Case reports of ventricular proarrhythmic effects in patients treated with flecainide for atrial fibrillation/flutter have included increased premature ventricular contractions (PVCs), VT, VF, and death.

As with other Class I agents, patients treated with flecainide for atrial flutter have been reported with 1:1 atrioventricular conduction due to slowing the atrial rate. A paradoxical increase in the ventricular rate also may occur in patients with atrial fibrillation who receive flecainide. Concomitant negative chronotropic therapy such as digoxin or beta-blockers may lower the risk of this complication.

Indications

For the prevention of PAF associated with disabling symptoms and paroxysmal supraventricular tachycardias (PSVT), including atrioventricular nodal reentrant tachycardia, atrioventricular reentrant tachycardia and other supraventricular tachycardias of unspecified mechanism associated with disabling symptoms in patients without structural heart disease.

Prevention of documented life-threatening ventricular arrhythmias, such as sustained ventricular tachycardia.

Not recommended in patients with less severe ventricular arrhythmias even if the patients are symptomatic (see Warnings). Because of proarrhythmic effects of flecainide (see Warnings), reserve use for patients in whom benefits outweigh risks.

Administration and Dosage

➤*Approved by the FDA:* 1985.

For patients with sustained ventricular tachycardia, initiate therapy in the hospital and monitor rhythm.

Flecainide has a long half-life (12 to 27 hours). Steady-state plasma levels in normal renal and hepatic function may not be achieved until 3 to 5 days of therapy at a given dose. Therefore, do not increase dosage more frequently than once every 4 days, since optimal effect may not be achieved during the first 2 to 3 days of therapy.

An occasional patient not adequately controlled by (or intolerant of) a dose given at 12 hour intervals may be dosed at 8 hour intervals.

Once the arrhythmia is controlled, it may be possible to reduce the dose, as necessary, to minimize side effects or effects on conduction.

➤*PSVT and PAF:* The recommended starting dose is 50 mg every 12 hours. Doses may be increased in increments of 50 mg twice daily every 4 days until efficacy is achieved. For PAF patients, a substantial increase in efficacy without a substantial increase in discontinuation for adverse experiences may be achieved by increasing the flecainide dose from 50 to 100 mg twice daily. The maximum recommended dose for patients with paroxysmal supraventricular arrhythmias is 300 mg/day.

FLECAINIDE ACETATE

▶*Sustained ventricular tachycardia:*

Initial dose – 100 mg every 12 hours. Increase in 50 mg increments twice daily every 4 days until effective. Most patients do not require > 150 mg every 12 hours (300 mg/day). Maximum dose is 400 mg/day.

Use of higher initial doses and more rapid dosage adjustments have resulted in an increased incidence of proarrhythmic events and CHF, particularly during the first few days of dosing (see Warnings). Therefore, a loading dose is not recommended.

▶*CHF or MI:* Use cautiously in patients with a history of CHF or myocardial dysfunction (see Warnings).

▶*Renal impairment:* In severe renal impairment (Ccr ≤ 35 mL/min/1.73 m²), the initial dosage is 100 mg once daily (or 50 mg twice daily). Frequent plasma level monitoring is required to guide dosage adjustments. In patients with less severe renal disease, initial dosage is 100 mg every 12 hours. Increase dosage cautiously at intervals > 4 days, observing the patient closely for signs of adverse cardiac effects or other toxicity. It may take > 4 days before a new steady-state plasma level is reached following a dosage change. Monitor plasma levels to guide dosage adjustments (see below).

▶*Transfer to flecainide:* Theoretically, when transferring patients from another antiarrhythmic to flecainide, allow at least 2 to 4 plasma half-lives to elapse for the drug being discontinued before starting flecainide at the usual dosage. Consider hospitalization of patients in whom withdrawal of a previous antiarrhythmic is likely to produce life-threatening arrhythmias.

▶*Administration with amiodarone:* When flecainide is given in the presence of amiodarone, reduce the usual flecainide dose by 50% and monitor the patient closely for adverse effects. Plasma level monitoring is strongly recommended to guide dosage with such combination therapy.

▶*Plasma level monitoring:* The majority of patients treated successfully had trough plasma levels between 0.2 and 1 mcg/mL. The probability of adverse experiences, especially cardiac, may increase with higher trough plasma levels, especially levels > 1 mcg/mL. Monitor trough plasma levels periodically, especially in patients with severe or moderate chronic renal failure or severe hepatic disease and CHF, as drug elimination may be slower.

Actions

▶*Pharmacology:* Flecainide has local anesthetic activity and belongs to the membrane stabilizing (Class I) group of antiarrhythmic agents; it has electrophysiologic effects characteristic of the IC class of antiarrhythmics.

Hemodynamic effects – Flecainide does not usually alter heart rate, although bradycardia and tachycardia have been reported occasionally.

Decreases in ejection fraction, consistent with a negative inotropic effect, have been observed after a single dose of 200 to 250 mg; both increases and decreases in ejection fraction have been encountered during multidose therapy at usual therapeutic doses (see Warnings).

Electrophysiology – Flecainide produces a dose-related decrease in intracardiac conduction in all parts of the heart, with the greatest effect on the His-Purkinje system (H–V conduction). Effects upon atrioventricular (AV) nodal conduction time and intra-atrial conduction times are less pronounced than those on the ventricle. Significant effects on refractory periods were observed only in the ventricle. Sinus node recovery times (corrected) are somewhat increased; this may be significant in sinus node dysfunction (see Warnings).

Flecainide causes a dose-related and plasma level-related decrease in single and multiple PVCs and can suppress recurrence of ventricular tachycardia. Plasma levels of 0.2 to 1 mcg/mL may be needed to obtain the maximal therapeutic effect; trough plasma levels in patients successfully treated for recurrent ventricular tachycardia were between 0.2 and 1 mcg/mL. Plasma levels > 0.7 to 1 mcg/mL are associated with a higher rate of cardiac adverse experiences (ie, conduction defects or bradycardia). The relationship of plasma levels to proarrhythmic events is not established, but dose reduction appears to lead to a reduced frequency and severity of such events.

▶*Pharmacokinetics:*

Absorption/Distribution – Oral absorption is nearly complete. Peak plasma levels are attained at about 3 hours (range, 1 to 6 hours). Flecainide does not undergo significant first-pass effect.

The plasma half-life averages 20 hours (range, 12 to 27 hours) after multiple oral doses. Steady-state levels are approached in 3 to 5 days; once at steady-state, no accumulation occurs during chronic therapy. Over the usual therapeutic range, plasma levels are approximately proportional to dose.

In patients with congestive heart failure (CHF; NYHA class III), the rate of flecainide elimination from plasma (mean half-life, 19 hours) is moderately slower than for healthy subjects (mean half-life, 14 hours).

Plasma protein binding is about 40% and is independent of plasma drug level over the range of 0.015 to about 3.4 mcg/mL.

Metabolism/Excretion – In vitro metabolic studies have confirmed that cytochrome P450 2D6 is involved in the metabolism of flecainide. About 30% of a single oral dose (range, 10% to 50%) is excreted in urine

unchanged. The two major urinary metabolites are meta-O-dealkylated flecainide (active, but ≈ ⅕ as potent) and the meta-O-dealkylated lactam (inactive). These two metabolites (primarily conjugated) account for most of the remaining portion of the dose. Several minor metabolites (≤ 3%) are also found in urine; 5% is excreted in feces.

Flecainide elimination depends on renal function. With increasing renal impairment, the extent of unchanged drug in urine is reduced and the half-life is prolonged. There is no simple relationship between creatinine clearance and the rate of flecainide elimination from plasma.

Hemodialysis removes only ≈ 1% of an oral dose as unchanged flecainide.

Contraindications

Preexisting second- or third-degree AV block, right bundle branch block when associated with a left hemiblock (bifascicular block), unless a pacemaker is present to sustain the cardiac rhythm if complete heart block occurs; recent MI (see Warnings); presence of cardiogenic shock; hypersensitivity to the drug.

Warnings

▶*Mortality:* Flecainide was included in the National Heart Lung and Blood Institute's Cardiac Arrhythmia Suppression Trial (CAST), a long-term multi-center, randomized, double-blind study in patients with asymptomatic non-life-threatening ventricular arrhythmias who had an MI > 6 days, but < 2 years previously. An excessive mortality or nonfatal cardiac arrest rate was seen in patients treated with flecainide compared with that seen in a carefully matched placebo-treated group. This rate was 16/315 (5.1%) for flecainide and 7/309 (2.3%) for its matched placebo. The average duration of treatment was 10 months.

▶*Ventricular pro-arrhythmic effects in patients with atrial fibrillation/flutter:* A review of the world literature revealed reports of 568 patients treated with oral flecainide for paroxysmal atrial fibrillation/flutter (PAF). Ventricular tachycardia was experienced in 0.4% (2/568) of these patients. Of 19 patients in the literature with chronic atrial fibrillation (CAF), 10.5% (2) experienced VT or VF. Flecainide is not recommended for use in patients with chronic atrial fibrillation. Case reports of ventricular proarrhythmic effects in patients treated with flecainide for atrial fibrillation/flutter have included increased PVCs, VT, VF and death.

As with other class I agents, patients treated with flecainide for atrial flutter have been reported with 1:1 atrioventricular conduction due to slowing the atrial rate. A paradoxical increase in the ventricular rate also may occur in patients with atrial fibrillation who receive flecainide. Concomitant negative chronotropic therapy such as digoxin or beta-blockers may lower the risk of this complication.

▶*Survival:* As with other antiarrhythmics, there is no evidence that flecainide favorably affects survival or the incidence of sudden death.

▶*Non-life-threatening ventricular arrhythmias:* The applicability of the CAST results to other populations (eg, those without recent infarction) is uncertain, but at present it is prudent to consider the risks of Class IC agents, coupled with the lack of any evidence of improved survival, generally unacceptable in patients whose ventricular arrhythmias are not life-threatening, even if the patients are experiencing unpleasant but not life-threatening symptoms or signs.

▶*Proarrhythmic effects:* Flecainide can cause new or worsened arrhythmias. Such proarrhythmic effects range from an increase in frequency of PVCs to the development of more severe ventricular tachycardia (eg, tachycardia that is more sustained or more resistant to conversion to sinus rhythm, with potentially fatal consequences. Three-fourths of proarrhythmic events were new or worsened ventricular tachyarrhythmias, the remainder being increased frequency of PVCs or new supraventricular arrhythmias.

In patients treated with flecainide for sustained ventricular tachycardia, 80% of proarrhythmic events occurred within 14 days of the onset of therapy. In studies of 225 patients with supraventricular arrhythmia, there were 9 (4%) proarrhythmic events, 8 of them in patients with paroxysmal atrial fibrillation. Of the 9, 7 were exacerbations of supraventricular arrhythmias, while 2 were ventricular arrhythmias, including one fatal case of VT/VF and one wide complex VT, both in patients with paroxysmal atrial fibrillation and known coronary artery disease.

It is uncertain if flecainide's risk of proarrhythmia is exaggerated in patients CAF, high ventricular rate or exercise. Wide complex tachycardia and ventricular fibrillation have been reported in two of 12 CAF patients undergoing maximal exercise tolerance testing. In patients with complex arrhythmias, it is difficult to distinguish a spontaneous variation in the underlying rhythm disorder from drug-induced worsening. As a result, the following occurrence rates are approximations.

Among patients treated for sustained ventricular tachycardia (who frequently also had heart failure, a low ejection fraction, a history of MI or cardiac arrest), the incidence of proarrhythmic events was 13% when dosage was initiated at 200 mg/day with slow upward titration, without exceeding 300 mg/day. In patients with *sustained* ventricular tachycardia using a higher initial dose (400 mg/day) the incidence of proarrhythmic events was 26%; moreover, in about 10%, proarrhythmic events were fatal. With lower initial doses, the incidence of fatal proarrhythmic events decreased to 0.5%.

FLECAINIDE ACETATE

The relatively high frequency of proarrhythmic events in patients with sustained ventricular tachycardia and serious underlying heart disease, and the need for titration and monitoring, requires that therapy of patients with sustained ventricular tachycardia be started in the hospital.

➤*Sick sinus syndrome:* Use only with extreme caution; the drug may cause sinus bradycardia, sinus pause or sinus arrest. The frequency probably increases with higher trough plasma levels, especially when they exceed 1 mcg/mL.

➤*Heart failure:* Flecainide has a negative inotropic effect and may cause or worsen CHF, particularly in patients with cardiomyopathy, preexisting severe heart failure (NYHA functional class III or IV) or low ejection fractions (< 30%). In patients with supraventricular arrhythmias, new or worsened CHF developed in 0.4% of patients. In patients with sustained ventricular tachycardia during a mean duration of 7.9 months of flecainide therapy, 6.3% developed new CHF. In patients with sustained ventricular tachycardia and a history of CHF in a mean duration of 5.4 months of therapy, 25.7% developed worsened CHF. Exacerbation of preexisting CHF occurred more commonly in studies including patients with Class III or IV failure than in studies which excluded such patients. Use cautiously in patients with a history of CHF or myocardial dysfunction. The initial dosage should be no more than 100 mg twice daily; monitor patients carefully. Give close attention to maintenance of cardiac function, including optimal digitalis, diuretic or other therapy. Where CHF has developed or worsened during treatment, the time of onset has ranged from a few hours to several months after starting therapy. Some patients who develop reduced myocardial function while on flecainide can continue with adjustment of digitalis or diuretics; others may require dosage reduction or discontinuation of flecainide. When feasible, monitor plasma flecainide levels. Keep trough plasma levels less than 0.7 to 1 mcg/mL.

➤*Cardiac conduction:* Flecainide slows cardiac conduction in most patients to produce dose-related increases in PR, QRS and QT intervals.

The PR interval increases an average of 25% (0.04 seconds) and as much as 118%. Approximately one-third of patients may develop new first-degree AV heart block (PR interval ≥ 0.2 seconds). The QRS complex increases an average of 25% (0.02 seconds) and as much as 150%. Many patients develop QRS complexes with a duration of ≥ 0.12 seconds. In one study, 4% of patients developed new bundle branch block. The degree of lengthening of PR and QRS intervals does not predict either efficacy or the development of cardiac adverse effects. In clinical trials, it was unusual for PR intervals to increase to ≥ 0.3 seconds, or for QRS intervals to increase to ≥ 0.18 seconds; thus, use caution and consider dose reductions. The QT interval widens about 8% but most (about 60% to 90%) is due to widening of the QRS duration. The JT interval (QT minus QRS) only widens about 4% on the average. Significant JT prolongation occurs in < 2% of patients. Rare cases of torsades de pointes-type arrhythmias have occurred.

Clinically significant conduction changes have been observed at these rates: Sinus node dysfunction such as sinus pause, sinus arrest and symptomatic bradycardia (1.2%), second-degree AV block (0.5%), and third-degree AV block (0.4%). If second-or third-degree AV block, or right bundle branch block associated with a left hemiblock occurs, discontinue therapy unless a ventricular pacemaker is in place to ensure an adequate ventricular rate.

➤*Electrolyte disturbance:* Hypokalemia or hyperkalemia may alter the effects of Class I antiarrhythmic drugs. Correct preexisting hypokalemia or hyperkalemia before administration.

➤*Effects on pacemaker thresholds:* Flecainide increases endocardial pacing thresholds and may suppress ventricular escape rhythms. Effects are reversible if flecainide is discontinued. Use with caution in patients with permanent pacemakers or temporary pacing electrodes. Do not administer to patients with existing poor thresholds or nonprogrammable pacemakers unless suitable pacing rescue is available.

Determine the pacing threshold in patients with pacemakers prior to instituting therapy, after 1 week of administration and at regular intervals thereafter. Generally, threshold changes are within the range of multiprogrammable pacemakers, and a doubling of either voltage or pulse width is usually sufficient to regain capture.

➤*Urinary pH:* Flecainide elimination is altered by urinary pH; alkalinization (as may occur in rare conditions such as renal tubular acidosis or strict vegetarian diet) decreases, and acidification increases flecainide renal excretion. These alterations in pH (outside a range of pH 5 to 7) may produce toxic or subtherapeutic plasma levels. See Drug Interactions.

➤*Hepatic function impairment:* Since flecainide elimination from plasma can be markedly slower in patients with significant hepatic impairment, do not use in such patients unless the potential benefits outweigh the risks. If used, frequent and early plasma level monitoring is required to guide dosage (see Plasma level monitoring in the Administration and Dosage section); make dosage increases very cautiously when plasma levels have plateaued (after > 4 days).

➤*Elderly:* From age 20 to 80, plasma levels are only slightly higher with advancing age; flecainide elimination from plasma is somewhat slower in elderly subjects than in younger subjects. Patients up to age 80 and above have been safely treated with usual doses.

➤*Pregnancy: Category C.* Flecainide had teratogenic and embryotoxic effects in one breed of rabbit when given in doses up to 35 mg/kg/day. There are no adequate and well controlled studies in pregnant women. Use during pregnancy only if potential benefits outweigh potential hazards to the fetus.

➤*Lactation:* Flecainide is excreted in breast milk in concentrations as high as 4 times (with average levels about 2.5 times) corresponding plasma levels; assuming a maternal plasma level at the top of the therapeutic range (1 mcg/mL), the calculated daily dose to a nursing infant (assuming about 700 mL breast milk over 24 hours) would be less than 3 mg. Because of the drug's potential for serious adverse effects in infants, determine whether to discontinue nursing or discontinue the drug, taking into account the importance of the drug to the mother.

➤*Children:* Safety and efficacy for use in children younger than 18 years of age have not been established.

In pediatric patients with structural heart disease, flecainide has been associated with cardiac arrest and sudden death. Flecainide should be started in the hospital with rhythm monitoring. Any use of flecainide in children should be directly supervised by a cardiologist skilled in the treatment of arrhythmias in children.

Drug Interactions

➤*CYP450 system:* Drugs that inhibit CYP2D6 (such as quinidine) may increase the plasma concentrations of flecainide in patients who are on chronic flecainide therapy, especially if these patients are extensive metabolizers.

Flecainide Drug Interactions			
Precipitant drug	Object drug*		Description
Amiodarone	Flecainide	↑	Flecainide plasma levels may be increased (see Administration and Dosage).
Cimetidine	Flecainide	↑	Flecainide plasma levels and half-life may be increased.
Cisapride	Flecainide	↑	The risk of life-threatening cardiac arrhythmias, including torsades de pointes, may be increased due to possibly additive prolongation of the QT interval.
Flecainide	Cisapride		
Disopyramide	Flecainide	↑	Disopyramide has negative inotropic properties; do not use with flecainide unless benefits outweigh risks.
Propranolol	Flecainide	↑	Flecainide and propranolol levels were increased in healthy subjects. Negative inotropic effects were additive; effects on PR interval were less than additive.
Flecainide	Propranolol	↑	
Ritonavir	Flecainide	↑	Coadministration may produce large increases in serum flecainide concentrations. Ritonavir is contraindicated in patients receiving flecainide.
Urinary acidifiers	Flecainide	↓	Alterations in urinary excretion and plasma elimination of flecainide occur with changes in urinary pH (acidic urine increases elimination and decreases bioavailability; alkaline urine decreases elimination and increases bioavailability). See Warnings.
Urinary alkalinizers	Flecainide	↑	
Verapamil	Flecainide	↑	Verapamil has negative inotropic properties; do not use with flecainide unless benefits outweigh risks.
Flecainide	Digoxin	↑	Digoxin's absorption, peak concentration and bioavailability may be increased.

*↑ = Object drug increased. ↓ = Object drug decreased.

➤*Drug/Food interactions:* Milk may inhibit absorption in infants. A reduction in flecainide dosage should be considered when milk is removed from the diet of infants.

Adverse Reactions

Most frequent – Dizziness (18.9%), including lightheadedness, faintness, unsteadiness and near syncope; dyspnea (10.3%); headache (9.6%); nausea (8.9%); fatigue (7.7%); palpitation (6.1%); chest pain (5.4%); asthenia (4.9%); tremor (4.7%); constipation (4.4%); edema (3.5%); abdominal pain (3.3%).

➤*Cardiovascular:* New or worsened arrhythmias (see Warnings); episodes of unresuscitatable VT or ventricular fibrillation (cardiac arrest); new or worsened CHF (see Warnings); second-degree (0.5%) or third-degree (0.4%) AV block; sinus bradycardia, sinus pause or sinus arrest (1.2%) (see Warnings); tachycardia (1% to 3%); angina pectoris, bradycardia, hypertension, hypotension (< 1%).

FLECAINIDE ACETATE

In post-MI patients with asymptomatic PVCs and non-sustained ventricular tachycardia, flecainide therapy was associated with a 5.1% rate of death and non-fatal cardiac arrest, compared with a 2.3% rate in a matched placebo group (see Warnings).

➤*CNS:* Hypoesthesia, paresthesia, paresis, ataxia, flushing, increased sweating, vertigo, syncope, somnolence, tinnitus, anxiety, insomnia, depression, malaise (1% to 3%); twitching, weakness, convulsions, neuropathy, speech disorder, stupor, amnesia, confusion, euphoria, depersonalization, morbid dreams, apathy (< 1%).

➤*Dermatologic:* Rash (1% to 3%); urticaria, exfoliative dermatitis, pruritus, alopecia (< 1%).

➤*GI:* Vomiting, diarrhea, dyspepsia, anorexia (1% to 3%); flatulence, change in taste, dry mouth (< 1%).

➤*GU:* Impotence, decreased libido, polyuria, urinary retention (< 1%).

➤*Hematologic:* Leukopenia, thrombocytopenia (< 1%).

➤*Ophthalmic:* Visual disturbances including blurred vision, difficulty in focusing, spots before eyes (15.9%); diplopia (1% to 3%); eye pain/irritation, photophobia, nystagmus (< 1%).

➤*Miscellaneous:* Fever (1% to 3%); swollen lips, tongue and mouth, arthralgia, bronchospasm, myalgia (< 1%).

Overdosage

➤*Symptoms:* Animal studies suggest that the following events might occur with overdosage: Lengthening of the PR interval; increase in the QRS duration, QT interval and amplitude of the T wave; reduction in heart rate and myocardial contractility; conduction disturbances; hypotension; death from respiratory failure or asystole.

➤*Treatment:* Treatment should be supportive and may include the following: Removal of unabsorbed drug from the GI tract (charcoal instillation appears to be effective in lowering flecainide plasma concentrations, even after an interval of 90 minutes from ingestion of flecainide); inotropic agents or cardiac stimulants such as dopamine, dobutamine or isoproterenol; mechanical ventilation; circulatory assists such as intra-aortic balloon pumping; transvenous pacing in the event of conduction block. Because of the drug's long plasma half-life (12 to 27 hours) and the possibility of nonlinear elimination kinetics at very high doses, these supportive treatments may need to be continued for extended periods of time. Since flecainide elimination is much slower when urine is very alkaline (pH ≥ 8), theoretically, acidification of urine to promote drug excretion may be beneficial in overdose cases with very alkaline urine. There is no evidence that acidification from normal urinary pH increases excretion. Hemodialysis is not effective. Refer to General Management of Acute Overdosage.

Patient Information

Take as prescribed; serious heart disturbances can result from missing doses, and serious side effects can result from increasing or decreasing doses without supervision.

MEXILETINE HCl

Rx	**Mexitil** (Boehringer Ingelheim)	**Capsules:** 150 mg	(BI 66). Red and caramel. In 100s and UD 100s.
		200 mg	(BI 67). Red. In 100s and UD 100s.
		250 mg	(BI 68). Red and aqua. In 100s and UD 100s.

Refer to the general introductory discussion concerning Antiarrhythmic Agents.

WARNING

Mortality: In the National Heart, Lung and Blood Institute's Cardiac Arrhythmia Suppression Trial (CAST), a long-term, multicentered, randomized, double-blind study in patients with asymptomatic non-life-threatening ventricular arrhythmias who had an MI more than 6 days but less than 2 years previously, an excessive mortality or non-fatal cardiac arrest rate was seen in patients treated with encainide or flecainide (7.7%) compared with that seen in patients assigned to matched placebo-treated groups (3%). The average duration of treatment with encainide or flecainide in this study was 10 months.

The applicability of these results to other populations (eg, those without recent MI) is uncertain. Considering the known proarrhythmic properties of mexiletine and the lack of evidence of improved survival for any antiarrhythmic drug in patients without life-threatening arrhythmias, the use of mexiletine as well as other antiarrhythmic agents should be reserved for patients with life-threatening ventricular arrhythmia.

Indications

Treatment of documented, life-threatening ventricular arrhythmias, such as sustained ventricular tachycardia. Because of the proarrhythmic effects of mexiletine, use with lesser arrhythmias is generally not recommended.

Administration and Dosage

➤*Approved by the FDA:* December 30, 1985.

Individualize dosage. Administer with food or antacids.

Perform clinical and ECG evaluation as needed to determine whether the desired antiarrhythmic effect has been obtained and to guide titration and dose adjustment.

➤*Initial dose:* 200 mg every 8 hours when rapid control of arrhythmia is not essential, with a minimum of 2 to 3 days between adjustments. Adjust dose in 50 or 100 mg increments.

Control can be achieved in most patients with 200 to 300 mg given every 8 hours. If satisfactory response is not achieved at 300 mg every 8 hours, and the patient tolerates mexiletine well, try 400 mg every 8 hours. The severity of CNS side effects increases with total daily dose; do not exceed 1200 mg/day.

➤*Renal/hepatic function impairment:* In general, patients with renal failure will require the usual doses of mexiletine. Patients with severe liver disease, however, may require lower doses and must be monitored closely. Similarly, marked right-sided CHF can reduce hepatic metabolism and reduce the dose needed.

➤*Loading dose:* When rapid control of ventricular arrhythmia is essential, administer an initial loading dose of 400 mg, followed by a 200 mg dose in 8 hours. Onset of therapeutic effect is usually observed within 30 minutes to 2 hours.

➤*Twice-daily dosage:* If adequate suppression is achieved on a dose of ≤ 300 mg every 8 hours, the same total daily dose may be given in divided doses every 12 hours with monitoring. The dose may be adjusted to a maximum of 450 mg every 12 hours.

➤*Transferring to mexiletine:* When transferring from other Class I oral antiarrhythmics to mexiletine, based on theoretical considerations, initiate with a 200 mg dose, and titrate to response as described above, 6 to 12 hours after the last dose of quinidine sulfate, 3 to 6 hours after the last dose of procainamide, 6 to 12 hours after the last disopyramide dose or 8 to 12 hours after the last tocainide dose.

Hospitalize patients in whom withdrawal of the previous antiarrhythmic agent is likely to produce life-threatening arrhythmias.

When transferring from lidocaine to mexiletine, stop the lidocaine infusion when the first oral dose of mexiletine is administered. Maintain the IV line until suppression of the arrhythmia appears satisfactory. Consider the similarity of adverse effects of lidocaine and mexiletine and the additive potential.

Actions

➤*Pharmacology:*

Mechanism – Structurally like lidocaine, mexiletine inhibits the inward sodium current, thus reducing the rate of rise of the action potential, Phase 0. Mexiletine decreases the effective refractory period (ERP) in Purkinje fibers. The decrease in ERP is of lesser magnitude than the decrease in action potential duration (APD), with a resulting increase in ERP/APD ratio.

Hemodynamic effects – Small decreases in cardiac output and increases in systemic vascular resistance have occurred, with no significant negative inotropic effect. Blood pressure and pulse rate remain essentially unchanged. Mild depression of myocardial function has been observed following IV mexiletine (dosage form not available in the US) in patients with cardiac disease.

Electrophysiology – Mexiletine is a local anesthetic and a Class IB antiarrhythmic compound with electrophysiologic properties similar to lidocaine. In patients with normal conduction systems, mexiletine has minimal effect on cardiac impulse generation and propagation. In clinical trials, no development of second- or third-degree AV block was observed. It did not prolong ventricular depolarization (QRS duration) or repolarization (QT intervals). Theoretically, mexiletine may be useful in treating ventricular arrhythmias associated with a prolonged QT interval. In patients with preexisting conduction defects, depression of the sinus rate, prolongation of sinus node recovery time, decreased conduction velocity and increased ERP of the intraventricular conduction system have occasionally been observed.

Among the patients entered into studies, about 30% in each treatment group had a ≥ 70% reduction in PVC count, and about 40% failed to complete the 3 month studies because of adverse effects. Follow-up of patients has demonstrated continued effectiveness in long-term use.

➤*Pharmacokinetics:*

Absorption/Distribution – Mexiletine is well absorbed (≈ 90%) from the GI tract. The absorption rate is reduced in clinical situations (such as acute MI) in which gastric emptying time is increased. Narcotics, atropine and magnesium-aluminum hydroxide may slow absorption;

MEXILETINE HCl

metoclopramide may accelerate absorption (see Drug Interactions). The first-pass metabolism of mexiletine is low.

Peak blood levels are reached in 2 to 3 hours. The therapeutic range is approximately 0.5 to 2 mcg/mL. An increase in the frequency of CNS adverse effects has been observed when plasma levels exceed 2 mcg/mL. Plasma levels within the therapeutic range can be attained with either 2 or 3 times daily dosing, but peak to trough differences are greater with the twice-daily regimen. It is 50% to 60% bound to plasma protein with a volume of distribution of 5 to 7 L/kg.

Metabolism/Excretion – Mexiletine is metabolized in the liver primarily by CYP2D6, although it is a substrate for CYP1A2. The most active minor metabolite is N-methylmexiletine, which is < 20% as potent as mexiletine. Urinary excretion of N-methylmexiletine is < 0.5%.

In healthy subjects, the elimination half-life is 10 to 12 hours. Hepatic impairment prolongs it to a mean of 25 hours. Little change in half-life occurs with reduced renal function. In eight patients with creatinine clearance < 10 mL/min, the mean plasma elimination half-life was 15.7 hours; in seven patients with creatinine clearance between 11 and 40 mL/min, the mean half-life was 13.4 hours.

Approximately 10% is excreted unchanged by the kidney. Urinary acidification accelerates excretion, while alkalinization retards it (see Drug Interactions).

Special populations –

Hepatic function impairment: Hepatic impairment prolongs the elimination half-life of mexiletine. In 8 patients with moderate to severe liver disease, the mean half-life was approximately 25 hours.

Contraindications

Cardiogenic shock; preexisting second- or third-degree AV block (if no pacemaker).

Warnings

➤*Proarrhythmia:* Mexiletine can worsen arrhythmias; it is uncommon in patients with less serious arrhythmias (frequent premature beats or nonsustained ventricular tachycardia) but is of greater concern in patients with life-threatening arrhythmias, such as sustained ventricular tachycardia. In patients with such arrhythmias subjected to programmed electrical stimulation or to exercise provocation, 10% to 15% of patients had exacerbation of the arrhythmia, a rate not greater than that of other agents.

➤*Survival:* Antiarrhythmic drugs have not been shown to enhance survival in patients with ventricular arrhythmias.

➤*Initial therapy:* As with other antiarrhythmics, initiate therapy in the hospital.

➤*Mortality:* In the National Heart, Lung and Blood Institute's Cardiac Arrhythmia Suppression Trial (CAST), a long-term, multicentered, randomized, double-blind study in patients with asymptomatic non-life-threatening ventricular arrhythmias who had experienced MIs more than 6 days but less than 2 years previously, an excessive mortality or non-fatal cardiac arrest rate was seen in patients treated with encainide or flecainide (7.7%) compared with patients assigned to matched placebo-treated groups (3%). The average duration of treatment with encainide or flecainide in this study was 10 months.

The applicability of these results to other populations (eg, those without recent MI) is uncertain. Considering the known proarrhythmic properties of mexiletine and the lack of evidence of improved survival for any antiarrhythmic drug in patients without life-threatening arrhythmias, the use of mexiletine as well as other antiarrhythmic agents should be reserved for patients with life-threatening ventricular arrhythmia.

➤*Hepatic function impairment:* Since mexiletine is metabolized in the liver, and hepatic impairment prolongs the elimination half-life, carefully monitor patients with liver disease. Observe caution in patients with hepatic dysfunction secondary to CHF.

Abnormal liver function tests have been reported, some in the first few weeks of therapy with mexiletine. Most have occurred along with CHF or ischemia; their relationship to mexiletine has not been established.

➤*Pregnancy: Category C.* Mexiletine freely crosses the placenta. There are no adequate and well controlled studies in pregnant women. Use during pregnancy only if the potential benefits outweigh the potential hazards to the fetus.

➤*Lactation:* Mexiletine appears in breast milk in concentrations similar to those in plasma. If mexiletine is essential, consider alternative infant feeding.

➤*Children:* Safety and efficacy in children have not been established.

Precautions

➤*Cardiovascular effects:* If a ventricular pacemaker is operative, patients with second- or third-degree heart block may be treated with mexiletine if continuously monitored. Some patients with preexisting first-degree AV block were treated with mexiletine; none developed second- or third-degree AV block. Exercise caution in such patients or in patients with preexisting sinus node dysfunction or intraventricular conduction abnormalities.

Use with caution in patients with hypotension and severe CHF.

➤*AST elevation and liver injury:* Elevations of AST more than 3 times the upper limit of normal occurred in about 1% of both mexiletine-treated and control patients. Approximately 2% of patients in the mexiletine compassionate use program had elevations of AST at least 3 times the upper limit of normal. These elevations were frequently associated with CHF, acute MI, blood transfusions and other medications. These elevations were often asymptomatic and transient and usually not associated with elevated bilirubin levels and usually did not require discontinuation of therapy. Marked elevations of AST (more than 1000 U/L) were seen before death in four patients with end-stage cardiac disease (severe CHF, cardiogenic shock).

Rare instances of severe liver injury, including hepatic necrosis, have been reported. Carefully evaluate patients in whom an abnormal liver test has occurred, or who have signs or symptoms suggesting liver dysfunction. If persistent or worsening elevation of hepatic enzymes is detected, consider discontinuing therapy.

➤*Hematologic effects:* Among 10,867 patients treated with mexiletine in the compassionate use program, marked leukopenia (neutrophils less than 1000/mm³) or agranulocytosis were seen in 0.06%; milder depressions of leukocytes were seen in 0.08% and thrombocytopenia was observed in 0.16%. Many of these patients were seriously ill and were receiving concomitant medications with known hematologic adverse effects. Rechallenge with mexiletine in several cases was negative. If significant hematologic changes are observed, carefully evaluate the patient and, if warranted, discontinue mexiletine. Blood counts usually return to normal within 1 month of discontinuation.

➤*CNS effects:* Convulsions occurred in about 2 of 1000 patients. Of these patients, 28% discontinued therapy. Convulsions occurred in patients with and without a history of seizures. Use with caution in patients with a known seizure disorder.

➤*Urinary pH:* Avoid concurrent drugs or diets which may markedly alter urinary pH. Minor fluctuations in urinary pH associated with normal diet do not affect mexiletine excretion. See Drug Interactions.

Drug Interactions

➤*CYP450 system:* Because mexiletine is a substrate for CYP2D6 and CYP1A2, inhibition or induction of either of these enzymes would be expected to alter mexiletine concentrations.

Mexiletine Drug Interactions			
Precipitant drug	Object drug*		Description
Aluminum-Magnesium Hydroxide Atropine Narcotics	Mexiletine	↓	Mexiletine absorption may be slowed.
Cimetidine	Mexiletine	↔	Cimetidine may increase or decrease mexiletine plasma levels.
Fluvoxamine	Mexiletine	↑	The clearance of mexiletine was decreased by 38% following coadministration with fluvoxamine, a CYP1A2 inhibitor.
Hydantoins	Mexiletine	↓	Increased mexiletine clearance leading to lower steady-state plasma levels may occur.
Metoclopramide	Mexiletine	↑	Mexiletine absorption may be accelerated.
Propafenone	Mexiletine	↑	Mexiletine plasma concentrations may be elevated in extensive metabolizers due to propafenone inhibiting the metabolism (CYP2D6) of mexiletine. When mexiletine is initiated, slowly titrate the dose.
Rifampin	Mexiletine	↓	Increased mexiletine clearance leading to lower steady-state plasma levels may occur.
Urinary acidifiers	Mexiletine	↓	Renal clearance of mexiletine is related to urinary pH. In acidic urine, mexiletine clearance may be increased.
Urinary alkalinizers	Mexiletine	↑	Renal clearance of mexiletine is related to urinary pH. In alkaline urine, mexiletine clearance may be decreased.
Mexiletine	Caffeine	↑	Clearance of caffeine may be decreased by 50%
Mexiletine	Theophylline	↑	Serum theophylline levels may be increased; increased pharmacologic and toxic effects may occur.

* ↑ = Object drug increased. ↓ = Object drug decreased. ↔ = Undetermined clinical effect.

MEXILETINE HCl

Adverse Reactions

Dosages in controlled studies ranged from 600 to 1200 mg/day; some patients (8%) in the compassionate use program were treated with 1600 to 3200 mg/day. In the controlled trials, the most frequent adverse reactions were upper GI distress (41%), tremor (12.6%), lightheadedness (10.5%) and coordination difficulties (10.2%). These reactions were generally not serious, dose-related, and reversible if the dosage was reduced, if the drug was taken with food or antacids or if it was discontinued. However, they still led to therapy discontinuation in 40%.

➤*Cardiovascular:* Palpitations (4.3% to 7.5%); chest pain (2.6% to 7.5%); increased ventricular arrhythmias/PVCs (1% to 1.9%); angina/angina-like pain (0.3% to 1.7%); CHF (< 1%); syncope, hypotension (0.6%); bradycardia (0.4%); edema, AV block/conduction disturbances, hot flashes (0.2%); atrial arrhythmias, hypertension, cardiogenic shock (0.1%).

➤*CNS:* Dizziness/lightheadedness (18.9% to 26.4%); tremor (13.2%); nervousness (5% to 11.3%); coordination difficulties (≈ 9.7%); changes in sleep habits (≈ 7.5%); headache, blurred vision/visual disturbances (5.7% to 7.5%); paresthesias/numbness (2.4% to 3.8%); weakness (1.9% to 5%); fatigue (1.9% to 3.8%); speech difficulties (2.6%); confusion/clouded sensorium (1.9% to 2.6%); tinnitus (1.9% to 2.4%); depression (2.4%); short-term memory loss (0.9%); hallucinations and other psychological changes, malaise (0.3%); psychosis and convulsions/seizures (0.2%); loss of consciousness (0.06%).

➤*GI:* Nausea/vomiting/heartburn (≈ 40%); diarrhea (5.2%); constipation (4%); dry mouth (2.8%); changes in appetite (2.6%); abdominal pain/cramps/discomfort (1.2%); pharyngitis (< 1%); altered taste (0.5%); salivary changes (0.4%); dysphagia (0.2%); oral mucous membrane changes (0.1%); peptic ulcer (0.08%); upper GI bleeding (0.07%); esophageal ulceration (0.01%).

➤*Lab test abnormalities:* Abnormal liver function tests (0.5%); positive ANA, thrombocytopenia (0.2%); leukopenia, including neutropenia and agranulocytosis (0.1%); myelofibrosis (0.02%).

➤*Miscellaneous:* Rash (3.8% to 4.2%); nonspecific edema (3.8%); dyspnea/respiratory (3.3% to 5.7%); arthralgia (1.7%); fever (1.2%); diaphoresis (0.6%); hair loss, impotence/decreased libido (0.4%); urinary hesitancy/retention (0.2%); hiccoughs, dry skin, laryngeal/pharyngeal changes (0.1%); SLE syndrome (0.04%).

Myelofibrosis was reported in two patients; one was receiving long-term thiotepa therapy and the other had pretreatment myeloid abnormalities.

Exfoliative dermatitis and Stevens-Johnson syndrome have occurred rarely.

Postmarketing – There have been isolated, spontaneous reports of pulmonary changes including pulmonary infiltration and pulmonary fibrosis during mexiletine therapy with or without other drugs or diseases that are known to produce pulmonary toxicity. A causal relationship to mexiletine therapy has not been established. In addition, there have been isolated reports of drowsiness, nystagmus, ataxia, dyspepsia, hypersensitivity reaction, and exacerbation of CHF in patients with pre-existing compromised ventricular function. There have been rare reports of pancreatitis associated with mexiletine treatment.

Overdosage

➤*Symptoms:* Clinical findings associated with mexiletine hydrochloride overdosage have included drowsiness, confusion, nausea, hypotension, sinus bradycardia, paresthesia, seizures, bundle branch block, AV heart block, asystole, ventricular tachyarrhythmia, including ventricular fibrillation, cardiovascular collapse and coma. The lowest known dose in a fatality case was 4.4 g with postmortem serum mexiletine level of 34 to 37 mcg/mL. Patients have recovered from ingestion of 4 to 18 g mexiletine.

➤*Treatment:* There is no specific antidote for mexiletine. Management of mexiletine overdosage includes general supportive measures, close observation and monitoring of vital signs. In addition, the use of pharmacologic interventions (eg, pressor agents, atropine, or anticonvulsants) or transvenous cardiac pacing is suggested, depending on the patient's clinical condition. Refer to General Management of Acute Overdosage.

Patient Information

Take medication with food or an antacid.

Adverse effects such as nausea, vomiting, heartburn, diarrhea, constipation, dizziness, tremor, nervousness, coordination difficulties, changes in sleep habits, headache, visual disturbances, tingling/numbness, weakness, ringing in the ears and palpitations/chest pain may occur. Notify physician if they become bothersome.

Notify physician if signs of liver injury or blood cell damage occur, such as unexplained general tiredness, jaundice, fever or sore throat.

Avoid changes in diet that could drastically acidify or alkalinize the urine.

PROPAFENONE HCl

Rx	**Propafenone** (Various, eg, Watson)	**Tablets:** 150 mg	In 100s and 500s.
Rx	**Rythmol** (Reliant)		(150). White, scored. Film coated. In 100s and UD 100s.
Rx	**Propafenone** (Various, eg, Watson)	225 mg	In 100s and 500s.
Rx	**Rythmol** (Reliant)		(225). Tan, scored. Film coated. In 100s and UD 100s.
Rx	**Propafenone** (Various, eg, Ethex, Mutual, URL)	300 mg	In 100s.
Rx	**Rythmol** (Reliant)		(300). White, scored. Film coated. In 100s and UD 100s.
Rx	**Rythmol SR** (Reliant)	**Capsules, extended-release:** 225 mg	(a 225). White. In 100s.
		325 mg	(a 325). White. In 100s.
		425 ng	(a 425). White. In 100s.

Refer to the general introductory discussion concerning Antiarrhythmic Agents.

WARNING

In the National Heart, Lung, and Blood Institute's Cardiac Arrhythmia Suppression Trial (CAST), a long-term, multi-center, randomized, double-blind study in patients with asymptomatic non-life-threatening ventricular arrhythmias who had an MI more than 6 days but less than 2 years previously, an increased rate of death or reversed cardiac arrest rate (7.7%) was seen in patients treated with encainide or flecainide (Class 1C antiarrhythmics) compared with that seen in patients assigned to placebo (3%). The average duration of treatment with encainide or flecainide in this study was 10 months.

The applicability of the CAST results to other populations (eg, those without recent MI) or other antiarrhythmic drugs is uncertain, but at present, it is prudent to consider any 1C antiarrhythmic to have a significant risk in patients with structural heart disease. Given the lack of any evidence that these drugs improve survival, antiarrhythmic agents should generally be avoided in patients with non-life-threatening ventricular arrhythmias, even if the patients are experiencing unpleasant, but not life-threatening symptoms or signs.

Indications

➤*Atrial fibrillation/flutter:*

Immediate-release (IR) – To prolong the time to recurrence of paroxysmal atrial fibrillation/flutter associated with disabling symptoms in patients without structural heart disease.

Some patients with atrial flutter treated with propafenone have developed 1:1 conduction, producing an increase in ventricular rate. Concomitant treatment with drugs that increase the functional AV refractory period is recommended.

Extended-release (ER) – To prolong the time to recurrence of symptomatic atrial fibrillation in patients with structural heart disease.

The use of propafenone in patients with chronic atrial fibrillation has not been evaluated. Do not use propafenone to control ventricular rate during atrial fibrillation.

➤*Paroxysmal supraventricular tachycardia (PSVT) (IR only):* To prolong the time to recurrence of PSVT associated with disabling symptoms in patients without structural heart disease.

➤*Ventricular arrhythmias (IR only):* For the treatment of ventricular arrhythmias, such as sustained ventricular tachycardia, that are life-threatening. Because of the proarrhythmic effects of propafenone, its use with lesser ventricular arrhythmias is not recommended, even if patients are symptomatic, and reserve any use of the drug for patients in whom the potential benefits outweigh the risks.

Propafenone, like other antiarrhythmic drugs, has not been shown to enhance survival in patients with ventricular or atrial arrhythmias.

Administration and Dosage

➤*Approved by the FDA:* 1989.

➤*IR:* Individually titrate on the basis of response and tolerance. Initiate with 150 mg every 8 hours (450 mg/day). Dosage may be increased at a minimum of 3- to 4-day intervals to 225 mg every 8 hours (675 mg/day) and, if necessary, to 300 mg every 8 hours (900 mg/day). The safety and efficacy of dosages exceeding 900 mg/day have not been established. In those patients in whom significant widening of the QRS complex or second- or third-degree AV block occurs, consider dose reduction.

PROPAFENONE HCl

As with other antiarrhythmics, in the elderly or patients with marked previous myocardial damage, increase dose more gradually during initial treatment phase.

➤SR: Individually titrate on the basis of response and tolerance. Therapy should be initiated with 225 mg given every 12 hours. Dosage may be increased at a minimum of 5-day intervals to 325 mg given every 12 hours. If additional therapeutic effect is needed, the dose may be increased to 425 mg given every 12 hours.

In patients with hepatic impairment or having significant widening of the QRS complex or second or third degree AV block, dose reduction should be considered.

The SR capsules can be taken with or without food. Do not crush or further divide the contents of the capsule.

Actions

➤Pharmacology: Propafenone is a Class IC antiarrhythmic with local anesthetic effects and direct stabilizing action on myocardial membranes. Propafenone's electrophysiological effect manifests itself in a reduction of upstroke velocity (Phase 0) of the monophasic action potential. In Purkinje fibers, and to a lesser extent myocardial fibers, propafenone reduces fast inward current carried by sodium ions. Diastolic excitability threshold is increased and effective refractory period prolonged. Propafenone reduces spontaneous automaticity and depresses triggered activity.

Propafenone has beta-sympatholytic activity at about 1/50 the potency of propranolol in animals and a beta-adrenergic blocking potency (per mg) about 1/40 that of propranolol in man. In clinical trials, resting heart rate decreases of about 8% were noted at the higher end of the therapeutic plasma concentration range. At very high concentrations in vitro, propafenone can inhibit the slow inward current carried by calcium but this calcium antagonist effect probably does not contribute to antiarrhythmic efficacy. Propafenone has local anesthetic activity approximately equal to procaine.

Propafenone causes a dose- and concentration-related decrease in rate of single and multiple PVCs and can suppress recurrence of ventricular tachycardia. Based on percent of patients attaining substantial (80% to 90%) suppression of ventricular ectopic activity, it appears trough levels of 0.2 to 1.5 mcg/mL can provide good suppression, with higher concentrations giving a greater rate of good response.

Mean Changes in ECG Intervals Produced by Propafenone[1]								
	Total daily dose							
	337.5 mg		450 mg		675 mg		900 mg	
Interval	msec	%	msec	%	msec	%	msec	%
RR	−14.5	−1.8	30.6	3.8	31.5	3.9	41.7	5.1
PR	3.6	2.1	19.1	11.6	28.9	17.8	35.6	21.9
QRS	5.6	6.4	5.5	6.1	7.7	8.4	15.6	17.3
QTc	2.7	0.7	−7.5	−1.8	5	1.2	14.7	3.7

[1] In any individual patient, ECG changes in the table cannot be readily used to predict efficacy or plasma concentration.

Hemodynamic effects – Sympathetic stimulation may be a vital component supporting circulatory function in patients with congestive heart failure (CHF), and its inhibition by the beta blockade produced by propafenone may in itself aggravate CHF.

Like other Class IC antiarrhythmics, propafenone exerts a negative inotropic effect on the myocardium. Cardiac catheterization studies in patients with moderately impaired ventricular function (mean CI = 2.61 L/min/m²) utilizing IV propafenone infusions (2 mg/kg over 10 min plus 2 mg/min for 30 min) that gave mean plasma levels of 3 mcg/mL (well above the therapeutic range of 0.2 to 1.5 mcg/mL) showed significant increases in pulmonary capillary wedge pressure, systemic and pulmonary vascular resistances and depression of cardiac output and index.

Electrophysiology – In electrophysiology studies in patients with ventricular tachycardia, propafenone prolongs atrioventricular (AV) conduction while having little or no effect on sinus node function. Both AV nodal conduction time (AH interval) and His-Purkinje conduction time (HV interval) are prolonged. Propafenone has little or no effect on the atrial functional refractory period, but AV nodal functional and effective refractory periods are prolonged. In patients with Wolff-Parkinson-White syndrome (WPW), propafenone reduces conduction and increases the effective refractory period of the accessory pathway in both directions. Propafenone slows conduction and consequently produces dose-related changes in the PR interval and QRS duration. QTc interval does not change.

➤Pharmacokinetics:

Absorption/Distribution – Propafenone is nearly completely absorbed after oral administration with peak plasma levels occurring approximately 3.5 hours after administration in most individuals. It exhibits extensive first-pass metabolism resulting in a dose-dependent and dosage-form-dependent absolute bioavailability (eg, a 150 mg tablet had absolute bioavailability of 3.4%, a 300 mg tablet 10.6% and 300 mg solution 21.4%). Bioavailability increases further at doses above those recommended. Propafenone follows a nonlinear pharmaco-

kinetic disposition presumably due to saturation of first-pass hepatic metabolism as the liver is exposed to higher concentrations of propafenone and shows a very high degree of interindividual variability. For example, for a threefold increase in daily dose from 300 to 900 mg/day, there is a tenfold increase in steady-state plasma concentration.

Metabolism/Excretion – There are two genetically determined patterns of propafenone metabolism. In > 90% of patients, the drug is rapidly and extensively metabolized with an elimination half-life of 2 to 10 hours. These patients metabolize propafenone into two active metabolites: 5-hydroxypropafenone (formed by CYP2D6) and N-depropylpropafenone (formed by CYP3A4 and CYP1A2). In vitro, these metabolites have antiarrhythmic activity comparable to propafenone, but in man they both are usually present in concentrations less than 20% of propafenone. Nine additional metabolites have been identified, most in only trace amounts. The saturable hydroxylation pathway is responsible for the nonlinear pharmacokinetic disposition.

In fewer than 10% of patients, propafenone metabolism is slower because the 5-hydroxy metabolite is not formed or is minimally formed. The estimated propafenone elimination half-life ranges from 10 to 32 hours. In these patients, the N-depropylpropafenone is present in quantities comparable to the levels measured in extensive metabolizers. In slow metabolizers, propafenone pharmacokinetics are linear.

There are significant differences in plasma concentrations of propafenone in slow and extensive metabolizers, the former achieving concentrations 1.5 to 2 times those of the extensive metabolizers at daily doses of 675 to 900 mg/day. At low doses the differences are greater, with slow metabolizers attaining concentrations more than 5 times those of extensive metabolizers. Because the difference decreases at high doses and is mitigated by the lack of the active 5-hydroxy metabolite in the slow metabolizers, and because steady-state conditions are achieved after 4 to 5 days of dosing, the recommended dosing regimen is the same for all patients. Titrate dosage carefully with close attention to clinical and ECG evidence of toxicity. In addition, the beta-blocking action of propafenone appears to be enhanced in slow metabolizers.

Special populations –

Hepatic function impairment: Bioavailability increases and the clearance of propafenone is reduced and the elimination half-life increased in patients with significant hepatic dysfunction (see Warnings).

Contraindications

Uncontrolled CHF; cardiogenic shock; sinoatrial, AV and intraventricular disorders of impulse generation or conduction (eg, sick sinus node syndrome, AV block) in the absence of an artificial pacemaker; bradycardia; marked hypotension; bronchospastic disorders; manifest electrolyte imbalance; hypersensitivity to the drug.

Warnings

➤Mortality: In the National Heart, Lung and Blood Institute's Cardiac Arrhythmia Suppression Trial (CAST), a long-term, multicenter, randomized, double-blind study in patients with asymptomatic non-life-threatening ventricular ectopy who had an MI more than 6 days but less than 2 years previously, and demonstrated mild to moderate left ventricular dysfunction, an excessive mortality or non-fatal cardiac arrest rate was seen in patients treated with encainide or flecainide (7.7%) compared with that seen in patients assigned to carefully matched placebo-treated groups (3%). The average duration of treatment with encainide or flecainide in this study was 10 months.

The applicability of these results to other populations (eg, those without recent MI) and to other antiarrhythmic drugs is uncertain, but at present it is prudent to consider any IC antiarrhythmic to have a significant risk in patients with structural heart disease. Given the lack of any evidence that these drugs improve survival, antiarrhythmic agents should generally be avoided in patients with non-life-threatening ventricular arrhythmias, even if the patients are experiencing unpleasant, but not life-threatening, symptoms or signs.

➤Proarrhythmic effects: Propafenone, like other antiarrhythmic agents, may cause new or worsened arrhythmias. Such proarrhythmic effects range from an increase in frequency of PVCs to the development of more severe ventricular tachycardia, ventricular fibrillation or torsades de pointes (ie, tachycardia that is more sustained or more rapid), which may lead to fatal consequences. It may also worsen premature ventricular contractions or supraventricular arrhythmias, and it may prolong the QT interval. It is therefore essential that each patient be evaluated electrocardiographically and clinically prior to, and during therapy to determine whether response to propafenone supports continued use. Because propafenone prolongs the QRS interval in the electrocardiogram, changes in the QT interval are difficult to interpret.

Overall in clinical trials, 4.7% of all patients had new or worsened ventricular arrhythmia possibly representing a proarrhythmic event. Of the patients who had worsening of VT (4%), 92% had a history of VT or VT/VF, 71% had coronary artery disease and 68% had a prior MI. The incidence of proarrhythmia in patients with less serious or benign arrhythmias, which include patients with an increase in frequency of PVCs, was 1.6%. Although most proarrhythmic events occurred during the first week of therapy, late events also were seen and the CAST study suggests that an increased risk is present throughout treatment.

In the 474 patient US multicenter trial in patients with symptomatic supraventricular tachycardia (SVT), 1.9% of these patients experienced

PROPAFENONE HCl

ventricular tachycardia (VT) or ventricular fibrillation (VF) during the study. However, in 4 of the 9 patients, the ventricular tachycardia was of atrial origin. Six of the 9 patients that developed ventricular arrhythmias did so within 14 days of onset of therapy. About 2.3% of all patients had a recurrence of SVT during the study which could have been a change in the patients' arrhythmia behavior or could represent a proarrhythmic event. Case reports in patients treated with propafenone for atrial fibrillation/flutter have included increased PVCs, VT, VF, and death.

➤*Non-life-threatening arrhythmias:* Use of propafenone is not recommended in patients with less severe ventricular arrhythmias, even if the patients are symptomatic.

➤*Survival:* There is no evidence from controlled trials that the use of propafenone favorably affects survival or the incidence of sudden death.

➤*Nonallergic bronchospasm (eg, chronic bronchitis, emphysema):* In general, these patients should not receive propafenone or other agents with beta-adrenergic blocking activity.

➤*Congestive heart failure (CHF):* New or worsened CHF has occurred in 3.7% of patients with ventricular arrhythmia; of those, 0.9% were probably or definitely related to propafenone. Of the patients with CHF probably related to propafenone, 80% had preexisting heart failure and 85% had coronary artery disease. CHF attributable to propafenone developed rarely (< 0.2%) in patients who had no previous history of CHF.

As propafenone exerts both beta blockade and a (dose-related) negative inotropic effect on cardiac muscle, patients with CHF should be fully compensated before receiving propafenone. If CHF worsens, discontinue propafenone unless CHF is due to the cardiac arrhythmia and, if indicated, restart at a lower dosage only after adequate cardiac compensation has been established.

➤*Conduction disturbances:* Propafenone slows AV conduction and also causes first degree AV block. Average PR interval prolongation and increases in QRS duration are closely correlated with dosage increases and concomitant increases in propafenone plasma concentrations. The incidence of first-, second- and third-degree AV block observed in 2127 ventricular arrhythmia patients was 2.5%, 0.6% and 0.2%, respectively. Development of second- or third-degree AV block requires a reduction in dosage or discontinuation of propafenone. Bundle branch block (1.2%) and intraventricular conduction delay (1.1%) have occurred in patients receiving propafenone. Bradycardia has also occurred (1.5%). Experience in patients with sick sinus node syndrome is limited and these patients should not be treated with propafenone.

Propafenone should not be given to patients with atrioventricular and intraventricular conduction defects in the absence of a pacemaker (see Contraindications).

➤*Effects on pacemaker threshold:* Pacing and sensing thresholds of artificial pacemakers may be altered. Monitor and program pacemakers accordingly during therapy.

➤*Hematologic disturbances:* Agranulocytosis (fever, chills, weakness, and neutropenia) has been reported in patients receiving propafenone. Generally, the agranulocytosis occurred within the first 2 months of propafenone therapy and upon discontinuation of therapy, the white count usually normalized by 14 days. Unexplained fever and/or decrease in white cell count, particularly during the first 3 months of therapy, warrants consideration of possible agranulocytosis/granulocytopenia. Instruct patients to promptly report the development of any signs of infection such as fever, sore throat or chills.

➤*Renal function impairment:* A considerable percentage of propafenone metabolites (18.5% to 38% of the dose/48 hours) are excreted in the urine. Administer cautiously to patients with impaired renal function. Carefully monitor for signs of overdosage.

➤*Hepatic function impairment:* Propafenone is highly metabolized by the liver; administer cautiously to patients with impaired hepatic function. Severe liver dysfunction increases the bioavailability of propafenone to approximately 70%, compared to 3% to 40% for patients with normal liver function; the mean half-life is approximately 9 hours. The dose of propafenone should be approximately 20% to 30% of the dose given to patients with normal hepatic function. Carefully monitor for excessive pharmacological effects.

➤*Fertility impairment:* IV propafenone decreases spermatogenesis in rabbits, dogs and monkeys. These effects were reversible, were not found following oral dosing and were seen only at lethal or sublethal dose levels.

➤*Elderly:* Because of the possible increased risk of impaired hepatic or renal function in this age group, use with caution. The effective dose may be lower in these patients.

➤*Pregnancy: Category C.* Propafenone is embryotoxic in rabbits and rats when given in doses 3 and 6 times, respectively, the maximum recommended human dose. There are no adequate and well controlled studies in pregnant women. Use during pregnancy only if the potential benefit justifies the potential risk to the fetus.

➤*Lactation:* Propafenone is excreted in breast milk. Decide whether to discontinue nursing or to discontinue the drug, taking into account the importance of the drug to the mother.

➤*Children:* The safety and efficacy of propafenone in children have not been established.

Precautions

➤*Elevated ANA titers:* Positive ANA titers have occurred. They have been reversible upon cessation of treatment and may disappear even with continued therapy. These laboratory findings were usually not associated with clinical symptoms, but there is one case of drug-induced lupus erythematosus (positive rechallenge); it resolved completely upon therapy discontinuation. Carefully evaluate patients who develop an abnormal ANA test and, if persistent or worsening elevation of ANA titers is detected, consider discontinuing therapy.

➤*Renal / Hepatic changes:* Renal changes have been observed in the rat following 6 months of oral administration of propafenone at doses of 180 and 360 mg/kg/day (2 to 4 times the maximum recommended human dose). Both inflammatory and noninflammatory changes in the renal tubules with accompanying interstitial nephritis were observed. These lesions were reversible in that they were not found in rats treated at these dosage levels and allowed to recover for 6 weeks. Fatty degenerative changes of the liver were found in rats following chronic administration of propafenone at dose levels 3 times the maximum recommended human dose.

➤*Neuromuscular dysfunction:* Exacerbation of myasthenia gravis has been reported during propafenone therapy.

Drug Interactions

➤*CYP 450 system:* Drugs that inhibit CYP2D6, CYP1A2, and CYP3A4 might lead to increased plasma levels of propafenone. When propafenone is administered with inhibitors of these enzymes, closely monitor patients and adjust dose accordingly.

Propafenone Drug Interactions			
Precipitant drug	Object drug *		Description
Anesthetics, local	Propafenone	↑	Concurrent use (ie, during pacemaker implantations, surgery or dental use) may increase the risks of CNS side effects.
Cimetidine	Propafenone	↑	The maximum propafenone concentration may be increased, possibly resulting in increased pharmacologic effects.
Cisapride	Propafenone	↑	The risk of life-threatening cardiac arrhythmias, including torsades de pointes, may be increased due to possibly additive prolongation of the QT interval.
Propafenone	Cisapride		
Quinidine	Propafenone	↑	Serum propafenone levels may be increased in rapid, extensive metabolizers of the drug, possibly increasing the pharmacologic effects.
Rifamycins	Propafenone	↓	Increased propafenone clearance may occur, resulting in decreased plasma levels and a possible loss of therapeutic effect.
Ritonavir	Propafenone	↑	Coadministration may produce large increases in serum propafenone concentrations. Ritonavir is contraindicated in patients receiving propafenone.
SSRIs (eg, fluoxetine)	Propafenone	↑	Plasma propafenone levels may be elevated. Certain SSRIs may inhibit the metabolism (CYP2D6) of propafenone.
Propafenone	Anticoagulants	↑	Increased warfarin plasma levels and prothrombin time may occur.
Propafenone	Beta blockers	↑	The plasma levels and pharmacologic effects of beta blockers metabolized by the liver may be increased.
Propafenone	Cyclosporine	↑	Increased whole blood cyclosporine trough levels and decreased renal function may occur.
Propafenone	Desipramine	↑	Coadministration may result in elevated serum desipramine levels.
Propafenone	Digoxin	↑	Serum digoxin levels may be increased, resulting in toxicity.
Propafenone	Mexiletine	↑	Mexiletine plasma concentrations may be elevated in extensive metabolizers due to propafenone inhibiting the metabolism (CYP2D6) of mexiletine.
Propafenone	Theophylline	↑	Propafenone may increase theophylline concentrations, possibly resulting in toxicity.

* ↑ = Object drug increased. ↓ = Object drug decreased.

PROPAFENONE HCl

➤ *Drug/Food interactions:* Although food increased the peak blood level and bioavailability of propafenone in a single dose study, food did not change bioavailability significantly during multiple dose administration.

Adverse Reactions

Propafenone Adverse Reactions (%)[a]							
	Incidence by total daily dose					Incidence vs placebo	
Adverse reaction	450 mg (n = 1430)	600 mg (n = 1337)	≥ 900 mg (n = 1333)	Total incidence (n = 2127)	% of patients who discontinued	Propafenone (n = 247)	Placebo (n = 111)
Cardiovascular							
Angina	1.7	2.1	3.2	4.6	0.5	1.2	—
Atrial fibrillation	0.7	0.7	0.5	1.2	0.4	—	—
AV block, first-degree	0.8	1.2	2.1	2.5	0.3	4.5	0.9
AV block, second-degree	—	—	—	—	—	1.2	—
Bradycardia	0.5	0.8	1.1	1.5	0.5	—	—
Bundle branch block	0.3	0.7	1	1.2	0.5	1.2	—
Chest pain	0.5	0.7	1.4	1.8	0.2	—	—
CHF	0.8	2.2	2.6	3.7	1.4	—	—
Hypotension	0.1	0.5	1	1.1	0.4	—	—
Intraventricular conduction delay	0.2	0.7	0.9	1.1	0.1	4	—
Palpitations	0.6	1.6	2.6	3.4	0.5	2.4	0.9
Proarrhythmia	2	2.1	2.9	4.7	4.7	1.2	—
PVCs	0.6	0.6	1.1	1.5	0.1	—	—
QRS duration, increased	0.5	0.9	1.7	1.9	0.5	—	—
Syncope	0.8	1.3	1.4	2.2	0.7	—	—
Ventricular tachycardia	1.4	1.6	2.9	3.4	1.2	—	—
CNS							
Anorexia	0.5	0.7	1.6	1.7	0.4	1.6	0.9
Anxiety	0.7	0.5	0.9	1.5	0.6	2	1.8
Ataxia	0.3	0.6	1.5	1.6	0.2	—	—
Dizziness	3.6	6.6	11	12.5	2.4	6.5	5.4
Drowsiness	0.6	0.5	0.7	1.2	0.2	—	—
Fatigue	1.8	2.8	4.1	6	1	—	—
Headache	1.5	2.5	2.8	4.5	1	4.5	4.5
Insomnia	0.3	1.3	0.7	1.5	0.3	—	—
Loss of balance	—	—	—	—	—	1.2	—
Tremor	0.3	0.8	1.1	1.4	0.3	—	—
GI							
Abdominal pain/ cramps	0.8	0.9	1.1	1.7	0.4	—	—
Constipation	2	4.1	5.3	7.2	0.5	4	—
Diarrhea	0.5	1.6	1.7	2.5	0.6	1.2	0.9
Dry mouth	0.9	1	1.4	2.4	0.2	2	0.9
Dyspepsia	1.3	1.7	2.5	3.4	0.9	—	—
Flatulence	0.3	0.7	0.9	1.2	0.1	1.2	—
Nausea/vomiting	2.4	6.1	8.9	10.7	3.4	2.8	0.9
Unusual taste	2.5	4.9	6.3	8.8	0.7	7.3	0.9
Other							
Blurred vision	0.6	2.4	3.1	3.8	0.8	2	0.9
Diaphoresis	0.6	0.4	1.1	1.4	0.3	—	—
Dyspnea	2.2	2.3	3.6	5.3	1.6	2	2.7
Edema	0.6	0.4	1	1.4	0.2	—	—
Pain, joints	0.2	0.4	0.9	1	0.1	—	—

Propafenone Adverse Reactions (%)[a]							
	Incidence by total daily dose					Incidence vs placebo	
Adverse reaction	450 mg (n = 1430)	600 mg (n = 1337)	≥ 900 mg (n = 1333)	Total incidence (n = 2127)	% of patients who discontinued	Propafenone (n = 247)	Placebo (n = 111)
Rash	0.6	1.4	1.9	2.6	0.8	—	—
Weakness	0.6	1.6	1.7	2.4	0.7	—	—

[a] Data are pooled from separate studies and are not necessarily comparable.

Adverse reactions occur most frequently in the GI, cardiovascular and CNS. About 20% of patients discontinued treatment due to adverse reactions. The most common events were dizziness, unusual taste, first-degree AV block, intraventricular conduction delay, nausea or vomiting and constipation. Headache was common, but not increased compared to placebo.

The most common adverse reactions appeared to be dose-related, especially dizziness, nausea or vomiting, unusual taste, constipation and blurred vision. Some less common reactions may also have been dose-related, such as first degree AV block, CHF, dyspepsia and weakness.

In addition to the reactions listed in the table, the following adverse reactions were reported (< 1%) either in clinical trials or in marketing experience (causal relationship not determined).

➤ *Cardiovascular:* Atrial flutter; AV dissociation; cardiac arrest; flushing; hot flashes; sick sinus syndrome; sinus pause or arrest; supraventricular tachycardia; prolongation of the PR and QRS intervals.

➤ *CNS:* Abnormal dreams, speech or vision; apnea; coma; confusion; depression; memory loss; numbness; paresthesias; psychosis/mania; seizures (0.3%); tinnitus; unusual smell sensation; vertigo.

➤ *GI:* Cholestasis (0.1%); elevated liver enzymes (alkaline phosphatase, serum transaminases) (0.2%); gastroenteritis, hepatitis (0.03%). A number of patients with liver abnormalities associated with propafenone therapy have been reported in postmarketing experience. Some appeared due to hepatocellular injury, some were cholestatic and some showed a mixed picture.

➤ *Hematologic:* Agranulocytosis; anemia; bruising; granulocytopenia; increased bleeding time; leukopenia; purpura; thrombocytopenia.

➤ *Miscellaneous:* Alopecia; eye irritation; hyponatremia/inappropriate ADH secretion; impotence; increased glucose; kidney failure; positive ANA (0.7%); lupus erythematosus; muscle cramps; muscle weakness; nephrotic syndrome; pain; pruritus.

Overdosage

➤ *Symptoms:* The following symptoms are usually most severe within 3 hours of ingestion may include hypotension, somnolence, bradycardia, intra-atrial and intraventricular conduction disturbances, and rarely convulsions and high grade ventricular arrhythmias.

➤ *Treatment:* Defibrillation as well as infusion of dopamine and isoproterenol have been effective in controlling rhythm and blood pressure. Convulsions have been alleviated with IV diazepam. General supportive measures such as ventilatory assistance and cardiopulmonary resuscitation may be necessary. Refer to General Management of Acute Overdosage. Hemodialysis does not appear to alter drug clearance.

Patient Information

Palpitations, chest pain, blurred or abnormal vision, or difficult breathing may occur. Notify the physician if these become bothersome.

Notify the physician if signs of infection develop such as fever, sore throat, chills or unusual bruising or bleeding.

Be aware of signs of overdosage or toxicity such as hypotension, excessive drowsiness, decreased heart rate or abnormal heartbeat.

BRETYLIUM TOSYLATE

Rx	Bretylium Tosylate in 5% Dextrose (Various, eg, Abbott)	Injection: 2 mg/mL (500 mg/vial)	In 250 mL vials.
		4 mg/mL (1000 mg/vial)	In 250 mL vials.
Rx	Bretylium Tosylate (Various)	Injection: 50 mg/mL	In 10 mL amps, vials and syringes.

Refer to the general introductory discussion concerning Antiarrhythmic Agents.

Indications

For prophylaxis and therapy of ventricular fibrillation.

In the treatment of life-threatening ventricular arrhythmias (ie, ventricular tachycardia) which have failed to respond to first-line antiarrhythmic agents (eg, lidocaine).

➤ *Unlabeled uses:* Bretylium is a second-line agent following lidocaine in the protocol for advanced cardiac life support during CPR. For resistant VF and VT (after lidocaine, defibrillation and procainamide failures), give bretylium 5 to 10 mg/kg IV; repeat as needed up to 30 mg/kg; use a bolus every 15 to 30 minutes, infusion 1 to 2 mg/min.

For life-threatening arrhythmia use an undiluted infusion of 1 g/250 mL.

Administration and Dosage

➤ *Approved by the FDA:* July 1978.

For short-term use only.

Keep patient supine during therapy or closely observe for postural hypotension. The optimal dose has not been determined. Dosages > 40 mg/kg/day have been used without apparent adverse effect. As soon as possible, and when indicated, change patient to an oral antiarrhythmic agent for maintenance therapy.

➤ *Immediate life-threatening ventricular arrhythmias:* Administer undiluted, 5 mg/kg by rapid IV injection. If ventricular fibrillation

BRETYLIUM TOSYLATE

persists, increase dosage to 10 mg/kg and repeat as necessary.

➤*Maintenance:* For continuous suppression, administer the diluted solution by continuous IV infusion at 1 to 2 mg/minute. Alternatively, infuse the diluted solution at a dosage of 5 to 10 mg/kg over > 8 minutes, every 6 hours.

➤*Other ventricular arrhythmias:* IV – Dilute before administration. Administer 5 to 10 mg/kg by IV infusion over > 8 minutes. More rapid infusion may cause nausea and vomiting. Give subsequent doses at 1 to 2–hour intervals if the arrhythmia persists. For maintenance therapy, the same dosage may be administered every 6 hours, or a constant infusion of 1 to 2 mg/min may be given.

IM – 5 to 10 mg/kg undiluted. Do not dilute prior to injection. Give subsequent doses at 1 to 2–hour intervals if the arrhythmia persists. Thereafter, maintain with same dosage every 6 to 8 hours.

Do not give > 5 mL in any one site. Do not inject into or near a major nerve; vary injection sites. Repeated injection into the same site may cause atrophy and necrosis of muscle tissue, fibrosis, vascular degeneration and inflammatory changes.

➤*Children:* The following dosages have been suggested.

Acute ventricular fibrillation – 5 mg/kg/dose IV, followed by 10 mg/kg at 15 to 30–minute intervals, maximum total dose 30 mg/kg.

Maintenance – 5 to 10 mg/kg/dose every 6 hours.

Other ventricular arrhythmias – 5 to 10 mg/kg/dose every 6 hours.

➤*Dilution and administration rates for continuous infusion:* Dilute bretylium using the following table and administer as a constant infusion of 1 to 2 mg/min.

Administration Rates for Continuous Infusion Maintenance Bretylium Therapy						
Preparation				Administration		
Amount of bretylium	Volume of IV fluid[1] (mL)	Final volume (mL)	Final conc. (mg/mL)	Dose (mg/min)	Micro-drops per min	mL/hr
500 mg (10 mL)[2]	50[2]	60[2]	8.3[2]	1	7	7
				1.5	11	11
				2	14	14
2 g (40 mL)	500	540	3.7	1	16	16
1 g (20 mL)	250	270	3.7	1.5	24	24
				2	32	32
1 g (20 mL)	500	520	1.9	1	32	32
500 mg (10 mL)	250	260	1.9	1.5	47	47
				2	63	63

[1] May be either Dextrose or Sodium Chloride Injection, USP.
[2] For fluid restricted patients.

➤*IV compatibility:* Bretylium is compatible with the following: 5% Dextrose Injection; 5% Dextrose in 0.45% Sodium Chloride; 5% Dextrose in 0.9% Sodium Chloride; 5% Dextrose in Lactated Ringer's; 0.9% Sodium Chloride; 5% Sodium Bicarbonate; 20% Mannitol; ⅙ M Sodium Lactate; Lactated Ringer's; Calcium Chloride (54.4 mEq/L) in 5% Dextrose; Potassium Chloride (40 mEq/L) in 5% Dextrose.

Actions

➤*Pharmacology:* Bretylium tosylate inhibits norepinephrine release by depressing adrenergic nerve terminal excitability, inducing a chemical sympathectomy-like state. Catecholamine stores are not depleted, but the drug causes an early release of norepinephrine from the adrenergic postganglionic nerve terminals. Therefore, transient catecholamine effects on myocardium (tachycardia) and on peripheral vascular resistance (rise in blood pressure) are often seen shortly after use. Subsequently, bretylium blocks the release of norepinephrine in response to neuron stimulation. Peripheral adrenergic blockade causes orthostatic hypotension but has less effect on supine blood pressure. It has a positive inotropic effect on the myocardium.

Electrophysiology – The mechanisms of action are not established. The following actions have been demonstrated in animals: (1) Increase in ventricular fibrillation threshold; (2) increase in action potential duration and effective refractory period without changes in heart rate; (3) little effect on the rate of rise or amplitude of the cardiac action potential (Phase 0) or in resting membrane potential (Phase 4) in normal myocardium. However, when cell injury slows rate of rise, decreases amplitude and lowers resting membrane potential, bretylium transiently restores these parameters toward normal; (4) decrease in disparity in action potential duration between normal and infarcted regions; (5) increase in impulse formation and spontaneous firing rate of pacemaker tissue, and in ventricular conduction velocity.

The restoration of injured myocardial cell electrophysiology toward normal, as well as the increase of the action potential duration and effective refractory period, without changing their ratio, may help suppress reentry of aberrant impulses and decrease induced dispersion of local excitable states.

Hemodynamic effects – The mild increase in arterial pressure, followed by a modest decrease, remain within normal limits. Pulmonary artery pressure, pulmonary capillary wedge pressure, right atrial pressure, cardiac index, stroke volume index, and stroke work index are not significantly changed.

➤*Pharmacokinetics:* Peak plasma concentration and peak hypotensive effects are seen within 1 hour of IM administration. However, suppression of premature ventricular beats is not maximal until 6 to 9 hours after dosing, when mean plasma concentration declines to less than one half of peak level. Antifibrillatory effects occur within minutes of an IV injection. Suppression of ventricular tachycardia and other ventricular arrhythmias develops more slowly, usually 20 minutes to 2 hours after parenteral administration.

The terminal half-life ranges from 6.9 to 8.1 hours. In 2 patients with creatinine clearances of 1 and 21 mL/min, half-lives were 31.5 and 16 hours, respectively. During dialysis, a 2-fold increase in clearance occurs. The drug is eliminated intact by the kidneys. Approximately 70% to 80% of an IM dose is excreted in the urine during the first 24 hours, with an additional 10% excreted over the next 3 days.

Warnings

➤*Limited use:* Limit use to intensive care units, coronary care units, or other facilities with equipment and personnel for constant cardiac and blood pressure monitoring.

➤*Hypotension:* Postural hypotension occurs regularly in ≈ 50% of patients while they are supine, manifested by dizziness, lightheadedness, vertigo, or faintness. Hypotension may occur at doses lower than those needed to suppress arrhythmias. Keep patients supine until tolerance develops. Tolerance occurs unpredictably, but may be present after several days. Hypotension with supine systolic pressure > 75 mmHg need not be treated unless symptomatic. If supine systolic pressure falls below 75 mmHg, infuse dopamine or norepinephrine to increase blood pressure; use dilute solution and monitor blood pressure closely because pressor effects are enhanced by bretylium. Perform volume expansion with blood or plasma and correct dehydration where appropriate.

➤*Transient hypertension and increased frequency of arrhythmias:* Because of the initial release of norepinephrine from adrenergic postganglionic nerve terminals, transient hypertension and increased frequency of arrhythmias may occur.

➤*Fixed cardiac output:* Avoid use with fixed cardiac output (ie, severe aortic stenosis or severe pulmonary hypertension) since severe hypotension may result from a fall in peripheral resistance without a compensatory increase in cardiac output. If survival is threatened by arrhythmia, the drug may be used, but give vasoconstrictive catecholamines (eg, norepinephrine) promptly if severe hypotension occurs.

➤*Renal function impairment:* Since the drug is excreted principally via the kidneys, increase the dosage interval in patients with impaired renal function.

➤*Pregnancy: Category C.* Reduced uterine blood flow with fetal hypoxia (caused by bradycardia) is a potential risk. It is not known whether bretylium tosylate can cause harm when administered to a pregnant woman or can affect reproduction capacity. Give to a pregnant woman only if clearly needed.

➤*Children:* Safety and efficacy for use in children have not been established. It has been administered to a limited number of pediatric patients, but such use has been inadequate to define proper dosage and limitations (see Administration and Dosage).

Drug Interactions

Bretylium Drug Interactions			
Precipitant drug	Object drug*		Description
Bretylium	Catecholamines	↑	The pressor effects of catecholamines (eg, dopamine, norepinephrine) are enhanced by bretylium. When catecholamines are administered, use dilute solutions and closely monitor blood pressure (see Warnings).
Bretylium	Digoxin	↑	Digitalis toxicity may be aggravated by the initial release of norepinephrine caused by bretylium. When a life-threatening cardiac arrhythmia occurs, use bretylium only if the etiology of the arrhythmia does not appear to be digitalis toxicity and if other antiarrhythmic drugs are not effective. Avoid simultaneous initiation of therapy.

* ↑ = Object drug increased

Adverse Reactions

➤*Cardiovascular:* Hypotension and postural hypotension (most frequent; see Warnings); bradycardia, increased premature ventricular contractions, transient hypertension, initial increase in arrhythmias, precipitation of angina, sensation of substernal pressure (0.1% to 0.2%).

➤*CNS:* Vertigo, dizziness, lightheadedness, syncope (0.7%).

➤*GI:* Nausea and vomiting, primarily after rapid IV administration (3%).

BRETYLIUM TOSYLATE

Overdosage

➤*Symptoms:* With life-threatening arrhythmias, underdosing with bretylium probably presents a greater risk to the patient than potential overdosage. However, 1 case of accidental overdose occurred in which a rapidly injected IV bolus of 30 mg/kg was given instead of an intended 10 mg/kg dose during an episode of ventricular tachycardia. Marked hypertension resulted, followed by protracted refractory hypotension. The patient died 18 hours later in asystole, complicated by renal failure and aspiration pneumonitis. Bretylium serum levels were 8000 ng/mL.

The exaggerated hemodynamic response was attributed to the rapid injection of a very large dose while some effective circulation was still present. Neither the total dose nor the serum levels observed in this patient are in themselves associated with toxicity. Total doses of 30 mg/kg are not unusual and do not cause toxicity when given incrementally during cardiopulmonary resuscitation procedures. Similarly, patients maintained on chronic bretylium tosylate therapy have had documented serum levels of 12,000 ng/mL. These levels were achieved after sequential dosage increases over time with no apparent ill effects.

➤*Treatment:* If bretylium is overdosed and symptoms of toxicity develop, give nitroprusside or consider another short-acting IV antihypertensive agent. Do not use long-acting drugs that might potentiate subsequent hypotensive effects of bretylium. Treat hypotension with appropriate fluid therapy and pressor agents such as dopamine or norepinephrine. Dialysis is probably not useful in treating bretylium overdose.

AMIODARONE HCl

Rx	Pacerone (Upsher Smith)	Tablets: 100 mg	Lactose. (P US 144). In 30s and UD 100s.
Rx	Amiodarone HCl (Various, eg, Eon Labs, Teva)	Tablets: 200 mg	In 60s, 100s, 250s, 500s, and UD 100s.
Rx	Cordarone (Wyeth-Ayerst)		Lactose. (C 200 WYETH 4188). Pink, scored, convex. In 60s and UD 100s.
Rx	Pacerone (Upsher Smith)		Lactose. (P$_{200}$ U-S 0147). Pink, scored. In 60s, 90s, 500s, and UD 100s.
Rx	Pacerone (Upsher Smith)	Tablets: 400 mg	Lactose. (P$_{400}$ 01 45). Light yellow, oval, scored. In 30s, 100s, 500s, and UD 100s.
Rx	Amiodarone HCl (Various, eg, American Pharm Partners, Faulding)	Injection: 50 mg/mL	May contain benzyl alcohol. In 3 mL vials and amps.
Rx	Cordarone (Wyeth-Ayerst)		20.2 mg/mL benzyl alcohol. In 3 mL amps.

Refer to the general introductory discussion concerning Antiarrhythmic Agents.

WARNING

Life threatening arrhythmias: Use amiodarone only in patients with the indicated life-threatening arrhythmias because its use is accompanied by substantial toxicity.

Potentially fatal toxicities: Potentially fatal toxicities, the most important of which is pulmonary toxicity (hypersensitivity pneumonitis or interstitial/alveolar pneumonitis) that has resulted in clinically manifested disease in some patients with ventricular arrhythmias and as abnormal diffusion capacity without symptoms in a much higher percentage of patients. Pulmonary toxicity has been fatal ≈ 10% of the time. Overt liver disease can occur and has been fatal in a few cases. Like other antiarrhythmics, amiodarone can exacerbate the arrhythmia (eg, by making the arrhythmia less well tolerated or more difficult to reverse). Significant heart block or sinus bradycardia has also been seen. Although the frequency of such proarrhythmic events does not appear greater with amiodarone than with many other agents used in this population, the effects are prolonged when they occur (see Warnings).

Indications

➤*Ventricular arrhythmias:*

Oral – Only for treatment of the following documented life-threatening recurrent ventricular arrhythmias that do not respond to documented adequate doses of other antiarrhythmics or when alternative agents are not tolerated:

1.) Recurrent ventricular fibrillation (VF).
2.) Recurrent hemodynamically unstable ventricular tachycardia (VT).

Parenteral – Initiation of treatment and prophylaxis of frequently recurring VF and hemodynamically unstable VT in patients refractory to other therapy. It can also be used to treat patients with VT/VF for whom oral amiodarone is indicated, but who are unable to take oral medication.

➤*Unlabeled uses:* Amiodarone has shown effectiveness for conversion of atrial fibrillation and maintenance of sinus rhythm. It also appears to be useful in treating supraventricular tachycardia, and IV amiodarone has shown effectiveness in the treatment of AV nodal reentry tachycardia.

Administration and Dosage

➤*Approved by the FDA:* December 27, 1985.

➤*Oral:* To ensure that an antiarrhythmic effect will be observed without waiting several months, loading doses are required. Individual patient titration is suggested.

Because of the food effect on absorption, administer amiodarone consistently with regard to meals.

Life-threatening ventricular arrhythmias (eg, ventricular fibrillation or hemodynamically unstable ventricular tachycardia) –

Amiodarone Dosage Suggestions			
	Loading dose (daily)	Adjustment and maintenance dose (daily)	
Ventricular arrhythmias	1 to 3 weeks 800 to 1600 mg	≈ 1 month 600 to 800 mg	usual maintenance 400 mg

Closely monitor patients during the loading phase, particularly until risk of recurrent ventricular tachycardia or fibrillation has abated. Because of the serious nature of the arrhythmia and the lack of predictable time course of effect, administer the loading dose in a hospital. Loading doses of 800 to 1600 mg/day are required for 1 to 3 weeks (occasionally longer) until initial therapeutic response occurs. Administer in divided doses with meals for total daily doses of ≥ 1000 mg or when GI intolerance occurs. If side effects become excessive, reduce the dose. Elimination of recurrence of ventricular fibrillation and tachycardia usually occurs within 1 to 3 weeks, along with reduction in complex and total ventricular ectopic beats.

When starting therapy, attempt to gradually discontinue prior antiarrhythmic drugs. When adequate arrhythmia control is achieved or if side effects become prominent, reduce dose to 600 to 800 mg/day for 1 month and then to the maintenance dose, usually 400 mg/day. Some patients may require larger maintenance doses, up to 600 mg/day, and some can be controlled on lower doses. The drug may be administered as a single daily dose, or in patients with severe GI intolerance, as a twice daily dose.

Use the lowest effective dose to prevent the occurrence of side effects. In all instances, be guided by the severity of the patient's arrhythmia and response to therapy. Plasma concentrations may be helpful in evaluating nonresponsiveness or unexpectedly severe toxicity. When dosage adjustments are necessary, closely monitor the patient for an extended time because of the long and variable half-life and the difficulty in predicting the time required to attain a new steady-state drug level.

Concurrent antiarrhythmic agents – In general, reserve the combination of amiodarone with other antiarrhythmic therapy for patients with life-threatening arrhythmias who are incompletely responsive to a single agent or incompletely responsive to amiodarone. During transfer to amiodarone, reduce the dose levels of previously administered agents by 30% to 50% several days after the addition of amiodarone when arrhythmia suppression should be beginning. Review the continued need for the other antiarrhythmic agent after the effects of amiodarone have been established and attempt discontinuation. If the treatment is continued, carefully monitor these patients for adverse effects, especially conduction disturbances and exacerbation of tachyarrhythmias. In amiodarone-treated patients who require additional antiarrhythmic therapy, the initial dose of such agents should be approximately half of the usual recommended dose.

➤*Parenteral:* Amiodarone shows considerable interindividual variation in response. Thus, although a starting dose adequate to suppress life-threatening arrhythmias is needed, close monitoring with adjustment of dose as needed is essential. The recommended starting dose of amiodarone IV is ≈ 1000 mg over the first 24 hours of therapy, delivered by the following infusion regimen.

Amiodarone IV Dose Recommendations During the First 24 Hours	
Loading infusions	
First rapid	150 mg over the *first* 10 minutes (15 mg/min). Add 3 mL amiodarone IV (150 mg) to 100 mL D5W (concentration = 1.5 mg/mL). Infuse 100 mL over 10 minutes.
Followed by slow	360 mg over the *next* 6 hours (1 mg/min). Add 18 mL amiodarone IV (900 mg) to 500 mL D5W (concentration = 1.8 mg/mL).
Maintenance infusion	540 mg over the *remaining* 18 hours (0.5 mg/min). Decrease the rate of the slow loading infusion to 0.5 mg/min.

AMIODARONE HCl

After the first 24 hours, continue the maintenance infusion rate of 0.5 mg/min (720 mg/24 hrs) utilizing a concentration of 1 to 6 mg/mL. Give amiodarone IV concentrations > 2 mg/mL via a central venous catheter. In the event of breakthrough episodes of VF or hemodynamically unstable VT, 150 mg supplemental infusions of amiodarone IV mixed in 100 mL D5W may be given. Administer such infusions over 10 minutes to minimize the potential for hypotension. The rate of the maintenance infusion may be increased to achieve effective arrhythmia suppression.

The first 24-hour dose may be individualized for each patient; however, in controlled clinical trials, mean daily doses > 2100 mg were associated with an increased risk of hypotension. The initial infusion rate should not exceed 30 mg/min.

Based on experience from clinical studies, a maintenance infusion of ≤ 0.5 mg/min can be cautiously continued for 2 to 3 weeks regardless of patient's age, renal function, or left ventricular function. There is limited experience in patients receiving amiodarone IV for > 3 weeks.

Administration – Surface properties of solutions containing injectable amiodarone are altered such that drop size may be reduced. This reduction may lead to underdosage of the patient by ≤ 30%. If drop counter infusion sets are used, amiodarone must be delivered by a volumetric infusion pump.

When possible, administer amiodarone IV through a central venous catheter for that purpose. Use an in-line filter during administration.

Amiodarone IV concentrations > 3 mg/mL in D5W have been associated with a high incidence of peripheral vein phlebitis; however, concentrations of ≤ 2.5 mg/mL appear to be less irritating. Therefore, for infusions > 1 hour, amiodarone IV concentrations should not exceed 2 mg/mL unless a central venous catheter is used.

Admixture incompatibility – Amiodarone IV in D5W, in a concentration of 4 mg/mL, forms a precipitate and is incompatible with the following drugs: Aminophylline, cefamandole, cefazolin, mezlocillin, heparin (no amiodarone concentration stated), and sodium bicarbonate (amiodarone concentration of 3 mg/mL).

➤*IV to oral transition:* During or after treatment with IV amiodarone, patients may be transferred to oral amiodarone therapy. Use IV amiodarone for acute treatment until the patient's ventricular arrhythmias are stabilized. Most patients require this therapy for 48 to 96 hours, but IV amiodarone may be given safely for longer periods if necessary. The optimal dose for changing from IV to oral administration will depend on the dose already administered, as well as the bioavailability of oral amiodarone. When changing to oral therapy, clinical monitoring is recommended, particularly for elderly patients.

The following table provides suggested doses of oral amiodarone to be initiated after varying durations of IV administration. These recommendations are made on the basis of a comparable total body amount of amiodarone delivered by the IV and oral routes, based on 50% bioavailability of oral amiodarone.

Recommendations for Oral Amiodarone Dosage After IV Infusion	
Duration of amiodarone IV infusions[1]	Initial daily dose of oral amiodarone
< 1 week	800 to 1600 mg
1 to 3 weeks	600 to 800 mg
> 3 weeks[2]	400 mg

[1] Assuming a 720 mg/day infusion (0.5 mg/min).
[2] Amiodarone IV is not intended for maintenance treatment.

➤*Storage/Stability:* Store at room temperature ≈ 25°C (77°F). Protect from light (amiodarone IV does not need to be protected from light during administration).

Amiodarone IV infusions exceeding 2 hours must be administered in glass or polyolefin bottles containing D5W.

Amiodarone adsorbs to polyvinyl chloride (PVC) tubing, and the clinical trial dose administration schedule was designed to account for this adsorption. Clinical trials were conducted using PVC tubing; therefore its use is recommended. The concentrations and rates of infusion provided in Administration and Dosage reflect doses identified in these studies. It is important that the recommended infusion regimen be followed closely.

Amiodarone IV has been found to leach out plasticizers, including DEHP (di-–ethylhexyl]phthalate) from IV tubing (including PVC tubing). The degree of leaching increases when infusing amiodarone IV at higher concentrations and lower flow rates than recommended.

Amiodarone Solution Stability			
Solution	Concentration (mg/mL)	Container	Comments
5% Dextrose in Water (D5W)	1 to 6	PVC	Physically compatible, with amiodarone loss < 10% at 2 hours
5% Dextrose in Water (D5W)	1 to 6	Polyolefin, glass	Physically compatible, with no amiodarone loss at 24 hours

Actions

➤*Pharmacology:* Amiodarone possesses electrophysiologic characteristics of all 4 Vaughan Williams classes but has predominantly Class III antiarrhythmic effects. This may be caused by ≥ 2 major properties: Prolongation of myocardial cell-action potential duration, refractory period and noncompetitive α- and β-adrenergic inhibition.

Like Class I drugs, amiodarone blocks sodium channels at rapid pacing frequencies, and like Class II drugs, it exerts a noncompetitive antisympathetic action. One of its main effects with prolonged administration is to lengthen the cardiac action potential, a Class III effect. The negative chronotropic effect of amiodarone in nodal tissues is similar to the effect of class IV drugs. In addition to blocking sodium channels, amiodarone blocks myocardial potassium channels, which contributes to the slowing of conduction and the prolongation of refractoriness. The antisympathetic action and the block of calcium and potassium channels are responsible for the negative dromotropic effects on the sinus node and for the slowing of conduction and prolongation of refractoriness in the atrioventricular (AV) node. Its vasodilatory action can decrease cardiac workload and, consequently, myocardial oxygen consumption.

IV administration prolongs intranodal conduction and refractoriness of the AV node but, unlike oral dosing, has little or no effect on sinus cycle length, refractoriness of the right atrium and right ventricle, repolarization, intraventricular conduction, and intranodal conduction. These differences between oral and IV administration suggest that the initial acute effects of amiodarone IV may be predominantly focused on the AV node, causing an intranodal conduction delay and increased nodal refractoriness caused by slow channel blockade (Class IV activity) and noncompetitive adrenergic antagonism (Class II activity).

Hemodynamics – After IV use, amiodarone relaxes vascular smooth muscle, reduces peripheral vascular resistance (afterload) and slightly increases cardiac index. However, after oral dosing it produces no significant change in left ventricular ejection fraction (LVEF), even in patients with depressed LVEF. After acute IV dosing, it may have a mild negative inotropic effect.

Electrophysiology – Amiodarone increases the cardiac refractory period without influencing resting membrane potential, except in automatic cells where slope of prepotential is reduced, generally reducing automaticity. These electrophysiologic effects are reflected in decreased sinus rate of 15% to 20%, increased PR and QT intervals of ≈ 10%, development of U-waves, and changes in T-wave contour. These changes should not require discontinuation, although amiodarone can cause marked sinus bradycardia or sinus arrest and heart block. Rarely, QT prolongation has been associated with worsening of arrhythmia (see Warnings).

➤*Pharmacokinetics:*

Absorption – Following oral administration, amiodarone is slowly and variably absorbed; bioavailability is ≈ 50%. Maximum plasma concentrations are attained 3 to 7 hours after a single dose. Steady-state plasma concentrations, at a constant oral dosing, are reached in an average of 265 days. Although electrophysiologic effects can be seen within hours after an IV dose, effects on abnormal rhythms are not seen before 2 to 3 days and usually require 1 to 3 weeks, even when a loading dose is used. There is no well-established relationship of plasma concentration to effectiveness, but it does appear that concentrations between 1 and 2.5 mg/L are effective with acceptable toxicity. Plasma concentrations with chronic dosing at 100 to 600 mg/day are approximately dose-proportional, with a mean 0.5 mg/L increase for each 100 mg/day. Food increases the rate and extent of absorption.

Peak serum concentrations after single 5 mg/kg 15 minute IV infusions in healthy subjects range between 5 and 41 mg/L. Peak concentrations after 10 minute infusions of 150 mg in patients with ventricular fibrillation (VF) or hemodynamically unstable ventricular tachycardia (VT) range between 7 and 26 mg/L. Because of rapid distribution, serum concentrations decline to 10% of peak values within 30 to 45 minutes after the end of the infusion. After 48 hours of continued infusions (125, 500, or 1000 mg/day) plus supplemental (150 mg) infusions (for recurrent arrhythmias), amiodarone mean serum concentrations between 0.7 to 1.4 mg/L are observed.

Distribution – Amiodarone has a very large but variable volume of distribution, averaging ≈ 60 L/kg, because of extensive accumulation in various sites, especially adipose tissue and highly perfused organs (eg, liver, lung, spleen). One major metabolite, desethylamiodarone (DEA), accumulates to an even greater extent in almost all tissues. The pharmacological activity of this metabolite is unknown. Amiodarone and its metabolite have a limited transplacental transfer (10% to 50%). They have been detected in breast milk (see Warnings). The drug is highly protein bound (≈ 96%).

Metabolism – DEA is the major metabolite of amiodarone. DEA serum concentrations > 0.05 mg/L are not usually seen until after several days of continuous infusion but with prolonged therapy reach approximately the same concentration as amiodarone. The enzymes responsible for the N-deethylation are believed to be the cytochrome P450 3A (CYP3A) subfamily, principally CYP3A4.

Excretion – Amiodarone has biphasic elimination with an initial one-half reduction of plasma levels after 2.5 to 10 days. A much slower ter-

AMIODARONE HCl

minal plasma-elimination phase shows a mean half-life of the parent compound of ≈ 53 days. For the metabolite, the mean half-life is ≈ 61 days. The main route of elimination is via hepatic excretion into bile. The drug has a very low plasma clearance with negligible renal excretion; it does not appear necessary to modify dose in patients with renal, hepatic, or cardiac abnormalities. Neither amiodarone nor its metabolite is dialyzable.

Contraindications

Hypersensitivity to the drug or any of its components.

➤*Oral:* Severe sinus-node dysfunction causing marked sinus bradycardia; second- and third-degree AV block; when episodes of bradycardia have caused syncope (except when used in conjunction with a pacemaker).

➤*Parenteral:* Marked sinus bradycardia; second- and third-degree AV block unless a functioning pacemaker is available; cardiogenic shock.

Warnings

➤*Potentially fatal toxicities:* Amiodarone has several potentially fatal toxicities, the most important of which is pulmonary toxicity (hypersensitivity pneumonitis or interstitial/alveolar pneumonitis) that has resulted in clinically manifest disease at rates as high as 10% to 17% in some series of patients with ventricular arrhythmias given doses around 400 mg/day, and as abnormal diffusion capacity without symptoms in a much higher percentage of patients. Pulmonary toxicity has been fatal ≈ 10% of the time. Liver injury is common with amiodarone, but is usually mild and evidenced only by abnormal liver enzymes. Overt liver disease can occur and has been fatal in a few cases. Like other antiarrhythmics, amiodarone can exacerbate the arrhythmia by making it less well tolerated or more difficult to reverse. This has occurred in 2% to 5% of patients in various series, and significant heart block or sinus bradycardia has been seen in 2% to 5%. Although the frequency of such proarrhythmic events does not appear greater with amiodarone than with many other agents used in this population, the effects are prolonged when they occur.

➤*Life-threatening arrhythmias:* Amiodarone is intended for use only in patients with the indicated life-threatening arrhythmias because its use is accompanied by substantial toxicity.

High-risk patients – Even in patients at high risk of arrhythmic death, in whom the toxicity of amiodarone is an acceptable risk, amiodarone poses major management problems that could be life-threatening in a population at risk of sudden death, so make every effort to use alternative agents first.

The difficulty of using amiodarone effectively and safely poses a significant risk to patients. Because absorption and elimination are variable, maintenance dose selection is difficult, and it is not unusual to require dosage decrease or treatment discontinuation. The time at which a previously controlled life-threatening arrhythmia will recur after discontinuation or dose adjustment is unpredictable, ranging from weeks to months. The patient is obviously at great risk during this time and may need prolonged hospitalization. Attempts to substitute other antiarrhythmic agents when amiodarone must be stopped is difficult because of the gradual changing amiodarone body burden. A similar problem exists when amiodarone is not effective; it still poses the risk of an interaction with whatever subsequent treatment is tried.

Survival – There is no evidence that amiodarone favorably affects survival. Refer to the Antiarrhythmic Agents introduction.

➤*Ophthalmologic effects:* Cases of optic neuropathy or optic neuritis, usually resulting in visual impairment, have occurred in patients treated with amiodarone. In some cases, visual impairment has progressed to permanent blindness. Optic neuropathy or neuritis may occur at any time following initiation of therapy. A causal relationship to the drug has not been clearly established.

If symptoms of visual impairment appear, prompt ophthalmic examination is recommended. Appearance of optic neuropathy or neuritis calls for reevaluation of therapy. Regular ophthalmic examination, including fundoscopy and slit-lamp examination, is recommended during administration of amiodarone. Corneal microdeposits appear in virtually all adults treated with amiodarone. They are usually discernible only by slit-lamp examination but give rise to symptoms such as visual halos or blurred vision in as many as 10% of patients. Corneal microdeposits are reversible upon reduction of dose or drug discontinuation. Asymptomatic microdeposits are not a reason to reduce dose or stop treatment. Some patients develop photophobia and dry eyes. Vision is rarely affected, and drug discontinuation is rarely needed.

➤*Pulmonary toxicity:*

Oral – Amiodarone may cause a clinical syndrome of cough and progressive dyspnea accompanied by functional, radiographic, gallium-scan, and pathological data consistent with pulmonary toxicity. The frequency varies from 2% to 17%; fatalities, secondary to pulmonary toxicity, occur in ≈ 10% of cases. However, in patients with life-threatening arrhythmias, discontinuation of therapy because of suspected drug-induced pulmonary toxicity should be undertaken with caution, as the most common cause of death in these patients is sudden cardiac death. Make every effort to rule out other causes of respiratory impairment (eg, CHF with Swan-Ganz catheterization if necessary, respiratory infection, pulmonary embolism, malignancy) before discontinuing

amiodarone. In addition, bronchoalveolar lavage, transbronchial lung biopsy, or open lung biopsy may be necessary to confirm the diagnosis, especially in cases where no acceptable alternative therapy is available.

Any new respiratory symptom suggests pulmonary toxicity; therefore, repeat and evaluate the history, physical exam, chest x-ray, gallium scan, and pulmonary function tests (with diffusion capacity). In some cases, rechallenge at a lower dose has not resulted in return of interstitial/alveolar pneumonitis. A 15% decrease in diffusion capacity has a high sensitivity but only a moderate specificity for pulmonary toxicity; as the decrease in diffusion capacity approaches 30%, the sensitivity decreases, but the specificity increases.

Preexisting pulmonary disease does not appear to increase the risk of developing pulmonary toxicity; however, these patients have a poorer prognosis if pulmonary toxicity does develop.

Hypersensitivity pneumonitis: Hypersensitivity pneumonitis usually appears earlier in the course of therapy, and rechallenging these patients results in a more rapid recurrence of greater severity. Bronchoalveolar lavage is the procedure of choice to confirm this diagnosis, which can be made when a T-suppressor/cytotoxic (CD8-positive) lymphocytosis is noted. Institute steroid therapy and discontinue amiodarone therapy.

Interstitial/Alveolar pneumonitis: Interstitial/alveolar pneumonitis may result from the release of oxygen radicals or phospholipidosis and is characterized by findings of diffuse alveolar damage, interstitial pneumonitis, or fibrosis in lung biopsy specimens. Phospholipidosis (foamy cells, foamy macrophages), caused by inhibition of phospholipase, will be present in most cases of amiodarone-induced pulmonary toxicity; however, these changes are also present in ≈ 50% of patients. Use these cells as markers of therapy but not as evidence of toxicity. A diagnosis of amiodarone-induced interstitial/alveolar pneumonitis should lead, at a minimum, to dose reduction or, preferably, to withdrawal of amiodarone to establish reversibility, especially if other acceptable antiarrhythmic therapies are available. Where these measures have been instituted, a reduction in symptoms of amiodarone-induced pulmonary toxicity was usually noted within the first week, and a clinical improvement was greatest in the first 2 to 3 weeks. Chest x-ray changes usually resolve within 2 to 4 months.

According to some experts, steroids may prove beneficial. Prednisone in doses of 40 to 60 mg/day or equivalent doses of other steroids have been given and tapered over the course of several weeks depending on the condition of the patient. In some cases, rechallenge with amiodarone at a lower dose has not resulted in return of toxicity. Recent reports suggest that the use of lower loading and maintenance doses of amiodarone are associated with a decreased incidence of amiodarone-induced pulmonary toxicity.

If a diagnosis of amiodarone-induced hypersensitivity pneumonitis is made, discontinue amiodarone and institute steroid treatment. If a diagnosis of amiodarone-induced interstitial/alveolar pneumonitis is made, institute steroid therapy, and discontinue amiodarone or, at a minimum, reduce dosage, because some cases may resolve. In some patients, rechallenge at a lower dose has not resulted in return of interstitial/alveolar pneumonitis; however, in some patients (perhaps because of severe alveolar damage), the pulmonary lesions have not been reversible.

Parenteral –

ARDS: 2% of patients were reported to have adult respiratory distress syndrome (ARDS) during clinical studies. This clinical and radiographic picture can arise after a variety of lung injuries, such as those resulting from trauma, shock, prolonged cardiopulmonary resuscitation, and aspiration pneumonitis, conditions present in many of the patients enrolled in the clinical studies. It is not possible to determine what role, if any, amiodarone IV played in causing or exacerbating the pulmonary disorder in those patients.

Pulmonary fibrosis: Only 1 of more than 1000 patients treated with amiodarone IV in clinical studies developed pulmonary fibrosis. In that patient, the condition was diagnosed 3 months after treatment with amiodarone IV, during which time she received oral amiodarone.

➤*Cardiac effects:*

Proarrhythmia – Amiodarone can cause serious exacerbation of the presenting arrhythmia, a risk that may be enhanced by concomitant antiarrhythmics. Exacerbation has included new ventricular fibrillation, incessant ventricular tachycardia, increased resistance to cardioversion, and polymorphic ventricular tachycardia associated with QT prolongation (torsades de pointes). Amiodarone has caused symptomatic bradycardia or sinus arrest with suppression of escape foci in 2% to 4% of patients.

Bradycardia/AV block – Drug-related bradycardia occurred in 5% of 1836 patients in clinical trials while they were receiving amiodarone IV for life-threatening VT/VF; it was not dose-related. Treat bradycardia by slowing the infusion rate or discontinuing amiodarone IV. In some patients, inserting a pacemaker is required. Treat patients with a known predisposition to bradycardia or AV block with amiodarone IV in a setting where a temporary pacemaker is available.

Hypotension – Hypotension is the most common adverse effect seen with amiodarone IV. Clinically significant hypotension during infusions was seen most often in the first several hours and was not dose-related, but appeared to be related to the rate of infusion. Treat hypotension initially by slowing the infusion; additional standard therapy may be

AMIODARONE HCl

needed, including the following: Vasopressor drugs, positive inotropic agents, and volume expansion. Monitor the initial rate of infusion closely, and do not exceed that prescribed in Administration and Dosage.

➤*Surgery:*

Volatile anesthetic agents – Close perioperative monitoring is recommended in patients undergoing general anesthesia who are on amiodarone therapy as they may be more sensitive to the myocardial depressant and conduction effects of halogenated inhalational anesthetics.

Hypotension postbypass – Rare occasions of hypotension upon discontinuation of cardiopulmonary bypass during open-heart surgery in patients receiving amiodarone have been reported. The relationship of this effect to amiodarone therapy is unknown.

ARDS – Postoperatively, occurrences of ARDS have been reported in patients receiving amiodarone therapy who have undergone either cardiac or noncardiac surgery. Although patients usually respond well to vigorous respiratory therapy, in rare instances the outcome has been fatal. Until further studies have been performed, closely monitor FiO_2 and the determinants of oxygen delivery to the tissues (eg, SaO_2, PaO_2) in patients on amiodarone.

➤*CNS effects:* Neurologic problems (20% to 40%) are rarely a reason to stop therapy and may respond to dose reductions.

➤*GI effects:* GI complaints occur in ≈ 25% of patients but rarely require discontinuation of drug. These commonly occur during high-dose administration (eg, loading dose) and usually respond to dose reduction or divided doses.

➤*Hepatic effects:*

Oral – Elevated hepatic enzyme levels are frequent and, in most cases, asymptomatic. Regularly monitor liver enzymes in patients on relatively high maintenance doses. If the increase exceeds 3 times normal, or doubles in a patient with an elevated baseline, consider discontinuation or dosage reduction. When a biopsy has been done, histology has resembled that of alcoholic hepatitis or cirrhosis. Hepatic failure has rarely caused death.

Parenteral – Elevations of blood hepatic enzyme values (ALT, AST, and GGT) are seen commonly in patients with immediately life-threatening VT/VF. Interpreting elevated AST activity can be difficult because the values may be elevated in patients who have had recent MI, CHF, or multiple electrical defibrillations. In 81% of patients with baseline and on-therapy data available, the liver enzyme elevations either improved during therapy or remained at baseline levels. Baseline abnormalities in hepatic enzymes are not a contraindication to treatment.

Two cases of fatal hepatocellular necrosis after treatment with amiodarone IV have occurred. The patients were treated for atrial arrhythmias with an initial infusion rate much higher than recommended (1500 mg over 5 hours). Because these episodes of hepatic necrosis may have been caused by the rapid rate of infusion with possible rate-related hypotension, monitor the initial rate of infusion closely, and do not exceed that prescribed in Administration and Dosage.

In patients with life-threatening arrhythmias, weigh the potential risk of hepatic injury against the potential benefit of therapy. Monitor carefully for evidence of progressive hepatic injury. Give consideration to reducing the rate of administration or withdrawing amiodarone IV in such cases.

➤*Carcinogenesis:* Amiodarone caused a statistically significant, dose-related increase in the incidence of thyroid tumors (follicular adenoma or carcinoma in rats).

➤*Fertility impairment:* Amiodarone also reduced fertility of male and female rats at a dose of 90 mg/kg/day (1.4 times the highest recommended human maintenance dose).

➤*Elderly:* Healthy subjects > 65 years of age show lower clearances of amiodarone than younger subjects (100 vs 150 mL/kg/hr) and an increase in half-life (from ≈ 20 to 47 days). Clinical studies of amiodarone tablets did not include sufficient numbers of subjects ≥ 65 years of age to determine whether they respond differently from younger subjects. Other reported clinical experience has not identified differences in responses between the elderly and younger patients. In general, dose selection for an elderly patient should be cautious, usually starting at the low end of the dosing range, reflecting the greater frequency of decreased hepatic, renal, or cardiac function, and of concomitant disease or other drug therapy.

➤*Pregnancy: Category D.*

Oral – Amiodarone has been embryotoxic (increased fetal resorption and growth retardation) in the rat.

Amiodarone can cause fetal harm when administered to a pregnant woman. Although its use is uncommon, there have been some reports of congenital goiter/hypothyroidism and hyperthyroidism. If amiodarone is used during pregnancy or if the patient becomes pregnant while taking amiodarone, apprise the patient of the potential hazard to the fetus. Use only if the potential benefits outweigh the potential hazards to the fetus.

➤*Lactation:* Amiodarone is excreted in breast milk. Nursing offspring of lactating rats given amiodarone are less viable and have reduced body-weight gains. Therefore, when amiodarone therapy is indicated, advise the mother to discontinue nursing.

➤*Children:* Safety and efficacy for use in children have not been established; therefore, amiodarone is not recommended in children. There have been reports of fatal "gasping syndrome" in neonates (children < 1 month of age) following the administration of IV solutions containing the preservative benzyl alcohol. Symptoms include a striking onset of gasping respiration, hypotension, bradycardia, and cardiovascular collapse.

Precautions

➤*Monitoring:* Perform baseline chest x-rays and pulmonary function tests, including diffusion capacity before therapy initiation. Repeat a history, physical exam, and chest x-ray every 3 to 6 months.

Monitor thyroid function at baseline and periodically during therapy, particularly in the elderly and in any patient with a history of thyroid nodules, goiter, or other thyroid dysfunction.

Perform regular ophthalmic examination, including fundoscopy and slit-lamp examination, during administration of amiodarone.

Monitor liver enzymes on a regular basis.

Closely monitor FiO_2 and the determinants of oxygen delivery to the tissues (eg, SaO_2, PaO_2) in patients on amiodarone.

➤*Long-term use:* There has been limited experience in patients receiving amiodarone IV longer than 3 weeks.

➤*Thyroid abnormalities:* Amiodarone inhibits peripheral conversion of thyroxine (T_4) to triiodothyronine (T_3), prompting increased T_4 levels, increased levels of inactive reverse T_3, and decreased levels of T_3. It is also a potential source of large amounts of inorganic iodine. Because of its release of inorganic iodine, or maybe for other reasons, amiodarone can cause hypothyroidism or hyperthyroidism. Monitor thyroid function at baseline and periodically during therapy, particularly in the elderly and in any patient with a history of thyroid nodules, goiter, or other thyroid dysfunction. Because of the slow elimination of amiodarone and its metabolites, high plasma iodide levels, altered thyroid function, and abnormal thyroid function tests may persist for several weeks or even months following amiodarone withdrawal.

Hypothyroidism – Hypothyroidism is best managed by dose reduction or thyroid hormone supplement. Individualize therapy and discontinue amiodarone if necessary.

Hyperthyroidism – Hyperthyroidism usually poses a greater hazard to the patient than hypothyroidism because of the possibility of arrhythmia breakthrough or aggravation. If any new signs of arrhythmia appear, consider the possibility of hyperthyroidism. Aggressive medical treatment is indicated, including, if possible, dose reduction or withdrawal of amiodarone. The institution of antithyroid drugs, beta-adrenergic blockers, or temporary corticosteroid therapy may be necessary. The action of antithyroid drugs may be especially delayed in amiodarone-induced thyrotoxicosis because of substantial quantities of preformed thyroid hormones stored in the gland. Radioactive iodine therapy is contraindicated because of the low radioiodine uptake associated with amiodarone-induced hyperthyroidism. Experience with thyroid surgery in this setting is extremely limited, and this form of therapy runs the theoretical risk of inducing thyroid storm. Amiodarone-induced hyperthyroidism may be followed by a transient period of hypothyroidism.

➤*Electrolyte disturbances:* Antiarrhythmics may be ineffective or arrhythmogenic in patients with hypokalemia; correct potassium or magnesium deficiency before therapy begins as these disorders can exaggerate the degree of QTc prolongation and increase the potential for torsades de pointes. Give special attention to electrolyte and acid-base balance in patients experiencing severe or prolonged diarrhea or in patients receiving concomitant diuretics.

➤*Benzyl alcohol:* Benzyl alcohol, contained in some of these products as a preservative, has been associated with a fatal "gasping syndrome" in premature infants.

➤*Photosensitivity:* Amiodarone has induced photosensitization in ≈ 10% of patients; some protection may be afforded by sun-barrier creams or protective clothing. During long-term treatment, a blue-gray discoloration of the exposed skin may occur. The risk may be increased in patients of fair complexion or those with excessive sun exposure and may be related to cumulative dose and duration of therapy. This is slowly and, occasionally, incompletely reversible on discontinuation of drug but is of cosmetic importance only.

Drug Interactions

In view of the long and variable half-life of amiodarone, potential for drug interactions exists not only with concomitant medication, but also with drugs given after discontinuation of amiodarone.

The following interactions occurred with oral administration unless otherwise noted.

AMIODARONE HCl

Amiodarone Drug Interactions			
Precipitant drug	Object drug*		Description
Amiodarone	Anticoagulants	↑	Prothrombin time (PT) may increase. Potentiation of antico-agulant response is almost always seen in patients receiving amiodarone and can result in seri-ous or fatal bleeding. A 30% to 50% anticoagulant dose reduction is typically required. Onset is 3 to 4 days and may persist for months after amiodarone discon-tinuation. Closely monitor PT.
Amiodarone	Beta blockers	↑	Effects of beta blockers eliminated by hepatic metabolism may be increased. Because amiodarone has weak beta blocking activity, concomitant use can increase risk of hypotension and bradycardia.
Amiodarone	Calcium channel blockers	↑	Amiodarone inhibits AV conduc-tion and decreases myocardial contractility; increased risk of AV block with verapamil or diltiazem or hypotension with any calcium blocker may occur.
Amiodarone	Cisapride	↑	Risk of life-threatening cardiac arrhythmias, including torsades de pointes, may be increased because of possibly additive pro-longation of the QT interval.
Amiodarone	Cyclosporine	↑	Concomitant use has produced persistently elevated plasma cyclosporine levels resulting in elevated creatinine despite reduc-tion in dose of cyclosporine.
Amiodarone	Dextromethor-phan	↑	Chronic use (> 2 weeks) of amio-darone administration impairs metabolism of dextromethor-phan.
Amiodarone	Digoxin	↑	Amiodarone may increase digoxin serum concentrations by ≥ 70%. On initiation of amio-darone, review the need for digi-talis therapy and reduce the dose by ≈ 50% or discontinue. If treat-ment is continued, closely moni-tor serum levels.
Amiodarone	Disopyramide	↑	Increases QT prolongation and possible arrhythmias.
Amiodarone	Fentanyl	↑	May cause hypotension, bradycar-dia, decreased cardiac output.
Amiodarone	Flecainide	↑	Increased plasma flecainide levels may occur. Reduce the dose of flecainide needed to maintain therapeutic plasma concentra-tions.
Amiodarone	Hydantoins Phenytoin	↑	Chronic use (> 2 weeks) of amio-darone impairs metabolism of phenytoin. Increased hydantoin concentrations with symptoms of toxicity may occur. Also, amio-darone serum levels may be decreased.
Hydantoins Phenytoin	Amiodarone	↓	
Amiodarone	Lidocaine	↑	Sinus bradycardia was seen in a patient receiving oral amiodarone who was given lidocaine for local anesthesia. A seizure associated with increased IV lidocaine con-centrations was observed in 1 patient.
Amiodarone	Methotrexate	↑	Chronic use (> 2 weeks) of amio-darone impairs metabolism of methotrexate. Methotrexate toxic-ity may be increased.
Amiodarone	Procainamide	↑	Increased procainamide or NAPA serum levels may occur (55% and 33%, respectively).
Amiodarone	Quinidine	↑	Quinidine levels may be increased by 33%, producing potentially fatal cardiac dysrhythmias.
Amiodarone	Theophylline	↑	Increased theophylline levels with toxicity may occur. Effects may not be seen for ≥ 1 week of con-comitant therapy and may persist for an extended period after amiodarone discontinuation.

Amiodarone Drug Interactions			
Precipitant drug	Object drug*		Description
Cholestyramine	Amiodarone	↓	Increased enterohepatic elimina-tion of amiodarone and reduced serum levels and half-life may occur.
Cimetidine	Amiodarone	↑	Increased serum amiodarone levels may occur.
Fluoroquino-lones Sparfloxacin Gatifloxacin Moxifloxacin Grepafloxacin	Amiodarone	↑	Risk of life-threatening cardiac arrhythmias, including torsades de pointes, may be increased.
Rifamycins	Amiodarone	↓	Serum concentrations of amio-darone and its active metabolite may be decreased, reducing its pharmacologic effect.
Ritonavir	Amiodarone	↑	Large increases in amiodarone concentrations may occur, increasing the risk of amiodarone toxicity.

* ↑ = Object drug increased.   ↓ = Object drug decreased.

➤*Drug/Lab test interactions:* Amiodarone alters the results of thy-roid function tests, causing an increase in serum T_4 and serum reverse T_3 levels and a decline in serum T_3 levels. Despite these biochemical changes, most patients remain clinically euthyroid (see Precautions). Elevations in liver enzymes (ALT and AST) can occur.

Adverse Reactions

➤*Oral:* Adverse reactions, common in most patients treated with amiodarone for ventricular arrhythmias with relatively large doses (≥ 400 mg/day), occur in ≈ 75% of patients and cause discontinuation in 7% to 18%. Most effects appear more frequently with treatment beyond 6 months, although rates appear relatively constant beyond 1 year. Reactions most frequently requiring discontinuation include the follow-ing: Pulmonary infiltrates or fibrosis, paroxysmal ventricular tachycar-dia, CHF, elevation of liver enzymes.

Cardiovascular – Bradycardia, cardiac arrhythmias (see Warnings), SA node dysfunction, CHF (1% to 3%); hypotension (< 1%; see Warn-ings).

CNS – Malaise, fatigue, tremor/abnormal involuntary movements, lack of coordination, abnormal gait/ataxia, dizziness, paresthesias (4% to 9%); decreased libido, insomnia, headache, sleep disturbances (1% to 3%); peripheral neuropathy (see Warnings).

Dermatologic – Photosensitivity (10%; see Precautions); solar derma-titis (4% to 9%); blue discoloration of skin (see Precautions), rash, spon-taneous ecchymosis, alopecia (< 1%).

GI – Nausea, vomiting (10% to 33%); constipation, anorexia (4% to 9%); abdominal pain, abnormal salivation (1% to 3%; see Warnings).

Hepatic – Abnormal liver function tests (4% to 9%; see Warnings); nonspecific hepatic disorders (1% to 3%); hepatitis, cholestatic hepa-titis, cirrhosis (rare).

Special senses – Visual disturbances (4% to 9%); abnormal taste and smell (1% to 3%); optic neuritis; optic neuropathy; permanent blind-ness; papilledema; corneal degeneration; eye discomfort; scotoma; lens opacities; macular degeneration; photophobia; dry eyes; visual halos (see Warnings).

Miscellaneous – Pulmonary inflammation or fibrosis (4% to 9%; see Warnings); hypothyroidism and hyperthyroidism (see Precautions), edema, coagulation abnormalities, flushing (1% to 3%); epididymitis, vasculitis, pseudotumor cerebri, thrombocytopenia, angioedema.

➤*Parenteral:* The most important adverse effects were hypotension, asystole/cardiac arrest/electromechanical dissociation (EMD), cardio-genic shock, CHF, bradycardia, liver function test abnormalities, VT, and AV block. Overall, treatment was discontinued for ≈ 9% of the patients because of adverse effects. The most common adverse effects leading to discontinuation of IV therapy were hypotension (1.6%), asys-tole/cardiac arrest/EMD (1.2%), VT (1.1%), and cardiogenic shock (1%).

IV Amiodarone Adverse Reactions (%)			
Adverse reaction	Controlled studies (n = 814)	Open label studies (n = 1022)	Total (n = 1836)
Abnormal liver function tests	4.2	2.8	3.4
Bradycardia	6	4	4.9
Cardiac arrest	3.5	2.5	2.9
CHF	2.2	2	2.1
Fever	2.9	1.2	2
Hypotension	20.2	12	15.6
Nausea	3.5	4.2	3.9
Ventricular tachycardia	1.8	2.9	2.4

AMIODARONE HCl

Other adverse reactions include the following:

Cardiovascular – Atrial fibrillation, nodal arrhythmia, prolonged QT interval, sinus bradycardia, VF (< 2%).

GI – Diarrhea, vomiting (< 2%).

Miscellaneous – Abnormal kidney function, lung edema, respiratory disorder, shock, Stevens-Johnson syndrome, thrombocytopenia (< 2%).

Overdosage

➤*Symptoms:* There have been a few reported cases of oral overdose in which 3 to 8 g of the drug were taken. There were no deaths or permanent sequelae. The most likely effects of an inadvertent overdose of amiodarone are hypotension, cardiogenic shock, bradycardia, AV block, and hepatotoxicity.

➤*Treatment:* Include usual supportive measures in treatment. Refer to General Management of Acute Overdosage. In addition, monitor the patient's cardiac rhythm and blood pressure; if bradycardia occurs, use a β-adrenergic agonist or a pacemaker. Treat hypotension with inadequate tissue perfusion by using positive inotropic or vasopressor agents. Neither amiodarone nor its metabolite is dialyzable.

Patient Information

Photosensitization (photoallergy or phototoxicity) may occur; therefore, caution patients to take protective measures (ie, sunscreens, protective clothing) against exposure to sunlight or ultraviolet light (eg, tanning beds) until tolerance is determined.

Because of the food effect on absorption, instruct patients to take amiodarone consistently with regard to meals.

ADENOSINE

Rx	Adenocard (Fujisawa)	Injection: 3 mg/mL	NaCl 9 mg/mL. Preservative free. In 2 mL vials and 2 and 5 mL syringes.

Refer to the general introductory discussion concerning Antiarrhythmic Agents. For information on the symptomatic relief of vericose veins, refer to the Adenosine Phosphate monograph in the CNS chapter.

Indications

➤*Paroxysmal supraventricular tachycardia (PSVT):* Conversion to sinus rhythm of PSVT, including that associated with accessory bypass tracts (Wolff-Parkinson-White [W-P-W] syndrome). When clinically advisable, attempt appropriate vagal maneuvers (eg, Valsalva maneuver) prior to use.

➤*Unlabeled uses:* Adenosine has been used in the noninvasive assessment of patients with suspected coronary artery disease in conjunction with [201]thallium tomography; results are similar to assessment with IV dipyridamole.

Administration and Dosage

➤*Approved by the FDA:* October 1989.

For rapid bolus IV use only. To be certain the solution reaches the systemic circulation, administer either directly into a vein or, if given into an IV line, as proximal as possible and follow with a rapid saline flush.

➤*Adult:*

Initial dose – 6 mg as a rapid IV bolus (administered over a 1 to 2 second period).

Repeat administration – If the first dose does not result in elimination of the supraventricular tachycardia within 1 to 2 minutes, give 12 mg as a rapid IV bolus. Repeat 12 mg dose a second time if required.

➤*Children:* The dosages used in neonates, infants, children, and adolescents were equivalent to those administered to adults on a weight basis.

< 50 kg –
  Initial dose: 0.05 to 0.1 mg/kg as a rapid IV bolus given either centrally or peripherally. A saline flush should follow.
  Repeat administration: If conversion of PSVT does not occur within 1 to 2 minutes, additional bolus injections of adenosine can be administered at incrementally higher doses, increasing the amount given by 0.05 to 0.1 mg/kg. Follow each bolus with a saline flush. Continue this process until sinus rhythm is established or a maximum single dose of 0.3 mg/kg is used.

≥ 50 kg – Administer the adult dose.

Doses > 12 mg are not recommended.

➤*Storage/Stability:* Store at room temperature 15° to 30°C (59° to 86°F). Do not refrigerate as crystallization may occur. If this occurs, let crystals warm to room temperature. The solution must be clear at the time of use. Discard unused portion.

Actions

➤*Pharmacology:* Adenosine slows conduction time through the AV node, can interrupt the re-entry pathways through the AV node, and can restore normal sinus rhythm in patients with PSVT, including PSVT associated with W-P-W syndrome.

Adenosine is antagonized competitively by methylxanthines such as caffeine and theophylline and potentiated by blockers of nucleoside transport such as dipyridamole (see Drug Interactions). Adenosine is not blocked by atropine.

The usual IV bolus dose of 6 or 12 mg will not have systemic hemodynamic effects. When larger doses are given by infusion, adenosine decreases blood pressure by decreasing peripheral resistance.

➤*Pharmacokinetics:* IV adenosine is rapidly removed from the circulation. Following an IV bolus, adenosine is taken up by erythrocytes and vascular endothelial cells. Adenosine is primarily metabolized to inosine and adenosine monophosphate (AMP). Half-life of AMP is estimated to be < 10 seconds.

➤*Clinical trials:* In controlled studies, bolus doses of 3, 6, 9, and 12 mg were studied. A cumulative 60% of patients with PSVT had converted to normal sinus rhythm within 1 minute after an IV bolus dose of 6 mg (some converted on 3 mg and failures were given 6 mg), and a cumulative 92% converted after a bolus dose of 12 mg. From 7% to 16% of patients converted after 1 to 4 placebo bolus injections.

Similar results were seen in a variety of patient subsets, including those using or not using digoxin, those with W-P-W syndrome, blacks, whites, and Hispanics.

Contraindications

Second- or third-degree AV block (except in patients with a functioning artificial pacemaker); sinus node disease, such as sick sinus syndrome or symptomatic bradycardia (except in patients with a functioning artificial pacemaker); known hypersensitivity to adenosine.

Warnings

➤*Heart block:* Adenosine decreases conduction through the AV node and may produce a short-lasting first-, second- or third-degree heart block. Institute appropriate therapy as needed. Patients who develop high-level block on 1 dose of adenosine should not be given additional doses. Because of the very short half-life, these effects are generally self-limiting.

Transient or prolonged episodes of asystole have been reported with fatal outcomes in some cases. Rarely, ventricular fibrillation has been reported following adenosine administration, including resuscitated and fatal events. In most instances, these cases were associated with the concomitant use of digoxin and, less frequently, with digoxin and verapamil. Although no causal relationship or drug-drug interaction has been established, use adenosine with caution in patients receiving digoxin or digoxin and verapamil in combination. Appropriate resuscitative measures should be made available.

➤*Arrhythmias:* At the time of conversion to normal sinus rhythm, a variety of new rhythms may appear on the ECG. They generally last only a few seconds without intervention and may take the form of premature ventricular contractions, atrial premature contractions, sinus bradycardia, sinus tachycardia, skipped beats, and varying degrees of AV nodal block. Such findings were seen in 55% of patients.

➤*Treatment of other arrhythmias:* Adenosine is not effective in converting rhythms other than PSVT, such as atrial flutter, atrial fibrillation, or ventricular tachycardia to normal sinus rhythm. Use in such patients has not resulted in adverse consequences.

➤*Ventricular response:* In the presence of atrial flutter or atrial fibrillation, a transient modest slowing of ventricular response may occur immediately following use.

➤*Bronchoconstriction:* Adenosine administered by inhalation has been reported to cause bronchoconstriction in asthmatic patients, presumably due to mast cell degranulation and histamine release. These effects have not been observed in normal subjects. Adenosine has been administered to a limited number of patients with asthma and mild-to-moderate exacerbation of their symptoms has been reported. Respiratory compromise has occurred using adenosine infusion in patients with obstructive pulmonary disease. Use adenosine with caution in patients with obstructive lung disease not associated with bronchoconstriction (eg, emphysema, bronchitis) and avoid use in patients with bronchoconstriction or bronchospasm (eg, asthma). Discontinue adenosine in any patient who develops severe respiratory difficulties.

➤*Mutagenesis:* Adenosine, like other nucleosides at millimolar concentrations present for several doubling times of cells in culture, is known to produce a variety of chromosomal alterations.

➤*Elderly:* Use adenosine with caution in geriatric patients because this population may have a diminished cardiac function, nodal dysfunction, concomitant diseases, or drug therapy that may alter hemodynamic function and produce severe bradycardia or AV block.

➤*Pregnancy: Category C.* As adenosine is a naturally occurring material, widely dispersed throughout the body, no fetal effects would be anticipated. However, because it is not known whether the drug can cause fetal harm when administered to pregnant women, use during pregnancy only if clearly needed.

ADENOSINE

Drug Interactions

Adenosine Drug Interactions			
Precipitant drug	Object drug*		Description
Carbamazepine	Adenosine	↑	Carbamazepine may increase the degree of heart block produced by other agents. As the primary effect of adenosine is to decrease conduction through the AV node, higher degrees of heart block may be produced in the presence of carbamazepine.
Dipyridamole	Adenosine	↑	The effects of adenosine are potentiated. Thus, smaller doses of adenosine may be effective in the presence of dipyridamole.
Methylxanthines (eg, caffeine, theophylline)	Adenosine	↓	The effects of adenosine are antagonized. In the presence of methylxanthines, larger doses of adenosine may be required or adenosine may be ineffective.
Adenosine	Digoxin Verapamil	↑	The use of adenosine with digoxin and verapamil may rarely be associated with ventricular fibrillation.

* ↑ = Object drug increased.   ↓ = Object drug decreased.

Adverse Reactions

➤*Cardiovascular:* Facial flushing (18%); headache (2%); sweating, palpitations, chest pain, hypotension (< 1%); prolonged asystole; ventricular fibrillation; ventricular tachycardia; transient increase in blood pressure; bradycardia; atrial fibrillation (postmarket).

➤*CNS:* Lightheadedness (2%); dizziness, tingling in arms, numbness (1%); apprehension, blurred vision, burning sensation, heaviness in arms, neck/back pain (< 1%).

➤*GI:* Nausea (3%); metallic taste, tightness in throat, pressure in groin (< 1%).

➤*Respiratory:* Shortness of breath/dyspnea (12%); chest pressure (7%); hyperventilation, head pressure (< 1%); bronchospasm (postmarket).

Overdosage

Adverse effects are generally rapidly self-limiting. Individualize treatment of prolonged adverse effects and direct toward the specific effect. Methylxanthines are competitive antagonists of adenosine (see Drug Interactions). Refer to General Management of Acute Overdosage.

DOFETILIDE

Rx	Tikosyn (Pfizer)	**Capsules:** 125 mcg	(TKN 125 PFIZER). Light orange/white. In 14s, 60s, and UD 40s.
		250 mcg	(TKN 250 PFIZER). Peach. In 14s, 60s, and UD 40s.
		500 mcg	(TKN 500 PFIZER). Peach/white. In 14s, 60s, and UD 40s.

WARNING

To minimize the risk of induced arrhythmia, place patients initiated or reinitiated on dofetilide in a facility that can provide calculations of Ccr, continuous electrocardiographic (ECG) monitoring, and cardiac resuscitation for a minimum of 3 days. Dofetilide is available only to hospitals and prescribers who have received appropriate dofetilide dosing and treatment initiation education (see Administration and Dosage).

Indications

➤*Conversion of atrial fibrillation/atrial flutter (AF/AFl):* For the conversion of AF/AFl to normal sinus rhythm. Dofetilide has not been shown to be effective in patients with paroxysmal atrial fibrillation.

➤*Maintenance of normal sinus rhythm (delay in AF/AFl recurrence):* For the maintenance of normal sinus rhythm (delay in time to recurrence of AF/AFl) in patients with AF/AFl of > 1 week duration who have been converted to normal sinus rhythm. Reserve dofetilide for patients in whom AF/AFl is highly symptomatic because of life-threatening ventricular arrhythmias.

➤*Unlabeled uses:* Ventricular arrhythmias (inconclusive data).

Administration and Dosage

➤*Approved by the FDA:* October 1, 1999.

Dofetilide is only available to hospitals and prescribers who receive dosing and treatment initiation education through the *Tikosyn* education program. For more information, call 877-TIKOSYN.

➤*Dosage initiation:* Therapy with dofetilide must be initiated (and, if necessary, reinitiated) in a setting that provides continuous ECG monitoring and in the presence of personnel trained in the management of serious ventricular arrhythmias for a minimum of 3 days. Do not discharge patients within 12 hours of electrical or pharmacological conversion to normal sinus rhythm.

Anticoagulate patients with atrial fibrillation according to usual medical practice prior to electrical or pharmacological cardioversion. Anticoagulant therapy may be continued after cardioversion according to usual medical practice for the treatment of people with atrial fibrillation. Correct hypokalemia before initiation of dofetilide therapy.

Step 1, ECG assessment – Prior to administration of the first dose, the QTc must be determined using an average of 5 to 10 beats. If the QTc is > 440 msec (500 msec in patients with ventricular conduction abnormalities), dofetilide is contraindicated. Do not use if heart rate is < 60 bpm. Patients with heart rates < 50 bpm have not been studied.

Step 2, calculation of Ccr – Prior to the administration of the first dose, the patient's Ccr must be calculated using the following formulas:

$$\text{Males:} \quad \frac{\text{Weight (kg)} \times (140 - \text{age})}{72 \times \text{serum creatinine (mg/dL)}} = \text{Ccr}$$

Females: $0.85 \times$ above value

Step 3, starting dose – The starting dose of dofetilide is determined as follows:

Starting Dose of Dofetilide	
Calculated Ccr	Dofetilide dose
> 60 mL/min	500 mcg twice daily
40 to 60 mL/min	250 mcg twice daily
20 to < 40 mL/min	125 mcg twice daily
< 20 mL/min	Dofetilide is contraindicated in these patients

Step 4 – Administer the adjusted dofetilide dose based on Ccr and begin continuous ECG monitoring.

Step 5 – At 2 to 3 hours after administering the first dose of dofetilide, determine the QTc. If the QTc has increased by > 15% compared with the baseline established in Step 1 or if the QTc is > 500 msec (550 msec in patients with ventricular conduction abnormalities), adjust subsequent dosing as follows:

Subsequent Dofetilide Dosing	
If starting dose based on Ccr is:	Then the adjusted dose (for QTc prolongation) is:
500 mcg twice daily	250 mcg twice daily
250 mcg twice daily	125 mcg twice daily
125 mcg twice daily	125 mcg once a day

Step 6 – At 2 to 3 hours after each subsequent dose of dofetilide, determine the QTc (for in-hospital doses 2 to 5). No further down-titration of dofetilide based on QTc is recommended.

Note: Discontinue dofetilide if at any time after the second dose of dofetilide is given, the QTc is > 500 msec (550 msec in patients with ventricular conduction abnormalities).

Step 7 – Patients are to be continuously monitored by ECG for a minimum of 3 days or for a minimum of 12 hours after electrical or pharmacological conversion to normal sinus rhythm, whichever is greater.

In general, antiarrhythmic therapy for AF/AFl aims to prolong the time in normal sinus rhythm. Recurrence is expected in some patients.

➤*Monitoring:* Reevaluate renal function and QTc every 3 months or as medically warranted. Discontinue dofetilide if QTc is > 500 msec (550 msec in patients with ventricular conduction abnormalities), and carefully monitor until QTc returns to baseline levels. If renal function deteriorates, adjust dose as described in Dosage Initiation: Step 3.

➤*Consideration of a lower dose:* The highest dose of 500 mcg twice daily of dofetilide as modified by the dosing initiation led to greater effectiveness than lower doses of 125 or 250 mcg twice daily as modified. However, the risk of torsades de pointes (TdP) is related to dose as well as to patient characteristics. Physicians, in consultation with their patients, may therefore in some cases choose doses lower than determined by the algorithm. It is critically important that if at any time this lower dose is increased, the patient needs to be rehospitalized for

DOFETILIDE

3days. Previous toleration of higher doses does not eliminate the need for rehospitalization.

Maximum dose – The maximum recommended dose in patients with a calculated Ccr > 60 mL/min is 500 mcg twice daily; doses > 500 mcg twice daily have been associated with an increased incidence of torsades de pointes.

➤*Cardioversion:* Do not consider electrical conversion if patients do not convert to normal sinus rhythm within 24 hours of initiation of dofetilide therapy. Monitor patients continuing on dofetilide after successful electrical cardioversion by electrocardiography for 12 hours post cardioversion or a minimum of 3 days after initiation of dofetilide therapy, whichever is greater.

➤*Switching from Class I or other Class III antiarrhythmic therapy:* Withdraw previous antiarrhythmic therapy before initiating dofetilide therapy under careful monitoring for a minimum of 3 plasma half-lives. Do not initiate dofetilide following amiodarone therapy until amiodarone plasma levels are < 0.3 mcg/mL or until amiodarone has been withdrawn for ≥ 3 months.

➤*Storage/Stability:* Protect from moisture and humidity. Dispense in tight containers.

Actions

➤*Pharmacology:* Dofetilide shows Vaughan Williams Class III antiarrhythmic activity. The mechanism of action is blockade of the cardiac ion channel carrying the rapid component of the delayed rectifier potassium currents, I_{Kr}. At concentrations covering several orders of magnitude, dofetilide blocks only I_{Kr} with no relevant block of the other repolarizing potassium currents (eg, I_{Ks}, I_{K1}). At clinically relevant concentrations, dofetilide has no effect on sodium channels (associated with Class I effect), adrenergic alpha-receptors, or adrenergic beta-receptors.

Electrophysiology – Dofetilide increases the monophasic action potential duration in a predictable, concentration-dependent manner, primarily caused by delayed repolarization. This effect, and the related increase in effective refractory period, is observed in the atria and ventricles in both resting and paced electrophysiology studies. The increase in QT interval observed on the surface ECG is a result of prolongation of both effective and functional refractory periods in the His-Purkinje system and the ventricles.

Dofetilide did not influence cardiac conduction velocity and sinus node function in a variety of studies in patients with or without structural heart disease. This is consistent with a lack of effect of dofetilide on the PR interval and QRS width in patients with preexisting heart block or sick sinus syndrome.

Dofetilide terminates induced reentrant tachyarrhythmias (eg, atrial fibrillation/flutter, ventricular tachycardia) and prevents their reinduction. Dofetilide does not increase the electrical energy required to convert electrically induced ventricular fibrillation, and it significantly reduces the defibrillation threshold in patients with ventricular tachycardia and ventricular fibrillation undergoing implantation of a cardioverter-defibrillator device.

Hemodynamics – In hemodynamic studies, dofetilide had no effect on cardiac output, cardiac index, stroke volume index, or systemic vascular resistance in patients with ventricular tachycardia, mild-to-moderate CHF or angina, and either normal or low left ventricular ejection fraction. There was no evidence of a negative inotropic effect related to dofetilide therapy in patients with atrial fibrillation. There was no increase in heart failure in patients with significant left ventricular dysfunction. In the overall clinical program, dofetilide did not affect blood pressure and decreased heart rate by 4 to 6 bpm.

➤*Pharmacokinetics:*

Absorption/Distribution – The oral bioavailability of dofetilide is > 90%, with maximal plasma concentrations occurring at ≈ 2 to 3 hours in the fasted state. Oral bioavailability is unaffected by food or antacids. Steady-state plasma concentrations are attained within 2 to 3 days, with an accumulation index of 1.5 to 2. Plasma concentrations are dose-proportional. Plasma-protein binding of dofetilide is 60% to 70%, is independent of plasma concentration, and is unaffected by renal impairment. Volume of distribution if 3 L/kg.

Metabolism – In vitro studies with human liver microsomes show that dofetilide may be metabolized by CYP3A4, but it has a low affinity for this isoenzyme. Metabolites are formed by N-dealkylation and N-oxidation. There are no quantifiable metabolites circulating in plasma, but 5 metabolites have been identified in the urine.

Excretion – The terminal half-life of dofetilide is ≈ 10 hours. Approximately 80% of a single dose of dofetilide is excreted in the urine, of which ≈ 80% is excreted as unchanged dofetilide with the remaining 20% consisting of inactive or minimally active metabolites. Elimination is by cationic renal secretion. Renal elimination involves glomerular filtration and active tubular secretion.

Special populations –

Renal function impairment: In volunteers with varying degrees of renal impairment and patients with arrhythmias, the clearance of dofetilide decreases with decreasing Ccr. As a result, the half-life of dofetilide is longer in patients with lower Ccr. Because increase in QT

interval and the risk of ventricular arrhythmias are directly related to plasma concentrations of dofetilide, dosage adjustment based on calculated Ccr is critically important (see Administration and Dosage). Patients with severe renal impairment (Ccr < 20 mL/min) were not included in clinical or pharmacokinetic studies (see Contraindications).

Hepatic function impairment: There was no clinically significant alteration in the pharmacokinetics of dofetilide in volunteers with mild-to-moderate hepatic impairment (Child-Pugh Class A and B) compared with age- and weight-matched healthy volunteers. Patients with severe hepatic impairment were not studied.

Gender: A population pharmacokinetic analysis showed that women have ≈ 12% to 18% lower dofetilide oral clearances than men (14% to 22% greater plasma dofetilide levels) after correction for weight and Ccr. In females, as in males, renal function was the single most important factor influencing dofetilide clearance.

Contraindications

Congenital or acquired long QT syndromes; hypersensitivity to the drug; severe renal impairment (calculated Ccr < 20 mL/min); concomitant use of verapamil or the cation transport system inhibitor cimetidine, trimethoprim (alone or in combination with sulfamethoxazole), or ketoconazole. In addition, do not use other known inhibitors of the renal cation transport system such as prochlorperazine and megestrol in patients on dofetilide. Do not use in patients with a baseline QT interval or QTc > 440 msec (500 msec in patients with ventricular conduction abnormalities).

Warnings

➤*Ventricular arrhythmia:* Dofetilide can cause serious ventricular arrhythmias, primarily TdP type ventricular tachycardia, a polymorphic ventricular tachycardia associated with QT interval prolongation.

QT prolongation – QT interval prolongation is directly related to dofetilide plasma concentration. Factors such as reduced Ccr or certain dofetilide drug interactions will increase dofetilide plasma concentration. A linear relationship between mean QTc increase and dofetilide dose has also been demonstrated in patients with renal impairment, ischemic heart disease, and supraventricular and ventricular arrhythmias. The probability of a patient remaining in sinus rhythm at 6 months increased in an approximately linear fashion with an increasing dose of dofetilide.

TdP – The risk of TdP may be reduced by controlling the plasma concentration through adjustment of the initial dofetilide dose according to Ccr and by monitoring the ECG for excessive increases in the QT interval. In the supraventricular arrhythmia population (patients with AF and other supraventricular arrhythmias), the overall incidence of TdP was 0.8%. There were no cases of TdP on placebo (see Adverse Reactions).

Mortality – Because of the small number of events, an excess mortality due to dofetilide cannot be ruled out with confidence in the pooled survival analysis of placebo-controlled trials in patients with supraventricular arrhythmias. However, in 2 large placebo-controlled mortality studies in patients with significant heart disease, there were no more deaths in dofetilide-treated patients than in patients given placebo (see Adverse Reactions).

➤*Gender:* Female patients consituted 32% of the patients in the placebo-controlled trials of dofetilide. As with other drugs that cause TdP, dofetilide was associated with a greater risk of TdP in female patients than in male patients. During the dofetilide clinical development program, the risk of TdP in females was ≈ 3 times the risk in males. Unlike TdP, the incidence of other ventricular arrhythmias was similar in female patients receiving dofetilide and patients receiving placebo. Although no study specifically investigated this risk, in posthoc analyses, no increased mortality was observed in females on dofetilide compared with females on placebo.

➤*Renal function impairment:* The overall systemic clearance of dofetilide is decreased and plasma concentration increased with decreasing Ccr. The dose of dofetilide must be adjusted based on Ccr (see Administration and Dosage). There is no information about the effectiveness of hemodialysis in removing dofetilide from plasma.

➤*Hepatic function impairment:* After adjustment for Ccr, no additional dose adjustment is required for patients with mild or moderate hepatic impairment. Patients with severe hepatic impairment have not been studied; use caution.

➤*Fertility impairment:* Increased incidences of testicular atrophy and epididymal oligospermia and a reduction in testicular weight were observed in rats. Reduced testicular weight and increased incidence of testicular atrophy were also consistent findings in dogs and mice. The no effect doses for these findings in chronic administration studies in these 3 species (3, 0.1, and 6 mg/kg/day) were associated with mean dofetilide AUCs that were ≈ 4, 1.3, and 3 times the maximum likely human AUC, respectively.

➤*Elderly:* Of the total number of patients in clinical studies of dofetilide, 46% were 65 to 89 years of age. No overall differences in safety, effect on QTc, or effectiveness were observed between elderly and younger patients.

➤*Pregnancy:* Category C. Dofetilide adversely affects in utero growth and survival of rats and mice when administered orally during oraganogenesis at doses of ≥ 2 mg/kg/day. Other than an increased inci-

DOFETILIDE

dence of nonossified fifth metacarpal and the occurrence of hydroureter and hydronephroses at doses as low as 1 mg/kg/day in the rat, structural anomalies associated with drug treatment were not observed in either species at doses < 2 mg/kg/day. The clearest drug-effect associations were for sternebral and vertebral anomalies in both species; cleft palate, adactyly, levocardia, dilation of cerebral ventricles, hydroureter, hydronephroses, and unossified metacarpal in the rat; and increased incidence of unossified calcaneum in the mouse. The "no observed adverse effect dose" in both species was 0.5 mg/kg/day. The mean dofetilide AUCs (0 to 24 hours) at this dose in the rat and mouse are estimated to be about equal to the maximum likely human AUC and about half the likely human AUC, respectively.

There are no adequate and well-controlled studies in pregnant women. Therefore, administer dofetilide to pregnant women only when the benefit to the patient justifies the potential risk to the fetus.

▶*Lactation:* There is no information on the presence of dofetilide in breast milk. Advise patients not to breastfeed an infant if they are taking dofetilide.

▶*Children:* The safety and efficacy of dofetilide in children < 18 years of age have not been established.

Precautions

▶*Cardiac conduction disturbances:* Animal and human studies have not shown any adverse effects of dofetilide on conduction velocity. No effect on AV nodal conduction following dofetilide treatment was noted in healthy volunteers and in patients with first degree heart block. Dofetilide has been used safely in conjunction with pacemakers.

▶*Electrolyte disturbances:* Hypokalemia or hypomagnesemia may occur with administration of potassium-depleting diuretics, increasing the potential for TdP. Maintain potassium levels within the normal range prior to administration of dofetilide and in the normal range during administation of dofetilide.

Drug Interactions

▶*Discontinuation prior to administration of potentially interacting drugs:* Allow a washout period of ≥ 2 days if dofetilide needs to be discontinued to allow dosing of potentially interacting drugs.

▶*Drug-drug interactions:* Because there is a linear relationship between dofetilide plasma concentration and QTc, concomitant drugs that interfere with the metabolism or renal elimination of dofetilide may increase the risk of arrhythmia (TdP). Dofetilide is eliminated by cationic renal secretion, and 3 inhibitors of this process have been shown to increase systemic dofetilide exposure. The magnitude of the effect on renal elimination by cimetidine, trimethoprim, and ketoconazole (all contraindicated concomitant uses with dofetilide) suggests that all renal cation transport inhibitors should be contraindicated.

▶*CYP 450:* Dofetilide is metabolized to a small extent by the CYP3A4 isoenzyme of the cytochrome P450 system. Inhibitors of the CYP3A4 isoenzyme may increase systemic dofetilide exposure. Use caution when coadministering inhibitors of this isoenzyme (eg, macrolide antibiotics, azole antifungal agents, protease inhibitors, serotonin reuptake inhibitors, amiodarone, cannabinoids, diltiazem, grapefruit juice, nefazadone, norfloxacin, quinine, zafirlukast) with dofetilide as they can potentially increase dofetilide levels. Dofetilide is not an inhibitor of CYP3A4 nor of other cytochrome P450 isoenzymes and is not expected to increase levels of drugs metabolized by CYP3A4.

Dofetilide Drug Interactions			
Precipitant	Object*		Description
Amiloride Metformin Megestrol Prochlorperazine Triamterene	Dofetilide	↑	Inhibitors of dofetilide elimination of renal cationic secretion are contraindicated. Use caution when coadministering drugs actively secreted via cationic secretion as they might increase dofetilide levels.
Antiarrhythmic agents (Class I or Class III)	Dofetilide	↑	Withhold Class I or Class III antiarrhythmic agents for ≥ 3 plasma half-lives prior to dofetilide dosing.
Bepridil Certain oral macrolides Cisapride Phenothiazines Tricyclic antidepressants	Dofetilide	↑	Administration of drugs that prolong the QT interval have not been studied in conjunction with dofetilide administration and are not recommended for coadministration.
Cimetidine	Dofetilide	↑	Concomitant use of cimetidine is contraindicated. Cimetidine increased dofetilide plasma levels by 58%. Use omeprazole, ranitidine, or antacids as an alternative to cimetidine.
Digoxin	Dofetilide	↔	A higher occurrence of torsades de pointes was associated in patients concomitantly administered digoxin with dofetilide.

Dofetilide Drug Interactions			
Precipitant	Object*		Description
Ketoconazole	Dofetilide	↑	Concomitant use of ketoconazole is contraindicated. Ketoconazole increased dofetilide C_{max} and AUC by 53% and 41% in males and 97% and 69% in females, respectively.
Potassium-depleting diuretics	Dofetilide	↑	Hypokalemia or hypomagnesemia may occur with administration of potassium-depleting diuretics, increasing the potential for torsades de pointes. Potassium levels should be within normal range prior to administration of dofetilide and maintained in the normal range during dofetilide administration.
Trimethoprim Trimethoprim/ sulfamethoxazole	Dofetilide	↑	Concomitant use of trimethoprim alone or in combination with sulfamethoxazole is contraindicated. Coadministration increased dofetilide AUC by 103% and C_{max} by 93%
Verapamil	Dofetilide	↑	Concomitant use of verapamil is contraindicated. Dofetilide peak plasma concentrations increased by 42% when coadministered with verapamil, although overall exposure to dofetilide was not significantly increased. Concomitant administration was associated with a higher occurrence of torsades de pointes.

* ↑ = Object drug increased.   ↔ = Undetermined clinical effect.

▶*Drug/Food interactions:* Grapefruit juice can potentially increase dofetilide levels.

Adverse Reactions

In studies of patients with supraventricular arrhythmias, 8.7% of patients in the dofetilide groups were discontinued from clinical trials because of adverse events compared with 8% in the placebo groups. The most frequent reason for discontinuation (> 1%) was ventricular tachycardia (2% on dofetilide vs 1.3% on placebo). The most frequent adverse events were headache, chest pain, and dizziness.

Dofetilide Adverse Reactions in Patients with Supraventricular Arrythmias (> 2%)		
Adverse reaction	Dofetilide (n = 1346)	Placebo (n = 677)
Headache	11	9
Chest pain	10	7
Dizziness	8	6
Respiratory tract infection	7	5
Dyspnea	6	5
Nausea	5	4
Flu syndrome	4	2
Insomnia	4	3
Accidental injury	3	1
Back pain	3	2
Diarrhea	3	2
Rash	3	2
Abdominal pain	3	2

Adverse events reported at a rate > 2%, but no more frequently on dofetilide than on placebo, were the following: Angina pectoris, anxiety, arthralgia, asthenia, atrial fibrillation, complications (application, injection, incision, insertion, or device), hypertension, pain, palpitation, peripheral edema, supraventricular tachycardia, sweating, urinary tract infection, ventricular tachycardia.

The following adverse events have been reported with a frequency of ≤ 2% and numerically more frequently with dofetilide than placebo in patients with supraventricular arrhythmias: Angioedema, bradycardia, cerebral ischemia, cerebrovascular accident, edema, facial paralysis, flaccid paralysis, heart arrest, increased cough, liver damage, migraine, myocardial infarct, paralysis, paresthesia, sudden death, syncope.

▶*Serious arrhythmias and conduction disturbances:* TdP is the only arrhythmia that showed a dose-response relationship to dofetilide treatment. It did not occur in placebo-treated patients. The incidence of TdP in patients with supraventricular arrhythmias was 0.8% (11/1346). The incidence of TdP in patients who were dosed according to the recommended dosing regimen was 0.8% (4/525).

DOFETILIDE

Incidence of Serious Arrhythmias and Conduction Disturbances in Patients with Supraventricular Arrhythmias Receiving Dofetilide (%)

Arrhythmia event	Dofetilide dose				Placebo
	< 250 mcg BID (n = 217)	250 mcg BID (n = 388)	> 250 to 500 mcg BID (n = 703)	> 500 mcg BID (n = 38)	(n = 677)
Ventricular arrhythmias[1,2]	3.7	2.6	3.4	14.8	2.7
Ventricular fibrillation	0	0.3	0.4	2.6	0.1
Ventricular tachycardia[2]	3.7	2.6	3.3	13.2	2.5
Torsades de pointes	0	0.3	0.9	10.5	0
Various forms of block					
AV block	0.9	1.5	0.4	0	0.3
Bundle branch block	0	0.5	0.1	0	0.1
Heart block	0	0.5	0.1	0	0.1

[1] Patients with > 1 arrhythmia are counted only once in this category.
[2] Ventricular arrhythmias and ventricular tachycardia include all cases of TdP.

A total of 1511 patients were exposed to dofetilide for 1757 patient years. The incidence of TdP was 3.3% in CHF patients and 0.9% in patients with a recent MI.

The rate of TdP was reduced when patients were dosed according to their renal function, as shown in the following table.

Incidence of Torsades de Pointes Before and After Introduction of Dofetilide Dosing According to Renal Function (%)

Population	Total	Before	After
Supraventricular arrhythmias (n = 1346)	0.8	3.1	0.4
Moderate-to-severe CHF (n = 762)	3.3	4.7	2.9
Recent MI (n = 749)	0.9	3	0.6
Atrial fibrillation (n = 249)	1.6	0	1.9

The majority of the episodes of TdP occurred within the first 3 days of dofetilide therapy.

Incidence of Serious Arrhythmias and Conduction Disturbances in Patients with Atrial Fibrillation Receiving Dofetilide (%)

	Dofetilide (n = 249)	Placebo (n = 257)
Ventricular arrhythmias[1,2]	14.5	13.6
Ventricular fibrillation	4.8	3.1
Ventricular tachycardia[2]	12.4	11.3
Torsades de pointes	1.6	0
Various forms of block		
AV block	0.8	2.7
(Left) bundle branch block	0	0.4
Heart block	1.2	0.8

[1] Patients with > 1 arrhythmia are counted only once in this category.
[2] Ventricular arrhythmias and ventricular tachycardia include all cases of TdP.

Mortality – In a pooled survival analysis of patients in the supraventricular arrhythmia population (low prevalence of structural heart disease), deaths occurred in 0.9% of patients receiving dofetilide and 0.4% in the placebo group. Adjusted for duration of therapy, primary diagnosis, age, gender, and prevalence of structural heart disease, the point estimate of the hazard ratio for the pooled studies was 1.1 (95% CI: 0.3, 4.3). The CHF and MI trials examined mortality in patients with structural heart disease (ejection fraction ≤ 35%). In these large, double-blind studies, deaths occurred in 36% of dofetilide patients and 37% of placebo patients. One-year mortality on dofetilide was 31% vs 32% on placebo in an analysis of 506 patients with AF/AFl at baseline.

Overdosage

Dofetilide overdose was rare in clinical studies; there were 2 reported cases of dofetilide overdose in the oral clinical program. One patient received very high multiples of the recommended dose (28 capsules), was treated with gastric aspiration 30 minutes later, and experienced no events. One patient inadvertently received two 500 mcg doses 1 hour apart and experienced ventricular fibrillation and cardiac arrest 2 hours after the second dose.

➤*Symptoms:* The most prominent manifestation of overdosage is likely to be excessive prolongation of the QT interval. In the supraventricular arrhythmia population, only 38 patients received doses > 500 mcg twice daily, all of whom received 750 mcg twice daily regardless of Ccr. In this very small patient population, the incidence of TdP was 10.5% (4/38 patients), and the incidence of new ventricular fibrillation was 2.6% (1/38 patients).

➤*Treatment:* There is no known antidote to dofetilide. Therefore, treatment of overdose is symptomatic and supportive. In cases of overdose, initiate cardiac monitoring. Charcoal slurry may be given soon after overdose but has been useful only when given within 15 minutes of dofetilide administration. Treatment of TdP or overdose may include administration of isoproterenol infusion, with or without cardiac pacing. Administration of IV magnesium sulfate may be effective in the management of TdP. Continue close medical monitoring and supervision until the QT interval returns to normal levels.

Isoproterenol infusion into anesthetized dogs with cardiac pacing rapidly attenuates the dofetilide-induced prolongation of atrial and ventricular effective refractory periods in a dose-dependent manner. Magnesium sulfate, administered prophylactically either IV or orally in a dog model, was effective in the prevention of dofetilide-induced TdP ventricular tachycardia. Similarly, in humans, IV magnesium sulfate may terminate TdP, regardless of cause.

Patient Information

Prior to initiation of dofetilide therapy, advise the patient to read the patient package insert and reread it each time therapy is renewed in case the patient's status has changed. Fully instruct the patient on the need for compliance with the recommended dosing of dofetilide, the potential for drug interactions, and the need for periodic monitoring of QTc and renal function to minimize the risk of serious abnormal rhythms.

Instruct patients to notify their health care providers of any change in OTC, prescription, or supplement use. If a patient is hospitalized or is prescribed a new medication for any condition, the patient must inform the health care provider of ongoing dofetilide therapy.

Instruct patients to immediately report symptoms associated with altered electrolyte balance, such as excessive or prolonged diarrhea, sweating, vomiting, appetite loss, or thirst to their health care provider.

Instruct patients not to double the next dose if a dose is missed. Take the next dose at the usual time.

Indications

Calcium Channel Blocking Agents – Summary of Indications[1]

Indications ✔ = labeled X = unlabeled	Amlodipine	Diltiazem	Diltiazem SR	Diltiazem ER	Diltiazem IV	Felodipine	Isradipine	Nicardipine	Nicardipine SR	Nicardipine IV	Nifedipine	Nifedipine ER	Nimodipine	Nisoldipine	Verapamil	Verapamil SR	Verapamil ER	Verapamil IV
Angina pectoris																		
Vasospastic	✔	✔		✔							✔	✔[2]			✔		✔[3]	
Chronic stable	✔	✔		✔				✔			✔	✔[2]			✔		✔[3]	
Unstable															✔		✔[3]	
Hypertension	✔		✔	✔		✔	✔	✔	✔	✔		✔		✔	✔	✔	✔	
Subarachnoid hemorrhage													✔					
Atrial fibrillation/flutter					✔													✔
Paroxysmal supraventricular tachycardia					✔										✔[4]			✔
Unlabeled uses																		
Prevention of migraine headaches		X													X			
Pulmonary hypertension	X	X			X						X							
Raynaud's phenomenon	X	X			X		X				X							
Preterm labor											X							
Hypertrophic cardiomyopathy															X			

[1] For more detailed information, see the information below and individual drug monographs.
[2] Except *Adalat CC*.
[3] *Covera-HS* only.
[4] For prophylaxis of repetitive paroxysmal supraventricular tachycardia.

➤*Vasospastic (Prinzmetal's or variant) angina (amlodipine, diltiazem immediate-release [IR] and extended-release [ER], nifedipine IR and ER [except Adalat CC], verapamil IR and ER [Covera-HS only]):* Treatment of spontaneous coronary artery spasm presenting as Prinzmetal's variant angina (resting angina with ST segment elevation during attacks).

➤*Chronic stable (classic effort-associated) angina (amlodipine, diltiazem IR and ER, nicardipine, nifedipine IR and ER [except Adalat CC], verapamil IR and ER [Covera-HS only]):* For the treatment of chronic stable angina, alone or in combination with other antianginals.

➤*Unstable angina at rest:* Verapamil IR and ER (*Covera-HS* only).

➤*Hypertension:* Amlodipine, diltiazem sustained-release (SR) and ER, felodipine, isradipine, nicardipine IR and SR, nicardipine IV, nifedipine ER, nisoldipine, and oral verapamil.

➤*Subarachnoid hemorrhage (SAH) (nimodipine only):* For the improvement of neurological outcome by reducing the incidence and severity of ischemic deficits in patients with subarachnoid hemorrhage from ruptured intracranial berry aneurysms regardless of their post-ictus neurological condition (ie, Hunt and Hess Grades I to V).

➤*Paroxysmal supraventricular tachycardias (PSVT) (diltiazem IV and verapamil IV):* Rapid conversion of PSVT to sinus rhythm.

➤*Prophylaxis of repetitive PSVT:* Verapamil IR.

➤*Atrial fibrillation/flutter (diltiazem IV and verapamil IV):* For temporary control of rapid ventricular rate in atrial fibrillation or atrial flutter.

Actions

➤*Pharmacology:* In specialized automatic and conducting cells in the heart, calcium is involved in genesis of action potential. In contractile cells of the myocardium, it links excitation to contraction and controls energy storage and use. Systemic and coronary arteries are influenced by movement of calcium across cell membranes of vascular smooth muscle. Contractile processes of cardiac and vascular smooth muscle depend upon movement of extracellular calcium ions into these cells through specific ion channels.

The calcium channel blockers (ie, slow channel blockers, calcium antagonists), share the ability to inhibit movement of calcium ions across the cell membrane. The effects on the cardiovascular system include depression of mechanical contraction of myocardial and smooth muscle and depression of both impulse formation (automaticity) and conduction velocity. Calcium channel blockers are classified by structure as follows: Diphenylalkylamines – **verapamil**; benzothiazepines – **diltiazem**; dihydropyridines – **amlodipine, felodipine, isradipine, nicardipine, nifedipine, nimodipine, nisoldipine**.

Although these agents are similar in that they all act on the slow (calcium) channel, they have different degrees of selectivity in their effects on vascular smooth muscle, myocardium, or specialized conduction and pacemaker tissues. The resulting clinical effects depend on the direct activity of the drug, reflex physiological responses (primarily β-adrenergic response to vasodilation), and the patient's cardiovascular status.

This heterogeneity of the calcium blockers, in part, determines their clinical application and the different side effects produced by each agent.

In animals, **nimodipine** had a greater effect on cerebral arteries than on other arteries, possibly because it is highly lipophilic. While studies show a favorable effect on severity of neurological deficits caused by cerebral vasospasm following SAH, there is no arteriographic evidence that the drug prevents or relieves spasm of these arteries. Therefore, the actual mechanism of action is unknown.

Hemodynamic – (See Pharmacokinetics table.) These agents dilate the coronary arteries and arterioles in normal and ischemic regions and inhibit coronary artery spasm. This increases myocardial oxygen delivery in patients with coronary artery spasm and vasospastic (Prinzmetal's or variant) angina.

The drugs reduce arterial blood pressure at rest and with exercise by dilating peripheral arterioles and reducing total peripheral resistance (afterload) against which the heart works. This reduces myocardial energy consumption and oxygen requirements and probably accounts for the efficacy in chronic stable angina.

These agents exhibit a negative inotropic effect, but this is rare because of reflex responses to vasodilation. In patients with normal ventricular function, there may be a small increase in cardiac index without major effects on ejection fraction or left ventricular end diastolic pressure or volume (LVEDP or LVEDV). Usual **verapamil** IV doses may slightly increase left ventricular filling pressure. Acute worsening of heart failure may be seen when **verapamil** is used in moderate to severe cardiac dysfunction. In patients with impaired ventricular function, most acute studies have shown some increase in ejection fraction and reduction in left ventricular filling pressure. **Nicardipine** use in coronary artery disease and normal or moderately abnormal left ventricular function significantly increased ejection fraction and cardiac output with no significant change or a small decrease in LVEDP. Administration of a single dose of **nisoldipine** leads to decreased systemic vascular resistance and blood pressure with a transient increase in heart rate.

Electrophysiology – **Verapamil** slows AV conduction and prolongs the effective refractory period (ERP) within the AV node in a rate-related manner, thus reducing ventricular rate because of atrial flutter or atrial fibrillation. By interrupting re-entry at the AV node, verapamil can restore normal sinus rhythm in patients with PSVT, including Wolff-Parkinson-White (W-P-W) syndrome. It can interfere with sinus node impulse generation and induce sinus arrest or sinoatrial block in patients with sick sinus syndrome. AV block can occur in patients without pre-existing conduction defects. Verapamil decreases the frequency of episodes of PSVT. Verapamil may shorten the antegrade ERP of the accessory bypass tracts. It does not alter the normal atrial action potential or intraventricular conduction time, but it depresses amplitude, velocity of depolarization, and conduction in depressed atrial fibers.

Patients with supraventricular tachycardia convert to normal sinus rhythm within 10 minutes after verapamil IV (approximately 60% to 80%). About 70% of patients with atrial flutter or fibrillation with a fast ventricular rate respond with a decrease in heart rate of at least 20%. Conversion of atrial flutter or fibrillation to sinus rhythm is uncommon (about 10%) after verapamil and may reflect the spontaneous conversion rate. Slowing of the ventricular rate in patients with atrial fibrillation/flutter lasts 30 to 60 minutes after a single injection.

Because a small fraction (less than 1%) of patients treated with verapamil have life-threatening adverse responses, the initial use of verapamil injection should, if possible, be in a treatment setting with monitoring and resuscitation facilities, including D.C.-cardioversion capability. As familiarity with the patient's response is gained, use in an office setting may be acceptable.

Diltiazem decreases SA and AV conduction in isolated tissues. Diltiazem IV in doses of 20 mg prolongs AH conduction time and AV node functional and effective refractory periods by approximately 20%. Diltiazem-associated prolongation of the AH interval is not more pronounced in patients with first-degree heart block. In patients with sick sinus syndrome, diltiazem significantly prolongs sinus cycle length (up to 50%).

➤*Pharmacokinetics:*

Calcium Channel Blocking Agents: Pharmacokinetics*

	Parameters	Amlodipine	Diltiazem	Felodipine	Isradipine	Nicardipine	Nifedipine	Nimodipine	Nisoldipine	Verapamil
Pharmacokinetics	Extent of absorption (oral) (%)	nd	nd	≈ 100	90-95	≈ 100	100	nd	nd	> 90
	Absolute bioavailability (oral) (%)	64-90	40	≈ 20	15-24	≈ 35	45-75 (IR) 84-89 (ER)	≈ 13	≈ 5	20-35 (IR)
	Volume of distribution	nd	≈ 305 L (IV)	10 L/kg	3 L/kg	8.3 L/kg (IV)	nd	nd	nd	nd
	T_{max} (h)	6-12	2-4 (IR) 10-14 (ER) 6-11 (SR)	2.5-5	1.5 (IR) 7-18 (CR)	0.5-2 (IR) 1-4 (SR)	0.5 (IR) 6 (ER)	1	6-12	1-2 (IR) ≈ 11 (ER) ≈ 7-9 (SR)
	Protein binding (%)	93	70-80	> 99	95	> 95	92-98	> 95	> 99	≈ 90
	Metabolism	Hepatic	Hepatic	Hepatic	Hepatic	Hepatic	Hepatic	Hepatic	Hepatic	Hepatic
	Major metabolites	90% converted to inactive	Desacetyl-diltiazem[1]	6 inactive	Mono acids and cyclic lactone[2]	nd	Inactive	Numerous, inactive	5 major urinary metabolites	Norverapamil[3]
	Half-life, elimination (h)	30-50	3-4.5 (IR) 4-9.5 (ER) 5-7 (SR) ≈ 3.4 (IV)	11-16	8	2-4	≈ 2 (IR) ≈ 7 (ER)	≈ 8-9[4]	7-12	2.8-7.4[5] 4.5-12[6] ≈ 12 (SR) 2-5 (IV)
	Clearance, systemic	nd	≈ 65 L/h (IV)	≈ 0.8 L/min	1.4 L/min	0.4 L/h•kg (IV)	nd	nd	nd	nd
	Excreted unchanged in urine (%)	10	2-4	±	0	< 1	< 0.1	< 1	trace	3-4
	Excreted in urine (%)	nd	nd	70	60-65	60 (oral) 49 (IV)	60-80	nd	60-80	≈ 70
	Excreted in feces (%)	nd	nd	10	25-30	35 (oral) 43 (IV)	15	nd	nd	≥ 16
ECG Changes	Heart rate	±	0-↓	↑↑	↑	↑↑	0-↑		±	±
	QRS complex	0	nd	0	0	0	nd		0	nd
	PR interval	0	↑	0	0	0	nd		0	↑
	QT interval	0	nd	0	↑	↑	nd		0	nd
Hemodynamics	Myocardial contractility	0-↓	0-↓	0-↓	↓	0-↓	0-↓	na	0-↓	↓↓
	Cardiac output/index	↑	0-↑	nd	↑	↑↑	↑		nd	±
	Peripheral vascular resistance	↓↓	↓↓[7]	↓↓[7]	↓↓	↓↓↓	↓↓↓		↓↓[10]	↓↓

* ↑↑↑ or ↓↓↓ = pronounced effect; ↑↑ or ↓↓ = moderate effect; ↑ or ↓ = slight effect; ± = negligible amount or effect; nd = no data; na = not applicable.
[1] 25% to 50% as potent a coronary vasodilator as diltiazem; plasma levels are 10% to 20% of the parent drug.
[2] Of 6 metabolites identified, accounting for > 75%.
[3] Major metabolite; cardiovascular activity is ≈ 20% that of verapamil.
[4] Earlier elimination rates are much more rapid, equivalent to a half-life of 1 to 2 hours.
[5] After single doses.
[6] After repetitive doses.
[7] Dose-related.

Contraindications

Hypersensitivity to the drug; in patients with known hypersensitivity to dihydropyridine calcium channel blockers (**nisoldipine**); sick sinus syndrome or second- or third-degree AV block except with a functioning pacemaker, hypotension less than 90 mmHg systolic (**diltiazem**, and **verapamil**).

➤*Diltiazem:* Acute MI and pulmonary congestion documented by x-ray on admission.

Injectable –
• Sick sinus syndrome except in the presence of a functioning ventricular pacemaker.
• Second- or third-degree AV block except in the presence of a functioning ventricular pacemaker.
• Severe hypotension or cardiogenic shock.
• Hypersensitivity to the drug.
• IV diltiazem and IV beta-blockers should not be administered together or in close proximity (within a few hours).

• Atrial fibrillation or atrial flutter associated with an accessory bypass tract such as in W-P-W syndrome or short PR syndrome.
• Initial use of injectable forms of diltiazem should be, if possible, in a setting where monitoring and resuscitation capabilities, including DC cardioversion/defibrillation, are present. Once familiarity of the patient's response is established, use in an office setting may be acceptable.
• Ventricular tachycardia.
• In newborns, because of the presence of benzyl alcohol (*Cardizem Lyo-Ject Syringe* only).

➤*Nicardipine:* Advanced aortic stenosis.

➤*Verapamil:* Severe left ventricular dysfunction; cardiogenic shock and severe CHF, unless secondary to a supraventricular tachycardia amenable to verapamil therapy, and in patients with atrial flutter or atrial fibrillation and an accessory bypass tract.

Verapamil IV –
• Severe hypotension or cardiogenic shock.
• Second- or third-degree AV block (except in patients with a functioning artificial ventricular pacemaker).

- Sick sinus syndrome (except in patients with a functioning artificial ventricular pacemaker).
- Severe CHF (unless secondary to a supraventricular tachycardia amenable to verapamil therapy).
- IV β-adrenergic blocking agents. IV verapamil and IV beta-adrenergic blocking drugs should not be administered in close proximity to each other (within a few hours) because both may have a depressant effect on myocardial contractility and AV conduction (see Drug Interactions).
- Patients with atrial flutter or atrial fibrillation and an accessory bypass tract (eg, W-P-W, Lown-Ganong-Levine [L-G-L] syndromes) are at risk to develop ventricular tachyarrhythmia, including ventricular fibrillation if verapamil is administered. Therefore, the use of verapamil in these patients is contraindicated.
- Ventricular tachycardia. Patients with wide-complex ventricular tachycardia (QRS greater than or equal to 0.12 sec) can result in marked hemodynamic deterioration and ventricular fibrillation.
- Known hypersensitivity.

Warnings

➤*Hypotension:* Hypotension, usually modest and well tolerated, occasionally may occur during initial titration or with dosage increases, and may be more common in patients taking concomitant β-blockers. Hypotensive episodes may be caused by excess vasodilation induced by **nifedipine** or by direct cardiodepressor effects of **verapamil** and **diltiazem**. Nifedipine has the greatest effect on vascular smooth muscle; therefore, incidence of adverse reactions resulting from vasodilation (eg, headache, flushing) is greater. Because **amlodipine**-induced hypotension is gradual in onset, acute hypotension rarely has been reported. Nonetheless, exercise caution when administering amlodipine as with any other peripheral vasodilator, particularly in patients with severe aortic stenosis.

Systolic pressure less than 90 mmHg or diastolic pressure less than 60 mmHg was seen in 5% to 10% of patients with supraventricular tachycardia and in about 10% of the patients with atrial flutter/fibrillation who were given IV **verapamil**.

Carefully monitor blood pressure during initial administration and titration. Closely observe patients already taking antihypertensives.

➤*CHF:* CHF has developed rarely, usually in patients receiving a β-blocker, after beginning **nifedipine**. Patients with tight aortic stenosis may be at greater risk, as the unloading effect would be of less benefit to these patients because of their fixed impedance to flow across the aortic valve.

Isradipine – Exercise caution when using isradipine in CHF, particularly in combination with a beta-blocker.

Nisoldipine – Exercise caution when using nisoldipine in patients with heart failure or compromised ventricular function, particularly in combination with a beta-blocker.

Verapamil – Verapamil has a negative inotropic effect that is usually compensated by its afterload reduction (decreased systemic vascular resistance) properties without a net impairment of ventricular performance. In clinical studies with oral **verapamil**, 1.8% developed CHF or pulmonary edema. Avoid verapamil in patients with severe left ventricular dysfunction (ie, ejection fraction less than 30%) or moderate to severe symptoms of cardiac failure and in patients with any degree of ventricular dysfunction if they are receiving a β-adrenergic blocker. Control patients with milder ventricular dysfunction, if possible, with digitalis or diuretics before verapamil treatment.

Use **diltiazem**, **nicardipine**, **nisoldipine**, **felodipine**, and **amlodipine** with caution in CHF patients.

➤*Cardiac conduction:* **Verapamil** IV slows AV nodal conduction and SA nodes; it rarely produces second- or third-degree AV block, bradycardia, and in extreme cases, asystole. This is more likely to occur in patients with sick sinus syndrome (which is more common in older patients). Asystole in patients other than those with sick sinus syndrome is usually of short duration (a few seconds or less), with spontaneous return to AV nodal or normal sinus rhythm.

Oral **verapamil** may lead to first-degree AV block and transient bradycardia, sometimes accompanied by nodal escape rhythms. PR-interval prolongation is correlated with verapamil plasma concentrations especially during the early titration phase of therapy. Higher degrees of AV block are infrequent (0.8%). Marked first-degree block or progressive development to second- or third-degree AV block requires dose reduction or discontinuation of verapamil and institution of appropriate therapy, depending on the clinical situation.

Patients with atrial flutter/fibrillation and an accessory AV pathway may develop increased antegrade conduction, producing a very rapid ventricular response or ventricular fibrillation after receiving IV verapamil (or digitalis). Although a risk of this occurring with oral verapamil has not been established, such patients receiving oral verapamil may be at risk and its use in these patients is contraindicated (see Contraindications). Treatment is usually D.C. cardioversion.

Diltiazem prolongs AV node refractory periods without significantly prolonging sinus node recovery time, except in sick sinus syndrome. This may rarely result in abnormally slow heart rates (particularly in sick sinus syndrome) or second- or third-degree AV block. Concomitant use with β-adrenergic blockers or digitalis may be additive on cardiac conduction. A patient with Prinzmetal's angina developed periods of asystole (2 to 5 seconds) after 60 mg diltiazem. If high-degree AV block occurs in sinus rhythm, discontinue diltiazem IV and institute appropriate supportive measures.

➤*Premature ventricular contractions (PVCs):* During conversion or marked reduction in ventricular rate, benign complexes of unusual appearance (sometimes resembling PVCs) may occur after **verapamil** IV. Similar complexes of no clinical significance occur during spontaneous conversion of supraventricular tachycardia after D.C. cardioversion and other therapy. These complexes appear to have no clinical significance.

➤*Hypertrophic cardiomyopathy:* Serious adverse effects were seen in 120 patients with hypertrophic cardiomyopathy (most refractory or intolerant to propranolol) who received oral **verapamil** at doses up to 720 mg/day. Three patients died with pulmonary edema; all had severe left ventricular outflow obstruction and a history of left ventricular dysfunction. Eight had pulmonary edema or severe hypotension; most had abnormally high (greater than 20 mmHg) pulmonary wedge pressure and a marked left ventricular outflow obstruction. Coadministration of quinidine preceded the severe hypotension in 3 of the 8 patients (2 of whom developed pulmonary edema). Sinus bradycardia occurred in 11%, second-degree AV block in 4% and sinus arrest in 2%. Most adverse effects responded to dose reduction; discontinuation of verapamil was rare.

➤*Antiplatelet effects:* Calcium channel blockers, alone and with aspirin, have caused inhibition of platelet function. Episodes of bruising, petechiae, and bleeding have occurred.

Nifedipine – Decreases platelet aggregation in vitro. Limited clinical studies have demonstrated a moderate but statistically significant decrease in platelet aggregation and increase in bleeding time in some patients. This is thought to be a function of inhibition of calcium transport across the platelet membrane.

➤*Withdrawal syndrome:* Abrupt withdrawal of calcium channel blockers may cause increased frequency and duration of chest pain. The rebound angina is probably the result of the increased flow of calcium into cells causing coronary arteries to spasm. Gradually taper the dose under medical supervision. Results of other studies do not support the occurrence of a withdrawal syndrome; however, caution is still warranted when discontinuing these agents.

➤*β-blocker withdrawal:* Patients recently withdrawn from β-blockers may develop a withdrawal syndrome with increased angina, probably related to increased sensitivity to catecholamines. Initiation of **nifedipine** will not prevent this occurrence and might exacerbate it by provoking reflex catecholamine release. Taper β-blockers rather than stopping them abruptly before beginning nifedipine.

Nicardipine – Gradually reduce β-blocker dose over 8 to 10 days with coadministration.

➤*Hepatic function impairment:* Patients with hepatic impairment (liver cirrhosis) have a longer disposition half-life and higher bioavailability of **nifedipine** than healthy volunteers. Protein binding may be greatly reduced in patients with renal or hepatic impairment.

Because **verapamil** is highly metabolized by the liver, it should be administered cautiously to patients with impaired hepatic function. Severe liver dysfunction prolongs the elimination half-life of verapamil to about 14 to 16 hours; therefore, administer approximately 30% of the dose given to patients with normal liver function to these patients. Carefully monitor for abnormal prolongation of the PR interval or other signs of excessive pharmacologic effects.

Bioavailability of nifedipine is increased in hepatic cirrhosis. With **nifedipine** IV, half-life and volume of distribution are increased and plasma protein binding is decreased. Carefully monitor for abnormal prolongation of the PR interval and other signs of excessive pharmacologic effects.

Because **amlodipine**, **diltiazem**, **nicardipine**, **felodipine**, **nisoldipine**, and **nimodipine** are extensively metabolized by the liver, use with caution in impaired hepatic function or reduced hepatic blood flow. In severe liver disease, elevated nicardipine blood levels (4-fold increase in AUC) and prolonged half-life (19 hours) occurred; patients on nimodipine had an approximately doubled maximum drug concentration. Consider decreasing the dose of calcium channel blockers and monitor drug response (ie, blood pressure, PR interval) in cirrhosis patients.

➤*Renal function impairment:* The pharmacokinetics of **diltiazem** in patients with impaired renal function are similar to the pharmacokinetic profile of patients with normal renal function. However, caution is still advised. About 70% of a dose of **verapamil** is excreted as metabolites in the urine. Administer verapamil cautiously to patients with impaired renal function. Carefully monitor these patients for abnormal prolongation of the PR interval or other signs of overdosage (see Overdosage). Effects of single IV doses should not increase, although duration may be prolonged.

Nicardipine – Mean plasma concentrations, AUC, and maximum concentration were approximately 2-fold higher in patients with mild renal impairment. Doses must be adjusted.

Nifedipine – Although nifedipine has been used safely in patients with renal dysfunction and has exerted a beneficial effect in certain cases, rare, reversible elevations in BUN and serum creatinine have occurred in patients with pre-existing chronic renal insufficiency. The relationship to therapy is uncertain in most cases but probable in some.

➤*Increased angina:* About 7% of patients developed increased frequency, duration or severity of angina on starting **nicardipine** or at the time of dosage increases. Rarely, patients, particularly those who have severe obstructive coronary artery disease have developed increased frequency, duration, or severity of angina or acute MI on starting **nifedipine** or at the time of dosage increase. The mechanism of these effects have not been established.

➤*Increased intracranial pressure:* **Verapamil** IV has increased intracranial pressure in patients with supratentorial tumors at the time of anesthesia induction. Use with caution and perform appropriate monitoring.

➤*Duchenne's muscular dystrophy:* **Verapamil** may decrease neuromuscular transmission in patients with Duchenne's muscular dystrophy, and prolong recovery from the neuromuscular blocking agent vecuronium. It may be necessary to decrease dosage of verapamil when administering it to patients with attenuated neuromuscular transmission. Verapamil IV can precipitate respiratory muscle failure in these patients; therefore, use with caution.

➤*Carcinogenesis:* Rats treated with **nicardipine** showed a dose-dependent increase in thyroid hyperplasia and neoplasia (follicular adenoma carcinoma), possibly linked to a nicardipine-induced reduction in plasma thyroxine levels with a consequent increase in thyroid stimulating hormone (TSH) plasma levels. In rats given **nimodipine**, a higher incidence of adenocarcinoma of the uterus and Leydig-cell adenoma of testes occurred. In rats given **isradipine** or **felodipine**, there were dose-dependent increases in benign Leydig cell tumors and testicular hyperplasia.

➤*Elderly:* Make dose selection for an elderly patient with caution, usually starting at the low end of the dosing range, reflecting the greater frequency of decreased hepatic, renal, or cardiac function and of concomitant disease or other drug therapy.

➤*Pregnancy:* Category C. Teratogenic and embryotoxic effects have been demonstrated in small animals, usually at doses higher than the usual human dosage. There are no well-controlled studies in pregnant women. Use during pregnancy only when clearly needed and when potential benefits outweigh potential hazards to the fetus.

Amlodipine – Significantly decreased litter size (by about 50%) and significantly increased the number of intrauterine deaths (about 5-fold) in rats administered 10 mg/kg amlodipine for 14 days before mating and throughout mating and gestation. Gestation period and duration of labor is also prolonged.

Diltiazem – Doses given at 4 to 10 times the human dose resulted in embryo and fetal death and skeletal abnormalities; incidence of stillbirths was increased at 20 or more times the human dose.

Felodipine – In rabbits, doses 0.8 to 8 times the maximum dosage resulted in digital anomalies (dose-related) in the fetuses, and a prolongation of parturition with difficult labor and increased frequency of fetal and early postnatal deaths occurred in rats. Significant enlargement of the mammary glands also occurred in pregnant rabbits.

Isradipine – There was a significant reduction in maternal weight gain in rats with a dose 150 times the maximum recommended human dose (MRHD). Decrements in maternal body weight gain and increased fetal resorptions occurred in rabbits following doses 2.5, 7.5, and 25 times the MRHD. Also, reduced maternal body weight gain during late pregnancy in rats was associated with reduced birth weights and decreased peri- and postnatal pup survival.

Nicardipine – Nicardipine was embryocidal in animals at 150 mg/kg/day but not 25 to 50 times the human dose. However, dystocia, reduced birth weights, reduced neonatal survival, and reduced neonatal weight gain occurred at 50 times the human dose.

Nifedipine – Nifedipine administration was associated with a variety of embryotoxic, placentotoxic, and fetotoxic effects, including stunted fetuses (rats, mice, rabbits), rib deformities (mice), cleft palate (mice), small placentas, and underdeveloped chorionic villi (monkeys), embryonic and fetal deaths (rats, mice, rabbits), and prolonged pregnancy/decreased neonatal survival (rats; not evaluated on other species). On a mg/kg basis, all of the doses associated with teratogenic, embryotoxic, or fetotoxic effects in animals were higher (3.5 to 42 times) than the MRHD of 120 mg/day. The doses associated with placentotoxic effect in monkeys were equivalent to or lower than the MRHD on a mg/m^2 basis.

Nimodipine – In animals, nimodipine has resulted in malformations and stunted fetuses at doses of 1 and 10 mg/kg/day but not at 3 mg/kg/day in 1 study. Doses of 30 to 100 mg/kg/day resulted in stunted fetuses, still-births, and higher incidences of skeletal variation.

Nisoldipine – Nisoldipine was fetotoxic but not teratogenic in rats and rabbits at doses resulting in maternal toxicity (reduced maternal body weight gain). In pregnant rats, increased fetal resorption (postimplantation loss) was observed at 100 mg/kg/day and decreased fetal weight was observed at both 30 and 100 mg/kg/day. These doses are, respectively, about 5 and 16 times the MRHD when compared on a mg/m^2 basis. In pregnant rabbits, decreased fetal and placental weights were observed at a dose of 30 mg/kg/day, about 10 times the MRHD when compared on a mg/m^2 basis. In a study in which pregnant monkeys (both treated and control) had high rates of abortion and mortality, the only surviving fetus from a group exposed to a maternal dose of 100 mg nisoldipine/kg/day (about 30 times the MRHD when compared on a mg/m^2 basis) presented with forelimb and vertebral abnormalities not previously seen in control monkeys of the same strain.

Verapamil, oral – Oral verapamil in rats with doses 1.5 and 6 times the human dose was embryocidal and retarded fetal growth and development, probably due to reduced weight gains in dams. Verapamil crosses the placenta and can be detected in umbilical vein blood at delivery.

➤*Lactation:* **Verapamil**, **diltiazem**, and **nifedipine** are excreted in breast milk. One report suggests that diltiazem concentrations in breast milk may approximate serum levels. Significant concentrations of **nicardipine** and **nimodipine** appear in maternal milk of rats. It is not known if nimodipine, **isradipine, amlodipine, nisoldipine**, or **felodipine** are excreted in breast milk. Discontinue nursing while taking amlodipine, diltiazem, nicardipine, verapamil, or nimodipine. If using felodipine, isradipine, nifedipine, or nisoldipine, decide whether to discontinue nursing or discontinue the drug, taking into account the importance of the drug to the mother.

➤*Children:* Safety and efficacy of oral **verapamil, diltiazem, felodipine, amlodipine, nicardipine, nifedipine, nisoldipine**, and **isradipine** have not been established. Use of *Procardia* in the pediatric population is not recommended.

Controlled studies of IV **verapamil** have not been conducted in pediatric patients, but uncontrolled experience indicates that results of treatment are similar to those in adults. Patients under 6 months of age may not respond to IV verapamil; this resistance may be related to a developmental difference of AV node responsiveness. However, in rare instances, severe hemodynamic side effects, some of them fatal, have occurred following IV verapamil administration in neonates and infants. Therefore, use caution when administering verapamil to this group of pediatric patients. The most commonly used single doses in patients up to 12 months of age have ranged from 0.1 to 0.2 mg/kg of body weight, while in patients 1 to 15 years of age, the most commonly used single doses ranged from 0.1 to 0.3 mg/kg of body weight. Most of the patients received the lower dose of 0.1 mg/kg once, but in some cases, the dose was repeated once or twice every 10 to 30 minutes.

Precautions

➤*Acute hepatic injury:* In rare instances, symptoms consistent with acute hepatic injury, as well as significant elevations in enzymes such as alkaline phosphatase, CPK, LDH, AST, and ALT have occurred with oral **diltiazem** and **nifedipine**. The potential for acute hepatic injury exists following administration of IV diltiazem. These were reversible on drug discontinuation. Drug relationship was uncertain in most cases, but probable in some. These laboratory abnormalities rarely have been associated with clinical symptoms; however, cholestasis with or without jaundice has occurred with nifedipine. Rare instances of allergic hepatitis also occurred with nifedipine.

Elevations of transaminases with and without concomitant elevations in alkaline phosphatase and bilirubin have occurred with **verapamil**. Elevations sometimes have been transient and may disappear with continued verapamil treatment. Several cases of hepatocellular injury related to verapamil have been proven by rechallenge; half of these cases had clinical symptoms (malaise, fever, or right upper quadrant pain) in addition to elevations of AST, ALT, and alkaline phosphatase. Periodically monitor liver function in patients treated with verapamil.

Isolated cases of elevated LDH, alkaline phosphatase, and ALT levels have occurred rarely with **nimodipine.**

➤*Edema:* Mild to moderate peripheral edema, typically associated with arterial vasodilation and not caused by left ventricular dysfunction, occurs in 10% to about 30% of patients receiving **nifedipine**. It occurs primarily in the lower extremities and usually responds to diuretic therapy. With patients whose angina is complicated by CHF, differentiate this peripheral edema from the effects of increasing left ventricular dysfunction.

Peripheral edema, generally mild and not associated with generalized fluid retention, may occur with **felodipine** within 2 to 3 weeks of therapy initiation. The incidence is both age- and dose-dependent, with frequency ranging from about 10% in patients under 50 years of age taking 5 mg/day to about 30% in patients over 60 years of age taking 20 mg/day.

Drug Interactions

➤*CYP450:* CYP3A4 has a major role in the metabolism of all the calcium channel blockers. Inducers and inhibitors of CYP3A4 can affect the metabolism of the dihydropyridines as well as **verapamil** and **diltiazem**. In general, diltiazem and verapamil inhibit other CYP3A4 substrates (eg, midazolam, carbamazepine), whereas the dihydropyridines do not.

Calcium Channel Blocker Drug Interactions			
Precipitant drug	Object drug*		Description
Amiodarone	Calcium channel blockers–Diltiazem, verapamil	↑	Coadministration may result in cardiotoxicity with bradycardia and decreased cardiac output. Monitor closely.
Azole antifungals	Calcium channel blockers–Nisoldipine	↑	Serum nisoldipine concentrations may be elevated. If coadministration cannot be avoided, observe clinical response, monitor cardiovascular status, and adjust nisoldipine dose accordingly.
Azole antifungals–Itraconazole	Calcium channel blockers–Felodipine, isradipine, nifedipine	↑	Serum concentrations of the calcium channel blocker may be increased. Observe clinical response, monitor cardiovascular status, and adjust calcium channel blocker dose accordingly.
Barbiturates	Calcium channel blockers–Felodipine, nifedipine, verapamil	↓	Pharmacologic effects of the calcium channel blocker may be decreased.
Beta-blockers	Calcium channel blockers	↑	Coadministration may cause additive or synergistic effects. Diltiazem, isradipine, nicardipine, nifedipine, and verapamil may inhibit the metabolism of certain beta-blockers. Monitor cardiac function and adjust dosages as needed.
Calcium channel blockers–Diltiazem, isradipine, nicardipine, nifedipine, verapamil	Beta-blockers		
Calcium salts	Calcium channel blockers–Verapamil	↓	Clinical effects and toxicities of verapamil may be reversed by calcium.
Carbamazepine, Oxcarbazepine	Calcium channel blockers–Felodipine	↓	Pharmacologic effects of felodipine may be decreased. Patients may require higher doses of felodipine.
Cisapride	Calcium channel blockers–Nifedipine	↑	Cisapride may increase nifedipine serum concentrations. Monitor closely and adjust dose of nifedipine as needed.
Cyclosporine	Calcium channel blockers–Nifedipine, felodipine	↑	Pharmacologic and toxic effects of nifedipine or felodipine may be increased. Cyclosporine levels and toxicity may be increased when given concurrently with diltiazem, felodipine, nicardipine, or verapamil. However, verapamil may be nephroprotective when given before cyclosporine. Monitor cyclosporine levels and adjust the dose as needed.
Calcium channel blockers–Diltiazem, felodipine, nicardipine, verapamil	Cyclosporine		
Erythromycin	Calcium channel blockers–Felodipine	↑	Coadministration may increase the effects of felodipine. Monitor cardiovascular status closely and adjust felodipine dose as needed.
H₂ antagonists–Cimetidine, ranitidine	Calcium channel blockers–Diltiazem, felodipine, isradipine, nicardipine, nifedipine, nimodipine, nisoldipine, verapamil	↑	Serum concentrations of the calcium channel blocker may be increased when given concurrently with cimetidine. Ranitidine also has been shown to affect diltiazem concentrations. Monitor cardiovascular status closely. Adjust dose as needed.
Hydantoins (eg, phenytoin)	Calcium channel blockers–Felodipine, nisoldipine, verapamil	↓	The pharmacologic effects of the calcium channel blocker may be decreased. Monitor cardiovascular status closely. Adjust dose as needed.
Melatonin	Calcium channel blockers–Nifedipine	↓	Concurrent use may decrease the antihypertensive effects of nifedipine.
Nafcillin	Calcium channel blockers–Nifedipine	↓	Nafcillin administration results in a large reduction in the plasma concentration of nifedipine; loss of efficacy is likely to result. Nafcillin would be expected to reduce the plasma concentrations of other calcium channel blockers as well. Avoid coadministration.
Quinupristin/Dalfopristin	Calcium channel blockers–Nifedipine	↑	Concurrent use may increase the plasma concentration of nifedipine. The metabolism of other calcium channel blockers would likely be reduced by quinupristin/dalfopristin.
Rifampin	Calcium channel blockers–Diltiazem, isradipine, nicardipine, nifedipine, verapamil	↓	Coadministration may decrease the therapeutic effects of the calcium channel blocker. Monitor cardiovascular status closely. Adjust dose as needed.
St. John's Wort	Calcium channel blockers–Nifedipine	↓	Coadministration may reduce the plasma concentration of nifedipine. The metabolism of other calcium channel blockers would likely be increased by St. John's Wort as well.
Valproic acid	Calcium channel blockers–Nimodipine	↑	Valproic acid increases the AUC of nimodipine with no effect on the elimination half-life. Monitor closely.
Calcium channel blockers	Anesthetics	↑	Calcium channel blockers may potentiate the cardiac effects and vascular dilation associated with anesthetics. Severe hypotension has been reported during fentanyl anesthesia with concomitant use of a beta blocker and a calcium channel blocker. Titrate doses carefully.
Calcium channel blockers–Verapamil	Antiarrhythmic agents–Disopyramide, flecainide	↑	Concomitant use of verapamil and flecainide may have additive effects. Until data on possible interactions between verapamil and disopyramide are obtained, the manufacturer recommends not administering disopyramide within 48 h before or 24 h after verapamil administration.
Calcium channel blockers–Verapamil	Antineoplastics-Doxorubicin	↑	Verapamil appears to increase doxorubicin serum concentrations.
Antineoplastics	Calcium channel blockers–Verapamil	↓	The absorption of verapamil can be reduced by the cyclophosphamide, oncovin, procarbazine, prednisone (COPP) and the vindesine, adriamycin, cisplatin (VAC) drug regimens.
Calcium channel blockers–Diltiazem, verapamil	Benzodiazepines–Midazolam, triazolam	↑	Effects of certain benzodiazepines may be increased.
Calcium channel blockers–Diltiazem, verapamil	Buspirone	↑	Coadministration may increase the effects of buspirone. Monitor closely and adjust buspirone dose as needed.
Calcium channel blockers–Diltiazem, verapamil	Carbamazepine	↑	Serum carbamazepine concentrations may be increased. Monitor serum levels and adjust dosage as necessary.
Calcium channel blockers–Nifedipine	Calcium channel blockers–Diltiazem	↑	Diltiazem increases nifedipine plasma concentrations and nifedipine increases diltiazem plasma concentrations.
Calcium channel blockers–Diltiazem	Calcium channel blockers–Nifedipine		
Calcium channel blockers–Diltiazem, nifedipine, verapamil	Digoxin	↑	Serum digoxin concentrations may be elevated, causing increased toxicity. Coadministration with diltiazem or nifedipine has produced conflicting reports. Monitor digoxin levels and adjust the dose as needed.
Calcium channel blockers–Verapamil	Dofetilide	↑	Concurrent use may increase dofetilide plasma concentration with increased risk of ventricular arrhythmias. Coadministration is contraindicated.
Calcium channel blockers–Verapamil	Ethanol	↑	Verapamil may cause increased and prolonged CNS effects of ethanol.

			Calcium Channel Blocker Drug Interactions		

Precipitant drug	Object drug*		Description
Calcium channel blockers– Diltiazem, verapamil	HMG-CoA reductase inhibitors	↑	Plasma concentrations of certain HMG-CoA reductase inhibitors (eg, atorvastatin) may be elevated. If coadministration cannot be avoided, administer a conservative dose of the HMG-CoA reductase inhibitor.
Calcium channel blockers– Isradipine	Lovastatin	↓	Plasma concentrations of lovastatin may be reduced, decreasing pharmacologic effect. Monitor clinical response and adjust therapy as needed.
Calcium channel blockers– Diltiazem, verapamil	Imipramine	↑	Coadministration increases imipramine serum concentrations.
Calcium channel blockers– Diltiazem, verapamil	Lithium	↑↓	Coadministration with verapamil has caused a reduction in lithium levels and toxicity. Coadministration with diltiazem has caused neurotoxicity.
Calcium channel blockers– Diltiazem	Methylprednisolone	↑	Pharmacologic and toxic effects of methylprednisolone may be increased.
Calcium channel blockers– Diltiazem	Moricizine	↑	Concurrent use may increase moricizine concentrations, while moricizine may decrease diltiazem concentrations.
Moricizine	Calcium channel blockers– Diltiazem	↓	
Calcium channel blockers– Verapamil	Nondepolarizing muscle relaxants	↑	Nondepolarizing muscle relaxant effects may be enhanced. Respiratory depression may be prolonged. Avoid concurrent use if possible.
Calcium channel blockers– Verapamil	Prazosin	↑	Concurrent use may increase serum prazosin concentrations and may increase the sensitivity to prazosin-induced postural hypotension.
Calcium channel blockers– Diltiazem, verapamil	Quinidine	↑	Coadministration may increase the therapeutic and adverse effects of quinidine. Use quinidine with verapamil only when no other alternative exists. Closely monitor quinidine serum levels and cardiac effects. Quinidine decreased the AUC of nisoldipine by 26% but not the peak concentration.
Quinidine	Calcium channel blockers– Nisoldipine	↓	
Calcium channel blockers– Nifedipine	Quinidine	↓	Serum levels and actions of quinidine may be decreased. Serum concentrations and actions of nifedipine may be increased.
Quinidine	Calcium channel blockers– Nifedipine	↑	
Calcium channel blockers– Diltiazem, verapamil	Sirolimus	↑	Coadministration may increase sirolimus plasma concentrations.
Calcium channel blockers– Diltiazem, nifedipine, verapamil	Tacrolimus	↑	Tacrolimus levels may be elevated, increasing toxicity. Monitor serum levels and adjust dosage as needed.
Calcium channel blockers– Diltiazem, verapamil	Theophyllines	↑	Pharmacologic and toxic effects of theophyllines may be increased. Monitor serum levels and adjust dosage as needed.
Calcium channel blockers– Nifedipine	Vincristine	↑	Vincristine levels may be elevated, possibly increasing toxicity.

* ↑ = Object drug increased. ↓ = Object drug decreased.

▶*Drug/Food interactions:* Grapefruit juice may increase the serum concentrations of **felodipine, nicardipine, nifedipine, nisoldipine, verapamil,** and possibly **amlodipine.**

Diltiazem – Administration of certain diltiazem ER products with a high-fat breakfast increased AUC and C_{max}.

Felodipine – When administered with either a high fat or carbohydrate diet, felodipine C_{max} is increased by approximately 60%; AUC is unchanged. Coadministration with grapefruit juice resulted in more than a 2-fold increase in the AUC and C_{max} but no prolongation in the half-life of felodipine.

Isradipine – Administration with food significantly increases isradipine's time to peak by about an hour but has no effect on the AUC. Food has been shown to decrease the extent of bioavailability of isradipine CR by up to 25%.

Nicardipine – When nicardipine was administered 1 or 3 hours after a high-fat meal, the mean C_{max} and AUC were lower (20% to 30%) than when given to fasting subjects. When nicardipine SR was administered with a high-fat breakfast, mean C_{max} was 45% lower, AUC was 25% lower, and trough levels were 75% higher than when given in the fasting state.

Nifedipine – When *Adalat CC* was given immediately after a high-fat meal in healthy volunteers, there was an average increase of 60% in the peak plasma concentration, a prolongation in the time to peak concentration, but no significant change in the AUC. Coadministration of nifedipine with grapefruit juice resulted in up to a 2-fold increase in AUC and C_{max}. Avoid coadministration.

Nimodipine – Nimodipine administration following a standard breakfast resulted in a 68% lower peak plasma concentration and 38% lower bioavailability relative to dosing under fasted conditions.

Nisoldipine – Food with a high-fat content had a pronounced effect on the release of nisoldipine from the coat-core formulation and resulted in a significant increase in C_{max} by up to 300%. However, total exposure was decreased about 25%, presumably because more of the drug was released proximally. Avoid concomitant intake of a high-fat meal with nisoldipine ER. Do not administer nisoldipine with grapefruit juice, as this has been shown to result in a mean increase in C_{max} of about 3-fold (ranging up to 7-fold) and AUC of almost 2-fold (ranging up to 5-fold).

Verapamil – Administration of verapamil SR with food produced decreased AUC but a narrower peak-to-trough ratio.

Adverse Reactions

Calcium Channel Blocker Adverse Reactions (%)[*]

	Adverse Reactions	Amlodipine	Diltiazem Oral (IV)[1]	Felodipine	Isradipine[1]	Nicardipine Oral (IV)[1]	Nifedipine[1]	Nimodipine	Nisoldipine	Verapamil Oral (IV)[1]
Cardiovascular	Angina/Angina pectoris		< 2	0.5-1.5		†	≤ 1			≤ 1
	Angina increased					5.6[2]	≤ 1			
	Arrhythmia	≤ 1	< 2 (1[3])	0.5-1.5			≤ 1			
	Arrhythmia, ventricular		< 1				< 0.5			
	Atrial fibrillation	≤ 1	1.4		≤ 1		< 1		≤ 1	
	AV block (1°, 2°, or 3°)		≤ 7.6 (< 1)			(†)			≤ 1	0.8-1.7
	Bradycardia	≤ 1	≤ 6 (< 1)				< 1	≤ 1		1.4 (1.2)
	Chest pain	≤ 1	< 1	0.5-1.5	≤ 2.7	(0.7)	≤ 3		2	≤ 1
	CHF		< 2 (< 1)					< 1	≤ 1	1.8
	Edema	1.8-14.6[4]	≤ 6 (< 1)		3.5-35.9[2]	0.6-1	10-30[2]	≤ 1.2[2]		1.7-3
	ECG abnormalities		≤ 4.1			0.6 (1.4)		≤ 1.4		2
	Facial edema			0.5-1.5			≤ 1		≤ 1	
	Hypertension		< 1			(0.7)		< 1	≤ 1	1.7
	Hypotension	≤ 1	< 2	0.5-1.5	≤ 1	† (5.6)	< 1	≤ 8.1[2]	≤ 1	0.7-2.5
	Hypotension, postural	≤ 1	< 1			≤ 0.9 (1.4)	< 1		≤ 1	0.4
	Hypotension, symptomatic		(3.2)							(1.5)
	MI		< 1	0.5-1.5	≤ 1				≤ 1	≤ 1
	Palpitations	0.7-4.5[2]	≤ 2	0.4-2.5	1-5.1[2]	2.8-4.1	≤ 7	< 1	3	≤ 1
	Peripheral edema		2-15 (4.3)	2-17.4		(†)	7-29[2]		7-29[2]	3.7
	Sinus bradycardia		< 1							
	Supraventricular tachycardia					(0.7)			≤ 1	
	Syncope	≤ 1	< 2 (< 1)	0.5-1.5	≤ 1	0.8 (0.7)	≤ 1		≤ 1	≤ 1
	Tachycardia	≤ 1	< 2	0.5-1.5	≤ 3.4	0.8-3.4 (3.5)	≤ 1	≤ 1.4		
	Vasculitis	≤ 1								≤ 1
	Vasodilation		≤ 3			4.7-5.5 (0.7)			4	
	Ventricular extrasystoles	≤ 0.1	≤ 2			† (1.4)			≤ 1	
	Ventricular tachycardia	≤ 1	(< 1)			† (0.7)				
CNS	Abnormal dreams	≤ 1	< 2			0.4			≤ 1	
	Amnesia	≤ 0.1	< 2						≤ 1	
	Anxiety/Anxiety disorders	≤ 1		0.5-1.5		†	≤ 1		≤ 1	
	Asthenia	1-2	≤ 4 (< 1)	2.2-3.9		0.9-5.8 (0.7)	≤ 4			2
	Ataxia	≤ 0.1					≤ 1		≤ 1	
	Confusion					† (†)	< 1		≤ 1	≤ 1
	Depression	≤ 1	< 2	0.5-1.5	≤ 1	†	≤ 1	≤ 1.4	≤ 1	(†)
	Dizziness/Lightheadedness	≤ 3.4[2]	≤ 10 (< 1)	2.7-3.7	3.4-8	1.6-6.9 (1.4)	4-27	< 1	3-10[2]	3-4.7 (1.2)
	Drowsiness				≤ 1					
	Equilibrium disturbances						≤ 2			≤ 1
	Fatigue/Lethargy	4.5[2]			≤ 8.5[2]		4-5.9			1.7-4.5
	Headache	7.3	≤ 12 (< 1)	10.6-14.7	10.3-22	6.2-8.2	10-23	≤ 4.1[2]	22	2.2-12.1 (1.2)
	Hypesthesia	≤ 1				(0.7)	≤ 1		≤ 1	
	Insomnia	≤ 1	< 2	0.5-1.5	≤ 1	0.6	< 3		≤ 1	≤ 1
	Malaise	≤ 1	< 1			0.6	≤ 1		≤ 1	
	Migraine	≤ 0.1					≤ 1		≤ 1	
	Nervousness	≤ 1	≤ 2	0.5-1.5	≤ 1	0.6	≤ 7		≤ 1	
	Paresthesia	≤ 1	< 2 (< 1)	1.2-1.6	≤ 1	1 (0.7)	≤ 3		≤ 1	≤ 1
	Shakiness/Jitteriness						≤ 2			≤ 1
	Sleep disturbances						≤ 2			1.4
	Somnolence	1.3-1.6[4]	< 2	0.5-1.5		1.1-1.4	< 3		≤ 1	≤ 1
	Tremor	≤ 1	< 2			0.6	≤ 8		≤ 1	
	Vertigo	≤ 1	< 1			†	≤ 3		≤ 1	(†)
	Weakness				≤ 1.2		10-12			

	Adverse Reactions	Amlodipine	Diltiazem Oral (IV)[1]	Felodipine	Isradipine[1]	Nicardipine Oral (IV)[1]	Nifedipine[1]	Nimodipine	Nisoldipine	Verapamil Oral (IV)[1]
Dermatologic	Acne							≤ 1.4	≤ 1	
	Dermatitis	≤ 0.1	≤ 1				≤ 2			
	Erythema multiforme	≤ 1	< 1							≤ 1
	Hair loss	≤ 0.1	†				≤ 1		≤ 1	≤ 1
	Injection site reactions		(3.9)			(1.4)				
	Leukocytoclastic vasculitis		†	0.5						
	Pruritus	1-2	< 2 (< 1)		≤ 1		< 3	< 1	≤ 1	
	Rash	1-2	≤ 2	0.2-2	≤ 2.6	0.4-1.2	≤ 3	≤ 2.4	≤ 2	≤ 2.4
	Rash maculopapular	≤ 1							≤ 1	
	Stevens-Johnson syndrome		†				< 0.5			≤ 1
	Urticaria	≤ 0.1	< 1	0.5-1.5	≤ 1		≤ 2		≤ 1	≤ 1 (†)
GI	Abdominal discomfort	1.6	1	0.5-1.5	≤ 5.1	(0.7)	< 3			(0.6)
	Abdominal distention		≤ 2		1.2					
	Acid regurgitation			0.5-1.5						
	Anorexia	≤ 1	< 2						≤ 1	
	Appetite increase	≤ 0.1							≤ 1	
	Constipation	≤ 1	≤ 3.6 (< 1)	0.3-1.5	≤ 3.8	0.6	≤ 3.3			3.9-11.7
	Diarrhea	≤ 1	≤ 2	0.5-1.5	≤ 3.4		< 3	≤ 4.2	≤ 1	≤ 2.4
	Dry mouth	≤ 1	< 2 (< 1)	0.5-1.5	≤ 1	0.4-1.4	< 3		≤ 1	≤ 1
	Dysgeusia	≤ 0.1	< 2				≤ 1		≤ 1	
	Dysphagia	≤ 1							≤ 1	
	Dyspepsia	1-2	≤ 6	0.5-3.9		0.8-1.5 (†)	< 3		≤ 1	2.5-2.7
	Flatulence	≤ 1	< 1	0.5-1.5			< 3		≤ 1	
	Gastritis	≤ 0.1							≤ 1	
	GI distress									≤ 1
	GI hemorrhage		< 1				< 1	< 1	≤ 1	
	Gingival hyperplasia	≤ 1	†	< 0.5			≤ 1		≤ 1	≤ 1
	Nausea	2.9[2]	≤ 2.2 (< 1)	1-1.7	1-5.1	1.9-2.2 (4.9)	2-11	0.6-1.4	2	1.7-2.7 (0.9)
	Thirst	≤ 1	< 2							
	Vomiting	≤ 1	≤ 2 (< 1)	0.5-1.5	≤ 1.3	0.4-0.6 (4.9)	≤ 1	< 1		
GU	Decreased libido			0.5-1.5	≤ 1		≤ 1		≤ 1	
	Dysuria	≤ 0.1		0.5-1.5			≤ 1		≤ 1	
	Gynecomastia		< 2	0.5-1.5			< 0.5		≤ 1	
	Hematuria					(0.7)	≤ 1		≤ 1	
	Impotence		≤ 2	0.5-1.5	≤ 1	†	≤ 3		≤ 1	≤ 1
	Nocturia	≤ 1	< 2		≤ 1	0.4	≤ 1		≤ 1	
	Polyuria	≤ 1	< 2	0.5-1.5		(1.4)	< 3			
	Sexual difficulties	≤ 2	< 2				≤ 2			
	Urinary frequency	≤ 1		0.5-1.5	1.3-3.4	≤ 0.6 (†)	≤ 3		≤ 1	≤ 1
Hematologic	Anemia			0.5-1.5			< 0.5	< 1	≤ 1	
	Ecchymosis								≤ 1	≤ 1
	Leukopenia	≤ 1	†		≤ 1		< 0.5		≤ 1	
	Petechiae		< 2						≤ 1	
	Purpura	≤ 1	< 1				≤ 1			≤ 1
	Thrombocytopenia	≤ 1	†			(†)	< 0.5	< 1		
Musculoskeletal	Arthralgia	≤ 1	1.4	0.5-1.5		†	< 3		≤ 1	≤ 1
	Arthritis						< 1		≤ 1	
	Back pain	≤ 1	1.7-2.9	0.5-1.5			≤ 1			
	Hypertonia	≤ 0.1	< 1			(†)	≤ 1		≤ 1	
	Leg cramps				≤ 1		≤ 3		≤ 1	
	Leg pain			0.5-1.5			≤ 3			
	Muscle cramps	1-2	< 2	0.5-1.5			≤ 8	≤ 1.4		≤ 1
	Myalgia	≤ 1	≤ 2.3	0.5-1.5		1	≤ 1		≤ 1	1.1
	Neck pain		< 1			(†)	< 1			
	Rigors	≤ 1					≤ 1			

Calcium Channel Blocker Adverse Reactions (%)[*]

	Adverse Reactions	Amlodipine	Diltiazem Oral (IV)[1]	Felodipine	Isradipine[1]	Nicardipine Oral (IV)[1]	Nifedipine[1]	Nimodipine	Nisoldipine	Verapamil Oral (IV)[1]
Respiratory	Bronchitis		≤ 4	0.5-1.5						
	Cough	≤ 0.1		0.8-1.7	≤ 1		≤ 6			
	Cough increased		1-3				< 1		≤ 1	
	Dyspnea	1-2	≤ 6 (< 1)	0.5-1.5	≤ 3.4	0.6 (0.7)	≤ 6	≤ 1.2	≤ 1	1.4
	Epistaxis	≤ 1	< 2	0.5-1.5			≤ 3		≤ 1	
	Nasal congestion		< 2				≤ 6			
	Pharyngitis		1.4-6	0.5-1.5			< 1		≤ 5	3
	Respiratory disorder		< 1			(†)	≤ 1			
	Respiratory infection			0.5-1.5			≤ 1			
	Rhinitis	≤ 0.1	≤ 9.6			†			≤ 1	2.7
	Sinusitis		2	0.5-1.5		†	≤ 1		≤ 3	3
	Upper respiratory infection			0.7-3.9			≤ 1			5.4
	Wheezing						6	< 1		
Special senses	Abnormal vision	≤ 1				†	≤ 1		≤ 1	
	Amblyopia		(< 1)				< 1		≤ 1	
	Blurred vision		< 1			†	≤ 2			≤ 1
	Conjunctivitis	≤ 1				(†)			≤ 1	
	Tinnitus	≤ 1	< 2			† (†)	≤ 1		≤ 1	≤ 1
Miscellaneous	Accidental injury		≤ 1.3							1.5
	Angioedema	≤ 1		0.5-1.5			≤ 0.5			
	Chills						≤ 2		≤ 1	
	Fever		< 1			(†)	≤ 2		≤ 1	
	Flu-like illness/syndrome/symptoms		≤ 2.3	0.5-1.5					≤ 1	3.7
	Flushing	0.7-4.5[4]	≤ 3 (1.7)	3.9-6.9	1.2-5.1[2]	5.6-9.7	≤ 25	≤ 2.1		0.6-0.8
	Gout		1-2				≤ 1		≤ 1	
	Hot flashes					†	≤ 1			
	Hyperglycemia	≤ 1	< 2							
	Infection		≤ 6			†				12.1
	Pain	≤ 1	≤ 6			0.6	< 3			
	Sore throat					†	6			
	Sweating		< 1 (< 1)			(1.4)	≤ 2	< 1	≤ 1	≤ 1
	Sweating increased	≤ 1				0.6	≤ 1			(†)
	Weight gain	≤ 1	< 2				≤ 1		≤ 1	
	Weight loss						< 1		≤ 1	

[*] Data are pooled from separate studies and are not necessarily comparable.
[1] Includes data for SR/ER form.
[2] Dose-related.
[3] Functional rhythm or isorhythmic dissociation.
[4] Dose-related and higher in females.
†Occurs, no incidence reported.

In addition to the adverse effects listed in the table, the following have been reported:

Amlodipine – Peripheral ischemia, peripheral neuropathy, rash erythematous, pancreatitis, micturition disorder, postural dizziness, depersonalization, allergic reaction, hot flushes, arthrosis, diplopia, eye pain (less than or equal to 1%); cardiac failure, pulse irregularity, skin discoloration/dryness, twitching, cold/clammy skin, apathy, agitation, loose stools, parosmia, muscle weakness, abnormal visual accommodation, xerophthalmia (less than or equal to 0.1%).

Diltiazem – Asymptomatic hypotension (4.3%); bundle branch block, hallucination, personality change, photosensitivity, gait abnormalities, crystalluria, osteoarticular pain, neck rigidity, hyperuricemia, albuminuria (less than 2%); arthrosis (1%); eye irritation, pallor, phlebitis, tooth disorder, eructation, skin hypertrophy (nevus), cystitis, kidney calculus, dysmenorrhea, pyelonephritis, urinary tract infection, eye hemorrhage, ophthalmitis, otitis media, sinus pause, sinus node dysfunction, ventricular fibrillation, kidney failure, respiratory distress, contact dermatitis, stomach ulcers, colitis, neuropathy, myocardial ischemia, vaginitis, prostate disease, bursitis, bone pain, lymphadenopathy, ear pain, bigeminal extrasystole, asystole, atrial flutter (less than 1%).

Felodipine – Sneezing (less than or equal to 1.6%); rhinorrhea (0.2% to 1.6%); premature beats, irritability, erythema, urinary urgency, visual disturbances, influenza, arm/foot/hip/knee pain, contusion (0.5% to 1.5%); warm sensation (less than or equal to 1.5%).

Isradipine – Foot cramps, shortness of breath, ventricular fibrillation, numbness, tingling, transient ischemic attack, stroke, hyperhidrosis, visual disturbance, throat discomfort (less than or equal to 1%).

Nicardipine – Pedal edema (4.4% to 8%); hemopericardium, hypokalemia, intracranial hemorrhage, injection site pain (0.7%); ST segment depression, inverted T wave, deep-vein thrombophlebitis, hypophosphatemia, ear disorder, allergic reaction, peripheral vascular disorder, hyperkinesia, atypical chest pain (rare).

Nifedipine – Giddiness (27%); heat sensation (4% to 25%); muscle tremor (8%); heartburn (11%); mood changes (less than or equal to 7%); transient hypotension (5%); abdominal cramps, joint stiffness; muscle inflammation, chest congestion (less than or equal to 2%); periorbital edema, eructation, GI reflux, melena, abnormal lacrimation, breast pain (less than or equal to 1%); cellulitis, pelvic pain, cardiac arrest, extrasystole, phlebitis, cutaneous angiectases, esophagitis, lymphadenopathy, rales, diplopia, kidney calculus, breast engorgement (less than 1%); erythromelalgia, allergenic hepatitis, arthritis with ANA (+), transient blindness, exfoliative dermatitis, toxic epidermal necrolysis, paranoia, psychiatric disturbances (less than 0.5%). Very rarely, therapy was associated with an increase in anginal pain, possibly caused by associated hypotension. Transient unilateral loss of vision also occurred.

In a subgroup of approximately 250 patients with a diagnosis of CHF as well as angina pectoris (about 10% of the total patient population), dizziness or lightheadedness, peripheral edema, headache, or flushing each occurred in 1 in 8 patients. Hypotension occurred in about 1 in 20 patients. Syncope occurred in approximately 1 patient in 250. MI or symptoms of CHF each occurred in about 1 patient in 15. Atrial or ventricular dysrhythmias each occurred in approximately 1 patient in 150.

Nimodipine – GI symptoms (less than or equal to 2.4%); rebound vasospasm, jaundice, hyponatremia, disseminated intravascular coagulation, deep-vein thrombosis, neurological deterioration, phenytoin toxicity, decreased platelet count, hepatitis, hematoma (less than 1%).

Nisoldipine – Cellulitis, cerebrovascular accident, jugular venous distension, systolic ejection murmur, venous insufficiency, colitis, glossitis, hepatomegaly, melena, mouth ulceration, diabetes mellitus, thyroiditis, hypokalemia, increased serum creatine kinase, increased nonprotein nitrogen, myasthenia, myositis, blepharitis, ear pain, glaucoma, itchy eyes, keratoconjunctivitis, otitis media, retinal detachment, watery eyes, temporary unilateral loss of vision, vitreous floater, increased BUN and serum creatinine, vaginal hemorrhage, vaginitis, tenosynovitis, abnormal thinking, cerebral ischemia, end inspiratory wheeze and fine rales, laryngitis, pleural effusion, dry skin, herpes simplex, herpes zoster, pustular rash, skin discoloration, skin ulcer, fungal dermatitis, exfoliative dermatitis, T wave abnormalities on ECG (flattening, inversion, nonspecific changes), asthma (less than or equal to 1%); chest tightness (rare).

Verapamil – Allergy aggravated (less than or equal to 2%); ankle edema (1.4%); pulmonary edema (1.8%); severe tachycardia (1%); atrioventricular dissociation, claudication, cerebrovascular accident, psychotic symptoms, exanthema, hyperkeratosis, macules, galactorrhea/hyperprolactinemia, spotty menstruation, bruising (less than or equal to 1%); broncho/laryngeal spasm, itch (rare); rotary nystagmus, sleepiness, muscle fatigue, seizures during injection (occasional); respiratory failure (low frequency).

In clinical trials related to the control of ventricular response in digitalized patients who had atrial fibrillation or flutter, ventricular rates below 50 at rest occurred in 15% of patients and asymptomatic hypotension occurred in 5% of patients.

➤*Lab test abnormalities:* Rare, usually transient, but occasionally significant elevations of enzymes such as alkaline phosphatase, CPK, LDH, AST, and ALT have occurred with **diltiazem** and **nifedipine** (see Precautions). **Felodipine** patients experienced an ALT increase of 0.5% to 1.5%. Positive direct Coombs' test with or without hemolytic anemia has occurred with **nifedipine**. Abnormal liver function test (1.2%), isolated cases of decreased platelet counts (0.3%), and elevated nonfasting serum glucose (0.4%), LDH (0.4%), alkaline phosphatase (0.2%), and ALT (0.2%) have occurred rarely with **nimodipine**. Abnormal liver function tests have occurred with **nisoldipine**, elevated liver function tests have occurred with **isradipine**, elevated liver enzymes occurred with **verapamil** (1.4%), and abnormal liver chemistries were reported with **nicardipine**.

➤*Postmarketing experience:*

Amlodipine – Jaundice and hepatic enzyme elevations (mostly consistent with cholestasis or hepatitis), in some cases severe enough to require hospitalization, have been reported in association with use of amlodipine.

Diltiazem – Infrequently reported postmarketing events include the following: Allergic reactions; alopecia; asystole; angioedema; erythema multiforme; Stevens-Johnson syndrome; toxic epidermal necrolysis; extrapyramidal symptoms; gingival hyperplasia; hemolytic anemia; increased bleeding time; leukopenia; purpura; retinopathy; thrombocytopenia; generalized rash; leukocytoclastic vasculitis; exfoliative dermatitis.

Nifedipine – There have been rare reports of the following: Toxic epidermal necrolysis; exfoliative dermatitis; Stevens-Johnson syndrome; and photosensitivity reactions.

Nisoldipine – Systemic hypersensitivity reaction has been reported very rarely, which may include 1 or more of the following: Angioedema, shortness of breath, tachycardia, chest tightness, hypotension, rash.

Overdosage

➤*Symptoms:* Symptoms of overdosage include marked and prolonged hypotension and bradycardia, both of which may result in decreased cardiac output. Junctional rhythms and second- or third-degree AV block may be seen. Death has occurred. Toxic **diltiazem** blood levels in man are not known, but there have been 29 reports of diltiazem overdose in doses ranging from less than 1 to 10.8 g. Sixteen of these reports involved multiple drug ingestions.

Ingestion of 900 mg of **nifedipine** IR and 4800 mg **nifedipine** ER in 2 patients resulted in dizziness, palpitations, flushing, nervousness, loss of consciousness, nausea, vomiting, generalized edema, and profound hypotension. One patient had sinus bradycardia and varying degrees of AV block. Both patients recovered. Significant hyperglycemia was seen initially in the nifedipine IR patient, but plasma glucose levels rapidly normalized without further treatment.

One patient ingested 250 mg **amlodipine** and was asymptomatic. Another patient ingested 120 mg, underwent gastric lavage, and remained normotensive. A third patient took 105 mg and had hypotension (90/50 mmHg), which normalized following plasma expansion. A 19 month old ingested 30 mg (2 mg/kg) and had no evidence of hypotension but had a heart rate of 180 bpm.

➤*Treatment:* If the patient is seen shortly after oral ingestion, employ lavage, activated charcoal, and cathartics. Treatment is supportive. Refer to General Management of Acute Overdosage. Beta-adrenergic agonists and IV calcium have been used effectively. Treat cardiac failure with inotropic agents (isoproterenol, dopamine, or dobutamine) and diuretics. In patients with hypertrophic cardiomyopathy, use α-adrenergic agents (phenylephrine HCl or metaraminol bitartrate) to maintain blood pressure; avoid isoproterenol and norepinephrine. Monitor cardiac and respiratory function; elevate the extremities. Because these agents are highly protein bound, dialysis is not likely to help. Verapamil cannot be removed by hemodialysis.

Calcium Channel Blocker Overdosage: Suggested Treatment of Acute Cardiovascular Adverse Reactions*		
Adverse reaction	Proven effective treatment[1]	Supportive treatment
Symptomatic hypotension requiring treatment	Dopamine Calcium chloride Isoproterenol HCl Metaraminol bitartrate Norepinephrine bitartrate	IV fluids Trendelenburg position
Bradycardia, AV block, h asystole	Atropine Calcium chloride Cardiac pacing Isoproterenol HCl Norepinephrine bitartrate	IV fluids
Rapid ventricular rate (caused by antegrade conduction in flutter/fibrillation with W-P-W or L-G-L syndromes)	D.C. cardioversion Lidocaine Procainamide	IV fluids

* Actual treatment and dosage should depend on the severity of the clinical situation and the judgment and experience of the treating physician.
[1] Drug therapy is administered IV.

Patient Information

Notify physician if any of the following occur: Irregular heart beat, shortness of breath, swelling of the hands and feet, pronounced dizziness, constipation, nausea, or hypotension.

➤*Diltiazem (Dilacor XR):* Swallow whole; do not open, crush, or chew.

➤*Felodipine:* Swallow whole; do not crush or chew.

Mild gingival hyperplasia has occurred; good dental hygiene decreases its incidence and severity.

➤*Isradipine:* Swallow controlled-release tablets whole. Do not chew, divide, or crush. The empty tablet shell is eliminated in the stool.

➤*Nifedipine ER:* Swallow whole; do not chew, divide, or crush. Take *Adalat CC* on an empty stomach. An empty tablet may appear in the stool; this is no cause for concern.

➤*Nisoldipine:* Nisoldipine is an extended-release tablet; swallow whole. Do not chew, divide, or crush the tablet. Do not administer with a high-fat meal. Grapefruit juice, which has been shown to increase significantly the bioavailability of nisoldipine and other dihydropyridine-type calcium channel blockers, should not be taken with nisoldipine.

➤*Verapamil ER / SR:* Do not crush or chew the contents of the pellet-filled capsule. When the sprinkle method of administration is prescribed, explain to patients the details of proper technique. Swallow *Covera-HS* tablets whole; do not break, crush, or chew. The patient should not be concerned if they occasionally observe this outer shell in their stool as it passes from the body.

NISOLDIPINE

Rx	Sular (First Horizon)	Tablets, extended-release: 10 mg	Lactose. (891 ZENECA 10). Oyster. Film-coated. In 100s.
		20 mg	Lactose. (892 ZENECA 20). Yellow cream. Film-coated. In 100s and UD 100s.
		30 mg	Lactose. (893 ZENECA 30). Mustard. Film-coated. In 100s and UD 100s.
		40 mg	Lactose. (894 ZENECA 40). Burnt orange. Film-coated. In 100s.

For complete prescribing information, refer to the Calcium Channel Blockers group monograph.

Indications

➤*Hypertension:* Treatment of hypertension, alone or in combination with other antihypertensive agents.

Administration and Dosage

➤*Approved by the FDA:* February 2, 1995.

Administer orally once daily. Administration with a high-fat meal can lead to excessive peak drug concentration and should be avoided. Avoid grapefruit products before and after dosing. Nisoldipine is an extended-release dosage form; swallow whole, do not bite, divide, or crush.

Adjust the dosage to each patient's needs. Initiate therapy with 20 mg orally once daily, then increase by 10 mg/week, or longer intervals, to attain adequate control of blood pressure. The usual maintenance dosage is 20 to 40 mg once daily. Blood pressure response increases over the 10 to 60 mg daily dose range, but adverse event rates also increase.

NISOLDIPINE

Doses beyond 60 mg once daily are not recommended. Nisoldipine has been used safely with diuretics, ACE inhibitors, and beta-blocking agents.

➤*Elderly/Hepatic function impairment:* Patients over 65 years of age or patients with impaired liver function are expected to develop higher plasma concentrations of nisoldipine. Monitor blood pressure closely during any dosage adjustment. A starting dose not exceeding 10 mg daily is recommended in these patient groups.

➤*Storage/Stability:* Protect from light and moisture. Store at controlled room temperature, 20° to 25°C (68° to 77°F). Dispense in tight, light-resistant containers.

NIFEDIPINE

Rx	**Nifedipine** (Mylan)	**Tablets, extended-release:** 30 mg	In 100s and 300s.
Rx	**Adalat CC** (Bayer)		Lactose. (30 ADALAT CC). Pink. Film-coated. In 100s and UD 100s.
Rx	**Afeditab CR** (Watson)		(ELN 30). Brick red. In 100s.
Rx	**Nifediac CC** (Teva)		(B 30). Mustard yellow. Film coated. In 100s, 300s, and 1000s.
Rx	**Nifedical XL** (Teva)		Lactose. (B 30). Reddish brown. Film-coated. In 100s and 300s.
Rx	**Procardia XL** (Pfizer)		(PROCARDIA XL 30). Rose pink. Film-coated. In 100s, 300s, 5000s, and UD 100s.
Rx	**Nifedipine** (Mylan)	**Tablets, extended-release:** 60 mg	In 100s and 300s.
Rx	**Adalat CC** (Bayer)		Lactose. (60 ADALAT CC). Salmon. Film-coated. In 100s and UD 100s.
Rx	**Afeditab CR** (Watson)		(ELN 60). Brick red. In 100s.
Rx	**Nifediac CC** (Teva)		Lactose. (B 60). Mustard yellow. Film coated. In 100s, 300s, and 1000s.
Rx	**Nifedical XL** (Teva)		Lactose. (B 60). Reddish brown. Film-coated. In 100s and 300s.
Rx	**Procardia XL** (Pfizer)		(PROCARDIA XL 60). Rose pink. Film-coated. In 100s, 300s, 5000s, and UD 100s.
Rx	**Nifedipine** (Mylan)	**Tablets, extended-release:** 90 mg	In 100s.
Rx	**Adalat CC** (Bayer)		Lactose. (90 ADALAT CC). Dark red. Film-coated. In 100s and UD 100s.
Rx	**Nifediac CC** (Teva)		Lactose. (B 90). Yellow. Film coated. In 100s.
Rx	**Procardia XL** (Pfizer)		(PROCARDIA XL 90). Rose pink. Film-coated. In 100s and UD 100s.
Rx	**Nifedipine** (Various, eg, Purepac)	**Capsules:** 10 mg	May be liquid-filled. In 100s and 300s.
Rx	**Adalat** (Bayer)		Saccharin. (Adalat 10). Orange. In 100s, 300s, and UD 100s.
Rx	**Procardia** (Pfizer)		Liquid-filled. Saccharin. (PROCARDIA PFIZER 260). In 100s and 300s.
Rx	**Nifedipine** (Various, eg, Major, Purepac)	**Capsules:** 20 mg	May be liquid-filled. In 100s and 300s.
Rx	**Adalat** (Bayer)		(Adalat 20). Orange/Light brown. In 100s, 300s, and UD 100s.
Rx	**Procardia** (Pfizer)		Liquid-filled. (PROCARDIA 20 PFIZER 261). In 100s.

For complete prescribing information, refer to the Calcium Channel Blockers group monograph.

Indications

➤*Vasospastic angina (except Adalat CC):* For the management of vasospastic angina confirmed by any of the following criteria: 1) Classical pattern of angina at rest accompanied by ST segment elevation; 2) angina or coronary artery spasm provoked by ergonovine; or 3) angiographically demonstrated coronary artery spasm. In patients who have had angiography, the presence of significant fixed obstructive disease is not incompatible with the diagnosis of vasospastic angina, provided that the above criteria are satisfied. Also may be used when clinical presentation suggests a vasospastic component, but where vasospasm has not been confirmed (eg, where pain has a variable threshold on exertion, or in unstable angina where electrocardiographic findings are compatible with intermittent vasospasm, or when angina is refractory to nitrates or adequate doses of beta blockers).

➤*Chronic stable angina (except Adalat CC):* Classic effort-associated angina without vasospasm in patients who remain symptomatic despite adequate doses of beta blockers or organic nitrates or who cannot tolerate those agents.

➤*Hypertension:* Extended-release only. May be used alone or in combination with other antihypertensive agents.

Administration and Dosage

Individualize dosage. Excessive doses can result in hypotension. Avoid coadministration of nifedipine with grapefruit juice.

➤*Capsules:*

Dosage – 10 mg 3 times/day; swallow whole. Usual range is 10 to 20 mg 3 times/day. Some patients, especially those with coronary artery spasm, respond only to higher doses, more frequent administration, or both. In such patients, 20 to 30 mg 3 or 4 times/day may be effective. Doses above 120 mg/day are rarely necessary. More than 180 mg/day is not recommended.

Titrate throughout 7 to 14 days to assess response to each dose level; monitor blood pressure before proceeding to higher doses. If symptoms warrant, titrate more rapidly, but assess frequently based on physical activity level, attack frequency, and sublingual nitroglycerin consumption. Increase dose from 10 to 20 mg 3 times/day, and then 30 mg 3 times/day throughout 3 days.

Hospitalized patients – In hospitalized patients under close observation, the dose may be increased in 10 mg increments throughout 4- to 6-hour periods as required to control pain and arrhythmias caused by ischemia. A single dose should rarely exceed 30 mg.

➤*Tablets, extended-release:* Take care when dispensing nifedipine to assure the extended-release doseform has been prescribed. Swallow whole; do not bite or divide tablet.

Procardia XL and Nifedical XL – 30 or 60 mg once daily. Titrate over a 7- to 14-day period. Titration may proceed more rapidly if the patient is frequently assessed. Titration to doses above 120 mg is not recommended.

Angina patients maintained on the nifedipine capsule formulation may be switched to the extended-release tablet at the nearest equivalent total daily dose. Experience with doses greater than 90 mg in angina is limited; therefore, use with caution and only when clinically warranted.

Adalat CC (hypertension) – Administer once daily on an empty stomach. In general, titrate over a 7- to 14-day period, starting with 30 mg once daily. Base upward titration on therapeutic efficacy and safety. Usual maintenance dose is 30 to 60 mg once daily. Titration to doses above 90 mg/day is not recommended.

➤*Discontinuation:* No "rebound effect" has been observed upon discontinuation of nifedipine. However, if discontinuation of nifedipine is necessary, sound clinical practice suggests the dosage be decreased gradually with close physician supervision.

➤*Concomitant drug therapy:* Concomitant drug therapy with β-blockers may be beneficial in chronic stable angina; however, the effects of concurrent treatment cannot be predicted, especially in patients with compromised left ventricular function or cardiac conduction abnormalities. Closely monitor blood pressure because severe hypotension can occur.

Long-acting nitrates may be safely coadministered but no controlled studies have evaluated the antianginal effectiveness of this combination. Sublingual nitroglycerin may be taken to control acute angina, particularly during nifedipine titration.

➤*Storage/Stability:*

Capsules – Store at controlled room temperature 15° to 25°C (59° to 77°F). Protect from light, moisture, and humidity. Prevent freezing; capsules may be liquid-filled. Replace cap tightly after each opening.

Tablets – Store below 30°C (86°F). Protect from moisture and humidity.

NICARDIPINE HCl

Rx	Nicardipine HCl (Various, eg Mylan)	Capsules: 20 mg	In 90s and 500s.
Rx	Cardene (Roche)		(CARDENE 20 mg ROCHE). White. In 100s and 500s.
Rx	Nicardipine HCl (Various, eg Mylan)	Capsules: 30 mg	In 90s and 500s.
Rx	Cardene (Roche)		(CARDENE 30 mg ROCHE). Lt. blue. In 100s and 500s.
Rx	Cardene SR (Roche)	Capsules, sustained-release: 30 mg	Lactose. (CARDENE SR 30 mg ROCHE). Pink. In 60s and 200s.
		45 mg	Lactose. (CARDENE SR 45 mg ROCHE). Powder blue. In 60s and 200s.
		60 mg	Lactose. (CARDENE SR 60 mg ROCHE). Light blue/white. In 60s.
Rx	Cardene I.V. (ESP Pharma)	Injection: 2.5 mg/mL	48 mg sorbitol. In 10 mL amps.

For complete prescribing information, refer to the Calcium Channel Blockers group monograph.

Indications

➤*Oral:*

Chronic stable (effort-associated) angina (immediate-release only) – Use alone or with beta blockers.

Hypertension (immediate- and sustained-release) – Management of hypertension alone or with other antihypertensives. In administering immediate-release nicardipine, be aware of the relatively large peak to trough differences in blood pressure (BP) effect.

➤*Parenteral:* Short-term treatment of hypertension when oral therapy is not feasible or desirable. For prolonged control of BP, transfer patients to oral medication as soon as possible.

Administration and Dosage

➤*Approved by the FDA:* December 1988.

➤*Oral:*

Angina (immediate-release only) – Individualize dosage. Usual initial dose is 20 mg 3 times/day (range, 20 to 40 mg 3 times/day). Allow at least 3 days before increasing dose to ensure achievement of steady-state plasma drug concentrations.

Hypertension – Individualize dosage.

Immediate-release: Initial dose is 20 mg 3 times daily (range, 20 to 40 mg 3 times daily). The maximum BP-lowering effect occurs approximately 1 to 2 hours after dosing. To assess adequacy of response, measure BP 8 hours after dosing. Because of nicardipine's prominent peak effects, measure BP 1 to 2 hours after dosing, particularly during initiation of therapy. Allow at least 3 days before increasing the dose to ensure achievement of steady-state plasma drug concentrations.

Sustained-release: Initial dose is 30 mg twice daily. Effective doses have ranged from 30 to 60 mg twice daily. The maximum BP-lowering effect at steady state is sustained from 2 to 6 hours after dosing. When initiating therapy or increasing the dose, measure BP 2 to 4 hours after the first dose or dose increase, as well as at the end of a dosing interval.

The total daily dose of immediate-release nicardipine may not be a useful guide in judging the effective dose of the sustained-release form. Titrate patients currently receiving the immediate-release form with the sustained-release form starting at their current total daily dose of immediate-release nicardipine, then re-examine to assess adequacy of BP control.

Concomitant use with other antianginal agents (immediate-release) – Sublingual nitroglycerin may be taken as required to abort acute anginal attacks during therapy. May be safely coadministered with short- and long-acting nitrates and with beta-blockers.

Concomitant use with other antihypertensive agents (immediate- and sustained-release) – May be safely coadministered with thiazide diuretics and beta-blockers.

Renal impairment – Titrate dose beginning with 20 mg 3 times a day (immediate-release) or 30 mg twice daily (sustained-release).

Hepatic impairment – Starting dose is 20 mg twice a day (immediate-release) with individual titration, maintaining the twice a day schedule.

CHF – Caution is advised when titrating dosage in patients with CHF (immediate- and sustained-release).

➤*Parenteral:* Intended for IV use. Individualize dosage based on severity of hypertension and response of patient during dosing. Monitor BP both during and after the infusion; avoid too-rapid or excessive reduction in systolic or diastolic pressure during parenteral treatment.

Dosage –

As a substitute for oral nicardipine: The IV infusion rate required to produce an average plasma concentration equivalent to a given oral dose at steady state is shown in the following table:

Equivalent Nicardipine Doses: Oral vs IV Infusion	
Oral dose	Equivalent IV infusion rate
20 mg q 8 h	0.5 mg/h
30 mg q 8 h	1.2 mg/h
40 mg q 8 h	2.2 mg/h

Initiation in a drug-free patient: The time course of BP decrease is dependent on the initial rate of infusion and the frequency of dosage adjustment. Administer by slow continuous infusion at a concentration of 0.1 mg/mL. With constant infusion, BP begins to fall within minutes. It reaches about 50% of its ultimate decrease in about 45 minutes and does not reach final steady state for about 50 hours.

When treating acute hypertensive episodes in patients with chronic hypertension, discontinuation of infusion is followed by a 50% offset of action in 30 ± 7 minutes but plasma levels of drug and gradually decreasing antihypertensive effects exist for about 50 hours.

• *Titration* – For gradual reduction in BP, initiate therapy at 50 mL/h (5 mg/h). If desired BP reduction is not achieved at this dose, the infusion rate may be increased by 25 mL/h (2.5 mg/h) every 15 minutes up to a maximum of 150 mL/h (15 mg/h) until desired reduction of BP is achieved. For more rapid reduction of BP, initiate at 50 mL/h (5 mg/h). If desired BP reduction is not achieved at this dose, the infusion rate may be increased by 25 mL/h (2.5 mg/h) every 5 minutes up to a maximum of 150 mL/h (15 mg/h) until desired reduction of BP is achieved. Following achievement of the BP goal, decrease the infusion rate to 30 mL/h (3 mg/h).

• *Maintenance* – Adjust rate of infusion to maintain desired response.

Conditions requiring infusion adjustment:

• *Hypotension or tachycardia* – If there is concern of impending hypotension or tachycardia, discontinue the infusion. When BP has stabilized, infusion may be restarted at low doses (eg, 30 to 50 mL/h [3 to 5 mg/h]) and adjusted to maintain desired BP.

• *Infusion site changes* – Continue IV use as long as BP control is needed. Change the infusion site every 12 hours if administered via peripheral vein.

• *Cardiac/Renal/Hepatic function impairment* – Use caution when titrating in patients with CHF or renal or hepatic function impairment.

Transfer to oral antihypertensives: If treatment includes transfer to an oral antihypertensive other than nicardipine, generally initiate therapy upon discontinuation of the infusion. If oral nicardipine is to be used, administer the first dose of a 3 times daily regimen 1 hour prior to discontinuation of the infusion.

Preparation of infusion: Ampules must be diluted before infusion.

• *Dilution* – Administer by slow continuous IV infusion at a concentration of 0.1 mg/mL. Dilute each ampule (25 mg) with 240 mL compatible IV fluid resulting in 250 mL of solution at a concentration of 0.1 mg/mL.

• *Admixture compatibility* – Nicardipine for IV use is compatible and stable in glass or polyvinyl chloride containers for 24 hours at controlled room temperature with the following: Dextrose 5% Injection; Dextrose 5% and Sodium Chloride 0.45% or 0.9% Injection; Dextrose 5% with Potassium 40 mEq; Sodium Chloride 0.45% or 0.9% Injection.

• *Admixture incompatibility* – Nicardipine IV is not compatible with Sodium Bicarbonate 5% Injection or Lactated Ringer's Injection.

➤*Storage/Stability:*

Oral – Store capsules at 15° to 30°C (59° to 86°F) in light-resistant containers.

Parenteral – Store ampules at controlled room temperature, 20° to 25°C (68° to 77°F). Freezing does not adversely affect the product. Avoid exposure to elevated temperature. The diluted solution is stable for 24 hours at room temperature. Protect from light. Store ampule in carton until used.

ISRADIPINE

Rx	DynaCirc CR (Reliant)	Tablets, controlled-release: 5 mg	(DynaCirc CR 5). Lt. pink. Film-coated. In 30s and 100s.
		10 mg	(DynaCirc CR 10). Beige. Film-coated. In 30s and 100s.
Rx	DynaCirc (Reliant)	Capsules: 2.5 mg[1]	Lactose. (DynaCirc 2.5). White. In 60s and 100s.
		5 mg[1]	Lactose. (DynaCirc 5). Lt. pink. In 60s and 100s.

[1] May contain benzyl alcohol and parabens.

For complete prescribing information, refer to the Calcium Channel Blockers group monograph.

Indications

➤*Hypertension:* For the management of hypertension, alone or concurrently with thiazide-type diuretics.

Administration and Dosage

➤*Approved by the FDA:* December 1990.

Individualize dosage.

➤*DynaCirc:* The recommended initial dose is 2.5 mg twice daily alone or in combination with a thiazide diuretic. An antihypertensive response usually occurs within 2 to 3 hours; maximal response may require 2 to 4 weeks. If a satisfactory reduction in blood pressure (BP) does not occur after this period, the dose may be adjusted in increments of 5 mg/day at 2- to 4-week intervals up to a maximum of 20 mg/day. However, most patients show no additional response to doses above 10 mg/day and adverse effects are increased in frequency above 10 mg/day.

➤*DynaCirc CR:* Recommended initial dose is 5 mg once daily alone or in combination with a thiazide diuretic. An antihypertensive response usually occurs within 2 hours with the peak antihypertensive response occurring 8 to 10 hours postdose; BP reduction is maintained for at least 24 hours following drug administration. If necessary, the dose may be adjusted in increments of 5 mg at 2- to 4-week intervals up to a maximum dose of 20 mg/day. Adverse experiences are increased in frequency above 10 mg/day.

Swallow controlled-release tablets whole; do not bite or divide.

➤*Special populations:* The bioavailability of isradipine (increased AUC) is increased in elderly patients (above 65 years of age), patients with hepatic functional impairment, and patients with mild renal impairment. Ordinarily, the starting dose for these patients should be 2.5 mg twice daily (immediate-release) or 5 mg once daily (controlled-release).

➤*Storage/Stability:* Store below 30°C (86°F) in a tight container. Protect from from light, moisture, and humidity.

NIMODIPINE

Rx	Nimotop (Bayer)	Capsules, liquid-filled: 30 mg	(NIMOTOP). Ivory. In UD 30s and 100s.

For complete prescribing information, refer to the Calcium Channel Blockers group monograph.

Indications

➤*Subarachnoid hemorrhage (SAH):* For the improvement of neurological outcome by reducing the incidence and severity of ischemic deficits in patients with SAH from ruptured intracranial berry aneurysms regardless of their postictus neurological condition (ie, Hunt and Hess Grades I to V).

Administration and Dosage

➤*Approved by the FDA:* December 1988.

Commence therapy within 96 hours of the SAH, using 60 mg (two 30 mg capsules) every 4 hours for 21 consecutive days.

If the capsule cannot be swallowed (eg, time of surgery, unconscious patient), make a hole in both ends of the capsule with an 18-gauge needle and extract the contents into a syringe. Empty the contents into the patient's in situ nasogastric tube and wash down the tube with 30 mL normal saline. The contents of the nimodipine capsule must not be administered by IV injection or other parenteral routes.

➤*Hepatic function impairment:* Patients with hepatic cirrhosis have substantially reduced clearance and approximately doubled C_{max}. Reduce dosage to 30 mg every 4 hours with close monitoring of blood pressure and heart rate.

➤*Storage/Stability:* Store in original foil package at 25°C (77°F); excursions permitted to 15° to 30°C (59° to 86°F). Protect from freezing and light.

FELODIPINE

Rx	Plendil (AstraZeneca)	Tablets, extended release: 2.5 mg	Lactose. (PLENDIL 450). Sage green. In 30s, 100s, and UD 100s.
		5 mg	Lactose. (PLENDIL 451). Lt. red-brown. In 30s, 100s, and UD 100s.
		10 mg	Lactose. (PLENDIL 452). Red-brown. In 30s, 100s, and UD 100s.

For complete prescribing information, refer to the Calcium Channel Blockers group monograph.

Indications

➤*Hypertension:* For the treatment of hypertension, alone or concomitantly with other antihypertensives.

Administration and Dosage

➤*Approved by the FDA:* August 1991.

The recommended starting dose is 5 mg once daily. Depending on the patient's response, the dosage can be decreased to 2.5 mg or increased to 10 mg once daily. These adjustments generally should occur at intervals of not less than 2 weeks. The recommended dosage range is 2.5 to 10 mg once daily. In clinical trials, doses above 10 mg daily increased blood pressure (BP) response but a large increase in the rate of periph-

eral edema and other vasodilatory adverse events. Modification of the recommended dosage usually is not required in renal impairment.

Take without food or with a light meal. Swallow whole; do not crush or chew.

➤*Elderly:* Patients over 65 years are likely to develop higher plasma felodipine concentrations. In general, dose selection for an elderly patient should be cautious, usually starting at the low end of the dosing range (2.5 mg daily). Closely monitor BP during dosage adjustment.

➤*Liver function impairment:* Patients with impaired liver function may have elevated plasma drug concentrations and may respond to lower doses; closely monitor BP during dosage adjustment of felodipine.

➤*Storage/Stability:* Store below 30°C (86°F). Keep container tightly closed. Protect from light.

AMLODIPINE

Rx	Norvasc (Pfizer)	Tablets: 2.5 mg	(NORVASC 2.5). White, diamond shape. In 90s and 100s.
Rx	Amvaz (Reddy)		(R 176). Off-white. In 90s and 500s.
Rx	Norvasc (Pfizer)	Tablets: 5 mg	(NORVASC 5). White, elongated octagon. In 90s, 100s, 300s, and UD 100s.
Rx	Amvaz (Reddy)		(R 177). White to off-white. In 90s, 500s, and UD 7s.
Rx	Norvasc (Pfizer)	Tablets: 10 mg	(NORVASC 10). White. In 90s, 100s, and UD 100s.
Rx	Amvaz (Reddy)		(R 178). White to off-white, oval. In 90s, 500s, and UD 7s.

For complete prescribing information, refer to the Calcium Channel Blockers group monograph.

Indications

➤*Hypertension:* For the treatment of hypertension, alone or in combination with other antihypertensives.

➤*Chronic stable angina:* For treatment of chronic stable angina, alone or in combination with other antianginals.

➤*Vasospastic (Prinzmetal's or variant) angina:* Confirmed or suspected vasospastic angina, alone or in combination with other antianginals.

Administration and Dosage

➤*Approved by the FDA:* July 31, 1992.

➤*Hypertension:* Individualize dosage. Usual dose is 5 mg once daily. Maximum dose is 10 mg once daily. Small, fragile, or elderly patients or patients with hepatic insufficiency may be started on 2.5 mg once daily; this dose also may be used when adding amlodipine to other antihypertensive therapy. In general, titrate over 7 to 14 days; proceed more rapidly if clinically warranted with frequent assessment of the patient.

➤*Angina (chronic stable or vasospastic):* 5 to 10 mg, using the lower dose for elderly and patients with hepatic insufficiency. Most patients require 10 mg.

AMLODIPINE

➤*Coadministration with other antihypertensive or antianginal drugs:* Amlodipine has been administered safely with thiazides, ACE inhibitors, beta-blockers, long-acting nitrates, or sublingual nitroglycerin.

➤*Storage/Stability:* Store at controlled room temperature, 15° to 30°C (59° to 86°F). Dispense in tight, light-resistant containers.

DILTIAZEM HCl

Rx	Diltiazem HCl (Various, eg, Mylan, Teva, Watson)	Tablets: 30 mg	May contain lactose or methylparaben. In 100s, 500s, and 1000s.
Rx	Cardizem (Biovail)		Lactose, methylparaben. (MARION 1771). Green. In 100s, 500s and UD 100s.
Rx	Diltiazem HCl (Various, eg, Mylan, Teva, Watson)	Tablets: 60 mg	May contain lactose or methylparaben. In 100s, 500s, and 1000s.
Rx	Cardizem (Biovail)		Lactose, methylparaben. (MARION 17 72). Yellow, scored. In 100s, 500s, and UD 100s.
Rx	Diltiazem HCl (Various, eg, Mylan, Teva, Watson)	Tablets: 90 mg	May contain lactose or methylparaben. In 100s, 500s, and 1000s.
Rx	Cardizem (Biovail)		Lactose, methylparaben. (CARDIZEM 90 mg). Green, scored. In 100s and UD 100s.
Rx	Diltiazem HCl (Various, eg, Mylan, Teva, Watson)	Tablets: 120 mg	May contain lactose or methylparaben. In 100s, 500s, and 1000s.
Rx	Cardizem (Biovail)		Lactose, methylparaben. (CARDIZEM 120 mg). Yellow, scored. In 100s and UD 100s.
Rx	Cardizem LA (Biovail)	Tablets, extended-release: 120 mg	Sucrose. (B 120 mg). White, capsule-shaped. In 7s, 30s, 90s, and 1000s.
		180 mg	Sucrose. (B 180 mg). White, capsule-shaped. In 7s, 30s, 90s, and 1000s.
		240 mg	Sucrose. (B 240 mg). White, capsule-shaped. In 7s, 30s, 90s, and 1000s.
		300 mg	Sucrose. (B 300 mg). White, capsule-shaped. In 7s, 30s, 90s, and 1000s.
		360 mg	Sucrose. (B 360 mg). White, capsule-shaped. In 7s, 30s, 90s, and 1000s.
		420 mg	Sucrose. (B 420 mg). White, capsule-shaped. In 7s, 30s, 90s, and 1000s.
Rx	Diltiazem HCl Extended Release (Various, eg, Mylan, Teva)	Capsules, extended-release:[a] 60 mg	May contain sucrose or sugar spheres. In 100s.
Rx	Diltiazem HCl Extended Release (Various, eg, Mylan, Teva)	Capsules, extended-release:[a] 90 mg	May contain sucrose or sugar spheres. In 100s.
Rx	Diltiazem HCl Extended Release (Various, eg, Apotex Corp., Mylan, Purepac, Teva)	Capsules, extended-release:[a] 120 mg	May contain sucrose or sugar spheres. In 30s, 90s, 100s, 500s, and 1000s.
Rx	Cardizem CD (Biovail)		Sucrose. (cardizem CD 120 mg). Lt. turquoise blue. In 30s, 90s, and UD 100s.
Rx	Cartia XT (Andrx)		Sucrose. (Andrx 597 120 mg). White/Orange. In 30s, 90s, 500s, and 1000s.
Rx	Dilacor XR (Watson)		(A Dilacor XR 120 mg). Pink/Flesh. In 100s and 500s.
Rx	Diltia XT (Andrx)		Lactose. (Andrx 548 120 mg). White. In 100s, 500s, and 1000s.
Rx	Taztia XT (Andrx)		(ANDRX 696 120 mg). Pink. In 30s and 90s.
Rx	Tiazac (Forest)		Sucrose. (Tiazac 120). Lavender. In 7s, 30s, 90s, and 1000s.
Rx	Diltiazem HCl Extended Release (Various, eg, Apotex Corp., Purepac, Teva)	Capsules, extended-release:[a] 180 mg	May contain sucrose or sugar spheres. In 30s, 90s, 100s, 500s, and 1000s.
Rx	Cardizem CD (Biovail)		Sucrose. (cardizem CD 180 mg). Lt. turquoise blue/Blue. In 30s, 90s, and UD 100s.
Rx	Cartia XT (Andrx)		Sucrose. (Andrx 598 180 mg). Yellow/Orange. In 30s, 90s, 500s, and 1000s.
Rx	Dilacor XR (Watson)		(A Dilacor XR 180 mg). Lavender/Flesh. In 100s and 500s.
Rx	Diltia XT (Andrx)		Lactose. (Andrx 549 180 mg). Gray/White. In 100s, 500s, and 1000s.
Rx	Taztia XT (Andrx)		(ANDRX 697 180 mg). Lt. blue/Buff. In 30s and 90s.
Rx	Tiazac (Forest)		Sucrose. (Tiazac 180). White/Blue-green. In 7s, 30s, 90s, and 1000s.
Rx	Diltiazem HCl Extended Release (Various, eg, Apotex Corp., Purepac, Teva)	Capsules, extended-release:[a] 240 mg	May contain sucrose or sugar spheres. In 30s, 90s, 100s, 500s, and 1000s.
Rx	Cardizem CD (Biovail)		Sucrose. (cardizem CD 240 mg). Blue. In 30s, 90s, and UD 100s.
Rx	Cartia XT (Andrx)		Sucrose. (Andrx 599 240 mg). Lt. brown/Orange. In 30s, 90s, 500s, and 1000s.
Rx	Dilacor XR (Watson)		(A Dilacor XR 240 mg). Lt. blue/Flesh. In 100s and 500s.
Rx	Diltia XT (Andrx)		Lactose. (Andrx 550 240 mg). Gray. In 100s, 500s, and 1000s.
Rx	Taztia XT (Andrx)		(ANDRX 698 240 mg). Pink/Lt. blue. In 30s and 90s.
Rx	Tiazac (Forest)		Sucrose. (Tiazac 240). Blue-green/Lavender. In 7s, 30s, 90s, and 1000s.
Rx	Diltiazem HCl Extended Release (Various, eg, Purepac, Teva)	Capsules, extended-release:[a] 300 mg	May contain sucrose or sugar spheres. In 30s, 90s, 500s, and 1000s.
Rx	Cardizem CD (Biovail)		Sucrose. (cardizem CD 300 mg). Lt. gray/Blue. In 30s, 90s, and UD 100s.
Rx	Cartia XT (Andrx)		Sucrose. (Andrx 600 300 mg). Orange. In 30s, 90s, 500s, and 1000s.
Rx	Taztia XT (Andrx)		(ANDRX 699 300 mg). Pink/Buff. In 30s and 90s.
Rx	Tiazac (Forest)		Sucrose. (Tiazac 300). White/Lavender. In 7s, 30s, 90s, and 1000s.
Rx	Diltiazem HCl (Various, eg, Inwood)	Capsules, extended-release:[a] 360 mg	In 90s.
Rx	Cardizem CD (Biovail)		Sucrose. (cardizem CD 360 mg). Lt. blue/White. In 90s.
Rx	Taztia XT (Andrx)		(ANDRX 700 360 mg). Lt. blue. In 30s and 90s.
Rx	Tiazac (Forest)		Sucrose. (Tiazac 360). Blue-green. In 7s, 30s, 90s, and 1000s.

DILTIAZEM HCl

Rx	Tiazac (Forest)	Capsules, extended-release:[a] 420 mg	Sucrose. (Tiazac 420). White. In 7s, 30s, 90s, and 1000s.
Rx	Cardizem SR (Biovail)	Capsules, sustained-release:[a] 60 mg	Sucrose. (CARDIZEM SR 60 mg). Ivory/Brown. In 100s.
		90 mg	Sucrose. (CARDIZEM SR 90 mg). Gold/Brown. In 100s.
		120 mg	Sucrose. (CARDIZEM SR 120 mg). Caramel/Brown. In 100s.
Rx	Diltiazem HCl (Various, eg, Apotex, Baxter, Bedford, Bertek)	Injection: 5 mg/mL	In 5, 10, and 25 mL vials.
Rx	Cardizem (Biovail)		In 5 and 10 mL single-use vials.
Rx	Cardizem (Biovail)	Powder for injection: 25 mg	Single-use containers. Carton of 6 Lyo-Ject syringes with diluent.

[a] Note: The terms "extended-release" and "sustained-release" sometimes are used interchangeably.

For complete prescribing information, refer to the Calcium Channel Blockers group monograph.

Indications

➤*Oral:* Angina pectoris caused by coronary artery spasm.

Chronic stable angina (classic effort-associated angina).

Hypertension (extended- and sustained-release only).

➤*Parenteral:*

Atrial fibrillation or flutter – Temporary control of rapid ventricular rate in atrial fibrillation or atrial flutter. It should not be used in patients with atrial fibrillation or atrial flutter associated with an accessory bypass tract such as in Wolff-Parkinson-White (WPW) syndrome or short PR syndrome.

Paroxysmal supraventricular tachycardia – Rapid conversion of paroxysmal supraventricular tachycardias (PSVT) to sinus rhythm. This includes atrioventricular (AV) nodal re-entrant tachycardias and reciprocating tachycardias associated with an extranodal accessory pathway such as WPW syndrome or short PR syndrome.

Administration and Dosage

➤*Approved by the FDA:* 1982.

➤*Immediate-release tablets:* Individualize dosage. Start with 30 mg 4 times/day before meals and at bedtime; gradually increase dosage (given in divided doses 3 or 4 times/day) at 1- to 2-day intervals until optimum response is obtained. Although individual patients may respond to any dosage level, the average optimum dosage range appears to be 180 to 360 mg/day.

➤*Extended-release tablets:*

Cardizem LA – Intended for once daily administration. Patients treated with diltiazem alone or in combination with other medications may be switched safely to once daily extended-release diltiazem tablets at the nearest equivalent total daily dose. However, subsequent titration to higher or lower doses may be necessary and should be initiated as clinically warranted.

Swallow tablets whole; do not crush or chew. Take tablets at about the same time once every day, either in the morning or at bedtime.

Hypertension: Individualize dosage. When used as monotherapy, starting dose usually is 180 to 240 mg once daily; some patients may respond to lower doses. Maximum antihypertensive effect usually is observed by 14 days of chronic therapy; therefore, schedule dosage adjustments accordingly. May be titrated to a maximum dose of 540 mg daily.

Angina: Individualize dosage. Initial dose of 180 mg may be increased at intervals of 7 to 14 days if adequate response is not obtained. Doses above 360 mg appear not to confer any additional benefit.

➤*Extended-release capsules:* Hypertensive or anginal patients treated with other formulations of diltiazem can be switched safely to extended-release diltiazem at the nearest equivalent total daily dose. However, subsequent titration to higher or lower doses may be necessary and should be initiated as clinically indicated.

Hypertension – Individualize dosage. Start with 60 to 120 mg twice daily or 180 to 240 mg once daily. Maximum antihypertensive effect is usually observed by 14 days of chronic therapy; therefore, schedule dosage adjustments accordingly. Optimum dosage range is 240 to 360 mg/day, but some patients may respond to lower doses. Individual patients may respond to higher doses of up to 480 mg once daily.

Angina – Individualize dosage. Start with 120 or 180 mg once daily. Individual patients may respond to higher doses of up to 480 mg once daily. When necessary, carry titration out over 7 to 14 days.

Cardizem CD and Cartia XT –

Hypertension: 180 to 240 mg once daily; some patients may respond to lower doses. Maximum antihypertensive effect is usually achieved by 14 days of chronic therapy; therefore, adjust dosage accordingly. Usual range is 240 to 360 mg once daily; some patients may respond to higher doses up to 480 mg once daily. Doses up to 540 mg have been studied in clinical trials. The incidence of side effects increases as the dose increases, with first-degree AV block, dizziness, and sinus bradycardia bearing the strongest relationship to dose.

Angina: Start with 120 or 180 mg once daily. Some patients may respond to higher doses of up to 480 mg once daily. When necessary, titration may be carried out over a 7- to 14-day period.

Dilacor XR and Diltia XT –

Hypertension: 180 to 240 mg once daily; adjust dose as needed. Individual patients, particularly those 60 years of age and older, may respond to a lower dose of 120 mg. Usual range is 180 to 480 mg once daily. Although current clinical experience with the 540 mg dose is limited, the dose may be increased to 540 mg with little or no increased risk of adverse reactions. Do not exceed 540 mg once daily. May be used alone or in combination with other antihypertensive medications, such as diuretics.

Angina: Start with a dose of 120 mg once daily. Titrate to doses of up to 480 mg once daily. When necessary, titration may be carried out over a 7- to 14-day period.

Administration: Administration in the morning on an empty stomach is recommended. Do not open, chew, or crush the capsules; swallow whole.

Tiazac –

Hypertension: Usual starting doses are 120 to 240 mg once daily. Maximum antihypertensive effect is usually observed by 14 days of chronic therapy; therefore, schedule dosage adjustments accordingly. The usual dosage range is 120 to 540 mg once daily. Current clinical experience with 540 mg dose is limited. May be used alone or in combination with other antihypertensive medications.

Angina: Start with a dose of 120 to 180 mg once daily. Patients may respond to higher doses of up to 540 mg once daily. When necessary titration should be carried out over 7 to 14 days.

➤*Sustained-release capsules:*

Cardizem SR – Start with 60 to 120 mg twice daily. Adjust dosage when maximum antihypertensive effect is achieved (usually by 14 days of chronic therapy). Optimum dosage range is 240 to 360 mg/day, but some patients may respond to lower doses. May be used alone or in combination with other antihypertensive medications, such as diuretics.

➤*Parenteral:*

Direct IV single injections (bolus) – The initial dose is 0.25 mg/kg as a bolus administered over 2 minutes (20 mg is a reasonable dose for the average patient). If response is inadequate, a second dose may be administered after 15 minutes. The second bolus dose should be 0.35 mg/kg administered over 2 minutes (25 mg is a reasonable dose for the average patient). Individualize subsequent IV bolus doses. Dose patients with low body weights on a mg/kg basis. Some patients may respond to an initial dose of 0.15 mg/kg, although duration of action may be shorter.

Continuous IV infusion – For continued reduction of the heart rate (up to 24 hours) in patients with atrial fibrillation or atrial flutter, an IV infusion may be administered. Immediately following bolus administration of 20 mg (0.25 mg/kg) or 25 mg (0.35 mg/kg) and reduction of heart rate, begin an IV infusion. The recommended initial infusion rate is 10 mg/h. Some patients may maintain response to an initial rate of 5 mg/h. The infusion rate may be increased in 5 mg/h increments up to 15 mg/h as needed, if further reduction in heart rate is required. The infusion may be maintained for up to 24 hours. Therefore, infusion duration longer than 24 hours and infusion rates exceeding 15 mg/h are not recommended.

Dilution – For continuous IV infusion, aseptically transfer the appropriate quantity (see table) to the desired volume of either normal saline, D5W, or D5W/0.45% NaCl. Mix thoroughly. Use within 24 hours. Keep refrigerated until use.

Dilution of Diltiazem Injection or *Cardizem Lyo-Ject*				
Diluent volume (mL)	Quantity of diltiazem injection or *Cardizem Lyo-Ject* to add	Final concentration (mg/mL)	Dose[a] (mg/h)	Infusion rate (mL/h)
100	125 mg (25 mL)	1	10 15	10 15
250	250 mg (50 mL)	0.83	10 15	12 18
500	250 mg (50 mL)	0.45	10 15	22 33

[a] 5 mg/h may be appropriate for some patients.

DILTIAZEM HCl

	Dilution of *Cardizem Monovial*				
Diluent volume (mL)	Quantity of *Cardizem Monovial* to add	Final concentration (mg/mL)	Dose[a] (mg/h)	Infusion rate (mL/h)	
100	100 mg (1 *Monovial*)	1	10 15	10 15	
250	200 mg (2 *Monovials*)	0.8	10 15	12.5 18.8	
500	200 mg (2 *Monovials*)	0.4	10 15	25 37.5	

[a] 5 mg/h may be appropriate for some patients.

Admixture compatibility / incompatibility – Diltiazem is physically compatible and chemically stable in the following parenteral solutions for at least 24 hours when stored in glass or PVC bags at controlled room temperature (15° to 30°C; 59° to 86°F) or refrigerated (2° to 8°C; 36° to 46°F): 5% dextrose injection; 0.9% sodium chloride injection; 5% dextrose and 0.45% sodium chloride injection.

Diltiazem is incompatible when mixed with furosemide solution.

Physical incompatibilities – Because of potential physical incompatibilities, it is recommended that diltiazem injection, *Cardizem Lyo-Ject* syringe, or *Cardizem Monovial* not be mixed with any other drugs in the same container. If possible, it is recommended that diltiazem injection, *Cardizem Lyo-Ject* syringe, or *Cardizem Monovial* not be coinfused in the same IV line.

Diltiazem injection / Cardizem Lyo-Ject syringe: Physical incompatibilities (eg, precipitate formation or cloudiness) were observed when diltiazem injection or *Cardizem Lyo-Ject* syringe was infused in the same IV line with the following drugs: acetazolamide, acyclovir, aminophylline, ampicillin, ampicillin sodium/sulbactam sodium, cefamandole, cefoperazone, diazepam, furosemide, hydrocortisone sodium succinate, insulin (regular, 100 units/mL), methylprednisolone sodium succinate, mezlocillin, nafcillin, phenytoin, rifampin, and sodium bicarbonate. NOTE: *Cardizem Lyo-Ject* syringe was found to be compatible with insulin (regular, 100 units/mL).

Cardizem Monovial: Physical incompatibilities (eg, precipitate formation or cloudiness) were observed when *Cardizem Monovial* at a concentration of 1 mg/mL diluted with normal saline was infused in the same IV line with the following drugs: acetazolamide, acyclovir, cefoperazone sodium, furosemide, phenytoin, and rifampin. NOTE: *Cardizem Monovial* at a concentration of 1 mg/mL diluted in normal saline was infused in the same IV line and was found to be compatible with the following drugs: aminophylline, ampicillin sodium, ampicillin sodium/sulbactam sodium, cefamandole, hydrocortisone sodium succinate, regular insulin (100 units/mL), methylprednisolone sodium succinate, mezlocillin sodium, nafcillin sodium, and sodium bicarbonate.

►*Concomitant therapy:* Concomitant therapy with β-blockers or digitalis is usually well tolerated, but the effects of coadministration cannot be predicted, especially in patients with left ventricular dysfunction or cardiac conduction abnormalities. Use caution in titrating dosages for patients with impaired renal or hepatic function.

Sublingual nitroglycerin may be taken as required to abort acute anginal attacks. Diltiazem may be used safely with short-acting and long-acting nitrates, but no controlled studies have evaluated the antianginal efficacy of this combination.

An additive antihypertensive effect occurs when diltiazem is coadministered with other antihypertensives. Adjust the dose of diltiazem or the concomitant antihypertensive accordingly.

►*Storage / Stability:*
Oral –
Cardizem CD and Cardizem LA: Store at 25°C (77°F); excursions permitted to 15° to 30°C (59° to 86°F). Avoid excessive humidity.
Tiazac: Store at controlled room temperature 20° to 25°C (68° to 77°F). Avoid excessive humidity.
Other oral doseforms: Store at controlled room temperature 15° to 30°C (59° to 86°F). Protect from light. Dispense in tight, light-resistant containers using a child-resistant closure. Avoid excessive humidity.

Parenteral –
Diltiazem injection: Store injection under refrigeration at 2° to 8°C (36° to 46°F). Do not freeze. May be stored at room temperature for up to 1 month; destroy after 1 month at room temperature. Discard unused portion of single-use containers.
Cardizem Lyo-Ject and Cardizem Monovial: Store at room temperature 15° to 30°C (59° to 86°F). Do not freeze. Reconstituted material is stable for 24 hours at controlled room temperature. Discard unused portion (*Cardizem Lyo-Ject* only).

VERAPAMIL HCl

Rx	**Verapamil HCl** (Various, eg, Geneva, Major, Watson)	**Tablets:** 40 mg	May contain lactose. In 30s, 100s, 500s, and 1000s.
Rx	**Calan** (Searle)		Lactose. (CALAN 40). Pink. Film-coated. In 100s.
Rx	**Verapamil HCl** (Various, eg, Geneva, Ivax, Major, Mylan, Watson)	**Tablets:** 80 mg	May contain lactose. In 100s, 250s, 500s, 1000s, 7000s, and UD 100s.
Rx	**Calan** (Searle)		Lactose. (CALAN 80). Peach, oval, scored. Film-coated. In 100s, 500s, and 1000s.
Rx	**Verapamil HCl** (Various, eg, Geneva, Ivax, Major, Mylan, Watson)	**Tablets:** 120 mg	May contain lactose. In 100s, 250s, 500s, 1000s, 4000s, and UD 100s.
Rx	**Calan** (Searle)		Lactose. (CALAN 120). Brown, oval, scored. Film-coated. In 100s and 1000s.
Rx	**Verapamil HCl Extended Release** (Various, eg, Ivax, Mylan)	**Tablets, extended-release:**[1] 120 mg	In 100s.
Rx	**Verapamil HCl Extended Release** (Various, eg, Ivax, Mylan)	**Tablets, extended-release:**[1] 180 mg	In 100s and 500s.
Rx	**Covera-HS** (Searle)		(COVERA-HS 2011). Lavender. Film-coated. In 100s and UD 100s.
Rx	**Verapamil HCl Extended Release** (Various, eg, Ivax, Mylan)	**Tablets, extended-release:**[1] 240 mg	In 100s and 500s.
Rx	**Covera-HS** (Searle)		(COVERA-HS 2021). Pale yellow. Film-coated. In 100s and UD 100s.
Rx	**Calan SR** (Searle)	**Tablets, sustained-release:**[1] 120 mg	(CALAN SR 120). Lt. violet, oval. Film-coated. In 100s and UD 100s.
Rx	**Isoptin SR** (Abbott)		(KNOLL 120 SR). Lt. violet, oval. Film-coated. In 100s.
Rx	**Calan SR** (Searle)	**Tablets, sustained-release:**[1] 180 mg	(CALAN SR 180). Lt. pink, oval, scored. Film-coated. In 100s and UD 100s.
Rx	**Isoptin SR** (Abbott)		(ISOPTIN SR 180 MG). Lt. pink, oval, scored. Film-coated. In 100s.
Rx	**Calan SR** (Searle)	**Tablets, sustained-release:**[1] 240 mg	(CALAN SR 240). Lt. green, capsule shape, scored. Film-coated. In 100s, 500s, and UD 100s.
Rx	**Isoptin SR** (Abbott)		(ISOPTIN SR). Lt. green, capsule shape, scored. Film-coated. In 100s and 500s.
Rx	**Verapamil HCl Extended Release** (Various, eg, Mylan, Teva, UDL)	**Capsules, extended-release:**[1] 120 mg	May be pellet-filled. May contain sugar. In 100s, 500s, and UD 100s.
		180 mg	May be pellet-filled. May contain sugar. In 100s, 500s, and UD 100s.
		240 mg	May be pellet-filled. May contain sugar. In 100s, 500s, and UD 80s.
Rx	**Verelan PM** (Schwarz Pharma)	**Capsules, extended-release:**[1] 100 mg	Sugar. (SCHWARZ 4085/100 mg). White/Amethyst. In 100s.
		200 mg	Sugar. (SCHWARz 4086 200 mg). Amethyst. In 100s.
		300 mg	Sugar. (SCHWARz 4087 300 mg). Lavender/Amethyst. In 100s.

VERAPAMIL HCl

Rx	Verelan (Schwarz Pharma)	Capsules, sustained-release:[1] 120 mg	Pellet-filled. Sugar, parabens. (SCHWARZ 2490 VERELAN 120 mg). Yellow. In 100s.
		180 mg	Pellet-filled. Sugar, parabens. (SCHWARZ 2489 VERELAN 180 mg). Lt. gray/yellow. In 100s.
		240 mg	Pellet-filled. Sugar, parabens. (SCHWARz 2491 VERELAN 240 mg). Dk. blue/yellow. In 100s.
		360 mg	Pellet-filled. Sugar, parabens. (SCHWARz 2495 VERELAN 360 mg). Lavender/Yellow. In 100s.
Rx	Verapamil HCl (Various, eg, Abbott, American Regent)	Injection: 2.5 mg/mL	May contain sodium chloride. In 2 and 4 mL vials, amps, and syringes. Also in 2 mL fill in single-use, 2 mL *Carpuject* syringe; and 2 mL fill in single-use 2 mL *Carpuject Interlink* syringe.

[1] Note: The terms "extended-release" and "sustained-release" sometimes are used interchangeably.

For complete prescribing information, refer to the Calcium Channel Blockers group monograph.

Indications

➤*Oral:*

Immediate-release:

Angina: Treatment of vasospastic (Prinzmetal's variant), chronic stable (classic effort-associated) and unstable (crescendo, preinfarction) angina.

Arrhythmias: With digitalis to control ventricular rate at rest and during stress in chronic atrial flutter or fibrillation. May use for prophylaxis of repetitive paroxysmal supraventricular tachycardia (PSVT).

Hypertension: Treatment of essential hypertension.

Sustained-release/Extended-release – For management of hypertension and angina (*Covera-HS* only).

➤*Parenteral:*

Supraventricular tachycardias – Rapid conversion to sinus rhythm of PSVTs, including those associated with accessory bypass tracts (Wolff-Parkinson-White [W-P-W] and Lown-Ganong-Levine [L-G-L] syndromes). When clinically advisable, attempt appropriate vagal maneuvers (eg, Valsalva maneuver) prior to verapamil administration.

Atrial flutter or fibrillation – Temporary control of rapid ventricular rate in atrial flutter or atrial fibrillation except when the atrial flutter and/or atrial fibrillation are associated with accessory bypass tracts (W-P-W and LGL syndromes).

Administration and Dosage

Avoid verapamil in patients with severe left ventricular dysfunction (eg, ejection fractions less than 30%) or moderate to severe symptoms of cardiac failure and in patients with any degree of ventricular dysfunction if they are receiving a beta-adrenergic blocker. If possible, control patients with milder ventricular dysfunction with optimum doses of digitalis or diuretics before verapamil treatment.

Individualize dosage. Do not exceed 480 mg/day; safety and efficacy are not established. Half-life increases during chronic use; maximum response may be delayed.

➤*Immediate-release:*

Angina – Usual dose is 80 to 120 mg 3 times/day. However, 40 mg 3 times a day may be warranted in patients who have increased response to verapamil (eg, decreased hepatic function, elderly). Base upward titration on safety and efficacy evaluated approximately 8 hours after dosing. Dosage may be increased daily (eg, unstable angina) or weekly until optimum clinical response is obtained.

Arrhythmias – Dosage range in digitalized patients with chronic atrial fibrillation is 240 to 320 mg/day in divided doses 3 or 4 times/day. Dosage range for prophylaxis of PSVT (nondigitalized patients) is 240 to 480 mg/day in divided doses 3 or 4 times/day. Maximum effects will be apparent during the first 48 hours of therapy.

Hypertension – The usual initial monotherapy dose is 80 mg 3 times/day (240 mg/day). Daily dosages of 360 and 480 mg have been used, but there is no evidence that dosages beyond 360 mg provide added effect. Consider beginning titration at 40 mg 3 times/day in patients who might respond to lower doses (eg, elderly people or those of small stature). Antihypertensive effects are evident within the first week of therapy. Base upward titration on therapeutic efficacy, assessed at the end of the dosing interval.

➤*Extended-release:* Individualize the dose by titration. When administered at bedtime, office evaluation of blood pressure (BP) during morning and early afternoon hours is essentially a measure of peak effect. The usual evaluation of trough effect, which sometimes might be needed to evaluate the appropriateness of any given dose, would be just prior to bedtime. Swallow whole; do not chew, break, or crush the tablets.

Capsules – The usual daily dose is 240 mg once daily in the morning. However, initial doses of 120 mg/day may be warranted in patients who may have an increased response to verapamil (eg, elderly people, those of small stature). Base upward titration on therapeutic efficacy and safety evaluated approximately 24 hours after dosing. The antihypertensive effects of extended-release verapamil are evident within the first week of therapy.

If adequate response is not obtained with 120 mg verapamil, the dose may be titrated upward in the following manner:
   180 mg in the morning,
   240 mg in the morning,
   360 mg in the morning,
   480 mg in the morning.

Tablets – Initiate therapy with 180 mg given in the morning. Lower initial doses of 120 mg/day may be warranted in patients who may have an increased response to verapamil (eg, elderly people or those of small stature). Base upward titration on therapeutic efficacy and safety evaluated weekly and approximately 24 hours after the previous dose. The antihypertensive effects of extended-release verapamil tablets are evident within the first week of therapy.

If adequate response is not obtained with 180 mg verapamil extended-release tablets, the dose may be titrated upward in the following manner:
   240 mg each morning,
   180 mg each morning plus 180 mg each evening; or 240 mg each morning plus 120 mg each evening,
   240 mg every 12 hours.

Covera-HS tablets – Initiate therapy with 180 mg/day at bedtime. Clinical trials explored dose ranges between 180 and 540 mg given at bedtime and found effects to persist throughout the dosing interval.

If an adequate response is not obtained with 180 mg, the dose may be titrated upward in the following manner:
   240 mg each evening,
   360 mg each evening (2 × 180 mg),
   480 mg each evening (2 × 240 mg).

Verelan PM – Usual daily dose is 200 mg/day at bedtime. In rare instances, initial doses of 100 mg/day may be warranted in patients who have an increased response to verapamil (eg, impaired or hepatic function, elderly, people of small stature). Base upward titration on safety and efficacy evaluated approximately 24 hours after dosing. Antihypertensive effects are evident within the first week of therapy.

If an adequate response is not obtained with 200 mg, the dose may be titrated upward in the following manner:
   300 each evening,
   400 mg each evening (2 × 200 mg).

➤*Sustained-release:* Individualize the dose by titration. Dose of 120 mg/day may be warranted in patients who may have increased response (eg, elderly or people of small stature). Antihypertensive effects are evident within the first week. When switching from the immediate-release formulation, total daily dose (in mg) may remain the same.

Calan SR and Isoptin SR – Initiate therapy with 180 mg given in the morning with food. Base upward titration on safety and efficacy evaluated weekly and approximately 24 hours after the previous dose.

Sustained release characteristics are not altered when the tablet is divided in half.

If adequate response is not obtained with 180 mg, the dose may be titrated upward in the following manner:
   240 each morning,
   180 mg each morning plus 180 each evening, or 240 mg each morning plus 120 mg each evening,
   240 mg every 12 hours.

Verelan – Usual daily dose is 240 mg once daily in the morning. Base upward titration on safety and efficacy evaluated approximately 24 hours after dosing.

If adequate response is not obtained with 120 mg, the dose may be titrated upward in the following manner:
   180 mg in the morning,
   240 mg in the morning,
   360 mg in the morning,
   480 mg in the morning.

Pellet-filled capsules – Do not chew or crush the contents of the capsule. Pellet-filled capsules also may be administered by carefully opening the capsule and sprinkling the pellets on a spoonful of applesauce. Swallow the applesauce immediately without chewing and follow with a glass of cool water to ensure complete swallowing of the pellets. The applesauce used should not be hot, and it should be soft enough to be

VERAPAMIL HCl

swallowed without chewing. Use any pellet/applesauce mixture immediately and do not store for future use. Subdividing the contents of the capsule is not recommended.

➤*Parenteral:* For IV use only. Give as slow IV injection over at least 2 minutes under continuous ECG and BP monitoring. A small fraction (less than 1%) of patients may have life-threatening adverse responses (rapid ventricular rate in atrial flutter/fibrillation, and an accessory bypass tract, marked hypotension or extreme bradycardia/asystole); monitor initial use of IV verapamil and have resuscitation facilities available, including D.C. cardioversion capability. As familiarity with patient's response is gained, use in an office setting may be acceptable.

Initial dose – 5 to 10 mg (0.075 to 0.15 mg/kg) as an IV bolus over at least 2 minutes.

Repeat dose – 10 mg (0.15 mg/kg) 30 minutes after the first dose if the initial response is not adequate.

Older patients – Give over at least 3 minutes to minimize risk of unwanted drug effects.

Children –

0 to 1 year: 0.1 to 0.2 mg/kg (usual single dose range, 0.75 to 2 mg) as an IV bolus over at least 2 minutes (under continuous ECG monitoring).

1 to 15 years: 0.1 to 0.3 mg/kg (usual single dose range, 2 to 5 mg) IV bolus over at least 2 minutes. Do not exceed 5 mg.

Repeat dose: Repeat above dose 30 minutes after the first dose if the initial response is not adequate (under continuous ECG monitoring).

Do not exceed a single dose of 10 mg in patients 1 to 15 years of age.

Incompatibility – A crystalline precipitate immediately forms when verapamil is administered into an infusion line containing sodium bicarbonate. A milky white precipitate forms when verapamil is given by IV push into the same line being used for nafcillin infusion.

For stability reasons, this product is not recommended for dilution with sodium lactate injection in polyvinyl chloride bags. Verapamil is physically compatible and chemically stable for at least 24 hours at 25°C (77°F) protected from light in most common large volume parenteral solutions. Avoid admixing IV verapamil with albumin, amphotericin B, hydralazine HCl, aminophylline, and trimethoprim/sulfamethoxazole. Verapamil will precipitate in any solution with a pH above 6.

➤*Concomitant therapy:* Concomitant therapy with oral beta-adrenergic blocking agents may be beneficial in certain patients with chronic stable angina or hypertension, but available information is not sufficient to predict with confidence the effects of concurrent treatment in patients with left ventricular dysfunction or cardiac conduction abnormalities.

➤*Storage/Stability:* Store at controlled room temperature 15° to 30°C (59° to 86°F). Protect from light.

Extended-release tablets (Covera-HS, Verelan) – Store at controlled room temperature 20° to 25°C (68° to 77°F).

Oral – Dispense in tight, light-resistant container. Protect from moisture.

Parenteral – Discard any unused amount of solution.

Nitrates

Indications

➤*Acute angina (nitroglycerin-sublingual, transmucosal or translingual spray; isosorbide dinitrate-sublingual; amyl nitrite):* For relief of acute anginal episodes; prophylaxis prior to events likely to provoke an attack. Because of the more rapid relief of chest pain with sublingual nitroglycerin, limit the use of sublingual isosorbide dinitrate for aborting an acute anginal attack in patients intolerant or unresponsive to sublingual nitroglycerin.

➤*Angina prophylaxis (nitroglycerin-topical, transdermal, translingual spray, transmucosal and oral sustained release; isosorbide dinitrate; isosorbide mononitrate; erythrityl tetranitrate; pentaerythritol tetranitrate):* Prophylaxis and long-term management of recurrent angina.

➤*Nitroglycerin IV:* Control of blood pressure in perioperative hypertension associated with surgical procedures, especially cardiovascular procedures, such as endotracheal intubation, anesthesia, skin incision, sternotomy, cardiac bypass and in the immediate postsurgical period.

Congestive heart failure (CHF) associated with acute MI; treatment of angina pectoris unresponsive to organic nitrates or β-blockers; production of controlled hypotension during surgical procedures.

➤*Unlabeled uses:* Sublingual and topical nitroglycerin and oral nitrates have been used to reduce cardiac workload in patients with acute MI and in CHF.

Nitroglycerin ointment has been used as adjunctive treatment of Raynaud's disease and other peripheral vascular diseases. A synergistic effect (reduced platelet deposition and increased platelet survival) occurred when isosorbide dinitrate (40 mg/day) and prostaglandin E_1 (5 ng/kg/min for 6 hours) were used in patients with peripheral vascular disease. It may also be beneficial as an aid to venous cannulation in children < 1 year of age using a dose of 0.4 to 0.8 mg.

IV nitroglycerin (5 to 100 mcg/min infusion) may be used in the treatment of hypertensive crisis, specifically in patients who have hypertension with angina or MI.

Refer to the individual drug monographs for FDA labeled indications.

Actions

➤*Pharmacology:* Relaxation of vascular smooth muscle via stimulation of intracellular cyclic guanosine monophosphate production is the principal pharmacologic action of nitrates. Although venous effects predominate, nitroglycerin produces a dose-dependent dilation of both arterial and venous beds. Dilation of the postcapillary vessels, including large veins, promotes peripheral pooling of blood and decreases venous return to the heart, reducing left ventricular end-diastolic pressure (preload). Arteriolar relaxation reduces systemic vascular resistance and arterial pressure (afterload). Myocardial oxygen consumption or demand (as measured by the pressure-rate product, tension-time index and stroke-work index) is decreased by both arterial and venous effects of nitroglycerin, and a more favorable supply-demand ratio is achieved. In coronary circulation, the nitrates redistribute circulating blood flow along collateral channels, improving perfusion to the ischemic myocardium. While the large epicardial coronary arteries are also dilated by nitroglycerin, the extent to which this action contributes to relief of exertional angina is unclear.

Therapeutic doses reduce systolic, diastolic and mean arterial blood pressure. Effective coronary perfusion pressure is usually maintained, but can be compromised if blood pressure falls excessively or increased heart rate decreases diastolic filling time. Elevated central venous and pulmonary capillary wedge pressures (PCWP), pulmonary vascular resistance and systemic vascular resistance are also reduced. Reflex tachycardia may occur, presumably in response to decreased blood pressure. Cardiac index may be increased, decreased or unchanged. Patients with elevated left ventricular filling pressure and systemic vascular resistance values with a depressed cardiac index are likely to have improved cardiac index. When filling pressures and cardiac index are normal, cardiac index may be slightly reduced by nitrates.

➤*Pharmacokinetics:*

Doseform, Onset and Duration of Available Nitrates			
Nitrates	Dosage form	Onset (minutes)	Duration
Amyl nitrite	Inhalant	0.5	3 to 5 min
Nitroglycerin	IV	1 to 2	3 to 5 min
	Sublingual	1 to 3	30 to 60 min
	Translingual spray	2	30 to 60 min
	Transmucosal tablet	1 to 2	3 to 5 hours[1]
	Oral, sustained release	20 to 45	3 to 8 hours
	Topical ointment	30 to 60	2 to 12 hours[2]
	Transdermal	30 to 60	up to 24 hours[3]
Isosorbide dinitrate	Sublingual	2 to 5	1 to 3 hours
	Oral	20 to 40	4 to 6 hours
	Oral, sustained release	up to 4 hours	6 to 8 hours

Doseform, Onset and Duration of Available Nitrates			
Nitrates	Dosage form	Onset (minutes)	Duration
Isosorbide mono- nitrate	Oral	30 to 60	nd[4]

[1] A significant antianginal effect can persist for 5 hours if the tablet has not completely dissolved by this time.
[2] Depends on total amount used per unit of surface area.
[3] Tolerance may develop after 12 hours (see Precautions, Administration and Dosage).
[4] nd = No data.

Nitroglycerin, isosorbide dinitrate and erythrityl tetranitrate are readily absorbed from the sublingual mucosa. Nitroglycerin is also absorbed through the skin. Nitroglycerin ointments and transdermal systems provide a gradual release of the drug which reaches target organs before hepatic inactivation.

Nitroglycerin has a short half-life, estimated at 1 to 4 minutes, resulting in a low plasma concentration after IV infusion. At plasma concentrations between 50 and 500 ng/mL, plasma protein binding of nitroglycerin is approximately 60%.

Nitrates are metabolized in the liver by nitrate reductase. Although less potent as vasodilators, the two active major metabolites, 1,2 and 1,3 dinitroglycerols, have longer plasma half-lives than the parent compound and appear in substantial concentration; therefore, they may be responsible for some of the pharmacologic activity. Dinitrates are further metabolized to inactive mononitrates. Isosorbide dinitrate, however, is metabolized to 2- and 5-mononitrates, which are both active and accumulate more than the parent drug with long-term therapy, and ultimately to glycerol and CO_2. Since isosorbide mononitrate is a major active metabolite of isosorbide dinitrate, and since most of the clinical activity of the dinitrate is attributable to the mononitrate, isosorbide mononitrate is now available as a single entity product.

Extensive first-pass deactivation follows GI absorption. Hepatic reductase activity may be saturated by some oral nitroglycerin doses, resulting in prolonged pharmacologic effects.

Approximately one-third of an inhaled dose of amyl nitrite is excreted in the urine.

Contraindications

Hypersensitivity or idiosyncrasy to nitrates; severe anemia; closed angle glaucoma; postural hypotension; early MI (sublingual nitroglycerin); head trauma or cerebral hemorrhage (since these drugs may increase intracranial pressure); allergy to adhesives (transdermal).

➤*Amyl nitrite:* Pregnancy (see Warnings).

➤*Nitroglycerin IV:* Hypotension or uncorrected hypovolemia, since IV use in such states could produce severe hypotension or shock; inadequate cerebral circulation; increased intracranial pressure; constrictive pericarditis; pericardial tamponade.

Warnings

➤*MI:* Data supporting the use of nitrates during the early days of the acute phase of MI are insufficient to establish safety. In acute MI, use nitrates only under close clinical observation and with hemodynamic monitoring. In general, a long-acting form should not be used because its effects are difficult to terminate rapidly should excessive hypotension or tachycardia develop. The effects of isosorbide mononitrate are difficult to terminate rapidly; avoid use in patients with acute MI or CHF.

➤*Arcing:* A cardioverter/defibrillator should not be discharged through a paddle electrode that overlies a transdermal nitroglycerin system. The arcing that may be seen in this situation is harmless in itself, but it may be associated with local current concentration that can cause damage to the paddles and burns to the patient.

➤*Postural hypotension:* May occur, even with small doses. Transient episodes of dizziness, weakness, syncope or other signs of cerebral ischemia due to postural hypotension may develop following administration, particularly if the patient is standing immobile. Alcohol accentuates this reaction. Use measures which facilitate venous return (eg, head-low posture, deep breathing, movements of the extremities) to hasten recovery. Fatalities have occurred.

➤*Angina:* Nitrates may aggravate angina caused by hypertrophic cardiomyopathy.

➤*Nitroglycerin IV:* The available preparations differ in concentration or volume per vial or ampule. When switching from one product to another, pay attention to the dilution, dosage and administration instructions. Some of these products contain alcohol and propylene glycol; safety for intracoronary injection has not been established.

Absorption – Nitroglycerin readily migrates into many plastics. To avoid absorption of nitroglycerin into plastic parenteral solution containers, dilute and store only in glass parenteral solution bottles. Since some filters also absorb nitroglycerin, avoid if possible (see IV Administration and Dosage).

Hepatic or renal disease, severe – Use with caution.

Hypotension – Avoid excessive prolonged hypotension, because of possible deleterious effects on the brain, heart, liver and kidney from poor perfusion and the attendant risk of ischemia, thrombosis and altered organ function. Paradoxical bradycardia and increased angina pectoris may accompany nitroglycerin-induced hypotension. Use with caution in subjects who may have volume depletion from diuretics or in those with low systolic blood pressure (eg, < 90 mmHg). Patients with normal or low PCWP are especially sensitive to the hypotensive effects of IV nitroglycerin. A fall in PCWP precedes the onset of arterial hypotension; the PCWP is thus a useful guide to safe titration of the drug.

Alcohol intoxication – Has developed in patients on high-dose IV nitroglycerin. Consider this complication when administering high doses for prolonged periods.

➤*Sublingual nitroglycerin:* Absorption is dependent on salivary secretion. Dry mouth (including drug-induced dry mouth) decreases absorption.

➤*Transdermal nitroglycerin:* Not for immediate relief of anginal attacks.

➤*Pregnancy: Category C.* Safety for use is not established. Use only when clearly needed and when potential benefits outweigh potential hazards to the fetus.

Category X (amyl nitrite) – Because it markedly reduces systemic blood pressure and blood flow on the maternal side of the placenta, amyl nitrite can cause harm to the fetus when it is administered to a pregnant woman.

➤*Lactation:* It is not known whether nitrates are excreted in breast milk. Exercise caution when administering to a nursing woman.

Because of the potential for serious adverse reactions in nursing infants from **amyl nitrite**, decide whether to discontinue nursing or to discontinue the drug, taking into account the importance of the drug to the mother.

➤*Children:* Safety and efficacy for use in children have not been established.

Precautions

➤*Tolerance:* Tolerance to vascular and antianginal effects of nitrates may develop. Several well controlled clinical trials have used exercise testing to assess the antianginal efficacy of continuously delivered nitrates. In the large majority of these trials, active agents were indistinguishable from placebo after 24 hours or less of continuous therapy. Attempts to overcome nitrate tolerance by dose escalation even to doses far in excess of those used acutely, have consistently failed. Only after nitrates had been absent from the body for several hours was their antianginal efficacy restored.

The use of a low-nitrate or nitrate-free period should be part of the therapeutic strategy. Tolerance may be altered with short periods (10 to 12 hours) of nitrate withdrawal. Minimize tolerance by using smallest effective dose, by using pulse therapy (intermittent dosing) or by alternating with other coronary vasodilators. It is generally recommended to take the last daily dose of a short-acting agent no later than 7 pm. Administering short-acting isosorbide dinitrate 2 or 3 times daily instead of 4, sustained-release isosorbide dinitrate once daily or an eccentric regimen of twice daily at 8 am and 2 pm, giving the two daily doses of isosorbide mononitrate 7 hours apart (creating a 17 hour gap between second dose of each day and first dose of next day) or using nitroglycerin transdermal patches for only 12 hours during the day (see Nitroglycerin Transdermal Administration and Dosage), may reduce the possibility of tolerance developing. Although further studies are necessary, administration of acetylcysteine may reverse tolerance to nitroglycerin in patients in whom complete tolerance has developed. Nitrates that appear least likely to be associated with tolerance are the short-acting formulations (eg, sublingual, translingual spray), with the exception of the IV form. The transmucosal formulation also appears to be associated with minimal tolerance.

Controlled clinical trial data suggest that the intermittent use of nitrates is associated with decreased exercise tolerance, in comparison to placebo, during the last part of the nitrate-free interval; the clinical relevance of this observation is unknown, but consider the possibility of increased frequency or severity of angina during the nitrate-free interval. Further investigations of the tolerance phenomenon and best regimen are ongoing. A final evaluation of the effectiveness of the product will be announced by the FDA.

If patients generally experience anginal episodes at night, the use of a beta blocker or calcium channel blocker during this interval may be beneficial. Patients who generally experience anginal episodes during the day do not appear to be at significant risk with a nightly nitrate-poor period.

➤*Glaucoma:* Intraocular pressure may be increased; therefore, caution is required in administering to patients with glaucoma.

➤*Excessive dosage:* Excessive dosage may produce severe headache. Lowering the dose and using analgesics will help control the headaches, which diminish or disappear as therapy continues. Discontinue the drug if blurred vision or dry mouth occurs.

➤*Volume depletion/hypotension:* Severe hypotension (particularly with upright posture) may occur with even small doses of isosorbide mononitrate. Exercise caution in patients who may be volume depleted

or hypotensive for any reason. Hypotension may be accompanied by paradoxical bradycardia and increased angina pectoris.

➤*Withdrawal:* In terminating treatment of angina, gradually reduce the dosage to prevent withdrawal reactions.

➤*Drug abuse and dependence:* Amyl nitrite is abused for sexual stimulation. The effect of inhalation is almost instantaneous, causing lightheadedness, dizziness and euphoria.

Drug Interactions

Nitrate Drug Interactions

Precipitant drug	Object drug*		Description
Alcohol	Nitrates	↑	Severe hypotension and cardiovascular collapse may occur.
Aspirin	Nitrates	↑	Increased nitrate serum concentrations and actions may occur.
Calcium channel blockers	Nitrates	↑	Marked symptomatic orthostatic hypotension may occur. Dosage adjustment of either agent may be necessary.
Dihydroergotamine	Nitrates	⟷	Increased bioavailability of dihydroergotamine with resultant increase in mean standing systolic blood pressure, or functional antagonism between these agents, decreasing the antianginal effects.
Nitroglycerin	Heparin	↓	Pharmacologic effects of heparin may be decreased; data conflict.

* ↑ = Object drug increased. ↓ = Object drug decreased. ⟷ = Undetermined clinical effect.

➤*Drug/Lab test interactions:* Nitrates may interfere with *Zlatkis-Zak* color reaction causing false report of decreased serum cholesterol.

Adverse Reactions

➤*Cardiovascular:* Tachycardia; retrosternal discomfort; palpitations; hypotension (sometimes with paradoxical bradycardia and increased angina pectoris); syncope; collapse; crescendo angina; rebound hypertension; arrhythmias; atrial fibrillation; premature ventricular contractions; postural hypotension.

➤*CNS:* Headache which may be severe and persistent (up to 50%); apprehension; restlessness; weakness; vertigo; dizziness; agitation; anxiety; confusion; insomnia; nervousness; nightmares; dyscoordination; hypoesthesia; hypokinesia.

➤*Dermatologic:* Drug rash or exfoliative dermatitis; cutaneous vasodilation with flushing; crusty skin lesions; pruritus; rash.

Contact dermatitis from **transdermal nitroglycerin** may occur. The transdermal delivery system itself, not the nitroglycerin molecule, may be responsible.

Nitroglycerin ointment may cause topical allergic reactions; erythematous, vesicular and pruritic lesions; anaphylactoid reactions characterized by oral mucosal and conjunctival edema.

Sublingual nitroglycerin tablets may cause a local burning or tingling sensation in the oral cavity at the point of dissolution. Absence of this effect does not indicate loss of potency; some older patients may not experience this effect. The stabilized tablets may be less likely to produce these sensations.

➤*GI:* Nausea; vomiting; diarrhea; dyspepsia; involuntary passing of urine and feces; abdominal pain; tenesmus; tooth disorder.

➤*GU:* Dysuria; impotence; urinary frequency.

➤*Musculoskeletal:* Arthralgia.

➤*Respiratory:* Bronchitis; pneumonia; upper respiratory tract infection.

➤*Miscellaneous:* Muscle twitching; pallor; perspiration; cold sweat; hemolytic anemia; asthenia; blurred vision; diplopia; edema; malaise; neck stiffness; rigors; increased appetite. Allergic responses, resulting in itching or wheezing and tracheobronchitis have occurred.

Methemoglobinemia – Case reports of clinically significant methemoglobinemia are rare at conventional doses of nitrates. Formation of methemoglobin is dose-related and in the case of genetic abnormalities of hemoglobin that favor methemoglobin formation, even conventional doses of nitrates could produce harmful concentrations of methemoglobin. Treat with high-flow oxygen and administer methylene blue slowly at a dose of 0.2 mL/kg (1 to 2 mg/kg) IV. Refer to the methylene blue monograph in Antidotes Section.

Overdosage

➤*Symptoms:* Toxic effects may result from inhalation of the drug as dust, by ingestion or by excessive absorption through the intact skin or mucous membranes. Prolonged contact will produce skin eruptions. Signs and symptoms result primarily from vasodilation and methemoglobinemia. Manifestations include hypotension, tachycardia, flushing, perspiring skin (later becoming cold and cyanotic), headache, vertigo, palpitations, visual disturbances, diaphoresis, dizziness, syncope, nausea, vomiting (possibly with colic and bloody diarrhea), anorexia, initial hyperpnea, dyspnea and slow breathing, slow pulse (dicrotic and intermittent), heart block, increased intracranial pressure with cerebral symptoms of confusion, moderate fever and paralysis. Tissue hypoxia due to methemoglobinemia can lead to cyanosis, metabolic acidosis, coma, convulsions and death due to cardiovascular collapse.

➤*Treatment:* If nitrates are ingested, induce emesis or perform gastric lavage followed by charcoal administration; however, nitrates are usually rapidly and completely absorbed. Keep patient recumbent in shock position and comfortably warm or temporarily terminate the infusion until the patient's condition stabilizes. Gastric lavage may be of use if the medication has only recently been swallowed. Passive movement of the extremities may aid venous return. Administer oxygen and artificial ventilation if necessary. Monitor methemoglobin levels as indicated.

Treat severe hypotension and reflex tachycardia by elevating the legs and administering IV fluids. Since the duration of the hemodynamic effects following IV nitroglycerin administration is quite short, additional corrective measures are usually not required. However, if indicated, consider an IV α-adrenergic agonist (eg, phenylephrine, methoxamine). Treat methemoglobinemia (see Adverse Reactions).

Epinephrine is ineffective in reversing the severe hypotensive events associated with overdosage; epinephrine and related compounds are contraindicated in overdosage.

Patient Information

Avoid alcohol.

➤*Brand interchange:* Do not change from one brand of this drug to another without consulting your pharmacist or physician. Products manufactured by different companies may not be equally effective.

May cause headache, dizziness or flushing. Notify physician if blurred vision, dry mouth or persistent headache occurs. In patients who get headaches, the headaches may be a marker of the drug's activity. Patients should not try to avoid headaches by altering the treatment schedule, since loss of headache may be associated with simultaneous loss of efficacy. Aspirin or acetaminophen may be used for relief.

Take oral nitrates on an empty stomach with a glass of water.

Carefully follow the prescribed schedule of dosing.

Keep tablets and capsules in original container. Keep container closed tightly.

➤*Inhalants:* Use when lying down only. Highly flammable; do not use where it might be ignited. Use in a well ventilated room.

➤*Sublingual tablets:* Dissolve tablet under tongue; do not swallow. A lack of burning or stinging sensation does not indicate a loss of potency. Use when seated. Take at the first sign of an anginal attack before severe pain develops. If angina is not relieved in 5 minutes, dissolve a second tablet under the tongue. If pain is not relieved within another 5 minutes, dissolve a third tablet. If pain continues or intensifies, notify physician immediately or report to the nearest emergency room.

➤*Translingual spray:* Spray onto or under tongue. Do not inhale spray.

➤*Transmucosal tablets:* Place under the upper lip or in a buccal pouch (between cheek and gum). Allow to dissolve slowly over a 3- to 5-hour period. Do not chew or swallow tablets. Release of nitroglycerin begins immediately upon contact with the mucosa and will continue until the tablet dissolves. Time to dissolution increases as patients familiarize themselves with the tablet's presence. Rate of dissolution may be increased by touching the tablet with the tongue or drinking hot liquids.

➤*Sustained release nitroglycerin:* Swallow whole; do not chew. Not for sublingual use.

➤*Topical ointment:* Patient instructions are available with products. Spread a thin layer on skin using applicator or dose-measuring papers; do not use fingers; do not rub or massage. Keep tube tightly closed.

➤*Transdermal nitroglycerin:* Patient instructions are available with products. Advise patients that there is enough residual nitroglycerin in discarded patches that they are a potential hazard to children and pets. Use caution when discarding.

ISOSORBIDE MONONITRATE, ORAL

Rx	**Isosorbide Mononitrate** (Various, eg, Purepac)	**Tablets:** 10 mg	Lactose. In 100s.
Rx	**Monoket** (Schwarz Pharma)		Lactose. (10 SCHWARz 610). White, scored. In 60s, 100s, 180s and UD 100s.
Rx	**ISMO** (ESP Pharma)	**Tablets:** 20 mg	(ISMO 20W). Orange. Film coated. In 100s, UD 100s.
Rx	**Isosorbide Mononitrate** (eg, Purepac, Teva)		Lactose. In 100s and 500s.
Rx	**Monoket** (Schwarz Pharma)		Lactose. (20 SCHWARz 620). White, scored. In 60s, 100s, 180s and UD 100s.
Rx	**Isosorbide Mononitrate** (Various, eg, Ethex, Kremers Urban)	**Tablets, extended release:** 30 mg	In 100s and UD 100s.
Rx	**Imdur** (Key)		(IM DUR 30 30). Rose colored. Scored. In 30s, 100s and UD 100s.
Rx	**Isosorbide Mononitrate** (Various, eg, Ethex, Kremers Urban, Schwarz Pharma)	**Tablets, extended release:** 60 mg	In 100s and UD 100s.
Rx	**Imdur** (Key)		(IM DUR 60 60). Yellow, scored. In 30s, 100s and UD 100s.
Rx	**Isotrate ER** (Apothecon)		(WC 176). Lactose. White, scored. In 100s and 500s.
Rx	**Isosorbide Mononitrate** (Various, eg, Ethex, Kremers Urban)	**Tablets, extended release:** 120 mg	In 100s and UD 100s.
Rx	**Imdur** (Key)		(IMDUR 120). White. In 30s, 100s and UD 100s.

For complete prescribing information, refer to the Nitrates group monograph.

Indications

➤*Angina pectoris:* Prevention of angina pectoris; not to abort acute anginal episodes.

Administration and Dosage

➤*Approved by the FDA:* December 1991.

➤*Tablets:* 20 mg twice daily, with the two doses given 7 hours apart. A starting dose of 5 mg (½ tablet of the 10 mg dosing strength) might be appropriate for persons of particularly small stature, but should be

increased to at least 10 mg by the second or third day of therapy. Suggested regimen is to give first dose on awakening and second dose 7 hours later. The asymmetric dosing regimen provides a daily nitrate-free interval to minimize the development of tolerance.

➤*Tablets, extended release:* Initially, 30 mg (given as ½ of a 60 mg tablet) or 60 mg (one tablet) once daily. After several days, the dosage may be increased to 120 mg (given as two 60 mg tablets) once daily. Rarely 240 mg may be required. Suggested regimen is to give in the morning on arising. Do not crush or chew extended release tablets, and swallow them with a half glassful of liquid.

ISOSORBIDE DINITRATE, SUBLINGUAL AND CHEWABLE

Rx	**Isosorbide Dinitrate** (Various, eg, Major, Moore, Parmed, Rugby, Schein)	**Tablets, sublingual:** 2.5 mg	In 100s, 500s, 1000s and UD 100s.
Rx	**Isordil** (Wyeth-Ayerst)		Lactose. (2.5 W). Yellow. In 500s and Redipak 100s.
Rx	**Isosorbide Dinitrate** (Various, eg, Major, Moore, Parmed, Rugby, Schein, URL)	**Tablets, sublingual:** 5 mg	In 100s, 1000s and UD 100s.
Rx	**Isordil** (Wyeth-Ayerst)		Lactose. (5 W). Pink. In 500s and Redipak 100s.

ISOSORBIDE DINITRATE, SUBLINGUAL AND CHEWABLE

Rx	**Isosorbide Dinitrate** (Various, eg, Major)	**Tablets, sublingual:** 10 mg	In 100s and 1000s.
Rx	**Isordil** (Wyeth-Ayerst)		Lactose. (10 WYETH). White. In 100s.
Rx	**Sorbitrate** (Zeneca)	**Tablets, chewable:** 5 mg	(S 810). Sugar. Green, scored. In 100s and 500s.
Rx	**Sorbitrate** (Zeneca)	**Tablets, chewable:** 10 mg	(S 815). Sugar. Yellow, scored. In 100s.

For complete prescribing information, refer to the Nitrates group monograph.

Indications

➤*Angina:* Treatment and prevention of angina pectoris.

Administration and Dosage

➤*Angina pectoris:* Usual starting dose is 2.5 to 5 mg for sublingual tablets and 5 mg for chewable tablets. Titrate upward until angina is relieved or side effects limit the dose.

➤*Acute prophylaxis:* 5 to 10 mg sublingual or chewable tablets every 2 to 3 hours. Limit use of sublingual or chewable isosorbide dinitrate for aborting an acute anginal attack in patients intolerant of or unresponsive to sublingual nitroglycerin.

Do not crush or chew sublingual tablets; do not crush chewable tablets before administering.

ISOSORBIDE DINITRATE, ORAL

Rx	**Isosorbide Dinitrate** (Various, eg, Geneva, Goldline, Major, Moore, Par, Parmed, Rugby, Schein, UDL, URL)	**Tablets:** 5 mg	In 100s, 1000s and UD 100s.
Rx	**Isordil Titradose** (Biovail)		Lactose. (WYETH 4152). Pink, scored. In 100s, 500s, 1000s and Redipak 100s.
Rx	**Sorbitrate** (Zeneca)		Lactose. (S 770). Green, scored. Oval. In 100s, 500s and UD 100s.
Rx	**Isosorbide Dinitrate** (Various, eg, Geneva, Goldline, Major, Moore, Par, Parmed, Rugby, Schein, UDL, URL)	**Tablets:** 10 mg	In 100s, 500s, 1000s and UD 100s.
Rx	**Isordil Titradose** (Biovail)		Lactose. (WYETH 4153). White, scored. In 100s, 500s, 1000s and Redipak 100s.
Rx	**Sorbitrate** (Zeneca)		Lactose. (S 780). Yellow, scored. Oval. In 100s, 500s and UD 100s.
Rx	**Isosorbide Dinitrate** (Various, eg, Geneva, Goldline, Major, Moore, Par, Parmed, Rugby, Schein, UDL, URL)	**Tablets:** 20 mg	In 90s, 100s, 120s, 180s, 240s, 360s, 500s, 1000s and UD 100s.
Rx	**Isordil Titradose** (Biovail)		Lactose. (WYETH 4154). Green, scored. In 100s and Redipak 100s.
Rx	**Sorbitrate** (Zeneca)		Lactose. (S 820). Blue, scored. Oval. In 100s and UD 100s.
Rx	**Isosorbide Dinitrate** (Various, eg, Major, Moore, Par, Parmed, Rugby, URL)	**Tablets:** 30 mg	In 100s, 500s, 1000s and UD 100s.
Rx	**Isordil Titradose** (Biovail)		Lactose. (WYETH 4159). Blue, scored. In 100s, 500s and Redipak 100s.
Rx	**Sorbitrate** (Zeneca)		Lactose. (S 773). White, scored. Oval. In 100s and UD 100s.
Rx	**Isordil Titradose** (Biovail)	**Tablets:** 40 mg	Lactose. (WYETH 4192). Light green, scored. In 100s and Redipak 100s.
Rx	**Sorbitrate** (Zeneca)		Lactose. (S 774) Light blue, scored. Oval. In 100s and UD 100s.
Rx	**Isochron** (Forest)	**Tablets, extended release:** 40 mg	In 100s.
Rx	**Isosorbide Dinitrate** (Various, eg, Geneva, Goldline, Major, Parmed, URL)	**Tablets, sustained release:** 40 mg	In 90s, 100s, 250s, 1000s and UD 100s.
Rx	**Dilatrate-SR** (Schwarz Pharma)	**Capsules, sustained release:** 40 mg	(SCHWARZ 0920). Pink/opaque. In 60s and 100s.

For complete prescribing information, refer to the Nitrates group monograph.

Indications

➤*Angina:* Treatment and prevention of angina pectoris; not to abort acute anginal episodes.

Administration and Dosage

➤*Tablets:* Initial dose is 5 to 20 mg; maintenance dose is 10 to 40 mg every 6 hours.

➤*Sustained release:* The initial dose is 40 mg; maintenance controlled release dose is 40 to 80 mg every 8 to 12 hours. Do not crush or chew these preparations.

➤*Tolerance:* Tolerance to these agents may develop. Consider administering the short-acting preparations 2 or 3 times daily (last dose no later than 7 pm) and the sustained release preparations once daily or twice daily at 8 am and 2 pm. See Precautions.

NITROGLYCERIN, INTRAVENOUS

Rx	**Nitroglycerin** (Various, eg, American Regent, Goldline)	**Injection:** 5 mg/mL	In 5 and 10 mL vials.
Rx	**Nitro-Bid IV** (Hoechst Marion Roussel)		In 1, 5 and 10 mL vials.[1]
Rx	**Nitroglycerin in 5% Dextrose** (Various, eg, Abbott, Baxter)	**Injection solution:** 25 mg	In 250 mL.
		50 mg	In 250 and 500 mL.
		100 mg	In 250 mL.
		200 mg	In 500 mL.

[1] With 45 mg propylene glycol per mL.

For complete prescribing information, refer to the Nitrates group monograph.

Indications

Control of blood pressure in perioperative hypertension (ie, associated with endotracheal intubation, anesthesia, skin incision, sternotomy, cardiac bypass) and in the immediate postsurgical period.

Congestive heart failure associated with acute myocardial infarction.

Angina pectoris unresponsive to recommended doses of organic nitrates or β-blockers.

To produce controlled hypotension during surgical procedures.

Administration and Dosage

➤*Preparation of infusion:* Not for direct IV injection. Dilute in D5W or 0.9% NaCl Injection prior to infusion. Do not mix with other drugs. Base infusion concentration on patient's fluid requirements and expected duration of infusion. Preparations differ in concentration and volume per vial. Refer to manufacturers' package literature for dilution recommendations for specific products.

➤*Administration sets:* Use only with glass IV bottles and administration set provided. Total amount of nitroglycerin (40% to 80%) in the final diluted solution for infusion could be adsorbed by PVC tubing of IV administration sets in general use. Greater adsorption occurs with low flow rates, high concentrations and long tubing. Although rate of loss is

NITROGLYCERIN, INTRAVENOUS

highest during early administration (when flow rates are lowest), the loss is neither constant nor self-limiting; consequently, no simple calculation or correction can convert theoretical infusion rate (based on concentration of solution) to actual delivery rate. Manufacturers have developed non-PVC infusion tubing in which nitroglycerin loss is < 5%. Use IV sets provided by manufacturers or use similar infusion sets.

Infusion pumps may fail to occlude the non-PVC infusion sets completely because non-PVC tubing is less pliable than standard PVC tubing. Excessive flow at low infusion rate settings may result, causing alarms or unregulated gravity flow when the infusion pump is stopped. This could lead to overinfusion of nitroglycerin.

➤*Dosage requirements:* Initially, 5 mcg/min delivered through an infusion pump. Titrate to the clinical situation, initially in 5 mcg/min increments with increases every 3 to 5 minutes until some response is noted. If no response occurs at 20 mcg/min, use increments of 10 to 20 mcg/min. Once a partial blood pressure response is observed, reduce the dose and lengthen the interval between increments.

Some patients with normal or low left ventricular filling pressure or PCWP (eg, angina patients without other complications) may be hypersensitive and may respond fully to doses as small as 5 mcg/min. Titrate carefully and monitor closely.

There is no fixed optimum dose. Continuously monitor physiologic parameters (eg, blood pressure, heart rate) and other measurements (eg, PCWP) to achieve correct dose. Maintain adequate blood and coronary perfusion pressures.

➤*Storage/Stability:* Protect from freezing and light.

NITROGLYCERIN, SUBLINGUAL

Rx	**Nitroglycerin** (Various, eg, Endo, Konec)	**Tablets, sublingual:** 0.3 mg (1/200 gr)	In 100s.
Rx	**NitroQuick** (Ethex)		ETH 3 Lactose. In 100s.
Rx	**Nitrostat** (Parke-Davis)		Lactose, sucrose. In 100s.
Rx	**NitroTab** (Able)		Lactose. (N 3). In 100s.
Rx	**Nitroglycerin** (Various, eg, Endo, Konec)	0.4 mg (1/150 gr)	In 25s and 100s.
Rx	**NitroQuick** (Ethex)		4 ETH Lactose. In 25s and 100s.
Rx	**Nitrostat** (Parke-Davis)		Lactose, sucrose. (N 4). In 100s.
Rx	**NitroTab** (Able)		Lactose. In 100s.
Rx	**Nitroglycerin** (Various, eg, Endo, Konec)	0.6 mg (1/100 gr)	In 100s.
Rx	**NitroQuick** (Ethex)		Lactose. In 100s.
Rx	**Nitrostat** (Parke-Davis)		Lactose, sucrose. In 100s.
Rx	**NitroTab** (Able)		Lactose. In 100s.

For complete prescribing information, refer to the Nitrates group monograph.

Indications

➤*Angina pectoris:* Acute relief of an attack or acute prophylaxis of angina pectoris due to coronary artery disease.

Administration and Dosage

Dissolve 1 tablet under tongue or in buccal pouch (between cheek and gum) at first sign of an acute anginal attack. Repeat approximately every 5 minutes until relief is obtained. Take no more than 3 tablets in 15 minutes. If pain continues, notify physician immediately. May be used prophylactically 5 to 10 minutes prior to activities that might precipitate an acute attack.

The patient should rest during administration, preferably in the sitting position.

➤*Storage/Stability:* Dispense in the original container; store at room temperature. Protect from moisture. The stabilized sublingual tablets are less subject to potency loss than the previous conventional sublingual tablets. Unused tablets should be discarded 6 months after the original bottle is opened.

NITROGLYCERIN, TRANSLINGUAL

Rx	**Nitrolingual** (Horizon)	**Aerosol spray, translingual:** 0.4 mg/metered dose	In 14.48 g (200 metered doses). In 1s.

For complete prescribing information, refer to the Nitrates group monograph.

Indications

➤*Angina pectoris:* Acute relief of an attack or prophylaxis of angina pectoris due to coronary artery disease.

Administration and Dosage

At the onset of attack, spray 1 or 2 metered doses onto or under the tongue. No more than 3 metered doses are recommended within 15 minutes. If chest pain persists, seek prompt medical attention. May use prophylactically 5 to 10 minutes prior to engaging in activities that might precipitate an acute attack. Do not inhale spray.

NITROGLYCERIN, TRANSMUCOSAL

Rx	**Nitrogard** (Forest)	**Tablets, buccal, controlled release:** 2 mg	(2). Off-white. In 100s and UD 100s.
		3 mg	(3). Off-white. In 100s and UD 100s.

For complete prescribing information, refer to the Nitrates group monograph.

Indications

➤*Angina pectoris:* Treatment and prevention of angina pectoris due to coronary artery disease.

Administration and Dosage

Insert 1 mg every 3 to 5 hours during waking hours. Place tablet between lip and gum above incisors, or between cheek and gum.

NITROGLYCERIN, SUSTAINED RELEASE

Rx	**Nitroglycerin** (Various, eg, Dixon-Shane, Goldline, Major, Moore, Rugby, URL, Vitarine)	**Capsules, sustained release:** 2.5 mg	In 60s, 100s, and UD 60s and 100s.
Rx	**Nitro-Time** (Time-Cap Labs)		Lactose, sucrose. (TCL-1221). Pink/clear. In 60s, 90s, and 100s.
Rx	**Nitroglycerin** (Various, eg, Dixon-Shane, Goldline, Major, Moore, Rugby, URL, Vitarine)	**Capsules, sustained release:** 6.5 mg	In 60s, 100s, and UD 100s.
Rx	**Nitro-Time** (Time-Cap Labs)		Lactose, sucrose. (TCL-1222). Blue/yellow. In 60s, 90s, and 100s.
Rx	**Nitroglycerin** (Various, eg, Dixon-Shane, Major, Moore, Rugby, URL, Vitarine)	**Capsules, sustained release:** 9 mg	In 30s, 60s, 100s, and UD 100s.
Rx	**Nitro-Time** (Time-Cap Labs)		Lactose, sucrose. (TCL-1223). Green/yellow. In 60s, 90s, and 100s.

For complete prescribing information, refer to the Nitrates group monograph.

Indications

➤*Angina pectoris:* Prevention of angina pectoris. "Possibly effective" for the management, prophylaxis, or treatment of anginal attacks.

Administration and Dosage

The usual starting dose is 2.5 or 2.6 mg, 3 or 4 times daily. Titrate upward to an effective dose until side effects limit the dose. The dose generally may be increased by 2.5 or 2.6 mg increments 2 to 4 times daily over a period of days or weeks. Doses as high as 26 mg given 4 times daily have been reported effective.

NITROGLYCERIN, SUSTAINED RELEASE

Give the smallest effective dose 2 to 4 times daily. Monitor blood pressure at initiation of therapy or dosage change.

Tolerance may develop. Consider administering on a reduced schedule (once or twice daily). See Precautions.

Capsules must be swallowed; not for chewing or sublingual use.

NITROGLYCERIN TRANSDERMAL SYSTEMS

	Product/Distributor	Release Rate (mg/hr)	Surface Area (cm²)	Total NTG Content (mg)	How Supplied
Rx	**Minitran** (3M Pharm.)	0.1	3.3	9	In 33s.
Rx	**Nitro-Dur** (Key)	0.1	5	20	In 30s and 100s, UD 30s and 100s.
Rx	**Transderm-Nitro** (Summit)	0.1	5	12.5	In 30s and UD 30s and 100s.
Rx	**Nitroglycerin Transdermal** (Various, eg, Goldline, Major, Moore, Mylan, Parmed, Schein)	0.2	6 - 10[1]	16 - 62.5[1]	In 30s.
Rx	**Minitran** (3M Pharm.)	0.2	6.7	18	In 33s.
Rx	**Nitrek** (Bertek)	0.2	8	22.4	In 30s.
Rx	**Nitro-Dur** (Key)	0.2	10	40	In 30s, 100s and UD 30s and 100s.
Rx	**Transderm-Nitro** (Summit)	0.2	10	25	In 30s and UD 30s and 100s.
Rx	**Deponit** (Schwarz Pharma)	0.2	16	16	In 30s and 100s.
Rx	**Nitro-Dur** (Key)	0.3	15	60	In 30s, 100s and UD 30s and 100s.
Rx	**Nitroglycerin Transdermal** (Various, eg, Goldline, Major, Moore, Mylan, Parmed, Schein)	0.4	13 - 20[1]	32 - 125[1]	In 30s.
Rx	**Minitran** (3M Pharm.)	0.4	13.3	36	In 33s.
Rx	**Nitrek** (Bertek)	0.4	16	44.8	In 30s.
Rx	**Nitro-Dur** (Key)	0.4	20	80	In 30s, 100s and UD 30s and 100s.
Rx	**Transderm-Nitro** (Summit)	0.4	20	50	In 30s and UD 30s and 100s.
Rx	**Deponit** (Schwarz Pharma)	0.4	32	32	In 30s and 100s.
Rx	**Nitroglycerin Transdermal** (Various, eg, Goldline, Major, Mylan, Parmed, Rugby)	0.6	20 - 30[1]	75 - 187.5[1]	In 30s.
Rx	**Minitran** (3M Pharm.)	0.6	20	54	In 33s.
Rx	**Nitrek** (Bertek)	0.6	24	67.2	In 30s.
Rx	**Nitro-Dur** (Key)	0.6	30	120	In 30s and 100s.
Rx	**Transderm-Nitro** (Summit)	0.6	30	75	In 30s.
Rx	**Nitro-Dur** (Key)	0.8	40	160	In 30s, 100s and UD 30s and 100s.
Rx	**Transderm-Nitro** (Summit)	0.8	40	100	In 30s and UD 30s.

[1] Various systems have the same release rates but variable surface areas and NTG contents.

For complete prescribing information, refer to the Nitrates group monograph.

Indications

➤*Angina pectoris:* Prevention of angina pectoris due to coronary artery disease.

Administration and Dosage

Transdermal systems are continuously absorbed into systemic circulation from a pad applied to skin.

Patient instructions for application are provided with products.

Apply once daily to a skin site free of hair and not subject to excessive movement. Do not apply to distal parts of extremities. Avoid areas with cuts or irritations.

Individualize dosage. Titrate dose as needed for optimum effect.

➤*Starting dose:* 0.2 to 0.4 mg/hr. Doses between 0.4 and 0.8 mg/hr have shown continued effectiveness for 10 to 12 hours daily for at least 1 month of intermittent administration. Although the minimum nitrate-free interval has not been defined, data show that a nitrate-free interval of 10 to 12 hours is sufficient. Thus, an appropriate dosing schedule would include a daily "patch-on" period of 12 to 14 hours and a "patch-off" period of 10 to 12 hours. Tolerance is a major factor limiting efficacy when the system is used continuously for > 12 hours each day.

These products differ in delivery system mechanism. The most important common denominator is amount of drug released per hour. However, a wide range of patient variability has been seen in bioavailability studies. The skin is a major factor influencing absorption rate; physical exercise and elevated ambient temperatures (eg, sauna) may increase the absorption. Other factors are related to the patient's preference and product differences: Ease of application and removal, adhesiveness, comfort, size and appearance.

Nitrate tolerance may be more likely with higher dosages, longer acting products or more frequent dosing. Transdermal systems release nitroglycerin at a constant rate and maintain steady-state plasma concentration; thus, tolerance may occur (see Precautions and Administration and Dosage).

NITROGLYCERIN, TOPICAL

Rx	**Nitroglycerin** (Various, eg, Fougera, IDE, Parmed)	**Ointment:** 2% in a lanolin-petrolatum base	In 30 and 60 g tubes.
Rx	**Nitro-Bid** (Hoechst Marion Roussel)		In 20 and 60 g tubes and UD 1 g (100s).

For complete prescribing information, refer to the Nitrates group monograph.

Indications

➤*Angina:* Prevention and treatment of angina pectoris due to coronary artery disease.

Administration and Dosage

➤*Usual therapeutic dose:* 1 to 2 inches (25 to 50 mm) every 8 hours, up to 4 to 5 inches (100 to 125 mm) every 4 hours. Start with ½ inch (12.5 mm) every 8 hours; increase by ½ inch with each application to achieve desired effects. The greatest attainable decrease in resting blood pressure not associated with clinical hypotension, especially during orthostasis, indicates optimal dosage.

To apply ointment, use the applicator or dose-measuring paper to spread in a thin uniform layer over at least a 2¼ x 3½ inch area. The ointment may be applied to the chest or back.

One inch (25 mm) of ointment contains ≈ 15 mg nitroglycerin.

AMYL NITRITE

Rx	Amyl Nitrite (Various, eg, Goldline, Moore)	Inhalant: 0.3 mL	In 12s.
Rx	Amyl Nitrite Aspirols (Lilly)		In 12s.
Rx	Amyl Nitrite Vaporole (B-W)		In 12s.

For complete prescribing information, refer to the Nitrates group monograph.

Indications

Relief of angina pectoris.

Administration and Dosage

Usual adult dose is 0.3 mL by inhalation, as required.

Crush the capsule and wave under the nose; 1 to 6 inhalations from one capsule are usually sufficient to produce the desired effect. May repeat in 3 to 5 minutes.

▶ *Storage / Stability:* Protect from light. Store in a cool place, 15° to 30°C (59° to 86°F).

ISOXSUPRINE HCl

Rx	Isoxsuprine HCl (Various)	Tablets: 10 mg	In 60s, 100s, 500s, 1000s and UD 100s.
Rx	Vasodilan (Mead Johnson)		(10 MJ 543). In 100s, 1000s and UD 1000s.
Rx	Voxsuprine (Major)		In 100s, 250s, 1000s and UD 100s.
Rx	Isoxsuprine HCl (Various)	Tablets: 20 mg	In 60s, 100s, 500s, 1000s and UD 100s.
Rx	Vasodilan (Mead Johnson)		(20 MJ 544). In 100s and 1000s.
Rx	Voxsuprine (Major)		In 100s, 250s, 1000s and UD 100s.

For complete prescribing information, refer to the Antihypertensives Treatment Guidelines in the Appendix.

Indications

➤*"Possibly effective"*: For relief of symptoms associated with cerebral vascular insufficiency; peripheral vascular disease of arteriosclerosis obliterans, thromboangitis obliterans (Buerger's disease) and Raynaud's disease.

➤*Unlabeled uses:* Isoxsuprine has been used in the treatment of dysmenorrhea and threatened premature labor (see Warnings), but efficacy has not been established.

Administration and Dosage

10 to 20 mg, 3 or 4 times daily.

Actions

➤*Pharmacology:* Isoxsuprine is a vasodilator that acts primarily on blood vessels within skeletal muscle. In healthy subjects, resting blood flow in skeletal muscle is increased; cutaneous blood flow is usually not affected. Isoxsuprine is an α-adrenoreceptor antagonist with β-adrenoreceptor stimulating properties; however, vasodilation is not blocked by propranolol. Isoxsuprine may act directly on vascular smooth muscle. The drug also causes cardiac stimulation (increased contractility, heart rate and cardiac output) and uterine relaxation. At high doses, it lowers blood viscosity and inhibits platelet aggregation.

Contraindications

Immediately postpartum; in the presence of arterial bleeding.

Warnings

➤*Rash:* If rash appears, discontinue use. A causal relationship is not established.

➤*Pregnancy: Category C.* There are no reports of isoxsuprine causing congenital defects. Hypotension, hypocalcemia, hypoglycemia, ileus, tachycardia and death have occurred when cord serum levels are > 10 ng/mL.

Pulmonary edema has been reported in mothers treated with β-stimulants. Isoxsuprine is neither approved nor recommended for the treatment of premature labor; more selective agents are available (see the Ritodrine monograph in the Endocrine and Metabolic Agents chapter).

Adverse Reactions

➤*Cardiovascular:* Hypotension; tachycardia; chest pain.

➤*GI:* Nausea; vomiting; abdominal distress.

➤*Miscellaneous:* Dizziness; weakness; severe rash (see Warnings).

Patient Information

May cause palpitations or skin rash. Notify physician if these symptoms become particularly bothersome.

If dizziness (orthostatic hypotension) occurs, avoid sudden changes in posture.

PAPAVERINE HCl

Rx	Papaverine HCl (Various)	Capsules, timed release: 150 mg	In 100s and 1000s.
Rx	Pavagen TD (Rugby)		In 100s, 500s and 1000s.
Rx	Papaverine HCl (Various)	Injection: 30 mg/mL	In 2 mL vials and 10 mL multiple-dose vials.

For complete prescribing information, refer to the Antihypertensives Treatment Guidelines in the Appendix.

Indications

➤*Ischemia:* For relief of cerebral and peripheral ischemia associated with arterial spasm and myocardial ischemia complicated by arrhythmias.

Administration and Dosage

150 mg every 12 hours. In difficult cases, increase to 150 mg every 8 hours, or 300 mg every 12 hours.

Actions

➤*Pharmacology:* Papaverine directly relaxes the tonus of various smooth muscle, especially when it has been spasmodically contracted. It relaxes the smooth musculature of the larger blood vessels, especially coronary, systemic peripheral and pulmonary arteries. Vasodilation may be related to its ability to inhibit cyclic nucleotide phosphodiesterase, thus increasing levels of intracellular cyclic AMP. During administration, the muscle cell is not paralyzed and still responds to drugs and other stimuli causing contraction. The antispasmodic effect is direct and unrelated to muscle innervation. It has little effect on the CNS, although very large doses tend to produce some sedation and sleepiness. In certain situations, mild respiratory stimulation can be observed because of stimulation of carotid and aortic body chemoreceptors.

Possibly because of its direct vasodilating action on cerebral blood vessels, papaverine increases cerebral blood flow and decreases cerebral vascular resistance in healthy subjects; oxygen consumption is unaltered. These effects have been used to explain the reported benefits in cerebral vascular encephalopathy.

Papaverine acts on the heart to depress conduction and irritability and to prolong the refractory period of the myocardium, which provide the basis for its clinical trial in abrogating atrial and ventricular premature systoles and ominous ventricular arrhythmias. The coronary vasodilator action could be an additional factor of therapeutic value when such rhythms are secondary to insufficiency or occlusion of the coronary arteries.

➤*Pharmacokinetics:*

Absorption/Distribution – Oral bioavailability is ≈ 54%. Peak plasma levels occur 1 to 2 hours after a dose.

Metabolism/Excretion – Papaverine is metabolized in the liver. Although estimates of its biologic half-life vary widely, reasonably constant plasma levels can be maintained after 4 days with regular administration at 6-hour intervals. The drug is excreted in the urine in an inactive form.

Contraindications

Large doses can depress atrioventricular and intraventricular conduction and thereby produce serious arrhythmias (see Warnings).

Warnings

➤*Cardiac:* Large doses can depress AV and intraventricular conduction and thereby produce serious arrhythmias. When conduction is depressed, it may produce transient ectopy of ventricular origin, either premature beats or paroxysmal tachycardia.

In patients with acute coronary thrombosis, the occurrence of ventricular cardiac arrhythmias is serious and requires measures designed to decrease myocardial irritability.

➤*Hepatic toxicity:* Chronic hepatitis, as evidenced by an increase in serum bilirubin and serum glutamic transaminase, has been reported in three cases following long-term papaverine therapy. One patient had jaundice, and another had abnormal liver function on biopsy.

➤*Pregnancy: Category C.* Safety for use during pregnancy has not been established. Use only when clearly needed and when the potential benefits outweigh the potential hazards to the fetus.

➤*Lactation:* It is not known whether this drug is excreted in breast milk. Safety for use in the nursing mother has not been established.

➤*Children:* Safety and efficacy for use in children have not been established.

Precautions

➤*Glaucoma:* Use with caution in patients with glaucoma.

Drug Interactions

➤*Levodopa:* Loss of control of Parkinson's disease may occur following the introduction of papaverine. Although the mechanism is unknown, papaverine may block dopamine receptors in the striatum.

Adverse Reactions

➤*Cardiovascular:* Increase in heart rate and depth of respiration; slight increase in blood pressure.

➤*CNS:* Vertigo; drowsiness; excessive sedation; headache.

➤*GI:* Nausea; abdominal distress; anorexia; constipation; diarrhea.

PAPAVERINE HCl

➤*Miscellaneous:* Sweating; flushing of face; skin rash; malaise; hepatic hypersensitivity; chronic hepatitis (see Warnings).

Overdosage

➤*Ingestion:* Injestion of > 10 times the usual therapeutic dose has not resulted in untoward effects; however, a single dose of 0.1 to 0.5 g/kg could be fatal to an adult.

➤*Acute poisoning:*

Symptoms – Drowsiness, weakness, nystagmus, diplopia, incoordination and lassitude, progressing to coma with cyanosis and respiratory depression.

Treatment – To delay drug absorption, give tap water, milk or activated charcoal; then evacuate stomach contents by gastric lavage or emesis, followed by catharsis. If coma and respiratory depression occur, take appropriate measures. Hemodialysis has been suggested. Maintain blood pressure. Avoid concurrent administration of other depressant drugs.

➤*Chronic poisoning:*

Symptoms – Drowsiness, depression, weakness, anxiety, ataxia, headache, blurred vision, gastric upset and pruritic skin rashes characterized by urticaria or erythematous macular eruptions. Any of the formed elements of the blood may be decreased in number.

Treatment – Discontinue medication at the onset of any unusual symptoms or abnormal hematologic findings. Severe hypotension may occur. Recovery should occur, except in patients with aplastic anemia.

Patient Information

May cause dizziness (hypotension) or drowsiness; use caution when driving or performing other tasks requiring alertness, coordination or physical dexterity. Alcohol may intensify these effects.

May cause flushing, sweating, headache, tiredness, jaundice, skin rash, nausea, anorexia, abdominal distress, constipation or diarrhea. Notify physician if these effects become pronounced.

HYDRALAZINE HCl

Rx	Hydralazine (Various, eg, Camall, Goldline, Rugby, Schein)	**Tablets:** 10 mg	In 100s, 1000s and UD 100s.
Rx	Apresoline (Novartis)		Lactose. Yellow. In 100s and 1200s.
Rx	Hydralazine (Various, eg, Camall, Goldline, Rugby)	**Tablets:** 25 mg	In 100s, 1000s and UD 100s.
Rx	Apresoline (Novartis)		Blue. In 100s and 1000s.
Rx	Hydralazine (Various, eg, Camall, Goldline, Rugby)	**Tablets:** 50 mg	In 100s, 1000s and UD 100s.
Rx	Apresoline (Novartis)		Lactose. Light blue. In 100s and 1000s.
Rx	Hydralazine (Various, eg, Camall, Goldline, Rugby)	**Tablets:** 100 mg	In 100s and 1000s.
Rx	Apresoline (Novartis)		Tartrazine. Peach. In 100s.
Rx	Hydralazine (Solopak)	**Injection:** 20 mg per mL	In 1 mL vials.

For complete prescribing information, refer to the Antihypertensives Treatment Guidelines in the Appendix.

Indications

➤*Oral:* Essential hypertension, alone or in combination with other agents.

➤*Parenteral:* Severe essential hypertension when the drug cannot be given orally or when the need to lower blood pressure is urgent.

➤*Unlabeled uses:* Hydralazine in doses up to 800 mg 3 times daily has been effective in reducing afterload in the treatment of congestive heart failure (CHF), severe aortic insufficiency and after valve replacement.

Administration and Dosage

The bioavailability of hydralazine tablets is enhanced by the concurrent ingestion of food.

➤*Initiate therapy:* Gradually increase dosages; individualize dosage. Start with 10 mg 4 times daily for the first 2 to 4 days, increase to 25 mg 4 times daily for the balance of the first week.

➤*Second and subsequent weeks:* Increase dosage to 50 mg 4 times daily.

➤*Maintenance:* Adjust dosage to lowest effective level. Twice daily dosage may be adequate. In a few resistant patients, up to 300 mg/day may be required for a significant antihypertensive effect. In such cases, consider a lower dosage of hydralazine combined with a thiazide and/or reserpine or a beta blocker. However, when combining therapy, individual titration is essential to ensure the lowest possible therapeutic dose of each drug.

Children – 0.75 mg/kg/day initially in 4 divided doses. Dosage may be increased gradually over the next 3 to 4 weeks to a maximum of 7.5 mg/kg or 200 mg daily.

➤*Parenteral:* Therapy in the hospitalized patient may be initiated IV or IM. Use parenterally only when the drug cannot be given orally. Usual dose is 20 to 40 mg, repeated as necessary. Certain patients (especially those with marked renal damage) may require a lower dose. Check blood pressure frequently; it may begin to fall within a few minutes after injection; average maximal decrease occurs in 10 to 80 minutes. Where there is a previously existing increased intracranial pressure, lowering the blood pressure may increase cerebral ischemia. Most patients can transfer to the oral form in 24 to 48 hrs.

Children – 0.1 to 0.2 mg/kg/dose every 4 to 6 hours as needed.

Eclampsia – Hydralazine is the drug of choice. A dose of 5 to 10 mg every 20 minutes as an IV bolus has been recommended. If there is no effect after 20 mg, try another agent.

➤*Storage/Stability:* Use hydralazine injection as quickly as possible after drawing through a needle into a syringe. Hydralazine changes color after contact with a metal filter.

Actions

➤*Pharmacology:* Hydralazine exerts a peripheral vasodilating effect through a direct relaxation of vascular smooth muscle. Hydralazine, by altering cellular calcium metabolism, interferes with the calcium movements within the vascular smooth muscle that are responsible for initiating or maintaining the contractile state.

The peripheral vasodilating effect of hydralazine results in decreased arterial blood pressure (diastolic more than systolic); decreased peripheral vascular resistance; and an increased heart rate, stroke volume and cardiac output. The preferential dilation of arterioles, as compared to veins, minimizes postural hypotension and promotes the increase in cardiac output. Hydralazine usually increases the renin activity in plasma, presumably as a result of increased secretion of renin by the renal juxtaglomerular cells in response to reflex sympathetic discharge. This increase in renin activity leads to the production of angiotensin II, which then causes stimulation of aldosterone and consequent sodium reabsorption. The drug also maintains or increases renal and cerebral blood flow. Because of the reflex increases in cardiac function, hydralazine is commonly used in combination with a drug which inhibits sympathetic activity (ie, beta blockers, clonidine, methyldopa).

➤*Pharmacokinetics:* Hydralazine is rapidly absorbed after oral use. Half-life is 3 to 7 hours. Protein binding is 87%, and bioavailability is 30% to 50%. Plasma levels vary widely among individuals. Peak plasma concentrations occur 1 to 2 hours after ingestion; duration of action is 6 to 12 hours. Hypotensive effects are seen 10 to 20 minutes after parenteral use and last 2 to 4 hours. Hydralazine is subject to polymorphic acetylation; slow acetylators generally have higher plasma levels of hydralazine and require lower doses to maintain control of blood pressure. Hydralazine undergoes extensive hepatic metabolism; it is excreted in the urine as active drug (12% to 14%) and metabolites.

Contraindications

Hypersensitivity to hydralazine; coronary artery disease; mitral valvular rheumatic heart disease.

Warnings

➤*Lupus erythematosus:* Hydralazine may produce a clinical picture simulating systemic lupus erythematosus (eg, arthralgia, dermatoses, fever, splenomegaly) including glomerulonephritis. Symptoms usually regress when the drug is discontinued, but residual effects have been detected years later. Long-term treatment with steroids may be necessary. Lupus occurs more frequently in "slow acetylators". The syndrome usually occurs after at least 6 months of continuous therapy. Although hydralazine-induced lupus may develop in patients on low doses, the likelihood increases with larger doses and with long duration of therapy. In one study, hydralazine use for 3 years duration resulted in drug-induced lupus in 5.4% of patients on 100 mg/day, 10.4% on 200 mg/day, and no patients on 50 mg/day. It is also more common in women and whites vs men and blacks, respectively.

Perform complete blood counts and antinuclear antibody (ANA) titer determinations before and during prolonged therapy, even in the asymptomatic patient. These studies are also indicated if the patient develops arthralgia, fever, chest pain, continued malaise or other unexplained signs or symptoms. If the ANA titer reaction is positive, carefully weigh benefits to be derived from hydralazine.

➤*Renal function impairment:* In hypertensive patients with normal kidneys who are treated with hydralazine, there is evidence of increased renal blood flow and a maintenance of glomerular filtration

HYDRALAZINE HCl

rate. Renal function may improve where control values were below normal prior to administration. Use with caution in patients with advanced renal damage.

➤*Pregnancy: Category C.* Studies in mice indicate that high doses of hydralazine are teratogenic (cleft palate and facial and cranial bone malformations). There are no adequate and well controlled studies in pregnant women. Safety for use during pregnancy has not been established. Use only when the potential benefits outweigh potential hazards to the fetus.

Thrombocytopenia, leukopenia, petechial bleeding and hematomas have been reported in newborns of females taking hydralazine. Symptoms resolved spontaneously within 1 to 3 weeks.

➤*Lactation:* Hydralazine is excreted in breast milk. Exercise caution when administering to a nursing woman. Hydralazine is compatible with breastfeeding according to the American Academy of Pediatrics.

➤*Children:* Safety and efficacy for use in children have not been established in controlled clinical trials, although there is experience with use in children (see Administration and Dosage).

Precautions

➤*Cardiovascular:* The "hyperdynamic" circulation caused by hydralazine may accentuate specific cardiovascular inadequacies (eg, increased pulmonary artery pressure in patients with mitral valvular disease). It may reduce the pressor responses to epinephrine. Postural hypotension may result from hydralazine but is less common than with ganglionic blocking agents. Use with caution in patients with cerebral vascular accidents.

Coronary artery disease – Myocardial stimulation produced by hydralazine can cause anginal attacks and ECG changes of myocardial ischemia. The drug has been implicated in the production of myocardial infarction. Use with caution in patients with suspected coronary artery disease.

Pulmonary hypertension – Use hydralazine with caution in patients with pulmonary hypertension. Severe hypotension may result. Monitor carefully.

Lipids – Hydralazine may cause some decrease in total cholesterol.

➤*Peripheral neuritis:* As evidenced by paresthesias, numbness and tingling, has been observed. Evidence suggests an antipyridoxine effect; add pyridoxine to the regimen if symptoms develop.

➤*Hematologic effects:* Blood dyscrasias consisting of reduction in hemoglobin and red cell count, leukopenia, agranulocytosis and purpura have been reported. If such abnormalities develop, discontinue therapy. Periodic blood counts are advised.

➤*Tartrazine sensitivity:* Some of these products contain tartrazine, which may cause allergic-type reactions (including bronchial asthma) in susceptible individuals. Although the incidence of tartrazine sensitivity in the general population is low, it is frequently seen in patients who also have aspirin hypersensitivity. Specific products containing tartrazine are identified in the product listings.

Drug Interactions

Hydralazine Drug Interactions

Precipitant drug	Object drug*		Description
Beta blockers Metoprolol Propranolol	Hydralazine	↑	Serum levels of either drug may be increased by concurrent use.
Hydralazine	Beta blockers Metoprolol Propranolol	↑	
Indomethacin	Hydralazine	↓	The pharmacologic effects of hydralazine may be decreased.

* ↑ = Object drug increased. ↓ = Object drug decreased.

➤*Drug/Food interactions:* Administration with food results in higher plasma hydralazine levels.

Adverse Reactions

Adverse reactions with hydralazine are usually reversible when dosage is reduced. However, it may be necessary to discontinue the drug.

➤*Cardiovascular:* Palpitations; tachycardia; angina pectoris.

➤*CNS:* Peripheral neuritis evidenced by paresthesia, numbness and tingling (see Precautions); headache; dizziness; tremors; psychotic reactions characterized by depression, disorientation or anxiety.

➤*GI:* Constipation; paralytic ileus; nausea; vomiting; diarrhea.

➤*Hematologic:* Blood dyscrasias, consisting of reduction in hemoglobin and RBC, leukopenia, agranulocytosis and purpura (see Precautions); lymphadenopathy; splenomegaly.

➤*Hypersensitivity:* Rash; urticaria; pruritus; fever; chills; arthralgia; eosinophilia; hepatitis (rare).

➤*Ophthalmic:* Lacrimation; conjunctivitis.

➤*Miscellaneous:* Nasal congestion; flushing; edema; muscle cramps; hypotension; paradoxical pressor response; dyspnea; urination difficulty; anorexia; lupus-like syndrome (see Warnings); hoarseness due to drug-induced lupus. The incidence of toxic reactions, particularly the LE syndrome, is high in the group of patients receiving large doses of hydralazine. (See Warnings.)

Overdosage

No deaths due to acute poisoning have been reported. Highest known dose survived in adults is 10 g orally.

➤*Symptoms:* Hypotension, tachycardia, headache and generalized skin flushing. Complications can include myocardial ischemia and subsequent myocardial infarction, cardiac arrhythmias and profound shock.

➤*Treatment:* There is no specific antidote. Evacuate gastric contents, prevent aspiration and protect the airway; instill activated charcoal slurry, if possible. These manipulations may have to be omitted or carried out after cardiovascular status has been stabilized, since they might precipitate cardiac arrhythmias or increase the depth of shock.

Cardiovascular support is of primary importance. Treat shock with volume expanders without vasopressors. If necessary, use a vasopressor that is least likely to precipitate or aggravate cardiac arrhythmias. Tachycardia responds to beta blockers. Digitalization may be necessary. Monitor renal function and support as required.

No experience has been reported with extracorporeal or peritoneal dialysis.

Patient Information

Take with meals.

Notify physician of any unexplained prolonged general tiredness or fever, muscle or joint aching or chest pain.

MINOXIDIL

Rx	**Minoxidil** (Various, eg, Elkins-Sinn, PAR, Southwood, URL, Watson)	**Tablets:** 2.5 mg		In 100s, 500s, and 1000s.
Rx	**Loniten** (Upjohn)			Lactose. (U 121 2½ mg). Scored. In 100s.
Rx	**Minoxidil** (Various, eg, Major, PAR, Southwood, URL, Watson)	**Tablets:** 10 mg		In 100s, 500s and 1000s.
Rx	**Loniten** (Upjohn)			Lactose. (LONITEN 10). Scored. In 100s.

For complete prescribing information, refer to the Antihypertensives Treatment Guidelines in the Appendix.

> ## WARNING
>
> Minoxidil may produce serious adverse effects. It can cause pericardial effusion, occasionally progressing to tamponade, and it can exacerbate angina pectoris. Reserve for hypertensive patients who do not respond adequately to maximum therapeutic doses of a diuretic and 2 other antihypertensive agents.
>
> In experimental animals, minoxidil caused several kinds of myocardial lesions and other adverse cardiac effects (see Warnings).
>
> Administer under close supervision, usually concomitantly with a β-adrenergic blocking agent, to prevent tachycardia and increased myocardial workload. Usually, it must be given with a diuretic, frequently one acting in the ascending limb of the loop of Henle to prevent serious fluid accumulation. When first administering minoxidil, hospitalize and monitor patients with malignant hypertension and those already receiving guanethidine (see Drug Interactions) to avoid too rapid or large orthostatic decreases in blood pressure.

Indications

➤*Severe hypertension:* Severe hypertension that is symptomatic or associated with target organ damage, and is not manageable with maximum therapeutic doses of a diuretic plus 2 other antihypertensives. Use in milder degrees of hypertension is not recommended because the benefit-risk ratio in such patients has not been defined.

Topical minoxidil is used for the treatment of male pattern baldness (alopecia androgenetica) of the vertex of the scalp (see Minoxidil Topical Solution monograph in the Dermatological Agents chapter). Use of the tablets, in any formulation, to promote hair growth is not an approved use. Effects of extemporaneous formulations and dosages have not been shown to be safe and effective.

Administration and Dosage

➤*Approved by the FDA:* October 1979.

➤*Adults and children (over 12 years of age):* Initial dosage is 5 mg/day as a single dose. Daily dosage can be increased to 10, 20, then 40 mg in single or divided doses if required. Effective range is usually 10 to 40 mg/day. Maximum dosage is 100 mg/day.

➤*Children (less than 12 years of age):* Initial dosage is 0.2 mg/kg/day as a single dose. Dose may be increased in 50 to 100% increments until optimum blood pressure control is achieved. Effective range is usually 0.25 to 1 mg/kg/day. Maximum dosage is 50 mg daily. Experience in children is limited, particularly in infants; monitor closely. Titrate carefully for optimal effects.

➤*Dose frequency:* The magnitude of within-day fluctuation of arterial pressure during therapy is directly proportional to the extent of pressure reduction. If supine diastolic pressure has been reduced less than 30 mm Hg, administer the drug only once a day; if reduced more than 30 mm Hg, divide the daily dosage into 2 equal parts.

➤*Dosage adjustment intervals:* Must be carefully titrated and adjusted at at 3-day intervals or more because full response to a given dose is not attained until then. If more rapid management is required, adjustments can be made every 6 hours with careful monitoring.

➤*Concomitant drug therapy:*

Diuretics – Use minoxidil with a diuretic in patients relying on renal function for maintaining salt and water balance. Diuretics have been used at the following dosages when starting minoxidil therapy: hydrochlorothiazide (50 mg twice daily) or other thiazides at equally effective doses; chlorthalidone (50 to 100 mg/day); furosemide (40 mg twice daily). If excessive salt and water retention results in a weight gain of more than 2.3 kg (5 lb), change diuretic therapy to furosemide. In furosemide-treated patients, increase dosage in accordance with their needs.

Beta-blockers/Other sympathetic nervous system suppressants – When beginning therapy, the β-blocker dosage should be equal to 80 to 160 mg/day propranolol in divided doses. If β-blockers are contraindicated, use methyldopa 250 to 750 mg twice daily; give for at least 24 hours before starting minoxidil due to delay in onset. Clonidine may also be used to prevent tachycardia induced by minoxidil; usual dosage is 0.1 to 0.2 mg twice daily.

Sympathetic nervous system suppressants may not completely prevent a heart rate increase, but usually prevent tachycardia. Typically, patients receiving a β-blocker prior to minoxidil have bradycardia; expect an increase in heart rate toward normal when minoxidil is added. Simultaneous treatment with minoxidil and a β-blocker or other sympathetic nervous system suppressant causes little change in heart rate, since their opposing cardiac effects usually nullify each other.

➤*Storage/Stability:* Store *Loniten* at controlled room temperature of 20° to 25°C (68° to 77°F); store minoxidil at controlled room temperature of 15° to 30°C (59° to 86°F).

Actions

➤*Pharmacology:* Minoxidil is a direct-acting peripheral vasodilator. It does not interfere with vasomotor reflexes; therefore, it does not produce orthostatic hypotension. The drug does not affect CNS function.

Because it causes peripheral vasodilation, minoxidil elicits a reduction of peripheral arteriolar resistance. This action, with the associated fall in blood pressure, triggers sympathetic, vagal inhibitory, and renal homeostatic mechanisms, including an increase in renin secretion, which leads to increased cardiac rate and output, and salt and water retention. These adverse effects can usually be minimized by coadministration of a diuretic and a β-adrenergic blocking agent or other sympathetic nervous system suppressant.

Antihypertensive effects – Minoxidil reduces elevated systolic and diastolic blood pressure by decreasing peripheral vascular resistance. The blood pressure response to minoxidil is dose-related and proportional to the extent of hypertension. In humans, forearm and renal vascular resistance decline; forearm blood flow increases while renal blood flow and glomerular filtration rate (GFR) are preserved.

When used in severely hypertensive patients resistant to other therapy, frequently with an accompanying diuretic and β-adrenergic blocker, minoxidil decreased the blood pressure and reversed encephalopathy and retinopathy. The drug reduced supine diastolic blood pressure by 20 mm Hg, or by 90 mm Hg or less in approximately 75% of the patients studied.

➤*Pharmacokinetics:*

Absorption/Distribution – Minoxidil is not protein bound and is at least 90% absorbed from the GI tract. Plasma levels of the parent drug reach a maximum within the first hour and decline rapidly thereafter.

Onset/Duration: The extent and time course of blood pressure reduction by minoxidil do not correspond closely to its plasma concentration. After an effective single oral dose, blood pressure usually starts to decline within 30 minutes, reaches a minimum between 2 and 3 hours and recovers at a linear rate of about 30% per day. The total duration of effect is approximately 75 hours.

When minoxidil is administered chronically once or twice a day, the time required to achieve maximum effect on blood pressure is inversely related to the size of the dose. Thus, maximum effect is achieved on 10 mg/day within 7 days, on 20 mg/day within 5 days, and on 40 mg/day within 3 days.

Metabolism/Excretion – Predominantly by conjugation with glucuronic acid, 90% is metabolized. Metabolites exert much less pharmacologic effect than minoxidil itself; all are excreted principally in the urine. Renal clearance corresponds to the GFR. Minoxidil and its metabolites are hemodialyzable. Average plasma half-life is 4.2 hours.

Contraindications

Hypersensitivity to any component of the product; pheochromocytoma (because the drug may stimulate secretion of catecholamines from the tumor through its antihypertensive action).

Warnings

➤*Mild hypertension:* Because of potential for serious adverse effects, use in milder degrees of hypertension is not recommended; benefit-risk ratio in such patients is not defined.

➤*Cardiac lesions:*

Animal toxicology – Minoxidil has produced cardiac lesions in animals in general, including grossly visible hemorrhagic lesions of the atrium, epicardium, endocardium, and walls of small arteries and arterioles; necrosis of papillary muscles and subendocardial areas of left ventricle. Cardiac hypertrophy and dilation occurred but was partly reversed by diuretics in monkeys, suggesting increased heart weight may be related to fluid overload. In a 1-year dog study, serosanguinous pericardial fluid was noted.

Human toxicology – Autopsies of 150 patients who died from various causes who had also received minoxidil did not reveal right atrial or other hemorrhagic pathology of the kind seen in dogs. Instances of necrotic areas in papillary muscles were seen, but occurred in the presence of known pre-existing ischemic heart disease and did not appear different from or more common than lesions in patients never exposed to minoxidil.

MINOXIDIL

➤*ECG changes:* Rarely, a large negative amplitude of the T wave may encroach upon the ST segment, but the ST segment is not independently altered. These changes usually disappear with continuance of treatment and revert to the pretreatment state if therapy is discontinued. No symptoms, alterations in blood cell counts or plasma enzyme concentrations, or signs of myocardial damage have been noted. Long-term treatment of patients manifesting such changes has provided no evidence of deteriorating cardiac function. At present, the changes appear to be nonspecific and without identifiable clinical significance.

➤*Fluid and electrolyte balance:* Monitor fluid and electrolyte balance and body weight. Give with a diuretic to prevent fluid retention and possible CHF; a loop diuretic is usually required. If used without a diuretic, retention of several hundred mEq salt and corresponding volumes of water can occur in a few days, leading to increased plasma and interstitial fluid volume and local or generalized edema. Diuretics alone or with restricted salt intake usually minimize fluid retention, but reversible edema developed in approximately 10% of nondialysis patients so treated. Ascites has also occurred. Diuretic effectiveness is limited by impaired renal function. Condition of patients with pre-existing CHF occasionally deteriorates due to fluid retention, but because of the fall in blood pressure (afterload reduction), more than twice as many improve than worsen.

Refractory fluid retention rarely requires discontinuation of minoxidil. Under close medical supervision, it may be possible to resolve refractory salt retention by discontinuing the drug for 1 or 2 days, and then resuming treatment in conjunction with vigorous diuretic therapy.

➤*Tachycardia/Angina:* Minoxidil increases heart rate; this can be prevented by coadministration of a β-adrenergic blocking drug or other sympathetic nervous system suppressants (eg, clonidine, methyldopa). The ability of β-adrenergic blocking agents to minimize papillary muscle lesions in animals is further reason for such concomitant use.

In addition, angina may worsen or appear for the first time during treatment, probably because of the increased oxygen demands associated with increased heart rate and cardiac output. This can usually be prevented by sympathetic blockade or β-adrenergic blocking drugs.

➤*Pericardial effusion:* Occasionally with tamponade, it has occurred in about 3% of treated patients not on dialysis, especially those with inadequate or compromised renal function. Many cases were associated with connective tissue disease, the uremic syndrome, CHF, or fluid retention, but were instances in which these potential causes of effusion were not present. Observe patients closely for signs of pericardial disorder. Perform echocardiographic studies if suspicion arises. More vigorous diuretic therapy, dialysis, pericardiocentesis, or surgery may be required. If the effusion persists, consider drug withdrawal.

➤*Hazard of rapid control of blood pressure:* Too rapid control of very severe blood pressure elevation can precipitate syncope, cerebrovascular accidents, MI, and ischemia of special sense organs with resulting decrease or loss of vision or hearing. Patients with compromised circulation or cryoglobulinemia may also suffer ischemic episodes of affected organs. Although such events have not been unequivocally associated with minoxidil use, experience is limited.

Hospitalize any patient with malignant hypertension during initial treatment to assure that blood pressure is not falling more rapidly than intended.

➤*Hemodilution:* Hematocrit, hemoglobin, and erythrocyte count usually fall about 7% initially and then recover to pretreatment levels.

➤*Hypersensitivity reactions:* Manifested as a skin rash, hypersensitivity reactions occur in fewer than 1% of patients and rare reports of bullous eruptions and Stevens-Johnson syndrome. Deciding whether the drug should be discontinued depends on treatment alternatives.

➤*Renal function impairment:* Renal failure or dialysis patients may require smaller doses; closely supervise to prevent precipitation of cardiac failure or exacerbation of renal failure.

➤*Carcinogenesis:* Dietary administration of minoxidil to mice for up to 2 years was associated with an increased incidence of malignant lymphomas in females at all dose levels (10, 25, and 63 mg/kg/day) and an increased incidence of hepatic nodules in males (63 mg/kg/day). There was no effect of dietary minoxidil on the incidence of malignant liver tumors.

➤*Fertility impairment:* In rats given 1or 5 times the maximum recommended human dose, there was a dose-dependent reduction in conception rate.

➤*Elderly:* Clinical studies did not include sufficient numbers of subjects 65 years of age and older to determine whether they respond differently from younger subjects. Other reported clinical experience has not identified differences in responses between elderly and younger patients. In general, dose selection for an elderly patient should be cautious, usually starting at the low end of the dosing range, reflecting the greater frequency of decreased hepatic, renal, or cardiac function, and of concomitant disease or other drug therapy.

➤*Pregnancy:* Category C. Minoxidil reduced conception rate and increased fetal absorption in small animals when administered at 5 times the human dose. There are no adequate and well-controlled studies in pregnant women. Use only when clearly needed and when potential benefits outweigh potential hazards to the fetus.

➤*Lactation:* Safety for use in the nursing mother has not been established. Minoxidil is excreted in breast milk; do not nurse while taking minoxidil.

➤*Children:* Use in children is limited, particularly in infants. The recommendations under Administration and Dosage are only a rough guide; careful titration is essential.

Precautions

➤*Monitoring:* Monitor initially and periodically thereafter body weight, blood pressure, fluid, and electrolyte balance; signs and symptoms of pericardial effusion; ECG changes; CBC; alkaline phosphatase; renal function tests.

➤*Myocardial infarction:* Minoxidil has not been used in patients who have had an MI within the preceding month. A reduction in arterial pressure with the drug might further limit blood flow to the myocardium, although this might be compensated by decreased oxygen demand because of lower blood pressure.

➤*Hypertrichosis:* Elongation, thickening, and enhanced pigmentation of fine body hair develops within 3- to 6-weeks after starting therapy in approximately 80% of patients. It is usually first noticed on the temples, between the eyebrows, between the hairline and the eyebrows, or in the sideburn area of the upper lateral cheek, later extending to the back, arms, legs, and scalp. Upon discontinuation of the drug, new hair growth stops, but 1- to 6-months may be required for restoration to pretreatment appearance.

No endocrine abnormalities have been found to explain the abnormal hair growth; thus, it is hypertrichosis without virilism. Inform patients (especially children and women) about this effect before therapy.

➤*Lab test abnormalities:* Repeat tests that are abnormal at initiation of minoxidil therapy (eg, urinalysis, renal function tests, ECG, chest x-ray, echocardiogram) to ascertain whether improvement or deterioration is occurring under therapy. Initially, perform such tests frequently, at 1- to 3-month intervals, and as stabilization occurs, at 6- to 12-month intervals.

Drug Interactions

➤*Guanethidine:* Although minoxidil does not cause orthostatic hypotension, use in patients on guanethidine can result in profound orthostatic effects. If possible, discontinue guanethidine well before minoxidil is instituted. If this is not possible, start minoxidil in the hospital and institutionalize the patient until severity of effects are no longer present or the patient has learned to avoid activities that provoke them.

Adverse Reactions

➤*Cardiovascular:* Pericardial effusion and occasionally with tamponade (3%). Changes in direction and magnitude of T waves occur (approximately 60%). (See Warnings).

➤*GI:* Nausea; vomiting.

➤*Hematologic:* Initially, hematocrit, hemoglobin, and erythrocyte count usually fall about 7%, and then recover to pretreatment levels. Thrombocytopenia and leukopenia (WBC fewer than 3000/mm^3) have been reported rarely.

➤*Hypersensitivity:* Rashes including bullous eruptions (rare) and Stevens-Johnson syndrome. (See Warnings.)

➤*Lab test abnormalities:* Alkaline phosphatase increased varyingly without other evidence of liver or bone abnormality. Serum creatinine increased an average of 6% and BUN slightly more, but later declined to pretreatment levels.

➤*Miscellaneous:* Temporary edema (7%); breast tenderness (fewer than 1%).

Hypertrichosis – Elongation, thickening, and enhanced pigmentation of fine body hair develops within 3- to 6-weeks after starting therapy in approximately 80% of patients (see Precautions).

Overdosage

➤*Symptoms:* Exaggerated hypotension is likely in association with residual sympathetic nervous system blockade from previous therapy (guanethidine-like effects or alpha-adrenergic blockade), which prevents compensatory maintenance of blood pressure.

➤*Treatment:* Administer normal saline IV to maintain blood pressure and facilitate urine formation. Avoid sympathomimetics (eg, norepinephrine, epinephrine) with excessive cardiac stimulating action. Phenylephrine, angiotensin II, vasopressin, and dopamine reverse hypotension due to minoxidil, but use only in underperfusion of a vital organ.

Radioimmunoassay can determine plasma concentration. However, due to blood level variations, it is difficult to establish a warning level. At 100 mg/day, peak blood levels of 1641 and 2441 ng/mL were seen in two patients. Regard an increase greater than 2000 ng/mL as overdosage unless the patient has taken no more than the maximum dose.

MINOXIDIL

Patient Information

Patient package insert is available with product.

Minoxidil is usually taken with at least 2 other antihypertensive medications. Take all medications as prescribed; do not discontinue any except on advice of physician.

Enhanced growth and darkening of fine body hair (approximately 80% of patients) may occur; however, do not stop medication without consulting physician.

Notify physician immediately if any of the following occur: Heart rate increase of 20 bpm or more over normal; rapid weight gain of more than 5 pounds (2.3 kg); unusual swelling of extremities, face, or abdomen; breathing difficulty, especially when lying down; new or aggravated angina symptoms (chest, arm, or shoulder pain); severe indigestion; dizziness, lightheadedness, or fainting.

Nausea or vomiting may occur.

EPOPROSTENOL SODIUM (PGI$_2$; PGX; Prostacyclin)

Rx	Flolan (GlaxoWellcome)	**Powder for reconstitution:** 0.5 mg	Mannitol, NaCl. In 17 mL.
		1.5 mg	Mannitol, NaCl. In 17 mL.

For complete prescribing information, refer to the Antihypertensives Treatment Guidelines in the Appendix.

Indications

➤*Pulmonary hypertension:* Long-term IV treatment of primary pulmonary hypertension in NYHA Class III and Class IV patients (see Clinical Trials).

Administration and Dosage

➤*Approved by the FDA:* September 20, 1995.

➤*Acute dose ranging:* Determine the initial chronic infusion rate of epoprostenol using an acute dose-ranging procedure (see Precautions). In clinical trials, the mean maximum dose that did not elicit dose-limiting pharmacologic effects was 8.6 ng/kg/min.

➤*Continuous chronic infusion:* Administer chronic continous infusion through a central venous catheter. Temporary peripheral IV infusions may be used until central access is established. Initiate chronic infusions at 4 ng/kg/min less than the maximum-tolerated infusion (MTI) rate determined during acute dose ranging. If the MTI rate is < 5 ng/kg/min, start the chronic infusion at one-half the MTI rate. During clinical trials, the mean initial chronic infusion rate was 5 ng/kg/min.

➤*Dosage adjustments:*

Increments – Base changes in the chronic infusion rate on persistence, recurrence or worsening of the patient's symptoms of PPH and the occurrence of adverse events due to excessive doses. Expect increases from the initial chronic dose.

Consider increments in dose if symptoms of PPH persist or recur after improving. Increase the infusion by 1 to 2 ng/kg/min increments at intervals sufficient to allow assessment of clinical response; these intervals should be at least 15 minutes. Observe the patient and monitor standing and supine blood pressure and heart rate for several hours to ensure that the new dose is tolerated.

Decrements – During chronic infusion, the occurrence of dose-related pharmacological events similar to those observed during acute dose ranging may necessitate a decrease in infusion rate, but the adverse event may occasionally resolve without dosage adjustment. Gradually make 2 ng/kg/min decrements every 15 minutes or longer until the dose-limiting effects resolve. Avoid abrupt withdrawal or sudden large reductions in infusion rates.

In patients receiving lung transplants, doses of epoprostenol were tapered after the initiation of cardiopulmonary bypass.

➤*Administration:* Epoprostenol is administered by continuous IV infusion via a central venous catheter using an ambulatory infusion pump. During dose-ranging, epoprostenol sodium may be administered peripherally.

The ambulatory infusion pump used to administer epoprostenol should be: (1) Small and light weight; (2) able to adjust infusion rates in 2 ng/kg/min increments; (3) equipped with occlusion, end of infusion and low battery alarms; (4) accurate to ± 6% of the programmed rate; and (5) positive pressure driven (continuous or pulsating) with intervals between pulses not exceeding 3 minutes at infusion rates. The reservoir should be made of polyvinyl chloride, polypropylene or glass.

➤*Reconstitution: Important note:* Reconstituted solutions of epoprostenol must not be diluted or administered with other parenteral solutions or medications.

To make 100 mL solution with a final concentration of –

3000 ng/mL: Dissolve contents of one 0.5 mg vial with 5 mL diluent; withdraw 3 mL and add sufficient diluent to make 100 mL.

5000 ng/mL: Dissolve contents of one 0.5 mg vial with 5 mL diluent; withdraw entire contents and add sufficient diluent to make a total of 100 mL.

10,000 ng/mL: Dissolve contents of two 0.5 mg vials each with 5 mL diluent; withdraw entire contents and add sufficient diluent to make a total of 100 mL.

15,000 ng/mL: Dissolve contents of one 1.5 mg vial with 5 mL diluent; withdraw entire contents and add sufficient diluent to make a total of 100 mL.

Infusion rates – Calculated using the following formula:

$$\text{Infusion rate (mL/hr)} = \frac{[\text{Dose (ng/kg/min)} \times \text{Weight (kg)} \times 60]}{\text{final concentration (ng/mL)}}$$

The following table provides infusion delivery rates for doses ≤ 16 ng/kg/min based on patient weight, drug delivery rate and concentration of the solution to be used. This table may be used to select the most appropriate concentration of epoprostenol that will result in an infusion rate between the minimum and maximum flow rates of the infusion pump and that will allow the desired duration of infusion.

Infusion Rates for Epoprostenol (mL/hr)								
Dose or drug delivery rate (ng/kg/min)								
Patient weight (kg)	2	4	6	8	10	12	14	16
Concentration = 3000 ng/mL								
10	-	-	1.2	1.6	2	2.4	2.8	3.2
20	-	1.6	2.4	3.2	4	4.8	5.6	6.4
30	1.2	2.4	3.6	4.8	6	7.2	8.4	9.6
40	1.6	3.2	4.8	6.4	8	9.6	11.2	12.8
50	2	4	6	8	10	12	14	16
60	2.4	4.8	7.2	9.6	12	14.4	16.8	19.2
70	2.8	5.6	8.4	11.2	14	16.8	19.6	22.4
80	3.2	6.4	9.6	12.8	16	19.2	22.4	25.6
90	3.6	7.2	10.8	14.4	18	21.6	25.2	28.8
100	4	8	12	16	20	24	28	32
Concentration = 5000 ng/mL								
10	-	-	-	1	1.2	1.4	1.7	1.9
20	-	1	1.4	1.9	2.4	2.9	3.4	3.8
30	-	1.4	2.2	2.9	3.6	4.3	5	5.8
40	1	1.9	2.9	3.8	4.8	5.8	6.7	7.7
50	1.2	2.4	3.6	4.8	6	7.2	8.4	9.6
60	1.4	2.9	4.3	5.8	7.2	8.6	10.1	11.5
70	1.7	3.4	5	6.7	8.4	10.1	11.8	13.4
80	1.9	3.8	5.8	7.7	9.6	11.5	13.4	15.4
90	2.2	4.3	6.5	8.6	10.8	13	15.1	17.3
100	2.4	4.8	7.2	9.6	12	14.4	16.8	19.2
Concentration = 10,000 ng/mL								
10	-	-	-	-	-	-	-	-
20	-	-	-	1	1.2	1.4	1.7	1.9
30	-	-	1.1	1.4	1.8	2.2	2.5	2.9
40	-	1	1.4	1.9	2.4	2.9	3.4	3.8
50	-	1.2	1.8	2.4	3	3.6	4.2	4.8
60	-	1.4	2.2	2.9	3.6	4.3	5	5.8
70	-	1.7	2.5	3.4	4.2	5	5.9	6.7
80	-	1.9	2.9	3.8	4.8	5.8	6.7	7.7
90	-	2.2	3.2	4.3	5.4	6.5	7.6	8.6
100	-	2.4	3.6	4.8	6	7.2	8.4	9.6
Concentration = 15,000 ng/mL								
10	-	-	-	-	-	-	-	-
20	-	-	-	-	-	-	-	-
30	-	-	-	1	1.2	1.4	1.7	1.9
40	-	-	1	1.3	1.6	1.9	2.2	2.6
50	-	-	1.2	1.6	2	2.4	2.8	3.2
60	-	1	1.4	1.9	2.4	2.9	3.4	3.8
70	-	1.1	1.7	2.2	2.8	3.4	3.9	4.5
80	-	1.3	1.9	2.6	3.2	3.8	4.5	5.1
90	-	1.4	2.2	2.9	3.6	4.3	5	5.8
100	-	1.6	2.4	3.2	4	4.8	5.6	6.4

➤*Storage/Stability:* Store unopened vials at 15° to 25°C (59° to 77°F). Protect from light. Protect reconstituted solutions of epoprostenol from light and refrigerate at 2° to 8°C (36° to 46°F) for ≤ 40 hours. Do not freeze. Discard any solution that has been frozen. Discard any solution if it has been refrigerated for > 48 hours.

A single reservoir of reconstitued solution can be administered at room temperature for a duration of 8 hours or it can be used with a cold pouch and administered ≤ 24 hours with the use of two frozen 6 oz gel

EPOPROSTENOL SODIUM (PGI₂; PGX; Prostacyclin)

packs. Insulate solution from temperatures > 25°C (77°F) and < 0°C (32°F). Do not expose to direct sunlight.

Actions

►*Pharmacology:* Epoprostenol has two major pharmacological actions: (1) Direct vasodilation of pulmonary and systemic arterial vascular beds, and (2) inhibition of platelet aggregation. In animals, the vasodilatory effects reduce right and left ventricular afterload and increase cardiac output and stroke volume (SV). The effect on heart rate in animals varies with dose. At low doses, there is vagally mediated bradycardia, but at higher doses, epoprostenol causes reflex tachycardia in response to direct vasodilation and hypotension. No major effects on cardiac conduction have been observed. Additional pharmacologic effects in animals are bonchodilation, inhibition of gastric acid secretion and decreased gastric emptying.

Hematologic – Acute IV infusion for ≤ 15 minutes in patients with secondary and primary pulmonary hypertension produces dose-related increases in cardiac index (CI) and SV, and dose-related decreases in pulmonary vascular resistance (PVR), total pulmonary resistance (TPR) and mean systemic arterial pressure (mSAP). The effects of epoprostenol on mean pulmonary artery pressure (mPAP) in patients with primary pulmonary hypertension (PPH) were variable and minor.

►*Pharmacokinetics:* Epoprostenol is rapidly hydrolyzed at neutral pH in blood and is also subject to enzymatic degradation.

The in vitro half-life in human blood at 37°C (98°F) and pH 7.4 is ≈ 6 minutes; the in vivo half-life is therefore expected to be ≤ 6 minutes. The in vitro pharmacologic half-life in human plasma, based on inhibition of platelet aggregation, was similar for males and females.

Epoprostenol is metabolized to two primary metabolites: 6–keto-PGF1a (formed by spontaneous degradation) and 6,1 5–diketo-13,14–dihydro-PGF1a (enzymatically formed), both of which have pharmacological activity orders of magnitued less than epoprostenol in animal test systems.

►*Clinical trials:* Exercise capacity, as measured by the 6 minute walk test, improved significantly in patients receiving continuous IV epoprostenol plus standard therapy for 8 or 12 weeks compared with those receiving standard therapy alone. Improvements were apparent the first week of therapy. Increases in exercise capacity were accompanied by significant improvement in dyspnea and fatigue, as measured by the Congestive Heart Failure Questionnaire and the Dyspnea Fatigue Index.

Survival was improved in NYHA functional Class III and Class IV PPH patients treated with epoprostenol for 12 weeks in a multicenter, open, randomized, parallel study. At the end of the treament period, 8 of 40 patients receiving standard therapy alone died, wheras none of the 41 patients receiving epoprostenol died.

Contraindications

Chronic use in patients with CHF due to severe left ventricular systolic dysfunction; hypersensitivity to the drug or to structurally related compounds.

Warnings

►*Reconstitution:* Epoprostenol must be reconstituted only as directed using sterile diluent for epoprostenol. Epoprostenol must not be reconstituted or mixed with any other parenteral medications or solutions prior to or during administration.

►*Abrupt withdrawal:* Abrupt withdrawal (including interruptions in drug delivery) or sudden large reductions in dosage may result in symptoms associated with rebound pulmonary hypertension, including dyspnea, dizziness and asthenia. In clinical trials, one Class III PPH patient's death was judged attributable to the interruption of epoprostenol. Avoid abrupt withdrawal.

►*Pulmonary edema:* Some patients with primary pulmonary hypertension have developed pulmonary edema during dose ranging, which may be associated with pulmonary veno-occlusive disease. Epoprostenol should not be used chronically in patients who develop pulmonary edema during dose ranging.

►*Elderly:* In general, dose selection for an elderly patient should be cautious, reflecting the greater frequency of decreased hepatic, renal or cardiac function and of concomitant disease or other drug therapy.

►*Pregnancy: Category B.* There are no adequate and well controlled studies in pregnant women. Use during pregnancy only if clearly needed.

►*Lactation:* It is not known whether this drug is excreted in breast milk. Exercise caution when epoprostenol is administered to a nursing woman.

►*Children:* Safety and efficacy have not been established.

Precautions

►*Diagnosis:* Carefully establish the diagnosis of PPH by standard clinical tests to exclude secondary causes of pulmonary hypertension.

►*Dose ranging:* Although dose ranging in clinical trials was performed during right heart catheterization employing a pulmonary artery catheter, in uncontrolled studies, acute dose ranging was performed without cardiac catheterization. Carefully weigh the risk of cardiac catheterization in patients with PPH against the potential benefits. During acute dose ranging, asymptomatic increases in pulmonary artery pressure coincident with increases in cardiac output occurred rarely. In such cases, consider dose reduction, but such an increase does not imply that chronic treatment is contraindicated.

►*Chronic use:* Epoprostenol is delivered continuously on an ambulatory basis through a permanent indwelling central venous catheter. Unless contraindicated, administer anticoagulant therapy to PPH patients to reduce the risk of pulmonary thromboembolism or systemic embolism through a patent foramen ovale. Base the decision to initiate therapy with epoprostenol on the understanding that there is a high likelihood that IV therapy will be needed for prolonged periods, possibly years.

Based on clinical trials, the acute hemodynamic response to epoprostenol did not correlate well with improvement in exercise tolerance of survival during chronic use. Adjust dosage during chronic use at the first sign of recurrence or worsening of symptoms attributable to PPH or the occurrence of adverse events associated with epoprostenol (see Administration and Dosage).

Drug Interactions

Epoprostenol Drug Interactions			
Precipitant drug	Object drug*		Description
Epoprostenol	Diuretics Vasodilators	↑	Coadministration could cause additional reductions in blood pressure.
Epoprostenol	Antiplatelet agents Anticoagulants	↑	Coadministration can increase the risk of bleeding, although this did not occur in clinical trials.

* ↑ = Object drug increased.

Adverse Reactions

During clinical trials, adverse reactions were classified as follows: (1) Occurring during acute dose ranging, (2) occurring during chronic dosing and (3) association with the drug delivery system.

►*Miscellaneous:*

Acute dose ranging – During acute dose ranging, epoprostenol was administered in 2 ng/kg/min increments until the patients developed symptomatic intolerance. The adverse reactions that limited further increases in dose were generally related to the major pharmacologic effect of epoprostenol, vasodilation.

Epoprostenol Adverse Reactions (n = 391)	
Adverse reaction	Incidence
Flushing	58
Headache	49
Nausea/Vomiting	32
Hypotension	16
Anxiety, nervousness, agitation	11
Chest pain	11
Dizziness	8
Bradycardia	5
Abdominal pain	5
Musculoskeletal pain	3
Dyspnea	2
Back pain	2
Sweating	1
Dyspepsia	1
Hypesthesia/Paresthesia	1
Tachycardia	1

Drug delivery system – Local infection (21%); pain at the injection site (13%); sepsis (once); infections (14%). The rate was higher than reported in patients using chronic indwelling central venous catheters to administer parenteral nutrition, but lower than reported in oncology patients using these catheters. Malfunctions in the delivery system resulting in an inadvertent bolus of or a reduction in epoprostenol were associated with symptoms related to excess or insufficient epoprostenol, respectively.

Chronic administration – Interpretation of adverse events is complicated by the clinical features of PPH, which are similar to some of the pharmacologic effects of epoprostenol (eg, dizziness, syncope). Adverse events probably related to the underlying disease include dyspnea, fatigue, chest pain, right ventricular failure and pallor. Several adverse reactions, on the other hand, can clearly be attributed to epoprostenol. These include headache, jaw pain, flushing, diarrhea, nausea and vomiting, flu-like symptoms and anxiety/nervousness. Thrombocytopenia

EPOPROSTENOL SODIUM (PGI₂; PGX; Prostacyclin)

has also been reported. In an effort to separate the adverse effects of the drug from the adverse effects of the underlying disease, the following table lists adverse events that occurred at a rate at least 10% difference in the two groups in controlled trials.

Adverse Reactions Regardless of Attribution Occurring with ≥ 10% Difference Between Epoprostenol and Standard Therapy Alone (%)		
Adverse reaction	Epoprostenol (n = 52)	Standard therapy (n = 54)
Occurrence more common with epoprostenol		
Cardiovascular		
Tachycardia	35	24
Flushing	42	2
GI		
Diarrhea	37	6
Nausea/Vomiting	67	48
Musculoskeletal		
Jaw pain	54	0
Myalgia	44	31
Non-specific musculoskeletal pain	35	15
CNS		
Anxiety/Nervousness/Tremor	21	9
Dizziness	83	70
Headache	83	33
Hypesthesia, hyperesthesia, paresthesia	12	2
Miscellaneous		
Chills/Fever/Sepsis/ Flu-like symptoms	25	11
Occurrence more common with standard therapy		
Cardiovascular		
Heart failure	31	52
Syncope	13	24
Shock	0	13
Respiratory		
Hypoxia	25	37

Adverse Reactions Regardless of Attribution Occurring With < 10% Difference Between Epoprostenol and Standard Therapy Alone (%)		
Adverse reaction	Epoprostenol (n = 52)	Standard therapy (n = 54)
Cardiovascular		
Angina pectoris	19	20
Arrhythmia	27	20
Bradycardia	15	9
Supraventricular tachycardia	8	0
Pallor	21	30
Cyanosis	31	39
Palpitation	63	61
Cerebrovascular accident	4	0
Hemorrhage	19	11
Hypotension	27	31
Myocardial ischemia	2	6

Adverse Reactions Regardless of Attribution Occurring With < 10% Difference Between Epoprostenol and Standard Therapy Alone (%)		
Adverse reaction	Epoprostenol (n = 52)	Standard therapy (n = 54)
GI		
Abdominal pain	27	31
Anorexia	25	30
Ascites	12	17
Constipation	6	2
Metabolic		
Edema	60	63
Hypokalemia	6	4
Weight reduction	27	24
Weight gain	6	4
Musculoskeletal		
Arthralgia	6	0
Bone pain	0	4
Chest pain	67	65
CNS		
Confusion	6	11
Convulsion	4	0
Depression	37	44
Insomnia	4	4
Respiratory		
Cough increase	38	46
Dyspnea	90	85
Epistaxis	4	2
Pleural effusion	4	2
Dermatologic		
Pruritus	4	0
Rash	10	13
Sweating	15	20
Special senses		
Amblyopia	8	4
Vision abnormality	4	0
Miscellaneous		
Asthenia	87	81

Overdosage

Signs and symptoms of excessive doses of epoprostenol during clinical trials are the expected dose-limiting pharmacologic effects of epoprostenol, including flushing, headache, hypotension, tachycardia, nausea, vomiting and diarrhea. Treatment will ordinarily require dose reduction of epoprostenol. One patient vomited and became unconscious with an initially unrecordable blood pressure. Epoprostenol was discontinued and the patient regained consciousness within seconds.

Single IV doses (2703 and 27,027 times the recommended acute phase human dose) were lethal to mice and rats, respectively. Symptoms of acute toxicity were hypoactiviy, ataxia, loss of righting reflex, deep slow breathing and hypothermia.

Patient Information

Patients receiving epoprostenol should receive the following information: The drug is infused continuously through a permanent indwelling central venous catheter via a small, portable infusion pump. Thus, therapy with epoprostenol requires commitment by the patient to drug reconstitution, drug administration and care of the permanent central venous catheter. Brief interruptions in the delivery of epoprostenol may result in rapid symptomatic deterioration. Base the decision to receive epoprostenol for PPH on the understanding that there is a high likelihood that therapy with epoprostenol will be needed for prolonged periods, possibly years.

ETHAVERINE HCl

Rx	**Ethaquin** (B.F. Ascher)	**Tablets:** 100 mg	In 100s, 500s and 1000s.
Rx	**Ethatab** (Whitby)		(Glaxo 281). Yellow. In 100s and UD 100s.
Rx	**Ethavex-100** (Econo Med)		(Ethavex). Scored. In 100s and 1000s.

For complete prescribing information, refer to the Antihypertensives Treatment Guidelines in the Appendix.

Indications

Peripheral and cerebral vascular insufficiency associated with arterial spasm; as a smooth muscle spasmolytic in spastic conditions of the GI and GU tracts. Data are not conclusive to show ethaverine to be effective in the conditions for which it is presently labeled.

Administration and Dosage

100 mg 3 times daily. May be increased to 200 mg 3 times daily. It is most effective when given early in course of vascular disorder. Long-term therapy is required.

Actions

➤*Pharmacology:* Ethaverine is closely related to papaverine and has similar actions and uses (see Papaverine monograph).

Contraindications

Complete atrioventricular dissociation.

Warnings

➤*Pregnancy:* Safety for use during pregnancy has not been established. Do not use in pregnant women unless essential to the welfare of the patient.

➤*Lactation:* Safety for use in the nursing mother has not been established. Do not use in women of childbearing age unless essential to the welfare of the patient.

Precautions

➤*Glaucoma:* Administer with caution to patients with glaucoma.

Adverse Reactions

Nausea; anorexia; abdominal distress; dryness of the throat; hypotension; malaise; vertigo; headache; lassitude; drowsiness; flushing; sweating; respiratory depression; cardiac depression; cardiac arrhythmia.

Patient Information

May cause dizziness (hypotension) or drowsiness; use caution when driving or performing other tasks requiring alertness.

May cause flushing, sweating, headache, tiredness, rash, nausea, anorexia, abdominal distress or diarrhea. Notify physician if these symptoms become pronounced.

PERIPHERAL VASODILATOR COMBINATIONS

Rx	**Lipo-Nicin/100 mg** (ICN Pharm)	**Tablets:** 100 mg niacin, 75 mg niacinamide, 150 mg vitamin C, 25 mg B_1, 2 mg B_2 and 10 mg B_6. *Dose:* 1 tablet daily.	Blue. In 100s.
Rx	**Lipo-Nicin/300 mg** (ICN Pharm)	**Capsules, timed release:** 300 mg niacin, 150 mg vitamin C, 25 mg B_1, 2 mg B_2 and 10 mg B_6. *Dose:* 1 capsule daily.	Clear. In 100s.

In these combinations: *NIACIN* (see Vitamins monograph) is used for its vasodilating action.

Human B-Type Natriuretic Peptide

NESIRITIDE

| *Rx* | **Natrecor** (Scios) | **Powder for injection, lyophilized:** 1.58 mg | Mannitol. In 1.5 mg single-use vials. |

Indications

▶*Acutely decompensated CHF:* For the IV treatment of patients with acutely decompensated CHF who have dyspnea at rest or with minimal activity. In this population, the use of nesiritide reduced pulmonary capillary wedge pressure and improved dyspnea.

Administration and Dosage

▶*Approved by the FDA:* August 10, 2001.

For IV use only. There is limited exposure with administering nesiritide for > 48 hours. Monitor blood pressure closely during nesiritide administration.

▶*Dosage:* The recommended dose of nesiritide is an IV bolus of 2 mcg/kg followed by a continous infusion at a dose of 0.01 mcg/kg/min. Do not initiate nesiritide at a dose greater than the recommended dose.

Prime the IV tubing with an infusion of 25 mL prior to connecting to the patient's vascular access port and prior to administering the bolus or starting the infusion.

Bolus followed by infusion – After preparation of the infusion bag, as described previously, withdraw the bolus volume (see table below) from the nesiritide infusion bag and administer it over ≈ 60 seconds through an IV port in the tubing. Immediately following the administration of the bolus, infuse nesiritide at a flow rate of 0.1 mL/kg/hr. This will deliver a nesiritide infusion dose of 0.01 mcg/kg/min.

To calculate the appropriate bolus volume and infusion flow rate to deliver a 0.01 mcg/kg/min dose, use the following formulas (or refer to the following dosing table).

Bolus volume (mL) = 0.33 × patient weight (kg)

Infusion flow rate (mL/hr) = 0.1 × patient weight (kg)

Nesiritide Weight-Adjusted Bolus Volume and Infusion Flow Rate (2 mcg/kg Bolus Followed by a 0.01 mcg/kg/min Dose)		
Patient weight (kg)	Volume of bolus (mL)	Rate of infusion (mL/hr)
60	20	6
70	23.3	7
80	26.7	8
90	30	9
100	33.3	10
110	36.7	11

▶*Preparation of infusion:*
1.) Reconstitute one 1.5 mg vial of nesiritide by adding 5 mL of diluent removed from a prefilled 250 mL plastic IV bag containing the diluent of choice. The following preservative-free diluents are recommended for reconstitution: 5% Dextrose Injection, 0.9% Sodium Chloride Injection, 5% Dextrose and 0.45% Sodium Chloride Injection, or 5% Dextrose and 0.2% Sodium Chloride Injection.
2.) Do not shake the vial. Rock the vial gently so that all surfaces, including the stopper, are in contact with the diluent to ensure complete reconstitution. Use only a clear, essentially colorless solution.
3.) Withdraw the entire contents of the reconstituted vial and add to the 250 mL plastic IV bag. This will yield a solution with a nesiritide concentration of ≈ 6 mcg/mL. Invert the IV bag several times to ensure complete mixing of the solution.
4.) Use the reconstituted solution within 24 hours, as nesiritide contains no antimicrobial preservative. Parenteral drug products should be inspected visually for particulate matter and discoloration prior to administration whenever solution and container permit.

▶*Dosage adjustments:* If hypotension occurs during nesiritide administration, reduce or discontinue the dose and start other measures to support blood pressure (eg, IV fluids, changes in body position). In the Vasodilation in the Management of Acute Congestive Heart Failure (VMAC) trial, when symptomatic hypotension occurred, nesiritide was discontinued and could be subsequently restarted at a dose that was reduced by 30% (with no bolus administration) once the patient was stabilized. Because hypotension caused by nesiritide may be prolonged (up to hours), a period of observation may be necessary before restarting the drug.

In the VMAC trial, there was limited experience with increasing the dose above the recommended dose (23 patients, all of whom had central hemodynamic monitoring). In those patients, the infusion dose was increased by 0.005 mcg/kg/min (preceded by a bolus of 1 mcg/kg), no more frequently than every 3 hours up to a maximum dose of 0.03 mcg/kg/min. Nesiritide should not be titrated at frequent intervals as is done with other IV agents that have a shorter half-life.

▶*Admixture incompatibilities:* Nesiritide is physically and chemically incompatible with injectable formulations of heparin, insulin, ethacrynate sodium, bumetanide, enalaprilat, hydralazine, and furosemide. Do not coadminister these drugs as infusions with nesiritide through the same IV catheter. The preservative sodium metabisulfite is incompatible with nesiritide. Do not administer injectable drugs that contain sodium metabisulfite in the same infusion line as nesiritide. The catheter must be flushed between administration of nesiritide and incompatible drugs.

Nesiritide binds to heparin and, therefore, could bind to the heparin lining of a heparin-coated catheter, decreasing the amount of nesiritide delivered to the patient for some period of time. Therefore, do not administer nesiritide through a central heparin-coated catheter. Concomitant administration of a heparin infusion through a separate catheter is acceptable.

▶*Storage / Stability:* Store nesiritide at controlled room temperature (20° to 25°C; 68° to 77°F); excursions permitted to 15° to 30°C (59° to 86°F), or refrigerated (2° to 8°C; 36° to 46°F). Reconstituted vials may be left at controlled room temperature (20° to 25°C; 68° to 77°F) or may be refrigerated (2° to 8°C; 36° to 46°F) for ≤ 24 hours. Keep in carton until time of use.

Actions

▶*Pharmacology:* Nesiritide is a human B-type natriuretic peptide (hBNP) and is manufactured from *Escherichia coli* using recombinant DNA technology. Human BNP binds to the particulate guanylate cyclase receptor of vascular smooth muscle and endothelial cells, leading to increased intracellular concentrations of guanosine 3'5'-cyclic monophosphate (cGMP) and smooth muscle cell relaxation. Cyclic GMP serves as a second messenger to dilate veins and arteries. Nesiritide has been shown to relax isolated human arterial and venous tissue preparations that were precontracted with either endothelin-1 or the alpha-adrenergic agonist phenylephrine.

In human studies, nesiritide produced dose-dependent reductions in pulmonary capillary wedge pressure (PCWP) and systemic arterial pressure in patients with heart failure.

In animals, nesiritide had no effect on cardiac contractility or on measures of cardiac electrophysiology such as atrial and ventricular effective refractory times or atrioventricular node conduction.

▶*Pharmacokinetics:* In patients with CHF, nesiritide administered IV by infusion or bolus exhibits biphasic disposition from the plasma. The mean terminal elimination half-life ($t_{1/2}$) of nesiritide is ≈ 18 minutes and was associated with ≈ ⅔ of the area-under-the-curve (AUC). The mean initial elimination phase was estimated to be ≈ 2 minutes. In these patients, the mean volume of distribution of the central compartment (Vc) of nesiritide was estimated to be 0.073 L/kg, the mean steady-state volume of distribution (V_{ss}) was 0.19 L/kg, and the mean clearance (CL) was ≈ 9.2 mL/min/kg. At steady-state, plasma BNP levels increase from baseline endogenous levels by ≈ 3-fold to 6-fold with nesiritide infusion doses ranging from 0.01 to 0.03 mcg/kg/min.

Human BNP is cleared from the circulation via the following 3 independent mechanisms, in order of decreasing importance:
1.) Binding to cell surface clearance receptors with subsequent cellular internalization and lysosomal proteolysis;
2.) proteolytic cleavage of the peptide by endopeptidases, such as neutral endopeptidase, which are present on the vascular lumenal surface; and
3.) renal filtration.

Pharmacodynamics – The recommended dosing regimen of nesiritide is a 2 mcg/kg IV bolus followed by an IV infusion dose of 0.01 mcg/kg/min. With this dosing regimen, 60% of the 3-hour effect on PCWP reduction is achieved within 15 minutes after the bolus, reaching 95% of the 3-hour effect within 1 hour. Approximately 70% of the 3-hour effect on SBP reduction is reached within 15 minutes. The pharmacodynamic half-life of the onset and offset of the hemodynamic effect of nesiritide is longer than what the pharmacokinetic half-life of 18 minutes would predict.

▶*Clinical trials:* The VMAC trial was a randomized, double-blind study of 489 patients (246 patients requiring a right heart catheter, 243 patients without a right heart catheter) who required hospitalization for management of shortness of breath at rest because of acutely decompensated CHF. The study compared the effects of nesiritide, placebo, and IV nitroglycerin when added to background therapy (IV and oral diuretics, non-IV cardiac medications, dobutamine, and dopamine).

In the VMAC study, patients receiving nesiritide reported greater improvement in their dyspnea at 3 hours than patients receiving placebo (p = 0.034).

The following table summarizes the changes in the VMAC trial in PCWP and other measures during the first 3 hours.

Nesiritide Mean Hemodynamic Change from Baseline			
Effects at 3 hours	Placebo (n = 62)	Nitroglycerin (n = 60)	Nesiritide (n = 124)
Pulmonary capillary wedge pressure (mmHg)	-2	-3.8	-5.8[1]
Right atrial pressure (mmHg)	0	-2.6	-3.1[1]
Cardiac index (L/min/M²)	0	0.2	0.1

NESIRITIDE

Nesiritide Mean Hemodynamic Change from Baseline			
Effects at 3 hours	Placebo (n = 62)	Nitroglycerin (n = 60)	Nesiritide (n = 124)
Mean pulmonary artery pressure (mmHg)	-1.1	-2.5	-5.4[1]
Systemic vascular resistance (dynes*sec*cm^{-5})	-44	-105	-144
Systolic blood pressure[2] (mmHg)	-2.5	-5.7[1]	-5.6[1]

[1] $p < 0.05$ compared with placebo.
[2] Based on all treated subjects: Placebo (n = 142), nitroglycerin (n = 143), nesiritide (n = 204).

Contraindications

Hypersensitivity to any of the product's components. Nesiritide should not be used as primary therapy for patients with cardiogenic shock or in patients with a systolic blood pressure < 90 mmHg.

Warnings

➤*Cardiac:* Avoid administration of nesiritide in patients suspected of having, or known to have, low cardiac filling pressures. Nesiritide is not recommended for patients for whom vasodilating agents are not appropriate, such as patients with significant valvular stenosis, restrictive or obstructive cardiomyopathy, constrictive pericarditis, pericardial tamponade, or other conditions in which cardiac output is dependent upon venous return, or for patients suspected to have low cardiac filling pressures.

➤*Hypotension:* Nesiritide may cause hypotension. In the VMAC trial, in patients given the recommended dose (2 mcg/kg bolus followed by a 0.01 mcg/kg/min infusion) or the adjustable dose, the incidence of symptomatic hypotension in the first 24 hours was similar for nesiritide (4%) and IV nitroglycerin (5%). When hypotension occurred, however, the duration of symptomatic hypotension was longer with nesiritide (mean duration was 2.2 hours) than with nitroglycerin (mean duration was 0.7 hours). In earlier trials, when nesiritide was initiated at doses higher than the 2 mcg/kg bolus followed by a 0.01 mcg/kg/min infusion (eg, 0.015 and 0.03 mcg/kg/min preceded by a small bolus), there were more hypotensive episodes and these episodes were of greater intensity and duration. They were also more often symptomatic and more likely to require medical intervention. Administer nesiritide only in settings where blood pressure can be monitored closely and reduce the dose or discontinue the drug in patients who develop hypotension. The rate of symptomatic hypotension may be increased in patients with a blood pressure < 100 mmHg at baseline; nesiritide should be used cautiously in these patients. The potential for hypotension may be increased by combining nesiritide with other drugs that may cause hypotension. For example, in the VMAC trial, in patients treated with either nesiritide or nitroglycerin therapy, the frequency of symptomatic hypotension in patients who received an oral ACE inhibitor was 6%, compared with a frequency of symptomatic hypotension of 1% in patients who did not receive an oral ACE inhibitor.

➤*Hypersensitivity reactions:* Parenteral administration of protein pharmaceuticals or *E. coli*-derived products should be attended by appropriate precautions in case of an allergic or untoward reaction. No serious allergic or anaphylactic reactions have been reported with nesiritide.

➤*Renal function impairment:* Nesiritide may affect renal function in susceptible individuals. In patients with severe heart failure whose renal function may depend on the activity of the renin-angiotensin-aldosterone system, treatment with nesiritide may be associated with azotemia. When nesiritide was initiated at doses > 0.01 mcg/kg/min (0.015 and 0.03 mcg/kg/min), there was an increased rate of elevated serum creatinine over baseline, compared with standard therapies, although the rate of acute renal failure and need for dialysis was not increased. In the 30-day follow-up period in the VMAC trial, 5 patients in the nitroglycerin group (2%) and 9 patients in the nesiritide group (3%) required first-time dialysis.

➤*Pregnancy:* Category C. It is not known whether nesiritide can cause fetal harm when administered to a pregnant woman or can affect reproductive capacity. Use nesiritide in pregnancy only if the potential benefit justifies any potential risk to the fetus.

➤*Lactation:* It is not known whether this drug is excreted in human milk. Therefore, exercise caution when nesiritide is administered to a nursing woman.

➤*Children:* The safety and effectiveness of nesiritide in pediatric patients has not been established.

Drug Interactions

➤*ACE inhibitors:* Concomitant therapy may cause an increase in symptomatic hypotension.

Adverse Reactions

Adverse events that occurred with ≥ 3% frequency during the first 24 hours of nesiritide infusion are shown in the following table.

Nesiritide Adverse Reactions (≥ 3%)					
	VMAC trial		Other long infusion trials		
Adverse event	Nitroglycerin (n = 216)	Nesiritide recommended dose (n = 273)	Control[1] (n = 256)	Nesiritide mcg/kg/min 0.015 (n = 253)	0.03 (n = 246)
Cardiovascular					
Hypotension	12	11	8	22	35
Symptomatic hypotension	5	4	3	11	17
Asymptomatic hypotension	8	8	5	12	20
Ventricular tachycardia (VT)	5	3	10	10	4
Nonsustained VT	5	3	9	9	4
Ventricular extrasystoles	1	3	6	4	4
Angina pectoris	2	2	2	6	6
Bradycardia	< 1	1	< 1	3	5
CNS					
Headache	20	8	9	9	7
Insomnia	4	2	3	6	6
Dizziness	2	3	3	6	5
Anxiety	3	3	1	3	2
GI					
Nausea	6	4	5	9	13
Vomiting	2	1	1	2	4
Miscellaneous					
Abdominal pain	5	1	4	2	3
Back pain	3	4	2	2	1

[1] Includes dobutamine, milrinone, nitroglycerin, placebo, dopamine, nitroprusside, or amrinone.

➤*Reactions ≥ 1%:* Adverse events that are not listed in the above table that occurred in ≥ 1% of patients who received any of the above nesiritide doses included the following:

Cardiovascular – Tachycardia, atrial fibrillation, AV node conduction abnormalities.

CNS – Confusion, paresthesia, somnolence, tremor.

Dermatologic – Sweating, pruritus, rash.

Respiratory – Increased cough, hemoptysis, apnea.

Miscellaneous – Catheter pain, fever, injection site reaction, increased creatinine, leg cramps, amblyopia, anemia.

➤*Lab test abnormalities:* In the PRECEDENT trial, the incidence of elevations in serum creatinine to > 0.5 mg/dL above baseline through day 14 was higher in the nesiritide 0.015 mcg/kg/min group (17%) and the nesiritide 0.03 mcg/kg/min group (19%) than with standard therapy (11%). In the VMAC trial, through day 30, the incidence of elevations in creatinine to > 0.5 mg/dL above baseline was 28% and 21% in the nesiritide (2 mcg/kg bolus followed by 0.01 mcg/kg/min) and nitroglycerin groups, respectively.

Overdosage

No data are available with respect to overdosage in humans. The expected reaction would be excessive hypotension, which should be treated with drug discontinuation or reduction and appropriate measures.

Endothelin Receptor Antagonist

BOSENTAN

Rx	Tracleer (Actelion Pharm.)	Tablets: 62.5 mg	(62.5). Orange/White. Film-coated. In 60s.
		125 mg	(125). Orange/White. Film-coated. In 60s.

WARNING

Use of bosentan requires attention to 2 significant concerns: Potential for serious liver injury and potential damage to a fetus.

Warning:

Potential liver injury – Bosentan causes at least 3-fold (upper limit of normal; ULN) elevation of liver aminotransferases (ALT and AST) in approximately 11% of patients, accompanied by elevated bilirubin in a small number of cases. Because these changes are a marker for potential serious liver injury, serum aminotransferase levels must be measured prior to initiation of treatment and then monthly (see Warnings). To date, in a setting of close monitoring, elevations have been reversible within a few days to 9 weeks, either spontaneously or after dose reduction or discontinuation and without sequelae.

Elevations in aminotransferases require close attention. Avoid bosentan in patients with elevated aminotransferases (greater than 3 × ULN) at baseline because monitoring liver injury may be more difficult.

If liver aminotranferase elevations are accompanied by clinical symptoms of liver injury (eg, nausea, vomiting, fever, abdominal pain, jaundice, or unusual lethargy or fatigue) or increases in bilirubin greater than or equal to 2 × ULN, stop treatment. There is no experience with the re-introduction of bosentan in these circumstances.

Contraindication:

Pregnancy – Bosentan is very likely to produce major birth defects if used by pregnant women, as this effect has been seen consistently when it is administered to animals. Therefore, pregnancy must be excluded before the start of treatment with bosentan and prevented thereafter by the use of a reliable method of contraception. Hormonal contraceptives, including oral, injectable, and implantable contraceptives should not be used as the sole means of contraception because these may not be effective in patients receiving bosentan. Obtain monthly pregnancy tests.

Because of potential liver injury and in an effort to make the chance of fetal exposure to bosentan as small as possible, bosentan may be prescribed only through the *Tracleer* Access Program by calling (866) 228-3546. Adverse events can also be reported directly via this number.

Indications

➤*Pulmonary arterial hypertension (PAH):* For the treatment of PAH in patients with WHO Class III or IV symptoms, to improve exercise ability and decrease the rate of clinical worsening.

➤*Unlabeled uses:* Possible improvement of microcirculatory blood flow in splanchnic organs during septic shock.

Administration and Dosage

➤*Approved by the FDA:* November 20, 2001.

Initiate bosentan treatment at a dose of 62.5 mg twice daily for 4 weeks and then increase to the maintenance dose of 125 mg twice daily. Doses more than 125 mg twice daily did not appear to confer additional benefit sufficient to offset the increased risk of liver injury.

In patients with a body weight less than 40 kg but who are older than 12 years of age, the recommended initial and maintenance dose is 62.5 mg twice daily.

Administer tablets in the morning and evening with or without food.

Dosage Adjustment and Monitoring in Patients Developing Aminotransferase Abnormalities with Bosentan	
ALT/AST levels	Treatment and monitoring recommendations
> 3 and ≤ 5 × ULN	Confirm by another aminotransferase test; if confirmed, reduce the daily dose or interrupt treatment and monitor aminotransferase levels at least every 2 weeks. If the aminotransferase levels return to pretreatment values, continue or reintroduce the treatment as appropriate.
> 5 and ≤ 8 × ULN	Confirm by another aminotransferase test; if confirmed, stop treatment and monitor aminotransferase levels at least every 2 weeks. Once the aminotransferase levels return to pretreatment values, consider reintroduction of the treatment.
> 8 × ULN	Stop treatment and do not consider bosentan reintroduction. There is no experience with reintroduction of bosentan in these circumstances.

If liver aminotransferase elevations are accompanied by clinical symptoms of liver injury (eg, nausea, vomiting, fever, abdominal pain, jaundice, unusual lethargy or fatigue) or increases in bilirubin at least 2 × ULN, stop treatment. There is no experience with the reintroduction of bosentan in these circumstances.

➤*Treatment discontinuation:* There is limited experience with abrupt discontinuation of bosentan. No evidence for acute rebound has been observed. Nevertheless, to avoid the potential for clinical deterioration, consider gradual dose reduction (62.5 mg twice daily for 3 to 7 days).

➤*Storage/Stability:* Store at 20° to 25°C (68° to 77°F). Excursions are permitted between 15° and 30°C (59° and 86°F).

Actions

➤*Pharmacology:* Bosentan is the first of a new drug class, an endothelin receptor antagonist. Endothelin-1 (ET-1) is a neurohormone, the effects of which are mediated by binding to ET_A and ET_B receptors in the endothelium and vascular smooth muscle. ET-1 concentrations are elevated in plasma and lung tissue of patients with PAH, suggesting a pathogenic role for ET-1 in this disease. Bosentan is a specific and competitive antagonist at endothelin receptor types ET_A and ET_B. Bosentan has a slightly higher affinity for ET_A receptors than for ET_B receptors.

➤*Pharmacokinetics:*

Absorption/Distribution – The absolute bioavailability of bosentan in healthy volunteers is approximately 50% and is unaffected by food. The volume of distribution is approximately 18 L. Bosentan is highly bound (more than 98%) to plasma proteins, mainly albumin. Bosentan does not penetrate into erythrocytes. After oral administration, maximum plasma concentrations of bosentan are attained within 3 to 5 hours.

Metabolism/Excretion – Bosentan has 3 metabolites, 1 of which is pharmacologically active and may contribute 10% to 20% of the effect of bosentan. Bosentan is an inducer of CYP2C9 and CYP3A4 and possibly also of CYP2C19. Total clearance after a single IV dose is about 8 L/hr. Upon multiple dosing, plasma concentrations decrease gradually to 50% to 65% of those seen after single dose administration, probably the effect of auto-induction of the metabolizing liver enzymes. Steady state is reached within 3 to 5 days. Bosentan is eliminated by biliary excretion following metabolism in the liver. Less than 3% of an administered oral dose is recovered in urine. The terminal elimination half-life is approximately 5 hours. Pharmacokinetics of bosentan were not studied in patients with PAH, but exposure is expected to be greater in such patients because increased (30% to 40%) bosentan exposure was observed in patients with severe chronic heart failure.

Special populations –

Hepatic function impairment, preexisting: The influence of liver impairment on the pharmacokinetics of bosentan has not been evaluated, but in vitro and in vivo evidence showing extensive hepatic metabolism of bosentan suggests that liver impairment would significantly increase exposure of bosentan. Exercise caution during the use of bosentan in patients with mildly impaired liver function. Generally avoid bosentan in patients with moderate or severe liver abnormalities and/or elevated aminotransferases greater than 3 × ULN.

Renal function impairment: In patients with severe renal impairment (Ccr 15 to 30 mL/min), plasma concentrations of bosentan were essentially unchanged and plasma concentrations of the 3 metabolites were increased approximately 2-fold compared with people with normal renal function. These differences do not appear to be clinically important.

Contraindications

Pregnancy (see Warnings); coadministration with cyclosporine A, glyburide (see Drug Interactions); hypersensitivity to bosentan or any component of the medication.

Warnings

➤*Hepatotoxicity:* Elevations in ALT or AST by greater than 3 × ULN were observed in 11% of bosentan-treated patients (N = 658) compared with 2% of placebo-treated patients (N = 280). Three-fold increases were seen in 12% of 95 PAH patients on 125 mg twice daily and 14% of 70 PAH patients on 250 mg twice daily. Eight-fold increases were seen in 2% of PAH patients on 125 mg twice daily and 7% of PAH patients on 250 mg twice daily. Bilirubin increases to at least 3 × ULN were associated with aminotransferase increases in 0.3% of patients treated with bosentan.

The combination of hepatocellular injury (increases in aminotransferases of greater than 3 × ULN) and increases in total bilirubin (at least 3 × ULN) is a marker for potential serious liver injury.

Elevations of AST and/or ALT associated with bosentan are dose-dependent, occur early and late in treatment, usually progress slowly and are typically asymptomatic, and to date have been reversible after treat-

BOSENTAN

ment interruption or cessation. These aminotransferase elevations may reverse spontaneously while continuing treatment with bosentan.

Liver aminotransferase levels must be measured prior to initiation of treatment and then monthly. If elevated aminotransferase levels are seen, changes in monitoring and treatment must be initiated. If liver aminotransferase elevations are accompanied by clinical symptoms of liver injury (eg, nausea, vomiting, fever, abdominal pain, jaundice, unusual lethargy or fatigue) or increases in bilirubin at least $2 \times$ ULN, stop treatment. There is no experience with the reintroduction of bosentan in these circumstances.

➤ *Hepatic function impairment:* Liver aminotransferase levels must be measured prior to initiation of treatment and then monthly. Generally avoid bosentan in patients with moderate or severe liver impairment. In addition, generally avoid bosentan in patients with elevated aminotransferases (greater than $3 \times$ ULN) because monitoring liver injury in these patients may be more difficult.

There are no specific data to guide dosing in hepatically impaired patients. Exercise caution in patients with mildly impaired liver function. Generally avoid bosentan in patients with moderate or severe liver impairment.

➤ *Carcinogenesis:* Two years of dietary administration of bosentan to mice produced an increased incidence of hepatocellular adenomas and carcinomas in males at doses as low as 450 mg/kg/day (approximately 8 times the maximum recommended human dose [MRHD] of 125 mg twice daily on a mg/m² basis. In the same study, doses more than 2000 mg/kg/day (approximately 32 times the MRHD) were associated with an increased incidence of colon adenomas in males and females. In rats, dietary administration of bosentan for 2 years was associated with an increased incidence of brain astrocytomas in males at doses as low as 500 mg/kg/day (approximately 16 times the MRHD).

➤ *Fertility impairment:* Many endothelin receptor antagonists have profound effects on the histology and function of the testes in animals. These drugs have been shown to induce atrophy of the seminiferous tubules of the testes and to reduce sperm counts and male fertility in rats when administered for more than 10 weeks. Where studied, testicular tubular atrophy and decreases in male fertility observed with endothelin receptor antagonists appear irreversible.

An increased incidence of testicular tubular atrophy was observed in rats given bosentan orally at doses as low as 125 mg/kg/day (approximately 4 times the MRHD and the lowest doses tested) for 2 years but not at doses as high as 1500 mg/kg/day (approximately 50 times the MRHD) for 6 months. Effects on sperm count and motility were evaluated only in the much shorter duration fertility studies in which males had been exposed to the drug for 4 to 6 weeks.

There are no data on the effects of bosentan or other endothelin receptor antagonists on testicular function in humans.

➤ *Elderly:* Clinical experience with bosentan in subjects at least 65 years of age has not included a sufficient number of such subjects to identify a difference in response between elderly and younger patients.

In general, exercise caution in dose selection for elderly patients given the greater frequency of decreased hepatic, renal, or cardiac function, and of concomitant disease or other drug therapy in this age group.

➤ *Pregnancy: Category X.* Bosentan is expected to cause fetal harm if administered to pregnant women. Bosentan was teratogenic in rats given oral doses at least 60 mg/kg/day (twice the maximum recommended human oral dose of 125 mg twice daily on a mg/m² basis). In an embryo-fetal toxicity study in rats, bosentan showed dose-dependent teratogenic effects, including malformations of the head, mouth, face, and large blood vessels. Bosentan increased stillbirths and pup mortality at oral doses of 60 and 300 mg/kg/day (2 and 10 times, respectively, the MRHD on a mg/m² basis). Although birth defects were not observed in rabbits given oral doses of up to 1500 mg/kg/day, plasma concentrations of bosentan in rabbits were lower than those reached in the rat. The similarity of malformations induced by bosentan and those observed in endothelin-1 knockout mice and in animals treated with other endothelin receptor antagonists indicates that teratogenicity is a class effect of these drugs. There are no data on the use of bosentan in pregnant women.

Pregnancy must be excluded before the start of treatment with bosentan and prevented thereafter by use of reliable contraception. Hormonal contraceptives, including oral, injectable, and implantable contraceptives may not be reliable in the presence of bosentan and should not be used as the sole contraceptive method in patients receiving bosentan (see Drug Interactions). Input from a gynecologist or similar expert on adequate contraception should be sought as needed.

Start bosentan only in patients known not to be pregnant. For female patients of childbearing potential, a prescription for bosentan should not be issued by the prescriber unless the patient assures the prescriber that she is not sexually active or provides negative results from a urine or serum pregnancy test performed during the first 5 days of a normal menstrual period and at least 11 days after the last unprotected act of sexual intercourse.

Obtain monthly follow-up urine or serum pregnancy tests in women of childbearing potential taking bosentan. Advise the patient that if there is any delay in onset of menses or any other reason to suspect pregnancy, she must notify the physician immediately for pregnancy testing. If the pregnancy test is positive, the physician and patient must discuss the risk to the pregnancy and to the fetus.

➤ *Lactation:* It is not known whether this drug is excreted in human milk. Because many drugs are excreted in human milk, breastfeeding while taking bosentan is not recommended.

➤ *Children:* Safety and efficacy in pediatric patients have not been established.

Precautions

➤ *Monitoring:* Obtain monthly follow-up urine or serum pregnancy tests in women of childbearing potential taking bosentan.

Liver aminotransferase levels must be measured prior to initiation of treatment and then monthly. If elevated aminotransferase levels are seen, changes in monitoring and treatment must be initiated.

Monitor hemoglobin levels after 1 and 3 months of treatment and then every 3 months.

➤ *Hematologic:* Treatment with bosentan caused a dose-related decrease in hemoglobin and hematocrit. Monitor hemoglobin levels after 1 and 3 months of treatment and then every 3 months. The overall mean decrease in hemoglobin concentration for bosentan-treated patients was 0.9 g/dL (change to end of treatment). Most of this decrease of hemoglobin concentration was detected during the first few weeks of bosentan treatment and levels stabilized by 4 to 12 weeks of bosentan treatment.

In placebo-controlled studies of all uses of bosentan, marked decreases in hemoglobin (more than 15% decrease from baseline resulting in values less than 11 g/dL) were observed in 6% of bosentan-treated patients and 3% of placebo-treated patients. In patients with PAH treated with doses of 125 and 250 mg twice daily marked decreases in hemoglobin occurred in 3% compared with 1% in placebo-treated patients.

A decrease in hemoglobin concentration by at least 1 g/dL was observed in 57% of bosentan-treated patients as compared with 29% of placebo-treated patients. In 80% of those patients whose hemoglobin decreased by at least 1 g/dL, the decrease occurred during the first 6 weeks of bosentan treatment.

During the course of treatment the hemoglobin concentration remained within normal limits in 68% of bosentan-treated patients compared with 76% of placebo patients.

The explanation for the change in hemoglobin is not known, but it does not appear to be hemorrhage or hemolysis. If a marked decrease in hemoglobin concentration occurs, undertake further evaluation to determine the cause and need for specific treatment.

Drug Interactions

➤ *CYP450 isoenzymes:* Bosentan is metabolized by CYP2C9 and CYP3A4. Inhibition of these isoenzymes may increase the plasma concentration of bosentan. Bosentan is an inducer of CYP3A4 and CYP2C9. Consequently, plasma concentrations of drugs metabolized by these 2 isoenzymes will be decreased when bosentan is coadministered. Bosentan had no relevant inhibitory effect on any CYP isoenzymes tested (CYP1A2, CYP2C9, CYP2C19, CYP2D6, CYP3A4). Consequently, bosentan is not expected to increase the plasma concentrations of drugs metabolized by these enzymes.

Bosentan Drug Interactions			
Precipitant drug	Object drug*		Description
Cyclosporine A	Bosentan	↑	Coadministration increased bosentan trough concentrations by ≈ 30-fold and steady-state concentrations by 3- to 4-fold. Cyclosporine A plasma concentrations decreased by ≈ 50%. Coadministration is contraindicated.
Bosentan	Cyclosporine A	↓	
Glyburide	Bosentan	↓	Glyburide plasma concentrations were decreased by ≈ 40% when administered with bosentan, whereas the plasma concentrations of bosentan were also decreased by ≈ 30%. However, coadministration is contraindicated because an increased risk of elevated liver aminotransferases was also observed in patients receiving concomitant therapy.
Bosentan	Glyburide		
Ketoconazole	Bosentan	↑	Coadministration increased bosentan plasma concentrations by ≈ 2-fold. No dosage adjustment of bosentan is necessary, but consider increased effects of bosentan.

Endothelin Receptor Antagonist

BOSENTAN

Bosentan Drug Interactions			
Precipitant drug	Object drug*		Description
Bosentan	Hormonal contraceptives (including oral, injectable, and implantable)	↓	Many of these drugs are metabolized by CYP3A4. There is a possibility of contraception failure when bosentan is coadministered. Women should not rely on hormonal contraception alone when taking bosentan.
Bosentan	Simvastatin and other statins	↓	The plasma concentrations of simvastatin and its metabolite decreased by ≈ 50% when coadministered with bosentan. Bosentan is also expected to reduce plasma concentrations of other statins significantly metabolized by CYP3A4 (ie, lovastatin, atorvastatin). Monitor cholesterol levels and adjust statin dose accordingly.
Bosentan	Warfarin	↓	Coadministration decreased the plasma concentrations of S-warfarin and R-warfarin by 29% and 38%, respectively. Clinically relevant changes in INR or warfarin dose were not seen in patients with PAH during clinical trials.

* ↑ = Object drug increased.   ↓ = Object drug decreased.

Adverse Reactions

In placebo-controlled studies of bosentan in pulmonary arterial hypertension and for other diseases (primarily chronic heart failure), a total of 677 patients were treated with bosentan at daily doses ranging from 100 to 2000 mg and 288 patients were treated with placebo. The duration of treatment ranged from 4 weeks to 6 months. For the adverse drug reactions that occurred in at least 3% of bosentan-treated patients, the only ones that occurred more frequently on bosentan than on placebo (at least a 2% difference) were headache (16% vs 13%), flushing (7% vs 2%), abnormal hepatic function (6% vs 2%), leg edema (5% vs 1%), and anemia (3% vs 1%).

Adverse Reactions in ≥ 3% of Bosentan Patients Treated with 125 to 250 mg Twice Daily		
Adverse reaction[1]	Bosentan (N = 165)	Placebo (N = 80)
Headache	22	20
Nasopharyngitis	11	8
Flushing	9	5
Abnormal hepatic function	8	3
Edema, lower limb	8	5
Hypotension	7	4
Palpitations	5	1
Dyspepsia	4	0
Edema	4	3
Fatigue	4	1
Pruritus	4	0

[1] Only AEs with onset from start of treatment to 1 calendar day after end of treatment are included. All reported events (at least 3%) are included except those too general to be informative, and those not reasonably associated with the use of the drug because they were associated with the condition being treated or are very common in the treated population.

► *Lab test abnormalities:* Increased liver aminotransferases (see Warning Box and Warnings); decreased hemoglobin and hematocrit (see Precautions).

Overdosage

Bosentan has been given as a single dose of up to 2400 mg in healthy volunteers or up to 2000 mg/day for 2 months in patients without any major clinical consequences. The most common side effect was headache of mild to moderate intensity. In the cyclosporine A interaction study, in which doses of 500 and 1000 mg twice daily of bosentan were given concomitantly with cyclosporine A, trough plasma concentrations of bosentan increased 30-fold, resulting in severe headaches, nausea, and vomiting, but no serious adverse events. Mild decreases in blood pressure and increases in heart rate were observed.

There is no specific experience of overdosage with bosentan beyond the doses described above. Massive overdosage may result in pronounced hypotension requiring active cardiovascular support.

Patient Information

Advise patients to consult the medication guide on the safe use of bosentan.

The physician should discuss with the patient the importance of monthly monitoring of serum aminotransferases and urine or serum pregnancy testing and of avoidance of pregnancy. The physician should discuss options for effective contraception and measures to prevent pregnancy with their female patients. Input from a gynecologist or similar expert on adequate contraception should be sought as needed.

Beta-Adrenergic Blocking Agents

Indications

➤*Hypertension (all except esmolol and sotalol):* Used alone as initial drug choice or in combination with other drugs, particularly a thiazide diuretic. Not indicated for treatment of hypertensive emergencies.

➤*Angina pectoris (nadolol, propranolol, atenolol, metoprolol):* Long-term management.

➤*Hypertrophic subaortic stenosis (propranolol):* Useful in managing exertional or other stress-induced angina, palpitations, and syncope. Improves exercise performance. Efficacy appears to be caused by reduction of elevated outflow pressure gradient that is exacerbated by beta receptor stimulation. Clinical improvement may be temporary.

➤*Cardiac arrhythmias (acebutolol, esmolol, propranolol, sotalol):* Use acebutolol for ventricular premature beats only. Use sotalol for documented life-threatening ventricular arrhythmias, such as sustained ventricular tachycardia.

Supraventricular arrhythmias (propranolol) – Paroxysmal atrial tachycardias, particularly those arrhythmias induced by catecholamines or digitalis or associated with the Wolff-Parkinson-White syndrome (see Warnings); persistent sinus tachycardia that is noncompensatory and impairs the well-being of the patient.

Tachycardias and arrhythmias caused by thyrotoxicosis when they cause distress or increased hazard and when immediate effect is necessary as adjunctive, short-term (2 to 4 weeks) therapy. May be used with, but not in place of, specific therapy.

Persistent atrial extrasystoles that impair the well-being of the patient and do not respond to conventional measures. Atrial flutter and fibrillation when ventricular rate cannot be controlled by digitalis alone, or when digitalis is contraindicated.

Supraventricular tachycardia (esmolol) – Rapid control of ventricular rate in patients with atrial fibrillation or atrial flutter in perioperative, postoperative, or other emergent circumstances in which short-term control of ventricular rate with a short-acting agent is desirable.

Sinus tachycardia (esmolol) – Noncompensatory sinus tachycardia in which the rapid heart rate requires intervention. Esmolol is not intended for use in chronic settings where transfer to another agent is anticipated.

Intraoperative and postoperative tachycardia and hypertension (esmolol) – Treatment of tachycardia and hypertension that may occur during induction and tracheal intubation, during surgery, on emergence from anesthesia, and in the postoperative period, when in the physician's judgment such specific intervention is indicated.

Ventricular tachycardias (propranolol) – In ventricular tachycardias, with the exception of those induced by catecholamines or digitalis, propranolol is not the drug of first choice. In critical situations when cardioversion techniques or other drugs are not indicated or are ineffective, propranolol may be considered.

Persistent premature ventricular extrasystoles that impair the well-being of the patient and do not respond to conventional measures.

Tachyarrhythmias of digitalis intoxication (propranolol) – If it is persistent following discontinuation of digitalis and correction of electrolyte abnormalities, tachyarrhythmias are usually reversible with oral propranolol. Severe bradycardia may occur. Reserve IV propranolol for life-threatening arrhythmias. Temporary maintenance with oral therapy may be indicated.

Resistant tachyarrhythmias caused by excessive catecholamine action during anesthesia (propranolol) – All general inhalation anesthetics produce some degree of myocardial depression; therefore, use propranolol with extreme caution.

Maintenance of normal sinus rhythm (sotalol) – In patients with highly symptomatic atrial fibrillation/atrial flutter (AFIB/AFL) who are currently in sinus rhythm (*Betapace AF* only).

➤*MI (propranolol, timolol):* Indicated in clinically stable patients who have survived the acute phase of an MI to reduce cardiovascular mortality and risk of reinfarction. Initiate treatment within 1 to 4 weeks after infarction.

Metoprolol and atenolol – Both are also indicated in the treatment of hemodynamically stable patients with definite or suspected acute MI. Treatment can be initiated as soon as the patient's clinical condition allows or within 3 to 10 days of the acute event.

➤*CHF (metoprolol):* Treatment of stable, symptomatic (NYHA Class II or III) heart failure of ischemic, hypertensive, or cardiomyopathic origin (*Toprol-XL* 25 mg only). Studied in patients already receiving ACE inhibitors, diuretics, and, in the majority of cases, digitalis. In this population, *Toprol-XL* decreased the rate of mortality plus hospitalization, largely through a reduction in cardiovascular mortality and hospitalizations for heart failure.

➤*Pheochromocytoma (propranolol):* After primary treatment with an alpha-adrenergic blocking agent has been instituted, propranolol may be useful as adjunctive therapy if the control of tachycardia becomes necessary before or during surgery.

With inoperable or metastatic pheochromocytoma, propranolol may be useful as an adjunct to the management of symptoms caused by excessive beta receptor stimulation.

➤*Migraine (propranolol, timolol):* For the prophylaxis of common migraine headache.

➤*Essential tremor (propranolol):* For the management of familial or hereditary essential tremor consisting of involuntary, rhythmic, and oscillatory movements. Propranolol causes a reduction in the tremor amplitude but not in the tremor frequency. It is not indicated for the treatment of tremor associated with Parkinsonism.

➤*Unlabeled uses:* The agents listed have been evaluated for use in the following conditions:

Akathisia (antipsychotic-induced) – Propranolol (30 to 120 mg/day), metoprolol (50 to 400 mg/day).

Atrial fibrillation (rapid heart rate control) – Metoprolol (2.5 to 5 mg IV bolus over 2 minutes, up to 3 doses).

Atrial fibrillation (maintenance heart rate control) – Metoprolol (25 to 100 mg twice daily).

Angina (stable) – Acebutolol, bisoprolol.

Angina (unstable) – Atenolol (5 mg over 5 minutes IV, up to 3 doses; 25 to 100 mg/day orally), esmolol (500 mcg/kg bolus and infusion of 10 to 200 mcg/kg/minute), metoprolol (5 mg over 5 minutes IV, up to 3 doses; 25 to 100 mg twice daily orally).

CHF (stable) – Immediate-release metoprolol (initial dose of 12.5 mg twice daily, increase to up to 50 mg twice daily), bisoprolol (initial dose of 2.5 mg daily, increase to up to 10 mg daily).

Generalized anxiety disorder – Propranolol (initial dose of 10 mg twice daily; maximum daily dose is 360 mg).

Hypertensive crises – Esmolol (loading dose of 500 mcg/kg over 1 minute, followed by infusion at 25 to 50 mcg/kg/min, which may be increased by 25 mcg/kg/min every 10 to 20 minutes until the desired response is obtained; maximum dose is 300 mcg/kg/min).

Hyperthyroidism adjunctive therapy – Propranolol and nadolol may provide symptomatic improvement until euthyroid state is achieved.

Migraine prophylaxis – Atenolol (50 to 200 mg/day), metoprolol (100 to 200 mg/day), and nadolol (40 to 240 mg/day).

Parkinsonian tremor – Propranolol SR (initial dose of 60 mg in the morning; may be increased up to 160 mg/day); nadolol.

Prevention of variceal bleeding caused by portal hypertension – Propranolol (initial dose of 40 mg twice daily; average maintenance dose is 160 mg/day), nadolol (80 mg/day), atenolol, timolol, metoprolol.

Beta-Adrenergic Blocking Agents – Summary of Indications[1]												
Indications ✔= labeled x = unlabeled	Acebutolol	Atenolol	Betaxolol	Bisoprolol	Carteolol	Esmolol	Metoprolol[2]	Nadolol	Penbutolol	Pindolol	Propranolol[2]	Sotalol	Timolol
Hypertension	✔	✔	✔	✔	✔		✔	✔	✔	✔	✔		✔
Angina pectoris		✔					✔	✔			✔		
Cardiac arrhythmias													
Supraventricular arrhythmias/tachycardias						✔					✔		
Sinus tachycardia						✔							
Intraoperative and postoperative tachycardia and hypertension						✔							
Ventricular arrhythmias/tachycardias											✔	✔[3]	
Premature ventricular contractions (PVCs)	✔										✔		
Digitalis-induced tachyarrhythmias											✔		

Beta-Adrenergic Blocking Agents

Beta-Adrenergic Blocking Agents – Summary of Indications[1]

Indications ✔ = labeled x = unlabeled	Acebutolol	Atenolol	Betaxolol	Bisoprolol	Carteolol	Esmolol	Metoprolol[2]	Nadolol	Penbutolol	Pindolol	Propranolol[2]	Sotalol	Timolol
Resistant tachyarrhythmias (during anesthesia)											✔		
Atrial ectopy							x						
Maintenance of normal sinus rhythm												✔	
MI		✔					✔				✔		✔
CHF (stable)[4]				x			✔[5]						
Pheochromocytoma											✔		
Migraine prophylaxis		x					x	x			✔		✔
Hypertrophic subaortic stenosis											✔		
Parkinsonian tremors								x			x[6]		
Akathisia, antipsychotic-induced							x				x		
Variceal bleeding in portal hypertension		x					x	x			x		x
Atrial fibrillation													
Rapid heart rate control							x						
Maintenance heart rate control							x						
Generalized anxiety disorder											x		
Angina													
Stable	x			x									
Unstable		x				x	x						

[1] For more detailed information, see preceding Indications and individual monographs.
[2] Includes long-acting formulation.
[3] Not *Betapace AF.*
[4] See Precautions or Warnings.
[5] *Toprol-XL* 25 mg only.
[6] Sustained-release only.

Actions

➤*Pharmacology:*

Pharmacologic/Pharmacokinetic Properties of Beta-Adrenergic Blocking Agents

0 – none + – low ++ – moderate +++ – high Drug	Adrenergic-receptor blocking activity		Membrane stabilizing activity	Intrinsic sympathomimetic activity	Lipid solubility	Extent of absorption (%)	Absolute oral bioavailability (%)	Half-life (hrs)	Protein binding (%)	Metabolism/Excretion
Acebutolol	β_1[1]		+[2]	+	Low	90	20-60	3-4	26	Hepatic; renal excretion 30% to 40%; nonrenal excretion 50% to 60% (bile; intestinal wall)
Atenolol	β_1[1]		0	0	Low	50	50-60	6-7	6-16	≈ 50% excreted unchanged in feces
Betaxolol	β_1[1]		+	0	Low	≈ 100	89	14-22	≈ 50	Hepatic; > 80% recovered in urine, 15% unchanged
Bisoprolol	β_1[1]		0	0	Low	≥ 90	80	9-12	≈ 30	≈ 50% excreted unchanged in urine, remainder as inactive metabolites; < 2% excreted in feces.
Esmolol	β_1[1]		0	0	Low	na[3]	na[3]	0.15	55	Rapid metabolism by esterases in cytosol of red blood cells
Metoprolol	β_1[1]		0[2]	0	Moderate	≈ 100	40-50	3-7	12	Hepatic; renal excretion, < 5% unchanged
Metoprolol, long-acting							77[4]			
Carteolol	β_1	β_2	0	++	Low	85	85	6	23-30	50% to 70% excreted unchanged in urine
Nadolol	β_1	β_2	0	0	Low	30	30-50	20-24	30	Urine, unchanged
Penbutolol	β_1	β_2	0	+	High	≈ 100	≈ 100	≈ 5	80-98	Hepatic (conjugation, oxidation); renal excretion of metabolites (17% as conjugate)
Pindolol	β_1	β_2	0	+++	Low	> 95	≈ 100	3-4[5]	40	Urinary excretion of metabolites (60% to 65%) and unchanged drug (35% to 40%)
Propranolol	β_1	β_2	++	0	High	< 90	30	3-5	90	Hepatic; < 1% excreted unchanged in urine
Propranolol, long-acting							9-18	8-11		
Sotalol	β_1	β_2	0	0	Low	nd[6]	90-100	12	0	Not metabolized; excreted unchanged in urine
Timolol	β_1	β_2	0	0	Low to moderate	90	75	4	< 10	Hepatic; urinary excretion of metabolites and unchanged drug

[1] Inhibits β_2 receptors (bronchial and vascular) at higher doses.
[2] Detectable only at doses much greater than required for beta blockade.
[3] Not applicable (available IV only).
[4] Average bioavailability; not absolute.
[5] In elderly hypertensive patients with normal renal function, t½ variable: 7 to 15 hours.
[6] No data.

Beta-adrenergic receptor blocking agents compete with beta-adrenergic agonists for available beta receptor sites. Propranolol, nadolol, timolol, penbutolol, carteolol, sotalol, and pindolol inhibit both the β_1 receptors (located chiefly in myocardium, kidney, and eye) and β_2 receptors (located chiefly in adipose tissue, pancreas, liver, and smooth and skeletal muscle), inhibiting the chronotropic, inotropic, and vasodilator responses to β-adrenergic stimulation. Metoprolol, acebutolol, bisopro-lol, esmolol, betaxolol, and atenolol are cardioselective and preferentially inhibit β_1 receptors.

Propranolol and, to a lesser extent, acebutolol and betaxolol, exert a quinidine-like (anesthetic) membrane action (membrane stabilizing activity; MSA), which affects cardiac action potential. Pindolol, carteo-lol, penbutolol, and acebutolol have intrinsic sympathomimetic activity (ISA) in therapeutic dosage ranges. ISA or partial agonist activity is mediated directly at adrenergic receptor sites and may be blocked by

Beta-Adrenergic Blocking Agents

other β antagonists. ISA is manifested by a smaller reduction in resting cardiac output and resting heart rate (4 to 8 beats per minute [BPM]) than is seen with drugs lacking ISA; clinical significance has not been evaluated and there is no evidence that exercise cardiac output is less affected by pindolol.

➤*Pharmacokinetics:*

Absorption – Systemic bioavailability following oral administration of metoprolol, acebutolol, timolol, and propranolol is low because of significant first-pass hepatic metabolism. Pindolol, sotalol, and carteolol have no significant first-pass effect; first-pass metabolism of bisoprolol is ≈ 20%. Ingestion with food enhances the bioavailability of propranolol and metoprolol, and reduces the absorption of sotalol; this effect is not noted with nadolol, carteolol, pindolol, bisoprolol, or betaxolol.

Distribution – There is no simple correlation between dose or plasma level and therapeutic effect; the dose-sensitivity range observed in clinical practice is wide because sympathetic tone varies widely among individuals. There is no reliable test to estimate sympathetic tone or to determine whether total β-blockade has been achieved; proper dosage requires titration. There appear to be significant correlations between acebutolol plasma levels and both the reduction in resting heart rate and the percent of β-blockade of exercise-induced tachycardia.

Metoprolol and propranolol readily enter the CNS. Because of their high water solubility, sotalol, acebutolol, carteolol, nadolol, and atenolol do not pass the blood-brain barrier; these drugs may have a lower incidence of CNS side effects.

➤*Clinical trials:* Clinical response to β-blockade includes slowing of sinus heart rate, depressed AV conduction, decreased cardiac output, and reduction of systolic and diastolic blood pressure at rest and on exercise, reduction of supine and standing blood pressure, inhibition of isoproterenol-induced tachycardia, and reduction of reflex orthostatic tachycardia. β-adrenergic receptor blockade is useful in conditions (eg, angina, hypertension) in which, because of pathologic or functional changes, sympathetic activity is detrimental to the patient. Also, in some situations, sympathetic stimulation is vital: In patients with severely damaged hearts, adequate ventricular function is maintained by virtue of sympathetic drive, which should be preserved. β-adrenergic blockade may worsen AV block by preventing necessary facilitating effects of sympathetic activity on conduction.

β₂-adrenergic blockade results in passive bronchial constriction by interfering with endogenous adrenergic bronchodilator activity in patients subject to bronchospasm and may also interfere with exogenous bronchodilators. Although **pindolol** does not eliminate sympathetic tone entirely, there is no controlled evidence that it is safer than other agents or is less likely to cause conditions such as heart failure, heart block, or bronchospasm.

Hypertension – β-blockers decrease standing and supine blood pressure. They are effective antihypertensives when used alone or with other antihypertensives. Although not established, several mechanisms have been proposed: Competitive antagonism of catecholamines at peripheral (non-CNS) adrenergic neuron sites (especially cardiac) leading to decreased cardiac output; a central effect leading to reduced sympathetic outflow to the periphery; blockade of the beta-adrenergic receptors responsible for renin release from the kidneys. These mechanisms appear less likely for **pindolol** than other β-blockers in view of the modest effect on resting cardiac output and its inconsistent effect on plasma renin activity. **Propranolol** may cause a small increase in serum potassium concentration when used in the treatment of hypertension.

Angina – May reduce myocardial oxygen requirements by blocking catecholamine-induced increases in heart rate, systolic blood pressure and velocity, and extent of myocardial contraction. Oxygen requirements may be increased by increasing left ventricular fiber length, end diastolic pressure, and systolic ejection period. Net physiologic effect of β-adrenergic blockade is advantageous and is manifested during exercise by delayed onset of pain and increased work capacity.

Arrhythmias – **Propranolol** and **acebutolol** prolong the effective refractory period of the AV node and slow AV conduction.

MI – The precise mechanism by which beta-blockers exert their beneficial effects is unclear. These drugs reduce myocardial oxygen demand by lowering heart rate and blood pressure, which has a protective effect on jeopardized ischemic myocardial tissue. Beta blockers also seem to attenuate the malignancy of ventricular ectopy, possibly by altering the biological milieu in which these arrhythmias occur. Improvements in mortality probably result from reductions in cardiac rupture, reinfarction, ventricular fibrillation, and a reduced predilection for plaque rupture.

Migraine – The mechanism has not been established. Beta-adrenergic receptors have been demonstrated in the pial vessels of the brain.

Antitremor – The specific mechanism has not been established, but β₂ receptors may be involved. A central effect is also possible.

Contraindications

Sinus bradycardia; greater than first-degree heart block; cardiogenic shock; CHF unless secondary to a tachyarrhythmia treatable with β-blockers; overt cardiac failure; hypersensitivity to β-blocking agents.

➤*Acebutolol, carteolol:* Persistently severe bradycardia.

➤*Propranolol, nadolol, timolol, penbutolol, carteolol, sotalol, and pindolol:* Bronchial asthma, including severe chronic obstructive pulmonary disease.

➤*Metoprolol:* Treatment of MI in patients with a heart rate < 45 BPM; significant heart block greater than first-degree (PR interval ≥ 0.24 sec); systolic blood pressure < 100 mmHg; moderate to severe cardiac failure.

➤*Sotalol:* Congenital or acquired long QT syndromes.

Warnings

➤*Mortality:* The National Heart Lung and Blood Institute conducted the Cardiac Arrhythmia Suppression Trial (CAST-I), a long-term, multicenter, randomized, double-blind study in patients with asymptomatic non-life-threatening ventricular ectopy who had an MI > 6 days but < 2 years previously. An excessive mortality or nonfatal cardiac arrest was seen in patients treated with encainide or flecainide (56/730) compared with that seen in patients assigned to matched placebo-treated groups (22/725), and a similar excess has been seen with moricizine. The average duration of treatment with encainide or flecainide in this study was 10 months.

CAST-II originally was designed as a blinded, randomized trial divided into a 14-day exposure phase to evaluate the risk of initiating treatment with moricizine after MI, and a long-term phase to evaluate survival after MI. The study was stopped early because the first 14-day period of treatment with moricizine after MI was associated with excess mortality, as compared with no treatment or placebo. As with the antiarrhythmic agents used in CAST-I, the use of moricizine to reduce mortality after MI is not only ineffective, but also harmful.

The applicability of these results to other populations (eg, those without recent MI) and to other than Class I antiarrhythmic agents is uncertain. **Sotalol** is devoid of Class I effects, and in a large controlled trial in patients with a recent MI who did not necessarily have ventricular arrhythmias, sotalol did not produce increased mortality at doses up to 320 mg/day. Conversely, in the large postinfarction study using a nontitrated initial dose of 320 mg once daily and in a second small randomized trial in high-risk postinfarction patients treated with high doses (320 mg twice daily), there have been suggestions of an excess of early sudden deaths.

➤*Proarrhythmia:* Like other antiarrhythmic agents, sotalol can provoke new or worsened ventricular arrhythmias in some patients, including sustained ventricular tachycardia or ventricular fibrillation, with potentially fatal consequences. Because of its effect on cardiac repolarization (QTc interval prolongation), torsades de pointes (a polymorphic ventricular tachycardia with prolongation of the QT interval and a shifting electrical axis) is the most common form of proarrhythmia associated with sotalol, occurring in about 4% of high-risk (history of sustained ventricular tachycardia/ventricular fibrillation [VT/VF]) patients. The risk of torsades de pointes progressively increases with prolongation of the QT interval and is worsened also by reduction in heart rate and reduction in serum potassium.

Overall, 4.3% of patients experienced a new or worsened ventricular arrhythmia. Of this 4.3%, there was new or worsened sustained ventricular tachycardia in ≈ 1% of patients and torsades de pointes in 2.4%. Additionally, in ≈ 1% of patients, deaths were considered possibly drug-related and may have been associated with proarrhythmic events. In patients with a history of sustained ventricular tachycardia, the incidence of torsades de pointes was 4% and worsened VT ≈ 1%; in patients with other, less serious, ventricular and supraventricular arrhythmias, the incidence of torsades de pointes was 1% and 1.4%, respectively. Torsade de pointes arrhythmias were dose-related.

In addition to dose and presence of sustained VT, other risk factors for torsades de pointes were gender (females had a higher incidence), excessive prolongation of the QTc interval, and history of cardiomegaly or CHF. Patients with sustained ventricular tachycardia and a history of CHF appear to have the highest risk for serious proarrhythmia (7%). Of the patients experiencing torsades de pointes, ≈ ⅔ spontaneously reverted to their baseline rhythm. The others were either converted electrically (D/C cardioversion or overdrive pacing) or treated with other drugs. Although **sotalol** therapy was discontinued in most patients experiencing torsades de pointes, 17% were continued on a lower dose. Nonetheless, use with particular caution if the QTc is > 500 msec on-therapy and give serious consideration to reducing the dose or discontinuing therapy when the QTc exceeds 550 msec. However, because of the multiple risk factors associated with torsades de pointes, exercise caution regardless of the QTc interval.

Proarrhythmic events must be anticipated not only on initiating sotalol therapy, but with every upward dose adjustment. Proarrhythmic events most often occur within 7 days of initiating therapy or of an increase in dose; 75% of serious proarrhythmias (torsades de pointes and worsened VT) occurred within 7 days of initiating therapy, while 60% of such events occurred within 3 days of initiation or a dosage change. Initiating therapy at 80 mg twice daily with gradual upward dose titration and appropriate evaluations for efficacy and safety prior to dose escalation, should reduce the risk of proarrhythmia. Avoiding excessive accumulation of sotalol in patients with diminished renal function, by appropriate dose reduction, should also reduce the risk of proarrhythmia (see Administration and Dosage).

➤*Cardiac failure:* Sympathetic stimulation is a vital component supporting circulatory function in CHF, and β-blockade carries the potential hazard of further depressing myocardial contractility and precipitating more severe failure. Administer cautiously in hypertensive patients who have CHF controlled by digitalis and diuretics. β-blockers do not abolish the inotropic action of digitalis on heart muscle. Digitalis and β-blockers slow AV conduction. If cardiac failure persists, withdraw β-blocker therapy.

Although cardiac failure rarely occurs in properly selected patients, advise patients to consult a physician at the first sign or symptom of impending CHF or unexplained respiratory symptoms.

In patients without a history of cardiac failure, continued myocardial depression can lead to cardiac failure. At the first sign or symptom of impending cardiac failure, fully digitalize patients or treat with diuretics and closely observe the response. If cardiac failure continues, withdraw therapy (gradually, if possible).

Studies suggest that in certain patients with CHF, beta blockers may result in symptomatic and hemodynamic improvements. β₁ selective agents are the drugs of choice; start with a low dose and titrate upward. They should not be used as routine therapy nor for acute heart failure. In these studies, most patients had idiopathic dilated cardiomyopathy. Further study is needed to identify patients most likely to benefit from therapy as well as the appropriate drug.

➤*Wolff-Parkinson-White syndrome:* In several cases, the tachycardia was replaced by a severe bradycardia requiring a demand pacemaker after **propranolol** administration with as little as 5 mg.

➤*Abrupt withdrawal:* The occurrence of a β-blocker withdrawal syndrome is controversial. However, hypersensitivity to catecholamines has been observed in patients withdrawn from β-blocker therapy. Exacerbation of angina, MI, ventricular arrhythmias, and death have occurred after abrupt discontinuation of therapy. When discontinuing chronically administered β-blocking agents, particularly in patients with ischemic heart disease, reduce dosage gradually over 1 to 2 weeks and carefully monitor the patient. If therapy with an alternative β-adrenergic blocker is desired, the patient may be transferred directly to comparable doses of another agent without interrupting β-blocking therapy. If angina markedly worsens or acute coronary insufficiency develops, reinstitute administration promptly, at least temporarily, and employ other measures to manage unstable angina.

Because coronary artery disease may be unrecognized, do not discontinue therapy abruptly, even in patients treated only for hypertension, as abrupt withdrawal may result in transient symptoms (eg, tremulousness, sweating, palpitations, headache, malaise).

It has been suggested that β-adrenergic blockers may be discontinued abruptly during acute MI if indicated because the withdrawal phenomenon is not a major clinical problem in these patients.

➤*Peripheral vascular disease:* Treatment with β-antagonists reduces cardiac output and can precipitate or aggravate the symptoms of arterial insufficiency in patients with peripheral or mesenteric vascular disease. Exercise caution with such patients and observe closely for evidence of progression of arterial obstruction.

➤*Nonallergic bronchospasm (eg, chronic bronchitis, emphysema):* In general, do not administer β-blockers to patients with bronchospastic diseases. Administer **nadolol, timolol, penbutolol, propranolol, sotalol, carteolol,** and **pindolol** with caution, because they may block bronchodilation produced by endogenous or exogenous catecholamine stimulation of β₂ receptors.

Because of their relative β₁ selectivity, low doses of **metoprolol, acebutolol, betaxalol, bisoprolol,** and **atenolol** may be used with caution in patients with bronchospastic disease who do not respond to, or cannot tolerate, other antihypertensive treatment. Because β₁ selectivity is not absolute, use the lowest possible dose of a β₂-stimulating agent. It may be advisable initially to administer in smaller divided doses, instead of larger doses twice daily, to avoid the higher plasma levels associated with the longer dosing interval. **Esmolol** may also be used with caution in patients with asthma if an IV agent is required.

Because it is unknown to what extent β₂-stimulating agents may exacerbate myocardial ischemia and the extent of infarction, β-blockers should not be used prophylactically. If bronchospasm not related to CHF occurs, discontinue β-blockers. A theophylline derivative or a β₂ agonist may be administered cautiously, depending on the clinical condition of the patient. Both theophylline derivatives and β₂ agonists may produce serious cardiac arrhythmias.

➤*Bradycardia:*

Metoprolol – Metoprolol produces a decrease in sinus heart rate in most patients; this decrease is greatest among patients with high initial heart rates and least among patients with low initial heart rates. Acute MI (particularly inferior infarction) may, in itself, produce significant lowering of the sinus rate. If the sinus rate decreases to < 40 BPM, particularly if associated with lowered cardiac output, give IV atropine (0.25 to 0.5 mg). If treatment with atropine is not success-

ful, discontinue metoprolol and consider cautious administration of isoproterenol or installation of a cardiac pacemaker.

➤*Pheochromocytoma:* It is hazardous to use **propranolol** or **atenolol** unless α-adrenergic blocking drugs are already in use, because this would predispose to serious blood pressure elevation. Blocking only the peripheral dilator (β) action of epinephrine leaves its constrictor (α) action unopposed. In the event of hemorrhage or shock, there is a disadvantage in having both β and α blockade; the combination prevents the increase in heart rate and peripheral vasoconstriction needed to maintain blood pressure.

➤*Sinus bradycardia (heart rate < 50 bpm):* This occurred in 13% of patients receiving **sotalol** in clinical trials, and led to discontinuation in about 3%. Bradycardia itself increases risk of torsades de pointes. Sinus pause, sinus arrest, and sinus node dysfunction occur in < 1% of patients. Incidence of 2nd- or 3rd- degree AV block is ≈ 1%.

➤*Electrolyte disturbances:* Do not use **sotalol** in patients with hypokalemia or hypomagnesemia prior to correction of imbalance, as these conditions can exaggerate the degree of QT prolongation and increase the potential for torsades de pointes. Give special attention to electrolyte and acid-base balance in patients experiencing severe or prolonged diarrhea or patients receiving concomitant diuretic drugs.

➤*Hypotension:* If hypotension (systolic blood pressure ≤ 90 mmHg) occurs, discontinue drug and carefully assess patient's hemodynamic status and extent of myocardial damage. Invasive monitoring of central venous, pulmonary capillary wedge, and arterial pressures may be required. Institute fluids, positive inotropic agents, balloon counterpulsation or other appropriate therapy. If hypotension is associated with sinus bradycardia or AV block, direct treatment at reversing these.

In clinical trials, 20% to 50% of patients treated with **esmolol** have had hypotension, generally defined as systolic pressure < 90 mmHg or diastolic pressure < 50 mmHg. About 12% of the patients have been symptomatic (mainly diaphoresis or dizziness). Hypotension can occur at any dose, but is dose-related; therefore, doses > 200 mcg/kg/min are not recommended. Closely monitor patients, especially if pretreatment blood pressure is low. Decrease of dose or termination of infusion reverses hypotension, usually within 30 minutes.

➤*Anaphylaxis:* Anaphylaxis has occurred and may include symptoms such as profound hypotension, bradycardia with or without AV nodal block, severe sustained bronchospasm, hives, and angioedema. Deaths have occurred. Refer to Management of Acute Hypersensitivity Reactions.However, patients have been resistant to conventional therapy, especially epinephrine. Aggressive therapy may be required.

➤*Anesthesia and major surgery:* Necessity, or desirability, of withdrawing β-blockers prior to major surgery is controversial. β-blockade impairs the heart's ability to respond to β-adrenergically mediated reflex stimuli. While this might help prevent arrhythmic response, risk of excessive myocardial depression during general anesthesia may be enhanced, and difficulty restarting and maintaining heart beat has occurred. If β-blockers are withdrawn, allow several days between the last dose and anesthesia. If treatment is continued, take particular care when using anesthetics that depress the myocardium, such as ether, cyclopropane and trichlorethylene; use the lowest possible β-blocker doses. Others may recommend withdrawal of β-blockers well before surgery takes place.

In the event of emergency surgery, effects of β-blockers can be reversed by β-receptor agonists (eg, isoproterenol, dopamine, dobutamine, norepinephrine).

➤*AV block:* **Metoprolol** slows AV conduction and may produce significant first (PR interval ≥ 0.26 sec), second, or third-degree heart block. Acute MI also produces heart block.

If heart block occurs, discontinue metoprolol and give IV atropine (0.25 to 0.5 mg). If treatment with atropine is not successful, consider cautious administration of isoproterenol or installation of a cardiac pacemaker.

➤*Sick sinus syndrome:* Use **sotalol** only with extreme caution in patients with sick sinus syndrome associated with symptomatic arrhythmias because it may cause sinus bradycardia, sinus pauses, or sinus arrest.

➤*Concomitant use of calcium channel blockers (atenolol):* Bradycardia and heart block can occur and the left ventricular end diastolic pressure can rise when beta-blockers are administered with verapamil or diltiazem. Patients with preexisting conduction abnormalities or left ventricular dysfunction are particularly susceptible.

➤*Recent acute MI (sotalol):* Sotalol can be used safely and effectively in the long-term treatment of life-threatening ventricular arrhythmias following an MI. However, experience in the use of sotalol to treat cardiac arrhythmias in the early phase of recovery from acute MI is limited and at least at high initial doses is not reassuring. In the first 2 weeks post-MI, caution is advised and careful dose titration is especially important, particularly in patients with markedly impaired ventricular function.

➤*Intraoperative and postoperative tachycardia and hypertension:* Do not use esmolol as the treatment for hypertension in patients in whom the increased blood pressure is primarily caused by the vaso-

Beta-Adrenergic Blocking Agents

constriction associated with hypothermia.

➤*Renal/Hepatic function impairment:* Use with caution. **Timolol's** half-life is essentially unchanged in moderate renal insufficiency; however, marked hypotensive responses have been seen in patients with marked renal impairment undergoing dialysis. Dosage reduction may be necessary in impaired renal or hepatic function.

Because **nadolol, carteolol, sotalol,** and **atenolol** are eliminated primarily by the kidney, half-life increases in renal failure; dosage adjustments are necessary (see Administration and Dosage). **Bisoprolol's** half-life is increased in patients with creatinine clearance < 40 mL/min and in cirrhosis; adjust dosage. Although **acebutolol** is excreted through the GI tract, the active metabolite, diacetolol, is eliminated primarily by the kidney; reduce daily acebutolol dose (see Administration and Dosage). Administer **esmolol** with caution in impaired renal function because its acid metabolite is primarily excreted unchanged by the kidney. Elimination half-life of the acid metabolite was prolonged 10-fold and plasma level was considerably elevated in end-stage renal disease. Poor renal function has only minor effects on **pindolol** clearance, but poor hepatic function may cause pindolol blood levels to increase substantially. Expect **penbutolol** conjugate accumulation upon multiple dosing in renal insufficiency. **Metoprolol's** systemic availability and half-life in renal failure do not differ significantly from those in normal subjects; dosage reduction is usually not needed. **Betaxolol** is primarily metabolized in the liver to metabolites that are inactive and then excreted by the kidneys; clearance is somewhat reduced in patients with renal failure but little changed in patients with hepatic disease. Reduce dosage in patients with severe renal impairment and those on dialysis; dosage reductions have not routinely been necessary in hepatic insufficiency.

➤*Pregnancy:* Category D (**atenolol**). Atenolol can cause fetal harm when administered to a pregnant woman. Atenolol crosses the placental barrier and appears in cord blood. Administration of atenolol, starting in the second trimester of pregnancy, has been associated with the birth of infants that are small for gestational age. No studies have been performed on the use of atenolol in the first trimester and the possibility of fetal injury cannot be excluded.

Category C (**betaxolol, esmolol, metoprolol, nadolol, timolol, propranolol, penbutolol, carteolol, bisoprolol**). Embryotoxic effects have been demonstrated in animals at doses 5 to 600 times higher than the maximum recommended doses in humans.

Category B (**acebutolol, pindolol, sotalol**). Acebutolol and its major metabolite, diacetolol, cross the placenta. Neonates of mothers who received acebutolol during pregnancy have reduced birth weight and decreased blood pressure and heart rate. Sotalol crosses the placenta and is found in amniotic fluid; subnormal birth weight has occurred.

Safety for use during pregnancy has not been established. Use only when clearly needed and when the potential benefits outweigh the potential hazards to the fetus.

Although cases of teratogenicity in humans have not been reported, problems have occurred during delivery. These include the following: Neonatal bradycardia, hypoglycemia and apnea, low Apgar scores, maternal and fetal bradycardia, hypothermia, oliguria, poor peripheral perfusion, and small birth weight infants (caused by chronic therapy). Some of the effects on the neonate may last up to 72 hours postpartum.

➤*Lactation:* **Propranolol, pindolol, timolol, sotalol, betaxalol,** and **nadolol** are excreted in breast milk. **Acebutolol** and diacetolol (its major metabolite) appear in breast milk with a milk:plasma ratio of 7.1 and 12.2, respectively. **Metoprolol** is excreted in breast milk in very small quantities; an infant consuming 1 L of breast milk would receive a dose of < 1 mg of the drug. **Atenolol** is excreted in breast milk at a ratio of 1.5 to 6.8. In one patient, the peak atenolol milk:plasma ratio was 3.6 and the estimated infant dose (maternal dose, 100 mg/day) was 0.13 mg/feeding (75 mL). Another infant developed cyanosis and 2 incidences of bradycardia following maternal atenolol ingestion (100 mg/day). Small amounts of **bisoprolol** (< 2% of the dose) are detected in the breast milk of rats; it is not known if it is excreted in human breast milk. Betaxolol is excreted in sufficient amounts to have pharmacological effects in the infant. It is not known if **penbutolol, carteolol,** or **esmolol** are excreted in breast milk. Nursing should not be undertaken by mothers receiving these drugs.

➤*Children:* Safety and efficacy for use in children have not been established.

IV administration of **propranolol** is not recommended in children; however, oral propranolol has been used (see Administration and Dosage).

Precautions

➤*Diabetes/Hypoglycemia:* β-adrenergic blockade may blunt premonitory signs and symptoms (eg, pulse rate, tachycardia, blood pressure changes) of acute hypoglycemia, but other manifestations such as dizziness and sweating may not be significantly affected. Hypoglycemic attacks may be accompanied by a precipitous elevation of blood pressure in patients on **propranolol**. Nonselective β-blockers may potentiate insulin-induced hypoglycemia. This is less likely with cardioselective agents. **Atenolol** does not potentiate insulin-induced hypoglycemia and, unlike nonselective β-blockers, does not delay recovery of blood glucose to normal levels.

Use with caution in diabetic patients, especially those with labile diabetes. β blockade reduces the release of insulin in response to hyperglycemia; it may be necessary to adjust the dose of antidiabetic drugs. Propranolol therapy, particularly in infants and children, diabetic or not, has been associated with hypoglycemia, especially during fasting as in preparation for surgery. Hypoglycemia also has been found after this type of drug therapy and prolonged physical exertion and has occurred in renal insufficiency, both during dialysis and sporadically, in patients on propranolol.

➤*Thyrotoxicosis:* β-adrenergic blockers may mask clinical signs (eg, tachycardia) of developing or continuing hyperthyroidism. Abrupt withdrawal may exacerbate symptoms of hyperthyroidism, including thyroid storm; therefore, monitor closely and withdraw the drug slowly.

Propranolol may change thyroid-function tests, increasing T_4 and reverse T_3, and decreasing T_3.

➤*Serum lipid concentrations:* Although study results conflict, β-blockers may alter serum lipids including an increase in the concentration of total triglycerides, total cholesterol and LDL and VLDL cholesterol, and a decrease in the concentration of HDL cholesterol; however, this finding is not clinically significant. Other studies suggest **pindolol** does not significantly alter serum lipid concentrations and **acebutolol** actually lowers total and LDL cholesterol levels; **carteolol** and **bisoprolol** did not significantly alter total cholesterol and triglycerides. Further studies are needed.

➤*Muscle weakness:* β-blockade has potentiated muscle weakness consistent with certain myasthenic symptoms (eg, diplopia, ptosis, generalized weakness). **Timolol** rarely increased muscle weakness in some patients with myasthenia gravis or myasthenic symptoms.

Drug Interactions

Beta-Blocker Drug Interactions			
Precipitant drug	Object drug*		Description
Aluminum salts Barbiturates Calcium salts Cholestyramine Colestipol Penicillins (ampicillin) Rifampin	β-blockers	↓	The bioavailability and plasma levels of certain β-blockers may be decreased by these agents, possibly resulting in a decreased pharmacologic effect.
Calcium channel blockers	β-blockers	↑	Pharmacologic effects of β-blockers as well as nifedipine and verapamil may be synergistic or additive. Diltiazem and nicardipine may decrease the metabolism of certain beta blockers, thus increasing the pharmacologic effects.
Cimetidine	β-blockers Metoprolol Propranolol	↑	Pharmacokinetic parameters of β-blockers metabolized by cytochrome P450 may be altered by cimetidine; pharmacodynamic effects may be increased.
Contraceptives, oral	β-blockers	↑	Bioavailability and plasma levels of certain β-blockers may be increased.
Diphenhydramine	β-blockers	↑	Diphenhydramine may increase plasma concentrations and cardiovascular effects of certain β-blockers through inhibition of CYP2D6-mediated metabolism.
Flecainide	β-blockers	↑	The bioavailability of either agent may be increased, possibly increasing the pharmacologic effects.
β-blockers	Flecainide		
Haloperidol	β-blockers Propranolol	↑	Pharmacologic effects (hypotensive episodes) of both drugs may be increased.
β-blockers Propranolol	Haloperidol		
Hydralazine	β-blockers Metoprolol Propranolol	↑	Serum levels and, hence, pharmacologic effects of β-blockers and hydralazine may be enhanced.
β-blockers Metoprolol Propranolol	Hydralazine		
Hydroxychloroquine	β-blockers	↑	Plasma concentrations and cardiovascular effects of certain β-blockers may be increased because hydroxychloroquine inhibits the CYP2D6-mediated β-blocker metabolism.
Loop diuretics	β-blockers Propranolol	↑	Propranolol plasma levels and cardiovascular effects may be enhanced. Atenolol was not affected.

Beta-Adrenergic Blocking Agents

Beta-Blocker Drug Interactions			
Precipitant drug	Object drug*		Description
MAO inhibitors	β-blockers Metoprolol Nadolol	↑	Bradycardia may develop during concurrent use.
NSAIDs Salicylates Sulfinpyrazone	β-blockers	↓	NSAIDs, salicylates, and sulfinpyrazone may inhibit the synthesis of prostaglandins involved in the antihypertensive activity of β-blockers.
Phenothiazines	β-blockers Propranolol		Propranolol bioavailability and plasma levels and phenothiazine plasma levels may be increased, possibly resulting in increased effects.
β-blockers Propranolol	Phenothiazines		
Propafenone	β-blockers Metoprolol Propranolol	↑	Plasma levels of β-blockers metabolized by the liver may be increased.
Quinidine	β-blockers	↑	Plasma β-blocker levels may be increased in "extensive metabolizers," possibly resulting in increased effects.
Quinolones Ciprofloxacin	β-blockers	↑	Bioavailability of β-blockers metabolized by cytochrome P450 may be increased.
SSRIs	β-blockers Metoprolol Propranolol	↑	Certain SSRIs may inhibit the metabolism (CYP2D6) of certain β-blockers, leading to excessive β-blockade.
Thioamines	β-blockers Metoprolol Propranolol	↑	The pharmacokinetics of the β-blockers may be altered, increasing the pharmacologic effects.
Thyroid hormones	β-blockers Metoprolol Propranolol	↓	The actions of certain β-blockers may be impaired when the hypothyroid patient is converted to the euthyroid state.
β-blockers Propranolol	Anticoagulants	↑	Propranolol may increase the anticoagulant effect of warfarin.
β-blockers Metoprolol Propranolol	Benzodiazepines	↑	Effects of certain benzodiazepines may be increased by lipophilic β-blockers. Atenolol does not interact.
β-blockers	Clonidine	↑	Life-threatening and fatal increases in blood pressure have occurred after discontinuation of clonidine in patients receiving a β-blocker or after simultaneous withdrawal.
β-blockers	Disopyramide	⟷	Difficult to predict; disopyramide clearance may be decreased; adverse effects may occur (eg, sinus bradycardia, hypotension) or there may be no occurrence of synergistic or additive negative inotropic effects.
β-blockers	Epinephrine	↑	Nonselective β-blockade allows alpha receptor effects of epinephrine to predominate. Increasing vascular resistance leads to initial hypertensive episode followed by bradycardia.
β-blockers	Ergot alkaloids	↑	Peripheral ischemia manifested by cold extremities, possible peripheral gangrene may develop due to ergot alkaloid-mediated vasoconstriction and β-blocker-mediated blockade of peripheral β$_2$ receptors, allowing for unopposed ergot action.
β-blockers Propranolol	Gabapentin	↑	Gabapentin adverse reactions may be increased.
β-blockers	Lidocaine	↑	Increased lidocaine levels may occur, resulting in toxicity.
β-blockers	Nondepolarizing muscle relaxants	⟷	β-blockers may potentiate, counteract, delay, or have no effect on the actions of the nondepolarizing muscle relaxants.
β-blockers	Prazosin	↑	Concurrent administration may increase the postural hypotension produced by prazosin.
β-blockers	Sulfonylureas	↓	Hypoglycemic effects of sulfonylureas may be attenuated.

Beta-Blocker Drug Interactions			
Precipitant drug	Object drug*		Description
β-blockers Nonselective	Theophylline	⟷	Reduced elimination of theophylline may occur. Pharmacologic antagonism can also be expected, thus reducing the effects of one or both agents. Cardioselective agents may be preferred.

* ↑ = Object drug increased. ↓ = Object drug decreased. ⟷ = Undetermined clinical effect.

➤*Drug/Lab test interactions:* These agents may produce hypoglycemia and interfere with **glucose** or **insulin** tolerance tests. **Propranolol** and **betaxolol** may interfere with the glaucoma screening test because of a reduction in intraocular pressure.

➤*Drug/Food interactions:* Food enhances the bioavailability of **metoprolol** and **propranolol**; food does not enhance the bioavailability of **nadolol**, **bisoprolol**, or **pindolol**. The rate of **carteolol** and **penbutolol** absorption is slowed by the presence of food; however, extent of absorption is not appreciably affected. **Sotalol** absorption is reduced ≈ 20% by a standard meal.

Adverse Reactions

Most adverse effects are mild and transient and rarely require withdrawal of therapy.

➤*Cardiovascular:* Bradycardia; torsades de pointes and other serious new ventricular arrhythmias (see Warnings); cardiovascular disorder; automatic implantable cardioverter/defibrillator (AICD) discharge; development of mitral regurgitation; cardiac reinfarction; total cardiac arrest; nonfatal cardiac arrest; cardiogenic shock; development of ventricular septal defect; chest pain; hypertension; hypotension (including asymptomatic and orthostatic); peripheral ischemia; flushing; worsening of angina and arterial insufficiency; shortness of breath; peripheral vascular insufficiency (cold extremities, paresthesia of hands); arterial insufficiency; claudication (including intermittent); heart failure; CHF; sinoatrial block; cerebral vascular accident; edema; pulmonary edema; vasodilation; presyncope and syncope; tachycardia (including ventricular); palpitations; conduction disturbances; first-, second- and third-degree heart block; intensification of AV block; abnormal ECG; bundle branch block plus major axis deviation; supraventricular tachycardia (including atrial fibrillation and flutter); angina pectoris; AV block; MI; thrombosis; cerebrovascular disorder; leg cramps; thrombophlebitis; disturbance rhythm atrial; disturbance rhythm subjective; diaphoresis; proarrhythmia; peripheral vascular disorder.

➤*CNS:* Dizziness; vertigo; tiredness/fatigue; headache; mental depression (lassitude, weakness); peripheral neuropathy; paralysis; paresthesias; hypesthesia; hyperesthesia; lethargy; anxiety; nervousness; diminished concentration/memory; somnolence; restlessness; insomnia; sleep disturbances; nightmares; bizarre or many dreams; sedation; change in behavior; altered consciousness; mood change; slightly clouded sensorium; incoordination; reversible mental depression progressing to catatonia; hallucinations; an acute reversible syndrome characterized by disorientation of time and place, short-term memory loss, emotional lability, decreased performance on neuropsychometrics, slurred speech, tinnitus and lightheadedness; increase in signs and symptoms of myasthenia gravis; ataxia; neuralgia; neuropathy; numbness; stupor; abnormal thinking; amnesia; impaired concentration; confusion; seizures; local weakness; stroke.

It has been suggested that the more lipophilic the β-blocker, the higher the CNS penetration and subsequent incidence of adverse CNS effects. These effects may improve or disappear when a less lipophilic agent is substituted.

➤*Dermatologic:* Rash; pruritus; skin irritation; increased pigmentation; sweating/hyperhidrosis; alopecia (including reversible); dry skin; psoriasis (often reversible); acne; eczema; flushing; exfoliative dermatitis; peripheral skin necrosis; psoriasiform rash or exacerbation of psoriasis; erythematous rash; hypertrichosis; skin disorders; erythema, skin discoloration; burning at infusion site; thrombophlebitis; local skin necrosis; cutaneous vasculitis.

➤*Endocrine:* Hyperglycemia; hypoglycemia; unstable diabetes.

➤*GI:* Gastric/epigastric pain; flatulence; gastritis; constipation; nausea; diarrhea; colon problem; dry mouth; vomiting; heartburn; appetite disorder; anorexia; bloating; abdominal discomfort/pain; mesenteric arterial thrombosis; ischemic colitis; retroperitoneal fibrosis; hepatomegaly; dyspepsia; taste distortion; elevated liver enzymes (see Lab Test Abnormalities); elevated bilirubin; acute hepatitis with jaundice; GI disorder; increased appetite; mouth ulceration; rectal disorders; dysphagia; abnormal taste; taste loss; abdominal distension; taste perversion; digestive tract disorders; taste abnormalities; indigestion.

➤*GU:* Sexual dysfunction; impotence or decreased libido; dysuria; nocturia; pollakiuria; urinary retention or frequency; urinary tract infection; cystitis; renal colic; GU disorder; renal failure; cystitis; micturition disorder; oliguria; proteinuria; abnormal renal function; renal pain; menstrual disorders; prostatitis.

Beta-Adrenergic Blocking Agents

➤*Hematologic:* Agranulocytosis; nonthrombocytopenic or thrombocytopenic purpura; bleeding; thrombocytopenia; eosinophilia; leukopenia; pulmonary emboli; hyperlipidemia; anemia; leukocytosis; lymphadenopathy; purpura.

➤*Hypersensitivity:* Pharyngitis; photosensitivity reaction; erythematous rash; fever combined with aching and sore throat; laryngospasm; respiratory distress; angioedema; anaphylaxis (see Warnings).

➤*Lab test abnormalities:* **Propranolol** may elevate blood urea levels in patients with severe heart disease. **Propranolol** and **metoprolol** may cause elevated serum transaminase, alkaline phosphatase, and LDH. **Timolol** may produce slight increases in BUN, serum potassium, and serum uric acid, and slight decreases in hemoglobin and hematocrit and HDL cholesterol; however, these alterations are not progressive and are not associated with clinical manifestations. Increases in liver function tests have been reported.

Minor persistent elevations in AST and ALT have occurred in 7% of patients treated with **pindolol**, but progressive elevations were not observed and liver injury has not been reported. Alkaline phosphatase, LDH, and uric acid are also elevated on rare occasions. The significance of this is unknown. Elevations of AST and ALT of 1 to 2 times normal have occurred with **bisoprolol** (3.9% to 6.2%). Small increases in uric acid, creatinine, BUN, serum potassium, glucose, and phosphorus, and decreases in WBC and platelets have also occurred, although they were generally not of clinical importance. Liver abnormalities (increased AST and ALT) have occurred in a small number of patients receiving **acebutolol**.

The development of antinuclear antibodies (ANA) has been associated with β-blocker therapy. Symptoms of arthralgia and myalgias were infrequent and reversed upon drug discontinuation.

➤*Musculoskeletal:* Joint pain; arthralgia; muscle cramps/pain; back/neck pain; arthritis; twitching/tremor; localized pain; extremity pain; myalgia; pain; shoulder pain; joint disorder; arthropathy; tendonitis; chest pain; muscle cramps.

➤*Ophthalmic:* Eye irritation/discomfort; visual disturbances; dry/burning eyes; blurred vision; conjunctivitis; ocular pain/pressure; abnormal lacrimation; ptosis; eye disorder; abnormal vision; blepharitis; ocular hemorrhage; iritis; cataract; scotoma; diplopia.

➤*Respiratory:* Bronchospasm; dyspnea; cough; bronchial obstruction; rales; wheeziness; nasal stuffiness; pharyngitis; rhonchi; laryngospasm with respiratory distress; asthma; rhinitis; sinusitis; pulmonary problem; upper respiratory tract problem; cold symptoms; flu symptoms; bronchitis; lung disorder; cough; epistaxis; pneumonia; tracheobronchitis.

➤*Miscellaneous:* Facial swelling; weight gain; weight loss; decreased exercise tolerance; lupus syndrome and lupus-like reactions; Peyronie's disease; Raynaud's phenomenon; speech disorder; rigors; earache; gout; asthenia; malaise; infection; fever; death; tinnitus; injury; salivation; sweating; allergy; breast pain; breast fibroadenosis; labyrinth disorders; deafness; acidosis; diabetes; hypercholesterolemia; hyperglycemia; hyperkalemia; hyperlipemia; hyperuricemia; hypokalemia; thirst; cold sensation; systemic lupus erythmatosus (rarely); speech disorder; midscapular pain; pemphigoid rash; hypertensive reaction in patients with pheochromocytoma.

Overdosage

➤*Symptoms:* Bradycardia, hypotension, low-output cardiac failure, and cardiogenic shock are the most common effects of beta-blocker intoxication.

Cardiovascular – Asystole; tachycardia (partial agonists); prolonged QT interval (sotalol); prolonged QRS complex (membrane-stabilizing agents); ventricular dysrhythmias (membrane-stabilizing agents, sotalol); hypotension; hypertension (partial agonists); bradycardia; AV block.

CNS – Seizures; coma; depressed level of consciousness.

GI – Mesenteric ischemia; esophageal spasms.

Metabolic – Hyperkalemia; hypoglycemia.

Respiratory – Apnea; cyanosis; respiratory depression; bronchospasm.

Miscellaneous – Renal failure.

➤*Treatment:* Perform evaluation of the "ABCs" (airway, breathing, and circulation) as well as rapid assessment of serum glucose levels with correction of hypoglycemia using IV glucagon. Early ventilatory control is essential in addition to chest radiography, serum electrolytes, and arterial blood gases. Administer activated charcoal to all patients and perform gastric lavage in patients who present within 1 to 2 hours after ingestion. In patients who ingest sustained-release preparations, consider whole-bowel irrigation with polyethylene glycol solution. Treat seizures with initial administration of benzodiazepines. Use barbiturates if benzodiazepines are ineffective. **Atenolol, acebutolol, sotalol,** and **nadolol** are the only beta-blockers that can successfully be removed by hemodialysis. Although rare, bronchospasm should be treated with β-agonists. Parenteral ephinephrine may be required in severe cases. See Management of Acute Overdosage.

Other treatments for cardiovascular complications include the following:

1.) *Catecholamine agents:* Epinephrine had the greatest effect of all agents. High-dose isoproterenol and dopamine also have been used for β-blocker toxicity.
2.) *Phosphodiesterase inhibitors:* A positive inotropic effect without an increase in myocardial oxygen demand has been shown in the canine model using amrinone. Milrinone, aminophylline, and theophylline also have been employed for β-blocker toxicity.
3.) *Atropine:* Atropine is the least effective agent in the treatment of β-blocker toxicity, although it is the most frequently used. The lack of effect of a 1 mg dose of atropine may be diagnostic for β-blocker poisoning.
4.) *Pacing:* External cardiac pacing or transvenous pacing is often attempted to treat β-blocker-induced bradycardia; however, it may be ineffective. Overdrive pacing may be necessary in cases of torsades de pointes associated with sotalol intoxication.
5.) *Intra-aortic balloon pump:* If other measures fail, insertion of an intra-aortic balloon pump may restore perfusion.

Patient Information

Do not discontinue medication abruptly, except on advice of physician. Sudden cessation of therapy may precipitate or exacerbate angina.

Consult pharmacist or physician before using other products that may contain α-adrenergic stimulants (eg, nasal decongestants, *otc* cold preparations).

Notify physician if symptoms of CHF occur (eg, difficult breathing, especially on exertion or when lying down; night cough; swelling of the extremities).

Notify physician if any of the following occur: Slow pulse rate, dizziness, lightheadedness, confusion or depression, skin rash, fever, sore throat, unusual bleeding or bruising.

May produce drowsiness, dizziness, lightheadedness, blurred vision; patient should observe caution while driving or performing other tasks requiring alertness, coordination, or physical dexterity.

➤*Diabetics:* These agents may mask signs of hypoglycemia or alter blood glucose levels.

➤*Propranolol and metoprolol:* Food may enhance bioavailability; take at the same time each day.

➤*Nadolol, pindolol, acebutolol, atenolol, carteolol, bisoprolol, betaxolol, and penbutolol:* May be taken without regard to meals.

➤*Sotalol:* Food may reduce absorption. Take on an empty stomach.

ATENOLOL

Rx	**Atenolol** (Various, eg, Geneva, ESI Lederle, Mutual, Mylan, Teva, UDL, URL)	**Tablets:** 25 mg	In 100s, 500s, 1000s, *Robot Ready* 25s, and UD 100s.
Rx	**Tenormin** (AstraZeneca)		(T 107). White. In 100s.
Rx	**Atenolol** (Various, eg, Danbury, ESI Lederle, Mutual, Mylan, Schein, Teva, URL)	**Tablets:** 50 mg	In 100s and 1000s.
Rx	**Tenormin** (AstraZeneca)		(Tenormin 105). White, scored. In 100s, 1000s, and UD 100s.
Rx	**Atenolol** (Various, eg, Danbury, ESI Lederle, Mutual, Mylan, Schein, Teva, URL)	**Tablets:** 100 mg	In 100s and 1000s.
Rx	**Tenormin** (AstraZeneca)		(Tenormin 101). White. In 100s and UD 100s.

For complete prescribing information, refer to the Beta-Adrenergic Blocking Agents group monograph.

Indications

➤*Angina pectoris:* Long-term management of angina pectoris caused by coronary atherosclerosis.

➤*Hypertension:* Used alone or with other antihypertensive agents.

➤*MI:* Indicated for use in acute MI.

Administration and Dosage

➤*Approved by the FDA:* August 1981.

➤*Hypertension (oral):*

Initial dosage – 50 mg once daily, used alone or in combination with other antihypertensive agents. The full effect of this dose will usually be seen within 1 to 2 weeks. If an optimal response is not achieved, increase to 100 mg/day. Dosage > 100 mg/day is unlikely to produce any further benefit.

ATENOLOL

►*Angina pectoris (oral):*

Initial dosage – 50 mg/day. If an optimal response is not achieved within 1 week, increase to 100 mg/day. Some patients may require 200 mg/day for optimal effect.

With once-daily dosing, 24-hour control is achieved by giving doses larger than necessary to achieve an immediate maximum effect. The maximum early effect on exercise tolerance occurs with doses of 50 to 100 mg, but the effect at 24 hours is attenuated, averaging ≈ 50% to 75% of that with once-daily doses of 200 mg.

►*Acute MI:*

IV – Initiate treatment as soon as possible after the patient's arrival in the hospital and after eligibility is established. Begin treatment with 5 mg over 5 minutes followed by another 5 mg IV injection 10 minutes later. Dilutions in Dextrose Injection, Sodium Chloride Injection, or Sodium Chloride and Dextrose Injection may be used. These admixtures are stable for 48 hours if not used immediately.

Oral – In patients who tolerate the full 10 mg IV dose, initiate 50 mg tablets 10 minutes after the last IV dose, followed by another 50 mg dose 12 hours later. Thereafter, administer 100 mg/day or 50 mg twice daily for a further 6 to 9 days or until discharged from the hospital. If bradycardia or hypotension requiring treatment or any other untoward effects occur, discontinue atenolol. (See full prescribing information prior to initiating therapy with atenolol tablets.)

If there is any question concerning the use of IV atenolol, eliminate the IV administration and use the tablets at a dosage of 100 mg once daily or 50 mg twice daily for ≥ 7 days.

►*Elderly/Renal function impairment:* Dosage adjustment is required since atenolol is excreted via the kidneys. No significant accumulation occurs until creatinine clearance falls below 35 mL/min/1.73 m². The following maximum oral dosages are recommended:

Atenolol Dosage Adjustment in Severe Renal Impairment		
Creatinine clearance (mL/min/1.73 m²)	Elimination half-life (hrs)	Maximum dosage
15-35	16-27	50 mg/day
< 15	> 27	25 mg/day

►*Hemodialysis:* Give 25 or 50 mg after each dialysis; administer under hospital supervision as marked decreases in blood pressure can occur.

►*Storage/Stability:* Store at controlled room temperature, 20° to 25°C (68° to 77°F). Dispense in well-closed, light-resistant containers.

ESMOLOL HCl

Rx	**Esmolol** (Baxter)	**Injection:** 10 mg/mL	Preservative free. In 10 mL vials.
Rx	**Brevibloc** (Baxter)		In 10 mL vials.
Rx	**Brevibloc Double Strength** (Baxter)	**Injection:** 20 mg/mL	Preservative free. In ready-to-use 5 mL vials and 100 mL bags.
Rx	**Brevibloc** (Baxter)	**Injection:** 250 mg/mL	25% alcohol. In 10 mL amps.[1]

[1] With 25% propylene glycol.

For complete prescribing information, refer to the Beta-Adrenergic Blocking Agents group monograph.

Indications

►*Supraventricular tachycardia:* For rapid control of ventricular rate in patients with atrial fibrillation or atrial flutter in perioperative, postoperative, or other emergent circumstances where short-term control of ventricular rate with a short-acting agent is desirable. Esmolol is not intended for use in chronic settings where transfer to another agent is anticipated.

►*Noncompensatory sinus tachycardia:* When rapid heart rate requires specific intervention.

►*Intraoperative and postoperative tachycardia and hypertension:* For treatment of tachycardia and hypertension that occur during induction and tracheal intubation, during surgery, on emergence from anesthesia, and in the postoperative period, when in the physician's judgment such specific intervention is indicated.

Administration and Dosage

►*Approved by the FDA:* December 31, 1986.

►*Supraventricular tachycardia:* 50 to 200 mcg/kg/min; average dose is 100 mcg/kg/min, although dosages as low as 25 mcg/kg/min have been adequate. Dosages as high as 300 mcg/kg/min provide little added effect and an increased rate of adverse effects, and are not recommended. Individualize dosage by titration in which each step consists of a loading dose followed by a maintenance dose.

To initiate treatment, administer a loading dose infusion of 500 mcg/kg/min for 1 minute followed by a 4-minute maintenance infusion of 50 mcg/kg/min. If adequate therapeutic effect is not observed within 5 minutes, repeat loading dose and follow with maintenance infusion increased to 100 mcg/kg/min. Continue titration procedure, repeating loading infusion, increasing maintenance infusion by increments of 50 mcg/kg/min (for 4 minutes). As desired heart rate or a safety endpoint (eg, lowered blood pressure) is approached, omit loading infusion and titrate the maintenance dosage up or down to endpoint. Also, if desired, increase interval between titration steps from 5 to 10 minutes.

This specific dosage regimen has not been intraoperatively studied. Because of the time required for titration, it may not be optimal for intraoperative use.

The safety of dosages > 300 mcg/kg/min has not been studied.

In the event of an adverse reaction, reduce dosage or discontinue the drug. If a local infusion site reaction develops, use an alternative site. Avoid butterfly needles.

Dosage in Supraventricular Tachycardia				
Time	Loading dose (over 1 minute)		Maintenance dose (over 4 minutes)	
(minutes)	mcg/kg/min	mg/kg/min	mcg/kg/min	mg/kg/min
0 to 1	500	0.5		
1 to 5			50	0.05
5 to 6	500	0.5		
6 to 10			100	0.1

Dosage in Supraventricular Tachycardia				
Time	Loading dose (over 1 minute)		Maintenance dose (over 4 minutes)	
(minutes)	mcg/kg/min	mg/kg/min	mcg/kg/min	mg/kg/min
10 to 11	500	0.5		
11 to 15			150	0.15
15 to 16	—			
16 to 20			200[1]	0.2[1]
20 to (24 hours)			Maintenance dose titrated to heart rate or other clinical endpoint	

[1] As the desired heart rate or endpoint is approached, the loading infusion may be omitted and the maintenance infusion titrated to 300 mcg/kg/min (0.3 mg/kg/min) or downward as appropriate. Maintenance dosages > 200 mcg/kg/min (0.2 mg/kg/min) have not been shown to have significantly increased benefits. The interval between titration steps may be increased.

►*Transfer to alternative agents:* After achieving adequate heart rate control and stable clinical status, transition to alternative antiarrhythmic agents (eg, propranolol, digoxin, verapamil) may be accomplished. A recommended dosage guideline is propranolol 10 to 20 mg every 4 to 6 hours, digoxin 0.125 to 0.5 mg every 6 hours (orally or IV), or verapamil 80 mg every 6 hours. However, consider labeling instructions for the agent selected.

Reduce the dosage of esmolol as follows: 30 minutes after the first dose of the alternative agent, reduce esmolol infusion rate by 50%. Following the second dose of the alternative agent, monitor patient's response and, if satisfactory control is maintained for the first hour, discontinue esmolol infusion.

►*Intraoperative and postoperative tachycardia and hypertension:* In the intraoperative and postoperative settings, it is not always advisable to slowly titrate the dose of esmolol to a therapeutic effect. Therefore, 2 dosing options are presented: Immediate control dosing and a gradual control when the physician has time to titrate.

Immediate control – For intraoperative treatment of tachycardia and hypertension, give an 80 mg (≈ 1 mg/kg) bolus dose over 30 seconds followed by a 150 mcg/kg/min infusion, if necessary. Adjust the infusion rate as required up to 300 mcg/kg/min to maintain desired heart rate or blood pressure.

Gradual control – For postoperative tachycardia and hypertension, the dosing schedule is the same as that used in supraventricular tachycardia. To initiate treatment, administer a loading dosage infusion of 500 mcg/kg/min for 1 minute followed by a 4-minute maintenance infusion of 50 mcg/kg/min. If an adequate therapeutic effect is not observed within 5 minutes, repeat the same loading dosage and follow with a maintenance infusion increased to 100 mcg/kg/min (see Supraventricular tachycardia).

►*Withdrawal effects:* These may occur with abrupt withdrawal of β-blockers following chronic use in patients with coronary artery disease (CAD) (see Warnings), but these have not been reported with esmolol. However, use caution when abruptly discontinuing esmolol infusions.

The use of esmolol infusions up to 24 hours has been well documented. Limited data indicate that esmolol is well tolerated up to 48 hours.

Beta-Adrenergic Blocking Agents

ESMOLOL HCl

►*Preparation of solution:*

250 mg/mL amp – Aseptically prepare a 10 mg/mL infusion by adding two 2500 mg ampuls to a 500 mL container or one 2500 mg ampul to a 250 mL container of one of the IV fluids listed below (see Compatibility/Stability). This yields a final concentration of 10 mg/mL. The diluted solution is stable for ≥ 24 hours at room temperature. Esmolol has been well tolerated when administered via a central vein.

The 250 mg/mL strength is concentrated, and is not for direct IV injection; dilute prior to infusion. Do not mix with sodium bicarbonate. Do not mix with other drugs prior to dilution in a suitable IV fluid.

10 mg/mL – This dosage form is prediluted to provide a ready-to-use 10 mg/mL concentration. It may be used to administer an esmolol loading dose infusion by hand-held syringe while the maintenance infusion is being prepared.

►*Compatibility/Stability:* Esmolol, at a final concentration of 10 mg/mL, is compatible with the following solutions and is stable for ≥ 24 hours at controlled room temperature or under refrigeration: 5% Dextrose Injection; 5% Dextrose in Lactated Ringer's Injection; 5% Dextrose in Ringer's Injection; 5% Dextrose and 0.9% or 0.45% Sodium Chloride Injection; Lactated Ringer's Injection; Potassium Chloride (40 mEq/L) in 5% Dextrose Injection; 0.9% or 0.45% Sodium Chloride Injection.

Esmolol is *not* compatible with 5% Sodium Bicarbonate Injection.

►*Storage/Stability:* Store at controlled room temperature 15° to 30°C; 59° to 86°F. Freezing does not adversely affect the product, but avoid exposure to elevated temperatures.

BETAXOLOL HCl

Rx	Kerlone (Sanofi)	Tablets: 10 mg	Lactose. (KERLONE 10). White, scored. Film-coated. In 100s.
		20 mg	Lactose. (KERLONE 20 β). White. Film-coated. In 100s.

For complete prescribing information, refer to the Beta-Adrenergic Blocking Agents group monograph.

Indications

►*Hypertension:* Management of hypertension, used alone or concomitantly with other antihypertensive agents, particularly thiazide-type diuretics.

Administration and Dosage

►*Approved by the FDA:* October 27, 1989.

►*Initial dose:* 10 mg once daily, alone or added to diuretic therapy. The full antihypertensive effect is usually seen within 7 to 14 days; if the desired response is not achieved, the dose can be doubled. Increasing the dose > 20 mg has not produced a statistically significant additional antihypertensive effect; however, the 40 mg dose is well tolerated. Anticipate an increased effect (reduction) on heart rate with increasing dosage. If monotherapy with betaxolol does not produce the desired response, consider the addition of a diuretic agent or other antihypertensive. To discontinue treatment, gradually withdraw betaxolol over 2 weeks. Carefully observe patients and advise them to limit physical activity to a minimum.

►*Elderly:* Consider reducing the starting dose to 5 mg.

►*Renal function impairment:* In patients with renal impairment, clearance of betaxolol declines with decreasing renal function.

In patients with severe renal impairment and those undergoing dialysis, the initial dose is 5 mg once daily. If the desired response is not achieved, dosage may be increased by 5 mg/day increments every 2 weeks to a maximum dose of 20 mg/day.

►*Storage/Stability:* Store at controlled room temperature, 15° to 25°C (59° to 77°F).

PENBUTOLOL SULFATE

Rx	Levatol (Schwarz Pharma)	Tablets: 20 mg	(RC22). Yellow, scored, capsule shape. In 100s.

For complete prescribing information, refer to the Beta-Adrenergic Blocking Agents group monograph.

Indications

►*Hypertension:* Treatment of mild-to-moderate arterial hypertension. Used alone or in combination with other antihypertensive agents.

Administration and Dosage

►*Approved by the FDA:* January 5, 1989.

Usual starting and maintenance dose, used alone or with other antihypertensive agents (eg, thiazide diuretics) is 20 mg once daily.

Doses of 40 to 80 mg have been well tolerated but have not shown greater antihypertensive effect. Full effect of a 20 or 40 mg dose is seen by the end of 2 weeks. A dose of 10 mg also lowers blood pressure, but the full effect is not seen for 4 to 6 weeks.

►*Storage/Stability:* Store at controlled room temperature 15° to 30°C (59° to 86°F). Keep tightly closed and protected from light.

CARTEOLOL HCl

Rx	Cartrol (Abbott)	Tablets: 2.5 mg	Lactose. Gray. In 100s.
		5 mg	Lactose. White. In 100s.

For complete prescribing information, refer to the Beta-Adrenergic Blocking Agents group monograph.

Indications

►*Hypertension:* Used alone or in combination with other antihypertensive agents.

Administration and Dosage

►*Approved by the FDA:* December 28, 1988.

►*Initial:* 2.5 mg as a single daily dose, either alone or with a diuretic. If adequate response is not achieved, gradually increase to 5 and 10 mg as single daily doses. Doses > 10 mg/day are unlikely to produce further benefit and may decrease response.

►*Maintenance:* 2.5 or 5 mg once daily.

►*Renal function impairment:* Individualize dosage.

Carteolol Dosage Interval in Renal Impairment	
Creatinine clearance (mL/min)	Dosage interval (hrs)
> 60	24
20 to 60	48
< 20	72

►*Storage/Stability:* Store at controlled room temperature, 15° to 30°C (59° to 86°F).

BISOPROLOL FUMARATE

Rx	Bisoprolol Fumarate (Eon)	Tablets: 5 mg	In 30s and 100s.
Rx	Zebeta (Barr)		(B1 LL). Pink, scored, heart shape, biconvex. Film-coated. In 30s.
Rx	Bisoprolol Fumarate (Eon)	10 mg	In 30s and 100s.
Rx	Zebeta (Barr)		(B3 LL). White, heart shape, biconvex. Film-coated. In 30s.

For complete prescribing information, refer to the Beta-Adrenergic Blocking Agents group monograph.

Indications

►*Hypertension:* Used alone or in combination with other antihypertensive agents.

Administration and Dosage

►*Approved by the FDA:* July 31, 1992.

Individualize dosage. May be given without regard to meals.

►*Initial dose:* 5 mg once daily. In some patients, 2.5 mg may be appropriate. If the antihypertensive effect of 5 mg is inadequate, the dose may be increased to 10 mg and then, if necessary, to 20 mg once daily.

►*Renal/Hepatic function impairment:* In patients with renal dysfunction (creatinine clearance < 40 mL/min) or hepatic impairment (hepatitis or cirrhosis), use an initial daily dose of 2.5 mg and use caution in dose titration. Since limited data suggest that bisoprolol is not dialyzable, drug replacement is not necessary in patients undergoing hemodialysis.

►*Elderly:* Dose adjustment is not necessary unless there is also significant renal or hepatic dysfunction.

►*Storage/Stability:* Store at controlled room temperature 15° to 30°C (59° to 86°C).

Beta-Adrenergic Blocking Agents

PINDOLOL

Rx	**Pindolol** (Various, eg, Mutual, Mylan, URL, Watson)	**Tablets:** 5 mg	In 100s, 500s, and 1000s.
Rx	**Visken** (Novartis)		(Visken 5 V). White, heart shape. In 100s.
Rx	**Pindolol** (Various, eg, Mutual, Mylan, URL, Watson)	**Tablets:** 10 mg	In 100s, 500s, and 1000s.
Rx	**Visken** (Novartis)		(Visken 10 V). White, heart shape. In 100s.

For complete prescribing information, refer to the Beta-Adrenergic Blocking Agents group monograph.

Indications

➤*Hypertension:* Management of hypertension, used alone or with other antihypertensive agents, particularly with a thiazide-type diuretic.

Administration and Dosage

➤*Approved by the FDA:* September 3, 1982.

Individualize dosage.

➤*Initial dose:* 5 mg twice daily, alone or with other antihypertensive agents. The antihypertensive response usually occurs within the first week of treatment. However, maximal response may occur within 2 weeks or, occasionally, longer. If a satisfactory reduction in blood pressure does not occur within 3 to 4 weeks, adjust dose in increments of 10 mg/day at 3- to 4-week intervals, to a maximum of 60 mg/day.

➤*Storage/Stability:* Store and dispense below 86°F (30°C) in a tight, light-resistant container.

METOPROLOL

Rx	**Metoprolol Tartrate** (Various, eg, Caraco, Mylan)	**Tablets:** 25 mg	In 30s, 90s, 100s, and 1000s.
Rx	**Metoprolol Tartrate** (Various, eg, Mylan, Qualit-est, Teva, URL, Watson)	**Tablets:** 50 mg	In 100s and 1000s.
Rx	**Lopressor** (Novartis)		Lactose. (GEIGY 51 51). Pink, scored, capsule shape, biconvex. In 100s, 1000s, and UD 100s.
Rx	**Metoprolol Tartrate** (Various, eg, Mylan, Qualit-est, Teva, URL, Watson)	**Tablets:** 100 mg	In 100s and 1000s.
Rx	**Lopressor** (Novartis)		Lactose. (GEIGY 71 71). Light blue, scored, capsule shape, biconvex. In 100s and 1000s.
Rx	**Toprol XL** (AstraZeneca)	**Tablets, extended-release:** 25 mg (23.75 mg metoprolol succinate equivalent to 25 mg metoprolol tartrate)	(AB). White, scored, oval, biconvex. Film-coated. In 100s.
		50 mg (47.5 mg metoprolol succinate equivalent to 50 mg metoprolol tartrate)	(A mo). White, scored, biconvex. Film-coated. In 100s.
		100 mg (95 mg metoprolol succinate equivalent to 100 mg metoprolol tartrate)	(A ms). White, scored, biconvex. Film-coated. In 100s.
		200 mg (190 mg metoprolol succinate equivalent to 200 mg metoprolol tartrate)	(A my). White, scored, oval, biconvex. Film-coated. In 100s.
Rx	**Metoprolol Tartrate** (Abbott)	**Injection:** 1 mg/mL	In amps, *Carpuject* sterile cartridge units with Interlink System Cannula, and *Carpuject* sterile cartridge units with Luer-Lock.
Rx	**Lopressor** (Novartis)		In 5 mL amps.

For complete prescribing information, refer to the Beta-Adrenergic Blocking Agents group monograph.

Indications

➤*Hypertension:* Used alone or in combination with other antihypertensive agents.

➤*Angina pectoris:* See Administration and Dosage section.

➤*MI:* Immediate-release tablets and injection.

➤*CHF:* Treatment of stable, symptomatic (NYHA Class II or III) heart failure of ischemic, hypertensive, or cardiomyopathic origin (*Toprol-XL* **25 mg only**).

Administration and Dosage

➤*Approved by the FDA:* August 1978.

➤*Tablets (immediate-release) and injection:* Individualize dosage; take at the same time each day.

Hypertension –

Initial dosage: 100 mg/day in single or divided doses, used alone or added to a diuretic and taken with or immediately following meals. The dosage may be increased at weekly (or longer) intervals until optimum blood pressure reduction is achieved. In general, the maximum effect of any given dosage level will be apparent after 1 week of therapy.

Maintenance dose: 100 to 450 mg/day. Dosages > 450 mg/day have not been studied. While once-daily dosing is effective and can maintain a reduction in blood pressure throughout the day, lower doses (especially 100 mg) may not maintain a full effect at the end of the 24-hour period; larger or more frequent daily doses may be required. Measure blood pressure near the end of the dosing interval to determine whether satisfactory control is being maintained.

Angina pectoris –

Initial dosage: 100 mg/day in 2 divided doses. Dosage may be gradually increased at weekly intervals until optimum clinical response is obtained or a pronounced slowing of heart rate occurs. Effective dosage range is 100 to 400 mg/day. Dosages > 400 mg/day have not been studied. If treatment is to be discontinued, reduce dosage gradually over 1 to 2 weeks.

MI –

Early treatment: During the early phase of definite or suspected acute MI, initiate treatment as soon as possible after the patient's arrival in a coronary care or similar unit immediately after the patient is hemodynamically stable.

Administer 3 IV bolus injections of 5 mg each, at ≈ 2 minute intervals. During IV administration, carefully monitor blood pressure, heart rate, and ECG.

In patients who tolerate the full IV dose (15 mg), give 50 mg orally every 6 hours 15 minutes after the last IV dose and continue for 48 hours. Thereafter, administer a maintenance dosage of 100 mg twice daily.

In patients who do not tolerate the full IV dose, start with 25 or 50 mg orally every 6 hours (depending on the degree of intolerance) 15 minutes after the last IV dose or as soon as the clinical condition allows. In patients with severe intolerance, discontinue treatment.

Late treatment: Patients who have contraindications to early treatment, who do not tolerate the full early treatment, and in whom therapy is delayed for any other reason should be started at 100 mg orally, twice daily, as soon as their clinical condition allows. Continue for ≥ 3 months. Although the efficacy beyond 3 months has not been conclusively established, data from studies with other beta blockers suggest that treatment continue for 1 to 3 years.

➤*Tablets, extended-release:* The extended-release tablets are for once-daily administration. When switching from immediate-release metoprolol tablets to extended-release, use the same total daily dose. Individualize dosage; titration may be needed in some patients. (*Toprol XL* tablets are scored and can be divided. Whole or half tablets should be swallowed and not chewed or crushed.)

Hypertension – The usual initial dosage is 50 to 100 mg/day in a single dose whether used alone or added to a diuretic. The dosage may be increased at weekly (or longer) intervals until optimum blood pressure reduction is achieved. In general, the maximum effect of any given dosage level will be apparent after 1 week of therapy. Dosages > 400 mg/day have not been studied.

Angina pectoris – Individualize dosage. The usual initial dosage is 100 mg/day in a single dose. The dosage may be gradually increased at weekly intervals until optimum clinical response has been obtained or there is a pronounced slowing of the heart rate. Dosages > 400 mg/day have not been studied. If treatment is to be discontinued, reduce dosage gradually over a period of 1 to 2 weeks.

METOPROLOL

CHF – Dosage must be individualized and closely monitored during up-titration. Prior to initiation of therapy, stabilize the dosing of diuretics, ACE inhibitors, and digitalis (if used). The recommended starting dose is 25 mg once daily for 2 weeks in patients with NYHA Class II heart failure and 12.5 mg once daily in patients with more severe heart failure. Then double the dose every 2 weeks to the highest dosage level tolerated by the patient or up to 200 mg. If transient worsening of heart failure occurs, it may be treated with increased dose of diuretics, and it may be necessary to lower the dose of metoprolol or temporarily discontinue it. The dose should not be increased until symptoms of worsening heart failure have been stabilized; initial difficulty with titration should not preclude later attempts to introduce metoprolol. If heart failure patients experience symptomatic bradycardia, reduce the dose.

➤*Storage / Stability:* Store at 25°C (77°F). Excursions permitted to 15° to 30°C (59° to 86°F). Do not freeze. Protect from moisture. Store in a tight, light-resistant container.

TIMOLOL MALEATE

Rx	**Timolol Maleate** (Various, eg, Mylan)	**Tablets:** 5 mg		In 100s.
Rx	**Blocadren** (Merck)			(MSD 59 BLOCADREN). Light blue. In 100s.
Rx	**Timolol Maleate** (Various, eg, Mylan)	**Tablets:** 10 mg		In 100s.
Rx	**Timolol Maleate** (Various, eg, Mylan)	**Tablets:** 20 mg		In 100s.
Rx	**Blocadren** (Merck)			(MSD 437 BLOCADREN). Light blue, scored, capsule shape. In 100s.

For complete prescribing information, refer to the Beta-Adrenergic Blocking Agents group monograph.

Indications

➤*Hypertension:* Used alone or in combination with other antihypertensive agents, especially thiazide-type diuretics.

➤*MI:* For clinically stable survivors of acute MI, to reduce cardiovascular mortality, and the risk of reinfarction.

➤*Migraine prophylaxis:* For prophylaxis of migraines.

Administration and Dosage

➤*Approved by the FDA:* August 1978.

➤*Hypertension:*
Initial dosage – 10 mg twice daily used alone or added to a diuretic.

Maintenance dosage – 20 to 40 mg/day. Titrate, depending on blood pressure and heart rate. Increases to a maximum of 60 mg/day divided into 2 doses may be necessary. There should be an interval of at least 7 days between dosage increases.

➤*MI:* Long-term prophylactic use in patients who have survived the acute phase of an MI — 10 mg twice daily.

➤*Migraine:* Initial dosage is 10 mg twice daily. During maintenance therapy, the 20 mg daily dosage may be given as a single dose. Total daily dosage may be increased to a maximum of 30 mg in divided doses or decreased to 10 mg once daily depending on clinical response and tolerability. Discontinue if a satisfactory response is not obtained after 6 to 8 weeks of the maximum daily dosage.

➤*Storage / Stability:* Store at controlled room temperature, 15° to 30°C (59° to 86°F). Keep container tightly closed. Protect from light.

SOTALOL HCl

Rx	**Sotalol HCl** (Various, eg, Eon, Global, Par, Teva)	**Tablets:** 80 mg		Lactose. In 100s, 500s, and 1000s.
Rx	**Betapace** (Berlex)			Lactose. (Betapace 80 mg). Light blue, scored, capsule shape. In 100s and UD 100s.
Rx	**Sotalol HCl** (Various, eg, Eon, Global, Par, Teva)	**Tablets:** 120 mg		Lactose. In 100s, 500s, and 1000s.
Rx	**Betapace** (Berlex)			Lactose. (Betapace 120 mg). Light blue, scored, capsule shape. In 100s and UD 100s.
Rx	**Sotalol HCl** (Various, eg, Eon, Global, Par, Teva)	**Tablets:** 160 mg		Lactose. In 100s, 500s, and 1000s.
Rx	**Betapace** (Berlex)			Lactose. (Betapace 160 mg). Light blue, scored, capsule shape. In 100s and UD 100s.
Rx	**Sotalol HCl** (Various, eg, Eon, Global, Par, Teva)	**Tablets:** 240 mg		Lactose. In 100s, 500s, and 1000s.
Rx	**Betapace** (Berlex)			Lactose. (Betapace 240 mg). Light blue, scored, capsule shape. In 100s and UD 100s.
Rx	**Sotalol HCl AF** (Apotex)	**Tablets:** 80 mg		(APO AF 80). White to off-white, capsule shape, scored. In 100s.
Rx	**Betapace AF** (Berlex)			Lactose. (80 mg/BERLEX). White, scored, capsule shape. In UD 60s and 100s.
Rx	**Sotalol HCl AF** (Apotex)	**Tablets:** 120 mg		(APO AF 120). White to off-white, capsule shape, scored. In 100s.
Rx	**Betapace AF** (Berlex)			Lactose. (120 mg/BERLEX). White, scored, capsule shape. In UD 60s and 100s.
Rx	**Sotalol HCl AF** (Apotex)	**Tablets:** 160 mg		(APO AF 160). White to off-white, capsule shape, scored. In 100s.
Rx	**Betapace AF** (Berlex)			Lactose. (160 mg/BERLEX). White, scored, capsule shape. In UD 60s and 100s.

For complete prescribing information, refer to the Beta-Adrenergic Blocking Agents group monograph.

WARNING

To minimize the risk of induced arrhythmia, patients initiated or reinitiated on *Betapace* or *Betapace AF* should be placed for a minimum of 3 days (on their maintenance dose) in a facility that can provide cardiac resuscitation, continuous electrocardiographic monitoring, and calculations of creatinine clearance. For detailed instructions regarding dose selection and special cautions for people with renal impairment, see Administration and Dosage.

Do not substitute *Betapace* for *Betapace AF* because of significant differences in labeling (eg, patient package insert, dosing administration, and safety information).

Indications

➤*Sotalol:*
Ventricular arrhythmias – Treatment of documented ventricular arrhythmias, such as sustained ventricular tachycardia, that are life-threatening. Because of the proarrhythmic effects, including a 1.5% to 2% rate of torsades de pointes or new VT/VF in patients with either NSVT or supraventricular arrhythmias, its use in patients with less severe arrhythmias, even if the patients are symptomatic, is generally not recommended. Avoid treatment of patients with asymptomatic ventricular premature contractions.

➤*Betapace AF:*
Maintenance of normal sinus rhythm – Maintenance of normal sinus rhythm (delay in time to recurrence of atrial fibrillation/atrial flutter [AFIB/AFL]) in patients with symptomatic AFIB/AFL who are currently in sinus rhythm. Because *Betapace AF* can cause life-threatening ventricular arrhythmias, reserve its use for patients in whom AFIB/AFL is highly symptomatic. Do not give this product to patients with paroxysmal AFIB/AFL that is easily reversed (eg, by Valsalva maneuver).

➤*Betapace:* *Betapace* is not approved for AFIB/AFL indication and should not be substituted for *Betapace AF*. *Betapace AF* is distributed with a patient package insert that is appropriate for patients with AFIB/AFL.

Administration and Dosage

➤*Approved by the FDA:* October 30, 1992.

➤*Betapace:* The recommended initial dose is 80 mg twice daily. This dose may be increased if necessary, after appropriate evaluation, to 240 or 320 mg/day (120 to 160 mg twice daily). In most patients, a therapeutic response is obtained at a total daily dose of 160 to 320 mg/day, given in 2 or 3 divided doses. Some patients with life-threatening refractory ventricular arrhythmias may require doses as high as 480 to

SOTALOL HCl

640 mg/day; however, only use these doses when the potential benefit outweighs the increased risk of adverse events, in particular proarrhythmia. Because of the long terminal elimination half-life of sotalol, dosing on more than a twice-daily regimen is usually not necessary.

Adjust dosage gradually, allowing 3 days between dosing increments in order to attain steady-state plasma concentrations, and to allow monitoring of QT intervals. Graded dose adjustment will help prevent the usage of doses that are higher than necessary to control the arrhythmia.

Initiate and increase doses in a hospital with facilities for cardiac rhythm monitoring and assessment. Administer only after appropriate clinical assessment and individualize the dosage for each patient on the basis of therapeutic response and tolerance. Proarrhythmic events can occur not only at initiation of therapy, but also with each upward dosage adjustment.

Renal function impairment – Because sotalol is excreted predominantly in urine and its terminal elimination half-life is prolonged in conditions of renal impairment, modify the dosing interval (time between divided doses) when creatinine clearance is < 60 mL/min according to the following table.

Sotalol Dosing Interval in Renal Impairment	
Creatinine clearance (mL/min)	Dosing interval[1] (hours)
≥ 60	12
30 to 59	24
10 to 29	36 to 48
< 10	Individualize dose

[1] The initial dose of 80 mg and subsequent doses should be administered at these intervals. See following paragraph for dosage escalations.

Dose escalations in renal impairment should be done after administration of ≥ 5 to 6 doses at appropriate intervals (see above table).

Exercise extreme caution in the use of sotalol in patients with renal failure undergoing hemodialysis. The half-life of sotalol is prolonged (≤ 69 hours) in anuric patients. However, sotalol can be partly removed by dialysis with subsequent partial rebound in concentrations when dialysis is completed. Both safety (eg, heart rate, QT interval) and efficacy (eg, arrhythmia control) must be closely monitored.

➤*Betapace AF:* Therapy with *Betapace AF* must be initiated (and if necessary, titrated) in a setting that provides continuous ECG monitoring and in the presence of personnel trained in the management of serious ventricular arrhythmias. Patients should continue to be monitored in this way for a minimum of 3 days on the maintenance dose. In addition, do not discharge patients within 12 hours of electrical or pharmacological conversion to normal sinus rhythm.

The QT interval is used to determine patient eligibility for *Betapace AF* treatment and for monitoring safety during treatment. The baseline QT interval must be ≤ 450 msec in order for a patient to be started on *Betapace AF* therapy. During initiation and titration, monitor the QT interval 2 to 4 hours after each dose. If the QT interval prolongs to ≥ 500 msec, the dose must be reduced or the drug discontinued.

The dose of *Betapace AF* must be individualized according to creatinine clearance. Modify the dosing interval according to the following table.

Betapace AF Dosing Interval in Renal Impairment	
Creatinine clearance (mL/min)	Dosing interval (hours)
> 60	12
40 to 60	24
< 40	Contraindicated

The recommended initial dose of *Betapace AF* is 80 mg and is initiated as shown in the dosing algorithm described below. The 80 mg dose can be titrated upward to 120 mg during initial hospitalization or after discharge on 80 mg in the event of recurrence, by rehospitalization and repeating the same steps used during the initiation of therapy (see Upward Titration of Dose).

Patients with atrial fibrillation should be anticoagulated according to usual medical practice. Hypokalemia should be corrected before initiation of *Betapace AF* therapy (see Warnings).

Patients to be discharged on *Betapace AF* therapy from an inpatient setting should have an adequate supply of *Betapace AF* to allow uninterrupted therapy until the patient can fill a *Betapace AF* prescription.

Initiation of therapy –
1.) Electrocardiographic assessment: Prior to administration of the first dose, the QT interval must be determined using an average of 5 beats. If the baseline QT is > 450 msec (JT ≥ 330 msec if QRS over 100 msec), *Betapace AF* is contraindicated.
2.) Prior to the administration of the first dose, the patient's creatinine clearance should be calculated.
3.) Starting dose: The starting dose of *Betapace AF* is 80 mg twice daily if the creatinine clearance is > 60 mL/min, and 80 mg once daily if the creatinine clearance is 40 to 60 mL/min. If the creatinine clearance is < 40 mL/min, *Betapace AF* is contraindicated.
4.) Administer the appropriate daily dose of *Betapace AF* and begin continuous ECG monitoring with QT interval measurements 2 to 4 hours after each dose.
5.) If the 80 mg dose level is tolerated and the QT interval remains < 500 msec after ≥ 3 days (after 5 or 6 doses if patient is receiving once daily dosing), the patient can be discharged. Alternatively, during hospitalization, the dose can be increased to 120 mg twice daily and the patient followed for 3 days on this dose (followed for 5 or 6 doses if the patient is receiving once-daily doses).

Upward titration of dose – If the 80 mg dose level (given once or twice daily depending upon the creatinine clearance) does not reduce the frequency of relapses of AFIB/AFL and is tolerated without excessive QT interval prolongation (ie, ≥ 520 msec), the dose level may be increased to 120 mg (once or twice daily depending on the creatinine clearance). As proarrhythmic events can occur not only at initiation of therapy, but also with each upward dosage adjustment, steps 2 through 5 used during initiation of *Betapace AF* therapy should be followed when increasing the dose level. In a US multicenter dose-response study, a 120 mg dose (once or twice daily) was found to be the most effective in prolonging the time to ECG-documented symptomatic recurrence of AFIB/AFL. If the 120 mg dose does not reduce the frequency of early relapse of AFIB/AFL and is tolerated without excessive QT interval prolongation (≥ 520 msec), an increase to 160 mg (once or twice daily depending on the creatinine clearance) can be considered. Steps 2 through 5 used during the initiation of therapy should be used again to introduce such an increase.

Maintenance of Betapace AF therapy – Regularly re-evaluate renal function and QT if medically warranted. If QT is ≥ 520 msec (JT ≥ 430 msec if QRS is > 100 msec), reduce the dose of *Betapace AF* therapy and carefully monitor patients until QT returns to < 520 msec. If the QT interval is ≥ 520 msec while on the lowest maintenance dose level (80 mg), discontinue the drug. If renal function deteriorates, reduce the daily dose in half by administering the drug once daily as described in Initiation of Therapy, step 3.

Special considerations – The maximum recommended dose in patients with a calculated creatinine clearance > 60 mL/min is 160 mg twice daily; doses > 160 mg twice daily have been associated with an increased incidence of torsades de pointes and are not recommended.

A patient who misses a dose should not double the next dose. The next dose should be taken at the usual time.

➤*Transfer to sotalol from other antiarrhythmic therapy:* Before starting sotalol, generally withdraw previous antiarrhythmic therapy under careful monitoring for a minimum of 2 to 3 plasma half-lives if the patient's clinical condition permits. Treatment has been initiated in some patients receiving IV lidocaine without ill effect. After discontinuation of amiodarone, do not initiate sotalol until the QT interval is normalized.

➤*Transfer to Betapace AF from Betapace:* Patients with a history of symptomatic AFIB/AFL who are currently receiving *Betapace* for the maintenance of normal sinus rhythm should be transferred to *Betapace AF* because of the significant differences in labeling (ie, patient package insert for *Betapace AF*, dosing, administration, and safety information).

➤*Storage/Stability:* Store at 25°C; excursions permitted between 15° and 30°C.

ACEBUTOLOL HCl

Rx	**Acebutolol HCl** (Various, eg, Mylan, Watson)	**Capsules:** 200 mg	In 100s and 1000s.
Rx	**Sectral** (ESP Pharma)		(Wyeth 4177 Sectral 200). Purple/orange. In 100s and *Redipak* 100s.
Rx	**Acebutolol HCl** (Various, eg, ESI Lederle, Mylan, Watson)	**Capsules:** 400 mg	In 100s and 1000s.
	Sectral (ESP Pharma)		(Wyeth 4179 Sectral 400). Brown/orange. In 100s.

For complete prescribing information, refer to the Beta-Adrenergic Blocking Agents group monograph.

Indications

➤*Hypertension:* Used alone or in combination with other antihypertensive agents.

➤*Ventricular arrhythmias:* Management of ventricular premature beats.

Administration and Dosage

➤*Approved by the FDA:* December 28, 1984.

➤*Hypertension:*

Initial dose – 400 mg in uncomplicated mild-to-moderate hypertension. May be given in a single daily dose, but 200 mg twice daily may be required for adequate control. Optimal response usually occurs with 400 to 800 mg/day (range, 200 to 1200 mg/day given twice daily). The

Beta-Adrenergic Blocking Agents

ACEBUTOLOL HCl

drug may be combined with another antihypertensive agent. As dosage is increased, β_1-selectivity diminishes.

➤*Ventricular arrhythmia:*

Initial dose – 400 mg (200 mg twice daily). Increase dosage gradually until optimal response is obtained, usually 600 to 1200 mg/day. To discontinue treatment, gradually reduce dosage over 2 weeks.

➤*Elderly:* Since bioavailability increases about 2-fold, older patients may require lower maintenance doses. Avoid doses > 800 mg/day.

➤*Renal/Hepatic function impairment:* Reduce the daily dose by 50% when creatinine clearance is < 50 mL/min. Reduce by 75% when it is < 25 mL/min. Use cautiously in impaired hepatic function.

➤*Storage/Stability:* Keep tightly closed. Store at room temperature 25°C (77°F). Protect from light.

NADOLOL

Rx	**Nadolol** (Various, eg, Apothecon, Mylan, UDL)	**Tablets**: 20 mg	In 100s and UD 100s.
Rx	**Corgard** (Monarch)		(CORGARD 20 BL 232). Scored. In 100s and *Unimatic* 100s.
Rx	**Nadolol** (Various, eg, Apothecon, Mylan, UDL, Zenith)	**Tablets**: 40 mg	In 100s, 1000s, and UD 100s.
Rx	**Corgard** (Monarch)		(CORGARD 40 BL 208). Scored. In 100s, 1000s, and *Unimatic* 100s.
Rx	**Nadolol** (Various, eg, Apothecon, Mylan, UDL, Zenith)	**Tablets**: 80 mg	In 30s, 100s, 500s, 1000s, and UD 100s.
Rx	**Corgard** (Monarch)		(CORGARD 80 BL 241). Scored. In 100s, 1000s, and *Unimatic* 100s.
Rx	**Nadolol** (Various, eg, Apothecon, Zenith)	**Tablets**: 120 mg	In 100s, 500s, and 1000s.
Rx	**Corgard** (Monarch)		(CORGARD 120 MG BL 208). Scored. In 100s and 1000s.
Rx	**Nadolol** (Various, eg, Apothecon, Zenith)	**Tablets**: 160 mg	In 100s, 500s, and 1000s.
Rx	**Corgard** (Monarch)		(246). Scored. In 100s.

For complete prescribing information, refer to the Beta-Adrenergic Blocking Agents group monograph.

Indications

➤*Angina pectoris:* Long-term management.

➤*Hypertension:* Used alone or in combination with other antihypertensive agents.

Administration and Dosage

➤*Approved by the FDA:* December 1979.

Individualize dosage. May be given without regard to meals.

➤*Angina pectoris:*

Initial – 40 mg once daily. Gradually increase dosage in 40 to 80 mg increments at 3 to 7 day intervals until optimum clinical response is obtained or there is pronounced slowing of the heart rate.

Maintenance dose – Usual dose is 40 or 80 mg once daily. Up to 160 or 240 mg once daily may be needed.

The safety and efficacy of dosages exceeding 240 mg/day have not been established. To discontinue, reduce dosage gradually over 1 to 2 weeks.

➤*Hypertension:*

Initial – 40 mg once daily, alone or in addition to diuretic therapy. Gradually increase dosage in 40 to 80 mg increments until optimum blood pressure reduction is achieved.

Maintenance dose – Usual dose is 40 or 80 mg once daily. Up to 240 or 320 mg once daily may be needed.

➤*Renal function impairment:* Nadolol is excreted principally by the kidneys and, although nonrenal elimination does occur, dosage adjustments are necessary in patients with renal impairment. The following dosage intervals are recommended.

Nadolol Dosage Adjustment in Renal Failure	
Creatinine clearance (mL/min/1.73 m²)	Dosage interval (hours)
> 50	24
31 to 50	24 to 36
10 to 30	24 to 48
< 10	40 to 60

➤*Storage/Stability:* Store at room temperature; avoid excessive heat. Protect from light. Keep bottle tightly closed.

PROPRANOLOL HCl

Rx	**Propranolol HCl** (Various, eg, Mylan, Schein, Watson)	**Tablets**: 10 mg	In 100s, 500s, 1000s, 5000s, and UD 100s.
Rx	**Inderal** (Wyeth-Ayerst)		(I INDERAL 10). Orange, scored, hexagonal. In 100s, 1000s, 5000s, and UD 100s.
Rx	**Propranolol HCl** (Various, eg, Mylan, Schein, Watson)	**Tablets**: 20 mg	In 100s, 500s, 1000s, 5000s, and UD 100s.
Rx	**Inderal** (Wyeth-Ayerst)		(I INDERAL 20). Blue, scored, hexagonal. In 100s, 1000s, 5000s, and UD 100s.
Rx	**Propranolol HCl** (Various, eg, Mylan, Schein, Watson)	**Tablets**: 40 mg	In 100s, 500s, 1000s, 5000s, and UD 100s.
Rx	**Inderal** (Wyeth-Ayerst)		(I INDERAL 40). Green, scored, hexagonal. In 100s, 1000s, 5000s, and UD 100s.
Rx	**Propranolol HCl** (Various, eg, Mylan, Watson)	**Tablets**: 60 mg	In 100s, 500s, and UD 100s.
Rx	**Inderal** (Wyeth-Ayerst)		(I INDERAL 60). Pink, scored, hexagonal. In 100s and 1000s.
Rx	**Propranolol HCl** (Various, eg, Mylan, Schein)	**Tablets**: 80 mg	In 100s, 500s, 1000s, and UD 100s.
Rx	**Inderal** (Wyeth-Ayerst)		(I INDERAL 80). Yellow, scored, hexagonal. In 100s, 1000s, and 5000s.
Rx	**Propranolol HCl** (Various, eg, Qualitest, Watson)	**Tablets**: 90 mg	In 100s and 500s.
Rx	**Propranolol HCl** (Various, eg, ESI Lederle)	**Capsules, extended-release**: 60 mg	In 100s and 1000s.
Rx	**Inderal LA** (Wyeth-Ayerst)		(INDERAL LA 60). White/light blue. In 100s and 1000s.
Rx	**Propranolol HCl** (Various, eg, ESI Lederle)	**Capsules, extended-release**: 80 mg	In 100s and 1000s.
Rx	**Inderal LA** (Wyeth-Ayerst)		(INDERAL LA 80). Light blue. In 100s, 1000s, and UD 100s.
Rx	**InnoPran XL** (Reliant)		Sugar spheres. (80 RD201). Gray/White. In 30s, 100s, 500s, and UD 100s.
Rx	**Propranolol HCl** (Various, eg, ESI Lederle)	**Capsules, extended-release**: 120 mg	In 100s and 1000s.
Rx	**Inderal LA** (Wyeth-Ayerst)		(INDERAL LA 120). Light blue/Dark blue. In 100s, 1000s, and UD 100s.
Rx	**InnoPran XL** (Reliant)		Sugar spheres. (120 RD201). Gray/off-white. In 30s, 100s, 500s, and UD 100s.
Rx	**Propranolol HCl** (Various, eg, ESI Lederle)	**Capsules, extended-release**: 160 mg	In 100s.
Rx	**Inderal LA** (Wyeth-Ayerst)		(INDERAL LA 160). Dark blue. In 100s, 1000s, and UD 100s.

Beta-Adrenergic Blocking Agents

PROPRANOLOL HCl

Rx sf	Propranolol HCl (Roxane)	Solution, oral: 4 mg/mL	Parabens, saccharin, sorbitol. Dye free. Strawberry-mint flavor. In 500 mL and UD 5 mL patient cups (40s).
		8 mg/mL	Parabens, saccharin, sorbitol. Dye free. Strawberry-mint flavor. In 500 mL.
Rx sf	Propranolol Intensol (Roxane)	Oral solution, concentrated: 80 mg/mL	Alcohol and dye free. In 30 mL with dropper.
Rx	Propranolol HCl (Various, eg, Bedford)	Injection: 1 mg/mL	In 1 mL vials.
Rx	Inderal (Wyeth-Ayerst)		In 1 mL amps.

For complete prescribing information, refer to the Beta-Adrenergic Blocking Agents group monograph.

Indications

➤*Cardiac arrhythmias (except ER):* Supraventricular, ventricular, tachyarrhythmias of digitalis intoxication, and resistant tachyarrhythmias caused by excessive catecholamine action during anesthesia.

➤*MI (except ER):* For treatment of MI.

➤*Hypertrophic subaortic stenosis (except InnoPran XL):* Especially for treatment of exertional or other stress-induced angina, palpitations, and syncope.

➤*Pheochromocytoma (except ER):* As adjunctive therapy following primary treatment with an alpha-adrenergic blocker.

➤*Hypertension:* Used alone or in combination with other antihypertensive agents.

➤*Migraine prophylaxis (except Innopran XL):* For prophylaxis of migraines.

➤*Angina pectoris (except Innopran XL):* When caused by coronary atherosclerosis.

➤*Essential tremor (except ER):* Familial or hereditary.

Administration and Dosage

➤*Approved by the FDA:* November 1967.

Adult Propranolol Dosage Based on Indication			
Indication	Initial dosage	Usual range	Maximum daily dose
Arrhythmias		10-30 mg tid-qid (given ac and hs)	
Hypertension	40 mg bid or 80 mg once daily (ER)	120-240 mg/day (given bid-tid) or 80-160 mg once daily (ER)	640 mg
Angina	80 mg once daily (ER)	80-320 mg bid, tid, qid or 160 mg once daily (ER)	320 mg
MI		180-240 mg/day (given bid or tid)	240 mg
Hypertrophic subaortic stenosis		20-40 mg tid-qid (given ac and hs) or 80-160 mg once daily (ER)	
Pheochromocytoma		60 mg/day × 3 days preoperatively (in divided doses)	
Inoperable tumor		30 mg/day (in divided doses)	
Migraine	80 mg/day once daily (ER) or in divided doses	160-240 mg once daily (ER) or in divided doses	240 mg
Essential tremor	40 mg bid	120 mg/day	320 mg

➤*Hypertension:* The time course of full blood pressure response ranges from a few days to several weeks. While twice-daily dosing is effective and can maintain a reduction in blood pressure throughout the day, some patients, especially with lower doses, may experience a modest blood pressure rise toward the end of the 12-hour dosing interval. Evaluate by measuring blood pressure near the end of the dosing interval. If control is inadequate, a larger dose or 3 times daily dosing may achieve better control.

Extended-release capsules – The extended-release capsule should be administered once daily. Administer *InnoPran XL* at bedtime (approximately 10 pm) consistently either on an empty stomach or with food. The starting dose is 80 mg but dosage should be individualized and titration will be needed to a dose of 120 mg or higher. Doses of *InnoPran XL* above 120 mg had no additional effects on blood pressure. The time needed for full antihypertensive response is variable, but is usually achieved within 2 to 3 weeks.

➤*Angina pectoris:* Increased exercise tolerance and reduced ischemic changes in the ECG occur with twice daily, three times daily, or 4 times daily dosing.

Extended-release capsules – Gradually increase initial dosage at 3 to 7 day intervals until optimum response is obtained.

➤*MI:* The safety and efficacy of daily dosages > 240 mg for prevention of cardiac mortality have not been established. Higher dosages may be needed to effectively treat coexisting diseases such as angina or hypertension.

➤*Pheochromocytoma:* Administer concomitantly with an α-adrenergic blocking agent.

➤*Migraine:* Increase dosage gradually to achieve optimum migraine prophylaxis. If a satisfactory response is not obtained within 4 to 6 weeks after reaching the maximum dose, discontinue therapy. Withdraw gradually over several weeks.

➤*Parenteral:* Reserve IV use for life-threatening arrhythmias or those occurring under anesthesia.

Usual dose – 1 to 3 mg under careful monitoring (eg, central venous pressure, ECG). Do not exceed 1 mg/min to avoid lowering blood pressure and causing cardiac standstill. Allow sufficient time for the drug to reach site of action, particularly when slow circulation is present. If necessary, give a second dose after 2 minutes. Thereafter, do not give additional drug in < 4 hours. Do not give additional propranolol after the desired alteration in rate and/or rhythm is achieved. Transfer to oral therapy as soon as possible. IV use has not been evaluated adequately in managing hypertensive emergencies.

➤*Pediatrics:* IV use is not recommended; however, an unlabeled dose of 0.01 to 0.1 mg/kg/dose to a maximum of 1 mg/dose by slow infusion over 5 minutes has been used for arrhythmias.

Oral dosage for treating hypertension requires titration, beginning with a 1 mg/kg/day dosage regimen (ie, 0.5 mg/kg twice daily). May be increased at 3- to 5-day intervals to a maximum of 16 mg/kg/day.

The usual pediatric dosage range is 2 to 4 mg/kg/day in 2 equally divided doses (ie, 1 to 2 mg/kg twice daily). Dosage calculated by weight generally produces plasma levels in a therapeutic range similar to that in adults. Doses based on body surface area are not recommended since they usually result in plasma levels above the mean adult therapeutic range. Do not use doses > 16 mg/kg/day. To discontinue treatment, gradually decrease dose over 1 to 2 weeks. Data on use of extended-release capsules in this age group are too limited to permit adequate directions for use.

➤*Concentrated oral solution:* Mix with liquid or semi-solid food such as water, juices, soda or soda-like beverages, applesauce, and puddings. Draw into the dropper the amount prescribed for a single dose. Then squeeze the dropper contents into a liquid or semi-solid food. Stir the liquid or food gently for a few seconds. The entire amount of the mixture, of drug and liquid or drug and food, should be consumed immediately. Do not store for future use.

➤*Storage/Stability:* Store at controlled room temperature, 20° to 25°C (68° to 77°F). Protect from light, moisture, freezing, and excessive heat. Store in tight, light-resistant containers.

Alpha/Beta-Adrenergic Blocking Agents

LABETALOL HCl

Rx	**Labetalol HCl** (Various, eg, Apothecon, Eon, Ivax, Mutual, UDL, URL, Watson)	**Tablets:** 100 mg	In 30s, 100s, 250s, 500s, and 1000s.
Rx	**Trandate** (Faro Pharmaceuticals, Inc.)		(Trandate 100). Lt. orange, scored. Film-coated. In 100s, 500s, and UD 100s.
Rx	**Labetalol HCl** (Various, eg, Apothecon, Eon, Ivax, Mutual, UDL, URL, Watson)	**Tablets:** 200 mg	In 30s, 100s, 250s, 500s, and 1000s.
Rx	**Trandate** (Faro Pharmaceuticals, Inc.)		(Trandate 200). White, scored. Film-coated. In 100s, 500s, and UD 100s.
Rx	**Labetalol HCl** (Various, eg, Apothecon, Eon, Ivax, Mutual, Teva, URL, Watson)	**Tablets:** 300 mg	In 30s, 100s, 250s, 500s, and 1000s.
Rx	**Trandate** (Faro Pharmaceuticals, Inc.)		(Trandate 300). Peach, scored. Film-coated. In 100s, 500s, and UD 100s.
Rx	**Labetalol HCl** (Various, eg, Apothecon, Bedford Labs)	**Injection:** 5 mg/mL[1]	Dextrose, EDTA, parabens. In 20 and 40 mL multidose vials.
Rx	**Normodyne** (Key)		Dextrose, EDTA, parabens. In 20 mL multidose vials and 4 and 8 mL prefilled syringes.
Rx	**Trandate** (Faro Pharmaceuticals, Inc.)		In 20 and 40 mL multidose vials.

[1] With 0.1 mg EDTA and 0.8 mg methylparaben and 0.1 mg propylparaben.

Indications

►*Hypertension:*

Oral – Hypertension, alone or with other agents, especially thiazide and loop diuretics.

Parenteral – For control of blood pressure (BP) in severe hypertension.

►*Unlabeled uses:* Labetalol has effectively lowered BP and relieved symptoms in patients with pheochromocytoma; higher IV doses may be required. However, paradoxical hypertensive responses have occurred; therefore, use caution when administering labetalol.

Labetalol has been used in clonidine withdrawal hypertension.

Administration and Dosage

►*Oral:*

Initial dose – Individualize dosage. 100 mg twice daily, alone or added to a diuretic. After 2 or 3 days, using standing BP as an indicator, titrate dosage in increments of 100 mg twice daily, every 2 or 3 days. Full antihypertensive effect is usually seen within the first 1 to 3 hours of initial dose or dose increment.

Maintenance dose – 200 to 400 mg twice daily. Patients with severe hypertension may require 1.2 to 2.4 g/day. Should side effects (principally nausea or dizziness) occur with twice-daily dosing, the same total daily dose given 3 times/day may improve tolerability. Titration increments should not exceed 200 mg twice/day.

When transferring patients from other antihypertensives, introduce labetalol and progressively decrease dosage of existing therapy.

Elderly: Elderly patients will generally require lower maintenance dosages.

►*Parenteral:* For IV use. Individualize dosage. Keep patients supine during injection. Establish patient's ability to tolerate upright position before permitting ambulation.

Repeated IV injection – Initially, 20 mg (0.25 mg/kg for an 80 kg patient) slowly over 2 minutes. Measure supine BP immediately before and at 5 and 10 minutes after injection. Additional injections of 40 or 80 mg can be given at 10-minute intervals until a desired supine BP is achieved or a total of 300 mg has been injected. The maximum effect usually occurs within 5 minutes of each injection.

Slow continuous infusion – Dilute contents with IV fluids listed below. Two methods are: Add 200 mg to 160 mL of IV fluid to prepare 1 mg/mL solution at a rate of 2 mL/min (2 mg/min). Or, add 200 mg to 250 mL of an IV fluid to prepare 2 mg/3 mL solution; give at a rate of 3 mL/min (2 mg/min). Adjust infusion rate according to BP response. Use a controlled administration device. Continue infusion until satisfactory response is obtained; then discontinue infusion and start oral labetalol. Effective cumulative IV dose range is 50 to 200 mg, up to 300 mg.

►*Transfer to oral dosing (hospitalized patients):* Begin oral dosing when supine diastolic BP begins to rise. Recommended initial dose is 200 mg, then 200 or 400 mg, 6 to 12 hours later, depending on BP response. Thereafter, proceed as follows:

Labetalol Oral Titration Regimen for Inpatients	
Regimen	Daily Dose[1]
200 mg bid	400 mg
400 mg bid	800 mg
800 mg bid	1600 mg
1200 mg bid	2400 mg

[1] Total daily dose may be given in 3 divided doses.

While in the hospital, the dosage of labetalol may be increased at 1-day intervals to achieve the desired blood pressure reduction.

►*IV admixture compatibility/incompatibility:* At final concentrations of 1.25 to 3.75 mg/mL, labetalol is compatible and stable for 24 hours with the following parenteral solutions: Ringer's; Lactated Ringer's; 5% Dextrose and Ringer's; 5% Lactated Ringer's and 5% Dextrose; 5% Dextrose; 0.9% Sodium Chloride; 5% Dextrose and 0.2% Sodium Chloride; 2.5% Dextrose and 0.45% Sodium Chloride; 5% Dextrose and 0.9% Sodium Chloride; and 5% Dextrose and 0.33% Sodium Chloride. Labetalol is *not* compatible with 5% Sodium Bicarbonate Injection, furosemide, or other products that are alkaline.

►*Storage/Stability:* Store tablets and injection between 2° and 30°C (36° and 86°F). Protect the injection from light.

Actions

►*Pharmacology:* Labetalol combines both selective, competitive postsynaptic α_1-adrenergic blocking and nonselective, competitive β-adrenergic blocking activity. The ratios of α- to β-blockade are ≈ 1:3 and 1:7 after oral and IV use, respectively.

The α- and β-blocking actions decrease BP. Because of α_1-receptor blocking activity, standing BP is lowered more than supine, and symptoms of postural hypotension, including rare instances of syncope, can occur. In dose-related fashion, labetalol blunts exercise-induced increases in BP and heart rate. Pulmonary circulation during exercise is not affected.

Labetalol produces dose-related falls in BP without reflex tachycardia or significant reduction in heart rate. Hemodynamic effects are variable including small, nonsignificant changes in cardiac output and small decreases in total peripheral resistance. Elevated plasma renin levels are reduced. Doses that control hypertension do not affect renal function in patients with mild to severe hypertension and normal renal function.

Although β-adrenergic receptor blockade is useful in angina and hypertension, sympathetic stimulation is vital in some situations. For example, in patients with severely damaged hearts, adequate ventricular function may depend on sympathetic drive. β-blockade may worsen AV block by preventing the necessary facilitating effects of sympathetic activity on conduction. β_2-blockade results in passive bronchial constriction by interfering with endogenous adrenergic bronchodilator activity in patients subject to bronchospasm and may also interfere with exogenous bronchodilators in such patients.

Single oral doses in coronary artery disease patients had no significant effect on sinus rate, intraventricular conduction, or QRS duration. AV conduction time may be modestly prolonged. IV doses slightly prolonged AV nodal conduction time and atrial effective refractory period with small heart rate changes. Effects on AV nodal refractoriness were inconsistent.

►*Pharmacokinetics:*

Absorption/Distribution – Oral labetalol is completely absorbed; peak plasma levels occur in 1 to 2 hours. Steady-state plasma levels during repetitive dosing are reached by approximately the third day. The peak effects of single oral doses occur within 2 to 4 hours. The duration of effect depends upon dose, lasting 8 to 12 hours. The maximum, steady-state BP response upon oral, twice-daily dosing occurs within 24 to 72 hours. The maximum effect of each IV injection of labetalol at each dose level occurs within 5 minutes. Following discontinuation of IV therapy, BP rose gradually and progressively, approaching pretreatment baseline values in 16 to 18 hours. Because of an extensive first-pass effect, absolute bioavailability is 25%; this is increased by food and in the elderly. Protein binding is ≈ 50%. Labetalol is moderately lipid-soluble and crosses the placenta.

Metabolism/Excretion – Metabolism is mainly through conjugation to glucuronide metabolites, which are excreted in urine and in feces (via bile). Elimination half-life following oral and IV use is 6 to 8 hours and 5.5 hours, respectively. About 70% of the maximum beta-blocking effect is present for 5 hours after the administration of a single oral dose of 400 mg, with suggestion that ≈ 40% remains at 8 hours. In decreased hepatic or renal function, elimination half-life is not altered; however, the relative bioavailability in hepatically impaired patients is increased because of decreased "first-pass" metabolism. Total body

Alpha/Beta-Adrenergic Blocking Agents

LABETALOL HCl

clearance is ≈ 33 mL/min/kg. About 55% to 60% of a dose appears in urine as conjugates or unchanged drug in the first 24 hours. Neither hemodialysis nor peritoneal dialysis removes a significant amount of drug (< 1%).

Contraindications

Bronchial asthma; overt cardiac failure; greater than first-degree heart block; cardiogenic shock; severe bradycardia.

Warnings

➤*Cardiac failure:* Sympathetic stimulation is a vital component supporting circulatory function in CHF. β-blockade carries a potential hazard of further depressing myocardial contractility and precipitating more severe failure. Avoid use in overt CHF, although labetalol can be used with caution in patients with a history of heart failure who are well-compensated. CHF has been observed in patients receiving labetalol. Labetalol does not abolish the inotropic action of digitalis on heart muscle.

➤*Surgery:* Several deaths have occurred when labetalol injection was used during surgery, including when used in cases to control bleeding.

A synergism between labetalol and halothane anesthesia has been shown.

Withdrawing β-blockers prior to major surgery is controversial. Protracted severe hypotension and difficulty restarting or maintaining heartbeat have occurred with β-blockers; labetalol has not been evaluated in this setting.

➤*Patients without history of cardiac failure (latent cardiac insufficiency):* Continued depression of myocardium with β-blockers can lead to cardiac failure. At first sign or symptom of impending cardiac failure, fully digitalize or give diuretic; observe closely. If cardiac failure continues, withdraw (gradually, if possible).

➤*Withdrawal:* Angina has not been reported upon discontinuation. However, hypersensitivity to catecholamines has been seen in patients withdrawn from β-blockers. Exacerbation of angina and, in some cases, MI and ventricular dysrhythmias have occurred after abrupt discontinuation of such therapy. Abrupt withdrawal of these agents in patients without coronary artery disease has resulted in transient symptoms, including tremulousness, sweating, palpitation, headache, and malaise. When discontinuing chronic labetalol, particularly in ischemic heart disease, gradually reduce dosage over 1 to 2 weeks and carefully monitor. Do not discontinue abruptly, even in patients treated only for hypertension. In the absence of overt angina, when discontinuation is planned, carefully observe patient and advise to limit physical activity. If angina markedly worsens or acute coronary insufficiency develops, reinstitute promptly, at least temporarily, and take other measures.

➤*Nonallergic bronchospasm (eg, chronic bronchitis and emphysema):* Patients with bronchospastic disease should not receive β-blockers. However, labetalol may be used with caution in patients who do not respond to, or cannot tolerate, other antihypertensive agents. Use the smallest effective dose.

➤*Diabetes mellitus and hypoglycemia:* β-blockade may prevent the appearance of premonitory signs and symptoms (eg, tachycardia) of acute hypoglycemia. β-blockade also reduces insulin release in response to hyperglycemia; it may be necessary to adjust antidiabetic drug dose.

➤*Rapid decreases of BP:* Observe caution when reducing severely elevated BP. Although not reported with IV labetalol, adverse reactions, including cerebral infarction, optic nerve infarction, angina, and ischemic changes in the ECG have been reported with other agents when severely elevated BP was reduced over several hours to as long as 1 or 2 days. Achieve desired BP lowering over as long as possible.

➤*Hepatic toxicity:* Jaundice or hepatic dysfunction have rarely been associated with labetalol. Stop labetalol immediately if a patient develops jaundice or laboratory evidence of liver injury. Both have been reversible upon discontinuation. Hepatic necrosis and death have occurred. Injury has occurred after short- and long-term treatment and may be slowly progressive, despite minimal symptomatology.

➤*Hypersensitivity reactions:* While taking β-blockers, patients with a history of severe anaphylactic reaction to a variety of allergens may be more reactive to repeated challenge, either accidental, diagnostic, or therapeutic. Such patients may be unresponsive to the usual doses of epinephrine used to treat allergic reaction.

➤*Hepatic function impairment:* Use with caution; drug metabolism may be diminished. The relative bioavailability in hepatically impaired patients is increased because of decreased "first-pass" metabolism.

➤*Elderly:* As in the general population, some elderly patients ≥ 60 years of age have experienced orthostatic hypotension, dizziness, or lightheadedness during treatment with labetalol.

➤*Pregnancy:* Category C. There are no adequate and well-controlled studies in pregnant women. Use during pregnancy only if the potential benefits outweigh the potential hazards to the fetus.

Hypotension, bradycardia, hypoglycemia, and respiratory depression have occurred in infants of mothers who were treated with labetalol for hypertension during pregnancy.

Labor and delivery – Labetalol did not appear to affect the usual course of labor and delivery when given to pregnant hypertensive patients.

➤*Lactation:* Small amounts of labetalol (0.004% of the maternal dose) are excreted in breast milk. Exercise caution in nursing women.

➤*Children:* Safety and efficacy for use in children have not been established.

Precautions

➤*Monitoring:* Periodic determination of suitable hepatic laboratory tests would be appropriate. Perform appropriate laboratory testing at the first symptom/sign of liver dysfunction (eg, pruritus, dark urine, persistent anorexia, jaundice, right upper quadrant tenderness, or unexplained "flu-like" symptoms).

In patients with concomitant illnesses, such as impaired renal function, monitor appropriate tests.

Monitor the BP during and after completion of the infusion of IV injections. Avoid rapid or excessive falls in either systolic or diastolic BP during IV treatment. In patients with excessive systolic hypertension, use the decrease in systolic pressure as an indicator of effectiveness in addition to the response of the diastolic pressure.

➤*Hypotension:* Following oral administration, postural hypotension has been transient and is uncommon (2%) when the recommended starting dose and titration increments are closely followed. Symptomatic postural hypotension is most likely to occur 2 to 4 hours after a dose, especially following a large initial dose or upon large changes in dose. It is likely to occur if patients are tilted or allowed to assume the upright position within 3 hours of receiving labetalol injection (incidence 58%). Establish patient's ability to tolerate upright position before permitting ambulation.

Drug Interactions

Labetalol HCl Drug Interactions			
Precipitant drug	Object drug *		Description
Labetalol	Beta-adrenergic agonist	↓	Labetalol can blunt the bronchodilator effect of these drugs in patients with bronchospasm; a greater than normal dose of β-agonist bronchodilators may be required.
Labetalol	Calcium channel blockers (diphenylalkylamines)	↔	Take care if labetalol is used concomitantly with calcium antagonists of the verapamil type.
Labetalol	Nitroglycerin	↓	Labetalol blunts reflex tachycardia that nitroglycerin may produce without preventing its hypotensive effect; additional antihypertensive effects may occur.
Labetalol	Tricyclic antidepressants	↔	Coadministration resulted in an increased incidence of tremor.
Cimetidine	Labetalol	↑	Cimetidine increased the bioavailability of oral labetalol.
Glutethimide	Labetalol	↓	Glutethimide may decrease the pharmacologic effects of labetalol by inducing microsomal enzymes. This may occur several days after glutethimide discontinuation.
Halothane	Labetalol	↑	Synergistic adverse effects on cardiovascular hemodynamics may occur with concurrent IV labetalol, resulting in significant myocardial depression. During controlled hypotensive anesthesia, do not use high halothane concentrations (≥ 3%). If interaction occurs, reduce halothane dose to rapidly reverse symptoms.
Labetalol	Halothane		

* ↑ = Object drug increased. ↓ = Object drug decreased. ↔ = Undetermined clinical effect.

Alpha/Beta-Adrenergic Blocking Agents

LABETALOL HCl

➤*Drug/Lab test interactions:* Presence of a labetalol metabolite in urine may falsely increase urinary catecholamine levels when measured by a nonspecific trihydroxyindole reaction. In screening labetalol patients for pheochromocytoma, use specific radioenzymatic or high performance liquid chromatography assay techniques.

There have been reversible increases of serum transaminases in 4% of patients treated with labetalol and tested, and more rarely, reversible increases in blood urea.

Labetalol has produced a false-positive test for amphetamine when screening urine for the presence of drugs.

Adverse Reactions

Labetalol is usually well tolerated. Most adverse effects have been mild and transient. With oral labetalol, most occur early in the course of treatment. Discontinuation was required in 7% of all patients in controlled clinical trials.

➤*Oral:*

CNS – Fatigue; headache; drowsiness; paresthesias; rare instances of syncope.

Dermatologic – Rashes such as generalized maculopapular, lichenoid, urticarial; bullous lichen planus; psoriaform; facial erythema; reversible alopecia.

GI – Diarrhea; cholestasis with or without jaundice; reversible increases in serum transaminases.

GU – Ejaculation failure; impotence; priapism; difficulty in micturition; acute urinary bladder retention; Peyronie's disease.

Musculoskeletal – Asthenia; muscle cramps; toxic myopathy.

Respiratory – Dyspnea; bronchospasm.

Miscellaneous – Systemic lupus erythematosus; positive antinuclear factor; antimitochondrial antibodies; edema; nasal stuffiness; fever; vision abnormality; dry eyes.

➤*Parenteral:*

Cardiovascular – Ventricular arrhythmias.

CNS – Hypesthesia; somnolence/yawning.

Renal – Transient increases in BUN and serum creatinine associated with drops in BP, generally in patients with prior renal insufficiency.

Miscellaneous – Pruritus; flushing; wheezing.

➤*Oral and parenteral:*

CNS – Dizziness; tingling of scalp/skin; vertigo.

GI – Nausea; vomiting; dyspepsia; taste distortion.

Miscellaneous – Postural hypotension; increased sweating.

➤*Adverse effects not listed above have been reported with other β-adrenergic blockers:*

Cardiovascular – Intensification of AV block. See Contraindications.

CNS – Mental depression progressing to catatonia; acute reversible syndrome characterized by disorientation for time/place, short-term memory loss, emotional lability, clouded sensorium and decreased performance on neuropsychometrics.

GI – Mesenteric artery thrombosis; ischemic colitis.

Hematologic – Agranulocytosis; thrombocytopenic/nonthrombocytopenic purpura.

Hypersensitivity – Fever with aching and sore throat; laryngospasm; respiratory distress.

Overdosage

➤*Symptoms:* Excessive hypotension (posture-sensitive); excessive bradycardia.

➤*Treatment:* Institute gastric lavage or induce emesis to remove drug after oral ingestion. Place patient in supine position; raise legs if necessary. Employ these as needed:

Excessive bradycardia – Administer atropine or epinephrine.

Cardiac failure – Administer a digitalis glycoside and a diuretic. Dopamine or dobutamine also may be useful.

Hypotension – Administer vasopressors. Norepinephrine may be the drug of choice.

Bronchospasm – Administer epinephrine or an aerosolized β$_2$-agonist.

Seizures – Administer diazepam.

In severe β-blocker overdose resulting in hypotension or bradycardia, glucagon has been effective in large doses (5 to 10 mg rapidly over 30 seconds, followed by continuous infusion of 5 mg/hr; reduce as patient improves).

Neither hemodialysis nor peritoneal dialysis removes a significant amount of labetalol from the general circulation (< 1%).

Patient Information

Do not discontinue medication except on advice of a physician.

Consult physician at any sign of impending cardiac failure.

Transient scalp tingling may occur, especially when treatment is initiated.

CARVEDILOL

Rx	Coreg (GlaxoSmithKline)	**Tablets:** 3.125 mg	Lactose, sucrose. (39 SB). White, oval. Film-coated. In 100s.
		6.25 mg	Lactose, sucrose. (4140 SB). White, oval. Film-coated. In 100s.
		12.5 mg	Lactose, sucrose. (4141 SB). White, oval. Film-coated. In 100s.
		25 mg	Lactose, sucrose. (4142 SB). White, oval. Film-coated. In 100s.

Indications

➤*Essential hypertension:* Management of essential hypertension. Carvedilol can be used alone or in combination with other antihypertensive agents, especially thiazide-type diuretics.

➤*Congestive heart failure (CHF):* For the treatment of mild to severe heart failure of ischemic or cardiomyopathic origin, usually in addition to diuretics, ACE inhibitors, and digitalis, to increase survival and reduce the risk of hospitalization.

➤*Left ventricular dysfunction (LVD) following MI:* To reduce cardiovascular mortality in clinically stable patients who have survived the acute phase of a MI and have a left ventricular ejection fraction of 40% or less (with or without symptomatic heart failure).

➤*Unlabeled uses:* Treatment of angina pectoris.

Administration and Dosage

➤*Approved by the FDA:* September 14, 1995.

➤*Hypertension:* Take with food to slow the rate of absorption and reduce the incidence of orthostatic effects. The recommended starting dose is 6.25 mg twice daily. If this dose is tolerated, using standing systolic pressure measured about 1 hour after dosing as a guide, maintain the dose for 7 to 14 days, and then increase to 12.5 mg twice daily, if needed, based on trough BP, again using standing systolic pressure 1 hour after dosing as a guide for tolerance. Also maintain this dose for 7 to 14 days and then adjust upward to 25 mg twice daily if tolerated and needed. The full antihypertensive effect of carvedilol is seen within 7 to 14 days. Do not exceed total daily dose of 50 mg.

Addition of a diuretic to carvedilol or carvedilol to a diuretic can be expected to produce additive effects and exaggerate the orthostatic component of carvedilol action.

➤*CHF:* Dosage must be individualized. Take carvedilol with food to slow the rate of absorption. Closely monitor during up-titration. Prior to initiation of carvedilol, it is recommended that fluid retention be minimized.

The recommended starting dose of carvedilol is 3.125 mg twice daily for 2 weeks. If this dose is tolerated, it can then be increased to 6.25, 12.5, and 25 mg twice daily over successive intervals of at least 2 weeks. Maintain patients on lower doses if higher doses are not tolerated. A maximum dose of 50 mg twice daily has been administered to patients weighing over 85 kg (187 lbs) with mild to moderate heart failure.

Advise patients that initiation of treatment and (to a lesser extent) dosage increases may be associated with transient symptoms of dizziness or lightheadedness (and rarely syncope) within the first hour after dosing. Thus, during these periods, avoid situations such as driving or hazardous tasks, where symptoms could result in injury. In addition, vasodilatory symptoms often do not require treatment, but it may be useful to separate the time of dosing of carvedilol from that of the ACE inhibitor or to temporarily reduce the dose of the ACE inhibitor. Do not increase the dose of carvedilol until symptoms of worsening heart failure or vasodilation have been stabilized.

Treat fluid retention (with or without transient worsening heart failure symptoms) with an increase in the dose of diuretics.

Reduce the dose of carvedilol if patients experience bradycardia (heart rate less than 55 beats/minute).

Episodes of dizziness or fluid retention during initiation of carvedilol can generally be managed without discontinuation of treatment and do not preclude subsequent successful titration of, or a favorable response to, carvedilol.

➤*LVD following MI:* Dosage must be individualized and monitored during up-titration. Treatment with carvedilol may be started as an inpatient or outpatient and started after the patient is hemodynamically stable and fluid retention has been minimized. It is recommended that carvedilol be started at 6.25 mg twice daily and increased after 3 to 10 days, based on tolerability to 12.5 mg twice daily, then again to

CARVEDILOL

the target dose of 25 mg twice daily. A lower starting dose may be used (3.125 mg twice daily) and/or, the rate of up-titration may be slowed if clinically indicated (eg, because of low BP, heart rate, fluid retention). Maintain patients on lower doses if higher doses are not tolerated. The recommended dosing regimen need not be altered in patients who received treatment with an IV or oral β-blocker during the acute phase of the MI.

➤*Discontinuation:* Because carvedilol has β-blocking activity, do not discontinue abruptly. Severe exacerbation of angina and the occurrence of MI and ventricular arrhythmias have been reported. Instead, discontinue over 1 or 2 weeks.

➤*Storage/Stability:* Store below 30°C (86°F). Protect from moisture.

Actions

➤*Pharmacology:* Carvedilol is a racemic mixture in which nonselective β-adrenoreceptor blocking activity is present in the S(-) enantiomer and α-adrenergic blocking activity is present in both R(+) and S(-) enantiomers at equal potency. Carvedilol has no intrinsic sympathomimetic activity.

Carvedilol (1) reduces cardiac ouput, (2) reduces exercise- and/or isoproterenol-induced tachycardia, and (3) reduces reflex orthostatic tachycardia. Significant β-adrenoreceptor blocking effect is usually seen within 1 hour of drug administration. The mechanism by which β-blockade produces an antihypertensive effect has not been established.

Carvedilol also (1) attenuates the pressor effects of phenylephrine, (2) causes vasodilation, and (3) reduces peripheral vascular resistance. These effects contribute to the reduction of BP and usually are seen within 30 minutes of drug administration. Because of the α₁-receptor blocking activity of carvedilol, BP is lowered more in the standing than in the supine position, and symptoms of postural hypotension (1.8%), including rare instances of syncope, can occur.

When postural hypotension has occurred, it has been transient and is uncommon when administered with food at the recommended starting dose and titration increments are closely followed.

In hypertensive patients with normal renal function, therapeutic doses of carvedilol decreased renal vascular resistance with no change in glomerular filtration rate or renal plasma flow. Changes in excretion of sodium, potassium, uric acid, and phosphorus in hypertensive patients with normal renal function were similar after carvedilol and placebo.

Carvedilol has little effect on plasma catecholamines, plasma aldosterone, or electrolyte levels, but it does significantly reduce plasma renin activity when given for at least 4 weeks. It also increases levels of atrial natriuretic peptide.

➤*Pharmacokinetics:*

Absorption/Distribution – Carvedilol is rapidly and extensively absorbed following oral administration, with absolute bioavailability of approximately 25% to 35% because of a significant degree of first-pass metabolism. Plasma concentrations achieved are proportional to the oral dose administered. When administered with food, the rate of absorption is slowed, as evidenced by a delay in the time to reach peak plasma levels, with no significant difference in extent of bioavailability.

Carvedilol is more than 98% bound to plasma proteins (primarily albumin). It has a steady-state volume of distribution of approximately 115 L, indicating substantial distribution into extravascular tissues.

Metabolism/Excretion – Carvedilol is extensively metabolized. Following oral administration in healthy volunteers, carvedilol accounted for approximately 7% of the total in plasma as measured by AUC. Carvedilol is metabolized primarily by aromatic ring oxidation and glucuronidation. The oxidative metabolites are further metabolized by conjugation via glucuronidation and sulfation. The metabolites of carvedilol are excreted primarily via bile into the feces. Less than 2% of the dose was excreted unchanged in the urine. Demethylation and hydroxylation at the phenol ring produce 3 active metabolites with β-receptor blocking activity. Based on preclinical studies, the 4'-hydroxyphenyl metabolite is approximately 13 times more potent than carvedilol for β-blockade.

Compared to carvedilol, the 3 active metabolites exhibit weak vasodilating activity. Plasma concentrations of the active metabolites are about 10% of those observed for carvedilol and have pharmacokinetics similar to the parent.

Carvedilol undergoes stereoselective first-pass metabolism with plasma levels of R(+)-carvedilol approximately 2 to 3 times higher than S(-)-carvedilol following oral administration in healthy subjects. The mean apparent terminal elimination half-lives for R(+)-carvedilol range from 5 to 9 hours vs 7 to 11 hours for the S(-)-enantiomer.

The primary P450 enzymes responsible for the metabolism of both R(+)- and S(-)-carvedilol are CYP2D6 and CYP2C9, and to a lesser extent CYP3A4, 2C19, 1A2, and 2E1.

Carvedilol is subject to the effects of genetic polymorphism with poor metabolizers of debrisoquin (a marker for cytochrome P450 2D6) exhibiting 2- to 3-fold higher plasma concentrations of R(+)-carvedilol compared with extensive metabolizers. In contrast, plasma levels of S(-)-

carvedilol are increased only about 20% to 25% in poor metabolizers, indicating this enantiomer is metabolized to a lesser extent by cytochrome P450 than R(+)-carvedilol.

Following oral administration, the apparent mean terminal elimination half-life generally ranges from 7 to 10 hours. Plasma clearance ranges from 500 to 700 mL/min.

Special populations –

Elderly: Plasma levels of carvedilol average approximately 50% higher in the elderly compared with younger subjects.

Hepatic function impairment: Patients with cirrhotic liver disease exhibit significantly higher concentrations of carvedilol (approximately 4- to 7-fold) following single-dose therapy (see Warnings).

CHF: Steady-state plasma concentrations of carvedilol and its enantiomers increased proportionally over the 6.25 to 50 mg dose range in patients with CHF. Compared with healthy subjects, CHF patients had increased mean AUC and C_max values for carvedilol and its enantiomers, with up to 50% to 100% higher values observed in 6 patients with New York Heart Association (NYHA) class IV heart failure.

Renal function impairment: Although carvedilol is metabolized primarily by the liver, plasma concentrations have been reported to be increased in patients with renal impairment. Based on mean AUC data, approximately 40% to 50% higher plasma concentrations were observed in hypertensive patients with moderate to severe renal impairment, compared with a control group of hypertensive patients with normal renal function. However, the ranges of AUC values were similar for both groups. Changes in mean peak plasma levels were less pronounced, approximately 12% to 26% higher in patients with impaired renal function.

Consistent with its high degree of plasma protein binding, carvedilol does not appear to be cleared significantly by hemodialysis.

Contraindications

Patients with decompensated cardiac failure requiring the use of IV inotropic therapy (such patients should first be weaned from IV therapy before initiating carvedilol); bronchial asthma (see Warnings) or related bronchospastic conditions; second- or third-degree AV block; sick sinus syndrome or severe bradycardia (unless a permanent pacemaker is in place); cardiogenic shock; clinically manifest hepatic impairment; hypersensitivity to the drug.

Warnings

➤*Abrupt withdrawal:* Because carvedilol has β-blocking activity, do not discontinue abruptly. Severe exacerbation of angina and the occurrence of MI and ventricular arrhythmias have been reported. Instead, discontinue over 1 or 2 weeks.

➤*Bronchial asthma:* Two cases of death from status asthmaticus have occurred in patients receiving single doses of carvedilol.

➤*Bronchospasm, nonallergic (eg, chronic bronchitis, emphysema):* In general, do not give β-blockers to patients with bronchospastic diseease. However, carvedilol may be used with caution in patients who do not respond to, or cannot tolerate, other antihypertensive agents. If carvedilol is used, it is prudent to use the smallest effective dose so that inhibition of endogenous or exogenous β-agonists is minimized.

➤*Hepatotoxicity:* Mild hepatocellular injury, confirmed by rechallenge, has occurred rarely with carvedilol therapy. In controlled studies of hypertensive patients, the incidence of liver function abnormalities reported as adverse experiences was 1.1% in patients receiving carvedilol and 0.9% with placebo. One patient receiving carvedilol in a placebo-controlled trial withdrew because of abnormal hepatic function. Hepatic injury has been reversible and has occurred after short- and/or long-term therapy with minimal clinical symptomatology. No deaths caused by liver function abnormalities have been reported.

At the first symptom/sign of liver dysfunction (eg, pruritus, dark urine, persistent anorexia, jaundice, right upper quadrant tenderness, unexplained flu-like symptoms) perform laboratory testing. If the patient has laboratory evidence of liver injury or jaundice, stop therapy and do not restart.

➤*Hypotension and postural hypotension:* These occurred in 9.7% and syncope in 3.4% of CHF patients receiving carvedilol, compared with 3.6% and 2.5% of placebo patients, respectively. The risk for these events was highest during the first 30 days of dosing, corresponding to the up-titration period and was a cause for discontinuation of therapy in 0.7% of carvedilol patients, compared with 0.4% of placebo patients.

Postural hypotension occurred in 1.8% and syncope in 0.1% of patients, especially following the initial dose or at the time of dose increase. Postural hypotension or syncope was a cause for discontinuation of therapy in 1% of patients.

➤*Peripheral vascular disease:* β-blockers can precipitate or aggravate symptoms of arterial insufficiency in patients with peripheral vascular disease. Exercise caution in such individuals.

➤*Anesthesia and major surgery:* If carvedilol treatment is to be continued perioperatively, take particular care when anesthetic agents that depress myocardial function (eg, ether, cyclopropane, trichloroethylene) are used. See Overdosage for information on treatment of brady-

CARVEDILOL

cardia and hypertension.

➤*Diabetes and hypoglycemia:* β-blockers may mask some of the manifestations of hypoglycemia, particularly tachycardia. Nonselective β-blockers may potentiate insulin-induced hypoglycemia and delay recovery of serum glucose levels. Caution patients subject to spontaneous hypoglycemia, or diabetic patients receiving insulin or oral hypoglycemic agents, about these possibilities. In CHF patients with diabetes, carvedilol therapy may lead to worsening hyperglycemia, which responds to intensification of hypoglycemic therapy. It is recommended that blood glucose be monitored when carvedilol dosing is initiated, adjusted, or discontinued.

➤*Thyrotoxicosis:* β-adrenergic blockade may mask clinical signs of hyperthyroidism, such as tachycardia. Abrupt withdrawal of β-blockade may be followed by an exacerbation of the symptoms of hyperthyroidism or may precipitate thyroid storm.

➤*Pheochromocytoma:* In patients with pheochromocytoma, initiate an α-blocking agent prior to the use of any β-blocking agent. Although carvedilol has α- and β-blocking pharmacologic activities, there has been no experience with its use in this condition. Therefore, use caution in administering carvedilol to patients suspected of having pheochromocytoma.

➤*Prinzmetal variant angina:* Agents with nonselective β-blocking activity may provoke chest pain in patients with Prinzmetal variant angina. There has been no clinical experience with carvedilol in these patients, although the α-blocking activity may prevent such symptoms. However, take caution in the administration of carvedilol to patients suspected of having Prinzmetal variant angina.

➤*Cardiac failure:* Worsening cardiac failure or fluid retention may occur during up-titration of carvedilol. If such symptoms occur, increase diuretics and do not advance the carvedilol dose until clinical stability resumes. Occasionally, it is necessary to lower the carvedilol dose or temporarily discontinue it. Such episodes do not preclude subsequent successful titration of carvedilol.

➤*Hypersensitivity reactions:* While taking β-blockers, patients with a history of severe anaphylactic reaction to a variety of allergens may be more reactive to repeated challenge, either accidental, diagnostic, or therapeutic. Such patients may be unresponsive to the usual doses of epinephrine used to treat allergic reaction.

➤*Renal function impairment:* Rarely, use of carvedilol in patients with CHF has resulted in deterioration of renal function. Patients at risk appear to be those with low BP (systolic BP less than 100 mm Hg), ischemic heart disease, diffuse vascular disease, and/or underlying renal insufficiency. Renal function returned to baseline when carvedilol was stopped. In patients with these risk factors, it is recommended that renal function be monitored during up-titration of carvedilol and the drug discontinued or dosage reduced if worsening of renal function occurs.

➤*Hepatic function impairment:* Use of carvedilol in patients with clinically manifested hepatic impairment is not recommended.

➤*Carcinogenesis:* At doses of at least 200 mg/kg/day (at least 32 times the maximum recommended human dose [MRHD] as mg/m^2), carvedilol was toxic to adult rats (sedation, reduced weight gain) and was associated with a reduced number of successful matings, prolonged mating time, significantly fewer corpora lutea and implants per dam and complete resorption of 18% of the litters. The no-observed-effect dose level for overt toxicity and impairment of fertility was 60 mg/kg/day (10 times the MRHD as mg/m^2).

➤*Elderly:* Plasma levels of carvedilol average 50% higher in elderly vs younger subjects. There were no notable differences in efficacy or the incidence of adverse events between older and younger patients. With the exception of dizziness (8.8% in the elderly vs 6% in younger patients), there were no events for which the incidence in the elderly exceeded that in the younger population by greater than 2%.

➤*Pregnancy:* Category C. Studies performed in pregnant rats and rabbits given carvedilol revealed increased postimplantation loss in rats and rabbits. In the rats, there was also a decrease in fetal body weight at the maternally toxic dose of 300 mg/kg/day, which was accompanied by an elevation in the frequency of fetuses with delayed skeletal development (missing or stunted 13th rib). There are no adequate and well-controlled studies in pregnant women. Use during pregnancy only if the potential benefit justifies the potential risk to the fetus.

➤*Lactation:* It is not known whether this drug is excreted in breast milk. In rats, carvedilol or its metabolites (as well as other β-blockers) cross the placental barrier and are excreted in breast milk. There was increased mortality at 1 week postpartum in neonates from rats during the last trimester through day 22 of lactation. Because of the potential for serious adverse reactions in breastfed infants from β-blockers, especially bradycardia, decide whether to discontinue breastfeeding or to discontinue the drug, taking into account the importance of the drug to the mother. The effects of other α- and β-blocking agents have included perinatal and neonatal distress.

➤*Children:* Safety and efficacy in patients younger than 18 years of age have not been established.

Precautions

➤*Monitoring:* At the first symptom/sign of liver dysfunction (eg, pruritus, dark urine, persistent anorexia, jaundice, right upper quadrant tenderness, unexplained flu-like symptoms) perform laboratory testing. If the patient has laboratory evidence of liver injury or jaundice, stop therapy and do not restart.

➤*Cardiovascular effects:* In clinical trials, carvedilol caused bradycardia in about 2% of hypertensive patients, 9% of CHF patients, and 6.5% of MI patients with LVD. If pulse rate drops below 55 beats/minute, reduce the dosage.

To decrease the likelihood of syncope or excessive hypotension, initiate treatment with 3.125 mg twice daily for CHF patients and 6.25 mg twice daily for hypertensive patients. Then, slowly increase dosage and always take the drug with food. During initiation of therapy, caution the patient to avoid situations such as driving or hazardous tasks where injury could result should syncope occur.

➤*Photosensitivity:* Photosensitivity may occur; therefore, caution patients to take protective measures (ie, sunscreens, protective clothing) against exposure to ultraviolet light or sunlight until tolerance is determined.

Drug Interactions

➤*CYP450:* Because carvedilol undergoes substantial oxidative metabolism, the metabolism and pharmacokinetics of carvedilol may be affected by induction or inhibition of cytochrome P450 enzymes.

Interactions of carvedilol with strong inhibitors of CYP2D6 (eg, quinidine, fluoxetine, paroxetine, propafenone) have not been studied, but these drugs would be expected to increase blood levels of the R(+) enantiomer of carvedilol. Retrospective analysis of side effects in clinical trials showed that poor 2D6 metabolizers had a higher rate of dizziness during up-titration, presumably resulting from vasodilating effects of the higher concentrations of the α-blocking R(+) enantiomer.

Carvedilol Drug Interactions

Precipitant drug	Object drug*		Description
Carvedilol	Antidiabetic agents	↑	Agents with β-blocking properties may enhance the blood sugar-reducing effect of insulin and oral hypoglycemics. In patients taking insulin or oral hypoglycemics, regular monitoring of blood glucose is recommended.
Carvedilol	Calcium channel blockers (diltiazem, verapamil)	↑	Isolated cases of conduction disturbance (rarely with hemodynamic compromise) have been observed when carvedilol is coadministered with diltiazem. As with other agents with β-blocking properties, if carvedilol is to be administered orally with calcium channel blockers of the verapamil or diltiazem type, it is recommended that ECG and BP be monitored.
Carvedilol	Catecholamine-depleting agents (eg, reserpine)	↑	Closely observe patients taking agents with β-blocking properties and a drug that can deplete catecholamines for signs of hypotension or severe bradycardia.
Carvedilol	Clonidine	↑	Concomitant administration of clonidine with agents with β-blocking properties may potentiate BP and heart-rate-lowering effects. When concomitant treatment with agents with β-blocking properties and clonidine is to be terminated, discontinue the β-blocking agent first. Clonidine therapy can then be discontinued several days later by gradually decreasing the dosage.
Carvedilol	Cyclosporine	↑	Coadministration of carvedilol and cyclosporine may cause an increase in mean trough cyclosporine concentrations. Monitor cyclosporine concentrations closely after carvedilol initiation and adjust cyclosporine dose as appropriate.
Carvedilol	Digoxin	↑	Digoxin concentrations are increased by ≈ 15% during concurrent use. Therefore, increased monitoring of digoxin is recommended when initiating, adjusting, or discontinuing carvedilol.
Cimetidine	Carvedilol	↑	Cimetidine increased carvedilol AUC by ≈ 30% but caused no change in C_{max}.

Alpha/Beta-Adrenergic Blocking Agents

CARVEDILOL

Carvedilol Drug Interactions			
Precipitant drug	Object drug*		Description
Rifampin	Carvedilol	↓	Rifampin reduced AUC and C_{max} of carvedilol by ≈ 70%.
SSRIs (eg, fluoxetine, paroxetine)	Carvedilol	↑	Certain selective serotonin reuptake inhibitors (SSRIs) may inhibit metabolism of some beta blockers; possible excessive beta blockade (bradycardia) may occur. Monitor cardiac function during coadministration.
Diphenhydramine	Carvedilol	↑	Diphenhydramine may inhibit carvedilol metabolism, resulting in increased plasma concentrations and cardiovascular effects of carvedilol.
Carvedilol	Disopyramide	↑	Clearance of disopyramide may be decreased by carvedilol, resulting in increased adverse effects (eg, sinus bradycardia, hypotension). Monitor patients closely during coadministration.
Hydroxychloroquine	Carvedilol	↑	Hydroxychloroquine may inhibit metabolism of carvedilol, resulting in increased plasma concentrations and cardiovascular effects. Monitor patients when hydroxychloroquine is started or stopped.

* ↑ = Object drug increased. ↓ = Object drug decreased.

➤*Drug/Food interactions:* When taken with food, rate of absorption is slowed but extent of bioavailability is not affected. Taking with food minimizes the risk of orthostatic hypotension.

Adverse Reactions

➤*Hypertension:* In general, carvedilol is well tolerated at doses up to 50 mg/day. Most adverse events reported were of mild to moderate severity. In clinical trials directly comparing carvedilol monotherapy in doses up to 50 mg with placebo, 4.9% of carvedilol patients discontinued for adverse events vs 5.2% of placebo patients. Discontinuations were more common in the carvedilol group for postural hypotension (1% vs 0%). The overall incidence of adverse events increased with increasing doses of carvedilol. For individual adverse events, this could only be distinguished for dizziness, which increased in frequency from 2% to 5% as the total daily dose increased from 6.25 to 50 mg.

In addition to the following table, abdominal pain, back pain, chest pain, dependent edema, dyspepsia, dyspnea, fatigue, headache, injury, nausea, pain, rhinitis, sinusitis, somnolence, and upper respiratory tract infection were also reported, but rates were equal or greater in placebo-treated patients.

Carvedilol Adverse Reactions in Hypertension Trials (≥ 1%)		
Adverse reaction	Carvedilol (n = 1142)	Placebo (n = 462)
Cardiovascular		
Bradycardia	2	-
Postural hypotension	2	-
Peripheral edema	1	-
CNS		
Dizziness	6	5
Insomnia	2	1
Miscellaneous		
Diarrhea	2	1
Pharyngitis	2	1
UTI	2	1
Viral infection	2	1
Hypertriglyceridemia	1	-
Thrombocytopenia	1	-

➤*CHF:* In addition to the events in the following table, chest pain, injury, cardiac failure, abdominal pain, gout, insomnia, depression, anemia, viral infection, and dyspnea were also reported, but rates were equal or greater in placebo-treated patients.

Carvedilol Adverse Reactions in CHF Trials (%)				
	Mild to moderate HF		Severe HF	
Adverse reaction	Carvedilol (n = 765)	Placebo (n = 437)	Carvedilol (n = 1156)	Placebo (n = 1133)
Cardiovascular				
Bradycardia	9	1	10	3
Hypotension	9	3	14	8
Syncope	3	3	8	5
Angina pectoris	2	3	6	4

Carvedilol Adverse Reactions in CHF Trials (%)				
	Mild to moderate HF		Severe HF	
Adverse reaction	Carvedilol (n = 765)	Placebo (n = 437)	Carvedilol (n = 1156)	Placebo (n = 1133)
CNS				
Dizziness	32	19	24	17
Headache	8	7	5	3
GI				
Diarrhea	12	6	5	3
Nausea	9	5	4	3
Vomiting	6	4	1	2
Metabolic				
Hyperglycemia	12	8	5	3
Weight increase	10	7	12	11
BUN increase	6	5	-	-
NPN increase[1]	6	5	-	-
Hypercholesteremia	4	3	1	1
Peripheral edema	2	1	7	6
Respiratory				
Sinusitis	5	4	2	1
Bronchitis	5	4	5	5
Upper respiratory tract infection	18	18	14	13
Cough increased	8	9	5	4
Rales	4	4	4	2
Miscellaneous				
Asthenia	7	7	11	9
Fatigue	24	22	-	-
Pain	9	8	1	1
Arthralgia	6	5	1	1
Digoxin level increased	5	4	2	1
Vision abnormal	5	2		
Edema				
Generalized	5	3	6	5
Dependent	4	2	-	-

[1] NPN = Nonprotein nitrogen.

➤*The following were reported in greater than 1% up to 3% of patients:*

Cardiovascular – Fluid overload; postural hypotension; aggravated angina pectoris; AV block; palpitation; hypertension.

CNS – Hypethesia; vertigo; paresthesia.

GI – Melena; periodontitis.

GU – Renal insufficiency; albuminuria; hematuria.

Hematologic – Prothrombin decreased; purpura; thrombocytopenia.

Hepatic – ALT increased; AST increased.

Metabolic/Nutritional – Hyperuricemia; hypoglycemia; hyponatremia; increased alkaline phosphatase; glycosuria; hypervolemia; diabetes mellitus; GGT increased; weight loss; hyperkalemia; creatinine increased.

Miscellaneous – Allergy; malaise; hypovolemia; fever; leg edema; infection; back pain; muscle cramps; somnolence; infection; impotence; blurred vision.

➤*Postmarketing:* Aplastic anemia has been reported rarely and only when carvedilol was administered concomitantly with other medications associated with the event.

➤*The following adverse events were reported in patients with hypertension or CHF (greater than 0.1% to less than or equal to 1%):*

Cardiovascular – Peripheral ischemia; tachycardia.

CNS – Hypokinesia; nervousness; sleep disorder; aggravated depression; impaired concentration; abnormal thinking; paroniria; emotional lability.

Dermatologic – Pruritus; rash erythematous; rash maculopapular; rash psoriaform; photosensitivity reaction.

GI – Bilirubinemia; increased hepatic enzymes (0.2% of hypertension patients and 0.4% of CHF patients were discontinued from therapy because of increases in hepatic enzymes).

GU – Micturition frequency increased.

Hematologic – Anemia; leukopenia.

Metabolic/Nutritional – Hypokalemia; hypertriglyceridemia.

Miscellaneous – Dry mouth; sweating increased; decreased libido; asthma; tinnitus.

Alpha/Beta-Adrenergic Blocking Agents

CARVEDILOL

The following events were reported in 0.1% or less of patients and are potentially important: Complete AV block; bundle branch block; myocardial ischemia; cerebrovascular disorder; convulsions; migraine; neuralgia; paresis; anaphylactoid reaction; alopecia; exfoliative dermatitis; amnesia; GI hemorrhage; bronchospasm; pulmonary edema; decreased hearing; respiratory alkalosis; increased BUN; decreased HDL; pancytopenia; atypical lymphocytes.

Left ventricular dysfunction following MI – Adverse events reported in more than 3% of the patients were dyspnea, anemia, and lung edema. Hypertension and MI were also reported, but rates were equal or greater in placebo-treated patients. Adverse events reported with a frequency of more than 1% but not more than 3% were flu syndrome, cerebrovascular accident, peripheral vascular disorder, hypotonia, depression, GI, arthritis, gout, and UTI.

Overdosage

➤*Symptoms:* Overdosage may cause severe hypotension, bradycardia, cardiac insufficiency, cardiogenic shock, and cardiac arrest. Respiratory problems, bronchospasms, vomiting, lapses of consciousness, and generalized seizures also may occur.

➤*Treatment:* Place the patient in a supine position and, when necessary, keep under observation and treat under intensive care conditions. Gastric lavage or pharmacologically induced emesis may be used shortly after ingestion. The following agents may be administered.

For excessive bradycardia – Atropine 2 mg IV.

To support cardiovascular function – Glucagon 5 to 10 mg IV rapidly over 30 seconds, followed by a continuous infusion of 5 mg/hr; sympathomimetics (eg, dobutamine, isoproterenol, adrenaline) at doses according to body weight and effect.

If peripheral vasodilation dominates, it may be necessary to administer epinephrine or norepinephrine with continuous monitoring of circulatory conditions. For therapy-resistant bradycardia, perform pacemaker therapy. For bronchospasm, give β-sympathomimetics (as aerosol or IV) or aminophylline IV. In the event of seizures, slow IV injection of diazepam or clonazepam is recommended.

In the event of severe intoxication where there are symptoms of shock, treatment with antidotes must be continued for a sufficiently long period of time consistent with the 7- to 10-hour half-life of carvedilol.

Patient Information

Do not interrupt or discontinue using carvedilol without a physician's advice.

Advise CHF patients to consult their physician if they experience signs or symptoms of worsening CHF (eg, weight gain, increasing shortness of breath).

A drop in BP may be experienced when standing, resulting in dizziness and, rarely, fainting. Patients should sit or lie down when these symptoms of lowered BP occur. If experiencing dizziness or faintness, consult a physician about adjusting the dosage. Avoid driving or hazardous tasks if experiencing dizziness or fatigue.

Take with food.

Diabetic patients should report any changes in blood sugar levels to their physician.

Contact lens wearers may experience decreased lacrimation.

May cause photosensitivity. Avoid prolonged exposure to the sun and other ultraviolet light. Use sunscreens and wear protective clothing until tolerance is determined.

Antiadrenergic Agents — Centrally Acting

METHYLDOPA AND METHYLDOPATE HCl

Rx	Methyldopa (Various, eg, Ivax, Mylan)	**Tablets**: 250 mg methyldopa	May contain EDTA. In 100s, 500s, 1000s, and UD 100s.
Rx	Methyldopa (Various, eg, Ivax, Mylan)	**Tablets**: 500 mg methyldopa	May contain EDTA. In 100s, 500s, and UD 100s.
Rx	Methyldopate HCl (Various, eg, Abbott, American Regent)	**Injection**: 50 mg methyldopate HCl/mL	May contain sulfites,[1] EDTA. In single-dose vials and *ADD-vantage* vials.

[1] Refer to individual product package insert for sulfite content.

For complete prescribing information, refer to the Antihypertensives Treatment Guidelines in the Appendix.

Indications

➤*Hypertension:* Treatment of hypertension.

➤*Hypertensive crises:* Methyldopate HCl may be used to initiate treatment of hypertensive crises; however, because of its slow onset of action, other agents may be preferred for rapid reduction of blood pressure (BP).

Methyldopa is not recommended for the treatment of patients with pheochromocytoma.

➤*Unlabeled uses:* Hypertension in pregnancy.

Administration and Dosage

➤*Oral:*

Adults –

Initial therapy: 250 mg 2 or 3 times/day in the first 48 hours. Adjust dosage at intervals of not less than 2 days until an adequate response is achieved. To minimize sedation, increase dosage in the evening. By adjustment of dosage, morning hypotension may be prevented without sacrificing control of afternoon blood pressure.

Maintenance therapy: 500 mg to 2 g/day in 2 to 4 doses. The maximum recommended daily dosage is 3 g. Once an effective dosage range is attained, a smooth blood pressure response occurs in most patients in 12 to 24 hours.

Children – Individualize dosage. Initial oral dosage is based on 10 mg/kg/day in 2 to 4 doses. The maximum daily dosage is 65 mg/kg or 3 g, whichever is less.

Concomitant drug therapy – When methyldopa is given with antihypertensives other than thiazides, limit the initial dosage to 500 mg/day in divided doses; when added to a thiazide, the dosage of thiazide need not be changed.

➤*IV:* Add the desired dose to 100 mL of 5% dextrose or give in 5% dextrose injection in a concentration of 10 mg/mL. Administer over 30 to 60 minutes. When control has been obtained, substitute oral therapy starting with the same parenteral dosage schedule.

Adults – 250 to 500 mg every 6 hours as required (maximum 1 g every 6 hours).

Children – 20 to 40 mg/kg/day in divided doses every 6 hours. The maximum daily dosage is 65 mg/kg or 3 g, whichever is less.

➤*Tolerance:* Tolerance may occur, usually between the second and third month of therapy. Adding a diuretic or increasing the dosage of methyldopa frequently restores blood pressure control. A thiazide is recommended if therapy was not started with a thiazide or if effective control of blood pressure cannot be maintained on 2 g/day methyldopa.

➤*Discontinuation:* Methyldopa has a relatively short duration of action; therefore, withdrawal is followed by return of hypertension, usually within 48 hours. This is not complicated by a overshoot of BP.

➤*Renal function impairment:* Methyldopa is largely excreted by the kidneys; patients with impaired renal function may respond to smaller doses.

➤*Storage/Stability:* Store tablets and vials at controlled room temperature (15° to 30°C [59° to 86°F]). Dispense tablets in a well-closed container; use child-resistant closure.

Actions

➤*Pharmacology:* The mechanism of action of methyldopa has not been conclusively demonstrated but is probably because of the drug's metabolism to alpha-methylnorepinephrine, which lowers arterial pressure by the stimulation of central inhibitory α-adrenergic receptors, false neurotransmission, and/or reduction of plasma renin activity. Methyldopa causes a net reduction in tissue concentrations of serotonin, dopamine, norepinephrine, and epinephrine.

Methyldopa reduces standing and supine BP. It usually produces highly effective lowering of supine pressure with infrequent symptomatic postural hypotension. Exercise hypotension and diurnal BP variations rarely occur.

Methyldopate HCl, the ethyl ester of methyldopa HCl, is pharmacologically equivalent.

➤*Pharmacokinetics:*

Absorption/Distribution – Following oral administration, methyldopa is variably absorbed. The mean bioavailability is approximately 50%. Methyldopa crosses the blood-brain barrier and is converted in the CNS to active alpha-methylnoradrenaline. Methyldopa crosses the placental barrier and appears in cord blood and breast milk. A decrease in BP occurs within 4 to 6 hours following IV or oral administration and lasts 10 to 16 hours or 12 to 24 hours, respectively.

Metabolism/Excretion – Methyldopa is extensively metabolized. Approximately 17% of a dose of methyldopate HCl appears in plasma as free methyldopa. The average T_{max} is 2 hours. The total volume of distribution is about 0.6 L/kg. Approximately 70% (oral) and approximately 49% (IV) of the drug that is absorbed is excreted in the urine as methyldopa and its mono-O-sulfate conjugate. The renal clearance is approximately 130 mL/min (oral) and approximately 156 mL/min (IV) in healthy subjects and is diminished in renal insufficiency. After oral doses, excretion is essentially complete in 36 hours. Biphasic elimination occurs after IV and oral administration; the half-life of the alpha-phase is approximately 0.21 hours and the beta-phase approximately 1.28 hours in healthy subjects. Methyldopa is less than 20% bound to plasma proteins. The drug is removed by dialysis.

Contraindications

Active hepatic disease, such as acute hepatitis or active cirrhosis; if previous methyldopa therapy has been associated with liver disorders (see Warnings); coadministration with monoamine oxidase inhibitors (MAOIs) (see Drug Interactions); hypersensitivity to any component of these formulations, including sulfites.

Warnings

➤*Positive Coombs' test/hemolytic anemia:* It is important to recognize that a positive Coombs' test, hemolytic anemia, and liver disorders may occur with methyldopa therapy. The rare occurrences of hemolytic anemia or liver disorders could lead to potentially fatal complications unless properly recognized and managed.

With prolonged therapy, 10% to 20% of patients develop a positive direct Coombs' test, usually between 6 and 12 months of therapy. The lowest incidence reported was at a dosage of 1 g/day or less. This is associated rarely with hemolytic anemia, which could lead to potentially fatal complications and is difficult to predict. Prior existence or development of a positive direct Coombs' test is not a contraindication to methyldopa, but if it develops during therapy, determine whether hemolytic anemia exists and whether the positive Coombs' test may be a problem. For example, in addition to a positive direct Coombs' test there is less often a positive indirect Coombs' test that may interfere with cross-matching of blood.

Perform baseline and periodic blood counts (hematocrit, hemoglobin, or red cell count) to detect hemolytic anemia. A direct Coombs' test may be useful before therapy and at 6 and 12 months later. If Coombs'-positive hemolytic anemia occurs, discontinue methyldopa; anemia usually remits promptly. If not, corticosteroids may be given; consider other causes. If hemolytic anemia is related to methyldopa, do not reinstitute.

When methyldopa produces a positive Coombs' test alone or with hemolytic anemia, the red cell is usually coated with IgG gamma globulin. The positive Coombs' test may not revert to normal until weeks to months after methyldopa is stopped.

➤*Blood transfusions:* Should the need for transfusion arise in a patient receiving methyldopa, perform both a direct and indirect Coombs' test. In the absence of hemolytic anemia, usually only the direct Coombs' test will be positive. A positive direct Coombs' test alone will not interfere with typing or cross-matching. If the indirect Coombs' test is also positive, problems may arise in the major cross-match and the assistance of a hematologist or transfusion expert will be needed.

➤*Edema/Weight gain:* Some patients taking methyldopa experience clinical edema or weight gain, which may be controlled by use of a diuretic. Do not continue methyldopa if edema progresses or signs of heart failure appear.

➤*Hepatic toxicity:* Fever has occasionally occurred within the first 3 weeks of therapy, sometimes associated with eosinophilia or abnormalities in 1 or more liver function tests (eg, alkaline phosphatase, AST, ALT, bilirubin, prothrombin time). Jaundice with or without fever may occur, usually within the first 2 to 3 months of therapy. In some patients, the findings are consistent with cholestasis. In others, the findings are consistent with hepatitis and hepatocellular injury. Fatal hepatic necrosis has been reported rarely. These hepatic changes may represent hypersensitivity reactions. If fever, abnormalities in liver function tests or jaundice appear, discontinue therapy; temperature and abnormalities in liver function revert to normal when the drug is discontinued. Do not reinstitute methyldopa in such patients.

The incidence of severe cytotoxic injury is estimated to be less than 0.1% to 0.5%.

METHYLDOPA AND METHYLDOPATE HCl

▶*Hematologic disorders:* Rarely, a reversible reduction of the white blood cell (WBC) count with a primary effect on granulocytes has been seen but promptly returns to normal upon drug discontinuation. Rare cases of granulocytopenia have been reported. WBC returned to normal after drug discontinuation. Reversible thrombocytopenia occurs rarely.

▶*Renal function impairment:* Methyldopa and its metabolites accumulate in renal failure. There is a marked accumulation of unidentified metabolites in renal failure patients, which may explain the strong and prolonged hypotensive action of methyldopa in these patients.

Hypertension has recurred occasionally after dialysis in patients given methyldopa because the drug is removed by this procedure.

▶*Hepatic function impairment:* Use with caution in patients with previous liver disease or dysfunction.

▶*Elderly:* Syncope in older patients may be related to an increased sensitivity and advanced arteriosclerotic vascular disease. This may be avoided with lower doses.

▶*Pregnancy:* Category B (oral). Category C (IV). Methyldopa crosses the placenta and achieves fetal concentrations similar to the maternal serum. No unusual adverse reactions or obvious teratogenic effects have been reported despite rather wide use during pregnancy. Neonates born to mothers receiving methyldopa have demonstrated a decreased systolic blood pressure of 4 to 5 mm Hg for 2 days after delivery, compared with controls.

It also is not known whether methyldopate HCl can affect reproduction capacity or can cause fetal harm when given to a pregnant woman only.

Published reports of the use of methyldopa during all trimesters indicate that if this drug is used during pregnancy, the possibility of fetal harm appears remote. Use only when clearly needed and when potential benefits outweigh the potential hazards to the fetus.

▶*Lactation:* Methyldopa is excreted in breast milk in small amounts. After 750 to 2000 mg/day, milk levels of free and conjugated methyldopa ranged from 0.1 to 0.9 mcg/mL. The American Academy of Pediatrics considers methyldopa to be compatible with breastfeeding.

▶*Children:* See Administration and Dosage.

Precautions

▶*Monitoring:* Blood count, Coombs' tests, and liver function tests are recommended before initiating therapy and at periodic intervals. Perform periodic determinations of hepatic function, particularly during the first 6 to 12 weeks of therapy or when an unexplained fever occurs.

▶*Paradoxical pressor response:* This has been reported with IV administration of methyldopate HCl.

▶*Involuntary choreoathetotic movements:* Involuntary choreoathetotic movements have been observed rarely in patients with severe bilateral cerebrovascular disease. Should these occur, discontinue methyldopa therapy.

▶*Sedation:* Usually transient, sedation may occur during initial therapy or whenever the dose is increased.

▶*Urine discoloration:* Rarely, when urine is exposed to air after voiding, it may darken because of breakdown of methyldopa or its metabolites.

▶*Sulfite sensitivity:* Some of these products contain sulfites that may cause allergic-type reactions, including anaphylactic symptoms and life-threatening or less severe asthmatic episodes in certain susceptible persons. The overall prevalence of sulfite sensitivity in the general population is unknown and probably low; it is seen more frequently in asthmatic than in nonasthmatic people.

Drug Interactions

Methyldopa Drug Interactions			
Precipitant drug	Object drug*		Description
Methyldopa	Anesthetics	↑	Reduced doses of anesthetics may be required. Hypotension during anesthesia can be controlled by vasopressors because adrenergic receptors remain sensitive.
Methyldopa	Haloperidol	↑	Methyldopa may potentiate the antipsychotic effects of haloperidol or the combination may produce psychosis.
Methyldopa	Levodopa	↑	Blood-pressure-lowering effects of methyldopa may be potentiated by levodopa. Central effects of levodopa in Parkinson's disease may be potentiated by methyldopa.
Levodopa	Methyldopa	↑	
Methyldopa	Lithium	↑	Lithium toxicity characterized by GI symptoms, polyuria, muscle weakness, lethargy, and tremor has been reported following methyldopa coadministration.
Methyldopa	MAOIs	↑	Metabolites of methyldopa stimulate release of endogenous catecholamines that are usually metabolized by MAOIs, thereby leading to excessive sympathetic stimulation. Coadministration is contraindicated.
Methyldopa	Phenothiazines	↑	Serious elevations in blood pressure may occur.
Methyldopa	Sympathomimetics	↑	Methyldopa may potentiate the pressor effects of sympathomimetics and lead to hypertension.
Beta-blockers, nonselective (eg, propranolol)	Methyldopa	↑	Nonselective beta blockers and methyldopa rarely may cause a hypertensive crisis.
Ferrous sulfate or gluconate	Methyldopa	↓	A decrease in the bioavailability of methyldopa when it is ingested with ferrous sulfate or ferrous gluconate has been demonstrated.

* ↑ = Object drug increased. ↓ = Object drug decreased.

▶*Drug/Lab test interactions:* Methyldopa may interfere with tests for the following: Urinary uric acid by phosphotungstate method; serum creatinine by alkaline picrate method; AST by colorimetric methods. Interference with spectrophotometric methods for AST analysis is not reported.

Because methyldopa causes fluorescence in urine samples at the same wave lengths as catecholamines, falsely high levels of urinary catecholamines may occur and will interfere with the diagnosis of pheochromocytoma. Methyldopa does not interfere with measurement of vanillylmandelic acid (VMA) by methods converting VMA to vanillin.

Adverse Reactions

▶*Cardiovascular:* Bradycardia; prolonged carotid sinus hypersensitivity; aggravation of angina pectoris; CHF; paradoxical pressor response with IV use; pericarditis; myocarditis; vasculitis; orthostatic hypotension; edema and weight gain usually relieved by a diuretic. Discontinue methyldopa if edema progresses or signs of heart failure appear.

▶*CNS:* Sedation, usually transient, may occur during initial therapy or whenever the dose is increased; headache, asthenia, or weakness (may be early, transient symptoms); dizziness; lightheadedness; symptoms of cerebrovascular insufficiency; paresthesias; parkinsonism; Bell palsy; decreased mental acuity; involuntary choreoathetotic movements; psychic disturbances, including nightmares and reversible mild psychoses or depression.

▶*Dermatologic:* Rash; toxic epidermal necrolysis.

▶*Endocrine:* Breast enlargement; gynecomastia; lactation; hyperprolactinemia; amenorrhea.

▶*GI:* Nausea; vomiting; distention; constipation; flatus; diarrhea; colitis; dry mouth; sore or "black" tongue; pancreatitis; sialoadenitis.

▶*GU:* Impotence; decreased libido.

▶*Hematologic:* Positive Coombs' test, hemolytic anemia (see Warnings); bone marrow depression; leukopenia; granulocytopenia; thrombocytopenia; eosinophilia; positive tests for antinuclear antibody, lupus erythematosus cells, and rheumatoid factor.

▶*Hepatic:* Abnormal liver function tests; jaundice; hepatitis, liver disorders (see Warnings).

▶*Hypersensitivity:* Drug-related fever; lupus-like syndrome.

▶*Miscellaneous:* Nasal stuffiness; rise in BUN; arthralgia with or without joint swelling; myalgia.

Overdosage

▶*Symptoms:* Sedation; acute hypotension; weakness; bradycardia; dizziness; lightheadedness; constipation; distention; flatus; diarrhea; nausea; vomiting and other responses attributable to brain and GI malfunction.

▶*Treatment:* Employ gastric lavage or emesis and general supportive measures when ingestion is recent. When ingestion has been earlier, infusions may be helpful to promote urinary excretion. Otherwise, management includes special attention to cardiac rate and output, blood volume, electrolyte imbalance, paralytic ileus, urinary function, and cerebral activity. Refer to General Management of Acute Overdosage. Sympathomimetic drugs (eg, norepinephrine, epinephrine,

METHYLDOPA AND METHYLDOPATE HCl

metaraminol bitartrate) may be indicated. In severe cases, consider hemodialysis.

The oral LD_{50} of methyldopa is greater than 1.5 g/kg in the mouse and the rat. The acute IV LD_{50} of methyldopate HCl in the mouse is 321 mg/kg.

CLONIDINE HCl

For complete prescribing information, refer to the Antihypertensives Treatment Guidelines in the Appendix.

Indications

Injectable clonidine is used for severe pain in cancer patients. For further information, refer to the Clonidine monograph in the Central Analgesics section.

Patient Information

When urine is exposed to air after voiding, it may darken.

➤*Hypertension:* Treatment of hypertension; may be used alone or concomitantly with other antihypertensive agents.

➤*Unlabeled uses:* Clonidine has been evaluated for use in several conditions, see chart below.

Clonidine Unlabeled Uses	
Use	Dosage[1]
Alcohol withdrawal	300 to 600 mcg every 6 hours
Atrial fibrillation	75 mcg oral single dose or twice daily; alone or with digoxin
Attention deficit hyperactivity disorder	5 mcg/kg/day for 8 weeks
Constitutional growth delay in children	37.5 to 150 mcg/m²/day
Cyclosporine-associated nephrotoxicity	100 to 200 mcg/day transdermal
Diabetic diarrhea	100 to 600 mcg every 12 hours or 300 mcg/24-hr patch (1 to 2 patches/week)
Gilles de la Tourette's syndrome	150 to 200 mcg/day
Hyperhidrosis	250 mcg 3 to 5 times/day
Hypertensive "urgencies" (diastolic> 120 mmHg)	Initially 100 to 200 mcg, followed by 50 to 100 mcg/hour to a maximum of 800 mcg
Mania	Unknown
Menopausal flushing	100 to 400 mcg/day or 100 mcg/24-hr patch
Methadone/opiate detoxification	15 to 16 mcg/kg/day
Pheochromocytoma diagnosis (overnight clonidine suppression test)	300 mcg
Postherpetic neuralgia	200 mcg/day
Psychosis in schizophrenic patients	≤ 900 mcg/day
Reduction of allergen-induced inflammatory reactions in patients with extrinsic asthma	150 mcg for 3 days or 75 mcg/1.5 mL saline; inhalation
Restless leg syndrome	100 to 300 mcg/day; up to 900 mcg/day
Smoking cessation facilitation	150 to 400 mcg/day or 200 mcg/24-hour patch
Ulcerative colitis	300 mcg 3 times a day

[1] Dosage given as oral unless otherwise specified.

Actions

➤*Pharmacology:* Clonidine, an imidazoline derivative, is a central α-adrenergic stimulant that inhibits sympathetic cardio-accelerator and vasoconstrictor centers. Initially, clonidine stimulates peripheral α-adrenergic receptors producing transient vasoconstriction. Stimulation of α-adrenergic receptors in the brain stem results in reduced sympathetic outflow from the CNS and a decrease in peripheral resistance, renal vascular resistance, heart rate and blood pressure. Renal blood flow and glomerular filtration rate remain essentially unchanged.

Orthostatic effects are mild and infrequent. The drug does not alter normal hemodynamic responses to exercise. Acute studies have demonstrated a moderate reduction (15% to 20%) of cardiac output in the supine position with no change in the peripheral resistance, while at a 45° tilt there is a smaller reduction in cardiac output and a decrease of peripheral resistance. During long-term therapy, cardiac output tends to return to control values while peripheral resistance remains decreased. The coadministration of a diuretic enhances antihypertensive efficacy of clonidine.

Plasma renin activity and excretion of aldosterone and catecholamines is reduced. Clonidine acutely stimulates growth hormone release in children and adults, but does not produce a chronic elevation of growth hormone with long-term use.

➤*Pharmacokinetics:* Blood pressure declines within 30 to 60 minutes after an oral dose. The peak plasma level occurs in ≈ 3 to 5 hours with a plasma half-life of 12 to 16 hours and an elimination half-life of 6 to 24 hours. About 50% of the absorbed dose is metabolized in the liver. In patients with impaired renal function, half-life increases up to 41 hours. About 40% to 60% of the absorbed dose is recovered in the urine as unchanged drug in 24 hours.

Transdermal System – The system, a 0.2 mm thick film with four layers, contains a drug reservoir of clonidine, released at an approximately constant rate for 7 days. A microporous polypropylene membrane controls rate of delivery from system to skin.

Therapeutic plasma levels are achieved 2 to 3 days after initial application. Application of a new system at weekly intervals continuously maintains therapeutic plasma concentrations. When system is removed (and not replaced), therapeutic plasma clonidine levels persist for ≈ 8 hours and then decline slowly over several days; blood pressure returns gradually to pretreatment levels.

Contraindications

Hypersensitivity to clonidine or any component of adhesive layer of transdermal system.

Warnings

➤*Special risk patients:* Use with caution in patients with severe coronary insufficiency, conduction disturbances, recent MI or cerebrovascular disease.

➤*Tolerance:* Tolerance may develop, necessitating a re-evaluation of therapy.

➤*Blood pressure control:* In rare instances, loss of blood pressure control has been reported in patients using transdermal clonidine.

➤*Defibrillation or cardioversion:* Remove the transdermal clonidine systems before attempting defibrillation or cardioversion because of the potential for altered electrical conductivity that may increase the risk of arcing, a phenomenon associated with the use of defibrillators.

➤*Renal function impairment:* Use with caution in patients with chronic renal failure.

➤*Pregnancy: Category C.* Clonidine crosses the placenta, resulting in a cord:maternal ratio of 0.89 with mean amniotic fluid concentrations of 1.5 ng/mL following a mean maternal dose of 330 mcg/day. Also, the plasma levels in the newborn are approximately half the maternal levels. There are no adequate and well controlled studies in pregnant women. Use clonidine in pregnancy only if clearly needed.

➤*Lactation:* Clonidine is excreted in breast milk; following a 150 mcg oral dose, milk concentrations of 1.5 ng/mL may be achieved (milk: plasma ratio 1.5). Clinical significance is unknown. Exercise caution when administering to a nursing woman.

➤*Children:* Safety and efficacy for use in children have not been established.

Precautions

➤*Rebound hypertension:* Do not discontinue therapy without consulting a physician (see also Step-Down Therapy for Antihypertensives in the Treatment Guidelines section of the Appendix). Discontinue therapy by reducing the dose gradually over 2 to 4 days to avoid a rapid rise in blood pressure. Abrupt withdrawal of clonidine may result in subjective symptoms such as nervousness, agitation, headache, confusion, tremor and elevated catecholamine concentrations in the plasma,

Antiadrenergic Agents — Centrally Acting

CLONIDINE HCl

but such occurrences have usually been associated with previous administration of high oral doses (exceeding 1.2 mg/day) or with continuation of concomitant β-blocker therapy. Tachycardia, rebound hypertension, flushing, nausea, vomiting and cardiac arrhythmias have also occurred. The risk may be dose-related and may be increased with multiple drug therapy. Rare instances of hypertensive encephalopathy, cerebrovascular accidents and death have been reported after abrupt cessation of therapy.

If an excessive rise in blood pressure occurs, it can be reversed by resumption of therapy or by IV phentolamine, phenoxybenzamine or prazosin. Direct vasodilators and captopril have also been used. If therapy is to be discontinued in patients receiving β-blockers and clonidine concurrently, discontinue β-blockers several days before the gradual withdrawal of clonidine.

➤*Ophthalmologic effects:* Perform periodic eye examinations because retinal degeneration has been noted in animal studies.

➤*Perioperative use:* Continue administration of clonidine to within 4 hours of surgery and resume as soon as possible thereafter. Do not interrupt transdermal clonidine during the surgical period. Carefully monitor blood pressure and institute appropriate measures to control it as necessary. If transdermal therapy is started during the perioperative period, note that therapeutic plasma levels are not achieved until 2 to 3 days after initial application.

➤*Sensitization to transdermal clonidine:* In patients who have developed localized contact sensitization to transdermal clonidine, substitution of oral clonidine therapy may be associated with development of a generalized skin rash. In patients who develop an allergic reaction to transdermal clonidine that extends beyond the local patch site (such as generalized skin rash, urticaria or angioedema) oral clonidine substitution may elicit a similar reaction.

Drug Interactions

Clonidine Drug Interactions			
Precipitant drug	Object drug*		Description
Clonidine	Levodopa	↓	The effectiveness of levodopa may be reduced.
Beta-adrenergic blocking agents	Clonidine	↑	Attenuation or reversal of antihypertensive effect and potentially life-threatening increases in blood pressure.
Prazosin	Clonidine	↓	The antihypertensive effectiveness of clonidine may be decreased.
Tricyclic antidepressants	Clonidine	↓	Tricyclic antidepressants may block antihypertensive effects of clonidine and possibly life-threatening elevations in blood pressure may occur.
Verapamil	Clonidine	↑	Synergistic pharmacologic and toxic effects, possibly causing atrioventricular (AV) block and severe hypotension.

* ↑ = Object drug increased. ↓ = Object drug decreased.

Adverse Reactions

Most common – Dry mouth (40%); drowsiness (33%); dizziness (16%); sedation, constipation (10%).

➤*Cardiovascular:* Syncope; congestive heart failure; orthostatic symptoms; palpitations, tachycardia and bradycardia; Raynaud's phenomenon; ECG abnormalities (eg, sinus node arrest) manifested as Wenckebach period or ventricular trigeminy; conduction disturbances, arrhythmias, sinus bradycardia and atrioventricular block (rare).

➤*CNS:* Dreams or nightmares; insomnia; hallucinations; delirium; nervousness; agitation; restlessness; anxiety; depression; headache.

➤*Dermatologic:* Rash; angioneurotic edema; hives; urticaria; alopecia; pruritus.

➤*GI:* Abdominal pain; anorexia; malaise; nausea; vomiting; mild transient abnormalities in liver function tests; hepatitis; parotitis (rare).

➤*GU:* Impotence; decreased sexual activity/loss of libido; nocturia, difficulty in micturition and urinary retention.

➤*Hematologic:* Thrombocytopenia (rare).

➤*Metabolic:* Weight gain; transient elevation of blood glucose or serum creatine phosphokinase (rare); gynecomastia.

➤*Musculoskeletal:* Weakness; fatigue; muscle or joint pain; cramps of the lower limbs.

➤*Miscellaneous:* Increased sensitivity to alcohol; dryness, itching or burning of the eyes; dryness of the nasal mucosa; pallor; fever; weakly positive Coombs' test; discontinuation syndrome; blurred vision.

➤*Transdermal system:* The most frequent systemic reactions were dry mouth and drowsiness. The following have also been reported:

Cardiovascular – Chest pain; cerebrovascular accident; increases in blood pressure.

CNS – Fatigue; headache; lethargy; sedation; insomnia; nervousness; dizziness; irritability.

Dermatologic – Transient localized skin reactions; pruritus; erythema, allergic contact sensitization and contact dermatitis; localized vesiculation; hyperpigmentation; edema; excoriation; burning; papules; throbbing; blanching; generalized macular rash; maculopapular skin rash; urticaria; angioedema of the face and tongue.

GI – Constipation; nausea; change in taste; dry throat.

GU – Impotence/sexual dysfunction.

Overdosage

➤*Symptoms:* Bradycardia; hypotension; CNS depression; respiratory depression; apnea; hypothermia; miosis; coma; seizures; lethargy; agitation; irritability; vomiting; hypoventilation; reversible cardiac conduction defects; arrhythmias; transient hypertension; profound hypotension; weakness; somnolence; diminished or absent reflexes.

In a patient who ingested 100 mg clonidine, plasma levels were 60 ng/mL (1 hour), 190 ng/mL (1.5 hours), 370 ng/mL (2 hours) and 120 ng/mL (5.5 and 6.5 hours). The patient developed hypertension followed by hypotension, bradycardia, apnea, hallucinations, semicoma and premature ventricular contractions. The patient fully recovered after intensive treatment.

Because children commonly have GI illnesses that lead to vomiting, they may be particularly susceptible to hypertensive episodes resulting from abrupt inability to take medication.

➤*Treatment:* Induction of emesis is usually not recommended because of the rapid onset of CNS depression. Establish respiration if necessary, perform gastric lavage and administer activated charcoal. A saline cathartic (magnesium sulfate) will increase the rate of transport through the GI tract. Routine hemodialysis is of limited benefit because a maximum of 5% of circulating clonidine is removed.

Atropine sulfate may be useful for treatment of persistent bradycardia and hypotension with dopamine infusion in addition to IV fluids.

Hypertension has been treated with IV furosemide or diazoxide or α-blocking agents such as phentolamine. Tolazoline, an α-blocker, in IV doses of 10 mg at 30 minute intervals may reverse clonidine's effects if other efforts fail. Naloxone may be a useful adjunct for the management of clonidine-induced respiratory depression, hypotension or coma.

Patient Information

Advise patients who engage in potentially hazardous activities, such as operating machinery or driving, of potential sedative side effects.

Caution patients against interruption of clonidine therapy without a physician's advice.

Antiadrenergic Agents — Centrally Acting

CLONIDINE HCl — ORAL

Rx	**Clonidine** (Various, eg, Geneva, Mylan, UDL)	**Tablets:** 0.1 mg		In 100s, 500s, 1000s and UD 100s.
Rx	**Catapres** (Boehringer Ingelheim)			(BI-6). Tan, scored. In 100s, 1000s and UD 100s.
Rx	**Clonidine** (Various, eg, Geneva, Mylan, UDL)	**Tablets:** 0.2 mg		In 100s, 500s, 1000s and UD 100s.
Rx	**Catapres** (Boehringer Ingelheim)			(BI-7). Orange, scored. In 100s, 1000s and UD 100s.
Rx	**Clonidine** (Various, eg, Geneva, Mylan, UDL)	**Tablets:** 0.3 mg		In 100s and UD 100s.
Rx	**Catapres** (Boehringer Ingelheim)			(BI-11). Peach, scored. In 100s.

Administration and Dosage

Individualize dosage.

➤*Initial dose:* 100 mcg twice daily. Elderly patients may benefit from a lower initial dose.

➤*Maintenance dose:* Continue increments of 100 mcg/day at weekly intervals until the desired response is achieved; most common range is 200 to 600 mcg/day given in divided doses. The maximum dose is 2400 mcg/day. Minimize sedative effects by slowly increasing the daily dosage and giving the majority of the daily dose at bedtime.

➤*Children:* 50 to 400 mcg orally twice a day.

➤*Unlabeled route of administration:* Sublingual clonidine, using a dosage of 200 to 400 mcg/day, may be effective in hypertensive patients unable to take oral medication. Onset occurs within 30 to 60 minutes and blood pressure appears to be maintained on a twice-daily regimen.

➤*Renal function impairment:* Adjust dosage according to degree of renal impairment and carefully monitor patients. Because only a minimal amount of clonidine is removed during hemodialysis, there is no need to give supplemental clonidine following dialysis.

CLONIDINE HCl — TRANSDERMAL

	Product/Distributor	Release Rate (mg/24 hr)	Surface Area (cm²)	Total Clonidine Content (mg)	How Supplied
Rx	**Catapres-TTS-1** (Boehringer Ingelheim)	0.1	3.5	2.5	Mineral oil. In 12s.
Rx	**Catapres-TTS-2** (Boehringer Ingelheim)	0.2	7	5	Mineral oil. In 12s.
Rx	**Catapres-TTS-3** (Boehringer Ingelheim)	0.3	10.5	7.5	Mineral oil. In 4s.

Administration and Dosage

Apply to a hairless area of intact skin on upper arm or torso once every 7 days. Use a different skin site from the previous application. If the system loosens during the 7-day period, apply the adhesive overlay directly over the system to ensure good adhesion.

For initial therapy, start with the 0.1 mg system. If, after 1 or 2 weeks, desired blood pressure reduction is not achieved, add another 0.1 mg system or use a larger system. Dosage greater than two 0.3 mg systems usually does not improve efficacy. Note that the antihypertensive effect of the system may not commence until 2 to 3 days after application. Therefore, when substituting the transdermal system in patients on prior antihypertensive therapy, a gradual reduction of prior drug dosage is advised. Previous antihypertensive treatment may have to be continued, particularly in patients with severe hypertension.

GUANFACINE HCl

Rx	**Tenex** (ESP Pharma)	**Tablets:** 1 mg	Lactose. (1 AHR Tenex). Light pink. Diamond shape. In 100s, 500s and *Dis-Co* 100s.
		2 mg	Lactose. (2 AHR Tenex). Yellow. Diamond shape. In 100s.

For complete prescribing information, refer to the Antihypertensives Treatment Guidelines in the Appendix.

Indications

➤*Hypertension:* Management of hypertension, alone or in combination with other antihypertensives, especially thiazide-type diuretics.

➤*Unlabeled uses:* Guanfacine (0.03 to 1.5 mg/day) may be beneficial in ameliorating withdrawal symptoms when discontinuing heroin usage.

In a small study, guanfacine (1 mg/day for 12 weeks) significantly reduced the frequency of migraine headache and reduced nausea and vomiting.

Administration and Dosage

The recommended dose, alone or with other antihypertensives, is 1 mg/day given at bedtime to minimize daytime somnolence. If 1 mg does not produce a satisfactory result after 3 to 4 weeks of therapy, doses of 2 mg may be given, although most of the drug's effect is seen at 1 mg. The frequency of rebound hypertension is low, but it can occur. When rebound occurs, it does so after 2 to 4 days, which is delayed compared with clonidine HCl. This is consistent with the longer half-life of guanfacine. In most cases, after abrupt withdrawal of guanfacine, blood pressure returns to pretreatment levels slowly (within 2 to 4 days) without ill effects.

Higher daily doses have been used, but adverse reactions increase significantly with doses > 3 mg/day.

Actions

➤*Pharmacology:* Guanfacine is a centrally acting oral antihypertensive with α_2-adrenoreceptor agonist properties. Its principal mechanism of action appears to be stimulation of central α_2-adrenergic receptors. Guanfacine reduces sympathetic nerve impulses from the vasomotor center to the heart and blood vessels, resulting in a decrease in peripheral vascular resistance and a reduction in heart rate.

Hematologic – The decrease in blood pressure observed after single dose or long-term oral treatment with guanfacine was accompanied by a significant decrease in peripheral resistance and a slight reduction in heart rate (5 bpm). Cardiac output under conditions of rest or exercise was not altered by guanfacine.

Guanfacine lowered elevated plasma renin activity and plasma catecholamine levels in hypertensive patients, but this does not correlate with individual blood pressure responses. Growth hormone secretion was stimulated with single oral doses of 2 and 4 mg. Long-term use had no effect on growth hormone levels. Guanfacine had no effect on plasma aldosterone. A slight but insignificant decrease in plasma volume occurred after 1 month of guanfacine therapy. There were no changes in mean body weight or electrolytes.

➤*Pharmacokinetics:*

Absorption / Distribution – Relative to a 3 mg IV dose, the absolute oral bioavailability of guanfacine is about 80%. Peak plasma concentrations occur from 1 to 4 hours with an average of 2.6 hours after single oral doses or at steady state. The area under the concentration time-curve increases linearly with the dose.

The drug is ≈ 70% bound to plasma proteins, independent of drug concentration. The whole body volume of distribution is high (mean, 6.3 L/kg), which suggests high distribution of drug to tissues.

Metabolism / Excretion – In individuals with normal renal function, the average elimination half-life is approximately 17 hours (range, 10 to 30 hours). Younger patients tend to have shorter elimination half-lives (13 to 14 hours) while older patients tend to have half-lives at the upper end of the range. Steady-state blood levels were attained within 4 days in most subjects. Guanfacine and its metabolites are excreted primarily in the urine. Approximately 50% (40% to 75%) of the dose is eliminated in the urine as unchanged drug; the remainder is eliminated mostly as conjugates of metabolites produced by oxidative metabolism of the aromatic ring. The guanfacine to creatinine clearance ratio is > 1, suggesting that tubular secretion of drug occurs.

➤*Clinical trials:* The dose-response relationship for blood pressure and adverse effects of guanfacine given once daily as monotherapy has been evaluated in patients with mild to moderate hypertension. Patients were randomized to placebo or to 0.5, 1, 2, 3 or 5 mg guanfacine. A positive effect was not observed overall until doses of 2 mg were reached, although responses in white patients were seen at 1 mg; 24 hour effectiveness of 1 to 3 mg doses was documented using 24 hour ambulatory monitoring. While the 5 mg dose added an incremental increase in effectiveness, it caused an unacceptable increase in adverse reactions.

In patients with mild to moderate hypertension receiving a thiazide-type diuretic and guanfacine at bedtime, blood pressure response can persist for 24 hours after a single dose. Observed mean changes from baseline indicate similarity of response for placebo and the 0.5 mg dose. Doses of 1, 2 and 3 mg resulted in decreased blood pressure in the sitting position with no real differences among the three doses.

Antiadrenergic Agents — Centrally Acting

GUANFACINE HCl

While most of guanfacine's efficacy was present at 1 mg, adverse reactions at this dose were not clearly distinguishable from those associated with placebo. Adverse reactions were clearly present at 2 and 3 mg (see Adverse Reactions).

In another study of guanfacine and chlorthalidone, a significant decrease in blood pressure was maintained for a full 24 hours after dosing. While there was no significant difference between the 12 and 24 hour blood pressure readings, the fall in blood pressure at 24 hours was numerically smaller, suggesting possible escape of blood pressure in some patients and the need for individualization of therapy.

In a double-blind, randomized trial, either guanfacine or clonidine was given at recommended doses with 25 mg chlorthalidone for 24 weeks and then abruptly discontinued. Results showed equal degrees of blood pressure reduction with the two drugs; there was no tendency for blood pressure to increase despite maintenance of the same daily dose of the two drugs. Signs and symptoms of rebound phenomena were infrequent upon discontinuation of either drug. Abrupt withdrawal of clonidine produced a rapid return of diastolic and, especially, systolic blood pressure to approximately pretreatment levels, with occasional values significantly greater than baseline. Guanfacine withdrawal produced a more gradual increase to pretreatment levels, but also with occasional values significantly greater than baseline.

Contraindications

Hypersensitivity to guanfacine.

Warnings

➤*Renal function impairment:* Guanfacine clearance in patients with varying degrees of renal insufficiency is reduced, but drug plasma levels are only slightly increased compared to patients with normal renal function. Use the low end of the dosing range in patients with renal impairment. Patients on dialysis can be given usual doses of guanfacine, since the drug is poorly dialyzed.

➤*Pregnancy: Category B.* Administration to rats and rabbits at doses 200 and 100 times the maximum recommended human dose, respectively, were associated with reduced fetal survival and maternal toxicity. Guanfacine crosses the placenta in rats. There are no adequate and well controlled studies in pregnant women. Use during pregnancy only if clearly needed.

Labor and delivery – Not recommended in the treatment of acute hypertension associated with toxemia of pregnancy.

➤*Lactation:* Guanfacine is excreted in breast milk of rats. It is not known whether guanfacine is excreted in human breast milk. Use caution when administering to a nursing mother.

➤*Children:* Safety and efficacy in children < 12 years of age have not been demonstrated. Therefore, use in this age group is not recommended.

Precautions

➤*Special risk patients:* Use guanfacine with caution in patients with severe coronary insufficiency, recent myocardial infarction, cerebrovascular disease or chronic renal or hepatic failure.

➤*Sedation:* Like other centrally active oral α_2-adrenergic agonists, guanfacine causes sedation or drowsiness, especially when beginning therapy. These symptoms are dose-related. When used with other centrally active depressants (eg, phenothiazines, barbiturates, benzodiazepines), consider the potential for additive sedative effects.

➤*Rebound:* Abrupt cessation of therapy with centrally active oral α_2-adrenergic agonists may be associated with increases in plasma and urinary catecholamines, symptoms of nervousness and anxiety and, less commonly, increases in blood pressure to levels significantly greater than those prior to therapy.

The frequency of rebound hypertension is low, but when rebound occurs, it does so after 2 to 4 days, which is delayed compared with clonidine. This is consistent with guanfacine's longer half-life. In most cases, after abrupt withdrawal of guanfacine, blood pressure returns to pretreatment levels slowly (in 2 to 4 days) without ill effects.

Adverse Reactions

Adverse reactions are similar to those of other central α_2-adrenoreceptor agonists: Dry mouth; sedation (somnolence); weakness (asthenia); dizziness; constipation; impotence. While the reactions are common, most are mild and tend to disappear on continued dosing. The most common reasons for discontinuing therapy with guanfacine, either alone or in combination with chlorthalidone, were as follows: Dry mouth; somnolence; dizziness; fatigue; weakness; constipation; headache; impotence; insomnia; syncope; urinary incontinence; conjunctivitis; paresthesia; dermatitis; confusion; depression; palpitations.

The most commonly observed adverse reactions during guanfacine therapy showed a dose relationship from 0.5 to 3 mg.

Guanfacine Adverse Reactions (%)					
Adverse reaction	Placebo (n = 59)	0.5 mg (n = 60)	1 mg (n = 61)	2 mg (n = 60)	3 mg (n = 59)
Dry mouth	0	10	10	42	54
Somnolence	8	5	10	13	39
Asthenia	0	2	3	7	3
Dizziness	8	12	2	8	15
Headache	8	13	7	5	3
Impotence	0	0	0	7	3
Constipation	0	2	0	5	15
Fatigue	2	2	5	8	10

In another study of guanfacine in combination with chlorthalidone, the guanfacine dose was adjusted upward to 3 mg/day in 1 mg increments at 3 week intervals (ie, more similar to ordinary clinical use). The most common reactions were: Dry mouth (47%); constipation (16%); fatigue (12%); somnolence (10%); asthenia, dizziness (6%); headache, insomnia (4%).

In the clonidine/guanfacine comparisons, the most common adverse reactions were as follows:

Guanfacine vs Clonidine Adverse Reactions		
Adverse reaction	Guanfacine (n = 279)	Clonidine (n = 278)
Dry mouth	30%	37%
Somnolence	21%	35%
Dizziness	11%	8%
Constipation	10%	5%
Fatigue	9%	8%
Headache	4%	4%
Insomnia	4%	3%

Adverse reactions occurring in patients in the three controlled trials with a diuretic and in post-marketing surveillance (monotherapy or with other antihypertensives) were as follows:

➤*Cardiovascular:* Bradycardia; palpitations; substernal pain; chest pain; syncope; tachycardia; cardiac fibrillation, CHF, heart block, MI (rare).

➤*CNS:* Amnesia; confusion; depression; insomnia; decreased libido; paresthesias; vertigo; agitation; anxiety; malaise; nervousness; tremor.

➤*Dermatologic:* Dermatitis; pruritus; purpura; sweating; skin rash with exfoliation; alopecia; rash.

➤*GI:* Abdominal pain; diarrhea; dyspepsia; dysphagia; nausea; constipation.

➤*GU:* Testicular disorder; urinary incontinence/frequency; impotence; nocturia.

➤*Musculoskeletal:* Leg cramps; hypokinesia; arthralgia; leg pain; myalgia.

➤*Special senses:* Rhinitis; taste perversion/alterations in taste; tinnitus; conjunctivitis; iritis; vision disturbance; blurred vision.

➤*Miscellaneous:* Paresis; dyspnea; abnormal liver function tests; edema; asthenia; acute renal failure, cerebrovascular accident (rare).

Overdosage

➤*Symptoms:* Drowsiness, lethargy, bradycardia and hypotension have been observed. A 25-year-old female intentionally ingested 60 mg guanfacine. She presented with severe drowsiness and bradycardia of 45 bpm. Gastric lavage was performed and an infusion of isoproterenol (0.8 mg in 12 hours) was administered. She recovered quickly and without sequelae.

➤*Treatment:* Gastric lavage and supportive therapy, as appropriate. Guanfacine is not dialyzable in clinically significant amounts (2.4%).

Patient Information

May produce drowsiness or dizziness; observe caution while driving, operating dangerous machinery or performing other tasks requiring alertness, coordination or physical dexterity.

Warn patients that tolerance for alcohol and other CNS depressants may be diminished.

Advise patients not to discontinue therapy abruptly.

Medication should be taken at bedtime.

Antiadrenergic Agents — Centrally Acting

GUANABENZ ACETATE

Rx	Guanabenz Acetate (Various, eg, Ivax, Watson)	**Tablets:** 4 mg	In 100s and 500s.
Rx	Wytensin (Wyeth-Ayerst)		(Wyeth 73/W4). Orange. In 100s, 500s and Redipak 100s.
Rx	Guanabenz Acetate (Various, eg, Ivax, Watson)	8 mg	In 100s and 500s.
Rx	Wytensin (Wyeth-Ayerst)		(Wyeth 74/W8). Gray, scored. In 100s.

For complete prescribing information, refer to the Antihypertensives Treatment Guidelines in the Appendix.

Indications

➤*Hypertension:* Treatment of hypertension, alone or with a thiazide diuretic.

Administration and Dosage

➤*Initial dose:* Individualize dosage. Begin dosing with 4 mg twice a day, whether used alone or with a thiazide diuretic; increase in increments of 4 to 8 mg/day every 1 to 2 weeks. The maximum dose studied was 32 mg twice daily; doses this high are rarely needed.

Actions

➤*Pharmacology:* Guanabenz is an orally active central α_2-adrenergic agonist. Its antihypertensive action appears mediated via stimulation of central α-adrenergic receptors, resulting in decreased sympathetic outflow from the brain.

The acute antihypertensive effect occurs without major changes in peripheral resistance, but its chronic effect appears to be a decrease in peripheral resistance. Blood pressure decreases in both the supine and standing positions without alterations of normal postural mechanisms, so that postural hypotension has not been observed. Guanabenz decreases pulse rate by about five beats per minute. Cardiac output and left ventricular ejection fraction are unchanged during long-term therapy.

During long-term administration, a small decrease in serum cholesterol and total triglycerides occurs without affecting high density lipoprotein.

Plasma norepinephrine, serum dopamine beta-hydroxylase and plasma renin activity decrease during chronic administration.

➤*Pharmacokinetics:*

Absorption/Distribution – About 75% of an oral dose is absorbed and metabolized. The onset of action begins within 60 minutes after a single oral dose. Peak plasma concentrations of unchanged drug occur between 2 and 5 hours. The effect of meals on the absorption of guanabenz has not been studied.

Metabolism/Excretion – The average half-life is ≈ 6 hours. The effect of a single dose is reduced appreciably 6 to 8 hours after administration, and blood pressure approaches baseline values within 12 hours. The site(s) of metabolism have not been determined, but < 1% of unchanged drug is recovered in the urine.

Renal/Hepatic function impairment – The disposition of orally administered guanabenz is altered in patients with alcohol-induced liver disease or renal impairment. Mean plasma concentrations of guanabenz were higher in hepatic impaired patients than in healthy subjects. In renal impaired patients, half-life is prolonged and clearance decreased, especially in patients on hemodialysis. The clinical significance of these findings is unknown.

➤*Clinical trials:* With effective control of blood pressure in hypertensive patients, guanabenz has not demonstrated any significant effect on glomerular filtration rate, renal blood flow, body fluid volume or body weight. Similarly, a decrease in blood pressure and a natriuresis (5% to 240% increase in sodium excretion) occurred in hypertensive subjects 24 hours after salt loading following a single oral dose of guanabenz. After 7 consecutive days of administration and effective blood pressure control, no significant change in glomerular filtration rate, renal blood flow or body weight was observed. However, in clinical trials of 6 to 30 months duration, hypertensive patients with effective blood pressure control by guanabenz lost 1 to 4 pounds of body weight. The mechanism of this weight loss has not been established. Tolerance to the antihypertensive effect has not been observed.

Contraindications

Sensitivity to guanabenz.

Warnings

➤*Renal/Hepatic function impairment:* Use with caution in patients with severe hepatic or renal failure. The disposition of oral guanabenz is altered modestly.

➤*Pregnancy:* Category C. Guanabenz may have adverse fetal effects when administered to pregnant women. A teratology study in mice has indicated a possible increase in skeletal abnormalities when guanabenz is given orally at doses of 3 to 6 times maximum recommended human dose. Increased fetal loss has been observed after oral guanabenz administration to pregnant rats (14 mg/kg) and rabbits (20 mg/kg). Rats have shown slightly decreased live-birth indices, decreased fetal survival rate, and decreased pup body weight at oral doses of 6.4 and 9.6 mg/kg. There are no adequate, well controlled studies in pregnant women. Use during pregnancy only if the potential benefit justifies the potential risk to the fetus.

➤*Lactation:* No information is available on excretion in breast milk; therefore, do not administer to nursing mothers.

➤*Children:* Safety and efficacy for use in children < 12 years of age have not been demonstrated; therefore, use in this age group is not recommended.

Precautions

➤*Monitoring:* Monitor blood pressure carefully in patients with coexisting hypertension and chronic hepatic dysfunction or renal impairment.

➤*Sedation:* Guanabenz causes sedation or drowsiness in a large fraction of patients.

➤*Rebound:* Sudden cessation of therapy with central α-agonists like guanabenz may rarely result in "overshoot" hypertension and more commonly produces an increase in serum catecholamines and subjective symptomatology.

➤*Special risk:* Use with caution in patients with severe coronary insufficiency, recent myocardial infarction or cerebrovascular disease.

➤*Lab test abnormalities:* During long-term administration, there is a small decrease in serum cholesterol and total triglycerides; no change in high density lipoprotein occurs.

Rarely, a nonprogressive increase in liver enzymes has been observed, although there is no clinical evidence of hepatic disease.

Drug Interactions

➤*CNS depressants:* When guanabenz is used with centrally active depressants, (eg, phenothiazines, barbiturates and benzodiazepines), consider the potential for additive sedative effects.

Adverse Reactions

Side effects appear to be dose-related.

➤*Most common (at doses of 16 mg daily):*

Miscellaneous – Drowsiness/sedation (20% to 39%; however, the 20% incidence was observed in patients taking 8 mg daily); dry mouth (28% to 38%); dizziness (12% to 17%); weakness (10%); headache (5%).

These effects led to treatment discontinuation ≈ 15% of the time.

➤*Other adverse effects reported, but not distinguishable from placebo effects (≤ 3%):*

Cardiovascular – Chest pain; edema; arrhythmias; palpitations; atrioventricular dysfunction, AV block (rare).

CNS – Anxiety; ataxia; depression; sleep disturbances.

Dermatologic – Rash; pruritus.

GI – Nausea; epigastric pain; diarrhea; vomiting; constipation; abdominal discomfort.

GU – Urinary frequency; disturbances of sexual function.

Musculoskeletal – Aches in extremities; muscle aches.

Miscellaneous – Gynecomastia; taste disorders; dyspnea; nasal congestion; blurred vision.

Overdosage

➤*Symptoms:* Overdose has been reported in children. Symptoms included hypotension, somnolence, lethargy, irritability, miosis and bradycardia. Treatment results in complete and uneventful recovery.

➤*Treatment:* Institute supportive treatment while the drug is being eliminated from the body and until the patient is no longer symptomatic. Monitor vital signs and fluid balance. Gastric lavage, activated charcoal, ipecac, fluid, pressor agents and atropine have been used successfully to treat guanabenz overdose. Maintain an adequate airway and, if indicated, institute assisted respiration. There are no data regarding dialyzability of guanabenz. Refer to General Management of Acute Overdosage.

Patient Information

Use caution when operating dangerous machinery or driving motor vehicles until it is determined that drowsiness or dizziness is not manifested from taking guanabenz.

Tolerance for alcohol and other CNS depressants may be diminished.

Advise patients not to discontinue therapy abruptly.

RESERPINE

Rx	**Reserpine** (Various, eg, Eon, Moore, Rugby)	**Tablets**: 0.1 mg	In 100s, 1000s and 5000s.
Rx	**Reserpine** (Various, eg, Eon, Moore, Rugby, URL)	**Tablets**: 0.25 mg	In 100s, 1000s and 5000s.

For complete prescribing information, refer to the Antihypertensives Treatment Guidelines in the Appendix.

Indications

➤*Hypertension:* Mild essential hypertension.

Adjunctive therapy with other antihypertensive agents in more severe forms of hypertension.

➤*Psychotic states:* Relief of symptoms in agitated psychotic states (eg, schizophrenia), primarily in those individuals unable to tolerate phenothiazine derivatives or in those who also require antihypertensive medication.

Administration and Dosage

➤*Hypertension:* In the average patient not receiving other antihypertensive agents, the usual initial dosage is 0.5 mg daily for 1 or 2 weeks. For maintenance, reduce to 0.1 to 0.25 mg daily. Use higher dosages cautiously because occurrence of serious mental depression and other side affects may increase considerably.

➤*Psychiatric disorders:* The usual initial dosage is 0.5 mg daily, but may range from 0.1 to 1 mg. Adjust dosage upward or downward according to the patient's response.

➤*Children:* Reserpine is not recommended for use in children. If it is be used in treating a child, the usual recommended starting dose is 20 mcg/kg daily. The maximum recommended dose is 0.25 mg (total) daily.

Actions

➤*Pharmacology:* Reserpine depletes stores of catecholamine and 5-hydroxytryptamine in many organs, including the brain and adrenal medulla. Most of its pharmacological effects have been attributed to this action. Depletion is slower and less complete in the adrenal medulla than in other tissues. The depression of sympathetic nerve function results in a decreased heart rate and a lowering of arterial blood pressure. The sedative and tranquilizing properties of reserpine are thought to be related to depletion of catecholamine and 5-hydroxytryptamine from the brain.

➤*Pharmacokinetics:* Reserpine is characterized by slow onset of action and sustained effects. Both cardiovascular and CNS effects may persist for a period of time following withdrawal of the drug.

Mean maximum plasma levels of 1.54 ng/mL were attained after a median of 3.5 hours in six healthy subjects receiving a single oral 1 mg dose. Bioavailability was ≈ 50% of that of a corresponding IV dose. Plasma levels of reserpine after IV administration declined with a mean half-life of 33 hours. Reserpine is extensively bound (96%) to plasma proteins. No definitive studies on the metabolism of reserpine have been made.

Contraindications

Hypersensitivity; mental depression or history of mental depression (especially with suicidal tendencies); active peptic ulcer; ulcerative colitis; patients receiving electroconvulsive therapy.

Warnings

➤*Depression:* Exercise extreme caution in treating patients with a history of mental depression. Reserpine may cause mental depression.

Recognition of depression may be difficult, because this condition may often be disguised by somatic complaints (masked depression). Discontinue the drug at first signs of depression (eg, despondency, early morning insomnia, loss of appetite, impotence or self-deprecation). Drug-induced depression may persist for several months after drug withdrawal and may be severe enough to result in suicide.

➤*Ulcers:* Since reserpine increases GI motility and secretion, use cautiously in patients with a history of peptic ulcer, ulcerative colitis or gallstones (biliary colic may be precipitated).

➤*Cardiovascular effects:* Preoperative withdrawal of reserpine does not assure that circulatory instability will not occur. It is important that the anesthesiologist be aware of the patient's drug intake and consider this in the overall management, since hypotension has occurred in patients receiving reserpine. Anticholinergic or adrenergic drugs (eg, metaraminol, norepinephrine) have been employed to treat adverse vagocirculatory effects.

➤*Renal function impairment:* Exercise caution when treating hypertensive patients with renal insufficiency, since they adjust poorly to lowered blood pressure levels.

➤*Carcinogenesis:* Reserpine is an animal tumorigen, causing an increased incidence of mammary fibroadenomas in female mice, malignant tumors of the seminal vesicles in male mice and malignant adrenal medullary tumors in male rats. The breast neoplasms are thought to be related to reserpine's prolactin-elevating effect. The extent to which these findings indicate a risk to humans is uncertain. Tissue culture experiments show that about 33% of human breast tumors are prolactin-dependent, a factor of considerable importance if the use of the drug is contemplated in a patient with previously detected breast cancer. The possibility of an increased risk of breast cancer in reserpine users has been studied extensively; however, no firm conclusion has emerged. Although a few epidemiologic studies have suggested a slightly increased risk (less than two-fold in all studies except one in women who have used reserpine), other studies of generally similar design have not confirmed this.

➤*Pregnancy:* Category C. There are no adequate and well controlled studies of reserpine in pregnant women. Reserpine crosses the placental barrier. Increased respiratory tract secretions, nasal congestion, cyanosis and anorexia may occur in neonates of reserpine-treated mothers. Use during pregnancy only if the potential benefit justifies the potential risk to the fetus.

➤*Lactation:* Reserpine is excreted in breast milk. Increased respiratory tract secretions, nasal congestion, cyanosis and anorexia may occur in breastfed infants. Because of the potential for adverse reactions in nursing infants and the potential for tumorigenicity, decide whether to discontinue nursing or to discontinue the drug, taking into account the importance of the drug to the mother.

➤*Children:* Safety and efficacy have not been established by means of controlled clinical trials, although there is experience with the use of reserpine in children (see Administration and Dosage). Because of adverse effects such as emotional depression and lability, sedation and stuffy nose, reserpine is not usually recommended as a Step-2 drug in the treatment of hypertension in children.

Drug Interactions

Reserpine Drug Interactions			
Precipitant drug	Object drug*		Description
MAO inhibitors	Reserpine	↔	Avoid MAO inhibitors or use with extreme caution.
Tricyclic antidepressants	Reserpine	↓	Concurrent use may decrease the antihypertensive effect of reserpine.
Reserpine	Digitalis glycosides Quinidine	↑	Use reserpine cautiously with digitalis and quinidine, since cardiac arrhythmias have occurred.
Reserpine	Sympathomimetics, direct-acting	↑	Closely monitor concurrent use of reserpine and direct- or indirect-acting sympathomimetics. The action of direct-acting amines (eg, epinephrine, isoproterenol, phenylephrine, metaraminol) may be prolonged when given to patients taking reserpine. The action of indirect-acting amines (eg, ephedrine, tyramine, amphetamines) is inhibited.
	Sympathomimetics, indirect-acting	↓	

* ↑ = Object drug increased. ↓ = Object drug decreased. ↔ = Undetermined clinical effect.

Adverse Reactions

The following adverse reactions are listed in decreasing order of severity, not frequency.

➤*Cardiovascular:* Arrhythmias (particularly when used concurrently with digitalis or quinidine); syncope; angina-like symptoms; bradycardia; edema.

➤*CNS:* Parkinsonian syndrome and other extrapyramidal tract symptoms (rare); dizziness; headache; paradoxical anxiety; depression; nervousness; nightmares; dull sensorium; drowsiness.

➤*GI:* Vomiting; diarrhea; nausea; anorexia; dryness of mouth; hypersecretion.

➤*GU:* Pseudolactation; impotence; dysuria; gynecomastia; decreased libido; breast engorgement.

➤*Respiratory:* Dyspnea; epistaxis; nasal congestion.

➤*Special senses:* Deafness; optic atrophy; glaucoma; uveitis; conjunctival injection.

➤*Miscellaneous:* Hypersensitivity reactions: Purpura, rash, pruritus; weight gain; muscular aches.

Antiadrenergic Agents — Peripherally Acting

RESERPINE

Overdosage

➤*Symptoms:* No deaths due to acute poisoning with reserpine have been reported. Highest known doses survived: Children, 1000 mg (age and sex not specified), young children, 200 mg (20-month-old boy). The clinical picture of acute poisoning is characterized chiefly by signs and symptoms due to the reflex parasympathomimetic effect of reserpine.

Impairment of consciousness may occur and may range from drowsiness to coma, depending on the severity of overdosage. Flushing of the skin, conjunctival injection and pupillary constriction are to be expected. Hypotension, hypothermia, central respiratory depression and bradycardia may develop in cases of severe overdosage. Increased salivary secretion, gastric secretion and diarrhea may also occur.

➤*Treatment:* There is no specific antidote. Evacuate stomach contents, taking adequate precautions against aspiration and for protection of the airway. Activated charcoal slurry should be instilled.

Treat the effects of reserpine overdosage symptomatically. If hypotension is severe enough to require treatment with a vasopressor, use one having a direct action upon vascular smooth muscle (eg, phenylephrine, norepinephrine, metaraminol). Since reserpine is long-acting, observe the patient carefully for at least 72 hours, and administer treatment as required.

Patient Information

Inform patients of possible side effects and advise them to take the medication regularly and continuously as directed.

GUANETHIDINE MONOSULFATE

Rx	Ismelin (Ciba)	Tablets: 10 mg	(Ciba 49). Yellow, scored. In 100s.
		25 mg	(Ciba 103). White, scored. In 100s.

For complete prescribing information, refer to the Antihypertensives Treatment Guidelines in the Appendix.

> ### WARNING
>
> Orthostatic hypotension can occur frequently; inform patients about this potential hazard. Fainting spells may occur unless the patient is forewarned to sit or lie down with the onset of dizziness or weakness. Postural hypotension is most marked in the morning and is accentuated by hot weather, alcohol or exercise. Dizziness or weakness may be particularly bothersome during the initial period of dosage adjustment and with postural changes, such as arising in the morning. The potential occurrence of these symptoms may require alteration of daily activity. Caution the patient to avoid sudden or prolonged standing or exercise while taking the drug.

Indications

➤*Moderate and severe hypertension:* Either alone or as an adjunct.

➤*Renal hypertension:* Including that secondary to pyelonephritis, renal amyloidosis and renal artery stenosis.

Administration and Dosage

➤*Ambulatory patients:* Begin with 10 mg daily. Increase dosage gradually and do not increase more often than every 5 to 7 days (eg, visit 1, 10 mg/day; visit 2, 20 mg/day; visit 3, 30 or 37.5 mg/day; visit 4, 50 mg/day; visit 5 and subsequent, may increase by 12.5 or 25 mg if necessary). Take blood pressure in the supine position, after standing for 10 minutes and immediately after exercise if feasible. Increase dosage only if there has been *no* decrease in standing blood pressure from the previous levels. The average dose is 25 to 50 mg once daily. Reduce dosage in any of the following: Normal supine pressure, excessive orthostatic fall in pressure, severe diarrhea.

➤*Hospitalized patients:*

Initial dose – 25 to 50 mg; increase by 25 or 50 mg/day or every other day as indicated. This higher dosage is possible because hospitalized patients can be watched carefully. Unless absolutely impossible, take the standing blood pressure regularly. Do not discharge patients from the hospital until the effect of the drug on the standing blood pressure is known.

Loading dose (for severe hypertension) – Guanethidine is given 3 times daily at 6 hour intervals over 1 to 3 days; the nighttime dose is omitted. Once blood pressure is normalized, determine the daily maintenance dosage. Take the standing blood pressure regularly. Do not discharge patients from the hospital until the effect of the drug on the standing blood pressure is known. Advise patients about orthostatic hypotension and warn them not to get out of bed without help during dosage adjustment.

➤*Children:*

Initial dose – 0.2 mg/kg/24 hr (6 mg/m^2/24 hr) as a single oral dose.

Increment – 0.2 mg/kg/24 hr every 7 to 10 days.

Maximum – 3 mg/kg/24 hr.

➤*Combination therapy:* Thiazide diuretics enhance the effectiveness of guanethidine and may reduce the incidence of edema. When thiazide diuretics are added to the regimen, it is usually necessary to reduce the guanethidine dosage. After control is established, reduce dosage of all drugs to the lowest effective level.

If ganglionic blockers have not been discontinued before guanethidine is started, gradually withdraw them to prevent a spiking blood pressure response during the transfer period.

Actions

➤*Pharmacology:* Guanethidine inhibits or interferes with the release or distribution of the chemical mediator (presumably norepinephrine) at the sympathetic neuroeffector junction. In contrast to ganglionic blocking agents, the drug suppresses equally the responses mediated by α and β-adrenergic receptors but does not produce parasympathetic blockade. Since sympathetic blockade results in modest decreases in peripheral resistance and cardiac output, guanethidine lowers blood pressure in the supine position. It further reduces blood pressure by decreasing the degree of vasoconstriction which normally results from reflex sympathetic nervous activity on assumption of the upright posture, thus reducing the venous return and cardiac output more. The inhibition of sympathetic venoconstrictive mechanisms results in venous pooling of blood. Therefore, the effect is especially pronounced when the patient is standing. Both the systolic and diastolic pressures are reduced.

➤*Pharmacokinetics:* Guanethidine is incompletely absorbed, about 3% to 50% on oral administration. It is actively transported into adrenergic neurons. Adrenergic blockade occurs with a minimum plasma concentration of 8 ng/mL with doses of 10 to 50 mg/day at steady state. Guanethidine is partially metabolized by the liver to three metabolites (less active than the parent); parent drug and metabolites are excreted primarily in the urine. The drug is eliminated slowly because of extensive tissue binding. Renal clearance is 56 mL/min. Because of its long half-life (4 to 8 days), the drug accumulates slowly. Up to 2 weeks may be required to adequately evaluate the response to daily administration.

Contraindications

Known or suspected pheochromocytoma; hypersensitivity to guanethidine; frank congestive heart failure (CHF) not due to hypertension; use of MAO inhibitors (see Drug Interactions).

Warnings

➤*Potency:* This is a potent drug; its use can lead to serious clinical problems.

➤*Orthostatic hypotension:* Orthostatic hypotension can occur frequently. Dizziness or weakness may be particularly bothersome during the initial dosage period and with postural changes. (See Warning Box.)

➤*Preoperative withdrawal:* Recommended 2 weeks prior to surgery to reduce the possibility of vascular collapse and cardiac arrest during anesthesia. During emergency surgery, administer preanesthetic and anesthetic agents cautiously in reduced dosages. Have oxygen, atropine, vasopressors and adequate solutions for volume replacement ready for immediate use to counteract vascular collapse. *Use vasopressors only with extreme caution,* since guanethidine augments responsiveness to exogenously administered norepinephrine and vasopressors with respect to blood pressure and their propensity for the production of cardiac arrhythmias.

➤*Fever:* Fever reduces dosage requirements.

➤*Bronchial asthma:* Patients with bronchial asthma require special consideration as they are more apt to be hypersensitive to catecholamine depletion and their condition may be aggravated.

➤*Renal function impairment:* Use very cautiously in hypertensive patients with renal disease and nitrogen retention or rising BUN levels, since decreased blood pressure may further compromise renal function.

➤*Fertility impairment:* Inhibition of ejaculation has occurred. This effect, which is attributable to the sympathetic blockade caused by the drug, is reversible several weeks after discontinuation of the drug. Erectile potency is usually retained.

➤*Pregnancy: Category C.* Safety for use during pregnancy has not been established. Use only when clearly needed and when the potential benefits outweigh the potential hazards to the fetus.

➤*Lactation:* Guanethidine is excreted in breast milk. Because of the potential for serious adverse reactions in nursing infants, discontinue nursing or discontinue the drug, taking into account the importance of the drug to the mother.

➤*Children:* Safety and efficacy for use in children have not been established.

GUANETHIDINE MONOSULFATE

Precautions

➤*Cumulative effects:* The effects of guanethidine are cumulative; initial doses should be small and increased gradually in small increments.

➤*Sodium retention:* To minimize sodium retention and compensatory fluid retention, guanethidine is usually used with a thiazide diuretic.

➤*Cardiovascular disease:* Use very cautiously in hypertensive patients with coronary disease with insufficiency or recent myocardial infarction, and in cerebral vascular disease, especially with encephalopathy.

Use with great caution in patients with severe cardiac failure, since guanethidine may interfere with the adrenergic compensation in producing circulatory adjustment in patients with CHF. Both digitalis and guanethidine slow the heart rate.

In patients with incipient cardiac decompensation, monitor weight gain or edema, which may be averted by a concomitant thiazide.

➤*Peptic ulcer:* Use cautiously in patients with a history of peptic ulcer or other disorders which may be aggravated by a relative increase in parasympathetic tone.

Drug Interactions

Guanethidine Drug Interactions			
Precipitant drug	Object drug*		Description
Anorexiants	Guanethidine	↓	The hypotensive effects of guanethidine may be reversed.
Haloperidol	Guanethidine	↓	Haloperidol antagonizes the hypotensive effect of guanethidine.
Methylphenidate	Guanethidine	↓	Hypotensive effects of guanethidine may be impaired. Arrhythmias were reported in one case.
Minoxidil	Guanethidine	↑	Administration of minoxidil to patients on guanethidine can result in profound orthostatic effects. Discontinue guanethidine well before minoxidil is begun, if possible. If not possible, hospitalize the patient when starting minoxidil.
MAO inhibitors	Guanethidine	↓	Discontinue MAOIs at least 1 week before starting guanethidine therapy; the combination may decrease the effects of guanethidine.
Phenothiazines	Guanethidine	↓	The hypotensive effect of guanethidine is inhibited.
Sympathomimetics	Guanethidine	↓	The hypotensive effect of guanethidine may be reversed. Also, guanethidine potentiates the effects of the direct-acting sympathomimetics.
Guanethidine	Sympathomimetics	↑	
Thioxanthenes	Guanethidine	↓	The hypotensive effect of guanethidine is antagonized.
Tricyclic antidepressants	Guanethidine	↓	The hypotensive action of guanethidine is inhibited.

* ↑ = Object drug increased. ↓ = Object drug decreased.

Adverse Reactions

➤*Cardiovascular:* Bradycardia; fluid retention; edema with occasional development of CHF; angina.

➤*CNS:* Dizziness; weakness; lassitude; syncope resulting from either postural or exertional hypotension; fatigue; muscle tremor; mental depression; chest paresthesias; ptosis of the lids; blurred vision.

➤*GI:* Nausea; vomiting; dry mouth; parotid tenderness; diarrhea (may be severe and necessitate discontinuance of the medication); increase in bowel movements.

➤*GU:* Inhibition of ejaculation (see Warnings); rise in BUN; nocturia; urinary incontinence; priapism, impotence (rare).

➤*Hematologic:* Anemia, thrombocytopenia, leukopenia (rare).

➤*Respiratory:* Dyspnea; nasal congestion; asthma in susceptible individuals.

➤*Miscellaneous:* Myalgia; weight gain; dermatitis; scalp hair loss.

Overdosage

➤*Symptoms:* Postural hypotension and bradycardia are most likely to occur; diarrhea, possibly severe, may also occur. Unconsciousness is unlikely if adequate blood pressure and cerebral perfusion can be maintained.

➤*Treatment:* There is no specific antidote. Consider gastric lavage, activated charcoal and laxatives if conditions permit. In previously normotensive patients, treatment has consisted essentially of keeping the patient supine. Homeostatic control usually returns over 72 hours.

In previously hypertensive patients, particularly those with impaired cardiac reserve or other cardiovascular-renal disease, intensive treatment may be required to support vital functions or to control cardiac irregularities. Maintain the supine position if vasopressors are required; guanethidine may increase responsiveness to blood pressure rise and occurrence of cardiac arrhythmias. Administer atropine for sinus bradycardia.

Treat severe or persistent diarrhea symptomatically.

Monitor cardiovascular and renal function for a few days.

Patient Information

Notify physician of severe diarrhea, frequent dizziness or fainting.

GUANADREL

Rx	Hylorel (Fisons)	Tablets: 10 mg	(Hylorel 10). Light orange, scored. In 100s.

For complete prescribing information, refer to the Antihypertensives Treatment Guidelines in the Appendix..

Indications

Treatment of hypertension in patients not responding adequately to a thiazide-type diuretic. Add to a diuretic regimen for optimum blood pressure control.

Administration and Dosage

Individualize dosage. The usual starting dosage is 10 mg/day, which can be given as 5 mg 2 times daily by breaking the 10 mg tablet. Most patients will require a daily dosage of 20 to 75 mg, usually in twice daily doses. For larger doses, 3 or 4 times daily dosing may be needed. Adjust the dosage weekly or monthly until blood pressure is controlled.

With long-term therapy, some tolerance may occur and the dosage may have to be increased. Because guanadrel has a substantial orthostatic effect, monitor both supine and standing pressures, especially while adjusting dosage.

➤*Renal function impairment:* Adjust dosage. For initial therapy, reduce dosage to 5 mg every 24 hours in patients with Ccr 30 to 60 mL/min. For patients with Ccr < 30 mL/min, increase the interval to 48 hours. Cautiously make dosage increases at intervals ≥ 7 days for moderate renal insufficiency and ≥ 14 days for severe insufficiency.

Actions

➤*Pharmacology:* Guanadrel, structurally and pharmacologically similar to guanethidine, inhibits sympathetic vasoconstriction by inhibiting norepinephrine release from neuronal storage sites in response to nerve stimulation. Depletion of norepinephrine causes a relaxation of vascular smooth muscle which decreases total peripheral resistance and venous return. A hypotensive effect results, greater in the standing than in the supine position by about 10 mmHg systolic and 3.5 mmHg diastolic. The drug does not inhibit parasympathetic nerve function nor does it enter the CNS.

Guanadrel begins to decrease blood pressure within 2 hours and produces maximal decreases in 4 to 6 hours. No significant change in cardiac output accompanies the blood pressure decline in normal individuals. Heart rate is also decreased by about 5 beats/minute. Fluid retention occurs, particularly when guanadrel is not accompanied by a diuretic.

Guanadrel causes increased sensitivity to circulating norepinephrine, probably by preventing uptake of norepinephrine by adrenergic neurons. Thus it is dangerous in the presence of excess norepinephrine (eg, pheochromocytoma).

➤*Pharmacokinetics:*

Absorption – It is rapidly absorbed after oral administration. Plasma concentrations generally peak 1.5 to 2 hours after ingestion. Protein binding is < 20%.

Metabolism/Excretion – Half-life is about 10 hours, but individual variability is great. Approximately 85% of the drug is eliminated in the urine. Urinary excretion is about 85% complete within 24 hours; about 40% of a dose is excreted unchanged.

➤*Clinical trials:* Patients with initial supine blood pressures averaging 160 to 170/105 to 110 mmHg have decreases in blood pressure of 20

GUANADREL

to 25/15 to 20 mmHg in the standing position. Guanethidine and guanadrel are similar in effectiveness while methyldopa has a larger effect on supine systolic pressure. Side effects of guanadrel and guanethidine are generally similar while methyldopa has more CNS effects (depression, drowsiness) but fewer orthostatic effects and less diarrhea.

Contraindications

Known or suspected pheochromocytoma; concurrently with, or within 1 week of MAOIs; hypersensitivity to guanadrel; frank CHF.

Warnings

➤*Orthostatic hypotension:* Orthostatic hypotension and its consequences (dizziness, weakness) are frequent. Rarely, fainting upon standing or exercise occurs. Careful instructions to the patient can minimize symptoms; supine blood pressure is not an adequate assessment of guanadrel's effects. Patients with known regional vascular disease (cerebral, coronary) are at particular risk from marked orthostatic hypotension. Avoid hypotensive episodes even if this requires a poorer degree of blood pressure control.

➤*Surgery:* To reduce the possibility of vascular collapse during anesthesia, discontinue guanadrel 48 to 72 hours before elective surgery. If emergency surgery is required, cautiously administer preanesthetic and anesthetic agents in reduced dosage. Use vasopressors cautiously, as guanadrel can enhance the pressor response and increase arrhythmogenicity.

➤*Asthma:* Special care is needed in patients with bronchial asthma, as it may be aggravated by catecholamine depletion and sympathomimetic amines may interfere with the hypotensive effect of guanadrel.

➤*Renal function impairment:* As renal function declines, apparent total body clearance and renal and apparent nonrenal clearances decrease, and the terminal elimination half-life is prolonged. Dosage adjustments may be necessary, especially in patients with Ccr < 60 mL/min (see Administration and Dosage).

➤*Fertility impairment:* In rats, suppressed libido and reduced fertility were noted at 100 mg/kg/day (12 times the maximum human dose).

➤*Pregnancy:* Category B. There are no adequate and well-controlled studies in pregnant women. Use only when clearly needed and when the potential benefits outweigh the potential hazards to the fetus.

➤*Lactation:* It is not known if guanadrel is excreted in breast milk. Because of the potential for serious adverse reactions in the nursing infant, decide whether to discontinue nursing or to discontinue the drug, taking into account the importance of the drug to the mother.

➤*Children:* Safety and efficacy for use in children have not been established.

Precautions

➤*Salt and water retention:* Retention of salt and water may occur. Patients with CHF have not been studied, but guanadrel could interfere with the adrenergic mechanisms.

➤*Peptic ulcer:* Use guanadrel cautiously in patients with a history of peptic ulcer, which could be aggravated by a relative increase in parasympathetic tone.

Drug Interactions

Guanadrel Drug Interactions			
Precipitant drug	Object drug*		Description
Beta blockers	Guanadrel	↑	The effects of guanadrel may be potentiated, causing excessive postural hypotension and bradycardia.
Phenothiazines	Guanadrel	↓	The effects of guanadrel may be reversed.
Sympathomimetics	Guanadrel	↓	The hypotensive effect of guanadrel may be reversed. Also, guanadrel may potentiate the effects of the direct-acting sympathomimetics.
Guanadrel	Sympathomimetics	↑	
Tricyclic antidepressants (TCAs)	Guanadrel	↓	TCAs may block the norepinephrine-depleting effect and the blood pressure-lowering effect of guanadrel. Use caution with concomitant use. If the TCA is discontinued abruptly, an enhanced effect of guanadrel may occur.
Vasodilators	Guanadrel	↑	Concomitant use may increase the potential for symptomatic orthostatic hypotension and generally is not recommended.

*↑ = Object drug increased. ↓ = Object drug decreased.

Adverse Reactions

The following table displays the frequency of side effects that are generally higher during the first 8 weeks of therapy. Approximately 3.6% of patients withdrew from guanadrel therapy because of untoward effects.

Adverse Reactions of Antiadrenergic Drugs (%)			
Adverse reaction	Guanadrel (n = 1544)	Methyldopa (n = 743)	Guanethidine (n = 330)
Cardiovascular			
Palpitations	30	35	25
Chest pain	28	37	27
CNS			
Fatigue	64	76	57
Headache	58	69	50
Faintness (orthostatic/other)	47-49	41-46	45-48
Drowsiness	45	64	29
Visual disturbances	29	35	26
Paresthesias	25	35	16
Confusion	15	23	11
Psychological problems	4	5	4
Depression	2	4	2
Sleep disorders	2	2	3
Syncope	< 1	< 1	2
GI			
Increased bowel movements	31	28	36
Gas pain/indigestion	24-32	31-40	19-29
Constipation	21	29	20
Anorexia	19	23	18
Glossitis	8	11	5
Nausea/vomiting	4	5	4
Dry mouth, dry throat	2	4	< 1
Abdominal distress or pain	2	2	2
GU			
Nocturia	48	52	42
Urination urgency or frequency	34	40	28
Peripheral edema	29	37	23
Ejaculation disturbances	18	21	22
Impotence	5	12	7
Hematuria	2	4	2
Respiratory			
Shortness of breath on exertion	46	53	49
Coughing	27	36	22
Shortness of breath at rest	18	22	17
Miscellaneous			
Excessive weight gain/loss	42-44	51-54	42
Aching limbs	43	52	34
Leg cramps - nighttime	26	33	21
Leg cramps - daytime	21	26	20
Backache or neckache	2	1	2
Joint pain or inflammation	2	2	2

Overdosage

➤*Symptoms:* Marked dizziness and blurred vision related to postural hypotension progressing to syncope on standing. The patient should lie down until these symptoms subside.

➤*Treatment:* If excessive hypotension occurs and persists despite conservative treatment, a vasoconstrictor such as phenylephrine may be needed. Monitor carefully for hypersensitivity.

Patient Information

The medication may cause orthostatic hypotension; sit or lie down immediately at the onset of dizziness or weakness to prevent loss of consciousness. Postural hypotension is worst in the morning and upon arising and may be exaggerated by alcohol, fever, hot weather, prolonged standing, or exercise.

Do not take any prescription or OTC medications, especially medications for treatment of colds, allergy, or asthma, without the advice of a physician or pharmacist.

ALPHA-$_1$-ADRENERGIC BLOCKERS

Indications

▶*Hypertension:* For the treatment of hypertension, alone or in combination with other antihypertensive agents (except **tamsulosin**).

▶*Benign prostatic hyperplasia (BPH):*
Terazosin – Treatment of symptomatic BPH.

Doxazosin – Treatment of urinary outflow obstruction and obstructive symptoms (hesitation, intermittency, dribbling, weak urinary stream, incomplete emptying of the bladder) and irritative symptoms (nocturia, daytime frequency, urgency, burning) associated with BPH.

Tamsulosin – Treatment of the signs and symptoms of BPH.

▶*Unlabeled uses:*
Prazosin – Treatment of BPH.

Terazosin – Symptomatic treatment of chronic abacterial prostatitis.

Actions

▶*Pharmacology:* **Doxazosin**, **prazosin**, and **terazosin** selectively block alpha-$_1$-adrenergic receptors. This blockade causes a reduction in systemic vascular resistance, thus causing an antihypertensive effect. The degree of smooth muscle tone in the prostate and bladder neck is mediated by the alpha-$_1$-adrenergic receptor, which is present in high density in the prostatic stroma, prostatic capsule, and bladder neck. Blockade of the alpha-$_1$-adrenergic receptor decreases urethral resistance and may relieve the obstruction and improve urine flow and BPH symptoms.

Tamsulosin selectively inhibits the alpha-$_{1A}$-adrenergic receptor. Approximately 70% of the alpha-$_1$-adrenergic receptors in human prostate are of the alpha-$_{1A}$ subtype. Tamsulosin is not intended for use as an antihypertensive drug.

Doxazosin causes maximum reductions in blood pressure 2 to 6 hours after dosing, which is associated with a small increase in standing heart rate. Doxazosin has a greater effect on blood pressure and heart rate in the standing position.

Prazosin lowers blood pressure in the supine and standing positions. This effect is most pronounced on the diastolic blood pressure. The antihypertensive action usually is not accompanied by a reflex tachycardia.

Terazosin decreases blood pressure gradually within 15 minutes following oral administration. Terazosin treatment in normotensive men with BPH did not result in a clinically significant blood pressure-lowering effect.

▶*Pharmacokinetics:* Enterohepatic recycling of **doxazosin** is suggested by secondary peaking of plasma concentrations. Plasma elimination of doxazosin is biphasic. After morning dosing of doxazosin, the AUC was 11% less than after evening dosing and the time to peak concentration after evening dosing occurred significantly later than after morning dosing (5.6 vs 3.5 hours).

Terazosin undergoes minimal hepatic first-pass metabolism and nearly all the circulating dose is in the form of the parent drug.

The mean steady-state apparent volume of distribution of **tamsulosin** after IV administration was 16 L, which is suggestive of distribution into extracellular fluids in the body. Tamsulosin is widely distributed to most tissues. The cytochrome P450 enzymes that primarily catalyze the Phase I metabolism of tamsulosin have not been conclusively identified. The metabolites of tamsulosin undergo extensive conjugation to glucuronide or sulfate prior to renal excretion.

Pharmacokinetics of Alpha-$_1$-Adrenergic Blockers				
Parameter	Prazosin	Terazosin	Doxazosin	Tamsulosin
Oral bioavailability	nd	nd	≈ 65%	> 90% (fasting state)
T$_{max}$	≈ 3 h	≈ 1 h	≈ 2 to 3 h	4 to 5 h (fasting state) 6 to 7 h (fed state)
Protein binding	High	90% to 94%	≈ 98%	94% to 99%[1]
Metabolism	Extensively metabolized, primarily by demethylation and conjugation	nd	First-pass metabolism; extensively metabolized by the liver, mainly by O-demethylation or hydroxylation	CYP450
Half-life, elimination	2 to 3 h	≈ 12 h	≈ 22 h	9 to 15 h

Pharmacokinetics of Alpha-$_1$-Adrenergic Blockers				
Parameter	Prazosin	Terazosin	Doxazosin	Tamsulosin
Excretion	Bile and feces	Urine (≈ 40%)[2] Feces (≈ 60%)[3]	Urine (≈ 9%) Feces (≈ 63%)[4]	Urine (76%) Feces (21%)

nd = no data.
[1] Primarily bound to alpha-$_1$ acid glycoprotein.
[2] Approximately 10% of an oral dose is excreted as parent drug in the urine.
[3] Approximately 20% of an oral dose is excreted as parent drug in the feces.
[4] 4.8% of the dose is excreted as unchanged drug in the feces and a trace amount is excreted in the urine as unchanged drug.

Special populations –
Elderly: In patients 70 years of age and older taking **terazosin**, plasma clearance decreased by 31.7%, compared with younger patients. For **tamsulosin**, a 40% higher AUC in those 55 to 75 years of age was seen compared with younger subjects.

Hepatic function impairment: Administration of a single 2 mg dose of doxazosin to patients with cirrhosis (Child-Pugh Class A) showed a 40% increase in exposure to **doxazosin**.

Contraindications

Hypersensitivity to quinazolines (eg, **doxazosin**, **prazosin**, **tamsulosin**, **terazosin**) or to any components of the products.

Warnings

▶*"First-dose" effect and orthostatic hypotension:* **Prazosin**, **terazosin**, **doxazosin**, and **tamsulosin**, like other α-adrenergic blocking agents, can cause marked hypotension (especially postural hypotension) and syncope with sudden loss of consciousness with the first few doses. Anticipate a similar effect if therapy is interrupted for more than a few doses, if dosage is increased rapidly, or if another antihypertensive drug is introduced. Syncope is due to an excessive postural hypotensive effect, although the syncopal episode has occasionally been preceded by severe supraventricular tachycardia with heart rates of 120 to 160 beats per minute.

The "first-dose" phenomenon may be minimized by limiting the initial dose to 1 mg of **terazosin** or **prazosin** (given at bedtime) or **doxazosin**. Slowly increase dosage of these drugs. Add additional antihypertensives with caution. Caution patients to avoid situations where injury could result should syncope occur during initiation of therapy. Hypotension may develop in patients also receiving a β-adrenergic blocker.

If syncope occurs, place patient in recumbent position and treat supportively. More common than loss of consciousness are dizziness and lightheadedness.

Syncopal episodes have usually occurred within 30 to 90 minutes of the initial dose of **prazosin**; the incidence is approximately 1% with an initial dose of 2 mg or greater. Syncope occurred in about 1% of **terazosin** patients and was not necessarily associated with early doses. There is evidence that the orthostatic effect of terazosin is greater, even in chronic use, shortly after dosing. Syncope occurred in 0.7% of **doxazosin** patients with dose titration every 1 to 2 weeks; none of these events were reported at the starting dose of 1 mg and 1.2% occurred at 16 mg/day. Other symptoms of lowered blood pressure (eg, dizziness, lightheadedness palpitations) are more common, occurring in approximately 28% of terazosin patients and up to 23% of doxazosin patients (approximately 2% of doxazosin patients discontinued therapy).

▶*Priapism:* Rarely (probably less frequently than once in every several thousand patients), alpha-$_1$ antagonists have been associated with priapism (painful penile erection, sustained for hours and unrelieved by sexual intercourse or masturbation). Because this condition can lead to permanent impotence if not promptly treated, patients must be advised about the seriousness of the condition.

▶*Hepatic function impairment:* Administer **doxazosin** with caution to patients with evidence of impaired hepatic function or to patients receiving drugs known to influence hepatic metabolism.

▶*Fertility impairment:* Reduced fertility occurred in male rats treated with **doxazosin** 20 mg/kg/day. The effect was reversible within 2 weeks of drug withdrawal. Nine of 39 male rats failed to sire a litter after **terazosin** 30 to 120 mg/kg/day. Testicular atrophy also has occurred in rats and dogs receiving terazosin or **prazosin**. Studies in rats revealed significantly reduced fertility in males dosed with single or multiple daily doses of 300 mg/kg/day of **tamsulosin** (AUC exposure in rats about 50 times the human exposure with the maximum therapeutic dose). The effects on fertility were reversible, showing improvement by 3 days after a single dose and 4 weeks after multiple dosing. Effects on fertility in males were completely reversed within 9 weeks of discontinuation of multiple dosing. Multiple doses of 10 and 100 mg/kg/day tamsulosin (⅕ and 16 times the anticipated human AUC exposure) did not significantly alter fertility in male rats. Studies in female rats revealed significant reductions in fertility after single or multiple dosing with 300 mg/kg/day of the R-isomer or racemic mixture of tamsulosin, respectively.

Antiadrenergic Agents — Peripherally Acting

ALPHA-₁-ADRENERGIC BLOCKERS

➤*Pregnancy:* Category C (**prazosin**, **terazosin**, **doxazosin**). *Category B* (**tamsulosin**). A doxazosin dosage of 82 mg/kg/day in rabbits was associated with reduced fetal survival. In rats, maternal doxazosin doses 8 times the human AUC exposure (12 mg/day) delayed postnatal development. Terazosin doses 280 times the maximum recommended human dose in rats resulted in fetal resorptions; increased fetal resorptions, decreased fetal weight, and increased number of supernumerary ribs occurred with doses 60 times the maximum recommended human dose. Significantly more rat pups died in the group dosed with terazosin (more than 75 times the maximum recommended human dose) vs controls.

There are no adequate and well-controlled studies in pregnant women. Safety for use during pregnancy has not been established. Use only when clearly needed and when the potential benefits outweigh the potential hazards to the fetus. **Tamsulosin** is not indicated for use in women.

➤*Lactation:* **Doxazosin** accumulates in breast milk of lactating rats following a single 1 mg/kg dose with a maximum concentration about 20 times greater than the maternal plasma concentration. It is not known whether **terazosin** or **tamsulosin** are excreted in breast milk. Tamsulosin is not indicated for use in women. **Prazosin** is excreted in small amounts in breast milk. Exercise caution when administering these drugs to a nursing woman.

➤*Children:* Safety and efficacy for use in children have not been established.

Precautions

➤*Hemodilution:* Small but statistically significant decreases in hematocrit, hemoglobin, white blood cells, total protein, and albumin were observed in controlled clinical trials with **terazosin**. These laboratory findings suggest the possibility of hemodilution.

➤*Leukopenia/Neutropenia:* In hypertensive patients receiving **doxazosin**, mean WBC and neutrophil counts were decreased by 2.4% and 1%, respectively, compared with placebo, a phenomenon seen with other alpha blocking drugs. In BPH patients, the incidence of clinically significant WBC abnormalities was 0.4%. No patients became symptomatic as a result of the low counts. WBCs and neutrophil counts returned to normal after drug discontinuation.

➤*Weight gain:* There was a tendency for patients to gain weight during **terazosin** therapy. In placebo-controlled monotherapy trials, male and female patients receiving terazosin gained a mean of 0.8 and 1 kg, respectively, compared with losses of 0.1 and 0.5 kg, respectively, in the placebo group. Patients receiving **doxazosin** gained a mean of 0.6 kg compared with a mean loss of 0.1 kg for placebo patients.

➤*Cholesterol:* During controlled clinical studies, patients receiving **terazosin** monotherapy had a small but statistically significant decrease (3%) in total cholesterol and the combined LDL and VLDL fractions. No significant changes were observed in HDL fraction and triglycerides. In clinical trials involving normocholesterolemic patients, **doxazosin** reduced total serum cholesterol by 2% to 3% and LDL by 4%, and increased HDL to total cholesterol ratio by 4%. The clinical significance is unknown.

➤*Cardiotoxicity:* An increased incidence of myocardial necrosis or fibrosis occurred in rats and mice following 6 to 18 months of **doxazosin** 40 to 80 mg/kg/day. There is no evidence that similar lesions occur in humans.

➤*Prostatic cancer:* Carcinoma of the prostate and BPH cause many of the same symptoms and frequently co-exist. Therefore, examine patients thought to have BPH prior to starting **terazosin** therapy to rule out prostate carcinoma.

Drug Interactions

Alpha-₁- Antiadrenergic Blocker Drug Interactions			
Precipitant drug	Object drug*		Description
Alcohol	Alpha-₁-adrenergic blockers	↑	Coadministration may cause increased risk of hypotension. Advise patients to avoid alcohol.
Beta blockers	Alpha-₁-adrenergic blockers Prazosin	↑	Beta blockers may enhance the acute postural hypotensive reaction following the first dose of prazosin; terazosin and doxazosin have been combined with beta blockers with no adverse reaction.
Cimetidine	Alpha-₁-adrenergic blockers Tamsulosin	↑	Cimetidine decreased the clearance of tamsulosin 26% and increased the AUC 44%. Use with caution.
Indomethacin	Alpha-₁-adrenergic blockers Prazosin	↓	The antihypertensive action of prazosin may be decreased. No interaction occurred in patients receiving doxazosin, terazosin, and NSAIDs.
Verapamil	Alpha-₁-adrenergic blockers Prazosin Terazosin	↑	Verapamil appears to increase serum prazosin levels and may increase the sensitivity to prazosin-induced postural hypotension. Verapamil increased terazosin AUC 24%, C_{max} 25%, and C_{min} 32% and decreased T_{max} 0.5 h.
Alpha₁-adrenergic blockers Prazosin	Clonidine	↓	The antihypertensive effect of clonidine may be decreased.

* ↑ = Object drug increased. ↓ = Object drug decreased.

➤*Drug/Lab test interactions:* In a study of 5 patients given **prazosin** 12 to 24 mg/day for 10 to 14 days, there was an average increase of 42% in the urinary metabolite of norepinephrine and an average increase in urinary vanillylmandelic acid (VMA) of 17%. Therefore, false-positive results may occur in screening tests for pheochromocytoma in patients who are being treated with **prazosin**. If an elevated VMA is found, discontinue prazosin and retest the patient after 1 month.

Doxazosin and **terazosin** do not affect plasma concentrations of prostate specific antigen (PSA) in patients treated for up to 3 years (doxazosin), 2 years (terazosin), or 1 year (**tamsulosin**).

➤*Drug/Food interactions:* Administration of **terazosin** capsules immediately after meals delayed T_{max} by about 40 minutes. For **tamsulosin**, the T_{max} is reached by 4 to 5 hours under fasting conditions and by 6 to 7 hours after administration with food. Taking tamsulosin under fasted conditions results in a 30% increase in AUC and 40% to 70% increase in C_{max} compared with fed conditions.

Adverse Reactions

	Alpha-₁-Adrenergic Blocker Adverse Reactions (%)[1]						
	Hypertension			BPH			
Adverse Reaction	Prazosin	Terazosin	Doxazosin	Terazosin	Doxazosin	Tamsulosin 0.4 mg	Tamsulosin 0.8 mg
Cardiovascular							
Palpitations	5.3	4.3	2	0.9	1.2	-	-
Postural hypotension/ hypotension	1 to 4	1.3	0.3 to 1	0.6 to 3.9	0.3 to 1.7	0.2	0.4
Tachycardia	< 1	1.9	0.3	-	0.9	-	-
Arrhythmia	-	≥ 1	1	-	-	-	-
Chest pain	-	≥ 1	2	-	1.2	4	4.1
Vasodilation	-	≥ 1	-	-	-	-	-
Syncope	1 to 4	-	0.5 to 1	0.6	0.5	0.2	0.4
Peripheral ischemia	-	-	0.3	-	-	-	-
Angina pectoris	-	-	< 0.5	-	0.6	-	-
CNS							
Depression	1 to 4	0.3	1	-	-	-	-
Dizziness	10.3	19.3	19	9.1	15.6[2]	14.9	17.1
Decreased libido/ sexual dysfunction	-	0.6	2	-	0.8	1	2
Nervousness	1 to 4	2.3	2	-	-	-	-
Paresthesia	< 1	2.9	1	-	-	-	-
Somnolence	-	5.4	5	3.6	3	3	4.3
Anxiety	-	≥ 1	-	-	1.1	-	-
Insomnia	-	≥ 1	1	-	1.2	2.4	1.4
Asthenia	≈ 7	11.3[3]	1 to 12	7.4[3]	-	7.8	8.5

ALPHA-$_1$-ADRENERGIC BLOCKERS

Alpha-$_1$-Adrenergic Blocker Adverse Reactions (%)[1]						
	Hypertension			BPH		
Adverse Reaction	Prazosin	Terazosin	Doxazosin	Terazosin	Doxazosin	Tamsulosin 0.4 mg	Tamsulosin 0.8 mg
Fatigue	-	-	-	-	8	-	-
Drowsiness	7.6	-	-	-		-	-
Ataxia	-	-	1	-		-	-
Hypertonia	-	-	1	-		-	-
Hallucinations	< 1	-	-	-		-	-
Kinetic disorders	-	-	1	-		-	-
Dermatologic							
Pruritus	< 1	≥ 1	1	-	-	-	-
Rash	1 to 4	≥ 1	1	-	-	-	-
Sweating	-	≥ 1	0.5 to 1	-	1.1	-	-
Alopecia/Lichen planus	< 1	-	< 0.5	-	-	-	-
GI							
Nausea	4.9	4.4	3	1.7	1.5	2.6	3.9
Vomiting	1 to 4	≥ 1	≤ 2	-	1.4	-	-
Dry mouth	1 to 4	≥ 1	-	-	-	-	-
Diarrhea	1 to 4	≥ 1	2	-	2.3	6.2	4.3
Constipation	1 to 4	≥ 1	1	-	-	-	-
Abdominal discomfort/pain	< 1	≥ 1	0	-	2.4	-	-
Flatulence	-	≥ 1	1	-	-	-	-
Liver function abnormalities	< 1	-	-	-	-	-	-
Pancreatitis	< 1	-	-	-	-	-	-
Tooth disorder	-	-	-	-	-	1.2	2
Dyspepsia	-	≥ 1	1	-	1.7	-	-
GU							
Impotence	< 1	1.2	-	1.6	1.1	-	-
Urinary frequency	1 to 4	≥ 1	0	-	-	-	-
Urinary tract infection	-	≥ 1	-	1.3	1.4	-	-
Incontinence	< 1	≥ 1[4]	1	-	-	-	-
Polyuria	-	-	2	-	-	-	-
Priapism	< 1	-	-	-	-	-	-
Abnormal ejaculation	-	-	-	-	-	8.4	18.1
Dysuria	-	-	-	-	0.5	-	-
Musculoskeletal							
Shoulder/Neck/Back/ Extremity pain	-	1 to 3.5	-	-	-	7	8.3
Arthritis, joint disorder/muscle pain, gout, cramps	-	≥ 1	1	-	-	-	-
Arthralgia	< 1	≥ 1	1	-	-	-	-
Myalgia	-	≥ 1	1	-	-	-	-
Muscle weakness	-	-	1	-	-	-	-
Respiratory							
Dyspnea	1 to 4	3.1	1	1.7	2.6	-	-
Nasal congestion	1 to 4	5.9	-	1.9	-	-	-
Sinusitis	-	2.6	< 0.5	-	-	2.2	3.7
Bronchitis/Cold symptoms/bronchospasm	-	≥ 1	< 0.5	-	-	-	-
Epistaxis	1 to 4	≥ 1	1	-	-	-	-
Flu symptoms	-	≥ 1	< 0.5	2.4	1.1	-	-
Increased cough	-	≥ 1	< 0.5	-	-	3.4	4.5
Pharyngitis/Rhinitis	-	≥ 1	< 0.5/3	1.9	< 0.5	5.8/13.1	5.1/17.9
Special senses							
Blurred vision/ amblyopia	1 to 4	1.6	-	1.3	-	-	-
Abnormal vision	-	≥ 1	2	0.6	1.4	-	-
Conjunctivitis, reddened sclera/eye pain	1 to 4	≥ 1	1	-	-	-	-
Tinnitus	< 1	≥ 1	1	-	-	-	-
Vertigo	1 to 4	-	2	1.4	-	0.6	1
Amblyopia	-	-	-	1.3	-	0.2	2
Miscellaneous							
Headache	7.8	16.2	14	4.9	9.9	19.3	21.1
Edema	1 to 4	0.9	4	-	2.7	-	-
Peripheral edema	-	5.5	-	0.9	-	-	-
Weight gain	-	0.5	0.5 to 1	0.5	-	-	-
Facial edema	-	≥ 1	1	-	-	-	-
Fever	< 1	≥ 1	< 0.5	-	-	-	-
Flushing	-	-	1	-	-	-	-
Diaphoresis	< 1	-	-	-	-	-	-
Positive ANA titer	< 1	-	-	-	-	-	-
Infection	-	-	< 0.5	-	-	9	10.8
Pain	-	-	2	-	2	-	-

Antiadrenergic Agents — Peripherally Acting

ALPHA-₁-ADRENERGIC BLOCKERS

	Alpha-₁-Adrenergic Blocker Adverse Reactions (%)[1]						
	Hypertension			BPH			
Adverse Reaction	Prazosin	Terazosin	Doxazosin	Terazosin	Doxazosin	Tamsulosin 0.4 mg	Tamsulosin 0.8 mg
Lack of energy	6.9	-	-	-	-	-	-
Weakness	6.5	-	-	-	-	-	-
Fatigue/Malaise	-	-	12	-	-	-	-
Gout	-	≥ 1	-	-	-	-	-

[1] Data are pooled from separate studies and are not necessarily comparable.
[2] Includes vertigo.

[3] Includes weakness, tiredness, lassitude, and fatigue.
[4] Primarily reported in postmenopausal women.

➤*Doxazosin (hypertension):*
Cardiovascular – MI, cerebrovascular accident (fewer than 0.5%).
CNS – Hypesthesia, agitation (0.5% to 1%); paresis, tremor, twitching, confusion, migraine, impaired concentration, paroniria, amnesia, emotional lability, abnormal thinking, depersonalization (fewer than 0.5%).
Dermatologic – Dry skin, eczema (fewer than 0.5%).
GI – Increased appetite, anorexia, fecal incontinence, gastroenteritis (fewer than 0.5%).
GU – Breast pain, renal calculus (fewer than 0.5%).
Hematologic – Lymphadenopathy, purpura (fewer than 0.5%).
Metabolic / Nutritional – Thirst, gout, hypokalemia (fewer than 0.5%).
Special senses – Parosmia, earache, taste perversion, photophobia, abnormal lacrimation (fewer than 0.5%).
Miscellaneous – Pallor, hot flushes, fever/rigors, decreased weight (fewer than 0.5%).

➤*Postmarketing:*
Cardiovascular –
Prazosin: Angina pectoris, hypotension, bradycardia.
CNS –
Prazosin: Flushing, insomnia.
GU –
Doxazosin: Priapism, gynecomastia, hematuria, micturition disorder, micturition frequency, nocturia.
Hematologic –
Doxazosin: Leukopenia, thrombocytopenia.
Hepatic –
Doxazosin: Hepatitis, hepatitis cholestatic.
Miscellaneous –
Doxazosin: Allergic reaction, urticaria, bronchospasm aggravated, vomiting, hypesthesia, bradycardia.
Prazosin: Allergic reaction, asthenia, malaise, pain, gynecomastia, urticaria, vascuiltis, eye pain.
Tamsulosin: Allergic-type reactions (eg, skin rash, pruritus, angioedema of the tongue, lips, and face, urticaria) have been reported with positive rechallenge in some cases; priapism (rare); palpitations, constipation, vomiting (infrequent).

Terazosin: Allergic reactions, including anaphylaxis; priapism; thrombocytopenia; atrial fibrillation.

Overdosage

➤*Symptoms:* Accidental ingestion of at least 50 mg **prazosin** in a 2-year-old child produced profound drowsiness and depressed reflexes. No decrease in blood pressure was noted. Recovery was uneventful.

Several cases of **doxazosin** overdose have been reported (doses ranging from 1 to 40 mg in children and 60 to 70 mg in adults). All children made full recoveries. One adult developed hypotension that responded to fluid therapy. The other adult (with chronic renal failure, epilepsy, and depression) died; death was attributed to a grand mal seizure resulting from hypotension. The most likely manifestation of overdosage would be hypotension.

One patient reported an overdose of thirty 0.4 mg **tamsulosin** capsules. Following the ingestion of the capsules, the patient reported a severe headache.

➤*Treatment:* Restore blood pressure and normalize heart rate by keeping the patient supine. Treat shock with volume expanders. If necessary, use vasopressors and monitor and support renal function. These drugs are highly protein bound; dialysis may not be of benefit. Refer to General Management of Acute Overdosage.

Patient Information

Inform patients of the possibility of syncopal and orthostatic symptoms, especially at the initiation of therapy. Avoid driving or hazardous tasks for 12 to 24 hours after the first dose, after a dosage increase, and after interruption of therapy when treatment is resumed. Use caution when rising from a sitting or lying position. If dizziness or palpitations are bothersome, contact the physician for possible dose adjustment. These effects also may occur if patients drink alcohol, stand for long periods of time, or exercise, or if the weather is hot.

Drowsiness or somnolence may occur. Use caution when driving or operating heavy machinery.

Advise patients about the possibility of priapism as a result of treatment with alpha-₁ antagonists. Let patients know that this adverse event is very rare. If they experience priapism, advise them to bring it to immediate medical attention because, if not treated promptly, it can lead to permanent erectile dysfunction (impotence).

Advise patients not to crush, chew, or open **tamsulosin** capsules.

PRAZOSIN HCl

Rx	**Prazosin HCl** (Various, eg, Ivax)	**Capsules:** 1 mg (as base)	In 100s, 250s, 500s, and 1000s.
Rx	**Minipress** (Pfizer)		(431). White. In 250s.
Rx	**Prazosin HCl** (Various, eg, Ivax)	**Capsules:** 2 mg (as base)	In 100s, 250s, 500s, and 1000s.
Rx	**Minipress** (Pfizer)		(437). Pink/white. In 250s.
Rx	**Prazosin HCl** (Various, eg, Ivax)	**Capsules:** 5 mg (as base)	In 100s, 250s, and 500s.
Rx	**Minipress** (Pfizer)		(438). Blue/white. In 250s.

For complete prescribing information, refer to the Antihypertensives Treatment Guidelines in the Appendix and the Alpha-₁-Adrenergic Blockers group monograph.

Indications

➤*Hypertension:* Alone or in combination with other antihypertensive agents such as diuretics or beta blockers.

Administration and Dosage

Individualize dosage.

➤*Initial dose:* 1 mg 2 or 3 times daily.

➤*Maintenance dose:* Dosages may be increased slowly to 20 mg/day in divided doses; 6 to 15 mg/day in divided doses is used most commonly. Doses above 20 mg usually do not increase efficacy; however, a few patients may benefit from up to 40 mg/day. After initial adjustment, some patients can be maintained on a twice-daily regimen.

➤*Concomitant therapy:* When adding a diuretic or other antihypertensive, reduce dosage to 1 or 2 mg 3 times/day, then retitrate.

➤*Storage / Stability:* Store at controlled room temperature 15° to 30°C (59° to 86°F).

Antiadrenergic Agents — Peripherally Acting

TERAZOSIN HCl

Rx	Terazosin HCl (Geneva)	**Tablets:** 1 mg (as base)	In 100s and 1000s.
		2 mg (as base)	In 100s and 1000s.
		5 mg (as base)	In 100s and 1000s.
		10 mg (as base)	In 100s and 1000s.
Rx	Terazosin HCl (Various, eg, Apotex, Geneva, Teva)	**Capsules:** 1 mg (as base)	May contain lactose. In 100s and 500s.
Rx	Hytrin (Abbott)		Parabens. (HH). Grey. In 100s and UD 100s.
Rx	Terazosin HCl (Various, eg, Apotex, Geneva, Teva)	2 mg (as base)	May contain lactose. In 100s and 500s.
Rx	Hytrin (Abbott)		Parabens. (HY). Yellow. In 100s and UD 100s.
Rx	Terazosin HCl (Various, eg, Apotex, Geneva, Teva)	5 mg (as base)	May contain lactose. In 100s and 500s.
Rx	Hytrin (Abbott)		Parabens. (HK). Red. In 100s and UD 100s.
Rx	Terazosin HCl (Various, eg, Apotex, Geneva, Teva)	10 mg (as base)	May contain lactose. In 100s and 500s.
Rx	Hytrin (Abbott)		Parabens. (HN). Blue. In 100s. and UD 100s

For complete prescribing information, refer to the Antihypertensives Treatment Guidelines in the Appendix and the Alpha-$_1$-Adrenergic Blockers group monograph.

Indications

➤*Hypertension:* Alone or in combination with other antihypertensives such as diuretics or beta blockers.

➤*Benign prostatic hyperplasia (BPH):* Treatment of symptomatic BPH.

Administration and Dosage

➤*Approved by the FDA:* August 7, 1987.

Closely monitor patients to minimize the risk of severe hypotensive response. If terazosin is discontinued for several days or longer, reinstitute therapy using the initial dosing regimen.

➤*Hypertension:* Adjust dose and the dose interval (12 or 24 hours) individually. The following is a guide.

Initial dose – 1 mg at bedtime for all patients. Do not exceed this dose. Strictly observe initial dosing regimen to minimize severe hypotensive effects.

Subsequent doses – Slowly increase the dose to achieve the desired blood pressure response. The recommended dose range is 1 to 5 mg once daily; however, some patients may benefit from doses as high as 20 mg/day. Doses above 20 mg do not appear to provide further blood pressure effect, and doses above 40 mg have not been studied. Monitor blood pres-sure at the end of the dosing interval to be sure control is maintained. Measure blood pressure 2 to 3 hours after dosing to see if the maximum and minimum responses are similar, and to evaluate symptoms such as dizziness or palpitations. If response is substantially diminished at 24 hours, consider an increased dose or a twice-daily regimen.

➤*Benign prostatic hyperplasia:*

Initial dose – 1 mg at bedtime is the starting dose for all patients; do not exceed as an initial dose.

Subsequent doses – Increase the dose in a stepwise fashion to 2, 5 or 10 mg once daily to achieve desired improvement of symptoms or flow rates. Doses of 10 mg once daily are generally required for the clinical response; therefore, treatment with 10 mg for a minimum of 4 to 6 weeks may be required to assess whether a beneficial response has been achieved. Some patients may not achieve a clinical response. Although some patients have responded to 20 mg daily, there was an insufficient number of patients to draw definitive conclusions about this dose. There is insufficient data to support the use of doses above 20 mg in patients who do not respond.

➤*Concomitant therapy:* Observe caution when terazosin is administered concomitantly with other antihypertensive agents (especially verapamil) to avoid the possibility of significant hypotension. When adding an antihypertensive agent, dosage reduction and retitration may be necessary.

➤*Storage/Stability:* Store at controlled room temperature 20° to 25°C (68° to 77°F). Protect from light and moisture.

DOXAZOSIN MESYLATE

Rx	Doxazosin Mesylate (Various, eg, Apotex, Ethex, Ivax, Mylan, Teva)	**Tablets:** 1 mg (as base)	May contain lactose. In 100s, 500s, 1000s, and UD 100s.
Rx	Cardura (Pfizer)		Lactose. (Cardura 1 mg). White. In 100s and UD 100s.
Rx	Doxazosin Mesylate (Various, eg, Apotex, Ethex, Ivax, Mylan, Teva)	**Tablets:** 2 mg (as base)	May contain lactose. In 100s, 500s, 1000s, and UD 100s.
Rx	Cardura (Pfizer)		Lactose. (Cardura 2 mg). Yellow. In 100s and UD 100s.
Rx	Doxazosin Mesylate (Various, eg, Apotex, Ethex, Ivax, Mylan, Teva)	**Tablets:** 4 mg (as base)	May contain lactose. In 100s, 500s, 1000s, and UD 100s.
Rx	Cardura (Pfizer)		Lactose. (Cardura 4 mg). Orange. In 100s and UD 100s.
Rx	Doxazosin Mesylate (Various, eg, Apotex, Ethex, Ivax, Mylan, Teva)	**Tablets:** 8 mg (as base)	May contain lactose. In 100s, 500s, 1000s, and UD 100s.
Rx	Cardura (Pfizer)		Lactose. (Cardura 8 mg). Green. In 100s and UD 100s.

For complete prescribing information, refer to the Antihypertensives Treatment Guidelines in the Appendix and the Alpha-$_1$-Adrenergic Blockers group monograph.

Indications

➤*Hypertension:* Alone or in combination with other antihypertensive agents such as diuretics, beta blockers, calcium channel blockers, or ACE inhibitors for the treatment of hypertension.

➤*Benign prostatic hyperplasia (BPH):* For treatment of both urinary outflow obstruction and obstructive and irritative symptoms associated with BPH. Doxazosin may be used in all BPH patients whether hypertensive or normotensive.

Administration and Dosage

➤*Approved by the FDA:* November 2, 1990.

Individualize dosage. Initial dosage for hypertension or BPH is 1 mg once daily in the morning or evening. This starting dose is intended to minimize the frequency of postural hypotension and first dose syncope associated with doxazosin. Postural effects are most likely to occur between 2 and 6 hours after a dose. Therefore, take blood pressure measurements during this time period after the first dose and with each increase in dose. If doxazosin is discontinued for several days, restart therapy using the initial dosing regimen.

➤*Hypertension:* 1 to 16 mg once daily.

Initial dosage – 1 mg once daily.

Maintenance dose – Depending on standing blood pressure response (measured 2 to 6 hours postdose and 24 hours postdose), dosage may be increased to 2 mg and thereafter, if necessary, to 4, 8, and 16 mg to achieve the desired reduction in blood pressure. Increases in dose beyond 4 mg increase the likelihood of excessive postural effects (eg, syncope, postural dizziness/vertigo, postural hypotension). At a titrated dose of 16 mg once daily, the frequency of postural effects is approximately 12% compared with 3% for placebo.

➤*BPH:* 1 to 8 mg once daily.

Initial dosage – 1 mg once daily.

Maintenance dose – Depending on the urodynamics and BPH symptomatology, dosage may then be increased to 2 mg and thereafter to 4 and 8 mg once daily, the maximum recommended dose for BPH. The recommended titration interval is 1 to 2 weeks. Evaluate blood pressure routinely.

➤*Storage/Stability:* Store below 30°C (86°F).

TAMSULOSIN HCl

Rx	**Flomax** (Boehringer Ingelheim)	**Capsules:** 0.4 mg	(Flomax 0.4 mg BI 58). Olive green/orange. In 100s and 1000s.

For complete prescribing information, refer to the Antihypertensives Treatment Guidelines in the Appendix and to the Alpha-$_1$-Adrenergic Blockers group monograph.

Indications

➤*Benign prostatic hyperplasia (BPH):* For the treatment of the signs and symptoms of BPH.

Administration and Dosage

➤*Approved by the FDA:* April 15, 1997.

The recommended dose is 0.4 mg once daily, administered approximately 30 minutes following the same meal each day. Do not crush, chew, or open the capsules.

For those patients who fail to respond to the 0.4 mg dose after 2 to 4 weeks of dosing, the dose can be increased to 0.8 mg once daily. If administration is discontinued or interrupted for several days at either the 0.4 or 0.8 mg dose, start therapy again with the 0.4 mg once daily dose.

➤*Storage/Stability:* Store at 25°C (77°F); excursions permitted to 15° to 30°C (59° to 86°F).

ALFUZOSIN HCl

Rx	**Uroxatral** (Sanofi-Syntholabo)	**Tablets, extended-release:** 10 mg	Mannitol. (X10). White, yellow. In 30s. 100s, and UD 100s.

For complete prescribing information, refer to the Antihypertensives Treatment Guidelines in the Appendix and the Alpha-$_1$-Adrenergic Blockers group monograph.

Indications

➤*Benign prostatic hyperplasia (BPH):* Treatment of the signs and symptoms of BPH.

Administration and Dosage

➤*Approved by the FDA:* June 12, 2003.

The recommended dosage is one 10 mg alfuzosin HCl extended-release tablet daily to be taken immediately after the same meal each day. Do not chew or crush tablets.

➤*Storage/Stability:* Store at 25°C (77°F); excursions permitted to 15° to 30°C (59° to 86°F).

MECAMYLAMINE HCl

Rx	**Inversine** (Targacept[1])	**Tablets:** 2.5 mg	Lactose. (LBS01). Yellow. In 100s.

[1] Targacept, Inc., 200 East First St., Suite 300, Winston-Salem, NC 27101-4165; (336) 480-2100, fax (336) 480-2107.

Refer to the general discussion of these products in the Antihypertensives Treatment Guidelines in the Appendix.

Indications

➤*Severe hypertension:* For moderately severe to severe essential hypertension; uncomplicated malignant hypertension.

Administration and Dosage

➤*Dosage:* Start with 2.5 mg twice daily. Adjust dosage in increments of 2.5 mg at intervals of not less than 2 days until the desired blood pressure response occurs (a dosage just under that which causes signs of mild postural hypotension).

The average total daily dosage is 25 mg, usually in 3 divided doses. However, as little as 2.5 mg/day may be sufficient. A range of 2 to 4 or more doses may be required in severe cases when smooth control is difficult to obtain. In severe or urgent cases, larger increments at shorter intervals may be needed. Partial tolerance may develop, requiring an increase in dosage.

Administration after meals may cause a more gradual absorption and smoother control of blood pressure. The timing of doses in relation to meals should be consistent. Because blood pressure response is increased in the early morning, give larger dose at noon and in the evening. The morning dose should be relatively small or may be omitted.

➤*Blood pressure monitoring:* Determine the initial and maintenance dosage by blood pressure readings in the erect position at the time of maximal drug effect, as well as by other signs and symptoms of orthostatic hypotension.

Limit the effective maintenance dose to that which causes slight faintness or dizziness in the erect posture. If the patient or a relative can use a sphygmomanometer or another blood-pressure monitoring device, instructions may be given to reduce or omit a dose if readings fall below a designated level or if faintness or lightheadedness occurs. However, do not institute any changes without consulting a physician.

➤*Concomitant antihypertensive therapy:* Reduce the dosage of other agents, as well as that of mecamylamine, to avoid excessive hypotension. However, continue thiazides in usual dosage while decreasing mecamylamine by at least 50%.

Actions

➤*Pharmacology:* Mecamylamine is a potent, oral ganglionic blocker. Although the antihypertensive effect is predominantly orthostatic, the supine blood pressure is also significantly reduced.

➤*Pharmacokinetics:* Mecamylamine is almost completely absorbed from the GI tract. It has a gradual onset of action (0.5 to 2 hours) and a long-lasting effect (6 to 12 hours or more). It crosses the placental and blood-brain barriers. It is slowly excreted unchanged in the urine. The rate of renal elimination is markedly influenced by urinary pH. Alkalinization of urine reduces, and acidification promotes, renal excretion of mecamylamine.

Contraindications

Coronary insufficiency or recent MI; uremia; patients receiving antibiotics and sulfonamides with ganglionic blockers; glaucoma; organic pyloric stenosis; hypersensitivity to mecamylamine; mild, moderate, or labile hypertension; uncooperative patients.

Warnings

➤*CNS effects:* Mecamylamine readily penetrates into the brain and may produce CNS effects. Tremor, choreiform movements, mental aberrations, and convulsions occur rarely, but most often with large doses, especially in patients with cerebral or renal insufficiency.

➤*Discontinuation of therapy:* When mecamylamine is suddenly discontinued, hypertension returns. This may occur abruptly and may cause fatal cerebral vascular accidents or acute CHF. Withdraw drug gradually and substitute other antihypertensive therapy. The effects of mecamylamine can last from hours to days after therapy is discontinued.

➤*Renal/Cardiovascular function:* Evaluate the patient's condition, particularly renal and cardiovascular function. Give with great discretion, if at all, when renal insufficiency is manifested by a rising or elevated BUN. When renal, cerebral, or coronary blood flow is deficient, avoid any additional impairment that might result from hypotension. Use with caution in patients with marked cerebral and coronary arteriosclerosis or after a recent cerebral vascular accident.

➤*Pregnancy: Category C.* Mecamylamine crosses the placenta. It is not known whether mecamylamine can cause fetal harm when given to a pregnant woman. Give to a pregnant woman only if clearly needed.

➤*Lactation:* Because of the potential for serious adverse reactions in nursing infants, discontinue nursing or discontinue the drug, taking into account the importance of the drug to the mother.

➤*Children:* Safety and efficacy in pediatric patients have not been established.

Precautions

➤*Potentiation of effects:* The action of mecamylamine may be potentiated by the following: Excessive heat; fever; infection; hemorrhage; pregnancy; anesthesia; surgery; vigorous exercise; other antihypertensive drugs; alcohol; salt depletion resulting from diminished intake or increased excretion caused by diarrhea, vomiting, excessive sweating, or diuretics. During therapy, do not restrict sodium intake; if necessary, adjust the dosage.

➤*Urinary retention:* Urinary retention may occur; use caution in patients with prostatic hypertrophy, bladder neck obstruction, and urethral stricture.

Drug Interactions

➤*Antibiotics and sulfonamides:* Generally, do not treat patients receiving antibiotics and sulfonamides with ganglion blockers.

➤*Anesthesia, other antihypertensives, alcohol:* Concomitant use may potentiate the action of mecamylamine.

Adverse Reactions

➤*Cardiovascular:* Orthostatic dizziness; syncope; postural hypotension.

➤*CNS:* Weakness; fatigue; sedation; paresthesia; tremor; choreiform movements; mental aberrations; convulsions.

➤*GI:* Anorexia; dry mouth; glossitis; nausea; vomiting; constipation (sometimes preceded by small, frequent, liquid stools); ileus.

Frequent loose bowel movements with abdominal distention and decreased borborygmi may be the first signs of paralytic ileus. Discontinue the drug immediately and take remedial steps.

➤*GU:* Decreased libido; impotence; urinary retention.

➤*Respiratory:* Interstitial pulmonary edema; fibrosis.

➤*Special senses:* Dilated pupils; blurred vision.

Overdosage

➤*Symptoms:* Signs of overdosage include the following: Hypotension (which may progress to peripheral vascular collapse); postural hypotension; nausea; vomiting; diarrhea; constipation; paralytic ileus; urinary retention; dizziness; anxiety; dry mouth; mydriasis; blurred vision; palpitations. A rise in intraocular pressure may occur.

➤*Treatment:* Pressor amines may be used to counteract excessive hypotension. Because patients treated with ganglionic blockers are more than normally reactive to pressor amines, use small doses to avoid excessive response.

Patient Information

Take after meals. Use consistent timing of doses in relation to meals.

Mecamylamine may cause dizziness, lightheadedness, or fainting, especially when rising from a lying or sitting position. This effect may be increased by alcoholic beverages, exercise, or hot weather. Arising slowly may alleviate such symptoms.

Angiotensin-Converting Enzyme Inhibitors

WARNING

Pregnancy: When used in pregnancy during the second and third trimesters, angiotensin-converting enzyme inhibitors (ACEIs) can cause injury to and even death in the developing fetus. When pregnancy is detected, discontinue the ACEI as soon as possible (see Warnings). Refer to the general discussion of these products in the Antihypertensives Introduction.

Indications

Refer to individual monographs for specific indications.

ACEI Indications

Indications	Benazepril	Captopril	Enalapril	Enalaprilat	Fosinopril	Lisinopril	Moexipril	Perindopril	Quinapril	Ramipril	Trandolapril
Hypertension	✔	✔	✔	✔	✔	✔	✔	✔	✔	✔	✔
Heart failure		✔	✔		✔	✔			✔	✔¹	✔¹
Left ventricular dysfunction, post-MI		✔									✔
Left ventricular dysfunction, asymptomatic			✔								
Improve survival post-MI						✔					
Reduce risk of MI, stroke, and death from cardiovascular causes										✔	
Diabetic nephropathy		✔									

¹ Following MI.

➤*Hypertension:* The ACEIs are effective alone and in combination with other antihypertensives, especially thiazide-type diuretics. Blood pressure-lowering effects of ACEIs and thiazides are approximately additive.

Per JNC 7 guidelines†, use thiazide-type diuretics as initial therapy for most patients with hypertension, either alone or in combination with 1 or the other classes (eg, ACEIs).

➤*Heart failure:* **Captopril**, **enalapril**, **fosinopril**, **lisinopril**, and **quinapril** are indicated in the treatment of (congestive) heart failure, usually in combination with diuretics and/or digitalis. **Ramipril** and **trandolapril** are indicated in stable patients who are symptomatic from CHF within the first few days after sustaining acute MI.

➤*Left ventricular dysfunction:* **Enalapril** is indicated to treat clinically stable asymptomatic patients with left ventricular dysfunction (ejection fraction 35% or less). It has been shown to decrease the rate of developing overt heart failure and decrease the incidence of hospitalization for heart failure.

Captopril is indicated to improve survival following MI in clinically stable patients with left ventricular dysfunction manifested as an ejection fraction of 40% or less and to reduce the incidence of overt heart failure and subsequent hospitalizations for CHF in these patients.

Trandolapril is indicated in stable patients who have evidence of left ventricular systolic dysfunction (identified by wall motion abnormalities).

➤*MI:* **Lisinopril** is indicated in the treatment of hemodynamically stable patients within 24 hours of acute MI to improve survival.

➤*Reduction in risk of MI, stroke, and death from cardiovascular causes:* **Ramipril** is indicated in patients 55 years of age or older who are at high risk of developing a major cardiovascular event because of a history of coronary artery disease, stroke, peripheral vascular disease, or diabetes that is accompanied by at least 1 other cardiovascular risk factor (eg, hypertension, elevated total cholesterol levels, low HDL levels, cigarette smoking, documented microalbuminuria), to reduce the risk of MI, stroke, or death from cardiovascular causes.

➤*Diabetic nephropathy:* **Captopril** is indicated for the treatment of diabetic nephropathy (proteinuria over 500 mg/day) in patients with type 1 insulin-dependent diabetes mellitus and retinopathy. Captopril decreases the rate of progression of renal insufficiency and development of serious adverse clinical outcomes (death or need for renal transplantation or dialysis).

➤*Unlabeled uses:*
JNC 7 guidelines – Per JNC 7 guidelines, ACEIs have been shown in clinical trials to be beneficial in the following: Heart failure, post MI, high coronary disease risk, diabetes, chronic kidney disease, and recurrent stroke prevention.

Stroke prevention – **Perindopril**, alone and in combination with a diuretic, has been shown to reduce the risk of stroke among hypertensive and nonhypertensive individuals with a history of stroke or transient ischemic attack.

Migraine prophylaxis – One clinical study showed **lisinopril** to be effective as a prophylactic treatment of migraine.

Diabetic nephropathy – Other ACEIs (eg, **enalapril**, **ramipril**) have been shown to be effective in the treatment of diabetic nephropathy in normotensive patients.

Nondiabetic nephropathy – **Ramipril** and **benazepril** have shown favorable effects on the progression of nondiabetic nephropathy.

Bartter syndrome – ACEIs may be of benefit in the management of Bartter syndrome.

Renovascular hypertension – ACEIs have shown effectiveness in the treatment of renovascular hypertension.

Hypertensive emergencies/urgencies – **Enalaprilat** (1.25 mg IV over 5 minutes every 6 hours; titrate by 1.25 mg increments up to a maximum dose of 5 mg) may be useful in the management of hypertensive emergencies. **Captopril** (25 to 50 mg at 1- or 2-hour intervals) may be useful for hypertensive urgencies.

Scleroderma renal crisis – Prompt treatment of scleroderma renal crisis with ACEIs may reverse acute renal failure.

Hypertension in children (**Captopril**) – For infants, consider initial captopril doses of 0.15 to 0.3 mg/kg/dose followed by upward titration as needed. For children, consider initial doses of 0.3 to 0.5 mg/kg/dose given every 8 hours, followed by upward titration as needed. The maximum captopril dose is 6 mg/kg/day in divided doses.

Actions

➤*Pharmacology:* The ACEIs appear to act primarily through suppression of the renin-angiotensin-aldosterone system. Based on chemical structure, they can be classified into 3 groups: Sulfhydryl-containing (**captopril**); dicarbocyl-containing (**enalapril**, **lisinopril**, **benazepril**, **quinapril**, **moexipril**, **perindopril**, **trandolapril**, **ramipril**); and phosphorus-containing (**fosinopril**).

Synthesized by the kidneys, renin is released into the circulation where it acts on angiotensinogen to produce angiotensin I, a relatively inactive decapeptide. Angiotensin I is then converted by the angiotensin-converting enzyme (ACE) to angiotensin II, a potent endogenous vasoconstrictor that also stimulates aldosterone secretion from the adrenal cortex, contributing to sodium and fluid retention. ACEIs prevent the conversion of angiotensin I to angiotensin II by inhibiting ACE; they do not alter pressor responses to other agents.

Inhibiting ACE results in decreased plasma angiotensin II and increased plasma renin activity (PRA), the latter resulting from loss of negative feedback on renin release caused by reduction in angiotensin II. This leads to decreased aldosterone secretion, resulting in small increases in serum potassium along with sodium and fluid loss.

Increased prostaglandin synthesis also may play a role in the antihypertensive action of ACEI. ACE is identical to bradykininase (kininase II); thus, ACEIs can increase bradykinin levels. Because bradykinin stimulates prostaglandin biosynthesis, these peptides may contribute to the pharmacological effects of ACEIs.

The ACEIs produce a reduction of peripheral arterial resistance in hypertensive patients, an increase in cardiac output, and little or no change in heart rate. Renal blood flow increases, but glomerular filtration rate (GFR) is usually unchanged.

Blood pressure reduction may be progressive. To achieve maximal effects, several weeks of therapy may be required. Blood pressure-lowering effects of ACEIs and thiazide-type diuretics are additive, but captopril and β-blockers have a less than additive effect. Standing and supine blood pressures are lowered to about the same extent. Orthostatic effects and tachycardia are infrequent but may occur in volume- or salt-depleted patients. Abrupt withdrawal is not associated with a rapid increase in blood pressure.

The ACEIs are antihypertensive even in low-renin hypertensives. They are antihypertensive in all races studied, but black hypertensives (usually low-renin hypertensives) show a smaller average response to monotherapy than nonblacks.

Some ACEIs have demonstrated a beneficial effect on the severity of heart failure and an improvement in maximal exercise tolerance in patients with heart failure. In these patients, ACEIs significantly decrease peripheral (systemic vascular) resistance, blood pressure

† Chobanian AV, Bakris GI, Black HR, et al, and the National High Blood Pressure Education Program Coordinating Committee. The Seventh Report of the Joint National Committee on Prevention, Detection, Evaluation, and Treatment of High Blood Pressure: the JNC 7 report. *JAMA.* 2003;289:2560-2572. http://www.nhlbi.nih.gov/guidelines/hypertension/express.pdf

Angiotensin-Converting Enzyme Inhibitors

(afterload), pulmonary capillary wedge pressure (preload), and pulmonary vascular resistance, and increase cardiac output and exercise tolerance time. These effects occur after the first dose and persist for the duration of therapy.

➤*Pharmacokinetics:*

Absorption/Distribution – The presence of food in the GI tract reduces the absorption of **captopril** by about 30% to 40%. Food intake also reduces **moexipril** C_{max} 70% to 80% and AUC 40% to 50%. Therefore, take captopril and moexipril 1 hour before meals (see Drug Interactions).

Animal studies indicate that **benazepril** (and metabolites), **enalapril**, **lisinopril**, captopril, and **perindopril** cross the blood-brain barrier poorly, if at all. **Enalaprilat**, **fosinopril**/fosinoprilat, and **quinapril** do not cross the blood-brain barrier.

Metabolism/Excretion – With the exception of **captopril** and **lisinopril**, most of the ACEIs are prodrugs that are rapidly converted to their active metabolites following oral administration.

The effective half-lives for accumulation are as follows: 10 to 11 hours for benazeprilat, 11 hours for enalaprilat, 11.5 hours for fosinoprilat, 12 hours for lisinopril, 12 hours for moexiprilat, and 3 hours for quinaprilat.

Pharmacokinetics of the Active Moieties of ACEIs

ACEI	Onset (h)	Peak effect (h)	Duration (h)	Bioavailability (%)	T_{max} (h)	Protein binding	Effect of food on absorption	Active metabolite	Elimination half-life (h)	Routes of elimination
Benazepril	1	2-4	24	≥ 37	0.5-1 (1-4)[1,2]	≈ 96.7% (≈ 95.3%)[1]	slows absorption	benazeprilat		renal (20%)[1] bile (11%-12%)[1]
Captopril	≤ 0.5	1-1.5	6-10 (dose-related)	≥ 75	1	≈ 25%-30%	absorption reduced by ≈ 30%-40%		< 2	renal (> 95%)
Enalapril	1	4-6	≥ 24	≈ 60	1 (3-4)[1]		none	enalaprilat		renal feces
Enalaprilat	0.25	1-4	≈ 6	na			na			renal (> 90%)
Fosinopril	1	2-6	24	≈ 36	3	99.4%[1]	slows absorption	fosinoprilat	≈ 12[1]	renal (≈ 50%) feces (≈ 50%)
Lisinopril	1	6	24	≈ 25	7	none	none			renal (100%)
Moexipril	≈ 1	3-6	24	≈ 13	≈ 1.5[1]	≈ 50%[1]	markedly reduced	moexiprilat	2-9[1]	renal (13%) feces (53%)
Perindopril				≈ 75	≈ 1 (3-7)[1]	≈ 60% (10%-20%)[1]	reduces bioavailability of metabolite	perindoprilat	≈ 0.8-1 (3-10)[1]	renal
Quinapril	≤ 1	2-4	24	≥ 60	1 (≈ 2)[1]	≈ 97%	moderately reduced	quinaprilat	≈ 2[1]	renal
Ramipril	1-2	3-6	24	≥ 50-60	1 (2-4)[1]	≈ 73% (≈ 56%)[1]	slows absorption	ramiprilat	9-18[1]	renal (60%) feces (40%)
Trandolapril		4-8	24	≈ 10 (70)[1]	1 (4-10)[1]	≈ 80%	slows absorption	trandolaprilat	≈ 6 (10)[1]	renal (≈ 33%) feces (≈ 66%)

na – Not applicable.
[1] Active metabolite.
[2] 1 to 2 hours in fasting state and 2 to 4 hours in nonfasting state.

Special populations –

Hepatic function impairment:

• *Fosinopril* – In patients with hepatic insufficiency (alcoholic or biliary cirrhosis), the rate of hydrolysis of fosinopril may be slowed. The apparent total body clearance of fosinoprilat is approximately one half of that in patients with normal hepatic function.

• *Moexipril* – In patients with mild to moderate cirrhosis given single 15 mg doses, the C_{max} of moexipril was increased by about 50% and the AUC increased by about 120%, while the C_{max} for moexiprilat was decreased by about 50% and the AUC increase by about 300%.

• *Perindopril* – The bioavailability of perindoprilat is increased, and plasma concentrations were about 50% higher than those with normal liver function.

• *Quinapril* – Quinaprilat concentrations are reduced in patients with alcoholic cirrhosis because of impaired deesterification of quinapril.

• *Ramipril* – The metabolism of ramipril to ramiprilat appears to be slowed, and plasma ramipril levels are increased about 3-fold.

• *Trandolapril* – Following oral administration in patients with mild to moderate alcoholic cirrhosis, plasma concentrations of trandolapril and trandolaprilat were, respectively, 9- and 2-fold greater than in healthy subjects, but inhibition of ACE activity was not affected.

Renal function impairment:

• *Benazepril* – In patients with Ccr 30 mL/min or less, peak benazeprilat levels and the initial (alpha phase) half-life increase, and the time to steady state may be delayed. In patients with renal failure, biliary clearance may compensate to an extent.

• *Captopril* – Excretion rates are reduced and retention of captopril occurs in patients with impaired renal function. Captopril can be removed by hemodialysis.

• *Enalapril/Enalaprilat* – With GFR of 30 mL/min or less, peak and trough enalaprilat levels increase, T_{max} increases, and time to steady state may be delayed. Enalaprilat is dialyzable at the rate of 62 mL/min.

• *Fosinopril* – In patients with end-stage renal disease (Ccr less than 10 mL/min), the total body clearance of fosinoprilat is approximately one half of that in patients with normal renal function. Fosinopril is not well dialyzed.

• *Lisinopril* – Impaired renal function (GFR less than 30 mL/min) decreases lisinopril elimination, increases peak and trough levels, increases T_{max}, and time to attain steady state is prolonged. Lisinopril can be removed by hemodialysis.

• *Moexipril* – The effective elimination half-life and AUC of moexipril and moexiprilat are increased with decreasing renal function. At Ccr in the range of 10 to 40 mL/min, the half-life of moexiprilat is increased by a factor of 3 to 4.

• *Perindopril* – Perindoprilat AUC increases with decreasing renal function. At Ccr of 30 to 80 mL/min, AUC is about double that of 100 mL/min. When Ccr drops below 30 mL/min, AUC increases more markedly. Perindopril dialysis clearance ranges from 41.7 to 76.7 mL/min and perindoprilat dialysis clearance ranges from 37.4 to 91 mL/min.

• *Quinapril* – The half-life of quinaprilat increases as Ccr decreases. There is a linear correlation between plasma quinaprilat clearance and Ccr. Chronic hemodialysis or continuous ambulatory peritoneal dialysis has little or no effect on the elimination of quinapril and quinaprilat.

• *Ramipril* – In patients with Ccr less than 40 mL/min, peak levels of ramiprilat are approximately doubled, and trough levels may be as much as 5 times higher. In multiple dose regimens, the ramiprilat AUC is 3 to 4 times as large as it is in patients with normal renal function.

• *Trandolapril* – The plasma concentrations of trandolapril and trandolaprilat are approximately 2-fold greater and renal clearance is reduced by about 85% in patients with Ccr below 30 mL/min and in patients on hemodialysis.

Elderly:

• *Lisinopril* – Older patients have (approximately doubled) higher blood levels and AUC than younger patients.

• *Moexipril* – The AUC and C_{max} of moexiprilat is about 30% greater than in younger subjects.

• *Perindopril* – Plasma concentrations of perindopril and perindoprilat in patients older than 70 years of age are approximately twice those observed in younger patients.

• *Quinapril* – Elimination of quinaprilat may be reduced in patients 65 years of age and older.

• *Ramipril* – Peak ramiprilat levels and AUC are higher in older patients.

• *Trandolapril* – The plasma concentration of trandolapril is increased in elderly hypertensive patients, but the plasma concentration of trandolaprilat and inhibition of ACE activity are similar in elderly and young hypertensive patients.

Heart failure:

• *Fosinopril* – The effective half-life of fosinoprilat was 14 hours.

• *Perindopril* – Perindoprilat clearance is reduced in CHF patients, resulting in 40% higher-dose interval AUC.

• *Quinapril* – Elimination of quinaprilat may be reduced in patients with heart failure.

Contraindications

Hypersensitivity to these products and in patients with a history of angioedema related to previous treatment with an ACEI; in patients with hereditary or idiopathic angioedema (**enalapril**, **enalaprilat**, **lisinopril**).

Warnings

➤*Hematologic effects:* Neutropenia (less than 1000/mm³) with myeloid hypoplasia resulted from use of **captopril**. About half of the neutropenic patients developed systemic or oral cavity infections or other features of agranulocytosis. The risk of neutropenia is dependent on the patient's clinical status. In hypertension with normal renal function (serum creatinine less than 1.6 mg/dL, no collagen vascular disease [eg, systemic lupus erythematosus, scleroderma], neutropenia occurred in 1 patient in more than 8600 exposed. In patients with some degree of renal failure (serum creatinine at least 1.6 mg/dL) but no collagen vascular disease, the risk of neutropenia was about 1 in 500. Daily doses of captopril were relatively high. Concomitant allopurinol and captopril have been associated with neutropenia (see Drug Interactions). In collagen vascular diseases and impaired renal function, neutropenia has occurred in 3.7% of patients. In heart failure, the same risk factors for neutropenia appear present; about half of cases had serum creatinine at least 1.6 mg/dL, and more than 75% also were on procainamide.

Neutropenia usually has been detected within 3 months after captopril initiation. Bone marrow examinations consistently showed myeloid hypoplasia, frequently accompanied by erythroid hypoplasia and decreased numbers of megakaryocytes (eg, hypoplastic bone marrow, pancytopenia); anemia and thrombocytopenia were sometimes seen. In general, neutrophils returned to normal about 2 weeks after captopril was discontinued; serious infections were limited to clinically complex patients. About 13% of neutropenia cases were fatal, but almost all were in patients with serious illness having collagen vascular disease, renal failure, heart failure, immunosuppressant therapy, or a combination of these factors. Discontinuation of captopril and other drugs has generally led to prompt return of the normal WBC count; upon confirmation of neutropenia, withdraw the drug and closely observe the patient.

Neutropenia/leukopenia/agranulocytosis has occurred rarely with **enalapril** or **lisinopril** and in 1 patient on **quinapril**; a causal relationship cannot be excluded. Data are insufficient to show that **moexipril**, **perindopril**, **ramipril**, **benazepril**, **trandolapril**, or **fosinopril** do not cause agranulocytosis at similar rates. Periodically monitor WBC counts.

➤*Anaphylactoid and possibly related reactions:* Presumably because ACEIs affect the metabolism of eicosanoids and polypeptides, including endogenous bradykinin, patients receiving ACEIs may be subject to a variety of adverse reactions, some of them serious.

Angioedema – Angioedema has occurred in patients treated with ACEIs. It may occur at any time during treatment with **enalapril** (0.2%); **captopril**, **lisinopril**, **perindopril**, **quinapril** (0.1%); **trandolapril** (0.13%); **benazepril** (about 0.5%); **moexipril** (less than 0.5%); **ramipril** (0.3%); or **fosinopril** (0.2% to 1%). Angioedema of the face, extremities, lips, mucous membranes, tongue, glottis, or larynx has occurred. In instances where swelling has been confined to the face and lips, the condition has generally resolved without treatment, although antihistamines have been useful in relieving symptoms. Angioedema associated with laryngeal edema may be fatal. If laryngeal stridor or angioedema of the face, tongue, larynx, or glottis occurs and appears likely to cause airway obstruction, discontinue treatment and institute appropriate therapy (eg, epinephrine solution 1:1000 SC) immediately. Use with extreme caution in patients with hereditary angioedema (caused by a deficiency of C1 esterase inhibitor). Intestinal angioedema has been reported in patients treated with ACEIs. These patients presented with abdominal pain (with or without nausea or vomiting); in some cases there was no history of facial angioedema and C1 esterase levels were normal. The angioedema was diagnosed by procedures including abdominal CT scan or ultrasound, or at surgery, and symptoms resolved after stopping the ACE inhibitor. Include intestinal angioedema in the differential diagnosis of patients on ACE inhibitors presenting with abdominal pain. Symptoms resolved after stopping ACEIs. Patients with a history of angioedema unrelated to ACEI therapy may be at increased risk of angioedema while receiving an ACEI. Black patients receiving ACE inhibitor monotherapy have been reported to have a higher incidence of angioedema compared with non-blacks.

Anaphylactoid reactions during desensitization – Two patients undergoing desensitizing treatment with hymenoptera venom while receiving ACEIs sustained life-threatening anaphylactoid reactions. In the same patients, these reactions were avoided when ACEIs were temporarily withheld, but they reappeared upon inadvertent rechallenge.

Anaphylactoid reactions during membrane exposure – Anaphylactoid reactions have been reported in patients dialyzed with high-flux membranes and treated concomitantly with an ACEI. In such patients,

immediately stop dialysis and initiate aggressive therapy for anaphylactoid reactions. Symptoms have not been relieved by antihistamines in these situations. Consider a different type of dialysis membrane or a different class of medication. Anaphylactoid reactions also have occurred in patients undergoing low-density lipoprotein apheresis with dextran sulfate absorption.

➤*Proteinuria:* Total urinary proteins of more than 1 g/day were seen in about 0.7% of **captopril** patients. About 90% of affected patients showed evidence of prior renal disease or received relatively high doses of captopril (more than 150 mg/day) or both. Nephrotic syndrome occurred in approximately one fifth of these cases. In most cases, proteinuria cleared within 6 months, regardless of whether captopril was continued; creatinine and BUN were seldom altered.

➤*Hypotension:*

First-dose effect – ACEIs may cause a profound fall in blood pressure following the first dose. Excessive hypotension is rare in uncomplicated hypertensive patients, but is possible with ACEI use in severely salt/volume depleted people such as those treated vigorously with diuretics or patients on dialysis. Patients at risk for excessive hypotension, sometimes associated with oliguria or progressive azotemia, and rarely with acute renal failure and/or death, include those with the following conditions or characteristics: Heart failure, hyponatremia, high-dose diuretic therapy, recent intensive diuresis or increase in diuretic dose, renal dialysis, or severe volume and/or salt depletion. Correct volume and/or salt depletion before initiating treatment. Excessive perspiration, dehydration, vomiting, and/or diarrhea may also lead to an excessive fall in blood pressure because of reduction in fluid volume.

Minimize the possibility of hypotension either by discontinuing the diuretic or by increasing salt intake about 1 week prior to initiating ACEIs, or initiate with small doses. Alternatively, provide medical supervision for at least 2 hours after the initial dose and until blood pressure has stabilized for at least an additional hour.

A transient hypotensive response is not a contraindication for further doses of these agents, which usually can be given without difficulty once the blood pressure has stabilized. If excessive hypotension occurs, place patient in supine position and, if necessary, give normal saline IV. A dose reduction or discontinuation of the ACEI or concomitant diuretic may be necessary.

Heart failure – In heart failure where the blood pressure was either normal or low, transient decreases in mean blood pressure more than 20% occurred in about half of patients taking **captopril**. Transient hypotension may occur after the first several doses. This effect is usually well tolerated, and it is asymptomatic or produces brief, mild light-headedness. It rarely has been associated with arrhythmia or conduction defects. Start therapy under close medical supervision. Follow patients closely for the first 2 weeks and whenever the dose of ACEI or diuretic is increased. Also follow patients with ischemic heart, aortic stenosis, or cerebrovascular disease in whom an excessive fall in blood pressure could result in MI or cerebrovascular accident.

Hypotension is not a reason to discontinue the ACEI. Some decrease in systemic blood pressure is common and desirable in heart failure. The magnitude of the decrease is greatest early in treatment, stabilizes within 1 to 2 weeks, and generally returns to pretreatment levels without a decrease in efficacy within 2 months.

Acute MI – In a study, patients with an acute MI had a higher incidence of persistent hypotension (systolic blood pressure less than 90 mm Hg for more than 1 hour) when treated with **lisinopril**. Treatment must not be initiated in acute MI patients at risk of further serious hemodynamic deterioration after treatment with a vasodilator (eg, systolic blood pressure of 100 mm Hg or lower) or cardiogenic shock.

➤*Hepatic failure:* Rarely ACEIs have been associated with a syndrome that starts with cholestatic jaundice and progresses to fulminant hepatic necrosis and (sometimes) death. The mechanism of this syndrome is not understood. Patients receiving ACEIs who develop jaundice or marked elevations of hepatic enzymes should discontinue the ACEI and receive appropriate medical follow-up.

➤*Renal function impairment:* Some hypertensive patients with unilateral or bilateral renal artery stenosis have developed increases in BUN and serum creatinine after reduction of blood pressure (20% of patients with **enalapril**). Monitor renal function in such patients during the first few weeks of therapy. Dosage reduction and/or discontinuation of the ACEI and/or diuretic may be required. For some patients, it may not be possible to normalize blood pressure and maintain adequate renal perfusion.

About 20% of heart failure patients develop stable elevations of BUN and serum creatinine more than 20% above normal or baseline with long-term **captopril**. Less than 5% of patients, generally those with severe pre-existing renal disease, require treatment discontinuation; subsequent improvement probably relies on the severity of underlying renal disease.

In patients with severe CHF whose renal function may depend on the activity of the renin-angiotensin-aldosterone system, treatment with ACEIs may be associated with oliguria and/or progressive azotemia and, rarely, with acute renal failure and/or death.

Angiotensin-Converting Enzyme Inhibitors

Some hypertensive or heart failure patients with no apparent pre-existing renal vascular disease have developed increases in BUN and serum creatinine; these are usually minor and transient, especially when the ACEI was given with a diuretic. This is more likely to occur in patients with pre-existing renal impairment. Dosage adjustment and/or discontinuation of the diuretic and/or ACEI may be required. However, captopril has shown renal protective effects in hypertensive patients with some renal dysfunction.

Impaired renal function decreases **lisinopril** elimination, which is excreted principally through the kidneys, but this decrease becomes clinically important only when the GFR is less than 30 mL/min. The elimination half-life of quinaprilat increases as creatinine clearance decreases. Dosage adjustment may be necessary for **quinapril, benazepril, ramipril, captopril, trandolapril, moexipril, enalapril, perindopril**, and **lisinopril**. Impaired renal function decreases total clearance of fosinoprilat and approximately doubles the AUC. However, in general, no dosing adjustment is needed (see Pharmacokinetics).

➤*Hepatic function impairment:* Patients with impaired liver function could develop markedly elevated plasma levels of unchanged **fosinopril, moexipril**, or **ramipril**. No formal pharmacokinetic studies with ramipril have been done in hypertensive patients with impaired liver function. In patients with alcoholic or biliary cirrhosis, the rate, but not extent, of fosinopril hydrolysis was reduced; the total body clearance of fosinoprilat was decreased and AUC approximately doubled. Quinaprilat concentrations are reduced in patients with alcoholic cirrhosis caused by impaired deesterification of **quinapril**. Consider lower **trandolapril** doses in patients with mild to moderate alcoholic cirrhosis; plasma concentrations of trandolapril and trandolaprilat were increased. Perindoprilat plasma concentrations may be elevated.

➤*Elderly:* Elderly patients may have higher blood levels and AUC of **lisinopril**, ramiprilat, **perindopril**, quinaprilat, and moexiprilat. This may relate to decreased renal function rather than to age itself. No overall differences in effectiveness or safety were observed between elderly patients receiving **trandolapril, fosinopril**, or **benazepril**; however, greater sensitivity of some older individuals cannot be ruled out.

➤*Pregnancy:* Category C (first trimester); Category D (second and third trimesters). ACEIs can cause fetal and neonatal morbidity and death when administered to pregnant women. Several dozen cases have been reported in the world literature. When pregnancy is detected, discontinue ACEIs as soon as possible.

The use of ACEIs during the second and third trimesters of pregnancy has been associated with fetal and neonatal injury, including hypotension, neonatal skull hypoplasia, anuria, reversible or irreversible renal failure, and death. Oligohydramnios also has occurred, presumably resulting from decreased fetal renal function; oligohydramnios in this setting has been associated with fetal limb contractures, craniofacial deformation, and hypoplastic lung development. Prematurity, intrauterine growth retardation, and patent ductus arteriosus also have been reported, although it is not clear whether these occurrences were caused by the ACEI exposure.

These adverse effects do not appear to have resulted from intrauterine ACEI exposure that has been limited to the first trimester. Inform mothers whose embryos and fetuses are exposed to ACEIs only during the first trimester. Nonetheless, when patients become pregnant, make every effort to discontinue the use of the ACEI as soon as possible.

Rarely (probably less often than 1 in every 1000 pregnancies), no alternative to ACEIs will be found. In these rare cases, apprise the mother of the potential hazards to the fetus, and perform serial ultrasound examinations to assess the intra-amniotic environment.

If oligohydramnios is observed, discontinue the ACEI unless it is considered lifesaving for the mother. Contraction stress testing, a non-stress test, or biophysical profiling may be appropriate, depending on the week of pregnancy. However, patients and physicians should be aware that oligohydramnios may not appear until after the fetus has sustained irreversible injury.

Closely observe infants with histories of in utero exposure to ACEIs for hypotension, oliguria, and hyperkalemia. If oliguria occurs, direct attention toward support of blood pressure and renal perfusion. Exchange transfusion or dialysis may be required as a means of reversing hypotension or substituting for disordered renal function. Some of these agents may be removed from neonatal circulation by exchange transfusion or dialysis (see Overdosage); however, limited experience has not shown that such removal is central to the treatment of these infants.

➤*Lactation:* Several ACEIs have been detected in breast milk. Do not administer **trandolapril, captopril, benazepril, fosinopril, enalapril, quinapril**, or **ramipril** to nursing mothers. It is not known whether **lisinopril, moexipril**, or **perindopril** are excreted in breast milk. Because of the potential for serious adverse effects, exercise caution when these drugs are administered to nursing women. Decide whether to discontinue nursing or discontinue the drug, taking into account the importance of the drug to the mother.

➤*Children:* Safety and efficacy have not been established. However, there is limited experience with the use of **captopril** in children. Dos-

age, on a weight basis, was comparable to or less than that used in adults. Infants, especially newborns, may be more susceptible to the adverse hemodynamic effects of captopril. Excessive, prolonged, and unpredictable decreases in blood pressure and associated complications, including oliguria and seizures, have occurred. Use captopril in children only when other measures for controlling blood pressure have not been effective.

Antihypertensive effects of **enalapril** have been established in hypertensive pediatric patients 1 month to 16 years of age and with **lisinopril** in patients 6 to 16 years of age. Enalapril and lisinopril are not recommended in neonates and in pediatric patients with GFR less than 30 mL/min/1.73 m^2, because no data is available.

Precautions

➤*Monitoring:* Patients with impaired renal function should have WBCs and differential counts monitored prior to starting treatment and at approximately 2-week intervals for about 3 months, then periodically. Consider periodic monitoring of WBCs in patients with collagen vascular disease and renal disease.

➤*Hyperkalemia:* Elevated serum potassium (at least 0.5 mEq/L greater than the upper limit of normal) was observed in 0.4% of hypertensive patients given **trandolapril**; 1.4% with **perindopril**; about 1% of hypertensive patients given **benazepril, enalapril, ramipril**, or **moexipril**; about 2% of patients receiving **lisinopril** or **quinapril**, about 2.6% of hypertensive patients given **fosinopril**, and about 4.8% of CHF patients given lisinopril. In most cases, these were resolved despite continued therapy. Hyperkalemia was a cause of therapy discontinuation in 0.28% of hypertensive patients on enalapril, about 0.1% with lisinopril and fosinopril, less than 0.1% with quinapril, no patients on ramipril and trandolapril, 2% of type 1 diabetics with proteinuria receiving **captopril**, 0.6% of heart failure patients on lisinopril, and 0.1% of MI patients on lisinopril. Risk factors for development of hyperkalemia may include renal insufficiency, diabetes mellitus, and concomitant use of agents that increase serum potassium (eg, potassium-sparing diuretics, potassium supplements, and/or potassium-containing salt substitutes).

➤*Valvular stenosis:* Theoretically, patients with aortic stenosis might be at risk of decreased coronary perfusion when treated with vasodilators, because they do not develop as much afterload reduction as others. Use with caution in patients with obstruction in the outflow tract of the left ventricle (eg, aortic stenosis, hypertrophic cardiomyopathy).

➤*Surgery/Anesthesia:* In patients undergoing major surgery or during anesthesia with agents that produce hypotension, ACEIs will block angiotensin II formation secondary to compensatory renin release. Hypotension can be corrected by volume expansion.

➤*Cough:* Chronic cough has occurred with the use of all ACEIs, presumably caused by the inhibition of the degradation of endogenous bradykinin. Characteristically, the cough is nonproductive, persistent, and resolves within 1 to 7 days (but can take as long as 2 weeks) after therapy discontinuation. Consider ACEI-induced cough as part of the differential diagnosis of cough.

The cough appears to have a higher incidence in women. The incidence of cough, although still reported as 0.5% to 3% by some manufacturers, appears to range from 5% to 25% and has been reported to be as high as 39%, resulting in discontinuation rates as high as 15%. The use of sulindac, diclofenac, indomethacin, nifedipine, cromolyn, or nebulized bupivacaine may be effective in managing cough; although, this is only based on a small number of patients. Further study is needed.

➤*Photosensitivity:* Photosensitization may occur; therefore, caution patients to take protective measures (ie, sunscreens, protective clothing) against exposure to ultraviolet light or sunlight until tolerance is determined.

Drug Interactions

ACEI Drug Interactions			
Precipitant drug	Object drug*		Description
Antacids (eg, aluminum and magnesium hydroxide, simethicone)	ACEIs	↓	Bioavailability of ACEIs may be decreased. May be more likely with **captopril** and **fosinopril**. Separate the administration times by 1 to 2 hours if an interaction is suspected.
Capsaicin	ACEIs	↑	Capsaicin may cause or exacerbate coughing associated with ACEI treatment and vice versa.
Diuretics	ACEIs	↑	Possible excessive reduction in blood pressure, especially in those patients with intravascular volume depletion, can occur. Consider discontinuing the diuretic or increasing salt intake prior to initiation of treatment with an ACEI. If this is not possible, consider reduction of initial ACEI dose.

Angiotensin-Converting Enzyme Inhibitors

ACEI Drug Interactions			
Precipitant drug	Object drug*		Description
Iron salts	ACEIs Captopril	↓	Oral iron preparations may reduce captopril blood levels. Separate administration by at least 2 hours.
NSAIDS (eg, indomethacin, aspirin)	ACEIs	↓	This combination reduced hypotensive effects of ACEIs. More prominent in low-renin or volume-dependent hypertensive patients; concomitant use may further deteriorate renal function.
Rifampin	ACEIs Enalapril	↓	Pharmacologic effects of enalapril may be decreased.
ACEIs Captopril	Allopurinol	↑	A higher risk of hypersensitivity reaction is possible when these drugs are given concurrently.
ACEIs	Digoxin	↑↓	Plasma levels of digoxin may be increased or decreased, possibly because of altered renal clearance. Monitor digoxin plasma levels.
ACEIs	Diuretics (eg, loop diuretics)	↓	The effects of loop diuretics may be decreased; possible inhibition of angiotensin II production by the ACEI.
ACEIs	Lithium	↑	Increased serum lithium levels and symptoms of toxicity may occur; monitor lithium levels frequently.
ACEIs	Hypoglycemic agents/insulin	↑	Rarely, hypoglycemia has been reported during concomitant therapy. Monitor symptoms of hypoglycemia during initiation of therapy.

ACEI Drug Interactions			
Precipitant drug	Object drug*		Description
ACEIs	Potassium preparations/ Potassium-sparing diuretics	↑	Coadministration may result in elevated serum potassium concentrations. Use with caution; monitor potassium levels and renal function frequently.
ACEIs Quinapril	Tetracycline	↓	Tetracycline absorption was reduced 28% to 37%, possibly caused by the high magnesium content of quinapril tablets.

* ↑ = Object drug increased. ↓ = Object drug decreased.

▶*Drug / Lab test interactions:* **Captopril** may cause a false-positive urine test for acetone.

Fosinopril may cause a false-low measurement of serum digoxin levels with the *Digi-Tab RIA Kit for Digoxin.* Other kits, such as the *Coat-A-Count RIA Kit,* may be used.

▶*Drug / Food interactions:* Food significantly reduces the absorption of **captopril** 30% to 40%. Administer captopril 1 hour before meals. Food intake reduces the C_{max} and AUC of **moexipril** about 70% and 40%, respectively, after a low-fat breakfast and 80% and 50%, respectively, after a high-fat breakfast; take moexipril in the fasting state and administer 1 hour before meals. Food reduces the biotransformation of **perindopril** to the active metabolite perindoprilat by approximately 43%, resulting in a reduction in the plasma ACE inhibition curve of approximately 20%. The rate and extent of **quinapril** absorption are diminished moderately (about 25% to 30%) when administered during a high-fat meal. The rate, but not extent, of **ramipril**, **fosinopril**, and **trandolapril** absorption is reduced by food. Food does not reduce the GI absorption of **benazepril**, **enalapril**, and **lisinopril**.

Adverse Reactions

Adverse Reactions Shared by the ACEIs[1] (%)										
✔ = Reported; no incidence given. Adverse reactions	Benazepril	Captopril	Enalapril/Enalaprilat	Fosinopril	Lisinopril	Moexipril	Perindopril	Quinapril	Ramipril	Trandolapril
Cardiovascular										
Angina pectoris	< 1	0.2-0.3	1.5	0.2-1		< 1		< 0.5	< 1-3	
Bradycardia			0.5-1	0.4-1	0.3-1				< 1	0.3-4.7
Cardiac arrest		✔[2]	0.5-1	✔	0.3-1		✔		< 1	
Cerebrovascular accident		✔[2]	0.5-1	0.2-1	0.3-1	< 1	0.2	< 0.5	< 1	
Chest pain		1	2.1	0.2-2.2	3.4	> 1	2.4	2.4	< 1	0.3-1
Hypotension[3]	0.3	✔	0.9-6.7	0.2-4.4	1.2-9.7	0.51	0.3-1	2.9	0.5-11	0.3-11
MI		0.2-0.3	0.5- 1.2	0.2-1	0.3-1	< 1	0.3-1	< 0.5	< 1	
Orthostatic hypotension/effects	0.4	✔[2]	1.2-2.2	≤ 1.2-1.9	0.3- 1.2	0.51	0.3-1	< 0.5	2	
Palpitations	< 1	1	0.5-1	0.2-1	0.3-1	< 1	0.9-1.1	0.5-1	< 1	0.3-1
Peripheral edema	< 1				0.3-1	> 1				
Rhythm disturbances		✔[2]	0.5-1	≤ 0.2-1.4		< 1		< 0.5		
Tachycardia		1	0.5-1	0.4-1	0.3-1			0.5-1	< 1	
CNS										
Anxiety	< 1					< 1	0.3-1		< 1	0.3-1
Ataxia		✔[2]	0.5-1		0.3-1					
Confusion		✔[2]	0.5-1	0.2-1	0.3-1					
Depression		✔[2]	0.5-1	0.4-1			2	0.5-1	< 1	
Dizziness	3.6		0.5-7.9	1.6-11.9	5.4-11.8	4.3	8.2	3.9-7.7	1.9-4	1.3-23
Fatigue	2.4		0.5-3	≥ 1	2.5	2.4		2.6	2	
Headache	6.2		1.8-5.2	≥ 1	4.4-5.7	> 1	23.8	1.7		
Insomnia/Sleep disturbances	< 1		0.5-1	0.2-1	0.3-1	< 1	2.5	0.5-1	< 1	0.3-1
Malaise					0.3-1	< 1	0.3-1	0.5-1	< 1	
Nervousness	< 1	✔[2]	0.5-1		0.3-1	< 1	1.1	0.5-1	< 1	
Paresthesias	< 1		0.5-1	0.2-1	0.3-1		2.3	0.5-1	< 1	0.3-1
Peripheral edema	< 1				> 1					
Somnolence/Drowsiness	1.6	✔[2]	0.5-1	0.2-1	0.3-1	< 1	1.3	0.5-1	< 1	0.3-1
Vertigo			1.6	0.2-1	0.2		0.3-1	0.5-1	< 1-2	0.3-1
Dermatologic										
Alopecia	< 1		0.5-1		0.3-1	< 1		0.5-1		

Angiotensin-Converting Enzyme Inhibitors

Adverse Reactions Shared by the ACEls[1] (%)

✔ = Reported; no incidence given. Adverse reactions	Benazepril	Captopril	Enalapril/Enalaprilat	Fosinopril	Lisinopril	Moexipril	Perindopril	Quinapril	Ramipril	Trandolapril
Diaphoresis/Sweating	< 1		0.5-1	0.2-1	0.3-1	< 1	0.3-1	0.5-1	< 1	
Erythema multiforme		✔[2]	0.5-1				0.3-1		< 1	
Exfoliative dermatitis		✔[2]	0.5-1	✔			✔	< 0.5		
Flushing	< 1	0.2-0.5	0.5-1	0.2-1	0.3-1	1.6				0.3-1
Pemphigus/Pemphigoid	< 1	✔	0.5-1		0.3-1			0.5-1		0.3-1
Photosensitivity	< 1	✔	0.5-1	0.2-1	0.3-1	< 1		< 0.5	< 1	
Pruritus	< 1	2	0.5-1	0.2-1		< 1	0.3-1	0.5-1	< 1	0.3-1
Rash	< 1	4-7	0.5-1.4	0.2-1	0.01-1.7	1.6	2.3	1.4	< 1	0.3-1
Stevens-Johnson syndrome	< 1	✔[2]	0.5-1		rare				< 1	
Toxic epidermal necrolysis			0.5-1		rare				< 1	
Urticaria			0.5-1	0.2-1	0.3-1	< 1		< 1	< 1	
GI										
Abdominal pain			1.6	0.2-1	2.2	< 1	2.7	1	< 1	0.3-1
Anorexia			0.5-1						< 1	
Constipation	< 1		0.5-1	0.2-1	0.3-1	< 1	0.3-1	0.5-1	< 1	0.3-1
Diarrhea			1.4-2.1	> 1	2.7-3.7	3.1	4.3	1.7	≤ 1	0.3-1
Dry mouth			0.5-1	0.2-1	0.3-1	< 1	0.3-1	0.5-1	< 1	
Dysgeusia		2-4								
Dyspepsia		✔[2]	0.5-1		0.3-1	> 1	0.3-1.9	< 0.5	< 1	0.3-6.4
Hepatitis		✔[2]	0.5-1	0.2-1	0.3-1	< 1		< 0.5	< 1	
Nausea	1.3		1.3-1.4	1.2-2.2	2	> 1	2.3	2.4	2	
Pancreatitis	< 1	✔[2]	0.5-1	0.2-1	0.3-1	< 1	✔	< 0.5	< 1	0.3-1
Vomiting	< 1		1.3	1.2-2.2	0.3-1.1	< 1	1.5	2.4	2	0.3-1
GU										
Decreased libido	< 1			0.2-1	0.4					0.3-1
Impotence	< 1	✔[2]	0.5-1		1			0.5-1	< 1	0.3-1
Oliguria		0.1-0.2	0.5-1		0.3-1	< 1				
UTI	< 1		1.3		0.3-1		2.8	0.5-1		
Musculoskeletal										
Arthralgia	< 1	✔	✔	0.2-1	0.3-1	< 1	0.3-1	0.5-1	< 1	
Arthritis	< 1		✔	✔	0.3-1		1		< 1	
Muscle cramps			0.5-1	0.2-1	0.5					0.3-1
Myalgia	< 1	✔[2]	✔	0.2-1	0.3-1	1.3	0.3-1.1		< 1	4.7
Respiratory										
Asthma	< 1	✔	0.5-1		0.3-1					
Bronchitis	< 1		1.3		0.3-1		0.3-1			
Bronchospasm		✔[2]	0.5-1	0.2-1	0.3-1	< 1				
Cough[4]	1.2	0.5-2	1.3-2.2	2.2-9.7	0.5-3.5	6.1	6-12	2-4.3	8	1.9-35
Dyspnea	< 1		1.3	≥ 1	0.3-1	< 1	0.3-1		< 1	0.3-1
Pharyngitis				0.2-1	0.3-1	1.8	3.3	0.5-1		
Rhinitis		✔[2]		0.2-1	0.3-1	> 1	4.8			
Sinusitis	< 1			0.2-1	0.3-1	> 1	0.6-5.2			
Upper respiratory tract infection			0.5-1	2.2	1.5-2.1	> 1	8.6		✔	0.3-1
Miscellaneous										
Anemia[5]	✔	≤ 0.2		✔	0.3-1	< 1		< 0.5	< 1	
Angioedema[3]	0.5	0.1	✔	0.2-1	0.1	< 1	0.1	0.1	0.3	0.13
Asthenia	< 1	✔[2]	1.1-1.6		1.3		7.9		2	3.3
Blurred vision		✔[2]	0.5-1		0.3-1					
Eosinophilia		✔	✔	✔	0.3-1				< 1	
Fever		✔	0.5-1	0.4-1	0.3-1		0.3-1.5		< 1	
Syncope	0.1	✔[2]	0.5-2.2	0.2-1	0.3-1.8	0.51	0.3-1	0.5-1	< 1-2	5.9
Tinnitus			0.5-1	0.2-1	0.3-1	< 1	1.5		< 1	
Vasculitis		✔	✔		0.3-1		✔		< 1	

[1] Data are pooled from separate studies and are not necessarily comparable. Data included for both hypertension and heart failure indications.
[2] Postmarketing.
[3] See Warnings or Precautions.

[4] See Precautions. Although still reported at 0.5% to 3% by some manufacturers, the incidence appears to range from 5% to 25% and has been reported to be as high as 39%.
[5] Including aplastic and hemolytic.

➤*Cardiovascular:*

Benazepril – Postural dizziness (1.5%); postural hypotension (0.4%); ECG changes (rare).

Captopril – Raynaud syndrome, CHF (0.2% to 0.3%).

Enalapril – Pulmonary embolism and infarction, pulmonary edema, atrial fibrillation, Raynaud phenomenon (0.5 to 1%).

Fosinopril – Hypertensive crisis, claudication, hypertension, conduction disorder, cerebral infarction, sudden death, cardiorespiratory arrest, shock, transient ischemic attacks (0.2% to 1%).

Lisinopril – Ventricular/atrial tachycardia; pulmonary embolism, premature ventricular contractions, pulmonary infarction, paroxysmal nocturnal dyspnea, decreased blood pressure, chest discomfort, atrial fibrillation, arrhythmias, transient ischemic attack (0.3 to 1%); postinfarction angina (0.3%).

Perindopril – Abnormal ECG (1.8%); ventricular extrasystole, vasodilation, abnormal conduction, heart murmur (0.3% to 1%).

Quinapril – Vasodilation (0.5% to 1%); heart failure, hypertensive crisis, cardiogenic shock (less than 0.5%).

Ramipril – CHF, arrhythmia, transient ischemic attack (less than 1%).

Trandolapril – Stroke (3.3%); cardiogenic shock (3.8%); first-degree AV block (0.3% to 1%).

➤*CNS:*

Enalapril – Peripheral neuropathy, dream abnormality, dysesthesia (0.5% to 1%).

Fosinopril – Memory disturbance, tremor, mood change, numbness, behavior change (0.2% to 1%).

Lisinopril – Stroke, memory impairment, tremor, irritability, hypersomnia, peripheral neuropathy, spasm (0.3% to 1%).

Moexipril – Mood changes (less than 1%).

Perindopril – Migraine, amnesia, psychosexual disorder (0.3% to 1%).

Ramipril – Amnesia, convulsions, hearing loss, neuralgia, neuropathy, tremor, vision disturbances (less than 1%); angioneurotic edema (0.3%).

➤*Dermatologic:*

Benazepril – Dermatitis (less than 1%).

Captopril – Rash, often with pruritus and sometimes with fever, arthralgia, and eosinophilia occurred in 4 to 7 of 100 patients, usually during the first 4 weeks of therapy. It is usually maculopapular and rarely urticarial. The rash is usually mild and disappears within a few days of dosage reduction, short-term treatment with an antihistaminic agent, and/or discontinuing therapy; remission may occur even if captopril is continued. Between 7% and 10% of patients with rash have shown an eosinophilia and/or positive ANA titers. Pallor (0.2% to 0.5%).

Enalapril – Herpes zoster (0.5% to 1%).

Lisinopril – Erythema, herpes zoster, skin lesions, skin infections (0.3% to 1%).

Perindopril – Skin infection, tinea, dry skin, erythema, fever blisters (0.3% to 1%); purpura (0.1%).

Quinapril – Dermatopolymyositis (less than 0.5%).

Ramipril – Purpura, onycholysis (less than 1%).

➤*GI:*

Benazepril – Gastritis, melena (less than 1%).

Captopril – Weight loss may be associated with taste loss; taste impairment is reversible and usually self-limited (2 to 3 months) even with continuous administration (2% to 4%).

Enalapril – Hepatic failure, stomatitis, ileus, taste alterations, melena, glossitis (0.5% to 1%).

Fosinopril – Dysphagia, abdominal distention, flatulence, heartburn, appetite/weight change, hepatomegaly (0.2% to 1%); hepatic failure, jaundice (hepatocellular or cholestatic).

Lisinopril – Flatulence, gastritis, heartburn, GI cramps, weight loss/gain, taste disturbances, hepatocellular/cholestatic jaundice (0.3% to 1%).

Moexipril – Appetite/Weight change, taste alterations (less than 1%).

Perindopril – Flatulence (1%); dry mucous membranes, appetite increased, gastroenteritis (0.3% to 1%).

Quinapril – GI hemorrhage (less than 0.5%); flatulence, dry throat (0.5% to 1%).

Ramipril – Abdominal pain occurs sometimes with enzyme changes suggesting pancreatitis; dysphagia, gastroenteritis, increased salivation, taste disturbance (less than 1%).

Trandolapril – Gastritis (4.2%); abdominal distention (0.3% to 1%).

➤*Hematologic:* Small decreases in hemoglobin and/or hematocrit have been attributed to many ACEIs but are rarely of clinical importance unless another cause of anemia coexists.

Benazepril – Thrombocytopenia, hemolytic anemia, leukopenia (less than 1%).

Captopril – Neutropenia/agranulocytosis (see Warnings). Cases of anemia, thrombocytopenia, and pancytopenia have been reported.

Enalapril – Neutropenia, thrombocytopenia, bone marrow suppression (0.5% to 1%); hemolytic anemia, including cases of hemolysis in patients with G-6-PD deficiency, has been reported.

Fosinopril – Lymphadenopathy (0.2% to 1%); neutropenia, leukopenia.

Lisinopril – Rare cases of bone marrow depression, hemolytic anemia, leukopenia/neutropenia, thrombocytopenia.

Perindopril – Hematoma, ecchymosis (0.3% to 1%); leukopenia, neutropenia (0.1%).

Quinapril – Hemolytic anemia, agranulocytosis, thrombocytopenia (less than 0.5%).

Ramipril – Pancytopenia, hemolytic anemia, thrombocytopenia (less than 1%); leukopenia (rare).

Trandolapril – Decreased leukocytes, decreased neutrophils, low lymphocytes, thrombocytopenia (0.3% to 1%).

➤*Lab test abnormalities:* Hyperkalemia (see Precautions); hyponatremia, elevated liver transaminases and serum bilirubin.

Benazepril – Elevations in uric acid and blood glucose.

Captopril – Elevation of alkaline phosphatase.

Fosinopril – Elevations of LDH and alkaline phosphatase.

Moexipril – Elevations of uric acid (rare).

Perindopril – Triglyceride increase (1.3%); potassium decrease, uric acid increase, alkaline phosphatase increase, cholesterol increase, glucose increase (0.3% to 1%).

Ramipril – Elevations of uric acid and blood glucose (rare).

Trandolapril – Elevated serum uric acid (15%).

➤*Respiratory:* Eosinophilic pneumonitis has been attributed to many ACEIs.

Enalapril – Rhinorrhea, sore throat, hoarseness, pulmonary infiltrates (0.5% to 1%).

Fosinopril – Pleuritic chest pain, tracheobronchitis, abnormal breathing, sinus abnormalities (0.4% to 1%); laryngitis/hoarseness, epistaxis (0.2% to 1%); a symptom-complex of cough, bronchospasm, and eosinophilia has been observed in 2 patients.

Lisinopril – Common cold (1.1%); nasal congestion (0.4%); influenza (0.3%); malignant lung neoplasms, hemoptysis, pulmonary infiltrates, pleural effusion, wheezing, orthopnea, painful respiration, epistaxis, laryngitis, rhinorrhea, pneumonia, pharyngeal pain (0.3% to 1%).

Perindopril – Posterior nasal drip, rhinorrhea, throat disorder, sneezing, epistaxis, hoarseness (0.3% to 1%); pulmonary fibrosis (less than 0.1%).

Trandolapril – Epistaxis, throat inflammation (0.3% to 1%).

➤*Renal:* Elevation, usually transient and minor, in serum creatinine and BUN (see Warnings).

Benazepril – Proteinuria (rare; see Warnings).

Captopril – Proteinuria (1%; see Warnings); renal insufficiency, renal failure, nephrotic syndrome, polyuria, urinary frequency (0.1% to 0.2%).

Enalapril – Renal failure, renal dysfunction (0.5% to 1%).

Fosinopril – Renal insufficiency, urinary frequency, abnormal urination, kidney pain (0.2% to 1%).

Lisinopril – Renal dysfunction (2%); acute renal failure, anuria, uremia, progressive azotemia, pyelonephritis, dysuria (0.3% to 1%).

Moexipril – Urinary frequency (more than 1%); renal insufficiency (less than 1%).

Perindopril – Proteinuria (1% to 1.5%); kidney stone, urinary frequency, urinary retention, hematuria (0.3% to 1%).

Quinapril – Acute renal failure, worsening renal failure (less than 0.5%).

Ramipril – Abnormal kidney function (1%); proteinuria (rare).

➤*Miscellaneous:* Anaphylactoid reactions have occurred (see Warnings).

A symptom complex has occurred and may include the following: Positive ANA, elevated ESR, arthralgia, arthritis, myalgia/myositis, fever, interstitial nephritis, vasculitis, rash, eosinophilia, serositis, leukocytosis, photosensitivity, other dermatologic manifestations.

Benazepril – Hypertonia, infection (less than 1%).

Enalapril – Anosmia, conjunctivitis, dry eyes, tearing, flank pain, gynecomastia, myositis, serositis (0.5% to 1%).

Fosinopril – Musculoskeletal pain (0.2% to 3.3%); weakness (1.4%); edema, vision/taste disturbance, eye irritation, sexual dysfunction, hyperhidrosis, fall, gout, influenza, cold sensation, pain, swelling/weakness of extremities, abnormal vocalization, abnormal urination, kidney pain, weight gain, muscle ache (0.2% to 1%).

Lisinopril – Neck/hip/leg/knee/arm/joint/shoulder/low back pain, gout, lumbago, fluid overload, dehydration, diabetes mellitus, chills, virus infection, pain, pelvic/flank pain, edema, facial edema, visual loss, diplopia, photophobia, breast pain (0.3% to 1%).

Moexipril – Flu syndrome (3.1%); pain, urinary frequency (more than 1%).

Quinapril – Back pain (0.5% to 1.2%); amblyopia, viral infections, edema (0.5% to 1%); agranulocytosis (less than 0.5%).

Perindopril – Back pain (5.8% or less); low extremity pain (4.7%); edema (3.9%); injury (2.3%); viral infection (0.3% to 3.4%); upper extremity pain (0.2% to 2.8%); hypertonia (0.2% to 2.7%); seasonal allergy (2%); ear infection (1.3% or less); neck pain, male sexual dysfunction (1.4%); joint pain, menstrual disorder (1.1%); pain, cold/hot sensation, chills, fluid retention, facial edema, vaginitis, flank pain, gout, conjunctivitis, earache (0.3% to 1%).

Ramipril – Flu syndrome, edema, epistaxis, weight gain, hypoglycemia (less than 1%).

Trandolapril – Hypocalcemia (4.7%); intermittent claudication (3.8%); edema, extremity pain, gout (0.3% to 1%).

Postmarketing –
    Captopril: Anaphylactoid reactions; gynecomastia; cerebrovascular insufficiency; bullous pemphigus; glossitis; jaundice; hepatitis, including rare cases of necrosis; cholestasis; symptomatic hyponatremia; myasthenia; eosinophilic pneumonitis.

Overdosage

➤*Symptoms:* Hypotension is most common. Systolic blood pressures of 95 and 80 mm Hg have occurred following **lisinopril** and **captopril** overdoses, respectively. One reported case of **perindopril** overdose developed hypothermia and circulatory arrest, then died following ingestion of up to 180 mg.

➤*Treatment:* Treatment includes usual supportive measures. Refer to General Management of Acute Overdosage. The primary concern is correction of hypotension. Volume expansion with an IV infusion of normal saline is the treatment of choice to restore blood pressure.

Captopril, **enalaprilat**, trandolaprilat, **lisinopril**, and **perindopril** may be removed by hemodialysis. There are inadequate data concerning the efficacy of removing captopril by hemodialysis in neonates and children. Enalaprilat has been removed from neonatal circulation by peritoneal dialysis. **Benazepril** is only slightly dialyzable, but dialysis might be considered in overdosed patients with severely impaired renal function. It is not known if **ramipril**, **moexipril**, or ramiprilat are removed by hemodialysis. Hemodialysis and peritoneal dialysis have little effect on the elimination of **fosinoprilat**, **quinapril**, and quinaprilat. Use caution with concurrent use of ACEIs and polyacrylonitrile dialyzers because of the possibility of severe, sudden, and sometimes fatal reactions. Stop the dialysis immediately and begin measures to treat anaphylactoid reactions.

Patient Information

Apprise female patients of childbearing age about the consequences of second and third trimester exposure to ACEIs and that these consequences do not appear to have resulted from intrauterine ACEI exposure limited to the first trimester. Ask these patients to report pregnancies to their physicians as soon as possible.

Take **captopril** and **moexipril** 1 hour before meals.

Stop taking the drug and notify physician if any of the following occur: Sore throat, fever, swelling of hands or feet, irregular heartbeat, chest pains, signs of angioedema (eg, swelling of face, eyes, lips, tongue, difficulty swallowing or breathing, hoarseness).

Excessive perspiration, dehydration, vomiting, and diarrhea may lead to a fall in blood pressure.

May cause dizziness, fainting, or lightheadedness, especially during the first days of therapy; avoid sudden changes in posture. If actual syncope occurs, discontinue drug until physician has been contacted. Heart failure patients should avoid rapid increases in physical activity.

May cause rash or impaired taste perception. Notify physician if these persist.

Do not use potassium supplements or salt substitutes containing potassium without consulting a physician.

A persistent dry cough may occur and usually does not subside unless the medication is stopped. If this effect becomes bothersome, consult a physician.

Advise patients planning to undergo any surgery and/or anesthesia to inform their physician that they are taking an ACEI that has a long duration of action.

BENAZEPRIL HCl

Rx	**Benazepril HCl** (Various, eg, Ivax, Teva)	**Tablets:** 5 mg	May contain lactose, maltodextrin. In 100s, 500s, and 1000s.
	Lotensin (Novartis)		Lactose, castor oil. (LOTENSIN 5). Light yellow. In 100s.
	Benazepril HCl (Various, eg, Ivax, Teva)	10 mg	May contain lactose, maltodextrin. In 100s, 500s, 1000s, 2500s, 5000s, and UD 100s.
	Lotensin (Novartis)		Lactose, castor oil. (LOTENSIN 20). Pink. In 100s.
	Benazepril HCl (Various, eg, Ivax, Teva)	20 mg	May contain lactose, maltodextrin. In 100s, 500s, 1000s, 2500s, 5000s, and UD 100s.
	Lotensin (Novartis)		Lactose, castor oil. (LOTENSIN 10). Dark yellow. In 100s.
	Benazepril HCl (Various, eg, Ivax, Teva)	40 mg	May contain lactose, maltodextrin. In 100s, 500s, 1000s, 2500s, 5000s, and UD 100s..
	Lotensin (Novartis)		Lactose. (LOTENSIN 40). Dark rose. In 100s.

For complete prescribing information, refer to the Angiotensin-Converting Enzyme Inhibitors group monograph.

WARNING

When used in pregnancy during the second and third trimesters, ACEIs can cause injury and even death to the developing fetus. When pregnancy is detected, discontinue benazepril as soon as possible (see Warnings).

Indications

➤*Hypertension:* For the treatment of hypertension, alone or in combination with thiazide diuretics.

Administration and Dosage

➤*Approved by the FDA:* June 1991.

➤*Initial dose:* 10 mg once daily for patients not receiving a diuretic.

➤*Maintenance dosage:* 20 to 40 mg/day as a single dose or 2 equally divided doses. The divided regimen is more effective in controlling trough (predosing) blood pressure. Base dosage adjustment on peak (2 to 6 hours after dosing) and trough responses. If a once-daily regimen does not give adequate trough response, consider an increase in dosage or divided administration. A dose of 80 mg gives an increased response; experience is limited. Total daily doses above 80 mg have not been evaluated. If blood pressure is not controlled with benazepril alone, add a diuretic.

➤*Concomitant diuretics:* Symptomatic hypotension may follow the initial dose of benazepril. To reduce this likelihood, discontinue the diuretic 2 to 3 days prior to benazepril therapy. If blood pressure is not controlled, resume diuretic therapy. If the diuretic cannot be discontinued, use an initial dose of 5 mg benazepril.

➤*Renal function impairment:* 5 mg once daily in patients with Ccr less than 30 mL/min/1.73 m^2 (serum creatinine more than 3 mg/dL). Dosage may be titrated upward until blood pressure is controlled or to a maximum of 40 mg/day.

➤*Storage/Stability:* Do not store above 30°C (86°F). Protect from moisture. Dispense in a tight container.

Angiotensin-Converting Enzyme Inhibitors

CAPTOPRIL

Rx	Captopril (Various, eg, Geneva, Mylan, Teva, UDL, Watson, West-Ward)	Tablets: 12.5 mg	In 100s, 500s, 1000s, 5000s, UD 100s, and blister 600s.
Rx	Capoten (Bristol-Myers Squibb)		Lactose. White, oval. In 100s, 1000s, and UD 100s.
Rx	Captopril (Various, eg, Geneva, Mylan, Teva, UDL, Watson, West-Ward)	Tablets: 25 mg	In 100s, 500s, 1000s, 5000s, UD 100s, and blister 600s.
Rx	Capoten (Bristol-Myers Squibb)		Lactose. White, rounded square, quadrisected. In 100s, 1000s, and UD 100s.
Rx	Captopril (Various, eg, Geneva, Mylan, Teva, UDL, Watson, West-Ward)	Tablets: 50 mg	In 100s, 500s, 1000s, 5000s, UD 100s, and blister 600s.
Rx	Capoten (Bristol-Myers Squibb)		Lactose. White, oval. In 100s, 1000s, and UD 100s.
Rx	Captopril (Various, eg, Geneva, Mylan, Teva, UDL, Watson, West-Ward)	Tablets: 100 mg	In 100s, 500s,1000s, UD 100s, and blister 600s.
Rx	Capoten (Bristol-Myers Squibb)		Lactose. White, oval. In 100s.

For complete prescribing information, refer to the Angiotensin-Converting Enzyme Inhibitors group monograph.

> ### WARNING
>
> When used in pregnancy during the second and third trimesters, ACEIs can cause injury and even death to the developing fetus. When pregnancy is detected, discontinue captopril as soon as possible (see Warnings).

Indications

➤*Hypertension:* For the treatment of hypertension, alone or with other antihypertensive agents, especially thiazide-type diuretics. The blood pressure-lowering effects of captopril and thiazides are approximately additive.

Captopril may be used as initial therapy for patients with normal renal function. In patients with impaired renal function, particularly those with collagen vascular disease, reserve captopril for hypertensive patients who have either developed unacceptable side effects on other drugs or have failed to respond satisfactorily to drug combinations.

➤*Heart failure:* For the treatment of CHF usually in combination with diuretics and digitalis. The beneficial effect of captopril in heart failure does not require the presence of digitalis; however, most controlled clinical trial experience with captopril has been in patients receiving digitalis, as well as diuretic treatment.

➤*Left ventricular dysfunction (LVD) post-MI:* To improve survival following MI in clinically stable patients with LVD manifested as ejection fraction up to 40% and to reduce the incidence of overt heart failure and subsequent hospitalizations for CHF in these patients.

➤*Diabetic nephropathy:* For the treatment of diabetic nephropathy (proteinuria more than 500 mg/day) in patients with type 1 insulin-dependent diabetes mellitus and retinopathy.

Administration and Dosage

➤*Approved by the FDA:* 1981.

Individualize dosage. Administer 1 hour before meals.

➤*Hypertension:*

Initial dose – 25 mg 2 or 3 times/day. If possible, discontinue previous antihypertensive drug regimen 1 week before starting captopril. If satisfactory blood pressure reduction is not achieved after 1 or 2 weeks, increase to 50 mg 2 or 3 times/day. Dosage usually does not exceed 50 mg 3 times/day. If blood pressure is not controlled after 1 or 2 weeks at this dose (and patient is not already on a diuretic), add a modest dose of a thiazide diuretic (eg, 25 mg/day hydrochlorothiazide). Increase diuretic dose at 1- to 2-week intervals until highest usual antihypertensive dose is reached. Sodium restriction may be beneficial when captopril is used alone.

If further blood pressure reduction is required, dosage may be increased to 100 mg 2 or 3 times/day and then, if necessary, to 150 mg 2 or 3 times/day (while continuing diuretic). Usual dosage is 25 to 150 mg 2 or 3 times/day. Per JNC 7 guidelines, the usual dose is 25 to 100 mg/day. Do not exceed 450 mg/day.

Accelerated or malignant hypertension – When temporary discontinuation of current antihypertensive therapy is not practical or desirable, or when prompt titration to more normotensive blood pressure levels is indicated, continue diuretic but stop current medication and promptly initiate captopril at 25 mg 2 or 3 times/day under close supervision. Increase dose every 24 hours or less until a satisfactory response is obtained or the maximum dose is reached. In this regimen, a more potent diuretic (eg, furosemide) may be indicated. Beta blockers may be used with captopril, but the effects are less than additive.

➤*Heart failure:* Consider recent diuretic therapy and the possibility of severe salt/volume depletion. In patients with normal or low blood pressure who have been vigorously treated with diuretics and who may be hyponatremic and/or hypovolemic, a starting dose of 6.25 or 12.5 mg 3 times/day may minimize the magnitude or duration of the hypotensive effect. Titrate to usual daily dosage within the next several days.

Usual initial dosage is 25 mg 3 times/day. After 50 mg 3 times/day is reached, delay further dosage increases where possible, for at least 2 weeks to determine if a satisfactory response occurs. Most patients have had a satisfactory clinical improvement at 50 or 100 mg 3 times/day. Do not exceed a daily dose of 450 mg. Generally, use captopril in conjunction with a diuretic and digitalis.

➤*LVD post-MI:* Therapy may be initiated as early as 3 days after an MI. After a single 6.25 mg dose, initiate at 12.5 mg 3 times/day, then increase to 25 mg 3 times/day during the next several days and to a target dose of 50 mg 3 times/day over the next several weeks as tolerated. Other post-MI therapies (eg, thrombolytics, aspirin, beta blockers) may be used concurrently.

➤*Diabetic nephropathy:* Recommended dosage for long-term use is 25 mg 3 times/day. Other antihypertensives (eg, diuretics, beta blockers, centrally acting agents, vasodilators) may be used in conjunction with captopril if additional therapy is required to further lower blood pressure.

➤*Renal function impairment:* Excretion is reduced in patients with impaired renal function; these patients may respond to smaller or less frequent doses. Accordingly, reduce initial daily dosage and use smaller increments for titration, which should be quite slow (1- to 2-week intervals). After the desired therapeutic effect is achieved, slowly back-titrate to the minimal effective dose. When concomitant diuretic therapy is required, a loop diuretic (eg, furosemide), rather than a thiazide diuretic, is preferred in patients with severe renal impairment.

➤*Storage/Stability:* Do not store above 30°C (86°F). Keep bottle tightly closed (protect from moisture).

ENALAPRIL MALEATE

Rx	Enalapril Maleate (Various, eg, Geneva, Mylan, Teva, Watson)	Tablets: 2.5 mg	In 100s and 1000s.
Rx	Vasotec (Biovail)		Lactose. (VASOTEC MSD 14). Yellow, barrel-shape, scored. In 100s, 1000s, 10,000s, unit-of-use 90s, and UD 100s.
Rx	Enalapril Maleate (Various, eg, Geneva, Mylan, Teva, Watson)	Tablets: 5 mg	In 100s and 1000s.
Rx	Vasotec (Biovail)		Lactose. (MSD 712 VASOTEC). White, barrel-shape, scored. In 100s, 1000s,10,000s, unit-of-use 90s, and UD 100s.
Rx	Enalapril Maleate (Various, eg, Geneva, Mylan, Teva, Watson)	Tablets: 10 mg	In 100s and 1000s.
Rx	Vasotec (Biovail)		Lactose. (MSD 713 VASOTEC). Salmon, barrel-shape. In 100s, 1000s, 10,000s, unit-of-use 90s, and UD 100s.
Rx	Enalapril Maleate (Various, eg, Geneva, Mylan, Teva, Watson)	Tablets: 20 mg	In 100s and 1000s.
Rx	Vasotec (Biovail)		Lactose. (MSD 714 VASOTEC). Peach, barrel-shape. In 100s, 1000s, 10,000s, unit-of-use 90s, and UD 100s.
Rx	Enalaprilat (Various, eg, Abbott, Baxter, Bedford	Injection: 1.25 mg enalaprilat/mL	In 1 and 2 mL vials.

ENALAPRIL MALEATE

For complete prescribing information, refer to the Angiotensin-Converting Enzyme Inhibitors group monograph.

WARNING

When used in pregnancy during the second and third trimesters, ACEIs can cause injury and even death to the developing fetus. When pregnancy is detected, discontinue enalapril and enalaprilat injection as soon as possible (see Warnings).

Indications

➤*Hypertension:* For the treatment of hypertension, alone or in combination with other antihypertensive agents, especially thiazide-type diuretics. The blood pressure-lowering effects of enalapril and thiazides are approximately additive.

IV – For the treatment of hypertension when oral therapy is not practical.

➤*Heart failure (oral only):* For the treatment of symptomatic CHF, usually in combination with diuretics and digitalis.

➤*Asymptomatic left ventricular dysfunction (LVD) (oral only):* In clinically stable asymptomatic patients with LVD (ejection fraction up to 35%), enalapril decreases the rate of development of overt heart failure and decreases the incidence of hospitalization for heart failure.

Administration and Dosage

➤*Approved by the FDA:* December 24, 1985.

➤*Oral:*

Hypertension – Initial dosage is 5 mg once a day for patients not on diuretics. Adjust dosage according to blood pressure response. The usual dosage range is 10 to 40 mg/day as a single dose or in 2 divided doses. Per JNC 7 guidelines, the usual dose is 2.5 to 40 mg/day. In some patients treated once daily, the antihypertensive effect may diminish toward the end of the dosing interval. In such patients, consider an increase in dosage or twice-daily administration. If blood pressure is not controlled with enalapril alone, a diuretic may be added.

Concomitant diuretics: Symptomatic hypotension occasionally may occur following the initial dose of enalapril. If possible, discontinue the diuretic for 2 to 3 days before beginning enalapril to reduce the likelihood of hypotension. If blood pressure is not controlled with enalapril alone, diuretics may be resumed.

If the diuretic cannot be discontinued, give an initial dose of 2.5 mg. Keep patient under medical supervision for at least 2 hours and until blood pressure has stabilized for at least an additional hour.

Renal function impairment: Titrate the dosage upward until blood pressure is controlled or until a maximum dosage of 40 mg/day is reached. Use an initial dosage of 5 mg/day in normal renal function and mild impairment (Ccr more than 30 mL/min, serum creatinine up to 3 mg/dL); 2.5 mg/day in moderate to severe renal impairment (Ccr 30 mL/min or less, serum creatinine 3 mg/dL or more); 2.5 mg on the day of dialysis in dialysis patients (adjust dosage on nondialysis days based on blood pressure response).

Heart failure – As adjunctive therapy with diuretics and digitalis, the recommended starting dose is 2.5 mg. After the initial dose, observe the patient for at least 2 hours and until blood pressure has stabilized for at least an additional hour. If possible, reduce the dose of the diuretic, which may diminish the likelihood of hypotension. The appearance of hypotension after the initial enalapril dose does not preclude subsequent careful dose titration with the drug, following effective management of the hypotension. The recommended therapeutic dosing range for the treatment of heart failure is 2.5 to 20 mg/day given twice daily. Titrate doses upward as tolerated over a period of a few days or weeks. The maximum daily dose is 40 mg in divided doses.

Asymptomatic LVD: 2.5 mg twice daily, titrated as tolerated to the targeted daily dose of 20 mg in divided doses. After the initial dose, observe the patient for at least 2 hours and until blood pressure has stabilized for at least an additional hour. If possible, reduce the dose of any concomitant diuretic to diminish the likelihood of hypotension. The appearance of hypotension after the initial enalapril dose does not preclude subsequent careful dose titration with the drug, following effective management of the hypotension.

Renal function impairment in heart failure or hyponatremia: In patients with serum sodium less than 130 mEq/L or with serum creatinine more than 1.6 mg/dL, initiate at 2.5 mg/day under close supervision. The dose may be increased to 2.5 mg twice daily, then 5 mg twice daily and higher as needed, usually at intervals of 4 days or more if, at the time of dosage adjustment, there is not excessive hypotension or significant deterioration of renal function. The maximum daily dose is 40 mg

Pediatric hypertensive patients – The usual recommended starting dose is 0.08 mg/kg (up to 5 mg) once daily. Adjust dosage according to blood pressure response. Doses above 0.58 mg/kg (or in excess of 40 mg) have not been studied in pediatric patients.

Enalapril is not recommended in neonates and in pediatric patients with glomerular filtration rate less than 30 mL/min/1.73 m² as no data are available.

Preparation of suspension (for 200 mL of a 1 mg/mL suspension) – Add 50 mL of *Bicitra* to a polyethylene terephthalate (PET) bottle containing ten 20 mg tablets of enalapril, and shake for at least 2 minutes. Let concentrate stand for 60 minutes. Following the 60-minute hold time, shake the concentrate for an additional minute. Add 150 mL of *Ora-Sweet SF* to the concentrate in the PET bottle, and shake the suspension to disperse the ingredients.

➤*Parenteral (enalaprilat):* For IV administration only.

Hypertension – 1.25 mg every 6 hours IV over 5 minutes. A clinical response is usually seen within 15 minutes. Peak effects after the first dose may not occur for up to 4 hours. The peak effects of subsequent doses may exceed those of the first.

No dosage regimen has clearly shown to be more effective in treating hypertension than 1.25 mg every 6 hours. However, doses as high as 5 mg every 6 hours were well tolerated for up to 36 hours. There is inadequate experience with doses more than 20 mg/day. Patients have received enalaprilat for as long as 7 days.

The dose for patients being converted to IV from oral therapy is 1.25 mg every 6 hours. For conversion from IV to oral therapy, the recommended initial dose is 5 mg once daily.

Concomitant diuretics: Starting dose for hypertension is 0.625 mg IV over 5 minutes. Clinical response is usually seen within 15 minutes. Peak effects after the first dose may not occur for up to 4 hours, although most of the effect is usually apparent within the first hour. If there is inadequate clinical response after 1 hour, repeat the 0.625 mg dose. Give additional doses of 1.25 mg at 6-hour intervals.

For conversion from IV to oral therapy, the recommended initial dosage of enalapril maleate tablets for patients who have responded to 0.625 mg enalaprilat every 6 hours is 2.5 mg/day with subsequent dosage adjustment as necessary.

High-risk patients – Hypertensive patients at risk of excessive hypotension include those with the following concurrent conditions or characteristics: Heart failure, hyponatremia, high-dose diuretic therapy, recent intensive diuresis or increase in diuretic dose, renal dialysis, or severe volume or salt depletion of any etiology. Single doses of enalaprilat as low as 0.2 mg have produced excessive hypotension in normotensive patients with these diagnoses. Because of the potential for an extreme hypotensive response in these patients, initiate therapy under very close medical supervision. The starting dose should be no greater than 0.625 mg administered IV over a period of 5 minutes or more and preferably longer (up to 1 hour).

Renal function impairment – Administer 1.25 mg every 6 hours for patients with Ccr more than 30 mL/min (serum creatinine about 3 mg/dL). For Ccr 30 mL/min or less (serum creatinine 3 mg/dL or more), the initial dose is 0.625 mg. If there is inadequate clinical response after 1 hour, the 0.625 mg dose may be repeated. May give additional 1.25 mg doses at 6-hour intervals. For dialysis patients, the initial dose is 0.625 mg or less administered over 5 minutes or more preferably longer (up to 1 hour).

For conversion from IV to oral therapy, the recommended initial dose of enalapril maleate tablets is 5 mg once daily for patients with Ccr more than 30 mL/min and 2.5 mg once daily for patients with Ccr 30 mL/min or less. Then, adjust dosage according to blood pressure response.

Administration – Give as a slow IV infusion, as indicated above, over 5 minutes or more. It may be used as provided or diluted with up to 50 mL of a compatible diluent.

➤*Storage/Stability:*

Tablets – Store below 30°C (86°F) and avoid transient temperatures more than 50°C (122°F). Keep container tightly closed. Protect from moisture. Dispense in tight container if package is subdivided.

Suspension – Refrigerate the suspension at 2° to 8°C (36° to 46°F). The suspension can be stored for up to 30 days. Shake the suspension before each use.

IV – Store below 30°C (86°F). Enalaprilat as supplied and mixed with the following IV diluents has been found to maintain full activity for 24 hours at room temperature: 5% dextrose injection; 0.9% sodium chloride injection; 0.9% sodium chloride injection in 5% dextrose; 5% dextrose in Lactated Ringer's injection; *McGaw Isolyte E.*

FOSINOPRIL SODIUM

Rx	Fosinopril Sodium (Teva)	Tablets: 10 mg	Isopropyl alcohol, lactose. (9 3 72 22). White to off-white, rectangular, scored. In 90s and 1000s.
Rx	Monopril (Bristol-Myers Squibb)		Lactose. (BMS MONOPRIL 10). White to off-white, biconvex flat-end, diamond shape, scored. In 90s and 1000s.
Rx	Fosinopril Sodium (Teva)	Tablets: 20 mg	Isopropyl alcohol, lactose. (93 7223). White to off-white, capsule shape, scored. In 90s and 1000s.
Rx	Monopril (Bristol-Myers Squibb)		Lactose. (BMS MONOPRIL 20). White to off-white, oval. In 90s, 1000s, and UD 100s.
Rx	Fosinopril Sodium (Teva)	Tablets: 40 mg	Isopropyl alcohol, lactose. (93 7224). White to off-white, round, scored. In 90s and 1000s.
Rx	Monopril (Bristol-Myers Squibb)		Lactose. (BMS MONOPRIL 40). White to off-white, biconvex hexagonal. In 90s.

For complete prescribing information, refer to the Angiotensin-Converting Enzyme Inhibitors group monograph.

WARNING

When used in pregnancy during the second and third trimesters, ACEIs can cause injury and even death to the developing fetus. When pregnancy is detected, discontinue fosinopril as soon as possible (see Warnings).

Indications

►*Hypertension:* For the treatment of hypertension, alone or in combination with thiazide diuretics.

►*Heart failure:* For the management of heart failure as adjunctive therapy when added to conventional therapy, including diuretics with or without digitalis.

Administration and Dosage

►*Approved by the FDA:* 1991.

►*Hypertension:*

Initial dosage – 10 mg once daily. Adjust according to blood pressure response at peak (2 to 6 hours) and trough (about 24 hours after dosing) blood levels.

Maintenance dosage – Usual range needed to maintain a response is 20 to 40 mg/day, but some patients appear to have a further response to 80 mg. In some patients treated with once-daily dosing, the antihypertensive effect may diminish toward the end of the dosing interval. If trough response is inadequate, consider dividing the daily dose. If blood pressure is not adequately controlled with fosinopril alone, a diuretic may be added.

Concomitant diuretics – Symptomatic hypotension may occur following the initial dose. To reduce the likelihood of this effect, discontinue the diuretic 2 to 3 days prior to beginning fosinopril if possible. If blood pressure is not controlled, resume diuretic therapy. If diuretic cannot be discontinued, use an initial dose of 10 mg fosinopril.

►*Heart failure:* Digitalis is not required for fosinopril to manifest improvements in exercise tolerance and symptoms. Most placebo controlled clinical trial experience has been with digitalis and diuretics present as background therapy.

The usual starting dose of fosinopril is 10 mg once daily. Following the initial dose, observe the patient under medical supervision for at least 2 hours for the presence of hypotension or orthostasis and, if either is present, until blood pressure stabilizes. An initial dose of 5 mg is preferred in heart failure patients with moderate to severe renal failure or in those who have been vigorously diuresed.

Increase dosage over a several-week period to a dose that is maximal and tolerated but not exceeding 40 mg once daily. The usual effective dosage range is 20 to 40 mg once daily.

The appearance of hypotension, orthostasis, or azotemia early in dose titration should not preclude further careful dose titration. Consider reducing the dose of concomitant diuretic.

►*Renal function impairment:* In impaired renal function, the total body clearance of fosinoprilat is about 50% slower than that in normal renal function. Because hepatobiliary elimination partially compensates for diminished renal elimination, the total body clearance of fosinoprilat does not differ appreciably with any degree of renal insufficiency (Ccr less than 80 mL/min/1.73 m^2), including end-stage renal failure (Ccr less than 10 mL/min/1.73 m^2). This relative constancy of body clearance of active fosinoprilat, resulting from the dual route of elimination, permits use of the usual dose in any degree of renal impairment.

►*Storage/Stability:* Store at 25°C (77°F); excursions permitted to 15° to 30°C (59° to 86°F). Protect from moisture by keeping bottle tightly closed.

LISINOPRIL

Rx	Lisinopril (Various, eg, Apotex, Geneva, Mylan, Teva, Watson)	Tablets: 2.5 mg	In 100s, 500s, and 1000s.
Rx	Prinivil (Merck)		Mannitol. (MSD 15). White, flat-faced, beveled edge. In unit-of-use 30s, 100s, and UD 100s.
Rx	Zestril (AstraZeneca)		Mannitol. (ZESTRIL 2½ 135). White. In 100s.
Rx	Lisinopril (Various, eg, Apotex, Geneva, Mylan, Teva, Watson)	Tablets: 5 mg	In 100s and 1000s.
Rx	Prinivil (Merck)		Mannitol. (MSD 19 PRINIVIL). White, shield shape, scored. In 1000s, 10,000s, unit-of-use 90s and 100s, UD 100s, and blister pack 31s.
Rx	Zestril (AstraZeneca)		Mannitol. (ZESTRIL 130). Pink, capsule shape, bisected. In 100s and UD 100s.
Rx	Lisinopril (Various, eg, Apotex, Geneva, Mylan, Teva, Watson)	Tablets: 10 mg	In 100s and 1000s.
Rx	Prinivil (Merck)		Mannitol. (MSD 106 PRINIVIL). Light yellow, shield shape. In 1000s, 10,000s, unit-of-use 30s, 90s, 100s, UD 100s, and blister pack 31s.
Rx	Zestril (AstraZeneca)		Mannitol. (ZESTRIL 10 131). Pink. In 100s and UD 100s.
Rx	Lisinopril (Various, eg, Apotex, Geneva, Mylan, Teva, Watson)	Tablets: 20 mg	In 100s and 1000s.
Rx	Prinivil (Merck)		Mannitol. (MSD 207 PRINIVIL). Peach, shield shape. In 1000s, 10,000s, unit-of-use 30s, 90s, and 100s, UD 100s, and blister pack 31s.
Rx	Zestril (AstraZeneca)		Mannitol. (ZESTRIL 20 132). Red. In 100s and UD 100s.
Rx	Lisinopril (Various, eg, Apotex, Geneva, Mylan, Teva, Watson)	Tablets: 30 mg	In 100s, 500s, and 1000s.
Rx	Zestril (AstraZeneca)		Mannitol. (ZESTRIL 30 133). Red. In 100s.
Rx	Lisinopril (Various, eg, Apotex, Geneva, Mylan, Teva, Watson)	Tablets: 40 mg	In 100s, 500s, 1000s, and UD 100s.
Rx	Prinivil (Merck)		Mannitol. (MSD 237 Prinivil). Rose red, shield shape. In unit-of-use 100s.
Rx	Zestril (AstraZeneca)		Mannitol. (ZESTRIL 40 134). Yellow. In 100s.

For complete prescribing information, refer to the Angiotensin-Converting Enzyme Inhibitors group monograph.

LISINOPRIL

WARNING

When used in pregnancy during the second and third trimesters, ACEIs can cause injury and even death to the developing fetus. When pregnancy is detected, discontinue lisinopril as soon as possible (see Warnings).

Indications

➤*Hypertension:* For the treatment of hypertension. May be used alone as initial therapy or concomitantly with other classes of antihypertensive agents.

➤*Heart failure:* As adjunctive therapy in the management of heart failure in patients not responding adequately to diuretics and digitalis.

➤*Acute MI:* For the treatment of hemodynamically stable patients within 24 hours of acute MI to improve survival. Patients should receive, as appropriate, the standard recommended treatments such as thrombolytics, aspirin, and beta blockers.

Administration and Dosage

➤*Approved by the FDA:* December 29, 1987.

➤*Hypertension:*

Initial therapy – 10 mg once daily in patients with uncomplicated essential hypertension not on diuretic therapy. Usual once daily dosage range is 20 to 40 mg/day. Antihypertensive effect may diminish toward the end of the dosing interval most commonly with a dose of 10 mg/day. Measure blood pressure just prior to dosing to determine whether satisfactory control is being maintained for 24 hours. If it is not, consider an increase in dose. Doses up to 80 mg have been used but do not appear to give a greater effect. If blood pressure is not controlled with lisinopril alone, a low dose of a diuretic may be added (eg, 12.5 mg hydrochlorothiazide). After addition of a diuretic, it may be possible to reduce the dose of lisinopril.

Renal function impairment – Initiate lisinopril daily dosage according to the following chart. For hypertension, titrate dosage upward until blood pressure is controlled or to a maximum of 40 mg/day.

Lisinopril Dosage in Renal Impairment			
Renal status	Creatinine clearance (mL/min)	Serum creatinine (mg/dL)	Initial dose (mg/day)
Normal function to mild impairment	> 30	≤ 3	10
Moderate to severe impairment	≥ 10 to ≤ 30	≥ 3	5
Dialysis patients	< 10	—	2.5[1]

[1] Adjust dosage or dosing interval depending on the blood pressure response.

Concomitant diuretics – Symptomatic hypotension may occur occasionally following the initial dose of lisinopril. If possible, discontinue the diuretic for 2 to 3 days before beginning therapy with lisinopril to reduce the likelihood of hypotension (see Warnings). If the patient's blood pressure is not controlled with lisinopril alone, resume diuretic therapy as above. If the diuretic cannot be discontinued, use an initial dose of 5 mg and monitor for at least 2 hours and until blood pressure has stabilized for at least an additional hour.

➤*Heart failure:*

Initial dose – 5 mg once daily with diuretics and digitalis. When initiating treatment, give under medical observation, especially in patients with low blood pressure (systolic less than 100 mm Hg). The mean peak blood pressure lowering occurs 6 to 8 hours after dosing. Continue observation until blood pressure is stable. If possible, reduce concomitant diuretic dose to help minimize hypovolemia, which may contribute to hypotension. Appearance of hypotension after the initial dose does not preclude subsequent careful dose titration following effective hypotension management. The usual effective dosage range is 5 to 20 mg/day as a single dose.

Renal function impairment or hyponatremia – In patients with heart failure who have hyponatremia (serum sodium less than 130 mEq/L) or moderate to severe renal impairment (Ccr 30 mL/min or less or serum creatinine more than 3 mg/dL), initiate at a dose of 2.5 mg once daily under close supervision.

➤*Acute MI:* In hemodynamically stable patients, the first dose is 5 mg within 24 hours of the onset of symptoms of acute MI, followed by 5 mg after 24 hours, 10 mg after 48 hours, and then 10 mg once daily. Continue dosing for 6 weeks. Patients should receive, as appropriate, the standard recommended treatments such as thrombolytics, aspirin, and beta blockers. Give a lower 2.5 mg dose to patients with a low systolic blood pressure (120 mm Hg or less) when treatment is started or during the first 3 days after the infarct. If hypotension occurs (systolic blood pressure 100 mm Hg or less), a daily maintenance dose of 5 mg may be given with temporary reductions to 2.5 mg if needed. If prolonged hypotension occurs (systolic blood pressure less than 90 mm Hg for less than 1 hour), withdraw lisinopril. For patients who develop symptoms of heart failure, see Administration and Dosage for heart failure.

Renal function impairment – In acute MI, initiate lisinopril with caution in patients with evidence of renal dysfunction, defined as serum creatinine concentration exceeding 2 mg/dL.

➤*Elderly:* In general, blood pressure response and adverse experiences are similar in younger and older patients given similar doses of lisinopril. However, maximum blood levels and AUC are doubled in older patients. Make dosage adjustments with particular caution.

➤*Pediatric hypertensive patients 6 years of age and older:* The usual recommended starting dose is 0.07 mg/kg once daily (up to 5 mg total). Adjust dose according to blood pressure response. Doses above 0.61 mg/kg (or in excess of 40 mg) have not been studied in pediatric patients. Lisinopril is not recommended in pediatric patients less than 6 years of age or in pediatric patients with glomerular filtration rate less than 30 mL/min/1.73 m^2.

➤*Preparation of suspension (for 200 mL of a 1 mg/mL suspension):* Add 10 mL of purified water to a polyethylene terephthalate (PET) bottle containing ten 20 mg tablets of lisinopril and shake for at least 1 minute. Add 30 mL of *Bicitra* diluent and 160 mL of *Ora-Sweet SF* to the concentrate in the PET bottle, and gently shake for several seconds to disperse the ingredients. Store the suspension at or below 25°C (77°F) for up to 4 weeks. Shake the suspension before each use.

➤*Storage/Stability:* Store at controlled room temperature 15° to 30°C (59° to 86°F), and protect from moisture.

MOEXIPRIL HCl

Rx	**Moexipril HCl** (Teva)	**Tablets:** 7.5 mg	Lactose. (17). Pink, oval. Film-coated. In 100s.
Rx	**Univasc** (Schwarz Pharma)		Lactose. (707 SP 7.5). Pink, scored. Film-coated. In 100s and unit-of-use 90s.
Rx	**Moexipril HCl** (Teva)	**Tablets:** 15 mg	Lactose. (5150 93). Pink, oval. Film-coated. In 100s.
Rx	**Univasc** (Schwarz Pharma)		Lactose. (715 SP 15). Salmon, scored. Film-coated. In 100s and unit-of-use 90s.

For complete prescribing information, refer to the Angiotensin-Converting Enzyme Inhibitors group monograph.

WARNING

When used in pregnancy during the second and third trimesters, ACEIs can cause injury and death to the developing fetus. When pregnancy is detected, discontinue moexipril as soon as possible (see Warnings).

Indications

➤*Hypertension:* For the treatment of hypertension, alone or in combination with thiazide diuretics.

Administration and Dosage

➤*Approved by the FDA:* April 19, 1995.

➤*Initial dosage:* In patients not receiving diuretics, 7.5 mg 1 hour prior to a meal once daily. Adjust according to blood pressure response. The antihypertensive effect may diminish towards the end of the dosing interval. Measure blood pressure just prior to dosing to determine whether satisfactory blood pressure control is obtained. If control is not adequate, increase the dose or divide the dosing.

➤*Maintenance dosage:* 7.5 to 30 mg/day in 1 or 2 divided doses, 1 hour before meals. Total daily dosages greater than 60 mg/day have not been studied in hypertensive patients.

➤*Concomitant diuretics:* Symptomatic hypotension may occur after the initial dose of moexipril. To reduce risk of this effect, discontinue diuretic 2 to 3 days prior to beginning moexipril, if possible. If blood pressure is not controlled, resume diuretic therapy. If diuretic cannot be discontinued, use an initial dose of 3.75 mg moexipril.

➤*Renal function impairment:* Cautiously use an initial dose of 3.75 mg once daily in patients with Ccr up to 40 mL/min/1.73 m^2. Dosage may be titrated upward to a maximum of 15 mg/day.

➤*Storage/Stability:* Store tightly closed at controlled room temperature (20° to 25°C; 68° to 77°F). Protect from excessive moisture.

Angiotensin-Converting Enzyme Inhibitors

PERINDOPRIL ERBUMINE

Rx	Aceon (Solvay Pharm.)	Tablets: 2 mg	Lactose. (ACN 2 SLV SLV). White, oblong, scored. In 100s.
		4 mg	Lactose. (ACN 4 SLV SLV). Pink, oblong, scored. In 100s.
		8 mg	Lactose. (ACN 8 SLV SLV). Salmon, oblong, scored. In 100s.

For complete prescribing information, refer to the Angiotensin-Converting Enzyme Inhibitors group monograph.

WARNING

When used in pregnancy during the second and third trimesters, ACEIs can cause injury and even death to the developing fetus. When pregnancy is detected, discontinue perindopril as soon as possible (see Warnings).

Indications

➤*Hypertension:* For the treatment of patients with essential hypertension. It may be used alone or given with other classes of antihypertensives, especially thiazide diuretics.

Administration and Dosage

➤*Approved by the FDA:* December 1993.

➤*Use in uncomplicated hypertensive patients:* In patients with essential hypertension, the recommended initial dose is 4 mg once daily. The dosage may be titrated upward until blood pressure, when measured just before the next dose, is controlled or to a maximum of 16 mg/day. The usual maintenance dose range is 4 to 8 mg administered as a single daily dose. It also may be administered in 2 divided doses. When once-daily dosing was compared with twice-daily dosing in clinical studies, the twice-daily regimen generally was slightly superior, but not by more than about 0.5 to 1 mm Hg.

➤*Elderly:* As in younger patients, the recommended initial dosages for the elderly (older than 65 years of age) is 4 mg/day in 1 or 2 divided doses. The daily dosage may be titrated upward until blood pressure, when measured just before the next dose, is controlled, but experience with perindopril is limited in the elderly at doses exceeding 8 mg. Administer dosages above 8 mg cautiously and under close medical supervision.

➤*Concomitant diuretics:* If blood pressure is not adequately controlled with perindopril alone, a diuretic may be added. In patients currently being treated with a diuretic, symptomatic hypotension occasionally can occur following the initial dose of perindopril. To reduce likelihood of such a reaction, the diuretic should, if possible, be discontinued 2 to 3 days prior to beginning perindopril therapy. Then, if blood pressure is not controlled with perindopril alone, resume the diuretic.

If the diuretic cannot be discontinued, use an initial dose of 2 to 4 mg/day in 1 or 2 divided doses with careful medical supervision for several hours and until blood pressure has stabilized. Titrate the dosage as described above.

➤*Renal function impairment:* Perindoprilat elimination is decreased in renally impaired patients, with a marked increase in accumulation when Ccr drops below 30 mL/min. In patients with Ccr below 30 mL/min, safety and efficacy have not been established. For patients with lesser degrees of impairment (Ccr above 30 mL/min), the initial dosage should be 2 mg/day, and dosage should not exceed 8 mg/day because of limited clinical experience. During dialysis, perindopril is removed with the same clearance as in patients with normal renal function.

➤*Storage/Stability:* Store at controlled room temperature 20° to 25°C (68° to 77°F). Protect from moisture.

QUINAPRIL HCl

Rx	Accupril (Pfizer)	Tablets: 5 mg	Lactose. (PD 527 5). Brown, elliptical, scored. Film-coated. In 90s and UD 100s.
		10 mg	Lactose. (PD 530 10). Brown, triangular. Film-coated. In 90s and UD 100s.
		20 mg	Lactose. (PD 532 20). Brown. Film-coated. In 90s and UD 100s.
		40 mg	Lactose. (PD 535 40). Brown, elliptical. Film-coated. In 90s.

For complete prescribing information, refer to the Angiotensin-Converting Enzyme Inhibitors group monograph.

WARNING

When used in pregnancy during the second and third trimesters, ACEIs can cause injury and even death to the developing fetus. When pregnancy is detected, discontinue quinapril as soon as possible (see Warnings).

Indications

➤*Hypertension:* For the treatment of hypertension, alone or in combination with thiazide diuretics.

➤*Heart failure:* As adjunctive therapy in the management of heart failure when added to conventional therapy including diuretics and/or digitalis.

Administration and Dosage

➤*Approved by the FDA:* November 1991.

➤*Hypertension:*

Initial dose – 10 or 20 mg once daily for patients not on diuretics. Adjust according to blood pressure response at peak (2 to 6 hours) and trough (predose) blood levels. Adjust dosage at intervals of 2 weeks or more.

Maintenance dosage – Most patients require 20, 40, or 80 mg/day as a single dose or in 2 equally divided doses. Per JNC 7 guidelines, the usual dose is 10 to 40 mg/day. With once-daily dosing, the antihypertensive effect may diminish toward the end of the dosing interval; an increase in dosage or twice-daily administration may be warranted. In general, doses of 40 to 80 mg and divided doses give a somewhat greater effect at the end of the dosing interval.

Concomitant diuretics – If blood pressure is not adequately controlled with quinapril monotherapy, a diuretic may be added. In patients currently being treated with a diuretic, symptomatic hypotension may occur following the initial dose of quinapril. To reduce the likelihood of this effect, discontinue the diuretic 2 to 3 days prior to quinapril therapy if possible. If blood pressure is not controlled, resume diuretic therapy. If the diuretic cannot be discontinued, use an initial dose of 5 mg quinapril with careful supervision for several hours until blood pressure stabilizes.

Elderly (65 years of age and older) – 10 mg once daily followed by titration to the optimal response (see above).

Renal function impairment – Initial dose is 10 mg with Ccr above 60 mL/min, 5 mg with Ccr 30 to 60 mL/min, or 2.5 mg with Ccr 10 to 30 mL/min. There are insufficient data for dosage recommendation in patients with Ccr less than 10 mL/min.

Patients should subsequently have their dosage titrated (as directed above) to the optimal response.

➤*Heart failure:* The recommended starting dose is 5 mg twice daily. This dose may improve symptoms of heart failure, but increases in exercise duration have generally required higher doses. Therefore, if the initial dose is well tolerated, titrate dosage at weekly intervals until an effective dose, usually 20 to 40 mg/day given in 2 equally divided doses, is reached or undesirable hypotension, orthostasis, or azotemia prohibit reaching this dose.

Following the initial dose, observe the patient under medical supervision for at least 2 hours for the presence of hypotension or orthostasis and, if present, until blood pressure stabilizes. The appearance of hypotension, orthostasis, or azotemia early in dose titration should not preclude further careful dose titration. Consider reducing the dose of concomitant diuretics.

Renal function impairment or hyponatremia – Quinapril elimination is dependent on the level of renal function. In patients with heart failure and renal impairment, the recommended initial dose is 5 mg with Ccr above 30 mL/min or 2.5 mg with Ccr 10 to 30 mL/min. There are insufficient data for dosage recommendation in patients with Ccr less than 10 mL/min.

If the initial dose is well tolerated, quinapril may be given the following day as a twice-daily regimen. In the absence of excessive hypotension or significant deterioration of renal function, the dose may be increased at weekly intervals based on clinical and hemodynamic response.

➤*Storage/Stability:* Store at controlled room temperature 15° to 30°C (59° to 86°F). Protect from light.

RAMIPRIL

Rx	Altace (Monarch)	Capsules: 1.25 mg	Gelatin. Yellow. In 100s and UD 100s.
		2.5 mg	Gelatin. Orange. In 100s, 500s, 1000s, UD 100s, and bulk pack 5000s.
		5 mg	Gelatin. Red. In 100s, 500s, 1000s, UD 100s, and bulk pack 5000s.
		10 mg	Gelatin. Blue. In 100s, 500s, and 1000s.

For complete prescribing information, refer to the Angiotensin-Converting Enzyme Inhibitors group monograph.

WARNING

When used in pregnancy during the second and third trimesters, ACEIs can cause injury and even death to the developing fetus. When pregnancy is detected, discontinue ramipril as soon as possible (see Warnings).

Indications

▶*Reduction in risk of MI, stroke, and death from cardiovascular causes:* In patients 55 years of age and older at high risk of developing a major cardiovascular event because of a history of coronary artery disease, stroke, peripheral vascular disease, or diabetes that is accompanied by at least 1 other cardiovascular risk factor (eg, hypertension, elevated total cholesterol levels, low HDL levels, cigarette smoking, documented microalbuminuria), to reduce the risk of MI, stroke, or death from cardiovascular causes. Can also be used in addition to other needed treatment (eg, antihypertensive, antiplatelet, or lipid-lowering therapy).

▶*Hypertension:* For the treatment of hypertension, alone or in combination with thiazide diuretics.

▶*Heart failure post-MI:* For stable patients who have shown clinical signs of CHF within the first few days after sustaining acute MI.

Administration and Dosage

▶*Approved by the FDA:* January 28, 1991.

Blood pressure decreases associated with any dose of ramipril depend, in part, on the presence or absence of volume depletion (eg, past and current diuretic use) or the presence or absence of renal artery stenosis. If such circumstances are suspected to be present, the initial starting dose should be 1.25 mg once daily.

▶*Reduction in risk of MI, stroke, and death from cardiovascular causes:*

Initial dose – 2.5 mg once daily for 1 week, 5 mg once daily for the next 3 weeks, and then increased as tolerated to maintenance dose.

Maintenance dosage – 10 mg once daily. If the patient is hypertensive or recently post-MI, it also can be given as a divided dose.

▶*Hypertension:*

Initial dose – 2.5 mg once daily in patients not receiving a diuretic. Adjust according to blood pressure response.

Maintenance dosage – 2.5 to 20 mg/day as a single dose or in 2 equally divided doses. If the antihypertensive effect diminishes at the end of the dosing interval with once-daily use, consider twice-daily administration or an increase in dosage. If blood pressure is not controlled with ramipril alone, a diuretic can be added.

▶*Heart failure post-MI:* Starting dose is 2.5 mg twice daily (5 mg/day). A patient who becomes hypotensive at this dose may be switched to 1.25 mg twice daily, and after 1 week at the starting dose, titrate patients (if tolerated) toward a target dose of 5 mg twice daily, with dosage increases being about 3 weeks apart. After the initial dose, observe the patient for at least 2 hours and until blood pressure has stabilized for at least an additional hour. If possible, reduce the dose of any concomitant diuretic.

▶*Renal function impairment:* In patients with Ccr of 40 mL/min/1.73 m^2 or less (serum creatinine approximately 2.5 mg/dL or more) doses only 25% of those normally used should be expected to induce full therapeutic levels of ramiprilat.

Hypertension – Start with 1.25 mg once daily. Dosage may be titrated upward until blood pressure is controlled or to a maximum of 5 mg/day.

Heart failure post-MI – Start with 1.25 mg once daily. The dose may be increased to 1.25 mg twice daily and up to a maximum dose of 2.5 mg twice daily depending upon clinical response and tolerability.

▶*Concomitant diuretics:* Symptomatic hypotension may occur after the initial dose of ramipril. To reduce the likelihood of this effect, discontinue diuretic 2 to 3 days prior to beginning ramipril if possible. If blood pressure is not controlled, resume diuretic therapy. If the diuretic cannot be discontinued, use an initial dose of 1.25 mg ramipril.

▶*Administration:* Ramipril capsules are usually swallowed whole. However, the capsules may be opened and the contents sprinkled on a small amount (about 4 oz) of applesauce or mixed in 4 oz apple juice or water. The mixture should be consumed in its entirety.

▶*Storage / Stability:* Store at controlled room temperature (59° to 86°F).

Pre-prepared mixtures can be stored for up to 24 hours at room temperature or for up to 48 hours under refrigeration.

TRANDOLAPRIL

Rx	Mavik (Abbott)	Tablets: 1 mg	Lactose. (FT). Salmon, scored. In 100s and UD 100s.
		2 mg	Lactose. (FX). Yellow. In 100s and UD 100s.
		4 mg	Lactose. (FZ). Rose. In 100s and UD 100s.

For complete prescribing information, refer to the Angiotensin-Converting Enzyme Inhibitors group monograph.

WARNING

When used in pregnancy during the second and third trimesters, ACEIs can cause injury and even death to the developing fetus. When pregnancy is detected, discontinue trandolapril as soon as possible (see Warnings).

Indications

▶*Hypertension:* For the treatment of hypertension, alone or in combination with other antihypertensive medications, such as hydrochlorothiazide.

▶*Heart failure post-MI/left-ventricular dysfunction post-MI:* For stable patients who have evidence of left-ventricular systolic dysfunction (identified by wall motion abnormalities) or who are symptomatic from CHF within the first few days after sustaining acute MI.

Administration and Dosage

▶*Approved by the FDA:* April 26, 1996.

▶*Hypertension:*

Initial dose – 1 mg/day (2 mg/day in black patients) for patients not receiving a diuretic. Adjust dosage according to the blood pressure response. Make dosage adjustments at intervals of at least 1 week. Most patients have required dosages of 2 to 4 mg/day. There is little experience with doses more than 8 mg.

Maintenance dose – Patients inadequately treated with once-daily dosing at 4 mg may be treated with twice-daily dosing. If blood pressure is not adequately controlled with trandolapril monotherapy, a diuretic may be added.

Concomitant diuretics – In patients being treated with a diuretic, symptomatic hypotension occasionally can occur following the initial dose of trandolapril. To reduce the likelihood of hypotension, discontinue the diuretic 2 to 3 days prior to beginning therapy with trandolapril if possible. If blood pressure is not controlled with trandolapril alone, resume diuretic therapy. If the diuretic cannot be discontinued, give an initial dose of 0.5 mg trandolapril with careful medical supervision for several hours until blood pressure has stabilized. Titrate dosage as described above to optimal response.

▶*Heart failure post-MI or left-ventricular dysfunction post-MI:* The recommended starting dosage is 1 mg/day. Following the initial dose, titrate patients (as tolerated) toward a target dosage of 4 mg/day. If a 4 mg dose is not tolerated, patients can continue therapy with the greatest tolerated dose.

▶*Renal / hepatic function impairment:* For patients with a Ccr less than 30 mL/min or with hepatic cirrhosis, the recommended starting dosage is 0.5 mg/day. Titrate dosage as described above to optimal response.

▶*Storage / Stability:* Store at controlled room temperature (20° to 25°C; 68° to 77°F).

Angiotensin II Receptor Antagonists

Indications

➤*Hypertension:* For the treatment of hypertension, alone or in combination with other antihypertensive agents.

➤*Nephropathy in type 2 diabetics (losartan and irbesartan):* For the treatment of diabetic nephropathy with an elevated serum creatinine and proteinuria (urinary albumin to creatinine ratio 300 mg/g or more with losartan; greater than 300 mg/day with irbesartan) in patients with type 2 diabetes and a history of hypertension. In this population, losartan and irbesartan reduce the rate of progression of nephropathy as measured by the occurrence of doubling of serum creatinine or end stage renal disease (need for dialysis or renal transplantation).

➤*Heart failure (valsartan):* For the treatment of heart failure (NYHA class II to IV) in patients who are intolerant of angiotensin-converting enzyme inhibitors (ACEIs).

➤*Hypertension with left ventricular hypertrophy (losartan):* To reduce the risk of stroke in patients with hypertension and left ventricular hypertrophy, but there is evidence that this benefit does not apply to black patients.

Actions

➤*Pharmacology:* **Candesartan, eprosartan, irbesartan, losartan, olmesartan, telmisartan,** and **valsartan** are angiotensin II receptor (type AT$_1$) antagonists. Angiotensin II (formed from angiotensin I in a reaction catalyzed by angiotensin-converting enzyme [ACE; kininase II]) is a potent vasoconstrictor, the primary vasoactive hormone of the renin-angiotensin system, and an important component in the pathophysiology of hypertension. Its effects are vasoconstriction, stimulation of synthesis and release of aldosterone, cardiac stimulation, and renal re-absorption of sodium. AIIRAs block the vasoconstrictor and aldosterone-secreting effects of angiotensin II by selectively blocking the binding of angiotensin II to the AT$_1$ receptor in many tissues (eg, vascular smooth muscle, adrenal gland). There is also an AT$_2$ receptor in many tissues, but it is not known to be associated with cardiovascular homeostasis. AIIRAs have much greater affinity (greater than 10,000-fold, candesartan; 1000 times greater, eprosartan; greater than 8500-fold, irbesartan; approximately 1000-fold, losartan; greater than 12,500-fold, olmesartan; greater than 3000-fold, telmisartan; approximately 20,000-fold, valsartan) for the AT$_1$ than for the AT$_2$ receptor and do not exhibit any agonist activity. In vitro binding studies indicate that losartan is a reversible, competitive inhibitor of the AT$_1$ receptor. The active metabolite is 10 to 40 times more potent by weight than losartan and appears to be a reversible, non-competitive inhibitor of the AT$_1$ receptor. The primary metabolite of valsartan is essentially inactive with an affinity for the AT$_1$ receptor approximately 1/200 of valsartan itself.

AIIRAs do not inhibit ACE (kininase II, the enzyme that converts angiotensin I to angiotensin II and degrades bradykinin), nor do they bind to or block other hormone receptors or ion channels known to be important in cardiovascular regulation.

AIIRAs inhibit the pressor effect of angiotensin II (as well as angiotensin I) infusions. Removal of the negative feedback of angiotensin II causes a 2- to 3-fold rise in plasma renin activity and a consequent rise in angiotensin II plasma concentration in hypertensive patients. The resulting increased plasma renin activity and angiotensin II circulating levels are insufficient to alter the effects of AIIRAs on blood pressure. AIIRAs do not affect the response to bradykinin, whereas ACE inhibitors do increase the response. AIIRAs have very little effect on serum potassium. There was a small uricosuric effect with losartan leading to a minimal decrease in serum uric acid (mean decrease less than 0.4 mg/dL) during chronic oral administration.

➤*Pharmacokinetics:*

Angiotensin II Antagonist Pharmacokinetics

Parameters	Candesartan	Eprosartan	Irbesartan	Losartan (metabolite)[1]	Olmesartan	Telmisartan	Valsartan
Bioavailability	≈ 15%	≈ 13%	60% to 80%	≈ 33%	≈ 26%	42%/58% (40 mg/160 mg)	≈ 25%
Food effect (AUC/C$_{max}$)	no effect	↓< 25%	no effect	↓10%/↓14%	no effect	↓6%/↓20% (40 mg AUC/ 160 mg AUC)	↓40%/↓50%
Plasma bound	> 99%	≈ 98%	90%	98.7% (99.8%)	99%	> 99.5%	95%
T$_{max}$	3 to 4 hr	1 to 2 hr	1.5 to 2 hr	1 hr (3 to 4 hr)	1 to 2 hr	0.5 to 1 hr	2 to 4 hr
Volume of distribution	0.13 L/kg	308 L	53 to 93 L	≈ 34 L (≈ 12 L)	≈ 17L	≈ 500 L	17 L[2]
Converted to metabolites	minor	minor	< 20%	≈ 14%	none	≈ 11%	≈ 20%
Metabolism	O-deethylation	glucuronidation	CYP2C9	CYP2C9; CYP3A4	none	conjugation	unknown
Terminal half-life	≈ 9 hr	5 to 9 hr	11 to 15 hr	≈ 2 hr (6 to 9 hr)	≈ 13 hr	≈ 24 hr	≈ 6 hr[2]
Total plasma clearance	0.37 mL/min/kg	≈ 130 mL/min[2]	157 to 176 mL/min	≈ 600 mL/min (≈ 50 mL/min)	1.3 L/h	> 800 mL/min	≈ 2 L/hr[2]
Renal clearance	0.19 mL/min/kg	≈30 to 40 mL/min	3 to 3.5 mL/min	≈ 75 mL/min (≈ 25 mL/min)	0.6 L/h	nd[3]	≈ 0.62 L/hr[2]
Recovered in the urine	≈ 33%	≈ 7%	≈ 20%	≈ 45/≈ 35% (IV/oral)	35% to 50%	0.91%/ 0.49% (IV/oral)	≈ 13%
Recovered in the feces	≈ 67%	≈ 90%	≈ 80%	≈ 50/≈ 60% (IV/oral)	50% to 65%	> 97%	≈ 83%

[1] Active.
[2] IV dosing.
[3] nd = no data

AIIRAs do not accumulate in plasma upon repeated once-daily dosing.

Losartan undergoes substantial first-pass metabolism and is converted to an active carboxylic acid metabolite (14% of dose) that is responsible for most of the angiotensin II receptor antagonism. Cytochrome P450 2C9 and 3A4 isozymes are involved in losartan's biotransformation.

The enzyme(s) responsible for **valsartan** metabolism have not been identified but do seem to be cytochrome P450 isozymes.

In vitro studies of **irbesartan** oxidation by cytochrome P450 isoenzymes indicated irbesartan was oxidized primarily by 2C9; metabolism by 3A4 was negligible. Irbesartan was neither metabolized by, nor did it substantially induce or inhibit, isoenzymes commonly associated with drug metabolism (1A1, 1A2, 2A6, 2B6, 2D6, 2E1). There was no induction or inhibition of 3A4.

Telmisartan is metabolized by conjugation to form a pharmacologically inactive acylglucuronide; the glucuronide of the parent compound is the only metabolite that has been identified in human plasma and urine. After a single dose, the glucuronide represents approximately 11% of the measured radioactivity in plasma. The cytochrome P450 isoenzymes are not involved in the metabolism of telmisartan.

Candesartan is rapidly and completely bioactivated by ester hydrolysis during absorption from the GI tract to candesartan, a selective AT$_1$ subtype angiotensin II receptor antagonist. Candesartan is mainly excreted unchanged in urine and feces (via bile). It undergoes minor hepatic metabolism by O-deethylation to an inactive metabolite. Candesartan and its inactive metabolite do not accumulate in serum upon repeated once-daily dosing.

Olmesartan shows linear pharmacokinetics following single oral doses of up to 320 mg and multiple oral doses of up to 80 mg. Steady-state levels are achieved within 3 to 5 days, and no accumulation in plasma occurs with once-daily dosing. Following the rapid and complete conversion of olmesartan medoxomil to olmesartan during absorption, there is virtually no further metabolism of olmesartan. Olmesartan crossed the blood-brain barrier poorly, if at all. It passed across the placental barrier in rats and was distributed to the fetus. It was distributed to milk at low levels in rats.

Absolute bioavailability following a single 300 mg oral dose of **eprosartan** is approximately 13%. Eprosartan plasma concentrations peak at 1 to 2 hours after an oral dose in the fasted state. Plasma concentrations of eprosartan increase in a slightly less than dose-proportional manner over the 100 to 800 mg dose range. The terminal elimination half-life following oral administration is typically 5 to 9 hours.

Contraindications

Hypersensitivity to any component of these products.

Warnings

➤*Hypotension / Volume- or salt-depleted patients:* In patients who are intravascularly volume-depleted (eg, those treated with diuretics), symptomatic hypotension may occur. Correct these conditions prior to administration or start treatment under close medical supervision with a reduced dose.

If hypotension occurs, place the patient in the supine position and, if necessary, give an IV infusion of normal saline. A transient hypotensive response is not a contraindication to further treatment, which usually can be continued once the blood pressure has stabilized.

➤*Race:* Losartan was effective in reducing blood pressure regardless of race, although the effect was somewhat less in black patients (usually a low-renin population). In healthy black subjects, **irbesartan** AUC values were approximately 25% greater than in whites; there were no differences in C_{max} values.

➤*Gender:* Plasma concentrations of **telmisartan** are generally 2 to 3 times higher in females than in males. However, in clinical trials, no significant increases in blood pressure response or in the incidence of orthostatic hypotension were found in women. No dosage adjustment is necessary.

➤*Cough:* In trials where **valsartan** was compared with an ACE inhibitor with or without placebo, the incidence of dry cough was significantly greater in the ACE inhibitor group (7.9%) than in the groups who received valsartan (2.6%) or placebo (1.5%). In patients who had dry cough when previously receiving ACE inhibitors, the incidences of cough in patients who received AIIRAs, hydrochlorothiazide, or lisinopril were approximately 20%, approximately 19%, and 69%, respectively.

There was no significant difference in the incidence of cough between **losartan**, **olmesartan**, **eprosartan**, or **telmisartan** and placebo. **Irbesartan** use was not associated with an increased incidence of dry cough, as is typically associated with ACE inhibitor use.

➤*Renal function impairment:* As a consequence of inhibiting the renin-angiotensin-aldosterone system, changes in renal function may be anticipated in susceptible individuals. In patients whose renal function may depend on the activity of the renin-angiotensin-aldosterone system (eg, patients with severe CHF), treatment with ACE inhibitors and angiotensin receptor antagonists has been associated with oliguria or progressive azotemia and rarely, with acute renal failure or death. In studies of ACE inhibitors in patients with unilateral or bilateral renal artery stenosis, increases in serum creatinine or BUN have been reported. AIIRAs would be expected to behave similarly. In some patients, these effects were reversible upon discontinuation of therapy. No dosage adjustment is necessary for patients with renal impairment unless they are volume-depleted.

Losartan – Plasma concentrations of losartan are not altered in patients with Ccr above 30 mL/min. In patients with lower Ccr, AUCs are about 50% greater and they are doubled in hemodialysis patients. Plasma concentrations of the active metabolite are not significantly altered in patients with renal impairment or in hemodialysis patients.

Valsartan – There is no apparent correlation between renal function (measured by Ccr) and exposure (measured by AUC) to valsartan in patients with different degrees of renal impairment. Consequently, dose adjustment is not required in patients with mild to moderate renal dysfunction. No studies have been performed in patients with severe impairment of renal function (Ccr less than 10 mL/min). Valsartan is not removed from plasma by hemodialysis. In the case of severe renal disease, exercise care with valsartan dosing.

In a 4-day trial of valsartan in 12 patients with unilateral renal artery stenosis, no significant increases in serum creatinine or BUN were observed. There has been no long-term use of valsartan in patients with unilateral or bilateral renal artery stenosis, but anticipate an effect similar to that seen with ACE inhibitors.

Irbesartan – The pharmacokinetics of irbesartan are not altered in patients with renal impairment or in patients on hemodialysis. Irbesartan is not removed by hemodialysis.

Candesartan – In hypertensive patients with renal insufficiency, serum concentrations of candesartan were elevated. After repeated dosing, the AUC and C_{max} were approximately doubled in patients with severe renal impairment (Ccr less than 30 mL/min/1.73 m^2) compared with patients with normal kidney function. The pharmacokinetics of candesartan in hypertensive patients undergoing hemodialysis are similar to those in hypertensive patients with severe renal impairment. Candesartan cannot be removed by hemodialysis. No initial dosage adjustment is necessary in patients with renal insufficiency.

Telmisartan – Renal excretion does not contribute to telmisartan clearance. Based on modest experience in patients with mild-to-moderate renal impairment (Ccr of 30 to 80 mL/min), mean clearance approximately 50 mL/min), no dosage adjustment is necessary in patients with decreased renal function. Telmisartan is not removed from blood by hemofiltration.

Eprosartan – Following administration of 600 mg once daily, there was an almost 2-fold increase in AUC and a 50% and 30% increase in C_{max} in moderate and severe renal impairment. The unbound eprosartan fractions increased by 35% and 59% in patients with moderate and severe renal impairment. No initial dosing adjustment is generally necessary in patients with moderate and severe renal impairment, with maximum dose not exceeding 600 mg daily. Eprosartan was poorly removed by hemodialysis (CL_{HD} less than 1 L/hr).

➤*Hepatic function impairment:*

Candesartan – No differences in the pharmacokinetics were observed in patients with mild to moderate chronic liver disease. No initial dosage adjustment is necessary in patients with mild hepatic disease.

Irbesartan – The pharmacokinetics of irbesartan following repeated oral administration were not significantly affected in patients with mild to moderate cirrhosis of the liver. No dosage adjustment is necessary in patients with hepatic insufficiency.

Losartan – Following administration in patients with mild to moderate alcoholic cirrhosis of the liver, plasma concentrations of losartan and its active metabolite were, respectively, 5 times and about 1.7 times those in young male volunteers. Compared with healthy subjects, the total plasma clearance in patients with hepatic insufficiency was about 50% lower and the oral bioavailability was about 2 times higher. A lower starting dose is recommended for patients with a history of hepatic impairment.

Based on pharmacokinetic data that demonstrate significantly increased plasma concentrations of losartan in cirrhotic patients, consider a lower dose for patients with impaired hepatic function.

Olmesartan – Increases in $AUC_{0-\infty}$ and C_{max} were observed in patients with moderate hepatic impairment compared with those in matched controls, with an increase in AUC of about 60%.

Telmisartan – As the majority of telmisartan is eliminated by biliary excretion, patients with biliary obstructive disorders or hepatic insufficiency can be expected to have reduced clearance. Use telmisartan with caution in these patients. In patients with hepatic insufficiency, plasma concentrations of telmisartan are increased, and absolute bioavailability approaches 100%.

Valsartan – On average, patients with mild to moderate chronic liver disease have twice the exposure (measured by AUC values) to valsartan of healthy volunteers (matched by age, sex, and weight). In general, no dosage adjustment is needed in patients with mild to moderate liver disease. However, exercise care in this patient population.

As the majority of valsartan is eliminated in the bile, patients with mild to moderate hepatic impairment, including patients with biliary obstructive disorders, showed lower valsartan clearance (higher AUCs). Exercise care in administering valsartan to these patients.

Eprosartan – Eprosartan AUC (but not C_{max}) values increased, on average, by approximately 40% in men with decreased hepatic function compared with healthy men after a single 100 mg oral dose of eprosartan. The extent of eprosartan plasma protein binding was not influenced by hepatic dysfunction. No dosage adjustment is necessary for patients with hepatic impairment.

➤*Carcinogenesis:* Female rats given the highest dose (270 mg/kg/day) of **losartan** had a slightly higher incidence of pancreatic acinar adenoma.

➤*Fertility impairment:* The administration of toxic dosage levels of **losartan** in female rats was associated with a significant decrease in the number of corpora lutea/female, implants/female, and live fetuses/female at C-section. At 100 mg/kg/day only a decrease in the number of corpora lutea/female was observed. Fertility and reproductive performance in male rats were not affected.

➤*Elderly:* No dosage adjustment is necessary when initiating AIIRAs in the elderly. No overall differences in effectiveness or safety of **candesartan**, **irbesartan**, **losartan**, **olmesartan**, **eprosartan**, or **telmisartan** were observed between elderly patients and younger patients, but greater sensitivity of some older individuals cannot be ruled out.

Based on the pooled data from randomized trials, the decrease in diastolic blood pressure and systolic blood pressure with eprosartan was slightly less in patients 65 years of age and older compared with younger patients. Adverse experiences were similar in younger and older patients.

➤*Pregnancy: Category C* (first trimester); *Category D* (second and third trimesters).

Fetal / Neonatal morbidity / mortality – Drugs that act directly on the renin-angiotensin system can cause fetal and neonatal morbidity and death when administered to pregnant women. Several dozen cases have been reported in patients who were taking ACE inhibitors. When pregnancy is detected, discontinue AIIRAs as soon as possible.

The use of drugs that act directly on the renin-angiotensin system during the second and third trimesters of pregnancy has been associated with fetal and neonatal injury, including hypotension, neonatal skull hypoplasia, anuria, reversible or irreversible renal failure, and death. Oligohydramnios has also been reported, presumably resulting from decreased fetal renal function; oligohydramnios, in this setting, has

Angiotensin II Receptor Antagonists

been associated with fetal limb contractures, craniofacial deformation, and hypoplastic lung development. Prematurity, intrauterine growth retardation, and patent ductus arteriosus have also occurred, although it is not clear whether these occurrences were caused by exposure to the drug. These adverse effects do not appear to have resulted from intrauterine drug exposure in the first trimester.

Inform mothers whose embryos and fetuses are exposed to an AIIRA only during the first trimester. Nonetheless, when patients become pregnant, physicians should have the patient discontinue the use of AIIRAs as soon as possible.

Rarely (probably less often than once in every 1000 pregnancies), no alternative to an AIIRA will be found. In these rare cases, apprise the mother of the potential hazards to her fetus, and perform serial ultrasound examinations to assess the intra-amniotic environment.

If oligohydramnios is observed, discontinue the drug unless it is considered life-saving for the mother. Contraction stress testing (CST), a nonstress test (NST), or biophysical profiling (BPP) may be appropriate, depending on the week of pregnancy. However, patients and physicians should be aware that oligohydramnios may not appear until after the fetus has sustained irreversible injury.

Closely observe infants with histories of in utero exposure to an AIIRA for hypotension, oliguria, and hyperkalemia. If oliguria occurs, direct attention toward support of blood pressure and renal perfusion. Exchange transfusion or dialysis may be required as means of reversing hypotension or substituting for disordered renal function.

Candesartan – Oral doses of 10 mg/kg/day or greater of candesartan administered to pregnant rats during late gestation and continued through lactation were associated with reduced survival and an increased incidence of hydronephrosis in the offspring. The 10 mg/kg/day dose in rats is approximately 2.8 times the maximum recommended human dose (MRHD) of 32 mg on a mg/m^2 basis (comparison assumes human body weight of 50 kg). Candesartan given to pregnant rabbits at an oral dose of 3 mg/kg/day (approximately 1.7 times the MRHD on a mg/m^2 basis) caused maternal toxicity (decreased body weight and death) but, in surviving dams, had no adverse effects on fetal survival, fetal weight, or external, visceral, or skeletal development. No maternal toxicity or adverse effects on fetal development were observed when oral doses up to 1000 mg/kg/day of candesartan (approximately 138 times the MRHD on a mg/m^2 basis) were administered to pregnant mice.

Eprosartan – Eprosartan has been shown to produce maternal and fetal toxicities (maternal and fetal mortality, low maternal body weight and food consumption, resorptions, abortions, and litter loss) in pregnant rabbits given oral doses as low as 10 mg/kg/day of eprosartan. No maternal or fetal adverse effects were observed at 3 mg/kg/day; this oral dose yielded a systemic exposure (AUC) to unbound eprosartan 0.8 times that achieved in humans given 400 mg twice daily. No adverse effects on in utero or postnatal development and maturation of offspring were observed when eprosartan was administered to pregnant rats at oral doses up to 1000 mg/kg/day of eprosartan (the 1000 mg/kg/day dose in nonpregnant rats yielded systemic exposure to unbound eprosartan approximately 0.6 times the exposure achieved in humans given 400 mg twice daily).

Irbesartan – When pregnant rats were dosed with irbesartan from day 0 to day 20 of gestation (oral doses of 50, 180, and 650 mg/kg/day), increased incidences of renal pelvic cavitation, hydroureter, or absence of renal papilla were observed in fetuses at doses of at least 50 mg/kg/day (approximately equivalent to the MRHD, 300 mg/day, on a body surface area basis). Subcutaneous edema was observed in fetuses at doses of at least 180 mg/kg/day (about 4 times the MRHD on a body surface area basis). As these abnormalities were not observed in rats in which irbesartan exposure (oral doses of 50, 150, and 450 mg/kg/day) was limited to gestation days 6 to 15, they appear to reflect late gestational effects of the drug. In pregnant rabbits, oral doses of 30 mg/kg/day of irbesartan were associated with maternal mortality and abortion. Surviving females receiving this dose (about 1.5 times the MRHD on a body surface area basis) had a slight increase in early resorptions and a corresponding decrease in live fetuses. Irbesartan was found to cross the placental barrier in rats and rabbits.

Radioactivity was present in the rat and rabbit fetus during late gestation and in rat milk following oral doses of radiolabeled irbesartan.

Losartan – Losartan has been shown to produce adverse effects in rat fetuses and neonates, including decreased body weight, delayed physical and behavioral development, mortality, and renal toxicity. With the exception of neonatal weight gain (which was affected at doses as low as 10 mg/kg/day), doses associated with these effects exceeded 25 mg/kg/day (approximately 3 times the MRHD of 100 mg on a mg/m^2 basis). These findings are attributed to drug exposure in late gestation and during lactation. Significant levels of losartan and its active metabolite were shown to be present in rat fetal plasma during late gestation and in rat milk.

Telmisartan – In rabbits, embryolethality associated with maternal toxicity (reduced body weight gain and food consumption) was observed at 45 mg/kg/day of telmisartan (about 6.4 times the MRHD of 80 mg on a mg/m^2 basis). In rats, maternally toxic (reduction in body weight gain and food consumption) telmisartan doses of 15 mg/kg/day (about

1.9 times the MRHD on a mg/m^2 basis), administered during late gestation and lactation, were observed to produce adverse effects in neonates, including reduced viability, low birth weight, delayed maturation, and decreased weight gain. Telmisartan has been shown to be present in rat fetuses during late gestation and in rat milk. The no-observed-effect doses for developmental toxicity in rats and rabbits, 5 and 15 mg/kg/day, respectively, are about 0.64 and 3.7 times, on a mg/m^2 basis, the MRHD of telmisartan (80 mg/day).

➤*Lactation:* AIIRAs were present in rat milk. It is not known if AIIRAs are excreted in human breast milk. Because of the potential for adverse effects on the nursing infant, decide whether to discontinue nursing or discontinue the drug, taking into account the importance of the drug to the mother.

➤*Children:* Safety and efficacy have not been established.

Precautions

➤*Potassium supplements:* Tell patients receiving **losartan** not to use potassium supplements or salt substitutes containing potassium without consulting the prescribing physician.

➤*Lab test abnormalities:*

Liver function tests – Occasional elevations (more than 150% in **valsartan**-treated patients) of liver enzymes or serum bilirubin have occurred. Three patients (less than 0.1%) treated with valsartan discontinued treatment for elevated liver chemistries. Minor elevations of ALT, AST, and alkaline phosphatase occurred for comparable percentages of patients taking **eprosartan** or placebo in controlled clinical trials.

Creatinine/Blood urea nitrogen (BUN) – Minor increases in BUN or serum creatinine were observed infrequently with **candesartan**, in less than 0.1% of patients with essential hypertension treated with **losartan** alone, in 0.8% of patients taking **valsartan**, less than 0.7% with **irbesartan**, and 0.6% and 1.3%, respectively, of patients taking **eprosartan**. At least a 0.5 mg/dL rise in creatinine was observed in 0.4% of **telmisartan** patients compared with 0.3% of placebo patients.

Hemoglobin and hematocrit – A greater than 2 g/dL decrease in hemoglobin was observed in 0.8% of **telmisartan** patients compared with 0.3% of placebo patients. No patients discontinued therapy because of anemia.

Small decreases in hemoglobin and hematocrit occurred frequently in patients treated with **losartan** alone but were rarely of clinical importance.

Decreases of more than 20% in hemoglobin and hematocrit were observed in 0.4% and 0.8%, respectively, of **valsartan** patients, vs 0.1% and 0.1% with placebo. One valsartan patient discontinued treatment for microcytic anemia. Neutropenia was observed in 1.9% of patients treated with valsartan and 0.8% of patients treated with placebo.

Mean decreases in hemoglobin of 0.2 g/dL were observed in 0.2% of patients receiving **irbesartan**. Neutropenia (less than 1000 cells/mm^3) occurred at similar frequencies (0.3%).

Small decreases in hemoglobin and hematocrit (mean decreases of approximately 0.2 g/dL and 0.5 volume percent, respectively) were observed in patients treated with **candesartan** alone but were rarely of clinical importance. Anemia, leukopenia, and thrombocytopenia were associated with withdrawal of 1 patient each from clinical trials.

A greater than 20% decrease in hemoglobin was observed in 0.1% of patients taking **eprosartan**. Leukopenia (WBC count of up to 3×10^3/mm^3) occurred in 0.3% of patients taking eprosartan and in 0.3% of patients given placebo in controlled clinical trials. Neutropenia (neutrophil count of up to 1.5×10^3/mm^3) occurred in 1.3% of patients taking eprosartan and in 1.4% of patients given placebo in controlled clinical trials. Thrombocytopenia (platelet count of up to 100×10^9/L) occurred in 0.3% of patients taking eprosartan (1 patient) and in no patient given placebo in controlled clinical trials. Four patients receiving eprosartan in clinical trials were withdrawn for thrombocytopenia.

Small decreases in hemoglobin and hematocrit (mean decreases of approximately 0.3 g/dL and 0.3 volume percent, respectively) were observed with **olmesartan**.

Serum potassium – Increases of more than 20% in serum potassium were observed in 4.4% of **valsartan**-treated patients vs 2.9% of placebo-treated patients.

A small increase (mean increase of 0.1 mEq/L) was observed in patients treated with **candesartan** alone but was rarely of clinical importance. One patient from a CHF trial was withdrawn for hyperkalemia (serum potassium, 7.5 mEq/L). This patient was also receiving spironolactone.

A potassium value of at least 5.6 mmol/L occurred in 0.9% of patients taking **eprosartan** and 0.3% of patients given placebo in controlled clinical trials. One patient was withdrawn from clinical trials for hyperkalemia and 3 for hypokalemia.

Hyperuricemia – Hyperuricemia was rarely found (0.6% with **candesartan** vs 0.5% with placebo).

Angiotensin II Receptor Antagonists

Drug Interactions

Angiotensin II Receptor Antagonist Drug Interactions

Precipitant drug	Object drug[*]		Description
Cimetidine	Losartan	↑	Coadministration led to an increase of ≈ 18% in AUC of losartan but did not affect the pharmacokinetics of its active metabolite.
Fluconazole	Losartan	↑	Fluconazole may inhibit the metabolism of losartan (CYP2C9), causing increased antihypertensive and adverse effects. Fluconazole did not affect the pharmacokinetics of eprosartan.
Indomethacin	Losartan	↓	The hypotensive effect of losartan may be reduced.
Phenobarbital	Losartan	↓	Coadministration led to a reduction of ≈ 20% in the AUC of losartan and its active metabolite.
Rifamycins	Losartan	↓	Rifamycins may increase the metabolism of losartan, thereby decreasing antihypertensive effects.
Telmisartan	Digoxin	↑	Median increases in digoxin peak plasma concentration (49%) and in trough concentration (20%) were seen with coadministration.
Telmisartan	Warfarin	↔	Telmisartan administered for 10 days slightly decreased the mean warfarin trough plasma concentration; this decrease did not result in a change in the International Normalized Ratio.

[*] ↑ = Object drug increased. ↓ = Object drug decreased.
↔ = Undetermined clinical effect.

▶*CYP450:* In vitro studies show significant inhibition of the formation of the active metabolite of **losartan** by inhibitors of cytochrome P450 3A4 (eg, ketoconazole, troleandomycin) or P450 2C9 (sulfaphenazole). The pharmacodynamic consequences of concomitant use of losartan and these inhibitors have not been examined.

In vitro studies show significant inhibition of the formation of oxidized **irbesartan** metabolites with the known cytochrome CYP2C9 substrates/inhibitors, tolbutamide, and nifedipine. However, clinical consequences were negligible.

▶*Potassium:* As with other drugs that block angiotensin II or its effects, concomitant use of potassium-sparing diuretics (eg, spironolactone, triamterene, amiloride), potassium supplements, or salt substitutes containing potassium may lead to increases in serum potassium.

▶*Drug/Food interactions:* A meal has only minor effects on **losartan** AUC or on the AUC of the metabolite (about 10% decrease). Food decreases **valsartan**'s C_{max} by 50% and its AUC by 40%. Food slightly reduces the bioavailability of **telmisartan**, with an AUC reduction of about 6% with the 40 mg tablet and about 20% after a 160 mg dose. Food does not affect the bioavailability of **irbesartan**, **olmesartan**, or **candesartan**. Administering **eprosartan** with food delays absorption and causes variable changes (less than 25%) in C_{max} and AUC values that do not appear clinically important.

Adverse Reactions

In general, treatment with AIIRAs is well tolerated. In controlled clinical trials, discontinuation of therapy because of adverse reactions was required in 2.3% of patients treated with **losartan** or **valsartan**, 2.4% with **olmesartan** and **candesartan**, 2.8% with **telmisartan**, 3.3% with **irbesartan**, and 4% with **eprosartan** vs 3.7%, 2%, 2.7%, 3.4%, 6.1%, 4.5%, and 6.5%, respectively, given placebo.

Angiotensin II Receptor Antagonist Adverse Reactions (%)[1]

Adverse reaction	Candesartan (n = 2350)	Eprosartan (n = 1202)	Irbesartan (n = 1965)	Losartan (n = 1075)	Olmesartan (n = 3278)	Telmisartan (n = 1455)	Valsartan (n = 2316)
CNS							
Dizziness	4	≥ 1	≥ 1	3.5	3	1	> 1
Insomnia	-	< 1	-	1.4	> 0.5	> 0.3	> 0.2
Headache	≥ 1	≥ 1	≥ 1	≥ 1	> 1	1	> 1
Fatigue	> 1	2	4	-	> 0.5	1	2
Anxiety/Nervousness	≥ 0.5	< 1	≥ 1	< 1	-	> 0.3	> 0.2
Depression	≥ 0.5	1	< 1	< 1	-	> 0.3	-
GI							
Diarrhea	> 1	≥ 1	3	2.4	> 1	3	> 1
Dyspepsia/Heartburn	≥ 0.5	≥ 1	2	1.3	> 0.5	1	> 0.2
Nausea/Vomiting	> 1	< 1	≥ 1	≥ 1	-	1	> 1
Abdominal pain	> 1	2	≥ 1	≥ 1	> 0.5	1	2
Musculoskeletal							
Arthralgia	> 1	2	-	< 1	> 0.5	> 0.3	> 1
Pain[2]	3	< 1	≥ 1	1 to 1.8	> 1	1 to 3	> 0.2
Muscle cramp	-	-	-	1.1	-	-	> 0.2
Myalgia	≥ 0.5	≥ 1	-	1	> 0.5	1	> 0.2
Trauma	-	-	2	-	-	-	-
Respiratory							
Upper respiratory tract infection	6	8	9	7.9	> 1	7	> 1
Cough[3]	> 1	4	2.8	3.4	-	1	> 1
Nasal congestion	-	-	-	2	-	-	-
Sinus disorder	-	-	≥ 1	1.5	-	-	-
Sinusitis	> 1	≥ 1	-	1	> 1	3	> 1
Pharyngitis	2	4	≥ 1	≥ 1	> 1	1	> 1
Rhinitis	2	4	≥ 1	< 1	> 1	> 0.3	> 1
Influenza/Influenza-like symptoms	-	< 1	≥ 1	< 1	> 1	1	-
Bronchitis	> 1	≥ 1	-	< 1	> 1	> 0.3	-
Miscellaneous							
Viral infection	-	2	-	-	-	-	3
Edema	-	≥ 1	≥ 1	≥ 1	-	-	> 1
Chest pain	> 1	≥ 1	≥ 1	≥ 1	> 0.5	1	-
Rash	≥ 0.5	< 1	≥ 1	< 1	> 0.5	> 0.3	> 0.2
Tachycardia	≥ 0.5	< 1	≥ 1	< 1	> 0.5	> 0.3	-
Urinary tract infection	-	4	≥ 1	< 1	> 0.5	1	-
Peripheral edema	> 1	-	-	-	> 0.5	1	-
Albuminuria	> 1	< 1	-	-	-	-	-
Hypertension	-	-	-	-	-	1	-
Hypertriglyceridemia	≥ 0.5	1	-	-	> 1	-	-
Creatine phosphokinase increased	≥ 0.5	< 1	-	-	> 1	-	-
Hyperglycemia	≥ 0.5	< 1	-	-	> 1	-	-
Hematuria	≥ 0.5	< 1	-	-	> 1	-	-
Inflicted injury	-	2	-	-	> 1	-	-

[1] Data are pooled from separate studies and are not necessarily comparable.
[2] This includes back and leg pain.
[3] See Warnings.

➤*Candesartan:*

Cardiovascular – Palpitation (at least 0.5%).

CNS – Paresthesia, vertigo, somnolence (at least 0.5%).

Metabolic/Nutritional – Hyperuricemia (at least 0.5%).

Miscellaneous – Asthenia, fever, epistaxis, dyspnea, sweating increased, gastroenteritis (at least 0.5%).

Other reported events observed less frequently included angina pectoris, MI, and angioedema.

Adverse reactions occurred at about the same rates in men and women, older and younger patients, and black and nonblack patients.

Postmarketing experience: Abnormal hepatic function, hepatitis, neutropenia, leukopenia, agranulocytosis, pruritus, urticaria.

➤*Eprosartan:*

Cardiovascular – Angina pectoris, bradycardia, abnormal ECG, specific abnormal ECG, extrasystoles, atrial fibrillation, hypotension (including orthostatic hypotension), palpitations (less than 1%).

CNS – Ataxia, migraine, neuritis, nervousness, paresthesia, somnolence, tremor, vertigo (less than 1%).

Dermatologic – Eczema, furunculosis, pruritus, maculopapular rash, increased sweating (less than 1%).

GI – Anorexia, constipation, dry mouth, esophagitis, flatulence, gastritis, gastroenteritis, gingivitis, periodontitis, toothache (less than 1%).

GU – Cystitis, micturition frequency, polyuria, renal calculus, urinary incontinence (less than 1%).

Hematologic – Anemia, purpura (less than 1%).

Hepatic – Increased ALT and AST (less than 1%).

Metabolic/Nutritional – Diabetes mellitus, glycosuria, gout, hypercholesterolemia, hyperkalemia, hypokalemia, hyponatremia (less than 1%).

Musculoskeletal – Arthritis, aggravated arthritis, arthrosis, skeletal pain, tendinitis (less than 1%).

Respiratory – Asthma, epistaxis (less than 1%).

Special senses – Conjunctivitis, abnormal vision, xerophthalmia, tinnitus (less than 1%).

Miscellaneous – Alcohol intolerance, asthenia, substernal chest pain, peripheral edema, fever, hot flushes, malaise, rigors, herpes simplex, otitis externa, otitis media, leg cramps, peripheral ischemia (less than 1%).

Facial edema was reported in 5 patients receiving eprosartan. Angioedema has been reported with other AIIRAs.

➤*Irbesartan:*

Cardiovascular – Flushing, hypertension, cardiac murmur, MI, angina pectoris, arrhythmic/conduction disorder, cardio-respiratory arrest, heart failure, hypertensive crisis (less than 1%).

CNS – Sleep disturbance, numbness, somnolence, emotional disturbance, paresthesia, tremor, transient ischemic attack, cerebrovascular accident (less than 1%).

Dermatologic – Pruritus, dermatitis, ecchymosis, face erythema, urticaria (less than 1%).

Endocrine – Sexual dysfunction, libido change, gout (less than 1%).

GI – Constipation, oral lesion, gastroenteritis, flatulence, abdominal distention (less than 1%).

GU – Abnormal urination, prostate disorder (less than 1%).

Musculoskeletal – Extremity swelling, muscle cramp, arthritis, muscle ache, musculoskeletal chest pain, joint stiffness, bursitis, muscle weakness (less than 1%).

Respiratory – Epistaxis, tracheobronchitis, congestion, pulmonary congestion, dyspnea, wheezing (less than 1%).

Special senses – Vision disturbance, hearing abnormality, ear infection, ear pain, conjunctivitis, other eye disturbance, eyelid abnormality, ear abnormality (less than 1%).

Miscellaneous – Fever, chills, facial edema, upper extremity edema (less than 1%).

The incidence of hypotension or orthostatic hypotension was low in irbesartan-treated patients (0.4%), unrelated to dosage, and similar to the incidence among placebo-treated patients (0.2%). Dizziness, syncope, and vertigo were reported with equal or less frequency in patients receiving irbesartan compared with placebo.

Postmarketing experience: Urticaria, angioedema (involving swelling of the face, lips, pharynx, or tongue), increased liver function tests, jaundice. Hyperkalemia has been reported rarely.

➤*Losartan:*

Cardiovascular – Angina pectoris, second degree AV block, CVA, hypotension, MI, arrhythmias including atrial fibrillation, palpitation, sinus bradycardia, ventricular tachycardia, ventricular fibrillation (less than 1%).

CNS – Anxiety disorder, ataxia, confusion, dream abnormality, hypesthesia, decreased libido, memory impairment, migraine, paresthesia, peripheral neuropathy, panic disorder, sleep disorder, somnolence, tremor, vertigo (less than 1%).

Dermatologic – Alopecia, dermatitis, dry skin, ecchymosis, erythema, flushing, photosensitivity, pruritus, sweating, urticaria (less than 1%).

GI – Anorexia, constipation, dental pain, dry mouth, flatulence, gastritis (less than 1%).

GU – Impotence, nocturia, urinary frequency (less than 1%).

Musculoskeletal – Arm pain, hip pain, joint swelling, knee pain, shoulder pain, stiffness, arthritis, fibromyalgia, muscle weakness (less than 1%).

Respiratory – Dyspnea, pharyngeal discomfort, epistaxis, respiratory congestion (less than 1%).

Special senses – Blurred vision, burning/stinging in the eye, conjunctivitis, taste perversion, tinnitus, decrease in visual acuity (less than 1%).

Miscellaneous – Asthenia/fatigue (at least 1%); facial edema, fever, orthostatic effects, syncope, anemia, gout (less than 1%).

A patient with known hypersensitivity to aspirin and penicillin, when treated with losartan, was withdrawn from the study because of swelling of the lips and eyelids and facial rash, reported as angioedema, which returned to normal 5 days after therapy was discontinued.

Superficial peeling of palms and hemolysis was reported in 1 subject.

Postmarketing experience: Hepatitis (rare); dry cough (including positive rechallenges), hyperkalemia, hyponatremia. Angioedema, including swelling of the larynx and glottis, causing airway obstruction or swelling of the face, lips, pharynx, or tongue has been reported rarely in patients treated with losartan; some of these patients previously experienced angioedema with other drugs including ACE inhibitors. Vasculitis, including Henoch-Schönlein purpura, has been reported. Anaphylactic reactions have been reported.

➤*Olmesartan:*

GI – Gastroenteritis, nausea (greater than 0.5%).

Metabolic/Nutritional – Hypercholesterolemia, hyperlipemia, hyperuricemia (greater than 0.5%).

Musculoskeletal – Arthritis, skeletal pain (greater than 0.5%).

Miscellaneous – Pain, vertigo (greater than 0.5%).

Facial edema was reported in 5 patients receiving olmesartan. Angioedema has been reported with other AIIRAs.

➤*Telmisartan:*

Cardiovascular – Palpitation, dependent edema, angina pectoris, leg edema, abnormal ECG (more than 0.3%).

CNS – Somnolence, migraine, vertigo, paresthesia, involuntary muscle contractions, hypesthesia (greater than 0.3%).

Dermatologic – Dermatitis, eczema, pruritus (greater than 0.3%).

GI – Flatulence, constipation, gastritis, vomiting, dry mouth, hemorrhoids, gastroenteritis, enteritis, gastroesophageal reflux, toothache, nonspecific GI disorders (greater than 0.3%).

GU – Micturition frequency, cystitis (greater than 0.3%).

Metabolic – Gout, hypercholesterolemia, diabetes mellitus (greater than 0.3%).

Musculoskeletal – Arthritis, leg cramps (greater than 0.3%).

Respiratory – Asthma, dyspnea, epistaxis (greater than 0.3%).

Special senses – Abnormal vision, conjunctivitis, tinnitus, earache (greater than 0.3%).

Miscellaneous – Impotence, increased sweating, flushing, allergy, fever, leg pain, malaise, infection, fungal infection, abscess, otitis media, cerebrovascular disorder (greater than 0.3%).

A single case of angioedema was reported (among a total of 3781 patients treated with telmisartan).

➤*Valsartan:*

CNS – Paresthesia, somnolence (greater than 0.2%).

GU – Constipation, dry mouth, flatulence (greater than 0.2%).

Miscellaneous – Allergic reaction, asthenia, palpitations, dyspnea, vertigo, impotence, pruritus (greater than 0.2%).

Other reported events seen less frequently in clinical trials included chest pain, syncope, anorexia, vomiting, and angioedema.

Dose-related orthostatic effects were seen in less than 1% of patients. An increase in the incidence of dizziness was observed in patients treated with 320 mg valsartan (8%) compared with 10 to 160 mg (2% to 4%).

Postmarketing experience: Hepatitis (very rare), elevated liver enzymes, angioedema (rare), impaired renal function, hyperkalemia, alopecia.

Overdosage

Limited data are available. The most likely manifestation of overdosage with an AIIRA would be hypotension, dizziness, and tachycardia; bradycardia could occur from parasympathetic (vagal) stimulation. If symptomatic hypotension should occur, institute supportive treatment. Refer to General Management of Acute Overdosage. AIIRAs cannot be removed by hemodialysis.

Patient Information

Tell patients of childbearing age about the consequences of second- and third-trimester exposure to drugs that act on the renin-angiotensin system, and tell them that these consequences do not appear to have resulted from intrauterine drug exposure that has been limited to the first trimester. Ask these patients to report pregnancies to their physicians as soon as possible.

LOSARTAN POTASSIUM

Rx	Cozaar (Merck)	Tablets: 25 mg	Lactose, 2.12 mg potassium. (MRK 951). Lt. green, teardrop shape. Film-coated. In unit-of-use 90s and 100s and UD 100s.
		50 mg	Lactose, 4.24 mg potassium. (MRK 952 COZAAR). Green, teardrop shape. Film-coated. In 1000s, unit-of-use 30s, 90s, and 100s, and UD 100s.
		100 mg	Lactose, 8.48 mg potassium. (960 MRK). Dk. green, teardrop shape. Film-coated. In unit-of-use 30s and 100s and UD 100s.

For complete prescribing information, refer to the Angiotensin II Receptor Antagonists group monograph.

> ### WARNING
>
> When used in pregnancy during the second and third trimesters, drugs that act directly on the renin-angiotensin system can cause injury and even death to the developing fetus. When pregnancy is detected, discontinue losartan as soon as possible.

Indications

➤*Hypertension:* Treatment of hypertension alone or in combination with other antihypertensive agents.

➤*Hypertensive patients with left ventricular hypertrophy:* Used to reduce the risk of stroke in patients with hypertension and left ventricular hypertrophy, but there is evidence that this benefit does not apply to black patients.

➤*Nephropathy in type 2 diabetic patients:* Treatment of diabetic nephropathy with an elevated serum creatinine and proteinuria (urinary albumin to creatinine ratio greater than or equal to 300 mg/g) in patients with type 2 diabetes and a history of hypertension. In this population, losartan reduces the rate of progression of nephropathy as measured by the occurrence of doubling of serum creatinine or end stage renal disease (need for dialysis or renal transplantation).

Administration and Dosage

➤*Approved by the FDA:* April 14, 1995.

➤*Hypertension:* Dosing must be individualized. The usual starting dose is 50 mg once daily with or without food, with 25 mg used in patients with possible depletion of intravascular volume (eg, patients treated with diuretics) and patients with a history of hepatic impairment. Losartan can be administered once or twice daily with total daily doses ranging from 25 to 100 mg. If the antihypertensive effect measured at trough using once-daily dosing is inadequate, a twice-daily regimen at the same total daily dose or an increase in dose may give a more satisfactory response. The effect of losartan is substantially present within 1 week but in some studies the maximal effect occurred in 3 to 6 weeks.

Losartan may be administered with other antihypertensive agents. If blood pressure is not controlled by losartan alone, a low dose of a diuretic may be added. Hydrochlorothiazide has an additive effect.

➤*Hypertensive patients with left ventricular hypertrophy:* The usual starting dose is 50 mg of losartan once daily. Add hydrochlorothiazide 12.5 mg/day and/or increase the dose of losartan to 100 mg once daily followed by an increase in hydrochlorothiazide to 25 mg once daily based on blood pressure response.

➤*Nephropathy in type 2 diabetic patients:* The usual starting dose is 50 mg once daily. Increase the dose to 100 mg once daily based on blood pressure response. Losartan may be administered with insulin and other commonly used hypoglycemic agents (eg, sulfonylureas, glitazones, glucosidase inhibitors).

➤*Storage/Stability:* Store at 25°C (77°F); excursions permitted to 15° to 30°C (59° to 86°F). Keep container tightly closed. Protect from light.

VALSARTAN

Rx	Diovan (Novartis)	Tablets: 40 mg	(NVR DO). Yellow. In 30s and UD 100s.
		80 mg	(NVR DV). Pale red, almond shape. In 100s and UD 100s.
		160 mg	(NVR DX). Gray-orange, almond shape. In 100s and UD 100s.
		320 mg	(NVR DXL). Dark grayish violet, almond shape. In 100s and UD 100s.

For complete prescribing information, refer to the Angiotensin II Receptor Antagonists group monograph.

> ### WARNING
>
> When used in pregnancy during the second and third trimesters, drugs that act directly on the renin-angiotensin system can cause injury and even death to the developing fetus. When pregnancy is detected, discontinue valsartan as soon as possible.

Indications

➤*Hypertension:* Treatment of hypertension alone or in combination with other antihypertensive agents.

➤*Heart failure:* Treatment of heart failure (NYHA class II to IV) in patients who are intolerant of angiotensin-converting enzyme (ACE) inhibitors.

Administration and Dosage

➤*Approved by the FDA:* December 23, 1996.

➤*Hypertension:* The recommended starting dose is 80 or 160 mg once daily, with or without food, when used as monotherapy in patients who are not volume-depleted. Patients requiring greater reductions may be started at the higher dose. Valsartan may be used over a dose range of 80 to 320 mg once daily. The antihypertensive effect is substantially present within 2 weeks and maximal reduction is generally attained after 4 weeks. If additional antihypertensive effect is required, the dosage may be increased to a maximum of 320 mg or a diuretic may be added. Adding a diuretic has a greater effect than dose increases beyond 80 mg. Valsartan may be administered with other antihypertensive agents.

➤*Heart failure:* The recommended starting dose of valsartan is 40 mg twice daily. Up-titration to 80 and 160 mg twice daily should be done to the highest dose, as tolerated by the patient. Consider reducing the dose of concomitant diuretics. The maximum daily dose administered in clinical trials was 320 mg in divided doses. Concomitant use with an ACE inhibitor and a beta blocker is not recommended.

➤*Hepatic/Renal function impairment:* Exercise care when dosing patients with severe hepatic or renal function impairment.

➤*Storage/Stability:* Store at 25°C (77°F); excursions permitted to 15° to 30°C (59° to 86°F). Protect from moisture. Dispense in a tight container.

Angiotensin II Receptor Antagonists

IRBESARTAN

Rx	Avapro (Bristol-Myers Squibb Sanofi-Synthelabo Partnership)	Tablets: 75 mg	Lactose. (2771). White to off-white, oval. In 30s and 90s.
		150 mg	Lactose. (2772). White to off-white, oval. In 30s, 90s, 500s, and UD 100s.
		300 mg	Lactose. (2773). White to off-white, oval. In 30s, 90s, and 500s.

For complete prescribing information, refer to the Angiotensin II Receptor Antagonists group monograph.

> **WARNING**
>
> When used in pregnancy during the second and third trimesters, drugs that act directly on the renin-angiotensin system can cause injury and even death to the developing fetus. When pregnancy is detected, discontinue irbesartan as soon as possible.

Indications

➤*Hypertension:* Treatment of hypertension alone or in combination with other antihypertensive agents.

➤*Nephropathy in type 2 diabetic patients:* Treatment of diabetic nephropathy with an elevated serum creatinine and proteinuria (greater than 300 mg/day) in patients with type 2 diabetes and hypertension. In this population, irbesartan reduces the rate of progression of nephropathy as measured by the occurrence of doubling of serum creatinine or end-stage renal disease (need for dialysis or renal transplantation).

Administration and Dosage

➤*Approved by the FDA:* September 30, 1997.

➤*Hypertension:* The recommended initial dosage is 150 mg once daily with or without food. Patients may be titrated to 300 mg once daily.

Irbesartan may be administered with other antihypertensive agents. A low dose of a diuretic may be added if blood pressure is not controlled by irbesartan alone. Hydrochlorothiazide has an additive effect. Patients not adequately treated by the maximum dose of 300 mg once daily are unlikely to derive additional benefit from a higher dose or twice-daily dosing.

➤*Nephropathy in type 2 diabetic patients:* The recommended target maintenance dose is 300 mg once daily. There are no data on the clinical effects of lower doses of irbesartan on diabetic nephropathy.

➤*Children less than 6 years of age:* Safety and efficacy have not been established.

➤*Children 6 to 12 years of age:* An initial dose of 75 mg once daily is reasonable. Titrate patients requiring further reduction in blood pressure to 150 mg once daily.

➤*Adolescents 13 to 16 years of age:* An initial dose of 150 mg once daily is reasonable. Titrate patients requiring further reduction in blood pressure to 300 mg once daily. Higher doses are not recommended.

➤*Volume- and salt-depleted patients:* A lower initial dose of 75 mg is recommended in patients with depletion of intravascular volume or salt (eg, patients treated vigorously with diuretics or on hemodialysis).

➤*Storage/Stability:* Store between 15° and 30°C (59° and 86°F).

CANDESARTAN CILEXETIL

Rx	Atacand (AstraZeneca)	Tablets: 4 mg	Lactose. (ACF 004). White to off-white. In unit-of-use 30s.
		8 mg	Lactose. (ACG 008). Lt. pink. In unit-of-use 30s.
		16 mg	Lactose. (ACH 016). Pink. In unit-of-use 30s and 90s and UD 100s.
		32 mg	Lactose. (ACL 032). Pink. In unit-of-use 30s and 90s and UD 100s.

For complete prescribing information, refer to the Angiotensin II Receptor Antagonists group monograph.

> **WARNING**
>
> When used in pregnancy during the second and third trimesters, drugs that act directly on the renin-angiotensin system can cause injury and even death to the developing fetus. When pregnancy is detected, discontinue candesartan as soon as possible.

Indications

➤*Hypertension:* Treatment of hypertension alone or in combination with other antihypertensive agents.

Administration and Dosage

➤*Approved by the FDA:* June 4, 1998.

Individualize dosage. Administer with or without food. Blood pressure response is dose-related over the range of 2 to 32 mg. The usual recom-

mended starting dose is 16 mg once daily when used as monotherapy in patients who are not volume-depleted. Candesartan can be administered once or twice daily with total daily doses ranging from 8 to 32 mg. Larger doses do not appear to have a greater effect; there is relatively little experience with such doses. Most of the antihypertensive effect is present within 2 weeks; maximal blood pressure reduction generally is obtained within 4 to 6 weeks of treatment. If blood pressure is not controlled by candesartan alone, a diuretic may be added. Candesartan may be administered with other antihypertensive agents.

➤*Volume-depleted patients:* For patients with possible intravascular volume depletion (eg, patients treated with diuretics, particularly those with impaired renal function), initiate candesartan under close medical supervision and consider administering a lower dose.

➤*Storage/Stability:* Store at 25°C (77°F); excursions permitted to 15° to 30°C (59° to 86°F). Keep container tightly closed.

TELMISARTAN

Rx	Micardis (Boehringer Ingelheim)	Tablets: 20 mg	Sorbitol. (50H). White. In blister pack 28s.
		40 mg	Sorbitol. (51H). White, oblong. In blister pack 28s.
		80 mg	Sorbitol. (52H). White, oblong. In blister pack 28s.

For complete prescribing information, refer to the Angiotensin II Receptor Antagonists group monograph.

> **WARNING**
>
> When used in pregnancy during the second and third trimesters, drugs that act directly on the renin-angiotensin system can cause injury and even death to the developing fetus. When pregnancy is detected, discontinue telmisartan as soon as possible.

Indications

➤*Hypertension:* Treatment of hypertension alone or in combination with other antihypertensive agents.

Administration and Dosage

➤*Approved by the FDA:* November 10, 1998.

Individualize dosage. The usual starting dose is 40 mg once daily. Blood pressure response is dose-related over the range of 20 to 80 mg. May be administered with or without food. May be administered with other antihypertensive agents. Most of the antihypertensive effect is apparent within 2 weeks; maximal reduction is generally attained after 4 weeks. When additional blood pressure reduction beyond that achieved with 80 mg is required, a diuretic may be added.

➤*Special risk patients:* Patients on dialysis may develop orthostatic hypotension; monitor blood pressure closely. Initiate treatment under close medical supervision for patients with biliary obstructive disorders or hepatic insufficiency. Correct the condition of patients with depletion of intravascular volume or initiate therapy under close supervision.

➤*Storage/Stability:* Store at 25°C (77°F); excursions permitted to 15° to 30°C (59° to 86°F). Do not remove tablets from blisters until immediately before administration.

EPROSARTAN MESYLATE

Rx	**Teveten** (Biovail)	**Tablets:** 400 mg	Lactose. (SOLVAY 5044). Pink, oval. Film-coated. In 100s.
		600 mg	Lactose. (SOLVAY 5046). White, capsule shape. Film-coated. In 100s.

For complete prescribing information, refer to the Angiotensin II Receptor Antagonists group monograph.

WARNING

When used in pregnancy during the second and third trimesters, drugs that act directly on the renin-angiotensin system can cause injury and even death to the developing fetus. When pregnancy is detected, discontinue use of eprosartan as soon as possible.

Indications

➤*Hypertension:* Treatment of hypertension alone or in combination with other antihypertensives, such as diuretics and calcium channel blockers.

Administration and Dosage

➤*Approved by the FDA:* October 22, 1999.

The usual recommended starting dosage is 600 mg once daily with or without food when used as monotherapy in patients who are not volume-depleted. Eprosartan also can be administered once or twice daily with total daily doses ranging from 400 to 800 mg. There is limited experience with doses beyond 800 mg/day.

If the antihypertensive effect measured at trough using once-daily dosing is inadequate, a twice-daily regimen at the same total daily dose or an increase in dose may give a more satisfactory response. Achievement of maximum blood pressure reduction in most patients may take 2 to 3 weeks.

Eprosartan may be used in combination with other antihypertensive agents, such as thiazide diuretics or calcium channel blockers, if an additional blood-pressure-lowering effect is required. Discontinuation of treatment with eprosartan does not lead to a rapid rebound increase in blood pressure.

➤*Elderly and hepatic/renal function impairment:* No initial dosage adjustment is necessary for elderly or hepatically impaired patients, or those with renal impairment. No initial dosing adjustment is generally necessary in patients with moderate and severe renal impairment, with maximum dose not exceeding 600 mg/day.

➤*Storage/Stability:* Store at controlled room temperature 20° to 25°C (68° to 77°F).

OLMESARTAN MEDOXOMIL

Rx	**Benicar** (Sankyo Pharma)	**Tablets:** 5 mg	Lactose. (Sankyo C12). Yellow. Film-coated. In 30s.
		20 mg	Lactose. (Sankyo C14). White. Film-coated. In 30s, 90s, and blister card 100s.
		40 mg	Lactose. (Sankyo C15). White, oval. Film-coated. In 30s, 90s, and blister card 100s.

For complete prescribing information, refer to the Angiotensin II Receptor Antagonists group monograph.

WARNING

When used in pregnancy during the second and third trimesters, drugs that act directly on the renin-angiotensin system can cause injury and even death to the developing fetus. When pregnancy is detected, discontinue olmesartan as soon as possible.

Indications

➤*Hypertension:* Treatment of hypertension alone or in combination with other antihypertensive agents.

Administration and Dosage

➤*Approved by the FDA:* April 26, 2002.

Dosage must be individualized. The usual recommended starting dose is 20 mg once daily with or without food when used as monotherapy in patients who are not volume-contracted. For patients requiring further reduction in blood pressure after 2 weeks of therapy, the dose may be increased to 40 mg. Doses above 40 mg do not appear to have greater effect. Twice-daily dosing offers no advantage over the same total dose given once daily.

If blood pressure is not controlled by olmesartan alone, a diuretic may be added. Olmesartan may be administered with other antihypertensive agents.

➤*Volume-depleted patients:* For patients with possible depletion of intravascular volume (eg, patients treated with diuretics, particularly those with impaired renal function), initiate olmesartan under close medical supervision and consider using a lower starting dose.

➤*Storage/Stability:* Store at 20° to 25°C (68° to 77°F).

EPLERENONE

Rx	**Inspra** (Pfizer)	**Tablets**: 25 mg	Lactose. (Pfizer NSR/25). Yellow, diamond shape. Film-coated. In 30s, 90s, and unit doses.
		50 mg	Lactose. (Pfizer NSR/50). Yellow, diamond shape. Film-coated. In 30s and 90s.

Indications

➤*Congestive heart failure (CHF) post-myocardial infarction (MI):* To improve survival of stable patients with left ventricular systolic dysfunction (ejection fraction 40% or less) and clinical evidence of CHF after an acute MI.

➤*Hypertension:* For the treatment of hypertension alone or in combination with other antihypertensive agents.

➤*Unlabeled uses:* Possible therapy used alone or in combination with an angiotensin-converting enzyme inhibitor (ACEI) for reducing left ventricular hypertrophy (LVH); as adjunctive therapy in diabetic hypertensives with microalbuminuria.

Administration and Dosage

➤*Approved by the FDA:* September 30, 2002.

Eplerenone may be administered with or without food.

➤*CHF post-MI:* 50 mg once daily. Initiate treatment at 25 mg once daily and titrate to the target dose of 50 mg once daily, preferably within 4 weeks as tolerated by the patient.

Eplerenone Dose Adjustment in CHF

Serum potassium (mEq/L)	Action	Dose adjustment
< 5	Increase	25 mg every other day to 25 mg qd 25 mg qd to 50 mg qd
5 to 5.4	Maintain	No adjustment
5.5 to 5.9	Decrease	50 mg qd to 25 mg qd 25 mg qd to 25 mg every other day 25 mg every other day to withhold
≥ 6	Withhold	—

Following withholding eplerenone because of serum potassium 6 mEq/L or more, eplerenone can be restarted at a dose of 25 mg every other day when serum potassium levels have fallen below 5.5 mEq/L. Measure serum potassium before initiating eplerenone therapy, within the first week, and at 1 month after the start of treatment or dose adjustment. Periodically assess serum potassium thereafter. Factors such as patient characteristics and serum potassium levels may indicate that additional monitoring is appropriate.

➤*Hypertension:* 50 mg administered once daily. Eplerenone may be used alone or in combination with other antihypertensive agents. The full therapeutic effect is apparent within 4 weeks. For patients with an inadequate blood pressure response to 50 mg once daily, increase the dosage to 50 mg twice daily. Higher dosages are not recommended because they have no greater effect on blood pressure than 100 mg or because they are associated with an increased risk of hyperkalemia.

Concomitant medication – For patients receiving weak CYP3A4 inhibitors (eg, erythromycin, saquinavir, verapamil, fluconazole), reduce the starting dose to 25 mg once daily.

➤*Storage/Stability:* Store at 25°C (77°F); excursions permitted to 15° to 30°C (59° to 86°F).

Actions

➤*Pharmacology:* Eplerenone binds to the mineralocorticoid receptor and blocks the binding of aldosterone, a component of the renin-angiotensin-aldosterone system (RAAS). Aldosterone synthesis, which occurs primarily in the adrenal gland, is modulated by multiple factors, including angiotensin II and non-RAAS mediators such as adrenocorticotropic hormone (ACTH) and potassium. Aldosterone binds to mineralocorticoid receptors in epithelial (eg, kidney) and nonepithelial (eg, heart, blood vessels, brain) tissues and increases blood pressure through induction of sodium reabsorption and possibly other mechanisms.

Eplerenone produces sustained increases in plasma renin and serum aldosterone, consistent with inhibition of the negative regulatory feedback of aldosterone on renin secretion. The resulting increased plasma renin activity and aldosterone circulating levels do not overcome the effect of eplerenone.

Eplerenone has relative selectivity in binding to recombinant human mineralocorticoid receptors compared with its binding to recombinant human glucocorticoid, progesterone, and androgen receptors.

➤*Pharmacokinetics:*

Absorption – Mean peak plasma concentrations of eplerenone are reached approximately 1.5 hours following oral administration. The absolute bioavailability of eplerenone is unknown. Both C_{max} and AUC are dose proportional for doses of 25 to 100 mg and less than proportional at doses above 100 mg. Steady state is reached within 2 days. Absorption is not affected by food.

Distribution – The plasma protein binding of eplerenone is approximately 50% and is primarily bound to alpha 1-acid glycoproteins. The apparent volume of distribution at steady state ranged from 43 to 90 L. Eplerenone does not preferentially bind to red blood cells.

Metabolism – Eplerenone metabolism is primarily mediated via CYP3A4. No active metabolites of eplerenone have been identified in human plasma. Inhibitors of CYP3A4 (eg, ketoconazole, saquinavir) increase blood levels of eplerenone.

Excretion – Less than 5% of an eplerenone dose is recovered as unchanged drug in the urine and feces. Following a single oral dose, approximately 32% of the dose was excreted in the feces and approximately 67% was excreted in the urine. The elimination half-life of eplerenone is approximately 4 to 6 hours. The apparent plasma clearance is approximately 10 L/h.

Special populations –

Elderly: At steady state, elderly subjects (65 years of age and older) had increases in C_{max} (22%) and AUC (45%) compared with younger subjects (18 to 45 years of age).

Race: At steady state, C_{max} was 19% lower and AUC was 26% lower in blacks.

Renal function impairment: The pharmacokinetics of eplerenone were evaluated in patients with varying degrees of renal insufficiency and in patients undergoing hemodialysis. Compared with control subjects, steady-state AUC and C_{max} increased 38% and 24%, respectively, in patients with severe renal impairment and decreased 26% and 3%, respectively, in patients undergoing hemodialysis. No correlation was observed between plasma clearance of eplerenone and creatinine clearance (Ccr). Eplerenone is not removed by hemodialysis.

Hepatic function impairment: The pharmacokinetics of 400 mg eplerenone have been investigated in patients with moderate (Child-Pugh class B) hepatic impairment and compared with normal subjects. Steady-state C_{max} and AUC of eplerenone increased 3.6% and 42%, respectively.

Heart failure: The pharmacokinetics of 50 mg eplerenone were evaluated in 8 patients with heart failure (NYHA classification II-IV) and 8 matched (gender, age, weight) healthy controls. Compared with the controls, steady state AUC and C_{max} in patients with stable heart failure were 38% and 30% higher, respectively.

Contraindications

All patients with the following conditions: Serum potassium greater than 5.5 mEq/L at initiation; Ccr 30 mL/min or less; concomitant use with the following potent CYP3A4 inhibitors: Ketoconazole, itraconazole, nefazodone, troleandomycin, clarithromycin, ritonavir, and nelfinavir.

Also contraindicated for the treatment of hypertension in patients with the following conditions: Type 2 diabetes with microalbuminuria; serum creatinine greater than 2 mg/dL in males or greater than 1.8 mg/dL in females; Ccr less than 50 mL/min; concomitant use of potassium supplements or potassium-sparing diuretics (amiloride, spironolactone, or triamterene).

Warnings

➤*Hyperkalemia:* The principal risk of eplerenone is hyperkalemia. Hyperkalemia can cause serious, sometimes fatal arrhythmias. This risk can be minimized by patient selection, avoidance of certain concomitant treatments, dose reduction of eplerenone, and monitoring. The rates of hyperkalemia increase with declining renal function. Treat patients with CHF post-MI who have serum creatinine levels greater than 2 mg/dL (males) or greater than 1.8 mg/dL (females), patients who have Ccr 50 mL/min or less, and diabetic patients with CHF post-MI, including those with proteinuria, with caution.

➤*Hepatic function impairment:* In 16 subjects with mild to moderate hepatic impairment who received 400 mg of eplerenone, no elevations of serum potassium above 5.5 mEq/L were observed. The mean increase in serum potassium was 0.12 mEq/L in patients with hepatic impairment and 0.13 mEq/L in normal controls. The use of eplerenone in patients with severe hepatic impairment has not been evaluated.

➤*Carcinogenesis:* Statistically significant increases in benign thyroid tumors were observed after 2 years in male and female rats when administered eplerenone 250 mg/kg/day (highest dose tested) and in male rats only at 75 mg/kg/day. These dosages provided systemic AUC exposures approximately 2 to 12 times higher than the average human therapeutic exposure at 100 mg/day. Repeat dose administration of eplerenone to rats increases the hepatic conjugation and clearance of thyroxin, which results in increased levels of TSH by a compensatory mechanism. Drugs that have produced thyroid tumors by this rodent-specific mechanism have not shown a similar effect in humans.

➤*Fertility impairment:* Male rats treated with eplerenone 1000 mg/kg/day for 10 weeks (AUC 17 times that at the 100 mg/day human therapeutic dose) had decreased weights of seminal vesicles and epi-

EPLERENONE

didymides and slightly decreased fertility. Dogs administered eplerenone at dosages of 15 mg/kg/day and higher (AUC 5 times that at the 100 mg/day human therapeutic dose) had dose-related prostate atrophy. The prostate atrophy was reversible after daily treatment for 1 year at 100 mg/kg/day. Dogs with prostate atrophy showed no decline in libido, sexual performance, or semen quality. Testicular weight and histology were not affected by eplerenone in any test animal species at any dosage.

➤*Pregnancy:* Category B. There are no adequate and well-controlled studies in pregnant women. Use during pregnancy only if the potential benefit justifies the potential risk to the fetus.

Embryo-fetal development studies were conducted with doses up to 1000 mg/kg/day in rats and 300 mg/kg/day in rabbits (exposures up to 32 and 31 times the human AUC for the 100 mg/day therapeutic dose, respectively). No teratogenic effects were seen in rats or rabbits, although decreased body weight in maternal rabbits and increased rabbit fetal resorptions and postimplantation loss were observed at the highest administered dosage. Because animal reproduction studies are not always predictive of human response, use eplerenone during pregnancy only if clearly needed.

➤*Lactation:* The excretion of eplerenone in human breast milk after oral administration is unknown. Because many drugs are excreted in human milk and because of the unknown potential for adverse effects on the nursing infant, decide whether to discontinue nursing or discontinue the drug, taking into account the importance of the drug to the mother.

➤*Children:* Safety and efficacy have not been established in pediatric patients.

Precautions

➤*Monitoring:* Measure serum potassium before initiating therapy, within the first week, and at 1 month after the start of treatment or dose adjustment; assess periodically thereafter.

Drug Interactions

Eplerenone Drug Interactions			
Precipitant drug	Object drug*		Description
ACE inhibitors Angiotensin II antagonists	Eplerenone	↑	Increased risk of hyperkalemia with coadministration.
CYP3A4 inhibitors	Eplerenone	↑	Coadministration of potent inhibitors (eg, ketoconazole) resulted in increased exposure of about 5-fold; less potent inhibitors yielded about a 2-fold increase (see Administration and Dosage and Contraindications).
NSAIDs	Eplerenone	↑↓	Coadministration of NSAIDs with other potassium-sparing antihypertensives may cause decreased antihypertensive effect and results in severe hyperkalemia in patients with impaired renal function.
St. John's wort	Eplerenone	↓	Approximately 30% decrease in eplerenone AUC.
Eplerenone	Lithium	↑	Coadministration of lithium with diuretics and ACE inhibitors may lead to lithium toxicity; frequently monitor serum lithium levels if coadministered with eplerenone.

* ↑ = Object drug increased. ↓ = Object drug decreased.

➤*Drug/Food interactions:* Coadministration with grapefruit juice produced a small increase (about 25%) in exposure.

Adverse Reactions

➤*CHF post-MI:* Discontinuations caused by hyperkalemia or abnormal renal function were less than 1% in both groups.

Eplerenone Adverse Reactions in CHF Post-MI Patients (%)		
Adverse reaction	Eplerenone (n = 3307)	Placebo (n = 3301)
GU		
Abnormal vaginal bleeding	0.4	0.4
Gynecomastia (males)	0.4	0.5
Mastodynia (males)	0.1	0.1
Metabolic		
Hyperkalemia	3.4	2
Hypokalemia	0.6	1.6
Increased creatinine	2.4	1.5
Increased creatinine (> 0.5 mg/dL)	6.5	4.9

Hypokalemia (< 3.5 mEq/L) or Hyperkalemia (> 5.5 or ≥ 6 mEq/L) in CHF Post-MI Patients (%)		
Potassium (mEq/L)	Eplerenone (n = 3251)	Placebo (n = 3237)
< 3.5	8.4	13.1
> 5.5	15.6	11.2
≥ 6	5.5	3.9

Hyperkalemia (> 5.5 mEq/L) by Baseline Ccr in CHF Post-MI Patients (%)		
Baseline Ccr	Eplerenone	Placebo
≤ 30 mL/min	31.5	22.6
31 to 50 mL/min	24.1	12.7
51 to 70 mL/min	16.9	13.1
> 70 mL/min	10.8	8.7

Hyperkalemia (> 5.5 mEq/L) by Proteinuria and History of Diabetes in CHF Post-MI Patients (%)[1]		
	Eplerenone	Placebo
Proteinuria, no diabetes	16	11
Diabetes, no proteinuria	18	13
Proteinuria and diabetes	26	16

[1] Diabetes assessed as positive medical history at baseline; proteinuria assessed by positive dipstick urinalysis at baseline.

➤*Hypertension:* Eplerenone has been evaluated for safety in 3091 patients treated for hypertension. A total of 690 patients were treated for over 6 months and 106 patients were treated for over 1 year.

The most common reasons for discontinuation of eplerenone were angina pectoris/MI, dizziness, headache, and increased gamma glutamyl transpeptidase (GGT).

Adverse Reactions in Patients Treated with Eplerenone vs Placebo (%)[1]		
Adverse reaction	Eplerenone (25 to 400 mg)	Placebo
GI		
Abdominal pain	1	0
Diarrhea	2	1
Metabolic		
Hypercholesterolemia	1[2]	0
Hyperkalemia (> 5.5 mEq/L)	≤ 8.7[2]	≤ 1
Hypertriglyceridemia	1[3]	0
Hyponatremia (< 135 mEq/L)	2.3	0.6
Increased ALT (3 × ULN[3])	0.01[2]	0.003
Increased ALT (5 × ULN[3])	0.002[2]	0.003
Increased BUN (> 30 mg/dL)	0.5[2]	0
Increased serum creatinine (> 2 mg/dL)	0.2[2]	0
Increased uric acid (> 9 mg/dL)	0.3	0
Miscellaneous		
Albuminuria	1	0
Coughing	2	1
Dizziness	3	2
Fatigue	2	1
Influenza-like symptoms	2	1

[1] Data are pooled from separate studies and are not necessarily comparable.
[2] Dose-dependent.
[3] ULN = upper limit of normal.

EPLERENONE

Sex Hormone Related Adverse Events with Eplerenone in Hypertension Patients (%)				
	Rates in males			Rates in females
	Gyneco-mastia	Masto-dynia	Either	Abnormal vaginal bleeding
All controlled studies	0.5	0.8	1	0.6
Controlled studies lasting ≥ 6 months	0.7	1.3	1.6	0.8
Open label, long-term study	1	0.3	1	2.1

Metabolic –

Hyperkalemia: Patients with both type 2 diabetes and microalbuminuria are at increased risk of developing persistent hyperkalemia. In a study in such patients taking 200 mg eplerenone, the frequencies of maximum serum potassium levels greater than 5.5 mEq/L were 33% with eplerenone given alone and 38% when eplerenone was given with enalapril.

Rates of hyperkalemia increased with decreasing renal function. In all studies, serum potassium elevations greater than 5.5 mEq/L were observed in 10.4% of patients treated with eplerenone with baseline calculated Ccr less than 70 mL/min, 5.6% of patients with baseline Ccr of 70 to 100 mL/min, and 2.6% of patients with baseline Ccr of greater than 100 mL/min.

Overdosage

➤*Symptoms:* No cases of human overdosage with eplerenone have been reported. The most likely manifestation of human overdosage would be hypotension or hyperkalemia.

➤*Treatment:* Eplerenone cannot be removed by hemodialysis. Eplerenone binds extensively to charcoal. If symptomatic hypotension occurs, institute supportive treatment. If hyperkalemia develops, initiate standard treatment.

Patient Information

Inform patients receiving eplerenone not to use potassium supplements, salt substitutes containing potassium, or contraindicated drugs without consulting the prescribing physician.

ANTIHYPERTENSIVE COMBINATIONS

ANTIHYPERTENSIVE COMBINATIONS
Content given per capsule or tablet.

	Product and Distributor	Diuretic	Other Content	How Supplied
Rx	Renese-R Tablets (Pfizer)	2 mg polythiazide	0.25 mg reserpine	Lactose. (Pfizer 446). Blue, scored. In 100s and 1000s.
Rx	Chlorothiazide/Reserpine Tablets (Various, eg, Mylan)	500 mg chlorothiazide	0.125 mg reserpine	In 100s.
Rx	Chloroserpine Tablets (Rugby)	250 mg chlorothiazide	0.125 mg reserpine	In 100s and 1000s.
Rx	Hydrochlorothiazide/Reserpine Tablets (Various)	50 mg hydrochlorothiazide	0.125 mg reserpine	In 100s and 1000s.
Rx	Hydro-Serp Tablets (Rugby)			In 1000s.
Rx	Hydroserpine #2 Tablets (Various, eg, Rugby)			In 100s, 250s, 400s and 1000s.
Rx	Hydrochlorothiazide/Reserpine Tablets (Various)	25 mg hydrochlorothiazide	0.125 mg reserpine	In 100s and 1000s.
Rx	Hydroserpine #1 Tablets (Various, eg, Rugby)			In 100s and 1000s.
Rx	Salutensin-Demi (Shire)	25 mg hydroflumethiazide	0.125 mg reserpine	Lactose, sucrose. Yellow. In 100s.
Rx	Salutensin Tablets (Roberts)	50 mg hydroflumethiazide	0.125 mg reserpine	Lactose, sucrose. (BL S1)Green. In 100s and 1000s.
Rx	Diutensen-R Tablets (Wallace)	2.5 mg methyclothiazide	0.1 mg reserpine	White, pink. Mottled. In 100s, 500s and 5000s.
Rx	Metatensin #4 Tablets (Hoechst Marion Roussel)	4 mg trichlormethiazide	0.1 mg reserpine	Lactose. (Merrell 65) Lavender. In 100s.
Rx	Rauwolfia/Bendroflumethiazide Tablets (Various, eg, Rugby)	4 mg bendroflumethiazide	50 mg powdered rauwolfia serpentina	In 100s.
Rx	Rauzide Tablets (B-M Squibb)			In 100s.
Rx	Hydrap-ES Tablets (Parmed)	15 mg hydrochlorothiazide	0.1 mg reserpine 25 mg hydralazine HCl	(CC124). Salmon pink. In 100s, 500s, 1000s.
Rx	Ser-Ap-Es Tablets (Novartis)			Lactose, sucrose. (71). Salmon pink. In 100s and 1000s.
Rx	Tri-Hydroserpine Tablets (Rugby)			In 100s and 1000s.
Rx	Hydrochlorothiazide/Hydralazine Caps (Various, eg, Moore, Zenith-Goldline)	50 mg hydrochlorothiazide	50 mg hydralazine HCl	In 100s, 500s and 1000s.
Rx	Apresazide 50/50 Capsules (Novartis)			Parabens. Pink, white. In 100s.
Rx	Hydrochlorothiazide/Hydralazine Caps (Various, eg, Moore, Zenith-Goldline)	25 mg hydrochlorothiazide	25 mg hydralazine HCl	In 100s, 500s and 1000s.
Rx	Apresazide 25/25 Capsules (Novartis)			Parabens. Lt. blue, white. In 100s.
Rx	Atenolol/Chlorthalidone Tablets (Various, eg, Zenith-Goldline)	25 mg chlorthalidone	100 mg atenolol	In 50s, 100s, 250s, 500s, and 1000s.
Rx	Tenoretic 100 Tablets (Zeneca)			(ICI 117). White, scored. In 100s.
Rx	Atenolol/Chlorthalidone Tablets (Various, eg, Zenith-Goldline)	25 mg chlorthalidone	50 mg atenolol	In 50s, 100s, 250s, 500s, and 1000s.
Rx	Tenoretic 50 Tablets (Zeneca)			(ICI 115). White, scored. In 100s.
Rx	Corzide Tablets 80/5 (Monarch)	5 mg bendroflumethiazide	80 mg nadolol	Lactose. (CORZIDE 80/5 BL 284). In 100s.
Rx	Corzide Tablets 40/5 (Monarch)	5 mg bendroflumethiazide	40 mg nadolol	Lactose. (CORZIDE 40/5 BL 283). In 100s.
Rx	Bisoprolol Fumarate and Hydrochlorothiazide Tablets (Various, eg, ESI Lederle, Mylan, Purepac, Ivax)	6.25 mg hydrochlorothiazide	2.5 mg bisoprolol fumarate	In 100s, 500s, and 1000s.
Rx	Ziac Tablets (Barr			(LL B 12). In 30s and 100s.
Rx	Bisoprolol Fumarate and Hydrochlorothiazide Tablets (Various, eg, ESI Lederle, Mylan, Purepac, Ivax)	6.25 mg hydrochlorothiazide	5 mg bisoprolol fumarate	In 100s, 500s, and 1000s.
Rx	Ziac Tablets (Barr			(LL B 13). In 30s and 100s.
Rx	Bisoprolol Fumarate and Hydrochlorothiazide Tablets (Various, eg, ESI Lederle, Mylan, Purepac, Ivax)	6.25 mg hydrochlorothiazide	10 mg bisoprolol fumarate	In 30s, 100s, 500s, and 1000s.
Rx	Ziac Tablets (Barr)			(LL B 14). In 30s.
Rx	Timolide 10-25 Tablets (Merck)	25 mg hydrochlorothiazide	10 mg timolol maleate	(TIMOLIDE MSD 67). In 100s.
Rx	Propranolol/Hydrochlorothiazide Tablets (Various, eg, Mylan)	25 mg hydrochlorothiazide	80 mg propranolol HCl	In 100s and 1000s.
Rx	Inderide 80/25 Tablets (Wyeth-Ayerst)			Lactose. (Inderide 80/25). In 100s.
Rx	Propranolol/Hydrochlorothiazide Tablets (Various, eg, Mylan)	25 mg hydrochlorothiazide	40 mg propranolol HCl	In 100s.
Rx	Inderide 40/25 Tablets (Wyeth-Ayerst)			Lactose. (Inderide 40/25). In 100s, 1000s and UD 100s.
Rx	Methyldopa and Hydrochlorothiazide Tablets (Various, eg, Rugby)	50 mg hydrochlorothiazide	500 mg methyldopa	In 100s, 250s and 500s.
Rx	Aldoril D50 Tablets (Merck)			(MSD 935 ALDORIL). White. Oval. Film coated. In 100s.

ANTIHYPERTENSIVE COMBINATIONS

	Product and Distributor	Diuretic	Other Content	How Supplied
Rx	Methyldopa/Hydrochlorothiazide Tablets (Various, eg, Rugby)	30 mg hydrochlorothiazide	500 mg methyldopa	In 100s, 250s and 500s.
Rx	Aldoril D30 Tablets (Merck)			(MSD 694 ALDORIL). Salmon. Oval. Film coated. In 100s.
Rx	Methyldopa/Hydrochlorothiazide Tablets (Various, eg, Goldline, Mylan, Rugby)	25 mg hydrochlorothiazide	250 mg methyldopa	In 100s, 500s, 1000s and UD 100s.
Rx	Aldoril-25 Tablets (Merck)			(MSD 456 ALDORIL). White. Film coated. In 100s, 1000s and UD 100s.
Rx	Methyldopa/Hydrochlorothiazide Tablets (Various, eg, Mylan, Zenith-Goldline)	15 mg hydrochlorothiazide	250 mg methyldopa	In 100s, 500s, 1000s and UD 100s.
Rx	Aldoril-15 Tablets (Merck)			(MSD 423 ALDORIL). Salmon. Film coated. In 100s and 1000s.
Rx	Lopressor HCT 100/50 Tablets (Geigy)	50 mg hydrochlorothiazide	100 mg metoprolol tartrate	Lactose, sucrose. (GEIGY 73 73). White, yellow, scored. Capsule shape. In 100s.
Rx	Lopressor HCT 100/25 Tablets (Geigy)	25 mg hydrochlorothiazide	100 mg metoprolol tartrate	Lactose, sucrose. (GEIGY 53 53). White, pink, scored. Capsule shape. In 100s.
Rx	Lopressor HCT 50/25 Tablets (Geigy)	25 mg hydrochlorothiazide	50 mg metoprolol tartrate	Lactose, sucrose. (GEIGY 35 35). White, blue, scored. Capsule shape. In 100s.
Rx	Captopril and Hydrochlorothiazide Tablets (Teva)	25 mg hydrochlorothiazide	50 mg captopril	In 100s and 1000s.
Rx	Capozide 50/25 Tablets (B-M Squibb)			(CAPOZIDE 50/25). Peach. Biconvex, oval. In 100s.
Rx	Captopril and Hydrochlorothiazide Tablets (Teva)	25 mg hydrochlorothiazide	25 mg captopril	In 100s and 1000s.
Rx	Capozide 25/25 Tablets (B-M Squibb)			(CAPOZIDE 25/25). Peach, scored. Biconvex, square. In 100s.
Rx	Captopril and Hydrochlorothiazide Tablets (Teva)	15 mg hydrochlorothiazide	50 mg captopril	In 100s and 1000s.
Rx	Capozide 50/15 Tablets (B-M Squibb)			(CAPOZIDE 50/15). White, orange, mottled, scored. Oval. In 100s.
Rx	Captopril and Hydrochlorothiazide Tablets (Teva)	15 mg hydrochlorothiazide	25 mg captopril	In 100s and 1000s.
Rx	Capozide 25/15 Tablets (B-M Squibb)			(CAPOZIDE 25/15). White, orange, mottled, scored. Biconvex, square. In 100s.
Rx	Benazepril HCl/Hydrochlorothiazide Tablets (Sandoz)	25 mg hydrochlorothiazide	20 mg benazepril	Castor oil, lactose. (GG 367). Red. In 100s.
Rx	Lotensin HCT Tablets 20/25 (Novartis)			Lactose. (LOTENSIN HCT 75 75). Red, scored. Oblong. In 100s and Accu-Pak 100s.
Rx	Benazepril HCl/Hydrochlorothiazide Tablets (Sandoz)	12.5 mg hydrochlorothiazide	20 mg benazepril	Castor oil, lactose. (GG 366). Grayish-violet. In 100s.
Rx	Lotensin HCT Tablets 20/12.5 (Novartis)			Lactose. (LOTENSIN HCT 74 74). Grayish-violet, scored. Oblong. In 100s and Accu-Pak 100s.
Rx	Benazepril HCl/Hydrochlorothiazide Tablets (Sandoz)	12.5 mg hydrochlorothiazide	10 mg benazepril	Castor oil, lactose. (GG 365). Light pink. In 100s.
Rx	Lotensin HCT Tablets 10/12.5 (Novartis)			Lactose. (LOTENSIN HCT 72 72). Lt. pink, scored. Oblong. In 100s and Accu-Pak 100s.
Rx	Accuretic (Parke-Davis)	12.5 mg hydrochlorothiazide	10 mg quinapril HCl	Lactose. (PD 222). Pink, scored elliptical, biconvex. Film-coated. In 30s.
		12.5 mg hydrochlorothiazide	20 mg quinapril HCl	Lactose. (PD 220). Pink, scored triangular. Film-coated. In 30s.
		25 mg hydrochlorothiazide	20 mg quinapril.	Lactose. (PD 223). Pink, scored round, biconvex. Film-coated. In 30s.
Rx	Teveten HCT (Biovail)	12.5 mg hydrochlorothiazide	600 mg eprosartan	Lactose. (SOLVAY 5147). Butterscotch, capsule shape. Film-coated. In 100s.
Rx	Teveten HCT (Biovail)	25 mg hydrochlorothiazide	600 mg eprosartan	Lactose. (SOLVAY 5150). Brick red, capsule shape. Film-coated. In 100s.
Rx	Avalide (Bristol-Myers Squibb)	12.5 mg hydrochlorothiazide	150 mg irbesartan	Lactose. (2775). Peach, biconvex. Oval. In 30s, 90s, 500s, and blister pack 100s.
Rx	Avalide (Bristol-Myers Squibb)	12.5 mg hydrochlorothiazide	300 mg irbesartan	Lactose. (2776). Peach, biconvex. Oval. In 30s, 90s, 500s, and blister pack 100s.
Rx	Micardis HCT Tablets (Boehringer Ingelheim)	12.5 mg hydrochlorothiazide	40 mg telmisartan	Sorbitol, lactose. (H4). Bilayered (red and white to off-white), oblong. In blister pack 28s.
		12.5 mg hydrochlorothiazide	80 mg telmisartan	Sorbitol, lactose. (H8). Bilayered (red and white to off-white), oblong. In blister pack 28s.
Rx	Benazepril HCl/Hydrochlorothiazide (Sandoz)	6.25 mg hydrochlorothiazide	5 mg benazepril	Lactose. (GG 364). White. In 100s.
Rx	Lotensin HCT Tablets 5/6.25 (Novartis)			Lactose. (C-G 57LOTENSIN HCT 57 57). White, scored. Oblong. In 100s and Accu-Pak 100s.

ANTIHYPERTENSIVE COMBINATIONS

	Product and Distributor	Diuretic	Other Content	How Supplied
Rx	Enalapril Maleate/Hydrochlorothiazide Tablets (Eon)	25 mg hydrochlorothiazide	10 mg enalapril maleate	Lactose. (E 172). Salmon. In 100s and 1000s.
Rx	Vaseretic 10-25 Tablets (Biovail)			(VASERETIC MSD 720). Red. In 100s.
Rx	Enalapril Maleate/Hydrochlorothiazide Tablets (Eon)	12.5 mg hydrochlorothiazide	5 mg enalapril maleate	Lactose. (E 151). Green. In 100s and 1000s.
Rx	Vaseretic 5-12.5 Tablets (Biovail)			Lactose. (MSD 173). Square-capsule shape. In unit-of-use 100s.
Rx	Lisinopril/Hydrochlorothiazide Tablets (Various, eg, Geneva, Ivax)	25 mg hydrochlorothiazide	20 mg lisinopril	In 100s, 500s, 1000s, and UD 100s.
Rx	Prinzide 25 Tablets (Merck)			(MSD 142 PRINZIDE). In 30s and 100s.
Rx	Zestoretic Tablets (Zeneca)			(Stuart 145 Zestoretic). Peach. Biconvex. In 100s.
Rx	Lisinopril/Hydrochlorothiazide Tablets (Various, eg, Geneva, Ivax)	12.5 mg hydrochlorothiazide	20 mg lisinopril	In 100s, 500s, 1000s, and UD 100s.
Rx	Prinzide 12.5 Tablets (Merck)			(MSD 140 PRINZIDE). In 30s and 100s.
Rx	Zestoretic Tablets (Zeneca)			(Stuart 142 Zestoretic). White. Biconvex. In 100s.
Rx	Lisinopril/Hydrochlorothiazide Tablets (Various, eg, Geneva, Ivax)	12.5 mg hydrochlorothiazide	10 mg lisinopril	In 100s, 500s, 1000s, and UD 100s.
Rx	Prinzide Tablets (Merck)			(MSD 145 PRINZIDE). In 30s and 100s.
Rx	Zestoretic Tablets (Zeneca)			(Stuart 141). Peach. Biconvex. In 100s.
Rx	Clorpres Tablets (Bertek)	15 mg chlorthalidone	0.3 mg clonidine HCl	(M72). Yellow, scored. In 100s.
Rx	Combipres 0.3 Tablets (Boehringer Ingelheim)			Lactose, parabens. (BI 10). White, scored. Oval. In 100s.
Rx	Clorpres Tablets (Bertek)	15 mg chlorthalidone	0.2 mg clonidine HCl	(M27). Yellow, scored. In 100s.
Rx	Combipres 0.2 Tablets (Boehringer Ingelheim)			Lactose, parabens. (BI 9). Blue, scored. Oval. In 100s and 1000s.
Rx	Clorpres Tablets (Bertek)	15 mg chlorthalidone	0.1 mg clonidine HCl	(M1). Yellow, scored. In 100s.
Rx	Combipres 0.1 Tablets (Boehringer Ingelheim)			Lactose, parabens. (BI 8). Pink, scored. Oval. In 100s and 1000s.
Rx	Minizide 5 Capsules (Pfizer)	0.5 mg polythiazide	5 mg prazosin HCl	(436). Blue-green, blue. In 100s.
Rx	Minizide 2 Capsules (Pfizer)	0.5 mg polythiazide	2 mg prazosin HCl	(432). Blue-green, pink. In 100s.
Rx	Minizide 1 Capsules (Pfizer)	0.5 mg polythiazide	1 mg prazosin HCl	(430). Blue-green. In 100s.
Rx	Hyzaar Tablets (Merck)	12.5 mg hydrochlorothiazide	50 mg losartan potassium, 4.24 mg potassium	Lactose. (MRK 717 HYZAAR). Yellow. Teardrop shape. Film coated. In 30s, 90s, 100s and UD 100s.
Rx	Hyzaar Tablets (Merck)	25 mg hydrochlorothiazide	100 mg losartan potassium, 8.48 mg potassium	Lactose. (MRK 747 HYZAAR). Lt. yellow. Teardrop shape. Film-coated. In unit-of-use 30s and 100s and UD 100s.
Rx	Lotrel Capsules (Novartis)		2.5 mg amlodipine, 10 mg benazepril HCl	(LOTREL 2255). White/gold bands. In 100s.
			5 mg amlodipine, 10 mg benazepril HCl	(LOTREL 2260). Lt. brown/white bands. In 100s.
			5 mg amlodipine, 20 mg benazepril HCl	(LOTREL 2265). Pink/white bands. In 100s.
			10 mg amlodipine, 20 mg benazepril HCl	Lactose. (Lotrel 0364). Purple. In 100s.
Rx	Lexxel Extended-Release Tablets (Astra Pharm)		5 mg enalapril maleate, 2.5 mg felodipine	Lactose. (LEXXEL2, 5-2.5). White, biconvex. Film-coated. In unit-of-use 30s and UD 100s.
			5 mg enalapril maleate, 5 mg felodipine	Lactose. (LEXXEL 1, 5-5). White, biconvex. Film-coated. In unit-of-use 30s, 100s and UD 100s.
Rx	Uniretic Tablets (Schwarz)	25 mg hydrochlorothiazide	15 mg moexipril HCl	Lactose. (725 S P). In 100s.
		12.5 mg hydrochlorothiazide	15 mg moexipril HCl	(720 SP). White, oval, scored. Film coated. In 100s.
		12.5 mg hydrochlorothiazide	7.5 mg moexipril	Lactose. (712 S P). In 100s.
Rx	Diovan HCT Tablets (Novartis)	12.5 mg hydrochlorothiazide	80 mg valsartan	(CG HGH). Lt. orange. Talc. In 100s, 4000s, and UD 100s.
		12.5 mg hydrochlorothiazide	160 mg valsartan	(CG HHH). Dk. red. Talc. In 100s, 4000s, and UD 100s.
		25 mg hydrochlorothiazide	160 mg valsartan	Talc. (NVR HXH). Brown orange, ovaloid. In 100s and UD 100s.

ANTIHYPERTENSIVE COMBINATIONS

ANTIHYPERTENSIVE COMBINATIONS

	Product and Distributor	Diuretic	Other Content	How Supplied
Rx	**Benicar HCT** (Sankyo Pharma)	12.5 mg hydrochlorothiazide	20 mg olmesartan medoxomil	Lactose. (Sankyo C22). Reddish-yellow. Film-coated. In 30s, 90s, 1000s, and blister cards of 10.
		12.5 mg hydrochlorothiazide	40 mg olmesartan medoxomil	Lactose. (Sankyo C23). Reddish-yellow, oval. Film-coated. In 30s, 90s, 1000s, and blister cards of 10.
		25 mg hydrochlorothiazide	40 mg olmesartan medoxomil	Lactose. (Sankyo C25). Pink, oval. Film-coated. In 30s, 90s, 1000s, and blister cards of 10.
Rx	**Atacand HCT** (AstraZeneca)	12.5 mg hydrochlorothiazide	16 mg candesartan cilexetil	Lactose. (ACS 162). Peach, oval. Biconvex. In 1000s, UD 100s, and unit-of-use 30s and 90s.
		12.5 mg hydrochlorothiazide	32 mg candesartan cilexetil	Lactose. (ACJ 322). Yellow, oval. Biconvex. In 1000s, UD 100s, and unit-of-use 30s and 90s.
Rx	**Tarka Tablets** (Abbott)		1 mg trandolapril/240 mg verapamil	Lactose. (242 TARKA). White, oval, film-coated. In 100s.
			2 mg trandolapril/180 mg verapamil	Lactose. (182 TARKA). Pink, oval, film-coated. In 100s.
			2 mg trandolapril/240 mg verapamil	Lactose. (242 TARKA). Gold, oval. Film-coated. In 100s.
			4 mg trandolapril/240 mg verapamil	Lactose. (244). Reddish-brown, oval, film-coated. In 100s.
Rx	**Monopril-HCT** (Bristol-Myers Squibb)	12.5 mg hydrochlorothiazide	10 mg fosinopril sodium	Lactose. (1492). Peach. In 100s.
		12.5 mg hydrochlorothiazide	20 mg fosinopril sodium	Lactose. (1493). Peach, bisected. In 100s.

PHENTOLAMINE

Rx   **Phentolamine Mesylate for Injection** (Bedford)   **Powder for Injection:** 5 mg (as mesylate)   Mannitol. In 2 mL vials.

Indications

➤*Pheochromocytoma:* Prevention or control of hypertensive episodes that may occur in a patient with pheochromocytoma as a result of stress or manipulation during preoperative preparation and surgical excision.

Pharmacological test for pheochromocytoma (not the method of choice; see Warnings).

➤*Dermal necrosis:* Prevention and treatment of dermal necrosis and sloughing following IV administration or extravasation of norepinephrine or dopamine.

➤*Unlabeled uses:* Phentolamine has been used to treat hypertensive crises secondary to MAO inhibitor/sympathomimetic amine interactions and rebound hypertension on withdrawal of clonidine, propranolol or other antihypertensives. It has also been used in combination with papaverine as an intracavernous injection for impotence.

Administration and Dosage

➤*Prevention or control of hypertensive episodes in pheochromocytoma:* For use in preoperative reduction of elevated blood pressure, inject 5 mg (1 mg for children) IV or IM 1 or 2 hours before surgery. Repeat if necessary. During surgery, administer 5 mg for adults (1 mg for children) IV as indicated to help prevent or control paroxysms of hypertension, tachycardia, respiratory depression, convulsions or other effects of epinephrine intoxication.

Postoperatively, norepinephrine may be given to control hypotension which may follow complete removal of pheochromocytoma.

➤*Prevention and treatment of dermal necrosis and sloughing following IV administration or extravasation of norepinephrine* : For prevention, add 10 mg to each liter of solution containing norepinephrine. The pressor effect of norepinephrine is not affected. For treatment, inject 5 to 10 mg in 10 mL saline into the extravasation area ≤ 12 hours. For children, use 0.1 to 0.2 mg/kg up to a maximum of 10 mg.

➤*Diagnosis of pheochromocytoma (phentolamine blocking test):* Withhold sedatives, analgesics and all other medication not considered essential for at least 24 hours (preferably 48 to 72 hours) prior to the test. Withhold antihypertensive drugs until blood pressure returns to the untreated, hypertensive level. Do not perform the test on normotensive patients. Keep patient at rest in supine position throughout the test, preferably in a quiet, darkened room. Delay injection until blood pressure is stabilized, as evidenced by blood pressure readings taken every 10 minutes for at least 30 minutes.

IV test – Although a 5 mg test dose (1 mg for children) has been recommended, a 2.5 mg test dose will produce fewer false-positive tests and may minimize dangerous drops in blood pressure in patients with pheochromocytoma. If the 2.5 mg dose is negative, perform a 5 mg test before considering the test negative. Dissolve 5 mg phentolamine mesylate in 1 mL Sterile Water for Injection. Insert the syringe needle into a vein and delay injection until pressor response to venipuncture has subsided. Inject rapidly. Record blood pressure immediately, at 30 second intervals for the first 3 minutes, then at 60 second intervals for the next 7 minutes.

Positive response: Suggestive of pheochromocytoma, positive response is indicated by a drop in blood pressure of more than 35 mmHg systolic and 25 mmHg diastolic pressure. A typical positive response is a pressure reduction of 60 mmHg systolic and 25 mmHg diastolic. Maximal decrease in pressure is usually evident within 2 minutes after injection. Return to preinjection pressure commonly occurs within 15 to 30 minutes, but may return more rapidly. If blood pressure falls to a dangerous level, treat patient as outlined in the Overdosage section. Always confirm a positive response by other diagnostic procedures, preferably the measurement of urinary catecholamines or their metabolites.

Negative response: Indicated when the blood pressure is unchanged, negative response is elevated or is reduced less than 35 mmHg systolic and 25 mmHg diastolic after injection. A negative response may not exclude the diagnosis of pheochromocytoma, especially in patients with paroxysmal hypertension in whom the incidence of false-negative response is high.

IM test – Preparation is the same as for the IV test. Adult dosage is 5 mg IM; for children it is 3 mg. Record blood pressure every 5 minutes for 30 to 45 minutes following IM injection. Positive response is indicated by a drop in blood pressure of 35 mmHg systolic and 25 mmHg diastolic or greater within 20 minutes following injection.

Reliability – The test is most reliable in patients with sustained hypertension and least reliable in those with paroxysmal hypertension. False-positive tests may occur in patients with hypertension without pheochromocytoma.

➤*Storage/Stability:* Store between 15° to 30°C (59° to 86°F). Use reconstituted solution upon preparation; do not store.

Actions

➤*Pharmacology:* Phentolamine, an α-adrenergic blocking agent, blocks presynaptic (α_2) and postsynaptic (α_1) α-adrenergic receptors. It is a competitive antagonist of endogenous and exogenous α-active agents. It also acts on both the arterial tree and venous bed. Thus, total peripheral resistance is lowered and venous return to the heart is diminished. Phentolamine also causes cardiac stimulation.

Phentolamine has an immediate onset and a short duration of action.

Contraindications

Myocardial infarction, coronary insufficiency, angina or other evidence suggestive of coronary artery disease. Hypersensitivity to phentolamine or related compounds.

Warnings

Myocardial infarction, cerebrovascular spasm and cerebrovascular occlusion have followed phentolamine administration, usually in association with marked hypotensive episodes with shock-like states which occasionally follow parenteral use.

For screening tests in patients with hypertension, the generally available urinary assay of catecholamines or other biochemical assays have largely supplanted phentolamine and other pharmacological tests. None of the chemical or pharmacological tests are infallible in the diagnosis of pheochromocytoma. The phentolamine test is not the procedure of choice; reserve for cases in which additional confirmatory evidence is necessary and consider the risks involved.

➤*Pregnancy and Lactation:* Safety for use during pregnancy or lactation has not been established. Use only when clearly needed and when the potential benefits outweigh the potential hazards to the fetus or nursing infant.

Precautions

Tachycardia and cardiac arrhythmias may occur with phentolamine use. When possible, defer use of cardiac glycosides until cardiac rhythm returns to normal.

Drug Interactions

➤*Epinephrine and ephedrine:* The vasoconstricting and hypertensive effects of these drugs are antagonized by phentolamine.

Adverse Reactions

Acute and prolonged hypotensive episodes; tachycardia; cardiac arrhythmias.

Weakness; dizziness; flushing; orthostatic hypotension; nasal stuffiness; nausea; vomiting; diarrhea.

Overdosage

If blood pressure drops to a dangerous level or other evidence of shock occurs, treat vigorously and promptly. Include IV infusion of norepinephrine, titrated to maintain normal blood pressure. Epinephrine is contraindicated because it stimulates both α- and β-receptors; since α-receptors are blocked, the net effect of epinephrine administration is vasodilation and a further drop in blood pressure (epinephrine reversal).

PHENOXYBENZAMINE HCl

Rx   **Dibenzyline** (Wellspring)   **Capsules:** 10mg   (SKF E33). Red. In 100s

Indications

➤*Pheochromocytoma:* To control episodes of hypertension and sweating. If tachycardia is excessive, it may also be necessary to use a beta-blocker concomitantly.

➤*Unlabeled uses:* Phenoxybenzamine (5 to 60 mg/day) has shown efficacy in micturition disorders resulting from neurogenic bladder, functional outlet obstruction, and partial prastatic obstruction.

Administration and Dosage

Individualize dosage. Slowly increase small intial doses until the desired effect is obtained or side effects become troublesome. Observe patient before increasing dosage. Increase to a point where symptom-atic relief or objective improvement are obtained, but not so high that blockade side effects become troublesome.

Initially, 10 mg twice a day. Increase dosage every other day until optimal dosage is obtained as judged by blood pressure control. Usual dosage range is 20 mg to 40 mg, 2 or 3 times daily. In children, give 1 to 2 mg/kg/day, divided every 6 to 8 hours.

Actions

➤*Pharmacology:* An irreversible alpha-adrenergic receptor (both pre- and postsynaptic) blocking agent which can produce and maintain "chemical sympathectomy." It increases blood flow to skin, mucosa, and abdominal viscera, and lowers supine and standing blood pressures. It has no effect on the parasympathetic system.

PHENOXYBENZAMINE HCl

➤*Pharmacokinetics:* Absorption from the GI tract is incomplete (20% to 30%)

Contraindications

Conditions where a fall in blood pressure may be undesirable.

Warnings

➤*Concomitant therapy:* Phenoxybenzamine-induced alpha-adrenergic blockade leaves beta-adrenergic receptors unopposed. Compounds that stimulate both types of receptors (ie, epinephrine) may produce an exaggerated hypotensive response and tachycardia.

Phenoxybenzamine has shown in vitro mutagenic activity in the Ames test and in the mouse lymphoma assay. In animals, repeated intraperitoneal phenoxybenzamine resulted in peritoneal sarcomes; chronic oral dosing produced malignant GI tract tumors. Clinical significance is not established. Nevertheless, consider these results in determining benefit-to-risk ratio.

Precautions

Administer with caution to patients with marked cerebral or coronary arteriosclerosis or renal damage. Adrenergic blocking effects may aggravate respiratory infections.

Adverse Reactions

Nasal congestion, miosis, postural hypotension, tachycardia, and inhibition of ejaculation may occur. They vary according to degree of adrenergic blockade, and tend to decrease as therapy continues. GI irritation, drowsiness, and fatigue also occur.

Overdosage

➤*Symptoms:* Symptoms may include postural hypotension resulting in dizziness or fainting; tachycardia, particularly postural; vomiting; lethargy; shock. These are largely due to blockage of the sympathetic nervous system and of the circulating epinephrine.

➤*Treatment:* Discontinue the drug. Treat circulatory failure, if present. In mild overdosage, recumbent position with legs elevated usually restores cerebral circulation. In more severe cases, institute measures to combat shock. Usual pressor agents are not effective. Do not use epinephrine (see Warnings). The patient may have to be kept flat 24 hours or more as drug's effect is prolonged. Leg bandages and an abdominal binder may shorten disability period. May use norepinephrine IV to combat severe hypotension; it primarily stimulates alpha receptors. Although phenoxybenzamine is an alpha blocker, sufficient norepinephrine will overcome this effect.

Patient Information

Avoid alcoholic beverages.

If dizziness (postural hypotension) occurs, avoid sudden changes in posture.

Medication may cause nasal congestion and constricted pupils. Inhibition of ejaculation may occur, but generally decreases with continued therapy.

Avoid cough, cold, or allergy medications containing sympathomimetics, except on professional recommendation.

METYROSINE

| Rx | Demser (MSD) | Capsules: 250 mg | (MSD 690 DEMSER). Two-tone blue. In 100s. |

Indications

➤*Pheochromocytoma:* Preoperative preparation of patients; management when surgery is contraindicated; chronic treatment of malignant pheochromocytoma.

Not recommended for the control of essential hypertension.

Administration and Dosage

➤*Adults and children over 12:* Initial dosage is 250 mg 4 times daily. This may be increased by 250 to 500 mg every day to a maximum of 4 g/day in divided doses. When used for preoperative preparation, give the optimally effective dosage for at least 5 to 7 days (between 2 and 3 g/day); titrate by monitoring clinical symptoms and catecholamine excretion. In hypertensive patients, titrate dosage to achieve normal blood pressure and control of clinical symptoms. In normotensive patients, titrate dosage to reduce urinary metanephrines or vanillylmandelic acid by ≥ 50%.

Use in children under 12 years of age is limited and a dosage schedule cannot be given.

If patients are not adequately controlled by metyrosine, add an alpha-adrenergic blocker (phenoxybenzamine).

Actions

➤*Pharmacology:* Metyrosine inhibits tyrosine hydroxylase, which catalyzes the first transformation in catecholamine biosynthesis, ie, the conversion of tyrosine to dihydroxyphenylalanine (DOPA). Because this is the rate-limiting step, hydroxylase blockade results in decreased endogenous levels of catecholamines, usually measured as decreased urinary excretion of catecholamines and their metabolites.

In patients with pheochromocytoma who produce excessive amounts of norepinephrine and epinephrine, 1 to 4 g/day has reduced catecholamine biosynthesis from about 35% to 80%, as measured by the total excretion of catecholamines and their metabolites (metanephrine and vanillylmandelic acid). The maximum biochemical effect usually occurs within 2 to 3 days; the urinary concentration of catecholamines and their metabolites usually returns to pretreatment levels within 3 to 4 days after discontinuation. In some patients, the total excretion of catecholamines and catecholamine metabolites may be lowered to normal or near normal levels (< 10 mg/24 hours). In most patients treatment duration has been 2 to 8 weeks, but several patients have received metyrosine for periods of 1 to 10 years.

Most patients on metyrosine experience decreased frequency and severity of hypertensive attacks with headache, nausea, sweating and tachycardia. In patients who respond, blood pressure decreases progressively during the first 2 days; after withdrawal, it usually increases gradually to pretreatment values in 2 to 3 days.

➤*Pharmacokinetics:* Metyrosine is well absorbed from the GI tract. Approximately 53% to 88% (mean 69%) is recovered in the urine as unchanged drug following maintenance oral dosages of 600 to 4000 mg/24 hours. Less than 1% of administered drug is recovered as catechol metabolites. These metabolites are probably not present in sufficient amounts to contribute to the biochemical effects of metyrosine. The quantities excreted, however, are sufficient to interfere with accurate determination of urinary catecholamines determined by routine techniques.

The plasma half-life over 8 hours after single oral doses was 3.4 to 3.7 hours in three patients.

Contraindications

Hypersensitivity to metyrosine.

Warnings

➤*Maintain fluid volume during and after surgery:* When metyrosine is used preoperatively, especially with alpha-adrenergic blocking drugs, maintain adequate intravascular volume intraoperatively (especially after tumor removal) and post-operatively to avoid hypotension and decreased perfusion of vital organs resulting from vasodilatation and expanded volume capacity. After tumor removal, large volumes of plasma may be needed to maintain blood and central venous pressure.

Life-threatening arrhythmias may occur during anesthesia and surgery and may require treatment with a beta blocker or lidocaine. During surgery, monitor blood pressure and ECG continuously.

➤*Intraoperative effects:* While the preoperative use of metyrosine is thought to decrease intraoperative problems with blood pressure control, it does not eliminate the danger of hypertensive crises or arrhythmias during manipulation of the tumor. Phentolamine, an alpha-adrenergic blocking drug, may be needed.

➤*Renal/Hepatic function impairment:* Use with caution.

➤*Pregnancy:* Category C. Safety for use during pregnancy has not been established. Use only when clearly needed and when the potential benefits outweigh the potential hazards to the fetus.

➤*Lactation:* It is not known whether metyrosine is excreted in breast milk. Safety for use in the nursing mother has not been established.

➤*Children:* Safety and efficacy for use in children under 12 years of age have not been established.

Precautions

➤*Long-term use:* Human experience is limited and chronic animal studies have not been performed. Therefore, perform laboratory tests periodically in patients requiring prolonged metyrosine use, and observe caution with patients with impaired hepatic or renal function.

➤*Metyrosine crystalluria and urolithiasis:* Both have been found in dogs treated at doses similar to those used in humans; crystalluria has also been observed in a few patients. To minimize this risk, maintain sufficient water intake to achieve a daily urine volume of 2000 mL or more, particularly with doses greater than 2 g/day. Routinely examine the urine. Metyrosine will crystallize as needles or rods. If crystalluria occurs, further increase fluid intake; if it persists, reduce dosage or discontinue use.

Drug Interactions

➤*Phenothiazines or haloperidol:* Extrapyramidal effects of these drugs may be potentiated due to inhibition of catecholamine synthesis by metyrosine.

➤*Drug/Lab test interactions:* Spurious increases in urinary catecholamines may be observed due to the presence of metyrosine metabolites.

METYROSINE

Adverse Reactions

➤*CNS:* Sedation is most common, moderate to severe at low and high dosages. Sedative effects begin within the first 24 hours of therapy, are maximal after 2 to 3 days and tend to wane during the next few days. Sedation usually is not obvious after 1 week unless the dosage is increased, but at dosages greater than 2 g/day, some degree of sedation or fatigue may persist.

In most patients who experience sedation, temporary changes in sleep pattern (insomnia lasting 2 or 3 days; feelings of increased alertness and ambition) occur following drug withdrawal. Even those not experiencing sedation may report symptoms of psychic stimulation when the drug is discontinued.

Headache is reported infrequently.

Extrapyramidal signs – Drooling, speech difficulty and tremor (10%), occasionally accompanied by trismus and frank parkinsonism.

Anxiety and psychic disturbances – Depression, hallucinations, disorientation and confusion may be dose-dependent and may disappear with dosage reduction.

➤*GI:* Diarrhea (10%) may be severe. May need antidiarrheals if drug is continued. Infrequent – Decreased salivation, dry mouth, nausea, vomiting, abdominal pain.

➤*GU:* Infrequent – Impotence or failure to ejaculate. Crystalluria, transient dysuria and hematuria.

➤*Miscellaneous:* Infrequent – Slight breast swelling, galactorrhea, nasal stuffiness, eosinophilia, anemia, thrombocytopenia, thrombocytosis, increased AST, peripheral edema; hypersensitivity reactions such as urticaria and pharyngeal edema (rare).

Overdosage

Signs of metyrosine overdosage include those central nervous system effects observed in some patients even at low dosages.

At doses exceeding 2 g/day, some degree of sedation or feeling of fatigue may persist. Doses 2 to 4 g/day can result in anxiety or agitated depression, neuromuscular effects (including fine tremor of the hands, gross tremor of the trunk, tightening of the jaw with trismus), diarrhea and decreased salivation with dry mouth.

Reducing dose or discontinuing treatment causes these symptoms to disappear.

Patient Information

Maintain a daily liberal fluid intake.

Avoid alcohol or other CNS depressants.

May cause drowsiness; use caution while performing tasks requiring alertness.

Notify physician if any of the following occur: Drooling, speech difficulty, tremors, disorientation, diarrhea, painful urination.

NITROPRUSSIDE SODIUM

Rx	Sodium Nitroprusside (Elkins-Sinn)	Powder for Injection: 50 mg per vial	In single dose 5 mL vials.
Rx	Nitropress (Abbott)		In single dose 2 mL Fliptop Vials.

WARNING

After reconstitution, nitroprusside is not suitable for direct injection. The reconstituted solution must be further diluted in 5% Dextrose Injection before infusion (see Administration and Dosage).

Nitroprusside can cause precipitous decreases in blood pressure (see Administration and Dosage). In patients not properly monitored, these decreases can lead to irreversible ischemic injuries or death. Use only when available equipment and personnel allow blood pressure to be continuously monitored.

Except when used briefly or at low (< 2 mcg/kg/min) infusion rates, nitroprusside injection gives rise to important quantities of cyanide ion, which can reach toxic, potentially lethal levels (see Warnings). The usual dose rate is 0.5 to 10 mcg/kg/min, but infusion at the maximum dose rates should never last > 10 minutes. If blood pressure has not been adequately controlled after 10 minutes of infusion at the maximum rate, terminate administration immediately.

Although acid-base balance and venous oxygen concentration should be monitored and may indicate cyanide toxicity, these laboratory tests provide imperfect guidance.

Indications

In addition to the agents listed in this section, parenteral forms of methyldopa and hydralazine are also indicated for use in malignant hypertension.

➤*Hypertensive crises:* Immediate reduction of blood pressure of patients in hypertensive crises. Administer concomitant longer-acting antihypertensive medication so that the duration of treatment with nitroprusside can be minimized.

➤*Bleeding reduction during surgery:* Production of controlled hypotension in order to reduce bleeding during surgery.

➤*Acute congestive heart failure (CHF):* For use in acute congestive heart failure.

➤*Unlabeled uses:* Myocardial infarction with coadministration of dopamine; left ventricular failure with coadministration of oxygen, morphine and a loop diuretic.

Administration and Dosage

➤*Reconstitution:* Dissolve the contents of a 50 mg vial in 2 to 3 mL Dextrose in Water or Sterile Water for Injection. Depending on the desired concentration, the initially reconstituted solution containing 50 mg must be further diluted in 250 to 1000 mL 5% Dextrose Injection.

➤*Verification of the chemical integrity of the product:* Nitroprusside solution can be inactivated by reactions with trace contaminants. Products of these reactions are often blue, green or red, much brighter than the faint brownish color of unreacted nitroprusside. Do not use discolored solutions, or solutions with particulate matter visible.

➤*Admixture compatibility:* Esmolol and nitroprusside are compatible for at least 24 hours in 5% Dextrose Injection at room temperature and protected from light.

➤*CHF:* Nitroprusside can be titrated by increasing the infusion rate until measured cardiac output is no longer increasing, systemic blood pressure cannot be further reduced without compromising the perfusion of vital organs or the maximum recommended infusion rate has been reached, whichever comes earliest.

➤*Avoidance of excessive hypotension:* While the average effective rate in adults and children is about 3 mcg/kg/min, some patients will become dangerously hypotensive when they receive nitroprusside at this rate. Therefore, start at a very low rate (0.3 mcg/kg/min), with gradual upward titration every few minutes until the desired effect is achieved or the maximum recommended infusion rate (10 mcg/kg/min) has been reached.

Because nitroprusside's hypotensive effect is very rapid in onset and in dissipation, small variations in infusion rate can lead to wide, undesirable variations in blood pressure. Do not infuse through ordinary IV apparatus regulated only by gravity and mechanical clamps. Use only an infusion pump, preferably a volumetric pump.

Because nitroprusside can induce essentially unlimited blood pressure reduction, the blood pressure of a patient receiving this drug must be continuously monitored, using either a continually reinflated sphygmomanometer or (preferably) an intra-arterial pressure sensor.

➤*Infusion rates:* The table below shows the infusion rates for adults and children of various weights corresponding to the recommended initial and maximal doses (0.3 mcg/kg/min and 10 mcg/kg/min, respectively). Some of the listed infusion rates are so slow or so rapid as to be impractical, and these practicalities must be considered when the concentration to be used is selected. Note that when the concentration used in a given patient is changed, the tubing is still filled with a solution at the previous concentration.

Infusion Rates to Achieve Initial (0.3 mcg/kg/min) and Maximal (10 mcg/kg/min) Dosing of Nitroprusside								
		Nitroprusside concentration						
		200 mcg/mL		100 mcg/mL		50 mcg/mL		
		Infusion rate (mL/hr)		Infusion rate (mL/hr)		Infusion rate (mL/hr)		
Patient weight								
kg	lbs	Initial	Maximal	Initial	Maximal	Initial	Maximal	
10	22	1	30	2	60	4	120	
20	44	2	60	4	120	7	240	
30	66	3	90	5	180	11	360	
40	88	4	120	7	240	14	480	
50	110	5	150	9	300	18	600	
60	132	5	180	11	360	22	720	
70	154	6	210	13	420	25	840	
80	176	7	240	14	480	29	960	
90	198	8	270	16	540	32	1080	
100	220	9	300	18	600	36	1200	

➤*Avoidance of cyanide toxicity:* When > 500 mcg/kg nitroprusside is administered faster than 2 mcg/kg/min, cyanide is generated faster than the unaided patient can eliminate it (see Warnings).

➤*Consideration of methemoglobinemia and thiocyanate toxicity:* Rare patients receiving > 10 mg/kg of nitroprusside will develop methemoglobinemia; other patients, especially those with impaired renal function, will predictably develop thiocyanate toxicity after prolonged, rapid infusions. Test patients for these toxicities.

➤*Storage/Stability:* Protect the diluted solution from light by promptly wrapping with the supplied opaque sleeve, aluminum foil or other opaque material. It is not necessary to cover the infusion drip chamber or the tubing.

Store at room temperature 15° to 30°C (59° to 86°F).

If properly protected from light, the freshly reconstituted and diluted solution is stable for 24 hours.

Actions

➤*Pharmacology:* Nitroprusside is a potent IV antihypertensive agent. The principal pharmacological action of nitroprusside is relaxation of vascular smooth muscle and consequent dilation of peripheral arteries and veins. Other smooth muscle (eg, uterus, duodenum) is not affected. Nitroprusside is more active on veins than on arteries, but this selectivity is much less marked than that of nitroglycerin. Dilation of the veins promotes peripheral pooling of blood and decreases venous return to the heart, thereby reducing left ventricular end-diastolic pressure and pulmonary capillary wedge pressure (preload). Arteriolar relaxation reduces systemic vascular resistance, systolic arterial pressure and mean arterial pressure (afterload). Dilation of the coronary arteries also occurs.

In association with the decrease in blood pressure, nitroprusside administered IV to hypertensive and normotensive patients produces slight increases in heart rate and a variable effect on cardiac output. In hypertensive patients, moderate doses induce renal vasodilation roughly proportional to the decrease in systemic blood pressure, so there is no appreciable change in renal blood flow or glomerular filtration rate.

In normotensive subjects, acute reduction of mean arterial pressure to 60 to 75 mmHg by infusion of nitroprusside caused a significant increase in renin activity. In the same study, 10 renovascular-hypertensive patients given nitroprusside had significant increases in renin release from the involved kidney at mean arterial pressures of 90 to 137 mmHg.

The hypotensive effect of nitroprusside is seen within 1 to 2 minutes after the start of an adequate infusion, and it dissipates almost as rapidly after an infusion is discontinued. The effect is augmented by ganglionic blocking agents and inhaled anesthetics.

NITROPRUSSIDE SODIUM

➤*Pharmacokinetics:* Infused nitroprusside is rapidly distributed to a volume that is approximately coextensive with the extracellular space. The drug is cleared from this volume by intraerythrocytic reaction with hemoglobin (HgB), and nitroprusside's resulting circulatory half-life is about 2 minutes.

The products of the nitroprusside/HgB reaction are cyanmethemoglobin (cyanmetHgB) and cyanide ion (CN⁻). Safe use of nitroprusside injection must be guided by knowledge of the further metabolism of these products. The essential features of nitroprusside metabolism are: One molecule of nitroprusside is metabolized by combination with HgB to produce one molecule of cyanmethemoglobin and four CN⁻ ions; methemoglobin, obtained from HgB, can sequester cyanide as cyanmethemoglobin; thiosulfate reacts with cyanide to produce thiocyanate (SCN⁻); thiocyanate is eliminated in the urine; cyanide, not otherwise removed, binds to cytochromes; cyanide is much more toxic than methemoglobin or thiocyanate.

When the Fe⁺⁺⁺ of cytochromes is bound to cyanide, the cytochromes are unable to participate in oxidative metabolism. In this situation, cells may be able to provide for their energy needs by utilizing anaerobic pathways, but they thereby generate an increasing body burden of lactic acid. Other cells may be unable to utilize these alternate pathways, and they may die hypoxic deaths.

When CN⁻ is infused or generated within the bloodstream, essentially all of it is bound to methemoglobin until intraerythrocytic methemoglobin has been saturated. At healthy steady state, most people have < 1% of their HgB in the form of methemoglobin. Nitroprusside metabolism can lead to methemoglobin formation (a) through dissociation of cyanmethemeglobin formed in the original reaction of nitroprusside with HgB and (b) by direct oxidation of HgB by the released nitroso group. Relatively large quantities of nitroprusside, however, are required to produce significant methemoglobinemia.

When thiosulfate is supplied only by normal physiologic mechanisms, conversion of CN⁻ to SCN⁻ generally proceeds at about 1 mcg/kg/min. This rate of CN⁻ clearance corresponds to steady-state processing of a nitroprusside infusion of slightly > 2 mcg/kg/min. CN⁻ accumulates when nitroprusside infusions exceed this rate.

In patients with normal renal function, clearance of SCN⁻ is primarily renal, with a half-life of about 3 days. In renal failure, the half-life can be doubled or tripled.

➤*Clinical trials:* Nitroprusside has a prompt hypotensive effect, at least initially, in all populations. With increasing rates of infusion, nitroprusside lowers blood pressure without an observed limit of effect. The hypotensive effect of nitroprusside is also associated with reduced blood loss in a variety of major surgical procedures.

In patients with acute congestive heart failure and increased peripheral vascular resistance, administration of nitroprusside causes reductions in peripheral resistance, increases in cardiac output and reductions in left ventricular filling pressure.

Many trials have verified the clinical significance of the metabolic pathways described above. In patients receiving unopposed infusions of nitroprusside, cyanide and thiocyanate levels have increased with increasing rates of nitroprusside infusion. Mild to moderate metabolic acidosis has usually accompanied higher cyanide levels, but peak base deficits have lagged behind the peak cyanide levels by ≥ 1 hour.

Progressive tachyphylaxis to the hypotensive effects of nitroprusside has occurred in several trials and numerous case reports. This tachyphylaxis has frequently been attributed to concomitant cyanide toxicity; however, this is unproven and the mechanism of tachyphylaxis to nitroprusside remains unknown.

Contraindications

Treatment of compensatory hypertension, where the primary hemodynamic lesion is aortic coarctation or arteriovenous shunting; to produce hypotension during surgery in patients with known inadequate cerebral circulation or in moribund patients (A.S.A. Class 5E) coming to emergency surgery; patients with congenital (Leber's) optic atrophy or with tobacco amblyopia (these rare conditions are probably associated with defective or absent rhodanase and patients with unusually high cyanide/thiocyanate ratios); acute CHF associated with reduced peripheral vascular resistance such as high-output heart failure that may be seen in endotoxic sepsis.

Warnings

➤*Excessive hypotension:* Small transient excesses in the infusion rate of nitroprusside can result in excessive hypotension, sometimes to levels so low as to compromise the perfusion of vital organs. These hemodynamic changes may lead to a variety of associated symptoms (see Adverse Reactions). Nitroprusside-induced hypotension will be self-limited within 1 to 10 minutes after discontinuation of the infusion; during these few minutes, it may be helpful to put the patient into a head-down (Trendelenburg) position to maximize venous return. If hypotension persists more than a few minutes after discontinuation of the infusion, nitroprusside is not the cause, and the true cause must be sought.

➤*Cyanide toxicity:* Nitroprusside infusions at rates > 2 mcg/kg/min generate CN⁻ faster than the body can normally dispose of it. (When sodium thiosulfate is given, the body's capacity for CN⁻ elimination is greatly increased.) Methemoglobin normally present in the body can buffer a certain amount of CN⁻, but the capacity of this system is exhausted by the CN⁻ produced from about 500 mcg/kg nitroprusside. This amount of nitroprusside is administered in < 1 hour when the drug is administered at 10 mcg/kg/min (the maximum recommended rate). Thereafter, the toxic effects of CN⁻ may be rapid, serious and even lethal.

The true rates of clinically important cyanide toxicity cannot be assessed from spontaneous reports or published data. Most patients reported to have experienced such toxicity have received relatively prolonged infusions, and the only patients whose deaths have been unequivocally attributed to nitroprusside-induced cyanide toxicity have been patients who had received nitroprusside infusions at rates much greater than those now recommended (30 to 120 mcg/kg/min). Elevated cyanide levels, metabolic acidosis and marked clinical deterioration, however, have occasionally been reported in patients who received infusions at recommended rates for only a few hours and even, in one case, for only 35 minutes. In some of these cases, infusion of sodium thiosulfate caused dramatic clinical improvement, supporting the diagnosis of cyanide toxicity.

Cyanide toxicity may manifest itself as venous hyperoxemia with bright red venous blood, as cells become unable to extract the oxygen delivered to them; metabolic (lactic) acidosis; air hunger; confusion; death. Cyanide toxicity due to causes other than nitroprusside has been associated with angina pectoris and myocardial infarction, ataxia, seizures and stroke, and other diffuse ischemic damage.

➤*Hypertensive patients:* Hypertensive patients and patients concomitantly receiving other antihypertensive medications may be more sensitive to the effects of nitroprusside.

➤*Methemoglobinemia:* Nitroprusside infusions can cause sequestration of hemoglobin as methemoglobin. The back-conversion process is normally rapid, and clinically significant methemoglobinemia (> 10%) is only seen rarely. Even patients congenitally incapable of back-converting methemoglobin should demonstrate 10% methemoglobinemia only after they have received about 10 mg/kg nitroprusside; a patient receiving nitroprusside at the maximum recommended rate (10 mcg/kg/min) would take > 16 hours to reach this total accumulated dose.

Methemoglobin levels can be measured by most clinical laboratories. Suspect the diagnosis in patients who have received > 10 mg/kg of nitroprusside and who exhibit signs of impaired oxygen delivery despite adequate cardiac output and adequate arterial pO₂. Classically, methemoglobinemic blood is described as chocolate brown, without color change on exposure to air.

When methemoglobinemia is diagnosed, the treatment of choice is 1 to 2 mg/kg of methylene blue, administered IV over several minutes. In patients likely to have substantial amounts of cyanide bound to methemoglobin as cyanmethemoglobin, treatment of methemoglobinemia with methylene blue must be undertaken with extreme caution.

➤*Thiocyanate toxicity:* Most of the cyanide produced during metabolism of nitroprusside is eliminated in the form of thiocyanate. When cyanide elimination is accelerated by the co-infusion of thiosulfate, thiocyanate production is increased. Thiocyanate is mildly neurotoxic (eg, tinnitus, miosis, hyperreflexia) at serum levels of 1 mmol/L (60 mg/L). Thiocyanate toxicity is life-threatening when levels are 3 or 4 times higher (200 mg/L).

The steady-state thiocyanate level after prolonged infusions of nitroprusside is increased with increased infusion rate, and the half-time of accumulation is 3 to 4 days. To keep the steady-state thiocyanate level < 1 mmol/L, a prolonged infusion should not be more rapid than 3 mcg/kg/min; in anuric patients, the corresponding limit is just 1 mcg/kg/min. When prolonged infusions are more rapid than these, measure thiocyanate levels daily.

Physiologic maneuvers (eg, those that alter the pH of the urine) are not known to increase the elimination of thiocyanate. Thiocyanate clearance rates during dialysis, on the other hand, can approach the blood flow rate of the dialyzer.

Thiocyanate interferes with iodine uptake by the thyroid.

➤*Hepatic function impairment:* Since cyanide is metabolized by hepatic enzymes, it may accumulate in patients with severe liver impairment. Therefore, use with caution in patients with hepatic insufficiency.

➤*Elderly:* Use special caution as elderly patients may be more sensitive to the hypotensive effects of the drug.

➤*Pregnancy: Category C.* In three studies in pregnant ewes, nitroprusside crossed the placental barrier. Fetal cyanide levels were dose-related to maternal levels of nitroprusside. The metabolic transformation of nitroprusside given to pregnant ewes led to fatal levels of cyanide in the fetuses. The infusion of 25 mcg/kg/min nitroprusside for 1 hour in pregnant ewes resulted in the death of all fetuses. There are no adequate or well controlled studies in pregnant women. It is not known whether nitroprusside can cause fetal harm when administered to a pregnant woman or can affect reproductive capacity. Give to a pregnant woman only if clearly needed.

NITROPRUSSIDE SODIUM

The effects of administering sodium thiosulfate in pregnancy, either by itself or as a co-infusion with sodium nitroprusside, are completely unknown.

➤*Lactation:* It is not known whether nitroprusside and its metabolites are excreted in breast milk. Because of the potential for serious adverse reactions in nursing infants, decide whether to discontinue nursing or to discontinue the drug, taking into account the importance of the drug to the mother.

➤*Children:* See Administration and Dosage.

Precautions

➤*Monitoring:* The cyanide-level assay is technically difficult, and cyanide levels in body fluids other than packed red blood cells are difficult to interpret. Cyanide toxicity will lead to lactic acidosis and venous hyperoxemia, but these findings may not be present until ≥ 1 hour after the cyanide capacity of the body's red-cell mass has been exhausted.

➤*Intracranial pressure:* Like other vasodilators, nitroprusside can cause increases in intracranial pressure. In patients whose intracranial pressure is already elevated, use only with extreme caution.

➤*Anesthesia:* When nitroprusside (or any other vasodilator) is used for controlled hypotension during anesthesia, the patient's capacity to compensate for anemia and hypovolemia may be diminished. If possible, correct pre-existing anemia and hypovolemia prior to use.

Hypotensive anesthetic techniques may also cause abnormalities of the pulmonary ventilation/perfusion ratio. Patients intolerant of these abnormalities may require a higher fraction of inspired oxygen.

Exercise extreme caution in patients who are especially poor surgical risks (A.S.A. Classes 4 and 4E).

Adverse Reactions

➤*Cardiovascular:* Bradycardia; ECG changes; tachycardia.

➤*Hematologic:* Decreased platelet aggregation; methemoglobinemia (see Warnings).

➤*Miscellaneous:* Thiocyanate toxicity (see Warnings); flushing; venous streaking; irritation at the infusion site; rash; hypothyroidism; ileus; increased intracranial pressure (see Precautions).

Rapid blood pressure reduction – Abdominal pain, apprehension, diaphoresis, dizziness, headache, muscle twitching, nausea, palpitations, restlessness, retching and retrosternal discomfort have been noted when the blood pressure was reduced too rapidly. Symptoms quickly disappeared when the infusion was slowed or discontinued, and they did not reappear with a continued (or resumed) slower infusion.

Overdosage

➤*Symptoms:* Toxicity has occurred at doses well below the recommended maximum infusion rate of 10 mcg/kg/min. Overdosage of nitroprusside can be manifested as excessive hypotension, cyanide toxicity or as thiocyanate toxicity (see Warnings).

The acute IV mean lethal doses (LD50) of nitroprusside in rabbits, dogs, mice and rats are 2.8, 5, 8.4 and 11.2 mg/kg, respectively.

➤*Treatment:* Measure cyanide levels and blood gases for venous hyperoxemia or acidosis. Acidosis may not appear until > 1 hour after the appearance of dangerous cyanide levels; do not wait for laboratory tests. Reasonable suspicion of cyanide toxicity is adequate grounds for initiation of treatment.

Treatment of cyanide toxicity consists of: Discontinuing the administration of nitroprusside; providing a buffer for cyanide by using sodium nitrite to convert as much HgB into methemoglobin as the patient can safely tolerate; and then infusing sodium thiosulfate in sufficient quantity to convert the cyanide into thiocyanate.

The medications for treatment are contained in commercially available cyanide antidote kits. Alternatively, discrete stocks of medications can be used. Hemodialysis is ineffective in removal of cyanide, but it will eliminate most thiocyanate.

Antidote kits – Cyanide antidote kits contain both amyl nitrite and sodium nitrite for induction of methemoglobinemia. The amyl nitrite is supplied in the form of inhalant ampules, for use where IV administration of sodium nitrite may be delayed. In a patient who already has a patent IV line, use of amyl nitrite confers no benefit that is not provided by infusion of sodium nitrite.

Nitrite-thiosulfate regimen – Sodium nitrite is available in a 3% solution; inject 4 to 6 mg/kg (about 0.2 mL/kg) over 2 to 4 minutes. This dose converts about 10% of the patient's HgB into methemoglobin; this level of methemoglobinemia is not associated with any important hazard of its own. The nitrite infusion may cause transient vasodilation and hypotension, and this hypotension must, if it occurs, be routinely managed.

Immediately after infusion of the sodium nitrite, infuse sodium thiosulfate. This agent is available in 10% and 25% solutions, and the recommended dose is 150 to 200 mg/kg; a typical adult dose is 50 mL of the 25% solution. Thiosulfate treatment of an acutely cyanide-toxic patient will raise thiocyanate levels, but not to a dangerous degree.

The nitrite-thiosulfate regimen may be repeated, at half the original doses, after 2 hours.

Hydroxocobalamin – No concrete guidelines have been developed for hydroxocobalamin.
  Prophylactically during surgery: Doses of 25 mg/hr for 4 hours.
  Treatment: A dose of 4 to 5 g of hydroxocobalamin alone, or a combination of 8 g of sodium thiosulfate and 4 g of hydroxocobalamin.

DIAZOXIDE, PARENTERAL

Rx	Hyperstat IV (Schering)	Injection: 15 mg/mL	In 20 mL amps.

Indications

➤*Severe hypertension:* Emergency reduction of blood pressure; short-term use in severe, nonmalignant and malignant hypertension in hospitalized adults and in acute severe hypertension in hospitalized children when an urgent decrease of diastolic pressure is required. Institute treatment with oral agents as soon as the hypertensive emergency is controlled.

Administration and Dosage

Diazoxide injection was originally recommended for use by bolus administration of 300 mg. However, recent studies have shown that minibolus administration is as effective in reducing blood pressure, and therefore, it is the recommended dosage.

During and immediately following injection, the patient should remain supine. Administer only into a peripheral vein. The dose is given IV in ≤ 30 seconds. Do not give IM, SC or into body cavities. The solution's alkalinity is irritating to tissue; avoid extravasation. SC administration has produced inflammation and pain without subsequent necrosis. If SC leakage occurs, treat with warm compresses and rest.

➤*Adults:* Administer undiluted and rapidly by IV injections of 1 to 3 mg/kg, up to a maximum of 150 mg in a single injection. This dose may be repeated at 5 to 15 minute intervals until a satisfactory reduction in blood pressure has been achieved (diastolic pressure < 100 mmHg).

This method of administration of diazoxide is as effective as bolus administration of 300 mg, but usually reduces blood pressure more gradually, perhaps lessening the circulatory and neurological risks associated with acute hypotension.

➤*Repeated administration:* Repeated administration at intervals of 4 to 24 hours will usually maintain the blood pressure below pretreatment levels until oral antihypertensive medication can be instituted. Adjust the interval between injections by the duration of the response to each injection. It is usually unnecessary to continue treatment for > 4 to 5 days; do not use for > 10 days.

➤*Monitor:* Monitor the blood pressure closely until it has stabilized. Thereafter, hourly measurements will indicate any unusual response. Further decreases in blood pressure at ≥ 30 minutes after injection may be due to causes other than diazoxide. Have the patient remain recumbent for at least 1 hour after injection. In ambulatory patients, measure the blood pressure with the patient standing before ending surveillance.

➤*Concomitant diuretic therapy:* Because repeated administration can lead to sodium and water retention, a diuretic may be necessary for maximal blood pressure reduction and to avoid congestive failure.

➤*Storage/Stability:* Protect from light/freezing. Store between 2° to 30°C (36° to 86°F).

Actions

➤*Pharmacology:* Diazoxide, a nondiuretic antihypertensive, is structurally related to the thiazides. It promptly reduces blood pressure by relaxing smooth muscle in the peripheral arterioles. Increases in heart rate and in cardiac output occur as blood pressure is reduced. Coronary blood flow is maintained. Renal blood flow is increased after an initial decrease. Transient hyperglycemia occurs in the majority of patients.

➤*Pharmacokinetics:* Diazoxide is extensively bound to serum protein (> 90%) and may therefore displace other highly protein-bound agents. The plasma half-life is 28 ± 8.3 hours. The duration of antihypertensive effect varies, but is generally < 12 hours.

Generally, hypotensive effects begin within 1 min, maximum effects occurring within 2 to 5 min. Blood pressure increases gradually over the next 20 minutes, and then more slowly over the next 3 to 15 hours.

Contraindications

Treatment of compensatory hypertension, such as that associated with aortic coarctation or arteriovenous shunt; dissecting aortic aneurysm; hypersensitivity to diazoxide, thiazides or to other sulfonamide derivatives.

Warnings

➤*Myocardial lesions in animals:* Diazoxide IV in dogs induces subendocardial necrosis and necrosis of papillary muscles. These lesions,

DIAZOXIDE, PARENTERAL

which are also produced by other vasodilators (eg, hydralazine, minoxidil) and catecholamines, are presumed to be related to anoxia from reflex tachycardia and decreased blood pressure.

➤*Rapid decrease in blood pressure:* Observe caution when reducing severely elevated blood pressure. Use only the 150 mg minibolus. The 300 mg IV dose of diazoxide is less predictable and less controllable and has been associated with angina and with myocardial and cerebral infarction. Optic nerve infarction was reported when a 100 mmHg reduction in diastolic pressure occurred over 10 minutes following a single 300 mg bolus. In one prospective trial conducted in patients with severe hypertension and coexistent coronary artery disease, a 50% incidence of ischemic changes in the ECG was observed following single 300 mg bolus injections of diazoxide. Achieve the desired blood pressure over as long a period of time as is compatible. At least several hours and preferably 1 or 2 days is tentatively recommended.

Improved safety with equal efficacy can be achieved by giving diazoxide as a minibolus dose (see Administration and Dosage) until diastolic blood pressure < 100 mmHg is achieved. If hypotension severe enough to require therapy results, it usually responds to the Trendelenberg maneuver. If necessary, administer sympathomimetics such as dopamine or norepinephrine. Special attention is required in diabetes mellitus and if salt and water retention present serious problems.

Transient hyperglycemia occurs in the majority of patients, but usually requires treatment only in patients with diabetes mellitus; it will respond to the usual management including insulin. Monitor blood glucose levels, especially in patients with diabetes and in those requiring multiple injections of diazoxide. Cataracts have been observed in a few animals receiving repeated daily doses of IV diazoxide.

➤*Fluid and electrolyte balance:* Diazoxide causes sodium retention; repeat injections may precipitate edema and CHF. This retention responds to diuretic agents if adequate renal function exists. Coadministered thiazides may potentiate diazoxide's antihypertensive, hyperglycemic and hyperuricemic actions (see Drug Interactions). Increased extracellular fluid volume may cause treatment failure in nonresponsive patients.

➤*Pheochromocytoma:* Diazoxide is ineffective against hypertension due to pheochromocytoma.

➤*Pregnancy: Category C.* Safety for use is not established. Diazoxide crosses the placenta and appears in cord blood. It reduces fetal or pup survival, and reduces fetal growth in rats, rabbits and dogs at daily doses of 30, 21 or 10 mg/kg, respectively. In rats treated at term, doses of ≥ 10 mg/kg prolonged parturition.

If given prior to delivery, it may produce fetal or neonatal hyperbilirubinemia, thrombocytopenia, altered carbohydrate metabolism and other adverse reactions.

Labor and delivery – Not for use during pregnancy. IV administration during labor may stop uterine contractions, requiring administration of an oxytocic agent. An episode of maternal hypotension and fetal bradycardia occurred in a patient in labor who received both reserpine and hydralazine prior to administration of diazoxide. Neonatal hyperglycemia following intrapartum use of diazoxide IV occurred.

➤*Lactation:* Information is not available concerning the passage of diazoxide in breast milk. Decide whether to discontinue nursing or to discontinue the drug, taking into account the importance of the drug to the mother.

Precautions

➤*Monitoring:* Diazoxide requires close and frequent blood pressure monitoring; it may cause hypotension requiring treatment with sympathomimetic drugs. Use diazoxide primarily in the hospital and where facilities exist to treat such untoward reactions.

Perform appropriate diagnostic laboratory tests prior to, during and following diazoxide injection. Tests include: Hematologic (hematocrit, hemoglobin, white blood cell and platelet counts); metabolic (glucose, uric acid, total protein, albumin); electrolyte (sodium, potassium) and osmolality; renal function (creatinine, urine-protein); ECG.

➤*Special risk:* Use with care in patients with impaired cerebral or cardiac circulation, in whom abrupt reductions in blood pressure might be detrimental or in whom mild tachycardia or decreased blood perfusion may be deleterious. Avoid prolonged hypotension so as not to aggravate preexisting renal failure.

Drug Interactions

Since diazoxide is highly protein bound, it can be expected to displace other highly protein-bound agents (eg, warfarin), resulting in higher blood levels of these agents.

Diazoxide (Parenteral) Drug Interactions			
Precipitant drug	Object drug*		Description
Diazoxide	Hydantoins	↓	Serum hydantoin levels may be decreased, possibly resulting in decreased anticonvulsant action.
Diazoxide	Sulfonylureas	↓	Addition of diazoxide to sulfonylurea therapy could destabilize the patient, resulting in hyperglycemia.
Thiazide diuretics	Diazoxide	↑	Coadministration may potentiate the hyperuricemic and antihypertensive effects of diazoxide.

* ↑ = Object drug increased. ↓ = Object drug decreased.

➤*Drug/Lab test interactions:* Hyperglycemic and hyperuricemic effects of diazoxide preclude assessment of these metabolic states. Increased renin secretion, IgG concentrations and decreased cortisol secretion have occurred. Diazoxide inhibits glucagon-stimulated insulin release and will cause a false-negative insulin response to glucagon.

Adverse Reactions

The following adverse reactions were reported with rapid IV bolus administration of 300 mg diazoxide. The currently recommended minibolus dosing regimen may result in similar adverse effects, but with less frequency and severity. The most common adverse reactions were: Hypotension (7%); nausea, vomiting (4%); dizziness, weakness (2%). Additional adverse reactions were as follows:

➤*Cardiovascular:* Sodium and water retention after repeated injections, especially important in patients with impaired cardiac reserve; hypotension to shock levels; myocardial ischemia, usually transient and manifested by angina, atrial and ventricular arrhythmias and marked ECG changes, but occasionally leading to myocardial infarction; optic nerve infarction following too rapid decrease in severely elevated blood pressure; supraventricular tachycardia; palpitations; bradycardia; chest discomfort or nonanginal chest tightness.

➤*CNS:* Cerebral ischemia, usually transient, but occasionally leading to infarction and manifested by unconsciousness, convulsions, paralysis, confusion or focal neurological deficit such as numbness of the hands; vasodilative phenomena (eg, orthostatic hypotension), sweating, flushing and generalized or localized sensations of warmth; transient neurological findings secondary to alteration in regional blood flow to the brain, such as headache (sometimes throbbing), dizziness, lightheadedness, sleepiness (also reported as lethargy, somnolence or drowsiness), euphoria or "funny feeling," ringing in the ears and momentary hearing loss; weakness of short duration; apprehension; anxiety; malaise; blurred vision.

➤*GI:* Acute pancreatitis (rare); nausea; vomiting; abdominal discomfort; anorexia; alterations in taste; parotid swelling; salivation; dry mouth; ileus; constipation; diarrhea.

➤*Miscellaneous:* Hyperglycemia in diabetic patients after repeated injections; hyperosmolar coma in an infant; transient hyperglycemia in nondiabetic patients; transient retention of nitrogenous wastes; respiratory findings secondary to smooth muscle relaxation, such as dyspnea, cough and choking sensation; warmth or pain along injected vein; cellulitis without sloughing or phlebitis at injection site of extravasation; back pain and increased nocturia; lacrimation; hypersensitivity reactions; papilledema induced by plasma volume expansion secondary to the administration of diazoxide in a patient who had received 11 injections (300 mg/dose) over a 22 day period; transient cataract in an infant; hirsutism; decreased libido.

Overdosage

Overdosage may cause hypotension that can usually be controlled with the Trendelenburg maneuver. If necessary, sympathomimetic agents, such as dopamine or norepinephrine, may be administered. Failure of blood pressure to rise in response to such agents suggests that the hypotension may not have been caused by diazoxide. Excessive hyperglycemia will respond to conventional therapy of hyperglycemia. Diazoxide may be removed from blood by hemodialysis.

FENOLDOPAM MESYLATE

Rx	Corlopam (Neurex)	Injection, concentrate: 10 mg/mL	Sodium metabisulfite. In 5 mL single-dose ampules.
Rx	Fenoldopam Mesylate (Baxter)	Injection: 10 mg/mL	Sodium metabisulfite. In 1 and 2 mL single-dose ampules.

Indications

▶*Hypertensive emergency:* In-hospital, short-term (≤ 48 hours) management of severe hypertension when rapid, but quickly reversible, emergency reduction of blood pressure is clinically indicated, including malignant hypertension with deteriorating end-organ function.

Administration and Dosage

▶*Approved by the FDA:* September 23, 1997.

Administer by continuous IV infusion. Do not use a bolus dose. Avoid hypotension and rapid decreases in blood pressure. Titrate the initial dose upward or downward, no more frequently than every 15 minutes (and less frequently as goal pressure is approached) to achieve the desired therapeutic effect. The recommended increments for titration are 0.05 to 0.1 mcg/kg/min.

The optimal magnitude and rate of bp reduction in acutely hypertensive patients have not been rigorously determined, but both delay and too rapid decreases appear undesirable in sick patients. Doses < 0.1 mcg/kg/min have very modest effects and appear only marginally useful in this population. As the initial dose increases, there is a greater and more rapid bp reduction. Lower initial doses (0.03 to 0.1 mcg/kg/min) titrated slowly have been associated with less reflex tachycardia than higher initial doses (≥ 0.3 mcg/kg/min). In clinical trials, doses from 0.01 to 1.6 mcg/kg/min have been studied. Most of the effect of a given infusion rate is attained in 15 minutes. The following pharmacodynamic effects and corresponding infusion rates may serve as a guide in selecting an initial dose.

Pharmacodynamic Effects of Fenoldopam in Hypertensive Emergency Patients				
	Infusion rate mcg/kg/min			
Time point and pharmacodynamic parameters	0.01 (n = 25)	0.03 (n = 24)	0.1 (n = 22)	0.3 (n = 23)
Pre-infusion baseline				
Systolic BP	210 ± 21	208 ± 26	205 ± 24	211 ± 17
Diastolic BP	136 ± 16	135 ± 11	133 ± 14	136 ± 15
Heart rate	87 ± 20	84 ± 14	81 ± 19	80 ± 14
15 minutes of infusion[1]				
Systolic BP	-5 ± 4	-7 ± 4	-16 ± 4	-19 ± 4
Diastolic BP	-5 ± 3	-8 ± 3	-12 ± 2	-21 ± 2
Heart rate	-2 ± 3	1 ± 1	2 ± 1	11 ± 2
30 minutes of infusion[1]				
Systolic BP	-6 ± 4	-11 ± 4	-21 ± 3	-16 ± 4
Diastolic BP	-10 ± 3	-12 ± 3	-17 ± 3	-20 ± 2
Heart rate	-2 ± 3	-1 ± 1	3 ± 2	12 ± 3

[1] Mean change from baseline ± SE.

▶*Infusion rates:* The drug dose rate must be individualized according to body weight and according to the desired speed and extent of pharmacodynamic effect. The following table provides the calculated infusion volume in mL/min for a range of drug doses and body weights. Administer the infusion using a calibrated mechanical infusion pump that can accurately and reliably deliver the desired infusion rate.

Fenoldopam Infusion Rates (mL/min) to Achieve a Given Drug Dose Rate (mcg/kg/min)					
	0.025 mcg/kg/min	0.05 mcg/kg/min	0.1 mcg/kg/min	0.2 mcg/kg/min	0.3 mcg/kg/min
Body weight (kg)	Infusion rates (mL/min)				
40	0.025	0.05	0.1	0.2	0.3
50	0.031	0.06	0.13	0.25	0.38
60	0.038	0.08	0.15	0.3	0.45
70	0.044	0.09	0.18	0.35	0.53
80	0.05	0.1	0.2	0.4	0.6
90	0.056	0.11	0.23	0.45	0.68
100	0.063	0.13	0.25	0.5	0.75
110	0.069	0.14	0.28	0.55	0.83
120	0.075	0.15	0.3	0.6	0.9
130	0.081	0.16	0.33	0.65	0.98
140	0.088	0.18	0.35	0.7	1.05
150	0.094	0.19	0.38	0.75	1.13

The infusion can be abruptly discontinued or gradually tapered prior to discontinuation. Transition to oral therapy with another agent can begin at any time after bp is stable during fenoldopam infusion. Avoid concomitant use of beta blockers (see Warnings). Patients have received IV fenoldopam for ≤ 48 hours.

▶*Preparation of infusion solution:* Contents of ampules must be diluted before infusion. Each ampule is for single use only.

▶*Dilution* – The fenoldopam injection ampule concentrate must be diluted in 0.9% Sodium Chloride Injection or 5% Dextrose Injection for a final concentration of 40 mcg/mL: Add 4 mL of concentrate (40 mg of drug) to 1000 mL; 2 mL of concentrate (20 mg) to 500 mL; 1 mL of concentrate (10 mg) to 250 mL.

▶*Storage/Stability:* Store ampules at 2° to 30°C (36° to 86°F). The diluted solution is stable under normal ambient light and temperature conditions for ≤ 24 hours. Discard diluted solution that is not used within 24 hours of preparation.

Actions

▶*Pharmacology:* Fenoldopam is a rapid-acting vasodilator. It is an agonist for D_1–like dopamine receptors and binds with moderate affinity to α_2-adrenoceptors. It has no significant affinity for D_2–like receptors, α_1 and β adrenoceptors, $5HT_1$ and $5HT_2$ receptors, or muscarinic receptors. Fenoldopam is a racemic mixture with the R-isomer responsible for the biological activity. The R-isomer has ≈ 250–fold higher affinity for D_1–like receptors than does the S-isomer.

In animals, fenoldopam has vasodilating effects in coronary, renal, mesenteric and peripheral arteries. All vascular beds, however, do not respond uniformly. Vasodilating effects have been demonstrated in renal efferent and afferent arterioles. In humans, increases in renal blood flow were demonstrated in hypertensive and healthy subjects treated with IV fenoldopam but no beneficial renal effects have been shown in patients with heart failure, hepatic or severe renal disease.

▶*Pharmacokinetics:*

Absorption/Distribution – Administered as a constant infusion at a rate of 0.01 to 1.6 mcg/kg/min, fenoldopam produces steady-state plasma concentrations proportional to infusion rates. The elimination half-life is ≈ 5 minutes in mild to moderate hypertensives, with little difference between the R (active) and S isomers. Steady state concentrations are attained in ≈ 20 minutes (4 half-lives) and are similar in normotensive subjects and in patients with mild to moderate hypertension or hypertensive emergencies.

Clearance of parent (active) fenoldopam is not altered in patients with end-stage renal disease on continuous ambulatory peritoneal dialysis (CAPD) and is not affected on average, in severe hepatic failure. The effects of hemodialysis on the pharmacokinetics of fenoldopam have not been evaluated.

Metabolism/Excretion – Elimination is largely by conjugation, without participation of cytochrome P450 enzymes. The principal routes of conjugation are methylation, glucuronidation and sulfation. Animal data indicate that the metabolites are inactive. Approximately 90% of infused fenoldopam is eliminated in urine, 10% in feces, with only 4% of the dose excreted unchanged.

▶*Clinical trials:* In a multicenter comparison of four infusion rates, fenoldopam was administered as constant rate infusions of 0.01, 0.03, 0.1 and 0.3 mcg/kg/min for ≤ 24 hours to 94 patients experiencing hypertensive emergencies (defined as DBP ≥ 120 mmHg with evidence of compromise of end-organ function involving the cardiovascular, renal, cerebral or retinal systems). Infusion rates could be doubled after 1 hour if clinically indicated. Dose-related, rapid-onset decreases in systolic and diastolic blood pressures and increases in heart rate were observed. Table sample data after 15 and 30 minutes of infusion are in Administration and Dosage.

In two trials, 236 severely hypertensive patients (DBP ≥ 120 mmHg) with or without end-organ compromise received either fenoldopam or nitroprusside. Response rates were 79% in the fenoldopam group and 77% in the nitroprusside group. Response required a decline in supine DBP to < 110 mmHg if the baseline was between 120 and 150 mmHg, inclusive, or by ≥ 40 mmHg if the baseline was ≥ 150 mmHg. Patients were titrated to the desired effect. For fenoldopam, the dose ranged from 0.1 to 1.5 mcg/kg/min; for nitroprusside, the dose ranged from 1 to 8 mcg/kg/min. Most of the effect seen at 1 hour is present at 15 minutes. The additional effect seen after 1 hour occurs in all groups and may not be drug-related.

Warnings

▶*Beta blockers:* Use of beta blockers in conjunction with fenoldopam has not been studied in hypertensive patients; if possible, avoid concomitant use. If the drugs are used together exercise caution because unexpected hypotension could result from beta blocker inhibition of the reflex response to fenoldopam.

An increased incidence and degree of severity of fibro-osseous lesion of the sternum occurred in female mice treated for 24 months with high-dose fenoldopam (50 mg/kg/day reduced to 25 mg/kg/day on day 209) with those in the middle- (25 mg/kg/day) and high-dose groups exhibiting a higher incidence and degree of severity of chronic nephritis. Rats dosed at 10 or 20 mg/kg/day for 24 months exhibited a higher incidence of hyperplasia of collecting duct epithelium at the tip of the renal papilla.

FENOLDOPAM MESYLATE

In the in vitro chromosomal aberration assay with chinese hamster ovary cells, fenoldopam was associated with dose-dependent increases in chromosomal aberrations, and in the proportion of aberrant metaphases.

►*Pregnancy: Category B*. Doses of 12.5 to 200 mg/kg/day and 6.25 to 25 mg/kg/day in rats and rabbits revealed maternal toxicity at the highest doses. There are no well-controlled studies in pregnant women. Use in pregnancy only if clearly needed.

►*Lactation:* Fenoldopam is excreted in milk of rats. It is not known whether it is excreted in human milk. Use caution when administering to a nursing woman.

►*Children:* Safety and efficacy have not been established.

Precautions

►*Monitoring:* Monitor blood pressure and heart rate at frequent intervals, typically every 15 minutes to avoid hypotension and rapid decreases of blood pressure.

►*Intraocular pressure (IOP):* Administer to patients with glaucoma or intraocular hypertension with caution. In a study of 12 patients with open-angle glaucoma or ocular hypertension (mean baseline IOP was 29.2 mmHg; range, 22 to 33 mmHg), infusion of fenoldopam at escalating doses from 0.05 to 0.5 mcg/kg/min over a 3.5 hour period caused a dose-dependent increase in IOP. At peak effect, IOP was raised by a mean of 6.5 mmHg (range -2 to +8.5 mmHg, corrected for placebo effect). Upon discontinuation of fenoldopam infusion, IOP returned to baseline in 2 hours.

►*Tachycardia:* Fenoldopam causes dose-related tachycardia, particularly with infusion rates > 0.1 mcg/kg/min. Tachycardia diminishes over time but remains substantial at higher doses.

►*Hypotension:* Fenoldopam may occasionally produce a symptomatic hypotension; close monitoring of blood pressure during administration is essential. It is particulary important to avoid systemic hypotension when administering the drug to patients who have sustained an acute cerebral infarction or hemorrhage.

►*Hypokalemia:* Decreases in serum potassium occasionally to values < 3 mEq/L were observed after < 6 hours of fenoldopam infusion. It is not clear if the hypokalemia reflects a pressure natriuresis with enhanced potassium-sodium exchange or a direct drug effect. During clinical trials, electrolytes were monitored at intervals of 6 hours. Hypokalemia was treated with either oral or IV potassium supplementation. Patient management should include appropriate attention to serum electrolytes.

►*Sulfite sensitivity:* Fenoldopam contains sodium metabisulfite, a sulfite that may cause allergic-type reactions including anaphylactic symptoms and life-threatening or less severe asthmatic episodes in certain susceptible people. The overall prevalence of sulfite sensitivity in the general population is unknown and probably low. Sulfite sensitivity is seen more frequently in asthmatic than in nonasthmatic people.

Adverse Reactions

Fenoldopam causes a dose-related fall in blood pressure and increase in heart rate (see Precautions). In controlled studies of severe hypertension in patients with end-organ damage, 3% withdrew because of excessive falls in blood pressure. Increased heart rate could lead to ischemic cardiac events or worsened heart failure, although these events have not been observed. The most common events (> 5%) reported with fenoldopam use are headache, flushing, nausea and hypotension.

Fenoldopam Adverse Reactions (# of patients)						
	Fenoldopam doses (mcg/kg/min)					
Adverse reaction	Placebo (n = 7)	0.01 (n = 26)	0.03 - 0.04 (n = 31)	0.1 (n = 28)	0.3 - 0.4 (n = 29)	0.6 - 0.8 (n = 11)
Cardiovascular						
ST-T abnormalities	0	2	4	0	1	0
Flushing	0	0	0	0	1	3
Hypotension	0	0	0	2	0	2
Postural hypotension	0	2	0	0	0	0
Tachycardia	0	0	0	0	0	2
CNS						
Nervousness/ anxiety	0	0	1	0	0	2
Insomnia	0	2	0	0	0	0
Dizziness	0	1	1	2	2	0
GI						
Nausea	0	3	0	3	5	4
Vomiting	0	2	0	2	1	2
Abdominal pain/fullness	0	2	0	0	2	1
Constipation	0	0	0	0	0	2
Diarrhea	0	0	0	0	2	0
Metabolic/ Nutritional						
Increased creatinine	0	0	2	0	0	0
Hypokalemia	0	2	2	0	1	0
Miscellaneous						
Back pain	0	1	0	1	2	2
Headache	1	5	4	7	8	6
Injection site reaction	0	1	3	0	3	2
Nasal congestion	0	0	0	0	0	2
Sweating	0	0	0	1	1	2
Urinary tract infection	0	2	0	1	0	0

Additional adverse reactions (0.5% to 5%) are as follows:

►*Cardiovascular:* Extrasystoles; palpitations; bradycardia; heart failure; ischemic heart disease; myocardial infarction; angina pectoris.

►*Hematologic/Lymphatic:* Leukocytosis; bleeding.

►*Metabolic:* Elevated BUN, serum glucose, transaminase, LDH.

►*Respiratory:* Dyspnea; upper respiratory tract disorder.

►*Miscellaneous:* Non-specific chest pain; pyrexia; oliguria; limb cramp.

Overdosage

Intentional fenoldopam overdosage has not been reported. The most likely reaction would be excessive hypotension which should be treated with drug discontinuation and appropriate supportive measures.

Lowering cholesterol levels can arrest or reverse atherosclerosis in all vascular beds and can significantly decrease the morbidity and mortality associated with atherosclerosis. Each 10% reduction in cholesterol levels is associated with ≈ 20% to 30% reduction in the incidence of coronary heart disease. Hyperlipidemia, particularly elevated serum cholesterol and low-density lipoprotein (LDL) levels, is a risk factor in the development of atherosclerotic cardiovascular disease.

Individually assess potential benefits and risks of therapy. The cornerstone of treatment in primary hyperlipidemia is diet restriction and weight reduction. Limit or eliminate alcohol intake. Use drug therapy in conjunction with diet and after maximal efforts to control serum lipids by diet alone prove unsatisfactory, when tolerance to or compliance with diet is poor, or when hyperlipidemia is severe and risk of complications is high. Treat contributory diseases such as hypothyroidism or diabetes mellitus.

Elevated blood cholesterol levels are a major cause of coronary artery disease. Lowering these levels (specifically, LDL cholesterol) will reduce the risk of heart attacks caused by coronary heart disease (CHD).

►*Risk Factors:* Positive risk factors for CHD (other than high LDL) include: Age (men ≥ 45 years of age; women ≥ 55 years of age or women who go through premature menopause without estrogen replacement therapy); family history of premature CHD; smoking; hypertension (> 140/90 mmHg); low HDL cholesterol (< 35 mg/dL); obesity (> 30% overweight); and diabetes mellitus. Physical inactivity is not listed but should also be considered.

►*Negative:* Negative risk factors include: High HDL cholesterol (≥ 60 mg/dL); subtract one risk factor if the patient's HDL is at this level.

All Americans (except children < 2 years old) should adopt a diet that reduces total dietary fat, decreases intake of saturated fat, increases intake of polyunsaturated fat, and reduces daily cholesterol intake to ≤ 250 to 300 mg.

The following treatments guidelines are provided by the National Cholesterol Education Program Expert Panel on Detection, Evaluation and Treatment of High Blood Cholesterol in Adults ≥ 20 years of age.

Classification of Total and HDL-Cholesterol Levels (Adults ≥ 20 years of Age)	
Level (mg/dL) (mmol/L)	Classification
< 200 (5.2)	desirable
200-239 (5.2 - 6.2)	borderline-high
≥ 240 (6.2)	high
HDL < 35 (0.9)	low

1.) Total blood cholesterol < 200 mg/dL: HDL ≥ 35 mg/dL, repeat total cholesterol and HDL measurements within 5 years or with physical exam; provide education on general population eating pattern, physical activity, and risk factor education. HDL < 35 mg/dL, do lipoprotein analysis; base further action on LDL levels.
2.) Total blood cholesterol 200 to 239 mg/dL: HDL ≥ 35 mg/dL and < 2 risk factors, provide information on dietary modification, physical activity, and risk factor reduction; re-evaluate in 1 to 2 years, repeat total and HDL cholesterol measurements, and reinforce nutrition and physical activity education. HDL < 35 mg/dL or ≥ 2 risk factors, analyze lipoprotein; base further action on LDL levels.
3.) Total blood cholesterol ≥ 240 mg/dL: Analyze lipoprotein; base further action on LDL levels.

Classification of LDL-Cholesterol Levels	
Level (mg/dL) (mmol/L)	Classification
< 130 (3.4)	desirable
130 -159 (3.4 - 4.1)	borderline-high
≥ 160 (4.1)	high

1.) LDL ≥ 160 mg/dL without CHD and with < 2 risk factors: Dietary treatment.
2.) LDL ≥ 130 mg/dL without CHD and with ≥ 2 risk factors: Dietary treatment.
3.) LDL ≥ 190 mg/dL without CHD and with < 2 other risk factors, or LDL ≥ 160 mg/dL without CHD and with ≥ 2 other risk factors: Drug treatment.

►*Hyperlipidemias:* Elevation of serum cholesterol, triglycerides, or both is characteristic of hyperlipidemias. Differentiation of the specific biochemical abnormality requires identification of specific lipoprotein fractions in the serum. Lipoproteins transport serum lipids and are identified by their density and electrophoretic mobility. Chylomicrons are the largest and least dense of the lipoproteins, followed in order of increasing density and decreasing size by very low density lipoproteins (VLDL or pre-β), intermediate low density lipoproteins (ILDL or broad-β), low density lipoproteins (LDL or β) and high density lipoproteins (HDL or α). Triglycerides are transported primarily by chylomicrons and VLDL; the predominant cholesterol transporting lipoprotein is LDL.

Elevations and treatment associated with each type of hyperlipidemia follow:

Hyperlipidemias and Their Treatment[1]						
Hyperlipidemia type	I	IIa	IIb	III	IV	V
Lipids						
Cholesterol	N-⇧	↑	↑	N-↑	N-⇧	N-↑
Triglycerides	↑	N	↑	N-↑	↑	↑
Lipoproteins						
Chylomicrons	↑	N	N	N	N	↑
VLDL (pre-β)	N-⇧	N-↓	↑	N-⇧	↑	↑
ILDL (broad-β)[2]				↑		
LDL (β)	↓	↑	↑	↑	N-⇩	↓
HDL (α)	↓	N	N	N	N-⇩	↓
Treatment	Diet	Diet HMG-CoA reductase inhibitors Bile acid sequestrants Nicotinic acid	Diet HMG-CoA reductase inhibitors Bile acid sequestrants[3] Gemfibrozil[4] Nicotinic acid	Diet Nicotinic acid Gemfibrozil	Diet Gemfibrozil Nicotinic acid Fenofibrate	Diet Gemfibrozil Nicotinic acid[5] Fenofibrate

[1] N = normal ↑ = increase ↓ = decrease ⇧ = slight increase ⇩ = slight decrease
[2] An abnormal lipoprotein.
[3] Particularly useful if hypercholesterolemia predominates.
[4] In patients with inadequate response to weight loss, bile acid sequestrants, nicotinic acid.
[5] Norethindrone acetate (women) and oxandrolone (men) are effective, but use is not FDA-approved.

The following table summarizes the effects of the various antihyperlipidemic drugs on serum lipids and lipoproteins:

Antihyperlipidemic Drug Effects[1]					
	Lipids		Lipoproteins		
Drug	Cholesterol	Triglycerides	VLDL (pre-β)	LDL (β)	HDL
Atorvastatin	↓	↓	↓	↓	↑
Cerivastatin	↓	↓	↓	↓	↑
Cholestyramine	↓	→↑	→↑	↓	→↑
Colestipol	↓	→↑	↑	↓	→↑
Fenofibrate	↓	↓	↓	↑	↑
Fluvastatin	↓	↓	↓	↓	↑
Gemfibrozil	↓	↓	↓	→↓	↑
Lovastatin	↓	↓	↓	↓	↑
Nicotinic acid	↓	↓	↓	↓	↑
Pravastatin	↓	↓	↓	↓	↑
Simvastatin	↓	↓	↓	↓	↑

[1] ↓ = decrease ↑ = increase → = unchanged

➤*General considerations:*
1.) Define the type of hyperlipoproteinemia, and establish baseline serum cholesterol and triglyceride levels.
2.) Institute a trial of diet, weight reduction and physical activity, which are extremely important elements of therapy for high blood cholesterol. Remind patients to restrict their dietary intake of cholesterol and saturated fats and to adhere to prescribed dietary regimens. Drug therapy does not reduce the importance of adhering to diet.
3.) Carefully monitor the patient during treatment, including serum cholesterol and triglyceride levels.
4.) Consider failure of cholesterol level to fall or a significant rise in triglyceride level as indications to discontinue medication.

➤*Dietary treatment:* Reducing elevated cholesterol levels and maintaining adequate nutrition is the aim of dietary therapy. Step I and Step II diets are specifically designed to progressively reduce saturated fatty acids and cholesterol intake and promote weight loss in overweight individuals by eliminating excess total calories and increasing physical activity.

Step I – Total fat intake ≤ 30% of calories; saturated fatty acid intake < 8% to 10% of calories; cholesterol intake < 300 mg/day. Measure serum total cholesterol and adherence to diet at 4 to 6 weeks and at 3 months. If cholesterol and LDL level goals are met, monitor quarterly the first year and twice a year thereafter. If response is insufficient, proceed to Step II.

Step II – Saturated fatty acid intake < 7% of calories; cholesterol intake < 200 mg/day. Measure serum total cholesterol and adherence to diet at 4 to 6 weeks and at 3 months. Begin long-term monitoring if goal has been met. Consider drug therapy if goal has not been attained. Carry out intensive diet therapy and counseling for ≥ 6 months before starting drug therapy. Continue dietary treatment during drug treatment.

➤*Drug treatment:* **Cholestyramine** and **colestipol** are used to lower cholesterol. HMG-CoA reductase inhibitors, **gemfibrozil**, **nicotinic acid**, and **fenofibrate** are used to lower both cholesterol and triglycerides. Gemfibrozil and fenofibrate lower serum triglycerides much more effectively than cholesterol levels. When both cholesterol and triglycerides are elevated, treatment of the hypertriglyceridemia should take precedence. When hypercholesterolemia is treated first, an exacerbation of the hypertriglyceridemia may occur. Serum cholesterol often falls to normal levels without specific therapy following treatment of the hypertriglyceridemia.

First choice – Drugs of first choice include HMG-CoA reductase inhibitors, gemfibrozil or nicotinic acid. Measure LDL-cholesterol levels at 4 to 6 weeks and at 3 months. The target LDL level for treatment is ≤ 130 mg/dL. If the response is adequate, monitor every 4 months; if inadequate, switch to another agent or use a combination of two drugs. Refer patients who fail to respond to combination therapy to a lipid disorder specialist.

Estrogen – Estrogen replacement therapy can be considered in postmenopausal women with high serum cholesterol because estrogens have been shown to reduce total and LDL- and raise HDL-cholesterol levels.

Combination therapy – Because drug therapy of different hyperlipoproteinemias involves different mechanisms and pharmacologic actions, consider a combined drug regimen in stubborn cases. However, experience with combination therapy is limited. The coadministration of a bile acid sequestrant with either nicotinic acid or an HMG-CoA reductase inhibitor can lower LDL-cholesterol levels by ≥ 40% to 50%. Use HMG-CoA reductase inhibitors and gemfibrozil concomitantly with caution because of the risks of myopathy, rhabdomyolysis and acute renal failure.

Bile Acid Sequestrants

Refer to general discussions on these agents in Antihyperlipidemic Agents Introduction.

Indications

➤*Hyperlipoproteinemia:* Adjunctive therapy for the reduction of elevated serum cholesterol in patients with primary hypercholesterolemia (elevated LDL) who do not respond adequately to diet.

These agents may lower elevated cholesterol in patients who also have hypertriglyceridemia, but they are not indicated where hypertriglyceridemia is the abnormality of most concern.

➤*Biliary obstruction (cholestyramine only):* Relief of pruritus associated with partial biliary obstruction.

➤*Unlabeled uses:* **Cholestyramine** *in vitro* binds the toxin produced by *Clostridium difficile*, the causative organism of antibiotic-induced pseudomembranous colitis, with variable success. It is also effective in bile salt-mediated and postvagotomy diarrhea.

Cholestyramine has been used in the treatment of chlordecone *(Kepone)* pesticide poisoning. By binding chlordecone in the intestine, cholestyramine inhibits its enterohepatic recirculation, increases fecal excretion and accelerates elimination from the body.

Cholestyramine and **colestipol** have been used in the treatment of digitalis toxicity (see Cardiac Glycosides monograph).

Cholestyramine may be useful with thyroid hormone overdose.

Administration and Dosage

➤*Concomitant therapy:* Preliminary evidence suggests that the cholesterol-lowering effects of these agents and an HMG-CoA reductase inhibitor are additive. In addition, this combined effect may be useful in treating severe and refractory forms of hypercholesterolemia. Additive effects on LDL-cholesterol are also seen with combined cholestyramine and nicotinic acid therapy.

Actions

➤*Pharmacology:* Cholesterol is the major (and probably the sole) precursor of bile acids. During normal digestion, bile acids are secreted via the bile from the liver and gallbladder into the intestines to emulsify the fat and lipid materials in food, thus facilitating absorption. A major portion of the bile acids secreted is reabsorbed from the intestines and returned via the portal circulation to the liver, thus, completing the enterohepatic cycle.

Bile acid sequestering resins bind bile acids in the intestine to form an insoluble complex that is excreted in the feces. This results in a partial removal of bile acids from the enterohepatic circulation, preventing their absorption. Because these agents are anion-exchange resins, the chloride anions of the resin are replaced by other anions. These agents are hydrophilic but insoluble in water. They remain unchanged in the GI tract and are not absorbed.

The increased fecal loss of bile acids leads to increased oxidation of cholesterol to bile acids and a decrease in LDL and serum cholesterol levels. In humans, these drugs increase the hepatic synthesis of cholesterol, but plasma cholesterol levels fall secondary to an increased rate of clearance of cholesterol-rich lipoproteins from the plasma. Serum triglyceride levels may increase.

The fall in LDL concentration is apparent in 4 to 7 days. The decline in serum cholesterol is usually evident by 1 month. When the resins are discontinued, serum cholesterol usually returns to baseline within 1 month. Cholesterol may rise even with continued use; determine serum levels periodically.

When bile secretion is partially blocked, serum bile acid concentration rises. In patients with partial biliary obstruction, reduction of serum bile acid levels by cholestyramine reduces bile acid deposits in the dermal tissues with a resultant decrease in pruritus.

Contraindications

Hypersensitivity to bile acid sequestering resins or any components of the products; complete biliary obstruction.

Warnings

➤*Powder:* Avoid accidental inhalation or esophageal distress, do not take dry. Mix with fluids.

➤*Calcified material:* Calcified material has been observed in the biliary tree and the gall bladder; however, this may be due to liver disease and may not be drug-related. One patient experienced biliary colic on each of three occasions on which he took **cholestyramine**. Another patient, diagnosed as having an acute abdominal symptom complex, showed a "pasty mass" in the transverse colon on x-ray.

➤*Carcinogenesis:* The incidence of intestinal tumors in studies was greater in cholestyramine-treated rats than in controls. The total incidence of fatal and nonfatal neoplasms was similar in both treatment groups. Various alimentary system cancers were more prevalent with **cholestyramine**.

➤*Pregnancy:* These agents are not absorbed systemically, and are not expected to cause fetal harm when administered during pregnancy in recommended doses. Interference with fat-soluble vitamin absorption may be detrimental even with supplementation. No adverse fetal effects were observed when **cholestyramine** was used for the treatment of cholestasis of pregnancy.

➤*Lactation:* Exercise caution when administering to a nursing woman. The possible lack of proper vitamin absorption may have an effect on nursing infants.

➤*Children:* Dosage schedules have not been established. The effects of long-term administration and effectiveness in maintaining lowered cholesterol levels are unknown.

A 10-month-old baby with biliary atresia had an impaction presumed to be due to **cholestyramine** (9 g/day for 3 days). She died of acute intestinal sepsis.

Precautions

➤*Monitoring:* Determine serum cholesterol levels frequently during the first few months of therapy and periodically thereafter. Periodically measure serum triglyceride levels to detect significant changes.

➤*Diet:* Before instituting therapy, vigorously attempt to control serum cholesterol by an appropriate dietary regimen and weight reduction.

➤*Contributing diseases:* Investigate and treat diseases contributing to increased blood cholesterol before starting therapy (eg, hypothyroidism, diabetes mellitus, nephrotic syndrome, dysproteinemias, obstructive liver disease). Cholesterol reduction should occur during the first month of therapy. Continue therapy to sustain cholesterol reduction. If adequate reduction is not attained, discontinue therapy.

➤*Malabsorption:* Because they sequester bile acids, these resins may interfere with normal fat absorption and digestion and may prevent absorption of fat-soluble vitamins such as A, D, E, K and folic acid. With long-term therapy, supplemental vitamins A and D may be given in a water-miscible form or administered parenterally.

Chronic use may increase bleeding tendencies due to hypoprothrombinemia associated with vitamin K deficiency. This usually responds promptly to parenteral vitamin K_1; prevent recurrences by giving oral vitamin K_1.

➤*Reduced folate:* Reduction of serum or red cell folate has been reported over long-term administration of **cholestyramine**. Consider supplementation with folic acid.

➤*Hyperchloremic acidosis:* Prolonged use of chloride anion-exchange resins may cause hyperchloremic acidosis, especially in younger and smaller patients where relative dosage may be higher.

➤*Constipation:* These agents may produce or severely worsen preexisting constipation. Fecal impaction may occur and hemorrhoids may be aggravated. Avoid constipation in patients with symptomatic coronary artery disease. Most instances of constipation are mild, transient and controlled with standard treatment. Some patients require decreased dosage or discontinuation of therapy. Predisposing factors are high dose and age > 60 years. A laxative, stool softener or increased fluid and fiber intake may be helpful.

Drug Interactions

Bile Acid Sequestrant (BAS) Drug Interactions			
Precipitant drug	Object drug*		Description
BAS	Anticoagulants	↓	Cholestyramine may decrease anticoagulant effect.
BAS	Diclofenac	↓	The AUC and C_{max} of NSAIDs may be reduced.
BAS	Gemfibrozil	↓	Bioavailability may be reduced by colestipol.
BAS	Iopanoic acid	↓	Cholestyramine's apparent high affinity for iopanoic acid caused an abnormal cholecystography.
BAS	Mycophenolate	↓	≈ 40% decrease in AUC by cholestyramine.
BAS	Piroxicam	↓	Elimination may be enhanced by cholestyramine.
BAS	Thyroid hormones	↓	Possible loss of efficacy of thyroid and potential hypothyroidism with concurrent cholestyramine.
BAS	Ursodiol	↓	Cholestyramine and colestipol may interfere with the action of ursodiol by reducing its absorption.
BAS	Vitamins A, D, E, K	↓	Malabsorption may occur during administration of bile acid sequestrants (see Precautions).

*↓ = Object drug decreased.

Binding in the GI tract may delay or reduce the absorption of concomitant oral medication. Take other drugs at least 1 hour before or 4 to 6 hours after these agents. Discontinuation of a resin could pose a hazard if a potentially toxic, significantly bound drug has been titrated to a maintenance level while on the resin.

BAS Drug Interactions (Decreased Serum Levels or GI Absorption)		
Aspirin	Hydrocortisone	Phosphate supplements
Clindamycin	Imipramine	Propranolol
Clofibrate	Methyldopa	Tetracyclines
Digitalis glycosides	Nicotinic acid (niacin)	Thiazide diuretics
Furosemide	Penicillin G	Tolbutamide
Glipizide	Phenytoin	

Adverse Reactions

➤*GI:*

Most common – Constipation at times is severe and is occasionally accompanied by fecal impaction (see Warnings). Hemorrhoids may be aggravated.

Less frequent – Abdominal pain/distention/cramping; GI bleeding; bloating; flatulence; nausea; vomiting; diarrhea; loose stools; indigestion; heartburn; anorexia; steatorrhea; rectal bleeding/pain; black stools; hemorrhoidal bleeding; bleeding duodenal ulcer; peptic ulceration; ulcer attack; GI irritation; dysphagia; dental bleeding; dental caries; hiccoughs; sour taste; pancreatitis; diverticulitis; cholecystitis; cholelithiasis; impaction (rare).

➤*Cardiovascular:* Chest pain, angina, tachycardia (infrequent).

➤*CNS:* Headache (eg, migraine and sinus); anxiety; vertigo; dizziness; lightheadedness; insomnia; fatigue; tinnitus; syncope; drowsiness; femoral nerve pain; paresthesia.

➤*Hematologic:* Increased prothrombin time; ecchymosis; anemia.

➤*Hypersensitivity:* Urticaria; dermatitis; asthma; wheezing; rash.

➤*Musculoskeletal:* Backache; muscle/joint pains; arthritis.

➤*Renal:* Hematuria; dysuria; burnt odor to urine; diuresis.

➤*Miscellaneous:* Uveitis; fatigue; weight loss/gain; increased libido; swollen glands; edema; weakness; shortness of breath; swelling of hands/feet.

Bleeding tendencies due to hypoprothrombinemia (vitamin K deficiency); vitamin A (one case of night blindness) and D deficiencies; rash and irritation of the skin, tongue and perianal area; hyperchloremic acidosis in children (see Precautions); osteoporosis; calcified material in biliary tree and gall bladder (see Warnings).

➤*Lab test abnormalities:*

Colestipol – Transient, modest elevations of AST, ALT, and alkaline phosphatase.

Cholestyramine – Liver function abnormalities.

Overdosage

The chief potential harm would be GI tract obstruction. Location and degree of obstruction and status of gut motility determine treatment. Overdosage has been reported in a patient taking 150% of the maximum recommended daily dose of **cholestyramine** for several weeks; no ill effects were reported.

Patient Information

Medication is usually taken before meals.

Do not take the powder in dry form; mix with beverages, highly fluid soups, cereals, or pulpy fruits (see Administration and Dosage in individual monographs).

Swallow **colestipol** tablets whole; do not cut, crush, or chew.

Medication may interfere with absorption of concomitant drugs. Take other drugs 1 hour before or 4 to 6 hours after **cholestyramine** or **colestipol** (see Drug Interactions).

Constipation, flatulence, nausea, and heartburn may occur and may disappear with continued therapy. Notify physician if these effects become bothersome or if unusual bleeding (eg, from the gums or rectum) occurs.

Bile Acid Sequestrants

CHOLESTYRAMINE

Rx	**Cholestyramine** (Various, eg, Eon, Novopharm)	**Powder for suspension:** 4 g anhydrous cholestyramine resin/9 g powder	In 9 g packets (42s and 60s) and 378 g cans.
Rx	**LoCHOLEST** (Warner Chilcott)		Fructose, sorbitol, sucrose. Strawberry flavor. In 9 g pouches (60s) and 378 g cans.
Rx	**Questran** (Par)		Sucrose. In 378 g cans and 9 g single-dose packets (60s).
Rx	**Cholestyramine Light** (Various, eg, Eon, Novopharm)	**Powder for suspension:** 4 g anhydrous cholestyramine resin/dose	In 5 and 5.7 g packets (60s) and 210, 231, and 239 g cans.
Rx	**LoCHOLEST Light** (Warner Chilcott)	**Powder for suspension:** 4 g anhydrous cholestyramine resin/5.7 g powder	Aspartame, fructose, mannitol, sorbitol, 3.93 mg phenylalanine/g. Strawberry flavor. In 5.7 g pouches (60s) and 239.4 g cans.
Rx	**Prevalite** (Upsher Smith)	**Powder for suspension:** 4 g anhydrous cholestyramine resin/5.5 g powder	Aspartame, 14.1 mg phenylalanine/5.5 g. Orange flavor. In 5.5 g packets (42s and 60s) and 231 g cans (42 doses).
Rx	**Questran Light** (Par)	**Powder:** 4 g anhydrous cholestyramine resin/6.4 g powder	Maltodextrin, aspartame, 28 mg phenylalanine/6.4 g. Orange vanilla flavor. In 6.4 g packets (60s).

For complete prescribing information, refer to the Bile Acid Sequestrants group monograph.

Administration and Dosage

➤*Adults:* 4 g 1 to 2 times daily. Individualize dosage.

➤*Preparation:* Mix the contents of 1 powder packet or 1 level scoopful with 60 to 180 mL (2 to 6 fl oz) water or noncarbonated beverage. Do not take in dry form. Always mix with water or other fluids, highly fluid soups, or pulpy fruits, such as applesauce or crushed pineapple.

➤*Maintenance:* 2 to 4 packets or full scoops daily (8 to 16 g anhydrous cholestyramine resin) divided into 2 doses. Increase dose gradually, with periodic assessment of lipid/lipoprotein levels at intervals of ≥ 4 weeks. The maximum recommended daily dose is 6 packets or scoopfuls. Recommended administration time is at mealtime; may be modified to avoid interference with absorption of concomitant medications. Although the recommended dosing schedule is twice daily, cholestyramine may be administered in 1 to 6 doses/day.

COLESTIPOL HCl

Rx	**Colestid** (Pharmacia)	**Tablets:** 1 g	(U). Yellow, elliptical. In 120s and 500s.
		Granules: 5 g colestipol HCl/dose	*Unflavored:* In 300 and 500 g bottles and 5 g packets (30s and 90s).
		5 g colestipol HCl/7.5 g powder	*Flavored:* Aspartame, mannitol. Orange flavor. In 450 g bottles (60 doses) and 7.5 g packets (60s).

For complete prescribing information, refer to the Bile Acid Sequestrants group monograph.

Administration and Dosage

➤*Granules:*

Adults – 5 to 30 g/day given once or in divided doses. The starting dose is 5 g once or twice daily with a daily increment of 5 g at 1- or 2-month intervals.

Preparation – Mix in liquids, soups, cereals, or pulpy fruits. Do not take dry. Add the prescribed amount to a glassful (≥ 90 mL) of liquid; stir until completely mixed. Colestipol will not dissolve. May also mix with carbonated beverages slowly stirred in a large glass. Rinse glass with a small amount of additional beverage to ensure that all the medication is taken.

➤*Tablets:* 2 to 16 g/day given once or in divided doses. The starting dose is 2 g once or twice daily. Dosage increases of 2 g, once or twice daily, should occur at 1- or 2-month intervals. Periodically assess lipid/lipoprotein levels. If the desired effect is not obtained at recommended dose, consider combined therapy or alternate treatment.

Swallow tablets whole, one at a time; do not cut, chew, or crush. The tablets may be taken with plenty of water or other appropriate fluids.

COLESEVELAM HCl

Rx	**WelChol** (Sankyo Pharma)	**Tablets:** 625 mg	(Sankyo C01). Off-white. In 24s and 180s.

For complete prescribing information, refer to the Bile Acid Sequestrants group monograph.

Indications

➤*Elevated LDL cholesterol:* As adjunctive therapy to diet and exercise used alone or in combination with an HMG-CoA reductase inhibitor to reduce elevated LDL cholesterol in patients with primary hypercholesterolemia (Fredrickson type IIa).

Administration and Dosage

➤*Approved by the FDA:* May 30, 2000.

Take with a liquid.

➤*Monotherapy:* Starting dose is 3 tablets taken twice daily with meals or 6 tablets once daily with a meal. The dose can be increased to 7 tablets depending on desired therapeutic effect.

➤*Combination therapy:* For maximum therapeutic effect in combination with an HMG-CoA reductase inhibitor, the recommended dose of colesevelam is 3 tablets taken twice daily with meals or 6 tablets taken once daily with a meal. Doses of 4 to 6 tablets/day have been shown to be safe and effective when coadministered with an HMG-CoA reductase inhibitor or when the 2 drugs are dosed apart.

➤*Storage/Stability:* Store at room temperature (25°C; 77°F); excursions permitted to 15° to 30°C (59° to 86°F). Protect from moisture.

HMG-CoA Reductase Inhibitors

Refer to the general discussion of these products in the Antihyperlipidemic Agents Introduction.

Indications

Refer to individual product monographs for specific indications.

➤*Antihyperlipidemics:* Use HMG-CoA reductase inhibitors in addition to a diet restricted in saturated fat and cholesterol when diet and other nonpharmacological therapies alone have produced inadequate responses.

HMG-CoA Reductase Inhibitor Indications						
Indication	Atorvastatin	Fluvastatin	Lovastatin	Pravastatin	Rosuvastatin	Simvastatin
Heterozygous familial hypercholesterolemia in adolescents	✓		✓[a]	✓		✓
Homozygous familial hyperlipidemia	✓				✓	✓
Hypertriglyceridemia[b]	✓[c]			✓[c]	✓[c]	✓[c]
Mixed dyslipidemia	✓[d]	✓[d]	✓[d,e]	✓[d]	✓[d]	✓[d]
Primary dysbetalipoproteinemia	✓[f]			✓[f]		✓[f]
Primary hypercholesterolemia	✓[g]	✓[g]	✓[g]	✓[g]	✓[g]	✓[g]
Primary prevention of coronary events			✓	✓		✓
Secondary prevention of cardiovascular event(s)		✓	✓	✓		✓

[a] Immediate-release only.
[b] Not indicated in hypertriglyceridemia patients with low or normal LDL despite elevated total cholesterol.
[c] Includes Fredrickson type IV.
[d] Includes Fredrickson types IIa and IIb.
[e] Extended-release only.
[f] Includes Fredrickson type III.
[g] Includes heterozygous familial and nonfamilial hypercholesterolemia.

Before initiating treatment with HMG-CoA reductase inhibitors, exclude secondary causes of hypercholesterolemia (eg, poorly controlled hypothyroidism, nephrotic syndrome, dysproteinemias, obstructive liver disease, other drug therapy, alcoholism). Perform a lipid profile to measure total cholesterol (total-C), LDL cholesterol (LDL-C), HDL cholesterol (HDL-C), and triglycerides (TG). Estimate LDL-C in patients with TG less than 400 mg/dL (less than 4.5 mmol/L) using the following equation: LDL-C = total-C − (⅕TG + HDL-C). Determine LDL-C by ultracentrifugation for patients with TG greater than 400 mg/dL because this equation is less accurate.

Actions

➤*Pharmacology:* These agents, also referred to as the statins, competitively inhibit 3-hydroxy-3-methyl-glutaryl-coenzyme A (HMG-CoA) reductase, the enzyme that catalyzes the conversion of HMG-CoA to mevalonate. This conversion is an early rate-limiting step in cholesterol biosynthesis. By inhibiting this enzyme, statins markedly reduce plasma concentrations of LDL and total cholesterol and to a lesser extent Apo-B and triglycerides and increase levels of HDL cholesterol. The mechanism of the LDL-lowering effect may involve both reduction of VLDL concentration and induction of the LDL receptor, leading to reduced production and/or increased catabolism of LDL. **Lovastatin** and **simvastatin** are inactive lactone prodrugs that are rapidly hydrolyzed to their active beta-hydroxyacid forms. The other statins are administered in their active forms.

These agents are highly effective in reducing total cholesterol and LDL in heterozygous familial and nonfamilial forms of hypercholesterolemia and mixed hyperlipidemia. A marked response was seen within 1 to 2 weeks, and the maximum therapeutic response occurred within 4 to 6 weeks. The response was maintained during therapy. In studies of some agents, single daily doses given in the evening were more effective than in the morning, perhaps because cholesterol is synthesized mainly at night.

➤*Pharmacokinetics:*

Pharmacokinetics of HMG-CoA Reductase Inhibitors						
Drug	Bioavailability	Excretion	t½ (h)	Major metabolites	Protein binding	Effects of renal/hepatic impairment
Atorvastatin	≈ 14% absolute bioavailability; first-pass metabolism (CYP3A4)	< 2% (urine)	≈ 14[a]	Metabolized to ortho- and parahydroxylated derivatives (activity equivalent to parent)	≥ 98%	Plasma levels not affected by renal disease; markedly increased with chronic alcoholic liver disease.
Fluvastatin	98% absorbed; absolute bioavailability 24%; saturable first-pass metabolism (CYP2C9); mean relative bioavailibility is ≈ 29%for XR[b] compared with IR[c]	≈ 5% (urine) ≈ 90% (feces)	< 3 (IR) ≈ 9 (XR)	Hydroxylated metabolites (active, do not circulate systemically)	98%	Potential drug accumulation with hepatic insufficiency.
Lovastatin	≈ 30% absorbed; extensive first-pass metabolism (CYP3A4); < 5% of oral dose reaches general circulation as active inhibitors; bioavailability for XR was 190% compared with IR	10% (urine) 83% (feces)	3 to 4 (IR)	Beta-hydroxyacid; 6′-hydroxy derivative; 2 additional active metabolites	> 95%	Increased plasma concentration with severe renal disease.
Pravastatin	34% absorbed; absolute bioavailability 17%; extensive first-pass metabolism; plasma levels may not correlate with efficacy	≈ 20% (urine) 70% (feces)	77[d]	Major degradation product: 3α-hydroxy isomeric metabolite (1/10 to 1/40 activity of parent)	≈ 50%	Potential drug accumulation with renal or hepatic insufficiency. Mean AUC varied 18-fold in cirrhotic patients and peak values varied 47-fold.
Rosuvastatin	absolute biovailabilty ≈ 20%; not extensively metabolized (≈ 10%; CYP2C9)	90% (feces)	19	N-desmethyl rosuvastatin (≈ ⅙ to ½ activity of parent)	88%	Increased plasma concentrations with severe renal impairment and hepatic disease.
Simvastatin	≈ 85% absorbed; extensive first-pass metabolism (CYP3A4); < 5% of oral dose reaches general circulation	13% (urine) 60% (feces)	—	Beta-hydroxyacid; 6′-hydroxy, 6′-hydroxymethyl, 6′-exomethylene derivatives	≈ 95%	Higher systemic exposure may occur in hepatic and severe renal insufficiency.

[a] For unmetabolized atorvastatin only. The t½ is 20 to 30 hours for the active metabolites.
[b] XR = extended-release.
[c] IR = immediate-release.
[d] Parent plus metabolites.

➤*Clinical trials:*

Lipid-Lowering Properties of HMG-CoA Reductase Inhibitors in Placebo- and Active-Controlled Trials[a]					
Lipid/Lipoprotein[b]	TC	LDL	HDL	Apo-B	TG
Drugs	Mean Changes from Baseline (%)				
Atorvastatin					
10 mg	(−) 25 to 37	(−) 27 to 39	(+) 6 to 14	(−) 27 to 32	(−) 17 to 41
20 mg	(−) 33 to 35	(−) 30 to 43	(+) 9 to 11	(−) 35	(−) 26 to 39
40 mg	(−) 37	(−) 50	(+) 6	(−) 42	(−) 29
80 mg	(−) 44 to 58	(−) 41 to 60	(+) 5 to 7.5	(−) 50	(−) 37 to 53

HMG-CoA Reductase Inhibitors

Lipid-Lowering Properties of HMG-CoA Reductase Inhibitors in Placebo- and Active-Controlled Trials[a]

Lipid/Lipoprotein[b]	TC	LDL	HDL	Apo-B	TG
Drugs	Mean Changes from Baseline (%)				
Fluvastatin					
20 mg	(−) 16 to 17	(−) 22 to 25	(+) 2 to 6	(−) 19	(−) 12 to 17
40 mg	(−) 18 to 19	(−) 24 to 31	(+) 4 to 8	(−) 18	(−) 14 to 20
80 mg (IR)	(−) 27	(−) 34 to 36	(+) 4 to 9	(−) 28	(−) 18 to 23
80 mg (ER)	(−) 25	(−) 33 to 38	(+) 7 to 11	(−) 27	(−) 19 to 25
Lovastatin (IR)					
10 mg	(−) 16	(−) 21	(+) 5		(−) 10
20 mg	(−) 17 to 19	(−) 24 to 28	(+) 6 to 8	NA	(−) 7 to 10
40 mg	(−) 22 to 27	(−) 30 to 34	(+) 2 to 9		(−) 6 to 21
80 mg	(−) 29 to 34	(−) 40 to 42	(+) 8 to 10		(−) 19 to 27
Lovastatin (ER)					
10 mg	(−) 18	(−) 24	(+) 9		(−) 17
20 mg	(−) 21	(−) 30	(+) 12	NA	(−) 13
40 mg	(−) 25	(−) 35	(+) 13		(−) 10
60 mg	(−) 29	(−) 40	(+) 12		(−) 25
Pravastatin					
10 mg	(−) 16	(−) 22	(+) 7	NA	(−) 15
20 mg	(−) 21 to 24	(−) 26 to 32	(+) 1 to 2	(−) 23	(−) 10 to 11
40 mg	(−) 13 to 33	(−) 21 to 41	(+) 5 to 14	(−) 18	(−) 12 to 24
80 mg	(−) 27	(−) 37	(+) 3	NA	(−) 19
Rosuvastatin					
5 mg	(−) 24 to 33	(−) 28 to 45	(+) 3 to 13	(−) 38	(−) 21 to 35
10 mg	(−) 36 to 40	(−) 45 to 52	(+) 8 to 14	(−) 42	(−) 10 to 37
20 mg	(−) 34 to 40	(−) 31 to 55	(+) 8 to 22	(−) 46	(−) 23 to 37
40 mg	(−) 40 to 46	(−) 43 to 63	(+) 10 to 17	(−) 54	(−) 28 to 43
Simvastatin					
5 mg	(−) 19	(−) 26	(+) 10	NA	(−) 12
10 mg	(−) 23	(−) 30	(+) 12	NA	(−) 15
20 mg	(−) 28	(−) 38	(+) 8	NA	(−) 19
40 mg	(−) 25 to 50	(−) 28 to 50	(+) 7 to 13	(−) 32	(−) 8 to 41
80 mg	(−) 31 to 52	(−) 36 to 51	(+) 7 to 16	NA	(−) 24 to 38

* NA = not available, (−) = decrease, (+) = increase.
[a] Includes all studies regardless of indication. Data are pooled from different studies and are not necessarily comparable.

[b] TC = total cholesterol, LDL = low-density lipoprotein cholesterol, HDL = high-density lipoprotein cholesterol, Apo-B = apolipoprotein B, TG = triglyceride.

HMG-CoA reductase inhibitor vs cholestyramine – **Lovastatin** 40 and 80 mg/day was compared with cholestyramine 24 g daily in a randomized open parallel study. Lovastatin decreased total cholesterol 27% and 34% from baseline with the 40 and 80 mg/day doses, respectively, versus a 17% decrease with cholestyramine. Lovastatin 40 and 80 mg/day also reduced LDL by 32% and 42%, respectively, versus 23% with cholestyramine. There was no difference seen in HDL increases between the two drugs.

Patients treated with **pravastatin** in combination with cholestyramine had at least 50% reductions in LDL. Pravastatin attenuated cholestyramine-induced increases in triglyceride levels, which are of unknown clinical significance.

Atherosclerosis – In the Familial Atherosclerosis Treatment Study, **lovastatin** or niacin in combination with a bile acid sequestrant for 2.5 years in hyperlipidemic subjects significantly reduced the frequency of progression and increased the frequency of regression of coronary atherosclerotic lesions compared with diet and, in some cases, low-dose resin.

HMG-CoA reductase inhibitors vs HMG-CoA reductase inhibitors – Atorvastatin 10 mg was compared with lovastatin 20 mg, pravastatin 20 mg, and simvastatin 10 mg in three separate trials. In the first trial atorvastatin decreased total cholesterol, LDL, and TG by 27%, 36%, and 17% versus 19%, 27%, and 6%, respectively, with lovastatin from baseline. In the second trial, atorvastatin lowered total cholesterol, LDL, and TG by 25%, 35%, and 17% versus 17%, 23%, and 9%, respectively, with pravastatin. In the third trial, atorvastatin decreased total cholesterol, LDL, and TG by 29%, 37%, and 23% from baseline versus 24%, 30%, and 15%, respectively, with simvastatin.

In a multi-center trial rosuvastatin was compared with atorvastatin, simvastatin, and pravastatin. Rosuvastatin 10 mg reduced LDL-C significantly more than atorvastatin 10 mg; pravastatin 10, 20, 40 mg; and simvastatin 10, 20, and 40 mg (*P* < 0.002). Rosuvastatin 20 mg reduced LDL-C significantly more than atorvastatin 20 and 40 mg; pravastatin 20 and 40 mg; and simvastatin 20, 40, and 80 mg (*P* < 0.002). Rosuvastatin 40 mg reduced LDL-C significantly more than atorvastatin 40 mg; pravastatin 40 mg; and simvastatin 40 and 80 mg (*P* < 0.002). See the following table.

Change in LDL-C from Baseline (%)

	10 mg	20 mg	40 mg	80 mg
Rosuvastatin	− 46	− 52	− 55	−
Atorvastatin	− 37	− 43	− 48	− 51
Pravastatin	− 20	− 24	− 30	−
Simvastatin	− 28	− 35	− 39	− 46

Contraindications

Hypersensitivity to any component of these products; active liver disease or unexplained persistent elevated liver function tests; pregnancy, lactation (see Warnings).

Warnings

➤*Skeletal muscle effects:* All statins have been associated with myalgia, myopathy (ie, muscle pain, tenderness, or weakness with creatine phosphokinase [CPK] values above 10 times the ULN), and rhabdomyolysis. Uncomplicated myalgia has been reported with drugs in this class. Myopathy sometimes takes the form of rhabdomyolysis with or without acute renal failure secondary to myoglobinuria, and rare fatalities have occurred. Factors that may predispose patients to myopathy with HMG-CoA reductase inhibitors include advanced age (65 years of age or older), hypothyroidism, and renal insufficiency. The risk of myopathy/rhabdomyolysis is dose-related and also increases when statins are given concomitantly with other drugs that inhibit their metabolism (eg, cyclosporine, erythromycin, or azole antifungals) or other drugs that can cause myopathy when given alone (eg, fibrates or lipid-lowering doses of niacin). Generally avoid concomitant use of these agents with statins. If combination use is being considered, carefully weigh the benefit against the potential risks of these combinations. For dosage adjustments refer to individual product monographs. See also Drug Interactions.

Consider myopathy in any patient with diffuse myalgias, muscle tenderness or weakness, and/or marked CPK elevation. Advise patients to promptly report muscle pain, tenderness, or weakness, particularly with malaise or fever. Discontinue the drug if markedly elevated CPK levels occur or if myopathy is diagnosed or suspected.

Consider temporarily withholding or discontinuing drug therapy in any patient with an acute, serious condition suggestive of a myopathy or with a risk factor predisposing them to the development of renal failure secondary to rhabdomyolysis, including the following: Severe acute infection; sepsis; hypotension; major surgery; trauma; severe metabolic, endocrine, or electrolyte disorders; uncontrolled seizures.

➤*Endocrine effects:* Statins interfere with cholesterol synthesis and lower circulating cholesterol levels and, as such, might theoretically blunt adrenal or gonadal steroid hormone production. Small declines in total testosterone with no commensurate elevation in LH have been noted with the use of **fluvastatin**. **Pravastatin** showed inconsistent results with regard to possible effects on basal steroid hormone levels; **atorvastatin**, **lovastatin**, **rosuvastatin**, and **simvastatin** did not reduce basal plasma cortisol concentration or basal plasma testosterone concentration or impair adrenal reserve. Appropriately evaluate patients who display clinical evidence of endocrine dysfunction. Exercise caution when administering HMG-CoA reductase inhibitors with drugs that affect steroid levels or activity, such as ketoconazole, spironolactone, and cimetidine.

➤*CNS effects:* In animals, CNS vascular lesions characterized by perivascular hemorrhage, edema, mononuclear cell infiltration of perivascular spaces and other similar CNS vascular lesions have been observed with drugs in this class.

➤*Hyperlipidemia, secondary causes:* Prior to initiating therapy, exclude secondary causes of hyperlipidemia (eg, poorly controlled hypothyroidism, nephrotic syndrome, dysproteinemias, obstructive liver disease, other drug therapy, alcoholism) and measure total-C, HDL-C, and triglycerides.

➤*Hypersensitivity reactions:* An apparent hypersensitivity syndrome has occurred rarely with drugs in this class (see Adverse Reactions). Refer to Management of Acute Hypersensitivity Reactions.

➤*Renal function impairment:* A single 20 mg dose of **pravastatin** was given to patients with varying degrees of renal impairment. Although no effect on pravastatin or its 3α-hydroxy-isomeric metabolite was observed, a small increase in mean AUC values and half-life was seen for the inactive hydroxylation metabolite. Closely monitor patients with renal impairment. Higher systemic exposure of **simvastatin** may occur in severe renal insufficiency. Plasma concentrations after a single dose of **lovastatin** were approximately 2-fold higher in patients with severe renal insufficiency. Plasma concentrations of **rosuvastatin** increased to a clinically significant extent (about 3-fold) in patients with severe renal impairment. Consider a dose reduction for patients on 40 mg rosuvastatin therapy with unexplained persistent proteinuria during routine urinalysis testing.

➤*Hepatic function impairment:* Use with caution in patients who consume substantial quantities of alcohol, who have a history of liver disease, or have signs suggestive of liver disease. Active liver disease or unexplained persistent transaminase elevations are contraindications for the use of HMG-CoA reductase inhibitors (see Contraindications).

Marked persistent increases (greater than 3 times ULN occurring on 2 or more occasions) in serum transaminases have occurred. The incidence of these abnormalities with **lovastatin** was 0.1%, 0.9%, and 1.5% for 20, 40, and 80 mg, respectively. The incidence of these abnormalities with **rosuvastatin** was 0.4%, 0%, 0%, and 0.1% for 5, 10, 20, and 40 mg respectively. The incidence of these abnormalities with **fluvastatin** was 0.2%, 1.5%, and 2.7% with 20, 40, and 80 mg, respectively. The incidence of these abnormalities with **pravastatin** was less than 1.2%. The incidence of these abnormalities with simvastatin was 0.9% and 2.1% for 40 and 80 mg, respectively. The incidence of these abnormalities with **atorvastatin** was 0.2%, 0.2%, 0.6% and 2.3% for 10, 20, 40 and 80 mg, respectively. When the drug was interrupted or discontinued or the dosage was reduced, transaminase levels usually fell slowly to pretreatment levels. In pravastatin-treated patients, abnormalities did not appear to be related to treatment duration and were not associated with cholestasis.

For **lovastatin** it is recommended that liver function tests (LFTs) be performed before the initiation of treatment, 6 and 12 weeks after initiation of therapy or elevation in dose, and periodically (eg, semiannually) thereafter. For **rosuvastatin**, **fluvastatin**, and **atorvastatin**, it is recommended that LFTs be performed prior to and at 12 weeks following both the initiation of therapy and any elevation in dose, and periodically (eg, semiannually) thereafter. For **pravastatin** and **simvastatin**, perform LFTs prior to the initiation of therapy, prior to elevation of dose, and when otherwise clinically indicated. For patients titrated to the 80 mg dose of simvastatin, perform LFTs prior to titration, 3 months after titration to the 80 mg dose, and periodically thereafter (eg, semiannually) for the first year of treatment. Liver enzyme changes generally occur in the first 3 months of treatment with atorvastatin, fluvastatin, or rosuvastatin and within 3 to 12 months of starting lovastatin or simvastatin. Monitor patients who develop increased transaminase levels until the abnormalities resolve. If an increase in ALT or AST greater than 3 times ULN persists, reduce dose or withdraw therapy.

➤*Carcinogenesis:* Significantly increased incidence of uterine stromal polyps was observed in female rats given 80 mg/kg/day **rosuvastatin**. In mice, increased incidence of hepatocellular adenoma and carcinoma was observed at 200 mg/kg/day.

In mice, a statistically significant increase in the incidence of hepatocellular carcinomas and adenomas was observed in **lovastatin** doses of 500 mg/kg/day. In addition, an increase in the incidence of papilloma in nonglandular stomach mucosa was seen in mice.

Rats given **pravastatin** doses of 100 mg/kg showed an increased incidence of hepatocellular carcinomas in males (approximately 12 times the human dose of 80 mg based on body surface area). In mice, 250 and 500 mg/kg resulted in a significant increase in the incidence of lung adenomas in treated females (approximately 15- and 23-times the human dose of 80 mg based on AUC, respectively).

In mice receiving **simvastatin** (25, 100, and 400 mg/kg/day), the incidence of liver carcinoma and adenoma and lung adenoma was significantly increased. In female rats receiving simvastatin at levels approximately 11 times higher than in humans given 80 mg simvastatin based on AUC, there was a statistically significant increase in thyroid follicular adenomas.

In rats given **fluvastatin** doses of 6, 9, and 18 to 24 mg/kg/day (approximately 9 to 35 times the mean human drug levels after a 40 mg dose), a low incidence of forestomach squamous papillomas and 1 forestomach carcinoma was considered to reflect prolonged hyperplasia induced by direct contact exposure to fluvastatin rather than to systemic effects. An increased incidence of thyroid follicular cell adenomas and carcinomas occurred in males after 18 to 24 mg/kg/day. In contrast with other HMG-CoA reductase inhibitors, no hepatic adenomas or carcinomas were observed.

The carcinogenicity study with fluvastatin conducted in mice at dose levels of 0.3, 15, and 30 mg/kg/day revealed, as in rats, a statistically significant increase in forestomach squamous cell papillomas in males and females at 30 mg/kg/day and females at 15 mg/kg/day. These treatment levels represented plasma drug levels of approximately 0.05, 2, and 7 times the mean human plasma drug concentration after a 40 mg oral dose.

In rats at dose levels of 10, 30, and 100 mg/kg/day of **atorvastatin**, 2 rare muscle tumors were found in high-dose females. In one, there was a rhabdomyosarcoma and, in another, there was a fibrosarcoma. A study in mice given 100, 200, or 400 mg/kg/day found a significant increase in liver adenomas in high-dose males and liver carcinomas in high-dose females.

➤*Fertility impairment:* Drug-related testicular atrophy, decreased spermatogenesis, spermatocytic degeneration, and giant cell formation were seen in dogs given **lovastatin** 20 mg/kg/day and in dogs given **simvastatin** 10 mg/kg/day.

There was decreased fertility in male rats treated with simvastatin 25 mg/kg for 34 weeks.

Spermatidic giant cells were seen in testicles of dogs treated with **rosuvastatin** 30 mg/kg/day. This effect also was seen in monkeys as well as vacuolation of seminiferous tubular epithelium with doses of 30 mg/kg/day.

There was aplasia and aspermia in the epididymis of 2 of 10 rats treated with 100 mg/kg/day of **atorvastatin** for 3 months (16 times the human AUC at the 80 mg dose); testis weights were significantly lower at 30 and 100 mg/kg and epididymal weight was lower at 100 mg/kg. Male rats given 100 mg/kg/day for 11 weeks prior to mating had decreased sperm motility, spermatid head concentration, and increased abnormal sperm. Atorvastatin caused no adverse effects on semen parameters, or reproductive organ histopathology in dogs given doses of 10, 40, or 120 mg/kg for 2 years.

Seminal vesicles and testes were small in hamsters treated with **fluvastatin** for 3 months at 20 mg/kg/day (approximately 3 times the 40 mg human daily dose based on surface area, mg/m²). There was tubular degeneration and aspermatogenesis in testes as well as vesiculitis of seminal vesicles. Vesiculitis of seminal vesicles and edema of the testes were also seen in rats treated for 2 years at 18 mg/kg/day (approximately 4 times the human C_{max} achieved with a 40 mg daily dose).

➤*Elderly:* For the general patient population, plasma concentrations of **fluvastatin** do not vary either as a function of age or gender, but in patients older than 70 years of age, the AUC of **lovastatin** immediate-release, **simvastatin**, and **pravastatin** is increased. Elderly patients (65 years of age and older) demonstrated a greater treatment response to LDL-C, total-C, and LDL/HDL ratio than patients younger than 65 years of age with fluvastatin. The safety and efficacy of **atorvastatin**, **rosuvastatin**, and lovastatin extended-release in patients 70 years of age and older were similar to those of patients younger than 70 years of age.

➤*Pregnancy:* Category X. Contraindicated during pregnancy. Congenital anomalies and/or skeletal malformations have occurred in animals. There are no data in pregnant women. However, because HMG-CoA reductase inhibitors can decrease synthesis of cholesterol and possibly other products of the cholesterol biosynthesis pathway, they may cause fetal harm when given to pregnant women. Give to women of childbearing age only if they are highly unlikely to conceive and have been informed of potential hazards. If a patient becomes pregnant while on the drug, immediately discontinue the drug and apprise her of the potential hazard to the fetus.

➤*Lactation:* Atorvastatin is excreted in the milk of rats and is likely to be excreted in breast milk; it is not known whether lovastatin, simvastatin, and rosuvastatin are excreted in breast milk;a small amount of pravastatin is excreted in breast milk; fluvastatin is present in breast milk in a 2:1 ratio (milk:plasma). Because of the potential for serious adverse reactions in nursing infants, caution women taking these drugs not to nurse their infants.

➤*Children:* Atorvastatin, simvastatin, and lovastatin are indicated for treatment of patients 10 to 17 years of age with heterozygous familial hypercholesterolemia. Pravastatin is indicated for the treatment of patients 8 to 18 years of age with heterozygous familial hypercholesterolemia. Safety and efficacy have not been established for atorvastatin, simvastatin, and lovastatin in prepubertal patients and patients younger than 10 years of age. Safety and efficacy have not been established in patients younger than 8 years of age for pravastatin. Safety and efficacy have not been established in patients younger than 18 years of age for fluvastatin. Safety and efficacy of rosuvastatin have not been established in pediatric patients.

Precautions

➤*Monitoring:* For lovastatin, perform LFTs before initiating therapy, at 6 and 12 weeks after initiation of therapy or after dose elevation, and periodically thereafter (approximately 6-month intervals). For rosuvastatin, fluvastatin, and atorvastatin, it is recommended that LFTs be performed prior to and at 12 weeks following both the initiation of therapy and any elevation in dose, and periodically (eg, semiannually) thereafter. For pravastatin and simvastatin, perform LFTs prior to the initiation of therapy, prior to elevation of dose, and when otherwise clinically indicated. For patients titrated to the 80 mg dose of simvastatin, perform LFTs prior to titration, 3 months after titration to the 80 mg dose, and periodically thereafter (eg, semiannually) for the first year of treatment. Pay special attention to patients who develop elevated serum transaminase levels. If transaminase levels progress, particularly if they rise to 3 times the ULN and are persistent, discontinue the drug.

Because HMG-CoA reductase inhibitors may increase CPK and transaminase levels, consider this in the differential diagnosis of chest pain in patients treated with these agents.

➤*Diet:* Before instituting therapy, attempt to control hypercholesterolemia with diet, exercise, and weight reduction in obese patients. Treat underlying medical problems.

➤*Ophthalmologic effects:* There was a high prevalence of baseline lenticular opacities in the patient population included in the early clinical trials with lovastatin. During these trials, new opacities appeared in both the lovastatin and placebo groups. There was no clinically significant change in visual acuity in the patients who had new opacities reported nor was any patient, including those with opacities noted at baseline, discontinued from therapy because of a decrease in visual acuity.

A 3-year, double-blind study found no clinically significant differences between lovastatin and placebo groups in the incidence, type, or progression of lenticular opacities.

➤*Homozygous familial hypercholesterolemia:* HMG-CoA reductase inhibitors are reported to be less effective in patients with rare homozygous familial hypercholesterolemia, possibly because these patients have few functional LDL receptors.

Drug Interactions

➤*CYP450 system:* Atorvastatin, lovastatin, and simvastatin are primarily metabolized by CYP3A4; they may interact with CYP3A4 inhibitors (eg, itraconazole, erythromycin, protease inhibitors, nefazodone, cyclosporine) thereby increasing the risk of myopathy by reducing the elimination of the HMG-CoA reductase inhibitors.

Fluvastatin is primarily metabolized by CYP2C9; it may interact with CYP2C9 inhibitors. Data indicate that pravastatin and rosuvastatin are not metabolized by CYP3A4 to a clinically significant extent.

➤*Drugs that may cause myopathy:* The risk of myopathy is increased by the following lipid-lowering drugs that can cause myopathy when given alone: Gemfibrozil, other fibrates, and niacin (at least 1 g/day).

HMG-CoA Reductase Inhibitor Drug Interactions			
Precipitant drug	Object drug*		Description
Amiodarone	HMG-CoA reductase inhibitors Lovastatin Simvastatin	↑	Increased risk of myopathy with concomitant use. See Administration and Dosage of the individual monographs for dosing recommendations.
Antacids	HMG-CoA reductase inhibitors Rosuvastatin Atorvastatin	↓	Coadministration with *Maalox TC* suspension decreased atorvastatin levels by ≈ 35%; LDL-C reduction was not altered. Coadministration of rosuvastatin and an aluminum/magnesium combination antacid decreased rosuvastatin levels by 54%. Administer antacids at least 2 hours after rosuvastatin.
Azole antifungals (eg, itraconazole ketoconazole)	HMG-CoA reductase inhibitors	↑	Coadministration increased lovastatin levels ≈ 20-fold in healthy volunteers. Temporarily interrupt or consider reducing the dose of HMG-CoA reductase inhibitors if systemic azole antifungals are needed. The risk of myopathy is increased. Pravastatin and rosuvastatin levels are affected the least.
Bile acid sequestrants (BAS) (eg, colestipol, cholestyramine)	HMG-CoA reductase inhibitors	↓	The HMG-CoA reductase inhibitor may adsorb to the BAS, reducing the GI absorption of the HMG-CoA reductase inhibitor. A decrease in pravastatin (40% to 50%) and lovastatin bioavailability may occur. Take pravastatin 1 hour before or 4 hours after BAS. Coadministration of cholestyramine with fluvastatin resulted in decreased AUC and C_{max}. Take fluvastatin 4 hours after cholestyramine. Plasma levels of atorvastatin decreased ≈ 25% with coadministration with colestipol.
Cimetidine Ranitidine Omeprazole	HMG-CoA reductase inhibitors Fluvastatin	↑	Coadministration results in a significant increase in fluvastatin C_{max} (43% to 70%) and AUC (24% to 33%), with an 18% to 23% decrease in plasma clearance.
Cyclosporine	HMG-CoA reductase inhibitors Rosuvastatin	↑	Concurrent administration increases risk of severe myopathy or rhabdomyolysis. If coadministration cannot be avoided, consider decreasing HMG-CoA reductase inhibitor dose. See Administration and Dosage of the individual monographs for dosing information.
Diltiazem	HMG-CoA reductase inhibitors Atorvastatin Lovastatin Simvastatin	↑	Coadministration may result in elevated plasma levels of the HMG-CoA reductase inhibitor, increasing the risk of myopathy.
Fibric acid derivatives (eg, gemfibrozil)	HMG-CoA reductase inhibitors	↑	Severe myopathy or rhabdomyolysis reported with lovastatin. Urinary excretion and protein binding of pravastatin may be decreased. Avoid concurrent use. Coadministration increases the risk of myopathy. Concurrent use of gemfibrozil with pravastatin is not recommended. See Administration and Dosage of the individual monographs for dosing recommendations.
Glyburide	HMG-CoA reductase inhibitors Fluvastatin	↑	Coadministration increased glyburide C_{max}, AUC, and half life approximately 50%, 69%, and 121%, respectively. Coadministration also led to an increase in fluvastatin C_{max} and AUC by 44% and 51%, respectively. Monitor patients.
HMG-CoA reductase inhibitors Fluvastatin	Glyburide		
Isradipine	HMG-CoA reductase inhibitors Lovastatin	↓	Isradipine may increase clearance of lovastatin and its metabolites by increasing hepatic blood flow.

HMG-CoA Reductase Inhibitors

HMG-CoA Reductase Inhibitor Drug Interactions			
Precipitant drug	Object drug*		Description

Amiodarone	HMG-CoA reductase inhibitors
	  Lovastatin
	  Simvastatin
		↑	Increased risk of myopathy with concomitant use. See Administration and Dosage of the individual monographs for dosing recommendations.

Macrolides
  Erythromycin
  Clarithromycin
	HMG-CoA reductase inhibitors
	  Atorvastatin
	  Lovastatin
	  Simvastatin
		↑	Coadministration increases the risk of severe myopathy or rhabdomyolysis. **Atorvastatin** plasma levels increased by ≈ 40%.

Nefazodone	HMG-CoA reductase inhibitors
	  Atorvastatin
	  Lovastatin
	  Simvastatin
		↑	Increased risk of myopathy with concomitant use.

Niacin (nicotinic acid)	HMG-CoA reductase inhibitors	↑	Concurrent administration increases risk of severe myopathy or rhabdomyolysis.
Phenytoin	HMG-CoA reductase inhibitors Fluvastatin	↑	A single dose of extended release phenytoin 300 mg increased mean steady-state fluvastatin C_{max} by 27% and AUC by 40% and fluvastatin increased the mean phenytoin C_{max} by 5% and AUC by 20%. Monitor patients.
HMG-CoA reductase inhibitors Fluvastatin	Phenytoin		
Propranolol	HMG-CoA reductase inhibitors Simvastatin	↔	Concomitant administration resulted in a significant decrease in simvastatin C_{max}, but no change in AUC.

Protease Inhibitors (eg, nelfinavir, ritonavir)	HMG-CoA reductase inhibitors
	  Atorvastatin
	  Lovastatin
	  Simvastatin
		↑	Concomitant use may result in elevated plasma levels, increasing the risk of myopathy. Nelfinavir is contraindicated in patients taking lovastatin or simvastatin.

Protease Inhibitors
  Ritonavir
  Saquinavir
	HMG-CoA reductase inhibitors
	  Pravastatin
		↓	Concomitant use may result in decreased pravastatin plasma levels, possibly decreasing efficacy.

Rifampin	HMG-CoA reductase inhibitors
	  Fluvastatin
	  Simvastatin
		↓	Coadministration may cause a decrease in fluvastatin C_{max} and AUC and an increase in plasma clearance.

St. John's wort	HMG-CoA reductase inhibitors
	  Lovastatin
	  Simvastatin
		↓	Coadministration may result in decreased HMG-CoA reductase inhibitor plasma levels, possibly decreasing efficacy.

Verapamil	HMG-CoA reductase inhibitors
	  Atorvastatin
	  Lovastatin
	  Simvastatin
		↑	Increased risk of myopathy with concomitant use. See Administration and Dosage of the individual monographs for dosing recommendations.

HMG-CoA reductase inhibitors Fluvastatin	Diclofenac	↑	Coadministration increased the mean diclofenac C_{max} and AUC by 60% and 25%, respectively.

HMG-CoA reductase inhibitors
  Atorvastatin
  Fluvastatin
  Simvastatin
	Digoxin	↑	Slight elevation in digoxin levels possible. Concomitant multiple doses of **atorvastatin** and digoxin increased steady-state digoxin levels by ≈ 20%. A 40 mg **fluvastatin** dose demonstrated an 11% increase in digoxin C_{max} and a slight increase in digoxin urinary clearance. Monitor digoxin patients appropriately.

HMG-CoA reductase inhibitors
  Atorvastatin
  Rosuvastatin
	Oral contraceptives	↑	Coadministration with atorvastatin increased AUC for norethindrone and ethinyl estradiol by ≈ 30% and 20%, respectively.

HMG-CoA reductase inhibitors
  Fluvastatin
  Lovastatin
  Rosuvastatin
  Simvastatin
	Warfarin	↑	Increased INR has been demonstrated with concomitant use of lovastatin, simvastatin, rosuvastatin, and fluvastatin. Bleeding also has been reported in a few patients concomitantly receiving lovastatin. Atorvastatin and pravastatin had no clinically significant effect on PT when given with warfarin.

* ↑ = Object drug increased. ↓ = Object drug decreased. ↔ = Undetermined clinical effect.

▶*Drug/Food interactions:* Administration of **rosuvastatin** with food decreased the rate of drug absorption by 20% as assessed by C_{max} but there was no effect on the extent of absorption as assessed by AUC. Rosuvastatin may be given with or without food.

Under fasting conditions, **lovastatin** levels are approximately ⅔ of those found when given immediately after meals; take lovastatin with meals.

Food reduces systemic bioavailability of **pravastatin**, but lipid-lowering effects of the drug are similar when taken with, or 1 hour prior to, meals; pravastatin may be taken without regard to meals.

Simvastatin levels are similar when administered in a fasting state or with food; simvastatin may be taken without regard to meals.

No therapeutic differences were evident when **fluvastatin** was administered with food compared with 4 hours postprandially. Fluvastatin may be taken without regard to meals.

LDL-C reduction is similar whether **atorvastatin** is given with or without food anytime of day. Plasma atorvastatin concentrations are lower (approximately 30% for C_{max} and AUC) following evening drug administration compared with morning. Food decreases the rate and extent of drug absorption by approximately 25% and 9%, respectively.

Grapefruit juice – Coadministration with large quantities of grapefruit juice (at least 1 quart daily) may result in increased plasma levels of lovastatin, simvastatin, or atorvastatin, increasing the risk of myopathy. Avoid concurrent use.

Adverse Reactions

These agents are generally well tolerated; adverse reactions are usually mild and transient.

In placebo-controlled trials, more than 2% of **atorvastatin**-treated patients, 1% of **fluvastatin**-treated patients, and 1.7% of **pravastatin**-treated patients discontinued treatment because of adverse events; the most common reasons for discontinuation of pravastatin were asymptomatic serum transaminase increases and mild, non-specific GI complaints.

HMG-CoA Reductase Inhibitor Adverse Reactions (%)[a]						
Adverse reaction	Atorvastatin	Fluvastatin[b]	Lovastatin[b]	Pravastatin[c]	Rosuvastatin (n = 744)	Simvastatin
CNS						
Asthenia	2.2 - 3.8	—	1.2 - 3	—	2.7	1.6
Depression	< 2	—	—	—	≥ 2	—
Dizziness	≥ 2	1.9 - 2.2	0.5 - 2	3.3	≥ 2	—
Headache	2.5 - 16.7	4.7 - 8.9	2.1 - 7	6.2	5.5	3.5
Insomnia	≥ 2	0.9 - 2.7	0.5 - 1	< 1	≥ 2	—
Paresthesia	< 2	—	0.5 - 1	< 1	≥ 2	—
GI						
Abdominal pain/cramps	2.1 - 3.8	3.7 - 4.9	2 - 2.5	5.4	≥ 2	0.9 - 3.2
Acid regurgitation	—	—	0.5 - 1	—	—	—
Constipation	1.1 - 2.5	2.3 - 3.1	2 - 3.5	4	≥ 2	2.3
Diarrhea	2.7 - 5.3	3.5 - 4.9	2.2 - 3	6.2	3.4	0.5 - 1.9
Dry mouth	—	—	0.5 - 1	—	—	—
Dysgeusia	—	—	0.8	—	—	—
Dyspepsia	1.3 - 2.8	3.5 - 7.9	1 - 1.6	—	3.4	1.1
Flatulence	1.1 - 2.8	1.4 - 2.6	3.7 - 4.5	3.3	≥ 1	0.9 - 1.9
Gastroenteritis	< 2	—	—	—	≥ 2	—
Heartburn	—	—	1.6	2.9	—	—
Nausea/Vomiting	≥ 2/< 2	2.5 - 3.2	1.9 - 2.5/0.5 - 1	7.3	3.4/≥ 1	0.4 - 1.3
Tooth disorder	—	1.4 - 2.1	—	—	≥ 1	—
GU						
Urinary abnormality	—	—	—	2.4	—	—
Urinary tract infection	≥ 2	1.6 - 2.7	2 - 3	—	2.3	—
Musculoskeletal						
Arthralgia	2 - 5.1	1.3 - 4	0.5 - 1	—	≥ 2	—
Arthritis	≥ 2	1.3 - 2.1	—	—	≥ 2	—
Back pain	1.1 - 3.8	5.7	5	—	2.6	—
Leg pain	< 2	—	0.5 - 1	—	—	—
Localized pain	—	—	0.5 - 1	10	—	—
Muscle cramps/pain	—	—	0.6 - 1.1	—	—	—
Myalgia	1.3 - 5.6	3.8 - 5	1.8 - 3	2.7	2.8	1.2
Shoulder pain	—	—	0.5 - 1	—	—	—
Respiratory						
Bronchitis	≥ 2	1.8 -7.6	—	—	≥ 2	—
Common cold	—	—	—	7	≥ 2	—
Cough	—	1.9 - 2.4	—	2.6	≥ 2	—
Pharyngitis	1.3 - 2.5	2.4 - 3.8	—	—	—	—
Rhinitis	≥ 2	1.5 - 4.7	—	4	2.2	—
Sinusitis	2.5 - 6.4	2.6 - 3.5	4 - 6	—	2	—
Upper respiratory tract infection	—	12.5 - 16.2	—	—	—	2.1
Miscellaneous						
Accidental trauma	1.3 - 4.2	4.2 - 5.1	4 - 6	—	≥ 2	—
Allergy	0.9 - 2.8	1 - 2.3	—	< 1	—	—
Alopecia	< 2	—	0.5 - 1	< 1	—	—
Blurred vision/eye irritation	—	—	0.9 - 1.2	—	—	—
Chest pain	≥ 2	—	0.5 - 1	3.7	≥ 2	—
Fatigue	—	1.6 - 2.7	—	3.8	—	—
Flu syndrome	2.2 - 3.2	5.1 -7.1	5	2.4	2.3	—
Hypertension	< 2	—	—	—	≥ 2	—
Infection	2.8 - 10.3	—	11 - 16	—	≥ 2	—
Pain	—	—	3 - 5	—	≥ 2	—
Peripheral edema	≥ 2	—	—	—	≥ 2	—
Rash/Pruritus	1.1 - 3.9/< 2	1.6 - 2.3	0.8 - 1.3/0.5 - 1	4/< 1	≥ 2/≥ 1	0.6/0.5

[a] All events. Data are pooled from separate studies and are not necessarily comparable.
[b] Immediate-release and extended-release combined.
[c] Includes short-term and long-term studies.

The following adverse effects have also been reported with drugs in this class (includes postmarketing).

➤*Cardiovascular:* Angina pectoris; arrhythmia; palpitation; phlebitis; postural hypotension; syncope; vasodilation.

➤*CNS:* Abnormal dreams; anxiety; dysfunction of certain cranial nerves (eg, alteration of taste, impairment of extraocular movement, facial paresis); emotional lability; facial paralysis; hyperkinesia; hypertonia; hypesthesia; incoordination; memory loss; migraine; peripheral nerve palsy; peripheral neuropathy; psychic disturbances; somnolence; torticollis; tremor; vertigo.

➤*Dermatologic:* Acne; contact dermatitis; eczema; seborrhea; skin ulcer; sweating; urticaria; various skin changes (eg, nodules, discoloration, dryness of skin/mucous membranes, changes in hair/nails).

➤*GI:* Anorexia; biliary pain; cheilitis; cholestatic jaundice; cirrhosis; colitis; duodenal ulcer; dysphagia; enteritis; eructation; esophagitis; fatty change in liver; fulminant hepatic necrosis; gastritis; glossitis; gum hemorrhage; hemorrhage; hepatitis, including chronic active hepatitis; hepatoma; increased appetite; melena; pancreatitis; periodontal abscess; rectal mouth ulceration; stomach ulcer; stomatitis; tenesmus; ulcerative stomach.

➤*GU:* Abnormal ejaculation; albuminuria; breast enlargement; cystitis; dysuria; epididymitis; erectile dysfunction; fibrocystic breast; gynecomastia; hematuria; impotence; kidney calculus; loss of libido; metrorrhagia; nocturia; nephritis; renal failure; urinary frequency, incontinence, retention, and urgency; vaginal or uterine hemorrhage.

➤*Hematologic / Lymphatic:* Anemia; ecchymosis; lymphadenopathy; petechiae; thrombocytopenia.

➤*Hypersensitivity:* An apparent hypersensitivity syndrome has been reported rarely including 1 or more of the following features: Anaphylaxis; angioedema; arthritis; asthenia; chills; dermatomyositis; dyspnea; eosinophilia; erythema multiforme (eg, Stevens-Johnson syndrome); erythrocyte sedimentation rate (ESR) increase; fever; flushing; hemolytic anemia; leukopenia; lupus erythematosus-like syndrome; malaise; photosensitivity; polymyalgia rheumatica; positive antinuclear antibody (ANA); purpura; thrombocytopenia; toxic epidermal necrolysis; urticaria; vasculitis.

➤*Metabolic / Nutritional:* Diabetes mellitus; gout; hyperglycemia; hypoglycemia; increased CPK; weight gain.

➤*Musculoskeletal:* Bursitis; myalgia; myasthenia; myopathy; myositis; pathological fracture; rhabdomyolysis (see Warnings); tendinous contracture; tenosynovitis.

➤*Ophthalmic:* Amblyopia; dry eyes; eye hemorrhage; glaucoma; ophthalmoplegia; progression of cataracts (lens opacities; see Precautions); refraction disorder.

➤*Respiratory:* Asthma; dyspnea; epistaxis; pneumonia.

➤*Special senses:* Deafness; parosmia; taste loss; taste perversion; tinnitus.

➤*Miscellaneous:* Face edema; fever; generalized edema; malaise; neck rigidity; neck pain; pelvic pain; photosensitivity reaction.

➤*Lab test abnormalities:* Alkaline phosphatase and bilirubin; CPK (11% with **lovastatin**, levels at least twice normal); γ-glutamyl transpeptidase; increased serum transaminases (AST, ALT); liver function test abnormalities; thyroid function test abnormalities.

Overdosage

➤*Symptoms:* Five healthy volunteers received up to 200 mg **lovastatin** as a single dose without clinically significant adverse events. A few cases of accidental overdosage have been reported; no patients had any specific symptoms, and all recovered without sequelae. Maximum dose was 5 to 6 g.

The maximum single oral dose of **fluvastatin** capsules received by healthy volunteers was 80 mg. No clinically significant adverse experiences were seen at this dose. The maximum dose administered with an extended-release formulation was 640 mg for 2 weeks. This dose was not well tolerated and produced a variety of GI complaints and an increase in transaminase values.

A few cases of overdosage with **simvastatin** have occurred; no patients had any specific symptoms; all recovered without sequelae. The maximum dose taken was 3.6 g.

➤*Treatment:* Treat symptomatically and institute supportive measures as required. Refer to General Management of Acute Overdosage. The dialyzability of these agents and their metabolites is unknown.

There is no specific treatment for HMG-CoA reductase inhibitor overdosage. Because of extensive drug binding to plasma proteins, hemodialysis is not expected to significantly enhance atorvastatin clearance. Hemodialysis does not significantly enhance rosuvastatin clearance.

Patient Information

May cause photosensitivity (sensitivity to sunlight). Avoid prolonged exposure to the sun and other ultraviolet light. Use sunscreens and wear protective clothing until tolerance is determined.

If patient becomes pregnant, discontinue the drug immediately to avoid harmful effects in the developing fetus.

Promptly report unexplained muscle pain, tenderness, or weakness, especially if accompanied by fever or malaise.

Follow dietary and exercise recommendations.

Take **lovastatin** with meals; **fluvastatin, pravastatin, simvastatin, atorvastatin,** and **rosuvastatin** may be taken without regard to meals.

Advise patients to swallow lovastatin ER tablets whole; do not chew, crush, or cut.

When patients are taking rosuvastatin with an aluminum and magnesium hydroxide combination antacid, advise the patient to take the antacid at least 2 hours after rosuvastatin administration.

Advise patients to inform a physician of any medications they are taking before taking any new ones.

LOVASTATIN (Mevinolin)

Rx	**Lovastatin** (Various, eg, Eon, Mylan, Purepac, Teva)	**Tablets:** 10 mg	May contain lactose. In 30s, 60s, 100s, 500s, and 1000s.
Rx	**Mevacor** (Merck)		Lactose. (MSD 730 MEVACOR). Peach, octagonal. In unit-of-use 60s.
Rx	**Lovastatin** (Various, eg, Eon, Mylan, Purepac, Teva)	**Tablets:** 20 mg	May contain lactose. In 30s, 60s, 90s, 100s, 500s, and 1000s.
Rx	**Mevacor** (Merck)		Lactose. (MSD 731 MEVACOR). Lt. blue, octagonal. In 1000s, 10,000s, unit-of-use 60s and 90s, and UD 100s.
Rx	**Lovastatin** (Various, eg, Eon, Mylan, Purepac, Teva)	**Tablets:** 40 mg	May contain lactose. In 30s, 60s, 90s, 100s, 500s, and 1000s.
Rx	**Mevacor** (Merck)		Lactose. (MSD 732 MEVACOR). Green, octagonal. In 1000s, 10,000s, and unit-of-use 60s and 90s.
Rx	**Altoprev** (Andrx)	**Tablets, extended-release:** 10 mg	Sugar, lactose. (10). Dk. orange. In 30s.
		20 mg	Sugar, lactose. (20). Orange. In 30s.
		40 mg	Sugar, lactose. (40). Peach. In 30s.
		60 mg	Sugar, lactose. (60). Lt. peach. In 30s.

For complete prescribing information, refer to the HMG-CoA Reductase Inhibitors group monograph.

Indications

➤*Hypercholesterolemia (immediate-release only):* An adjunct to diet for the reduction of elevated total and LDL cholesterol levels in patients with primary hypercholesterolemia (types IIa and IIb), when the response to a diet restricted in saturated fat and cholesterol and to other nonpharmacological measures alone has been inadequate.

➤*Coronary heart disease (CHD):* To slow the progression of coronary atherosclerosis in patients with CHD as part of a treatment strategy to lower total and LDL cholesterol to target levels.

➤*Primary prevention of CHD:* In individuals without symptomatic cardiovascular disease, average to moderately elevated total cholesterol and LDL cholesterol, and below-average HDL cholesterol, lovastatin is indicated to reduce risk of MI, unstable angina, and coronary revascularization procedures.

➤*Adolescents 10 to 17 years of age with heterozygous familial hypercholesterolemia (immediate-release only):* As an adjunct to diet to reduce total and LDL cholesterol and Apo-B levels in adolescent boys and girls who are at least 1 year postmenarche, 10 to 17 years of age, with heterozygous familial hypercholesterolemia if after an adequate trial of diet therapy LDL cholesterol remains greater than 189 mg/dL or if LDL cholesterol remains greater than 160 mg/dL and there is a positive family history of premature cardiovascular disease or 2 or more other cardiovascular disease risk factors are present in the adolescent patient.

➤*Hyperlipidemia (extended-release only):* As an adjunct to diet for the reduction of elevated total and LDL cholesterol, Apo-B, and triglycerides and to increase HDL cholesterol in patients with primary hypercholesterolemia (heterozygous familial and nonfamilial) and mixed dyslipidemia (Fredrickson types IIa and IIb) when the response to diet restricted in saturated fat and cholesterol and to other nonpharmacological measures alone has been inadequate.

Administration and Dosage

➤*Approved by the FDA:* August 13, 1987.

Place the patient on a standard cholesterol-lowering diet before starting lovastatin and continue on this diet during treatment. Give immediate-release tablets once/day with evening meal and give extended-release tablets once/day in evening at bedtime.

➤*Adults:*

Immediate-release – Usual recommended starting dose is 20 mg once/day with the evening meal. Recommended dosage range is 10 to 80 mg/day in a single or 2 divided doses. Individualize dose according to the recommended goal of therapy. Start patients requiring reductions

in LDL cholesterol of 20% or more to achieve their goal on 20 mg/day of lovastatin. Consider a starting dose of 10 mg for patients requiring smaller reductions. Adjust at intervals of 4 weeks or more. Maximum dose is 80 mg/day. Monitor cholesterol levels periodically and consider reducing the dosage of lovastatin if cholesterol levels fall significantly below the targeted range.

Extended-release – Usual recommended starting dose is 20, 40, or 60 mg once/day given in the evening at bedtime. The recommended dosing range is 10 to 60 mg/day in single doses. Individualize dose according to the recommended goal of therapy. A starting dose of 10 mg may be considered for patients requiring smaller reductions. Adjust at intervals of 4 weeks or more. Swallow whole; do not chew or crush.

Monitor cholesterol levels periodically and consider reducing the dosage of the extended-release tablets if cholesterol levels fall significantly below the targeted range.

➤*Adolescents 10 to 17 years of age with heterozygous familial hypercholesterolemia (immediate-release only):* The recommended dosing range is 10 to 40 mg/day; the maximum recommended dose is 40 mg/day. Individualize dosage according to the recommended goal of therapy. Start patients requiring reductions in LDL cholesterol of 20% or more to achieve their goal on 20 mg/day of lovastatin. Consider a starting dose of 10 mg for patients requiring smaller reductions. Adjust at intervals of 4 weeks or more.

➤*Concomitant lipid-lowering therapy:* Lovastatin immediate-release is effective alone or when used concomitantly with bile acid sequestrants. Generally avoid use of lovastatin extended-release with fibrates or niacin. However, if lovastatin is used in combination with gemfibrozil, other fibrates, or lipid-lowering doses (1 g/day or more) of niacin, the dose of lovastatin generally should not exceed 20 mg/day as the risk of myopathy increases at higher doses.

➤*Concomitant cyclosporine:* Initiate lovastatin at 10 mg/day in patients taking cyclosporine. Maximum dose is 20 mg/day as the risk of myopathy increases at higher doses.

➤*Concomitant amiodarone or verapamil:* In patients taking amiodarone or verapamil concomitantly with lovastatin, the dose should not exceed 40 mg/day.

➤*Renal function impairment:* In patients with severe renal insufficiency (Ccr less than 30 mL/min), carefully consider dosage increases above 20 mg/day and, if deemed necessary, implement cautiously.

➤*Storage/Stability:*

Immediate-release – Store between 5° and 30°C (41° and 86°F). Protect from light and store in a well-closed, light-resistant container.

Extended-release – Store at controlled room temperature 20° to 25°C (68° to 77°F). Avoid excessive heat and humidity.

SIMVASTATIN

Rx	**Zocor** (Merck)	**Tablets:** 5 mg	Lactose. (MSD 726 ZOCOR). Buff, shield shape. Film-coated. In 1000s, unit-of-use 30s, 60s, and 90s, and UD 100s.
		10 mg	Lactose. (MSD 735 ZOCOR). Peach, shield shape. Film-coated. In 1000s, 10,000s, unit-of-use 30s and 90s, and UD 100s.
		20 mg	Lactose. (MSD 740 ZOCOR). Tan, shield shape. Film-coated. In 1000s, 10,000s, unit-of-use 30s, 60s, and 90s, and UD 100s.
		40 mg	Lactose. (MSD 749 ZOCOR). Brick red, shield shape. Film-coated. In 1000s, unit-of-use 30s, 60s, and 90s, and UD 100s.
		80 mg	Lactose. (543 80). Brick red, capsule shape. Film-coated. In 1000s, unit-of-use 30s, 60s, and 90s, and UD 100s.

For complete prescribing information, refer to the HMG-CoA Reductase Inhibitors group monograph.

Indications

➤*Adolescents 10 to 17 years of age with heterozygous familial hypercholesterolemia:* As an adjunct to diet to reduce total and LDL cholesterol and Apo-B levels in adolescent boys and girls who are at

least 1 year postmenarche, 10 to 17 years of age, with heterozygous familial hypercholesterolemia if after an adequate trial of diet therapy LDL cholesterol remains 190 mg/dL or greater or LDL cholesterol remains 160 mg/dL or greater and there is a positive family history of premature cardiovascular disease or 2 or more other cardiovascular disease risk factors are present in the adolescent patient.

SIMVASTATIN

➤*Hyperlipidemia:* To reduce elevated total and LDL cholesterol, Apo-B, and triglyceride levels; to increase HDL cholesterol in patients with primary hypercholesterolemia (heterozygous familial and nonfamilial) and mixed dyslipidemia (Fredrickson types IIa and IIb); treatment of hypertriglyceridemia (Fredrickson type IV hyperlipidemia); primary dysbetalipoproteinemia (Fredrickson type III hyperlipidemia); to reduce total and LDL cholesterol in homozygous familial hypercholesterolemia as an adjunct to other lipid-lowering treatments (eg, LDL apheresis) or if such treatments are unavailable.

➤*Primary and secondary prevention of coronary events:* In patients at high risk of coronary events because of existing coronary heart disease, diabetes, peripheral vessel disease, history of stroke or other cerebrovascular disease, to reduce the risk of total mortality by reducing coronary death; to reduce the risk of nonfatal MI and stroke; to reduce the need for coronary and noncoronary revascularization procedures.

Administration and Dosage

➤*Approved by the FDA:* December 23, 1991.

Place patient on a standard cholesterol-lowering diet. In patients with CHD or at high risk of CHD, simvastatin can be started simultaneously with diet. Individualize the dosage according to the goals of therapy and the patient's response.

➤*Dose:* The recommended usual starting dose is 20 to 40 mg once a day in the evening. For patients at high risk for a CHD event because of existing CHD, diabetes, peripheral vessel disease, history of stroke or other cerebrovascular disease, the recommended starting dose is 40 mg/day. Perform lipid determinations after 4 weeks of therapy and periodically thereafter.

➤*Homozygous familial hypercholesterolemia:* The recommended dosage is 40 mg/day in the evening or 80 mg/day in 3 divided doses of 20 mg, 20 mg, and an evening dose of 40 mg. Use simvastatin as an adjunct to other lipid-lowering treatments (eg, LDL apheresis) in these patients or if such treatments are unavailable.

➤*Adolescents 10 to 17 years of age with heterozygous familial hypercholesterolemia:* Usual recommended starting dose is 10 mg once a day in the evening. The recommended dosing range is 10 to 40 mg/day; maximum dose is 40 mg/day. Individualize dose according to recommended goal of therapy. Adjust at intervals of 4 weeks or more.

➤*Concomitant cyclosporine:* In patients taking cyclosporine concomitantly with simvastatin, begin therapy with 5 mg/day; do not exceed 10 mg/day.

➤*Concomitant amiodarone or verapamil:* In patients taking amiodarone or verapamil concomitantly with simvastatin, the dose should not exceed 20 mg/day.

➤*Concomitant lipid-lowering therapy:* Simvastatin is effective alone or when used concomitantly with bile acid sequestrants. The combined use of simvastatin with gemfibrozil should be avoided unless the benefit of further alteration in lipid levels is likely to outweigh the increased risk of this drug combination. However, if simvastatin is used in combination with gemfibrozil, the dose of simvastatin generally should not exceed 10 mg/day. Use with caution with other fibrates or lipid-lowering doses (1 g/day or more) of niacin.

➤*Renal function impairment:* Exercise caution when simvastatin is administered to patients with severe renal insufficiency. Initiate therapy in such patients with 5 mg/day and monitor closely.

➤*Storage/Stability:* Store between 5° and 30°C (41° and 86°F).

PRAVASTATIN SODIUM

Rx	Pravachol (Bristol-Myers Squibb)	Tablets: 10 mg	Lactose. (P PRAVACHOL 10). Pink-to-peach, rectangular. In 90s.
		20 mg	Lactose. (P PRAVACHOL 20). Yellow, rectangular. In 90s, 1000s, and UD 100s.
		40 mg	Lactose, FD & C Blue No 1. (P PRAVACHOL 40). Green, rectangular. In 90s and UD 100s.
		80 mg	Lactose. (BMS 80). Yellow, oval. In 90s and 500s.

For complete prescribing information, refer to the HMG-CoA Reductase Inhibitors group monograph.

Indications

➤*Primary prevention of coronary events:* In hypercholesterolemic patients without clinically evident coronary heart disease (CHD), to reduce the risk of MI; to reduce the risk of undergoing myocardial revascularization procedures; to reduce the risk of cardiovascular mortality with no increase in death from noncardiovascular causes.

➤*Secondary prevention of cardiovascular events:* In patients with clinically evident CHD, to reduce the risk of total mortality by reducing coronary death, MI, undergoing myocardial revascularization procedures, stroke, and stroke/transient ischemic attack, and slow the progression of coronary atherosclerosis.

➤*Hyperlipidemia:* As an adjunct to diet for the reduction of elevated total and LDL cholesterol, Apo-B, and triglyceride levels and to increase HDL cholesterol in patients with primary hypercholesterolemia and mixed dyslipidemia (Fredrickson types IIa and IIb). As adjunctive therapy to diet for the treatment of patients with elevated serum triglyceride levels (Fredrickson type IV). For the treatment of patients with primary dysbetalipoproteinemia (Fredrickson type III) who do not respond adequately to diet.

➤*Adolescents (8 years of age and older) with heterozygous familial hypercholesterolemia:* As an adjunct to diet and lifestyle modification for treatment of heterozygous familial hypercholesterolemia in children and adolescents 8 years of age and older if after an adequate trial of diet LDL-C remains 190 mg/dL or greater or LDL-C remains 160 mg/dL or greater AND there is a positive family history of premature cardiovascular disease or 2 or more other CVD risk factors are present in the patient.

Administration and Dosage

➤*Approved by the FDA:* October 31, 1991.

Place the patient on a standard cholesterol-lowering diet before starting pravastatin, and continue on this diet during treatment.

Pravastatin can be administered as a single dose at any time of the day, with or without food. Because the maximal effect of a given dose is seen within 4 weeks, perform periodic lipid determinations at this time and adjust dosage according to the patient's response to therapy and established treatment guidelines.

➤*Adults:* The recommended starting dose is 40 mg once/day. If a daily dose of 40 mg does not achieve desired cholesterol levels, 80 mg once/day is recommended.

➤*Pediatric patients:*

Children 8 to 13 years of age – 20 mg once daily. Doses greater than 20 mg have not been studied in this patient population.

Adolescents 14 to 18 years of age – The recommended starting dose is 40 mg once daily. Doses greater than 40 mg have not been studied in this patient population.

Re-evaluate children and adolescents treated with pravastatin in adulthood and make appropriate changes to their cholesterol-lowering regimen to achieve adult goals for LDL-C.

➤*Concomitant immunosuppressants:* In patients taking immunosuppressive drugs such as cyclosporine concomitantly with pravastatin, begin therapy with pravastatin 10 mg once/day at bedtime and titrate to higher doses with caution. Most patients treated with this combination received a maximum pravastatin dose of 20 mg/day.

➤*Concomitant lipid-lowering therapy:* The lipid-lowering effects of pravastatin on total and LDL cholesterol are enhanced when combined with a bile acid binding resin. When administering a bile acid binding resin (eg, cholestyramine, colestipol) and pravastatin, give pravastatin either 1 hour or more before or at least 4 hours following the resin. Avoid the combined use of pravastatin and fibrates unless the benefit of further alterations in lipid levels is likely to outweigh the increased risk of this drug combination.

➤*Renal/Hepatic function impairment:* Use a starting dose of 10 mg/day in significant renal or hepatic function impairment.

➤*Storage/Stability:* Store at 25°C (77°F); excursions permitted to 15° to 30°C (59° to 86°F). Keep tightly closed; protect from light and moisture.

HMG-CoA Reductase Inhibitors

ROSUVASTATIN CALCIUM

Rx	**Crestor** (AstraZeneca)	**Tablets:** 5 mg (as base)	Lactose. (ZD4522 5). Yellow. In 90s.
		10 mg (as base)	Lactose. (ZD4522 10). Pink. In 90s and UD 100s.
		20 mg (as base)	Lactose. (ZD4522 20). Pink. In 90s and UD 100s.
		40 mg (as base)	Lactose. (ZD4522 40). Pink, oval. In 30s and UD 100s.

For complete prescribing information, refer to the HMG-CoA Reductase Inhibitors group monograph.

Indications

➤*Hyperlipidemia:* As an adjunct to diet to reduce elevated total cholesterol, LDL cholesterol, Apo-B, non-HDL cholesterol, and triglyceride (TG) levels and to increase HDL-C in patients with primary hypercholesterolemia (heterozygous familial and nonfamilial) and mixed dyslipidemia (Fredrickson type IIa and IIb); as an adjunct to diet for the treatment of patients with elevated serum TG levels (Fredrickson type IV); to reduce LDL-C, total-C, and Apo-B in patients with homozygous familial hypercholesteroldemia (FH) as an adjunct to other lipid-lowering treatments (eg, LDL apheresis) or if such treatments are unavailable.

Administration and Dosage

➤*Approved by the FDA:* August 12, 2003

Place the patient on a standard cholesterol-lowering diet before starting rosuvastatin and continue on this diet during treatment. Rosuvastatin can be administered as a single dose at any time of day, with or without food.

➤*Hypercholesterolemia (heterozygous familial and nonfamilial) and mixed dyslipidemia (Fredrickson type IIa and IIb):* The dose range for rosuvastatin is 5 to 40 mg once daily. Individualize rosuvastatin therapy according to goal of therapy and response. The usual recommended starting dose of rosuvastatin is 10 mg once daily. Initiation of therapy with 5 mg once daily may be considered for patients requiring less aggressive LDL-C reductions or who have predisposing factors for myopathy. For patients with marked hypercholesterolemia (LDL-C greater than 190 mg/dL) and aggressive lipid targets, consider a 20 mg starting dose. Reserve the 40 mg dose of rosuvastatin for those patients who have not achieved goal LDL-C at 20 mg. After initiation and/or upon titration of rosuvastatin, analyze lipid levels within 2 to 4 weeks and adjust dosage accordingly.

➤*Homozygous FH:* The recommended starting dose of rosuvastatin is 20 mg once daily. The maximum recommended daily dose is 40 mg. Use as an adjunct to other lipid-lowering treatments (eg, LDL apheresis) or if such treatments are unavailable. Estimate response to therapy from pre-apheresis LDL-C levels.

➤*Concomitant cyclosporine:* In patients taking cyclosporine, limit rosuvastatin therapy to 5 mg once daily.

➤*Concomitant lipid-lowering therapy:* The effect of rosuvastatin on LDL-C and total-C may be enhanced when used in combination with a bile acid-binding resin. If rosuvastatin is used in combination with gemfibrozil, limit the dose of rosuvastatin to 10 mg once daily.

➤*Renal insufficiency:* No modification of dosage is necessary for patients with mild to moderate renal insufficiency. For patients with severe renal impairment (Ccr less than 30 mL/min/1.73 m^2) not on hemodialysis, start dosing at 5 mg once daily. Do not exceed 10 mg once daily.

Consider a dose reduction for patients on 40 mg rosuvastatin therapy with unexplained persistent proteinuria during routine urinalysis testing.

➤*Storage/Stability:* Store at controlled room temperature 20° to 25°C (68° to 77°F). Protect from moisture.

FLUVASTATIN SODIUM

Rx	**Lescol** (Novartis)	**Capsules:** 20 mg (as base)	Benzyl alcohol, parabens, EDTA. (20 LESCOL). Brown/Light brown. In 30s and 100s.
		40 mg (as base)	Benzyl alcohol, parabens, EDTA. (40 LESCOL). Brown/Gold. In 30s and 100s.
Rx	**Lescol XL** (Novartis)	**Tablets, extended-release:** 80 mg (as base)	(Lescol XL 80). Yellow. Film-coated. In 30s and 100s.

For complete prescribing information, refer to the HMG-CoA Reductase Inhibitors group monograph.

Indications

➤*Hyperlipidemia:* As an adjunct to diet to reduce elevated total and LDL cholesterol levels, Apo-B, and triglyceride levels and to increase HDL cholesterol levels in patients with primary hypercholesterolemia and mixed dyslipidemia (Fredrickson type IIa and IIb) whose response to dietary restriction of saturated fat and cholesterol and other non-pharmacological measures has not been adequate.

➤*Secondary prevention of coronary events:* To reduce the risk of undergoing coronary revascularization procedures in patients with coronary heart disease; to slow the progression of coronary atherosclerosis in patients with coronary heart disease as part of a treatment strategy to lower total and LDL cholesterol to target levels.

Administration and Dosage

➤*Approved by the FDA:* December 31, 1993.

Place the patient on a standard cholesterol-lowering diet before receiving fluvastatin and continue on this diet during treatment. May be taken without regard to meals.

➤*Dose:* For patients requiring LDL cholesterol reduction to a goal of 25% or more, the recommended starting dose is 40 mg daily as 1 capsule, or 40 mg twice daily, or 80 mg daily as 1 extended-release tablet administered as a single dose in the evening. For patients requiring LDL cholesterol reduction to a goal of less than 25%, a starting dose of 20 mg may be used. The recommended dosing range is 20 to 80 mg/day. Because the maximal reductions in LDL cholesterol of a given dose are seen within 4 weeks, perform periodic lipid determinations and adjust dosage according to the patient's response to therapy and established treatment guidelines. The therapeutic effect of fluvastatin is maintained with prolonged administration.

➤*Concomitant lipid-lowering therapy:* Lipid-lowering effects on total cholesterol and LDL cholesterol are additive when immediate-release fluvastatin is combined with a bile-acid-binding resin or niacin. When administering a bile-acid resin (eg, cholestyramine) and fluvastatin, administer fluvastatin at bedtime, at least 2 hours following the resin to avoid a significant interaction because of drug binding to resin.

➤*Renal function impairment:* Because fluvastatin is cleared hepatically with less than 6% of the administered dose excreted in the urine, dose adjustments for mild to moderate renal impairment are not necessary. Fluvastatin has not been studied at doses greater than 40 mg in patients with severe renal impairment; exercise caution when treating such patients at higher doses.

➤*Storage/Stability:* Store at 25°C (77°F); excursions permitted to 15° to 30°C (59° to 86°F). Dispense in a tight container and protect from light.

ATORVASTATIN CALCIUM

Rx	**Lipitor** (Pfizer)	**Tablets:** 10 mg (as base)	Lactose. (PD 155 10). White, elliptical. Film-coated. In 90s, 5000s, and UD 100s.
		20 mg (as base)	Lactose. (PD 156 20). White, elliptical. Film-coated. In 90s, 5000s, and UD 100s.
		40 mg (as base)	Lactose. (PD 157 40). White, elliptical. Film-coated. In 90s and 500s.
		80 mg (as base)	Lactose. (PD 158 80). White, elliptical. Film-coated. In 90s and 500s.

For complete prescribing information, refer to the HMG-CoA Reductase Inhibitors group monograph.

Indications

➤*Hypercholesterolemia (heterozygous familial and nonfamilial) and mixed dyslipidemia (Fredrickson type IIa and IIb):* As an adjunct to diet to reduce elevated total and LDL cholesterol, Apo-B, and triglyceride (TG) levels, and to increase HDL cholesterol in patients with primary hypercholesterolemia (heterozygous familial and nonfamilial) and mixed dyslipidemia (Fredrickson type IIa and IIb).

➤*Homozygous familial hypercholesterolemia (FH):* To reduce total and LDL cholesterol in patients with homozygous FH as an adjunct to other lipid-lowering treatments (eg, LDL apheresis) or if such treatments are unavailable.

➤*Dysbetalipoproteinemia:* For the treatment of patients with primary dysbetalipoproteinemia (Fredrickson type III) who do not respond adequately to diet.

➤*Elevated serum TG:* As an adjunct to diet for the treatment of patients with elevated serum TG levels (Fredrickson type IV).

➤*Adolescents (10 to 17 years of age) with heterozygous FH:* As an adjunct to diet to reduce total and LDL cholesterol and Apo-B levels in boys and postmenarchal girls 10 to 17 years of age with heterozygous FH if, after an adequate trial of diet therapy, LDL cholesterol remains 190 mg/dL or greater or LDL remains 160 mg/dL or greater AND there is a positive family history of premature cardiovascular disease (CVD) or 2 or more other CVD risk factors are present in the pediatric patient.

Administration and Dosage

➤*Approved by the FDA:* December 17, 1996.

Place the patient on a standard cholesterol-lowering diet before receiving atorvastatin, and continue on this diet during atorvastatin treatment.

➤*Hypercholesterolemia (heterozygous familial and nonfamilial) and mixed dyslipidemia (Fredrickson type IIa and IIb):* The recommended starting dose is 10 or 20 mg once daily. Patients who require a large reduction in LDL cholesterol (more than 45%) may be started at 40 mg once daily. The dosage range is 10 to 80 mg administered as a single dose once daily, at any time of the day, with or without food. Individualize therapy according to goal of therapy and response. After initiation and/or upon titration of atorvastatin, analyze lipid levels within 2 to 4 weeks and adjust dosage accordingly. Because the goal of treatment is to lower LDL cholesterol, the National Cholesterol Education Program recommends that LDL cholesterol levels be used to initiate and assess treatment response. Use total cholesterol to monitor therapy only if LDL cholesterol levels are not available.

➤*Heterozygous FH in pediatric patients (10 to 17 years of age):* Recommended starting dose is 10 mg/day; the maximum recommended dose is 20 mg/day. Individualize doses according to recommended goal of therapy. Make adjustments at intervals of 4 weeks or more.

➤*Homozygous FH:* The recommended dosage is 10 to 80 mg/day. Use atorvastatin as an adjunct to other lipid-lowering treatments (eg, LDL apheresis) in these patients or if such treatments are unavailable.

➤*Concomitant lipid-lowering therapy:* Atorvastatin may be used in combination with a bile-acid-binding resin for additive effect. Generally, avoid the combination of HMG-CoA reductase inhibitors and fibrates (eg, gemfibrozil).

➤*Storage/Stability:* Store at controlled room temperature 20° to 25°C (68° to 77°F).

GEMFIBROZIL

Rx	**Gemfibrozil** (Various, eg, Apotex, Mylan, UDL, Warner Chilcott)	**Tablets:** 600 mg	In 60s, 500s, blister pack 25s, and UD 100s.
Rx	**Lopid** (Parke-Davis)		(LOPID P-D 737). Parabens. White, scored, elliptical. Film coated. In 60s, 500s, and UD 100s.

Refer to the general discussion of these products in the Antihyperlipidemic Agents Introduction.

Indications

►*Hypertriglyceridemia:* Adjunctive therapy to diet in adult patients with very high elevations of serum triglyceride levels (Types IV and V hyperlipidemia) who present a risk of pancreatitis and who do not respond to diet. Consider therapy for those with triglyceride elevations between 1000 and 2000 mg/dL, and who have a history of pancreatitis or of recurrent abdominal pain typical of pancreatitis.

►*Reducing coronary heart disease risk:* Adjunctive therapy to diet. Consider gemfibrozil therapy in those Type IIb patients without history of or symptoms of existing coronary heart disease who have low HDL-cholesterol levels in addition to elevated LDL-cholesterol and triglyceride levels and who have not responded to weight loss, dietary therapy, exercise, and other pharmacologic agents (eg, bile acid sequestrants, nicotinic acid).

Administration and Dosage

►*Adults:* 1200 mg/daily in 2 divided doses 30 minutes before the morning and evening meal.

Actions

►*Pharmacology:* Gemfibrozil is a fibric acid derivative that decreases serum triglycerides and very low density lipoprotein (VLDL) cholesterol, and increases HDL cholesterol. Modest decreases in total and LDL cholesterol may be observed, except in Type IV hyperlipoproteinemia patients who often experience a rise in LDL, and in Type IIb patients who experience minimal effects on LDL levels but usually show significant increases in HDL.

Gemfibrozil inhibits peripheral lipolysis and decreases the hepatic extraction of free fatty acids, thus reducing hepatic triglyceride production. Gemfibrozil also inhibits synthesis and increases clearance of VLDL carrier apolipoprotein B, decreasing in VLDL production. The mechanism for increased HDL levels is unknown.

The drug may, in addition to elevating HDL cholesterol, reduce incorporation of long-chain fatty acids into newly formed triglycerides, accelerate turnover and removal of cholesterol from the liver, and increase excretion of cholesterol in the feces.

►*Pharmacokinetics:*

Absorption/Distribution – Gemfibrozil is well absorbed from the GI tract. Peak levels occur in 1 to 2 hours and appear proportional to the dose without accumulating after multiple doses.

Metabolism/Excretion – Gemfibrozil mainly undergoes oxidation to form a hydroxymethyl and a carboxyl metabolite. The plasma half-life is 1.5 hours following multiple doses. Biological half-life is considerably longer, due to enterohepatic circulation and reabsorbtion in the GI tract. Excretion is ≈ 70% urinary, mostly as the glucuronide conjugate, with < 2% excreted as unchanged drug; 6% is fecal.

►*Clinical trials:* In a 5-year trial with 4081 male patients between the ages of 40 and 55, gemfibrozil therapy was associated with significant reductions in total plasma triglycerides and a significant increase in HDL. Moderate reductions in total plasma cholesterol and LDL were observed for the gemfibrozil treatment group as a whole. The study involved subjects with serum non-HDL-cholesterol of > 200 mg/dL and no previous history of CHD. The gemfibrozil group experienced a 34% reduction in serious coronary events (sudden cardiac deaths plus fatal and nonfatal MIs) compared with placebo. There was a 37% reduction in nonfatal MI. The greatest reduction in the incidence of serious coronary events occurred in Type IIb patients who had elevations of both LDL and total plasma triglycerides. The mean increase in HDL among the Type IIb patients in this study was 12.6%.

Contraindications

Hepatic or severe renal dysfunction, including primary biliary cirrhosis; preexisting gallbladder disease (see Warnings); hypersensitivity to gemfibrozil.

Warnings

►*Cholelithiasis:* Gemfibrozil may increase cholesterol excretion into the bile, leading to cholelithiasis. If cholelithiasis is suspected, perform gallbladder studies. Discontinue therapy if gallstones are found.

►*Skeletal muscle effects:* Concomitant therapy with gemfibrozil and lovastatin has been associated with rhabdomyolysis, markedly elevated creatine kinase (CK) levels and myoglobinuria, frequently leading to acute renal failure. In patients with an unsatisfactory lipid response to either drug alone, any potential benefit of lovastatin and gemfibrozil coadministration does not outweigh the risks of severe myopathy, rhabdomyolysis, and acute renal failure (see Drug Interactions).

►*Myositis* – The use of fibrates alone, including gemfibrozil, may occasionally be associated with myositis. Promptly evaluate patients complaining of muscle pain, tenderness, or weakness for myositis, including serum CK level determination. Periodic monitoring of CK may not prevent the occurrence of severe myopathy and kidney damage. If myositis is suspected or diagnosed, withdraw therapy.

►*Renal function impairment:* There have been reports of worsening renal insufficiency upon the addition of gemfibrozil therapy in individuals with baseline plasma creatinine > 2 mg/dL. In such patients, consider the use of alternative therapy against the risks and benefits of a lower dose of gemfibrozil.

►*Mutagenesis:* Long-term administration of high doses (≈ 1 and 10 times the human dose) of gemfibrozil in rats was associated with an increased incidence of benign liver nodules, liver carcinomas and benign Leydig cell tumors; subcapsular unilateral and bilateral cataracts also occurred.

►*Fertility impairment:* Administration of ≈ 0.6 and 2 times the human dose to male rats for 10 weeks resulted in a dose-related decrease of fertility. This effect was reversed after a drug-free period of ≈ 8 weeks, and it was not transmitted to their offspring.

►*Pregnancy: Category C.* There are no adequate and well-controlled studies in pregnant women. Use during pregnancy only when the benefit clearly outweighs the possible risk to the fetus.

►*Lactation:* It is not known whether this drug is excreted in breast milk. Because many drugs are excreted in breast milk and because of the potential for tumorigenicity shown for gemfibrozil in animal studies, a decision should be made whether to discontinue nursing or to discontinue the drug, taking into account the importance of the drug to the mother.

►*Children:* Safety and efficacy in children have not been established.

Precautions

►*Monitoring:* Perform adequate pretreatment laboratory studies. Obtain periodic determinations of serum lipids during administration. Withdraw the drug after 3 months if response is inadequate.

Hematologic – Mild hemoglobin, hematocrit, and WBC decreases have been observed but have stabilized during long-term administration. Rarely, severe anemia, leukopenia, thrombocytopenia, and bone marrow hypoplasia may occur. Perform periodic blood counts during the first 12 months of administration.

Hepatotoxicity – Abnormal elevations of AST, ALT, LDH, bilirubin, and alkaline phosphatase have occurred and are usually reversible on drug discontinuation. Perform periodic liver function studies and terminate therapy if abnormalities persist.

Blood glucose – Gemfibrozil has a moderate hyperglycemic effect. Carefully monitor blood glucose levels during therapy.

►*Estrogen therapy:* Estrogen therapy is sometimes associated with rises in plasma triglycerides, especially in subjects with familial hypertriglyceridemia. Discontinuation of estrogen may obviate the need for specific drug therapy of hypertriglyceridemia.

Drug Interactions

Gemfibrozil Drug Interactions			
Precipitant drug	Object drug*		Description
Gemfibrozil	Anticoagulants	↑	Gemfibrozil may enhance the pharmacologic effects of these agents. If this combination cannot be avoided, observe for signs of bleeding and monitor prothrombin time.
Gemfibrozil	Cyclosporine	↓	Pharmacologic effect may be decreased. Monitor whole blood cyclosporine concentrations. Adjust the dose of cyclosporine as indicated and observe the patient for signs of toxicity or rejection when gemfibrozil therapy is stopped or started.
Gemfibrozil	HMG-CoA reductase inhibitors	↑	Rhabdomyolysis has been associated with the administration of HMG-CoA reductase inhibitors and gemfibrozil. If combined use cannot be evaded, frequently monitor for symptoms and signs of rhabdomyolysis and myopathy.

Fibric Acid Derivatives

GEMFIBROZIL

Gemfibrozil Drug Interactions			
Precipitant drug	Object drug*		Description
Gemfibrozil	Sulfonylureas	↑	Increased hypoglycemic effects may occur. Monitor blood glucose levels when gemfibrozil is stopped or started from the treatment regimen. Adjust glyburide dose accordingly.

* ↑ = Object drug increased.   ↓ = Object drug decreased.

Adverse Reactions

Clofibrate and gemfibrozil have chemical, clinical, and pharmacological similarities; the adverse findings with clofibrate may also apply to gemfibrozil.

➤*Cardiovascular:* Atrial fibrillation (0.7%).

➤*CNS:* Fatigue (3.8%); vertigo (1.5%); headache (1.2%); paresthesia; hypesthesia.

➤*Dermatologic:* Eczema (1.9%); rash (1.7%).

➤*GI:* Dyspepsia (19.6%); abdominal pain (9.8%); diarrhea (7.2%); nausea/vomiting (2.5%); constipation (1.4%); acute appendicitis (1.2%).

➤*Special senses:* Taste perversion.

➤*Other (drug relationship probable or not established):*
CNS – Dizziness; somnolence; peripheral neuritis; decreased libido; depression; headache; confusion; convulsions; syncope.

Cardiovascular – Intracerebral hemorrhage; peripheral vascular disease; extrasystoles.

Dermatologic – Exfoliative dermatitis; dermatitis; pruritus; alopecia.

GI – Cholestatic jaundice; pancreatitis; hepatoma; colitis.

GU – Impotence; decreased male fertility; renal dysfunction.

Hematologic – Anemia; leukopenia; bone marrow hypoplasia; eosinophilia; thrombocytopenia.

Immunologic – Angioedema; laryngeal edema; urticaria; anaphylaxis; lupus-like syndrome; vasculitis.

Lab test abnormalities – Liver function abnormalities (increased AST, ALT, LDH, CK, bilirubin, alkaline phosphatase); positive antinuclear antibody.

Musculoskeletal – Myopathy; myasthenia; myalgia; painful extremities; arthralgia; synovitis; rhabdomyolysis.

Special senses – Blurred vision; retinal edema; cataracts.

Miscellaneous – Weight loss; viral and bacterial infection (common cold, cough, and urinary tract infections).

Overdosage

Institute symptomatic supportive measures. Refer to General Management of Acute Overdosage.

Patient Information

Medication may cause abdominal or epigastric pain, diarrhea, nausea, or vomiting. Notify physician if these become pronounced.

FENOFIBRATE

Rx	**Tricor** (Abbott)	**Tablets:** 54 mg		Lactose. (TA). Yellow. In 90s.
		160 mg		Lactose. (TC). White. In 90s.
Rx	**Lofibra** (Gate)	**Capsules:** 67 mg		Micronized. Lactose. (N 240 67). Pink. In 100s.
Rx	**Fenofibrate** (Teva)	**Capsules:** 134 mg		Micronized. Lactose. (N 411 134). Lt. blue. In 100s.
Rx	**Lofibra** (Gate)			Micronized. Lactose. (N 411 134). Lt. blue. In 100s.
Rx	**Lofibra** (Gate)	**Capsules:** 200 mg		Micronized. Lactose. (N 412 200). Orange. In 100s.

Refer to the general discussion of these agents in the Antihyperlipidemic Agents introduction.

Indications

➤*Hypercholesterolemia:* Adjunctive therapy to diet for the reduction of LDL-C, total-C, triglycerides, and apolipoprotein B (apo B) and to increase HDL-C in adult patients with primary hypercholesterolemia or mixed dyslipidemia (Fredrickson Types IIa and IIb). Use lipid-altering agents in addition to a diet restricted in saturated fat and cholesterol when response to diet and nonpharmacological interventions alone has been inadequate.

➤*Hypertriglyceridemia:* Adjunctive therapy to diet for treatment of adult patients with hypertriglyceridemia (Fredrickson Types IV and V hyperlipidemia).

➤*Unlabeled uses:* Polymetabolic syndrome X.

Administration and Dosage

➤*Approved by the FDA:* February 13, 1998.

Place patients on an appropriate lipid-lowering diet before receiving fenofibrate and continue this diet during treatment. Give with meals, thereby optimizing the bioavailability of the medication.

➤*Primary hypercholesterolemia/mixed hyperlipidemia:* For the treatment of adult patients with primary hypercholesterolemia or mixed hyperlipidemia, the initial dose of fenofibrate is 160 mg/day.

➤*Hypertriglyceridemia:* For adult patients with hypertriglyceridemia, the initial dose is 54 to 160 mg/day. Individualize dosage according to patient response and adjust if necessary following repeat lipid determinations at 4- to 8-week intervals. The maximum dose is 160 mg/day.

Monitor lipid levels periodically and give consideration to reducing the dosage if lipid levels fall significantly below the targeted range.

➤*Renal function impairment:* Initiate treament with fenofibrate at a dose of 54 mg/day in patients with impaired renal function, and increase only after evaluation of the effects on renal function and lipid levels at this dose.

➤*Elderly:* In the elderly, limit the initial dose to 54 mg/day.

➤*Storage/Stability:* Store at controlled room temperature 15° to 30°C (59° to 86°F). Keep out of the reach of children. Protect from moisture.

Actions

➤*Pharmacology:* Fenofibric acid, the active metabolite of fenofibrate, produces reductions in total cholesterol, LDL cholesterol, apo B, total triglycerides, and triglyceride rich lipoprotein (VLDL) in treated patients. In addition, treatment with fenofibrate results in increases in high density lipoprotein (HDL) and apoproteins apoAI and apoAII.

Through its mechanism, fenofibrate increases lipolysis and elimination of triglyceride-rich particles from plasma by activating lipoprotein lipase and reducing production of apoprotein C-III (an inhibitor of lipoprotein lipase activity). The resulting fall in triglycerides produces an alteration in the size and composition of LDL from small, dense particles (which are thought to be atherogenic because of their susceptibility to oxidation), to large buoyant particles. These larger particles have a greater affinity for cholesterol receptors and are catabolized rapidly.

Fenofibrate also reduces serum uric acid levels in hyperuricemic and healthy individuals by increasing the urinary excretion of uric acid.

➤*Pharmacokinetics:*

Absorption/Distribution – Fenofibrate is well absorbed from the GI tract; absorption is increased when administered with food. Peak plasma levels of fenofibric acid occur within 6 to 8 hours after administration, and steady-state plasma levels are achieved within 5 days of dosing. Accumulation following multiple doses does not occur. Serum protein binding is approximately 99%.

Metabolism – Fenofibrate is rapidly hydrolyzed by esterases to the active metabolite, fenofibric acid; no unchanged fenofibrate is detected in plasma. Fenofibric acid is primarily conjugated with glucuronic acid and then excreted in urine. A small amount of fenofibric acid is reduced at the carbonyl moiety to a benzhydrol metabolite, which is, in turn, conjugated with glucuronic acid and excreted in urine.

Excretion – Fenofibrate is eliminated with a half-life of 20 hours, allowing once-daily administration. It is mainly excreted in urine in the form of metabolites, primarily fenofibric acid and fenofibric acid glucuronide; about 60% of the dose appears in urine and 25% in feces.

Contraindications

Hepatic or severe renal dysfunction, including primary biliary cirrhosis, and patients with unexplained persistent liver function abnormality; preexisting gallbladder disease (see Warnings); hypersensitivity to fenofibrate.

Warnings

➤*Pancreatitis:* This has been reported in patients taking fenofibrate, gemfibrozil, and clofibrate. This occurrence may represent a failure of efficacy in patients with severe hypertriglyceridemia, a direct drug effect, or a secondary phenomenon mediated through biliary tract stone or sludge formation and obstruction of the common bile duct.

Improving glycemic control in diabetic patients showing fasting chylomicronemia will usually reduce fasting triglycerides and eliminate chylomicronemia, thereby obviating the need for pharmacologic intervention.

➤*Cholelithiasis:* Fenofibrate, like clofibrate and gemfibrozil, may increase cholesterol excretion into the bile, leading to cholelithiasis. If cholelithiasis is suspected, gallbladder studies are indicated. Discon-

FENOFIBRATE

tinue therapy if gallstones are found.

➤*Skeletal muscle effects:* The use of fibrates alone, including fenofibrate, may occasionally be associated with myopathy. Treatment with drugs of the fibrate class has been associated on rare occasions with rhabdomyolysis, usually in patients with impaired renal function. Consider myopathy in any patient with diffuse myalgias, muscle tenderness or weakness, or marked elevations of creatine phosphokinase levels.

Advise patients to promptly report unexplained muscle pain, tenderness, or weakness, particularly if accompanied by malaise or fever. Assess CPK levels in patients reporting these symptoms and discontinue therapy if markedly elevated CPK levels occur or myopathy is diagnosed.

➤*Hypersensitivity reactions:* Acute hypersensitivity reactions including severe skin rashes requiring patient hospitalization and treatment with steroids have occurred very rarely during treatment with fenofibrate, including rare spontaneous reports of Stevens-Johnson syndrome and toxic epidermal necrolysis. Urticaria was seen in 1.1% vs 0% and rash in 1.4% vs 0.8% of fenofibrate and placebo patients, respectively, in controlled trials. Refer to Management of Acute Hypersensitivity Reactions.

➤*Renal function impairment:* In patients with Ccr less than 50 mL/min, the rate of clearance of fenofibric acid was greatly reduced, and it accumulated during chronic dosage. However, in patients with Ccr 50 to 90 mL/min, the oral clearance and the oral volume of distribution of fenofibric acid are increased compared with healthy adults (2.1 L/hr and 95 L vs 1.1 L/hr and 30 L, respectively). Therefore, minimize the dosage in patients who have Ccr less than 50 mL/min.

➤*Hepatic function impairment:* Fenofibrate is associated with increases in serum transaminases (AST or ALT). Increases to more than 3 times the upper limit of normal (ULN) occurred in 5.3% of patients taking fenofibrate.

When transaminase determinations were followed either after discontinuation of treatment or during continued treatment, a return to normal limits was usually observed. In an 8-week dose-ranging study, the incidence of ALT or AST elevations to at least 3 times the ULN was 13% in patients receiving dosages equivalent to 107 to 160 mg fenofibrate per day and was 0% in those receiving dosages equivalent to 54 mg or less or placebo. Hepatocellular, chronic active, and cholestatic hepatitis associated with fenofibrate therapy have been reported after exposures of weeks to several years. In extremely rare cases, cirrhosis has been reported in association with chronic active hepatitis. Perform regular periodic monitoring of liver function (see Precautions).

➤*Carcinogenesis:* The incidence of liver carcinoma, pancreatic carcinomas, pancreatic adenomas, and benign testicular interstitial cell tumors was increased in 24-month rat studies at doses from 0.3 to 6 times the maximum recommended human dose.

A comparative carcinogenicity study was done in rats comparing 3 drugs: Fenofibrate, clofibrate, and gemfibrozil. Pancreatic acinar adenomas were increased in males and females on fenofibrate; hepatocellular carcinoma and pancreatic acinar adenomas were increased in males and hepatic neoplastic nodules in females treated with clofibrate; hepatic neoplastic nodules were increased in males and females treated with gemfibrozil while testicular interstitial cell tumors were increased in males on all 3 drugs.

Electron microscopy studies have demonstrated peroxisomal proliferation following fenofibrate administration to the rat. An adequate study to test for peroxisome proliferation has not been done, but changes in peroxisome morphology and numbers have been observed in humans after treatment with other members of the fibrate class when liver biopsies were compared before and after treatment in the same individual.

➤*Elderly:* Fenofibric acid is known to be substantially excreted by the kidney, and the risk of adverse reactions to this drug may be greater in patients with impaired renal function. Because elderly patients are more likely to have decreased renal function, take care in dose selection.

➤*Pregnancy: Category C.* Fenofibrate is embryocidal and teratogenic in rats when given in doses 7 to 10 times the maximum recommended human dose and embryocidal in rabbits when given at 9 times the maximum recommended human dose. There are no adequate and well-controlled studies in pregnant women. Use during pregnancy only if the potential benefit justifies the potential risk to the fetus.

➤*Lactation:* Fenofibrate should not be used in nursing mothers. Because of the potential for tumorigenicity seen in animal studies, a decision should be made whether to discontinue nursing or discontinue the drug.

➤*Children:* Safety and efficacy in children have not been established.

Precautions

➤*Monitoring:* Obtain periodic determination of serum lipids during initial therapy in order to establish the lowest effective dose of fenofibrate. Withdraw therapy in patients who do not have an adequate response after 2 months of treatment with the maximum recommended dose of 160 mg/day. Also, perform liver function tests regularly.

➤*Initial therapy:* Ascertain that lipid levels are consistently abnormal before instituting fenofibrate therapy. Make every attempt to control serum lipids with appropriate diet, exercise, weight loss in obese patients, and control of any medical problems (eg, diabetes mellitus, hypothyroidism) that are contributing to the lipid abnormalities. If possible, discontinue or change medications known to exacerbate hypertriglyceridemia (eg, beta blockers, thiazides, estrogens) prior to consideration of triglyceride-lowering drug therapy.

➤*Hematologic changes:* Mild-to-moderate hemoglobin, hematocrit, and white blood cell decreases have been observed in patients following initiation of fenofibrate therapy. However, these levels stabilize during long-term administration. Extremely rare spontaneous reports of thrombocytopenia and agranulocytosis have been received during postmarketing surveillance outside of the US. Periodic blood counts are recommended during the first 12 months of fenofibrate administration.

Drug Interactions

Fenofibrate Drug Interactions			
Precipitant drug	Object drug*		Description
Fenofibrate	Anticoagulants	↑	Potentiation of coumarin-type anticoagulants has been observed with prolongation of the prothrombin time/INR. Frequent prothrombin time/INR determinations and anticoagulant dosage reduction are advisable.
Fenofibrate	Cyclosporine	↑	Coadministration may lead to increased risk of nephrotoxicity. Carefully consider the benefits and risks of using fenofibrate with immunosuppressants and other potentially nephrotoxic agents, and employ the lowest effective dose.
Fenofibrate	HMG-CoA reductase inhibitors	↑	The combined use of fenofibrate and HMG-CoA reductase inhibitors has been associated with rhabdomyolysis, marked elevated creatine kinase (CK) levels, and myoglobinuria, leading in a high proportion of cases to acute renal failure. Avoid this drug combination unless the benefit of further alterations in lipid levels is likely to outweigh the increased risk of this drug combination.
Bile acid sequestrants	Fenofibrate	↓	Because bile acid sequestrants may bind other drugs given concurrently, patients should take fenofibrate ≥ 1 hour before or 4 to 6 hours after a bile acid binding resin to avoid impeding its absorption.

* ↑ = Object drug increased.   ↓ = Object drug decreased.

➤*Drug/Food interactions:* The absorption of fenofibrate is increased by approximately 35% when administered with food compared with fasting conditions.

Adverse Reactions

Adverse events led to discontinuation of treatment in 5% of patients treated with fenofibrate and in 3% treated with placebo. Increases in liver function tests were the most frequent events causing discontinuation (1.6%) of fenofibrate treatment.

Fenofibrate Adverse Reactions (%)		
Adverse reaction	Fenofibrate[1] (n = 439)	Placebo (n = 365)
GI		
Diarrhea	2.3	4.1
Nausea	2.3	1.9
Constipation	2.1	1.4
Lab test abnormalities		
Liver function tests abnormal	7.5[2]	1.4
ALT increased	3	1.6
Creatine phosphokinase increased	3	1.4
AST increased	3.4[2]	0.5
Respiratory		
Respiratory disorder	6.2	5.5
Rhinitis	2.3	1.1

FENOFIBRATE

Fenofibrate Adverse Reactions (%)		
Adverse reaction	Fenofibrate[1] (n = 439)	Placebo (n = 365)
Miscellaneous		
Abdominal pain	4.6	4.4
Back pain	3.4	2.5
Headache	3.2	2.7
Asthenia	2.1	3
Flu syndrome	2.1	2.7

[1] Dosage equivalent to 200 mg fenofibrate.
[2] Significantly different from placebo.

Additional adverse events reported by at least 3 patients in placebo-controlled trials or reported in other controlled or open trials, regardless of causality, are listed below.

➤*Cardiovascular:* Angina pectoris; hypertension; vasodilation; coronary artery disorder; abnormal electrocardiogram; ventricular extrasystoles; MI; peripheral vascular disorder; migraine; varicose vein; cardiovascular disorder; hypotension; palpitation; vascular disorder; arrhythmia; phlebitis; tachycardia; extrasystoles; atrial fibrillation.

➤*CNS:* Dizziness; insomnia; depression; vertigo; decreased libido; anxiety; paresthesia; dry mouth; hypertonia; nervousness; neuralgia; somnolence.

➤*Dermatologic:* Rash; pruritus; eczema; herpes zoster; urticaria; acne; sweating; fungal dermatitis; skin disorder; alopecia; contact dermatitis; herpes simplex; maculopapular rash; nail disorder; skin ulcer.

➤*GI:* Dyspepsia; flatulence; nausea; increased appetite; gastroenteritis; cholelithiasis; rectal disorder; esophagitis; gastritis; colitis; tooth disorder; vomiting; anorexia; GI disorder; duodenal ulcer; nausea/vomiting; peptic ulcer; rectal hemorrhage; liver fatty deposit; cholecystitis; eructation; increased gamma glutamyl transpeptidase; diarrhea.

➤*GU:* Urinary frequency; prostatic disorder; dysuria; kidney function abnormal; urolithiasis; gynecomastia; unintended pregnancy; vaginal moniliasis; cystitis.

➤*Hematologic/Lymphatic:* Anemia; leukopenia; ecchymosis; eosinophilia; lymphadenopathy; thrombocytopenia.

➤*Metabolic/Nutritional:* Creatinine increased; weight gain; hypoglycemia; gout; weight loss; edema; hyperuricemia; peripheral edema.

➤*Musculoskeletal:* Myositis; myalgia; arthralgia; arthritis; tenosynovitis; joint disorder; arthrosis; leg cramps; bursitis; myasthenia.

➤*Respiratory:* Pharyngitis; bronchitis; cough increased; dyspnea; asthma; pneumonia; laryngitis; sinusitis.

➤*Special senses:* Conjunctivitis; eye disorder; amblyopia; ear pain; otitis media; abnormal vision; cataract specified; refraction disorder.

➤*Miscellaneous:* Chest pain; pain (unspecified); infection; malaise; allergic reaction; cyst; hernia; fever; photosensitivity reaction; accidental injury; diabetes mellitus.

Overdosage

If indicated, elimination of unabsorbed drug should be achieved by emesis or gastric lavage; observe usual precautions to maintain the airway. Because fenofibrate is highly bound to plasma proteins, do not consider hemodialysis. Refer to General Management of Acute Overdosage.

NIACIN (Nicotinic acid)

Rx	Niacor (Upsher-Smith)	**Tablets:** 500 mg	Lactose. (W 901). White, scored. In 100s.
Rx	Niaspan (Kos Pharmaceuticals)	**Tablets, extended-release:** 500 mg	(KOS/500). Off-white, capsule shape. In 100s.
		750 mg	(KOS/750). Off-white, capsule shape. In 100s.
		1000 mg	(KOS/1000). Off-white, capsule shape. In 100s.

Refer to the general discussion of these products in the Antihyperlipidemic Agents Introduction. The following is an abbreviated monograph for nicotinic acid. For complete prescribing information (eg, adverse reactions), refer to the Niacin monograph in the Nutritionals chapter.

Indications

▶*Hyperlipidemia:* Adjunctive therapy for treatment in adult patients with very high serum triglyceride levels (Types IV and V hyperlipidemia) who present a risk of pancreatitis and who do not respond adequately to dietary control.

Administration and Dosage

▶*Extended-release:* 500 mg at bedtime for 1 to 4 weeks, then 1000 mg at bedtime during weeks 5 to 8. After week 8, titrate to patient response and tolerance. If response to 1000 mg/day is inadequate, increase dose to 1500 mg/day; may subsequently increase dose to 2000 mg/day. Do not increase daily dose more than 500 mg in a 4-week period. Doses exceeding 2000 mg/day are not recommended.

▶*Immediate-release:* Adult dosage is 1 to 2 g given 2 to 3 times/day. Individualize the dose according to patient response. Initiate therapy at 250 mg as a single dose following the evening meal. The frequency of dosing and total daily dose may be increased every 4 to 7 days until the desired LDL or triglyceride level is achieved or the first-level therapeutic dose of 1.5 to 2 g/day is reached. If hyperlipidemia is not adequately controlled after 2 months at this level, increase dosage at 2- to 4-week intervals to 3 g/day (1 g 3 times/day). Do not exceed 6 g/day.

▶*Storage/Stability:*

Niacor – Store at controlled room temperature, 15° to 30°C (59° to 86°F).

Niaspan – Store at room temperature, 20° to 25°C (68° to 77°F).

Actions

▶*Pharmacology:* Nicotinic acid (but not nicotinamide) in gram doses produces an average 10% to 20% reduction in total and LDL cholesterol, a 30% to 70% reduction in triglycerides, and an average 20% to 35% increase in HDL cholesterol. Nicotinic acid also decreases serum levels of apolipoprotein B-100, the major component of VLDL and LDL fractions. The mechanism by which nicotinic acid exerts these effects is not entirely understood but may involve several actions, including a decrease in esterification of hepatic triglycerides. The effect of nicotinic acid-induced changes in lipids/lipoproteins on cardiovascular morbidity and mortality in individuals without pre-existing coronary disease has not been established.

▶*Pharmacokinetics:* The drug is rapidly absorbed from the GI tract. At a 1 g dose, peak plasma concentrations of 15 to 30 mcg/mL are reached within 30 to 60 minutes. About 88% of the immediate-release nicotinic acid oral dose is eliminated by the kidneys as unchanged drug and nicotinuric acid. Following single and multiple doses, approximately 60% to 76% of the niacin dose administered as extended-release niacin (nicotinic acid) was recovered in urine as niacin and metabolites. The elimination half-life ranges from 20 to 45 minutes.

Contraindications

Hepatic dysfunction; active peptic ulcer; arterial bleeding; hypersensitivity to niacin.

Warnings

▶*Hepatic dysfunction:* Cases of severe hepatic toxicity, including fulminant hepatic necrosis have occurred in patients who have substituted sustained-release (modified-release, timed-release) nicotinic acid products for immediate-release (crystalline) nicotinic acid at equivalent doses.

Perform liver function tests on all patients during therapy with nicotinic acid. Monitor serum transaminase levels, including ALT and AST, before treatment begins, every 6 to 12 weeks for the first year, and periodically thereafter (at approximately 6-month intervals). Pay special attention to patients who develop elevated serum transaminase levels; in these patients, repeat measurements promptly and then perform them more frequently. Discontinue the drug if the transaminase levels show evidence of progression, particularly if they rise to 3 times the upper limit of normal and are persistent or if they are associated with symptoms of nausea, fever, or malaise. Consider liver biopsy if elevations persist beyond discontinuation.

▶*Skeletal muscle effects:* Rare cases of rhabdomyolysis have been associated with coadministration of lipid-altering doses (1 g/day or greater) of nicotinic acid and HMG-CoA reductase inhibitors. Physicians contemplating combined therapy with HMG-CoA reductase inhibitors and nicotinic acid should weigh the potential benefits and risks and monitor patients for signs and symptoms of muscle pain, tenderness, or weakness, particularly during the initial months of therapy and during any periods of upward dosage titration. Consider periodic serum creatine phosphokinase (CPK) and potassium determinations in such situations, although there is no assurance that such monitoring will prevent the occurrence of severe myopathy.

▶*Flushing:* When flushing is distressing or persistent, 325 mg aspirin given 30 minutes before each scheduled dose of nicotinic acid or slow upward dose adjustment may help ameliorate this reaction. Do not drink hot liquids with or immediately after administration; this increases flushing.

Patient Information

Cutaneous flushing and a sensation of warmth, especially of the face and upper body, may occur. Itching or tingling and headache also may occur. These effects are transient and usually subside with continued therapy.

May cause GI upset; take with meals.

Swallow extended-release products whole; do not break, crush, or chew.

If dizziness occurs, avoid sudden changes in posture.

Avoid ingestion of alcohol or hot drinks around the time of nicotinic acid administration to minimize flushing.

Diabetic patients should notify their physician if there is a change in blood glucose while taking nicotinic acid.

Advise patients to notify their physician if taking vitamins or other nutritional supplements containing niacin or other related compounds such as nicotinamide.

EZETIMIBE

Rx	Zetia (Merck/Schering-Plough)	**Tablets:** 10 mg	Lactose. (414). Capsule shape. In 30s, 90s, 500s, and UD 100s.

Indications

▶*Primary hypercholesterolemia:*

Monotherapy – Administered alone as adjunctive therapy to diet for the reduction of elevated total cholesterol (total-C), low density lipoprotein cholesterol (LDL-C), and apolipoprotein B (Apo B) in patients with primary (heterozygous familial and nonfamilial) hypercholesterolemia.

Combination therapy with HMG-CoA reductase inhibitors – In combination with an HMG-CoA reductase inhibitor as adjunctive therapy to diet for the reduction of elevated total-C, LDL-C, and Apo B in patients with primary (heterozygous familial and nonfamilial) hypercholesterolemia.

▶*Homozygous familial hypercholesterolemia (HoFH):* With atorvastatin or simvastatin for the reduction of elevated total-C and LDL-C levels in patients with HoFH as an adjunct to other lipid-lowering treatments (eg, LDL apheresis) or if such treatments are unavailable.

▶*Homozygous sitosterolemia:* As adjunctive therapy to diet for the reduction of elevated sitosterol and campesterol levels in patients with homozygous familial sitosterolemia.

Therapy with lipid-altering agents should be a component of multiple-risk-factor intervention in individuals at increased risk for atherosclerotic vascular disease caused by hypercholesterolemia. Use lipid-altering agents in addition to an appropriate diet (including restriction of saturated fat and cholesterol) and when the response to diet and other nonpharmacological measures is inadequate.

Administration and Dosage

▶*Approved by the FDA:* October 25, 2002.

The patient should be placed on a standard cholesterol-lowering diet before receiving ezetimibe and continue on this diet during ezetimibe treatment.

▶*Dose:* The recommended dose of ezetimibe is 10 mg once daily. Ezetimibe can be administered with or without food.

▶*Coadministration with HMG-CoA reductase inhibitors:* Ezetimibe may be administered with an HMG-CoA reductase inhibitor for incremental effect. For convenience, the daily dose of ezetimibe may be taken at the same time as the HMG-CoA reductase inhibitor, according to the dosing recommendations for the HMG-CoA reductase inhibitor.

▶*Coadministration with bile acid sequestrants:* Dosing of ezetimibe should occur at least 2 hours before or at least 4 hours after administration of a bile acid sequestrant.

EZETIMIBE

▶*Storage/Stability:* Store at 25°C (77°F); excursions permitted to 15° to 30°C (59° to 86°F). Protect from moisture.

Actions

▶*Pharmacology:* Ezetimibe reduces total-C, LDL-C, Apo B, and triglycerides (TG), and increases HDL-C in patients with hypercholesterolemia. Ezetimibe reduces blood cholesterol by inhibiting the absorption of cholesterol by the small intestine. In a 2-week clinical study in 18 hypercholesterolemic patients, ezetimibe inhibited intestinal cholesterol absorption by 54%, compared with placebo. Ezetimibe had no clinically meaningful effect on the plasma concentrations of the fat-soluble vitamins A, D, and E (in a study of 113 patients), and did not impair adrenocortical steroid hormone production (in a study of 118 patients).

The cholesterol content of the liver is derived predominantly from 3 sources. The liver can synthesize cholesterol, take up cholesterol from the blood from circulating lipoproteins, or take up cholesterol absorbed by the small intestine. Intestinal cholesterol is derived primarily from cholesterol secreted in the bile and from dietary cholesterol.

Ezetimibe has a mechanism of action that differs from those of other classes of cholesterol-reducing compounds (ie, HMG-CoA reductase inhibitors, bile acid sequestrants [resins], fibric acid derivatives, plant stanols). Ezetimibe does not inhibit cholesterol synthesis in the liver or increase bile acid excretion. Instead, ezetimibe localizes and appears to act at the brush border of the small intestine and inhibits the absorption of cholesterol, leading to a decrease in the delivery of intestinal cholesterol to the liver. This causes a reduction of hepatic cholesterol stores and an increase in clearance of cholesterol from the blood; this distinct mechanism is complementary to that of HMG-CoA reductase inhibitors.

▶*Pharmacokinetics:*

Absorption – After oral administration, ezetimibe is absorbed and extensively conjugated to a pharmacologically active phenolic glucuronide (ezetimibe-glucuronide). After a single 10 mg dose of ezetimibe to fasted adults, mean ezetimibe peak plasma concentrations (C_{max}) of 3.4 to 5.5 ng/mL were attained within 4 to 12 hours (T_{max}). Ezetimibe-glucuronide mean C_{max} values of 45 to 71 ng/mL were achieved between 1 and 2 hours (T_{max}). There was no substantial deviation from dose proportionality between 5 and 20 mg. The absolute bioavailability of ezetimibe cannot be determined, as the compound is virtually insoluble in aqueous media suitable for injection. Ezetimibe has variable bioavailability; the coefficient of variation, based on intersubject variability, was 35% to 60% for area under the curve (AUC) values.

Distribution – Ezetimibe and ezetimibe-glucuronide are highly bound (greater than 90%) to human plasma proteins.

Metabolism/Excretion – Ezetimibe is primarily metabolized in the small intestine and liver via glucuronide conjugation (a phase II reaction) with subsequent biliary and renal excretion. Minimal oxidative metabolism (a phase I reaction) has been observed in all species evaluated.

In humans, ezetimibe is rapidly metabolized to ezetimibe-glucuronide. Ezetimibe and ezetimibe-glucuronide are the major drug-derived compounds detected in plasma, constituting approximately 10% to 20% and 80% to 90% of the total drug in plasma, respectively. Both ezetimibe and ezetimibe-glucuronide are slowly eliminated from plasma with a half-life of approximately 22 hours for both ezetimibe and ezetimibe-glucuronide. Plasma concentration-time profiles exhibit multiple peaks, suggesting enterohepatic recycling.

Following oral administration of ^{14}C-ezetimibe (20 mg) to human subjects, total ezetimibe (ezetimibe plus ezetimibe-glucuronide) accounted for approximately 93% of the total radioactivity in plasma. After 48 hours, there were no detectable levels of radioactivity in the plasma.

Approximately 78% and 11% of the administered radioactivity were recovered in the feces and urine, respectively, over a 10-day collection period. Ezetimibe was the major component in the feces and accounted for 69% of the administered dose, while ezetimibe-glucuronide was the major component in urine and accounted for 9% of the administered dose.

Special populations –

Elderly: In a multiple-dose study with ezetimibe given 10 mg once daily for 10 days, plasma concentrations for total ezetimibe were about 2-fold higher in older (65 years of age and older) healthy subjects compared with younger subjects.

Gender: In a multiple-dose study with ezetimibe given 10 mg once daily for 10 days, plasma concentrations for total ezetimibe were slightly higher (less than 20%) in women than in men.

Hepatic function impairment: After a single 10 mg dose of ezetimibe, the mean AUC for total ezetimibe was increased approximately 1.7-fold in patients with mild hepatic insufficiency (Child-Pugh score 5 to 6) compared with healthy subjects. The mean AUC values for total ezetimibe and ezetimibe were increased approximately 3- to 4-fold and 5- to 6-fold, respectively, in patients with moderate (Child-Pugh score 7 to 9) or severe hepatic impairment (Child-Pugh score 10 to 15). In a 14-day, multiple-dose study (10 mg daily) in patients with moderate hepatic insufficiency, the mean AUC values for total ezetimibe and ezetimibe were increased approximately 4-fold on day 1 and day 14 compared

with healthy subjects. Because of the unknown effects of the increased exposure to ezetimibe in patients with moderate or severe hepatic insufficiency, ezetimibe is not recommended in these patients.

Renal function impairment: After a single 10 mg dose of ezetimibe in patients with severe renal disease (n = 8; mean Ccr less than or equal to 30 mL/min/1.73 m²), the mean AUC values for total ezetimibe, ezetimibe-glucuronide, and ezetimibe were increased approximately 1.5-fold, compared with healthy subjects (n = 9).

Contraindications

Hypersensitivity to any component of the medication.

The combination of ezetimibe with an HMG-CoA reductase inhibitor is contraindicated in patients with active liver disease or unexplained persistent elevations in serum transaminases.

All HMG-CoA reductase inhibitors are contraindicated in pregnant and nursing women. When ezetimibe is administered with an HMG-CoA reductase inhibitor in a woman of childbearing potential, refer to the pregnancy category and product labeling for the HMG-CoA reductase inhibitor (see Warnings).

Warnings

▶*Hyperlipidemia, secondary causes:* Prior to initiating therapy with ezetimibe, exclude or, if appropriate, treat secondary causes for dyslipidemia (eg, diabetes, hypothyroidism, obstructive liver disease, chronic renal failure, and drugs that increase LDL-C and decrease HDL-C [progestins, anabolic steroids, and corticosteroids]). Perform a lipid profile to measure total-C, LDL-C, HDL-C, and TG. For TG levels greater than 400 mg/dL (greater than 4.5 mmol/L), determine LDL-C concentrations by ultracentrifugation.

▶*Hepatic function impairment:* Because of the unknown effects of the increased exposure to ezetimibe in patients with moderate to severe hepatic insufficiency, ezetimibe is not recommended in these patients.

▶*Pregnancy: Category C.* There are no adequate and well-controlled studies of ezetimibe in pregnant women. Use ezetimibe during pregnancy only if the potential benefit justifies the potential risk to the fetus.

In oral (gavage) embryo-fetal development studies of ezetimibe conducted in rats and rabbits during organogenesis, there was no evidence of embryolethal effects at the doses tested (250, 500, 1000 mg/kg/day). In rats, increased incidences of common fetal skeletal findings (extra pair of thoracic ribs, unossified cervical vertebral centra, shortened ribs) were observed at 1000 mg/kg/day (approximately 10 times the human exposure at 10 mg daily based on AUC_{0-24h} for total ezetimibe). In rabbits treated with ezetimibe, an increased incidence of extra thoracic ribs was observed at 1000 mg/kg/day (150 times the human exposure at 10 mg daily based on AUC_{0-24h} for total ezetimibe). Ezetimibe crossed the placenta when pregnant rats and rabbits were given multiple oral doses.

Multiple-dose studies of ezetimibe given in combination with HMG-CoA reductase inhibitors (statins) in rats and rabbits during organogenesis result in higher ezetimibe and statin exposures. Reproductive findings occur at lower doses in combination therapy compared with monotherapy.

All HMG-CoA reductase inhibitors are contraindicated in pregnant and nursing women. When ezetimibe is administered with an HMG-CoA reductase inhibitor in a woman of childbearing potential, refer to the pregnancy category and package labeling for the HMG-CoA reductase inhibitor (see Contraindications).

▶*Lactation:* In rat studies, exposure to total ezetimibe in nursing pups was up to half of that observed in maternal plasma. It is not known whether ezetimibe is excreted in human breast milk; therefore, do not use ezetimibe in nursing mothers unless the potential benefit justifies the potential risk to the infant.

▶*Children:* Treatment experience with ezetimibe in the pediatric population is limited to 4 patients (9 to 17 years of age) in the sitosterolemia study and 5 patients (11 to 17 years of age) in the HoFH study. Treatment with ezetimibe in children (under 10 years of age) is not recommended.

Precautions

▶*Monitoring:* When ezetimibe is coadministered with an HMG-CoA reductase inhibitor, perform liver function tests at initiation of therapy and according to the recommendations of the HMG-CoA reductase inhibitor. At the time of hospitalization for an acute coronary event, take lipid measures on admission or within 24 hours. These values can guide the physician on initiation of LDL-lowering therapy before or at discharge.

▶*Liver enzymes:* In controlled clinical monotherapy studies, the incidence of consecutive elevations (greater than or equal to 3 times the upper limit of normal [ULN]) in serum transaminases was similar between ezetimibe (0.5%) and placebo (0.3%).

In controlled clinical combination studies of ezetimibe initiated concurrently with an HMG-CoA reductase inhibitor, the incidence of consecutive elevations (greater than or equal to 3 times the ULN) in serum transaminases was 1.3% for patients treated with ezetimibe administered with HMG-CoA reductase inhibitors and 0.4% for patients treated with HMG-CoA reductase inhibitors alone. These elevations in trans-

EZETIMIBE

aminases were generally asymptomatic, not associated with cholestasis, and returned to baseline after discontinuation of therapy or with continued treatment. When ezetimibe is coadministered with an HMG-CoA reductase inhibitor, perform liver function tests at initiation of therapy and according to the recommendations of the HMG-CoA reductase inhibitor.

►*Skeletal muscle effects:* In clinical trials, there was no excess of myopathy or rhabdomyolysis associated with ezetimibe compared with the relevant control arm (placebo or HMG-CoA reductase inhibitor alone). However, myopathy and rhabdomyolysis are known adverse reactions to HMG-CoA reductase inhibitors and other lipid-lowering drugs. In clinical trials, the incidence of creatine phosphokinase greater than 10 times the ULN was 0.2% for ezetimibe vs 0.1% for placebo, and 0.1% for ezetimibe coadministered with an HMG-CoA reductase inhibitor vs 0.4% for HMG-CoA reductase inhibitors alone.

Drug Interactions

Ezetimibe Drug Interactions

Precipitant drug	Object drug*		Description
Antacids	Ezetimibe	↓	Administration of an aluminum- and magnesium-containing antacid decreased the C_{max} of ezetimibe 30% but had no significant effect on the AUC.
Cholestyramine	Ezetimibe	↓	Coadministration decreased the mean AUC of ezetimibe ≈ 55%. The incremental LDL-C reduction caused by adding ezetimibe to cholestyramine may be reduced.
Fibric acid derivatives Fenofibrate Gemfibrozil	Ezetimibe	↑	Coadministration of ezetimibe with fenofibrate or gemfibrozil increased the total ezetimibe concentration 1.5- and 1.7-fold, respectively. Because fibrates may increase cholesterol excretion into the bile, leading to cholelithiasis, and ezetimibe was shown in animal studies to increase cholesterol in the gallbladder bile, concomitant use is not recommended until use in patients is studied.
Cyclosporine	Ezetimibe	↑	Total ezetimibe level increased 12-fold in 1 transplant patient receiving multiple medications, including cyclosporine. Monitor closely.

* ↑ = Object drug increased.   ↓ = Object drug decreased.

►*Drug/Food interactions:* Coadministration with food (high-fat or nonfat meals) had no effect on the extent of absorption of ezetimibe when administered as ezetimibe 10 mg tablets. The C_{max} value of ezetimibe was increased 38% with consumption of high-fat meals. Ezetimibe may be administered with or without food.

Adverse Reactions

Ezetimibe Monotherapy Adverse Reactions (%)

Adverse reaction	Ezetimibe 10 mg (n = 1691)	Placebo (n = 795)
GI		
Abdominal pain	3	2.8
Diarrhea	3.7	3
Musculoskeletal		
Arthralgia	3.8	3.4
Back pain	4.1	3.9
Respiratory		
Coughing	2.3	2.1
Pharyngitis	2.3	2.1
Sinusitis	3.6	2.8
Miscellaneous		
Fatigue	2.2	1.8
Viral infection	2.2	1.8

The frequency of less common adverse events was comparable between ezetimibe and placebo.

Ezetimibe/HMG-CoA Reductase Inhibitors (Statin) Combination Adverse Reactions (%)[1]

Adverse reaction	Ezetimibe 10 mg (n = 262)	All statins[2] (n = 936)	Ezetimibe + all statins[2] (n = 925)	Placebo (n = 259)
CNS				
Dizziness	2.7	1.4	1.8	1.2
Headache	8	7.3	6.3	5.4
GI				
Abdominal pain	2.7	3.1	3.5	2.3
Diarrhea	3.4	2.9	2.8	1.5
Musculoskeletal				
Arthralgia	3.8	4.3	3.4	2.3
Back pain	3.4	3.7	4.3	3.5
Myalgia	5	4.1	4.5	4.6
Respiratory				
Pharyngitis	3.1	2.5	2.3	1.9
Sinusitis	4.6	3.6	3.5	1.9
Upper respiratory tract infection	13	13.6	11.8	10.8
Miscellaneous				
Chest pain	3.4	2	1.8	1.2
Fatigue	1.9	1.4	2.8	1.9

[1] Includes 4 placebo-controlled combination studies in which ezetimibe was initiated concurrently with an HMG-CoA reductase inhibitor.
[2] All statins = all doses of all HMG-CoA reductase inhibitors.

Overdosage

No cases of overdosage with ezetimibe have been reported. Administration of ezetimibe 50 mg/day to 15 subjects for up to 14 days was generally well tolerated. In the event of an overdosage, use symptomatic and supportive measures.

AMLODIPINE BESYLATE/ATORVASTATIN CALCIUM

Rx	**Caduet** (Pfizer)	**Tablets:** 5 mg amlodipine besylate/10 mg atorvastatin calcium (as base)	Calcium carbonate. (Pfizer CDT 051). White. Film coated. In 30s.
		5 mg amlodipine besylate/20 mg atorvastatin calcium (as base)	Calcium carbonate. (Pfizer CDT 052). White. Film coated. In 30s.
		5 mg amlodipine besylate/40 mg atorvastatin calcium (as base)	Calcium carbonate. (Pfizer CDT 054). White. Film coated. In 30s.
		5 mg amlodipine besylate/80 mg atorvastatin calcium (as base)	Calcium carbonate. (Pfizer CDT 058). White. Film coated. In 30s.
		10 mg amlodipine besylate/10 mg atorvastatin calcium (as base)	Calcium carbonate. (Pfizer CDT 101). Blue. Film coated. In 30s.
		10 mg amlodipine besylate/20 mg atorvastatin calcium (as base)	Calcium carbonate. (Pfizer CDT 102). Blue. Film coated. In 30s.
		10 mg amlodipine besylate/40 mg atorvastatin calcium (as base)	Calcium carbonate. (Pfizer CDT 104). Blue. Film coated. In 30s.
		10 mg amlodipine besylate/80 mg atorvastatin calcium (as base)	Calcium carbonate. (Pfizer CDT 108). Blue. Film coated. In 30s.

For additional prescribing information, refer to the individual monographs for Amlodipine and Atorvastatin Calcium.

Indications

Indicated in patients for whom treatment with both amlodipine and atorvastatin is appropriate.

➤*Amlodipine:* For the treatment of hypertension, chronic stable angina, and confirmed or suspected vasospastic angina (Prinzmetal or Variant angina).

➤*Atorvastatin:* As an adjunct to diet to reduce elevated total-cholesterol (C), LDL-C, apo B, and triglyceride (TG) levels and to increase HDL-C in patients with primary hypercholesterolemia (heterozygous familial and nonfamilial) and mixed dyslipidemia (Fredrickson types IIa and IIb); as an adjunct to diet for the treatment of patients with elevated serum TG levels (Fredrickson type IV); for the treatment of patients with primary dysbetalipoproteinemia (Fredrickson type III); to reduce total-C and LDL-C in patients with homozygous familial hypercholesterolemia as an adjunct to other lipid-lowering treatments (eg, LDL apheresis) or if such treatments are unavailable; to reduce total-C, LDL-C, and apo B levels in boys and postmenarchal girls (10 to 17 years of age with heterozygous familial hypercholesterolemia).

Administration and Dosage

➤*Approved by the FDA:* January 30, 2004.

Individualize dosage. Lipid-altering agents should be used in addition to a diet restricted in saturated fat and cholesterol, only when the response to diet and other nonpharmacological measures has been inadequate.

Amlodipine/Atorvastatin may be substituted for its individually titrated components. Patients may be given the equivalent dose of amlodipine/atorvastatin or a dose of amlodipine/atorvastatin with increased amounts of amlodipine, atorvastatin, or both for additional antianginal effects, blood pressure lowering, or lipid-lowering effect.

As initial therapy for one indication and continuation of treatment of the other, the recommended starting dose of amlodipine/atorvastatin should be selected based on the continuation of the component being used and the recommended starting dose of the added monotherapy. The maximum dose of the amlodipine component is 10 mg once daily. The maximum dose of the atorvastatin component is 80 mg/day.

➤*Concomitant therapy:* Atorvastatin may be used in combination with a bile acid-binding resin for additive effect. The combination of HMG-CoA reductase inhibitors and fibrates generally should be avoided.

➤*Storage / Stability:* Store at 25°C (77°F); excursions permitted to 15° to 30°C (59° to 86°F).

ASPIRIN/PRAVASTATIN

Rx	**Pravigard PAC** (Bristol-Myers Squibb)	**Tablets:** 81 mg aspirin (buffered)/20 mg pravastatin	Mineral oil (aspirin tablets), lactose (**Pravachol** tablets). Aspirin tablets: Buffered. (b). White, oval. Film coated. **Pravachol** tablets: (P PRAVACHOL 20). Yellow, rectangular. (In blister pack 5s).
		81 mg aspirin (buffered)/40 mg pravastatin	Mineral oil (aspirin tablets), lactose (**Pravachol** tablets). Aspirin tablets: Buffered. (b). White, oval. Film coated. **Pravachol** tablets: (P PRAVACHOL 40). Green, rectangular. (In blister pack 5s).
		81 mg aspirin (buffered)/80 mg pravastatin	Mineral oil (aspirin tablets), lactose (**Pravachol** tablets). Aspirin tablets: Buffered. (b). White, oval. Film coated. **Pravachol** tablets: (BMS 80). Yellow, oval. (In blister pack 5s).
		325 mg aspirin (buffered)/20 mg pravastatin	Mineral oil (aspirin tablets), lactose (**Pravachol** tablets). Aspirin tablets: (B). White. Film coated. **Pravachol** tablets: (P PRAVACHOL 20). Yellow, rectangular. (In blister pack 5s).
		325 mg aspirin (buffered)/40 mg pravastatin	Mineral oil (aspirin tablets), lactose (**Pravachol** tablets). Aspirin tablets: (B). White. Film coated. **Pravachol** tablets: (P PRAVACHOL 40). Green, rectangular. (In blister pack 5s).
		325 mg aspirin (buffered)/80 mg pravastatin	Mineral oil (aspirin tablets), lactose (**Pravachol** tablets). Aspirin tablets: (B). White. Film coated. **Pravachol** tablets: (BMS 80). Yellow, oval. (In blister pack 5s).

For additional prescribing information, refer to the HMG-CoA reductase inhibitors and Salicylates monographs.

Indications

For patients in whom treatment with both pravastatin and buffered aspirin is appropriate. As described in the labeling for pravastatin and buffered aspirin, both components of this product are indicated to reduce the occurrence of cardiovascular events, including death, MI, or stroke, in patients who have clinical evidence of cardiovascular and/or cerebrovascular disease. Place patients receiving treatment with this product on a standard cholesterol-lowering diet and continue on this diet during treatment.

Administration and Dosage

➤*Approved by the FDA:* June 24, 2003.

The recommended daily dose is 40 mg pravastatin with either 81 or 325 mg aspirin. If a daily dose of 40 mg pravastatin does not achieve desired cholesterol levels, 80 mg once daily (with 81 or 325 mg aspirin) is recommended. Some people may require lower doses of pravastatin, and this product is available also with 20 mg pravastatin. The daily dose can be taken any time of day with or without food. Because of the aspirin component, take the dose with a full glass of water unless the patient is fluid restricted.

➤*Hepatic function impairment:* Avoid use in patients with severe hepatic insufficiency.

➤*Renal function impairment:* Avoid use in patients with severe renal insufficiency.

➤*Pravastatin:* The recommended starting dose is 40 mg once/day. Pravastatin can be administered as a single dose, at any time of the day, with or without food. The maximal effect of a given dose is seen within 4 weeks. If a daily dose of 40 mg does not achieve desired cholesterol levels, 80 mg once/day is recommended.

Lower doses are recommended in some patients. A starting dose of 10 mg/day is recommended in patients with a history of significant renal or hepatic dysfunction. In patients taking immunosuppressive drugs such as cyclosporine concomitantly with pravastatin, begin therapy with 10 mg pravastatin once/day at bedtime and perform titration to higher doses with caution. Generally, do not exceed a 20 mg/day dose of pravastatin in those patients receiving concurrent immunosuppressive therapy.

➤*Aspirin:* Take each dose of aspirin with a full glass of water unless the patient is fluid restricted.

Prevention of recurrent MI or treatment of chronic stable angina pectoris – 81 or 325 mg once/day. Continue therapy indefinitely.

Ischemic stroke and TIA – 81 or 325 mg once/day. Continue therapy indefinitely.

ASPIRIN/PRAVASTATIN

Revascularization procedures –

CABG: 325 mg/day starting 6 hours postprocedure. Continue therapy for 1 year postprocedure.

Carotid endarterectomy: Doses of 81 mg once/day to 650 mg twice daily, started presurgery, are recommended. Continue therapy indefinitely.

►*Storage/Stability:* Store at 20° to 25°C (68° to 77°F); excursions permitted to 15° to 30°C (59° to 86°F).

NIACIN (EXTENDED RELEASE)/LOVASTATIN

Rx	Advicor (Kos)	Tablets: 500/20 mg	(KOS 502). Lt. yellow, capsule shape. In 30s, 90s, and 180s.
		750/20 mg	(KOS 752). Lt. orange, capsule shape. In 30s, 90s, and 180s.
		1000/20 mg	(KOS 1002). Dk. pink/lt. purple, capsule shape. In 30s, 90s, and 180s.

Refer to the general discussion of these products in the Antihyperlipidemic Agents Introduction.

Indications

►*Primary hypercholesterolemia/mixed dyslipidemia:* For the treatment of primary hypercholesterolemia (heterozygous familial and nonfamilial) and mixed dyslipidemia (Frederickson Types IIa and IIb) in the following: Patients treated with lovastatin who require further TG-lowering or HDL-raising who may benefit from having niacin added to their regimen; patients treated with niacin who require further LDL-lowering who may benefit from having lovastatin added to their regimen.

Administration and Dosage

The usual recommended starting dose for extended-release niacin tablets is 500 mg at bedtime. Niacin extended-release tablets must be titrated and the dose should not be increased by more than 500 mg every 4 weeks up to a maximum dose of 2000 mg/day, to reduce the incidence and severity of side effects. Patients already receiving a stable dose of niacin extended-release tablets may be switched directly to a niacin-equivalent dose of niacin extended-release/lovastatin tablets.

The usual recommended starting dose of lovastatin is 20 mg once/day. Make dose adjustments at intervals of 4 weeks or more. Patients already receiving a stable dose of lovastatin may receive concomitant dosage titration with niacin extended-release tablets, and switch to niacin extended-release/lovastatin tablets once a stable dose of niacin extended-release tablets has been reached.

Flushing of the skin may be reduced in frequency or severity by pretreatment with aspirin (taken up to approximately 30 minutes prior to niacin extended-release/lovastatin tablets dose) or other nonsteroidal anti-inflammatory drugs. Flushing, pruritus, and GI distress also are greatly reduced by slowly increasing the dose of niacin and avoiding administration on an empty stomach.

Equivalent doses of niacin extended-release/lovastatin tablets may be substituted for equivalent doses of niacin extended-release tablets but should not be substituted for other modified-release (sustained- or timed-release) niacin preparations or immediate-release (crystalline) niacin preparations. Patients previously receiving niacin products other than niacin extended-release tablets should be started on niacin extended-release tablets with the recommended niacin extended-release tablets titration schedule, and the dose should subsequently be individualized based on patient response.

Take niacin extended-release/lovastatin tablets at bedtime, with a low-fat snack, and individualize dose according to patient response.

Take whole; do not break, chew, or crush before swallowing. Do not increase the dose by more than 500 mg/day (based on the niacin extended release component) every 4 weeks. The lowest dose of niacin extended-release/lovastatin tablets is 500/20 mg. Doses greater than 2000/40 mg/day are not recommended. If therapy is discontinued for an extended period (greater than 7 days), begin reinstitution of therapy with the lowest dose.

►*Storage/Stability:* Store at room temperature (20° to 25°C; 68° to 77°F).

➤*Shock:* Shock is a state of inadequate tissue perfusion. It can be caused by, or cause, a decreased supply of, or an increased demand for, oxygen and nutrients. The imbalance between supply and demand interferes with normal cellular function. Widespread cellular dysfunction can result in death. Inadequate tissue perfusion can occur even if cardiac output, peripheral resistance, and other factors that determine blood pressure (eg, blood volume) are normal or elevated. Therefore, hypotension need not be present for the patient to be in shock.

Shock produces various physiologic responses. Some, such as lactic acidosis, occur as a direct result of tissue hypoperfusion. Others, such as catecholamine release, also serve to compensate for the absolute or relative reduction in tissue perfusion. The systemic responses to shock can be beneficial in the early stages and classically consist of an increase in circulating catecholamines, vasodilation, and increased vascular permeability. These early responses produce a "hyperdynamic" state, which may be referred to as "warm" shock, so named because blood flow to the skin and extremities is still maintained. If left uncorrected, however, these responses become counterproductive and contribute to the relentless progression of the shock state. Profound vascular decompensation occurs, which is associated with a further loss of blood flow to the vital organs, skin, and extremities. Thus, more advanced shock is "cold" shock.

➤*Clinical manifestations:* Clinical manifestations of shock are variable and nonspecific. In addition, underlying or concurrent disease states, drug therapy, and patient age may alter the response to hypoperfusion. Signs and symptoms of shock include:

Skin – Pallor, cyanosis, cold and clammy, sweating.

CNS – Agitation, confusion, disorientation, coma.

Cardiovascular – Tachycardia, arrhythmias, wide pulse pressure, gallop rhythm, hypotension.

Pulmonary – Tachypnea, pulmonary edema.

Renal – Oliguria (< 0.5 mL/kg/hr).

Metabolic – Acidosis, hypoglycemia or hyperglycemia.

➤*Causes:* The causes of shock are varied. Despite the etiology, advanced shock tends to follow a common clinical course. However, identifying the underlying cause may assist in the selection of general supportive therapy and is essential for selecting specific therapy.

➤*Types of shock:*

Hypovolemic shock – Hypovolemic shock occurs when intravascular volume is reduced by > 15% to 25%. The volume loss can be absolute (eg, hemorrhage, fluid loss due to burns, diarrhea or vomiting, excess diuresis, diabetes) or relative (eg, sequestration of body fluids, capillary leak).

Cardiogenic shock – Cardiogenic shock occurs when the heart is unable to deliver an adequate cardiac output to maintain vital organ perfusion. This can be caused by an acute MI, sustained ventricular arrhythmias, severe cardiomyopathy, or CHF.

Septic shock – Septic shock occurs as a result of circulatory insufficiency associated with overwhelming infection.

Obstructive shock – Obstructive shock occurs when obstruction of blood flow results in inadequate tissue perfusion. Massive pulmonary embolism, pericardial tamponade, restrictive pericarditis, and severe cardiac valve dysfunction can reduce blood flow enough to produce shock.

Neurogenic shock – An uncommon form of shock that occurs as a result of blockade of neurohumoral outflow. The neurohumoral blockade may be induced by pharmacologic agents (eg, spinal anesthesia) or by direct injury to the spinal cord.

Other causes of shock – Other causes include anaphylaxis, hypoglycemia, hypothyroidism and hypoadrenalism (ie, Addison's disease).

➤*Management:* Management of shock is aimed at providing basic life support (eg, airway, breathing, circulation) while attempting to correct the underlying cause. Antibiotics, inotropes, hormones (eg, insulin, thyroid) and other agents may be used to treat the underlying disease states in the shock patient. However, initial pharmacologic interventions are primarily aimed at supporting the circulation.

Blood pressure is a function of the peripheral vascular resistance and the cardiac output. Cardiac output is determined by the heart rate and stroke volume. The stroke volume is a function of the contractile state of the heart and the volume of blood in the ventricle available to be pumped out (ie, preload). Manipulation of any of these parameters can produce a change in blood pressure.

Fluids – Relative or absolute volume depletion occurs in most shock states, especially in the early or "warm" phase in which vasodilation is prominent. Adequate volume repletion is necessary to maintain cardiac output, urine flow, and the integrity of the microcirculation. Attempts to support the circulation with vasopressors or inotropes will be unsuccessful if the intravascular volume is depleted.

The choice of fluids is probably irrelevant in the early stages. Although whole blood might be preferred for the patient with hemorrhagic shock, the delay in availability of blood products often negates any advantage. There is no clear superiority of crystalloids or colloids in emergency fluid resuscitation. Hydroxyethyl starch and the dextrans are also suitable plasma volume expanders.

Vasopressors – Sympathomimetic agents are used in shock to treat hypoperfusion in normovolemic patients and in patients unresponsive to whole blood or plasma volume expanders. These agents increase myocardial contractility, constrict capacitance vessels, and dilate resistance vessels. In cardiogenic shock or advanced shock from other causes associated with a low cardiac output, they may be combined with vasodilators (eg, nitroprusside, nitroglycerin) to maintain blood pressure while the vasodilator improves myocardial performance. Nitroprusside is used to reduce preload and afterload and improve cardiac output. Nitroglycerin directly relaxes the venous vasculature and decreases preload.

Pharmacology – Sympathomimetic agents produce α-adrenergic stimulation (vasoconstriction), β_1-adrenergic stimulation (increase myocardial contractility, heart rate, automaticity, and AV conduction), and β_2-adrenergic activity (peripheral vasodilation). Dopamine also causes vasodilation of the renal and mesenteric, cerebral and coronary beds by dopaminergic receptor activation. Adrenergic agents are useful in improving hemodynamic status by improving myocardial contractility and increasing heart rate, which results in increased cardiac output. Peripheral resistance is increased by vasoconstriction. Increased cardiac output and increased peripheral resistance increase blood pressure. The relative activity and predominance of these actions result in a number of hemodynamic responses which may affect coronary perfusion, renal perfusion, cardiac output, total peripheral resistance and blood pressure. These actions are summarized in the Sites of Action/Hemodynamic Response table. The actual response of an individual patient will depend largely on clinical status at time of administration.

Other drugs – A number of other drug classes have been used as supportive therapy in shock patients. However, with the exception of vasodilator treatment of cardiogenic shock, none of these treatments appear superior to vasopressor therapy. These drugs include: Opiate antagonists, prostaglandin inhibitors, corticosteroids, and thyrotropin-releasing hormone.

Monitoring – The monitoring of shock patients and their response to drugs requires special vigilance. Monitor heart rate, blood pressure, and ECG continuously. Record urine output and fluid intake frequently. Due to rapid and life-threatening changes that can occur in the hemodynamically unstable patient, optimal drug selection, dose titration, and management is probably best achieved with the use of invasive hemodynamic monitoring. Monitoring of central venous pressures via a central venous catheter will provide an estimation of the patient's fluid status by approximating the diastolic pressure of the right ventricle. When warranted, additional hemodynamic data can be obtained through the use of a pulmonary artery catheter (ie, Swan-Ganz). Changes in the pulmonary artery wedge pressure (a measure of left ventricular end diastolic volume), cardiac output, and peripheral vascular resistance can be monitored and therapy adjusted accordingly.

Administration – Administration should only be via the IV route using a large-bore, free-flowing IV in the antecubital vein or a central vein because of unpredictable absorption. Small IVs in the extremities are both unreliable and unsafe for vasopressor administration. Frequent monitoring of the IV sites for extravasation injury is essential when vasopressor agents are being used.

Prolonged, high-dose therapy – Prolonged, high-dose therapy can produce cyanosis and tissue necrosis of distal extremities. The principle of using the lowest dose that produces an adequate response for the shortest period of time is very important when using these agents.

Plasma volume depletion – Prolonged use of vasopressors may result in plasma volume depletion; this should be corrected by appropriate fluid and electrolyte replacement therapy. If plasma volumes are not corrected, hypotension may recur when these drugs are discontinued. Blood pressure may be maintained at the risk of severe peripheral vasoconstriction with diminution in blood flow and tissue perfusion.

Acidosis – Acidosis lessens the response to vasopressors; therefore, correct acidosis if it exists or develops during the course of vasopressor therapy.

Avoid continuous IV therapy – Acute tolerance develops during continuous IV administration. High concentration/low volume (250 mL) vasopressor solutions administered with the aid of an infusion control device allows for maximum dosing flexibility since fluids and drugs can be regulated independently, and the development of tolerance is minimized.

Effects of Vasopressors Used in Shock

| | | SITES OF ACTION | | | | HEMODYNAMIC RESPONSE | | | | |
| | | HEART | | BLOOD VESSELS | | | | | | |
+++ pronounced effect ++ moderate effect + slight effect 0 no effect ↑ increase ↓ decrease		Contractility (Inotropic) β_1	SA Node Rate (Chronotropic) β_1	Vasoconstriction β_1	Vasodilatation α	Renal Perfusion	Cardiac Output	Total Peripheral Resistance	Blood Pressure	β_2
Inotropic	Isoproterenol	+++	+++	0	+++	↑[1] or ↓[2]	↑	↓	↑[3]↓[4]
	Dobutamine	+++	0 to +[5]	0 to +[5]	+	0	↑	↓	↑
	Dopamine	+++	+ to ++[5]	+ to +++[5]	0 to +[6]	↑[5]	↑	↓[5] or ↑	0 to ↑
Mixed	Epinephrine	+++	+++	+++[5]	++[5]	↓	↑	↓	↑[3]↓[4]
	Norepinephrine	++	++[7]	+++	0	↓	0 or ↓	↑	↑
	Ephedrine	++	++	+	0 to +	↓	↑	↑ or ↓	↑
	Mephentermine	+	+	+	++	↑ or ↓	↑	0 to ↑	↑
Pressors	Metaraminol	+	+	++	0	↓	↓	↑	↑
	Methoxamine	0	0[7]	+++	0	↓	0 or ↓	↑	↑
	Phenylephrine	0	0[7]	+++	0	↓	↓	↑	↑

[1] Cardiogenic or septicemic shock.
[2] Normotensive patient.
[3] Systolic effect.
[4] Diastolic effect.

[5] Effects are dose dependent.
[6] Dilates renal and splanchnic beds via dopaminergic effect at doses < 10 mcg/kg/min.
[7] Decreased heart rate may result from reflex mechanisms.

Common Dilutions and Infusion Rates for Selected Drugs Used in Shock

Drug	Usual Dilution for IV Infusion	Infusion Rate
Isoproterenol	2 mg (10 mL) in 500 mL D5W (4 mcg/mL) or 1 mg (5 mL) in 250 mL D5W	5 mcg/min
Dobutamine	250 mg in 250 to 500 mL NS or D5W (500 to 1000 mcg/mL)	2.5 to 15 mcg/kg/min
Dopamine	200 to 800 mg in 250 to 500 mL NS or D5W (400 to 3200 mcg/mL)	Low dose – 2.5 to 10 mcg/kg/min High dose – 20 to 50 mcg/kg/min
Norepinephrine	4 mg in 250 mL of D5W (16 mcg/mL)	Initial: 8 to 12 mcg/min Maintenance: 2 to 4 mcg/min

ISOPROTERENOL HCl

Rx	Isoproterenol (Various, eg, Abbott)	Injection: 1:5000 solution (0.2 mg per mL)[1]	In 5 and 10 mL vials.
Rx	Isuprel (Sanofi Winthrop)		In 1 and 5 mL amps.
Rx	Isuprel (Sanofi Winthrop)	Injection: 1:50,000 (0.02 mg/mL)[1]	In 10 mL w/needle.

[1] With sodium metabisulfite.

Refer to the general discussion of these products in the Vasopressors Used in Shock group monograph.

Indications

▶*Hypovolemic and septic shock:* As an adjunct to fluid and electrolyte replacement therapy and the use of other drugs and procedures in the treatment of hypovolemic and septic shock, low cardiac output (hypoperfusion) states, congestive heart failure and cardiogenic shock.

▶*Heart block and Adams-Stokes attacks:* For mild or transient episodes of heart block that do not require electric shock or pacemaker therapy.

For serious episodes of heart block and Adams-Stokes attacks (except when caused by ventricular tachycardia or fibrillation).

▶*Cardiac arrest:* For use in cardiac arrest until electric shock or pacemaker therapy, the treatments of choice, are available.

▶*Bronchospasm:* For use in bronchospasm occurring during anesthesia.

Administration and Dosage

▶*Parenteral:* Start isoproterenol 1:50,000 at the lowest recommended dose and gradually increase rate of administration while carefully monitoring the patient.

The usual route of administration is by IV injection or infusion. In an emergency, administer the drug by intracardiac injection. If time is not of utmost importance, initial therapy by IM or SC injection may be used. See Dosage for Adults with Heart Block, Adams-Stokes Attacks and Cardiac Arrest chart below.

There are no well controlled studies in children to establish appropriate dosing; however, the American Heart Association recommends an initial infusion rate of 0.1 mcg/kg/min, with the usual range being 0.1 mcg/kg/min to 1 mcg/kg/min.

Dosage for Adults with Heart Block, Adams - Stokes Attacks and Cardiac Arrest

Route	Dilution	Initial Dose	Subsequent Dose Range
IV injection	Dilute 1 mL of 1:5000 solution (0.2 mg) to 10 mL with Sodium Chloride or 5% Dextrose Injection	0.02 to 0.06 mg (1 to 3 mL of diluted solution)	0.01 to 0.2 mg (0.5 to 10 mL of diluted solution)
IV infusion	Dilute 10 mL of 1:5000 solution (2 mg) in 500 mL of D5W or dilute 5 mL of 1:5000 solution (1 mg) in 250 mL of D5W	5 mcg/min (1.25 mL/min of diluted solution)	
IM	Undiluted 1:5000 solution	0.2 mg (1 mL)	0.02 to 1 mg (0.1 to 5 mL)
SC	Undiluted 1:5000 solution	0.2 mg (1 mL)	0.15 to 0.2 mg (0.75 to 1 mL)
Intracardiac	Undiluted 1:5000 solution	0.02 mg (0.1 mL)	

ISOPROTERENOL HCl

➤*Storage/Stability:* Store at room temperature 15° to 30°C (59° to 86°F). Protect from light. Do not use if solution is pinkish to brownish in color.

Actions

➤*Pharmacology:* Isoproterenol has beta₁- and beta₂-adrenergic receptor activity. Primary actions are on the beta receptors of the heart and smooth muscle of the bronchi, skeletal muscle and vasculature and alimentary tract. Isoproterenol relaxes most smooth muscles, with the most pronounced effect on the bronchial and GI smooth muscle. It produces marked relaxation in the smaller bronchi and may even dilate the trachea and main bronchi past the resting diameter.

Hematologic – The positive inotropic and chronotropic actions of the drug increase minute blood flow. There is an increase in heart rate, an approximately unchanged stroke volume, and an increase in ejection velocity. The rate of discharge of cardiac pacemakers is increased with isoproterenol injection. Venous return to the heart is increased through a decreased compliance of the venous bed. Systemic resistance and pulmonary vascular resistance are decreased, and there is an increase in coronary and renal blood flow. Systolic blood pressure may increase and diastolic blood pressure may decrease. Mean arterial blood pressure is usually unchanged or reduced. The peripheral and coronary vasodilating effects of the drug may aid tissue perfusion.

➤*Pharmacokinetics:* Onset of activity is immediate after IV administration; duration is brief, 1 to 2 hours and < 1 hour.

Contraindications

Tachyarrhythmias; tachycardia or heart block caused by digitalis intoxication; ventricular arrhythmias which require inotropic therapy; angina pectoris.

Warnings

➤*Cardiogenic shock:* Isoproterenol injection, by increasing myocardial oxygen requirements while decreasing effective coronary perfusion, may have a deleterious effect on the injured or failing heart. Its use as the initial agent in treating cardiogenic shock following myocardial infarction is discouraged. However, when a low arterial pressure has been elevated by other means, isoproterenol hydrochloride injection may produce beneficial hemodynamic and metabolic effects.

➤*Heart block:* In a few patients, presumably with organic disease of the AV node and its branches, isoproterenol has paradoxically worsened heart block or precipitated Adams-Stokes attacks during normal sinus rhythm or transient heart block.

➤*Pregnancy: Category C.* It is not known whether isoproterenol can cause fetal harm when administered to a pregnant woman or can affect reproduction capacity. Use only when needed and when benefits outweigh potential hazards to the fetus.

➤*Lactation:* It is not known whether isoproterenol is excreted in breast milk. Exercise caution when administering to a nursing woman.

Precautions

➤*Hypovolemia:* Use is not a substitute for the replacement of blood, plasma, fluids and electrolytes, which should be restored promptly when loss has occurred. Hypovolemia should be corrected by suitable volume expanders before treatment with isoproterenol. Adequate filling of the intravascular compartment by suitable volume expanders is of primary importance in most cases of shock, and should precede the administration of vasoactive drugs. In patients with normal cardiac function, determination of central venous pressure is a reliable guide during volume replacement. If evidence of hypoperfusion persists after adequate volume replacement, give isoproterenol injection. Monitor systemic blood pressure, heart rate, urine flow, ECG; also monitor response to therapy by frequent determination of central venous pressure and blood gases. Closely observe patients in shock during administration.

➤*Cardiovascular disorders:* Use with caution in patients with coronary artery disease, coronary insufficiency, diabetes or hyperthyroidism and in patients sensitive to sympathomimetic amines.

➤*Cardiac effects:* If heart rate exceeds 110 beats/min, it may be advisable to decrease the infusion rate or temporarily discontinue the infusion. Determinations of cardiac output and circulation time may also be helpful. Take appropriate measures to ensure adequate ventilation. Pay careful attention to acid-base balance and to correction of electrolyte disturbances. In cases of shock associated with bacteremia, suitable antimicrobial therapy is, of course, imperative. Doses sufficient to increase heart rate to more than 130 beats/min may induce ventricular arrhythmia. Such increases in heart rate will also tend to increase cardiac work and oxygen requirements which may adversely affect the failing heart or the heart with a significant degree of arteriosclerosis. If precordial distress or anginal-type pain occurs, discontinue the drug immediately.

➤*Sulfite sensitivity:* Some of these products contain sulfites that may cause allergic-type reactions (including anaphylactic symptoms and life-threatening or less severe asthmatic episodes) in certain susceptible persons. The overall prevalence of sulfite sensitivity in the general population is unknown and probably low. It is seen more frequently in asthmatic or atopic nonasthmatic persons.

Drug Interactions

Isoproterenol Drug Interactions			
Precipitant drug	Object drug *		Description
Bretylium	Isoproterenol	↑	Bretylium potentiates the action of vasopressors on adrenergic receptors, possibly resulting in arrhythmias.
Guanethidine	Isoproterenol	↑	Guanethidine may increase the pressor response of the direct-acting vasopressors, possibly resulting in severe hypertension.
Halogenated hydrocarbon anesthetics	Isoproterenol	↑	Halogenated hydrocarbon anesthetics may sensitize the myocardium to the effects of catecholamines. Use of vasopressors may lead to serious arrhythmias; use with caution.
Oxytocic drugs	Isoproterenol	↑	In obstetrics, if vasopressor drugs are used either to correct hypotension or added to the local anesthetic solution, some oxytocic drugs may cause severe persistent hypertension.
Tricyclic antidepressants	Isoproterenol	↑	The pressor response of the direct-acting vasopressors may be potentiated by these agents; use with caution.

* ↑ = Object drug increased.

Adverse Reactions

➤*Cardiovascular:* Tachycardia; palpitations; hypertension; hypotension; ventricular arrhythmias; tachyarrhythmias; precordial distress; angina.

➤*CNS:* Flushing of the skin; sweating; mild tremors; nervousness; headache; dizziness; weakness.

➤*GI:* Nausea; vomiting.

Overdosage

➤*Symptoms:* Excessive doses in animals or man may result in cardiac enlargement and focal myocarditis. Cases of accidental overdosage are evidenced by tachycardia or other arrhythmias, palpitations, angina, hypotension or hypertension.

➤*Treatment:* Reduce rate of administration or discontinue isoproterenol until patient's condition stabilizes. Monitor blood pressure, pulse, respiration and EKG.

DOBUTAMINE

Rx	Dobutamine HCl (Various, eg, Abbott)	Injection: 12.5 mg/mL	May contain sulfites. In 20 mL vials.
Rx	Dobutrex (Lilly)		In 20 mL vials.[1]

[1] With 0.24 mg sodium bisulfite.

Refer to the general discussion of these products in the Vasopressors Used in Shock group monograph.

Indications

➤*Cardiac decompensation:* Inotropic support in the short-term treatment of adults with cardiac decompensation due to depressed contractility, resulting either from organic heart disease or from cardiac surgical procedures.

In patients who have atrial fibrillation with rapid ventricular response, use a digitalis preparation prior to instituting therapy with dobutamine.

➤*Unlabeled uses:* Doses of dobutamine 2 and 7.75 mcg/kg/min infused for 10 minutes each have been used investigationally in 12 children with congenital heart disease undergoing diagnostic cardiac catheterization. The drug appears effective in augmenting cardiovascular function in children, and no adverse effects were noted.

Administration and Dosage

➤*Rate of administration:* The rate of infusion needed to increase cardiac output usually ranges from 2.5 to 10 mcg/kg/min. On rare occasions, infusion rates up to 40 mcg/kg/min have been required. A metering device is recommended for controlling the rate of drug administration.

Adjust rate of administration and duration of therapy according to patient response, as determined by heart rate, presence of ectopic activity, blood pressure, urine flow, and, when possible, measurement of central venous or pulmonary wedge pressure and cardiac output.

Concentrations up to 5000 mcg/mL have been administered (250 mg/50 mL). Determine the final volume administered by the fluid requirements of the patient.

DOBUTAMINE

Infusion Rates of Various Dilutions of Dobutamine			
Desired Delivery Rate (mcg/kg/min)	Infusion Rate (mL/kg/min)		
	250 mcg/mL	500 mcg/mL	1000 mcg/mL
2.5	0.01	0.005	0.0025
5	0.02	0.01	0.005
7.5	0.03	0.015	0.0075
10	0.04	0.02	0.01
12.5	0.05	0.025	0.0125
15	0.06	0.03	0.015

▶*Admixture incompatibility:* Incompatible with alkaline solutions; do not mix with products such as 5% Sodium Bicarbonate Injection. Do not use dobutamine in conjunction with other agents or diluents containing both sodium bisulfite and ethanol. Dobutamine is also physically incompatible with hydrocortisone sodium succinate; cefazolin; cefamandole; neutral cephalothin; penicillin; sodium ethacrynate; sodium heparin.

▶*Admixture compatibility:* Dobutamine is compatible when administered through common tubing with dopamine, lidocaine, tobramycin, verapamil, nitroprusside, potassium chloride and protamine sulfate.

▶*Preparation of solution:* Reconstituted solution must be further diluted to at least 50 mL prior to administration in 5% Dextrose Injection, 5% Dextrose and 0.45% Sodium Chloride Injection, 5% Dextrose and 0.9% Sodium Chloride Injection, 10% Dextrose Injection, *Isolyte M* with 5% Dextrose Injection, Lactated Ringer's Injection, 5% Dextrose in Lactated Ringer's Injection, *Normosol-M* in D5-W, 20% *Osmitrol* in Water for Injection, 0.9% Sodium Chloride Injection or Sodium Lactate Injection.

Freezing is not recommended due to possible crystallization.

▶*Storage/Stability:* Store at room temperature 15° to 30°C (59° to 86°F). After dilution (in glass or *Viaflex* containers), the solution is stable for 24 hours at room temperature. Use IV solutions within 24 hours. Solutions containing dobutamine may exhibit a pink color that, if present, will increase with time. This color change is due to slight oxidation of the drug, but there is no significant loss of potency during the time periods stated above.

Actions

▶*Pharmacology:* Dobutamine is chemically related to dopamine. Its primary activity results from stimulation of the $beta_1$ receptors of the heart while producing comparatively mild chronotropic, hypertensive, arrhythmogenic and vasodilative effects. It has minor $alpha_1$ (vasoconstrictor) and $beta_2$ (vasodilator) effects. It does not cause the release of endogenous norepinephrine, as does dopamine.

Hematologic – In patients with depressed cardiac function, both dobutamine and isoproterenol increase the cardiac output to a similar degree. With dobutamine, this increase is usually not accompanied by marked increases in heart rate (although tachycardia is occasionally observed), and the cardiac stroke volume is usually increased. In contrast, isoproterenol increases the cardiac index primarily by increasing the heart rate while stroke volume changes little or declines. Dobutamine produces less increase in heart rate and less decrease in peripheral vascular resistance for a given inotropic effect than does isoproterenol.

Facilitation of atrioventricular conduction has been observed in human electrophysiologic studies and in patients with atrial fibrillation.

Systemic vascular resistance is usually decreased; occasionally, minimal vasoconstriction has been observed.

▶*Pharmacokinetics:*

Metabolism/Excretion – Routes of metabolism are methylation of the catechol and conjugation. The plasma half-life of dobutamine is two minutes. In urine, the major excretion products are the conjugates of dobutamine and the inactive 3-O-methyl dobutamine.

Onset – The onset of action is within 1 to 2 minutes; however, as much as 10 minutes may be required to obtain the peak effect of a particular infusion rate.

▶*Clinical trials:* Most clinical experience with dobutamine is short-term, up to several hours in duration. In the limited number of patients who were studied for 24, 48 and 72 hours, a persistent increase in cardiac output occurred in some, whereas the output of others returned toward baseline values.

Alteration of synaptic concentrations of catecholamines with either reserpine or tricyclic antidepressants does not alter the actions of dobutamine in animals, which indicates that the actions of dobutamine are not dependent on presynaptic mechanisms.

Contraindications

Idiopathic hypertrophic subaortic stenosis (IHSS); hypersensitivity to dobutamine.

Warnings

▶*Increase in heart rate or blood pressure:* Dobutamine may cause a marked increase in heart rate or blood pressure, especially systolic pressure. Approximately 10% of patients in clinical studies have had

rate increases of 30 beats/min or more, and about 7.5% have had a ≥ 50 mmHg increase in systolic pressure. Usually, reduction of dosage promptly reverses these effects. Because the drug facilitates atrioventricular conduction, patients with atrial fibrillation are at risk of developing rapid ventricular response. Patients with preexisting hypertension appear to face an increased risk of developing an exaggerated pressor response.

▶*Hypotension:* Precipitous decreases in blood pressure have occasionally been associated with dobutamine therapy. Decreasing the dose or discontinuing the infusion typically results in rapid return of blood pressure to baseline values. However, in rare cases, intervention may be required and reversibility may not be immediate.

▶*Ectopic activity:* Dobutamine may precipitate or exacerbate ventricular ectopic activity, but it rarely has caused ventricular tachycardia.

▶*Hypersensitivity reactions:* These may occasionally include skin rash, pruritus of the scalp, fever, eosinophilia and bronchospasm.

▶*Long-term safety:* Infusions ≤ 72 hours have revealed no adverse effects other than those seen with infusions of shorter duration.

▶*Pregnancy: Category B.* Dobutamine has not been administered to pregnant women; use only when clearly needed and when the potential benefits outweigh the potential hazards to the fetus.

▶*Children:* Safety and efficacy for use in children have not been established.

Precautions

▶*Monitoring:* Continuously monitor ECG and blood pressure. Monitor pulmonary wedge pressure and cardiac output whenever possible.

▶*Hypovolemia:* Use is not a substitute for the replacement of blood, plasma, fluids and electrolytes, which should be restored promptly when loss has occurred.

Correct hypovolemia with suitable volume expanders before treatment is instituted.

▶*Ineffective:* Ineffective in the presence of marked mechanical obstruction, such as severe valvular aortic stenosis.

▶*Usage following acute myocardial infarction:* Clinical experience following myocardial infarction has been insufficient to establish the safety of the drug for this use. Any agent that increases contractile force and heart rate may increase the size of an infarction by intensifying ischemia.

▶*Sulfite sensitivity:* This product contains sulfites which may cause allergic-type reactions including anaphylactic symptoms and life-threatening or less severe asthmatic episodes in certain susceptible persons. The overall prevalence of sulfite sensitivity in the general population is unknown and probably low. Sulfite sensitivity is seen more frequently in asthmatic or atopic nonasthmatics.

Drug Interactions

Dobutamine Drug Interactions			
Precipitant drug	Object drug*		Description
Bretylium	Dobutamine	↑	Bretylium may potentiate the action of vasopressors on adrenergic receptors, possibly resulting in arrhythmias.
Guanethidine	Dobutamine	↑	Guanethidine may increase the pressor response of the direct-acting vasopressors, possibly resulting in severe hypertension.
Halogenated hydrocarbon anesthetics	Dobutamine	↑	Halogenated hydrocarbon anesthetics may sensitize the myocardium to the effects of catecholamines. Use of vasopressors may lead to serious arrhythmias; use with extreme caution.
Oxytocic drugs	Dobutamine	↑	In obstetrics, if vasopressor drugs are used either to correct hypotension or added to local anesthetic solutions, some oxytocic drugs may cause severe persistent hypertension.
Tricyclic antidepressants	Dobutamine	↑	The pressor response of the direct-acting vasopressors may be potentiated by these agents; use with caution.

* ↑ = Object drug increased.

Adverse Reactions

▶*Cardiovascular:* Increased heart rate, blood pressure, ventricular ectopic activity (see Warnings); hypotension; premature ventricular beats (≈ 5%; dose-related).

▶*Miscellaneous:* Uncommon, 1% to 3%: Nausea; headache; anginal pain; nonspecific chest pain; palpitations; shortness of breath.

Injection site reactions – Phlebitis and local inflammatory changes have occurred following inadvertent infiltration.

DOBUTAMINE

Overdosage

▶*Symptoms:* Excessive alteration of blood pressure, anorexia, nausea, vomiting, tremore, anxiety, palpitations, headache, shortness of breath, anginal and nonspecific chest pain, myocardial ischemia, ventricular fibrillation or tachycardia

▶*Treatment:* Reduce the rate of administration or temporarily discontinue until condition stabilizes. Establish an airway and ensure oxygenation and ventilation. Initiate resuscitative measures promptly. Severe ventricular tachyarrhythmias may be successfully treated with propranolol or lidocaine.

DOPAMINE HCl

Rx	**Dopamine HCl** (Various, eg, American Regent, Astra, ESI)	**Injection:** 40 mg/mL	In 5 mL amps, 5, 10 and 20 mL vials and 5 and 10 mL syringes.
Rx	**Dopamine HCl** (Abbott)		In 5 mL and 10 mL Pintop vials, Fliptop vials and additive syringes.[1]
Rx	**Dopamine HCl** (Various, eg, American Regent, Astra, ESI)	**Injection:** 80 mg/mL	In 5 mL amps; 5 and 20 mL vials and 10 mL syringes.
Rx	**Dopamine HCl** (Abbott)		In 10 mL/[1]
Rx	**Dopamine HCl** (Various)	**Injection:** 160 mg/mL	In 5 mL vials.
Rx	**Dopamine HCl in 5% Dextrose** (Abbott)	**Injection:** 80 mg/100 mL (0.8 mg/mL)[2]	In 250 and 500 mL.
		160 mg/100 mL (1.6 mg/mL)[2]	In 250 and 500 mL.
		320 mg/100 mL (3.2 mg/mL)[2]	In 250 mL.

[1] With 9 mg sodium metabisulfite.
[2] With 50 mg sodium metabisulfite.

Refer to the general discussion of these products in the Vasopressors Used in Shock group monograph.

Indications

▶*Hemodynamic imbalances:* Correction of hemodynamic imbalances in shock syndrome due to myocardial infarction, trauma, endotoxic septicemia, open heart surgery, renal failure, and chronic cardiac decompensation as in congestive failure.

Patients most likely to respond adequately are those in whom physiological parameters such as urine flow, myocardial function and blood pressure have not profoundly deteriorated. The shorter the time between onset of signs and symptoms of shock and initiation of therapy with volume correction and dopamine, the better the prognosis.

▶*Unlabeled uses:* Chronic obstructive pulmonary disease (COPD) (4 mcg/kg/min); congestive heart failure (CHF) (2 to 5 mcg/kg/min); respiratory distress syndrome (RDS) in infants (starting at 5 mcg/kg/min).

Administration and Dosage

This is a potent drug; dilute before use if not prediluted.

▶*Rate of administration:* After dilution, administer IV. A metering device is essential for controlling the rate of flow. Titrate each patient to the desired hemodynamic or renal response with dopamine. In titrating to the desired increase in systolic blood pressure, the optimum dosage rate for renal response may be exceeded, thus necessitating a reduction in rate after the hemodynamic condition is stabilized.

Administration at rates > 50 mcg/kg/min have been used safely in advanced circulatory decompensation states.

▶*Suggested regimen:* When appropriate, increase blood volume with whole blood or plasma until central venous pressure is 10 to 15 cm water, or pulmonary wedge pressure is 14 to 18 mm Hg.

Begin administration of diluted solution at doses of 2 to 5 mcg/kg/min in patients likely to respond to modest increments of cardiac contractility and renal perfusion.

In more seriously ill patients, begin administration of diluted solution at doses of 5 mcg/kg/min and increase gradually using 5 to 10 mcg/kg/min increments, up to a rate of 20 to 50 mcg/kg/min, as needed. If doses in excess of 50 mcg/kg/min are required, check urine output frequently. If urine flow decreases in the absence of hypotension, consider reduction of dosage. More than 50% of patients are satisfactorily maintained on doses < 20 mcg/kg/min. In patients who do not respond to these doses, additional increments may be employed.

Treatment of all patients requires constant evaluation of therapy in terms of the blood volume, augmentation of cardiac contractility, and distribution of peripheral perfusion. Pay particular attention to diminution of established urine flow rate, increasing tachycardia or development of new dysrhythmias.

As with all potent drugs, take care to avoid inadvertent administration of a bolus of drug.

▶*Preparation of solution:* Add 200 to 400 mg dopamine to 250 to 500 mL of one of the following IV solutions: Sodium Chloride Injection, 5% Dextrose Injection, 5% Dextrose and 0.9% Sodium Chloride Injection, 5% Dextrose and 0.45% Sodium Chloride Solution, 5% Dextrose and Lactated Ringer's Solution, Sodium Lactate (⅙ Molar) Injection, Lactated Ringer's Injection.

Admixture incompatibilities – Do not add to 5% Sodium Bicarbonate or other alkaline IV solutions, oxidizing agents or iron salts since the drug is inactivated in alkaline solution.

▶*Storage/Stability:* Protect from light. Do not use if solution is discolored. Store at room temperature, 15° to 30°C (59° to 86°F).

Stable for a minimum of 24 hours after dilution; however, dilute just prior to administration.

Actions

▶*Pharmacology:* Dopamine is an endogenous catecholamine and a precursor of norepinephrine. It acts both directly and indirectly (releases norepinephrine stores) on alpha and beta$_1$ receptors and has dopaminergic effects.

Beta$_1$ actions produce an inotropic effect on the myocardium resulting in increased cardiac output. Dopamine causes less increase in myocardial oxygen consumption than isoproterenol and is usually not associated with a tachyarrhythmia. Systolic and pulse pressure usually increase with either no effect or a slight increase in diastolic pressure.

Total peripheral resistance (α effects) at low and intermediate therapeutic doses is usually unchanged. Blood flow to peripheral vascular beds may decrease while mesenteric flow increases. Dopamine dilates the renal and mesenteric vasculature presumably by activation of a dopaminergic receptor. This action is accompanied by increases in GFR, renal blood flow, and sodium excretion. An increase in urinary output produced by dopamine is usually not associated with a decrease in osmolality of the urine. The dopaminergic effect is overridden by alpha-adrenergic activity at higher doses of dopamine (> 10 mcg/kg/min).

Organ perfusion – Urine flow appears to be one of the better monitoring parameters of vital organ perfusion. Also, observe the patient for signs of reversal of confusion or comatose condition. Loss of pallor, increase in toe temperature or adequacy of nail bed capillary filling may also be used as indices of adequate dosage.

Renal function – When dopamine is given before urine flow has decreased to levels ≈ 0.3 mL/minute, prognosis is more favorable. Nevertheless, in oliguric or anuric patients, administration has resulted in an increase in urine flow which has reached normal levels. Dopamine may also increase urine flow in patients whose output is within normal limits, thus reducing preexisting fluid accumulation. Above those optimal doses, urine flow may decrease, necessitating dosage reduction. Coadministration of dopamine and diuretic agents may produce an additive or potentiating effect.

Cardiac output – Increased cardiac output is related to dopamine's direct inotropic effect on the myocardium, and at low or moderate doses appears to be related to a favorable prognosis. Increase in cardiac output has been associated with either static or decreased systemic vascular resistance (SVR). Low or moderate increments in cardiac output is believed to be a reflection of differential effects on specific vascular beds, with increased resistance in peripheral vascular beds (eg, femoral) and concomitant decreases in mesenteric and renal vascular beds. Redistribution of blood flow parallels these changes so that an increase in cardiac output is accompanied by an increase in mesenteric and renal blood flow; often the renal fraction of the total cardiac output has been found to increase. Increase in cardiac output produced by dopamine is not associated with substantial decreases in SVR.

Blood pressure – Manage hypotension due to inadequate cardiac output with low to moderate doses, which have little effect on SVR. At high doses, alpha-adrenergic activity is more prominent and may correct hypotension due to diminished SVR.

Prognosis is better in patients whose blood pressure and urine flow have not undergone extreme deterioration. Administer dopamine as soon as a definite trend toward decreased systolic and diastolic pressure becomes apparent.

▶*Pharmacokinetics:*

Absorption/Distribution – Dopamine has an onset of action within 5 minutes, a plasma half-life of ≈ 2 minutes and a duration of action of less than 10 minutes. The drug is widely distributed in the body but does not cross the blood-brain barrier.

Metabolism/Excretion – Dopamine is metabolized in the liver, kidney, and plasma by MAO and catechol-O-methyltransferase to inactive compounds. About 25% is taken up into specialized neurosecretory vesicles (the adrenergic nerve terminals), where it is hydroxylated to

DOPAMINE HCl

form norepinephrine. About 80% is excreted in the urine within 24 hours, primarily as HVA and its sulfate and glucuronide conjugates and as 3,4-dihydroxy-phenylacetic acid. A small portion is excreted unchanged.

Contraindications

Pheochromocytoma; uncorrected tachyarrhythmias or ventricular fibrillation.

Warnings

➤*Polyuria:* Doses ≤ 3 mcg/kg/min have been shown to improve kidney function.

➤*Pregnancy: Category C.* Animal studies have revealed no evidence of teratogenic effects. In 1 study, administration of dopamine to pregnant rats resulted in a decreased survival rate of the newborn and a potential for cataract formation in the survivors. There are no adequate and well-controlled studies in pregnant women and it is not known if dopamine crosses the placental barrier. The drug may be used in pregnant women when the expected benefit outweighs the potential risk to the fetus.

➤*Lactation:* It is not known whether this drug is excreted in breast milk. Because many drugs are excreted in breast milk, exercise caution when administering to a nursing woman.

➤*Children:* Safety and efficacy for use in children have not been established. It has been used in a limited number of pediatric patients, but such use has been inadequate to fully define proper dosage and use.

Precautions

➤*Monitoring:* Close monitoring of urine flow, cardiac output, pulmonary wedge pressure, and blood pressure during infusion is necessary.

➤*Hypovolemia:* Prior to treatment with dopamine, correct hypovolemia with whole blood or plasma as indicated. Monitoring of central venous pressure or left ventricular filling pressure may be helpful in detecting and treating hypovolemia.

➤*Decreased pulse pressure:* If a disproportionate rise in the diastolic pressure (a marked decrease in pulse pressure) is observed in patients receiving dopamine, decrease infusion rate and observe patient carefully for further evidence of predominant vasoconstriction, unless such an effect is desired.

➤*Occlusive vascular disease:* Closely monitor patients with a history of occlusive vascular disease (eg, arteriosclerosis, arterial embolism, Raynaud's disease, cold injury, frostbite, diabetic endarteritis, Buerger's disease) for any changes in color or temperature of the skin of the extremities. If a change occurs and is thought to be the result of compromised circulation to the extremities, weigh the benefits of continued dopamine infusion against the risk of possible necrosis. This condition may be reversed by either decreasing the rate of infusion or discontinuing the drug.

➤*Extravasation:* Infuse into a large vein to prevent extravasation. Extravasation may cause necrosis and sloughing of surrounding tissue. Large veins of the antecubital fossa are preferred to veins in the hand or ankle. Monitor the infusion site closely for free flow.

Antidote for extravasation – To prevent sloughing and necrosis in ischemic areas, infiltrate area as soon as possible with 10 to 15 mL 0.9% Sodium Chloride solution containing 5 to 10 mg phentolamine. Use a syringe with a fine hypodermic needle and infiltrate liberally throughout the ischemic area. Sympathetic blockade with phentolamine causes immediate and conspicuous local hyperemic changes if the area is infiltrated within 12 hours.

➤*Discontinuation:* When discontinuing the infusion, gradually decrease the dose of dopamine because sudden cessation may result in marked hypotension.

➤*Sulfite sensitivity:* Some of these products contain sulfites that may cause allergic-type reactions including anaphylactic symptoms and life-threatening or less severe asthmatic episodes in certain susceptible people. The overall prevalence of sulfite sensitivity in the general popu-

lation is unknown and probably low. It is seen more frequently in asthmatic or atopic nonasthmatic people.

Drug Interactions

Dopamine Drug Interactions			
Precipitant drug	Object drug*		Description
Dopamine	Guanethidine	↓	The antihypertensive effects of guanethidine may be partially or totally reversed by the mixed-acting sympathomimetics.
Halogenated hydrocarbon anesthetics	Dopamine	↑	Halogenated hydrocarbon anesthetics may sensitize the myocardium to the effects of catecholamines. Use of vasopressors may lead to serious arrhythmias; use with extreme caution.
Monoamine oxidase inhibitors (MAOIs)	Dopamine	↑	MAOIs increase the pressor response to dopamine by 6- to 20-fold. Dopamine is metabolized by MAOIs, and inhibition of this enzyme prolongs and potentiates the effect of dopamine. This interaction also may occur with furazolidone, an antimicrobial with MAOI activity. Avoid these combinations; if given inadvertently and hypertension occurs, administer phentolamine.
Oxytocic drugs	Dopamine	↑	In obstetrics, if vasopressor drugs are used to correct hypotension or are added to the local anesthetic solution, some oxytocics may cause severe persistent hypertension.
Dopamine	Phenytoin	↓	Concomitant infusion of dopamine has been reported to lead to seizures, severe hypotension, and bradycardia. If necessary, discontinue phenytoin and provide supportive treatment.
Tricyclic antidepressants	Dopamine	↓	The pressor response of the mixed-acting vasopressors may be decreased by these agents; a higher dose of the sympathomimetic may be necessary.

* ↑ = Object drug increased. ↓ = Object drug decreased.

Adverse Reactions

Most frequent – Ectopic beats; nausea and vomiting; tachycardia; anginal pain; palpitation; dyspnea; headache; hypotension; vasoconstriction.

Infrequent – Aberrant conduction; bradycardia; piloerection; widened QRS complex; azotemia; elevated presssure.

High doses may cause dilated pupils and ventricular arrhythmia.

Gangrene has occurred when high doses were administered for prolonged periods and in patients with occlusive vascular disease receiving low doses of dopamine. An isolated case of gangrene in a neonate has occurred.

Overdosage

➤*Symptoms:* Accidental overdosage is manifested by excessive blood pressure elevation.

➤*Treatment:* Reduce rate of administration or temporarily discontinue until patient's condition is stabilized. Because duration of action is quite short, no additional remedial measures are usually necessary. If these measures fail to stabilize the patient's condition, consider using the short-acting alpha-adrenergic blocking agent, phentolamine.

EPINEPHRINE

Rx	**Epinephrine** (Abbott)	**Solution:** 1:1000 (1 mg/mL)	In 1 mL amps[1]
Rx	**EpiPen** (Dey)		In 0.3 mL single-dose auto-injectors.[2]
Rx	**Adrenalin Chloride** (Monarch)	**Solution:** 1:1000 (1 mg/mL as HCl)	In 1 mL amps[3] and 30 mL *Steri-vials*.[4]
Rx	**EpiPen Jr** (Dey)	**Solution:** 1:2000 (0.5 mg/mL)	In 0.3 mL single-dose auto-injectors.[2]
Rx	**Epinephrine** (Abbott)	**Solution:** 1:10,000 (0.1 mg/mL)	In 10 mL single-dose *Abboject* prefilled syringes with either 18-G 3.5 inch or 21-G 1.5 inch needles, in 10 mL single-dose *Abboject* prefilled *LifeShield* syringes,[5] and in 10 mL vials.

[1] With 0.9 mg sodium metabisulfite and 9 mg sodium chloride per mL.
[2] With 0.5 mg sodium metabisulfite and 1.8 mg sodium chloride.
[3] With not more than 0.1% sodium bisulfite.
[4] With 0.5% chlorobutanol and not more than 0.15% sodium bisulfite.
[5] With 0.46 mg sodium metabisulfite and 8.16 mg sodium chloride per mL.

Refer to the general discussion of these products in the Vasopressors Used in Shock group monograph. See also Bronchodilators in the Respiratory Agents chapter and Agents for Glaucoma in the Ophthalmic and Otic Agents chapter.

Indications

➤*Injection:* In acute attacks of ventricular standstill, apply physical measures first. When external cardiac compression and attempts to restore the circulation by electrical defibrillation or use of a pacemaker fail, intracardiac puncture and intramyocardial injection of epineph-

EPINEPHRINE

rine may be effective. However, this method of administration should only be employed as a last resort and by personnel skilled in intracardiac injection technique.

Treatment and prophylaxis of cardiac arrest and attacks of transitory atrioventricular (AV) heart block with syncopal seizures (Stokes-Adams syndrome).

Epinephrine also is used as a hemostatic agent, and to treat mucosal congestion of hay fever, rhinitis, and acute sinusitis; to relieve bronchial asthmatic paroxysms; in syncope caused by complete heart block or carotid sinus hypersensitivity; for symptomatic relief of serum sickness, urticaria, and angioneurotic edema; for resuscitation in cardiac arrest following anesthetic accidents; in simple (open-angle) glaucoma; for relaxation of uterine musculature and to inhibit uterine contractions; to prolong the action of regional and local anesthetics; acute hypersensitivity (anaphylactoid reactions to drugs, animal serums, insect stings, and other allergens); treatment of acute asthmatic attacks to relieve bronchospasm not controlled by inhalation or SC administration of other solutions of the drug.

➤*Unlabeled uses:* Endoscopic injection therapy with epinephrine or a mixture of epinephrine and saline has been shown to be a safe and effective hemostatic option in the management of acute lower GI bleeding.

Administration and Dosage

➤*Solution (1:1000):* 0.2 to 1 mL (mg) SC or IM. Start with a small dose and increase if required. SC is the preferred route of administration. If given IM, avoid injection into the buttocks.

➤*Solution (1:10,000):* Administer by IV injection or, in cardiac arrest, by intracardiac injection into the left ventricular chamber or via endotracheal tube directly into the bronchial tree.

➤*Hypersensitivity / Bronchospasm:*

Adults – The IV dose for hypersensitivity reactions or to relieve bronchospasm usually ranges from 0.1 to 0.25 mg, injected slowly.

Pediatrics – Neonates may be given a dose of 0.01 mg/kg body weight. For the infant, 0.05 mg is an adequate initial dose and this may be repeated at 20- to 30-minute intervals in the management of asthma attacks. Administer 0.01 mg/kg or 0.3 mg/m^2 to a maximum of 0.5 mg SC, repeated every 4 hours if required.

EpiPen or EpiPen Jr – For a patient experiencing anaphylaxis, the patient is to inject the delivered dose IM into the anterolateral aspect of the thigh, through clothing if necessary. *EpiPen Jr*, which provides a dosage of 0.15 mg, may be more appropriate for patients weighing less than 30 kg. Each auto-injector contains a single dose of epinephrine. With severe, persistent anaphylaxis, repeat injections with an additional *EpiPen* may be necessary.

➤*Cardiac arrest:* 0.5 mg (0.5 mL of 1:1000 solution) diluted to 10 mL with sodium chloride injection or 0.5 to 1 mg (5 to 10 mL of 1:10,000 solution) can be administered IV or intracardially. During a resuscitation effort, give 0.5 mg (5 mL of 1:10,000 solution) IV every 5 minutes. Intracardiac dose usually ranges from 0.3 to 0.5 mg (3 to 5 mL of 1:10,000 solution). Follow intracardiac administration with external cardiac massage to permit the drug to enter coronary circulation. Alternatively, if the patient has been intubated, epinephrine can be injected via the endotracheal tube directly into the bronchial tree at the same dosage as for IV injection.

Use epinephrine secondarily to unsuccessful attempts with physical or electromechanical methods.

➤*Ophthalmological use:* To produce conjunctival decongestion, to control hemorrhage, produce mydriasis, and reduce intraocular pressure, use a concentration of 1:10,000 (0.1 mg/mL) to 1:1000 (1 mg/mL).

➤*Regional anesthesia:* A final concentration of 1:20,000 is recommended for infiltration injection, nerve block, caudal, or other epidural blocks. From 0.3 to 0.4 mg of epinephrine (0.3 to 0.4 mL of 1:1000 solution) may be mixed with spinal anesthetic agents.

➤*Intraspinal use:* Usual dose is 0.2 to 0.4 mL added to anesthetic spinal fluid mixture (may prolong anesthetic action by limiting absorption).

➤*Use with local anesthetics:* Epinephrine 1:100,000 (0.01 mg/mL) to 1:200,000 (0.05 mg/mL) is the usual concentration employed with local anesthetics.

➤*Storage / Stability:* Store at room temperature 15° to 30°C (59° to 86°F). Protect the solution from light, extreme heat, and freezing. Do not remove ampules or syringes from carton until ready to use. Discard unused portion.

Actions

➤*Pharmacology:* The actions of epinephrine resemble the effects of stimulation of adrenergic nerves. To a variable degree, it acts on both alpha and beta receptor sites of sympathetic effector cells. Its most prominent actions are on the beta receptors of the heart and of vascular and other smooth muscle. When given by rapid IV injection, epinephrine produces a rapid rise in blood pressure (mainly systolic); it produces direct stimulation of cardiac muscle, which increases the strength of ventricular contraction; it increases the heart rate; and it constricts the arterioles in the skin, mucosa, and splanchnic areas of circulation.

When given by slow IV injection, epinephrine usually produces a moderate rise in systolic and a fall in diastolic pressure. Although some increase in pulse pressure occurs, there is usually no great elevation in mean blood pressure. The compensatory reflex mechanisms that cause a pronounced increase in blood pressure do not antagonize the direct cardiac actions of epinephrine as much as with catecholamines that have a predominant action on alpha receptors.

Total peripheral resistance decreases by action of epinephrine on beta receptors of the skeletal muscle vasculature, and blood flow is thereby enhanced. Usually, this vasodilator effect predominates so that the modest rise in systolic pressure that follows slow injection or absorption is the result of direct cardiac stimulation and increase in cardiac output.

Epinephrine relaxes the smooth muscle of the bronchi and iris and is a physiologic antagonist of histamine. The drug also increases blood sugar and liver glycogenolysis.

➤*Pharmacokinetics:* IV injection produces an immediate and intensified response. Following IV injection, epinephrine disappears rapidly from the blood stream. Given SC or IM, epinephrine has a rapid onset and short duration of action.

The drug becomes fixed in the tissues and is inactivated chiefly by enzymatic transformation to metanephrine or normetanephrine, either of which is subsequently conjugated and excreted in the urine in the form of sulfates and glucuronides. Either sequence results in the formation of 3-methoxy-4-hydroxy-mandelic acid (vanillyl-mandelic acid; VMA), which is also detectable in the urine.

The larger portion of injected doses is excreted in the urine as inactivated compounds and the remainder either partly unchanged or conjugated.

Contraindications

Hypersensitivity to the drug, any component, or sympathomimetic amines. Narrow-angle (congestive) glaucoma; shock (nonanaphylactic); during general anesthesia with halogenated hydrocarbons or cyclopropane; individuals with organic brain damage; with local anesthesia for injection of certain areas (eg, fingers, toes) because of the danger of vasoconstriction producing sloughing of tissue; in labor because it may delay the second stage; in cardiac dilation and coronary insufficiency.

Epinephrine should not ordinarily be used in those cases where vasopressor drugs may be contraindicated (eg, in thyrotoxicosis, diabetes, obstetrics when maternal blood pressure is in excess of 130/80, hypertension, other cardiovascular disorders).

Warnings

➤*Use with caution in the following:* Elderly patients; cardiovascular disease; cardiac arrhythmias; hypertension; diabetes; hyperthyroidism; psychoneurotic individuals; bronchial asthma and emphysema with degenerative heart disease; thyrotoxicosis.

➤*Cardiovascular effects:* Inadvertently induced high arterial blood pressure may result in angina pectoris, aortic rupture, or cerebral hemorrhage.

Epinephrine may induce potentially serious cardiac arrhythmias in patients not suffering from heart disease and in patients with organic heart disease or who are receiving drugs that sensitize the myocardium.

➤*Pulmonary edema:* May result in fatalities because of the peripheral constriction and cardiac stimulation produced.

➤*Renal function impairment:* Initially, epinephrine administered parenterally may produce constriction of renal blood vessels and decreased urine formation.

➤*Pregnancy: Category C.* Epinephrine is teratogenic in small animals when given in doses about 25 times the human dose. There are no adequate and well-controlled studies in pregnant women. Use during pregnancy only if the potential benefit justifies the potential risk to the fetus.

Labor and delivery – Parenteral administration of epinephrine, if used to support blood pressure during low or other spinal anesthesia for delivery, can cause acceleration of fetal heart rate and should not be used in obstetrics when maternal blood pressure exceeds 130/80 mm Hg.

➤*Lactation:* It is not known if this drug is excreted in breast milk. Decide whether to discontinue nursing or to discontinue the drug, taking into account the importance of the drug to the mother.

➤*Children:* Epinephrine may be given safely to pediatric patients at a dosage appropriate to body weight.

Precautions

➤*Fibrillation:* Although epinephrine can produce ventricular fibrillation, its actions in restoring electrical activity in asystole and in enhancing defibrillation are well documented. However, use with caution in patients with ventricular fibrillation.

In patients with prefibrillatory rhythm, IV epinephrine must be used with extreme caution because of its excitatory action on the heart. Because the myocardium is sensitized to the drug by many anesthetic

EPINEPHRINE

agents, epinephrine may convert asystole to ventricular fibrillation if used in the treatment of anesthetic cardiac accidents.

➤*Sulfite sensitivity:* Sulfites may cause allergic-type reactions (eg, hives, itching, wheezing, anaphylaxis) in certain susceptible persons. Although the overall prevalence of sulfite sensitivity in the general population is probably low, it is seen more frequently in asthmatics or in atopic nonasthmatic persons. Specific products containing sulfites are identified in the product listings.

Drug Interactions

Epinephrine Drug Interactions			
Precipitant drug	Object drug *		Description
Alpha-adrenergic blockers (eg, phentolamine)	Epinephrine	↓	The vasoconstricting and hypertensive effects are antagonized by alpha-adrenergic blocking drugs.
Beta-adrenergic blockers, nonspecific	Epinephrine	↑	Coadministration allows alpha-receptor effects of epinephrine to predominate, causing hypertension and reflex bradycardia.
Cardiac glycosides	Epinephrine	↑	Cardiac glycosides may sensitize the myocardium to the actions of sympathomimetics.
Chlorpromazine	Epinephrine	↓	Chlorpromazine may reverse the pressor effects of epinephrine.
Diuretic drugs	Epinephrine	↓	Diuretic agents may decrease vascular response to pressor drugs such as epinephrine.
Furazolidone	Epinephrine	↑	Furazolidone may increase the pressor sensitivity to epinephrine, possibly resulting in hypertension. Avoid coadministration if possible.
Halogenated hydrocarbon anesthetics, cyclopropane	Epinephrine	↑	Halogenated hydrocarbon anesthetics and cyclopropane may sensitize the myocardium to the effects of epinephrine and may lead to serious arrhythmias; use with extreme caution.
Levothyroxine Antihistamines (eg, chlorpheniramine, tripelennamine, diphenhydramine)	Epinephrine	↑	The pressor response of the direct-acting vasopressors may be potentiated by these agents; use with caution.
Monoamine oxidase inhibitors (MAOIs)	Epinephrine	↑	Although coadministration of an MAOI with an indirect- or mixed-acting sympathomimetic may cause severe headache, hypertension, high fever, and hypertensive crisis, direct-acting sympathomimetics (eg, epinephrine) appear to interact minimally.
Methyldopa	Epinephrine	↑	Coadministration may result in increased pressor response, possibly resulting in hypertension.

Epinephrine Drug Interactions			
Precipitant drug	Object drug *		Description
Oxytocic drugs	Epinephrine	↑	Coadministration may result in hypertension.
Reserpine	Epinephrine	↑	Reserpine may potentiate the pressor response of epinephrine, resulting in hypertension.
Sympathomimetic drugs (eg, isoproterenol)	Epinephrine	↑	Do not coadminister epinephrine with other sympathomimetic drugs because of possible additive effects and increased toxicity. Combined effects may induce serious cardiac arrhythmias. They may be administered alternately when the preceding effect of other such drugs has subsided.
Tricyclic antidepressants	Epinephrine	↑	The pressor response of the direct-acting vasopressors may be potentiated by these agents; use with caution.
Epinephrine	Guanethidine	↓	Epinephrine may antagonize the effects of guanethidine, resulting in decreased antihypertensive effect and requiring increased dosage of guanethidine.

* ↑ = Object drug increased. ↓ = Object drug decreased.

Adverse Reactions

➤*Cardiovascular:* Anginal pain in patients with angina pectoris; palpitations; tachycardia. Cardiac arrhythmias and excessive rise in blood pressure may occur with therapeutic doses or inadvertent overdosage.

➤*Local:* Repeated local injections can result in necrosis from vascular constriction at injection sites.

➤*Systemic:* Cerebral hemorrhage; hemiplegia; subarachnoid hemorrhage; anxiety; restlessness; throbbing headache; tremor; weakness; dizziness; pallor; respiratory difficulty; nervousness; apprehension; sweating; nausea; vomiting; "epinephrine-fastness" with prolonged use.

➤*Miscellaneous:*

Transient and minor – Anxiety, headache, fear, and palpitations often occur with therapeutic doses, especially in hyperthyroid individuals.

Overdosage

➤*Symptoms:* Erroneous administration of large doses of epinephrine may lead to precordial distress, vomiting, headache, and dyspnea, as well as unusually elevated blood pressure, which may result in cerebrovascular hemorrhage.

➤*Treatment:* Most toxic effects can be counteracted by injection of an α-adrenergic blocker and a β-adrenergic blocker. In the event of a sharp rise in blood pressure, rapid acting vasodilators such as the nitrites, or α-adrenergic blocking agents can counteract the marked pressor effects.

If an epinephrine overdose induces pulmonary edema, treatment consists of a rapidly acting vasodilator such as nitrites or α-adrenergic blocking drugs.

NOREPINEPHRINE BITARTRATE (Levarterenol)

Rx	**Norepinehprine Bitartrate** (Abbott)	Injection: 1 mg (as base)/mL	In 4 mL amps.[1]
Rx	**Levophed** (Abbott)		In 4 mL amps.[2]

[1] Contains 0.46 mg sodium metabisulfite and 8.2 mg sodium chloride.

[2] Contains ≤ 2 mg metabisulfite.

Refer to the general discussion of these products in the Vasopressors Used in Shock group monograph.

Indications

Restoration of blood pressure in controlling certain acute hypotensive states (eg, pheochromocytomectomy, sympathectomy, poliomyelitis, spinal anesthesia, MI, septicemia, blood transfusion, drug reactions), and as an adjunct in the treatment of cardiac arrest and profound hypotension.

Administration and Dosage

➤*Restoration of blood pressure in acute hypotensive states:* Always correct blood volume depletion as fully as possible before any vasopressor is administered. When, as an emergency measure, intra-aortic pressures must be maintained to prevent cerebral or coronary artery ischemia, norepinephrine can be administered before and concurrently with blood volume replacement.

Average IV dosage – Add 4 mL of the solution to 1000 mL of 5% Dextrose Solution (4 mcg base/mL). Avoid a catheter tie-in technique as this promotes stasis. After observing the response to an initial dose of 2 to 3 mL (from 8 to 12 mcg of base) per minute, adjust the rate of flow to establish and maintain a low normal blood pressure (usually 80 to 100 mm Hg systolic) sufficient to maintain the circulation to vital organs. In previously hypertensive patients, raise the blood pressure no higher

than 40 mm Hg below the pre-existing systolic pressure. The average maintenance dose ranges from 0.5 to 1 mL (2 to 4 mcg of base) per minute.

Dosage adjustments – Great individual variation in the dose occurs; titrate dosage according to patient response. Occasionally, enormous daily doses (as high as 68 mg base) may be necessary if the patient remains hypotensive, but occult blood volume depletion should always be suspected and corrected when present. Central venous pressure monitoring is usually helpful.

If large fluid volumes are needed at a flow rate involving an excessive dose of the pressor agent per unit of time, use a solution more diluted than 4 mcg/mL. When large fluid volumes are undesirable, a larger concentration may be administered.

Duration of therapy – Continue the infusion until adequate blood pressure and tissue perfusion are maintained without therapy. Reduce infusion gradually, avoiding abrupt withdrawal. In some cases of vascular collapse caused by acute MI, treatment was required for up to 6 days.

➤*Adjunctive treatment in cardiac arrest:* Usually administered IV during cardiac resuscitation to restore and maintain an adequate blood pressure after an effective heartbeat and ventilation have been established. The powerful β-adrenergic stimulating action is also thought to

NOREPINEPHRINE BITARTRATE (Levarterenol)

increase the strength and effectiveness of systolic contractions once they occur.

➤*Diluent:* Administer in 5% Dextrose Solution in Distilled Water or 5% Dextrose in Saline Solution. These fluids containing dextrose are protection against significant loss of potency due to oxidation. Administration in saline solution alone is not recommended. If indicated, administer whole blood or plasma separately (for example, by use of a Y–tube and individual flasks if given simultaneously).

➤*Storage / Stability:* Store at room temperature. Protect from light.

Actions

➤*Pharmacology:* A powerful peripheral vasoconstrictor acting on arterial and venous beds (α-adrenergic action) and as a potent inotropic stimulator of the heart (β₁ action). Coronary vasodilation occurs secondary to enhanced myocardial contractility. These actions result in an increase in systemic blood pressure and coronary artery blood flow. Cardiac output will vary in response to systemic hypertension, but is usually increased in hypotension when the blood pressure is raised to an optimal level. Venous return is increased and the heart tends to resume a more normal rate and rhythm than in the hypotensive state.

In hypotension that persists after correction of blood volume deficits, norepinephrine helps raise the blood pressure to an optimal level and establish a more adequate circulation.

➤*Pharmacokinetics:* Norepinephrine is ineffective orally; SC absorption is poor. It is rapidly inactivated by catechol-O-methyltransferase and monoamine oxidase. Negligible amounts are normally found in urine. When given by IV infusion, the onset is rapid; duration is 1 to 2 minutes following discontinuation of infusion.

Contraindications

Do not give to patients who are hypotensive from blood volume deficits, except as an emergency measure to maintain coronary and cerebral artery perfusion until blood volume replacement therapy can be completed. If continuously administered to maintain blood pressure in the absence of blood volume replacement, the following may occur: Severe peripheral and visceral vasoconstriction, decreased renal perfusion and urine output, poor systemic blood flow despite "normal" blood pressure, tissue hypoxia, and lactic acidosis.

Do not give to patients with mesenteric or peripheral vascular thrombosis (because of the risk of increasing ischemia and extending the area of infarction) unless use is necessary as a life-saving procedure.

Use of norepinephrine during cyclopropane and halothane anesthesia is generally considered contraindicated because of the risk of producing ventricular tachycardia or fibrillation. The same type of cardiac arrhythmias may result from use in patients with profound hypoxia or hypercarbia.

Warnings

➤*Pregnancy: Category C.* Animal reproduction studies have not been conducted with norepinephrine. It also is not known whether this drug can cause fetal harm when administered to a pregnant woman or can affect reproduction capacity. Give norepinephrine to a pregnant woman only if clearly needed.

➤*Lactation:* It is not known whether this drug is excreted in breast milk. Because many drugs are excreted in breast milk, exercise caution when administering norepinephrine to a nursing woman.

➤*Children:* Safety and efficacy in children have not been established.

Precautions

➤*Hypovolemia:* Use is not a substitute for the replacement of blood, plasma, fluids, and electrolytes, which should be restored promptly when loss has occurred.

➤*Avoid hypertension:* Because of its potency and varying response to pressor substances, dangerously high blood pressure may be produced with overdoses. Monitor blood pressure every 2 minutes from the time administration is started until desired blood pressure is obtained, then every 5 minutes if administration is continued. Constantly watch flow rate. Never leave patient unattended during infusion. Headache may be a symptom of hypertension caused by overdosage.

➤*Infusion site:* Whenever possible, infuse into a large vein, particularly an antecubital vein, to minimize necrosis of the overlying skin from prolonged vasoconstriction. The femoral vein also may be an acceptable route of administration. Avoid a catheter tie-in technique, if possible, because the obstruction to blood flow around the tubing may cause stasis and increased local concentration of the drug. Occlusive vascular diseases (ie, atherosclerosis, arteriosclerosis, diabetic endarteritis, Buerger's disease) are more likely to occur in the lower extremity; therefore, avoid the veins of the leg in elderly patients or in those suffering from such disorders.

➤*Extravasation:* Infuse into a large vein, preferably of the antecubital fossa, to prevent extravasation. Extravasation may cause necrosis and sloughing of surrounding tissue. Monitor the infusion site closely for free flow.

Blanching along the course of the infused vein, sometimes without obvious extravasation, has been attributed to vasa vasorum constriction with increased permeability of the vein wall, permitting some leakage. This may rarely progress to superficial slough, particularly during infusion into leg veins in elderly patients or in those suffering from obliterative vascular disease. Hence, if blanching occurs, consider changing the infusion site at intervals to allow the effects of local vasoconstriction to subside.

Antidote for extravasation – To prevent sloughing and necrosis in ischemic areas, infiltrate area as soon as possible with 10 to 15 mL of saline solution containing 5 to 10 mg of phentolamine. Use a syringe with a fine hypodermic needle and infiltrate liberally throughout the ischemic area. Sympathetic blockade with phentolamine causes immediate and conspicuous local hyperemic changes if the area is infiltrated within 12 hours.

Phentolamine (5 to 10 mg) added directly to the infusion may also be an effective antidote against sloughing should extravasation occur, whereas the systemic vasopressor activity of norepinephrine is not impaired. Sympathetic nerve block has also been suggested.

The incidence of thrombosis in the infused vein and perivenous reactions and necrosis may be reduced if heparin is added to the infusion solution in an amount to supply 100 to 200 units/hour.

➤*Sulfite sensitivity:* Some of these products contain sulfites that may cause allergic-type reactions (including anaphylactic symptoms and life-threatening or less severe asthmatic episodes) in certain susceptible persons. The overall prevalence of sulfite sensitivity in the general population is unknown and probably low. It is seen more frequently in asthmatic or atopic nonasthmatic persons.

Drug Interactions

Norepinephrine Drug Interactions			
Precipitant drug	Object drug*		Description
Bretylium	Norepinephrine	↑	Bretylium may potentiate the action of vasopressors on adrenergic receptors, possibly resulting in arrhythmias.
Guanethidine	Norepinephrine	↑	Guanethidine may increase the pressor response of the direct-acting vasopressors, possibly resulting in severe hypertension.
Halogenated hydrocarbon anesthetics	Norepinephrine	↑	Halogenated hydrocarbon anesthetics may sensitize the myocardium to the effects of catecholamines. Use of vasopressors may lead to serious arrhythmias; use with extreme caution.
Oxytocic drugs	Norepinephrine	↑	In obstetrics, if vasopressor drugs are used either to correct hypotension or are added to the local anesthetic solution, some oxytocics may cause severe persistent hypertension.
Tricyclic antidepressants	Norepinephrine	↑	The pressor response of the direct-acting vasopressors may be potentiated by these agents; use with caution.
Monoamine oxidase inhibitors (MAOIs)	Norepinephrine	↑	Severe, prolonged hypertension may result.

* ↑ = Object drug increased.

Adverse Reactions

➤*Cardiovascular:* Norepinephrine's therapeutic index is four times that of epinephrine. Bradycardia sometimes occurs, probably as a reflex result of a rise in blood pressure; arrhythmias. Headache may indicate overdosage and extreme hypertension.

➤*CNS:* Anxiety; transient headache.

➤*Miscellaneous:* Ischemic injury due to potent vasoconstrictor action and tissue hypoxia; respiratory difficulty; extravasation necrosis at injection site. Gangrene has been reported in a lower extremity when the drug was infused into an ankle vein.

Overdosage

➤*Symptoms:* Overdosage may also result in headache, severe hypertension, reflex bradycardia, marked increase in peripheral resistance and decreased cardiac output. Prolonged administration of any potent vasopressor may result in plasma volume depletion.

➤*Treatment:* Correct by appropriate fluid and electrolyte replacement therapy. If plasma volumes are not corrected, hypotension may recur when norepinephrine is discontinued or blood pressure may be maintained at the risk of severe peripheral vasoconstriction with diminution in blood flow and tissue perfusion.

EPHEDRINE

Rx	**Ephedrine Sulfate** (Various, eg, UDL)	**Injection:** 50 mg/mL	In 1 mL single-dose vials
Rx	**Ephedrine Sulfate** (Abbott)		Preservative free. In 1 mL single-dose amps.

Refer to the general discussion of these products in the Vasopressors Used in Shock group monograph.

Indications

►*Hypotensive states:* To combat acute hypotensive states, especially those associated with spinal anesthesia; Stokes-Adams syndrome with complete heart block; a CNS stimulant in narcolepsy and depressive states; occasionally, acute bronchospasm. Also used in enuresis and myasthenia gravis.

As a pressor agent in hypotensive states following sympathectomy or following overdosage with ganglionic-blocking agents, antiadrenergic agents, veratrum alkaloids, or other drugs used for lowering blood pressure in the treatment of arterial hypertension.

Administration and Dosage

May be adminstered SC, IM or slow IV.

►*Adults:* The usual dose is 25 to 50 mg. Absorption by the IM route is more rapid than by SC injection. The IV route may be used if an immediate effect is desired. Also, 5 to 25 mg may be administered by slow IV push. Additional doses may be given at 5 to 10 minute intervals.

►*Pediatric dose:* 16.7 mg/m² SC or IM every 4 to 6 hours.

►*Labor:* Administer only sufficient dosage to maintain blood pressure at or below 130/80 mmHg.

►*Acute attacks of asthma:* Administer the smallest effective dose (0.25 to 0.5 mL).

►*Storage / Stability:* Ephedrine is subject to oxidation. Protect against exposure to light. Do not administer unless solution is clear. Discard unused portion.

Actions

►*Pharmacology:* Ephedrine is a potent sympathomimetic that stimulates both alpha and beta receptors and has clinical uses related to both actions. Its peripheral actions, which it owes in part to the release of epinephrine, simulate responses that are obtained when adrenergic nerves are stimulated. These include an increase in blood pressure, stimulation of heart muscle, constriction of arterioles, relaxation of the smooth muscle of the bronchi and GI tract, and dilation of the pupils. In the bladder, relaxation of the detrusor muscle is not prominent, but the tone of the trigone and vesicle sphincter is increased.

CNS – Ephedrine also has a potent effect on the CNS. It stimulates the cerebral cortex and subcortical centers.

Cardiovascular – The cardiovascular responses include moderate tachycardia, unchanged or augmented stroke volume, enhanced cardiac output, variable alterations in peripheral resistance, and, usually, a rise in blood pressure. The action of ephedrine is more prominent on the heart than on the blood vessels. Ephedrine increases the flow of coronary, cerebral and muscle blood.

Metabolic – Hepatic glycogenolysis is increased by ephedrine, but not as much as by epinephrine; usual doses are unlikely to produce hyperglycemia. Ephedrine increases oxygen consumption and metabolic rate, probably by central stimulation.

Myasthenia gravis – Administration of ephedrine produces a real but modest increase in motor power. The exact mechanism by which ephedrine affects skeletal muscle contraction is unknown.

►*Pharmacokinetics:* Ephedrine is rapidly and completely absorbed following parenteral injection. Onset of action by the IM route is more rapid (within 10 to 20 minutes) than by SC injection. Pressor and cardiac responses to ephedrine persist for up to 60 minutes following IM or SC administration of 25 to 50 mg.

Small amounts of ephedrine are slowly metabolized in the liver. The drug and its metabolites are excreted in the urine, mostly as unchanged ephedrine. Rate and percentage of urinary excretion is dependent on urinary pH which is increased by acidification of the urine. Elimination half-life of the drug is ≈ 3 hours when the urine is acidified to a pH of 5 and ≈ 6 hours when urinary pH is 6.3.

Contraindications

Hypersensitivity to the drug; angle closure glaucoma; patients anesthetized with cyclopropane or halothane (these agents may sensitize the heart to the arrhythmic action of sympathomimetic drugs); cases where vasopressor drugs are contraindicated (ie, thyrotoxicosis, diabetes, obstetrics where maternal blood pressure is in excess of 130/80 mmHg, hypertension and other cardiovascular disorders).

Warnings

►*Hypertension:* Ephedrine may cause hypertension resulting in intracranial hemorrhage, anginal pain in patients with coronary insufficiency or ischemic heart disease, or potentially fatal arrhythmias in patients with organic heart disease or who are receiving drugs that sensitize the myocardium.

►*Labor and delivery:* Parenteral administration of ephedrine to maintain blood pressure during low or other spinal anesthesia for delivery can cause acceleration of fetal heart rate and should not be used in obstetrics when maternal blood pressure exceeds 130/80 mmHg. It is not known what effect ephedrine may have on the newborn or on the child's later growth and development when administered to the mother just before or during labor.

►*Renal function impairment:* Initially, parenteral ephedrine may produce constriction of renal blood vessels and decreased urine formation.

►*Pregnancy: Category C.* It is unknown whether ephedrine can cause fetal harm when administered to a pregnant woman or can affect reproduction capacity. Give to a pregnant woman only if clearly needed.

►*Lactation:* Ephedrine is excreted in breast milk. Use by nursing mothers is not recommended.

Precautions

►*Cautious administration:* Administer with caution in patients with heart disease; coronary insufficiency; cardiac arrhythmias; angina pectoris; diabetes; hyperthyroidism; prostatic hypertrophy; hypertension; unstable vasomotor system or in patients on digitalis.

►*Prolonged use:* Prolonged use may produce a syndrome resembling an anxiety state.

Prolonged abuse of ephedrine can lead to symptoms of paranoid schizophrenia (eg, tachycardia, poor nutrition and hygiene, fever, cold sweat and dilated pupils).

►*Tolerance:* Although tolerance to ephedrine develops, addiction does not occur. Temporary cessation of medication restores the patient's original response to the drug.

►*Hypovolemia:* Use is not a substitute for the replacement of blood, plasma, fluids and electrolytes, which should be restored promptly when loss has occurred.

Drug Interactions

Ephedrine Drug Interactions			
Precipitant drug	Object drug *		Description
Ephedrine	Guanethidine	↓	The antihypertensive effects of guanethidine may be partially or totally reversed by the mixed-acting sympathomimetics.
Halogenated hydrocarbons	Ephedrine	↑	Halogenated anesthetics may sensitize the myocardium to the effects of catecholamines. Use of vasopressors may lead to serious arrhythmias; use with extreme caution.
Monoamine oxidase inhibitors (MAOIs)	Ephedrine	↑	MAOIs increase the pressor response to mixed-acting vasopressors. Possible hypertensive crisis and intracranial hemorrhage may occur. This interaction may also occur with **furazolidone,** an antimicrobial with MAO inhibitor activity. Avoid this combination; if given inadvertently and hypertension occurs, administer phentolamine.
Oxytocic drugs	Ephedrine	↑	In obstetrics, if vasopressor drugs are used either to correct hypotension or added to the local anesthetic solution, some oxytocic drugs may cause severe persistent hypertension.
Tricyclic antidepressants	Ephedrine	↓	The pressor response of the mixed-acting vasopressors may be decreased; a higher dose of the sympathomimetic may be necessary.

* ↑ = Object drug increased. ↓ = Object drug decreased.

Adverse Reactions

►*Cardiovascular:* Palpitation; tachycardia; precordial pain; cardiac arrhythmias.

►*CNS:* Headache; insomnia; sweating; nervousness; vertigo; confusion; delirium; restlessness; anxiety; tension; tremor; weakness; dizziness; hallucinations.

►*GI:* Nausea; vomiting; anorexia.

►*GU:* Vesical sphincter spasm resulting in difficult and painful urination; urinary retention may develop in males with prostatism.

EPHEDRINE

➤*Miscellaneous:* Respiratory difficulty; pallor.

Overdosage

➤*Symptoms:* The principal manifestation of ephedrine poisoning is convulsions. The following have occurred in acute poisoning: Nausea, vomiting, chills, cyanosis, irritability, nervousness, fever, suicidal behavior, tachycardia, dilated pupils, blurred vision, opisthotonos, spasms, convulsions, pulmonary edema, gasping respirations, coma and respiratory failure. Initially, the patient may have marked hypertension, followed later by hypotension accompanied by anuria. Large doses may lead to personality changes, with a psychological craving for the drug. Chronic use of ephedrine can also cause symptoms of tension and anxiety progressing to psychosis.

➤*Treatment:* Discontinue the drug. Remove the drug from the stomach by ipecac emesis, followed by activated charcoal or airway protected gastric lavage in depressed or hyperactive patients. If respirations are shallow or cyanosis is present, administer artificial respiration. Vasopressors are contraindicated. In cardiovascular collapse, maintain blood pressure.

For hypertension, 5 mg phentolamine mesylate diluted in saline may be administered slowly IV, or 100 mg may be given orally. Convulsions may be controlled by diazepam or paraldehyde. Cool applications and dexamethasone, 1 mg/kg, administered slowly IV, will control pyrexia.

MEPHENTERMINE SULFATE

Rx	**Wyamine Sulfate** (Wyeth-Ayerst)	**Injection:** 30 mg/mL	Parabens. In 10 mL.

Refer to the general discussion of these products in the Vasopressors Used in Shock group monograph.

Indications

Treatment of hypotension secondary to ganglionic blockade and that occurring with spinal anesthesia.

Although not recommended as corrective therapy for shock of hypotension secondary to hemorrhage, it may be used as an emergency measure to maintain blood pressure until blood or blood substitutes become available.

Administration and Dosage

Can be administered IM without irritation or abnormal tissue reaction. Injection of an undiluted parenteral solution containing 30 mg/mL, or a continuous infusion of a 1 mg/mL solution in 5% Dextrose in Water, directly into the vein, is the preferable route for treatment of shock. IV administration of undiluted mephentermine does not produce irritation and no untoward reaction will develop should extravasation occur.

➤*Shock and hypotension:* Dosage used in treatment of shock and hypotension is based on experimental observation that 0.5 mg/kg produces a positive inotropic action.

➤*Prevention of hypotension attendant to spinal anesthesia:* Administer 30 to 45 mg IM 10 to 20 minutes prior to anesthesia, operation or termination of the procedure.

➤*Hypotension following spinal anesthesia:* Administer 30 to 45 mg IV in a single injection. Repeat doses of 30 mg as necessary to maintain blood pressure. An immediate response and maintenance of blood pressure can be accomplished by the continuous IV infusion of a 0.1% solution of mephentermine in 5% Dextrose in Water (1 mg/mL). Regulate flow and duration of therapy according to patient response.

➤*Hypotension secondary to spinal anesthesia:* Administer an initial dose of 15 mg of mephentermine IV. This dose may be repeated if the response is not adequate.

➤*Treatment of shock following hemorrhage:* Although not recommended, the continuous IV infusion of a 0.1% solution of mephentermine in 5% Dextrose in Water may be useful in maintaining blood pressure until whole blood replacement can be accomplished.

➤*Preparation of IV solution:* The 0.1% solution can be prepared in the approximate concentration (0.115%) by adding 10 or 20 mL of mephentermine, 30 mg/mL, to 250 or 500 mL of 5% Dextrose in Water, respectively.

➤*Storage / Stability:* Store at room temperature, ≈ 25°C (77°F).

Actions

➤*Pharmacology:* Mephentermine sulfate is a mixed-acting sympathomimetic amine that acts both directly and indirectly (ie, releases norepinephrine). The increase in blood pressure produced by mephentermine is probably due primarily to an increase in cardiac output resulting from enhanced cardiac contraction; to a lesser degree, an increase in peripheral resistance due to peripheral vasoconstriction may also contribute to the elevation in blood pressure.

Mephentermine is metabolized in the liver by N-demethylation to normephentermine (or phentermine) with subsequent p–hydroxylation to p-hydroxynormephentermine (or p-hydroxyphentermine).

➤*Pharmacokinetics:* The duration of action is prolonged. Pressor response is evident 5 to 15 minutes after IM injection and has a duration of 1 to 2 hours. Following IV administration, the pressor response is almost immediate and persists for 15 to 30 minutes after the drug is discontinued.

The excretion rate of the drug and its metaboites is more rapid in an acidic urine and is only slightly influenced by urine output.

Contraindications

Hypersensitivity to the drug; hypotension induced by chlorpromazine, as the sympathomimetic amines will act to potentiate, rather than correct, the hypotension secondary to the adrenolytic effects of chlorpromazine; in combination with any MAOI (see Drug Interactions).

Warnings

➤*Cardiovascular disease:* Use mephentermine with caution in patients with known cardiovascular disease, and in chronically ill patients, as action on the cardiovascular system may be profound.

➤*Pregnancy: Category C.* Safety for use during pregnancy or in women of childbearing potential has not been established. Use only when clearly needed and when the potential benefits outweigh the potential hazards to the fetus. Mephentermine sulfate may increase uterine contractions especially during the third trimester of pregnancy.

➤*Lactation:* Safety for use during nursing has not been established. Use only when the potential benefits outweigh the potential hazards to the nursing infant.

➤*Children:* Safety and effectiveness have not been established.

Precautions

➤*Hypovolemia:* Use is not a substitute for the replacement of blood, plasma, fluids and electrolytes, which should be restored promptly when loss has occurred (ie, during or after surgery).

➤*Hemorrhagic shock:* Use with caution in treatment of shock secondary to hemorrhage. For effective emergency treatment, infuse 300 to 600 mg mephentermine in D5W. This will maintain blood pressure until volume replacement is accomplished.

➤*Hyperthyroidism:* Increased responsiveness to vasopressor agents may be seen.

➤*Hypertensive patients:* Administer with care to hypertensives.

Drug Interactions

Mephentermine Drug Interactions			
Precipitant drug	Object drug*		Description
Mephentermine	Guanethidine Reserpine	↓	The antihypertensive effects of guanethidine may be partially or totally reversed by the mixed-acting sympathomimetics.
Halogenated hydrocarbon anesthetics	Mephentermine	↑	Halogenated hydrocarbon anesthetics may sensitize the myocardium to the effects of catecholamines. Use of vasopressors may lead to serious arrhythmias; use with extreme caution.
Monoamine oxidase (MAO) inhibitors	Mephentermine	↑	MAOIs increase the pressor response to mixed-acting vasopressors. Possible hypertensive crisis and intracranial hemorrhage may occur. This interaction may also occur with **furazolidone**, an antimicrobial with MAO inhibitor activity. Avoid this combination; if given inadvertently and hypertension occurs, administer phentolamine.
Oxytocic drugs	Mephentermine	↑	In obstetrics, if vasopressor drugs are used either to correct hypotension or are added to the local anesthetic solution, some oxytocics may cause severe persistent hypertension.
Tricyclic antidepressants	Mephentermine	↓	The pressor response of the mixed-acting vasopressors may be decreased by these agents; a higher dose of the sympathomimetic may be necessary.

* ↑ = Object drug increased. ↓ = Object drug decreased.

Adverse Reactions

Side effects following administration are minimal and result from the central stimulatory effects. Following recommended doses, an occasional patient may display signs of anxiety. Cardiac arrhythmias may be produced and blood pressure may be raised excessively, particularly in patients with heart disease.

MEPHENTERMINE SULFATE

Overdosage

▶*Symptoms:* Effects of overdosage are an extension of the pharmacological activity of mephentermine. Cardiac contractility, cardiac output, systolic and diastolic blood pressure are usually raised. Other symptoms include hyperexcitability, prolonged wakefulness, weeping, incoherence, convulsions, flushing, tremor and hallucinations.

▶*Treatment:* Therapy of overdosage is symptomatic and supportive. Treat convulsions or cardiac arhythmias promptly if they occur. Because arrhythmias produced by mephentermine sulfate may be due to excessive beta-adrenergic stimulation, consider a beta-blocking agent such as propranolol.

METARAMINOL

Rx	Aramine (Merck)	Injection: 10 mg per mL (1%, as bitartrate)	In 10 mL vials.[1]

[1] With 0.15% methylparaben, 0.02% propylparaben and 0.2% sodium bisulfite.

Refer to the general discussion of these products in the Vasopressors Used in Shock group monograph.

Indications

Prevention and treatment of the acute hypotensive state occurring with spinal anesthesia; adjunctive treatment of hypotension due to hemorrhage; reactions to medications; surgical complications; shock associated with brain damage due to trauma or tumor.

▶*Probably effective:* As an adjunct in the treatment of hypotension due to cardiogenic shock or septicemia.

Administration and Dosage

May be given IM, SC or IV. Because the maximum effect is not immediately apparent, allow at least 10 minutes to elapse before increasing the dose. When the vasopressor is discontinued, observe the patient carefully so that therapy can be reinitiated promptly if the blood pressure falls too rapidly. The response to vasopressors may be poor in patients with coexistent shock and acidosis. Established methods of shock management and other measures directed to the specific cause of the shock state should also be employed.

▶*IM or SC injection (prevention of hypotension):* The recommended dose is 2 to 10 mg.

▶*IV infusion (adjunctive treatment of hypotension):* The recommended dose is 15 to 100 mg in 250 or 500 mL of Sodium Chloride Injection or 5% Dextrose Injection; adjust the rate of infusion to maintain the blood pressure at the desired level. Higher concentrations, 150 to 500 mg in 250 or 500 mL of infusion fluid, have been used. The concentration of drug in the infusion fluid may be adjusted depending on the patient's need for fluid replacement.

▶*Direct IV injection:* In severe shock, give by direct IV injection. The suggested dose is 0.5 to 5 mg, followed by an infusion of 15 to 100 mg in 250 to 500 mL of infusion fluid.

▶*Unlabeled route of administration:*

Endotracheal tube – If IV access is not available, the drug may be injected via the endotracheal tube. Perform five rapid insufflations; forcefully expel 5 mg diluted to a volume of 10 mL into the endotracheal tube; follow with five quick insufflations.

▶*Children:* 0.01 mg/kg as a single dose or a solution of 1 mg/25 mL in dextrose or saline.

▶*Admixture compatibility:* In addition to Sodium Chloride Injection and 5% Dextrose Injection, the following infusion solutions were found physically and chemically compatible with metaraminol when 5 mL (10 mg/mL) was added to 500 mL of infusion solution: Ringer's Injection, Lactated Ringer's Injection, 5% Dextran in Saline, *Normosol-R* pH 7.4, *Normosol-M* in 5% Dextrose Injection.

▶*Storage/Stability:* Avoid storage at temperatures below -20°C (-4°F) and above 40°C (104°F). Infusion solutions should be used within 24 hours.

Actions

▶*Pharmacology:* A potent sympathomimetic amine that increases both systolic and diastolic blood pressure, primarily by vasoconstriction; this effect is usually accompanied by a marked reflex bradycardia. Metaraminol has a direct effect on alpha-adrenergic receptors. It does not depend on release of norepinephrine but it has indirect activity. Prolonged infusions can deplete norepinephrine from sympathetic nerve endings. Repeated use may result in an overall diminution of sympathetic activity.

Renal, coronary and cerebral blood flow are a function of perfusion pressure and regional resistance. In most instances of cardiogenic shock, the beneficial effect of sympathomimetic amines is their positive inotropic effect. In patients with insufficient or failing vasoconstriction, there is additional advantage to the peripheral action of metaraminol, but in most patients with shock, vasoconstriction is adequate and any further increase is unnecessary. Therefore, blood flow to vital organs may decrease with metaraminol if regional resistance increases excessively. It increases cardiac output in hypotensive patients.

Metaraminol increases venous tone, causes pulmonary vasoconstriction and elevates pulmonary pressure even when cardiac output is reduced.

Pressor effect is decreased, but not reversed, by alpha-adrenergic blocking agents. When pressor responses are due primarily to vasoconstriction, cardiac stimulation may play a small role. Although uncommon, tachyphylaxis and a fall in blood pressure may occur with repeated use.

▶*Pharmacokinetics:* The pressor effect begins 1 to 2 minutes after IV infusion, ≈ 10 minutes after IM injection and 5 to 20 minutes after SC injection. The effect lasts from ≈ 20 minutes to 1 hour.

Contraindications

Do not use with cyclopropane or halothane anesthesia, unless clinical circumstances demand such use (see Drug Interactions); hypersensitivity to metaraminol.

Warnings

▶*Cardiac effects:* Metaraminol may cause cardiac arrhythmias. This may be particularly dangerous in patients with myocardial infarction or in patients who have received anesthetics that sensitize the heart to catecholamines (ie, cyclopropane, halothane, etc).

Prolonged administration may reduce the venous return and cardiac output and increase the work load of the heart.

▶*Pregnancy: Category C.* It is not known whether metaraminol can cause fetal harm when given to a pregnant woman or can affect reproductive capacity. Give metaraminol to a pregnant woman only if clearly needed.

▶*Lactation:* It is not known whether this drug is secreted in breast milk. Because many drugs are secreted in breast milk, exercise caution when giving metaraminol to a nursing woman.

▶*Children:* Safety and effectiveness have not been established.

Precautions

In heart or thyroid disease, hypertension or diabetes.

▶*Hypovolemia:* Use is not a substitute for the replacement of blood, plasma, fluids and electrolytes, which should be restored promptly when loss has occurred.

▶*Vasoconstriction:* When vasopressor amines are used for long periods, the resulting vasoconstriction may prevent adequate expansion of circulating volume and may perpetuate the shock state. Measurement of central venous pressure is useful in assessment of plasma volume. Therefore, employ blood or plasma volume expanders when circulating volume is decreased.

▶*Hypertension:* Avoid excessive blood pressure response. Rapidly induced hypertensive responses have been reported to cause acute pulmonary edema, arrhythmias and cardiac arrest.

▶*Cirrhosis:* Treat patients with cirrhosis cautiously and with adequate restoration of electrolytes if diuresis ensues. Fatal ventricular arrhythmia has been reported in one patient with Laennec's cirrhosis while receiving the drug. In several instances, ventricular extrasystoles that appeared during infusion subsided promptly when the rate of infusion was reduced.

▶*Cumulative effects:* Because of its prolonged action, a cumulative effect is possible, and with an excessive vasopressor response there may be a prolonged elevation of blood pressure, even with discontinuation. It is important to make frequent assessments of the blood pressure, particularly when administering IV.

▶*Extravasation:* Exercise care when selecting the site of administration of this drug, particularly when given by the IV route. The use of larger veins (the antecubital fossa or the thigh) is preferred. Avoid those of the ankle or dorsum of the hand, especially in patients with peripheral vascular disease, diabetes mellitus, Buerger's disease or hypercoagulability states. Extravasation may cause abscess formation, tissue necrosis and sloughing of surrounding tissue. Monitor the infusion site closely for free flow. Discontinue the infusion immediately if infiltration or thrombosis occurs.

Antidote for extravasation – To prevent sloughing and necrosis in ischemic areas, infiltrate area as soon as possible with 10 to 15 mL saline solution containing 5 to 10 mg phentolamine. Use a syringe with a fine hypodermic needle and infiltrate liberally throughout the ischemic area. Sympathetic blockade with phentolamine causes immediate and conspicuous local hyperemic changes if the area is infiltrated within 12 hours.

▶*Malaria:* Sympathomimetic amines may provoke a relapse in patients with a history of malaria.

▶*Sulfite sensitivity:* Some of these products contain sulfites that may cause allergic-type reaction (including anaphylactic symptoms and life-threatening or less severe asthmatic episodes) in certain susceptible persons. The overall prevalence of sulfite sensitivity in the general population is unknown and probably low. It is seen more frequently in asthmatic or atopic nonasthmatic persons.

METARAMINOL

Drug Interactions

Metaraminol Drug Interactions			
Precipitant drug	Object drug*		Description
Metaraminol	Guanethidine	↓	The antihypertensive effects of guanethidine may be partially or totally reversed by the mixed-acting sympathomimetics.
Digitalis glyco-sids	Metaraminol	↑	Use metaraminol with caution in digitalized patients, because the combination of digitalis and sympathomimetic amines may cause ectopic arrhythmias.
Halogenated hydrocarbon anesthetics	Metaraminol	↑	Halogenated hydrocarbon anesthetics may sensitize the myocardium to the effects of catecholamines. Use of vasopressors may lead to serious arrhythmias; use with extreme caution.
Monoamine oxidase (MAO) inhibitors	Metaraminol	↑	MAOIs increase the pressor response to mixed-acting vasopressors. Possible hypertensive crisis and intracranial hemorrhage may occur. This interaction may also occur with furazolidone, an antimicrobial with MAO inhibitor activity. Avoid this combination; if given inadvertently and hypertension occurs, administer phentolamine.
Oxytocic drugs	Metaraminol	↑	If vasopressor drugs are used in obstetrics to correct hypotension or added to the local anesthetic solution, some oxytocic drugs may cause severe persistent hypertension.

Metaraminol Drug Interactions			
Precipitant drug	Object drug*		Description
Tricyclic antide-pressants	Metaraminol	↓	The pressor response of the mixed-acting vasopressors may be decreased by these agents; a higher dose of the sympathomimetic may be necessary.

* ↑ = Object drug increased. ↓ = Object drug decreased.

Adverse Reactions

➤*Cardiovascular:* Sympathomimetic amines may cause sinus or ventricular tachycardia, or other arrhythmias, especially in patients with MI. Hypertension, hypotension following cessation of the drug, cardiac arrhythmias, cardiac arrest and palpitation have occurred.

➤*Miscellaneous:* Headache; flushing; sweating; tremors; dizziness; nausea; apprehension; abscess formation; tissue necrosis; sloughing at injection site.

Overdosage

Overdosage with metaraminol may cause convulsions, severe hypertension, headache, constricting sensation in the chest, nausea, vomiting, euphoria, diaphresis, pulmonary edema, tachycardia, bradycardia, sinus arrhythmia, atrial or ventricular arrhythmias, myocardial infarction, cardiac arrest, cerebral hemorrhage or cardiac arrhythmias. Patients with hyperthyroidism or hypertension are particularly sensitive to these effects. An appropriate antiarrhythmic agent may also be required.

PHENYLEPHRINE HCl

Rx	**Phenylephrine HCl** (Various, eg, American Regent)	**Injection:** 1% (10 mg/mL)	In 1 and 5 mL vials.
Rx	**Neo-Synephrine** (Sanofi Winthrop)		In 1 mL Uni-Nest amps.[1]

[1] With sodium bisulfite.

Refer to the general discussion of these products in the Vasopressors Used in Shock group monograph.

Indications

Treatment of vascular failure in shock, shock-like states, drug-induced hypotension, or hypersensitivity; to overcome paroxysmal supraventricular tachycardia; to prolong spinal anesthesia; as a vasoconstrictor in regional analgesia; to maintain an adequate level of blood pressure during spinal and inhalation anesthesia.

Administration and Dosage

Inject SC, IM, slow IV or in dilute solution as a continuous IV infusion. In patients with paroxysmal supraventricular tachycardia and, if indicated, in case of emergency, administer directly IV. Adjust dose according to the pressor response.

Phenylephrine Dosage Calculations		
Dose required (mg)	Phenylephrine 1% (mL)	Diluted phenylephrine[1] 0.1% (mL)
0.1	—	0.1
0.2	—	0.2
0.5	—	0.5
1	0.1	—
5	0.5	—
10	1	—

[1] For convenience in intermittent IV administration, dilute 1 mL phenylephrine 1% with 9 mL Sterile Water for Injection, USP.

➤*Mild or moderate hypotension:*

SC or IM – 2 to 5 mg (range, 1 to 10 mg). Do not exceed an initial dose of 5 mg. A 5 mg IM dose should raise blood pressure for 1 to 2 hours.

IV – 0.2 mg (range, 0.1 to 0.5 mg). Do not exceed an initial dose of 0.5 mg. Do not repeat injections more often than every 10 to 15 minutes. A 0.5 mg IV dose should elevate the pressure for ≈ 15 minutes.

To prepare a 0.1% solution of phenylephrine (0.1 mg/0.1 mL), dilute 1 mL of 1% solution with 9 mL Sterile Water for Injection.

➤*Severe hypotension and shock including drug-related hypotension:* Correct blood volume depletion as completely as possible before any vasopressor is administered. When intraaortic pressures must be maintained as an emergency measure to prevent cerebral or coronary artery ischemia, phenylephrine can be administered before and concurrently with blood volume replacement.

Hypotension and occasionally severe shock may result from overdosage or idiosyncratic reactions following administration of certain drugs, especially adrenergic and ganglionic blocking agents, rauwolfia, veratrum alkaloids and phenothiazine derivatives. Patients who receive a phenothiazine as preoperative medication are especially susceptible. As an adjunct in the management of such episodes, phenylephrine is a suitable agent for restoring blood pressure.

Higher initial and maintenance doses are required in patients with persistent or untreated severe hypotension or shock. Hypotension produced by powerful peripheral adrenergic blocking agents (chlorpromazine) or pheochromocytomectomy may also require more intensive therapy.

➤*Continuous infusion:* Add 10 mg to 250 or 500 mL of Dextrose Injection or Sodium Chloride Injection (providing a 1:25,000 or 1:50,000 dilution). To raise the blood pressure rapidly, start the infusion at ≈ 100 to 180 mcg/minute (based on 20 drops/mL, this would be 50 to 90 or 100 to 180 drops/minute). When the blood pressure is stabilized (at a low normal level for the individual), a maintenance rate of 40 to 60 mcg/minute usually suffices (based on 20 drops/mL, this would be 20 to 30 or 40 to 60 drops/minute). If the drop size of the infusion system varies from 20 drops/mL, adjust the dose accordingly.

If a prompt initial vasopressor response is not obtained, add additional increments of the drug (≥ 10 mg) to the infusion bottle. Adjust the flow rate until the desired blood pressure level is obtained. (A more potent vasopressor, such as norepinephrine, may be required.) Avoid hypertension. Check blood pressure frequently. Headache or bradycardia may indicate hypertension. Arrhythmias are rare.

➤*Spinal anesthesia:*

Hypotension – Administer SC or IM 3 or 4 minutes before injection of the spinal anesthetic. The total requirement for high anesthetic levels is usually 3 mg and, for lower levels, 2 mg. For hypotensive emergencies during spinal anesthesia, phenylephrine may be injected IV beginning with a dose of 0.2 mg. Any subsequent dose should not exceed the previous dose by > 0.1 to 0.2 mg; do not administer > 0.5 mg in a single dose.

Pediatric dose – To combat hypotension during spinal anesthesia in children, administer 0.5 to 1 mg/25 lbs, SC or IM.

Prolongation of spinal anesthesia – The addition of 2 to 5 mg phenylephrine to the anesthetic solution increases the duration of motor block by as much as 50% without an increase in the incidence of complications (eg, nausea, vomiting or blood pressure disturbances).

➤*Vasoconstrictor for regional analgesia:* Concentrations about 10 times those of epinephrine are recommended. The optimum strength is 1:20,000 (made by adding 1 mg phenylephrine to every 20 mL of local

PHENYLEPHRINE HCl

anesthetic solution). Some pressor responses may be expected when ≥ 2 mg are injected.

➤*Paroxysmal supraventricular tachycardia:* Rapid IV injection (within 20 to 30 seconds) is recommended; do not exceed an initial dose of 0.5 mg. Subsequent doses, which are determined by the initial blood pressure response, should not exceed the preceding dose by > 0.1 to 0.2 mg, and should never exceed 1 mg.

➤*Storage/Stability:* Protect from light.

Actions

➤*Pharmacology:* Phenylephrine is a powerful postsynaptic alpha-receptor stimulant with little effect on the beta receptors of the heart.

The predominant actions of phenylephrine are on the cardiovascular system. Parenteral administration causes a rise in systolic and diastolic pressures due to peripheral vasoconstriction. Accompanying the pressor response to phenylephrine is a marked reflex bradycardia that can be blocked by atropine; after atropine, large doses of the drug increase the heart rate only slightly. Cardiac output is slightly decreased, and peripheral resistance is considerably increased. Circulation time is slightly prolonged, and venous pressure is slightly increased; venous constriction is not marked. Most vascular beds are constricted; renal, splanchnic, cutaneous and limb blood flows are reduced, but coronary blood flow is increased. Pulmonary vessels are constricted, and pulmonary arterial pressure is raised.

The drug is a powerful vasoconstrictor with properties similar to those of norepinephrine but almost completely lacking the chronotropic and inotropic actions on the heart. Cardiac irregularities are seen rarely, even with large doses. In contrast to epinephrine and ephedrine, phenylephrine produces longer lasting vasoconstriction, a reflex bradycardia and increases the stroke output, producing no disturbance in the rhythm of the pulse.

In therapeutic doses, it produces little if any stimulation of either the spinal cord or cerebrum. An advantage is that repeated injections produce comparable effects.

Contraindications

Hypersensitivity to the drug; severe hypertension; ventricular tachycardia.

Warnings

➤*Pregnancy: Category C.* Safety for use during pregnancy has not been established. Use only when clearly needed and when the potential benefits outweigh the potential hazards to the fetus.

Labor and delivery – If used in conjunction with **oxytocic drugs**, the pressor effect of sympathomimetic pressor amines is potentiated.

➤*Lactation:* It is not known whether this drug is excreted in breast milk. Safety for use in the nursing mother has not been established. Because many drugs are excreted in breast milk, exercise caution when administering to a nursing woman.

Precautions

➤*Caution:* Use with extreme caution in elderly patients, patients with hyperthyroidism, bradycardia, partial heart block, myocardial disease or severe arteriosclerosis.

➤*Hypovolemia:* Use is not a substitute for the replacement of blood, plasma, fluids and electrolytes, which should be restored promptly when loss has occurred.

➤*Extravasation:* When infused, large veins of the antecubital fossa are preferred to veins in the hand or ankle to prevent extravasation. Extravasation may cause necrosis and sloughing of surrounding tissue. Monitor the infusion site closely for free flow.

Antidote for extravasation – To prevent sloughing and necrosis in ischemic areas, infiltrate area as soon as possible with 10 to 15 mL saline solution containing 5 to 10 mg phentolamine. Use a syringe with a fine hypodermic needle and infiltrate liberally throughout the ischemic area. Sympathetic blockade with phentolamine causes immediate and conspicuous local hyperemic changes if the area is infiltrated within 12 hours.

➤*Sulfite sensitivity:* Some of these products contain sulfites that may cause allergic-type reactions (including anaphylactic symptoms and life-threatening or less severe asthmatic episodes) in certain susceptible persons. The overall prevalence of sulfite sensitivity in the general population is unknown and probably low. It is seen more frequently in asthmatic or atopic nonasthmatic persons.

Drug Interactions

Phenylephrine Drug Interactions			
Precipitant drug	Object drug *		Description
Bretylium	Phenylephrine	↑	Bretylium may potentiate the action of vasopressors on adrenergic receptors, possibly resulting in arrhythmias.
Guanethidine	Phenylephrine	↑	Guanethidine may increase the pressor response of the direct-acting vasopressors, possibly resulting in severe hypertension.
Halogenated hydrocarbon anesthetics	Phenylephrine	↑	Halogenated hydrocarbon anesthetics may sensitize the myocardium to the effects of catecholamines. Use of vasopressors may lead to serious arrhythmias; use with extreme caution.
Monoamine oxidase inhibitors (MAOIs)	Phenylephrine	↑	MAOIs may significantly enhance the adrenergic effects of phenylephrine, and its pressor response may be increased 2- to 3-fold. Phenylephrine is metabolized by gut and liver MAO. This interaction may also occur with furazolidone, an antimicrobial with MAOI activity. Avoid this combination; if given inadvertently and hypertension occurs, administer phentolamine.
Oxytocic drugs	Phenylephrine	↑	If vasopressors are used in obstetrics to correct hypotension or are added to the local anesthetic solution, some oxytocics may cause severe persistent hypertension.
Tricyclic antidepressants	Phenylephrine	↔	Tricyclic antidepressants have both increased and decreased the sensitivity to IV phenylephrine.

* ↑ = Object drug increased. ↔ = Undetermined clinical effect.

Adverse Reactions

➤*Miscellaneous:* Headache; reflex bradycardia; excitability; restlessness; arrhythmias (rare).

Overdosage

➤*Symptoms:* Ventricular extrasystoles; short paroxysms of ventricular tachycardia; sensation of fullness in the head; tingling of the extremities.

➤*Treatment:* Relieve an excessive elevation of blood pressure by an α-adrenergic blocking agent (ie, phentolamine).

MIDODRINE HCl

Rx	ProAmatine (Shire)	Tablets: 2.5 mg	(RPC 2.5 003). White, scored. In 100s.
		5 mg	(RPC 5 004). Orange, scored. In 100s.
		10 mg	(RPC 10 007). Blue, scored. In 100s.

WARNING

Because midodrine can cause marked elevation of supine BP, use only in patients whose lives are considerably impaired despite standard clinical care. The indication for use of midodrine in the treatment of symptomatic orthostatic hypotension is based primarily on a change in a surrogate marker of effectiveness, an increase in systolic BP measured 1 minute after standing, a surrogate marker considered likely to correspond to a clinical benefit. Clinical benefits of midodrine, principally improved ability to carry out activities of daily living, have not been verified.

Indications

➤*Orthostatic hypotension (OH):* For the treatment of symptomatic OH. Use only in patients whose lives are considerably impaired despite standard clinical care.

➤*Unlabeled uses:* Management of stress urinary incontinence, treatment of retrograde ejaculation (used IV).

Administration and Dosage

➤*Approved by the FDA:* September 6, 1996.

The recommended dose of midodrine is 10 mg, 3 times/day. Have patient take dose during the daytime hours when upright, pursuing daily activities. A suggested dosing schedule of approximately 4-hour intervals is as follows: Shortly before or upon arising in the morning, midday, and late afternoon (not later than 6 pm). Doses may be given in 3-hour intervals, if required, to control symptoms. Do not give midodrine after the evening meal or less than 4 hours before bedtime. Because of the risk of supine hypertension, continue midodrine only in patients who appear to attain symptomatic improvement during initial treatment.

➤*Renal function impairment:* Starting dose is 2.5 mg (see Warnings).

➤*Storage/Stability:* Store at 25°C (77°F). Excursions permitted to 15° to 30°C (59° to 86°F).

Actions

➤*Pharmacology:* Midodrine is a prodrug. It forms an active metabolite by deglycination, desglymidodrine, that is an alpha₁ agonist, and exerts its actions via activation of the alpha-adrenergic receptors of the arteriolar and venous vasculature, producing an increase in vascular tone and an elevation of BP.

Administration of midodrine results in a rise in standing, sitting, and supine systolic and diastolic BP in patients with orthostatic hypotension of various etiologies. Standing systolic BP is elevated by about 15 to 30 mm Hg at 1 hour after a 10 mg dose of midodrine with some effect persisting for 2 to 3 hours.

➤*Pharmacokinetics:*

Absorption/Distribution – The plasma levels of the prodrug peak after about half an hour and decline with a half-life of approximately 25 minutes, while the metabolite reaches peak blood concentrations approximately 1 to 2 hours after a dose of midodrine and has a half-life of approximately 3 to 4 hours. The absolute bioavailability of midodrine is 93%. Neither midodrine nor desglymidodrine is significantly bound to plasma proteins. Desglymidodrine diffuses poorly across the blood-brain barrier.

Metabolism – It appears that deglycination of midodrine to desglymidodrine takes place in many tissues, and both compounds are metabolized in part by the liver.

Renal – Renal elimination of midodrine is insignificant. The renal clearance of desglymidodrine is 385 mL/min, approximately 80% by active renal secretion. It is possible that it occurs by the base-secreting pathway responsible for the secretion of other drugs that are bases (see Drug Interactions).

Contraindications

Severe organic heart disease; acute renal disease; urinary retention; pheochromocytoma; thyrotoxicosis; persistent and excessive supine hypertension (see Warnings).

Warnings

➤*Supine hypertension:* The most potentially serious adverse reaction associated with midodrine is supine hypertension. Systolic pressure of about 200 mm Hg was seen overall in about 13.4% of patients given 10 mg of midodrine. Systolic elevations of this degree were most likely to be observed in patients with relatively elevated pre-treatment systolic BPs (mean 170 mm Hg). Use of midodrine in such patients is not recommended. Sitting BPs were also elevated by midodrine therapy. Monitor supine and sitting BPs in patients beginning maintenance on midodrine.

Supine hypertension can often be controlled by preventing the patient from becoming fully supine (eg, sleeping with the head of the bed elevated).

➤*Urinary retention:* Use midodrine cautiously in patients with urinary retention problems because desglymidodrine acts on the alpha-adrenergic receptors of the bladder neck.

➤*Renal function impairment:* Desglymidodrine is eliminated via the kidneys, and higher blood levels would be expected in such patients. Use midodrine with caution in patients with renal impairment, a lower starting dose may be necessary (see Administration and Dosage). Assess renal function prior to initial use of midodrine.

➤*Hepatic function impairment:* Use midodrine with caution in patients with hepatic impairment, as the liver has a role in the metabolism of midodrine.

➤*Pregnancy: Category C.* Midodrine increased the rate of embryo resorption, reduced fetal body weight in rats and rabbits, and decreased fetal survival in rabbits when given in doses 13 (rat) and 7 (rabbit) times the maximum human dose based on body surface area (mg/m²). There are no adequate and well-controlled studies in pregnant women. Use midodrine during pregnancy only if the potential benefit justifies the potential risk to the fetus.

➤*Lactation:* It is not known whether this drug is excreted in breast milk. Because many drugs are excreted in breast milk, exercise caution when administering to a nursing woman.

➤*Children:* Safety and effectiveness in pediatric patients have not been established.

Precautions

➤*Monitoring:* Evaluate renal and hepatic function prior to initiating therapy and subsequently, as appropriate.

Monitor supine and sitting BPs in patients beginning maintenance on midodrine.

Monitor BP carefully when midodrine is used concomitantly with other agents that cause vasoconstriction.

➤*Heart rate:* A slight slowing of the heart rate may occur after administration of midodrine, primarily because of vagal reflex. If any signs or symptoms suggesting bradycardia (pulse slowing, increased dizziness, syncope) occur, discontinue midodrine and re-evaluate.

➤*Special risk:* Use midodrine with caution in patients with orthostatic hypotension who are also diabetic, those with a history of visual problem, or who are taking fludrocortisone acetate (see Drug Interactions), which is known to cause an increase in intraocular pressure and glaucoma.

Drug Interactions

Midodrine Drug Interactions			
Precipitant drug	Object drug*		Description
Alpha-adrenergic blocking agent (eg, prazosin, terazosin, doxazosin)	Midodrine	↓	Alpha-adrenergic antagonist agents can antagonize the effects of midodrine.
Metformin, H₂ antagonists, procainamide, triamterene, flecainide, quinidine	Midodrine	↔	There may be a potential for interactions with these drugs (see Actions).
Phenylephrine, pseudoephedrine, ephedrine, dihydroergotamine	Midodrine	↑	The use of drugs that stimulate alpha-adrenergic agonists may enhance or potentiate the pressor effects of midodrine.
Midodrine	Cardiac glycosides, psycho-pharmacologics, beta-blockers	↑	When coadministered with midodrine, cardiac glycosides, psycho-pharmacologic agents, or beta-blockers may enhance or precipitate bradycardia, A-V block, or arrhythmia (see Precautions).
Midodrine	Steroid therapy (eg, fludrocortisone)	↑	Concomitant use may increase the risk of supine hypertension. Reduce the dose of fludrocortisone or decrease the salt intake prior to initiation of treatment with midodrine. Fludrocortisone also causes an increase in intraocular pressure and glaucoma (see Precautions).

* ↑ = Object drug increased. ↓ = Object drug decreased. ↔ = Undetermined clinical effect.

MIDODRINE HCl

Adverse Reactions

The most frequent adverse reactions were as follows: supine and sitting hypertension; paresthesia and pruritus, mainly of the scalp; goosebumps; chills; urinary urge; urinary retention; urinary frequency.

The most potentially serious adverse reaction associated with midodrine therapy is supine hypertension.

Midodrine Adverse Events (%)		
Adverse reaction	Placebo n = 88	Midodrine n = 82
Paresthesia[1]	4.5	18.3
Piloerection	0	13.4
Dysuria[2]	0	13.4
Pruritus[3]	2.3	12.2
Supine hypertension[4]	0	7.3
Chills	0	4.9
Pain[5]	0	4.9
Rash	1.1	2.4

[1] Includes hyperesthesia and scalp paresthesia.
[2] Includes dysuria (1), increased urinary frequency (2), impaired urination (1), urinary retention (5), urinary urgency (2).
[3] Includes scalp pruritus.
[4] Includes patients who experienced an increase in supine hypertension.
[5] Includes abdominal pain and pain increase.

►*Miscellaneous:*
Less frequent – Headache; feeling of pressure/fullness in the head; vasodilation/flushing face; confusion/abnormal thinking; dry mouth; nervousness/anxiety; rash.

Rare – Visual field defect; dizziness; skin hyperesthesia; insomnia; somnolence; erythema multiforme; canker sore; dry skin; dysuria; impaired urination; asthenia; backache; pyrosis; nausea; GI distress; flatulence; leg cramps.

Overdosage

►*Symptoms:* The symptoms of overdose may include hypertension, piloerection (goosebumps), a sensation of coldness and urinary retention.

There are 2 reported cases of overdosage with midodrine, both in young males. They ingested between 205 and 250 mg of midodrine, and both recovered without sequelae.

►*Treatment:* Emesis and administration of alpha-sympatholytic drugs (eg, phentolamine). Desglymidodrine is dialyzable.

Patient Information

Caution patient to report symptoms of supine hypertension immediately. Symptoms may include cardiac awareness, pounding in the ears, headache, blurred vision, etc. Advise patient to discontinue the medication immediately if supine hypertension persists.

Caution patients about certain OTC products, such as cold remedies and diet aids, that can elevate BP.

Advise patients to avoid taking the dose if they are to be supine for any length of time. Advise patients to take the last dose 3 to 4 hours before bedtime to minimize night time hypertension.

SODIUM POLYSTYRENE SULFONATE

Rx	SPS (Carolina Medical Products Co.)	**Suspension:** 15 g per 60 mL. Sodium content 1.5 g (65 mEq).	With 21.5 mL sorbitol solution (equivalent to 20 g sorbitol) and 0.3% alcohol per 60 mL, propylene glycol, sodium saccharin and methyl- and propylparabens. Cherry flavor. In 120, 480 mL, and UD 60 mL.
Rx	Sodium Polystyrene Sulfonate (Roxane)	**Suspension:** 15 g per 60 mL.	With 14.1 g sorbitol and 0.1% alcohol per 60 mL. In 60, 120, 200, and 500 mL.
Rx	Kayexalate (Sanofi Winthrop)	**Powder:** Finely powdered sodium polystyrene sulfonate. Sodium content ≈ 100 mg (4.1 mEq) per g.	In 1 lb jars.
Rx	Kionex (Paddock)	**Powder:** Finely ground sodium polystyrene sulfonate (4 level tsp = ≈ 15 g). Sodium content ≈ 100 mg (4.1 mEq) per g.	In 454 g.

Indications

➤*Hyperkalemia:* Treatment of hyperkalemia.

Administration and Dosage

Individualize dosage.

➤*Oral:*

Adults – The average dose is 15 to 60 g, best provided by administering 15 g, 1 to 4 times daily.

Children – In smaller children and infants, employ lower doses by using the exchange ratio of 1 mEq potassium per gram of resin as the basis for calculation. A dose of approximately 1 g/kg every 6 hours has been recommended.

➤*Oral suspension (powdered formula):* Give each dose as a suspension in water, or for greater palatability, in syrup. The amount of fluid usually ranges from 20 to 100 mL, depending on the dose, or 3 to 4 mL/g resin. Use sorbitol to combat constipation.

➤*Nasogastric tube:* The resin may be introduced into the stomach through a plastic tube and, if desired, mixed with a diet appropriate for a patient with renal failure.

A sodium polystyrene sulfonate candy has been used successfully.†

➤*Enema:* Although less effective, the resin may be given in a daily enema consisting (for adults) of 30 to 50 g every 6 hours. After an initial cleansing enema, insert a soft, large (French 28) rubber tube into the rectum for a distance of about 20 cm, with the tip well into the sigmoid colon, and tape in place. Suspend the resin in the appropriate amount of aqueous vehicle (eg, 100 mL sorbitol or 20% Dextrose in Water) at body temperature and introduce by gravity, while the particles are kept in suspension by stirring. Flush the suspension with 50 or 100 mL of fluid (to make a total fluid of 150 to 200 mL) and then clamp the tube and leave in place. If back leakage occurs, elevate the hips on pillows or assume a knee-chest position temporarily. A somewhat thicker suspension may be used, but take care that no paste is formed, because the latter has a greatly reduced exchange surface and will be ineffective if deposited in the rectal ampulla. Keep the suspension in the sigmoid colon for several hours, if possible. Retention times of at least 30 minutes have been recommended. Then, irrigate the colon with a nonsodium-containing solution at body temperature to remove the resin. Two quarts of flushing solution may be necessary. Drain the returns constantly through a Y-tube connection.

➤*Preparation and storage:* Store at 15° to 30°C (59° to 86°F). Dispense in tight containers. Store repackaged product in refrigerator and use within 14 days of repackaging. Freshly prepare suspensions; do not store beyond 24 hours. Do not heat since this may alter the exchange properties of the resin.

Actions

➤*Pharmacology:* Sodium polystyrene sulfonate is a cation exchange resin used for the reduction of elevated potassium levels. As the resin passes along the intestine, or is retained in the colon after administration by enema, the sodium ions are partially released and are replaced by potassium ions. This action occurs primarily in the large intestine. The efficiency of this process is limited and unpredictable. Although the exchange capacity in vitro approximates 3.1 mEq potassium per gram, in vivo it is approximately 33%, or 1 mEq potassium per gram; however, the range is so large that electrolyte balance must be monitored. Onset of action after oral administration ranges from 2 to 12 hours, and is longer after rectal administration.

Warnings

➤*Severe hyperkalemia:* Since effective lowering of serum potassium may take hours to days, treatment with this drug alone may be insufficient to rapidly correct severe hyperkalemia associated with states of rapid tissue breakdown (eg, burns, renal failure) or hyperkalemia so marked as to constitute a medical emergency. Consider other definitive measures, including the use of IV calcium to antagonize the effects of hyperkalemia on the heart, IV sodium bicarbonate or glucose and insulin to cause an intracellular shift of potassium, or dialysis.

➤*Hypokalemia:* Serious potassium deficiency can occur. Carefully control by frequent serum potassium determinations within each 24-hour period. Since intracellular potassium deficiency is not always reflected by serum potassium levels, determine the level at which treatment should be discontinued based on the patient's clinical condition and ECG. Early clinical signs of severe hypokalemia include irritable confusion and delayed thought processes. It is often associated with a lengthened QT interval, widening, flattening or inversion of the T wave and prominent U waves. Cardiac arrhythmias may occur, such as premature atrial, nodal and ventricular contractions, and supraventricular and ventricular tachycardias. Toxic effects of digitalis are likely to be exaggerated. Severe muscle weakness, at times extending into paralysis, may also occur.

➤*Electrolyte imbalance:* Sodium polystyrene sulfonate is not totally selective for potassium, and small amounts of other cations (magnesium and calcium) can also be lost during treatment. Accordingly, monitor patients for all applicable electrolyte disturbances.

Precautions

➤*Sodium:* Use caution when administering to patients who cannot tolerate even a small increase in sodium loads (ie, severe congestive heart failure, severe hypertension, marked edema). One gram contains 100 mg (4.1 mEq) sodium, with about one-third being delivered to the body. Compensatory restriction of sodium intake from other sources may be indicated.

➤*Constipation:* Constipation, if it occurs, is treated with 10 to 20 mL of 70% sorbitol every 2 hours or as needed to produce one or two watery stools daily. This measure also reduces any tendency toward fecal impaction.

Drug Interactions

➤*Antacids/Laxatives:* Systemic alkalosis has occurred after cation exchange resins were administered orally in combination with nonabsorbable cation donating antacids and laxatives (eg, magnesium hydroxide, aluminum carbonate). Do not administer magnesium hydroxide with sodium polystyrene sulfonate. A grand mal seizure has occurred in one patient with chronic hypocalcemia of renal failure who was given sodium polystyrene sulfonate with magnesium hydroxide as a laxative. The simultaneous oral administration of sodium polystyrene sulfonate with these drugs may reduce the resin's potassium exchange capability. The effects of this interaction have only been demonstrated in patients with renal failure.

Adverse Reactions

➤*Electrolyte disturbance:* Hypokalemia; hypocalcemia; sodium retention.

➤*GI:* Gastric irritation; anorexia, nausea, vomiting and constipation may occur, especially with high doses. Occasionally, diarrhea develops. Large doses in elderly individuals may cause fecal impaction, which may be obviated through use of the resin in enemas. Intestinal obstruction, due to concretions of aluminum hydroxide when used in combination with sodium polystyrene sulfonate, has occurred.

† *Am J Hosp Pharm.* 1978;35:1034-1035.

EDETATE DISODIUM

Rx	**Edetate Disodium** (Various, eg, McGuff, Schein)	**Injection:** 150 mg/mL	In 20 mL vials.
Rx	**Endrate** (Abbott)		In 20 mL amps.

WARNING

Use of this drug is recommended only when the severity of the clinical condition justifies the aggressive measures associated with this type of therapy.

Indications

➤*Hypercalcemia:* Emergency treatment of hypercalcemia.

➤*Ventricular arrhythmias:* Control of ventricular arrhythmias associated with digitalis toxicity.

➤*Unlabeled uses:*

Chelation treatment – Chelation treatment is not indicated for atherosclerotic vascular diseases. Although it has been advocated for these diseases (eg, coronary artery disease, cerebrovascular disease, peripheral vascular disease) based on the theory of decalcification of atherosclerotic plaques, both the proposed explanations of pathogenesis and mechanism of action are suspect. In addition, edetate disodium (EDTA) is not innocuous. The medical community generally agrees that chelation therapy is not an acceptable treatment for atherosclerotic vascular diseases.

Administration and Dosage

➤*Adults:* Administer 50 mg/kg/day to a maximum dose of 3 g in 24 hours. Dissolve dose in 500 mL of 5% Dextrose Injection or 0.9% Sodium Chloride Injection. Infuse over ≥ 3 hours and do not exceed the patient's cardiac reserve. A suggested regimen includes five consecutive daily doses followed by 2 days without medication; repeat this regimen as necessary, up to 15 doses.

➤*Children:* Administer 40 mg/kg/day (18 mg/lb/day) to a maximum dose of 70 mg/kg/day. Dissolve in a sufficient volume of 5% Dextrose Injection or 0.9% Sodium Chloride Injection to bring the final concentration to not more than 3%. Infuse over ≥ 3 hours; do not exceed the patient's cardiac reserve.

➤*Storage/Stability:* Store at room temperature.

Actions

➤*Pharmacokinetics:* EDTA forms chelates with many divalent and trivalent metals. Because of its affinity for calcium, EDTA will lower serum calcium levels during IV infusion. Slow infusion may cause mobilization of extracirculatory calcium stores. The chelate formed is excreted in the urine. EDTA exerts a negative inotropic effect on the heart.

Additionally, EDTA forms chelates with other polyvalent metals, thus increasing urinary excretion of magnesium, zinc and other trace elements. It does not chelate with potassium, but may reduce the serum level; increased potassium excretion may occur.

Contraindications

Anuria; hypersensitivity to any component of the preparation.

Warnings

➤*Rapid IV infusion:* Rapid IV infusion or a high serum concentration of EDTA may cause a precipitous drop in serum calcium and may result in death. Toxicity depends on total dosage and rate of administration. Do not exceed recommended dosage and rates of administration.

➤*Dilution:* Dilution before infusion is necessary because of EDTA's irritant effect on the tissues and because of the danger of serious side effects.

➤*Calcium:* The oxalate method of determining serum calcium tends to give low readings in the presence of EDTA; modification (eg, acidifying the sample) or use of a different method may be required for accuracy. The least interference will be noted immediately before a subsequent dose is administered.

➤*Hypokalemia:* Use with caution in patients with clinical or subclinical potassium deficiency; monitor serum potassium levels and ECG changes.

➤*Diabetics:* Blood sugar and insulin requirements may be lower in insulin-dependent diabetics.

➤*Hypomagnesemia:* Consider the possibility of hypomagnesemia during prolonged therapy.

➤*Renal function impairment:* Prior to treatment, assess renal excretory function; perform periodic BUN and creatinine determinations and daily urinalysis during treatment.

➤*Pregnancy: Category C.* Safety for use during pregnancy has not been established. Use only when clearly needed and when the potential benefits outweigh the potential hazards to the fetus.

➤*Lactation:* Safety for use during breastfeeding has not been established.

Precautions

➤*Monitoring:* Because of the possibility of inducing an electrolyte imbalance during treatment, perform appropriate laboratory determinations to evaluate cardiac status. Repeat as often as clinically indicated, particularly in patients with ventricular arrhythmia and those with a history of seizures or intracranial lesions. If clinical evidence suggests any disturbance of liver function during treatment, perform appropriate laboratory determinations; withdraw drug if required.

➤*Postural hypotension:* After infusion, have the patient remain supine for a short time because of the possibility of postural hypotension.

➤*Cardiac effects:* Consider the possibility of an adverse effect on myocardial contractility when administering the drug to patients with heart disease. Use this drug cautiously in patients with limited cardiac reserve or incipient congestive failure.

Adverse Reactions

➤*CNS:* Transient circumoral paresthesia, numbness and headache.

➤*GI:* Nausea, vomiting and diarrhea (fairly common).

➤*Miscellaneous:* Transient drop in systolic and diastolic blood pressure; thrombophlebitis; febrile reactions; hyperuricemia; anemia; exfoliative dermatitis; other toxic skin and mucous membrane reactions. Nephrotoxicity and damage to the reticuloendothelial system with hemorrhagic tendencies have been reported with excessive dosages.

Overdosage

Because EDTA may produce a precipitous drop in serum calcium, have an IV calcium salt (such as calcium gluconate) available. Exercise extreme caution in the use of IV calcium in the treatment of tetany, especially in digitalized patients, because the action of the drug and the replacement of calcium ions may produce a reversal of the desired digitalis effect.

CARDIOPLEGIC SOLUTION

Rx   **Plegisol** (Abbott)   **Solution:** 17.6 mg calcium chloride dihydrate, 325.3 mg magnesium chloride hexahydrate, 119.3 mg potassium chloride and 643 mg sodium chloride per 100 mL (approx. 260 mOsm/L)   In single dose 1000 mL flexible plastic container.

Indications

With ischemia and hypothermia, induces cardiac arrest during open heart surgery.

Administration and Dosage

The following information is a guide:

Following institution of cardiopulmonary bypass at perfusate temperatures of 28° to 30°C, (82° to 86°F) and cross-clamping of the ascending aorta, administer the buffered solution by rapid infusion into the aortic root. The initial rate of infusion may be 300 mL/m^2/minute (about 540 mL/min in a 1.8 meter, 70 kg adult with 1.8 square meters of surface area) given for 2 to 4 minutes. Concurrent external cooling (regional hypothermia of the pericardium) may be accomplished by instilling a refrigerated (4°C) physiologic solution such as *Normosol-R* (balanced electrolyte replacement solution) or Ringer's Injection into the chest cavity. If myocardial electromechanical activity persists or recurs, the solution may be reinfused at a rate of 300 mL/m^2/min for 2 minutes. Repeat every 20 to 30 minutes or sooner if myocardial temperature rises above 15° to 20°C or returning cardiac activity is observed. The regional hypothermia solution around the heart also may be replenished continuously or periodically in order to maintain adequate hypothermia. Suction may be used to remove warmed infusates. An implanted thermistor probe may be used to monitor myocardial temperature.

The volumes of solution instilled into the aortic root may vary depending on the duration or type of open heart surgical procedure.

➤*Preparation of solution:* The solution contains no preservatives and is intended only for a single operative procedure. After adjusting pH with sodium bicarbonate, extemporaneous alternative buffering is not recommended. Discard the unused portion.

Add 10 mL (840 mg) of 8.4% Sodium Bicarbonate Injection (10 mEq each of sodium and bicarbonate) to each 1000 mL of the cardioplegic solution just prior to administration to adjust pH to approximately 7.8 when measured at room temperature. Use of any other Sodium Bicarbonate Injection may not achieve this pH due to the varying pH's of Sodium Bicarbonate Injections. Cool the buffered solution with added sodium bicarbonate to 4°C prior to administration and use within 24 hours of mixing.

➤*Admixture incompatibility:* Additives may be incompatible. Consult with pharmacist, if possible. When introducing additives, use aseptic technique, mix thoroughly and do not store.

➤*Storage / Stability:* Store at 25°C (77°F); however, brief exposure up to 40°C (104°F) does not adversely affect the product. Protect from freezing and extreme heat.

Actions

➤*Pharmacology:* Cardioplegic solution with added sodium bicarbonate, when cooled and instilled into the coronary artery vasculature, causes prompt arrest of cardiac electromechanical activity, combats intracellular ion losses and buffers ischemic acidosis. When used with hypothermia and ischemia, the action may be characterized as cold ischemic potassium-induced cardioplegia. This provides a quiet, relaxed heart and bloodless field of operation. The component electrolytes and their physiologic effects are listed below:

➤*Pharmacokinetics:*

Calcium (Ca^{++}) ion – Maintains integrity of cell membrane to ensure against calcium paradox during reperfusion.

Magnesium (Mg^{++}) ion – May help stabilize the myocardial membrane by inhibiting a myosin phosphorylase, which protects adenosine triphosphate (ATP) reserves for postischemic activity. The protective effects of magnesium and potassium are additive.

Potassium (K^{++}) ion – Causes prompt cessation of mechanical myocardial contractile activity. The immediacy of the arrest thus preserves energy supplies for postischemic contractile activity in diastole.

Chloride (Cl-) and sodium (Na$^+$) ions – Sodium is essential to maintain ionic integrity of myocardial tissue. Chloride ions maintain the electroneutrality of the solution and have no specific role in the production of cardiac arrest.

Bicarbonate (HCO$_3$-) anion – Acts as a buffer to render the solution slightly alkaline and compensate for the metabolic acidosis that accompanies ischemia.

Contraindications

Do not administer without the addition of 8.4% Sodium Bicarbonate Injection.

Not for IV injection; only for instillation into cardiac vasculature.

Warnings

Only those trained to perform open heart surgery should use this solution. It is intended only for use during cardiopulmonary bypass when the coronary circulation is isolated from the systemic circulation.

Right heart venting is recommended. If large volumes of cardioplegic solution are infused and allowed to return to the heart lung machine without any venting from the right heart, plasma magnesium and potassium levels may rise. Development of severe hypotension and metabolic acidosis while on bypass has occurred when large volumes (8 to 10 L) of solution are instilled and allowed to enter the pump and then the systemic circulation.

➤*Pregnancy: Category C.* Safety for use during pregnancy has not been established. Use only when clearly needed and when the potential benefits outweigh the potential hazards to the fetus.

Precautions

Monitor myocardial temperature during surgery to maintain hypothermia.

Continuous ECG monitoring of myocardial activity during the procedure is essential.

Appropriate equipment to defibrillate the heart following cardioplegia and inotropic agents during postoperative recovery should be readily available.

Do not administer unless solution is clear and container is undamaged.

Adverse Reactions

Potential hazards of open heart surgery include myocardial infarction, ECG abnormalities and arrhythmias, including ventricular fibrillation. Spontaneous recovery may be delayed or absent when circulation is restored. Defibrillation by electric shock may be required to restore normal cardiac function.

Overdosage

Overzealous instillation may result in unnecessary dilatation of the myocardial vasculature and leakage into the perivascular myocardium, possibly causing tissue edema.

ALPROSTADIL (Prostaglandin E₁; PGE₁)

| *Rx* | **Prostin VR Pediatric** (Upjohn) | **Injection:** 500 mcg/mL[1] | In 1 mL amps. |

[1] In 1 mL dehydrated alcohol.

WARNING

Apnea occurs in about 10% to 12% of neonates with congenital heart defects treated with alprostadil. Apnea is most often seen in neonates weighing less than 2 kg at birth and usually appears during the first hour of drug infusion. Monitor respiratory status throughout treatment; have ventilatory assistance immediately available.

Indications

For palliative, not definitive, therapy to temporarily maintain the patency of the ductus arteriosus until corrective or palliative surgery can be performed in neonates who have congenital heart defects and who depend upon the patent ductus for survival. Such defects include pulmonary atresia or stenosis, tricuspid atresia, tetralogy of Fallot, interruption of the aortic arch, coarctation of the aorta or transposition of the great vessels with or without other defects.

Administration and Dosage

The preferred administration route is continuous IV infusion into a large vein. Alternatively, the drug may be administered through an umbilical artery catheter placed at the ductal opening. Increases in blood pO₂ have been the same by either route.

Begin infusion with 0.05 to 0.1 mcg/kg/minute. A starting dose of 0.1 mcg/kg/min is recommended; however, adequate clinical response has been reported using a starting dose of 0.05 mcg/kg/min. After a therapeutic response is achieved (increased pO₂ in infants with restricted pulmonary blood flow or increased systemic blood pressure and blood pH in infants with restricted systemic blood flow), reduce the infusion rate to the lowest dosage that maintains the response. This may be accomplished by reducing the dosage from 0.1 to 0.05 to 0.025 to 0.01 mcg/kg/minute. If response to 0.05 mcg/kg/minute is inadequate, dosage can be increased up to 0.4 mcg/kg/minute, although in general, higher infusion rates do not produce greater effects.

➤*Preparation of solution:* Dilute 500 mcg alprostadil with Sodium Chloride Injection or Dextrose Injection. Dilute to volumes appropriate for the pump delivery system available. Discard and prepare fresh infusion solutions every 24 hours.

Sample Dilutions and Infusion Rates to Provide a Dosage of 0.1 mcg/kg/min		
Add 500 mcg alprostadil to:	Approximate concentration of resulting solution (mcg/mL)	Infusion rate (mL/min/kg)
250 mL	2	0.05
100 mL	5	0.02
50 mL	10	0.01
25 mL	20	0.005

➤*Storage/Stability:* Refrigerate at 2° to 8°C (35° to 46°F).

Actions

➤*Pharmacology:* Alprostadil (prostaglandin E₁) produces vasodilation, inhibits platelet aggregation and stimulates intestinal and uterine smooth muscle; IV doses of 1 to 10 mcg/kg lower the blood pressure in mammals by decreasing peripheral resistance. Reflex increases in cardiac output and rate accompany the reduction in blood pressure.

Smooth muscle of the ductus arteriosus, especially sensitive to alprostadil, relaxes in the presence of the drug. These effects are beneficial in infants who have congenital defects which restrict the pulmonary or systemic blood flow and who depend on a patent ductus arteriosus for adequate blood oxygenation and lower body perfusion.

In infants with restricted pulmonary blood flow, about 50% responded to alprostadil infusion with at least 10 mmHg increase in blood pO₂ (mean increase about 14 mmHg and mean increase in oxygen saturation about 23%). In general, patients who responded best had low pretreatment blood pO₂ and were 4 days old or less.

The increase in blood oxygenation is inversely proportional to pretreatment pO₂ values; patients with a low pO₂ respond best, and patients with a pO₂ ≥ 40 mmHg usually have little response.

In infants with restricted systemic blood flow, alprostadil often increased pH in those with acidosis. It also increased systemic blood pressure and decreased the ratio of pulmonary artery pressure to aortic pressure.

➤*Pharmacokinetics:* Alprostadil is rapidly metabolized. As much as 80% may be metabolized in one pass through the lungs, primarily by oxidation. Metabolites are excreted primarily by the kidneys, and excretion is essentially complete within 24 hours. No unchanged alprostadil has been found in the urine, and there is no evidence of tissue retention.

Contraindications

None known.

Warnings

Administer only by trained personnel in facilities that provide pediatric intensive care.

Precautions

➤*Monitoring:* Arterial pressure should be monitored intermittently by umbilical artery catheter, auscultation or with a Doppler transducer. If arterial pressure falls significantly, decrease the infusion rate immediately.

In infants with restricted pulmonary blood flow, measure efficacy of alprostadil by monitoring blood oxygenation. To measure efficacy in infants with restricted systemic blood flow, monitor systemic blood pressure and blood pH.

➤*Skeletal effects:* Cortical proliferation of the long bones has been observed in infants during long-term infusions of alprostadil. This regressed after drug withdrawal.

➤*Duration of infusion:* Infuse for the shortest time and at the lowest dose that will produce the desired effects. Weigh the risks of long-term infusion against the possible benefits that critically ill infants may derive from its administration.

➤*Hemostatic effects:* Because alprostadil inhibits platelet aggregation, use cautiously in neonates with bleeding tendencies.

➤*Respiratory distress syndrome:* Do not use alprostadil in respiratory distress syndrome. Make a differential diagnosis between respiratory distress syndrome (hyaline membrane disease) and cyanotic heart disease (restricted pulmonary blood flow). If full diagnostic facilities are not immediately available, cyanosis (pO₂ less than 40 mmHg) and restricted pulmonary blood flow apparent on an X-ray are appropriate indicators of congenital heart defects.

Adverse Reactions

➤*Cardiovascular:* Flushing (10%, more common after intra-arterial dosing); bradycardia (7%); hypotension (4%); tachycardia (3%); cardiac arrest, edema (1%); congestive heart failure, hyperemia, second degree heart block, shock, spasm of the right ventricle infundibulum, supraventricular tachycardia and ventricular fibrillation (< 1%).

➤*CNS:* Fever (14%); seizures (4%); cerebral bleeding, hyperextension of the neck, hyperirritability, hypothermia, jitteriness, lethargy and stiffness (< 1%).

➤*GI:* Diarrhea (2%); gastric regurgitation and hyperbilirubinemia (< 1%).

➤*Hematologic:* Disseminated intravascular coagulation (1%); anemia, bleeding and thrombocytopenia (< 1%).

➤*Renal:* Anuria and hematuria (< 1%).

➤*Respiratory:* Apnea (12%); bradypnea, bronchial wheezing, hypercapnia, respiratory depression, respiratory distress and tachypnea (< 1%).

➤*Miscellaneous:* Sepsis (2%); hypokalemia (1%); peritonitis, hypoglycemia and hyperkalemia (< 1%); cortical proliferation of the long bones.

Overdosage

➤*Symptoms:* Apnea, bradycardia, pyrexia, hypotension and flushing.

➤*Treatment:* If apnea or bradycardia occurs, discontinue infusion and provide appropriate medical treatment. Use caution in restarting the infusion. If pyrexia or hypotension occurs, reduce the infusion rate until symptoms subside. Flushing is usually a result of incorrect intra-arterial catheter placement; reposition catheter.

INDOMETHACIN SODIUM TRIHYDRATE

| *Rx* | **Indocin I.V.** (Merck) | **Powder for Injection:** 1 mg (as sodium trihydrate) | In single dose vials. |

Indications

For closure of a hemodynamically significant patent ductus arteriosus in premature infants weighing between 500 and 1750 g if, after 48 hours, usual medical management is ineffective. Clinical evidence of a hemodynamically significant patent ductus arteriosus should be present (ie, respiratory distress, a continuous murmur, a hyperactive precordium, cardiomegaly and pulmonary plethora on chest x–ray).

➤*Unlabeled uses:* Indomethacin IV has been used prophylactically to reduce the incidence of symptomatic patent ductus arteriosus in premature infants with a high probability of developing this condition; a single dose of 0.2 mg/kg 24 hours after birth has been used. However, no study has shown a significant decrease in neonatal morbidity.

Administration and Dosage

For IV use only.

A course of therapy is defined as 3 IV doses given at 12 to 24 hour intervals.

➤*Renal impairment:* If anuria or marked oliguria (urinary output < 0.6 mL/kg/hr) is evident at the scheduled time of the second or third dose, do not give additional doses until laboratory studies indicate that renal function has returned to normal.

Dosage According to Age			
	Dose (mg/kg)		
Age at 1st dose	1st	2nd	3rd
< 48 hours	0.2	0.1	0.1
2-7 days	0.2	0.2	0.2
> 7 days	0.2	0.25	0.25

If the ductus arteriosus closes or is significantly reduced in size after 48 hours or more from completion of the first course, no further doses are necessary. If the ductus arteriosus reopens, a second course of 1 to 3 doses may be given, each dose separated by a 12 to 24 hour interval as described above.

If the infant remains unresponsive to therapy after 2 courses, surgery may be necessary. If severe adverse reactions occur, stop the drug.

➤*Preparation of solution:* Prepare with 1 to 2 mL of Sodium Chloride Injection 0.9% or Water for Injection. All diluents should be preservative free (ie, without benzyl alcohol). If 1 mL of diluent is used, the concentration of indomethacin ≈ 0.1 mg/0.1 mL; if 2 mL of diluent is used, the concentration of the solution ≈ 0.05 mg/0.1 mL. Discard any unused portion of the solution. Prepare a fresh solution just prior to each administration. Once reconstituted, inject IV over 5 to 10 seconds.

Further dilution with IV infusion solutions is not recommended.

Actions

➤*Pharmacology:* Indomethacin sodium trihydrate is an injectable formulation of indomethacin used for closure of a patent ductus arteriosus in premature infants. Indomethacin is a potent inhibitor of prostaglandin synthesis, both in vitro and in vivo. The exact mechanism of action through which indomethacin causes closure of a patent ductus arteriosus is unknown, but it is believed to be through inhibition of prostaglandin synthesis.

In double-blind, placebo controlled studies of 460 preterm infants who weighed < 1750 g, those treated with IV indomethacin had a 75% to 80% closure rate, thus avoiding surgery.

➤*Pharmacokinetics:* Plasma half-life is variable among premature infants and varies inversely with postnatal age and weight. In a study of 28 infants, the plasma half-life of those less than 7 days old averaged 20 hours; in infants older than 7 days, the mean plasma half-life was 12 hours. The mean plasma half-life was 21 hours in infants weighing < 1000 g and 15 hours in those weighing > 1000 g.

Following IV administration in adults, indomethacin is eliminated via renal excretion, metabolism and biliary excretion, and it undergoes appreciable enterohepatic circulation. The mean plasma half-life of indomethacin is 4.5 hours; in the absence of enterohepatic circulation, it is 90 minutes.

Contraindications

Proven or suspected untreated infection; bleeding, especially active intracranial hemorrhage or GI bleeding; thrombocytopenia; coagulation defects; necrotizing enterocolitis; significant renal impairment; congenital heart disease patients in whom patency of the ductus arteriosus is necessary for satisfactory pulmonary or systemic blood flow (eg, pulmonary atresia, severe tetralogy of Fallot, severe coarctation of aorta).

Warnings

➤*GI effects:* Minor GI bleeding (ie, chemical detection of blood in the stool) has been reported.

➤*Hemorrhage:* Prematurity per se is associated with an increased incidence of spontaneous intraventricular hemorrhage. Indomethacin may inhibit platelet aggregation and increase the potential for intraventricular bleeding.

➤*Electrolyte balance:* Indomethacin may suppress water excretion to a greater extent than sodium excretion. Perform serum electrolyte determinations and monitor renal function during therapy.

➤*Renal function impairment:* Indomethacin may cause significant reduction in urine output (50% or more) with concomitant elevations of BUN and creatinine and reductions in glomerular filtration rate and creatinine clearance. In most infants, these effects are transient and disappear with cessation of therapy. Indomethacin may precipitate renal insufficiency, including acute renal failure, especially in infants with other conditions that may adversely affect renal function during therapy.

When significant suppression of urine volume occurs after a dose, do not give additional doses until urine output returns to normal levels.

Precautions

➤*Infection:* Indomethacin may mask the usual signs and symptoms of infection. Use with extra care in the presence of existing controlled infection.

➤*Hepatic effects:* Severe hepatic reactions have been reported in adults treated chronically with oral indomethacin. If clinical signs and symptoms consistent with liver disease develop in the neonate, or if systemic manifestations occur, discontinue the drug.

Avoid extravascular injection or leakage; the solution may irritate tissue.

Drug Interactions

➤*Aminoglycosides:* In one study of premature infants treated with indomethacin IV and also receiving either gentamicin or amikacin, both peak and trough levels of these aminoglycosides were significantly elevated.

➤*Digitalis:* In premature infants, the half-life of digitalis may be further prolonged, due to reduced renal function during therapy with indomethacin.

Frequent ECGs and serum digitalis levels may be required to prevent or detect digitalis toxicity early.

➤*Furosemide:* Indomethacin may blunt furosemide's natriuretic effect; this is attributed to inhibition of prostaglandin synthesis. In 19 premature infants with patent ductus arteriosus, infants receiving both agents had significantly higher urinary output, higher levels of sodium and chloride excretion and higher glomerular filtration rates than did infants receiving indomethacin alone. Data suggest furosemide helped to maintain renal function in the premature infant when indomethacin was added.

Adverse Reactions

Coagulation – Decreased platelet aggregation. There was greater incidence of bleeding problems (ie, gross or microscopic bleeding into the GI tract, oozing from skin after needle stick, pulmonary hemorrhage, disseminated intravascular coagulopathy).

➤*Renal:* Renal dysfunction in 41% of infants, including one or more of the following: Oliguria; reduced urine sodium, chloride or potassium, urine osmolality, free water clearance or glomerular filtration rate; elevated serum creatinine or BUN; uremia.

➤*Cardiovascular:* Pulmonary hypertension.

➤*GI:* GI bleeding (3% to 9%); vomiting, abdominal distention, transient ileus, localized perforation of small or large intestines (1% to 3%).

➤*Metabolic:* Hyponatremia; elevated serum potassium (3% to 9%); hypoglycemia, fluid retention (1% to 3%).

➤*The following adverse reactions have also been reported in infants treated with indomethacin; however, a causal relationship has not been established:*

Cardiovascular – Intracranial bleeding (3% to 9%); bradycardia (< 3%).

Respiratory – Apnea; exacerbation of preexisting pulmonary infection.

Metabolic – Acidosis/alkalosis.

GI – Necrotizing enterocolitis.

Ophthalmic – Retrolental fibroplasia (3% to 9%).

Additional adverse reactions have been reported with oral indomethacin. Relevance to the preterm neonate receiving indomethacin IV is unknown.

Indications

Treatment of small, uncomplicated varicose veins of the lower extremities.

Sclerosing agents may be useful as a supplement to venous ligation to obliterate residual varicosed veins or in patients who have conditions which increase the risk of surgery. Ineffective sclerotherapy may decrease the potential success of later surgery.

➤*Morrhuate sodium:* This has been used for the treatment of internal hemorrhoids; there is no substantial evidence for this indication.

➤*Unlabeled uses:* Sclerosing agents have been used to treat esophageal varices, introduced via a flexible fiberoptic esophagoscope.

Actions

➤*Pharmacology:* These agents are mild sclerosing drugs used in the treatment of varicose veins. They produce their effect by irritation and inflammation of the venous intimal endothelium and formation of a thrombus. This blood clot occludes the injected vein and fibrous tissue develops, resulting in the obliteration of the vein.

Morrhuate sodium is a mixture of the sodium salts of the saturated and unsaturated fatty acids of cod liver oil.

Contraindications

Hypersensitivity to any component of these drugs; acute superficial thrombophlebitis; underlying arterial disease; varicosities caused by abdominal and pelvic tumors; uncontrolled diabetes mellitus; sepsis; blood dyscrasia; thyrotoxicosis; tuberculosis; neoplasms; asthma; acute respiratory or skin diseases; any condition which causes the patient to be bedridden; extensive injection treatment in patients who are severely debilitated or senile; an unusual local reaction at the injection site or any systemic reaction; persistent occlusion of deep veins.

Delay treatment if there is any acute local or systemic infection, including infected ulcers.

Do not use if there is significant valvular or deep venous incompetence.

Warnings

➤*Anaphylactoid and allergic reactions:* Anaphylactoid and allergic reactions have occurred. Anaphylactoid reactions may occur within a few minutes after the injection and are most likely to occur when therapy is reinstituted after several weeks. Refer to Management of Acute Hypersensitivity Reactions.

➤*Pregnancy:* Safety for use during pregnancy has not been established. Use only when clearly needed and when the potential benefits outweigh the potential hazards to the fetus.

Precautions

Do not undertake sclerotherapy for the treatment of varicosities unless valvular competency and deep vein patency and competency are determined. Perform the Trendelenburg test, Perthes' test and angiography. Because of the danger of extension of thrombosis into the deep veins, perform a thorough preinjection evaluation for valvular competence and slowly inject a small amount (not more than 2 mL) of the preparation into the varicosity. Necrosis may result from direct injection of sclerosing agents.

Initially treat most patients with symptomatic primary varicosed veins with compression stockings. If this treatment is inadequate, surgery may be required.

For IV use only. Inadvertent intra-arterial injection may result in severe ischemic damage.

Adverse Reactions

➤*Local:* Burning; cramping sensations; urticaria; tissue sloughing and necrosis may occur with extravasation (morrhuate).

➤*Hypersensitivity:* Dizziness; weakness; vascular collapse; asthma; respiratory depression; GI disturbances (ie, nausea and vomiting); urticaria (see Warnings) (rare).

➤*Miscellaneous:* Postoperative sloughing can occur.

Pulmonary embolism has occurred. Drowsiness and headache may occur rarely with morrhuate.

ETHANOLAMINE OLEATE

| *Rx* | **Ethamolin**
(Questcor) | Injection: 5% | In 2 mL amps.[1] |

[1] With 2% benzyl alcohol.

Refer to the general discussion of these products in the Sclerosing Agents group monograph.

Indications

Treatment of patients with esophageal varices that have recently bled, to prevent rebleeding.

Not indicated for the treatment of patients with esophageal varices that have not bled.

Administration and Dosage

Local ethanolamine oleate injection sclerotherapy of esophageal varices should be performed by physicians who are familiar with an acceptable technique.

➤*IV dose:* Usual IV dose is 1.5 to 5 mL per varix.

➤*Maximum total dose per treatment session:* Should not exceed 20 mL or 0.4 mL/kg for a 50 kg patient. Patients with significant liver dysfunction (Child Class C) or concomitant cardiopulmonary disease should usually receive less than the recommended maximum dose.

Submucosal injections are not recommended as they are reportedly more likely to result in ulceration at the site of injection.

To obliterate the varix, injections may be made at the time of the acute bleeding espisode and then after 1 week, 6 weeks, 3 months and 6 months as indicated.

➤*Storage / Stability:* Store at controlled room temperature 15° to 30°C (59° to 86°F). Protect from light.

Actions

➤*Pharmacology:* Ethanolamine oleate is a mild sclerosing agent. When injected IV, it acts primarily by irritation of the intimal endothelium of the vein and produces a sterile dose-related inflammatory response. This results in fibrosis and occlusion of the vein. Ethanolamine oleate also rapidly diffuses through the venous wall and produces a dose-related extravascular inflammatory reaction.

The oleic acid component of ethanolamine oleate is responsible for the inflammatory response, and may also activate coagulation in vivo by release of tissue factor and activation of Hageman factor. The ethanolamine component, however, may inhibit fibrin clot formation by chelating calcium, so that a procoagulant action of ethanolamine oleate has not been demonstrated.

➤*Pharmacokinetics:* Ethanolamine oleate disappears from the injection site within 5 minutes via the portal vein. When volumes larger than 20 mL are injected, some ethanolamine oleate also flows into the azygos vein through the periesophageal vein. Within 4 days after injection, there is neutrophil infiltration of the esophageal wall and hemorrhage within 6 days. Granulation tissue is first seen at 10 days, red

thrombi obliterating the varices by 20 days, and sclerosis of the varices by 2½ months. Sclerosis of esophageal varices will be a delayed rather than an immediate effect of the drug.

In dogs, ethanolamine oleate 1 mL/kg injected into the right atrium over 1 minute increases extravascular lung water. The concentration of ethanolamine oleate reaching the lung in human treatment will be less than in the dog studies, but pleural effusions, pulmonary edema, pulmonary infiltration and pneumonitis have occurred. Minimize the total per session dose, especially in those with concomitant cardiopulmonary disease.

Contraindications

Hypersensitivity to ethanolamine, oleic acid or ethanolamine oleate.

Warnings

Sclerotherapy with ethanolamine oleate has no beneficial effect upon portal hypertension, the cause of esophageal varices, so that recanalization and collateralization may occur, necessitating reinjection.

➤*Varicosities of the leg:* Use of ethanolamine oleate injection is not supported by adequately controlled clinical trials and is not recommended.

➤*Hypersensitivity reactions:* Fatal anaphylactic shock was reported following injection of a larger than normal volume of ethanolamine oleate injection into a male who had a known allergic disposition. There are only three reports of anaphylaxis. Be prepared to treat anaphylaxis appropriately. In emergencies, administer 0.25 mL of a 1:1000 IV solution of epinephrine (0.25 mg); control allergic reactions with antihistamines. Have epinephrine 1:1000 immediately available. Refer to Management of Acute Hypersensitivity Reactions.

➤*Pregnancy: Category C.* It is not known whether ethanolamine oleate injection can cause fetal harm when administered to a pregnant woman or can affect reproduction capacity. Give to pregnant women only if clearly needed.

➤*Lactation:* It is not known whether this drug is excreted in breast milk. Exercise caution when ethanolamine oleate is administered to a nursing woman.

➤*Children:* Safety and efficacy in children have not been established. In one study, 21 children with esophageal varices were treated with ethanolamine oleate via an endotracheal tube using 2 to 5 mL injection per varix to a maximum of 20 mL. Variceal obliteration occurred in 18 of the children.

Precautions

➤*Renal failure:* Acute renal failure with spontaneous recovery followed injections of 15 to 20 mL in two women.

➤*Severe injection necrosis:* Severe injection necrosis may result from direct injection of sclerosing agents, especially if excessive vol-

ETHANOLAMINE OLEATE

umes are used. At least one fatal case of extensive esophageal necrosis and death has occurred. The drug should be administered by physicians who are familiar with an acceptable injection technique.

➤*Child Class C:* These patients are more likely to develop esophageal ulceration than those in Classes A and B. Complications of ulceration, necrosis and delayed esophageal perforation appear to occur more frequently when ethanolamine oleate is injected submucosally. This route is not recommended.

➤*Concomitant cardiorespiratory disease:* Careful monitoring and minimization of the total dose per session is recommended.

➤*Fatal aspiration pneumonia:* Has occurred in elderly patients undergoing esophageal variceal sclerotherapy with ethanolamine oleate. It appears to be procedure-related rather than drug-related, but as aspiration of blood or stomach contents is not uncommon in patients with bleeding esophageal varices, take special precautions to prevent its occurrence, especially in the elderly and critically ill subjects.

Adverse Reactions

The frequency of complications/adverse events per injection session was 13%.

Most common – Pleural effusion/infiltration (2.1%); esophageal ulcer (2.1%); pyrexia (1.8%); retrosternal pain (1.6%); esophageal stricture (1.3%); pneumonia (1.2%).

Local esophageal reactions – Pleural effusion/infiltration (2.1%); esophageal ulcer (2.1%); esophageal stricture (1.3%); esophagitis, tearing of the esophagus, sloughing of the mucosa overlying the injected varix, necrosis, periesophageal abscess and perforation (0.1% to 0.4%) (see Precautions). These complications appear to be dependent upon the dose and the patient's clinical state.

➤*Miscellaneous:* Pyrexia (1.8%); retrosternal pain (1.6%); fatal aspiration pneumonia (see Precautions); pneumonia (1.2%); bacteremia; anaphylactic shock (see Warnings); acute renal failure with spontaneous recovery (see Precautions). Spinal cord paralysis due to occlusion of the anterior spinal artery has been reported in one child 8 hours after ethanolamine oleate sclerotherapy.

Overdosage

Overdosage of ethanolamine oleate injection can result in severe intramural necrosis of the esophagus; complications have resulted in death. The minimum lethal dose of ethanolamine oleate injection administered IV to rabbits is 130 mg/kg.

MORRHUATE SODIUM

Rx	**Morrhuate Sodium** (Pasadena Research Labs)	**Injection:** 50 mg/mL	In 30 mL multiple use vials.
Rx	**Scleromate** (Palisades Pharm.)		In 5 mL amps, 10 mL vials, 10 mL fill in 20 mL vials.

Complete prescribing information for these products begins in the Sclerosing Agents group monograph.

Administration and Dosage

For IV use only. Avoid extravasation. Dosage depends on the size and degree of varicosity.

➤*To determine possible sensitivity:* 0.25 to 1 mL of 5% injection into a varicosity 24 hours before administration of a large dose.

➤*Usual adult dose for obliteration of small or medium veins:* 50 to 100 mg (1 to 2 mL). *For large veins:* 150 to 250 mg (3 to 5 mL). The drug may be given as multiple injections at one time or in single doses. Therapy may be repeated at 5 to 7 day intervals, according to the patient's response.

Following injection, the vein promptly becomes hard and swollen for 2 to 4 inches, depending on the size and response of the vein. After

24 hours, the vein is hard and slightly tender to the touch (with little or no periphlebitis). The skin around the injection becomes light-bronze; this color usually disappears quickly. An aching sensation and feeling of stiffness usually occurs and lasts approximately 48 hours.

When small veins are injected, or the injection solution is cold, or when solid matter has separated in the solution, warm the ampul or vial by immersing in hot water. The solution should become clear on warming; use only a clear solution that contains no solid matter. Because the solution froths easily, use a large bore needle to fill the syringe; however, use a small bore needle for the injection.

➤*Storage / Stability:* Store below 40°C (104°F); refrigerate preferably between 15° and 30°C (59° and 86°F).

PHENAZOPYRIDINE HCl (Phenylazo Diamino Pyridine HCl)

otc	**Azo-Standard** (Alcon)	**Tablets:** 95 mg	(W). In 30s.
otc	**Prodium** (Breckenridge)		In 12s and 30s.
Rx	**Phenazopyridine HCl** (Various, eg, Moore, Parmed, URL)	**Tablets:** 100 mg	In 100s, 1000s and UD 100s.
otc	**Baridium** (Pfeiffer)		In 32s.
Rx	**Geridium** (Goldline)		Burgundy. Sugar coated. In 100s and 1000s.
Rx	**Pyridiate** (Rugby)		In 100s.
Rx	**Pyridium** (Parke-Davis)		Sucrose, lactose. (WC 180). Maroon. In 100s, 1000s and UD 100s.
Rx	**Urogesic** (Edwards)		In 100s.
Rx	**UTI Relief** (Consumers Choice Systems)	**Tablets:** 97.2 mg	In 12s.
Rx	**Pyridium Plus** (Warner Chilcott)	**Tablets:** 150 mg	0.3 mg hyoscyamine HBr, 15 mg butabarbital. Lactose. (WC 182). Dk. Maroon. Coated. In 30s and 100s.
Rx	**Phenazopyridine HCl** (Various, eg, Moore, Parmed, URL)	**Tablets:** 200 mg	In 100s, 1000s and UD 100s.
Rx	**Geridium** (Goldline)		Burgundy. Sugar coated. In 100s.
Rx	**Pyridium** (Parke-Davis)		Sucrose, lactose. (P-D 181). Maroon. In 100s, 1000s and UD 100s.

Urinary analgesics in combination with urinary anti-infectives are listed in the Anti-Infectives chapter.

Indications

▶*Symptomatic relief:* Symptomatic relief of pain, burning, urgency, frequency and other discomforts arising from irritation of the lower urinary tract mucosa caused by infection, trauma, surgery, endoscopic procedures or passage of sounds or catheters. Its analgesic action may reduce or eliminate the need for systemic analgesics or narcotics.

Administration and Dosage

Do not use chronically to treat undiagnosed pain of the urinary tract. Such use could lead to serious delays in appropriate diagnosis and treatment. This product treats painful symptoms but does not treat the source or cause of the disorder causing the pain.

▶*Adults:* 200 mg 3 times/day after meals. Do not administer for > 2 days when used concomitantly with an antibacterial agent for the treatment of UTI.

▶*Children (6 to 12 years):* 12 mg/kg/day divided into three oral doses for 2 days.

▶*Storage/Stability:* Store at controlled room temperature 15° to 30°C (59° to 86°F).

Actions

▶*Pharmacology:* Phenazopyridine, an azo dye, is excreted in the urine where it exerts a topical analgesic effect on urinary tract mucosa; therefore, use only for relief of symptoms. Its mechanism of action is unknown. Phenazopyridine is compatible with antibacterial therapy and can help relieve pain and discomfort before antibacterial therapy controls the infection.

▶*Pharmacokinetics:* Phenazopyridine is rapidly excreted by the kidneys; 65% is excreted unchanged in urine.

Contraindications

Hypersensitivity to phenazopyridine; renal insufficiency.

Warnings

▶*Carcinogenesis:* Long-term administration of phenazopyridine has induced neoplasia in rats (large intestine) and mice (liver).

▶*Pregnancy: Category B.* There are no adequate and well controlled studies in pregnant women. Use during pregnancy only if clearly needed.

▶*Lactation:* No information is available on the appearance of this drug or its metabolites in breast milk.

▶*Children:* Do not give to children < 12 years of age unless directed by physician.

Precautions

▶*Skin/sclera discoloration:* A yellowish tinge of the skin or sclera may indicate accumulation because of impaired renal excretion; discontinue therapy if this occurs.

▶*Duration of therapy:* Treatment of a urinary tract infection (UTI) with phenazopyridine should not exceed 2 days because there is a lack of evidence that the combined administration of phenazopyridine and an antibacterial provides greater benefit than administration of the antibacterial alone after 2 days.

Drug Interactions

▶*Drug/Lab test interactions:* As an azo dye, phenazopyridine may interfere with urinalysis based on spectrometry or color reactions.

Adverse Reactions

Headache; rash; pruritus; occasional GI disturbances; anaphylactoid-like reaction; methemoglobinemia; hemolytic anemia; renal and hepatic toxicity (usually at overdosage levels); staining of contact lenses.

Overdosage

▶*Symptoms:* Exceeding the recommended dose in patients with good renal function or administering the usual dose to patients with impaired renal function (common in elderly patients), may lead to increased serum levels and toxic reactions. Methemoglobinemia generally follows a massive, acute overdose. Oxidative Heinz body hemolytic anemia may occur, and "bite cells" (degmacytes) may be present in chronic overdosage. Red blood cell G-6-PD deficiency may predispose the patient to hemolysis. Renal and hepatic impairment and failure, usually because of hypersensitivity, may also occur.

▶*Treatment:* Methylene blue 1 to 2 mg/kg IV (see individual monograph) or 100 to 200 mg ascorbic acid orally should cause prompt reduction of methemoglobinemia and disappearance of cyanosis. Refer to General Management of Acute Overdosage.

Patient Information

May cause GI upset; take after meals.

May cause a reddish orange discoloration of the urine and may stain fabric. This is not abnormal and represents no cause for alarm. Staining of contact lenses has also occurred.

Do not use long-term to treat undiagnosed urinary tract pain. This product treats painful symptoms but not the source or cause of the pain.

PENTOSAN POLYSULFATE SODIUM

Rx	**Elmiron** (Baker Norton)	**Capsule:** 100 mg	(BNP7600). White. In 100s.

Indications

▶*Interstitial cystitis:* The relief of bladder pain or discomfort associated with interstitial cystitis.

Administration and Dosage

The recommended dose of pentosan polysulfate sodium is 300 mg/day taken as one 100 mg capsule orally 3 times daily. Take with water ≥ 1 hour before or 2 hours after meals.

▶*Storage/Stability:* Store at controlled room temperature 15° to 30°C (59° to 86°F).

Actions

▶*Pharmacology:* Pentosan polysulfate sodium is a low molecular weight heparin-like compound. It has anticoagulant and fibrinolytic effects. The mechanism of action of pentosan polysulfate sodium in interstitial cystitis is not known. Pentosan polysulfate adheres to the bladder wall mucosal membrane and may act as a buffer to control cell permeability preventing irritating solutes in the urine from reaching the cells.

▶*Pharmacokinetics:*

Absorption – Pentosan polysulfate sodium absorption is ≈ 3% of the administered dose.

Distribution – Pentosan polysulfate sodium distributes to the uroepithelium of the GU tract with lesser amounts found in the liver, spleen, lung, skin, periosteum and bone marrow. Erythrocyte penetration is low in animals.

Metabolism – Sixty-eight percent of the dose at ≈ 1 hour after IV administration undergoes partial desulfation in the liver and spleen. Partial depolymerization occurs in the kidney. Both the desulfation and depolymerization can be saturated with continued dosing.

Excretion – The elimination half-life of pentosan polysulfate sodium has a mean value at 24 hours after IV injection of 40 mg. The elimination half-life in urine following oral pentosan polysulfate sodium is 4.8 hours for the unchanged drug. Urinary excretion averages 3.5% of the administered dose. After multiple doses of pentosan polysulfate sodium, urine excretion of radioactivity averaged 11% of the administered dose.

PENTOSAN POLYSULFATE SODIUM

▶*Clinical trials:* Unblinded evaluations of 2499 patients were made every 3 months for the patients' rating of overall change in pain in comparison to baseline and for the difference calculated in "pain/discomfort" scores. At baseline, pain/discomfort scores for the 2499 patients were severe or unbearable in 60%, moderate in 33% and mild or none in 7% of patients. At 3 months, 722/2499 (29%) of the patients originally in the study had pain scores that improved by one or two categories. By 6 months, in the 892 patients who continued taking pentosan polysulfate sodium, an additional 116/2499 (5%) of patients had improved pain scores. After 6 months, the percent of patients who reported the first onset of pain relief was < 1.5% of patients who originally entered in the study.

Contraindications

Hypersensitivity to the drug, structurally related compounds or excipients.

Warnings

▶*Alopecia:* Alopecia is associated with pentosan polysulfate sodium and with heparin products. Alopecia may begin within the first 4 weeks of treatment. Ninety-seven percent of the cases of alopecia reported were alopecia areata, limited to a single area on the scalp.

▶*Anticoagulant effects:* Pentosan polysulfate sodium is a weak anticoagulant (1/15 the activity of heparin). It inhibits the generation of factor Xa in plasma and inhibits thrombin-induced platelet aggregation in human platelet-rich plasma ex vivo. Bleeding complications of ecchymosis, epistaxis and gum hemorrhage have been reported. Evaluate patients undergoing invasive procedures or having signs/symptoms of underlying coagulopathy or other increased risk of bleeding (because of other therapies such as coumarin anticoagulants, heparin, t-PA, streptokinase or high dose aspirin) for hemorrhage. Also evaluate patients with diseases such as aneurysms, thrombocytopenia, hemophilia, GI ulcerations, polyps or diverticula before starting pentosan polysulfate sodium.

▶*Hepatic/Splenic function impairment:* Pentosan is desulfated by both the liver and the spleen. The extent to which hepatic insufficiency or splenic disorders may increase the bioavailability of the parent or active metabolites of pentosan polysulfate sodium is not known. Exercise caution when using pentosan polysulfate sodium in these patients. (Increases in PTT and PT [< 1% for both] or thrombocytopenia [0.2%] were noted).

▶*Hepatotoxicity:* Mildly (< 2.5 × normal) elevated transaminase, alkaline phosphatase, γ-glutamyl transpeptidase and lactic dehydrogenase occurred in 1.2% of patients. The increases usually appeared 3 to 12 months after the start of pentosan polysulfate sodium therapy and were not associated with jaundice or other clinical signs or symptoms. These abnormalities are usually transient, may remain essentially unchanged or may rarely progress with continued use.

▶*Pregnancy: Category B.* Animal studies did not reveal evidence of impaired fertility or harm to the fetus from pentosan polysulfate sodium. Adequate and well controlled studies have not been performed in pregnant women. Because animal studies are not always predictive of human response, use this drug in pregnancy only if clearly needed.

▶*Lactation:* It is not known whether this drug is excreted in breast milk. Exercise caution when pentosan polysulfate sodium is administered to a nursing woman.

▶*Children:* Safety and effectiveness in patients < 16 years old have not been established.

Precautions

▶*Monitoring:* Reassess patients after 3 months. If improvement has not occurred and if limiting adverse events are not present, pentosan polysulfate sodium may be continued for another 3 months.

▶*Thrombocytopenia:* A similar product that was given subcutaneously, sublingually or intramuscularly (and not initially metabolized by the liver) is associated with delayed immunoallergic thrombocytopenia with symptoms of thrombosis and hemorrhage. Exercise caution when using pentosan polysulfate sodium in patients who have a history of heparin-induced thrombocytopenia.

Adverse Reactions

▶*CNS:* Headache (3%); severe emotional liability/depression (2%); dizziness (1%); insomnia (≤ 1%).

▶*Dermatologic:* Alopecia (4%); rash (3%); pruritus, urticaria (≤ 1%).

▶*GI:* Diarrhea, nausea (4%); abdominal pain, dyspepsia (2%); anorexia, colitis, constipation, esophagitis, flatulence, gastritis, gum hemorrhage, mouth ulcer, vomiting (≤ 1%).

▶*Hematologic:* Increased partial thromboplastin time, increased prothrombin time, anemia, ecchymosis, leukopenia, thrombocytopenia (≤ 1%).

▶*Hypersensitivity:* Allergic reaction, photosensitivity (≤ 1%).

▶*Respiratory:* Epistaxis, dyspnea, pharyngitis, rhinitis (≤ 1%).

▶*Special senses:* Amblyopia, conjunctivitis, optic neuritis, retinal hemorrhage, tinnitus (≤ 1%).

▶*Miscellaneous:* Liver function abnormalities (1%; see Warnings).

Overdosage

Overdose has not been reported. Based upon the pharmacodynamics of the drug, toxicity is likely to be reflected as anticoagulation, bleeding, thrombocytopenia, liver function abnormalities and gastric distress. In the event of acute overdosage, give the patient gastric lavage if possible, carefully observe and give symptomatic and supportive treatment.

Patient Information

Patients should take the drug as prescribed, in the dosage prescribed and no more frequently than prescribed. Remind patients that pentosan polysulfate sodium has a weak anticoagulant effect. This effect may increase bleeding times.

DIMETHYL SULFOXIDE (DMSO)

| *Rx* | **Rimso-50** (Research Industries) | **Solution:** 50% aqueous solution | In 50 ml. |

Indications

▶*Interstitial cystitis:* For the symptomatic relief of interstitial cystitis.

▶*Unlabeled uses:* Dimethyl sulfoxide (DMSO) has been used in the topical treatment of musculoskeletal injuries and collagen diseases and the enhancement of percutaneous absorption of other drugs.

Other topical systemic uses include: Scleroderma; arthritis; tendinitis; bursitis; breast and prostate malignancies; retinitis pigmentosa; herpes virus infections; head and spinal cord injury; stroke. Some reports claim limited extravasation injury and enhanced antineoplastic activity when DMSO is used with some chemotherapy agents. It has been used in renal amyloidosis.

Administration and Dosage

Not for IM or IV injection.

Instill 50 ml DMSO solution directly into the bladder by catheter or asepto syringe and allow to remain for 15 minutes. Apply an analgesic lubricant gel, such as lidocaine jelly, to the urethra prior to inserting the catheter to avoid spasm. The medication is expelled by spontaneous voiding. Repeat every 2 weeks until maximum symptomatic relief is obtained. Thereafter, increase time intervals between treatments.

To reduce bladder spasm, administer oral analgesics or suppositories containing belladonna and opium prior to instillation. In patients with severe interstitial cystitis and very sensitive bladders, perform the initial treatment, and possibly the second and third (depending on patient response), under anesthesia (saddle block has been suggested).

▶*Storage/Stability:* Protect from strong light. Store at room temperature 15° to 30°C (59° to 86°F).

Actions

▶*Pharmacology:* DMSO is a clear, colorless liquid that is miscible with water and most organic solvents. Its broad range of pharmacological properties include: Anti-inflammatory action, membrane penetration, antifungal activity, cryoprotective effects for living cells and tissues, dissolution of collagen, nerve blockade, diuresis, cholinesterase inhibition, vasodilation and muscle relaxation.

▶*Pharmacokinetics:* Following topical application, DMSO is absorbed and widely distributed in tissue and body fluids. It is metabolized to dimethyl sulfone and dimethyl sulfide; DMSO and dimethyl sulfone are excreted in the urine and feces. DMSO is eliminated through the breath and skin and is responsible for the characteristic garlic odor. Unchanged DMSO has a half-life of 12 to 15 hours. Dimethyl sulfone can persist in serum > 2 weeks after a single intravesical instillation. No residual accumulation of DMSO has occurred after treatment for protracted periods of time.

Warnings

DMSO is available in a variety of forms not intended for human use (eg, veterinary and industrial solvents). Discourage human use of such products because of their unknown purity. Because of its cutaneous transport characteristics, impurities and contaminants may be systemically absorbed from topical use.

▶*Urinary tract infections, bacterial:* There is no clinical evidence of effectiveness in the treatment of bacterial urinary tract infections.

▶*Ocular lens:* In monkeys, dogs and rats, chronic administration of DMSO produces changes in the refractive index of the ocular lens and causes opacities. Although no ophthalmic changes have been observed in patients receiving therapy for cystitis, eye examinations are advisable before and after therapy.

▶*Hypersensitivity reactions:* DMSO can liberate histamine; hypersensitivity reactions may occur with topical administration. If anaphylactoid symptoms develop, institute appropriate therapy. Refer to Management of Acute Hypersensitivity Reactions.

▶*Pregnancy: Category C.* Safety for use during pregnancy has not been established. Use only when clearly needed and when the potential benefits outweigh the potential hazards to the fetus.

High intraperitoneal doses of DMSO caused teratogenesis in small animals, but oral or topical doses did not. Two studies in rabbits using large topical doses produced conflicting reproductive results.

DIMETHYL SULFOXIDE (DMSO)

➤*Lactation:* It is not known whether this drug is excreted in breast milk. Exercise caution when administering to a nursing woman.

➤*Children:* Safety and efficacy for use in children have not been established.

Precautions

➤*Monitoring:* Perform liver and renal function tests and complete blood counts every 6 months.

➤*Ophthalmic effects:* Lens opacities and changes in the refractive index have been seen in animals given chronic high doses of DMSO. Perform full eye evaluations, including slit-lamp examinations, prior to and periodically during treatment.

➤*Intravesical instillation:* Intravesical instillation may be harmful to patients with urinary tract malignancy because of DMSO-induced vasodilation.

➤*Garlic-like taste:* Garlic-like taste may occur within a few minutes after instillation. This taste may last several hours; odor on the breath and skin may remain for 72 hours.

➤*Transient chemical cystitis:* Transient chemical cystitis has followed instillation of DMSO. Moderately severe discomfort on administration usually becomes less prominent with repeated use.

Drug Interactions

➤*DMSO:* DMSO administration may decrease the formation of the active metabolite of **sulindac**, possibly resulting in a decreased therapeutic effect. A severe peripheral neuropathy has also occurred when topical DMSO was used concurrently with sulindac.

Adverse Reactions

Sedation (52%); nausea (32%); headache (42%); dizziness (18%); burning or aching eyes (9%); vomiting (6%); local dermatitis (3.5%); garlic-like breath, transient chemical cystitis (see Precautions); erythema; itching; burning; discomfort; blistering; maceration; scaling; dermatitis; burning on urination; transient disturbance of color perception; photophobia; flu syndrome; diarrhea; weight loss and gain; sore throat; cough; anorexia.

Overdosage

In case of accidental oral ingestion, induce emesis. Additional measures that may be considered are gastric lavage, activated charcoal and forced diuresis. Refer to General Management of Acute Overdosage.

Patient Information

A garlic-like taste may be noted within a few minutes of administration; odor on the breath and skin may be present and remain for up to 72 hours.

CELLULOSE SODIUM PHOSPHATE

Rx	**Calcibind** (Mission)	**Powder:** Inorganic phosphate content 31% to 36% and sodium content ≈ 11%	In 300 g bulk powder.

Indications

➤*Absorptive hypercalciuria Type* I: Absorptive hypercalciuria Type I with recurrent calcium oxalate or calcium phosphate nephrolithiasis. Appropriate use of CSP substantially reduces the incidence of new stone formation. Do not expect causes of hypercalciuria other than hyperabsorption to respond to CSP.

Characteristics of absorptive hypercalciuria Type I – Recurrent passage or formation of calcium oxalate or calcium phosphate renal stones; no evidence of bone disease; normal serum calcium and phosphorus; increased intestinal calcium absorption; hypercalciuria; normal urinary calcium during fasting; normal parathyroid function; and lack of renal "leak" or excessive skeletal mobilization of calculi.

Absorptive hypercalciuria Type II – Absorptive hypercalciuria Type II is identical, except it can be eliminated by a low-calcium diet.

Administration and Dosage

Initial dose of CSP is 15 g/day (5 g with each meal) in patients with urinary calcium > 300 mg/day (on moderate calcium-restricted diet). When urinary calcium declines to < 150 mg/day, reduce to 10 g/day (5 g with supper, 2.5 g with each remaining meal). Begin patients with controlled urinary calcium on moderate calcium-restricted diet < 300 mg/day (but > 200 mg/day) on 10 g/day.

Suspend each dose of CSP (powder) in a glass of water, soft drink or fruit juice; ingest within 30 minutes of a meal. Do not take with magnesium gluconate. The amount of bound dietary calcium is considerably reduced when CSP is administered > 1 hour after a meal. Base the initial and maintenance doses of CSP on measurements of 24-hour urinary calcium excretion.

➤*Concomitant magnesium supplements:* The dose of oral magnesium supplements, given as magnesium gluconate, depends upon the dose of CSP. Those receiving 15 g CSP/day should take 1.5 g of magnesium gluconate before breakfast and again at bedtime (separately from CSP). Those taking 10 g CSP/day should take 1 g of magnesium gluconate twice a day. To avoid binding of magnesium by CSP, give supplemental magnesium ≥ 1 hour before or after a dose of CSP.

➤*Storage/Stability:* Store in a dry place at room temperature 15° to 30°C (59° to 86°F).

Actions

➤*Pharmacology:* Cellulose Sodium Phosphate (CSP), a synthetic compound made by phosphorylation of cellulose, is insoluble in water and is nonabsorbable. CSP has excellent ion exchange properties, the sodium ion exchanging for calcium. When taken orally, CSP binds calcium; the complex of calcium and cellulose phosphate is then excreted in feces.

CSP alters urinary composition of calcium, magnesium (Mg), phosphate and oxalate by affecting their absorption in the intestinal tract. When given orally with meals, CSP binds dietary and secreted calcium and reduces urinary calcium by ≈ 50 mg/5 g of CSP. It also binds dietary magnesium and lowers urinary magnesium. Oral magnesium supplementation given separately from CSP partially overcomes this effect.

CSP administration increases urinary phosphorus and oxalate. The usual rise in urinary phosphorus of 150 to 250 mg/15 g of CSP largely reflects the hydrolysis of 7% to 30% of CSP in the intestinal tract and absorption of released phosphorus. An increase in urinary oxalate occurs. Because CSP binds divalent cations, the cations are not available to complex oxalate and limit its absorption. The rise in urinary oxalate may be largely prevented by moderate dietary oxalate restriction and a modest dose of CSP (10 to 15 g/day).

The marked reduction in urinary calcium, with only slightly increased urinary phosphorus and oxalate, leads to a reduction in urinary saturation and propensity for spontaneous nucleation of calcium oxalate and calcium phosphate (brushite).

CSP apparently does not alter the metabolism of trace metals because it does not significantly change the serum concentration of copper (Cu), zinc (Zn) or iron (Fe).

Contraindications

Primary or secondary hyperparathyroidism, including renal hypercalciuria (renal calcium leak); hypomagnesemic states (serum Mg < 1.5 mg/dl); osteoporosis, osteomalacia, osteitis; hypocalcemic states (eg, hypoparathyroidism, intestinal malabsorption); normal or low intestinal absorption and renal excretion of calcium; enteric hyperoxaluria.

Do not use in patients with high fasting urinary calcium or hypophosphatemia, unless a high skeletal mobilization of calcium can be excluded.

Warnings

➤*Congestive Heart Failure (CHF) or ascites:* The sodium contained in CSP (35 to 48 mEq exchangeable sodium per 15 g CSP) may represent a hazard.

➤*Pregnancy: Category C.* Safety for use during pregnancy has not been established. Because of the increased dietary calcium requirement in pregnant women, use only when clearly needed and when the potential benefits outweigh potential hazards to the fetus.

➤*Children:* Because of the increased requirement for dietary calcium in growing children, the use of CSP in children < 16 years of age is not recommended.

Precautions

➤*Parathyroid effects:* By inhibiting intestinal calcium absorption, CSP may stimulate parathyroid function, leading to hyperparathyroid hormone levels. Monitor parathyroid hormone levels. CSP treatment can maintain parathyroid function within normal limits if it is used only in absorptive hypercalciuria Type I at a dosage just sufficient to restore normal calcium absorption but not sufficient to cause subnormal absorption.

➤*Long-term use:* Complications that may potentially develop during long-term use include hyperoxaluria and hypomagnesiuria, which would negate the beneficial effect of hypocalciuria on new stone formation; magnesium depletion; depletion of trace metals (Cu, Zn, Fe). Minimize effects by restricting the use of CSP to only absorptive hypercalciuria Type I; take precautionary measures by monitoring serum Ca, Mg, Cu, Zn, Fe and parathyroid hormone, and perform complete blood counts every 3 to 6 months.

Repeat borderline values for parathyroid hormone and calcium promptly. Obtain serum PTH at least once between the first 2 weeks to 3 months; adjust or stop treatment if serum PTH rises above normal. If there is an inadequate hypocalciuric response to CSP treatment (a reduction in urinary calcium of < 30 mg/5 g of CSP) while patients are maintained on moderate calcium and sodium restriction, discontinue treatment. Consider cessation of treatment if urinary oxalate exceeds 55 mg/day on moderate dietary oxalate restriction.

➤*Dietary measures:* Moderate calcium intake; avoid dairy products. Moderately restrict dietary oxalate by avoiding spinach (and similar dark greens), rhubarb, chocolate and brewed tea. Avoid vitamin C supplementation because of its potential metabolism to oxalate. Discourage a high sodium intake to achieve an intake of < 150 mEq/day. Encourage fluid intake to achieve a minimum urine output of 2 L/day.

Adverse Reactions

➤*GI:* Poor taste of the drug; loose bowel movements; diarrhea; dyspepsia.

ALPROSTADIL (Prostaglandin E₁; PGE₁)

Rx	**Caverject** (Pharmacia & Upjohn)	**Injection, aqueous:** 10 mcg/mL	In 1 mL ampules and kit.[1]
		20 mcg/mL	In 1 mL ampules and kit.[1]
		40 mcg/2 mL	In 2 mL ampules and kit.[1]
Rx	**Caverject** (Pharmacia & Upjohn)	**Powder for injection, lyophilized:** 5 mcg/mL (after reconstitution)	With 8.4 mg benzyl alcohol and lactose. In vials with diluent syringes.
		10 mcg/mL (after reconstitution)	With 8.4 mg benzyl alcohol and lactose. In vials and vials with diluent syringes.
		20 mcg/mL (after reconstitution)	With 8.4 mg benzyl alcohol and lactose. In vials and vials with diluent syringes.
		40 mcg/mL (after reconstitution)	With 8.4 mg benzyl alcohol and lactose. In vials with diluent syringes.
Rx	**Caverject Impulse** (Pharmacia & Upjohn)	**Powder for injection, lyophilized:** 10 mcg/0.5 mL (after reconstitution)[2]	With 4.45 mg benzyl alcohol and lactose. In blister tray.[3]
		20 mcg/0.5 mL (after reconstitution)[4]	With 4.45 mg benzyl alcohol and lactose. In blister tray.[3]
Rx	**Edex** (Schwarz Pharma)	**Powder for injection, lyophilized:** 5 mcg/mL (after reconstitution)	Lactose. In single-dose vials and kit.[5]
		10 mcg/mL (after reconstitution)	Lactose. In single-dose vials and kit.[5]
		20 mcg/mL (after reconstitution)	Lactose. In single-dose vials and kit.[5]
		40 mcg/mL (after reconstitution)	Lactose. In single-dose vials and kit.[5]
Rx	**Muse** (Vivus)	**Pellet:** 125 mcg	In individual foil pouches.
		250 mcg	In individual foil pouches.
		500 mcg	In individual foil pouches.
		1000 mcg	In individual foil pouches.

[1] Kit contains 2 mL *Luer-lock* syringe, 2 one-half inch needles (one 27-gauge and one 30-gauge), alcohol swab.
[2] Amounts can be delivered in increments of 10 mcg/0.5 mL, 2.5 mcg/0.125 mL, 5 mcg/ 0.25 mL, or 7.5 mcg/0.375 mL.
[3] Blister tray contains 1 dual chamber syringe system, 1 needle, 2 alcohol swabs.

[4] Amounts can be delivered in increments of 20 mcg/0.5 mL, 5 mcg/0.125 mL, 10 mcg/ 0.25 mL, or 15 mcg/0.375 mL.
[5] Kit contains prefilled syringe (with 1.2 mL of 0.9% sodium chloride), plunger rod, 2 one-half inch needles (one 27-gauge and one 30-gauge), 2 alcohol swabs, tape.

For information on the use of alprostadil for patent ductus arteriosus, refer to the specific monograph in the Cardiovasculars chapter.

Indications

►*Erectile dysfunction:* Treatment of erectile dysfunction caused by neurogenic, vasculogenic, psychogenic, or mixed etiology.

Intracavernosal (Caverject only) – Intracavernosal alprostadil may be a useful adjunct to other diagnostic tests in the diagnosis of erectile dysfunction.

►*Unlabeled uses:* Critical limb ischemia, peripheral arterial disease, Raynaud disease, and peripheral angiography.

Administration and Dosage

►*Approved by the FDA:* July 6, 1995.

For use in men only. Individualize the dose for each patient by careful titration under physician supervision. In general, always employ the lowest possible effective dose. For specific administration techniques, refer to the patient information material provided with each product.

►*Intracavernosal:* A ½-inch, 27- to 30-gauge needle is generally recommended.

The first alprostadil injections must be done at the physician's office by medically trained personnel. Self-injection therapy by the patient can be started only after the patient is properly instructed and well-trained in the self-injection technique. The physician should make a careful assessment of the patient's skills and competence with this procedure. The injection site is usually along the dorso-lateral aspect of the proximal third of the penis. Avoid visible veins. Alternate the side of the penis that is injected and the site of injection.

The dose of alprostadil that is selected for self-injection treatment should provide the patient with an erection that is satisfactory for sexual intercourse and that is maintained for no longer than 1 hour. If the duration of erection is more than 1 hour, reduce the dose. Initiate self-injection therapy for use at home at the dose that was determined in the physician's office; however, make dose adjustments, if required, only after consultation with the physician. Adjust the dose in accordance with the titration guidelines described below. The effectiveness for long-term use of up to 6 months has been documented in an uncontrolled, self-injection study. The mean dose at the end of 6 months was 20.7 mcg.

Exercise careful and continuous follow-up of the patient while in the self-injection program. This is especially true for the initial self-injections because adjustments in the dose of alprostadil may be needed. The recommended frequency of injection is no more than 3 times weekly, with at least 24 hours between each dose. The reconstituted vial of alprostadil is intended for single use only; discard after use. Instruct the user in the proper disposal of the syringe, needle, and vial.

While on self-injection treatment, it is recommended that the patient visit the prescribing physician's office every 3 months. At that time, assess the efficacy and safety of the therapy and adjust the dose, if needed.

Initial titration – The patient must stay in the physician's office until complete detumescence occurs. If there is no response, then the next higher dose may be given within 1 hour. If there is a response, then wait at least 1 day before the next dose is given.

Erectile dysfunction of vasculogenic, psychogenic, or mixed etiology: Initiate dosage titration at 2.5 mcg. If there is a partial response, the dose may be increased by 2.5 mcg to a dose of 5 mcg within 1 hour. Do not give more than 2 doses within a 24-hour period during initial titration. If additional titration is required, doses in increments of 5 to 10 mcg may be given at least 24 hours apart until the dose that produces an erection suitable for intercourse and not exceeding a duration of 1 hour is reached. If there is no response to the initial 2.5 mcg dose, the second dose may be increased to 7.5 mcg within 1 hour. Do not give more than 2 doses within a 24-hour period during initial titration. If additional titration is required, doses in increments of 5 to 10 mcg may be given at least 24 hours apart.

Erectile dysfunction of pure neurogenic etiology (spinal cord injury): Initiate dosage titration at 1.25 mcg. The dose may be increased by 1.25 mcg to a dose of 2.5 mcg within 1 hour. Do not give more than 2 doses within a 24-hour period during initial titration. If additional titration is required, a dose of 5 mcg may be given during the next 24 hours. Thereafter, doses in increments of 5 mcg may be given at least 24 hours apart until the dose that produces an erection suitable for intercourse and does not exceed a duration of 1 hour is reached.

Adjunct to the diagnosis of erectile dysfunction (Caverject only) – In the simplest diagnostic test for erectile dysfunction (pharmacologic testing), patients are monitored for the occurrence of an erection after an intracavernosal injection of alprostadil. Extensions of this testing are the use of alprostadil as an adjunct to laboratory investigations, such as duplex or *Doppler* imaging, [133]*Xenon* washout tests, radioisotope penogram, and penile arteriography to allow visualization and assessment of penile vasculature. For these tests, use a single dose of alprostadil that induces a rigid erection.

Solution preparation –
   Caverject:
• *Dual chamber system* – Attach needle to device. Hold device with needle pointing upward and the plunger rod in the extended position. Turn the plunger rod slowly clockwise until it stops; this mixes the diluent and alprostadil powder. Turn the device upside down a couple of times to ensure it is completely mixed. Holding device upright, remove protective needle cap, and press the plunger rod as far as it will go. Slowly turn the end of the plunger rod clockwise to choose the dose. The number in the window is the dose in mcg.
• *Powder for injection* – Insert needle into diluent vial and draw out 1 mL diluent. Inject the 1 mL of diluent into the vial within the powder; do not remove the needle after injecting diluent. Gently swirl; do not shake the vial until all powder has dissolved. Draw out the appropriate amount of alprostadil and expel any air in the syringe.
• *Aqueous injection* – Remove ampule from wrapping and allow to warm to room temperature. Once at room temperature, vigorously shake the ampule for at least 30 seconds. After opening the ampule, immediately transfer the contents to a syringe and use promptly. Discard any remaining alprostadil in the syringe or ampule.
   Edex: Dissolve powder with 1.2 mL of 0.9% sodium chloride. Administer immediately over 5 to 10 minutes. Discard any unused portion.

►*Intraurethral:* Administer as needed to achieve an erection. The onset of effect is within 5 to 10 minutes after administration. The duration of effect is approximately 30 to 60 minutes. A medical professional should instruct each patient on proper technique for administering alprostadil prior to self-administration. The maximum frequency of use is no more than 2 systems per 24-hour period.

ALPROSTADIL (Prostaglandin E$_1$; PGE$_1$)

Initiation of therapy – Titrate dose under the supervision of a physician to test a patient's responsiveness to alprostadil, to demonstrate proper administration technique, and to monitor for evidence of hypotension. Individually titrate patients to the lowest dose that is sufficient for sexual intercourse. If necessary, increase the dose (or decrease) on separate occasions in a stepwise manner until the patient achieves an erection that is sufficient for sexual intercourse.

►*Storage/Stability:*

Aqueous injection – Store frozen at -20° to -10°C (-4° to 14°F) until dispensed. After dispensing, store in a freezer at -20°to -10°C (-4° to 14°F) for up to 3 months. During this 3-month period, the injection may be moved to and kept in a refrigerator at 2° to 8°C (36° to 46°F) for up to 7 days. Once refrigerated, it must be used within 7 days or discarded; do not refreeze. Once removed from the foil wrapping, use the solution in the ampule immediately after allowing it to warm to room temperature or discard. Use opened ampules immediately; do not store.

Caverject powder for injection vial – Store the 5, 10, and 20 mcg strengths at or below 25°C (77°F); excursions permitted to 15° to 30°C (59° to 86°F). Store the 40 mcg strength at 2° to 8°C (36° to 46°F) until dispensed. After dispensing, the 40 mcg strength may be stored at or below 25°C (77°F) for 3 months or until expiration date, whichever occurs first. Use the reconstituted solution within 24 hours when stored at or below 25°C (77°F); do not refrigerate or freeze.

Edex powder for injection – Store at controlled room temperature 15° to 30°C (59° to 86°F).

Intraurethral – Store unopened foil pouches in a refrigerator at 2° to 8°C (36° to 46°F). Do not expose to temperatures above 30°C (86°F). May be kept at room temperature (below 30°C [86°F]) for up to 14 days prior to use.

Actions

►*Pharmacology:* Alprostadil has a wide variety of pharmacological actions; vasodilation and inhibition of platelet aggregation are among the most notable of these effects. In animals, alprostadil relaxed retractor penis and corpus cavernosum urethrae. Alprostadil also relaxed isolated preparations of human corpus cavernosum and spongiosum, as well as cavernous arterial segments contracted by either noradrenaline or PGF$_{2\alpha}$ in vitro. In pigtail monkeys, alprostadil increased cavernous arterial blood flow. The degree and duration of cavernous smooth muscle relaxation in this animal was dose-dependent.

Alprostadil induces erection by relaxation of trabecular smooth muscle and by dilation of cavernosal arteries. This leads to expansion of lacunar spaces and entrapment of blood by compressing the venules against the tunica albuginea, a process referred to as the corporal veno-occlusive mechanism.

►*Pharmacokinetics:*

Absorption – For the treatment of erectile dysfunction, alprostadil is administered by injection into the corpora cavernosa or inserted intraurethrally.

Intracavernosal: Following intracavernosal injection of 20 mcg, mean peripheral plasma concentrations at 30 and 60 minutes after injection (89 and 102 pcg/mL, respectively) were not significantly greater than baseline levels of endogenous alprostadil (96 pcg/mL).

Intraurethral: Intraurethral administration is preceded by urination, and the residual urine disperses the medicated pellet, permitting alprostadil to be absorbed by the urethral mucosa. Once it is absorbed from the urethra, it is transported throughout the erectile bodies by communicating vessels between the corpus spongiosum and corpora cavernosa and is able to induce vasodilation of the targeted vascular beds. The transurethral absorption of alprostadil after administration is biphasic. Initial absorption is rapid, with approximately 80% of an administered dose absorbed within 10 minutes. The mean time to the maximum plasma PGE$_1$ concentration after a 1000 mcg intraurethral dose is approximately 16 minutes.

In 10 volunteers, endogenous PGE$_1$ levels in the ejaculate averaged 31 mcg (range, 0 to 161 mcg). In these same volunteers, an average of 123 mcg of additional PGE$_1$ (range, 30 to 369 mcg) was present in the ejaculate obtained 10 minutes after the highest dose (1000 mcg) of alprostadil. The mean total endogenous PGE content (PGE$_1$, PGE$_2$, 19-OH-PGE$_1$ and 19-OH-PGE$_2$) of the ejaculate in these subjects was 444 mcg (range, 0 to 1423 mcg).

Distribution –

Intracavernosal: Alprostadil is bound in plasma primarily to albumin (81%) and to a lesser extent to α-globulin IV-4 fraction (55%).

Intraurethral: Following intraurethral administration, alprostadil is absorbed from the urethral mucosa into the corpus spongiosum. A portion of the administered dose is transported to the corpora cavernosa through collateral vessels, while the remainder passes into the pelvic venous circulation through veins draining the corpus spongiosum. The half-life is short, varying between 30 seconds and 10 minutes. Peripheral venous plasma levels of PGE$_1$ are low or undetectable (less than 2 pg/mL) after administration. The mean maximum plasma PGE$_1$ concentration following administration of the highest dose of alprostadil (1000 mcg) was barely detectable (11.4 pg/mL). In a study of 14 subjects, the plasma PGE$_1$ level was shown to be undetectable within 60 minutes of alprostadil administration in most subjects.

Metabolism – Alprostadil is rapidly converted to compounds that are further metabolized prior to excretion. Following IV administration, approximately 80% of circulating alprostadil is metabolized in one pass through the lungs by enzymatic oxidation of the 15-hydroxyl group to 15-keto-PGE$_1$. The near-complete pulmonary first-pass metabolism of PGE$_1$ is the primary factor influencing the systemic pharmacokinetics of alprostadil and is a reason that peripheral venous plasma levels of PGE$_1$ are low or undetectable following alprostadil administration. The enzyme catalyzing this process has been isolated from many tissues in the lower GU tract including the urethra, prostate, and corpus cavernosum. 15-keto-PGE$_1$ retains little (1% to 2%) of the biological activity of PGE$_1$. 15-keto-PGE$_1$ is rapidly reduced to form the most abundant metabolite in plasma, 13,14-dihydro,15-keto PGE$_1$(DHK-PGE$_1$), which is biologically inactive. The majority of DHK-PGE$_1$ is further metabolized to smaller prostaglandin remnants that are cleared primarily by the kidney and liver.

Excretion – The metabolites of alprostadil are excreted primarily by the kidney, with almost 90% of an administered IV dose excreted in urine within 24 hours postdose. The remainder of the dose is excreted in the feces. There is no evidence of tissue retention of alprostadil or its metabolites following IV use.

Special populations –

Hepatic function impairment: In a study, 120 mcg alprostadil was administered by IV infusion over 2 hours. The mean C$_{max}$ value of PGE$_1$ in hepatically impaired patients was 96% higher than in healthy volunteers. Mean C$_{max}$ values of both 15-keto-PGE$_0$ and PGE$_0$ increased 65% as compared with those in healthy volunteers. The terminal half-lives were similar between the 2 groups.

Renal function impairment: In a study of patients with end-stage renal disease undergoing hemodialysis, 120 mcg alprostadil was administered by IV infusion over 2 hours. The mean C$_{max}$ value of PGE$_1$ in renally impaired patients was 37% lower as compared with that in healthy volunteers, whereas mean C$_{max}$ values of 15-keto-PGE$_0$ and PGE$_0$ in these patients increased 104% and 145%, respectively, as compared with those in healthy volunteers. The terminal half-lives were similar between the 2 groups.

Contraindications

Hypersensitivity to the drug; conditions that might predispose patients to priapism (eg, sickle cell anemia or trait, multiple myeloma, leukemia); patients with anatomical deformation of the penis (eg, angulation, cavernosal fibrosis, Peyronie disease); patients with penile implants (intracavernosal); use in women, children, or newborns (see Warnings); use in men for whom sexual activity is inadvisable or contraindicated; for sexual intercourse with a pregnant woman unless the couple uses a condom barrier.

►*Intraurethral:* Urethral stricture; balanitis; severe hypospadias; patients with acute or chronic urethritis; thrombocythemia; polycythemia.

Warnings

►*Priapism:* Prolonged erection (lasting more than 4 to 6 or fewer hours) and priapism (erection lasting more than 6 hours) have occurred in 4% and 0.4% of patients using alprostadil for up to 18 months, respectively. Pharmacologic intervention and/or aspiration of blood from the corpora cavernosum was required in some cases. To minimize the chances of prolonged erection or priapism, titrate slowly to the lowest effective dose. Instruct the patient to immediately report to his physician or, if unavailable, to seek immediate medical assistance for any erection that persists for more than 4 hours. Treat priapism according to established medical practice. In the majority of cases, spontaneous detumescence occurs. If priapism is not treated immediately, penile tissue damage and permanent loss of potency may result.

►*Penile fibrosis:* The overall incidence of penile fibrosis, including Peyronie disease, was 3%. In one self-injection clinical study where duration of use was up to 24 months, the incidence of fibrosis was 7.8%. Regular follow-up of patients, with careful examination of the penis, is strongly recommended to detect signs of penile fibrosis. Discontinue treatment in patients who develop penile angulation, cavernosal fibrosis, or Peyronie disease.

►*Penile pain:* Penile pain after intracavernosal administration was reported by 37% of patients at least once in clinical studies of up to 18 months in duration. In the majority of the cases, penile pain was rated mild or moderate in intensity; 3% discontinued treatment because of penile pain. The frequency of penile pain was 2% in 294 patients who received 1 to 3 injections of placebo.

►*Hematoma/Ecchymosis:* In most cases, hematoma/ecchymosis was judged to be a complication of a faulty injection technique. Accordingly, proper instruction of the patient in self-injection is of importance to minimize the potential for this.

►*Hemodynamic changes:* Hemodynamic changes, manifested as decreases in blood pressure and increases in pulse rate, principally at doses greater than 20 mcg, were observed during clinical studies and appeared to be dose-dependent. Only 3 patients discontinued treatment because of symptomatic hypotension.

►*Erectile dysfunction:* Diagnose and treat underlying treatable medical causes of erectile dysfunction prior to initiation of therapy.

ALPROSTADIL (Prostaglandin E$_1$; PGE$_1$)

▶*Pulmonary disease:* The pulmonary extraction of alprostadil following intravascular administration was reduced by 15% in patients with acute respiratory distress syndrome (ARDS) compared with a control group of patients with normal respiratory function who were undergoing cardiopulmonary bypass surgery. Pulmonary clearance was found to vary as a function of cardiac output and pulmonary intrinsic clearance in a group of 14 patients with ARDS or at risk of developing ARDS following trauma or sepsis. In this study, the extraction efficiency of alprostadil ranged from subnormal (11%) to normal (90%), with an overall mean of 67%.

▶*Pregnancy: Category C.* Alprostadil has been shown to be embryotoxic (decreased fetal weight) when administered as a SC bolus to pregnant rats at doses as low as 500 mcg/kg/day. Doses of 2000 mcg/kg/day resulted in increased resorptions, reduced numbers of live fetuses, increased incidence of visceral and skeletal variations (primarily left umbilical artery and generalized reduction in ossification of the entire skeleton), and gross visceral and skeletal malformations (primarily edema, hydrocephaly, anophthalmia/microphthalmia, and skeletal anomalies). The latter dose produced maternal toxicity (ataxia, lethargy, diarrhea, and retarded body weight gain). When administered by continuous IV infusion, evidence of embryotoxicity (decreased fetal weight gain and increased incidence of hydroureter) was observed at 2000 mcg/kg/day, a dose that also was associated with a decrease in maternal weight gain. Do not use for sexual intercourse with a pregnant woman unless the couple uses a condom barrier (see Contraindications).

▶*Children:* Not indicated for use in newborns or children. However, alprostadil (*Prostin VR Pediatric*) is used in newborns to maintain the patency of the ductus arteriosus in neonates with congenital heart defects (see specific monograph).

Precautions

▶*Monitoring:* During in-clinic dosing, monitor for symptoms of hypotension.

Drug Interactions

Alprostadil Drug Interactions			
Precipitant drug	Object drug*		Description
Alprostadil	Anticoagulants	↑	Patients on anticoagulants (eg, warfarin, heparin) may have increased propensity for bleeding after intracavernosal injection. Coadministration with heparin resulted in a 140% and 120% increase in PTT and TT, respectively. Use caution with coadministration.
Alprostadil	Vasoactive agents	↔	The safety and efficacy of combinations of alprostadil and other vasoactive agents have not been systematically studied. Therefore, the use of such combinations is not recommended.

* ↑ = Object drug increased. ↔ = Undetermined clinical effect.

Adverse Reactions

▶*Local:*

Local Adverse Reactions with Alprostadil (%)		
Adverse reaction	Intracavernosal	Intraurethral
Penile pain[1]	37	36
Urethral pain	-	13
Urethral burning	-	12
Urethral bleeding/spotting	< 1	3
Bleeding	15	-
Penile angulation	7	-
Prolonged erection	4	-
Penile fibrosis	3 to 5	-
Penis disorder[2]	3	-
Hematoma	3 to 5	-
Ecchymosis	2 to 4	-
Cavernous body fibrosis	2	-
Peyronie disease	1	-
Penile rash	1	-
Penile edema	1	-
Priapism	< 1	-
Balanitis	< 1	-
Penile warmth	< 1	-
Painful erection	< 1	-
Abnormal ejaculation	< 1	-
Injection site reaction[3]	< 1	-

[1] (*Edex* only) – Includes penile pain during injection (29%), during erection (35%), and after erection (30%).
[2] Includes numbness, yeast infection, irritation, sensitivity, phimosis, pruritus, erythema, venous leak, penile skin tear, strange feeling of penis, discoloration of penile head, itch at tip of penis.
[3] Includes hemorrhage, inflammation, itching, swelling, and edema.

▶*Systemic:*

Systemic Adverse Reactions with Alprostadil (%)		
Adverse reaction	Intracavernosal	Intraurethral
Cardiovascular		
Abnormal ECG	1	-
Hypertension	2	-
Hypotension	< 1	3
MI	1	-
Peripheral vascular disorder	< 1	-
Supraventricular extrasystoles	< 1	-
Vasodilation	< 1	-
Vasovagal reactions	< 1	-
CNS		
Headache	2	3
Dizziness	1	4
Fainting	1	0.4
Dermatological		
Nonapplication site pruritus	< 1	-
Rash	< 1	-
Skin disorder	1	-
Skin neoplasm	< 1	-
GU		
Hematuria	< 1	-
Impaired urination	< 1	-
Inguinal hernia	1	-
Prostatic disorder[1]	1 to 2	-
Scrotal disorder/edema	< 1	-
Testicular pain	< 1 to 1	5
Urinary frequency/urgency	< 1	-
Metabolic		
Hypertriglyceridemia	2	-
Hypercholesterolemia	1	-
Hyperglycemia	1	-
Respiratory		
Respiratory tract infection	4 to 5	3
Flu syndrome	2 to 3	4
Sinusitis	1 to 2	-
Rhinitis	2	2
Nasal congestion	1	-
Cough	1	-
Miscellaneous		
Abnormal vision	1	-
Accidental injury	-	3
Back pain	1 to 2	2
Diaphoresis	< 1	-
Dry mouth	< 1	-
Faulty injection technique[2]	6	-
Hypesthesia	< 1	-
Infection	2	-
Leg cramps	< 1 to 1	-
Localized pain[3]	2	-
Mydriasis	< 1	-
Nausea	< 1	-
Nongeneralized weakness	< 1	-
Pain	2	3
Pelvic pain	< 1	2
Serum creatinine increased	< 1	-
Trauma[4]	2	-

[1] Prostatitis, pain, hypertrophy, enlargement.
[2] Examples include injection into glans penis, urethra, or SC.
[3] Pain in various anatomical structures other than injection site.
[4] Injuries, fractures, abrasions, lacerations, dislocations.

▶*Female partners (Muse only):* The most common drug-related adverse event reported by female partners during clinical studies was vaginal burning/itching (5.8%). It is unknown whether this adverse event experienced by female partners was a result of the medication or a result of resuming sexual intercourse.

Overdosage

If overdose of alprostadil occurs, the patient should be under medical supervision until any systemic effects have resolved and/or until penile detumescence has occurred. Symptomatic treatment of any systemic symptoms would be appropriate.

Patient Information

Patient instructions for administration are included in each package of alprostadil.

The patient should not change the dose of alprostadil established in the physician's office without consulting the physician. The patient may expect an erection to occur within 5 to 20 minutes.

Do not use intraurethral alprostadil if the partner is pregnant unless the couple uses a condom barrier.

ALPROSTADIL (Prostaglandin E₁; PGE₁)

Instruct patient to report any penile redness, swelling, tenderness, or curvature of the erect penis.

Advise patients to seek medical assistance if an erection persists for longer than 4 hours.

Inform patients that the use of alprostadil offers no protection from the transmission of HIV.

YOHIMBINE HCl

Rx	**Yohimbine HCl** (Various, eg, Eon)	**Tablets:** 5.4 mg	May contain lactose. In 100s, 500s, and 1000s.
Rx	**Aphrodyne** (Star)		(APHRODYNE). Aqua, scored. In 100s and 1000s.
Rx	**Yocon** (Glenwood)		In 100s and 1000s.

Indications

Yohimbine has no FDA sanctioned indications.

▶*Unlabeled uses:* Sympatholytic and mydriatic. It may have activity as an aphrodisiac.

Impotence – Impotence has been successfully treated with yohimbine in male patients with vascular or diabetic origins and psychogenic origins (18 mg/day).

Orthostatic hypotension – Orthostatic hypotension may be favorably affected by yohimbine.

Administration and Dosage

▶*Male erectile impotence:* Experimental dosage has been 1 tablet (5.4 mg) 3 times/day. Occasional side effects reported with this dosage are nausea, dizziness, or nervousness. If side effects occur, reduce to one-half tablet 3 times/day, followed by gradual increases to 1 tablet 3 times/day. Results of therapy greater than 10 weeks are not known.

▶*Storage/Stability:* Store at controlled room temperature 15° to 30°C (59° to 86°F).

Actions

▶*Pharmacology:* Yohimbine, an indolalkylamine alkaloid, has chemical similarity to reserpine. It is the principal alkaloid of the bark of the *Corynanthe yohimbi* tree and also is found in *Rauwolfia serpentina* (L) Benth.

Yohimbine blocks presynaptic α_2-adrenergic receptors. Its peripheral autonomic nervous system effect is to increase parasympathetic (cholinergic) and decrease sympathetic (adrenergic) activity. In male sexual performance, erection is linked to cholinergic activity and α_2-adrenergic blockade, which theoretically results in increased penile blood inflow, decreased outflow, or both. Yohimbine exerts a stimulating action on mood and may increase anxiety. Such actions appear to require high doses. Yohimbine has a mild antidiuretic action, probably via stimulation of hypothalmic centers and release of posterior pituitary hormone.

Its action on peripheral blood vessels resembles that of reserpine, though it is weaker and of shorter duration. The drug reportedly exerts no significant influence on cardiac stimulation.

▶*Pharmacokinetics:*

Absorption/Distribution – Oral absorption appears to be extremely rapid, with a mean T_{max} of less than 1 hour. The low bioavailability of approximately 30% is thought to be caused by first-pass metabolism rather than poor absorption. The mean distribution half-life is less than 30 minutes, and the mean apparent volume of distribution ranged from 24.6 to 226 L. Approximately 82% of yohimbine is bound to plasma proteins.

Metabolism/Excretion – Yohimbine undergoes extensive first-pass metabolism that results in poor but highly variable bioavailability. It also undergoes extensive biotransformation in the liver and extrahepatic sites, and at least 2 hydroxylated metabolites have been identified. After single-dose administration, the terminal half-life of yohimbine is 0.25 to 2.5 hours. The active metabolite (11-hydroxy-yohimbine) has a longer elimination half-life of 6 hours. Less than 1% of the yohimbine dose is recovered in the urine as unchanged drug.

Contraindications

Renal disease; hypersensitivity to any component.

Warnings

▶*Special risk patients:* Not for use in geriatric, psychiatric, or cardio-renal patients with a history of gastric or duodenal ulcer. Generally, not for use in females.

▶*Pregnancy:* Do not use during pregnancy.

▶*Children:* Do not use in children.

Drug Interactions

▶*Antidepressants:* Do not use with yohimbine.

Adverse Reactions

Yohimbine readily penetrates the CNS and produces a complex pattern of responses in lower doses than those required to produce peripheral α-adrenergic blockade. These include antidiuresis and central excitation including elevated blood pressure and heart rate, increased motor activity, nervousness, irritability, and tremor. Dizziness, nausea, headache, and skin flushing have been reported.

Overdosage

Yohimbine may be toxic if ingested in high doses. The drug causes severe hypotension, abdominal distress, and weakness. Larger doses may cause CNS stimulation and paralysis.

Phosphodiesterase Type 5 Inhibitors

Indications

►*Erectile dysfunction:* For the treatment of erectile dysfunction.

►*Unlabeled uses:* The use of **sildenafil** in women with sexual dysfunction has been evaluated in small clinical trials. The results are quite mixed with many studies unable to demonstrate efficacy.

Actions

►*Pharmacology:* **Sildenafil**, **tadalafil**, and **vardenafil** are selective inhibitors of phosphodiesterase type 5 (PDE5). The physiologic mechanism of penile erection involves release of nitric oxide (NO) in the corpus cavernosum during sexual stimulation. NO activates the enzyme guanylate cyclase, resulting in increased synthesis of cyclic guanosine monophosphate (cGMP) in the smooth muscle cells of the corpus cavernosum. The cGMP, in turn, triggers smooth muscle relaxation, allowing increased blood flow into the penis, resulting in erection. Sildenafil, tadalafil, and vardenafil enhance the effects of NO by inhibiting PDE5 that is responsible for the degradation of cGMP in the smooth muscle cells of the corpus cavernosum. Because sexual stimulation is required to initiate the local release of NO, the inhibition of PDE5 by sildenafil, tadalafil, or vardenafil has no effect in the absence of sexual stimulation.

PDE5 also is found in lower concentrations in other tissues, including platelets, vascular and visceral smooth muscle, and skeletal muscle. In these tissues, inhibition of PDE5 may be the basis for the enhanced platelet antiaggregatory activity of NO, inhibition of platelet thrombus formation, and peripheral arterial-venous dilation.

Sildenafil is more potent on PDE5 than on other known phosphodiesterases (over 10-fold for PDE6, over 80-fold for PDE1, over 700-fold for PDE2, PDE3, PDE4, PDE7, PDE8, PDE9, PDE10, and PDE11). The approximate 4000-fold selectivity for PDE5 vs PDE3 is important because PDE3 is involved in the control of cardiac contractility. Sildenafil is only about 10-fold as potent for PDE5 compared with PDE6, an enzyme found in the retina. This lower selectivity is thought to be the basis for abnormalities related to color vision observed with higher doses or plasma levels.

In vitro studies have shown that the effect of tadalafil is more potent on PDE5 than on other phosphodiesterases. These studies have shown that tadalafil is more than 10,000-fold more potent for PDE5 than for PDE1, PDE2, PDE4, and PDE7 enzymes, which are found in the heart, brain, blood vessels, liver, leukocytes, skeletal muscle, and other organs. Tadalafil is more than 10,000-fold more potent for PDE5 than for PDE3, an enzyme found in the heart and blood vessels. Additionally, tadalafil is 700-fold more potent for PDE5 than for PDE6, which is found in the retina and is responsible for phototransduction. Tadalafil is more than 9,000-fold more potent for PDE5 than for PDE8, PDE9, PDE10, and 14-fold more potent for PDE5 than for PDE11A1, an enzyme found in human skeletal muscle. Tadalafil inhibits human recombinant PDE11A1 activity at concentrations within the therapeutic range. The physiological role and clinical consequence of PDE11 inhibition in humans have not been defined.

The inhibitory effect of vardenafil is more selective on PDE5 than for other known phosphodiesterases (more than 15-fold relative to PDE6, more than 130-fold relative to PDE1, more than 300-fold relative to PDE11, and more than 1000-fold relative to PDE2, PDE3, PDE4, PDE7, PDE8, PDE9, and PDE10).

Effects on blood pressure [BP] –
Sildenafil: Single oral doses of 100 mg sildenafil produced a mean maximum decrease of 8.4/5.5 mm Hg in healthy volunteers. The decrease in BP was most notable approximately 1 to 2 hours after dosing and was not different than placebo at 8 hours. Similar effects on BP were noted with 25, 50, and 100 mg sildenafil. Larger effects were recorded among patients receiving concomitant nitrates.

Vardenafil: In a clinical pharmacology study of patients with erectile dysfunction, single doses of 20 mg vardenafil caused a mean maximum decrease in supine BP of 7 mm Hg systolic and 8 mm Hg diastolic (compared with placebo), accompanied by a mean maximum increase in heart rate of 4 beats/minute. The maximum decrease in BP occurred between 1 and 4 hours after dosing. Following multiple dosing for 31 days, similar BP responses were observed on day 31 and day 1.

►*Pharmacokinetics:*
Absorption / Distribution –

Phosphodiesterase Type 5 Inhibitors Pharmacokinetics			
Parameters	Sildenafil	Tadalafil	Vardenafil
Bioavailability	≈ 40%	Not determined	≈ 15%
T_{max}	0.5 to 2 h (median, 1 h)[a]	0.5 to 6 h (median, 2 h)[b]	0.5 to 2 h (median, 1 h)[c]
Effect of food (high-fat meal)	C_{max} reduced by 29% T_{max} increased by 1 h	No effect	C_{max} reduced by 18% to 50%
Onset of action	≈ 30 min	≈ 30 min	≈ 20 min[d]
Maximum effect	no data	no data	45 to 90 min[d]
Duration of action	≥ 4 h	36 h	< 5 h

Phosphodiesterase Type 5 Inhibitors Pharmacokinetics			
Parameters	Sildenafil	Tadalafil	Vardenafil
Volume of distribution[e]	105 L	≈ 63 L	208 L
Protein binding[f]	≈ 96%	94%	≈ 95%
Metabolism	CYP3A4 (major) CYP2C9 (minor)	CYP3A4	CYP3A4 (major) CYP3A5, CYP2C isoforms (minor)
Active metabolite	Yes[g]	No	Yes[h]
Terminal half-life	≈ 4 h	17.5 h	4 to 5 h
Excretion	Feces (≈ 80%) Urine (≈ 13%)	Feces (≈ 61%) Urine (≈ 36%)	Feces (≈ 91% to 95%) Urine (≈ 2% to 6%)
Clearance	no data	2.5 L/h	56 L/h

[a] Oral dosing in the fasted state.
[b] Single oral dose.
[c] Single oral dose of 20 mg; fasted state.
[d] Based on animal studies.
[e] At steady state.
[f] For parent drug and major circulating metabolite.
[g] Accounts for approximately 20% of sildenafil's pharmacologic activity.
[h] Accounts for approximately 7% of vardenafil's pharmacologic activity.

Sildenafil and **vardenafil** are rapidly absorbed. The pharmacokinetics of sildenafil and vardenafil are dose-proportional over the recommended dose range. Protein binding for both drugs is independent of total drug concentrations.

Based on measurements of sildenafil in semen of healthy volunteers 90 minutes after dosing, less than 0.001% of the administered dose may appear in the semen of patients. Following a single oral dose of 20 mg vardenafil in healthy volunteers, a mean of 0.00018% of the administered dose was obtained in semen 90 minutes after dosing. Less than 0.0005% of the administered dose appeared in the semen of healthy subjects.

Metabolism / Excretion – **Sildenafil**, **tadalafil**, and **vardenafil** are cleared predominantly by the CYP3A4 (major route), 3A5 (major route; vardenafil), and CYP2C9 (minor route; sildenafil and vardenafil) hepatic microsomal isoenzymes. Sildenafil is converted into an active metabolite by N-desmethylation and is further metabolized. This metabolite has a PDE selectivity profile similar to sildenafil and an in vitro potency for PDE5 approximately 50% of the parent drug. Plasma concentrations of this metabolite are approximately 40% of those seen for sildenafil, so that the metabolite accounts for approximately 20% of sildenafil's pharmacologic effects. Both sildenafil and the metabolite have terminal half-lives of approximately 4 hours. The major circulating metabolite of vardenafil, M1, results from desethylation at the piperazine moiety of vardenafil. M1 is subject to further metabolism. The plasma concentration of M1 is approximately 26% that of the parent compound. M1 accounts for approximately 7% of total pharmacologic activity. Tadalafil is predominantly metabolized by CYP 3A4 to a catechol metabolite. The catechol metabolite undergoes extensive methylation and glucuronidation to form the methylcatechol and methylcatechol glucuronide conjugate, respectively. The major circulating metabolite is the methylcatechol glucuronide. In vitro data suggests that metabolites are not expected to be pharmacologically active at observed metabolite concentrations.

Special populations:
• *Elderly –* Healthy elderly volunteers (65 years of age and older) had a reduced clearance of **sildenafil**, with free plasma concentrations approximately 40% greater than those seen in healthy younger volunteers (18 to 45 years of age). In a study of healthy elderly (65 years of age and older) and younger (18 to 45 years of age) males, mean C_{max} and AUC of **vardenafil** were 34% and 52% higher, respectively, in elderly males. Healthy male elderly subjects (65 years of age and older) had a lower oral clearance of **tadalafil**, resulting in 25% higher exposure (AUC) with no effect on C_{max} relative to that observed in healthy subjects 19 to 45 years of age.

• *Renal function impairment –* In volunteers with severe (Ccr 30 mL/min or less) renal impairment, **sildenafil** clearance was reduced, resulting in approximately double the AUC and C_{max} compared with age-matched volunteers with no renal impairment. In the moderate (Ccr 30 to 50 mL/min) or severe (Ccr less than 30 mL/min) renal impairment groups, the AUC of **vardenafil** was 20% to 30% higher compared with that observed in a control group with normal (Ccr greater than 80 mL/min) renal function. In studies using single-dose **tadalafil** (5 to 10 mg), tadalafil exposure (AUC) doubled in subjects with mild (Ccr 51 to 80 mL/min) or moderate (Ccr 31 to 50 mL/min) renal insufficiency. In subjects with end-stage renal disease on hemodialysis, there was a 2-fold increase in C_{max} and 2.7- to 4.1-fold increase in AUC following single-dose administration of 10 or 20 mg tadalafil.

• *Hepatic function impairment –* In volunteers with hepatic cirrhosis (Child-Pugh A and B), **sildenafil** clearance was reduced, resulting in increases in AUC (84%) and C_{max} (47%) compared with age-matched volunteers with no hepatic impairment. In volunteers with mild hepatic impairment (Child-Pugh A), the C_{max} and AUC following a 10 mg **vardenafil** dose were increased by 22% and 17%, respectively, compared with healthy control subjects. In volunteers with moderate hepatic impairment (Child-Pugh B), the C_{max} and AUC following a 10 mg vardenafil dose were increased by 130% and 160%, respectively, compared with healthy control subjects.

Contraindications

Hypersensitivity to any component of the tablet; administration with nitrates (either regularly and/or intermittently) and nitric oxide donors because of the potentiation of hypotension (see Drug Interactions); coadministration with alpha-blockers (**vardenafil** only); coadministration with alpha-blockers other than 0.4 mg/day tamsulosin (**tadalafil** only).

Warnings

➤*Priapism:* Prolonged erections more than 4 hours and priapism (painful erections more than 6 hours in duration) have been reported infrequently for this class of compounds. In the event of an erection that persists more than 4 hours, whether painful or not, advise the patient to seek immediate medical assistance. If priapism is not treated immediately, penile tissue damage and permanent loss of potency may result.

➤*Cardiovascular effects:* There is a potential for cardiac risk associated with sexual activity. Treatments for erectile dysfunction, including these agents, generally should not be used in men for whom sexual activity is inadvisable because of their underlying cardiovascular status. Consider the cardiovascular status of patients to determine whether patients with underlying cardiovascular disease could be adversely affected by vasodilatory effects (eg, transient decreases in BP) of these drugs, especially in combination with sexual activity.

Patients with the following underlying conditions can be particularly sensitive to the actions of vasodilators, including **sildenafil**, **tadalafil**, and **vardenafil**: Those with left ventricular outflow obstruction (eg, aortic stenosis, idiopathic hypertrophic subaortic stenosis) and those with severely impaired autonomic control of BP.

There are no controlled clinical data on the safety or efficacy of sildenafil in patients who have suffered an MI, stroke, or life-threatening arrhythmia within the last 6 months; patients with resting hypotension (BP less than 90/50 mm Hg) or hypertension (BP greater than 170/110 mm Hg); or patients with cardiac failure or coronary artery disease causing unstable angina. Use caution when prescribing sildenafil in these groups. Use of vardenafil is not recommended in these patients.

The following groups of patients with cardiovascular disease were not included in clinical safety and efficacy trials for tadalafil, and, therefore, the use of tadalafil is not recommended in these groups until further information is available:
• Patients with an MI within the last 90 days
• patients with unstable angina or angina occurring during sexual intercourse
• patients with New York Heart Association Class 2 or greater heart failure in the last 6 months
• patients with uncontrolled arrhythmias, hypotension (BP less than 90/50 mm Hg), or uncontrolled hypertension (BP greater than 170/100 mm Hg)
• patients with a stroke within the last 6 months.

Sildenafil – Serious cardiovascular, cerebrovascular, and vascular events, including MI, sudden cardiac death, ventricular arrhythmia, cerebrovascular hemorrhage, transient ischemic attack, hypertension, subarachnoid and intracerebral hemorrhages, and pulmonary hemorrhage have been reported postmarketing in temporal association with sildenafil. Most of these patients had preexisting cardiovascular risk factors. Many of these events were reported to occur during or shortly after sexual activity, and a few were reported to occur shortly after the use of sildenafil without sexual activity. Others were reported to have occurred hours to days after sildenafil use and sexual activity. It is not possible to determine whether these events are directly related to sildenafil, to sexual activity, to the patient's underlying cardiovascular disease, to a combination of these factors, or to other factors.

Postmarketing data from late March through mid-November 1998 indicate 130 US patients have died after being prescribed sildenafil. Of the 130 US patients, 3 had strokes and 77 had cardiovascular events (41 with definite or suspected MI, 27 with cardiac arrest, 6 with cardiac symptoms, and 3 with coronary artery disease). Thirty-four percent of these patients died or had onset of symptoms leading to death within 4 to 5 hours of sildenafil use (including 27 during or immediately after sexual intercourse). Ninety (70%) of these patients had at least 1 risk factor reported for cardiovascular or cerebrovascular disease.

Tadalafil – The effect of a single dose of 100 mg tadalafil on the QT interval was evaluated at the time of peak tadalafil concentration in a randomized, double-blind, placebo, and active (IV ibutilide)-controlled crossover study in 90 healthy males 18 to 53 years of age. The mean change in QT_c (Friderica QT correction) for tadalafil, relative to placebo, was 3.5 msec. The mean change in QT_c (individual QT correction) for tadalafil, relative to placebo, was 2.8 msec. In this study, the mean increase in heart rate associated with a 100 mg dose of tadalafil compared with placebo was 3.1 beats/minute.

Vardenafil –

Congenital or acquired QT prolongation: In a study of the effects of vardenafil on QT interval in 59 healthy males, therapeutic (10 mg) and supratherapeutic (80 mg) doses of vardenafil and the active control moxifloxacin (400 mg) produced similar increases in QTc interval. Consider this observation in clinical decisions when prescribing vardenafil. Patients with congenital QT prolongation and those taking Class IA (eg, quinidine, procainamide) or Class III (eg, amiodarone, sotalol) antiarrhythmic medications should avoid using vardenafil.

➤*Renal function impairment:* In volunteers with severe renal impairment (Ccr 30 mL/min or less), **sildenafil** clearance was reduced, resulting in approximately double the AUC and C_{max}. Consider an initial dose of 25 mg sildenafil in these patients. There is no clinical data on the safety or efficacy of **vardenafil** in patients with end-stage renal disease requiring dialysis, and therefore, its use is not recommended.

Limit **tadalafil** to 5 mg not more than once daily in patients with severe renal insufficiency or end-stage renal disease. The starting dose in patients with a moderate degree of renal insufficiency should be 5 mg not more than once daily, and the maximum dose should be limited to 10 mg not more than once in every 48 hours. No dose adjustment is required in patients with mild renal insufficiency.

In patients with moderate (Ccr 30 to 50 mL/min) to severe (Ccr less than 30 mL/min) renal impairment, the AUC of vardenafil was 20% to 30% higher compared with that observed in a control group with normal renal function (Ccr more than 80 mL/min). No dosage adjustment for vardenafil is required.

➤*Hepatic function impairment:* In volunteers with hepatic cirrhosis, **sildenafil** clearance was reduced, resulting in increases in AUC (84%) and C_{max} (47%). Consider an initial sildenafil dose of 25 mg in these patients. In patients with mild or moderate hepatic impairment, do not exceed a 10 mg dose of **tadalafil**. Because of insufficient information in patients with severe hepatic impairment, use in these patients is not recommended. In volunteers with mild hepatic impairment (Child-Pugh A), the C_{max} and AUC following a 10 mg **vardenafil** dose were increased by 22% and 17%, respectively, compared with healthy control subjects. In volunteers with moderate hepatic impairment (Child-Pugh B), the C_{max} and AUC following a 10 mg vardenafil dose were increased by 130% and 160%, respectively, compared with healthy control subjects. Consequently, a starting dose of 5 mg is recommended for patients with moderate hepatic impairment, and the maximum dose should not exceed 10 mg. Vardenafil has not been evaluated in patients with severe (Child-Pugh C) hepatic impairment and its use is not recommended in these patients.

➤*Fertility impairment:* In beagle dogs given **tadalafil** daily for 3 to 12 months, there was treatment-related nonreversible degeneration and atrophy of the seminiferous tubular epithelium in the testes in 20% to 100% of the dogs that resulted in a decrease in spermatogenesis in 40% to 75% of the dogs at doses of 10 mg/kg/day or more.

➤*Elderly:* Healthy elderly volunteers (65 years of age and older) had reduced **sildenafil** clearance with free plasma concentrations approximately 40% greater than those in healthy younger volunteers 18 to 45 years of age. Consider an initial sildenafil dose of 25 mg in these patients. Healthy male elderly subjects (65 years of age and older) had a lower oral clearance of **tadalafil**, resulting in 25% higher exposure (AUC) with no effect on C_{max} relative to that observed in healthy subjects 19 to 45 years of age. In a study of healthy elderly (65 years of age and older) and younger (18 to 45 years of age) males, mean C_{max} and AUC of **vardenafil** were 34% and 52% higher, respectively, in elderly males. Consequently, consider a lower starting dose of vardenafil (5 mg) in patients 65 years of age and older.

➤*Pregnancy: Category B.* These agents are not indicated for use in women. There are no adequate and well-controlled studies of these agents in pregnant women. **Tadalafil** and/or its metabolites cross the placenta, resulting in fetal exposure in rats. In a rat prenatal and postnatal development study at doses of 60, 200, and 1000 mg/kg tadalafil, there was a reduction in postnatal survival of pups. Retarded physical development of pups in the absence of maternal effects was observed following maternal exposure to 1 and 8 mg/kg **vardenafil**, possibly because of vasodilation and/or secretion of the drug into milk. The number of living pups born to rats exposed pre- and postnatally was reduced at 60 mg/kg/day.

➤*Lactation:* These agents are not indicated for use in women. **Tadalafil** and/or its metabolites were secreted into the milk in lactating rats at concentrations approximately 2.4-fold greater than found in the plasma. **Vardenafil** was secreted into the milk of lactating rats at concentrations approximately 10-fold greater than found in plasma. Following a single oral dose of 3 mg/kg, 3.3% of the administered dose was excreted into the milk within 24 hours. It is not known if the drugs are excreted in human breast milk.

➤*Children:* These agents are not indicated for use in newborns or children.

Precautions

➤*Erectile dysfunction:* Undertake thorough medical history and physical examination to diagnose erectile dysfunction, determine potential underlying causes, and identify appropriate treatment.

Phosphodiesterase Type 5 Inhibitors

The safety and efficacy of combinations of **sildenafil**, **tadalafil**, or **vardenafil** with other treatments for erectile dysfunction have not been studied. Therefore, the use of such combinations is not recommended.

➤*Deformation of penis:* Use agents for the treatment of erectile dysfunction with caution in patients with anatomical deformation of the penis (eg, angulation, cavernosal fibrosis, or Peyronie disease) or in patients who have conditions that may predispose them to priapism (eg, sickle cell anemia, multiple myeloma, or leukemia).

➤*Bleeding disorders:* **Sildenafil**, **tadalafil**, or **vardenafil** have no effect on bleeding time when taken alone or with aspirin. In vitro studies with human platelets indicate that sildenafil potentiates the antiaggregatory effect of sodium nitroprusside (a nitric oxide donor). In rabbits, the combination of heparin and sildenafil had an additive effect on bleeding time, but this interaction has not been studied in humans. There is no safety information on the administration of sildenafil, tadalafil, or vardenafil to patients with bleeding disorders or active peptic ulceration.

➤*Visual disturbances:* Single oral doses of phosphodiesterase inhibitors have demonstrated transient, dose-related impairment of color discrimination (blue/green), with peak effects near the time of peak plasma levels. The findings were most evident 1 hour after administration, diminishing but still present 6 hours after administration. This finding is consistent with the inhibition of PDE6, which is involved in phototransduction in the retina. An evaluation of visual function at **sildenafil** and **tadalafil** doses up to twice the maximum recommended dose revealed no effects on visual acuity, intraocular pressure, or pupillometry. In a single-dose study of 25 healthy males, 40 mg **vardenafil**, twice the maximum daily recommended dose, did not alter visual acuity, intraocular pressure, or fundoscopic and slit lamp findings.

➤*Retinitis pigmentosa:* A minority of patients with retinitis pigmentosa have genetic disorders of retinal phosphodiesterases. There is no safety information on the administration of **sildenafil**, **tadalafil**, or **vardenafil** to patients with known hereditary degenerative retinal disorders, including retinitis pigmentosa. Therefore, administer with caution to these patients.

Drug Interactions

➤*CYP450 system:* PDE5 inhibitors are metabolized principally by the cytochrome P450 (CYP) isoforms 3A4 (major route), 3A5 (major route; **vardenafil**), and 2C9 (minor route; **sildenafil**, vardenafil). Therefore, inhibitors of these isoenzymes may increase PDE5 inhibitor concentrations and inducers of these isoenzymes may decrease PDE5 inhibitor concentrations. See the Administration and Dosage sections of the individual monographs for dosing recommendations.

PDE5 Inhibitor Drug Interactions			
Precipitant drug	Object drug[*]		Description
Alcohol	PDE5 inhibitors	↑	Alcohol and PDE5 inhibitors are mild systemic vasodilators. Substantial consumption of alcohol in combination with a PDE5 inhibitor may produce decreases in BP, postural dizziness, and orthostatic hypotension. Sildenafil did not potentiate the hypotensive effect of alcohol at maximum blood alcohol levels of 0.08%.
Alpha-blockers (eg, doxazosin, terazosin)	PDE5 inhibitors	↑	Coadministration of vardenafil with alpha-blockers is contraindicated because of the possibility of significant hypotension. Tadalafil also is contraindicated with alpha-blockers other than 0.4 mg/day tamsulosin. Sildenafil, when given with doxazosin, has lead to symptomatic hypotension. Sildenafil dose modifications are recommended (see Administration and Dosage).
PDE5 inhibitors	Alpha-blockers (eg, doxazosin, terazosin)		
Amlodipine	PDE5 inhibitors Sildenafil Tadalafil	↑	Coadministration of sildenafil and amlodipine produced an additional mean reduction of 8 mm Hg systolic and 7 mm Hg diastolic BP. Amlodipine administered with tadalafil reduced mean supine systolic/diastolic BP by 3/2 mm Hg.
PDE5 inhibitors Sildenafil Tadalafil	Amlodipine		
Angiotensin II receptor blockers	PDE5 inhibitors Tadalafil	↑	Concomitant administration of tadalafil and an angiotensin II receptor blocker produced a mean reduction in supine systolic/diastolic BP of 8/4 mm Hg.
PDE5 inhibitors Tadalafil	Angiotensin II receptor blockers		
Antacids	PDE5 inhibitors Tadalafil	↓	Simultaneous administration of tadalafil with an antacid (magnesium hydroxide/aluminum hydroxide) reduced the rate of tadalafil absorption without altering the AUC.

PDE5 Inhibitor Drug Interactions			
Precipitant drug	Object drug[*]		Description
Bendroflumethiazide	PDE5 inhibitors Tadalafil	↑	Coadministration of tadalafil and bendroflumethiazide produced a mean reduction in supine systolic/diastolic BP of 6/4 mm Hg.
PDE5 inhibitors Tadalafil	Bendroflumethiazide		
Beta-blockers, (nonspecific)	PDE5 inhibitors Sildenafil	↑	The AUC of sildenafil's active metabolite, N-desmethyl sildenafil, was increased 102% by nonspecific beta-blockers. This effect is not expected to be of clinical consequence.
Cimetidine	PDE5 inhibitors Sildenafil	↑	Coadministration yielded a 56% increase in plasma sildenafil concentrations.
Diuretics	PDE5 inhibitors Sildenafil	↑	The AUC of sildenafil's active metabolite, N-desmethyl sildenafil, was increased 62% by loop and potassium-sparing diuretics. This effect is not expected to be of clinical consequence.
Enalapril	PDE5 inhibitors Tadalafil	↑	Coadmnistration of tadalafil and enalapril produced a mean reduction in supine systolic/diastolic BP of 4/1 mm Hg.
PDE5 inhibitors Tadalafil	Enalapril		
Ketoconazole Itraconazole	PDE5 inhibitors	↑	Ketoconazole and itraconazole are CYP3A4 inhibitors and, therefore, would reduce sildenafil and vardenafil clearance. Concurrent use of ketoconazole and vardenafil produced a 10-fold increase in vardenafil AUC and a 4-fold increase in C_{max}. Dose adjustments are recommended (see Administration and Dosage).
Macrolides (eg, erythromycin)	PDE5 inhibitors	↑	Coadministration of sildenafil and erythromycin (CYP3A4 inhibitor) resulted in a 182% increase in sildenafil systemic exposure. Erythromycin produced a 4-fold increase in vardenafil AUC and a 3-fold increase in C_{max}. Also consider interactions with clarithromycin and troleandomycin. Azithromycin had no effect on sildenafil pharmacokinetics (see Administration and Dosage).
Metoprolol	PDE5 inhibitors Tadalafil	↑	Coadministration of tadalafil and metoprolol produced a mean reduction in supine systolic/diastolic BP of 5/3 mm Hg.
PDE5 inhibitors Tadalafil	Metoprolol		
Nifedipine	PDE5 inhibitors Vardenafil	↑	Coadministration of vardenafil and nifedipine produced an additional mean reduction of 6 mm Hg systolic and 5 mm Hg diastolic BP.
PDE5 inhibitors Vardenafil	Nifedipine		
Nitrates (eg, isosorbide dinitrate, nitroglycerin)	PDE5 inhibitors	↑	Concomitant use is contraindicated. Phosphodiesterase inhibitors potentiate the vasodilatory effect of circulating nitric oxide, resulting in a significant and potentially fatal drop in BP.
PDE5 inhibitors	Nitrates (eg, isosorbide dinitrate, nitroglycerin)		
Protease inhibitors (eg, ritonavir, indinavir, saquinavir)	PDE5 inhibitors	↑	When coadministered with a protease inhibitor, the PDE5 inhibitor plasma concentrations may be elevated, resulting in severe and potentially fatal hypotension. Dose modifications are recommended (see Administration and Dosage). Concomitant use of vardenafil with ritonavir or indinavir may lead to a decrease in the protease inhibitor plasma levels.
PDE5 inhibitors Vardenafil	Protease inhibitors (eg, ritonavir, indinavir)	↓	
Rifampin	PDE5 inhibitors Sildenafil Tadalafil	↓	Rifampin and other CYP3A4 inhibitors increased sildenafil and tadalafil clearance.
Tacrolimus	PDE5 inhibitors Sildenafil	↑	Sildenafil plasma concentrations may be elevated, increasing risk of side effects.

[*] ↑ = Object drug increased.   ↓ = Object drug decreased.

Phosphodiesterase Type 5 Inhibitors

➤*Drug/Food interactions:* Although specific interactions have not been studied, grapefruit juice (CYP3A4 inhibitor) would likely increase PDE5 inhibitor exposure. When taken with a high-fat meal, the rate of **sildenafil** absorption is reduced, with a mean delay in T_{max} of 60 minutes and a mean reduction in C_{max} of 29%. High-fat meals caused a reduction in C_{max} of **vardenafil** by 18% to 50%.

Adverse Reactions

	Phosphodiesterase Type 5 Inhibitors Adverse Reactions (%)[a]				
	Sildenafil	Vardenafil	Tadalafil		
			5 mg	10 mg	20 mg
Adverse reaction	(n = 734)[b]	(n = 2203)[c]	(N = 151)	(N = 394)	(N = 635)
CNS					
Dizziness	2	2	—	—	—
Headache	16	15	11	11	15
GI					
Diarrhea	3	< 2	—	—	—
Dyspepsia	7	4	4	8	10
Nausea	—	2	—	—	—
Respiratory					
Nasal congestion	4	—	2	3	3
Rhinitis	—	9	—	—	—
Sinusitis	< 2	3	—	—	—
Miscellaneous					
Abnormal vision[d]	3	< 2	—	—	—
Accidental injury	< 2	3	—	—	—
Back pain	< 2[e]	< 2	3	5	6
Flu syndrome	< 2[e]	3	—	—	—
Flushing[f]	10	11	2	3	3
Increased creatine kinase	—	2	—	—	—
Limb pain	—	—	1	3	3
Myalgia	—	—	1	4	3
Rash	2	—	—	—	—
Urinary tract infection	3	—	—	—	—

[a] Data are pooled from separate studies and are not necessarily comparable.
[b] PRN flexible-dose studies.
[c] Fixed and flexible-dose studies. Flexible-dose studies started all patients at 10 mg vardenafil and allowed decrease in dose to 5 mg or increase in dose to 20 mg based on side effects and efficacy.
[d] Mild and transient, predominantly color tinge to vision, but also increased sensitivity to light or blurred vision. Only 1 patient discontinued because of abnormal vision.
[e] Incidence is equally common to placebo.
[f] The term flushing includes facial flushing and flushing.

In fixed-dose studies, dyspepsia (17%) and abnormal vision (11%) were more common at the 100 mg **sildenafil** dose than at lower doses.

Placebo-controlled trials suggested a dose effect in the incidence of some adverse events (headache, flushing, dyspepsia, nausea, rhinitis) over the 5, 10, and 20 mg doses of **vardenafil**.

The following adverse reactions were reported in less than 2% of patients.

➤*Cardiovascular:* Angina pectoris, chest pain, hypotension, palpitation, postural hypotension, syncope, tachycardia.

Sildenafil – Abnormal ECG, AV block, cardiac arrest, cardiomyopathy, cerebral thrombosis, heart failure, myocardial ischemia.

Tadalafil – Hypertension, MI.

Vardenafil – Hypertension, MI, myocardial ischemia.

➤*CNS:* Hypesthesia, insomnia, paresthesia, somnolence, vertigo.

Sildenafil – Abnormal dreams, ataxia, depression, hypertonia, migraine, neuralgia, neuropathy, reflexes decreased, tremor.

Tadalafil – Dizziness.

Vardenafil – Hypertonia.

➤*Dermatologic:* Pruritus, sweating.

Sildenafil – Contact dermatitis, exfoliative dermatitis, herpes simplex, photosensitivity reaction, skin ulcer, urticaria.

Tadalafil – Rash.

Vardenafil – Photosensitivity reaction, rash.

➤*GI:* Abnormal liver function tests, dry mouth, dysphagia, esophagitis, gastritis, vomiting.

Sildenafil – Abdominal pain, colitis, gastroenteritis, gingivitis, glossitis, rectal hemorrhage, stomatitis.

Tadalafil – Diarrhea, gastroesophageal reflux, GGTP increased, loose stools, nausea, upper abdominal pain.

Vardenafil – Abdominal pain, gastroesophageal reflux, GGTP increased.

➤*GU:*
Sildenafil – Abnormal ejaculation, anorgasmia, breast enlargement, cystitis, genital edema, nocturia, urinary frequency, urinary incontinence.

Tadalafil – Erection increased, spontaneous penile erection.

Vardenafil – Abnormal ejaculation, priapism (including prolonged or painful erections).

➤*Hematologic:*
Sildenafil – Anemia, leukopenia.

➤*Metabolic/Nutritional:*
Sildenafil – Edema, gout, hyperglycemia, hypernatremia, hyperuricemia, hypoglycemia reaction, peripheral edema, thirst, unstable diabetes.

➤*Musculoskeletal:*
Sildenafil – Arthritis, arthrosis, bone pain, myalgia, myasthenia, synovitis, tendon rupture, tenosynovitis.

Tadalafil – Arthralgia, neck pain.

In **tadalafil** clinical pharmacology trials, back pain or myalgia generally occurred 12 to 24 hours after dosing and typically resolved within 48 hours. The back pain/myalgia associated with tadalafil treatment was characterized by diffuse bilateral lower lumbar, gluteal, thigh, or thoracolumbar muscular discomfort and was exacerbated by recumbancy. In general, pain was reported as mild or moderate in severity and resolved without medical treatment, but severe back pain was reported infrequently (less than 5% of all reports). When medical treatment was necessary, acetaminophen or nonsteroidal anti-inflammatory drugs were generally effective; however, in a small percentage of subjects who required treatment, a mild narcotic (eg, codeine) was used. Overall, approximately 0.5% of all tadalafil-treated subjects discontinued treatment as a consequence of back pain/myalgia. Diagnostic testing, including measures for inflammation, muscle injury, or renal damage revealed no evidence of medically significant underlying pathology.

Vardenafil – Arthralgia, myalgia, neck pain.

➤*Respiratory:* Dyspnea, pharyngitis.

Sildenafil – Asthma, bronchitis, cough increased, laryngitis, sputum increased.

Tadalafil – Epistaxis.

Vardenafil – Epistaxis.

➤*Special senses:* Conjunctivitis, eye pain.

Sildenafil – Cataract, deafness, dry eyes, ear pain, eye hemorrhage, mydriasis, photophobia, tinnitus.

Tadalafil – Blurred vision, conjunctival hyperemia, eyelid swelling, lacrimation increased; changes in color vision (less than 0.1%).

Vardenafil – Chromatopsia, dim vision, glaucoma, photophobia, tinnitus, watery eyes.

➤*Miscellaneous:* Asthenia, face edema, pain.

Sildenafil – Accidental fall, allergic reaction, chills, shock.

Tadalafil – Fatigue.

Vardenafil – Anaphylactic reaction (including laryngeal edema).

➤*Postmarketing:*
Sildenafil – Anxiety, diplopia, epistaxis, hematuria, increased intraocular pressure, ocular burning, ocular redness or bloodshot appearance, ocular swelling/pressure, paramacular edema, priapism, prolonged erection, retinal vascular disease or bleeding, seizure, temporary vision loss/decreased vision, vitreous detachment/traction.

Overdosage

In studies with healthy volunteers of single doses up to 800 mg **sildenafil**, adverse events were similar to those seen at lower doses, but incidence rates were increased. The maximum dose of **vardenafil** for which human data are available is a single 120 mg dose administered to 8 healthy male volunteers. The majority of these subjects experienced reversible back pain/myalgia and/or abnormal vision. Single doses up to 500 mg **tadalafil** have been given to healthy subjects, and multiple daily doses up to 100 mg have been given to patients. Adverse events were similar to those seen at lower doses. In cases of overdose, adopt standard supportive measures as required. Refer to General Management of Acute Overdosage. Renal dialysis is not expected to accelerate clearance as these drugs are highly bound to plasma proteins and are not significantly eliminated in urine.

Patient Information

Discuss with patients the contraindication of these agents with concurrent organic nitrates. Concomitant use with nitrates could cause BP to suddenly drop to an unsafe level, resulting in dizziness, syncope, or even heart attack or stroke.

Discuss with patients the potential cardiac risk of sexual activity in patients with preexisting cardiovascular risk factors. Advise patients who experience symptoms (eg, angina pectoris, dizziness, nausea) upon initiation of sexual activity to refrain from further activity and discuss the episode with their physician.

These agents offer no protection against sexually transmitted diseases. Consider counseling patients about the protective measures necessary to guard against sexually transmitted diseases, including the human immunodeficiency virus (HIV).

Advise patients that these agents have no effect in the absence of sexual stimulation. Sexual stimulation is required for an erection to occur after taking these agents.

Warn patients to seek immediate medical attention if erections last for more than 4 hours.

Advise patients to contact the prescribing physician if new medications that may interact with these agents are prescribed by another healthcare provider.

Advise patients not to take more than once per day.

Inform patients that substantial consumption of alcohol (eg, 5 units or greater) in combination with a PDE5 inhibitor can increase the potential for orthostatic signs and symptoms, including increase in heart rate, decrease in standing BP, dizziness, and headache.

➤*Alpha-blockers:*
Sildenafil – Advise patients that simultaneous administration of sildenafil doses above 25 mg and an alpha-blocker may lead to symptomatic hypotension in some patients. Therefore, advise patients not to take sildenafil doses above 25 mg within 4 hours of taking an alpha-blocker.

Tadalafil, vardenafil – Concomitant use of tadalafil or vardenafil with alpha-blockers (other than 0.4 mg tamsulosin with tadalafil) is contraindicated because coadministration can produce hypotension.

SILDENAFIL CITRATE

Rx	Viagra (Pfizer)	Tablets: 25 mg	Lactose. (VGR25 PFIZER). Blue, rounded-diamond shape. Film-coated. In 30s.
		50 mg	Lactose. (VGR50 PFIZER). Blue, rounded-diamond shape. Film-coated. In 30s and 100s.
		100 mg	Lactose. (VGR100 PFIZER). Blue, rounded-diamond shape. Film-coated. In 30s and 100s.

For complete prescribing information, refer to the Phosphodiesterase Type 5 Inhibitors group monograph.

Indications

➤*Erectile dysfunction:* For the treatment of erectile dysfunction.

Administration and Dosage

➤*Approved by the FDA:* March 27, 1998.

For most patients, the recommended dose is 50 mg taken as needed approximately 1 hour before sexual activity. However, sildenafil may be taken anywhere from 4 hours to 30 minutes before sexual activity. Based on effectiveness and tolerance, the dose may be increased to a maximum recommended dose of 100 mg or decreased to 25 mg. The maximum recommended dosing frequency is once per day.

➤*Dosage adjustment:* The following factors are associated with increased plasma levels of sildenafil: Older than 65 years of age (40% increase in AUC), hepatic impairment (eg, cirrhosis, 80%), severe renal impairment (Ccr under 30 mL/min, 100%), and concomitant use of potent cytochrome P450 3A4 inhibitors (eg, erythromycin, ketoconazole, itraconazole, saquinavir). Because higher plasma levels may increase the efficacy and incidence of adverse events, consider a starting dose of 25 mg in these patients.

Concomitant use with protease inhibitors – Do not exceed a maximum single dose of 25 mg sildenafil within a 48-hour period.

Concomitant use with alpha-blockers – Do not take 50 or 100 mg doses of sildenafil within 4 hours of alpha-blocker administration. A dose of 25 mg sildenafil may be taken at any time.

➤*Storage/Stability:* Store at 25°C (77°F); excursions permitted to 15° to 30°C (59° to 86°F).

TADALAFIL

Rx	Cialis (Lilly)	Tablets: 5 mg	Lactose. (C 5). Yellow, almond shape. Film-coated. In 30s.
		10 mg	Lactose. (C 10). Yellow, almond shape. Film-coated. In 30s.
		20 mg	Lactose. (C 20). Yellow, almond shape. Film-coated. In 30s.

For complete prescribing information, refer to the Phosphodiesterase Type 5 Inhibitors group monograph.

Indications

➤*Erectile dysfunction:* For the treatment of erectile dysfunction.

Administration and Dosage

➤*Approved by the FDA:* November 21, 2003.

The recommended starting dose in most patients is 10 mg taken prior to anticipated sexual activity. The dose may be increased to 20 mg or decreased to 5 mg, based on individual efficacy and tolerability. The maximum recommended dosing frequency is once daily in most patients. Tadalafil may be taken without regard to food.

Tadalafil was shown to improve erectile function compared with placebo up to 36 hours following dosing. Therefore, take this into consideration when advising patients on optimal use of tadalafil.

➤*Renal function impairment:* For patients with moderate (Ccr 31 to 50 mL/min) renal insufficiency, a starting dose of 5 mg not more than once daily is recommended, and the maximum dose is limited to 10 mg not more than once every 48 hours. For patients with severe (Ccr less than 30 mL/min) renal insufficiency on hemodialysis, the maximum recommended dose is 5 mg.

➤*Hepatic function impairment:* In mild or moderate hepatic impairment (Child-Pugh class A or B), do not exceed 10 mg once daily. In severe hepatic impairment (Child-Pugh class C), the use of tadalafil is not recommended.

➤*Concomitant medications:* For patients taking concomitant potent inhibitors of CYP3A4 (eg, ketoconazole, ritonavir), the maximum recommended dose of tadalafil is 10 mg, not to exceed once every 72 hours.

Concomitant use of nitrates in any form and alpha-adrenergic blockers (other than 0.4 mg once-daily tamsulosin) is contraindicated.

➤*Storage/Stability:* Store at 25°C (77°F); excursions permitted to 15° to 30°C (59° to 86°F).

VARDENAFIL HCl

Rx	Levitra (Bayer)	Tablets: 2.5 mg	(BAYER 2.5). Orange. Film-coated. In 30s.
		5 mg	(BAYER 5). Orange. Film-coated. In 30s.
		10 mg	(BAYER 10). Orange. Film-coated. In 6s and 30s.
		20 mg	(BAYER 20). Orange. Film-coated. In 6s and 30s.

For complete prescribing information, refer to the Phosphodiesterase Type 5 Inhibitors group monograph.

Indications

➤*Erectile dysfunction:* For the treatment of erectile dysfunction.

Administration and Dosage

➤*Approved by the FDA:* August 19, 2003.

For most patients, the recommended starting dose is 10 mg taken approximately 60 minutes before sexual activity. The dose may be increased to a maximum recommended dose of 20 mg or decreased to 5 mg based on efficacy and side effects. The maximum recommended dosing frequency is once daily. Vardenafil can be taken with or without food. Sexual stimulation is required for response to treatment.

➤*Elderly:* Consider a starting dose of 5 mg in patients 65 years of age and older.

➤*Hepatic function impairment:* Vardenafil clearance is reduced in patients with moderate hepatic impairment (Child-Pugh B); a starting dose of 5 mg is recommended. Do not exceed a maximum dose of 10 mg. Vardenafil has not been evaluated in patients with severe hepatic impairment (Child-Pugh C).

➤*Concomitant medications:* The dosage of vardenafil may require adjustment in patients receiving certain CYP3A4 inhibitors (eg, ketoconazole, itraconazole, ritonavir, indinavir, erythromycin). For ritonavir, do not exceed a single dose of 2.5 mg vardenafil in a 72-hour period. For indinavir, 400 mg/day ketoconazole, and 400 mg/day itraconazole, do not exceed a single dose of 2.5 mg vardenafil in a 24-hour period. For 200 mg/day ketoconazole, 200 mg/day itraconazole, and erythromycin, do not exceed a single dose of 5 mg vardenafil in a 24-hour period.

➤*Storage/Stability:* Store at 25°C (77°F); excursions permitted to 15° to 30°C (59° to 86°F).

ACETOHYDROXAMIC ACID (AHA)

Rx	Lithostat (Mission)	**Tablets:** 250 mg	(Mission MPC 500). White. In unit-of-use 100s.

Indications

➤*Chronic urea-splitting urinary infection, adjunctive therapy:* Do not use in lieu of curative surgical treatment (for patients with stones) or antimicrobial treatment. Long-term treatment may be warranted to maintain urease inhibition as long as urea-splitting infection is present.

Administration and Dosage

➤*Adults:* 250 mg, 3 to 4 times a day for a total dose of 10 to 15 mg/kg/day. The recommended starting dose is 12 mg/kg/day, administered at 6- to 8-hour intervals on an empty stomach. The maximum daily dose is ≤ 1.5 g.

➤*Children:* Initial dose is 10 mg/kg/day. Monitor clinical condition and hematologic status; dosage titration may be required.

➤*Renal function impairment:* Patients with serum creatinine of > 1.8 mg/dl should take no more than 1 g/day, dosed at 12-hour intervals. Further dosage reductions to prevent accumulation may be desirable. Do not treat patients with advanced (eg, serum creatinine > 2.5 mg/dl) renal insufficiency.

Actions

➤*Pharmacology:* Acetohydroxamic acid (AHA) reversibly inhibits the bacterial enzyme urease, thereby inhibiting the hydrolysis of urea and production of ammonia in urine infected with urea-splitting organisms. The reduced ammonia levels and decreased pH enhance the effectiveness of antimicrobial agents and increase the cure rate of these infections. AHA does not acidify urine directly, nor does it have a direct antibacterial effect.

In patients with urea-splitting urinary infections (often accompanied by struvite stone disease) that are recalcitrant to other management, AHA reduces the pathologically elevated urinary ammonia and pH levels.

➤*Pharmacokinetics:*

Absorption/Distribution – AHA is well absorbed from the GI tract after oral administration; peak blood levels occur 0.25 to 1 hour after a given dose; it is distributed throughout body water. AHA chelates with dietary iron. Treat concomitant hypochromic anemia with intramuscular iron.

Excretion – From 36% to 65% of the drug is excreted unchanged in the urine and provides the therapeutic effect, but the concentration of AHA in urine that is necessary to inhibit urease is incompletely delineated. Concentrations as low as 8 mcg/ml may be beneficial; expect higher concentrations (eg, 30 mcg/ml) to provide more complete urease inhibition. Plasma half-life of AHA is ≈ 5 to 10 hours with normal renal function and is prolonged in patients with reduced renal function.

Contraindications

In patients whose physical state and disease are amenable to surgery or antimicrobial agents, whose urine is infected by nonurease-producing organisms and whose renal function is poor (eg, serum creatinine > 2.5 mg/dl or Ccr < 20 ml/min) and in females without a satisfactory method of contraception whose urinary infections can be controlled by culture-specific oral antimicrobial agents; pregnancy.

Warnings

➤*Coombs-negative hemolytic anemia:* Coombs-negative hemolytic anemia has occurred. GI upset characterized by nausea, vomiting, anorexia and generalized malaise have accompanied the most severe forms of hemolytic anemia. Approximately 3% of patients developed hemolytic anemia of sufficient magnitude to interrupt treatment. Approximately 15% of patients on AHA have had only laboratory findings of an anemia. However, most patients developed a mild reticulocytosis. The untoward reactions have reverted to normal following treatment cessation. A complete blood count, including reticulocytes, is recommended after 2 weeks of treatment. If reticulocyte count is > 6%, reduce dosage. Perform a CBC and reticulocyte count at 3-month intervals for the treatment duration.

➤*Hematologic effects:* Bone marrow depression (leukopenia, anemia and thrombocytopenia) has occurred in animals receiving large doses of AHA but has not been seen in humans. Its bone marrow suppression is probably related to its ability to inhibit DNA synthesis, but anemia could also be related to depletion of iron stores. Hemolysis, with a decrease in the circulating RBCs, hemoglobin and hematocrit, has been noted. Platelet or white blood cell abnormalities have not been noted, but clinical monitoring is recommended.

➤*Renal function impairment:* Because AHA is eliminated primarily by the kidneys, closely monitor patients and reduce daily dose to avoid excessive drug accumulation.

➤*Hepatic function impairment:* Abnormalities have not been reported, but close monitoring is recommended because a derivative of AHA has caused significant liver dysfunction.

➤*Carcinogenesis:* Acetamide, a metabolite of AHA, caused hepatocellular carcinoma in rats at doses 1500 times the human dose.

➤*Mutagenesis:* AHA is cytotoxic and was positive for mutagenicity in the Ames test.

➤*Pregnancy: Category X.* May cause fetal harm when administered to a pregnant woman. AHA was teratogenic (retarded or clubbed rear leg at ≥ 750 mg/kg and exencephaly and encephalocele at 1500 mg/kg) when given to rats. Do not use in women who are or who may become pregnant. If a patient becomes pregnant while taking this drug, inform her of the potential hazard to the fetus.

➤*Lactation:* It is not known if AHA is secreted in breast milk. Discontinue nursing or the drug, taking into account the importance of the drug to the mother.

➤*Children:* Children with chronic, recalcitrant, urea-splitting urinary infection may benefit from AHA. Dosage has not been established; although, 10 mg/kg/day, taken in 2 or 3 divided doses for up to 1 year, has been tolerated. Monitor patients.

Drug Interactions

AHA Drug Interactions			
Precipitant drug	Object drug*		Description
Alcoholic beverages	AHA	↑	Alcoholic beverages taken with AHA have caused rash
AHA	Heavy metals	↓	AHA chelates heavy metals, notably iron. The absorption of iron and AHA from the intestinal lumen may be reduced when both drugs are taken concomitantly. When iron is indicated, administer IM.

* ↑ = Object drug increased. ↓ = Object drug decreased.

Adverse Reactions

Of 150 patients treated, most for > 1 year, adverse reactions have occurred in ≤ 30%. Adverse reactions seem more prevalent in patients with preexisting thrombophlebitis, phlebothrombosis or advanced degrees of renal insufficiency. The risk of adverse reactions is highest during the first year of treatment. Chronic treatment does not seem to increase risk or severity of adverse reactions.

➤*Cardiovascular:* Superficial phlebitis involving the lower extremities. One patient developed deep vein thrombosis of the lower extremities. All resolved following therapy.

Embolic phenomena were reported in three patients taking AHA; this resolved following discontinuation of AHA and implementation of medical therapy. Several patients have resumed AHA treatment without ill effect. Palpitations have also been reported.

➤*CNS:* Mild headaches (≈ 30%) during the first 48 hours of treatment respond to oral salicylate analgesics and usually disappear spontaneously.

Depression, anxiety, nervousness, malaise and tremulousness (20% to 25%). In most patients, the symptoms were mild and transitory; however, in ≈ 6%, symptoms warranted interruption or discontinuation of treatment.

➤*Dermatologic:* Nonpruritic, macular skin rash in the upper extremities and on the face have occurred when AHA has been taken long-term and usually concomitantly with alcohol. The rash commonly appears 30 to 45 minutes after ingestion of alcohol, may be associated with a general sensation of warmth and disappears spontaneously in 30 to 60 minutes. In some patients, the rash may warrant drug discontinuation. Alopecia has been reported.

➤*GI:* Nausea, vomiting, anorexia (20% to 25%). In most, symptoms were mild, transitory and did not interrupt treatment.

➤*Hematologic:* A mild reticulocytosis (5% to 6%) without anemia is even more prevalent than anemia. The laboratory findings are occasionally accompanied by malaise, lethargy, fatigue and GI symptoms that improve following cessation of treatment. Hematological abnormalities are more prevalent in patients with advanced renal failure (see Warnings).

Overdosage

➤*Symptoms:* Mild overdosages resulting in hemolysis have occurred occasionally with reduced renal function after several weeks or months of continuous treatment.

Acute deliberate overdosage has not occurred, but would be expected to induce the following: Anorexia, malaise, lethargy, diminished sense of well being, tremulousness, anxiety, nausea and vomiting. Laboratory findings are likely to include an elevated reticulocyte count and a severe hemolytic reaction requiring hospitalization, symptomatic treatment and possibly blood transfusions. Anticipate concomitant reduction in platelets or white blood cells.

➤*Treatment:* Cessation of treatment, monitoring of hematologic status, symptomatic treatment and blood transfusions as required. The drug is probably dialyzable but has not been clinically tested. Refer to General Management of Acute Overdosage.

NEOMYCIN AND POLYMYXIN B IRRIGANT

Rx	**Neosporin G.U. Irrigant** (GlaxoWellcome)	**Solution:** 40 mg neomycin (as sulfate) and 200,000 units poly- myxin B sulfate/ml	In 1 ml amps (10s and 50s) and 20 ml multidose vials.[1]

[1] With methylparaben.

Indications

➤*Urinary bladder irrigant:* Continuous irrigant or rinse for short-term use (up to 10 days) in the urinary bladder of abacteriuric patients to help prevent bacteriuria and gram-negative rod bacteremia associated with the use of indwelling catheters.

Administration and Dosage

Not for injection.

For use with catheter systems permitting continuous irrigation of the urinary bladder: Add 1 ml irrigant to 1 L isotonic saline solution. Connect the container to the inflow lumen of the three-way catheter. Connect the outflow lumen via a sterile disposable plastic tube to a disposable plastic collection bag.

Adjust flow rate to 1 L/24 hours. If the patient's urine output exceeds 2 L/day, increase flow rate to 2 L/24 hours.

The rinse of the bladder must be continuous. Do not interrupt the inflow or rinse solution for more than a few minutes.

Actions

➤*Pharmacology:* Polymyxin B sulfate is bactericidal to most gram-negative bacilli, particularly against *Pseudomonas* infections. Neomycin sulfate is bactericidal against a wide range of gram-negative organisms including *Proteus vulgaris* and gram-positive organisms.

When used topically, these drugs are rarely irritating.

Contraindications

Hypersensitivity to any component.

Precautions

➤*Recent UT surgery:* Safety and efficacy have not been established for use in patients with recent lower urinary tract surgery.

➤*Neomycin toxicity:* Neomycin is nephrotoxic and ototoxic, particularly when given parenterally in higher than recommended doses. Cases of nephrotoxicity or ototoxicity have been reported following its topical use for extensive burns and wound irrigation. Although the possibility of these reactions is remote with use of the minimal amount in bladder irrigations, such reactions may occur if irrigations are continued beyond the recommended maximum of 10 days; observe caution.

➤*Superinfection:* Use of antibiotics (especially prolonged or repeated therapy) may result in bacterial or fungal overgrowth of nonsusceptible organisms. Such overgrowth may lead to a secondary infection. Appropriate measures should be taken if superinfection occurs.

Adverse Reactions

The prevalence of neomycin hypersensitivity has increased; however, topical application to mucous membranes rarely results in local or systemic reactions.

CITRIC ACID, GLUCONO-DELTA-LACTONE AND MAGNESIUM CARBONATE IRRIGANT (Hemiacidrin)

Rx	**Renacidin** (Guardian)	**Powder for Solution:** 156 to 171 g citric acid (anhydrous), 21 to 30 g d-gluconic acid (as lactone) w/75 to 87 g purified magnesium hydroxycarbonate, 9 to 15 g magnesium acid citrate, 2 to 6 g Ca (as carbonate) and 17 to 21 g water (combined & free)/300 g bottle	In 150 g.
		Solution: 6.602 g citric acid (anhydrous), 0.198 g glucono-delta-lactone, 3.177 g magnesium carbonate and 0.023 g benzoic acid/100 ml	In 500 ml.

Indications

➤*Solution:* Local irrigation for dissolution of renal calculi composed of apatite (a calcium carbonate-phosphate compound) or struvite (magnesium ammonium phosphates) in patients who are not candidates for surgical removal of the calculi.

As adjunctive therapy to dissolve residual apatite or struvite calculi and fragments after surgery or to achieve partial dissolution of renal calculi to facilitate surgical removal.

For dissolution of bladder calculi of the struvite or apatite variety by local intermittent irrigation through a urethral catheter or cystostomy catheter as an alternative or adjunct to surgical procedures.

For use as an intermittent irrigating solution to prevent or minimize encrustations of indwelling urinary tract catheters.

➤*Powder for solution:* For use in preparing solutions for irrigating indwelling urethral catheters and the urinary bladder, to dissolve or prevent formation of calcifications.

➤*Unlabeled uses:* Hemiacidrin has been used as a renal pelvis irrigation, with meticulous attention to intrapelvic pressure and urosepsis.

Administration and Dosage

➤*Solution:*

Renal calculi – It is essential that patients be free from urinary tract infections prior to initiating chemolytic therapy. A nephrostomy tube is placed at surgery or percutaneously to permit lavage of the calculi. A single catheter may be sufficient if the calculus is not obstructing the ureter or ureteropelvic junction. In patients with an obstructed ureter, a retrograde catheter can be placed through the ureter to the renal pelvis via a cystoscope. This second catheter is used to irrigate the calculus while the percutaneous nephrostomy tube is used for drainage. Pressure measurements are made under fluoroscopy to assure that 2 to 3 ml/min can be infused without causing pain, pyelovenous or pyelotubular backflow or manometric evidence of elevated pressure within the collecting system.

For postoperative patients, irrigation should not be started before the fourth or fifth postoperative day. Irrigation of the renal pelvis is begun with sterile saline only after a sterile urine has been demonstrated. The saline is infused at a rate of 60 ml/hr initially, and the rate is increased until pain or an elevated pressure (25 cm H_2O) appears, or until a maximum flow rate of 120 ml/hr is achieved. Inspect the site of insertion for leakage. If leakage occurs, the irrigation is discontinued temporarily to allow for complete healing around the nephrostomy tube.

If no leakage or flank pain occurs, start irrigation with hemiacidrin with a flow rate equal to maximum rate achieved with the saline solution. Place a clamp on the inflow tube and instruct patients and nursing personnel to stop the irrigating solution whenever pain develops. Nursing personnel who are responsible for performing the irrigation must be instructed concerning location of the nephrostomy tube(s) and direction of flow of irrigating solution to ensure against misconnection of inflowing and egress tubes. Perform nephrostomograms periodically to assure proper placement of catheter tip and to assess efficacy. If stones fail to change size after several days of adequate irrigation, discontinue the procedure.

Upon demonstration of complete dissolution of the calculus, the inflow tube is clamped and left in place for a few days to ensure that no obstruction exists, after which time the nephrostomy tube is removed.

Bladder calculi – Chemolysis of bladder calculi is used as an alternative to cystoscopic or surgical removal of the stones in patients who refuse surgery or cystoscopic removal or in whom these procedures constitute an unwarranted risk. Following appropriate studies to evaluate possible vesicoureteral reflux, 30 ml of hemiacidrin is instilled through a urinary catheter into the bladder and the catheter is clamped for 30 to 60 minutes. The clamp is then released and the bladder is drained. This is repeated 4 to 6 times a day. A continuous drip through a 3-way Foley catheter is an alternative means of dissolving bladder stones. In the presence of bladder spasm and associated high pressure reflux, all precautions required for irrigation of the renal pelvis must be observed.

Indwelling urinary tract catheter encrustation – Periodic instillation of hemiacidrin is indicated to minimize or prevent encrustation of indwelling catheters which frequently results in plugging of the catheter and discomfort to the patient. This is accomplished by instilling 30 ml of the solution through the catheter and then clamping the catheter for 10 minutes, after which the clamp is removed to allow drainage of the bladder. This process is repeated 3 times a day.

➤*Powder for solution:* Irrigating indwelling catheters – Administer as a 10% solution (sterile) in distilled water. Irrigation is carried out with 30 to 60 ml 2 to 3 times daily by means of a rubber syringe.

➤*Preparation of the solution:* Always add powder to the water; do not add water to the powder when preparing solutions.

Dissolve the contents of one 300 g bottle in 3000 ml of sterile distilled water, or any smaller quantity of powder in the proportionately smaller amount of water. Since powder may be reactive upon addition to water, add slowly to the water, with constant agitation, in a container larger than that which the amount of solution actually requires. Do not stopper or cap the container during preparation. Thoroughly mix the solution for as long as possible (up to 15 to 20 minutes). This can be achieved through the use of a mechanical mixer where available. Solutions often vary in color from almost colorless to a definite clear yellow solution.

After thorough mixing, filter the solution through a coarse filter to remove any undissolved matter. Alternatively, if desired, allow the solution to stand and decant. (A 10% solution was filtered after 24 hours and the residue dried at 105°C for 8 hours, then weighed. The weight of the residue equalled 0.008% of the solution.)

The residue which may be noted on a filter consists primarily of the insolubles present in the original magnesium hydroxycarbonate, which has about 0.03% to 0.05% acid insolubles in the form of a small amount of silica (or calcium, as the silicate) and iron oxides which remain undissolved when the solution is prepared. It may be yellow or even brown or black in color.

CITRIC ACID, GLUCONO-DELTA-LACTONE AND MAGNESIUM CARBONATE IRRIGANT (Hemiacidrin)

➤*Storage/Stability:*

Solution – Minimize exposure of hemiacidrin to heat or cold. Store at controlled room temperature (15° to 30°C; 59° to 86°F). Avoid excessive heat or cold (keep from freezing). Brief exposure to temperatures of up to 40°C (104°F) or temperatures down to 5°C (41°F) does not adversely affect the product.

Actions

➤*Pharmacology:* The action of hemiacidrin on susceptible apatite calculi results from an exchange of magnesium from the irrigating solution for the insoluble calcium contained in the stone matrix or calcification. The magnesium salts thereby formed are soluble in the gluconocitrate irrigating solution resulting in the dissolution of the calculus. Struvite calculi are composed mainly of magnesium ammonium phosphates which are solubilized by hemiacidrin due to its acidic pH.

Hemiacidrin is not effective for dissolution of calcium oxalate, uric acid or cysteine stones.

Contraindications

➤*Solution:* Urinary tract infections (see Warnings); presence of demonstrable urinary tract extravasation.

➤*Powder for solution:* Biliary calculi; therapy or preventive therapy above the ureteral-vesical junction, therefore contraindicated for use with ureteral catheters, nephrostomy or pyelostomy tubes or renal lavage for dissolving calculi.

Warnings

➤*Urinary tract infection:* Stop the drug immediately if patient develops fever, urinary tract infection, signs and symptoms consistent with urinary tract infection, persistent flank pain, or if hypermagnesemia or elevated serum creatinine develops.

Urea-splitting bacteria reside within struvite and apatite stones which therefore serve as a source of infection. Dissolution therapy with hemiacidrin in the presence of an infected urinary tract may lead to sepsis and death. Obtain urine specimens for culture prior to initiating chemolytic therapy of the renal pelvis. Institute appropriate antibiotic therapy to treat any infection detected. A sterile urine must be present prior to initiating therapy. An infected stone can serve as a continual source for infection; therefore, continue antibiotic therapy throughout the course of dissolution therapy.

➤*Severe hypermagnesemia:* Severe hypermagnesemia has occurred. Use caution when irrigating the renal pelvis of patients with impaired renal function. Observe patients for early signs and symptoms of hypermagnesemia including nausea, lethargy, confusion and hypotension. Severe hypermagnesemia may result in hyporeflexia, dyspnea, apnea, coma, cardiac arrest and subsequent death. Monitor serum magnesium levels and evaluate deep tendon reflexes. Treatment of hypermagnesemia should include discontinuation of hemiacidrin followed by therapy with IV calcium gluconate, fluids and diuresis in severe cases.

➤*Not indicated:* Not indicated for dissolution of calcium oxalate, uric acid or cysteine calculi.

➤*Pregnancy: Category C.* It is not known whether hemiacidrin can cause fetal harm when administered to a pregnant woman or can affect reproduction capacity. Give to a pregnant woman only if clearly needed.

➤*Lactation:* Magnesium is known to be excreted into breast milk. However, it is not known whether hemiacidrin is excreted in breast milk. Exercise caution when hemiacidrin is administered to a nursing woman.

Precautions

➤*Vesicoureteral reflux:* Vesicoureteral reflux frequently occurs in patients with indwelling urethral or cystostomy catheters. Cystogram prior to initiation of hemiacidrin is essential for such patients. If reflux is demonstrated, all precautions recommended for renal pelvis irrigation must be taken.

➤*Catheter care:* Hospitalization is prolonged for days to weeks when chemolytic therapy is used in lieu of, or following, surgery. Reserve this therapy for selected patients. Care must be taken during chemolysis of renal calculi with hemiacidrin to maintain the patency of the irrigating catheter. Calculus fragments and debris may obstruct the outflow catheter. Continued irrigation under those circumstances leads to increased intrapelvic pressure with a danger of tissue damage or absorption of the irrigating solution. Catheter outflow blockage may be prevented by flushing the catheter with saline and repositioning of the catheter. Frequent monitoring of the system should be performed by a nurse, an aide or any person with sufficient skills to be able to detect any problems with the patency of the catheter. At the first sign of obstruction, discontinue the irrigation and disconnect the system.

➤*Intrapelvic pressures:* Intrapelvic pressures must be maintained at or below 25 cm of water. The preferred method of pressure control is the insertion of an open Y connection pop-off valve into the infusion line allowing immediate decompression if pressure exceeds 25 cm of water. An alternative method has been proposed to direct or stop the flow of the irrigating solution to prevent increased intrapelvic pressure: Placement of a pinch clamp on the inflow line which can be used by the patient or nurse to stop the irrigation at the first sign of flank pain. However, extreme caution must be taken when relying on cooperation of the patient. Patients may not be sufficiently alert to detect signs and symptoms of outflow obstruction. This is especially true in elderly patients, sedated patients or those with severe neurological dysfunction with varying degrees of sensory loss or motor paralysis.

➤*Monitoring:* Throughout the course of therapy, monitor patients to ensure safety. Obtain serum creatinine phosphate and magnesium every few days. Collect urine specimens for culture and antibacterial sensitivity every 3 days or less and at the first sign of fever. Stop the irrigation if any culture exhibits growth and initiate appropriate antibacterial therapy. The irrigation may be started again after a course of antibacterial therapy upon demonstration of a sterile urine. Struvite calculi frequently contain bacteria within the stone; therefore, continue antibacterial therapy throughout the course of dissolution therapy. Hypermagnesemia or an elevated serum creatinine level are indications to halt the irrigation until they return to pre-irrigation levels. Evidence of severe urothelial edema on X-ray is also an indication for temporarily halting the irrigation until the complication resolves.

Drug Interactions

➤*Magnesium-containing medications:* Concurrent use may contribute to production of hypermagnesemia and is not recommended.

Adverse Reactions

Solution – The most common adverse reaction in selected case series is transient flank pain which occurs in most patients. Additional reactions include: Urothelial ulceration or edema (13%); fever (20% but up to 40% in some case series); urinary tract infection, back pain, dysuria, transient hematuria, nausea, hypermagnesemia, hyperphosphatemia, elevated serum creatinine, candidiasis, bladder irritability (1% to 10%); septicemia, ileus, vomiting, thrombophlebitis (< 1%). Death from sepsis has occurred.

Powder for solution – Occasional temporary pain or burning sensation from this procedure; discontinue use if this occurs.

Hexitol Irrigants

Indications

In transurethral prostatic resection or other transurethral surgical procedures.

Administration and Dosage

Do not use unless solution is clear and seal unbroken. Use as required for irrigation.

➤*Storage / Stability:* Promptly use the contents of opened containers; discard unused portions of the solution. Do not warm > 66°C (150°F). Protect from freezing and avoid storage > 40°C (104°F).

Actions

➤*Pharmacology:* Hexitol irrigants are nonelectrolytic and nonhemolytic urologic irrigation solutions. The amount of solution absorbed intravascularly during transurethral prostatic surgery is variable and depends primarily on the extent and duration of the surgery. Mannitol is confined to the extracellular space, only slightly metabolized, rapidly excreted in the urine and is, therefore, an effective osmotic diuretic. The sorbitol-containing products will be metabolized to carbon dioxide (70%) and dextrose (30%) or excreted by the kidneys.

Contraindications

Anuria; injection.

Warnings

Use caution in significant cardiopulmonary or renal dysfunction (see Precautions).

➤*Systemic effects:* Irrigating fluids used during transurethral prostatectomy may enter the systemic circulation in relatively large volumes. Therefore, the irrigation solution must be considered as a systemic drug. The osmotic diuresis it may produce can significantly alter cardiopulmonary and renal dynamics.

➤*Diabetes mellitus:* Hyperglycemia from metabolism of sorbitol may occur in patients with diabetes mellitus.

➤*Sorbitol solution:* Use with caution in patients unable to metabolize sorbitol rapidly enough to avoid the development of hyperosmolar states.

Precautions

➤*Cardiovascular effects:* Carefully evalute cardiovascular status of the patient, particularly one with cardiac disease, before and during transurethral prostatic resection when mannitol irrigant is used. The quantity of fluid absorbed into systemic circulation may cause expansion of extracellular fluid, leading to fulminating CHF.

➤*Fluid and electrolyte balance:* Systemic absorption of the solutions may cause a shift of sodium-free intracellular fluid into the extracellular compartment, lowering serum sodium concentration and aggravating any preexisting hyponatremia.

A significant diuresis resulting from the irrigating solution may obscure and intensify inadequate hydration or hypovolemia. Excessive loss of water and electrolytes may lead to hypernatremia.

Adverse Reactions

Since significant systemic absorption occurs, the potential for systemic effects must be considered. The following effects have been noted from intravenous infusion:

➤*Cardiovascular:* Pulmonary congestion; hypotension; tachycardia; angina-like pains; thrombophlebitis.

➤*Electrolyte disturbance:* Acidosis; electrolyte loss; marked diuresis; urinary retention; edema; dry mouth; thirst; dehydration.

➤*Miscellaneous:* Blurred vision; convulsions; nausea; vomiting; rhinitis; chills; vertigo; backache; urticaria; diarrhea.

Additional reactions associated with sorbitol solution include slight increases in postoperative serum glucose and inhibition of intestinal absorption of vitamin B_{12}.

MANNITOL

Rx	**Resectisol** (Kendall McGaw)	**Solution:** 5 g/100 ml in distilled water (275 mOsm/L)	In 2000 ml.

For complete prescribing information, refer to the Hexitol Irrigants group monograph.

SORBITOL

Rx	**Sorbitol** (Kendall McGaw)	**Solution:** 3.3% (183 mOsm/L)	In 2000 ml.
Rx	**Sorbitol** (Travenol)	**Solution:** 3% (165 mOsm/L)	In 1500 and 3000 ml.

For complete prescribing information, refer to the Hexitol Irrigants group monograph.

MANNITOL AND SORBITOL

Rx	**Sorbitol-Mannitol** (Abbott)	**Solution:** 0.54 g mannitol and 2.7 g sorbitol/100 ml (178 mOsm/L)	In 1500 and 3000 ml.

For complete prescribing information, refer to the Hexitol Irrigants group monograph.

SUBY'S SOLUTION G

Rx	**Suby's Solution G** (Various, eg, Abbott, Travenol)	**Solution:** 3.24 g citric acid (monohydrate), 0.43 g sodium carbonate (anhydrous) and 0.38 g magnesium oxide (anhydrous) per 100 ml	In 1000 ml.

Indications

To dissolve phosphatic calculi or incrustations in the bladder and urethra; to irrigate the bladder and urethra with an acidic solution.

Administration and Dosage

Not for IV, SC or IM injection.

Administer 1 to 3 liters daily by intermittent irrigation or by tidal instillation and drainage to allow continuous irrigation of the bladder for periods of several hours. Intermittent irrigation of the bladder (after the manner of intermittent peritoneal dialysis) may be preferred to promote more prolonged contact of the irrigation with bladder stones; tidal (continuous in and out flow) irrigation may be less efficient and require larger amounts of irrigation fluid.

Use contents of opened container promptly to minimize the possibility of bacterial growth or pyrogen formation. Do not use solution unless clear and seal is intact. Discard unused portion.

Contraindications

Do not use in presence of fulminating bladder infections, bleeding, ulcerations or other open wounds.

Not for injection into body tissue.

Not for irrigation during transurethral surgical procedures.

These solutions are conductive; do not use in the presence of electrical instrumentation.

Warnings

For use in irrigation of the lower urinary tract only.

Not recommended for dissolving phosphate calculi in the renal pelvis because of the risk of creating back pressure that may reactivate an existing pyelonephritis.

Do not use solution to replace other indicated measures including correction of underlying metabolic disorders, surgical intervention and treatment of infection.

▶*Pregnancy: Category C.* It is not known whether this irrigation solution can cause fetal harm when given to a pregnant woman or can affect reproduction capacity. Administer to a pregnant woman only if clearly needed.

Precautions

Avoid reflux of the solution up the ureters into the renal pelvis. Repeated or continuous use may cause bleeding. Solution is irritating to urethra; after each treatment, irrigate with sterile saline or water.

Four cases of sudden death were reported during lavage therapy with a similarly acting solution. The autopsy indicated that calcium phosphate sludge resulting from dissolving stone is a severe irritant to the renal pelvis and is probably absorbed to some degree as evidenced by a terminal serum phosphorus of three times the normal level in one case. Disintegration of calculi into phosphate sludge by acids might form a variety of toxic compounds in small quantities. Since pyelonephritis accompanies renal calculus disease in many cases, pyelorenal backflow of chemicals may aggravate the infectious process causing progression to a severe toxemia.

Adverse Reactions

Discomfort or pain due to bladder irritation during irrigation. In the presence of undetected mucosal lesions, irrigation may initiate bleeding from the bladder.

ACETIC ACID FOR IRRIGATION

Rx	**Acetic Acid for Irrigation** (Various, eg, Abbott, Baxter, Kendall McGaw)	**Solution:** 0.25%	In 250, 500 and 1000 ml.

Indications

For bladder irrigation.

GLYCINE (AMINOACETIC ACID) FOR IRRIGATION

Rx	**Glycine for Irrigation** (Various, eg, Abbott, Baxter, Kendall McGaw)	**Solution:** 1.5%	In 1500, 2000, 3000, 4000 and 5000 ml.

Indications

For urological irrigation.

SODIUM CHLORIDE FOR IRRIGATION

Rx	**Sodium Chloride for Irrigation** (Various, eg, Abbott, Baxter, Kendall McGaw)	**Solution (Isotonic):** 0.9%	In 150, 250, 500, 1000, 1500, 2000 and 4000 ml.
Rx	**Sodium Chloride for Irrigation** (Various, eg, Abbott, Baxter)	**Solution (Hypotonic):** 0.45%	In 500, 1000 and 1500 ml.

Indications

For use as an irrigating solution.

STERILE WATER FOR IRRIGATION

Rx	**Sterile Water for Irrigation** (Various, eg, Abbott, Baxter, Kendall McGaw)		In 250, 500, 1000, 2000 and 4000 ml.

Indications

For use as an irrigating solution.

CYSTEAMINE BITARTRATE

Rx	**Cystagon** (Mylan)	**Capsules:** 50 mg (as cysteamine bitartrate)	(Cysta 50 Mylan). White. In 100s and 500s.
		150 mg (as cysteamine bitartrate)	(Cystagon 150 Mylan). White. In 100s and 500s.

Indications

➤*Nephropathic cystinosis:* Management in children and adults.

Administration and Dosage

➤*Approved by the FDA:* August 15, 1994.

➤*Initial dose:* For the management of nephropathic cystinosis, initiate therapy promptly once the diagnosis is confirmed (ie, increased white cell cystine). Start new patients on ¼ to ⅙ of the maintenance dose of cysteamine. The dose should then be raised gradually over 4 to 6 weeks to avoid intolerance.

➤*Maintenance:* The recommended cysteamine maintenance dose for children up to age 12 years is 1.3 g/m^2/day of the free base, given in 4 divided doses. Intact cysteamine capsules should not be administered to children under the age of ≈ 6 years due to the risk of aspiration. Cysteamine capsules may be administered to children under the age of ≈ 6 years by sprinkling the capsule contents over food. Patients > 12 years of age and > 110 lbs should receive 2 g/day, in 4 divided doses.

When cysteamine is well tolerated, the goal of therapy is to keep leukocyte cystine levels < 1 nmol/½ cystine/mg protein 5 to 6 hours following administration of cysteamine. Patients with poorer tolerability still receive significant benefit if white cell cystine levels are < 2 nmol/½ cystine/mg protein. The cysteamine dose can be increased to a maximum of 1.95 g/m^2/day to achieve this level. The dose of 1.95 g/m^2/day has been associated with an increased rate of withdrawal from treatment due to intolerance and an increased incidence of adverse events.

Cystinotic patients taking cysteamine HCl or phosphocysteamine solutions may be transferred to equimolar doses of cysteamine bitartrate capsules.

The recommended maintenance dose of 1.3 g/m^2/day can be approximated by administering cysteamine according to the following table, which takes surface area as well as weight into consideration.

Cysteamine Maintenance Dose	
Weight (lbs)	Cysteamine free base every 6 hours (mg)
0-10	100
11-20	150
21-30	200
31-40	250
41-50	300
51-70	350
71-90	400
91-110	450
> 110	500

Patients > 12 years of age and > 110 lbs should receive 2 g/day given in 4 divided doses as a starting maintenance dose. This dose should be reached after 4 to 6 weeks of incremental dosage increases as stated above. The dose should be raised if the leukocyte cystine level remains > 2 nmol/½ cystine/mg/protein.

Obtain leukocyte cystine measurements, taken 5 to 6 hours after dose administration, for new patients after the maintenance dose is achieved. Patients being transferred from cysteamine HCl or phosphocysteamine solutions to capsules should have their white cell cystine levels measured in 2 weeks, and thereafter every 3 months to assess optimal dosage as described above.

If cysteamine is poorly tolerated initially due to GI tract symptoms or transient skin rashes, temporarily stop therapy, then reinstitute at a lower dose and gradually increase to the proper dose.

Actions

➤*Pharmacology:* Cysteamine is a cystine-depleting agent that lowers the cystine content of cells in patients with cystinosis, an inherited defect of lysosomal transport. Cysteamine is an aminothiol that participates within lysosomes in a thiol-disulfide interchange reaction converting cystine into cysteine and cysteine-cysteamine mixed disulfide, both of which can exit the lysosome in patients with cystinosis.

Cystinosis is an autosomal recessive inborn error of metabolism in which the transport of cystine out of lysosomes is abnormal; in the nephropathic form, accumulation of cystine and formation of crystals damage various organs, especially the kidney, leading to renal tubular Fanconi syndrome and progressive glomerular failure, with end-stage renal failure by the end of the first decade of life. In four studies of cystinosis patients, renal death (need for transplant or dialysis) occurred at a median age of < 10 years. Patients with cystinosis also experience growth failure, rickets and photophobia due to cystine deposits in the cornea. With time, most organs are damaged, including the retina, muscles and CNS. There are ≈ 200 pretransplant cystinosis patients in the US with nephropathic cystinosis.

Healthy individuals and those heterozygous for cystinosis have white cell cystine levels of < 0.2 and usually < 1 nmol/½ cystine/mg protein, respectively. Individuals with nephropathic cystinosis have elevations of white cell cystine > 2 nmol/½ cystine/mg protein. White cell cystine is monitored in these patients to determine adequacy of dosing. In the Long Term Study (see Clinical trials) entry white cell cystine levels were 3.73 nmol/½ cystine/mg protein (range, 0.13 to 19.80) and were maintained close to 1 nmol/½ cystine/mg protein with a cysteamine dose range of 1.3 to 1.95 g/m^2/day. There are ≈ 200 pretransplant cystinosis patients in the US with nephropathic cystinosis.

➤*Clinical trials:* The National Collaborative Cysteamine Study (NCCS) treated 94 children with nephropathic cystinosis with increasing doses of cysteamine HCl (mean dose, 54 mg/kg/day) to attain white cell cystine levels of < 2 nmol/½ cystine/mg protein 5 to 6 hours postdose, and compared their outcome with a historical control group (n = 17). The principal measures of effectiveness were serum creatinine, calculated creatinine clearance (Ccr) and growth (height).

The average median white cell cystine level attained during treatment was 1.7 ± 0.2 nmol/½ cystine/mg protein. Twelve of the 94 cysteamine-treated patients required early dialysis or renal transplant. Median follow-up of cysteamine patients was > 32 months and 20% were followed > 5 years. Among cysteamine patients, glomerular function was maintained over time despite the longer period of treatment and follow-up. Placebo treated patients, in contrast, experienced a gradual rise in serum creatinine. Patients on treatment maintained growth (did not show increasing growth failure compared to healthy individuals) although growth velocity did not increase enough to allow patients to catch up to age norms. Calculated Ccr was evaluated for two groups, one with poor and one with good white cell cystine depletion. The final mean Ccr of the good depletion group was 20.8 ml/min/1.73 m^2 greater than the mean for the poor depletion group.

The Long Term Study, initiated in 1988, used cysteamine HCl and phosphocysteamine in 46 patients who completed the NCCS (averaging 6.5 years of treatment) and 93 new patients. Patients had cystinosis diagnosed by elevated white cell cystine (mean, 3.63 nmol/½ cystine/mg protein). New patients and 46 continuing patients were required to have serum creatinine < 3 and 4 mg/dl, respectively. Patients were randomized to doses of 1.3 or 1.95 g/m^2/day. Doses could be increased if white cell cystine levels were ≈ 2 nmol/½ cystine/mg protein and lowered due to intolerance.

White cell cystine levels averaged 1.72 ± 1.65 and 1.86 ± 0.92 nmol/½ cystine/mg protein in the 1.3 and 1.95 g/m^2/day groups, respectively. In new patients, serum creatinine was essentially unchanged over the period of follow-up (≈ 50% followed for 24 months) and phosphocysteamine and cysteamine HCl had similar effects. The long-term follow-up group (almost 80% were followed at least 2 years) had essentially no change in renal function. Both groups maintained height (although they did not catch up from baseline). There was no apparent difference between the two doses.

Contraindications

Hypersensitivity to cysteamine or penicillamine.

Warnings

➤*Rash:* If a skin rash develops, withhold cysteamine until the rash clears. Cysteamine may be restarted at a lower dose under close supervision, then slowly titrated to the therapeutic dose. If a severe skin rash develops such as erythema multiforme bullosa or toxic epidermal necrolysis, cysteamine should not be readministered.

➤*CNS symptoms:* CNS symptoms, such as seizures, lethargy, somnolence, depression and encephalopathy have been associated with cysteamine. If CNS symptoms develop, carefully evaluate the patient and adjust the dose as necessary. Neurological complications have been described in some cystinotic patients not on cysteamine treatment. This may be a manifestation of the primary disorder. Patients should not engage in hazardous activities until the effects of cysteamine on mental performance are known.

➤*Fertility impairment:* At an oral dose of 375 mg/kg/day (1.7 times the recommended human dose), cysteamine reduced the fertility of rats and offspring survival.

➤*Pregnancy:* Category C. It is not known whether cysteamine can cause fetal harm when administered to a pregnant woman. Use only when clearly needed and when the potential benefits outweigh the potential hazards to the fetus.

➤*Lactation:* It is not known whether cysteamine is excreted in breast milk. Because of the manifested potential of cysteamine for developmental toxicity in suckling rat pups when it was administered to their lactating mothers at an oral dose of 375 mg/kg/day, decide whether to discontinue nursing or to discontinue the drug, taking into account the importance of the drug to the mother.

➤*Children:* The safety and efficacy of cysteamine for cystinotic children have been established. Initiate therapy as soon as the diagnosis of nephropathic cystinosis has been confirmed.

CYSEAMINE BITARTRATE

Precautions

►*Monitoring:* Cysteamine has occasionally been associated with reversible leukopenia and abnormal liver function studies. Therefore, monitor blood counts and liver function studies.

Leukocyte cystine measurements are useful to determine adequate dosage and compliance. When measured 5 to 6 hours after cysteamine administration, the goal should be a level < 1 nmol/½ cystine/mg protein. In some patients with poorer tolerability for cysteamine, patients may still receive benefit with a white cell cystine level of < 2 nmol/½ cystine/mg protein. Measurements should be done every 3 months, more frequently when patients are transferred from cysteamine HCl or phosphocysteamine solutions to cysteamine bitartrate.

►*GI symptoms:* GI symptoms, including nausea, vomiting, anorexia and abdominal pain (sometimes severe), have been associated with cysteamine. If these develop, therapy may have to be interrupted and the dose adjusted. A dose of 1.95 g/m²/day (≈ 80 to 90 mg/kg/day) was associated with an increased number of withdrawals from treatment due to intolerance and an increased incidence of adverse events.

►*Concurrent therapy:* Cysteamine can be administered with electrolyte and mineral replacements necessary for management of the Fanconi syndrome as well as vitamin D and thyroid hormone.

Adverse Reactions

In three clinical trials, cysteamine or phosphocysteamine have been administered to 246 children with cystinosis. Causality of side effects is sometimes difficult to determine because adverse effects may result from the underlying disease.

Adverse reactions or intolerance leading to cessation of treatment occurred in 8% of patients in the US studies. Withdrawals due to intolerance, vomiting associated with medication, anorexia, lethargy and fever appeared dose-related, occurring more frequently in those patients receiving 1.95 vs 1.3 g/m²/day.

The most frequent adverse reactions seen involve the GI (see Precautions) and central nervous systems (see Warnings). These are especially prominent at the initiation of therapy. Temporarily suspending treatment, then gradual reintroduction may be effective in improving tolerance. The most common events (> 5%) were vomiting (35%), anorexia (31%), fever (22%), diarrhea (16%), lethargy (11%) and rash (7%).

Other adverse reactions are as follows:

►*CNS:* Somnolence; encephalopathy; headache; seizures; ataxia; confusion; tremor; hyperkinesia; decreased hearing; dizziness; jitteriness.

►*GI:* Nausea; bad breath; abdominal pain; dyspepsia; constipation; gastroenteritis; duodenitis; duodenal ulceration.

►*Psychiatric:* Nervousness; abnormal thinking; depression; emotional lability; hallucinations; nightmares.

►*Miscellaneous:* Abnormal liver function; anemia; leukopenia; dehydration; hypertension; urticaria.

Overdosage

►*Symptoms:* A single oral dose of 660 mg/kg was lethal to rats. Symptoms of acute toxicity were reduction of motor activity and generalized hemorrhage in the GI tract and kidneys. One case of massive human overdosage has been reported. The patient immediately vomited the drug and did not develop any symptoms.

►*Treatment:* Should overdose occur, appropriately support the respiratory and cardiovascular systems. No specific antidote is known. Refer to General Management of Acute Overdosage. Hemodialysis may be considered since cysteamine is poorly bound to plasma proteins.

TIOPRONIN

Rx	**Thiola** (Mission)	**Tablets:** 100 mg	(Mission SS 121). White. Sugar coated. In 100s.

Indications

►*Kidney stones:* Prevention of cystine (kidney) stone formation in patients with severe homozygous cystinuria with urinary cystine > 500 mg/day, who are resistant to treatment with conservative measures of high fluid intake, alkali and diet modification or who have adverse reactions to d-penicillamine.

Administration and Dosage

Attempt a conservative treatment program first. Provide ≥ 3 L of fluid, including two glasses with each meal and at bedtime. Advise the patient to awake at night to urinate and to drink two more glasses of fluids before returning to bed. Consume additional fluids if there is excessive sweating or intestinal fluid loss. Seek a minimum urine output of 2 L/day on a consistent basis. Provide a modest amount of alkali in order to maintain urinary pH at a high normal range (6.5 to 7).

►*Adverse reactions to d-penicillamine:* Patients who previously manifested adverse reactions to d-penicillamine are more likely to experience adverse reactions to tiopronin than patients who take tiopronin for the first time. A close supervision with a careful monitoring of potential side effects is mandatory during tiopronin treatment. Advise patients to report promptly any symptoms suggesting toxicity. Discontinue treatment if severe toxicity develops.

Excessive alkali therapy is not advisable. When urinary pH increases> 7 with alkali therapy, calcium phosphate nephrolithiasis may ensue because of the enhanced urinary supersaturation of hydroxyapatite in an alkaline environment. Potassium alkali are advantageous over sodium alkali because they do not cause hypercalciuria and are less likely to cause the complication of calcium stones.

In patients who continue to form cystine stones on the above conservative program, tiopronin may be added. Tiopronin may also be substituted for d-penicillamine in patients who have developed toxicity to the latter drug. In both situations, continue the conservative treatment program.

Base tiopronin dosage on the amount required to reduce urinary cystine concentration to below its solubility limit (generally < 250 mg/L). The extent of the decline in cystine excretion is generally dosage dependent.

►*Initial adult dosage:* 800 mg/day in adults with cystine stones; average dose is 1000 mg/day. However, some patients require less.

►*Children:* Initial dosage may be based on 15 mg/kg/day. Measure urinary cystine 1 month after treatment and every 3 months thereafter. Readjust dosage depending on urinary cystine value. Whenever possible, give in divided doses 3 times/day ≥ 1 hour before or 2 hours after meals.

In patients with severe toxicity to d-penicillamine, initiate tiopronin at a lower dosage.

Actions

►*Pharmacology:* Tiopronin is an active reducing and complexing thiol compound for the prevention of cystine (kidney) stone formation. It undergoes thiol-disulfide exchange with cystine to form a mixed disulfide of tiopronin-cysteine; a water-soluble mixed disulfide is formed and the amount of sparingly soluble cystine is reduced.

Cystine stones typically occur in ≈ 10,000 people in the US who are homozygous for cystinuria. These people excrete abnormal amounts of cystine in urine, as well as excessive amounts of other dibasic amino acids (eg, lysine, arginine, ornithine). They also show varying intestinal transport defects for these same amino acids. Stone formation is the result of poor aqueous solubility of cystine and is determined primarily by the urinary supersaturation of cystine. Thus, cystine stones, theoretically, form whenever urinary cystine concentration exceeds the solubility limit. Cystine solubility in urine is pH-dependent and ranges from 170 to 300 mg/L at pH 5, 190 to 400 mg/L at pH 7, and 220 to 500 mg/L at pH 7.5.

The goal of therapy is to reduce urinary cystine concentration below its solubility limit. It may be accomplished by dietary means to reduce cystine synthesis and by a high fluid intake to increase urine volume and thereby lower cystine concentration. These conservative measures alone may be ineffective. In some homozygous patients with severe cystinuria, d-penicillamine has been used as an additional therapy. However, d-penicillamine treatment is frequently accompanied by adverse reactions.

►*Pharmacokinetics:* Up to 48% of a dose appears in urine during the first 4 hours and up to 78% by 72 hours. Thus, in patients with cystinuria, a sufficient amount of tiopronin or its active metabolites could appear in urine to react with cystine, lowering cystine excretion.

The decrement in urinary cystine produced by tiopronin is generally proportional to the dose. A reduction in urinary cystine of 250 to 350 mg/day and 500 mg/day at a dosage of 1 and 2 g/day, respectively, might be expected. Tiopronin causes a sustained reduction in cystine excretion without loss of effectiveness. It has a rapid onset and offset of action, showing a fall in cystine excretion on the first day of administration and a rise on the first day of drug withdrawal.

►*Clinical trials:*
Versus penicillamine – A multiclinic trial involving 66 cystinuric patients indicated that tiopronin is associated with fewer or less severe adverse reactions than d-penicillamine. Among those stopping d-penicillamine because of toxicity, 64.7% could take tiopronin. In those without a history of d-penicillamine treatment, only 5.9% developed reactions of sufficient severity to require tiopronin withdrawal.

Contraindications

History of agranulocytosis, aplastic anemia or thrombocytopenia on this medication; pregnancy, lactation (see Warnings).

Warnings

►*Fatalities:* Fatalities from tiopronin are possible (but not reported), as has been reported with d-penicillamine from such complications as aplastic anemia, agranulocytosis, thrombocytopenia, Goodpasture's syndrome or myasthenia gravis.

►*Hepatotoxicity:* Jaundice and abnormal liver function tests have been reported during tiopronin therapy for non-cystinuric conditions. A direct cause-and-effect relationship, based upon these foreign reports, has not been established. Monitor patients carefully. If any abnormali-

TIOPRONIN

ties are noted, discontinue the drug and treat the patient with appropriate measures.

▶*Hematologic:* Leukopenia of the granulocytic series may develop without eosinophilia. Thrombocytopenia may be immunologic in origin or idiosyncratic. The reduction in peripheral blood white count to < 3500/mm^3 or in platelet count to < 100,000/mm^3 mandates cessation of therapy. Instruct patients to report promptly any symptom or sign of these hematological abnormalities, such as fever, sore throat, chills, bleeding or easy bruising.

▶*Proteinuria:* Proteinuria, sometimes sufficiently severe to cause nephrotic syndrome, may develop from membranous glomerulopathy. Closely observe patients.

▶*Complications:* Complications (rare) have occurred during d-penicillamine therapy and could occur during tiopronin treatment. Stop therapy if the following occurs: Abnormal urinary findings with hemoptysis and pulmonary infiltrates suggestive of Goodpasture's syndrome; appearance of myasthenic syndrome or myasthenia gravis; development of pemphigus-type reactions. Steroid treatment may be necessary.

▶*Drug fever:* Drug fever may develop, usually during the first month of therapy; discontinue until the fever subsides. Treatment may be reinstated at a small dose, with a gradual increase in dosage until the desired level is achieved.

▶*Rash:* Generalized rash (erythematous, maculopapular or morbilliform) accompanied by pruritis may develop during the first few months of treatment. It may be controlled by antihistamine therapy, typically recedes when tiopronin is discontinued and seldom recurs when tiopronin is restarted at a lower dosage. Less commonly, rash may appear late in treatment (after > 6 months). Usually located on the trunk, the late rash is associated with intense pruritis, recedes slowly after discontinuing treatment and usually recurs upon resumption of treatment.

▶*Lupus erythematous-like reaction:* Lupus erythematous-like reaction manifested by fever, arthralgia and lymphadenopathy may develop. It may be associated with a positive antinuclear antibody test, but not necessarily with nephropathy. It may require discontinuation of treatment.

▶*Pregnancy: Category C.* Skeletal defects and cleft palates occur in the fetus when d-penicillamine is given to pregnant rats at 10 times the dose recommended for humans. A similar teratogenicity might be expected for tiopronin. There are no adequate and well controlled studies in pregnant women. Use during pregnancy is contraindicated except in those with severe cystinuria.

▶*Lactation:* Because tiopronin may be excreted in breast milk and because of potential serious adverse reactions of nursing infants, advise mothers taking tiopronin not to nurse.

▶*Children:* Safety and effectiveness in children < 9 years old have not been established.

Precautions

▶*Monitoring:* Monitoring tests are recommended, including the following: Peripheral blood counts, direct platelet count, hemoglobin, serum albumin, liver function tests, 24-hour urinary protein and routine urinalysis at 3- to 6-month intervals during treatment. In order to assess the effect on stone disease, monitor urinary cystine frequently during the first 6 months when the optimum dose schedule is being determined and at 6-month intervals thereafter. Abdominal roentgenogram (KUB) is advised yearly to monitor the size and appearance of stone(s).

▶*Wrinkling and friability of skin:* Wrinkling and friability of skin usually occurs after long-term treatment and results from the effect of tiopronin on collagen.

▶*Hypoguesia:* Hypoguesia, often self-limiting, may develop as the result of trace metal chelation by tiopronin.

▶*Vitamin B$_6$ deficiency:* Vitamin B$_6$ deficiency is uncommonly associated with tiopronin treatment, unlike during d-penicillamine therapy.

Adverse Reactions

▶*Dermatologic:* Rash, lupus erythematous-like reaction, pruritis, wrinkling, friability (see Precautions and Warnings).

▶*GI:* Nausea, emesis, diarrhea or soft stools, anorexia, abdominal pain, bloating or flatus ($\approx$ 17%).

▶*Hematologic:* Increased bleeding, anemia, leukopenia, thrombocytopenia, eosinophilia ($\approx$ 4%).

▶*Hypersensitivity:* Laryngeal edema, dyspnea, respiratory distress, fever, chills, arthralgia, weakness, fatigue, myalgia, adenopathy ($\approx$ 4%).

▶*Renal:* Proteinuria, nephrotic syndrome, hematuria ($\approx$ 1%).

▶*Respiratory:* Bronchiolitis, hemoptysis, pulmonary infiltrates, dyspnea ($\approx$ 2%). Despite this apparent reduced toxicity to tiopronin relative to d-penicillamine, tiopronin treatment may potentially be associated with all adverse reactions reported with d-penicillamine.

These reactions are more likely to develop during tiopronin therapy among patients who have previously shown toxicity to d-penicillamine.

▶*Miscellaneous:* Drug fever (see Warnings), hypoguesia, vitamin B$_6$ deficiency (rare) (see Precautions), jaundice, abnormal liver function tests, myasthenic syndrome ($\approx$ 2%); impairment in taste and smell ($\approx$ 4%).

PENICILLAMINE

Rx	Cuprimine (Merck)	Capsules: 125 mg	Lactose. (MSD 672). Opaque yellow and gray. In 100s.
		250 mg	Lactose. (MSD 602). Ivory. In 100s.
Rx	Depen (Wallace)	Tablets, titratable: 250 mg	Lactose, EDTA. (37-4401). White. Scored. Oval. In 100s.

Indications

▶*Rheumatoid arthritis:* Because penicillamine can cause severe adverse reactions, restrict its use in rheumatoid arthritis to patients who have severe, active disease and who have failed to respond to an adequate trial of conventional therapy. Carefully consider the benefit-to-risk ratio. Use other measures, such as rest, physiotherapy, salicylates and corticosteroids, when indicated in conjunction with the drug.

▶*Wilson's disease (hepatolenticular degeneration):* Wilson's disease is an abnormality in copper metabolism. As a result, copper is deposited in several organs and produces pathologic effects most prominently seen in brain, liver, kidneys and eyes. Penicillamine is a copper-chelating agent intended to promote excretion of copper deposited in tissues.

▶*Cystinuria:* Cystinuria is characterized by excessive urinary excretion of dibasic amino acids, including arginine, lysine, ornithine and cystine. Stone formation is the only known pathology in cystinuria.

Penicillamine may be used as additional therapy, when conventional measures (eg, dilution and alkalinization of the urine, methionine restricted diet) are inadequate to control recurrent stone formation.

▶*Unlabeled uses:* The benefits of penicillamine's copper-chelating and immunological effects have been investigated for use in the treatment of primary biliary cirrhosis. Doses of 600 to 900 mg/day have been used with both success and failure. Some data suggest that penicillamine may be beneficial in scleroderma.

Administration and Dosage

Give penicillamine on an empty stomach $\geq$ 1 hour before meals or 2 hours after meals and $\geq$ 1 hour apart from any other drug, food or milk.

▶*Wilson's disease:* Initial dosage is 1 g/day for children or adults. This may be increased, as indicated by the urinary copper analyses, but it is seldom necessary to exceed 2 g/day. In patients who cannot tolerate 1 g/day initially, initiating dosage with 250 mg/day and increasing gradually allows closer control of the drug.

Determine optimal dosage by measuring urinary copper excretion. Quantitatively analyze for copper before and soon after initiating therapy. Perform 24-hour urinary copper analysis every 3 months for duration of therapy. The patient probably will be in a negative copper balance of 0.5 to 1 mg copper present in a 24-hour urine collection.

▶*Cystinuria:* Adult dosage – 2 g/day (range 1 to 4 g/day).

Pediatric dosage – 30 mg/kg/day in 4 divided doses. If 4 equal doses are not feasible, give the larger portion at bedtime. If adverse reactions necessitate a reduction in dosage, it is important to retain the bedtime dose. Initiating dosage with 250 mg/day, and increasing gradually, allows closer control of the drug and may reduce the incidence of adverse reactions.

Patients should drink about a pint of fluid at bedtime and another pint once during the night when urine is more concentrated and more acidic than during the day. The greater the fluid intake, the lower the dosage of penicillamine required.

Individualize dosage to limit cystine excretion to 100 to 200 mg/day in those with no history of stones, and below 100 mg/day in those who have had stone formation or pain. Consider the inherent tubular defect and the patient's size, age and rate of growth, as well as diet and water intake.

Rheumatoid arthritis – 2 or 3 months may be required before a clinical response is noted.

When treatment has been interrupted because of adverse reactions or other reasons, cautiously reintroduce the drug at a lower dosage and increase slowly.

Initial therapy – A single daily dose of 125 or 250 mg. Thereafter, increase dose at 1- to 3-month intervals by 125 or 250 mg/day as patient response and tolerance indicate. If satisfactory remission is achieved, continue the dose. If there is no improvement and if there are no signs of potentially serious toxicity after 2 to 3 months with doses of 500 to 750 mg/day, continue increases of 250 mg/day at 2- to 3-month intervals until satisfactory remission occurs or toxicity develops. If there is no discernible improvement after 3 to 4 months of treatment

PENICILLAMINE

with 1 to 1.5 g/day, assume the patient will not respond and discontinue the drug.

Maintenance therapy – Individualize dosage. Many patients respond to ≤ 500 to 750 mg/day. Changes in dosage level may not be reflected clinically or in the erythrocyte sedimentation rate for 2 to 3 months after each adjustment. Some patients will subsequently require an increase in dosage to achieve maximal disease suppression. In patients who respond but who evidence incomplete disease suppression after the first 6 to 9 months of treatment, increase daily dosage by 125 or 250 mg/day at 3-month intervals. Dosage > 1 g/day is unusual, but up to 1.5 g/day has been required.

Management of exacerbations – Following an initial good response, some patients may experience a self-limited exacerbation of disease activity that can subside within 12 weeks. They are usually controlled by adding nonsteroidal anti-inflammatory drugs. Consider an increase in maintenance dose only if the patient has demonstrated a true "escape" phenomenon (as evidenced by failure of the flare to subside within this time period).

Migratory polyarthralgia – Migratory polyarthralgia due to penicillamine is extremely difficult to differentiate from an exacerbation of the rheumatoid arthritis. Discontinuation or substantial reduction in dosage for several weeks will usually determine which of these processes is responsible for the arthralgia.

Duration of therapy – Duration of therapy has not been determined. If the patient has been in remission for ≥ 6 months, attempt a gradual, stepwise dosage reduction in decrements of 125 or 250 mg/day at ≈ 3-month intervals.

Concomitant drug therapy – See Drug Interactions. Salicylates, other nonsteroidal anti-inflammatory drugs or systemic corticosteroids may be continued when penicillamine is initiated. After improvement begins, analgesic and anti-inflammatory drugs may be discontinued slowly as symptoms permit. Months of penicillamine treatment may be required before steroids can be completely eliminated.

Dosage frequency – Dosages ≤ 500 mg/day can be given as a single daily dose. Dosages > 500 mg/day should be administered in divided doses.

➤*Alternative dosage forms:*

Elixir 50 mg/ml – Dissolve 48 capsules in 100 ml of water. Filter and stir in 100 ml of cherry syrup and 30 ml of alcohol. Bring the volume up to 240 ml with water. Shake well and store in the refrigerator.

Suppositories 750 mg – Melt 51 g of cocoa butter. Dissolve 150 capsules in the cocoa butter. Pour the mixture into a pre-lubricated suppository mold. Freeze, then store in the refrigerator.

➤*Storage/Stability:* Store at room temperature 15° to 30°C (59° to 86°F). Protect from moisture.

Actions

➤*Pharmacology:*

Rheumatoid arthritis – The mechanism of action of penicillamine in rheumatoid arthritis is unknown. Penicillamine markedly lowers IgM rheumatoid factor, but produces no significant depression in absolute levels of serum immunoglobulins; it dissociates macroglobulins (rheumatoid factor). The drug may decrease cell-mediated immune response by selectively inhibiting T-lymphocyte function. Penicillamine may also act as an anti-inflammatory agent by inhibiting release of lysosomal enzymes and oxygen radicals protecting lymphocytes from the harmful effects of hydrogen peroxide formed at inflammatory sites.

The onset of therapeutic response may not be seen for 2 or 3 months in those patients who respond. The optimum duration of therapy has not been determined. If remissions occur, they may last from months to years, but usually require continued treatment (see Administration and Dosage).

Wilson's disease: Penicillamine is a chelating agent that removes excess copper in patients with Wilson's disease. From in vitro studies that indicate that one atom of copper combines with two molecules of penicillamine, it would appear that 1 g penicillamine should be followed by the excretion of ≈ 200 mg of copper; however, the actual amount excreted is ≈ 1% of this. Noticeable improvement may not occur for 1 to 3 months. Occasionally, neurologic symptoms become worse during initiation of therapy.

Two types of patients require treatment for Wilson's disease:
  1.) The symptomatic and
  2.) the asymptomatic in whom it can be assumed the disease will develop in the future if the patient is not treated.

Cystinuria: Penicillamine reduces excess cystine excretion in cystinuria. Penicillamine with conventional therapy decreases crystalluria and stone formation and may decrease the size of or dissolve existing stones. This is done, at least in part, by disulfide interchange between penicillamine and cystine, resulting in a substance more soluble than cystine and readily excreted.

Poisoning: Penicillamine also forms soluble complexes with iron, mercury, lead and arsenic which are readily excreted by the kidneys. The drug may be used to treat poisoning by these metals.

➤*Pharmacokinetics:* It is well absorbed from the GI tract after oral administration (40% to 70%); peak plasma levels occur in 1 to 3 hours.

Take on an empty stomach, ≥ 1 hour before meals or 2 hours after meals, and ≥ 1 hour apart from any other drug, food or milk. This permits maximum absorption and reduces the likelihood or inactivation by metal binding in the GI tract.

Most (80%) of the plasma penicillamine is protein bound, primarily to albumin. Penicillamine is rapidly excreted in the urine (≈ 42.1 in 24 hours); 50% is excreted in the feces. Metabolites may be detected in the urine for up to 3 months after stopping the drug. Half-life ranges are 1.7 to 3.2 hours (average 2.1 hours).

Contraindications

History of penicillamine-related aplastic anemia or agranulocytosis; rheumatoid arthritis patients with a history or other evidence of renal insufficiency (because of the potential for causing renal damage); pregnancy (see Warnings); breastfeeding.

Warnings

➤*Fatalities:* Penicillamine has been associated with fatalities due to aplastic anemia, agranulocytosis, thrombocytopenia, sideroblastic anemia, Goodpasture's syndrome and myasthenia gravis.

➤*Hematologic:* Leukopenia (2%) and thrombocytopenia (4%) have occurred. A reduction in WBC < 3500, neutrophils < 2000/mm³, or monocytes > 500/mm³ mandate permanent withdrawal of therapy. Thrombocytopenia may be idiosyncratic, with decreased or absent megakaryocytes in marrow, when it is part of an aplastic anemia. In other cases, thrombocytopenia is presumably on an immune basis since the number of megakaryocytes in the marrow has been normal or sometimes increased. Platelet count < 100,000, even in the absence of clinical bleeding, or a progressive fall in either platelet count or WBC in three successive determinations, even though values are still in the normal range, requires at least temporary cessation of therapy.

➤*Hepatotoxicity:* Penicillamine has been associated with a mild elevation of hepatic enzymes that usually returns to normal even with continuation of the drug.

➤*Lupus erythematosus:* Certain patients will develop a positive antinuclear antibody (ANA) test and some may show a lupus erythematosus-like syndrome similar to other drug-induced lupus, but it is not associated with hypocomplementemia and may be present without nephropathy. A positive ANA test does not mandate drug discontinuance; however, a lupus erythematosus-like syndrome may develop later.

➤*Oral ulcerations:* Oral ulcerations may develop which may have the appearance of aphthous stomatitis; it usually recurs on rechallenge but often clears on a lower dosage. Although rare, cheilosis, glossitis and gingivostomatitis have been reported. They are frequently dose-related and may preclude further increase in dosage or require drug discontinuation.

➤*Hypogeusia:* Hypogeusia occurs in 25% to 33% of patients, except for a lesser incidence in Wilson's disease (4%). Most cases are established within 6 weeks, but most commonly resolve in 2 to 6 months despite continued treatment. Total loss of taste has occurred.

➤*Hypoglycemia:* Hypoglycemia has been reported in 4 patients receiving penicillamine therapy for rheumatoid arthritis. The mechanism of hypoglycemia is unknown. Two insulin-dependent diabetic patients experienced nighttime hypoglycemia after the addition of penicillamine. Both patients required a reduction in their insulin dosage.

Two nondiabetic patients who had never received insulin or oral hypoglycemics developed anti-insulin antibodies. In these patients, penicillamine was suspected to be responsible for the antibody formation because it has been known to induce autoimmune complexes (see Warnings).

➤*Autoimmune syndromes:* Autoimmune syndromes, which may be caused by penicillamine, include polymyositis, diffuse alveolitis and dermatomyositis and the following:

Goodpasture's syndrome – Goodpasture's syndrome is rare. Development of abnormal urinary findings associated with hemoptysis and pulmonary infiltrates on X-ray requires immediate drug cessation.

Obliterative bronchiolitis – Obliterative bronchiolitis has been reported rarely. Caution the patient to report immediately pulmonary symptoms such as exertional dyspnea or unexplained cough or wheezing. Consider pulmonary function studies at this time.

Myasthenic syndrome – Myasthenic syndrome sometimes progressing to myasthenia gravis has been reported. Ptosis and diplopia, with weakness of the extraocular muscles, are often early signs of myasthenia. In most cases, symptoms have receded after withdrawal of the drug.

Pemphigus vulgaris – Pemphigus vulgaris and pemphigus foliaceous are reported most frequently, usually as a late complication of therapy. The seborrhea-like characteristics of pemphigus foliaceous may obscure an early diagnosis. When pemphigus is suspected, discontinue penicillamine. Treatment has consisted of high doses of corticosteroids alone or, in some cases, concomitantly with an immunosuppressant. Treatment may be required for only a few weeks or months but may need to be continued for more than a year.

➤*Sensitivity reactions:* Once instituted for Wilson's disease or cystinuria, continue treatment with penicillamine on a daily basis. Interruptions for even a few days have been followed by sensitivity reactions after reinstitution of therapy.

PENICILLAMINE

►*Cross-sensitivity:* Cross-sensitivity may theoretically appear in patients allergic to penicillin. Reactions from contamination of penicillamine by trace amounts of penicillin have been eliminated now that penicillamine is produced synthetically rather than as a degradation product of penicillin.

►*Hypersensitivity reactions:* Allergic reactions occur in ≈ ⅓ of patients. They are more common at the start of treatment, and occur as generalized rashes or drug fever. Discontinue treatment and reinstitute at a low dosage such as 250 mg/day, with gradual increases. Administering prednisolone 20 mg/day for the first few weeks of penicillamine therapy reduces the severity of these reactions. Antihistamines may control pruritus.

Drug fever – Drug fever may appear in some patients, usually in the second to third week of therapy; it is sometimes accompanied by a macular cutaneous eruption.

In patients with Wilson's disease or cystinuria, because no alternative treatment is available, temporarily discontinue penicillamine until the reaction subsides. Reinstitute therapy with a small dose and gradually increase until the desired dosage is attained. Systemic steroid therapy may be necessary, and is usually helpful, in patients who develop toxic reactions a second or third time.

In rheumatoid arthritis patients, discontinue penicillamine and try another therapeutic alternative since the febrile reaction will recur in a high percentage of patients upon readministration.

Dermatologic: Observe the skin and mucous membranes for allergic reactions. Skin rashes (44% to 50%) are the most frequent adverse reactions. Early rash occurs during the first few months of treatment and is more common. It is usually a generalized pruritic, erythematous, maculopapular or morbilliform rash and resembles the allergic rash seen with other drugs. It usually disappears within days after stopping penicillamine and seldom recurs when the drug is restarted at a lower dosage. Pruritus and early rash are often controlled by antihistamine coadministration.

A late rash: A late rash is less commonly seen, usually after ≥ 6 months treatment, and requires drug discontinuation. It usually appears on the trunk, is accompanied by intense pruritus, and is usually unresponsive to topical corticosteroids. It may take weeks to disappear after penicillamine is stopped and usually recurs if the drug is restarted.

Pemphigoid rash: Pemphigoid rash the most serious dermatologic adverse reaction occurs most often after > 6 to 9 months of penicillamine. From 1 to 2 months may be required for resolution. Do not rechallenge patient.

The appearance of a drug eruption accompanied by fever, arthralgia, lymphadenopathy, or other allergic manifestations usually requires drug discontinuation.

►*Renal function impairment:* Proteinuria or hematuria may develop and may be a warning sign of membranous glomerulopathy which can progress to a nephrotic syndrome. In some patients, proteinuria disappears with continued therapy; in others, penicillamine must be discontinued. When proteinuria or hematuria develops, ascertain whether it is a sign of drug-induced glomerulopathy or is unrelated to penicillamine. History of proteinuria secondary to gold therapy may be a risk factor for penicillamine proteinuria.

Cautiously continue penicillamine in rheumatoid arthritis patients developing moderate degrees of proteinuria; obtain quantitative 24 hour urinary protein determinations at 1- to 2-week intervals. Do not increase dosage. If proteinuria exceeds 1 g/24 hours, or progressively increases, discontinue drug or reduce dosage. Proteinuria has cleared after dosage reduction. One year or more may be required for any urinary abnormalities to disappear after penicillamine has been discontinued.

In patients with Wilson's disease or cystinuria, the risks of continued penicillamine therapy in patients manifesting potentially serious urinary abnormalities must be weighed against the expected therapeutic benefits.

►*Pregnancy:* In 89 known pregnancies, penicillamine was given throughout and three infants had birth defects deemed attributable to the drug. All infants exhibited cutis laxia; one had hypotonia, hyperflexion of hips and shoulders, pyloric stenosis, vein fragility and varicosities; another showed growth retardation, hernia, perforated bowel and simian crease. The latter two died.

Use only when clearly needed and when the potential benefits outweigh the potential hazards to the fetus. Inform women of childbearing potential or who are pregnant of the possible hazards of penicillamine to the developing fetus and advise them to report promptly any missed menstrual periods or other indications of possible pregnancy.

►*Lactation:* Safety has not been established. (See Contraindications.)

►*Children:* The efficacy of penicillamine in juvenile rheumatoid arthritis has not been established.

Precautions

►*Dietary supplementation:* Because of their dietary restriction, give patients with Wilson's disease, cystinuria and rheumatoid arthritis whose nutrition is impaired 25 mg/day of pyridoxine during therapy,

since penicillamine increases the requirement for this vitamin. In Wilson's disease, multivitamin preparations must be copper free. Do not give mineral supplements; they may block response to penicillamine.

Iron deficiency may develop, especially in children and in menstruating women. If necessary, give iron in short courses. A period of 2 hours should elapse between administration of penicillamine and iron, since orally administered iron reduces the effects of penicillamine.

►*Collagen and elastin:* Effects of penicillamine on collagen and elastin make it advisable to consider a reduction in dosage to 250 mg/day when surgery is contemplated. Delay full therapy until wound healing is complete.

Penicillamine causes an increase in the amount of soluble collagen. This may cause increased skin friability at sites subject to pressure or trauma, such as shoulders, elbows, knees, toes and buttocks. Extravasations of blood may occur and may appear as purpuric areas, with external bleeding if the skin is broken, or as vesicles containing dark blood. Neither type is progressive. Therapy with penicillamine may be continued in the presence of the lesions. They may not recur if dosage is reduced. Other related effects are excessive wrinkling of the skin and development of small, white papules at venipuncture and surgical sites.

►*Monitoring:* When indicated, monitor drug toxicity or efficacy through urinalysis. In rheumatoid arthritis patients, discontinue the drug if unexplained gross hematuria or persistent microscopic hematuria develops. Perform liver function tests every 6 months for the duration of therapy because of rare reports of intrahepatic cholestasis and toxic hepatitis, and an annual X-ray for renal stones.

Because of the potential for serious adverse hematological and renal reactions, monitor white and differential blood cell count, hemoglobin determination, and direct platelet count every 2 weeks for the first 6 months of penicillamine therapy and monthly thereafter.

Drug Interactions

Penicillamine Drug Interactions

Precipitant drug	Object drug*		Description
Penicillamine	Digoxin	↓	Digoxin serum levels may be reduced, possibly decreasing its pharmacological effects. The digoxin dose may need to be increased.
Penicillamine	Gold therapy, antimalarial or cytotoxic drugs, oxyphenbutazone or pheylbutazone	↑	Do not use these drugs in patients who are concurrently receiving penicillamine. These drugs are associated with similar serious hematologic and renal reactions.
Penicillamine	Gold salts	↑	Patients who have had **gold salt** therapy discontinued due to a major toxic reaction may be at greater risk of serious adverse reactions with penicillamine, but not necessarily of the same type. However, this is controversial.
Antacids	Penicillamine	↓	The absorption of penicillamine is decreased by 66% with coadministration of antacids.
Iron salts	Penicillamine	↓	The absorption of penicillamine is decreased by 35% with coadministration of iron salts.

* ↑ = Object drug increased. ↓ = Object drug decreased.

►*Drug/Food interactions:* The absorption of penicillamine is decreased by 52% when taken with food.

Adverse Reactions

Penicillamine has a high incidence (> 50%) of untoward reactions, some of which are potentially fatal. Medical supervision throughout administration is mandatory.

►*CNS:* Tinnitus; myasthenia gravis; polyradiculopathy (rare); peripheral sensory and motor neuropathies (including polyradiculoneuropathy). Muscular weakness may or may not occur with the peripheral neuropathies. Reversible optic neuritis with racemic penicillamine (may be related to pyridoxine deficiency).

►*GI:* Anorexia, epigastric pain, nausea, vomiting or occasional diarrhea (17%); blunting, diminution or total loss of taste perception (12%); intrahepatic cholestasis and toxic hepatitis (rare); cheilosis, glossitis and gingivostomatitis (rare); stomatitis; reactivated peptic ulcer; hepatic dysfunction; pancreatitis; increased serum alkaline phosphatase and lactic dehydrogenase (LDH), positive cephalin flocculation and thymol turbidity tests; oral ulcerations; colitis; altered taste perception.

►*Hematologic:* Thrombocytopenia (4%); leukopenia (2%); bone marrow depression; sideroblastic anemia.

Thrombotic thrombocytopenic purpura, hemolytic anemia, red cell aplasia, monocytosis, leukocytosis, eosinophilia and thrombocytosis (see Warnings).

There have been reports associating penicillamine with leukemia; a cause-and-effect relationship has not been established.

PENICILLAMINE

▶*Hypersensitivity:* Generalized pruritus, early and late rashes (5% to 50%); lupus erythematosus-like syndrome (2%), similar to other drug-induced lupus; pemphigoid-type reactions; drug eruptions (may be accompanied by fever, arthralgia or lymphadenopathy); urticaria and exfoliative dermatitis; thyroiditis and hypoglycemia (extremely rare); migratory polyarthralgia, often with objective synovitis; polymyositis (some fatal); Goodpasture's syndrome (a severe and ultimately fatal glomerular nephritis associated with intra-alveolar hemorrhage); allergic alveolitis; obliterative bronchiolitis.

▶*Renal:* Proteinuria (6%) or hematuria which may progress to the nephrotic syndrome as a result of an immune complex membranous glomerulopathy.

▶*Miscellaneous:*
Rare – Thrombophlebitis; hyperpyrexia; falling hair or alopecia; lichen planus; myasthenia gravis; dermatomyositis; mammary hyperplasia; elastosis perforans serpiginosa; toxic epidermal necrolysis; anetoderma (cutaneous macular atrophy); fatal renal vasculitis; interstitial pneumonitis and pulmonary fibrosis; bronchial asthma; hot flashes.

Increased skin friability, excessive wrinkling of skin and development of small white papules at venipuncture and surgical sites have been reported. Penicillamine toxicity may be twice as common in elderly patients. The drug's chelating action may cause increased excretion of other heavy metals (eg, zinc, mercury, lead).

Patient Information

Take on an empty stomach, 1 hour before or 2 hours after meals and at least 1 hour apart from any other drug, food or milk.

Patients with cystinuria should drink copious amounts of water.

Notify physician if skin rash, unusual bruising or bleeding, sore throat, exertional dyspnea, unexplained coughing/wheezing, fever, chills, or other unusual effects occur.

Urinary alkalinizing agents are bases or salts of bases that increase the excretion of free base in the urine, effectively raising the urinary pH.

Used to correct acidosis in renal tubular disorders and to minimize uric acid crystallization as adjuvants to uricosuric agents in gout. Urine alkalinization increases solubility of sulfonamides and the renal elimination of phenobarbital.

SODIUM BICARBONATE

otc	**Sodium Bicarbonate** (Various eg, Rugby, URL)	**Tablets:** 325 mg	In 1000s.
		650 mg	In 1000s.
		Powder	In 120 g.

For information on parenteral sodium bicarbonate, refer to the monograph in the Nutrients and Nutritionals chapter.

Administration and Dosage

One gram of sodium bicarbonate provides 11.9 mEq of sodium and bicarbonate.

➤*Dosage:* 325 mg to 2 g, up to 4 times daily. The maximum daily intake is 15 g (240 mEq) in patients < 60 years old and 8 g (120 mEq) in those ≥ 60 years old.

Contraindications

Use cautiously in edema, CHF, liver cirrhosis and low-salt diets.

Precautions

➤*Use cautiously:* Use cautiously in toxemia of pregnancy or renal impairment.

➤*Prolonged therapy:* Prolonged therapy may lead to systemic alkalosis.

POTASSIUM CITRATE

Rx	**Urocit-K** (Mission)	**Tablets:** 5 mEq	(Mission MPC 600). In 100s.
		10 mEq	In 100s.

For complete prescribing information on citrate and citric acid, see monograph in the Nutrients and Nutritionals chapter.

Administration and Dosage

➤*Severe hypocitruria:* 60 mEq/day (20 mEq 3 times/day or 15 mEq 4 times/day with meals or ≤ 30 minutes after meals).

➤*Mild-to-moderate hypocitruria:* 30 mEq/day (10 mEq 3 times/day with meals).

Do not exceed 100 mEq/day.

POTASSIUM CITRATE COMBINATIONS

Rx	**Citrolith** (Beach Pharm.)	**Tablets:** 50 mg potassium citrate and 950 mg sodium citrate	(Beach 1136). In 100s & 500s.
Rx	**Polycitra** (Willen)	**Syrup:** 550 mg potassium citrate, 500 mg sodium citrate, 334 mg citric acid/5 ml. (1 mEq K, 1 mEq Na per ml; equiv. to 2 mEq bicarbonate)	Alcohol free. In 120 and 480 ml.
Rx sf	**Polycitra-LC** (Willen)	**Solution:** 550 mg K citrate, 500 mg sodium citrate, 334 mg citric acid/5 ml. (1 mEq K, 1 mEq Na per ml; equiv. to 2 mEq bicarbonate)	Alcohol free. In 120 and 480 ml.
Rx sf	**Polycitra-K** (Willen)	**Solution:** 1100 mg potassium citrate, 334 mg citric acid/5 ml. (2 mEq K/ml; equiv. to 2 mEq bicarbonate)	Alcohol free. In 120 and 480 ml.
		Crystals for Reconstitution: 3300 mg K citrate, 1002 mg citric acid per UD packet (equiv. to 30 mEq bicarb.)	Alcohol free. In single dose packets.

For complete prescribing information on citrate and citric acid, see monograph in the Nutrients and Nutritionals chapter.

Administration and Dosage

➤*Liquids:* 15 to 20 ml 4 times daily usually maintains a urinary pH of 7 to 7.6 for 24 hours; 10 to 15 ml 4 times daily usually maintains a urinary pH of 6.5 to 7.4.

Adults – 15 to 30 ml 4 times daily, after meals and at bedtime, diluted with water.

Children – 5 to 15 ml 4 times daily, after meals and at bedtime, diluted with water.

➤*Tablets:* 1 to 4 tablets with a full glass of water, after meals and at bedtime.

SODIUM CITRATE AND CITRIC ACID SOLUTION (Shohl's Solution, Modified)

Rx sf	**Bicitra** (Alza Corp.)	**Solution:** 500 mg sodium citrate/334 mg citric acid per 5 ml (1 mEq sodium equiv. to 1 mEq bicarbonate/ml)	Grape flavored. In 120 and 473 ml and UD 15 and 30 ml.
Rx	**Oracit** (Carolina Medical Products)	**Solution:** 490 mg sodium citrate/640 mg citric acid per 5 ml (1 mEq sodium equiv. to 1 mEq bicarbonate/ml)	In 500 ml and UD 15 and 30 ml.

Administration and Dosage

➤*Systemic alkalinization:*

Adults – 10 to 30 ml diluted in 30 to 90 ml water, after meals and at bedtime.

Children (> 2 years old) – 5 to 15 ml diluted in 30 to 90 ml water, after meals and at bedtime. Consult physician for use in children < 2 years old.

➤*Neutralizing buffer:* 15 ml diluted in 15 ml water, as a single dose.

AMMONIUM CHLORIDE

otc	Ammonium Cl (Various)	Tablets: 500 mg	In 100s and 1000s.
		Tablets, enteric coated: 486 mg	In 100s.

For information on parenteral ammonium chloride, refer to the monograph in the Nutrients and Nutritionals chapter.

Indications

Used as a diuretic or systemic and urinary acidifying agent.

Administration and Dosage

Usual dose is 1 to 2 g every four to six hours.

Contraindications

Markedly impaired renal or hepatic function.

Adverse Reactions

Gastric irritation; nausea; vomiting; acidosis with large doses.

Overdosage

▶*Symptoms:* Nausea, vomiting, thirst, headache, hyperventilation and progressive drowsiness leading to profound acidosis and hypokalemia.

▶*Treatment:* Correct acidosis and electrolyte loss by administering IV sodium bicarbonate or sodium lactate. Hypokalemia may be treated by oral potassium salts.

ASCORBIC ACID

Indications

Ascorbic acid is frequently used as a urinary acidifier; its efficacy is controversial.

Administration and Dosage

For dosage guidelines refer to the Ascorbic Acid monograph in Nutrients and Nutritional Agents.

Acid Phosphates

Indications

To acidify the urine and lower urinary calcium concentration.

Increases the antibacterial activity of methenamine.

Reduces odor and rash caused by ammoniacal urine.

Contraindications

Renal insufficiency (< 30% of normal), infected magnesium ammonium phosphate stones, hyperphosphatemia and hyperkalemia. Also use with caution if potassium regulation is desired. Use sodium acid phosphate cautiously in patients on sodium restriction.

Warnings

➤*Concurrent potassium supplementation:* Consider potassium content of these products. Decrease supplemental potassium dosage to avoid hyperkalemia.

➤*Pregnancy: Category C.* Safe use during pregnancy is not established. Use only when clearly needed and when potential benefits outweigh potential hazards to the fetus.

➤*Lactation:* Safety for use in the nursing mother has not been established. It is not known whether this drug is excreted in breast milk. Exercise caution when administering to a nursing woman.

Precautions

➤*Exercise caution in the following conditions:* Cardiac disease (particularly digitalized patients), Addison's disease, acute dehydration, severe renal insufficiency or chronic renal disease, extensive tissue breakdown (such as severe burns), myotonia congenita, cardiac failure, cirrhosis of the liver or severe hepatic disease, peripheral and pulmonary edema, hypernatremia, hypertension, toxemia of pregnancy, hypoparathyroidism, acute pancreatitis and rickets.

➤*Lab test abnormalities:* Carefully monitor renal function and serum electrolytes (calcium, phosphorus, potassium) at periodic intervals during phosphate therapy if required. High serum phosphate levels increase incidence of extraskeletal calcification.

Drug Interactions

Acid Phosphate Drug Interactions			
Precipitant drug	Object drug*		Description
Acid phosphates	Salicylates	↑	Acidified urine reduces excretion of salicylates and may lead to salicylate toxicity.

Acid Phosphate Drug Interactions			
Precipitant drug	Object drug*		Description
Antacids	Acid phosphates	↓	Antacids containing magnesium, calcium or aluminum in conjunction with phosphate preparations may bind the phosphate and prevent absorption.
Antihypertensives; Corticosteroids	Acid phosphates	↑	Antihypertensives, especially diazoxide, guanethidine, hydralazine, methyldopa or rauwolfia alkaloids; or corticosteroids, especially mineralocorticoids or corticotropin; used concurrently with sodium phosphate may result in hypernatremia.
Potassium-containing medications	Acid phosphates	↑	Potassium-containing medications or potassium-sparing diuretics may cause hyperkalemia when used concurrently with potassium salts. Perform periodic serum potassium level determinations.

* ↑ = Object drug increased. ↓ = Object drug decreased.

Adverse Reactions

Mild laxation may occur; it usually subsides with dosage reduction. If it persists, discontinue use. Abdominal discomfort, diarrhea, nausea and vomiting may occur.

Less frequent – Fast or irregular heartbeat, dizziness, headache, mental confusion, seizures, weakness or heaviness of legs, unusual tiredness, muscle cramps, numbness, tingling, pain or weakness in hands or feet, numbness or tingling around lips, shortness of breath or troubled breathing, swelling of feet or legs, unusual weight gain, low urine output, thirst, bone and joint pain.

Patient Information

Notify physician if abdominal pain, nausea or vomiting occurs.

Warn patients with kidney stones of the possibility of passing old stones when phosphate therapy is started.

Advise patients to avoid antacids containing aluminum, calcium or magnesium which may prevent phosphate absorption.

To assure against GI injury associated with oral ingestion of concentrated potassium salt preparations, instruct patients to dissolve tablets completely in an appropriate amount of water before taking.

POTASSIUM ACID PHOSPHATE

Rx	**K-Phos Original** (Beach)	**Tablets:** 500 mg (contains 3.7 mEq potassium)	Sodium free. (Beach 1111). White, scored. In 100s and 500s.

For complete prescribing information, refer to the Acid Phosphates group monograph.

Administration and Dosage

1 g dissolved in 180 to 240 ml water 4 times daily with meals and at bedtime. For best results, soak tablets in water for 2 to 5 minutes. Stir vigorously and swallow.

POTASSIUM ACID PHOSPHATE AND SODIUM ACID PHOSPHATE

Rx	**K-Phos Neutral** (Beach)	**Tablets:** 852 mg dibasic sodium phosphate anhydrous, 155 mg monobasic potassium phosphate and 130 mg monobasic sodium phosphate monohydrate (contains 1.1 mEq potassium and 13.0 mEq sodium)	(Beach 1125). White, film coated. In 100s and 500s.
Rx	**K-Phos M.F.** (Beach)	**Tablets:** 155 mg potassium acid phosphate and 350 mg sodium acid phosphate (contains 1.1 mEq potassium and 2.9 mEq sodium)	(Beach 1135). White, scored. In 100s and 500s.
Rx	**K-Phos No. 2** (Beach)	**Tablets:** 305 mg potassium acid phosphate and 700 mg sodium acid phosphate (contains 2.3 mEq potassium and 5.8 mEq sodium)	(Beach 1134). Brown. In 100s and 500s.

For complete prescribing information, refer to the Acid Phosphates group monograph.

Administration and Dosage

1 to 2 tablets 4 times daily with a full glass of water. When the urine is difficult to acidify, administer 1 tablet every 2 hours. Do not exceed 8 tablets in 24 hours.

In addition to the GI anticholinergics (refer to the Gastrointestinal Agents chapter), many of which are recommended for urologic conditions, the following agents are indicated specifically for urologic disorders. Urinary anticholinergics in combination with urinary anti-infective agents are listed in the Anti-Infectives, Systemic chapter. Urinary anticholinergics in combination with urinary analgesics also are available.

FLAVOXATE HCl

| Rx | Flavoxate (Global) | Tablets: 100 mg | (G 181). Off-white. Film-coated. In 100s. |
| Rx | Urispas (Ortho-McNeil) | | Castor oil. (URISPAS SKF). White. Film-coated. In UD 100s. |

Indications

For the symptomatic relief of dysuria, urgency, nocturia, suprapubic pain, frequency, and incontinence as may occur in cystitis, prostatitis, urethritis, urethrocystitis/urethrotrigonitis.

Not indicated for definitive treatment but is compatible with drugs used to treat urinary tract infections.

Administration and Dosage

➤*Adults and children over 12 years of age:* 100 or 200 mg 3 or 4 times/day. Reduce the dose when symptoms improve.

➤*Storage / Stability:* Store between 15° and 30°C (59° and 86°F).

Actions

➤*Pharmacology:* Flavoxate counteracts smooth muscle spasm of the urinary tract and exerts its effect directly on the muscle.

Contraindications

Pyloric or duodenal obstruction; obstructive intestinal lesions or ileus; achalasia; GI hemorrhage; obstructive uropathies of the lower urinary tract.

Warnings

➤*Glaucoma:* Give cautiously in patients with suspected glaucoma.

➤*Pregnancy: Category B.* There are no well-controlled studies in pregnant women. Use during pregnancy only when clearly needed.

➤*Lactation:* It is not known whether this drug is excreted in breast milk. Use caution when flavoxate is administered to a nursing woman.

➤*Children:* Safety and efficacy in children under 12 years of age have not been established.

Adverse Reactions

➤*Cardiovascular:* Tachycardia; palpitations.

➤*CNS:* Nervousness; vertigo; headache; drowsiness; mental confusion (especially in the elderly).

➤*GI:* Nausea; vomiting; dry mouth.

➤*Hypersensitivity:* Hyperpyrexia; urticaria and other dermatoses; eosinophilia.

➤*Special senses:* Blurred vision; increased ocular tension; disturbance in eye accommodation.

➤*Miscellaneous:* Dysuria; leukopenia.

Overdosage

The oral LD_{50} for flavoxate in rats is 4273 mg/kg. The oral LD_{50} for flavoxate in mice is 1837 mg/kg. It is not known whether flavoxate is dialyzable.

Patient Information

Inform patients that if drowsiness and blurred vision occur to not operate a motor vehicle or machinery or participate in activities where alertness is required.

OXYBUTYNIN CHLORIDE

Rx	Oxybutynin Chloride (Various, eg, Dixon-Shane, Goldline, Pliva, Sidmak, UDL, Watson)	Tablets: 5 mg	In 100s, 500s, 1000s, blister pack 25s, and UD 100s.
Rx	Ditropan (ALZA)		Lactose. (DITROPAN 92 00). Blue, scored. In 100s, 1000s, and UD 100s.
Rx	Ditropan XL (ALZA)	Tablets, extended-release: 5 mg	Lactose. (5 XL). Pale yellow. In 100s.
		10 mg	Lactose. (10 XL). Pink. In 100s.
		15 mg	Lactose. (15 XL). Gray. In 100s.
Rx	Oxybutynin Chloride (Various, eg, Apotex, Cypress, Morton Grove)	Syrup: 5 mg/5 mL	In 473 mL.
Rx	Ditropan (ALZA)		Sorbitol, sucrose, methylparaben. In 473 mL.
Rx	Oxytrol (Watson)	Transdermal system: 36 mg of oxybutynin delivering 3.9 mg oxybutynin per day.	(OXYTROL). 39 cm² system. In patient calendar boxes of 8 systems.

Indications

➤*Bladder instability / Overactive bladder:* For the relief of symptoms of bladder instability/treatment of overactive bladder associated with voiding in patients with uninhibited and reflex neurogenic bladder (eg, urgency, frequency, urinary leakage, urge incontinence, dysuria).

Administration and Dosage

➤*Immediate-release tablets and syrup:*

Adults – 5 mg (tablets or syrup) 2 or 3 times/day. Maximum dose is 5 mg 4 times/day.

Children (over 5 years of age) – 5 mg (tablets or syrup) 2 times/day. Maximum dose is 5 mg 3 times/day.

➤*Extended-release (ER) tablets:* 5 mg once daily. Dosage may be adjusted in 5 mg increments to achieve a balance of efficacy and tolerability (up to a maximum of 30 mg/day). Dosage adjustments may proceed at approximately weekly intervals.

The ER tablets may be administered with or without food and must be swallowed whole with the aid of liquids and not be chewed, divided, or crushed.

➤*Transdermal system:* Apply system to dry, intact skin on the abdomen, hip, or buttock. Select a new application site with each new system to avoid reapplication to the same site within 7 days.

The dose is one 3.9 mg/day system applied twice weekly (every 3 to 4 days).

➤*Storage / Stability:* Store at controlled room temperature 15° to 30°C (59° to 86°F). Dispense in a tight, light-resistant container.

Actions

➤*Pharmacology:* Oxybutynin exerts direct antispasmodic effect on smooth muscle and inhibits the muscarinic action of acetylcholine on smooth muscle. It exhibits one fifth of the anticholinergic activity of atropine but 4 to 10 times the antispasmodic activity. No blocking effects occur at skeletal neuromuscular junctions or autonomic ganglia (antinicotinic effects).

In patients with conditions characterized by involuntary bladder contractions, oxybutynin increases vesical capacity, diminishes frequency of uninhibited contractions of the detrusor muscle, and delays initial desire to void. Oxybutynin thus decreases urgency and the frequency of incontinent episodes and voluntary urination.

Oxybutynin is well tolerated in patients administered the drug from 30 days to 2 years.

➤*Pharmacokinetics:*

Absorption –

ER tablets: Following the first dose of oxybutynin ER tablets, oxybutynin plasma concentrations rise for 4 to 6 hours; thereafter, steady concentrations are maintained for up to 24 hours, minimizing fluctuations between peak and trough concentrations associated with oxybutynin.

The relative bioavailabilities of R- and S-oxybutynin from oxybutynin ER are 156% and 187%, respectively, compared with oxybutynin.

Mean R- and S-Oxybutynin Pharmacokinetic Parameters Following a Single Dose of 10 mg Oxybutynin ER (n = 43)		
Parameters	R-Oxybutynin	S-Oxybutynin
C_{max} (ng/mL)	1	1.8
T_{max} (h)	12.7	11.8
$t_{1/2}$ (h)	13.2	12.4
$AUC_{(0-48)}$ (ng·h/mL)	18.4	34.2
AUC_{inf} (ng·h/mL)	21.3	39.5

Steady-state oxybutynin plasma concentrations are achieved by day 3 of repeated oxybutynin ER dosing, with no observed drug accumulation or change in oxybutynin and desethyloxybutynin pharmacokinetic parameters.

Transdermal system: Following application of the first 3.9 mg/day transdermal system, oxybutynin plasma concentration increases for approximately 24 to 48 hours, reaching average maximum concentrations of 3 to 4 ng/mL. Thereafter, steady concentrations are maintained for up to 96 hours. Absorption of oxybutynin is bioequivalent when oxybutynin transdermal system is applied to the abdomen, buttocks, or hip.

OXYBUTYNIN CHLORIDE

Mean (SD) Oxybutynin Pharmacokinetic Parameters from Single and Multiple Dose Studies in Healthy Volunteers after Oxybutynin Transdermal System Application on the Abdomen				
Dosing	C_{max} (ng/mL)	T_{max}^{1} (h)	C_{avg} (ng/mL)	AUC (ng/mL × h)
Single	3 (0.8)	48	—	245 (59)[2]
	3.4 (1.1)	36	—	279 (99)[2]
Multiple	6.6 (2.4)	10	4.2 (1.1)	408 (108)[3]
	4.2 (1)	28	3.1 (0.7)	259 (57)[4]

[1] T_{max} given as median.
[2] AUC_{inf}.
[3] AUC_{0-96}.
[4] AUC_{0-84}.

Distribution –

ER tablets: Plasma concentrations of oxybutynin decline biexponentially following IV or oral administration. The volume of distribution is 193 L after IV administration of 5 mg oxybutynin chloride.

Transdermal system: Oxybutynin is widely distributed in body tissues following systemic absorption. The volume of distribution was estimated to be 193 L after IV administration of 5 mg oxybutynin chloride.

Metabolism – Oxybutynin is metabolized primarily by the cytochrome P450 enzyme systems, particularly CYP 3A4 found mostly in the liver and gut wall. Its metabolic products include phenylcyclohexylglycolic acid, which is pharmacologically inactive, and desethyloxybutynin, which is pharmacologically active.

ER tablets: Following oxybutynin ER administration, plasma concentrations of R- and S-desethyloxybutynin are 73% and 92%, respectively, of concentrations observed with oxybutynin.

Transdermal system: Transdermal administration of oxybutynin bypasses the first-pass GI and hepatic metabolism, reducing the formation of the N-desethyl metabolite. Only small amounts of CYP 3A4 are found in skin, limiting presystemic metabolism during transdermal absorption. The resulting plasma concentration AUC ratio of N-desethyl metabolite to parent compound following multiple oxybutynin transdermal applications was 1.3:1.

Excretion – Oxybutynin is extensively metabolized by the liver, with less than 0.1% of the administered dose excreted unchanged in the urine. Also, less than 0.1% of the administered dose is excreted as the metabolite desethyloxybutynin.

Adhesion of transdermal system – Adhesion was periodically evaluated during the phase 3 studies. Of the 4746 oxybutynin transdermal system evaluations in the phase 3 trials, 20 (0.4%) were observed at clinic visits to have become completely detached and 35 (0.7%) became partially detached during routine clinic use. Similar to the pharmacokinetic studies, more than 98% of the systems evaluated in the phase 3 studies were assessed as being 75% or more attached and thus would be expected to perform as anticipated.

Contraindications

Urinary retention; untreated angle-closure glaucoma; untreated narrow anterior chamber angles; partial or complete GI obstruction or retention; paralytic ileus; intestinal atony in the elderly or debilitated; megacolon; toxic megacolon complicating ulcerative colitis; severe colitis; myasthenia gravis; obstructive uropathy; unstable cardiovascular status in acute hemorrhage; hypersensitivity to the drug or any component of the product.

Warnings

➤*Heat prostration:* When administered in the presence of high environmental temperature, heat prostration (fever and heat stroke) may occur because of decreased sweating.

➤*Diarrhea:* Diarrhea may be an early symptom of incomplete intestinal obstruction, especially in patients with ileostomy or colostomy; in this instance, treatment with oxybutynin would be inappropriate and possibly harmful.

➤*GI disorders:* Doses administered to patients with ulcerative colitis may suppress GI motility and produce paralytic ileus and precipitate or aggravate toxic megacolon.

Because of the risk of gastric retention, administer ER tablets with caution to patients with GI obstructive disorders.

The ER tablets and transdermal system, like other anticholinergic drugs, may decrease GI motility and should be used with caution in patients with conditions such as ulcerative colitis, intestinal atony, and myasthenia gravis.

Use the ER tablets and transdermal system with caution in patients who have gastroesophageal reflux or who are concurrently taking drugs (such as bisphosphonates) that can cause or exacerbate esophagitis.

As with other nondeformable material, use caution when administering the ER tablets and to patients with pre-existing severe GI narrowing (pathologic or iatrogenic). There have been rare reports of obstructive symptoms in patients with known strictures in association with the ingestion of other drugs in nondeformable controlled-release formulations.

➤*Urinary retention:* Administer ER tablets with caution to patients with clinically significant bladder outflow obstruction because of the risk of urinary retention.

➤*Renal/Hepatic function impairment:* Use ER tablets with caution in patients with hepatic or renal impairment.

➤*Pregnancy: Category B.* Safety for use during pregnancy has not been established. Use only when clearly needed and when the potential benefits outweigh the potential hazards to the fetus.

➤*Lactation:* It is not known whether this drug is excreted in breast milk. Exercise caution when administering to a nursing woman.

➤*Children:* Safety and efficacy in children (under 5 years of age for immediate-release tablets/syrup) have not been established.

Precautions

➤*Use with caution:* Use with caution in the elderly and patients with autonomic neuropathy and hepatic or renal disease.

➤*Cardiac and other effects:* Symptoms of hyperthyroidism, coronary heart disease, CHF, cardiac arrhythmias, tachycardia, hypertension, hiatal hernia, and prostatic hypertrophy may be aggravated.

➤*Hazardous tasks:* Patients should use caution while driving or performing other tasks requiring alertness, coordination, or physical dexterity. Alcohol or other sedative drugs may enhance the drowsiness caused by oxybutynin.

Drug Interactions

Oxybutynin Drug Interactions			
Precipitant drug	Object drug*		Description
Oxybutynin	Anticholinergic agents	↑	Concomitant use may increase the frequency and/or severity of anticholinergic-like effects. Anticholinergic agents may potentially alter the absorption of some concomitantly administered drugs because of anticholinergic effects on GI motility.
Anticholinergic agents	Oxybutynin		
Oxybutynin	Beta blockers Atenolol	↑	The bioavailability of atenolol may be increased. If an increase in beta blockade is suspected, tailoring the beta blocker dose downward may be necessary.
Oxybutynin	Digoxin	↑	Serum levels of digoxin administered as slow-dissolution oral tablets may be increased and actions enhanced. Serum level monitoring may assist in tailoring dosage. Problems may be avoided with use of digoxin elixir or capsules.
Oxybutynin	Haloperidol	↔	Effects are variable. Use oxybutynin only when clearly needed. Routinely monitor these patients; discontinue anticholinergic or tailor haloperidol if necessary.
Oxybutynin	Phenothiazines	↓	Pharmacologic/therapeutic actions of phenothiazines may be decreased by anticholinergics. Tailor the phenothiazine dose as needed.
Amantadine	Oxybutynin	↑	Anticholinergic side effects may be increased. Decrease the dose of oxybutynin during coadministration. Monitor patient response and adjust the dose accordingly.

* ↑ = Object drug increased. ↓ = Object drug decreased. ↔ = Undetermined clinical effect.

Adverse Reactions

➤*Immediate-release tablets and syrup:*

Cardiovascular – Palpitations; tachycardia; vasodilation.

CNS – Dizziness; drowsiness; hallucinations; insomnia; restlessness.

Dermatologic – Decreased sweating; rash.

GI – Constipation; decreased GI motility; dry mouth; nausea.

GU – Urinary hesitancy and retention.

Ophthalmic – Amblyopia; cycloplegia; decreased lacrimation; mydriasis.

Miscellaneous – Asthenia; impotence; suppression of lactation.

OXYBUTYNIN CHLORIDE
➤*ER tablets:*

Oxybutynin ER Tablet Adverse Reactions (≥ 5%)	
Adverse reaction	ER 5 to 30 mg/day (n = 429)
CNS	
Somnolence	11.9
Headache	9.8
Dizziness	6.3
GI	
Dry mouth	60.8
Constipation	13.1
Diarrhea	9.1
Nausea	8.9
Dyspepsia	6.8
Special senses	
Blurred vision	7.7
Dry eyes	6.1
Miscellaneous	
Asthenia	6.8
Pain	6.8
Rhinitis	5.6
Urinary tract infection	5.1

The discontinuation rate for all adverse events was 6.8%. The most frequent adverse event causing early discontinuation of study medication was nausea (1.9%), while discontinuation due to dry mouth was 1.2%.

➤*ER tablets (2% to less than 5%):*
Cardiovascular – Hypertension; palpitation; vasodilation.

CNS – Insomnia; nervousness; confusion.

Dermatologic – Dry skin; rash.

GI – Flatulence; gastroesophageal reflux.

GU – Impaired urination (hesitancy); increased postvoid residual volume; urinary retention; cystitis.

Respiratory – Upper respiratory tract infection; cough; sinusitis; bronchitis; dry nasal and sinus mucous membranes; pharyngitis.

Miscellaneous – Abdominal pain; accidental injury; back pain; flu syndrome; arthritis.

➤*Transdermal system:* The safety of oxybutynin transdermal system was evaluated in a total of 417 patients who participated in 2 phase 3 clinical efficacy and safety studies and an open-label extension. Additional safety information was collected in phase 1 and phase 2 trials. In the 2 pivotal studies, a total of 246 patients received oxybutynin transdermal system during the 12-week treatment periods. A total of 411 patients entered the open-label extension and of those, 65 patients and 52 patients received oxybutynin transdermal system for at least 24 weeks and at least 36 weeks, respectively.

No deaths were reported during treatment. No serious adverse events related to treatment were reported.

Adverse events reported in the pivotal trials are summarized in the table below.

Adverse Events in Oxybutynin Transdermal System Patients (≥ 2%)[1]		
Adverse reaction[2]	*Oxytrol* (3.9 mg/day) (N = 246)	Placebo (N = 249)
Application site pruritus	14 to 16.8	4.3 to 6.1
Dry mouth	4.1 to 9.6	1.7 to 8.3
Application site erythema	5.6 to 8.3	1.7 to 2.3
Application site vesicles	3.2	0
Diarrhea	3.2	2.3
Dysuria	2.4	0
Constipation	3.3	0
Application site rash	3.3	0.9
Application site macules	2.5	0

Adverse Events in Oxybutynin Transdermal System Patients (≥ 2%)[1]		
Adverse reaction[2]	*Oxytrol* (3.9 mg/day) (N = 246)	Placebo (N = 249)
Abnormal vision	2.5	0

[1] Combination of study 1 and study 2.
[2] Includes adverse events judged by the investigator as possibly, probably, or definitely treatment-related.

Other adverse events reported by more than 1% of oxybutynin transdermal system-treated patients, and judged by the investigator to be possibly, probably, or definitely related to treatment include: Abdominal pain, nausea, flatulence, fatigue, somnolence, headache, flushing, rash, application site burning, and back pain.

Most treatment-related adverse events were described as mild or moderate in intensity. Severe application site reactions were reported by 6.4% of oxybutynin transdermal system-treated patients in Study 1 and 5% of oxybutynin transdermal system-treated patients in Study 2.

Treatment-related adverse events that resulted in discontinuation were reported by 11.2% of oxybutynin transdermal system-treated patients in study 1 and 10.7% of oxybutynin transdermal system-treated patients in study 2. Most of these were secondary to application site reaction. In the 2 pivotal studies, no patient discontinued oxybutynin transdermal system treatment due to dry mouth.

In the open-label extension, the most common treatment-related adverse events were application site pruritus, application site erythema, and dry mouth.

Overdosage
➤*Symptoms:* Signs of CNS excitation (eg, restlessness, tremor, irritability, convulsions, delirium, hallucinations); flushing; fever; nausea; vomiting; tachycardia; hypotension or hypertension; respiratory failure; paralysis; coma; dehydration; cardiac arrhythmias; and urinary retention.

Ingestion of 100 mg oxybutynin chloride in association with alcohol was reported in a 13-year-old boy who experienced memory loss, and a 34-year-old woman who developed stupor, followed by disorientation and agitation on awakening, dilated pupils, dry skin, cardiac arrhythmia, and retention of urine. Both patients fully recovered with symptomatic treatment.

Plasma concentration of oxybutynin declines within 1 to 2 hours after removal of transdermal systems.

➤*Treatment:* Treatment should be symptomatic and supportive and should be monitored for 24 hours. Maintain respiration and induce emesis or perform gastric lavage (emesis is contraindicated in a precomatose, convulsive, or psychotic state). Activated charcoal may be administered as well as a cathartic. Physostigmine may be considered to reverse symptoms of anticholinergic intoxication. Treat hyperpyrexia symptomatically with ice bags or other cold applications and alcohol sponges. Refer to General Management of Acute Overdosage.

Patient Information
Inform patients that heat prostration (fever and heat stroke because of decreased sweating) can occur when anticholinergics such as oxybutynin chloride are administered in the presence of high environmental temperature.

Inform patients that oxybutynin ER should be swallowed whole with liquids and not chewed, divided, or crushed. The medication is contained within a nonabsorbable shell designed to release the drug at a controlled rate. The tablet shell is eliminated from the body; patients should not be concerned if they occasionally notice in their stool something that looks like a tablet.

May cause drowsiness, dizziness, or blurred vision; alcohol or sedatives may enhance drowsiness. Observe caution while driving or performing other tasks requiring alertness, coordination, or physical dexterity.

May cause dry mouth.

Apply the oxybutynin transdermal system to dry, intact skin on the abdomen, hip, or buttock. Have the patient select a new application site with each new system to avoid reapplication to the same site within 7 days. Details on use of the system are explained in the patient information leaflet that should be dispensed with the product.

TOLTERODINE TARTRATE

Rx	Detrol (Pfizer)	**Tablets:** 1 mg	(TO). White. Film-coated. In 60s, 500s, and UD 140s.
		2 mg	(DT). White. Film-coated. In 60s, 500s, and UD 140s.
Rx	Detrol LA (Pfizer)	**Capsules, extended-release:** 2 mg	Sucrose. (2). Blue-green. In 30s, 90s, 500s, and UD blister 100s.
		4 mg	Sucrose. (4). Blue. In 30s, 90s, 500s, and UD blister 100s.

Indications

➤*Overactive bladder:* Treatment of patients with an overactive bladder with symptoms of urinary frequency, urgency, or urge incontinence.

Administration and Dosage

➤*Approved by the FDA:* March 25, 1998.

➤*Immediate-release:* The initial recommended dose is 2 mg twice daily. The dose may be lowered to 1 mg twice daily based on individual response and tolerability. For patients with significantly reduced hepatic function or who are currently taking drugs that are inhibitors of cytochrome P450 3A4, the recommended dose is 1 mg twice daily (see Drug Interactions).

➤*Extended-release (ER):* The recommended dose is 4 mg once daily taken with liquids and swallowed whole. The dose may be lowered to 2 mg daily based on individual response and tolerability; however, limited efficacy data is available for the 2 mg capsules.

For patients with significantly reduced hepatic or renal function or who are currently taking drugs that are potent inhibitors of CYP3A4, the recommended dose of the ER capsules is 2 mg daily.

➤*Storage/Stability:* Store at 15° to 30°C (59° to 86°F). Protect from light.

Actions

➤*Pharmacology:* Tolterodine is a competitive muscarinic receptor antagonist for overactive bladder. Urinary bladder contraction and salivation are mediated via cholinergic muscarinic receptors.

After oral administration, tolterodine is metabolized in the liver, resulting in the formation of the 5-hydroxymethyl derivative, a major active metabolite. The 5-hydroxymethyl metabolite, which exhibits antimuscarinic activity similar to that of tolterodine, contributes significantly to the therapeutic effect. Tolterodine and the 5-hydroxymethyl metabolite exhibit a high specificity for muscarinic receptors, and both show negligible activity or affinity for other neurotransmitter receptors and other potential cellular targets, such as calcium channels.

Tolterodine has a pronounced effect on bladder function in healthy volunteers. The main effects following a 6.4 mg single dose of tolterodine were an increase in residual urine reflecting an incomplete emptying of the bladder and a decrease in detrusor pressure. These findings are consistent with a potent antimuscarinic action on the lower urinary tract.

➤*Pharmacokinetics:*

Absorption – Tolterodine is rapidly absorbed; ≥ 77% is absorbed, but absolute bioavailability is highly variable (10% to 74%). Maximum steady-state serum concentrations (C_{max}) typically occur within 1 to 2 hours. The pharmacokinetics of tolterodine are dose-proportional over the range of 1 to 4 mg.

Distribution – Tolterodine is highly bound to plasma proteins, primarily α_1-acid glycoprotein. The 5-hydroxymethyl metabolite is not extensively protein bound, with unbound fraction concentrations averaging ≈ 36%. The blood-to-serum ratio of tolterodine and the 5-hydroxymethyl metabolite averages 0.6 and 0.8, respectively, indicating that these compounds do not distribute extensively into erythrocytes.

Metabolism – Tolterodine undergoes extensive and variable first-pass hepatic metabolism following oral dosing. The primary metabolic route involves the oxidation of the 5-methyl group mediated by the cytochrome P450 2D6 leading to the formation of an active 5-hydroxymethyl metabolite. Further metabolism leads to formation of the 5-carboxylic acid and N-dealkylated 5-carboxylic acid metabolites, which account for ≈ 51% and ≈ 29% of the metabolites recovered in the urine, respectively.

Variability in metabolism: A subset (≈ 7%) of the population is devoid of CYP2D6, the enzyme responsible for the formation of the 5-hydroxymethyl metabolite of tolterodine. The identified pathway of metabolism for these individuals ("poor metabolizers") is by dealkylation via cytochrome P450 3A4 (CYP3A4) to N-dealkylated tolterodine. The remainder of the population is referred to as "extensive metabolizers." Pharmacokinetic studies revealed that tolterodine is metabolized at a slower rate in poor metabolizers than in extensive metabolizers; this results in significantly higher serum concentrations of tolterodine and in negligible concentrations of the 5-hydroxymethyl metabolite.

Excretion – Following a 5 mg oral dose in healthy volunteers, 77% was recovered in urine and 17% was recovered in feces. Less than 1% (< 2.5% in poor metabolizers) of the dose was recovered as intact tolterodine, and 5% to 14% (< 1% in poor metabolizers) was recovered as the active 5-hydroxymethyl metabolite.

Special populations –

Renal insufficiency: Renal impairment can significantly alter the disposition of immediate-release tolterodine and its metabolites. Exposure

levels of other metabolites of tolterodine (eg, tolterodine acid, N-dealkylated tolterodine acid, N-dealkylated tolterodine, and N-dealkylated hydroxy tolterodine) were significantly higher (10- to 30-fold) in renally impaired patients compared with healthy volunteers. The recommended dose for patients with significantly reduced renal function is 2 mg/day (see Warnings).

Hepatic function impairment: Liver impairment can significantly alter the disposition of tolterodine. In a study conducted in cirrhotic patients, the elimination half-life of tolterodine was longer in cirrhotic patients (mean, 8.7 hours) than in healthy, young, and elderly volunteers, respectively (mean, 2 to 4 hours). The clearance of oral tolterodine was substantially lower in cirrhotic patients (≈ 1.1 L/hr/kg) than in the healthy volunteers (≈ 5.7 L/hr/kg). Patients with significantly reduced hepatic function should not receive doses > 1 mg twice daily (see Warnings).

Contraindications

Urinary retention; gastric retention; uncontrolled narrow-angle glaucoma; hypersensitivity to the drug or its ingredients.

Warnings

➤*Renal/Hepatic function impairment:* Patients with significantly reduced hepatic function should not receive doses > 1 mg twice daily (> 2 mg/day for ER capsules). Treat patients with renal impairment with caution.

➤*Pregnancy: Category C.* When given at doses of 30 to 40 mg/kg/day, tolterodine has been shown to cause embryolethality, reduce fetal weight, and increase the incidence of fetal abnormalities (ie, cleft palate, digital abnormalities, intra-abdominal hemorrhage, and various skeletal abnormalities, primarily reduced ossification) in mice. At these doses, AUC values were ≈ 20- to 25-fold higher than in humans. There are no studies of tolterodine in pregnant women. Use during pregnancy only if the potential benefit to the mother justifies the potential risk to the fetus.

➤*Lactation:* Tolterodine is excreted into the milk of mice. Offspring of female mice treated with tolterodine 20 mg/kg/day during the lactation period had slightly reduced body-weight gain. The offspring regained the weight during the maturation phase. It is not known whether tolterodine is excreted in human breast milk; therefore, discontinue administration during nursing.

➤*Children:* Safety and efficacy have not been established.

Precautions

➤*Urinary/Gastric retention:* Administer with caution to patients with clinically significant bladder outflow obstruction because of the risk of urinary retention and to patients with GI obstructive disorders, such as pyloric stenosis, because of the risk of gastric retention.

➤*Controlled narrow-angle glaucoma:* Use with caution in patients being treated for narrow-angle glaucoma.

Drug Interactions

➤*Fluoxetine:* Fluoxetine is a potent inhibitor of cytochrome P450 2D6 activity. A 4.8-fold increase in tolterodine AUC, a 52% decrease in C_{max}, and a 20% decrease in AUC of the 5-hydroxymethyl metabolite were observed with coadministration. The sums of unbound serum concentrations of tolterodine and the 5-hydroxymethyl metabolite are only 25% higher during the interaction. No dose adjustment is required when tolterodine and fluoxetine are coadministered.

➤*Cytochrome P450:*

3A4 inhibitors – Patients receiving cytochrome P450 3A4 inhibitors, such as macrolide antibiotics (erythromycin and clarithromycin), antifungal agents (ketoconazole, itraconazole, and miconazole), or cyclosporine or vinblastine should not receive doses of tolterodine > 1 mg twice daily (> 2 mg daily for ER capsules).

2D6 – Tolterodine is not expected to influence the pharmacokinetics of drugs that are metabolized by cytochrome P450 2D6, such as flecainide, vinblastine, carbamazepine, and tricyclic antidepressants.

➤*Drug/Food interactions:* Food intake increases the bioavailability of tolterodine (average increase 53%) and does not affect the levels of the 5-hydroxymethyl metabolite in extensive metabolizers. This change is not expected to be a safety concern and adjustment of dose is not needed.

Adverse Reactions

➤*Immediate-release:*

Miscellaneous – The most common adverse events were dry mouth, headache, constipation, vertigo/dizziness, and abdominal pain. Dry mouth, constipation, abnormal vision (accommodation abnormalities), urinary retention, and xerophthalmia are expected side effects of antimuscarinic agents.

TOLTERODINE TARTRATE

Dry mouth was the most frequently reported adverse event, occurring in 34.8% of patients treated with tolterodine and 9.8% of placebo-treated patients; 1% of patients treated with tolterodine discontinued treatment because of dry mouth.

The frequency of discontinuation caused by adverse events was highest during the first 4 weeks of treatment. Of patients treated with tolterodine 2 mg twice daily, 7% discontinued treatment because of adverse events. The most common adverse events leading to discontinuation were dizziness and headache.

Tolterodine Immediate-Release Adverse Reactions (> 1%)	
Adverse reaction	Tolterodine 2 mg bid (n = 986)
CNS	
Headache	7
Vertigo/Dizziness	5
Somnolence	3
GI	
Dry mouth	35
Abdominal pain	5
Constipation	7
Diarrhea	4
Dyspepsia	4
Ophthalmic	
Vision abnormal (including accommodation)	2
Xerophthalmia	3
Miscellaneous	
Arthralgia	2
Chest pain	2
Fatigue	4
Flu-like symptoms	3
Dysuria	2
Infection	1
Weight gain	1
Dry skin	1

➤*Extended-release:*

Miscellaneous – Adverse reactions were reported in 52% (n = 263) of patients receiving ER tolterodine and in 49% (n = 247) of patients receiving placebo. The most common adverse events reported by patients receiving ER tolterodine were dry mouth, headache, constipation, and abdominal pain. Dry mouth was the most frequently reported adverse event for patients treated with ER tolterodine, occurring in 23.4% of patients treated with ER tolterodine and 7.7% of placebo-treated patients. Dry mouth, constipation, abnormal vision (accommodation abnormalities), urinary retention, and dry eyes are expected side effects of antimuscarinic agents. A serious adverse event was reported by 1.4% (n = 7) of patients receiving ER tolterodine and by 3.6% (n = 18) of patients receiving placebo.

The frequency of discontinuation because of adverse events was highest during the first 4 weeks of treatment. Similar percentages of patients treated with ER tolterodine or placebo discontinued treatment because of adverse events. Dry mouth was reported as an adverse event in 2.4% (n = 12) of patients treated with ER tolterodine and in 1.2% (n = 6) of patients treated with placebo.

The following table lists the adverse events reported in ≥ 1% of patients treated with ER tolterodine 4 mg once daily in the 12-week study. The adverse events were reported regardless of causality.

Tolterodine ER Adverse Reactions (≥ 1%)	
Adverse reaction	ER Tolterodine (n = 505)
CNS	
Headache	6
Somnolence	3
Dizziness	2
Anxiety	1
GI	
Dry mouth	23
Constipation	6
Abdominal pain	4
Dyspepsia	3
Ophthalmic	
Xerophthalmia	3
Vision abnormal	1
Miscellaneous	
Fatigue	2
Sinusitis	2
Dysuria	1

Postmarketing: The following events have been reported in association with tolterodine use in clinical practice: Anaphylactoid reactions, tachycardia, and peripheral edema. Because these spontaneously reported events are from the worldwide postmarketing experience, the frequency of events and the role of tolterodine in their causation can not reliably be determined.

Overdosage

➤*Symptoms:* A 27-month-old child who ingested 5 to 7 tablets of tolterodine 2 mg was treated with a suspension of activated charcoal and was hospitalized overnight with symptoms of dry mouth. The child fully recovered.

➤*Treatment:* Overdosage with tolterodine can potentially result in severe central anticholinergic effects and should be treated accordingly.

ECG monitoring is recommended in the event of overdosage. In dogs, changes in the QT interval (slight prolongation of 10% to 20%) were observed at a suprapharmacologic dose of 4.5 mg/kg, which is ≈ 68 times higher than the recommended human dose. In clinical trials of healthy volunteers and patients, QT interval prolongation was not observed at doses ≤ 4 mg twice daily of tolterodine (higher doses were not evaluated).

Patient Information

Inform patients that antimuscarinic agents such as tolterodine may produce blurred vision, dizziness, or drowsiness.

TROSPIUM CHLORIDE

Rx	**Sanctura** (Odyssey, Indevus)	**Tablets:** 20 mg	Lactose, sucrose. Brownish yellow, biconvex. Glossy-coated. In 60s, 500s, and blister 14s.

Indications

➤*Overactive bladder:* For the treatment of overactive bladder with symptoms of urge urinary incontinence, urgency, and urinary frequency.

Administration and Dosage

➤*Approved by the FDA:* May 28, 2004.

The recommended dose is 20 mg twice daily. Dose at least 1 hour before meals or give on an empty stomach.

➤*Renal function impairment:* For patients with severe renal impairment (creatinine clearance [Ccr] less than 30 mL/min), the recommended dose is 20 mg once daily at bedtime.

➤*Elderly:* In elderly patients, 75 years of age and older, dose may be titrated down to 20 mg once daily based upon tolerability.

➤*Storage/Stability:* Store at controlled room temperature 20° to 25°C (68° to 77°F).

Actions

➤*Pharmacology:* Trospium is an antispasmodic, antimuscarinic agent. Trospium antagonizes the effect of acetylcholine on muscarinic receptors in cholinergically innervated organs. Its parasympatholytic action reduces the tonus of smooth muscle in the bladder. Receptor assays showed that trospium has negligible affinity for nicotinic receptors as compared with muscarinic receptors at concentrations obtained from therapeutic doses. Trospium increases maximum cystometric bladder capacity and volume at first detrusor contraction.

➤*Pharmacokinetics:*

Absorption – After oral administration, less than 10% of the dose is absorbed. Mean absolute bioavailability of a 20 mg dose is 9.6% (range, 4% to 16.1%). Peak plasma concentrations (C_{max}) occur between 5 to 6 hours postdose. Mean C_{max} increases greater than dose-proportionally; a 3-fold and 4-fold increase in C_{max} was observed for dose increases from 20 to 40 mg and from 20 to 60 mg, respectively. Mean area under the plasma concentration-time curve (AUC) exhibits dose linearity for single doses up to 60 mg. Trospium exhibits diurnal variability in exposure with a decrease in C_{max} and AUC of up to 59% and 33%, respectively, for evening relative to morning doses.

Distribution – Protein binding ranged from 50% to 85% when therapeutic concentration levels (0.5 to 50 ng/mL) were incubated with human serum in vitro. The majority of trospium is distributed in plasma. The apparent volume of distribution for a 20 mg oral dose is 395 (± 140) L.

Metabolism – The metabolic pathway of trospium in humans has not been fully defined. Of the 10% of the dose absorbed, metabolites account for approximately 40% of the excreted dose following oral administration. The major metabolic pathway is hypothesized as ester hydrolysis with subsequent conjugation of benzylic acid to form azoniaspironortropanol with glucuronic acid. Cytochrome P450 is not expected to contribute significantly to the elimination of trospium.

Excretion – The plasma half-life for trospium following oral administration is approximately 20 hours. After administration of oral trospium, the majority of the dose (85.2%) was recovered in feces and a smaller amount (5.8%) was recovered in urine; 60% of the radioactivity excreted in urine was unchanged trospium. The mean renal clearance for trospium (29.07 L/h) is 4-fold higher than average glomerular filtration rate, indicating that active tubular secretion is a major route of elimination for trospium. There may be competition for elimination with other compounds that also are renally eliminated (see Drug Interactions).

Trospium Mean Pharmacokinetic Parameter Estimates for a Single 20 mg Dose in Healthy Volunteers			
C_{max} (ng/mL)	$AUC_{0-\infty}$ (ng/mL·h)	T_{max} (h)	$t\frac{1}{2}$ (h)
3.5	36.4	5.3	18.3

Special populations –

Gender: Studies comparing the pharmacokinetics in different genders had conflicting results. When a single 40 mg trospium dose was administered to 16 elderly subjects, exposure was 45% lower in elderly females compared with elderly males. When 20 mg trospium was dosed twice daily for 4 days to 6 elderly males and 6 elderly females (60 to 75 years of age), AUC and C_{max} were 26% and 68% higher, respectively, in females without hormone replacement therapy than in males.

Renal function impairment: Severe renal impairment significantly altered the disposition of trospium. A 4.5-fold and 2-fold increase in mean $AUC_{0-\infty}$ and C_{max}, respectively, and the appearance of an additional elimination phase with a long half-life (approximately 33 hours) was detected in patients with severe renal insufficiency (Ccr less than 30 mL/min) compared with healthy, nearly age-matched subjects. The different pharmacokinetic behavior of trospium in patients with severe renal insufficiency necessitates adjustment of dosage frequency. The pharmacokinetics of trospium have not been studied in people with mild or moderate renal impairment (Ccr from 30 to 80 mL/min) (see Administration and Dosage).

Hepatic function impairment: C_{max} increased 12% and 63% in subjects with mild and moderate hepatic impairment, respectively, compared with healthy subjects. AUC was similar. Use caution when administering trospium to patients with moderate and severe hepatic dysfunction.

Contraindications

Patients with urinary retention, gastric retention, or uncontrolled narrow-angle glaucoma and patients at risk for these conditions; hypersensitivity to the drug or its ingredients.

Warnings

➤*Renal function impairment:* Dose modification is recommended in patients with severe renal insufficiency (Ccr less than 30 mL/min). In such patients, administer trospium as 20 mg once daily at bedtime (see Administration and Dosage).

➤*Hepatic function impairment:* Use caution when administering trospium in patients with moderate or severe hepatic dysfunction (see Special Populations in Pharmacokinetics).

➤*Elderly:* In 2 studies, the incidence of commonly reported anticholinergic adverse events in patients treated with trospium (including dry mouth, constipation, dyspepsia, UTI, and urinary retention) was higher in patients 75 years of age and older as compared with younger patients. This effect may be related to an enhanced sensitivity to anticholinergic agents in this patient population (see Administration and Dosage).

➤*Pregnancy: Category C.* Trospium has been shown to cause maternal toxicity in rats and a decrease in fetal survival in rats administered approximately 10 times the expected clinical exposure (AUC). There are no adequate and well-controlled studies in pregnant women. Use during pregnancy only if the potential benefit justifies the potential risk to the fetus.

➤*Lactation:* Trospium (2 mg/kg orally and 50 mcg/kg IV) was excreted, to a limited extent (less than 1%), into the milk of lactating rats. The activity observed in the milk was primarily from the parent compound. It is not known whether this drug is excreted in human milk. Exercise caution when administering trospium to a nursing mother. Use during lactation only if the potential benefit justifies the potential risk to the newborn.

➤*Children:* Safety and efficacy in pediatric patients have not been established.

Precautions

➤*Cardiac effects:* Asymptomatic, nonspecific T-wave inversions were observed in 1 study more often in subjects receiving trospium than in subjects receiving moxifloxacin or placebo following 5 days of treatment. This finding was not observed during routine safety monitoring in 2 other placebo-controlled clinical trials in 591 trospium-treated overactive bladder patients. The clinical significance of T-wave inversion in this study is unknown. Trospium is associated with an increase in heart rate that correlates with increasing plasma concentrations. In the study described above, trospium demonstrated a mean increase in heart rate compared with placebo of 9.1 beats/min for the 20 mg dose and of 18 beats/min for the 100 mg dose. In the 2 US placebo-controlled trials in patients with overactive bladder, the mean increase in heart rate compared with placebo in study 1 was observed to be 3 beats/min and in study 2 was 4 beats/min.

➤*Decreased GI motility:* Administer trospium with caution to patients with obstructive GI disorders because of the risk of gastric retention (see Contraindications). Trospium, like other anticholinergic drugs, may decrease GI motility. Use caution in patients with conditions such as ulcerative colitis, intestinal atony, and myasthenia gravis.

➤*Narrow-angle glaucoma:* In patients being treated for narrow-angle glaucoma, only use trospium if the potential benefits outweigh the risks and, in that circumstance, only with careful monitoring.

➤*Risk of urinary retention:* Administer trospium with caution to patients with clinically significant bladder outflow obstruction because of the risk of urinary retention.

Drug Interactions

➤*Anticholinergic agents:* The concomitant use of trospium with other anticholinergic agents that produce dry mouth, constipation, and other anticholinergic pharmacological effects may increase the frequency and/or severity of such effects. Anticholinergic agents potentially may alter the absorption of some concomitantly administered drugs because of anticholinergic effects on GI motility.

➤*Drugs eliminated by active tubular secretion:* Although studies to assess drug-drug interactions with trospium have not been conducted, trospium has the potential for pharmacokinetic interactions with other drugs that are eliminated by active tubular secretion (eg, digoxin, procainamide, pancuronium, morphine, vancomycin, metformin, and tenofovir). Coadministration of trospium with drugs that are

TROSPIUM CHLORIDE

eliminated by active tubular secretion may increase the serum concentration of trospium and/or the coadministered drug because of competition for this elimination pathway. Careful patient monitoring is recommended in patients receiving such drugs.

➤*Drug/Food interactions:* Administration with a high-fat meal resulted in reduced absorption, with AUC and C_{max} values 70% to 80% lower than those obtained when trospium was administered while fasting. Therefore, it is recommended that trospium be taken at least 1 hour prior to meals or on an empty stomach.

Adverse Reactions

In all placebo-controlled trials combined, the incidence of serious adverse events was 2.9% among patients receiving 20 mg trospium twice daily and 1.5% among patients receiving placebo. Of these, 0.2% and 0.3% were judged to be at least possibly related to treatment with trospium or placebo, respectively, by the investigator.

The 2 most common adverse events reported by patients receiving 20 mg trospium twice daily were dry mouth and constipation. The single most frequently reported adverse event for trospium, dry mouth, occurred in 20.1% of trospium-treated patients and 5.8% of patients receiving placebo. In the 2 phase 3 US studies, dry mouth led to discontinuation in 1.9% of patients treated with 20 mg trospium twice daily. For the patients who reported dry mouth, most had their first occurrence within the first month of treatment.

Trospium Adverse Reactions (≥ 1%)		
Adverse reaction	Trospium 20 mg twice daily (N = 591)	Placebo (N = 590)
GI		
Abdominal pain, upper	1.5	1.2
Constipation	9.6	4.6
Constipation, aggravated	1.4	0.8
Dry mouth	20.1	5.8
Dyspepsia	1.2	0.3
Flatulence	1.2	0.8
Miscellaneous		
Dry eyes, not otherwise specified	1.2	0.3
Fatigue	1.9	1.4
Headache	4.2	2
Urinary retention	1.2	0.3

Other adverse events from the phase 3 US placebo-controlled trials judged possibly related to treatment with trospium by the investigator, occurring in at least 0.5% of trospium-treated patients, and more common with trospium than placebo were the following: abdominal distention, dry skin, dry throat, dysgeusia, tachycardia (not otherwise specified), vision blurred, and vomiting (not otherwise specified). During controlled clinical studies, one event of angioneurotic edema was reported.

➤*Postmarketing:* Additional spontaneous adverse events, regardless of relationship to drug, reported from marketing experience with trospium include the following: anaphylactic reaction, chest pains, gastritis, hallucinations and delirium, "hypertensive crisis", palpitations, rhabdomyolysis, Stevens-Johnson syndrome, supraventricular tachycardia, syncope, and vision abnormal.

Overdosage

➤*Symptoms:* A 7-month-old baby experienced tachycardia and mydriasis after administration of a single dose of 10 mg trospium given by a sibling. The baby's weight was reported as 5 kg. Following admission into the hospital and approximately 1 hour after ingestion of the trospium, medicinal charcoal was administered for detoxification. While hospitalized, the baby experienced mydriasis and tachycardia up to 230 beats/min. Therapeutic intervention was not deemed necessary. The baby was discharged as completely recovered the following day.

➤*Treatment:* Overdosage with trospium may result in severe anticholinergic effects. Treatment should be provided according to symptoms and supportive care. In the event of overdosage, electrocardiogram monitoring is recommended.

Patient Information

Inform patients that anticholinergic agents, such as trospium, may produce clinically significant adverse effects related to anticholinergic pharmacological activity. For example, heat prostration (fever and heat stroke caused by decreased sweating) can occur when anticholinergics such as trospium are used in a hot environment.

Advise patients to exercise caution because anticholinergics such as trospium may produce dizziness or blurred vision. Alcohol may enhance the drowsiness caused by anticholinergic agents.

Instruct patients to take trospium 1 hour prior to meals or on an empty stomach. If a dose is skipped, advise patients to take their next dose 1 hour prior to their next meal.

BETHANECHOL CHLORIDE

Rx	**Bethanechol Chloride** (Various, eg, Goldline, Ivax, Qualitest, UDL)	**Tablets:** 5 mg	In 100s, 1000s, and UD 100s.
Rx	**Bethanechol Chloride** (Various, eg, Goldline, Ivax, Qualitest, UDL)	10 mg	In 100s, 250s, 1000s, and UD 100s.
Rx	**Bethanechol Chloride** (Various, eg, Goldline, Ivax, Qualitest, UDL)	25 mg	In 100s, 250s, 1000s, and UD 100s.
Rx	**Urecholine** (Odyssey)		Lactose. (OP 704). Yellow, scored. In 100s.
Rx	**Bethanechol Chloride** (Various, eg, Goldline, Ivax, Qualitest, UDL)	50 mg	In 100s, 500s, 1000s, and UD 100s.

Indications

➤*Urinary retention:* Acute postoperative and postpartum nonobstructive (functional) urinary retention and neurogenic atony of the urinary bladder with retention.

➤*Unlabeled uses:* Bethanechol has been used in adults for treatment (25 mg 4 times/day) and diagnosis (two 50 mcg/kg SC doses 15 minutes apart) of reflux esophagitis. In infants and children, an oral dosage of 3 mg/m²/dose 3 times/day has been used for gastroesophageal reflux.

Administration and Dosage

Individualize dose and route. Preferably, administer when the stomach is empty. If taken soon after eating, nausea and vomiting may occur.

➤*Oral:*

Adults – 10 to 50 mg 3 to 4 times/day. The minimum effective dose is determined by giving 5 or 10 mg initially; repeat the same amount hourly to a maximum of 50 mg until satisfactory response occurs.

➤*SC:* Do not give IV or IM (see Warnings). Usual dose is 5 mg; some patients respond to as little as 2.5 mg. The minimum effective dose is determined by injecting 2.5 mg initially and repeating the same amount at 15- to 30-minute intervals to a maximum of 4 doses until satisfactory response is obtained, unless disturbing reactions appear. The minimum effective dose may be repeated 3 or 4 times/day as required.

Rarely, single doses up to 10 mg are required. Such large doses may cause severe reactions; use only after determining that single doses of 2.5 to 5 mg are not sufficient.

If necessary, drug effects can be abolished promptly by atropine.

➤*Storage/Stability:* Store tablets in a tightly closed container at room temperature 15° to 30°C (59° to 86°F). Avoid storage > 40°C (104°F). Avoid storage of injection at < -20°C (-4°F) and > 40°C (104°F).

Actions

➤*Pharmacology:* Bethanechol is an ester of a choline-like compound. It acts principally by stimulating the parasympathetic nervous system. It increases the tone of the detrusor urinae muscle, usually producing a contraction strong enough to initiate micturition and empty the bladder. It stimulates gastric motility, increases gastric tone, and often restores impaired rhythmic peristalsis.

When spontaneous stimulation of the parasympathetic system is reduced and therapeutic intervention is necessary, acetylcholine can be given, but it is rapidly hydrolyzed by cholinesterase and its effects are transient. Bethanechol is not destroyed by cholinesterase and its effects are more prolonged than those of acetylcholine.

Bethanechol has prominent muscarinic action and slight or no nicotinic action. Doses that stimulate micturition and defecation and increase peristalsis do not ordinarily stimulate ganglia or voluntary muscles. Therapeutic test doses in healthy human subjects have little effect on heart rate, blood pressure, or peripheral circulation.

➤*Pharmacokinetics:* Effects appear ≤ 30 to 90 minutes after oral administration. Usual duration is 1 hour, although large doses (eg, 300 to 400 mg) may persist for ≤ 6 hours. SC administration is usually effective in 5 to 15 minutes.

A clinical study was conducted on the relative efficacy of oral and SC bethanechol on the stretch response of bladder muscle in patients with urinary retention. A 5 mg SC dose stimulated a response that was more rapid in onset and of larger magnitude than an oral dose of 50, 100, or 200 mg. However, the oral doses had a longer duration of effect than the SC dose. Although the 50 mg oral dose caused little change in intravesical pressure, this dose is effective in the rehabilitation of patients with decompensated bladders.

Contraindications

Hypersensitivity to bethanechol; hyperthyroidism; peptic ulcer; latent or active bronchial asthma; pronounced bradycardia; atrioventricular conduction defects; vasomotor instability; coronary artery disease; epilepsy; parkinsonism; coronary occlusion; hypotension; hypertension; when the strength or integrity of the GI or bladder wall is in question or in the presence of mechanical obstruction; when increased muscular activity of the GI tract or urinary bladder might prove harmful, as following recent urinary bladder surgery, GI resection, and anastomosis, or when there is possible GI obstruction; bladder neck obstruction; spastic GI disturbances; acute inflammatory lesions of the GI tract; peritonitis; marked vagotonia.

Warnings

➤*Parenteral dosage form:* For SC injection only; do not give IM or IV. Violent symptoms of cholinergic overstimulation, such as circulatory collapse, fall in blood pressure, abdominal cramps, bloody diarrhea, shock, or sudden cardiac arrest are likely if given IM or IV. These symptoms occur rarely after SC injection and may occur in cases of hypersensitivity or overdosage.

➤*Pregnancy:* Category C. It is not known whether bethanechol can cause fetal harm when administered to a pregnant woman or can affect reproduction capacity. Give to a pregnant woman only if clearly needed.

➤*Lactation:* It is not known whether this drug is excreted in breast milk. Because of the potential for serious adverse reactions, decide whether to discontinue nursing or discontinue the drug, taking into account the importance of the drug to the mother.

➤*Children:* Safety and efficacy have not been established. See Unlabeled uses.

Precautions

➤*Reflux infection:* In urinary retention, if the sphincter fails to relax as bethanechol contracts the bladder, urine may be forced up the ureter into the kidney pelvis. If there is bacteriuria, this may cause reflux infection.

➤*Tartrazine sensitivity:* Some of these products contain tartrazine, which may cause allergic-type reactions (including bronchial asthma) in susceptible individuals. Although the incidence of sensitivity is low, it is frequently seen in patients who also have aspirin hypersensitivity. Specific products containing tartrazine are identified in the product listing.

Drug Interactions

Bethanechol Chloride			
Precipitant drug	Object drug*		Description
Cholinergic drugs	Bethanechol	↑	Additive effects may occur, particularly with cholinesterase inhibitors.
Ganglionic blocking compounds	Bethanechol	↑	A critical fall in blood pressure may occur that is usually preceded by severe abdominal symptoms.
Quinidine Procainamide	Bethanechol	↑	Quinidine or procainamide may antagonize cholinergic effects of bethanechol.

*↑ = Object drug increased.

Adverse Reactions

Adverse reactions are rare following oral administration of bethanechol but are more common following SC injection. Adverse reactions are more likely to occur when dosage is increased.

➤*Cardiovascular:* Fall in blood pressure with reflex tachycardia; vasomotor response.

➤*Dermatologic:* Flushing producing a feeling of warmth; sensation of heat about the face; sweating.

➤*GI:* Abdominal cramps or discomfort; colicky pain; nausea; belching; diarrhea; borborygmi (rumbling/gurgling of stomach); salivation.

➤*Respiratory:* Bronchial constriction; asthmatic attacks.

➤*Special senses:* Lacrimation; miosis.

➤*Miscellaneous:* Malaise; urinary urgency; headache.

Overdosage

➤*Symptoms:* Early signs of overdosage are abdominal discomfort, salivation, flushing of the skin ("hot feeling"), sweating, nausea and vomiting.

➤*Treatment:* Atropine is a specific antidote. The recommended dose for adults is 0.6 mg. Repeat doses may be given every 2 hours according to clinical response.

The recommended dosage in infants and children ≤ 12 years of age is 0.01 mg/kg repeated every 2 hours as needed until the desired effect is obtained or adverse effects of atropine preclude further usage. The maximum single dose should not exceed 0.4 mg.

BETHANECHOL CHLORIDE

Subcutaneous injection of atropine is preferred except in emergencies when the IV route may be used. When administering bethanechol SC, always have a syringe containing atropine available.

Patient Information

To avoid nausea and vomiting, take 1 hour before or 2 hours after meals. If taken soon after eating, nausea and vomiting may occur.

May cause abdominal discomfort, salivation, sweating or flushing; notify physician if these effects are pronounced.

Dizziness, lightheadedness or fainting may occur, especially when getting up from a lying or sitting position.

NEOSTIGMINE METHYLSULFATE

Rx	**Prostigmin** (ICN)	**Injection:** 1:4000 (0.25 mg/mL)	In 1 mL amps.[1]
Rx	**Neostigmine Methylsulfate** (Various, eg, American Pharmaceutical Partners, American Regent Labs, Baxter)	**Injection:** 1:2000 (0.5 mg/mL)	In 1, 2, and 10 mL vials and 10 mL multidose vials.
Rx	**Prostigmin** (ICN)		In 1 mL amps[1] and 10 mL multidose vials.[2]
Rx	**Neostigmine Methylsulfate** (Various, eg, American Pharmaceutical Partners, American Regent Labs, Baxter)	**Injection:** 1:1000 (1 mg/mL)	In 10 mL multidose vials.
Rx	**Prostigmin** (ICN)		In 10 mL multidose vials.[2]

[1] With 0.2% methyl- and propylparabens.
[2] With 0.45% phenol and 0.2 mg sodium acetate.

Indications

➤*Urinary retention:* For the prevention and treatment of postoperative distention and urinary retention.

➤*Antidote for neuromuscular blocking agents:* As an antidote for nondepolarizing neuromuscular blocking agents (eg, tubocurarine, metocurine, gallamine, pancuronium) after surgery (refer to the Anticholinesterase Muscle Stimulant monograph).

➤*Myasthenia gravis:* For symptomatic control of myasthenia gravis when oral therapy is impractical (refer to the Anticholinesterase Muscle Stimulant monograph).

➤*Unlabeled uses:* For the treatment of acute colonic pseudo-obstruction in patients who failed conventional therapy; as an adjunct to postoperative analgesia.

Administration and Dosage

➤*Prevention of postoperative distention and urinary retention:* 1 mL of the 1:4000 solution (0.25 mg) SC or IM as soon as possible after operation; repeat every 4 to 6 hours for 2 or 3 days.

➤*Treatment of postoperative distention:* 1 mL of the 1:2000 solution (0.5 mg) SC or IM, as required.

➤*Treatment of urinary retention:* 1 mL of the 1:2000 solution (0.5 mg) SC or IM. If urination does not occur within 1 hour, catheterize the patient. After the patient has voided or the bladder is emptied, continue 0.5 mg injections every 3 hours for at least 5 injections.

➤*Storage/Stability:* Store at controlled room temperature (15° to 30°C; 59° to 86°F). Protect from light. Keep in carton until ready to use.

Actions

➤*Pharmacology:* Neostigmine inhibits acetylcholine hydrolysis by competing for attachment to acetylcholinesterase at sites of cholinergic transmission. It enhances cholinergic action by facilitating the transmission of impulses across neuromuscular junctions. It also has a direct cholinomimetic effect on skeletal muscle and possibly on autonomic ganglion cells and neurons of the CNS.

➤*Pharmacokinetics:*

Absorption/Distribution – Neostigmine is poorly absorbed orally. Following IM administration, the drug is rapidly absorbed and eliminated. Serum albumin binding ranges from 15% to 25%.

Metabolism/Excretion – Neostigmine undergoes hydrolysis by cholinesterase and is metabolized by microsomal enzymes in the liver. Approximately 80% is eliminated in the urine within 24 hours, with approximately 50% as the unchanged drug and 30% as metabolites. Following IV administration, plasma half life is 47 to 60 minutes (mean, 53 minutes).

Onset/Duration – Clinical effects usually begin within 20 to 30 minutes after IM injection and last 2.5 to 4 hours.

Contraindications

Hypersensitivity to neostigmine; peritonitis; mechanical obstruction of the intestinal or urinary tract.

Warnings

➤*Special risk patients:* Use with caution in patients with epilepsy, bronchial asthma, bradycardia, recent coronary occlusion, vagotonia, hyperthyroidism, cardiac arrhythmias, or peptic ulcer.

➤*Concomitant atropine administration:* When large doses are administered, the prior or simultaneous injection of atropine sulfate may be advisable. Use separate syringes for neostigmine and atropine.

➤*Hypersensitivity reactions:* Have atropine and antishock medication immediately available. Refer to Management of Acute Hypersensitivity Reactions.

➤*Pregnancy: Category C.* There are no adequate or well-controlled studies. It is not known whether neostigmine can cause fetal harm when administered to a pregnant woman or can affect reproductive capacity. Anticholinesterase drugs may cause uterine irritability and induce premature labor when given IV to pregnant women near term. Give to a pregnant woman only if clearly needed.

➤*Lactation:* It is not known whether neostigmine is excreted in breast milk. Because of the potential for serious adverse reactions in nursing infants, decide whether to discontinue nursing or to discontinue the drug, taking into account the importance of the drug to the mother.

➤*Children:* Safety and efficacy for use in children have not been established.

Drug Interactions

Neostigmine Drug Interactions			
Precipitant drug	Object drug*		Description
Aminoglycoside antibiotics (eg, neomycin, streptomycin, kanamycin)	Neostigmine	↑	Aminoglycoside antibiotics have a mild but definite nondepolarizing blocking action that may accentuate neuromuscular block.
Antiarrhythmic agents	Neostigmine	↓	May interfere with neuromuscular transmission. Use cautiously, if at all, in patients with myasthenia gravis. The neostigmine dose may have to be increased accordingly.
Corticosteroids	Neostigmine	↓	Corticosteroids may decrease the anticholinesterase effects of neostigmine. Profound muscular depression has occurred.
Local and general anesthetics	Neostigmine	↓	May interfere with neuromuscular transmission. Use cautiously, if at all, in patients with myasthenia gravis. The neostigmine dose may have to be increased accordingly.
Neostigmine	Depolarizing muscle relaxants (eg, succinylcholine, decamethonium)	↑/↓	Neostigmine may prolong or antagonize the neuromuscular blocking effects of these drugs.

* ↑ = Object drug increased.   ↓ = Object drug decreased.

Adverse Reactions

Side effects generally are caused by exaggerated pharmacological effects; salivation and fasciculation are the most common.

➤*Cardiovascular:* Cardiac arrest, cardiac arrhythmias (AV block and nodal rhythm, bradycardia, tachycardia), hypotension, nonspecific EKG changes, syncope.

➤*CNS:* Convulsions, dizziness, drowsiness, dysarthria, headache, loss of consciousness, miosis.

➤*Dermatologic:* Rash, urticaria.

➤*GI:* Bowel cramps, diarrhea, emesis, flatulence, increased peristalsis, nausea.

➤*Musculoskeletal:* Arthralgia, muscle cramps and spasms.

➤*Respiratory:* Bronchospasm; dyspnea; increased oral, pharyngeal, and bronchial secretions; respiratory arrest; respiratory depression.

➤*Miscellaneous:* Allergic reactions, anaphylaxis, diaphoresis, flushing, urinary frequency, visual changes, weakness.

NEOSTIGMINE METHYLSULFATE

Overdosage

▶*Symptoms:* Overdosage may result in cholinergic crisis, characterized by increasing muscle weakness. This, through involvement of respiratory muscles, may lead to death.

▶*Treatment:* Cholinergic crisis calls for the prompt withdrawal of all drugs of this type and the immediate use of atropine (see Anticholinergics/Antispasmodics in the Gastrointestinal chapter).

Atropine also may be used to abolish or minimize GI side effects or other muscarinic reactions; such use can lead to inadvertent induction of cholinergic crisis by masking signs of overdosage.

Patient Information

Instruct patients to notify their health care provider if diarrhea, difficulty breathing, increased salivary secretions, irregular heart beat, muscle weakness, nausea, severe abdominal pain, sweating, or vomiting occurs.

SEVELAMER HCl

Rx	**Renagel** (Genzyme)	**Tablets:** 400 mg (on an anhydrous basis)	(RENAGEL 400). Oval. Film-coated. In 360s.
		800 mg (on an anhydrous basis)	(RENAGEL 800). Oval. Film-coated. In 180s

Indications

➤*Hyperphosphatemia:* For the reduction of serum phosphorus in patients with end-stage renal disease (ESRD).

The safety and efficacy of sevelamer in ESRD patients who are not on hemodialysis have not been studied. In hemodialysis patients, sevelamer decreases the incidence of hypercalcemic episodes relative to patients on calcium acetate treatment.

Administration and Dosage

➤*Approved by the FDA:* October 30, 1998.

➤*Patients not taking a phosphate binder:* The recommended starting dose is 800 to 1600 mg, which can be administered as 1 to 2 sevelamer 800 mg tablets, two to four 400 mg tablets, or 2 to 4 capsules with each meal based on serum phosphorus level.

Sevelamer Starting Dose for Patients Not Taking a Phosphate Binder		
Serum phosphorus	Sevelamer 800 mg	Sevelamer 400 mg tablets or capsules
> 6 and < 7.5 mg/dL	1 tablet 3 times/day with meals	2 tablets or capsules 3 times/day with meals
≥ 7.5 mg and < 9 mg/dL	2 tablets 3 times/day with meals	3 tablets or capsules 3 times/day with meals
≥ 9 mg/dL	2 tablets 3 times/day with meals	4 tablets or capsules 3 times/day with meals

➤*Patients switching from calcium acetate:* In 84 ESRD patients on hemodialysis, a similar reduction in serum phosphorus was seen with equivalent doses (mg for mg) of sevelamer and calcium acetate.

Starting Dose for Patients Switching from Calcium Acetate to Sevelamer		
Calcium acetate 667 mg (tablets/meal)	Sevelamer 800 mg (tablets/meal)	Sevelamer 400 mg or capsules (tablets or capsules/meal)
1 tablet	1 tablet	2 tablets or capsules
2 tablets	2 tablets	3 tablets or capsules
3 tablets	3 tablets	5 tablets or capsules

➤*Dose titration:* Adjust dosage based on the serum phosphorus concentration with a goal of lowering serum phosphorus to 6 mg/dL or less. The dose may be increased or decreased by 1 tablet or capsule/meal at 2-week intervals as necessary. The average dose in phase 3 clinical trials was 4 capsules (403 mg) per meal. The maximum dose studied was 10 sevelamer capsules/meal (the equivalent of five 800 mg tablets/meal or ten 400 mg tablets/meal).

Sevelamer Dose Titration Guideline	
Serum phosphorus	Sevelamer dose
> 6 mg/dL	Increase 1 tablet/capsule per meal at 2-week intervals
3.5 to 6 mg/dL	Maintain current dose
< 3.5 mg/dL	Decrease 1 tablet/capsule per meal

➤*Storage/Stability:* Store at 25°C (77°F); excursions permitted to 15° to 30°C (59° to 86°F). Protect from moisture.

Actions

➤*Pharmacology:* Sevelamer is a polymeric phosphate binder for oral administration. Patients with ESRD retain phosphorus and can develop hyperphosphatemia. High serum phosphorus can precipitate serum calcium, resulting in ectopic calcification. When the product of serum calcium and phosphorus concentrations (Ca × P) exceeds 66, there is an increased risk of ectopic calcification. Hyperphosphatemia plays a role in the development of secondary hyperparathyroidism in renal insufficiency. An increase in parathyroid hormone (PTH) levels is characteristic of patients with chronic renal failure. Increased PTH levels can lead to osteitis fibrosa. A decrease in serum phosphorus may decrease serum PTH levels.

Treatment of hyperphosphatemia includes reduction in dietary intake of phosphate, inhibition of intestinal phosphate absorption with phosphate binders, and removal of phosphate with dialysis. Sevelamer taken with meals has been shown to decrease serum phosphorus concentrations in patients with ESRD who are on hemodialysis. Because sevelamer does not contain aluminum, it does not cause aluminum intoxication. Sevelamer also lowers low-density lipoprotein (LDL) and total serum cholesterol levels.

➤*Pharmacokinetics:* A mass-balance study in 16 healthy males and females showed that sevelamer is not systemically absorbed. No absorption studies have been performed in patients with renal disease.

➤*Clinical trials:* A crossover study of sevelamer and calcium acetate in 84 ESRD patients on hemodialysis who were hyperphosphatemic (serum phosphorus greater than 6 mg/dL) revealed that both agents significantly decreased mean serum phosphorus levels. The proportion of patients achieving a given level of serum phosphorus lowering was comparable between the 2 treatment groups (eg, about half the patients in each group had a decrease of at least 2 mg/dL at endpoint).

During calcium acetate treatment, 22% of patients developed serum calcium 11 mg/dL or greater on at least 1 occasion vs 5% for sevelamer. Thus, the risk of developing hypercalcemia was less with sevelamer compared with calcium acetate. Mean LDL cholesterol and mean total cholesterol declined significantly on sevelamer treatment (−24% and −15%, respectively) while no change occurred with calcium acetate.

Contraindications

Hypophosphatemia; bowel obstruction; known hypersensitivity to sevelamer or any of its constituents.

Warnings

➤*Mutagenesis:* In an in vitro mammalian cytogenetics test with metabolic activation, sevelamer caused a statistically significant increase in structural chromosome aberrations.

➤*Pregnancy: Category C.* In rats, at doses of 1.5 and 4.5 g/kg/day (approximately 15 and 45 times the recommended human dose based on mg/kg), sevelamer caused reduced or irregular ossification of fetal bones, probably because of a reduced absorption of fat-soluble vitamin D. In rabbits, sevelamer slightly increased prenatal mortality because of an increased incidence of early resorptions at a dose of 1 g/kg/day (approximately 10 times the recommended human dose based on mg/kg). Vitamin and other nutrient requirements are increased in pregnancy. The effect of sevelamer on the absorption of vitamins and other nutrients has not been studied in pregnant women. There are no adequate and well-controlled studies in pregnant women.

➤*Lactation:* There are no adequate and well-controlled studies in nursing mothers.

➤*Children:* The safety and efficacy have not been established.

Precautions

➤*Monitoring:* Monitor serum calcium, bicarbonate, and chloride levels. Sevelamer does not contain calcium or alkali supplementation.

➤*GI disorders:* The safety and efficacy of sevelamer in patients with dysphagia, swallowing disorders, severe GI motility disorders, or major GI tract surgery have not been established. Consequently, exercise caution when sevelamer is used in these patients.

➤*Vitamin deficiencies:* In preclinical studies in rats and dogs, sevelamer reduced vitamin D, E, K, and folic acid levels at doses of 6 to 100 times the recommended human dose. In clinical trials, there was no evidence of reduction in serum levels of vitamins in patients who were supplemented with multivitamins.

Drug Interactions

There is a possibility that sevelamer may bind concomitantly administered drugs and decrease their bioavailability. When alterations in blood levels of an oral drug can produce a clinically significant effect on safety or efficacy, administer the drug at least 1 hour before or 3 hours after sevelamer. Take special precautions when prescribing sevelamer to patients taking antiarrhythmic or antiseizure agents.

Adverse Reactions

In a placebo-controlled study with a 2-week treatment duration, adverse events with sevelamer (n = 24) were similar to those with placebo (n = 12).

Adverse Reactions of Sevelamer vs Calcium Acetate (%)		
Adverse reaction	Sevelamer (N = 82)	Calcium acetate (N = 82)
Cardiovascular	29	35
Hypertension	9	10
Hypotension	11	12
Thrombosis	10	6
GI	34	28
Diarrhea	16	10
Dyspepsia	11	4
Vomiting	12	5
Respiratory	10	22
Cough increased	4	11
Miscellaneous	44	46
Headache	10	11
Infection	15	11
Pain	13	16

SEVELAMER HCl

In a long-term, open-label extension trial, adverse events possibly related to sevelamer that were not dose-related, included: Nausea (7%); dyspepsia (5%); diarrhea, flatulence (4%); constipation (2%).

Overdosage

Sevelamer has been given to healthy volunteers in doses up to 14 g/day for 8 days with no adverse effects. There are no reported overdosages; systemic toxicity risk is low because sevelamer is not absorbed.

Patient Information

Inform patients to take sevelamer with meals and adhere to their prescribed diets.

Instruct patients to space doses of concomitant medications by at least 1 hour before or 3 hours after sevelamer.

Because the contents of sevelamer expand in water, instruct patients not to chew or take tablets and capsules apart prior to administration.

Vaginal Antifungal Agents

Indications

➤*Candidiasis:* Local treatment of vulvovaginal candidiasis (eg, moniliasis, vaginal yeast infection).

Actions

➤*Pharmacology:* Treatment of vaginal candidiasis (moniliasis) is complicated by a high recurrence rate because of the ubiquitous nature of *Candida albicans* and non-albicans species of *Candida.* Predisposing factors include diabetes, antibiotics, pregnancy, corticosteroids, oral contraceptives containing 75 to 150 mcg of estrogen, intrauterine devices, and decreased host immunity (eg, HIV).

Agents approved for local treatment of vulvovaginal candidiasis include **nystatin** (a polyene antibiotic), the imidazoles (**butoconazole, clotrimazole, miconazole, tioconazole**), and **terconazole** (a triazole derivative).

Nystatin and imidazoles – Nystatin and imidazoles bind to sterols in the cell membrane of the fungus with a resultant change in membrane permeability allowing leakage of intracellular components.

Terconazole – Terconazole's exact pharmacologic mode of action is uncertain. It may exert antifungal activity by disruption of normal fungal cell membrane permeability.

➤*Pharmacokinetics:*

Butoconazole – Approximately 1.7% is absorbed after vaginal administration. Peak plasma levels (13.6 to 18.6 ng/mL) of the drug and its metabolites were attained between 12 and 24 hours.

Terconazole – Following daily intravaginal administration of 0.8% terconazole 40 mg (0.8% cream × 5 g) for 7 days to healthy humans, plasma concentrations were low and gradually rose to a daily peak (mean of 5.9 ng/mL) at 6.6 hours. Following oral (30 mg) administration of terconazole, the harmonic half-life of elimination from the blood for the parent terconazole was 6.9 hours (range, 4 to 11.3). Terconazole is extensively metabolized. In vitro, terconazole is highly protein bound (94.9%) and the degree of binding is independent of the drug concentration.

Nystatin – Nystatin is not absorbed from intact skin or mucous membranes.

➤*Microbiology:* **Miconazole** is active against susceptible strains of *Trichophyton* spp., *Epidermophyton* spp., *Candida albicans*, and *Microsporium* spp. **Clotrimazole, tioconazole, nystatin, terconazole,** and **butoconazole** are active against *Candida* spp. (*Candida albicans*). Other pathogens commonly associated with vulvovaginitis (*Trichomonas* and *Gardnerella vaginalis*) do not respond to these antifungal agents.

Contraindications

Hypersensitivity to specific drug or component of the product.

Warnings

➤*Diagnosis:* It is important that vaginal infections be differentiated, as bacterial vaginosis, trichomoniasis, and vulvovaginal candidiasis may produce common symptoms. The diagnosis of vulvovaginitis (*Trichomonas vaginalis* and *Haemophilus vaginalis*) may be confirmed prior to therapy by KOH smears or cultures. This does not apply to *otc* use of these agents, which requires self-diagnosis by the patient.

➤*OTC products:*

Other conditions – If abdominal pain, fever, or offensive-smelling vaginal discharge is present, do not use these products. If there is no improvement within 3 to 7 days, stop using these products. Consult a doctor, a condition more serious than a yeast infection may be present.

Vaginal itch/discomfort – Patients should consult a physician before using these products if it is their first experience with vaginal itch and discomfort.

Recurrent infections – For patients with frequently recurrent candidal vaginitis, it is important to consider factors that predispose to infection. The discontinuation of oral contraceptives decreases the frequency of yeast vaginitis for many women. Eliminating nylon and tight-fitting garments can also be helpful. Many diabetic patients with poor glycemic control have recurring yeast vaginitis. Patients with recurrent yeast vaginitis should be tested for HIV.

➤*Pregnancy:* Category A – **nystatin;** *Category B* – **clotrimazole, nystatin**†; *Category C* – **butoconazole, terconazole, miconazole.** During pregnancy, use of a vaginal applicator may be contraindicated; manual insertion of vaginal tablets may be preferred. Use only on advice of physician.

Because small amounts of these drugs may be absorbed from the vagina, use during the first trimester only when essential. Use of **butoconazole** during the second and third trimesters has been approved. Possible exposure of the fetus through direct transfer of **terconazole**

from an irritated vagina to the fetus by diffusion across amniotic membranes may occur.

➤*Lactation:* Because nystatin is poorly absorbed, if at all, serum and milk levels would not occur with **nystatin.** It is not known whether the other drugs are excreted in breast milk. Safety for use during lactation has not been established. Exercise caution or temporarily discontinue nursing during administration.

Terconazole – Because of the potential for adverse reactions in nursing infants from terconazole, decide whether to discontinue nursing or to discontinue the drug, taking into account the importance of the drug to the mother.

➤*Children:* Safety and efficacy have not been established with **butoconazole, terconazole, nystatin,** and **miconazole** (*Monistat Dual-Pak* only). Safety and efficacy have not been established in children < 12 years of age with **clotrimazole, tioconazole,** and **miconazole.**

Precautions

➤*For vaginal use only:* Do not use creams in mouth or eyes.

➤*Irritation:* If irritation, sensitization, fever, chills, or flu-like symtoms occur, discontinue use.

➤*Chronic or recurrent candidiasis:* Chronic or recurrent candidiasis may be a symptom of unrecognized diabetes mellitus or a damaged immune system (including HIV infection). A persistently resistant infection may actually be caused by reinfection; evaluate sources of reinfection.

➤*Refractory patients:* If there is lack of response, repeat microbiological studies to confirm diagnosis and rule out other pathogens before reinstituting antifungal therapy.

Drug Interactions

➤*Miconazole:* Concomitant use of warfarin and miconazole intravaginal cream and suppository may cause an increase in PT, INR, and bleeding. Monitor appropriately.

Adverse Reactions

Irritation; sensitization; vulvovaginal burning.

Clotrimazole – Skin irritation with symptoms of redness, itching, burning, blistering, peeling, urticaria, or skin fissures.

Miconazole – Burning, irritation, pruritus, discharge, edema, and pain have occurred at the administration site. Other adverse reactions include GI cramping, nausea, and headache. Genital erythema, vaginal tenderness, dysuria, allergic reaction, dry mouth, flatulence, perianal burning, pelvic cramping, rash, urticaria, skin irritation, periorbital edema, and conjunctival pruritus occurred in < 1% of patients in trials.

Butoconazole – Vulvar/vaginal burning, itching, soreness and swelling, pelvic or abdominal pain or cramping, or a combination of 2 or more of these symptoms.

Terconazole – Headache (21% to 26%); dysmenorrhea (6%); pain of the female genitalia (5%); body pain (2.1%); abdominal pain (3.4%); fever (1% to 1.7%); chills (0.4%); vulvovaginal burning (5.2%); itching (2.3%); irritation (3.1%). Most frequent reason for discontinuing therapy was vulvovaginal itching (0.6% to 0.7%).

Photosensitivity reactions may occur following repeated dermal application under conditions of filtered artificial ultraviolet light.

Tioconazole – Vaginal swelling or redness; difficult or burning urination; headache; abdominal pain/cramping; upper respiratory tract infection.

Patient Information

Patient instructions are enclosed with product. Patients should carefully read *otc* product labeling.

Open applicator just prior to administration to prevent contamination. Clean reusable applicators after use with mild soap solution and rinse thoroughly with water.

Insert high into the vagina (except during pregnancy).

Complete full course of therapy. Use continuously, even during menstrual period.

Notify physician if burning or irritation, skin rash, or hives occur.

Refrain from sexual intercourse.

Use sanitary napkin or minipad to prevent staining of clothing. Do not use a tampon.

The base used in some of these formulations may interact with (weaken) certain latex products such as condoms, diaphragms, or vaginal spermicides. Concurrent use (within 72 hours) is not recommended. The effect is temporary and occurs only during treatment.

---

† Briggs GG, et al. *Drugs in Pregnancy and Lactation* 5th ed.

Vaginal Antifungal Agents

CLOTRIMAZOLE

otc	**Clotrimazole** (Various, eg, Taro)	**Vaginal suppositories:** 200 mg	In 3s with applicator.
otc	**Gyne-Lotrimin 3** (Schering-Plough)		In 3s with applicator.
otc	**Clotrimazole** (Various, eg, Taro)	**Vaginal cream:** 2%	In 21 g tube with 3 disposable applicators.
otc	**Gyne-Lotrimin 3** (Schering-Plough)		Benzyl alcohol. In 21 g tube with 3 disposable applicators.
otc	**Clotrimazole** (Various, eg, Alpharma, Major, Warrick)	**Vaginal cream:** 1%	In 15, 30, and 45 g with applicator(s).
otc	**Mycelex-7** (Bayer)		Benzyl alcohol, cetostearyl alcohol. In 45 g with 1 applicator or 45 g with 7 disposable applicators.
otc	**Gyne-Lotrimin 7** (Schering-Plough)		In 45 g with 1 applicator, 45 g with 7 applicators, or 45 g with 7 pre-filled applicators.
otc	**Mycelex-7 Combination Pack** (Bayer)	**Vaginal suppositories:** 100 mg	Lactose, povidone. In 7s with applicator.
		Topical cream: 1%	Benzyl alcohol, cetostearyl alcohol. Polysorbate 80. In 7 g tubes.
otc	**Clotrimazole Combination Pack** (Various, eg, Taro)	**Vaginal suppositories:** 200 mg	In 3s with applicator.
		Topical cream: 1%	In tubes.
otc	**Gyne-Lotrimin 3 Combination Pack** (Schering-Plough)	**Vaginal suppositories:** 200 mg	Lactose. In 3s with applicator.
		Topical cream: 1%	Benzyl alcohol, cetyl stearyl alcohol. In 7 g tubes.

Refer to the general discussion of these products in the Vaginal Antifungal agents group monograph. For information on oral and topical clotrimazole, refer to individual monographs.

Indications

➤*Yeast infections:* For the treatment of vaginal yeast infections (candidiasis).

Administration and Dosage

➤*Suppositories:* Insert 1 suppository intravaginally at bedtime for 3 consecutive days (200 mg).

➤*Cream:*
Intravaginal – Insert 1 applicatorful a day, preferably at bedtime, for 3 to 7 consecutive days.
Topical – Apply to affected areas twice daily (morning and evening) for 7 consecutive days or as needed.

MICONAZOLE NITRATE

otc	**Monistat-7** (Advanced Care Products)	**Vaginal suppositories:** 100 mg	In 7s with applicator.
otc	**Miconazole 7** (Rugby)		Hydrogenated vegetable oil base. In 7s with applicator.
otc	**Monistat** (Advanced Care Products)	**Topical cream:** 2%	In 9 g tubes.
otc	**Miconazole Nitrate** (Various, eg, Alpharma, E. Fougera, G & W Labs, Major, Rugby, Taro)	**Vaginal cream:** 2%	In 15, 30, and 45 g with applicator(s).
otc	**Femizol-M** (Lake Consumer Products)		In 45 g with applicator.
otc	**Monistat 7** (Advanced Care Products)		In 35 and 45 g tubes with 1 applicator or 7 *Ultraslim* disposable applicators, or in 7 prefilled applicators with 5 g cream.
otc	**Monistat 3** (Advanced Care Products)		In 3 prefilled applicators.
Rx	**Monistat Dual-Pak** (Personal Products Co.)	**Vaginal suppositories:** 1200 mg	Petrolatum base with parafin. In 1s with applicator.
		Topical cream: 2%	Steryl and cetyl alcohol. In 9 g tubes.
otc	**M-Zole 3 Combination Pack** (Alpharma)	**Vaginal suppositories:** 200 mg	Hydrogenated vegetable oil. In 3s with reusable applicator or 3 disposable applicators.
		Topical cream: 2%	In 9 g tubes.
otc	**Monistat 3 Combination Pack** (Advanced Care Products)	**Vaginal suppositories:** 200 mg	In 3s with 1 reusable applicator or 3 disposable applicators.
		Topical cream: 2%	In tubes.
otc	**Monistat 7 Combination Pack** (Advanced Care Products)	**Vaginal suppositories:** 100 mg	In 7s with 1 applicator.
		Topical cream: 2%	In tubes.
otc	**M-Zole 7 Dual Pack** (Alpharma)	**Vaginal suppositories:** 100 mg	Mineral oil. In 7s with 1 applicator.
		Topical cream: 2%	In 9 g tubes.

Refer to the general discussion of these products in the Vaginal Antifungal Agents group monograph. For information on topical miconazole, refer to the monograph in the Dermatologicals chapter.

Indications

➤*Suppositories:* For the treatment of vulvovaginal candidiasis (moniliasis).

➤*Cream:* For the relief of external vulvar itching and irritation associated with a yeast infection.

Administration and Dosage

➤*Suppositories:* Insert 1 suppository intravaginally once daily at bedtime for 1 day (1200 mg), 3 consecutive days (200 mg), or 7 consecutive days (100 mg).

➤*Cream:*
Intravaginal – Insert 1 applicatorful intravaginally once daily at bedtime for 3 to 7 days.
Topical – Apply to affected areas twice daily (morning and evening) for up to 7 days or as needed.
Repeat course if necessary, after ruling out other pathogens.

➤*Storage/Stability:* Store at 15° to 30°C (59° to 86°F).

Vaginal Antifungal Agents

TIOCONAZOLE

otc	**Vagistat-1** (Bristol-Myers Squibb)	**Vaginal ointment:** 6.5%	White petrolatum. In 300 mg prefilled, single-dose applicator.
otc	**Monistat 1** (Advanced Care Products)		In 4.6 g prefilled, single-dose applicator.

Refer to the general discussion of these products in the Vaginal Antifungal Agents group monograph.

Indications

➤*Yeast infections:* For the treatment of recurrent vaginal yeast infections (candidiasis).

Administration and Dosage

➤*Single dose:* Insert 1 applicatorful intravaginally just prior to bedtime.

NYSTATIN

Rx	**Nystatin** (Various, eg, Goldline)	**Vaginal tablets:** 100,000 units	In 15s and 30s with applicator(s).

Refer to the general discussion of these products in the Vaginal Antifungal Agents group monograph. For information on oral nystatin suspension and troches for oral candidiasis, oral nystatin tablets for intestinal candidiasis, and topical nystatin, refer to the individual monographs.

Indications

➤*Yeast infections:* For the treatment of vulvovaginal candidiasis (moniliasis).

Administration and Dosage

The usual dosage is 1 tablet inserted high in the vagina by means of applicator daily for 2 weeks.

Symptomatic relief may occur in a few days; continue full course of treatment.

➤*Storage/Stability:* Store at 15° to 30°C (59° to 86°F).

TERCONAZOLE

Rx	**Terconazole** (Various, eg, Taro, Watson)	**Vaginal cream:** 0.4%	Alcohols. In 45 g tubes.
	Terazol 7 (Ortho-McNeil)		Cetyl alcohol, stearyl alcohol. In 45 g tube with 1 measured-dose applicator.
Rx	**Terconazole** (Various, eg, Taro, Watson)	**Vaginal cream:** 0.8%	Alcohols. In 20 g tubes.
	Terazol 3 (Ortho-McNeil)		In 20 g tube with 1 measured-dose applicator.
Rx	**Terazol 3** (Ortho-McNeil)	**Vaginal suppositories:** 80 mg	Coconut oil/palm kernel oil. Elliptically shaped, white to off-white. In 2.5 g. In 3s.

Refer to the general discussion of these products in the Vaginal Antifungal Agents group monograph.

Indications

➤*Yeast infections:* For the local treatment of vulvovaginal candidiasis (moniliasis).

Administration and Dosage

➤*Suppositories:* Administer 1 suppository intravaginally once daily at bedtime for 3 consecutive days.

➤*Cream:*

0.4% – Administer one applicatorful (5 g) intravaginally once daily at bedtime for 7 consecutive days.

0.8% – Administer one applicatorful (5 g) intravaginally once daily at bedtime for 3 consecutive days.

Before prescribing another course of therapy, reconfirm diagnosis by smears or cultures and rule out other pathogens commonly associated with vulvovaginitis. The therapeutic effect of terconazole is not affected by menstruation.

BUTOCONAZOLE NITRATE

Rx	**Gynazole·1** (Ther-Rx)	**Vaginal cream:** 2%	EDTA, parabens, mineral oil. In 5 g prefilled, single-dose applicator (1s).
otc	**Mycelex-3** (Bayer)		Cetyl and stearyl alcohol, parabens, mineral oil. In 3 prefilled, single-dose applicators, or in 20 g with 3 disposable applicators.

Refer to the general discussion of these products in the Vaginal Antifungal Agents group monograph.

Indications

➤*Yeast infections:* For the treatment of vulvovaginal infections caused by *Candida albicans*.

Administration and Dosage

The recommended dose is 1 applicatorful of cream intravaginally once (*Gynazole•1*); or insert 1 applicatorful a day, preferably at bedtime for 3 consecutive days.

➤*Storage/Stability:* Do not store > 30°C (86°F). Avoid excessive heat and freezing.

CLINDAMYCIN PHOSPHATE

Rx	Cleocin (Pfizer)	Cream: 2%	Benzyl alcohol, cetostearyl alcohol, mineral oil. In 40 g tube with 7 disposable applicators.
		Suppositories: 100 mg (as base)	In cartons of 3 with applicator.

Indications

➤*Bacterial vaginosis:* For the treatment of bacterial vaginosis (formerly referred to as *Haemophilus* vaginitis, *Gardnerella* vaginitis, nonspecific vaginitis, *Corynebacterium* vaginitis, or anaerobic vaginosis) in nonpregnant women.

Cream only – Clindamycin cream can be used to treat pregnant women during the second and third trimester.

Administration and Dosage

For vaginal use only.

➤*Cream:* One applicatorful (5 g containing approximately 100 mg clindamycin) intravaginally, preferably at bedtime, for 3 or 7 consecutive days in nonpregnant women and for 7 consecutive days in pregnant women.

➤*Suppositories:* One suppository (containing clindamycin equivalent to 100 mg clindamycin/2.5 g suppository) intravaginally/day, preferably at bedtime, for 3 consecutive days.

➤*Storage/Stability:*

Cream – Store at controlled room temperature 20° to 25°C (68° to 77°F). Protect from freezing.

Suppositories – Store at 25°C (77°F); excursions permitted to 15° to 30°C (59° to 86°F). Avoid heat over 30°C (86°F) and high humidity.

Actions

➤*Pharmacology:* Clindamycin is a water soluble ester of the semisynthetic antibiotic produced by a 7(S)-chloro-substitution of the 7(R)-hydroxyl group of the parent antibiotic lincomycin. Clindamycin inhibits bacterial protein synthesis at the level of the bacterial ribosome. The antibiotic binds preferentially to the 50S ribosomal subunit and affects the process of peptide chain initiation. Although clindamycin is inactive in vitro, rapid in vivo hydrolysis converts this compound to the antibacterially active clindamycin.

➤*Pharmacokinetics:*

Cream – Following a once-daily intravaginal dose of 100 mg clindamycin vaginal cream administered to 6 healthy female volunteers for 7 days, approximately 5% of the administered dose was absorbed systemically. The peak serum clindamycin concentration averaged 18 and 25 ng/mL on day 1 and day 7, respectively. These peak concentrations were attained approximately 10 hours postdosing.

Following a once-daily intravaginal dose of 100 mg clindamycin vaginal cream administered for 7 consecutive days to 5 women with bacterial vaginosis, absorption was slower and less variable than that observed in healthy females. Approximately 5% of the dose was absorbed systemically. The peak serum clindamycin concentration averaged 13 and 16 ng/mL on day 1 and day 7, respectively. These peak concentrations were attained approximately 14 hours postdosing.

There was little or no systemic accumulation of clindamycin after repeated vaginal dosing of clindamycin vaginal cream. The systemic half life was 1.5 to 2.6 hours.

Suppositories – Systemic absorption of clindamycin was estimated following an intravaginal dose of 1 clindamycin suppository (equivalent to 100 mg clindamycin) administered once daily to 11 healthy female volunteers for 3 days. Approximately 30% of the administered dose was absorbed systemically on day 3 of dosing based on AUC. The mean AUC following day 3 of the suppository dosing was 3.2 mcg•h/mL. The C_{max} observed on day 3 of the suppository dosing averaged 0.27 mcg/mL and was observed approximately 5 hours after dosing. The mean apparent elimination half life after the suppository dosing was 11 hours and is considered to be limited by the absorption rate.

➤*Microbiology:* Clindamycin is active in vitro against most strains of the following organisms that have been reported to be associated with bacterial vaginosis: *Bacteroides* spp., *Gardnerella vaginalis*; *Mobiluncus* spp.; *Mycoplasma hominis*; *Peptostreptococcus* spp.

Contraindications

Hypersensitivity to clindamycin, lincomycin, or any components of the products; regional enteritis; ulcerative colitis; "antibiotic-associated" colitis.

Warnings

➤*Pseudomembranous colitis:* Pseudomembranous colitis has been reported with nearly all antibacterial agents, including clindamycin, and may range in severity from mild to life-threatening. Orally and parenterally administered clindamycin has been associated with severe colitis that may end fatally. Diarrhea, bloody diarrhea, and colitis (including pseudomembranous colitis) have been reported with the use of orally and parenterally administered clindamycin as well as with topical (dermal) formulations of clindamycin. Therefore, it is important to consider this diagnosis in patients who present with diarrhea subse-

quent to the administration of clindamycin, even when administered by the vaginal route, because approximately 5% (cream) and 30% (suppository) of the clindamycin dose is systemically absorbed from the vagina.

Treatment with antibacterial agents alters the normal flora of the colon and may permit overgrowth of clostridia. Studies indicate that a toxin produced by *Clostridium difficile* is a primary cause of "antibiotic-associated" colitis.

After the diagnosis of pseudomembranous colitis has been established, initiate therapeutic measures. Mild cases of pseudomembranous colitis usually respond to discontinuation of the drug alone. In moderate to severe cases, give consideration to management with fluids and electrolytes, protein supplementation, and treatment with an antibacterial drug clinically effective against *C. difficile* colitis.

Onset of pseudomembranous colitis symptoms may occur during or after antimicrobial treatment.

➤*Mineral oil/oleaginous base:* The cream contains mineral oil and the suppositories contain an oleaginous base, both which can weaken latex or rubber products such as condoms or vaginal contraceptive diaphragms. Use of such products within 72 hours following treatment with clindamycin is not recommended.

➤*Diagnosis:* A clinical diagnosis of bacterial vaginosis is usually defined by the presence of a homogeneous vaginal discharge that has a pH of greater than 4.5, emits a "fishy" amine odor when mixed with a 10% KOH solution, and contains clue cells on microscopic examination. Gram's stain results consistent with a diagnosis of bacterial vaginosis include markedly reduced or absent *Lactobacillus* morphology, predominance of *Gardnerella* morphotype, and absent or few white blood cells.

Rule out other pathogens commonly associated with vulvovaginitis (eg, *Trichomonas vaginalis*, *Chlamydia trachomatis*, *Neisseria gonorrhoeae*, *Candida albicans*, and herpes simplex virus).

➤*Pregnancy:* Category B. Clindamycin cream has been studied in pregnant women during the second trimester. In women treated for 7 days, abnormal labor was reported in 1.1% of patients who received clindamycin cream compared with 0.5% of patients who received placebo. There are no adequate and well-controlled studies in pregnant women during the first trimester of pregnancy treated with clindamycin cream; there are no adequate and well-controlled studies in pregnant women treated with clindamycin suppositories. Use during pregnancy only if clearly needed.

➤*Lactation:* It is not known if clindamycin is excreted in breast milk following the use of vaginally administered clindamycin. However, clindamycin has been detected in breast milk after oral or parenteral administration. Because of the potential for serious adverse reactions in nursing infants, decide whether to discontinue nursing or discontinue the drug, taking into account the importance of the drug to the mother.

➤*Children:* Safety and efficacy in children have not been established.

Precautions

➤*For intravaginal use only:* Avoid contact with the eyes. Clindamycin contains ingredients that will cause burning and irritation of the eye. In the event of accidental contact, rinse the eye with copious amounts of cool tap water.

➤*Overgrowth of nonsusceptible organisms:* The use of clindamycin may result in the overgrowth of nonsusceptible organisms, particularly yeasts, in the vagina. In studies using clindamycin suppositories, treatment-related moniliasis was reported in 2.7% of women patients and vaginitis in 3.6%. In women who received clindamycin cream treatment for 3 days, *C. albicans* was reported in 8.8% and vaginitis in 9% of patients; in the 7-day treatment, *C. albicans* was detected in 10.5% and vaginitis in 10.7% of patients.

Drug Interactions

➤*Neuromuscular blocking agents:* Clindamycin has been shown to have neuromuscular blocking properties that may enhance the action of other neuromuscular blocking agents; use with caution in patients receiving such agents.

Adverse Reactions

➤*Cream:*

Nonpregnant women – In clinical trials involving nonpregnant women, 1.8% of 600 patients who received treatment with clindamycin cream for 3 days and 2.7% of 1325 patients who received treatment for 7 days discontinued therapy because of drug-related adverse events. Medical events judged to be related, probably related, possibly related, or of unknown relationship to vaginally administered clindamycin cream were reported for 20.7% of the patients receiving treatment for 3 days and 21.3% of the patients receiving treatment for 7 days.

CLINDAMYCIN PHOSPHATE

Adverse Events Occurring in ≥ 1% of Nonpregnant Patients Receiving Clindamycin Cream		
	Clindamycin cream	
Adverse reaction	3 day (n = 600)	7 day (n = 1325)
GU		
Trichomonal vaginitis	0	1.3
Vaginal moniliasis	7.7	10.4
Vulvovaginal disorder	3.2	5.3
Vulvovaginitis	6	4.4
Miscellaneous		
Moniliasis (body)	1.3	0.2

Other adverse events (less than 1%):
- *CNS* – Dizziness, headache, vertigo.
- *Dermatologic* – Erythema, maculopapular rash, moniliasis, pruritus (nonapplication site), rash, urticaria.
- *GI* – Abdominal cramps, constipation, diarrhea, dyspepsia, flatulence, generalized abdominal pain, GI disorder, localized abdominal pain, nausea, vomiting.
- *GU* – Endometriosis, menstrual disorder, metrorrhagia, urinary tract infection, vaginal discharge, vaginal pain, vaginitis/vaginal infection.
- *Respiratory* – Epistaxis.
- *Miscellaneous* – Allergic reaction, bacterial infection, fungal infection, halitosis, hyperthyroidism, inflammatory swelling, taste perversion.

Pregnant women – In a clinical trial involving pregnant women during the second trimester, 1.7% of 180 patients who received treatment for 7 days discontinued therapy because of drug-related adverse events. Medical events judged to be related, probably related, possibly related, or of unknown relationship to vaginally administered clindamycin cream were reported for 22.8% of pregnant patients.

Adverse Events Occurring in ≥ 1% of Pregnant Patients Receiving Clindamycin Cream or Placebo		
	Clindamycin cream	Placebo
Adverse reaction	7 day (n = 180)	7 day (n = 184)
GU		
Abnormal labor	1.1	0.5
Vaginal moniliasis	13.3	7.1
Vulvovaginal disorder	6.7	7.1
Miscellaneous		
Fungal infection	1.7	0
Pruritus, nonapplication site	1.1	0

Other adverse events (less than 1%):
- *Dermatologic* – Erythema, pruritus (topical application site).
- *GU* – Dysuria, metrorrhagia, trichomonal vaginitis, vaginal pain.
- *Miscellaneous* – Upper respiratory infection.

➤*Suppositories:* In clinical trials involving nonpregnant women, 3 of 589 (0.5%) patients who received treatment with clindamycin suppositories discontinued therapy because of drug-related adverse events. Adverse events judged to have a reasonable possibility of having been caused by clindamycin suppositories were reported for 10.5% of patients. Events reported by 1% or more of patients receiving clindamycin suppositories were as follows:

GU – Vulvovaginal disorder (3.4%), vaginal pain (1.9%), vaginal moniliasis (1.5%).

Miscellaneous – Fungal infection (1%).

Other adverse events (less than 1%) –
Dermatologic: Application-site pain, application-site pruritus, nonapplication-site pruritus, rash.
GI: Abdominal cramps, diarrhea, localized abdominal pain, nausea, vomiting.
GU: Dysuria, menstrual disorder, pyelonephritis, vaginal discharge, vaginitis/vaginal infection.
Miscellaneous: Fever, flank pain, generalized pain, headache, localized edema, moniliasis.

➤*Other clindamycin formulations:* Clindamycin vaginal cream and suppositories afford minimal peak serum levels and systemic exposure of clindamycin compared with 100 mg oral clindamycin dosing. Although these lower levels of exposure are less likely to produce the common reactions seen with oral clindamycin, the possibility of these and other reactions cannot be excluded presently. Refer to the Clindamycin and Lincomycin monographs in the Anti-Infectives chapter.

Overdosage

Vaginally applied cream or suppositories could be absorbed in sufficient amounts to produce systemic effects.

Patient Information

Instruct patients not to engage in vaginal intercourse or use other vaginal products (eg, tampons, douches) during treatment with this product.

Advise patients that the cream contains mineral oil and the suppositories contain an oleaginous base, both which can weaken latex or rubber products such as condoms or vaginal contraceptive diaphragms. Use of such products within 72 hours following treatment with clindamycin is not recommended.

METRONIDAZOLE

Rx	**MetroGel-Vaginal** (3M)	**Gel:** 0.75%	EDTA, parabens. In 70 g tube with 5 applicators.

Metronidazole is also available for topical and systemic use. For further information, refer to the individual monographs in the Anti-infectives chapter and the Dermatological Agents chapter.

Indications

➤*Bacterial vaginosis:* For the treatment of bacterial vaginosis (formerly referred to as *Haemophilus* vaginitis, *Gardnerella* vaginitis, nonspecific vaginitis, *Corynebacterium* vaginitis, or anaerobic vaginosis).

Administration and Dosage

One applicatorful (approximately 5 g containing approximately 37.5 mg metronidazole) intravaginally once or twice daily for 5 days. For once-a-day dosing, administer at bedtime.

➤*Storage/Stability:* Store at controlled room temperature 15° to 30°C (59° to 86°F). Protect from freezing.

Actions

➤*Pharmacology:* Metronidazole, a member of the imidazole class, is classified therapeutically as an antiprotozoal and antibacterial agent. The intracellular target of action of metronidazole on anaerobes are largely unknown. The 5-nitro group of metronidazole is reduced by metabolically active anaerobes, and studies have demonstrated that the reduced form of the drug interacts with bacterial DNA. However, it is not clear whether interaction with DNA alone is an important component in the bactericidal action of metronidazole.

➤*Pharmacokinetics:*
Healthy subjects – A single intravaginal 5 g dose of metronidazole vaginal gel (equivalent to 37.5 mg metronidazole) to 12 healthy subjects resulted in a mean maximum serum metronidazole concentration of 237 ng/mL (range, 152 to 368 ng/mL). This is approximately 2% of the mean maximum serum metronidazole concentration reported in the same subjects administered a single oral 500 mg dose of metronidazole (mean C_{max} = 12,785 ng/mL; range, 10,013 to 17,400 ng/mL). These peak concentrations were obtained 6 to 12 hours after dosing with metronidazole vaginal gel and 1 to 3 hours after dosing with oral metronidazole.

The extent of exposure (AUC) of metronidazole, when administered as a single intravaginal 5 g dose was approximately 4% of the AUC of a single oral 500 mg dose (4977 ng•h/mL and approximately 125,000 ng•h/mL, respectively). When administered vaginally, absorption was approximately half that of an equivalent oral dose.

Patients with bacterial vaginosis – Single and multiple 5 g doses of metronidazole vaginal gel to 4 patients with bacterial vaginosis resulted in a mean maximum serum metronidazole concentration of 214 ng/mL on day 1 and 294 ng/mL on day 5. Steady-state metronidazole serum concentrations following oral dosages of 400 to 500 mg twice daily have been reported to range from 6000 to 20,000 ng/mL.

➤*Microbiology:* Metronidazole is active in vitro against most strains of the following organisms that have been reported to be associated with bacterial vaginosis: *Bacteroides* sp.; *Gardnerella vaginalis*; *Mobiluncus* sp.; *Peptostreptococcus* sp.

Contraindications

Hypersensitivity to metronidazole, parabens, or other ingredients of the formulation or other nitroimidazole derivatives.

Warnings

➤*Convulsive seizures and peripheral neuropathy:* Convulsive seizures and peripheral neuropathy, the latter characterized mainly by numbness or paresthesia of an extremity, have been reported in patients treated with oral or IV metronidazole. The appearance of abnormal neurologic signs demands the prompt discontinuation of metronidazole vaginal gel therapy. Administer with caution to patients with CNS diseases.

➤*Psychotic reactions:* Psychotic reactions have been reported in alcoholic patients who were using oral metronidazole and disulfiram concurrently. Do not administer metronidazole vaginal gel to patients who have taken disulfiram within the last 2 weeks.

METRONIDAZOLE

➤*Diagnosis:* A clinical diagnosis of bacterial vaginosis is usually defined by the presence of a homogeneous vaginal discharge that has a pH of greater than 4.5, emits a "fishy" amine odor when mixed with a 10% KOH solution, and contains clue cells on microscopic examination. Gram's stain results consistent with a diagnosis of bacterial vaginosis include markedly reduced or absent *Lactobacillus* morphology, predominance of *Gardnerella* morphotype, and absent or few white blood cells.

Rule out other pathogens commonly associated with vulvovaginitis (eg, *Trichomonas vaginalis, Chlamydia trachomatis, Neisseria gonorrheae, Candida albicans,* herpes simplex virus).

➤*Hepatic function impairment:* Patients with severe hepatic disease metabolize metronidazole slowly. This results in the accumulation of metronidazole and its metabolites in the plasma. Accordingly, administer metronidazole vaginal gel cautiously in these patients.

➤*Carcinogenesis:* Metronidazole has shown evidence of carcinogenic activity in a number of studies involving chronic oral administration in mice and rats.

➤*Pregnancy:* Category B. Metronidazole crosses the placental barrier and rapidly enters the fetal circulation. There are no adequate and well-controlled studies in pregnant women. Use during pregnancy only if clearly needed.

➤*Lactation:* Specific studies of metronidazole levels in breast milk following intravaginally administered metronidazole have not been performed. However, metronidazole is secreted in breast milk in concentrations similar to those found in plasma following oral administration. Decide whether to discontinue nursing or to discontinue the drug, taking into account the importance of the drug to the mother.

➤*Children:* Safety and efficacy in children have not been established.

Precautions

➤*Vaginal candidiasis:* Known or previously unrecognized vaginal candidiasis may present more prominent symptoms during metronidazole vaginal gel therapy; approximately 6% to 10% of patients developed symptomatic *Candida* vaginitis during or immediately after therapy.

➤*For intravaginal use only:* Avoid contact with the eyes. Metronidazole vaginal gel contains ingredients that may cause burning and irritation of the eye. In the event of accidental contact with the eye, rinse with copious amounts of cool tap water.

Drug Interactions

Metronidazole Vaginal Gel Interactions			
Precipitant drug	Object drug*		Description
Cimetidine	Metronidazole	↑	Use of cimetidine with oral metronidazole may prolong the half-life and decrease plasma clearance of metronidazole. Consider this possibility with the vaginal gel.
Metronidazole	Anticoagulants	↑	Oral metronidazole may potentiate the anticoagulant effect of warfarin, resulting in a prolongation of prothrombin time. Consider this possibility with the vaginal gel.
Metronidazole	Disulfiram	↑	Concurrent use may result in acute psychosis or a confusional state. Do not administer vaginal gel to patients who have taken disulfiram within the last 2 weeks.
Metronidazole	Ethanol	↑	Disulfiram-like reaction to alcohol has occurred with oral metronidazole. Consider the possibility of such a reaction with the vaginal gel.

Metronidazole Vaginal Gel Interactions			
Precipitant drug	Object drug*		Description
Metronidazole	Lithium	↑	In patients stabilized on relatively high doses of lithium, short-term oral metronidazole therapy has been associated with elevation of serum lithium levels and, in a few cases, signs of lithium toxicity. Consider this possibility with the vaginal gel.

* ↑ = Object drug increased.

➤*Drug/Lab test interactions:* Metronidazole may interfere with certain types of determinations of serum chemistry values, such as AST, ALT, LDH, triglycerides, and glucose hexokinase; values of zero may be observed.

Adverse Reactions

In a randomized, single-blind clinical trial of 505 nonpregnant women who received metronidazole vaginal gel once or twice/day, 2 patients (1 from each regimen) discontinued therapy early because of drug-related adverse events. One patient discontinued the drug because of moderate abdominal cramping and loose stools, while the other patient discontinued the drug because of mild vaginal burning. These symptoms resolved after discontinuation of the drug.

Medical events judged to be related, probably related, or possibly related to administration of metronidazole vaginal gel once or twice/day were reported for 39% (195/505) of patients.

➤*CNS:* Headache (5%); dizziness (2%); depression, fatigue (less than 1%).

➤*Dermatologic:* Generalized itching or rash (less than 1%).

➤*GI:* GI discomfort (7%); nausea and/or vomiting (4%); unusual taste (2%); decreased appetite, diarrhea/loose stools (1%); abdominal bloating/gas, dry mouth, thirst (less than 1%).

➤*GU:* Vaginal discharge (12%); symptomatic *Candida* cervicitis/vaginitis (10%); vulva/vaginal irritative symptoms (9%); pelvic discomfort (3%); darkened urine (less than 1%).

➤*Miscellaneous:* Unspecified cramping (1%).

Other metronidazole formulations – Other effects that have been reported in association with the use of topical (dermal) formulations of metronidazole include skin irritation, transient skin erythema, and mild skin dryness and burning (2% or less).

Metronidazole vaginal gel affords minimal peak serum levels and systemic exposure of metronidazole compared with 500 mg oral dosing. Although these lower levels of exposure are less likely to produce the common reactions seen with oral metronidazole, the possibility of these and other reactions cannot be excluded. Refer to the Metronidazole Oral monograph in the Anti-Infectives chapter.

Overdosage

Vaginally applied metronidazole gel could be absorbed in sufficient amounts to produce systemic effects (see Warnings).

Patient Information

Caution patients about drinking alcohol while being treated with metronidazole vaginal gel. While blood levels are significantly lower than with usual doses of oral metronidazole, a possible interaction with alcohol cannot be excluded.

Instruct patients not to engage in vaginal intercourse during treatment with this product.

Advise patients that this medicine is to be used intravaginally only.

MISCELLANEOUS VAGINAL PREPARATIONS

otc	**Lubrin** (Kenwood/Bradley)	**Inserts:** Caprylic/capric trigylceride, glycerin *Indication:* Prolonged lubrication for sexual intercourse. *Dosage:* 1 intravaginally 5 to 30 minutes before intercourse. Allow 5 to 10 minutes for insert to dissolve.	In 5s and 12s.
otc	**Vaginex** (Quality Health)	**Cream:** Tripelennamine HCl *Indication:* Temporary relief of external vaginal irritation. *Dosage:* Apply externally 3 or 4 times a day.	In 30 and 300 g.
otc	**Replens** (Warner Lambert)	**Gel:** Glycerin, mineral oil, methylparaben *Indication:* Replenishes vaginal moisture. *Dosage:* Apply intravaginally.	In 3 and 8 pre-filled applicators.
otc	**Astroglide** (BioFilm)	**Gel:** Glycerin, propylene glycol, parabens *Indication:* Vaginal lubricant. *Dosage:* Apply externally or internally.	In 66.5 ml bottle and 5 ml travel packets.
otc	**Lubricating Jelly** (Taro)	**Jelly:** Glycerin, propylene glycol *Indication:* Provides additional vaginal moisture. *Dosage:* Apply as needed.	In 60 and 125 g.
otc	**K-Y** (Johnson & Johnson)	**Jelly:** Glycerin, hydroxyethyl cellulose, methylparaben *Indication:* Vaginal lubricant *Dosage:* Apply as needed.	Sterile or regular. In 12, 60 and 120 g.
otc	**Surgel** (Ulmer)	**Gel:** Propylene glycol, glycerin *Indication:* Vaginal lubricant.	In 120 and 240 ml and 1 gal.
Rx	**Fem pH** (Pharmics)	**Vaginal jelly:** 0.9% glacial acetic acid, 0.025% oxyquinoline sulfate, glycerin, lactic acid, PEG 4500 *Indication:* Adjunctive therapy when restoration and maintenance of vaginal acidity is desirable *Dosage:* 1 applicatorful administered intravaginally morning and evening.	In 50 g with applicator.
otc	**Trimo-San** (Milex)	**Jelly:** 0.025% oxyquinoline sulfate, 0.7% sodium borate, 0.1% sodium lauryl sulfate, glycerin, methylparaben *Indication:* Controls odor-causing bacteria. Helps maintain normal vaginal pH 4. *Dosage:* ½ applicator 2 or 3 times per week.	In 120 g with applicator.
Rx	**Amino-Cerv pH 5.5** (Milex)	**Cream:** 8.34% urea, 0.5% sodium propionate, 0.83% methionine, 0.35% cystine, 0.83% inositol *Indications:* Treatment of mild cervicitis and postpartum cervicitis/cervical tears, postconization and for postsurgical procedures. *Dosage:* See manufacturer's information.	Water miscible base. In 82.5 g with applicator. Buffered to pH 5.5 in water-miscible creme base.
otc	**Yeast X** (Fleet)	**Suppositories:** Pulsatilla 28× *Indication:* Relieves vaginal irritation, itching and burning. *Dosage:* One suppository daily as needed.	In 12s with applicator.
otc	**Norforms** (Fleet)	**Suppositories:** PEG-18, PEG-32, PEG-20 stearate, methylparaben *Indication:* Feminine deodorant. *Dosage:* One suppository daily as needed.	In 12s and 24s with applicator.
otc	**Moist Again** (Lake)	**Gel:** Aloe vera, EDTA, methylparaben, glycerin *Indication:* Vaginal lubricant. *Dosage:* Apply as needed.	In 70.8 g.
otc	**H-R Lubricating Jelly** (Carter-Wallace)	**Jelly:** Hydroxypropyl, methylcellulose, parabens *Indication:* Vaginal lubricant. *Dosage:* Apply as needed.	In 150 g.
otc	**Vagi·Gard Maximum Strength** (Lake)	**Cream:** 20% benzocaine, 3% resorcinol, methylparaben, sodium sulfite, EDTA, mineral oil *Indication:* Relieves external vaginal irritation, itching and burning. *Dosage:* Apply externally 3 to 4 times/day.	In 45 g.
otc	**Vagi·Gard Advanced Sensitive Formula** (Lake)	**Cream:** 5% benzocaine, 2% resorcinol, methylparaben, sodium sulfite, EDTA, mineral oil *Indication:* Relieves external vaginal irritation, itching and burning. *Dosage:* Apply externally 3 to 4 times/day.	In 45 g.
otc	**UTI Feminine Hygiene Pack** (Consumers Choice Systems)	**Kit:** *Indication:* For temporary relief of minor irritations and burning. *Dosage:* Apply to the affected area ≤ 3 to 4 times daily.	
		Wipes: Polysorbate 20, EDTA, methylparabens.	In 20s.
		Cream: Oat beta glucan, aloe. Cetyl alcohol, cetearyl alchol, EDTA, parabens.	In 15 g.
otc	**Yeast·Gard** (Lake)	**Suppositories:** Pulsatilla 28×, *Candida albicans* 28× *Indication:* Relieves vaginal irritation, itching and burning. *Dosage:* One suppository daily for 7 days.	In 15s with applicator.
otc	**WHF Lubricating Gel** (Lake)	**Gel:** Chlorhexidine gluconate, methylparaben, glycerin *Indication:* Relieves vaginal dryness. *Dosage:* Apply as needed.	In 113.4 g tube and 3 g individual packets.
otc	**Massengill Feminine Cleansing Wash** (SmithKline Beecham)	**Liquid:** Sodium laureth sulfate, sodium oleth sulfate, magnesium oleth sulfate, PEG-120 methyl glucose dioleate, parabens *Indication:* Vaginal cleansing. *Dosage:* Apply externally.	In 240 ml.
otc	**Vagisil** (Combe)	**Powder:** Cornstarch, aloe, mineral oil, magnesium stearate, silica, benzethonium chloride, fragrance *Indication:* Absorbs moisture. *Dosage:* Apply externally.	In 198 and 312 g.
otc	**Maxilube** (Mission)	**Jelly:** Water, silicone oil, glycerin, carbomer 934, triethanolamine, sodium lauryl sulfate, parabens *Indication:* Vaginal lubricant.	In 90 and 150 g.
Rx	**Aci-jel** (Ortho-McNeil)	**Jelly:** 0.921% glacial acetic acid, 0.025% oxyquinoline sulfate, 0.7% ricinoleic acid, 5% glycerin. Propylparaben, egg albumen. *Indication:* For restoration and maintenance of vaginal activity.	In 85 g tube with applicator.

DOUCHE PRODUCTS

otc	**Massengill Douche** (SK-Beecham)	**Powder:** Ammonium alum, phenol, methyl salicylate, eucalyptus oil, menthol, thymol, PEG-8	In 120, 240, 480 and 660 g jar and UD Packettes (10s and 12s).
otc	**Trichotine Douche** (Reed & Carnrick)	**Powder:** Sodium lauryl sulfate, sodium perborate, monohydrate silica	In 150 and 360 g.
Rx	**Vagisec Douche** (Schmid)	**Solution:** Polyoxyethylene nonyl phenol, EDTA	In 120 ml.
otc	**Trichotine Douche** (Reed & Carnrick)	**Solution:** Sodium lauryl sulfate, sodium borate, 8% SD alcohol 23-A, EDTA	In 120 and 240 ml.
otc	**Massengill Baking Soda Freshness** (SK-Beecham)	**Solution:** Sodium bicarbonate	In 180 ml.
otc	**Yeast-Gard Medicated Douche** (Lake)	**Concentrate:** 10% povidone-iodine	In 240 ml.
otc	**Massengill Medicated Douche w/Cepticin** (SK-Beecham)	**Liquid concentrate:** 12% povidone-iodine	In 120 and 240 ml.
otc	**Yeast-Gard Medicated Disposable Douche Premix** (Lake Pharm)	**Solution:** Octoxynol-9, lactic acid, sodium lactate, sodium benzoate, aloe vera	In 180 ml twin-pack.
otc	**Massengill Medicated Disposable Douche w/Cepticin** (SK-Beecham)	**Solution:** 10% povidone-iodine (0.30% when diluted)	In 5 ml vial w/180 ml bottle of sanitized water.
otc	**Summer's Eve Medicated Disposable Douche** (Fleet)	**Solution:** 0.30% povidone-iodine when reconstituted	In 135 ml (1s and 2s).
otc	**Yeast-Gard Medicated Disposable Douche** (Lake)		In 180 ml twin-pack w/two 5.4 ml medicated douche concentrate packets.
otc	**Summer's Eve Disposable Douche** (Fleet)	**Solution, regular:** Citric acid, sodium benzoate	In 135 ml (1s, 2s and 4s).
		Solution, scented: Citric acid, octoxynol 9, sodium benzoate, EDTA	In herbal, musk and white flowers scents. In 135 ml (1s, 2s and 4s).
otc	**Summer's Eve Post–Menstrual Disposable Douche** (Fleet)	**Solution:** Sodium lauryl sulfate, parabens, monosodium and disodium phosphates, EDTA	In 135 ml (2s).
otc	**Feminique Disposable Douche** (Schmid)	**Solution:** Vinegar	In 180 ml (2s).
otc	**Massengill Disposable Douche** (SK-Beecham)		In 180 ml.
otc	**Massengill Vinegar & Water Extra Mild** (SK-Beecham)		Preservative free. In 180 ml.
otc	**Summer's Eve Disposable Douche** (Fleet)		In 135 ml (1s and 2s).
otc	**Summer's Eve Disposable Douche Extra Cleansing** (Fleet)	**Solution:** Vinegar, sodium chloride, benzoic acid	In 135 ml (1s, 2s and 4s).
otc	**Massengill Vinegar & Water Extra Cleansing with Puraclean** (SK-Beecham)	**Solution:** Vinegar, cetylpyridinium chloride, diazolidinyl urea, EDTA	In 180 ml.

Indications

Vaginal douches are for general cleansing of the vaginal and perineal areas; for deodorizing; for relief of itching, burning and edema; for removing vaginal secretions or discharge or for altering vaginal acidity.

➤*Povidone-iodine, cetylpyridinium chloride, eucalyptol, menthol, oxyquinoline sulfate, phenol, sodium perborate, and thymol:* Povidone-iodine, cetylpyridinium chloride, eucalyptol, menthol, oxyquinoline sulfate, phenol, sodium perborate, and thymol may have antiseptic or germicidal activity.

Povidine-iodine also relieves minor irritation. It may be absorbed from the vagina; advise patients with thyroid disorders and pregnant patients to avoid iodine-containing douches.

➤*Eucalyptol, menthol, phenol, methyl salicylate, and thymol:* Eucalyptol, menthol, phenol, methyl salicylate, and thymol are counterirritants used for their anesthetic or antipruritic effects.

➤*Ammonium alum:* Ammonium alum is an astringent that reduces local edema and inflammation; high concentrations can be irritating.

➤*Docusate sodium, octoxynol 9, alkyl aryl sulfonate, sodium lauryl sulfate, and benzalkonium chloride:* Docusate sodium, octoxynol 9, alkyl aryl sulfonate, sodium lauryl sulfate, and benzalkonium chloride are surfactants that facilitate douche spread over vaginal mucosa.

➤*Sodium perborate, sodium bicarbonate, lactic acid, sodium acetate, and citric acid:* Sodium perborate, sodium bicarbonate, lactic acid, sodium acetate, and citric acid affect pH.

Patient Information

Consult manufacturers' recommendations for proper dilution and use of these products.

Vaginal douches are not contraceptive agents.

Douche no sooner than 6 hours after use of a vaginal spermicide.

If irritation occurs, discontinue use.

If infection or disease is suspected, consult physician.

Spermicides

Actions

▶*Pharmacology:* Topical contraceptive agents provide spermicidal action, which is generally reliable when properly used, either in conjunction with a vaginal diaphragm or as the sole method of contraception. These agents are generally less effective than oral contraceptives. To minimize the potential for conception, follow directions for use carefully.

Condom use and STD – The CDC advises the use of condoms to prevent sexually transmitted diseases (STD). If used properly, condoms help prevent infection by *Chlamydia trachomatis*, *Ureaplasma urealyticum*, *Trichomonas vaginalis*, *Candida albicans*, herpes simplex 1 and 2 (when lesions are on penis or female genital area), human papilloma virus, *Treponema pallidum*, *Haemophilus ducreyi* and AIDS.

Nonoxynol 9 – Nonoxynol 9 helps to inhibit a variety of sexually transmissible organisims, including those responsible for gonorrhea, chlamydial infection, candidiasis, genital herpes, syphilis, trichomoniasis and AIDS.

The following table gives ranges of pregnancy rates reported for various means of contraception. Efficacy in most cases depends greatly upon degree of compliance and user reliability. No other contraceptive drug or device except levonorgestrel implant and medroxyprogesterone injection approaches the efficacy of the combined oral contraceptives.

Pregnancy Rates for Various Means of Contraception (%)[1]		
Method of contraception	Lowest expected[2]	Typical[3]
Oral Contraceptives		3
Combined	0.1	nd[4]
Progestin only	0.5	nd
Mechanical/Chemical		
Levonorgestrel implant	0.2	0.2
Medroxyprogesterone injection	0.3	0.3
IUD		
Progesterone	2	nd
Copper T 380A	0.8	nd
Condom		
Without spermicide	2	12
With spermicide[5]	1.8	4-6
Spermicide alone	3	21
Diaphragm (with spermicidal cream or gel)	6	18
Female condom	2-4	12-25

Pregnancy Rates for Various Means of Contraception (%)[1]		
Method of contraception	Lowest expected[2]	Typical[3]
Periodic abstinence (ie, rhythm; all methods)	1-9	20
Sterility		
Vasectomy	0.1	0.15
Tubal ligation	0.2	0.4
No contraception	85	85

[1] During first year of continuous use.
[2] Best guess of percentage expected to experience an accidental pregnancy among couples who initiate a method and use it consistently and correctly.
[3] A "typical" couple who initiates a method and experiences an accidental pregnancy.
[4] nd = no data.
[5] Used as a separate product (not in condom package).

Warnings

▶*Sensitivity:* Should sensitivity to the ingredients or irritation of the vagina or penis develop, discontinue use and consult your physician.

▶*Pregnancy:* Controversy surrounds the relationship between the use of vaginal spermicides during pregnancy and congenital malformations. One 1981 study has suggested an association between vaginal spermicides and congenital anomalies (eg, limb-reduction deformities, neoplasms, chromosomal abnormalities). However, many other studies do not support these findings and several of the authors of the 1981 study agree that a causal association is unlikely. The FDA concurs with the Advisory Committee on Fertility and Maternal Health Drugs that there is currently no need for a labeling revision of spermicidal products.

Patient Information

Consult manufacturers' recommendations for proper use of these products. The following general principles should be noted:

Apply at least 10 minutes, but not more than 1 hour before intercourse to ensure effectiveness.

Apply high in the vagina, near the cervix.

Reapply prior to each time intercourse takes place.

Allow suppositories adequate time to disperse.

Do not douche for 6 to 8 hours after intercourse. Premature douching may dilute the spermicide, remove few sperm and may propel sperm into the uterus.

MISCELLANEOUS SPERMICIDES

otc	**Delfen Contraceptive** (Advanced Care)	**Vaginal Foam:** 12.5% nonoxynol 9	In 20 g w/applicator and 42 g refills.
otc	**Conceptrol Disposable Contraceptive** (Advanced Care)	**Vaginal Gel:** 4% nonoxynol 9	In 2.7 g prefilled applications (6s and 10s).
otc	**Semicid** (Whitehall)	**Suppositories:** 100 mg nonoxynol 9	Methylparaben. In 9s and 18s.
otc	**VCF** (Apothecus)	**Vaginal Film:** 28% nonoxynol 9	Glycerin, alcohol. In 3s, 6s and 12s.

For complete prescribing information, see the Spermicides group monograph.

SPERMICIDES USED WITH A VAGINAL DIAPHRAGM

otc	**Gynol II Contraceptive** (Advanced Care)	**Gel:** 2% nonoxynol 9	In 75 g w/applicator and 75 and 114 g refills.
otc	**Shur-Seal** (Milex)	**Gel:** 2% nonoxynol 9	In 24 UD gel paks.
otc	**K-Y Plus** (Johnson & Johnson)	**Gel:** 2.2% nonoxynol 9	Methylparaben. In 113 g.
otc	**Advantage 24** (Women's Health Institute)	**Gel:** 3.5% nonoxynol 9	Mineral oil, glycerin, parabens, palm oil, sorbic acid. In 3s and 6s (1.5 g each) with applicators.
otc	**Gynol II Extra Strength Contraceptive** (Advanced Care)	**Jelly:** 3% nonoxynol 9	In 75 g and 114 g.

For complete prescribing information, see the Spermicides group monograph.

Administration and Dosage

The following products are for use in conjunction with a vaginal diaphragm.

SPERMICIDE-CONTAINING CONDOMS

otc	**Excita Extra** (Schmid)	**Condom:** 8% nonoxynol 9	Ribbed. In 3s, 12s and 36s.
otc	**Sheik Elite** (Schmid)		In 3s, 12s. 24s and 36s

For complete prescribing information, see the Spermicides group monograph.

Actions

▶*Pharmacology:* A latex condom with a lubricant containing the spermicide nonoxynol 9. The combination of barrier protection combined with the spermicide improves contraceptive effectiveness over traditional condoms.

Thiazides and Related Diuretics

Indications

▶*Edema:* Adjunctive therapy in edema associated with congestive heart failure (CHF), hepatic cirrhosis and corticosteroid and estrogen therapy. Useful in edema due to renal dysfunction (ie, nephrotic syndrome, acute glomerulonephritis, chronic renal failure).

Indapamide – Indapamide alone is indicated for edema associated with CHF.

Metolazone, rapidly acting (Mykrox) – Metolazone, rapidly acting (*Mykrox*) has not been evaluated for the treatment of CHF or fluid retention due to renal or hepatic disease, and the correct dosage for these conditions and other edematous states has not been established. Since a safe and effective diuretic dose has not been established, do not use *Mykrox* when diuresis is desired.

▶*Hypertension:* As the sole therapeutic agent or to enhance other antihypertensive drugs in more severe forms of hypertension.

▶*Unlabeled uses:*

Calcium nephrolithiasis – Thiazide diuretics have been used alone and in combination with amiloride or allopurinol to prevent formation and recurrence of calcium nephrolithiasis in hypercalciuric and normal calciuric patients. Thiazides correct hypercalciuria, reduce urinary saturation, enhance inhibitor activity against spontaneous nucleation of both calcium oxalate and brushite, and restore normal parathyroid function and intestinal calcium absorption. Doses of hydrochlorothiazide 50 or 100 mg daily, trichloromethiazide 4 mg/day, chlorthalidone 50 mg/day and indapamide 2.5 mg/day have been used.

Osteoporosis – Thiazide diuretics may be useful in reducing the incidence of osteoporosis in postmenopausal women, either alone or in combination with calcium or estrogen. Further studies are necessary to confirm this use. Although data conflict, use of thiazides in older patients may be associated with a reduced risk of hip fracture.

Diabetes insipidus – Thiazide diuretics reduce urine volume by 30% to 50%. They constitute the mainstay of therapy for nephrogenic diabetes insipidus.

Administration and Dosage

▶*Edema:* Intermittent therapy may be advantageous. With administration every other day, or on a 3- to 5-day per week schedule, electrolyte imbalance is less likely.

▶*Hypertension:* Reduce dosage of other agents as soon as thiazides are added to the regimen to prevent excessive hypotension. As blood pressure falls, a further reduction in dosage may be necessary.

▶*Renal impairment:* If the patient has a creatinine clearance < 40 to 50 ml/min, a glomerular filtration rate < 25 ml/min or is not responsive to thiazides, a loop diuretic may be more effective. **Metolazone** is the only thiazide-like diuretic that may produce diuresis in patients with GFR < 20 ml/min. Indapamide may also be effective in patients with renal function impairment.

▶*Concomitant administration:* Concurrent metolazone and furosemide (and probably other loop diuretics) have been used in the management of patients refractory to furosemide or other diuretics administered alone due to their synergistic effect on diuresis (see Drug Interactions). Metolazone 2.5 to 10 mg is added to the therapy, and the dose is doubled every 24 hours until the desired response is achieved. Decrease the furosemide dose if synergism occurs with the first dose of metolazone. Hydrochlorothiazide (50 mg) may be used and may be safer because of its shorter action. This effect has also been noted with other thiazides in combination with other loop diuretics.

Actions

▶*Pharmacology:* Thiazide diuretics increase the urinary excretion of sodium and chloride in approximately equivalent amounts. They inhibit reabsorption of sodium and chloride in the cortical thick ascending limb of the loop of Henle and the early distal tubules. Many of these compounds possess some degree of carbonic anhydrase inhibition activity (metolazone has no activity) due to the sulfonamide moiety; however, this is unlikely to be encountered clinically. Other common actions include the following: Increased potassium and bicarbonate excretion, decreased calcium excretion and uric acid retention. At maximal therapeutic dosages all thiazides are approximately equal in diuretic efficacy, but metolazone may be more effective in patients with impaired renal function. Metolazone and quinethazone (quinazoline derivatives), chlorthalidone (a phthalimidine derivative) and indapamide (an indoline) are included here because of their structural and pharmacological similarities to the thiazides.

The exact antihypertensive mechanism of the thiazides is unknown, although sodium depletion appears to be of primary importance. During initial therapy, cardiac output decreases and extracellular volume diminishes. With chronic therapy, cardiac output normalizes, peripheral vascular resistance falls, and there is a persistent small reduction in extracellular volume.

In hypertensive patients, daily doses of indapamide have no appreciable cardiac inotropic or chronotropic effect, and little or no effect on glomerular filtration rate or renal plasma flow. The drug decreases peripheral resistance, with little or no effect on cardiac output, rate or rhythm. Indapamide had an antihypertensive effect in patients with varying degrees of renal impairment, although in general, diuretic effects declined as renal function decreased.

▶*Pharmacokinetics:* The antihypertensive action requires several days to produce effects. Administration for up to 2 to 4 weeks is usually required for optimal therapeutic effect. The duration of the antihypertensive effect of the thiazides is sufficiently long to adequately control blood pressure with a single daily dose. Despite extensive use of diuretics, pharmacokinetic data are limited. It is important to emphasize the lack of relationship between plasma levels and diuretic effect.

Pharmacokinetics of Thiazides and Related Diuretics

Diuretic	Onset (hours)	Peak (hours)	Duration (hours)	Equivalent dose (mg)	Percent absorbed	Half-life (hours)
Bendroflumethiazide	2	4	16 to 12	5	≈ 100	3 to 3.9
Benzthiazide	2	4 to 6	16 to 18	50	nd[1]	nd[1]
Chlorothiazide	2[2]	4[2]	16 to 12	500	10 to 21[3]	0.75 to 2
Chlorthalidone	2 to 3	2 to 6	24 to 72	50	64[3]	40
Hydrochlorothiazide	2	4 to 6	16 to 12	50	65 to 75	5.6 to 14.8
Hydroflumethiazide	2	4	16 to 12	50	50	≈ 17
Indapamide	1 to 2	within 2	up to 36	2.5	93	≈ 14
Methyclothiazide	2	6	24	5	nd[1]	nd[1]
Metolazone[4]	1	2	12 to 24	5	65	nd[1]
Polythiazide	2	6	24 to 48	2	nd[1]	25.7
Quinethazone	2	6	18 to 24	50	nd[1]	nd[1]
Trichlormethiazide	2	6	24	2	nd[1]	2.3 to 7.3

[1] nd = No data.
[2] Following IV use, onset of action is 15 minutes; peak occurs in 30 minutes.
[3] Bioavailability may be dose-dependent.
[4] *Mykrox*: Peak plasma concentrations reached in 2 to 4 hrs, t½ ≈ 14 hrs.

Contraindications

Anuria; renal decompensation; hypersensitivity to thiazides or related diuretics or sulfonamide-derived drugs; hepatic coma or precoma (**metolazone**).

Warnings

▶*Parenteral use:* Use IV **chlorothiazide** only when patients are unable to take oral medication or in an emergency. In infants and children, IV use is not recommended.

Avoid simultaneous administration of chlorothiazide with whole blood or its derivatives.

▶*Lupus erythematosus:* Lupus erythematosus exacerbation or activation has occurred.

▶*Hypersensitivity reactions:* Hypersensitivity reactions may occur in patients with or without a history of allergy or bronchial asthma; cross-sensitivity with sulfonamides may also occur. Have epinephrine 1:1000 immediately available. Refer to Management of Acute Hypersensitivity Reactions.

▶*Renal function impairment:* Use with caution in severe renal disease since these agents may precipitate azotemia. Cumulative effects of the drug may develop in patients with impaired renal function. Monitor renal function periodically. If progressive renal impairment becomes evident, indicated by a rising nonprotein nitrogen (NPN) or BUN, consider withholding or discontinuing therapy. If the patient has a creatinine clearance < 40 to 50 ml/min, a glomerular filtration rate (GFR) < 25 ml/min or is not responsive to thiazides, a loop diuretic may be more effective. **Metolazone** is the only thiazide-like diuretic that may produce diuresis in patients with GFR < 20 ml/min. Indapamide may also be useful in patients with impaired renal function.

Thiazides and Related Diuretics

►*Hepatic function impairment:* Use with caution since minor alterations of fluid and electrolyte balance may precipitate hepatic coma.

►*Pregnancy: Category B* (**chlorothiazide, chlorthalidone, hydrochlorothiazide, indapamide, metolazone**); *Category C* (**bendroflumethiazide, benzthiazide, hydroflumethiazide, methyclothiazide, trichlormethiazide**). Routine use during normal pregnancy is inappropriate. Diuretics decrease plasma volume and can decrease placental perfusion. Diuretics do not prevent development of toxemia, nor are they useful in the treatment of toxemia.

Thiazides are indicated in pregnancy when edema is due to pathologic causes, just as they are in the absence of pregnancy. Dependent edema in pregnancy, resulting from restriction of venous return by the gravid uterus, is not properly treated by the use of diuretics. In rare instances, hypervolemia during normal pregnancy results in edema that may cause extreme discomfort that is not relieved by rest; a short course of diuretics may provide relief.

Thiazides cross the placental barrier and appear in cord blood. Use only when clearly needed and when potential benefits outweigh the potential hazards to the fetus. These hazards include fetal or neonatal jaundice, thrombocytopenia, hemolytic anemia, electrolyte imbalances and hypoglycemia.

►*Lactation:* Thiazides may appear in breast milk. **Chlorthalidone** has a low milk to plasma ratio of 0.05. Discontinue nursing or the drug taking into account the importance of the drug to the mother.

►*Children:* **Bendroflumethiazide, benzthiazide, chlorthalidone, hydrochlorothiazide, methyclothiazide, metolazone, hydroflumethiazide, trichlormethiazide** – Safety and efficacy have not been established. **Metolazone** is not recommended for use in children. In infants and children, IV use of **chlorothiazide** has been limited and is generally not recommended.

Precautions

►*Fluid/electrolyte balance:* Perform initial and periodic determinations of serum electrolytes, BUN, uric acid and glucose. Observe patients for clinical signs of fluid or electrolyte imbalance (eg, hyponatremia, hypochloremic alkalosis, hypokalemia, hypomagnesemia, changes in serum and urinary calcium). Serum and urine electrolyte determinations are particularly important in patients vomiting excessively or receiving parenteral fluids, in patients subject to electrolyte imbalance (including those with heart failure, kidney disease and cirrhosis), and in patients on a salt restricted diet. Warning signs of imbalance include the following: Dry mouth, thirst, weakness, lethargy, drowsiness, restlessness, muscle pains or cramps, confusion, seizures, muscular fatigue, hypotension, oliguria, tachycardia and GI disturbances.

Hypokalemia – Hypokalemia may develop (with consequent weakness, cramps, cardiac dysrhythmias) during concomitant corticosteroids, ACTH and especially with brisk diuresis, with severe liver disease or cirrhosis, vomiting or diarrhea, or after prolonged therapy. Inadequate oral electrolyte intake also contributes to hypokalemia. Hypokalemia may cause cardiac arrhythmias and sensitize or exaggerate the heart's response to toxic effects of digitalis (eg, increased ventricular irritability). Avoid or treat hypokalemia by using potassium-sparing diuretics, potassium supplements or foods with high potassium content. Hypokalemia is a particular hazard in digitalized patients or patients who have or have had a ventricular arrhythmia; dangerous or fatal arrhythmias may be precipitated. Hypokalemia is dose-related.

Hyponatremia/Hypochloremia – A chloride deficit is generally mild and usually does not require specific treatment, except in extraordinary circumstances (as in liver or renal disease). However, treatment of metabolic or hypochloremic alkalosis may require chloride replacement. Dilutional hyponatremia may occur in edematous patients in hot weather; appropriate therapy is water restriction, rather than salt administration, except in rare life-threatening instances. Thiazide-induced hyponatremia has been associated with death and neurologic damage in elderly patients. CNS manifestations include seizures, coma and extensor-plantar response. Infrequently, severe hyponatremia accompanied by hypokalemia has occurred with recommended **indapamide** doses, primarily in elderly females.

Rarely, the rapid onset of severe hyponatremia or hypokalemia has occurred following initial doses of thiazide and non-thiazide diuretics. When symptoms consistent with electrolyte imbalance appear rapidly, discontinue the drug and initiate supportive measures immediately. Parenteral electrolytes may be required.

Hypomagnesemia – Thiazide diuretics have been shown to increase urinary excretion of magnesium, resulting in hypomagnesemia.

Hypercalcemia – Calcium excretion may be decreased by thiazide diuretics. Thiazides may cause a slight intermittent elevation of serum calcium in the absence of calcium metabolism disorders. Serum calcium levels return to normal upon discontinuation. Pathologic changes in the parathyroid glands with hypercalcemia and hypophosphatemia may occur in a few patients on prolonged thiazide therapy. Marked hypercalcemia may be evidence of hidden hyperparathyroidism. Common complications of hyperparathyroidism such as renal lithiasis, bone resorption and peptic ulceration are not seen. Discontinue thiazides before performing parathyroid function tests.

Hyperuricemia – Hyperuricemia may occur or acute gout may be precipitated in certain patients receiving thiazides, even in those patients without a history of gouty attacks. Hyperuricemia with infrequent gouty attacks may occur in patients with a history of gout. Monitor serum uric acid concentrations periodically during treatment. One report suggests that it is not necessary to lower uric acid levels with pharmacologic measures in patients receiving thiazide diuretics who are without renal damage or history of gout. Serum uric acid increased by an average of 1 mg/dl in patients on **indapamide**.

Glucose tolerance – Hyperglycemia may occur with thiazide diuretics. Insulin or oral hypoglycemic agent dosage requirements in diabetic patients may be altered. Latent diabetes mellitus may become manifest during thiazide diuretic administration; diabetic complications may occur. Monitor serum glucose concentrations (see Drug Interactions). Administration time (ie, morning vs evening) may influence glucose tolerance; in a small study, blood glucose levels were higher when trichlormethiazide was taken in the evening.

►*Post-sympathectomy:* Antihypertensive effects may be enhanced in the postsympathectomy patient.

►*Lipids:* Use thiazides with caution in patients with moderate or high cholesterol concentrations and in patients with elevated triglyceride levels. Thiazides may cause increased concentrations of total serum cholesterol, total triglycerides and LDL (but not HDL) in some patients, although these appear to return to pretreatment levels with long-term therapy. **Indapamide** does not appear to increase serum cholesterol.

►*Photosensitivity:* Photosensitization may occur; therefore, caution patients to take protective measures (ie, sunscreens, protective clothing) against exposure to ultraviolet light and/or sunlight until tolerance is determined.

►*Tartrazine sensitivity:* Some of these products contain tartrazine (FD&C yellow #5), which may cause allergic-type reactions (including bronchial asthma) in susceptible individuals. Although the incidence of sensitivity is low, it is frequently seen in patients who also have aspirin hypersensitivity. Specific products containing tartrazine are identified in the product listings.

Drug Interactions

Thiazides and Related Diuretic Drug Interactions			
Precipitant drug	Object drug*		Description
Thiazides	Allopurinol	↑	Concurrent use may increase the incidence of hypersensitivity reactions to allopurinol.
Thiazides	Anesthetics	↑	Effects of these drugs may be potentiated by thiazide administration; dosage adjustments may be required. Monitor and correct fluid and electrolyte imbalance prior to surgery if feasible.
Thiazides	Anticoagulants	↓	Anticoagulant effects may be diminished.
Thiazides	Antigout agents	↓	Since thiazide diuretics may raise blood uric acid levels, dosage adjustment of antigout agents may be necessary.
Thiazides	Antineoplastics	↑	Thiazides may prolong antineoplastic-induced leukopenia.
Thiazides	Calcium salts	↑	Hypercalcemia resulting from renal tubular reabsorption or bone release of calcium may be amplified by exogenous calcium.
Thiazides	Diazoxide	↑	Hyperglycemia, often with symptoms and similar to frank diabetes, may occur.
Thiazides	Digitalis glycosides	↑	Diuretic-induced hypokalemia and hypomagnesemia may precipitate digitalis-induced arrhythmias.
Thiazides	Lithium	↑	Thiazides may induce lithium toxicity by decreasing its renal excretion. However, they have been used together for therapeutic reasons and can be coadministered safely with close lithium level monitoring.
Thiazides	Loop diuretics	↑	Both groups have synergistic effects that may result in profound diuresis and serious electrolyte abnormalities. Certain combinations have been used therapeutically in patients refractory to furosemide (see Administration and Dosage).
Thiazides	Methyldopa	↑	There have been rare occurrences of hemolytic anemia with concomitant use.

Thiazides and Related Diuretic Drug Interactions

Precipitant drug	Object drug[*]		Description
Thiazides	Nondepolarizing muscle relaxants	↑	Neuromuscular blocking effects may be increased; respiratory depression may be prolonged.
Thiazides	Sulfonylureas insulin	↓	Thiazides increase fasting blood glucose and may decrease sulfonylurea hypoglycemia. Hyponatremia may also occur. The dosage may need to be adjusted.
Thiazides	Vitamin D	↑	The biological actions of vitamin D may be enhanced. Hypercalcemia could manifest.
Amphotericin B, Corticosteroids	Thiazides	↑	Electrolyte depletion may be intensified, particularly hypokalemia. Monitor potassium levels.
Anticholinergics	Thiazides	↑	Anticholinergics may substantially increase thiazide diuretic absorption.
Bile acid sequestrants (cholestyramine, colestipol)	Thiazides	↓	Bile acid sequestrants bind thiazides and reduce their absorption from the GI tract by up to 85%. Thiazides should be given ≥ 2 hours before the resin.
Methenamines	Thiazides	↓	Possible decreased effectiveness of thiazides due to the alkalinization of urine.
NSAIDs	Thiazides	↓	Some NSAIDs (particularly indomethacin) may reduce the diuretic, natriuretic and antihypertensive effects of thiazide diuretics. Observe closely to determine if the desired diuretic effects are obtained. Sulindac may enhance the diuretic effect.

[*] ↑ = Object drug increased. ↓ = Object drug decreased

➤ *Drug/Lab test interactions:* Thiazides may decrease serum PBI levels without signs of thyroid disturbance. Thiazides may also cause diagnostic interference of serum electrolyte levels, blood and urine glucose levels (usually only in patients with a predisposition to glucose intolerance), serum bilirubin levels (by displacement from albumin binding), and serum uric acid levels. In uremic patients, serum magnesium levels may be increased. **Bendroflumethiazide** and **trichlormethiazide** may interfere with the **phenolsulfonphthalein test** due to decreased excretion. In the **phentolamine** and **tyramine tests**, bendroflumethiazide may produce false-negative and trichlormethiazide may produce false-positive results.

Adverse Reactions

Adverse Reactions of Thiazides and Related Diuretics

Adverse reaction	Bendroflumethiazide	Benzthiazide	Chlorothiazide	Chlorthalidone	Hydrochlorothiazide	Hydroflumethiazide	Indapamide	Methyclothiazide	Metolazone	Polythiazide	Quinethazone	Trichlormethiazide
Cardiovascular												
Hypotension			✓			✓						
Orthostatic hypotension	✓	✓	✓		✓	✓	< 5%	✓	< 2%[1]	✓	✓	✓
Palpitations							< 5%		< 2%[2]			✓
CNS												
Dizziness/Lightheadedness	✓	✓	✓	✓	✓	✓	≥ 5%	✓	10%[2]	✓	✓	✓
Vertigo	✓		✓	✓	✓	✓	< 5%		✓[3]	✓	✓	✓
Headache	✓	✓	✓	✓	✓	✓	≥ 5%	✓	9%[2]	✓	✓	✓
Paresthesias	✓	✓	✓	✓	✓	✓		✓	✓[3]			✓
Xanthopsia	✓	✓	✓	✓	✓	✓		✓				
Weakness	✓	✓	✓	✓	✓	✓	≥ 5%	✓	< 2%[2]			
Restlessness/Insomnia	✓	✓	✓	✓	✓	✓	< 5%	✓	✓[3]			
Drowsiness							< 5%		✓[3]			✓
Fatigue/Lethargy/Malaise/Lassitude							≥ 5%		4%[2]			✓
Anxiety							≥ 5%		< 2%[3]			
Depression							< 5%		< 2%[2]			✓
Nervousness							≥ 5%		< 2%[2]			
Blurred vision (may be transient)	✓		✓		✓	✓	< 5%	✓	✓[3]			
GI												
Anorexia	✓	✓	✓	✓	✓	✓	< 5%	✓	✓[3]	✓	✓	✓
Gastric irritation/epigastric distress	✓	✓	✓	✓	✓	✓	< 5%	✓		✓	✓	✓
Nausea	✓	✓	✓	✓	✓	✓	< 5%	✓	< 2%[2]	✓	✓	✓
Vomiting	✓	✓	✓	✓	✓	✓	< 5%	✓	< 2%[2]	✓	✓	✓
Abdominal pain/cramping/bloating	✓	✓	✓	✓	✓	✓	< 5%	✓	< 2%[2]			
Diarrhea	✓	✓	✓	✓	✓	✓	< 5%	✓	< 2%[2]			✓
Constipation	✓	✓	✓	✓	✓	✓	< 5%	✓	< 2%[2]			✓
Jaundice (intrahepatic/cholestatic)	✓	✓	✓	✓	✓	✓		✓	✓[3]	✓	✓	✓
Pancreatitis	✓		✓		✓	✓		✓	✓[3]	✓	✓	✓
Sialadenitis	✓		✓		✓	✓		✓		✓	✓	✓
Hepatitis	✓								✓[3]			
Dry mouth							< 5%		< 2%[1]			
GU												
Nocturia							< 5%		< 2%[1]			
Impotence/Reduced libido	✓	✓	✓	✓	✓	✓	< 5%	✓	< 2%[2]	✓	✓	✓
Renal failure/dysfunction							✓		✓			
Interstitial nephritis							✓					
Hematologic:												
Leukopenia	✓	✓	✓	✓	✓	✓		✓	✓[3]	✓	✓	✓
Thrombocytopenia	✓	✓	✓	✓	✓	✓		✓	✓[3]	✓	✓	✓
Agranulocytosis	✓	✓	✓	✓	✓	✓		✓	✓[3]	✓	✓	✓
Aplastic/Hypoplastic anemia	✓	✓	✓	✓	✓	✓		✓	✓[3]	✓	✓	✓
Hemolytic anemia	✓		✓		✓	✓		✓				
Dermatologic												
Purpura	✓	✓	✓	✓	✓	✓		✓	✓[3]	✓	✓	✓
Photosensitivity/Photosensitivity dermatitis	✓	✓	✓	✓	✓	✓		✓	✓[3]	✓	✓	✓
Rash	✓	✓	✓	✓	✓	✓	< 5%	✓	< 2%[2]	✓	✓	✓
Urticaria	✓	✓	✓	✓	✓	✓		✓	✓[3]	✓	✓	✓
Necrotizing angiitis, vasculitis, cutaneous vasculitis	✓	✓	✓	✓	✓	✓	< 5%	✓	✓[2]	✓	✓	✓
Fever	✓		✓		✓	✓		✓				
Anaphylactic reactions	✓		✓		✓[4]	✓		✓				
Pruritus	✓						< 5%		< 2%[1]			
Alopecia		✓[5]			✓							
Exfoliative dermatitis/toxic epidermal necrolysis	✓	✓[5]	✓		✓							
Erythema multiforme, Stevens-Johnson syndrome		✓[5]			✓			✓				
Metabolic												
Hyperglycemia	✓	✓	✓	✓	✓	✓	< 5%	✓	✓[3]	✓	✓	✓
Glycosuria	✓	✓	✓	✓	✓	✓	< 5%	✓	✓[3]	✓	✓	✓
Hyperuricemia	✓	✓	✓	✓	✓	✓	< 5%	✓		✓[3]		✓
Electrolyte imbalance								✓		✓		
Miscellaneous												
Respiratory distress (including pneumonitis/pulmonary edema)	✓		✓		✓	✓						
Muscle cramp/spasm	✓	✓	✓	✓	✓	✓	≥ 5%	✓	6%[2]			✓

[1] Rapidly acting doseform only.
[2] Percentage of occurrence refers to rapidly acting doseform; however, this adverse reaction also occurred with the slow-acting doseform.
[3] Slow-acting doseform only.
[4] Possibly with life-threatening anaphylactic shock.
[5] IV doseform.

Whenever adverse reactions are moderate or severe, reducing the thiazide dosage or withdrawing therapy will generally reverse the effect.

➤ *Cardiovascular:*

Hydrochlorothiazide – Allergic myocarditis.

Indapamide – Premature ventricular contractions, irregular heartbeat (< 5%).

Metolazone –
   Rapidly acting: Chest pain (precordial pain; 3%); cold extremities, edema (< 2%).

Slow-acting: Venous thrombosis; chest pain; excessive volume depletion; hemoconcentration.

➤**CNS:**

Indapamide – Loss of energy, numbness of extremities, tension, irritability, agitation (> 5%); tingling of extremities (< 5%).

Metolazone –
  Slow-acting: Syncope, neuropathy.
  Rapidly acting: Weird feeling, neuropathy (< 2%).

➤**GI:** Cholecystitis (possible increased risk in patients with gallstones).

Metolazone –
  Rapidly acting: Bitter taste (< 2%).

➤**GU:**

Bendroflumethiazide – Allergic glomerulonephritis.

Chlorothiazide IV – Hematuria.

Indapamide – Frequent urination, polyuria (< 5%).

➤**Dermatologic:**

Bendroflumethiazide – Ecchymosis.

Indapamide – Hives (< 5%).

Metolazone –
  Rapidly acting: Dry skin (< 2%).

Trichlormethiazide – Lichenoid dermatitis.

➤**Musculoskeletal:**

Metolazone – Joint pain; back pain (rapidly acting; < 2%); swelling (slow-acting).

➤**Respiratory:**

Indapamide – Rhinorrhea (< 5%).

Metolazone –
  Rapidly acting: Cough, epistaxis, sinus congestion, sore throat (< 2%).

Trichlormethiazide – Dyspnea.

➤**Miscellaneous:** Neutropenia.

Bendroflumethiazide – Metabolic acidosis in diabetics.

Indapamide – Flushing, weight loss (< 5%).

Methyclothiazide – Inappropriate ADH secretion.

Metolazone –
  Slow-acting: Chills; acute gouty attack.
  Rapidly acting: Eye itching, tinnitus (< 2%).

➤**Lab test abnormalities:** Hypercalcemia; hypokalemia; hyponatremia; hypomagnesemia; hypochloremia; hypochloremic alkalosis; hypophosphatemia; increase in BUN; elevation of creatinine; decreased serum PBI levels.

Clinical hypokalemia – Clinical hypokalemia occurred in 3% and 7% of patients given **indapamide** 2.5 mg and 5 mg, respectively.

Increases in plasma levels of total cholesterol, triglycerides and LDL cholesterol have been associated with thiazide diuretics (see Precautions).

Fluid/electrolyte imbalance – There are isolated reports of nonedematous individuals developing severe fluid and electrolyte derangements after only brief exposure to normal doses of thiazides. This condition is usually manifested as severe dilutional hyponatremia, hypokalemia and hypochloremia. It may be due to inappropriately increased ADH secretion and appears to be idiosyncratic. Potassium replacement is apparently the most important therapy along with removal of the offending drug.

Overdosage

➤*Symptoms:* Changes due to plasma volume depletion (eg, orthostatic hypotension, dizziness, drowsiness, syncope, electrolyte abnormalities, hemoconcentration, hemodynamic changes); signs of potassium deficiency (eg, confusion, dizziness, muscular weakness, and GI disturbances); nausea; vomiting. In severe instances, hypotension and depressed respiration may occur. Lethargy of varying degrees may progress to coma within a few hours, with minimal depression of respiration and cardiovascular function and without significant serum electrolyte changes or dehydration. GI irritation and hypermotility, temporary BUN elevation, CNS effects, cardiac abnormalities and seizures have also been reported, especially in patients with compromised renal function.

➤*Treatment:* Perform gastric lavage or induce emesis; give activated charcoal. Prevent aspiration. Avoid cathartics since electrolyte and fluid loss may be enhanced. GI effects are usually of short duration, but may require symptomatic treatment. Monitor serum electrolyte levels and renal function. Maintain hydration, electrolyte balance, respiration and cardiovascular-renal function. Asymptomatic hyperuricemia usually responds to fluids, but if clinical gout is suspected, indomethacin may be started. Support respiration and cardiac circulation if hypotension and depressed respiration occur. Refer to General Management of Acute Overdosage. Dialysis is unlikely to be effective.

Patient Information

May cause GI upset; may be taken with food or milk.

Drug will initially increase urination, which should subside after a few weeks; take early during the day or as directed.

Notify physician if muscle pain, weakness or cramps, nausea, vomiting, restlessness, excessive thirst, tiredness, drowsiness, increased heart rate or pulse, diarrhea or dizziness occurs.

May cause photosensitivity (sensitivity to sunlight). Avoid prolonged exposure to the sun and other ultraviolet light. Use sunscreens and wear protective clothing until tolerance is determined.

May increase blood sugar levels in diabetics.

Do not drink alcohol or take other medications without physician's approval; this includes nonprescription medicines for appetite control, asthma, colds, cough, hay fever or sinus.

Do not interrupt, discontinue or adjust the dose even if feeling well. Follow physician's instructions regarding missed dose.

May cause gout attacks. Contact physician if significant sudden joint pain occurs.

CHLOROTHIAZIDE

Rx	**Chlorothiazide** (Various, eg, Major, Mylan)	**Tablets:** 250 mg	In 100s and 250s.
Rx	**Diuril** (Merck)		Lactose. (MSD 214). White, scored. In 100s and 1000s.
Rx	**Chlorothiazide** (Various, eg, Goldline, Mylan)	**Tablets:** 500 mg	In 100s, 500s, 1000s and UD 100s.
Rx	**Diurigen** (Goldline)		In 100s and 1000s.
Rx	**Diuril** (Merck)		Lactose. (MSD 432). White, scored. In 100s, 1000s, 5000s and UD 100s.
Rx	**Diuril** (Merck)	**Oral Suspension:** 250 mg per 5 ml	0.5% alcohol, saccharin, 0.12% methylparaben, 0.02% propylparaben, 0.1% benzoic acid, sucrose. In 237 ml.
Rx	**Diuril** (Merck)	**Powder for Injection, lyophilized:** 500 mg (as sodium)	0.25 g mannitol. In 20 ml vials.

For complete prescribing information, refer to the Thiazides and Related Diuretics group monograph.

Administration and Dosage

➤**Adults:**

Edema – 0.5 to 1 g once or twice a day, orally or IV. Reserve IV route for patients unable to take oral medication or for emergency situations.

Many patients with edema respond to intermittent therapy (administration on alternate days or on 3 to 5 days each week). With an intermittent schedule, excessive response and undesirable electrolyte imbalance are less likely to occur.

Hypertension (oral forms only) – Starting dose is 0.5 to 1 g/day as a single or divided dose. Adjust dosage according to the blood pressure response. Rarely, some patients may require up to 2 g/day in divided doses.

➤*Infants and children:*

Oral – 22 mg/kg/day (10 mg/lb/day) in 2 doses. Infants < 6 months may require up to 33 mg/kg/day (15 mg/lb/day) in 2 doses.

On this basis, infants up to 2 years of age may be given 125 to 375 mg daily in 2 doses. Children from 2 to 12 years of age may be given 375 mg to 1 g daily in 2 doses.

IV use is not generally recommended.

➤*Preparation of parenteral solution:* Add 18 ml of sterile water for injection to the vial to prepare an isotonic solution. Never add < 18 ml. Discard unused solution after 24 hours. The solution is compatible with dextrose or sodium chloride solutions for IV infusion. Avoid simultaneous administration with whole blood or its derivatives. Extravasation must be rigidly avoided. Do not give SC or IM.

HYDROCHLOROTHIAZIDE

Rx	**Hydrochlorothiazide** (Various, eg, Major, Schein, Zenith)	**Tablets**: 25 mg	In 30s, 100s, 500s, 1000s, 5000s, UD 32s and UD 100s.
Rx	**Esidrix** (Ciba)		Lactose, sucrose. (Ciba 22). Pink, scored. In 100s.
Rx	**HydroDIURIL** (Merck)		Lactose. (MSD 42). Peach, scored. In 100s and 1000s.
Rx	**Hydro-Par** (Parmed)		Peach, scored. In 1000s.
Rx	**Oretic** (Abbott)		Lactose. (ORETIC). White. In 100s, 1000s and UD 100s.
Rx	**Hydrochlorothiazide** (Various, eg, Danbury, Schein, Zenith)	**Tablets**: 50 mg	In 30s, 100s, 500s, 1000s, 5000s and UD 100s.
Rx	**Esidrix** (Ciba)		Lactose, sucrose. (Ciba 46). Yellow, scored. In 100s and consumer pack 360s and 720s.
Rx	**Ezide** (Econo Med)		In 100s and 1000s.
Rx	**Hydro-Par** (Parmed)		In 1000s and 5000s.
Rx	**Hydrochlorothiazide** (Various, eg, Schein)	**Tablets**: 100 mg	In 30s, 100s, 250s, 500s, 1000s and UD 100s.
Rx	**Hydrochlorothiazide** (Various, eg, Mylan, Watson)	**Capsules**: 12.5 mg	In 100s and 500s.
Rx	**Microzide Capsules** (Watson)		Lactose. (Microzide 12.5). Light teal/teal. In 100s.
Rx	**Hydrochlorothiazide** (Roxane)	**Solution**: 50 mg per 5 ml	Saccharin. Mint flavor. In 500 ml.

For complete prescribing information, refer to the Thiazides and Related Diuretics group monograph.

Administration and Dosage

➤*Edema:*

Initial – 25 to 200 mg daily for several days, or until dry weight is attained.

Maintenance – 25 to 100 mg daily or intermittently. Refractory patients may require up to 200 mg daily.

➤*Hypertension:*
Initial – 12.5 to 50 mg daily as a single dose. Doses > 50 mg are often associated with marked reductions in serum potassium. Patients usually do not require doses > 50 mg daily when combined with other antihypertensives.

Infants and children – Usual dosage is 2.2 mg/kg (1 mg/lb) daily in two doses. Pediatric patients with hypertension only rarely will benefit from doses > 50 mg daily.

Infants (< 6 months): Up to 3.3 mg/kg (1.5 mg/lb) daily in two doses.
Infants (6 months to 2 years of age): 12.5 to 37.5 mg daily in two doses. Base dosage on body weight.
Children (2 to 12 years of age): 37.5 to 100 mg daily in two doses. Base dosage on body weight.

BENDROFLUMETHIAZIDE

Rx	**Naturetin** (Princeton)	**Tablets**: 5 mg	(606). Green, scored. In 100s.
		10 mg	(618). Orange, scored. In 100s.

For complete prescribing information, see Thiazides and Related Diuretics group monograph.

Administration and Dosage

➤*Edema:* 5 mg once daily, preferably in the morning.
Initial – Up to 20 mg once daily or divided into 2 doses.

Maintenance – 2.5 to 5 mg daily. Intermittent therapy may be advantageous in many patients. By giving the preparation every other day or on a 3 to 5 day per week schedule, electrolyte imbalance is still possible but less likely.

➤*Hypertension:*
Initial – 5 to 20 mg daily.
Maintenance – 2.5 to 15 mg/day.

METHYCLOTHIAZIDE

Rx	**Methyclothiazide** (Various, eg, Schein, Zenith)	**Tablets**: 2.5 mg	In 100s and 1000s.
Rx	**Methyclothiazide** (Various, eg, Geneva, Parmed, Zenith)	**Tablets**: 5 mg	In 1000s.
Rx	**Aquatensen** (Wallace)		(Wallace 153). Peach, scored. Convex. Rectangular. In 100s, 500s.
Rx	**Enduron** (Abbott)		(Enduron). Salmon. Square. In 100s, 1000s, 5000s and *Abbo-Pac* 100s.

For complete prescribing information, see Thiazides and Related Diuretics group monograph.

Administration and Dosage

➤*Edema (adults):* 2.5 to 10 mg once daily. Maximum effective single dose is 10 mg.

➤*Hypertension (adults):* 2.5 to 5 mg once daily. If blood pressure control is not satisfactory after 8 to 12 weeks with 5 mg once daily, add another antihypertensive.

INDAPAMIDE

Rx	**Indapamide** (Various, eg, Major, Mylan, Purepac, Teva, Watson, Zenith)	**Tablets**: 1.25 mg	In 100s, 500s, and 1000s.
Rx	**Lozol** (Rhone-Poulenc Rorer)		(R 7). Orange. Octagonal. Film coated. In 100s.
Rx	**Lozol** (Rhone-Poulenc Rorer)	2.5 mg	(R 8). White. Octagonal. Film coated. In 100s, 1000s and UD 100s.

For complete prescribing information, see Thiazides and Related Diuretics group monograph.

Administration and Dosage

➤*Edema of congestive heart failure:*
Adults – 2.5 mg as a single daily dose in the morning. If response is not satisfactory after 1 week, increase to 5 mg once daily.

➤*Hypertension:*
Adults – 1.25 mg as a single daily dose taken in the morning. If the response to 1.25 mg is not satisfactory after 4 weeks, increase the daily dose to 2.5 mg taken once daily. If the response to 2.5 mg is not satisfactory after 4 weeks, the daily dose may be increased to 5 mg taken once daily, but consider adding another antihypertensive. If the antihypertensive response is insufficient, combine with other antihypertensives. Reduce the usual dose of other agents by 50% during initial combination therapy. Further dosage adjustments may be necessary.

In general, doses ≥ 5 mg have not provided additional effects on blood pressure or heart failure, but are associated with a greater degree of hypokalemia. There is little experience with doses > 5 mg once daily.

TRICHLORMETHIAZIDE

Rx	**Trichlormethiazide** (Various)	**Tablets:** 4 mg	In 100s and 1000s.
Rx	**Diurese** (American Urologicals)		In 100s and 1000s.
Rx	**Metahydrin** (Hoechst Marion Roussel)		Tartrazine. (Merrell 63). Aqua. In 100s.
Rx	**Naqua** (Schering)		(S AHH or 547). Aqua. In 1000s.

For complete prescribing information, refer to the Thiazides and Related Diuretics group monograph.

Administration and Dosage

➤*Edema:* 2 to 4 mg once daily.

➤*Hypertension:* 2 to 4 mg once daily.

In initiating therapy, doses may be given twice daily.

METOLAZONE

Rx	**Mykrox** (Fisons)	**Tablets:** 0.5 mg	(MYKROX). White. In 100s.
Rx	**Metolazone** (Various, eg, Eon, Mylan)	**Tablets:** 2.5 mg	In 100s and 1000s.
Rx	**Zaroxolyn** (Fisons)		(2 1/2 Zaroxolyn). Pink. In 100s, 1000s and UD 100s.
Rx	**Metolazone** (Various, eg, Eon)	**Tablets:** 5 mg	In 100s.
Rx	**Zaroxolyn** (Fisons)		(5 Zaroxolyn). Blue. In 100s, 1000s and UD 100s.
Rx	**Metolazone** (Various, eg, Eon)	**Tablets:** 10 mg	In 100s.
Rx	**Zaroxolyn** (Fisons)		(10 Zaroxolyn). Yellow. In 100s, 1000s and UD 100s.

For complete prescribing information, refer to the Thiazides and Related Diuretics group monograph.

Administration and Dosage

Individualize dosage.

➤*Zaroxolyn:*

Mild-to-moderate essential hypertension – 2.5 to 5 mg once daily.

Edema of renal disease – 5 to 20 mg once daily.

Edema of cardiac failure – 5 to 20 mg once daily.

➤*Mykrox:*

Mild-to-moderate hypertension – 0.5 mg as a single daily dose taken in the morning. If response is inadequate, increase the dose to 1 mg daily.

Do not increase dosage if blood pressure is not controlled with 1 mg. Rather, add another antihypertensive agent with a different mechanism of action.

➤*Brand interchange:* The metolazone formulations are not bioequivalent or therapeutically equivalent at the same doses. *Mykrox* is more rapidly and completely bioavailable. Do not interchange brands.

If switching patients currently on *Zaroxolyn* to *Mykrox*, determine the dose by titration starting at 0.5 mg once daily and increasing to 1 mg once daily if needed.

CHLORTHALIDONE

Rx	**Thalitone** (Monarch)	**Tablets:** 15 mg	Lactose. (M 024). White. Kidney shaped. In 100s.
Rx	**Chlorthalidone** (Various, eg, Geneva, Goldline)	**Tablets:** 25 mg	In 100s, 1000s.
Rx	**Thalitone** (Monarch)		Lactose. (HTI/76). White, scored. Kidney shape. In 100s.
Rx	**Chlorthalidone** (Various, eg, Geneva, Goldline, Major, Schein)	**Tablets:** 50 mg	In 100s, 250s, and 1000s.
Rx	**Chlorthalidone** (Various, eg, Goldline, Schein)	**Tablets:** 100 mg	In 100s, 500s and 1000s.
Rx	**Hygroton** (RPR)		(RPR 21). White, scored. In 100s.

For complete prescribing information, refer to the Thiazides and Related Diuretics group monograph.

Administration and Dosage

Individualize dosage. Initiate therapy at lowest possible dose. Give a single dose with food in the morning. Maintenance doses may be lower than initial doses.

➤*Edema:* Initiate therapy with 50 to 100 mg (*Thalitone*, 30 to 60 mg) daily, or 100 mg (*Thalitone*, 60 mg) on alternate days. Some patients may require 150 or 200 mg (*Thalitone*, 90 to 120 mg) at these intervals, or 120 mg *Thalitone* daily. Dosages above this level, however, do not usually create a greater response.

➤*Hypertension:* Initiate therapy with a single daily dose of 25 mg (*Thalitone*, 15 mg). If response is insufficient after a suitable trial, increase to 50 mg (*Thalitone*, increase from 30 to 50 mg). For additional control, increase dosage to 100 mg once daily (except *Thalitone*) or add a second antihypertensive. Increases in serum uric acid and decreases in serum potassium are dose-related over the 25 to 100 mg/day (*Thalitone*, 15 to 50 mg/day) range.

Note – Doses > 25 mg/day are likely to potentiate potassium excretion, but provide no further benefit in sodium excretion or blood pressure reduction.

WARNING

These agents are potent diuretics; excess amounts can lead to a profound diuresis with water and electrolyte depletion. Careful medical supervision is required and dosage must be individualized.

Indications

➤*Edema:* Edema associated with CHF, hepatic cirrhosis and renal disease, including the nephrotic syndrome. Particularly useful when greater diuretic potential is desired.

Parenteral administration is indicated when a rapid onset of diuresis is desired (eg, acute pulmonary edema), when GI absorption is impaired or when oral use is not practical for any reason. As soon as it is practical, replace with oral therapy.

➤*Hypertension (furosemide, oral; torsemide, oral):* Alone or in combination with other antihypertensive drugs. Hypertensive patients who are inadequately controlled with thiazides may not be adequately controlled with furosemide alone.

➤*Ethacrynic acid: Ascites:* Short-term management of ascites due to malignancy, idiopathic edema and lymphedema.

Congenital heart disease, nephrotic syndrome – Short-term management of hospitalized pediatric patients, other than infants.

Pulmonary edema, acute – Adjunctive therapy.

➤*Unlabeled uses:* Ethacrynic acid is being investigated for the treatment of glaucoma; a single injection into the eye may reduce intraocular pressure for a week or more. Further study is needed.

Bumetanide 1 mg may be beneficial in the treatment of adult nocturia; it is not effective in males with prostatic hypertrophy.

Administration and Dosage

Individualize therapy. Reserve parenteral use for when oral medication is not practical or in emergency situations. Replace with oral therapy as soon as practical.

➤*Concomitant administration:* Concurrent metolazone and furosemide have been used in the management of patients refractory to furosemide or other diuretics due to their synergistic effect on diuresis. Metolazone 2.5 to 10 mg is added to the therapy, and the dose is doubled every 24 hours until the desired response is achieved. Decrease the furosemide dose if the synergism occurs with the first dose of metolazone. Hydrochlorothiazide (50 mg) may be used and may be safer because of its shorter action. This effect has also been noted with other thiazides in combination with other loop diuretics.

Actions

➤*Pharmacology:* Furosemide and ethacrynic acid inhibit primarily reabsorption of sodium and chloride, not only in proximal and distal tubules, but also the loop of Henle. High efficacy is largely due to unique site of action. Action on distal tubule is independent of any inhibitory effect on carbonic anhydrase or aldosterone.

In contrast, bumetanide is more chloruretic than natriuretic and may have an additional action in the proximal tubule; it does not appear to act on the distal tubule.

Torsemide acts from within the lumen of the thick ascending portion of the loop of Henle, where it inhibits the $Na^+/K^+/2Cl^-$-carrier system; effects in other segments of the nephron have not been demonstrated. Diuretic activity thus correlates better with the rate of drug excretion in urine than with the blood concentration. Torsemide increases the urinary excretion of sodium, chloride, and water, but does not significantly alter glomerular filtration rate, renal plasma flow or acid-base balance.

Because ethacrynic acid inhibits the reabsorption of filtered sodium to a much greater proportion than most other diuretics, it may be effective in many patients with significant degrees of renal insufficiency.

➤*Pharmacokinetics:* These agents are metabolized and excreted primarily through the urine. Protein binding of these agents exceeds 90%. Furosemide is metabolized ≈ 30% to 40%, and its urinary excretion is 60% to 70%. Significantly more furosemide is excreted in urine after IV injection than after the tablet or oral solution. Recent evidence suggests that furosemide glucuronide is the only, or at least the major, biotransformation product of furosemide.

Oral administration of bumetanide revealed that 81% was excreted in urine, 45% of it as unchanged drug. Bumetanide increases potassium excretion in a dose-related fashion; it also decreases uric acid excretion and increases serum uric acid. Urinary and biliary metabolites are formed by oxidation of the N-butyl side chain. Biliary excretion of bumetanide amounted to only 2% of the administered dose.

Torsemide is cleared from the circulation by both hepatic metabolism (≈ 80% of total clearance) and excretion into the urine (≈ 20% of total clearance). The major metabolite in humans is the carboxylic acid derivative, which is biologically inactive. Two of the lesser metabolites possess some diuretic activity, but for practical purposes metabolism terminates the action of the drug. Most renal clearance occurs via active secretion of the drug by the proximal tubules into tubular urine. Simultaneous food intake delays the time to C_{max} by about 30 minutes, but overall bioavailability and diuretic activity are unchanged.

Pharmacokinetic Parameters of the Loop Diuretics

Diuretic	Bioavailability (%)	Half-life (min)	Onset of action (min)	Peak (min)	Duration (hr)	Dosage (mg)	Relative potency	Doses/day
Furosemide								
Oral	60-64[1]	≈ 120[2]	within 60	60-120[4]	6-8	20-80	1	1-2
IV or IM			within 5[3]	30	2	20-40	1	
Ethacrynic acid								
Oral	≈100	60	within 30	120	6-8	50-100	0.6-0.8	1-2
IV			within 5	15-30	2	50	0.6-0.8	1-2
Bumetanide								
Oral	72-96	60-90[5]	30-60	60-120	4-6	0.5-2	≈ 40	1
IV			within minutes	15-30	0.5-1	0.5-1	≈ 40	1-3
Torsemide								
Oral	≈ 80	210	within 60	60-120	6-8	5-20	2-4	1
IV			within 10	within 60	6-8	5-20	2-4	1

[1] Decreased in uremia and nephrosis.
[2] Prolonged in renal failure, uremia and in neonates.
[3] Somewhat delayed after IM administration.
[4] Decreased in CHF.
[5] Prolonged in renal disease.

Contraindications

Anuria; hypersensitivity to these compounds or to sulfonylureas; infants (ethacrynic acid); patients with hepatic coma or in states of severe electrolyte depletion until the condition is improved or corrected (bumetanide).

Warnings

➤*Dehydration:* Excessive diuresis may result in dehydration and reduction in blood volume with circulatory collapse and the possibility of vascular thrombosis and embolism, particularly in elderly patients.

➤*Hepatic cirrhosis and ascites:* In these patients, sudden alterations of electrolyte balance may precipitate hepatic encephalopathy and coma. Do not institute therapy until the basic condition is improved. Initiate therapy in the hospital with small doses and careful monitoring. Supplemental potassium chloride and, if required, an aldosterone antagonist help to prevent hypokalemia and metabolic alkalosis.

➤*Ototoxicity:* Tinnitus, reversible and irreversible hearing impairment, deafness and vertigo with a sense of fullness in the ears have been reported. Deafness is usually reversible and of short duration (1 to 24 hours); however, irreversible hearing impairment has occurred. Usually, ototoxicity is associated with rapid injection, with severe renal impairment, with doses several times the usual dose and with concurrent use with other ototoxic drugs.

➤*Systemic lupus erythematosus:* Systemic lupus erythematosus may be exacerbated or activated.

➤*Diarrhea:* In a few patients, ethacrynic acid has produced severe, watery diarrhea. If this occurs, discontinue the drug and do not readminister.

Because of the amount of sorbitol in the **furosemide** solution vehicle, the possibility of diarrhea, especially in children, exists when higher dosages are given.

Thrombocytopenia – Since there have been rare spontaneous reports of thrombocytopenia with **bumetanide,** observe regularly for possible occurrence.

▶*Hypersensitivity reactions:* Patients with known sulfonamide sensitivity may show allergic reactions to **furosemide, torsemide** or **bumetanide.** Bumetanide use following instances of allergic reactions to furosemide suggests a lack of cross-sensitivity. Refer to Management of Acute Hypersensitivity Reactions.

▶*Renal function impairment:* If increasing azotemia, oliguria or reversible increases in BUN or creatinine occur during treatment of severe progressive renal disease, discontinue therapy.

If high-dose parenteral **furosemide** therapy is used, controlled IV infusion is advisable. For adults, an infusion rate ≤ 4 mg/min has been used.

▶*Pregnancy: Category B* (ethacrynic acid, torsemide); *Category C* (furosemide, bumetanide). There are no adequate and well controlled studies in pregnant women. Use only when clearly needed and when the potential benefits outweigh the potential hazards to the fetus.

Furosemide – Furosemide caused unexplained maternal deaths and abortions in rabbits when 25 to 100 mg/kg (2 to 8 times the maximum recommended human dose) was administered. No pregnant rabbits survived a dose of 100 mg/kg. Data indicate that fetal lethality can precede maternal deaths. Studies in mice and rabbits showed an increased incidence of fetal hydronephrosis. Since furosemide may increase the incidence of patent ductus arteriosus in preterm infants with respiratory-distress syndrome (see Children), use caution when administering before delivery.

Bumetanide – Bumetanide appears to be nonteratogenic, but has a slight embryocidal effect in rats when given in doses of 3400 times the maximum human therapeutic dose and in rabbits at doses of 3.4 times the maximum human therapeutic dose. In rabbits, a decrease in litter size and an increase in resorption rate were noted at oral doses 3.4 to 10 times the maximum human therapeutic dose.

Torsemide – Fetal and maternal toxicity (decrease in average body weight, increase in fetal resorption and delayed fetal ossification) occurred in rabbits and rats.

▶*Lactation:* **Furosemide** appears in breast milk; such transfer of **ethacrynic acid, torsemide** and **bumetanide** is unknown. Because of the potential for adverse reactions in nursing infants, decide whether to discontinue nursing or to discontinue the drug, taking into account the importance of the drug to the mother.

▶*Children:* Safety and efficacy for use of **torsemide** in children, **bumetanide** in children < 18 years old, and **ethacrynic acid** in infants (oral) and children (IV) have not been established.

Furosemide – Furosemide stimulates renal synthesis of prostaglandin E_2 and may increase the incidence of patent ductus arteriosus when given in the first few weeks of life, to premature infants with respiratory-distress syndrome. Renal calcifications (from barely visible on x–ray to staghorn) have occurred in some severely premature infants treated with IV furosemide for edema due to patent ductus arteriosus and hyaline membrane disease. Concurrent use of chlorothiazide has reportedly decreased hypercalciuria and dissolved some calculi.

Precautions

▶*Monitoring:* Observe for blood dyscrasias, liver or kidney damage or idiosyncratic reactions. Perform frequent serum electrolyte, calcium, glucose, uric acid, CO_2, creatinine and BUN determinations during the first few months of therapy and periodically thereafter (see Electrolyte imbalance and Laboratory test abnormalities).

▶*Cardiovascular effects:* Too vigorous a diuresis, as evidenced by rapid and excessive weight loss, may induce an acute hypotensive episode. In elderly cardiac patients, avoid rapid contraction of plasma volume and the resultant hemoconcentration to prevent thromboembolic episodes, such as cerebral vascular thromboses and pulmonary emboli.

▶*Electrolyte imbalance:* Electrolyte imbalance may occur, especially in patients receiving high doses with restricted salt intake. Perform periodic determinations of serum electrolytes. Observe patients for signs of fluid or electrolyte imbalance (eg, hyponatremia, hypochloremic alkalosis, hypokalemia, hypomagnesemia, hypocalcemia). Digitalis therapy may exaggerate metabolic effects of hypokalemia with reference to myocardial activity. Serum and urine electrolyte determinations are important in patients who are vomiting excessively, in patients who are receiving parenteral fluids, corticosteroids or ACTH, during brisk diuresis or when cirrhosis is present. Warning signs are dryness of mouth, thirst, anorexia, weakness, lethargy, drowsiness, restlessness, muscle pains or cramps, muscle fatigue, tetany (rarely), hypotension, oliguria, tachycardia, arrhythmia and GI disturbances (eg, nausea/vomiting).

Profound electrolyte and water loss may be avoided by weighing the patient periodically, adjusting dosage, initiating treatment with small doses and using the drugs intermittently. When excessive diuresis occurs, withdraw the drugs until homeostasis is restored. If excessive electrolyte loss occurs, reduce dosage or withdraw the drug temporarily.

Hypokalemia – Hypokalemia prevention requires particular attention to the following: Patients receiving digitalis and diuretics for CHF, hepatic cirrhosis and ascites; in aldosterone excess with normal renal function; potassium-losing nephropathy; certain diarrheal states; or where hypokalemia is an added risk to the patient (eg, history of ventricular arrhythmias).

Possible drug-related deaths occurred with **ethacrynic acid** in critically ill patients refractory to other diuretics. There are two categories: Patients with severe myocardial disease who received digitalis and developed acute hypokalemia with fatal arrhythmia; or patients with severely decompensated hepatic cirrhosis with ascites, with or without encephalopathy, who had electrolyte imbalances and died because of intensification of the electrolyte defect. Liberalization of salt intake and supplementary potassium are often necessary.

Hypomagnesemia – Loop diuretics increase the urinary excretion of magnesium.

Hypocalcemia – Serum calcium levels may be lowered (rare cases of tetany have occurred).

▶*Gastric hemorrhage:* **Ethacrynic acid** may increase the risk of gastric hemorrhage associated with corticosteroid treatment.

▶*Hyperuricemia:* Asymptomatic hyperuricemia can occur, and rarely, gout may be precipitated. Reversible elevations of BUN may be seen, usually in association with dehydration, particularly in patients with renal insufficiency. Serum creatinine may also be increased.

▶*Glucose:* Increases in blood glucose and alterations in glucose tolerance tests (fasting and 2 hour postprandial sugar) have been observed. Rare cases of precipitation of diabetes mellitus have occurred. Although these effects have not been reported with **bumetanide**, the possibility of an effect on glucose metabolism exists.

▶*Lipids:* Increases in LDL and total cholesterol and triglycerides with minor decreases in HDL cholesterol may occur.

▶*Photosensitivity:* Photosensitization (photoallergy or phototoxicity) may occur; therefore, caution patients to take protective measures (ie, sunscreens, protective clothing) against exposure to sunlight or ultraviolet light (eg, tanning beds) until tolerance is determined.

Drug Interactions

Loop Diuretic Drug Interactions			
Precipitant drug	Object drug*		Description
Loop diuretics	Aminoglycosides	↑	Auditory toxicity appears to be increased with concurrent use. Hearing loss of varying degrees may occur.
Loop diuretics	Anticoagulants	↑	Anticoagulant activity may be enhanced.
Loop diuretics Furosemide	Beta blockers Propranolol	↑	Plasma levels of propranolol may be increased.
Loop diuretics	Chloral hydrate	↑	Although rare, transient diaphoresis, hot flashes, hypertension, tachycardia, weakness and nausea may occur with concurrent use.
Loop diuretics	Digitalis glycosides	↑	Diuretic-induced electrolyte disturbances may predispose to digitalis-induced arrhythmias.
Loop diuretics	Lithium	↑	Possible increased plasma lithium levels and toxicity.
Loop diuretics	Nondepolarizing muscle relaxants	↔	The actions of the muscle relaxants may be antagonized or potentiated, perhaps dependent on the loop diuretic dosage.
Loop diuretics	Sulfonylureas	↓	Loop diuretics may decrease glucose tolerance, resulting in hyperglycemia in patients previously well controlled on sulfonylureas.
Loop diuretics	Theophyllines	↔	The actions of theophyllines may be altered, enhanced or inhibited.
Charcoal	Loop diuretics Furosemide	↓	Charcoal can reduce the absorption of furosemide. Depending on the clinical situation, this will reduce its effectiveness or toxicity.
Cisplatin	Loop diuretics	↑	Additive ototoxicity may occur.
Clofibrate	Loop diuretics Furosemide	↑	An exaggerated diuretic response may occur.
Hydantoins Phenytoin	Loop diuretics Furosemide	↓	Hydantoins may reduce the diuretic effects of furosemide.
NSAIDs	Loop diuretics	↓	Effects of the loop diuretics may be decreased.
Probenecid	Loop diuretics	↓	The actions of the loop diuretics may be reduced.

Loop Diuretic Drug Interactions			
Precipitant drug	Object drug*		Description
Salicylates	Loop diuretics	↓	The diuretic response may be impaired in patients with cirrhosis and ascites.
Thiazide diuretics	Loop diuretics	↑	Both groups have synergistic effects that may result in profound diuresis and serious electrolyte abnormalities (see Administration and Dosage).

* ↑ = Object drug increased. ↓ = Object drug decreased. ↔= Undetermined clinical effect.

➤*Drug/Food interactions:* The bioavailability of **furosemide** is decreased and its degree of diuresis reduced when administered with food.

Adverse Reactions

➤*Furosemide:*

GI – Anorexia; nausea; vomiting; diarrhea; oral and gastric irritation; cramping; constipation; pancreatitis; jaundice; ischemic hepatitis.

CNS – Vertigo; headache; blurred vision; hearing loss; dizziness; paresthesia; xanthopsia; restlessness; fever.

Hematologic – Anemia; leukopenia; purpura; aplastic anemia; thrombocytopenia; agranulocytosis.

Dermatologic – Photosensitivity; urticaria; pruritus; necrotizing angiitis (vasculitis, cutaneous vasculitis); interstitial nephritis; exfoliative dermatitis; erythema multiforme; rash; occasionally, local irritation and pain with parenteral use.

Cardiovascular – Orthostatic hypotension; thrombophlebitis; chronic aortitis.

Miscellaneous – Glycosuria; muscle spasm; weakness; urinary bladder spasm; hyperuricemia; hyperglycemia.

➤*Ethacrynic acid:*

GI – Anorexia; nausea; vomiting; diarrhea; pancreatitis (acute); jaundice; discomfort; pain; sudden watery, profuse diarrhea; GI bleeding; dysphagia.

Hematologic – Severe neutropenia has occurred in a few critically ill patients also receiving agents known to produce this effect. Rare instances of Henoch-Schoenlein purpura have occurred in patients with rheumatic heart disease. Thrombocytopenia; agranulocytosis.

Miscellaneous – Fever; chills; hematuria; apprehension; confusion; fatigue; malaise; acute gout; sense of fullness in the ears; abnormal liver function tests in seriously ill patients on multiple drug therapy that included ethacrynic acid (rare); vertigo; headache; blurred vision; tinnitus; hearing loss (irreversible); rash; occasionally, local irritation and pain have occurred with parenteral use; hyperuricemia; hyperglycemia. Acute symptomatic hypoglycemia with convulsions occurred in two uremic patients who received doses above those recommended.

➤*Bumetanide:*

CNS – Asterixis; encephalopathy with preexisting liver disease; impaired hearing; ear discomfort; vertigo; headache; dizziness.

GI – Upset stomach; dry mouth; nausea; vomiting; diarrhea; pain.

GU – Premature ejaculation; difficulty maintaining erection; renal failure.

Musculoskeletal – Weakness; arthritic pain; pain; muscle cramps; fatigue.

Cardiovascular – Hypotension; ECG changes; chest pain.

Miscellaneous – Hives; pruritus; itching; dehydration; sweating; hyperventilation; nipple tenderness; rash; thrombocytopenia.

Lab test abnormalities – Diuresis rarely (≤ 1%) accompanied by changes in LDH, total serum bilirubin, serum proteins, AST, ALT, alkaline phosphatase, cholesterol and creatinine clearance; deviations in hemoglobin, prothrombin time, hematocrit, WBC, platelet counts and differential counts; increases in urinary glucose and protein; hyperuricemia; hypochloremia; hypokalemia; azotemia; hyponatremia; increased serum creatinine; hyperglycemia; variations in phosphorus, CO_2 content, bicarbonate and calcium (see Precautions).

➤*Torsemide:*

CNS – Headache (7.3%); dizziness (3.2%); asthenia (2%); insomnia (1.2%); nervousness (1.1%); syncope.

GI – Diarrhea (2%); constipation, nausea (1.8%); dyspepsia (1.6%); edema (1.1%); GI hemorrhage; rectal bleeding.

Cardiovascular – ECG abnormality (2%); sore throat (1.6%); chest pain (1.2%); atrial fibrillation; hypotension; ventricular tachycardia; shunt thrombosis.

Respiratory – Rhinitis (2.8%); cough increase (2%).

Musculoskeletal – arthralgia (1.8%); myalgia (1.6%).

Lab test abnormalities – Hyperglycemia; hyperuricemia; hypokalemia; hypovolemia.

Miscellaneous – Excessive urination (6.7%); rash.

Overdosage

➤*Symptoms:* Acute profound water loss, volume and electrolyte depletion, dehydration, reduction of blood volume, and circulatory collapse with a possibility of vascular thrombosis and embolism. Electrolyte depletion may be manifested by weakness, dizziness, mental confusion, anorexia, lethargy, vomiting and cramps.

➤*Treatment:* Replace fluid and electrolyte losses by careful monitoring of the urine and electrolyte output and serum electrolyte levels. Assure adequate drainage in urinary bladder outlet obstruction (such as prostatic hypertrophy). Hemodialysis does not accelerate furosemide or torsemide elimination. Induce emesis or perform gastric lavage. If required, give oxygen or artificial respiration. Treatment includes supportive measures. Refer to General Management of Acute Overdosage.

Patient Information

May cause GI upset; take with food or milk (see Drug Interactions). Torsemide may be given without regard to meals.

Drug will increase urination; take early in the day.

Notify physician if muscle weakness, cramps, nausea or dizziness occurs.

Orthostatic hypotension may occur; get up slowly.

➤*Diabetes mellitus patients:* May increase blood glucose levels, affecting urine glucose tests.

➤*Photosensitivity:* Photosensitivity may occur in some patients. Caution patients to take protective measures (ie, sunscreens, protective clothing) against exposure to ultraviolet light or sunlight.

➤*Hypertensive patients:* Hypertensive patients should avoid medications that may increase blood pressure, including *otc* products for appetite suppression and cold symptoms.

FUROSEMIDE

Rx	**Furosemide** (Various, eg, Danbury, Geneva, Major, Mylan, Parmed, Roxane, Schein, Zenith)	**Tablets:** 20 mg	In 100s, 500s, 1000s and UD 100s.
Rx	**Lasix** (Aventis)		Lactose. (Lasix Hoechst). White. Oval. In 100s, 500s, 1000s and UD 100s.
Rx	**Furosemide** (Various, eg, Danbury, Geneva, Major, Mylan, Parmed, Roxane, Schein, Zenith)	**Tablets:** 40 mg	In 60s, 100s, 500s and 1000s and UD 100s.
Rx	**Lasix** (Aventis)		Lactose. (Lasix 40). White, scored. In 500s, 1000s, UD 100s and unit-of-use 100s.
Rx	**Furosemide** (Various, eg, Danbury, Geneva, Mylan, Parmed, Roxane, Schein)	**Tablets:** 80 mg	In 100s, 500s, 1000s and UD 100s.
Rx	**Lasix** (Aventis)		Lactose. (Lasix 80). White. In 50s, 500s and UD 100s.
Rx	**Furosemide** (Various, eg, Geneva, Roxane)	**Oral Solution:** 10 mg/ml	In 60 and 120 ml.
Rx	**Furosemide** (Roxane)	**Oral Solution:** 40 mg/5 ml	Pineapple/peach flavor. In 500 ml and UD 5 & 10 ml.
Rx	**Furosemide** (Various, eg, American Regent, Sanofi Winthrop)	**Injection:** 10 mg/ml	In 10 ml and 2, 4, and 10 ml single-dose vials.

For complete prescribing information, refer to the Loop Diuretics group monograph.

Loop Diuretics

FUROSEMIDE

Administration and Dosage

➤*Oral:*

Edema – 20 to 80 mg/day as a single dose. Ordinarily, prompt diuresis ensues. Depending on response, administer a second dose 6 to 8 hours later. If response is not satisfactory, increase by increments of 20 or 40 mg, no sooner than 6 to 8 hours after previous dose, until desired diuresis occurs. This dose should then be given once or twice daily (eg, at 8 am and 2 pm). Dosage may be titrated up to 600 mg/day in patients with severe edema.

Mobilization of edema may be most efficiently and safely accomplished with an intermittent dosage schedule; the drug is given 2 to 4 consecutive days each week. With doses > 80 mg/day, clinical and laboratory observations are advisable.

Hypertension – 40 mg twice a day; adjust according to response. If the patient does not respond, add other antihypertensive agents. Observe blood pressure changes when used with other antihypertensives, especially during initial therapy. Reduce dosage of other agents by ≥ 50% as soon as furosemide is added to prevent excessive drop in blood pressure. As blood pressure falls, reduce dose or discontinue other antihypertensives.

Infants and children – 2 mg/kg. If diuresis is unsatisfactory, increase by 1 or 2 mg/kg, no sooner than 6 to 8 hours after previous dose. Doses > 6 mg/kg are not recommended. For maintenance therapy, adjust dose to the minimum effective level. A dose range of 0.5 to 2 mg/kg twice daily has also been recommended.

CHF and chronic renal failure – It has been suggested that doses as high as 2 to 2.5 g/day or more are well tolerated and effective in these patients.

➤*Parenteral:*

Edema –

Initial dose: 20 to 40 mg IM or IV. Give the IV injection slowly (1 to 2 minutes); ordinarily, prompt diuresis ensues. If needed, another dose may be given in the same manner 2 hours later. The dose may be raised by 20 mg and given no sooner than 2 hours after previous dose, until desired diuretic effect is obtained. This dose should then be given once or twice daily. Administer high-dose parenteral therapy as a controlled infusion at a rate ≤ 4 mg/min.

Acute pulmonary edema – The usual initial dose is 40 mg IV (over 1 to 2 minutes). If response is not satisfactory within 1 hour, increase to 80 mg IV (over 1 to 2 minutes). Additional therapy (eg, digitalis, oxygen) may be given concomitantly.

Infants and children – 1 mg/kg IV or IM given slowly under close supervision. If diuretic response after the initial dose is not satisfactory, increase the dosage by 1 mg/kg, no sooner than 2 hours after previous dose, until desired effect is obtained. Doses > 6 mg/kg are not recommended.

CHF and chronic renal failure – It has been suggested that doses as high as 2 to 2.5 g/day or more are well tolerated and effective in these patients. For IV bolus injections, the maximum should not exceed 1 g/day given over 30 minutes.

IV incompatibility – Furosemide is a mildly buffered alkaline solution; do not mix with highly acidic solutions of pH < 5.5. Sodium Chloride injection, Lactated Ringer's Injection and 5% Dextrose Injection have been used after pH has been adjusted when necessary. A precipitate formed when furosemide was admixed with gentamicin, netilmicin or milrinone in 5% Dextrose or 0.9% Sodium Chloride, but not with amikacin, kanamycin or tobramycin. Furosemide admixed with cefoperazone sodium in 5% Dextrose is stable for 2 days at 25°C (77°F) and 5 days at 4°C (39°F).

➤*Storage/Stability:* Exposure to light may cause slight discoloration; do not dispense discolored tablets or use discolored injection. Store injection and oral solution at room temperature (15° to 30°C; 59° to 86°F)

BUMETANIDE

Rx	**Bumex** (Roche)	**Tablets:** 0.5 mg	Lactose. (Roche Bumex 0.5). Green, scored. In 100s, 500s and UD 100s.
		1 mg	Lactose. (Roche Bumex 1). Yellow, scored. In 100s, 500s and UD 100s.
		2 mg	Lactose. (Roche Bumex 2). Peach, scored. In 100s and UD 100s.
Rx	**Bumetanide** (Various, eg, Bedford, Hoffman-LaRoche, Sanofi Winthrop)	**Injection:** 0.25 mg per ml	In 2 ml amps, 2, 4 and 10 ml vials and 4 ml fill in 5 ml vials.

[1] With 0.01% EDTA and 1% benzyl alcohol.

For complete prescribing information, refer to the Loop Diuretics group monograph.

Administration and Dosage

Because cross-sensitivity with furosemide is rare, bumetanide can be substituted at about a 1:40 ratio of bumetanide to furosemide in patients allergic to furosemide.

➤*Oral:* 0.5 to 2 mg/day, given as a single dose. If diuretic response is not adequate, give a second or third dose at 4- to 5-hour intervals, up to a maximum daily dose of 10 mg. An intermittent dose schedule, given on alternate days or for 3 to 4 days with rest periods of 1 to 2 days in between, is the safest and most effective method for the continued control of edema. In patients with hepatic failure, keep the dose to a minimum, and if necessary, increase the dose carefully.

➤*Parenteral:* Reserve for patients in whom GI absorption may be impaired or in whom oral administration is not practical.

Initially, 0.5 to 1 mg IV or IM. Administer IV over a period of 1 to 2 minutes. If the initial response is insufficient, give a second or third dose at intervals of 2 to 3 hours; do not exceed a daily dosage of 10 mg. End parenteral treatment and start oral treatment as soon as possible.

➤*Renal function impairment:* In patients with severe chronic renal insufficiency, a continuous infusion of bumetanide (12 mg over 12 hours) may be more effective and less toxic than intermittent bolus therapy.

➤*Storage/Stability:* Bumetanide injection with 5% Dextrose in Water, 0.9% Sodium Chloride and Lactated Ringer's solution in glass and plasticized PVC (*Viaflex*) containers have no significant absorption effects or loss due to drug degradation. However, freshly prepare solutions and use within 24 hours.

ETHACRYNIC ACID

Rx	**Edecrin** (Merck)	**Tablets:** 25 mg	Lactose. (MSD 65). White, scored. Capsule shape. In 100s.
		50 mg	Lactose. (MSD 90). Green, scored. Capsule shape. In 100s.
Rx	**Edecrin Sodium** (Merck)	**Powder for Injection:** 50 mg (as ethacrynate sodium) per vial	In 50 ml vials for reconstitution.[1]

[1] With 62.5 mg mannitol and 0.1 mg thimerosal.

For complete prescribing information, refer to the Loop Diuretics group monograph.

Administration and Dosage

➤*Oral:*

Initial therapy – Give minimally effective dose (usually, 50 to 200 mg daily) on a continuous or intermittent dosage schedule to produce gradual weight loss of 2.2 to 4.4 kg/day (1 to 2 lb/day). Adjust dose in 25 to 50 mg increments. Higher doses, up to 200 mg twice daily, achieved gradually, are most often required in patients with severe, refractory edema.

Children – Initial dose is 25 mg. Make careful increments of 25 mg to achieve maintenance. Dosage for infants has not been established.

Maintenance therapy – Administer intermittently after an effective diuresis is obtained using an alternate daily schedule or more prolonged periods of diuretic therapy interspersed with rest periods. This allows time to correct any electrolyte imbalance and may provide a more efficient diuretic response. The chloruretic effect may cause retention of bicarbonate and metabolic alkalosis. Correct by giving chloride

(ammonium chloride or arginine chloride). Do not give ammonium chloride to cirrhotic patients.

Concomitant diuretic therapy – Ethacrynic acid has additive effects when used with other diuretics; therefore, use an initial dose of 25 mg and dose changes of 25 mg increments to avoid electrolyte depletion.

➤*Parenteral:* Do not give SC or IM because of local pain and irritation. The usual IV dose for the average adult is 50 mg, or 0.5 to 1 mg/kg. Give slowly through the tubing of a running infusion or by direct IV injection over several minutes. Usually, only one dose is necessary; occasionally, a second dose may be required; use a new injection site to avoid thrombophlebitis. A single IV dose, not exceeding 100 mg, has been used. Insufficient pediatric experience precludes recommendation for this age group.

Preparation of solution – Add 50 ml of 5% Dextrose Injection or Sodium Chloride Injection to vial. Dextrose 5% solutions may have a low pH (< 5); the resulting solution may be hazy or opalescent. Use of such a solution is not recommended. Do not mix this solution with whole blood or its derivatives. Discard unused reconstituted solution after 24 hours.

Loop Diuretics

TORSEMIDE

Rx	Torsemide (Teva)	Tablets: 5 mg	Lactose. In 100s.
Rx	Demadex (Roche)		Lactose. (102 5). White, scored. Oval. In UD 100s.
Rx	Torsemide (Teva)	10 mg	Lactose. In 100s.
Rx	Demadex (Roche)		Lactose. (103 10). White, scored. Oval. In UD 100s.
Rx	Torsemide (Teva)	20 mg	Lactose. In 100s.
Rx	Demadex (Roche)		Lactose. (104 20). White, scored. Oval. In UD 100s.
Rx	Torsemide (Teva)	100 mg	Lactose. In 100s.
Rx	Demadex (Roche)		Lactose. (105 100). White, scored. Capsule shape. In UD 100s.
Rx	Demadex (Roche)	Injection: 10 mg/ml	In 2 and 5 ml amps.

For complete prescribing information, refer to the Loop Diuretics group monograph.

Administration and Dosage

➤*Approved by the FDA:* August 23, 1993.

Torsemide may be given at any time in relation to a meal.

Because of high bioavailability, oral and IV doses are therapeutically equivalent, so patients may be switched to and from the IV form with no change in dose. Administer the IV injection slowly over a period of 2 minutes.

➤*Congestive heart failure:* The usual initial dose is 10 or 20 mg once daily oral or IV. If the diuretic response is inadequate, titrate the dose upward by approximately doubling until the desired diuretic response is obtained. Single doses > 200 mg have not been adequately studied.

➤*Chronic renal failure:* The usual initial dose is 20 mg once daily oral or IV. If the diuretic response is inadequate, titrate the dose upward by approximately doubling until the desired diuretic response is obtained. Single doses > 200 mg have not been adequately studied.

➤*Hepatic cirrhosis:* The usual initial dose is 5 or 10 mg once daily oral or IV, administered together with an aldosterone antagonist or a potassium-sparing diuretic. If the diuretic response is inadequate, titrate the dose upward by approximately doubling until the desired diuretic response is obtained. Single doses > 40 mg have not been adequately studied.

➤*Hypertension:* The usual initial dose is 5 mg once daily. If the 5 mg dose does not provide adequate reduction in blood pressure within 4 to 6 weeks, the dose may be increased to 10 mg once daily. If the response to 10 mg is insufficient, add an additional antihypertensive agent to the treatment regimen.

➤*Elderly:* Special dosage adjustment is not necessary.

Potassium-Sparing Diuretics

Actions

▶*Pharmacology:* In the kidney, potassium is filtered at the glomerulus and then absorbed parallel to sodium throughout the proximal tubule and thick ascending limb of the loop of Henle, so that only minor amounts reach the distal convoluted tubule. As a result, potassium appearing in urine is secreted at the distal tubule and collecting duct. The potassium-sparing diuretics interfere with sodium reabsorption at the distal tubule, thus decreasing potassium secretion. They exert a weak diuretic and antihypertensive effect when used alone. Their major use is to enhance the action and counteract the kaliuretic effect of thiazide and loop diuretics.

Spironolactone – Spironolactone, a competitive inhibitor of aldosterone, binds to aldosterone receptors of the distal tubule and prevents the formation of a protein important in sodium transport. The dose of spironolactone required to produce an effect varies according to the amount of aldosterone present. It is effective in primary and secondary hyperaldosteronism. Spironolactone is effective in lowering systolic and diastolic blood pressure in both primary hyperaldosteronism and essential hypertension, although aldosterone secretion may be normal in benign essential hypertension. In addition, spironolactone interferes with testosterone synthesis and may increase peripheral conversion of testosterone to estradiol. This action may be responsible for endocrine abnormalities occasionally noted with therapy.

Amiloride/Triamterene – Amiloride and triamterene not only inhibit sodium reabsorption induced by aldosterone, but they also inhibit basal sodium reabsorption. They are not aldosterone antagonists, but act directly on the renal distal tubule, cortical collecting tubule and collecting duct. They induce a reversal of polarity of the transtubular electrical-potential difference and inhibit active transport of sodium and potassium. Amiloride may inhibit sodium, potassium-ATPase. Amiloride decreases the enhanced urinary excretion of magnesium that occurs when a thiazide or loop diuretic is used alone; it also decreases calcium excretion.

Potassium-Sparing Diuretics: Pharmacological and Pharmacokinetic Properties			
Parameters	Amiloride	Spironolactone	Triamterene
Pharmacology			
Tubular site of action	Proximal = distal	Distal	Distal
Mechanism of action	Na+, K+–ATPase inhibition; Na+/H+ exchange mechanism inhibition (proximal tubule)	Aldosterone antagonism	Membrane effect
Action:			
Onset (hours)	2	24 to 48	2 to 4
Peak (hours)	6 to 10	48 to 72	6 to 8
Duration (hours)	24	48 to 72	12 to 16
Pharmacokinetics			
Bioavailability	15% to 25%	> 90%	30% to 70%
Protein binding	23%	≥ 98%[1]	50% to 67%
Half-life (hours)	6 to 9	20[2]	3
Active metabolites	none	canrenone	hydroxytriamterene sulfate
Peak plasma levels (hours)	3 to 4	canrenone: 2 to 4[3]	3
Excreted unchanged in urine	≈ 50%[4]	_[4]	≈ 21%
Daily dose (mg)	5 to 20	25 to 400	200 to 300

[1] Canrenone > 98%.
[2] 10 to 35 hours for canrenone.
[3] 40% excreted in stool within 72 hours.
[4] Metabolites primarily excreted in urine, but also in bile.

AMILORIDE HCl

Rx	**Midamor** (Merck)	**Tablets:** 5 mg	(MSD 92). Yellow. Diamond shape. In 100s.

Refer to the general discussion of these agents in the Potassium-Sparing Diuretics introduction.

Indications

Adjunctive treatment with thiazide or loop diuretics in congestive heart failure (CHF) or hypertension to help restore normal serum potassium in patients who develop hypokalemia on the kaliuretic diuretic; prevent hypokalemia in patients who would be at particular risk if hypokalemia were to develop (eg, digitalized patients or patients with significant cardiac arrhythmias).

▶*Unlabeled uses:* Amiloride (10 to 20 mg/day) may be useful in reducing lithium-induced polyuria without increasing lithium levels as is seen with thiazide diuretics.

Aerosolized amiloride (drug dissolved in 0.3% saline delivered by nebulizer) appears to slow the progression of pulmonary function reduction in adults with cystic fibrosis.

Administration and Dosage

Administer with food.

▶*Concomitant therapy:* Add amiloride 5 mg/day to the usual antihypertensive or diuretic dosage of a kaliuretic diuretic. Increase dosage to 10 mg/day, if necessary; doses> 10 mg are usually not needed. If persistent hypokalemia is documented with 10 mg, increase the dose to 15 mg, then 20 mg, with careful titration of the dose and careful monitoring of electrolytes.

In patients with CHF, potassium loss may decrease after an initial diuresis; reevaluate the need or dosage for amiloride. Maintenance therapy may be intermittent.

▶*Single drug therapy:* The starting dose is 5 mg/day. Increase to 10 mg/day, if necessary; doses > 10 mg are usually not needed. If persistent hypokalemia is documented with 10 mg, increase the dose to 15 mg, then 20 mg, with careful monitoring of electrolytes.

Contraindications

Hypersensitivity to amiloride; serum potassium > 5.5 mEq/L; antikaliuretic therapy or potassium supplementation (see Drug Interactions); renal function impairment (see Warnings); patients receiving spironolactone or triamterene.

Warnings

▶*Hyperkalemia:* Amiloride may cause hyperkalemia (serum potassium > 5.5 mEq/L), which, if uncorrected, is potentially fatal. Hyperkalemia occurs commonly (≈ 10%) when amiloride is used alone. This incidence is greater in patients with renal impairment, diabetes mellitus (with or without recognized renal insufficiency) and in the elderly. When amiloride is used concomitantly with a thiazide diuretic in patients without these complications, the risk of hyperkalemia is reduced to ≈ 1% to 2%. Monitor serum potassium carefully, particularly when amiloride is first introduced, at the time of diuretic dosage adjustments and during any illness that could affect renal function.

Symptoms – Symptoms of hyperkalemia include paresthesias, muscular weakness, fatigue, flaccid paralysis of the extremities, bradycardia, shock, and ECG abnormalities. The ECG in hyperkalemia is characterized primarily by tall, peaked T waves or elevations from previous tracings. There may also be lowering of the R wave, increased depth of the S wave, widening or disappearance of the P wave, progressive widening of the QRS complex, prolongation of the PR interval, and ST depression. Mild hyperkalemia is not usually associated with an abnormal ECG.

Treatment – Discontinue the drug immediately. Monitor ECG and serum potassium levels. If serum potassium exceeds 6.5 mEq/L, take active measures to reduce it, including IV sodium bicarbonate solution or oral or parenteral glucose with rapid-acting insulin. If needed, give sodium polystyrene sulfonate orally or by enema. Persistent hyperkalemia may require dialysis.

▶*Diabetes mellitus:* Hyperkalemia has occurred with the use of amiloride, even in patients without evidence of diabetic nephropathy. If possible, avoid use of amiloride in diabetic patients. If it is used, moni

AMILORIDE HCl

tor serum electrolytes and renal function frequently. Discontinue use ≥ 3 days before glucose tolerance testing.

➤*Metabolic or respiratory acidosis:* Cautiously institute amiloride in severely ill patients in whom respiratory or metabolic acidosis may occur, such as patients with cardiopulmonary disease or poorly controlled diabetes. Monitor acid-base balance frequently. Shifts in acid-base balance alter the ratio of extracellular/intracellular potassium; the development of acidosis may be associated with rapid increases in serum potassium.

➤*Renal function impairment:* Anuria, acute or chronic renal insufficiency and evidence of diabetic nephropathy are contraindications because potassium retention is accentuated and may result in the rapid development of hyperkalemia. Do not give to patients with evidence of renal impairment (BUN > 30 mg/dl or serum creatinine > 1.5 mg/dl) or diabetes mellitus without continuous monitoring of serum electrolytes, creatinine and BUN levels.

➤*Hepatic function impairment:* In patients with preexisting severe liver disease, hepatic encephalopathy, manifested by tremors, confusion and coma, and increased jaundice, may occur in association with amiloride. Because amiloride is not metabolized by the liver, drug accumulation is not anticipated in patients with hepatic dysfunction, but accumulation can occur if hepatorenal syndrome develops.

➤*Pregnancy: Category B.* There are no adequate and well controlled studies in pregnant women. Safety for use during pregnancy has not been established. Use only when clearly needed and when the potential benefits outweigh the potential hazards to the fetus. See also discussion of thiazide diuretic use during pregnancy.

➤*Lactation:* It is not known whether amiloride is excreted in breast milk. In rats, amiloride is excreted in milk in concentrations higher than those found in blood. Because of the potential for serious adverse reactions in nursing infants, decide whether to discontinue nursing or to discontinue the drug, taking into account the importance of the drug to the mother.

➤*Children:* Safety and efficacy for use in children have not been established.

Precautions

➤*Electrolyte imbalance and BUN increases:* Hyponatremia and hypochloremia may occur when amiloride is used with other diuretics. Increases in BUN levels usually accompany vigorous fluid elimination, especially when diuretic therapy is used in seriously ill patients, such as those who have hepatic cirrhosis with ascites and metabolic alkalosis, or those with resistant edema. Carefully monitor serum electrolytes and BUN levels.

Drug Interactions

Amiloride Drug Interactions			
Precipitant drug	Object drug*		Description
Amiloride	Digoxin	↓	In six healthy subjects, amiloride increased the renal clearance and decreased the nonrenal clearance of digoxin. It also appeared to decrease the inotropic effect of digoxin.
Amiloride	Potassium preparations	↑	Concurrent administration may result in severe hyperkalemia, possibly with cardiac arrhythmias or cardiac arrest. Avoid concomitant use.

Amiloride Drug Interactions			
Precipitant drug	Object drug*		Description
ACE inhibitors	Amiloride	↑	Use of ACE inhibitors may result in elevated serum potassium concentration. Concurrent use with amiloride may lead to significant hyperkalemia.
NSAIDs	Amiloride	↓	NSAIDs may reduce the therapeutic effect of amiloride. Also, since indomethocin may be associated with increased potassium levels, consider this effect when amiloride is used concurrently.

* ↑ = Object drug increased. ↓ = Object drug decreased.

Adverse Reactions

➤*Cardiovascular:* Angina pectoris, orthostatic hypotension, arrhythmia, palpitations (≤ 1%).

➤*CNS:* Headache (3% to 8%); dizziness, encephalopathy (> 1% to < 3%); paresthesia, tremors, vertigo, nervousness, mental confusion, insomnia, decreased libido, depression, somnolence (≤ 1%).

➤*Dermatologic:* Skin rash, itching, pruritus, alopecia (≤ 1%).

➤*GI:* Nausea, anorexia, diarrhea, vomiting (3% to 8%); abdominal pain, gas pain, appetite changes, constipation (> 1% to < 3%); jaundice, GI bleeding, GI disturbance, abdominal fullness, thirst, dry mouth, heartburn, flatulence, dyspepsia (≤ 1%); activation of probable preexisting peptic ulcer; abnormal liver function.

➤*GU:* Impotence (> 1% to < 3%); polyuria, dysuria, urinary frequency, bladder spasms (≤ 1%).

➤*Hematologic:* Aplastic anemia; neutropenia.

➤*Metabolic:* Elevated serum potassium levels > 5.5 mEq/L (> 1% to < 3%).

➤*Musculoskeletal:* Weakness, fatigue, muscle cramps (> 1% to < 3%); joint/back/chest pain, neck or shoulder ache, pain of the extremities (≤ 1%).

➤*Respiratory:* Cough, dyspnea (> 1% to < 3%); shortness of breath (≤ 1%).

➤*Special senses:* Visual disturbances, nasal congestion, tinnitus, increased intraocular pressure (≤ 1%).

Overdosage

➤*Symptoms:* The most likely signs are dehydration and electrolyte imbalance.

➤*Treatment:* Discontinue therapy and observe patient closely. Induce emesis or perform gastric lavage. Treatment is symptomatic and supportive. Refer to General Management of Acute Overdosage. If hyperkalemia occurs, reduce the serum potassium levels (see Warnings). It is not known whether amiloride is dialyzable.

Patient Information

May cause GI upset; take with food.

Notify physician if any of the following occurs: Muscular weakness, fatigue, muscle cramps.

May cause dizziness, headache or visual disturbances; observe caution while driving or performing other tasks requiring alertness, coordination or physical dexterity.

Avoid large quantities of potassium rich food.

SPIRONOLACTONE

Rx	Spironolactone (Various, eg, Geneva, Mylan, Parmed)	Tablets: 25 mg	In 100s, 250s, 500s and 1000s.
Rx	Aldactone (Searle)		(Searle 1001 Aldactone 25). Lt. yellow. Film coated. In 100s, 500s, 1000s, 2500s and UD 100s.
Rx	Aldactone (Searle)	Tablets: 50 mg	(Searle 1041 Aldactone 50). Lt. orange, scored. Oval. Film coated. In 100s and UD 100s.
Rx	Aldactone (Searle)	Tablets: 100 mg	(Searle 1031 Aldactone 100). Peach, scored. Film coated. In 100s and UD 100s.

Refer to the general discussion of these agents in the Potassium-Sparing Diuretics introduction.

WARNING

Spironolactone has been shown to be a tumorigen in chronic toxicity studies in rats (see Warnings). Use only in those conditions described in the Indications section. Avoid unnecessary use of the drug.

Indications

➤*Primary hyperaldosteronism:* Diagnosis of primary hyperaldosteronism.

Short-term preoperative treatment of patients with primary hyperaldosteronism.

Long-term maintenance therapy for patients with discrete aldosterone-producing adrenal adenomas who are poor operative risks, or who decline surgery.

Long-term maintenance therapy for patients with bilateral micronodular or macronodular adrenal hyperplasia (idiopathic hyperaldosteronism).

➤*Edematous conditions when other therapies are inappropriate or inadequate:*

CHF – Management of edema and sodium retention; also indicated with digitalis.

SPIRONOLACTONE

Cirrhosis of the liver accompanied by edema or ascites – For maintenance therapy in conjunction with bed rest and the restriction of fluid and sodium.

Nephrotic syndrome – For nephrotic syndrome.

➤*Essential hypertension:* Essential hypertension usually in combination with other drugs.

➤*Hypokalemia:* Hypokalemia and the prophylaxis of hypokalemia in patients taking digitalis.

➤*Unlabeled uses:* Spironolactone has been used in the treatment of hirsutism (50 to 200 mg/day) due to its antiandrogenic properties. One study suggested that a lower dosage (50 mg twice daily on days 4 through 21 of the menstrual cycle) may help minimize the risk of metrorrhagia that occurs with higher doses.

Symptoms of premenstrual syndrome (PMS) have been relieved at a dosage of 25 mg 4 times daily beginning on day 14 of the menstrual cycle.

The combination of spironolactone (2 mg/kg/day) and testolactone (20 to 40 mg/kg/day) for at least 6 months may be effective for short-term treatment of familial male precocious puberty.

Spironolactone 100 mg/day appears effective in short-term treatment of acne vulgaris.

Administration and Dosage

Spironolactone may be administered in single or divided doses.

➤*Diagnosis of primary hyperaldosteronism:* As an initial diagnostic measure to provide presumptive evidence of primary hyperaldosteronism in patients on normal diets, as follows:

Long test – 400 mg/day for 3 to 4 weeks. Correction of hypokalemia and hypertension provides presumptive evidence for diagnosis of primary hyperaldosteronism.

Short test – 400 mg/day for 4 days. If serum potassium increases, but decreases when spironolactone is discontinued, consider a presumptive diagnosis of primary hyperaldosteronism.

➤*Maintenance therapy for hyperaldosteronism:* 100 to 400 mg daily in preparation for surgery. For patients unsuitable for surgery, employ the drug for long-term maintenance therapy at lowest possible dose.

➤*Edema:*

Adults (CHF, hepatic cirrhosis, nephrotic syndrome) – Initially, 100 mg/day (range, 25 to 200 mg/day). When given as the sole diuretic agent, continue for ≥ 5 days at the initial dosage level, then adjust to the optimal level. If after 5 days an adequate diuretic response has not occurred, add a second diuretic, which acts more proximally in the renal tubule. Because of the additive effect of spironolactone with such diuretics, an enhanced diuresis usually begins on the first day of combined treatment; combined therapy is indicated when more rapid diuresis is desired. Spironolactone dosage should remain unchanged when other diuretic therapy is added.

Children – 3.3 mg/kg/day (1.5 mg/lb/day) administered in single or divided doses.

➤*Essential hypertension:*

Adults – Initially, 50 to 100 mg/day in single or divided doses. May also be combined with diuretics, which act more proximally, and with other antihypertensive agents. Continue treatment for ≥ 2 weeks since the maximal response may not occur sooner. Individualize dosage.

Children – A dose of 1 to 2 mg/kg twice daily has been recommended.

➤*Hypokalemia:* 25 to 100 mg/day. Useful in treating diuretic-induced hypokalemia when oral potassium supplements or other potassium-sparing regimens are considered inappropriate.

Contraindications

Anuria; acute renal insufficiency; significant impairment of renal function; hyperkalemia; patients receiving amiloride or triamterene.

Warnings

➤*Hyperkalemia:* Carefully evaluate patients for possible fluid and electrolyte balance disturbances. Hyperkalemia may occur with impaired renal function or excessive potassium intake and can cause cardiac irregularities which may be fatal. No potassium supplement should ordinarily be given with spironolactone.

Treat hyperkalemia – Treat hyperkalemia promptly by rapid IV glucose (20% to 50%) and regular insulin, using 0.25 to 0.5 units of insulin/g of glucose. This is a temporary measure to be repeated as required. Treatment of hyperkalemia may also include: IV calcium to antagonize effects on the heart; bicarbonate if patient is acidotic; or sodium polystyrene sulfonate exchange resin to remove potassium. Discontinue spironolactone and restrict potassium intake (including dietary potassium).

➤*Renal function impairment:* Use of spironolactone may cause a transient elevation of BUN, especially in patients with preexisting renal impairment. The drug may cause mild acidosis.

➤*Carcinogenesis:* Spironolactone was a tumorigen in chronic toxicity studies in rats. At 25 to 250 times the usual human dose, there was a significant dose-related increase in benign adenomas of the thyroid and testes, in malignant mammary tumors and in proliferative changes in the liver. At 500 mg/kg, the effects included hepatocytomegaly, hyperplastic liver nodules and hepatocellular carcinoma. A dose-related (> 20 mg/kg/day) incidence of myelocytic leukemia was observed in rats fed daily doses of potassium canrenoate. In the rat, myelocytic leukemia and hepatic, thyroid, testicular and mammary tumors were observed.

➤*Pregnancy:* Spironolactone or its metabolites may cross the placental barrier. Feminization occurs in male rat fetuses. Weigh anticipated benefit against possible hazard to the fetus. See also discussion of thiazide diuretic use during pregnancy.

➤*Lactation:* Canrenone, a metabolite of spironolactone, appears in breast milk. The estimated maximum dose to the infant is ≈ 0.2% of the mother's daily dose. Labeling suggests an alternative method of infant feeding when using spironolactone; however, the American Academy of Pediatrics considers the drug to be compatible with breastfeeding.

Precautions

➤*Hyponatremia:* Hyponatremia may be caused or aggravated by spironolactone, especially in combination with other diuretics. Symptoms include dry mouth, thirst, lethargy, and drowsiness.

➤*Gynecomastia:* Gynecomastia may develop and appears to be related to both dosage and duration of therapy. It is normally reversible when therapy is discontinued; however, in rare instances, some breast enlargement may persist.

➤*Reversible hyperchloremic metabolic acidosis:* Reversible hyperchloremic metabolic acidosis usually in association with hyperkalemia, occurs in some patients with decompensated hepatic cirrhosis, even in the presence of normal renal function.

Drug Interactions

Spironolactone Drug Interactions			
Precipitant drug	Object drug*		Description
Spironolactone	Anticoagulants	↓	The hypoprothrombinemic effect may be decreased.
Spironolactone	Digitalis glycosides	↔	The interaction is complex and difficult to predict. Spironolactone increases the half-life of digoxin and can decrease its clearance. This may result in increased serum digoxin levels and subsequent toxicity. In addition, the drug may attenuate the inotropic action of digoxin. Spironolactone decreases and increases digitoxin's elimination half-life.
Spironolactone	Mitotane	↓	One patient failed to respond to mitotane while receiving concurrent spironolactone. Mitotane toxicity developed when the drug was discontinued.
Spironolactone	Potassium preparations	↑	Concurrent administration may result in hyperkalemia, possibly with cardiac arrhythmias or cardiac arrest. Avoid concomitant use.
ACE inhibitors	Spironolactone	↑	Use of ACE inhibitors may elevate serum potassium. Concurrent use with spironolactone may lead to significant hyperkalemia.
Salicylates	Spironolactone	↓	The diuretic effect of spironolactone may be decreased by concurrent salicylate use, possibly due to reduced tubular secretion of canrenone; this interaction is dose-dependent. The antihypertensive action does not appear altered.

* ↑ = Object drug increased ↓ = Object drug decreased ↔ = Undetermined clinical effect

➤*Drug/Lab test interactions:* Spironolactone and its metabolites can interfere with the radioimmunoassay for measuring **digoxin**, resulting in falsely elevated serum digoxin values.

➤*Drug/Food interactions:* The administration of spironolactone with food appears to increase its absorption. In one study, the AUC and maximum serum concentration of spironolactone were significantly increased by food.

Adverse Reactions

Adverse reactions are usually reversible upon discontinuation of the drug.

➤*CNS:* Drowsiness; lethargy; headache; mental confusion; ataxia.

➤*Dermatologic:* Maculopapular or erythematous cutaneous eruptions; urticaria.

SPIRONOLACTONE

➤*Endocrine:* Inability to achieve or maintain erection; gynecomastia; irregular menses or amenorrhea; postmenopausal bleeding; hirsutism; deepening of the voice.

➤*GI:* Cramping; diarrhea; gastric bleeding; ulceration; gastritis; vomiting.

➤*Miscellaneous:* Drug fever; hyperchloremic metabolic acidosis in decompensated hepatic cirrhosis; carcinoma of the breast; agranulocytosis.

May produce drowsiness, lack of coordination and mental confusion; observe caution while driving or performing other tasks requiring alertness, coordination or physical dexterity.

May cause GI cramping, diarrhea, lethargy, thirst, headache, skin rash, menstrual abnormalities, deepening of the voice and breast enlargement in men. Notify physician if these effects occur.

TRIAMTERENE

| Rx | Dyrenium (SmithKline Beecham) | **Capsules:** 50 mg | (Dyrenium 50). Red. In 100s and UD 100s. |
| | | 100 mg | (Dyrenium 100). Red. In 100s, 1000s and UD 100s. |

Refer to the general discussion of these agents in the Potassium-Sparing Diuretics introduction.

Indications

➤*Edema:* Edema associated with congestive heart failure (CHF), hepatic cirrhosis and the nephrotic syndrome; steroid-induced edema, idiopathic edema and edema due to secondary hyperaldosteronism.

May be used alone or with other diuretics, either for additive diuretic effect or antikaliuretic (potassium-sparing) effect. It promotes increased diuresis in patients resistant or only partially responsive to other diuretics because of secondary hyperaldosteronism.

Administration and Dosage

Individualize dosage.

When used alone, the usual starting dose is 100 mg twice/daily after meals. When combined with other diuretics or antihypertensives, decrease the total daily dosage of each agent initially, and then adjust to the patient's needs. Do not exceed 300 mg/day.

Contraindications

Patients receiving spironolactone or amiloride; anuria; severe hepatic disease; hyperkalemia (see Warnings); hypersensitivity to triamterene; severe or progressive kidney disease or dysfunction, with the possible exception of nephrosis; preexisting elevated serum potassium (impaired renal function, azotemia) or patients who develop hyperkalemia while on triamterene.

Warnings

➤*Hyperkalemia:* Abnormal elevation of serum potassium levels (≥ 5.5 mEq/L) can occur. Hyperkalemia is more likely to occur in patients with renal impairment and diabetes (even without evidence of renal impairment), and in the elderly or severely ill. Since uncorrected hyperkalemia may be fatal, serum potassium levels must be monitored at frequent intervals especially when dosages are changed or with any illness that may influence renal function.

Hyperkalemia rarely occurs in patients with adequate urinary output, but is possible if large doses are used for long periods of time; if it occurs, withdraw triamterene. Normal adult serum potassium range is 3.5 to 5 mEq/L. Treat levels persistently > 6 mEq/L. Neonate levels are higher than adult levels. Serum potassium levels do not necessarily indicate true body potassium concentration. A rise in plasma pH may cause a decrease in plasma potassium concentration and an increase in the intracellular potassium concentration. Patients who receive intensive or prolonged therapy may experience a rebound kaliuresis upon abrupt withdrawal. Gradually withdraw triamterene in such patients.

When triamterene is added to other diuretic therapy, or when patients are switched to triamterene from other diuretics, discontinue potassium supplementation.

If hyperkalemia is present or suspected, obtain an ECG. If the ECG shows no widening of the QRS or arrhythmia in the presence of hyperkalemia, discontinue triamterene and any potassium supplementation and substitute a thiazide alone. Sodium polystyrene sulfonate may be administered to enhance excess potassium excretion. The presence of a widened QRS complex or arrhythmia in association with hyperkalemia requires prompt additional therapy. For tachyarrhythmia, infuse 44 mEq of sodium bicarbonate or 10 ml of 10% calcium gluconate or calcium chloride over several minutes. For asystole, bradycardia or AV block, transvenous pacing is also recommended.

The effect of calcium and sodium bicarbonate is transient. Repeat as required. Remove excess potassium by dialysis or oral or rectal administration of sodium polystyrene sulfonate. Infusion of glucose and insulin are also used to treat hyperkalemia.

The following agents, given with triamterene, may cause hyperkalemia especially in patients with renal insufficiency: Blood from blood bank (may contain up to 30 mEq of potassium per liter of plasma or up to 65 mEq per liter of whole blood when stored for > 10 days); low-salt milk (may contain up to 60 mEq of potassium per liter); potassium-containing medications (such as parenteral penicillin G potassium); salt substitutes (most contain substantial amounts of potassium).

➤*Hypersensitivity reactions:* Monitor patients regularly for blood dyscrasias, liver damage or other idiosyncratic reactions.

➤*Renal function impairment:* Perform periodic BUN and serum potassium determinations to check kidney function, especially in patients with suspected or confirmed renal insufficiency and in elderly or diabetic patients; diabetic patients with nephropathy are especially prone to develop hyperkalemia.

➤*Hepatic function impairment:* Triamterene is extensively metabolized in the liver. One study showed that the clearance of triamterene is markedly decreased in patients with cirrhosis and ascites. However, the overall diuretic response may not be affected.

➤*Pregnancy: Category B.* Triamterene crosses the placental barrier and appears in the cord blood of animals; this may occur in humans. No congenital defects have been noted when used during pregnancy. There are no adequate and well controlled studies in pregnant women. Use only when clearly needed and when the potential benefits outweigh the potential hazards to the fetus. See also discussion of thiazide diuretic use during pregnancy.

➤*Lactation:* Triamterene appears in the milk of animals receiving the drug; this may occur in humans. If the drug is essential, the patient should stop nursing.

➤*Children:* Safety and efficacy have not been established.

Precautions

➤*Electrolyte imbalance:* In CHF, renal disease or cirrhosis, electrolyte imbalance may be aggravated or caused by diuretics. The use of full doses of a diuretic when salt intake is restricted can result in a low salt syndrome.

Triamterene can cause mild nitrogen retention which is reversible upon withdrawal; this is seldom observed with intermittent therapy.

➤*Renal stones:* Triamterene has been found in renal stones with other usual calculus components. Therefore, use cautiously in patients with histories of stone formation.

➤*Hematologic effects:* Triamterene is a weak folic acid antagonist. Since cirrhotics with splenomegaly may have marked variations in hematological status, it may contribute to the appearance of megaloblastosis in cases where folic acid stores have been depleted. Perform periodic blood studies in these patients.

➤*Metabolic acidosis:* Triamterene may cause decreasing alkali reserve with a possibility of metabolic acidosis.

➤*Diabetes mellitus:* Triamterene may raise blood glucose levels for adult-onset diabetes; dosage adjustments of hypoglycemic agents may be necessary. Concurrent use with chlorpropamide may increase the risk of severe hyponatremia.

➤*Photosensitivity:* Photosensitization (photoallergy or phototoxicity) may occur; therefore, caution patients to take protective measures (ie, sunscreens, protective clothing) against exposure to sunlight or ultraviolet light (eg, tanning beds) until tolerance is determined.

Drug Interactions

Triamterene Drug Interactions			
Precipitant drug	Object drug*		Description
Triamterene	Amantadine	↑	Amantadine plasma levels may increase and urinary excretion may decrease, possibly increasing the risk for developing adverse effects.
Triamterene	Potassium preparations	↑	Concurrent administration may result in severe hyperkalemia, possibly with cardiac arrhythmias or cardiac arrest. Avoid concomitant use.
ACE inhibitors	Triamterene	↑	Use of ACE inhibitors may elevate serum potassium. Concurrent use with triamterene may lead to significant hyperkalemia.
Cimetidine	Triamterene	↑	Cimetidine may increase the bioavailability and decrease the renal clearance and hydroxylation of triamterene.

TRIAMTERENE

Triamterene Drug Interactions			
Precipitant drug	Object drug*		Description
Indomethacin	Triamterene	↑	Rapid progress into acute renal failure has occurred with concurrent use. Use this combination only when clearly needed.

* ↑ = Object drug increased

➤*Drug/Lab test interactions:* Triamterene and **quinidine** have similar fluorescence spectra; thus, triamterene will interfere with the fluorescent measurement of quinidine serum levels.

Adverse Reactions

➤*GI:* Diarrhea; nausea; vomiting; jaundice; liver enzyme abnormalities. Nausea can usually be prevented by giving the drug after meals.

➤*Hematologic:* Thrombocytopenia; megaloblastic anemia.

➤*Renal:* Azotemia; elevated BUN and creatinine. Triamterene has been found in renal stones (see Precautions).

Interstitial nephritis – Interstitial nephritis has been reported rarely in patients on a hydrochlorothiazide/triamterene combination and with triamterene alone. Onset was immediate to 10 weeks after initiation of therapy; resolution began upon discontinuation of the drug.

In patients predisposed to gouty arthritis, serum uric acid levels may increase.

➤*Miscellaneous:* Electrolyte inbalance (see Precautions); hyperkalemia (see Warnings); weakness; fatigue; dizziness; hypokalemia; headache; dry mouth; anaphylaxis; photosensitivity; rash.

Overdosage

➤*Symptoms:* Electrolyte imbalance is the major concern, particularly hyperkalemia (see Warnings). Other symptoms may include nausea, vomiting, other GI disturbances and weakness. Hypotension may occur. Triamterene may induce reversible acute renal failure.

➤*Treatment:* Induce immediate evacuation of the stomach through emesis and gastric lavage. Carefully evaluate electrolyte and fluid balance. Dialysis may be of some benefit. Treatment includes usual supportive measures. Refer to General Management of Acute Overdosage.

Patient Information

May cause GI upset; take after meals.

May cause weakness, headache, nausea, vomiting and dry mouth; notify physician if these become severe or persistent.

Notify physician if fever, sore throat, mouth sores, or unusual bleeding or bruising occurs.

Avoid prolonged exposure to sunlight; photosensitivity may occur.

If single daily dose is prescribed, take in morning to minimize effect of increased frequency of urination on nighttime sleep.

If dose is missed, do not take more than prescribed dose at next dosing interval.

Carbonic Anhydrase Inhibitors

Indications

➤*Glaucoma:* For adjunctive treatment of chronic simple (open-angle) glaucoma and secondary glaucoma; preoperatively in acute angle-closure glaucoma when delay of surgery is desired to lower intraocular pressure (IOP).

➤*Acetazolamide:*

Tablets, sustained release capsules and injection – For the prevention or amelioration of symptoms associated with acute mountain sickness in climbers attempting rapid ascent and in those who are susceptible to acute mountain sickness despite gradual ascent.

Tablets and injection only – For adjunctive treatment of edema due to CHF, drug-induced edema and centrencephalic epilepsy (petit mal, unlocalized seizures).

Actions

➤*Pharmacology:* These agents are nonbacteriostatic sulfonamides that inhibit the enzyme carbonic anhydrase. This action reduces the rate of aqueous humor formation, resulting in decreased IOP. This action is independent of systemic acid-base balance.

By inhibiting hydrogen ion secretion by the renal tubule, these agents cause increased excretion of sodium, potassium, bicarbonate and water, thus producing an alkaline diuresis. Carbonic anhydrase inhibitors cause some decrease in renal blood flow and glomerular filtration rate. Redistribution of flow to the renal cortex occurs. These changes are mild and unrelated to diuretic activity.

Evidence seems to indicate that **acetazolamide** has utility as an adjuvant in the treatment of certain dysfunctions of the CNS (eg, epilepsy). Inhibition of carbonic anhydrase in this area appears to retard abnormal, paroxysmal, excessive discharge from CNS neurons.

➤*Pharmacokinetics:*

Pharmacokinetics of Carbonic Anhydrase Inhibitors				
Carbonic anhydrase inhibitor	IOP Lowering Effects			Relative inhibitor potency
	Onset (hours)	Peak effect (hours)	Duration (hours)	
Dichlorphenamide	within 1	2 to 4	6 to 12	30
Acetazolamide				
Tablets	1 to 1.5	1 to 4	8 to 12	1
Sustained-release capsules	2	3 to 6	18 to 24	
Injection (IV)	2 min	15 min	4 to 5	
Methazolamide	2 to 4	6 to 8	10 to 18	–[1]

[1] Quantitative data not available; reported to be more active than acetazolamide.

Methazolamide – Peak plasma concentrations for the 25, 50 and 100 mg twice daily regimens were 2.5, 5.1 and 10.7 mcg/ml, respectively. Approximately 55% is bound to plasma proteins. The mean steady-state plasma elimination half-life is ≈ 14 hours. At steady state ≈ 25% of the dose is recovered unchanged in the urine. Renal clearance accounts for 20% to 25% of the total clearance of drug. After repeated dosing, methazolamide accumulates to steady-state concentrations in 7 days.

Contraindications

Hypersensitivity to these agents; depressed sodium or potassium serum levels; marked kidney and liver disease or dysfunction; suprarenal gland failure; hyperchloremic acidosis; adrenocortical insufficiency; severe pulmonary obstruction with inability to increase alveolar ventilation since acidosis may be increased (**dichlorphenamide**); cirrhosis (**acetazolamide, methazolamide**); long-term use in chronic noncongestive angle-closure glaucoma, since organic closure of the angle may occur while worsening glaucoma is masked by lowered IOP.

Warnings

➤*Hepatic function impairment:* Use of **methazolamide** in this condition could precipitate hepatic coma.

➤*Pregnancy: Category C.* Animal studies with some of these drugs have demonstrated teratogenicity (skeletal anomalies). Do not use during pregnancy, especially during the first trimester, unless the potential benefits outweigh the potential hazards.

➤*Lactation:* Safety for use in the nursing mother has not been established. It is not known whether all carbonic anhydrase inhibitors are excreted in breast milk. **Acetazolamide** appeared in breast milk of a patient taking 500 mg twice/day. However, the infant ingested only 0.06% of the dose, an amount unlikely to cause adverse effects.

➤*Children:* Safety and efficacy for use in children have not been established.

Precautions

➤*Monitoring:* Monitor for hematologic reactions common to sulfonamides. Obtain baseline CBC and platelet counts before therapy and at regular intervals during therapy.

Hypokalemia – Hypokalemia may develop when severe cirrhosis is present, during concomitant use of steroids or ACTH, and with interference with adequate oral electrolyte intake. Hypokalemia can sensi-

tize or exaggerate the response of the heart to the toxic effects of digitalis (eg, increased ventricular irritability). Hypokalemia may be avoided or treated with potassium supplements or foods with a high potassium content.

➤*Dose increases:* Increasing the dose of **acetazolamide** does not increase diuresis and may increase drowsiness or paresthesia; it often results in decreased diuresis. However, very large doses have been given with other diuretics to promote diuresis in complete refractory failure.

➤*Pulmonary conditions:* Use **dichlorphenamide** with caution in patients with severe degrees of respiratory acidosis. These drugs may precipitate or aggravate acidosis. Use with caution in patients with pulmonary obstruction or emphysema when alveolar ventilation may be impaired.

➤*Cross-sensitivity:* Cross-sensitivity between antibacterial sulfonamides and sulfonamide derivative diuretics, including acetazolamide and various thiazides, has been reported.

Drug Interactions

Carbonic Anhydrase Inhibitor (CAI) Drug Interactions			
Precipitant drug	Object drug[*]		Description
Acetazolamide	Cyclosporine	↑	Increased trough cyclosporine levels with possible nephrotoxicity and neurotoxicity may occur.
Acetazolamide	Primidone	↓	Primidone serum and urine concentrations may be decreased.
CAIs	Salicylates	↑	Concurrent use may result in accumulation and toxicity of the CAI, including CNS depression and metabolic acidosis. Also, CAI-induced acidosis may allow increased CNS penetration by salicylates.
Salicylates	CAIs	↑	
Diflunisal	CAIs	↑	Concurrent use may result in a significant decrease in intraocular pressure; the effect may be less pronounced with methazolamide. Increased side effects may also occur.

[*] ↑ = Object drug increased ↓ = Object drug decreased

Adverse Reactions

Sulfonamide-type adverse reactions may occur (see Systemic Sulfonamides monograph in the Anti-Infectives chapter).

➤*CNS:* Convulsions; weakness; malaise; fatigue; nervousness; drowsiness; depression; dizziness; disorientation; confusion; ataxia; tremor; tinnitus; headache; lassitude; flaccid paralysis; paresthesias of the extremities.

➤*Dermatologic:* Urticaria; pruritus; skin eruptions; rash (including erythema multiforme, Stevens-Johnson syndrome, toxic epidermal necrolysis); photosensitivity.

➤*GI:* Melena; anorexia; nausea; vomiting; constipation; taste alteration; diarrhea.

➤*Hematologic:* Bone marrow depression; thrombocytopenia; thrombocytopenic purpura; hemolytic anemia; leukopenia; pancytopenia; agranulocytosis.

➤*Renal:* Hematuria; glycosuria; urinary frequency; renal colic; renal calculi; crystalluria; polyuria; phosphaturia.

➤*Miscellaneous:* Weight loss; fever; acidosis (usually corrected with bicarbonate); decreased/absent libido; impotence; electrolyte imbalance; hepatic insufficiency; transient myopia.

Overdosage

➤*Symptoms:* Symptoms of overdosage or toxicity may include drowsiness, anorexia, nausea, vomiting, dizziness, paresthesias, ataxia, tremor and tinnitus.

➤*Treatment:* In the event of overdosage, induce emesis or perform gastric lavage. The electrolyte disturbance most likely to be encountered from overdosage is hyperchloremic acidosis that may respond to bicarbonate administration. Potassium supplementation may be required. Observe carefully; give supportive treatment.

Patient Information

If GI upset occurs, take with food.

Avoid prolonged exposure to sunlight or sunlamps; may cause photosensitivity.

May cause drowsiness; observe caution while driving or performing other tasks requiring alertness, coordination or physical dexterity.

Notify physician if sore throat, fever, unusual bleeding or bruising, tingling or tremors in the hands or feet, flank or loin pain, or skin rash occurs.

Carbonic Anhydrase Inhibitors

ACETAZOLAMIDE

Rx	**Acetazolamide** (Various, eg, Mutual, URL)	**Tablets:** 125 mg	In 50s, 100s, and 250s.
Rx	**Acetazolamide** (Various, eg, Qualitest, Schein, URL)	**Tablets:** 250 mg	In 100s, 500s, 1000s and UD 100s.
Rx	**Dazamide** (Major)		In 100s, 250s, 1000s and UD 100s.
Rx	**Diamox** (Wyeth-Ayerst)		(Diamox 250 D2 LL). White, scored. In 1000s and UD 100s.
Rx	**Diamox Sequels** (Barr)	**Capsules, sustained-release:** 500 mg	(Diamox D3). Orange. In 30s and 100s.
Rx	**Acetazolamide** (Various, eg, Bedford Labs)	**Powder for Injection, lyophilized:** 500 mg	In vials.

For complete prescribing information, see Carbonic Anhydrase Inhibitor monograph.

Administration and Dosage

➤*Chronic simple (open-angle) glaucoma:*
Adults – 250 mg to 1 g/day, usually in divided doses for amounts > 250 mg. Dosage > 1 g daily does not usually increase the effect.

➤*Secondary glaucoma and preoperative treatment of acute congestive (closed-angle) glaucoma:*
Adults –
  Short-term therapy: 250 mg every 4 hours or 250 mg twice daily.
  Acute cases: 500 mg followed by 125 or 250 mg every 4 hours.

IV therapy may be used for rapid relief of increased intraocular pressure. A complementary effect occurs when used with miotics or mydriatics.
Children –
  Parenteral: 5 to 10 mg/kg/dose, IM or IV, every 6 hours.
  Oral: 10 to 15 mg/kg/day in divided doses, every 6 to 8 hours.

➤*Diuresis in congestive heart failure:*
Adults – Initially, 250 to 375 mg (5 mg/kg) once daily in the morning. If, after an initial response, the patient stops losing edema fluid, do not increase the dose; allow for kidney recovery by skipping medication for a day. Best diuretic results occur when given on alternate days, or for 2 days alternating with a day of rest. Failures in therapy may result from overdosage or from too frequent dosages.

➤*Drug-induced edema:* Most effective if given every other day or for 2 days alternating with a day of rest.
Adults – 250 to 375 mg once daily for 1 or 2 days.
Children – 5 mg/kg/dose, oral or IV, once daily in the morning.

➤*Epilepsy:*
Adults and Children – 8 to 30 mg/kg/day in divided doses. The optimum range is 375 to 1000 mg daily. When given in combination with other anticonvulsants, the starting dose is 250 mg once daily.

It is not clearly known whether the beneficial effects observed in epilepsy are due to direct inhibition of carbonic anhydrase in the CNS or whether they are due to the slight degree of acidosis produced by the divided dosage. The best results to date have been seen in petit mal in children. Good results, however, have been seen in patients, both children and adult, in other types of seizures such as grand mal, mixed seizure patterns, myoclonic jerk patterns.

➤*Acute mountain sickness:* 500 to 1000 mg/day, in divided doses of tablets or sustained release capsules. For rapid ascent (ie, in rescue or military operations), use the higher dose (1000 mg). If possible, initiate dosing 24 to 48 hours before ascent and continue for 48 hours while at high altitude, or longer as needed to control symptoms.

➤*Sustained release:* May be used twice daily, but is only indicated for use in glaucoma and acute mountain sickness.

➤*Parenteral:* Direct IV administration is preferred; IM administration is painful because of the alkaline pH of the solution.

➤*Preparation and storage of parenteral solution:* Reconstitute each 500 mg vial with ≥ 5 ml of Sterile Water for Injection. Reconstituted solutions retain potency for 1 week if refrigerated. However, since this product contains no preservative, use within 24 hours of reconstitution.

➤*Oral liquid dose form:* If required, acetazolamide tablets may be crushed and suspended in a cherry, chocolate, raspberry or other sweet syrup. Do not use a vehicle with alcohol or glycerin. Alternatively, one tablet can be submerged in 10 ml of hot water and added to 10 ml of honey or syrup. When prepared in a 70% sorbitol solution with a pH of 4 to 5 and stored in amber glass bottles, the suspension is stable for ≥ 2 to 3 months at temperatures < 30°C (86°F).

METHAZOLAMIDE

Rx	**Methazolamide** (Various, eg, Mikart)	**Tablets:** 25 mg	In 100s.
		50 mg	In 100s.

For complete prescribing information, refer to the Carbonic Anhydrase Inhibitor group monograph.

Administration and Dosage

➤*Glaucoma:* 50 to 100 mg 2 or 3 times daily. May be used with miotic and osmotic agents.

DIURETIC COMBINATIONS

Rx	**Amiloride/ Hydrochlorothiazide-** (Various, eg, Goldline, Warner Chilcott)	**Tablets:** 5 mg amiloride HCl and 50 mg hydrochlorothiazide	In 100s, 500s and 1000s.
Rx	**Moduretic** (Merck)		Lactose. (917). Peach, scored. Diamond shape. In 100s and UD 100s.
Rx	**Spironolactone/ Hydrochlorothiazide** (Various, eg, Danbury, Goldline, Mylan)	**Tablets:** 25 mg spironolactone and 25 mg hydrochlorothiazide	In 100s, 250s, 500s and 1000s.
Rx	**Aldactazide** (Searle)		(Searle 1011 Aldactazide 25). Tan. Film coated. In 100s, 500s, 1000s and UD 100s.
Rx	**Aldactazide** (Searle)	**Tablets:** 50 mg spironolactone and 50 mg hydrochlorothiazide	(Searle 1021 Aldactazide 50). Tan, scored. In 100s and UD 100s.
Rx	**Triamterene/ Hydrochlorothiazide** (Various, eg, Geneva)	**Tablets:** 37.5 mg triamterene and 25 mg hydrochlorothiazide	In 100s, 500s and 1000s.
Rx	**Maxzide-25MG** (Bertek)		(Maxzide LL M9). Lt. green, scored. Bow-tie shape. In 100s, UD 100s.
Rx	**Triamterene/Hydrochlorothiazide** (Duramed)	**Capsules:** 37.5 mg triamterene and 25 mg hydrochlorothiazide	Lactose. (DPI/488). White. In 1000s.
Rx	**Dyazide** (SmithKline Beecham)		Lactose. (Dyazide). Red and white. In 1000s, unit-of-use 100s and UD 100s.
Rx	**Triamterene/Hydrochlorothiazide-** (Various, eg, Geneva, Goldline, Zenith)	**Capsules:** 50 mg triamterene and 25 mg hydrochlorothiazide	In 100s and 1000s.
Rx	**Triamterene/Hydrochlorothiazide-** (Various, eg, Barr, Danbury, Geneva, Goldline, Major, Schein, UDL, Warner Chilcott)	**Tablets:** 75 mg triamterene and 50 mg hydrochlorothiazide	In 100s, 250s, 500s, 1000s, and UD 100s.
Rx	**Maxzide** (Bertek)		(Maxzide LL M8). Lt. yellow, scored. Bow-tie shape. In 100s, 500s, UD 100s.

For complete information concerning the components of the combined diuretic products, consult the appropriate drug monographs in the Diuretics section.

Administration and Dosage

Fixed-dose combination drugs are not indicated for initial therapy of edema or hypertension; they require therapy titrated to the individual patient. If the fixed combination represents the determined dosage, its use may be more convenient in patient management. The treatment of hypertension and edema is not static; reevaluate as conditions in each patient warrant.

Dosage for each combination/strength varies. Refer to labeling for specific guidelines.

➤*Amiloride/Hydrochlorothiazide:* 1 to 2 tablets daily with meals.

➤*Spironolactone/Hydrochlorothiazide:*
25 mg/25 mg – 1 to 8 tablets daily.
50 mg/50 mg – 1 to 4 tablets daily.

➤*Triamterene/Hydrochlorothiazide:*
37.5 mg/25 mg – 1 or 2 tablets/capsules daily.
50 mg/25 mg – 1 or 2 capsules twice daily after meals.
75 mg/50 mg – 1 tablet daily.

Actions

➤*Pharmacology:* The combination of a thiazide and a potassium-sparing diuretic provides additive diuretic activity and antihypertensive effects through different mechanisms of action and also minimizes the potassium depletion characteristics of thiazides.

Precautions

➤*Triamterene/Hydrochlorothiazide:*
Bioavailability – Use caution when changing to another triamterene/hydrochlorothiazide combination product. Combination products are not equivalent.

Osmotic Diuretics

Actions

➤*Pharmacology:* Osmotic agents induce diuresis by elevating the osmolarity of the glomerular filtrate, thereby hindering the tubular reabsorption of water. Excretion of sodium and chloride is increased. These agents are freely filtered at the glomerulus; poorly reabsorbed by the renal tubule; not secreted by the tubule; relatively pharmacologically inert; usually resistant to metabolic alteration (except glycerin). Activity in the kidneys depends on the concentration of osmotically active particles in solution.

The main indication for osmotic diuretics (primarily mannitol) is prophylaxis of acute renal failure in conditions in which glomerular filtration is greatly reduced (ie, severe trauma, cardiovascular operations). By maintaining a flow of dilute urine, damage to the nephron by high concentrations of toxic solute does not occur. They are also employed to reduce intracranial pressure and elevated intraocular pressure. In the eyes, these agents act by creating an osmotic gradient between the plasma and ocular fluids.

Mannitol is the most widely used osmotic diuretic. The other agents include urea, glycerin and isosorbide. For specific approved indications, refer to individual drug monographs.

➤*Pharmacokinetics:* **Mannitol** is only slightly metabolized, while the rest is freely filtered by the glomeruli and excreted intact in urine. About 7% is reabsorbed by the renal tubules. Approximately 90% of an injected dose is recovered in urine after 24 hours. In severe renal insufficiency, the rate of mannitol excretion is greatly reduced; retained mannitol may increase extracellular tonicity, expand the extracellular fluid and induce an apparent hyponatremia with increased serum osmolality.

Osmotic Diuretics Pharmacokinetics

Diuretic	Route	Onset (min)	Peak (hrs)	Duration (hrs)	Half-life	Metabolized (%)	Ocular penetration	Distribution
Glycerin	PO	10-30	1-1.5	4-5	30-45 minutes	80	poor	E[1]
Isosorbide	PO	10-30	1-1.5	5-6	5-9.5 hrs	0	good	TBW[2]
Mannitol	IV	30-60	1	6-8	15-100 minutes	7-10	very poor	E[1]
Urea	IV	30-45	1	5-6	-	-	good	TBW[2]

[1] E = extracellular water   [2] TBW = total body water

MANNITOL

Rx	**Osmitrol** (Baxter)	**Injection:** 5%		In 1000 ml.
		10%		In 500 and 1000 ml.
		15%		In 500 ml.
		20%		In 250 and 500 ml.
Rx	**Mannitol** (Various, eg, American Regent,IMS, Pasadena)	**Injection:** 25%		In 50 ml.

Refer to the general discussion of these agents in the Osmotic Diuretics Introduction.

Indications

➤*Therapeutic:* To promote diuresis in the prevention or treatment of the oliguric phase of acute renal failure before irreversible renal failure becomes established.

Reduction of intracranial pressure and treatment of cerebral edema by reducing brain mass.

Reduction of elevated intraocular pressure when the pressure cannot be lowered by other means.

To promote urinary excretion of toxic substances.

➤*Urologic irrigation (2.5% only):* Irrigation in transurethral prostatic resection or other transurethral surgical procedures.

Administration and Dosage

Administer by IV infusion only. Individualize concentration and rate of administration. The usual adult dose ranges from 20 to 200 g/24 hours; in most instances, an adequate response will be achieved with 50 to 100 g/24 hours. Adjust the administration rate to maintain a urine flow of ≥ 30 to 50 ml/hour.

➤*Test dose:* For patients with marked oliguria or inadequate renal function, give 0.2 g/kg (about 50 ml of a 25% solution, 75 ml of a 20% solution, or 100 ml of a 15% solution) infused over 3 to 5 minutes. If urine flow does not increase, administer a second test dose. If response is inadequate, reevaluate the patient.

➤*Prevention of acute renal failure (oliguria):*
Adults – 50 to 100 g as a 5% to 25% solution during cardiovascular and other types of surgery.

➤*Treatment of oliguria:*
Adults – 50 to 100 g of a 15% to 25% solution.

➤*Reduction of intracranial pressure and brain mass:* 1.5 to 2 g/kg as a 15% to 25% solution, infused over 30 to 60 minutes, to reduce brain mass before or after neurosurgery. Evaluate the circulatory and renal reserve, fluid and electrolyte balance, body weight, and total input and output before and after mannitol infusion. Reduced cerebrospinal fluid pressure may be observed within 15 minutes after starting infusion.

➤*Reduction of intraocular pressure:* 1.5 to 2 g/kg, as a 20% solution (7.5 to 10 ml/kg) or as a 15% solution (10 to 13 ml/kg) over a period as short as 30 minutes. When used preoperatively, administer 1 to 1.5 hours before surgery to achieve maximal effect.

➤*Adjunctive therapy to promote diuresis in intoxications:* The concentration depends on the fluid requirement and urinary output of the patient. Give IV fluids and electrolytes to replace losses. If benefits are not seen after 200 g mannitol, discontinue the infusion.

➤*Urologic irrigation:* Use 2.5% solution. The use of 2.5% mannitol solution minimizes hemolytic effect of water alone, the entrance of hemolyzed blood into the circulation, and the resulting hemoglobinemia which is considered a major factor in producing serious renal complications.

Dilution of mannitol – Add contents of two 50 ml vials (25% mannitol) to 900 ml sterile water for injection.

➤*Preparation of solution:* When exposed to low temperatures, mannitol solution may crystallize. Concentrations > 15% have a greater tendency to crystallize. If crystals are observed, warm the bottle in a hot water bath, a dry heat oven or autoclave, then cool to body temperature or less before administering.

When infusing concentrated mannitol, the administration set should include a filter.

Contraindications

Anuria due to severe renal disease; severe pulmonary congestion or frank pulmonary edema; active intracranial bleeding except during craniotomy; severe dehydration; progressive renal damage or dysfunction after instituting mannitol therapy, including increasing oliguria and azotemia; progressive heart failure or pulmonary congestion after mannitol therapy.

Warnings

➤*Fluid and electrolyte imbalance:* By sustaining diuresis, mannitol may obscure and intensify inadequate hydration or hypovolemia. Excessive loss of water and electrolytes may lead to serious imbalances. Loss of water in excess of electrolytes can cause hypernatremia. Shift of sodium free intracellular fluid into the extracellular compartment following mannitol infusion may lower serum sodium concentration and aggravate preexisting hyponatremia. Also, movement of potassium ions from intracellular to extracellular space may cause hyperkalemia. Electrolyte measurements, including sodium and potassium, are therefore of vital importance in monitoring mannitol infusion.

➤*Renal function impairment:* Use a test dose (see Administration and Dosage); try a second test dose if there is an inadequate response, but do not attempt > 2 test doses.

If urine output continues to decline during infusion, closely review the patient's clinical status and suspend mannitol infusion, if necessary. Accumulation of mannitol may result in overexpansion of the extracellular fluid which may intensify existing or latent CHF.

Osmotic nephrosis, a reversible vacuolization of the tubules of unknown clinical significance, may proceed to severe irreversible nephrosis; monitor renal function closely.

➤*Pregnancy: Category C.* It is not known whether mannitol can cause fetal harm when administered to a pregnant woman or can affect reproduction capacity. Give to a pregnant woman only if clearly needed.

MANNITOL

➤*Lactation:* It is not known whether this drug is excreted in breast milk; exercise caution when administering to a nursing woman.

➤*Children:* Safety and efficacy for patients ≤ 12 years of age has not been established.

Precautions

➤*CHF:* Carefully evaluate cardiovascular status before rapid administration of mannitol since sudden expansion of the extracellular fluid may lead to fulminating CHF.

➤*Hypovolemia:* By sustaining diuresis, mannitol may obscure and intensify inadequate hydration or hypovolemia.

➤*Pseudoagglutination:* Do not give electrolyte free mannitol solutions with blood. If blood is given simultaneously, add ≥ 20 mEq of sodium chloride to each liter of mannitol solution to avoid pseudoagglutination.

➤*Hemoconcentration:* The obligatory diuretic response following rapid infusion of 15%, 20% or 25% mannitol may further aggravate pre-existing hemoconcentration.

Adverse Reactions

➤*Cardiovascular:* Edema; thrombophlebitis; hypotension; hypertension; tachycardia; angina-like chest pains; CHF.

➤*CNS:* Headache; blurred vision; convulsions; dizziness.

➤*GI:* Nausea; vomiting; diarrhea.

➤*Renal:* Urinary retention; osmotic nephrosis.

➤*Metabolic:* Fluid and electrolyte imbalance; acidosis; electrolyte loss; dehydration.

➤*Miscellaneous:* Pulmonary congestion; dry mouth; thirst; rhinitis; local pain; skin necrosis; chills; urticaria; fever.

Overdosage

➤*Symptoms:* Larger than recommended doses may result in increased electrolyte excretion, particularly sodium, chloride and potassium. Sodium depletion can result in orthostatic tachycardia or hypotension and decreased central venous pressure. Chloride metabolism closely follows that of sodium. Potassium deficit can impair neuromuscular function and cause intestinal dilation and ileus. If urine flow is inadequate, pulmonary edema or water intoxication may occur. Other symptoms include hypotension, polyuria that rapidly converts to oliguria, stupor, convulsions, hyperosmolality, hyponatremia.

➤*Treatment:* Discontinue infusion immediately. Institute supportive measures to correct fluid and electrolyte imbalances. Hemodialysis is beneficial to clear mannitol and reduce serum osmolality.

UREA

Rx	Ureaphil (Abbott)	Injection: 40 g per 150 ml	In single-dose containers.

Refer to the general discussion of these agents in the Osmotic Diuretics Introduction.

Indications

The 30% solution is used to reduce intracranial pressure (in the control of cerebral edema) and intraocular pressure.

➤*Unlabeled uses:* Intra-amniotic injection has been used to induce abortion.

Administration and Dosage

Administer as a 30% solution by slow IV infusion, at a rate not to exceed 4 ml/minute.

An isosmotic concentration of dextrose or invert sugar is administered with urea to prevent the hemolysis produced by pure solutions of urea.

Do not exceed 120 g/day.

➤*Adults:* 1 to 1.5 g/kg (0.45 to 0.68 g/lb).

➤*Children:* 0.5 to 1.5 g/kg. In children up to 2 years of age, as little as 0.1 g/kg may be adequate.

➤*Preparation of solution:* For 135 ml of a 30% solution of sterile urea, mix the contents of one 40 g vial with 105 ml of 5% or 10% Dextrose Injection or Invert Sugar. Each ml of a 30% solution provides 300 mg of urea. Use fresh solution; discard any unused portion within 24 hours after reconstitution.

Contraindications

Severely impaired renal function; active intracranial bleeding; marked dehydration; frank liver failure; infusion into veins of the lower extremities of elderly patients (phlebitis and thrombosis of superficial and deep veins may occur).

Warnings

➤*Electrolyte imbalance:* Urea may cause depletion of electrolytes that can result in hyponatremia and hypokalemia.

➤*Extravasation:* Extravasation of the solution at the injection site may cause local reactions ranging from mild irritation to tissue necrosis.

➤*Renal function impairment:* Administer with caution. Mild elevation of BUN does not preclude its use. Perform frequent laboratory studies; determine if renal function is adequate to eliminate the infused urea and that produced endogenously.

Patients exhibiting a temporary reduction in urine volume are generally able to maintain a satisfactory elimination of urea. However, if diuresis does not follow the injection of urea in such patients within 6 to 12 hours, withdraw the drug pending further evaluation of renal function.

To ensure bladder emptying, use an indwelling urethral catheter in comatose patients.

➤*Hepatic function impairment:* Administer with caution in patients with liver impairment, since there may be a significant rise in blood ammonia levels.

➤*Pregnancy: Category C.* Safety for use during pregnancy has not been established. Use only when clearly needed and when the potential benefits outweigh the potential hazards to the fetus.

➤*Lactation:* It is not known whether this drug is excreted in breast milk. Exercise caution when administering to a nursing mother.

Precautions

➤*Intracranial bleeding:* Arterial oozing has been reported when intracranial surgery is performed on patients following treatment with urea; however, this has not been a significant problem. Do not use in the presence of active intracranial bleeding unless such use is preliminary to prompt surgical intervention to control hemorrhage. Reduction of brain edema induced by urea may result in reactivation of intracranial bleeding.

➤*Rapid IV administration:* Rapid IV administration of hypertonic solutions of urea may be associated with hemolysis as well as a direct effect on the cerebral vasomotor centers that may result in increased capillary bleeding. Do not exceed an infusion rate of 4 ml/minute.

➤*Blood loss:* Urea may temporarily maintain circulatory volume and blood pressure in spite of considerable blood loss. Consequently, when excessive blood loss occurs within a short period of time, blood replacement should be adequate and simultaneous with the infusion of urea. Do not administer urea through the same administration set that blood is being infused. Hypothermia, when used with urea infusion, may increase the risk of venous thrombosis and hemoglobinuria.

Drug Interactions

➤*Lithium:* Urea may increase the renal excretion of lithium, thereby decreasing its effects.

Adverse Reactions

No serious reactions have been noted when solutions are infused slowly, provided renal function is not seriously impaired and there is no active intracranial bleeding. If an adverse reaction occurs, discontinue the infusion, evaluate the patient and institute appropriate therapy; save the remainder of the fluid for examination.

The following reactions have occurred: Headaches (similar to those following lumbar puncture); nausea; vomiting; syncope; disorientation; transient agitated confusional state (less frequent); chemical phlebitis and thrombosis near the injection site (infrequent).

Reactions that may occur because of the reconstituted solution or the technique of administration include the following: Febrile response; infection at the injection site; venous thrombosis or phlebitis extending from the injection site; extravasation; hypervolemia.

Overdosage

In the event of overdosage, as reflected by unusually elevated blood urea nitrogen (BUN) levels, discontinue the drug, evaluate the patient and institute corrective measures.

GLYCERIN (Glycerol)

| *Rx* | **Osmoglyn** (Alcon) | **Solution:** 50% (0.6 g glycerin/ml) | Lime flavor. In 220 ml. |

Refer to the general discussion of these agents in the Osmotic Diuretics Introduction.

Indications

➤*Glaucoma:* To interrupt acute attacks.

➤*Prior to and after ocular surgery:* Where reduction of intraocular pressure is indicated.

➤*Unlabeled uses:* Glycerin has also been given by the IV route (with proper preparation) to lower intraocular and intracranial pressure.

Administration and Dosage

1 to 2 g/kg, 1 to 1.5 hours prior to surgery.

Actions

➤*Pharmacology:* An oral osmotic agent for reducing intraocular pressure. It adds to the tonicity of the blood until metabolized and eliminated by the kidneys. Maximal reduction of intraocular pressure will occur 1 hour after glycerin administration. The effect will last ≈ 5 hours.

Contraindications

Well established anuria; severe dehydration; frank or impending acute pulmonary edema; severe cardiac decompensation; hypersensitivity to any of the ingredients.

Warnings

➤*Route of administration:* For oral use only; not for injection.

➤*Pregnancy:* Category C. Safety for use during pregnancy has not been established. Use only when clearly needed and when the potential benefits outweigh the potential hazards to the fetus.

Precautions

➤*Urinary retention:* Avoid acute urinary retention in the preoperative period. Continued use may result in weight gain.

➤*Special risk:* Use cautiously in hypervolemia, confused mental states, congestive heart disease, diabetic patients, severely dehydrated individuals and cardiac, renal or hepatic disease.

Adverse Reactions

Nausea, vomiting, headache, confusion and disorientation may occur. Severe dehydration, cardiac arrhythmias or hyperosmolar nonketotic coma which can result in death have been reported.

ISOSORBIDE

| *Rx* | **Ismotic** (Alcon) | **Solution:** 45% (100 g per 220 ml) | With 4.6 mEq sodium and 0.9 mEq potassium per 220 ml. Alcohol, saccharin, sorbitol. Vanilla-mint flavor. In 220 ml. |

Refer to the general discussion of these agents in the Osmotic Diuretics Introduction.

Indications

For the short-term reduction of intraocular pressure prior to and after intraocular surgery.

May be used to interrupt an acute attack of glaucoma. Use where less risk of nausea and vomiting than that posed by other oral hyperosmotic agents is needed.

Administration and Dosage

For oral use only.

➤*Initial dose:* 1.5 g/kg (equivalent to 1.5 ml/lb).

➤*Dose range:* 1 to 3 g/kg 2 to 4 times a day as indicated.

Palatability may be improved if the medication is poured over cracked ice and sipped.

Contraindications

Well established anuria; severe dehydration; frank or impending acute pulmonary edema; severe cardiac decompensation; hypersensitivity to any component of this preparation.

Warnings

➤*Fluid/Electrolyte balance:* With repeated doses, maintain adequate fluid and electrolyte balance.

➤*Urinary output:* If urinary output continues to decrease, closely review the patient's clinical status. Accumulation may result in overexpansion of the extracellular fluid.

➤*Pregnancy:* Category B. There is no adequate information on whether this drug affects fertility in humans or has a teratogenic potential or other adverse fetal effect. Use during pregnancy only if clearly needed.

Precautions

➤*Repetitive doses:* Use repetitive doses with caution, particularly in patients with diseases associated with salt retention. Ensure that the patient's bladder has been emptied prior to surgery.

Adverse Reactions

Nausea; vomiting; headache; confusion; disorientation; gastric discomfort; thirst; hiccoughs; hypernatremia; hyperosmolarity; rash; irritability; syncope; lethargy; vertigo; dizziness; lightheadedness.

NONPRESCRIPTION DIURETICS

otc	**Maximum Strength Aqua•Ban** (Thompson Medical)	**Tablets:** 50 mg pamabrom	Lactose. In 30s.

Indications

For the relief of temporary water weight gain, bloating, swelling, or full feeling associated with the premenstrual and menstrual periods.

Administration and Dosage

Take 1 tablet 4 times/day. Do not take > 4 tablets in a 24-hour period.

Nonprescription diuretic products are promoted for the alleviation of menstrual discomfort. When taken 5 to 6 days before onset of menses, *otc* diuretics may help relieve symptoms related to water retention. These include excess water weight, bloating, swelling, painful breasts, cramps, and tension.

The most frequently used *otc* diuretic agents are ammonium chloride and caffeine. These agents are classified as Category I (generally recognized as safe and effective and not misbranded).

Sympathomimetics

Indications

►*Bronchodilation:* Relief of reversible bronchospasm associated with acute and chronic bronchial asthma, exercise-induced bronchospasm (EIB), bronchitis, emphysema, bronchiectasis, or other obstructive pulmonary diseases.

According to the National Asthma Education and Prevention Program's Expert Panel Report II, long-acting β_2 agonists (eg, **salmeterol**) are used concomitantly with anti-inflammatory medications for long-term control of symptoms, especially nocturnal symptoms. They also prevent EIB. Short-acting β_2 agonists (eg, **albuterol**, **bitolterol**, **pirbuterol**, **terbutaline**) are the therapy of choice for relief of acute symptoms and prevention of EIB.

Refer to individual monographs for indications of specific agents.

Actions

►*Pharmacology:* Sympathomimetic agents are used to produce bronchodilation. They relieve reversible bronchospasm by relaxing the smooth muscles of the bronchioles in conditions associated with asthma, bronchitis, emphysema, or bronchiectasis. Bronchodilation may additionally facilitate expectoration. Some agents are also used for other purposes. See monographs for Vasopressors Used in Shock, Nasal Decongestants, and Ophthalmic Vasoconstrictors/Mydriatics.

The pharmacologic actions of these agents include: Alpha-adrenergic stimulation (vasoconstriction, nasal decongestion, pressor effects); β_1-adrenergic stimulation (increased myocardial contractility and conduction); and β_2-adrenergic stimulation (bronchial dilation and vasodilation, enhancement of mucociliary clearance, inhibition of cholinergic neurotransmission). Beta-adrenergic drugs stimulate adenyl cyclase, the enzyme that catalyzes the formation of cyclic-3'5' adenosine monophosphate (cyclic AMP) from adenosine triphosphate (ATP). Cyclic AMP that is formed inhibits the release of mediators of immediate hypersensitivity from inflammatory cells, especially from mast cells and basophils. This increase of cyclic AMP leads to activation of protein kinase A, which inhibits the phosphorylation of myosin and lowers intracellular ionic calcium concentrations, resulting in relaxation.

Other adrenergic actions include alpha receptor-mediated contraction of GI and urinary sphincters; α receptor-mediated lipolysis; α and β receptor-mediated decrease in GI tone; and changes in renin secretion, uterine relaxation, hepatic glycogenolysis/gluconeogenesis, and pancreatic beta cell secretion.

The relative selectivity of action of sympathomimetic agents is the primary determinant of clinical usefulness; it can predict the most likely side effects. β_2 selective agents provide the greatest benefit with minimal side effects. Direct administration via inhalation provides prompt effects and minimizes systemic activity. These drugs also inhibit histamine release from mast cells, produce vasodilation, and increase ciliary motility. Bitolterol functions as a prodrug that must first be hydrolyzed by esterases in tissue and blood to its active moiety, colterol. Isoproterenol is one of the most potent bronchodilators available.

Sympathomimetic Bronchodilators: Pharmacologic Effects and Pharmacokinetic Properties

Sympatho-mimetic	Adrenergic receptor activity		β_2 potency[1]	Route	Onset (minutes)	Duration (hrs)
Salmeterol[2]	β_1	$< \beta_2$	0.5	Inh	within 20	12
Albuterol[2]	β_1	$< \beta_2$	2	PO	within 30	4-8
				Inh[3]	within 5	3-6
Bitolterol[2]	β_1	$< \beta_2$	5	Inh	2-4	5 ≥ 8
Isoetharine[2]	β_1	$< \beta_2$	6	Inh[3]	within 5	2-3
Metaproterenol[2]	β_1	$< \beta_2$	15	PO	≈ 30	4
				Inh[3]	5-30	1- ≥ 6
Pirbuterol[2]	β_1	$< \beta_2$	5	Inh	within 5	5
Terbutaline[2]	β_1	$< \beta_2$	4	PO	30	4-8
				SC	5-15	1.5-4
				Inh	5-30	3-6
Isoproterenol	β_1	β_2	1	IV	immediate	< 1
				Inh[3]	2-5	1-3
Ephedrine	α β_1	β_2	—	PO	15-60	3-5
				SC	> 20	≤ 1
				IM	10-20	≤ 1
				IV	immediate	—
Epinephrine	α β_1	β_2	—	SC	5-10	4-6
				IM	—	1-4
				Inh[3]	1-5	1-3

[1] Relative molar potency: 1 = most potent.
[2] These agents all have minor β_1 activity.
[3] May be administered via aerosol or bulb nebulizer or IPPB administration.

Contraindications

Hypersensitivity to any component (allergic reactions are rare); cardiac arrhythmias associated with tachycardia; angina, preexisiting cardiac arrhythmias associated with tachycardia, known hypersensitivity to sympathomimetic amines, and ventricular arrhythmias requiring inotropic therapy, tachycardia or heart block caused by digitalis intoxication (**isoproterenol**); patients with organic brain damage, local anesthesia of certain areas (eg, fingers, toes) because of the risk of tissue sloughing, labor, cardiac dilitation, coronary insufficiency, cerebral arteriosclerosis, organic heart disease (**epinephrine**); in those cases where vasopressors may be contraindicated; narrow-angle glaucoma, nonanaphylactic shock during general anesthesia with halogenated hydrocarbons or cyclopropane (**epinephrine**, **ephedrine**).

Warnings

►*Special risk patients:* Administer with caution to patients with diabetes mellitus, hyperthyroidism, prostatic hypertrophy (**ephedrine**) or history of seizures; elderly; psychoneurotic individuals, patients with long-standing bronchial asthma and emphysema who have developed degenerative heart disease (**epinephrine**).

In patients with status asthmaticus and abnormal blood gas tensions, improvement in vital capacity and blood gas tensions may not accompany apparent relief of bronchospasm following isoproterenol. Facilities for administering oxygen and ventilatory assistance are necessary.

Diabetes – Large doses of IV **albuterol** and IV **terbutaline** may aggravate preexisting diabetes mellitus and ketoacidosis. Relevance to the use of oral or inhaled albuterol and oral terbutaline is unknown. Diabetic patients receiving any of these agents may require an increase in dosage of insulin or oral hypoglycemic agents.

►*Cardiovascular effects:* Use with caution in patients with cardiovascular disorders including coronary insufficiency, ischemic heart disease, coronary artery disease, cardiac arrhythmias, CHF, and hypertension.

Beta-adrenergic agonists can produce significant cardiovascular effects measured by pulse rate, blood pressure, symptoms, or ECG changes (eg, flattening of T-waves, prolongation of the QTc interval, and ST-segment depression).

Isoproterenol doses sufficient to increase the heart rate > 130 bpm may increase the likelihood of inducing ventricular arrhythmias.

These agents may cause toxic symptoms through idiosyncratic response or overdosage. If cardiac rate increases sharply, angina patients may experience anginal pain until the cardiac rate decreases.

Patients who were administered **bitolterol** did not reveal a preferential $\beta_2$adrenergic effect. At doses that produced long duration of bronchodilator activity with a mean maximum bronchodilating effect of ≈ 40% increase in FEV$_1$ (forced expiratory volume in 1 second), a < 10 beat/minute mean maximum increase in heart rate was seen. The effect on the heart rate was transient and similar to the increases seen in the isoproterenol-treated patients in these studies.

Closely monitor patients receiving **epinephrine**. Inadvertently induced high arterial blood pressure may result in angina pectoris, aortic rupture, or cerebral hemorrhage. Cardiac arrhythmias develop in some individuals even after therapeutic doses. Epinephrine causes changes in the ECG even in healthy people, including a decrease in amplitude of the T-wave.

Ephedrine may cause hypertension resulting in intracranial hemorrhage. It may induce anginal pain in patients with coronary insufficiency or ischemic heart disease.

Large doses of inhaled or oral **salmeterol** (12 to 20 times the recommended dose) have been associated with clinically significant prolongation of the QTc interval, which has the potential for producing ventricular arrhythmias.

Significant changes in systolic and diastolic blood pressure can occur in some patients after use of any beta-adrenergic aerosol bronchodilator.

►*Paradoxical bronchospasm:* Occasional patients have developed severe paradoxical airway resistance with repeated, excessive use of inhalation preparations; the cause is unknown. Discontinue the drug immediately and institute alternative therapy because patients may not respond to other therapy until the drug is withdrawn.

►*Usual dose response:* Advise patients to contact a physician if they do not respond to their usual dose of a sympathomimetic amine.

Close supervision is recommended in patients requiring > 3 **isoproterenol** aerosolized treatments. Further therapy with the bronchodilator aerosol alone is inadvisable when 3 to 5 treatments within 6 to 12 hours produce minimal or no relief. Reduce **epinephrine** dose if bronchial irritation, nervousness, restlessness, or sleeplessness occurs. Do not continue to use epinephrine, but seek medical assistance immediately if symptoms are not relieved within 20 minutes or become worse.

►*CNS effects:* Sympathomimetics may produce CNS stimulation.

IV **albuterol** sulfate in animals has demonstrated that it crosses the blood-brain barrier and reaches brain concentrations of ≈ 5% of the plasma concentrations.

➤*Long-term use:* Prolonged use of **ephedrine** may produce a syndrome resembling an anxiety state. Many patients develop nervousness and a sedative may be needed. After prolonged use or overdosage, elevated serum lactic acid levels with severe metabolic acidosis have occurred, as have transient blood glucose elevations.

➤*Acute symptoms:* Do not use **salmeterol** to treat acute asthma symptoms. If the patient's short-acting, inhaled β₂-agonist becomes less effective (eg, the patient needs more inhalations than usual), obtain medical evaluation immediately. Increasing its use in this situation is inappropriate. Do not use salmeterol more frequently than twice daily (morning and evening) at the recommended dose. When prescribing salmeterol, provide patients with a short-acting, inhaled β₂-agonist (eg, albuterol) for treatment of symptoms that occur despite regular twice-daily (morning and evening) use of salmeterol.

Asthma may deteriorate acutely over a period of hours or chronically over several days. In this setting, increased use of inhaled, short-acting β₂-agonists is a marker of destabilization of asthma and requires re-evaluation of the patient. Consider alternative treatment regimens, especially inhaled or systemic corticosteroids. If the patient uses ≥ 4 inhalations/day of a short-acting β₂-agonist on a regular basis, or if > 1 canister (200 inhalations per canister) is used in an 8-week period, have the patient see the physician for re-evaluation of treatment.

Use with short-acting β₂-agonists – When patients begin treatment with **salmeterol**, advise those who have been taking short-acting, inhaled β₂-agonists on a regular daily basis to discontinue their regular daily dosing regimen, and clearly instruct them to use short-acting, inhaled β₂-agonists only for symptomatic relief if they develop asthma symptoms while taking salmeterol.

➤*Morbidity/Mortality:* It was previously suggested that an increased risk of death or near death from asthma may be associated with the regular use of inhaled beta agonists. Another study demonstrated that patients with mild intermittent asthma were neither harmed nor did they benefit from regularly scheduled daily use of short-acting inhaled beta agonists. However, regularly scheduled, daily use of beta agonists is not recommended.

Excessive use of inhalants – Deaths from excessive use of inhaled sympathomimetics have been reported; the exact cause is unknown, but cardiac arrest following an unexpected severe acute asthmatic crisis and subsequent hypoxia is suspected.

➤*Overdosage/IV injection:* Overdosage or inadvertent IV injection of conventional SC **epinephrine** doses may cause extremely elevated arterial pressure, which may result in cerebrovascular hemorrhage, particularly in elderly patients; severe peripheral constriction and cardiac stimulation resulting in pulmonary arterial hypertension and potentially fatal pulmonary edema; and ventricular hyperirritability, which may result in death from ventricular fibrillation. Epinephrine is rapidly inactivated in the body, and treatment is primarily supportive. If necessary, pressor effects may be counteracted by rapidly acting vasodilators or alpha-adrenergic blocking drugs. If prolonged hypotension follows such measures, it may be necessary to administer another pressor drug, such as norepinephrine. If an epinephrine overdose induces pulmonary edema that interferes with respiration, treatment consists of a rapidly acting alpha-adrenergic blocking drug (eg, phentolamine) or intermittent positive-pressure respiration. Transient bradycardia followed by tachycardia may also result, and these may be accompanied by potentially fatal cardiac arrhythmias. Ventricular, premature contractions may appear within 1 minute after injection and may be followed by multifocal, ventricular tachycardia (prefibrillation rhythm). Subsidence of the ventricular effects may be followed by atrial tachycardia and occasionally by AV block. Treatment of arrhythmias consists of administration of a beta-adrenergic blocking drug, such as propranolol. Overdosage sometimes also results in extreme pallor and coldness of skin, metabolic acidosis, and kidney failure. Take suitable corrective measures.

➤*Respiratory depression:* When compressed oxygen is used as the aerosol propellant, determine the percentage of oxygen by the patient's individual requirements to avoid depression of respiratory drive.

➤*Hypersensitivity reactions:* Hypersensitivity (allergic) reactions can occur after administration of **bitolterol**, **albuterol**, **metaproterenol**, **terbutaline**, **ephedrine**, **salmeterol**, and possibly other bronchodilators. See Management of Acute Hypersensitivity Reactions.

➤*Carcinogenesis:* A significant increase in the incidence of leiomyomas of the mesovarium and ovarian cysts has been demonstrated with **albuterol** and **terbutaline** in animal studies. **Salmeterol** caused a dose-related increase in the incidence of smooth muscle hyperplasia and cystic glandular hyperplasia of the uterus in mice.

➤*Elderly:* Lower doses may be required because of increased sympathomimetic sensitivity. Observe special caution when using in elderly patients who have concomitant cardiovascular disease that could be adversely affected by this class of drug. Based on available data, no adjustment of **salmeterol** dosage in geriatric patients is warranted.

➤*Pregnancy:* Category B (**terbutaline**). Category C (**albuterol**, **bitolterol**, **ephedrine**, **epinephrine**, **isoetharine**, **isoproterenol**, **metaproterenol**, **salmeterol**, **pirbuterol**). Several of these agents are teratogenic and embryocidal in animal studies. There is no evidence

that these class effects in animals are relevant to use in humans. There are no adequate and well-controlled studies in pregnant women. Use only when clearly needed and when potential benefits outweigh potential hazards to the fetus.

Labor and delivery – Use of β₂-active sympathomimetics inhibits uterine contractions. Adverse reactions include increased heart rate, transient hyperglycemia, hypokalemia, cardiac arrhythmias, pulmonary edema, cerebral and myocardial ischemia, and increased fetal heart rate and hypoglycemia in the neonate. Although these effects are unlikely with aerosol use, consider the potential for untoward effects.

Oral **albuterol** has the potential to delay preterm labor. There are no well-controlled studies that demonstrate that they stop preterm labor or prevent labor at term. Therefore, use cautiously in pregnant patients when given for relief of bronchospasm to avoid interference with uterine contractility. **Terbutaline** is not indicated for and is not used for the management of preterm labor. Maternal death has occurred with terbutaline and other drugs in this class.

Parenteral administration of **ephedrine** to maintain blood pressure during low or other spinal anesthesia for delivery can cause acceleration of fetal heart rate; do not use in obstetrics when maternal blood pressure exceeds 130/80.

➤*Lactation:* **Terbutaline**, **ephedrine**, and **epinephrine** are excreted in breast milk. It is not known whether other agents are excreted in breast milk. Decide whether to discontinue nursing or to discontinue the drug, taking into account the importance of the drug to the mother.

➤*Children:*

Inhalation – Safety and efficacy for use of **bitolterol**, **pirbuterol**, **isoetharine**, **salmeterol**, and **terbutaline** in children ≤ 12 years of age have not been established. **Albuterol** aerosol and inhalation powder in children < 4 years of age and **albuterol** solution for inhalation in children < 2 years of age have not been established. **Metaproterenol** may be used in children ≥ 6 years of age.

Injection – Parenteral **terbutaline** is not recommended for use in children < 12 years of age. Administer **epinephrine** with caution to infants and children. Syncope has occurred following administration to asthmatic children.

Oral – **Metaproterenol** is not recommended for use in children < 6 years of age. **Terbutaline** is not recommended for use in children < 12 years of age. Safety and efficacy have not been established for **albuterol** in children < 2 years of age (syrup) and < 6 years of age (tablets and extended release tablets).

In children, **ephedrine** is effective in the oral therapy of asthma. Because of its CNS-stimulating effect, it is rarely used alone. This effect is usually countered by an appropriate sedative; however, its rationale has been questioned.

Precautions

➤*Tolerance:* Tolerance may occur with prolonged use of sympathomimetic agents, but temporary cessation of the drug restores its original effectiveness.

➤*Hypokalemia:* Decreases in serum potassium levels have occurred, possibly through intracellular shunting, which can produce adverse cardiovascular effects. The decrease is usually transient, not requiring supplementation.

➤*Hyperglycemia:* **Isoproterenol** causes less hyperglycemia than does **epinephrine**. Isoproterenol and epinephrine are equally effective in stimulating the release of free fatty acids and energy production.

Glycogenolysis in the liver is increased by **ephedrine** but not as much as by **epinephrine**; usual doses of ephedrine are unlikely to produce hyperglycemia.

➤*Parkinson's disease:* **Epinephrine** may temporarily increase rigidity and tremor.

➤*Parenteral use:* Administer **epinephrine** with great caution and in carefully circumscribed quantities in areas of the body served by end arteries or with otherwise limited blood supply (eg, fingers, toes, nose, ears, genitals) or if peripheral vascular disease is present to avoid vasoconstriction-induced tissue sloughing.

➤*Combined therapy:* Concomitant use with other sympathomimetic agents is not recommended, as it may lead to deleterious cardiovascular effects. This does not preclude the judicious use of an adrenergic stimulant aerosol bronchodilator in patients receiving tablets. Do not give on a routine basis. If regular coadministration is required, consider alternative therapy.

Do not use ≥ 2 beta-adrenergic aerosol bronchodilators simultaneously because of the potential of additive effects.

Patients must be warned not to stop or reduce corticosteroid therapy without medical advice, even if they feel better when they are being treated with β₂ agonists. These agents are not to be used as a substitute for oral or inhaled corticosteroids.

➤*Sulfites:* Some of these products contain sulfites that may cause allergic-type reactions (including anaphylactic symptoms and life-threatening or less severe asthmatic episodes) in certain susceptible

Sympathomimetics

persons. The overall prevalence of sulfite sensitivity in the general population is unknown and probably low. It is seen more frequently in asthmatic or atopic nonasthmatic persons.

➤*Benzyl alcohol:* Benzyl alcohol, contained in some of these products as a preservative, has been associated with a fatal "gasping syndrome" in premature infants.

➤*Drug abuse and dependence:* Prolonged abuse of **ephedrine** can lead to symptoms of paranoid schizophrenia. Patients exhibit such signs as tachycardia, poor nutrition and hygiene, fever, cold sweat, and dilated pupils. Some measure of tolerance develops, but addiction does not occur. With all sympathomimetic aerosols, cardiac arrest and even death may be associated with abuse.

Drug Interactions

Most interactions listed apply to sympathomimetics when used as vasopressors; however, consider the interaction when using the bronchodilator sympathomimetics.

Sympathomimetic Bronchodilator Drug Interactions			
Precipitant drug	Object drug*		Description
Beta blockers	Sympatho-mimetics	↓	Concomitant use may inhibit cardiac, bronchodilating, and vasodilating effects. Severe bronchospasms may be produced in asthmatic patients taking **albuterol** or **salmeterol**. Consider cardioselective beta blockers, and use with caution if there are no alternatives to beta blocker therapy. With **epinephrine**, an initial hypertensive episode followed by bradycardia may occur.
Furazolidone	Sympatho-mimetics	↑	The pressor sensitivity to mixed-acting sympathomimetics (eg, **ephedrine**) may be increased. Direct-acting agents (eg, **epinephrine**) are not affected.
Guanethidine	Sympatho-mimetics		Guanethidine potentiates the effects of the direct-acting sympathomimetics (eg, **epinephrine**) and inhibits the effects of the mixed-acting agents (eg, **ephedrine**). Guanethidine hypotensive action may also be reversed, requiring increased guanethidine dosage.
	Direct	↑	
	Mixed	↓	
Sympatho-mimetics	Guanethidine	↓	
Methyldopa	Sympatho-mimetics	↑	Concurrent administration may result in an increased pressor response.
MAO inhibitors	Sympatho-mimetics	↑	Coadministration of MAO inhibitors and mixed-acting sympathomimetics (eg, **ephedrine**) may result in severe headache, hypertension, and hyperpyrexia, resulting in hypertensive crisis. MAO inhibitors also potentiate the actions of beta-adrenergic agonists on the vascular system. Direct-acting agents (eg, **epinephrine**) interact minimally. Avoid coadministration with sympathomimetics or within 2 weeks.
Oxytocic drugs (eg, ergonovine)	Sympatho-mimetics	↓	Concurrent administration may result in severe hypotension.

Sympathomimetic Bronchodilator Drug Interactions			
Precipitant drug	Object drug*		Description
Rauwolfia alkaloids	Sympatho-mimetics		Reserpine potentiates the pressor response of the direct-acting sympathomimetics (eg, **epinephrine**), which may result in hypertension. The pressor response of the mixed-acting agents (eg, **ephedrine**) is decreased.
	Direct	↑	
	Mixed	↓	
Tricyclic antidepressants (TCAs)	Sympatho-mimetics		TCAs potentiate the pressor response of direct-acting sympathomimetics (eg, **epinephrine**); dysrhythmias have occurred. The pressor response of mixed-acting agents (eg, **ephedrine**) is decreased. TCAs also potentiate the actions of beta-adrenergic agonists on the vascular system.
	Direct	↑	
	Mixed	↓	
Sympatho-mimetics	Theophylline	↔	Enhanced toxicity, particularly cardiotoxicity, has been noted. Decreased theophylline levels may occur. **Ephedrine** may cause theophylline toxicity.
General anesthetics (eg, halothane, cyclopropane) Cardiac glycosides	Isoproterenol Epinephrine Ephedrine	↑	The potential for the myocardium to be sensitized to the effects of sympathomimetic amines is increased. Arrhythmias may result with coadministration and may respond to beta blockers.
Alpha-adrenergic blockers (eg, phentolamine)	Ephedrine Epinephrine	↓	Vasoconstricting and hypertensive effects are antagonized.
Diuretics	Ephedrine Epinephrine	↓	Vascular response may be decreased.
Antihistamines	Epinephrine	↑	**Epinephrine** effects may be potentiated.
Ergot alkaloids Phenothiazines Nitrites	Epinephrine	↓	Pressor effects of epinephrine may be reversed.
Levothyroxine	Epinephrine	↑	**Epinephrine** effects may be potentiated.
Epinephrine	Insulin or oral hypoglycemic agents	↓	Diabetics may require an increased dose of the hypoglycemic agent.
Ergot alkaloids Isoproterenol	Isoproterenol Ergot alkaloids	↑	Coadministration may result in additive peripheral vasoconstriction.
Albuterol Salmeterol	Diuretics	↑	ECG changes and hypokalemia associated with these diuretics may worsen with coadministration.
Albuterol	Digoxin	↓	Digoxin serum levels may be decreased.

* ↑ = Object drug increased. ↓ = Object drug decreased. ↔ = Undetermined clinical effect.

➤*Drug/Lab test interactions:* **Isoproterenol** causes false elevations of bilirubin as measured in vitro by a sequential multiple analyzer. Isoproterenol inhalation may result in enough absorption of the drug to produce elevated urinary **epinephrine** values. Although small with standard doses, the effect is likely to increase with larger doses.

Adverse Reactions

Sympathomimetic Bronchodilator Adverse Reactions (%)[1]										
Adverse reaction	Salmeterol	Albuterol	Bitolterol	Isoetharine	Metaproterenol	Pirbuterol	Terbutaline	Isoproterenol	Ephedrine	Epinephrine
Cardiovascular										
Palpitations	1-3	< 1-10	1.5-3	✔[2]	0.3-4	1.3-1.7	≤ 23	< 5-22	✔	7.8-30
Tachycardia	1-3	1-10	< 3.7	✔	< 17	1.2-1.3	1.3-3	2-12	✔	≤ 2.6
Blood pressure changes/ hypertension		1-5	< 1	✔	0.3		< 1	2-5		✔
Chest tightness/pain/discomfort, angina		< 3	≤ 1.5		0.2	< 1.3	1.3-1.5	✔		≤ 2.6
PVCs, arrhythmias, skipped beats			0.5			< 1	≈ 4	< 1-3	✔	✔

Sympathomimetics

Sympathomimetic Bronchodilator Adverse Reactions (%)[1]

Adverse reaction	Salmeterol	Albuterol	Bitolterol	Isoetharine	Metaproterenol	Pirbuterol	Terbutaline	Isoproterenol	Ephedrine	Epinephrine
CNS										
Tremor	4	< 1-24.2	9-26.6	✔	1-33	1.3-6	< 5-38	< 15		16-18
Dizziness/vertigo	≥ 3	< 1-7	1-4	✔	1-4	0.6-1.2	1.3-10	1.5-5	✔	3.3-7.8
Shakiness/nervousness/tension	1-3	1-20	1.5-11.1	✔	2.6-14	4.5-7	< 5-31	< 15	✔	8.5-31
Weakness		< 2		✔	1.3	< 1	≤ 1.3	✔		1.6-2.6
Drowsiness		< 1			0.7		< 5-11.7	< 5		8.2-14
Restlessness		< 1		✔						✔
Hyperactivity/Hyperkinesia, excitement		1-20	< 1	✔		< 1		✔		
Headache	28	2-22	≤ 8.4	✔	≤ 4	1.3-2	7.8-10	1.5-10	✔	3.3-10
Insomnia		1-11	< 1	✔	1.8	< 1	✔	1.5	✔	✔
GI										
Nausea/Vomiting	1-3	2-15	≤ 3	✔	< 14	≤ 1.7	1.3-10	< 15	✔	1-11.5
Heartburn/GI distress/disorder	1-3	≤ 5			≤ 4		< 10	≤ 5-10		
Diarrhea	1-3	1			0.7	< 1.3				
Dry mouth		< 3			1.3	< 1.3				
Respiratory										
Cough	7	< 1-5	≤ 4.1		≤ 4	1.2		1-5		
Wheezing		≤ 1.5					✔	1.5		
Dyspnea		1.5	≤ 1				≤ 2	≤ 1.5		≤ 2
Bronchospasm		1-15.4	≤ 1.5					≤ 18		
Throat dryness/irritation, pharyngitis	≥ 3	≤ 6	2.5-5		≤ 4	< 1	✔	3.1		
Miscellaneous										
Flushing		< 1	< 1			< 1	≤ 2.4	✔		≤ 1.3
Sweating		< 1					≤ 2.4	✔	✔	✔
Anorexia/Appetite loss		1				< 1			✔	✔
Unusual/bad taste or taste/smell change		< 1			≤ 0.3	< 1	✔			

[1] Data pooled for all routes of administration, all age groups, from separate studies, and are not necessarily comparable.

[2] ✔ = Reported; no incidence given.

Adverse reactions are generally transient, and no cumulative effects have been reported. It is usually not necessary to discontinue treatment; however, in selected cases temporarily reduce dosage. After the reaction has subsided, increase dosage in small increments to optimal dosage. In addition to the table, other adverse reactions are as follows:

➤**Albuterol:**
CNS – CNS stimulation, malaise (1.5%); emotional lability, fatigue, nightmares, aggressive behavior (1%); lightheadedness, disturbed sleep, irritability (< 1%).

Respiratory – Bronchitis (1.5% to 4%); nasal congestion (1% to 2%); sputum increase (1.5%); epistaxis (1% to 3%); hoarseness (rare in adults; 2% in children 4 to 12 years old).

Miscellaneous – Increased appetite, stomachache (3%); muscle cramps (1% to 3%); pallor, conjunctivitis, anorexia, teeth discoloration, dyspepsia (1%); dilated pupils, epigastric pain, micturition difficulty, muscle spasm, voice changes (< 1%); urticaria, angioedema, rash, bronchospasm, oropharyngeal edema (rare with oral and inhaled albuterol). Rarely, erythema multiforme and Stevens-Johnson syndrome have been associated with the administration of albuterol sulfate syrup in children. There have been rare reports of GI obstruction in such patients in association with ingestion of products containing delivery systems similar to that contained in albuterol sulfate extended-release tablets.

➤**Bitolterol:**
Miscellaneous – Lightheadedness (6.8%). Elevations of AST, decrease in platelets and WBC counts and proteinuria (rare); clinical relevance or relationship is unknown. The overall incidence of cardiovascular effects was ≈ 5%.

➤**Ephedrine:** Precordial pain; contact dermatitis after topical application.

Parenteral: Vesical sphincter spasm from repeated injections resulting in difficult and painful urination; urinary retention in males with prostatism. Confusion, delirium, and hallucinations; cerebral hemorrhage.

➤**Epinephrine:** Anxiety; fear; pallor.
Parenteral: Cerebral hemorrhage; induce or aggravate psychomotor agitation; disorientation; impairment of memory; assaultive behavior; panic; hallucinations; suicidal or homicidal tendencies; schizophrenic-type thought disorders or paranoid delusions; hemiplegia; and subarachnoid and cerebral hemorrhage; direct vasoconstrictive effect on the renal circulation; syncope in children; temporary rigidity and tremor in Parkinson's disease patients; fatal ventricular fibrillation; occlusion of the central retinal artery, shock, and angina in coronary-artery disease; urticaria, wheal, and hemorrhage at injection site; pain at injection site (1.6% to 2.6%); local tissue necrosis from vascular constriction due to repeated injections at the same site.

➤**Isoetharine:**
Miscellaneous – Anxiety.

➤**Isoproterenol:**
Cardiovascular – Adams-Stokes attacks; cardiac arrest; hypotension; precordial ache/distress. In a few patients, presumably with organic disease of the AV node and its branches, isoproterenol has precipitated Adams-Stokes seizures during normal sinus rhythm or transient heart block.

Respiratory – Bronchitis (5%); sputum increase (1.5%); rebound bronchospasm; coronary insufficiency; paradoxical airway resistance; pulmonary edema.

➤**Metaproterenol:**
Respiratory – Asthma exacerbation (1% to 4%); hoarseness, nasal congestion (0.7%).

Miscellaneous – Rash (1.3%); backache, fatigue, skin reaction (0.7%).

➤*Pirbuterol:*

CNS – Anxiety, confusion, depression, fatigue, syncope (< 1%).

Dermatologic – Alopecia, edema, pruritus, rash, bruising (< 1%).

GI – Abdominal pain/cramps, glossitis, stomatitis (< 1%).

Miscellaneous – Hypotension, numbness in extremities, weight gain (< 1%).

➤*Salmeterol:*

Respiratory – Upper respiratory tract infection, nasopharyngitis (14%); nasal cavity/sinus disease (6%); sinus headache, lower respiratory tract infection (4%); allergic rhinitis (≥ 3%); rhinitis, laryngitis, tracheitis/bronchitis (1% to 3%).

Musculoskeletal – Joint/back pain, muscle cramp/contraction, myalgia/myositis, muscular soreness (1% to 3%).

Miscellaneous – Giddiness, influenza (≥ 3%); viral gastroenteritis, urticaria, dental pain, malaise/fatigue, rash/skin eruption, dysmenorrhea (1% to 3%).

➤*Terbutaline:*

Miscellaneous – ECG changes, such as sinus pause, atrial premature beats, AV block, ventricular premature beats, ST-T-wave depression, T-wave inversion, sinus bradycardia, and atrial escape beat with aberrant conduction; increased heart rate; muscle cramps; central stimulation; pain at injection site (0.5% to 2.6%); elevations in liver enzymes, seizures, and hypersensitivity vasculitis (rare).

Overdosage

➤*Inhalation:*

Symptoms – Exaggeration of the effects listed under Adverse Reactions can occur. Seizures, hypokalemia, anginal pain, hyperglycemia, hypotension, or hypertension may result. Clinically significant prolongation with QTc interval and cardiac arrest have been reported with use.

Treatment – Discontinue medication with general supportive measures. Monitor blood pressure and ECG. The judicious use of a cardioselective β-receptor blocker (ie, metoprolol, atenolol) is suggested, bearing in mind the danger of inducing an asthmatic attack. Dialysis is not appropriate.

➤*Systemic:*

Symptoms – Palpitations; tachycardia; transient arrhythmias; bradycardia; extrasystoles; heart block; angina; hyperglycemia and increased insulin levels followed by rebound hypoglycemia; hypokalemia; hypo- or hypertension; significant drop in blood pressure caused by peripheral vasodilation; fever; chills; cold perspiration; blanching of the skin; nausea; vomiting; mydriasis. Central actions produce insomnia, anxiety, nervousness, drowsiness, muscle cramps, headache, sweating, and tremor. Delirium, convulsions, collapse, and coma may occur.

The principal manifestation of **ephedrine** sulfate poisoning is convulsions. The following signs and symptoms may also occur: Initially, the patient may have hypertension, followed later by hypotension accompanied by anuria. Nausea, vomiting, chills, cyanosis, irritability, nervousness, fever, suicidal behavior, tachycardia, dilated pupils, blurred vision, opisthotonos, spasms, convulsions, pulmonary edema, gasping respirations, coma, and respiratory failure.

Treatment – Discontinue medication or reduce dosage. Emesis, gastric lavage, or charcoal may be useful following overdose with oral agents. If pronounced, a β-adrenergic blocker (propranolol) may be used, but consider the possibility of aggravation of airway obstruction; phentolamine may be used to block strong α-adrenergic actions. Treatment includes usual supportive measures. Monitor blood pressure, pulse respiration, and ECG. If respirations are shallow or cyanosis is present, administer artificial respiration. Vasopressors are contraindicated. In cardiovascular collapse, maintain blood pressure. For hypertension, 5 mg phentolamine mesylate diluted in saline may be administered slowly IV, or 100 mg may be given orally. Convulsions may be controlled by diazepam or paraldehyde. Cool applications and dexamethasone 1 mg/kg administered slowly IV may control pyrexia. Refer to General Management of Acute Overdosage.

Patient Information

➤*Inhalation:* Patient instructions are available with products. Many patients do not use metered-dose inhalers correctly, even after repeated instructions. Do not assume the patient understands the use of inhaled drugs and the proper administration technique. Use verbal instructions as well as an actual demonstration if possible. Repeat instructions at follow-up visits.

Thoroughly shake the inhaler with canister in place for 5 to 10 seconds; breathe out to the end of a normal breath. Hold the inhaler system upright; place the mouthpiece into the mouth, close the lips tightly or position mouthpiece 2 to 3 finger widths from open mouth, and tilt head back slightly. While activating the inhaler, take a slow, deep breath for 3 to 5 seconds; hold the breath for ≈ 10 seconds, and exhale slowly. Allow ≥ 1 minute between inhalations (puffs) if necessary. Allow ≥ 2 minutes between inhalations for **metaproterenol**. Rinse mouth with water after each use.

Do not exceed recommended dosage; excessive use may lead to adverse effects or loss of effectiveness. Do not stop or adjust the dose.

Do not change brands without consulting the physician or pharmacist.

Notify physician if treatment is less effective, symptoms worsen, or the need to use this product increases in frequency. Usual adverse events include palpitations, chest pain, rapid heart rate, and tremor or nervousness.

Isoproterenol – May cause the patient's saliva to turn pinkish red.

Salmeterol – Shake well before using. Salmeterol is not meant to relieve acute asthmatic symptoms, which should be treated with an inhaled, short-acting bronchodilator. The bronchodilator action usually lasts for ≥ 12 hours; therefore, do not use more often than every 12 hours. While using salmeterol, seek medical attention immediately if the short-acting bronchodilator treatment becomes less effective for symptom relief, if more inhalations than usual are needed, or if more than the maximum number of inhalations of short-acting bronchodilator treatment prescribed for a 24-hour period are needed. If the patient uses ≥ 4 inhalations/day of a short-acting β₂-agonist on a regular basis or if > 1 canister (200 inhalations/canister) is used in an 8-week period, have the patient see the physician for re-evaluation of treatment. When using salmeterol to prevent exercise-induced bronchospasm, administer the dose ≥ 30 to 60 minutes before exercise.

➤*Metered dose inhalers:* The contents of metered dose inhalers are under pressure. Do not puncture. Do not use or store near heat or open flame. Exposure to temperatures > 120°F may cause bursting. Never throw container into fire or incinerator. Keep out of reach of children. If unusual smell or taste is noted with use, discontinue use in consultation with physician.

Warn patients that adverse cardiovascular effects may occur (eg, palpitations, chest pain, rapid heart rate, tremor, nervousness).

➤*Proper nebulizer use:* Find a location where the patient can sit comfortably for 10 to 15 minutes. Plug in the compressor. Mix the medication as directed, or empty the prepared unit dose vials (UDVs) into the nebulizer. Do not mix different types of medications without permission from the physician or pharmacist. Assemble the mask or mouthpiece and connect the tubing from this to the port on the compressor. Sit in a comfortable, upright position. Put the mask over nose and mouth (make sure it fits properly so the mist does not flow up into eyes); or if using a mouthpiece, put it into mouth. Turn on the compressor. Take slow, deep breaths. If possible, hold breath for 10 seconds before slowly exhaling. Continue until medication chamber is empty. Wash mask with hot, soapy water. Rinse well and allow to air dry before re-use.

➤*Oral:* Do not exceed prescribed dosage. If GI upset occurs, take with food.

May cause nervousness, restlessness, insomnia (especially **ephedrine**); if these effects continue after reducing dosage, notify physician.

Notify physician if palpitations, tachycardia, chest pain, muscle tremors, dizziness, headache, flushing, or difficult urination (ephedrine) occurs or if breathing difficulty persists.

➤*Epinephrine injection:* In the event of a life-threatening situation, follow these steps immediately to administer epinephrine:

1.) Remove blue plastic needle cover. Hold syringe upright and push plunger to expel air and excess epinephrine (plunger will stop).
2.) Rotate rectangular plunger ¼ turn to the right. Plunger will align with slot in barrel of syringe. Wipe injection site with alcohol swab, if available.
3.) Insert needle straight into arm or thigh.
4.) Push plunger until it stops. Syringe will inject a 0.3 mL dose for adults and children > 12 years of age. *Children:* Syringe barrel has 0.1 mL graduations so that smaller doses can be measured. *Administer to infants to 2 years of age:* 0.05 to 0.1 mL; *2 to 6 years of age:* 0.15 mL; and *6 to 12 years of age:* 0.2 mL. Once initial injection has been administered, follow these additional steps.
5.) Contact physician, if possible.
6.) Prepare syringe for a possible second injection. Turn the rectangular plunger ¼ turn to the right to line up with rectangular slot in the syringe (a slight wiggling may aid the turning and alignment of the plunger).
7.) *The second injection:* If, after 10 minutes from the first injection, symptoms are not noticeably improved, a second injection is required. Dispose of syringe and remaining contents.
8.) Keep patient warm and avoid exertion.

LEVALBUTEROL HCl

Rx	Xopenex (Sepracor)	Solution for inhalation: 0.31 mg/3 mL (as base)	Preservative-free. Sulfuric acid. In UD 3 mL vials.
		0.63 mg/3 mL (as base)	Preservative-free. Sulfuric acid. In UD 3 mL vials.
		1.25 mg/3 mL (as base)	Preservative-free. Sulfuric acid. In UD 3 mL vials.

For complete prescribing information, refer to the Sympathomimetic Bronchodilator group monograph.

Indications

▶*Bronchospasm:* For the treatment or prevention of bronchospasm in adults, adolescents, and children 6 years of age and older with reversible obstructive airway disease.

Administration and Dosage

▶*Approved by the FDA:* March 25, 1999.

▶*Children 6 to 11 years of age:* 0.31 mg administered 3 times/day by nebulization. Do not exceed routine dosing of 0.63 mg 3 times/day.

▶*Adults and adolescents 12 years of age and older:* 0.63 mg administered 3 times/day (every 6 to 8 hours) by nebulization.

Patients 12 years of age and older with more severe asthma or patients who do not respond adequately to a dose of 0.63 mg levalbuterol may benefit from a dosage of 1.25 mg 3 times/day. Closely monitor patients receiving the higher dose for adverse systemic effects and balance the risks of such effects against the potential for improved efficacy.

The use of levalbuterol can be continued as medically indicated to control recurring bouts of bronchospasm. During this time, most patients gain optimal benefit from regular use of the inhalation solution.

If a previously effective dosage regimen fails to provide the expected relief, seek immediate medical advice because this is often a sign of seriously worsening asthma that requires reassessment of therapy.

▶*Administration:* The safety and efficacy of levalbuterol inhalation solution have been established in clinical trials when administered using the *PARI LC Jet* and the *PARI LC Plus* nebulizers, and the *PARI Master Dura-Neb 2000* and *Dura-Neb 3000* compressors. The safety and efficacy of levalbuterol inhalation solution when administered using other nebulizer systems have not been established.

Drug compatibility (physical and chemical), efficacy, and safety of levalbuterol solution for inhalation when mixed with other drugs in a nebulizer have not been established.

▶*Storage/Stability:* Store in the protective foil pouch between 20° and 25°C (68° and 77°F). Protect from light and excessive heat. Keep unopened vials in the foil pouch. Once the foil pouch is opened, use the vials within 2 weeks. If the individual vial is removed from the foil pouch and is not used immediately, protect from light and use within 1 week. Discard the vial if the solution is not colorless.

SALMETEROL XINAFOATE

Rx	Serevent Diskus (GlaxoSmithKline)	Powder for inhalation: 50 mcg (as base)	Lactose. In 60 blisters and institutional pack containing 28 blisters.

For complete prescribing information, refer to the Sympathomimetic Bronchodilator group monograph.

> **WARNING**
>
> Data from a large, placebo-controlled US study that compared the safety of salmeterol (*Serevent* inhalation aerosol) or placebo added to usual asthma therapy showed a small but significant increase in asthma-related deaths in patients receiving salmeterol (13 deaths out of 13,174 patients treated for 28 weeks) vs those on placebo (4 of 13,179). Subgroup analyses suggest the risk may be greater in black patients compared with white patients.

Indications

▶*Asthma/Bronchospasm:* For long-term, twice daily (morning and evening) administration in the maintenance treatment of asthma and in the prevention of bronchospasm in patients 4 years of age and older with reversible obstructive airway disease, including patients with symptoms of nocturnal asthma who require regular treatment with inhaled, short-acting β₂-agonists. Do not use in patients whose asthma can be managed by occasional use of short-acting, inhaled β₂-agonists. Salmeterol may be used alone or in combination with inhaled or systemic corticosteroid therapy.

▶*Chronic obstructive pulmonary disease (COPD):* Long-term, twice daily (morning and evening) administration in the maintenance treatment of bronchospasm associated with COPD (including emphysema and chronic bronchitis).

▶*Exercise-induced bronchospasm (EIB):* For the prevention of EIB in patients 4 years of age and older.

Administration and Dosage

▶*Approved by the FDA:* February 4, 1994.

▶*Asthma/Bronchospasm:* The usual dosage for adults and children 4 years of age and older is 1 inhalation (50 mcg) twice daily (morning and evening, approximately 12 hours apart).

If a previously effective dosage regimen fails to provide the usual response, immediately seek medical advice because this is often a sign of destabilization of asthma. Under these circumstances, re-evaluate the therapeutic regimen and consider additional therapeutic options, such as inhaled or systemic corticosteroids. If symptoms arise in the period between doses, use a short-acting, inhaled β₂-agonist for immediate relief.

To gain full therapeutic benefit, administer twice daily (morning and evening) in the treatment of reversible airway obstruction.

▶*COPD:* The usual dosage for adults is 1 inhalation (50 mcg) twice daily (morning and evening), approximately 12 hours apart.

▶*Prevention of EIB:* One inhalation at least 30 minutes before exercise protects patients against EIB. When used intermittently as needed for prevention of EIB, this protection may last up to 9 hours in adolescents and adults and up to 12 hours in patients 4 to 11 years of age. Do not use additional doses of salmeterol for 12 hours after the administration of this drug. In patients who are receiving salmeterol twice daily (morning and evening), do not use additional salmeterol for prevention of EIB. If this dose is not effective, consider other appropriate therapy for EIB.

▶*Administration:* Do not exhale into the inhalation device; only activate and use the inhalation device in a level, horizontal position. Do not use a spacer.

▶*Storage/Stability:* Store at controlled room temperature, 20° to 25°C (68° to 77°F), in a dry place away from direct heat or sunlight. Keep out of reach of children. Keep the device dry and never wash the mouthpiece or any part of the device. The inhalation device is not reusable; discard after every blister has been used (when the dose indicator reads "0") or 6 weeks after removal from the moisture-protective foil overwrap pouch, whichever comes first. Do not attempt to take the device apart.

ALBUTEROL

Rx	Albuterol (Various, eg, Mylan)	Tablets: 2 mg (as sulfate)	May contain lactose. In 100s, 500s, and 600s.
Rx	Proventil (Schering)		Lactose. (Proventil 2 252). White, scored. In 100s and 500s.
Rx	Albuterol (Various, eg, Mylan, UDL)	Tablets: 4 mg (as sulfate)	May contain lactose. In 100s, 500s, and 600s.
Rx	Proventil (Schering)		Lactose. (Proventil 4 573). White, scored. In 100s and 500s.
Rx	VoSpire ER (Odyssey)	Tablets, extended release: 4 mg (as sulfate)	(V 4). Green. In 100s.
Rx	VoSpire ER (Odyssey)	Tablets, extended release: 8 mg (as sulfate)	(V 8). White. In 100s.
Rx	Albuterol (Various, eg, Alpharma, Mylan, Teva)	Syrup: 2 mg (as sulfate)/5 mL	May contain sorbitol. In 473 mL.
Rx	Proventil (Schering)		Saccharin. Strawberry flavor. In 480 mL.

Sympathomimetics

ALBUTEROL

Rx	**Albuterol** (Various, eg, Andrx, Apothecon, Major, Sidmak, Warrick)	**Aerosol:** Delivers 90 mcg/actuation	In 6.8 g (≥ 80 inhalations) and 17 g (≥ 200 inhalations).
Rx	**Proventil** (Schering)		In 17 g (200 inhalations).
Rx	**Proventil HFA**[1] (Key)		In 6.7 g (200 inhalations). Contains no chlorofluorocarbons (CFCs).
Rx	**Ventolin HFA**[1] (GlaxoSmithKline)		In 18 g (200 inhalations). Contains no CFCs.
Rx	**Albuterol** (Various, eg, Alpharma, Dey, Ivax, Nephron)	**Solution for inhalation:** 0.083% (as sulfate)	In 3 mL UD vials.
Rx	**Proventil** (Schering)		In 3 mL UD vials.
Rx	**Albuterol** (Various, eg, Ivax, Nephron)	**Solution for inhalation:** 0.5% (as sulfate)	In 0.5 mL vials and 20 mL with dropper.
Rx	**Proventil** (Schering)		In 20 mL with dropper.
Rx	**AccuNeb** (Dey)	**Solution for inhalation:** 0.63 mg/3 mL (as sulfate)	Preservative-free. In 3 mL UD vials.
		1.25 mg/3 mL	Preservative-free. In 3 mL UD vials.

[1] As sulfate.

For complete prescribing information, refer to the Sympathomimetic Bronchodilator group monograph.

Indications

➤*Bronchospasm:* For relief and prevention of bronchospasm in patients with reversible obstructive airway disease; acute attacks of bronchospasm (inhalation solution); prevention of exercise-induced bronchospasm. Tablets are indicated for children ≥ 6 years of age; aerosol and inhalation powder are indicated for children ≥ 4 years of age (≥ 12 years of age for *Proventil*); syrup and solution for inhalation are indicated for children ≥ 2 years of age.

➤*Unlabeled uses:* Albuterol has been shown to be effective for treating hyperkalemia in patients with renal failure.

Administration and Dosage

➤*Inhalation aerosol:*

Adults and children ≥ 4 years of age (≥ 12 years of age for Proventil) – 2 inhalations every 4 to 6 hours. In some patients, 1 inhalation every 4 hours may be sufficient. More frequent administration or a larger number of inhalations is not recommended. If previously effective dosage fails to provide relief, this may be a marker of destabilization of asthma and requires re-evaluation of the patient and treatment regimen.

Maintenance therapy (Proventil only) – For maintenance therapy or to prevent exacerbation of bronchospasm, 2 inhalations 4 times/day should be sufficient.

Prevention of exercise-induced bronchospasm –

Adults and children ≥ 4 years of age (≥ 12 years of age for Proventil): 2 inhalations 15 minutes prior to exercise.

➤*Inhalation solution:*

Adults and children ≥ 12 years of age – 2.5 mg 3 to 4 times/day by nebulization. Dilute 0.5 mL of the 0.5% solution with 2.5 mL sterile normal saline. Deliver over ≈ 5 to 15 minutes.

Children 2 to 12 years of age (≥ 15 kg) – 2.5 mg (1 UD vial) 3 to 4 times/day by nebulization. Children weighing < 15 kg who require < 2.5 mg/dose (ie, less than a full UD vial) should use the 0.5% inhalation solution. Deliver over ≈ 5 to 15 minutes.

AccuNeb – The usual starting dosage for patients 2 to 12 years of age is 1.25 mg or 0.63 mg administered 3 or 4 times/day, as needed, by nebulization. More frequent administration is not recommended. Deliver over 5 to 15 minutes. *AccuNeb* has not been studied in the setting of acute attacks of bronchospasm.

➤*Tablets:*

Adults and children ≥ 12 years of age – Usual starting dosage is 2 or 4 mg 3 or 4 times/day. Do not exceed a total daily dose of 32 mg. Use doses > 4 mg 4 times/day only when the patient fails to respond. If a favorable response does not occur, cautiously increase stepwise, up to a maximum of 8 mg 4 times/day, as tolerated.

Children 6 to 12 years of age – Usual starting dosage is 2 mg 3 to 4 times/day. Do not exceed a total daily dose of 24 mg (given in divided doses). For those who fail to respond to the initial starting dosage, cautiously increase stepwise, but do not exceed 24 mg/day in divided doses.

Elderly and those sensitive to β-adrenergic stimulants – Start with 2 mg 3 or 4 times/day. If adequate bronchodilation is not obtained, increase dosage gradually to as much as 8 mg 3 or 4 times/day.

➤*Tablets, extended-release:*

Volmax –

Adults and children > 12 years of age: Usual recommended dose is 8 mg every 12 hours; in some patients, 4 mg every 12 hours may be sufficient. In unusual circumstances (eg, low adult body weight), initial doses may be 4 mg every 12 hours and progress to 8 mg every 12 hours according to response. The dose may be cautiously increased stepwise under physician supervision to a maximum of 32 mg/day in divided doses (eg, every 12 hours) if symptoms are not controlled.

Children 6 to 12 years of age: Usual recommended dose is 4 mg every 12 hours. The dose may be cautiously increased stepwise under physician supervision to a maximum of 24 mg/day in divided doses (eg, every 12 hours) if symptoms are not controlled.

Proventil Repetabs –

Adults and children > 12 years of age: The usual starting dose is 4 or 8 mg every 12 hours. Use doses > 8 mg twice/day when patients fail to respond to this dose. Increase the dose cautiously stepwise to a maximum of 16 mg twice daily as tolerated. Do not exceed total daily dose of 32 mg.

Children 6 to 12 years of age: The usual starting dose is 4 mg every 12 hours. Use doses > 4 mg twice a day when patients fail to respond to this dose. Increase the dose cautiously stepwise to a maximum of 12 mg twice daily as tolerated.

Switching to extended-release tablets – Patients maintained on regular-release albuterol can be switched to *Proventil Repetabs* or *Volmax* extended-release tablets. A 4 mg extended-release tablet every 12 hours is equivalent to a regular 2 mg tablet every 6 hours. Multiples of this regimen up to the maximum recommended dose also apply.

Do not crush or chew extended-release tablets.

➤*Syrup:*

Adults and children > 12 years of age – Usual starting dose is 2 or 4 mg (1 to 2 teaspoonfuls; 5 to 10 mL) 3 or 4 times/day. Give doses > 4 mg 4 times/day only when patient fails to respond. If a favorable response does not occur, cautiously increase, but do not exceed 8 mg 4 times/day.

Children (6 to 12 years of age) – Usual starting dose is 2 mg (1 teaspoonful; 5 mL) 3 or 4 times/day. If patient does not respond to 2 mg 4 times/day, cautiously increase stepwise. Do not exceed 24 mg/day in divided doses.

Children (2 to 6 years of age) – Initiate at 0.1 mg/kg 3 times/day. The starting dose should not exceed 2 mg 3 times/day. If the patient does not respond to the initial dose, increase stepwise to 0.2 mg/kg 3 times/day. Do not exceed 4 mg 3 times/day.

Elderly and those sensitive to β-adrenergic stimulation – Restrict initial dose to 2 mg (1 teaspoonful; 5 mL) 3 or 4 times/day.

Sympathomimetics

BITOLTEROL MESYLATE

Rx	**Tornalate** (Elan)	**Solution for inhalation:** 0.2%	In 10, 30, and 60 mL w/dropper.[1]

[1] With 25% alcohol and propylene glycol.

For complete prescribing information, refer to the Sympathomimetic Bronchodilator group monograph.

Indications

►*Asthma/Bronchospasm:* For prophylaxis and treatment of bronchial asthma and reversible bronchospasm. May be used with concurrent theophylline or steroid therapy.

Administration and Dosage

►*Solution for inhalation:* For adults and children > 12 years of age, administer during a 10- to 15-minute period. The treatment period can be adjusted by varying the amount of diluent (normal saline solution) placed in the nebulizer with the medication. The total volume (medication plus diluent) is usually adjusted to 2 to 4 mL.

Dosing Regimens for Bitolterol Solution for Inhalation 0.2%				
	Continuous flow nebulization		Intermittent flow nebulization	
Doses	Volume (mL)	Bitolterol (mg)	Volume (mL)	Bitolterol (mg)
Usual dose	1.25	2.5	0.5	1
Decreased dose	0.75	1.5	0.25	0.5
Increased dose	1.75	3.5	0.75	1.5

Up to 1 mL of solution for inhalation, 0.2% (2 mg) can be administered with the intermittent flow system to severely obstructed patients.

The usual frequency of treatments is 3 times/day. Treatments may be increased up to 4 times/day; however, the interval between treatments should be ≥ 4 hours. For some patients, 2 treatments a day may be adequate. Seek medical advice immediately if the previously effective dosage regimen fails to provide the usual relief as this is often a sign of seriously worsening asthma that would require reassessment of therapy.

Do not exceed the maximum daily dose of 8 mg with an intermittent flow nebulization system or 14 mg with a continuous flow nebulization system.

ISOETHARINE HCl

Rx	**Isoetharine** (Roxane)	**Solution for inhalation:** 1%	EDTA, parabens, sulfites. In 10 and 30 mL w/dropper.

For complete prescribing information, refer to the Sympathomimetic Bronchodilator group monograph.

Indications

►*Asthma/Bronchospasm:* For bronchial asthma and reversible bronchospasm that occurs with bronchitis and emphysema.

Administration and Dosage

Isoetharine Doses		
Method of administration	Usual dose	Range of dose of 1:3 dilution[1]
Hand bulb nebulizer	4 inhalations	3 to 7 inhalations undiluted
Oxygen aerosolization[2]	0.5 mL	1 to 2 mL
IPPB[3]	0.5 mL	1 to 4 mL

[1] Dilution of 1 part isoetharine plus 3 parts of normal saline solution.
[2] Administered with oxygen flow adjusted to 4 to 6 L/min over 15 to 20 minutes.
[3] IPPB = intermittent positive pressure breathing. Usually an inspiratory flow rate of 15 L/min at a cycling pressure of 15 cm H_2O is recommended. It may be necessary, according to patient and type of IPPB apparatus, to adjust flow rate to 6 to 30 L/min, cycling pressure to 10 to 15 cm H_2O, and further dilution according to the needs of the patient.

Usually, treatment does not need to be repeated more often than every 4 hours; although in severe cases, more frequent administration may be necessary.

►*Storage/Stability:* Do not use if discolored or contains a precipitate. Protect from light.

METAPROTERENOL SULFATE

Rx	**Alupent** (Boehringer Ingelheim)	**Aerosol:** Delivers 0.65 mg/actuation	In 7 g (100 inhalations) and 14 g canisters and refills (200 inhalations).
Rx	**Metaproterenol Sulfate** (Various, eg, Dey)	**Solution for inhalation:** 0.4%	May contain EDTA. In 2.5 mL UD vials.
Rx	**Alupent** (Boehringer Ingelheim)		EDTA. In 2.5 mL UD vials.[1]
Rx	**Metaproterenol Sulfate** (Various, eg, Dey)	**Solution for inhalation:** 0.6%	May contain EDTA. In 2.5 mL UD vials.
Rx	**Alupent** (Boehringer Ingelheim)		EDTA. In 2.5 mL UD vials.[1]
Rx	**Metaproterenol Sulfate** (Various)	**Solution for inhalation:** 5%	May contain EDTA, benzalkonium chloride. In 10 and 30 mL w/dropper.
Rx	**Alupent** (Boehringer Ingelheim)		EDTA, benzalkonium chloride. In 10 or 30 mL w/dropper.

[1] For use with an IPPB device.

For complete prescribing information, refer to the Sympathomimetic Bronchodilator group monograph.

Indications

►*Asthma/Bronchospasm:* For bronchial asthma and reversible bronchospasm that may occur in association with bronchitis and emphysema; treatment of acute asthmatic attacks in children ≥ 6 years of age (5% solution for inhalation *only*).

Administration and Dosage

►*Aerosol:* 2 to 3 inhalations every 3 to 4 hours. Do not exceed 12 inhalations/day. Not recommended for children < 12 years of age.

►*Solution for inhalation:* Usually, treatment does not need to be repeated more often than every 4 hours to relieve acute bronchospasm attacks. In chronic bronchospastic pulmonary diseases, give 3 to 4 times/day. A single dose of nebulized metaproterenol in the treatment of an acute attack of asthma may not completely abort an attack. Not recommended for children < 12 years of age.

Administer the unit-dose vial by oral inhalation using an intermittent positive pressure breathing (IPPB) device. The usual adult dose is

1 vial per nebulization treatment. Each 0.4% vial is equivalent to 0.2 mL of the 5% solution diluted to 2.5 mL with normal saline. Each 0.6% vial is equivalent to 0.3 mL of the 5% solution diluted to 2.5 mL with normal saline.

Dosage and Dilution for Metaproterenol Solutions for Inhalation 5%			
Administration	Usual dose	Range	Dilution
Adults and children ≥ 12 years of age			
Hand bulb nebulizer	10 inhalations	5 to 15 inhalations	No dilution
IPPB or nebulizer	0.3 mL	0.2 to 0.3 mL	In ≈ 2.5 mL saline or other diluent
Children 6 to 12 years of age			
Nebulizer	0.1 mL	0.1 to 0.2 mL	In saline to a total volume of 3 mL

►*Storage/Stability:* Store inhalant solution < 25°C (77°F). Protect from light. Do not use solution if it is darker than slightly yellow, pinkish, or if it contains a precipitate.

Sympathomimetics

PIRBUTEROL ACETATE

Rx	**Maxair Autohaler** (3M Pharm.)	**Aerosol:** Delivers 0.2 mg (as acetate)/actuation	In 2.8 g (80 inhalations) and 14 g (400 inhalations).

For complete prescribing information, refer to the Sympathomimetic Bronchodilator group monograph.

Indications

➤*Asthma/Bronchospasm:* For prevention and reversal of bronchospasm in patients with reversible bronchospasm including asthma. Use with or without concurrent theophylline or corticosteroid therapy.

Administration and Dosage

➤*Adults and children ≥ 12 years of age:* 2 inhalations (0.4 mg) repeated every 4 to 6 hours. One inhalation (0.2 mg) may be sufficient for some patients.

Do not exceed a total daily dose of 12 inhalations.

If previously effective dosage regimen fails to provide the usual relief, seek medical advice immediately as this is often a sign of seriously worsening asthma that would require reassessment of therapy.

TERBUTALINE SULFATE

Rx	**Terbutaline Sulfate** (Global)	**Tablets:** 2.5 mg	Oval. In 100s.
Rx	**Brethine** (Novartis)		Lactose. (Geigy 72). White, oval, scored. In 100s, 1000s, and UD 100s.
Rx	**Terbutaline Sulfate** (Global)	**Tablets:** 5 mg	In 100s.
Rx	**Brethine** (Novartis)		Lactose. (Geigy 105). White, scored. In 100s, 1000s, and UD 100s.
Rx	**Brethine** (Novartis)	**Injection:** 1 mg/mL	In 2 mL amp with 1 mL fill.

For complete prescribing information, refer to the Sympathomimetic Bronchodilator group monograph.

Indications

➤*Asthma/Bronchospasm:* For prevention and reversal of bronchospasm in patients ≥ 12 years of age with asthma and reversible bronchospasm associated with bronchitis and emphysema.

➤*Unlabeled uses:* As a tocolytic agent to treat preterm labor.

Administration and Dosage

➤*Oral:*

Adults > 15 years of age – 5 mg given at 6-hour intervals, 3 times/day during waking hours. If side effects are pronounced, dose may be reduced to 2.5 mg 3 times/day. Do not exceed 15 mg in 24 hours.

Children (12 to 15 years of age) – 2.5 mg 3 times/day. Not recommended for children < 12 years of age. Do not exceed 7.5 mg in 24 hours.

➤*Parenteral:* Usual dose is 0.25 mg SC into the lateral deltoid area. If significant improvement does not occur in 15 to 30 minutes, administer a second 0.25 mg dose. If a patient fails to respond to a second 0.25 mg dose within 15 to 30 minutes, consider other therapeutic measures. Do not exceed a total dose of 0.5 mg in 4 hours.

➤*Storage/Stability:* Store at controlled room temperature 15° to 30°C (59° to 86°F). Protect from light.

ISOPROTERENOL HCl

Rx	**Isoproterenol HCl** (ESI Lederle)	**Injection:** (1:5000 solution) 0.2 mg/mL	Sodium bisulfite. In 5 mL amps.
Rx	**Isuprel** (Abbott)		Sodium metabisulfite. In 1 and 5 mL amps.
Rx	**Isoproterenol HCl** (Abbott)	**Injection:** (1:50,000) 0.02 mg/mL	Sodium metabisulfite. In 10 mL prefilled syringes.

For complete prescribing information, refer to the Sympathomimetic Bronchodilator group monograph.

Indications

➤*Bronchospasm:* For bronchospasm during anesthesia.

Isoproterenol also is used as a vasopressor in shock. Refer to Vasopressors Used in Shock in the Cardiovascular Agents chapter.

Administration and Dosage

For the management of bronchospasm during anesthesia, dilute 1 mL (0.2 mg) of a 1:5000 solution to 10 mL with Sodium Chloride Injection or 5% Dextrose Injection, administer an initial dose of 0.01 to 0.02 mg (0.5 to 1 mL of diluted solution) IV, and repeat when necessary; or use a 1:50,000 solution undiluted and administer an initial dose of 0.01 to 0.02 mg (0.5 to 1 mL).

EPHEDRINE SULFATE

otc	**Ephedrine Sulfate** (West-Ward)	**Capsules:** 25 mg	In 100s.
Rx	**Ephedrine Sulfate** (Various, eg, Abbott, Bedford, Taylor)	**Injection:** 50 mg/mL	In 1 mL amps.

For complete prescribing information, refer to the Sympathomimetic Bronchodilator group monograph.

Indications

➤*Asthma/Bronchospasm:* Ephedrine sulfate injection is indicated in the treatment of allergic disorders, such as bronchial asthma and for the relief of acute bronchospasm. Oral ephedrine is indicated for temporary relief of shortness of breath, tightness of chest, wheezing, and for easing breathing in bronchial asthma.

Ephedrine is used also as a vasopressor in shock. Refer to Vasopressors Used in Shock in the Cardiovascular Agents chapter.

➤*Unlabeled uses:* Ephedrine has been used to treat narcolepsy and depression and to enhance physical and mental energy.

Administration and Dosage

➤*Oral:*

Adults and children ≥ 12 years of age – 12.5 to 25 mg every 4 hours, not to exceed 150 mg in 24 hours.

Children < 12 years of age – For use in children < 12 years of age, consult a physician.

➤*Parenteral:*

Adults – The usual parenteral dose is 25 to 50 mg (range, 10 to 50 mg) administered SC or IM, or 5 to 25 mg administered slowly IV repeated every 5 to 10 minutes, if necessary.

Children – The usual SC, IV, or IM dose is 0.5 to 0.75 mg/kg or 16.7 to 25 mg/m^2 every 4 to 6 hours.

Sympathomimetics

EPINEPHRINE

Rx	**Adrenalin Chloride Solution** (Monarch)	**Solution for inhalation:** 1:100 (10 mg/mL as HCl) solution	In 7.5 mL.[1]
Rx	**Adrenalin Chloride Solution** (Monarch)	**Topical solution:** 1:1000 (1 mg/mL as HCl) solution	In 30 mL.[2]
otc	**microNefrin** (Bird)	**Solution for inhalation:** 2.25% racepinephrine HCl (1.125% epinephrine base)	In 15 and 30 mL.[3]
otc	**Nephron** (Nephron)		In 15 mL.[3]
otc	**S2** (Nephron)		In 15 mL.[3]
otc	**Epinephrine Mist** (Various, eg, Alpharma, Major)	**Aerosol:** 0.22 mg epinephrine/spray	May contain alcohol. In 15 mL.
otc	**Primatene Mist** (Whitehall Robins)		34% alcohol. In 15 mL w/mouthpiece or 15 and 22.5 mL refills.
Rx	**Epinephrine** (Various, eg, Abbott, American Regent)	**Injection:** 1:1000 (1 mg/mL as HCl) solution	May contain sodium metabisulfite. In 1 mL amps.
Rx	**Adrenalin Chloride Solution** (Monarch)		In 1 mL amps[4] and 30 mL *Steri-vials.*[5]
Rx	**Epinephrine** (Abbott)	**Injection:** 1:10,000 (0.1 mg/mL) solution	In 10 mL prefilled syringe.[4]

[1] With benzethonium chloride and 0.2% sodium bisulfite.
[2] With chlorobutanol and 0.15% sodium bisulfite.
[3] With sodium bisulfite, potassium metabisulfite, chlorobutanol, benzoic acid, and propylene glycol.
[4] With sodium bisulfite.
[5] With sodium bisulfite and chlorobutanol.

For complete prescribing information, refer to the Sympathomimetic Bronchodilator group monograph. See also Vasopressors Used in Shock in the Cardiovascular Agents chapter.

Indications

➤*Inhalation:* For temporary relief of shortness of breath, tightness of chest, and wheezing of bronchial asthma; postintubation and infectious croup.

microNefrin – Chronic obstructive lung disease, chronic bronchitis, bronchiolitis, bronchial asthma, and other peripheral airway diseases; croup (postintubation and infectious).

➤*Topical solution:* For use as a nasal decongestant.

➤*Injection:* Epinephrine is used to relieve respiratory distress caused by bronchospasm, to provide rapid relief of hypersensitivity reactions to drugs and other allergens, and to prolong the action of anesthetics. Its cardiac effects may be of use in restoring cardiac rhythm in cardiac arrest from various causes, but it is not used in cardiac failure or in hemorrhagic, traumatic, or cardiogenic shock. Epinephrine is used as a hemostatic agent. It is also used in treating mucosal congestion of hay fever, rhinitis, and acute sinusitis; to relieve bronchial asthmatic paroxysms; in syncope caused by complete heart block or carotid sinus hypersensitivity; for symptomatic relief of serum sickness, urticaria, angioneurotic edema; for resuscitation in cardiac arrest following anesthetic accidents; in simple (open angle) glaucoma; for relaxation of uterine musculature and to inhibit uterine contractions. Epinephrine injection can be used to prolong the action of anesthetics used in local and regional anesthesia.

Administration and Dosage

Refer to specific product labeling for detailed administration and dosage information.

➤*Inhalation aerosol:* Start treatment at the first symptoms of bronchospasm. Individualize dosage.

Adults and children ≥ 4 years of age – Start with 1 inhalation, then wait ≥ 1 minute. If not relieved, use once more. Do not use again for ≥ 3 hours.

➤*Nebulization:*
Adults and children ≥ 4 years of age –
 Hand pump nebulizer: Place 0.5 mL (10 drops) of epinephrine into nebulizer reservoir. Place nebulizer nozzle into the partially opened mouth. Squeeze the bulb 1 to 3 times. Inhale deeply. Take 1 to 3 inhalations not more often than every 3 hours.
 Aerosol-nebulizer: Add 0.5 mL (≈ 10 drops) racemic epinephrine into nebulizer reservoir; add 3 mL of diluent or 0.2 to 0.4 mL (≈ 4 to 8 drops) of *microNefrin* to 4.6 to 4.8 mL water. Administer for 15 minutes every 3 to 4 hours. Supervise children during use.

➤*Children < 4 years of age:* Consult a physician.

➤*Topical solution:* Apply locally as drops or spray, or with a sterile swab, as required. See product labeling for dilution instructions.

➤*Injection:*
Solution (1:1000) –
 Adult dose: 0.2 to 1 mL (0.2 to 1 mg) SC (preferred) or IM.
 For infants and children: Give 0.01 mL/kg or 0.3 mL/m^2 (0.01 mg/kg or 0.3 mg/m^2) SC. Do not exceed 0.5 mL (0.5 mg) in a single pediatric dose. Repeat every 4 hours if necessary.

Solution (1:10,000) – The adult IV dose for hypersensitivity reactions or to relieve bronchospasm usually ranges from 0.1 to 0.25 mg (1 to 2.5 mL of 1:10,000 solution) injected slowly. Neonates may be given a dose of 0.01 mg/kg; for the infant, 0.05 mg is an adequate initial dose and this may be repeated at 20- to 30-minute intervals in the management of asthma attacks.

Alternatively, if the patient has been intubated, epinephrine can be injected via the endotracheal tube directly into the bronchial tree at the same dosage for IV injection. It is rapidly absorbed through the lung capillary bed.

FORMOTEROL FUMARATE

Rx	**Foradil Aerolizer** (Schering)	**Inhalation powder in capsules:** 12 mcg	(CG FXF). In blister pack 18s and 60s with *Aerolizer Inhaler.*[1]

[1] With 25 mg lactose as carrier.

For complete prescribing information, refer to the Sympathomimetic Bronchodilator group monograph.

Indications

➤*Asthma/Bronchospasm:* For long-term, twice-daily (morning and evening) administration in the maintenance treatment of asthma and in the prevention of bronchospasm in adults and children ≥ 5 years of age with reversible obstructive airway disease, including patients with symptoms of nocturnal asthma who require regular treatment with inhaled, short-acting, beta$_2$-agonists. It is not indicated for patients whose asthma can be managed by occasional use of inhaled, short-acting, beta$_2$-agonists.

➤*Prevention of exercise-induced bronchospasm (EIB):* For the acute prevention of EIB in adults and children ≥ 12 years of age when administered on an occasional, as-needed basis.

➤*Concomitant therapy:* Can be used concomitantly with short-acting beta$_2$-agonists, inhaled or systemic corticosteroids, and theophylline therapy. A satisfactory clinical response to formoterol does not eliminate the need for continued treatment with an anti-inflammatory.

➤*Chronic obstructive pulmonary disease (COPD):* For long-term, twice daily (morning and evening) administration in the maintenance of bronchoconstriction in patients with COPD including chronic bronchitis and emphysema.

Formoterol is not a substitute for inhaled or oral corticosteroids. Do not stop or reduce corticosteroids at the time formoterol is initiated.

Administration and Dosage

➤*Approved by the FDA:* February 16, 2001.

Administer formoterol capsules only by the oral inhalation route and only using the *Aerolizer Inhaler.* Do not ingest formoterol orally (eg, swallow). Always store formoterol capsules in the blister, and remove only immediately before use.

When beginning treatment with formoterol, instruct patients who have been taking inhaled, short-acting beta$_2$-agonists on a regular basis (eg, 4 times/day) to discontinue the regular use of these drugs and use them only for symptomatic relief of acute asthma symptoms.

➤*Asthma/Bronchospasm:* For adults and children ≥ 5 years of age, the usual dosage is the inhalation of the contents of one 12 mcg formoterol capsule every 12 hours using the *Aerolizer Inhaler.* The patient must not exhale into the device. The total daily dose of formoterol should not exceed 1 capsule twice daily (24 mcg total daily dose). More frequent administration or administration of a larger number of inhalations is not recommended. If symptoms arise between doses, take an inhaled short-acting beta$_2$-agonist for immediate relief.

Seek medical advice immediately if a previously effective dosage regimen fails to provide the usual response, as this is often a sign of destabilization of asthma. Under these circumstances, reevaluate the therapeutic regimen and consider additional therapeutic options, such as inhaled or systemic corticosteroids.

FORMOTEROL FUMARATE

➤*Prevention of EIB:* For adults and adolescents ≥ 12 years of age, the usual dosage is the inhalation of the contents of one 12 mcg formoterol capsule ≥ 15 minutes before exercise, administered on an occasional as-needed basis.

Do not use additional doses of formoterol for 12 hours after the administration of this drug. Regular, twice-daily dosing has not been studied in preventing EIB. Patients who are receiving formoterol twice daily for maintenance treatment of their asthma should not use additional doses for prevention of EIB and may require a short-acting bronchodilator.

➤*Maintenance treatment of COPD:* The usual dosage is the inhalation of the contents of one 12 mcg formoterol capsule every 12 hours using the *Aerolizer Inhaler.* A total daily dose of > 24 mcg is not recommended. If a previously effective dosage regimen fails to provide the usual response, seek medical advice immediately as this is often a sign of destabilization of COPD. Under these circumstances, re-evaluate the therapeutic regimen and consider additional therapeutic options.

➤*Storage/Stability:*

Prior to dispensing – Store in a refrigerator (2° to 8°C; 36° to 46°F).

After dispensing to patient – Store at 20° to 25°C (68° to 77°F). Protect from heat and moisture. Always store capsules in the blister and only remove from the blister immediately before use.

Always discard the capsules and *Aerolizer Inhaler* by the "Use by" date and always use the new *Aerolizer Inhaler* provided with each new prescription.

Diluents

SODIUM CHLORIDE

otc	**Sodium Chloride 0.45%** (Dey)	**Solution:** 0.45% sodium chloride	Preservative free. In single-use 3 and 5 mL vials.
otc	**Sodium Chloride 0.9%** (Dey)	**Solution:** 0.9% sodium chloride	Preservative free. In 3, 5, and 15 mL.
Rx	**Sodium Chloride** (Various, eg, Abbott, American Regent, ESI Lederle)	**Injection:** 0.9% sodium chloride	In 1, 2, 2.5, 5, 10, and 30 mL.[1]

[1] With 9 mg benzyl alcohol.

Indications

To dilute bronchodilator solutions for inhalation. Also for tracheal lavage. The parenteral preparation is indicated only for diluting or dissolving drugs for IV, IM, or SC injection, according to manufacturer's instructions of the drug to be administered.

Indications

Symptomatic relief or prevention of bronchial asthma and reversible bronchospasm associated with chronic bronchitis and emphysema.

➤*Unlabeled uses:* Treatment of apnea and bradycardia of prematurity. Doses of 2 mg/kg/day have been used to maintain serum concentrations between 3 and 5 mcg/mL.

Theophylline 300 mg/day was effective in reducing essential tremor in one study of 20 patients.

Theophylline 10 mg/kg/day may significantly improve pulmonary function and dyspnea in patients with chronic obstructive pulmonary disease.

Administration and Dosage

➤*Parenteral administration:* See theophylline and dextrose and aminophylline.

Individualize dosage. Base dosage adjustments on clinical response and improvement in pulmonary function with careful monitoring of serum levels. If possible, monitor serum levels to maintain levels in the therapeutic range of 10 to 20 mcg/mL. Levels > 20 mcg/mL may produce toxicity, and it may even occur with levels between 15 to 20 mcg/mL, particularly when factors known to reduce theophylline clearance are present (see Warnings). Once stabilized on a dosage, serum levels tend to remain constant. Data are available that indicate that the serum theophylline concentrations required to produce maximum physiologic benefit may fluctuate with the degree of bronchospasm present and are variable.

Calculate dosages on the basis of lean body weight, since theophylline does not distribute into fatty tissue. Regardless of salt used, dosages should be equivalent based on anhydrous theophylline content.

➤*Individualize frequency of dosing:* With immediate-release products, dosing every 6 hours generally is required, especially in children; intervals up to 8 hours may be satisfactory in adults. Some children and adults requiring higher than average doses (those having rapid rates of clearance; eg, half-lives < 6 hours) may be more effectively controlled during chronic therapy with sustained-release products. Determine dosage intervals to produce minimal fluctuations between peak and trough serum theophylline concentrations. Consider the absorption profile and the elimination rate. When converting from an immediate-release to a sustained-release product, the total daily dose should remain the same, and only the dosing interval adjusted.

➤*Acute symptoms requiring rapid theophyllinization in patients not receiving theophylline:* To achieve a rapid effect, an initial loading dose is required. Dosage recommendations are for theophylline anhydrous.

Dosage Guidelines for Rapid Theophyllinization[1]		
Patient group	Oral loading	Maintenance
Children 1 to 9 years of age	5 mg/kg	4 mg/kg q 6 hr
Children 9 to 16 years of age and young adult smokers	5 mg/kg	3 mg/kg q 6 hr
Otherwise healthy non-smoking adults	5 mg/kg	3 mg/kg q 8 hr
Older patients, patients with cor pulmonale	5 mg/kg	2 mg/kg q 8 hr
Patients with CHF	5 mg/kg	1 to 2 mg/kg q 12 hr

[1] In patients not receiving theophylline.

➤*Timed-release capsules:* These dosage forms gradually release the active medication so that the total daily dosage may be administered in 1 to 3 doses divided by 8 to 24 hours, depending on the patient's pharmacokinetic profile, thus reducing the number of daily doses required. In the following timed-release capsule product listings, the manufacturer's recommended average dosing intervals are presented in parentheses. Nevertheless, frequency of dosing must be individualized based on the absorption profile of the drug and the rate of elimination of the drug from the patient. These products are not necessarily interchangeable. If patients are switched from one brand to another,

➤*Infants (preterm to < 1 year):*

Theophylline Dosage Guidelines for Infants	
Age	Initial maintenance dose
Premature infants	
≤ 24 days postnatal	1 mg/kg q 12 hr
> 24 days postnatal	1.5 mg/kg q 12 hr
Infants (6 to 52 weeks)	(× age in weeks] + 5) × kg = 24 hr dose in mg
≤ 26 weeks	Divide into q 8 hr dosing
26 to 52 weeks	Divide into q 6 hr dosing

Guide final dosage by serum concentration after a steady state has been achieved.

➤*Acute symptoms requiring rapid theophyllinization in patients receiving theophylline:* Each 0.5 mg/kg theophylline administered as a loading dose will increase the serum theophylline concentration by ≈ 1 mcg/mL. Ideally, defer the loading dose if a serum theophylline concentration can be obtained rapidly.

If this is not possible, exercise clinical judgment. When there is sufficient respiratory distress to warrant a small risk, then 2.5 mg/kg of theophylline administered in rapidly absorbed form is likely to increase serum concentration by ≈ 5 mcg/mL. If the patient is not experiencing theophylline toxicity, this is unlikely to result in dangerous adverse effects. Maintenance doses are in the Dosage Guidelines table.

➤*Chronic therapy:* Slow clinical titration is generally preferred.

Initial dose – 16 mg/kg/24 hours or 400 mg/24 hours, whichever is less, of anhydrous theophylline in divided doses at 6 or 8 hour intervals.

Increasing dose – The above dosage may be increased in ≈ 25% increments at 3-day intervals so long as the drug is tolerated or until the maximum dose (indicated below) is reached.

➤*Maximum dose (where the serum concentration is not measured):* Do not attempt to maintain any dose that is not tolerated.

Maximum Daily Theophylline Dose Based on Age	
Age	Maximum daily dose[1]
1 to 9 years	24 mg/kg/day
9 to 12 years	20 mg/kg/day
12 to 16 years	18 mg/kg/day
> 16 years	13 mg/kg/day

[1] Not to exceed listed dose or 900 mg, whichever is less.

Exercise caution in younger children who cannot complain of minor side effects. Older adults and those with cor pulmonale, CHF, or liver disease may have unusually low dosage requirements; they may experience toxicity at the maximal dosages recommended.

➤*Measurement of serum theophylline concentrations during chronic therapy:* Measurement of serum theophylline concentrations during chronic therapy is recommended. Obtain the serum sample at the time of peak absorption, 1 to 2 hours after administration for immediate-release products and 5 to 9 hours after the morning dose for most sustained-release formulations. The patient must not miss doses during the previous 48 hours, and dosing intervals must have been reasonably typical during that period of time. The table below provides guidance to dosage adjustments based on serum theophylline level determinations:

Dosage Adjustment After Serum Theophylline Measurement		
If serum theophylline is:		Directions
Too low	5 to 10 mcg/mL	Increase dose by ≈ 25% at 3-day intervals until either the desired clinical response or serum concentration is achieved.[1]
Within desired range	10 to 20 mcg/mL	Maintain dosage if tolerated. Recheck serum theophylline concentration at 6 to 12 month intervals.[2]
Too high	20 to 25 mcg/mL	Decrease doses by ≈ 10%. Recheck serum theophylline concentration after 3 days.[2]
	25 to 30 mcg/mL	Skip next dose and decrease subsequent doses by about 25%. Recheck serum theophylline after 3 days.
	> 30 mcg/mL	Skip next 2 doses and decrease subsequent doses by 50%. Recheck serum theophylline after 3 days.

[1] The total daily dose may need to be administered at more frequent intervals if asthma symptoms occur repeatedly at the end of a dosing interval.

[2] Finer adjustments in dosage may be needed for some patients.

closely monitor their theophylline serum levels; serum concentrations may vary greatly following brand interchange.

Actions

➤*Pharmacology:* The methylxanthines (theophylline, its soluble salts and derivatives) directly relax the smooth muscle of the bronchi and pulmonary blood vessels, stimulate the CNS, induce diuresis, increase gastric acid secretion, reduce lower esophageal sphincter pressure, and inhibit uterine contractions. Theophylline is also a central respiratory stimulant. Aminophylline has a potent effect on diaphragmatic contractility in healthy people and may then be capable of reducing fatigability and thereby improve contractility in patients with chronic obstructive airway disease. The exact mode of action is unclear.

For many years, the proposed main mechanism of action of the xanthines was inhibition of phosphodiesterase, which results in an increase in cyclic adenosine monophosphate (cAMP). However, this effect is negligible at therapeutic concentrations. Other effects that appear to occur at therapeutic concentrations and may collectively play a role in the mechanism of the xanthines include the following: Inhibition of extracellular adenosine (which causes bronchoconstriction), although it is unlikely that this is a main mechanism; stimulation of endogenous catecholamines, although this also does not appear to be a major mechanism; antagonism of prostaglandins PGE_2 and $PGF_{2\alpha}$; direct effect on mobilization of intracellular calcium resulting in smooth muscle relaxation; beta-adrenergic agonist activity on the airways. None of these mechanisms have been proven.

➤*Pharmacokinetics:*

Absorption – Theophylline is well absorbed from oral liquids and uncoated plain tablets; maximal plasma concentrations are reached in 2 hours. Rectal absorption from suppositories is slow and erratic, the oral route is generally preferred. Enteric coated tablets and some sustained release dosage forms may be unreliably absorbed. Food may alter bioavailability and absorption pattern of some sustained release preparations; close monitoring is advised (see Drug Interactions).

Distribution – Average volume of distribution is 0.45 L/kg (range, 0.3 to 0.7 L/kg). Theophylline does not distribute into fatty tissue, but readily crosses the placenta and is excreted into breast milk. Approximately 40% is bound to plasma protein. Therapeutic serum levels generally range from 10 to 20 mcg/mL. Although some bronchodilatory effect occurs at lower concentrations, stabilization of hyperreactive airways is most evident at levels > 10 mcg/mL, and adverse effects are uncommon at levels < 20 mcg/mL. Once a patient is stabilized, serum levels tend to remain constant with the same dosage.

Metabolism / Excretion – Xanthines are biotransformed in the liver (85% to 90%) to 1, 3–dimethyluric acid, 3–methylxanthine and 1–methyluric acid; 3–methylxanthine accumulates in concentrations approximately 25% of those of theophylline.

Excretion is by the kidneys; < 15% of the drug is excreted unchanged. Elimination kinetics vary greatly. Plasma elimination half-life averages about 3 to 15 hours in adult nonsmokers, 4 to 5 hours in adult smokers (1 to 2 packs per day), 1 to 9 hours in children and 20 to 30 hours for premature neonates. In the neonate, theophylline is metabolized partially to caffeine. The premature neonate excretes about 50% unchanged theophylline and may accumulate the caffeine metabolite.

A prolonged half-life may occur in congestive heart failure, liver dysfunction, alcoholism, respiratory infections and patients receiving certain other drugs (see Drug Interactions). Total clearance appears relatively unaffected by renal failure.

Equivalent dose – Because of differing theophylline content, the various salts and derivatives are not equivalent on a weight basis. The table below indicates percentage of anhydrous theophylline and approximate equivalent dose of each compound. Product listings include anhydrous theophylline dosage equivalents.

Theophylline Content and Equivalent Dose of Various Theophylline Salts		
Theophylline salts	Theophylline %	Equivalent dose
Theophylline anhydrous	100	100 mg
Theophylline monohydrate	91	110 mg
Aminophylline anhydrous	86	116 mg
Aminophylline dihydrate	79	127 mg
Oxtriphylline	64	156 mg

Dyphylline – A chemical derivative of theophylline, it is not a theophylline salt as are the other agents. It is about one-tenth as potent as theophylline. Following oral administration, dyphylline is 68% to 82% bioavailable. Peak plasma concentrations are reached within 1 hour, and its half-life is 2 hours. The minimal effective therapeutic concentration is 12 mcg/mL. It is not metabolized to theophylline and 83% ± 5% is excreted unchanged in the urine.

Contraindications

Hypersensitivity to any xanthine; peptic ulcer; underlying seizure disorders (unless receiving appropriate anticonvulsant medication).

➤*Aminophylline:* Hypersensitivity to ethylenediamine.

➤*Aminophylline rectal suppositories:* Irritation or infection of rectum or lower colon.

Warnings

➤*Status asthmaticus:* This is a medical emergency and is not rapidly responsive to usual doses of conventional bronchodilators. Optimal therapy frequently requires both parenteral medication and close monitoring, preferably in an intensive care setting. Oral theophylline products alone are not appropriate for status asthmaticus.

➤*Toxicity:* Excessive doses may cause severe toxicity; monitor serum levels to assure maximum benefit with minimum risk. Incidence of toxicity increases significantly at serum levels > 20 mcg/mL (75% of

patients with levels > 25 mcg/mL). Serum levels > 20 mcg/mL are rare after appropriate use of recommended doses. However, if theophylline plasma clearance is reduced for any reason (eg, hepatic impairment; patients > 55 years old, particularly males and those with chronic lung disease; cardiac failure; sustained high fever; infants < 1 year old), even conventional doses may result in increased serum levels and potential toxicity. Frequently, such patients have markedly prolonged levels following drug discontinuation.

Serious side effects such as ventricular arrhythmias, convulsions or even death may appear as the first sign of toxicity without any previous warning. Less serious signs of toxicity (eg, nausea, restlessness) may occur frequently when initiating therapy, but are usually transient; when such signs are persistent during maintenance therapy, they are often associated with serum concentrations > 20 mcg/mL. Serious toxicity is not reliably preceded by less severe side effects.

➤*Cardiac effects:* Theophylline may cause dysrhythmias or worsen preexisting arrhythmias. Any significant change in cardiac rate or rhythm warrants monitoring and further investigation. Many patients who require theophylline may exhibit tachycardia due to underlying disease; the relationship to elevated serum theophylline concentrations may not be appreciated. Ventricular arrhythmias respond to lidocaine.

➤*Pregnancy: Category C.* It is not known whether theophylline can cause fetal harm when administered to a pregnant woman or can affect reproduction capacity. Give only if clearly needed. Theophylline has been found in cord serum and crosses the placenta; newborns may have therapeutic serum levels. Apnea has been associated with theophylline withdrawal in a neonate. Theophylline-related human congenital defects or malformations have not been reported.

➤*Lactation:* Theophylline distributes readily into breast milk with a milk:plasma ratio of 0.7 and may cause irritability or other signs of toxicity in nursing infants. Decide whether to discontinue nursing or to discontinue the drug, taking into account the importance of the drug to the mother.

➤*Children:* Sufficient numbers of infants < 1 year of age have not been studied in clinical trials to support use in this age group; however, there is evidence that the use of dosage recommendations for older infants and young children may result in the development of toxic serum levels. Carefully consider associated benefits and risks in this age group. (See Administration and Dosage and Unlabeled uses.)

Precautions

➤*Use with caution:* Cardiac disease; hypoxemia; hepatic disease; hypertension; congestive heart failure (CHF); alcoholism; elderly (particularly males); and neonates.

➤*GI effects:* Use cautiously in peptic ulcer. Local irritation may occur; centrally mediated GI effects may occur with serum levels > 20 mcg/mL. Reduced lower esophageal pressure may cause reflux, aspiration and worsening of airway obstruction.

➤*Alcohol:* The addition of alcohol in liquid formulations is not necessary for absorption and may be potentially harmful.

Drug Interactions

Agents that Decrease Theophylline Levels		
Aminoglutethimide	Rifampin	Carbamazepine[1]
Barbiturates	Smoking (cigarettes and marijuana)	Isoniazid[1]
Charcoal	Sulfinpyrazone	Loop diuretics[1]
Hydantoins[2]	Sympathomimetics (β-agonists)	
Ketoconazole	Thioamines[3]	

Agents that Increase Theophylline Levels		
Allopurinol	Disulfiram	Quinolones
Beta blockers (non-selective)	Ephedrine	Thiabendazole
Calcium channel blockers	Influenza virus vaccine	Thyroid hormones[4]
Cimetidine	Interferon	Carbamazepine[1]
Contraceptives, oral	Macrolides	Isoniazid[1]
Corticosteroids	Mexiletine	Loop diuretics[1]

[1] May increase or decrease theophylline levels.
[2] Decreased hydantoin levels may also occur.
[3] Increased theophylline clearance in hyperthyroid patients.
[4] Decreased theophylline clearance in hypothyroid patients.

➤*Benzodiazepines:* The sedative effects of benzodiazepines may be antagonized by theophyllines, although their pharmacokinetics do not appear to be altered. Coadministration may be beneficial in reversing sedation produced by benzodiazepines.

➤*Beta-agonists:* Acts synergistically with theophylline in vitro; an additive effect has also been demonstrated in vivo.

➤*Halothane:* Coadministration with theophylline has resulted in catecholamine-induced arrhythmias.

➤*Ketamine:* Coadministration with theophylline has resulted in extensor-type seizures.

➤*Lithium:* Plasma levels may be reduced by theophyllines.

➤*Nondepolarizing muscle relaxants:* A dose-dependent reversal of neuromuscular blockade by theophyllines may occur.

➤*Probenecid:* May increase the pharmacologic effects of dyphylline due to decreased dyphylline renal excretion.

➤*Propofol:* Theophyllines may antagonize the sedative effects of propofol.

➤*Ranitidine:* Case reports suggest that theophylline plasma levels may be increased by ranitidine, possibly increasing pharmacologic and toxic effcts. However, several controlled studies indicate that an interaction does not occur. It appears that if this interaction occurs, it is rare.

➤*Tetracyclines:* The incidence of theophylline adverse reactions may possibly be enhanced by concurrent tetracyclines.

➤*Drug / Lab test interactions:* Currently available analytical methods for measuring serum theophylline levels are specific, and metabolites and other drugs generally do not affect the results. However, be aware of the specific laboratory method used and whether other factors will interfere with the assay for theophylline.

➤*Drug / Food interactions:* Theophylline elimination is increased (half-life shortened) by a low carbohydrate, high protein diet and charcoal broiled beef (due to a high polycyclic carbon content). Conversely, elimination is decreased (prolonged half-life) by a high carbohydrate low protein diet. Food may alter the bioavailability and absorption pattern of certain sustained release preparations. Some sustained release preparations may be subject to rapid release of their contents when taken with food, resulting in toxicity. It appears that consistent administration in the fasting state allows predictability of effects.

Adverse Reactions

Adverse reactions/toxicity are uncommon at serum theophylline levels < 20 mcg/mL.

Levels > 20 mcg / mL – 75% of patients experience adverse reactions (eg, nausea, vomiting, diarrhea, headache, insomnia, irritability).

Levels > 35 mcg / mL – Hyperglycemia; hypotension; cardiac arrhythmias; tachycardia (> 10 mcg/mL in premature newborns); seizures; brain damage; death.

➤*Cardiovascular:* Palpitations; tachycardia; extrasystoles; hypotension; circulatory failure; life-threatening ventricular arrhythmias.

➤*CNS:* Irritability; restlessness; headache; insomnia; reflex hyperexcitability; muscle twitching; convulsions.

➤*GI:* Nausea; vomiting; epigastric pain; hematemesis; diarrhea; rectal irritation or bleeding (aminophylline suppositories). Therapeutic doses of theophylline may induce gastroesophageal reflux during sleep or while recumbent, increasing the potential for aspiration which can aggravate bronchospasm.

➤*Renal:* Proteinuria; potentiation of diuresis.

➤*Respiratory:* Tachypnea; respiratory arrest.

➤*Miscellaneous:* Fever; flushing; hyperglycemia; inappropriate antidiuretic hormone syndrome; rash; alopecia. Ethylenediamine in aminophylline can cause sensitivity reactions, including exfoliative dermatitis and urticaria.

Overdosage

➤*Symptoms:* Anorexia; nausea; vomiting; nervousness; insomnia; agitation; irritability; headache; tachycardia; extrasystoles; tachypnea; fasciculation; tonic/clonic convulsions. Convulsions or ventricular arrhythmias may be the first signs of toxicity. Hyperamylasemia, simulating pancreatitis, has also been noted. Other symptoms of intoxication are listed under Adverse Reactions.

Serious adverse effects are rare at serum theophylline concentrations < 20 mcg/mL. Between 20 and 40 mcg/mL, sinus tachycardia and cardiac arrhythmias occur. Above 40 mcg/mL, seizures and cardiorespiratory arrest can occur. However, convulsions and death have been reported at concentrations as low as 25 mcg/mL.

Acute overdosage appears to be better tolerated with the more serious reactions (eg, seizures) occurring with chronic overdosage (levels > 40 mcg/mL), but rarely in the acute situation unless levels exceed 100 mcg/mL. Also, symptoms such as hypokalemia, hypercalcemia, hyperglycemia and decreased serum bicarbonate concentrations occur more frequently with acute overdosage.

Overdosage with sustained release preparations may cause a dramatic increase in serum theophylline concentrations much later (≥ 12 hours) than the increases that occur with other preparations. Early treatment will help but not prevent these delayed elevated levels.

➤*Treatment:*

Treatment if seizure has not occurred – Induce vomiting, even if emesis has occurred spontaneously; ipecac syrup is preferred. However, do not induce emesis in patients with impaired consciousness. Take precautions against aspiration, especially in infants and children. If vomiting is unsuccessful or contraindicated, perform gastric lavage (of no value ≥ 1 hour post-ingestion). Administer a cathartic (particularly for sustained-release preparations; sorbitol may be useful) and activated charcoal. Prophylactic phenobarbital may increase the seizure threshold.

If seizure occurs – Establish an airway and administer oxygen. Administer IV diazepam 0.1 to 0.3 mg/kg, up to 10 mg. Monitor vital signs, maintain blood pressure and provide adequate hydration.

Post-seizure coma – Maintain airway and oxygenation. Perform intubation and lavage instead of inducing emesis. Introduce the cathartic and activated charcoal via a large bore gastric lavage tube. Provide full supportive care and adequate hydration while the drug is metabolized. If repeated oral activated charcoal is ineffective, charcoal hemoperfusion may be indicated.

Supportive care – Employ usual supportive measures. Refer to General Management of Acute Overdosage. Do not use stimulants (analeptic agents). Continuously monitor cardiac function. Verapamil has been used to treat atrial arrhythmias; lidocaine or procainamide may be used for ventricular arrhythmias. May need IV fluids to treat dehydration, acid-base imbalance and hypotension; the latter may also be treated with vasopressors. Apnea will require ventilatory support. Treat hyperpyrexia, especially in children, with tepid water sponge baths or a hypothermic blanket.

Monitor theophylline serum level until it falls below 20 mcg/mL because secondary rises of plasma theophylline may occur from redistribution, delayed absorption, etc; this has been reported with sustained release products.

Dialysis – Charcoal hemoperfusion rapidly removes theophylline and may be indicated when the serum concentration is > 60 mcg/mL, even in the absence of obvious toxicity. Forced diuresis, peritoneal dialysis and extracorporeal methods are inadequate. However, hemodialysis appears capable of removing ≈ 36% to 40% of serum theophylline.

"Gastric dialysis": With oral activated charcoal, 20 to 40 g every 4 hours until serum level is < 20 mcg/mL, may shorten half-life and speed removal, regardless of route. Mechanism may include enhancing drug concentration gradient into the GI lumen, a disruption of an enterohepatic recycling process or binding unabsorbed drug.

Patient Information

If GI upset occurs with liquid or non-sustained release forms, take with food.

Do NOT chew or crush enteric coated or sustained release tablets or capsules.

Take at the same time, with or without food, each day.

Notify physician if nausea, vomiting, insomnia, jitteriness, headache, rash, severe GI pain, restlessness, convulsions or irregular heartbeat occurs.

Avoid large amounts of caffeine-containing beverages, such as tea, coffee, cocoa and cola drinks or large amounts of chocolate; these products may increase side effects.

➤*Brand interchange:* Do not change from one brand to another without consulting your pharmacist or physician. Products manufactured by different companies may not be equally effective.

Individual doses are determined by response (decrease in symptoms). Blood levels must be checked regularly to avoid underdosing and overdosing. Do not change the dose of your medication without consulting your physician.

THEOPHYLLINE

Rx	**Theophylline** (Various)	**Tablets:** 100 mg	In 100s.
Rx	**Theolair** (3M Pharmaceuticals)	**Tablets:** 125 mg	(Riker 342). White, scored. In 100s.
Rx	**Theophylline** (Various)	**Tablets:** 200 mg	In 100s and 500s.
Rx	**Theophylline** (Various)	**Tablets:** 300 mg	In 100s, 500s and 1000s.
Rx	**Quibron-T Dividose** (Roberts)		(BL 512). Ivory. Triple scored. In 100s and 500s.
Rx	**Bronkodyl** (Winthrop)	**Capsules:** 100 mg	Brown and white. In 100s.
Rx	**Elixophyllin** (Forest)		Dye free. (Forest 642). In 100s.
Rx	**Bronkodyl** (Winthrop)	**Capsules:** 200 mg	Green and white. In 100s.
Rx	**Elixophyllin** (Forest)		Dye free. (Forest 643). In 100s and 500s.
Rx	**Accurbron** (Hoechst Marion Roussel)	**Syrup:** 150 mg per 15 mL (50 mg per 5 mL)	7.5% alcohol. Dye free. Saccharin, sorbitol, sugar. In pt.
Rx	**Theophylline** (Various, eg, Balan, Barre-National, Bioline, Geneva, Moore, Rugby, Schein, URL)	**Elixir:** 80 mg per 15 mL (26.7 mg per 5 mL)	In pt and gal and UD 15 and 30 mL.
Rx	**Asmalix** (Century)		20% alcohol. In gal.
Rx	**Elixomin** (Cenci)		20% alcohol. Orange raspberry flavor. In pt.
Rx	**Elixophyllin** (Forest)		20% alcohol. Saccharin. Mixed fruit flavor. In pt, qt and gal.
Rx sf	**Lanophyllin** (Lannett)		20% alcohol. In pt and gal.
Rx	**Theophylline Extended-Release** (Dey)	**Tablets, extended-release:** 100 mg	In 100s, 500s and 1000s.
		200 mg	In 100s, 500s and 1000s.
		300 mg	In 100s, 500s and 1000s.
Rx	**Slo-Phyllin Gyrocaps** (Rhone-Poulenc Rorer)	**Capsules, timed release (8 to 12 hours):** 60 mg	Sucrose. (WHR 1354). White. In 100s.
		125 mg	Sucrose. (WHR 1355). Brown. In 100s, 1000s and UD 100s.
		250 mg	Sucrose. (WHR 1356). Purple. In 100s, 1000s and UD 100s.
Rx	**Theo-24** (UCB Pharma)	**Capsules, timed release (24 hours):** 100 mg	(Theo-24 100 mg Searle 2832). Gold and clear. In 100s and UD 100s.
		200 mg	(Theo-24 200 mg Searle 2842). Orange and clear. In 100s, 500s and UD 100s.
		300 mg	(Theo-24 300 mg Searle 2852). Red and clear. In 100s, 500s and UD100s.
		Note: Patients receiving once daily doses ≥ 13 mg/kg or ≥ 900 mg (whichever is less) should avoid eating a high-fat-content morning meal or should take medication at least 1 hour before eating. If patient cannot comply with this regimen, place on alternative therapy.	
Rx	**Theophylline** (Various, eg, Mason, Parmed)	**Capsules, extended release:** 100 mg	In 100s.
		125 mg	In 100s.
		200 mg	In 100s.
		300 mg	In 100s.
Rx	**Theophylline SR** (Various, eg, Balan, Bioline, Geneva, Goldline, Major, Moore, Rugby, Sidmak)	**Tablets, timed release (12 to 24 hours):** 100 mg	In 100s and 500s.
		200 mg	In 100s, 500s, 1000s, UD 100s.
		300 mg	In 100s, 500s, 1000s, UD 100s.
Rx	**Theophylline** (Able)	**Tablets, extended release:** 400 mg	(A380). White to off-white, scored. In 30s, 100s, 500s, and 1,000s.
		600 mg	(A382). White to off-white, oval. In 30s, 100s, 500s, and 1,000s.
Rx	**Theochron** (Various, eg, Inwood, Lemmon)	**Tablets, extended release:** 100 mg	In 100s, 500s, 1000s.
		200 mg	In 100s, 500s, 1000s.
		300 mg	In 100s, 500s, 1000s.
Rx	**Theochron** (Forest)	**Tablets, extended release (12 to 24 hours):** 450 mg	(IL3614/450). Off-white, capsule shape, scored. In 100s, 500s, and 1000s.
Rx	**Quibron-T/SR Dividose** (Roberts)	**Tablets, timed release (8 to 12 hours):** 300 mg	White. Triple scored. In 100s and 500s.
Rx	**Theocron** (Inwood)	**Tablets, timed release (12 to 24 hours):** 100 mg	Dye free. (IL/3584). White, scored. Convex. In 100s, 500s, 1000s.
		200 mg	Dye free. (IL/3583). White, scored. Oval. In 100s, 500s, 1000s.
		300 mg	Dye free. (IL/3581). White, scored. Capsule shape. In 100s, 500s, 1000s.
Rx	**Uniphyl** (Purdue Frederick)	**Tablets, timed release (24 hours):** 400 mg	(PF U400). White, scored. In 100s, 500s, UD 100s.
		600 mg	(PF U600). White, scored. In 100s.

For complete prescribing information, refer to the Xanthine Derivatives group monograph.

Administration and Dosage

▶*Time-release capsules:* These dosage forms gradually release the active medication so that the total daily dosage may be administered in 1 to 3 doses divided by 8 to 24 hours, depending on the patient's pharmacokinetic profile, thus reducing the number of daily doses required. In the previous product listings, the manufacturer's recom-mended average dosing intervals are presented in parentheses. Nevertheless, frequency of dosing must be individualized, based on the absorption profile of the drug and the rate of elimination of the drug from the patient. These products are not necessarily interchangeable. If patients are switched from one brand to another, closely monitor their theophylline serum levels; serum concentrations may vary greatly following brand interchange.

Xanthine Derivatives

OXTRIPHYLLINE (Choline Theophyllinate) – 64% theophylline

Rx	**Oxtriphylline** (Various, eg, Bolar, Genetco, Goldline, Interstate, Major, Rugby)	**Tablets:** 100 mg (equiv. to 64 mg theophylline)	In 100s and 500s.
Rx	**Oxtriphylline** (Various, eg, Balan, Bioline, Bolar, Interstate, Major, Parmed, Rugby)	**Tablets:** 200 mg (equiv. to 127 mg theophylline)	In 100s, 500s and 1000s.
Rx	**Oxtriphylline** (Various, eg, Moore, PBI)	**Syrup, pediatric:** 50 mg (equiv. to 32 mg theophylline) per 5 mL	In pt.
Rx	**Oxtriphylline** (Various, eg, PBI, UDL)	**Elixir:** 100 mg (equiv. to 64 mg theophylline) per 5 mL	In pt and UD 5 and 10 mL.

For complete prescribing information, refer to the Xanthine Derivatives group monograph.

Administration and Dosage

➤*Adults:* 4.7 mg/kg every 8 hours.

➤*Children (9 to 16 years) and adult smokers:* 4.7 mg/kg every 6 hours.

➤*Children (1 to 9 years):* 6.2 mg/kg every 6 hours.

➤*Sustained action:* If total daily maintenance dosage is established at approximately 800 or 1200 mg, 1 sustained action tablet every 12 hours may be substituted.

THEOPHYLLINE AND DEXTROSE

Rx	**Theophylline and 5% Dextrose** (Abbott and Baxter)	**Injection:** 200 mg/container	In 50 mL (4 mg/mL) and 100 mL (2 mg/mL).
		400 mg/container	In 100 mL (4 mg/mL), 250 mL (1.6 mg/mL), 500 mL (0.8 mg/mL) and 1000 mL (0.4 mg/mL).
		800 mg/container	In 250 mL (3.2 mg/mL), 500 mL (1.6 mg/mL) and 1000 mL (0.8 mg/mL).

For complete prescribing information, refer to the Xanthine Derivative group monograph.

Administration and Dosage

Substitute oral therapy for IV theophylline as soon as adequate improvement is achieved.

See also aminophylline for parenteral administration guidelines, noting the difference of theophylline content.

➤*The following may be incompatible when mixed with theophylline in IV fluids:* Anileridine; ascorbic acid; chlorpromazine; codeine phosphate; corticotropin; dimenhydrinate; epinephrine HCl; erythromycin gluceptate; hydralazine; hydroxyzine HCl; insulin; levorphanol tartrate; meperidine; methadone; methicillin sodium; morphine sulfate; norepinephrine bitartrate; oxytetracycline; papaverine; penicillin G potassium; phenobarbital sodium; phenytoin sodium; procaine; prochlorperazine maleate; promazine; promethazine; tetracycline; vancomycin; vitamin B complex with C.

➤*Children:* Due to marked variation in theophylline metabolism, use this drug only if clearly needed in infants < 6 months of age.

AMINOPHYLLINE (Theophylline Ethylenediamine) – 79% theophylline

Rx	**Aminophylline** (Various, eg, Balan, Bioline, Geneva-Marsam, Goldline, Major, Roxane, Rugby, Searle, URL)	**Tablets:** 100 mg (equiv. to 79 mg theophylline)	Plain or enteric coated. In 100s, 1000s and UD 100s.
Rx	**Aminophylline** (Various, eg, Balan, Bioline, Geneva-Marsam, Goldline, Major, Moore, Roxane, Rugby, Searle, URL)	**Tablets:** 200 mg (equiv. to 158 mg theophylline)	Plain or enteric coated. In 100s, 1000s and UD 100s.
Rx	**Aminophylline** (Various, eg, Balan, Barre, Bioline, Major, PBI, Roxane, Rugby, URL)	**Oral Liquid:** 105 mg (equiv. to 90 mg theophylline) per 5 mL	In 240 and 500 mL.
Rx	**Aminophylline** (Various, eg, Abbott, American Regent, Elkins-Sinn, Moore, Solopak)	**Injection:** 250 mg (equiv. to 197 mg theophylline) per 10 mL. For IV use.	In 10 and 20 mL amps & vials & syringes.
Rx	**Aminophylline** (Various, eg, Rugby, Schein)	**Suppositories:** 250 mg (equiv. to 197.5 mg theophylline)	In 10s and 25s.
Rx	**Aminophylline** (Various, eg, Parmed, Rugby, Schein)	**Suppositories:** 500 mg (equiv. to 395 mg theophylline)	In 10s and 25s.

For complete prescribing information, refer to the Xanthine Derivative group monograph.

Administration and Dosage

For oral and rectal dosage, refer to the Equivalent Dosage table in Actions and to the Administration section in the Xanthine Derivatives group monograph.

For dosage in infants from preterm up to 8-week-old term infants, see Administration section in the Xanthine Derivatives group monograph.

➤*IV:* The loading dose may be infused into 100 to 200 mL of 5% Dextrose Injection or 0.9% Sodium Chloride Injection. Do not exceed 25 mg/min infusion rate.

➤*Parenteral administration:* Inject aminophylline slowly, not more than 25 mg/min, when given IV. Substitute oral therapy for IV aminophylline as soon as adequate improvement is achieved.

Loading dose –

In patients currently not receiving theophylline products: 6 mg/kg.

In patients currently receiving theophylline products: If possible, determine the time, amount, route of administration and form of last dose and defer loading dose if a serum concentration can be rapidly obtained. Each 0.5 mg/kg theophylline (0.6 mg/kg aminophylline) will increase the serum theophylline concentration by approximately 1 mcg/mL. When respiratory distress warrants a small risk, 2.5 mg/kg theophylline (3.1 mg/kg aminophylline IV) increases serum concentration by approximately 5 mcg/mL. If the patient is not experiencing theophylline toxicity, this is unlikely to result in dangerous side effects. The proper time to obtain blood to measure the peak serum level of theophylline after an IV loading dose is 15 to 30 minutes.

Maintenance infusions: Administer by a large volume infusion to deliver the desired amount of drug each hour. Aminophylline is compatible with most common IV solutions. Monitor serum theophylline concentrations to accurately maintain therapeutic concentrations and guide dosage adjustments.

Aminophylline Maintenance Infusion Rates (mg/kg/hr)		
Patient group	First 12 hours	Beyond 12 hours
Neonates to infants < 6 months old	Not recommended	
Children 6 months to 9 years of age	1.2	1
Children ages 9 to 16 years of age and young adult smokers	1	0.8
Otherwise healthy nonsmoking adults	0.7	0.5
Older patients and those with cor pulmonale	0.6	0.3
Patients with CHF, liver disease	0.5	0.1-0.2

➤*Compatibility:* Do not mix the following solutions with aminophylline in IV fluids: Anileridine HCl; ascorbic acid; chlorpromazine; codeine phosphate; dimenhydrinate; dobutamine HCl; epinephrine; erythromycin gluceptate; hydralazine; insulin; levorphanol tartrate; meperidine; methadone; methicillin; morphine sulfate; norepinephrine bitartrate; oxytetracycline; penicillin G potassium; phenobarbital; phenytoin; prochlorperazine; promazine; promethazine; tetracycline; vancomycin; verapamil; vitamin B complex with C.

DYPHYLLINE (Dihydroxypropyl Theophylline)

Rx	Dyphylline (Various, eg, Balan, Major)	**Tablets:** 200 mg	In 100s and 1000s.
Rx	Lufyllin (Wallace)		(Wallace 521). White, scored. Rectangular. In 100s, 1000s, 5000s and UD 100s.
Rx	Dyphylline (Various, eg, Balan, Major, URL)	**Tablets:** 400 mg	In 100s and 1000s.
Rx	Lufyllin-400 (Wallace)		(Wallace 731). White, scored. Capsule shape. In 100s, 1000s, 2500s and UD 100s.
Rx	Lufyllin (Wallace)	**Elixir:** 100 mg per 15 mL (33.3 mg/5 mL)	20% alcohol. White port wine, saccharin. In pt and gal.
Rx	Dilor (Savage)	**Elixir:** 160 mg per 15 mL (53.3 mg/5 mL)	18% alcohol. Saccharin, sorbitol, sucrose, parabens. Mint flavor. In pt and gal.
Rx	Dilor (Savage)	**Injection:** 250 mg per mL	In 2 mL amps.
Rx	Lufyllin (Wallace)		In 2 mL amps.

For complete prescribing information, refer to the Xanthine Derivatives group monograph.

Administration and Dosage

➤*Oral:*

Adults – Up to 15 mg/kg every 6 hours.

➤*IM:* (Not for IV administration.)

Adults – 250 to 500 mg injected slowly every 6 hours. Do not exceed 15 mg/kg every 6 hours.

Children – Safety and efficacy have not been established.

Actions

➤*Pharmacology:* Dyphylline is a derivative of theophylline; it is not a theophylline salt and is not metabolized to theophylline in vivo. Although dyphylline is 70% theophylline by molecular weight ratio, the amount of dyphylline equivalent to a given amount of theophylline is not known. Dyphylline may result in fewer side effects than theophylline salts, but blood levels and possibly activity are lower. Specific dyphylline serum levels may be used to monitor therapy; serum theophylline levels will NOT measure dyphylline. The minimal effective therapeutic concentration is 12 mcg/mL.

IPRATROPIUM BROMIDE

Rx	Ipratropium Bromide (Dey)	**Solution for Inhalation:** 0.02% (500 mcg per vial)	Preservative free. In 25 and 60 unit-dose vials (2.5 ml each).
Rx	Atrovent (Boehringer Ingelheim)	**Aerosol:** Each actuation delivers 18 mcg	In 14.7 g metered dose inhaler w/mouthpiece (200 inhalations).
Rx	Atrovent (Boehringer Ingelheim)	**Solution for Inhalation:** 0.02% (500 mcg per vial)	Preservative free. In 25 unit dose vials per foil pouch.
Rx	Ipratropium Bromide (Various, eg, Baush & Lomb, Roxane)	**Nasal spray:** 0.03%. Each spray delivers 21 mcg	In 30 mL with spray pump (345 sprays).
Rx	Atrovent (Boehringer Ingelheim)		In 30 mL bottles with spray pump (345 sprays).
Rx	Ipratropium Bromide (Various, eg, Bausch & Lamb, Roxane)	**Nasal spray:** 0.06%. Each spray delivers 42 mcg	In 15 mL with spray pump (165 sprays).
Rx	Atrovent (Boehringer Ingelheim)		In 15 mL bottles with spray pump (165 sprays).

Indications

➤*Bronchospasm (solution and aerosol):* As a bronchodilator for maintenance treatment of bronchospasm associated with COPD, including chronic bronchitis and emphysema.

➤*Rhinorrhea:*

Perennial rhinitis (0.03% nasal spray) – Symptomatic relief of rhinorrhea associated with allergic and nonallergic perennial rhinitis in patients ≥ 12 years of age.

Common cold (0.06% nasal spray) – Symptomatic relief of rhinorrhea associated with the common cold in patients ≥ 12 years of age.

Administration and Dosage

➤*Aerosol:* The usual dose is 2 inhalations (36 mcg) 4 times a day. Patients may take additional inhalations as required; however, do not exceed 12 inhalations in 24 hours.

➤*Solution:* The usual dose is 500 mcg (1 unit dose vial) administered 3 to 4 times a day by oral nebulization, with doses 6 to 8 hours apart. The solution can be mixed in the nebulizer with albuterol if used within 1 hour.

➤*Nasal spray:*

0.03% – The usual dose is 2 sprays (42 mcg) per nostril 2 or 3 times daily (total dose, 168 to 252 mcg/day). Optimum dosage varies.

0.06% – The recommended dose is 2 sprays (84 mcg) per nostril 3 or 4 times daily (total dose, 504 to 672 mcg/day). Optimum dosage varies.

The safety and efficacy of use beyond 4 days in patients with the common cold have not been established.

➤*Concomitant therapy:* Ipratropium has been used concomitantly with other drugs, including sympathomimetic bronchodilators, methylxanthines, steroids and cromolyn sodium, commonly used in the treatment of COPD, without adverse drug reactions.

➤*Storage/Stability:*

Aerosol – Store below 30°C (86°F); avoid excessive humidity.

Solution – Store between 15° and 30°C (59° and 86°F). Protect from light. Store unused vials in the foil pouch.

Nasal spray – Store tightly closed between 15° and 30°C (59° and 86°F). Avoid freezing.

Actions

➤*Pharmacology:* Ipratropium for oral inhalation is a synthetic quaternary anticholinergic (parasympatholytic) ammonium compound chemically related to atropine. It appears to inhibit vagally mediated reflexes by antagonizing the action of acetylcholine. Anticholinergics prevent the increases in intracellular concentrations of cyclic guanosine monophosphate (cyclic GMP), which are caused by interaction of acetylcholine with the muscarinic receptor on bronchial smooth muscle.

The bronchodilation following inhalation is primarily a local, site-specific effect. Much of an inhaled dose is swallowed as shown by fecal excretion studies.

Ipratropium has anti-secretory properties and when applied locally, inhibits secretions from the serous and seromucous glands lining the nasal mucosa.

➤*Pharmacokinetics:* Ipratropium is poorly absorbed into the systemic circulation from the nasal mucosa. Less than 20% of an 84 mcg per nostril dose is absorbed from the nasal mucosa, but the amount which is systematically absorbed from nasal administration exceeds the amount absorbed from either inhalation solution (2% of a 500 mcg dose) or inhalation aerosol (20% of a 36 mcg mouthpiece dose). Ipratropium is minimally bound (≤ 9% in vitro) to plasma albumin and α_1-acid glycoprotein. It is partially metabolized to inactive ester hydrolysis products. The elimination half-life is about 1.6 hours.

➤*Clinical trials:*

Bronchospasm – In controlled 90 day studies in patients with bronchospasm associated with chronic obstructive pulmonary disease (COPD) (chronic bronchitis and emphysema), significant improvements in pulmonary function (FEV_1 and $FEF_{25\%}$ to $_{75\%}$ increases of ≥ 15%) occurred within 15 minutes, reached a peak in 1 to 2 hours and persisted for 3 to 4 hours in most patients and up to 6 hours in some patients. In addition, significant increases in Forced Vital Capacity (FVC) occurred.

Rhinorrhea – In four controlled 4 and 8 week comparisons of ipratropium nasal spray 0.03% (42 mcg per nostril, 2 or 3 times daily), with its vehicle, in patients with allergic or nonallergic perennial rhinitis, there was a statistically significant decrease in the severity and duration of rhinorrhea with ipratropium throughout the entire study period. An effect was seen as early as the first day of therapy. There was no effect of ipratropium nasal spray 0.03% on degree of nasal congestion, sneezing or postnasal drip.

Contraindications

Hypersensitivity to ipratropium, atropine or its derivatives or to soya lecithin or related food products such as soy bean or peanut (inhalation aerosol).

Warnings

➤*Acute bronchospasm:* Use of itratropium as a single agent for relief of bronchospasm in acute COPD exacerbation has not been adequately studied.

➤*Special risk patients:* Use with caution in patients with narrow angle glaucoma, prostatic hypertrophy or bladder neck obstruction.

➤*Hypersensitivity reactions:* Immediate hypersensitivity reactions may occur after administration of ipratropium bromide, as demonstrated by rare cases of urticaria, angioedema, rash, bronchospasm and oropharyngeal edema.

➤*Pregnancy: Category B.* No adequate and well controlled studies have been conducted in pregnant women. Use during pregnancy only if clearly needed.

➤*Lactation:* It is not known whether this drug is excreted in breast milk. Although lipid-insoluble quaternary bases pass into breast milk, it is unlikely that ipratropium would reach the infant to an important extent, especially when taken by inhalation. However, exercise caution when administering to a nursing mother.

➤*Children:* Safety and efficacy in children < 12 years old have not been established.

Adverse Reactions

Inhalation aerosol – Cough (≈ 3% to 5.9%); dryness of the oropharynx (≈ 5%); nervousness (3.1%); irritation from aerosol (1.6% to ≈ 3%); dizziness, headache, GI distress, dry mouth, exacerbation of symptoms (1% to ≈ 3%); nausea (≈ 1% to 2.8%); palpitation (1.8%); rash (1.2%); blurred vision/difficulty in accommodation, drying of secretions (≈ 1%); urinary difficulty, fatigue, insomnia, hoarseness, tachycardia, paresthesias, drowsiness, coordination difficulty, itching, hives, flushing, alopecia, constipation, tremor, mucosal ulcers (< 1%).

Inhalation solution – Tachycardia, palpitations, eye pain, urinary retention, urinary tract infection, urticaria (< 3%). Headache, mouth dryness and aggravation of COPD symptoms were more common with ≥ 2000 mcg/day.

Anticholinergics

IPRATROPIUM BROMIDE

	Ipratropium Inhalation Solution Adverse Reactions (%)[1]				
Adverse Reaction	Albuterol (2.5 mg tid) (n = 205)	Ipratropium (500 mcg tid) (n = 219)	Ipratropium/ Albuterol (500 mcg tid/2.5 mg tid) (n = 100)	Ipratropium/ Metaproterenol (500 mcg tid/15 mg tid) (n =108)	Metaproterenol (15 mg tid) (n = 212)
CNS					
Dizziness	3.9	2.3	4	1.9	3.3
Insomnia	1	0.9	1	4.6	0.5
Tremor	1	0.9	0	8.3	7.1
Nervousness	1	0.5	1	6.5	4.7
GI					
Mouth dryness	2	3.2	3	1.9	0
Nausea	2.9	4.1	2	1.9	3.8
Constipation	1	0.9	1	3.7	0
Respiratory (lower)					
Coughing	5.4	4.6	6	6.5	8
Dyspnea	12.7	9.6	9	16.7	13.2
Bronchitis	16.6	14.6	20	15.7	24.5
Bronchospasm	5.4	2.3	5	4.6	2.8
Sputum increased	3.4	1.4	0	4.6	1.4
Respiratory disorder	2	0	4	6.5	6.1
Respiratory (upper)					
Upper respiratory tract infection	12.2	13.2	16	9.3	11.3
Pharyngitis	2.9	3.7	4	5.6	4.2
Rhinitis	2.4	2.3	0	1.9	4.2
Sinusitis	5.4	2.3	4	0.9	2.8
Miscellaneous					
Headache	6.3	6.4	9	6.5	5.2
Pain	2.9	4.1	5	0.9	3.3
Influenza-like symptoms	0.5	3.7	1	6.5	4.7
Back pain	2.4	3.2	0	1.9	1.9
Chest pain	2	3.2	1	5.6	4.2
Hypertension/Hypertension aggravated	1.5	0.9	4	0.9	1.9
Arthritis	0.5	0.9	3	0.9	1.4

[1] Data are pooled from separate studies and are not necessarily comparable.

Nasal spray (0.03%) – Headache, upper respiratory tract infection (9.8%); epistaxis (7% to 9%); pharyngitis (8.1%); nasal dryness (5.1%); miscellaneous nasal symptoms (3.1%); nausea (2.2%); nasal irritation, blood-tinged mucus (2%); dry mouth/throat, dizziness, ocular irritation, blurred vision, conjunctivitis, hoarseness, cough, taste perversion (< 2%).

Nasal spray (0.06%) – Epistaxis (8.2%); nasal dryness (4.8%); dry mouth/throat (1.4%); nasal congestion (1.1%); taste perversion, nasal burning, conjunctivitis, coughing, dizziness, hoarseness, palpitation, pharyngitis, tachycardia, thirst, tinnitus, blurred vision, urinary retention (< 1%).

➤*Allergic:* Allergic-type reactions such as skin rash, angioedema of the tongue, throat, lips, and face, urticaria (including giant urticaria), laryngospasm, and anaphylactic reactions have been reported. Many patients had a history of allergies with drugs or food, including soybeans.

Additional anticholinergic reactions – Those reported with ipratropium products included precipitation or worsening of narrow angle glaucoma, urinary retention, prostatic disorders, tachycardia, constipation, and bowel obstruction.

Overdosage

Acute overdosage by inhalation is unlikely.

Patient Information

Temporary blurred vision, precipitation or worsening of narrow-angle glaucoma, or eye pain may result if aerosol is sprayed into the eyes or solution comes into direct contact with the eyes. For the solution, use of a nebulizer with mouthpiece rather than face mask may be preferable to reduce the likelihood of the solution reaching the eyes.

Advise patients that the solution can be mixed in the nebulizer with albuterol if used within 1 hour. Compatibility data are not available with other drugs.

➤*Nasal spray:* Initial pump priming requires 7 actuations of the pump. If used regularly as recommended, no further priming is required. If not used for > 24 hours, the pump will require 2 actuations, or if not used for > 7 days, the pump will require 7 actuations to reprime.

TIOTROPIUM BROMIDE

Rx	Spiriva (Boehringer Ingelheim)	**Powder for inhalation:** 18 mcg (as base)	In blister packs containing 6 capsules with inhaler.

Indications

➤*Chronic obstructive pulmonary disease (COPD):* For the long-term, once-daily, maintenance treatment of bronchospasm associated with COPD, including chronic bronchitis and emphysema.

Administration and Dosage

➤*Approved by the FDA:* January 30, 2004.

➤*Dose:* Inhalation of the contents of 1 tiotropium capsule, once daily, with the *HandiHaler* inhalation device.

➤*Administration:* Tiotropium capsules are for inhalation only; do not swallow.

1.) Immediately before using the tiotropium dose, peel back the aluminum foil using the tab until 1 capsule is fully visible. Peel back the foil lidding only as far as the "STOP" line printed on the blister foil to prevent exposure of more than 1 capsule. Immediately use the drug after opening the packaging over an individual capsule or its effectiveness may be reduced.
2.) Open the dust cap of the *HandiHaler* by pulling it upwards, then open the mouthpiece.
3.) Place the capsule in the center chamber. It does not matter which end of the capsule is placed in the chamber.

4.) Firmly close the mouthpiece until a click is heard, leaving the dust cap open.
5.) Hold the *HandiHaler* device with the mouthpiece upwards, press the piercing button completely in once, and release. This makes holes in the capsules and allows the medication to be released.
6.) Breathe out completely. Do not breathe into the mouthpiece at any time.
7.) Raise the *HandiHaler* device to mouth and close lips tightly around the mouthpiece.
8.) Keep head in an upright position, and breathe in slowly and deeply but at a rate sufficient to hear the capsule vibrate. Breathe in until lungs are full, then hold breath as long as is comfortable. At the same time, take the *HandiHaler* device out of mouth. Resume normal breathing.
9.) To ensure getting the full dose of tiotropium, repeat this once again.
10.) After finishing taking the daily dose of tiotropium, open the mouthpiece again. Tip out the used capsule and dispose. Close the mouthpiece and dust cap for storage.

➤*Storage/Stability:* Store at 25°C (77°F); excursions permitted to 15° to 30°C (59° to 86°F). Do not expose capsules to extreme temperature or moisture. Do not store capsules in the *HandiHaler* device.

TIOTROPIUM BROMIDE

Actions

➤*Pharmacology:* Tiotropium is a long-acting, antimuscarinic agent, which is often referred to as an anticholinergic. It has similar affinity to the subtypes of muscarinic receptors M_1 to M_5. In the airways, it exhibits pharmacological effects through inhibition of M_3-receptors at the smooth muscle, leading to bronchodilation. In preclinical in vitro and in vivo studies, prevention of methacholine-induced bronchoconstriction effects were dose-dependent and lasted longer than 24 hours. The bronchodilation following inhalation of tiotropium is predominantly a site-specific effect.

➤*Pharmacokinetics:*

Absorption – Tiotropium is administered by dry powder inhalation. The majority of the delivered dose is deposited in the GI tract and, to a lesser extent, in the lung, the intended organ. Many of the pharmacokinetic data described here were obtained with higher doses than recommended for therapy.

Following dry powder inhalation by young healthy volunteers, the absolute bioavailability of 19.5% suggests that the fraction reaching the lung is highly bioavailable. It is expected from the chemical structure of the compound (quaternary ammonium compound) that tiotropium is poorly absorbed from the GI tract. Oral solutions of tiotropium have an absolute bioavailability of 2% to 3%. Maximum tiotropium plasma concentrations were observed 5 minutes after inhalation.

Distribution – Tiotropium shows a volume of distribution of 32 L/kg, indicating that the drug binds extensively to tissues. The drug is bound by 72% to plasma proteins. At steady state, peak tiotropium plasma levels in COPD patients were 17 to 19 pg/mL when measured 5 minutes after an 18 mcg dry powder inhalation dose and decreased rapidly in a multicompartmental manner. Steady-state trough plasma concentrations were 3 to 4 pg/mL. Local concentrations in the lung are not known, but the mode of administration suggests substantially higher concentrations in the lung. Studies in rats have shown that tiotropium does not readily penetrate the blood-brain barrier.

Metabolism – The extent of biotransformation appears to be small. Tiotropium, an ester, is nonenzymatically cleaved to the alcohol N-methylscopine and dithienylglycolic acid, neither of which bind to muscarinic receptors.

In vitro experiments with human liver microsomes and human hepatocytes suggest that a fraction of the administered dose (74% of an IV dose is excreted unchanged in the urine, leaving 25% for metabolism) is metabolized by cytochrome P450-dependent oxidation and subsequent glutathione conjugation to a variety of phase 2 metabolites. This enzymatic pathway can be inhibited by CYP450 2D6 and 3A4 inhibitors (eg, quinidine, ketoconazole, and gestodene). Thus, CYP450 2D6 and 3A4 are involved in the metabolic pathway that is responsible for elimination of a small part of the administered dose.

Excretion – The terminal elimination half-life of tiotropium is between 5 and 6 days following inhalation. Total clearance was 880 mL/min after an IV dose in young healthy volunteers with an inter-individual variability of 22%. IV administered tiotropium is mainly excreted unchanged in urine (74%). After dry powder inhalation, urinary excretion is 14% of the dose, the remainder being mainly nonabsorbed drug in the gut, which is eliminated via the feces. The renal clearance of tiotropium exceeds the creatinine clearance (Ccr), indicating active secretion into the urine. After chronic, once-daily inhalation by COPD patients, pharmacokinetic steady state was reached after 2 to 3 weeks with no accumulation thereafter.

Special populations –

Elderly: Advanced age was associated with a decrease of tiotropium renal clearance (326 mL/min in COPD patients younger than 58 years of age to 163 mL/min in COPD patients older than 70 years of age), which may be explained by decreased renal function. Tiotropium excretion in urine after inhalation decreased from 14% (young healthy volunteers) to approximately 7% (COPD patients). Plasma concentrations were numerically increased with advancing age within COPD patients (43% increase in AUC_{0-4} after dry powder inhalation), which was not significant when considered in relation to inter- and intra-individual variability.

Renal function impairment: Renal impairment was associated with increased plasma drug concentrations and reduced drug clearance after IV infusion and dry powder inhalation. Mild renal impairment (Ccr 50 to 80 mL/min), which often is seen in elderly patients, increased tiotropium plasma concentrations (39% increase in AUC_{0-4} after IV infusion). In COPD patients with moderate to severe renal impairment (Ccr less than 50 mL/min), the IV administration of tiotropium resulted in doubling of the plasma concentrations (82% increase in AUC_{0-4}), which was confirmed by plasma concentrations after dry powder inhalation.

Contraindications

History of hypersensitivity to atropine or its derivatives, including ipratropium, or to any component of the product.

Warnings

➤*Bronchospasm:* Tiotropium is intended as a once-daily maintenance treatment for COPD and is not indicated for the initial treatment of acute episodes of bronchospasm (ie, rescue therapy). Inhaled medicines, including tiotropium, may cause paradoxical bronchospasm. If this occurs, stop treatment with tiotropium and consider other treatments.

➤*QT prolongation:* In a multicenter, randomized, double-blind trial that enrolled 198 patients with COPD, the number of subjects with changes from baseline-corrected QT interval of 30 to 60 msec was higher in the tiotropium group as compared with placebo. No patients in either group had QT of more than 500 msec. Other clinical studies with tiotropium did not detect an effect of the drug on QTc intervals.

➤*Hypersensitivity reactions:* Immediate hypersensitivity reactions, including angioedema, may occur after administration of tiotropium. If such a reaction occurs, stop therapy at once and consider alternative treatment. Refer to Management of Acute Hypersensitivity Reactions.

➤*Renal function impairment:* Because tiotropium is a predominantly renally excreted drug, closely monitor patients with moderate to severe renal impairment (Ccr 50 mL/min or less) (see Pharmacokinetics).

➤*Elderly:* In the placebo-controlled studies, a higher frequency of dry mouth, constipation, and urinary tract infections was observed with increasing age in the tiotropium group.

➤*Pregnancy: Category C.* In rats, fetal resorption, litter loss, decreases in the number of live pups at birth and the mean pup weights, and a delay in pup sexual maturation were observed at inhalation tiotropium doses of at least 0.078 mg/kg (approximately 35 times the recommended human daily dose [RHDD] on a mg/m^2 basis). In rabbits, an increase in postimplantation loss was observed at an inhalation dose of 0.4 mg/kg/day (approximately 360 times the RHDD on a mg/m^2 basis). There are no adequate and well-controlled studies in pregnant women. Use during pregnancy only if the potential benefit justifies the potential risk to the fetus.

➤*Lactation:* Based on lactating rodent studies, tiotropium is excreted into breast milk. It is not known whether tiotropium is excreted in human milk. Exercise caution if administering to a nursing woman.

➤*Children:* The safety and efficacy of tiotropium in pediatric patients have not been established.

Precautions

➤*Special risk:* As an anticholinergic drug, tiotropium potentially may worsen signs and symptoms associated with narrow-angle glaucoma, prostatic hyperplasia, or bladder-neck obstruction; use with caution in patients with any of these conditions.

Drug Interactions

➤*Anticholinergic agents:* The coadministration of tiotropium with other anticholinergic-containing drugs (eg, ipratropium) has not been studied and, therefore, is not recommended.

Adverse Reactions

The most commonly reported adverse drug reaction was dry mouth. Dry mouth usually was mild and often resolved during continued treatment. Other reactions reported in individual patients and consistent with possible anticholinergic effects included blurred vision, constipation, glaucoma, increased heart rate, urinary difficulty, and urinary retention.

Tiotropium Adverse Reactions in 1-Year COPD Clinical Trials (%)				
	Placebo-controlled trials		Ipratropium-controlled trials	
Adverse reaction	Tiotropium (n = 550)	Placebo (n = 371)	Tiotropium (n = 356)	Ipratropium (n = 179)
GI				
Abdominal pain	5	3	6	6
Constipation	4	2	1	1
Dry mouth	16	3	12	6
Dyspepsia	6	5	1	1
Vomiting	4	2	1	2
Respiratory				
Epistaxis	4	2	1	1
Pharyngitis	9	7	7	3
Rhinitis	6	5	3	2
Sinusitis	11	9	3	2
Upper respiratory tract infection	41	37	43	35
Miscellaneous				
Accidents	13	11	5	8
Chest pain (non-specific)	7	5	5	2
Edema, dependent	5	4	3	5
Infection	4	3	1	3
Moniliasis	4	2	3	2
Myalgia	4	3	4	3
Rash	4	2	2	2
Urinary tract infection	7	5	4	2

TIOTROPIUM BROMIDE

➤*Cardiovascular:* Angina pectoris (including aggravated angina pectoris) (1% to 3%); atrial fibrillation, supraventricular tachycardia (less than 1%).

➤*CNS:* Depression, dysphonia, paresthesia (1% to 3%).

➤*GI:* Gastroesophageal reflux, GI disorder not otherwise specified, stomatitis (including ulcerative stomatitis) (1% to 3%).

➤*Metabolic:* Hypercholesterolemia, hyperglycemia (1% to 3%).

➤*Musculoskeletal:* Arthritis (at least 3%); skeletal pain (1% to 3%).

➤*Respiratory:* Coughing (at least 3%); laryngitis (1% to 3%).

➤*Miscellaneous:* Influenza-like symptoms (at least 3%); allergic reaction, cataract, herpes zoster, leg pain (1% to 3%); angioedema, urinary retention (less than 1%).

Postmarketing – Epistaxis, palpitations, pruritus, urticaria.

Overdosage

High doses of tiotropium may lead to anticholinergic signs and symptoms. However, there were no systemic anticholinergic adverse effects following a single inhaled dose of up to 282 mcg tiotropium in 6 healthy volunteers. In a study of 12 healthy volunteers, bilateral conjunctivitis and dry mouth were seen following repeated once-daily inhalation of 141 mcg tiotropium.

Acute intoxication by inadvertent oral ingestion of tiotropium capsules is unlikely because it is not well-absorbed systemically.

A case of overdose has been reported from postmarketing experience. A female patient was reported to have inhaled 30 capsules over a 2.5-day period and developed altered mental status, tremors, abdominal pain, and severe constipation. The patient was hospitalized, tiotropium was discontinued, and the constipation was treated with an enema. The patient recovered and was discharged on the same day.

Patient Information

It is important for patients to understand how to correctly administer tiotropium capsules using the *HandiHaler* inhalation device (see Administration and Dosage and Patient's Instructions for Use). Instruct patients to administer tiotropium capsules only via the *HandiHaler* device and not to use the *HandiHaler* device for administering other medications. Tiotropium capsules are not to be swallowed.

Instruct patients to store capsules in sealed blisters and only to remove them immediately before use. Advise patients to discard capsules inadvertently exposed to air (ie, not intended for immediate use).

Normally, during a 1-month period of use, the *HandiHaler* device does not need to be cleaned. However, if cleaning is needed, see the Patient's Instructions for Use.

Eye pain or discomfort, blurred vision, vision halos, or colored images in association with red eyes from conjunctival congestion and corneal edema may be signs of acute narrow-angle glaucoma. If any of these signs and symptoms develop, instruct patients to immediately consult a physician. Miotic eye drops alone are not considered to be effective treatment.

Instruct patients to take care not to allow the powder to enter into the eyes, as this may cause blurring of vision and pupil dilation.

Tiotropium is a once-daily maintenance bronchodilator; instruct patients not to use it for immediate relief of breathing problems (ie, as a rescue medication).

IPRATROPIUM BROMIDE AND ALBUTEROL SULFATE

| Rx | **Combivent** (Boehringer Ingelheim) | **Aerosol:** Each actuation delivers 18 mcg ipratropium bromide and 103 mcg albuterol sulfate (equiv. to 90 mcg albuterol base) | In 14.7 g metered dose inhaler w/mouthpiece (200 inhalations). |
| Rx | **DuoNeb** (Dey) | **Inhalation solution:** 0.5 mg ipratropium bromide and 3 mg albuterol sulfate (equiv. to 2.5 mg albuterol base) | In 3 mL unit-dose vials. In 30s and 60s. |

For complete prescribing information, refer to the individual Ipratropium Bromide and Albuterol monographs.

Indications

➤*Bronchospasm:* For use in patients with chronic obstructive pulmonary disease (COPD) on a regular aerosol bronchodilator who continue to have evidence of bronchospasm and require a second bronchodilator.

Administration and Dosage

➤*Approved by the FDA:* October 24, 1996.

➤*Combivent:* Shake well before using.

The recommended dose is 2 inhalations 4 times a day. Patients may take additional inhalations as required; however, advise the patient not to exceed 12 in 24 hours. It is recommended to "test spray" 3 times before using for the first time and in cases where the aerosol has not been used for> 24 hours.

➤*DuoNeb:* The recommended dose is one 3 mL vial administered 4 times/day via nebulization with up to 2 additional 3 mL doses allowed per day, if needed. Administer via jet nebulizer connected to an air compressor with an adequate air flow, equipped with mouthpiece or suitable face mask.

The use of these agents can be continued as medically indicated to control recurring bouts of bronchospasm. If a previously effective regimen fails to provide the usual relief, medical advice should be sought immediately, as this is often a sign of worsening COPD, which would require reassessment of therapy.

➤*Storage / Stability:* Store *Combivent* between 15° and 30°C (59° and 86°F). Avoid excessive humidity. For optimal results, the canister should be at room temperature before use. Store *DuoNeb* between 2° and 25°C (36° and 77°F). Protect from light.

ZAFIRLUKAST

Rx	Accolate (AstraZeneca)	Tablets: 10 mg	Lactose, povidone. (ACCOLATE 10 ZENECA). White. Film-coated. In 60s and UD 100s.
		20 mg	Lactose, povidone. (ACCOLATE 20 ZENECA). White. Film-coated. In 60s and UD 100s.

Indications

➤*Asthma:* Prophylaxis and chronic treatment of asthma in adults and children ≥ 5 years of age.

➤*Unlabeled uses:* Chronic urticaria.

Administration and Dosage

➤*Approved by the FDA:* September 26, 1996.

Because food reduces bioavailability of zafirlukast, take ≥ 1 hour before or 2 hours after meals.

➤*Adults and children ≥ 12 years of age:* The recommended dose of zafirlukast is 20 mg twice daily.

➤*Children 5 to 11 years of age:* The recommended dose of zafirlukast is 10 mg twice daily.

➤*Storage/Stability:* Store at controlled room temperature (20° to 25°C; 68° to 77°F). Protect from light and moisture. Dispense in original air-tight container.

Actions

➤*Pharmacology:* Zafirlukast is a selective and competitive leukotriene receptor antagonist (LTRA) of leukotriene D_4 and E_4 (LTD_4 and LTE_4), components of slow-reacting substance of anaphylaxis (SRSA). Cysteinyl leukotriene production and receptor occupation have been correlated with the pathophysiology of asthma, including airway edema, smooth muscle constriction and altered cellular activity associated with the inflammatory process, which contribute to the signs and symptoms of asthma.

In vitro studies demonstrated that zafirlukast antagonized the contractile activity of 3 leukotrienes (LTC_4, LTD_4, and LTE_4) in conducting airway smooth muscle.

Zafirlukast inhibits bronchoconstriction caused by several kinds of inhalational challenges. Pretreatment with single oral doses of zafirlukast inhibited bronchoconstriction caused by sulfur dioxide and cold air in patients with asthma. Pretreatment with single doses of zafirlukast attenuated the early- and late-phase reaction caused by inhalation of various antigens such as grass, cat dander, ragweed, and mixed antigens in patients with asthma. Zafirlukast also attenuated the increase in bronchial hyperresponsiveness to inhaled histamine that followed inhaled allergen challenge.

➤*Pharmacokinetics:*

Absorption/Distribution – Zafirlukast is rapidly absorbed following oral administration. Peak plasma concentrations are achieved 3 hours after dosing. Zafirlukast is > 99% bound to plasma proteins, predominantly albumin. Administration of zafirlukast with food reduced the mean bioavailability by ≈ 40%. The apparent steady-state volume of distribution is ≈ 70 L, suggesting moderate distribution into the tissues. Steady-state plasma concentrations of zafirlukast are proportional to the dose and predictable from single-dose pharmacokinetic data.

Metabolism/Excretion – Zafirlukast is extensively metabolized. The most common metabolic products are hydroxylated metabolites, which are excreted in the feces. Urinary excretion accounts for ≈ 10% of the dose and the remainder is excreted in the feces. Unmetabolized zafirlukast is not detected in urine. Liver microsomes that hydroxylate metabolites of zafirlukast are formed through the cytochrome P450 2C9 (CYP2C9) enzyme pathway. Additional in vitro studies utilizing human liver microsomes show that zafirlukast inhibits the CYP3A4 and CYP2C9 isoenzymes at concentrations close to the clinically achieved plasma concentrations. The metabolites of zafirlukast found in plasma are at least 90 times less potent as LTD_4 receptor antagonists than zafirlukast in a standard in vitro test of activity. The apparent oral clearance of zafirlukast is ≈ 20 L/h. Studies in the rat and dog suggest that biliary excretion is the primary route of excretion. The mean terminal elimination half-life of zafirlukast is ≈ 10 hours in healthy subjects and patients with asthma.

Special populations –

Elderly: In patients > 65 years of age, there is an ≈ 2- to 3-fold greater C_{max} and AUC compared with young adult patients.

Hepatic function impairment: In patients with hepatic impairment (biopsy-proven cirrhosis), there is a reduced clearance resulting in a 50% to 60% greater C_{max} and AUC compared with healthy subjects.

➤*Clinical trials:* In a study, the effect of zafirlukast on most efficacy parameters was comparable with the active control (1600 mcg inhaled cromolyn sodium 4 times/day) and superior to placebo at endpoint for decreasing rescue beta$_2$-agonist use. Improvement in asthma symptoms occurred within 1 week of initiating treatment with zafirlukast.

Contraindications

Hypersensitivity to zafirlukast or any of its inactive ingredients.

Warnings

➤*Acute asthma attacks:* Zafirlukast is not indicated for use in the reversal of bronchospasm in acute asthma attacks, including status asthmaticus. Therapy with zafirlukast can be continued during acute exacerbations of asthma.

➤*Infection:* An increased proportion of zafirlukast patients > 55 years of age reported infections as compared with placebo-treated patients. These infections were mostly mild or moderate in intensity and predominantly affected the respiratory tract. Infections occurred equally in both sexes, were dose-proportional to total milligrams of zafirlukast exposure, and were associated with coadministration of inhaled corticosteroids.

➤*Hypersensitivity reactions:* Hypersensitivity reactions, including urticaria, angioedema, and rashes, with or without blistering have been reported in association with zafirlukast therapy.

➤*Hepatic function impairment:* The clearance of zafirlukast is reduced in patients with biopsy-proven cirrhosis such that the C_{max} and AUC are ≈ 50% to 60% greater than those of healthy adults.

➤*Carcinogenesis:* Male mice given 300 mg/kg/day of zafirlukast had a greater incidence of hepatocellular adenomas; female mice at this dose showed a greater incidence of whole body histiocytic sarcomas. Male and female rats given 2000 mg/kg/day of zafirlukast had a greater incidence of urinary bladder transitional cell papillomas.

➤*Elderly:* The clearance of zafirlukast is reduced in elderly patients (≥ 65 years of age), such that C_{max} and AUC are ≈ 2- to 3-fold higher than those of younger adults.

➤*Pregnancy: Category B.* At 2000 mg/kg/day in rats, maternal toxicity and deaths were seen with increased incidence of early fetal resorption. Spontaneous abortions occurred in cynomolgus monkeys at a maternally toxic dose of 2000 mg/kg/day orally. There are no adequate and well-controlled trials in pregnant women. Because animal reproduction studies are not always predictive of human response, use zafirlukast during pregnancy only if clearly needed.

➤*Lactation:* Zafirlukast is excreted in breast milk. Following repeated 40 mg twice daily dosing in healthy women, average steady-state concentrations of zafirlukast in breast milk were 50 ng/mL compared with 255 ng/mL in plasma. Do not administer to nursing women.

➤*Children:* The safety and effectiveness of zafirlukast in patients < 5 years of age have not been established.

Precautions

➤*Hepatotoxicity:* Rarely, elevations of ≥ 1 liver enzyme have occurred in patients receiving zafirlukast in controlled clinical trials. In clinical trials, most of these have been observed at doses 4 times higher than the recommended dose. The following hepatic events (which have occurred predominantly in females) have been reported from postmarketing adverse event surveillance of patients who have received the recommended dose of zafirlukast (40 mg/day): Cases of symptomatic hepatitis (with or without hyperbilirubinemia) without other attributable cause; and, rarely, hyperbilirubinemia without other elevated liver function tests. In most, but not all, postmarketing reports, the patients' symptoms abated and the liver enzymes returned to healthy or near healthy after stopping zafirlukast. In rare cases, patients have progressed to hepatic failure.

If liver dysfunction is suspected based upon clinical signs or symptoms (eg, right upper quadrant abdominal pain, nausea, fatigue, lethargy, pruritus, jaundice, flu-like-symptoms, anorexia, enlarged liver), discontinue zafirlukast. Immediately measure liver function tests, in particular serum ALT, and manage the patient accordingly. If liver function tests are consistent with hepatic dysfunction, do not resume zafirlukast therapy.

➤*Eosinophilia:* In rare cases, patients on zafirlukast therapy may present with systemic eosinophilia, sometimes with clinical features of vasculitis consistent with Churg-Strauss syndrome, a condition that is often treated with systemic steroid therapy. These events usually, but not always, have been associated with the reduction of oral steroid therapy. Physicians should be alert to eosinophilia, vasculitic rash, worsening pulmonary symptoms, cardiac complications, or neuropathy presenting in their patients. A causal association between zafirlukast and these underlying conditions has not been established.

Drug Interactions

Because of zafirlukast's inhibition of cytochrome P450 2C9 and 3A4 isoenzymes, use caution with coadministration of drugs known to be metabolized by these isoenzymes.

ZAFIRLUKAST

Zafirlukast Drug Interactions			
Precipitant drug	Object drug*		Description
Aspirin	Zafirlukast	↑	Coadministration of zafirlukast with aspirin results in mean increased plasma levels of zafirlukast by ≈ 45%.
Erythromycin	Zafirlukast	↓	Coadministration of a single dose of zafirlukast with erythromycin to steady state results in decreased mean plasma levels of zafirlukast by ≈ 40% because of decreased zafirlukast bioavailability.
Theophylline	Zafirlukast	↓	Coadministration of zafirlukast at steady state with a single dose of a liquid theophylline preparation results in decreased mean plasma levels of zafirlukast by ≈ 30%, but no effects on plasma theophylline levels were observed.
Zafirlukast	Warfarin	↑	Coadministration of zafirlukast with warfarin results in a clinically significant increase in prothrombin time (PT). Closely monitor PT and adjust anticoagulant dose accordingly.

* ↑ = Object drug increased. ↓ = Object drug decreased.

➤*Drug / Food interactions:* The bioavailability of zafirlukast may be decreased when taken with food. Take zafirlukast ≥ 1 hour before or 2 hours after meals.

Adverse Reactions

➤*CNS:* Headache (12.9%); dizziness (1.6%).

➤*GI:* Nausea (3.1%); diarrhea (2.8%); abdominal pain (1.8%); vomiting (1.5%); dyspepsia (1.3%).

➤*Hypersensitivity:* Hypersensitivity reactions, including urticaria, angioedema, and rashes, with or without blistering, have occurred.

➤*Miscellaneous:* Infection (3.5%; see Warnings); pain (generalized, 1.9%); asthenia (1.8%); accidental injury, myalgia, fever (1.6%); back pain, ALT elevation (1.5%); agranulocytosis; bleeding; bruising; edema; arthralgia; eosinophilia (see Precautions).

Overdosage

No deaths occurred at oral zafirlukast doses of 2000 mg/kg in mice or rats and 500 mg/kg in dogs.

Overdosage with zafirlukast has been reported in 4 patients surviving reported doses as high as 200 mg. The predominant symptoms reported following zafirlukast overdose were rash and upset stomach. It is reasonable to employ the usual supportive measures in the event of an overdose.

Patient Information

Take regularly as prescribed, even during symptom-free periods.

Take zafirlukast ≥ 1 hour before or 2 hours after meals.

Do not use to treat acute episodes of asthma.

Advise patients to contact their physician immediately if they experience symptoms of hepatic dysfunction (eg, right upper quadrant abdominal pain, nausea, fatigue, lethargy, pruritus, jaundice, flu-like symptoms, anorexia).

Do not decrease the dose or stop taking any other antiasthma medications unless instructed by a physician.

Nursing women should not take zafirlukast.

MONTELUKAST SODIUM

Rx	Singulair (Merck)	Tablets: 10 mg (as base)	Lactose. (MRK 117 SINGULAIR). Beige, rounded square. Film-coated. In unit-of-use 30s and 90s and UD 100s.
		Tablets, chewable: 4 mg (as base)	Mannitol, aspartame, 0.674 mg phenylalanine. (MRK 711 SINGULAIR). Pink, oval. Cherry flavor. In unit-of-use 30s and 90s and UD 100s.
		5 mg (as base)	Mannitol, aspartame, 0.842 mg phenylalanine. (MRK 275 SINGULAIR). Pink. Cherry flavor. In unit-of-use 30s and 90s and UD 100s.
		Granules: 4 mg (as base)/packet	Mannitol. In 30 packets.

Indications

➤*Asthma:* Prophylaxis and chronic treatment of asthma in adults and pediatric patients 12 months of age and older.

➤*Seasonal allergic rhinitis:* Relief of symptoms of seasonal allergic rhinitis in adults and pediatric patients 2 years of age and older.

➤*Unlabeled uses:* Chronic urticaria, atopic dermatitis.

Administration and Dosage

➤*Approved by the FDA:* February 20, 1998.

For asthma, the dose should be taken in the evening. For seasonal allergic rhinitis, the time of administration may be individualized. Patients with combined asthma and seasonal allergic rhinitis should take only 1 tablet daily in the evening.

➤*Adults and adolescents 15 years of age and older:* One 10 mg tablet daily.

➤*Children 6 to 14 years of age:* One 5 mg chewable tablet daily.

➤*Children 2 to 5 years of age:* One 4 mg chewable tablet or one 4 mg oral granule packet daily.

➤*Children 12 to 23 months of age with asthma:* One packet of 4 mg granules daily taken in the evening.

➤*Administration of oral granules:* Montelukast 4 mg oral granules can be administered directly in the mouth or mixed with a spoonful of cold or room temperature soft foods; based on stability studies, use only applesauce, carrots, rice, or ice cream. Do not open the packet until ready to use. After opening the packet, the full dose (with or without mixing with food) must be administered within 15 minutes. If mixed with food, the oral granules must not be stored for future use. Discard any unused portion. Montelukast oral granules are not intended to be dissolved in liquid for administration. However, liquids may be taken subsequent to administration. The granules can be administered without regard to the time of meals.

➤*Storage / Stability:* Store at 25°C (77°F); excursions permitted to 15° to 30°C (59° to 86°F). Protect from moisture and light.

Actions

➤*Pharmacology:* Montelukast is a selective and orally active leukotriene receptor antagonist that inhibits the cysteinyl leukotriene (CysLT$_1$) receptor. It binds with high affinity and selectivity to the CysLT$_1$ receptor (in preference to other pharmacologically important airway receptors, such as the prostanoid, cholinergic, or beta-adrenergic receptor). Montelukast inhibits physiologic actions of LTD$_4$ at the CysLT$_1$ receptor without any agonist activity.

The cysteinyl leukotrienes (LTC$_4$, LTD$_4$, LTE$_4$) are products of arachidonic acid metabolism and are released from various cells, including mast cells and eosinophils. These eicosanoids bind to CysLT receptors found in the human airway. Cysteinyl leukotrienes and leukotriene receptor occupation have been correlated with the pathophysiology of asthma and allergic rhinitis.

Asthma – In asthma, leukotriene-mediated effects include airway edema, smooth muscle contraction, and altered cellular activity associated with the inflammatory process. In allergic rhinitis, CysLTs are released from the nasal mucosa after allergen exposure during early- and late-phase reactions and are associated with symptoms of allergic rhinitis.

Montelukast causes inhibition of airway CysLT$_1$ receptors as demonstrated by the ability to inhibit bronchoconstriction caused by inhaled LTD$_4$ in asthmatics. Doses as low as 5 mg cause substantial blockage of LTD$_4$-induced bronchoconstriction. In 1 study, montelukast inhibited early- and late-phase bronchoconstriction caused by antigen challenge by 75% and 57%, respectively.

Seasonal allergic rhinitis – In patients with seasonal allergic rhinitis 15 years of age and older who received montelukast, a mean increase of 0.2% in peripheral blood eosinophil counts was noted, compared with a mean increase of 12.5% in placebo-treated patients.

➤*Pharmacokinetics:*

Absorption – Montelukast is rapidly absorbed following oral administration. After administration of the 10 mg film-coated tablet to fasted adults, the mean peak plasma concentration (C$_{max}$) is achieved in 3 to 4 hours (T$_{max}$). The mean oral bioavailability is 64%. The oral bioavailability and C$_{max}$ are not influenced by a standard meal in the morning.

For the 5 mg chewable tablet, the mean C$_{max}$ is achieved in 2 to 2.5 hours after administration to adults in the fasted state. The mean oral bioavailability is 73% in the fasted state vs 63% when administered with a standard meal in the morning.

For the 4 mg chewable tablet, the mean C$_{max}$ is achieved 2 hours after administration in pediatric patients 2 to 5 years of age in the fasted state.

The 4 mg oral granule formulation is bioequivalent to the 4 mg chewable tablet when administered to adults in the fasted state. A high-fat meal in the morning did not affect the AUC of montelukast oral granules; however, the meal decreased C$_{max}$ by 35% and prolonged T$_{max}$ from approximately 2.3 hours to approximately 6.4 hours.

The comparative pharmacokinetics of montelukast when administered as two 5 mg chewable tablets vs one 10 mg film-coated tablet have not been evaluated.

MONTELUKAST SODIUM

Distribution – Montelukast is more than 99% bound to plasma proteins. The steady-state volume of distribution averages 8 to 11 L. Studies in rats indicate minimal distribution across the blood-brain barrier.

Metabolism – Montelukast is extensively metabolized. In vitro studies using human liver microsomes indicate that cytochromes P450 3A4 and 2C9 are involved in the metabolism of montelukast.

Excretion – The plasma clearance of montelukast averages 45 mL/min in healthy adults. Following an oral dose of radiolabeled montelukast, 86% of the radioactivity was recovered in 5-day fecal collections and less than 0.2% was recovered in urine. Coupled with estimates of montelukast oral bioavailability, this indicates that montelukast and its metabolites are excreted almost exclusively via the bile.

In several studies, the mean plasma half-life ranged from 2.7 to 5.5 hours in healthy young adults. The pharmacokinetics of montelukast are nearly linear for oral doses up to 50 mg. During once-daily dosing with 10 mg montelukast, there is little accumulation of the parent drug in plasma (14%).

Special populations –
Elderly: The plasma half-life of montelukast is slightly longer in the elderly. No dosage adjustment in the elderly is required.

Hepatic function impairment: Patients with mild to moderate hepatic insufficiency and clinical evidence of cirrhosis had evidence of decreased metabolism of montelukast resulting in 41% higher mean montelukast area under the plasma concentration curve (AUC) following a single 10 mg dose. The elimination of montelukast was slightly prolonged compared with that in healthy subjects (mean half-life, 7.4 hours). No dosage adjustment is required in patients with mild to moderate hepatic insufficiency.

Contraindications

Hypersensitivity to any component of this product.

Warnings

➤*Acute asthma attacks:* Montelukast is not indicated for use in the reversal of bronchospasm in acute asthma attacks, including status asthmaticus. Advise patients to have appropriate rescue medication available. Therapy with montelukast can be continued during acute exacerbations of asthma.

➤*Fertility impairment:* In fertility studies in female rats, montelukast produced reductions in fertility and fecundity indices at an oral dose of 200 mg/kg (estimated exposure was approximately 70 times the AUC for adults at the maximum recommended daily oral dose).

➤*Elderly:* No overall differences in safety or efficacy were observed between these subjects and younger subjects, but greater sensitivity of some older individuals cannot be ruled out. Plasma half-life is slightly longer in the elderly. No dosage adjustment is required.

➤*Pregnancy: Category B.* Montelukast crosses the placenta following oral dosing in rats and rabbits. There are no adequate and well-controlled studies in pregnant women. Use during pregnancy only if clearly needed.

Merck maintains a registry to monitor the pregnancy outcomes of pregnant women exposed to montelukast. Health care providers are encouraged to report any prenatal exposure to montelukast by calling the Pregnancy Registry at (800) 986-8999.

➤*Lactation:* Studies in rats have shown that montelukast is excreted in breast milk. It is not known if montelukast is excreted in human milk. Exercise caution when administering to a nursing mother.

➤*Children:* The safety and efficacy in pediatric patients below 12 months of age have not been established.

Precautions

➤*Exercise-induced bronchoconstriction:* Do not use montelukast as monotherapy for the treatment and management of exercise-induced bronchospasm. Patients who have exacerbations of asthma after exercise should continue to use their usual regimen of inhaled beta-agonists as prophylaxis and have a short-acting inhaled beta-agonist available for rescue.

➤*Concurrent corticosteroids:* While the dose of inhaled corticosteroid may be reduced gradually under medical supervision, do not abruptly substitute montelukast for inhaled or oral corticosteroids.

➤*Eosinophilia:* In rare cases, patients on therapy with montelukast may present with systemic eosinophilia, sometimes with clinical features of vasculitis consistent with Churg-Strauss syndrome, a condition that is often treated with systemic corticosteroid therapy. These events usually, but not always, have been associated with the reduction of oral corticosteroid therapy. Physicians should be alert to eosinophilia, vasculitic rash, worsening pulmonary symptoms, cardiac complications, and/or neuropathy in their patients. A causal association between montelukast and these conditions has not been established.

➤*Phenylketonurics:* Inform phenylketonuric patients that the 4 and 5 mg chewable tablets contain phenylalanine (a component of aspartame), 0.674 and 0.842 mg per tablet, respectively.

➤*Aspirin sensitivity:* Avoid aspirin and nonsteroidal anti-inflammatory drugs (NSAIDs) while taking montelukast in patients with known aspirin sensitivity. Although montelukast is effective in improving airway function in asthmatics with documented aspirin sensitivity, it has not been shown to truncate bronchoconstrictor response to aspirin and other NSAIDs in aspirin-sensitive asthmatic patients.

Drug Interactions

➤*CYP450 inducers:* Phenobarbital decreased the AUC of montelukast approximately 40% following a single 10 mg dose of montelukast. No dosage adjustment for montelukast is recommended. It is reasonable to employ appropriate clinical monitoring when potent cytochrome P450 enzyme inducers, such as phenobarbital or rifampin, are coadministered with montelukast.

Adverse Reactions

➤*Seasonal allergic rhinitis:*

Adults and adolescents 15 years of age and older – Montelukast has been evaluated for safety in 2199 adult and adolescent patients 15 years of age and older in clinical trials. Montelukast administered once daily in the morning or in the evening was generally well tolerated with a safety profile similar to that of placebo. In placebo-controlled clinical trials, the following event was reported with a frequency of 1% or more and at an incidence greater than placebo, regardless of causality assessment: Upper respiratory infection, 1.9% of patients receiving montelukast vs 1.5% of patients receiving placebo. The incidence of somnolence was similar to that of placebo in all studies.

Pediatric patients 2 to 14 years of age – Montelukast has been evaluated in 280 pediatric patients 2 to 14 years of age in a 2-week, multicenter, double-blind, placebo-controlled, parallel-group, safety study. Montelukast administered once daily in the evening was generally well tolerated with a safety profile similar to that of placebo. In this study, the following events occurred with a frequency of 2% or more and at an incidence greater than placebo, regardless of causality assessment: Headache, otitis media, pharyngitis, upper respiratory infection.

➤*Asthma:*
Adults and adolescents 15 years of age and older –

Montelukast Adverse Reactions (≥ 1%)		
Adverse reaction	Montelukast 10 mg/day (n = 1955)	Placebo (n = 1180)
CNS		
Headache	18.4	18.1
Dizziness	1.9	1.4
GI		
Abdominal pain	2.9	2.5
Dyspepsia	2.1	1.1
Gastroenteritis, infectious	1.5	0.5
Lab test abnormalities[1]		
ALT increased	2.1	2
AST increased	1.6	1.2
Pyuria	1	0.9
Respiratory		
Influenza	4.2	3.9
Cough	2.7	2.4
Congestion, nasal	1.6	1.3
Miscellaneous		
Asthenia/Fatigue	1.8	1.2
Dental pain	1.7	1
Rash	1.6	1.2
Fever	1.5	0.9
Trauma	1	0.8

[1] Number of patients tested (montelukast and placebo, respectively): ALT and AST, 1935, 1170; pyuria, 1924, 1159.

Children 6 to 14 years of age – In patients 6 to 14 years of age receiving montelukast, the following adverse events occurred with a frequency of 2% or more and more frequently than in pediatric patients who received placebo, regardless of causality assessment: Diarrhea; laryngitis; pharyngitis; nausea; otitis; sinusitis; viral infection; influenza; fever; dyspepsia.

Children 2 to 5 years of age – In patients 2 to 5 years of age receiving montelukast, the following events occurred with a frequency of 2% or more and more frequently than in pediatric patients who received placebo, regardless of causality assessment: Rhinorrhea; otitis; ear pain; rash; urticaria; fever; cough; abdominal pain; diarrhea; headache; sinusitis; influenza; gastroenteritis; eczema; varicella; pneumonia; dermatitis; conjunctivitis.

Children 12 to 23 months of age – In patients 12 to 23 months of age receiving montelukast, the following adverse events occurred with a frequency of 2% or more and more frequently than in patients receiving placebo, regardless of causality assessment: Upper respiratory infection; wheezing; otitis media; pharyngitis; tonsillitis; cough; rhinitis.

➤*Postmarketing experience:* The following additional adverse reactions have been reported in postmarketing use: Hypersensitivity reactions (eg, anaphylaxis, angioedema, pruritus, urticaria, and, very rarely, hepatic eosinophilic infiltration); dream abnormalities; hallucinations; drowsiness; irritability; agitation, including aggressive behav-

MONTELUKAST SODIUM

ior; restlessness; insomnia; nausea; vomiting; dyspepsia; diarrhea; arthralgia; myalgia, including muscle cramps; increased bleeding tendency, bruising; palpitations; edema; seizures, pancreatitis (very rare).

In rare cases, patients on therapy with montelukast for asthma may present with systemic eosinophilia (see Precautions).

Overdosage

➤*Symptoms:* No mortality occurred following single oral doses of montelukast up to 5000 mg/kg in mice (estimated exposure was approximately 250 times the AUC for adults and children at the maximum recommended daily oral dose) and rats (estimated exposure was approximately 170 times the AUC for adults and children at the maximum recommended daily oral dose). In chronic asthma studies, montelukast has been administered at doses up to 200 mg/day to patients for 22 weeks and, in short-term studies, up to 900 mg/day to patients for approximately 1 week without clinically important adverse experiences.

There have been reports of acute overdosage in pediatric patients in postmarketing experience and clinical studies of up to at least 150 mg/day with montelukast. The clinical and laboratory findings observed were consistent with the safety profile in adults and older pediatric patients. There were no adverse experiences reported in the majority of overdosage reports. The most frequent adverse experiences observed were thirst, somnolence, mydriasis, hyperkinesia, and abdominal pain.

➤*Treatment:* No specific information is available on the treatment of overdosage with montelukast. In the event of overdose, it is reasonable to employ the usual supportive measures: Remove unabsorbed material from the GI tract, employ clinical monitoring and institute supportive therapy, if required. Refer to General Management of Acute Overdosage. It is not known whether montelukast is removed by peritoneal dialysis or hemodialysis.

Patient Information

Advise patients to take montelukast daily as prescribed, even when they are asymptomatic, as well as during periods of worsening asthma, and to contact a physician if the asthma is not well controlled.

Advise patients that oral montelukast tablets are not for the treatment of acute asthma attacks. Patients need to have appropriate short-acting inhaled beta-agonist medication available to treat asthma exacerbations.

Advise patients using montelukast to seek medical attention if short-acting inhaled bronchodilators are needed more often than usual or if more than the maximum number of inhalations of short-acting bronchodilator treatment prescribed for a 24-hour period are needed.

Instruct patients receiving montelukast not to decrease the dose or to stop taking any other antiasthma medications unless instructed by a physician.

Instruct patients who have exacerbations of asthma after exercise to continue to use their usual regimen of inhaled beta-agonists as prophylaxis unless otherwise instructed by a physician. All patients should have a short-acting inhaled beta-agonist available for rescue.

Advise patients with known aspirin sensitivity to avoid aspirin and NSAIDs while taking montelukast.

➤*Chewable tablets:*

Phenylketonurics – Inform caregivers of phenylketonuric patients that the 4 and 5 mg chewable tablets contain phenylalanine (a component of aspartame), 0.674 and 0.842 mg per 4 and 5 mg chewable tablet, respectively.

ZILEUTON

| *Rx* | **Zyflo** (Abbott) | **Tablets:** 600 mg | (ZL 600). White. Oval. Film coated. In 120s. |

Indications

➤*Asthma:* The prophylaxis and chronic treatment of asthma in adults and children ≥ 12 years of age.

Administration and Dosage

The recommended dosage of zileuton for the symptomatic treatment of patients with asthma is one 600 mg tablet 4 times a day for a total daily dose of 2400 mg. For ease of administration, zileuton may be taken with meals and at bedtime.

Actions

➤*Pharmacology:* Zileuton is a specific inhibitor of 5–lipoxygenase and thus inhibits leukotriene (LTB$_1$, LTC$_1$, LTD$_1$ and LTE$_1$) formation. Both the R(+) and S(−) enantiomers are pharmacologically active as 5–lipoxygenase inhibitors. Leukotrienes are substances that induce numerous biological effects including augmentation of neutrophil and eosinophil migration, neutrophil and monocyte aggregation, leukocyte adhesion, increased capillary permeability and smooth muscle contraction. These effects contribute to inflammation, edema, mucus secretion and bronchoconstriction in the airways of asthmatic patients. Sulfido-peptide leukotrienes (LTC$_1$, LTD$_1$, LTE$_1$, also known as the slow-releasing substances of anaphylaxis) and LTB$_4$, a chemoattractant for neutrophils and eosinophils, can be measured in a number of biological fluids including bronchoalveolar lavage fluid (BALF) from asthmatic patients. Zileuton inhibits leukotriene-dependent smooth muscle contractions. Pretreatment with zileuton attenuated bronchoconstriction caused by cold air challenge in patients with asthma.

➤*Pharmacokinetics:*

Absorption – Zileuton is rapidly absorbed upon oral administration with a mean time to peak plasma concentration (T$_{max}$) of 1.7 hours and a mean peak level (C$_{max}$) of 4.98 mcg/ml. The absolute bioavailability of zileuton is unknown. Systemic exposure (mean AUC) following 600 mg zileuton administration is 19.2 mcg•hr/ml. Plasma concentrations of zileuton are proportional to dose, and steady-state levels are predictable from single-dose pharmacokinetic data.

Food: Administration of zileuton with food resulted in a small but statistically significant increase (27%) in zileuton C$_{max}$ without significant changes in the extent of absorption (AUC) or T$_{max}$. Therefore, zileuton can be administered with or without food.

Distribution – The apparent volume of distribution of zileuton is ≈ 1.2 L/kg. Zileuton is 93% bound to plasma proteins, primarily to albumin, with minor binding to alpha-acid glycoprotein.

Metabolism – Several zileuton metabolites have been identified in plasma and urine. These include two diastereomeric O-glucuronide conjugates (major metabolites) and an N-dehydroxylated metabolite of zileuton. The urinary excretion of the inactive N-dehydroxylated metabolite and unchanged zileuton each accounted for < 0.5% of the dose. Liver microsomes have shown that zileuton and its N-dehydroxylated metabolite can be oxidatively metabolized by the cytochrome P450 isoenzymes 1A2, 2C9 and 3A4 (CYP1A2, CYP2C9 and CYP3A4).

Excretion – Elimination of zileuton is predominantly via metabolism with a mean terminal half-life of 2.5 hours. Apparent oral clearance of zileuton is 7 ml/min/kg. Zileuton activity is primarily because of the parent drug. Orally administered zileuton is well absorbed into the systemic circulation with 94.5% and 2.2% of the dose recovered in urine and feces, respectively.

Elderly – Zileuton pharmacokinetics were similar in healthy elderly subjects (> 65 years) compared with healthy younger adults (18 to 40 years).

Hepatic function impairment – Zileuton is contraindicated in patients with active liver disease (see Contraindications and Precautions).

Renal function impairment – Zileuton pharmacokinetics were similar in healthy subjects and in subjects with mild, moderate and severe renal insufficiency. In subjects with renal failure requiring hemodialysis, pharmacokinetics were not altered by hemodialysis and a very small percentage of the administered zileuton dose (< 0.5%) was removed by hemodialysis. Therefore, dosing adjustment in patients with renal dysfunction or undergoing hemodialysis is not necessary.

➤*Clinical trials:* Two double-blind, parallel, placebo controlled, multicenter studies have established the efficacy of zileuton in the treatment of asthma. Three hundred seventy-three patients were enrolled in the 6–month, double-blind phase of study 1, and 401 patients were enrolled in the 3–month double-blind phase of study 2. In these studies, the patients were mild-to-moderate asthmatics who had a mean baseline FEV$_1$ of ≈ 2.3 liters and used inhaled beta-agonists as needed. In each study, patients were randomized to receive zileuton 400 mg four times daily, zileuton 600 mg four times daily or placebo. Only the zileuton 600 mg four times daily dosage regimen was shown to be effective by demonstrating statistically significant improvement across several parameters.

Contraindications

Active liver disease or transaminase elevations greater than or equal to three times the upper limit of normal (≥ 3×ULN); hypersensitivity to zileuton or any of its inactive ingredients.

Warnings

➤*Hepatotoxicity:* Elevations of one or more liver function tests may occur during zileuton therapy. These laboratory abnormalities may progress, remain unchanged or resolve with continued therapy. In a few cases, initial transaminase elevations were first noted after discontinuing treatment, usually within 2 weeks. The ALT test is considered the most sensitive indicator of liver injury. The frequency of ALT elevations (≥ 3×ULN) was ≥ 1.9%.

Sixty-one percent of ALT elevations occurred during the first 2 months of zileuton therapy. After 2 months of treatment, the rate of new ALT elevations ≥ 3×ULN stabilized at a mean of 0.3% per month for patients receiving zileuton plus usual asthma care compared with 0.11% per month for patients receiving usual asthma care alone. Of 61 zileuton plus usual asthma care patients with ALT elevations from 3 to 5×ULN, 32 patients (52%) had ALT values decrease to < 2×ULN while continuing zileuton therapy. Twenty-one of 61 patients (34%) had further increases in ALT levels to ≥ 5×ULN. In patients who discontinued zileuton, elevated ALT levels returned to < 2×ULN in an average of 32 days (range 1 to 111 days). The overall rate of ALT elevation ≥ 3×ULN was 3.2%. One patient developed symptomatic hepatitis with jaundice, which resolved upon discontinuation of therapy. An additional 3 patients with transaminase elevations developed mild hyperbilirubinemia that was < 3×ULN. There was no evidence of hypersensitivity or other alternative etiologies for these findings. In subset analyses, females > 65 years of age appeared to be at an increased risk for ALT elevations. Patients with preexisting transaminase elevations may also be at an increased risk for ALT elevations.

➤*Acute asthma attacks:* Zileuton is not indicated for use in the reversal of bronchospasm in acute asthma attacks, including status asthmaticus. Therapy with zileuton can be continued during acute exacerbations of asthma.

➤*Hematologic:* Occurrences of low white blood cell count (≤ 2.8 × 10^9/L) were observed in 1% of 1678 patients taking zileuton and 0.6% of 1056 patients taking placebo. These findings were transient, and the majority of cases returned toward normal or baseline with continued zileuton therapy. All remaining cases returned toward normal or baseline after discontinuation of zileuton. Similar findings were also noted in a long-term safety surveillance study of 2458 patients treated with zileuton plus usual asthma care versus 489 patients treated only with usual asthma care for ≤ 1 year. The clinical significance of these observations is unknown.

➤*Hepatic function impairment:* Because treatment with zileuton may result in increased hepatic transaminases, use with caution in patients who consume substantial quantities of alcohol or have a history of liver disease.

➤*Carcinogenesis:* Increases in the incidence of liver, kidney and vascular tumors in female mice and a trend towards an increase in the incidences of liver tumors in male mice were observed at 450 mg/kg/day.

➤*Pregnancy: Category C.* Developmental studies indicated adverse effects (reduced body weight and increased skeletal variations) in rats at an oral dose of 300 mg/kg/day. There are no adequate and well controlled studies in pregnant women. Use zileuton during pregnancy only if the potential benefit justifies the potential risk.

➤*Lactation:* Zileuton and its metabolites are excreted in rat milk. It is not known if zileuton is excreted in human breast milk. Decide whether to discontinue nursing or to discontinue the drug.

➤*Children:* The safety and effectiveness of zileuton in pediatric patients < 12 years of age have not been established.

Precautions

➤*Monitoring:* Evaluate hepatic transaminases at initiation of and during therapy with zileuton. Monitor serum ALT before treatment begins, once-a-month for the first 3 months, every 2 to 3 months for the remainder of the first year and periodically thereafter for patients receiving long-term zileuton therapy. If symptoms of liver dysfunction (right upper quadrant pain, nausea, fatigue, lethargy, pruritus, jaundice or "flu-like" symptoms) develop or transaminase elevations > 5 times the ULN occur, discontinue therapy and follow transaminase levels until normal.

Drug Interactions

Liver microsomes have shown that zileuton and its N-dehydroxylated metabolite can be oxidatively metabolized by the cytochrome P450 isoenzymes 1A2, 2C9 and 3A4. Therefore, use caution when prescribing a medication that inhibits any of these enzymes.

ZILEUTON

Zileuton Drug Interactions			
Precipitant Drug	Object Drug*		Description
Digoxin Oral Contraceptives Phenytoin Prednisone	Zileuton	↔	Coadministration have shown no significant interactions.
Zileuton	Propranolol	↑	Coadministration of zileuton and propranolol results in doubling of propranolol AUC and consequent increased beta blocker activity.
Zileuton	Theophylline	↑	Coadministration of zileuton and theophylline results in, on average, an approximate doubling of serum theophylline concentrations. Reduce theophylline dosage in these patients and monitor serum theophylline concentrations closely.
Zileuton	Warfarin	↑	Coadministration of zileuton and warfarin results in a clinically significant increase in prothrombin time (PT). Monitor PT closely.

*↑ = Object drug increased. ↔ = Undetermined clinical effect.

Adverse Reactions

Patients Experiencing Adverse Events with Zileuton (%)		
Body system/Event	Zileuton (n = 475)	Placebo (n = 491)
GI		
Dyspepsia	8.2	2.9
Nausea	5.5	3.7
Miscellaneous		
Headache	24.6	24
Pain (unspecified)	7.8	5.3
Abdominal pain	4.6	2.4
Asthenia	3.8	2.4
Accidental injury	3.4	2
ALT elevation[1]	12	0.2
Low white blood cell[1]	1	0.6
Myalgia	3.2	2.9
Discontinuation	9.7	8.4

[1] See Warnings.

Other adverse events (frequency > 1%): Arthralgia; chest pain; conjunctivitis; constipation; dizziness; fever; flatulence; hypertonia; insomnia; lymphadenopathy; malaise; neck pain/rigidity; nervousness; pruritus; somnolence; urinary tract infection; vaginitis; vomiting.

Overdosage

►Symptoms: The oral minimum lethal doses in mice and rats were 500 to 1000 and 300 to 1000 mg/kg in various preparations, respectively (providing> 3 and 9 times the systemic exposure achieved at the maximum recommended human daily oral dose, respectively). No deaths occurred, but nephritis was reported in dogs at an oral dose of 1000 mg/kg. Human experience of acute overdose with zileution is limited. A patient in a clinical trial took between 6.6 and 9 g of zileuton in a single dose. Vomiting was induced, and the patient recovered without sequelae.

►Treatment: Zileuton is not removed by dialysis. If an overdose occurs, treat the patient symptomatically and institute supportive measures as required. If indicated, achieve elimination of unabsorbed drug by emesis or gastric lavage; observe usual precautions to maintain the airway.

Patient Information

Inform patients that zileuton is indicated for the chronic treatment of asthma and should be taken regularly as prescribed even during symptom-free periods.

Zileuton is not a bronchodilator; do not use to treat acute episodes of asthma.

When taking zileuton, do not decrease the dose or stop taking any other antiasthma medications unless instructed by a physician.

While using zileuton, seek medical attention if short-acting bronchodilators are needed more often than usual or if more than the maximum number of inhalations of short-acting bronchodilator treatment prescribed for a 24–hour period are needed.

The most serious side effect of zileuton is elevation of liver enzymes. While taking zileuton, patients must have liver enzyme tests monitored on a regular basis. If patients experience signs or symptoms of liver dysfunction (right upper quadrant pain, nausea, fatigue, lethargy, pruritus, jaundice or "flu-like" symptoms), contact a physician immediately.

Zileuton can interact with other drugs. While taking zileuton, consult a doctor before starting or stopping any prescription or non-prescription medicines.

A patient leaflet is included with the tablets.

OMALIZUMAB

Rx	**Xolair** (Genentech)	**Powder for injection, lyophilized:** 202.5 mg (150 mg/1.2 mL after reconstitution)	Preservative free. 145.5 mg sucrose. In single-use 5 mL vials.

Indications

➤*Moderate to severe persistent asthma:* For adults and adolescents 12 years of age and older with moderate to severe persistent asthma who have a positive skin test or in vitro reactivity to a perennial aeroallergen and those symptoms are inadequately controlled with inhaled corticosteroids.

➤*Unlabeled uses:* Omalizumab may be beneficial in treating seasonal allergic rhinitis.

Administration and Dosage

➤*Approved by the FDA:* June 20, 2003.

Omalizumab 150 to 375 mg is administered SC every 2 or 4 weeks. Because the solution is slightly viscous, the injection may take 5 to 10 seconds to administer. Doses (mg) and dosing frequency are determined by serum total immunoglobulin E (IgE) level (units/mL), measured before the start of treatment, and body weight (kg). See the dose determination chart below for appropriate dose assignment. Doses of more than 150 mg are divided among more than 1 injection site to limit injections to not more than 150 mg per site.

Omalizumab Doses Administered by SC Injection Every 4 Weeks (mg)

Pretreatment serum IgE (units/mL)	Body weight (kg)			
	30 to 60	> 60 to 70	> 70 to 90	> 90 to 150
≥ 30 to 100	150	150	150	300
> 100 to 200	300	300	300	See next table
> 200 to 300	300	See next table	See next table	See next table

Omalizumab Doses Administered by SC Injection Every 2 Weeks (mg)

Pretreatment serum IgE (units/mL)	Body weight (kg)			
	30 to 60	> 60 to 70	> 70 to 90	> 90 to 150
> 100 to 200	See previous table	See previous table	See previous table	225
> 200 to 300	See previous table	225	225	300
> 300 to 400	225	225	300	Do not dose
> 400 to 500	300	300	375	Do not dose
> 500 to 600	300	375	Do not dose	Do not dose
> 600 to 700	375	Do not dose	Do not dose	Do not dose

➤*Dosage adjustment:* Total IgE levels are elevated during treatment and remain elevated for up to 1 year after the discontinuation of treatment. Therefore, retesting of IgE levels during omalizumab treatment cannot be used as a guide for dose determination. Base dose determination after treatment interruptions lasting less than 1 year on serum IgE levels obtained at the initial dose determination. Total serum IgE levels may be retested for dose determination if treatment with omalizumab has been interrupted for 1 year or more.

Adjust doses for significant changes in body weight.

➤*Preparation:* Prepare omalizumab for SC administration by using sterile water for injection only.

The lyophilized product takes 15 to 20 minutes to dissolve. The fully reconstituted product will appear clear or slightly opalescent and may have a few small bubbles or foam around the edge of the vial. The reconstituted product is somewhat viscous; in order to obtain the full 1.2 mL dose, all of the product must be withdrawn from the vial before expelling any air or excess solution from the syringe.
1.) Draw 1.4 mL sterile water for injection into a 3 mL syringe equipped with a 1 inch 18-gauge needle.
2.) Inject the sterile water for injection directly into the product.
3.) Keeping the vial upright, gently swirl the vial for approximately 1 minute to evenly wet the powder. Do not shake.
4.) Gently swirl the vial for 5 to 10 seconds approximately every 5 minutes in order to dissolve any remaining solids. There should be no visible gel-like particles in the solution. Some vials may take longer than 20 minutes to dissolve completely. Do not use if the contents do not dissolve completely by 40 minutes.
5.) Invert the vial for 15 seconds in order to allow the solution to drain toward the stopper. Using a new 3 mL syringe equipped with a 1 inch 18-gauge needle, insert the needle into the inverted vial. Before removing the needle from the vial, pull the plunger all the way back to the end of the syringe barrel in order to remove all of the solution from the inverted vial.
6.) Replace the 18-gauge needle with a 25-gauge needle for SC injection.
7.) Expel air, large bubbles, and any excess solution in order to obtain the required 1.2 mL dose.

Number of Injections and Total Injection Volumes for Asthma

Dose (mg)	Number of injections	Total volume injected (mL)*
150	1	1.2
225	2	1.8
300	2	2.4
375	3	3

* 1.2 mL maximum delivered volume per vial.

➤*Storage/Stability:* Ship omalizumab at controlled ambient temperature (30°C or lower 86°F or lower). Store omalizumab under refrigerated conditions (2° to 8°C; 36° to 46°F). Do not use beyond the expiration date stamped on carton.

Omalizumab is for single use only and contains no preservatives. The solution may be used for SC administration within 8 hours following reconstitution when stored in the vial at 2° to 8°C (36° to 46°F), or within 4 hours of reconstitution when stored at room temperature.

Protect reconstituted omalizumab vials from direct sunlight.

Actions

➤*Pharmacology:* Omalizumab is a recombinant DNA-derived humanized IgG1κ murine monoclonal antibody that selectively binds to human IgE. Omalizumab inhibits the binding of IgE to the high-affinity IgE receptor (FcεRI) on the surface of mast cells and basophils. Reduction in surface-bound IgE on FcεRI-bearing cells limits the degree of release of mediators of the allergic response. Treatment with omalizumab also reduces the number of FcεRI receptors on basophils in atopic patients.

In clinical studies, serum free IgE levels were reduced in a dose-dependent manner within 1 hour following the first dose and maintained between doses. Mean serum free IgE decrease was greater than 96% using recommended doses.

After discontinuation of omalizumab dosing, the omalizumab-induced increase in total IgE and decrease in free IgE were reversible, with no observed rebound in IgE levels after drug washout. Total IgE levels did not return to pretreatment levels for up to 1 year after discontinuation of omalizumab.

➤*Pharmacokinetics:*

Absorption/Distribution – After SC administration, omalizumab is absorbed with an average absolute bioavailability of 62%. Omalizumab was absorbed slowly, reaching peak serum concentrations after an average of 7 to 8 days. The pharmacokinetics of omalizumab are linear at doses greater than 0.5 mg/kg. Following multiple doses of omalizumab, areas under the serum concentration-time curve from day 0 to day 14 at steady state were up to 6-fold of those after the first dose.

The apparent volume of distribution following SC administration was approximately 78 mL/kg.

Metabolism/Excretion – Clearance of omalizumab involves IgG clearance processes as well as clearance via specific binding and complex formation with its target ligand, IgE. Liver elimination of IgG includes degradation in the liver reticuloendothelial system (RES) and endothelial cells. Intact IgG is also excreted in bile.

Omalizumab serum elimination half-life averaged 26 days, with apparent clearance averaging approximately 2.4 mL/kg/day. In addition, doubling body weight approximately doubled apparent clearance.

Contraindications

Severe hypersensitivity reaction to omalizumab.

Warnings

➤*Hypersensitivity reactions:* Anaphylaxis has occurred within 2 hours of the first or subsequent administration of omalizumab in fewer than 0.1% of patients without other identifiable allergic triggers. These events included urticaria and throat and/or tongue edema. Observe patients after injection of omalizumab; medications for the treatment of severe hypersensitivity reactions including anaphylaxis should be available. If a severe hypersensitivity reaction to omalizumab occurs, discontinue therapy.

➤*Carcinogenesis:* Malignant neoplasms were observed in 0.5% of omalizumab-treated patients compared with 0.2% of control patients in clinical studies of asthma and other allergic disorders. The observed malignancies in omalizumab-treated patients were a variety of types, with breast, nonmelanoma skin, prostate, melanoma, and parotid occurring more than once, and 5 other types occurring once each. The majority of patients were observed for less than 1 year. The impact of longer exposure to omalizumab or use in patients at higher risk for malignancy (eg, elderly, current smokers) is not known.

➤*Pregnancy: Category B.* There are no adequate and well-controlled studies in pregnant women. Use during pregnancy only if clearly needed.

OMALIZUMAB

➤*Lactation:* The excretion of omalizumab in milk was evaluated in female cynomolgus monkeys receiving SC doses of 75 mg/kg/week. Neonatal plasma levels of omalizumab after in utero exposure and 28 days of nursing were between 11% and 94% of the maternal plasma level. Milk levels of omalizumab were 1.5% of maternal blood concentration. While omalizumab presence in human milk has not been studied, IgG is excreted in human milk and therefore it is expected that omalizumab will be present in human milk. The potential for omalizumab absorption or harm to the infant are unknown; exercise caution when administering omalizumab to a nursing woman.

➤*Children:* Safety and effectiveness in pediatric patients younger than 12 years of age have not been established.

Precautions

➤*Acute exacerbations:* Omalizumab has not been shown to alleviate asthma exacerbations acutely and should not be used for the treatment of acute bronchospasm or status asthmaticus.

➤*Concomitant corticosteroid use:* Do not abruptly discontinue systemic or inhaled corticosteroids upon initiation of omalizumab therapy. Perform decreases in corticosteroids under the direct supervision of a physician. Decreases may need to be performed gradually.

➤*Serum IgE levels:* Serum total IgE levels increase following administration of omalizumab because of formation of omalizumab:IgE complexes. Elevated serum total IgE levels may persist for up to 1 year following discontinuation of omalizumab. Serum total IgE levels obtained less than 1 year following discontinuation may not reflect steady state free IgE levels and should not be used to reassess the dosing regimen.

➤*Immunogenicity:* Low titers of antibodies to omalizumab were detected in approximately less than 0.1% of patients treated with omalizumab.

Adverse Reactions

The most serious adverse reactions occurring in clinical studies with omalizumab are malignancies and anaphylaxis. The observed incidence of malignancy among omalizumab-treated patients was 0.5%. Anaphylactic reactions were rare but temporally associated with omalizumab administration.

The adverse reactions most commonly observed among patients treated with omalizumab included injection site reaction (45%), viral infections (23%), upper respiratory tract infection (20%), sinusitis (16%), headache (15%), and pharyngitis (11%). These were also the most frequently reported adverse reactions resulting in clinical intervention (eg, discontinuation of omalizumab or the need for concomitant medication to treat an adverse reaction).

Adverse Events More Frequent in Omalizumab-Treated Patients (≥ 1%)		
Adverse reaction	Omalizumab (n = 738)	Placebo (n = 717)
Dermatologic		
Pruritus	2	1
Dermatitis	2	1
Musculoskeletal		
Arthralgia	8	6
Fracture	2	1
Leg pain	4	2
Arm pain	2	1
Miscellaneous		
Pain	7	5
Fatigue	3	2
Dizziness	3	2
Earache	2	1

➤*Injection site reactions:* Injection site reactions of any severity occurred at a rate of 45% in omalizumab-treated patients compared with 43% in placebo-treated patients. The types of injection site reactions included: Bruising, redness, warmth, burning, stinging, itching, hive formation, pain, indurations, mass, and inflammation.

Severe injection site reactions occurred more frequently in omalizumab-treated patients compared with patients in the placebo group (12% vs 9%).

The majority of injection site reactions occurred within 1 hour postinjection, lasted fewer than 8 days, and generally decreased in frequency at subsequent dosing visits.

➤*Hypersensitivity:* Allergic symptoms, including urticaria, dermatitis, and pruritus were observed in patients treated with omalizumab. There were also 3 cases of anaphylaxis observed within 2 hours of omalizumab administration in which there were no other identifiable allergic triggers (see Warnings).

Overdosage

Single IV doses of up to 4000 mg have been administered to patients without evidence of dose-limiting toxicities. The highest cumulative dose administered to patients was 44,000 mg over a 20-week period, which was not associated with toxicities.

Patient Information

Inform patients receiving omalizumab to not decrease the dose of, or stop taking any other asthma medications unless otherwise instructed by their physicians.

Inform patients that they may not see immediate improvement in their asthma after beginning omalizumab therapy.

Corticosteroids

For additional information, refer to the general discussion of Systemic Glucocorticoids in the Endocrine and Metabolic Agents chapter.

WARNING

Adrenal insufficiency: Deaths caused by adrenal insufficiency have occurred in asthmatic patients during and after transfer from systemic corticosteroids to inhaled corticosteroids. After withdrawal from systemic corticosteroids, several months are required for recovery of hypothalamic-pituitary-adrenal (HPA) function. During this period of HPA suppression, patients may exhibit symptoms of adrenal insufficiency when exposed to trauma, surgery, or infections, particularly gastroenteritis or other conditions with acute electrolyte loss. Although inhaled glucocorticoids may control asthmatic symptoms during these episodes, they do not provide the necessary mineralocorticoid for the treatment of these emergencies. Patients previously maintained on ≥ 20 mg/day of prednisone (or equivalent) may be most susceptible, especially when their systemic corticosteroids have been almost completely withdrawn.

Stress/Severe asthma attack: During periods of stress or a severe asthmatic attack, have patients withdrawn from systemic corticosteroids resume them (in large doses) immediately and contact a physician. Have patients carry a warning card indicating that they may need supplementary systemic corticosteroids during such periods. To assess the risk of adrenal insufficiency in emergency situations, periodically perform routine adrenal cortical function tests, including measurement of early morning resting cortisol levels in all patients. An early morning resting cortisol level may be accepted as normal only if it falls at or near the normal mean level.

Indications

►*Asthma, chronic:* Maintenance and prophylactic treatment of asthma; includes patients who require systemic corticosteroids and may benefit from systemic dose reduction/elimination.

For specific labeled indications, refer to individual drug monographs.

Administration and Dosage

►*Comparative efficacy:* Specific dosage guidelines for individual agents are included in the product listings. The relative anti-inflammatory potency of inhaled corticosteroids are in the following order: Flunisolide = triamcinolone acetonide < beclomethasone dipropionate = budesonide < fluticasone. Current data only supports a difference in potency, not efficacy, among the inhaled corticosteroids. The principle advantage of more potent inhaled corticosteroids may be in improved patient compliance and acceptance.

Estimated Comparative Daily Dosages for Inhaled Corticosteroids (Adults)[1]

Drug	Low dose	Medium dose	High dose
Beclomethasone dipropionate	168 to 504 mcg	504 to 840 mcg	> 840 mcg
42 mcg/puff	4 to 12 puffs	12 to 20 puffs	> 20 puffs
84 mcg/puff	2 to 6 puffs	6 to 10 puffs	> 10 puffs
Budesonide *Turbuhaler*	200 to 400 mcg	400 to 600 mcg	> 600 mcg
200 mcg/dose	1 to 2 inhalations	2 to 3 inhalations	> 3 inhalations
Flunisolide	500 to 1000 mcg	1000 to 2000 mcg	> 2000 mcg
250 mcg/puff	2 to 4 puffs	4 to 8 puffs	> 8 puffs
Fluticasone	88 to 264 mcg	264 to 660 mcg	> 660 mcg
MDI:[2] 44, 110, 220 mcg/puff	2 to 6 puffs (44 mcg) or 2 puffs (110 mcg)	2 to 6 puffs (110 mcg)	> 6 puffs (110 mcg) or > 3 puffs (220 mcg)
DPI:[3] 50, 100, 250 mcg/puff	2 to 6 inhalations (50 mcg)	3 to 6 inhalations (100 mcg)	> 6 inhalations (100 mcg) or> 2 inhalations (250 mcg)
Triamcinolone acetonide	400 to 1000 mcg	1000 to 2000 mcg	> 2000 mcg
100 mcg/puff	4 to 10 puffs	10 to 20 puffs	> 20 puffs

[1] *Guidelines for the Diagnosis and Management of Asthma.* Expert Panel Report 2. National Institutes of Health. National Heart, Lung, and Blood Institute. February 1997. http://www.lungusa.org/asthma/astnhlbi.html

[2] MDI = Metered dose inhaler.
[3] DPI = Dry powder inhaler.

Estimated Comparative Daily Dosages for Inhaled Corticosteroids (Children)[1]

Drug	Low dose	Medium dose	High dose
Beclomethasone dipropionate (6 to 12 years of age)	84 to 336 mcg	336 to 672 mcg	> 672 mcg
42 mcg/puff	2 to 8 puffs	8 to 16 puffs	> 16 puffs
84 mcg/puff	1 to 4 puffs	4 to 8 puffs	> 8 puffs
Budesonide *Turbuhaler* (≥ 6 years of age)	100 to 200 mcg	200 to 400 mcg	> 400 mcg
200 mcg/dose		1 to 2 inhalations	> 2 inhalations
Flunisolide (6 to 15 years of age)	500 to 750 mcg	1000 to 1250 mcg	> 1250 mcg
250 mcg/puff	2 to 3 puffs	4 to 5 puffs	> 5 puffs
Fluticasone (≥ 12 years of age)	88 to 176 mcg	176 to 440 mcg	> 440 mcg
MDI:[2] 44, 110 mcg/puff	2 to 4 puffs (44 mcg)	4 to 10 puffs (44 mcg) or 2 to 4 puffs (110 mcg)	> 4 puffs (110 mcg)
DPI:[3] 50, 100, 250 mcg/dose	2 to 4 inhalations (50 mcg)	2 to 4 inhalations (100 mcg)	> 4 inhalations (100 mcg) or> 2 inhalations (250 mcg)
Triamcinolone acetonide (6 to 12 years of age)	400 to 800 mcg	800 to 1200 mcg	> 1200 mcg
100 mcg/puff	4 to 8 puffs	8 to 12 puffs	> 12 puffs

[1] *Guidelines for the Diagnosis and Management of Asthma.* Expert Panel Report 2. National Institutes of Health. National Heart, Lung, and Blood Institute. February 1997. http://www.lungusa.org/asthma/astnhlbi.html

[2] MDI = Metered dose inhaler.
[3] DPI = Dry powder inhaler.

►*Patients receiving concomitant systemic steroids:* Stabilize the patient's asthma before treatment is started. Initially, use inhaled corticosteroids concurrently with usual maintenance dose of systemic steroid. After ≈ 1 week, start gradual withdrawal of the systemic steroid by reducing the daily or alternate daily dose. Make the next reduction after 1 or 2 weeks, depending on response. These decrements should not exceed 2.5 mg prednisone or equivalent. A slow rate of withdrawal cannot be overemphasized.

During withdrawal, some patients may experience symptoms of steroid withdrawal (eg, joint or muscular pain, lassitude, depression) despite maintenance or even improvement of respiratory function. Encourage continuance with the inhaler, but observe for objective signs of adrenal insufficiency. If adrenal insufficiency occurs, increase the systemic steroid dose temporarily and continue further withdrawal more slowly.

During periods of stress or severe asthma attack, transfer patients may require supplementary systemic steroids (see Warning box).

Actions

►*Pharmacology:* Corticosteroids may have direct inhibitory effects on many cells involved in airway inflammation in asthma (eg, macrophages, T-lymphocytes, eosinophils, airway epithelial cells). In vitro, corticosteroids decrease cytokine-mediated survival of eosinophils, reducing the number of eosinophils in the circulation and airways of patients with asthma during corticosteroid therapy. While corticosteroids may not inhibit the release of mast cells in an allergic reaction, they do reduce the number of mast cells within the airway. Corticosteroids may also inhibit plasma exudation and the secretion of mucous in inflamed airways.

Inhaled corticosteroids have anti-inflammatory effects of the bronchial mucosa of asthma patients. Treatment with inhaled corticosteroids for 1 to 3 months results in a reduction in mast cells, macrophages, T-lymphocytes, and eosinophils in the epithelium and submucosa in the bronchioles. By reducing airway inflammation, inhaled corticosteroids lessen airway hyperresponsiveness in asthmatic adults and children. Long-term therapy reduces airway responsiveness to histamine cholinergic agonists, and allergens. Treatment also lowers responsiveness to exercise, fog, cold air, bradykinin, adenosine, and irritants. Inhaled corticosteroids make the airways less sensitive to these spasmogens and limits the maximal narrowing of the airway. Maximal effects of inhaled corticosteroid treatment may not be seen for several months.

►*Pharmacokinetics:*

Pharmacokinetics of Inhaled Corticosteroids

Parameters	Corticosteroids				
	Beclomethasone	Budesonide	Flunisolide	Fluticasone	Triamcinolone
Absorption Systemic bioavailability from lungs	≈ 20%	25%	40%	20	21.5%
Distribution Vd (L/kg)	NA	4.3	1.8	3.5	1.4
Protein binding	87%	85% to 90%	NA	91%	≈ 68%
Metabolism Site	liver (CYP3A)	liver (CYP3A)	liver	liver (CYP3A4)	mostly from liver, less extensively from the kidneys
Metabolites (Activity)	beclomethasone 17-mono-propionate (active), free beclomethasone (very weak anti-inflammatory effects)	16α-hydroxy-prednisolone and 6β-hydroxy-budesonide (< 1% of parent)	6β-OH (low corticosteroid potency)	17β-carboxylic acid (negligible in animal studies)	6β-hydroxy-triamcinolone acetonide, 21-carboxy-triamcinolone acetonide, and 21-carboxy-6β-hydroxytriamcinolone acetonide (less active than parent)
Excretion Site	feces, urine (< 10%)	urine (≈ 60%), feces	renal (50%), feces (40%)	feces, urine (< 0.02%)	urine (≈ 40%), feces (≈ 60%)
T½	2.8 hr	2.8 hr	≈ 1.8 hr	3.1 hr	1.5 hr

Contraindications

Relief of acute bronchospasm; primary treatment of status asthmaticus or other acute episodes of asthma when intensive measures are required; hypersensitivity to any ingredients.

►*Vanceril:* Relief of asthma that can be controlled by bronchodilators and other nonsteroid medications; in patients who require systemic corticosteroid treatment infrequently; treatment of nonasthmatic bronchitis.

Warnings

►*Infections:* Localized fungal infections with *Candida albicans* or *Aspergillus niger* have occurred in the mouth, pharynx, and occasionally the larynx. Positive cultures for oral *Candida* may be present in up to 34% to 75% of patients. Incidence of clinically apparent infection is low and may require treatment with appropriate antifungal therapy or discontinuance of inhaled steroid treatment. Actions that may minimize the problem include dose reduction, decreasing dose frequency, rinsing mouth after use, and use of an add-on spacer device.

Use inhaled corticosteroids with caution, if at all, in patients with active or quiescent tuberculous infection of the respiratory tract; untreated systemic fungal, bacterial, parasitic, or viral infection; or ocular herpes simplex.

►*Compromised immune systems:* People who are on drugs that suppress the immune system are more susceptible to infections than healthy individuals. For example, chickenpox and measles can have a more serious or even fatal course in nonimmune children or adults on corticosteroids. In such children or adults who have not had these diseases, take particular care to avoid exposure. How the dose, route, and duration of corticosteroid administration affect the risk of disseminated infection is unknown. The contribution of the underlying disease or prior corticosteroid treatment to the risk is also unknown. If exposed to chickenpox, prophylaxis with varicella-zoster immune globulin (VZIG) may be indicated. If exposed to measles, prophylaxis with pooled IM immunoglobulin (IG) may be indicated. If chickenpox develops, consider treatment with antiviral agents.

►*Acute asthma:* These products are not bronchodilators and are not for rapid relief of bronchospasm. Contact a physician immediately when asthmatic episodes do not respond to bronchodilators. Patients may require systemic corticosteroids.

There is no evidence that control of asthma can be achieved by inhaled corticosteroids in amounts greater than recommended doses.

►*Bronchospasm:* This may occur with an immediate increase in wheezing following dosing. If bronchospasm occurs following corticosteroid inhalation, treat immediately with a short-acting inhaled bronchodilator. Discontinue inhalation treatment, and institute an alternative treatment.

Instruct patients to contact their health care provider immediately when episodes of asthma do not respond to bronchodilators during treatment with corticosteroid inhalation. During such episodes, patients may require treatment with systemic corticosteroids.

►*Combination with prednisone:* Combination therapy of inhaled corticosteroids with systemic corticosteroids may increase the risk of HPA suppression compared to a therapeutic dose of either one alone. Use inhaled corticosteroids with caution in patients already receiving prednisone.

►*Replacement therapy:* Transfer from systemic steroid therapy may unmask allergic conditions previously suppressed (eg, rhinitis, conjunctivitis, eczema).

►*Pregnancy:* Category C; Category B (**budesonide** only). Glucocorticoids are teratogenic in rodents. Findings include cleft palate, internal hydrocephaly, and axial skeletal defects; CNS and cranial malformations were observed in monkeys. There are no adequate and well-controlled studies in pregnant women. Use these agents during pregnancy only if the benefit clearly justifies the potential risk to the fetus. Infants born of mothers who received substantial doses during pregnancy should be observed for adrenal insufficiency.

Budesonide – Studies of pregnant women have not shown that *Pulmicort Turbuhaler* increases the risk of abnormalities when administered during pregnancy. The results from a large population-based prospective cohort epidemiological study indicate no increased risk for congenital malformations from the use of inhaled budesonide during early pregnancy. Congenital malformations were studied in 2014 infants born to mothers reporting the use of inhaled budesonide for asthma in early pregnancy (usually 10 to 12 weeks after the last menstrual period), the period when most major organ malformations occur. The rate of recorded congenital malformations was similar compared with the general population rate (3.8% vs 3.5%, respectively). In addition, after exposure to inhaled budesonide, the number of infants born with orofacial clefts was similar to the expected number in the normal population (4 children vs 3.3, respectively).

►*Lactation:* Glucocorticoids are excreted in breast milk. It is unknown whether inhaled corticosteroids are excreted in breast milk. Decide whether to discontinue nursing or to discontinue the drug.

►*Children:* Insufficient information is available to warrant use in children < 6 years of age or < 12 with **fluticasone** and **beclomethasone**. Monitor growth in children and adolescents because there is evidence that oral corticosteroids may suppress growth in a dose-related fashion, particularly in higher doses for extended periods.

Precautions

►*Steroid withdrawal:* During withdrawal from oral steroids, some patients may experience symptoms of systemically active steroid withdrawal (eg, joint or muscular pain, lassitude, depression), despite maintenance or even improvement of respiratory function. Although steroid withdrawal effects are usually transient and not severe, severe and even fatal exacerbation of asthma can occur if the previous daily oral corticosteroid requirement had significantly exceeded 10 mg/day of prednisone or equivalent.

➤*HPA suppression:* In responsive patients, inhaled corticosteroids may permit control of asthmatic symptoms with less HPA suppression. Because these agents are absorbed and can be systemically active, the beneficial effects in minimizing or preventing HPA dysfunction may be expected only when recommended dosages are not exceeded. When administered in excessive doses or at recommended doses in a minority of susceptible patients, systemic corticosteroid effects (eg, hypercorticoidism, adrenal suppression) may occur. Slowly reduce or discontinue corticosteroid therapy when these events occur. Titrate patients to the lowest effective dose because of individual sensitivity to cortisol product effects. Carefully observe patients for evidence of systemic corticosteroid effects. Take particular care in observing patients postoperatively or during periods of stress for evidence of a decrease in adrenal function.

Flunisolide – Because of the possibility of higher systemic absorption, monitor patients using **flunisolide** for any evidence of systemic corticosteroid effect. If such changes occur, discontinue slowly, consistent with accepted procedures for discontinuing oral corticosteroids. When flunisolide is used chronically at 2 mg/day, monitor patients periodically for effects on the HPA axis.

➤*Glaucoma:* Rare instances of glaucoma, increased intraocular pressure, and cataracts have been reported following the inhaled administration of corticosteroids.

➤*Long-term effects:* The effects of long-term glucocorticoid inhalation are unknown. Although there is no clinical evidence of adverse effects, the local and systemic effects on developmental or immunologic processes in the mouth, pharynx, trachea, and lung are unknown.

There is no information about effects on acute, recurrent, or chronic pulmonary infection (including active or quiescent tuberculosis) or effects of long-term use on lung or other tissues. Use with caution (see Warnings).

➤*Pulmonary infiltrates:* Pulmonary infiltrates with eosinophilia may occur with **beclomethasone** or **flunisolide**. This may manifest because of systemic steroid withdrawal when inhalational agents are used, but a causative role for either agent or vehicle cannot be ruled out.

➤*Reduction in growth velocity:* A reduction in growth velocity in children may occur as a result of inadequate control of chronic diseases such as asthma or from corticosteroid use. Closely follow the growth of adolescents taking corticosteroids by any route, and weigh the benefits of corticosteroid therapy and asthma control against the possibility of growth suppression if an adolescent's growth appears slowed.

Drug Interactions

➤*Ketoconazole:* A potent inhibitor of cytochrome P450 3A4 may increase plasma levels of **budesonide** and **fluticasone** during concomitant dosing. The clinical significance is unknown. Use caution.

Adverse Reactions

Suppression of HPA function (see Warning Box; Warnings).

Inhaled Corticosteroids Adverse Reactions (%)							
	Beclomethasone dipropionate	Budesonide inhalation powder	Budesonide inhalation suspension	Flunisolide	Fluticasone propionate aerosol	Fluticasone propionate inhalation powder	Triamcinolone acetonide
Cardiovascular							
Tachycardia	< 2	—	—	1 to 3	—	—	—
Chest pain	< 2	—	1 to 3	3 to 9	—	—	—
CNS							
Headache	12[1] 22 to 27[2]	13 to 14	—	25	17 to 22	9 to 15	7 to 21
Migraine	< 2	1 to 3	—	—	—	1 to 3	—
Insomnia	< 2	1 to 3	—	1 to 3	—	—	—
Dermatological							
Eczema	< 2[2]	—	1 to 3	3 to 9	—	—	—
Pruritus	< 2[2]	—	1 to 3	3 to 9	—	—	—
Rash	Rare[1] < 2	—	< 1 to 4	3 to 9	1 to 3	—	1 to 3
GI							
Nausea	1[1] < 2	1 to 3	—	25	1 to 3	—	—
Dyspepsia	3 to 6[2]	1 to 4	—	1 to 3	1 to 3	—	—
Dry mouth	—	1 to 3	—	1 to 3	—	—	1 to 3
Oral candidiasis	—	2 to 4	—	3 to 9	2 to 5	3 to 11	1 to 3
Gastroenteritis	—	1 to 3	5	—	—	1 to 3	—
Vomiting	—	1 to 3	2 to 4	25	1 to 3	—	1 to 3
Diarrhea	< 2	—	2 to 4	10	1 to 3	< 4	1 to 3
Abdominal pain	—	1 to 3	2 to 3	3 to 9	—	1 to 3	1 to 3
Anorexia	—	—	1 to 3	3 to 9	—	—	—
GU							
Dysmenorrhea	1 to 3[1] < 4[2]	—	—	—	1 to 3	1 to 3	—
Menstrual disturbance	—	—	—	3 to 9	—	1 to 3	—
Hypersensitivity							
Urticaria	Rare[1] < 2	—	—	1 to 3	Rare	1 to 3	Rare
Angioedema	Rare[1]	—	—	—	Rare	Rare	—
Respiratory							
Upper respiratory tract infections	9[1] < 2	19 to 24	34 to 38	25	15 to 22	16 to 22	—
Pharyngitis	8[1] 11 to 14[2]	5 to 10	—	1 to 3	10 to 14	6 to 13	7 to 25
Rhinitis	6[1]	—	7 to 12	3 to 9	1 to 3	2 to 9	—
Sinusitis	3[1] 3 to 4[2]	2 to 11	—	3 to 9	3 to 6	4 to 6	2 to 9
Nasal congestion	5 to 6[2]	—	—	15	8 to 16	4 to 7	—
Coughing	1 to 3[1] 7 to 9[2]	—	5 to 9	3 to 9	—	—	—
Dysphonia	1 to 3[1] < 2[2]	—	1 to 3	—	3 to 8	< 1 to 6	—
Bronchospasm	Rare[1] < 2	—	—	—	Rare	—	—
Sneezing	2 to 3[2]	—	—	3 to 9	—	1 to 3	—

Corticosteroids

Inhaled Corticosteroids Adverse Reactions (%)

	Beclomethasone dipropionate	Budesonide inhalation powder	Budesonide inhalation suspension	Flunisolide	Fluticasone propionate aerosol	Fluticasone propionate inhalation powder	Triamcinolone acetonide
Epistaxis	—	—	2 to 4	1 to 3	—	1 to 3	—
Chest congestion	< 2	—	—	3 to 9	1 to 3	1 to 3	1 to 3
Bronchitis	< 2	—	—	1 to 3	1 to 3	1 to 4	—
Special senses							
Taste alteration	< 2	1 to 3	—	10	—	—	—
Otitis media	—	—	9 to 12	—	—	1 to 3	—
Ear infection	—	—	2 to 5	3 to 9	—	—	—
Conjunctivitis	—	—	< 1 to 4	—	—	1 to 3	—
Earache	< 2	—	1 to 3	1 to 3	—	1 to 3	—
Miscellaneous							
Infection, viral	5 to 8[2]	—	3 to 5	—	—	—	—
Weight changes	—	1 to 3	—	1 to 3	—	—	1 to 3
Back pain	1[1]	2 to 6	—	—	—	—	2 to 4
Influenza-like syndrome	< 1 to 3[2]	6 to 14	1 to 3	10	3 to 8	3 to 4	2 to 5
Pain	2[1] < 2	5	—	—	—	1 to 3	1 to 3
Fever	< 2	< 4	—	3 to 9	1 to 3	2 to 4	—
Infection	—	1 to 3	1 to 3	—	—	—	—

[1] *QVAR.*   [2] *Vanceril* (both strengths).

➤*Beclomethasone:*

Miscellaneous – Fatigue (2% to 3%); increased asthma symptoms (< 2% to 3%); rigors, rectal hemorrhage, lacrimation, arthralgia, depression, skin discoloration, UTI, lymphadenopathy, respiratory disorder (< 2%).

➤*Budesonide inhalation powder:*

Musculoskeletal – Fracture, myalgia, neck pain (1% to 3%).

Miscellaneous – Voice alteration (1% to 6%); ecchymosis, syncope, hypertonia (1% to 3%).

➤*Budesonide inhalation suspension:*

CNS – Hyperkinesias, emotional lability (1% to 3%).

Dermatologic – Pustular rash, contact dermatitis (1% to 3%).

Musculoskeletal – Fracture, myalgia (1% to 3%).

Special senses – Eye infection, otitis externa (1% to 3%).

Miscellaneous – Moniliasis (3% to 4%); allergic reaction, fatigue, stridor, cervical lymphadenopathy, purpura, herpes simplex (1% to 3%).

Postmarketing: Hypersensitivity reactions, symptoms of hypocorticism/hypercorticism, psychiatric symptoms including depression, aggressive reactions, irritability, anxiety and psychosis, bone disorders including avascular necrosis of the femoral head and osteoporosis (< 1%).

➤*Flunisolide:*

CNS – Dizziness, irritability, nervousness, shakiness (3% to 9%); anxiety, depression, faintness, fatigue, hyperactivity, hypoactivity, moodiness, numbness, vertigo (1% to 3%).

Dermatologic – Acne, hives (1% to 3%).

GI – Upset stomach (10%); heartburn (3% to 9%); constipation, gas, increased appetite (1% to 3%); abdominal fullness (< 1%).

Hematologic – Capillary fragility, enlarged lymph nodes (1% to 3%).

Respiratory – Sore throat (20%); cold symptoms (15%); runny nose, sinus congestion, sinus drainage, sinus infection, hoarseness, sputum, wheezing (3% to 9%); glossitis, mouth/throat irritation, phlegm, chest tightness, dyspnea, head stuffiness, laryngitis, nasal irritation, pleurisy, pneumonia, sinus discomfort (1% to 3%); shortness of breath (< 1%).

Special senses – Loss of smell (3% to 9%); blurred vision, eye discomfort, eye infection (1% to 3%).

Miscellaneous – Edema, palpitations (3% to 9%); chills, malaise, peripheral edema, sweating, weakness (1% to 3%).

➤*Fluticasone:*

CNS – Giddiness, nervousness (1% to 3%).

Respiratory – Nasal discharge (4% to 5%); allergic rhinitis (3% to 5%); pain in nasal sinus(es), laryngitis, acute nasopharyngitis, dyspnea, irritation caused by inhalant, tonsillitis (1% to 3%).

GI – Stomach disorder, gastroenteritis/colitis, abdominal discomfort, mouth/throat irritation (1% to 3%).

GU – Moniliasis, candidiasis of vagina, pelvic inflammatory disease, vaginitis/vulvovaginitis (1% to 3%).

Musculoskeletal – Back problems (< 1% to 4%); joint pain, sprain/strain, aches and pains, limb pain, muscular soreness, disorder/symptoms of neck (1% to 3%).

Special senses – Eye irritation, dental disorder, conjunctivitis (1% to 3%).

Miscellaneous – Dermatitis, rash/skin eruption, injury (1% to 3%).

Postmarketing: Throat soreness and irritation; hoarseness; aphonia; Cushingoid features; growth velocity reduction in children/adolescents; weight gain; hyperglycemia; restlessness; agitation; aggression; depression; immediate bronchospasm; asthma exacerbation; dyspnea; wheezing; chest tightness; cough; pruritus; contusions; ecchymosis; laryngitis; bronchospasm.

➤*Triamcinolone:*

GU – Cystitis, urinary tract infection, vaginal monilia (1% to 3%).

Musculoskeletal – Bursitis, myalgia, tenosynovitis (1% to 3%).

Respiratory – Hoarseness; cough; increased wheezing; irritated throat; dry throat; dry mouth; oral candidiasis.

Miscellaneous – Facial edema, photosensitivity, toothache, easy bruisability, steroid withdrawal symptoms, voice alteration (1% to 3%).

Overdosage

The potential for acute toxic effects following overdose of inhaled corticosteroids is low. Chronic overdosage may result in signs/symptoms of hypercorticoidism.

Patient Information

Patient instructions are available with each product.

Rinse mouth with water without swallowing after each dose to reduce the risk of oral candidiasis. If the infection develops, treat with appropriate therapy. Corticosteroid therapy may need to be interrupted.

Instruct patients whose systemic corticosteroids have been reduced or withdrawn to carry a warning card indicating the need for supplemental systemic steroids in the event of stress or severe asthmatic attack that is unresponsive to bronchodilators.

Advise patients not to stop therapy abruptly. If discontinuation is necessary, contact the physician.

This medication is intended for treatment of asthma. It does not contain medication intended to provide rapid relief of breathing difficulties during an asthma attack. It is very important that the medication is used regularly at the intervals recommended by doctor, and not as an emergency measure.

Warn people who are on immunosuppressant doses of corticosteroids to avoid exposure to chickenpox or measles. Advise patients to seek medical advice without delay if they are exposed.

Advise patients receiving bronchodilators (eg, albuterol) by inhalation to use the bronchodilator several minutes before the corticosteroid inhalant to enhance penetration of the steroid into the bronchial tree and reduce potential toxicity from the inhaled fluorocarbon propellants in the 2 aerosols.

Notify physician if sore throat or sore mouth occurs.

➤*Administration technique:* The success of these agents is a function of proper administration technique. The following guidelines may be useful:

Aerosol – Thoroughly shake the inhaler with canister in place; breathe out to the end of a normal breath. Hold the inhaler system upright; place the mouthpiece into the mouth and close the lips tightly. While activating the inhaler, take a slow, deep breath for 3 to 5 seconds, hold the breath for ≈ 10 seconds, and exhale slowly. Allow ≥ 1 minute between inhalations (puffs). Rinse the mouth with water after each use to help reduce dry mouth and hoarseness.

Corticosteroids

Inhaled powder – Hold inhaler upright, and twist the cover off. Twist the grip fully to the right as far as it will go, then twist it back. You will hear a click. Exhale; then place the mouthpiece between lips, slightly tilt head back, and inhale deeply and forcefully. Remove inhaler from mouth, and hold breath for ≈ 10 seconds. Allow ≥ 1 minute between inhalations (puffs). Rinse the mouth with water after each use to help reduce dry mouth and hoarseness.

BECLOMETHASONE DIPROPIONATE

| *Rx* | QVAR (IVAX) | Aerosol: 40 mcg/actuation | In 7.3 g canisters (100 actuations) with actuator. |
| | | 80 mcg/actuation | In 7.3 g canisters (100 actuations) with actuator. |

For complete prescribing information, refer to the Corticosteroids Respiratory Inhalant group monograph.

Indications

Not indicated for the relief of acute bronchospasm.

➤*Asthma, chronic:* In the maintenance treatment of asthma as prophylactic therapy in patients 5 years of age and older; for asthma patients who require systemic corticosteroid administration when adding an inhaled corticosteroid may reduce or eliminate the need for systemic corticosteroids.

Administration and Dosage

➤*Approved by the FDA:* May 1976.

Test aerosol by spraying 2 times into the air before first use and in cases where the product has not been used for over 10 days. Rinse mouth after inhalation.

The safety and efficacy in children less than 5 years of age have not been established.

The onset and degree of symptom relief will vary in individual patients. Improvement in asthma symptoms should be expected within the first or second week of starting treatment, but maximum benefit should not be expected until 3 to 4 weeks of therapy. For patients who do not respond adequately to the starting dose after 3 to 4 weeks of therapy, higher doses may provide additional asthma control. The safety and efficacy of beclomethasone when administered in excess of recommended doses have not been established.

The aerosol solution does not require shaking. Two actuations of the 40 mcg strength should provide a dose comparable to 1 actuation of the 80 mcg strength. The recommended dosage relative to CFC-based beclomethasone dipropionate (CFC-BDP) inhalation aerosols is lower because of differences in delivery characteristics between the products.

Recommended Doses in Patients ≥ 5 Years of Age		
Previous therapy	Recommended starting dose	Highest recommended dose
Adults and adolescents		
Bronchodilators alone	40 to 80 mcg twice daily	320 mcg twice daily
Inhaled corticosteroids	40 to 160 mcg twice daily	320 mcg twice daily
Children 5 to 11 years of age		
Bronchodilators alone	40 mcg twice daily	80 mcg twice daily
Inhaled corticosteroids	40 mcg twice daily	80 mcg twice daily

Titrate the dose downward over time to the lowest level that maintains proper asthma control. The aerosol may have a different taste and inhalation sensation than that of an inhaler containing CFC propellant.

➤*Patients not receiving systemic corticosteroids:* Follow the doses recommended above. In patients who respond to beclomethasone, improvement in pulmonary function is usually apparent within 1 to 4 weeks after the start of therapy. Once the desired effect is achieved, consider tapering to the lowest effective dose.

➤*Concomitant systemic corticosteroid therapy:* See Administration in group monograph.

➤*Storage/Stability:* Store at 25°C (77°F). Excursions permitted between 15° and 30°C (59° and 86°F). For optimal results, the canister should be at room temperature when used. Do not use actuator with any other inhalation drug product.

BUDESONIDE

Rx	Pulmicort Turbuhaler (AstraZeneca)	Powder: 200 mcg (each actuation delivers ≈ 160 mcg)/metered dose	(Pulmicort™ 200 mcg). In 200 dose *Turbuhaler*.
Rx	Pulmicort Respules (AstraZeneca)	Inhalation suspension: 0.25 mg/2 mL	EDTA. In single-dose envelopes. In 30s.
		0.5 mg/2 mL	EDTA. In single-dose envelopes. In 30s.

For complete prescribing information, refer to the Corticosteroids Respiratory Inhalant group monograph.

Indications

Not indicated for the relief of acute bronchospam.

➤*Turbuhaler:*

Asthma, chronic – For the maintenance treatment of asthma as prophylactic therapy in adults and children 6 years of age and older and for patients requiring oral corticosteroid therapy for asthma. Many of these patients may be able to reduce or eliminate their requirement for oral corticosteroids over time.

➤*Respules:*

Asthma, chronic – For the maintenance treatment of asthma and as prophylactic therapy in children 12 months to 8 years of age.

Administration and Dosage

➤*Turbuhaler:* Administer by the orally inhaled route in asthmatic patients 6 years of age and older. Individual patients will experience a variable onset and degree of symptom relief. Generally, budesonide has a relatively rapid onset of action for an inhaled corticosteroid. Improvement in asthma control following inhaled administration of budesonide can occur within 24 hours of treatment initiation, although maximum benefit may not be achieved for 1 to 2 weeks or longer. The safety and efficacy of budesonide when administered in excess of recommended doses have not been established.

➤*Respules:* Administer by the inhaled route via jet nebulizer connected to an air compressor in asthmatic patients 12 months to 8 years of age. Individual patients will experience a variable onset and degree of symptom relief. Improvement in asthma control following inhaled administration of budesonide can occur within 2 to 8 days of initiation of treatment, although maximum benefit may not be achieved for 4 to 6 weeks. The safety and efficacy of budesonide when administered in excess of recommended doses have not been established. In all patients, it is desirable to downward-titrate to the lowest effective dose once asthma stability is achieved. The recommended starting dose and highest recommended dose, based on prior asthma therapy, are listed in the following table.

Budesonide Recommended Starting Dose and Highest Recommended Dose		
Previous therapy	Recommended starting dose[1]	Highest recommended dose
Turbuhaler		
Adults		
Bronchodilators alone	200-400 mcg twice daily	400 mcg twice daily
Inhaled corticosteroids[2]	200-400 mcg twice daily	800 mcg twice daily
Oral corticosteroids	400-800 mcg twice daily	800 mcg twice daily
Children ≥ 6 years of age[3]		
Bronchodilators alone	200 mcg twice daily	400 mcg twice daily
Inhaled corticosteroids[2]	200 mcg twice daily	400 mcg twice daily
Oral corticosteroids	The highest recommended dose in children is 400 mcg twice daily.	
Respules		
Children 12 months to 8 years of age		
Bronchodilators alone	0.5 mg total daily dose administered either once or twice daily in divided doses	0.5 mg total daily dose

BUDESONIDE

Budesonide Recommended Starting Dose and Highest Recommended Dose		
Previous therapy	Recommended starting dose[1]	Highest recommended dose
Inhaled corticosteroids	0.5 mg total daily dose administered either once or twice daily in divided doses	1 mg total daily dose
Oral corticosteroids	1 mg total daily dose administered either as 0.5 mg twice daily or 1 mg once daily	1 mg total daily dose

[1] 200 mcg released with each actuation delivers ≈ 160 mcg from the mouthpiece to the patient (*Turbuhaler*).

[2] In patients with mild to moderate asthma who are well controlled on inhaled corticosteroids, dosing budesonide 200 mcg or 400 mcg once daily may be considered. Administer budesonide once daily either in the morning or evening.

[3] Insufficient information is available to warrant use in children less than 6 years of age.

►*Respules:* In symptomatic children not responding to nonsteroidal therapy, a starting dose of 0.25 mg once daily also may be considered.

If once-daily treatment with budesonide does not provide adequate control of asthma symptoms, increase the total daily dose or administer as a divided dose.

►*Patients not receiving systemic oral corticosteroids (Respules)*: Patients who require maintenance therapy of their asthma may benefit from treatment at the recommended doses above. Once the desired clinical effect is achieved, give consideration to tapering to the lowest effective dose. For the patients who do not respond adequately to the starting dose, give consideration to administering the total daily dose as a divided dose if a once-daily dosing schedule was followed. If necessary, higher doses up to the maximum recommended doses may provide additional asthma control.

►*Patients maintained on chronic oral corticosteroids:* Initially, use concurrently with the patient's usual maintenance dose of systemic corticosteroid. After approximately 1 week, gradual withdrawal of the systemic corticosteroid may be initiated by reducing the daily or alternate daily dose. Further incremental reductions may be made after an interval of 1 or 2 weeks, depending on patient response. Generally, these decrements should not exceed 25% of the prednisone dose or its equivalent. A slow rate of withdrawal is strongly recommended. During reduction of oral corticosteroids, monitor patients carefully for asthma instability, including objective measures of airway function, and for adrenal insufficiency. During withdrawal, some patients may experience symptoms of systemic corticosteroid withdrawal (eg, joint or muscular pain, lassitude, depression) despite maintenance or even improvement in pulmonary function. Encourage such patients to continue with treatment but monitor for objective signs of adrenal insufficiency. If evidence of adrenal insufficiency occurs, the systemic corticosteroid doses should be increased temporarily and thereafter,

withdrawal should continue more slowly. During periods of stress or a severe asthma attack, transfer patients may require supplementary treatment with systemic corticosteroids.

Turbuhaler – In all patients, it is desirable to titrate to the lowest effective dose once asthma stability is achieved.

Instruct patients to prime *Pulmicort Turbuhaler* prior to initial use and to inhale deeply and forcefully each time the unit is used. Rinsing the mouth after inhalation also is recommended.

Respules – Administer *Pulmicort Respules* via jet nebulizer connected to an air compressor with an adequate air flow, equipped with a mouthpiece or suitable face mask. Ultrasonic nebulizers are not suitable for the adequate administration of *Pulmicort Respules* and therefore, are not recommended.

The effects of mixing *Pulmicort Respules* with other nebulizable medications has not been adequately assessed; administer separately in the nebulizer.

►*Concomitant systemic steroid therapy:* See Administration in group monograph.

►*Storage/Stability:* Store *Pulmicort Turbuhaler* and *Pulmicort Respules* at room temperature 20° to 25°C (68° to 77°F). Store *Pulmicort Turbuhaler* in a tightly covered container in a dry place.

Respules – Store upright, protected from light. When an envelope has been opened, the shelf life of the unused *Pulmicort Respules* is 2 weeks when protected. After opening the aluminum foil envelope, return the unused *Pulmicort Respules* to the aluminum foil envelope to protect from light. Any opened *Pulmicort Respules* must be used promptly. Gently shake using a circular motion before use. Keep out of reach of children. Do not freeze.

FLUNISOLIDE

Rx	AeroBid (Forest)	**Aerosol:** ≈ 250 mcg/actuation	In canisters (100 metered doses).
Rx	AeroBid-M (Forest)		Menthol flavor. In canisters (100 metered doses).

For complete prescribing information, refer to the Corticosteroids Respiratory Inhalant group monograph.

WARNING

Particular care is needed in patients who are transferred from systemically active corticosteroids to flunisolide inhaler because deaths because of adrenal insufficiency have occurred in asthmatic patients during and after transfer from systemic corticosteroids to aerosol corticosteroids. After withdrawal from systemic corticosteroids, a number of months are required for recovery of hypothalamic-pituitary-adrenal (HPA) function. During this period of HPA suppression, patients may exhibit signs and symptoms of adrenal insufficiency when exposed to trauma, surgery, or infections, particularly gastroenteritis. Although flunisolide inhaler may provide control of asthmatic symptoms during these episodes, it does not provide the systemic steroid that is necessary for coping with these emergencies. During periods of stress or a severe asthmatic attack, instruct patients who have been withdrawn from systemic corticosteroids to resume systemic steroids (in large doses) immediately and to contact their physician for further instruction. Also instruct these patients to carry a warning card indicating that they may need supplementary systemic steroids during periods of stress or a severe asthma attack. To assess the risk of adrenal insufficiency in emergency situations, periodically perform routine tests of adrenal cortical function, including measurement of early morning resting cortisol levels, in all patients. An early morning resting cortisol level may be accepted as normal if it falls at or near the normal mean level.

Indications

►*Asthma, chronic:* For maintenance treatment of asthma as prophylactic therapy; for asthma patients who require systemic corticosteroids, where adding an inhaled corticosteroid may reduce or eliminate the need for systemic corticosteroids.

Administration and Dosage

►*Approved by the FDA:* August 17, 1984.

It is advised to rinse the mouth after inhalation.

►*Adults:* 2 inhalations (500 mcg) twice daily, morning and evening (total daily dose 1 mg). Do not exceed 4 inhalations twice daily (2 mg).

►*Children 6 to 15 years of age:* 2 inhalations twice daily (total daily dose 1 mg). Higher doses have not been studied. With chronic use, monitor children for growth and for effects on the HPA axis. Insufficient information is available to warrant use in children less than 6 years of age.

►*Patients not receiving systemic corticosteroids:* Follow above directions. In responsive patients, pulmonary function usually improves within 1 to 4 weeks.

►*Concomitant systemic corticosteroid therapy:* See Administration in group monograph.

►*Storage/Stability:* Do not puncture. Do not store or administer near heat or open flame because exposure to temperatures 49°C (120°F) or more may cause the container to explode. Do not throw container into fire or incinerator.

Corticosteroids

FLUTICASONE PROPIONATE

Rx	Flovent (GlaxoSmithKline)	**Aerosol:** 44 mcg/actuation	In 7.9 and 13 g canisters containing 60 and 120 metered doses, respectively, with propellants. With actuator.
		110 mcg/actuation	In 7.9 and 13 g canisters containing 60 and 120 metered doses, respectively, with propellants. With actuator.
		220 mcg/actuation	In 7.9 and 13 g canisters containing 60 and 120 metered doses, respectively, with propellants. With actuator.
Rx	Flovent Rotadisk (GlaxoSmithKline)	**Powder for inhalation:** 50 mcg/actuation	Lactose. In 4 blisters containing 15 *Rotadisks* with inhalation device.
		100 mcg/actuation	Lactose. In 4 blisters containing 15 *Rotadisks* with inhalation device.
		250 mcg/actuation	Lactose. In 4 blisters containing 15 *Rotadisks* with inhalation device.
Rx	Flovent Diskus (GlaxoSmithKline)	**Powder for inhalation:** 50 mcg/actuation	In inhalation device containing 28 or 60 blisters.
		100 mcg/actuation	In inhalation device containing 28 or 60 blisters.
		250 mcg/actuation	In inhalation device containing 28 or 60 blisters.

For complete prescribing information, refer to the Corticosteroids Respiratory Inhalant group monograph.

WARNING

Particular care is needed for patients who are transferred from systematically active corticosteroids to fluticasone propionate because deaths because of adrenal insufficiency have occurred in patients with asthma during and after transfer from systemic corticosteroids to less systemically available inhaled corticosteroids. After withdrawal from systemic corticosteroids, a number of months are required for recovery of hypothalamic-pituitary-adrenal (HPA) function.

Patients who have been previously maintained on 20 mg/day or more of prednisone (or its equivalent) may be most susceptible, particularly when their systemic corticosteroids have been almost completely withdrawn. During this period of HPA suppression, patients may exhibit signs and symptoms of adrenal insufficiency when exposed to trauma, surgery, or infection (particularly gastroenteritis) or other conditions associated with severe electrolyte loss. Although fluticasone propionate inhalation may provide control of asthma symptoms during these episodes, in recommended doses it supplies less than normal physiological amounts of glucocorticoid systemically and does not provide the mineralocorticoid activity that is necessary for coping with these emergencies.

During periods of stress or a severe asthma attack, patients who have been withdrawn from systemic corticosteroids should be instructed to resume oral corticosteroids (in large doses) immediately and to contact their physicians for further instruction. These patients should also be instructed to carry a warning card indicating that they may need supplementary systemic corticosteroids during periods of stress or a severe asthma attack.

Indications

➤*Asthma, chronic:* For the maintenance treatment of asthma as prophylactic therapy in patients 4 years of age and older (*Flovent Rotadisk* and *Flovent Diskus*) and 12 years of age and older (*Flovent*). Also indicated for patients requiring oral corticosteroid therapy for asthma. Many of these patients may be able to reduce or eliminate their requirement for oral corticosteroids over time.

Fluticasone is not indicated for relief of acute bronchospasm.

Administration and Dosage

➤*Approved by the FDA:* March 27, 1996.

Advise patients to rinse mouth after inhalation.

Individual patients will experience a variable time to onset and degree of symptom relief. Improvement can occur within 24 hours of beginning treatment, although maximum benefit may not be achieved for 1 to 2 weeks or longer.

After asthma stability has been achieved, titrate to the lowest effective dose to reduce side effect possibility. For patients not responding adequately to the starting dose after 2 weeks, higher doses may provide additional asthma control.

➤*Fluticasone aerosol:*

Recommended Doses for Fluticasone Aerosol

Previous therapy	Recommended starting dose	Highest recommended dose
Bronchodilators alone	88 mcg twice daily	440 mcg twice daily
Inhaled corticosteroids	88-220 mcg twice daily[1]	440 mcg twice daily
Oral corticosteroids	880 mcg twice daily	880 mcg twice daily

[1] Starting doses more than 88 mcg twice daily may be considered for patients with poorer asthma control or those who have previously required doses of inhaled corticosteroids that are in the higher range for that specific agent.

➤*Fluticasone powder:*

Recommended Doses for Fluticasone Powder

Previous therapy	Recommended starting dose	Highest recommended dose
Adults and adolescents		
Bronchodilators alone	100 mcg twice daily	500 mcg twice daily
Inhaled corticosteroids	100-250 mcg twice daily[1]	500 mcg twice daily
Oral corticosteroids	500[2]-1000 mcg twice daily	1000 mcg twice daily
Children 4 to 11 years of age		
Bronchodilators alone	50 mcg twice daily	100 mcg twice daily
Inhaled corticosteroids	50 mcg twice daily	100 mcg twice daily

[1] Starting doses more than 100 mcg twice daily for adults and adolescents and 50 mcg twice daily for children 4 to 11 years of age may be considered for patients with poorer asthma control or those who have previously required doses of inhaled corticosteroids that are in the higher range for that specific agent.
[2] Designated with the *Diskus*.

Concomitant systemic corticosteroid therapy – For patients currently receiving chronic oral corticosteroids, reduce prednisone no faster than 2.5 mg/day on a weekly basis, beginning after at least 1 week of aerosol therapy. Monitor patients for signs of asthma instability, including serial objective measures of airflow, and for signs of adrenal insufficiency. Decrease fluticasone dosage to the lowest effective dose once prednisone reduction is complete (see Administration in group monograph).

➤*Children:* Because individual responses may vary, children previously maintained on fluticasone propionate *Rotadisk* 50 or 100 mcg twice daily may require dosage adjustments upon transfer to the fluticasone propionate *Diskus*.

➤*Storage/Stability:* Shake well before using. Store aerosol between 2° and 30°C (36° and 86°F) and powder at 20° to 25°C (68° to 77°F) in a dry place. Store aerosol canister with nozzle end down. Do not spray in eyes. Do not puncture or incinerate aerosol canister. Store aerosol canister at room temperature before use. Protect from freezing and direct heat or sunlight. Use *Rotadisk* blisters within 2 months after opening the moisture-protective foil. The *Diskus* device is not reusable. Discard the *Diskus* device after 6 weeks (50 mcg strength) or 2 months (100 and 250 mcg strengths) after removal from the moisture-protective foil overwrap pouch or after all blisters have been used (when the dose indicator reads "0"), whichever comes first.

TRIAMCINOLONE ACETONIDE

Rx **Azmacort**   **Aerosol:** 100 mcg/actuation from spacer mouthpiece   In 20 g inhaler (60 mg triamcinolone acetonide) with actuator
(Aventis Pharm.)   (≥ 240 metered doses).

For complete prescribing information, refer to the Corticosteroids Respiratory Inhalant group monograph.

WARNING

Particular care is needed in patients who are transferred from systemically active corticosteroids to triamcinolone inhalation aerosol because deaths because of adrenal insufficiency have occurred in asthmatic patients during and after transfer from systemic corticosteroids to aerosolized steroids in recommended doses. After withdrawal from systemic corticosteroids, a number of months is usually required for recovery of hypothalamic-pituitary-adrenal (HPA) function. For some patients who have received large doses of oral steroids for long periods of time before therapy with triamcinolone is initiated, recovery may be delayed for 1 year or longer. During this period of HPA suppression, patients may exhibit signs and symptoms of adrenal insufficiency when exposed to trauma, surgery, or infections, particularly gastroenteritis or other conditions with acute electrolyte loss. Although triamcinolone may provide control of asthmatic symptoms during these episodes, in recommended doses it supplies only normal physiological amounts of corticosteroid systemically and does not provide the increased systemic steroid that is necessary for coping with these emergencies. During periods of stress or a severe asthmatic attack, patients who have been recently withdrawn from systemic corticosteroids should be instructed to resume systemic steroids (in large doses) immediately and to contact their physician for further instruction. Instruct these patients to carry a warning card indicating that they may need supplementary systemic steroids during periods of stress or a severe asthma attack.

Indications

➤*Asthma, chronic:* In the maintenance treatment of asthma as prophylactic therapy; for asthma patients who require systemic corticosteroids, where adding an inhaled corticosteroid may reduce or eliminate the need for the systemic corticosteroids.

Administration and Dosage

➤*Approved by the FDA:* April 23, 1982.

Rinsing the mouth after inhalation is advised. Different considerations must be given to the following goups of patients in order to obtain the full therapeutic benefit of triamcinolone inhalation aerosol.

Note: In all patients, it is desirable to titrate to the lowest effective dose once asthma stability had been achieved.

➤*Adults:* The usual dosage is 2 inhalations (200 mcg) 3 to 4 times a day or 4 inhalations (400 mcg) twice daily. Do not exceed a maximum daily intake of 16 inhalations (1600 mcg). Higher initial doses (12 to 16 inhalations/day) may be considered in patients with more severe asthma.

➤*Children 6 to 12 years of age:* The usual dosage is 1 or 2 inhalations (100 to 200 mcg) 3 to 4 times a day or 2 to 4 inhalations (200 to 400 mcg) twice daily. Do not exceed a maximum daily intake of 12 inhalations (1200 mcg). There is insufficient information to warrant use in children less than 6 years of age.

In patients who respond to triamcinolone, improvement in pulmonary function is usually apparent within 1 to 2 weeks after the initiation of therapy. Do not increase the prescribed dosage; contact physician if symptoms do not improve or if condition worsens.

➤*Patients not receiving systemic corticosteroids:* Follow above directions. In responsive patients, an improvement in pulmonary function is usually apparent within 1 to 2 weeks.

➤*Concomitant systemic corticosteroid therapy:* See Administration in group monograph.

➤*Storage / Stability:* For best results, keep the canister at room temperature before use. Shake well before using. Do not puncture. Do not use or store near heat or open flame; exposure to greater than 48.8°C (120°F) may cause bursting. Never throw canister into fire or incinerator.

For information on the systemic use of corticosteroids, refer to the Adrenal Cortical Steroids (glucocorticoids) monograph in the Endocrine and Metabolic Agents chapter.

Indications

See individual product listings for specific labeled indications.

Intranasal Steroids Indications						
	Beclomethasone	Budesonide	Flunisolide	Fluticasone	Mometasone	Triamcinolone
Nasal polyps	✔[a]	X[b]		X		
Nonallergic (vasomotor) rhinitis	✔			✔		
Perennial allergic rhinitis	✔	✔	✔	✔	✔	✔
Seasonal allergic rhinitis	✔	✔	✔	✔	✔[c]	✔
Recurrent chronic sinusitis[d]		X		X	X	

[a] ✔ = Approved uses.
[b] X = Unlabeled uses.
[c] Treatment and prophylaxis.
[d] As adjunctive therapy with an antibiotic and/or decongestant.

➤*Pharmacokinetics:*

Pharmacokinetics of Intranasal Steroids						
Parameters	Corticosteroids					
	Beclomethasone	Budesonide	Flunisolide	Fluticasone	Mometasone	Triamcinolone
Bioavailability	44%	≈ 34%	50%	< 2%	Virtually undetectable	Minimal
Vd	20 L, 424 L[a]	2 to 3 L/kg	NA[b]	4.2 L/kg[c]	NA	99.5 L[c]
Protein binding	87%	85% to 90%[d]	NA	91%[c]	98% to 99%[e]	NA
Site of metabolism		Liver (CYP3A)	Liver	Liver (CYP3A4)	Liver (CYP3A4)	Liver
Metabolites (activity)	17-monopropionate (active), free beclomethasone (very weak; prodrug)	16α-hydroxy-prednisolone and 6β-hydroxy-budesonide (< 1% of parent)	NA	17β-carboxylic acid (inactive)	6β-hydroxymometasone furoate	6β-hydroxy-triamcinolone acetonide, 21-carboxy-triamcinolone acetonide, and 21-carboxy-6β-hydroxy-triamcinolone acetonide (substantially < parent)
Excretion site	Feces (≈ 60%), urine (≈ 12%)[f]	Feces, urine (≈ 66%)	Feces (≈ 50%), urine (≈ 50%)	Feces (> 95%), urine (< 5%)[c]	Feces, urine	Feces (≈ 60%), urine (≈ 40%)
t½	0.5 h, 2.7 h[a,c]	2 to 3 h[c]	1 to 2 h	7.8 h[c]	5.8 h[c]	3.1 h

[a] Value for metabolite.
[b] Not available.
[c] Data from IV administration.
[d] Over a concentration range of 1 to 100 nmol/L.
[e] Over a concentration range of 5 to 500 ng/mL.
[f] Data from oral administration.

Special populations –

Hepatic function impairment: Reduced liver function may affect the elimination of corticosteroids. The systemic availability of oral **budesonide** was doubled by compromised liver function. The relevance of this finding to intranasal budesonide has not been established.

Children: Children had **budesonide** plasma concentrations approximately twice that observed in adults after intranasal administration primarily because of differences in weight.

Contraindications

Untreated localized infections involving the nasal mucosa (**flunisolide**); hypersensitivity to the drug or any component of the product.

Warnings

➤*Special senses:* Rare instances of wheezing, nasal septum perforation, cataracts, glaucoma, and increased intraocular pressure have been reported. Temporary or permanent loss of the sense of smell and taste has been reported with **flunisolide** use (see Adverse Reactions).

➤*Systemic corticosteroids:* The combined administration of alternate-day systemic prednisone with these products may increase the likelihood of HPA suppression. Therefore, use with caution in patients already on alternate-day prednisone.

Replacement of a systemic corticosteroid with intranasal corticosteroids can be accompanied by signs of adrenal insufficiency.

During withdrawal from oral corticosteroids, some patients may experience withdrawal symptoms (eg, joint or muscular pain, lassitude, depression). Carefully monitor patients previously treated with systemic corticosteroids for prolonged periods and then transferred to intranasal steroids to avoid acute adrenal insufficiency in response to stress. This is particularly important in patients who have asthma or

Administration and Dosage

Please refer to the individual monographs for specific dosing information.

Use intranasal steroids at regular intervals for optimal effect.

➤*Duration of therapy:* Although some symptomatic relief may be achieved sooner, maximum benefit may not be reached until at least 2 weeks of therapy. Generally do not continue use beyond 3 weeks in the absence of significant symptomatic improvement.

Actions

➤*Pharmacology:* These drugs have potent glucocorticoid and weak mineralocorticoid activity. The mechanisms responsible for the anti-inflammatory action of corticosteroids on the nasal mucosa are unknown. However, glucocorticoids have a wide range of inhibitory activities against multiple cell types (eg, mast cells, eosinophils, neutrophils, macrophages, lymphocytes) and mediators (eg, histamine, eicosanoids, leukotrienes, cytokines) involved in allergic and nonallergic/irritant-mediated inflammation. These agents, when administered topically in recommended doses, exert direct local anti-inflammatory effects with minimal systemic effects. Exceeding the recommended dose may result in systemic effects, including hypothalamic-pituitary-adrenal (HPA) function suppression.

other conditions where too rapid a decrease in systemic corticosteroids may cause a severe exacerbation of their symptoms.

➤*Excessive doses/sensitivity:* If recommended doses of intranasal **beclomethasone** are exceeded or if individuals are particularly sensitive or predisposed by virtue of recent systemic steroid therapy, symptoms of hypercorticism may occur, including, very rarely, menstrual irregularities, acneiform lesions, cataracts, and cushingoid features. If such changes occur, discontinue slowly, consistent with accepted procedures for discontinuing oral steroids. Avoid doses greater than recommended.

➤*Hypersensitivity reactions:* Rare cases of immediate and delayed hypersensitivity reactions, including angioedema, bronchospasm, rash, and urticaria have been reported after intranasal administration of corticosteroids. Refer to Management of Acute Hypersensitivity Reactions.

➤*Hepatic function impairment:* Reduced liver function may affect the elimination of corticosteroids. The systemic availability of oral **budesonide** was doubled by compromised liver function. The relevance of this finding to intranasal budesonide has not been established.

➤*Carcinogenesis:*

Flunisolide – Flunisolide was administered to mice at doses of 5, 50, and 500 mcg/kg/day and to rats at doses of 0.5, 1, and 2.5 mcg/kg/day. There was an increased incidence of benign pulmonary adenomas in mice but not rats. Female rats receiving the highest oral dose had an increased incidence of mammary adenocarcinoma compared with control rats.

Budesonide – Budesonide caused a significant increase in the incidence of gliomas and hepatocellular tumors in the male rats receiving an oral dose of 50 mcg/kg (approximately twice the maximum recommended daily intranasal dose in adults and children on a mcg/m^2 basis, respectively).

➤*Fertility impairment:*

Beclomethasone – In rats, beclomethasone caused decreased conception rates at an oral dose of 16 mg/kg (approximately 390 times the intranasal maximum recommended daily dose [MRDD] in adults on a mg/m^2 basis). There was no significant effect of beclomethasone on fertility in rats at oral doses of 1.6 mg/kg (approximately 40 times the intranasal MRDD in adults on a mg/m^2 basis). Inhibition of the estrous cycle in dogs was observed following oral dosing at 0.5 mg/kg (approximately 40 times the intranasal MRDD in adults on a mg/m^2 basis). No inhibition of the estrous cycle in dogs was seen following 12 months exposure at an estimated inhalation dose of 0.33 mg/kg (approximately 25 times the intranasal MRDD in adults on a mg/m^2 basis).

Budesonide – In rats at SC doses of 20 mcg/kg and above (less than the intranasal MRDD in adults on a mcg/m^2 basis), budesonide caused a decrease in prenatal viability and viability of the pups at birth and during lactation, along with a decrease in maternal body-weight gain. No such effects were noted at 5 mcg/kg (less than the intranasal MRDD in adults on a mcg/m^2 basis).

Flunisolide – Female rats receiving high doses of flunisolide (200 mcg/kg/day or 1180 mcg/m^2 body surface area) showed some evidence of impaired fertility.

Triamcinolone – Triamcinolone acetonide caused increased fetal resorptions and stillbirths and decreases in pup weight and survival at doses of 5 mcg/kg and above (approximately one fifth the intranasal MRDD in adults on a mcg/m^2 basis). Doses of 1 mcg/kg did not include the above mentioned effects.

➤*Elderly:* In general, use caution in dose selection for an elderly patient, starting at the low end of the dosing range, reflecting greater frequency of decreased hepatic, renal, or cardiac function, and concomitant disease or other drug therapy.

➤*Pregnancy:* Category C. There are no adequately controlled trials in pregnant women. However, animal studies have demonstrated teratogenic, fetotoxic, and embryocidal effects. Topical administration of recommended doses is unlikely to achieve significant systemic levels; however, use these agents during pregnancy only if the potential benefits outweigh the potential hazards to the fetus.

Carefully observe infants born of mothers who have received substantial doses of corticosteroids during pregnancy for signs of adrenal insufficiency.

➤*Lactation:* It is not known whether these drugs are excreted in breast milk. Because other corticosteroids are excreted in human milk, use caution when administering to nursing women.

➤*Children:*

Beclomethasone, budesonide, flunisolide, triamcinolone – Safety and efficacy for use in children younger than 6 years of age have not been established.

Fluticasone – Safety and efficacy for use in children younger than 4 years of age have not been established.

Mometasone – Safety and efficacy for use in children younger than 2 years of age have not been established.

Controlled clinical studies have shown that intranasal corticosteroids may cause a reduction in growth velocity in pediatric patients. This effect has been observed in the absence of laboratory evidence of HPA axis suppression, suggesting that growth velocity is a more sensitive indicator of systemic corticosteroid exposure in pediatric patients than some commonly used tests of HPA-axis function. The long-term effects of this reduction in growth velocity associated with intranasal corticosteroids, including the impact on final adult height, are unknown. The potential for "catch-up" growth following discontinuation of treatment with intranasal corticosteroids has not been adequately studied. Routinely monitor the growth of pediatric patients receiving intranasal corticosteroids (eg, via stadiometry). Weigh the potential growth effects of prolonged treatment against the clinical benefits obtained and the risks/benefits of treatment alternatives. To minimize the systemic effects of intranasal corticosteroids, titrate each patient to the lowest dose that effectively controls his/her symptoms.

Precautions

➤*Monitoring:* Routinely monitor the growth of pediatric patients receiving intranasal corticosteroids (eg, via stadiometry). Carefully monitor patients previously treated for prolonged periods with systemic corticosteroids and then transferred to topical corticosteroids for acute adrenal insufficiency in response to stress. Examine periodically for evidence of *Candida* infection or other signs of adverse effects on the nasal mucosa.

➤*Nasopharyngeal irritation:* If persistent nasopharyngeal irritation occurs, it may be an indication to stop therapy.

➤*Infections:* Localized infections of the nose and pharynx with *Candida albicans* have developed only rarely. When such an infection occurs, it may require treatment with appropriate local or systemic therapy and/or discontinuation of steroid treatment.

Use with caution, if at all, in patients with active or quiescent tuberculosis infections of the respiratory tract, or in untreated fungal, bacterial, or systemic viral infections, or ocular herpes simplex.

Individuals receiving immunosuppressant agents are more susceptible to infections than healthy individuals. For example, chickenpox and measles can have a more serious or fatal course in susceptible children or adults receiving immunosuppressant doses of corticosteroids. Take particular care to avoid exposure in children or adults who have not had these diseases or who have not been properly immunized. Prophylaxis with varicella-zoster immune globulin (VZIG) may be indicated if exposed to chickenpox. If an individual is exposed to measles, prophylaxis with pooled immunoglobulin may be indicated. Consider treatment with antiviral agents if chickenpox develops.

➤*Wound healing:* Because of the inhibitory effect of corticosteroids on wound healing, do not use nasal steroids in patients who have experienced recent nasal septal ulcers, recurrent epistaxis, or nasal surgery or trauma until healing has occurred.

➤*Vasoconstrictors:* In the presence of excessive nasal mucosa secretion or edema of the nasal mucosa, the drug may fail to reach the site of intended action. In such cases, use a nasal vasoconstrictor during the first 2 to 3 days of therapy.

➤*Systemic effects:* Although systemic effects are low when used in recommended dosage, HPA suppression and other systemic effects may occur, especially with excessive doses.

➤*Long-term treatment:* Examine patients periodically over several months or longer for possible changes in the nasal mucosa.

Drug Interactions

Intranasal Corticosteroid Drug Interactions			
Precipitant drug	Object drug*		Description
Cimetidine	Budesonide	↑	Coadministration caused a slight decrease in budesonide clearance and a corresponding increase in its oral bioavailability.
Inhibitors of CYP3A4 (eg, ketoconazole, itraconazole, clarithromycin, erythromycin, cimetidine, ritonavir)	Budesonide Fluticasone	↑	Concomitant administration may inhibit metabolism and increase systemic exposure of the intranasal steroid. After oral administration of ketoconazole, the mean plasma concentration of oral budesonide increased by more than 7-fold. Coadministration of oral ritonavir and intranasal fluticasone resulted in a significant increase in fluticasone plasma concentrations resulting in possible Cushing syndrome and adrenal suppression. Use with caution.

* ↑ = Object drug increased.

Adverse Reactions

Intranasal Corticosteroid Adverse Reactions (%)[a]							
Adverse reaction	Beclomethasone	Budesonide	Flunisolide (nasal solution)	Flunisolide (nasal spray)	Fluticasone	Mometasome	Triamcinolone
CNS							
Dizziness					1 to 3		
Headache	< 5		≤ 5		7 to 16	17 to 26	≥ 2
Lightheadedness	< 5						
GI							
Abdominal pain					1 to 3		
Diarrhea					1 to 3	2 to < 5	
Dyspepsia						2 to < 5	

Intranasal Steroids

Intranasal Corticosteroid Adverse Reactions (%)[a]							
Adverse reaction	Beclomethasone	Budesonide	Flunisolide (nasal solution)	Flunisolide (nasal spray)	Fluticasone	Mometasome	Triamcinolone
Nausea	< 5		≤ 5	> 1	3 to 5	2 to < 5	
Vomiting			≤ 5		3 to 5	1 to 5	≥ 2
Hypersensitivity reactions							
Anaphylaxis					Rare[b]	✔[b,c]	
Angioedema	Rare	Rare[b]			Rare[b]	✔[b]	
Bronchospasm	Rare				Rare[b]		
Dyspnea					Rare[b]		
Edema of face/tongue					Rare[b]		
Pruritus					Rare[b]		
Rash	Rare				Rare[b]		
Wheezing	Rare	Rare			Rare[b]	2 to < 5	
Urticaria	Rare				Rare[b]		
Respiratory							
Asthma symptoms					3 to 7	2 to < 5	≥ 2
Bronchitis					1 to 3	2 to < 5	
Bronchospasm		2					
Cough		2		> 1	4	7 to 13	2
Epistaxis	< 3	8	≤ 5[d]	3 to 9	6 to 7[d]	8 to 11[d]	3
Mild nasopharyngeal irritation	24						
Nasal burning/stinging			45	13	2 to 3	✔[b]	
Nasal dryness	✔			> 1			
Nasal irritation	✔	2	≤ 5		2 to 3	2 to < 5	
Nasal mucosal ulceration	Rare				Rare[b]	Rare	
Nasal septal perforation	Rare	Rare[b]	Rare	Rare	Rare[b]	Rare[b]	Rare
Nasal stuffiness/ congestion	< 3		≤ 5				
Rhinitis						2 to < 5	≥ 2
Pharyngitis		4		> 1	6 to 8	10 to 12	5
Rhinorrhea	< 3				1 to 3		
Sinusitis					≤ 1	4 to 5	≥ 2
Sneezing	4		≤ 5				
Throat discomfort (burning, itching, swelling, pain)		Rare[b]	≤ 5		Rare[b]		
Throat dryness/irritation	✔	Rare[b]			Rare[b]		
Upper respiratory tract infection						5 to 7	
Special senses							
Aftertaste				17			
Blurred vision					✔[b]		
Cataracts	Rare				Rare[b]		
Conjunctivitis					✔[b]	2 to < 5	
Dry/irritated eyes					✔[b]		
Earache						2 to < 5	
Glaucoma	Rare				Rare[b]		
Hoarseness				≤ 1	Rare[b]		
Increased intraocular pressure	Rare	Rare			Rare[b]	Rare	
Loss of taste/smell	Rare	Rare[b]	≤ 5	≤ 1	✔[b]	Rare[b]	
Otitis media						2 to < 5	≥ 2
Unpleasant taste/smell	✔						
Watery eyes	< 3		≤ 5				

Intranasal Steroids

Intranasal Corticosteroid Adverse Reactions (%)[a]

Adverse reaction	Beclomethasone	Budesonide	Flunisolide (nasal solution)	Flunisolide (nasal spray)	Fluticasone	Mometasone	Triamcinolone
Miscellaneous							
Aches and pains					1 to 3		
Arthralgia						2 to < 5	
Chest pain						2 to < 5	
Dysmenorrhea						1 to 5	
Fever					1 to 3		
Flu-like symptoms					1 to 3	2 to < 5	
Growth suppression	✔	✔			✔[b]		
Infection	Rare[e]	Rare[e]	Rare[e]	Rare[e]	Rare[e]	Rare[e]	Rare[e]
Myalgia						2 to < 5	
Palpitations		Rare[b]					
Viral infection						8 to 14	
Voice changes					Rare[b]		

[a] Data pooled from all age groups and from separate studies and are not necessarily comparable.
[b] Occurred during postmarketing.
[c] ✔ = Reported; no incidence given.
[d] Including bloody mucus.
[e] Localized infections of the nose and pharynx with *Candida albicans*.

Overdosage

Acute overdosage is unlikely with intranasal corticosteroids. However, chronic overdosage may occur and result in hypercorticism and adrenal suppression. If such symptoms occur, slowly discontinue intranasal corticosteroids consistent with accepted procedures for discontinuing oral steroid therapy.

Patient Information

Instruct patients to read the patient instructions provided with the product.

Advise patients that effects may not be immediate and not to exceed the recommended dosage. Benefit requires regular use and usually occurs within a few days. One to 2 weeks may pass before full effect is achieved.

Advise patients to contact their health care provider if symptoms worsen or do not improve by 3 weeks of treatment.

Instruct patients to clear nasal passages before use. If nasal passages are blocked, use of a topical nasal decongestant 5 to 10 minutes prior to administering the intranasal steroid may be beneficial.

Instruct patients to shake bottle gently before each use. Patients will also need to prime the pump the first time it is used and if it has not been used for more than a week.

Instruct patients to close the other nostril with a finger and tilt head slightly forward while using.

Advise patients to avoid blowing nose for at least 10 to 15 minutes after use.

Advise patients to avoid spraying into eyes or directly into nasal septum.

Advise patients not to use the bottle for more than the labeled number of sprays, even if the bottle is not completely empty.

Advise patients on immunosuppressant doses of corticosteroids to avoid exposure to chicken pox or measles and to seek medical advice if exposed.

Advise patients to contact their health care provider if they experience recurrent episodes of epistaxis or nasal septum discomfort.

FLUNISOLIDE

Rx	Flunisolide (Bausch & Lomb)	Solution: 0.025% (25 mcg/actuation)[a]	In 25 mL nasal pump dispenser (200 sprays/bottle).
Rx	Nasarel (Ivax Laboratories)	Spray: 0.025% (29 mcg/actuation)[b]	In 25 mL spray bottles (200 sprays/bottle) with meter pump and nasal adapter.

[a] With propylene glycol, polyethylene glycol 3350, benzalkonium chloride, EDTA.

[b] With 0.01% benzalkonium chloride, butylated hydroxytoluene, EDTA, polyethylene glycol 400, sorbitol.

For complete prescribing information, refer to the Intranasal Steroids group monograph.

Indications

►*Allergic rhinitis:* For the relief and management of nasal symptoms of seasonal and perennial allergic rhinitis.

Administration and Dosage

►*Approved by the FDA:* March 8, 1995.

Encourage patients with blocked nasal passages to use a decongestant just before administration to ensure adequate penetration of the spray. Advise patients to clear their nasal passages of secretions prior to use.

►*Adults:* 2 sprays in each nostril 2 times/day. The dose may be increased to 2 sprays in each nostril 3 times/day.

►*Children 6 to 14 years of age:* 1 spray in each nostril 3 times/day or 2 sprays in each nostril 2 times/day.

►*Maximum dose:*
Adults – 8 sprays in each nostril per day.
Children 6 to 14 years of age – 4 sprays in each nostril per day.

►*Maintenance dose:* After the desired clinical effect is obtained, reduce the maintenance dose to the smallest amount necessary to control symptoms. Some patients with perennial allergic rhinitis may be maintained on 1 spray in each nostril per day.

►*Duration:* Improvement in symptoms usually becomes apparent within a few days. However, relief may not occur in some patients for as long as 2 weeks. Do not use for more than 3 weeks in absence of significant symptomatic improvement.

►*Priming:* Before use, prime the nasal spray by pushing down on the pump 5 or 6 times until a fine mist appears. If the pump has not been used for 5 days or more, the spray must be primed again.

►*Storage/Stability:* Store between 15° and 30°C (59° and 86°F).

BECLOMETHASONE DIPROPIONATE

Rx	Beconase AQ (GlaxoSmithKline)	Spray: 0.042% (42 mcg/actuation)[a]	In 25 g bottles (180 metered doses per bottle) with metering atomizing pump and nasal adapter.

[a] With dextrose, polysorbate 80, benzalkonium chloride, 0.25% v/w phenylethyl alcohol.

For complete prescribing information, refer to the Intranasal Steroids group monograph.

Indications

►*Nasal polyps:* Prevention of recurrence of nasal polyps following surgical removal.

►*Rhinitis:* For the relief of symptoms of seasonal or perennial allergic and nonallergic (vasomotor) rhinitis.

Administration and Dosage

►*Approved by the FDA:* July 27, 1987.

In the presence of excessive nasal mucous secretion or edema of the nasal mucosa, advise patients to use a nasal vasoconstrictor during the first 2 or 3 days of therapy with the nasal spray.

►*Adults and children 12 years of age or older:* 1 or 2 nasal inhalations (42 to 84 mcg) in each nostril twice daily (total dose, 168 to 336 mcg/day).

►*Children 6 to 11 years of age:* Start with 1 nasal inhalation in each nostril twice daily (168 mcg). Patients not adequately responding

BECLOMETHASONE DIPROPIONATE

or those with more severe symptoms may use 2 sprays in each nostril twice daily (336 mcg/day).

➤*Maximum dosage:* 2 sprays in each nostril twice daily (336 mcg/day).

➤*Maintenance dose:* Once adequate control is achieved, decrease the dosage to 1 spray in each nostril twice daily.

➤*Duration:* Improvement of rhinitis symptoms usually becomes apparent within a few days after the start of therapy. However, symptomatic relief may not occur in some patients for as long as 2 weeks. Do not continue therapy beyond 3 weeks in the absence of significant

symptomatic improvement. Treatment of symptoms associated with nasal polyps may have to be continued for several weeks or more before a therapeutic result can be fully assessed. Recurrence of symptoms caused by polyps can occur after stopping treatment, depending on the severity of the disease.

➤*Priming:* Before use, prime the nasal spray by pushing down on the pump 6 times until a fine mist appears. If the pump has not been used for 7 days or more, the spray must be primed again.

➤*Storage/Stability:* Store between 15° and 30°C (59° and 86°F). Discard the bottle when the labeled number of actuations have been used. Shake well before use.

TRIAMCINOLONE ACETONIDE

Rx	Nasacort AQ (Aventis)	Spray: 55 mcg/actuation[a]	In 6.5 and 16.5 g bottles (providing 30 and 120 actuations, respectively) with metered-dose pump unit and nasal adapter.

[a] With polysorbate 80, dextrose, benzalkonium chloride, and EDTA.

For complete prescribing information, refer to the Intranasal Steroids group monograph.

Indications

➤*Allergic rhinitis:* Treatment of the nasal symptoms of seasonal and perennial allergic rhinitis in adults and children 6 years of age and older.

Administration and Dosage

➤*Approved by the FDA:* May 20, 1996.

➤*Adults and children 12 years of age and older:* 2 sprays in each nostril once daily (220 mcg/day).

➤*Children 6 to 11 years of age:* 1 spray in each nostril once daily (110 mcg/day).

➤*Maximum dose:* 2 sprays in each nostril once daily (220 mcg/day).

➤*Maintenance dose:* When the maximum benefit has been achieved and symptoms have been controlled, reduce the dose to 1 spray in each nostril once daily (110 mcg/day). Use the minimum effective dose to ensure continued control of symptoms. Greater symptom control may be achieved with regular scheduled use.

➤*Duration:* Improvement in symptoms may be seen within the first day of treatment, and generally, it takes 1 week of treatment to reach maximum benefit. Do not use for more than 3 weeks in absence of significant symptomatic improvement.

➤*Priming:* Before use, prime the nasal spray by pushing down on the actuator until a fine spray appears (5 pumps). If the pump has not been used for more than 14 days, the spray must be reprimed with 1 spray.

➤*Storage/Stability:* Store at controlled room temperature 20° to 25°C (68° to 77°F). Discard the bottle when the labeled number of actuations has been used, even if the bottle is not completely empty.

BUDESONIDE

Rx	Rhinocort Aqua (AstraZeneca)	Spray: 32 mcg/actuation[a]	In 8.6 g bottles (120 metered sprays) with metered-dose pump.

[a] Dextrose, polysorbate 80, EDTA.

For complete prescribing information, refer to the Intranasal Steroids group monograph.

Indications

➤*Allergic rhinitis:* Management of nasal symptoms of seasonal or perennial allergic rhinitis in adults and children 6 years of age and older.

Administration and Dosage

➤*Approved by the FDA:* February 21, 1994.

➤*Adults and children 6 years of age and older:* 1 spray in each nostril once daily (64 mcg/day). Some patients who do not achieve symptom control at the recommended starting dose may benefit from an increased dose.

➤*Maximum dose:*

Adults 12 years of age and older – 4 sprays in each nostril once daily (256 mcg/day).

Children younger than 12 years of age – 2 sprays in each nostril once daily (128 mcg/day).

➤*Maintenance dose:* After the desired clinical effect is obtained, reduce the maintenance dose to the smallest amount necessary to control symptoms.

➤*Duration:* Improvement of symptoms may be noticed within the first 10 hours or over 1 to 2 days. However, maximum benefit may not be achieved in some patients until approximately 2 weeks after initiation of treatment.

➤*Priming:* Prior to initial use, gently shake the container and prime the pump by actuating 8 times. If used daily, the pump does not need to be reprimed. If not used for 2 consecutive days, reprime with 1 spray or until a fine mist appears. If not used for more than 14 days, rinse the applicator and reprime with 2 sprays or until a fine mist appears.

➤*Storage/Stability:* Store at controlled room temperature, 20° to 25°C (68° to 77°F) with the valve up. Shake gently before use. Do not freeze. Protect from light. Discard the bottle after 120 sprays following initial priming.

FLUTICASONE PROPIONATE

Rx	Flonase (GlaxoSmithKline)	Spray: 50 mcg/actuation[a]	In 16 g (120 actuations) amber glass bottles with metering atomizing pump and nasal adapter.

[a] With dextrose, polysorbate 80, 0.02% w/w benzalkonium chloride, 0.25% w/w phenylethyl alcohol.

For complete prescribing information, refer to the Intranasal Steroids group monograph.

Indications

➤*Rhinitis:* Management of nasal symptoms of seasonal and perennial allergic and nonallergic rhinitis in adults and children 4 years of age and older.

Administration and Dosage

➤*Approved by the FDA:* October 19, 1994.

Inform patients to use fluticasone propionate at regular intervals for optimal effect.

➤*Adults:* 2 sprays in each nostril once daily (total daily dose, 200 mcg). The same dose divided into 100 mcg twice daily (ie, 8 am and 8 pm) is also effective.

➤*Adolescents and children 4 years of age and older:* 1 spray in each nostril (100 mcg) once daily. Patients not adequately responding to 100 mcg may use 2 sprays in each nostril (200 mcg).

➤*Maximum dose:* 2 sprays in each nostril (200 mcg/day).

➤*Maintenance dose:* After the first few days, patients may be able to reduce their dosage to 1 spray in each nostril (100 mcg) once daily for maintenance therapy. Some patients (12 years of age and older) with seasonal allergic rhinitis may find as-needed use of 200 mcg once daily effective for symptom control. Greater symptom control may be achieved with regular scheduled use.

➤*Priming:* Initially prime the pump with 6 actuations before use or after a period of non-use (1 week or more).

➤*Storage/Stability:* Store between 4° and 30°C (39° and 86°F). Discard the bottle when the labeled number of actuations has been used. Shake gently before use.

MOMETASONE FUROATE MONOHYDRATE

Rx	**Nasonex** (Schering)	**Spray:** 0.05% (50 mcg/actuation)[a]	In 17 g bottles (120 sprays) with metered-dose manual pump spray unit.

[a] Glycerin, 0.25% w/w phenylethyl alcohol, citric acid, benzalkonium chloride, polysorbate 80.

For complete prescribing information, refer to the Intranasal Steroids group monograph.

Indications

➤*Allergic rhinitis:* Treatment of the nasal symptoms of seasonal and perennial allergic rhinitis in adults and children 2 years of age and older; prophylaxis of nasal symptoms of seasonal allergic rhinitis in adults and adolescents 12 years of age and older.

Administration and Dosage

➤*Approved by the FDA:* October 1, 1997.

Use mometasone only once daily at a regular interval for optimal effect.

➤*Adults and children 12 years of age and older:* 2 sprays (50 mcg) in each nostril once daily (total daily dose, 200 mcg).

In patients with a known seasonal allergen that precipitates nasal symptoms of seasonal allergic rhinitis, prophylaxis with mometasone (200 mcg/day) is recommended 2 to 4 weeks prior to the anticipated start of the pollen season.

➤*Children 2 to 11 years of age:* 1 spray (50 mcg) in each nostril once daily (total daily dose, 100 mcg).

➤*Duration:* Improvement in nasal symptoms has been shown to occur within 11 hours to 2 days after the first dose. Maximum benefit is usually achieved within 1 to 2 weeks.

➤*Priming:* Prior to use, the pump must be primed by actuating 10 times or until a fine spray appears. The pump can be stored for up to 1 week without priming. If unused for more than 1 week, reprime by actuating 2 times or until a fine spray appears.

➤*Storage/Stability:* Store at 25°C (77°F); excursions permitted to 15° to 30°C (59° to 86°F). Protect from light. Avoid prolonged exposure to direct light when removed from its cardboard container. Brief exposure to light, as with normal use, is acceptable. Shake well before each use.

ACETYLCYSTEINE (N-Acetylcysteine)

Rx	**Acetylcysteine** (Various, Cetus, DuPont)	**Solution:** 10% (as sodium)	In 4, 10 and 30 ml vials.[1]
Rx	**Mucomyst** (Apothecon)		In 4, 10 and 30 ml vials.[1]
Rx	**Acetylcysteine** (Various, Cetus, Dey, DuPont)	**Solution:** 20% (as sodium)	In 4, 10, 30 and 100 ml vials.[1]
Rx	**Mucomyst** (Apothecon)		In 4, 10 and 30 ml vials.[1]

[1] May contain EDTA.

Indications

➤*Mucolytic:* Adjuvant therapy for abnormal, viscid, or inspissated mucus secretions in chronic bronchopulmonary disease (chronic emphysema, emphysema with bronchitis, chronic asthmatic bronchitis, tuberculosis, bronchiectasis, primary amyloidosis of lung).

• Acute bronchopulmonary disease (pneumonia, bronchitis, tracheobronchitis).
• Pulmonary complications of cystic fibrosis.
• Tracheostomy care.
• Pulmonary complications associated with surgery.
• Use during anesthesia.
• Posttraumatic chest conditions.
• Atelectasis due to mucus obstruction.
• Diagnostic bronchial studies (bronchograms, bronchospirometry, bronchial wedge catheterization).

➤*Antidote:* To prevent or lessen hepatic injury which may occur following ingestion of a potentially hepatotoxic quantity of acetaminophen. Initiate treatment as soon as possible after overdose and, in any case, within 24 hours of ingestion.

➤*Unlabeled uses:* As an ophthalmic solution to treat keratoconjunctivitis sicca (dry eye). It has been used as an enema to treat bowel obstruction due to meconium ileus or its equivalent.

Administration and Dosage

➤*Nebulization (face mask, mouth piece, tracheostomy):* 1 to 10 ml of the 20% solution or 2 to 20 ml of the 10% solution every 2 to 6 hours; the dose for most patients is 3 to 5 ml of the 20% solution or 6 to 10 ml of the 10% solution 3 to 4 times a day.

➤*Nebulization (tent, croupette):* Very large volumes are required, occasionally up to 300 ml during a treatment period. The dose is the volume of solution that will maintain a very heavy mist in the tent or croupette for the desired period. Administration for intermittent or continuous prolonged periods, including overnight, may be desirable.

➤*Instillation:*

Direct – 1 to 2 ml of a 10% to 20% solution as often as every hour.

Tracheostomy – 1 to 2 ml of a 10% to 20% solution every 1 to 4 hours by instillation into the tracheostomy.

May be introduced directly into a particular segment of the bronchopulmonary tree by inserting (under local anesthesia and direct vision) a plastic catheter into the trachea. Instill 2 to 5 ml of the 20% solution by a syringe connected to the catheter.

Percutaneous intratracheal catheter – 1 to 2 ml of the 20% solution or 2 to 4 ml of the 10% solution every 1 to 4 hours by a syringe attached to the catheter.

➤*Diagnostic bronchograms:* 2 or 3 administrations of 1 to 2 ml of the 20% solution or 2 to 4 ml of the 10% solution by nebulization or by instillation intratracheally, prior to the procedure.

➤*Preparation of solution:* The 20% solution may be diluted with either Sodium Chloride for Injection or Inhalation or Sterile Water for Injection or Inhalation. The 10% solution may be used undiluted. Refrigerate unused, undiluted solution and use within 96 hours.

➤*Equipment compatibility:* Certain materials in nebulization equipment react with acetylcysteine, especially certain metals (notably iron and copper) and rubber. Where materials may come into contact with acetylcysteine solution, use parts made of the following materials: Glass, plastic, aluminum, anodized aluminum, chromed metal, tantalum, sterling silver or stainless steel. Silver may become tarnished after exposure, but this is not harmful to the drug action or to the patient.

➤*Acetaminophen overdosage:* Administer acetylcysteine immediately if ≤ 24 hours have elapsed from the reported time of acetaminophen ingestion. Do not await results of assays for acetaminophen level before initiating treatment. In one study, acetylcysteine administered as long as 36 hours after the acetaminophen overdose was beneficial in some patients. The following procedures are recommended:

1.) Empty the stomach promptly by lavage or by inducing emesis with syrup of ipecac. Repeat the ipecac dose if emesis does not occur in 20 minutes.
2.) If activated charcoal has been administered, lavage before administering acetylcysteine. Activated charcoal may adsorb acetylcysteine, thereby reducing its effectiveness.
3.) Draw blood for acetaminophen plasma assay and for baseline AST, ALT, bilirubin, prothrombin time, creatinine, BUN, blood sugar and electrolytes. If an assay cannot be obtained or if the acetaminophen level is clearly in the toxic range, continue acetylcysteine for the full course of therapy. Monitor hepatic and renal function and electrolyte and fluid balance.
4.) Administer a 140 mg/kg loading dose of acetylcysteine.
5.) Administer the first maintenance dose (70 mg/kg) 4 hours after the loading dose. Repeat the maintenance dose at 4 hour intervals for a total of 17 doses unless the acetaminophen assay reveals a nontoxic level.
6.) If the patient vomits the loading dose or any maintenance dose within 1 hour of administration, repeat that dose.
7.) If the patient is persistently unable to retain the orally administered acetylcysteine, administer by duodenal intubation.
8.) Repeat AST, ALT, bilirubin, prothrombin time, creatinine, BUN, blood sugar and electrolytes daily if the acetaminophen plasma level is in the potentially toxic range.

Preparation of oral solution – Dilute the 20% solution with cola drinks or other soft drinks to a final concentration of 5% (see Dosage Guide table). If administered via gastric tube or Miller-Abbott tube, water may be used as the diluent. Prepare fresh dilutions and use within 1 hour. Remaining undiluted solutions in opened vials can be refrigerated up to 96 hours.

Acetaminophen assays – The acute ingestion of acetaminophen in quantities of ≥ 150 mg/kg may result in hepatic toxicity. However, the reported history of the quantity of a drug ingested as an overdose is often inaccurate and is not a reliable guide to antidotal therapy. Therefore, determine plasma or serum acetaminophen concentrations as early as possible, but no sooner than 4 hours following an acute overdose to assess the potential risk of hepatotoxicity. If an acetaminophen assay cannot be obtained, assume that the overdose is potentially toxic.

Interpretation of acetaminophen assays (refer to the following nomogram) – When results of the plasma acetaminophen assay are available, refer to the nomogram. Values above the solid line connecting 200 mcg/ml at 4 hours with 50 mcg/ml at 12 hours are associated with a possibility of hepatic toxicity if an antidote is not administered. Do not wait for assay results to begin treatment.

If the plasma level is above the broken line, continue with maintenance doses of acetylcysteine. It is better to err on the safe side; thus, the broken line is plotted 25% below the solid line which defines possible toxicity.

If the plasma level is below the broken line described above, there is minimal risk of hepatic toxicity and acetylcysteine treatment can be discontinued.

Estimating potential for hepatotoxicity – The following nomogram estimates the probability that plasma levels in relation to intervals postingestion will result in hepatotoxicity.

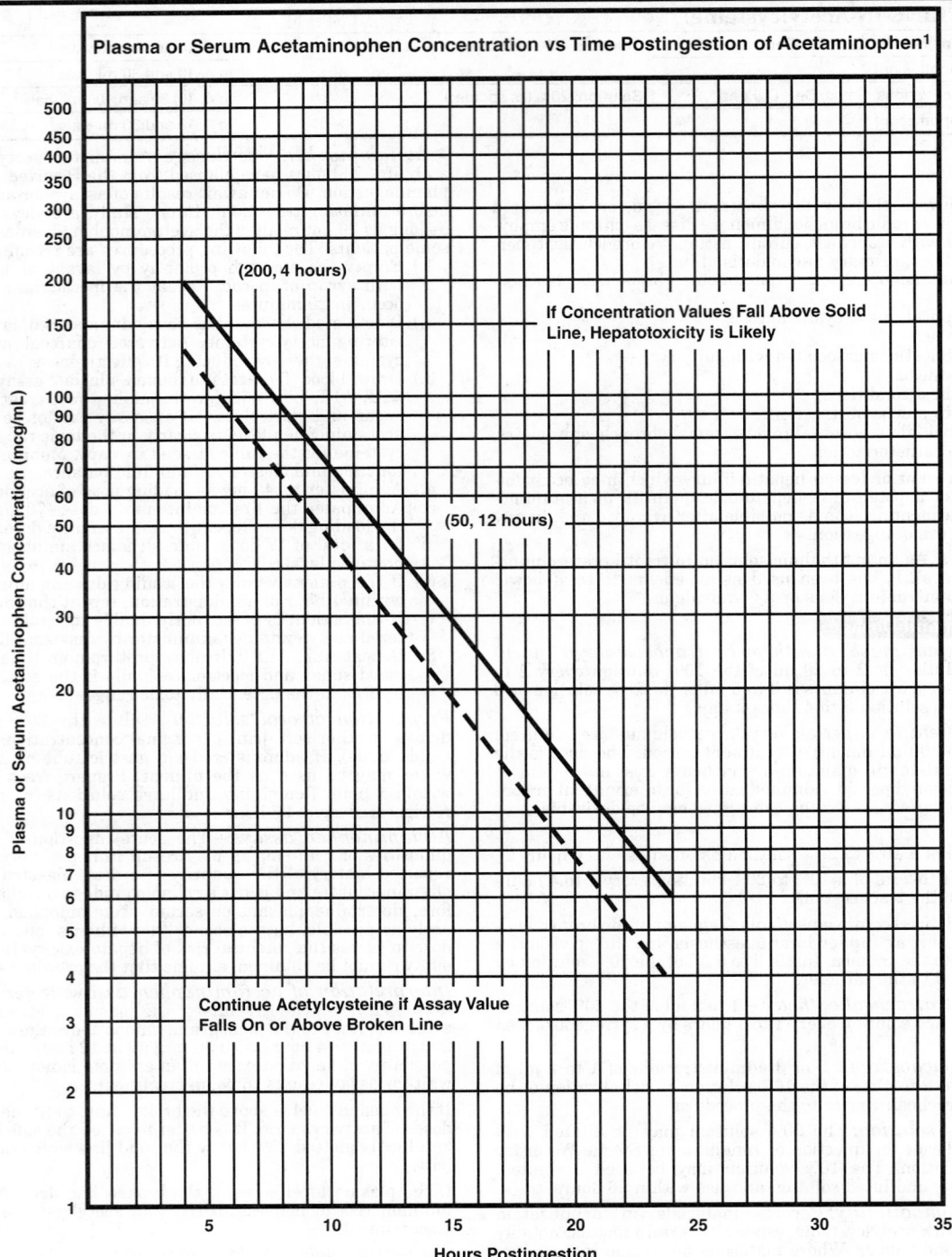

Plasma or Serum Acetaminophen Concentration vs Time Postingestion of Acetaminophen[1]

(200, 4 hours)

If Concentration Values Fall Above Solid Line, Hepatotoxicity is Likely

(50, 12 hours)

Continue Acetylcysteine if Assay Value Falls On or Above Broken Line

Plasma or Serum Acetaminophen Concentration (mcg/mL)

Hours Postingestion

[1] Adapted from Rumack and Matthews. *Pediatrics*. 1975;55:871-876.

ACETYLCYSTEINE (N-Acetylcysteine)

➤*Supportive treatment:* Maintain fluid and electrolyte balance. Treat as necessary for hypoglycemia. Administer vitamin K_1 if prothrombin time ratio exceeds 1.5; administer fresh frozen plasma if the prothrombin time ratio exceeds 3. Avoid diuretics and forced diuresis.

Acetylcysteine Dosage Guide and Preparation				
Loading dose (140 mg/kg)*				
Body weight		Acetylcysteine (g)	20% solution (ml)	Diluent (ml)	5% solution (ml)
(kg)	(lb)				
100-109	220-240	15	75	225	300
90-99	198-218	14	70	210	280
80-89	176-196	13	65	195	260
70-79	154-174	11	55	165	220
60-69	132-152	10	50	150	200
50-59	110-130	8	40	120	160
40-49	88-108	7	35	105	140
30-39	66-86	6	30	90	120
20-29	44-64	4	20	60	80
Maintenance dose (70 mg/kg)*				
(kg)	(lb)				
100-109	220-240	7.5	37	113	150
90-99	198-218	7	35	105	140
80-89	176-196	6.5	33	97	130
70-79	154-174	5.5	28	82	110
60-69	132-152	5	25	75	100
50-59	110-130	4	20	60	80
40-49	88-108	3.5	18	52	70
30-39	66-86	3	15	45	60
20-29	44-64	2	10	30	40

* If patient weighs < 20 kg (usually patients < 6 years of age), calculate the dose. Each ml of 20% solution contains 200 mg acetylcysteine. Add 3 ml of diluent to each ml of 20% solution. Do not decrease the proportion of diluent.

➤*Admixture incompatibility:* Tetracycline, chlortetracycline, oxytetracycline, erythromycin lactobionate, amphotericin B and sodium ampicillin are incompatible when mixed in the same solution with acetylcysteine. Administer from separate solutions. Iodized oil, chymotrypsin, trypsin and hydrogen peroxide are also incompatible.

Actions

➤*Pharmacology:* The viscosity of pulmonary mucus secretions depends on the concentration of mucoprotein in the secretory fluid, the presence of disulfide bonds between these macromolecules and, to a lesser extent, DNA. The mucolytic action of acetylcysteine is related to the sulfhydryl group in the molecule, which acts directly to split disulfide linkages between mucoprotein molecular complexes, resulting in depolymerization and a decrease in mucus viscosity. Its action is unaffected by the presence of DNA. The mucolytic activity of acetylcysteine increases with increasing pH. Significant mucolysis occurs between pH 7 and 9.

Acetylcysteine also reduces the extent of liver injury following acetaminophen overdose. It is thought that acetylcysteine protects the liver by maintaining or restoring glutathione levels, or by acting as an alternate substrate for conjugation with, and thus, detoxification of the reactive metabolite of acetaminophen.

➤*Pharmacokinetics:* Following a 200 to 400 mg oral dose, peak plasma concentrations of 0.35 to 4 mg/L are achieved within 1 to 2 hours. Protein binding is ≈ 50% 4 hours post-dose. Volume of distribution is 0.33 to 0.47 L/kg. The terminal half-life of reduced acetylcysteine is 6.25 hours. Approximately 70% of total body clearance is nonrenal.

Contraindications

Hypersensitivity to acetylcysteine. As an antidote, there are no contraindications.

Warnings

➤*Bronchial secretions:* An increased volume of liquefied bronchial secretions may occur; when cough is inadequate, maintain an open airway by mechanical suction if necessary. When there is a large mechanical block due to a foreign body or local accumulation, clear the airway by endotracheal aspiration, with or without bronchoscopy.

➤*Asthmatics:* Carefully observe asthmatics under treatment with acetylcysteine. If bronchospasm progresses, discontinue medication immediately.

➤*Antidotal use:*

Allergic effects – Generalized urticaria has been observed rarely. If this or other allergic symptoms appear, discontinue treatment unless it is deemed essential and the allergic symptoms can be otherwise controlled.

Hepatic effects – If encephalopathy due to hepatic failure occurs, discontinue treatment to avoid further administration of nitrogenous substances. No data indicate that acetylcysteine adversely influences hepatic failure, but this is theoretically possible.

Vomiting – Occasionally severe and persistent, it occurs as a symptom of acute acetaminophen overdose. Treatment with oral acetylcysteine may aggravate this. Evaluate patients at risk of gastric hemorrhage (eg, esophageal varices, peptic ulcers) concerning the risk of upper GI hemorrhage vs the risk of developing hepatic toxicity. Diluting acetylcysteine minimizes its propensity to aggravate vomiting.

➤*Pregnancy: Category B.* There are no adequate and well controlled studies in pregnant women. Use only when clearly needed.

➤*Lactation:* It is not known whether this drug is excreted in breast milk. Exercise caution when administering to a nursing woman.

Precautions

➤*Disagreeable odor:* Administration may initially produce a slight disagreeable odor which soon disappears.

➤*Face mask use:* A face mask may cause stickiness on the face after nebulization; remove with water.

➤*Solution color:* May change in the opened bottle, but this does not significantly impair the drug's safety or efficacy.

➤*Continued nebulization:* Continued acetylcysteine nebulization with a dry gas results in concentration of drug in the nebulizer due to evaporation. Extreme concentration may impede nebulization and drug delivery. Dilute with Sterile Water for Injection as concentration occurs.

Adverse Reactions

➤*Bronchospasm:* Clinically overt acetylcysteine-induced bronchospasm occurs infrequently and unpredictably even in patients with asthmatic bronchitis or bronchitis complicating bronchial asthma.

➤*Acquired sensitization:* Acetylcysteine sensitization has occurred rarely. Sensitization has been confirmed in several inhalation therapists who reported a history of dermal eruptions after frequent and extended exposure to acetylcysteine.

➤*Irritation to the tracheal and bronchial tracts:* This has occurred, and although hemoptysis has occurred in patients receiving acetylcysteine, such findings are not uncommon in patients with bronchopulmonary disease. A causal relationship has not been established.

➤*Antidotal use:* Large doses of oral acetylcysteine may result in nausea, vomiting and other GI symptoms. Rash (with or without mild fever), pruritus, angioedema, bronchospasm, tachycardia, hypotension and hypertension have occurred.

Other – Stomatitis; nausea; vomiting; fever; rhinorrhea; drowsiness; clamminess; chest tightness; bronchoconstriction.

DORNASE ALFA (Recombinant human deoxyribonuclease; DNase)

Rx	Pulmozyme (Genentech)	Solution for inhalation: 1 mg/ml	Preservative free. With 0.15 mg/ml calcium chloride dihydrate and 8.77 mg/ml sodium chloride. In 2.5 ml amps.

Indications

➤*Cystic fibrosis:* Daily administration in conjunction with standard therapies in the management of CF patients to reduce the frequency of respiratory infections requiring parenteral antibiotics and to improve pulmonary function.

Administration and Dosage

➤*Approved by the FDA:* December 30, 1993.

➤*Dosage:* The recommended dose for use in most CF patients is one 2.5 mg single-use amp inhaled once daily using a recommended nebulizer. Some patients may benefit from twice daily administration.

➤*Nebulizers:* Clinical trials have been performed with the following nebulizers and compressors: The disposable jet nebulizer *Hudson T Updraft* II and disposable jet nebulizer *Marquest Acorn* II in conjunction

with a *Pulmo-Aide* compressor, and the reusable *PARI LC Jet⁺* nebulizer, in conjunction with the *PARI PRONEB* compressor. Safety and efficacy have been demonstrated only with these recommended nebulizer systems. No clinical data are currently available that support the safety and efficacy of administration of dornase with other nebulizer systems. The patient should follow the manufacturer's instructions on the use and maintenance of the equipment. Do not dilute or mix dornase with other drugs in the nebulizer. Mixing of dornase with other drugs could lead to adverse physicochemical or functional changes in dornase or the admixed compound.

➤*Storage/Stability:* Store under refrigeration (2° to 8°C; 36° to 46°F). Protect amps from light. Do not use beyond the expiration date stamped on the amp. Store unused amps in their protective foil pouch under refrigeration.

Mucolytics

DORNASE ALFA (Recombinant human deoxyribonuclease; DNase)

Actions

➤*Pharmacology:* Dornase is a highly purified solution of recombinant human deoxyribonuclease I (rhDNase), an enzyme that selectively cleaves DNA. The protein is produced by genetically engineered Chinese Hamster Ovary (CHO) cells containing DNA encoding for the native human protein, deoxyribonuclease I (DNase). The purified glycoprotein contains 260 amino acids with an approximate molecular weight of 37,000 daltons. The primary amino acid sequence is identical to that of the native human enzyme. Dornase is administered by inhalation of an aerosol mist produced by a compressed air driven nebulizer system.

In cystic fibrosis (CF) patients, retention of viscous purulent secretions in the airways contributes both to reduced pulmonary function and to exacerbations of infection. Purulent pulmonary secretions contain very high concentrations of extracellular DNA released by degenerating leukocytes that accumulate in response to infection. In vitro, dornase hydrolyzes the DNA in sputum of CF patients and reduces sputum viscoelasticity.

➤*Pharmacokinetics:* When 2.5 mg dornase was administered by inhalation to 18 CF patients, mean sputum concentrations of 3 mcg/ml DNase were measurable within 15 minutes. Mean sputum concentrations declined to an average of 0.6 mcg/ml 2 hours following inhalation. Inhalation of up to 10 mg 3 times daily by four CF patients for 6 consecutive days did not result in a significant elevation of serum concentrations of DNase above normal endogenous levels. After administration of up to 2.5 mg dornase twice daily for 6 months to 321 CF patients, no accumulation of serum DNase was noted.

➤*Clinical trials:* In a large, randomized, placebo controlled trial, clinically stable CF patients (≥ 5 years of age) with baseline forced vital capacity (FVC) ≥ 40% of predicted, and receiving standard therapies for CF were treated with placebo (n = 325), 2.5 mg dornase once a day (n = 322) or 2.5 mg dornase twice a day (n = 321) for 6 months administered via a nebulizer. Both doses of dornase resulted in significant reductions compared with the placebo group in the number of patients experiencing respiratory tract infections requiring use of parenteral antibiotics. Administration of dornase reduced the relative risk of developing a respiratory tract infection by 27% and 29% for the daily dose and twice daily dose, respectively. The data suggest that the effects of dornase on respiratory tract infections in older patients (> 21 years) may be smaller than in younger patients, and that twice daily dosing may be required in the older patients. Patients with baseline FVC > 85% may also benefit from twice a day dosing. The reduced risk of respiratory infection observed in dornase–treated patients did not directly correlate with improvement in FEV_1 during the initial 2 weeks of therapy.

Within 8 days of the start of treatment with dornase, mean FEV_1 increased 7.9% in those treated once a day and 9% in those treated twice a day compared to the baseline values. The mean FEV_1 observed during long-term therapy increased 5.8% and 5.6% from baseline at the 2.5 mg daily dose level and 2.5 mg twice daily dose level, respectively. Placebo recipients did not show significant mean changes in pulmonary function testing. For patients ≥ 5 years of age with baseline FVC ≥ 40%, administration of dornase decreased the incidence of occurrence of first respiratory tract infection requiring parenteral antibiotics, and improved mean FEV_1 regardless of age or baseline FVC.

Incidence of First Respiratory Tract Infection Requiring Parenteral Antibiotics Following Dornase			
	Placebo (n = 325)	2.5 mg once daily (n = 322)	2.5 mg twice daily (n = 321)
Percent of patients infected	43%	34%	33%
Age			
5-20 years	42%	25%	28%
≥ 21 years	44%	48%	39%
Baseline FVC			
40-85% predicted	54%	41%	44%
> 85% predicted	27%	21%	14%

In other studies, dornase did not produce a pulmonary function benefit in short-term usage in patients with FVC < 40% of predicted. Studies are in progress to assess the impact of chronic use on pulmonary function and infection risk in this population. Clinical trials have indicated that dornase therapy can be continued or initiated during an acute respiratory exacerbation. Short-term studies demonstrated that doses in excess of 2.5 mg twice daily did not provide further improvement in FEV_1. Patients who have received the drug on a cyclical regimen (eg, 10 mg twice daily for 14 days, followed by a 14 day washout period) showed rapid improvement in FEV_1 with the initiation of each cycle and a return to baseline with each dornase withdrawal.

Contraindications

Hypersensitivity to dornase, Chinese Hamster Ovary cell products, or any component of the product.

Warnings

➤*Pregnancy:* Category B. There are no adequate and well controlled studies in pregnant women. Use this drug during pregnancy only if clearly needed.

➤*Lactation:* It is not known whether dornase is excreted in breast milk. Exercise caution when administering to a nursing woman.

➤*Children:* Safety and efficacy in children < 5 years of age have not been studied.

Precautions

➤*Administration:* Use in conjunction with standard therapies for CF. Safety and efficacy of daily administration have not been demonstrated in patients with FVC < 40% of predicted or for > 12 months.

Drug Interactions

Clinical trials have indicated that dornase can be effectively and safely used in conjunction with standard CF therapies including oral, inhaled and parenteral antibiotics, bronchodilators, enzyme supplements, vitamins, oral and inhaled corticosteroids and analgesics.

Adverse Reactions

Patients have been exposed to dornase for up to 12 months in clinical trials. Most adverse events were not more common on dornase than on placebo and probably reflected the sequelae of the underlying lung disease. In most cases, events that were increased were mild, transient in nature, and did not require alterations in dosing. Few patients experienced adverse events resulting in permanent discontinuation from dornase, and the discontinuation rate was similar for placebo (2%) and dornase (3%).

Dornase Adverse Reactions (%)			
Adverse event	Placebo (n=325)	Dornase once daily (n=322)	Dornase twice daily (n=321)
Voice alteration	7	12	16
Pharyngitis	33	36	40
Laryngitis	1	3	4
Rash	7	10	12
Chest pain	16	18	21
Conjunctivitis	2	4	5

Other adverse reactions reported include the following:

➤*GI:* Intestinal obstruction; gall bladder disease; liver disease; pancreatic disease.

➤*Metabolic/Nutritional:* Diabetes mellitus; hypoxia; weight loss.

➤*Respiratory:* Apnea; bronchiectasis; bronchitis; change in sputum; cough increase; dyspnea; hemoptysis; lung function decrease; nasal polyps; pneumonia; pneumothorax; rhinitis; sinusitis; sputum increase; wheeze.

➤*Miscellaneous:* Abdominal pain; asthenia; fever; flu syndrome; malaise; sepsis.

Death – Causes of death were consistent with progression of CF and included apnea, cardiac arrest, cardiopulmonary arrest, cor pulmonale, heart failure, massive hemoptysis, pneumonia, pneumothorax and respiratory failure.

Allergic reactions – Skin rash and urticaria have been observed, and were mild and transient in nature. Within all studies, a small percentage of patients developed serum antibodies to dornase (2% to 4%). None of these patients developed anaphylaxis, and the clinical significance of serum antibodies to dornase is unknown.

Overdosage

Cystic fibrosis patients have received up to 20 mg twice daily for up to 6 days and 10 mg twice daily intermittently (2 weeks on/2 weeks off drug) for 168 days. These doses were well tolerated.

Patient Information

Dornase must be stored in the refrigerator at 2° to 8°C (36° to 46°F) and protected from strong light. Keep refrigerated during transport and do not expose to room temperatures for a total time of 24 hours. Discard the solution if it is cloudy or discolored. Dornase contains no preservative and, once opened, the entire ampule must be used or discarded.

Instruct patients in the proper use and maintenance of the nebulizer and compressor system used in the delivery of the drug. Do not dilute or mix dornase with other drugs in the nebulizer. Mixing of dornase with other drugs could lead to adverse physicochemical or functional changes in dornase or the admixed compound.

CROMOLYN SODIUM (Disodium Cromoglycate)

Rx	Cromolyn Sodium (Various, eg, Alpharma, Dey)	Solution for inhalation: 20 mg/2 mL	In 60 and 120 UD vials or amps.
Rx	Intal (Aventis)	Solution for inhalation: 20 mg/2 mL	In 60 and 120 UD amps.
		Aerosol: 800 mcg/actuation	In 8.1 g (≥ 112 metered sprays) and 14.2 g (≥ 200 metered sprays).
otc	Nasalcrom (Pharmacia)	Nasal solution: 40 mg/mL[1] (Each actuation delivers 5.2 mg)	In 13 mL or 26 mL metered spray device.
Rx	Gastrocrom (Celltech)	Oral concentrate: 100 mg/5 mL	In 8 UD amps/foil pouch.

[1] With benzalkonium chloride and EDTA.

Indications

►*Bronchial asthma (inhalation solution, aerosol):* As prophylactic management of bronchial asthma. Cromolyn is given on a regular, daily basis in patients with frequent symptomatology requiring a continuous medication regimen.

►*Prevention of bronchospasm (inhalation solution, aerosol):* To prevent acute bronchospasm induced by exercise, toluene diisocyanate, environmental pollutants, and known antigens.

►*Allergic rhinitis (nasal solution):* To prevent and treat allergic rhinitis caused by airborne pollens from trees, grasses, or ragweed, and by mold, animals, and dust. To prevent and relieve the following nasal symptoms: Runny/itchy nose, sneezing, and allergic stuffy nose.

►*Mastocytosis (oral):* Improves diarrhea, flushing, headaches, vomiting, urticaria, abdominal pain, nausea, and itching in some patients.

►*Unlabeled uses:* Cromolyn has been used as an alternative therapy in refractory forms of chronic urticaria/angioedema. Oral cromolyn has been used for the treatment of food allergies and mucosal and serosal eosinophilic gastroenteritis.

Administration and Dosage

►*Approved by the FDA:* May 28, 1982.

►*Inhalation solution (adults and children at least 2 years of age):* Initially, 20 mg (1 amp/vial) administered by nebulization 4 times/day at regular intervals. The effectiveness of therapy depends upon administration at regular intervals.

Administer solution from a power-operated nebulizer having an adequate flow rate and equipped with a suitable face mask or mouthpiece. Hand operated nebulizers are not suitable.

Introduce cromolyn into the patient's therapeutic regimen when the acute episode has been controlled, the airway has been cleared, and the patient is able to inhale adequately.

Improvement ordinarily occurs within the first 4 weeks of administration, although some patients may demonstrate an immediate response. Efficacy is manifested by a decrease in the severity of clinical symptoms, or the need for concomitant therapy, or both.

Prevention of acute bronchospasm – Inhale 20 mg (1 amp/vial) administered by nebulization shortly before exposure to the precipitating factor.

►*Aerosol (adults and children at least 5 years of age):* For management of bronchial asthma, the usual starting dose is 2 metered sprays inhaled 4 times/day at regular intervals. Do not exceed this dose. Not all patients will respond to the recommended dose, and a lower dose may provide efficacy in younger patients.

Advise patients with chronic asthma that the effect of therapy is dependent upon its administration at regular intervals, as directed. Introduce therapy into the patient's therapeutic regimen when the acute episode has been controlled, the airway has been cleared, and the patient is able to inhale adequately.

Improvement ordinarily occurs within the first 4 weeks of administration, although some patients may demonstrate an immediate response. Efficacy is manifested by a decrease in the severity of clinical symptoms, or the need for concomitant therapy, or both.

Prevention of acute bronchospasm – The usual dose is inhalation of 2 metered dose sprays shortly (ie, 10 to 15 minutes but not more than 60 minutes) before exposure to the precipitating factor.

►*Nasal solution:*

Adults and children at least 2 years of age – 1 spray in each nostril 3 to 6 times daily at regular intervals every 4 to 6 hours. Maximum effects may not be seen for 1 to 2 weeks. Clear the nasal passages before administering the spray and inhale through the nose during administration (see Patient Information).

►*Oral:*

Adults (13 years of age or older) – 2 ampules 4 times/day 30 minutes before meals and at bedtime.

Children 2 to 12 years of age – 1 ampule 4 times/day 30 minutes before meals and at bedtime.

If satisfactory control of symptoms is not achieved within 2 to 3 weeks, the dosage may be increased; do not exceed 40 mg/kg/day.

The effect of therapy is dependent upon its administration at regular intervals as directed. Not for inhalation or injection.

Maintenance – Once a therapeutic response has been achieved, the dose may be reduced to the minimum required to maintain the patient with a lower degree of symptomatology. To prevent relapses, maintain the dosage.

Administer as a solution at least 30 minutes before meals and at bedtime after preparation according to the following directions.
1.) Break open and squeeze liquid contents of ampule(s) into a glass of water.
2.) Stir solution.
3.) Drink all of the liquid.

►*Nonsteroidal agents:* Add cromolyn (inhalation solution and aerosol) to the patient's existing treatment regimen (eg, bronchodilators). Concomitant medications may be decreased gradually when a clinical response to cromolyn is evident (approximately 2 to 4 weeks) and asthma is under good control. Titrate the frequency of cromolyn administration downward to the lowest effective level if concomitant medications are discontinued or required on no more than an as-needed basis. The usual decrease is from 4 to 3 ampules/vials per day for the nebulizer solution, or from 2 metered inhalations 4 times/day to 3 times/day to twice daily for the inhalation aerosol. Gradually reduce dosage to avoid asthma exacerbations. Clinical deterioration in these patients whose dosage has been decreased to less than 4 ampules/vials or 4 inhalations per day may require an increase in cromolyn dosage and the introduction of, or increase in, symptomatic medications.

►*Corticosteroids:* Continue concomitant corticosteroid treatment following the introduction of cromolyn (inhalation solution and aerosol). If the patient improves, attempt to decrease corticosteroid dosage. Even if the corticosteroid-dependent patient fails to improve following cromolyn use, attempt gradual tapering of steroid dosage while maintaining close patient supervision. Consider reinstituting steroid therapy for a patient subjected to significant stress (eg, a severe asthmatic attack, surgery, trauma, severe illness) while being treated or within 1 year (occasionally up to 2 years) after corticosteroid treatment has been terminated, in case of adrenocortical insufficiency. When respiratory function is impaired, as may occur in severe exacerbation of asthma, a temporary increase in the amount of corticosteroids or other agents may be required to regain control of the patient's asthma.

It is particularly important to exercise great care if for any reason cromolyn is withdrawn in cases where its use has permitted a reduction in the corticosteroid maintenance dose. In such cases, continued close supervision of the patient is essential because there may be a sudden reappearance of severe manifestations of asthma that will require immediate therapy and possible reintroduction of corticosteroids.

►*Compatibility:* Cromolyn nebulizer solution has demonstrated compatibility with 5% metaproterenol sulfate, 0.5% isoproterenol HCl, 1% isoetharine HCl, 2.25% epinephrine, 0.1% terbutaline sulfate, 0.02% ipratropium bromide, and 20% acetylcysteine solution for at least 1 hour after their admixture. It also was compatible with 0.6% and 5% metaproterenol sulfate, 0.2% atropine sulfate, 0.5% albuterol sulfate, and 0.9% sodium chloride solution for at least 90 minutes after their admixture. It is important to note that the stated medications may not be identical to the formulations currently marketed in the US.

►*Storage/Stability:*

Inhalation solution – Store at controlled room temperature 20° to 25°C (68° to 77°F). Protect from light. Do not use if the solution contains a precipitate or becomes discolored. Store ampules in foil pouch until ready to use.

Aerosol and nasal solution – Store at controlled room temperature 20° to 25°C (68° to 77°F). Do not puncture, incinerate, or place the aerosol near sources of heat. Protect nasal solution from light.

Oral concentrate – Store between 15° to 30°C (59° to 86°F). Protect from light. Do not use the concentrate if it contains a precipitate or becomes discolored. Store ampules in foil pouch until ready to use.

Actions

►*Pharmacology:* Cromolyn is an anti-inflammatory agent. It has no intrinsic bronchodilator, antihistaminic, vasoconstrictor, or glucocorticoid activity. In animal studies, cromolyn inhibits sensitized and mast cells degranulation that occurs after exposure to specific antigens. The drug inhibits the release of mediators, histamine, and SRS-A (the slow-reacting substance of anaphylaxis, a leukotriene) from the mast cell. Studies have demonstrated that cromolyn indirectly inhibits calcium

CROMOLYN SODIUM (Disodium Cromoglycate)

ions from entering the mast cell, resulting in the prevention of mediator release. Immediate and nonimmediate bronchoconstrictive reactions induced by the inhalation of antigens can be inhibited by cromolyn. Cromolyn also attenuates bronchospasms caused by exercise, toluene diisocyanate, aspirin, cold air, sulfur dioxide, and environmental pollutants. Cromolyn acts locally on the lung to which it is directly applied.

➤*Pharmacokinetics:* After inhalation, approximately 8% is absorbed from the lung and rapidly excreted unchanged in bile and urine. The remainder is either exhaled or deposited in the oropharynx, swallowed, and excreted via the alimentary tract.

Cromolyn is poorly absorbed from the GI tract. No more than 1% of an administered dose is absorbed after oral administration, the remainder being excreted in the feces. Very little absorption of cromolyn was seen after oral administration of 500 mg to each of 12 volunteers. From 0.28% to 0.5% of the administered dose was recovered in the first 24 hours of urinary excretion in 3 subjects. The mean urinary excretion over 24 hours in the remaining 9 subjects was 0.45%.

Contraindications

Hypersensitivity to cromolyn or to any ingredient contained in these products.

Warnings

➤*Acute asthma:* Cromolyn has no role in the treatment of acute asthma, especially status asthmaticus; it is a prophylactic drug with no benefit for acute situations.

➤*Hypersensitivity reactions:* Severe anaphylactic reactions may occur rarely with cromolyn. Refer to General Management of Acute Hypersensitivity Reactions.

➤*Renal/Hepatic function impairment:* In view of the biliary and renal routes of excretion, decrease the dose or discontinue the drug in these patients.

➤*Pregnancy: Category B.* There are no adequate and well-controlled studies in pregnant women. Use only when clearly needed. Animal studies have demonstrated adverse fetal effects (increased resorptions, decreased fetal weight) only at very high parenteral doses.

➤*Lactation:* It is not known whether this drug is excreted in human milk. Exercise caution when the drug is administered to a nursing woman.

➤*Children:*

Aerosol – Safety and efficacy in children less than 5 years of age have not been established.

Inhalation solution – Safety and efficacy in children less than 2 years of age have not been established.

Nasal – Do not use in children under 2 years of age unless directed by a physician.

Oral – In neonatal rats, cromolyn increased mortality at oral doses of 1000 mg/kg or greater. In term infants up to 6 months of age, data suggest the dose not exceed 20 mg/kg/day. Reserve use in children less than 2 years of age for patients with severe disease in which potential benefits clearly outweigh risks.

Precautions

➤*Bronchospasm/Cough:* Occasionally, patients experience cough or bronchospasm following inhalation and, at times, may not be able to continue treatment despite prior bronchodilator administration. Rarely, very severe bronchospasm has occurred.

➤*Asthma:* Symptoms may recur if drug is reduced below recommended dosage or discontinued.

➤*Eosinophilic pneumonia (pulmonary infiltrates with eosinophilia):* If this occurs during the course of therapy, discontinue the drug.

➤*Aerosol:* Because of the propellants in this preparation, use with caution in patients with coronary artery disease or cardiac arrhythmias.

Adverse Reactions

The most frequently reported adverse reactions attributed to cromolyn sodium (on the basis of recurrence following readministration) involve the respiratory tract and include bronchospasm (sometimes severe, associated with a precipitous fall in pulmonary function [FEV$_1$]), cough, laryngeal edema (rare), nasal congestion (sometimes severe), pharyngeal irritation, and wheezing.

➤*Aerosol:*

Frequent – Throat irritation or dryness; bad taste; cough; wheeze; nausea.

Infrequent –
CNS: Dizziness; headache.
GU: Dysuria; urinary frequency.
Hypersensitivity: Anaphylaxis; rash; urticaria; angioedema.
Special senses: Lacrimation; swollen parotid gland.

Miscellaneous: Joint swelling and pain; substernal burning; myopathy; pulmonary infiltrates with eosinophilia.

Rare (unclear if attributable to drug) –
CNS: Vertigo; drowsiness.
Dermatologic: Exfoliative dermatitis; photodermatitis.
Musculoskeletal: Myalgia; polymyositis.
Respiratory: Hemoptysis; sneezing; nasal itching; nasal bleeding; nasal burning.
Miscellaneous: Stomachache; anemia; hoarseness; nephrosis; liver disease; serum sickness; periarteritic vasculitis; pericarditis; peripheral neuritis.

➤*Inhalation solution:*
Miscellaneous – Cough; nasal congestion; wheezing; sneezing; nausea; drowsiness; nasal itching; epistaxis; nose burning; serum sickness; stomachache.

➤*Nasal solution:*
Miscellaneous – Sneezing; nasal stinging; nasal irritation.

➤*Oral concentrate:* Most of the adverse events reported in mastocytosis patients have been transient and could represent symptoms of the disease. The most frequently reported adverse events in mastocytosis patients who have received cromolyn during clinical studies were headache and diarrhea. Each occurred in 4 of 87 patients. Pruritus, nausea, and myalgia were each reported in 3 patients and abdominal pain, rash, and irritability in 2 patients. There was also one report of malaise.

Adverse events have been reported during studies in other clinical conditions and during foreign postmarketing surveillances. In most cases, these reports were incomplete and attribution to cromolyn was not determined.

Cardiovascular – Tachycardia; premature ventricular contractions (PVCs); palpitations.

CNS – Dizziness; headache; paresthesia; migraine; hypesthesia; convulsions; psychosis; anxiety; depression; hallucinations; behavior change; insomnia; nervousness.

Dermatologic – Pruritus; rash; flushing; urticaria/angioedema; erythema and burning; photosensitivity.

GI – Diarrhea; nausea; abdominal pain; constipation; dyspepsia; flatulence; glossitis; stomatitis; vomiting; dysphagia; esophagospasm.

Hematologic – Polycythemia; neutropenia; pancytopenia.

Musculoskeletal – Arthralgia; myalgia; leg stiffness/weakness.

Miscellaneous – Pharyngitis; dyspnea; fatigue; edema; unpleasant taste; chest pain; postprandial lightheadedness and lethargy; dysuria; urinary frequency; purpura; hepatic function test abnormal; tinnitus; lupus erythematosus syndrome.

Overdosage

There is no clinical syndrome associated with an overdosage of cromolyn. In several animal species, acute toxicity with cromolyn occurs only with very high exposure levels. No deaths occurred at the highest oral doses tested in mice, 8000 mg/kg (approximately 5100 and 2700 times the maximum recommended daily inhalation doses in adults and children, respectively, on a mg/m^2 basis) or in rats, 8000 mg/kg (approximately 10,000 and 5400 times the maximum recommended daily inhalation doses in adults and children, respectively, on a mg/m^2 basis).

Patient Information

➤*Nasal solution:* Stop using the nasal spray and consult the physician if any of the following occurs: Shortness of breath, wheezing, or chest tightness; hives or swelling of the mouth or throat; symptoms worsen; new symptoms emerge; there is no improvement within 2 weeks; product needed for more than 12 weeks. Other medications (eg, allergy medications) may be used safely with cromolyn nasal solution. Do not use to treat sinus infection, asthma, or cold symptoms.

Directions for use – Blow nose before administering spray. Hold pump with thumb at bottom and nozzle between fingers. If this is the first time using the pump, or if you have not used the pump for several days, spray in the air until you get a fine mist. Insert nozzle into nostril, spray upward while breathing in through the nose. Repeat in other nostril. Brief stinging or sneezing may occur right after use. Keep clean by wiping nozzle. If used more than 12 weeks, consult a physician.

➤*Aerosol:*
Directions for use – Take the cover off the mouthpiece. Shake the inhaler gently. Hold inhaler and breathe out slowly and fully, expelling as much air as possible. Do not breathe into the inhaler; it could clog the inhaler valve. Place the mouthpiece into your mouth, close your lips around it, and tilt your head back. Keep your tongue below the opening of the inhaler. While breathing in deeply and slowly through the mouth, fully depress the top of the metal canister with your index finger. Remove the inhaler from your mouth. Hold your breath for several seconds, then breathe out slowly. Keep track of the number of actuations used from each canister of cromolyn inhaler and discard the canister after 112 actuations from the 8.1 g canister or 200 actuations from the 14.2 g canister.

CROMOLYN SODIUM (Disodium Cromoglycate)

➤*Inhalation solution:* Do not swallow solution because it is poorly absorbed orally. Empty the ampule into a power-driven nebulizer as directed. Do not mix different types of medications without permission from your health care provider.

Directions for use – Squeeze the contents of the ampule into the solution container of your nebulizer. Once the nebulizer has been assembled and contains cromolyn inhalation solution, hold the mask close to the face and switch on the device. Breathe through the mouth

and out through the nose in a normal, relaxed manner. Nebulization should take approximately 5 to 10 minutes.

➤*Oral:* The effect of therapy depends upon administration at regular intervals as directed.

Take at least 30 minutes before meals and at bedtime. Break open ampule(s) and squeeze liquid contents into a glass of water. Stir solution and drink all of the liquid.

NEDOCROMIL SODIUM

Rx	Tilade (Monarch)	Aerosol: 1.75 mg/actuation	In 16.2 g canisters providing at least 104 metered inhalations. With mouthpiece.

Indications

➤*Asthma:* Maintenance therapy in the management of adult and pediatric patients 6 years of age and older with mild to moderate asthma.

Nedocromil is not indicated for the reversal of acute bronchospasm.

Administration and Dosage

➤*Approved by the FDA:* December 30, 1992.

➤*Asthma:* Two inhalations 4 times/day at regular intervals to provide 14 mg/day. In patients whose asthma is well controlled on this dosage (ie, patients who only need occasional inhaled or oral beta$_2$-agonists and who are not experiencing serious exacerbations), less frequent administration may be effective.

Nedocromil may be added to the patient's existing treatment regimen (eg, bronchodilators). When a clinical response to nedocromil is evident and if the asthma is under good control, attempt to decrease concomitant medication usage gradually.

Advise patients that the optimal effect of nedocromil therapy depends on its administration at regular intervals, even during symptom-free periods.

Each nedocromil inhaler canister must be primed with 3 actuations prior to the first use. If a canister remains unused for more than 7 days, then it should be reprimed with 3 actuations.

➤*Storage/Stability:* Store between 2° to 30°C (36° to 86°F). Do not freeze.

Actions

➤*Pharmacology:* Nedocromil is an inhaled anti-inflammatory agent for the preventive management of asthma. It inhibits the in vitro activation of, and mediator release from, a variety of inflammatory cell types associated with asthma (eg, eosinophils, neutrophils, macrophages, mast cells, monocytes, platelets). In vitro, nedocromil inhibits the release of mediators (eg, histamine, leukotriene C$_4$, prostaglandin D$_2$). Similar studies with human bronchoalveolar cells showed inhibition of histamine release from mast cells and beta-glucuronidase release from macrophages.

Nedocromil inhibits the development of early and late bronchoconstriction responses to inhaled antigens. The development of airway hyperresponsiveness to nonspecific bronchoconstrictors also was inhibited. Nedocromil reduced antigen-induced increases in airway microvasculature leakage when administered IV.

The drug acutely inhibits the bronchoconstrictor response to several kinds of challenge. Pretreatment with single doses inhibited the bronchoconstriction caused by sulfur dioxide, inhaled neurokinin A, various antigens, exercise, cold air, fog, and adenosine monophosphate.

Nedocromil has no bronchodilator, antihistamine, or corticosteroid activity, and when delivered by inhalation at the recommended dose, has no known systemic activity.

➤*Pharmacokinetics:* Systemic bioavailability of nedocromil administered as an inhaled aerosol is low. In a single-dose study of 20 healthy adult subjects who were administered a 3.5 mg dose, the mean AUC was 5 ng•h/mL and the mean C$_{max}$ was 1.6 ng/mL, attained approximately 28 minutes after dosing. The mean half-life was 3.3 hours. Urinary excretion over 12 hours averaged 3.4% of the administered dose, of which about 75% was excreted in the first 6 hours of dosing.

In a multiple-dose study, 6 healthy adult volunteers received a 3.5 mg single dose followed by 3.5 mg 4 times/day for 7 consecutive days. Accumulation of the drug was not observed. Following single- and multiple-dose inhalations, urinary excretion accounted for 5.6% and 12% of the drug administered, respectively. After IV administration, urinary excretion was approximately 70%. The absolute bioavailability was 8% for single- and 17% for multiple-inhaled doses.

Similarly, in a multiple-dose study of 12 asthmatic adult patients, each given a 3.5 mg single dose followed by 3.5 mg 4 times/day for 1 month, both single-dose and multiple-dose inhalations gave a mean high plasma

concentration of 2.8 ng/mL between 5 and 90 minutes, mean AUC of 5.6 ng•h/mL, and a mean terminal half-life of 1.5 hours. The mean 24-hour urinary excretion after either single- or multiple-dose administration represented approximately 5% of the administered dose.

Nedocromil is approximately 89% protein bound in human plasma over a concentration range of 0.5 to 50 mcg/mL. This binding is reversible. It is not metabolized after IV administration and is excreted unchanged.

➤*Clinical trials:* The effectiveness of nedocromil was compared with cromolyn sodium and placebo in an 8-week, double-blind, parallel group trial during which medication was given 4 times/day. Patients (N = 306) were randomized to treatment (103 nedocromil; 104 cromolyn sodium; 99 placebo). All patients were sustained-release theophylline-dependent and this drug was stopped prior to starting the test treatment. Efficacy was assessed on the basis of diary card symptom scores and FEV$_1$.

This study showed that nedocromil is effective in the management of symptoms and pulmonary function in primarily atopic mild to moderate asthmatics. Both active treatments were statistically significantly better than placebo for the primary efficacy variable (summary symptom score); nedocromil and cromolyn sodium were not significantly different for this parameter. However, a statistically significant difference favoring cromolyn sodium was seen for nighttime asthma and FEV$_1$.

In allergic asthmatics who are well controlled on cromolyn sodium, there is no evidence that the substitution of nedocromil for cromolyn sodium would confer additional benefit to the patient. Efficacy with one agent is not known to be predictive of efficacy with the other.

Contraindications

Hypersensitivity to nedocromil or other ingredients in the preparation.

Warnings

➤*Acute bronchospasm:* Nedocromil is not a bronchodilator and, therefore, should not be used for the reversal of acute bronchospasm, particularly status asthmaticus. Ordinarily, continue nedocromil during acute exacerbations unless the patient becomes intolerant to the use of inhaled dosage forms.

➤*Pregnancy:* Category B. There are no adequate and well-controlled studies in pregnant women. Use during pregnancy only if clearly needed.

➤*Lactation:* It is not known whether this drug is excreted in breast milk. Exercise caution when administering to a nursing woman.

➤*Children:* Safety and efficacy in children 6 through 11 years of age have been established in adequate and well-controlled clinical trials. The safety and efficacy of nedocromil in patients below 6 years of age have not been established.

Precautions

➤*Coughing/Bronchospasm:* As with other inhaled asthma medications, bronchospasm, which can be life-threatening, may occur immediately after administration. If this occurs, discontinue nedocromil and institute alternative therapy.

➤*Corticosteroids:* If systemic or inhaled corticosteroid therapy is reduced in patients receiving nedocromil, careful monitoring is necessary.

Adverse Reactions

Nedocromil is generally well tolerated. Of the 4400 patients who received 2 inhalations of nedocromil 4 times/day, 2632 were in placebo-controlled, parallel trials. Of these, 6% withdrew from the trials because of adverse events, compared with 5.7% of the 2446 patients who received placebo. The reasons for withdrawal were generally similar in the nedocromil and placebo-treated groups, except that patients withdrew because of bad taste statistically more frequently on nedocromil than on placebo. Headache reported as severe or very severe, some with nausea and ill feeling, was experienced by 1% of nedocromil patients and 0.7% of placebo patients.

Mast Cell Stabilizers

NEDOCROMIL SODIUM

Nedocromil Adverse Reactions				
	\% Experiencing adverse reaction		\% Withdrawing	
Adverse reaction	Nedocromil (N = 2632)	Placebo (N = 2402)	Nedocromil	Placebo
GI				
Nausea[1]	3.9	2.3	1.1	0.5
Vomiting[1]	2.5	1.6	0.2	0.3
Abdominal pain[1]	1.9	1.3	0.2	0.1
Dyspepsia	1.5	1.1	0.1	0.1
Diarrhea	1.3	1.2	0.1	0
Respiratory				
Coughing	8.9	10.2	1.1	1.2
Bronchospasm[2]	8.4	11.8	1.4	2
Pharyngitis	7.6	7.5	0.5	0.4
Rhinitis[1]	7.3	6	0.1	0.1
Upper respiratory infection	6.7	6.3	0.1	0.2
Sinusitis	3.3	4.1	1.1	0
Dyspnea	2.5	3.3	0.8	1
Sputum increased	1.5	1.4	0.1	0.2
Bronchitis	1.1	1.5	0.1	0.1
Respiratory disorder	0.8	1.1	0	0
Miscellaneous				
Unpleasant taste[1]	11.6	3.1	1.6	0
Headache	8.1	7.5	0.4	0.2
Chest pain	3.6	3.8	0.7	0.5
Fever	3.1	3.7	0.1	0.1
Viral infection	2.4	3.2	0.1	0.1
Conjunctivitis	1.1	0.7	0	0.1
Fatigue	1	0.8	0.2	0
Dizziness	0.8	1.3	0.1	0.2
Rash[2]	0.5	1.2	0.1	0

[1] Statistically significantly higher frequency on nedocromil (*P* < 0.05).
[2] Statistically significantly higher frequency on placebo (*P* < 0.05).

➤*Miscellaneous:* Arthritis; tremor; sensation of warmth (less than 1%).

In clinical trials with 2632 patients receiving nedocromil, 2 patients (0.08%) developed neutropenia and 3 patients (0.11%) developed leukopenia. Although it is unclear if these reactions were caused by nedocromil, in several cases these abnormal laboratory tests returned to normal when nedocromil was discontinued.

There have been reports of clinically significant elevation of hepatic transaminases (ALT and AST greater than 10 times the upper limit of the normal reference range in 1 patient) associated with the administration of nedocromil. It is unclear if these abnormal laboratory tests in asymptomatic patients were caused by nedocromil.

Postmarketing – Cases of bronchospasm immediatley following dosing with nedocromil have been reported. Isolated cases of pneumonitis with eosinophilia (PIE syndrome) and anaphylaxis also have been reported in which a relationship to the drug is undetermined.

Overdosage

Animal studies by several routes of administration (inhalation, oral, IV, SC) have demonstrated little potential for significant toxicity in humans from inhalation of high doses of nedocromil. Head shaking/tremor and salivation were observed in dogs following daily inhalation doses of 5 mg/kg and transient hypotension was detected following daily SC doses of 8 mg/kg. In addition, clonic convulsions were observed in dogs following daily inhalation doses of 20 mg/kg plus SC doses of 20 mg/kg giving peak plasma levels of 7.6 mcg/mL, some three orders of magnitude greater than peak plasma levels (2.5 ng/mL) of the human daily dose. Nedocromil does not pass the blood-brain barrier. Therefore, overdosage is unlikely to result in clinical manifestations requiring more than observation and discontinuation of the drug where appropriate.

Patient Information

An illustrated leaflet for the patient is included in each nedocromil pack.

Prime each nedocromil inhaler canister with 3 actuations prior to the first use. If a canister remains unused for more than 7 days, then reprime with 3 actuations.

Nedocromil must be used regularly to achieve benefit, even during symptom-free periods.

Nedocromil is not meant to relieve acute asthma symptoms. If symptoms do not improve or the condition worsens, do not increase the dosage; notify the physician immediately.

The full therapeutic effect of nedocromil may not be obtained for 1 week or longer after initiating treatment.

Because the therapeutic effect depends upon local delivery to the lungs, it is essential that patients be properly instructed in the correct method of use (see Patient Instructions for Use).

NITRIC OXIDE

Rx	**INOmax** (INO Therapeutics, Inc.)	**Gas:** 100 ppm	In 353 (delivered volume 344 L) and 1963 L (delivered volume 1918 L).
		800 ppm	In 353 (delivered volume 344 L) and 1963 L (delivered volume 1918 L).

Indications

➤*Neonates with hypoxic respiratory failure:* Nitric oxide, in conjunction with ventilatory support and other appropriate agents, is indicated for the treatment of term and near-term (> 34 weeks) neonates with hypoxic respiratory failure associated with clinical or echocardiographic evidence of pulmonary hypertension, where it improves oxygenation and reduces the need for extracorporeal membrane oxygenation.

➤*Unlabeled uses:* Reduce pulmonary artery pressure (PAP) and pulmonary vascular resistance during neonatal cardiac oprations; symptomatic treatment of hypoxemia or pulmonary hypertension due to allograft dysfunction subsequent to lung transplantation; adult respiratory distress syndrome (conflicting data).

Administration and Dosage

➤*Approved by the FDA:* December 23, 1999.

The recommended dose of nitric oxide is 20 ppm. Maintain treatment up to 14 days or until the underlying oxygen desaturation has resolved and the neonate is ready to be weaned from nitric oxide therapy.

An initial dose of 20 ppm was used in the clinical trials. In 1 study, patients whose oxygenation improved with 20 ppm were dose-reduced to 5 ppm as tolerated at the end of 4 hours of treatment. In another study, patients whose oxygenation failed to improve on 20 ppm could be increased to 80 ppm, but those patients did not then improve on the higher dose. Ordinarily, do not use doses > 20 ppm of nitric oxide as the risk of methemoglobinemia and elevated NO_2 levels increases significantly.

Use additional therapies to maximize oxygen delivery. In patients with collapsed alveoli, additional therapies might include surfactant and high frequency oscillatory ventilation.

The safety and effectiveness of inhaled nitric oxide have been established in a population receiving other therapies for hypoxic respiratory failure, including vasodilators, IV fluids, bicarbonate therapy, and mechanical ventilation. Different dose regimens for nitric oxide were used in the clinical studies.

Administer nitric oxide while monitoring for PaO_2, methemoglobin, and NO_2.

Nitric oxide must be delivered by a system that provides operator-determined concentrations of nitric oxide in the breathing gas, with a constant concentration throughout the respiratory cycle and that does not cause generation of excessive inhaled nitrogen dioxide. In the ventilated neonate, institute precise monitoring of inspired nitric oxide and NO_2 using a properly calibrated analysis device with alarms. Calibrate this system using a precisely defined calibration mixture of nitric oxide and nitrogen dioxide (eg, *INOcal*). Draw sample gas for analysis and measure oxygen levels before the Y-piece, proximal to the patient.

In the event of a system failure or a wall-outlet power failure, have a backup battery power supply and a reserve nitric oxide delivery system available.

Do not discontinue the nitric oxide dose abruptly, as it may result in an increase in PAP or worsening of blood oxygenation (PaO_2). Deterioration in oxygenation and elevation in PAP may also occur in children with no apparent response to nitric oxide. Discontinue/wean cautiously.

➤*Occupational exposure:* The exposure limit set by the Occupational Safety and Health Administration for nitric oxide is 25 ppm and 5 ppm for NO_2.

➤*Storage/Stability:* Store at 25°C (77°F).

Actions

➤*Pharmacology:* Nitric oxide is a compound produced by many cells of the body. It relaxes vascular smooth muscle by binding to the heme moiety of cytosolic guanylate cyclase, activating guanylate cyclase and increasing intracellular levels of cyclic guanosin 3′, 5′-monophosphate, which then leads to vasodilation. When inhaled, nitric oxide produces pulmonary vasodilation.

Inhaled nitric oxide appears to increase the partial pressure of arterial oxygen (PaO_2) by dilating pulmonary vessels in better ventilated areas of the lung, redistributing pulmonary blood flow away from lung regions with low ventilation/perfusion (V/Q) ratios toward regions with normal ratios.

Persistent pulmonary hypertension of the newborn (PPHN) occurs as a primary developmental defect or as a condition secondary to other diseases such as meconium aspiration syndrome (MAS), pneumonia, sepsis, hyaline membrane disease, congenital diaphragmatic hernia (CDH), and pulmonary hypoplasia. In these states, pulmonary vascular resistance (PVR) is high, which results in hypoxemia secondary to right-to-left shunting of blood through the patent ductus arteriosus and foramen ovale. In neonates with PPHN, inhaled nitric oxide improves oxygenation (as indicated by significant increase in PaO_2).

➤*Pharmacokinetics:*

Absorption – The pharmacokinetics of nitric oxide were studied in adults. Nitric oxide is absorbed systemically after inhalation. Most of it traverses the pulmonary capillary bed where it combines with hemoglobin that is 60% to 100% oxygen-saturated. At this level of oxygen saturation, nitric oxide combines predominantly with oxyhemoglobin to produce methemoglobin and nitrate. At low oxygen saturation, nitric oxide can combine with deoxyhemoglobin to transiently form nitrosyl-hemoglobin, which is converted to nitrogen oxides and methemoglobin upon exposure to oxygen.

Distribution – Within the pulmonary system, nitric oxide can combine with oxygen and water to produce nitrogen dioxide and nitrite, respectively, which interact with oxyhemoglobin to produce methemoglobin and nitrate. Thus, the end products of nitric oxide that enter the systemic circulation are predominantly methemoglobin and nitrate.

Metabolism – Methemoglobin disposition has been investigated as a function of time and nitric oxide exposure concentration in neonates with respiratory failure. The methemoglobin (MetHb) concentration-time profiles during the first 12 hours of exposure to 0, 5, 20, and 80 ppm of inhaled nitric oxide were studied. Methemoglobin concentrations increased during the first 8 hours of nitric oxide exposure. The mean methemoglobin level remained < 1% in the placebo group and in the 5 and 20 ppm nitric oxide groups, but reached ≈ 5% in the 80 ppm nitric oxide group. Methemoglobin levels > 7% were attained only in patients receiving 80 ppm, where they comprised 35% of the group. The average time to reach peak methemoglobin was 10 hours (median, 8 hours) in these 13 patients, but 1 patient did not exceed 7% until 40 hours.

Excretion – Nitrate has been identified as the predominant nitric oxide metabolite excreted in the urine, accounting for > 70% of the nitric oxide dose inhaled. Nitrate is cleared from the plasma by the kidney at rates approaching the glomerular filtration rate.

Contraindications

Treatment of neonates known to be dependent on right-to-left shunting of blood.

Warnings

➤*Abrupt withdrawal:* Abrupt discontinuation of nitric oxide may lead to worsening oxygenation and increasing PAP.

➤*Mutagenesis:* Nitric oxide has demonstrated genotoxicity in *Salmonella* (Ames Test), human lymphocytes, and after in vivo exposure in rats.

➤*Pregnancy: Category C.* It is not known whether nitric oxide can cause fetal harm when administered to a pregnant woman or can affect reproduction capacity. Nitric oxide is not intended for adults.

➤*Lactation:* Nitric oxide is not indicated for use in the adult population, including nursing mothers. It is not known whether nitric oxide is excreted in breast milk.

➤*Children:* Nitric oxide for inhalation has been studied in a neonatal population (up to 14 days of age). No information about its effectiveness in other age populations is available.

Precautions

➤*Lab test abnormalities:*

Methemoglobinemia – Methemoglobinemia increases with the dose of nitric oxide. In the clinical trials, maximum methemoglobin levels usually were reached ≈ 8 hours after initiation of inhalation, although methemoglobin levels have peaked as late as 40 hours following initiation of nitric oxide therapy. In 1 study, 13 of 37 (35%) of neonates treated with nitric oxide 80 ppm had methemoglobin levels exceeding 7%. Following discontinuation or reduction of nitric oxide the methemoglobin levels returned to baseline over a period of hours.

Elevated NO_2 levels – In 1 study, NO_2 levels were < 0.5 ppm when neonates were treated with placebo, 5 ppm, and 20 ppm nitric oxide over the first 48 hours. The 80 ppm group had a mean peak NO_2 level of 2.6 ppm.

Drug Interactions

A clinically significant interaction with other medications used in the treatment of hypoxic respiratory failure cannot be excluded based on the available data. In particular, although there are no data to evaluate the possibility, nitric oxide donor compounds, including sodium nitroprusside and nitroglycerin, may have an additive effect with nitric oxide on the risk of developing methemoglobinemia.

Adverse Reactions

From all controlled studies, ≥ 6 months of follow-up is available for 278 patients who received nitric oxide and 212 patients who received placebo. Among these patients, there was no evidence of an adverse effect of treatment or the need for rehospitalization, special medical services, pulmonary disease, or neurological sequelae.

NITRIC OXIDE

In 1 study, treatment groups were similar with respect to the incidence and severity of intracranial hemorrhage, Grade IV hemorrhage, periventricular leukomalacia, cerebral infarction, seizures requiring anticonvulsant therapy, pulmonary hemorrhage, or GI hemorrhage.

Nitric Oxide Adverse Events (> 5%)		
Adverse event	Inhaled NO (n = 97)	Placebo (n = 89)
Hypotension	13	10
Withdrawal symptoms	12	10
Atelectasis	9	9
Hematuria	8	6
Hyperglycemia	8	7
Sepsis	7	2
Infection	6	3

Nitric Oxide Adverse Events (> 5%)		
Adverse event	Inhaled NO (n = 97)	Placebo (n = 89)
Cellulitis	5	0
Stridor	5	3

Overdosage

►*Symptoms:* Overdosage with nitric oxide will be manifested by elevations in methemoglobin and NO_2. Elevated NO_2 may cause acute lung injury. Elevations in methemoglobinemia reduce the oxygen delivery capacity of the circulation.

►*Treatment:* In clinical studies, NO_2 levels > 3 ppm or methemoglobin levels > 7% were treated by reducing the dose of or discontinuing nitric oxide. Based upon the clinical situation, methemoglobinemia that does not resolve after reduction or discontinuation of therapy can be treated with IV vitamin C, IV methylene blue, or blood transfusion.

FLUTICASONE PROPIONATE/SALMETEROL

Rx	Advair Diskus (GlaxoSmithKline)	**Powder for inhalation:** 100 mcg fluticasone propionate, 50 mcg salmeterol[a]	Lactose. In 28 and 60 blisters in a disposable, purple-colored device.
		250 mcg fluticasone propionate, 50 mcg salmeterol[a]	Lactose. In 28 and 60 blisters in a disposable, purple-colored device.
		500 mcg fluticasone propionate, 50 mcg salmeterol[a]	Lactose. In 28 and 60 blisters in a disposable, purple-colored device.

[a] Supplied as 72.5 mcg salmeterol xinaforte, equivalent to 50 mcg base.

For complete prescribing information, please refer to the Corticosteroids and Sympathomimetics group monographs.

WARNING

Data from a large placebo-controlled US study that compared the safety of salmeterol or placebo added to usual asthma therapy showed a small but significant increase in asthma-related deaths in patients receiving salmeterol (13 deaths out of 13,174 patients treated for 28 weeks) vs those on placebo (4 of 13,179). Subgroup analyses suggest the risk may be greater in blacks compared with whites.

Indications

➤*Asthma, chronic:* For the long-term, twice-daily maintenance treatment of asthma in patients 4 years of age and older.

Not indicated for the relief of acute bronchospasm.

➤*Chronic obstructive pulmonary disease (COPD) associated with chronic bronchitis:* For the twice-daily maintenance treatment of airflow obstruction in patients with COPD associated with chronic bronchitis. Fluticasone propionate/salmeterol 250 mcg/50 mcg twice daily is the only approved dosage for the treatment of COPD associated with chronic bronchitis. Higher doses, including fluticasone propionate/salmeterol 500 mcg/50 mcg, are not recommended.

Administration and Dosage

➤*Approved by the FDA:* August 24, 2000.

Administer by the orally inhaled route only. The maximum recommended dose of fluticasone propionate/salmeterol is 500 mcg/50 mcg twice daily.

➤*Asthma, chronic:*

Adults and children 12 years of age and older – One inhalation twice daily (morning and evening, approximately 12 hours apart).

More frequent administration or a higher number of inhalations of the prescribed strength is not recommended because some patients are more likely to experience adverse effects with higher doses of salmeterol. The safety and efficacy of fluticasone propionate/salmeterol when administered in excess of recommended doses have not been established.

For all patients, titrate to the lowest effective strength after adequate asthma stability is achieved.

If symptoms arise in the period between doses, administer an inhaled, short-acting β_2-agonist for immediate relief.

Patients receiving fluticasone propionate/salmeterol twice daily should not use additional salmeterol or other inhaled, long-acting β_2-agonists (eg, formoterol) for prevention of exercise-induced bronchospasm or for any other reason.

Improvement in asthma control following inhaled administration of fluticasone propionate/salmeterol can occur within 30 minutes of beginning treatment, although maximum benefit may not be achieved for 1 week or longer after starting treatment. Individual patients will experience a variable time to onset and degree of symptom relief.

Replacing the current strength of fluticasone propionate/salmeterol with a higher strength may provide additional asthma control for patients who do not respond adequately to the starting dose after 2 weeks of therapy.

If a previously effective dosage regimen fails to provide adequate improvement in asthma control, reevaluate the therapeutic regimen and consider additional therapeutic options, such as replacing the current strength of fluticasone propionate/salmeterol with a higher strength, adding an additional inhaled corticosteroid, or initiating oral corticosteroids.

Advise patients to rinse mouth with water after inhalation without swallowing.

Patients not currently on an inhaled corticosteroid – A starting dose of fluticasone propionate/salmeterol 100 mcg/50 mcg twice daily is recommended for patients who are not currently on an inhaled corticosteroid and whose disease severity warrants treatment with 2 maintenance therapies, including patients on noncorticosteroid maintenance therapy.

Patients currently on an inhaled corticosteroid – The following table provides the recommended starting dose for patients currently on an inhaled corticosteroid.

Recommended Starting Doses of Fluticasone Propionate/Salmeterol for Arthritis Patients (Age ≥ 12) Taking Inhaled Corticosteroids		
Current daily dose of inhaled corticosteroid		Recommended strength and dosing schedule of fluticasone propionate/salmeterol
Beclomethasone dipropionate	≤ 420 mcg	100 mcg/50 mcg twice daily
	462 to 840 mcg	250 mcg/50 mcg twice daily
Budesonide	≤ 400 mcg	100 mcg/50 mcg twice daily
	800 to 1200 mcg	250 mcg/50 mcg twice daily
	1600 mcg[a]	500 mcg/50 mcg twice daily
Flunisolide	≤ 1000 mcg	100 mcg/50 mcg twice daily
	1250 to 2000 mcg	250 mcg/50 mcg twice daily
Fluticasone propionate inhalation aerosol	≤ 176 mcg	100 mcg/50 mcg twice daily
	440 mcg	250 mcg/50 mcg twice daily
	660 to 880 mcg[a]	500 mcg/50 mcg twice daily
Fluticasone propionate inhalation powder	≤ 200 mcg	100 mcg/50 mcg twice daily
	500 mcg	250 mcg/50 mcg twice daily
	1000 mcg[a]	500 mcg/50 mcg twice daily
Triamcinolone acetonide	≤ 1000 mcg	100 mcg/50 mcg twice daily
	1100 to 1600 mcg	250 mcg/50 mcg twice daily

[a] Do not use fluticasone propionate/salmeterol for transferring patients from systemic corticosteroid therapy.

Children 4 to 11 years of age – For patients 4 to 11 years of age who are symptomatic on an inhaled corticosteroid, the dosage is 1 inhalation of fluticasone propionate/salmeterol 100 mcg/50 mcg twice daily (morning and evening, approximately 12 hours apart).

➤*COPD associated with chronic bronchitis:* The dosage for adults is 1 inhalation (250 mcg/50 mcg) twice daily (morning and evening, approximately 12 hours apart).

Fluticasone propionate/salmeterol 250 mcg/50 mcg twice daily is the only approved dosage for the treatment of COPD associated with chronic bronchitis. Higher doses, including fluticasone propionate/salmeterol 500 mcg/50 mcg, are not recommended because no additional improvement in lung function was observed in clinical trials and higher doses of corticosteroids increase the risk of systemic effects. The benefit of treating patients with COPD associated with chronic bronchitis with fluticasone propionate/salmeterol 250 mcg/50 mcg for periods longer than 6 months has not been evaluated. Periodically reevaluate patients treated with fluticasone propionate/salmeterol 250 mcg/50 mcg for COPD associated with chronic bronchitis for periods longer than 6 months to assess the continuing benefits and potential risks of treatment.

If shortness of breath occurs in the period between doses, an inhaled, short-acting β_2-agonist should be taken for immediate relief.

Patients who are receiving fluticasone propionate/salmeterol twice daily should not use additional salmeterol or other inhaled, long-acting β_2-agonists (eg, formoterol) for the maintenance treatment of COPD or for any other reason.

➤*Storage/Stability:* Store at 20° to 25°C (68° to 77°F) in a dry place away from direct heat or sunlight. Keep out of the reach of children. The inhalation device is not reusable; therefore, discard 1 month after removal from the moisture-protective, foil overwrap pouch or after every blister has been used (when the dose indicator reads "0"), whichever comes first. Do not attempt to take the device apart.

Indications

➤*Oral:* For temporary relief of nasal congestion due to the common cold, hay fever or other upper respiratory allergies, and nasal congestion associated with sinusitis; to promote nasal or sinus drainage.

➤*Topical:* Symptomatic relief of nasal and nasopharyngeal mucosal congestion due to the common cold, sinusitis, hay fever or other upper respiratory allergies.

Administration and Dosage

Recommended Dosage Guidelines for Oral and Topical Nasal Decongestants (Dosage Maximum/24 h)[1]			
Drug and route	Adults ≥ 12 years of age	Children 6 to < 12 years of age	Children 2 to < 6 years of age
Ephedrine sulfate Topical Sprays	0.25%: 2 or 3 sprays in each nostril no more than q 4 h (6 doses/24 h)	0.25%: 1 or 2 sprays in each nostril no more than q 4 h (6 doses/24 h)	not recommended
Epinephrine HCl Topical	0.1%: Apply as drops or spray or with sterile swab as required	same as adults	not recommended
Naphazoline Topical Sprays	0.05%: 1 or 2 sprays in each nostril no more than q 6 h (4 doses/24 h)	not recommended	not recommended
Drops	0.05%: 1 or 2 drops in each nostril no more than q 6 h (4 doses/24 h)	not recommended	not recommended
Oxymetazoline HCl Topical Sprays	0.05%: 2 or 3 sprays in each nostril q 10 to 12 h (2 doses/24 h)	same as adults	not recommended
Phenylephrine HCl Oral	10-20 mg q 4 h (120 mg/24 h)	10 mg q 4 h (60 mg/24 h)	0.25% drops: 1 mL q 4 h (6 doses/24 h); (15 mg/24 h)
Topical Sprays	0.25%, 0.5%, 1%: 2 to 3 sprays in each nostril no more than q 4 h (6 doses/24 h)	0.25%: 2 to 3 sprays in each nostril no more than q 4 h (6 doses/24 h)	not recommended
Drops	0.25%, 0.5%, 1%: 2 to 3 drops in each nostril no more than q 4 h (6 doses/24 h)		0.125%: 2 to 3 drops in each nostril no more than q 4 h (6 doses/24 h)
Pseudoephedrine HCl Oral	60 mg q 4 to 6 h (240 mg/24 h)	30 mg q 4 to 6 h (120 mg/24 h)	15 mg q 4 to 6 h (60 mg/24 h)
Oral SR, CR	120 mg SR q 12 h or 240 mg CR q 24 h (240 mg/24 h)	not recommended	not recommended
Pseudoephedrine sulfate Oral ER	120 mg ER q 12 h (240 mg/24 h)	not recommended	not recommended
Tetrahydrozoline HCl Topical Sprays	0.1%: 3 to 4 sprays in each nostril prn, no more than q 3 h (8 doses/24 h)	same as adults	not recommended
Drops	0.1%: 2 to 4 drops in each nostril prn, no more than q 3 h (8 doses/24 h)	same as adults	0.05%: 2 to 3 drops in each nostril prn no more than q 3 h (8 doses/24 h)
Xylometazoline HCl Topical Sprays	0.1%: 1 to 3 sprays in each nostril q 8 to 10 h (3 doses/24 h)	0.05%: 1 spray in each nostril q 8 to 10 h (3 doses/24 h)	same dose for 2 to 12 years of age
Drops	0.1%: 2 to 3 drops in each nostril q 8 to 10 h (3 doses/24 h)	0.05%: 2 to 3 drops in each nostril q 8 to 10 h (3 doses/24 h)	same dose for 2 to 12 years of age

[1] Refer to manufacturer's directions. SR = sustained release; CR = controlled release; ER = extended release

Actions

➤*Pharmacology:* Drugs that cause vasoconstriction, such as decongestants, act on the adrenergic receptors in the nasal mucosa by affecting the blood vessels' sympathetic tone and provoking vasoconstriction. Available decongestants include noradrenaline releasers (eg, amphetamines, **pseudoephedrine**), alpha$_1$-adrenergic agonists (eg, **phenylephrine**), and alpha$_2$-adrenergic agonists (eg, **naphazoline**, **oxymetazoline**). Decongestants improve nasal ventilation by shrinking swollen nasal mucosa. Constriction in the mucous membranes results in their shrinkage; this promotes drainage, thus improving ventilation and the stuffy feeling.

Decongestants are sympathomimetic amines administered directly to swollen membranes (eg, via spray, drops) or systemically via the oral route. They are used in acute conditions such as hay fever, allergic rhinitis, vasomotor rhinitis, sinusitis, and the common cold to relieve membrane congestion.

Oral agents are not as effective as topical products, especially on an immediate basis, but generally have a longer duration of action, cause less local irritation, and are not associated with rebound congestion (rhinitis medicamentosa).

Contraindications

Monoamine oxidase inhibitor (MAOI) therapy; hypersensitivity.

➤*Oral:*

Sustained-release pseudoephedrine – Children < 12 years of age.

➤*Topical:*

Tetrahydrozoline – 0.1% solution in children < 6 years of age; 0.05% solution in infants < 2 years of age.

Systemic effects are less likely from topical use, but use caution in the conditions listed for oral agents. Adverse reactions are more likely with excessive use, in the elderly, and in children.

Warnings

➤*Special risk patients:* Administer with caution to patients with thyroid disease, diabetes, cardiovascular disease, coronary artery disease, hypertension, intraocular pressure, peripheral vascular disease, heart disease, or difficulty in urination due to enlargement of the prostate gland, unless directed by a physician. Rarely, some tablets may cause bowel obstruction or blockage, usually in people with severe narrowing of the bowel, esophagus, stomach, or intestine. If a patient has had obstruction or narrowing of the bowel, have him or her consult a physician before taking oral tablet products. Advise patients to contact their physician if they experience persistent abdominal pain or vomiting. As with any drug, if a patient is pregnant or nursing a baby, she should seek the advice of a health professional before using these products.

➤*Hypertension:* Hypertensive patients should use these products only with medical advice, as they may experience a change in blood pressure because of the added vasoconstriction. Studies suggest pseudoephedrine is the drug of choice. Sustained-action preparations may affect the cardiovascular system to a lesser degree.

➤*Excessive use:* Do not exceed recommended dosage. If nervousness, dizziness, or sleeplessness occur, discontinue use and have the patient consult a physician. Do not take topical products for > 3 days or oral products for > 7 days. If symptoms do not improve or are accompanied by a fever, the patient should consult a physician.

➤*Rebound congestion (rhinitis medicamentosa):* Following topical application, this may occur after the vasoconstriction subsides. Patients who increase the amount of drug and frequency of use may produce toxicity and perpetuate the rebound congestion.

Treatment – A simple but uncomfortable solution is to completely withdraw the topical medication. A more acceptable method is to gradually withdraw therapy by initially discontinuing the medication in one nostril, followed by total withdrawal. Substituting an oral decongestant for a topical one also may be useful.

➤*Elderly:* Patients ≥ 60 years of age are more likely to experience adverse reactions to sympathomimetics. Overdosage may cause hallucinations, convulsions, CNS depression, and death. Demonstrate safe use of a short-acting sympathomimetic before use of a sustained-action formulation in elderly patients.

➤*Pregnancy:* (*Category C* – **tetrahydrozoline**, **pseudoephedrine**, **phenylephrine**, **epinephrine**, **ephedrine**, **oxymetazoline**). It is not known whether these agents can cause fetal harm or affect reproduction capacity. Give only when clearly needed.

➤*Lactation:*

Oral preparations – Consult a physician before using.

Topical – It is not known if these agents are excreted in breast milk. Exercise caution when administering to a nursing woman.

➤*Children:* Use in children is product-specific. Refer to individual product listings.

Precautions

➤*Acute use:* Use topical decongestants only in acute states and not longer than 3 days. Use sparingly (especially the imidazolines) in all patients, particularly infants, children, and patients with cardiovascular disease.

➤*Stinging sensation:* Some individuals may experience a mild, transient stinging sensation after topical application.

➤*Sulfite sensitivity:* Some of the nasal decongestant products contain sulfites that may cause allergic-type reactions including anaphylactic symptoms and life-threatening or less severe asthmatic episodes in certain susceptible people. The overall prevalence of sulfite sensitivity in the general population is unknown but is probably low. Sulfite sensitivity is seen more frequently in asthmatic than in nonasthmatic people. Products containing sulfites are identified in the product listings.

Drug Interactions

Most interactions listed apply to sympathomimetics when used as vasopressors; however, consider the interaction when using the nasal decongestants.

Nasal Decongestant Drug Interactions			
Precipitant drug	Object drug*		Description
Beta blockers	Epinephrine	↑	An initial hypertensive episode followed by bradycardia may occur.
Furazolidone	Nasal decongestants	↑	The pressor sensitivity to mixed-acting agents (eg, ephedrine) may be increased. Direct-acting agents (eg, epinephrine) are not affected.
Guanethidine	Nasal decongestants		Guanethidine potentiates the effects of the direct-acting agents (eg, epinephrine) and inhibits the effects of the mixed-acting agents (eg, ephedrine). Guanethidine's hypotensive action also may be reversed.
	Direct	↑	
	Mixed	↓	
Nasal decongestants	Guanethidine	↓	
Methyldopa	Nasal decongestants	↑	Coadministration may result in an increased pressor response.
MAO inhibitors	Nasal decongestants	↑	Concurrent use of MAOIs and mixed-acting agents (eg, ephedrine) may result in severe headache, hypertension, and hyperpyrexia, possibly resulting in hypertensive crisis. Direct-acting agents (eg, epinephrine) interact minimally, if at all.
Rauwolfia alkaloids	Nasal decongestants		Reserpine potentiates the pressor response of direct-acting agents (eg, epinephrine), which may result in hypotension. The pressor response of mixed-acting agents (eg, ephedrine) is decreased.
	Direct	↑	
	Mixed	↓	
Tricyclic anti-depressants (TCAs)	Nasal decongestants		TCAs potentiate the pressor response of direct-acting agents (eg, epinephrine); dysrhythmias have occurred. The pressor response of mixed-acting agents (eg, ephedrine) is decreased.
	Direct	↑	
	Mixed	↓	
Urinary acidifiers	Nasal decongestants	↓	Acidification of the urine may increase the elimination of the nasal decongestant; therapeutic effects may be decreased. Conversely, urinary alkalinization may decrease the elimination of these agents, possibly increasing therapeutic or toxic effects.
Urinary alkalinizers		↑	

* ↑ = Object drug increased. ↓ = Object drug decreased.

Adverse Reactions

➤*Cardiovascular:* Arrhythmias; palpitations; tachycardia; transient hypertension; bradycardia.

➤*CNS:* Headache; lightheadedness; dizziness; drowsiness; tremor; insomnia; nervousness; restlessness; giddiness; psychological disturbances; prolonged psychosis (eg, paranoia, terror, delusions); weakness.

➤*GI:* Nausea; gastric irritation.

➤*Hypersensitivity:* Hypersensitivity reactions such as rash, urticaria, leukopenia, agranulocytosis, and thrombocytopenia may occur.

➤*Miscellaneous:* Orofacial dystonia; sweating; blepharospasm (eg, ocular irritation, tearing, photophobia); urinary retention may occur in patients with prostatic hypertrophy.

Topical use – Burning; stinging; sneezing; dryness; local irritation; rebound congestion.

Overdosage

➤*Symptoms:* Overdoses have caused hypertension, bradycardia, drowsiness, and rebound hypotension in adults; a shock-like syndrome with hypotension and bradycardia also may occur. In either case, the treatment of overdosage is usually that of watchful expectancy and general supportive measures. If possible, keep the patient warm and maintain fluid balance orally or parenterally, if necessary. Overdosage of **tetrahydrozoline** nasal solution may result in oversedation in young children.

➤*Treatment:* Treatment is supportive; in severe cases, IV phentolamine may be used. See General Management of Acute Overdosage.

Tetrahydrozoline – There is no known antidote. The use of stimulants is contraindicated. If respiratory rate drops to ≤ 10, administer oxygen and assist respiration. Monitor blood pressure to prevent hypotensive crisis.

Patient Information

Patients with hypertension, heart disease, or other cardiovascular diseases, thyroid disease, diabetes, or difficulty urinating due to an enlarged prostate should use these products only with medical advice.

➤*Topical:* Notify physician of insomnia, dizziness, weakness, tremor, or irregular heart beat.

Do not exceed recommended dosage and do not use longer than 3 days. If symptoms persist, contact the doctor. Frequent or prolonged use may cause nasal congestion to recur or worsen.

Stinging, burning, sneezing, increased nasal discharge, or drying of the nasal mucosa may occur.

Do not share container with other patients. Do not allow tip of container to touch the nasal passage. Discard after medication is no longer required.

Proper use – Spray – Keep head upright. Sniff hard for a few minutes after use.

Drops – Recline on a bed and hang your head over the edge; remain in this position for several minutes after using the drops, turning the head from side to side.

Inhalers – Warm in the hand before use. Wipe the inhaler after each use.

➤*Oral:* Do not exceed recommended dosage; higher doses may cause nervousness, dizziness, or sleeplessness.

If symptoms do not improve within 7 days or are accompanied by a high fever, consult physician before continuing use.

Arylalkylamines

PSEUDOEPHEDRINE SULFATE

otc	**Drixoral 12 Hour Non-Drowsy Formula** (Schering-Plough Healthcare)	**Tablets, extended-release:** 120 mg	Sugar, lactose, butylparabens. (DRIXORAL NDF). In 10s.

For complete prescribing information, refer to the Nasal Decongestants group monograph.

Indications

➤*Nasal congestion:* For temporary relief of nasal congestion due to the common cold, hay fever, or other upper respiratory allergies, and associated with sinusitis.

Administration and Dosage

➤*Adults and children (≥ 12 years of age):* 120 mg every 12 hours. Do not exceed 240 mg in 24 hours.

Do not crush or chew sustained release preparations.

PSEUDOEPHEDRINE HCl (d-Isoephedrine HCl)

otc	**Pseudoephedrine HCl** (Various, eg, Geneva, Roxane, Rugby)	**Tablets:** 30 mg	In 24s, 100s, 1000s, blister pack 100s.
otc	**Congestaid** (Zee Medical)		In 24s.
otc	**Genaphed** (Goldline)		In 24s.[1]
otc	**Medi-First Sinus Decongestant** (Textilease Medique[2])		In 100s and 250s.
otc	**Sudodrin** (Textilease Medique[2])		(FR4). In 250s, 250s, and 1000s.
otc	**Simply Stuffy** (McNeil Consumer)		In 24s.[1]
otc	**Sudafed Non-Drowsy, Maximum Strength** (Warner-Lambert Consumer)		(SU). In 24s, and 96s.[3]
otc	**Pseudoephedrine HCl** (Various, eg, Geneva, Roxane)	**Tablets:** 60 mg	In 100s, 1000s, and blister pack 100s.
otc	**Cenafed** (Century)		In 100s.

Arylalkylamines

PSEUDOEPHEDRINE HCl (d-Isoephedrine HCl)

otc	**Sudafed, Children's Non-Drowsy** (Warner-Lambert Consumer)	**Tablets, chewable:** 15 mg	Orange flavor. In 24s.[4]
otc	**Triaminic Allergy Congestion Softchews** (Novartis Consumer)		Orange flavor. In 18s.[5]
otc	**Sudafed Non-Drowsy 12 Hour Long-Acting** (Warner-Lambert Consumer)	**Tablets, extended-release:** 120 mg	Capsule shape. (SUDAFED 12 HOUR). In 10s.
otc	**Dimetapp, Maximum Strength 12-Hour Non-Drowsy Extentabs** (Whitehall-Robins)		Capsule shape. In 10s.
otc	**Efidac 24 Pseudoephedrine** (Hogil)	**Tablets, controlled-release:** 240 mg (immediate-release 60 mg, controlled-release 180 mg).	In 6s, 12s, and UD 1s.
otc	**Sudafed Non-Drowsy 24 Hour Long-Acting** (Warner-Lambert Consumer)		(SU-24). In 10s.
otc	**Sinustop** (Nature's Way)	**Capsules:** 60 mg	In 20s.[6]
otc	**Dimetapp, Maximum Strength, Non-Drowsy Liqui-Gels** (Whitehall-Robins)	**Capsules, softgel:** 30 mg	In 12s.[7]
otc	**Nasal Decongestant, Children's Non-Drowsy** (Various, eg, AmerisourceBergen[8])	**Liquid:** 15 mg/5 mL	In 118 mL.
otc	**Simply Stuffy** (McNeil-PPC)		Corn syrup, sucralose. Alcohol-free. Cherry berry flavor. In 120 mL.
otc	**Triaminic Allergy Congestion** (Novartis Consumer)		In 118 mL.[9]
otc sf	**Sudafed, Children's Non-Drowsy** (Warner-Lambert Consumer)		Alcohol free. Grape flavor. In 118 mL.[10]
otc	**Pseudoephedrine HCl** (Various, eg, Rugby)	**Liquid:** 30 mg/5 mL	In 120 and 473 mL.
otc	**Decofed Syrup** (Various)		In 118 and 473 mL.
otc	**Cenafed Syrup** (Century)		In 120 and 480 mL, and 3.8 L.[11]
otc	**Silfedrine, Children's** (Silarx)		In 118 and 237 mL.[12]
otc	**Nasal Decongestant Oral** (Various, eg, ProMetic)	**Drops:** 7.5 mg/0.8 mL	In 15 and 30 mL w/dropper.
otc	**Dimetapp Decongestant Pediatric** (Whitehall-Robins)		In 15 mL.[13]
otc	**Kid Kare** (Rugby)		Alcohol free. Cherry flavor. In 30 mL w/dropper.[14]
otc	**PediaCare Decongestant, Infants'** (Pharmacia Consumer)		Alcohol free. Fruit flavor. In 15 mL w/dropper.[15]

[1] With lactose.
[2] Textilease Medique Products, 900 Lively Blvd., Wood Dale, IL 60191; (630) 694-4100.
[3] With lactose, sucrose.
[4] With aspartame, mannitol, 0.78 mg phenylalanine.
[5] With aspartame, mannitol, sorbitol, sucrose, 17.5 mg phenylalanine.
[6] With echinacea purpura, ginger, goldenseal root.
[7] With mannitol, sorbitol.
[8] AmerisourceBergen, 1300 Morris Dr., Chesterbrook, PA 19087; (888)276-6034.

[9] With EDTA, sucrose, sorbitol.
[10] With EDTA, saccharin, sorbitol.
[11] With methylparaben.
[12] With methylparaben, saccharin, sucrose.
[13] With corn syrup, menthol, sorbitol, sucrose.
[14] With sorbitol, sugar.
[15] With sorbitol, sucrose.

For complete prescribing information, refer to the Nasal Decongestants group monograph.

Indications

▶*Nasal congestion:* Temporary relieves nasal congestion due to the common cold, hay fever, or other upper respiratory allergies, and nasal congestion associated with sinusitis; reduces swelling of nasal passages; relieves sinus pressure; promotes nasal or sinus drainage; restores freer breathing through the nose.

Administration and Dosage

▶*Adults (≥ 12 years of age):* 60 mg every 4 to 6 hours (120 mg sustained-release every 12 hours, 240 mg controlled-release every 24 hours). Do not exceed 240 mg in 24 hours.

▶*Children (6 to 12 years of age):* 30 mg every 4 to 6 hours. Do not exceed 120 mg in 24 hours.

Children (2 to 5 years of age) – 15 mg every 4 to 6 hours. Do not exceed 60 mg in 24 hours.

Children (< 2 years of age) – Consult a physician.

PHENYLEPHRINE HCl

Rx	**AH-chew D** (WE Pharm)	**Tablets, chewable:** 10 mg	(WE 07). Scored. Bubble gum flavor. In 100s.
otc	**Little Noses Gentle Formula, Infants & Children** (Vetco[1])	**Solution:** 0.125%	**Drops:** Alcohol free. In 15 mL w/dropper.[2]
otc	**Afrin Children's Pump Mist** (Schering-Plough Healthcare)	**Solution:** 0.25%	**Spray:** In 15 mL.[2]
otc	**Little Colds For Infants and Children** (Vetco[1])		**Oral drops:** Alcohol free. Grape flavor. In 30 mL w/dropper.[3]
otc	**Neo-Synephrine 4-Hour Mild Formula** (Bayer Corp.)		**Spray:** In 15 mL.[4]
otc	**Rhinall** (Scherer)		**Spray:** In 40 mL.[5]
			Drops: In 30 mL.[5]
otc	**Neo-Synephrine 4-Hour Regular Strength** (Bayer Corp.)	**Solution:** 0.5%	**Drops:** In 15 mL.[4]
			Spray: In 15 mL.[4]
otc	**Vicks Sinex Ultra Fine Mist** (Procter & Gamble)		**Spray:** In 14.7 mL.[6]
otc	**Phenylephrine HCl** (Various, eg, Rugby)	**Solution:** 1%	In 480 mL.
otc	**4-Way Fast Acting** (Bristol-Myers)		**Spray:** In 30 mL.[7]
otc	**Neo-Synephrine 4-Hour Extra Strength** (Bayer Corp.)		**Drops:** In 15 mL.[4]
			Spray: In 15 mL.[4]

[1] Vetco, 105 Baylis Road, Melville, NY 11747; (631)755-1155.
[2] With EDTA, benzalkonium chloride.
[3] With sorbitol, sucralose.
[4] With benzalkonium chloride, thimerosal.

[5] With chlorobutanol, sodium bisulfite, benzalkonium chloride.
[6] With benzalkonium chloride, camphor, EDTA, eucalyptol, menthol, tyloxapol.
[7] With benzalkonium chloride, boric acid, sodium borate.

For complete prescribing information, refer to the Nasal Decongestants group monograph.

Arylalkylamines

PHENYLEPHRINE HCl

Indications

➤*Nasal congestion:* For prompt, temporary relief of nasal congestion due to the common cold, sinusitis, hay fever, or other upper respiratory allergies, or associated with sinusitus.

Administration and Dosage

➤*Adults (≥ 12 years of age):* 2 to 3 sprays or drops in each nostril. Repeat every 3 to 4 hours (0.25% and 0.5%). The 1% solution should be repeated no more often than every 4 hours. Do not give to children < 12 years of age unless directed by a physician.

Orally – 1 or 2 tablets every 4 hours.

➤*Children (6 to < 12 years of age):*
0.25% – 2 to 3 sprays or drops in each nostril not more often than every 4 hours.

Orally – 1 tablet every 4 hours.

➤*Children (2 to < 6 years of age):*
0.25% oral drops – 1 dropperful (1 mL) by mouth every 4 hours not to exceed 6 doses in a 24-hour period.

0.125% – 2 or 3 drops into each nostril not more often than every 4 hours.

➤*Children (< 2 years of age):* Consult a physician.

EPINEPHRINE HCl

| *Rx* | **Adrenalin Chloride** (Monarch) | **Solution:** 1 mg/mL | In 30 mL.[1] |

[1] With chlorobutanol, sodium bisulfite.

For complete prescribing information, refer to the Nasal Decongestants group monograph.

Indications

Used to treat mucosal congestion of hay fever, rhinitis, and acute sinusitis.

Administration and Dosage

➤*Adults and children (≥ 6 years of age):* Apply locally as drops or spray, or with a sterile swab, as required.

EPHEDRINE SULFATE

| *otc* | **Pretz-D** (Parnell) | **Solution:** 0.25% | **Spray:** In 50 mL.[1] |

[1] With yerba santa.

For complete prescribing information, refer to the Nasal Decongestants group monograph.

Indications

For temporary relief of nasal congestion due to a cold, hay fever (allergic rhinitis), or associated with sinusitis. Reduces swelling of nasal passages and shrinks swollen membranes. Promotes nasal or sinus drainage, temporarily relieves sinus congestion and pressure.

Administration and Dosage

➤*Adults and children (≥ 12 years of age):* 2 or 3 sprays in each nostril no more than every 4 hours.

➤*Children (6 to 11 years of age):* 1 or 2 sprays in each nostril with adult supervision not more than every 4 hours.

Imidazolines

NAPHAZOLINE HCl

| *otc* | **Privine** (Heritage) | **Solution:** 0.05% | **Drops:** In 25 mL w/dropper.[1] |
| | | | **Spray:** In 20 mL.[1] |

[1] With benzalkonium chloride, EDTA.

For complete prescribing information, refer to the Nasal Decongestants group monograph.

Indications

➤*Nasal congestion:* For the temporary relief of nasal congestion due to the common cold, hay fever, or other upper respiratory allergies, or associated with sinusitis.

Administration and Dosage

➤*Adults and children (≥ 12 years of age):* 1 or 2 drops or sprays in each nostril no more than every 6 hours. Do not use in children < 12 years of age unless directed by physician.

Imidazolines

OXYMETAZOLINE HCl

		Solution: 0.05%	
otc	**Oxymetazoline HCl** (Various, eg, Alpharma, Clay Park, Thames)		**Spray:** In 15 and 30 mL.
otc	**12 Hour Nasal** (Various, eg, URL)		**Spray:** In 15 mL.
otc	**Twice-A-Day 12-Hour Nasal** (Major)		**Spray:** In 15 and 30 mL.[1]
otc	**Neo-Synephrine 12-Hour Extra Moisturizing** (Bayer Corp.)		**Spray:** In 15 mL.[2]
otc	**Neo-Synephrine 12-Hour** (Bayer Corp.)		**Spray:** In 15 mL.[2]
otc	**Duration** (Schering-Plough Healthcare)		**Spray:** In 30 mL.[3]
otc	**Afrin 12-Hour Original Pump Mist** (Schering-Plough Healthcare)		**Spray:** In 15 mL.[3]
otc	**Afrin 12-Hour Original** (Schering-Plough Healthcare)		**Spray:** In 15 mL. [3]
otc	**Afrin Severe Congestion with Menthol** (Schering-Plough Healthcare)		**Spray:** In 15 mL.[4]
otc	**Afrin Sinus with Vapornase** (Schering-Plough Healthcare)		**Spray:** In 15 mL. [4]
otc	**Afrin No-Drip 12-Hour** (Schering-Plough Healthcare)		**Spray:** In 15 mL.[5]
otc	**Afrin No-Drip 12-Hour Extra Moisturizing** (Schering-Plough Healthcare)		**Spray:** In 15 mL.[6]
otc	**Afrin No-Drip 12-Hour Severe Congestion with Menthol** (Schering-Plough Healthcare)		**Spray:** In 15 mL.[7]
otc	**Afrin No-Drip Sinus with Vapornase** (Schering-Plough Healthcare)		**Spray:** In 15 mL.[7]
otc	**Dristan 12-Hr Nasal** (Whitehall-Robins)		**Spray:** In 15 mL.[8]
otc	**Duramist Plus 12-Hr Decongestant** (Pfeiffer)		**Spray:** In 15 mL.[9]
otc	**Genasal** (Goldline)		**Spray:** In 15 and 30 mL.[10]
otc	**Nasal Decongestant, Maximum Strength** (Taro)		**Spray:** In 15 and 30 mL.
otc	**Nasal Relief** (Rugby)		**Spray:** In 15 mL.[11]
otc	**Nōstrilla 12-Hour** (Heritage)		**Spray:** In 15 mL metered pump spray.[12]
otc	**Vicks Sinex 12-Hour Long-Acting** (Procter & Gamble)		**Spray:** In 15 mL.[13]
otc	**Vicks Sinex 12-Hour Ultra Fine Mist for Sinus Relief** (Procter & Gamble)		**Spray:** In 15 mL.[14]

[1] With EDTA, benzalkonium chloride, benzyl alcohol.
[2] With benzalkonium chloride, phenylmercuric acetate, glycine, sorbitol, sodium chloride.
[3] With benzalkonium chloride, EDTA.
[4] With benzalkonium chloride, benzyl alcohol, camphor, EDTA, eucalyptol, menthol.
[5] With carboxymethylcellulose sodium, microcrystalline cellulose, benzalkonium chloride, benzyl alcohol, EDTA.
[6] With carboxymethylcellulose sodium, microcrystalline cellulose, benzalkonium chloride, benzyl alcohol, EDTA, glycerin.
[7] With carboxymethylcellulose sodium, microcrystalline cellulose, benzalkonium chloride, benzyl alcohol, camphor, EDTA, eucalyptol, menthol.

[8] With benzalkonium chloride, hydroxypropylmethylcellulose, thimerosal, sodium chloride.
[9] With benzalkonium chloride, EDTA, sodium chloride.
[10] With benzalkonium chloride, phenylmercuric acetate, sorbitol.
[11] With EDTA, phenylmercuric acetate, sodium chloride.
[12] With benzalkonium chloride, glycine, sorbitol.
[13] With benzalkonium chloride, camphor, chlorhexidine gluconate, EDTA, eucalyptol, menthol, sodium chloride, tyloxapol.
[14] With aromatic vapors (camphor, eucalyptus, menthol), tyloxapol, EDTA, benzalkonium chloride, sodium chloride.

For complete prescribing information, refer to the Nasal Decongestants group monograph.

Indications

►*Nasal congestion:* For the temporary relief of nasal congestion due to a cold, hay fever, or other upper respiratory allergies, or associated with sinusitis. Reduces swelling of nasal passages; shrinks swollen membranes. Temporarily restores freer breathing through the nose; temporarily relieves sinus congestion and pressure.

Administration and Dosage

►*Adults and children (≥ 6 years):* 2 or 3 sprays of 0.05% solution in each nostril twice daily, morning and evening, or every 10 to 12 hours. Do not exceed 2 doses in any 24-hour period.

TETRAHYDROZOLINE HCl

Rx	**Tyzine Pediatric** (Kenwood)	**Solution:** 0.05%	**Drops:** In 15 mL with dropper.[1]
Rx	**Tyzine** (Kenwood)	**Solution:** 0.1%	**Drops:** In 30 mL with dropper.[1]
			Spray: In 15 mL.[1]

[1] With benzalkonium chloride, EDTA.

For complete prescribing information, refer to the Nasal Decongestants group monograph.

Indications

►*Nasal decongestion:* For decongestion of nasal and nasopharyngeal mucosa.

Administration and Dosage

►*Adults and children (≥ 6 years of age):* 2 to 4 drops of 0.1% solution instilled in each nostril as needed, or 3 to 4 sprays in each nostril as needed, no more than every 3 hours.

►*Children (2 to 6 years of age):* 2 to 3 drops of 0.05% solution in each nostril as needed no more than every 3 hours.

Imidazolines

XYLOMETAZOLINE HCl

otc	**Otrivin Pediatric Nasal** (Novartis Consumer)	**Solution:** 0.05%	**Drops:** In 25 mL dropper bottle.[1]
otc	**Natru-Vent** (Boehringer Ingelheim Consumer Health)		**Spray:** Preservative free. In metered-dose pump spray bottles (100 sprays).[2]
otc	**Otrivin** (Novartis Consumer)	**Solution:** 0.1%	**Drops:** In 25 mL dropper bottle.[3]
			Spray: In 20 mL.[3]
otc	**Natru-Vent** (Boehringer Ingelheim Consumer Health)		**Spray:** Preservative free. In two 10 mL bottles.[2]

[1] With benzalkonium chloride, EDTA.
[2] With sorbitol.

[3] With benzalkonium chloride, sodium chloride, EDTA.

For complete prescribing information, refer to the Nasal Decongestants group monograph.

Indications

➤*Spray / Drops:* For the temporary relief of nasal congestion due to the common cold, hay fever, or other respiratory allergies.

➤*Pediatric drops:* For temporary relief of nasal and sinus congestion and pressure due to a cold.

Administration and Dosage

➤*Adults (≥ 12 years of age):* 2 to 3 drops or 1 to 3 sprays (0.1%) in each nostril every 8 to 10 hours. Do not give 0.1% solution to children < 12 years of age.

➤*Children (2 to 12 years of age):* 2 to 3 drops or 1 spray (0.05%) in each nostril every 8 to 10 hours. Do not exceed 3 doses in any 24-hour period.

NASAL DECONGESTANT COMBINATIONS

otc	**Dristan Fast Acting Formula** (Whitehall-Robins)	**Solution:** 0.5% phenylephrine HCl and 0.2% pheniramine maleate	**Spray:** In 15 mL.[1]

[1] With mannitol, sorbitol, benzalkonium chloride, benzyl alcohol.

For complete prescribing information, refer to the Nasal Decongestants group monograph.

In this combination: **PHENYLEPHRINE HCl** is a decongestant. **PHENIRAMINE MALEATE** is an antihistamine.

Indications

➤*Nasal congestion:* Relieves nasal congestion due to colds and sinusitis.

NASAL DECONGESTANT INHALERS

otc	**Benzedrex** (B.F. Ascher)	**Inhaler:** 250 mg propylhexedrine	In single plastic inhalers.[1]
otc	**Vicks Vapor Inhaler** (Procter & Gamble Consumer)	**Inhaler:** 50 mg levmetamfetamine	In single plastic inhalers.[2]

[1] With menthol, lavender oil.

[2] With camphor, lavender oil, menthol.

For complete prescribing information, refer to the Nasal Decongestants group monograph.

Indications

➤*Nasal congestion:* For the temporary relief of nasal congestion due to the common cold, hay fever, upper respiratory allergies, or sinusitis.

Administration and Dosage

➤*Adults and children (≥ 6 years of age):* 1 to 2 inhalations in each nostril (while blocking the other nostril) not more than every 2 hours. Do not exceed recommended dosage. Do not use these products for > 3 days. If symptoms persist beyond this time, consult physician.

NASAL PRODUCTS

otc	**Nasal Spray** (Various, eg, Ivax)	**Solution:** Sodium chloride	**Spray:** In 45 mL.
otc	**Pretz Moisturizing** (Parnell)		**Spray:** In 50 mL.[1]
otc	**Afrin Saline, Extra Moisturizing** (Schering-Plough HealthCare)		**Spray:** In 45 mL.[2]
otc	**Simply Saline** (Blairex)		**Spray:** In 44 mL.
otc	**Pretz Irrigation** (Parnell)		**Spray:** In 237 mL.[3]
otc	**SalineX** (Muro)	**Solution:** 0.4% sodium chloride	**Drops:** In 15 mL.[4]
			Mist: In 50 mL.[4]
otc	**Ayr Saline** (B.F. Ascher)	**Solution:** 0.65% sodium chloride	**Drops:** In 50 mL.[2]
			Mist: In 50 mL.[2]
			Gel: In 14 g.[5]
otc	**Breathe Free** (Thompson Medical)		**Spray:** In 45 mL.[6]
otc	**HuMist Moisturizing Mist** (Scherer)		**Spray:** In 45 mL.[7]
otc	**NaSal** (Bayer Corp.)		**Drops:** Alcohol free. In 15 mL.[8]
			Spray: Alcohol free. In 30 mL.[8]
otc	**Nasal Moist** (Blairex)		**Spray:** Alcohol free, dye free. In 45 mL.
			Mist pump: Alcohol free, dye free. In 15 mL.
			Gel: Alcohol free, dye free. In 28.5 g and unit-of-use 2 mL.[9]
otc	**Ocean** (Fleming and Co.)		**Spray:** In 45 and 473 mL.[6]
otc	**Mycinaire Saline Mist** (Pfieffer)		**Spray:** In 45 mL.[6]

NASAL PRODUCTS

otc	**Rhinaris Lubricating Mist** (Pharmascience)	**Solution:** 15% polyethylene glycol, 5% propylene glycol	**Spray:** In 30 mL.[10]
		Solution: 15% polyethylene glycol, 20% propylene glycol	**Gel:** In 28.35 g.[10]
otc	**Nasal·Ease with Zinc** (Health Care Products)	**Solution:** Zinc acetate	**Gel:** In 14.1 g.[11]
otc	**Nasal·Ease with Zinc Gluconate** (Health Care Products)	**Solution:** Zinc gluconate	**Spray:** In 30 mL.[12]

[1] With glycerin, yerba santa.
[2] With benzalkonium chloride, EDTA.
[3] With yerba santa.
[4] With benzalkonium chloride, propylene glycol, polyethylene glycol, EDTA.
[5] With aloe vera gel, glycerin, parabens.
[6] With benzalkonium chloride.

[7] With chlorobutanol.
[8] With benzalkonium chloride, thimerosal.
[9] With aloe vera.
[10] With benzalkonium chloride, sodium chloride.
[11] With aloe vera, calendula extract, parabens, glycerin, tocopherol acetate, EDTA.
[12] With sodium chloride, benzalkonium chloride, glycerin.

For complete prescribing information, refer to the Nasal Decongestants group monograph.

Indications

Can be used as a nasal wash for sinuses and to restore moisture, thin nasal secretions, and relieve dry, crusted, and inflamed nasal membranes due to colds, low humidity, nasal decongestant overuse, allergies, minor nose bleeds, winter dryness, air travel, pregnancy, oxygen therapy, chronic sinusitis, asthma, intranasal and endoscopic sinus surgery, and other irritations.

Administration and Dosage

➤*Spray / Drops:* 2 to 6 sprays/drops in each nostril every 2 hours, as often as needed, or as directed by a doctor. To spray, hold head in upright position and give short, firm squeezes in each nostril. For drops, tilt head back and hold bottle upside down.

➤*HuMist:* Use is suggested for adults ≥ 12 years of age.

➤*Rhinaris:*
Adults and children (> 2 years of age) – 1 or 2 sprays into each nostril every 4 hours as needed.

Nasal•Ease with Zinc Gluconate –
   Adults and children (≥ 4 years of age): 1 to 2 sprays/drops in each nostril 2 to 4 times/day. Discontinue use after 5 days.

➤*Gel:* Apply around nostrils, under nose, or in nostrils as needed to help relieve discomfort. Use at bedtime to prevent drying and crusting.

Rhinaris – Apply a small amount of gel into each nostril every 4 hours as needed.

ALPHA₁-PROTEINASE INHIBITOR (HUMAN)

Rx	**Aralast** (Baxter)	**Powder for injection, lyophilized:** 400 mg (≥ 16 mg alpha₁-PI/mL when reconstituted)	Preservative free. In single-dose vial[1] with 25 mL diluent.
		Powder for injection, lyophilized: 800 mg (≥ 16 mg alpha₁-PI/mL when reconstituted)	Preservative free. In single-dose vial[1] with 50 mL diluent.
Rx	**Prolastin** (Bayer)	**Powder for injection, lyophilized:** 500 mg (≥ 20 mg alpha₁-PI/mL when reconstituted)	Preservative free. In single-dose vial[2] with 20 mL diluent.
		Powder for injection, lyophilized: 1000 mg (≥ 20 mg alpha₁-PI/mL when reconstituted)	Preservative free. In single-dose vial[2] with 40 mL diluent.
Rx	**Zemaira** (Aventis)	**Powder for injection, lyophilized:** 1000 mg	Preservative free. In single-dose vial[3] with 20 mL diluent.

[1] With polyethylene glycol, sodium, and albumin. With total alpha₁-PI functional activity in mg stated on the label of each vial.

[2] With polyethylene glycol, sucrose, sodium, and small amounts of other plasma proteins. With total alpha₁-PI functional activity in mg as stated on the label of each vial.

[3] With sodium and mannitol. The specific activity is ≥ 0.7 mg of functional alpha₁-PI/mg of total protein. The total alpha₁-PI functional activity in mg is stated on the label of each vial.

Indications

➤*Congenital alpha₁-proteinase inhibitor (alpha₁-PI; alpha₁-antitrypsin) deficiency:* For chronic augmentation therapy in patients having congenital deficiency of alpha₁-PI with clinically evident emphysema.

Clinical data demonstrating the long-term effects of chronic augmentation or replacement therapy of individuals with alpha₁-PI are not available.

Aralast and *Zemaira* are not indicated as therapy for lung disease patients in whom congenital alpha₁-PI deficiency has not been established.

Prolastin is not indicated for use in patients other than those with PiZZ, PiZ(null), or Pi(null)(null) phenotypes.

Administration and Dosage

➤*Approved by the FDA:* December 2, 1987.

➤*Dosage:* The recommended dosage is 60 mg/kg/body weight administered once weekly by IV infusion.

➤*Administration:* For IV use only. Give at a rate of approximately 0.08 mL/kg/min as determined by the response and comfort of the patient. Administer *Zemaira* reconstituted solution through a filter. The infusion should take approximately 15 to 30 minutes to complete. If adverse events occur, reduce the rate or interrupt the infusion until the symptoms subside. The infusion may then be resumed at a rate tolerated by the subject.

➤*Functional activity:* Each vial of *Aralast* and *Prolastin* has the functional activity, as determined by inhibition of porcine pancreatic elastase, stated on the label of the bottle. *Zemaira*'s functional activity is determined by the capacity to neutralize human neutrophil elastase.

➤*Storage/Stability:* Give within 3 hours after reconstitution. Do not refrigerate after reconstitution. Give alone without mixing other agents or diluting solutions. Refrigerate at 2° to 8°C (35° to 46°F) or at temperatures not to exceed 25°C (77°F). Avoid freezing. Do not use after expiration date printed on the label. *Aralast* must be used within 1 month once removed from refrigeration. Discard partially used vials; do not save for future use.

Actions

➤*Pharmacology:* Alpha₁-PI functions in the lungs to inhibit serine proteases such as neutrophil elastase (NE), which is capable of degrading protein components of the alveolar walls and is chronically present in the lung. In the healthy lung, alpha₁-PI is thought to provide more than 90% of the anti-NE protection in the lower respiratory tract.

Alpha₁-PI deficiency is an autosomal, codominant, hereditary disorder characterized by low serum and lung levels of alpha₁-PI. Severe forms of the deficiency are frequently associated with slowly progressive, moderate to severe panacinar emphysema that most often manifests in the third to fourth decades of life, resulting in a significantly lower life expectancy. Individuals with alpha₁-PI deficiency have little protection against NE released by a chronic, low-level of neutrophils in their lower respiratory tract, resulting in a protease:protease inhibitor imbalance in the lung. The emphysema associated with alpha₁-PI deficiency is typically worse in the lower lung zones. It is believed to develop because there are insufficient amounts of alpha₁-PI in the lower respiratory tract to inhibit NE. This imbalance allows unopposed destruction of the connective tissue framework of the lung parenchyma.

➤*Pharmacokinetics:* In clinical studies of alpha₁-PI in 23 subjects with the PiZZ variant of congenital deficiency of alpha₁-antitrypsin deficiency and documented destructive lung disease, the mean in vivo recovery of alpha₁-PI was 4.2 mg (immunologic)/dL/mg (functional)/kg administered. Half-life of alpha₁-PI in vivo was approximately 4.5 days. Nineteen of the subjects received alpha₁-PI replacement therapy, 60 mg/kg/week for up to 26 weeks (average, 24 weeks). Blood levels of alpha₁-PI were maintained above 80 mg/dL. Within a few weeks, bronchoalveolar lavage studies demonstrated significantly increased levels of alpha₁-PI and functional antineutrophil elastase capacity in the epithelial lining fluid of the lower respiratory tract of the lungs.

In 18 subjects treated with a single dose (60 mg/kg) of *Zemaira*, the AUC and standard deviation (SD) were 144 mcM × day (SD 27), maximum serum concentration was 44.1 mcM (SD 10.8), clearance was 603 mL/day (SD 129), and terminal half-life was 5.1 days (SD 2.4).

➤*Clinical trials:* A clinical study was conducted to compare *Aralast* (test drug) with a commercially available preparation of alpha₁-PI (*Prolastin*). All subjects were to have been diagnosed as having congenital alpha₁-PI deficiency and emphysema but no alpha₁-PI augmentation therapy within the preceding 6 months. Twenty-eight subjects were randomized to receive *Aralast* or *Prolastin*, 60 mg/kg/week IV, for 10 consecutive weeks.

It was concluded that at a dose of 60 mg/kg/week administered IV, *Aralast* and *Prolastin* had similar effects in maintaining target serum alpha₁-PI trough levels and increasing antigenic levels of alpha₁-PI in epithelial lining fluid (ELF) with maintenance augmentation therapy.

In a double-blind, controlled clinical study to evaluate the safety and efficacy of *Zemaira*, 44 subjects were randomized to receive 60 mg/kg/week of either *Zemaira* or *Prolastin* for 10 weeks. After 10 weeks, all subjects received *Zemaira* for an additional 14 weeks. All subjects were followed for a total of 24 weeks to complete the safety evaluation. The mean trough serum alpha₁-PI levels at steady state (weeks 7 to 11) in the *Zemaira*-treated subjects were statistically equivalent to those in the *Prolastin*-treated subjects. Both groups were maintained above 11 mcM (80 mg/dL). The mean of the steady state trough serum antigenic alpha₁-PI level for *Zemaira*-treated subjects was 17.7 mcM and for *Prolastin*-treated subjects it was 19.1 mcM. The difference between the *Zemaira* and the *Prolastin* groups was not considered clinically significant and may be related to the higher specific activity of *Zemaira*.

Contraindications

In individuals with selective IgA deficiencies (IgA level less than 15 mg/dL) who have known antibody against IgA, because they may experience severe reactions, including anaphylaxis, to IgA that may be present.

➤*Zemaira:* Hypersensitivity to any of its components or a history of anaphylaxis or severe systemic response to alpha₁-PI products

Warnings

➤*Infectious transmission:* Because alpha₁-PI is derived from pooled human plasma, it may carry a risk of transmitting infectious agents (eg, viruses and, theoretically, the Creutzfeldt-Jakob disease [CJD] agent).

There is also the possibility that unknown infectious agents may be present in such products. Individuals who receive infusions of blood or plasma products may develop signs and/or symptoms of some viral infections, particularly hepatitis C. All infections thought by a physician possibly to have been transmitted by these products should be reported by the physician or other health care provider to Bayer Corporation for *Prolastin* (1-800-228-8371), to Baxter Healthcare Corporation for *Aralast* (1-888-675-2762 [US] or 1-323-225-9735 [international]), or to Aventis Behring for *Zemaira* (1-800-504-5434). Weigh the risks and benefits of the use of this product and discuss with the patient.

Prolastin has been heat-treated in solution at 60°C for 10 hours in order to reduce the potential for transmission of infectious disease. No cases of hepatitis B or hepatitis C have been recorded in individuals receiving *Prolastin*. However, as all individuals receive prophylaxis against hepatitis B, no conclusion can be drawn at this time regarding potential transmission of hepatitis B virus.

During clinical studies, no cases of hepatitis A, B, C, or HIV viral infections were reported with the use of *Zemaira*.

➤*Hypersensitivity reactions:* If anaphylactic or severe anaphylactoid reactions occur, discontinue infusion immediately. Epinephrine and other appropriate supportive therapy should be available for the treatment of any acute anaphylactic or anaphylactoid reaction.

ALPHA₁-PROTEINASE INHIBITOR (HUMAN)

➤*Pregnancy: Category C*. It is not known whether this drug can cause fetal harm when administered to a pregnant woman or can affect reproduction capacity. Use only when clearly needed and when the potential benefits outweigh the potential hazards to the fetus.

➤*Lactation:* It is not known whether alpha₁-PI is excreted in human milk. Because many drugs are excreted in human milk, exercise caution when administering alpha₁-PI to a nursing woman.

➤*Children:* Safety and efficacy in children have not been established.

Precautions

➤*Monitoring:* The "threshold" level of *Prolastin* in the serum believed to provide adequate antielastase activity in the lung of individuals with alpha₁-antitrypsin deficiency is 80 mg/mL (based on commercial standards for alpha₁-PI immunologic assay). However, assays of alpha₁-PI based on commercial standards measure antigenic activity of alpha₁-PI is expressed as actual functional activity (ie, actual capacity to neutralize porcine pancreatic elastase). As functional activity may be less than antigenic activity, serum levels of alpha₁-PI determined using commercial immunologic assays may not accurately reflect actual functional alpha₁-PI levels. Therefore, although it may be helpful to monitor serum levels of alpha₁-PI in individuals receiving *Prolastin* using currently available commercial assays of antigenic activity, do not use results of these assays to determine the required therapeutic dosage.

➤*Circulatory overload:* There will be an increase in plasma volume following IV administration of *Prolastin* and *Zemaira*. Use caution in patients at risk for circulatory overload.

➤*Hepatitis B immunization:* It is recommended that in preparation for receiving *Prolastin*, recipients be immunized against hepatitis B using a licensed hepatitis B vaccine. If it becomes necessary to treat an individual with *Prolastin*, and time is insufficient for adequate antibody response to vaccination, administer a single dose of hepatitis B immune globulin (human), 0.06 mL/kg/body weight, IM, at the time of administration of the initial dose of hepatitis B vaccine.

Adverse Reactions

➤*Prolastin:* Delayed fever (maximum temperature rise was 38.9°C, resolving spontaneously over 24 hours) occurring up to 12 hours following treatment (0.77%); light-headedness, dizziness (0.19%). Mild transient leukocytosis and dilutional anemia several hours after infusion have also been noted.

Postmarketing – Occasional reports of other flu-like symptoms, allergic-like reactions, chills, dyspnea, rash, tachycardia, and rarely, hypotension.

➤*Aralast:* Upper and lower respiratory tract infections (96.3%); COPD exacerbations, headache, somnolence (0.3%); chills, fever, vasodilation, dizziness, pruritus, rash, abnormal vision, chest pain, increased cough, dyspnea (0.1%).

ALT or AST elevations of at least 2 times the upper limit of normal (up to 3.7 times) were noted in 11.1% of subjects. Elevations were transient lasting 3 months or less.

➤*Zemaira:* Asthenia, injection site pain, dizziness, headache, paresthesia, pruritus (1%).

Summary of Adverse Reactions		
	Zemaira	*Prolastin*
Subject treated	89	32
Subjects with adverse events regardless of causality (%)	78	63
Subjects with related adverse events (%)	6	13
Subjects with related serious adverse events	0	0
Number of infusions	1296	160
Adverse events regardless of causality (rates per infusion)	298 (0.230)	83 (0.519)
Related adverse events (rates per infusion)	6 (0.005)	5 (0.03)

The frequencies of adverse events per infusion that were at least 0.4% in *Zemaira*-treated subjects, regardless of causality, were: Headache (2.5%); upper respiratory tract infection (1.6%); sinusitis (1.5%); injection site hemorrhage, sore throat (0.9%); bronchitis (0.8%); asthenia, fever (0.6%); pain, rhinitis, bronchospasm, chest pain (0.5%); increased cough, rash, infection (0.4%).

The following adverse events, regardless of causality, occurred at a rate of 0.2% to less than 0.4% per infusion: Abnormal pain; diarrhea; dizziness; ecchymosis; myalgia; pruritus; vasodilation; accidental injury; back pain; dyspepsia; dyspnea; hemorrhage; injection site reaction; lung disorder; migraine; nausea; paresthesia.

Diffuse interstitial lung disease was noted on a routine chest x-ray of 1 subject at week 24. Causality could not be determined.

In a retrospective analysis, during the 10-week blinded portion of the 24-week clinical study, 6 subjects (20%) of the 30 treated with *Zemaira* had a total of 7 exacerbations of their COPD. Nine subjects (64%) of the 14 treated with *Prolastin* had a total of 11 exacerbations of their COPD. The observed difference between groups was 44% (95% confidence interval from 8% to 70%). Over the entire 24-week treatment period of the 30 subjects in the *Zemaira* treatment group, 7 subjects (23%) had a total of 11 exacerbations of their COPD.

Patient Information

Inform patients of the early signs of hypersensitivity reactions including hives, generalized urticaria, tightness of the chest, dyspnea, wheezing, faintness, hypotension, and anaphylaxis. Advise patients to discontinue use of the product and contact their physician and/or seek immediate emergency care, depending on the severity of the reaction, if these symptoms occur.

As with all plasma-derived products, some viruses, such as parvovirus B19, are particularly difficult to remove or inactivate at this time. Parvovirus B19 may most seriously affect pregnant women and immunecompromised individuals. Symptoms of parvovirus B19 include fever, drowsiness, chills, and runny nose followed 2 weeks later by a rash and joint pain. Encourage patients to consult their physician if such symptoms occur.

BERACTANT (Natural Lung Surfactant)

Rx **Survanta**
(Ross Laboratories)

Suspension: 25 mg phospholipids per ml suspended in 0.9% sodium chloride solution.[1]

In single use vials containing 8 ml suspension.

[1] With 0.5 to 1.75 mg triglycerides, 1.4 to 3.5 mg free fatty acids and < 1 mg protein per ml.

Indications

Prevention and treatment ("rescue") of RDS (hyaline membrane disease) in premature infants. Beractant significantly reduces the incidence of RDS, mortality due to RDS and air leak complications.

➤*Prevention:* In premature infants < 1250 g birth weight or with evidence of surfactant deficiency, give beractant as soon as possible, preferably within 15 minutes of birth.

➤*Rescue:* To treat infants with RDS confirmed by x-ray and requiring mechanical ventilation, give beractant as soon as possible, preferably by 8 hours of age.

Administration and Dosage

For intratracheal administration only.

Marked improvements in oxygenation may occur within minutes of administration of beractant. Therefore, frequent and careful clinical observation and monitoring of systemic oxygenation are essential to avoid hyperoxia.

➤*Dosage:* Each dose of beractant is 100 mg of phospholipids/kg birth weight (4 ml/kg). The following table shows the total dosage for a range of birth weights.

Beractant Dosing Chart			
Weight (g)	Total dose (ml)	Weight (g)	Total dose (ml)
600-650	2.6	1301-1350	5.4
651-700	2.8	1351-1400	5.6
701-750	3	1401-1450	5.8
751-800	3.2	1451-1500	6
801-850	3.4	1501-1550	6.2
851-900	3.6	1551-1600	6.4
901-950	3.8	1601-1650	6.6
951-1000	4	1651-1700	6.8
1001-1050	4.2	1701-1750	7
1051-1100	4.4	1751-1800	7.2
1101-1150	4.6	1801-1850	7.4
1151-1200	4.8	1851-1900	7.6
1201-1250	5	1901-1950	7.8
1251-1300	5.2	1951-2000	8

Four doses can be administered in the first 48 hours of life; give doses no more frequently than every 6 hours.

➤*Preparation:* Inspect visually for discoloration prior to administration. The color of beractant is off-white to light brown. If settling occurs during storage, swirl the vial gently (do not shake) to redisperse. Some foaming at the surface may occur during handling and is inherent in the nature of the product.

Beractant is to be refrigerated (2° to 8°C; 36° to 46°F). Before administration, warm by standing at room temperature for at least 20 minutes or warm in the hand for at least 8 minutes. Artificial warming methods should not be used. If a prevention dose is to be given, begin preparation before the infant's birth.

Unopened, unused vials that have been warmed to room temperature may be returned to the refrigerator within 8 hours of warming and stored for future use. The drug should not be warmed and returned to the refrigerator more than once. Enter each single-use vial of beractant only once. Discard used vials with residual drug. Beractant does not require reconstitution or sonication before use.

➤*Dosing procedures:* Beractant is administered intratracheally by instillation through a 5 French end-hole catheter inserted into the infant's endotracheal tube with the tip of the catheter protruding just beyond the end of the endotracheal tube above the infant's carina. Before inserting the catheter through the endotracheal tube, shorten the length of the catheter. Do not instill beractant into a main-stem bronchus.

It is important to ensure homogenous distribution of beractant throughout the lungs. In the controlled clinical trials, each dose was divided into four quarter-doses. Each quarter-dose was administered with the infant in a different position. The sequence of positions was: Head and body inclined slightly down, head turned to the right; head and body inclined slightly down, head turned to the left; head and body inclined slightly up, head turned to the right; head and body inclined slightly up, head turned to the left.

➤*First dose:* Determine the total dose based on the infant's birth weight. Slowly withdraw the entire contents of the vial into a plastic syringe through a large-gauge needle (eg, at least 20 gauge). Do not filter beractant and avoid shaking.

Attach the premeasured 5 French end-hole catheter to the syringe. Fill the catheter with beractant and discard any excess through the catheter so that only the total dose to be given remains in the syringe.

Before administering beractant, assure proper placement and patency of the endotracheal tube. The endotracheal tube may be suctioned before administering beractant. Allow the infant to stabilize before proceeding with dosing.

Prevention strategy – Weigh, intubate and stabilize the infant. Administer the dose as soon as possible after birth, preferably within 15 minutes. Position the infant appropriately and gently inject the first quarter-dose through the catheter over 2 to 3 seconds.

After administration of the first quarter-dose, remove the catheter from the endotracheal tube. Manually ventilate with a hand-bag with sufficient oxygen to prevent cyanosis, at a rate of 60 breaths/minute, and sufficient positive pressure to provide adequate air exchange and chest wall excursion.

Rescue strategy – Give the first dose as soon as possible after the infant is placed on a ventilator for management of RDS. In the clinical trials, immediately before instilling the first quarter-dose, the infant's ventilator settings were changed to a rate of 60/minute, inspiratory time 0.5 second and FiO$_2$ 1.

Position the infant appropriately and gently inject the first quarter-dose through the catheter over 2 to 3 seconds. After administration of the first quarter-dose, remove the catheter from the endotracheal tube. Return the infant to the mechanical ventilator.

Both strategies – Ventilate the infant for at least 30 seconds or until stable. Reposition the infant for instillation of the next quarter-dose.

Instill the remaining quarter-doses using the same procedures. After instillation of each quarter-dose, remove the catheter and ventilate for at least 30 seconds or until the infant is stabilized. After instillation of the final quarter-dose, remove the catheter without flushing it. Do not suction the infant for 1 hour after dosing unless signs of significant airway obstruction occur.

After completion of the dosing procedure, resume usual ventilator management and clinical care.

➤*Repeat doses:* The dosage is also 100 mg phospholipids/kg and is based on the infant's birth weight. The infant should not be reweighed for determination of the dosage.

The need for additional doses is determined by evidence of continuing respiratory distress. Significant reductions in mortality due to RDS were observed in multiple-dose trials. Administer dose no sooner than 6 hours after the preceding dose if the infant remains intubated and requires at least 30% inspired oxygen to maintain a PaO$_2$ ≤ 80 torr.

Obtain radiographic confirmation of RDS before administering additional doses to those who received a prevention dose.

Prepare beractant and position the infant for administration of each quarter-dose as previously described. After instillation of each quarter-dose, remove the dosing catheter from the endotracheal tube and ventilate the infant for at least 30 seconds or until stable.

In clinical studies, ventilator settings used to administer repeat doses were different than those used for the first dose. For repeat doses, the FiO$_2$ was increased by 0.2 or an amount sufficient to prevent cyanosis. The ventilator delivered a rate of 30/minute with an inspiratory time < 1 second. If the infant's pretreatment rate was ≥ 30 it was left unchanged during instillation.

Manual hand-bag ventilation should not be used to administer repeat doses. During the dosing procedure, ventilatory settings may be adjusted at the discretion of the clinician to maintain appropriate oxygenation and ventilation. After completion of the dosing procedure, resume usual ventilator management and clinical care.

➤*Educational material:* Review of audiovisual instructional materials describing dosage and administration procedures is recommended before using beractant. Materials are available on request from Ross Laboratories.

➤*Storage/Stability:* Store unopened vials under refrigeration (2° to 8°C; 36° to 46°F). Protect from light. Store vials in carton until ready for use. Vials are for single use only. Upon opening, discard unused drug.

Actions

➤*Pharmacology:* Beractant is a sterile, non-pyrogenic pulmonary surfactant intended for intratracheal use only. It is a natural bovine lung extract containing phospholipids, neutral lipids, fatty acids and surfactant-associated proteins to which colfosceril palmitate (dipalmitoylphosphatidylcholine; DPPC), palmitic acid and tripalmitin are added to standardize the composition and to mimic surface-tension lowering properties of natural lung surfactant. Its protein content consists of two hydrophobic, low molecular weight, surfactant-associated proteins commonly known as SP-B and SP-C. It does not contain the hydrophilic, large molecular weight surfactant-associated protein known as SP-A.

Endogenous pulmonary surfactant lowers surface tension on alveolar surfaces during respiration and stabilizes the alveoli against collapse

BERACTANT (Natural Lung Surfactant)

at resting transpulmonary pressures. Deficiency of pulmonary surfactant causes respiratory distress syndrome (RDS) in premature infants. Beractant replenishes surfactant and restores surface activity to the lungs of these infants.

Beractant reproducibly lowers minimum surface tension to < 8 dynes/cm in vitro, restores pulmonary compliance to excised rat lungs artifically made surfactant-deficient in situ, and improves lung pressure-volume measurements, lung compliance, and oxygenation in premature rabbits and sheep in vivo.

➤*Pharmacokinetics:* Beractant is administered directly to the target organ, the lungs, where biophysical effects occur at the alveolar surface. In surfactant-deficient premature rabbits and lambs, alveolar clearance of the lipid components is rapid. Most of the dose becomes lung-associated within hours of administration, and the lipids enter endogenous surfactant pathways of reutilization and recycling. In surfactant-sufficient adult animals, clearance is more rapid than in premature and young animals. There is less reutilization and recycling of surfactant in adult animals.

➤*Clinical trials:* Each dose in all studies was 100 mg phospholipids/kg birth weight.

Prevention studies – In infants of 600 to 1250 g birth weight and 23 to 29 weeks estimated gestational age, a dose of beractant was given within 15 minutes of birth to prevent the development of RDS. Up to three additional doses in the first 48 hours, as often as every 6 hours, were given if RDS subsequently developed and infants required mechanical ventilation with an $FiO_2 \geq 0.3$.

Rescue studies – In infants of 600 to 1750 g birth weight with RDS requiring mechanical ventilation and an $FiO_2 \geq 0.4$, the initial dose of beractant was given after RDS developed and before 8 hours of age. Infants could receive up to three additional doses in the first 48 hours, as often as every 6 hours, if they required mechanical ventilation and an $FiO_2 \geq 0.3$.

Prevention/Rescue Studies with Beractant

Parameter	Prevention studies[1]		Rescue studies[1]	
	Beractant (n = 210)	Control (n = 220)	Beractant (n = 402)	Control (n = 396)
Incidence of RDS (%)	27.6 – 28.6	48.3 – 63.5	na[2]	na[2]
Death due to RDS (%)	1.1 – 2.5	10.5 – 19.5	6.4 – 11.6	18.1 – 22.3
Death or BPD due to RDS (%)	27.5 – 48.7	44.2 – 52.8	43.6 – 59.1	63.4 – 66.8
Death due to any cause (%)	7.6 – 16.5[3]	13.7 – 22.8	15.2 – 21.7	26.4 – 28.2
Air leaks[4] (%)	5.9 – 14.5	19.6 – 21.7	11.2 – 11.8	22.2 – 29.5
Pulmonary interstitial emphysema (%)	20.8 – 26.5	33.2 – 40	16.3 – 20.8	34 – 44.4

[1] Data pooled from two studies
[2] na = Not applicable
[3] In one study, no cause of death in the beractant group was significantly increased; the higher number of deaths in this group was due to the sum of all causes.
[4] Pneumothorax or pneumopericardium.

Marked improvements in oxygenation may occur within minutes of administration.

Significant improvements in the arterial-alveolar oxygen ratio (a/APO_2), FiO_2 and mean airway pressure (MAP) were sustained for 48 to 72 hours in beractant-treated infants in four single-dose and two multiple-dose rescue studies and in two multiple-dose prevention studies. In the single-dose prevention studies, the FiO_2 improved significantly.

Multiple-dose studies – In 605 (333 treated) of 916 surviving infants, there are trends for decreased cerebral palsy and need for supplemental oxygen in beractant infants. Wheezing at the time of examination tended to be more frequent among beractant infants, although there was no difference in bronchodilator therapy.

Warnings

➤*Intratracheal administration:* Administer only by instillation into the trachea (see Administration and Dosage).

➤*Oxygenation/lung compliance:* Beractant can rapidly affect oxygenation and lung compliance. Therefore, restrict its use to a highly supervised clinical setting with immediate availability of clinicians experienced with intubation, ventilator management and general care of premature infants. Frequently monitor infants receiving beractant with arterial or transcutaneous measurement of systemic oxygen and CO_2.

Transient episodes of bradycardia and decreased oxygen saturation have occurred during dosing. If these occur, stop the dosing procedure and initiate appropriate measures to alleviate the condition. After stabilization, resume the dosing procedure.

Precautions

➤*Rales and moist breath sounds:* These can occur transiently after administration. Endotracheal suctioning or other remedial action is not necessary unless clear-cut signs of airway obstruction are present.

➤*Nosocomial sepsis:* Increased probability of post-treatment nosocomial sepsis in beractant-treated infants was observed in controlled clinical trials. The increased risk for sepsis was not associated with increased mortality among these infants. The causative organisms were similar in treated and control infants.

Adverse Reactions

The most commonly reported adverse experiences were associated with the dosing procedure. In the multiple-dose controlled clinical trials, transient bradycardia occurred with 11.9% of doses. Oxygen desaturation occurred with 9.8% of doses.

Other reactions during the dosing procedure occurred with < 1% of doses and included: Endotracheal tube reflux; pallor; vasoconstriction; hypotension; endotracheal tube blockage; hypertension; hypocarbia; hypercarbia; apnea. No deaths occurred during the dosing procedure, and all reactions resolved with symptomatic treatment.

The occurrence of concurrent illnesses common in premature infants was evaluated in the controlled trials.

Concurrent Illnesses During Beractant Treatment (%)

Concurrent event	Beractant	Control
Patent ductus arteriosus	46.9	47.1
Intracranial hemorrhage	48.1	45.2
Severe intracranial hemorrhage	24.1	23.3
Pulmonary air leaks	10.9	24.7
Pulmonary interstitial emphysema	20.2	38.4
Necrotizing enterocolitis	6.1	5.3
Apnea	65.4	59.6
Severe apnea	46.1	42.5
Post-treatment sepsis	20.7	16.1
Post-treatment infection	10.2	9.1
Pulmonary hemorrhage	7.2	5.3

When all controlled studies were pooled, there was no difference in intracranial hemorrhage. However, in one of the single-dose rescue studies and one of the multiple-dose prevention studies, the rate of intracranial hemorrhage was significantly higher in beractant patients than control patients (63.3% vs 30.8% and 48.8% vs 34.2%, respectively).

Overdosage

➤*Symptoms:* Based on animal data, overdosage might result in acute airway obstruction. Rales and moist breath sounds can transiently occur after beractant is given, and do not indicate overdosage. Endotracheal suctioning or other remedial action is not required unless clear-cut signs of airway obstruction are present.

➤*Treatment:* Treatment should be symptomatic and supportive. Refer to General Management of Acute Overdosage.

CALFACTANT

Rx	Infasurf (Forest Pharmaceuticals)	Suspension, intratracheal: 35 mg phospholipids per ml suspended in 0.9% sodium chloride solution[1] and 0.65 mg proteins[2]	In single-use vials, containing 6 ml suspension.

[1] Including 26 mg phosphatidylcholine of which 16 mg is disaturated phosphatidylcholine.

[2] Including 0.26 mg of SP-B.

Indications

➤*Respiratory distress syndrome (RDS):* For the prevention of RDS in premature infants < 29 weeks of gestational age at high risk for RDS and for the treatment ("rescue") of premature infants ≤ 72 hours of age who develop RDS and require endotracheal intubation. Calfactant prophylaxis should be administered as soon as possible, preferably ≤ 30 minutes after birth.

Administration and Dosage

➤*Approved by the FDA:* July 1, 1998.

Data from controlled trials on the efficacy of calfactant are limited to doses of ≈ 100 mg phospholipid/kg and up to a total of 4 doses.

For intratracheal administration only. Administer through an endotracheal tube. Draw dose into a syringe from the single-use vial using a 20-gauge or larger needle; avoid excessive foaming. Administer under the supervision of clinicians experienced in the acute care of newborn infants with respiratory failure who require intubation. Rapid and substantial increases in blood oxygenation and improved lung compliance often follow calfactant instillation. Monitor closely following administration and adjust oxygen therapy and ventilator pressures appropriately.

➤*Directions for use:* Calfactant does not require reconstitution. Do NOT dilute or sonicate. Do NOT shake. Gently swirl or agitate the vial for redispersion. Visible flecks in the suspension and foaming at the surface are normal. Warming before administration is not necessary.

CALFACTANT

Unopened, unused vials that have warmed to room temperature can be returned to refrigerated storage within 24 hours for future use. Avoid repeated warming to room temperature.

➤*Prophylaxis of RDS at birth:* Instill a prophylactic dose of 3 ml/kg of birth weight as soon as possible after birth. Administer as 2 doses of 1.5 ml/kg each. Usually the immediate care and stabilization of the premature infant born with hypoxemia or bradycardia should precede calfactant prophylaxis.

➤*Treatment of RDS:* Instill 3 ml/kg of birth weight, administered as 2 doses of 1.5 ml/kg. Repeat doses of 3 ml/kg of birth weight, up to a total of 3 doses 12 hours apart, have been given.

➤*Dosing procedure:* Administer calfactant intratracheally through a side-port adapter into the endotracheal tube. Two attendants facilitate the dosing: 1 to instill the calfactant and the other to monitor the patient and assist in positioning. After each aliquot is instilled, position the infant with either the right or left side dependent. Administer while ventilation is continued over 20 to 30 breaths for each aliquot, with small bursts timed only during the inspiratory cycles. A pause followed by evaluation of the respiratory status and repositioning should separate the two aliquots.

Calfactant has been administered through a 5 French feeding catheter inserted into the endotracheal tube. The total dose was instilled in 4 equal aliquots with the catheter removed between each of the instillations and mechanical ventilation resumed for 0.5 to 2 minutes. Each of the aliquots was administered with the patient in 1 of 4 different positions (prone, supine, right and left lateral) to facilitate even distribution of the surfactant. Repeat doses were administered as early as 6 hours after the previous dose for a total of up to 4 doses if the infant was still intubated and required at least 30% inspired oxygen to maintain a $PaO_2 \le 80$ torr.

➤*Dosing precautions:* During administration of calfactant liquid suspension into the airway, infants often experience bradycardia, reflux of calfactant into the endotracheal tube, airway obstruction, cyanosis, dislodgement of the endotracheal tube or hypoventilation. If any of these events occur, interrupt administration and stabilize the infant's condition using appropriate interventions before resuming administration. Endotracheal suctioning or reintubation is sometimes needed when signs of airway obstruction are present during administration.

➤*Storage/Stability:* Refrigerate at 2° to 8°C (36° to 46°F) and protect from light. Vials are for single use only. After opening, discard unused drug. Unopened, unused vials that have warmed to room temperature can be returned to refrigerated storage within 24 hours for future use. Avoid repeated warming to room temperature.

Actions

➤*Pharmacology:* Calfactant is a lung surfactant intended for intratracheal instillation only. It is an extract of natural surfactant from calf lungs that includes phospholipids, neutral lipids and hydrophobic surfactant-associated proteins B and C (SP-B and SP-C).

Endogenous lung surfactant is essential for effective ventilation because it modifies alveolar surface tension thereby stabilizing the alveoli. Lung surfactant deficiency is the cause of RDS in premature infants. Calfactant restores surface activity to the lungs of these infants.

Calfactant adsorbs rapidly to the surface of the air:liquid interface and modifies surface tension similarly to natural lung surfactant. A minimum surface tension of ≤ 3 mN/m is produced in vitro by calfactant as measured on a pulsating bubble surfactometer. Ex vivo, calfactant restores the pressure volume mechanics and compliance of surfactant-deficient rat lungs. In vivo, calfactant improves lung compliance, respiratory gas exchange and survival in preterm lambs with profound surfactant deficiency.

➤*Pharmacokinetics:* No human studies of absorption, biotransformation, or excretion have been performed. The administration of calfactant into the lungs of adult rabbits results in the persistence of 50% of the dose in the lung alveolar lining and 25% in the lung tissue 24 hours later. Less than 5% is found in other organs. In premature lambs with lethal surfactant deficiency, < 30% of instilled calfactant is present in the lung lining after 24 hours.

Warnings

➤*Instillation:* Calfactant is intended for intratracheal use only.

➤*Transient episodes:* Reflux of calfactant into the endotracheal tube, cyanosis, bradycardia, or airway obstruction have occurred during the dosing procedures (see Adverse Reactions). These events require stopping calfactant administration and taking appropriate measures to alleviate the condition. After the patient is stable, dosing can proceed with appropriate monitoring.

Precautions

➤*Monitoring:* The administration of exogenous surfactants, including calfactant, often rapidly improves oxygenation and lung compliance. Following administration of calfactant, monitor patients carefully so that oxygen therapy and ventilatory support can be modified in response to changes in respiratory status.

Optimal care of premature infants at risk for RDS and newborn infants with RDS who need endotracheal intubation requires an acute care unit organized, staffed, equipped, and experienced with intubation, ventilator management, and general care of these patients.

➤*Intracranial ventricular effects:* An increased proportion of patients with both intraventricular hemorrhage (IVH) and periventricular leukomalacia (PVL) was observed in calfactant-treated infants in controlled trials. These observations were not associated with increased mortality.

Adverse Reactions

The most common adverse reactions associated with calfactant dosing procedures in the controlled trials were: Cyanosis (65%); airway obstruction (39%); bradycardia (34%); reflux of surfactant into the endotracheal tube (21%); requirement for manual ventilation (16%); reintubation (3%). These events were generally transient and not associated with serious complications or death.

The incidence of common complications of prematurity and RDS in the 4 controlled calfactant trials are presented in the table below. Prophylaxis and treatment study results for each surfactant are combined.

Common Complications of Prematurity and RDS in Controlled Trials (%)				
Complication	Calfactant (*Infasurf*) (n = 1001)	Colfosceril (*Exosurf Neonatal*) (n = 978)	Calfactant (*Infasurf*) (n = 553)	Beractant (*Survanta*) (n = 566)
Apnea	61	61	76	76
Patent ductus arteriosus	47	48	45	48
Intracranial hemorrhage	29	31	36	36
Severe intracranial hemorrhage[1]	12	10	9	7
IVH and PVL[2]	7	3	5	5
Sepsis	20	22	28	27
Pulmonary air leaks	12	22	15	15
Pulmonary interstitial emphysema	7	17	10	10
Pulmonary hemorrhage	7	7	7	6
Necrotizing enterocolitis	5	5	17	18

[1] Grade III and IV by the method of Papile.
[2] Combined incidence of intraventricular hemorrhage and periventricular leukomalacia.

Two-year follow-up data of neurodevelopmental outcomes in 415 infants enrolled at 5 centers that participated in the calfactant vs colfosceril controlled trials demonstrated significant developmental delays in equal percentages of calfactant and colfosceril patients.

Overdosage

There have been no reports of overdosage with calfactant. While there are no known adverse effects of excess lung surfactant, overdosage would result in overloading the lungs with an isotonic solution. Support ventilation until clearance of the liquid is accomplished.

PORACTANT ALFA (PORCINE ORIGIN)

Rx	Curosurf (Dey)	**Suspension, intratracheal:** 1.5 mL (120 mg phospholipids)	Preservative free. In single-use vials.
		3 mL (240 mg phospholipids)	

Indications

➤*Respiratory distress syndrome (RDS):* For the treatment (rescue) of RDS in premature infants.

➤*Unlabeled uses:* Prophylaxis for RDS; adult RDS due to viral pneumonia; HIV-infected infants with *Pneumocystis carinii* pneumonia; treatment in adult RDS following near drowning.

Administration and Dosage

➤*Approved by the FDA:* November 18, 1999.

➤*Dosage:* The initial dose of poractant is 2.5 mL/kg birth weight. Up to 2 subsequent doses of 1.25 mL/kg birth weight can be administered at 12-hour intervals if needed (ie, in infants who remain intubated and require mechanical ventilation and supplemental oxygen). The maximum recommended total dose (sum of the initial and up to 2 repeat doses) is 5 mL/kg.

Sufficient information is not available regarding the effects of administering initial doses of poractant other than 2.5 mL/kg (200 mg/kg), subsequent doses other than 1.25 mL/kg (100 mg/kg), administration of > 3 total doses, dosing more frequently than every 12 hours, or initiating therapy with poractant > 15 hours after diagnosing RDS. Adequate data are not available on the use of poractant in conjunction with experimental therapies of RDS (eg, high-frequency ventilation).

➤*Dosing procedures:* Before use, slowly warm the vial to room temperature and gently turn upside-down in order to obtain a uniform suspension. Do not shake.

PORACTANT ALFA (PORCINE ORIGIN)

Slowly withdraw the entire contents of the vial of poractant into a 3 or 5 mL plastic syringe through a large-gauge needle (eg, ≥ 20 gauge). Attach the pre-cut 8-cm 5 French catheter to the syringe. Fill the catheter with poractant. Discard excess poractant through the catheter so that only the total dose to be given remains in the syringe.

For intratracheal administration only. Administer by instillation through a 5 French end-hole catheter (cut to a standard length of 8 cm) inserted into the infant's endotracheal tube, with the tip positioned distally in the endotracheal tube. Do not extend the catheter tip beyond the distal tip of the endotracheal tube. Administer each dose of poractant as 2 aliquots, with each aliquot administered into 1 of the 2 main bronchi by positioning the infant with either the right or left side dependent.

Before administering poractant, assure proper placement and patency of the endotracheal tube. At the discretion of the clinician, the endotracheal tube may be suctioned before administering poractant. Allow the infant to stabilize before proceeding with dosing.

Immediately before poractant administration, change the infant's ventilator setting to a rate of 40 to 60 breaths/min, inspiratory time 0.5 seconds, and supplemental oxygen sufficient to maintain SaO_2 > 92%. Keep the infant in a neutral position (head and body in alignment without inclination). Briefly disconnect the endotracheal tube from the ventilator. Insert the pre-cut 5 French catheter into the endotracheal tube and instill the first aliquot (1.25 mL/kg birth weight) of poractant. Position the infant such that either the right or left side is dependent for this aliquot. After the first aliquot of surfactant is instilled, remove the catheter from the endotracheal tube and manually ventilate the infant with 100% oxygen at a rate of 40 to 60 breaths/min for 1 minute. When the infant is stable, reposition the infant such that the other side is dependent and administer the remaining aliquot using the same procedures. After instillation of the second aliquot, remove the catheter without flushing. Do not suction airways for 1 hour after surfactant instillation unless signs of significant airway obstruction occur.

After completion of the dosing procedure, resume usual ventilator management and clinical care. In the clinical trials, ventilator management was modifed to maintain a PaO_2 of about 55 mmHg, $PaCO_2$ of 35 to 45, and pH > 7.3.

➤*Dosing precautions:* Transient episodes of bradycardia, decreased oxygen saturation, reflux of the surfactant into the endotracheal tube, hypotension, and airway obstruction have occurred during the dosing procedure of poractant. These events require interrupting the administration of poractant and taking appropriate measures to alleviate the condition. After stabilization, dosing may resume with appropriate monitoring.

➤*Storage/Stability:* Store poractant in a refrigerator at 2° to 8°C (36° to 46°F). Unopened vials may be warmed to room temperature for up to 24 hours prior to use. Do not warm poractant to room temperature and return to the refrigerator more than once. Protect from light. Do not shake. Vials are for single use only. After opening the vial, discard the unused portion of the drug.

Actions

➤*Pharmacology:* Endogenous pulmonary surfactant reduces surface tension at the air-liquid interface of the alveoli during ventilation and stabilizes the alveoli against collapse at resting transpulmonary pressures. A deficiency of pulmonary surfactant in preterm infants results in RDS characterized by poor lung expansion, inadequate gas exchange, and a gradual collapse of the lungs (atelectasis). Poractant compensates for the deficiency of surfactant and restores surface activ-

ity to the lungs of these infants. Poractant reduces mortality and pneumothoraces associated with RDS.

➤*Pharmacokinetics:* In adult and newborn rabbits, ≈ 50% of the radiolabeled component was rapidly removed from the alveoli in the first 3 hours after single intratracheal administration of poractant-^{14}C-DPPC (dipalmitoylphosphatidylcholine). Of the total ^{14}C-DPPC recovered in newborn rabbits, < 0.6% was found in the serum, liver, kidneys, and brain, respectively, at 48 hours. The half-life in the lung appeared to be ≈ 25 hours in adult rabbits and 67 hours in newborn rabbits.

Precautions

➤*Monitoring:* The administration of exogenous surfactant, including poractant, can rapidly affect oxygenation and lung compliance. Therefore, infants receiving poractant should receive frequent clinical and laboratory assessments so that oxygen and ventilatory support can be modified to respond to respiratory changes.

Correction of acidosis, hypotension, anemia, hypoglycemia, and hypothermia is recommended prior to poractant administration.

Adverse Reactions

Transient adverse effects seen with the administration of poractant include bradycardia, hypotension, endotracheal tube blockage, and oxygen desaturation.

Complications of Prematurity: Poractant vs Control (%)		
Adverse reaction	Poractant alfa 2.5 mL/kg (200 mg/kg) (n = 78)	Control[1] (n = 66)
Acquired pneumonia	17	21
Acquired septicemia	14	18
Bronchopulmonary dysplasia	18	22
Intracranial hemorrhage	51	64
Patent ductus arteriosus	60	48
Pneumothorax	21	36
Pulmonary interstitial emphysema	21	38

[1] Control patients were disconnected from the ventilator and manually ventilated for 2 minutes. No surfactant was instilled.

Immunological studies have not demonstrated differences in levels of surfactant-anti-surfactant immune complexes and anti-poractant antibodies between patients treated with poractant and patients who received control treatment.

Follow-up – Seventy-six infants (45 treated with poractant) were evaluated at 1 year of age and 73 infants (44 treated with poractant) at 2 years of age. Data from follow-up evaluations for weight and length, persistent respiratory symptoms, incidence of cerebral palsy, visual impairment, or auditory impairment were similar between treatment groups. In 16 patients (10 treated with poractant and 6 controls) evaluated at 5.5 years of age, the developmental quotient, derived using the Griffiths Mental Developmental Scales, was similar between both groups.

Overdosage

➤*Treatment:* In the event of accidental overdosage, and only if there are clear clinical effects on the infant's respiration, ventilation, or oxygenation, aspirate as much of the suspension as possible and manage the infant with supportive treatment, with particular attention to fluid and electrolyte balance. Refer to General Management of Acute Overdosage.

Indications

As a group, these agents are used for the relief of manifestations of immediate-type hypersensitivity reactions. The varying degrees of anticholinergic, antihistaminic, and antimuscarinic activity make many antihistamines useful as sedatives, antiemetics, antitussives, antiparkinson agents, adjuncts to pre- or postoperative analgesic therapy, and agents to combat motion sickness. Refer to individual monographs on the following pages for specific indications.

➤*Unlabeled uses:* One study suggested the combination of an H_1 and H_2 antagonist may be useful in patients with chronic idiopathic urticaria who do not adequately respond to an H_1 antagonist alone.

Actions

➤*Pharmacology:*

Antihistamines: Dosage and Effects

Antihistamine	Dose[1] (mg)	Dosing interval[2] (hrs)	Sedative effects	Antihistaminic activity	Anticholinergic activity	Antiemetic effects
First-Generation (non-selective)						
Alkylamines						
Brompheniramine	4	4 to 6	+	+++	++	—
Chlorpheniramine	4	4 to 6	+	++	++	—
Dexchlorpheniramine	2	4 to 6	+	+++	++	—
Ethanolamines						
Clemastine	1	12	++	+ to ++	+++	++ to +++
Diphenhydramine	25 to 50	6 to 8	+++	+ to ++	+++	++ to +++
Phenothiazines						
Promethazine	12.5 to 25	6 to 24	+++	+++	+++	++++
Piperazines						
Hydroxyzine	25 to 100	4 to 8	+++	++ to +++	++	+++
Piperidines						
Azatadine	1 to 2	12	++	++	++	—
Cyproheptadine	4	8	+	++	++	—
Phenindamine	25	4 to 6	±	++	++	—
Second-Generation (peripherally selective)						
Phthalazinone						
Azelastine[3]	0.5	12	±	++ to +++	±	—
Piperazine						
Cetirizine	5 to 10	24	±	++ to +++	±	—
Piperidines						
Fexofenadine	60	12	±	—	±	—
Loratadine	10	24	±	++ to +++	±	—

* ++++ = very high, +++ = high, ++ = moderate, + = low, ± = low to none. — = No data.
[1] Usual single adult dose.
[2] For conventional dosage forms.
[3] Some effects may be enhanced or reduced as a result of administration via the nasal route.

Antihistamines are reversible, competitive H_1 receptor antagonists that reduce or prevent most of the physiologic effects that histamine normally induces at the H_1 receptor site. They do not prevent histamine release nor bind with histamine that has already been released. Antihistaminic effects include inhibition of respiratory, vascular, and GI smooth muscle constriction; decreased capillary permeability, which reduces the wheal, flare, and itch response; and decreased histamine-activated exocrine secretions (eg, salivary, lacrimal). Antihistamines with strong anticholinergic (atropine-like) properties also can potentiate the drying effect by suppressing cholinergically innervated exocrine glands. **First-generation antihistamines** bind nonselectively to central and peripheral H_1 receptors and can result in CNS stimulation or depression. CNS depression, which usually occurs with higher therapeutic doses, allows some of these agents to be used clinically for sedation. However, **second-generation antihistamines** are selective for peripheral H_1 receptors and, as a group, are less sedating. Several first-generation agents (eg, diphenhydramine, some piperazines, promethazine) with strong anticholinergic properties bind to central muscarinic receptors and produce antiemetic effects, decreasing nausea, vomiting, and motion sickness (see Antiemetic/Antivertigo agents). At doses much higher than that needed to antagonize histamine, a few agents (especially promethazine) exhibit local anesthetic effects. Some agents (eg, cyproheptadine, azatadine) also have antiserotonergic effects.

Switching from one class of antihistamines to another may restore responsiveness when a patient becomes refractory to the effects of a particular agent.

➤*Pharmacokinetics:*

First-generation agents – Pharmacokinetics of first-generation agents have not been extensively studied. With a few exceptions, these agents are well absorbed following oral administration, have an onset of action within 15 to 30 minutes, are maximal within 1 to 2 hours and have a duration of action of about 4 to 6 hours, although some are much longer acting (see Pharmacology table). Most are metabolized by the liver. Antihistamine metabolites and small amounts of unchanged drug are excreted in urine. Small amounts may be excreted in breast milk.

Second-generation agents – Intranasal administration of **azelastine** yields peak levels in 2 to 3 hours with an elimination half-life of 22 hours. Metabolism by the P450 system results in steady-state peak levels of a major active metabolite (desmethylazelastine), which are 20% to 50% of azelastine levels. The elimination half-life of the metabolite is predicted to be 54 hours. The major route of excretion is via feces.

The pharmacokinetics of the second-generation agents have been studied more thoroughly and are provided in the table below.

Pharmacokinetics of Peripherally Selective H_1 Antagonists

	Onset of action	T_{max} (hours)	Elimination $t\frac{1}{2}$ (hours)	Protein binding (%)	P450 metabolism	Food effect on absorption
Cetirizine	rapid	1	8.3	93	↓; 50% excreted unchanged	delayed 1.7 hours
Fexofenadine	rapid	2.6	14.4	60 to 70	↓↓; 95% excreted unchanged	—
Loratadine	rapid	1.3 to 2.5[1]	8.4 to 28[1]	97 (75)[2]	↑; 3A4, 2D6	delayed 1 hour

↑ = High, ↓ = Low, ↓↓ = Very low.
[1] All active constituents (parent drug and active metabolites).
[2] Active metabolite.
— = No data.

Contraindications

➤*First-generation antihistamines:* Hypersensitivity to specific or structurally related antihistamines; newborn or premature infants (see Warnings); nursing mothers (see Warnings); narrow-angle glaucoma; stenosing peptic ulcer; symptomatic prostatic hypertrophy; bladder neck obstruction; pyloroduodenal obstruction; monoamine oxidase inhibitor (MAOI) use (see Drug Interactions); elderly, debilitated patients (**cyproheptadine**).

➤*Second-generation antihistamines:* Hypersensitivity to specific or structurally related antihistamines.

Warnings

➤*Respiratory disease:* In general, antihistamines are not recommended to treat *lower* respiratory tract symptoms (eg, emphysema, chronic bronchitis, asthma) because their anticholinergic (drying) effects may thicken secretions and impair expectoration. However, several reports indicate antihistamines can be safely used in asthmatic patients with severe perennial allergic rhinitis without exacerbating the asthma.

➤*Pre- and postoperative adjunctive therapy:* Nonselective antihistamines may potentiate CNS depressants, such as narcotics, nonnarcotic analgesics, and barbiturates. Narcotic requirements may be reduced by as much as 50%. Reduce dosage appropriately when using antihistamines as pre- and postsurgical adjunctive therapy.

➤*Seizure threshold:* **Promethazine** may lower the seizure threshold; consider this when giving to people with known seizure disorders or when giving in combination with narcotics or local anesthetics that may also affect seizure threshold.

➤*Sleep apnea:* Avoid sedatives and CNS depressants in patients with a history of sleep apnea.

➤*Drug abuse:* Nonmedical parenteral use of concurrent **butorphanol** and **diphenhydramine** has also been reported.

➤*Hypersensitivity reactions:* Hypersensitivity reactions may occur, and any of the usual manifestations of drug allergy may develop. Have epinephrine 1:1000 immediately available. Refer to Management of Acute Hypersensitivity Reactions.

➤*Renal / Hepatic function impairment:* Use a lower initial dose of **loratadine** (10 mg every other day) in patients with renal or hepatic impairment.

➤*Elderly:* Antihistamines are more likely to cause dizziness, excessive sedation, syncope, toxic confusional states, and hypotension in patients ≥ 60 years of age and may also cause paradoxical stimulation. Dosage reduction may be required.

The phenothiazine side effects (extrapyramidal signs, especially parkinsonism, akathisia, and persistent dyskinesia) are more prone to develop in the elderly.

➤*Pregnancy:* (*Category B* – **chlorpheniramine, dexchlorpheniramine, diphenhydramine, brompheniramine, cetirizine, cyproheptadine, clemastine, azatadine, loratadine**; *Category C* – **azelastine, fexofenadine, hydroxyzine, promethazine**). Safety for use during pregnancy has not been established. Several possible associations with malformations have been found, but significance is unknown. Use only when clearly needed and when the potential benefits outweigh the potential hazards to the fetus. Do not use during the third trimester; newborn and premature infants may have severe reactions (eg, convulsions) to some antihistamines.

Reports of jaundice, hyperreflexia, and prolonged extrapyramidal symptoms occurred in infants whose mothers received phenothiazines during pregnancy. **Promethazine**, taken within 2 weeks of delivery, may inhibit newborn platelet aggregation.

➤*Lactation:* Although quantitative determinations of antihistaminic drugs in breast milk have not been reported, qualitative tests have documented the excretion of **diphenhydramine, cetirizine,** and **pyrilamine** in breast milk. **Loratadine** and its metabolite pass easily into breast milk and achieve concentrations that are equivalent to plasma levels with an AUC milk/AUC plasma ratio of 1.17 and 0.85, respectively. Because of the higher risk of adverse effects for infants generally, and for newborns and prematures in particular, antihistamine therapy is contraindicated in nursing mothers.

➤*Children:* Antihistamines may diminish mental alertness; conversely, they may occasionally produce excitation, particularly in the young child.

Avoid using **phenothiazines** in children with hepatic diseases, Reye's syndrome, a history of sleep apnea, or a family history of sudden infant death syndrome (SIDS).

Precautions

➤*Hematologic:* Use **promethazine** with caution in bone marrow depression. Leukopenia and agranulocytosis have been reported, usually when used with other toxic agents.

➤*Anticholinergic effects:* Antihistamines have varying degrees of atropine-like actions; use with caution in patients with a predisposition to urinary retention, history of bronchial asthma, increased intraocular pressure, hyperthyroidism, cardiovascular disease, or hypertension. Antihistamines may thicken bronchial secretions caused by anticholinergic properties and may inhibit expectoration and sinus drainage.

➤*Phenothiazines:* Use phenothiazines with caution in patients with cardiovascular disease, liver dysfunction, or ulcer disease. Promethazine has been associated with cholestatic jaundice.

Use cautiously in people with acute or chronic respiratory impairment, particularly children, because phenothiazines may suppress the cough

reflex. If hypotension occurs, epinephrine is not recommended because phenothiazines may reverse its usual pressor effect and cause a paradoxical further lowering of blood pressure. Because these drugs have an antiemetic action, they may obscure signs of intestinal obstruction, brain tumor, or overdosage of toxic drugs.

Phenothiazines elevate serum prolactin levels, which persist through chronic administration. Approximately ⅓ of breast cancers are prolactin-dependent in vitro, an important factor if these drugs are prescribed for a patient with a history of breast cancer. Although galactorrhea, amenorrhea, gynecomastia, and impotence have been reported, the clinical significance of elevated serum prolactin levels is unknown.

➤*Hazardous tasks:* Antihistamines have varying degrees of sedative effects and may cause drowsiness and reduce mental alertness; patients should not drive or perform other tasks requiring alertness, coordination, or physical dexterity. Supervise children who are taking antihistamines when they engage in potentially hazardous activities (eg, bicycle riding).

➤*Photosensitivity:* Photosensitization may occur; therefore, caution patients to take protective measures (eg, sunscreens, protective clothing) against exposure to ultraviolet light or sunlight until tolerance is determined.

Drug Interactions

Antihistamine Drug Interactions			
Precipitant drug	Object drug*		Description
Antihistamines	Alcohol, CNS depressants	↑	Additive CNS depressant effects may occur. This may be less likely with second-generation agents.
Ketoconazole	Loratadine	↑	Plasma levels (including metabolites) may be increased. No clinically relevant changes in loratadine safety profile.
Cimetidine	Azelastine Loratadine	↑	Concomitant use resulted in substantially increased plasma levels of loratadine and an increase of ≈ 65% in levels of orally administered azelastine.
Erythromycin	Loratadine	↑	Plasma levels (including metabolites) may be increased. No clinically relevant changes in loratadine safety profile.
MAO Inhibitors	Antihistamines	↑	MAOIs may prolong and intensify the anticholinergic and sedative effects of antihistamines; may cause hypotension and extrapyramidal reactions with phenothiazines and severe hypotension with dexchlorpheniramine.
Antihistamines	MAOIs	↑	

* ↑ = Object drug increased

See the Antipsychotic Agents monograph for a complete discussion of the drug interactions that relate to the phenothiazine antihistamine, promethazine.

➤*Drug / Lab test interactions:* **Diagnostic pregnancy tests** based on hCG may result in false-negative or false-positive interpretations in patients on promethazine. Increased **blood glucose tolerance** has occurred in promethazine patients.

Phenothiazines may increase **serum cholesterol, spinal fluid protein,** and **urinary urobilinogen levels;** decrease **protein bound iodine (PBI);** yield false-positive **urine bilirubin tests;** interfere with **urinary ketone** and **steroid determinations**.

Discontinue antihistamines ≈ 4 days prior to **skin testing procedures;** these drugs may prevent or diminish otherwise positive reactions to dermal reactivity indicators.

➤*Drug / Food interactions:* Food increased the AUC of **loratadine** by ≈ 40% and the metabolite by ≈ 15%; absorption was delayed by 1 hour; peak levels were unaffected. Although not expected to be clinically important, take on an empty stomach. The AUC of loratadine rapidly disintegrating tablets was increased by 26% when administered without water compared to water; peak levels were not significantly affected. Bioavailability was unaffected; dissolved remnants may be swallowed with or without water.

Systemic absorption of **cetirizine** was delayed by 1.7 hours, and peak plasma levels were decreased by 23%. However, cetirizine may be taken with or without food.

Adverse Reactions

➤*Allergic:* Peripheral, angioneurotic, and laryngeal edema; dermatitis; asthma; lupus erythematosus-like syndrome; urticaria; drug rash; anaphylactic shock; photosensitivity.

➤*Cardiovascular:* Postural hypotension; palpitations; bradycardia; tachycardia; reflex tachycardia; extrasystoles; faintness; hypertension; hypotension; venous thrombosis at injection site (**IV promethazine**); cardiac arrest; ECG changes, including blunting of T-waves and prolongation of the QT interval.

➤*CNS:* Drowsiness (often transient); sedation; dizziness; faintness; disturbed coordination (most frequent). Fatigue; lassitude; confusion; restlessness; excitation; tremor; grand mal seizures; headache; insomnia; euphoria; paresthesias; blurred vision; oculogyric crisis; torticollis; catatonic-like states; hallucinations; disorientation; tongue protrusion (usually in association with IV administration or excessive dosage); disturbing dreams/nightmares; pseudoschizophrenia; weakness; diplopia; vertigo; tinnitus; acute labyrinthitis; hysteria; neuritis; convulsions. Extrapyramidal reactions may occur with high doses; these reactions usually respond to dose reduction.

➤*GI:* Epigastric distress (most frequent, especially ethylenediamines); anorexia; increased appetite and weight gain; nausea; vomiting; diarrhea; constipation; stomatitis.

Nasal spray – Glossitis; ulcerative and aphthous stomatitis; increased ALT.

➤*GU:* Urinary frequency; dysuria; urinary retention; early menses; induced lactation; gynecomastia; inhibition of ejaculation.

➤*Hematologic:* Hemolytic anemia; hypoplastic anemia; aplastic anemia; thrombocytopenia; leukopenia; agranulocytosis; pancytopenia.

➤*Respiratory:* Thickening of bronchial secretions (most frequent); chest tightness; wheezing; nasal stuffiness; dry mouth, nose, and throat; sore throat; respiratory depression.

Nasal spray – Paroxysmal sneezing; rhinitis; epistaxis.

➤*Special senses:*

Nasal spray – Bitter taste (most frequent); conjunctivitis, eye abnormality, eye pain, watery eyes, taste loss, nasal burning.

➤*Miscellaneous:* Tingling, heaviness, and weakness of the hands; thrombocytopenic purpura; obstructive jaundice (usually reversible upon drug discontinuation); tissue necrosis following SC administration of IV promethazine; erythema; high or prolonged glucose tolerance curves; glycosuria; elevated spinal fluid proteins; elevation of plasma cholesterol levels; excessive perspiration; chills.

Nasal spray – Temporomandibular dislocation.

Adverse Events Greater Than Placebo for Peripherally Selective H₁ Antagonists (%)[1]				
Adverse reaction	Azelastine (n = 391)	Cetirizine (n = 2034)	Fexofenadine (n = 679)	Loratadine (n = 1926)
CNS				
Dizziness	2	2	—	—
Drowsiness/Somnolence	11.5	13.7	1.3	8
Fatigue	2.3	5.9	1.3	4
Headache	14.8	> 2	> 1	12
Weight increase	2	—	—	—
Ear, nose, throat				
Dry mouth, nose, throat	2.8	5	—	3
Pharyngitis	3.8	2	> 1	—
Epistaxis	2	—	—	—
GI				
Nausea, vomiting, abdominal distress, bowel changes	2.8	> 2	1.3 to 1.6	—
Miscellaneous				
Dysmenorrhea	—	—	1.5	—

[1] Data pooled from several studies and are not necessarily comparable.

➤*Phenothiazines:* These antihistamines infrequently cause typical phenothiazine adverse effects. See the Antipsychotic Agents monograph for a complete discussion.

Overdosage

➤*Symptoms:* Effects may vary from mild CNS depression (sedation, apnea, diminished mental alertness) and cardiovascular collapse to stimulation (insomnia, hallucinations, tremors, or convulsions), especially in children and geriatric patients. Profound hypotension, respiratory depression, unconsciousness, coma, and death may occur, particularly in infants and children. Convulsions rarely occur and indicate a poor prognosis. The convulsant dose lies near the lethal dose.

Toxic effects are seen within 30 minutes to 2 hours and result in drowsiness, dizziness, ataxia, tinnitus, blurred vision, and hypotension. Anticholinergic effects result in fixed dilated pupils, flushing, dry mouth, hyperthermia (especially in children), and fever. GI symptoms also may occur. Hyperpyrexia to 41.8°C (107°F) and acute oral and facial dystonic reactions have been reported.

Children often manifest CNS stimulation and may have hallucinations, toxic psychosis, delirium tremens, excitement, ataxia, incoordination, muscle twitching, athetosis, hyperthermia, cyanosis, convulsions, and hyperreflexia followed by postictal depression and cardiorespiratory arrest. Seizures resistant to therapy may follow and may be preceded by mild depression. A paradoxical reaction has been reported in children receiving single doses of 75 to 125 mg oral **promethazine,** characterized by hyperexcitability and nightmares. CNS stimulation in adults usually manifests as seizures. Marked cerebral irritation, resulting in jerking of muscles and possible convulsions, may be followed by deep stupor. Occasionally, respiratory depression, cardiovascular collapse, and death follows a latent period.

Less common findings include ECG changes, such as wandering pacemaker, prolonged QT interval, and nonspecific ST-T wave changes that disappear quickly. The EEG may show general cerebral dysrhythmia and diffuse delta wave activity that can persist after clinical recovery.

➤*Treatment:* Take adequate precautions to protect against aspiration, especially in infants and children. Administer activated charcoal as a slurry with water and a cathartic to minimize absorption. Correct acidosis and electrolyte imbalances. Do not induce emesis in unconscious patients. Gastric lavage is indicated within 3 hours after ingestion and even later if large amounts were taken. Isotonic or ½ isotonic saline is the lavage of choice, particularly for children. For adults, tap water can be used. Continue therapy directed at reversing the effects of timed-release medication and at supporting the patient. Hemoperfusion may be used in severe cases. **Cetirizine, fexofenadine,** and **loratadine** do not appear to be dialyzable. Refer to General Management of Acute Overdosage.

Hypotension is an early sign of impending cardiovascular collapse; treat vigorously using general supportive measures or specific vasopressor treatment (eg, norepinephrine, phenylephrine, dopamine). Avoid epinephrine; it may worsen hypotension. May use propranolol for refractory ventricular arrhythmias.

Administer 0.1 mg/kg IV diazepam slowly for convulsions; repeat as needed. IV physostigmine may reverse central anticholinergic effects. Use with caution. Avoid analeptics; they may cause convulsions. Depressant effects of **promethazine** are not reversed by naloxone.

Ice packs and cooling sponge baths, not alcohol, can help reduce a child's fever.

Patient Information

Inform physician of a history of glaucoma, peptic ulcer, urinary retention, or pregnancy before starting antihistamine therapy.

Some antihistamines may cause nervousness, insomnia, and dry mouth.

Some antihistamines may cause drowsiness or dizziness; observe caution while driving or performing other tasks requiring alertness, coordination, or physical dexterity. Avoid alcohol and other CNS depressants (eg, sedatives, hypnotics, tranquilizers, antianxiety agents).

Some antihistamines may cause GI upset; take with food.

Avoid prolonged exposure to sunlight; some agents may cause photosensitivity.

Do not crush or chew sustained release preparations.

➤*Phenothiazines:* Report any involuntary muscle movements or unusual sensitivity to sunlight.

Alkylamines, Nonselective

BROMPHENIRAMINE TANNATE

Rx	BrōveX CT (Athlon)	Tablets, chewable: 12 mg	Sucrose. (273). Yellow, oval, scored. Banana flavor. In 60s.
Rx	BrōveX (Athlon)	Oral suspension: 12 mg/5 mL	Methylparaben, saccharin, sucrose, tartrazine. Banana flavor. In 20 and 118 mL.

For complete prescribing information, refer to the Antihistamines group monograph.

Indications

▶*Allergies:* For the temporary relief of sneezing, itchy, watery eyes, itchy nose or throat, and runny nose caused by hay fever (allergic rhinitis), or other respiratory allergies.

Administration and Dosage

Administer the recommended dose every 12 hours. Shake suspension well before use.

▶*Adults and children 12 years of age and older:* 12 to 24 mg, not to exceed 48 mg in 24 hours.

▶*Children:*
6 to under 12 years of age – 6 to 12 mg, not to exceed 24 mg in 24 hours.

2 to under 6 years of age – 6 mg, not to exceed 12 mg in 24 hours.
12 months to 2 years –
  Oral suspension: 3 mg, not to exceed 6 mg in 24 hours. Dosage should be established by a physician for children under 12 months.
  Chewable tablets: Dosage should be established by a physician for children under 2 years of age.

▶*Storage/Stability:* Store at controlled room temperature, between 20° and 25°C (68° to 77°F). Dispense in a tight, light-resistant, and child-resistant container.

Precautions

▶*Tartrazine sensitivity:* This product contains tartrazine, which may cause allergic-type reactions (including bronchial asthma) in certain susceptible people. Although the overall incidence of tartrazine sensitivity in the general population is low, it is frequently seen in patients who also have aspirin hypersensitivity.

CHLORPHENIRAMINE MALEATE

otc	Chlorpheniramine Maleate (Various, eg, Contract Pharmacal, URL)	Tablets: 4 mg	In 24s, 100s, and 1000s.
otc	Aller-Chlor (Rugby)		In 24s and 1000s.
otc	Allergy (Major)		Lactose. In 24s and 100s.
otc	Allergy Relief (Zee Medical)		In 12s.
otc	Chlo-Amine (Hollister-Stier)	Tablets, chewable: 2 mg	Sugar. Orange flavor. In 96s.
otc	Chlor-Trimeton Allergy 8 Hour (Schering-Plough Healthcare)	Tablets, extended-release: 8 mg	(374). In 15s.
otc	Chlor-Trimeton Allergy 12 Hour (Schering-Plough Healthcare)	Tablets, extended-release: 12 mg	(009). In 10s.
otc	Efidac 24[1] (Hogil)	Tablets, extended-release: 16 mg	Mannitol. In 6s.
Rx	Chlorpheniramine Maleate (Various, eg, Qualitest)	Capsules, sustained-release: 8 mg	In 100s and 1000s.
Rx	Chlorpheniramine Maleate (Various, eg, Qualitest)	Capsules, sustained-release: 12 mg	In 100s and 1000s.
otc	Aller-Chlor (Rugby)	Syrup: 2 mg/5 mL	5% alcohol, parabens, sugar. In 118 mL.

[1] 4 mg immediate release, 12 mg controlled release.

For complete prescribing information, refer to the Antihistamines group monograph.

Indications

▶*Allergic rhinitis:* For the temporary relief of sneezing, itchy, watery eyes, itchy throat, and runny nose caused by hay fever and other upper respiratory allergies and the common cold.

Administration and Dosage

Individualize dosage.

▶*Tablets or syrup:*
Adults and children 12 years of age and older – 4 mg every 4 to 6 hours. Do not exceed 24 mg in 24 hours.
Children –
  6 to 12 years of age: 2 mg (break 4 mg tablets in half) every 4 to 6 hours. Do not exceed 12 mg in 24 hours.

Less than 6 years of age: Consult a doctor.
▶*Extended-release tablets:*
Adults and children 12 years of age and older – 8 mg every 8 to 12 hours or 12 mg every 12 hours. Do not exceed 24 mg in 24 hours.
Efidac –
  Adults and children 12 years of age and older: 16 mg with liquid every 24 hours. Do not exceed 16 mg in 24 hours. Swallow each tablet whole; do not divide, crush, chew, or dissolve.

▶*Sustained-release capsules:*
Adults and children 12 years of age and older – 8 or 12 mg every 12 hours, up to 16 to 24 mg/day.

Children 6 to 12 years of age – 8 mg at bedtime or during the day as indicated.

▶*Storage/Stability:* Store between 15° and 30°C (59° and 86°F).

DEXCHLORPHENIRAMINE MALEATE

Rx	Dexchlorpheniramine Maleate (Various, eg, Amide, URL)	Tablets, extended-release: 4 mg	In 100s and 1000s.
Rx	Dexchlorpheniramine Maleate (Various, eg, Amide, Breckenridge, URL)	Tablets, extended-release: 6 mg	In 100s and 1000s.

For complete prescribing information, refer to the Antihistamines group monograph.

Indications

▶*Hypersensitivity reactions, type I:* For the treatment of perennial and seasonal allergic rhinitis; vasomotor rhinitis; allergic conjunctivitis; mild, uncomplicated allergic skin manifestations of urticaria and angioedema; amelioration of allergic reactions to blood or plasma; dermographism; and adjunctive anaphylactic therapy.

Administration and Dosage

Individualize dosage.

▶*Adults and children 12 years of age and older:* 4 or 6 mg at bedtime or every 8 to 10 hours.

▶*Children 6 to 12 years of age:* 4 mg/day, preferably taken at bedtime.

▶*Storage/Stability:* Store between 2° and 30°C (36° and 86°F).

Alkylamines, Nonselective

TRIPROLIDINE HCl

Rx sf	Zymine (Vindex Pharmaceuticals)	Liquid: 1.25 mg/5 mL	Alcohol free. Apple flavor. In 15 and 473 mL.

For complete prescribing information, refer to the Antihistamines group monograph.

Indications

➤*Allergies:* For the symptomatic relief of perennial and seasonal allergic rhinitis, vasomotor rhinitis, allergic conjunctivitis caused by inhalant allergens and foods, and mild uncomplicated allergic skin manifestations of urticaria and angioedema.

Administration and Dosage

➤*Adults and children (12 years of age and older):* 10 mL every 4 to 6 hours, not to exceed 40 mL in 24 hours.

➤*Children:*

6 to 12 years of age – 5 mL every 4 to 6 hours, not to exceed 20 mL in 24 hours.

4 to 6 years of age – 3.75 mL every 4 to 6 hours, not to exceed 15 mL in 24 hours.

2 to 4 years of age – 2.5 mL every 4 to 6 hours, not to exceed 10 mL in 24 hours.

4 months to 2 years – 1.25 mL every 4 to 6 hours, not to exceed 5 mL in 24 hours.

➤*Storage/Stability:* Store between 15° to 30°C (59° to 86°F). Dispense in tight, light- and child-resistant containers.

Ethanolamines, Nonselective

CARBINOXAMINE MALEATE

Rx	Histex CT (Teamm Pharm[1])	Tablets, timed-release: 8 mg	(258). Blue, scored. Film-coated. In 30s and 100s.
Rx sf	Pediatex (Zyber Pharmaceuticals)	Liquid: 1.75 mg/5 mL	Alcohol and dye free. Cotton candy flavor. In 15 and 473 mL.
Rx sf	Histex Pd (Teamm Pharm[1])	Liquid: 4 mg/5 mL	Saccharin, sorbitol. Alcohol and dye free. Gum fruit flavor. In 473 mL.

[1] Teamm Pharmaceuticals, 3000 Aerial Center Parkway, Suite 110, Morrisville, NC 27560; 919-481-9020, 866-481-9020, fax 919-481-9311.

For complete prescribing information, refer to the Antihistamines group monograph.

Indications

➤*Allergic rhinitis:* For relief of nasal and nonnasal symptoms of seasonal and perennial allergic rhinitis.

Administration and Dosage

➤*Tablets:*

Adults and children 12 years of age and older – 1 tablet (8 mg) twice daily (every 12 hours).

Children 6 to 12 years of age – ½ tablet twice daily (every 12 hours).

The tablets are not recommended for children under 6 years of age. Tablets may be broken in half for ease of administration without affecting release of the medication, but should not be crushed or chewed prior to swallowing.

➤*Liquids:*

Histex Pd –

Adults and children 6 years of age and older: 5 mL 4 times/day.

Children:
• *18 months to 6 years of age* – 2.5 mL 4 times/day.
• *9 to 18 months of age* – 1.25 to 2.5 mL 4 times/day.

Pediatex –

Adults and children 6 years of age and older: 10 mL 4 times/day.

Children:
• *18 months to 6 years of age* – 5 mL 4 times/day.
• *9 to 18 months of age* – 3.75 to 5 mL 4 times/day.
• *6 to 9 months of age* – 3.75 mL 4 times/day.
• *3 to 6 months of age* – 2.5 mL 4 times/day.
• *1 to 3 months of age* – 1.25 mL 4 times/day.

➤*Storage/Stability:* Store between 15° and 30°C (59° to 86°F).

Warnings

➤*Pregnancy: Category C.* It is not known whether this product can cause fetal harm when administered to a pregnant woman or affect reproduction capacity. Administer to pregnant women only if clearly needed.

CLEMASTINE FUMARATE

otc	Clemastine Fumarate (Various, eg, Geneva)	Tablets: 1.34 mg as fumarate (equiv. to 1 mg clemastine)	In 100s.
otc	Dayhist-1 (Major)		Lactose. In 8s.
otc	Tavist Allergy (Novartis Consumer Health)		Lactose. (TAVIST ALLERGY). In 8s.
Rx	Clemastine Fumarate (Various, eg, Teva)	Tablets: 2.68 mg (equiv. to 2 mg clemastine)	In 100s.
Rx	Clemastine Fumarate (Various, eg, Apotex, Teva)	Syrup: 0.67 mg (equiv. to 0.5 mg clemastine)/5 mL	May contain alcohol. In 118 and 120.

For complete prescribing information, refer to the Antihistamines group monograph.

Indications

➤*Allergic rhinitis:* For the relief of symptoms associated with allergic rhinitis or other upper respiratory allergies, such as sneezing, rhinorrhea, pruritus, and lacrimation, in adults (tablets and syrup) and in children 6 to 12 years of age (syrup only).

➤*Urticaria/Angioedema:* For the relief of mild, uncomplicated allergic skin manifestations of urticaria and angioedema in adults (tablets and syrup) and in children 6 to 12 years of age (syrup only).

Administration and Dosage

Individualize dosage.

➤*Allergic rhinitis:*

Adults – 1.34 mg every 12 hours or twice daily. Dosage may be increased as needed. Do not exceed 8.04 mg/day for the syrup or 2.68 mg in 24 hours for the tablets.

Children 6 to 12 years of age (syrup only) – 0.67 mg twice daily. Dosage may be increased as needed. Single doses of up to 2.25 mg clemastine have been well tolerated. Do not exceed 4.02 mg/day.

➤*Urticaria/Angioedema:*

Adults – 2.68 mg twice daily, not to exceed 8.04 mg/day.

Children 6 to 12 years of age (syrup only) – 1.34 mg twice daily, not to exceed 4.02 mg/day.

➤*Storage/Stability:* Store between 15° and 30°C (59° to 86°F).

Ethanolamines, Nonselective

DIPHENHYDRAMINE HCl

otc	**Diphenhydramine** (Various, eg, Eon, Marlex)	**Tablets:** 25 mg	In 24s and 100s.
otc	**Banophen** (Major)		In 24s and 100s.
otc	**Genahist** (Goldline)		In 24s.
otc	**Benadryl Allergy Ultratabs** (Pfizer)		In 24s, 48s, and 100s.
otc	**Diphenhist Captabs** (Rugby)		Lactose. Capsule shape. In 100s.
otc	**AllerMax Caplets, Maximum Strength** (Pfeiffer)	**Tablets:** 50 mg	Lactose. In 24s.
otc	**Benadryl Allergy** (Pfizer)	**Tablets, chewable:** 12.5 mg	Aspartame, 4.2 mg phenylalanine. Grape flavor. In 24s.
otc/Rx[1]	**Diphenhydramine HCl** (Various, eg, Eon, Marlex, Major)	**Capsules:** 25 mg	In 24s, 100s, and 1000s.
otc	**Banophen** (Major)		In 24s and 100s.
otc	**Benadryl Allergy Kapseals** (Pfizer)		Lactose. In 24s and 48s.
otc	**Benadryl Dye-Free Allergy Liqui Gels** (Pfizer)		Sorbitol. In 24s.
otc	**Genahist** (Goldline)		Lactose, parabens. In 100s.
otc/Rx[1]	**Diphenhydramine HCl** (Various, eg, Eon, Major)	**Capsules:** 50 mg	In 100s and 1000s.
otc sf	**Genahist** (Goldline)	**Liquid:** 12.5 mg/5 mL	Alcohol free. Cherry flavor. In 118 mL.
otc sf	**Scot-Tussin Allergy Relief Formula Clear** (Scot-Tussin)		Menthol, parabens. Alcohol and dye free. Cherry-strawberry flavor. In 118 mL.
otc	**AllerMax** (Pfeiffer)		0.5% alcohol, glucose, saccharin, sorbitol, sucrose, menthol. Raspberry flavor. In 118 mL.
otc	**Benadryl Children's Allergy** (Pfizer)		Sugar. Alcohol free. Cherry flavor. In 118 and 236 mL.
otc sf	**Benadryl Children's Dye-Free Allergy** (Pfizer)		Saccharin, sorbitol. Alcohol free. Bubble gum flavor. In 118 mL.
otc	**Diphen AF** (Morton Grove)		Saccharin, sugar. Alcohol free. Cherry flavor. In 118, 237, and 473 mL.
otc	**Diphenhist** (Rugby)	**Oral solution:** 12.5 mg/5 mL	Saccharin, sucrose. Alcohol free. In 473 mL.
otc	**Banophen Allergy** (Major)	**Elixir:** 12.5 mg/5 mL	Sugar. In 118 mL.
otc	**Siladryl** (Silarx)		5.6% alcohol. Cherry flavor. In 118 mL.
Rx	**Tusstat** (Century)	**Syrup:** 12.5 mg/5 mL	5% alcohol. In 30, 118, and 473, and 3.8 L.
Rx	**Diphenhydramine HCl** (Various, eg, Abbott)	**Injection:** 50 mg/mL	In 1 mL fill in 2 mL cartridges.
Rx	**Benadryl** (Parke-Davis)		In 1 mL amps, 1 and 10 mL *Steri-vials*,[2] and 1 mL *Steri-dose* syringe.

[1] Products are available OTC or *Rx*, depending on product labeling.

[2] With benzethonium chloride.

For complete prescribing information, refer to the Antihistamines group monograph. For a complete listing of diphenhydramine sleep aids, see Nonprescription Sleep Aids in the CNS Agents chapter. For more information on Diphenhydramine as an Antitussive, see the Antitussive section of this chapter.

Indications

➤*Hypersensitivity reactions, type I:* Perennial and seasonal allergic rhinitis; vasomotor rhinitis and sneezing caused by the common cold; allergic conjunctivitis caused by inhalant allergens and foods; mild, uncomplicated allergic skin manifestations of urticaria and angioedema; amelioration of allergic reactions to blood or plasma in patients with a known history of such reactions; dermographism; as adjunctive anaphylactic therapy; for uncomplicated allergic conditions of the immediate type. Parenteral therapy also is indicated when oral therapy is impossible or contraindicated.

➤*Motion sickness (injection only):* For active treatment of motion sickness.

➤*Antiparkinsonism:* Parkinsonism in the elderly who are unable to tolerate more potent agents; mild cases of parkinsonism in other age groups; in other cases of parkinsonism in combination with centrally acting anticholinergic agents. Parenteral therapy is also indicated when oral therapy is impossible or contraindicated.

➤*Antitussive (syrup only):* Antitussive for control of coughs caused by colds or allergy.

➤*Unlabeled uses:* For antipsychotic-induced dystonia, diphenhydramine 50 mg IM or IV has been shown to be effective. Diphenhydramine also has been used as an antianxiety agent in doses of 25 to 200 mg/day.

Administration and Dosage

Individualize dosage.

➤*Hypersensitivity reactions, type I/Antiparkinsonism/Motion sickness:*

Oral –
Adults: 25 to 50 mg, every 4 to 6 hours. Maximum daily dosage is 300 mg.
Children 6 to under 12 years of age: 12.5 to 25 mg, every 4 to 6 hours. Maximum daily dosage is 150 mg.

Parenteral – Administer IV or deeply IM. The injectable form is indicated when the oral form is impractical.
Adults: 10 to 50 mg administered IV at a rate generally not exceeding 25 mg/min, or deep IM; 100 mg if required. Maximum daily dosage is 400 mg.
Children: 5 mg/kg/day or 150 mg/m^2/day. Maximum daily dosage is 300 mg divided into 4 doses administered IV at a rate generally not exceeding 25 mg/min, or deep IM.

➤*Antitussive (syrup only):*
Adults – 25 mg every 4 hours, not to exceed 150 mg in 24 hours.
Children –
6 to 12 years of age: 12.5 mg every 4 hours, not to exceed 75 mg in 24 hours.
2 to 6 years of age: 6.25 mg every 4 hours, not to exceed 25 mg in 24 hours.

➤*Storage/Stability:* Store at controlled room temperature, 15° to 30°C (59° to 86°F). Protect injection from freezing and light.

Phenothiazines, Nonselective

PROMETHAZINE HCl

Rx	**Phenergan** (Wyeth Labs)	**Tablets:** 12.5 mg	Lactose, saccharin. (Wyeth 19). Orange, scored. In 100s.
Rx	**Promethazine HCl** (Various, eg, Geneva)	**Tablets:** 25 mg	In 100s and 1000s.
Rx	**Phenergan** (Wyeth Labs)		Lactose, saccharin. (Wyeth 27). White, scored. In 100s and blister pack 100s.
Rx	**Promethazine HCl** (Various, eg, Geneva)	**Tablets:** 50 mg	In 100s.
Rx	**Phenergan** (Wyeth Labs)		Lactose. (Wyeth 227). Pink. In 100s.
Rx	**Promethazine HCl** (Various, eg, Morton Grove)	**Syrup:** 6.25 mg/5 mL	Alcohol. In 473 mL.
Rx	**Phenadoz** (Paddock)	**Suppositories:** 12.5 mg	Cocoa butter. In 12s.
Rx	**Phenergan** (Wyeth Labs)		Cocoa butter. In 12s.
Rx	**Promethazine HCl** (Alpharma)	**Suppositories:** 25 mg	Hard fat. In 12s.
Rx	**Phenadoz** (Paddock)		Cocoa butter. In 12s.
Rx	**Phenergan** (Wyeth Labs)		Cocoa butter. In 12s.
Rx	**Promethazine HCl** (Various, eg, Major)	**Suppositories:** 50 mg	In 12s.
Rx	**Phenergan** (Wyeth Labs)		Cocoa butter. In 12s.
Rx	**Promethazine HCl** (Various, eg, Abbott)	**Injection:** 25 mg/mL	May contain EDTA. In 1 mL amps.
Rx	**Phenergan** (Wyeth Labs)		EDTA, 0.25 mg/mL sodium metabisulfite. In 1 mL amps.
Rx	**Promethazine HCl** (Various, eg, Abbott)	**Injection:** 50 mg/mL	May contain EDTA. In 1 mL amps.
Rx	**Phenergan** (Wyeth Labs)		EDTA, 0.25 mg/mL sodium metabisulfite. In 1 mL amps.

For complete prescribing information, refer to the Antihistamines group monograph. For more information on Promethazine as an Antiemetic/Antivertigo agent, see the Antiemetic/Antivertigo monograph in the CNS Agents chapter.

Indications

➤*Hypersensitivity reactions, type* I: Perennial and seasonal allergic rhinitis; vasomotor rhinitis; allergic conjunctivitis caused by inhalant allergens and foods; mild, uncomplicated allergic skin manifestations of urticaria and angioedema; amelioration of allergic reactions to blood or plasma; dermographism; adjunctive anaphylactic therapy. Parenteral therapy is indicated when oral therapy is impossible or contraindicated.

➤*Sedation:* Preoperative, postoperative, or obstetric sedation; relief of apprehension and production of light sleep.

➤*Antiemetic:* Prevention and control of nausea and vomiting associated with certain types of anesthesia and surgery and in postoperative patients.

➤*Motion sickness (oral and rectal only):* Active and prophylactic treatment of motion sickness.

➤*Analgesia:* Adjunctive therapy for control of postoperative pain.

Administration and Dosage

The preferred parenteral route of administration is deep IM injection; properly administered IV doses are well tolerated, but this method is associated with increased hazard. IV administration should be at a concentration not to exceed 25 mg/mL at a rate no greater than 25 mg/min. Avoid SC and intra-arterial injection because tissue necrosis and gangrene can result.

Individualize dosage; after initiation, adjust to smallest effective dose.

➤*Hypersensitivity reactions, type* I:
Oral / Rectal – May be administered rectally or parenterally if the oral route is not feasible; however, resume oral administration as soon as possible if continued therapy is warranted.

Adults and children greater than 2 years of age: Usual dose is 25 mg at bedtime; 12.5 mg before meals and at bedtime may be given, if necessary. Single 25 mg doses at bedtime or 6.25 to 12.5 mg taken 3 times daily will usually suffice. The administration of promethazine HCl in 25 mg doses will control minor transfusion reactions of an allergic nature.

Parenteral –
Adults: 25 mg; may repeat dose within 2 hours if needed. Resume oral therapy as soon as patient's circumstances permit.

Children 2 years of age and older: Dose should not exceed half the adult dose.

➤*Sedation:*
Oral / Rectal – If used for preoperative sedation, administer the night before surgery to relieve apprehension and produce quiet sleep.

Adults: 25 to 50 mg at bedtime.

Children more than 2 years of age: 12.5 to 25 mg at bedtime.

Parenteral –
Adults: 25 to 50 mg at bedtime for nighttime sedation. Doses of 50 mg provide sedation and relieve apprehension during early stages of labor. When labor is definitely established, 25 to 75 mg (average dose, 50 mg) promethazine injection may be given IM or IV with an appropriately reduced dose of any desired narcotic. If necessary, promethazine injection with a reduced dose of analgesic may be repeated once or twice at 4-hour intervals. Do not exceed 100 mg/24 hours for patients in labor.

Children 2 to 12 years of age: Do not exceed half the adult dose.

➤*Antiemetic:*
Oral / Rectal –
Adults: Usual dose is 25 mg; doses of 12.5 to 25 mg may be repeated every 4 to 6 hours as needed for prophylaxis or treatment of active nausea/vomiting.

Children more than 2 years of age: Usual dose is 25 mg or 0.5 mg/lb; doses of 12.5 to 25 mg may be repeated every 4 to 6 hours as needed for prophylaxis or treatment of active nausea/vomiting. Adjust dose to the age, weight, and severity of condition for the patient being treated. Antiemetics are not recommended for treatment of uncomplicated vomiting in pediatric patients; limit use to prolonged vomiting of known etiology.

Parenteral –
Adults: Usual dose is 12.5 to 25 mg, may repeat every 4 hours as needed. If used postoperatively, reduce doses of concomitant analgesics or barbiturates accordingly.

Children 2 to 12 years of age: Do not exceed half the adult dose. Do not use when etiology of vomiting is unknown.

➤*Motion sickness (oral and rectal only):*
Adults – Usual dose is 25 mg twice daily; take first dose 30 to 60 minutes before anticipated travel; repeat 8 to 12 hours later if needed. On successive travel days, take 25 mg on rising and again before the evening meal.

Children more than 2 years of age – 12.5 to 25 mg twice daily.

➤*Pre- and postoperative use:*
Oral / Rectal –
Adults: For preoperative use, 25 to 50 mg administered with an appropriately reduced dose of narcotic or barbiturate and the required amount of a belladonna alkaloid.

Postoperative sedation and adjunctive use with analgesics may be obtained by the administration of 25 to 50 mg doses in adults.

Children more than 2 years of age: For preoperative use, 0.5 mg/lb in combination with an appropriately reduced dose of narcotic or barbiturate and the appropriate dose of an atropine-like drug.

Postoperative sedation and adjunctive use with analgesics may be obtained by the administration of 12.5 to 25 mg in children.

Parenteral –
Adults: 25 to 50 mg in combination with appropriately reduced doses of analgesics, hypnotics, and atropine-like drugs as appropriate.

Children 2 to 12 years of age: 0.5 mg/lb in combination with an appropriately reduced dose of narcotic or barbiturate and the appropriate dose of an atropine-like drug.

➤*Use in children:* Exercise caution when administering promethazine to pediatric patients 2 years of age and older because of the potential for fatal respiratory depression. Antiemetics are not recommended for treatment of uncomplicated vomiting in pediatric patients; limit use to prolonged vomiting of known etiology. The extrapyramidal symptoms that can occur secondary to promethazine administration may be confused with the CNS signs of undiagnosed primary disease (eg, encephalopathy, Reye's syndrome). Avoid the use of promethazine in pediatric patients whose signs and symptoms may suggest Reye's syndrome or other hepatic diseases.

➤*Storage / Stability:*
Tablets – Store at controlled room temperature 20° to 25°C (68° to 77°F). Protect from light and dispense in a tight, light-resistant container.

Syrup – Store at controlled room temperature 15° to 25°C (59° to 77°F).

Suppositories – Store refrigerated between 2° and 8°C (36° and 46°F).

Phenothiazines, Nonselective

PROMETHAZINE HCl

Dispense in a well-closed container.

Injection – Store at controlled room temperature 20° to 25°C (68° to 77°F). Protect from light. Keep covered in carton until time of use. Do not use if solution has developed color or contains a precipitate.

Contraindications

Comatose patients; CNS depression from large amounts of barbiturates, general anesthetics, tranquilizers, alcohol, narcotics, or narcotic analgesics; previous promethazine or phenothiazine hypersensitivity or idiosyncrasy; intra-arterial or SC injection. Antihistamines are contraindicated for use in the treatment of lower respiratory tract symptoms including asthma.

Piperazines, Nonselective

HYDROXYZINE

Rx	Hydroxyzine HCl (Various, eg, Sidmak, URL)	**Tablets:** 10 mg (as HCl)	In 100s, 500s, and 1000s.
Rx	Hydroxyzine HCl (Various, eg, Sidmak, URL)	**Tablets:** 25 mg (as HCl)	In 100s, 500s, and 1000s.
Rx	Hydroxyzine HCl (Various, eg, Sidmak, URL)	**Tablets:** 50 mg (as HCl)	In 100s, 500s, and 1000s.
Rx	Hydroxyzine Pamoate (Various, eg, Barr, IVAX, URL)	**Capsules:** 25 mg (as pamoate)[1]	In 100s, 500s, 1000s, and UD 100s.
Rx	Vistaril (Pfizer)		Sucrose. Two-tone green. In 100s.
Rx	Hydroxyzine Pamoate (Various, eg, Barr, IVAX, URL)	**Capsules:** 50 mg (as pamoate)[1]	In 100s, 500s, 1000s, and UD 100s.
Rx	Vistaril (Pfizer)		Sucrose. Green/white. In 100s.
Rx	Hydroxyzine Pamoate (Various, eg, Barr)	**Capsules:** 100 mg (as pamoate)[1]	In 100s, 500s, and 1000s.
Rx	Vistaril (Pfizer)		Sucrose. Green/gray. In 100s.
Rx	Hydroxyzine HCl (Various, eg, Alpharma, Hi-Tech Pharmacal, Morton Grove, URL)	**Syrup:** 10 mg/5 mL (as HCl)	May contain alcohol. In 118 and 473 mL.
Rx	Vistaril (Pfizer)	**Oral suspension:** 25 mg/5 mL (as pamoate)[1]	Sorbitol. Lemon flavor. In 120 and 473 mL.
Rx	Hydroxyzine HCl (Various, eg, Abbott, American Pharmaceutical Partners, American Regent)	**Injection:** 25 mg/mL (as HCl)	May contain benzyl alcohol. In 1 and 2 mL vials.
Rx	Hydroxyzine HCl (Various, eg, Abbott, American Pharmaceutical Partners, American Regent)	**Injection:** 50 mg/mL (as HCl)	May contain benzyl alcohol. In 1, 2, and 10 mL vials.

[1] Hydroxyzine pamoate is equivalent to hydroxyzine.

For complete prescribing information, refer to the Antihistamines group monograph and the individual monograph in Antianxiety Agents.

Indications

➤*Pruritus:* In the management of pruritus caused by allergic conditions such as chronic urticaria and atopic or contact dermatoses and in histamine-mediated pruritus; parenterally as adjunctive therapy in allergic conditions with strong emotional overlay, such as asthma, chronic urticaria, and pruritus.

➤*Sedation (oral only):* As a sedative when used as premedication and following general anesthesia.

➤*Analgesia, adjunctive therapy (parenteral only):* As adjunctive pre- and postoperative or pre- and postpartum medication to permit reduction in narcotic dosage.

➤*Antiemetic (parenteral only):* Effective in controlling nausea and vomiting, excluding nausea and vomiting associated with pregnancy.

In addition to the above listed indications, hydroxyzine is used for management of anxiety, tension, and psychomotor agitation in conditions of emotional stress. Refer to the individual monograph in Antianxiety Agents section for complete prescribing information.

Administration and Dosage

➤*Approved by the FDA:* April 1956.

Individualize dosage. Start patients on IM therapy only when indicated; maintain on oral therapy whenever possible.

Hydroxyzine injection is for deep IM administration only and may be given without further dilution. Avoid IV, SC, or intra-arterial administration. The preferred site of administration for adults is the upper, outer quadrant of the buttock or the mid-lateral thigh. For children, it is preferable to administer in the mid-lateral thigh; for infants and small children, use the periphery of the upper, outer quadrant of the gluteal region only when necessary, such as in burn patients, to minimize the possibility of damage to the sciatic nerve. The deltoid area should be used only if well developed such as in certain adults and older children, and then only with caution to avoid radial nerve injury. Do not make IM injections into the lower and mid-third of the upper arm.

➤*Pruritus:*
Oral –
  Adults: 25 mg 3 or 4 times/day.
  Children:
  • *More than 6 years of age* – 50 to 100 mg/day in divided doses.
  • *Less than 6 years of age* – 50 mg/day in divided doses.

Parenteral –
  Adults only: 25 mg 3 to 4 times/day.

➤*Sedation (oral only):*

Adults – 50 to 100 mg as premedication or following general anesthesia. Hydroxyzine may potentiate concomitant narcotics (eg, meperidine), nonnarcotic analgesics, and barbiturates; reduce dosages accordingly. Atropine and other belladonna alkaloids may be given as appropriate.

Children – 0.6 mg/kg.

➤*Antiemetic/Analgesia, adjunctive therapy (parenteral only):*

Adults – 25 to 100 mg IM as an antiemetic and as pre- and postoperative and pre- and postpartum adjunctive medication to permit reduction of narcotic dosage and control emesis. Reduce dosage of concomitant CNS depressants and narcotics by as much as 50%.

Children – 0.5 mg/lb body weight IM as an antiemetic and as pre- and postoperative adjunctive therapy to permit reduction of narcotic dosage and control emesis. Reduce dosage of concomitant CNS depressants and narcotics by as much as 50%.

➤*Storage/Stability:* Store injection below 86°F (30°C); protect from freezing.

Oral suspension – Shake vigorously until product is completely resuspended. Store oral dosage forms at controlled room temperature 15° to 30°C (59° to 86°F). Dispense in a tight, light-resistant container.

CYPROHEPTADINE HCl

Rx	Cyproheptadine HCl (Various, eg, Par, IVAX)	**Tablets:** 4 mg	In 100s and 1000s.
Rx	Cyproheptadine HCl (Various, eg, Alpharma)	**Syrup:** 2 mg/5 mL	Alcohol. In 473 mL.

For complete prescribing information, refer to the Antihistamines group monograph.

Indications

➤*Hypersensitivity reactions, type* I: Perennial and seasonal allergic rhinitis; vasomotor rhinitis; allergic conjunctivitis caused by inhalant allergens and foods; mild, uncomplicated allergic skin manifestations of urticaria and angioedema; amelioration of allergic reactions to blood or plasma; cold urticaria; dermographism; adjunctive anaphylactic therapy.

Administration and Dosage

➤*Approved by the FDA:* August 1961.

Individualize dosage.

➤*Adults:* 4 to 20 mg daily. Initiate therapy with 4 mg 3 times daily. Most patients require 12 to 16 mg/day and occasionally as much as 32 mg/day. Do not exceed 0.5 mg/kg/day.

➤*Children:* Calculate total daily dosage as approximately 0.25 mg/kg/day or 8 mg/m^2.

7 to 14 years of age – 4 mg 2 or 3 times daily. Do not exceed 16 mg/day.

2 to 6 years of age – 2 mg 2 or 3 times daily. Do not exceed 12 mg/day.

➤*Storage/Stability:* Store at controlled room temperature, 15° to 30°C (59° to 86°F), in a well-closed container.

PHENINDAMINE TARTRATE

otc	Nolahist (Amarin)	**Tablets:** 25 mg	Alcohol and dye free. In 24s and 100s.

For complete prescribing information, refer to the Antihistamines group monograph.

Indications

➤*Allergic rhinitis:* For the temporary relief of runny nose, sneezing, itching of the nose or throat, and itchy, watery eyes caused by hay fever or other upper respiratory allergic rhinitis.

Administration and Dosage

➤*Adults and children 12 years of age and older:* 25 mg every 4 to 6 hours. Do not exceed 150 mg in 24 hours.

➤*Children:*

6 to under 12 years of age – 12.5 mg (½ tablet) every 4 to 6 hours. Do not exceed 75 mg in 24 hours.

Less than 6 years of age – Consult a doctor.

➤*Storage/Stability:* Store at 15° to 30°C (59° to 86°F). Keep in a tight, light-resistant container.

AZELASTINE HCl

Rx	Astelin (Wallace Laboratories)	**Nasal spray:** 137 mcg/spray	Benzalkonium chloride, EDTA. 17 mg (100 metered sprays) per bottle. In 2s.

For complete prescribing information, refer to the Antihistamines group monograph.

Indications

➤*Seasonal allergic rhinitis:* For treatment of symptoms of seasonal allergic rhinitis, such as rhinorrhea, sneezing, and nasal pruritus in adults and children 5 years of age and older.

➤*Vasomotor rhinitis:* For treatment of the symptoms of vasomotor rhinitis, such as rhinorrhea, nasal congestion, and postnasal drip in adults and children 12 years of age and older.

Administration and Dosage

➤*Approved by the FDA:* October 1996.

Before initial use, replace the screw cap on the bottle with the pump unit and prime the delivery system with 4 sprays or until a fine mist appears. When 3 days or more have elapsed since last use, reprime the pump with 2 sprays or until a fine mist appears.

➤*Seasonal allergic rhinitis:*

Adults and children 12 years of age and older – 2 sprays per nostril twice daily.

Children 5 to 11 years of age – 1 spray per nostril twice daily.

➤*Vasomotor rhinitis:*

Adults and children 12 years of age and older – 2 sprays per nostril twice daily.

➤*Storage/Stability:* Store at controlled room temperature 20° to 25°C (68° to 77°F). Protect from freezing.

Piperazine, Peripherally-selective

CETIRIZINE HCl

Rx	Zyrtec (Pfizer)	Tablets: 5 mg	Lactose. (Zyrtec 5). White, rectangular. Film coated. In 100s.
		10 mg	Lactose. (Zyrtec 10). White, rectangular. Film coated. In 100s.
		Tablets, chewable: 5 mg	Lactose. (ZYRTEC C5). Purple. In 30s.
		10 mg	Lactose. (ZYRTEC C10). Purple. In 30s.
		Syrup: 5 mg/5 mL	Parabens, sugar. Banana-grape flavor. In 120 and 473 mL.

For complete prescribing information, refer to the Antihistamines group monograph.

Indications

➤*Seasonal allergic rhinitis:* For the relief of symptoms associated with seasonal allergic rhinitis caused by allergens such as ragweed, grass, and tree pollens in adults and children 2 years of age and older. Symptoms treated effectively include sneezing, rhinorrhea, nasal pruritus, ocular pruritus, tearing, and redness of the eyes.

➤*Perennial allergic rhinitis:* For the relief of symptoms associated with perennial allergic rhinitis caused by allergens such as dust mites, animal dander, and molds in adults and children 6 months of age and older. Symptoms treated effectively include sneezing, rhinorrhea, postnasal discharge, nasal pruritus, ocular pruritus, and tearing.

➤*Chronic idiopathic urticaria:* For the treatment of the uncomplicated skin manifestations of chronic idiopathic urticaria in adults and children 6 months of age and older. It significantly reduces the occurrence, severity, and duration of hives and significantly reduces pruritus.

Administration and Dosage

➤*Approved by the FDA:* December 12, 1995.

➤*Adults and children 12 years of age and older:* 5 or 10 mg once daily depending on symptom severity. May be given with or without food.

➤*Children:*

6 to 11 years of age – 5 or 10 mg once daily depending on symptom severity.

2 to 5 years of age – 2.5 mg once daily. The dosage in this age group can be increased to a maximum dose of 5 mg/day given as 5 mg once daily or as 2.5 mg given every 12 hours.

6 months up to 2 years of age – 2.5 mg once daily. The dose in children 12 to 23 months of age can be increased to a maximum dose of 5 mg/day given as 2.5 mg every 12 hours.

➤*Renal/Hepatic function impairment:* In patients 12 years of age and older with decreased renal function (Ccr 11 to 31 mL/min), hemodialysis patients (Ccr less than 7 mL/min), and in hepatically impaired patients, 5 mg once daily is recommended. Similarly, pediatric patients 6 to 11 years of age with impaired renal or hepatic function should use the lower recommended dose. Because of the difficulty in reliably administering doses of less than 2.5 mg of syrup and in the absence of pharmacokinetic and safety information in children below 6 years of age with impaired renal or hepatic function, its use in this impaired patient population is not recommended.

➤*Storage/Stability:* Store at 20° to 25°C (68° to 77°F); excursions permitted to 15° to 30°C (59° to 86°F). Syrup can also be refrigerated at 2° to 8°C (36° to 46°F).

Contraindications

In addition to those described in the group monograph, the use of cetirizine is contraindicated in patients with hypersensitivity to hydroxyzine.

Piperidines, Peripherally-selective

DESLORATADINE

Rx	Clarinex (Schering)	Tablets: 5 mg	Lactose. (C5). Lt. blue. Film coated. In 100s, 500s, unit-of-use 30s, and UD hospital pack 100s.
Rx	Clarinex RediTabs (Schering)	Tablets, rapidly disintegrating: 5 mg	Mannitol, aspartame, phenylalanine.[1] (C). Pink. Tutti frutti flavor. In 30s.

[1] Contains 1.75 mg phenylalanine per tablet.

For complete prescribing information, refer to the Antihistamines group monograph.

Indications

➤*Allergic rhinitis:* For the relief of the nasal and nonnasal symptoms of seasonal and perennial allergic rhinitis in patients 12 years of age and older.

➤*Chronic idiopathic urticaria:* Symptomatic relief of pruritus and reduction in the number and size of hives in patients 12 years of age and older.

Administration and Dosage

➤*Approved by the FDA:* December 21, 2001.

➤*Adults and children 12 years of age and older:* The recommended dose is 5 mg once daily. In patients with liver or renal impairment, a starting dose of one 5 mg tablet every other day is recommended based on pharmacokinetic data.

Place rapidly disintegrating tablets on the tongue immediately after opening the blister; tablet disintegration occurs rapidly. Administer with or without water.

➤*Storage/Stability:* Protect tablet unit-of-use packaging and UD hospital packs from excessive moisture. Store at 2° to 25°C (36° to 77°F). Heat sensitive; avoid exposure at or above 30°C (86°F).

Store disintegrating tablets at 25°C (77°F); excursions permitted between 15° to 30°C (59° to 86°F).

FEXOFENADINE HCl

Rx	Allegra (Aventis)	Tablets: 30 mg	(03 0088 or 03 E). Peach. Film-coated. In 100s and 500s.
		60 mg	(06 0088 or 06 E). Peach. Film-coated. In 100s, 500s, and blister pack 100s.
		180 mg	(018 0088 or 018 E). Peach. Film-coated. In 100s and 500s.
		Capsules: 60 mg	Lactose. (Allegra 60 mg). White opaque/pink opaque. In 60s, 100s, 500s, and blister pack 100s.

For complete prescribing information, refer to the Antihistamines group monograph.

Indications

➤*Seasonal allergic rhinitis:* For the relief of symptoms associated with seasonal allergic rhinitis in adults and children 6 years of age and older. Symptoms include sneezing; rhinorrhea; itchy nose, palate, and throat; and itchy, watery, and red eyes.

➤*Chronic idiopathic urticaria:* For the treatment of uncomplicated skin manifestations of chronic idiopathic urticaria in adults and children 6 years of age and older. It significantly reduces pruritus and the number of wheals.

Administration and Dosage

➤*Approved by the FDA:* July 25, 1995.

➤*Seasonal allergic rhinitis:*

Adults and children 12 years of age and older – 60 mg twice daily or 180 mg once daily.

Children 6 to 11 years of age – 30 mg twice daily.

➤*Chronic idiopathic urticaria:*

Adults and children 12 years of age and older – 60 mg twice daily.

Children 6 to 11 years of age – 30 mg twice daily.

➤*Renal function impairment:*

Adults and children 12 years of age and older – 60 mg once daily as a starting dose.

Children 6 to 11 years of age – 30 mg once daily as a starting dose.

➤*Storage/Stability:* Store capsules and tablets at controlled room temperature 20° to 25°C (68° to 77°F). Protect from excessive moisture.

Piperidines, Peripherally-selective

LORATADINE

otc	**Loratadine** (Geneva)	**Tablets:** 10 mg	In 100s.
otc	**Claritin** (Schering)		Lactose. (458/Claritin 10). White to off-white. In 100s and 500s, unit-of-use 30s, and UD 100s.
otc	**Claritin Non-Drowsy Allergy** (Schering-Plough)		In 10s and 20s.
otc	**Tavist ND** (Novartis)		Lactose. In 30s.
otc	**Alavert** (Wyeth Consumer)	**Tablets, orally disintegrating:** 10 mg	Aspartame, corn syrup, mannitol, 8.4 mg phenylalanine. In 12s, 24s, and 48s.
otc	**Claritin Reditabs** (Schering)	**Tablets, rapidly disintegrating:** 10 mg	Mannitol. (C). White to off-white. Mint flavor. In unit-of-use 30s.
otc	**Claritin** (Schering)	**Syrup:** 1 mg/mL	Sugar, EDTA. In 480 mL.

For complete prescribing information, refer to the Antihistamines group monograph.

Indications

➤*Allergic rhinitis:* For the relief of nasal and nonnasal symptoms of seasonal allergic rhinitis.

➤*Unlabeled uses:* For the treatment of chronic idiopathic urticaria in patients 2 years of age and older.

Administration and Dosage

➤*Approved by the FDA:* April 12, 1993.

➤*Adults and children 6 years of age and older:* 10 mg once daily.

➤*Children 2 to 5 years of age:* 5 mg (5 mL) syrup once daily.

➤*Hepatic/Renal function impairment (GFR less than 30 mL/min):*

Adults and children 6 years of age and older – 10 mg every other day as starting dose.

Children 2 to 5 years of age – 5 mg every other day as starting dose.

➤*Rapidly disintegrating tablets:* Place tablets on the tongue. Tablet disintegration occurs rapidly. Administer with or without water.

Use within 6 months of opening laminated foil pouch and immediately upon opening individual tablet blister.

➤*Storage/Stability:* Protect unit dose packs, unit-of-use packs, and rapidly disintegrating tablets from excessive moisture. Store tablets between 2° and 30°C (36° and 86°F). Store syrup and rapidly disintegrating tablets between 2° and 25°C (36° and 77°F).

ANTIHISTAMINE COMBINATIONS

ANTIHISTAMINE COMBINATIONS

Rx	**Poly-Histine** (Sanofi-Synthelabo)	**Elixir:** 4 mg phenyltoloxamine citrate, 4 mg pyrilamine maleate, 4 mg pheniramine maleate/5 mL	4% alcohol. Lemon-lime flavor. In 473 mL.

Indications

For perennial and seasonal allergic rhinitis; vasomotor rhinitis; allergic conjunctivitis caused by inhalant allergens and food; and mild, uncomplicated allergic skin manifestations of urticaria.

Administration and Dosage

➤*Adults 12 years of age and older:* 10 mL every 4 hours.

➤*Children:*

6 to 12 years of age – 5 mL every 4 hours.

2 to 6 years of age – 2.5 mL every 4 hours.

Under 2 years of age – Use only as directed by the physician.

➤*Storage/Stability:* Store at 25°C (77°F); excursions permitted to 15° to 30°C (59° to 86°F). Dispense in tight, light-resistant containers.

Precautions

Caution patients against mechanical activities requiring alertness, such as driving an automobile or working with machinery.

Adverse Reactions

Drowsiness, nervousness, dry mouth and throat, headaches, dizziness, paresthesia, and nausea.

BENZONATATE

Rx	**Benzonatate Softgels** (Various, eg, Inwood, Sidmak)	**Capsules:** 100 mg	In 100s and 500s.
Rx	**Tessalon Perles** (Forest)		Parabens. (T). Yellow. In 100s and 500s.
Rx	**Benzonatate Softgels** (Various, eg, Inwood)	**Capsules:** 200 mg	In 100s and 500s.
Rx	**Tessalon** (Forest)		Parabens. (0698). Yellow. In 100s and 500s.

Indications

Symptomatic relief of cough.

Administration and Dosage

➤*Adults and children 10 years of age and older:* 100 to 200 mg 3 times/day, up to 600 mg/day.

➤*Storage/Stability:* Store at controlled room temperature 15° to 30°C (59° to 86°F).

Actions

➤*Pharmacology:* Benzonatate is related to anesthetic agents of the para-amino-benzoic class (eg, tetracaine). It anesthetizes stretch receptors in respiratory passages, lungs, and pleura, dampening their activity, and reducing the cough reflex at its source. It has no inhibitory effect on the respiratory center in recommended dosage. Onset of action is 15 to 20 minutes; effects last 3 to 8 hours.

Contraindications

Hypersensitivity to benzonatate or related compounds (eg, tetracaine).

Warnings

➤*Behavior changes:* Isolated instances of bizarre behavior, including mental confusion and visual hallucinations, have been reported in patients taking benzonatate in combination with other prescribed drugs.

➤*Hypersensitivity reactions:* Severe hypersensitivity reactions (eg, bronchospasm, laryngospasm, cardiovascular collapse) have been reported that are possibly related to local anesthesia from sucking or chewing the capsule instead of swallowing it. Severe reactions have required intervention with vasopressor agents and supportive measures.

➤*Pregnancy: Category C.* It is not known whether the drug can cause fetal harm or can affect reproduction capacity. Give to a pregnant woman only if clearly needed.

➤*Lactation:* It is not known whether this drug is excreted in breast milk. Exercise caution when administering to a nursing woman.

➤*Children:* Safety and efficacy in children below 10 years of age have not been established.

Precautions

➤*CNS effects:* Benzonatate is chemically related to anesthetic agents of the para-amino-benzoic acid class (eg, procaine, tetracaine) and has been associated with adverse CNS effects possibly related to a prior sensitivity to related agents or interaction with concomitant medication.

➤*Local anesthesia:* Release of benzonatate in the mouth can produce a temporary local anesthesia of the oral mucosa and choking could occur. Swallow the capsules without chewing.

Adverse Reactions

Sedation; headache; dizziness; mental confusion; visual hallucinations; constipation; nausea; GI upset; pruritus; skin eruptions; nasal congestion; sensation of burning in the eyes; vague "chilly" sensation; chest numbness; hypersensitivity (eg, bronchospasm, laryngospasm, cardiovascular collapse; see Warnings).

Overdosage

Rare instances of deliberate or accidental overdose have resulted in death.

➤*Symptoms:* If capsules are chewed or dissolved in the mouth, oropharyngeal anesthesia will develop rapidly. CNS stimulation may cause restlessness and tremors that may proceed to clonic convulsions followed by profound CNS depression.

➤*Treatment:* Includes usual supportive measures. Refer to General Management of Acute Overdosage. Evacuate gastric contents and administer copious amounts of activated charcoal slurry. Even in the conscious patient, cough and gag reflexes may be so depressed as to necessitate protection against aspiration of gastric contents and orally administered materials.

Treat convulsions with IV short-acting barbiturate and titrate to the smallest effective dosage. Employ intensive support of respiration and cardiovascular-renal function if required. Do not use CNS stimulants.

Patient Information

Do not chew or suck capsules; swallow whole.

DEXTROMETHORPHAN HBr

otc	**Robitussin CoughGels** (Wyeth)	**Gelcaps:** 15 mg	Liquid-filled. Sorbitol. In 20s.
otc	**DexAlone** (DexGen)	**Gelcaps:** 30 mg	Liquid-filled. Sorbitol. In 30s.
otc	**Hold DM** (B. F. Ascher)	**Lozenges:** 5 mg	Sucrose, corn syrup. Original and cherry flavor. In 10s.
otc sf	**Scot-Tussin DM Cough Chasers** (Scot-tussin)		Peppermint oil, sorbitol. Dye-free. In 20s.
otc	**Trocal** (Textilease)	**Lozenges:** 7.5 mg	Cherry flavor. In 10s, 50s, and 500s.
otc	**Simply Cough** (McNeil-PPC)	**Liquid:** 5 mg/5 mL	Corn syrup, sucralose. Alcohol-free. Cherry berry flavor. In 120 mL.
otc sf	**Benylin Pediatric** (Pfizer)	**Liquid:** 7.5 mg/5 mL	Alcohol free. Saccharin, sorbitol. Grape flavor. In 118 mL.
otc	**Creo-Terpin** (Lee)	**Liquid:** 10 mg/15 mL (3.33 mg/5 mL)	Tartrazine, 25% alcohol, corn syrup, saccharin. In 120 mL.
otc sf	**Benylin Adult** (Pfizer)	**Liquid:** 15 mg/5 mL	Alcohol free. Saccharin, sorbitol. In 118 mL.
otc	**Robitussin Maximum Strength Cough** (Whitehall-Robins)		1.4% alcohol, glucose, corn syrup, saccharin. Cherry flavor. In 118 and 237 mL.
otc	**Vicks 44 Cough Relief** (Procter and Gamble)	**Liquid:** 10 mg/5 mL	31 mg sodium/15 mL, alcohol, corn syrup, saccharin. In 118 mL.
otc sf	**Robitussin Pediatric Cough** (Whitehall-Robins)	**Syrup:** 7.5 mg/5 mL	Alcohol free. Saccharin, sorbitol. Cherry flavor. In 118 mL.
otc	**Silphen DM** (Silarx)	**Syrup:** 10 mg/5 mL	5% alcohol, menthol, methylparaben, sucrose. In 118 mL.
otc	**Delsym** (Celltech)	**Oral suspension, extended-release:** Dextromethorphan polistirex equivalent to 30 mg dextromethorphan HBr/5mL.	0.26% alcohol and 5 mg sodium/5 mL, corn syrup, sucrose, parabens. Orange flavor. In 89 mL.

Indications

Temporarily relieves cough caused by minor throat and bronchial irritation as may occur with the common cold or inhaled irritants.

Administration and Dosage

➤*Gelcaps:*

Adults and children 12 years of age and older – 30 mg every 6 to 8 hours. Do not exceed 120 mg in 24 hours. Do not use in children less than 12 years of age.

DEXTROMETHORPHAN HBr

➤*Lozenges:*
Adults and children 12 years of age and older – 5 to 15 mg every 1 to 4 hours up to 120 mg/day.

Children 6 to under 12 years of age – 5 to 10 mg every 1 to 4 hours up to 60 mg/day. Do not give to children under 6 years of age unless directed by a physician.

➤*Liquid and syrup:*
Adults and children 12 years of age and older – 10 to 20 mg every 4 hours or 30 mg every 6 to 8 hours up to 120 mg/day.

Children –
6 to under 12 years of age: 15 mg every 6 to 8 hours up to 60 mg/day.
2 to under 6 years of age: 7.5 mg every 6 to 8 hours up to 30 mg/day.

➤*Extended-release suspension:*
Adults and children 12 years of age and older – 60 mg every 12 hours up to 120 mg/day.

Children –
6 to under 12 years of age: 30 mg every 12 hours up to 60 mg/day.
2 to under 6 years of age: 15 mg every 12 hours up to 30 mg/day.

➤*Storage/Stability:* Store at controlled room temperature (15° to 30°C; 59° to 86°F).

Actions

➤*Pharmacology:* Dextromethorphan is the d-isomer of the codeine analog of levorphanol; it lacks analgesic and addictive properties. Its cough suppressant action is due to a central action on the cough center in the medulla. Dextromethorphan 15 to 30 mg equals 8 to 15 mg codeine as an antitussive.

➤*Pharmacokinetics:* Dextromethorphan is rapidly absorbed from the GI tract. It undergoes metabolism in the liver and is then excreted in the urine as unchanged drug and demethylated metabolites.

Contraindications

Hypersensitivity to any component.

Warnings

➤*Use:* For persistent or chronic cough (eg, smoking, asthma, emphysema) or cough accompanied by excessive secretions, consult a doctor before use. If cough persists for more than 1 week, tends to recur, or is accompanied by fever, rash, or persistent headache, consult a physician. These could be signs of a serious condition.

➤*Pregnancy: Category C.*

➤*Lactation:* It is not known if dextromethorphan is excreted in breast milk.

Precautions

➤*Drug abuse and dependence:* Anecdotal reports of abuse of dextromethorphan-containing cough/cold products has increased, especially among teenagers. Additional data is needed before determining the abuse and dependency potential of dextromethorphan.

➤*Tartrazine sensitivity:* Some of these products contain tartrazine, which may cause allergic-type reactions (including bronchial asthma) in certain susceptible people. Although the overall incidence of tartrazine sensitivity in the general population is low, it is frequently seen in patients who also have aspirin hypersensitivity.

Drug Interactions

Dextromethorphan Drug Interactions			
Precipitant drug	Object drug *		Description
MAOIs	Dextromethorphan	↑	Hyperpyrexia, abnormal muscle movement, hypotension, coma, and death have been associated with concurrent use. Avoid coadministration and avoid use for 2 weeks after stopping the MAOI.
Quinidine	Dextromethorphan	↑	Plasma dextromethorphan levels may be elevated because of quinidine inhibiting the metabolism of dextromethrophan (via CYP 2D6). Increased toxic effects may develop. Reduce dose if needed.
Sibutramine	Dextromethorphan	↑	A "serotonin syndrome," including CNS irritability, motor weakness, shivering, myoclonus, and altered consciousness, may occur because of additive serotonergic effects. Coadministration is not recommended.

Adverse Reactions

Adverse reactions may include dizziness, drowsiness, and GI disturbances.

Overdosage

➤*Symptoms:*
Adults – Altered sensory perception; ataxia; slurred speech; dysphoria.

Children – Ataxia, respiratory depression; convulsions.

DIPHENHYDRAMINE HCl

otc	**AllerMax** (Pfeiffer)	**Liquid:** 12.5 mg/5 mL	0.5% alcohol, glucose, saccharin, sorbitol, sucrose, menthol. Raspberry flavor. In 118 mL.
otc/Rx[1]	**Hydramine Cough** (Various, eg, Alpharma)	**Syrup:** 12.5 mg/5 mL	May contain alcohol. In 473 mL.
otc	**Silphen Cough** (Silarx)		Menthol, parabens, sucrose, 5% alcohol. Strawberry flavor. In 118 mL.
Rx	**Tusstat** (Century)		5% alcohol. In 30, 120, 473, and 3.8 L.

[1] Products are available OTC or *Rx*, depending on product labeling.

Refer to the Antihistamines group monograph for complete prescribing information. Also refer to the Diphenhydramine HCl monograph in the Antihistamines section.

Indications

For the control of cough caused by colds, allergy, or bronchial irritation.

Administration and Dosage

➤*Adults:* 25 mg every 4 hours, not to exceed 150 mg in 24 hours.

➤*Children:*
6 to 12 years of age – 12.5 mg every 4 hours, not to exceed 75 mg in 24 hours.

2 to 6 years of age – 6.25 mg every 4 hours, not to exceed 25 mg in 24 hours.

➤*Storage/Stability:* Store at controlled room temperature (15° to 30°C; 59° to 86°F).

DEXTROMETHORPHAN HBr/BENZOCAINE

otc	**Cough-X** (B.F. Ascher)	**Lozenges:** 5 mg dextromethorphan and 2 mg benzocaine	Dye free. Menthol-eucalyptus flavor. In 9s.
otc	**Tetra-Formula** (Reese Pharm.)	**Lozenges:** 10 mg dextromethorphan HBr and 15 mg benzocaine	Sucrose, glucose, dextrose. In 10s.

For complete prescribing information, refer to the Dextromethorphan HBr and Benzocaine individual monographs.

Indications

Temporarily supresses cough caused by minor throat and bronchial irritants as may occur with the common cold. Also for the temporary relief of occasional minor irritation and sore throat.

Administration and Dosage

Do not exceed recommended dosage. Do not use for more than 2 days for sore throat or for more than 7 days for cough unless directed by a doctor. Do not use for persistent or chronic cough such as occurs with smoking, asthma, emphysema, or if cough is accompanied by excessive phlegm unless directed by a doctor. Allow lozenge to dissolve slowly in the mouth.

➤*Cough-X:*
Adults and children 6 years of age and older – One lozenge every 2 hours as needed, not to exceed 12 lozenges in 24 hours or as directed by a physician.

Children 2 to 6 years of age – One lozenge every 4 hours not to exceed 6 lozenges in 24 hours, or as directed by a physician.

In children, take care to prevent choking on lozenge.

➤*Tetra-Formula:*
Adults and children 6 years of age and older – Dissolve 1 lozenge slowly in the mouth; do not chew. May be repeated every 4 hours or as directed by a physician.

Children under 6 years of age – Consult a physician.

➤*Storage/Stability:* Store below 86°F and protect from moisture.

GUAIFENESIN (Glyceryl Guaiacolate)

otc	Hytuss (Hyrex)	**Tablets:** 100 mg	(HY). White, scored. In 100s and 1000s.
Rx	Guaifenesin (Various, eg, URL)	**Tablets:** 200 mg	In 100s.
Rx	Organidin NR (Medpointe)		Rose, scored. In 100s.
Rx	Allfen Jr (MCR American)	**Tablets:** 400 mg	Dye-free. (ALLFEN JR). Scored. In 100s.
otc	Mucinex (Adams)	**Tablets, extended-release:** 600 mg	Bi-layered. In 20s, 40s, and 500s.
otc	Hytuss 2X (Hyrex)	**Capsules:** 200 mg	EDTA, benzyl alcohol, FD&C Blue No. 1, parabens. In 100s.
otc	Guaifenesin (Various, eg, URL)	**Syrup:** 100 mg per 5 mL	In 473 mL.
otc	Altarussin (Altaire)		Alcohol-free. Corn syrup, menthol, saccharin. In 118 mL.
otc	Guiatuss (Various, eg, Goldline)		May contain corn syrup, saccharin, and menthol. In 118 mL.
otc sf	Diabetic Tussin (Health Care Products)	**Liquid:** 100 mg per 5 mL	Alcohol- and dye-free. 8.4 mg per 5 mL phenylalanine. Aspartame, menthol, methylparaben. In 118 mL.
Rx	Ganidin NR (Cypress)		In 473 mL.
Rx	Guaifenesin NR (Silarx)		Raspberry flavor. In 473 mL.
Rx	Organidin NR (Medpointe)		Saccharin, sorbitol. Raspberry flavor. In 473 mL.
otc	Robitussin (Wyeth)		Alcohol-free. Glucose, corn syrup, saccharin, menthol. In 118 and 237 mL.
otc	Siltussin DAS (Silarx)		Strawberry flavor. In 118 mL.
otc sf	Scot-Tussin Expectorant (Scot-Tussin)		Alcohol- and dye-free. Contains phenylalanine.[a] Aspartame, parabens, menthol. Grape flavor. In 118 mL.
otc	Siltussin SA (Silarx)		Strawberry flavor. In 118, 237, and 473 mL.
otc sf	Naldecon Senior EX (Sandoz)	**Liquid:** 200 mg per 5 mL	Alcohol-free. Sorbitol, saccharin. In 120 mL.

[a] Amount not specified.

Indications

➤*Expectorant:* For the temporary relief of coughs associated with respiratory tract infections and related conditions such as sinusitis, pharyngitis, bronchitis, and asthma when these conditions are complicated by tenacious mucus and/or mucus plugs and congestion. The drug is effective in productive as well as nonproductive cough, but it is of particular value in dry, nonproductive cough that tends to injure the mucous membranes of the air passages.

Administration and Dosage

➤*Immediate-release:*

Adults and children 12 years of age and older – 200 to 400 mg every 4 hours, not to exceed 2,400 mg/day.

Children –

  6 to 11 years of age: 100 to 200 mg every 4 hours, not to exceed 1,200 mg/day.

  2 to 5 years of age: 50 to 100 mg every 4 hours, not to exceed 600 mg/day.

  6 months to younger than 2 years of age: Individualize dosage. 25 to 50 mg every 4 hours, not to exceed 300 mg/day.

➤*Extended-release:* Do not crush, chew, or break tablet. Take with a full glass of water without regard to meals.

Adults and children 12 years of age and older – 600 to 1,200 mg every 12 hours, not to exceed 2,400 mg/day.

➤*Storage/Stability:* Store at controlled-room temperature between 15° and 30°C (59° and 86°F). Protect from light and moisture.

Actions

➤*Pharmacology:* Guaifenesin is an expectorant that increases respiratory tract fluid secretions and helps loosen phlegm and bronchial secretions. By reducing the viscosity of secretions, guaifenesin increases the efficiency of the mucociliary mechanism in removing accumulated secretions from the upper and lower airway.

➤*Pharmacokinetics:* Guaifenesin is readily absorbed from the GI tract and is rapidly metabolized and excreted in the urine. Guaifenesin has a plasma half-life of 1 hour. The major urinary metabolite is β-(2-methoxyphenoxy) lactic acid.

Contraindications

Hypersensitivity to guaifenesin or any other ingredients of the product.

Warnings

➤*Children: Allfen JR* tablets are not recommended for children younger than 6 years of age. *Scot-Tussin* liquid is not recommended for children younger than 2 years of age. *Naldecon Senior EX* and *Mucinex* are not recommended for children younger than 12 years of age.

➤*Persistent cough:* Not for persistent cough such as occurs with smoking, asthma, chronic bronchitis, or emphysema, or where cough is accompanied by excessive secretions. A persistent cough may indicate a serious condition. If cough persists for more than 1 week, tends to recur, or is accompanied by high fever, rash, or persistent headache, consult health care provider.

➤*Kidney stone formation:* Reports in the literature have suggested that consumption of large quantities of guaifenesin-containing medications may be associated with an increased risk of drug-induced kidney stone formation.

➤*Pregnancy: Category C.* It is not known whether guaifenesin can cause fetal harm when administered to a pregnant woman or can affect reproduction capacity. Give to a pregnant woman only if clearly needed.

➤*Lactation:* It is not known whether guaifenesin is excreted in human milk. Because many drugs are excreted in human milk, exercise caution when guaifenesin is administered to a nursing mother and decide whether to discontinue nursing or to discontinue the drug, taking into account the importance of the drug to the mother.

Drug Interactions

➤*Drug/Lab test interactions:* Guaifenesin may increase renal clearance for urate and thereby lower serum uric acid levels. Guaifenesin may produce an increase in urinary 5-hydroxyindoleacetic acid and may therefore interfere with the interpretation of this test for the diagnosis of carcinoid syndrome. It also may falsely elevate vanillylmandelic acid test for catechols. Discontinue administration of this drug 48 hours prior to the collection of urine specimens for such tests.

Adverse Reactions

Nausea and vomiting (most common but still infrequent); dizziness, headache, rash (including urticaria) (rarely reported).

Overdosage

Overdosage with guaifenesin is unlikely to produce serious toxic effects because of its wide margin of safety. When laboratory animals were administered guaifenesin in doses up to 5 g/kg by stomach tube, no toxicity resulted. Provide symptomatic and supportive treatment.

Patient Information

Advise patients not to crush, chew, or break extended-release tablets.

Advise patients to discontinue use and consult their health care provider if the cough lasts more than 7 days, returns, or is accompanied by fever, rash, or persistent headache.

IODINATED GLYCEROL

Rx	**Iophen** (Rugby)	**Tablets:** 30 mg (15 mg organically bound iodine)	In 100s.
Rx	**Iophen** (Various, eg, Barre-National, Genetco, Geneva, Major, Moore, Rugby)	**Elixir:** 60 mg (30 mg organically bound iodine) per 5 ml	In 120 and 480 ml.
Rx	**Par Glycerol** (Par)		21.75% alcohol, peppermint oil, corn syrup, saccharin. Caramel-mint flavor. In pt.
Rx	**R-Gen** (Goldline)		21.75% alcohol. In pt.
Rx	**Iophen** (Various, eg, Barre-National, Goldline, Major, Moore, Rugby)	**Solution:** 50 mg (25 mg organically bound iodine) per ml	In 30 ml.

Administration and Dosage

➤*Adults:* 60 mg 4 times/day.

➤*Children:* Up to half the adult dose, based on weight.

IODINE PRODUCTS

Rx	**Potassium Iodide** (Various, eg, Balan, Goldline, Harber)	**Solution:** 1 g potassium iodide per ml. **Dose:** 0.3 ml (300 mg) to 0.6 ml (600 mg) 3 or 4 times a day, diluted in water. Do not take more than 12 times a day.	In 30 and 240 ml and pt.
Rx sf	**Potassium Iodide** (Roxane)		In 30 and 240 ml.
Rx	**SSKI** (Upsher-Smith)		In 30 and 240 ml.
Rx	**Pima** (Fleming)	**Syrup:** 325 mg potassium iodide per 5 ml. **Dose:** Adults – 5 to 10 ml 3 times daily. Children – 2.5 to 5 ml 3 times daily.	Sugar. Black raspberry flavor. In pt and gal.

Indications

As expectorants in the symptomatic treatment of chronic pulmonary diseases where tenacious mucus complicates the problem, including bronchial asthma, chronic bronchitis, bronchiectasis and pulmonary emphysema. Also used as adjunctive treatment in respiratory tract conditions such as cystic fibrosis, chronic sinusitis and after surgery to help prevent atelectasis.

For other indications for iodine (including use in a radiation emergency), refer to the Iodine Products monograph in the Thyroid Drug section in the Endocrinologic and Metabolic Agents chapter.

Administration and Dosage

➤*Adult:* Initially, 300 to 1000 mg after meals, 2 or 3 times daily. If tolerated, optimal dose is 1 to 1.5 g 3 times a day.

➤*Children:* Half the adult dose of potassium iodide. See individual product inserts for dosage information.

Actions

➤*Pharmacology:* Iodides enhance the secretion of respiratory fluids, thus decreasing the mucus viscosity. In addition, iodides may stimulate breakdown of fibrinoid material in inflammatory exudates. Objective evidence of clinical efficacy is lacking. Because of the potential for adverse effects, other agents are usually preferred.

➤*Pharmacokinetics:* Iodide is absorbed as iodinated amino acids and distributed largely extracellularly. It accumulates in the thyroid gland, and its concentration is far greater in gastric and salivary secretions than in extracellular fluids. Most of plasma iodine is in the form of thyroid hormones. The kidney serves as the chief excretory organ.

Contraindications

Hypersensitivity to iodides.

➤*Potassium iodide:* Impaired renal function; acute bronchitis; hyperthyroidism; Addison's disease; acute dehydration; heat cramps; hyperkalemia; iodism; tuberculosis.

➤*Iodinated glycerol:* Pregnancy, newborns, and nursing mothers (see Warnings).

Warnings

➤*Thyroid disease history:* Use with caution or avoid use in these patients.

➤*GI effects:* Several reports of nonspecific small bowel lesions (stenosis with or without ulceration) have been associated with the administration of enteric-coated potassium salts. These lesions have caused obstruction, hemorrhage and perforation. Surgery was frequently required, and deaths have occurred. Administer coated potassium-containing formulations only when indicated and discontinue immediately if abdominal pain, distention, nausea, vomiting or GI bleeding occurs.

➤*Hypersensitivity reactions:* Occasionally, persons are markedly sensitive to iodides; use care during initial administration. Refer to Management of Acute Hypersensitivity Reactions.

➤*Pregnancy:* (*Category X* – iodinated glycerol; *Category D* – potassium iodide). The fetal thyroid begins to concentrate iodine in the 12th to 14th week of gestation. Use of inorganic iodides in pregnant women during this period and thereafter has rarely induced fetal goiter (with or without hypothyroidism) with the potential for airway obstruction. Fetal harm, abnormal thyroid function and goiter may occur when potassium iodide is administered to a pregnant woman. Because of the possible development of fetal goiter, if the drug is used during pregnancy or if the patient becomes pregnant during therapy, apprise the patient of the potential hazard.

➤*Lactation:* **Potassium iodide** is excreted in breast milk. Use by nursing mothers may cause skin rash and thyroid suppression in the infant. Do not give **iodinated glycerol** to a nursing mother.

➤*Children:* Safety and efficacy in children have not been established for **potassium iodide**. **Iodinated glycerol** is contraindicated in newborns.

Precautions

➤*Hypothyroidism:* In some patients, prolonged use of iodides can lead to hypothyroidism. In patients sensitive to iodides and in hyperthyroidism, iodine-induced goiter may occur. Concurrent use of antithyroid drugs may potentiate the hypothyroid effect of iodides.

➤*Cystic fibrosis:* Children with this disease appear to have an exaggerated susceptibility to the goitrogenic effect of iodides.

➤*Pulmonary tuberculosis:* Pulmonary tuberculosis is considered a contraindication to the use of iodides by some authorities; use with caution in such cases and in patients having Addison's disease, cardiac disease, hyperthyroidism, myotonia congenita or renal impairment.

➤*Acne:* Iodides may cause a flare-up of adolescent acne.

➤*Dermatitis:* Dermatitis and other reversible manifestations of iodism have occurred with chronic use of inorganic iodides. If skin rash appears, discontinue use.

Drug Interactions

➤*Lithium:* Lithium and other antithyroid drugs may potentiate the hypothyroid and goitrogenic effects of these medications if used concurrently.

➤*Potassium-containing medications and potassium-sparing diuretics:* These drugs may result in hyperkalemia and cardiac arrhythmias or cardiac arrest if used with potassium iodide products.

➤*Drug/Lab test interactions:* **Thyroid function tests** may be altered by iodide.

Adverse Reactions

Thyroid adenoma; goiter; myxedema. Hypersensitivity may be manifested by angioneurotic edema, cutaneous and mucosal hemorrhages and symptoms resembling serum sickness, such as fever, arthralgia, lymph node enlargement and eosinophilia.

➤*Miscellaneous:* GI bleeding; confusion; irregular heartbeat; numbness; tingling; pain or weakness in hands or feet; unusual tiredness; weakness or heaviness of legs; fever; swelling of neck or throat; thyroid gland enlargement, acute parotitis (rare).

Chronic iodine poisoning – This or iodism may occur during prolonged treatment. Symptoms include: Metallic taste; burning of mouth or throat; soreness of the mouth, teeth and gums; ulceration of mucous membranes; increased salivation; coryza; sneezing; swelling of the eyelids. Gastric disturbance, nausea, vomiting, epigastric pain and diarrhea are common. There may be a severe headache, productive cough, pulmonary edema and swelling and tenderness of the salivary glands. Acneiform skin lesions are seen in the seborrheic areas. Severe and sometimes fatal skin eruptions may develop. If iodism appears, withdraw the drug and institute appropriate supportive therapy.

Overdosage

Acute overdosage with iodinated glycerol is rare; there have been no reports of any serious problems.

Acute toxicity from potassium iodide is also rare. An occasional individual may show marked sensitivity which can occur immediately or hours after administration. Angioedema, laryngeal edema and cutaneous hemorrhages may occur. Symptoms disappear soon after drug dis-

IODINE PRODUCTS

continuation. Abundant fluid and salt intake helps eliminate iodide. Treat hyperkalemia immediately.

Patient Information

Discontinue use and notify physician if epigastric pain, skin rash, metallic taste, or nausea and vomiting occurs.

Combination products are frequently used in respiratory conditions. These products present two problems: (1) The patient may not need the components of the product; (2) the patient may need the components, but in different strengths or intervals.

➤**Product Selection Guidelines**: When recommending a respiratory combination product, consider the following guidelines.

Patient's data –
Symptoms: Pain, fever, congestion, runny nose, productive/nonproductive cough.
Patient's medical history/health: Age, allergy history, pregnancy, heart disease, hypertension, asthma, bronchitis, glaucoma, hyperthyroidism, diabetes, depression.
Drugs patient is currently taking: Other cold or allergy medications; medications for hypertension, diabetes, etc.

Do not exceed the recommended dosage. Do not take an *otc* product for > 7 days. If symptoms do not improve or are accompanied by fever, consult a physician.

Humidification of room air and adequate fluid intake (6 to 8 glasses/day) are important in treating cold symptoms.

Sulfite/Tartrazine sensitivity – Some of these products contain sulfites or tartrazine, which may cause allergic-type reactions (eg, hives, itching, wheezing, anaphylaxis) in certain susceptible persons. Although overall prevalence of sensitivity in general population is probably low, it is seen more frequently in asthmatics or in atopic nonasthmatic persons (sulfites) or in those with aspirin hypersensitivity (tartrazine).

Sugar free liquid products (sf) – The small amount of sugar in usual doses of medication is probably insignificant to the well controlled diabetic. However, consider the effects of alcohol and sympathomimetics in addition to the sugar content.

Sustained release formulations – Products with identical active ingredients are listed together. Due to formulation differences, do not consider them bioequivalent.

Dosage – Usually average adult dose. For children, consult package literature or physician.

➤**Groups**: These combination products are presented in groups based on the components of their formulations. Products with identical or similar ingredients are listed adjacent to each other, regardless of therapeutic claims, which may differ even for identical formulations. Pediatric preparations (those products intended mainly or exclusively for children) are grouped at the end of each respective section.

Antiasthmatic Combinations – These contain xanthine derivatives and sympathomimetics for bronchodilation. Many products also contain expectorants to facilitate mobilization of mucus.

    Xanthine Combinations
    Xanthine-Sympathomimetic Combinations

Upper Respiratory Combinations – These are used primarily for relief of symptoms associated with colds, upper respiratory tract infections and allergic conditions (eg, acute rhinitis, sinusitis).

    Decongestant Combinations
    Antihistamine and Analgesic Combinations
    Decongestant and Antihistamine Combinations
    Decongestant, Antihistamine and Analgesic Combinations
    Decongestant, Antihistamine and Anticholinergic Combinations

Cough Preparations – These include an antitussive or expectorant, but may also contain ingredients for relief of associated symptoms.

    Antitussive Combinations
    Expectorant Combinations
    Narcotic Antitussives with Expectorants
    Nonnarcotic Antitussives with Expectorants
    Antitussive and Expectorant Combinations

➤**Ingredients**: An FDA advisory review panel has proposed monographs for all *otc* cold, cough, allergy, bronchodilator and antihistamine products. In addition, the FDA proposes to classify *otc* drugs as "monograph conditions" (old Category I) and "nonmonograph conditions" (old Categories II and III). When using these combination products, consider the prescribing information for each ingredient.

Antihistamines – (See individual monograph). These are used for symptomatic relief from allergic rhinitis (hay fever) including runny nose, sneezing, itching of the nose or throat, and itchy and watery eyes. The anticholinergic effects of antihistamines may cause a thickening of bronchial secretions; therefore, these agents may be counterproductive in respiratory conditions characterized by congestion. Antihistamines may cause drowsiness.

Xanthines – (See individual monograph). These, primarily theophylline, relieve bronchial spasm by direct action on the bronchial smooth muscle in bronchospastic conditions such as asthma and chronic bronchitis. Product listings include anhydrous theophylline dosage equivalents. Some xanthine-containing combination products are available *otc*, but asthmatic patients should use them only under physician supervision.

Sympathomimetics – These are used for their α-adrenergic (vasoconstrictor/decongestant) or β$_2$-adrenergic (bronchodilator) effects.
Decongestants: Used for temporary relief of nasal congestion due to colds or allergy. Given orally, they are less effective than topical nasal decongestants, and they have a potential for systemic side effects. Frequent or prolonged topical use may lead to local irritation and rebound congestion.
Bronchodilators: Ephedrine common in these combinations, stimulates cardiac (β$_1$) receptors. Bronchodilation is weaker than with catecholamines; α-adrenergic effects may decrease congestion of mucous membranes. Other β-active agents are effective bronchodilators, but pseudoephedrine is not.

Narcotic antitussives – The antitussive dose is lower than that required for analgesia. Consider general precautions for the use of narcotics, including the potential for abuse, when using these products. See Narcotic Antitussive monograph for complete prescribing information. See also the Narcotic Agonist Analgesics monograph for complete information on the narcotics.
Codeine: 10 to 20 mg every 4 to 6 hours.
Hydrocodone (dihydrocodeinone): 5 to 10 mg every 6 to 8 hours.
Hydromorphone HCl: 2 mg every 4 hours.

Nonnarcotic antitussives – These decrease the cough reflex without inducing many of the common characteristics of narcotic preparations.
Dextromethorphan: 10 to 30 mg every 4 to 8 hours.
Diphenhydramine: 25 mg every 4 hours.
Carbetapentane: This has atropine-like and local anesthetic actions and suppresses cough reflex through selective depression of the medullary cough center.
  • *Dose –* 15 to 30 mg, 3 or 4 times daily.
Caramiphen edisylate: A weak anticholinergic and centrally acting antitussive.
  • *Dose –*
    Adults: 10 to 20 mg every 4 to 6 hours.
    Children (6 to 12): 5 to 10 mg q 4 to 6 h;
    Children (2 to 6): 2.5 to 5 mg q 4 to 6 h.

Expectorants – In the FDA's final monograph for *otc* expectorants, guaifenesin (see individual monograph) is the only agent approved for use as an expectorant. Guaifenesin may help loosen phlegm and thin bronchial secretions to rid the bronchial passageways of bothersome mucus, drain bronchial tubes or make coughs more productive. Humidification of room air and adequate fluid intake (6 to 8 glasses/day) are important therapeutic measures as well.
Dose:
  • *Adults –* 200 to 400 mg every 4 hours, not to exceed 2400 mg in 24 hours.
  • *Children –* Lower dosages are specified on labeling. Consult a physician for children < 2 years of age.

Other ingredients not upgraded by the FDA include: Ammonium chloride, beechwood creosote, benzoin preparations, camphor, eucalyptol/eucalyptus oil, iodines, ipecac syrup, menthol/peppermint oil, pine tar preparations, potassium guaiacolsulfonate, sodium citrate, squill preparations, terpin hydrate preparations, tolu preparations and turpentine oil. Products containing these ingredients must be reformulated.

Analgesics – These (eg, acetaminophen, aspirin, ibuprofen, sodium salicylate) are frequently included to treat headache, fever, muscle aches, pain. See individual monographs.

Anticholinergics – (See individual monograph). These are included for their drying effects on mucus secretions. This action may be beneficial in acute rhinorrhea; however, drying of respiratory secretions may lead to thickened mucus and more difficult expectoration. Traditionally, anticholinergics have been avoided in patients with asthma or chronic obstructive pulmonary disease (COPD); however, some patients respond well to these agents. Caution is still advised in this group.

An anticholinergic for oral inhalation is available as a bronchodilator for maintenance of bronchospasm associated with COPD, including chronic bronchitis and emphysema (see Ipratropium monograph).

The FDA has ruled that no anticholinergic product for *otc* use is recognized as safe and effective. Therefore, the products must be reapproved by new drug application (NDA) before November 10, 1986, or be regarded as misbranded (*Federal Register* 1985 Nov 8; 50:46582-87).

Papaverine HCl – (See individual monograph). This relaxes the smooth muscle of the bronchial tree.

Barbiturates – (See individual monograph). These are included for sedative effects as "correctives" with xanthines or sympathomimetics which may cause CNS stimulation. The sedative efficacy of low doses (eg, 8 mg phenobarbital) is questionable.

Caffeine – (See individual monograph). This is included for CNS stimulation to counteract antihistamine depression and to enhance concomitant analgesics.

ANTIASTHMATIC COMBINATIONS

XANTHINE COMBINATIONS, CAPSULES AND TABLETS
Content given per capsule or tablet.

	Product & Distributor	Xanthine[1]	Expectorant	Other	Average Adult Dose	How Supplied
Rx	**Quibron-300 Capsules** (Roberts)	300 mg theophylline	180 mg guaifenesin		16 mg/kg/day or 400 mg theophylline/day, in divided doses, q 6 to 8 h	(Roberts 068). Yellow and white. In 100s.
Rx	**Bronchial Capsules** (Various, eg, Moore)	150 mg theophylline	90 mg guaifenesin		16 mg/kg/day or 400 mg theophylline/day, in divided doses, q 6 to 8 h	In 100s and 1000s.
Rx	**Glyceryl-T Capsules** (Rugby)[2]	150 mg theophylline	90 mg guaifenesin		1 or 2 bid or tid	In 100s.
Rx	**Quibron Capsules** (BMS)	150 mg theophylline	90 mg guaifenesin		16 mg/kg/day or 400 mg theophylline/day, in divided doses, q 6 to 8 h	(M022). Yellow. In 100s, 1000s and UD 100s.
Rx	**Mudrane GG-2 Tablets** (ECR Pharm)	111 mg theophylline	100 mg guaifenesin		1 tid or qid	(GG 9533). Green, mottled. In 100s.
Rx	**Dyphylline & Guaifenesin** (Econolab)	200 mg dyphylline	200 mg guaifenesin		1 qid	In 100s.
Rx	**Dyflex-G Tablets** (Econo Med)	200 mg dyphylline	200 mg guaifenesin		1 or 2 qid	In 100s and 1000s.
Rx	**Dyline G.G. Tablets** (Seatrace)	200 mg dyphylline	200 mg guaifenesin		1 tid or qid	(0551 and 0123) Pink, scored. In 100s and 1000s.
Rx	**Lufyllin-GG Tablets** (Wallace)	200 mg dyphylline	200 mg guaifenesin		1 qid	(Wallace 541). Yellow, scored. In 100s, 3000s and UD 100s.
Rx	**Panfil G** (Pan American Labs)	200 mg dyphylline	100 mg guaifenesin		1 tid or qid after meals	Lactose. Orange/green. (PAL/0305). In 100s

[1] Theophylline content given as anhydrous unless otherwise specified. [2] Form of theophylline unknown.

Refer to the general discussion of these products in the Respiratory Combinations Introduction.

XANTHINE COMBINATIONS, LIQUIDS
Content given per 15 ml.

	Product & Distributor	Xanthine[1]	Expectorant	Other	Average Adult Dose	How Supplied
Rx	**Theolate Liquid** (Various, eg, Barre-National)	150 mg theophylline	90 mg guaifenesin		15 ml q 6 to 8 h	In 118 ml, pt and gal.
Rx	**Glyceryl-T Liquid** (Rugby)					In 480 ml.
Rx	**Synophylate-GG Syrup** (Central)	150 mg theophylline (300 mg theophylline sodium glycinate)	100 mg guaifenesin	10% alcohol. Saccharin, sorbitol, sucrose	3 mg theophylline/kg q 8 h	In pt and gal.
Rx sf	**Elixophyllin GG Liquid** (Forest)	100 mg theophylline	100 mg guaifenesin	Sorbitol	3 mg theophylline/kg q 8 h	Alcohol and dye free. In 237 and 473 ml.
Rx	**Theophylline KI Elixir** (Various, eg, Qualitest)[2]	80 mg theophylline	130 mg potassium iodide		3 mg theophylline/kg q 8 h	In 480 ml and gal.
Rx	**Elixophyllin-KI Elixir** (Forest)			Saccharin, sodium bisulfite, sucrose, anise oil		In 237 ml.
Rx	**Iophylline Elixir** (Various, eg, Major)[2]	120 mg theophylline	30 mg iodinated glycerol		15 to 30 ml tid	In 480 ml.
Rx	**Dilor-G Liquid** (Savage)	300 mg dyphylline	300 mg guaifenesin	Saccharin, sorbitol, sucrose, parabens	5 or 10 ml tid or qid	Alcohol free. Mint flavor. In pt and gal.
Rx	**Dyline-GG Liquid** (Seatrace)	300 mg dyphylline	300 mg guaifenesin	Menthol, parabens, saccharin, sorbitol, sucrose[2]	5 or 10 ml tid or qid	Peppermint flavor. In pt and gal.
Rx	**Panfil G** (Pan American Labs)	300 mg dyphylline	150 mg guaifenesin	Parabens, sorbitol, sucrose.	10 ml tid or qid	Vanilla flavor. In pints.
Rx	**Dyphylline-GG Elixir** (Various, eg, Barre-National, Goldline, Qualitest, Silarx)	100 mg dyphylline	100 mg guaifenesin	17% alcohol. Saccharin, sucrose	30 ml qid	In 473 ml.
Rx	**Lufyllin-GG Elixir** (Wallace)					Wine flavor. In pt and gal.

ANTIASTHMATIC COMBINATIONS

XANTHINE COMBINATIONS, LIQUIDS

	Product & Distributor	Xanthine[1]	Expectorant	Other	Average Adult Dose	How Supplied
Rx	**Brondelate Elixir** (Various, eg, Barre-National, CMC, Harber)[2]	192 mg theophylline (300 mg oxtriphylline)	150 mg guaifenesin		10 ml qid	In 480 ml and gal.
Rx	**Oxtriphylline and Guaifenesin Elixir** (Barre-National)			20% alcohol		Cherry flavor. In pt and gal.

[1] Theophylline content given as anhydrous unless otherwise specified. [2] May contain alcohol.

Refer to the general discussion of these products in the Respiratory Combinations Introduction.

XANTHINE-SYMPATHOMIMETIC COMBINATIONS, TABLETS
Content given per tablet.

	Product & Distributor	Xanthine[1]	Sympathomimetic	Expectorant	Other	Average Adult Dose	How Supplied
otc	**Theodrine Tablets** (Rugby)	120 mg theophylline[2]	22.5 mg ephedrine HCl			1 to 2 q 4 h up to 3 doses/day	In 1000s.
otc	**Tedrigen Tablets** (Goldline)				7.5 mg phenobarbital	1 to 2 q 4 h	In 100s and 1000s.
Rx	**Hydrophed Tablets** (Rugby)	130 mg theophylline	25 mg ephedrine sulfate		10 mg hydroxyzine HCl	1 bid to qid	In 100s and 1000s.
Rx	**Marax Tablets** (Roerig)						Dye free. Scored. M-shaped. In 100s and 500s.
Rx	**Mudrane GG Tablets** (ECR Pharm)	111 mg theophylline (130 mg aminophylline anhydrous)	16 mg ephedrine HCl	100 mg guaifenesin	8 mg phenobarbital	1 tid or qid	(GG 9551). Yellow, mottled, scored. In 100s.
Rx	**Mudrane Tablets** (ECR Pharm)	111 mg theophylline (130 mg aminophylline anhydrous)	16 mg ephedrine HCl	195 mg potassium iodide	8 mg phenobarbital	1 tid or qid	(9550). Yellow, scored. In 100s.
Rx	**Quadrinal Tablets** (Knoll)	65 mg theophylline (130 mg theophylline calcium salicylate)	24 mg ephedrine HCl	320 mg potassium iodide	24 mg phenobarbital	1 tid or qid	(14). White, scored. Biconvex. In 100s.
otc	**Primatene Dual Action Tablets** (Whitehall)	60 mg theophylline	12.5 mg ephedrine HCl	100 mg guaifenesin		2 q 4 h	In 24s.
Rx	**Lufyllin-EPG Tablets** (Wallace)	100 mg dyphylline	16 mg ephedrine HCl	200 mg guaifenesin	16 mg phenobarbital	1 to 2 q 6 h	In 100s.

[1] Theophylline content given as anhydrous unless otherwise specified. [2] Form of theophylline unknown.

Refer to the general discussion of these products in the Respiratory Combinations Introduction.

XANTHINE-SYMPATHOMIMETIC COMBINATIONS, LIQUIDS
Content given per 15 ml.

	Product & Distributor	Xanthine[1]	Sympathomimetic	Expectorant	Other	Average Adult Dose	How Supplied
Rx	**Lufyllin-EPG Elixir** (Wallace)	150 mg dyphylline	24 mg ephedrine HCl	300 mg guaifenesin	5.5% alcohol. 24 mg phenobarbital	10 to 20 ml q 6 h	In 480 ml.

[1] Theophylline content given as anhydrous unless otherwise specified.

Refer to the general discussion of these products in the Respiratory Combinations Introduction.

ANTIASTHMATIC COMBINATIONS

PEDIATRIC XANTHINE-SYMPATHOMIMETIC COMBINATIONS

Content given per 15 ml.

	Product & Distributor	Xanthine[1]	Sympathomimetic	Other	Average Adult Dose	How Supplied
Rx	**Theomax DF Syrup** (Various, eg, Barre-National)	97.5 mg theophylline	18.75 mg ephedrine sulfate	5% alcohol. 7.5 mg hydroxyzine HCl	*Children (> 5 yrs)* - 5 ml tid or qid *(2 to 5 yrs)* - 2.5 to 5 ml tid or qid	In pt and gal.
Rx	**Marax-DF Syrup** (Roerig)			7.5 mg hydroxyzine HCl, sucrose[2]	*Children (> 5 yrs)* - 5 ml tid or qid *(2 to 5 yrs)* - 2.5 to 5 ml tid or qid	In pt and gal.

[1] Theophylline content given as anhydrous unless otherwise specified.　　　[2] May contain alcohol.

Refer to the general discussion of these products in the Respiratory Combinations Introduction.

UPPER RESPIRATORY COMBINATIONS

DECONGESTANT AND ANALGESIC COMBINATIONS

Content given per capsule, tablet, or 5 mL.

	Product & Distributor	Decongestant	Analgesic	Average Adult Dose	Excipients & How Supplied
otc	Alka-Seltzer Plus Cold & Sinus Tablets (Bayer)	5 mg phenylephrine HCl	250 mg acetaminophen	2 q 4 h up to 8/day	4 mg phenylalanine, aspartame, acesulfame K, saccharin, sorbitol. In 20s.
otc	Cepacol Sore Throat Liquid[1] (J.B. Williams)	10 mg pseudoephedrine HCl	106.7 mg acetaminophen	30 mL q 4 to 6 h up to 120 mL/day	Alcohol free. Tartrazine, honey, saccharin, sorbitol. Honey flavor. 237 mL.
otc	Alka-Seltzer Plus Cold & Sinus Liqui-Gels[1] (Bayer)	30 mg pseudoephedrine HCl	325 mg acetaminophen	2 q 4 h up to 8/day	Liquid-filled. Sorbitol. (AS+ C&S). In 12s and 20s.
otc	Allerest Allergy & Sinus Relief Maximum Strength Tablets[1] (Heritage)			2 q 4 to 6 h up to 8/day	In 24s.
otc	Ornex No Drowsiness Tablets[1] (B.F. Ascher)				Capsule shape. In 24s and 48s.
otc	Phenapap Tablets[1] (Rugby)				In 100s.
otc	Sinutab Sinus Without Drowsiness Regular Strength Tablets (Warner-Lambert)			2 q 4 h up to 8/day	In 24s.
otc	Sudafed Cold & Sinus Non-Drowsy Liqui-Caps (Warner-Lambert)			2 q 4 to 6 h up to 8/day	Liquid-filled. Sorbitol. In 10s and 20s.
otc	Dilotab Tablets (Zee Medical)	30 mg pseudoephedrine HCl	500 mg acetaminophen	2 q 6 h up to 8/day	In 24s.
otc	Dristan Cold Non-Drowsy Maximum Strength Tablets (Whitehall-Robins)			2 q 6 h up to 8/day	Capsule shape. In 20s.
otc	Mapap Sinus Maximum Strength Geltabs (Major)			2 q 4 to 6 h up to 8/day	In 24s.
otc	Nasal Decongestant Sinus Non-Drowsy Tablets (Topco)			2 q 6 h up to 8/day	In 24s.
otc	Ornex No Drowsiness Maximum Strength Tablets (BF Ascher)				(ORNEX MAX). Capsule shape. In 24s and 48s.
otc	Sine-Off No-Drowsiness Formula Tablets (Hogil)				(SINE-OFF). Capsule shape. In 24s.
otc	Sinus-Relief Maximum Strength Tablets (Major)				Dextrose. Capsule shape. In 24s.
otc	Sinutab Sinus Without Drowsiness Maximum Strength Tablets (Warner-Lambert)				Round (tablet); capsule shape (caplet). In 24s and 48s.
otc	Sudafed Sinus Headache Non-Drowsy Tablets (Warner-Lambert)				Round (tablet); capsule shape (caplet). In 24s and 48s.
otc	SudoGest Sinus Maximum Strength Tablets (Major)				Dextrose. In 24s.
otc	Tavist Sinus Maximum Strength Tablets (Novartis)				Lactose, dextrose, methylparaben. (Tavist Sinus). Capsule shape. In 24s.
otc	Tylenol Sinus Non-Drowsy Maximum Strength Geltabs, Tablets, and Gelcaps (McNeil)			2 q 4 to 6 h up to 8/day	**Tablets:** (TYLENOL Sinus). Capsule shape. In 24s. **Geltabs:** Parabens. (TYLENOL SINUS). In 24s, 48s, and 60s. **Gelcaps:** Parabens. (TYLENOL SINUS). In 24s, 48s, and 60s.
otc	Advil Cold & Sinus Tablets (Whitehall-Robins)	30 mg pseudoephedrine HCl	200 mg ibuprofen	1 to 2 q 4 to 6 h up to 6/day	Parabens, sucrose. (ADVIL COLD & SINUS). Oval. In 40s.
otc	Advil Cold & Sinus Liqui-gels (Whitehall-Robins)				Sorbitol. In 16s and 32s.
otc	Advil Flu & Body Ache Tablets (Whitehall-Robins)				Parabens, sucrose. Capsule shape. In 20s.
otc	Dristan Sinus Tablets (Whitehall-Robins)				Parabens, sucrose. Oval. In 20s.
otc	Motrin Sinus Headache Tablets (McNeil)				(Motrin Sinus Headache). Capsule shape. In 20s.
otc	Aleve Cold & Sinus Tablets (Bayer)	120 mg pseudoephedrine HCl	220 mg naproxen sodium (200 mg naproxen)	1 q 12 h up to 2/day	Extended release. Lactose. Capsule shape. In 10s, 20s, and 40s.
otc	Aleve Sinus & Headache Tablets (Bayer)				Extended release. Lactose. Capsule shape. In 10s.

[1] This product also may be used in children; refer to package labeling for dosing.

For complete prescribing information, refer to the Respiratory Combinations Introduction.

UPPER RESPIRATORY COMBINATIONS

PEDIATRIC DECONGESTANT AND ANALGESIC COMBINATIONS
Content given per tablet, 5 mL (liquid), or 1 mL (drops).

	Product & Distributor	Decongestant	Analgesic	Average Dose	Excipients & How Supplied
otc	**Tylenol Infant's Cold Concentrated Drops** (McNeil)	9.375 mg/mL pseudoephedrine HCl	100 mg/mL acetaminophen	**2 to 3 yrs** - 1.6 mL q 4 to 6 h up to 6.4 mL/day	Alcohol free. Saccharin, corn syrup. Bubble-gum flavor. In 15 mL w/dropper.
otc	**Tylenol Children's Sinus Suspension** (McNeil)	15 mg pseudoephedrine HCl	160 mg acetaminophen	**6 to 11 yrs** - 10 mL q 4 to 6 h up to 40 mL/day; **2 to 5 yrs** - 5 mL q 4 to 6 h up to 20 mL/day	Acesulfame K, butylparaben, corn syrup, sorbitol. Fruit flavor. In 118 mL.
otc	**Triaminic Softchews Allergy Sinus & Headache Tablets** (Novartis)	15 mg pseudoephedrine HCl		**6 to 11 yrs** - 2 q 4 to 6 h up to 8/day; **2 to 5 yrs** - 1 q 4 to 6 h up to 4/day	11.2 mg phenylalanine, aspartame, mannitol, sorbitol, sucrose. Fruit-punch flavor. In 18s.
otc	**Children's Ibuprofen Cold Suspension** (Major)	15 mg pseudoephedrine HCl	100 mg ibuprofen/5 mL	**6 to 11 yrs** - 10 mL q 6 h up to 40 mL/day; **2 to 5 yrs** - 5 mL q 6 h up to 20 mL/day	Alcohol-free. Corn syrup. Berry flavor. In 120 mL.
otc	**Children's Advil Cold Suspension** (Whitehall-Robins)	15 mg pseudoephedrine HCl	100 mg ibuprofen	**6 to 11 yrs (48 to 95 lbs)** - 10 mL q 6 h up to 40 mL/day; **2 to 5 yrs (24 to 47 lbs)** - 5 mL q 6 h up to 20 mL/day	Sorbitol, sucrose. Alcohol free. Grape flavor. In 120 mL.
otc	**Motrin Children's Cold Suspension** (McNeil)			**6 to 11 yrs** - 10 mL q 6 h up to 40 mL/day; **2 to 5 yrs** - 5 mL q 6 h up to 20 mL/day	Acesulfame K, sucrose. Berry, dye free berry, or grape flavors. In 118 mL.

Refer to the general discussion of these products in the Respiratory Combinations Introduction. Some of the products in the previous Decongestant and Analgesic Combinations table also may be used in children.

UPPER RESPIRATORY COMBINATIONS

DECONGESTANT AND EXPECTORANT COMBINATIONS
Content given per capsule, tablet, or 5 mL.

	Product & Distributor	Decongestant	Expectorant	Other	Average Adult Dose	Excipients & How Supplied
Rx	Broncholate Syrup (Sanofi-Synthelabo)	6.25 mg ephedrine HCl	100 mg guaifenesin		10 to 20 mL q 4 h up to 120 mL/day	Orange flavor. In 473 mL.
Rx	KIE Syrup[1] (Laser)	8 mg ephedrine HCl	150 mg potassium iodide		10 to 15 mL q 4 to 6 h up to 60 mL/day	Saccharin, sorbitol, sucrose. Cherry flavor. In 473 mL.
otc	Mini Two-Way Action Tablets (BDI Pharm)	12.5 mg ephedrine HCl	200 mg guaifenesin		1 to 2 q 4 h up to 12/day	In 6s, 24s, and 60s.
otc	Primatene Tablets (Whitehall-Robins)				2 q 4 h up to 12/day	In 24s and 60s.
otc	Dynafed Asthma Relief Tablets (BDI Pharm)	25 mg ephedrine HCl	200 mg guaifenesin		½ to 1 q 4 h up to 6/day	In 60s.
otc	Mini Two-Way Action Tablets (BDI Pharm)					In 6s, 48s and 60s.
otc	Bronkaid Dual Action Tablets (Bayer)	25 mg ephedrine sulfate	400 mg guaifenesin		1 q 4 h up to 6/day	Capsule shape. In 24s.
otc	Rescon-GG Liquid[1] (Capellon)	5 mg phenylephrine HCl	100 mg guaifenesin		10 mL q 4 to 6 h up to 40 mL/day	Alcohol and dye free. Parabens, sorbitol, sugar. Cherry flavor. In 118 and 473 mL.
Rx sf	Entex Liquid[1] (Andrx)	7.5 mg phenylephrine HCl	100 mg guaifenesin		5 to 10 mL q 4 to 6 h up to 40 mL/day	Alcohol and dye free. Punch flavor. In 15 and 473 mL.
Rx	Guaifed-PD Capsules[1] (Verum Pharm)	7.5 mg phenylephrine HCl	200 mg guaifenesin		1 to 2 q 12 h	Extended release. Maltodextrin, parabens, sucrose. (GUAIFED 200-7.5 VERUM). Purple/White. In 30s and 100s.
Rx	Entex ER Capsules[1] (Andrx)	10 mg phenylephrine HCl	300 mg guaifenesin		1 or 2 q 12 h	Extended release. Maltodextrin, sucrose, parabens. (ENTEX ER 334). White. In 30s and 100s.
Rx	Guaifed Capsules[1] (Verum Pharm)	15 mg phenylephrine HCl	400 mg guaifenesin		1 q 12 h	Extended release. Maltodextrin, parabens, sucrose. (GUAIFED 400-15 VERUM). Purple/White. In 30s and 100s.
Rx	SINUvent PE Tablets[1] (WE Pharm)	15 mg phenylephrine HCl	600 mg guaifenesin		2 bid q 12 h	Extended release. (WE). Lt. green, capsule shape, scored. In 100s.
Rx	Endal Nasal Decongestant Tablets (PediaMed)	20 mg phenylephrine HCl	300 mg guaifenesin		2 q 12 h	Timed release. Capsule shape. In 100s.
Rx	Deconsal II Capsules (Carolina Pharmaceuticals)	20 mg phenylephrine HCl	375 mg guaifenesin		1 to 2 q 12 h up to 3/day	Extended-release. Sucrose. (CAROLINA PHARMA DECONSAL II). Blue, yellow opaque. In 30s and 100s.
Rx	GFN 600/Phenylephrine 20 Tablets[1] (Cypress)	20 mg phenylephrine HCl	600 mg guaifenesin		1 to 2 q 12 h up to 2/day	Dye free. (CYP 269). White, oval, scored. In 100s.
Rx	Liquibid-PD Tablets[1] (Capellon)	25 mg phenylephrine HCl	275 mg guaifenesin		1 or 2 q 12 h up to 4/day	Sustained release. White/Blue bilayered, triangular, scored. In 100s.
Rx	Entex LA Capsules[1] (Andrx)	30 mg phenylephrine HCl	400 mg guaifenesin		1 q 12 h up to 2/day	Extended release. Maltodextrin, sucrose. (ANDRX 333). Yellow and blue. In 100s.
Rx	Entex LA Tablets[1] (Andrx)	30 mg phenylephrine HCl	600 mg guaifenesin		1 q 12 h up to 2/day	Sustained release. Dye free. (ENTEX LA 330/330). White, oval, scored. In 100s.
Rx	PhenaVent LA Tablets (Ethex)	30 mg phenylephrine HCl	600 mg guaifenesin			(ETHEX 443). White to off-white, capsule shape. Film-coated. In 100s.
Rx	Liquibid-D Tablets[1] (Capellon)	40 mg phenylephrine HCl	600 mg guaifenesin		1 q 12 h	(LIQUIBID-D). White, oval, scored. In 100s.
Rx	Liquibid-D 1200 Tablets[1] (Capellon)	40 mg phenylephrine HCl	1200 mg guaifenesin		1 q 12 h	Sustained release. (1200). Lt. green, capsule shape, scored. Film coated. In 100s.
Rx	PhenaVent D Tablets (Ethex)					(ETHEX 444). White to off-white, capsule shape. Film-coated. In 100s.
otc	Guiatuss PE Liquid (Alpharma)	30 mg pseudoephedrine HCl	100 mg guaifenesin		10 mL q 4 h up to 40 mL/day	Alcohol free. Corn syrup, methylparaben, saccharin. Fruit mint flavor. In 118 mL.
otc	Robafen PE Liquid[1] (Major)					Alcohol free. Glucose, corn syrup, saccharin. In 118 mL.
otc	Robitussin PE Liquid[1] (Whitehall-Robins)					Corn syrup, glucose, saccharin. In 118 and 237 mL.
otc	Sudafed Non-Drowsy Non-Drying Sinus Liquid Caps (Warner-Lambert)	30 mg pseudoephedrine HCl	120 mg guaifenesin		2 q 4 h up to 8/day	Liquid filled. Sorbitol. In 24s.

UPPER RESPIRATORY COMBINATIONS

DECONGESTANT AND EXPECTORANT COMBINATIONS

	Product & Distributor[1]	Decongestant	Expectorant	Other	Average Adult Dose	Excipients & How Supplied
otc	Guaifed Syrup[1] (Muro)	30 mg pseudoephedrine HCl	200 mg guaifenesin		10 mL q 4 to 6 h up to 40 mL/day	Alcohol free. EDTA, menthol, saccharin, sorbitol, sucrose. Cherry flavor. In 473 mL.
otc	Robitussin Severe Congestion Liqui-Gels[1] (Whitehall-Robins)				2 q 4 h up to 8/day	Liquid filled. Mannitol, sorbitol. (AHR 8601). In 24s.
otc	Severe Congestion Tussin Softgels[1] (AmerisourceBergen)					Sorbitol. In 12s.
otc	Sinutab Non-Drying Liquid Caps (Warner-Lambert)					Liquid filled. Sorbitol. In 24s.
otc	Robitussin Cold Sinus & Congestion Tablets[1] (Whitehall-Robins)	30 mg pseudoephedrine HCl	200 mg guaifenesin	325 mg acetaminophen	2 q 4 h up to 8/day	Lactose. Capsule shape. In 20s.
otc	Tylenol Sinus Severe Congestion Tablets (McNeil)				2 q 4 to 6 h up to 8/day	Capsule shape. In 24s.
Rx	PanMist-S Syrup[1] (Pan American)	40 mg pseudoephedrine HCl	200 mg guaifenesin		≤ 10 mL qid	Alcohol free. Grape flavor. In 15 and 473 mL.
Rx	Coldmist JR Tablets[1] (Breckenridge)	45 mg pseudoephedrine HCl	600 mg guaifenesin		1 or 2 q 12 h	Sustained release. In 100s.
Rx	Profen II Tablets[1] (IVAX)	45 mg pseudoephedrine HCl	800 mg guaifenesin		1 to 1½ q 12 h up to 3/day	Extended release. (PROFEN-II 307). White, scored. In 100s.
Rx	Pseudoephedrine HCl/Guaifenesin SR Tablets[1] (URL)	48 mg pseudoephedrine HCl	595 mg guaifenesin		1 or 2 q 12 h up to 4/day	Extended release. (α 1891). White, capsule shape. In 100s.
Rx	PanMist JR Tablets[1] (Pan American)	58 mg pseudoephedrine HCl	600 mg guaifenesin		1 or 2 q 12 h	Extended release. (PAL 0768). White, capsule shape. Dye-free. In 100s.
Rx	Respa-1st Tablets[1] (Respa)	60 mg pseudoephedrine HCl	600 mg guaifenesin			Sustained release. (RESPA 87). White, scored. In 100s.
Rx	Respaire-60 SR Capsules[1] (Laser)	60 mg pseudoephedrine HCl	200 mg guaifenesin		2 q 12 h up to 4/day	Extended release. (LASER 0174). Green/clear. In 100s.
Rx	Versacaps Capsules[1] (Seatrace)	60 mg pseudoephedrine HCl	300 mg guaifenesin		1 q 12 h	Sustained release. Benzyl alcohol, EDTA, parabens, sucrose. In 100s.
otc	Congestac Tablets[1] (B.F. Ascher)	60 mg pseudoephedrine HCl	400 mg guaifenesin		1 q 4 to 6 h up to 4/day	(C). Capsule shape. In 12s and 24s.
otc	Refenesen Plus Severe Strength Cough & Cold Medicine Tablets (Reese)	60 mg pseudoephedrine HCl				Capsule shape. In 16s.
Rx	Zephrex Tablets[1] (Sanofi-Synthelabo)	60 mg pseudoephedrine HCl	500 mg guaifenesin		1 q 4 to 6 h	(Sanofi 460). Oval. Film coated. In 100s.
Rx	Sudal 60/500 Tablets[1] (Atley)	60 mg pseudoephedrine HCl	500 mg guaifenesin		1 to 2 q 12 h	Sustained release. (SUDAL 60 A P). White, capsule shape, scored. In 100s.
Rx	AMBI 60/580 Tablets[1] (AMBI)	60 mg pseudoephedrine HCl	580 mg guaifenesin		1 or 2 q 12 h up to 4/day	(AMBI 121). White, capsule shape. In 100s.
Rx	Maxifed-G Tablets[1] (MCR American)	60 mg pseudoephedrine HCl			1 or 2 q 12 h	(MAXIFED G 514). White, capsule shape. In 100s.
Rx	Guaifenesin/Pseudoephedrine HCl Tablets[1] (Major)	60 mg pseudoephedrine HCl	600 mg guaifenesin		1 or 2 q 12 h up to 4/day	Sustained release. In 100s.
Rx	AquatabD Dose Pack Tablets[1] (Adams)					Sustained release. (Adams 044). White, scored. In 56s.
Rx	Deconsal II Tablets[1] (Celltech)					Sustained release. (MEDEVA/017). Dark blue, scored. In 100s and 500s.
Rx	Durasal II Tablets[1] (Prasco)					Sustained release. (300). Mottled blue, capsule shape, scored. In 100s.
Rx	Guaifenex PSE 60 Tablets[1] (Ethex)					Extended release. Lactose. (ETHEX/214). Blue, scored. Capsule shape. In 100s.
Rx	Iosal II Tablets[1] (Iopharm)					Sustained release. In 100s.
Rx	G/P 1200/60 Tablets[1] (Cypress)	60 mg pseudoephedrine HCl	1200 mg guaifenesin		1 q 12 h up to 2/day	Sustained release. (CYP 272). White. In 100s.
Rx	AquatabD Tablets[1] (Adams)	75 mg pseudoephedrine HCl	1200 mg guaifenesin		1 q 12 h up to 2/day	Extended release. (Adams 068). Lt. green, oval, scored. In 100s.
Rx	Maxifed Tablets[1] (MCR American)	80 mg pseudoephedrine HCl	700 mg guaifenesin		1 to 1½ q 12 h	(MAXIFED/MCR 520). Green, capsule shape, scored. In 100s.
Rx	Coldmist LA Tablets[1] (Breckenridge)	80 mg pseudoephedrine HCl	800 mg guaifenesin		1 q 8 h up to 3/day	Extended release. (B-067). White, capsule shape. In 100s.
Rx	Pseudoephedrine HCl/Guaifenesin LA Tablets[1] (URL)	85 mg pseudoephedrine HCl	795 mg guaifenesin		1 q 12 h up to 3/day	Timed release. (NL 734). White, capsule shape. In 100s.
Rx	PanMist LA Tablets[1] (Pan American)					Extended release. (PAL 07/92). Pink with red specks, capsule shape. In 100s.
Rx	H 9600 SR Tablets[1] (Hawthorn)	90 mg pseudoephedrine HCl	600 mg guaifenesin		1 q 12 h	Sustained release. Dye-free. (HAW 301). Scored, capsule shape. In 100s.
Rx	Profen Forte Tablets[1] (IVAX)	90 mg pseudoephedrine HCl	800 mg guaifenesin		1 q 12 h up to 2/day	Extended release. (PROFEN FORTE 315). White, scored. In 100s.

UPPER RESPIRATORY COMBINATIONS

DECONGESTANT AND EXPECTORANT COMBINATIONS

	Product & Distributor	Decongestant	Expectorant	Other	Average Adult Dose	Excipients & How Supplied
Rx	**Dynex Tablets**[1] (Athlon)	90 mg pseudoephedrine HCl	1200 mg guaifenesin		1 q 12 h	Dye free. Sustained release. (DG 033). Scored. Capsule shape. In 30s and 100s.
Rx	**Pseudovent Capsules** (Ethex)					Sustained release. EDTA, methylparaben, sucrose. (ETHEX 016). White/clear. In 100s.
Rx	**Respaire-120 SR Capsules** (Laser)				1 q 12 h up to 2/day	Extended release. (LASER 0169). Orange/clear. In 100s.
Rx	**Entex PSE Capsules**[1] (Andrx)	120 mg pseudoephedrine HCl	400 mg guaifenesin		1 q 12 h up to 2/day	Extended-release. Maltodextrin, sucrose. (ANDRX 132). (B 366). White and blue. In 100s.
Rx sf	**GP-500 Tablets**[1] (Marnel)	120 mg pseudoephedrine HCl	500 mg guaifenesin		1 bid	Dye free. Sustained release. (GP-500). White, scored, capsule shape. In 100s.
Rx	**Nasatab LA Tablets**[1] (ECR Pharm)					Sustained release. (MX/225). White, scored, capsule shape. Film-coated. In 100s.
Rx	**Stamoist E Tablets**[1] (Huckaby)					Sustained release. (STAMOIST E). White, capsule shape, scored. Film-coated. In 100s.
Rx	**V-Dec-M Tablets**[1] (Seatrace)					Sustained release. (AM/PM). White, scored. In 12s and 100s.
Rx	**Touro LA Tablets** (Dartmouth)	120 mg pseudoephedrine HCl	525 mg guaifenesin		1 q 12 h	Sustained release. (DP636 TOURO LA). Capsule shape. In 100s.
Rx	**Entex PSE Tablets**[1] (Andrx)	120 mg pseudoephedrine HCl	600 mg guaifenesin		1 q 12 h	Sustained release. Sugar. (Entex PSE 032 032). Yellow, scored. In 100s.
Rx	**Guaifenex PSE 120 Tablets**[1] (Ethex)					Extended release. Dye free. (Ethex 208). White, capsule shape, scored. In 100s.
Rx	**GuaiMAX-D Tablets**[1] (Schwarz)					Extended release. (GUAIMAX-D SP 2055). White to off-white, capsule shape, scored. In 100s.
Rx	**Guaipax PSE Tablets**[1] (Eon)					Sustained release. (E784). White, scored, oval. In 100s, 250s, and 500s.
Rx	**Miraphen PSE Tablets**[1] (Major)					Sustained release. In 500s.
Rx	**Zephrex LA Tablets**[1] (Sanofi-Synthelabo)					Extended release. (Sanofi LA). Orange, oval. In 100s.
Rx	**GFN/PSE Tablets**[1] (Cypress)					Sustained release. (CYP 266). White. In 100s.
Rx	**Guaifenex GP Tablets** (Ethex)	120 mg pseudoephedrine HCl	1200 mg guaifenesin		1 q 12 h up to 2/day.	Extended release. Dye free. Lactose. (ETHEX 373). White, scored, oval. Film-coated. In 100s.

[1] This product also may be used in children; refer to package labeling for dosing.

Refer to the general discussion of these products in the Respiratory Combinations Introduction. Some of the products in the following Pediatric Decongestant Expectorant Combinations table also may be used in adults.

PEDIATRIC DECONGESTANT AND EXPECTORANT COMBINATIONS
Content given per capsule or 5 mL.

	Product & Distributor	Decongestant	Expectorant	Average Dose	Excipients & How Supplied
otc	**Thera-Hist Expectorant Chest Congestion Liquid** (Major)	15 mg pseudoephedrine HCl	50 mg guaifenesin	*6 to < 12 yrs* - 10 mL q 4 to 6 h up to 40 mL/day; *2 to < 6 yrs* - 5 mL q 4 to 6 h up to 20 mL/day	EDTA, sorbitol, sucrose. Citrus flavor. In 118 mL.
otc	**Triacting Liquid** (Various, eg, AmerisourceBergen, Topco)				May contain EDTA, sorbitol, or sucrose. In 118 mL.
otc	**Triaminic Chest Congestion Liquid** (Novartis)				EDTA, sorbitol, sucrose. Citrus flavor. In 118 mL.
Rx	**Pseudovent-PED Capsules**[1] (Ethex)	60 mg pseudoephedrine HCl	300 mg guaifenesin	*6 to 12 yrs* - 1 q 12 h	Sustained release. EDTA, parabens, sucrose. (ETHEX/015). Blue/clear. In 100s.

[1] This product also may be used in adults; refer to package labeling for dosing.

Refer to the general discussion of these products in the Respiratory Combinations Introduction. Some of the products in the previous Decongestant and Expectorant Combinations table also may be used in children.

UPPER RESPIRATORY COMBINATIONS

ANTIHISTAMINE AND ANALGESIC COMBINATIONS
Content given per capsule or tablet.

	Product & Distributor	Antihistamine	Analgesic	Average Adult Dose	Excipients & How Supplied
otc	Coricidin HBP Cold & Flu Tablets[1] (Schering-Plough)	2 mg chlorpheniramine maleate	325 mg acetaminophen	2 q 4 to 6 h up to 12/day	Sugar, lactose, butylparaben. In 24s.
otc	Percogesic Extra Strength Tablets (Medtech)	12.5 mg diphenhydramine HCl	500 mg acetaminophen	2 q 6 h up to 8/day	Dextrose. Capsule shape. In 40s.
otc	Tylenol Severe Allergy Tablets (McNeil)			2 q 4 to 6 h up to 8/day	Capsule shape. (TYLENOL Severe Allergy). In 24s.
otc	Tylenol PM Extra Strength Tablets, Gelcaps, and Geltabs (McNeil)	25 mg diphenhydramine HCl	500 mg acetaminophen	2 hs	Tablets: (TYLENOL PM). Capsule shape. In 24s, 50s, 100s, and 150s. Gelcaps: Parabens. (TYLENOL PM). In 50s. Geltabs: Parabens. (TYLENOL PM). In 50s and 100s.
Rx	Ed-Flex Capsules[1] (Edwards)	20 mg phenyltoloxamine citrate	300 mg acetaminophen 200 mg salicylamide	1 or 2 q 4 h up to 8/day	(ED-FLEX). Red. In 30s and 100s.
Rx	Duraxin Capsules[1] (Portal)	25 mg phenyltoloxamine citrate	325 mg acetaminophen 200 mg salicylamide	1 or 2 q 4 to 6 h up to 8/day	In 30s.
otc	Aceta-Gesic Tablets[1] (Rugby)	30 mg phenyltoloxamine citrate	325 mg acetaminophen	1 or 2 q 4 h up to 8/day	In 24s and 1000s.
otc	Major-gesic Tablets[1] (Major)				In 100s and 1000s.
otc	Percogesic Tablets[1] (Medtech)				Sucrose. (PERCOGESIC). In 24s, 50s, and 90s.
otc	Phenylgesic Tablets[1] (Ivax)				Orange. In 100s and 1000s.

[1] This product also may be used in children; refer to package labeling for dosing.

For complete prescribing information, refer to the Respiratory Combinations Introduction.

DECONGESTANT, ANTIHISTAMINE, AND EXPECTORANT COMBINATIONS
Content given per tablet or 5 mL.

	Product & Distributor	Decongestant	Antihistamine	Expectorant	Average Adult Dose	Excipients & How Supplied
Rx	Decolate Tablets (Wesley)	5 mg phenylephrine HCl	4 mg chlorpheniramine maleate	100 mg guaifenesin	1 tid or qid	In 1000s.
Rx	Polaramine Expectorant Liquid[1] (Schering)	20 mg pseudoephedrine sulfate	2 mg dexchlorpheniramine maleate	100 mg guaifenesin	5 to 10 mL tid or qid	7.2% alcohol, menthol, sorbitol, sugar. In 473 mL.

[1] This product also may be used in children; refer to package labeling for dosing instructions.

Refer to the general discussion of these products in the Respiratory Combinations Introduction.

PEDIATRIC DECONGESTANT, ANTIHISTAMINE, AND EXPECTORANT COMBINATIONS
Content given per 1 mL.

	Product & Distributor	Decongestant	Antihistamine	Expectorant	Average Dose	How Supplied
Rx	Donatussin Drops (Laser)	2 mg/mL phenylephrine HCl	1 mg/mL chlorpheniramine maleate	20 mg/mL guaifenesin	1 to 2 yrs - 1 to 2 mL q 4 to 6 h up to 8 mL/day; 6 mos to 1 yr - 0.6 to 1 mL q 4 to 6 h up to 4 mL/day; 3 to 6 mos - 0.3 to 0.6 mL q 4 to 6 h up to 2.4 mL/day; < 3 mos - 2 to 3 drops/month of age q 4 to 6 h up to 12 drops/day	Peach flavor. In 30 mL with dropper.

Refer to the general discussion of these products in the Respiratory Combinations Introduction. Some of the products in the previous Decongestant, Antihistamine, and Expectorant Combinations table also may be used in children.

UPPER RESPIRATORY COMBINATIONS

DECONGESTANTS AND ANTIHISTAMINES
Content given per capsule, tablet, or 5 mL.

	Product & Distributor	Decongestant	Antihistamine	Average Adult Dose	Excipients & How Supplied
Rx	Bromfed Capsules (Verum Pharm)	15 mg phenylephrine	12 mg brompheniramine maleate	1 q 12 h	Extended release. Parabens, sucrose. (BROMFED 12-15 VERUM). Purple/Clear. In 100s.
otc	Histatab Plus Tablets[1] (Century)	5 mg phenylephrine HCl	2 mg chlorpheniramine maleate	2 q 4 h up to 12/day	In 30s, 100s, and 1000s.
Rx	Ed A-Hist Liquid[1] (Edwards)	10 mg phenylephrine HCl	4 mg chlorpheniramine maleate	5 mL tid or qid	5% alcohol. Grape flavor. In 473 mL.
Rx	Ed A-Hist Tablets (Edwards)	20 mg phenylephrine HCl	8 mg chlorpheniramine maleate	1 q 12 h	Sustained release. (MAR-CPM). Lt brown. In 100s.
Rx	Promethazine HCl and Phenylephrine HCl Syrup[1] (Various, eg, Alpharma)	5 mg phenylephrine HCl	6.25 mg promethazine HCl	5 mL q 4 to 6 h up to 30 mL/day	7% alcohol. May contain sorbitol, sugar, parabens. In 118 and 473 mL and 3.8 L.
Rx	Phenergan VC Syrup[1] (Wyeth-Ayerst)	5 mg phenylephrine HCl			7% alcohol, saccharin. In 118 and 473 mL.
Rx	Prometh VC Plain Syrup[1] (Alpharma)				7% alcohol. In 3.8 L.
Rx	R-Tanna Tablets (Prasco)	25 mg phenylephrine tannate	9 mg chlorpheniramine tannate	1 or 2 q 12 h	(KL142). Mottled tan, capsule shape. In 100s.
Rx	AlleRx Suspension[1] (Adams)	5 mg phenylephrine tannate	2 mg chlorpheniramine tannate, 12.5 mg pyrilamine tannate	30 mL q 12 h	Methylparaben, saccharin, sucrose. Raspberry flavor. In 473 mL.
Rx	Dytan-D Chewable Tablets[1] (Hawthorn)	5 mg phenylephrine tannate	25 mg diphenhydramine tannate	1 to 2 q 12 h	Aspartame, sorbitol, 1.5 mg phenylalanine. (HAW 577). Blue, triangular, scored. Berry flavor. In 60s.
Rx	Viravan-S Suspension (PediaMed)	12.5 mg phenylephrine tannate	30 mg pyrilamine tannate	5 to 10 mL q 12 h	In 118 and 473 mL.
Rx	Viravan-T Chewable Tablets[1] (PediaMed)	25 mg phenylephrine tannate	30 mg pyrilamine tannate	1 q 12 h	Sugar, saccharin. (VIRAVAN). Mottled brown, scored. Dye-free. Grape flavor. In 100s.
Rx	Ryna-12 Tablets[1] (Wallace)	25 mg phenylephrine tannate	60 mg pyrilamine tannate	1 or 2 q 12 h	(WALLACE 673). Buff, capsule shape, scored. In 100s.
Rx	Semprex-D Capsules (Celltech)	60 mg pseudoephedrine HCl	8 mg acrivastine	1 q 4 to 6 h up to 4/day	Lactose. (MEDEVA SEMPREX-D). Dk green opaque/white opaque. In 100s.
otc	Bromfed Syrup (Muro)	30 mg pseudoephedrine HCl	2 mg brompheniramine maleate	10 mL q 4 to 6 h up to 40 mL/day	Saccharin, sorbitol, sucrose, methylparaben. Orange-lemon flavor. In 480 mL.
Rx	Brofed Liquid[1] (Marnel)	30 mg pseudoephedrine HCl	4 mg brompheniramine maleate	10 mL tid	Parabens, saccharin, sorbitol, sucrose, corn syrup, menthol. Mint flavor. In 473 mL.
Rx	Rondec Syrup[1] (Biovail)	45 mg pseudoephedrine HCl	4 mg brompheniramine maleate	5 mL qid	Saccharin, sorbitol. Cherry flavor. In 118 and 473 mL.
Rx	Lodrane 12 D Tablets[1] (ECR)	45 mg pseudoephedrine HCl	6 mg brompheniramine maleate	1 or 2 q 12 h	Extended release. (ECR 645). White, oval, scored. Dye free. In 100s.
Rx	Brompheniramine Maleate/Pseudoephedrine HCl Syrup[1] (Cypress)	60 mg pseudoephedrine HCl	4 mg brompheniramine maleate	5 mL qid	Saccharin, sorbitol. Raspberry flavor. In 473 mL.
Rx	Bromfed Tablets[1] (Muro)			1 q 4 h up to 6/day	Lactose. (MURO 4060). White, scored. In 100s.
Rx sf	Lodrane Liquid[1] (ECR)			5 mL q 4 to 6 h up to 20 mL/day	Alcohol and dye free. Cherry flavor. In 473 mL.
Rx	Touro Allergy Capsules[1] (Dartmouth)	60 mg pseudoephedrine HCl	5.75 mg brompheniramine maleate	1 or 2 q 12 h	Sustained release. Sucrose. Orange/clear. (TOURO ALLERGY). In 100s.
Rx	Lodrane LD Capsules[1] (ECR)	60 mg pseudoephedrine HCl	6 mg brompheniramine maleate	1 or 2 q 12 h	Dye free. (ECR 6006). Clear. In 100s.
Rx	Respahist Capsules[1] (Respa)			1 or 2 q 12 h up to 4/day	Sustained release. In 100s.
Rx	Histex SR Capsules (Teamm Pharm)[3]	120 mg pseudoephedrine HCl	10 mg brompheniramine maleate	1 q 12 h	Extended release. (SR 089). Peach/clear. In 30s and 100s.
Rx	Bromfenex Capsules (Ethex)	120 mg pseudoephedrine HCl	12 mg brompheniramine maleate	1 q 12 h	Extended release. Sucrose. (Ethex/019). Lt green/clear.In 100s.
Rx	ULTRAbrom Capsules (WE Pharm)				Extended release. In 100s and dispenser pack 10s.
Rx	Rondec Tablets[1] (Biovail)	60 mg pseudoephedrine HCl	4 mg carbinoxamine maleate	1 qid	Lactose. (D 22). Orange. In 100s and 500s.
Rx	Palgic-D Tablets[1] (Pan American)	80 mg pseudoephedrine HCl	8 mg carbinoxamine maleate	1 q 12 h	Extended release. Dye-free. (PAL 61/31). White, capsule shape, scored. In 100s.
Rx	Coldec D Tablets[1] (Breckenridge)	80 mg pseudoephedrine HCl	8 mg carbinoxamine maleate	1 q 12 h	White, capsule shape. In 100s.
Rx	Rondec-TR Tablets (Biovail)	120 mg pseudoephedrine HCl	8 mg carbinoxamine maleate	1 bid	Timed release. Dextrose, lactose. (D 25). Blue. In 100s.
Rx	Zyrtec-D 12 Hour Tablets (Pfizer)	120 mg pseudoephedrine HCl	5 mg cetirizine HCl	1 bid	Extended release. Lactose. (ZYRTEC-D). White, bilayered. In 100s.

DECONGESTANTS AND ANTIHISTAMINES

UPPER RESPIRATORY COMBINATIONS

	Product & Distributor	Decongestant	Antihistamine	Average Adult Dose	Excipients & How Supplied
Rx	PSE CPM[1] Tablets (Boca)	15 mg pseudoephedrine HCl	2 mg chlorpheniramine maleate	2 q 4 to 6 h;	Chewable. Aspartame, sugar. (BOCA 133). Purple, capsule shape, scored. Grape flavor. In 100s.
otc	Allerest Maximum Strength Tablets (Heritage Consumer Products)	30 mg pseudoephedrine HCl	2 mg chlorpheniramine maleate	2 q 4 to 6 h up to 8/day	In 24s.
Rx	Deconamine Syrup[1] (Kenwood)			5 to 10 mL tid or qid	Alcohol and dye free. Sorbitol, sucrose. Grape flavor. In 473 mL.
otc sf	Scot-Tussin Hayfebrol Liquid[1] (Scot-Tussin)			10 mL q 6 h up to 40 mL/day	Alcohol and dye free. Parabens, menthol. In 120 mL.
Rx	Histex Liquid[1] (Teamm Pharm[3])			10 mL q 4 to 6 h	Peach flavor. In 15, 29.6, and 473 mL.
otc sf	Ryna Liquid[1] (Wallace)			10 mL q 4 to 6 h up to 40 mL/day	Alcohol and dye free. Sorbitol, saccharin. In 118 mL.
Rx	Deconamine Tablets (Kenwood)	60 mg pseudoephedrine HCl	4 mg chlorpheniramine maleate	1 tid or qid	Lactose. (KENWOOD 184). White, scored. In 100s.
Rx	Kronofed-A Jr. Capsules (Ferndale)			1 q 12 h	Sustained release. (FL). In 100s and 500s.
otc	Sudafed Cold & Allergy Maximum Strength Tablets[1] (Warner-Lambert)			1 q 4 to 6 h up to 4/day	Lactose. In 24s.
Rx	Clorfed Tablets[1] (Stewart-Jackson)			1 to 2 q 12 h	Extended-release. (CLORFED). White, scored. In 100s.
Rx sf	Amerifed Liquid[1] (AMBI Pharm)	80 mg pseudoephedrine HCl	4 mg chlorpheniramine maleate	5 mL q 8 h up to 15 mL/day	Parabens, aspartame, phenylalanine. Alcohol free. Raspberry flavor. In 30 and 473 mL.
Rx	QDALL (Atley)	100 mg pseudoephedrine HCl	12 mg chlorpheniramine maleate	1 qd up to 2/day	Sucrose. (QD 112). Blue/Yellow. In 100s.
Rx	Chlorpheniramine Maleate/Pseudoephedrine HCl ER Capsules (Various, eg, Eon, Kremers Urban)	120 mg pseudoephedrine HCl	8 mg chlorpheniramine maleate	1 q 12 h	Extended release. May contain parabens and sucrose. In 100s, 250s, 500s, and 1000s.
Rx	Colfed-A Capsules (Breckenridge)				Extended release. Sucrose. (B-145). Blue/clear. In 100s.
Rx	Deconamine SR Capsules (Kenwood)				Sustained release. Sugar. (KENWOOD 181). Blue/yellow. In 100s, 500s, and 1000s.
Rx	Deconomed SR Capsules (Iopharm)				Sustained release. Sucrose, parabens. Blue/clear. In 100s and 500s.
Rx	Kronofed-A Capsules (Ferndale)				Sustained release. (FL). In 100s and 500s.
Rx	N D Clear Capsules (Seatrace)				Sustained release. Clear. In 100s and 1000s.
Rx	Rinade B.I.D. Capsules (Economed)			1 q 12 to 24 h up to 2/day	Extended release. Dye free. In 100s.
Rx	Time-Hist Capsules (MCR American)			1 q 12 h	Sustained release. (PT/026). Clear. In 100s.
Rx	Biohist-LA Tablets[1] (IVAX)	120 mg pseudoephedrine HCl	12 mg chlorpheniramine maleate	½ to 1 q 12 h	Sustained release. In 100s.
Rx	Histade Capsules (Breckenridge)			1 q 12 h	Sustained release. Sucrose. (B170). Red. In 100s.
otc	Benadryl Allergy & Sinus Fastmelt Dissolving Tablets (Warner-Lambert)	30 mg pseudoephedrine HCl	19 mg diphenhydramine citrate (12.5 mg diphenhydramine HCl)	2 q 4 to 6 h up to 8/day	4.6 mg phenylalanine, aspartame, mannitol. In 20s.
otc	Benadryl Allergy & Sinus Liquid[1] (Warner-Lambert)	30 mg pseudoephedrine HCl	12.5 mg diphenhydramine HCl	10 mL q 4 to 6 h up to 40 mL/day	Saccharin, sorbitol. Grape flavor. In 118 mL.
otc	Benadryl Allergy & Sinus Tablets (Warner-Lambert)	60 mg pseudoephedrine HCl	25 mg diphenhydramine HCl	1 q 4 to 6 h up to 4/day	In 24s.
Rx	Allegra-D Tablets (Aventis)	120 mg pseudoephedrine HCl	60 mg fexofenadine HCl	1 bid	Extended release. (Allegra-D). White, tan. Film-coated. Layered. In 60s, 100s, 500s, and blister pack 100s.
Rx	Quadra-Hist D Capsules (Ethex)	80 mg pseudoephedrine HCl	16 mg phenyltoloxamine citrate, 16 mg pyrilamine maleate, 16 mg pheniramine maleate	1 q 8 to 12 h	Extended release. Sucrose. (ETHEX/056). Opaque pink/white. In 100s.

UPPER RESPIRATORY COMBINATIONS

DECONGESTANTS AND ANTIHISTAMINES

	Product & Distributor	Decongestant	Antihistamine	Average Adult Dose	Excipients & How Supplied
otc	Triprolidine HCl w/Pseudoephedrine HCl Syrup[1] (Various, eg, Ivax)	30 mg pseudoephedrine HCl	1.25 mg triprolidine HCl	10 mL q 4 to 6 h up to 40 mL/day	In 118 mL.
otc	Allerfrim Syrup[1] (Rugby)			10 mL q 4 to 6 h up to 40 mL/day	Sucrose, methylparaben, sorbitol, corn syrup. In 118 and 473 mL.
otc	Aprodine Syrup[1] (Major)				In 118 mL.
otc	Silafed Syrup[1] (Silarx)	60 mg pseudoephedrine HCl	2.5 mg triprolidine HCl	10 mL q 4 h up to 40 mL/day	Methylparaben, sucrose, saccharin. In 118 and 237 mL.
otc	Actifed Cold & Allergy Tablets[1] (Warner-Lambert)			1 q 4 to 6 h up to 4/day	Sucrose, lactose. In 12s and 24s.
otc	Allerfrim Tablets[1] (Rugby)				Lactose. (Rugby). Scored. Film-coated. In 24s, 100s, and 1000s.
otc	Aprodine Tablets[1] (Major)				Lactose. In 24s.
otc	Cenafed Plus Tablets[1] (Century)				In 30s and 1000s.
otc	Genac Tablets[1] (Ivax)				Lactose. White. In 48s.
otc	Sudafed Sinus Nighttime Maximum Strength Tablets[1] (Warner-Lambert)				Lactose, sucrose. In 12s.
Rx	Trinalin Repetabs Tablets (Key)	120 mg pseudoephedrine sulfate	1 mg azatadine maleate	1 bid	Sustained release. Sugar, lactose, butylparaben. (TRINALIN 703). Coral. Sugar-coated. In 100s.
otc	Chlor-Trimeton Allergy-D 4 Hour Tablets[1] (Schering-Plough)	60 mg pseudoephedrine sulfate	4 mg chlorpheniramine maleate	1 q 4 to 6 h up to 4/day	Lactose. In 24s.
otc	Chlor-Trimeton Allergy-D 12 Hour Tablets (Schering-Plough)	120 mg pseudoephedrine sulfate	8 mg chlorpheniramine maleate	1 q 12 h up to 2/day	Butylparaben, sugar, lactose. (LA CTM D). In 24s.
Rx	Drixomed Tablets (Iopharm)	120 mg pseudoephedrine sulfate	6 mg dexbrompheniramine maleate	1 q 12 h up to 2/day	Sustained release. Green. In 100s and 500s.
otc	Drixoral Cold & Allergy Tablets (Schering-Plough)				Sugar, lactose, butylparaben. (DRIXORAL). In 10s.
otc	Claritin-D 12 Hour Tablets (Schering-Plough)	120 mg pseudoephedrine sulfate	5 mg loratadine	1 q 12 h	Extended release. Lactose, sugar, butylparaben. (CLARITIN-D). White. In 100s, unit of use 30s, and UD 100s.
otc	Alavert Allergy & Sinus D-12 Hour Tablets (Wyeth Consumer)			1 q 12 h up to 2/day	Extended release. Lactose. In 12s.
otc	Claritin-D 24 Hour Tablets (Schering-Plough)	240 mg pseudoephedrine sulfate	10 mg loratadine	1 q 24 h	Extended release. Sugar. (CLARITIN-D 24 HOUR). White, oval. In 100s and UD 100s.
Rx	C-PHED Tannate Suspension[1] (Morton Grove)	75 mg pseudoephedrine tannate	4.5 mg chlorpheniramine tannate	10 to 20 mL q 12 h up to 40 mL/day	Strawberry/banana flavor. In 118 mL.
Rx	CP-TANNIC Suspension[1] (Cypress)				Strawberry/banana flavor. In 473 mL.
Rx	Tanafed DP Suspension[1] (First Horizon)	75 mg pseudoephedrine tannate	2.5 mg dexchlorpheniramine tannate	10 to 20 mL q 12 h up to 40 mL/day	Methylparaben, saccharin, sucrose. Strawberry-banana flavor. In 20, 118, and 473 mL.

[1] This product also may be used in children; refer to package labeling for dosing.

Refer to the general discussion of these products in the Respiratory Combinations Introduction. Some of the products in the following Pediatric Decongestants and Antihistamines table also may be used in adults.

UPPER RESPIRATORY COMBINATIONS

PEDIATRIC DECONGESTANTS AND ANTIHISTAMINES
Content given per tablet, capsule, 5 mL (liquid), or 1 mL (drops).

	Product & Distributor	Decongestant	Antihistamine	Average Dose	Excipients & How Supplied
Rx	Bromfed-PD Capsules[1] (Verum Pharm)	7.5 mg phenylephrine HCl	6 mg brompheniramine maleate	6 to < 12 yrs - 1 q 12 h	Extended release. Parabens, sucrose. (BROMFED-PD 6-7.5 VERUM). Purple. In 100s.
Rx	Dallergy-JR Capsules[1] (Laser)	20 mg phenylephrine HCl	4 mg chlorpheniramine maleate	6 to 12 yrs - 1 q 12 h up to 2/day	Extended release. Sucrose. (DALLERGY JR Laser 176). Maize/Clear. In 100s.
Rx	Rescon-Jr. Tablets[1] (Capellon)			> 12 yrs - 1 or 2 q 12 h; 6 to 12 yrs - 1 q 12 h	Extended-release. (RESCON JR). Yellow and white, capsule shape, scored. In 100s.
Rx	Nuhist Suspension (Dayton)	5 mg phenylephrine tannate	4.5 mg chlorpheniramine tannate	> 6 yrs - 5 to 10 mL q 12 h; 2 to 6 yrs - 2.5 to 5 mL q 12 h; < 2 yrs - titrate dose	Methylparaben, saccharin, sucrose. In 473 mL.
Rx	Rhinatate-NF Pediatric Suspension (Major)			> 6 yrs - 5 to 10 mL q 12 h; 2 to 6 yrs - 2.5 to 5 mL q 12 h; < 2 yrs - titrate dose individually	Methylparaben, saccharin, sucrose. In 473 mL
Rx	R-Tanna S Pediatric Suspension (Prasco)				Methylparaben, saccharin, sucrose. Grape flavor. In 118 mL
Rx	Rynatan Pediatric Suspension (Wallace)				Tartrazine, methylparaben, saccharin, sucrose. Strawberry-currant flavor. In 473 mL.
Rx	Phenylephrine Tannate/Chlorpheniramine Tannate/Pyrilamine Tannate Pediatric Suspension (Duramed)	5 mg phenylephrine tannate	2 mg chlorpheniramine tannate, 12.5 mg pyrilamine tannate	> 6 yrs - 5 to 10 mL q 12 h; 2 to 6 yrs - 2.5 to 5 mL q 12 h; < 2 yrs - titrate dose individually	Methylparaben, saccharin, sucrose. Strawberry-blackberry-currant flavor. In 118 mL unit of use and 473 mL.
Rx	Rhinatate Pediatric Suspension (Major)				Methylparaben, saccharin, sucrose. Strawberry-blackberry-currant flavor. In 473 mL.
Rx	Triotann Pediatric Suspension (Prasco)				Methylparaben, saccharin, sucrose. Strawberry-blackberry-currant flavor. In 473 mL.
Rx	Triotann-S Pediatric Suspension (Duramed)				Methylparaben, saccharin, sucrose. Strawberry-blackberry-currant flavor. In 118 mL unit of use.
Rx	Duonate-12 Suspension (URL)	5 mg phenylephrine tannate	30 mg pyrilamine tannate	> 6 yrs - 5 to 10 mL q 12 h; 2 to 6 yrs - 2.5 to 5 mL q 12 h; < 2 yrs - titrate dose individually	In 118 mL unit of use with oral syringe.
Rx	P-Tanna 12 Suspension (Prasco)				Methylparaben, saccharin, sucrose. Strawberry-currant flavor. In 118 mL.
Rx	R-Tanna 12 Suspension (Duramed)				Saccharin, sucrose, methyparaben. Strawberry-currant flavor. In 118 mL unit of use with oral syringe.
Rx	Ryna-12 S Suspension (Wallace)				Methylparaben, saccharin, sucrose. Strawberry-currant flavor. In 118 mL unit of use with oral syringe.
Rx	Acculist Drops (PediaMed)	12.5 mg pseudoephedrine HCl	1 mg brompheniramine maleate	12 to 24 mos - 1 mL qid up to 4 mL/day; 6 to 12 mos - 0.75 mL qid up to 3 mL/day; 3 to 6 mos - 0.5 mL qid up to 2 mL/day; 1 to 3 mos - 0.25 mL qid up to 1 mL/day.	Saccharin, sorbitol. Cherry flavor. In 30 mL w/dropper.
otc	Bromanate Elixir (Alpharma)	15 mg pseudoephedrine HCl	1 mg brompheniramine maleate	6 to < 12 yrs - 10 mL q 4 h up to 40 mL/day	Alcohol free. Grape flavor. In 118, 237, and 473 mL.
otc	Dimaphen Elixir[1] (Major)			6 to < 12 yrs - 10 mL q 4 to 6 h up to 40 mL/day	Alcohol free. Saccharin, sorbitol. Grape flavor. In 118 and 237 mL
otc	Dimetapp Cold & Allergy Elixir[1] (Whitehall-Robins)			6 to < 12 yrs - 10 mL q 4 h up to 40 mL/day	Alcohol free. Corn syrup, saccharin, sorbitol. Grape flavor. In 118 and 237 mL.
Rx	Brompheniramine Maleate/Pseudoephedrine HCl Syrup (Cypress)	60 mg pseudoephedrine HCl	4 mg brompheniramine maleate	> 6 yrs - 5 mL qid; 2 to 6 yrs - 2.5 mL qid	Saccharin, sorbitol. Raspberry flavor. In 473 mL
Rx	Bromfenex PD Capsules[1] (Ethex)	60 mg pseudoephedrine HCl	6 mg brompheniramine maleate	6 to 12 yrs - 1 q 12 h	Extended release. Opaque green/clear. Sucrose. (Ethex/020). In 100s.
Rx	ULTRAbrom PD Capsules[1] (WE Pharm)				Extended release. (WE 04). Purple/clear. In 100s.
Rx	Rondec Oral Drops (Biovail)	15 mg pseudoephedrine HCl	1 mg carbinoxamine maleate	12 to 24 mos - 1 mL qid; 6 to 12 mos - 0.75 mL qid; 3 to 6 mos - 0.5 mL qid; 1 to 3 mos - 0.25 mL qid	Saccharin, sorbitol. Cherry flavor. In 30 mL w/dropper.

UPPER RESPIRATORY COMBINATIONS

PEDIATRIC DECONGESTANTS AND ANTIHISTAMINES

	Product & Distributor	Decongestant	Antihistamine	Average Dose	Excipients & How Supplied
Rx	**Palgic DS Syrup** (Pan American)	15 mg pseudoephedrine HCl	2 mg carbinoxamine maleate	≥ 6 yrs - 10 mL qid; 18 mos to 6 yrs - 5 mL qid; 9 to 18 mos - 3.75 to 5 mL qid; 6 to 9 mos - 3.75 mL qid; 3 to 6 mos - 2.5 mL qid; 1 to 3 mos - 1.25 mL qid	Strawberry/pineapple flavor. In 15 and 473 mL.
Rx sf	**Pediatex-D Liquid** (Zyber)	20 mg pseudoephedrine HCl	2 mg carbinoxamine maleate	≥ 6 yrs - 10 mL qid; 18 mos to 6 yrs - 5 mL qid; 9 to 18 mos - 3.75 to 5 mL qid; 6 to 9 mos - 3.75 mL qid; 3 to 6 mos - 2.5 mL qid; 1 to 3 mos - 1.25 mL qid	Alcohol and dye free. Cotton candy flavor. In 20 and 473 mL.
Rx	**Palgic DS Syrup** (Pan American)	25 mg pseudoephedrine HCl	2 mg carbinoxamine maleate	≥ 6 yrs - 10 mL qid; 18 mos to 6 yrs - 5 mL qid; 10 to 18 mos - 5 mL qid; 7 to 9 mos - 3.75 mL qid; 4 to 6 mos - 2.5 mL qid; 1 to 3 mos - 1.25 mL qid	Strawberry/pineapple flavor. In 15 and 475 mL.
Rx sf	**Carbinoxamine Oral Drops** (Morton Grove)			9 to 18 mos - 1 mL qid; 6 to 9 mos - 0.75 mL qid; 3 to 6 mos - 0.5 mL qid; 1 to 3 mos - 0.25 mL qid	Alcohol free. Parabens, sorbitol. Raspberry or fruit flavors. In 30 mL w/dropper.
Rx	**Cydec Oral Drops** (Cypress)				Raspberry flavor. In 30 mL.
Rx sf	**Carbinoxamine Syrup**[1] (Morton Grove)	60 mg pseudoephedrine HCl	4 mg carbinoxamine maleate	> 6 yrs - 5 mL qid; 18 mos to 6 yrs - 2.5 mL qid	Alcohol free. Parabens, sorbitol. Raspberry or fruit flavors. In 118, 237, and 473 mL.
otc	**PediaCare Children's Cold & Allergy Liquid** (Pharmacia)	15 mg pseudoephedrine HCl	1 mg chlorpheniramine maleate	6 to 11 yrs - 10 mL q 4 to 6 h up to 40 mL/day	Alcohol free. Corn syrup, sorbitol. Bubble-gum flavor. In 120 mL.
otc	**Thera-Hist Cold & Allergy Syrup** (Major)			6 to < 12 yrs - 10 mL q 4 to 6 h up to 40 mL/day	Sorbitol, sucrose. In 118 mL.
otc	**Tri-Acting Cold & Allergy Syrup** (Topco)				Alcohol free. Sorbitol, sucrose. Orange flavor. In 118 mL.
otc	**Triacting Cold & Allergy Liquid** (AmerisourceBergen)				Alcohol free. Sorbitol, sucrose. Orange flavor. In 118 mL.
otc	**Triaminic Cold & Allergy Liquid** (Novartis)				Alcohol free. Sorbitol, sucrose. Orange flavor. In 118 and 147 mL.
otc	**Triaminic Softchews Tablets** (Novartis)			6 to < 12 yrs - 2 q 4 to 6 h up to 8/day	17.5 mg phenylalanine, aspartame, mannitol, sucrose. Orange flavor. In 18s.
Rx	**Pediox Tablets**[1] (Atley)	15 mg pseudoephedrine HCl	2 mg chlorpheniramine maleate	6 to < 12 yrs - 1 q 4 to 6 h	Chewable. Aspartame, phenylalanine, mannitol, sorbitol, xylitol. Grape flavor. (15 2 P). Purple, scored. In 100s.
otc	**Benadryl Children's Allergy & Cold Fastmelt Tablets**[1] (Warner-Lambert)	30 mg pseudoephedrine HCl	19 mg diphenhydramine citrate (12.5 mg diphenhydramine HCl)	6 to < 12 yrs - 1 q 4 h up to 4/day	4.6 mg phenylalanine, aspartame, mannitol. In 20s.
otc sf	**Benadryl Children's Allergy & Sinus Liquid**[1] (Warner-Lambert)	30 mg pseudoephedrine HCl	12.5 mg diphenhydramine HCl	6 to < 12 yrs - 5 mL q 4 to 6 h up to 20 mL/day	Alcohol free. Saccharin, sorbitol. Grape flavor. In 118 mL.
Rx	**Quadra-Hist D PED Capsules** (Ethex)	40 mg pseudoephedrine HCl	8 mg phenyltoloxamine citrate, 8 mg pyrilamine maleate, 8 mg pheniramine maleate	6 to 12 yrs - 1 q 8 to 12 h	Extended release. Sucrose. (ETHEX/057). White opaque. In 100s.
Rx sf	**Chlorpheniramine Tannate/Pseudoephedrine Tannate Suspension** (Various, eg, URL)	75 mg pseudoephedrine tannate	4.5 mg chlorpheniramine tannate	6 to 12 yrs - 5 to 10 mL q 12 h up to 20 mL/day; 2 to 6 - 2.5 to 5 mL q 12 h up to 10 mL/day	Alcohol free. Strawberry/banana flavor. In 118 and 473 mL.

[1] This product also may be used in adults; refer to package labeling for dosing.

Refer to the general discussion of these products in the Respiratory Combinations Introduction. Some of the products in the previous Decongestants and Antihistamines table also may be used in children.

UPPER RESPIRATORY COMBINATIONS

DECONGESTANT, ANTIHISTAMINE, AND ANALGESIC COMBINATIONS
Content given per capsule, tablet, packet, or 5 mL.

	Product & Distributor	Decongestant	Antihistamine	Analgesic/Other	Average Adult Dose	Excipients & How Supplied
otc	Alka-Seltzer Plus Cold Medicine Effervescent Tablets (Bayer)	5 mg phenylephrine HCl	2 mg chlorpheniramine maleate	250 mg acetaminophen	2 tablets dissolved in 118 mL water q 4 h up to 8/day	Acesulfame K, aspartame, phenylalanine, saccharin, sorbitol. Original, orange, and cherry flavors. In 12s, 20s, 36s, and 48s.
otc	Decoduit Tablets (Wesley Pharmacal)	5 mg phenylephrine HCl	2 mg chlorpheniramine maleate	300 mg acetaminophen	2 q 4 to 6 h up to 12/day	In 1000s.
otc	Dristan Cold Multi-Symptom Formula Tablets (Whitehall Robins)	5 mg phenylephrine HCl	2 mg chlorpheniramine maleate	325 mg acetaminophen	2 q 4 h up to 12/day	In 20s, 40s, and 75s.
otc	Dryphen, Multi-Symptom Formula Tablets (Major)					In 40s.
otc sf	Scot-Tussin Original Clear 5-Action Cold and Allergy Formula Liquid[1] (Scot-Tussin)	4.2 mg phenylephrine HCl	13.3 mg pheniramine maleate	83.3 mg Na citrate, 83.3 mg Na salicylate, 25 mg caffeine citrate	5 mL q 3 to 4 h up to qid	Alcohol and dye free. Saccharin, parabens. Cherry-strawberry flavor. In 118 and 473 mL and 3.8 L.
otc	Scot-Tussin Original 5-Action Cold and Allergy Formula Syrup[1] (Scot-Tussin)					Alcohol free. Sugar, parabens, sorbitol. Grape flavor. In 118 and 473 mL and 3.8 L.
otc	Comtrex Acute Head Cold & Sinus Pressure Relief, Multi-Symptom Maximum Strength Tablets (Bristol-Myers Squibb)	30 mg pseudoephedrine HCl	2 mg brompheniramine maleate	500 mg acetaminophen	2 q 6 h up to 8/day	Parabens. In 24s.
otc	Alka-Seltzer Plus Cold Medicine Liqui-Gels[1] (Bayer)	30 mg pseudoephedrine HCl	2 mg chlorpheniramine maleate	325 mg acetaminophen	2 q 4 h up to 8/day	Liquid filled. Sorbitol. (AS+ COLD). In 12s and 20s.
otc	Kolephrin Tablets[1] (Pfeiffer)				2 q 4 to 6 h up to 8/day	Capsule shape. In 24s and 36s.
otc	Actifed Cold & Sinus Maximum Strength Tablets (Warner-Lambert)	30 mg pseudoephedrine HCl	2 mg chlorpheniramine maleate	500 mg acetaminophen	2 q 6 h up to 8/day	Capsule shape. In 20s.
otc	Comtrex Allergy-Sinus Treatment, Maximum Strength Tablets (Bristol-Myers Squibb)					Parabens. In 24s and 50s.
otc	Good Sense Maximum Strength Dose Sinus Tablets (Perrigo)					Capsule shape. In 24s.
otc	Good Sense Maximum Strength Pain Relief Allergy Sinus Gelcaps (Perrigo)					In 24s.
otc	Sine-Off Sinus Medicine Tablets (Hogil Pharm.)					Capsule shape. In 24s and 96s.
otc	Sinutab Sinus Allergy, Maximum Strength Tablets (Warner-Lambert)					Capsule shape. In 24s.
otc	Tylenol Allergy Sinus, Maximum Strength Tablets, Gelcaps, and Geltabs (McNeil Consumer Health)				2 q 4 to 6 h up to 8/day	**Tablets:** Capsule shape. In 24s and 48s. **Gelcaps:** (TYLENOL A/S). Parabens, EDTA. In 24s and 48s. **Geltabs:** (TYLENOL A/S). Parabens, EDTA. In 24s and 48s.
otc	Comtrex Flu Therapy & Fever Relief Day & Night, Multi-Symptom Maximum Strength Tablets (Bristol-Myers Squibb)	Day: 30 mg pseudoephedrine HCl / Night: 30 mg pseudoephedrine HCl	Night: 2 mg chlorpheniramine maleate	500 mg acetaminophen	Day: 2 q 6 h up to 4/day / Night: 2 hs ≥ 6 h after last daytime dose	Day: Orange, capsule shape. Night: Parabens. Green. In 24s (18 day; 6 night).
Rx	Simplet Tablets (Major)	60 mg pseudoephedrine HCl	4 mg chlorpheniramine maleate	500 mg acetaminophen	1 tid or qid	In 100s.
otc	Singlet for Adults Tablets (SmithKline Beecham Consumer)			650 mg acetaminophen	1 q 4 to 6 h up to 4/day	Sucrose. Capsule shape. In 100s.
otc	TheraFlu Flu and Cold Medicine Original Formula Powder (Novartis Consumer Health)				1 packet dissolved in 177 mL hot water q 4 to 6 h up to 4/day	Sucrose. In 6s.
otc	Triaminicin Cold, Allergy, Sinus Medicine Tablets (Novartis Consumer Health)				1 q 4 to 6 h up to 4/day	Lactose, methylparaben. In 24s.

UPPER RESPIRATORY COMBINATIONS

DECONGESTANT, ANTIHISTAMINE, AND ANALGESIC COMBINATIONS

	Product & Distributor	Decongestant	Antihistamine	Analgesic/Other	Average Adult Dose	Excipients & How Supplied
otc	TheraFlu Flu & Cold Medicine for Sore Throat, Maximum Strength Powder (Novartis Consumer Health)	60 mg pseudoephedrine HCl	4 mg chlorpheniramine maleate	1000 mg acetaminophen	1 packet dissolved in 177 mL hot water q 6 h up to 4/day	Sucrose, aspartame, 20 mg phenylalanine. Apple cinnamon flavor. In 6s.
otc	TheraFlu Flu & Sore Throat, Maximum Strength Powder (Novartis Consumer Health)					Acesulfame K, aspartame, sorbitol, sucrose. In 6s.
otc	TheraFlu Flu & Sore Throat Night Time, Maximum Strength Powder (Novartis Consumer Health)					Alcohol free. Acesulfame K, aspartame, 25 mg phenylalanine, sucrose. Apple cinnamon flavor. In 6s.
otc	Advil Allergy Sinus Tablets (Wyeth)	30 mg pseudoephedrine HCl	2 mg chlorpheniramine maleate	200 mg ibuprofen	1 q 4 to 6 h up to 6/day	Oval. In 10s and 20s.
otc	Tavist Allergy/Sinus/Headache Tablets (Novartis Consumer Health)	30 mg pseudoephedrine HCl	0.335 mg clemastine fumarate	500 mg acetaminophen	2 q 6 h up to 8/day	Methylparaben. Capsule shape. In 24s and 48s.
otc	Tylenol Allergy Sinus, Maximum Strength, Day and Night Formula Tablets(McNeil)	Day: 30 mg pseudoephedrine HCl	2 mg chlorpheniramine maleate	500 mg acetaminophen	2 q 4 to 6 h up to 8/day	Capsule shape. In 12s.
		Night: 30 mg pseudoephedrine HCl	25 mg diphenhydramine HCl	500 mg acetaminophen	2 q 4 to 6 h up to 8/day	Capsule shape. In 12s.
otc	Benadryl Allergy & Cold Tablets (Warner-Lambert)	30 mg pseudoephedrine HCl	12.5 mg diphenhydramine HCl	500 mg acetaminophen	2 q 6 h up to 8/day	(Benadryl Allergy/Cold). Capsule shape. In 24s.
otc	Benadryl Allergy & Sinus Headache Tablets and Gelcaps (Warner-Lambert)					(Benadryl). Capsule shape. In 24s and 48s.
otc	Benadryl Maximum Strength Severe Allergy & Sinus Headache Tablets (Warner-Lambert)	30 mg pseudoephedrine HCl	25 mg diphenhydramine HCl	500 mg acetaminophen	2 q 6 h up to 8/day	Capsule shape. In 20s.
otc	Sine-Off Night Time Formula Sinus, Cold, & Flu Medicine Geltabs (Hogil Pharm.)					Capsule shape. In 10s.
otc	Sudafed Maximum Strength Sinus Nighttime Plus Pain Relief Tablets (Warner-Lambert)					(SU NT). Capsule shape. In 20s.
otc	Tylenol Allergy Sinus NightTime, Maximum Strength Tablets (McNeil Consumer Healthcare)				2 hs	Capsule shape. In 24s.
otc	Tylenol Flu NightTime, Maximum Strength Gelcaps (McNeil Consumer Healthcare)				2 q 6 h up to 8/day	Parabens. In 24s.
otc	Tylenol Flu, Maximum Strength Gelcaps (McNeil Consumer Healthcare)				2 at bedtime; may repeat q 6 h up to 8/day.	Benzyl alcohol, castor oil, parabens. Capsule shape. In 12s.
otc	Contac Day & Night Allergy/Sinus Relief Tablets (SmithKline Beecham)	Day: 60 mg pseudoephedrine HCl / Night: 60 mg pseudoephedrine HCl	Night: 50 mg diphenhydramine HCl	650 mg acetaminophen / 650 mg acetaminophen	Day: 1 q 6 h / Night: 1 q 6 h (≤ 4/day in any combination)	Day: Capsule shape. White. Night: Capsule shape. Green. In 20s (15 day; 5 night).
otc	Tylenol Sinus NightTime, Maximum Strength Tablets (McNeil Consumer Healthcare)	30 mg pseudoephedrine HCl	6.25 mg doxylamine succinate	500 mg acetaminophen	2 q 4 to 6 h up to 8/day	Capsule shape. In 24s.
otc	Coricidin 'D' Cold, Flu, & Sinus Tablets[1] (Schering-Plough Healthcare Products)	30 mg pseudoephedrine sulfate	2 mg chlorpheniramine maleate	325 mg acetaminophen	2 q 4 to 6 h up to 8/day	Lactose. (Coricidin D). In 24s.
otc	Drixoral Allergy Sinus Tablets (Schering-Plough Healthcare Products)	60 mg pseudoephedrine sulfate	3 mg dexbrompheniramine maleate	500 mg acetaminophen	2 q 12 h up to 4/day	Extended release. Parabens. (DRIXORAL C + F)In 12s.

[1] This product also may be used in children; refer to package labeling for dosing.

Refer to the general discussion of these products in the Respiratory Combinations Introduction.

UPPER RESPIRATORY COMBINATIONS

PEDIATRIC DECONGESTANT, ANTIHISTAMINE, AND ANALGESIC COMBINATIONS

Content given per tablet or 5 mL.

Product & Distributor	Decongestant	Antihistamine	Analgesic	Average Dose	Excipients & How Supplied
otc **Tylenol Children's Cold Chewable Tablets** (McNeil Consumer Healthcare)	7.5 mg pseudoephedrine HCl	0.5 mg chlorpheniramine maleate	80 mg acetaminophen	**6 to 11 yrs** - 4 q 4 to 6 h up to 16/day	Aspartame, mannitol, 6 mg phenylalanine. Grape flavor. In 24s.
otc **Tylenol Children's Cold Liquid** (McNeil Consumer Healthcare)	15 mg pseudoephedrine HCl	1 mg chlorpheniramine maleate	160 mg acetaminophen	**6 to 11 yrs** - 10 mL q 4 to 6 h up to 40 mL/day	Sorbitol, sucrose. Alcohol free. Grape flavor. In 120 mL.

Refer to the general discussion of these products in the Respiratory Combinations Introduction. Some of the products in the previous Decongestant, Antihistamine, and Analgesic Combinations table also may be used in children.

UPPER RESPIRATORY COMBINATIONS

DECONGESTANT, ANTIHISTAMINE, AND ANTICHOLINERGIC COMBINATIONS
Content given per tablet or 5 mL.

	Product & Distributor	Decongestant	Antihistamine	Anticholinergic	Average Adult Dose	Excipients & How Supplied
Rx	Dallergy Syrup[1] (Laser)	10 mg phenylephrine HCl	2 mg chlorpheniramine maleate	0.625 mg methscopolamine nitrate	10 mL q 4 to 6 h up to 40 mL/day	In 473 mL.
Rx	AH-chew Tablets[1] (WE Pharm.)	10 mg phenylephrine HCl	2 mg chlorpheniramine maleate	1.25 mg methscopolamine nitrate		Chewable. (WE 03). Scored. Grape flavor. In 100s.
Rx	Dehistine Syrup[1] (Cypress)				10 mL q 4 to 6 h, up to 40 mL/day	Alcohol free. Root beer flavor. In 473 mL.
Rx	Duradryl Syrup[1] (Breckenridge Pharm.)				5 or 10 mL q 3 or 4 h	Corn syrup. In 473 mL.
Rx	Extendryl Chewable Tablets[1] (Fleming)				2 q 4 h up to 12/day	Tan, scored. Root beer flavor. In 100s and 1000s.
Rx	Extendryl Syrup[1] (Fleming)				10 mL q 4 h up to 40 mL/day	Rootbeer flavor. In 473 mL and 3.8 L.
Rx	Ex-Histine Syrup[1] (WE Pharm.)				10 mL q 4 to 6 h up to 40 mL/day	Rootbeer flavor. In 473 mL.
Rx	Dallergy Tablets[1] (Laser)	10 mg phenylephrine HCl	4 mg chlorpheniramine maleate	1.25 mg methscopolamine nitrate	1 q 4 to 6 h up to 4/day	(Laser Dallergy). Scored. In 100s.
Rx	Drihist SR Tablets[1] (Prasco)	20 mg phenylephrine HCl	8 mg chlorpheniramine maleate	2.5 mg methscopolamine nitrate	1 q 12 h	Sustained release. (110). White, capsule shape, scored. In 100s.
Rx	Extendryl SR Capsules (Fleming)					Sustained release. (F SR). Green/Red. In 100s and 1000s.
Rx	Hista-Vent DA Tablets[1] (Ethex)					Sustained release. (ETH 227). Brown, capsule shape. In 100s.
Rx	OMNIhist L.A. Tablets (WE Pharm.)					Sustained release. (WE 02). White, scored. In 100s.
Rx	Pre-Hist-D Tablets[1] (Marnel)					Sustained release. (MD CPM). White, scored. In 100s.
Rx	AeroHist Plus Tablets[1] (Aero)					Extended release. (2376 aero). White, capsule shape, scored. In 100s.
Rx	Rescon-MX Tablets (Capellon)	40 mg phenylephrine HCl	8 mg chlorpheniramine maleate	2.5 mg methscopolamine nitrate	1 q 12 h	Extended-release. (PHE). Green and white, capsule shape, scored. In 100s.
Rx	Dallergy Tablets[1] (Propst)	20 mg phenylephrine HCl	12 mg chlorpheniramine maleate	2.5 mg methscopolamine nitrate	1 q 12 h up to 2/day	Extended release. (DALLERGY 12H). White, capsule shape, scored. In 100s.
Rx	AccuHist LA Tablets (PediaMed)	20 mg phenylephrine HCl	8 mg chlorpheniramine maleate	0.19 mg hyoscyamine sulfate, 0.04 mg atropine sulfate, 0.01 mg scopolamine HBr	1 q 12 h up to 2/day	Sustained release. Lactose. (PROPST 010). White, capsule shape. In 100s and 500s.
Rx	Bellahist-D LA Tablets (Cypress)					Extended release. Alcohol and dye free. (CYP 449). Capsule shape, scored. In 100s.
Rx	Stahist Tablets (Huckaby)	25 mg phenylephrine HCl, 40 mg pseudoephedrine	8 mg chlorpheniramine maleate	0.19 mg hyoscyamine sulfate, 0.04 mg atropine sulfate, 0.01 mg scopolamine HBr	1 q 12 h	Sustained release. Dye free. In 100s.
Rx	AlleRx-D Tablets (Adams Labs)	120 mg pseudoephedrine HCl		2.5 mg methscopolamine nitrate	1 q 12 h up to 2/day	Controlled release. (Adams 006). Yellow, elongated, scored. In 60s.
Rx	PSE 120/MSC 2.5 Tablets (Cypress)					Sustained release. (CYP 281). White, scored. In 60s.
Rx	Pannaz S Syrup[1] (Pan American Labs)	15 mg pseudoephedrine HCl	2 mg carbinoxamine maleate	1.25 mg methscopolamine nitrate	5 to 10 mL qid	Blueberry flavor. In 15 and 473 mL.
Rx	Pannaz Tablets (Pan American Labs)	90 mg pseudoephedrine HCl	8 mg carbinoxamine maleate	2.5 mg methscopolamine nitrate	1 q 12 h up to 2/day	Extended release. (PAL 88). Light green, speckled. In 100s.
Rx	Durahist Tablets[1] (ProEthic)	60 mg pseudoephedrine HCl	8 mg chlorpheniramine maleate	1.25 mg methscopolamine nitrate	1 q 12 h up to 2/day	Sustained release. Talc. (PE 424). White, scored. In 100s.
Rx sf	Respa A.R. Tablets (Respa Pharm.)	90 mg pseudoephedrine HCl	8 mg chlorpheniramine maleate	0.024 mg belladonna alkaloids (atropine, hyoscyamine, scopolamine)	1 q 12 h	Dye free. In 100s.

UPPER RESPIRATORY COMBINATIONS

DECONGESTANT, ANTIHISTAMINE, AND ANTICHOLINERGIC COMBINATIONS

	Product & Distributor	Decongestant	Antihistamine	Anticholinergic	Average Adult Dose	Excipients & How Supplied
Rx	CPM 8/PSE 90/MSC 2.5 Tablets[1] (Cypress)	90 mg pseudoephedrine HCl	8 mg chlorpheniramine maleate	2.5 mg methscopolamine nitrate	1 q 12 hr up to 2/day	Sustained release. (CYP282). White, scored. In 100s.
Rx	Pannaz Tablets[1] (Pan American Labs)					Sustained release. (PAL 88). Lt. green, scored. In 100s.
Rx	Mescolor Tablets[1] (First Horizon)	120 mg pseudoephedrine HCl	8 mg chlorpheniramine maleate	2.5 mg methscopolamine nitrate	1 q 12 h up to 2/day	Sustained release. Dye free. (HP 15). White, scored. Film-coated. In 100s.
Rx	Rescon-MX Tablets[1] (Capellon)					Sustained release. (RES CON). Mottled green, scored. In 100s.
Rx	Xiral Tablets[1] (Hawthorn)					Sustained release. Dye free. (HAW 500). White, capsule shape, scored. In 100s.
Rx	AlleRx Dose Pack Tablets (Adams Labs.)	*Day:* 120 mg pseudoephedrine HCl		2.5 mg methscopolamine nitrate	1 am	*Day:* Controlled release. (Adams/006). Yellow, elongated, scored.
		Night:	8 mg chlorpheniramine maleate	2.5 mg methscopolamine nitrate	1 pm	*Night:* Controlled release. (Adams/007). Blue, elongated, scored. In 20s (10 day; 10 night).

[1] This product also may be used in children; refer to package labeling for dosing.

Refer to the general discussion of these products in the Respiratory Combinations Introduction.

PEDIATRIC DECONGESTANT, ANTIHISTAMINE, AND ANTICHOLINERGIC COMBINATIONS

Content given per capsule.

	Product & Distributor	Decongestant	Antihistamine	Anticholinergic	Average Dose	Excipients & How Supplied
Rx	Extendryl JR Capsules (Fleming)	10 mg phenylephrine HCl	4 mg chlorpheniramine maleate	1.25 mg methscopolamine nitrate	**6 to 12 yrs** - 1 q 12 h	(F JR). Green/Red. In 100s and 1000s.
Rx	AeroKid Syrup (Aero)					Glycerin, sorbitol, saccharin. Raspberry flavor. In 20, 120, and 480 mL.

Refer to the general discussion of these products in the Respiratory Combinations Introduction. Some of the products in the previous Decongestant, Antihistamine, and Anticholinergic Combinations monograph also may be used in children.

UPPER RESPIRATORY COMBINATIONS

ANTITUSSIVE COMBINATIONS
Content given per tablet, capsule, packet, pouch, or 5 mL.

	Product & Distributor	Antitussive	Antihistamine	Decongestant	Other	Average Adult Dose	Excipients & How Supplied
Rx	Tussizone-12 RF Suspension[1] (Mallinckrodt)	30 mg carbetapentane tannate	4 mg chlorpheniramine tannate			5 to 10 mL q 12 h	Tartrazine, methylparaben, saccharin, sucrose. Strawberry currant flavor. In 118 mL.
Rx	Tannic-12 Tablets (Cypress)	60 mg carbetapentane tannate	5 mg chlorpheniramine tannate			1 to 2 q 12 h	Dye free. (CYP 303). Tan, capsule shape, scored. In 100s.
Rx	Trionate Tablets (Breckenridge Pharm.)						(B072). Off-white, capsule shape. In 100s.
Rx	Tussi-12 Tablets (Wallace)						(Wallace 0681). Mauve, capsule shape, scored. In 100s.
Rx	Tussizone-12 RF Tablets (Mallinckrodt)						(0037 0681). Mauve, capsule shape, scored. In 100s.
Rx	Quad Tann Tablets (Breckenridge Pharm.)	60 mg carbetapentane tannate	5 mg chlorpheniramine tannate	10 mg phenylephrine tannate, 10 mg ephedrine tannate		1 to 2 q 12 h	(B-816). Beige, capsule shape. In 100s.
Rx	Rynatuss Tablets (Wallace)						(Wallace 717). Mauve, capsule shape, scored. In 100s, 500s, and 2000s.
Rx	C-Tanna 12D Suspension[1] (Prasco)	30 mg carbetapentane tannate	30 mg pyrilamine tannate	5 mg phenylephrine tannate		5 to 10 mL q 12 h	Glycerin, methylparaben, sucrose. Purple, strawberry flavor. In 118 mL.
Rx	Tussi-12D S Suspension[1] (Wallace)						Tartrazine, methylparaben, saccharin, sucrose. Strawberry-currant flavor. In 120 mL with oral syringe.
Rx	C-Tanna 12D Tablets[1] (Prasco)	60 mg carbetapentane tannate	40 mg pyrilamine tannate	10 mg phenylephrine tannate		1 or 2 q 12 h	Corn starch. (KL-165). Mottled pink, oval, scored. In 100s.
Rx	Tussi-12D Tablets[1] (Wallace)						(WALLACE 0692). Pink, capsule shape, scored. In 100s.
c-iii	Cycofed Syrup[1] (Cypress)	20 mg codeine phosphate		60 mg pseudoephedrine HCl		5 mL q 6 h up to 20 mL/day	Spearmint flavor. In 473 mL.
c-iii	Nucofed Syrup[1] (Monarch)						Alcohol free. Sorbitol, sucrose. Mint flavor. In 473 mL.
c-iii	Nucofed Capsules (Monarch)					1 q 6 h up to 4/day	Lactose. (M 018). Green/clear. In 60s.
c-v	Dihistine DH Elixir[1] (Alpharma)	10 mg codeine phosphate	2 mg chlorpheniramine maleate	30 mg pseudoephedrine HCl		10 mL q 4 to 6 h up to 40 mL/day	5% alcohol. In 118 and 473 mL and 3.8 L.
c-v	Decohistine DH Liquid (Morton Grove)					5 to 10 mL q 4 to 6 h up to 40 mL/day	5.8% alcohol, sugar, menthol, parabens, sorbitol. Grape/honey flavor. In 118 and 473 mL and 3.8 L.
c-v sf	Ryna-C Liquid[1] (Wallace)					10 mL q 4 to 6 h up to 40 mL/day	Alcohol and dye free. Saccharin, sorbitol. In 118 and 473 mL.
c-v	Prometh w/Codeine Cough Syrup[1] (Alpharma)	10 mg codeine phosphate	6.25 mg promethazine HCl			5 mL q 4 to 6 h up to 30 mL/day	7% alcohol, corn syrup, parabens, saccharin. In 118 mL.
c-v	Promethazine HCl w/Codeine Syrup[1] (Various, eg. Major, Morton Grove, URL)						In 118 and 473 mL.
c-v	Promethazine VC w/Codeine Cough Syrup[1] (URL)	10 mg codeine phosphate	6.25 mg promethazine HCl	5 mg phenylephrine HCl		5 mL q 4 to 6 h up to 30 mL/day	7.1% alcohol, EDTA, sugar, methylparaben. Cherry/raspberry flavor. In 473 mL.
c-v	Prometh VC w/Codeine Cough Syrup[1] (Alpharma)			5 mg phenylephrine HCl			7% alcohol, parabens, sugar, saccharin. In 118, 237, and 473 mL and 3.8 L.
c-v	Tricodene Cough & Cold Liquid[1] (Pfeiffer)	8.2 mg codeine phosphate	12.5 mg pyrilamine maleate			10 mL q 6 to 8 h up to 60 mL/day	In 120 mL.

ANTITUSSIVE COMBINATIONS

UPPER RESPIRATORY COMBINATIONS

	Product & Distributor	Antitussive	Antihistamine	Decongestant	Other	Average Adult Dose	Excipients & How Supplied
c-v	Codimal PH Syrup[1] (Schwarz)	10 mg codeine phosphate	8.33 mg pyrilamine maleate	5 mg phenylephrine HCl		10 mL q 4 to 6 h up to 60 mL/day	Alcohol free. Sucrose. In 118 and 473 mL.
c-v	Triacin-C Cough Syrup[1] (Alpharma)	10 mg codeine phosphate	1.25 mg triprolidine HCl	30 mg pseudoephedrine HCl		10 mL q 4 to 6 h up to 40 mL/day	4.3% alcohol, methylparaben. Caramel flavor. In 118 and 473 mL and 3.8 L.
otc	Dimetapp Long Acting Cough Plus Cold Syrup (Wyeth)	7.5 mg dextromethorphan HBr		15 mg pseudoephedrine HCl		20 mL qid up to 80 mL/day	Corn syrup, saccharin. Fruit punch flavor. In 118 mL.
otc	Robitussin Honey Cough & Cold Liquid (Whitehall-Robins)	10 mg dextromethorphan HBr		20 mg pseudoephedrine HCl		15 mL q 6 h up to 60 mL/day	Saccharin. In 118 mL.
otc	Top Care Maximum Strength Soothing Cough & Head Congestion Relief D Liquid[1] (Topco Assoc.)						5% alcohol, corn syrup, saccharin. Cherry flavor. In 118 mL.
otc	Vicks 44D Cough & Head Congestion Relief Liquid[1] (Procter & Gamble)						5% alcohol, saccharin, corn syrup. In 118 and 236 mL.
otc	Robitussin Maximum Strength Cough & Cold Syrup (Whitehall-Robins)	15 mg dextromethorphan HBr		30 mg pseudoephedrine HCl		10 mL q 6 h up to 40 mL/day	1.4% alcohol, corn syrup, saccharin, glucose. In 237 mL.
otc	666 Cold Preparation, Maximum Strength Liquid[1] (Monticello Drug Co.)	3.3 mg dextromethorphan HBr		10 mg pseudoephedrine HCl	108.3 mg acetaminophen	30 mL q 4 h up to 120 mL/day	Saccharin, sucrose. In 177 mL.
otc	Vicks DayQuil Multi-Symptom Cold/Flu Relief Liquid[1] (Procter & Gamble)						Saccharin, sucrose. In 177 mL.
otc	Robitussin Honey Flu Multi-Symptom Liquid (Whitehall-Robins)	6.6 mg dextromethorphan HBr		20 mg pseudoephedrine HCl	166.6 mg acetaminophen	15 mL q 4 h up to 60 mL/day	Saccharin, corn syrup, menthol. In 118 mL.
otc	Vicks DayQuil LiquiCaps Multi-Symptom Cold/Flu Relief Capsules[1] (Procter & Gamble)	10 mg dextromethorphan HBr		30 mg pseudoephedrine HCl	250 mg acetaminophen	2 q 4 h up to 8/day	Sorbitol. In 12s, 20s, and 36s.
otc	Alka-Seltzer Plus Cold & Flu Liqui-Gels[1] (Bayer)	10 mg dextromethorphan HBr		30 mg pseudoephedrine HCl	325 mg acetaminophen	2 q 4 h up to 8/day	Liquid filled. Sorbitol. In 12s.
otc	Alka-Seltzer Plus Liqui-Gels Flu Medicine[1] (Bayer)					2 q 4 h up to 8/day	Liquid filled. Sorbitol. In 12s.
otc	Histenol-Forte Tablets (Zee Medical)						In 24s.
otc	Tylenol Cold Non-Drowsy Formula Gelcaps and Tablets[1] (McNeil Consumer Healthcare)	15 mg dextromethorphan HBr		30 mg pseudoephedrine HCl	325 mg acetaminophen	2 q 6 h up to 8/day	Gelcaps: Parabens. (TYLENOL COLD). In 24s. Tablets: (TYLENOL Cold). Capsule shape. In 24s.
otc	Top Care Multi-Symptom Pain Relief Cold Tablets[1] (Topco Assoc.)						Capsule shape. In 24s.
otc	Comtrex Multi-Symptom Maximum Strength Non-Drowsy Cold & Cough Relief Tablets (Bristol-Myers)	15 mg dextromethorphan HBr		30 mg pseudoephedrine HCl	500 mg acetaminophen	2 q 6 h up to 8/day	Parabens. Capsule shape. In 24s.
otc	Thera-Flu Non-Drowsy Formula Maximum Strength Tablets (Novartis Consumer Healthcare)						Lactose, methylparaben. (Thera-Flu). Capsule shape. In 12s and 24s.
otc	Tylenol Flu Maximum Strength Non-Drowsy Gelcaps (McNeil Consumer Healthcare)						Parabens. (TYLENOL FLU). In 24s.
otc	Sudafed Non-Drowsy Severe Cold Formula Maximum Strength Tablets (Warner-Lambert)						(Sudafed SCF). In 24s.
otc	Robitussin Honey Flu Non-Drowsy Syrup (Whitehall-Robins)	20 mg dextromethorphan HBr		60 mg pseudoephedrine HCl	500 mg acetaminophen	1 pouch q 4 h in 4 to 177 mL of hot beverage (eg, tea)	Corn syrup, saccharin. In 6s.

ANTITUSSIVE COMBINATIONS

UPPER RESPIRATORY COMBINATIONS

	Product & Distributor	Antitussive	Antihistamine	Decongestant	Other	Average Adult Dose	Excipients & How Supplied
otc	Thera-Flu Non-Drowsy Flu, Cold & Cough Maximum Strength Powder (Novartis Consumer Healthcare)	30 mg dextromethorphan HBr		60 mg pseudoephedrine HCl	1000 mg acetaminophen	1 packet dissolved in 177 mL hot water q 6 h up to 4/day	Sucrose. Lemon flavor. In 6s and 12s.
otc	TheraFlu Severe Cold & Congestion Non-Drowsy, Maximum Strength Powder (Novartis Consumer Healthcare)						Acesulfame K, aspartame, 17 mg phenylalanine, sucrose. Lemon flavor. In 6s.
Rx sf	Alacol DM Syrup[1] (Ballay)	10 mg dextromethorphan HBr	2 mg brompheniramine maleate	5 mg phenylephrine HCl		10 mL q 4 h up to 60 mL/day	Saccharin, sorbitol. Alcohol free. Black raspberry flavor. In 473 mL.
Rx sf	Bromatane DX Syrup[1] (Ivax)	10 mg dextromethorphan HBr	2 mg brompheniramine maleate	30 mg pseudoephedrine HCl		10 mL q 4 to 6 h up to 40 mL/day	0.95% alcohol. In 473 mL.
Rx	Bromfed DM Cough Syrup[1] (Verum Pharm)					10 mL q 4 h up to 60 mL/day	Saccharin, sorbitol, sucrose, methylparaben. Cherry flavor. In 473 mL.
otc	Robitussin Allergy & Cough Liquid[1] (Whitehall-Robins)					10 mL q 4 h up to 40 mL/day	Alcohol and dye free. Saccharin, sorbitol. In 118 mL.
Rx	Carbodex DM Syrup[1] (Tri-Med)	15 mg dextromethorphan HBr	4 mg brompheniramine maleate	45 mg pseudoephedrine HCl		5 mL qid	Menthol, sorbitol. In 473 mL.
Rx	Carbofed DM Syrup[1] (Hi-Tech Pharmacal)						Sorbitol. Grape flavor. In 473 mL.
Rx	Rondec-DM Syrup[1] (BioVail)						Saccharin, sorbitol. Grape flavor. In 118 and 473 mL.
Rx sf	Coldec DM[1] (Silarx)	15 mg dextromethorphan HBr	4 mg brompheniramine maleate	60 mg pseudoephedrine HCl		5 mL qid	Alcohol free. Saccharin, sorbitol. Grape flavor. In 480 mL.
Rx	Rondamine DM Syrup[1] (Major)						< 0.2% alcohol. Grape flavor. In 120 and 473 mL and 3.8 L.
Rx sf	Sildec-DM Syrup[1] (Silarx)						Alcohol free. Saccharin, sorbitol. Grape flavor. In 473 mL.
Rx sf	Anaplex-DM Liquid[1] (ECR)	30 mg dextromethorphan HBr	4 mg brompheniramine maleate	60 mg pseudoephedrine HCl		5 mL q 4 to 6 h up to 20 mL/day	Alcohol and dye free. Fruit flavor. In 473 mL.
Rx	DMax Syrup[1] (Great Southern)	15 mg dextromethorphan HBr	4 mg carbinoxamine maleate	8 mg phenylephrine HCl		10 mL q 6 h up to 40 mL/day	Berry flavor. In 30 and 473 mL.
Rx	Balamine DM Syrup[1] (Ballay)	12.5 mg dextromethorphan HBr	4 mg carbinoxamine maleate	60 mg pseudoephedrine HCl		5 mL qid	Menthol. Grape flavor. In 473 mL.
Rx	Cydec-DM Syrup[1] (Cypress)	15 mg dextromethorphan HBr	4 mg carbinoxamine maleate	60 mg pseudoephedrine HCl		5 mL qid	Grape flavor. In 118 and 437 mL and 3.8 L.
Rx sf	Tussafed Syrup[1] (Everett)						Alcohol free. Menthol. Grape flavor. In 120 and 480 mL.
otc sf	Tricodene Sugar Free Liquid[1] (Pfeiffer)	10 mg dextromethorphan HBr	2 mg chlorpheniramine maleate			10 mL q 4 to 6 h up to 60 mL/day	Alcohol free. Sorbitol, mannitol, menthol, saccharin. In 120 mL.
otc sf	Scot-Tussin DM Liquid[1] (Scot-Tussin)	15 mg dextromethorphan HBr	2 mg chlorpheniramine maleate			10 mL q 6 to 8 h up to 40 mL/day	Alcohol and dye free. Parabens. In 118, 237, and 473 mL and 3.8 L.
otc	Coricidin HBP Cough & Cold Tablets (Schering-Plough Healthcare Products)	30 mg dextromethorphan HBr	4 mg chlorpheniramine maleate			1 q 6 h up to 4/day	Sugar. (C C + C). In 16s.
otc	Coricidin HBP Maximum Strength Flu Tablets (Schering-Plough Healthcare Products)	15 mg dextromethorphan HBr	2 mg chlorpheniramine maleate		500 mg acetaminophen	2 q 6 h up to 8/day	Lactose. In 20s.
otc	Alka-Seltzer Plus Flu Medicine Effervescent Tablets (Bayer)	15 mg dextromethorphan HBr	2 mg chlorpheniramine maleate		500 mg aspirin	2 dissolved in 118 mL water q 6 h up to 8/day	Acesulfame K, aspartame, 6.7 mg phenylalanine, mannitol, saccharin. Honey/orange flavor. In 20s.
otc	Father John's Medicine Plus Liquid (Oakhurst Co.)	1.66 mg dextromethorphan HBr	0.66 mg chlorpheniramine maleate	1.66 mg phenylephrine HCl		30 mL q 4 h up to 180 mL/day	Alcohol free. In 118 mL.
otc	Alka-Seltzer Plus Cold & Cough Medicine Effervescent Tablets (Bayer)	10 mg dextromethorphan HBr	2 mg chlorpheniramine maleate	5 mg phenylephrine HCl		2 dissolved in 118 mL water q 4 h up to 8/day	Aspartame, 11 mg phenylalanine, sorbitol. In 20s.

UPPER RESPIRATORY COMBINATIONS

ANTITUSSIVE COMBINATIONS

	Product & Distributor	Antitussive	Antihistamine	Decongestant	Other	Average Adult Dose	Excipients & How Supplied
Rx sf	Amerituss AD Liquid[1] (AMBI Pharm)	15 mg dextromethorphan HBr	3 mg chlorpheniramine maleate	10 mg phenylephrine HCl		10 mL q 6 h	Phenylalanine, aspartame. Alcohol free. In 473 mL.
Rx sf	Norel DM Liquid[1] (US Pharm)	15 mg dextromethorphan HBr	4 mg chlorpheniramine maleate	10 mg phenylephrine HCl		5 mL q 4 h up to 30 mL/day	Sorbitol. Alcohol and dye free. In 473 mL.
otc	Alka-Seltzer Plus Nose & Throat Effervescent Tablets (Bayer)	10 mg dextromethorphan HBr	2 mg chlorpheniramine maleate	5 mg phenylephrine HCl	250 mg acetaminophen	2 tablets fully dissolved in 120 mL water q 4 h up to 8 tablets/day	Acesulfame K, aspartame, maltodextrin, saccharin, sorbitol, 5.6 mg phenylalanine. Citrus blend flavor. In 20s.
otc	Robitussin PM Cough & Cold Liquid[1] (Wyeth Consumer)	7.5 mg dextromethorphan HBr	1 mg chlorpheniramine maleate	15 mg pseudoephedrine HCl		20 mL q 6 h up to 80 mL/day	Corn syrup, saccharin. Alcohol free. In 118 mL.
otc sf	Rescon-DM Liquid[1] (Capellon Pharm.)	10 mg dextromethorphan HBr	2 mg chlorpheniramine maleate	30 mg pseudoephedrine HCl		10 mL q 4 to 6 h up to 40 mL/day	Alcohol and dye free. In 118 and 473 mL.
otc	Robitussin Flu Liquid[1] (Whitehall-Robins)	5 mg dextromethorphan HBr	1 mg chlorpheniramine maleate	15 mg pseudoephedrine HCl	160 mg acetaminophen	20 mL q 4 h up to 80 mL/day	Alcohol free. In 118 mL.
otc	Vicks 44M Cough, Cold, & Flu Relief Liquid (Procter & Gamble)	7.5 mg dextromethorphan HBr	1 mg chlorpheniramine maleate	15 mg pseudoephedrine HCl	162.5 mg acetaminophen	20 mL q 6 h up to 80 mL/day	10% alcohol, corn syrup, saccharin. In 236 mL.
otc	Alka-Seltzer Plus Cold & Cough Liqui-Gels[1] (Bayer)	10 mg dextromethorphan HBr	2 mg chlorpheniramine maleate	30 mg pseudoephedrine HCl	325 mg acetaminophen	2 q 4 h up to 8/day	Liquid filled. Sorbitol. (AS+ C&C). In 12s and 20s.
otc	Kolephrin/DM Tablets[1] (Pfeiffer)	15 mg dextromethorphan HBr	2 mg chlorpheniramine maleate	30 mg pseudoephedrine HCl		2 q 4 to 6 h up to 8/day	Capsule shape. In 30s.
otc	Top Care Multi-Symptom Pain Relief Cold Tablets[1] (Topco Assoc.)	15 mg dextromethorphan HBr	2 mg chlorpheniramine maleate	30 mg pseudoephedrine HCl	325 mg acetaminophen	2 q 6 h up to 8/day	Capsule shape. In 24s.
otc	Tylenol Cold Complete Formula Tablets[1] (McNeil Consumer Healthcare)						Capsule shape. In 24s.
otc	Mapap Cold Formula Tablets[1] (Major)						In 24s.
otc	Contac Severe Cold & Flu Maximum Strength Tablets (SmithKline Beecham)	15 mg dextromethorphan HBr	2 mg chlorpheniramine maleate	30 mg pseudoephedrine HCl	500 mg acetaminophen	2 q 6 h up to 8/day	Capsule shape. In 30s.
otc	Comtrex Day & Night Cold & Cough Relief, Multi-Symptom Maximum Strength Tablets (Bristol-Myers Squibb)					Day: 2 q 6 h up to 4/day Night: 2 ≥ 6 h after day dose	Day: Capsule shape. In 24s (18 day; 6 night).
otc	Genacol Maximum Strength Cold & Flu Relief Tablets (Ivax)					2 q 6 h up to 8/day	In 50s.
otc	Comtrex Cough and Cold Relief, Multi-Symptom Maximum Strength Tablets[1] (Bristol-Myers Squibb)						Parabens. Capsule shape. In 24s.
otc	Cold Symptoms Relief Maximum Strength Tablets (Major)						In 24s.
otc	TheraFlu Maximum Strength NightTime Formula Flu, Cold, & Cough Medicine Tablets (Novartis Consumer Healthcare)						Lactose. Capsule shape. In 12s and 24s.
otc	Robitussin Honey Flu Nighttime Syrup (Whitehall-Robins)	20 mg dextromethorphan HBr	4 mg chlorpheniramine maleate	60 mg pseudoephedrine HCl	500 mg acetaminophen	1 pouch q 4 h in 4 to 177 mL of hot beverage (eg, tea) up to 4/day	Corn syrup, saccharin. In 6s.
otc	TheraFlu, Cold & Cough Powder (Novartis Consumer Healthcare)	20 mg dextromethorphan HBr	4 mg chlorpheniramine maleate	60 mg pseudoephedrine HCl	650 mg acetaminophen	1 packet dissolved in 177 mL hot water q 4 to 6 h up to 4/day	Sucrose. Lemon flavor. In 6s and 12s.
otc	TheraFlu Cold & Cough Night Time Powder (Novartis Consumer Healthcare)						Sucrose. Lemon flavor. In 6s.

UPPER RESPIRATORY COMBINATIONS

ANTITUSSIVE COMBINATIONS

Product & Distributor	Antitussive	Antihistamine	Decongestant	Other	Average Adult Dose	Excipients & How Supplied
otc **TheraFlu Flu, Cold, & Cough and Sore Throat, Maximum Strength Powder** (Novartis Consumer Healthcare)	30 mg dextromethorphan HBr	4 mg chlorpheniramine maleate	60 mg pseudoephedrine HCl	1000 mg acetaminophen	1 pack dissolved in 6 oz water q 4 to 6 h up to 4 doses/day	Aspartame, acesulfame K, phenylalanine, sucrose. Cherry flavor. In 6s.
otc **TheraFlu Flu & Cough Night Time, Maximum Strength Powder** (Novartis Consumer Healthcare)					1 pack dissolved in 177 mL hot water q 6 h up to 4/day	Acesulfame K, aspartame, 26 mg phenylalanine, saccharin, sucrose. Cherry flavor. In 6s.
otc **TheraFlu Flu, Cold, & Cough NightTime, Maximum Strength Powder** (Novartis Consumer Healthcare)						Sucrose. Lemon flavor. In 6 and 12 packs.
otc **TheraFlu Severe Cold & Congestion Night Time, Maximum Strength Powder** (Novartis Consumer Healthcare)						Sucrose. Lemon flavor. In 6s.
otc **Top Care Maximum Strength Flu, Cold, & Cough Medicine Night Time Powder** (Topco Assoc.)						Sucrose. Lemon flavor. In 6s.
otc **Contac Day & Night Cold & Flu Tablets** (SmithKline Beecham)	*Day:* 30 mg dextromethorphan HBr / *Night:*	*Night:* 50 mg diphenhydramine HCl	60 mg pseudoephedrine HCl / 60 mg pseudoephedrine HCl	650 mg acetaminophen / 650 mg acetaminophen	*Day:* 1 q 6 h / *Night:* 1 q 6 h / ≤ 4 in any combination per day	*Day:* Yellow, capsule shape. *Night:* Blue, capsule shape. In 20s (15 day; 5 night).
otc **Vicks NyQuil Cough Syrup**[1] (Procter & Gamble)	5 mg dextromethorphan HBr	2.1 mg doxylamine succinate			30 mL q 6 to 8 h up to 120 mL/day	Alcohol, corn syrup, saccharin. Cherry flavor. In 177 mL.
otc **Alka-Seltzer Plus Night-Time Cold Medicine Effervescent Tablets** (Bayer)	10 mg dextromethorphan HBr	6.25 mg doxylamine succinate	5 mg phenylephrine HCl		2 dissolved in 118 mL water hs or q 4 h up to 8/day	Acesulfame K, aspartame, 7.8 mg phenylalanine, sorbitol. In 20s.
otc **All-Nite Liquid** (Major)	5 mg dextromethorphan HBr	2.1 mg doxylamine succinate	10 mg pseudoephedrine HCl	167 mg acetaminophen	30 mL q 6 h up to 120 mL/day	10% alcohol, saccharin, corn syrup. Original and cherry flavors. In 177 mL.
otc **Nite Time Cold Formula for Adults Liquid** (Alpharma)					30 mL hs or q 6 h up to 120 mL/day	10% alcohol, saccharin, sucrose. In 296 mL.
otc **Tylenol Flu NightTime, Maximum Strength Liquid**[1] (McNeil Consumer Healthcare)					30 mL q 6 h up to 120 mL/day	Corn syrup, saccharin, sorbitol. In 237 mL.
otc **Vicks NyQuil Multi-Symptom Cold/Flu Relief Liquid** (Procter & Gamble)						10% alcohol, corn syrup, saccharin. Regular and cherry flavors. In 180, 300, and 420 mL.
otc **Top Care LiquiCaps Nite Time Multi-Symptom Cold/Flu Relief Capsules** (Topco Assoc.)	10 mg dextromethorphan HBr	6.25 mg doxylamine succinate	30 mg pseudoephedrine HCl	250 mg acetaminophen	2 q 4 h up to 8/day	Sorbitol. In 20s.
otc **Vicks NyQuil Multi-Symptom Cold & Flu Relief LiquiCaps Capsules** (Proctor & Gamble)						Sorbitol. (NyQuil). In 12s, 20s, and 36s.
otc **Alka-Seltzer Plus NightTime Cold Liqui-Gels** (Bayer)	10 mg dextromethorphan HBr	6.25 mg doxylamine succinate	30 mg pseudoephedrine HCl	325 mg acetaminophen	2 hs	Liquid filled. Alcohol free. Sorbitol. In 12s, 20s, and 36s.
Rx **Prometh w/Dextromethorphan Syrup**[1] (Alpharma)	15 mg dextromethorphan HBr	6.25 mg promethazine HCl			5 mL q 4 to 6 h up to 30 mL/day	7% alcohol, parabens, saccharin. Lemon/mint flavor. In 118, 237, and 473 mL and 3.8 L.
Rx **Promethazine w/Dextromethorphan Cough Syrup** (Morton Grove)						7.1% alcohol, saccharin. Pineapple flavor. In 118 and 473 mL.

UPPER RESPIRATORY COMBINATIONS

ANTITUSSIVE COMBINATIONS

	Product & Distributor	Antitussive	Antihistamine	Decongestant	Other	Average Adult Dose	Excipients & How Supplied
otc sf	Codal-DM Syrup[1] (Cypress)	10 mg dextromethorphan HBr	8.33 mg pyrilamine maleate	5 mg phenylephrine HCl		10 mL q 4 h up to 60 mL/day	Alcohol and dye free. In 473 mL.
otc sf	Codimal DM Syrup[1] (Schwarz)						Alcohol and dye free. Menthol, saccharin, sorbitol. In 120 and 473 mL and 3.8 L.
otc sf	Dicomal-DM Syrup[1] (Econolab)						Alcohol and dye free. Menthol, saccharin, sorbitol. In 473 mL.
otc	Robitussin Night Relief Liquid (Whitehall-Robins)	5 mg dextromethorphan HBr	8.3 mg pyrilamine maleate	10 mg pseudoephedrine HCl	108.3 mg acetaminophen,	30 mL hs or q 6 h up to 120 mL/day	Alcohol free. Saccharin, sorbitol. Cherry flavor. In 177 mL.
Rx	Tanafed DMX Suspension[1] (First Horizon)	25 mg dextromethorphan tannate	2.5 mg dexchlorpheniramine tannate	75 mg pseudoephedrine tannate		10 to 20 mL q 12 h up to 40 mL/day	Methylparaben, saccharin, sucrose. Cotton candy flavor. In 20, 118, and 473 mL.
c-v	Pancof PD Syrup[1] (Pan American)	3 mg dihydrocodeine bitartrate	2 mg chlorpheniramine maleate	7.5 mg phenylephrine HCl		5 to 10 mL q 4 to 6 h up to 40 mL/day	In 120 mL.
c-iii sf	Pancof Syrup[1] (Pan American)	7.5 mg dihydrocodeine bitartrate	2 mg chlorpheniramine maleate	15 mg pseudoephedrine HCl		5 to 10 mL q 4 to 6 h	Saccharin, sorbitol. Alcohol- and dye-free. In 473 mL.
c-iii	Hycodan Tablets[1] (Endo)	5 mg hydrocodone bitartrate			1.5 mg homatropine MBr	1 q 4 to 6 h up to 6/day	Lactose. (Hycodan). White, scored. In 100s.
c-iii	Hycodan Syrup[1] (Endo)					5 mL q 4 to 6 h up to 30 mL/day	Sorbitol, sugar, parabens. Cherry flavor. In 473 mL.
c-iii	Hydromet Syrup[1] (Alpharma)						Saccharin, sucrose, methylparaben. Cherry flavor. In 473 mL and 3.8 L.
c-iii	Hydromide Syrup[1] (Major)						< 0.1% alcohol. Cherry flavor. In 473 mL.
c-iii	Hydropane Syrup[1] (Watson)					5 mL q 4 to 6 h up to 30 mL/day	Parabens, sucrose. Cherry flavor. In 473 mL and 3.8 L.
c-iii	Tussigon Tablets[1] (Daniels)					1 q 4 to 6 h up to 6/day	(dp 082). Blue, scored. In 100s and 500s.
c-iii	Detussin Liquid[1] (Alpharma)	5 mg hydrocodone bitartrate		60 mg pseudoephedrine HCl		5 mL qid	5% alcohol, corn syrup, saccharin, methylparaben. Cherry flavor. In 473 mL.
c-iii	Histussin D Liquid[1] (Sanofi-Synthelabo)						In 473 mL.
c-iii	P-V-Tussin Tablets (Numark)					1 q 4 to 6 h up to 4/day	Lactose. (NUMARK 10/91). Orange, capsule shape, scored. In 100s.
c-iii sf	Anaplex HD Liquid[1] (ECR Pharmaceuticals)	1.7 mg hydrocodone bitartrate	2 mg brompheniramine maleate	30 mg pseudoephedrine HCl		10 mL tid or qid up to 40 mL/day	Alcohol and dye free. Strawberry flavor. In 118 and 473 mL.
c-iii	Hydrocodone Bitartrate 5 mg/Pseudo- ephedrine HCl 30 mg/Carbinoxamine Maleate 2 mg Liquid[1] (URL)	5 mg hydrocodone bitartrate	2 mg carbinoxamine maleate	30 mg pseudoephedrine HCl		5 to 10 mL q 4 to 6 h up to 30 mL/day	Alcohol free. In 473 mL.
c-iii sf	Histex HC Liquid[1] (Teamm Pharm)						Saccharin, sorbitol. Alcohol-free. Peach flavor. In 473 mL.
c-iii sf	S-T Forte 2 Liquid[1] (Scot-Tussin)	2.5 mg hydrocodone bitartrate	2 mg chlorpheniramine maleate			5 mL tid or qid up to 20 mL/day	Alcohol and dye free. Menthol, parabens. In 473 mL and 3.8 L.
c-iii	ED-TLC Liquid[1] (Edwards)	1.67 mg hydrocodone bitartrate	2 mg chlorpheniramine maleate	5 mg phenylephrine HCl		10 mL tid or qid	In 473 mL.
c-iii	Hydrocodone HD Liquid[1] (Morton Grove)					10 mL q 4 h up to 40 mL/day	Alcohol free. Sugar, menthol, parabens. Cherry flavor. In 236 and 473 mL.
c-iii sf	Endal HD (PediaMed)	2 mg hydrocodone bitartrate	12.5 mg diphenhydramine HCl	7.5 mg phenylephrine		10 mL q 4 h up to 40 mL/day	Alcohol free. Cherry flavor. In 473 mL.

ANTITUSSIVE COMBINATIONS

UPPER RESPIRATORY COMBINATIONS

Product & Distributor	Antitussive	Antihistamine	Decongestant	Other	Average Adult Dose	Excipients & How Supplied
c-iii sf Lortuss HC Liquid[1] (ProEthic)	3.75 mg hyrocodone bitartrate		7.5 mg phenylephrine		5 mL q 4 h up to 30 mL/day	Saccharin, sorbitol. Grape flavor. In 20 and 473 mL.
c-iii Endagen-HD Liquid[1] (Jones Pharma)	1.7 mg hydrocodone bitartrate	2 mg chlorpheniramine maleate	5 mg phenylephrine HCl		10 mL tid or qid	Cherry flavor. In 473 mL.
c-iii Vanex HD Liquid[1] (Abana)		2 mg chlorpheniramine maleate	5 mg phenylephrine HCl			Dye free. Cherry flavor. In 480 mL.
c-iii sf Hydro-PC Liquid[1] (Cypress)	2 mg hydrocodone bitartrate	2 mg chlorpheniramine maleate	5 mg phenylephrine HCl		10 mL q 4 h up to 40 mL/day	Strawberry flavor. In 473 mL.
c-iii Hydro-PC II Liquid[1] (Cypress)	2 mg hydrocodone bitartrate	2 mg chlorpheniramine maleate	7.5 mg phenylephrine HCl		10 mL q 4 h up to 40 mL/day	Strawberry flavor. In 473 mL.
c-iii sf Comtussin HC Syrup[1] (Econolab)	2.5 mg hydrocodone bitartrate	2 mg chlorpheniramine maleate	5 mg phenylephrine HCl		10 mL q 4 h up to 40 mL/day	Sorbitol, saccharin. In 473 mL
c-iii sf Cytuss HC Liquid[1] (Cypress)						In 473 mL.
c-iii sf Histussin HC Syrup[1] (Sanofi-Synthelabo)					5 mL up to qid	Alcohol free. Orange/pineapple flavor. In 473 mL.
c-iii sf Hydrocodone CP Syrup[1] (Morton Grove)					5 mL qid	Alcohol free. Saccharin, sorbitol. Fruit flavor. In 237 and 473 mL.
c-iii sf Histinex HC Syrup[1] (Ethex)					10 mL q 4 h up to 40 mL/day	Alcohol free. Saccharin, sorbitol. Fruit flavor. In 473 and 946 mL.
c-iii sf Atuss HC Liquid[1] (Atley)	2.5 mg hydrocodone bitartrate	2 mg chlorpheniramine maleate	10 mg phenylephrine HCl		10 mL q 4 h up to 40 mL/day	Menthol, sucrose. Cherry flavor. In 473 mL.
c-iii ED Tuss HC Syrup[1] (Edwards)	2.5 mg hydrocodone bitartrate	4 mg chlorpheniramine maleate	10 mg phenylephrine HCl		5 mL q 4 h up to 20 mL/day	5% alcohol, saccharin, sorbitol. Grape flavor. In 473 mL.
c-iii Maxi-Tuss HC Liquid[1] (MCR American Pharm.)					5 mL q 4 h up to 30 mL/day	In 473 mL.
c-iii sf Endal HD Plus Syrup[1] (PediaMed)	3.5 mg hydrocodone bitartrate	2 mg chlorpheniramine maleate	7.5 mg phenylephrine HCl		10 mL q 4 h up to 40 mL/day	Saccharin, sorbitol. Alcohol free. In 473 mL.
c-iii sf Z-Cof HC Syrup[1] (Zyber)	3.5 mg hydrocodone bitartrate	2.5 mg chlorpheniramine maleate	10 mg phenylephrine HCl		10 mL q 4 to 6 h up to 40 mL/day	Saccharin, sorbitol. Black raspberry flavor. In 473 mL.
c-iii sf Poly-Tussin Syrup[1] (Pharmakon)	5 mg hydrocodone bitartrate	2 mg chlorpheniramine maleate	5 mg phenylephrine HCl		5 to 10 mL q 4 h	Alcohol free. Saccharin, sorbitol. Raspberry flavor. In 473 mL.
c-iii Atuss MS Liquid[1] (Atley)	5 mg hydrocodone bitartrate	2 mg chlorpheniramine maleate	10 mg phenylephrine HCl		10 mL q 4 h up to 40 mL/day	Phenylalanine. Alcohol free. In 473 mL.
c-iii sf Hydron CP Liquid[1] (Cypress)						Menthol, sucrose. Pineapple/orange flavor. Alcohol-free. In 473 mL.
c-iii sf Maxi-Tuss HCX Liquid[1] (MCR American Pharmaceuticals)	6 mg hydrocodone bitartrate	2 mg chlorpheniramine maleate	12 mg phenylephrine HCl		5 mL q 4 h up to 30 mL/day	Saccharin, sorbitol. Pineapple-orange flavor. Alcohol-free. In 473 mL.
c-iii sf Histinex PV Syrup[1] (Ethex)	2.5 mg hydrocodone bitartrate	2 mg chlorpheniramine maleate	30 mg pseudoephedrine HCl		10 mL q 4 to 6 h up to 40 mL/day	Alcohol-free. In 480 mL.
c-iii Hyphed Liquid[1] (Cypress)		2 mg chlorpheniramine maleate				Alcohol free. Parabens, saccharin, sorbitol. Fruit flavor. In 473 mL.
c-iii P-V-Tussin Syrup[1] (Numark)						5% alcohol. Raspberry flavor. In 473 mL.
c-iii Tussend Syrup[1] (Monarch)						5% alcohol, glucose, parabens, saccharin, sorbitol, sucrose. Banana flavor. In 473 mL and 3.8 L.
c-iii sf Hydro-Tussin HC Syrup[1] (Ethex)	3 mg hydrocodone bitartrate	2 mg chlorpheniramine maleate	15 mg pseudoephedrine HCl		5 to 10 mL qid	5% alcohol, corn syrup, parabens, saccharin, sucrose. Banana flavor. In 473 mL.
c-iii sf Pancof-HC Liquid[1] (Pan American Labs)						Alcohol and dye free. In 473 mL. Alcohol and dye free. In 480 mL.
c-iii sf Hydron PSC Liquid[1] (Cypress)	5 mg hydrocodone bitartrate	2 mg chlorpheniramine maleate	30 mg pseudoephedrine HCl		5 mL tid or qid	Menthol, saccharin, sorbitol. Alcohol-free. Vanilla flavor. In 473 mL.

UPPER RESPIRATORY COMBINATIONS

ANTITUSSIVE COMBINATIONS

	Product & Distributor	Antitussive	Antihistamine	Decongestant	Other	Average Adult Dose	Excipients & How Supplied
c-iii	Tussend Tablets[1] (Monarch)	5 mg hydrocodone bitartrate	4 mg chlorpheniramine maleate	60 mg pseudoephedrine HCl		1 q 4 to 6 h up to 4/day	Lactose. (MPC100). Yellow, capsule shape, scored. In 100s.
c-iii sf	Statuss Green Liquid[1] (Huckaby)	2.5 mg hydrocodone bitartrate	2 mg chlorpheniramine maleate, 3.3 mg pyrilamine maleate	5 mg phenylephrine HCl, 3.3 mg pseudoephedrine HCl		10 mL q 4 to 6 h up to 40 mL/day	Alcohol free. In 473 mL.
c-iii	Tussionex Pennkinetic Suspension[1] (CellTech)	10 mg hydrocodone (as polistirex)	8 mg chlorpheniramine (as polistirex)			5 mL q 12 h up to 10 mL/day	Extended release. Alcohol free. Parabens, sucrose, corn syrup. In 473 mL.
c-iii	Notuss PD Liquid (Stewart-Jackson)	4 mg hydrocodone bitartrate	2 mg dexchlorpheniramine maleate	5 mg phenylephrine HCl		5 mL tid or qid up to 20 mg/day	Menthol, sorbitol, sugar. Grape flavor. In 473 mL.
c-iii sf	Hydro-DP Syrup[1] (Cypress)	2 mg hydrocodone bitartrate	12.5 mg diphenhydramine HCl	7.5 mg phenylephrine HCl		10 mL q 4 h up to 40 mL/day	Alcohol-free. Saccharin, sorbitol. Cherry flavor. In 118 and 473 mL.
c-iii	Codal-DH Syrup[1] (Cypress)	1.66 mg hydrocodone bitartrate	8.33 mg pyrilamine maleate	5 mg phenylephrine HCl		5 to 10 mL q 4 h	In 473 mL.
c-iii	Codimal DH Syrup[1] (Schwarz)						Alcohol free. Menthol, sucrose. In 118 and 473 mL.
c-iii	Dicomal-DH Syrup[1] (Econolab)						In 473 mL.

[1] This product also may be used in children; refer to package labeling for dosing.

For complete prescribing information, refer to the Respiratory Combinations introduction. Some of the products in the following Pediatric Antitussive Combinations table also may be used in adults.

UPPER RESPIRATORY COMBINATIONS

PEDIATRIC ANTITUSSIVE COMBINATIONS
Content given per tablet, 5 mL (liquid), or 1 mL (drops).

	Product & Distributor	Decongestant	Antihistamine	Antitussive	Other	Average Dose	Excipients & How Supplied
Rx	Tussi-12 S Suspension (Wallace)		4 mg chlorpheniramine tannate	30 mg carbetapentane tannate		> 6 yrs - 5 to 10 mL q 12 h; 2 to 6 yrs - 2.5 to 5 mL q 12 h	Methylparaben, saccharin, sucrose, tartrazine. Strawberry-currant flavor. in 118 mL with syringe.
Rx	DMax Pediatric Drops (Great Southern)	2 mg phenylephrine	2 mg carbinoxamine maleate	4 mg dextromethorphan HBr		1 to 3 mo - 2 to 3 drops/mo of age qid; 3 to 6 mo - 0.5 mL qid; 6 to 12 mo - 0.75 mL qid; 12 to 24 mo - 1 mL qid	Purple. Berry flavor. In 30 mL bottle with 1 mL dropper.
Rx	Tannic-12 Suspension (Cypress)	5 mg phenylephrine tannate	4 mg chlorpheniramine tannate	30 mg carbetapentane tannate		> 6 yrs - 5 to 10 mL q 12 h; 2 to 6 yrs - 2.5 to 5 mL q 12 h	Methylparaben, saccharin, sucrose. Strawberry flavor. In 473 mL.
Rx	Rynatuss Pediatric Suspension (Wallace)	5 mg phenylephrine tannate, 5 mg ephedrine tannate	4 mg chlorpheniramine tannate	30 mg carbetapentane tannate		> 6 yrs - 5 to 10 mL q 12 h; 2 to 6 yrs - 2.5 to 5 mL q 12 h	Tartrazine, methylparaben, saccharin, sucrose. Strawberry-currant flavor. In 237 and 473 mL.
Rx sf	Lortuss DM Liquid[1] (ProEthic)	7.5 mg phenylephrine HCl	2 mg brompheniramine maleate	15 mg dextromethorphan HBr		≥ 12 yrs - 10 mL q 6 h up to 40 mL/day; 6 to 12 yrs - 5 mL q 6 h up to 20 mL/day; < 6 yrs - consult a physician	Alcohol-free. Saccharin, sorbitol. Tutti-fruiti flavor. In 20 and 473 mL.
Rx	Viravan-DM Suspension (PediaMed)	12.5 mg phenylephrine	30 mg pyrilamine	25 mg dextromethorphan		6 to 12 yrs - 5 mL q 12 h; 2 to 6 yrs - 2.5 mL q 12 h	Methylparaben, sucralose, sucrose. Grape flavor. In 473 mL.
Rx	Viravan-DM Chewable Tablets (PediaMed)	25 mg phenylephrine	30 mg pyrilamine	25 mg dextromethorphan		6 to 12 yrs - ½ to 1 q 12 h; 2 to 6 yrs - ½ q 12 h	Sugar, sucralose. Dye free. (VIRAVAN-DM). Mottled brown, scored. Grape flavor. In 100s
otc	Dimetapp Decongestant Plus Cough Infant Drops (Whitehall-Robins)	9.375 mg/mL pseudoephedrine HCl		3.125 mg/mL dextromethorphan HBr		2 to 3 yrs - 1.6 mL q 4 to 6 h up to 6.4 mL/day	Alcohol free. Corn syrup, menthol, sucrose. Grape flavor. In 15 mL with dropper.
otc	Pedia Care Infants' Decongestant & Cough Drops (Pharmacia)						Alcohol free. Sorbitol. Cherry flavor. In 15 mL with dropper.
otc	Pedia Relief Decongestant Plus Cough Infants' Drops (Major)						Alcohol free. Sorbitol. Cherry flavor. In 15 mL with dropper.
otc	Tylenol Infants' Cold Decongestant & Fever Reducer Plus Cough Concentrated Drops (McNeil)	9.375 mg/mL pseudoephedrine HCl		3.125 mg/mL dextromethorphan HBr	100 mg/mL acetaminophen	2 to 3 yrs - 1.6 mL q 4 to 6 h up to 6.4 mL/day	Alcohol free. Acesulfame K, corn syrup. Cherry flavor. In 15 mL with dropper.
otc sf	Sudafed Children's Non-Drowsy Cold & Cough Liquid[1] (Warner-Lambert)	15 mg pseudoephedrine HCl		5 mg dextromethorphan HBr		6 to < 12 yrs - 10 mL q 4 h up to 40 mL/day; 2 to < 6 yrs - 5 mL q 4 h up to 20 mL/day	Alcohol-free. Saccharin, sorbitol. Cherry-berry flavor. In 118 mL.

UPPER RESPIRATORY COMBINATIONS

PEDIATRIC ANTITUSSIVE COMBINATIONS

	Product & Distributor	Decongestant	Antihistamine	Antitussive	Other	Average Dose	Excipients & How Supplied
otc	**Dimetapp Children's Non-Drowsy Flu Syrup**[1] (Whitehall-Robins)	15 mg pseudoephedrine HCl		5 mg dextromethorphan HBr	160 mg acetaminophen	*6 to < 12 yrs* - 10 mL q 4 h up to 40 mL/day; *2 to < 6 yrs* - 5 mL q 4 h up to 20 mL/day	Alcohol free. Corn syrup, saccharin, sorbitol. Fruit flavor. In 118 mL.
otc	**Triaminic Throat Pain & Cough Softchews Tablets**[1] (Novartis)					*6 to < 12 yrs* - 2 q 4 to 6 h up to qid; *2 to < 6 yrs* - 1 q 4 to 6 h up qid.	Aspartame, mannitol, 28.1 mg phenylalanine. Grape flavor. In 18s.
otc	**Pedia Care Children's Long-Lasting Cough Plus Cold Liquid** (Pharmacia)	15 mg pseudoephedrine HCl		7.5 mg dextromethorphan HBr		*6 to 11 yrs* - 10 mL q 6 to 8 h up to 40 mL/day; *2 to 5 yrs* - 5 mL q 6 to 8 h up to 20 mL/day	Alcohol free. Corn syrup, sorbitol. Grape flavor. In 120 mL.
otc	**Robitussin Pediatric Cough & Cold Formula Liquid**[1] (Whitehall-Robins)					*6 to < 12 yrs* - 10 mL q 6 h up to 40 mL/day; *2 to < 6 yrs* - 5 mL q 6 h up to 20 mL/day	Alcohol free. Corn syrup, saccharin. Fruit punch flavor. In 118 mL.
otc	**Triaminic AM Non-Drowsy Cough & Decongestant Liquid**[1] (Novartis)						EDTA, sorbitol, sucrose. Orange/Strawberry flavor. In 118 mL.
otc	**Triaminic Cough & Congestion Liquid** (Novartis)						Alcohol free. EDTA, sorbitol, sucrose. Orange strawberry flavor. In 118 mL.
otc	**Triaminic Cough & Sore Throat Liquid** (Novartis)	15 mg pseudoephedrine HCl		7.5 mg dextromethorphan HBr	160 mg acetaminophen	*6 to < 12 yrs* - 10 mL q 6 h up to 40 mL/day; *2 to < 6 yrs* - 5 mL q 6 h up to 20 mL/day	Alcohol free. EDTA, sucrose. Grape flavor. In 118 and 237 mL.
Rx sf	**AccuHist DM Pediatric Drops** (Pediamed)	15 mg pseudoephedrine HCl	1 mg brompheniramine maleate	4 mg dextromethorphan HBr		*12 to 24 mos* - 1 mL qid up to 4 mL/day; *6 to 12 mo* - 0.75 mL qid up to 3 mL/day; *3 to 6 mo* - 0.5 mL qid up to 2 mL/day; *1 to 3 mo* - 0.25 mL qid up to 1 mL/day.	Saccharin, sorbitol. Alcohol free. Grape flavor. In 30 mL.
Rx	**AccuHist PDX Drops** (PediaMed)	12.5 mg/mL pseudoephedrine HCl	1 mg/mL brompheniramine maleate	3 mg/mL dextromethorphan HBr		*12 to 24 mo* - 1 mL qid, up to 4 mL/day; *6 to 12 mo* - 0.75 mL qid, up to 3 mL/day; *3 to 6 mo* - 0.5 mL quid, up to 2 mL/day; *1 to 3 mo* - 0.25 mL qid, up to 1 mL/day.	Saccharin, sorbitol. Grape flavor. In 30 mL w/ dropper.

PEDIATRIC ANTITUSSIVE COMBINATIONS

UPPER RESPIRATORY COMBINATIONS

	Product & Distributor	Decongestant	Antihistamine	Antitussive	Other	Average Dose	Excipients & How Supplied
otc	Bromanate DM Cold & Cough Elixir[1] (Alpharma)	15 mg pseudoephedrine HCl	1 mg brompheniramine maleate	5 mg dextromethorphan HBr		*6 to < 12 yrs* - 5 mL q 4 h up to 30 mL/day	Alcohol free. Grape flavor. In 118 mL.
otc	Children's Elixir DM Cough & Cold Elixir[1] (AmerisourceBergen)					*6 to < 12 yrs* - 10 mL q 4 to 6 h up to 40 mL/day	Alcohol free. Saccharin, sorbitol. Grape flavor. In 118 mL.
otc	Dimaphen DM Cold & Cough Elixir[1] (Major)						Alcohol free. Saccharin, sorbitol. Grape flavor. In 118 mL.
otc	Dimetapp DM Children's Cold & Cough Elixir[1] (Whitehall-Robins)					*6 to < 12 yrs* - 10 mL q 4 h up to 40 mL/day	Alcohol free. Sorbitol, saccharin, corn syrup. Grape flavor. In 118 and 237 mL.
otc	Dimetapp Children's Nighttime Flu Syrup[1] (Whitehall-Robins)	15 mg pseudoephedrine HCl	1 mg brompheniramine maleate	5 mg dextromethorphan HBr	160 mg acetaminophen	*6 to < 12 yrs* - 10 mL q 4 h up to 40 mL/day	Alcohol free. Corn syrup, saccharin, sorbitol. Bubble gum flavor. In 118 mL.
Rx	C.P.-DM Drops (Hi-Tech)	15 mg/mL pseudoephedrine HCl	1 mg/mL carbinoxamine maleate	4 mg/mL dextromethorphan HBr		*12 to 24 mos* - 1 mL qid;	Saccharin, sorbitol. Grape flavor. In 30 mL with dropper.
Rx sf	Carbofed DM Oral Drops (Hi-Tech)					*6 to 12 mos* - 0.75 mL qid; *3 to 6 mos* -	Alcohol free. In 30 mL with dropper.
Rx	Rondec-DM Oral Drops (Biovail)					0.5 mL qid; *1 to 3 mos* -	Saccharin, sorbitol. Grape flavor. In 30 mL with dropper.
Rx	Andehist DM NR Oral Drops (Silarx)					0.25 mL qid.	Saccharin, sorbitol. Grape flavor. In 30 mL with dropper.
Rx	Carbodex DM Drops (Tri-Med)	15 mg/mL pseudoephedrine HCl	2 mg/mL carbinoxamine maleate	4 mg/mL dextromethorphan HBr		*9 to 18 mos* - 1 mL qid; *6 to 9 mos* - 0.75 mL qid; *3 to 6 mos* - 0.5 mL qid; *1 to 3 mos* - 0.25 mL qid.	In 30 mL.
Rx sf	Sildec-DM Oral Drops (Silarx)					*12 to 24 mos* - 1 mL qid; *6 to 12 mos* - 0.75 mL qid; *3 to 6 mos* - 0.5 mL qid; *1 to 3 mos* - 0.25 mL qid	Alcohol free. Saccharin, sorbitol. Grape flavor. In 30 mL with dropper.
Rx	Pediatex-DM Liquid[1] (Zyber Pharm)	15 mg pseudoephedrine HCl	2 mg carbinoxamine maleate	15 mg dextromethorphan HBr		*6 to 12 yrs* - 5 mL qid; *18 mos to 6 yrs* - 2.5 mL qid	Saccharin, sorbitol. Cotton candy flavor. In 20 and 473 mL.
Rx	Balamine DM Oral Drops (Ballay)	25 mg/mL pseudoephedrine HCl	2 mg/mL carbinoxamine maleate	3.5 mg/mL dextromethorphan HBr		*9 to 18 mos* - 1 mL qid; *6 to 9 mos* - 0.75 mL qid; *3 to 6 mos* - 0.5 mL qid; *1 to 3 mos* - 0.25 mL qid	Menthol. Grape flavor. In 30 mL with dropper.
Rx	Cydec-DM Drops (Cypress)	25 mg/mL pseudoephedrine HCl	2 mg/mL carbinoxamine maleate	4 mg/mL dextromethorphan HBr			Grape flavor. In 30 mL with dropper.
Rx	Balamine DM Syrup[1] (Ballay)	60 mg pseudoephedrine HCl	4 mg carbinoxamine maleate	12.5 mg dextromethorphan HBr		*≥ 6 yrs* - 5 mL qid; *18 mos to 6 yrs* - 2.5 mL qid	Menthol. Grape flavor. In 473 mL.

UPPER RESPIRATORY COMBINATIONS

PEDIATRIC ANTITUSSIVE COMBINATIONS

	Product & Distributor	Decongestant	Antihistamine	Antitussive	Other	Average Dose	Excipients & How Supplied
Rx	Cydec-DM Syrup[1] (Cypress)	60 mg pseudoephedrine HCl	4 mg carbinoxamine maleate	15 mg dextromethorphan HBr		≥ 6 yrs - 5 mL qid; 18 mos to 6 yrs - 2.5 mL qid	Grape flavor. In 118 and 473 mL and 3.8 L.
otc	Tylenol Children's Cold Plus Cough Chewable Tablets (McNeil)	7.5 mg pseudoephedrine HCl	0.5 mg chlorpheniramine maleate	2.5 mg dextromethorphan HBr	80 mg acetaminophen	6 to 11 yrs - 4 q 4 to 6 h up to 16/day	Aspartame, mannitol, 4 mg phenylalanine. (TYLENOL C/C TC/C). Cherry flavor. In 24s.
otc	All-Nite Children's Cold/Cough Relief Liquid[1] (Major)	10 mg pseudoephedrine HCl	0.67 mg chlorpheniramine maleate	5 mg dextromethorphan HBr		6 to 11 yrs - 15 mL q 6 h up to 60 mL/day	Sucrose. Cherry flavor. In 118 mL.
otc	Nite Time Children's Liquid[1] (Topco)						Alcohol free. Sucrose. Cherry flavor. In 118 mL.
otc	Vicks Children's NyQuil Cold/Cough Relief Liquid[1] (Procter & Gamble)						Alcohol free. Sucrose. Cherry flavor. In 118 mL.
otc	Vicks Pediatric 44M Cough & Cold Relief Liquid[1] (Procter & Gamble)						Alcohol free. Corn syrup, saccharin. Cherry flavor. In 115 mL.
otc	Kid Kare Children's Cough/Cold Liquid (Rugby)	15 mg pseudoephedrine HCl	1 mg chlorpheniramine maleate	5 mg dextromethorphan HBr		6 to 11 yrs - 10 mL q 4 to 6 h up to 40 mL/day	Alcohol free. Sorbitol, corn syrup. Cherry flavor. In 118 mL.
otc	Pedia Care Cough-Cold Liquid (Pharmacia)						Alcohol free. Corn syrup, sorbitol. Cherry flavor. In 118 mL.
otc	Pedia Care Multi-Symptom Cold Liquid (Pharmacia)						Alcohol free. Corn syrup, sorbitol. Cherry flavor. In 120 mL.
otc	Thera-Hist Cold & Cough Syrup[1] (Major)						Sorbitol, sucrose. Cherry flavor. In 118 mL.
otc	Tri-Acting Cold & Cough Syrup (Topco)						Alcohol free. Sorbitol, sucrose. Cherry flavor. In 118 mL.
otc	Triaminic Cold & Cough Liquid (Novartis)						Alcohol free. Sorbitol, sucrose. Cherry flavor. In 118 mL.
otc	PediaCare Children's Multi-Symptom Cold Chewable Tablets (Pharmacia)					6 to < 12 yrs - 2 q 4 to 6 h up to 8/day	Aspartame, phenylalanine, sucrose. Cherry Flavor. In 18s.
otc	Triaminic Cold & Cough Softchews Tablets[1] (Novartis)						Aspartame, mannitol, 17.7 mg phenylalanine, sucrose. (T2). Cherry flavor. In 18s.
otc	Triaminic Cough Softchews Tablets[1] (Novartis)						Aspartame, sucrose, 22.5 mg phenylalanine, mannitol. (T5). Strawberry flavor. In 18s.
otc	Tylenol Children's Cold Plus Cough Suspension (McNeil)	15 mg pseudoephedrine HCl	1 mg chlorpheniramine maleate	5 mg dextromethorphan HBr	160 mg acetaminophen	6 to 11 yrs - 10 mL q 4 to 6 h up to 40 mL/day	Alcohol free. Acesulfame K, butylparaben, corn syrup, sorbitol. Cherry flavor. In 120 mL.
otc	Pedia Care NightRest Cough & Cold Liquid (Pharmacia)	15 mg pseudoephedrine HCl	1 mg chlorpheniramine maleate	7.5 mg dextromethorphan HBr		6 to 11 yrs - 10 mL q 6 to 8 h up to 40 mL/day	Alcohol free. Corn syrup, sorbitol. Cherry flavor. In 120 mL.
otc	Robitussin Pediatric Night Relief Cough & Cold Liquid (Whitehall-Robins)					6 to < 12 yrs - 10 mL q 6 h up to 40 mL/day	Alcohol free. Corn syrup, saccharin. Fruit punch flavor. In 118 mL.
otc	Triaminic Cold & Night Time Cough Liquid (Novartis)						Alcohol free. Sorbitol, sucrose. Grape flavor. In 118 mL.
otc	Triaminic Cold, Cough & Fever Liquid (Novartis)	15 mg pseudoephedrine HCl	1 mg chlorpheniramine maleate	7.5 mg dextromethorphan HBr	160 mg acetaminophen	6 to < 12 yrs - 10 mL q 6 h up to 40 mL/day	Acesulfame K, EDTA, sucrose. Bubble gum flavor. In 118 mL.
otc	Tylenol Children's Flu Suspension (McNeil)					6 to 11 yrs - 10 mL q 6 to 8 h up to 40 mL/day	Alcohol free. Acesulfame K, butylparaben, corn syrup, sorbitol. Bubble gum flavor. In 120 mL.

UPPER RESPIRATORY COMBINATIONS

PEDIATRIC ANTITUSSIVE COMBINATIONS

Product & Distributor	Decongestant	Antihistamine	Antitussive	Other	Average Dose	Excipients & How Supplied
Rx **Atuss-12 DM Suspension, extended-re-lease**[1] (Atley)	30 mg pseudoephedrine HCl (as polistirex)	6 mg chlorpheniramine maleate (as polistirex)	30 mg/5 mL dextromethorphan HBr (as polistirex)		**6 to 12 yrs** - 2.5 to 5 mL q 12 h; **2 to 6 yrs** - 2.5 mL q 12 h.	Corn syrup, parabens. In 20 and 473 mL.

[1] This product also may be used in adults; refer to package labeling for dosing.

Refer to the general discussion of these products in the Respiratory Combinations Introduction. Some of the products in the previous Antitussive Combinations table also may be used in children.

908

ANTITUSSIVE AND EXPECTORANT COMBINATIONS
Content given per tablet, 5 mL, or packet.

	Product & Distributor	Antitussive	Expectorant	Decongestant	Antihistamine/Other	Average Adult Dose	Excipients & How Supplied
Rx	Levall Liquid[1] (Athlon Pharmaceuticals)	20 mg carbetapentane citrate	100 mg guaifenesin	15 mg phenylephrine HCl		5 mL q 4 to 6 h up to 20 mL/day	Alcohol free. Strawberry flavor. In 15 and 473 mL.
c-v	Dihistine Expectorant Liquid (Alpharma)	10 mg codeine phosphate	100 mg guaifenesin	30 mg pseudoephedrine HCl		10 mL q 4 h up to 40 mL/day	7.5% alcohol, saccharin, sorbitol, sucrose. In 473 mL.
c-v	Guiatuss DAC Liquid[1] (Various, eg, Alpharma, Ivax)						May contain alcohol. In 473 mL.
c-v sf	Halotussin DAC Syrup[1] (Watson Laboratories)						1.9% alcohol, saccharin, sorbitol. Cherry-raspberry flavor. In 480 mL.
c-v sf	Mytussin DAC Liquid[1] (Morton Grove Pharmaceuticals)						1.7% alcohol, menthol, saccharin, sorbitol. Strawberry-raspberry flavor. In 118 and 473 mL.
c-v	Novagest Expectorant with Codeine Liquid[1] (Major)						8.2% alcohol, sugar, menthol, parabens. In 118 and 473 mL.
c-iii	Nucofed Expectorant Syrup[1] (Monarch)	20 mg codeine phosphate	200 mg guaifenesin	60 mg pseudoephedrine HCl		5 mL q 6 h up to 20 mL/day	12.5% alcohol, saccharin, sucrose. Cherry flavor. In 473 mL.
c-iii	Nucotuss Expectorant Syrup[1] (Alpharma)						12.5% alcohol. In 473 mL.
c-v	Tussirex Syrup (Scot-Tussin)	10 mg codeine phosphate	83.3 mg sodium citrate	4.17 mg phenylephrine HCl	13.33 mg pheniramine maleate, 83.33 mg sodium salicylate, 25 mg caffeine citrate	5 mL tid	Alcohol and dye free. 0.17 mg menthol. In 473 mL and 3.8 L.
c-v sf	Tussirex Sugar Free Liquid (Scot-Tussin)						Alcohol and dye free. 0.17 mg menthol. In 30 and 473 mL and 3.8 L.
Rx	Donatussin Syrup[1] (Laser)	15 mg dextromethorphan HBr	100 mg guaifenesin	10 mg phenylephrine HCl	2 mg/5 mL chlorpheniramine maleate	10 mL q 6 h up to 40 mL/day	In 30, 115, and 473 mL.
Rx	Tussafed Ex Syrup[1] (Everett Laboratories)	30 mg dextromethorphan HBr	200 mg guaifenesin	10 mg phenylephrine HCl		5 mL qid	Alcohol free. EDTA, saccharin, sorbitol. Cherry-vanilla flavor. In 473 mL.
Rx	SINUtuss DM Tablets[1] (WE Pharm)	30 mg dextromethorphan HBr	600 mg guaifenesin	15 mg phenylephrine HCl		2 tablets bid	Dye-free. (WE 45). Capsule shape, scored. In 100s.
Rx sf	Lemotussin-DM Liquid[1] (Seneca)	7.5 mg dextromethorphan HBr	50 mg guaifenesin, 50 mg potassium guaiacolsulfonate		2 mg chlorpheniramine maleate	5 to 10 mL q 6 to 8 h	Parabens, saccharin, sorbitol. Alcohol free. In 473 mL.
otc	Guiatuss CF Syrup[1] (Alpharma)	10 mg dextromethorphan HBr	100 mg guaifenesin	30 mg pseudoephedrine HCl		10 mL q 4 h up to 40 mL/day	Alcohol free. Cherry flavor. In 120 mL.
otc	Robafen CF Syrup[1] (Major)						Alcohol free. Saccharin, sorbitol. In 118 and 237 mL.
otc	Robitussin CF Syrup[1] (Whitehall-Robins)						Alcohol free. Saccharin, sorbitol. In 355 mL.
otc	Comtrex Multi-Symptom Deep Chest Cold & Congestion Relief Softgels (Bristol-Myers Squibb)	10 mg dextromethorphan HBr	100 mg guaifenesin	30 mg pseudoephedrine HCl	250 mg acetaminophen	2 q 4 h up to 12/day	Sorbitol. In 24s.
otc	Robitussin Cold, Multi-Symptom Cold & Flu Softgels (Whitehall-Robins)					2 q 4 h up to 8/day	Sorbitol. (AHR 8602). In 12s.
otc	Sudafed Multi-Symptom Cold & Cough Liquid Caps (Warner-Lambert)						Sorbitol. (SMS). In 20s.
otc	Cold & Cough Tussin Softgels[1] (AmerisourceBergen)	10 mg dextromethorphan HBr	200 mg guaifenesin	30 mg pseudoephedrine HCl		2 q 4 h up to 8/day	Sorbitol. In 12s.
otc	Robitussin Cold, Cold & Cough Softgels[1] (Whitehall-Robins)						Sorbitol. (AHR 8600). In 12s and 20s.
otc	Robitussin Cold, Cold & Congestion Softgels and Tablets[1] (Whitehall-Robins)						Capsule shape. In 20s.

UPPER RESPIRATORY COMBINATIONS

ANTITUSSIVE AND EXPECTORANT COMBINATIONS

	Product & Distributor	Antitussive	Expectorant	Decongestant	Antihistamine/Other	Average Adult Dose	Excipients & How Supplied
otc	**Robitussin Cold, Multi-Symptom Cold & Flu Tablets**[1] (Whitehall-Robins)	10 mg dextromethorphan HBr	200 mg guaifenesin	30 mg pseudoephedrine HCl	325 mg acetaminophen	2 q 4 h up to 8/day	Capsule shape. In 20s.
Rx sf	**PanMist-DM Syrup**[1] (Pan American Laboratories)	15 mg dextromethorphan HBr	100 mg guaifenesin	40 mg pseudoephedrine HCl		Up to 10 mL tid or qid	Alcohol and dye free. Strawberry flavor. In 15 and 473 mL.
otc	**Tylenol Multi-Symptom Cold Severe Congestion Tablets**[1] (McNeil Consumer)	15 mg dextromethorphan HBr	200 mg guaifenesin	30 mg pseudoephedrine HCl	325 mg acetaminophen	2 q 6 to 8 h up to 8/day	Capsule shape. In 24s.
Rx sf	**Z-Cof DM Syrup**[1] (Zyber Pharmaceuticals)	15 mg dextromethorphan HBr	200 mg guaifenesin	40 mg pseudoephedrine HCl		10 mL bid or tid up to 30 mL/day	Alcohol free. Grape flavor. In 473 mL.
Rx	**Duraflu Tablets**[1] (ProEthic)	20 mg dextromethorphan HBr	200 mg guaifenesin	60 mg pseudoephedrine HCl	500 mg acetaminophen	1 qid up to 4/day	Dye-free. (PE 723). Scored. In 100s.
otc	**TheraFlu Maximum Strength Flu & Congestion Non-Drowsy Powder** (Novartis)	30 mg dextromethorphan HBr	400 mg guaifenesin	60 mg pseudoephedrine HCl	1000 mg acetaminophen	1 packet dissolved in 177 mL hot water q 6 h up to 4/day	Aspartame, 25 mg phenylalanine, sucrose. Honey lemon flavor. In 6s.
otc	**TheraFlu Maximum Strength Flu, Cold & Cough Powder** (Novartis)						Alcohol free. Aspartame, phenylalanine, sucrose. Honey lemon flavor. In 6s.
Rx	**GFN 550/PSE 60/DM 30 Tablets**[1] (Cypress)	30 mg dextromethorphan HBr	550 mg guaifenesin	60 mg pseudoephedrine HCl		1 to 2 q 12 h up to 4/day	Extended release. Dye-free. (CYP 28 7). In 100s.
Rx	**Touro CC Tablets**[1] (Dartmouth Pharmaceuticals)	30 mg dextromethorphan HBr	575 mg guaifenesin	60 mg pseudoephedrine HCl		1 or 2 q 12 h up to 4/day	Sustained release. Dye-free. (TOURO CC/DP). Capsule shape, scored. In 100s.
Rx	**Maxifed DM Tablets**[1] (MCR American Pharmaceutical)	30 mg dextromethorphan HBr	580 mg guaifenesin	60 mg pseudoephedrine HCl		1 to 2 q 12 h up to 4/day.	Extended release. Dye free. (MAXIFED DM). Capsule shape, scored. In 100s.
Rx	**AMBI 60/580/30 Tablets**[1] (AMBI)					1 to 2 q 12 h up to 4/day.	Extended release. Dye free. (AMBI/722). Capsule shape, scored. In 100s.
Rx	**GFN 600/PSE 60/DM 30 Tablets**[1] (Cypress)	30 mg dextromethorphan HBr	600 mg guaifenesin	60 mg pseudoephedrine HCl		1 to 2 q 12 h up to 4/day	Sustained release. Dye-free. White, capsule shape, scored. In 100s.
Rx	**Tussafed-LA Tablets**[1] (Everett)						Sustained release. Dye free. Capsule shape, scored. In 100s.
Rx	**Profen II DM Tablets**[1] (IVAX)	30 mg dextromethorphan HBr	800 mg guaifenesin	45 mg pseudoephedrine HCl		1 or 1½ q 12 h up to 3/day	Extended release. (PROFEN II DM). White, capsule shape, scored. In 100s.
Rx	**Medent-DM Tablets**[1] (Stewart-Jackson Pharmacal)	30 mg dextromethorphan HBr	800 mg guaifenesin	60 mg pseudoephedrine HCl		1 to 1½ q 12 h or 1 q 8 h up to 3/day	Sustained release. Dye free. (SJ/641). Oval, scored. In 100s.
Rx	**PanMist-DM Tablets**[1] (Pan American Laboratories)	32 mg dextromethorphan HBr	595 mg guaifenesin	48 mg pseudoephedrine HCl		1 or 2 q 12 h up to 4/day	Extended release. (PAL 07/59). Green, capsule shape, scored. In 100s.
Rx	**Maxifed DMX Tablets**[1] (MCR American Pharmaceutical)	40 mg dextromethorphan HBr	700 mg guaifenesin	80 mg pseudoephedrine HCl		½ to 1 ½ q 12 h up to 3/day	Extended release. In 100s.
Rx	**Humibid DM Capsules**[1] (Carolina Pharmaceuticals)[2]	50 mg dextromethorphan HBr	400 mg guaifenesin	200 mg potassium guaiacolsulfonate		1 q 12 h up to 2/day	Extended release. Sucrose. (HUMABID DM CAROLINA PHARMA). Lt. blue, white opaque. In 30s and 100s.
Rx	**Profen Forte DM Tablets**[1] (Ivax)	60 mg dextromethorphan HBr	800 mg guaifenesin	90 mg pseudoephedrine HCl		1 q 12 h up to 2/day	Sustained release. (PROFEN FORTE DM/316). White, capsule shape, scored. In 100s.
Rx	**MAXIPHEN DM Tablets**[1] (AMBI)	60 mg dextromethorphan HBr	1000 mg guaifenesin	40 mg phenylephrine HCl		1 q 12 h up to 2/day.	Extended-release. Dye-free. (Maxiphen DM). Capsule shape, scored. In 100s.
Rx	**Aquatab C Tablets** (Adams)	60 mg dextromethorphan HBr	1200 mg guaifenesin	60 mg pseudoephedrine HCl		1 q 12 h up to 2/day	Extended release. (Adams 063). Lt. yellow, oval, scored. In 100s.

UPPER RESPIRATORY COMBINATIONS

ANTITUSSIVE AND EXPECTORANT COMBINATIONS

	Product & Distributor	Antitussive	Expectorant	Decongestant	Antihistamine/ Other	Average Adult Dose	Excipients & How Supplied
Rx	GFN 1200/DM 60/PSE 120 Tablets (Cypress)	60 mg dextromethorphan HBr	1200 mg guaifenesin	120 mg pseudoephedrine HCl		1 q 12 h up to 2/day	Sustained release. Dye free. (CYP 273). White, capsule shape, scored. In 100s.
Rx	Pancof-EXP Syrup[1] (Pan American)	7.5 mg dihydrocodeine bitartrate	100 mg guaifenesin	15 mg pseudoephedrine		5 to 10 ml q 4 to 6 h	Saccharin, sorbitol, menthol. Alcohol- and dye-free. In 25 and 473 mL.
c-iii	Atuss-G Syrup[1] (Atley)	2 mg hydrocodone bitartrate	100 mg guaifenesin	10 mg phenylephrine HCl		10 mL q 4 h up to 40 mL/day	Menthol, saccharin, sucrose. Grape flavor. In 473 mL.
c-iii	Donatussin DC Syrup[1] (Laser)	2.5 mg hydrocodone bitartrate	50 mg guaifenesin	7.5 mg phenylephrine HCl		10 mL q 4 to 6 h up to 40 mL/day	Alcohol free. In 118 and 473 mL.
c-iii	Tussafed HC Syrup[1] (Everett Laboratories)					10 mL q 4 to 6 h up to 60 mL/day	Alcohol free. In 473 mL.
c-iii sf	Entex HC Liquid[1] (Andrx Laboratories)	5 mg hydrocodone bitartrate	100 mg guaifenesin	7.5 mg phenylephrine HCl		5 to 10 mL q 4 to 6 h up to 40 mL/day	Alcohol and dye free. Cherry flavor. In 15 and 473 mL.
c-iii sf	Levall 5.0 Liquid[1] (Athlon Pharmaceuticals)	5 mg hydrocodone bitartrate	100 mg guaifenesin	15 mg phenylephrine HCl		5 mL q 4 to 6 hr up to 20 mL/day	Alcohol free. Grape flavor. In 15 and 473 mL.
c-iii	ZTuss Expectorant Liquid[1] (Huckaby Pharmacal)	2.5 mg hydrocodone bitartrate	100 mg guaifenesin	15 mg pseudoephedrine HCl	2 mg chlorpheniramine maleate	10 mL q 4 to 6 h	Phenylalanine. In 473 mL.
c-iii	Hydro-Tussin HD Liquid[1] (Ethex)	2.5 mg hydrocodone bitartrate	100 mg guaifenesin	30 mg pseudoephedrine HCl		10 mL q 4 to 6 h	Alcohol free. Saccharin, sorbitol. In 473 mL.
c-iii	Su-Tuss HD Elixir[1] (Cypress)						5% alcohol. Fruit punch flavor. In 473 mL.
c-iii sf	Pancof-XP Liquid[1] (Pan American Labs)	3 mg hydrocodone bitartrate	100 mg guaifenesin	15 mg pseudoephedrine HCl		5 to 10 mL qid	Alcohol and dye free. In 473 mL.
c-iii sf	Protuss-D Liquid[1] (Horizon)	5 mg hydrocodone bitartrate	300 mg potassium guaiacolsulfonate	30 mg pseudoephedrine HCl		5 to 7.5 mL q 6 h	Alcohol and dye free. Saccharin, sorbitol. In 120 and 473 mL.

[1] This product may also be used in children; refer to package labeling for dosing.

Refer to the general discussion of these products in the Respiratory Combinations Introduction. Some of the products in the following Pediatric Antitussive and Expectorant Combinations table also may be used in adults.

[2] Carolina Pharmaceutical, Inc., 2500 Regency Parkway, Cary, NC 27511.

PEDIATRIC ANTITUSSIVE AND EXPECTORANT COMBINATIONS
Content given per 5 mL.

	Product & Distributor	Decongestant	Antihistamine	Antitussive	Expectorant	Dose	Excipients & How Supplied
Rx	AccuHist PDX Syrup[1] (PediaMed)	5 mg phenylephrine HCl	2 mg/5 mL brompheniramine maleate	5 mg dextromethorphan HBr	50 mg guaifenesin	**6 to < 12 yrs** - 5 mL q 4 to 6 h, up to 30 mL/day; **2 to < 6 yrs** - 2.5 mL q 4 to 6 h, up to 15 mL/day.	Sucrose. Grape flavor. In 473 mL.
c-v	Nucofed Pediatric Expectorant Syrup[1] (Monarch)	30 mg pseudoephedrine HCl		10 mg codeine phosphate	100 mg guaifenesin	**6 to < 12 yrs** - 5 mL q 6 h up to 20 mL/day; **2 to < 6 yrs** - 2.5 mL q 6 h up to 10 mL/day	6% alcohol, EDTA, saccharin, sucrose. Strawberry flavor. In 473 mL.
c-v	Nucotuss Pediatric Expectorant Syrup[1] (Alpharma)						6% alcohol. Strawberry flavor. In 473 mL.
otc	Robitussin Cough & Cold Infant Drops[1] (Whitehall-Robins)	6 mg/mL pseudoephedrine HCl		2 mg/mL dextromethorphan HBr	40 mg/mL guaifenesin	**2 to < 6 yrs** - 2.5 mL q 4 h up to 10 mL/day	Corn syrup, menthol, saccharin, sorbitol. In 30 mL.
Rx	AccuHist DM Pediatric Syrup[1] (PediaMed)	30 mg pseudoephedrine HCl	2 mg brompheniramine maleate	5 mg dextromethorphan HBr	50 mg guaifenesin	**6 to < 12 yrs** - 5 mL q 6 h up to 20 mL/day; **2 to < 6 yrs** - 2.5 mL q 6 h up to 10 mL/day	Corn syrup, sucrose. Alcohol free. Grape flavor. In 473 mL.

[1] This product also may be used in adults; refer to package labeling for dosing.

Refer to the general discussion of these products in the Respiratory Combinations Introduction. Some of the products in the previous Antitussive and Expectorant Combinations table also may be used in children.

UPPER RESPIRATORY COMBINATIONS

ANTITUSSIVES WITH EXPECTORANTS
Content given per tablet or 5 mL.

	Product & Distributor	Antitussive	Expectorant	Average Adult Dose	Excipients & How Supplied
c-v	**Cheracol Cough Syrup**[1] (Lee Pharmaceuticals)	10 mg codeine phosphate	100 mg guaifenesin	10 mL q 4 to 6 h up to 60 mL/day	4.75% alcohol, fructose, sucrose. In 60, 120, and 480 mL.
c-v sf	**Gani-Tuss NR Liquid**[1] (Various, eg, Cypress)			10 mL q 4 h up to 60 mL/day	Alcohol free. Raspberry flavor. In 120 and 473 mL.
c-v sf	**Guiatuss AC Syrup**[1] (Various, eg, Alpharma, Ivax)				3.5% alcohol. In 118 and 473 mL.
c-v sf	**Halotussin AC Liquid**[1] (Watson)				Alcohol free. Sorbitol, menthol, saccharin. In 118 and 480 mL and 3.8 L.
c-v sf	**Mytussin AC Cough Syrup**[1] (Morton Grove Pharmaceuticals)			5 to 10 mL q 4 to 6 h up to 60 mL/day	3.5% alcohol, menthol, saccharin, sorbitol. Fruit flavor. In 118, 237, and 473 mL.
c-v sf	**Romilar AC Liquid**[1] (Scot-Tussin)			10 mL q 4 h up to 60 mL/day	Alcohol and dye free. Menthol, aspartame, phenylalanine, parabens. In 473 mL.
c-v	**Tussi-Organidin NR Liquid**[1] (Wallace)				Saccharin, sorbitol. Raspberry flavor. In 473 mL.
c-v	**Tussi-Organidin-S NR Liquid**[1] (Wallace)				Saccharin, sorbitol. Raspberry flavor. In 118 mL unit-of-use container w/10 mL graduated syringe and fitment.
c-iii	**Codeine Phosphate and Guaifenesin Tablets** (Ethex)	10 mg codeine phosphate	300 mg guaifenesin	1 q 4 h up to 6/day	Sugar. (ETHEX 223). Red, oval. In 100s.
otc sf	**Benylin Expectorant Liquid**[1] (Warner Lambert)	5 mg dextromethorphan HBr	100 mg guaifenesin	20 mL q 6 to 8 h up to 80 mL/day	Alcohol free. Saccharin, sorbitol. Raspberry flavor. In 118 mL.
otc	**Vicks 44E Cough & Chest Congestion Relief Liquid**[1] (Procter & Gamble)	6.67 mg dextromethorphan HBr	66.7 mg guaifenesin	15 mL q 4 h up to 90 mL/day	5% alcohol, corn syrup, saccharin. In 118 and 236 mL.
otc	**Cheracol D Cough Formula Syrup**[1] (Lee Pharmaceuticals)	10 mg dextromethorphan HBr	100 mg guaifenesin	10 mL q 4 h up to 60 mL/day	4.75% alcohol, fructose, sucrose. In 118 and 177 mL.
otc	**Cheracol Plus Liquid**[1] (Lee Pharmaceuticals)				4.75% alcohol, fructose, sucrose. In 118 mL.
otc sf	**Diabetic Tussin DM Liquid**[1] (Health Care Products)				Alcohol and dye free. Aspartame, 8.4 mg phenylalanine, methylparaben, menthol. In 118 mL.
otc	**Extra Action Cough Syrup**[1] (Rugby)				Corn syrup, glucose, saccharin. In 118 mL.
Rx sf	**Gani-Tuss-DM NR Liquid**[1] (Cypress)				Alcohol free. Raspberry flavor. In 118 and 473 mL.
otc	**Genatuss DM Syrup**[1] (Ivax)				Alcohol free. Corn syrup, menthol, saccharin. In 118 mL.
otc	**Guaifenesin DM Syrup**[1] (UDL)				Alcohol free. Saccharin, sorbitol. In UD 5 and 10 mL.
Rx sf	**Guaifenesin-DM NR Liquid**[1] (Silarx)				Alcohol free. Methylparaben, saccharin, sorbitol. Raspberry flavor. In 118 and 473 mL and 3.8 L.
otc	**Guiatuss-DM Syrup**[1] (Various, eg, Alpharma, Ivax)				Alcohol free. May contain sucrose. In 118 and 237 mL.
otc	**Mytussin DM Syrup**[1] (Morton Grove Pharmaceuticals)			5 to 10 mL q 4 h up to 60 mL/day	Alcohol free. Sugar, menthol, saccharin. Cherry flavor. In 118 mL and 3.8 L.
otc sf	**Phanatuss DM Cough Syrup**[1] (Pharmakon Labs)			10 mL q 3 to 4 h up to 60 mL/day	Alcohol free. Parabens, saccharin, menthol. In 118 mL.
otc	**Robitussin-DM Liquid**[1] (Whitehall-Robins)			10 mL q 4 h up to 60 mL/day	Glucose, corn syrup, saccharin. In 118, 237, 360, and 473 mL.
otc sf	**Robitussin Sugar Free Cough Liquid**[1] (Whitehall-Robins)				Alcohol and dye free. Methylparaben, saccharin. In 118 mL.
otc	**Siltussin DM Cough Syrup**[1] (Silarx)				Alcohol free. Sucrose, saccharin, methylparaben. In 118 mL.
otc sf	**Tolu-Sed DM Liquid**[1] (Scherer)			5 to 10 mL q 4 h or 15 mL q 6 to 8 h up to 60 mL/day	10% alcohol. In 118 mL.
Rx	**Tussi-Organidin-DM NR Liquid**[1] (Wallace)			10 mL q 4 h up to 60 mL/day	Saccharin, sorbitol. Raspberry flavor. In 473 mL.

UPPER RESPIRATORY COMBINATIONS

ANTITUSSIVES WITH EXPECTORANTS

	Product & Distributor	Antitussive	Expectorant	Average Adult Dose	Excipients & How Supplied
otc	Kolephrin GG/DM Liquid[1] (Pfeiffer)	10 mg dextromethorphan HBr	150 mg guaifenesin	10 mL q 4 h up to 60 mL/day	Alcohol free. Glucose, saccharin, sucrose. Cherry flavor. In 118 mL.
Rx	Aquatab DMSyrup[1] (Adams)	10 mg dextromethorphan HBr	200 mg guaifenesin	5 to 10 mL q 4 h up to 60 mL/day	Acesulfame K, aspartame, menthol, methylparaben, phenylalanine. In 473 mL.
otc	Coricidin HBP Chest Congestion & Cough-Softgel Capsules (Schering-Plough)			1 or 2 q 4 h up to 12/day	Sorbitol. In 20s.
otc sf	Diabetic Tussin Maximum Strength DM Liquid[1] (Health Care Products)			10 mL q 4 h up to 60 mL/day	Alcohol and dye free. Aspartame, 8.4 mg phenylalanine, menthol, methylparaben. In 118 and 237 mL.
otc	Robitussin Cough & Congestion Formula Liquid[1] (Wyeth)				Alcohol free. Corn syrup, menthol, saccharin, sorbitol. In 118 mL.
otc	Tuss-DM Tablets[1] (Hyrex)			1 or 2 q 4 h up to 12/day	In 100s, 1000s, and UD 50s.
otc sf	Safe Tussin Liquid[1] (Kramer)	15 mg dextromethorphan HBr	100 mg guaifenesin	10 mL q 6 h up to 40 mL/day	Alcohol and dye free. Sorbitol, menthol. Mint flavor. In 120 mL.
otc sf	Scot-Tussin Senior Clear Liquid (Scot-tussin)	15 mg dextromethorphan HBr	200 mg guaifenesin	5 mL q 4 h up to 30 mL/day	Parabens, phenylalanine, menthol, aspartame. Alcohol free. In 118 mL.
Rx	Hydro-Tussin DM Liquid[1] (Ethex)	20 mg dextromethorphan HBr	200 mg guaifenesin	5 mL q 4 h up to 30 mL/day	Saccharin, sorbitol. In 473 mL.
Rx	Maxi-tuss DM Liquid[1] (MCR American Pharmaceuticals)				Glucose, menthol, parabens, saccharin. Black cherry flavor. In 473 mL.
Rx	SU-TUSS DM Liquid[1] (Cypress)				5% alcohol. Fruit flavor. In 473 mL.
Rx	Respa-DM Tablets[1] (Respa)	28 mg dextromethorphan HBr	600 mg guaifenesin	1 or 2 q 12 h up to 4/day	Sustained release. Dye free. (RESPA 78). Scored. In 100s.
Rx	Atuss-12 DX Suspension[1] (Atley)	Dextromethorphan polistirex (equivalent to 30 mg dextromethorphan HBr)	200 mg guaifenesin/5 mL	5 to 10 mL q 12 h	Extended release. Parabens, honey. Honey-lemon flavor. In 20 and 473 mL.
Rx	Dextromethorphan HBr/Guaifenesin Tablets[1] (URL)	30 mg dextromethorphan HBr	500 mg guaifenesin	1 or 2 q 12 h up to 4/day	Extended release. Dye-free. (NL 736). Capsule shape, scored. In 100s.
Rx	Sudal-DM Tablets[1] (Atley Pharmaceuticals)	30 mg dextromethorphan HBr	500 mg guaifenesin	1 or 2 q 12 h up to 4/day	Sustained release. Dye-free. (SUDAL DM/P). Scored. In 100s.
Rx	Touro DM Tablets[1] (Dartmouth)	30 mg dextromethorphan HBr	575 mg guaifenesin	1 or 2 q 12 h up to 4/day	Sustained release. (TOURO DM/DP311). Lt. blue, scored. In 100s.
Rx	Guaifenesin DM Tablets[1] (Prasco)	30 mg dextromethorphan HBr	600 mg guaifenesin	1 or 2 q 12 h up to 4/day	Extended release. (310). Green, capsule shape. In 100s.
Rx	Guaifenex DM Tablets[1] (Ethex)				Extended release. (Ethex/213). Green, capsule shape, scored. In 100s.
Rx	Guiadrine DM Tablets[1] (Breckenridge Pharmaceutical)				Sustained release. In 100s and 250s.
Rx	Iobid DM Tablets[1] (Iopharm)				Sustained release. In 100s.
Rx	Z-Cof LA Tablets[1] (Zyber)	30 mg dextromethorphan HBr	650 mg guaifenesin	1 or 2 q 12 h up to 4/day	Sustained release. (ZYBER 105). White, scored. In 100s.
Rx	GFN 1000/DM 50 Tablets[1] (Cypress)	50 mg dextromethorphan HBr	1000 mg guaifenesin	1 q 12 h up to 2/day	Extended release. (CYP 288). Capsule shape, scored. In 100s.
Rx	Allfen-DM Tablets[1] (MCR American Pharmaceuticals)	55 mg dextromethorphan HBr	1000 mg guaifenesin	1 q 12 h up to 2/day	Extended release. Dye-free. (ALLFEN DM). Scored. In 100s.
Rx	AMBI 1000/55 Tablets[1] (AMBI)			1 to 1.5 q 12 h or 1 q 8 h up to 3/day	Extended release. Dye Free (AMBI 120). Capsule shape, scored. In 100s.
Rx	Dex GG TR Tablets[1] (Boca Pharmacal)	60 mg dextromethorphan HBr	1000 mg guaifenesin	1 q 12 h up to 2/day	Extended release. (BOCA 122). White. In 100s.
Rx	GFN 1000/DM 60 Tablets[1] (Cypress)				Sustained release. (CYP 267). White, capsule shape, scored. In 100s.
Rx	Guaifenesin 1000 mg and Dextromethorphan HBr 60 mg LA Tablets[1] (URL Laboratories)				In 100s.
Rx	Muco-Fen DM Tablets[1] (Ivax)				Long-acting. Dye-free. (MUCOFEN DM). Scored. In 100s.

UPPER RESPIRATORY COMBINATIONS

ANTITUSSIVES WITH EXPECTORANTS

	Product & Distributor	Antitussive	Expectorant	Average Adult Dose	Excipients & How Supplied
Rx	Aquatab DM Tablets[1] (Adams)	60 mg dextromethorphan HBr	1200 mg guaifenesin	1 q 12 h up to 2/day	(Adams 002). Lt. blue, oval, scored. In 100s.
Rx	GFN 1200/DM 60 Tablets[1] (Cypress)				Sustained release. (CYP263). White, scored. In 100s.
Rx	TUSSI-bid Tablets[1] (Capellon Pharmaceuticals)				Sustained release. (L/DM). Mottled pink, capsule shape, scored. In 100s.
c-iii sf	Maxi-Tuss HCG Liquid[1] (MCR American Pharmaceutical)	6 mg hydrocodone bitartrate	200 mg/5 mL guaifenesin	5 to 10 mL pc and hs (not less than 4 h apart) up to 50 mL/day	Alcohol free. Aspartame, phenylalanine, parabens. In 480 mL.
c-iii sf	Pneumotussin 2.5 Cough Syrup[1] (ECR Pharmaceuticals)	2.5 mg hydrocodone bitartrate	200 mg guaifenesin	10 mL q 4 to 6 h	Alcohol and dye free. Cherry punch flavor. In 473 mL.
c-iii	Pneumotussin Tablets[1] (ECR Pharmaceuticals)	2.5 mg hydrocodone bitartrate	300 mg guaifenesin	1 or 2 q 4 to 6 h up to 8/day	Dye free. (ECR 2.5). White, capsule shape, scored. In 100s.
c-iii sf	Hydrocodone Bitartrate and Guaifenesin Liquid[1] (Various, eg, Ethex, Ivax, Kremers Urban, Watson)	5 mg hydrocodone bitartrate	100 mg guaifenesin	5 mL q 4 h pc and hs up to 30 mL/day	Alcohol and dye free. May contain menthol, parabens, sorbitol, saccharin. In 473 and 946 mL.
c-iii sf	Codiclear DH Syrup[1] (Schwarz Pharma)				Alcohol and dye free. Saccharin, sorbitol. In 118 and 473 mL.
c-iii	Hycosin Expectorant Syrup[1] (Alpharma)				10% alcohol, parabens, saccharin, saccharin, sorbitol, sucrose. Butterscotch flavor. In 473 mL.
c-iii	Hycotuss Expectorant Syrup[1] (Endo)				10% alcohol, saccharin, sorbitol, sugar, parabens. Butterscotch flavor. In 473 mL.
c-iii sf	Hydrocodone GF Syrup[1] (Morton Grove Pharmaceuticals)				Alcohol and dye free. Saccharin, sorbitol. Fruit flavor. In 237 and 473 mL.
c-iii sf	Kwelcof Liquid[1] (B.F. Ascher & Company)				Alcohol and dye free. Menthol, saccharin, sorbitol. Fruit flavor. In 473 mL.
c-iii sf	Vitussin Syrup[1] (Cypress)				Alcohol and dye free. Cherry flavor. In 473 mL.
c-iii sf	Atuss EX Syrup[1] (Atley Pharmaceuticals)	2.5 mg hydrocodone bitartrate	120 mg potassium guaiacolsulfonate	10 to 15 mL q 4 to 6 h up to 60 mL/day	Alcohol and dye free. Menthol, saccharin, sorbitol. Cherry flavor. In 473 mL.
c-iii sf	Hydron EX Liquid[1] (Cypress)				Saccharin, sorbitol. Alcohol-free. Cherry flavor. In 473 mL.
c-iii sf	Prolex DH Liquid[1] (Blansett Pharmacal)	4.5 mg hydrocodone bitartrate	300 mg potassium guaiacolsulfonate	5 to 7.5 mL qid	Alcohol free. Saccharin, sorbitol, menthol. Tropical fruit punch flavor. In 25, 118, and 473 mL.
c-iii sf	Hydron KGS Liquid[1] (Cypress)	5 mg hydrocodone bitartrate	300 mg potassium guaiacolsulfonate	5 to 7.5 mL qid	Alcohol free. Saccharin, sorbitol. Wild cherry flavor. In 473 mL.
c-iii sf	Protuss Liquid[1] (Horizon Pharmaceutical)				Alcohol free. Saccharin, sorbitol. Grape flavor. In 20, 118, and 473 mL.
c-iii sf	Marcof Expectorant Syrup[1] (Marnel)	5 mg hydrocodone bitartrate	350 mg potassium guaiacolsulfonate	5 mL q 4 h pc and hs up to 30 mL/day	Alcohol and dye free. Menthol, saccharin, sorbitol. In 473 mL.
c-ii	Dilaudid Cough Syrup (Knoll)	1 mg hydromorphone HCl	100 mg guaifenesin	5 mL q 3 to 4 h	5% alcohol. Peach flavor. In 473 mL.

[1] This product also may be used in children; refer to package labeling for dosing.

Refer to the general discussion of these products in the Respiratory Combinations Introduction. Some of the products in the following Pediatric Antitussives with Expectorant table also may be used in adults.

914

UPPER RESPIRATORY COMBINATIONS

PEDIATRIC ANTITUSSIVES WITH EXPECTORANTS

Content given per 5 mL (liquid) or 1 mL (drops).

	Product & Distributor	Antitussive	Expectorant	Average Dose	Excipients & How Supplied
otc	Robitussin DM Infant Drops (Whitehall-Robins)	2 mg/mL dextromethorphan HBr	40 mg/mL guaifenesin	2 to < 6 yrs - 2.5 mL q 4 h up to 15 mL/day	Alcohol free. Corn syrup, saccharin. Fruit punch flavor. In 30 mL with oral syringe.
otc	Vicks Pediatric 44e Cough & Chest Congestion Relief Liquid[1] (Procter & Gamble)	3.3 mg dextromethorphan HBr	33.3 mg guaifenesin	6 to 11 yrs - 15 mL q 4 h up to 90 mL/day; 2 to 5 yrs - 7.5 mL q 4 h up to 45 mL/day	Corn syrup, saccharin. Cherry flavor. In 118 mL.

[1] This product also may be used in adults; refer to package labeling for dosing.

Refer to the general discussion of these products in the Respiratory Combinations Introduction. Some of the products in the previous Antitussives with Expectorants table also may be used in children.

TOPICAL COMBINATIONS

	Product & Distributor	Ingredients	Excipients & How Supplied
otc	Nose Better Gel (Lee Pharm.)	0.5% allantoin, 0.75% camphor, 0.5% menthol	Lanolin, methylparaben. In 12.9 g.
otc	TheraPatch Vapor Patch for Kids Cough Suppressant (LecTec Corp.)	4.7% camphor, 2.6% menthol	Glycerin. Cherry scent. In 7s.
otc	Triaminic Vapor Patch for Cough (Novartis Consumer Health)		Glycerin. Cherry and menthol scents. In 6s.
otc	Mentholatum Cherry Chest Rub for Kids (Mentholatum Co.)	4.7% camphor, 2.6% menthol, 1.2% eucalyptus oil	Petrolatum. In 28 g.
otc	TheraFlu Vapor Stick (Novartis)	4.8% camphor, 2.6% menthol	Cetyl alcohol, eucalyptus oil, parabens. In herbal and menthol scents. In 51 g.
otc	TheraFlu Vapor Stick Cough & Muscle Aches (Novartis)		Cetyl alcohol, eucalyptus oil, parabens. In 51 g.
otc	Tom's of Maine Natural Cough & Cold Rub Cough Suppressant (Tom's of Maine)		In 92.4 g.
otc	Vicks VapoRub Cream (Procter & Gamble)	5.2% camphor, 2.8% menthol, 1.2% eucalyptus oil	Cetyl and stearyl alcohol, EDTA, glycerin, parabens. In 56 g.
otc	Mentholatum Ointment (Mentholatum Co.)	9% camphor, 1.3% menthol	Petrolatum. In 28 g.
otc	Breathe Right Children's Colds Nasal Strips (CNS Inc.)	Menthol	In 10s.
otc	Breathe Right Colds Nasal Strips (CNS Inc.)		In 10s.

CAFFEINE

otc	**Caffedrine** (Various, eg, Blairex)	**Tablets:** 200 mg	In 16s.
otc	**Maximum Strength NoDoz** (Bristol-Myers)		Sucrose. Caplet shape. Coated. In 36s.
otc	**Vivarin** (GlaxoSmithKline)		Dextrose. (V). Coated. In 16s, 24s, 40s, and 80s.
otc	**Keep Alert** (Magno-Humphries Labs.)		Caplet shape. In 60s.
otc	**357 HR Magnum** (BDI)		In 36s, 100s, and 500s.
otc	**Overtime** (BDI)		In 100s and 500s.
otc	**20-20** (BDI)		In 100s and 500s.
otc	**Valentine** (BDI)		In 100s and 500s.
otc	**Keep Going** (Block Drug Co.)		Caplet shape. In 4s.
otc	**Lucidex** (Xanodyne[2])	**Tablets, enteric coated:** 100 mg	In 24s.
otc	**.44 Magnum** (BDI)	**Capsules:** 200 mg	In 100s and 500s.
otc	**Molie** (BDI)		In 100s and 500s.
otc	**Fastlene** (BDI)		In 100s and 500s.
otc	**Enerjets** (Chilton Labs)	**Lozenges:** 75 mg	Sugar. Coffee, mocha mint, and "bitterscotch" flavors. In 10s.
Rx	**Cafcit** (Mead Johnson)	**Oral solution:** 20 mg/mL (caffeine citrate)[1]	Preservative free. In 3 mL vials.
		Injection: 20 mg/mL (caffeine citrate)[1]	Preservative free. In 3 mL vials.
Rx	**Caffeine and Sodium Benzoate** (Bedford)	**Injection:** 250 mg/mL (121 mg caffeine, 129 mg sodium benzoate)	In 2 mL single-use vials.
Rx	**Caffeine and Sodium Benzoate** (American Regent)	**Injection:** 250 mg/mL (125 mg caffeine, 125 mg sodium benzoate)	In 2 mL single-dose vials.

[1] 2 mg of caffeine citrate is equivalent to 1 mg caffeine base.

[2] Xanodyne Pharmacal, Inc., 7310 Turfway Rd., Suite 490, Florence, KY 41042; 877-XA-NODYNE, fax 859-371-6391; http://www.xanodyne.com.

Indications

►*Fatigue/drowsiness (oral):* As an aid in staying awake and restoring mental alertness.

►*Analgesia (oral):* As an adjuvant in analgesic formulations.

►*Apnea of prematurity (caffeine citrate [oral and injectable]):* For the short-term treatment of apnea of prematurity in infants between 28 and < 33 weeks gestational age.

►*Respiratory depression (caffeine and sodium benzoate injectable):* In conjunction with supportive measures to treat respiratory depression associated with overdosage with CNS depressants (eg, narcotic analgesics, alcohol). However, because of questionable benefit and transient action, most authorities believe caffeine and other analeptics should not be used in these conditions and recommend other supportive therapy.

►*Unlabeled uses:*

Atopic dermatitis – Topical treatment with 30% caffeine in a hydrophilic base or in a hydrocortisone cream produces improvement in pruritus, erythema, scaling, lichenification, oozing, and dermatitis. This may be related to caffeine's property of liberating water from epidermal and SC tissues, similar to urea.

Obesity – In combination with ephedrine, caffeine causes a modest, but significant, weight loss in obese individuals when energy intake is restricted over an extended period. This reflects a synergistic interaction as it is not seen with either agent alone.

Headache – Caffeine enhances the effect of ergotamine and may have direct actions on the extracranial vasculature or on trigeminal afferents in the treatment of migraine. Caffeine has been shown to effectively relieve headache resulting from lumbar puncture, and appears to produce an intrinsic analgesic effect in headaches of nonvascular origin.

Alcohol intoxication – For the treatment of excited or comatose alcoholic patients.

Postprandial hypotension – Postprandial decreases in blood pressure occur in elderly individuals, particularly after meals high in carbohydrates. Caffeine 250 mg, attenuated postprandial hypotension in a small number of patients.

Analeptic use of caffeine is strongly discouraged by most clinicians.

Administration and Dosage

►*Fatigue/drowsiness (oral):* 100 to 200 mg by mouth every 3 to 4 hours, as needed. Not recommended for children < 12 years of age.

►*Apnea of prematurity (caffeine citrate [oral and injectable]):* Prior to initiation of caffeine citrate, baseline serum levels of caffeine should be measured in infants previously treated with theophylline, since preterm infants metabolize theophylline to caffeine. Likewise, measure baseline serum levels of caffeine in infants born to mothers who consumed caffeine prior to delivery, since caffeine readily crosses the placenta.

The recommended loading dose and maintenance doses are as follows:

Caffeine Citrate Loading and Maintance Doses				
	Dose of caffeine citrate volume	Dose of caffeine citrate mg/kg	Route	Frequency
Loading dose	1 mL/kg	20 mg/kg	IV[1] (over 30 min)	1 time
Maintenance dose	0.25 mL/kg	5 mg/kg	IV[1] (over 10 min) or orally	Every 24 hrs[2]

[1] Using a syringe infusion pump.
[2] Beginning 24 hours after the loading dose.

Note that the dose of caffeine base is one-half the dose when expressed as caffeine citrate (eg, 20 mg of caffeine citrate is equivalent to 10 mg of caffeine base).

Serum concentrations of caffeine may need to be monitored periodically throughout treatment to avoid toxicity. Serious toxicity has been associated with serum levels > 50 mg/L.

►*Respiratory depression (caffeine and sodium benzoate injectable):* Administer 500 mg (≈ 250 mg anhydrous caffeine) IM or slow IV injection in emergency respiratory failure or a maximum single dose of 1 g (≈ 500 mg anhydrous caffeine). The usual and maximum safe dose is 500 mg; do not exceed 2.5 g/24 hours.

CAFFEINE

➤*Storage / Stability:*

Citrated caffeine parenteral solution –

Drug compatibility: Caffeine citrate injection, 20 mg/mL is chemically stable for 24 hours at room temperature when combined with the following test products: 5% Dextrose Injection; 50% Dextrose Injection; *Intralipid* 20% IV fat emulsion; *Aminosyn* 8.5% Crystalline Amino Acid Solution; Dopamine HCl Injection 40 mg/mL diluted to 0.6 mg/mL with 5% Dextrose Injection; 10% Calcium Gluconate Injection (0.465 mE q/Ca^{+2}/mL); heparin sodium injection 1000 units/mL diluted to 1 unit/mL with 5% Dextrose Injection; fentanyl citrate injection 50 mcg/mL diluted to 10 mcg/mL with 5% Dextrose Injection.

Actions

➤*Pharmacology:* Caffeine, a methylxanthine, exerts its pharmacological effects by increasing calcium permeability in sarcoplasmic reticulum, inhibiting phosphodiesterase promoting accumulation of cyclic AMP, and is a competitive, nonselective antagonist at adenosine A$_1$ and A$_{2A}$ receptors. Evidence suggests that adenosine receptor antagonism is the most important factor responsible for most pharmacological effects of methylxanthines in doses that are administered therapeutically or consumed in xanthine-containing beverages.

Caffeine is a potent stimulant of the CNS. Its cortical effects are milder and of shorter duration than those of the amphetamines. In slightly larger doses it stimulates medullary, vagal, vasomotor, and respiratory centers, promoting bradycardia, vasoconstriction and increased respiratory rate. Caffeine produces a positive inotropic effect on the myocardium and a positive chronotropic effect at the sinoatrial node, causing transient increases in heart rate, force of contraction, cardiac output, and heart work. In doses > 250 mg, the centrally mediated vagal effects of caffeine may be masked by increased sinus rates, tachycardia, extrasystoles, or other major ventricular arrhythmias. Caffeine constricts cerebral vasculature, but directly dilates peripheral blood vessels, decreasing peripheral vascular resistance. The latter effect (and possibly vagal cardiac stimulation) on blood pressure is offset by increased cardiac output (and possibly stimulation of the medullary vasomotor area). The overall effect of caffeine on heart rate and blood pressure depends on whether CNS or peripheral effects predominate.

Caffeine stimulates voluntary skeletal muscle, increasing the force of contraction and decreasing muscular fatigue. It also stimulates gastric acid secretion from parietal cells. Caffeine increases renal blood flow and glomerular filtration rate and decreases proximal tubular reabsorption of sodium and water, resulting in mild diuresis. It also stimulates glycogenolysis and lipolysis.

Long-term administration of caffeine results in an upregulation of A$_1$ receptors in the brain, as well as an enhanced sensitivity to adenosine analogs that have an affinity for A$_1$ receptors. Tolerance to the cardiovascular, CNS, and diuretic effects may develop. Differences in effects of caffeine on various organ systems may be observed in nonusers of caffeine vs habitual consumers. Acute ingestion of caffeine produces increases in systolic blood pressure, plasma catecholamines, plasma renin activity, and heart rate; chronic ingestion has little or no effect on these hemodynamic variables.

The amount of caffeine derived from dietary sources is given in the following table:

Caffeine Content from Various Sources		
Source	Serving size	Caffeine (mg)
Coffee:[1]		
Espresso	2 oz	120
Regular, brewed	5 to 8 oz	40 to 180
Instant	5 to 8 oz	30 to 120
Decaffeinated	5 to 8 oz	1 to 5
Tea:[1]		
Brewed	5 to 8 oz	20 to 110
Instant/Bags	5 to 8 oz	20 to 50
Soft drinks:		
Mountain Dew	12 oz	55
Coke	12 oz	47
Pepsi	12 oz	37
Slice	12 oz	11
Chocolate:		
Baking chocolate	1 oz	25 to 58
Milk chocolate	1 oz	1 to 15
Medications, otc:		
Analgesics	1 tablet	32 to 65
Cold combinations	1 tablet	30 to 65
Stimulants	1 tablet	75 to 200
Other:		
Guarana	1 g	25 to 50

[1] Depending on strength of brew and product.

➤*Pharmacokinetics:*

Absorption / Distribution – Caffeine is well absorbed orally (99%) and is widely distributed throughout the body. It is also absorbed through the skin. Absorption following rectal administration may be slow and erratic. Peak plasma levels of 5 to 25 mcg/mL are achieved 15 to 120 minutes after 250 mg. Protein binding is ≈ 17%. Caffeine readily crosses the blood-brain barrier and placenta; low concentrations are also present in breast milk. Therapeutic plasma concentrations are ≈ 6 to 13 mcg/mL; those > 20 mcg/mL may produce adverse effects. The lethal concentration is > 100 mcg/mL.

Metabolism / Excretion – Caffeine is metabolized in the liver and is excreted in the urine as methyluric acid, methylxanthine, and other metabolites with only ≈ 1% excreted unchanged. In the adult, plasma half-life ranges from 3 to 7 hours. Half-life is increased with smoking and is prolonged in pregnancy (≤ 18 hours), cirrhosis, and with concomitant use of some drugs (see Drug Interactions).

Neonates have a greatly reduced capacity to metabolize caffeine, and it is largely excreted unchanged in the urine until hepatic metabolism becomes significantly developed, usually at about 6 months of age. Elimination half-lives are ≈ 3 to 7 hours in adults but may be in excess of 100 hours in neonates. Preterm infants at birth exhibit half-lives of 65 to 103 hours; term infants at birth, 82 hours; 3- to 4-month-old infants, 14.4 hours; and 5- to 6-month-old infants, 2.6 hours. In newborns, plasma and cerebrospinal fluid levels are nearly identical.

Contraindications

Caffeine and sodium benzoate solution in neonates (see Warnings); hypersensitivity to any components.

Warnings

➤*Renal / Hepatic function impairment:* Administer caffeine citrate with caution in infants with impaired renal or hepatic function.

➤*Pregnancy: Category C.* Safety for use in pregnancy has not been established. Caffeine crosses the placenta and achieves fetal blood and tissue levels similar to maternal concentrations. Excessive caffeine intake (> 600 mg/day) has been weakly associated with increased fetal loss, low birth weight, premature deliveries, an increase in the incidence of fetal breathing activity and a significant fall in baseline fetal heart rate. Three cases of fetal arrhythmia have also been reported. However, when used in moderation, there is no association with these effects or congenital malformations. Caffeine causes birth defects in animals when administered at doses toxic to the mother.

➤*Lactation:* Caffeine appears in the breast milk of nursing mothers. Milk:plasma ratios of 0.5 and 0.76 have been reported. Approximately 1.3 to 3.1 mg of caffeine would be ingested by a nursing infant whose mother had 35 to 336 mg of oral caffeine.

➤*Children:* Serious metabolic disturbances in premature neonates given IV fluids with benzyl alcohol as a preservative have been attributed to the accumulation of the benzoic-acid metabolite of the benzyl alcohol. This risk led to the recommendation that caffeine and sodium benzoate injection should not be used in neonates. Benzoates can also displace bound bilirubin from albumin, putting neonates at risk of kernicterus.

Precautions

➤*Necrotizing enterocolitis:* Carefully monitor patients being treated with caffeine citrate for the development of necrotizing enterocolitis due to reports in the published literature that have raised a question regarding the possible association between the use of methylxanthines and development of necrotizing enterocolitis, although a causal relationship between methylxanthine use and necrotizing enterocolitis has not been established.

➤*Depression:* Too vigorous treatment with parenteral caffeine can produce further depression in the already depressed patient; therefore, do not exceed 1 g as a single dose of caffeine and sodium benzoate.

➤*GI effects:* Theophylline derivatives tend to relax the lower esophageal sphincter and increase gastric acid secretion. Caffeine-containing products may exacerbate duodenal ulcers. Caffeine may also considerably aggravate diarrhea in patients with irritable colon.

➤*Seizure disorder:* Caffeine is a CNS stimulant and in cases of caffeine overdose, seizures have been reported. Use caffeine citrate with caution in infants with seizure disorders.

➤*Cardiovascular disease:* Although no cases of cardiac toxicity were reported in the placebo-controlled trial, caffeine has been shown to increase heart rate, left ventricular output, and stroke volume in published studies. Therefore, use caffeine citrate with caution in infants with cardiovascular disease.

➤*Metabolic effects:* Caffeine stimulates glycogenolysis and lipolysis which increases free fatty acids and produces hyperglycemia. Caffeine also causes a release of catecholamines and increased metabolic activity.

➤*Bone mineral density:* Lifetime caffeinated coffee intake equivalent to 2 cups/day is associated with decreased bone density in older women (mean age, 72.7 years) who do not drink milk on a daily basis. In elderly women whose calcium balance was impaired (< 800 mg of calcium/day), high caffeine intake predisposed them to bone loss of the

CAFFEINE

hip. However, caffeine or coffee-induced calcium loss and bone loss are insignificant in the face of adequate calcium intake.

➤*Withdrawal:* Symptoms occur within 12 to 24 hours following cessation of chronic caffeine ingestion (as little as 100 mg of caffeine/day) and may endure up to 7 days. The most common symptom is headache, but other frequently reported reactions include fatigue, depression, anxiety, and insomnia.

Drug Interactions

Caffeine Drug Interactions			
Precipitant drug	Object drug*		Description
Allopurinol	Caffeine	↔	Allopurinol inhibits the conversion of caffeine metabolite methylxanthine to methyluric acid.
Cimetidine Contraceptives, oral Disulfiram Fluoroquinolones	Caffeine	↑	Caffeine hepatic metabolism may be impaired, resulting in decreased clearance and increased half-life. Consider avoiding caffeine consumption if excessive CNS or cardiovascular effects occur.
Mexiletine	Caffeine	↑	Concomitant administration reduced the elimination of caffeine by 30% to 50%.
Phenytoin	Caffeine	↓	Phenytoin decreases the half-life of caffeine and increases clearance. Concomitant administration results in lower caffeine levels.
Smoking	Caffeine	↓	Smoking induces hepatic metabolism and increases caffeine clearance.
Caffeine	Aspirin	↑	Caffeine appears to increase the GI absorption of aspirin, but does not appear to affect salicylate elimination.
Caffeine	Clozapine	↑	Caffeine may inhibit clozapine metabolism (P450 1A2), resulting in elevation of clozapine levels; possible increase in side effects may occur.
Caffeine	Lithium	↓	Caffeine may reduce serum lithium concentrations and may enhance renal clearance. Monitoring of serum lithium concentrations and adjustments in lithium dose may be necessary.
Caffeine	Theophylline	↑	Ingestion of caffeine (120 to 630 mg daily) can reduce theophylline clearance 23% and increase the elimination half-life. Serum theophylline levels may be increased. Advise patients to avoid drastic changes in daily caffeine intake.

* ↑ = Object drug increased. ↓ = Object drug decreased. ↔ = Undetermined clinical effect.

➤*Drug/Lab test interactions:* Caffeine produces false-positive elevations of serum urate as measured by the Bittner method. Caffeine also produces slight increases in urine levels of vanillylmandelic acid (VMA), catecholamines, and 5-hydroxyindoleacetic acid. Because high urine levels of VMA or catecholamines may result in false-positive diagnosis of pheochromocytoma or neuroblastoma, avoid caffeine intake during tests for these disorders.

➤*Drug/Food interactions:* Coffee and tea consumed with a meal or 1 hour after a meal significantly inhibits the absorption of dietary iron. Clinical significance has not been determined.

Adverse Reactions

➤*Cardiovascular:* Tachycardia; extrasystoles; palpitations; other cardiac arrhythmias.

➤*CNS:* Insomnia; restlessness; excitement; nervousness; tinnitus; scintillating scotoma; muscular tremor; headache; lightheadedness.

Large doses of caffeine also may produce agitation, a condition resembling anxiety neurosis, hyperesthesia, and muscle twitches.

➤*GI:* Nausea; vomiting; diarrhea; stomach pain.

➤*Miscellaneous:* Hypersensitivity (eg, dermatitis, rhinitis, bronchial asthma); urticaria; hyperglycemia; diuresis.

➤*Caffeine citrate:*

Dermatologic – Rash (8.7%); dry skin, skin breakdown (2.2%).

GI – Necrotizing enterocolitis (4.3%); gastritis, GI hemorrhage (2.2%).

Metabolic/Nutritional – Acidosis, healing abnormal (2.2%).

Respiratory – Dyspnea, lung edema (2.2%).

Miscellaneous – Feeding intolerance (8.7%); sepsis (4.3%); accidental injury, hemorrhage, cerebral hemorrhage, retinopathy of prematurity, kidney failure, disseminated intravascular coagulation (2.2%).

Overdosage

➤*Symptoms:* Ingestion of 15 to 30 mg/kg results in significant toxicity (vomiting, myoclonus, myocardial irritability, hematemesis). Oral doses of 5 to 50 g (mean, 10 g) have produced fatalities; the lethal dose is estimated to be 100 to 200 mg/kg. In adults, IV doses of 57 mg/kg have been fatal. Toxicity correlates to serum caffeine levels. Several cups of coffee may produce caffeine concentrations of 5 to 10 mcg/mL. Symptoms of agitation and myoclonus develop at levels of 5 to 10 mcg/mL; cardiac arrhythmias and seizures may develop at 50 to 100 mcg/mL. Caffeine concentrations as low as 80 mcg/mL up to 1560 mcg/mL have been associated with death, although patients with concentrations up to 200 mcg/mL have survived. Fatalities have also been observed after the use of coffee enemas as a homeopathic therapy. Other symptoms of caffeine overdose that may develop include opisthotonus, decerebrate posturing, generalized muscular hypertonicity, rhabdomyolysis with resultant renal failure, pulmonary edema, hyperglycemia, hypokalemia, leukocytosis, ketosis, and metabolic acidosis.

Infants and children – In one 5-year-old patient, death occurred following oral ingestion of ≈ 3 g. Signs and symptoms reported in the literature after caffeine overdose in preterm infants include fever, tachypnea, jitteriness, fine tremor of the extremities, hypertonia, opisthotonos, tonic-clonic movements, nonpurposeful jaw and lip movements, vomiting, hyperglycemia, elevated blood urea nitrogen, and elevated total leukocyte concentration. Seizures have also been reported. One case of caffeine overdose complicated by development of intraventricular hemorrhage and long-term neurological sequalae has been reported. No deaths associated with caffeine overdose have been reported in preterm infants.

➤*Treatment:* Primarily symptomatic and supportive. GI decontamination should include gastric lavage followed by activated charcoal. Control seizures with IV diazepam or phenobarbital. Caffeine levels have been shown to decrease after exchange transfusions. Even though not clearly established, indications for hemodialysis should include a caffeine serum concentration > 100 mcg/mL and life-threatening seizures or cardiac arrhythmias, regardless of serum concentration.

Patient Information

Do not exceed recommended dosage.

Advise pregnant women to limit their intake of caffeine and caffeine-containing beverages to a minimum.

Discontinue use if increased or abnormal heart rate, dizziness, or palpitations occur.

If fatigue or drowsiness persists or recurs, consult physician.

Not intended for use as a substitute for normal sleep.

➤*Caffeine citrate:* Discard any unused portion of the medication.

It is important that the dose be measured accurately (ie, with a 1 cc or other appropriate syringe).

Consult a physician if the baby continues to have apnea events; do not increase the dose without medical consultation.

Consult a physician if the baby begins to demonstrate signs of GI intolerance, such as abdominal distention, vomiting, or bloody stools or seems lethargic.

Analeptics

DOXAPRAM HCl

Rx	Doxapram HCl (Bedford)	Injection: 20 mg/mL	0.9% benzyl alcohol. In 20 mL multiple-dose vials.
Rx	Dopram (ESI Lederle Generics)		0.9% benzyl alcohol. In 20 mL multiple-dose vials.

Indications

➤*Postanesthesia:* When the possibility of airway obstruction or hypoxia have been eliminated, doxapram may be used to stimulate respiration in patients with drug-induced postanesthesia respiratory depression or apnea other than that due to muscle relaxants.

With simultaneous administration of oxygen to pharmacologically stimulate deep breathing in the "stir-up" regimen in the postoperative patient.

➤*Drug-induced CNS depression:* To stimulate respiration, hasten arousal, and encourage return of laryngopharyngeal reflexes in patients with mild-to-moderate respiratory and CNS depression due to overdosage. Exercise care to prevent vomiting and aspiration.

Controlled ventilation and standard supportive care for respiratory depression due to CNS overdose is safer, more reliable, and more effective than doxapram.

➤*Chronic pulmonary disease associated with acute hypercapnia:* As a temporary measure in hospitalized patients with acute respiratory insufficiency superimposed on chronic obstructive pulmonary disease (COPD). Use for a short period of time ($\approx$ 2 hours) to prevent elevation of arterial CO_2 tension during the administration of oxygen. Do not use in conjunction with mechanical ventilation.

➤*Unlabeled uses:*

Neonatal apnea (apnea of prematurity) – Doxapram has been used when methylxanthines have failed. Begin at 0.1 to 0.2 mg/kg/hour and increase up to 1.5 mg/kg/hr as needed.

Obstructive sleep apnea – Doxapram was found to decrease the length of sleep apneas.

Laryngospasm secondary to postoperative tracheal extubation – Doxapram has occasionally been reported to relieve laryngospasm.

Administration and Dosage

➤*Postanesthetic use (IV):* By IV injection (see table below); slow administration of the drug and careful observation of the patient during administration and for some time subsequently are advisable.

Doxapram Dosage for Postanesthetic Use (IV)						
	Recommended dosage		Maximum dose per single injection		Maximum total dose	
IV administration	mg/kg	mg/lb	mg/kg	mg/lb	mg/kg	mg/lb
Single injection	0.5 to 1	0.25 to 0.5	1.5	0.7	1.5	0.7
Repeat injections (5 min intervals)	0.5 to 1	0.25 to 0.5	1.5	0.7	2	1
Infusion	0.5 to 1	0.25 to 0.5	-	-	4	2

By infusion – Prepare the solution by adding 250 mg of doxapram (12.5 mL) to 250 mL of dextrose or saline solution. Initiate infusion at a rate of $\approx$ 5 mg/min until a satisfactory respiratory response is observed, and maintained at a rate of 1 to 3 mg/min. Adjust the rate of infusion to sustain the desired level of respiratory stimulation with a minimum of side effects. The recommended total dosage by infusion is 4 mg/kg (2 mg/lb), or $\approx$ 300 mg for the average adult.

➤*Management of drug-induced CNS depression:*

Doxapram Dosage for Drug-induced CNS Depression				
	Method 1 Priming dose single/ repeat IV injection		Method 2 Rate of intermittent IV infusion	
Level of depression	mg/kg	mg/lb	mg/kg/hr	mg/lb/hr
Mild[1]	1	0.5	1 to 2	0.5 to 1
Moderate[2]	2	1	2 to 3	1 to 1.5

[1] Class 0: Asleep, but can be aroused and can answer questions. Class 1: Comatose, will withdraw from painful stimuli, reflexes intact.

[2] Class 2: Comatose, will not withdraw from painful stimuli, reflexes intact. Class 3: Comatose, reflexes absent, no depression of circulation or respiration.

Using single or repeat single IV injections (method 1) – Give priming IV dose of 2 mg/kg (1 mg/lb) body weight and repeat in 5 minutes. Repeat every 1 to 2 hours until patient awakens. Watch for relapse into unconsciousness or development of respiratory depression, because doxapram does not affect the metabolism of CNS depressant drugs.

If relapse occurs, resume 1 to 2 hourly injections until arousal is sustained, or total maximum daily dose (3 g) is given. Allow patient to sleep until 24 hours has elapsed from first injection, using assisted or automatic respiration if necessary.

Repeat procedure the following day until patient breathes spontaneously and sustains desired level of consciousness, or until maximum dosage (3 g) is given. Administer repetitive doses only to patients who have shown response to the initial dose. Failure to respond appropri-

ately indicates the need for neurologic evaluation for a possible CNS source of sustained coma.

Intermittent IV infusion (method 2) – Give priming dose of 2 mg/kg (1 mg/lb) body weight. If patient awakens, watch for relapse; if no response, continue general supportive treatment for 1 to 2 hours and repeat doxapram. If some respiratory stimulation occurs, prepare IV infusion of 250 mg of doxapram (12.5 mL) in 250 mL of saline or dextrose solution. Deliver at a rate of 1 to 3 mg/min according to size of patient and depth of coma. Discontinue use at end of 2 hours or if patient begins to awaken.

Continue supportive treatment for 0.5 to 2 hours and repeat the steps following the priming dose as above. Do not exceed 3 g/day.

➤*Chronic obstructive pulmonary disease associated with acute hypercapnia:* Mix 400 mg in 180 mL of dextrose or Normal Saline solution (concentration of 2 mg/mL). Start infusion at 1 to 2 mg/min (0.5 to 1 mL/min); if indicated, increase to maximum of 3 mg/min. Determine arterial blood gases prior to administration and at least every 30 minutes during the 2 hours of infusion to ensure against development of CO_2 retention and acidosis. Altering oxygen concentration or flow rate may necessitate adjustment in doxapram infusion rate.

Predictable blood gas patterns are more readily established with continuous infusion. If the blood gases deteriorate, discontinue infusion. Additional infusions beyond the maximum 2 hour administration period are not recommended.

Preparation of solution – Doxapram is compatible with 5% and 10% Dextrose in Water or Normal Saline.

  Admixture incompatibility: Admixture of doxapram with alkaline solutions such as 2.5% thiopental sodium, bicarbonate, or aminophylline will result in precipitation or gas formation.

Actions

➤*Pharmacology:* Doxapram produces respiratory stimulation mediated through the peripheral carotid chemoreceptors. The respiratory stimulant action is manifested by an increase in tidal volume associated with a slight increase in respiratory rate. As the dosage is increased, the central respiratory centers in the medulla are stimulated with progressive stimulation of other parts of the brain and spinal cord.

A pressor response due to improved cardiac output rather than peripheral vasoconstriction may occur. If there is no cardiac impairment, the pressor effect is greater in hypovolemic than in normovolemic states. Following administration, an increased release of catecholamines has occurred.

Although opiate-induced respiratory depression is antagonized by doxapram, the analgesic effect is not affected.

➤*Pharmacokinetics:* The onset of respiratory stimulation following the recommended single IV injection usually occurs in 20 to 40 seconds, with peak effect at 1 to 2 minutes. The duration of effect varies from 5 to 12 minutes. Doxapram is extensively metabolized; metabolites and a small amount of unchanged drug are excreted in the urine. The plasma half-life ranges from 2.4 to 4.1 hours.

Contraindications

Hypersensitivity to the drug; newborns (product contains benzyl alcohol); epilepsy or other convulsive states; mechanical disorders of ventilation such as mechanical obstruction, muscle paresis, flail chest, pneumothorax, acute bronchial asthma, pulmonary fibrosis, or other conditions resulting in restriction of chest wall, muscles of respiration or alveolar expansion; head injury; cerebrovascular accident; significant cardiovascular impairment; severe hypertension.

Warnings

➤*Postanesthetic use:* Exercise the same consideration to preexisting disease states as in non-anesthetized individuals. Doxapram is neither an antagonist to muscle relaxant drugs nor a specific narcotic antagonist. Ensure adequacy of airway and oxygenation prior to use. Administer carefully and only under careful supervision to patients with hypermetabolic states such as hyperthyroidism or pheochromocytoma.

Because narcosis may recur after stimulation with doxapram, maintain close observation until patient has been fully alert for 30 minutes to 1 hour.

➤*Drug-induced CNS and respiratory depression:* Doxapram alone may not stimulate adequate spontaneous breathing or provide sufficient arousal in patients who are severely depressed either due to respiratory failure or to CNS depressant drugs. Use as an adjunct to established supportive measures and resuscitative techniques.

➤*COPD:* In an attempt to lower pCO_2, do not increase rate of infusion in severely ill patients because of the associated increased work in breathing. Do not use in conjunction with mechanical ventilation.

In some patients, arrhythmias in acute respiratory failure secondary to COPD are probably the result of hypoxia. Use with caution in these patients.

DOXAPRAM HCl

Obtain arterial blood gases prior to the initiation of doxapram infusion and oxygen administration, then at least every ½ hour. Doxapram administration does not diminish the need for careful patient monitoring or the need for supplemental oxygen in acute respiratory failure. Discontinue use if the arterial blood gases deteriorate and initiate mechanical ventilation.

➤*Pregnancy: Category B.* There are no adequate and well-controlled studies in pregnant women. Use during pregnancy only when clearly needed.

➤*Lactation:* It is not known whether this drug is excreted in breast milk. Exercise caution when administering to a nursing mother.

➤*Children:* Safety and efficacy for use in children < 12 years of age have not been established. The use of benzyl alcohol in newborns has been associated with metabolic, CNS, respiratory, circulatory, and renal dysfunction; however, doxapram has been used to treat apnea of prematurity (see Unlabeled Uses).

Precautions

➤*Administration:* Avoid vascular extravasation or use of a single injection site over an extended period; thrombophlebitis or local skin irritation may occur. Rapid infusion may result in hemolysis.

IV short-acting barbiturates, oxygen, and resuscitative equipment should be readily available to manage overdosage manifested by excessive CNS stimulation. Slow administration and careful observation of the patient during and following administration are advisable to ensure that the protective reflexes have been restored and to prevent possible posthyperventilation hypoventilation. Administer cautiously to patients receiving sympathomimetics or MAOIs, since an additive pressor effect may occur. An adequate airway is essential. Employ recommended dosages; do not exceed maximum total dosages. Use the minimum effective dosage to avoid side effects.

➤*Blood pressure:* Blood pressure increases are generally modest, but significant increases have occurred. Not recommended for use in severe hypertension. If sudden hypotension or dyspnea develop, discontinue use. Monitor blood pressure and deep tendon reflexes to prevent overdosage.

➤*Lowered pCO$_2$:* Lowered pCO$_2$ induced by hyperventilation produces cerebral vasoconstriction and slowing of the cerebral circulation.

➤*Benzyl alcohol:* Doxapram contains benzyl alcohol, which has been associated with a fatal "gasping syndrome" in premature infants.

Drug Interactions

Doxapram Drug Interactions			
Precipitant drug	Object drug*		Description
Doxapram	Anesthetics	↑	Because an increase in epinephrine release has been noted with doxapram, delay initiation of therapy for at least 10 minutes following discontinuance of anesthetics known to sensitize the myocardium to catecholamines.

Doxapram Drug Interactions			
Precipitant drug	Object drug*		Description
Doxapram	MAOIs	↑	Administer cautiously to patients receiving these drugs because an additive pressor effect may occur.
Doxapram	Muscle relaxants	↓	Doxapram may temporarily mask residual effects of muscle relaxants.
Doxapram	Sympathomimetics	↑	Administer cautiously to patients receiving these drugs because an additive pressor effect may occur.

* ↑ = Object drug increased. ↓ = Object drug decreased.

Adverse Reactions

➤*Cardiovascular:* Phlebitis; variations in heart rate; lowered T-waves; arrhythmias; chest pain; tightness in chest. A mild-to-moderate increase in blood pressure is commonly noted and may be of concern in patients with severe cardiovascular diseases (see Precautions).

➤*GI:* Nausea; vomiting; diarrhea; desire to defecate.

➤*GU:* Urinary retention; stimulation of urinary bladder with spontaneous voiding; elevation of BUN; albuminuria.

➤*Hematologic:* A decrease in hemoglobin, hematocrit, or red blood cell count has occurred in postoperative patients. In the presence of preexisting leukopenia, a further decrease in WBC has occurred following anesthesia and treatment with doxapram.

➤*Respiratory:* Cough; dyspnea; tachypnea; laryngospasm; bronchospasm; hiccoughs; rebound hypoventilation.

➤*Miscellaneous:*
Central and autonomic nervous systems – Headache; dizziness; apprehension; disorientation; pupillary dilatation; hyperactivity; convulsions; bilateral Babinski; involuntary movements; muscle spasticity; increased deep tendon reflexes; clonus; pyrexia; flushing; sweating; pruritus and paresthesia such as a feeling of warmth, burning or hot sensation, especially in the area of the genitalia and perineum.

Overdosage

➤*Symptoms:* Excessive pressor effect, tachycardia, skeletal muscle hyperactivity, and enhanced deep tendon reflexes may be early signs of overdosage. Evaluate blood pressure, pulse rate, and deep tendon reflexes periodically and adjust dosage or infusion rate accordingly.

➤*Treatment:* There is no specific antidote. Management should be symptomatic. Refer to General Management of Acute Overdosage. Convulsive seizures are unlikely at recommended dosages, but short-acting IV barbiturates, oxygen, and resuscitative equipment should be available. There is no evidence that doxapram is dialyzable. Due to the half-life of doxapram, it is unlikely that dialysis would be appropriate treatment for overdosage.

MODAFINIL

c-iv	**Provigil** (Cephalon)	**Tablets:** 100 mg		Lactose, talc. (PROVIGIL 100 MG). White, capsule-shape. In 100s.
		200 mg		Lactose, talc. (PROVIGIL 200 MG). White, scored, capsule-shape. In 100s.

Indications

➤*Narcolepsy:* To improve wakefulness in patients with excessive daytime sleepiness associated with narcolepsy.

Administration and Dosage

➤*Approved by the FDA:* December 24, 1998.

The dose of modafinil is 200 mg/day, given as a single dose in the morning. Doses of 400 mg/day, given as a single dose, have been well tolerated, but there is no consistent evidence that this dose confers additional benefit.

➤*Hepatic function impairment:* In patients with severe hepatic impairment, reduce the modafinil dose to 50% of that recommended for patients with normal hepatic function.

➤*Renal function impairment:* There is inadequate information to determine safety and efficacy of dosing in patients with severe renal impairment.

➤*Elderly:* In elderly patients, elimination of modafinil and its metabolites may be reduced as a consequence of aging. Therefore, give consideration to the use of lower doses in this population.

Actions

➤*Pharmacology:* Modafinil is a wakefulness-promoting agent for oral administration. The precise mechanism(s) through which modafinil promotes wakefulness is unknown. Modafinil has wake-promoting actions like sympathomimetic agents including amphetamine and methylphenidate, although the pharmacologic profile is not identical to that of sympathomimetic amines.

At pharmacologically relevant concentrations, modafinil does not bind to most potentially relevant receptors for sleep/wake regulation, including those for norepinephrine, serotonin, dopamine, GABA, adenosine, histamine-3, melatonin, or benzodiazepines. Modafinil also does not inhibit the activities of MAO-B or phosphodiesterases II-V.

Modafinil is not a direct- or indirect-acting dopamine receptor agonist. In vitro, modafinil binds to the dopamine reuptake site and causes an increase in extracellular dopamine, but no increase in dopamine release. In a preclinical model, the wakefulness induced by amphetamine, but not modafinil, is antagonized by the dopamine receptor antagonist haloperidol.

Modafinil does not appear to be a direct or indirect α_1-adrenergic agonist. Although modafinil-induced wakefulness can be attenuated by the α_1-adrenergic receptor antagonist prazosin, in assay systems known to be responsive to α-adrenergic agonists, modafinil has no activity. Modafinil does not display sympathomimetic activity in the rat vas deferens preparations. Unlike sympathomimetic agents, modafinil does not reduce cataplexy in narcoleptic canines and has minimal effects on cardiovascular and hemodynamic parameters.

In the cat, equal wakefulness-promoting doses of methylphenidate and amphetamine increased neuronal activation throughout the brain. Modafinil at an equivalent wakefulness-promoting dose selectively and prominently increased neuronal activation in more discrete regions of the brain. The relationship of this finding in cats to the effects of modafinil in humans is unknown.

In addition to its wakefulness-promoting effects and increased locomotor activity in animals, modafinil produces psychoactive and euphoric effects, alterations in mood, perception, and thinking, and feelings typi-

MODAFINIL

cal of other CNS stimulants in humans. Modafinil is reinforcing, as evidenced by its self-administration in monkeys previously trained to self-administer cocaine; modafinil was also partially discriminated as stimulant-like.

➤*Pharmacokinetics:*

Absorption/Distribution – Absorption is rapid, with peak plasma concentrations occurring at 2 to 4 hours. The bioavailability of modafinil is approximately equal to that of an aqueous suspension. Food has no effect on overall bioavailability; however, absorption may be delayed by ≈ 1 hour if taken with food.

Modafinil is well distributed in body tissue with an apparent volume of distribution (≈ 0.9 L/kg) larger than the volume of total body water (0.6 L/kg). In plasma, modafinil is moderately bound to plasma protein (≈ 60%, mainly to albumin).

Metabolism/Excretion – The major route of elimination (≈ 90%) is metabolism, primarily by the liver, with subsequent renal elimination of the metabolites. Urine alkalinization has no effect on the elimination of modafinil. Metabolism occurs through hydrolytic deamidation, S-oxidation, aromatic ring hydroxylation, and glucuronide conjugation. Less than 10% of an administered dose is excreted as the parent compound; 81% was recovered in 11 days post-dose, predominantly in the urine (80% vs 1% in the feces). The largest fraction of the drug in urine was modafinil acid, but ≥ 6 other metabolites were present in lower concentrations. Only 2 metabolites reach appreciable concentrations in plasma, modafinil acid and modafinil sulfone. These metabolites did not appear to contribute to the CNS-activating properties of modafinil. The effective elimination half-life of modafinil after multiple doses is ≈ 15 hours.

Modafinil shows a possible induction effect on its own metabolism after chronic administration of doses ≥ 400 mg/day. Induction of hepatic metabolizing enzymes, most importantly cytochrome P450 CYP3A4, has also been observed in vitro after incubation of primary cultures of human hepatocytes with modafinil.

Stereochemistry – Modafinil is a racemic compound whose enantiomers have different pharmacokinetics (eg, the half-life of the I-isomer is ≈ 3 times that of the d-isomer). The enantiomers do not interconvert. At steady state, total exposure to the I-isomer is ≈ 3 times that for the d-isomer. The trough concentration of circulating modafinil after once-daily dosing consists of 90% of the I-isomer and 10% of the d-isomer. The enantiomers of modafinil exhibit linear kinetics upon multiple dosing of 200 to 600 mg/day once daily in healthy volunteers. Apparent steady states of total modafinil and I-(-)-modafinil are reached after 2 to 4 days of dosing.

Special populations –

Age: A slight decrease (≈ 20%) in oral clearance of modafinil was observed in a single-dose study at 200 mg in 12 subjects with a mean age of 63 years (range, 53 to 72 years), but the change was considered unlikely to be clinically significant. In a multiple-dose study (300 mg/day) in 12 patients with a mean age of 82 years (range, 67 to 87 years), the mean levels of modafinil in plasma were ≈ 2 times those historically obtained in matched younger subjects. Because of potential effects from the multiple concomitant medications with which most of the patients were being treated, the apparent difference in modafinil pharmacokinetics may not be solely attributable to the effects of aging. However, the results suggest that the clearance of modafinil may be reduced in the elderly.

Renal function impairment: In a single-dose 200 mg modafinil study, severe chronic renal failure (creatinine clearance ≤ 20 ml/min) did not significantly influence the pharmacokinetics of modafinil, but exposure to modafinil acid (an inactive metabolite) was increased 9-fold.

Hepatic function impairment: Pharmacokinetics and metabolism were examined in patients with cirrhosis of the liver (n = 9). In these patients, the oral clearance of modafinil was decreased by ≈ 60% and the steady-state concentration was doubled compared to healthy patients. Reduce the modafinil dose in patients with severe hepatic impairment (see Administration and Dosage).

Contraindications

Hypersensitivity to modafinil.

Warnings

➤*Cardiovascular effects:* In clinical studies of modafinil, signs and symptoms including chest pain, palpitations, dyspnea, and transient ischemic T-wave changes on ECG were observed in 3 subjects in association with mitral valve prolapse or left ventricular hypertrophy. It is recommended that modafinil not be used in patients with a history of left ventricular hypertrophy or ischemic ECG changes, chest pain, arrhythmia, or other clinically significant manifestations of mitral valve prolapse in association with CNS stimulant use. Modafinil has not been evaluated or used to any appreciable extent in patients with a recent history of MI or unstable angina, and such patients should be treated with caution. Modafinil has not been systematically evaluated in patients with hypertension. Periodic monitoring of hypertensive patients may be appropriate.

➤*CNS effects:* One healthy male volunteer developed paranoid delusions and auditory hallucinations with multiple daily 600 mg doses of modafinil and sleep deprivation. There was no evidence of psychosis 36 hours after drug discontinuation. Exercise caution when modafinil is given to patients with a history of psychosis.

➤*Renal function impairment:* In patients with severe renal impairment (mean creatinine clearance 16.6 ml/min), a 200 mg single-dose of modafinil did not lead to increased exposure to modafinil but resulted in much higher exposure to the inactive metabolite, modafinil acid, than is seen in subjects with normal renal function. There is little information available about the safety of such levels of this metabolite.

➤*Hepatic function impairment:* In patients with severe hepatic impairment, with or without cirrhosis, administer modafinil at a reduced dose as modafinil clearance was decreased compared with that in healthy subjects (see Administration and Dosage).

➤*Elderly:* To the extent that elderly patients may have diminished renal or hepatic function, consider dosage reductions (see Administration and Dosage). Safety and efficacy in individuals > 65 years of age have not been established. Experience in a limited number of patients (n = 15) who were > 65 years of age in US clinical trials showed an incidence of adverse experiences similar to other age groups.

➤*Pregnancy: Category C.* Embryotoxicity was observed in the absence of maternal toxicity when rats received oral modafinil throughout the period of organogenesis. At a dose of 200 mg/kg/day (10 times the maximum recommended daily human dose [MRHD] of 200 mg on a mg/m^2 basis) there was an increase in resorption, hydronephrosis, and skeletal variations. The no-effect dose for these effects was 100 mg/kg/day (5 times the MRHD on a mg/m^2 basis). Although a threshold dose for embryotoxicity has been identified, the full spectrum of potential toxic effects on the fetus has not been characterized. There are no adequate and well-controlled trials with modafinil in pregnant women. Seven normal births occurred in patients who had received modafinil during pregnancy. Use during pregnancy only if the potential benefit outweighs the potential risk.

➤*Lactation:* It is not known whether modafinil or its metabolites are excreted in breast milk. Exercise caution when administering to a nursing woman.

➤*Children:* Safety and efficacy in individuals < 16 years of age have not been established.

Precautions

➤*Drug abuse and dependence:* In addition to its wakefulness-promoting effects and increased locomotor activity in animals, modafinil produces psychoactive and euphoric effects, alterations in mood, perception, and thinking, and feelings typical of other CNS stimulants in humans. In in vitro binding studies, modafinil binds to the dopamine reuptake site and causes an increase in extracellular dopamine but no increase in dopamine release. Modafinil is reinforcing, as evidenced by its self-administration in monkeys previously trained to self-administer cocaine. In some studies, modafinil was also partially discriminated as stimulant-like. Physicians should follow patients closely, especially those with a history of drug or stimulant (eg, methylphenidate, amphetamine, cocaine) abuse. Observe patients for signs of misuse or abuse (eg, incrementation of doses, drug-seeking behavior).

The abuse potential of modafinil (200, 400, and 800 mg) was assessed relative to methylphenidate (45 and 90 mg) in an inpatient study of individuals experienced with drugs of abuse. Results from this clinical study demonstrated that modafinil produced psychoactive and euphoric effects and feelings consistent with other scheduled CNS stimulants.

Withdrawal – The effects of modafinil withdrawal were monitored following 9 weeks of modafinil use in 1 US Phase 3 controlled clinical trial. No specific symptoms of withdrawal were observed during 14 days of observation although sleepiness returned in narcoleptic patients.

➤*Hazardous tasks:* Although modafinil has not been shown to produce functional impairment, any drug affecting the CNS may alter judgment, thinking, or motor skills. Caution patients about operating an automobile or other hazardous machinery until they are reasonably certain that modafinil therapy will not adversely affect their ability to engage in such activities.

Drug Interactions

➤*P450 systems:* In a controlled study in patients with narcolepsy, chronic dosing of modafinil at 400 mg/day once daily resulted in an ≈ 20% mean decrease in modafinil plasma trough concentrations by week 9, relative to those at week 3, suggesting that chronic administration might have caused induction of its metabolism. In addition, coadministration of potent inducers of CYP3A4 (eg, carbamazepine, phenobarbital, rifampin) or inhibitors of CYP3A4 (eg, ketoconazole, itraconazole) could alter the levels of modafinil because of the partial involvement of that enzyme in the metabolic elimination of the compound.

MODAFINIL

In in vitro studies, modafinil slightly induced CYP1A2, CYP2B6, and CYP3A4 in a concentration-dependent manner. Exercise caution when modafinil is coadministered with drugs that depend on these 3 enzymes for their clearance. Specifically, lower blood levels of such drugs could result. A modest induction of CYP3A4 by modafinil has been indicated; hence the clearance of CYP3A4 substrates such as cyclosporine or steroidal contraceptives and, to a lesser degree, theophylline may be increased.

In vitro studies showed that modafinil has little or no capacity to inhibit the major CYP enzymes except for CYP2C19, which is reversibly inhibited at pharmacologically relevant concentrations of modafinil. Drugs that are largely eliminated via CYP2C19 metabolism, such as diazepam, propranolol, and phenytoin may have prolonged elimination upon coadministration with modafinil and may require dosage reduction.

Modafinil Drug Interactions			
Precipitant drug	Object drug*		Description
MAOIs	Modafinil	↔	Use caution when administering MAO inhibitors and modafinil.
Methylphenidate	Modafinil	↓	Modafinil absorption may be delayed by ≈ 1 hour.
Modafinil	Clomipramine	↑	One incident of increased levels of clomipramine and its active metabolite desmethylclomipramine has been reported in a patient with narcolepsy during treatment with modafinil.
Modafinil	Cyclosporine	↓	After 1 month of 200 mg/day modafinil, cyclosporine blood levels were decreased by 50% in 1 patient.
Modafinil	Phenytoin	↑	Monitor patients receiving modafinil and phenytoin, a CYP2C9 substrate, for signs of phenytoin toxicity.
Modafinil	Contraceptives, oral	↓	The effectiveness of oral contraceptives may be reduced when used with modafinil. Alternative or concomitant methods of contraception are recommended for patients treated with modafinil and for 1 month after discontinuation of modafinil.
Modafinil	Tricyclic antidepressants	↑	In tricyclic-treated patients deficient in CYP2D6 (ie, poor debrisoquine metabolizers [7% to 10% of the white population; similar or lower in other populations]), the amount of metabolism by CYP2C19 may be substantially increased. Modafinil may cause plasma elevations of certain tricyclics (eg, clomipramine, desipramine) in these patients. A reduction in the dose of tricyclic agents might be needed.
Modafinil	Warfarin	↑	Monitoring of prothrombin times is suggested as a precaution for the first several months of coadministration of modafinil and warfarin, a CYP2C9 substrate, and thereafter whenever modafinil dosing is changed.

* ↑ = Object drug increased. ↓ = Object drug decreased. ↔ = Undetermined clinical effect.

➤Drug/Food interactions: Although food has no effect on overall modafinil bioavailability, absorption may be delayed by ≈ 1 hour.

Adverse Reactions

Modafinil is generally well tolerated. In controlled clinical trials, most adverse experiences were mild-to-moderate. The most commonly observed adverse events (≥ 5%) associated with the use of modafinil more frequently than placebo were headache, infection, nausea, nervousness, anxiety, and insomnia.

In US placebo-controlled Phase 3 clinical trials, 5% of the 369 patients who received modafinil discontinued therapy because of an adverse experience. The most frequent (≥ 1%) reasons for discontinuation that occurred at a higher rate for modafinil than placebo patients were headache, nausea, depression, and nervousness (1%).

Modafinil Adverse Reactions (≥ 1%) (%)		
Adverse reaction	Modafinil (n = 369)	Placebo (n = 185)
CNS		
Headache	50	40
Nervousness	8	6
Dizziness	5	4
Depression	4	3
Anxiety	4	1
Cataplexy	3	2
Insomnia	3	1
Paresthesia	3	1
Dyskinesia[1]	2	0
Hypertonia	2	0
Confusion	1	0
Amnesia	1	0
Emotional lability	1	0
Ataxia	1	0
Tremor	1	0
Cardiovascular		
Hypotension	2	1
Hypertension	2	0
Vasodilation	1	0
Arrhythmia	1	0
Syncope	1	0
Dermatologic		
Herpes simplex	1	0
Dry skin	1	0
GI		
Nausea	13	4
Diarrhea	8	4
Dry mouth	5	1
Anorexia	5	1
Abnormal liver function[2]	3	2
Vomiting	2	1
Mouth ulcer	1	0
Gingivitis	1	0
Thirst	1	0
GU		
Abnormal urine	1	0
Urinary retention	1	0
Abnormal ejaculation[3]	1	0
Metabolic/Nutritional		
Hyperglycemia	1	0
Albuminuria	1	0
Respiratory		
Rhinitis	11	8
Pharyngitis	6	3
Lung disorder	4	2
Dyspnea	2	1
Asthma	1	0
Epistaxis	1	0
Special senses		
Amblyopia	2	1
Abnormal vision	2	0
Miscellaneous		
Chest pain	2	1
Neck pain	2	1
Chills	2	0
Eosinophilia	2	0
Rigid neck	1	0
Fever/Chills	1	0
Joint disorder	1	0

[1] Oro-facial dyskinesias.
[2] Elevated liver enzymes.
[3] Incidence adjusted for gender.

➤Lab test abnormalities: Mean plasma levels of **gamma-glutamyl transferase (GGT)** were found to be higher following administration of modafinil but not placebo. However, few subjects (1%) had GGT elevations outside of the normal range. Shift of the modafinil-treated population to higher, but not clinically significantly abnormal, GGT values appeared to increase with time in the 9-week US Phase 3 clinical trials.

MODAFINIL

Although there were more abnormal **eosinophil** counts following modafinil administration than placebo in US Phase 1 and 2 studies, the difference does not appear to be clinically significant. Observed shifts were from normal to high.

Overdosage

➤*Symptoms:* A total of 151 doses of 1000 mg/day (5 times the MRHD of 200 mg) or more, have been recorded for 32 individuals. Doses of 4000 mg and 4500 mg were taken intentionally by 2 patients participating in foreign depression studies. In both cases, the adverse experiences observed were limited, expected, and not life-threatening, and the patients recovered fully by the following day. The adverse experiences included excitation or agitation, insomnia, and slight or moderate elevations in hemodynamic parameters. In neither of these cases nor in other instances of doses of > 1000 mg/day, including experience with up to 21 consecutive days of dosing at 1200 mg/day, were any unexpected effects or specific organ toxicities observed. Other observed high-dose effects in clinical studies have included anxiety, irritability, aggressiveness, confusion, nervousness, tremor, palpitations, sleep disturbances, nausea, diarrhea, and decreased prothrombin time.

➤*Treatment:* No specific antidote to the toxic effects of modafinil overdose has been identified to date. Manage such overdoses with primarily supportive care, including cardiovascular monitoring. If there are no contraindications, consider induced emesis or gastric lavage. There are no data to suggest the use of dialysis or urinary acidification or alkalinization in enhancing drug elimination. Refer to General Management of Acute Overdosage.

Patient Information

Advise patients to notify their physician if they become pregnant or intend to become pregnant during therapy. Caution patients regarding the potential increased risk of pregnancy when using oral, depot, or implantable contraceptives with and for 1 month after discontinuation of modafinil.

Advise patients to notify their physician if they are breastfeeding an infant.

Advise patients to inform their physician if they are taking or plan to take any prescription or *otc* drugs because of the potential for interactions between modafinil and other drugs.

Advise patients that the use of modafinil in combination with alcohol has not been studied. Advise patients that it is prudent to avoid alcohol while taking modafinil.

Advise patients to notify their physican if they develop a rash, hives, or a related allergic phenomenon.

Indications

➤*Narcolepsy:* To improve wakefulness in patients with excessive daytime sleepiness associated with narcolepsy.

➤*Attention deficit disorder with hyperactivity:* Indicated as an integral part of a total treatment program that includes other remedial measures (psychological, educational, social) for a stabilizing effect in children 3 to 16 years of age with a behavioral syndrome characterized by moderate to severe distractibility, short attention span, hyperactivity, emotional lability, and impulsivity. Do not diagnose this syndrome with finality when these symptoms are only of comparatively recent origin. Nonlocalizing (soft) neurological signs, learning disability, and abnormal EEG may be present and a diagnosis of CNS dysfunction may be warranted.

➤*Exogenous obesity:* As a short-term adjunct in a regimen of weight reduction based on caloric restriction, for patients refractory to alternative therapy (eg, repeated diets, group programs, other drugs). Weigh the limited usefulness against the possible risks inherent in use.

➤*Unlabeled uses:* Cocaine dependence treatment (**dextroamphetamine**), autism (**dextroamphetamine**).

Administration and Dosage

Administer at the lowest effective dosage and adjust individually. Avoid late evening doses, particularly with the long-acting form, because of the resulting insomnia.

When treating attention deficit disorder in children, occasionally interrupt drug administration to determine if there is a recurrence of behavioral symptoms sufficient to require continued therapy.

Actions

➤*Pharmacology:* Amphetamines are sympathomimetic amines with CNS stimulant activity. CNS effects are mediated by release of norepinephrine from central noradrenergic neurons. At higher doses, dopamine may be released in the mesolimbic system.

Peripheral alpha and beta activity includes elevation of systolic and diastolic blood pressures and weak bronchodilator and respiratory stimulant action. At therapeutic doses, the heart rate may be reflexly slowed; large doses may produce cardiac arrhythmias.

There is neither specific evidence that clearly establishes the mechanism whereby amphetamines produce mental and behavioral effects in children, nor conclusive evidence regarding how these effects relate to the condition of the CNS.

The site of action for appetite suppression is thought to be the lateral hypothalamic feeding center.

➤*Pharmacokinetics:* Amphetamine is metabolized in the liver by aromatic hydroxylation, N-dealkylation, and deamination.

Amphetamines are effective after oral administration and effects last for several hours.

Dextroamphetamine – Following administration of three 5 mg tablets, average maximal dextroamphetamine plasma concentrations (C_{max}) of 36.6 ng/mL were achieved at ≈ 3 hours. Following administration of one 15 mg sustained-release capsule, maximal dextroamphetamine plasma concentrations were obtained ≈ 8 hours after dosing. The average C_{max} was 23.5 ng/mL. The average plasma t½ was similar for the tablet and sustained-release capsule and was ≈ 12 hours.

Methamphetamine – Methamphetamine is rapidly absorbed from the GI tract. The biological half-life has been reported in the range of 4 to 5 hours. Excretion occurs primarily in the urine and is dependent on urine pH. Alkaline urine will increase the drug half-life significantly. Approximately 62% of an oral dose is eliminated in the urine within the first 24 hours with ≈ 33% as intact drug and the remainder as metabolites.

Amphetamine mixture – Following administration of immediate-release amphetamine mixture tablets, the peak plasma concentrations occurred in ≈ 3 hours for d-amphetamine and l-amphetamine.

The time to reach maximum plasma concentration (T_{max}) for extended-release amphetamine mixture capsules is ≈ 7 hours, which is ≈ 4 hours longer compared with the immediate-release formulation.

A single dose of 20 mg extended-release amphetamine mixture capsules provided comparable plasma concentration profiles of d-amphetamine and l-amphetamine with 10 mg immediate-release amphetamine mixture tablets twice daily administered 4 hours apart.

The mean elimination half-life is 1 hour shorter for d-amphetamine and 2 hours shorter for l-amphetamine in children 6 to 12 years of age compared with that of adults (t½ is 10 hours for d-amphetamine and 13 hours for l-amphetamine in adults and 9 and 11 hours, respectively, for children). Extended-release amphetamine mixture capsules demonstrate linear pharmacokinetics over the dose range of 10 to 30 mg. There is no unexpected accumulation at steady state.

Food does not affect the extent of absorption of extended-release amphetamine mixture capsules, but prolongs T_{max} by 2.5 hours (from 5.2 hours at fasted state to 7.7 hours after a high-fat meal). Opening the capsule and sprinkling the contents on applesauce results in comparable absorption to the intact capsule taken in the fasted state.

Special populations:
• *Children* – Children eliminated amphetamine faster than adults.
• *Gender* – Systemic exposure to amphetamine was 20% to 30% higher in women than in men because of the higher dose administered to women on a mg/kg body weight basis.

Contraindications

Advanced arteriosclerosis; symptomatic cardiovascular disease; moderate to severe hypertension; hyperthyroidism; known hypersensitivity or idiosyncrasy to the sympathomimetic amines; glaucoma; agitated states; history of drug abuse; during or within 14 days following administration of MAO inhibitors (hypertensive crises may result).

Warnings

➤*Tolerance:* When tolerance to the anorectic effect develops, do not exceed recommended dose in an attempt to increase the effect; rather, discontinue the drug.

➤*Drug dependence:* Amphetamines have been extensively abused. Tolerance, extreme psychological dependence, and severe social disability have occurred. Patients may increase the dosage to many times that recommended. Abrupt cessation following prolonged high dosage results in extreme fatigue, mental depression, and changes on the sleep EEG.

Manifestations of chronic intoxication – Severe dermatoses, marked insomnia, irritability, hyperactivity, and personality changes have occurred. Disorganization of thoughts, poor concentration, visual hallucinations, and compulsive behavior often occur. The most severe manifestation of chronic intoxication is psychosis, often clinically indistinguishable from paranoid schizophrenia. This is rare with oral amphetamines.

➤*Growth inhibition:* Decrements in the predicted growth (ie, weight gain or height) rate have been reported with the long-term use of stimulants in children. Therefore, carefully monitor patients requiring long-term therapy.

➤*Pregnancy: Category C.* Safety for use during pregnancy has not been established. Reproduction studies in mammals at many times the human dose have suggested an embryotoxic and teratogenic potential. Congenital defects associated with amphetamine use include cardiac abnormalities, bifidexencephaly, and biliary atresia. **Methamphetamine** has been shown to have teratogenic and embryocidal effects in mammals given high multiples of the human dose. There are no adequate and well-controlled studies in pregnant women. Use in women who are or who may become pregnant (especially those in the first trimester) only when clearly needed and when the potential benefits outweigh the potential hazards to the fetus.

Infants born to mothers dependent on amphetamines have an increased risk of premature delivery and low birth weight. Also, these infants may experience symptoms of withdrawal as demonstrated by dysphoria, including agitation and significant lassitude.

➤*Lactation:* Amphetamines are excreted in breast milk. Advise patients to discontinue nursing while taking amphetamines.

➤*Children:* Safety and efficacy have not been established for the use of amphetamines as anorectic agents in children < 12 years of age.

Amphetamine and **dextroamphetamine** are not recommended in children < 3 years of age for attention deficit disorder with hyperactivity. In psychotic children, amphetamines may exacerbate symptoms of behavior disturbance and thought disorder. Amphetamines may exacerbate motor and phonic tics and Tourette's syndrome. Therefore, clinical evaluation for tics and Tourette's syndrome in children and their families should precede use of stimulants.

Data are inadequate to determine whether chronic administration of amphetamines may be associated with growth inhibition; therefore, monitor growth during treatment and interrupt treatment in patients who are not growing or gaining weight as expected.

Long-term effects in children have not been well established.

Extended-release amphetamine mixture – Extended-release amphetamine mixture capsules are indicated for children ≥ 6 years of age. Effects in children 3 to 5 years of age have not been studied.

Precautions

➤*Hypertension:* Exercise caution in prescribing amphetamines for patients with even mild hypertension.

➤*Prescribe or dispense:* Prescribe or dispense the least amount feasible at one time to minimize the possibility of overdosage.

➤*Potentially hazardous tasks:* Amphetamines may impair the ability of the patient to engage in potentially hazardous activities such as operating machinery or vehicles; caution the patient accordingly.

➤*Attention deficit disorders:* Drug treatment is not indicated in all cases and should be considered only in light of the complete history and evaluation of the child. Amphetamine use should depend on the chronicity and severity of the child's symptoms and appropriateness for his/her age. Use should not depend solely on the presence of ≥ 1 of the behavioral characteristics.

When these symptoms are associated with acute stress reactions, amphetamine treatment is usually not indicated.

➤*Fatigue:* Do not use **methamphetamine** to combat fatigue or replace rest in normal people.

➤*Tartrazine sensitivity:* Some of these products contain tartrazine, which may cause allergic-type reactions (including bronchial asthma) in susceptible individuals. Although the incidence of tartrazine sensitivity in the general population is low, it is frequently seen in patients who also have aspirin hypersensitivity. Specific products containing tartrazine are identified in the product listings.

Drug Interactions

Insulin requirements in diabetes mellitus may be altered in association with the use of **methamphetamine** and the concomitant dietary regimen.

Amphetamine Drug Interactions			
Precipitant drug	Object drug*		Description
Furazolidone	Amphetamines	↑	Increased sensitivity to amphetamines may occur. If an interaction is suspected, monitor patient for signs and symptoms of amphetamine toxicity and reduce the amphetamine dose accordingly.
MAO inhibitors	Amphetamines	↑	Exaggerated pharmacologic effects from the amphetamines may occur. Avoid coadministration. The hypertensive reaction may occur for up to several weeks after discontinuing the MAO inhibitor.
SSRIs	Amphetamines	↑	Increased sensitivity to effect of sympathomimetics and increased risk of "serotonin syndrome" may occur. If these agents must be given concurrently, monitor the patient for increased signs and symptoms of CNS effects. Adjust therapy as needed.
Urinary acidifiers	Amphetamines	↓	The elimination of amphetamines is hastened with a concomitant reduction in their duration of action. No special precautions appear necessary. This interaction has been exploited therapeutically in the management of amphetamine overdose.
Urinary alkalinizers	Amphetamines	↑	Alkalinized urine may prolong the effects of amphetamines. Avoid agents that may alkalinize urine, particularly in overdose situations.
Amphetamines	Guanethidine	↓	Amphetamines may reverse the hypotensive effects of guanethidine. Monitor patients. If there is a loss of blood pressure control, stop the amphetamine or switch to alternative hypotensive therapy.

* ↑ = Object drug increased. ↓ = Object drug decreased.

➤*Drug/Lab test interactions:* Plasma **corticosteroid** levels may be increased. This increase is greatest in the evening. This should be considered if determination of plasma corticosteroid levels is desired in a person receiving amphetamines. **Urinary steroid** determinations may be altered by amphetamines.

Adverse Reactions

➤*Cardiovascular:* Palpitations; tachycardia; elevation of blood pressure; reflex decrease in heart rate; arrhythmias (at larger doses). There have been isolated reports of cardiomyopathy associated with chronic amphetamine use.

➤*CNS:* Overstimulation; restlessness; dizziness; insomnia; dyskinesia; euphoria; dysphoria; tremor; headache; changes in libido; psychotic episodes at recommended doses (rare). CNS stimulants have exacerbated Tourette's disorder and have exacerbated motor and phonic tics.

➤*GI:* Dry mouth; unpleasant taste; diarrhea; constipation; other GI disturbances. Anorexia and weight loss may occur as undesirable effects when amphetamines are used other than for their anorectic effect.

➤*Miscellaneous:* Urticaria; impotence; changes in libido; suppression of growth in children with long-term stimulant use.

Overdosage

➤*Symptoms:* Individual patient response to amphetamines varies widely. Manifestations of acute overdosage with amphetamines include the following: Restlessness; irritability; insomnia; tremor; hyperreflexia; rhabdomyolysis; rapid respiration; hyperpyrexia; assaultiveness; hallucinations; panic states; diaphoresis; mydriasis; flushing; hyperactivity; confusion; hypertension or hypotension; extrasystoles; tachypnea; fever; delirium; self-injury; marked hypertension; arrhythmias. Fatigue and depression usually follow the central stimulation. Cardiovascular effects include arrhythmias, hypertension or hypotension, and circulatory collapse. GI symptoms include nausea, vomiting, diarrhea, and abdominal cramps. Fatal poisoning usually is preceded by convulsions and coma.

➤*Treatment:* Consult with a certified poision control center for up-to-date guidance and advice. Treatment is largely symptomatic and includes gastric evacuation, although this is usually ineffective > 4 hours after ingestion. After emptying the stomach, administer activated charcoal and a cathartic. Acidification of the urine increases amphetamine excretion. Experience with hemodialysis and peritoneal dialysis is inadequate to permit recommendations.

If acute, severe hypertension complicates amphetamine overdosage, administration of IV phentolamine has been suggested. However, a gradual drop in blood pressure usually results from sufficient sedation. Chlorpromazine antagonizes the central stimulant effects of amphetamines and can be used to treat amphetamine intoxication.

Because much of the long-acting form of medication is coated for gradual release, direct therapy at reversing the effects of the ingested drug and at supporting the patient; continue until overdosage symptoms subside. Use saline cathartics to hasten the evacuation of pellets that have not released medication.

Amphetamine mixture – Consider the prolonged release of mixed amphetamine salts from extended-release amphetamine mixture capsules when treating patients with overdose.

Patient Information

Regardless of indication, administer amphetamines at the lowest effective dosage and individually adjust dosage. Avoid late evening doses because of the resulting insomnia.

Do not chew or crush sustained-release or long-acting tablets.

Do not increase dosage, except on physician's advice.

Amphetamines may impair the ability of the patient to engage in potentially hazardous activities such as operating machinery or vehicles; caution the patient accordingly.

May cause nervousness, restlessness, insomnia, dizziness, anorexia, dry mouth, and GI disturbances. Notify physician if these effects become pronounced.

DEXTROAMPHETAMINE SULFATE

c-ii	**Dextroamphetamine Sulfate** (Various, eg, Barr)	**Tablets:** 5 mg	In 100s.
c-ii	**Dexedrine** (GlaxoSmithKline)		Tartrazine, lactose, sucrose. (SKF E19). Orange, triangular, scored. In 100s.
c-ii	**DextroStat** (Shire Richwood)		Tartrazine, lactose, sucrose. (RP 51). Yellow, scored. In 100s, 500s, and 1000s.
c-ii	**Dextroamphetamine Sulfate** (Various, eg, Barr)	**Tablets:** 10 mg	In 100s.
c-ii	**DextroStat** (Shire Richwood)		Tartrazine, lactose, sucrose. (RP 52). Yellow, scored. In 100s and 500s.
c-ii	**Dextroamphetamine Sulfate** (Various, eg, Barr)	**Capsules, sustained-release:** 5 mg	In 100s.
c-ii	**Dexedrine Spansules** (Glaxo-SmithKline)		Sugar spheres. (5 mg 3512/5 mg SB). Clear and brown. In 100s.
c-ii	**Dextroamphetamine Sulfate** (Various, eg, Barr)	**Capsules, sustained-release:** 10 mg	In 100s.
c-ii	**Dexedrine Spansules** (Glaxo-SmithKline)		Sugar spheres. (10 mg 3513/10 mg SB). Clear and brown. In 100s.
c-ii	**Dextroamphetamine Sulfate** (Various, eg, Barr)	**Capsules, sustained-release:** 15 mg	In 100s.
c-ii	**Dexedrine Spansules** (Glaxo-SmithKline)		Sugar spheres. (15 mg 3514/15 mg SB). Clear/Brown. In 100s.

Complete prescribing information for these products begins in the Amphetamines group monograph.

Indications

➤*Narcolepsy:* To improve wakefulness in patients with excessive day-time sleepiness associated with narcolepsy.

➤*Attention deficit disorder with hyperactivity:* Indicated as an integral part of a total treatment program that includes other remedial measures (psychological, educational, social) for a stabilizing effect in children 3 to 16 years of age with a behavioral syndrome characterized by moderate to severe distractibility, short attention span, hyperactivity, emotional lability, and impulsivity. Do not diagnose this syndrome with finality when these symptoms are only of comparatively recent origin. Nonlocalizing (soft) neurological signs, learning disability, and abnormal EEG may be present and a diagnosis of CNS dysfunction may be warranted.

Administration and Dosage

➤*Narcolepsy:* 5 to 60 mg/day in divided doses.

Children (6 to 12 years of age) – Narcolepsy seldom occurs in children < 12 years of age. When it does, initial dose is 5 mg/day; increase in increments of 5 mg at weekly intervals until optimal response is obtained (maximum 60 mg/day).

Adults (≥ 12 years of age) – Start with 10 mg/day; raise in increments of 10 mg/day at weekly intervals. If adverse reactions appear (eg, insomnia, anorexia), reduce dose. Long-acting forms may be used for once-a-day dosage. With tablets, give first dose on awakening; give additional doses (1 or 2) at intervals of 4 to 6 hours.

➤*Attention deficit disorder in children:* Not recommended for children < 3 years of age.

Children (3 to 5 years of age) – 2.5 mg/day; increase in increments of 2.5 mg/day at weekly intervals until optimal response is obtained.

Children (≥ 6 years of age) – 5 mg once or twice daily; increase in increments of 5 mg/day at weekly intervals until optimal response is obtained. Dosage will rarely exceed 40 mg/day.

Long-acting forms may be used for once-a-day dosage. With tablets, give first dose on awakening; additional doses (1 or 2) may be given at intervals of 4 to 6 hours.

➤*Storage/Stability:* Dispense in a tight, light-resistant container. Store at 15° to 30°C (59° to 86°F).

METHAMPHETAMINE HCl (Desoxyephedrine HCl)

c-ii	**Methamphetamine HCl** (Able)	**Tablets:** 5 mg	Corn starch, lactose. (A 396). In 30s, 100s, 500s, and 1000s.
c-ii	**Desoxyn** (Abbott)		Lactose. (TE). White. In 100s.

For complete prescribing information for these products, refer to the Amphetamines general monograph.

Indications

➤*Attention deficit disorder with hyperactivity:* Indicated as an integral part of a total treatment program that includes other remedial measures (psychological, educational, social) for a stabilizing effect in children 3 to 16 years of age with a behavioral syndrome characterized by moderate to severe distractibility, short attention span, hyperactivity, emotional lability, and impulsivity. Do not diagnose this syndrome with finality when these symptoms are only of comparatively recent origin. Nonlocalizing (soft) neurological signs, learning disability, and abnormal EEG may be present and a diagnosis of CNS dysfunction may be warranted.

➤*Exogenous obesity:* As a short-term adjunct in a regimen of weight reduction based on caloric restriction, for patients refractory to alternative therapy (eg, repeated diets, group programs, other drugs). Weigh the limited usefulness against the possible risks inherent in use.

Administration and Dosage

➤*Attention deficit disorder in children:* Initially, 5 mg once or twice daily; increase in increments of 5 mg at weekly intervals until an optimum response is achieved. Usual effective dose is 20 to 25 mg/day.

Total daily dose may be given as conventional tablets in 2 divided doses. Where possible, interrupt drug administration to determine if there is a recurrence of behavioral symptoms sufficient to require continued therapy.

➤*Obesity:* 5 mg 30 minutes before each meal.

Treatment duration should not exceed a few weeks. Do not use in children < 12 years of age.

➤*Storage/Stability:* Store below 30°C (86°F).

AMPHETAMINE MIXTURES

c-ii	**Amphetamine Salt Combo** (Barr)	**Tablets:** 5 mg (1.25 mg dextroamphetamine sulfate, 1.25 mg dextroamphetamine saccharate, 1.25 mg amphetamine aspartate, 1.25 mg amphetamine sulfate)	(b 971 5). Blue, oval, scored. In 50s, 100s, and 500s.
c-ii	**Adderall** (Shire Richwood)		Lactose, sucrose. (AD 5). Blue, scored. In 100s.
c-ii	**Adderall** (Shire Richwood)	7.5 mg (1.875 mg dextroamphetamine sulfate, 1.875 mg dextroamphetamine saccharate, 1.875 mg amphetamine aspartate, 1.875 mg amphetamine sulfate)	Lactose, sucrose. (AD 7.5). Blue, scored. In 100s.
c-ii	**Amphetamine Salt Combo** (Barr)	10 mg (2.5 mg dextroamphetamine sulfate, 2.5 mg dextroamphetamine saccharate, 2.5 mg amphetamine aspartate, 2.5 mg amphetamine sulfate)	(b 972 1/0). Blue, oval, scored. In 50s, 100s, and 500s.
c-ii	**Adderall** (Shire Richwood)		Lactose, sucrose. (AD 10). Blue, scored. In 100s.
c-ii	**Adderall** (Shire Richwood)	12.5 mg (3.125 mg dextroamphetamine sulfate, 3.125 mg dextroamphetamine saccharate, 3.125 mg amphetamine aspartate, 3.125 mg amphetamine sulfate)	Lactose, sucrose. (AD 12.5). Orange, scored. In 100s.
c-ii	**Adderall** (Shire Richwood)	15 mg (3.75 mg dextroamphetamine sulfate, 3.75 mg dextroamphetamine saccharate, 3.75 mg amphetamine aspartate, 3.75 mg amphetamine sulfate)	Lactose, sucrose. (AD 15). Orange, scored. In 100s.

Amphetamines

AMPHETAMINE MIXTURES

c-ii	**Amphetamine Salt Combo** (Barr)	20 mg (5 mg dextroamphetamine sulfate, 5 mg dextroamphetamine saccharate, 5 mg amphetamine aspartate, 5 mg amphetamine sulfate)	(b 973 2/0). Peach, oval, scored. In 50s, 100s, and 500s.
c-ii	**Adderall** (Shire Richwood)		Lactose, sucrose. (AD 20). Orange, scored. In 100s.
c-ii	**Amphetamine Salt Combo** (Barr)	30 mg (7.5 mg dextroamphetamine sulfate, 7.5 mg dextroamphetamine saccharate, 7.5 mg amphetamine aspartate, 7.5 mg amphetamine sulfate)	(b 974 3/0). Peach, oval, scored. In 50s, 100s, and 500s.
c-ii	**Adderall** (Shire Richwood)		Lactose, sucrose. (AD 30). Orange, scored. In 100s.
c-ii	**Adderall XR** (Shire)	**Capsules:** 5 mg (1.25 mg dextroamphetamine saccharate, 1.25 mg amphetamine aspartate monohydrate, 1.25 mg dextroamphetamine sulfate, 1.25 mg amphetamine sulfate)	Sugar spheres, talc. (ADDERALL XR 5 mg). Clear/Blue. In 100s.
		10 mg (2.5 mg dextroamphetamine saccharate, 2.5 mg amphetamine aspartate monohydrate, 2.5 mg dextroamphetamine sulfate, 2.5 mg amphetamine sulfate)	Sugar spheres. (SHIRE 381 10 mg). Blue. In 100s.
		15 mg (3.75 mg dextroamphetamine saccharate, 3.75 mg amphetamine aspartate monohydrate, 3.75 mg dextroamphetamine sulfate, 3.75 mg amphetamine sulfate)	Sugar spheres, talc. (ADDERALL XR 15 mg). Blue/White. In 100s.
		20 mg (5 mg dextroamphetamine saccharate, 5 mg amphetamine aspartate monohydrate, 5 mg dextroamphetamine sulfate, 5 mg amphetamine sulfate)	Sugar spheres. (SHIRE 381 20 mg). Orange. In 100s.
		25 mg (6.25 mg dextroamphetamine saccharate, 6.25 mg amphetamine aspartate monohydrate, 6.25 mg dextroamphetamine sulfate, 6.25 mg amphetamine sulfate)	Sugar spheres, talc. (ADDERALL XR 25 mg). Orange/White. In 100s.
		30 mg (7.5 mg dextroamphetamine saccharate, 7.5 mg amphetamine aspartate monohydrate, 7.5 mg dextroamphetamine sulfate, 7.5 mg amphetamine sulfate)	Sugar spheres. (SHIRE 381 30 mg). Natural/Orange. In 100s.

For complete prescribing information for these products, refer to the Amphetamines group monograph.

Indications

➤*Narcolepsy:* To improve wakefulness in patients with excessive daytime sleepiness associated with narcolepsy.

➤*Attention deficit disorder with hyperactivity:* Indicated as an integral part of a total treatment program that includes other remedial measures (psychological, educational, social) for a stabilizing effect in children 3 to 16 years of age with a behavioral syndrome characterized by moderate to severe distractibility, short attention span, hyperactivity, emotional lability, and impulsivity. Do not diagnose this syndrome with finality when these symptoms are only of comparatively recent origin. Nonlocalizing (soft) neurological signs, learning disability, and abnormal EEG may be present and a diagnosis of CNS dysfunction may be warranted.

Administration and Dosage

These mixtures contain various salts of amphetamine and dextroamphetamine.

Regardless of indication, administer amphetamines at the lowest effective dosage and individually adjust dosage. Avoid late evening doses because of the resulting insomnia.

➤*Immediate-release tablets:*

Narcolepsy – 5 to 60 mg/day in divided doses.

Children (6 to 12 years of age): Narcolepsy seldom occurs in children < 12 years of age. When it does, initial dose is 5 mg/day; increase in increments of 5 mg at weekly intervals until optimal response is obtained (maximum 60 mg/day).

Adults (≥ 12 years of age): Start with 10 mg/day; raise in increments of 10 mg/day at weekly intervals. If adverse reactions appear (eg, insomnia or anorexia), reduce dose. Give first dose on awakening; additional doses (1 or 2) at intervals of 4 to 6 hours.

Attention deficit disorder in children – Not recommended for children < 3 years of age.

Children (3 to 5 years of age): 2.5 mg/day; increase in increments of 2.5 mg/day at weekly intervals until optimal response is obtained.

Children (≥ 6 years of age): 5 mg once or twice daily; increase in increments of 5 mg/day at weekly intervals until optimal response is obtained. Dosage will rarely exceed 40 mg/day.

Give first dose on awakening; additional doses (1 or 2) may be given at intervals of 4 to 6 hours.

➤*Extended-release capsules:* In children with attention deficit hyperactivity disorder (ADHD) who are ≥ 6 years of age and are starting treatment for the first time or switching from another medication, start with 10 mg once daily in the morning; daily dosage may be raised in increments of 10 mg at weekly intervals. Individualize dosage according to the needs and responses of the patient. Administer amphetamines at the lowest effective dosage. The maximum recommended dose is 30 mg/day; doses > 30 mg/day of extended-release amphetamine mixture capsules have not been studied.

Amphetamines are not recommended for children < 3 years of age. Extended-release amphetamine mixture capsules have not been studied in children < 6 years of age.

Extended-release amphetamine mixture capsules may be taken whole, or the capsule may be opened and the entire contents sprinkled on applesauce. If the patient is using the sprinkle administration method, the sprinkled applesauce should be consumed immediately; it should not be stored. Patients should take the applesauce with sprinkled beads in its entirety without chewing. The dose of a single capsule should not be divided. The contents of the entire capsule should be taken, and the patient should not take anything < 1 capsule/day.

Give extended-release amphetamine mixture capsules upon awakening. Avoid afternoon doses because of the potential for insomnia.

Where possible, occasionally interrupt drug administration to determine if there is a recurrence of behavioral symptoms sufficient to require continued therapy.

➤*Storage/Stability:* Dispense in a tight, light-resistant container. Store at 25°C (77°F); excursions permitted to 15° to 30°C (59° to 86°F).

DEXMETHYLPHENIDATE HCl

c-ii	**Focalin** (Novartis)	**Tablets:** 2.5 mg	Lactose. (D 2.5). Blue. In 100s.
		5 mg	Lactose. (D 5). Yellow. In 100s.
		10 mg	Lactose. (D 10). White. In 100s.

WARNING

Drug dependence: Give dexmethylphenidate cautiously to patients with a history of drug dependence or alcoholism. Chronic, abusive use can lead to marked tolerance and psychological dependence with varying degrees of abnormal behavior. Frank psychotic episodes can occur, especially with parenteral abuse. Careful supervision is required during drug withdrawal from abusive use because severe depression may occur. Withdrawal following chronic therapeutic use may unmask symptoms of the underlying disorder that may require follow-up.

Indications

➤*Attention deficit hyperactivity disorder (ADHD):* For the treatment of ADHD. Dexmethylphenidate is indicated as an integral part of a total treatment program for ADHD that may include other measures (eg, psychological, educational, social) for patients with this syndrome. Drug treatment may not be indicated for all patients with this syndrome. Stimulants are not intended for use in the patient who exhibits symptoms secondary to environmental factors or other primary psychiatric disorders, including psychosis.

The effectiveness of dexmethylphenidate > 6 weeks has not been systematically evaluated in controlled trials. Therefore, the physician who elects to use dexmethylphenidate for extended periods should periodically reevaluate the long-term usefulness of the drug for the individual patient.

Administration and Dosage

➤*Approved by the FDA:* November 13, 2001.

Administer twice daily, at least 4 hours apart, with or without food.

Individualize dosage according to the needs and responses of the patient.

➤*Patients new to methylphenidate:* The recommended starting dose of dexmethylphenidate for patients who are not currently taking racemic methylphenidate, or for patients who are on stimulants other than methylphenidate is 5 mg/day (2.5 mg twice daily).

Dosage may be adjusted in 2.5 to 5 mg increments to a maximum of 20 mg/day (10 mg twice daily). In general, dosage adjustments may proceed at approximately weekly intervals.

➤*Patients currently using methylphenidate:* For patients currently using methylphenidate, the recommended starting dose of dexmethylphenidate is half the dose of racemic methylphenidate. The maximum recommended dose is 20 mg/day (10 mg twice daily).

➤*Maintenance/Extended treatment:* It is generally agreed that pharmacological treatment of ADHD may be needed for extended periods. The physician who elects to use dexmethylphenidate for extended periods in patients with ADHD should periodically reevaluate the long-term usefulness of the drug for the individual patient with periods off medication to assess the patient's functioning without pharmacotherapy. Improvement may be sustained when the drug is either temporarily or permanently discontinued.

➤*Dose reduction and discontinuation:* If paradoxical aggravation of symptoms or other adverse events occur, reduce the dosage, or, if necessary, discontinue the drug.

If improvement is not observed after appropriate dosage adjustment over a 1-month period, discontinue the drug.

➤*Storage/Stability:* Store at 25°C (77°F); excursions permitted 15° to 30°C (59° to 86°F). Protect from light and moisture.

Actions

➤*Pharmacology:* Dexmethylphenidate HCl is a CNS stimulant. It is the more pharmacologically active enantiomer of the *d-* and *l-*enantiomers and is thought to block the reuptake of norepinephrine and dopamine into the presynaptic neuron and increase the release of these monoamines into the extraneuronal space. The mode of therapeutic action in ADHD is not known.

➤*Pharmacokinetics:*

Absorption – Dexmethylphenidate HCl is readily absorbed following oral administration. In patients with ADHD, plasma dexmethylphenidate concentrations increase rapidly, reaching a maximum in the fasted state at ≈ 1 to 1.5 hours postdose. No differences in the pharmacokinetics of dexmethylphenidate were noted following single and repeated twice-daily dosing, thus indicating no significant drug accumulation in children with ADHD.

When given to children as capsules in single doses of 2.5, 5, and 10 mg, C_{max} and AUC of dexmethylphenidate were proportional to dose. In the same study, plasma dexmethylphenidate levels were comparable to those achieved following single *dl-threo*-methylphenidate HCl doses given as capsules in twice the total milligram amount (equimolar with respect to dexmethylphenidate).

Food effects: In a single-dose study conducted in adults, coadministration of 2 × 10 mg dexmethylphenidate with a high fat breakfast resulted in a dexmethylphenidate t_{max} of 2.9 hours postdose as compared with 1.5 hours postdose when given in a fasting state. C_{max} and AUC were comparable in the fasted and nonfasted states.

Distribution – Plasma dexmethylphenidate concentrations in children decline exponentially following oral administration.

Metabolism – In humans, dexmethylphenidate is metabolized primarily to *d*-α-phenyl-piperidine acetic acid (also known as *d*-ritalinic acid) by de-esterification. This metabolite has little or no pharmacological activity.

In vitro studies showed that dexmethylphenidate did not inhibit cytochrome P450 isoenzymes.

Excretion – After oral dosing of radiolabeled racemic methylphenidate in humans, ≈ 90% of the radioactivity was recovered in urine. The main urinary metabolite was ritalinic acid, accountable for ≈ 80% of the dose.

The mean plasma elimination half-life of dexmethylphenidate is ≈ 2.2 hours.

Special populations –

Gender: Pharmacokinetic parameters were similar for boys and girls (mean age, 10 years).

Age: The pharmacokinetics of dexmethylphenidate after administration have not been studied in children < 6 years of age. When single doses of dexmethylphenidate were given to children between 6 and 12 years of age and healthy adult volunteers, C_{max} of dexmethylphenidate was similar; however, children showed somewhat lower AUCs compared with adults.

Renal insufficiency: Since very little unchanged drug is excreted in the urine, renal insufficiency is expected to have little effect on the pharmacokinetics of dexmethylphenidate.

Contraindications

Patients with marked anxiety, tension, and agitation, because the drug may aggravate these symptoms; hypersensitivity to methylphenidate or other components of the product; patients with glaucoma, motor tics, or with a family history or diagnosis of Tourette's syndrome; during treatment with monoamine oxidase inhibitors (MAOIs), and also within a minimum of 14 days following discontinuation of an MAOI (hypertensive crises may result).

Warnings

➤*Depression:* Do not use dexmethylphenidate to treat severe depression.

➤*Fatigue:* Do not use dexmethylphenidate for the prevention or treatment of normal fatigue states.

➤*Long-term suppression of growth:* Although a causal relationship has not been established, suppression of growth (eg, weight gain, height) has been reported with the long-term use of stimulants in children. Therefore, carefully monitor patients requiring long-term therapy. Patients who are not growing or gaining weight as expected should have their treatment interrupted.

➤*Psychosis:* In psychotic children, administration of methylphenidate may exacerbate symptoms of behavior disturbance and thought disorder.

➤*Seizures:* Methylphenidate may lower the convulsive threshold in patients with history of seizures, in patients with prior EEG abnormalities in the absence of a history of seizures, and, very rarely, in the absence of a history of seizures and no prior EEG evidence of seizures. In the presence of seizures, discontinue the drug.

➤*Hypertension and other cardiovascular conditions:* Use cautiously in patients with hypertension. Monitor blood pressure at appropriate intervals in all patients taking dexmethylphenidate, especially those with hypertension. Caution is indicated in treating patients whose underlying medical conditions might be compromised by increases in blood pressure or heart rate (eg, preexisting hypertension, heart failure, recent MI, hyperthyroidism).

➤*Visual disturbance:* Difficulties with accommodation and blurring of vision have been reported.

➤*Carcinogenesis:* Lifetime carcinogenicity studies have not been carried out with dexmethylphenidate. In a lifetime carcinogenicity study carried out in B6C3F1 mice, racemic methylphenidate caused an increase in hepatocellular adenomas and, in males only, an increase in hepatoblastomas at a daily dose of ≈ 60 mg/kg/day. The significance to these results to humans is unknown.

➤*Pregnancy: Category C.* When dexmethylphenidate was administered to rats throughout pregnancy and lactation at doses of up to 20 mg/kg/day, postweaning body weight gain was decreased in male offspring at the highest dose, but no other effects of postnatal development were observed. At the highest doses tested, plasma levels (AUCs)

DEXMETHYLPHENIDATE HCl

of dexmethylphenidate in pregnant rats and rabbits were ≈ 5 and 1 times, respectively, those in adults dosed with the maximum recommended human dose of 20 mg/day.

Adequate and well-controlled studies in pregnant women have not been conducted. Use dexmethylphenidate during pregnancy only if the potential benefit justifies the potential risk to the fetus.

➤*Lactation:* It is not known whether dexmethylphenidate is excreted in human milk. Because many drugs are excreted in human milk, exercise caution if dexmethylphenidate is administered to a nursing woman.

➤*Children:* The safety and efficacy of dexmethylphenidate in children < 6 years of age have not been established. Long-term effects of dexmethylphenidate in children have not been well established.

Precautions

➤*Monitoring:* Periodic CBC, differential, and platelet counts are advised during prolonged therapy.

Drug Interactions

Dexmethylphenidate Drug Interactions			
Precipitant drug	Object drug*		Description
Methylphenidate (racemic)	Antihypertensive agents	↓	Methylphenidate may decrease the effectiveness of drugs used to treat hypertension.
Dexmethylphenidate HCl	Pressor agents (eg, dopamine, epinephrine, phenylephrine)	↓	Because of possible effects on blood pressure, use dexmethylphenidate cautiously with pressor agents.
Methylphenidate (racemic)	Coumarin anticoagulants (eg, warfarin)	↑	Dexmethylphenidate HCl may inhibit the metabolism of warfarin-like drugs. It may be necessary to adjust the dosage or monitor coagulation times when starting or stopping therapy.
Methylphenidate (racemic)	Anticonvulsants (eg, phenobarbital, phenytoin, primidone)	↑	Downward dose adjustments of anticonvulsant therapy may be required when given concomitantly with methylphenidate.
Methylphenidate (racemic)	Tricyclic antidepressants (eg, amitriptyline)	↑	It may be necessary to adjust the dosage of antidepressant therapy when giving these agents concurrently.
Methylphenidate (racemic)	Selective serotonin reuptake inhibitors (SSRIs)	↑	Methylphenidate may inhibit the metabolism of SSRI antidepressants. It may be necessary to adjust the SSRI dose when given concomitantly with methylphenidate.
Methylphenidate (racemic)	Clonidine	↔	Serious adverse events have been reported in concomitant use with clonidine; however, no causality for the combination has been established.

* ↑ = Object drug increased. ↓ = Object drug decreased. ↔ = Undetermined clinical effect.

Adverse Reactions

Discontinuation of treatment – No dexmethylphenidate-treated patients discontinued because of adverse events in 2 placebo-controlled trials. Overall, 7.3% of dexmethylphenidate-treated children experienced an adverse event that resulted in discontinuation. The most common reasons for discontinuation were twitching (described as motor or vocal tics), anorexia, insomnia, and tachycardia (≈ 1% each).

Adverse reactions ≥ 5% – The following table enumerates treatment-emergent adverse events for 2 placebo-controlled, parallel group trials in children with ADHD at dexmethylphenidate doses of 5, 10, and 20 mg/day. The table includes only those events that occurred in ≥ 5% of patients treated with dexmethylphenidate where the incidence in patients treated with dexmethylphenidate was at least twice the incidence in placebo-treated patients.

Treatment-emergent Adverse Reactions[1] Occurring During Double-blind Treatment in Clinical Trials of Dexmethylphenidate (%)		
Adverse reaction	Dexmethylphenidate (n = 79)	Placebo (n = 82)
Abdominal pain	15	6
Anorexia	6	1
Fever	5	1
Nausea	9	1

[1] Events, regardless of causality, for which the incidence for patients treated with dexmethylphenidate was at least 5% and twice the incidence among placebo-treated patients. Incidence has been rounded to the nearest whole number.

Adverse reactions with other methylphenidate HCl products – Nervousness and insomnia are the most common adverse reactions reported with other methylphenidate products. In children, loss of appetite, abdominal pain, weight loss during prolonged therapy, insomnia, and tachycardia may occur more frequently; however, any of the other adverse reactions listed below may also occur.

➤*Cardiovascular:* Angina, arrhythmia, palpitations, pulse increased or decreased, blood pressure increased or decreased, cerebral arteritis or occlusion.

➤*CNS:* Dizziness, drowsiness, dyskinesia, headache, rare reports of Tourette's syndrome, toxic psychosis.

➤*Dermatologic:* Skin rash, urticaria, exfoliative dermatitis, erythema multiforme with histopathological findings of necrotizing vasculitis, thrombocytopenic purpura.

➤*Hematologic/Lymphatic:* Leukopenia, anemia.

➤*Hepatic:* Abnormal liver function, ranging from transaminase elevation to hepatic coma.

➤*Miscellaneous:* Nausea, fever, arthralgia, transient depressed mood, scalp hair loss.

Very rare reports of neuroleptic malignant syndrome (NMS) have been received and in most of these, patients were concurrently receiving therapies associated with NMS.

Overdosage

➤*Symptoms:* Signs and symptoms of acute methylphenidate overdosage, resulting principally from overstimulation of the CNS and from excessive sympathomimetic effects, may include the following: Vomiting, agitation, tremors, hyperreflexia, muscle twitching, convulsions (may be followed by coma), euphoria, confusion, hallucinations, delirium, sweating, flushing, headache, hyperpyrexia, tachycardia, palpitations, cardiac arrhythmias, hypertension, mydriasis, dryness of mucous membranes.

➤*Treatment:* Treatment consists of appropriate supportive measures. The patient must be protected against self-injury and against external stimuli that would aggravate overstimulation already present. Gastric contents may be evacuated by gastric lavage as indicated. Before performing gastric lavage, control agitation and seizures if present and protect the airway. Other measures to detoxify the gut include administration of activated charcoal and a cathartic. Intensive care must be provided to maintain adequate circulation and respiratory exchange; external cooling procedures may be required for hyperpyrexia.

Efficacy of peritoneal dialysis for dexmethylphenidate overdosage has not been established.

As with the management of all overdosage, consider the possibility of multiple drug ingestion. The physician may wish to consider contacting a poison control center for up-to-date information on the management of overdosage with methylphenidate.

Patient Information

To assure safe and effective use of dexmethylphenidate, discuss the information and instructions provided in the patient information section with patients.

METHYLPHENIDATE HCl

c-ii	**Methylphenidate HCl** (Various, eg, Able, Danbury, Qualitest)	**Tablets:** 5 mg	In 100s and 1000s.
c-ii	**Methylin** (Mallinckrodt)		Lactose, talc. Color-additive-free. (5 M). White. In 100s and 1000s.
c-ii	**Ritalin** (Novartis)		Lactose. (CIBA 7). Yellow. In 100s.
c-ii	**Methylphenidate HCl** (Various, eg, Able, Danbury, Qualitest)	**Tablets:** 10 mg	In 100s and 1000s.
c-ii	**Methylin** (Mallinckrodt)		Lactose, talc. Color-additive-free. (10 M). White, scored. In 100s and 1000s.
c-ii	**Ritalin** (Novartis)		Lactose. (CIBA 3). Pale green, scored. In 100s.
c-ii	**Methylphenidate HCl** (Various, eg, Able, Danbury, Qualitest)	**Tablets:** 20 mg	In 100s and 1000s.
c-ii	**Methylin** (Mallinckrodt)		Lactose, talc. Color-additive-free. (20 M). White, scored. In 100s and 1000s.
c-ii	**Ritalin** (Novartis)		Sucrose, talc. (CIBA 34). Pale yellow, scored. In 100s.
c-ii	**Methylin** (Mallinckrodt)	**Tablets, chewable:** 2.5 mg	Aspartame, 0.42 mg phenylalanine. (2.5 CHEW M). White to cream color, rounded square. Grape flavor. In 30s and 100s.
		5 mg	Aspartame, 0.84 mg phenylalanine. (5 CHEW M). White to cream color, rounded square. Grape flavor. In 30s, 100s, and 1000s.
		10 mg	Aspartame, 1.68 mg phenylalanine. (10 CHEW M). White to cream color, rounded square. Grape flavor. In 30s, 100s, and 1000s.
c-ii	**Metadate ER** (Celltech)[1]	**Tablets, extended-release:** 10 mg	Lactose. Color-additive-free. (561 MD). White, oval. In 100s.
c-ii	**Methylin ER** (Mallinckrodt)		Color-additive-free. (1423 M). White to off-white. In 100s.
c-ii	**Concerta** (McNeil)[2]	**Tablets, extended-release:** 18 mg	Lactose. (alza 18). Yellow. In 100s.
c-ii	**Methylphenidate HCl** (Various, eg, Danbury, Qualitest)	**Tablets, extended-release:** 20 mg	In 30s and 100s.
c-ii	**Metadate ER** (Celltech)[1]		Lactose. Color-additive-free. (562 MD). White. In 100s.
c-ii	**Methylin ER** (Mallinckrodt)		Color-additive-free. (1451 M). White to off-white. In 100s.
c-ii	**Concerta** (McNeil)[2]	**Tablets, extended-release:** 27 mg	Lactose. (alza 27). Gray. In 100s.
c-ii	**Concerta** (McNeil)[2]	**Tablets, extended-release:** 36 mg	Lactose. (alza 36). White. In 100s.
c-ii	**Concerta** (McNeil)[2]	**Tablets, extended-release:** 54 mg	Lactose. (alza 54). Brownish-red. In 100s.
c-ii	**Ritalin-SR** (Novartis)	**Tablets, sustained-release:** 20 mg	Lactose, alcohol, mineral oil. Color-additive-free. (CIBA 16). White. In 100s.
c-ii	**Metadate CD** (Celltech)[3]	**Capsules, extended-release:** 10 mg	Sugar spheres. (CELLTECH 574 10 mg). Green and white. In 100s.
c-ii	**Metadate CD** (Celltech)[3]	**Capsules, extended-release:** 20 mg	Sugar spheres. (CELLTECH 575 20 mg). Blue/white. In 30s, UD 100s.
c-ii	**Ritalin LA** (Novartis)[4]		Sugar spheres, talc. (NVR R20). White. In 100s.
c-ii	**Metadate CD** (Celltech)[3]	**Capsules, extended-release:** 30 mg	Sugar spheres. (CELLTECH 576 30 mg). Red brown/white. In 100s.
c-ii	**Ritalin LA** (Novartis)[4]		Sugar spheres, talc. (NVR R30). Yellow. In 100s.
c-ii	**Ritalin LA** (Novartis)[4]	**Capsules, extended-release:** 40 mg	Sugar spheres, talc. (NVR R40). Lt. brown. In 100s.

[1] Methylphenidate is incorporated into a (cetyl alcohol) wax matrix, allowing for the gradual diffusion of methylphenidate as it passes through the GI tract. The water-soluble ingredients (methylphenidate, lactose) are released gradually as the GI fluids penetrate the crevices of the tablet. Extended-release tablets may be used in place of the immediate-release tablets when the 8-hour dosage of *Metadate ER* tablets corresponds to the titrated 8-hour dosage of the immediate-release tablets.

[2] The initial dose of *Concerta* is released from the outer coating over 1 to 2 hours, and the remainder is released at a controlled rate over 10 hours. Therefore, the total methylphenidate dose is released over 12 hours. For the 18 mg tablet, 4 mg is released initially from the outer layer of the tablet, then 14 mg is released over 10 hours. For the 27 mg tablet, 6 mg is initially released and then 21 mg over 10 hours. For the 36 mg tablet, 8 mg is initially released and then 28 mg over 10 hours. For the 54 mg tablet, 12 mg is initially released and then 42 mg over 10 hours.

[3] The immediate-release beads comprise 30% of the total methylphenidate dose (ie, 6 mg of a 20 mg capsule) and provide the initial phase, rapid release of methylphenidate. The second set of beads provides the second, extended-release phase of methylphenidate, and comprise 70% of the total methylphenidate dose (ie, 14 mg from a 20 mg capsule).

[4] Extended-release formulation using *SODAS* technology, a bi-modal release delivery system. Fifty percent of the contents are immediate-release beads to provide rapid onset. The second half of the contents consists of delayed-release beads that are released approximately 4 hours after administration. This delivery system mimics twice-daily administration of immediate-release methylphenidate.

WARNING

Drug dependence: Give cautiously to emotionally unstable patients (eg, those with a history of drug dependence or alcoholism), because they may increase dosage on their own initiative.

Chronic abuse can lead to marked tolerance and psychic dependence with varying degrees of abnormal behavior. Frank psychotic episodes can occur, especially with parenteral abuse. Careful supervision is required during drug withdrawal, because severe depression and the effects of chronic overactivity can be unmasked. Long-term follow-up may be required because of basic personality disturbances.

Indications

➤*Attention deficit disorder (ADD)/attention deficit hyperactivity disorder (ADHD):* As part of a total treatment program in patients with a behavioral syndrome characterized by moderate to severe distractibility, short attention span, hyperactivity, emotional lability, and impulsivity.

Stimulants are not for the patient who exhibits symptoms secondary to environmental factors or primary psychiatric disorders, including psychosis. When symptoms are associated with acute stress reactions, methylphenidate usually is not indicated.

➤*Narcolepsy (Ritalin, Ritalin SR, Metadate ER, Methylin):* For the treatment of narcolepsy.

➤*Unlabeled uses:* Depression in medically ill (including stroke) elderly persons; alleviation of neurobehavioral symptoms after traumatic brain injury (mixed efficacy); improvement in pain control, sedation, or both in patients receiving opiates.

Administration and Dosage

➤*Adults:* Individualize dosage. Administer in divided doses 2 or 3 times daily, preferably 30 to 45 minutes before meals. Average dose is 20 to 30 mg/day. Dosage ranges from 10 to 15 mg/day up to 40 to 60 mg/day. In patients who are unable to sleep if medication is taken late in the day, take the last dose before 6 p.m.

➤*Children (6 years of age and older):* Individualize dosage. Start with small doses (eg, 5 mg twice daily before breakfast and lunch) with gradual increments of 5 to 10 mg/week. Daily dosage above 60 mg is not recommended. If improvement is not observed after dosage adjustment over 1 month, discontinue use. If paradoxical aggravation of symptoms or other adverse effects occur, reduce dosage or discontinue the drug.

➤*All patients:* Sustained-release (SR) and *Methylin ER* tablets have a duration of approximately 8 hours and may be used in place of regular tablets when the 8-hour dosage of the SR tablets and *Methylin ER* corresponds to the titrated 8-hour dosage of the regular tablets. SR and *Methylin ER* tablets must be swallowed whole, never crushed or chewed. Take the chewable tablets (child or adult dose) with at least 8 oz (a full glass; 240 mL) of water or other fluid. Taking this product without enough liquid may cause choking.

➤*Maintenance/Extended treatment:* Discontinue periodically to assess condition. Improvement may be sustained when the drug is

METHYLPHENIDATE HCl

either temporarily or permanently discontinued. Drug treatment should not and need not be indefinite and usually may be discontinued after puberty.

➤*Dose reduction and discontinuation:* If paradoxical aggravation of symptoms or other adverse events occur, reduce dosage or discontinue the drug.

If improvement is not observed after appropriate dosage adjustment over a 1-month period, discontinue the drug.

➤*Concerta:* Administer orally once daily in the morning with or without food. Advise patients to swallow the capsules whole with the aid of liquids, and not chew, divide, or crush them. Individualize dosage. The medication is contained within a nonabsorbable shell designed to release the drug at a controlled rate. The tablet shell, along with insoluble core components, is eliminated from the body; patients should not be concerned if they occasionally notice in their stool something that looks like a tablet.

Patients new to methylphenidate – The recommended starting dose for patients who are not currently taking methylphenidate or for patients who are on stimulants other than methylphenidate is 18 mg once daily. Dosage may be adjusted at weekly intervals to a maximum of 54 mg/day taken once daily in the morning.

Patients currently using methylphenidate – The recommended dose for patients currently taking methylphenidate twice daily, 3 times/day, or SR doses of 10 to 60 mg/day is provided in the following table. Dosing recommendations are based on current dose regimen and clinical judgment.

Dosage may be adjusted at weekly intervals to a maximum of 54 mg/day taken once daily in the morning.

Recommended Dose Conversion from Methylphenidate Regimens to *Concerta*	
Previous methylphenidate daily dose	Recommended *Concerta* dose
5 mg methylphenidate twice daily or 5 mg methylphenidate 3 times daily or 20 mg methylphenidate SR	18 mg every morning
10 mg methylphenidate twice daily or 10 mg methylphenidate 3 times daily or 40 mg methylphenidate SR	36 mg every morning
15 mg methylphenidate twice daily or 15 mg methylphenidate 3 times daily or 60 mg methylphenidate SR	54 mg every morning

A 27 mg dosage strength is available for physicians who wish to prescribe between the 18 and 36 mg dosages. In other methylphenidate regimens, use clinical judgment when selecting the starting dose. Daily dosage above 54 mg is not recommended.

➤*Metadate CD:* Administer once daily in the morning before breakfast. The capsules may be swallowed whole with the aid of liquids, or alternatively, the capsule may be opened and the capsule contents sprinkled onto a small amount (tablespoon) of applesauce and given immediately; do not store for future use. Drinking some fluids (eg, water) should follow the intake of the sprinkles with applesauce. The capsules and the capsule contents must not be crushed or chewed.

Sprinkle administration – Sprinkle onto a small amount of soft food (eg, applesauce). The entire capsule contents must be used as a single 20 mg dose. The dose cannot be split because the immediate-release and extended (continuous)-release beads (which comprise the capsule at a ratio of 30%:70% of the total dose, respectively), cannot be physically distinguished from one another. Administer the dose immediately after sprinkling. Do not store for future use. The beads contained within the capsules must not be crushed or chewed.

Initial treatment – 20 mg once daily. Adjust dosage in weekly 20 mg increments to a maximum of 60 mg/day taken once daily in the morning, depending upon tolerability and degree of efficacy. Daily dosage above 60 mg is not recommended.

➤*Ritalin LA:* Individualize dosage.

Initial treatment – The recommended starting dose is 20 mg once daily. Dosage may be adjusted in weekly 10 mg increments to a maximum of 60 mg/day taken once daily in the morning, depending on tolerability and degree of efficacy observed. Daily dosage above 60 mg is not recommended. When a lower initial dose is appropriate, patients may begin treatment with an immediate-release methylphenidate product at a lower dose. After titration to 10 mg twice daily, these patients may be switched to *Ritalin LA* according to the guidelines in the table below.

Patients currently using methylphenidate – The recommended dose for patients currently taking methylphenidate twice daily or SR is provided below. Dosing recommendations are based on current dose regimen and clinical judgment.

Ritalin LA Dosing Regimens in Current Methylphenidate Users	
Previous methylphenidate dose	Recommended *Ritalin LA* dose
10 mg bid or 20 mg methylphenidate SR	20 mg qd
15 mg methylphenidate bid	30 mg qd

Ritalin LA Dosing Regimens in Current Methylphenidate Users	
Previous methylphenidate dose	Recommended *Ritalin LA* dose
20 mg bid or 40 mg methylphenidate SR	40 mg qd
30 mg bid or 60 mg methylphenidate SR	60 mg qd

➤*Storage/Stability:* Keep out of reach of children.

Ritalin – Do not store above 30°C (86°F). Protect from light. Dispense in tight, light-resistant container.

Concerta, Metadate CD, and Ritalin LA – Store at 25°C (77°F); excursions permitted to 15° to 30°C (59° to 86°F). Protect from humidity. Store in tight container.

Metadate ER, Methylin, and Methylin ER – Store at room temperature, 15° to 30°C (59° to 86°F). Protect from moisture and light. Dispense in a tight, light-resistant container.

Actions

➤*Pharmacology:* A mild CNS stimulant with actions similar to the amphetamines. The exact mechanism of action is not fully understood but presumably activates the brain stem arousal system and cortex to produce its stimulant effect.

➤*Pharmacokinetics:* Methylphenidate is rapidly and well absorbed from the GI tract. Peak plasma levels occur in children in 4.7 hours for the SR tablets, 1 to 2 hours for the chewable tablets, and 1.9 hours for the regular tablets. The mean plasma half-life for methylphenidate HCl tablets and chewable tablets and *Concerta* tablets is approximately 3 to 3.5 hours. Plasma half-life for *Metadate CD* is reportedly 6.8 hours. About 80% of a dose is metabolized to ritalinic acid and excreted in urine. In adult patients who received SR and ER tablets, plasma concentrations of methylphenidate's major metabolite appear to be greater in females than in males. SR and ER tablets are more slowly but as extensively absorbed as regular tablets. Relative bioavailability of SR and ER tablets compared with the regular tablet was 105% in children and 101% in adults. In children, an average of 67% of an SR tablet dose was excreted vs 86% in adults.

The administration of the ER methylphenidate tablets with food resulted in a greater C_{max} and $AUC_{0\to\infty}$ than when administered in a fasting condition. The presence of food delayed the peak concentrations of the chewable tablets by approximately 1 hour (1.5 hours fasted and 2.4 hours fed). Overall, a high-fat meal increased the AUC of the chewable tablets by about 20% on average.

Pharmacokinetic and statistical analyses for a multiple-dose study demonstrated that TID administration of 2 *Metadate* 10 mg ER tablets met the requirements for bioequivalence to 1 methylphenidate SR 20 mg tablet when given every 8 hours. Pharmacokinetic parameters (ie, $AUC_{0\to\infty}$, T_{max}, C_{max}, C_{min}, C_{av}) demonstrated achievement of steady state following TID administration of 2 *Metadate* 10 mg ER tablets.

Contraindications

Marked anxiety, tension, and agitation because the drug may aggravate these symptoms; hypersensitivity to methylphenidate or other components of the product; glaucoma; motor tics or a family history or diagnosis of Tourette syndrome.

➤*Ritalin, Ritalin SR, Concerta, Metadate CD, Ritalin LA, Methylin chewable:* Concurrent treatment with monoamine oxidase inhibitors (MAOIs) and within a minimum of 14 days following discontinuation of an MAOI (hypertensive crisis may result).

Warnings

➤*Seizure disorders:* Methylphenidate may lower the convulsive threshold in patients with a history of seizures, with prior EEG abnormalities in absence of seizures and, very rarely, in the absence of history of seizures and no prior EEG evidence of seizures. Safe concomitant use with anticonvulsants has not been established. If seizures occur, discontinue the drug.

➤*GI obstruction:* Because the *Concerta* tablet is nondeformable and does not appreciably change in shape in the GI tract, do not administer to patients with pre-existing severe GI narrowing (pathologic or iatrogenic; eg, esophageal motility disorders, small bowel inflammatory disease, "short gut" syndrome because of adhesions or decreased transit time, past history of peritonitis, cystic fibrosis, chronic intestinal pseudo-obstruction, or Meckel's diverticulum). There have been rare reports of obstructive symptoms in patients with known strictures in association with the ingestion of other drugs in nondeformable controlled-release formulations. Because of the controlled-release design of the tablet, only use *Concerta* in patients who are able to swallow the tablet whole.

➤*Hypertension:* Use cautiously; monitor blood pressure in all patients, especially those with hypertension. Studies of methylphenidate have shown modest increases of resting pulse and systolic and diastolic blood pressure. Therefore, caution is indicated in treating patients whose underlying medical conditions might be compromised by increases in blood pressure or heart rate (eg, those with pre-existing hypertension, heart failure, recent MI, or hyperthyroidism).

➤*Severe depression:* Do not use methylphenidate for severe depression of either exogenous or endogenous origin.

METHYLPHENIDATE HCl

➤*Fatigue:* Do not use methylphenidate for the prevention or treatment of normal fatigue states.

➤*Long-term suppression of growth:* Suppression of growth has been reported with long-term use in children. Interrupt treatment for patients who are not growing or gaining weight as expected.

➤*Psychosis:* Methylphenidate may exacerbate symptoms of behavior disturbances and thought disorder.

➤*Visual disturbances:* Visual disturbances have occurred rarely. Difficulties with accommodation and blurring of vision have occurred.

➤*Carcinogenesis:* In a lifetime carcinogenicity study of mice, methylphenidate caused an increase in hepatocellular adenomas and, in males only, an increase in hepatoblastomas, at a daily dose of approximately 60 mg/kg/day. This dose is approximately 30 times the maximum recommended human dose on a mg/kg basis.

➤*Pregnancy: Category C.* Until more information is available, methylphenidate should not be prescribed for women of childbearing age unless, in the opinion of the physician, the potential benefits outweigh the possible risks. In the small numbers of patients reported who received methylphenidate during their pregnancy, no evidence of increased malformation rate was found. However, in a recently conducted study, methylphenidate has been shown to have teratogenic effects in rabbits when given in doses of 200 mg/kg/day, which is approximately 167 times and 78 times the maximum recommended human dose on a mg/kg and a mg/m^2 basis, respectively.

➤*Lactation:* It is not known whether methylphenidate is excreted in human milk. Because many drugs are excreted in human milk, exercise caution if methylphenidate is administered to a nursing woman.

➤*Children:* Do not use in children under 6 years of age because safety and efficacy have not been established. In psychotic children, the drug may exacerbate symptoms of behavior disturbance and thought disorder.

Safety and efficacy of long-term use in children are not established. Although a causal relationship has not been established, suppression of growth (eg, weight gain or height) has been reported with long-term use of stimulants in children. Carefully monitor patients on long-term therapy.

Precautions

➤*Monitoring:* Perform periodic CBC, differential, and platelet counts during prolonged therapy.

➤*Phenylketonurics:* Each 2.5 mg chewable tablet contains 0.42 mg phenylalanine; each 5 mg chewable tablet contains 0.84 mg phenylalanine; and each 10 mg chewable tablet contains 1.68 mg phenylalanine.

➤*Agitation:* Patients with an element of agitation may react adversely; discontinue therapy if necessary.

➤*Prescribing:* Drug treatment is not indicated in all cases of this behavioral syndrome; consider only in light of the complete history and evaluation of the child. The decision to prescribe methylphenidate should depend on the physician's assessment of the chronicity and severity of the child's symptoms and their appropriateness for his or her age. Prescription should not depend solely on the presence of 1 or more of the behavioral characteristics.

➤*Acute stress:* When symptoms are associated with acute stress reactions, treatment with methylphenidate usually is not indicated.

➤*Drug abuse and dependence:* Give cautiously to emotionally unstable patients (eg, those with a history of drug dependence or alcoholism), because they may increase dosage on their own initiative.

Chronic abuse can lead to marked tolerance and psychic dependence with varying degrees of abnormal behavior. Frank psychotic episodes can occur, especially with parenteral abuse. Careful supervision is required during drug withdrawal because severe depression, as well as the effects of chronic overactivity, can be unmasked. Long-term follow-up may be required because of the patient's basic personality disturbances.

Drug Interactions

Methylphenidate Drug Interactions			
Precipitant drug	Object drug*		Description
Methylphenidate	Anticonvulsants (eg, phenytoin, phenobarbital, primidone)	↑	Anticonvulsant levels may be increased, resulting in increased pharmacologic and toxic effects of the anticonvulsant.
Methylphenidate	Coumarin anticoagulants	↑	Human pharmacologic studies have shown that methylphenidate may inhibit the metabolism of coumarin anticoagulants.
Methylphenidate	Guanethidine	↓	Antihypertensive effect of guanethidine may be decreased by concurrent methylphenidate. Arrhythmias were reported in 1 case. Antiarrhythmics may be needed.

Methylphenidate Drug Interactions			
Precipitant drug	Object drug*		Description
Methylphenidate	Tricyclic antidepressants	↑	Coadministration may cause increased serum concentration of tricyclic antidepressants.
Methylphenidate	Selective serotonin reuptake inhibitors (SSRIs)	↑	Coadministration may cause an increased serum concentration of the SSRIs.
MAOIs	Methylphenidate	↑	Hypertensive crisis may result with coadministration. Monitor blood pressure during combined MAOI and methylphenidate use. This combination is contraindicated with *Ritalin, Ritalin SR, Metadate CD, Concerta,* and *Ritalin LA.*

* ↓ = Object drug decreased. ↑ = Object drug increased.

Adverse Reactions

➤*Methylphenidate (Ritalin, Ritalin SR, Metadate ER, Methylin, Methylin ER):*

Cardiovascular – Blood pressure and pulse changes, increased and decreased; tachycardia; angina; cardiac arrhythmias; palpitations.

CNS – Dizziness; headache; dyskinesia; drowsiness; Tourette syndrome (rare); toxic psychosis.

GI – Anorexia; nausea; abdominal pain; weight loss during prolonged therapy.

Hypersensitivity – Skin rash; urticaria; fever; arthralgia; exfoliative dermatitis; erythema multiforme with histopathological findings of necrotizing vasculitis; thrombocytopenic purpura.

Miscellaneous –

Most common: Nervousness and insomnia, usually controlled by reducing dosage and omitting the drug in the afternoon or evening.

Children: Loss of appetite, abdominal pain, weight loss during prolonged therapy, insomnia, and tachycardia may occur more frequently; however, any of the other adverse reactions listed above also may occur.

Other (causal relationship not established): Leukopenia and/or anemia; scalp hair loss; abnormal liver function, ranging from transaminase elevation to hepatic coma; cerebral arteritis and/or occlusion; transient depressed mood; neuroleptic malignant syndrome (very rare).

➤*Methylphenidate HCl extended-release tablets (Concerta):*

Discontinuation: Events associated with discontinuation in more than 1 patient included the following: Twitching (tics, 1.8%), anorexia (loss of appetite, 0.9%), aggravation reaction (0.7%), hostility (0.7%), insomnia (0.7%), somnolence (0.5%).

Other adverse events:

Concerta Adverse Reactions (%)		
Adverse event	Concerta (n = 106)	Placebo (n = 99)
CNS		
Dizziness	2	0
Insomnia	4	1
GI		
Vomiting	4	3
Anorexia (loss of appetite)	4	0
Respiratory		
Upper respiratory tract infection	8	5
Cough increased	4	2
Pharyngitis	4	3
Sinusitis	3	0
Miscellaneous		
Headache	14	10
Abdominal pain (stomachache)	7	1

In a long-term, uncontrolled study (407 children), the cumulative incidence of new onset of tics was 8% after 10 months of *Concerta* treatment.

➤*Methylphenidate HCl extended-release capsules:*
Metadate CD:

Metadate CD Adverse Reactions (%)		
Adverse event	Metadate CD (n = 188)	Placebo (n = 190)
Headache	12	8
Abdominal pain (stomachache)	7	4
Anorexia (appetite loss)	9	2
Insomnia	5	2

Ritalin LA:
• *Discontinuation* – Events associated with discontinuation in at least 1 patient included the following: Anger, hypomania, anxiety, depressed mood, fatigue, migraine, lethargy.

METHYLPHENIDATE HCl

• *Other adverse events* – Events with incidence greater than 5% included headache, insomnia, upper abdominal pain, decreased appetite, and anorexia; insomnia (3.1%).

Overdosage

➤*Symptoms:* Symptoms result principally from CNS overstimulation and excessive sympathomimetic effects and include the following: Vomiting; agitation; tremors; hyperreflexia; muscle twitching; convulsions (may be followed by coma); euphoria; confusion; hallucinations; delirium; sweating; flushing; headache; hyperpyrexia; tachycardia; palpitations; cardiac arrhythmias; hypertension; mydriasis; dry mucous membranes.

➤*Treatment:* Treatment consists of supportive measures. Protect the patient against self-injury and against external stimuli that would aggravate overstimulation. Gastric contents may be evacuated by gastric lavage. In severe intoxication, use a carefully titrated dosage of a short-acting barbiturate before gastric lavage. Other measures to detoxify the gut include administration of activated charcoal and a cathartic. Maintain adequate circulation and respiratory exchange; external cooling procedures may be required for hyperpyrexia. Efficacy of peritoneal dialysis or extracorporeal hemodialysis has not been established, but benefit is unlikely because of methylphenidate's large volume of distribution.

Consider the prolonged release of methylphenidate from *Metadate CD*, *Ritalin LA*, and *Concerta* when treating overdose. Consider the possibility of multiple drug ingestion. The physician may consider contacting a poison control center for up-to-date information on the management of overdosage with methylphenidate.

Patient Information

➤*Ritalin, Methylin:* Take last daily dose early in the evening (prior to 6 p.m.) to avoid insomnia. It is often recommended that methylphenidate be taken 30 to 45 minutes before meals.

➤*Metadate CD:* Instruct patient to take 1 dose in the morning before breakfast. Also instruct patient that the capsule may be swallowed whole or, alternatively, the capsule may be opened and the contents sprinkled onto a small amount (tablespoon) of applesauce and given immediately, and not stored for future use. The capsules and the capsule contents must not be crushed or chewed.

Discuss the information and instructions provided in the patient information leaflet with the patient.

➤*Ritalin LA:* Administer once daily in the morning. Capsules may be swallowed whole or opened and contents sprinkled onto a spoonful of cool applesauce and consumed immediately in its entirety. Capsules or contents should not be crushed, chewed, or divided.

➤*Chewable tablets:*

Choking – Taking the chewable tablets without adequate fluid may cause the tablets to swell and block your throat or esophagus and may cause choking. Do not take this product if you have difficulty in swallowing. If you experience chest pain, vomiting, or difficulty in swallowing or breathing after taking this product, seek immediate medical attention.

Directions – Take this product (child or adult dose) with at least 8 oz (a full glass; 240 mL) of water or other fluid. Taking this product without enough liquid may cause choking.

Phenylketonurics – These tablets contain phenylalanine.

PEMOLINE

c-iv	**Pemoline** (Apothecon, Mallinckrodt)	**Tablets:** 18.75 mg		Lactose. In 100s.
c-iv	**Cylert** (Abbott)			Lactose. (TH). White, scored. In 100s.
c-iv	**Pemoline** (Apothecon, Mallinckrodt)	**Tablets:** 37.5 mg		Lactose. In 100s.
c-iv	**Cylert** (Abbott)			Lactose. (TI). Orange, scored. In 100s.
c-iv	**Pemoline** (Apothecon, Mallinckrodt)	**Tablets:** 75 mg		Lactose. In 100s.
c-iv	**Cylert** (Abbott)			Lactose. (TJ). Tan, scored. In 100s.
c-iv	**Cylert** (Abbott)	**Tablets, chewable:** 37.5 mg		Mannitol. (TK). Orange, scored. In 100s.
c-iv	**PemADD CT** (Mallinckrodt)			(A 186). Peach, square, scored. In 100s.

WARNING

Because of its association with life-threatening hepatic failure, pemoline should not ordinarily be considered as first-line drug therapy for attention deficit hyperactivity disorder (ADHD). Because pemoline provides an observable symptomatic benefit, patients who fail to show substantial clinical benefit within 3 weeks of completing dose titration should be withdrawn from therapy.

Since pemoline's marketing in 1975, 15 cases of acute hepatic failure have been reported to the FDA. While the absolute number of reported cases is not large, the rate of reporting ranges from 4 to 17 times the rate expected in the general population. This estimate may be conservative because of underreporting and because the long latency between initiation of pemoline treatment and the occurrence of hepatic failure may limit recognition of the association. If only a portion of actual cases were recognized and reported, the risk could be substantially higher.

Of the 15 cases reported as of December 1998, 12 resulted in death or liver transplantation, usually within 4 weeks of the onset of signs and symptoms of liver failure. The earliest onset of hepatic abnormalities occurred 6 months after initiation of pemoline. Although some reports described dark urine and nonspecific prodromal symptoms (eg, anorexia, malaise, GI symptoms), in other reports it was not clear if any prodromol symptoms preceded the onset of jaundice.

Initiate treatment only in individuals without liver disease and with normal baseline liver function tests. It is not clear if baseline and periodic liver function testing are predictive of these instances of acute liver failure; however, it is believed that early detection of drug-induced hepatic injury along with immediate withdrawal of the suspect drug enhances the likelihood for recovery. Accordingly, the following liver monitoring program is recommended: Determine serum ALT levels at baseline and every 2 weeks thereafter. If pemoline therapy is discontinued and then restarted, perform liver function test monitoring at baseline and reinitiate at the frequency above.

Discontinue pemoline if serum ALT is increased to a clinically significant level or any increase ≥ 2 times the upper limit of normal, or if clinical signs and symptoms suggest liver failure.

The physician should obtain written informed consent from the patient prior to initiation of pemoline therapy.

Indications

➤*ADHD:* As part of a total treatment program in children with a behavioral syndrome characterized by moderate to severe distractibility, short attention span, hyperactivity, emotional lability, and impulsivity.

➤*Unlabeled uses:* Pemoline has been used in the treatment of narcolepsy, fatigue, and excessive daytime sleepiness.

Administration and Dosage

Administer as a single dose each morning. Recommended starting dose is 37.5 mg/day. Gradually increase at 1-week intervals using increments of 18.75 mg until desired response is obtained. Mean effective doses range from 56.25 to 75 mg/day. Maximum recommended dose is 112.5 mg/day.

Clinical improvement is gradual; significant benefit may not be evident until week 3 or 4 of administration.

Interrupt drug administration occasionally to determine if there is a recurrence of behavioral symptoms sufficient to require continued therapy.

Actions

➤*Pharmacology:* Pemoline is a CNS stimulant. Although structurally dissimilar from the amphetamines and methylphenidate, it has pharmacologic activity similar to that of other stimulants but with minimal sympathomimetic effects. Although the exact mechanism of action is unknown, pemoline may act through dopaminergic mechanisms.

➤*Pharmacokinetics:* Pemoline is rapidly absorbed from the GI tract. About 50% is protein bound. Peak serum levels occur within 2 to 4 hours after ingestion of a single dose. Serum half-life is ≈ 12 hours. Steady state is reached in ≈ 2 to 3 days. The drug is widely distributed throughout body tissues, including the brain. Pemoline is metabolized by the liver and is primarily excreted by the kidneys. About 50% is excreted unchanged; only minor fractions are present as metabolites.

Pemoline has a gradual onset of action. Using the recommended schedule of dosage titration, significant clinical benefit may not be evident until the third or fourth week of drug administration.

Contraindications

Hypersensitivity or idiosyncrasy to pemoline; hepatic insufficiency.

Warnings

➤*Renal function impairment:* Administer with caution to patients with significantly impaired renal function.

➤*Pregnancy:* Category B. There are no adequate and well-controlled studies in pregnant women. Use pemoline during pregnancy only if clearly needed. Studies in rats have shown an increased incidence of

PEMOLINE

stillbirths and cannibalization when pemoline was administered at a dose of 37.5 mg/kg/day. Postnatal survival was reduced at doses of 18.75 and 37.5 mg/kg/day.

➤*Lactation:* It is not known whether pemoline is excreted in breast milk. Exercise caution when administering pemoline to a nursing woman.

➤*Children:* Safety and efficacy in children < 6 years of age have not been established.

In psychotic children, administration may exacerbate symptoms of behavior disturbance and thought disorder. CNS stimulants, including pemoline, can precipitate motor and phonic tics and Tourette's syndrome. Therefore, clinical evaluation for tics and Tourette's syndrome in children and their families should precede use of stimulants.

Chronic administration may be associated with growth inhibition; therefore, monitor growth during treatment. Long-term effects in children have not been well established.

Treatment is not indicated in all cases of ADHD; consider therapy only in light of complete history and evaluation of the child. The decision to prescribe pemoline should depend on the assessment of the chronicity and severity of the child's symptoms and their appropriateness for his or her age, and not depend solely on the presence of ≥ 1 of the behavioral characteristics.

Precautions

➤*Hepatic effects:* Determine serum ALT levels at baseline, and every 2 weeks thereafter. If pemoline therapy is discontinued and then restarted, monitor liver function tests at baseline and reinitiate at the frequency above. Discontinue pemoline if serum ALT is increased to clinically significant levels or any increase ≥ 2 times the upper limit of normal, or if clinical signs and symptoms suggest liver failure.

➤*Drug abuse and dependence:* The pharmacologic similarity of pemoline to other psychostimulants with known dependence liability suggests that psychological or physical dependence might occur. There have been isolated reports of transient psychotic symptoms in adults after the long-term misuse of excessive oral doses. Give with caution to emotionally unstable patients who may increase the dosage on their own initiative.

Drug Interactions

Carefully monitor patients receiving pemoline with other drugs, especially drugs with CNS activity.

Decreased seizure threshold has been reported in patients receiving pemoline concomitantly with antiepileptic medications.

Adverse Reactions

If adverse reactions are significant or protracted, reduce dosage or discontinue drug.

Most frequent – Insomnia usually occurs early in therapy prior to optimum therapeutic response; it is often transient or responds to dosage reduction.

➤*CNS:* Convulsive seizures; Tourette's syndrome; hallucinations; dyskinetic movements of tongue, lips, face, and extremities; abnormal oculomotor function (eg, nystagmus, oculogyric crisis); mild depression; dizziness; increased irritability; headache; drowsiness.

➤*GI:* Anorexia with weight loss may occur during the first weeks. In most cases it is transient; weight gain usually resumes within 3 to 6 months; stomachache; nausea.

➤*GU:* A case of elevated acid phosphatase in association with prostatic enlargement occurred in a 63-year-old male who received pemoline for sleepiness. The acid phosphatase normalized with discontinuation of pemoline and was again elevated with rechallenge.

➤*Hepatic:* Hepatic dysfunction including elevated liver enzymes, hepatitis, jaundice, and fatal hepatic failure has occurred. Elevated liver enzymes are not rare and appear reversible upon drug discontinuance. Most patients with elevated liver enzymes were asymptomatic.

➤*Miscellaneous:* Growth suppression with long-term use of stimulants in children; skin rashes; aplastic anemia (rare).

Overdosage

➤*Symptoms:* Symptoms of acute overdosage result principally from CNS overstimulation and excessive sympathomimetic effects and include the following: Vomiting; agitation; tremors; hyperreflexia; muscle twitching; convulsions (may be followed by coma); euphoria; confusion; hallucinations; delirium; sweating; flushing; headache; hyperpyrexia; tachycardia; hypertension; mydriasis.

Other – Amphetamine toxicity includes euphoria, restlessness, excessive speech and motor activity, tremor, and insomnia; severe choreoathetosis with rhabdomyolysis have occurred.

➤*Treatment:* Treatment consists of appropriate supportive measures. Protect the patient against self-injury and external stimuli that would aggravate overstimulation already present. Gastric contents may be evacuated. Chlorpromazine is reported useful in decreasing CNS stimulation and sympathomimetic effects.

Efficacy of peritoneal dialysis or extracorporeal hemodialysis for pemoline overdosage is not established.

Patient Information

Advise patients to follow their doctors instructions for liver function tests prior to and during pemoline therapy.

Advise patients to be alert for signs and symptoms of liver dysfunction (eg, jaundice, anorexia, GI complaints, malaise) and to report them to their doctor immediately should they occur.

The physician prescribing pemoline should obtain written informed consent from patients prior to initiation of pemoline therapy.

Take daily dose in the morning.

Notify physician if insomnia occurs and persists.

Anorexiants

Indications

In addition to the nonamphetamine anorexiants included in this section, amphetamines are also used for short-term obesity therapy.

➤*Exogenous obesity:* As a short-term adjunct in a regimen of weight reduction based on caloric restriction. Measure the limited usefulness of these agents against their inherent risks. Refer to individual monographs for extended indications.

Actions

➤*Pharmacology:* Adrenergic agents (eg, **diethylpropion**, **benzphetamine**, **phendimetrazine**, **phentermine**) act by modulating central norepinephrine and dopamine receptors through the promotion of catecholamine release. Aside from phentermine, other adrenergic agents are infrequently used, perhaps because of the lack of long-term, well-controlled data or the fear of their potential abuse. Older adrenergic weight-loss drugs (eg, amphetamine, methamphetamine, phenmetrazine), which strongly engage in dopamine pathways, are no longer recommended because of the risk of their abuse.

➤*Pharmacokinetics:*

Distribution – **Diethylpropion** is rapidly absorbed from the GI tract after oral administration and is extensively metabolized through a complex pathway of biotransformation involving N-dealkylation and reduction. Many of these metabolites are biologically active and may participate in the therapeutic action of diethylpropion. Diethylpropion and its active metabolites are believed to cross the blood-brain barrier and the placenta, and are excreted mainly by the kidneys with 75% to 106% of the dose recovered in the urine within 48 hours after dosing. The plasma half-life of the aminoketone metabolites is ≈ 4 to 6 hours.

Excretion – Most of the drugs and their metabolites are excreted via the kidneys. The average half-lives for **phendimetrazine** are ≈ 1.9 hours for *Bontril PDM*, 9.8 hours for *Bontril*, and 3.7 hours for *Prelu-2*.

➤*Clinical trials:* Short-term clinical trials report greater weight loss in adult obese subjects treated with dietary management and anorexiants vs those treated with diet and placebo. The rate of weight loss is greatest in the first weeks of therapy and decreases in succeeding weeks. The amount of weight loss varies from trial to trial, and appears to be related, in part, to variables other than the drug prescribed, such as the investigator, the population treated, and the diet prescribed.

Because the longest reported trial involving **phentermine** was 36 weeks, the drug is indicated only for short-term treatment of obesity. Phentermine therapy should be limited to patients with a BMI of > 30 kg/m^2, or > 27 kg/m^2 if comorbidities exist.

Contraindications

Advanced arteriosclerosis; symptomatic cardiovascular disease; moderate-to-severe hypertension; hyperthyroidism; known hypersensitivity or idiosyncrasy to sympathomimetic amines; glaucoma; highly nervous or agitated states; history of drug abuse; during or within 14 days following the administration of MAO inhibitors (hypertensive crises may result); coadministration with other CNS stimulants.

➤*Pregnancy: Category X.* **Benzphetamine HCl** is contraindicated during pregnancy (see Warnings).

Warnings

➤*Tolerance:* Tolerance to the anorectic effects may develop within a few weeks. If tolerance to the anorectic effect develops, do not exceed the recommended dose in an attempt to increase the effect; rather, discontinue the drug.

➤*Other drugs:* These agents should not be used in combination with other anorectic agents, including prescribed drugs (eg, SSRIs [eg, fluoxetine, sertraline, fluvoxamine, paroxetine]), *otc* preparations, and herbal products. When using CNS-active agents, consider the possibility of adverse interactions with alcohol.

➤*Primary pulmonary hypertension (PPH):* PPH, a rare, frequently fatal disease of the lungs, has been reported to occur in patients receiving certain anorectic agents. The initial symptom of PPH is usually dyspnea. Other initial symptoms include the following: Angina pectoris, syncope, or lower extremity edema. Advise patients to report immediately any deterioration in exercise tolerance. Discontinue treatment in patients who develop new, unexplained symptoms of dyspnea, angina pectoris, syncope, or lower extremity edema.

➤*Valvular heart disease:* Serious regurgitant cardiac valvular disease, primarily affecting the mitral, aortic, or tricuspid valves, has been reported in otherwise healthy people who had taken certain anorectic agents in combination for weight loss. The etiology of these valvulopathies has not been established and their course in individuals after the drugs are stopped is not known.

➤*Pregnancy:* (*Category X* - Benzphetamine HCl. *Category B* - Diethylpropion. *Category C* - Phentermine, phendimetrazine). Safety for use during pregnancy has not been established. Use in women who are or who may become pregnant (especially those in the first trimester) only when clearly needed and when the potential benefits outweigh the potential hazards to the fetus.

In animal studies with **phendimetrazine**, conception rate was adversely affected, as well as survival and body weight of pups. Congenital malformations are associated with phendimetrazine use, but a causal relationship has not been proven. Animal and clinical studies have not shown a teratogenic potential for **diethylpropion**. Abuse of diethylpropion during pregnancy may result in withdrawal symptoms in the human neonate.

➤*Lactation:* Safety for use in the nursing mother has not been established. Amphetamines are excreted in human milk. Advise mothers taking amphetamines to refrain from nursing.

Diethylpropion and its metabolites are excreted in breast milk. Exercise caution when administering to a nursing woman.

➤*Children:* **Phendimetrazine** and **benzphetamine** are not recommended for use in children < 12 years of age. **Diethylpropion** is not recommended for use in pediatric patients < 16 years of age.

Phentermine – Safety and efficacy have not been established for *Adipex-P. Pro-Fast SA, ProFast HS,* and *Pro-Fast SR* are not recommended in patients < 12 years of age. *Ionamin* is not recommended in children < 16 years of age.

Precautions

➤*Psychological disturbances:* Psychological disturbances occurred in patients who received an anorectic agent together with a restrictive diet.

➤*Cardiovascular disease:* Exercise caution in prescribing amphetamines for patients with even mild hypertension.

➤*Dispensing:* The least amount feasible should be prescribed or dispensed at one time in order to minimize the possibility of overdosage.

➤*Convulsions:* Convulsions may increase in some epileptics receiving **diethylpropion**. Dose titration or drug discontinuance may be necessary.

➤*Diabetes:* Insulin requirements in diabetes mellitus may be altered in association with the use of anorexigenic drugs and the concomitant dietary restrictions.

➤*Drug abuse and dependence:* These drugs are chemically and pharmacologically related to the amphetamines, and have abuse potential. Intense psychological dependence and severe social dysfunction may occur. If this occurs, gradually reduce the dosage to avoid withdrawal symptoms (eg, extreme fatigue, sleep EEG changes, mental depression). Chronic intoxication is manifested by severe dermatoses, marked insomnia, irritability, hyperactivity, and personality changes. Psychosis, often clinically indistinguishable from schizophrenia, is the most severe manifestation.

➤*Hazardous tasks:* May produce dizziness, extreme fatigue, and depression after abrupt cessation of prolonged high-dosage therapy; patients should observe caution while driving or performing other tasks requiring alertness.

➤*Tartrazine sensitivity:* Some of these products contain tartrazine, which may cause allergic-type reactions (including bronchial asthma) in susceptible individuals. Although the incidence of tartrazine sensitivity in the general population is low, it is frequently seen in patients who also have aspirin hypersensitivity. Specific products containing tartrazine are identified in the product listings.

Drug Interactions

Phentermine may decrease the hypotensive effect of adrenergic neuron blocking drugs.

Anorexiant Drug Interactions			
Precipitant drug	Object drug*		Description
Furazolidone	Anorexiants	↑	MAO inhibitors may increase the pressor response to the anorexiants. Possible hypertensive crisis and intracranial hemorrhage may occur. This interaction may also occur with **furazolidone**, an antimicrobial with MAO inhibitor activity. Avoid this combination.
MAO inhibitors			
Selective serotonin reuptake inhibitors (SSRIs)	Anorexiants	↑	Increased sensitivity to effect of sympathomimetics and increased risk of "serotonin syndrome" may occur. Monitor patient for increased signs/symptoms of CNS effects.
Anorexiants	Guanethidine	↓	Anorexiants may decrease the hypotensive effect of guanethidine.
Anorexiants	Tricyclic antidepressants	↑	Amphetamines may enhance the effects of tricyclic antidepressants.

* ↑ = Object drug increased. ↓ = Object drug decreased.

Adverse Reactions

➤*Cardiovascular:* Palpitations; tachycardia; arrhythmias (including ventricular); precordial pain; primary pulmonary hypertension or regurgitant cardiac valvular disease; elevation of blood pressure. ECG changes have been reported with **diethylpropion**; valvulopathy has been reported with diethylpropion very rarely, but the causal relationship is unknown. Isolated reports of cardiomyopathy have been associated with chronic amphetamine use.

➤*CNS:* Overstimulation; cerebrovascular accident; nervousness; restlessness; dizziness; insomnia; malaise; anxiety; euphoria; drowsiness; depression; agitation; dysphoria; dyskinesia; tremor; headache; psychotic episodes (rare); agitation; jitteriness; depression following withdrawal of the drug. An increase in convulsive episodes occurred in a few epileptics.

➤*GI:* Dry mouth; unpleasant taste; nausea; vomiting; abdominal discomfort; diarrhea; GI disturbances; constipation; stomach pain.

➤*GU:* Dysuria; polyuria; urinary frequency; impotence; menstrual upset; gynecomastia; changes in libido.

➤*Hematologic:* Bone marrow depression; agranulocytosis; leukopenia.

➤*Hypersensitivity:* Urticaria; rash; erythema.

➤*Ophthalmic:* Mydriasis; blurred vision.

➤*Miscellaneous:* Hair loss; muscle pain; excessive sweating; ecchymosis; flushing; dyspnea.

Overdosage

➤*Symptoms:*

CNS – Restlessness; tremor; tachypnea; hyperreflexia; hyperpyrexia; rhabdomyolysis; confusion; belligerence; assaultiveness; hallucinations; panic states. Depression and fatigue usually follow central stimulation.

Convulsions, coma, and death may result.

Cardiovascular – Arrhythmias (tachycardia); hypertension or hypotension; circulatory collapse.

GI – Nausea; vomiting; diarrhea; abdominal cramps.

➤*Treatment:* Includes symptomatic and supportive therapy. Refer to Management of Acute Overdosage.

Sedate patient with a barbiturate or another sedative, and employ gastric lavage. Give activated charcoal if ingestion was recent.

Experience with hemodialysis or peritoneal dialysis is inadequate to permit recommendations.

Patient Information

May cause insomnia; avoid taking medication late in the day.

Caution patients about concomitant use of alcohol or other CNS-active drugs and anorectic agents.

Weight reduction requires strict adherence to dietary restriction.

Do not take more frequently than prescribed.

Notify physician if palpitations, nervousness, or dizziness occurs.

Medication may cause dry mouth and constipation; notify physician if these become pronounced.

May produce dizziness or blurred vision; observe caution while driving or performing other tasks requiring alertness.

These drugs should generally be taken on an empty stomach.

Do not crush or chew sustained-release products.

BENZPHETAMINE HCl

c-iii	**Didrex** (Pharmacia)	**Tablets:** 50 mg	Lactose, sorbitol. (DIDREX 50). Peach, scored. In 100s and 500s.

Complete prescribing information begins in the Anorexiants group monograph.

Indications

➤*Obesity:* For the management of exogenous obesity as a short-term adjunct (a few weeks) in a regimen of weight reduction based on caloric restriction. Weigh the limited usefulness of agents of this class against possible risks inherent in their use.

Administration and Dosage

Individualize dosage. Initiate dosage with 25 to 50 mg once daily; increase according to response. Dosage ranges from 25 to 50 mg, 1 to

3 times daily. A single daily dose is preferably given in the mid morning or mid afternoon, according to the patient's eating habits. In an occasional patient, it may be desirable to avoid late afternoon administration.

➤*Storage/Stability:* Store at controlled room temperature (20° to 25°C; 68° to 77°F).

DIETHYLPROPION HCl

c-iv	**Diethylpropion HCl** (Various, eg, Schein, Watson)	**Tablets:** 25 mg	In 100s.
c-iv	**Tenuate** (Aventis)		Lactose. (TENUATE 25 or MERRELL 697). White. In 100s.
c-iv	**Diethylpropion HCl** (Various, eg, Watson)	**Tablets, controlled release:** 75 mg	In 100s.
c-iv	**Tenuate Dospan** (Aventis)		Mannitol. (TENUATE 75 or MERRELL 698). White. In 100s and 250s.

Complete prescribing information begins in the Anorexiants group monograph.

Indications

➤*Obesity:* For the management of exogenous obesity as a short-term (a few weeks) in a regimen of weight reduction based on caloric restriction in patients with an initial body mass index (BMI) of ≥ 30 kg/m^2 and who have not responded to appropriate weight reducing regimen (diet or exercise) alone.

Diethylpropion is indicated for use as monotherapy only.

Administration and Dosage

➤*Immediate-release tablets:* 25 mg 3 times daily, 1 hour before meals, and in midevening if needed to overcome night hunger.

➤*Controlled-release tablets:* 75 mg once daily, in midmorning.

➤*Storage/Stability:* Keep tightly closed; store at room temperature, preferably < 30°C (< 86°F). Protect from excessive heat.

PHENDIMETRAZINE TARTRATE

c-iii	**Phendimetrazine** (Various, eg, Camall, Eon, Major, Schein)	**Tablets:** 35 mg	In 100s, 1000s, and 5000s.
c-iii	**Bontril PDM** (Amerin)		Sugar, isopropyl alcohol, lactose. (48 A). Green, white, and yellow layered; scored. In 100s and 1000s.
c-iii	**Bontril Slow-Release** (Amerin)	**Capsules, sustained release:** 105 mg	(A 047). Green/Yellow. In 100s.
c-iii	**Melfiat-105 Unicelles** (Numark)		Sucrose. (NUMARK 1082). Orange/Clear. In 100s.
c-iii	**Prelu-2** (Roxane)		Sucrose. Celery/Green. In 100s.

Complete prescribing information begins in the Anorexiants group monograph.

Indications

➤*Obesity:* For the management of exogenous obesity as a short-term adjunct (a few weeks) in a regimen of weight reduction based on caloric restriction. Measure the limited usefulness of this class against possible risk factors inherent in their use.

Administration and Dosage

➤*Immediate-release tablets:* 35 mg 2 or 3 times daily, 1 hour before meals.

Individualize dosage to obtain an adequate response with the lowest effective dosage. In some cases, ½ tablet (17.5 mg) per dose may be adequate. Dosage should not exceed 2 tablets 3 times/day.

➤*Sustained-release capsules:* 105 mg once daily in the morning 30 to 60 minutes before the morning meal.

➤*Storage/Stability:* Store at controlled room temperature (15° to 30°C; 59° to 86°F). Protect from moisture.

PHENTERMINE HCl

c-iv	**Phentermine HCl** (Various, eg, Camall)	**Tablets:** 8 mg	In 1000s.
c-iv	**Pro-Fast SA** (American Pharmaceuticals)		Lactose, tartrazine. In 100s.
c-iv	**Phentermine HCl** (Various, eg, Eon)	**Capsules:** 15 mg phentermine resin	In 100s and 1000s.
c-iv	**Ionamin** (Celltech)		Lactose. (Ionamin 15). Yellow/gray. In 100s and 400s.
c-iv	**Phentermine HCl** (Various, eg, Camall)	**Capsules:** 18.75 mg (equivalent to 15 mg phentermine base)	In 1000s.
c-iv	**Pro-Fast HS** (American Pharmaceuticals)		EDTA, benzyl alcohol, parabens. Gray/Yellow. In 100s.
c-iv	**Phentermine HCl** (Various, eg, Amide, Camall, Eon)	**Capsules:** 30 mg (equivalent to 24 mg phentermine base)	In 100s and 1000s.
c-iv	**Ionamin** (Celltech)	**Capsules:** 30 mg phentermine resin	Lactose. (Ionamin 30). Yellow. In 100s.
c-iv	**Phentermine HCl** (Various, eg, Amide, Camall, Purepac)	**Tablets:** 37.5 mg (equivalent to 30 mg phentermine base)	In 100s and 1000s.
c-iv	**Adipex-P** (Gate)		Lactose, sucrose. (ADIPEX-P 9 9). Blue/White, oblong, scored. In 30s, 100s, and 1000s.
c-iv	**Phentermine HCl** (Various, eg, Amide, Geneva, Ivax, Rugby, URL)	**Capsules:** 37.5 mg (equivalent to 30 mg phentermine base)	In 100s and 1000s.
c-iv	**Adipex-P** (Gate)		Lactose. (ADIPEX-P 37.5). Blue/White. In 100s.
c-iv	**Pro-Fast SR** (American Pharmaceuticals)		Sugar, tartrazine, EDTA, benzyl alcohol, parabens. Black/Yellow. In 100s.

Complete prescribing information begins in the Anorexiants group monograph.

Indications

▶*Obesity:* For short-term (a few weeks) adjunct in a regimen of weight reduction based on exercise, behavioral modification, and caloric restriction in the management of exogenous obesity for patients with an initial body mass index ≥ 30 kg/m^2 or ≥ 27 kg/m^2 in the presence of other risk factors (eg, hypertension, diabetes, hyperlipidemia).

Administration and Dosage

Individualize dosage.

Take 8 mg 3 times daily, ½ hour before meals, or 15 to 37.5 mg as a single daily dose before breakfast or 10 to 14 hours before bedtime.

Take *Pro-Fast HS* and *Pro-Fast SR* capsules ≈ 2 hours after breakfast for appetite control. Take *Adipex-P* capsules and tablets before breakfast or 1 to 2 hours after breakfast; the tablet dosage may be adjusted to the patient's need (ie, ½ tablet [18.75 mg] daily or 18.75 mg 2 times/day may be adequate).

Swallow *Ionamin* capsules whole.

Avoid late-evening medication because of the possibility of resulting insomnia.

▶*Storage/Stability:* Store at 15° to 30°C (59° to 86°F).

SIBUTRAMINE HCl

c-iv **Meridia** (Knoll)	**Capsules:** 5 mg	Lactose. (MERIDIA -5-). Blue/yellow. In 100s.
	10 mg	Lactose. (MERIDIA -10-). Blue/white. In 100s.
	15 mg	Lactose. (MERIDIA -15-). Yellow/white. In 100s.

Indications

➤*Obesity:* Management of obesity, including weight loss and maintenance of weight loss, in conjunction with a reduced calorie diet. Sibutramine is recommended for obese patients with an initial body mass index (BMI) ≥ 30 kg/m^2, or ≥ 27 kg/m^2 in the presence of other risk factors (eg, hypertension, diabetes, dyslipidemia). BMI is calculated by taking the patient's weight, in kilograms, and dividing by the patient's height, in meters, squared. Metric conversions are as follows: Pounds ÷ 2.2 = kilograms; inches x 0.0254 = meters.

Administration and Dosage

➤*Approved by the FDA:* November 22, 1997.

The recommended starting dose is 10 mg administered once daily with or without food. If there is inadequate weight loss, the dose may be titrated after 4 weeks to a total of 15 mg once daily. The 5 mg dose should be reserved for patients who do not tolerate the 10 mg dose. Take blood pressure and heart rate changes into account when making decisions regarding dose titration.

Doses > 15 mg daily are not recommended. In most of the clinical trials, sibutramine was given in the morning.

Analysis of numerous variables has indicated that ≈ 60% of patients who lose ≥ 4 lbs in the first 4 weeks of treatment with a given dose of sibutramine in combination with a reduced-calorie diet lose ≥ 5% (placebo-subtracted) of their initial body weight by the end of 6 months to 1 year of treatment on that dose. Conversely, ≈ 80% of patients who do not lose ≥ 4 lbs in the first 4 weeks of treatment with a given dose do not lose ≥ 5% (placebo-subtracted) of their initial body weight by the end of 6 months to 1 year of treatment on that dose. If a patient has not lost ≥ 4 lbs in the first 4 weeks of treatment, consider reevaluation of therapy, which may include increasing the dose or discontinuing sibutramine.

The safety and efficacy of sibutramine have not been determined beyond 2 years at this time.

➤*Storage/Stability:* Store at 15° to 30°C, 59° to 86°F. Protect capsules from heat and moisture. Dispense in tight, light-resistant container.

Actions

➤*Pharmacology:* Sibutramine produces its therapeutic effects by norepinephrine, serotonin, and dopamine reuptake inhibition. Sibutramine and its major pharmacologically active metabolites (M_1 and M_2) do not act via release of monoamines.

Sibutramine exerts its pharmacological actions predominantly via its secondary (M_1) and primary (M_2) amine metabolites. The parent compound, sibutramine, is a potent inhibitor of serotonin (5-hydroxytryptamine, 5-HT) and norepinephrine reuptake in vivo but not in vitro. However, metabolites M_1 and M_2 inhibit the reuptake of these neurotransmitters both in vitro and in vivo.

In human brain tissue, M_1 and M_2 also inhibit dopamine reuptake in vitro, but with ≈ 3-fold lower potency than for the reuptake inhibition of serotonin or norepinephrine.

A study using plasma samples taken from sibutramine-treated volunteers showed monoamine reuptake inhibition of norepinephrine > serotonin > dopamine; maximum inhibitions were norepinephrine = 73%, serotonin = 54%, and dopamine = 16%. Sibutramine, M_1, and M_2 exhibit no evidence of anticholinergic or antihistaminergic actions. These compounds also lack monoamine oxidase inhibitory activity.

➤*Pharmacokinetics:*

Absorption – Sibutramine is rapidly absorbed from the GI tract (T_{max}, 1.2 hours) following oral administration and undergoes extensive first-pass metabolism in the liver (oral clearance, 1750 L/hr; half-life, 1.1 hr) to form the pharmacologically active mono- and di-desmethyl metabolites M_1 and M_2. Peak plasma concentrations of M_1 and M_2 are reached within 3 to 4 hours. On average, ≥ 77% of a single oral dose of sibutramine is absorbed.

Effect of food: Administration of a single 20 mg dose of sibutramine with a standard breakfast resulted in reduced peak M_1 and M_2 concentrations (by 27% and 32%, respectively) and delayed the time to peak by ≈ 3 hours. However, the AUCs of M_1 and M_2 were not significantly altered.

Distribution – Radiolabeled studies in animals indicated rapid and extensive distribution into tissues: Highest concentrations of radiolabeled material were found in the eliminating organs, liver and kidney. In vitro, sibutramine, M_1, and M_2 are extensively bound (97%, 94%, and 94%, respectively) to human plasma proteins at plasma concentrations seen following therapeutic doses.

Metabolism – Sibutramine is metabolized in the liver principally by the cytochrome P450 (3A4) isoenzyme, to desmethyl metabolites, M_1

and M_2. These active metabolites are further metabolized by hydroxylation and conjugation to pharmacologically inactive metabolites, M_5 and M_6. Following oral radiolabeled sibutramine, essentially all of the peak radiolabeled material in plasma was accounted for by unchanged sibutramine (3%), M_1 (6%), M_2 (12%), M_5 (52%), and M_6 (27%).

M_1 and M_2 plasma concentrations reached steady state within 4 days of dosing and were ≈ 2-fold higher than following a single dose. The elimination half-lives of M_1 and M_2, 14 and 16 hours, respectively, were unchanged following repeated dosing.

Excretion – Approximately 85% (range, 68% to 95%) of a single oral dose was excreted in urine and feces over a 15-day collection period with the majority of the dose (77%) excreted in the urine. Major metabolites in urine were M_5 and M_6; unchanged sibutramine, M_1, and M_2 were not detected. The primary route of excretion for M_1 and M_2 is hepatic metabolism, and for M_5 and M_6 is renal excretion.

Special populations –

Geriatric: Plasma concentrations of M_1 and M_2 were similar between elderly (ages, 61 to 77) and young (ages, 19 to 30) subjects following a single 15 mg oral dose. Plasma concentrations of the inactive metabolites M_5 and M_6 were higher in the elderly; these differences are not likely to be of clinical significance.

Gender: Mean C_{max} and AUC of M_1 and M_2 were slightly higher (≤ 19% and ≤ 36%, respectively) in females than males. Somewhat higher steady-state trough plasma levels were observed in female obese patients from a large clinical efficacy trial. However, these differences are not likely to be of clinical significance. Dosage adjustment based upon the gender of a patient is not necessary.

Race: A trend towards higher concentrations in black patients over white patients was noted for M_1 and M_2. However, these differences are not considered to be of clinical significance.

Renal insufficiency: Because sibutramine and its active metabolites M_1 and M_2 are eliminated by hepatic metabolism, renal disease is unlikely to have a significant effect on their disposition. Elimination of the inactive metabolites M_5 and M_6, which are renally excreted, may be affected in this population. Do not use sibutramine in patients with severe renal impairment.

Hepatic insufficiency: In 12 patients with moderate hepatic impairment receiving a single 15 mg oral dose of sibutramine, the combined AUCs of M_1 and M_2 were increased by 24% compared with healthy subjects while M_5 and M_6 plasma concentrations were unchanged. The observed differences in M_1 and M_2 concentrations do not warrant dosage adjustments in patients with mild-to-moderate hepatic impairment. Do not use sibutramine in patients with severe hepatic dysfunction.

Contraindications

Patients receiving monoamine oxidase inhibitors (MAOIs; see Warnings); hypersensitivity to sibutramine or any of the active ingredients of sibutramine; patients with anorexia nervosa; patients taking other centrally acting appetite-suppressant drugs.

Warnings

➤*Blood pressure and pulse:* Sibutramine substantially increases blood pressure in some patients. Regular monitoring of blood pressure is required when prescribing sibutramine.

In placebo-controlled obesity studies, sibutramine 5 to 20 mg once daily was associated with mean increases in systolic and diastolic blood pressure of ≈ 1 to 3 mmHg relative to placebo, and with mean increases in pulse rate relative to placebo of ≈ 4 to 5 beats/minute (bpm). Larger increases were seen in some patients, particularly when therapy was initiated at the higher doses. In premarketing placebo-controlled obesity studies, 0.4% of patients treated were discontinued for hypertension (SBP ≥ 160 mmHg or DBP ≥ 95 mmHg), compared with 0.4% in the placebo group; 0.4% of patients treated with sibutramine were discontinued for tachycardia (pulse rate ≥ 100 bpm), compared with 0.1% in the placebo group. Measure blood pressure and pulse prior to starting therapy with sibutramine and monitor at regular intervals thereafter. For patients who experience a sustained increase in blood pressure or pulse rate while receiving sibutramine, consider either dose reduction or discontinuation. Give with caution to those patients with a history of hypertension, and do not give to patients with uncontrolled or poorly controlled hypertension.

Use caution – Use caution when prescribing sibutramine with other agents that may raise blood pressure or heart rate, including certain decongestants, cough, cold, and allergy medications that contain agents such as ephedrine or pseudoephedrine.

➤*Concurrent MAOIs:* Sibutramine is a norepinephrine, serotonin, and dopamine reuptake inhibitor and should not be used concomitantly with MAOIs (see Drug Interactions). There should be at least a 2-week interval after stopping MAOIs before starting treatment with sibutramine. Similarly, there should be at least a 2-week interval after stop-

SIBUTRAMINE HCl

ping sibutramine before starting treatment with MAOIs.

➤*Serotonin syndrome:* The rare, but serious, constellation of symptoms termed "serotonin syndrome" has also been reported with the concomitant use of selective serotonin reuptake inhibitors (SSRIs) and agents for migraine therapy (eg, sumatriptan, dihydroergotamine), certain opioids (eg, dextromethorphan, meperidine, pentazocine, fentanyl), lithium, or tryptophan. Serotonin syndrome has also occurred with the concomitant use of 2 serotonin reuptake inhibitors. The syndrome requires immediate medical attention and may include ≥ 1 of the following symptoms: Excitement, hypomania, restlessness, loss of consciousness, confusion, disorientation, anxiety, agitation, motor weakness, myoclonus, tremor, hemiballismus, hyperreflexia, ataxia, dysarthria, incoordination, hyperthermia, shivering, pupillary dilation, diaphoresis, emesis, and tachycardia. Because sibutramine inhibits serotonin reuptake, it should not be administered with other serotonergic agents such as those listed above.

➤*Concomitant cardiovascular disease:* Treatment with sibutramine has been associated with increases in heart rate or blood pressure. Therefore, it should not be used in patients with a history of coronary artery disease, CHF, arrhythmias, or stroke.

➤*Glaucoma:* Because sibutramine can cause mydriasis, use with caution in patients with narrow-angle glaucoma.

➤*Causes of obesity:* Exclude organic causes of obesity (eg, untreated hypothyroidism) before prescribing sibutramine.

➤*Renal/Hepatic function impairment:* Patients with severe renal impairment or severe hepatic dysfunction have not been systematically studied; therefore, do not use sibutramine in such patients.

➤*Fertility impairment:* In rats, at 13 times the human combined AUC, there was maternal toxicity, and the dams' nest-building behavior was impaired, leading to a higher incidence of perinatal mortality.

➤*Elderly:* In general, dose selection for an elderly patient should be cautious, reflecting the greater frequency of decreased hepatic, renal, or cardiac function; concomitant disease; or other drug therapy.

➤*Pregnancy: Category C.* In rabbits dosed at 3, 15, or 75 mg/kg/day, plasma AUCs greater than ≈ 5 times those following the human dose of 15 mg caused maternal toxicity. At markedly toxic doses, Dutch Belted rabbits had a slightly higher than control incidence of pups with a broad short snout, short rounded pinnae, short tail, and, in some, shorter thickened long bones in the limbs; at comparably high doses in New Zealand White rabbits, 1 study showed a slightly higher-than-control incidence of pups with cardiovascular anomalies, while a second study showed a lower incidence than in the control group.

No adequate and well-controlled studies have been conducted in pregnant women. The use of sibutramine is not recommended during pregnancy. Women of childbearing potential should use adequate contraception while taking this drug. Advise patients to notify their physician if they become pregnant or intend to become pregnant during therapy.

➤*Lactation:* It is not known whether sibutramine or its metabolites are excreted in breast milk. It is not recommended for use in nursing mothers. Advise patients to notify their physician if they are breast-feeding.

➤*Children:* The safety and efficacy in pediatric patients < 16 years of age have not been established.

Precautions

➤*Abuse/Physical and psychological dependence:* Physicians should carefully evaluate patients for history of drug abuse and follow such patients closely, observing them for signs of misuse or abuse (eg, drug development of tolerance, incrementation of doses, drug-seeking behavior).

➤*Primary pulmonary hypertension (PPH):* Certain centrally acting weight loss agents that cause release of serotonin from nerve terminals have been associated with PPH, a rare but lethal disease. In premarketing clinical studies, no cases of PPH have been reported with sibutramine. However, because of the low incidence of this disease in the underlying population, it is not known whether or not sibutramine may cause this disease.

➤*Seizures:* During premarketing testing, seizures were reported in < 0.1% of treated patients. Use cautiously in patients with a history of seizures; discontinue in any patient who develops seizures.

➤*Gallstones:* Weight loss can precipitate or exacerbate gallstone formation.

➤*Interference with cognitive and motor performance:* Although sibutramine did not affect psychomotor or cognitive performance in healthy volunteers, any CNS active drug has the potential to impair judgment, thinking or motor skills.

➤*Lab test abnormalities:* Abnormal liver function tests, including increases in AST, ALT, GGT, LDH, alkaline phosphatase, and bilirubin, were reported as adverse events in 1.6% of sibutramine-treated obese

patients vs 0.8% of placebo patients. In these studies, potentially clinically significant values (total bilirubin ≥ 2 mg/dL; ALT, AST, GGT, LDH, or alkaline phosphatase ≥ 3 times the upper limit of normal) occurred in 0% (alkaline phosphatase) to 0.6% (ALT) of the sibutramine-treated patients and in none of the placebo-treated patients. Abnormal values tended to be sporadic, often diminished with continued treatment and did not show a clear dose-response relationship.

Drug Interactions

See Warnings for more information.

Sibutramine Drug Interactions			
Precipitant drug	Object drug*		Description
Alcohol	Sibutramine	↑	Concomitant use of sibutramine and excess alcohol is not recommended.
Cimetidine	Sibutramine	↔	Concomitant administration resulted in small increases in combined sibutramine metabolites (M_1 and M_2), plasma C_{max} (3.4%), and AUC (7.3%); these differences are unlikely to be of clinical significance.
Erythromycin	Sibutramine	↔	Concomitant erythromycin resulted in small increases in sibutramine metabolites' AUC (< 14%) for M_1 and M_2. A small reduction in C_{max} for M_1 (11%) and a slight increase in C_{max} for M_2 (10%) were observed.
Ketoconazole	Sibutramine	↔	Concomitant administration resulted in moderate increases in sibutramine metabolites' AUC and C_{max} of 58% and 36% for M_1 and of 20% and 19% for M_2, respectively.
Sibutramine	Agents that may raise blood pressure or increase heart rate (see Description)	↑	These agents include decongestants, cough, cold, and allergy products that contain agents such as ephedrine or pseudoephedrine. Use caution when using concurrently with sibutramine. See Warnings.
Sibutramine	CNS-active drugs	↑	Caution is advised if the concomitant administration of sibutramine with other centrally acting drugs is indicated. See Warnings.
Sibutramine	MAOIs (eg, phenelzine, selegiline, tranylcypromine)	↑	In patients receiving MAOIs in combination with serotonergic agents (eg, fluoxetine, fluvoxamine, paroxetine, sertraline, venlafaxine), there have been reports of serious, sometimes fatal, reactions ("serotonin syndrome"; see Warnings). Because sibutramine inhibits serotonin reuptake, it should not be used concomitantly with an MAOI. At least 2 weeks should elapse between discontinuation of an MAOI and initiation of treatment with sibutramine. Similarly, ≥ 2 weeks should elapse between discontinuation of therapy and initiation of treatment with an MAOI.
Sibutramine	SSRIs, ergot alkaloids (eg, dihydroergotamine), lithium, certain opioids (eg, dextromethorphan, meperidine, pentazocine, fentanyl), 5-HT$_1$ receptor agonists (eg, sumatriptan, zolmitriptan), tryptophan	↑	The serotonergic effects of these agents may be additive. A "serotonin syndrome" may occur (see Warnings). Concomitant administration of these agents is not recommended. Carefully monitor patients if concurrent use cannot be avoided.

* ↑ = Object drug increased.   ↔ = Undetermined clinical effect.

➤*Drug/Food interactions:* Administration of a single 20 mg dose of sibutramine with a standard breakfast resulted in reduced peak M_1 and M_2 concentrations (by 27% and 32%, respectively) and delayed the time to peak by ≈ 3 hours. However, the AUCs of M_1 and M_2 were not significantly altered.

Adverse Reactions

In placebo-controlled studies, 9% of patients treated with sibutramine and 7% of patients treated with placebo withdrew for adverse events.

SIBUTRAMINE HCl

Sibutramine Adverse Reactions in Obese Patients (≥ 1%)		
Adverse reaction	Sibutramine (n = 2068)	Placebo (n = 884)
Cardiovascular		
Tachycardia	2.6	0.6
Vasodilation	2.4	0.9
Migraine	2.4	2
Hypertension/Increased BP	2.1	0.9
Palpitation	2	0.8
CNS		
Headache	30.3	18.6
Dry mouth	17.2	4.2
Insomnia	10.7	4.5
Dizziness	7	3.4
Nervousness	5.2	2.9
Anxiety	4.5	3.4
Depression	4.3	2.5
Paresthesia	2	0.5
Somnolence	1.7	0.9
CNS stimulation	1.5	0.5
Emotional lability	1.3	0.6
Dermatologic		
Rash	3.8	2.5
Sweating	2.5	0.9
Herpes simplex	1.3	1
Acne	1	0.8
GI		
Anorexia	13	3.5
Constipation	11.5	6
Increased appetite	8.7	2.7
Nausea	5.9	2.8
Dyspepsia	5	2.6
Gastritis	1.7	1.2
Vomiting	1.5	1.4
Rectal disorder	1.2	0.5
GU		
Dysmenorrhea	3.5	1.4
Urinary tract infection	2.3	2
Vaginal monilia	1.2	0.5
Metrorrhagia	1	0.8
Metabolic/Nutritional		
Thirst	1.7	0.9
Generalized edema	1.2	0.8
Musculoskeletal		
Arthralgia	5.9	5
Myalgia	1.9	1.1
Tenosynovitis	1.2	0.5
Joint disorder	1.1	0.6
Respiratory		
Rhinitis	10.2	7.1
Pharyngitis	10	8.4
Sinusitis	5	2.6
Cough increase	3.8	3.3
Laryngitis	1.3	0.9
Special senses		
Taste perversion	2.2	0.8
Ear disorder	1.7	0.9
Ear pain	1.1	0.7
Miscellaneous		
Back pain	8.2	5.5
Flu syndrome	8.2	5.8
Injury accident	5.9	4.1
Asthenia	5.9	5.3
Abdominal pain	4.5	3.6
Chest pain	1.8	1.2
Neck pain	1.6	1.1
Allergic reaction	1.5	0.8

The following additional adverse events were also reported.

➤*CNS:* Agitation, hypertonia, abnormal thinking (≥ 1).

➤*GI:* Diarrhea, flatulence, gastroenteritis, tooth disorder (≥ 1).

➤*Hematologic:* Ecchymosis (bruising) was observed in 0.7% of sibutramine-treated patients vs 0.2% with placebo. One patient had prolonged bleeding of a small amount that occurred during minor facial surgery. Sibutramine may have an effect on platelet function caused by its effect on serotonin uptake.

➤*Renal:* Acute interstitial nephritis (confirmed by biopsy) was reported in 1 obese patient receiving sibutramine. After discontinuation of the medication, dialysis and oral corticosteroids were administered; renal function normalized. The patient made a full recovery.

➤*Respiratory:* Bronchitis; dyspnea (≥ 1).

➤*Seizures:* See Precautions.

➤*Miscellaneous:* Fever; peripheral edema; arthritis; pruritus; amblyopia; leg cramps; menstrual disorder (≥ 1).

➤*Postmarketing:* Voluntary reports of adverse events temporally associated with the use of sibutramine are listed below. It is important to emphasize that although these events occurred during treatment with sibutramine, they may have no causal relationship with the drug. Obesity itself, concurrent disease states/risk factors, or weight reduction may be associated with an increased risk for some of these events: Abnormal dreams, abnormal ejaculation, abnormal gait, abnormal vision, alopecia, amnesia, anaphylactic shock, anaphylactoid reaction, anemia, anger, angina pectoris, arthrosis, atrial fibrillation, blurred vision, bursitis, cerebrovascular accident, chest pressure, chest tightness, cholecystitis, cholelithiasis, concentration impaired, confusion, CHF, depression aggravated, dermatitis, dry eye, duodenal ulcer, edema, epistaxis, eructation, eye pain, facial edema, GI hemorrhage, Gilles de la Tourette's syndrome, goiter, heart arrest, heart rate decreased, hematuria, hyperglycemia, hyperthyroidism, hypesthesia, hypoglycemia, hypothyroidism, impotence, increased intraocular pressure, increased salivation, increased urinary frequency, intestinal obstruction, leukopenia, libido decreased, libido increased, limb pain, lymphadenopathy, manic reaction, micturition difficulty, mood changes, mouth ulcer, MI, nasal congestion, nightmares, otitis externa, otitis media, petechiae, photosensitivity (eye), photosensitivity (skin), respiratory disorder, serotonin syndrome, short-term memory loss, speech disorder, stomach ulcer, sudden unexplained death, supraventricular tachycardia, syncope, thrombocytopenia, tinnitus, torsade de pointes, transient ischemic attack, tremor, twitch, urticaria, vascular headache, ventricular tachycardia, ventricular extrasystoles, ventricular fibrillation, vertigo, yawn.

Overdosage

➤*Symptoms:* Three cases of overdose have been reported. The first was in a 2-year-old child who ingested up to eight 10 mg capsules. No complications were observed during the overnight hospitalization, and the child was discharged the following day with no sequelae. The second report was a 30-year-old male who ingested ≈ 100 mg of sibutramine in an attempt to commit suicide. The patient suffered no adverse effects or ECG abnormalities postingestion. The third report was a 45-year-old who ingested 400 mg and was hospitalized for observation; a heart rate of 120 bpm was noted. He was discharged the next day with no apparent sequelae.

➤*Treatment:* There is no specific antidote to sibutramine. Treatment should consist of general measures employed in the management of overdosage: An airway should be established; cardiac and vital sign monitoring is recommended; general symptomatic and supportive measures should be instituted. Cautious use of β-blockers may be indicated to control elevated blood pressure or tachycardia. The benefits of forced diuresis and hemodialysis are unknown. Refer to General Management of Acute Overdosage.

Patient Information

Instruct patients to read the patient package insert before starting therapy with sibutramine and to reread it each time the prescription is renewed.

Discuss with patients any part of the package insert that is relevant to them. In particular, emphasize the importance of keeping appointments for follow-up visits.

Advise patients to notify their physician if they develop a rash, hives, or other allergic reactions.

Advise patients to inform their physician if they are taking, or plan to take, any prescription or *otc* drugs, especially weight-reducing agents, decongestants, antidepressants, cough suppressants, lithium, dihydroergotamine, sumatriptan, or tryptophan, because there is a potential for interactions.

Remind patients of the importance of having their blood pressure and pulse monitored at regular intervals.

Instruct patients not to take an extra capsules to "make up" for a missed dose.

Indications

Refer to individual product listings for specific indications.

➤*Analgesia/Anesthesia:* Relief or management of moderate-to-severe acute and chronic pain; preoperative medication; support of anesthesia; as analgesic adjuncts during anesthesia; obstetrical analgesia; as a primary anesthetic agent for the induction and maintenance of anesthesia with 100% oxygen (**sufentanil**, **alfentanil**); in patients undergoing major surgical procedures; relief of anxiety in patients with dyspnea associated with pulmonary edema secondary to acute left ventricular dysfunction; intrathecally or epidurally for pain relief for extended periods without attendant loss of motor, sensory, or sympathetic function; pain relief of MI (**morphine**); management of opiate dependence (**levomethadyl**); detoxification treatment of narcotic addiction and temporary maintenance treatment of narcotic addiction (**methadone**); to induce conscious sedation prior to a diagnostic or therapeutic procedure in hospital setting, as an anesthetic premedication in the operating room setting or to induce conscious sedation prior to diagnostic or therapeutic procedure (*Fentanyl Oralet*); for analgesic action of short duration during anesthetic periods, premedication, induction, and maintenance, and in the immediate postoperative period (**fentanyl** and **remifentanil**).

Used for their antitussive (**codeine**) and antidiarrheal (**opium**; see Antidiarrheal Combination products) effects.

Administration and Dosage

➤*Brompton's Cocktail:* Brompton's Cocktail or Mixture is an oral narcotic mixture used for chronic severe pain. The original formula contained heroin or **morphine** (10 mg), cocaine (10 mg), alcohol, chloroform water, and syrup; it was given on schedule as pain prophylaxis, rather than "as needed." Currently, "Brompton's Mixture" designates any alcoholic solution containing morphine and either cocaine or a phenothiazine. A single-entity narcotic (usually morphine) can be equally effective. Cocaine apparently does not add to the mixture's effectiveness; **methadone** has been recommended. Various adjunctive drugs, including aspirin or acetaminophen, tricyclic antidepressants, stimulants (eg, dextroamphetamine), and antihistamines (eg, dimenhydrinate), may be effective when given with a narcotic solution.

The use of Brompton's Cocktail established the value of regular administration of narcotic analgesics for chronic severe pain. Adjunctive drugs may benefit selected patients but "standard" combinations are not advocated.

Actions

➤*Pharmacology:* Narcotic analgesics are classified as agonists, mixed agonist-antagonists, or partial agonists by their activity at opioid receptors. There are 3 major classes of opioid receptors in the CNS designated mu (μ), kappa (κ), and delta (δ).

Consequences of the μ-receptor activation include analgesia, respiratory depression, miosis, reduced GI motility, and euphoria. κ receptors act primarily in the spinal cord and cause analgesia, dysphoria, and psychotomimetic effects. They also cause less intense miosis and respiratory depression than μ-receptor activation. The consequence of δ-receptor stimulation in human beings is unclear. In animals, relatively specific δ agonists (ie, pen 5 pencillamine) produce analgesia and positive reinforcing effects at supraspinal sites and anti-nociception for thermal stimuli at spinal sites. Morphine-like narcotic agonists have activity at the μ, κ, and δ receptors. Narcotic agonists include natural opium alkaloids (eg, morphine, codeine), semisynthetic analogs (eg, hydromorphone, oxymorphone, oxycodone), and synthetic compounds (eg, methadone, sufentanil, fentanyl, levorphanol).

Mixed *agonist-antagonist* drugs (eg, nalbuphine, pentazocine) have agonist activity at some receptors and antagonist activity at other receptors; also included are the *partial agonists* (eg, butorphanol, buprenorphine).

Narcotic antagonists – Narcotic antagonists (eg, naloxone) do not have agonist activity at any of the opioid receptor sites (see individual monographs). Antagonists block the opiate receptor, inhibit pharmacological activity of the agonist, and precipitate withdrawal in dependent patients. Opiate receptors in the CNS mediate analgesic activity. Narcotic agonists occupy the same receptors as endogenous opioid peptides (enkephalins or endorphins), and both may alter the central release of neurotransmitters from afferent nerves sensitive to noxious stimuli.

Secondary pharmacological effects – The narcotics have a variety of secondary pharmacological effects, including the following:

Cardiovascular: Peripheral vasodilation, reduced peripheral resistance, and inhibition of baroreceptors. Orthostatic hypotension and fainting may occur when the patient sits up.

CNS: Euphoria; drowsiness; apathy; mental confusion; alterations in mood; reduction in body temperature; feelings of relaxation; dysphoria. Nausea and vomiting are caused by direct stimulation of the emetic chemoreceptors located in the medulla. **Hydromorphone** increases CSF pressure.

Dermatologic: Histamine release, pruritus, flushing, and red eyes.

GI:
• *Stomach* – Decreases gastric motility, thus prolonging gastric emptying time. This may lead to esophageal reflux.
• *Small intestine* – Decreases biliary, pancreatic, and intestinal secretions and delays digestion of food in the small intestine. Resting tone increases and periodic spasms occur.
• *Large intestine* – Propulsive peristaltic waves in the colon are diminished and tone increases until it spasms. This, along with the inattention to the normal stimuli for defecation reflex, contribute to constipation.
• *Biliary tract* – The sphincter of Oddi constricts leading to epigastric distress or biliary colic.

GU: Increases smooth muscle tone in the urinary tract and can induce spasms. Urinary urgency and difficulty with urination may result.

Respiratory: Depressant effects first diminish tidal volume, then respiratory rate, because of reduced sensitivity of the respiratory center to carbon dioxide.
• *Cough* – Suppresses cough reflex by direct effect on cough center in the medulla.

Miscellaneous: **Hydromorphone** causes transient hyperglycemia; **codeine** causes release of antidiuretic hormone.

Comparative pharmacology is summarized below. Consider these comparisons as approximations that may vary widely among patients.

Narcotic Agonist Comparative Pharmacology[1]							
Drug	Analgesic	Antitussive	Constipation	Respiratory depression	Sedation	Emesis	Physical dependence
Phenanthrenes							
Codeine	+	+++	+	+	+	+	+
Hydrocodone	+	+++	nd[2]	+	nd[2]	nd[2]	+
Hydromorphone	++	+++	+	++	+	+	++
Levorphanol	++	++	++	++	++	+	++
Morphine	++	+++	++	++	++	+	++
Oxycodone	++	+++	++	++	++	++	++
Oxymorphone	++	+	++	+++	nd[2]	+++	+++
Phenylpiperidines							
Alfentanil	++	nd[2]	nd[2]	nd[2]	nd[2]	nd[2]	nd[2]
Fentanyl	++	nd[2]	nd[2]	+	nd[2]	+	nd[2]
Meperidine	++	+	+	++	+	+	++
Sufentanil	+++	nd[2]	nd[2]	nd[2]	nd[2]	nd[2]	nd[2]
Diphenylheptanes							
Levomethadyl	++	nd[2]	++	nd[2]	nd[2]	+	+
Methadone	++	++	++	++	+	+	+
Propoxyphene	+	nd[2]	nd[2]	+	+	+	+
Anilidopiperidines							
Remifentanil	+++	nd[2]	+	++	nd[2]	++	

[1] Table adapted from Catalano RB. The medical approach to management of pain caused by cancer. *Semin Oncol* 1975;2:379-92 and Reuler JB, et al. The chronic pain syndrome: Misconceptions and management. *Ann Intern Med* 1980;93:588-96.
[2] nd – No data available.

➤*Pharmacokinetics:* Administration IV is most reliable and rapid; IM or SC use may delay absorption and peak effect. Many agents undergo a significant first-pass effect. **Meperidine** is metabolized to normeperidine, a metabolite with significant pharmacologic activity. The half-life of normeperidine is 15 to 30 hours and accumulates with chronic dosing. Accumulation of this metabolite may lead to CNS excitation (eg, tremors, twitches, seizures).

Levomethadyl acetate HCl (LAAM) undergoes first-pass metabolism to its demethylated metabolite nor-LAAM, which is sequentially N-demethylated to dinor-LAAM. Both metabolites are active and contribute to the extent and duration of levomethadyl's clinical activity. Half-lives were ≈ 2 days for nor-LAAM and ≈ 4 days for dinor-LAAM.

Propoxyphene is metabolized in the liver to yield norpropoxyphene, which has a half-life of 30 to 36 hours. Norpropoxyphene has substantially less CNS-depressant effect than propoxyphene but a greater local anesthetic effect, which is similar to that of amitriptyline and antiarrhythmic agents, such as lidocaine and quinidine. The initial volume of distribution of **remifentanil** is ≈ 100 ml/kg. Remifentanil subsequently distributes into peripheral tissues with a steady-state volume of distribution of ≈ 350 ml/kg. These 2 distribution volumes generally correlate with total body weight (except in severely obese patients when they correlate better with ideal body weight [IBW]). Remifentanil is ≈ 70% bound to plasma proteins. Blood concentration decreases 50% (in 3 to 6 minutes) after a 1-minute infusion of remifentanil, or after prolonged continuous infusion because of rapid distribution and elimination processes, and is independent of duration of drug administration. Remifentanil depresses respiration in a dose-related fashion. The duration of action of remifentanil at a given dose does not increase with longer duration of administration because of lack of drug accumulation. Remifentanil clearance is reduced by ≈ 20% during hypothermic cardiopulmonary bypass.

Pharmacokinetic profiles are summarized in the following table using morphine as the standard:

Pharmacokinetics of Narcotic Agonist Analgesics[1]						
Drug	Onset (minutes)	Peak (hours)	Duration[2] (hours)	t½ (hours)	Approximate equi-analgesic doses[3] (mg)	
					Parenteral	Other
Alfentanil	immediate	nd[4]	nd[4]	1 to 2[5]	IM 0.4 to 0.8	nd[4]
Codeine	10 to 30	0.5 to 1	4 to 6	3	IM 120 to 130 SC 120	Oral 180 - 200[6]
Fentanyl	7 to 8	nd[4]	1 to 2	1.5 to 6	IM 0.1 to 0.2	Transdermal 25 mcg/hr
Hydrocodone	nd[4]	nd[4]	4 to 6	3.3 to 4.5	nd[4]	Oral 30
Hydromorphone	15 to 30	0.5 to 1	4 to 5	2 to 3	IM 1.3 to 1.5 SC 1 to 1.5	Oral 7.5
Levomethadyl	2 to 4 hrs	1.5 to 2	48 to 72	2 to 6 days	nd[4]	nd[4]
Levorphanol	30 to 90	0.5 to 1	6 to 8	11 to 16	IM 2 SC 2	Oral 4
Meperidine	10 to 45	0.5 to 1	2 to 4	3 to 4	IM 75 SC 75 to 100	Oral 300[6]
Methadone	30 to 60	0.5 to 1	4 to 6[7]	15 to 30	IM 10 SC 8 to 10	Oral 10 to 20
Morphine	15 to 60[8]	0.5 to 1	3 to 7	1.5 to 2	IM 10 SC 10	Oral 30 to 60
Oxycodone	15 to 30	1	4 to 6	nd[4]	IM 10 to 15 SC 10 to 15	Oral 30[6]
Oxymorphone	5 to 10	0.5 to 1	3 to 6	nd[4]	IM 1 SC 1 to 1.5	Rectal 5, 10
Propoxyphene (PO)	30 to 60	2 to 2.5	4 to 6	6 to 12	nd[4]	Oral 130[9]
Remifentanil	1	1 min	short[10]	≈ 3 to 10 min	nd[4]	nd[4]
Sufentanil	1.3 to 3[5]	nd[4]	nd[4]	2.5	IM 0.01 to 0.04	nd[4]

[1] Caution: Recommended doses do not apply for adult patients with body weight < 50 kg. Recommended doses do not apply to patients with renal or hepatic insufficiency or other conditions affecting drug metabolism and kinetics.
[2] After IV administration, peak effects may be more pronounced but duration is shorter. Duration of action may be longer with the oral route.
[3] Based on morphine 10 mg IM or SC. The initial dose of the new drug is given at ½ to ⅔ of the calculated dose because opioid-specific tolerance may occur, and the new drug may have more relative effectiveness (and more side effects) than the drug being discontinued.
[4] nd – No data available.
[5] Data based on IV administration.
[6] Starting doses lower (codeine, 30 mg; oxycodone, 5 mg; meperidine, 50 mg).
[7] Duration and half-life increase with repeated use because of cumulative effects.
[8] Data based on intrathecal or epidural administration.
[9] Starting doses lower (propoxyphene, 65 to 130 mg). In equimolar doses (100 mg of napsylate equals 65 mg of HCl).
[10] The duration of action does not increase with prolonged administration.

Contraindications

Hypersensitivity to narcotics; acute or severe bronchial asthma; upper airway obstruction; significant respiratory depression; in premature infants or during labor when delivery of a premature infant is anticipated.

➤*Morphine, epidural, or intrathecal:* Presence of infection at injection site; anticoagulant therapy; bleeding diathesis; parenterally administered corticosteroids within a 2-week period or other concomitant drug therapy or medical condition that would contraindicate the technique of epidural or intrathecal analgesia.

➤*Morphine, injection:* Heart failure secondary to chronic lung disease; cardiac arrhythmias; brain tumor; acute alcoholism; delirium tremens; idiosyncrasy to the drug. Because of its stimulating effect on the spinal cord, morphine should not be used in convulsive states (eg, status epilepticus, tetanus, strychnine poisoning).

➤*Morphine, immediate release oral solution:* Respiratory insufficiency; severe CNS depression; heart failure secondary to chronic lung disease; cardiac arrhythmias; increased intracranial or cerebrospinal pressure; head injuries; brain tumor; acute alcoholism; delirium tremens; convulsive disorders; after biliary tract surgery; suspected surgi-

cal abdomen; surgical anastomosis; idiosyncrasy to the drug; concomitantly with MAO inhibitors or within 14 days of such treatment.

➤*Levorphanol:* Acute alcoholism; increased intracranial pressure; respiratory depression; anoxia.

➤*Meperidine:* In patients taking monoamine oxidase inhibitors (MAOIs) or in those who have received such agents within 14 days.

➤*Hydromorphone:* In patients not already receiving large amounts of parenteral narcotics; patients with respiratory depression in the absence of resuscitative equipment; status asthmaticus; use as obstetrical analgesia; in the presence of an intracranial lesion associated with increased intracranial pressure; when ventilatory function is depressed (chronic obstructive pulmonary disease, cor pulmonale, emphysema, kyphoscoliosis, status asthmaticus).

➤*Fentanyl:*
Transdermal – Hypersensitivity to fentanyl and adhesives; in the management of acute or postoperative pain, including use in outpatient surgeries; in the management of mild or intermittent pain responsive to PRN or non-opioid therapy; in doses exceeding 25 mcg/hour at the initiation of opioid therapy; in children < 12 years of age or patients < 18 years of age who weigh < 50 kg, except in an authorized investigational research setting.

Transmucosal – In children who weigh < 10 kg; treatment of acute or chronic pain (safety for use in these patients have not been established); doses > 15 mcg/kg in children and > 5 mcg/kg in adults because of the excessive frequency of significant hypoventilation at higher doses; for use at home or in any other setting outside a hospital setting.

➤*Opium:* Opium tincture in children; diarrhea caused by poisoning until the toxic material has been eliminated.

➤*Oxycodone:* Hypercarbia; paralytic ileus.

➤*Oxymorphone:* Paralytic ileus; treatment of pulmonary edema secondary to a chemical respiratory irritant.

➤*Remifentanil:* Epidural or intrathecal administration.

Warnings

For important warnings associated with **methadone**, **levomethadyl**, **propoxyphene**, and transmucosal and transdermal **fentanyl**, refer to individual monographs.

➤*Suicide:* Do not prescribe **propoxyphene** for patients who are suicidal or addiction-prone. Many of the propoxyphene-related deaths have occurred in patients with histories of emotional disturbances, suicidal ideation, or suicide attempts as well as misuse of tranquilizers, alcohol, and other CNS-active drugs. Some deaths were a consequence of accidental ingestion of excessive quantities of propoxyphene alone or in combination with other drugs. Warn patients not to exceed dosage recommended by physician.

➤*Respiratory depression:* Narcotics may be expected to produce serious or potentially fatal respiratory depression if given in an excessive dose, too frequently, or in full dosage to compromised or vulnerable patients because the doses required to produce analgesia in the general clinical population may cause serious respiratory depression in vulnerable patients. Safe use of this potent opioid requires that the dose and dosage interval be individualized to each patient based on the severity of the pain, weight, age, diagnosis, and physical status of the patient, and the type and dose of concurrently administered medication.

Reduce the initial **levorphanol** dose by ≥ 50% when the drug is given to patients with any condition affecting respiratory reserve or in conjunction with other drugs affecting the respiratory center. Subsequent doses should then be individually titrated according to the patient's response. Respiratory depression produced by levorphanol can be reversed by naloxone, a specific antagonist. Respiratory depression in spontaneously breathing patients is generally managed by decreasing the rate of infusion of **remifentanil** by 50% or by temporarily discontinuing the infusion.

➤*CNS depressants:* Use with caution and in reduced dosage in patients concurrently receiving other narcotic analgesics, general anesthetics, phenothiazines, other tranquilizers, sedative-hypnotics (including barbiturates), tricyclic antidepressants, and other CNS depressants (including alcohol). Respiratory depression, hypotension, and profound sedation or coma may result.

➤*Head injury and increased intracranial pressure:* Narcotics may obscure the clinical course of patients with head injuries. The respiratory-depressant effects and the capacity to elevate CSF pressure may be markedly exaggerated in the presence of head injury, brain tumor, other intracranial lesions, or preexisting elevated intracranial pressure. Use with extreme caution and only if deemed essential.

➤*Administration:* **Sufentanil**, **fentanyl**, **remifentanil**, **alfentanil**, and **morphine sulfate** should be administered only by personnel specifically trained in the use of IV and epidural anesthetics and management of the respiratory effects of potent opioids.

An opioid antagonist, resuscitative and intubation equipment, and oxygen should be readily available.

Prior to catheter insertion, the physician should be familiar with patient conditions (such as infection at the injection site, bleeding diathesis, anticoagulant therapy) that call for special evaluation of the benefit vs risk potential.

➤*Parenteral therapy:* Give by very slow IV injection, preferably as a diluted solution. The patient should be lying down. Rapid IV injection increases the incidence of adverse reactions; respiratory depression, hypotension, apnea, circulatory collapse, cardiac arrest, and anaphylactoid reactions have occurred. Do not administer IV unless a narcotic antagonist and facilities for assisted or controlled respiration are available. Use caution when injecting SC or IM in chilled areas or in patients with hypotension or shock, because impaired perfusion may prevent complete absorption; with repeated injections, an excessive amount may be suddenly absorbed if normal circulation is reestablished.

Smooth muscle hypertonicity may result in biliary colic, difficulty in urination, and possible urinary retention requiring catheterization. Give consideration to inherent risks in urethral catheterization (eg, sepsis) when epidural or intrathecal administration is considered, especially in the perioperative period.

Hydrochlorides of opium alkaloids – Do not administer IV.

➤*Epidural administration:* Limit epidural or intrathecal administration of preservative free **morphine** and **sufentanil** to the lumbar area. Intrathecal use has been associated with a higher incidence of respiratory depression than epidural use.

Verify proper placement of the needle or catheter in the epidural space before injection of sufentanil or preservative free morphine to ensure that unintentional intravascular or intrathecal administration does not occur. Unintentional intravascular injection of sufentanil could result in a potentially serious overdose, including acute truncal muscular rigidity and apnea. Unintentional intrathecal injection of the full sufentanil/bupivacaine epidural doses and volume could produce effects of high spinal anesthesia, including prolonged paralysis and delayed recovery. If analgesia is inadequate, the placement and integrity of the catheter should be verified prior to the administration of any additional epidural medications. Administer sufentanil epidurally by slow injection.

➤*Maintenance of general anesthesia:* Administer continuous infusions only by an infusion device. Use IV bolus administration of **remifentanil** only during the maintenance of general anesthesia. In nonintubated patients, administer remifentanil doses over 30 to 60 seconds.

Interruption of infusion – Interruption of an infusion of **remifentanil** will result in rapid offset of effect. Rapid clearance and lack of drug accumulation result in rapid dissipation of respiratory-depressant and analgesic effects upon discontinuation of remifentanil at recommended doses. Precede discontinuation of an infusion of remifentanil with the establishment of adequate postoperative analgesia.

IV tubing – Make injections of **remifentanil** into IV tubing at or close to the venous cannula. Upon discontinuation of remifentanil, clear the IV tubing to prevent the inadvertent administration of remifentanil at a later point in time. Failure to adequately clear the IV tubing to remove residual remifentanil has been associated with respiratory depression, apnea, and muscle rigidity upon the administration of additional fluids or medications through the same IV tubing.

Do not administer remifentanil into the same IV tubing with blood because of potential inactivation by nonspecific esterases in blood products.

➤*Asthma and other respiratory conditions:* The use of bisulfites is contraindicated in asthmatics. Bisulfites and **morphine** may potentiate each other, preventing use by causing severe adverse reactions. Use with extreme caution in patients having an acute asthmatic attack, bronchial asthma, chronic obstructive pulmonary disease or cor pulmonale, a substantially decreased respiratory reserve, and preexisting respiratory depression, hypoxia, or hypercapnia. Even usual therapeutic doses of narcotics may decrease respiratory drive while simultaneously increasing airway resistance to the point of apnea. Reserve use for those whose conditions require endotracheal intubation and respiratory support or control of ventilation. In these patients, consider alternative non-opioid analgesics, and employ only under careful medical supervision at the lowest effective dose.

➤*Hypotensive effect:* Narcotic analgesics may cause severe hypotension in the postoperative patient or in individuals whose ability to maintain blood pressure has been compromised by a depleted blood volume, or coadministration of drugs such as phenothiazines or general anesthetics. In ambulatory patients, orthostatic hypotension may occur.

Observe patients with reduced circulating blood volume, impaired myocardial function, or on sympatholytic drugs carefully for orthostatic hypotension, particularly in transport.

➤*Renal / Hepatic function impairment:* Renal and hepatic dysfunction may cause a prolonged duration and cumulative effect. Administer with caution; smaller doses may be necessary.

Meperidine – In patients with renal dysfunction, normeperidine (an active metabolite of meperidine) may accumulate, resulting in increased CNS adverse reactions.

➤*Elderly:* Appropriately reduce the initial dose in elderly and debilitated patients. Consider the effect of the initial dose in determining supplemental doses. Use caution because opioids have the ability to depress respiration and reduce ventilatory drive to a clinically significant event.

The rate of **propoxyphene** metabolism may be reduced in some patients. Consider increased dosing intervals.

Because elderly, cachectic, or debilitated patients may have altered pharmacokinetics due to poor fat stores, muscle wasting, or altered clearance, do not start them on **transdermal fentanyl** doses > 25 mcg/hr unless they are already taking > 135 mg oral **morphine** per day or an equivalent dose of another opioid.

If **transmucosal fentanyl** is used in patients > 65 years of age, reduce the dose to 2.5 to 5 mcg/kg. Although studies in the elderly have not been conducted, elderly patients have been shown to be twice as sensitive as the younger population to the effects of the forms of fentanyl.

In 1 clincial trial, **alfentanil** doses required to produce anesthesia, as determined by appearance of delta waves in EEG, were 40% lower in geriatric patients than that needed in healthy young patients.

Remifentanil blood concentrations fell as rapidly after termination of administration in the elderly as in young adults.

While the effective biological half-life of remifentanil is unchanged, elderly patients have been shown to be twice as sensitive to the pharmacodynamic effects as younger patients. Decrease the recommended starting dose by 50% in patients > 65 years of age.

➤*Pregnancy:* Category C; Category B (oxycodone). Safety for use during pregnancy has not been established. There are no adequate and well-controlled studies in pregnant women. Use in pregnant women only if the potential benefits outweigh the possible risks.

The placental transfer of narcotics is rapid. Maternal addiction and neonatal effects following illicit use. Withdrawal symptoms include irritability, excessive crying, yawning, sneezing, increased respiratory rate, tremors, convulsions, hyperreflexia, fever, vomiting, increased stools, and diarrhea. Symptoms usually appear during the first days of life.

Some association between congenital defects and first trimester exposure to **codeine** has been reported. **Alfentanil** and **sufentanil** have an embryocidal effect in rats and rabbits when given in doses 2.5 times the upper human dose for 10 days to over 30 days. **Fentanyl** has been shown to impair fertility and to have an embryocidal effect in rats at doses 0.3 times the upper human dose for 12 days.

Levomethadyl is not recommended for use in pregnancy. Advise women who may become pregnant about the risks of therapy and the desirability of discontinuing levomethadyl prior to a planned pregnancy. Current regulations mandate monthly pregnancy tests in female patients of childbearing potential who are using levomethadyl. If a patient becomes pregnant while on levomethadyl, transfer her to **methadone** for the remainder of the pregnancy. If it appears wiser to continue a specific patient on levomethadyl, the physician should be alert to possible respiratory depression in the newborn and other perinatal complications.

Labor – Narcotics cross the placenta and can produce respiratory depression and psycho-physiologic effects in the neonate. Resuscitation may be required; have naloxone available. The use of epidurally administered **sufentanil** in combination with bupivacaine 0.125% with or without epinephrine is indicated for labor and delivery. Sufentanil is not recommended for IV use or in larger epidural doses during labor and delivery because of potential risks to the newborn after delivery. In a human clinical trial, the average maternal **remifentanil** concentrations were approximately twice those seen in the fetus. However, in some cases, fetal concentrations were similar to those in the mother. The umbilical arterio-venous ratio of remifentanil concentrations was ≈ 30%, suggesting metabolism of remifentanil in the neonate. The use of **alfentanil**, **levorphanol**, **oxycodone**, **hydromorphone**, and **fentanyl** is not recommended. Use of **levomethadyl** in labor and delivery is not recommended unless, in the opinion of the treating physician, the potential benefits outweigh the possible hazards. Do not use **methadone** for obstetrical analgesia. Its long duration of action increases the probability of neonatal respiratory depression. It has also been associated with low infant birthweight.

Therapeutic **morphine** and **codeine** doses have increased duration of labor.

➤*Lactation:* Most of these agents appear in breast milk, but effects on the infant may not be significant. Some recommend waiting 4 to 6 hours after use before breastfeeding. Withdrawal symptoms can occur in breastfeeding infants when maternal administration of an opioid-analgesic is stopped. Decide whether to discontinue nursing or to discontinue the drug, taking into account the importance of the drug to the mother.

Methadone – Methadone enters breast milk in concentrations approaching plasma levels (range, 0.17 to 5.6 mcg/ml) and may prevent withdrawal symptoms in addicted infants. **Meperidine** achieves an average milk:plasma ratio of > 1 (peak milk levels of 0.13 mcg/ml occur 2 hours after a 50 mg IM dose). Significant levels of **alfentanil** were found in breast milk 4 hours after administration of 60 mcg/kg. No detectable levels were found after 28 hours.

➤*Children:* Safety and efficacy of IV **sufentanil** and **remifentanil** in children < 2 years of age undergoing cardiovascular surgery have been documented in a limited number of cases. Safety and efficacy of **fentanyl (transmucosal and injection)** and remifentanil in children < 2 years of age are not established; fentanyl transmucosal is contraindicated in children who weigh < 10 kg; safety and effectiveness have not been established. Do not administer **fentanyl transdermal systems** to children < 12 years of age or patients < 18 years of age who weigh < 50 kg except in an authorized investigational research setting. There are no adequate data to support the use of **alfentanil** in children < 12 years of age. Use of **levomethadyl** or **levorphanol** is not recommended in those < 18 years of age. Safety and effectiveness of **oxymorphone** in children < 18 years of age have not been established. Methemoglobinemia has occurred rarely in premature neonates undergoing emergency anesthesia and surgery including combined use of **fentanyl**, pancuronium, and atropine; a cause-and-effect relationship has not been established. Hypotension has occurred in neonates with respiratory distress syndrome receiving alfentanil 20 mcg/kg.

Do not use **oxycodone** in children; **propoxyphene** use is not recommended in children. **Methadone** is not recommended as an analgesic in children; documented clinical experience is insufficient to establish suitable dosage regimens. Safety of **transdermal fentanyl, propoxyphene, morphine, opium**, and **hydromorphone** are not established in children.

Precautions

➤*Monitoring:* Because of the possibility of delayed respiratory depression, continue monitoring patients well after surgery. Monitor vital signs routinely. Continually monitor vital signs and oxygenation during the administration of **remifentanil**.

Patients receiving monitored anesthesia care (MAC) should be continuously monitored by people not involved in the conduct of the surgical or diagnostic procedure. Oxygen supplementation should be immediately available and provided where clinically indicated. Continuously monitor oxygen saturation. Observe the patient for early signs of hypotension, apnea, upper airway obstruction, or oxygen desaturation.

➤*Acute abdominal conditions:* Narcotics may obscure diagnosis or clinical course.

➤*Special risk patients:* Use caution and reduce initial dose in debilitated patients and in those suffering from conditions accompanied by hypoxia or hypercapnia when even moderate therapeutic doses may dangerously decrease pulmonary ventilation. Also exercise caution in patients sensitive to CNS depressants, including those with cardiovascular, pulmonary, renal, or hepatic disease; myxedema; convulsive disorders; increased intracranial or ocular pressure; acute alcoholism; delirium tremens; cerebral arteriosclerosis; fever; decreased respiratory reserve (eg, emphysema, severe obesity, asthma, chronic obstructive pulmonary disease or cor pulmonale, sleep apnea syndrome); inflammatory bowel disease; diarrhea secondary to poisoning until the toxin is eliminated; diarrhea secondary to pseudomembranous colitis; GI hemorrhage; bronchial asthma; hypothyroidism; kyphoscoliosis; Addison's disease; prostatic hypertrophy; urethral stricture; gallbladder disease or gallstones; recent GI or GU tract surgery; toxic psychosis.

In obese patients (> 20% above ideal body weight), determine the **alfentanil** and **sufentanil** dosage on the basis of ideal body weight.

Bradycardia – **Fentanyl, sufentanil, remifentanil**, and **alfentanil** may produce bradycardia, which may be treated with ephedrine or anticholinergic drugs, such as atropine or glycopyrrolate. Use caution when administering to patients with bradyarrhythmias.

➤*Skeletal muscle rigidity:* **Alfentanil, fentanyl**, and **sufentanil** may cause skeletal muscle rigidity, particularly of the truncal muscles. The incidence and severity of muscle rigidity is usually dose-related. Alfentanil, fentanyl, and sufentanil may produce muscular rigidity that involves all skeletal muscles, including those of the neck and extremities. The incidence may be reduced by 1) routine methods of administration of neuromuscular blocking agents for balanced opioid anesthesia; 2) administration of up to ¼ of the full paralyzing dose of a neuromuscular blocking agent just prior to administration of alfentanil, fentanyl, or sufentanil; following loss of consciousness, a full paralyzing dose of a neuromuscular blocking agent should be administered; or 3) simultaneous administration of alfentanil, fentanyl, or sufentanil and a full paralyzing dose of a neuromuscular blocking agent when alfentanil, fentanyl, or sufentanil is used in rapidly administered anesthetic dosages.

Skeletal muscle rigidity can be caused by **remifentanil** and is related to the dose and speed of administration. Remifentanil may cause chest wall rigidity (inability to ventilate) after single doses of > 1 mcg/kg administered over 30 to 60 seconds, or after infusion rates > 0.1 mcg/kg/min. Single doses of < 1 mcg/kg may cause chest wall rigidity when given concurrently with a continuous infusion of remifentanil.

Muscle rigidity seen during the use of remifentanil in spontaneously breathing patients may be treated by stopping or decreasing the rate of administration of remifentanil. Resolution of muscle rigidity after discontinuing the infusion of remifentanil occurs within minutes. In the case of life-threatening muscle rigidity, a rapid-onset neuromuscular blocker or naloxone may be administered.

➤*Supraventricular tachycardias:* Use with caution in atrial flutter and other supraventricular tachycardias; vagolytic action may increase the ventricular response rate.

➤*Cardiovascular effects:* Limit use of **levorphanol** in acute MI or in cardiac patients with myocardial dysfunction or coronary insufficiency because the effects of levorphanol on the work of the heart are unknown.

➤*Biliary surgery:* Use narcotic analgesics with caution in patients about to undergo surgery of the biliary tract because it may cause spasm of the sphincter of Oddi. **Levorphanol** has been shown to cause moderate to marked rises in pressure in the common bile duct when given in analgesic doses; it is not recommended for use in biliary surgery.

➤*Seizures:* Seizures may be aggravated or may occur in individuals without a history of convulsive disorders if dosage is substantially increased above recommended levels because of tolerance. Observe patients with known seizure disorders closely for **morphine**-induced seizure activity.

➤*Cough reflex:* Cough reflex is suppressed. Exercise caution when using narcotic analgesics postoperatively and in patients with pulmonary disease.

➤*Intraoperative awareness:* Intraoperative awareness has been reported in patients < 55 years of age when **remifentanil** has been administered with propofol infusion rates of ≤ 75 mcg/kg/min.

➤*Tolerance:* Some patients develop tolerance to the narcotic analgesic. This may occur after days or months of continuous therapy. The dose generally needs to be increased to obtain adequate analgesia.

Cross-tolerance is not complete. Switching to another narcotic agonist, starting with half the predicted equianalgesic dose, may circumvent the cross-tolerance.

➤*Drug abuse and dependence:* Narcotic analgesics have abuse potential. Psychological/physical dependence and physical tolerance/dependence may develop upon repeated use. Most patients who receive opiates for medical reasons do not develop dependence.

Narcotics can lead to physical dependence with prolonged use. Symptoms include increased tolerance to analgesic effect and complaints, pleas, demands, or manipulative actions shortly before next scheduled dose. Hospitalize patients to treat withdrawal.

Infants born to mothers physically dependent on narcotics will also be physically dependent and may exhibit respiratory difficulties and withdrawal symptoms.

Analysis of some deaths from overdose observed in the development of **levomethadyl** has shown that when levomethadyl is diverted into channels of abuse, the uninformed addict can become impatient with the slow onset of levomethadyl (2 to 4 hours) and take illicit drugs, resulting in a potentially lethal combined overdose when the peak levomethadyl effect develops. Because of these risks of diversion and accidental death, levomethadyl has been approved for use only when dispensed by a licensed facility and is not given in take-home doses.

Acute abstinence syndrome (withdrawal) – Severity is related to the degree of dependence, the abruptness of withdrawal, and the drug used. Generally, withdrawal symptoms develop at the time the next dose would ordinarily be given. For heroin and **morphine**, symptoms gradually increase in intensity, reach a maximum in 36 to 72 hours, and subside over 5 to 10 days. In contrast, **methadone** withdrawal is slower in onset, and the patient may not recover for 6 to 7 weeks. **Meperidine** withdrawal has often run its course within 4 to 5 days. **Hydrocodone** peaks at 48 to 72 hours. Withdrawal precipitated by narcotic antagonists is manifested by onset of symptoms within minutes and maximum intensity within 30 minutes.

Do not use a narcotic antagonist to detect dependence. If a narcotic antagonist must be used for serious respiratory depression in a physically dependent patient, give with extreme care, using ⅒ to ⅕ the usual initial dose.

With morphine, cerebral and spinal receptors may develop tolerance/dependence independently, as a function of local dosage. Take care to avert withdrawal in those patients who have been maintained on parenteral/oral narcotics when epidural or intrathecal administration is considered. Withdrawal may occur following chronic epidural or intrathecal administration, as well as the development of tolerance to morphine by these routes.

Symptoms of withdrawal –
  Early: Yawning; lacrimation; rhinorrhea; "yen sleep"; sweating.
  Intermediate: Mydriasis; piloerection; tachycardia; twitching; tremor; restlessness; irritability; anxiety; anorexia.
  Late: Muscle spasm; fever; nausea; diarrhea; vomiting; kicking movements; weakness; depression; body aches; weight loss; severe backache; abdominal and leg pains; abdominal and muscle cramps; hot and cold flashes; insomnia; intestinal spasm; coryza and repetitive sneezing; increase in body temperature, blood pressure, respiratory rate, and heart rate; spontaneous orgasm.

Patients may experience withdrawal symptoms (nasal congestion, abdominal symptoms, diarrhea, muscle aches, anxiety) over the 72-hour dosing interval if the dose of **levomethadyl** is too low.

Treatment – Primarily symptomatic and supportive; maintain proper fluid and electrolyte balance and administer a tranquilizer to suppress anxiety. Severe withdrawal symptoms may require narcotic replacement. Gradual withdrawal using successively smaller doses will minimize symptoms.

Methadone is not a tranquilizer; patients may react to problems and stresses with the same anxiety symptoms as others do. Do not confuse such symptoms with narcotic abstinence; do not treat anxiety by increasing the methadone dose.

During induction of methadone maintenance, patients being withdrawn from heroin may show withdrawal symptoms, which should be differentiated from methadone-induced side effects. During prolonged methadone use, side effects gradually disappear over several weeks. However, constipation and sweating often persist.

►*Hazardous tasks:* May produce drowsiness or dizziness. Patients should use caution while driving or performing other tasks requiring alertness, coordination, or physical dexterity.

►*Sulfite sensitivity:* May cause allergic-type reactions (eg, hives, itching, wheezing, anaphylaxis) in certain susceptible persons. Although the overall prevalence of sulfite sensitivity in the general population is probably low, it is seen more frequently in asthmatics or in atopic nonasthmatic persons. Specific products containing sulfites are identified in the product listings.

Drug Interactions

Narcotic Agonist Analgesics Drug Interactions			
Precipitant drug	Object drug*		Description
Agonist/Antagonist analgesics	Narcotic agonist analgesics	↓	Do not administer agonist/antagonist analgesics (eg, pentazocine, nalbuphine, butorphanol, dezocine, buprenorphine) to a patient who has received or is receiving a course of therapy with a pure agonist opioid analgesic such as **levorphanol** or **oxycodone**. In opioid-dependent patients, mixed agonist/antagonist analgesics may precipitate withdrawal symptoms.
Barbiturate anesthetics	Narcotic agonist analgesics	↑	Barbiturate anesthetics may increase the respiratory and CNS-depressant effects of the narcotics because of additive pharmacologic activity.
Chlorpromazine Thioridazine	Narcotic agonist analgesics	↑	Although the analgesic effect of narcotics may be potentiated, a higher incidence of toxic effects may occur. Avoid combination with **meperidine**.
MAOIs Furazolidone	Narcotic agonist analgesics	↑	MAOIs markedly potentiate the action of **morphine**. **Meperidine** has precipitated unpredictable, severe, occasionally fatal reactions in those concurrently receiving MAOIs or those who have received such agents within 14 days. The mechanism may be related to a preexisting hyperphenylalaninemia. Reactions have included coma, respiratory depression, cyanosis, and hypotension; in others, hyperexcitability, convulsions, tachycardia, hyperpyrexia, and hypertension have occurred. Use caution. If a narcotic is needed, perform a sensitivity test. Use hydrocortisone IV or prednisolone for severe reactions; use IV chlorpromazine in those with hypertension and hyperpyrexia. Value of narcotic antagonists for these reactions is unknown.
Antihistamines Chloral hydrate Glutethimide Methocarbamol	Morphine	↑	Depressant effects of morphine may be enhanced.
Amitriptyline	Morphine	↑	Monitor for increased CNS and respiratory depression when administered with morphine.
Charcoal	Propoxyphene	↓	Charcoal decreases the GI absorption of propoxyphene.
Cigarette smoking	Propoxyphene	↓	Cigarette smoking may induce liver enzymes responsible for the metabolism of propoxyphene; efficacy is reportedly decreased in smokers. Patients may increase the dosage to obtain adequate pain relief.
Cimetidine	Alfentanil Meperidine Methadone Morphine	↑	Monitor for increased respiratory and CNS depression (methadone, morphine, meperidine). Cimetidine reduces alfentanil clearance. Smaller alfentanil doses will be required with prolonged administration, and the duration of action of alfentanil may be extended. Concomitant administration of cimetidine and morphine has been reported to precipitate apnea, confusion, and muscle twitching in an isolated report.
Clomipramine	Morphine	↑	Monitor for increased CNS and respiratory depression when administered with morphine.
Diazepam	Alfentanil Fentanyl	↑	Diazepam may produce cardiovascular depression when given with high doses of fentanyl and alfentanil. Administration prior to or following high doses of alfentanil decreases blood pressure secondary to vasodilation; recovery may be prolonged.
Droperidol	Fentanyl	↑	May cause hypotension and decrease pulmonary arterial pressure.
Erythromycin	Alfentanil	↑	Concomitant use with alfentanil can significantly inhibit alfentanil clearance and may increase the risk of prolonged or delayed respiratory depression.
Fluvoxamine	Methadone	↑	Monitor for increased CNS depression when taken with methadone. Monitor for signs and symptoms of withdrawal when fluvoxamine is discontinued.
Hydantoins	Meperidine Methadone	↓	Hydantoins may decrease the pharmacologic effects of meperidine and methadone, possibly because of increased hepatic metabolism of the narcotic.
Nitrous oxide	Fentanyl Sufentanil	↑	Nitrous oxide may cause cardiovascular depression with high-dose sufentanil and fentanyl.
Nortriptyline	Morphine	↑	Monitor for increased CNS and respiratory depression when administered with morphine.
Protease inhibitors	Alfentanil Fentanyl Hydrocodone Meperidine Methadone Oxycodone Propoxyphene	↑	Avoid combination with meperidine and propoxyphene; monitor for increased CNS and respiratory depression with other agents (alfentanil, fentanyl, methadone, hydrocodone, oxycodone).
Rifampin	Methadone	↓	Rifampin may reduce methadone blood concentration, producing withdrawal symptoms. Mechanism may be due to increased methadone hepatic metabolism; enhanced microsomal drug-metabolized enzymes may influence drug disposition.
Methadone	Desipramine	↑	Desipramine blood levels have increased with concurrent methadone therapy.
Morphine Propoxyphene	Anticoagulants	↑	Propoxyphene and morphine may potentiate warfarin's anticoagulant effect and that of other anticoagulants. Potentiation of the hypoprothrombinemic effect of warfarin by propoxyphene may occur.
Propoxyphene	Carbamazepine	↑	Pharmacologic effects may increase when used with propoxyphene. Monitor serum carbamazepine levels and the patient for symptoms of toxicity.
Sufentanil	Beta blockers	↑	The incidence and degree of bradycardia and hypotension during induction of sufentanil may be greater in patients on chronic beta blocker therapy.
Sufentanil	Calcium channel blockers	↑	The incidence and degree of bradycardia and hypotension during induction of sufentanil may be greater in patients on chronic calcium channel blocker therapy.

* ↑ = Object drug increased. ↓ = Object drug decreased.

➤*Drug/Lab test interactions:* Narcotics may increase biliary tract pressure with resultant increases in plasma **amylase** or **lipase**; therefore, determinations of these levels may be unreliable for 24 hours after narcotic administration.

➤*Drug/Food interactions:* In 1 study, **morphine** oral solution after a high-fat meal increased morphine's area under the concentration-time curve 34% vs morphine in the fasting state.

Adverse Reactions

Major hazards – Respiratory depression; apnea; circulatory depression; respiratory arrest; coma; shock; cardiac arrest; hypoventilation.

Most cases of serious or fatal adverse events involving **levorphanol** reported to the manufacturer and the FDA have involved either the administration of large initial doses or too frequent doses of the drug to non-opioid-tolerant patients, or the simultaneous administration of levorphanol with other drugs affecting respiration. Reduce the initial levorphanol dose by approximately ≥ 50% when it is given to patients along with another drug affecting respiration.

Most frequent – Respiratory depression; skeletal muscle rigidity; apnea; bradycardia; lightheadedness; dizziness; sedation; nausea; vomiting; sweating. Symptoms are more prominent in ambulatory patients and in those without severe pain. Use lower doses in these patients. Some reactions may be alleviated if the ambulatory patient lies down.

➤*Cardiovascular:* Flushing; faintness; peripheral circulatory collapse; tachycardia; bradycardia; arrhythmia; palpitations; chest wall rigidity; hypertension; hypotension; orthostatic hypotension; syncope; cardiac arrest; shock; heart block; extrasystoles; pallor; ventricular extrasystole; bronchoconstriction; ECG changes consistent with myocardial ischemia; elevated CPK-MB level; asystole hypercarbia (**alfentanil**) and phlebitis following IV injection. Circulatory depression, peripheral circulatory collapse, and cardiac arrest have occurred after rapid IV **hydromorphone** injection.

Physicians should be alert to palpitations, syncope, or other symptoms suggestive of episodes of irregular cardiac rhythm in patients taking **levomethadyl** and should promptly evaluate such cases.

➤*CNS:* Euphoria; dysphoria; delirium; insomnia; agitation; anxiety; fear; hallucinations; disorientation; drowsiness; sedation; lethargy; mental and physical impairment; skeletal or uncoordinated movements; coma; mood changes; weakness; headache; mental cloudiness; blurred vision; diplopia; miosis; tremor; convulsions; psychic dependence; toxic psychoses; depression; increased intracranial pressure; hypesthesia; prolonged emergence from anesthesia; awareness under anesthesia without pain; rapid awakening from anesthesia; nightmares; nystagmus; twitch; amnesia; paranoid reaction; drug withdrawal; suicide attempt; hypokinesia; dyskinesia; hyperkinesia; speech disorder; abnormal gait; paresthesia; stupor; apathy. Injection near a nerve trunk may result in sensory-motor paralysis which is usually transitory.

Choreic movements have been induced by **methadone**. Seizures have occurred following **fentanyl** administration.

➤*GI:* Nausea; vomiting; diarrhea; cramps; abdominal pain; taste alterations; dry mouth; anorexia; constipation; biliary tract spasm; xerostomia; ileus; paralytic ileus; toxic megacolon in patients with inflammatory bowel disease; flatulence; dyspepsia; dysphagia; gastroesophageal reflux. Patients with chronic ulcerative colitis may have increased colonic motility; toxic dilatation occurred in acute ulcerative colitis.

Coadministration of anthraquinone laxatives (especially senna compounds) in an approximate dose of 187 mg senna concentrate per 120 mg codeine equivalent may counteract narcotic-induced constipation.

➤*GU:* Ureteral spasm and spasm of vesical sphincters; urinary retention or hesitancy; oliguria; antidiuretic effect; reduced libido or potency; kidney failure; difficulty urinating; impotence; difficult ejaculation; urinary incontinence; dysuria.

➤*Hypersensitivity:* Pruritus; urticaria; hives; facial swelling; itching; bronchospasm; laryngeal edema; laryngospasm; other skin rashes; edema; anaphylaxis; hemorrhagic urticaria (rare). Wheal and flare over the vein with IV injection may occur. Anaphylactoid reactions have occurred following IV administration. A case of **morphine**-induced thrombocytopenia has occurred.

➤*Lab test abnormalities:* Abnormal liver function tests with **propoxyphene**. Reversible thrombocytopenia has been described in a narcotics addict with chronic hepatitis.

➤*Miscellaneous:* Depression of cough reflex; interference with thermal regulation; chills; pain at injection site; local tissue irritation and induration following SC injection, particularly when repeated; skeletal muscle rigidity of neck and extremities; atelectasis; airway obstruction; asthma exacerbation; accommodation abnormality; myasthenia; sweating; rhinitis; cyanosis; postoperative pain; tearing; yawning; arthralgia; malaise; flu syndrome; hot flashes; shivering; hiccups; hemoptysis; pharyngitis; rhonchi; stridor; nasal congestion; pleural effusion; pulmonary edema; rales; bronchitis; rhinorrhea; abnormal liver function; hyperglycemia; electrolyte disorders; increased CPK level; anemia;

lymphopenia; leukocytosis; thrombocytopenia; bradypnea (**alfentanil** for MAC); reversible jaundice, including cholestatic jaundice (**propoxyphene**). **Sufentanil** may cause erythema and intraoperative muscle movement. Subacute painful myopathy has occurred following chronic **propoxyphene** overdosage.

Overdosage

In general, the shorter the onset and duration of action of the opiate, the greater the intensity and rapidity of symptom onset. Infants and children may be relatively more sensitive on a body weight basis. Elderly patients are comparatively intolerant.

➤*Symptoms:* In severe overdosage, mainly by the IV route, apnea, circulatory collapse, convulsions, cardiac arrest, pulmonary edema, and death may occur. The less severely poisoned patient often presents with a triad of CNS depression, miosis, and respiratory depression. Serious overdosage is characterized by respiratory depression, extreme somnolence progressing to stupor or coma, constricted pupils, skeletal muscle flaccidity, and cold and clammy skin. Hypotension, bradycardia, hypothermia, pulmonary edema, pneumonia, or shock occurs in ≤ 40% of patients.

➤*Treatment:* Employ supportive measures as indicated. Refer to General Management of Acute Overdosage. Give primary attention to reestablishment of adequate respiratory exchange; provide a patent airway and institute assisted or controlled ventilation; if depressed respiration is associated with muscular rigidity, use an IV neuromuscular blocker.

Administer a narcotic antagonist. Because the duration of action of most narcotics exceeds that of the narcotic antagonist, repeat the antagonist to maintain adequate respiration; keep the patient under surveillance. Do not give an antagonist in the absence of clinically significant respiratory or cardiovascular depression. Naloxone is the antagonist of choice (see individual monograph).

IV fluids and vasopressors for the treatment of hypotension and other supportive measures may be employed. Glycopyrrolate or atropine may be useful for the treatment of bradycardia or hypotension.

Respiratory depression may be delayed in onset up to 24 hours following epidural or intrathecal administration of **morphine**. In painful conditions, reversal of narcotic effect may result in acute onset of pain and release of catecholamines. Careful administration of naloxone may permit reversal of side effects without affecting analgesia. Parenteral administration of narcotics in patients receiving epidural or intrathecal morphine may result in overdosage.

In cases of oral overdose, evacuate the stomach by emesis or gastric lavage if treatment can be instituted within 2 hours following ingestion. Absorption of drugs from the GI tract may be decreased by giving activated charcoal which, in many cases, is more effective than emesis or lavage. Observe the patient for a rise in temperature or pulmonary complications that may require antibiotic therapy.

Forced diuresis, peritoneal dialysis, hemodialysis, or charcoal hemoperfusion have not been established as beneficial for a **codeine**, **methadone**, or **levomethadyl** overdosage. Dialysis is of little value in poisoning due to **propoxyphene**.

Patient Information

May cause drowsiness, dizziness, or blurring of vision; use caution while driving or performing other tasks requiring alertness, coordination, or physical dexterity.

Orthostatic hypotension may occur with the use of this medication, expecially in ambulatory patients. Patients should get up slowly from a sitting or lying position.

Do not take **levomethadyl** daily; daily use of the usual dose will lead to serious overdose.

Avoid alcohol and other CNS depressants.

If transferring from **levomethadyl** to **methadone**, wait 48 hours after the last dose of levomethadyl before ingesting the first dose of methadone or other narcotic.

Notify physician if nausea, vomiting, or constipation become prominent.

If GI upset occurs, these agents may be taken with food.

Notify physician if shortness of breath or difficulty in breathing occurs.

Do not adjust the dose without consulting the physician.

Consult physician if the patient is pregnant or planning to become pregnant.

Because of this drug's potential for abuse, protect it from theft and do not to give to anyone other than the individual for whom it was prescribed.

Do not discontinue the drug abruptly if therapy has lasted more than a few weeks. Consult physician.

Avoid exposing the **fentanyl transdermal** system application site to a direct external heat source. There is a potential for temperature-dependent increases in fentanyl release from the system.

ALFENTANIL HCl

c-ii	Alfenta (Taylor)	Injection: 500 mcg (as HCl)/ml	Preservative free. In 2, 5, 10, and 20 ml amps.

For complete prescribing information, refer to the Narcotic Agonist Analgesics group monograph.

Indications

►*Analgesic:* Analgesic adjunct given in incremental doses in the maintenance of anesthesia with barbiturate/nitrous oxide/oxygen.

Analgesic administered by continuous infusion with nitrous oxide/oxygen in the maintenance of general anesthesia.

►*Anesthetic:* Primary anesthetic for induction of anesthesia in general surgery when endotracheal intubation and mechanical ventilation are required.

►*Monitored anesthesia care (MAC):* Analgesic component for monitored anesthesia care.

Administration and Dosage

Individualize dosage and titrate to desired effect in each patient according to body weight, physical status, underlying pathological conditions, use of other drugs, and type and duration of surgical procedure and anesthesia. In obese patients (> 20% above ideal total body weight), determine dosage on the basis of lean body weight. Reduce dose in elderly or debilitated patients.

Monitor vital signs routinely.

►*Children (< 12 years of age):* Use is not recommended.

►*Premedication:* Individualize the selection of preanesthetic medications.

►*Neuromuscular blocking agents:* Neuromuscular blocking agents should be compatible with the patient's condition.

In patients administered anesthetic (induction) dosages, qualified personnel and adequate facilities are essential for the management of intraoperative and postoperative respiratory depression.

Use a tuberculin syringe or equivalent for accuracy in small volumes.

Alfentanil Dosage Range for Use During General Anesthesia				
Clinical status	≈ Duration of anesthesia	Induction (Initial dose)	Maintenance (Increments/Infusion)	Total dose
Spontaneously breathing/ Assisted ventilation	≤ 30 min	8-20 mcg/kg	3-5 mcg/kg every 5-20 min or 0.5-1 mcg/kg/min	8-40 mcg/kg
Assisted or controlled ventilation				
Incremental injection (to attenuate response to laryngoscopy and intubation)	30-60 min	20-50 mcg/kg	5-15 mcg/kg every 5-20 min	up to 75 mcg/kg
Continuous infusion[1] (to provide attenuation of response to intubation and incision)	> 45 min	50-75 mcg/kg	0.5-3 mcg/kg/min. Average infusion rate 1-1.5 mcg/kg/min	dependent on duration of procedure
Anesthetic induction (give slowly [over 3 min]). Reduce concentration of inhalation agents by 30%-50% for initial hour)	> 45 min	130-245 mcg/kg	0.5-1.5 mcg/kg/min or general anesthetic	dependent on duration of procedure
MAC (for sedated and responsive spontaneously breathing patients)	≤ 30 min	3-8 mcg/kg	3-5 mcg/kg every 5-20 min or 0.25 to 1 mcg/kg/min	3-40 mcg/kg

[1] 0.5 to 3 mcg/kg/min with nitrous oxide/oxygen in general surgery. Following anesthetic induction dose, reduce infusion rate requirements by 30% to 50% for the first hour of maintenance. Vital sign changes that indicate response to surgical stress or lightening of anesthesia may be controlled by increasing rate to a max of 4 mcg/kg/min or administering bolus doses of 7 mcg/kg. If changes are not controlled after 3 bolus doses given over 5 minutes, use a barbiturate, vasodilator, or inhalation agent. Always adjust infusion rates downward in the absence of these signs until there is some response to surgical stimulation. Rather than an increase in infusion rate, administer 7 mcg/kg bolus doses of alfentanil or a potent inhalation agent in response to signs of lightening of anesthesia within the last 15 minutes of surgery. Discontinue infusion ≥ 10 to 15 minutes prior to the end of surgery.

►*Admixture compatibility:* Physical and chemical compatibilities of alfentanil have been demonstrated in solution (concentration range, 25 to 80 mcg/ml) with Normal Saline, 5% Dextrose in Normal Saline, 5% Dextrose in Water, and Lactated Ringers.

CODEINE

c-ii	Codeine Sulfate (Various, eg, Roxane)	Tablets: 15 mg	In 100s and UD 100s.
		30 mg	In 100s and UD 100s.
		60 mg	In 100s and UD 100s.
c-ii	Codeine Phosphate (Roxane)	Solution, oral: 15 mg/5 ml	In 500 ml and UD 5 ml.
c-ii	Codeine Phosphate (Various, eg, ESI Lederle, Wyeth-Ayerst[1])	Injection: 30 mg	In 1 ml vials and 1 ml *Tubex*.
c-ii	Codeine Phosphate (Various, eg, ESI Lederle, Wyeth-Ayerst[2])	Injection: 60 mg	In 1 ml *Tubex*.

[1] With ≤ 1.5 mg sodium metabisulfite.

[2] With ≤ 2 mg sodium metabisulfite.

For complete prescribing information, refer to the Narcotic Agonist Analgesic group monograph.

Indications

Codeine is a narcotic analgesic and antitussive that resembles morphine pharmacologically but with milder actions. It is a less-potent antitussive than morphine on a weight basis; however, it is widely used as a cough suppressant because of its low incidence of adverse reactions at the usual antitussive dose. Codeine is ⅔ as effective orally as parenterally.

►*Pain/Cough:* Relief of mild-to-moderate pain and for coughing induced by chemical or mechanical irritation of the respiratory system.

Administration and Dosage

►*Analgesic:*

Adults – 15 to 60 mg every 4 to 6 hours, orally, IM, IV, or SC. Usual dose is 30 mg. Do not exceed 360 mg in 24 hours.

Children (≥ 1 year of age) – 0.5 mg/kg or 15 mg/m² of body surface every 4 to 6 hours SC, IM, or orally. Do not use IV in children.

►*Antitussive:* (See also Narcotic Antitussive monograph.)

Adults – 10 to 20 mg orally every 4 to 6 hours. Do not exceed 120 mg in 24 hours.

Children (6 to 12 years of age) – 5 to 10 mg orally every 4 to 6 hours. Do not exceed 60 mg in 24 hours.
 (2 to 6 years): 2.5 to 5 mg orally every 4 to 6 hours. Do not exceed 30 mg in 24 hours.

►*Storage/Stability:* Protect from light (injection).

FENTANYL

c-ii	Fentanyl (Various, eg, ESI Lederle, Schein)	Injection: 0.05 mg base (as citrate)/ml	In 2, 5, 10, and 20 ml amps; 20, 30, and 50 ml vials; and 2 and 5 ml *Carpujects*.
c-ii	Sublimaze (Taylor)		Preservative free. In 2, 5, 10, and 20 ml amps.

For complete prescribing information, refer to the Narcotic Agonist Analgesics group monograph.

Indications

►*Pain:* For analgesic action of short duration during anesthesia (premedication, induction, maintenance), and in the immediate postoperative period (recovery room) as needed.

For use as a narcotic analgesic supplement in general or regional anesthesia.

For administration with a neuroleptic such as droperidol (see monograph in the General Anesthetics section) as an anesthetic premedication, for induction of anesthesia, and as an adjunct in maintenance of general and regional anesthesia.

FENTANYL

For use as an anesthetic agent with oxygen in selected high-risk patients (open heart surgery or certain complicated neurological or orthopedic procedures).

Administration and Dosage

Individualize dosage. Monitor vital signs routinely.

➤*Concomitant anesthesia:* Certain forms of conduction anesthesia, such as spinal anesthesia and some peridural anesthetics, can alter respiration by blocking intercostal nerves. Fentanyl can also alter respiration through other mechanisms.

➤*Concomitant narcotic administration:* The respiratory depressant effect of fentanyl may persist longer than the analgesic effect. Consider the total dose of all narcotic analgesics used. Use narcotics in reduced doses initially, ¼ to ⅓ those usually recommended.

➤*Premedication:* 0.05 to 0.1 mg IM, 30 to 60 minutes prior to surgery.

➤*Adjunct to general anesthesia:*

Total low dose – 0.002 mg/kg in small doses for minor, painful surgical procedures and postoperative pain relief.

Maintenance low dose – 0.002 mg/kg. Infrequently needed in minor procedures.

Total moderate dose – 0.002 to 0.02 mg/kg. In addition to adequate analgesia, some abolition of the stress response should occur. Respiratory depression necessitates artificial ventilation and careful observation of postoperative ventilation.

Maintenance moderate dose – 0.002 to 0.02 mg/kg. Use 0.025 to 0.1 mg IV or IM when movement or changes in vital signs indicate surgical stress or lightening of analgesia.

Total high dose – 0.02 to 0.05 mg/kg. For "stress free" anesthesia. Use during open heart surgery and complicated neurosurgical and orthopedic procedures where surgery is prolonged and the stress response is detrimental. Inject with nitrous oxide/oxygen to attenuate the stress response. Postoperative ventilation and observation are required.

Maintenance high dose – 0.02 to 0.05 mg/kg. Ranging from 0.025 mg to half the initial loading dose. Individualize dosage. Administer when vital signs indicate surgical stress and lightening of analgesia.

➤*Adjunct to regional anesthesia:* 0.05 to 0.1 mg IM or slowly IV over 1 to 2 minutes as required.

➤*Postoperatively (recovery room):* 0.05 to 0.1 mg IM for the control of pain, tachypnea, and emergence delirium; repeat dose in 1 to 2 hours as needed.

➤*Children (2 to 12 years of age):* For induction and maintenance, a reduced dose as low as 2 to 3 mcg/kg is recommended. Safety and efficacy in children < 2 years of age have not been established.

➤*General anesthetic:* 0.05 to 0.1 mg/kg with oxygen and a muscle relaxant when attenuation of the responses to surgical stress is especially important. Up to 0.15 mg/kg may be necessary. It has been used for open heart surgery and other major surgical procedures to protect the myocardium from excess oxygen demand and for complicated neurological and orthopedic procedures.

➤*Storage / Stability:* Protect from light.

FENTANYL TRANSMUCOSAL SYSTEM

c-ii	**Actiq** (Cephalon)	**Lozenge on a stick:** 200 mcg	Sucrose, liquid glucose. Raspberry flavor. In 24s with gray carton/foil pouch.
		400 mcg	Sucrose, liquid glucose. Raspberry flavor. In 24s with blue carton/foil pouch.
		600 mcg	Sucrose, liquid glucose. Raspberry flavor. In 24s with orange carton/foil pouch.
		800 mcg	Sucrose, liquid glucose. Raspberry flavor. In 24s with purple carton/foil pouch.
		1200 mcg	Sucrose, liquid glucose. Raspberry flavor. In 24s with green carton/foil pouch.
		1600 mcg	Sucrose, liquid glucose. Raspberry flavor. In 24s with burgundy carton/foil pouch.

For complete prescribing information, refer to the Narcotic Agonist Analgesics group monograph.

WARNING

Fentanyl transmucosal contains the potent narcotic fentanyl citrate in a formulation that:

Fentanyl Oralet:
- Carries a risk of hypoventilation with its use that may result in death if not monitored by trained personnel supported by appropriate, immediately available equipment.
- Use only as an anesthetic premedication or for inducing conscious sedation prior to a diagnostic or therapeutic procedure in a monitored anesthesia care setting.
- Administer in hospital settings such as the operating room, emergency department, ICU, or other monitored anesthesia care settings in hospitals where there is immediate access to life support equipment, oxygen, facilities for endotracheal intubation, IV fluids, and opioid antagonists.
- Can only be used safely in patients being monitored by 1) direct visual observation by a health professional whose sole responsibility is observation of the patient and by 2) some means of measuring respiratory function such as pulse oximetry until the patient has completely recovered.
- Only administer by people specifically trained in the use of anesthetic drugs and the management of the respiratory effects of potent opioids, including respiratory and cardiac resuscitation of patients in the age group being treated. Such training must include the establishment and maintenance of a patent airway and assisted ventilation.
- Only use by health care practitioners instructed in the use of the product by the director of anesthesia of the institution in which the product will be used.
- Contraindicated for use at any other setting outside a hospital.

Fentanyl transmucosal use is contraindicated in:
- Children who weigh < 10 kg (22 lbs).
- Treatment of acute or chronic pain. The safety of this product for these indications has not been established.
- Doses > 15 mcg/kg in children, and in doses > 5 mcg/kg in adults. Because of the excessive frequency of significant hypoventilation at higher doses, the maximum dose any child or adult should receive is 400 mcg, regardless of weight.

Actiq:
- Indicated only for the management of breakthrough cancer pain in patients with malignancies already receiving and tolerant to opioid therapy for their underlying persistent cancer pain.
- It is contraindicated in the management of acute or postoperative pain. Because life-threatening hypoventilation could occur at any dose in patients not taking chronic opiates, do not use in opioid non-tolerant patients.
- Use only in the care of cancer patients and only by oncologists and pain specialists who are knowledgeable of and skilled in the use of Schedule II opioids to treat cancer pain.
- Instruct patients and their caregivers that this drug contains a medicine in an amount which can be fatal to a child. Keep all units out of reach of children, and discard opened units properly.

Indications

➤*Anesthesia (Fentanyl Oralet only):* Only indicated for use in a hospital setting 1) as an anesthetic premedication in the operating room setting or 2) to induce conscious sedation prior to a diagnostic or therapeutic procedure in other monitored anesthesia care settings in the hospital.

➤*Breakthrough cancer pain (Actiq only):* Only indicated for the management of breakthrough cancer pain in patients with malignancies who are already receiving and are tolerant to opioid therapy for their underlying persistent cancer pain. Patients considered opioid-tolerant are those who are taking ≥ 60 mg morphine/day, 50 mcg transdermal fentanyl/hour, or an equianalgesic dose of another opioid for ≥ 1 week.

Administration and Dosage

➤*Fentanyl Oralet:* Individualize doses based on the status of each patient, the clinical environment, and the desired therapeutic effect; reduce dosage in elderly, debilitated, or other vulnerable patients.

Some of the factors to be considered in determining an individualized dose are age, body weight, physical status, general condition and medi-

cal status, underlying pathological condition, use of other drugs, type of anesthesia to be used, and the type and length of the procedure.

Fentanyl transmucosal doses of 5 mcg/kg provide effects similar to usual doses of fentanyl given IM (0.75 to 1.25 mcg/kg). Larger doses have not been shown to increase efficacy. As with all opioids, reduce the dosage in vulnerable patients. The magnitude of the expected effect will vary from mild with doses of 5 mcg/kg to marked with doses of 15 mcg/kg. Adults should not receive doses > 5 mcg/kg (400 mcg), and most children who are not apprehensive at onset may be managed with the same 5 mcg/kg dose. Children apprehensive at onset and some younger children may need doses of 5 to 15 mcg/kg with an attendant increased risk of hypoventilation.

Children – Because of the excessive frequency of significant hypoventilation at higher doses, doses > 15 mcg/kg (maximum dose, 400 mcg) are contraindicated in children.

Selection of dosage strength is based on patient weight; a dose range of 5 to 15 mcg/kg is recommended. Premedication of children < 40 kg may require doses of 10 to 15 mcg/kg.

Pediatric Fentanyl Transmucosal (*Fentanyl Oralet*) Dosage Regimen		
Patient weight (kg)	5 to 10 mcg/kg	10 to 15 mcg/kg
< 10	contraindicated	contraindicated
10	100 mcg	100 mcg
15	100 mcg	200 mcg
20	100 or 200 mcg	200 or 300 mcg
25	200 mcg	300 mcg
30	300 mcg	300 or 400 mcg
35	300 mcg	400 mcg
≥ 40	400 mcg	use 400 mcg (see Adults)

Adults – Because of the excessive frequency of significant hypoventilation at higher doses, doses > 5 mcg/kg (maximum, 400 mcg) are contraindicated in adults.

Vulnerable patients – Consider selection of a lower dose for vulnerable patients (eg, patients with head injury, cardiovascular or pulmonary disease, hepatic disease, liver dysfunction). If signs of excessive opioid effects appear before the unit is consumed, immediately remove the dosage unit from the patient's mouth.

Elderly – If fentanyl transmucosal is to be used in patients > 65 years old, reduce the dose to 2.5 to 5 mcg/kg. Although studies in the elderly have not been conducted, elderly patients are twice as sensitive to the effects of other forms of fentanyl as the younger population. Like all potent opioid analgesics, fentanyl transmucosal can depress respiration and reduce ventilatory drive to a clinically significant extent.

Administration – Remove the foil overwrap just prior to administration. After the plastic overcap is removed, instruct the patient to place the fentanyl transmucosal unit in the mouth and to suck (not chew) it. Chewed or swallowed fentanyl contributes little to the peak concentration, but is responsible for a prolonged "tail" on the blood level profile as it is slowly absorbed.

Remove the unit using the handle after it is consumed or if the patient has achieved an adequate effect or shows signs of respiratory depression.

Place any remaining portion of the fentanyl transmucosal unit in the plastic overcap and dispose of the unit appropriately as required for Schedule II drugs.

Begin administration of the unit 20 to 40 minutes prior to the anticipated need for desired effect. Patients typically take 10 to 20 minutes for complete consumption. Peak effect occurs ≈ 20 to 30 minutes after the start of administration. If hypoventilation or some other adverse event occurs before the dosage unit is consumed, immediately remove the unit from the patient's mouth.

Advise health care professionals skilled in airway management and resuscitative measures to attend to the patient at all times. Administer only in monitored settings and by people specifically trained in the use of anesthetics and the management of the respiratory effects of potent opioids, including maintenance of a patent airway and assisted ventilation. Some means for measuring respiratory function, such as pulse oximetry, is recommended.

Safety and handling – Fentanyl transmucosal is supplied in individually sealed dosage forms that pose no known risk to health care providers having incidental dermal contact. Treat accidental dermal exposure by rinsing the affected area with cool water.

FENTANYL TRANSMUCOSAL SYSTEM

Disposal – Remove the drug matrix from the handle by grasping it with tissue paper, and separate the drug matrix from the handle using a twisting motion. Then flush the drug matrix down the toilet. If any drug matrix remains on the handle, it may be removed by placing the handle under warm running tap water until the remaining portion of the drug matrix is dissolved. Dispose of the drug-free handle according to institutional protocol. During the disposal process, avoid contact of the drug matrix with the skin, eyes, or mucous membranes. Wash hands thoroughly when finished. Disposal must be consistent with State and Federal regulations.

➤*Actiq:* Use has not been established with opioid-tolerant children < 16 years of age. Keep out of the reach of children.

Open the foil package immediately prior to product use. Place the unit in the patient's mouth between the cheek and lower gum, moving it from one side to the other using the handle. Instruct the patient to suck, not chew, the lozenge. A unit dose, if chewed and swallowed, might result in lower peak concentrations and lower bioavailability.

Instruct the patient to consume the lozenge over a 15-minute period. Longer or shorter consumption times may produce less efficacy than reported in clinical trials. If signs of excessive opioid effects appear before the unit is consumed, remove the drug matrix from the patient's mouth immediately and decrease future doses.

Dose titration – Initial dose to treat episodes of breakthrough cancer pain should be 200 mcg. Prescribe patients an initial titration supply of six 200 mcg units. Advise patients to use all units before increasing to a higher dose.

Redosing within a single episode: Until the appropriate dose is reached, it may be necessary to use an additional unit during a single episode. Redosing may start 15 minutes after the previous unit has been completed (30 minutes after the start of the previous unit). Do not give > 2 units for each individual breakthrough cancer pain episode while patients are in the titration phase and consuming units which individually may be subtherapeutic.

Increasing the dose: At each new dose during titration, prescribe 6 units of the titration. Evaluate each new dose used in the titration period over several episodes of breakthrough cancer pain (generally 1 to 2 days) to determine whether it provides adequate efficacy with acceptable side effects. The incidence of side effects is likely to be greater during this initial titration period compared to later, after the effective dose is determined.

Daily limit: Once a successful dose has been found (ie, an average episode is treated with a single unit), instruct patients to limit consumption to ≤ 4 units/day. If consumption increases to > 4 units/day, reevaluate the dose of the long-acting opioid for persistent cancer pain.

Discontinuation: A gradual downward titration is recommended for discontinuation because it is not known at what dose level the opioid may be discontinued without producing the signs and symptoms of abrupt withdrawal.

Safety and handling: Actiq is supplied in individually sealed child-resistant foil pouches. The amount of fentanyl contained in the drug can be lethal to a child. Keep out of the reach of children.

Disposal: See disposal of *Fentanyl Oralet.* Dispose of units remaining from a prescription as soon as they are no longer needed. Dispose of all units immediately after use. Partially consumed units represent a special risk because they are no longer protected by the child-resistant pouch, yet may contain enough medicine to be fatal to a child.

A temporary storage bottle is provided to be used in the event that a partially consumed unit cannot be disposed of promptly.

➤*Storage/Stability:* Protect from freezing and moisture. Do not store *Fentanyl Oralet* above 30°C (86°F) or *Actiq* above 25°C (77°F).

FENTANYL TRANSDERMAL SYSTEM

	Product/Distributor	Dose (mcg/hr)	System size (cm²)	Fentanyl content (mg)	How Supplied
c-ii	**Duragesic-25** (Janssen)	25	10	2.5	In cartons containing 5 individually packaged systems.[2]
c-ii	**Duragesic-50[1]** (Janssen)	50	20	5	
c-ii	**Duragesic-75[1]** (Janssen)	75	30	7.5	
c-ii	**Duragesic-100[1]** (Janssen)	100	40	10	

[1] For use only in opioid-tolerant patients.

[2] < 0.2 ml alcohol is released during use.

For complete prescribing information, refer to the Narcotic Agonist Analgesics group monograph.

WARNING

Because serious or life-threatening hypoventilation could occur, fentanyl transdermal is contraindicated:
- in the management of acute or postoperative pain, including use in out-patient surgeries.
- in the management of mild or intermittent pain responsive to PRN or non-opioid therapy.
- in doses exceeding 25 mcg/hr at the initiation of opioid therapy.

Do not administer fentanyl transdermal system to children < 12 years of age or patients < 18 years of age who weigh < 50 kg (110 lbs) except in an authorized investigational research setting.

Fentanyl transdermal system is indicated for treatment of chronic pain (such as that of malignancy) that:
- cannot be managed by lesser means such as acetaminophen-opioid combinations, nonsteroidal analgesics, or PRN dosing with short-acting opioids, and
- require continuous opioid administration.

Only use the 50, 75, and 100 mcg/hr doses in patients who are already on and are tolerant to opioid therapy.

Indications

➤*Pain:* Management of chronic pain in patients requiring continuous opioid analgesia for pain that cannot be managed by lesser means such as acetaminophen-opioid combinations, nonsteroidal analgesics, or PRN dosing with short-acting opioids.

In patients with chronic pain, it is possible to individually titrate the dose of the transdermal system to minimize the risk of adverse effects while providing analgesia. In properly selected patients, fentanyl transdermal system is a safe and effective alternative to other opioid regimens.

Administration and Dosage

Individualize dosage. The most important factor to be considered in determining the appropriate dose is the extent of preexisting opioid tolerance. Reduce initial doses in elderly or debilitated patients.

➤*Application:* Apply to nonirritated and nonirradiated skin on a flat surface, such as chest, back, flank, or upper arm. Clip (do not shave) hair at the application site prior to system application. If the site of application must be cleansed prior to application of the system, do so with clear water. Do not use soaps, oils, lotions, alcohol, or any other agents that might irritate the skin or alter its characteristics. Allow the skin to dry completely prior to system application.

Apply immediately upon removal from the sealed package. Do not alter the system (eg, cut) in any way prior to application. Firmly press the transdermal system in place with the palm of the hand for 30 seconds, making sure the contact is complete, especially around the edges.

Each system may be worn continuously for 72 hours. If analgesia for > 72 hours is required, apply a new system to a different skin site after removal of the previous transdermal system.

Keep out of the reach of children. Fold used systems so that the adhesive side of the system adheres to itself, then flush the system down the toilet immediately upon removal. Dispose of any systems remaining from a prescription as soon as they are no longer needed. Remove unused systems from their pouch and flush down the toilet.

➤*Dose selection:* In selecting an initial dose, give attention to 1) the daily dose, potency, and characteristics of the opioid the patient has been taking previously (eg, whether it is a pure agonist or mixed agonist-antagonist); 2) the reliability of the relative potency estimates used to calculate the dose needed (potency estimates may vary with the route of administration); 3) the degree of opioid tolerance, if any; 4) the general condition and medical status of the patient. Maintain each patient at the lowest dose providing acceptable pain control. Unless the patient has preexisting opioid tolerance, use the lowest dose, 25 mcg/hr, as the initial dose.

To convert patients from oral or parenteral opioids to the transdermal system, use the following methodology:
1.) Calculate the previous 24-hour analgesic requirement.
2.) Convert this amount to the equianalgesic oral morphine dose using the table in the Actions section of the Narcotic Agonist Analgesics group monograph.
3.) The following table displays the range of 24-hour oral and IM morphine doses that are approximately equivalent to each transdermal system dose. Use this table to find the calculated 24-hour morphine dose and the corresponding transdermal fentanyl dose. Initiate treatment using the recommended dose and titrate patients upwards until analgesic efficacy is attained. Upwards titration may be done no more frequently than 3 days after the initial dose; thereafter, it may be done no more frequently than every 6 days. For delivery rates in excess of 100 mcg/hr, multiple systems may be used.

Initial Fentanyl Transdermal Dose Based on Daily Oral Morphine Dose[1]		
Oral 24-hour morphine (mg/day)	IM 24-hour morphine (mg/day)	Fentanyl transdermal (mcg/hr)
45-134	8-22	25
135-224	23-37	50

FENTANYL TRANSDERMAL SYSTEM

Initial Fentanyl Transdermal Dose Based on Daily Oral Morphine Dose[1]		
Oral 24-hour morphine (mg/day)	IM 24-hour morphine (mg/day)	Fentanyl transdermal (mcg/hr)
225-314	38-52	75
315-404	53-67	100
405-494	68-82	125
495-584	83-97	150
585-674	98-112	175
675-764	113-127	200
765-854	128-142	225
855-944	143-157	250
945-1034	158-172	275
1035-1124	173-187	300

[1] Do not use this table to convert from fentanyl transdermal system to other therapies because this conversion to fentanyl is conservative. Use of this table for conversion to other analgesic therapies can overestimate the dose of the new agent. Overdosage of the new analgesic agent is possible.

The majority of patients are adequately maintained with transdermal fentanyl administered every 72 hours. A small number of patients may require systems to be applied every 48 hours. Because of the increase in serum fentanyl concentration over the first 24 hours following initial system application, the initial evaluation of the maximum analgesic effect cannot be made before 24 hours of wearing. The initial dosage may be increased after 3 days.

During the initial application, patients should use short-acting analgesics as needed until analgesic efficacy with the transdermal system is attained. Thereafter, some patients may still require periodic supplemental doses of other short-acting analgesics for breakthrough pain.

➤*Dose titration:* The recommended initial fentanyl transdermal dose based upon the daily oral morphine dose is conservative, and 50% of patients are likely to require a dose increase after initial application. The initial dosage may be increased after 3 days, based on the daily dose of supplemental analgesics required by the patient in the second or third day of the initial application.

It may take up to 6 days after increasing the dose for the patient to reach equilibrium on the new dose. Therefore, patients should wear a higher dose through 2 applications before any further increase in dosage is made on the basis of the average daily use of a supplemental analgesic.

Base appropriate dosage increments on the daily dose of supplementary opioids, using the ratio of 90 mg/24 hours of oral morphine to a 25 mcg/hour increase in transdermal fentanyl dose.

➤*Discontinuation:* Upon system removal, it takes ≥ 17 hours for the fentanyl serum concentration to fall by 50% after system removal. Titrate the dose of the new analgesic based on the patient's report of pain until adequate analgesia has been attained. For patients requiring discontinuation of opioids, a gradual downward titration is recommended because it is not known at what dose level the opioid may be discontinued without producing the signs and symptoms of abrupt withdrawal.

HYDROMORPHONE HCl

c-ii	**Hydromorphone HCl** (Various, eg, Endo, Roxane)	**Tablets:** 2 mg	In 100s and UD 100s.
c-ii	**Dilaudid** (Abbott)		(K 2). Orange. In 100s, 500s, and UD 100s.
c-ii	**Hydromorphone HCl** (Various, eg, Endo, Roxane)	**Tablets:** 4 mg	In 100s, 500s, and UD 100s.
c-ii	**Dilaudid** (Abbott)		(K 4). Yellow. In 100s, 500s, and UD 100s.
c-ii	**Hydromorphone HCl** (Various, eg, Roxane)	**Tablets:** 8 mg	In 100s.
c-ii	**Dilaudid** (Abbott)		Lactose, sodium bisulfite. (8 Knoll). White, scored. Triangular. In 100s.
c-ii	**Hydromorphone HCl** (Various, eg, Roxane)	**Liquid:** 5 mg/5 ml	In 120, 250, and 500 ml and 4 and 8 ml UD patient cups.
c-ii	**Dilaudid-5** (Abbott)		Parabens, sucrose, glycerin. May contain sodium bisulfite. In 473 ml.
c-ii	**Hydromorphone HCl** (Various, eg, Wyeth-Ayerst)	**Injection:** 1 mg/ml	In 1 ml fill in 2 ml *Tubex.*
c-ii	**Dilaudid** (Abbott)		In 1 ml amps.
c-ii	**Hydromorphone HCl** (Various, eg, ESI Lederle, Schein, Wyeth-Ayerst)	**Injection:** 2 mg/ml	In 1 and 20 ml vials and 1 ml fill in 2 ml *Tubex.*
c-ii	**Dilaudid** (Abbott)		In 1 ml amps and 20 ml vials.[1]
c-ii	**Hydromorphone HCl** (Various, eg, ESI Lederle, Wyeth-Ayerst)	**Injection:** 4 mg/ml	In 1 ml fill in 2 ml *Tubex.*
c-ii	**Dilaudid** (Abbott)		In 1 ml amps.
c-ii	**Hydromorphone HCl** (Schein)	**Injection:** 10 mg/ml	In 1 ml and 5 ml.
c-ii	**Dilaudid-HP** (Abbott)		0.2% sodium citrate, 0.2% citric acid. In 1 and 5 ml amps and 50 ml single-dose vials.
c-ii	**Dilaudid-HP** (Abbott)	**Powder for injection, lyophilized:** 250 mg (10 mg/ml after reconstitution)	In single-dose vials.
c-ii	**Hydromorphone HCl** (Paddock)	**Suppositories:** 3 mg	In 6s.
c-ii	**Dilaudid** (Abbott)		In 6s.

[1] With EDTA and methyl- and propylparabens.

For complete prescribing information, refer to the Narcotic Agonist Analgesics group monograph.

Indications

➤*Pain:* Relief of moderate to severe pain.

Administration and Dosage

➤*Oral:*

Tablet – 2 to 4 mg every 4 to 6 hours; ≥ 4 mg every 4 to 6 hours for more severe pain.

Liquid – 2.5 to 10 mg every 4 to 6 hours.

➤*Parenteral:* 1 to 2 mg SC or IM every 4 to 6 hours as needed. For severe pain, administer 3 to 4 mg every 4 to 6 hours as needed. May be given by slow IV injection over 2 to 3 minutes.

Only give the high-potency strength to patients tolerant of other narcotics.

➤*Rectal:* 3 mg every 6 to 8 hours or as directed by physician.

➤*Children:* Safety and efficacy have not been established.

➤*Storage:* Refrigerate suppositories.

LEVORPHANOL TARTRATE

c-ii	**Levorphanol Tartrate** (Roxane)	**Tablets:** 2 mg	(54 410). Lactose. White, scored. In 100s.
c-ii	**Levo-Dromoran** (ICN)		Lactose. Scored. In 100s.

For complete prescribing information, refer to the Narcotic Agonist Analgesics group monograph.

Indications

►*Pain (Levorphanol Tartrate only):* Management of pain where an opioid analgesic is appropriate.

►*Pain / Preoperative medication (Levo-Dromoran only):* Management of moderate-to-severe pain or as a preoperative medication where an opioid analgesic is appropriate.

Administration and Dosage

►*Approved by the FDA:* December 19, 1991.

►*Oral:* Recommended starting dose is 2 mg. Repeat in 6 to 8 hours (*Levo-Dromoran*) or 3 to 6 hours (*Levorphanol Tartrate*) as needed, provided the patient is assessed for signs of hypoventilation and excessive sedation.

Levo-Dromoran – If necessary, increase the dose to up to 3 mg every 6 to 8 hours, after adequate evaluation of the patient's response. Higher doses may be appropriate in opioid-tolerant patients. Adjust dosage according to the severity of the pain; the patient's age, weight, physical status, and underlying diseases; use of concomitant medications; and other factors.

The effective daily dosage range, depending on the severity of the pain, is 8 to 16 mg in 24 hours in the nontolerant patient. Total oral daily doses of > 6 to 12 mg in 24 hours are generally not recommended as starting doses in non-opioid-tolerant patients; lower total daily doses may be appropriate.

Levorphanol Tartrate – The effective daily dosage range, depending on the severity of the pain, is 8 to 16 mg in 24 hours in the nontolerant patient. Total oral daily doses of > 16 mg in 24 hours are generally not recommended as starting doses in non-opioid-tolerant patients

►*Chronic pain:* Individualize dosage. Because there is incomplete cross-tolerance among opioids, when converting a patient from morphine to levorphanol, begin the total daily dose of oral levorphanol at ≈ 1/15 to 1/12 of the total daily dose of oral morphine that such patients had previously required, and then adjust the dose to the patient's clinical response. If a patient is to be placed on fixed-schedule dosing (round-the-clock) with this drug, take care to allow adequate time after each dose change (≈ 72 hours) for the patient to reach a new steady state before a subsequent dose adjustment to avoid excessive sedation due to drug accumulation.

►*Perioperative period (Levo-Dromoran):* Levorphanol has been used for analgesic action during premedication and the postoperative period. Factors to be considered in determining the dosage include age, body weight, physical status, underlying pathological condition, use of other drugs, type of anesthesia used, the surgical procedure involved, and the severity of pain.

►*Premedication (Levo-Dromoran):* Individualize the preoperative medication dose. Two mg levorphanol is approximately equivalent to 10 to 15 mg of morphine or 100 mg of meperidine.

MEPERIDINE HCl

c-ii	**Meperidine HCl** (Various, eg, Amide, Barr, Mallinckrodt, Roxane, Watson, Wyeth-Ayerst)	**Tablets:** 50 mg	In 100s, 500s, 1000s, and UD 25s.
c-ii	**Demerol** (Sanofi-Synthelabo)		(W / D 35). White, scored, convex. In 100s, 500s, and UD 25s.
c-ii	**Meperidine HCl** (Various, eg, Amide, Barr, Mallinckrodt, Roxane, Watson)	**Tablets:** 100 mg	In 100s, 500s, and 1000s.
c-ii	**Demerol** (Sanofi-Synthelabo)		(W / D 37). White, convex. In 100s.
c-ii	**Meperidine HCl** (Roxane)	**Syrup:** 50 mg/5 mL	In 500 mL and UD 5 mL.
c-ii	**Demerol** (Sanofi-Synthelabo)		Glucose, saccharin. Alcohol free. Banana flavor. In pt.
c-ii	**Meperidine HCl** (Various, eg, Baxter, ESI Lederle, Wyeth-Ayerst)	**Injection:** 25 mg/mL	In 1 mL vials and 1 mL fill in 2 mL cartridge units.
c-ii	**Demerol** (Abbott)		In 1 mL *Carpuject* syringes.
c-ii	**Meperidine HCl** (Various, eg, Baxter, ESI Lederle)	**Injection:** 50 mg/mL	In 1 mL vials.
c-ii	**Demerol** (Abbott)		In 1, 1.5, and 2 mL amps, 30 mL vials, and 1 mL *Carpuject* syringes.
c-ii	**Meperidine HCl** (Various, eg, Baxter, ESI Lederle, Wyeth-Ayerst)	**Injection:** 75 mg/mL	In 1 mL vials and 1 mL fill in 2 mL cartridge units.
c-ii	**Demerol** (Abbott)		In 1 mL *Carpuject* syringes.
c-ii	**Meperidine HCl** (Various, eg, Baxter, ESI Lederle, Wyeth-Ayerst)	**Injection:** 100 mg/mL	In 1 mL vials and 20 mL vials.
c-ii	**Demerol** (Abbott)		In 1 mL amp, 20 mL vial, and 1 mL *Carpuject* syringes.

For complete prescribing information, refer to the Narcotic Agonist Analgesics group monograph.

Indications

►*Oral and parenteral:* Relief of moderate-to-severe pain.

►*Parenteral:* For preoperative medication, support of anesthesia, and obstetrical analgesia.

Administration and Dosage

►*Approved by the FDA:* November 1942.

►*Relief of pain:* Individualize dosage. While SC administration is suitable for occasional use, IM administration is preferred for repeated doses. If IV administration is required, decrease dosage and inject very slowly, preferably using a diluted solution. Meperidine is less effective when administered orally than when given parenterally. Reduce proportionately (usually by 25% to 50%) when administering concomitantly with phenothiazines and other tranquilizers.

Take each dose of the syrup in ½ glass of water; if taken undiluted, it may exert a slight topical anesthetic effect on mucous membranes.

Pain relief –

Adults: 50 to 150 mg IM, SC, or orally every 3 to 4 hours, as necessary.

Children: 1.1 to 1.75 mg/kg (0.5 to 0.8 mg/lb) IM, SC, or orally up to adult dose, every 3 or 4 hours, as necessary.

►*Preoperative medication:*

Adults – 50 to 100 mg IM or SC, 30 to 90 minutes before beginning anesthesia.

Children – 1.1 to 2.2 mg/kg (0.5 to 1 mg/lb) IM or SC, up to adult dose, 30 to 90 minutes before beginning anesthesia.

►*Support of anesthesia:* Meperidine may be administered in repeated doses diluted to 10 mg/mL by slow IV injection, or by continuous IV infusion of solution diluted to 1 mg/mL. Individualize dosage.

►*Obstetrical analgesia:* When pains become regular, administer 50 to 100 mg IM or SC; repeat at 1- to 3-hour intervals.

METHADONE HCl

c-ii	**Methadone HCl** (Roxane)	**Tablets**: 5 mg	In 100s and UD 100s.
c-ii	**Dolophine HCl** (Roxane)		(54 162). White, scored. In 100s and UD 25s.
c-ii	**Methadose** (Mallinckrodt)		(Methadose 5). White, scored. In 100s.
c-ii	**Methadone HCl** (Roxane)	**Tablets**: 10 mg	In 100s and UD 100s.
c-ii	**Dolophine HCl** (Roxane)		(54 549). White, scored. In 100s and UD 25s.
c-ii	**Methadose** (Mallinckrodt)		(Methadose 10). White, scored. In 100s.
c-ii	**Methadone HCl Diskets**[1] (Roxane)	**Tablets, dispersable**: 40 mg	In 100s.
c-ii	**Methadose**[2] (Mallinckrodt)		(Methadose 40). White, quadrisected. In 100s.
c-ii	**Methadone HCl** (Roxane)	**Solution, oral**: 5 mg/5 mL	8% alcohol, sorbitol. Citrus flavor. In 500 mL.
		10 mg/5 mL	8% alcohol, sorbitol. Citrus flavor. In 500 mL.
c-ii	**Methadone HCl**[1] (Various, eg, Roxane, UDL)	**Concentrate, oral**: 10 mg/mL	In 1 qt.
c-ii	**Methadone HCl Intensol** (Roxane)		In 30 mL with calibrated dropper.
c-ii	**Methadose**[1] (Mallinckrodt)		Cherry flavor. In 1 qt.
c-ii	**Methadone HCl** (aaiPharma)	**Injection**: 10 mg/mL	0.9% NaCl. In 20 mL vials.[2]
c-ii	**Methadone HCl**[1] (Various, eg, Mallinckrodt, Roxane)	**Powder**	In 50, 100, and 500 g.

[1] For detoxification and maintenance only.   [2] With 0.5% chlorobutanol.

For complete prescribing information, refer to the Narcotic Agonist Analgesics group monograph.

Indications

➤*Pain/Detoxification:* For relief of severe pain; detoxification and temporary maintenance treatment of narcotic addiction. Methadone is ineffective for the relief of general anxiety.

➤*Note:* If used to treat heroin dependence for > 3 weeks, the procedure passes from treatment of acute withdrawal syndrome (detoxification) to maintenance therapy. Maintenance may be undertaken only by approved methadone programs. This does not preclude maintenance treatment of addicts hospitalized for other conditions and who require temporary maintenance during the critical period of their stays or whose enrollment has been verified in a program approved for maintenance treatment with methadone.

Administration and Dosage

Oral methadone is ≈ ½ as potent as parenteral. Oral administration results in a delay of onset, a lower peak, and an increased duration of analgesic effect. Duration of effect increases with repeated use because of cumulative effects.

➤*Pain:*

Adults – 2.5 to 10 mg IM, SC, or orally every 3 or 4 hours as necessary. Adjust dosage according to the severity of pain and patient response. For exceptionally severe pain, or in those tolerant of narcotic analgesia, it may be necessary to exceed the usual recommended dosage. Injection IM is preferred for repeated doses; SC use may cause local irritation.

Children – Not for analgesic use because of insufficient documentation.

➤*Detoxification:* Detoxification treatment should not exceed 21 days and may not be repeated earlier than 4 weeks after completion of the preceding course.

Oral administration is preferred. However, if the patient is unable to ingest oral methadone, the parenteral form may be used.

Initially, a single dose of 15 to 20 mg will often suppress withdrawal symptoms. Provide additional methadone if withdrawal symptoms are not suppressed or if symptoms reappear. When patients are physically dependent on high doses, 40 mg/day in single or divided doses is usually an adequate stabilizing dose. Continue stabilization for 2 to 3 days, then gradually decrease the dose on a daily basis or at 2-day intervals. Provide a sufficient amount to keep withdrawal symptoms at a tolerable level. In hospitalized patients, a daily reduction of 20% of total daily dose may be tolerated and may cause little discomfort. In ambulatory patients, a somewhat slower schedule may be needed. If methadone is administered > 3 weeks, the procedure is considered to have progressed from detoxification or treatment of the acute withdrawal syndrome to maintenance treatment, even though the goal and intent may be eventual total withdrawal.

➤*Maintenance treatment:* Individualize dosage. Initial dosage should control abstinence symptoms following narcotic withdrawal, but should not cause sedation, respiratory depression, or other effects of acute intoxication. If patients have been heavy heroin users up to admission day, they may be given 20 mg methadone 4 to 8 hours after heroin is stopped or 40 mg in a single oral dose. If they enter treatment with little or no narcotic tolerance, initial dosage may be halved. When in doubt, use smaller dose. Keep the patient under observation. If abstinence symptoms are distressing, give additional 10 mg doses as needed. Adjust dosage as tolerated and required, up to 120 mg/day.

For a complete description of detoxification and maintenance regulations and dosage protocols, consult a local approved methadone program.

MORPHINE SULFATE

c-ii	**Morphine Sulfate** (Various, eg, Ethex, Roxane)	**Tablets**: 15 mg	In 100s and UD 100s.
c-ii	**MSIR** (Purdue Frederick)		Lactose. (PF MI 15). In 100s.
c-ii	**Morphine Sulfate** (Various, eg, Ethex, Roxane)	**Tablets**: 30 mg	In 100s and UD 100s.
c-ii	**MSIR** (Purdue Frederick)		Lactose. (PF MI 30). In 100s.
c-ii	**MS Contin** (Purdue Frederick)	**Tablets, controlled-release**: 15 mg	(PF M15). Blue. In 100s, 500s, and UD 25s.
c-ii	**Oramorph SR** (aaiPharma)		Lactose. (15). White. In 100s and blister pack 100s.
c-ii	**MS Contin** (Purdue Frederick)	**Tablets, controlled-release**: 30 mg	(PF M30). Lavender. In 50s, 100s, 250s, 500s, and UD 25s.
c-ii	**Oramorph SR** (aaiPharma)		Lactose. (30). White. In 100s and blister pack 100s.
c-ii	**MS Contin** (Purdue Frederick)	**Tablets, controlled-release**: 60 mg	(PF M 60). Orange. In 100s, 500s, and UD 25s.
c-ii	**Oramorph SR** (aaiPharma)		Lactose. (60). White. In 100s and blister pack 25s.
c-ii	**MS Contin** (Purdue Frederick)	**Tablets, controlled-release**: 100 mg	(PF 100). Gray. In 100s, 500s, and UD 25s.
c-ii	**Oramorph SR** (aaiPharma)		Lactose. (100). White. In 100s and UD 25s.
c-ii	**MS Contin** (Purdue Frederick)	**Tablets, controlled-release**: 200 mg	(PF 200). Green. Capsule shape. In 100s.
c-ii	**Morphine Sulfate** (Endo)	**Tablets, extended-release**: 15 mg	Lactose. (E652/15). Blue. In 100s and 500s.
		30 mg	Lactose. (E653/30). Green. In 100s and 500s.
		60 mg	Lactose. (E656/60). Orange, capsule shape. In 100s and 500s.
		100 mg	Lactose. (E658/100). Blue, capsule shape. In 100s and 500s.

MORPHINE SULFATE

c-ii	**Morphine Sulfate** (Ranbaxy)	**Tablets, soluble:** 10 mg	Lactose, sucrose. In 100s.
		15 mg	Lactose, sucrose. In 100s.
		30 mg	Lactose, sucrose. In 100s.
c-ii	**Avinza** (Ligand)	**Capsules, extended release:** 30 mg	Sugar starch spheres, talc. Yellow/White. (e 30 mg 505). In 100s.
		60 mg	Sugar starch spheres, talc. Bluish-green/white. (e 60 mg 506). In 100s.
		90 mg	Sugar starch spheres, talc. Red/White. (e 90 mg 507). In 100s.
		120 mg	Sugar starch spheres, talc. Blue-violet/white. (e 120 mg 508). In 100s.
c-ii	**Kadian** (Mayne Pharma)	**Capsules, sustained-release pellets:** 20 mg	Sucrose. (KADIAN 20 mg). Yellow. In 30s, 60s, and 100s.
		30 mg	Sucrose. (KADIAN 30 mg). Blue violet. In 30s, 60s, and 100s.
		50 mg	Sucrose. (KADIAN 50 mg). Blue. In 30s, 60s, and 100s.
		60 mg	Sucrose. (KADIAN 60 mg). Pink. In 30s, 60s, and 100s.
		100 mg	Sucrose. (KADIAN 100 mg). Green. In 30s, 60s, and 100s.
c-ii	**Morphine Sulfate** (Roxane)	**Solution:** 10 mg/5 mL	In 100 and 500 mL and UD 5 and 10 mL.
c-ii	**MSIR** (Various, eg, Ethex, Purdue Frederick)		EDTA. In 120 mL.
c-ii	**Morphine Sulfate** (Roxane)	**Solution:** 20 mg/5 mL	In 100 and 500 mL.
c-ii	**MSIR** (Purdue Frederick)		EDTA. In 120 mL.
c-ii	**Morphine Sulfate** (Ethex)	**Solution:** 20 mg/mL	Alcohol free. In 30, 120, and 240 mL.
c-ii	**MSIR** (Purdue Frederick)		EDTA. In 30 and 120 mL w/dropper.
c-ii	**Roxanol** (aaiPharma)		In 30 and 120 mL with calibrated dropper.
c-ii	**Roxanol T** (aaiPharma)		Flavored. In 30 and 120 mL with calibrated dropper.
c-ii	**Roxanol 100** (aaiPharma)	**Solution:** 100 mg/5 mL	In 240 mL with calibrated spoon.
c-ii	**Morphine Sulfate**[1] (Abbott)	**Injection:** 0.5 mg/mL	In 10 mL amps and vials.
c-ii	**Astramorph PF**[1] (AstraZeneca)		In 2 and 10 mL amps and 10 mL vials.
c-ii	**Duramorph**[1] (Baxter)		In 10 mL amps.
c-ii	**Morphine Sulfate** (Various, eg, Abbott,[1] ESI Lederle, Faulding)	**Injection:** 1 mg/mL	In 2, 30, and 60 mL vials and 10 mL amps and vials.
c-ii	**Astramorph PF**[1] (AstraZeneca)		In 2 and 10 mL amps and 10 mL vials.
c-ii	**Duramorph**[1] (Baxter)		In 10 mL amps.
c-ii	**Morphine Sulfate** (Various, eg, Abbott, Wyeth-Ayerst)	**Injection:** 2 mg/mL	In 30 mL vials and 1 mL syringes and *Tubex*.
c-ii	**Morphine Sulfate** (Various, eg, Abbott, Wyeth-Ayerst)	**Injection:** 4 mg/mL	In 1 and 2 mL disp. syringes and 1 mL *Tubex*.
c-ii	**Morphine Sulfate** (Various, eg, Baxter, Faulding)	**Injection:** 5 mg/mL	In 1 and 30 mL vials.
c-ii	**Morphine Sulfate** (Various, eg, Abbott, Baxter, ESI Lederle, Wyeth-Ayerst)	**Injection:** 8 mg/mL	In 1 mL vials, amps, and syringes and 1 mL fill in 2 mL *Tubex*, amps, and vials.
c-ii	**Morphine Sulfate** (Various, eg, Abbott, Baxter, ESI Lederle, Faulding[2])	**Injection:** 10 mg/mL	In 1 mL syringes, vials, amps, 10 and 30 mL vials, 30 mL syringes, and 1 mL fill in 2 mL *Tubex*, amps, and vials.
c-ii	**Infumorph 200**[1] (ESI Lederle)		In 20 mL (200 mg) amps.
c-ii	**DepoDur**[1] (Endo)	**Injection, extended-release liposomal:** 10 mg/mL	In 10 mg/1 mL, 15 mg/1.5 mL, and 20 mg/2 mL vials in cartons of 5.
c-ii	**Morphine Sulfate** (Various, eg, Abbott,[1] Baxter, ESI Lederle)	**Injection:** 15 mg/mL	In 1 mL amps and vials, 20 mL amps and vials, and 1 mL fill in 2 mL *Tubex*, amps, and vials.
c-ii	**Morphine Sulfate** (Various, eg, Abbott,[1] Faulding[2])	**Injection:** 25 mg/mL	In 4, 10, 20, 30, 40, and 50 mL syringes and 10, 20, and 40 mL vials.
c-ii	**Infumorph 500**[1] (ESI Lederle)		In 20 mL (500 mg) amps.
c-ii	**Morphine Sulfate** (Various, eg, Abbott,[1] Faulding[2])	**Injection:** 50 mg/mL	In 10, 20, 30, and 50 mL syringes and 20, 40, and 50 mL vials.
c-ii	**Morphine Sulfate** (Various, eg, G & W, Paddock)	**Rectal suppositories:** 5 mg	In 12s.
c-ii	**RMS** (Upsher-Smith)		In 12s.
c-ii	**Morphine Sulfate** (Various, eg, G & W, Paddock)	**Rectal suppositories:** 10 mg	In 12s
c-ii	**RMS** (Upsher-Smith)		In 12s.
c-ii	**Morphine Sulfate** (Various, eg, G & W, Paddock)	**Rectal suppositories:** 20 mg	In 12s.
c-ii	**RMS** (Upsher-Smith)		In 12s.
c-ii	**Morphine Sulfate** (Various, eg, G & W, Paddock)	**Rectal suppositories:** 30 mg	In 12s and 50s.
c-ii	**RMS** (Upsher-Smith)		In 12s.
c-ii	**Morphine Sulfate** (Paddock)	**Compounding powder**	In 25 g.

[1] Preservative free.

[2] Contains sulfites; for IV use only.

For complete prescribing information, refer to the Narcotic Agonist Analgesics group monograph.

Indications

Morphine is the principal opium alkaloid.

➤*Oral:*

Immediate-release tablets/solution – Relief of moderate-to-severe pain.

Controlled/Extended/Sustained-release tablets – Relief of moderate-to-severe pain in those who require opioid analgesics for more than a few days.

➤*Parenteral:*

IV – Relief of severe pain; pain of MI; used preoperatively to sedate the patient and allay apprehension, facilitate anesthesia induction, and reduce anesthetic dosage; control postoperative pain; relieve anxiety and reduce left ventricular work by reducing preload pressure; treatment of dyspnea associated with acute left ventricular failure and pulmonary edema; produce anesthesia for open-heart surgery.

MORPHINE SULFATE

SC/IM – Relief of severe pain; relieve preoperative apprehension; preoperative sedation; control postoperative pain; supplement to anesthesia; analgesia during labor; acute pulmonary edema; allay anxiety.

IV/Epidural/Intrathecal – Management of pain not responsive to nonnarcotic analgesics (*Duramorph, Astramorph PF; Infumorph* for continuous epidural/intrathecal use only).

➤*Rectal:* Severe acute and chronic pain.

Administration and Dosage

Morphine may suppress respiration in the elderly, those taking other CNS depressants, the very ill, and those patients with respiratory problems; therefore, lower doses may be required.

➤*Oral:*

Immediate-release – 5 to 30 mg (solution or tablets) every 4 hours or as directed by physician.

Controlled/Extended/Sustained-release – Swallow whole; do not break, chew, or crush. See below for sustained-release capsule administration.

  Initial therapy: There has been no evaluation of controlled/extended/sustained-release morphine as an initial opioid analgesic in the management of pain. Because it may be more difficult to titrate a patient to adequate analgesia using a controlled/extended/sustained-release morphine, it is ordinarily advisable to begin treatment using an immediate-release morphine formulation.

The *MS Contin* 200 mg tablet is for use only in opioid-tolerant patients requiring daily morphine-equivalent dosages of ≥ 400 mg. Reserve this strength for patients who have already been titrated to a stable analgesic regimen using lower strengths of *MS Contin* or other opioids. If *Kadian* is chosen, start with 20 mg in those who do not have a proven tolerance to opioids. Increase at a rate ≤ 20 mg every other day. Individualize dosage.

The daily dose of *Avinza* must be limited to a maximum of 1600 mg/day. *Avinza* doses of over 1600 mg/day contain a quantity of fumaric acid that has not been demonstrated to be safe, and which may result in serious renal toxicity. The 60, 90, and 120 mg capsules are for use only in opioid-tolerant patients.

  Conversion from conventional immediate-release oral morphine to controlled/extended/sustained-release oral morphine: Give ½ the total daily oral morphine dose every 12 hours; ⅓ the total daily oral morphine requirement every 8 hours (*MS Contin* and extended-release tablets only); or the full daily morphine dose every 24 hours (*Kadian* only). The 15 mg tablet should be used for initial conversion for patients whose total daily requirement is expected to be < 60 mg. The 30 mg tablet strength is recommended for patients with a daily morphine requirement of 60 to 120 mg. When the total daily dose is expected to be > 120 mg, the appropriate combination of tablet strengths should be employed.

  Conversion from parenteral morphine or other opioids (parenteral or oral) to controlled/extended/sustained-release: Particular care must be exercised in the conversion process. Because of uncertainty about, and intersubject variation in, relative estimates of opioid potency and cross-tolerance, initial dosing regimens should be conservative; that is, an underestimation of the 24-hour oral morphine requirement is preferred to an overestimate. To this end, initial individual doses should be estimated conservatively. In patients whose daily morphine requirements are expected to be ≤ 120 mg/day, the 30 mg tablet strength is recommended for the initial titration period. Once a stable dose regimen is reached, the patient can be converted to the 60 or 100 mg tablet strength, or appropriate combination of tablet strengths, if desired.

  Conversion from controlled/extended/sustained-release oral morphine to parenteral opioids: It is best to assume that the parenteral-to-oral potency is high. For example, to estimate the required 24-hour dose of morphine for IM use, one could employ a conversion of 1 mg morphine IM for every 6 mg of morphine as controlled-release tablet. Of course, the IM 24-hour dose would have to be divided by 6 and administered every 4 hours. This approach is recommended because it is least likely to cause overdose. For *Kadian*, initiate treatment at half the calculated equivalent parenteral dose. For example, to estimate the 24-hour dose of parenteral morphine for a patient taking *Kadian*, one would take the 24-hour *Kadian* dose, divide by an oral-to-parenteral conversion ratio of 3, divide the estimated 24-hour parenteral dose into 6 divided doses (for a 4-hour dosing interval), then halve this dose as an initial trial.

  Conversion of sustained-release (Kadian) to other controlled-release oral forms: Kadian is not bioequivalent to other controlled-release formulations. Conversion from *Kadian* to the same total daily dose may lead to either excessive sedation at peak or inadequate analgesia at trough; observe closely and adjust dosage as appropriate.

  Dosing adjustments: If signs of excessive opioid effects are observed early in a dosing interval, the next dose should be reduced. If this adjustment leads to inadequate analgesia (ie, "breakthrough" pain occurs late in the dosing interval), the dosing interval may be shortened. Alternatively, a supplemental dose of a short-acting analgesic may be given. As experience is gained, adjustments can be made to obtain an appropriate balance between pain relief, opioid side effects, and the convenience of the dosing schedule. It is recommended that the dosing interval never be extended beyond 12 hours because the administration of very large single doses may lead to acute overdose.

Sustained-release (Kadian) – Capsules may be opened and the entire contents sprinkled on a small amount of applesauce immediately prior to ingestion. The pellets in the capsules should not be chewed, crushed, or dissolved because of risk of overdose.

Open the capsule and sprinkle entire contents over ≈ 10 mL of water and flush with swirling through a prewetted 16 French gastrostomy tube fitted with funnel at the port end. Additional aliquots of water are used to transfer all pellets and to flush the tube. Do not attempt the administration of pellets through a nasogastric tube.

May be given once or twice daily.

➤*SC/IM:* Prepare soluble tablets in sterile water and filter through a 0.22 micron membrane filter.

Adults – 10 mg (range, 5 to 20 mg)/70 kg every 4 hours as needed.

Children – 0.05 to 0.2 mg/kg every 4 hours as needed. Do not exceed 10 to 15 mg/dose.

➤*IV:*

Adults – 2 to 10 mg/70 kg of body weight. A strength of 2.5 to 15 mg of morphine may be diluted in 4 to 5 mL of Water for Injection. Administer slowly over 4 to 5 minutes. Rapid IV use increases the incidence of adverse reactions (see Warnings). Do not administer IV unless a narcotic antagonist is immediately available.

Continuous IV infusion – 0.1 to 1 mg/mL in 5% Dextrose in Water by controlled-infusion device; higher concentrations have been used.

➤*Severe chronic pain associated with terminal cancer:* Prior to initiation of the morphine infusion (in concentrations between 0.2 to 1 mg/mL), a loading dose of ≥ 15 mg of morphine sulfate may be administered by IV push to alleviate pain.

The infusion dosage range is 0.8 to 80 mg/hr, though doses up to 144 mg/hr have been used. Thus, for the 1 mg/mL solution, the infusion may be run from 0.8 to 80 mg/hr, and for a 0.5 mg/mL solution, the infusion may be run from 1.6 to 160 mL/hr.

A constant infusion rate must be maintained with an infusion pump in order to assure proper dosage control. Take care to avoid overdosage (respiratory depression) or abrupt cessation of therapy, which may give rise to withdrawal symptoms.

➤*Open-heart surgery:* Administer large doses (0.5 to 3 mg/kg) of morphine IV as the sole anesthetic or with a suitable anesthetic agent. The patients are given oxygen and cardiovascular function is not depressed by morphine, as long as adequate ventilation is maintained.

➤*MI pain:* 8 to 15 mg administered parenterally. For very severe pain, additional smaller doses may be given every 3 to 4 hours as needed.

➤*Rectal:* 10 to 30 mg every 4 hours as needed or as directed by physician.

➤*Epidural (Duramorph, Astramorph PF):*

Adults – Initial injection of 5 mg in the lumbar region may provide satisfactory pain relief for up to 24 hours. If adequate pain relief is not achieved within 1 hour, carefully administer incremental doses of 1 to 2 mg at intervals sufficient to assess effectiveness. Give no more than 10 mg/24 hours.

For continuous infusion, an initial dose of 2 to 4 mg/24 hours is recommended. Further doses of 1 to 2 mg may be given if pain relief is not achieved initially.

Aged or debilitated patients – Administer with extreme caution (see Warnings). Doses < 5 mg may provide satisfactory pain relief for up to 24 hours.

Infumorph, Duramorph, Astramorph PF – Employ doses > 20 mg/day with caution since they may be associated with a higher likelihood of serious side effects. The starting dose must be individualized. The recommended initial epidural dose in patients who are not tolerant to opioids range from 3.5 to 7.5 mg/day. The usual starting dose for continuous epidural infusion, based upon limited data in patients who have some degree of opioid tolerance, is 4.5 to 10 mg/day. The dose requirements may increase significantly during treatment, frequently to 20 to 30 mg/day.

➤*Intrathecal:*

Adult – Intrathecal dosage is usually ⅒ that of epidural dosage. A single injection of 0.2 to 1 mg may provide satisfactory pain relief for up to 24 hours. (Caution: This is only 0.4 to 2 mL of the 0.5 mg/mL potency or 0.2 to 1 mL of the 1 mg/mL potency.) Do not inject intrathecally > 2 mL of the 0.5 mg/mL potency or 1 mL of the 1 mg/mL potency. Use in lumbar area only. Repeated intrathecal injections are not recommended. A constant IV infusion of 0.6 mg/hr naloxone for 24 hours after intrathecal injection may reduce incidence of potential side effects.

Infumorph – Familiarize with the continuous microinfusion device. To minimize risk from glass or other particles, the product must be filtered through ≤ 5 micron microfilter before injecting into the microinfusion device. If dilution is required, 0.9% NaCl injection is recommended. Individualize the starting dose. The recommended initial lumbar intrathecal dose range in patients with no tolerance to opioids is 0.2 to 1 mg/day. The published range of doses for individuals who have some degree of opioid tolerance varies from 1 to 10 mg/day. Limited experience with

MORPHINE SULFATE

continuous intrathecal infusion of morphine has shown that the daily doses have to be increased over time.

Aged or debilitated – Use extreme caution. Lower dose is usually satisfactory.

Repeat dosage – If pain recurs, consider alternative administration routes because experience with repeated doses by this route is limited.

➤*Intraventricular:* Currently available data indicate that this route of administration is effective in select patients with a short life expectancy and recalcitrant pain due to head and neck malignancies and tumors (eg, superior sulcus tumors, breast carcinoma) that affect the brachial plexus. One to 2 doses per day are generally administered.

OPIUM

c-ii	**Opium Tincture, Deodorized** (Ranbaxy)	**Liquid:** 10 mg anhydrous morphine equiv./mL	19% alcohol. In 120 mL and pt.
c-iii	**Paregoric** (Various, eg, Alpharma, Major)	**Liquid:** 2 mg anhydrous morphine equiv./5 mL	45% alcohol.[1] In pt.

[1] May also contain benzoic acid or camphor.

For complete prescribing information, refer to the Narcotic Agonist Analgesics group monograph.

Indications

➤*Diarrhea:* For treatment of diarrhea.

➤*Unlabeled uses:*

Neonatal abstinence syndrome – Treatment of opioid-related drug withdrawal (neonates). Diluted opium tincture is the preferred treatment for neonatal withdrawal in newborns. Paregoric contains benzoic acid (an oxidative product of benzyl alcohol), usually camphor, and other ingredients that may have potential toxic effects.

Management of short bowel syndrome – Used to slow gastric emptying and delay bowel transit time in short bowel syndrome.

Administration and Dosage

➤*Caution:* Opium tincture contains 25 times more morphine than paregoric. Do not confuse opium tincture with paregoric; this may lead to a potentially fatal overdose of morphine.

➤*Opium tincture:*

Adults – 0.6 mL (single dose < 1 mL) 4 times daily, maximum of 6 mL/day.

➤*Paregoric:*

Adults – 5 to 10 mL 1 to 4 times daily.

Children – 0.25 to 0.5 mL/kg 1 to 4 times daily.

Warnings

➤*Caution:* Opium tincture contains 25 times more morphine than paregoric. Do not confuse opium tincture with paregoric; this may lead to a potentially fatal overdose of morphine. It is best to dispense to the nursery diluted opium tincture that contains a concentration of morphine equivalent to the concentration in paregoric.

OXYCODONE HCl

c-ii	**Oxycodone HCl** (Various, eg, Amide, Ethex, Watson)	**Tablets:** 5 mg	In 100s, 500s, and UD 100s.
c-ii	**M-oxy** (Mallinckrodt)		(M-OXY 5). White, scored. In 100s.
c-ii	**Percolone** (Endo Laboratories)		(EPI 132 5). White, biconvex, scored. In 100s and UD 100s.
c-ii	**Roxicodone** (aaiPharma)		(54 582). White, scored. In 100s and UD 100s.
c-ii	**Endocodone** (Endo)		(Endo 657). White, biconvex, scored. In 100s.
c-ii	**Oxycodone HCl** (Endo)	**Tablets, extended-release:** 10 mg	(E702 10). White. Coated. In 30s and 500s.
c-ii	**OxyContin** (Purdue Pharma LP)		Lactose. (OC 10). White, convex. In 100s and UD 25s.
c-ii	**Oxycodone HCl** (Endo)	**Tablets, extended-release:** 20 mg	(E703 20). Pink. Coated. In 30s and 500s.
c-ii	**OxyContin** (Purdue Pharma LP)		Lactose. (OC 20). Pink, convex. In 100s and UD 25s.
c-ii	**Oxycodone HCl** (Endo)	**Tablets, extended-release:** 40 mg	(E705 40). Yellow. Coated. In 30s and 500s.
c-ii	**OxyContin** (Purdue Pharma LP)		Lactose. (OC 40). Yellow, convex. In 100s and UD 25s.
c-ii	**Oxycodone HCl** (Teva)	**Tablets, extended-release:** 80 mg[1]	Lactose. (93 33). Green, oval. Film-coated. In 100s.
c-ii	**OxyContin** (Purdue Pharma LP)		Lactose. (OC 80). Green, convex. In 100s and UD 25s.
c-ii	**OxyContin** (Purdue Pharma LP)	**Tablets, extended-release:** 160 mg[1]	Lactose. (OC 160). Blue, caplet shape, convex. In 100s and UD 25s.
c-ii	**Roxicodone** (aaiPharma)	**Tablets, immediate-release:** 15 mg	Lactose. (54 710). Green, scored. In 100s and UD 100s.
		30 mg	Lactose. (54 199). Blue, scored. In 100s and UD 100s.
c-ii	**Oxycodone HCl** (Ethex)	**Capsules, immediate-release:** 5 mg	Lactose. (Ethex 041). Buff/white. In 100s.
c-ii	**OxyIR** (Purdue Frederick)		Sucrose. (O-IR PF5mg). Beige/orange. In 100s.
c-ii	**Roxicodone** (aaiPharma)	**Solution, oral:** 5 mg/5 mL	Alcohol, sorbitol. In 500 mL and UD 5 mL.
c-ii	**Roxicodone Intensol** (aaiPharma)	**Solution, concentrate:** 20 mg/mL	In 30 mL with dropper.
c-ii	**Oxydose** (Ethex)		Saccharin, sorbitol. Berry flavor. In 30 mL with dropper.
c-ii	**OxyFAST** (Purdue Pharma LP)		Saccharin. In 30 mL with dropper.

[1] For use in opioid-tolerant patients only.

For complete prescribing information, refer to the Narcotic Agonist Analgesics group monograph.

OXYCODONE HCl

> ### WARNING
>
> Controlled-release oxycodone is an opioid agonist and a Schedule II controlled substance with an abuse liability similar to morphine.
>
> Oxycodone can be abused in a manner similar to other opioid agonists, legal or illicit. This should be considered when prescribing or dispensing oxycodone controlled-release tablets in situations where the physician or pharmacist is concerned about an increased risk of misuse, abuse, or diversion.
>
> Oxycodone controlled-release tablets are indicated for the management of moderate-to-severe pain when a continuous, around-the-clock analgesic is needed for an extended period of time.
>
> Oxycodone controlled-release tablets are not intended for use as a prn (as needed) analgesic.
>
> Oxycodone 80 and 160 mg controlled-release tablets are for use in opioid-tolerant patients only. These tablet strengths may cause fatal respiratory depression when administered to patients not previously exposed to opioids.
>
> Oxycodone controlled-release tablets are to be swallowed whole and are not to be broken, chewed, or crushed. Taking broken, chewed, or crushed oxycodone controlled-release tablets leads to rapid release and absorption of a potentially fatal dose of oxycodone.

Indications

➤*Pain:* Relief of moderate-to-severe pain.

Immediate-release tablets – Management of moderate-to-severe pain where use of an opioid analgesic is appropriate.

Controlled-release tablets – Management of moderate-to-severe pain when a continuous, around-the-clock analgesic is needed for an extended period of time. Not intended for use as a prn analgesic.

Individualize treatment in every case, initiating therapy at the appropriate point along a progression from nonopioid analgesics, such as nonsteroidal anti-inflammatory drugs (NSAIDs) and acetaminophen to opioids in a plan of pain management such as outlined by the World Health Organization, the Agency for Healthcare Research and Quality (formerly known as the Agency for Health Care Policy and Research), the Federation of State Medical Boards Model Guidelines, or the American Pain Society.

Not indicated for pain in the immediate postoperative period (the first 12 to 24 hours following surgery), or if the pain is mild or not expected to persist for an extended period of time. Oxycodone controlled-release tablets are only indicated for postoperative use if the patient is already receiving the drug prior to surgery or if the postoperative pain is expected to be moderate-to-severe and persist for an extended period of time. Individualize treatment, moving from parenteral to oral analgesics as appropriate.

➤*Unlabeled uses:* Postherpetic neuralgia (controlled-release).

Administration and Dosage

➤*Immediate-release tablets:*

Adults – 10 to 30 mg every 4 hours (5 mg every 6 hours for *OxyIR*, oxycodone immediate-release capsules, *Oxydose*, and *OxyFAST*) as needed. Individualize dosage.

OxyFAST and *Oxydose* 20 mg/mL solution are highly concentrated solutions. Take care in prescribing and dispensing this solution strength.

Children – Not recommended for use in children.

Immediate-release tablets are intended for the management of moderate-to-severe pain in patients who require treatment with an oral opioid analgesic. Individually adjust the dose according to severity of pain, patient response, and patient size. If the pain increases in severity, if analgesia is not adequate, or if tolerance occurs, a gradual increase in dosage may be required.

Start patients who have not been receiving opioid analgesics on immediate-release tablets in a dosing range of 5 to 15 mg every 4 to 6 hours as needed for pain. Titrate the dose based upon the individual patient's response to his/her initial dose of immediate-release tablets. Patients with chronic pain should have their dosage given on an around-the-clock basis to prevent the reoccurrence of pain rather than treating the pain after it has occurred. This dose can then be adjusted to an acceptable level of analgesia, taking into account side effects experienced by the patient.

For control of severe chronic pain, administer on a regularly scheduled basis, every 4 to 6 hours, at the lowest dosage level that will achieve adequate analgesia.

As with any potent opioid, it is critical to adjust the dosing regimen for each patient individually, taking into account the patient's prior analgesic treatment experience. Although it is not possible to list every condition that is important to the selection of the initial dose, give attention to the following:

1.) the daily dose, potency, and characteristics of a pure agonist or mixed agonist/antagonist the patient has been previously taking;

2.) the reliability of the relative potency estimate to calculate the dose of oxycodone needed;

3.) the degree of opioid tolerance;

4.) the general condition and medical status of the patient; and

5.) the balance between pain control and adverse experiences

Conversion from fixed-ratio opioid/acetaminophen, opioid/aspirin, or opioid/nonsteroidal combination drugs – When converting patients from fixed-ratio opioid/nonopioid drug regimens, a decision should be made whether or not to continue the nonopioid analgesic. If a decision is made to discontinue the use of the nonopioid analgesic, it may be necessary to titrate the dose of the immediate-release tablets in response to the level of analgesia and adverse effects afforded by the dosing regimen. If the nonopioid regimen is continued as a separate single entity agent, base the starting dose upon the most recent dose of opioid as a baseline for further titration of oxycodone. Gauge incremental increases according to side effects to an acceptable level of analgesia.

Patients currently on opioid therapy – If a patient has been receiving opioid-containing medications prior to taking immediate-release tablets, the potency of the prior opioid relative to oxycodone should be factored into the selection of the total daily dose (TDD) of oxycodone.

In converting patients from other opioids to immediate-release tablets, close observation and adjustment of dosage based upon the patient's response to immediate-release tablets is imperative. Administration of supplemental analgesia for breakthrough or incident pain and titration of the total daily dose of immediate-release tablets may be necessary, especially in patients who have disease states that are changing rapidly.

Maintenance of therapy – Continual reevaluation of the patient receiving immediate-release tablets is important, with special attention to the maintenance of pain control and the relative incidence of side effects associated with therapy. If the level of pain increases, make efforts to identify the source of increased pain while adjusting the dose as described above to decrease the level of pain.

During chronic therapy, especially for noncancer-related pain (or pain associated with other terminal illnessess), the continued need for the use of opioid analgesics should be reassessed as appropriate.

Cessation of therapy – When a patient no longer requires therapy with immediate-release tablets or other opioid analgesics for the treatment of pain, it is important that therapy be gradually discontinued over time to prevent the development of an opioid abstinence syndrome (narcotic withdrawal). In general, therapy can be decreased by 25% to 50% per day with careful monitoring for signs and symptoms of withdrawal. If the patient develops these signs or symptoms, the dose should be raised to the previous level and titrated down more slowly, either by increasing the interval between decreases, decreasing the amount of change in dose, or both. It is not known at what dose of immediate-release tablets that treatment may be discontinued without risk of the opioid abstinence syndrome.

➤*Controlled-release tablets:* Controlled-release oxycodone is an opioid agonist and a schedule II controlled substance with an abuse liability similar to morphine. Oxycodone, like morphine and other opioids used in analgesia, can be abused and is subject to criminal diversion.

Swallow tablets whole; do not break, chew, or crush. Taking broken, chewed, or crushed tablets could lead to the rapid release and absorption of a potentially fatal dose of oxycodone.

One 160 mg tablet is comparable to two 80 mg tablets when taken on an empty stomach. However, with a high-fat meal there is a 25% greater peak plasma concentration following one 160 mg tablet. Use dietary caution when patients are initially titrated to 160 mg tablets.

In treating pain, it is vital to assess the patient regularly and systematically. Regularly review therapy and adjust based upon the patient's own reports of pain and side effects and the health professional's clinical judgment.

Controlled-release tablets are intended for the management of moderate-to-severe pain when a continuous, around-the-clock analgesic is needed for an extended period of time. The controlled-release nature of the formulation allows it to be effectively administered every 12 hours. While symmetric (same AM and PM), around-the-clock, every-12-hour dosing is appropriate for the majority of patients, some patients may benefit from asymmetric (different dose given in AM than in PM) dosing, tailored to their pain pattern. It is usually appropriate to treat a patient with only 1 opioid for around-the-clock therapy.

Initial – It is critical to initiate the dosing regimen for each patient individually, taking into account the patient's prior opioid and nonopioid analgesic treatment. Give attention to the following:

1.) the general condition and medical status of the patient;

2.) the daily dose, potency, and kind of the analgesic(s) the patient has been taking;

3.) the reliability of the conversion estimate used to calculate the dose of oxycodone;

4.) the patient's opioid exposure and opioid tolerance (if any);

5.) special safety issues associated with conversion to controlled-release tablet doses at or exceeding 160 mg every 12 hours (see Special Instructions for Controlled-Release 80 and 160 mg Tablets); and

6.) the balance between pain control and adverse experiences.

OXYCODONE HCl

Take care to use low initial doses of controlled-release tablets in patients who are not already opioid tolerant, especially those who are receiving concurrent treatment with muscle relaxants, sedatives, or other CNS-active medications.

Patients not already taking opioids (opioid näive) – A reasonable starting dose for most patients who are opioid näive is 10 mg every 12 hours. If a nonopioid analgesic (eg, aspirin, acetaminophen, NSAID) is being provided, it may be continued.

Patients currently on opioid therapy –

1.) Using standard conversion ratio estimates (see table below), multiply the mg/day of the previous opioids by the appropriate multiplication factors to obtain the equivalent total daily dose of oral oxycodone.

2.) Divide this 24-hour oxycodone dose in half to obtain the twice a day (every 12 hours) dose of controlled-release tablets.

3.) Round down to a dose that is appropriate for the tablet strengths available (10, 20, 40, 80, and 160 mg tablets).

4.) Discontinue all other around-the-clock opioid drugs when controlled-release tablet therapy is initiated.

No fixed conversion ratio is likely to be satisfactory in all patients, especially patients receiving large opioid doses. The recommended doses shown in the following table are only a starting point, and close observation and frequent titration are indicated until patients are stable in the new therapy.

Multiplication Factors for Converting the Daily Dose of Prior Opioids to the Daily Dose of Oral Oxycodone[1]		
Mg/day prior opioid × factor = mg/day oral oxycodone		
	Oral prior opioid	Parenteral prior opioid
Oxycodone	1	—
Codeine	0.15	—
Fentanyl TTS	see below	see below
Hydrocodone	0.9	—
Hydromorphone	4	20
Levorphanol	7.5	15
Meperidine	0.1	0.4
Methadone	1.5	3
Morphine	0.5	3

[1] To be used only for conversion to oral oxycodone. For patients receiving high-dose parenteral opioids, a more conservative conversion is warranted. For example, for high-dose parenteral morphine, use 1.5 instead of 3 as a multiplication factor.

In all cases, supplemental analgesia (see below) should be made available in the form of immediate-release oral oxycodone or another suitable short-acting analgesic.

Controlled-release tablets can be safely used concomitantly with usual doses of nonopioid analgesics and analgesic adjuvants, provided care is taken to select a proper initial dose.

Conversion from transdermal fentanyl to controlled-release tablets – Eighteen hours following the removal of the transdermal fentanyl patch, treatment with controlled-release tablets can be initiated. Although there has been no systematic assessment of such conversion, a conservative oxycodone dose, ≈ 10 mg every 12 hours of controlled-release tablets, should be initially substituted for each 25 mcg/hr

fentanyl transdermal patch. Closely follow the patient for early titration as there is very limited clinical experience with this conversion.

Dosage individualization – Once therapy is initiated, pain relief and other opioid effects should be frequently assessed. Titrate patients to adequate effect (generally mild or no pain with the regular use of no more than 2 doses of supplemental analgesia per 24 hours). Rescue medication should be available (see Supplemental analgesia). Because steady-state plasma concentrations are approximated within 24 to 36 hours, dosage adjustment may be carried out every 1 to 2 days. It is most appropriate to increase the every 12 hour dose, not the dosing frequency. There is no clinical information on dosing intervals shorter than every 12 hours. As a guideline, except for the increase from 10 to 20 mg every 12 hours, the total daily oxycodone dose usually can be increased by 25% to 50% of the current dose at each increase.

If signs of excessive opioid-related adverse experiences are observed, the next dose may be reduced. If this adjustment leads to inadequate analgesia, a supplemental dose of immediate-release oxycodone may be given. Alternatively, nonopioid analgesic adjuvants may be employed. Make dose adjustments to obtain an appropriate balance between pain relief and opioid-related adverse experiences.

If significant adverse events occur before the therapeutic goal of mild or no pain is achieved, the events should be treated aggressively. Once adverse events are under control, upward titration should continue to an acceptable level of pain control.

During periods of changing analgesic requirements, including initial titration, frequent contact is recommended between physician, other members of the health care team, the patient, and the caregiver/family.

Special instructions for 80 and 160 mg controlled-release tablets – For use in opioid-tolerant patients only.

Controlled-release tablets, 80 and 160 mg, are for use only in opioid-tolerant patients requiring daily oxycodone equivalent dosages of ≥ 160 mg for the 80 mg tablet and ≥ 320 mg for the 160 mg tablet. Take care in the prescribing of this tablet strength. Instruct patients against use by individuals other than the patient for whom it was prescribed, as such inappropriate use may have severe medical consequences.

Supplemental analgesia – Most patients given around-the-clock therapy with controlled-release opioids will need to have immediate-release medication available for "rescue" from breakthrough pain or to prevent pain that occurs predictably during certain patient activities (incident pain).

Therapy maintenance – The intent of the titration period is to establish a patient-specific every-12-hour dosing that will maintain adequate analgesia with acceptable side effects for as long as pain relief is necessary. Should pain recur, the dose can be incrementally increased to reestablish pain control. The method of therapy adjustment outlined above should be employed to reestablish pain control.

During chronic therapy, especially for noncancer pain syndromes, the continued need for around-the-clock opioid therapy should be reassessed periodically (eg, every 6 to 12 months) as appropriate.

Therapy cessation – When the patient no longer requires therapy with the controlled-release tablets, taper doses gradually over several days to prevent signs and symptoms of withdrawal in the physically dependent patient.

Conversion from controlled-release tablets to parenteral opioids – To avoid overdose, follow conservative dose conversion ratios. For patients receiving high-dose parenteral opioids, a more conservative conversion is warranted.

OXYMORPHONE HCl

c-ii	Numorphan (Endo Laboratories)	Injection: 1 mg/mL	In 1 mL amps.
		1.5 mg/mL	In 10 mL multidose vials.[1]
		Suppositories: 5 mg	In 6s.

[1] With parabens.

For complete prescribing information, refer to the Narcotic Agonist Analgesics group monograph.

Indications

➤*Pain:* Relief of moderate-to-severe pain.

➤*Preoperative medication/anesthesia/anxiety:* Parenterally for preoperative medication, support of anesthesia, obstetrical analgesia, and for relief of anxiety in patients with dyspnea associated with pulmonary edema secondary to acute left ventricular dysfunction.

Administration and Dosage

➤*Approved by the FDA:* April 1959.

Use smaller doses of oxymorphone than those recommended below for debilitated and elderly patients and those with severe liver disease.

➤*IV:* Initially, 0.5 mg. In nondebilitated patients, the dose can be cautiously increased until satisfactory pain relief is obtained.

➤*SC or IM:* Initially, 1 to 1.5 mg every 4 to 6 hours, as needed. For analgesia during labor, give 0.5 to 1 mg IM.

➤*Rectal:* 5 mg every 4 to 6 hours, as needed. In nondebilitated patients, cautiously increase dose until pain relief is satisfactory.

➤*Children:* Safety for use in children < 18 years of age has not been established.

➤*Storage/Stability:* Refrigerate suppositories at 2° to 8°C (36° to 46°F). Protect injections from light; store at 15° to 30°C (59° to 86°F).

PROPOXYPHENE (Dextropropoxyphene)

c-iv	**Darvon-N** (Eli Lilly)	**Tablets:** 100 mg (as napsylate)	Lactose. (Lilly Darvon-N 100). Buff, elliptical. Film-coated. In 100s, 500s, and UD 100s.
c-iv	**Propoxyphene HCl** (Various, eg, Major, Mylan)	**Capsules:** 65 mg (as HCl)	In 100s, 500s, 1000s, and UD 100s.
c-iv	**Darvon Pulvules** (Eli Lilly)		(Lilly H03 Darvon). Opaque pink, parabola shape. In 100s, 500s, and UD 100s.

For complete prescribing information, refer to the the Narcotic Agonist Analgesics monograph.

WARNING

Fatalities:
- Do not prescribe propoxyphene for patients who are suicidal or addiction-prone.
- Prescribe propoxyphene with caution for patients taking tranquilizers or antidepressant drugs and patients who use alcohol in excess.
- Tell patients not to exceed the recommended dose and to limit alcohol intake.

Propoxyphene products in excessive doses, either alone or in combination with other CNS depressants (including alcohol), are a major cause of drug-related deaths. Fatalities within the first hour of overdosage are not uncommon. In a survey of deaths due to overdosage conducted in 1975, in ≈ 20% of fatal cases, death occurred within the first hour (5% within 15 minutes). Propoxyphene should not be taken in higher doses than those recommended by the physician. Judicious prescribing of propoxyphene is essential for safety. Consider nonnarcotic analgesics for depressed or suicidal patients. Do not prescribe propoxyphene for suicidal or addiction-prone patients. Caution patients about the concomitant use of propoxyphene products and alcohol because of potentially serious CNS-additive effects of these agents. Because of added CNS depressant effects, cautiously prescribe with concomitant sedatives, tranquilizers, muscle relaxants, antidepressants, or other CNS-depressant drugs. Advise patients of the additive depressant effects of these combinations.

Many propoxyphene-related deaths have occurred in patients with histories of emotional disturbances, suicidal ideation or attempts, or misuse of tranquilizers, alcohol, and other CNS-active drugs. Deaths have occurred as a consequence of the accidental ingestion of excessive quantities of propoxyphene alone or in combination with other drugs. Do not exceed the recommended dosage.

Indications

➤*Pain:* Relief of mild-to-moderate pain.

Administration and Dosage

Because of differences in molecular weight, 100 mg of propoxyphene napsylate is required to supply propoxyphene equivalent to 65 mg of the HCl. In hepatic or renal impairment, reduce total daily dosage.

➤*Propoxyphene HCl:*
Usual dose – 65 mg every 4 hours as needed. Do not exceed 390 mg/day.

➤*Propoxyphene napsylate:*
Usual dose – 100 mg every 4 hours as needed. Do not exceed 600 mg/day.

➤*Elderly:* Propoxyphene metabolism rate may be reduced in some patients. Consider increased dosing interval.

REMIFENTANIL HCl

c-ii	**Ultiva** (Abbott)	**Powder for injection, lyophilized:** 1 mg/mL (as HCl; after reconstitution)	Preservative free. In 3, 5, and 10 mL vials.

For complete prescribing information, refer to the Narcotic Agonist Analgesics group monograph.

Indications

➤*General anesthesia:* An analgesic agent for use during the induction and maintenance of general anesthesia for inpatient and outpatient procedures and for continuation as an analgesic into the immediate postoperative period under the direct supervision of an anesthesia practitioner in a postoperative anesthesia care unit or intensive care setting.

➤*Monitored anesthesia care:* An analgesic component of monitored anesthesia care.

Administration and Dosage

➤*Approved by the FDA:* July 12, 1996.

For IV use only. Individualize dosage.

Administer continuous infusions of remifentanil only by an infusion device. The injection site should be close to the venous cannula. Clear all IV tubing at the time of discontinuation of infusion.

➤*During general anesthesia:* Remifentanil is not recommended as the sole agent in general anesthesia because loss of consciousness cannot be assured and because of a high incidence of apnea, muscle rigidity, and tachycardia. Remifentanil is synergistic with other anesthetics and doses of thiopental, propofol, isoflurane, and midazolam have been reduced by up to 75% with the coadministration of remifentanil.

Remifentanil Dosing Guidelines: General Anesthesia and Continuing as an Analgesic into the Postoperative Care Unit or Intensive Care Setting			
Phase	Continuous IV infusion (mcg/kg/min)	Infusion dose range (mcg/kg/min)	Supplemental IV bolus dose (mcg/kg)
Induction of anesthesia (through intubation)	0.5 to 1[1]	NA[2]	NA[2]
Maintenance of anesthesia with:			
Nitrous oxide (66%)	0.4	0.1 to 2	1
Isoflurane (0.4 to 1.5 MAC)	0.25	0.05 to 2	1

Remifentanil Dosing Guidelines: General Anesthesia and Continuing as an Analgesic into the Postoperative Care Unit or Intensive Care Setting			
Phase	Continuous IV infusion (mcg/kg/min)	Infusion dose range (mcg/kg/min)	Supplemental IV bolus dose (mcg/kg)
Propofol (100 to 200 mcg/kg/min)	0.25	0.05 to 2	1
Continuation as an analgesic into the immediate postoperative period	0.1	0.025 to 0.2	Not recommended

[1] An initial dose of 1 mcg/kg may be administered over 30 to 60 seconds.
[2] No data available.

➤*During induction of anesthesia:* Administer at an infusion rate of 0.5 to 1 mcg/kg/min with a hypnotic or volatile agent for the induction of anesthesia. If endotracheal intubation is to occur < 8 minutes after the start of infusion of remifentanil, then an initial dose of 1 mcg/kg may be administered over 30 to 60 seconds.

➤*During maintenance of anesthesia:* After endotracheal intubation, decrease the infusion rate of remifentanil in accordance with the dosing guidelines in the table above. Due to the rapid onset and short duration of action of remifentanil, the rate of administration during anesthesia can be titrated upward in 25% to 100% increments or downward in 25% to 50% decrements every 2 to 5 minutes to attain the desired level of µ-opioid effect. In response to light anesthesia or transient episodes of intense surgical stress, supplemental bolus doses of 1 mcg/kg may be administered every 2 to 5 minutes. At infusion rates > 1 mcg/kg/min, consider increases in the concomitant anesthetic agents to increase the depth of anesthesia.

➤*Continuation as an analgesic into the immediate postoperative period under the direct supervision of an anesthesia practitioner:* Remifentanil infusions may be continued into the immediate postoperative period for select patients for whom later transition to longer-acting analgesics may be desired. The use of bolus injections of remifentanil to treat pain during the postoperative period is not recommended. When used as an IV analgesic in the immediate postoperative period, administer remifentanil initially by continuous infusion at a rate of 0.1 mcg/kg/min. The infusion rate may be adjusted every 5 minutes in 0.025 mcg/kg/min increments to balance the patient's level of analgesia and respiratory

REMIFENTANIL HCl

rate. Infusion rates > 0.2 mcg/kg/min are associated with respiratory depression (respiratory rate < 8 breaths/min).

➤*Guidelines for discontinuation:* Upon discontinuation of remifentanil, clear the IV tubing to prevent inadvertent administration at a later time.

Because of the rapid offset of action, no residual analgesic activity will be present within 5 to 10 minutes after discontinuation. For patients undergoing surgical procedures where postoperative pain is generally anticipated, administer alternative analgesics prior to discontinuation of remifentanil. The choice of analgesic should be appropriate for the patient's surgical procedure and the level of follow-up care (see Warnings).

➤*Analgesic component of monitored anesthesia care:* It is strongly recommended that supplemental oxygen be supplied whenever remifentanil is administered.

Remifentanil Dosing Guidelines - Monitored Anesthesia Care			
Method	Timing	Remifentanil	Remifentanil + 2 mg midazolam
Single IV dose	Given 90 seconds before local anesthetic	1 mcg/kg over 30 to 60 seconds	0.5 mcg/kg over 30 to 60 seconds
Continuous IV infusion	Beginning 5 minutes before local anesthetic	0.1 mcg/kg/min	0.05 mcg/kg/min
	After local anesthetic	0.05 mcg/kg/min (range: 0.025 to (0.2 mcg/kg/min)	0.025 mcg/kg/min (range: 0.025 to 0.2 mcg/kg/min)

➤*Single dose:* A single IV dose of 0.5 to 1 mcg/kg over 30 to 60 seconds may be given 90 seconds before the placement of the local or regional anesthetic block.

➤*Continuous infusion:* When used alone as an IV analgesic component of monitored anesthesia care, administer initially by continuous infusion at a rate of 0.1 mcg/kg/min beginning 5 minutes before placement of the local or regional anesthetic block.

Because of the risk for hypoventilation, decrease the infusion rate of remifentanil to 0.05 mcg/kg/min following placement of the block. Thereafter, rate adjustments of 0.025 mcg/kg/min at 5-minute intervals may be used to balance the patient's level of analgesia and respiratory rate. Rates > 0.2 mcg/kg/min are generally associated with repiratory depression (respiratory rates < 8 breaths/min).

Bolus doses of remifentanil administered simultaneously with a continuous infusion of remifentanil to spontaneously breathing patients are not recommended.

➤*Individualization of dosage:*
Elderly – Decrease the starting doses of remifentanil by 50% in elderly patients (> 65 years of age). Cautiously titrate to effect.

Children – The same doses (per kg) as adults are recommended for pediatric patients ≥ 2 years of age.

Obesity – Base the starting dose of remifentanil on ideal body weight (IBW) in obese patients (> 30% over their IBW).

➤*Preanesthetic medication:* The need for premedication and the choice of anesthetic agents must be individualized. In clinical studies, patients who received remifentanil frequently received a benzodiazepine premedication.

➤*Preparation for administration:* To reconstitute solution, add 1 mL of diluent per mg of remifentanil. Shake well to dissolve. When reconstituted as directed, the solution contains ≈ 1 mg of remifentanil activity per mL. Remifentanil should be diluted to a recommended final concentration of 25, 50, or 250 mcg/mL prior to administration. Do not administer remifentanil without dilution.

➤*Admixture compatibility and stability:* Remifentanil is stable for 24 hours at room temperature after reconstitution and further dilution to concentrations of 20 to 250 mcg/mL with the following IV fluids: Sterile Water for Injection; 5% Dextrose Injection; 5% Dextrose and 0.9% Sodium Chloride Injection; 0.9% Sodium Chloride Injection; 0.45% Sodium Chloride Injection; Lactated Ringers and 5% Dextrose Injection.

Remifentanil has been shown to be compatible with propofol when coadministered into a running IV administration set.

➤*Storage / Stability:* Store at 2° to 25°C (36° to 77°F).

Warnings

➤*Maintenance of general anesthesia:* Administer continuous infusions only by an infusion device. Use IV bolus administration of remifentanil only during the maintenance of general anesthesia. In nonintubated patients, administer remifentanil doses over 30 to 60 seconds.

Interruption of infusion – Interruption of an infusion of remifentanil will result in rapid offset of effect. Rapid clearance and lack of drug accumulation result in rapid dissipation of respiratory-depressant and analgesic effects upon discontinuation of remifentanil at recommended doses. Precede discontinuation of an infusion of remifentanil with the establishment of adequate postoperative analgesia.

IV tubing – Make injections of remifentanil into IV tubing at or close to the venous cannula. Upon discontinuation of remifentanil, clear the IV tubing to prevent the inadvertent administration of remifentanil at a later point in time. Failure to adequately clear the IV tubing to remove residual remifentanil has been associated with the appearance of respiratory depression, apnea, and muscle rigidity upon the administration of additional fluids or medications through the same IV tubing.

Do not administer remifentanil into the same IV tubing with blood because of potential inactivation by nonspecific esterases in blood products.

SUFENTANIL CITRATE

c-ii	Sufentanil Citrate (ESI Lederle)	Injection: 50 mcg (as citrate)/ml	In 1, 2, and 5 ml amps.
c-ii	Sufenta (Taylor)		Preservative free. In 1, 2, and 5 ml amps.

For complete prescribing information, refer to the Narcotic Agonist Analgesics group monograph.

Indications

➤*Analgesia:* Analgesic adjunct at dosages of up to 8 mcg/kg to maintain balanced general anesthesia in patients who are intubated and ventilated.

➤*Anesthetic:* A primary anesthetic agent at dosages ≥ 8 mcg/kg to induce and maintain anesthesia with 100% oxygen in patients undergoing major surgical procedures. In patients who are intubated and ventilated, such as cardiovascular surgery or neurosurgical procedures in the sitting position, to provide favorable myocardial and cerebral oxygen balance or when extended postoperative ventilation is anticipated.

➤*Epidural analgesic:* For epidural administration as an analgesic combined with low-dose bupivacaine, usually 12.5 mg per administration, during labor and vaginal delivery.

Administration and Dosage

Individualize dosage. In obese patients (> 20% above ideal total body weight), determine dosage on the basis of lean body weight. Reduce dosage in the elderly or debilitated. Monitor vital signs routinely.

For IV injection.

➤*Adult dosage range (analgesic dosages):*
Total dosage –
1 to 2 mcg/kg: Administer with nitrous oxide/oxygen in patients undergoing general surgery ≤ 8 hours in which endotracheal intubation and mechanical ventilation are required. Expected duration of anesthesia is 1 to 2 hours.

• *Maintenance* – 10 to 25 mcg (0.2 to 0.5 ml) in increments as needed for surgical stress or lightening of analgesia. Individualize supplemental dosages. Adjust maintenance infusion rates based upon the induction dose of sufentanil so that the total dose does not exceed 1 mcg/kg/hr of expected surgical time.
2 to 8 mcg/kg: Administer with nitrous oxide/oxygen in more complicated major surgical procedures in which endotracheal intubation and

mechanical ventilation are required. Provides some attenuation of sympathetic reflex activity in response to surgical stimuli, hemodynamic stability, and relatively rapid recovery. Expected duration of anesthesia is 2 to 8 hours.

• *Maintenance* – 10 to 50 mcg (0.2 to 1 ml) in increments as needed for stress or lightening of analgesia. Individualize supplemental dosages. Adjust maintenance infusion rates based upon the induction dose of sufentanil so that the total dose does not exceed 1 mcg/kg/hr of expected surgical time.

8 to 30 mcg/kg (anesthetic doses): Administer with 100% oxygen and a muscle relaxant. Sufentanil produces sleep at doses ≥ 8 mcg/kg and maintains a deep level of anesthesia without additional agents. At doses of up to 25 mcg/kg, catecholamine release is attenuated; 25 to 30 mcg/kg blocks sympathetic responses including catecholamine release. Use high doses in patients undergoing major surgical procedures in which endotracheal intubation and mechanical ventilation are required (eg, cardiovascular surgery and neurosurgery in the sitting position). Postoperative observation is essential and postoperative mechanical ventilation may be required because of extended postoperative respiratory depression. Titrate dosage to individual patient response.

• *Maintenance* – 0.5 to 10 mcg/kg for surgical stress, such as incision, sternotomy, or cardiopulmonary bypass. Base the maintenance infusion rate for sufentanil upon the induction dose so that the total dose for the procedure does not exceed 30 mcg/kg.

➤*Epidural use in labor and delivery:* 10 to 15 mcg administered with 10 ml bupivacaine 0.125% with or without epinephrine. Mix sufentanil and bupivacaine together before administration. Doses can be repeated twice (for a total of 3 doses) at ≥ 1-hour intervals until delivery.

Administer sufentanil by slow injection. Closely monitor respiration following each administration of an epidural injection of sufentanil.

➤*Children (< 12 years of age):* For induction and maintenance of anesthesia in children undergoing cardiovascular surgery, a dose of 10 to 25 mcg/kg administered with 100% oxygen is recommended. Supplemental doses of up to 25 to 50 mcg are recommended for maintenance.

TRAMADOL HCl

Rx	**Tramadol** (Various, eg, Caraco, Eon, Ivax, Mallinckrodt, Purepac, Watson)	**Tablets:** 50 mg	In 100s, 500s, and 1000s.
Rx	**Ultram** (Ortho-McNeil)		Lactose. (Ultram 659). White, capsule shape, scored. Film-coated. In 100s, 500s, and UD 100s.

Indications

➤*Pain:* Management of moderate to moderately severe pain.

Administration and Dosage

➤*Approved by the FDA:* March 3, 1995.

Individualize dose based on the lowest effective dose. Starting at the lowest possible dose and titrating upward as needed has resulted in increased tolerability and fewer discontinuations. Can be administered without regard to meals.

For moderate to moderately severe chronic pain not requiring rapid onset of analgesic effect, administer 25 mg/day in the morning and titrate in 25 mg increments as separate doses every 3 days to reach 100 mg/day (25 mg 4 times/day). Thereafter, increase the dose by 50 mg as tolerated every 3 days to reach 200 mg/day (50 mg 4 times/day). After titration, administer 50 to 100 mg every 4 to 6 hours as needed for pain relief. Do not exceed 400 mg/day.

For patients requiring rapid onset of analgesic relief and for whom the benefits outweigh the risk of discontinuation due to adverse effects associated with higher initial doses, administer 50 to 100 mg every 4 to 6 hours as needed, not to exceed 400 mg/day.

➤*Elderly:* Use caution when selecting a dose for patients over 65 years of age; start at the low end of the dosing range. Do not exceed 300 mg/day in patients 75 years of age and older.

➤*Renal function impairment:* In patients with a Ccr less than 30 mL/min, increase the dosing interval to 12 hours, with a maximum daily dose of 200 mg. Because hemodialysis only removes 7% of an administered dose, dialysis patients can receive their regular dose on the day of dialysis.

➤*Hepatic function impairment:* The recommended dose for patients with cirrhosis is 50 mg every 12 hours.

➤*Storage/Stability:* Dispense in a tight container. Store at 25°C (77°F); excursions permitted to 15 to 30°C (59 to 86°F).

Actions

➤*Pharmacology:* Tramadol is a centrally acting synthetic opioid analgesic compound. Although its mode of action is not completely understood, from animal tests at least 2 complementary mechanisms appear applicable: Binding to μ-opioid receptors and inhibition of reuptake of norepinephrine and serotonin. Tramadol derives opioid activity from low affinity binding of the parent compound to μ-opioid receptors and higher affinity binding of the *O*-desmethyl metabolite (M1). In animal models, M1 is up to 6 times more potent than tramadol in producing analgesia and 200 times more potent in μ-opioid binding. The relative contribution of both tramadol and M1 to human analgesia is dependent upon the plasma concentrations of each compound.

Tramadol-induced antinociception is only partially antagonized by the opiate antagonist naloxone in animal tests. In addition, tramadol inhibits reuptake of norepinephrine and serotonin in vitro, as have some other opioid analgesics. These latter mechanisms may contribute independently to the overall analgesic profile of tramadol. Onset of analgesia is evident within 1 hour after administration and reaches a peak in approximately 2 to 3 hours. The duration of analgesia is about 6 hours.

Apart from analgesia, tramadol may produce a constellation of symptoms (eg, dizziness, somnolence, nausea, constipation, sweating, pruritus) similar to that of other opioids. In contrast to morphine, tramadol has not been shown to cause histamine release. At therapeutic doses, tramadol has no effect on heart rate, left ventricular function, or cardiac index. Orthostatic changes in blood pressure have been observed.

➤*Pharmacokinetics:*

Absorption – Tramadol is rapidly and almost completely absorbed after oral administration. The mean absolute bioavailability of a 100 mg oral dose is about 75%. Administration with food does not significantly affect its rate or extent of absorption; therefore, it can be administered without regard to meals. The mean peak plasma concentration is about 308 ng/mL and occurs at approximately 2 hours after a single 100 mg oral dose in healthy subjects. At this dose, the mean peak plasma concentration of M1 is about 55 ng/mL and occurs approximately 3 hours postdose. The separate [+]- and [-]-enantiomers of tramadol generally follow a parallel time course in plasma following single and multiple doses although small differences (approximately 10%) exist in the absolute amount of each enantiomer present.

Steady state is achieved of both tramadol and M1 after 2 days with a 4 times daily dosing regimen. The plasma half-life of tramadol following single and multiple dosing was 6 and 7 hours, respectively.

Distribution – The volume of distribution was 2.6 and 2.9 L/kg in male and female subjects, respectively, following a 100 mg IV dose. Binding to human plasma proteins is approximately 20% and appears to be independent of concentration up to 10 mcg/mL. Saturation of plasma protein binding occurs only at concentrations outside the clinically relevant range.

Metabolism – Tramadol is extensively metabolized after oral administration. The major metabolic pathways appear to be *N*- and *O*-demethylation and glucuronidation or sulfation in the liver. Only one metabolite, M1, is pharmacologically active. Production of M1 is dependent on the CYP2D6 isoenzyme of cytochrome P-450. Approximately 7% of the population has reduced activity of the CYP2D6 isoenzyme of cytochrome P-450. These individuals are "poor metabolizers" of debrisoquine, dextromethorphan, and tricyclic antidepressants, among other drugs. Based on a population PK analysis of phase 1 studies in healthy subjects, concentrations of tramadol were approximately 20% higher in "poor metabolizers" vs "extensive metabolizers," while M1 concentrations were 40% lower.

Excretion – Approximately 30% of the dose is excreted in the urine as unchanged drug, whereas 60% of the dose is excreted as metabolites. The remainder is excreted either as unidentified or as unextractable metabolites. The mean terminal plasma elimination half-lives of racemic tramadol and racemic M1 are 6.3 ± 1.4 and 7.4 ± 1.4 hours, respectively. The plasma elimination half-life of tramadol increased from approximately 6 to 7 hours upon multiple dosing.

Renal function impairment: Renal function impairment results in a decreased rate and extent of excretion of tramadol and its active metabolite, M1. In patients with creatinine clearances of less than 30 mL/min, adjustment of the dosing regimen is recommended (see Administration and Dosage). The total amount of tramadol and M1 removed during a 4-hour dialysis period is less than 7% of the administered dose.

Hepatic function impairment: Metabolism of tramadol and M1 is reduced in patients with advanced cirrhosis of the liver, resulting in a larger area under the serum concentration-time curve for tramadol and longer tramadol and M1 elimination half-lives (13 and 19 hours, respectively). In cirrhotic patients, adjustment of the dosing regimen is recommended (see Administration and Dosage).

Elderly: In subjects older than 75 years of age, maximum serum concentrations are slightly elevated (208 vs 162 ng/mL) and the elimination half-life is slightly prolonged (7 vs 6 hours) compared with subjects 65 to 75 years of age. Adjustment of the daily dose is recommended for patients older than 75 years of age (see Administration and Dosage).

Gender: The absolute bioavailability of tramadol was 73% in males and 79% in females. The plasma clearance was 6.4 mL/min/kg in males and 5.7 in females following a 100 mg IV dose. Following a single oral dose, and after adjusting for body weight, females had a 12% higher peak tramadol concentration and a 35% higher area under the concentration-time curve compared to males. This difference may not be of any clinical significance.

➤*Clinical trials:* Tramadol has been given in single oral doses of 50, 75, and 100 mg to patients with pain following surgical procedures and pain following oral surgery (extraction of impacted molars).

Following oral surgery, pain relief was demonstrated in some patients at single doses of 50 and 75 mg. A dose of 100 mg tended to provide analgesia superior to codeine sulfate 60 mg, but it was not as effective as the combination of aspirin 650 mg/codeine phosphate 60 mg.

Patients with chronic conditions entered a double-blind phase of 1 to 3 months. Average daily doses of approximately 250 mg tramadol in divided doses produced analgesia comparable with 5 doses of acetaminophen 300 mg/codeine phosphate 30 mg daily, 5 doses of aspirin 325 mg/codeine phosphate 30 mg daily, and with 2 to 3 doses of acetaminophen 500 mg/oxycodone HCl 5 mg daily.

Contraindications

Hypersensitivity to tramadol or any other component of this product or opioids; in any situation where opioids are contraindicated, including acute intoxication with any of the following: Alcohol, hypnotics, centrally acting analgesics, opioids or psychotropic drugs, narcotics.

Warnings

➤*Seizure:* Seizures have been reported in patients receiving tramadol within the recommended dosage range. Spontaneous postmarketing reports indicate the seizure risk is increased with doses above the recommended range. Concomitant use with selective serotonin reuptake inhibitors (SSRIs), tricyclic compounds (eg, TCAs, cyclobenzaprine, promethazine), or other opioids also increases the risk of seizures. Administration of tramadol with neuroleptics, MAO inhibitors (see Warnings), or other drugs that reduce the seizure threshold may also enhance the seizure risk. Risk of convulsions may also increase in patients with epilepsy, those with a history of seizures, or in patients with a recognized risk for seizure (eg, head trauma, metabolic disorders, alcohol and drug withdrawal, CNS infections). In a tramadol overdose, naloxone administration may also increase the risk of seizure (see Overdosage).

TRAMADOL HCl

►*Concomitant CNS depressants and SSRIs:* Use with caution and in reduced dosages when administering to patients receiving CNS depressants such as alcohol, opioids, anesthetic agents, narcotics, phenothiazines, tranquilizers, or sedative hypnotics.

►*Concomitant MAO inhibitors:* Use with great caution in patients taking MAO inhibitors. Animal studies have shown increased deaths with combined administration. Concomitant use of tramadol with MAO inhibitors or SSRIs increases the risk of adverse events, including seizure and serotonin syndrome.

►*Withdrawal:* Withdrawal symptoms may occur if tramadol is discontinued abruptly. These symptoms may include: Anxiety, sweating, insomnia, rigors, pain, nausea, tremors, diarrhea, upper respiratory symptoms, piloerection, and rarely hallucinations. Clinical experience suggests that withdrawal symptoms may be relieved by reinstitution of therapy followed by a gradual, tapered dose reduction of the medication combined with symptomatic support.

►*Hypersensitivity reactions:* Serious and rarely fatal anaphylactoid reactions have been reported in patients receiving therapy with tramadol. When these events do occur it is often following the first dose. Other reported allergic reactions include pruritus, hives, bronchospasm, angioedema, toxic epidermal necrolysis, and Stevens-Johnson syndrome. Patients with a history of anaphylactoid reactions to codeine and other opioids may be at increased risk and therefore should not receive tramadol (see Contraindications).

►*Renal/Hepatic function impairment:* Impaired renal function results in a decreased rate and extent of excretion of tramadol and its active metabolite, M1. In patients with creatinine clearances less than 30 mL/min, dosing reduction is recommended (see Administration and Dosage).

Metabolism of tramadol and M1 is reduced in patients with advanced cirrhosis of the liver. In cirrhotic patients, dosing reduction is recommended (see Administration and Dosage).

With the prolonged half-life in these conditions, achievement of steady state is delayed, so that it may take several days for elevated plasma concentrations to develop.

►*Carcinogenesis:* A slight, but statistically significant, increase in 2 common murine tumors, pulmonary and hepatic, was observed in a mouse carcinogenicity study, particularly in aged mice. Mice were dosed orally up to 30 mg/kg (90 mg/m^2 or 0.36 times the maximum daily human dosage of 246 mg/m^2) for approximately 2 years.

►*Mutagenesis:* Weakly mutagenic results occurred in the presence of metabolic activation in the mouse lymphoma assay and micronucleus test in rats.

►*Elderly:* Use caution when selecting a dose for an elderly patient, start at the low end of the dosing range, to account for the greater frequency of decreased hepatic, renal, or cardiac function and of concomitant disease or other drug therapy. Daily doses greater than 300 mg are not recommended in patients over 75 years of age (see Administration and Dosage). Patients older than 75 years of age had slightly elevated serum concentrations and a slightly prolonged elimination half-life (see Actions). Patients over 75 years of age also experienced more treatment-limiting adverse events during clinical trials, as compared with those less than 65 years of age. Constipation resulted in the discontinuation of treatment in 10% of those over 75 years of age.

►*Pregnancy:* Category C. Tramadol is embryotoxic and fetotoxic in mice (360 mg/m^2), rats (150 mg/m^2), and rabbits (900 mg/m^2) at maternally toxic doses 3 to 15 times the maximum human dose or higher. These dosages on a mg/m^2 basis are 1.4, greater than or equal to 0.6, and greater than or equal to 3.6 times the maximum daily human dosage (246 mg/m^2) respectively. Embryo and fetal toxicity consisted primarily of decreased fetal weights, skeletal ossification and increased supernumerary ribs at maternally toxic dose levels. Transient delays in developmental or behavioral parameters were also seen in pups from rat dams allowed to deliver. Embryo and fetal lethality were reported only in one rabbit study at 300 mg/kg (3600 mg/m^2).

In peri- and postnatal studies in rats, progeny of dams receiving oral (gavage) dose levels of 50 mg/kg or more had decreased weights, and pup survival was decreased early in lactation at 80 mg/kg.

Do not use in pregnant women prior to or during labor unless the potential benefits outweigh the risks. Safe use in pregnancy has not been established. Tramadol has been shown to cross the placenta. The mean ratio of serum tramadol in the umbilical veins compared to maternal veins was 0.83 for 40 women given tramadol during labor. Chronic use during pregnancy may lead to physical dependence and

postpartum withdrawal symptoms in the newborn. There are no adequate and well controlled studies in pregnant women. Neonatal seizures, neonatal withdrawal syndrome, fetal death, and stillbirth have been reported during postmarketing. Use during pregnancy only if the potential benefit justifies the risk to the fetus.

►*Lactation:* Both tramadol and its active metabolite, M1, are excreted into human milk. Tramadol is not recommended for obstetrical preoperative medication or for postdelivery analgesia in nursing mothers because its safety in infants and newborns has not been studied. Following a single IV 100 mg dose, the cumulative excretion in breast milk within 16 hours postdose was 100 mcg of tramadol (0.1% of the maternal dose) and 27 mcg of M1.

►*Children:* Not recommended in children because safety and efficacy in patients less than 16 years of age have not been established.

Precautions

►*Respiratory depression:* Administer tramadol cautiously in patients at risk for repiratory depression. In these patients, consider alternative nonopioid analgesics. When large doses of tramadol are administered with anesthetic medications or alcohol, respiratory depression may result. Treat respiratory depression as an overdose (see Overdosage).

►*Increased intracranial pressure or head trauma:* Use with caution in patients with increased intracranial pressure or head injury. Pupillary changes (miosis) from tramadol may obscure the existence, extent, or course of intracranial pathology. Clinicians should also maintain a high index of suspicion for adverse drug reactions when evaluating altered mental status in these patients if they are receiving tramadol.

►*Acute abdominal conditions:* Tramadol may complicate the clinical assessment of patients with acute abdominal conditions.

►*Drug abuse and dependence:* Tramadol may induce psychic and physical dependence of the morphine-type (μ-opioid). Dependence and abuse, including drug-seeking behavior and taking illicit actions to obtain the drug are not limited to those patients with prior history of opioid dependence. The risk in patients with substance abuse has been observed to be higher. Do not use in opioid-dependent patients. Tramadol has been shown to reinitiate physical dependence in some patients who have been previously dependent on other opioids. Tramadol is associated with craving and tolerance development.

►*Hazardous tasks:* Tramadol may impair the mental and/or physical abilities required for the performance of potentially hazardous tasks such as driving a car or operating machinery. Caution the patient using this drug accordingly.

Drug Interactions

Tramadol Drug Interactions			
Precipitant drug	Object drug*		Description
Carbamazepine	Tramadol	↓	Coadministration causes a significant increase in tramadol metabolism and therefore may result in reduced analgesic effect.
Quinidine	Tramadol	↔	Quinidine selectively inhibits CYP2D6, therefore coadministration results in increased tramadol concentrations and decreased M1 concentrations. The clinical consequences of these findings are unknown.
SSRIs	Tramadol	↑	Serotonin syndrome may occur, use concurrently with caution as tramadol inhibits norepinephrine and serotonin reuptake.
Tramadol	SSRIs		
MAO inhibitors	Tramadol	↑	Use concurrently with caution as tramadol inhibits norepinephrine and serotonin reuptake.
Tramadol	MAO inhibitors		
Tramadol	Warfarin	↑	The oral anticoagulant effect of warfarin may be increased. Carefully monitor coagulation values and adjust dose as needed when tramadol is initiated or discontinued.
Tramadol	Digoxin	↑	Rare reports of digoxin toxicity have been reported in postmarketing surveillance.

* ↓ = Object drug decreased. ↑ = Object drug increased. ↔ = Undetermined clinical effect.

TRAMADOL HCl

Adverse Reactions

Tramadol was administered to 550 patients during the double-blind or open-label extension periods in US studies of chronic nonmalignant pain. The following table reports the cumulative incidence rate of adverse reactions by 7, 30, and 90 days for the most frequent reactions (5% or more by 7 days). The most frequently reported events were in the CNS and GI system. Although the reactions listed in the table are felt to be probably related to tramadol administration, the reported rates also include some events that may have been caused by underlying disease or concomitant medication. The overall incidence rates of adverse experiences in these trials were similar for tramadol and the active control groups, (acetaminophen 300 mg with codeine phosphate 30 mg), and aspirin 325 mg with codeine phosphate 30 mg. However, the rates of withdrawals because of adverse events appeared to be higher in the tramadol groups.

Cumulative Incidence of Tramadol Adverse Reactions (%)			
Adverse reaction	Up to 7 days	Up to 30 days	Up to 90 days
Dizziness/Vertigo	26	31	33
Nausea	24	34	40
Constipation	24	38	46
Headache	18	26	32
Somnolence	16	23	25
Vomiting	9	13	17
Pruritus	8	10	11
CNS stimula tion[1]	7	11	14
Asthenia	6	11	12
Sweating	6	7	9
Dyspepsia	5	9	13
Dry mouth	5	9	10
Diarrhea	5	6	10

[1] CNS stimulation is a composite of nervousness, anxiety, agitation, tremor, spasticity, euphoria, emotional lability, and hallucinations.

➤*Cardiovascular:* Vasodilation (1% to less than 5%); syncope, orthostatic hypotension, tachycardia (less than 1%); abnormal ECG; hypertension; hypotension; myocardial ischemia; palpitations; pulmonary edema; pulmonary embolism.

➤*CNS:* Anxiety, confusion, coordination disturbance, euphoria, nervousness, sleep disorder (1% to less than 5%); abnormal gait, amnesia, cognitive dysfunction, depression, difficulty in concentration, hallucinations, paresthesia, seizure (see Warnings), tremor (less than 1%); migraine; speech disorders.

➤*Dermatologic:* Rash (1% to less than 5%); Stevens-Johnson syndrome/toxic epidermal necrolysis, urticaria, vesicles (less than 1%).

➤*GI:* Abdominal pain, anorexia, flatulence (1% to less than 5%); GI bleeding; hepatitis; liver failure; stomatitis.

➤*GU:* Urinary retention/frequency, menopausal symptoms (1% to less than 5%); dysuria, menstrual disorder (less than 1%).

➤*Special senses:* Miosis, visual disturbance (1% to less than 5%); dysgeusia (less than 1%); cataracts; deafness; tinnitus.

➤*Lab test abnormalities:* Creatinine increase; elevated liver enzymes; hemoglobin decrease; proteinuria.

➤*Miscellaneous:* Hypertonia, malaise (1% to less than 5%); accidental injury, allergic reaction, anaphylaxis, death, dyspnea, serotonin syndrome (mental status change, hyperreflexia, fever, shivering, tremor, agitation, diaphoresis, seizures, and coma), suicidal tendency, weight loss (less than 1%).

Overdosage

➤*Symptoms:* Serious potential consequences of overdosage are respiratory depression, lethargy, coma, seizure, cardiac arrest, and death (see Warnings). Fatalities have been reported in postmarketing in association with both intentional and unintentional overdose with tramadol.

➤*Treatment:* In treating an overdose, give primary attention to maintaining adequate ventilation along with general supportive treatment. While naloxone will reverse some symptoms caused by overdosage with tramadol, the risk of seizures is also increased with naloxone administration. In animals convulsions following the administration of toxic doses of tramadol could be suppressed with barbiturates or benzodiazepines but were increased with naloxone. Naloxone administration did not change the lethality of an overdose in mice. Hemodialysis is not expected to be helpful in an overdose because it removes less than 7% of the administered dose in a 4-hour dialysis period.

Patient Information

Tramadol may impair mental or physical abilities or coordination required for the performance of potentially hazardous tasks such as driving a car or operating machinery.

Instruct patients not to take with products containing alcohol.

Instruct patients to use caution when taking tramadol with other medications such as tranquilizers, hypnotics, or other opiate-containing analgesics.

NARCOTIC ANALGESIC COMBINATIONS

Content given per tablet, capsule, 5 mL oral solution, and mL injection, or suppository.

	Product and Distributor	Narcotic	Acetaminophen	Aspirin	Other Content	Average Adult Dose	How Supplied
c-v	Acetaminophen w/Codeine Oral Solution[1] (Various, eg., Morton Grove, Roxane)	12 mg codeine phosphate	120 mg			15 mL q 4 h	In 120 mL, pt and gal.
c-v	Capital w/Codeine Suspension (Carnrick)						Fruit punch flavor. In 473 mL.
c-v	Tylenol w/Codeine Elixir (McNeil)				7% alcohol, saccharin, sucrose		Cherry flavor. In 480 mL.
c-iii	Acetaminophen w/Codeine Tablets (Various, eg, Lemmon)	15 mg codeine phosphate	300 mg			1 to 4 q 4 h	In 100s and 1000s.
c-iii	Tylenol w/Codeine No. 2 Tablets (McNeil)				Sodium metabisulfite		(McNeil Tylenol Codeine 2). White. In 100s and UD 500s.
c-iii	Acetaminophen w/Codeine Tablets (Various, eg, Lemmon, Moore, Purepac, Roxane)	30 mg codeine phosphate	300 mg			0.5 to 2 q 4 h	In 100s, 1000s and UD 100s.
c-iii	Aceta w/Codeine Tablets (Century)					1 tid	In 100s and 1000s.
c-iii	Tylenol w/Codeine No. 3 Tablets (McNeil)	30 mg codeine phosphate			Sodium metabisulfite	0.5 to 2 q 4 h	(McNeil Tylenol Codeine 3). White. In 100s, 500s, 1000s and UD 500s.
c-iii	Fioricet w/Codeine Capsules (Watson)	30 mg codeine phosphate	325 mg		40 mg caffeine, 50 mg butalbital	1 or 2 q 4 h up to 6/day	(Fioricet codeine). Dark blue/gray. In 100s and ControlPak 25s.
c-iii	Aspirin w/Codeine No. 3 Tablets (Various, eg, Goldline, Moore, Schein, URL, Zenith)	30 mg codeine phosphate		325 mg		1 or 2 q 4 h	In 100s and 1000s.
c-iii	Empirin w/Codeine No. 3 Tablets (GlaxoWellcome)						(Empirin 3). White. In 100s, 500s, 1000s and Dispenserpak 25s.
c-iii	Ascomp with Codeine Capsules (Breckenridge)	30 mg codeine phosphate		325 mg	40 mg caffeine, 50 mg butalbital	1 or 2 q 4 h up to 6/day	In 100s and 500s.
c-iii	Fiorinal w/Codeine Capsules (Novartis)						(F-C Sandoz 78-107). Blue/yellow. In 100s and ControlPak 25s.
c-iii	Acetaminophen w/Codeine Tabs (Various, eg, Lemmon, Moore, Purepac)	60 mg codeine phosphate	300 mg			1 q 4 h	In 100s, 500s, 1000s.
c-iii	Tylenol w/Codeine No. 4 Tablets (McNeil)	60 mg codeine phosphate			Sodium metabisulfite		(McNeil Tylenol Codeine 4). White. In 100s, 500s, and UD 500s.
c-iii	Aspirin w/Codeine No. 4 Tablets (Various, eg, Goldline, Major, Moore, Rugby, URL, Zenith)			325 mg		1 q 4 h	In 100s, 500s and 1000s.
c-iii	Empirin w/Codeine No. 4 Tablets (GlaxoWellcome)						(Empirin 4). White. In 100s, 500s and Dispenserpak 25s.
c-iii	Hydrocodone Bitartrate and Ibuprofen (Teva)	7.5 mg hydrocodone bitartrate			200 mg ibuprofen	1 q 4 to 6 h up to 5/day	Lactose. (5161). White. Film-coated. In 100s.
c-iii	Vicoprofen Tablets (Abbott)						(VP). White. Convex. Film coated. In 100s, 500s and UD 100s.
c-iii	Lortab Elixir (Whitby)	2.5 mg hydrocodone bitartrate	167 mg		7% alcohol, saccharin, sorbitol, sucrose, parabens	15 mL q 4 to 6 h up to 6/day	Tropical fruit punch flavor. In 473 mL.
c-iii	Hydrocodone Bitartrate and Acetaminophen Elixir (Various, eg, Mallinckrodt, Pharmaceutical Associates)				7% alcohol.	15 mL q 4 to 6 h up to 90 mL/day	In 473 mL.
c-iii	Lortab 2.5/500 Tablets (Whitby)	2.5 mg hydrocodone bitartrate	500 mg		Sucrose	1 or 2 q 4 to 6 h up to 8/day	(Whitby/901). White/pink specks. In 100s and 500s.

NARCOTIC ANALGESIC COMBINATIONS

	Product and Distributor	Narcotic	Aspirin	Acetaminophen	Other Content	Average Adult Dose	How Supplied
c-iii	**Anexsia Tablets** (Andrx)	5 mg hydrocodone bitartrate		325 mg		1 or 2 q 4 to 6 hr as needed up to 12/day	(M365). White, capsule shape, scored. In 100s and 1000s.
c-iii	**Norco 5/325 Tablets** (Watson)	5 mg hydrocodone bitartrate			Sucrose	1 to 2 q t to 6 hr	(Watson 913). White with orange specks, scored, capsule shape. In 100s and 500s.
c-iii	**Zydone Tablets** (Endo)	5 mg hydrocodone bitartrate		400 mg		1 or 2 q 4 to 6 h up to 8/day	(E5). Yellow, convex. Octagonal shape. In 100s, 500s, and UD 100s.
c-iii	**Hydrocodone Bitartrate & Acetaminophen Caps** (Various, eg, Goldline, Rugby)	5 mg hydrocodone bitartrate		500 mg		1 or 2 q 4 to 6 h up to 8/day	In 100s and 500s.
c-iii	**Hydrocodone Bitartrate and Acetaminophen Tablets** (Various, eg, Geneva, Goldline, Moore, Rugby, Watson)						In 100s and 500s.
c-iii	**Bancap HC Capsules** (Forest)						(Forest 610A). Yellow/orange. In 100s and 500s.
c-iii	**Ceta-Plus Capsules** (Seatrace)						(Seatrace). White. In 100s.
c-iii	**Co-Gesic Tablets** (Central)						(500-5) White, scored. Oval. In 100s and 500s.
c-iii	**Hydrocet Capsules** (Carnrick)						(C 8657). Blue/white. In 100s.
c-iii	**Hydrogesic Capsules** (Edwards)	5 mg hydrocodone bitartrate		500 mg		1 or 2 q 4 to 6 h up to 8/day	In 100s.
c-iii	**Hy-Phen Tablets** (B.F. Ascher)						(225-450). White, scored. Capsule shape. In 100s.
c-iii	**Margesic H Capsules** (Marnel)						(Margesic H). Gray/lavender. In 100s.
c-iii	**Lorcet-HD Capsules** (UAD)						(1120). Maroon. In 100s.
c-iii	**Lortab 5/500 Tablets** (Whitby)				Sugar		(UCB 902). White w/blue specks, scored. Capsule shape. In 100s, 500s and UD 100s.
c-iii	**Anexsia 5/500 Tablets** (Mallinckrodt)						(BMP 207). White, scored. In 100s.
c-iii	**Panacet 5/500 Tablets** (ECR Pharm)						(ECR 0141). White, scored. Oval. In 100s.
c-iii	**Stagesic Capsules** (Huckaby)	5 mg hydrocodone bitartrate		500 mg	Parabens	1 to 2 q 4 to 6 h up to 8/day	(Stagesic). White. In 100s.
c-iii	**T-Gesic Capsules** (T.E. Williams)					1 to 2 q 6 to 8 h	(T-Gesic/TEW). White. In 100s.
c-iii	**Vicodin Tablets** (Abbott)					1 or 2 q 4 to 6 h up to 8/day	(Vicodin). White, scored. Capsule shape. In 100s, 500s and UD 100s.
c-iii	**Anexsia Tablets** (Andrx)	7.5 mg hydrocodone bitartrate		325 mg		1 q 4 to 6 hr as needed up to 8/day	(M366). White, oval. In 100s and 1000s.
c-iii	**Zydone Tablets** (Endo)	7.5 mg hydrocodone bitartrate		400 mg		1 q 4 to 6 h up to 6/day	(E 7.5). Blue, convex. Octagonal shape. In 100s, 500s, and UD 100s.
c-iii	**Lortab 7.5/500 Tablets** (Whitby)	7.5 mg hydrocodone bitartrate		500 mg	Sucrose	1 q 4 to 6 h	(Whitby/903). White w/green specks, scored. Capsule shape. In 100s, 500s and UD 100s.
c-iii	**Hydrocodone with Acetaminophen Tablets** (Various, eg, Watson)						In 100s and 500s.
c-iii	**Anexsia 7.5/650 Tablets** (Mallinckrodt)	7.5 mg hydrocodone bitartrate		650 mg		1 q 4 to 6 h	(BMP 188). Peach, scored. Capsule shape. In 100s.
c-iii	**Lorcet Plus Tablets** (UAD)						(U 201). White, scored. Capsule shape. In 100s, 500s and UD 100s.
c-iii	**Hydrocodone Bitartrate/Acetaminophen Caplets** (Various, eg, King Pharm)						In 100s and 500s.

NARCOTIC ANALGESIC COMBINATIONS

NARCOTIC ANALGESIC COMBINATIONS

	Product and Distributor	Narcotic	Acetaminophen	Aspirin	Other Content	Average Adult Dose	How Supplied
c-iii	Vicodin ES Tablets (Abbott)	7.5 mg hydrocodone bitartrate	750 mg			1 q 4 to 6 h up to 5/day	(Vicodin ES). White, scored. Oval. In 100s and UD 100s.
c-iii	Hydrocodone with Acetaminophen Tablets (Various, eg, Barr, Geneva, Mallinckrodt, Royce, URL, Zenith Goldline)					1 q 4 to 6 h up to 6/day	In 100s, 500s, and 1000s.
c-iii	Hydrocodone Bitartrate and Acetaminophen (Mallinckrodt)	10 mg hydrocodone bitartrate	325 mg				(M367). White, oval, bisected. In 100s, 500s, and UD 100s.
c-iii	Norco Tablets (Watson Labs)					1 q 4 to 6 h up to 6/day	(NORCO 539). Yellow, bisected. Capsule shape. In 100s and 500s.
c-iii	Zydone Tablets (Endo)	10 mg hydrocodone bitartrate	400 mg			1 q 4 to 6 h up to 6/day	(E 10). Red, convex. Octagonal shape. In 100s, 500s, and UD 100s.
c-iii	Lortab 10/500 Tablets (UCB Pharma)	10 mg hydrocodone bitartrate	500 mg			1 q 4 to 6 h up to 6/day	(UCB/910). Pink. Capsule shape. In 100s and 500s.
c-iii	Hydrocodone Bitartrate and Acetaminophen Tablets (Various, eg, Barr, Mallinckrodt, Qualitest, Watson)						
c-iii	Hydrocodone Bitartrate and Acetaminophen Tablets (Major)	10 mg hydrocodone bitartrate	650 mg		In 500s.	1 q 4 to 6 h up to 6/day	
c-iii	Lorcet 10/650 Tablets (UAD)	10 mg hydrocodone bitartrate	650 mg			1 q 4 to 6 h	(UAD 6350). Light blue, scored. Capsule shape. In 20s, 100s and UD 100s.
c-iii	Hydrocodone Bitartrate and Acetaminophen Tablets (Various, eg, Inwood, Mallinckrodt)	10 mg hydrocodone bitartrate	660 mg			1 q 4 to 6 h up to 6/day	In 100s and 500s.
c-iii	Anexsia 10/660 Tablets (Mallinckrodt)					1 q 4 to 6 h	(KPI 3). White, scored. Capsule shape. In 100s and 1000s.
c-iii	Vicodin HP Tablets (Abbott)						(Vicodin HP). White, scored. Oval. In 100s.
c-iii	Maxidone (Watson)	10 mg hydrocodone bitartrate	750 mg		Lactose.	1 q 4 to 6 hr, up to 5/day.	(Maxidone 634). Yellow, capsule shape, scored. In 100s and 500s.
c-iii	Alor 5/500 Tablets (Atley)	5 mg hydrocodone bitartrate		500 mg		1 to 2 q 4 to 6 h up to 8/day	(AP Alor). In 100s.
c-iii	Lortab ASA Tablets (Whitby)					1 or 2 q 4 to 6 h	Pink, scored. In 100s.
c-iii	Panasal 5/500 Tablets (E.C. Robins)					1 or 2 q 4 to 6 h up to 8/day	(ECR 0131). Pink, mottled, scored. In 100s.
c-iii	Panlor DC (Pan American Labs)	16 mg dihydrocodeine bitartrate	356.4 mg		30 mg caffeine	2 q 4 h	(PAL/0016). Red. In 100s.
c-iii	Synalgos-DC Capsules (Wyeth-Ayerst)	16 mg dihydrocodeine bitartrate		356.4 mg	30 mg caffeine	2 q 4 h	(Wyeth 4191). Blue/gray. In 100s and 500s.
c-iii	Panlor SS Tablets (Pan American Labs)	32 mg dihydrocodeine bitartrate	712.8 mg		60 mg caffeine		(PAL 032). Lavender, oval, scored. In 100s.
c-ii	Acetaminophen with Oxycodone Tablets (Various, eg, Goldline, Major)	5 mg oxycodone HCl	325 mg			1 q 6 h	In 100s, 500s 1000s and UD 25s.
c-ii	Endocet Tablets (Endo Labs.)	5 mg oxycodone HCl	325 mg			1 q 6 h	(Endo 602). White. In 100s and 500s.
c-ii	Percocet Tablets (Du Pont)	5 mg oxycodone HCl	325 mg			1 q 6 h	(Percocet 5). In 100s, 500s and UD 100s.
c-ii	Roxicet Tablets (Roxane)						(54 543). White, scored. In 100s, 500s and UD 100s.
c-ii	Roxicet Oral Solution (Roxane)				0.4% alcohol, EDTA, saccharin, sucrose	5 mL q 6 h	In 500 mL and UD 5 mL.

NARCOTIC ANALGESIC COMBINATIONS

	Product and Distributor	Narcotic	Acetaminophen	Aspirin	Other Content	Average Adult Dose	How Supplied
c-ii	**Oxycodone with Acetaminophen Capsules** (Various, eg, Goldline, Major, Schein)	5 mg oxycodone HCl	500 mg			1 q 6 h	In 100s, 500s, 1000s and UD 25s.
c-ii	Roxicet 5/500 Caplets (Roxane)						(54 730). White, scored. In 100s and UD 100s.
	Roxilox Capsules (Roxane)						(HD532). In 100s.
	Tylox Capsules (McNeil)				Sodium metabisulfite		(Tylox McNeil). Red. In 100s and UD 100s.
c-ii	Endocet Tablets (Endo)	7.5 mg oxycodone HCl	325 mg			1 q 6 h prn, not to exceed 8 tablets daily	(E700 7.5/325). Peach, capsule shape. In 100s and 500s.
c-ii	Percocet (Endo)	7.5 mg oxycodone HCl	500 mg			1 q 6 h	(PERCOCET 7.5). Peach, capsule shape. In 100s and 500s.
c-ii	Endocet Tablets (Endo)	10 mg oxycodone	325 mg			1 q 6 h prn, not to exceed 6 tablets daily	(E712 10/325). Yellow, oval. In 100s and 500s.
c-ii	Percocet (Endo)	10 mg oxycodone HCl	325 mg			1 q 6 h	In 100s, 500s, and UD 100s.
c-ii	Percocet (Endo)	10 mg oxycodone HCl	650 mg			1 q 6 h	(PERCOCET 10). Yellow, oval. In 100s and 500s.
c-ii	Percocet (Endo)	2.5 mg oxycodone HCl	325 mg				(PERCOCET 2.5). Pink, oval. In 500s and UD 100s.
c-ii	Percodan-Demi Tablets (Du Pont)	2.25 mg oxycodone HCl, 0.19 mg oxycodone terephthalate		325 mg		1 or 2 q 6 h	White, scored. In 100s.
c-ii	Oxycodone with Aspirin Tablets (Various, eg, Goldline)	4.5 mg oxycodone HCl, 0.38 mg oxycodone terephthalate		325 mg		1 q 6 h	In 100s, 500s, 1000s and UD 25s.
c-ii	Percodan Tablets (DuPont)						Yellow, scored. In 500s, 1000s, and UD 250s.
c-ii	Roxiprin Tablets (Roxane)						(54 902). White, scored. In 100s, 1000s and UD 100s.
c-iv	Propoxyphene Napsylate and Acetaminophen Tablets (Various, eg, Moore)	50 mg propoxyphene napsylate	325 mg			2 q 4 h	In 100s, 500s, 550s, 1000s and UD 100s.
c-iv	Darvocet-N 50 Tablets (aaiPharma)	50 mg propoxyphene napsylate	325 mg			2 q 4 h	(Lilly Darvocet-N 50). Orange. In RxPak 100s, 500s and UD 100s.
c-iv	Darvocet A500 (aaiPharma)	100 mg propoxyphene napsylate	500 mg				Film-coated. In 100s.
c-iv	Propoxyphene Napsylate and Acetaminophen Tablets (Various, eg, Zenith)	100 mg propoxyphene napsylate	650 mg			1 q 4 h	In 30s, 50s, 100s, 500s, 1000s and UD 100s.
c-iv	Darvocet-N 100 Tablets (aaiPharma)						(Darvocet-N 100). Orange. In RxPak 100s, 500s, UD 100s, UD 500s and RN 500s.
c-iv	Propoxyphene HCl w/Acetaminophen Tablets (Various, eg, Moore, Mylan)	65 mg propoxyphene HCl	650 mg			1 q 4 h	In 500s.
c-iv	Darvon Compound-32 Pulvules (Lilly)	32 mg propoxyphene HCl		389 mg	32.4 mg caffeine	1 q 4 h	(DARVON COMP). Pink. In 100s.
c-iv	Darvon Compound-65 Pulvules (Lilly)	65 mg propoxyphene HCl		389 mg	32.4 mg caffeine	1 q 4 h	Red/gray. Lilly 3111 DARVON COMP. 65. In 500s and RxPak 100s.
c-ii	B & O Supprettes No. 15A Suppositories (PolyMedica)	30 mg powdered opium			16.2 mg powdered belladonna extract. Polyethylene glycol/Polysorbate 60 base	1 or 2/day	Scored. In 12s.

NARCOTIC ANALGESIC COMBINATIONS

	Product and Distributor	Narcotic	Acetaminophen	Aspirin	Other Content	Average Adult Dose	How Supplied
c-ii	**Opium and Belladonna Suppositories** (Wyeth-Ayerst)	60 mg powdered opium			15 mg belladonna extract. Cocoa butter base	1 or 2/day	In 20s.
c-ii	**B & O Supprettes No. 16A Suppositories** (PolyMedica)				16.2 mg powdered belladonna extract. Polyethylene glycol/Polysorbate 60 base	1 or 2/day	Scored. In 12s.

[1] May contain alcohol.

Ingredients

Components of these combinations include the following (see individual monographs):

➤ *NARCOTIC ANALGESICS:* Codeine, hydrocodone bitartrate, dihydrocodeine bitartrate, opium, oxycodone terephthalate, meperidine HCl, oxycodone HCl, propoxyphene HCl, propoxyphene napsylate.

➤ *NONNARCOTIC ANALGESICS:* Acetaminophen and salicylates.

➤ *CAFFEINE:* Caffeine, a traditional component of many analgesic formulations, may be beneficial in certain vascular headaches.

➤ *BARBITURATES:* Barbiturates are used for their sedative effects.

➤ *PROMETHAZINE HCl:* Promethazine HCl (a phenothiazine derivative with antihistaminic properties), used for its sedative effect.

➤ *BELLADONNA ALKALOIDS:* Belladonna alkaloids are used as antispasmodics.

Precautions

➤ *Sulfite sensitivity:* Some of these products contain sulfites that may cause allergic-type reactions (eg, hives, itching, wheezing, anaphylaxis) in certain susceptible people. Although the overall prevalence of sulfite sensitivity in the general population is probably low, it is seen more frequently in asthmatics or in atopic nonasthmatic people. Specific products containing sulfites are identified in the product listing.

Mixed narcotic agonist-antagonists (pentazocine, butorphanol, and nalbuphine) are primarily κ-opioid receptor agonists and μ-opioid receptor antagonists. They produce analgesia in nontolerant patients but may precipitate withdrawal in those dependent on morphine-like drugs.

A partial agonist analgesic (buprenorphine) is an antagonist at the κ-opioid receptor but is a partial agonist at the μ-opioid receptor. It may also precipitate withdrawal effects in those dependent on morphine-like drugs, but to a lesser degree than mixed agonist-antagonists. Partial agonists also produce less psychotomimetic effects that are seen with mixed agonist-antagonists.

Narcotic Agonist-Antagonist Pharmacokinetics

Agonist/Antagonist		Onset (min)	Peak (min)	Duration (h)	Equivalent dose[1] (mg)	Relative antagonist activity
Buprenorphine	IM	15	60	≥ 6	0.3	Equipotent with naloxone
	IV[2]	-	-			
Butorphanol	IM	≤ 15	30-60	3-4	2	More potent than pentazocine, but less than naloxone
	IV	Few min	30-60	3-4		
	Nasal	≤ 15	60-120	4-5		
Nalbuphine	SC/IM	< 15	60	3-6	10	10 times that of pentazocine
	IV	2-3	nd			
Pentazocine	SC/IM	15-20	15-60	4-6	30	Weak
	IV	2-3	nd	nd		
	Oral	15-30	nd	≥ 3		

* nd – no data

[1] Parenteral dose equivalent to 10 mg morphine.
[2] When given IV, the time to onset and peak effect are shortened

BUPRENORPHINE HCl

c-iii	**Subutex** (Reckitt Benckiser)	**Tablets, sublingual:** 2 mg (as base)	Lactose. White, oval. In 30s.
		8 mg (as base)	Lactose. White, oval. In 30s.
c-iii	**Buprenorphine HCl** (Abbott)	**Injection:** 0.324 mg (equiv. to 0.3 mg buprenorphine)/mL	In 1 mL *Carpuject*.[1]
c-iii	**Buprenex** (Reckitt Benckiser)		In 1 mL amps.[1]

[1] With 50 mg anhydrous dextrose.

Refer to the general discussion in the Narcotic Agonist-Antagonist Analgesic introduction.

Indications

➤*Tablets:* Treatment of opioid dependence.

➤*Injection:* Relief of moderate to severe pain.

➤*Note:* Under the Drug Addiction Treatment Act of 2000 (DATA) codified at 21 U.S.C. 823 (g), prescription use of buprenorphine sublingual tablets in the treatment of opioid dependence is limited to physicians who meet certain qualifying requirements and have notified the Secretary of Health and Human Services (HHS) of their intent to prescribe this product for the treatment of opioid dependence.

Administration and Dosage

➤*Tablets:* Buprenorphine tablets are administered sublingually as a single daily dose in the range of 12 to 16 mg/day. When taken sublingually, buprenorphine and buprenorphine/naloxone have similar clinical effects and are interchangeable. Buprenorphine tablets contain no naloxone and are preferred for use during induction. Following induction, buprenorphine/naloxone, because of the presence of naloxone, is preferred when clinical use includes unsupervised administration. Limit the use of buprenorphine for unsupervised administration to those patients who cannot tolerate buprenorphine/naloxone (eg, those patients who have been shown to be hypersensitive to naloxone).

Administration – Place tablets under the tongue until they are dissolved. For doses requiring the use of more than 2 tablets, patients are advised to place all the tablets at once or, alternatively (if they cannot fit in more than 2 tablets comfortably), place 2 tablets at a time under the tongue. Either way, the patient should continue to hold the tablets under the tongue until they dissolve; swallowing the tablets reduces the bioavailability of the drug. To ensure consistency in bioavailability, patients should follow the same manner of dosing with continued use of the product.

Induction – Prior to induction, consider the type of opioid dependence (ie, long- or short-acting opioid), the time since last opioid use, and the degree or level of opioid dependence. To avoid precipitating withdrawal, undertake induction with buprenorphine when objective and clear signs of withdrawal are evident.

In a 1-month study of buprenorphine/naloxone tablets, induction was conducted with buprenorphine tablets. Patients received 8 mg buprenorphine on day 1 and 16 mg on day 2. From day 3 onward, patients received buprenorphine/naloxone tablets at the same buprenorphine dose as day 2. Induction in the studies of buprenorphine solution was accomplished over 3 to 4 days, depending on the target dose. In some studies, gradual induction over several days led to a high rate of drop-out of buprenorphine patients during the induction period. Therefore, it is recommended that an adequate maintenance dose, titrated to clinical effectiveness, should be achieved as rapidly as possible to prevent undue opioid withdrawal symptoms.

Patients taking heroin or other short-acting opioids: At treatment initiation, administer the dose of buprenorphine at least 4 hours after the patient last used opioids or, preferably, when early signs of withdrawal appear.

Patients taking methadone or other long-acting opioids: There is little controlled experience with the transfer of methadone-maintained patients to buprenorphine. Available evidence suggests that withdrawal symptoms are possible during induction of buprenorphine treatment. Withdrawal appears more likely in patients maintained on higher doses of methadone (more than 30 mg) and when the first buprenorphine dose is administered shortly after the last methadone dose.

Maintenance – Buprenorphine/Naloxone is the preferred medication for maintenance treatment because of the presence of naloxone in the formulation.

Adjusting the dose until the maintenance dose is achieved: Clinical studies have shown that 16 mg of buprenorphine or buprenorphine/naloxone is a clinically effective dose compared with placebo and indicate that doses as low as 12 mg may be effective in some patients.

Reducing dosage and stopping treatment – Make the decision to discontinue therapy with buprenorphine or buprenorphine/naloxone after a period of maintenance or brief stabilization as part of a comprehensive treatment plan. Gradual and abrupt discontinuation have been used but no controlled trials have been undertaken to determine the best method of dose taper at the end of treatment.

➤*Injection:*

Patients 13 years of age and older – 0.3 mg (1 mL) deep IM or slow IV (over at least 2 minutes), at up to 6-hour intervals, as needed. Repeat once (up to 0.3 mg) if required, 30 to 60 minutes after initial dosage, giving consideration to previous dose pharmacokinetics; use thereafter only as needed. In high-risk patients (eg, elderly, debilitated, presence of respiratory disease) and/or in patients where other CNS depressants are present, such as in the immediate postoperative period, reduce dose by approximately one half. Exercise extra caution with the IV route of administration, particularly with the initial dose.

Occasionally, it may be necessary to give single doses up to 0.6 mg to adults depending on the severity of the pain and the response of the patient. This dose should only be given IM and only to adult patients who are not in a high-risk category. Data are insufficient to recommend single doses greater than 0.6 mg for long-term use.

Children – Buprenorphine has been used in children 2 to 12 years of age at doses between 2 and 6 mcg/kg of body weight given every 4 to 6 hours. There is insufficient experience to recommend a dose in infants below 2 years of age, single doses greater than 6 mcg/kg of body weight, or the use of a repeat or second dose at 30 to 60 minutes (such as is used in adults). Because there is some evidence that not all children clear buprenorphine faster than adults, do not undertake fixed interval or round-the-clock dosing until the proper inter-dose interval has been established by clinical observation of the child. Physicians should recognize that, as with adults, some pediatric patients may not need to be remedicated for 6 to 8 hours.

➤*Storage/Stability:*

Injection – Store at controlled room temperature (15° to 30°C; 59° to 86°F). Avoid excessive heat (over 40°C or 104°F), and protect from prolonged exposure to light. Do not freeze.

Tablets – Store at 25°C (77°F). Excursions permitted to 15° to 30°C (59° to 86°F).

BUPRENORPHINE HCl

Actions

➤*Pharmacology:* Buprenorphine is a partial agonist at the μ-opioid receptor and an antagonist at the κ-opioid receptor. Buprenorphine is an opioid analgesic derived from thebaine; a 0.3 mg parenteral dose is approximately equivalent to 10 mg morphine in analgesic and respiratory depressant effects in adults. Buprenorphine exerts its analgesic effect via high affinity binding to μ subclass opiate receptors in the CNS. Although buprenorphine may be classified as a partial agonist, under the conditions of recommended use it behaves very much like classical μ agonists such as morphine. Buprenorphine has a very slow rate of dissociation from its receptor. This could account for its longer duration of action than morphine, the unpredictability of its reversal by opioid antagonists, and its low level of manifest physical dependence.

Its narcotic antagonist activity is approximately equipotent to naloxone.

Physiological effects – Buprenorphine in IV (2, 4, 8, 12, and 16 mg) and sublingual (12 mg) doses have been administered to nondependent subjects to examine cardiovascular, respiratory, and subjective effects at doses comparable with those used for treatment of opioid dependence. Compared with placebo, there were no statistically significant differences among any of the treatment conditions for blood pressure, heart rate, respiratory rate, O_2 saturation, or skin temperature across time. Systolic blood pressure was higher in the 8 mg group than placebo (3 hour AUC values). Minimum and maximum effects were similar across all treatments. Subjects remained responsive to low voice and responded to computer prompts. Some subjects showed irritability, but no other changes were observed.

Cardiovascular – Buprenorphine may cause a decrease or, rarely, an increase in pulse rate and blood pressure in some patients.

Respiratory effects – A therapeutic dose of 0.3 mg buprenorphine IV can decrease respiratory rate similarly to an equianalgesic dose of morphine (10 mg).

The respiratory effects of sublingual buprenorphine were compared with the effects of methadone in a double-blind, parallel group, dose-ranging comparison of single doses of buprenorphine sublingual solution (1, 2, 4, 8, 16, or 32 mg) and oral methadone (15, 30, 45, or 60 mg) in nondependent, opioid-experienced volunteers. In this study, hypoventilation not requiring medical intervention was reported more frequently after buprenorphine doses of 4 mg and higher than after methadone. Both drugs decreased O_2 saturation to the same degree.

➤*Pharmacokinetics:*

Absorption/Distribution – Plasma levels of buprenorphine increased with the sublingual dose of buprenorphine. Both C_{max} and AUC increased in a linear fashion with the increase in dose (in the range of 4 to 16 mg), although the increase was not directly dose-proportional. The C_{max} of buprenorphine tablets 16 mg was about 5.47 ng/mL and the AUC_{0-48} is about 32.63 h•ng/mL. Plasma protein binding is about 96%, primarily to alpha and beta globulin.

Metabolism – Buprenorphine undergoes N-dealkylation to norbuprenorphine and glucuronidation. The N-dealkylation pathway is mediated by cytochrome P-450 3A4 isozyme. Norbuprenorphine, an active metabolite, can further undergo glucuronidation.

Excretion – A mass balance study of buprenorphine showed complete recovery of radiolabel in urine (30%) and feces (69%) collected up to 11 days after dosing. Almost all of the dose was accounted for in terms of buprenorphine, norbuprenorphine, and 2 unidentified buprenorphine metabolites. In urine, most of buprenorphine and norbuprenorphine was conjugated (buprenorphine, 1% free and 9.4% conjugated; norbuprenorphine, 2.7% free and 11% conjugated). In feces, almost all of the buprenorphine and norbuprenorphine were free (buprenorphine, 33% free and 5% conjugated; norbuprenorphine, 21% free and 2% conjugated). Buprenorphine has a mean elimination half-life from plasma of 37 hours.

Pharmacodynamics – Onset of analgesic effect occurs 15 minutes after IM injection, peaks in 1 hour, and persists for 6 hours or longer. When given IV, the time to onset and peak is shortened.

Special populations –
Hepatic function impairment: The effect of hepatic impairment on the pharmacokinetics of buprenorphine is unknown. Because it is extensively metabolized, the plasma levels will be expected to be higher in patients with moderate and severe hepatic impairment. Therefore, in patients with hepatic impairment, adjust dosage and observe patients for symptoms of precipitated opioid withdrawal.

Contraindications

Hypersensitivity to buprenorphine.

Warnings

➤*Narcotic-dependent patients:* Because of the narcotic antagonist activity of buprenorphine, use in physically dependent individuals may result in withdrawal effects. The drug may not be substituted in acutely dependent narcotic addicts because of its antagonist component.

➤*Respiratory depression:* Significant respiratory depression has been associated with buprenorphine, particularly by the IV route. A number of deaths have occurred when addicts have intravenously misused buprenorphine, usually with benzodiazepines concomitantly. Deaths also have been reported in association with concomitant administration of buprenorphine with other depressants, such as alcohol or other opioids. Warn patients of the potential danger of the self-administration of benzodiazepines or other depressants while under treatment with buprenorphine.

As with other potent opioids, clinically significant respiratory depression may occur within the recommended dose range in patients receiving therapeutic doses of buprenorphine. Use buprenorphine with caution in patients with compromised respiratory function (eg, COPD, cor pulmonale, decreased respiratory reserve, hypoxia, hypercapnia, preexisting respiratory depression). Particular caution is advised if buprenorphine is administered to patients taking or recently receiving drugs with CNS/respiratory depressant effects. In patients with the physical and/or pharmacological risk factors above, reduce the dose by approximately one half.

Naloxone may not be effective in reversing the respiratory depression produced by buprenorphine. Therefore, as with other potent opioids, the primary management of overdose should be the re-establishment of adequate ventilation with mechanical assistance of respiration, if required.

➤*Head injury/increased intracranial pressure:* Buprenorphine may elevate cerebrospinal fluid (CSF) pressure; use with caution in head injury, intracranial lesions, and other states where CSF pressure may be increased. Buprenorphine can produce miosis and changes in consciousness levels that may interfere with patient evaluation.

➤*Hepatitis:* Cases of cytolytic hepatitis and hepatitis with jaundice have been observed in the addict population receiving buprenorphine both in clinical trials and in postmarketing adverse event reports. The spectrum of abnormalities ranges from transient asymptomatic elevations in hepatic transaminases to case reports of hepatic failure, hepatic necrosis, hepatorenal syndrome, and hepatic encephalopathy. In many cases, the presence of pre-existing liver enzyme abnormalities, infection with hepatitis B or hepatitis C virus, concomitant usage of other potentially hepatotoxic drugs, and ongoing injecting drug use may have played a causative or contributory role. In other cases, insufficient data were available to determine the etiology of the abnormality. The possibility exists that buprenorphine had a causative or contributory role in the development of the hepatic abnormality in some cases. Measurements of liver function tests prior to initiation of treatment is recommended to establish a baseline. Periodic monitoring of liver function tests during treatment is also recommended. A biological and etiological evaluation is recommended when a hepatic event is suspected. Depending on the case, carefully discontinue the drug to prevent withdrawal symptoms and a return to illicit drug use, and initiate strict monitoring of the patient.

➤*Allergic reactions:* Cases of acute and chronic hypersensitivity to buprenorphine have been reported in clinical trials and in the postmarketing experience. The most common signs and symptoms include rash, hives, and pruritus. Cases of bronchospasm, angioneurotic edema, and anaphylactic shock have been reported. A history of hypersensitivity to buprenorphine is a contraindication to buprenorphine or buprenorphine/naloxone use.

➤*Hepatic function impairment:* Buprenorphine is metabolized by the liver; the activity may be increased and/or extended in those individuals with impaired hepatic function or those receiving other agents known to decrease hepatic clearance.

The effect of hepatic impairment on the pharmacokinetics of buprenorphine is unknown. Because it is extensively metabolized, the plasma levels will be expected to be higher in patients with moderate and severe hepatic impairment. Therefore, adjust dosage and watch patients for symptoms of precipitated opioid withdrawal.

➤*Carcinogenesis:* Buprenorphine was administered in the diet to rats at doses of 0.6, 5.5, and 56 mg/kg/day (estimated exposure was approximately 0.4, 3, and 35 times the recommended human daily sublingual dose of 16 mg on a mg/m² basis) for 27 months. Statistically significant dose-related increases in testicular interstitial (Leydig's) cell tumors occurred, according to the trend test adjusted for survival. Pairwise comparison of the high dose against control failed to show statistical significance.

➤*Mutagenesis:* Buprenorphine was studied in a series of tests utilizing gene, chromosome, and DNA interactions in both prokaryotic and eukaryotic systems. Results were equivocal in the Ames test, negative in studies in 2 laboratories, but positive for frame shift mutation at a high dose (5 mg/plate) in a third study. Results were positive in the Green-Tweets (*Escherichia coli*) survival test, positive in a DNA synthesis inhibition (DSI) test with testicular tissue from mice, for both in vivo and in vitro incorporation of [3H]thymidine, and positive in an unscheduled DNA synthesis (UDS) test using testicular cells from mice.

➤*Fertility impairment:* Dietary administration of buprenorphine/naloxone in the rat at dose levels of 500 ppm or greater (equivalent to approximately 47 mg/kg/day or greater; estimated exposure was approximately 28 times the recommended human daily sublingual dose of 16 mg on a mg/m² basis) produced a reduction in fertility demonstrated by reduced female conception rates.

➤*Pregnancy: Category C.* Following oral administration to the rat, dose-related postimplantation losses, evidenced by increases in the

BUPRENORPHINE HCl

numbers of early resorptions with consequent reductions in the numbers of fetuses, were observed at doses of 10 mg/kg/day or greater (estimated exposure was approximately 6 times the recommended human daily sublingual dose of 16 mg on a mg/m^2 basis). In the rabbit, increased postimplantation losses occurred at an oral dose of 40 mg/kg/day. Following IM administration in the rat and rabbit, postimplantation losses, as evidenced by decreases in live fetuses and increases in resorptions, occurred at 30 mg/kg/day.

Significant increases in skeletal abnormalities (eg, extra thoracic vertebra or thoraco-lumbar ribs) were noted in rats after SC administration of 1 mg/kg/day and up (estimated exposure was approximately 0.6 times the recommended human daily sublingual dose of 16 mg on a mg/m^2 basis or approximately 9.5 times the recommended human daily dose of 1.2 mg on a mg/m^2 basis) but were not observed at oral doses up to 160 mg/kg/day.

In rabbits, buprenorphine produced statistically significant preimplantation losses at oral doses of 1 mg/kg/day or greater and postimplantation losses that were statistically significant at IV doses of 0.2 mg/kg/day or greater (estimated exposure was approximately 0.3 times the recommended human daily sublingual dose of 16 mg on a mg/m^2 basis).

Dystocia was noted in pregnant rats treated with IM buprenorphine 5 mg/kg/day (approximately 3 times the recommended human daily sublingual dose of 16 mg on a mg/m^2 basis). Both fertility and peri- and postnatal development studies with buprenorphine in rats indicated increases in neonatal mortality after oral doses of 0.8 mg/kg/day and up (approximately 0.5 times the recommended human daily sublingual dose of 16 mg on a mg/m^2 basis), after IM doses of 0.5 mg/kg/day and up (approximately 0.3 times the recommended human daily sublingual dose of 16 mg on a mg/m^2 basis), and after SC doses of 0.1 mg/kg/day and up (approximately 0.06 times the recommended human daily sublingual dose of 16 mg on a mg/m^2 basis). Delays in the occurrence of righting reflex and startle response were noted in rat pups at an oral dose of 80 mg/kg/day (approximately 50 times the recommended human daily sublingual dose of 16 mg on a mg/m^2 basis).

Neonatal withdrawal has been reported in the infants of women treated with buprenorphine during pregnancy. From postmarketing reports, the time to onset of neonatal withdrawal symptoms ranged from day 1 to day 8 of life with most occurring on day 1. Adverse events associated with neonatal withdrawal syndrome include hypertonia, neonatal tremor, neonatal agitation, and myoclonus. There have been rare reports of convulsions and in one case, apnea and bradycardia also were reported

There are no adequate and well-controlled studies of buprenorphine or buprenorphine/naloxone in pregnant women. Use only if the potential benefits outweigh the potential hazards to the fetus.

➤*Lactation:* An apparent lack of milk production during general reproduction studies with buprenorphine in rats caused decreased viability and lactation indices. Use of high doses of sublingual buprenorphine in pregnant women showed that buprenorphine passes into the mother's milk. Therefore, breastfeeding is not advised in mothers treated with buprenorphine or buprenorphine/naloxone.

➤*Children:* The safety and effectiveness of buprenorphine injection have been established for children between 2 and 12 years of age.

Buprenorphine tablets and buprenorphine/naloxone are not recommended for use in pediatric patients. Safety and effectiveness in patients below 16 years of age have not been established.

Precautions

➤*Use with caution in the following:* Elderly or debilitated; severe impairment of hepatic, pulmonary, or renal function; myxedema or hypothyroidism; adrenal cortical insufficiency (eg, Addison's disease); CNS depression or coma; toxic psychoses; prostatic hypertrophy or urethral stricture; acute alcoholism; delirium tremens or kyphoscoliosis.

➤*Biliary tract dysfunction:* Buprenorphine increases intracholedochal pressure to a similar degree as other opiates; administer with caution.

➤*Acute abdominal conditions:* As with other μ-opioid receptor agonists, the administration of buprenorphine or buprenorphine/naloxone may obscure the diagnosis or clinical course of patients with acute abdominal conditions.

➤*Drug abuse and dependence:* Buprenorphine is a partial agonist at the μ-opioid receptor and chronic administration produces dependence of the opioid type, characterized by moderate withdrawal upon abrupt discontinuation or rapid taper. The withdrawal syndrome is milder than seen with full agonists, and may be delayed in onset.

Neonatal withdrawal has been reported in the infants of women treated with buprenorphine during pregnancy.

➤*Hazardous tasks:* May cause dizziness or drowsiness; observe caution while driving or performing other tasks requiring alertness.

Buprenorphine may impair the mental or physical abilities required for the performance of potentially dangerous tasks, such as driving a car or operating machinery, especially during drug induction and dose adjustment. Caution patients about operating hazardous machinery, including automobiles, until they are reasonably certain that buprenorphine therapy does not adversely affect their ability to engage in such activi-

ties. Like other opioids, buprenorphine may produce orthostatic hypotension in ambulatory patients.

Drug Interactions

Buprenorphine HCl Drug Interactions			
Precipitant drug	Object drug*		Description
Barbiturate anesthetics	Buprenorphine	↑	Barbiturate anesthetics may increase the respiratory and CNS depression of buprenorphine because of additive pharmacologic activity.
Benzodiazepines	Buprenorphine	↑	Coma and death have been associated with the concomitant IV misuse of buprenorphine and benzodiazepines by addicts.
CNS depressants (eg, narcotic analgesics, general anesthetics, benzodiazepines, phenothiazines, other tranquilizers, sedative/hypnotics, other CNS depressants including alcohol)	Buprenorphine	↑	Patients receiving both agents may exhibit increased CNS depression. When combined therapy is contemplated, consider reduction of the dose of one or both agents.
CYP3A4 inducers (eg, phenobarbital, carbamazepine, phenytoin, rifampin)	Buprenorphine	↓	Although not investigated, it is recommended to closely monitor patients when buprenorphine is coadministered with a CYP3A4 inducer. May cause possible increased clearance.
CYP3A4 inhibitors (ie, azole antifungals, macrolide antibiotics, protease inhibitors)	Buprenorphine	↑	Coadministration may increase buprenorphine plasma concentrations. Buprenorphine dosage adjustment may be required.
MAO inhibitors	Buprenorphine	↔	Exercise caution. Specific information is not available.

*↑ = Object drug increased. ↓ = Object drug decreased. ↔ = Undetermined clinical effect.

Adverse Reactions

➤*Buprenorphine injection:*

Cardiovascular – Hypotension (1% to 5%); hypertension, tachycardia, bradycardia, Wenckebach block (less than 1%).

CNS – Sedation (67%); dizziness/vertigo (5% to 10%); headache (1% to 5%); confusion, dreaming, psychosis, euphoria, weakness/fatigue, nervousness, slurred speech, paresthesia, depression (less than 1%); malaise, hallucinations, depersonalization, coma, tremor (infrequent); dysphoria/agitation, convulsions/lack of muscle coordination (rare).

Dermatologic – Sweating (1% to 5%); pruritus, injection site reaction (less than 1%); rash, pallor (infrequent); urticaria (rare).

GI – Nausea (5% to 10%); nausea/vomiting (1% to 5%); constipation, dry mouth (less than 1%); dyspepsia, flatulence (infrequent); loss of appetite, diarrhea (rare).

Ophthalmic – Miosis (1% to 5%); blurred vision, diplopia, conjunctivitis, visual abnormalities (less than 1%); amblyopia (infrequent).

Respiratory – Hypoventilation (1% to 5%); dyspnea, cyanosis (less than 1%); apnea (infrequent).

Miscellaneous – Urinary retention, flushing/warmth, chills/cold, tinnitus (less than 1%).

➤*Buprenorphine tablets:*

Buprenorphine Adverse Events In a 4-Week Study (≥ 5%)		
Adverse event	Buprenorphine tablets 16 mg/day (N = 103)	Placebo (N = 107)
CNS		
Headache	29.1	22.4
Insomnia	21.4	15.9
GI		
Nausea	13.6	11.2
Abdominal pain	11.7	6.5
Vomiting	7.8	4.7
Constipation	7.8	2.8
Diarrhea	4.9	15
Miscellaneous		
Asthenia	4.9	6.5
Chills	7.8	7.5
Infection	11.7	6.5
Pain	18.4	18.7
Back pain	7.8	11.2

BUPRENORPHINE HCl

Buprenorphine Adverse Events In a 4-Week Study (≥ 5%)		
Adverse event	Buprenorphine tablets 16 mg/day (N = 103)	Placebo (N = 107)
Withdrawal syndrome	18.4	37.4
Vasodilation	3.9	6.5
Rhinitis	9.7	13.1
Sweating	12.6	10.3

Overdosage

➤*Symptoms:* Although the antagonist activity of buprenorphine may become manifest at doses somewhat higher than the recommended therapeutic range, doses in the recommended therapeutic range may produce clinically significant respiratory depression in certain circumstances (see Warnings). Manifestations of acute overdose include pinpoint pupils, sedation, hypotension, respiratory depression, and death.

➤*Treatment:* Carefully monitor cardiac and respiratory status. Establish a patent airway and institute assisted or controlled ventilation. Employ oxygen, IV fluids, vasopressors, and other supportive measures as indicated. Refer to General Management of Acute Overdosage. The primary management of overdose is mechanical assistance of respiration. Naloxone may not be effective in reversing respiratory depression produced by buprenorphine.

High doses of naloxone HCl, 10 to 35 mg/70 kg, may be of limited value in the management of buprenorphine overdose. Doxapram (a respiratory stimulant) also has been used.

Patient Information

Patients should inform their family members that, in the event of emergency, the treating physician or emergency room staff should be informed that the patient is physically dependent on narcotics and that the patient is being treated with buprenorphine or buprenorphine/naloxone tablets.

Caution patients that a serious overdose and death may occur if benzodiazepines, sedatives, tranquilizers, antidepressants, or alcohol are taken at the same time as buprenorphine.

Buprenorphine may impair the mental or physical abilities required for the performance of potentially dangerous tasks, such as driving a car or operating machinery, especially during drug induction and dose adjustment. Caution patients about operating hazardous machinery, including automobiles, until they are reasonably certain that buprenorphine therapy does not adversely affect their ability to engage in such activities. Like other opioids, buprenorphine may produce orthostatic hypotension in ambulatory patients.

Patients should consult their physician if other prescription medications currently are being used or are prescribed for future use.

Do not exceed prescribed dosage. Avoid alcohol and benzodiazepines.

BUPRENORPHINE HCl COMBINATIONS

c-iii	**Suboxone** (Reckitt Benckiser)	**Tablets, sublingual:** 2 mg buprenorphine base/ 0.5 mg naloxone	Lactose, acesulfame K. Orange, hexagonal. Lemon/Lime flavor. In 30s.
		8 mg buprenorphine base/2 mg naloxone	Lactose, acesulfame K. Orange, hexagonal. Lemon/Lime flavor. In 30s.

Refer to the general discussion in the Narcotic Agonist-Antagonist Analgesic introduction and the Buprenorphine and Naloxone monographs.

Indications

➤*Opioid dependence:* Treatment of opioid dependence.

Administration and Dosage

➤*Approved by the FDA:* October 8, 2002.

Buprenorphine/naloxone tablets are administered sublingually as a single daily dose in the range of 12 to 16 mg/day. When taken sublingually, buprenorphine and buprenorphine/naloxone have similar clinical effects and are interchangeable. Buprenorphine tablets contain no naloxone and are preferred for use during induction. Following induction, buprenorphine/naloxone, because of the presence of naloxone, is preferred when clinical use includes unsupervised administration. Limit the use of buprenorphine for unsupervised administration to those patients who cannot tolerate buprenorphine/naloxone (eg, those patients who have been shown to be hypersensitive to naloxone).

➤*Administration:* Place tablets under the tongue until they are dissolved. For doses requiring the use of more than 2 tablets, patients are advised to place all the tablets at once or, alternatively (if they cannot fit in more than 2 tablets comfortably), place 2 tablets at a time under the tongue. Either way, the patient should continue to hold the tablets under the tongue until they dissolve; swallowing the tablets reduces the bioavailability of the drug. To ensure consistency in bioavailability, patients should follow the same manner of dosing with continued use of the product.

➤*Induction:* Prior to induction, consider the type of opioid dependence (ie, long- or short-acting opioid), the time since last opioid use, and the degree or level of opioid dependence. To avoid precipitating withdrawal, undertake induction with buprenorphine when objective and clear signs of withdrawal are evident.

In a 1-month study of buprenorphine/naloxone tablets, induction was conducted with buprenorphine tablets. Patients received 8 mg buprenorphine on day 1 and 16 mg on day 2. From day 3 onward, patients received buprenorphine/naloxone tablets at the same buprenorphine dose as day 2. Induction in the studies of buprenorphine solution was accomplished over 3 to 4 days, depending on the target dose. In some studies, gradual induction over several days led to a high rate of dropout of buprenorphine patients during the induction period. Therefore, it is recommended that an adequate maintenance dose, titrated to clinical effectiveness, should be achieved as rapidly as possible to prevent undue opioid withdrawal symptoms.

Patients taking heroin or other short-acting opioids – At treatment initiation, administer the dose of buprenorphine at least 4 hours after the patient last used opioids or, preferably, when early signs of withdrawal appear.

Patients on methadone or other long-acting opioids – There is little controlled experience with the transfer of methadone-maintained patients to buprenorphine. Available evidence suggests that withdrawal symptoms are possible during induction of buprenorphine treatment. Withdrawal appears more likely in patients maintained on higher doses of methadone (more than 30 mg) and when the first buprenorphine dose is administered shortly after the last methadone dose.

➤*Maintenance:* Buprenorphine/Naloxone is the preferred medication for maintenance treatment because of the presence of naloxone in the formulation.

Adjusting the dose until the maintenance dose is achieved – The recommended target dose of buprenorphine/naloxone is 16 mg/day. Clinical studies have shown that 16 mg buprenorphine or buprenorphine/naloxone is a clinically effective dose compared with placebo and indicate that doses as low as 12 mg may be effective in some patients. Progressively adjust the dosage of buprenorphine/naloxone in increments/decrements of 2 or 4 mg to a level that holds the patient in treatment and suppresses opioid withdrawal effects. This is likely to be in the range of 4 to 24 mg/day, depending on the individual.

➤*Reducing dosage and stopping treatment:* Make the decision to discontinue therapy with buprenorphine/naloxone after a period of maintenance or brief stabilization as part of a comprehensive treatment plan. Gradual and abrupt discontinuation have been used, but no controlled trials have been undertaken to determine the best method of dose taper at the end of treatment.

➤*Storage/Stability:* Store at 25°C (77°F). Excursions permitted to 15° to 30°C (59° to 86°F).

Contraindications

Do not administer to patients who have been shown to be hypersensitive to buprenorphine or naloxone.

Warnings

➤*Opioid withdrawal effects:* Because it contains naloxone, buprenorphine/naloxone is highly likely to produce marked and intense withdrawal symptoms if misused parenterally by individuals dependent on opioid agonists (eg, heroin, morphine, methadone). Sublingually, buprenorphine/naloxone may cause opioid withdrawal symptoms in these people if administered before the agonist effects of the opioid have subsided.

BUTORPHANOL TARTRATE

c-iv	**Butorphanol Tartrate** (Various, eg, Abbott, Apotex, Baxter, Bedford, Bertek, Novaplus)	**Injection:** 1 mg/mL[1]	In 2 mL vials.
c-iv	**Stadol** (Bristol-Myers Squibb)		In 1 mL vials.
c-iv	**Butorphanol Tartrate** (Various, eg, Abbott, Apotex, Baxter, Bedford, Bertek, Novaplus)	**Injection:** 2 mg/mL[1]	In 1 and 2 mL vials.
c-iv	**Stadol** (Bristol-Myers Squibb)		In 1, 2 and 10[2] mL vials.
c-iv	**Butorphanol Tartrate** (Various, eg, Mylan, Roxane)	**Nasal spray:** 10 mg/mL	In 2.5 mL.
c-iv	**Stadol NS** (Bristol-Myers Squibb)		In 2.5 mL metered-dose spray pump. Delivers an average of 14 to 15 doses.[3]

[1] 1 mg of tartrate salt is equal to 0.68 mg base.
[2] With 0.1 mg/mL benzethonium chloride.

[3] If not used for ≥ 48 hours, the unit must be reprimed. With repriming before each dose, the unit will deliver ≈ 8 to 10 doses.

Refer to the general discussion in the Narcotic Agonist-Antagonist Analgesic introduction.

Indications

➤*Parenteral/Nasal:* Management of pain (including postoperative analgesia).

In clinical trials, nasal butorphanol was effective in the treatment of migraine headache pain.

➤*Parenteral:* For preoperative or preanesthetic medication; to supplement balanced anesthesia; for relief of pain during labor.

Administration and Dosage

➤*Pain:*

IV – 1 mg (dosage range, 0.5 to 2 mg) repeated every 3 to 4 hours as necessary.

IM – 2 mg (dosage range, 1 to 4 mg) every 3 to 4 hours as necessary in patients who will be able to remain recumbent. Do not exceed single doses of 4 mg.

Nasal – 1 mg (1 spray in 1 nostril). If adequate pain relief is not achieved within 60 to 90 minutes, an additional 1 mg dose may be given. The initial 2 dose sequence may be repeated in 3 to 4 hours as needed. Depending on the pain severity, an initial 2 mg dose (1 spray in each nostril) may be used in patients who will be able to remain recumbent. Do not give additional 2 mg doses for 3 to 4 hours.

➤*Preoperative/Preanesthetic use:* Individualize dosage. Usual dose is 2 mg IM 60 to 90 minutes before surgery.

➤*Balanced anesthesia:* 2 mg IV shortly before induction or 0.5 to 1 mg IV in increments during anesthesia. The increment may be up to 0.06 mg/kg depending on previous drugs administered. The total dose will vary, but patients seldom require < 4 mg or > 12.5 mg.

➤*Labor:* 1 to 2 mg IV or IM in patients at full term in early labor; repeat after 4 hours.

➤*Children:* Not recommended in children < 18 years of age.

➤*Elderly:*

Parenteral – Use one half the usual dose at twice the usual interval. Base subsequent doses and intervals on patient response.

Nasal – 1 mg initially. Allow 90 to 120 minutes to elapse before deciding whether a second 1 mg dose is needed.

➤*Renal/Hepatic function impairment:* Increase the initial dosage interval to 6 to 8 hours. Determine subsequent doses by patient response.

Actions

➤*Pharmacology:* Butorphanol is a potent analgesic with both narcotic agonist and antagonist effects. The analgesic potency on a weight basis appears to be 3.5 to 7 times that of morphine, 30 to 40 times that of meperidine, and 20 times that of pentazocine. The exact mechanism of action is unknown. Narcotic antagonist analgesics may exert their analgesic effect via a CNS mechanism, perhaps subcortical, in the limbic system.

Narcotic antagonist activity – Butorphanol's narcotic antagonist activity is ≈ 30 times that of pentazocine and 1/40 that of naloxone.

Effect on respiration – A parenteral dose of 2 to 3 mg butorphanol produces analgesia and respiratory depression approximately equal to that of 10 mg morphine or 80 mg meperidine. However, butorphanol appears to have a ceiling effect at 30 to 60 mcg/kg in the degree of respiratory depression produced; it is reversible by naloxone.

Cardiovascular effects – Hemodynamic changes after IV administration, similar to those seen with pentazocine, include increased pulmonary artery pressure, pulmonary wedge pressure, left ventricular end-diastolic pressure, systemic arterial pressure, pulmonary vascular resistance, and increased cardiac workload.

➤*Pharmacokinetics:*

Butorphanol Pharmacokinetics Based on Route of Administration			
Parameter	IV	IM	Nasal
Onset (min)	rapid	10-15	within 15
Peak (h)	0.5-1	0.5-1	1-2
Duration (h)	3-4	3-4	4-5
Half-life (h)	2.1-8.8	-	2.9-9.2
AUC (h•ng/mL)	4.4-13	-	0.3-10.3

Butorphanol is extensively metabolized in the liver. The major metabolite is hydroxybutorphanol; norbutorphanol is produced in small amounts. The elimination half-life of hydroxybutorphanol may be greater than the parent compound. Elimination occurs in the urine (70% to 80%) and feces (≈ 15%). In the urine, ≈ 5% is excreted unchanged, 49% as hydroxybutorphanol and < 5% as norbutorphanol. Elimination half-life is increased in the elderly and in patients with decreased creatinine clearance. Protein binding is ≈ 80%.

Contraindications

Hypersensitivity to butorphanol or any components of the products.

Warnings

➤*Physically dependent narcotic:* Physically dependent narcotic patients should not receive butorphanol prior to detoxification; it may precipitate withdrawal. However, there is some controversy about whether butorphanol can induce withdrawal in opioid-dependent patients based on its relative action/inaction at various opiate receptors; specifically, whether it has antagonistic action at the μ receptor.

➤*Head injury and increased intracranial pressure:* Butorphanol, like other potent analgesics, may elevate cerebrospinal fluid pressure; use in cases of head injury can produce effects (eg, miosis) that may obscure the clinical course of these patients. Use with extreme caution and only if essential.

➤*Cardiovascular disease:* Butorphanol increases the cardiac workload; limit its use in acute MI or in ventricular dysfunction or coronary insufficiency to those situations where the benefits outweigh the risk.

Severe hypertension has occurred rarely. Discontinue butorphanol and treat the hypertension. Naltrexone has also been effective.

➤*Renal/Hepatic function impairment:* The drug is metabolized in the liver and excreted by the kidneys; increase the dosage interval (see Administration and Dosage).

➤*Elderly:* The mean half-life of butorphanol is increased by 25% (to > 6 hours) in patients > 65 years of age. Elderly patients may be more sensitive to its side effects, especially dizziness.

➤*Pregnancy:* Category C. Safety for use during pregnancy prior to 37 weeks of gestation has not been established. Prolonged use during gestation may result in neonatal withdrawal. At term, butorphanol rapidly crosses the placenta. Use only when clearly needed and when potential benefits outweigh potential hazards to the fetus.

Labor and delivery – Butorphanol injection may be used during labor (see Administration and Dosage). Reports of infant respiratory distress/apnea following butorphanol use during labor have been associated with administration of a dose ≤ 2 hours prior to delivery, use of multiple doses, use with additional analgesic or sedative drugs or use in preterm pregnancies. In 119 patients, 1 mg IV during labor was associated with transient (10 to 90 minutes) sinusoidal fetal heart rate patterns but was not associated with adverse neonatal outcomes. Use with caution in the presence of an abnormal fetal heart rate pattern.

Nasal spray is not recommended during labor/delivery.

➤*Lactation:* Butorphanol appears in breast milk following the injectable route; assume the drug will appear in breast milk following the nasal route as well. The amount an infant would receive is probably clinically insignificant (estimated at 4 mcg/L of milk using 2 mg IM 4 times daily).

➤*Children:* Safety and efficacy for use in children < 18 years of age have not been established. Not recommended for use in this age group.

BUTORPHANOL TARTRATE

Precautions

➤*Respiratory conditions:* Butorphanol causes some respiratory depression. Administer with caution and in low dosage to patients with respiratory depression, severely limited respiratory reserve, bronchial asthma, obstructive respiratory conditions or cyanosis.

➤*Drug abuse and dependence:* Although butorphanol has low physical dependence liability, exercise care in administering to emotionally unstable patients and to those prone to drug misuse and abuse. Abuse has been reported, sometimes in combination with diphenhydramine. A distinct withdrawal syndrome developed upon discontinuation of the drug.

➤*Hazardous tasks:* May cause dizziness or drowsiness; observe caution while driving or performing other tasks requiring alertness, coordination or physical dexterity.

Drug Interactions

➤*Barbiturate anesthetics:* Barbiturate anesthetics may increase the respiratory and CNS depression of butorphanol because of additive pharmacologic activity.

Adverse Reactions

➤*Parenteral/Nasal:*

Cardiovascular – Hypotension (< 1%).

CNS – Somnolence (43%); dizziness (19%); confusion (3% to 9%); anxiety, euphoria, floating feeling, nervousness, paresthesia (≥ 1%); abnormal dreams, agitation, dysphoria, hallucinations, hostility, drug dependence (< 1%).

Dermatologic – Sweating/Clammy (3% to 9%); pruritus (≥ 1%); rash/hives (< 1%).

GI – Nausea/Vomiting (13%); dry mouth (3% to 9%); stomach pain (≥ 1%).

Miscellaneous – Asthenia/Lethargy, headache (3% to 9%); blurred vision, sensation of heat (≥ 1%); impaired urination (< 1%).

➤*Nasal:*

Cardiovascular – Vasodilation (3% to 9%); palpitations (≥ 1%); hypertension (< 1%).

CNS – Insomnia (11%); tremor (≥ 1%); convulsion, delusions, depression (< 1%).

GI – Anorexia, constipation (3% to 9%).

Respiratory – Nasal congestion (13%); dyspnea, epistaxis, nasal irritation, pharyngitis, rhinitis, sinus congestion, upper respiratory tract infection (3% to 9%); bronchitis, cough, sinusitis (≥ 1%); apnea, shallow breathing (< 1%).

Special senses – Tinnitus, unpleasant taste (3% to 9%); ear pain (≥ 1%).

Miscellaneous – Edema (< 1%).

Overdosage

➤*Symptoms:* Overdosage could produce some respiratory depression and variable cardiovascular and CNS effects.

➤*Treatment:* Immediate treatment for suspected overdosage is IV naloxone (see individual monograph). Constantly evaluate the respiratory and cardiac status. Institute appropriate supportive measures (eg, oxygen, IV fluids, vasopressors, assisted or controlled respiration). Refer to General Management of Acute Overdosage.

Patient Information

May cause drowsiness; observe caution while driving or performing other tasks requiring alertness, coordination or physical dexterity.

Do not use alcohol or other CNS depressant drugs concurrently.

Instruct patients on the proper use of the nasal spray.

NALBUPHINE HCl

Rx	**Nalbuphine HCl** (Various, eg, Bioline, DuPont Critical Care, Goldline, Moore, Quad, Rugby, Schein, VHA Supply)	**Injection:** 10 mg/ml		In 1 and 10 ml vials.
Rx	**Nubain**[1] (DuPont)			In 1ml amps[2] and 10 ml vials.
Rx	**Nalbuphine HCl** (Various, eg, Bioline, DuPont Critical Care, Goldline, Moore, Quad, Rugby, Schein, VHA Supply)	**Injection:** 20 mg/ml		In 1 and 10 ml vials.
Rx	**Nubain**[1] (DuPont)			In 1ml amps[2], 10 ml vials and 1 ml disp. syringe.

[1] With 0.1% sodium metabisulfite and methyl— and propylparabens.

[2] This size also available as sulfite/paraben-free.

Refer to the general discussion in the Narcotic Agonist-Antagonist Analgesic introduction.

Indications

Relief of moderate to severe pain.

For preoperative analgesia, as a supplement to balanced analgesia, to surgical and postsurgical anesthesia and for obstetrical analgesia during labor and delivery.

Administration and Dosage

➤*Adults:* Usual dose is 10 mg/70 kg administered SC, IM or IV every 3 to 6 hours as necessary. Individualize dosage. In nontolerant individuals, the recommended single maximum dose is 20 mg, with a maximum total daily dose of 160 mg.

➤*Patients dependent of narcotics:* Patients dependent of narcotics may experience withdrawal symptoms upon the administration of nalbuphine. If unduly troublesome, control by slow IV administration of small increments of morphine until relief occurs. If the previous analgesic was morphine, meperidine, codeine or another narcotic with similar duration of activity, administer ¼ the anticipated nalbuphine dose initially. Observe for signs of withdrawal. If untoward symptoms do not occur, progressively increase doses at appropriate intervals until analgesia is obtained.

Actions

➤*Pharmacology:* Nalbuphine, a potent analgesic with narcotic agonist and antagonist actions, has a chemical structure similar to phenanthrene derivatives, oxymorphone and naloxone. Its analgesic potency is essentially equivalent to that of morphine and ≈ 3 times that of pentazocine on a milligram basis. Unlike the other agonist-antagonists, nalbuphine does not significantly increase pulmonary artery pressure or systemic vascular resistance or cardiac work.

➤*Pharmacokinetics:* Onset of action occurs within 2 to 3 minutes after IV administration, and in < 15 minutes following SC or IM injection. Nalbuphine is metabolized in the liver; plasma half-life is 5 hours. The duration of analgesic activity ranges from 3 to 6 hours. Aproximately 7% is excreted unchanged in the urine.

The narcotic antagonist activity of nalbuphine is 10 times that of pentazocine.

Contraindications

Hypersensitivity to nalbuphine.

Warnings

➤*Head injury and increased intracranial pressure:* The possible respiratory depressant effects and the potential of potent analgesics to elevate cerebrospinal fluid pressure may be markedly exaggerated in the presence of head injury, intracranial lesions or a preexisting increase in intracranial pressure. Potent analgesics can produce effects that may obscure the clinical course of patients with head injuries. Therefore, use with extreme caution and only if deemed essential.

➤*Renal/Hepatic function impairment:* The drug is metabolized in the liver and excreted by the kidneys; patients with renal or liver dysfunction may overreact to customary doses. Therefore, use with caution and administer in reduced amounts.

➤*Pregnancy:* Safe use in pregnancy has not been established. Prolonged use during pregnancy could result in neonatal withdrawal. Administer to pregnant women only when the potential benefits outweigh the possible hazards.

Labor and delivery – May produce respiratory depression in the neonate. Use with caution in women delivering premature infants.

➤*Children:* Clinical experience not available; not recommended in patients < 18 years of age.

Precautions

➤*Respiratory depression:* At the usual adult dose of 10 mg/70 kg, nalbuphine causes respiratory depression approximately equal to that produced by equal doses of morphine. However, in contrast to morphine, nalbuphine exhibits a ceiling effect; increases in dosage beyond 30 mg produce no further respiratory depression. Respiratory depression induced by nalbuphine can be reversed by naloxone. Administer with caution at low doses to patients with impaired respiration (eg, from other medication, uremia, bronchial asthma, severe infection, cyanosis or respiratory obstructions).

➤*Myocardial infarction:* Use with caution in patients with myocardial infarction who have nausea or vomiting.

➤*Biliary tract surgery:* Use with caution in patients about to undergo biliary tract surgery because it may cause spasm of the sphincter of Oddi.

➤*Drug abuse and dependence:* Nalbuphine's low abuse potential is less than codeine and propoxyphene. Psychological and physical dependence and tolerance may follow nalbuphine abuse. Cautiously prescribe to emotionally unstable patients or to individuals with a history of narcotic abuse.

NALBUPHINE HCl

Abrupt discontinuation after prolonged use has been followed by symptoms of narcotic withdrawal.

▶*Hazardous tasks:* May produce drowsiness. Observe caution while driving or performing other tasks requiring alertness, coordination or physical dexterity.

▶*Sulfite sensitivity:* May cause allergic-type reactions (eg, hives, itching, wheezing, anaphylaxis) in certain susceptible people. Although the overall prevalence of sulfite sensitivity in the general population is probably low, it is seen more frequently in asthmatics or in atopic non-asthmatic people. Specific products containing sulfites are identified in the product listings.

Drug Interactions

▶*Barbiturate anesthetics:* Barbiturate anesthetics may increase the respiratory and CNS depression of nalbuphine because of additive pharmacologic activity.

Adverse Reactions

Most frequent – Sedation (36%).

Less frequent – Sweaty/clammy feeling (9%); nausea/vomiting (6%); dizziness/vertigo (5%); dry mouth (4%); headache (3%).

▶*Other adverse reactions (≤ 1%):*

Cardiovascular – Hypertension; hypotension; bradycardia; tachycardia, pulmonary edema.

CNS – Nervousness; depression; restlessness; crying; floating feeling; hostility; unusual dreams; confusion; faintness; hallucinations; euphoria; dysphoria; feeling of heaviness; numbness; tingling; unreality. The incidence of psychotomimetic effects (unreality, depersonalization, delusions, dysphoria, hallucinations) is less than with pentazocine.

Dermatologic – Itching; burning; urticaria.

GI – Cramps; dyspepsia; bitter taste.

Respiratory – Respiratory depression; dyspnea; asthma.

Miscellaneous – Speech difficulty; urinary urgency; blurred vision; flushing; warmth.

Overdosage

▶*Symptoms:* The administration of single doses of 72 mg nalbuphine SC to 8 normal subjects resulted primarily in symptoms of sleepiness and mild dysphoria.

▶*Treatment:* The immediate IV administration of naloxone is a specific antidote (see individual monograph). Treatment includes usual supportive measures. Refer to General Management of Acute Overdosage.

Patient Information

May cause drowsiness; observe caution while driving or performing other tasks requiring alertness.

PENTAZOCINE

c-iv	Talwin (Abbott Hospital Products)	Injection: 30 mg (as lactate)/ml	In 10 ml vials[1], 1 ml *Uni-Amps,* 1 ml *Uni-Nest* amps and 1 and 2 ml fill in 2 ml *Carpuject.*[2]

[1] With 2 mg acetone sodium bisulfite and 1 mg methylparaben per ml.   [2] With 1 mg acetone sodium bisulfite.

Refer to the general discussion in the Narcotic Agonist-Antagonist Analgesic introduction.

Indications

▶*Oral and parenteral:* Relief of moderate to severe pain.

▶*Parenteral:* For preoperative or preanesthetic medication; supplement to surgical anesthesia.

Administration and Dosage

▶*Parenteral:*

Adults – 30 mg IM, SC or IV; may repeat every 3 to 4 hours. Doses in excess of 30 mg IV or 60 mg IM or SC are not recommended. Do not exceed a total daily dosage of 360 mg.

Use SC only when necessary; severe tissue damage is possible at injection sites. When frequent injections are needed, administer IM, constantly rotating injection sites.

Patients in labor – A single 30 mg IM dose is most common. A 20 mg IV dose, given 2 or 3 times at 2 to 3 hour intervals, has resulted in adequate pain relief when contractions become regular.

Children (< 12 years of age) – Clinical experience is limited; use is not recommended.

Admixture incompatibility – Do not mix pentazocine in the same syringe with soluble barbiturates because precipitation will occur.

Actions

▶*Pharmacology:* Pentazocine, a potent analgesic, weakly antagonizes the effects of morphine, meperidine and other opiates at the μ-opioid receptor. Pentazocine, presumed to exert its agonistic actions at the kappa (κ) and sigma (ς) opioid receptors, may precipitate withdrawal symptoms in patients taking narcotic analgesics regularly. In addition, it produces incomplete reversal of cardiovascular, respiratory and behavioral depression induced by morphine and meperidine. Pentazocine also has sedative activity. Parenterally, 30 mg is usually as effective as 10 mg morphine or 75 to 100 mg meperidine. Orally, a 50 mg dose is equivalent to 60 mg codeine.

▶*Pharmacokinetics:* Pentazocine is well absorbed from the GI tract and from SC and IM sites. However, it undergoes extensive first-pass hepatic metabolism. Oral bioavailability is < 20%, and was increased 3-fold in cirrhotic patients. Concentrations in plasma coincide closely with onset, intensity and duration of analgesia. Pentazocine passes into fetal circulation. It is excreted via the kidney, < 5% unchanged.

Contraindications

Hypersensitivity to pentazocine or any product component.

Warnings

▶*"Ts and Blues":* Injection IV of oral preparations of **pentazocine** (*Talwin,* "Ts") and **tripelennamine** (PBZ, "Blues"), an H₁-blocking antihistamine, has become a common form of drug abuse. The combination is used as a "substitute" for heroin. The tablets are dissolved in tap water, filtered and injected IV.

The most frequent and serious complication of IV "Ts and Blues" addiction is pulmonary disease, due to occlusion of pulmonary arteries and arterioles with unsterile particles of cellulose and talc used as tablet binders. The occlusion leads to granulomatous foreign body reactions, infections, increased pulmonary artery resistance and pulmonary hypertension. Neurologic complications from IV injection of "Ts and Blues" include seizures, strokes and CNS infections. The replacement of oral pentazocine with the pentazocine/naloxone combination may decrease the popularity of this mixture. A few cases of abuse involving pentazocine/naloxone combination and tripelennamine have been reported, however.

▶*Tissue damage:* Severe sclerosis of skin, subcutaneous tissues and underlying muscle has occurred at injection sites following multiple doses of pentazocine lactate. Rotate injection sites; IM may be tolerated better than SC.

▶*Head injury and increased intracranial pressure:* Pentazocine can produce effects which may obscure the clinical course of head injury patients. The potential for elevating cerebrospinal fluid pressure may be attributed to CO₂ retention due to the respiratory depressant effects of the drug. These effects may be exaggerated in the presence of head injury, other intracranial lesions or a preexisting increase in intracranial pressure. Use with extreme caution and only if essential.

▶*Myocardial infarction (MI):* Exercise caution in the IV use of pentazocine for patients with acute MI accompanied by hypertension or left ventricular failure. Pentazocine IV elevates systemic and pulmonary arterial pressure, systemic vascular resistance and left ventricular end-diastolic pressure, causing increased cardiac workload. Use the oral form with caution in MI patients who have nausea or vomiting.

▶*Acute CNS manifestations:* Patients receiving therapeutic doses have experienced hallucinations (usually visual), disorientation and confusion which have cleared spontaneously. If the drug is reinstituted, acute CNS manifestations may recur.

Seizures have occurred with the use of pentazocine.

▶*Renal / Hepatic function impairment:* The drug is metabolized in the liver and excreted by the kidney; administer with caution to patients with such impairment. Extensive liver disease predisposes to greater side effects (eg, marked apprehension, anxiety, dizziness, drowsiness), and may be the result of decreased drug metabolism.

▶*Pregnancy: Category C.* Pentazocine rapidly crosses the placenta with cord blood levels 40% to 70% of maternal serum levels. Chronic maternal ingestion of pentazocine may result in neonatal withdrawal symptoms. Mothers addicted to "Ts and Blues" have lower birth weight infants who have problems similar to infants born of other narcotic addicted mothers. Safe use during pregnancy has not been established. Administer only when the benefits outweigh the hazards.

Labor – Patients receiving pentazocine during labor have experienced no adverse effects other than those that occur with commonly used analgesics. Use with caution in women delivering premature infants.

▶*Lactation:* Safety for use in the nursing mother has not been established.

▶*Children:* Safety and efficacy in children < 12 years of age have not been established.

Precautions

▶*Respiratory conditions:* Use caution and low dosage in patients with respiratory depression (eg, from other medication, uremia, severe infection), severely limited respiratory reserve, severe bronchial asthma, obstructive respiratory conditions, cyanosis.

PENTAZOCINE

➤*Biliary tract pressure elevation:* Biliary tract pressure elevation generally occurs for varying periods following narcotic use. However, some evidence suggests pentazocine causes little or no elevation in biliary tract pressures. Clinical significance of these findings is unknown.

➤*Patients receiving narcotics:* Pentazocine is a mild narcotic antagonist. Some patients previously given narcotics, including methadone for the daily treatment of narcotic dependence, have experienced withdrawal symptoms after receiving pentazocine.

➤*Drug abuse and dependence:* Exercise special care in prescribing to emotionally unstable patients and to those with history of drug abuse; closely supervise when therapy exceeds 4 or 5 days. Psychological and physical dependence have occurred in such patients and, rarely, in patients without history of drug abuse. Abrupt discontinuation after extended use has resulted in withdrawal symptoms. If more than minor difficulty is encountered, reinstitute parenteral pentazocine with gradual withdrawal. Avoid substituting methadone or other narcotics in pentazocine abstinence syndrome.

➤*Hazardous tasks:* May produce sedation, dizziness and occasional euphoria; observe caution while driving or performing other tasks requiring alertness, coordination or physical dexterity.

➤*Sulfite sensitivity:* May cause allergic-type reactions (eg, hives, itching, wheezing, anaphylaxis) in certain susceptible people. Although the overall prevalence of sulfite sensitivity in the general population is probably low, it is seen more frequently in asthmatics or in atopic non-asthmatic people.

Drug Interactions

Pentazocine Drug Interactions			
Precipitant drug	Object drug*		Description
Pentazocine	Alcohol	↑	Due to the potential for increased CNS depressant effects, use cautiously in patients currently receiving pentazocine.
Barbiturate anesthetics	Pentazocine	↑	Barbiturate anesthetics may increase the respiratory and CNS depression of pentazocine because of additive pharmacologic activity.

* ↑ = Object drug increased. ↓ = Object drug decreased.

Adverse Reactions

Most common – Nausea; dizziness or lightheadedness; vomiting; euphoria.

➤*Cardiovascular:* Hypotension; decrease in blood pressure; tachycardia; circulatory depression; shock; hypertension.

➤*CNS:* Sedation; headache; weakness or faintness; depression; disturbed dreams; insomnia; syncope; hallucinations; tremor; irritability; excitement; tinnitus; disorientation; confusion (see Warnings).

➤*Dermatologic:* Soft tissue induration; nodules; cutaneous depression; ulceration (sloughing); severe sclerosis of the skin, subcutaneous tissues and, rarely, underlying muscle at the injection site; diaphoresis; stinging on injection; flushed skin; dermatitis; pruritus; toxic epidermal necrolysis.

➤*GI:* Constipation; cramps; abdominal distress; anorexia; diarrhea; dry mouth; taste alteration.

➤*Hematologic:* Depression of white blood cells (especially granulocytes), usually reversible; moderate transient eosinophilia.

➤*Hypersensitivity:* Edema of the face; sweating; anaphylactic reaction; rash; urticaria.

➤*Ophthalmic:* Blurred vision; focusing difficulty; nystagmus; diplopia; miosis.

➤*Respiratory:* Respiratory depression; dyspnea; transient apnea in newborns whose mothers received parenteral pentazocine during labor.

➤*Miscellaneous:* Urinary retention; paresthesia; chills; neuromuscular and psychiatric muscle tremors; alterations in rate or strength of uterine contractions during labor (parenteral form).

Overdosage

➤*Symptoms:* The clinical picture of overdosage has not been well defined. High doses produce marked respiratory depression, increased blood pressure and tachycardia.

➤*Treatment:* Employ oxygen, IV fluids, vasopressors and other supportive measures, as indicated. Consider assisted or controlled ventilation. For respiratory depression, parenteral naloxone is a specific and effective antagonist (see individual monograph).

Refer to General Management of Acute Overdosage.

Patient Information

May cause drowsiness; observe caution while driving or performing other tasks requiring alertness, coordination or physical dexterity.

Avoid alcohol and other CNS depressants.

Notify physician if skin rash, confusion or disorientation occurs.

PENTAZOCINE COMBINATIONS

c-iv	**Talwin Compound** (Sanofi Winthrop)	**Tablets:** 12.5 mg (as HCl) and 325 mg aspirin	White. In 100s.
c-iv	**Pentazocine HCl and Acetaminophen** (Watson)	**Tablets:** 25 mg (as HCl) and 650 mg acetaminophen	(396 25 650). Aqua, capsule shape. In 100s, 500s, and 1000s.
c-iv	**Talacen** (Sanofi Winthrop)		Sodium metabisulfite. (Winthrop T37). Blue, scored. In 100s and UD 250s.
c-iv	**Pentazocine and Naloxone HCl** (Royce)	**Tablets:** 50 mg (as HCl) and 0.5 mg naloxone HCl	In 100s, 500s and 1000s.
c-iv	**Talwin NX** (Sanofi Winthrop)		(T51). Yellow, scored. Oblong. In 100s and UD 250s.

Refer to the general discussion in the Narcotic Agonist-Antagonist Analgesic introduction. For complete prescribing information, refer to the Pentazocine monograph.

WARNING

Talwin Nx: Talwin Nx is intended for oral use only. Severe, potentially lethal reactions (eg, pulmonary emboli, vascular occlusion, ulceration and abscesses, withdrawal symptoms in narcotic-dependent individuals) may result from misuse of this drug by injection or in combination with other substances.

Administration and Dosage

➤*Adults:*

Pentazocine and aspirin – 2 tablets 3 or 4 times daily.

Pentazocine and acetaminophen – 1 tablet every 4 hours, up to 6 tablets per day.

Pentazocine and naloxone – Initially, 50 mg every 3 or 4 hours; increase to 100 mg if necessary. Do not exceed a total daily dosage of 600 mg. When anti-inflammatory or antipyretic effects are desired in addition to analgesia, aspirin can be administered concomitantly.

Pentazocine tablets are intended for oral use only. Severe, potentially lethal reactions may result from misuse by injection or when combined with other substances. Oral pentazocine tablets contain 0.5 mg naloxone, a narcotic antagonist, to aid in elimination of the abuse potential.

➤*Children:* Clinical experience is limited; not recommended for children < 12 years of age.

Actions

➤*Pharmacology:*

Talwin NX – *Talwin NX* tablets, which contain naloxone, produce analgesic effects when administered orally because naloxone has poor bioavailability. Injected IV (an unintended use), naloxone will block the pharmacologic effects of pentazocine, producing withdrawal symptoms in opioid-dependent individuals.

CLONIDINE HCl

Rx	**Duraclon** (aaiPharma)	**Injection:** 100 mcg/ml	Preservative-free. In 10 ml vials.
		500 mcg/ml	Preservative-free. In 10 ml vials.

Clonidine is also used orally as an antihypertensive. For further information, refer to the Clonidine monograph in the Antihypertensives section.

WARNING

Epidural clonidine is not recommended for obstetrical, post-partum or peri-operative pain management. The risk of hemodynamic instability, especially hypotension and bradycardia, from epidural clonidine may be unacceptable in these patients. However, in a rare obstetrical, postpartum or perioperative patient, potential benefits may outweigh the possible risks.

Clonidine injection is a centrallyacting analgesic solution for use in continuous epidural infusion devices.

Clonidine is an imidazole derivative and exists as a mesomeric compound.

Indications

➤*Severe pain:* Clonidine is indicated in combination with opiates for the treatment of severe pain in cancer patients that is not adequately relieved by opioid analgesics alone. Epidural clonidine is more likely to be effective in patients with neuropathic pain than somatic or visceral pain.

Administration and Dosage

The recommended starting dose of clonidine for continuous epidural infusion is 30 mcg/hr. Although dosage may be titrated up or down depending on pain relief and occurrence of adverse events, experience with dosage rates > 40 mcg/hr is limited.

Clonidine must not be used with a preservative.

➤*Storage/Stability:* Store at controlled room temperature 15° to 30°C (59° to 86°F). Discard unused portion.

Actions

➤*Pharmacology:* Epidurally administered clonidine produces dose-dependent analgesia not antagonized by opiate antagonists. The analgesia is limited to the body regions innervated by the spinal segments where analgesic concentrations of clonidine are present. Clonidine is thought to produce analgesia at presynaptic and postjunctional alpha-2-adrenoceptors in the spinal cord by preventing pain signal transmission to the brain.

➤*Pharmacokinetics:*

Distribution – Following a 10 minute IV infusion of 300 mcg clonidine to 5 male volunteers, plasma clonidine levels showed an initial rapid distribution phase (mean half–life of 11 minutes) followed by a slower elimination phase (half–life of 9 hours) over 24 hours. Clonidine's total body clearance (CL) was 219 ml/min.

Following a 700 mcg clonidine epidural dose given over 5 minutes to 4 male and 5 female volunteers, peak clonidine plasma levels (4.4 ng/ml) were obtained in 19 minutes. Following sample collection for 24 hours, the plasma elimination half-life was determined to be 22 hours. CL was 190 ml/min. In cerebral spinal fluid (CSF), peak clonidine levels (418 ng/ml) were achieved in 26 minutes. The clonidine CSF elimination half-life was 1.3 hours when samples were collected for 6 hours. Compared with men, women had a lower mean plasma clearance, longer mean plasma half-life and higher mean peak level of clonidine in both plasma and CSF.

In cancer patients who received 14 days of clonidine epidural infusion (rate = 30 mcg/hr) plus morphine by patient-controlled analgesia (PCA), steady-state clonidine plasma concentrations of 2.2 and 2.4 ng/ml were obtained on dosing days 7 and 14, respectively. CL was 279 and 272 ml/min on these days. CSF concentrations were not determined in these patients.

Clonidine is highly lipid soluble and readily distributes into extravascular sites including the CNS. Clonidine's volume of distribution is 2.1 L/kg. The binding of clonidine to plasma protein is primarily to albumin and varies between 20% and 40% in vitro. Epidurally administered clonidine readily partitions into plasma via the epidural veins and attains systemic concentrations (0.5 to 2.0 ng/ml) that are associated with a hypotensive effect mediated by the central nervous system.

Metabolism – Clonidine metabolism follows minor pathways with the major metabolite p-hydroxyclonidine present at < 10% of the concentration of unchanged drug in the urine.

Excretion – Following an IV dose of clonidine, 72% of the administered dose was excreted within 96 hours in urine, of which 40% to 50% was unchanged clonidine. Renal clearance for clonidine was determined to be 133 ml/min.

Renal function impairment: In a study in which clonidine was given to subjects with varying degrees of kidney function, elimination half-lives varied (17.5 to 41 hours) as a function of creatinine clearance. In subjects undergoing hemodialysis, only 5% of body clonidine stores was removed.

➤*Clinical trials:* In a double-blind, randomized study of cancer patients with severe intractable pain below the C4 dermatome not controlled by morphine, 38 patients were randomized to an epidural infusion of clonidine plus epidural morphine, and 47 subjects received epidural placebo plus epidural morphine. Successful analgesia, defined as a decrease in either morphine use or Visual Analog Score (VAS) pain, was significantly more common with epidural clonidine than placebo (45% vs 21%).

Contraindications

Patients with a history of sensitivity or allergic reactions to clonidine; in the presence of an injection site infection; in patients on anticoagulant therapy; patients with a bleeding diathesis; administration above the C4 dermatome because there are no adequate safety data to support such use.

Warnings

➤*Postoperative or obstetrical analgesia:* Epidural clonidine is not recommended for obstetrical, postpartum or perioperative pain management. The risk of hemodynamic instability, especially hypotension and bradycardia, from epidural clonidine may be unacceptable in these patients.

➤*Hypotension:* Because severe hypotension may follow clonidine administration, use with caution in all patients. It is not recommended in most patients with severe cardiovascular disease or in those who are otherwise hemodynamically unstable. Balance the benefit of administration in these patients against the potential risks resulting from hypotension.

Monitor vital signs frequently, especially during the first few days of epidural clonidine therapy. When clonidine is infused into the upper thoracic spinal segments, more pronounced decreases in blood pressure may be seen.

Clonidine decreases sympathetic outflow from the CNS resulting in decreases in peripheral resistance, renal vascular resistance, heart rate and blood pressure. However, in the absence of profound hypotension, renal blood flow and glomerular filtration rate remain essentially unchanged.

Most episodes of hypotension occur within the first 4 days after beginning epidural clonidine. However, hypotensive episodes may occur throughout the trial duration. There was a tendency for these episodes to occur more commonly in women and in those with higher serum clonidine levels. Patients experiencing hypotension also tended to weigh less than those who did not experience hypotension. The hypotension usually responded to IV fluids and, if necessary, parenteral ephedrine. Severe hypotension may occur even if IV fluid pretreatment is given.

➤*Withdrawal:* Sudden cessation of clonidine treatment, regardless of the route of administration, has, in some cases, resulted in symptoms such as nervousness, agitation, headache and tremor, accompanied or followed by a rapid rise in blood pressure. The likelihood of such reactions appears to be greater after administration of higher doses or with concomitant beta-blocker treatment. Special caution is therefore advised in these situations. Rare instances of hypertensive encephalopathy, cerebrovascular accidents and death have been reported after abrupt clonidine withdrawal. Patients with a history of hypertension or other underlying cardiovascular conditions may be at particular risk of the consequences of abrupt discontinuation of clonidine.

When discontinuing therapy with epidural clonidine, the physician should reduce the dose gradually over 2 to 4 days to avoid withdrawal symptoms.

An excessive rise in blood pressure following discontinuation of epidural clonidine can be treated by administration of clonidine or by IV phentolamine. If therapy is to be discontinued in patients receiving a beta-blocker and clonidine concurrently, discontinue the beta-blocker several days before the gradual discontinuation of epidural clonidine.

➤*Catheter-related infection:* Implantable epidural catheters are associated with a risk of catheter-related infections, including meningitis and epidural abscess. Eighteen percent of subjects discontinued this study as a result of catheter-related problems (eg, infections, accidental dislodging), and one subject developed meningitis, possibly as a result of a catheter-related infection. Evaluation of fever in a patient receiving epidural clonidine should include the possibility of a catheter-related infection such as meningitis or epidural abscess.

➤*Renal function impairment:* Adjust dosage according to the degree of renal impairment, and monitor patients carefully. Because only a minimal amount of clonidine is removed during routine hemodialysis, there is no need to give supplemental clonidine following dialysis.

➤*Pregnancy:* Category C. Clonidine readily crosses the placenta and its concentrations are equal in maternal and umbilical cord plasma; amniotic fluid concentrations can be 4 times those found in serum. There are no adequate and well controlled studies in pregnant women during early gestation when organ formation takes place. Use epidural clonidine during pregnancy only if the potential benefits justify the

CLONIDINE HCl

potential risk to the fetus.

Labor and delivery – Clonidine during labor has demonstrated no apparent adverse effects on the infant at the time of delivery. However, these studies did not monitor the infants for hemodynamic effects in the days following delivery. There are no adequate controlled clinical trials evaluating the safety, efficacy and dosing of clonidine in obstetrical settings. Because maternal perfusion of the placenta is critically dependent on blood pressure, use of clonidine as an analgesic during labor and delivery is not indicated.

➤*Lactation:* Concentrations of clonidine in human breast milk are approximately twice those found in maternal plasma. Exercise caution when clonidine is administered to a nursing woman.

➤*Children:* Restrict the use of clonidine to pediatric patients with severe intractable pain from malignancy that is unresponsive to epidural or spinal opiates or other more conventional analgesic techniques. Select the starting dose on a per kilogram basis (0.5 mcg/kg/hour) and cautiously adjust based on the clinical response.

Precautions

➤*Monitoring:* Closely monitor patients receiving epidural clonidine from a continuous infusion device for the first few days to assess their response.

➤*Cardiac effects:* Clonidine frequently causes decreases in heart rate. Symptomatic bradycardia can be treated with atropine. Rarely, atrioventricular block greater than first degree has been reported. Clonidine does not alter the hemodynamic response to exercise but may mask the increase in heart rate associated with hypovolemia.

➤*Respiratory depression and sedation:* Clonidine administration may result in sedation through the activation of alpha-adrenoceptors in the brainstem. High clonidine doses cause sedation and ventilatory abnormalities that are usually mild. Tolerance to these effects can develop with chronic administration. These effects have been reported with bolus doses.

➤*Depression:* Depression has been seen in a small percentage of patients treated with oral or transdermal clonidine. Depression commonly occurs in cancer patients and may be exacerbated by clonidine treatment. Monitor for the signs and symptoms of depression, especially in patients with a known history of affective disorders.

➤*Pain:* Clonidine is most effective in well-localized, "neuropathic" pain that is characterized as electrical, burning or shooting in nature and is localized to a dermatomal or peripheral nerve distribution. It may be less effective or ineffective in the treatment of pain that is diffuse, poorly localized or visceral in origin.

➤*Hazardous tasks:* May produce drowsiness; patients should observe caution while driving or performing other tasks requiring alertness, coordination, or physical dexterity.

Drug Interactions

Clonidine Drug Interactions			
Precipitant drug	Object drug*		Description
Beta blockers	Clonidine	↑	Beta blockers may exacerbate the hypertensive response seen with clonidine withdrawal. Also, because of the potential for additive effects such as bradycardia and AV block, use caution in patients receiving clonidine with agents known to affect sinus node function or AV nodal conduction (eg, digitalis, calcium channel blockers, beta blockers).
Fluphenazine	Clonidine	↑	There is one reported case of a patient with acute delirium associated with the simultaneous use of fluphenazine and oral clonidine. Symptoms resolved when clonidine was withdrawn and recurred when the patient was rechallenged with clonidine.
Narcotic analgesics	Clonidine	↑	Narcotic analgesics may potentiate the hypotensive effects of clonidine.
Tricyclic antidepressants	Clonidine	↓	Tricyclic antidepressants may antagonize the hypotensive effects of clonidine. The effects of tricyclic antidepressants on clonidine's analgesic actions are not known.
Clonidine	Alcohol/ barbiturates	↑	Clonidine may potentiate the CNS-depressive effect of alcohol, barbiturates or other sedating drugs.

Clonidine Drug Interactions			
Precipitant drug	Object drug*		Description
Clonidine	Local anesthetics	↑	Epidural clonidine may prolong the duration of pharmacologic effects of epidural local anesthetics, including sensory and motor blockade.

* ↑ = Object drug increased. ↓ = Object drug decreased.

Adverse Reactions

The following adverse events may be related to administration of either clonidine or morphine.

Clonidine Adverse Reactions		
Adverse Events	Clonidine (%)	Placebo (%)
Total number of patients who experienced ≥ 1 adverse event	97.4	80.5
Hypotension	44.8	10.6
Postural hypotension	31.6	0
Dry mouth	13.2	8.5
Nausea	13.2	21.3
Somnolence	13.2	21.3
Dizziness	13.2	4.3
Confusion	13.2	10.6
Vomiting	10.5	14.9
Nausea/Vomiting	7.9	2.1
Sweating	5.3	0
Anxiety	11	2
Chest pain	5.3	0
Hallucination	5.3	2.1
Tinnitus	5.3	0
Constipation	6	4.3
Tachycardia	2.6	4.3
Hypoventilation	2.6	4.3
Urinary tract infection	22	nd[1]
Dyspnea	6	nd
Infection	6	nd
Asthenia	5	nd
Hyperaesthesia	5	nd
Pain	5	nd
Skin ulcer	5	nd
Decreased heart rate	†[2]	nd
Rebound hypertension	11	nd

[1] nd = No data.
[2] † = Occurs, but the incidence is unknown.

The following adverse reactions have also been reported with the use of any dosage form of clonidine. In many cases patients were receiving concomitant medication and a causal relationship has not been established. For more adverse reactions, refer to the oral clonidine monograph in the antihypertensives section.

➤*CNS:* Cerebrovascular accidents, other behavioral changes (rare).

➤*GI:* Hepatitis, parotitis, ileus and pseudo-obstruction, abdominal pain (rare).

➤*Metabolic:* Transient elevation of serum phosphatase (rare).

➤*Miscellaneous:* Thrombocytopenia, syncope, blurred vision (rare); withdrawal syndrome (1%).

Overdosage

The largest overdose reported to date involved a 28-year-old white male who ingested 100 mg clonidine powder. This patient developed hypertension followed by hypotension, bradycardia, apnea, hallucinations, semicoma and premature ventricular contractions. The patient fully recovered after intensive treatment. Plasma clonidine levels were 60 ng/ml after 1 hour, 190 ng/ml after 1.5 hours, 370 ng/ml after 2 hours and 120 ng/ml after 5.5 and 6.5 hours. In mice and rats, the oral LD50 of clonidine is 206 and 465 mg/kg, respectively.

➤*Symptoms:* Hypertension may develop early and may be followed by hypotension, bradycardia, respiratory depression, hypothermia, drowsiness, decreased or absent reflexes, irritability and miosis. With large oral overdoses, reversible cardiac conduction defects or arrhythmias, apnea, coma and seizures have been reported. As little as 100 mcg of oral clonidine has produced signs of toxicity in pediatric patients.

CLONIDINE HCl

➤*Treatment:* There is no specific antidote for clonidine overdosage. Supportive care may include atropine sulfate for bradycardia, IV fluids or vasopressor agents for hypotension. Hypertension associated with overdosage has been treated with IV furosemide, diazoxide or alpha-blocking agents such as phentolamine. Naloxone may be a useful adjunct in the treatment of clonidine-induced respiratory depression, hypotension or coma; monitor blood pressure because the administration of naloxone has occasionally resulted in paradoxical hypertension. Tolazoline administration has yielded inconsistent results and is not recommended as first-line therapy. Dialysis is not likely to significantly enhance clonidine elimination.

Patient Information

Warn patients of the risks of rebound hypertension. Patients should not discontinue clonidine except under the supervision of a physician. Patients should notify their physician immediately if clonidine administration is inadvertently interrupted for any reason.

Advise patients who engage in potentially hazardous activities, such as operating machinery or driving, of the potential sedative and hypotensive effects of epidural clonidine.

Inform patients that sedative effects may be increased by CNS-depressing drugs and that opiates may increase hypotensive effects.

ACETAMINOPHEN (N-Acetyl-P-Aminophenol, APAP)

otc	**FeverAll, Infants** (Alpharma)	**Suppositories:** 80 mg	In 6s.
otc	**Acetaminophen** (Various, eg, Goldline, Moore, Rugby)	**Suppositories:** 120 mg	In 12s.
otc	**FeverAll** (Alpharma)		In 12s.
otc	**Acephen** (G & W Labs)		In 6s, 12s and UD 12s, 50s and 100s.
otc	**FeverAll, Children's** (Alpharma)		In 6s.
otc	**Neopap** (PolyMedica)	**Suppositories:** 125 mg	In 12s.
otc	**Acetaminophen** (Harber)	**Suppositories:** 300 mg	In 12s.
otc	**Acetaminophen** (Various, eg, Rugby)	**Suppositories:** 325 mg	In 12s.
otc	**FeverAll** (Alpharma)		In 12s.
otc	**Acephen** (G & W Labs)		In 6s, 12s, 50s and 100s.
otc	**FeverAll, Junior Strength** (Alpharma)		In 6s.
otc	**Acetaminophen** (Various, eg, Goldline, Moore, Rugby)	**Suppositories:** 650 mg	In 12s.
otc	**FeverAll** (Alpharma)		In 12s.
otc	**Acephen** (G & W Labs)		In 12s, 500s and UD 50s and 100s.
otc	**Acetaminophen** (Various, eg, Moore, Rugby, Schein)	**Tablets, chewable:** 80 mg	In 30s, and 100s.
otc	**Apacet** (Parmed)		In 30s.
otc	**Children's Dynafed Jr.** (BDI)		(44 185). Fruit flavor. In 36s.
otc	**Genapap, Children's** (Goldline)		Fruit flavor. Saccharin free. In 30s.
otc	**Children's Māpap** (Major)		3 mg phenylalanine, aspartame, mannitol, sucrose. Grape, fruit splash flavors. In 30s.
otc	**Children's Tylenol Soft Chews** (McNeil-CPC)		Aspartame. Grape and fruit flavors. In 30s.
otc sf	**Panadol, Children's** (SmithKline Beecham)		(P). Scored. Fruit flavor. In 30s.
otc	**Tempra 3** (Mead Johnson Nutritional)		In 30s.
otc	**Tylenol, Children's** (McNeil-CPC)		(Tylenol 80). Scored. Fruit, bubble gum or grape flavor. In 30s, 48s and 96s.
otc	**Tylenol Junior Strength** (McNeil-CPC)	**Tablets, chewable:** 160 mg	Aspartame (6 mg phenylalanine). (TYLENOL 160). Grape and fruit flavors. In 24s.
otc	**Acetaminophen** (Various, eg, Geneva, Moore, Roxane, Rugby, Schein)	**Tablets:** 325 mg	In 50s, 100s, 1000s and UD 100s.
otc	**Aceta** (Century)		In 100s and 1000s.
otc	**Genapap** (Goldline)		In 100s.
otc	**Genebs** (Goldline)		In 100s.
otc	**Mapap Regular Strength** (Major)		Scored. In 100s, 1000s and UD 100s.
otc	**Maranox** (C.S. Dent)		In 8s.
otc	**Meda Tab** (Circle)		In 100s.
otc	**Tapanol Regular Strength** (Circle)		In 100s and 250s.
otc	**Tylenol Caplets** (McNeil-CPC)		In 24s, 50s and 100s.
otc	**Tylenol Regular Strength Tablets** (McNeil-CPC)		(TYLENOL 325). In 24s, 50s, 100s and 200s.
otc	**Acetaminophen** (Various, eg, Geneva, Moore)	**Tablets:** 500 mg	In 100s, 1000s and UD 100s.
otc	**Aceta** (Century)		In 100s and 1000s.
otc	**Aspirin Free Anacin Maximum Strength** (Whitehall)		In 60s.
otc	**Extra Strength Dynafed E.X.** (BDI)		In 36s.
otc	**Genebs Extra Strength** (Goldline)		In 100s.
otc	**Mapap Extra Strength** (Major)		In 30s, 60s, 100s, 200s, 1000s and UD 100s.
otc	**Panadol** (SmithKline Beecham)		(P 500). In 30s and 60s.
otc	**Redutemp** (Inter. Ethical Labs)		In 60s.
otc	**Tapanol Extra Strength** (Republic)		In 100s.
otc	**Tylenol Extra Strength** (McNeil-CPC)		(TYLENOL 500). In 100s.
otc	**UN-Aspirin Extra Strength** (Zee Medical)		In 24s.
otc	**Acetaminophen** (Roxane)	**Tablets:** 650 mg	In 1000s and UD 100s.
otc	**Tylenol Arthritis** (McNeil-CPC)	**Tablets, extended release:** 650 mg	(TYLENOL ER). Caplet-shaped. In 100s.
otc sf	**Panadol, Junior Strength** (Sterling Health)	**Caplets:** 160 mg	In 30s.
otc	**Aspirin Free Pain Relief** (Hudson)	**Caplets:** 500 mg	In 100s.
otc	**Genapap Extra Strength** (Goldline)		In 50s and 100s.
otc	**Genebs Extra Strength** (Goldline)		In 100s.
otc	**Panadol** (SmithKline Beecham)		(P 500). In 24s.
otc	**Tapanol Extra Strength** (Republic)		In 50s, 100s and 175s.
otc	**Tylenol Extended Relief** (McNeil-CPC)	**Caplets:** 650 mg	(Tylenol ER). In 100s.
otc	**Tylenol 8 Hour** (McNeil)	**Caplets, extended-release:** 650 mg	Polyvinyl alcohol, povidone. In 24s, 50s, 100s, and 150s.

ACETAMINOPHEN (N-Acetyl-P-Aminophenol, APAP)

otc	**Aspirin Free Anacin Maximum Strength** (Whitehall)	**Gelcaps:** 500 mg	(AF Anacin). In 100s.
otc	**Tapanol Extra Strength** (Republic)		In 100s and 175s.
otc	**Tylenol Extra Strength** (McNeil-CPC)		Gelatin coated. (TYLENOL 500). In 24s, 50s and 100s.
otc	**Tylenol 8 Hour** (McNeil)	**Geltabs, extended-release:** 650 mg	Benzyl alcohol, EDTA, parabens, povidone. In 20s, 40s, and 80s.
otc	**Acetaminophen** (Various, eg, Moore)	**Capsules:** 500 mg	In 50s, 100s and 1000s.
otc	**Meda Cap** (Circle)		In 100s.
otc	**Silapap, Children's** (Silarx)	**Elixir:** 80 mg/2.5 ml	Alcohol-free. In 237 ml.
otc	**Ridenol** (R.I.D.)	**Elixir:** 80 mg/5 ml	In 120 ml.
otc	**Acetaminophen** (Various, eg, Pharm. Assoc. Inc)	**Elixir:** 120 mg/5 ml	In UD 27 ml (100s).
otc	**Aceta** (Century)		In 120 ml and gal.
otc	**Oraphen-PD** (Great Southern)		In 120 ml.
otc	**Acetaminophen** (Various, eg, Goldline, Rugby, Schein)	**Elixir:** 160 mg/5 ml	In 118 and 120 ml, pt and gal.
otc	**Apra** (Altaire)		Alcohol-free. Sorbitol, sucrosee. Grape flavor. In 118 mL.
otc	**Genapap, Children's** (Goldline)		In 120 ml.
otc	**Mapap, Children's** (Major)		Alcohol free. Cherry flavor. In 120 ml.
otc	**Tylenol, Children's** (McNeil-CPC)		Alcohol free. Sorbitol, sucrose, butylparaben, corn syrup. Cherry flavor. In 60 and 120 ml.
otc	**Dolono** (R.I.D)		Alcohol free. Sorbitol, sucrose. Cherry flavor. In 120 mL.
otc	**Acetaminophen** (Various, eg, Roxane, UDL Labs)	**Liquid:** 160 mg/5 ml	In 120 and 500 ml and UD 100s.
otc *sf*	**Panadol, Children's** (SmithKline Beecham)		Alcohol free. Saccharin, sorbitol. Fruit flavor. In 59 and 118 ml.
otc	**Tempra 2 Syrup** (Mead Johnson Nutritional)		In 120 ml.
otc	**Acetaminophen** (Various, eg, Goldline)	**Liquid:** 500 mg/15 ml	In 237 ml.
otc	**Tylenol Extra Strength** (McNeil-CPC)		7% alcohol. Sorbitol, sucrose. Mint flavor. In 240 ml with dosage cup.
otc	**Acetaminophen Drops** (Various, eg, Bioline, Moore, Schein)	**Solution:** 100 mg/ml	In 15 ml.
otc	**Apacet** (Parmed)		In 15 ml.
otc	**Genapap, Infants' Drops** (Goldline)		Alcohol free. Fruit flavor. In 15 ml w/0.8 ml dropper.
otc	**Infantaire Drops** (Altaire)		In 15 and 30 mL.
otc	**Mapap Infant Drops** (Major)		Alcohol free. Fruit flavor. In 15 and 30 ml.
otc *sf*	**Panadol, Infants' Drops** (SmithKline Beecham)		Alcohol free. Saccharin. Fruit flavor. In 14.8 ml with 0.8 ml dropper.
otc	**Silapap, Infants** (Silarx)		Alcohol free. Fruit flavor. In 15 ml with dropper.
otc	**Tempra 1** (Mead Johnson Nutritional)		In 15 ml.
otc	**Tylenol, Infants' Drops** (McNeil-CPC)		Alcohol free. Saccharin, butylparaben, corn syrup, sorbitol. Fruit flavor. In 7.5 ml and in 30 ml w/0.8 ml dropper.

Indications

An analgesic-antipyretic in the presence of aspirin allergy, patients with blood coagulation disorders who are being treated with oral anticoagulants, bleeding diatheses (eg, hemophilia), upper GI disease (eg, ulcer, gastritis, hiatal hernia) and gouty arthritis; a variety of arthritic and rheumatic conditions involving musculoskeletal pain, as well as in other painful disorders; headache; pain associated with earache, teething, tonsillectomy, menstruation; toothache; diseases accompanied by discomfort and fever such as the common cold, "flu" and other bacterial or viral infections.

►*Unlabeled uses:* Prophylactic acetaminophen use in children receiving DTP vaccination appears to decrease incidence of fever and injection site pain. A dose immediately following vaccination and every 4 to 6 hours thereafter for 48 to 72 hours is suggested.

Administration and Dosage

►*Oral:*

Adults – 325 to 650 mg every 4 to 6 hrs, or 1 g 3 to 4 times/day. Do not exceed 4 g/day.

Tylenol 8 hour: 1300 mg every 8 hours. Swallow whole; do not crush, chew, or dissolve. Do not take more than 3900 mg in 24 hours. Do not use for more than 10 days unless directed by a doctor.

Children – May repeat doses every 4 hours; do not exceed 5 doses in 24 hours.

Acetaminophen Dosage for Children			
Age	Dosage (mg)	Age	Dosage (mg)
0-3 months	40	6-8 years	320
4-11 months	80	9-10 years	400
1-< 2 years	120	11 years	480
2-3 years	160	12-14 years	640
4-5 years	240	> 14 years	650

A 10 to 15 mg/kg/dose schedule has also been recommended.

Tylenol 8 hour: Ask a physician.

►*Suppositories:*

Adults – 650 mg every 4 to 6 hrs. Give no more than 4 g in 24 hours.

Children –

(*3 to 11 months*): 80 mg every 6 hours.

(*1 to 3 years*): 80 mg every 4 hours.

(*3 to 6 years*): 120 to 125 mg every 4 to 6 hours. Give ≤ 720 mg in 24 hrs.

(*6 to 12 years*): 325 mg every 4 to 6 hours. Give ≤ 2.6 g in 24 hours.

►*Storage/Stability:* Store suppositories below 27°C (80°F) or refrigerate.

Store tablets and oral solutions at 15° to 30°C (59° to 86°F).

Actions

►*Pharmacology:* Acetaminophen (APAP) is the active metabolite of phenacetin and acetanilid.

The site and mechanism of the analgesic effect is unclear. APAP reduces fever by a direct action on the hypothalamic heat-regulating centers, which increases dissipation of body heat (via vasodilation and sweating). The action of endogenous pyrogen on heat-regulating centers is inhibited. APAP is almost as potent as aspirin in inhibiting prostaglandin synthetase in the CNS, but its peripheral inhibition of prostaglandin synthesis is minimal, which may account for its lack of clinically significant antirheumatic or anti-inflammatory effects.

Generally, antipyretic and analgesic effects of APAP and aspirin are comparable. Aspirin is clearly superior to APAP for pain of inflammatory origin. APAP does not inhibit platelet aggregation, affect prothrombin response or produce GI ulceration.

►*Pharmacokinetics:*

Absorption – Absorption of acetaminophen is rapid and almost complete from the GI tract. Peak plasma concentrations occur within 0.5 to 2 hours, with slightly faster absorption of liquid preparations. With overdosage, absorption is complete in 4 hours.

ACETAMINOPHEN (N-Acetyl-P-Aminophenol, APAP)

Distribution – Serum protein binding varies from 20% to 50% at toxic concentrations.

Metabolism/Excretion – The half-life in plasma is ≈ 2 hours. Acetaminophen is relatively uniformly distributed throughout most body fluids. Binding of the drug to plasma proteins is variable; only 20% to 50% may be bound at the concentrations encountered during acute intoxication. Ninety percent to 100% of the drug is recovered in the urine within the first day, primarily after hepatic conjugation with glucuronic acid (≈ 60%), sulfuric acid (≈ 35%) or cysteine (≈ 3%); small amounts of hydroxylated and deacetylated metabolites also have been detected.

Acetaminophen is extensively metabolized and excreted in urine primarily as inactive glucuronate and sulfate conjugates (94%). About 4% is metabolized via cytochrome P450 oxidase to a toxic metabolite normally detoxified by preferential conjugation with cellular glutathione and excreted in urine as conjugates of cysteine and mercapturic acid. When APAP is used chronically or taken acutely in large doses, glutathione stores are depleted and hepatic necrosis may occur; 2% is excreted unchanged. Half-life is slightly prolonged in neonates and in cirrhotics.

Contraindications

Hypersensitivity to acetaminophen.

Warnings

➤*Dosage:* Do not exceed recommended dosage.

➤*Hepatotoxicity:* Hepatotoxicity and severe hepatic failure occurred in chronic alcoholics following therapeutic doses. The hepatotoxicity is believed to be caused by induction of hepatic microsomal enzymes resulting in an increase in toxic metabolites or by the reduced amount of glutathione responsible for conjugating toxic metabolites. A safe dose for a chronic alcohol abuser has not been determined. Caution chronic alcoholics to limit acetaminophen intake to ≤ 2 g/day.

➤*Hypersensitivity reactions:* If a sensitivity reaction occurs, discontinue use.

➤*Pregnancy: Category B.* Acetaminophen crosses the placenta. It is routinely used during all stages of pregnancy; when used in therapeutic doses, it appears safe for short-term use. Continuous high daily dosage probably caused severe anemia in a mother, and the neonate had fatal kidney disease. Although there is no evidence of a relationship between acetaminophen ingestion and congenital malformations, 3 cases of congenital hip dislocation may have been associated with acetaminophen.

➤*Lactation:* Acetaminophen is excreted in breast milk in low concentrations with reported milk:plasma ratios of 0.91 to 1.42 at 1 and 12 hours, respectively. No adverse effects in nursing infants were reported.

➤*Children:* Consult physician for use > 5 days (children), > 10 days (adults) or > 3 days for fever (adults and children).

Precautions

➤*Severe or recurrent pain or high or continued fever:* Severe or recurrent pain or high or continued fever may indicate serious illness. If pain persists for > 5 days or if redness or swelling is present, consult physician.

Drug Interactions

The potential hepatotoxicity of APAP may be increased by large doses or long-term administration of the following agents because of hepatic microsomal enzyme induction. The therapeutic effects of APAP may also be decreased.
- Barbiturates
- Carbamazepine
- Hydantoins
- Isoniazid
- Rifampin
- Sulfinpyrazone

Acetaminophen Drug Interactions			
Precipitant drug	Object drug*		Description
Alcohol, ethyl	APAP	↑	Hepatotoxicity has occurred in chronic alcoholics following various dose levels (moderate to excessive) of acetaminophen.
Anticholinergics	APAP	↓	The onset of acetaminophen effect may be delayed or decreased slightly, but the ultimate pharmacological effect is not significantly affected by anticholinergics.
Beta blockers, propranolol	APAP	↑	Propranolol appears to inhibit the enzyme systems responsible for the glucuronidation and oxidation of acetaminophen. Therefore, the pharmacologic effects of acetaminophen may be increased.
Charcoal, activated	APAP	↓	Reduces acetaminophen absorption when administered as soon as possible after overdose.

Acetaminophen Drug Interactions			
Precipitant drug	Object drug*		Description
Contraceptives, oral	APAP	↓	Increase in glucuronidation resulting in increased plasma clearance and a decreased half-life of acetaminophen.
Probenecid	APAP	↑	Probenecid may increase the therapeutic effectiveness of acetaminophen slightly.
APAP	Lamotrigine	↓	Serum lamotrigine concentrations may be reduced, producing a decrease in therapeutic effects.
APAP	Loop diuretics	↓	The effects of the loop diuretic may be decreased because APAP may decrease renal prostaglandin excretion and decrease plasma renin activity.
APAP	Zidovudine	↓	The pharmacologic effects of zidovudine may be decreased because of enhanced nonhepatic or renal clearance of zidovudine.

* ↑ = Object drug increased. ↓ = Object drug decreased.

➤*Drug/Lab test interactions:* Acetaminophen may interfere with home blood glucose measurement systems; decreases of > 20% in mean glucose values may be noted. This effect appears to be drug, concentration and system dependent.

Adverse Reactions

➤*Hematologic:* Hemolytic anemia; neutropenia; leukopenia; pancytopenia; thrombocytopenia.

➤*Hypersensitivity:* Skin eruptions; urticarial and erythematous skin reactions; fever.

➤*Miscellaneous:* Hypoglycemic coma; jaundice.

Overdosage

➤*Symptoms:* Acute poisoning may be manifested by nausea, vomiting, drowsiness, confusion, liver tenderness, low blood pressure, cardiac arrhythmias, jaundice and acute hepatic and renal failure. These occur within the first 24 hours and may persist for ≥ 1 week. Death has occurred because of liver necrosis. Acute renal failure may also occur. However, there are often no specific early symptoms or signs.

The course of APAP poisoning is divided into 4 stages (postingestion time):

Stage 1: (12-24 hours) – Nausea, vomiting, diaphoresis, anorexia;

Stage 2: (24-48 hours) – Clinically improved; AST, ALT, bilirubin and prothrombin levels begin to rise;

Stage 3: (72-96 hours) – Peak hepatotoxicity; AST of 20,000 not unusual;

Stage 4: (7-8 days) – Recovery.

Hepatotoxicity – Hepatotoxicity may result. The minimal toxic dose is 10 g (140 mg/kg), but liver damage has occurred with a single 5.85 g dose; ≥ 20 to 25 g are potentially fatal. Children appear less susceptible to toxicity than adults because they have less capacity for glucuronidation metabolism. Initial signs of toxicity may include nausea, vomiting, anorexia, malaise, diaphoresis, abdominal pain and diarrhea. Hepatotoxicity usually is not apparent for 48 to 72 hours. If an acute dose of ≥ 150 mg/kg was ingested, or if the dose cannot be determined, obtain a serum acetaminophen assay after 4 hours following ingestion. If in the toxic range, obtain liver function studies and repeat at 24-hour intervals. Hepatic failure may lead to encephalopathy, coma and death.

Plasma acetaminophen levels > 300 mcg/ml at 4 hours postingestion were associated with hepatic damage in 90% of patients; minimal hepatic damage is anticipated if plasma levels at 4 hours are < 120 mcg/ml or < 30 mcg/ml at 12 hours after ingestion.

Chronic excessive use (> 4 g/day) eventually may lead to transient hepatotoxicity. The kidneys may undergo tubular necrosis; the myocardium may be damaged.

➤*Treatment:* Perform gastric lavage in all cases, preferably within 4 hours of ingestion.

Refer also to General Management of Acute Overdosage.

Oral **N-acetylcysteine** is a specific antidote for APAP toxicity. Administration IV can cause anaphylaxis. If patient vomits within 1 hour of administration of **N-acetylcysteine,** repeat the dose. Refer to the Acetylcysteine monograph in the Respiratory Drugs chapter for complete prescribing information and for a specific nomogram to guide treatment.

Patient Information

Severe or recurrent pain or high or continued fever may indicate serious illness. If pain persists for > 5 days or if redness or swelling is present, consult physician.

Do not exceed the recommended dosage. Consult physician for use > 5 days (children), > 10 days (adults) or > 3 days for fever (adults and children).

Indications

Mild to moderate pain; fever; various inflammatory conditions such as rheumatic fever, rheumatoid arthritis and osteoarthritis.

➤*Aspirin:* Aspirin, for reducing the risk of recurrent transient ischemic attacks (TIAs) or stroke in men who have had transient ischemia of the brain due to fibrin platelet emboli. It has not been effective in women and is of no benefit for completed strokes.

➤*Aspirin:* Aspirin, to reduce the risk of death or nonfatal myocardial infarction (MI) in patients with previous infarction or unstable angina pectoris.

➤*Unlabeled uses:* Possible effect of long-term aspirin-like analgesics to prevent cataract formation is being studied. Dipyridamole is often added to aspirin to prevent MI and stroke, but data do not show improved antithrombotic aspirin efficacy during coadministration. Low-dose aspirin may help prevent toxemia of pregnancy and may be beneficial in pregnant women with inadequate uteroplacental blood flow (eg, systemic lupus erythematosus). Further studies are needed. See Warnings.

Actions

➤*Pharmacology:* The salicylates have analgesic, antipyretic and anti-inflammatory effects. **Aspirin** and other salicylic acid derivatives are hydrolyzed to salicylic acid. Salicylamide and **diflunisal** are structurally related, but are not true salicylates because they are not hydrolyzed to salicylic acid.

Salicylates have analgesic, antipyretic, anti-inflammatory and antirheumatic effects. The pharmacological effects of these agents are qualitatively similar. Salicylates lower elevated body temperature through vasodilation of peripheral vessels, thus enhancing dissipation of excess heat. The anti-inflammatory and analgesic activity may be mediated through inhibition of the prostaglandin synthetase enzyme complex.

Aspirin – Aspirin differs from the other agents in this group in that it more potently inhibits prostaglandin synthesis, has greater anti-inflammatory effects and irreversibly inhibits platelet aggregation. The aspirin molecule's acetyl group is believed to account for these differences. Aspirin inhibits prostaglandin production by acetylating cyclo-oxygenase, the initial enzyme in the prostaglandin biosynthesis pathway.

Irreversible inhibition of platelet aggregation (aspirin) – Single analgesic aspirin doses prolong bleeding time. Acetylation of platelet cyclo-oxygenase prevents synthesis of thromboxane A_2, a prostaglandin derivative, which is a potent vasoconstrictor and inducer of platelet aggregation and platelet release reaction. Aspirin (no other salicylates) inhibits platelet aggregation for the life of the platelet (7 to 10 days).

Aspirin has shown some success as an antiplatelet agent in patients with thromboembolic disease. Low doses of aspirin inhibit platelet aggregation and may be more effective than higher doses. Larger doses inhibit cyclo-oxygenase in arterial walls, interfering with prostacyclin production, a potent vasodilator and inhibitor of platelet aggregation. Combinations of dipyridamole or sulfinpyrazone with aspirin have been recommended for antithrombotic action for prophylaxis in various high risk situations (ie, coronary bypass graft patency, total hip replacement).

Myocardial infarction (MI) – **Aspirin** use in MI patients was associated with ≈ 20% reduction in risk of subsequent death and nonfatal reinfarction, a median absolute decrease of 3% from the 12% to 22% event rates with placebo. Daily aspirin dosage in post-MI studies was 300 mg in one and 900 to 1500 mg in five. In aspirin-treated unstable angina patients (325 mg/day), reduction in risk was about 50%, a reduction in event rate of 5% from the 10% rate with placebo over the 12-week study.

In the Aspirin Myocardial Infarction Study (AMIS) trial, 1 g/day was associated with small increases in systolic BP (average, 1.5 to 2.1 mmHg) and diastolic BP (0.5 to 0.6 mmHg). Uric acid levels and BUN increased by < 1 mg/dl.

In the Second International Study of Infarct Survival (ISIS-2) trial, patients who received a combination of aspirin (160 mg/day) and streptokinase after the onset of suspected acute MI had significantly fewer reinfarctions, strokes and deaths than those patients who received placebo. Also, the combination was significantly better than either drug alone; their separate effects on vascular deaths appeared additive.

Other pharmacological actions – Inhibition of prothrombin synthesis and prolonged prothrombin time are clinically significant only after large doses (≥ 6 g/day). Doses > 3 to 5 g/day have a uricosuric effect; low doses (< 2 g/day) decrease uric acid secretion.

➤*Pharmacokinetics:*

Absorption/Distribution – Salicylates are rapidly and completely absorbed after oral use. Bioavailability is dependent on the dosage form, presence of food, gastric emptying time, gastric pH, presence of antacids or buffering agents and particle size. Bioavailability of some enteric coated products may be erratic. Food slows the absorption of salicylates. Absorption from rectal suppositories is slower, resulting in lower salicylate levels. **Aspirin** is partially hydrolyzed to salicylic acid during absorption and is distributed to all body tissues and fluids, including fetal tissues, breast milk and CNS. Highest concentrations are found in plasma, liver, renal cortex, heart and lungs. Protein binding of salicylates is concentration-dependent. At low therapeutic concentrations (100 mcg/ml), ≈ 90% is bound; at higher plasma concentrations (400 mcg/ml), 76% is bound. Signs of salicylism (eg, tinnitus) occur at serum levels > 200 mcg/ml; severe toxic effects may occur at levels > 400 mcg/ml (see Adverse Reactions).

Metabolism/Excretion – Salicylic acid is eliminated by renal excretion and by oxidation and conjugation of metabolites. **Aspirin** has a half-life of ≈ 15 to 20 minutes. Salicylic acid has a half-life of 2 to 3 hours at low doses; at higher doses, it may exceed 20 hours. In therapeutic anti-inflammatory doses, half-life ranges from 6 to 12 hours. Plasma salicylate levels increase disproportionately as dosage is increased. Elimination is determined by zero order kinetics. Renal excretion of unchanged drug depends upon urine pH. As urinary pH changes from 5 to 8, renal clearance of free ionized salicylate increases from 2% to 3% of amount excreted to > 80%.

Contraindications

Hypersensitivity to salicylates or nonsteroidal anti-inflammatory drugs (NSAIDs). Use extreme caution in patients with history of adverse reactions to salicylates. Cross-sensitivity may exist between aspirin and other NSAIDs which inhibit prostaglandin synthesis, and aspirin and tartrazine. Aspirin cross-sensitivity does not appear to occur with sodium salicylate, salicylamide or choline salicylate. Aspirin hypersensitivity is more prevalent in those with asthma, nasal polyposis, chronic urticaria.

In hemophilia, bleeding ulcers and hemorrhagic states.

➤*Magnesium salicylate:* Magnesium salicylate in advanced chronic renal insufficiency due to magnesium retention.

Warnings

➤*Reye's syndrome:*

Salicylate association – Use of salicylates, particularly **aspirin**, in children or teenagers with influenza or chickenpox may be associated with development of Reye's syndrome. This rare, acute, life-threatening condition is characterized by vomiting, lethargy and belligerence that may progress to delirium and coma. Mortality rate is 20% to 30%; permanent brain damage has been reported in survivors.

A causal relationship is controversial, but CDC, FDA, American Academy of Pediatrics' Committee on Infectious Diseases and Surgeon General advise against salicylate use in children and teens with influenza or chickenpox. (See Warning Box.)

➤*Otic effects:* Discontinue use if dizziness, ringing in ears (tinnitus) or impaired hearing occurs. Tinnitus probably represents blood salicylic acid levels reaching or exceeding the upper limit of the therapeutic range. It is a helpful guide to dose titration. Temporary hearing loss disappears gradually upon discontinuation of the drug.

➤*Use in surgical patients:* Avoid **aspirin**, if possible, for 1 week prior to surgery because of the possibility of postoperative bleeding.

➤*Hypersensitivity reactions:* **Aspirin** intolerance, manifested by acute bronchospasm, generalized urticaria/angioedema, severe rhinitis or shock occurs in 4% to 19% of asthmatics. Symptoms occur within 3 hours after ingestion. The aspirin triad consists of the association of asthma, nasal polyps and aspirin intolerance. Have epinephrine 1:1000 immediately available. Refer to Management of Acute Hypersensitivity Reactions.

Foods – Foods may contribute to a reaction. Some foods with 6 mg/100 g salicylate include curry powder, paprika, licorice, Benedictine liqueur, prunes, raisins, tea, gherkins. A typical American diet contains 10 to 200 mg/day salicylate.

Desensitization – Desensitization has been successfully induced and maintained. Perform in hospital; generally maintain with one **aspirin**/day. Any NSAID can maintain desensitization. However, if maintenance is interrupted, sensitivity will reappear (2 to 5 days).

➤*Hepatic function impairment:* Use caution in liver damage, pre-existing hypoprothrombinemia and vitamin K deficiency. Reversible hepatic encephalopathy occurred in a chronic alcoholic with cirrhosis who took ASA 5 g/day for osteoarthritis. Aspirin-induced hepatotoxicity occurred after therapeutic doses for rheumatoid arthritis.

➤*Pregnancy: Category D* (aspirin); *Category C* (salsalate, magnesium salicylate). **Aspirin** may produce adverse maternal effects: Anemia, ante- or postpartum hemorrhage, prolonged gestation and labor. Salicylates readily cross the placenta. By inhibiting prostaglandin synthesis, salicylates may cause constriction of ductus arteriosus, and, possibly, other untoward fetal effects. Maternal aspirin use during later stages of pregnancy may cause adverse fetal effects: Low birth weight, increased incidence of intracranial hemorrhage in premature infants, stillbirths, neonatal death. Salicylates may be teratogens. Avoid use during pregnancy, especially in third trimester.

➤*Lactation:* Salicylates are excreted in breast milk in low concentrations, producing peak milk levels ranging from 1.1 to 10 mcg/ml. Adverse effects on platelet function in the nursing infant have not been reported, but are a potential risk.

➤*Children:* Safety and efficacy of **magnesium salicylate** or **salsalate** have not been established. Administration of **aspirin** to children (including teenagers) with acute febrile illness has been associated with the development of Reye's syndrome. Dehydrated febrile children appear more prone to salicylate intoxication.

Precautions

➤*Renal effects:* Use with caution in chronic renal insufficiency; **aspirin** may cause a transient decrease in renal function, and may aggravate chronic kidney diseases (rare).

In patients with renal impairment, take precautions when administering **magnesium salicylate**. Discontinue other drugs containing magnesium and monitor serum magnesium levels if dosage levels of magnesium salicylate are high.

➤*GI effects:* Use caution in those intolerant to salicylate because of GI irritation, and in gastric ulcers, peptic ulcer, mild diabetes, gout, erosive gastritis or bleeding tendencies. **Salsalate** and **choline salicylate** may cause less GI irritation than **aspirin**.

Although fecal blood loss is less with enteric coated aspirin than with uncoated, give enteric coated aspirin with caution to patients with GI distress, ulcer or bleeding problems. Occult GI bleeding occurs in many patients but is not correlated with gastric distress. The amount of blood lost is usually clinically insignificant (average, 2.5 ml), but with prolonged use, it may result in iron deficiency anemia. Patients developing peptic ulcers while taking salicylates for rheumatic disease have healed during treatment with cimetidine and antacids despite continued salicylate use. In addition, although acute aspirin use results in mucosal lesions, only 20% to 25% of those on chronic aspirin for rheumatism develop mucosal injury.

➤*Hematologic effects:* **Aspirin** interferes with hemostasis. Avoid use if patients have severe anemia, history of blood coagulation defects, or take anticoagulants (see Drug Interactions).

➤*Long-term therapy:* To avoid potentially toxic concentrations, warn patients on long-term therapy not to take other salicylates (nonprescription analgesics, etc).

Periodically monitor plasma salicylic acid concentrations during long-term treatment to aid maintenance of therapeutic levels (100 to 300 mcg/ml). Toxic manifestations are not usually seen until concentrations exceed 300 mcg/ml. Monitor urinary pH regularly; sudden acidification, as from pH 6.5 to 5.5, can double the plasma level, resulting in toxicity.

➤*Salicylism:* Salicylism may require dosage adjustment.

➤*Controlled release aspirin:* Controlled release aspirin, because of its relatively long onset of action, is not recommended for antipyresis or short-term analgesia. Not recommended in children > 12; contraindicated in all children with fever accompanied by dehydration.

➤*Benzyl alcohol:* Some of these products contain the preservative benzyl alcohol, which has been associated with a fatal "gasping syndrome" in premature infants.

➤*Tartrazine sensitivity:* Some of these products contain tartrazine, which may cause allergic-type reactions (including bronchial asthma) in susceptible individuals. Although the incidence of tartrazine sensitivity in the general population is low, it is frequently seen in patients who also have aspirin hypersensitivity. Specific products containing tartrazine are identified in the product listings.

Drug Interactions

Salicylate Drug Interactions			
Precipitant drug	Object drug*		Description
Alcohol	Salicylates	↑	The risk of GI ulceration increases when salicylates are given concomitantly. Ingestion of alcohol during salicylate therapy may also prolong bleeding time.
Ammonium chloride	Salicylates	↑	Urinary acidifiers decrease salicylate excretion.
Ascorbic acid			
Methionine			
Antacids	Salicylates	↓	Antacids and urinary alkalinizers may decrease the pharmacologic effects of salicylates. Urinary alkalinization increases the renal excretion of salicylic acid due to decreased tubular reabsorption of un-ionized drug. The magnitude of the antacid interaction depends on the agent, dose and pretreatment urine pH.
Urinary alkalinizers			
Carbonic anhydrase inhibitors	Salicylates	↑	Salicylate intoxication has occurred after coadministration of these agents. However, salicylic acid renal elimination may be increased if urine is kept alkaline. Conversely, salicylates may displace acetazolamide from protein binding sites resulting in toxicity. Further study is needed.
Salicylates	Carbonic anhydrase inhibitors		
Charcoal, activated	Aspirin	↓	Coadministration decreases aspirin absorption, depending on charcoal dose and interval between ingestion. May be useful (see Overdosage).
Corticosteroids	Salicylates	↓	Corticosteroids increase salicylate clearance and decrease serum levels.
Nizatidine	Salicylates	↑	Increased serum salicylate levels have occurred in patients receiving high dose aspirin (3.9 g/day) and concurrent nizatidine.
Aspirin	Anticoagulants, oral	↑	Therapeutic aspirin has an additive hypoprothrombinemic effect. Impaired platelet function may prolong bleeding time. Use caution.
Anticoagulants, oral	Aspirin		
Aspirin	Heparin	↑	Aspirin can increase bleeding risk in heparin anticoagulated patients.
Aspirin	Nitroglycerin	↑	Nitroglycerin, when taken with aspirin, may result in unexpected hypotension. Data are limited. If hypotension occurs, reduce the nitroglycerin dose.
Aspirin	NSAIDs	↓	Aspirin may decrease NSAID serum concentrations. Concomitant use offers no advantage and may significantly increase incidence of GI effects.
Aspirin	Valproic acid	↑	Aspirin displaces the drug from its protein-binding sites and may decrease its total body clearance, thus increasing the pharmacologic effects.
Salicylates	Angiotensin-converting enzyme inhibitors	↓	Antihypertensive effectiveness of these agents may be decreased by concurrent salicylate administration, possibly due to prostaglandin inhibition. Consider discontinuing salicylates if problems occur.
Salicylates	Beta-adrenergic blockers	↓	Beta-adrenergic blockers may have their antihypertensive action blunted by concurrent salicylate administration, possibly due to prostaglandin inhibition. Consider discontinuing salicylates if problems occur.
Salicylates	Loop diuretics	↓	Loop diuretics may be less effective when given with salicylates in patients with compromised renal function or with cirrhosis with ascites; however, data conflict.
Salicylates	Methotrexate	↑	Salicylates increase drug levels causing toxicity by interfering with protein binding and renal elimination of the antimetabolite.
Salicylates	Probenecid	↓	Salicylates antagonize the uricosuric effect of probenecid and sulfinpyrazone. While salicylates in large doses (> 3 g/day) have a uricosuric effect, smaller amounts may reduce the uricosuric effect of these agents.
	Sulfinpyrazone		
Salicylates	Spironolactone	↓	Salicylates may inhibit the diuretic effects; antihypertensive action does not appear altered. Effects depend on the dose of spironolactone.
Salicylates	Sulfonylureas	↑	Salicylates in doses > 2 g/day have a hypoglycemic action, perhaps by altering pancreatic beta cell function. They may potentiate the glucose-lowering effect of these drugs.
	Insulin		

* ↑ = Object drug increased. ↓ = Object drug decreased.

► *Drug/Lab test interactions:* Salicylates compete with thyroid hormone for binding sites on thyroid binding pre-albumin and possibly thyroid-binding globulin resulting in increases in **protein bound iodine (PBI)**. Salicylates probably do not interfere with T_3 resin uptake.

Serum uric acid – Serum uric acid levels are elevated by salicylate levels < 10 mg/dl and decreased by levels > 10 mg/dl. Combined **phenylbutazone** and salicylates decrease uric acid excretion and may increase serum uric acid by an average of 2 mg/dl.

Salicylates in moderate to large (anti-inflammatory) doses cause false-negative readings for **urine glucose** by the glucose oxidase method and false-positive readings by the copper reduction method.

Salicylates in the urine interfere with **5–HIAA** determinations by fluorescent methods, but not by the nitrosonaphthol colorimetric method.

Salicylates in the urine interact with **urinary ketone** determinations by the ferric chloride (Gerhardt) method producing a reddish color.

Large doses may decrease urinary excretion of **PSP (phenolsulfonphthalein)**.

Salicylates in the urine result in falsely elevated **VMA (vanillylmandelic acid)** with most tests, but falsely decrease VMA determinations by the Pisano method.

Adverse Reactions

► *Dermatologic:* Hives, rashes and angioedema may occur, especially in patients suffering from chronic urticaria.

► *GI:* Nausea, dyspepsia (5% to 25%), heartburn, epigastric discomfort, anorexia, acute reversible hepatotoxicity, massive GI bleeding and occult blood loss may occur. Aspirin may potentiate peptic ulcer.

Chronic aspirin use may cause persistent iron deficiency anemia.

► *Hematologic:* Prolongation of bleeding time, leukopenia, thrombocytopenia, purpura, decreased plasma iron concentration, shortened erythrocyte survival time.

► *Hepatic:* High aspirin doses reportedly produced reversible hepatic dysfunction.

► *Miscellaneous:* Fever, thirst, dimness of vision.

Allergic reactions – Allergic and anaphylactic reactions were noted when hypersensitive individuals took aspirin. Fatal anaphylactic shock, while not common, has been reported.

Aspirin intolerance – Aspirin intolerance, manifested by exacerbation of bronchospasm and rhinitis, may occur in patients with a history of nasal polyps, asthma or rhinitis. The mechanism of this intolerance may be the result of aspirin-induced shunting of prostaglandin synthesis to the lipoxygenase pathway and liberation of leukotrienes, ie, slow-reacting substance of anaphylaxis.

Salicylism – Mild "salicylism" may occur after repeated use of large doses and consists of dizziness, tinnitus (manifested as musical perceptions in one patient), difficulty hearing, nausea, vomiting, diarrhea, mental confusion, CNS depression, headache, sweating, hyperventilation and lassitude. Salicylate serum concentrations correlate with pharmacological actions and adverse effects observed. See table below:

Serum Salicylate: Clinical Correlations		
Serum salicylate concentration (mcg/ml)	Desired effects	Adverse effects/ intoxication
≈ 100	Antiplatelet Antipyresis Analgesia	GI intolerance and bleeding, hypersensitivity, hemostatic defects
150-300	Anti-inflammatory	Mild salicylism
250-400	Treatment of rheumatic fever	Nausea/vomiting, hyperventilation, salicylism, flushing, sweating, thirst, headache, diarrhea, and tachycardia

Serum Salicylate: Clinical Correlations		
Serum salicylate concentration (mcg/ml)	Desired effects	Adverse effects/ intoxication
> 400-500		Respiratory alkalosis, hemorrhage, excitement, confusion, asterixis, pulmonary edema, convulsions, tetany, metabolic acidosis, fever, coma, cardiovascular collapse, renal and respiratory failure

Overdosage

► *Symptoms:*
Acute lethal dose (approximate) –
  Adults: 10 to 30 g.
  Children: 4 g.

Respiratory alkalosis is seen initially in acute salicylate ingestions. Hyperpnea and tachypnea occur as a result of increased CO_2 production and a direct stimulatory effect of salicylate on the respiratory center. Other symptoms may include nausea, vomiting, hypokalemia, tinnitus, neurologic abnormalities (eg, disorientation, irritability, hallucinations, lethargy, stupor, coma, seizures), dehydration, hyperthermia, hyperventilation, hyperactivity, thrombocytopenia, platelet dysfunction, hypoprothrombinemia, increased capillary fragility and other hematologic abnormalities. Symptoms may progress quickly to depression, coma, respiratory failure and collapse. Although blood glucose is usually normal or slightly elevated, hypoglycemia may occur with chronic toxicity or in late acute toxicity. A mixed respiratory alkalosis and metabolic acidosis may also develop.

Chronic salicylate toxicity may occur when > 100 mg/kg/day is ingested for 2 or more days. It is more difficult to recognize and is associated with increased morbidity and mortality. Compared to acute poisoning, hyperventilation, dehydration, systemic acidosis and severe CNS manifestations occur more frequently.

► *Treatment:* Initial treatment includes induction of emesis or gastric lavage to remove any unabsorbed drug from the stomach. Activated charcoal diminishes salicylate absorption, most effectively if given within 2 hours after ingestion. Monitor salicylate levels, acid-base and fluid and electrolyte balance. Further therapy is largely supportive. Refer to General Management of Acute Overdosage. Reduce hyperthermia; treat severe convulsions with diazepam. Forced alkaline diuresis will enhance renal excretion of salicylates. Hemodialysis is very efficient in eliminating salicylate, but use only in patients who are severely poisoned, and in those with noncardiogenic pulmonary edema, severe CNS symptoms, renal failure, acidosis refractory to conservative therapy or clinical deterioration despite other therapies. Rarely, IV vitamin K may be indicated to correct hypoprothrombinemia.

Patient Information

May cause GI upset; take with food or after meals.

Do not crush or chew sustained release preparations.

Take with a full glass of water (240 ml) to reduce the risk of lodging medication in the esophagus.

Patients allergic to tartrazine dye should avoid **aspirin**.

Notify physician if ringing in ears or persistent GI pain occurs.

Do not use **aspirin** if it has a strong vinegar-like odor.

ASPIRIN (Acetylsalicylic Acid; ASA)

otc	**Bayer Children's Aspirin** (Bayer)	**Tablets, chewable:** 81 mg	Saccharin. (BAYER BAYER BAYER BAYER). Orange flavor. In 36s.
otc	**St. Joseph Adult Chewable Aspirin** (Schering-Plough)		Saccharin. (SJ). Orange flavor. In 36s.
otc	**Aspergum** (Schering-Plough)	**Gum tablets:** 227.5 mg	Chewable. Glucose, saccharin, sugar. Orange or cherry flavor. In 16s, 40s.
otc	**Aspirin** (Various, eg, Moore, Parmed, Rugby, URL, Warner-C)	**Tablets:** 325 mg	In 100s, 200s, 250s, 500s and 1000s.
otc	**Genuine Bayer Aspirin Caplets** (Bayer)		**Caplets:** (BAYER BAYER BAYER BAYER). Film coated. In 50s, 100s and 200s.
otc	**Empirin** (GlaxoWellcome)		(Tabloid brand). White. In 50s, 100s and 250s.
otc	**Aspirin** (URL)	**Tablets:** 500 mg	In 100s.
otc	**Arthritis Foundation Pain Reliever** (McNeil-CPC)		In 50s.
otc	**Maximum Bayer Aspirin Tablets and Caplets** (Bayer)		**Tablets:** Film coated. In 30s, 60s and 100s.
			Caplets: Film coated. In 30s and 60s.
otc	**Norwich Extra-Strength** (Procter & Gamble)		In 150s.

ASPIRIN (Acetylsalicylic Acid; ASA)

otc	Ecotrin Adult Low Strength (SmithKline Beecham)	Tablets, enteric coated: 81 mg	Tartrazine. (ECOTRIN LOW). In 36s.
otc	Halfprin 81 (Kramer)		In 90s.
otc	Heartline (BDI)		In 36s.
otc	½ Halfprin (Kramer)	Tablets, enteric coated: 165 mg	Red. In 60s and 200s.
otc	Aspirin (Various, eg, Geneva, Major, Moore, Parmed, Rugby, URL)	Tablets, enteric coated: 325 mg	In 30s, 60s, 90s, 100s, 1000s and UD 100s.
otc	Ecotrin Tablets and Caplets (SmithKline Beecham)		Tablets: (Ecotrin Reg). In 100s, 250s and 1000s.
			Caplets: (Ecotrin Reg). In 100s.
otc	Ecotrin Maximum Strength Caplets (SmithKline Beecham)	Tablets, enteric coated: 500 mg	Caplets: (Ecotrin Max). In 60s.
otc	Extra Strength Bayer Enteric 500 Aspirin (Bayer)		(Bayer 500). In 60s.
otc	Aspirin (Various, eg, Moore, Rugby)	Tablets, enteric coated: 650 mg	In 100s and 1000s.
otc	Extended Release Bayer 8-Hour Caplets (Bayer)	Tablets, extended release: 650 mg	White, scored. In 50s.
Rx	ZORprin (Boots)	Tablets, controlled release: 800 mg	(BA57). White. Elongated. In 100s.
otc	Bayer Low Adult Strength (Bayer)	Tablets, delayed release: 81 mg	Lactose. (81). In 120s.
otc	Aspirin (Various, eg, Goldline, Moore, Rugby, URL)	Suppositories[1]: 120 mg	In 12s.
		200 mg	In 12s.
		300 mg	In 12s.
		600 mg	In 12s and 100s.

[1] Refrigerate.

For complete prescribing information, refer to the Salicylates group monograph.

Administration and Dosage

➤*Minor aches and pains:* 325 to 650 mg every 4 hours as needed. Some extra strength (500 mg) products suggest 500 mg every 3 hours or 1000 mg every 6 hours.

➤*Arthritis, other rheumatic conditions (eg, osteoarthritis):* 3.2 to 6 g/day in divided doses.

Juvenile rheumatoid arthritis – 60 to 110 mg/kg/day in divided doses (every 6 to 8 hours). When starting at lower doses (eg, 60 mg/kg/day), may increase by 20 mg/kg/day after 5 to 7 days, followed by 10 mg/kg/day after another 5 to 7 days.

Maintain a serum salicylate level of 150 to 300 mcg/ml.

➤*Acute rheumatic fever:*

Adults – 5 to 8 g/day, initially.

Children – 100 mg/kg/day for 2 weeks, then 75 mg/kg/day for 4 to 6 weeks.

Therapeutic salicylate level – Therapeutic salicylate level is 150 to 300 mcg/ml.

➤*Transient ischemic attacks in men:* 1300 mg/day in divided doses (650 mg 2 times daily, or 325 mg 4 times daily). One study indicated that a dose of 300 mg/day is as effective as the larger dose and may be associated with fewer side effects.

➤*Myocardial infarction prophylaxis:* 300 or 325 mg/day. This use applies to solid oral doseforms (buffered and plain) and to buffered aspirin in solution.

➤*Children:*

Analgesic/antipyretic dosage – 10 to 15 mg/kg/dose every 4 hours (see table), up to 60 to 80 mg/kg/day. Do not use in children or teenagers with chickenpox or flu symptoms due to the possibility of Reye's syndrome (see Warnings). Dosage recommendations by age and weight are as follows:

Recommended Aspirin Dosage in Children					
Age (years)	Weight		Dosage (mg every 4 hours)	No. of 81 mg tablets (every 4 hours)	No. of 325 mg tablets (every 4 hours)
	lbs	kg			
2-3	24-35	10.6-15.9	162	2	½
4-5	36-47	16-21.4	243	3	
6-8	48-59	21.5-26.8	324	4	1
9-10	60-71	26.9-32.3	405	5	
11	72-95	32.4-43.2	486	6	1½
12-14	≥ 96	≥ 43.3	648	8	2

Kawasaki disease (mucocutaneous lymph node syndrome) – For acute febrile period, 80 to 180 mg/kg/day; very high doses may be needed to achieve therapeutic levels. After the fever resolves, dosage may be adjusted to 10 mg/kg/day.

ASPIRIN (Acetylsalicylic Acid; ASA), BUFFERED

otc	Tri-Buffered Bufferin Tablets and Caplets (Bristol-Myers Squibb)	Tablets: 325 mg with calcium carbonate, magnesium oxide and magnesium carbonate	Tablets: (B). White. In 12s, 36s, 60s, 100s, 200s, 275s, 1000s.
			Caplets: (B). White, scored. In 36s, 60s and 100s.
otc	Buffered Aspirin (Various, eg, Geneva, Goldline, Major, Moore, Rugby, UDL, URL)	Tablets: 325 mg with buffers	In 100s, 500s, 1000s and UD 100s and 200s.
otc	Bayer Buffered Aspirin (Bayer)		(Bayer Buffered). In 100s.
otc	Asprimox (Invamed)	Caplets: 325 mg with buffers	In 100s and 500s.
otc	Asprimox Extra Protection for Arthritis Pain (Invamed)		In 100s and 500s.
otc	Adprin-B (Pfeiffer)	Tablets, coated: 325 mg with calcium carbonate, magnesium carbonate and magnesium oxide	In 130s.
otc	Asprimox (Invamed)	Tablets, coated: 325 mg with 75 mg aluminum hydroxide, 75 mg magnesium hydroxide and calcium carbonate	Capsule shape. In 100s and 500s.
otc	Magnaprin (Rugby)	Tablets, coated: 325 mg with 50 mg magnesium hydroxide, 50 mg aluminum hydroxide and calcium carbonate	Film coated. In 100s and 500s.
otc	Ascriptin (Rhone-Poulenc Rorer)		(Ascriptin). In 60s.
otc	Ascriptin A/D (Rhone-Poulenc Rorer)	Tablets, coated: 325 mg with 75 mg magnesium hydroxide, 75 mg aluminum hydroxide and calcium carbonate	(AP Ascriptin). Capsule shape. In 225s.
otc	Magnaprin Arthritis Strength Captabs (Rugby)		Capsule shape. In 100s and 500s.
otc	Bufferin (Bristol-Myers)	Tablets, coated: 325 mg with 158 mg calcium carbonate, 63 mg magnesium oxide and 34 mg magnesium carbonate	(B). In 12s, 36s, 60s, 100s, 200s and UD 150s.

ASPIRIN (Acetylsalicylic Acid; ASA), BUFFERED

otc	**Extra Strength Bayer Plus Caplets** (Bayer)	**Tablets:** 500 mg with calcium carbonate, magnesium carbonate and magnesium oxide	In 30s and 60s.
otc	**Ascriptin Extra Strength** (Rhone-Poulenc Rorer)	**Tablets, coated:** 500 mg with 80 mg magnesium hydroxide, 80 mg aluminum hydroxide and calcium carbonate	Capsule shape. In 50s.
otc	**Arthritis Pain Formula** (Whitehall)	**Tablets:** 500 mg with 100 mg magnesium hydroxide and 27 mg aluminum hydroxide	Capsule shape. In 40s, 100s, and 175s.
otc	**Alka-Seltzer with Aspirin** (Bayer)	**Tablets, effervescent:** 325 mg with 1.9 g sodium bicarbonate and 1 g citric acid per dry tablet, 567 mg sodium/tablet	In 12s, 24s, 36s, 72s, 96s, and 100s.
otc	**Alka-Seltzer with Aspirin (Flavored)** (Bayer)	**Tablets, effervescent:** 325 mg with 1.7 g sodium bicarbonate and 1.2 g citric acid per dry tablet, 506 mg sodium/tablet	Saccharin and flavoring. In 12s, 24s and 36s.
otc	**Alka-Seltzer Extra Strength with Aspirin** (Bayer)	**Tablet, effervescent:** 500 mg with 1.9 g sodium bicarbonate and 1 g citric acid	In 12s and 24s.
otc	**Asprimox Extra Protection for Arthritis Pain** (Invamed)	**Tablets :** 325 mg with 75 mg aluminum hydroxide, 75 mg magnesium hydroxide and calcium carbonate	Capsule shape. In 100s and 500s.

Complete prescribing information for these products begins in the Salicylates monograph.

Administration and Dosage

The addition of small amounts of antacids may decrease GI irritation and increase the dissolution and absorption rates of these products.

CHOLINE SALICYLATE

otc	**Arthropan** (Purdue Frederick)	**Liquid:** 870 mg/5 mL	Menthol. Mint flavor. In 240 mL.

Complete prescribing information for these products begins in the Salicylates monograph.

Administration and Dosage

Has fewer GI side effects than aspirin.

►*Adults and children (> 12 years):* 870 mg every 3 to 4 hours; maximum 6 times/day. Rheumatoid arthritis patients may start with 5 to 10 ml, up to 4 times/day.

DIFLUNISAL

Rx	**Diflunisal** (Various, eg, Lemmon, West Point Pharma)	**Tablets:** 250 mg	In 100s, 500s and unit-of-use 60s.
Rx	**Dolobid** (MSD)		(MSD 675). Peach. Film coated. In unit-of-use 60s and UD 100s.
Rx	**Diflunisal** (Various, eg, Lemmon, West Point Pharma)	**Tablets:** 500 mg	In 100s, 500s and unit-of-use 60s.
Rx	**Dolobid** (MSD)		(MSD 697). In UD 100s and unit-of-use 60s.

Indications

Acute or long-term symptomatic treatment of mild to moderate pain, rheumatoid arthritis and osteoarthritis.

Administration and Dosage

►*Mild to moderate pain:* Initially, 1 g, followed by 500 mg every 8 to 12 hours. A lower dosage may be appropriate; for example, 500 mg initially, followed by 250 mg every 8 to 12 hours.

►*Osteoarthritis/rheumatoid arthritis:* 500 mg to 1 g daily in 2 divided doses. Individualize dosage. Do not exceed maintenance doses higher than 1.5 g daily.

Actions

►*Pharmacology:* Diflunisal, a salicylic acid derivative, is a nonsteroidal, peripherally acting, nonnarcotic analgesic with anti-inflammatory and antipyretic properties. Chemically, it differs from aspirin and is not metabolized to salicylic acid. Its mechanisms are unknown. Diflunisal is a prostaglandin synthetase inhibitor.

►*Pharmacokinetics:*

Absorption/Distribution – Diflunisal is rapidly and completely absorbed following oral administration; peak plasma concentrations occur between 2 to 3 hours, producing significant analgesia within 1 hour and maximum analgesia within 2 to 3 hours. The first dose tends to have a slower onset of pain relief than other drugs achieving comparable peak effects. Time required to achieve steady-state increases with dosage, from 3 to 4 days with 125 mg twice daily to 7 to 9 days with 500 mg twice daily, because of its long half-life and nonlinear pharmacokinetics. An initial loading dose shortens the time to reach steady-state levels; 2 to 3 days of observation are necessary for evaluating changes in treatment regimens if a loading dose is not used. More than 99% is bound to plasma proteins.

Metabolism – Concentration-dependent pharmacokinetics prevail; doubling the dosage more than doubles drug accumulation. The plasma half-life of diflunisal is 8 to 12 hours; it increases in renal impairment. The drug is excreted in the urine as glucuronide conjugates which account for about 90% of the dose. Less than 5% is recovered in the feces.

►*Clinical trials:* Diflunisal 500 mg is comparable in analgesic efficacy but produces longer lasting responses than aspirin 650 mg, acetaminophen 600 to 650 mg and acetaminophen 650 mg with propoxyphene napsylate 100 mg. Diflunisal 1 g is comparable in analgesic efficacy to acetaminophen 600 mg with codeine 60 mg. Patients treated with diflunisal generally continue to have a good analgesic effect 8 to 12 hours after dosing.

Osteoarthritis – Diflunisal 500 or 750 mg daily was as effective as aspirin 2 or 3 g daily, and produced a lower overall incidence of GI disturbances, dizziness, edema and tinnitus.

Rheumatoid arthritis – In controlled clinical trials, diflunisal's effectiveness was established for both acute exacerbations and long-term management of rheumatoid arthritis. Activity was demonstrated by clinical improvement in the signs and symptoms of disease activity.

Diflunisal has been compared to aspirin in several controlled trials. Diflunisal dosages of 500 mg to 1 g daily have been comparable to aspirin dosages of 2 to 4 g daily for 8 to 12 weeks (up to 52 weeks in open-label extensions). Patients also generally experienced less GI effects, tinnitus, hearing loss and dyspepsia with diflunisal.

In two double-blind multicenter studies of 12 weeks' duration, diflunisal 500 or 750 mg daily was compared to ibuprofen 1.6 or 2.4 g daily or naproxen 750 mg daily; they were comparable in effectiveness and tolerability. The naproxen study was extended to 48 weeks on an open-label basis; diflunisal continued to be effective and generally well tolerated.

In patients with rheumatoid arthritis, diflunisal and gold salts may be used in combination at their usual dosage levels. The combination does not alter the course of the underlying disease but usually results in additional symptomatic relief.

Antipyretic activity – Diflunisal is not recommended for use as an antipyretic agent. In single 250, 500 or 750 mg doses, the drug produced measurable, but not clinically useful, decreases in temperature in patients with fever; however, it may mask fever in some patients, particularly with chronic or high doses.

Uricosuric effect – An increase in the renal clearance of uric acid and a decrease in serum uric acid occurred with diflunisal doses of 500 or 750 mg daily. Patients on long-term diflunisal therapy, 500 mg or 1 g daily, showed prompt and consistent reduction in mean serum uric acid levels, as much as 1.4 mg%. It is not known whether diflunisal interferes with the activity of other uricosuric agents.

Effect on platelet function – As an inhibitor of prostaglandin synthetase, diflunisal has a dose-related effect on platelet function and bleeding time. At 2 g daily, diflunisal inhibits platelet function. In contrast to aspirin, these effects were reversible because of the absence of the acetyl group. Bleeding time was only slightly increased at 1 g daily; at 2 g daily, a greater increase occurred.

Effect on fecal blood loss – Effect on fecal blood loss was not significantly different from placebo at a dose of 1 g daily. Diflunisal 2 g daily caused a statistically significant increase in fecal blood loss, but only one-half that associated with aspirin 2.6 g daily.

Contraindications

Hypersensitivity to diflunisal.

Patients in whom acute asthmatic attacks, urticaria or rhinitis are precipitated by aspirin or other nonsteroidal anti-inflammatory drugs.

DIFLUNISAL

Warnings

►*Peptic ulceration and GI bleeding:* Peptic ulceration and GI bleeding have been reported. Fatalities occurred rarely. In patients with active GI bleeding or an active peptic ulcer, weigh the benefits of therapy against possible hazards; institute an appropriate ulcer treatment regimen and monitor progress. When administered to patients with a history of GI disease, monitor closely.

►*Renal function impairment:* Because diflunisal is eliminated primarily by the kidneys, monitor patients with significant renal impairment; use a lower daily dosage.

►*Pregnancy: Category C.* Safety for use during pregnancy has not been established. Use during the first two trimesters only if the potential benefits outweigh the unknown potential hazards to the fetus. Because of the known effect of this drug class on the fetal cardiovascular system (closure of ductus arteriosus), use during the third trimester is not recommended.

►*Lactation:* Diflunisal is excreted in breast milk in concentrations 2% to 7% of that in plasma. Because of the potential for adverse reactions in nursing infants, discontinue either nursing or the drug.

►*Children:* Use in children < 12 years of age is not recommended. Safety and efficacy in infants and children have not been established.

Precautions

►*Platelet function and bleeding time:* Platelet function and bleeding time are inhibited by diflunisal at higher doses.

►*Ophthalmologic effects:* Ophthalmologic effects have been reported with these agents; perform ophthalmologic studies in patients who develop eye complaints during treatment.

►*Peripheral edema:* Peripheral edema has been observed. Use with caution in patients with compromised cardiac function, hypertension or other conditions predisposing to fluid retention.

►*Acetylsalicylic acid:* Acetylsalicylic acid has been associated with Reye's syndrome. Because diflunisal is a salicylic acid derivative, the possibility of its association with Reye's syndrome cannot be excluded.

►*Lab test abnormalities:* Borderline elevations of liver tests may occur in up to 15% of patients. These abnormalities may progress, may remain essentially unchanged or may be transient with continued therapy. Meaningful (3 times the upper limit of normal) elevations of ALT or AST occurred in < 1% of patients.

A patient with signs or symptoms suggesting liver dysfunction, or with an abnormal liver test, should be evaluated for evidence of development of more severe hepatic reactions. Severe hepatic reactions, including jaundice, have occurred with diflunisal and other NSAIDs. Although such reactions are rare, if abnormal liver tests persist or worsen, if clinical signs and symptoms consistent with liver disease develop, or if systemic manifestations occur (eg, eosinophilia, rash), discontinue drug; liver reactions can be fatal.

Drug Interactions

Diflunisal Drug Interactions			
Precipitant drug	Object drug*		Description
Diflunisal	Acetaminophen	↑	Administration of diflunisal resulted in ≈ 50% increased acetaminophen plasma levels. Acetaminophen had no effect on diflunisal plasma levels.
Diflunisal	Anticoagulants, oral	↑	Coadministration of diflunisal may increase hypoprothrombinemic effects of anticoagulants. Diflunisal competitively displaces coumarins from protein-binding sites. Monitor prothrombin time during and for several days after coadministration. Adjust dosage of oral anticoagulants as required.
Diflunisal	Hydrochlorothiazide	↑	Coadministration of diflunisal resulted in significantly increased plasma levels of hydrochlorothiazide. Diflunisal decreased the hyperuricemic effects of hydrochlorothiazide.

Diflunisal Drug Interactions			
Precipitant drug	Object drug*		Description
Diflunisal	Indomethacin	↑	Administration of diflunisal decreased renal clearance and significantly increased plasma levels of indomethacin. The combined use has also been associated with fatal GI hemorrhage.
Diflunisal	Sulindac	↓	Administration of diflunisal resulted in lowering of the plasma levels of the active sulindac sulfide metabolite by ≈ ⅓.

* ↑ = Object drug increased. ↓ = Object drug decreased.

Adverse Reactions

Listed below are adverse reactions reported in 1314 patients who received long-term treatment (24 to 96 weeks). In general, the adverse reactions listed below were 2 to 14 times less frequent in 1113 patients who received short-term treatment.

►*Incidence < 1% to 9% (causal relationship known):*
CNS – Headache (3% to 9%); dizziness, somnolence, insomnia (1% to 3%); vertigo, nervousness, depression, hallucinations, confusion, disorientation, lightheadedness, paresthesias (< 1%).

Dermatologic – Rash (3% to 9%); pruritus, sweating, dry mucous membranes, stomatitis, erythema multiforme, Stevens-Johnson syndrome, toxic epidermal necrolysis, exfoliative dermatitis, photosensitivity, urticaria (< 1%).

GI – Nausea, dyspepsia, GI pain, diarrhea (3% to 9%); vomiting, constipation, flatulence (1% to 3%); peptic ulcer, GI bleeding/perforation, anorexia, eructation, cholestasis, jaundice (sometimes with fever), gastritis, hepatitis, abnormal liver function tests (< 1%).

GU – Dysuria, renal impairment (including renal failure), interstitial nephritis, hematuria, proteinuria (< 1%).

Hypersensitivity –
(< 1%): Acute anaphylactic reaction with bronchospasm. A potentially life-threatening apparent hypersensitivity syndrome was reported. This multisystem syndrome includes constitutional symptoms (fever, chills) and cutaneous findings. It may involve major organs (changes in liver function, jaundice, leukopenia, thrombocytopenia, eosinophilia, renal impairment including renal failure) and less specific findings (adenitis, arthralgia, arthritis, malaise, anorexia, disorientation).

Miscellaneous – Fatigue/tiredness, tinnitus (1% to 3%); asthenia, edema, thrombocytopenia, agranulocytosis (rare), transient visual disturbances including blurred vision (< 1%).

►*Incidence < 1% (causal relationship unknown):*
Miscellaneous – Dyspnea; muscle cramps; palpitations; syncope; chest pain.

Overdosage

►*Symptoms:* Cases of overdosage have occurred and deaths have been reported. Most patients recovered without permanent sequelae. The most common signs and symptoms were drowsiness, vomiting, nausea, diarrhea, hyperventilation, tachycardia, sweating, tinnitus, disorientation, stupor and coma. Diminished urine output and cardiorespiratory arrest have also been reported.

The lowest fatal dosage was 15 g without any other drugs. In a mixed drug overdose, ingestion of 7.5 g diflunisal resulted in death.

►*Treatment:* Treatment is symptomatic and supportive. Empty the stomach by inducing vomiting or by gastric lavage. Refer to General Management of Acute Overdosage. Because of high degree of protein binding, hemodialysis may not be effective.

Patient Information

May cause GI upset; may be taken with water, milk or meals.

Do not take **aspirin** or **acetaminophen** with diflunisal, except on professional advice.

Swallow tablets whole; do not crush or chew.

MAGNESIUM SALICYLATE

otc	**Backache Maximum Strength Relief** (B-M Squibb)	**Caplets:** 467 mg (as tetrahydrate)	Film coated. In 24s and 50s.
Rx	**Novasal** (US Pharmaceutical)	**Tablet:** 600 mg (as tetrahydrate)	(0700/US). Light red, oval, scored. Film-coated. In 100s.
otc	**Extra Strength Doan's** (Ciba Consumer)	**Caplets:** 500 mg	(DOAN'S). In 24s and 48s.
otc	**Bayer Select Maximum Strength Backache** (Bayer)	**Caplets:** 580 mg (as tetrahydrate)	In 24s and 50s.
otc	**Momentum Muscular Backache Formula** (Whitehall)	**Caplets:** 580 mg (as tetrahydrate, equivalent to 467 mg magnesium salicylate anhydrous)	(MSM). In 48s.
Rx	**Magan** (Adria)	**Tablets:** 545 mg	(Adria 412). Pink. In 100s and 500s.
Rx	**Mobidin** (Ascher)	**Tablets:** 600 mg	(0310). Yellow, scored. In 100s and 500s.

Complete prescribing information for these products begins in the Salicylates monograph.

Administration and Dosage

A sodium free salicylate derivative that may have a low incidence of GI upset. The product labeling and dosage are expressed as magnesium salicylate anhydrous. The possibility of magnesium toxicity exists in people with renal insufficiency.

Usual dose is 650 mg every 4 hours or 1090 mg, 3 times a day. May increase to 3.6 to 4.8 g/day in 3 or 4 divided doses.

Safety and efficacy for use in children have not been established.

SALICYLATE COMBINATIONS

Rx	**Choline Magnesium Trisalicylate** (Various, eg, Sidmak, Zenith Goldline)	**Tablets:** 500 mg salicylate (as 293 mg choline salicylate, 362 mg Mg salicylate)	(SL 528). Yellow, scored. Film coated, capsule shape. In 100s and 500s.
		750 mg salicylate (as 440 mg choline salicylate, 544 mg Mg salicylate)	(SL 529). Blue, scored. Film coated, capsule shape. In 100s and 500s.
		1000 mg salicylate (as 587 mg choline salicylate, 725 mg Mg salicylate)	(SL 530). Pink, scored. Capsule shape, film coated. In 100s and 500s.
Rx	**Choline Magnesium Trisalicylate** (Various, eg, Cypress)	**Liquid:** 500 mg salicylate (as 293 mg choline salicylate, 362 mg Mg salicylate)/5 ml	In 237 ml.

Complete prescribing information for these products begins in the Salicylates monograph.

SALSALATE (Salicylsalicylic Acid)

Rx	**Salsalate** (Various, eg, Geneva, Goldline, Major, Moore, Rugby, URL, Vitarine)	**Tablets:** 500 mg	In 100s, 500s and UD 100s.
Rx	**Amigesic** (Amide)		(A 019). Yellow or blue. Film coated. In 100s and 500s.
Rx	**Argesic-SA** (Econo Med)		In 100s.
Rx	**Salflex** (Carnrick)		Dye free. (C 8671). White. Film coated. In 100s.
Rx	**Salsitab** (Upsher-Smith)		(500). Blue. Film coated. In 100s, 500s and UD 100s.
Rx	**Salsalate** (Various, eg, Copley, Geneva, Goldline, Major, Moore, Rugby, URL, Vitarine)	**Tablets:** 750 mg	In 100s, 500s and UD 100s.
Rx	**Amigesic Caplets** (Amide)		(A0 10). Yellow or blue, scored. Film coated, Capsule shaped. In 100s and 500s.
Rx	**Artha-G** (T.E. Williams)		(Artha-G). Lavender, scored. In 120s.
Rx	**Marthritic** (Marnel)		In 100s.
Rx	**Salsitab** (Upsher-Smith)		(750). Blue, scored. Film coated. In 100s, 500s and UD 100s.
Rx	**Salflex** (Carnrick)		Dye free. (C 8672). White, scored. Film coated. In 100s and 500s.

Complete prescribing information for these products begins in the Salicylates monograph.

Administration and Dosage

After absorption, the drug is partially hydrolyzed into two molecules of salicylic acid. Insoluble in gastric secretions, it is not absorbed until it reaches the small intestine.

Usual adult dose is 3000 mg/day given in divided doses.

SODIUM SALICYLATE

otc	**Sodium Salicylate** (Various, eg, Moore, Rugby)	**Tablets, enteric coated:** 325 mg	In 100s.
otc	**Sodium Salicylate** (Various, eg, Moore, Rugby)	**Tablets, enteric coated:** 650 mg	In 100s, 500s and 1000s.

Complete prescribing information for these products begins in the Salicylates monograph.

Administration and Dosage

Less effective than an equal dose of aspirin in reducing pain or fever. Patients hypersensitive to aspirin may be able to tolerate sodium salicylate. Platelets are not affected; however, prothrombin time is increased. Each gram contains 6.25 mEq sodium.

Usual dose is 325 to 650 mg every 4 hours.

SODIUM THIOSALICYLATE

Rx	**Sodium Thiosalicylate** (Various)	**Injection:** 50 mg/ml	In 30 ml vials and 2 ml amps.
Rx	**Rexolate** (Hyrex)		In 30 ml vials.

Complete prescribing information for these products begins in the Salicylates monograph.

Administration and Dosage

Intramuscular administration is preferred.

➤*Acute gout:* 100 mg every 3 to 4 hrs for 2 days, then 100 mg/day until asymptomatic.

➤*Muscular pain, musculoskeletal disturbances:* 50 to 100 mg/day or on alternate days.

➤*Rheumatic fever:* 100 to 150 mg every 4 to 8 hours for 3 days, then reduce to 100 mg twice daily. Continue until patient is asymptomatic.

NONNARCOTIC ANALGESIC COMBINATIONS

Content given per capsule, tablet, or packet.

NONNARCOTIC ANALGESIC COMBINATIONS

	Product and Distributor	Acetaminophen	Aspirin	Other Analgesics	Caffeine	Other Content	How Supplied
otc	**Painaid Tablets** (Zee Medical)	110 mg	162 mg	152 mg salicylamide	32.4 mg		In 24s.
otc	**Saleto Tablets** (Mallard)	115 mg	210 mg	65 mg salicylamide	16 mg		Pink. In 100s, 1000s, and *Sani-Pak* 1000s.
otc	**FemBack Caplets** (CCA Laboratories)	150 mg		150 mg salicylamide		44 mg phenyl-toloxamine citrate	Coated. In 24s.
otc	**Vanquish Caplets** (Bayer)	194 mg	227 mg		33 mg	50 mg magnesium hydroxide, 25 mg aluminum hydroxide	(Vanquish). In 60s and 100s.
otc	**Excedrin Migraine** (Bristol-Myers Squibb)	250 mg	250 mg		65 mg		(E). In 50s and 100s.
otc	**Excedrin Extra Strength Caplets, Tablets, and Geltabs** (Bristol-Myers Squibb)						**Caplets:** Saccharin. (E). In 24s, 50s, 100s, 175s, and 275s. **Tablets:** Saccharin. (E). In 24s, 50s, 100s, 175s, and 275s. **Geltabs:** Saccharin. In 24s, 40s, and 80s.
otc	**Painaid BRF Back Relief Formula Tablets** (Zee Medical)			250 mg magnesium salicylate tetrahydrate			In 24s.
otc	**Painaid ESF Extra-Strength Formula Tablets** (Zee Medical)		250 mg		65 mg		In 24s.
otc	**Pamprin Maximum Pain Relief Caplets** (Chattem)			250 mg magnesium salicylate		25 mg pamabrom	In 16s and 32s.
otc	**Summit Extra Strength Caplets** (Pfeiffer Pharmaceuticals)		250 mg		65 mg		Coated. In 50s.
otc	**Goody's Extra Strength Headache Powder** (Goody's Pharmaceuticals)	260 mg	520 mg		32.5 mg		Lactose. In 2s, 6s, 24s, and 50s.
Rx	**Duraxin Capsules** (Portal)	325 mg		200 mg salicylamide		25 mg phenyl-toloxamine citrate	In 30s.
otc	**Goody's Body Pain Powder** (Goody's Pharmaceuticals)		500 mg				Lactose. In 6s and 24s.
otc	**Aceta-Gesic** (Rugby)			150 mg salicylamide		30 mg phenyl-toloxamine citrate	In 24s, 100s, and 1000s.
Rx	**Levacet Tablets** (Pharmakon)	400 mg	400 mg	150 mg salicylamide	40 mg	50 mg phenyl-toloxamine citrate	(LEVACET). Yellow, capsule shape. In 50s.

NONNARCOTIC ANALGESIC COMBINATIONS

	Product and Distributor	Acetaminophen	Aspirin	Other Analgesics	Caffeine	Other Content	How Supplied
otc	**Excedrin Tension Headache Geltabs** and **Caplets** (Bristol-Myers Squibb)	500 mg			65 mg		**Geltabs:** Parabens. In 50s and 100s. **Caplets:** Parabens. Capsule shape. In 50s and 100s.
otc	**Excedrin Aspirin Free Geltabs** and **Caplets** (Bristol-Myers Squibb)				65 mg		**Geltabs:** (AF Excedrin). In 24s, 50s, and 100s. **Caplets:** Saccharin, parabens. (AFE). In 24s, 50s, and 100s.
otc	**Excedrin QuickTabs** (Bristol-Myers Squibb)				65 mg		Mannitol, sucralose. Spearmint and peppermint flavors. In 16s and 32s.
otc	**Premsyn PMS Caplets** (Chattem)					25 mg pamabrom, 15 mg pyrilamine maleate	In 20s and 40s.
otc	**Vitelle Lurline PMS Tablets** (Fielding)					25 mg pamabrom, 50 mg pyridoxine HCl	In 50s.
otc	**Pamprin Multi-Symptom Maximum Strength Caplets** and **Tablets** (Chattem)					25 mg pamabrom, 15 mg pyrilamine maleate	**Caplets:** (PAMPRIN). In 24s and 48s. **Tablets:** (PAMPRIN). In 12s, 24s, and 48s.
otc	**Midol Maximum Strength Menstrual Caplets** and **Gelcaps** (Bayer)				60 mg	15 mg pyrilamine maleate	**Caplets:** (Midol MENSTRUAL). In 8s and 24s. **Gelcaps:** EDTA. In 24s.
otc	**Midol Maxiumum Strength PMS Caplets** and **Gelcaps** (Bayer)					25 mg pamabrom, 15 mg pyrilamine maleate	**Caplets:** (MIDOL). In 24s. **Gelcaps:** EDTA. In 24s.
otc	**Fem-1 Tablets** (BDI)					25 mg pamabrom	In 16s.
otc	**Painaid PMF Premenstrual Formula Tablets** (Zee Medical)					25 mg pamabrom	In 24s.
Rx	**Flextra-DS Tablets** (Poly Pharm)					50 mg phenyltoloxamine citrate	In 100s.
otc	**Anacin Aspirin Free Maximum Strength Tablets** (Whitehall)						**Tablets:** In 30s, 60s, 100s, and 750s.
otc	**APAP-Plus Tablets** (Textilease Medique Products Co.)				65 mg		In 100s, 200s, and 500s.
otc	**Midol Teen Maximum Strength Caplets** (Bayer)					25 mg pamabrom	(Midol TEEN). In 24s.
otc	**Anacin Aspirin Free Extra Strength Tablets** (Whitehall)						In 60s.
otc	**Women's Tylenol Multi-Symptom Menstrual Relief Caplets** (McNeil Consumer)					25 mg pamabrom	In 24s.
Rx	**Hyflex-650 Tablets** (Breckenridge)	650 mg				60 mg phenyltoloxamine citrate	(B/064). Red, scored. In 100s.
Rx	**Ultracet Tablets** (Ortho-McNeil)	325 mg				37.5 mg tramadol HCl	(O-M 650). Yellow, capsule shape. Film-coated. In 20s, 100s, 500s, and UD 100s.
c-iv	**Micrainin Tablets** (Wallace)		325 mg			200 mg meprobamate	(Wallace 37-0120). Capsule-shape. White/orange. In 100s.

NONNARCOTIC ANALGESIC COMBINATIONS

NONNARCOTIC ANALGESIC COMBINATIONS

	Product and Distributor	Acetaminophen	Aspirin	Caffeine	Other Analgesics	Other Content	How Supplied
otc	**Anacin Caplets and Tablets** (Whitehall)		400 mg	32 mg			**Caplets:** In 100s. **Tablets:** Coated. In 30s, 50s, 100s, 200s, and 300s.
otc	**P-A-C Analgesic Tablets** (Lee Pharmaceuticals)						In 100s and 1000s.
otc	**Anacin Maximum Strength Tablets** (Whitehall)		500 mg	32 mg			In 20s, 40s, and 75s.
otc	**Bayer Extra Strength Back & Body Pain** (Bayer)			32.5 mg			Capsule shape. In 50s and 100s.
otc	**Bayer PM Extra Strength Aspirin Plus Sleep Aid Caplet** (Bayer)					25 mg diphenhydramine HCl	(BAYER PM). In 24s.
otc	**Bayer Plus Extra Strength** (Bayer)					250 mg calcium carbonate	In 50s.
otc	**BC Powder Original Formula** (Block)		650 mg	33.3 mg	195 mg salicylamide		Lactose. In 50s.
otc	**BC Powder Arthritis Strength** (Block)		742 mg	38 mg	222 mg salicylamide		Lactose. In 50s.
otc	**Mobigesic Tablets** (BF Ascher)				325 mg magnesium salicylate anhydrous	30 mg phenyltoloxamine citrate	In 18s, 50s, and 100s.
Rx	**Magsal Tablets** (U.S. Pharm)				600 mg magnesium salicylate tetrahydrate	25 mg phenyltoloxamine dihydrogen citrate	(0321/US). Green, oval. In 100s.

Indications

Components of these combinations include the following (see individual monographs):

NONNARCOTIC ANALGESICS: Acetaminophen, aspirin, salicylates, salicylamide.

BARBITURATES, MEPROBAMATE, and ANTIHISTAMINES: (eg, pyrilamine, diphenhydramine, phenyltoloxamine) are used for their sedative effects.

ANTACIDS: (eg, calcium carbonate, magnesium hydroxide, aluminum hydroxide) are used to minimize gastric upset from salicylates.

CAFFEINE, a traditional component of many analgesic formulations, may be beneficial in certain vascular headaches.

PAMABROM is used as a diuretic.

AMINOBENZOATE retards the conjugation of salicylic acid and prolongs the action of salicylates.

Other components listed, but not contributing to the analgesic properties of these products include: Pyridoxine HCl.

Administration and Dosage

▶Dose: The average adult dose is 1 or 2 capsules or tablets or 1 powder packet every 2 to 6 hours as needed for pain. Each product varies; for complete prescribing information, refer to the product label/packaging information.

NONNARCOTIC ANALGESICS WITH BARBITURATES

Rx	**Butalbital, Acetaminophen, and Caffeine Tablets** (Various, eg, Major, Schein, Teva, Zenith Goldline)	**Tablets:** 325 mg acetaminophen, 40 mg caffeine, 50 mg butalbital	In 30s, 50s, 100s, 500s, 1000s, and UD 100s.
Rx	**Americet** (MCR American)		In 100s.
Rx	**Esgic** (Forest)		(535-11). White, scored. Capsule shape. In 100s.
Rx	**Fioricet** (Novartis)		(Fioricet). Light blue. In 100s, 500s, and UD 100s.
Rx	**Repan** (Everett)		(162E305). White. In 100s.
Rx	**Margesic** (Marnel)	**Capsules:** 325 mg acetaminophen, 40 mg caffeine, 50 mg butalbital	(Margesic/Mar). White. In 100s.
Rx	**Triad** (UAD Laboratories)		(TRIAD/UAD 905). White. In 100s.
Rx	**Esgic** (Gilbert Laboratories)		(535-12). White. In 100s.
Rx	**Medigesic** (US Pharm Corp)		(US/US). White. In 100s.
c-iii	**Butalbital, Aspirin, and Caffeine Capsules** (Various, eg, Lannett, Major)	**Capsules:** 325 mg aspirin, 40 mg caffeine, 50 mg butalbital	In 100s and 1000s.
c-iii	**Butalbital Compound** (Various, eg, Qualitest)		In 100s.
c-iii	**Fiorinal** (Novartis)		Benzyl alcohol, EDTA, parabens. (Fiorinal 78-103). Lime green/green. In 100s, 500s, and UD 25s.
Rx	**Phrenilin** (Carnrick)	**Tablets:** 325 mg acetaminophen, 50 mg butalbital	(C 8650). Violet, scored. In 100s and 500s.
Rx	**Marten-Tab** (Marnel)		(MIA/106). White. Capsule shape. In 100s.
Rx	**Butalbital, Acetaminophen, and Caffeine Tablets** (Various, eg, Able, Inwood, Major, Qualitest, URL, West-Ward)	**Tablets:** 500 mg acetaminophen, 40 mg caffeine, 50 mg butalbital	In 100s and 500s.
Rx	**Esgic-Plus** (Forest)		(Forest 678). White, scored. Capsule shape. In 100s and 500s.
Rx	**Esgic-Plus** (Forest)	**Capsules:** 500 mg acetaminophen, 40 mg caffeine, 50 mg butalbital	(Forest 0372/Esgic Plus). Red. In 20s, 100s, and 500s.
Rx	**Axocet** (Savage)	**Tablets:** 650 mg acetaminophen, 50 mg butalbital	(0389). Blue, capsule shape. In 100s.
Rx	**Bupap** (ECR Pharmaceuticals)		(59010/240). Blue, scored. Capsule shape. In 100s.
Rx	**Dolgic** (Athlon[1])		(MIA/112). Blue. Capsule shape. In 100s.
Rx	**Promacet** (MCR American)		In 100s.
Rx	**Repan CF** (Everett Labs)		(EVERETT 166). Blue, scored. Capsule shape. In 100s.
Rx	**Sedapap** (Merz Pharmaceuticals)		(MP 392). White. Capsule shape. In 100s.
Rx	**Phrenilin Forte** (Carnrick)	**Capsules:** 650 mg acetaminophen, 50 mg butalbital	Benzyl alcohol, parabens, EDTA. (C 8656). Amethyst. In 100s and 500s.
Rx	**Tencon** (International Ethical Labs)		In 100s.
Rx	**Butex Forte** (Athlon[1])		Benzyl alcohol, EDTA, parabens. (Butex Forte/070). White. In 100s.
Rx	**Bucet** (Forest)		Benzyl alcohol, EDTA, parabens. (Bucet/UAD 307). White. In 20s, 100s, and 500s.
c-iii	**Butalbital, Aspirin, and Caffeine Tablets** (Various, eg, Purepac, Schein, Zenith Goldline)	**Tablets:** 325 mg aspirin, 40 mg caffeine, 50 mg butalbital	In 30s, 50s, 100s, 500s, 1000s, and UD 100s.
c-iii	**Butalbital Compound** (Various, eg, Qualitest)		In 100s and 1000s.

[1] Athlon Pharmaceuticals, Inc., P. O. Box 3181, Ridgeland, MS 39158; (601) 899–5714.

For complete prescribing information, refer to the individual component drug monographs.

Administration and Dosage

➤*Adults:* 1 or 2 every 4 hours, as needed.

Precautions

➤*Benzyl alcohol:* Some of these products contain the preservative benzyl alcohol, which has been associated with a fatal "gasping syndrome" in premature infants.

DICLOFENAC SODIUM AND MISOPROSTOL

Rx	**Arthrotec** (Pharmacia)	**Tablets:**[1] 50 mg diclofenac sodium/200 mcg misoprostol	Lactose. (AAAA50 SEARLE 1411). White to off-white. Film-coated. In 60s, 90s, and UD 100s.
		75 mg diclofenac sodium/200 mcg misoprostol	Lactose. (AAAA75 SEARLE 1421). White to off-white. Film-coated. In 60s and UD 100s.

[1] Each tablet consists of an enteric-coated core containing diclofenac sodium surrounded by an outer mantle containing misoprostol.

This is an abbreviated monograph. For complete prescribing information, refer to the NSAID and misoprostol monographs.

WARNING

The administration of this product by any route is contraindicated in pregnant women because its misoprostol component can cause abortion.

Reports, primarily from Brazil, of congenital anomalies and fetal death subsequent to use of misoprostol alone, as an abortifacient, have been received.

Patients must be advised of the abortifacient property and warned not to give the drug to others.

Uterine rupture has been reported when misoprostol was administered intravaginally in pregnant women to induce labor or to induce abortion beyond the first trimester of pregnancy.

Uterine perforation has been reported following administration of combined vaginal and oral misoprostol in pregnant women to induce abortion. In each of these reported cases, the gestational age of the pregnancies was unknown.

Do not use in women with childbearing potential unless the patient requires nonsteroidal anti-inflammatory drug (NSAID) therapy and is at high risk of developing gastric or duodenal ulceration or of developing complications from gastric or duodenal ulcers associated with the use of the NSAID. In such patients, this drug may be prescribed if the patient:
• Had a negative serum pregnancy test within 2 weeks prior to beginning therapy;
• is capable of complying with effective contraceptive measures;
• has received both oral and written warnings of the hazards of misoprostol, the risk of possible contraception failure, and the danger to other women of childbearing potential should the drug be taken by mistake;
• will begin using this product only on the second or third day of the next normal menstrual period.

Indications

➤*Arthritis:* Treatment of the signs and symptoms of osteoarthritis or rheumatoid arthritis in patients at high risk of developing NSAID-induced gastric and duodenal ulcers and their complications.

Administration and Dosage

➤*Approved by the FDA:* December 1997.

Swallow tablets whole; do not chew, crush, or dissolve. May be taken with meals to minimize GI effects. This fixed combination product is not appropriate for patients who would not receive the appropriate dose of both ingredients.

➤*Osteoarthritis:* The recommended dose for maximal GI mucosal protection is 50 mg diclofenac/200 mcg misoprostol 3 times daily. For patients who experience intolerance, 50 mg/200 mcg or 75 mg/200 mcg twice daily can be used, but are less effective in preventing ulcers.

➤*Rheumatoid arthritis:* Recommended dose is 50 mg diclofenac/200 mcg misoprostol 3 or 4 times daily. For patients who experience intolerance, 50 mg/200 mcg or 75 mg/200 mcg twice daily can be used, but are less effective in preventing ulcers.

➤*Special dosing considerations:* For gastric ulcer prevention, 200 mcg 3 and 4 times daily are therapeutically equivalent, but more protective than the twice-daily regimen. For duodenal ulcer prevention, 4 times daily is more protective than the 2- or 3-times daily regimens. However, the 4-times daily regimen is less tolerated.

Dosages may be individualized using the separate products (misoprostol and diclofenac), after which the patient may be changed to the appropriate combination diclofenac/misoprostol dose. If clinically indicated, misoprostol cotherapy with diclofenac/misoprostol, or use of the individual components to optimize the misoprostol dose, or frequency of administration may be appropriate. The total dose of misoprostol should not exceed 800 mcg/day, and do not administer more than 200 mcg of misoprostol at any one time. Doses of diclofenac higher than 150 mg/day in osteoarthritis or higher than 225 mg/day in rheumatoid arthritis are not recommended.

➤*Storage/Stability:* Store at or below 25°C (77°F) in a dry area.

Actions

➤*Pharmacology:* This product is a combination containing diclofenac sodium, an NSAID with analgesic properties, and misoprostol, a GI mucosal protective prostaglandin E_1 analog. Diclofenac sodium has anti-inflammatory, analgesic, and antipyretic properties. The mechanism of action of diclofenac, like other NSAIDs, is not completely understood, but may be related to prostaglandin synthetase inhibition.

A deficiency of prostaglandins within the gastric and duodenal mucosa may lead to diminishing bicarbonate and mucus secretion and may contribute to the mucosal damage caused by NSAIDs.

Misoprostol is a synthetic prostaglandin E_1 analog with gastric antisecretory and (in animals) mucosal protective properties. It can increase bicarbonate and mucus production, but in humans this has been shown at doses of 200 mcg and above that are also antisecretory. Therefore, it is not possible to tell whether the ability of misoprostol to prevent gastric and duodenal ulcers is the result of its antisecretory effect, its mucosal protective effect, or both.

➤*Pharmacokinetics:* The pharmacokinetics following oral administration of a single dose or multiple doses of diclofenac/misoprostol to healthy subjects under fasted conditions are similar to the pharmacokinetics of the 2 individual components. Food decreases the multiple-dose bioavailability profile of both formulations.

Contraindications

Hypersensitivity to diclofenac, misoprostol, or other prostaglandins; patients who have experienced asthma, urticaria, or other allergic-type reactions after taking aspirin or other NSAIDs; severe, rarely fatal, anaphylactic-like reactions to diclofenac sodium have been reported; pregnancy (see Black Box Warning).

Warnings

➤*Pregnancy: Category X* (see Black Box Warnings). Contraindicated in pregnancy. One case of amniotic fluid embolism, which resulted in maternal and fetal death, has been reported with use of misoprostol during pregnancy. Severe vaginal bleeding, retained placenta, shock, fetal bradycardia, and pelvic pain also have been reported. These women were administered misoprostol vaginally and/or orally over a range of doses.

Misoprostol may endanger pregnancy (may cause miscarriage) and thereby cause harm to the fetus when administered to a pregnant woman. Misoprostol produces uterine contractions, uterine bleeding, and expulsion of the products of conception. Miscarriages caused by misoprostol may be incomplete.

The diclofenac sodium component, like other NSAIDs, which are prostaglandin-inhibiting drugs, may affect the fetal cardiovascular system causing premature closure of the ductus arteriosus. NSAIDs may also inhibit uterine contractions.

Patients should avoid pregnancy during treatment and for 1 month or through 1 menstrual cycle after discontinuation.

➤*Lactation:* Diclofenac sodium is found in the milk of breastfeeding mothers. It is unlikely that misoprostol is excreted into breast milk because the drug is rapidly metabolized by the body. Excretion of the active metabolite (misoprostol acid) into breast milk is possible but has not been studied. Because of the potential for serious adverse reactions in nursing infants, this product is not recommended during breastfeeding.

➤*Children:* Safety and efficacy in pediatric patients have not been established.

Adverse Reactions

➤*GI:* GI disorders had the highest reported incidence in patients receiving diclofenac/misoprostol. These events were generally minor, but led to discontinuation of therapy in 9% of patients on diclofenac/misoprostol and 5% on diclofenac.

GI Adverse Reactions: Diclofenac/Misoprostol vs Diclofenac (%)		
GI disorder	Diclofenac/Misoprostol	Diclofenac
Abdominal pain	21	15
Diarrhea	19	11
Dyspepsia	14	11
Nausea	11	6
Flatulence	9	4

Diarrhea and abdominal pain developed early in the course of therapy and were usually self-limited (resolved after 2 to 7 days). Rare instances of profound diarrhea leading to severe dehydration have been reported in patients receiving misoprostol. Monitor patients with an underlying condition (eg, inflammatory bowel disease, dehydration) carefully if this product is prescribed. The incidence of diarrhea can be minimized by administering diclofenac/misoprostol with food and by avoiding coadministration with magnesium-containing antacids.

Patient Information

Advise patients to report any signs or symptoms of GI ulceration or bleeding, skin rash, weight gain, or swelling. Advise patients to stop therapy and seek immediate medical attention if signs of liver toxicity

DICLOFENAC SODIUM AND MISOPROSTOL

occur (eg, nausea, fatigue, lethargy, itching, jaundice, right upper quadrant tenderness, "flu-like" symptoms).

Do not take this product if pregnant, and avoid becoming pregnant while taking this medicine and for at least 1 month or through 1 menstrual cycle after discontinuation. If pregnancy occurs during diclofenac/misoprostol therapy, stop taking the drug and contact the physician immediately.

Diarrhea, abdominal pain, upset stomach, and nausea may develop during the first few weeks of therapy and stop after about a week with continued treatment. To minimize diarrhea, take with meals and avoid antacids containing magnesium (if needed, use one containing aluminum or calcium instead). If difficulty persists (more than 7 days), or if experiencing severe diarrhea, cramping, or nausea, call the physician.

Swallow tablets whole. Do not chew, crush, or dissolve.

NAPROXEN AND LANSOPRAZOLE

Rx	**Prevacid NapraPAC 375**[1] (TAP Pharmaceuticals)	**Tablets:** 375 mg naproxen	(NPR LE 375). Pink, oval. In blister cards.
		Capsules, delayed release: 15 mg lansoprazole	Sucrose, FD&C Blue No.1. (PREVACID 15). Pink/green. In blister cards.
Rx	**Prevacid NapraPAC 500**[1] (TAP Pharmaceuticals)	**Tablets:** 500 mg naproxen	(NPR LE 500). Yellow, capsule shape. In blister cards.
		Capsules, delayed release: 15 mg lansoprazole	Sucrose, FD&C Blue No.1. (PREVACID 15). Pink/green. In blister cards.

[1] In weekly (7-day) blister cards containing 14 *Naprosyn* tablets and 7 *Prevacid* capsules and in 1-month administration packs containing 4 weekly blister cards.

For complete prescribing information, refer to the Proton Pump Inhibitors and the Nonsteroidal Anti-Inflammatory Agents group monographs.

Indications

➤*Nonsteroidal anti-inflammatory drug (NSAID)-associated gastric ulcers:* For reducing the risk of NSAID-associated gastric ulcers in patients with a history of documented gastric ulcer who require the use of an NSAID for treatment of the signs and symptoms of rheumatoid arthritis, osteoarthritis, and ankylosing spondylitis.

Administration and Dosage

Each daily dose consists of one 15 mg lansoprazole capsule and 2 of either 375 or 500 mg naproxen tablets. Take the lansoprazole capsule and 1 of the naproxen tablets before eating in the morning with a glass of water. Take the second naproxen tablet in the evening with a glass of water. The maximum daily naproxen dose of naproxen/lansoprazole is 1000 mg.

Swallow lansoprazole delayed-release capsules whole. Do not chew or crush.

➤*Dosage adjustment:* For naproxen/lansoprazole, no adjustment of the 15 mg lansoprazole component is necessary in patients with renal insufficiency or for the elderly. However, consider dose adjustment for the naproxen component for patients with renal insufficiency, liver disease, or the elderly.

➤*Storage / Stability:* Store at 25°C (77°F); excursion permitted to 15° to 30°C (59° to 86°F). Protect from light and moisture. Store and dispense in original container.

Indications

NSAIDs: Summary of Indications

Legend: ✔ -Labeled X- Unlabeled

Indications	Celecoxib	Diclofenac potassium	Diclofenac sodium/Diclofenac sodium XR	Etodolac	Fenoprofen	Flurbiprofen	Ibuprofen	Indomethacin	Indomethacin SR	Ketoprofen	Ketoprofen SR	Ketorolac	Meclofenamate	Mefenamic acid	Meloxicam	Nabumetone	Naproxen	Oxaprozin	Piroxicam	Rofecoxib	Sulindac	Tolmetin	Valdecoxib
Rheumatoid arthritis (RA)	✔	✔	✔	✔	✔	✔	✔	✔	✔	✔	✔		✔			✔	✔	✔	✔	✔	✔	✔	✔
Osteoarthritis (OA)	✔	✔	✔	✔	✔	✔	✔	✔	✔	✔	✔				✔	✔	✔	✔	✔	✔	✔	✔	✔
Ankylosing spondylitis		✔	✔[1]	X		X		✔	✔								✔				✔		
Mild to moderate pain				✔	✔		✔						✔	✔[2]						✔			
Pain	✔	✔								✔		✔[3]					✔						
Primary dysmenorrhea	✔	✔				X	✔			✔			✔	✔			✔		X	✔			✔
Juvenile RA		X	X	X				X									✔	X			X	✔	
Tendinitis				X				✔	✔								✔				✔		
Bursitis				X				✔	✔								✔				✔		
Acute painful shoulder			X	X				✔	✔												✔		
Acute gout				X		X		✔									✔				✔		
Fever							✔[4]																
Familial adenomatous polyposis (FAP)	✔																						
Sunburn								X[5]															
Migraine																							
Abortive (acute attack)					X	X						X	X	X			X						
Prophylactic			X			X	X	X		X			X				X						
Menstrual						X		X		X			X	X			X						
Cluster headache								X															
Polyhydramnios								X															
Acne vulgaris, resistant						X																	
Menorrhagia													X										
Premenstrual syndrome														X			X						
Cystoid macular edema								X[5]															
Closure of persistent patent ductus arteriosus								✔[6]															

[1] Sodium only, not sodium XR.
[2] Therapy not to exceed 1 week.
[3] Therapy not to exceed 5 days.
[4] In children only.
[5] Topical formulation.
[6] IV formulation only.

►*Rheumatoid arthritis (RA) (except **ketorolac, mefenamic acid,** and **meloxicam**) and osteoarthritis (OA) (except **ketorolac** and **mefenamic acid**):* Relief of signs and symptoms; treatment of acute flares and exacerbation; long-term management.

Concomitant therapy – Concomitant therapy with other second-line drugs (eg, gold salts) demonstrates additional therapeutic benefit. Whether they can be used with partially effective doses of corticosteroids for a "steroid-sparing" effect and result in greater improvement is not established.

Use with salicylates is not recommended; greater benefit is not achieved, and the potential for adverse reactions is increased. The use of aspirin with nonsteroidal anti-inflammatory agents (NSAIDs) may cause a decrease in blood levels of the nonaspirin drug.

*Juvenile RA (**tolmetin, naproxen**) –* For the treatment of juvenile RA.

►*Mild to moderate pain (**diclofenac potassium, etodolac, fenoprofen, ibuprofen, ketoprofen, ketorolac, meclofenamate, mefenamic acid, naproxen, naproxen sodium, rofecoxib**):* Postextraction dental pain, postsurgical episiotomy pain, and soft tissue athletic injuries.

►*Primary dysmenorrhea:* **Celecoxib, diclofenac potassium, ibuprofen, ketoprofen, mefenamic acid, naproxen, naproxen sodium, rofecoxib, valdecoxib.**

►*Idiopathic heavy menstrual blood loss:* **Meclofenamate.**

►*Unlabeled uses:* Selected NSAIDs have been used in the treatment of juvenile RA, symptomatic treatment of sunburn, and for various migraine headaches. For other uses, refer to the Summary of Indications table.

Actions

►*Pharmacology:* Clinically, there are no clear guidelines to assist in selecting the most appropriate agent. Base selection on clinical experience, patient convenience, side effects, and cost.

NSAIDs exhibit antipyretic, analgesic, and anti-inflammatory activities. The major mechanism of therapeutic effects is believed to result from inhibition of prostaglandin synthesis. NSAIDs inhibit cyclooxygenase (COX), the enzyme that catalyzes the synthesis of cyclic endoperoxides from arachidonic acid to form prostaglandins. In the gastric mucosa, prostaglandins decrease gastric acid synthesis, stimulate the production of glutathione that scavenges superoxides, promote the generation of a protective barrier of mucus and bicarbonate, and promote adequate blood flow to the gastric mucosal cells. Prostaglandin in the kidneys modulates intrarenal plasma flow and electrolyte balance.

Two COX isoenzymes have been identified: COX-1 and COX-2. COX-1, expressed constitutively, is synthesized continuously and is present in all tissues and cell types, most notably in platelets, endothelial cells, the GI tract, renal microvasculature, glomerulus, and collecting ducts. COX-1 is important for homeostatic maintenance, such as platelet aggregation, the regulation of blood flow in the kidney and stomach, and the regulation of gastric acid secretion. Inhibition of COX-1 activity is considered a major contributor to NSAID GI toxicity. COX-2 is considered an inducible isoenzyme, although there is some constitutive expression in the kidney, brain, bone, female reproductive system, neoplasias, and GI tract. The function of the COX-2 isoenzyme is induced during pain and inflammatory stimuli.

Many NSAIDs inhibit both COX-1 and COX-2. Most NSAIDs are mainly COX-1 selective (eg, **aspirin, ketoprofen, indomethacin, piroxicam, sulindac**). Others are considered slightly selective for COX-1 (eg, **ibuprofen, naproxen, diclofenac**) and others may be considered slightly selective for COX-2 (eg, **etodolac, nabumetone, meloxicam**). The mechanism of action of **celecoxib, rofecoxib,** and **valdecoxib** is primarily selective inhibition of COX-2; at therapeutic concentrations, the COX-1 isoenzyme is not inhibited, thus GI toxicity may be decreased.

Other mechanisms that may contribute to NSAID anti-inflammatory activity include the reduction of superoxide radicals, induction of apoptosis, inhibition of adhesion molecule expression, decrease of nitric oxide synthase, decrease of proinflammatory cytokine levels (tumor necrosis factor-α, interleukin-1), modification of lymphocyte activity, and alteration of cellular membrane functions.

Central analgesic activity has been demonstrated in animal pain models by some NSAIDs such as diclofenac, ibuprofen, indomethacin, and ketoprofen. This may be because of the interference of prostaglandin formation or with transmitters or modulators in the nociceptive system. Other proposals include the central action mediated by opioid peptides, inhibition of serotonin release, or inhibition of excitatory amino acids or N-methyl-D-aspartate receptors. Antipyretic activity of NSAIDs is because of the inhibition of prostaglandin E_2 (PGE_2) synthesis in circumventricular organs in and near the preoptic hypothalamic area. Infections, tissue damage, inflammation, graft rejection, malignancies, and other disease states enhance the formation of cytokines that increase PGE_2 production. PGE_2 triggers the hypothalamus to promote increases in heat generation and decreases in heat loss.

RA – No one NSAID has demonstrated a clear advantage for the treatment of RA. Individual patients have demonstrated variability in response to certain NSAIDs. Anti-inflammatory activity is shown by reduced joint swelling, reduced pain, reduced duration of morning stiffness and disease activity, increased mobility, and by enhanced functional capacity (demonstrated by an increase in grip strength, delay in time-to-onset of fatigue, and a decrease in time to walk 50 feet).

OA – Improvement is demonstrated by increased range of motion and a reduction in the following: Tenderness with pressure, pain in motion and at rest, night pain, stiffness and swelling, overall disease activity, and by increased range of motion. There is no data to suggest superiority of one NSAID over another as therapy for OA in terms of efficacy and toxicity. NSAIDs for OA are to be used intermittently if possible during painful episodes and prescribed at the minimum effective dose to reduce the potential of renal and GI toxicities. Do not use **indomethacin** chronically because of its greater toxicity profile and its potential for accelerating progression of OA.

Acute gouty arthritis, ankylosing spondylitis – Relief of pain; reduced fever, swelling, redness, and tenderness; and increased range of motion have occurred with treatment of NSAIDs.

Dysmenorrhea – Excess prostaglandins may produce uterine hyperactivity. These agents reduce elevated prostaglandin levels in menstrual fluid and reduce resting and active intrauterine pressure, as well as frequency of uterine contractions. Probable mechanism of action is to inhibit prostaglandin synthesis rather than provide analgesia.

➤*Pharmacokinetics:*

Absorption/Distribution – NSAIDs are rapidly and almost completely absorbed. **Naproxen sodium** is more rapidly absorbed than the **naproxen** formulation and is used when more prompt relief is desired. **Diclofenac potassium** is formulated to release diclofenac in the stomach. **Diclofenac sodium** resists dissolution in the low pH of gastric fluid but allows a rapid release of the drug in the higher-pH environment in the duodenum. In general, food delays absorption but does not significantly affect total amount absorbed. However, the rate of absorption of **meclofenamic acid** decreased by 26% and C_{max} was delayed by 3 hours when administered 0.5 hours after a meal. In general, administer NSAIDs with meals to minimize GI effects. Some NSAIDs can be given with an aluminum and magnesium hydroxide antacid, which does not affect absorption. All NSAIDs are highly protein bound (> 90%). Because **diclofenac** is enteric coated, its time to peak levels are delayed despite its relatively short half-life.

Metabolism/Excretion – Most NSAIDs have negligible hepatic metabolism, except for **etodolac**, **ketorolac**, **nabumetone**, **oxaprozin**, and **meloxicam**. **Celecoxib** and **mefenamic acid** undergo metabolism via cytochrome P450 2C9 isoenzymes. Excretion is via the kidney, primarily as metabolites. **Valdecoxib** undergoes extensive hepatic metabolism involving both P450 isoenzymes (3A4 and 2C9) and non-P450-dependent pathways (eg, glucuronidation). **Sulindac** and **nabumetone** are inactive prodrugs converted by the liver to active metabolites.

Pharmacokinetic Parameters/Maximum Dosage Recommendations of NSAIDs

NSAID	Bioavailability (%)	Half-life (hours)	Volume of distribution	Clearance	Peak (hours)	Protein binding (%)	Renal elimination (%)	Fecal elimination (%)
Acetic acids								
Diclofenac	50 to 60	2	0.1 to 0.2 L/kg	350 mL/min	2	> 99	65	-
Indomethacin	98	4.5	0.29 L/kg	0.084 L/hr/kg	2	90	60	33
Sulindac	90	7.8	NS[1]	≈ 2.71 L/hr	2 to 4	> 93	50	25
Tolmetin	NS[1]	2 to 7	NS[1]	NS[1]	0.5 to 1	NS[1]	≈ 100	-
COX-2 inhibitors								
Celecoxib	NS[1]	11	400 L	27.7 L/hr	3	97	27	57
Rofecoxib	93	17	91 L	120 to 141 mL/min	2 to 3	87	72	14
Valdecoxib	83	8 to 11	≈ 86 L	≈ 6 L/hr	≈ 3	≈ 98	≈ 90	< 5
Fenamates								
Meclofenamate	≈ 100	1.3	23 L	206 mL/min	0.5 to 2	> 99	70	30
Mefenamic acid	NS[1]	2	1.06 L/kg	21.23 L/hr	2 to 4	> 90	52	20
Naphthylalkanones								
Nambumetone	> 80	22.5	0.1 to 0.2 L/kg	26.1 mL/min	9 to 12	> 99	80	9
Oxicams								
Piroxicam	NS[1]	50	0.15 L/kg	0.002 to 0.003 L/kg/hr	3 to 5	98.5	NS[1]	NS[1]
Meloxicam	89	15 to 20	10 L	7 to 9 mL/min	4 to 5	99.4	50	50
Propionic acids								
Fenoprofen	NS[1]	3	NS[1]	NS[1]	2	99	90	-
Flurbiprofen	NS[1]	5.7	0.1 to 0.2 L/kg	1.13 L/hr	≈ 1.5	> 99	> 70	-
Ibuprofen	> 80	1.8 to 2	0.15 L/kg	≈ 3 to 3.5 L/hr	1 to 2	99	45 to 79	-
Ketoprofen	90	2.1	0.1 L/kg	6.9 L/hr	0.5 to 2	> 99	80	-
Ketoprofen ER	90	5.4	0.1 L/kg	6.8 L/hr	6 to 7	> 99	80	-
Naproxen	95	12 to 17	0.16 L/kg	0.13 mL/min/kg	2 to 4	> 99	95	-
Oxaprozin	95	42 to 50	10 to 12.5 L	0.25 to 0.34 L/hr	3 to 5	> 99	65	35
Pyranocarboxylic acid								
Etodolac	≥ 80	7.3	0.362 L/kg	47 mL/hr/kg	≈ 1.5	> 99	72	16

Pharmacokinetic Parameters/Maximum Dosage Recommendations of NSAIDs								
NSAID	Bioavailability (%)	Half-life (hours)	Volume of distribution	Clearance	Peak (hours)	Protein binding (%)	Renal elimination (%)	Fecal elimination (%)
Pyrrolizine carboxylic acid								
Ketorolac	100	5 to 6	≈ 0.2 L/kg	≈ 0.025 L/hr/kg	2 to 3	99	91	6

[1] NS = Not studied.

Contraindications

Hypersensitivity to the drug or any components.

➤*NSAID hypersensitivity:* Because of potential cross-sensitivity to other NSAIDs, do not give these agents to patients in whom aspirin or other NSAIDs have induced symptoms of asthma, rhinitis, urticaria, nasal polyps, angioedema, bronchospasm, and other symptoms of allergic or anaphylactoid reactions. Severe, rarely fatal anaphylactic-like and asthmatic reactions have been reported in such patients receiving NSAIDs.

➤*Fenoprofen or mefenamic acid:* Pre-existing renal disease.

➤*Mefenamic acid:* Active ulceration or chronic inflammation of either the upper or lower GI tract.

➤*Indomethacin suppositories:* History of proctitis or recent rectal bleeding.

➤*Celecoxib:* Hypersensitivity to sulfonamides.

➤*Ketorolac:* Active peptic ulcer disease; recent GI bleeding or perforation; a history of peptic ulcer disease or GI bleeding; advanced renal impairment or patients at risk for renal failure because of volume depletion; labor and delivery because, through its prostaglandin synthesis inhibitory effect, it may adversely affect fetal circulation and inhibit uterine contractions, thus increasing the risk of uterine hemorrhage; nursing mothers because of the potential adverse effects of prostaglandin-inhibiting drugs on neonates; previously demonstrated hypersensitivity to ketorolac tromethamine, allergic manifestations to aspirin or other NSAIDs; as prophylactic analgesic before any major surgery; intraoperatively when hemostasis is critical because of the increased risk of bleeding; suspected or confirmed cerebrovascular bleeding, hemorrhagic diathesis, incomplete hemostasis and those at high risk of bleeding; patients currently receiving ASA or NSAIDs because of the cumulative risks of inducing NSAID-related adverse events; for neuraxial (epidural or intrathecal) administration because of its alcohol content; concomitant use with probenecid.

Warnings

➤*GI effects:* Serious GI toxicity such as inflammation, bleeding, ulceration and perforation of the stomach, small, or large intestine, can occur at any time, with or without warning symptoms, in patients treated chronically with NSAID therapy. Although minor upper GI problems (eg, dyspepsia) are common, usually developing early in therapy, remain alert for ulceration and bleeding in patients treated chronically with NSAIDs even in the absence of previous GI tract symptoms. In patients observed in clinical trials of several months to 2 years duration, symptomatic upper GI ulcers, gross bleeding, or perforation occurred in ≈ 1% of patients treated for 3 to 6 months, and in ≈ 2% to 4% of patients treated for 1 year. These trends continue, thus increasing the likelihood of developing a serious GI event at some time during the course of therapy. However, even short-term therapy is not without risk. In patients receiving **nabumetone**, the incidence of peptic ulcers was 0.3% at 3 to 6 months, 0.5% at 1 year, and 0.8% at 2 years. Only 1 in 5 patients who develop a serious upper GI adverse event on NSAID therapy is symptomatic. Inform patients about the signs or symptoms of serious GI toxicity and what steps to take if they occur.

Studies have shown that patients with a history of peptic ulcer disease or GI bleeding and who use NSAIDs, have a greater than 10-fold risk for developing a GI bleed than patients with neither of these risk factors. In addition, treatment with oral corticosteroids or anticoagulants, longer duration of NSAID therapy, smoking, alcoholism, older age, and poor general health status contribute to an increased risk for a GI bleed. High-dose NSAIDs probably carry a greater risk of these reactions, although controlled clinical trials generally do not show this. In considering the use of relatively large doses (within the recommended dosage range), sufficient benefit should offset the potential increased risk of GI toxicity. To minimize the potential risk for an adverse GI event, use the lowest effective dose for the shortest possible duration. For high-risk patients, consider alternate therapies that do not involve NSAIDs.

Ketorolac is contraindicated in patients with previously documented peptic ulcers and GI bleeding. In patients with active peptic ulcer and active RA, attempt to treat the arthritis with nonulcerogenic drugs. Fatalities have occurred. GI bleeding is associated with higher morbidity and mortality in patients acutely ill with other conditions, the elderly, and patients with hemorrhagic disorders. In patients with active GI bleeding or an active peptic ulcer, institute an appropriate ulcer regimen, and have the physician weigh the benefits of therapy with the NSAID against possible hazards, and carefully monitor the patient's progress. When the NSAID is given to patients with a history of upper or lower GI tract disease, it should be given under close supervison and only after consulting the Adverse Reactions section.

Do not give **indomethacin** to patients with active GI lesions or a history of recurrent GI lesions unless the high risk is warranted and patients can be monitored closely. To reduce GI effects, give NSAIDs after meals, with food, or with antacids (does not apply to enteric-coated **diclofenac**).

Higher doses of **meloxicam** (eg, chronic daily 30 mg doses) were associated with increased risk of serious GI effects. Do not exceed daily doses of 15 mg.

If diarrhea occurs with **mefenamic acid** or diarrhea, GI irritation, and abdominal pain occur with **meclofenamate**, reduce dosage or temporarily discontinue use. Some patients may be unable to tolerate further therapy with these agents.

➤*CNS effects:* **Indomethacin** may aggravate depression or other psychiatric disturbances, epilepsy, and parkinsonism; use with considerable caution. If severe CNS adverse reactions develop, discontinue the drug. Some of these agents also may cause headaches (highest incidence with **fenoprofen**, **indomethacin**, **ketorolac**, and **celecoxib**). If headache persists despite dosage reduction, discontinue use.

➤*Hypersensitivity reactions:* A potentially fatal apparent hypersensitivity syndrome has occurred with **sulindac**; this syndrome may include constitutional symptoms, cutaneous findings, involvement of major organs, conjunctivitis, or other less specific findings. The clinical picture of hypersensitivity reactions may vary from vasomotor rhinitis, urticaria, and angioedema to serious bronchoconstriction and, in some cases, anaphylactic shock. This may be because of an allergic immunological hypersensitivity reaction or a pseudoallergic reaction characterized by mast-cell degranulation by complement components, histamine liberation by drugs, and interference with endogenous eicosanoid biosynthesis. The former mechanism appears to be responsible for the anaphylactic shock or urticaria that may develop after taking amidopyrine or noramidopyrine, the latter for the bronchoconstriction encountered after ingestion of aspirin, noramidopyrine, or of aminophenazone and other pyrazole drugs.

Rarely, fever and other evidence of hypersensitivity, including abnormalities in ≥ 1 liver function tests and severe skin reactions, have occurred during therapy with sulindac. Fatalities have occurred in these patients. Hepatitis, jaundice, or both, with or without fever, may occur usually within the first 1 to 3 months of therapy. Consider determination of liver function whenever a patient on therapy with sulindac develops unexplained fever, rash, or other dermatologic reactions or constitutional symptoms. If unexplained fever or other evidence of hypersensitivity occurs, discontinue therapy with sulindac. The elevated temperature and abnormalities in liver function caused by sulindac characteristically have reverted to normal after discontinuation of therapy. Administration of sulindac should not be reinstituted in such patients.

Anaphylactoid reactions – Anaphylactoid reactions have occurred in patients without known exposure to NSAIDs, but they typically occur in asthmatic patients who experience rhinitis with or without nasal polyps, or who exhibit severe, potentially fatal bronchospasm after taking aspirin or other NSAIDs. Anaphylactoid reactions have occurred in patients with aspirin hypersensitivity and in patients who discontinued **tolmetin**, then restarted it. These reactions appear to occur more often with tolmetin than other NSAIDs not structurally related but data conflict. Refer to Management of Acute Hypersensitivity Reactions.

➤*Renal function impairment:* NSAID metabolites are eliminated primarily by kidneys; use with caution in those with renal function impairment. Assess renal function before and during therapy. Monitor serum creatinine or creatinine clearance. Reduce dosage to avoid excessive accumulation.

In cases of advanced kidney disease, treatment with **piroxicam** and **meloxicam** and **valdecoxib** is not recommended. However, if NSAID therapy must be initiated, close monitoring of the patient's kidney function is advisable. **Sulindac** metabolites have been reported rarely as the major or a minor component in renal stones in association with other calculus components. Use sulindac with caution in patients with a history of renal lithiasis and keep patients well hydrated while receiving the drug.

➤*Hepatic function impairment:* **Naproxen** may exhibit an increase in unbound fraction and a reduced clearance of free drug in cirrhotic liver patients, suggesting an increased potential for toxicity in this group; consider reducing the dose. Also, **sulindac** AUC may increase in patients with cirrhosis because of altered sulfide formation/metabolism. Disposition of total and free **etodolac** is not altered in patients with compensated hepatic cirrhosis. Effects of hepatic disease on other NSAIDs is unknown. Use caution in patients with impaired hepatic function or history of liver disease.

In patients treated with a single 15 mg dose of **meloxicam**, there was no marked difference in plasma concentrations in patients with mild and moderate hepatic impairment compared with healthy subjects. Protein binding of meloxicam was not affected by hepatic insufficiency. No dose adjustment is needed in patients with mild to moderate hepatic insufficiency; patients with severe hepatic impairment have not been adequately studied.

Valdecoxib plasma concentrations are significantly increased (130%) in patients with moderate (Child-Pugh Class B) hepatic impairment. In clinical trials, doses of valdecoxib above those recommended have been associated with fluid retention. The use of valdecoxib in patients with severe hepatic impairment (Child-Pugh Class C) is not recommended.

➤*Elderly:* Age appears to increase the possibility of adverse reactions to NSAIDs. The risk of serious ulcer disease is increased in elderly patients (> 65 years of age) taking NSAIDs; this risk appears to increase with the dose. Use with greater care and begin with reduced dosages. In **nabumetone**- and **valdecoxib**-treated patients, no differences in overall efficacy and safety were observed between older and younger patients. **Ketorolac** is cleared more slowly by the elderly; use caution and reduce dosage.

➤*Pregnancy: Category B* (**ketoprofen, naproxen, naproxen sodium, flurbiprofen, diclofenac, fenoprofen, ibuprofen, indomethacin, meclofenamate, sulindac**). *Category C* (**etodolac, ketorolac, mefenamic acid, meloxicam, nabumetone, oxaprozin, tolmetin, piroxicam, rofecoxib, celecoxib, valdecoxib**). All NSAIDs are *Category D* if used in the third trimester or near delivery.

Safety for use during pregnancy has not been established; use is not recommended. There are no adequate and well-controlled studies in pregnant women. An increased incidence of dystocia, increased postimplantation loss, decreased pup survival, increased length of delivery time, embryolethality, septal heart defects, stillbirth, and delayed parturition occurred in animals. Agents that inhibit prostaglandin synthesis may cause closure of the ductus arteriosus and other untoward effects to the fetus. GI tract toxicity increased in pregnant women in the last trimester. Some NSAIDs may prolong pregnancy if given before onset of labor.

The known effects of drugs of this class on the human fetus during the third trimester of pregnancy include: Constriction of the ductus arteriosus prenatally, tricuspid incompetence, and pulmonary hypertension; nonclosure of the ductus arteriosus postnatally, which may be resistant to medical management; myocardial degenerative changes, platelet dysfunction with resultant bleeding, intracranial bleeding, renal dysfunction or failure, renal injury/dysgenesis that may result in prolonged or permanent renal failure, oligohydramnios, GI bleeding or perforation, and increased risk of necrotizing enterocolitis. Avoid during pregnancy, especially in the third trimester.

➤*Lactation:* Most NSAIDs are excreted in breast milk. **Naproxen** appears at ≈ 1% of maternal serum concentration. In 10 healthy women, recovery of **flurbiprofen** in breast milk accounted for 0.05% (range, 0.03% to 0.07%) of a 100 mg dose; average peak concentration in milk was 0.09 mcg/mL. **Ibuprofen** was not detected in breast milk of 12 women who had ingested 400 mg every 6 hours over 24 hours. **Ketorolac** was detected in breast milk at a maximum milk-to-plasma ratio of 0.037. In general, do not use in nursing mothers because of effects on the infant's cardiovascular system.

➤*Children:* **Mefenamic acid** and **meclofenamate** are not recommended in children < 14 years of age. Safety and efficacy of **meloxicam** and **valdecoxib** use have not been established in children < 18 years of age. **Indomethacin's** safety is not established in children; not recommended in children ≤ 14 years of age, except in circumstances that warrant the risk. When using indomethacin in children ≥ 2 years of age, closely monitor liver function. Hepatotoxicity, including fatalities, has occurred in children with juvenile RA. Suggested starting dose is 2 mg/kg/day in divided doses. Do not exceed 4 mg/kg/day or 150 to 200 mg/day, whichever is less. As symptoms subside, reduce dosage or discontinue drug. For use of IV indomethacin in premature infants, see Agents for Patent Ductus Arteriosus. **Tolmetin** and **naproxen** are the only agents labeled for juvenile RA, although studies are being conducted with other agents. Safety and efficacy of tolmetin and naproxen in infants < 2 years of age are not established. Safety and efficacy of other NSAIDs in children are not established.

Precautions

➤*Monitoring:* Serious GI tract ulceration and bleeding can occur without warning. Follow chronically treated patients for signs and symptoms of ulceration and bleeding; inform them of the importance of this follow-up (see Warnings).

Monitor transaminases and other hepatic enzymes in patients treated with NSAIDs. For patients on **diclofenac** therapy, it is recommended that a determination from lab results be made within 4 weeks of initiating therapy and at intervals thereafter. If clinical signs and symptoms consistent with liver disease develop, or if systemic manifestations occur (eg, eosinophilia, rash) and abnormal liver tests are detected, persist, or worsen, discontinue diclofenac immediately.

➤*Corticosteroid use:* NSAIDs cannot be expected to be a substitute for corticosteroids or to treat corticosteroid insufficiency. Abrupt discontinuation of corticosteroids may lead to disease exacerbation.

➤*Functional class IV RA patients (incapacitated, largely or wholly bedridden, confined to wheelchair):* Safety and efficacy are not established.

➤*Steroid dosage:* If corticosteroid dosage is reduced or eliminated during NSAID therapy, reduce dosage slowly and observe patient closely for evidence of adverse effects, including adrenal insufficiency and exacerbation of symptoms (see Adrenalcortical Steroids, Glucocorticoids monograph).

➤*Porphyria:* Avoid the use of NSAIDs in patients with hepatic porphyria. To date, 1 patient has been described in whom **diclofenac** probably triggered a clinical attack of porphyria. The postulated mechanism demonstrated in rats for causing such attacks by diclofenac, as well as some other NSAIDs, is through stimulation of the porphyria precursor delta-aminolevulinic acid (ALA).

➤*Aseptic meningitis:* Aseptic meningitis with fever and coma has been observed on rare occasions in patients on NSAIDs therapy. Although it is probably more likely to occur in patients with systemic lupus erythematosus (SLE) and related connective tissue diseases, it has been reported in patients who do not have an underlying chronic disease. If signs or symptoms of meningitis develop in a patient on NSAID therapy, consider the possibility of it being related to the NSAID.

➤*Platelet aggregation:* NSAIDs can inhibit platelet aggregation; the effect is reversible, quantitatively less, and of shorter duration than that seen with aspirin. These agents prolong bleeding time (within normal range) in healthy subjects. This may be exaggerated in patients with underlying hemostatic defects; use with caution and carefully monitor in people with intrinsic coagulation defects and in those on anticoagulant therapy.

➤*Pre-existing asthma:* About 10% of patients with asthma may have aspirin-sensitive asthma. The use of aspirin in patients with aspirin-sensitive asthma has been associated with severe bronchospasm, which can be fatal. Because cross reactivity, including bronchospasm, between aspirin and other NSAIDs has been reported in such aspirin-sensitive patients, do not administer NSAIDs to patients with this form of aspirin sensitivity, and use the drug with caution in patients with preexisting asthma.

➤*Hematologic effects:* Decreased hemoglobin or hematocrit levels have rarely required discontinuation. Anemia may be because of fluid retention, GI blood loss, or an incompletely described effect upon erythropoiesis. If anemia is suspected in patients on long-term therapy, determine hemoglobin and hematocrit values. Frequently determine hemoglobin values in patients with initial values ≤ 10 g/dL who are to receive long-term therapy.

Patients on long-term treatments should have their CBC and a chemistry profile checked periodically. Low white blood cell counts occur rarely, are transient, and usually return to normal while therapy continues. Persistent leukopenia, granulocytopenia, or thrombocytopenia warrants further evaluation and may require discontinuing the drug.

Postoperative hematomas and other signs of wound bleeding have occurred with perioperative IM use of **ketorolac**. Exercise caution when administering pre- or intraoperatively and when administering perioperatively if strict hemostasis is critical.

➤*Cardiovascular effects:* May cause fluid retention and peripheral edema. Use caution in compromised cardiac function, hypertension, in patients on chronic diuretic therapy, or other conditions predisposing to fluid retention. Agents may be associated with significant deterioration of circulatory hemodynamics in severe heart failure and hyponatremia, presumably because of inhibition of prostaglandin-dependent compensatory mechanisms.

➤*Ophthalmologic effects:* Perform ophthalmological studies in patients who develop eye complaints during therapy. Effects include blurred or diminished vision, scotomata, changes in color vision, corneal deposits, and retinal disturbances, including maculas. Discontinue therapy if ocular changes are noted. Blurred vision may be significant and warrants thorough examination, including central visual fields and color vision testing. These changes may be asymptomatic; perform periodic examinations in patients on prolonged therapy.

➤*Infection:* NSAIDs may mask the usual signs of infection. Use with extra care in the presence of existing controlled infection. The pharmacologic activity of NSAIDs in reducing inflammation and possibly fever may diminish the utility of these diagnostic signs in detecting complications of presumed noninfectious, painful conditions.

➤*Renal effects:* Acute renal insufficiency, interstitial nephritis with hematuria, nephrotic syndrome, proteinuria, hyperkalemia, hyponatremia, renal papillary necrosis, and other renal medullary changes may occur.

Long-term administration of NSAIDs has resulted in renal papillary necrosis and other renal medullary changes. Renal toxicity also has been seen in patients in whom renal prostaglandins have a compensatory role in the maintenance of renal perfusion. In these patients, administration of NSAIDs may cause dose-dependent reduction in prostaglandin formation and, secondarily, in renal blood flow, which may precipitate overt renal decompensation. Patients at greatest risk of this reaction are those with impaired renal function, heart failure, liver dysfunction, those taking diuretics and ACE inhibitors, and the elderly. Discontinuation of NSAID therapy is usually followed by recovery to the pretreatment state.

Exercise caution when initiating treatment with NSAIDs in patients with considerable dehydration. It is advisable to rehydrate patients first and then start therapy with NSAIDs. Correct hypovolemia before treatment with **ketorolac** is initiated. They are not recommended in patients with pre-existing kidney disease.

Acute renal insufficiency – Patients with pre-existing renal disease or compromised renal perfusion are at greatest risk for acute renal insufficiency. A form of renal toxicity seen in patients with prerenal conditions leads to reduced renal blood flow or blood volume. NSAID use may cause a dose-dependent reduction in prostaglandin formation and precipitate overt renal decompensation. Patients at greatest risk are the elderly; premature infants; those with heart failure, renal or hepatic dysfunction, SLE, chronic glomerulonephritis, dehydration, diabetes mellitus, or impaired renal function; those taking ACE inhibitors; septicemia; pyelonephritis; concomitant use of any nephrotoxic drug; extracellular volume depletion from any cause; and those on diuretics. Recovery usually follows discontinuation.

Those patients at high risk who chronically take NSAIDs should have renal function monitored if they have signs or symptoms that may be consistent with mild azotemia (eg, malaise, fatigue, loss of appetite). Patients occasionally may develop some elevation of serum creatinine and BUN levels without any signs and symptoms. There may also be substantial proteinuria and, on renal biopsy, electron microscopy has shown foot process fusion and T-lymphocyte infiltration in the renal interstitium.

Interstitial nephritis – Interstitial nephritis has occurred with increased frequency in patients receiving NSAIDs and may be due to altered prostaglandin metabolism.

GU tract problems have occurred in patients taking **fenoprofen**, most frequently, dysuria, cystitis, hematuria, interstitial nephritis, and nephrotic syndrome. This may be preceded by fever, rash, arthralgia, oliguria, and azotemia, and may progress to anuria. Rapid recovery followed early recognition and drug withdrawal.

Hyperkalemia – Another potentially serious NSAID-induced renal electrolyte abnormality is hyperkalemia. NSAIDs tend to blunt prostaglandin-mediated renin release, leading to diminished aldosterone formation and, hence, decreased potassium excretion. NSAIDs can augment sodium and chloride reabsorption within the renal tubule in the setting of diminished glomerular filtration rate by opposing natriuretic and diuretic prostaglandins. This decreases the delivery of intraluminal sodium for sodium-potassium exchange at the distal nephron.

Papillary necrosis – Papillary necrosis may present as an acute or chronic form of NSAID nephropathy in the setting of massive NSAID overdose in a dehydrated patient with preexisting normal renal function. The chronic form is associated with analgesic-abuse nephropathy.

➤*Hepatic effects:* Borderline liver function test elevations may occur in ≈ 15% of patients and may progress, remain essentially unchanged,

or become transient with continued therapy. The ALT test is probably the most sensitive indicator of liver dysfunction. Meaningful (≥ 3 times upper limit of normal) AST or ALT elevations occurred in ≈ 1% of patients. If symptoms or signs suggesting liver dysfunction, or an abnormal test occurs, evaluate for more severe hepatic reactions. Severe reactions, including jaundice and fatal fulminant hepatitis, liver necrosis, and hepatic failure have occurred rarely, some with fatal outcomes. Evaluate a patient with symptoms and signs suggesting liver dysfunction, or in whom an abnormal liver test has occurred, for evidence of the development of more severe hepatic reactions while on therapy with NSAIDs. If an NSAID is to be used in the presence of impaired liver function, it must be done under strict observation. Discontinue treatment if abnormal tests persist or worsen, if clinical signs and symptoms consistent with liver disease develop, or if systemic manifestations occur (eg, eosinophilia, rash).

➤*Pancreatitis:* Pancreatitis has occurred in patients receiving **sulindac**. If pancreatitis is suspected, discontinue the drug, start supportive therapy, and monitor closely (eg, serum and urine amylase, amylase/creatinine clearance ratio, electrolytes, serum calcium, glucose, lipase). Check for other causes of pancreatitis as well as for conditions that mimic pancreatitis.

➤*Auditory effects:* Perform periodic auditory function tests during chronic **fenoprofen** therapy in patients with impaired hearing.

➤*Heavy menstrual blood loss evaluation:* Prior to prescribing **meclofenamate** for heavy blood flow and primary dysmenorrhea, make a thorough risk/benefit assessment that takes into account the results described in the clinical pharmacology section. It is recommended that meclofenamate treatment not be prescribed for heavy menstrual flow without establishing its idiopathic nature. Fully evaluate spotting or bleeding between cycles and do not treat with meclofenamate. Worsening of menstrual blood loss or excessive blood loss failing to respond to meclofenamate should also be evaluated by an appropriate work-up and not treated with meclofenamate.

➤*Dermatologic effects:* A combination of dermatologic and allergic signs and symptoms suggestive of serum sickness have occasionally occurred in conjunction with the use of **piroxicam**. These include arthralgias, pruritus, fever, fatigue, and rash including vesiculobullous reactions and exfoliative dermatitis.

➤*Concomitant NSAID therapy:* Do not use **naproxen sodium** and **naproxen** concomitantly; both drugs circulate as naproxen anion.

Do not use **diclofenac** immediate-release, delayed-release, and extended-release tablets concomitantly with other diclofenac-containing products because they also circulate in plasma as diclofenac anion.

➤*Photosensitivity:* Photosensitivity may occur; caution patients to take protective measures (ie, sunscreens, protective clothing) against UV or sunlight until tolerance is determined.

Drug Interactions

➤*Cytochrome P450:* Exercise caution when coadministering **celecoxib** and **mefenamic acid** with drugs known to inhibit the isoenzyme 2C9.

NSAID Drug Interactions			
Precipitant drug	Object drug*		Description
Bisphosphonates	NSAIDs	↑	Risk of gastric ulceration may be increased. Use cautiously.
Cholestyramine	NSAIDs	↓	The effects of NSAIDs may be decreased. Cholestyramine has enhanced piroxicam and meloxicam plasma clearance and decreased the GI absorption of NSAIDs.
Cimetidine	NSAIDs	↔	NSAID plasma concentrations may be increased or decreased by cimetidine; some studies report no effect. Also, indomethacin and sulindac have increased ranitidine and cimetidine bioavailability.
Colestipol	NSAIDs	↓	The effects of diclofenac may be decreased because colestipol may interfere with the absorption of diclofenac, thereby reducing bioavailability.
Diflunisal	NSAIDs Indomethacin	↑	Diflunisal may decrease the renal clearance and significantly increase indomethacin plasma concentrations that may produce toxicity.
Dimethyl sulfoxide (DMSO)	NSAIDs Sulindac	↓	DMSO may decrease the formation of the active metabolite of sulindac, possibly resulting in a decreased therapeutic effect. Also, topical DMSO with sulindac has resulted in severe peripheral neuropathy.
Fluconazole	NSAIDs Celecoxib Valdecoxib	↑	Increase in celecoxib plasma concentration may occur because of inhibition of celecoxib metabolism. May increase valdecoxib AUC also.
Ketoconazole	NSAIDs Valdecoxib	↑	May increase valdecoxib AUC.
Phenobarbital	NSAIDs Fenoprofen	↓	Phenobarbital, an enzyme inducer, may decrease fenoprofen half-life. Dosage adjustments of fenoprofen may be required if phenobarbital is added or withdrawn.
Phenylbutazone	NSAIDs Etodolac	↑	Phenylbutazone can increase by approximately 80% the free fraction of etodolac. Coadministration is not recommended.
Probenecid	NSAIDs	↑	Probenecid may increase the concentrations and possibly the toxicity of NSAIDs. Do not use ketorolac and probenecid concomitantly.
Rifampin	NSAIDs Rofecoxib	↓	Coadministration of rofecoxib with rifampin may produce a decrease in rofecoxib plasma concentrations.
Ritonavir	NSAIDs Piroxicam	↑	Ritonavir may increase the concentrations and possibly the toxicity of piroxicam by inhibiting its metabolism.
Salicylates	NSAIDs	↓	Plasma concentrations of NSAIDs may be decreased by salicylates. Avoid concurrent use because it offers no therapeutic advantage and may significantly increase the incidence of GI effects.

NSAID Drug Interactions			
Precipitant drug	Object drug*		Description
Salicylates	NSAIDs Ketorolac	↑	Increased risk of serious ketorolac-related side effects may occur. Salicylates may displace ketorolac from protein binding sites and may produce possible synergistic side effects. Ketorolac is contraindicated in patients receiving aspirin.
Sulcralfate	NSAIDs	↓	The effects of diclofenac may be decreased, possibly because of decreased absorption. Sucralfate does not appear to alter ketoprofen or naproxen bioavailability.
NSAIDs	ACE inhibitors	↓	Antihypertensive effects of captopril may be blunted or completely abolished by indomethacin. Other reports suggest that NSAIDs may diminish the antihypertensive effect of ACE inhibitors.
NSAIDs	Aminoglycosides	↑	Aminoglycoside plasma concentrations may be elevated in premature infants because of NSAIDs reducing the glomerular filtration rate. Reduce aminoglycoside dose prior to NSAID initiation and monitor serum aminoglycoside levels and renal function.
NSAIDs	Anticoagulants	↑	Coadministration may prolong prothrombin time (PT). Also consider the effects NSAIDs have on platelet function and gastric mucosa. Monitor PT and patients closely, especially the first few days, and instruct patients to watch for signs and symptoms of bleeding.
NSAIDs	Beta blockers	↓	The antihypertensive effect of beta blockers may be impaired, possibly because of NSAID inhibition of renal prostaglandin synthesis, thereby allowing unopposed pressor systems to produce hypertension. Avoid using this combination if possible. Monitor blood pressure and adjust beta blocker dose as needed. Consider using a non-interacting NSAID (eg, sulindac).
NSAIDs Cyclosporine	Cyclosporine NSAIDs	↑	Nephrotoxicity of both agents may be increased.
NSAIDs Valdecoxib	Dextromethorphan	↑	Coadministration may increase dextromethorphan plasma levels.
NSAIDs Ibuprofen Indomethacin	Digoxin	↑	Ibuprofen and indomethacin may increase digoxin serum levels.
NSAIDs Indomethacin	Dipyridamole	↑	Indomethacin and dipyridamole coadministration may augment water retention.
NSAIDs	Diuretics	↓	Effects of diuretics may be decreased.
NSAIDs	Hydantoins	↑	Serum phenytoin levels may be increased, resulting in an increase in pharmacologic and toxic effects of phenytoin.
NSAIDs	Lithium	↑	Serum lithium levels may be increased; however, sulindac has no effect or may decrease lithium levels. Monitor for signs of lithium toxicity.
NSAIDs	Methotrexate	↑	The risks of methotrexate toxicity (eg, stomatitis, bone marrow suppression, nephrotoxicity) may be increased. At higher than recommended doses, rofecoxib may increase the methotrexate plasma concentrations. Celecoxib and meloxicam did not have a significant effect on methotrexate pharmacokinetics.
NSAIDs Indomethacin	Penicillamine	↑	Indomethacin may increase the bioavailability of penicillamine.
NSAIDs Indomethacin Diclofenac	Potassium-sparing diuretics	↓	Effects of potassium-diuretics may be decreased. Coadministration may increase serum potassium levels.
NSAIDs Rofecoxib	Theophylline	↑	Coadministration may increase plasma theophylline concentrations. Monitor plasma concentrations closely.
NSAIDs	Thiazide diuretics	↔	Decreased antihypertensive and diuretic action of thiazides may occur with concurrent indomethacin. Naproxen also has been implicated. Sulindac may enhance the effects of thiazides.

*↑ = Object drug increased. ↓ = Object drug decreased. ↔ = Undetermined clinical effect.

▶*Drug/Lab test interactions:* **Naproxen** use may result in increased urinary values for 17-ketogenic steroids because of an interaction between naproxen or its metabolites with m-dinitro-benzene used in this assay. Although 17-hydroxycorticosteroid measurements (Porter-Silber test) do not appear to be artificially altered, temporarily discontinue naproxen therapy 72 hours before adrenal function tests are performed. Naproxen may interfere with some urinary assays of 5-hydroxy indoleacetic acid.

Tolmetin – Tolmetin metabolites in urine give positive tests for proteinuria using acid precipitation tests (eg, **sulfosalicylic acid**). Use commercially available dye-impregnated reagent strips.

Mefenamic acid – A false-positive reaction for urinary bile, using the diazo tablet test, may result. If biliuria is suspected, use other procedures (ie, the Harrison spot test).

Fenoprofen – Amerlex-M kit assay values of total and free triiodothyronine in patients on fenoprofen have been reported as falsely elevated on the basis of a chemical cross-reaction that directly interferes with the assay. Thyroid-stimulating hormone, total thyroxine, and thyrotropin-releasing hormone response are not affected.

Oxaprozin – False-positive urine immunoassay screening tests for benzodiazepines have been reported in patients taking oxaprozin. This is because of the lack of specificity of the screening tests. False-positive test results may be expected for several days following discontinuation of oxaprozin therapy. Confirmatory tests, such as gas chromatography/mass spectrometry, will distinguish oxaprozin from benzodiazepines.

NSAIDs, by decreasing platelet adhesion and aggregation, can prolong bleeding time ≈ 3 to 4 minutes.

▶*Drug/Food interactions:* Administration of **tolmetin** with milk had no effect on peak-plasma tolmetin concentration, but decreased total tolmetin bioavailability by 16%. When tolmetin was taken immediately after a meal, peak plasma concentrations were reduced by 50%, while total bioavailability was again decreased by 16%. Peak concentration of **etodolac** is reduced by ≈ 50% and the time to peak is increased by 1.4 to 3.8 hours following administration with food; however, the extent of absorption is not affected. Food may reduce the rate of absorption of **oxaprozin**, but the extent is unchanged.

Adverse Reactions

NSAIDs Adverse Reactions (%)[1]

	Adverse reaction	Celecoxib	Diclofenac	Etodolac	Fenoprofen	Flurbiprofen	Ibuprofen	Indomethacin	Ketoprofen	Ketorolac	Meclofenamate	Mefenamic acid	Meloxicam	Nabumetone	Naproxen	Oxaprozin	Piroxicam	Rofecoxib	Sulindac	Tolmetin	Valdecoxib
Cardiovascular	Palpitations	<2	<1	<1	2.5		<1	<1	<1	<1	<1	<1	<2	<1	1-3	<1	<1	<2	<1		<2
	Hypertension		<1	<1		<1	<1	<1	<1	1-3		<1	<2	<1			<1	3.5-10	<1	3-9	1.6-2.1
	MI	<2	<1	<1		<1			<1			<1	<2	<1			<1	<0.1			<0.1
	Tachycardia	<2	<1		<1			<1	<1			<1	<2				<1	<2			<2
	CHF	<0.1	<1	<1			<1	<1	<1			<1			<1		<1	<0.1	<1	<1	<2
	Arrhythmia		<1			<1	<1[2]	<1	<1			<1	<2	<1			<1		<1		<2
	Angina/Angina pectoris	<2				<1							<2	<1				<2			<2
	CVA	<0.1	<1			<1												<0.1			
	Pulmonary embolism	<0.1				<1												<0.1			<0.1
	Syncope	<0.1		<1				<1		<1		<1	<2				<1	<2	<1		<0.1
	Vasculitis	<0.1		<1[3]								<1	<2	<1		<1					
	Flushing		<1	<1				<1										<2			
	Hypotension		<1					<1				<1	<2				<1				<2
CNS	Headache	15.8	3-9	<1	8.7	3-9	1-3	11.7	3-9	17	3-9	1-10	2.4-8.3	3-9	3-9		1-10	4.7	3-9	3-9	4.8-8.5
	Dizziness	2	1-3	3-9	6.5	1-3	3-9	3-9	1-3	7	3-9	1-10	1.1-3.8	3-9	3-9		1-10	3	3-9	3-9	2.6-2.7
	Asthenia/malaise	<2	<1	3-9	1-5.4					<1	<1	<1	<2	<1	<1	<1	<1	2.2		3-9	<2
	Depression	<2	<1	1-3	<1		<1	1-3		<1	<1	<1	<2	<1	<1		<1	<2		1-3	<2
	Nervousness	<2		1-3	5.7	1-3	1-3	<1		<1			<1	<2	1-3		<1		1-3		<2
	Somnolence	<2		<1	8.5		<1	1-3					<1	<2	1-3		<1	<2	<1		<2
	Tremor		<1		2.2					<1			<1	<2	<1		<1				<2
	Confusion			<1	1.4	<1	<1	<1	<1				<1	<2	<1		<1	<0.1			<2
	Fatigue	<2			1.7			1-3			<1		<2	1-3				2.2			<2
	Drowsiness		<1					<1	6			<1			3-9		<1			1-3	
	Insomnia	2.3	<1	<1			<1	<1	<1	<1	<1	<1	≤3.6	1-3	<1		<1	<2	<1		<2
	Lightheadedness							<1							1-3						
	Vertigo	<2						1-3	<1	<1			2	<1	1-3		<1	<2	<1		<2
	CNS inhibition[4]															1-3					
	CNS inhibition or excitation					1-3[5]			3-9[6]												
	Paresthesia	<2	<1	<1		<1	<1	<1	<1	<1	<1	<1	<2	<1			<1	<2	<1		<2
	Anxiety	<2	<1					<1				<1	<2	<1			<1	<2			<2
	Hypesthesia	<2																<2			<2
	Migraine	<2								<1								<2			<2
	Aseptic meningitis		<1					<1[7]		<1					<1			<0.1	<1		
	Convulsions		<1			<1		<1			<1	<2					<1		<1		<0.1
	Hypertonia	<2				<1															<2
	Hallucinations							<1		<1	<1	<1					<1	<0.1			
	Abnormal dreams/dream abnormalities							<1		<1		<1	<2				<1		<1		
Dermatologic	Rash	2.2	1-3	1-3	3.7	1-3	3-9	<1	1-3	1-3	3-9	1-10	0.3-3	3-9	<1	3-9	1-10	<2	3-9		1.4-2.1
	Pruritus	<2	1-3	1-3	4.2	<1	1-3	<1	<1	1-3	1-3	1-10	≤2.4	3-9	3-9	<1	1-10	<2	1-3		<2
	Increased sweating	<2	<1	<1	4.6	<1		<1	<1	1-3		<1	<2	1-3	1-3		<1	<2			<2
	Skin eruptions														3-9						
	Urticaria	<2	<1	<1	<1	<1	<1	<1	<1	<1	1-3	<1	<2	<1	<1	<1	<1	<2		<1	<2
	Skin irritation																			1-3	
	Alopecia/Loss of hair	<2	<1	<1	<1	<1	<1	<1		<1		<1	<2	<1	<1	<1	<1	<2		<1	<2
	Photosensitivity/Photo-sensitivity reaction	<2	<1	<1		<1				<1		<1	<2	<1	<1[8]	<1				<1	<2
	Erythema multiforme	<0.1	<1[9]	<1			<1	<1	<1		<1		<0.1	<1	<1	<1	<1			<1	<1
	Stevens-Johnson syndrome	<0.1	<1	<1	<1		<1	<1	<1		<1	<1	<0.1	<1	<1	<1	<1	<0.1	<1		
	Toxic epidermal necrolysis/Lyell's syndrome	<0.1			<1	<1	<1	<1	<1				<0.1	<1		<1		<0.1	<1	<1	
	Exfoliative dermatitis	<0.1	<1		<1	<1		<1	<1		<1	<1				<1	<1		<1		
	Bullous eruption/rash		<1						<1				<2	<1							
	Eczema		<1			<1		<1													<2

NSAIDs Adverse Reactions (%)[1]

_GI_

Adverse reaction	Celecoxib	Diclofenac	Etodolac	Fenoprofen	Flurbiprofen	Ibuprofen	Indomethacin	Ketoprofen	Ketorolac	Meclofenamate	Mefenamic acid	Meloxicam	Nabumetone	Naproxen	Oxaprozin	Piroxicam	Rofecoxib	Sulindac	Tolmetin	Valdecoxib
Abdominal pain or cramps	4.1	3-9	3-9	2	3-9	1-3	1-3	3-9		3-9	1-10	1.9-4.7	12	3-9	1-3	1-10	3.4	10 (pain) 1-3 (cramps)	3-9	7-8.2
Abdominal distension		1-3					<1											<2		
Diarrhea	5.6	3-9	3-9	1.8	3-9	1-3	1-3	3-9	7	10-33	1-10	1.9-7.8	14	1-3	3-9	1-10	6.5	3-9	3-9	5.4-6
Nausea	3.5	3-9	3-9	7.7	3-9	3-9	3-9	3-9	12	11	1-10	2.4-7.2	3-9	3-9	3-9	1-10	5.2	3-9	11	6.3-7
Vomiting	<2	<1	1-3	2.6	1-3			1-3	1-3		1-10	0.6-2.6	1-3	<1	1-3	1-10	<2		3-9	<2
Nausea and vomiting						1-3	1-3			11										
Constipation	<2	3-9	1-3	7	1-3	1-3	1-3	3-9	1-3	1-3	1-10	0.8-2.6	3-9	3-9	3-9	1-10	<2	3-9	1-3	<2
Flatulence	2.2	1-3	3-9	<1	1-3	1-3	<1	3-9	1-3	3-9	1-10	0.4-3.2	3-9		1-3	1-10	<2	1-3	3-9	2.9-3.5
Peptic ulcer bleed		1-3	<1			<1							<2		<1					
Dyspepsia/Indigestion	8.8	3-9	10	10.3	3-9	1-3	3-9	11	12		1-10	3.8-9.5	13	1-3	3-9	1-10	3.5	3-9	3-9	7.9-8.7
Gastritis	<2		1-3	<1	<1	<1		<1	<1		<1	<2	1-3			<1	<2	<1	1-3	<2
Melena	<2	<1	1-3				<1	<1			<1	<2	<1	<1		<1				
GI bleeding	<0.1	0.6		<1	1-3	<1					<1	<2	<1	<1	<1		<0.1	<1	<1	<0.1
Epigastric/GI pain							3-9		13											
Heartburn							3-9			3-9	1-10			3-9		1-10	4.2			
Abdominal/GI distress						1-3	1-3								1-3				3-9	
Bloating						1-3	<1													1.9-2.1
GI fullness						1-3			1-3											
Stomatitis	<2					<1		1-3	1-3	1-3	<1		1-3	1-3	<1	<1		<1	<1	<2
Anorexia/Decreased appetite	<2		<1	<1			1-3	<1	1-3	<1			<1		1-3	1-10		1-3		
Positive stool guaiac					<1								3-9							
Dry mouth	<2	<1	<1	<1	<1	<1		<1	<1		<1	<2	1-3			<1	<2			<2
Gross bleeding/ perforation											1-10					1-10				
Epigastric discomfort																		3.8		
Peptic ulcer		0.6	<1	<1	<1		<1	<1		1-3	1-10	<2	<1		<1	1-10	<0.1	<1	<1	<2
Hepatitis	<0.1	<1	<1		<1	<1		<1			<1	<2			<1	<1	<0.1	<1	<1	<2
Jaundice	<0.1	<1	<1	<1		<1		<1			<1	<0.1	<1	<1	<1	<1	<0.1	<1[10]		
Pancreatitis	<0.1	<1[11]	<1	<1		<1		<1			<1	<2	<1	<1	<1	<1	<0.1	<1		
Colitis		<1	<1		<1					<1		<2		<1			<1			<2
Hematemesis							<1	<1			<1	<2		<1		<1				<2
Appetite increase	<2							<1	<1			<2	<1							<2
Eructation	<2		<1					<1	<1		<1	<2	<1			<1				<2
Esophagitis	<2		<1[12]								<1	<2				<1		<2		<2
Gastroenteritis	<2						<1							<1				<2	<1	<2
Liver failure	<0.1		<1								<1	<0.1	<1			<1	<0.1	<1		
Appetite change		<1				<1					<1					<1	<2			
Rectal bleeding/hemorrhage							<1	<1	<1		<1			<1	<1	<1				
Glossitis											<1			<1		<1			<1	

NSAIDs Adverse Reactions (%)[1]

System	Adverse reaction	Celecoxib	Diclofenac	Etodolac	Fenoprofen	Flurbiprofen	Ibuprofen	Indomethacin	Ketoprofen	Ketorolac	Meclofenamate	Mefenamic acid	Meloxicam	Nabumetone	Naproxen	Oxaprozin	Piroxicam	Rofecoxib	Sulindac	Tolmetin	Valdecoxib
GU	Dysuria	<2		1-3	<1							<1		<1		1-3	<1	<2	<1	<1	<2
	Urinary frequency/Polyuria	<2	<1	1-3			<1	<1		<1		<1	0.1-2.4			1-3	<1				<2
	Urinary tract infection/symptoms	<2				3-9			1-3				0.3-6.9					2.8		1-3	<2
	Renal function impairment/insufficiency/abnormal			<1				<1	3-9			1-10				<1	1-10		<1		
	Hematuria	<2	<1	<1	<1	<1	<1	<1	<1	<1		<1	<2	<1	<1	<1	<1		<1	<1	<2
	Interstitial nephritis/acute interstitial nephritis	<0.1	<1	<1	<1	<1		<1	<1			<1	<0.1	<1	<1	<1	<1	<0.1	<1		
	Renal failure			<1	<1	<1		<1	<1	<1		<1	<2	<1	<1				<1	<1	
	Albuminuria	<2											<2	<1							<2
	Cystitis	<2		<1	<1		<1					<1					<1	<2			<2
	Menstrual disorder/disturbance	<2				<1										<1		<2			<2
	Renal calculi/stones	<2		<1											<1				<1		<0.1
	Acute renal failure	<0.1	<1				<1									<1		<0.1			<0.1
	Azotemia		<1		<1		<1								<1						
	Impotence		<1						<1						<1						<2
	Nephrotic syndrome		<1					<1							<1	<1	<1	<1	<1		
	Oliguria		<1	<1						<1		<1					<1				
	Papillary necrosis/renal papillary necrosis		<1	<1	<1		<1								<1						
	Proteinuria		<1					<1		<1		<1					<1		<1	<1	
	Vaginal bleeding/hemorrhage	<2	<1			<1		<1							<1				<1		<2
	Gynecomastia						<1	<1	<1										<1		
Hematologic/Lymphatic	Purpura		<1		<1			<1	1-3			<1	<2		1-3		<1		<1	<1	
	Ecchymoses	<2		<1		<1		<1				<1			3-9	<1	<1		<1		<2
	Anemia	<2		<1				<1		<1		1-10	≤4.1	<1		<1	1-10				<2
	Agranulocytosis	<0.1	<1	<1	<1		<1	<1	<1		<1	<1	<0.1		<1	<1	<1	<0.1	<1	<1	
	Leukopenia	<0.1	<1	<1		<1		<1			<1	<1	<2	<1	<1	<1	<1	<0.1	<1		<2
	Thrombocytopenia	<0.1	<1	<1	<1	<1	<1[13]		<1			<1	<2	<1	<1	<1	<1	<0.1	<1	<1	<2
	Hemolytic anemia		<1	<1	<1	<1	<1	<1			<1	<1			<1		<1		<1	<1	
	Aplastic anemia	<0.1	<1		<1	<1	<1	<1				<1			<1		<1		<1		
	Pancytopenia	<0.1		<1	<1							<1				<1	<1				<0.1
	Eosinophilia		<1			<1	<1			<1	<1	<1				<1	<1				<2
	Neutropenia		<1				<1			<1									<1		
	Lymphadenopathy				<1	<1						<1				<1				<1	<2
Hypersensitivity	Anaphylaxis or anaphylactic/anaphylactoid reaction	<0.1	<1	<1[14]	<1	<1	<1	<1	<1			<1	<0.1[15]	<1	<1	<1	<1	<0.1	<1	<1	
	Angioedema/Angioneurotic edema	<0.1	<1	<1	<1	<1	<1	<1				<1	<2	<1	<1			<1	<0.1	<1	
	Allergy/Allergic reaction	<2		<1					<1				<2					<2			<2
	Serum sickness							<1								<1	<1			<1	
Lab test abnormalities	ALT or AST elevations	<2	2		<1								<2								<2
	Liver test abnormalities/elevations		3-9	<1		1-3	<1				<1	1-10			<1	<1	<1	1-10		<1	<1
	BUN increased	<2		<1				<1	3-9				<2							1-3	<2
	Bleeding time increased			<1								1-10					1-10				
	Hemoglobin and hematocrit decreases		<1			<1	<1				<1									1-3	
	Creatinine increase	<2		<1									<2								<2

NSAIDs Adverse Reactions (%)[1]

	Adverse reaction	Celecoxib	Diclofenac	Etodolac	Fenoprofen	Flurbiprofen	Ibuprofen	Indomethacin	Ketoprofen	Ketorolac	Meclofenamate	Mefenamic acid	Meloxicam	Nabumetone	Naproxen	Oxaprozin	Piroxicam	Rofecoxib	Sulindac	Tolmetin	Valdecoxib
Metabolic/Nutritional	Fluid retention		1-3					1-3	<1									<2			
	Peripheral edema	2.1			5													<2			2.4-3
	Edema	< 2		<1		3-9	1-3	<1	3-9	4	1-3	1-10	0.5-4.5[16]	3-9	3-9	<1	1-10		1-3	3-9	<2
	Body weight changes		<1			1-3		<1				<1	<2			<1	<1			3-9	<2
	Thirst			<1				<1							1-3						<2
	Lower extremity edema																	3.7			
	Hyperglycemia	<2		<1[17]				<1				<1		<1	<1		<1		<1		<2
	Hyperkalemia					<1		<1							<1		<1	<0.1	<1		<2
	Hypokalemia	<2													<1						<2
	Weight gain	<2						<1	<1						<1			<2			
Musculoskeletal	Arthralgia	<2											≤5.3					<2			< 2
	Myalgia	<2							<1						<1			<2			1.9-2
	Muscle weakness							<1							<1			<2	<1		
Respiratory	Dyspnea	<2	<1	<1	2.8	<1		<1	<1	<1		<1	<2	<1	3-9		<1	< 2	<1		<2
	Upper respiratory infection	8.1			1.5								≤8.3			<1		8.5			5.7-6.7
	Rhinitis	2		<1		1-3	<1		<1	<1											<2
	Pharyngitis	2.3		<1				<1					0.6-3.2					<2			<2
	Sinusitis	5		<1												<1		2.7			1.8-2.6
	Bronchitis	<2		<1		<1												2			<2
	Coughing	<2							<1				0.2-2.4	<1				<2			<2
	Epistaxis	<2	<1			<1		<1	<1	<1	<1						<1	<2	<1	<1	<2
	Asthma		<1	<1		<1		<1				<1	<2	<1			<1	<2			
	Pneumonia	<2										<1					<1	<2			<2
	Bronchospasm	<2						<1		<1			<2				<0.1		<1		<2
	Pulmonary edema					<1			<1	<1							<0.1				<0.1
Special senses	Tinnitus	<2	1-3	1-3	4.5	1-3	1-3	1-3	1-3	<1	1-3	1-10	<2	3-9	3-9	1-3	1-10	<2	1-3	1-3	<2
	Hearing disturbances							<1							1-3						
	Blurred vision	<2	<1	1-3	2.2			<1		<1	<1	<1				<1	<1	<2	<1		<2
	Visual disturbances/ changes			<1		1-3		1-3						<1	1-3				<1	1-3	
	Conjunctivitis	<2		<1									<2		<1	<1	<1	<2			<2
	Hearing loss/impairment	<1[18]			1.6			<1	<1	<1	<1					<1	<1	<1		<1	
	Diplopia		<1		<1			<1	<1												
	Taste disorder/perversion/ disturbance/alteration/ changes	<2	<1	<1		<1			<1			<1	<2	<1		<1					<2
Miscellaneous	Chills			1-3		<1			<1					<1	<1			<2			<2
	Fever	<2		1-3	<1	<1		<1		<1		<1	<2	<1	<1		<1	<2		<1	<2
	Back pain	2.8											0.4-3					2.5			1.6-2.7
	Injury, accidental	2.9																			3.7-4
	Influenza-like disease/ symptoms	<2											4.5-5.8				<1	2.9			2-2.2
	Pain	<2						<1					0.9-5.2					<2			<2
	Accident, household												3.2-4.5								
	Fall												≤2.6								
	Chest pain	<2	<1					<1										<2		1-3	<2
	Infection			<1					<1	<1		<1					<1	<2			
	Face edema	<2						<1					<2								<2

[1] Data are pooled from separate studies and are not necessarily comparable.
[2] Sinus tachycardia, sinus bradycardia.
[3] Including necrotizing and allergic.
[4] CNS inhibition (depression, sedation, somnolence, or confusion).
[5] CNS stimulation (eg, anxiety, insomnia, reflexes increased, tremor) or CNS inhibition (eg, amnesia, asthenia, somnolence, malaise, depression).
[6] CNS inhibition (eg, somnolence, malaise, depression) or CNS excitation (eg, insomnia, nervousness, dreams).
[7] With fever and coma.
[8] Resembling porphyria cutanea tarda.
[9] Erythema multiforme major.
[10] Sometimes with fever.
[11] With or without concomitant hepatitis.
[12] With or without stricture or cardiospasm.
[13] With or without purpura.
[14] Anaphylactic/Anaphylactoid reaction (including shock).
[15] Including shock.
[16] Edema, dependent edema, peripheral edema, and leg edema combined.
[17] In previously uncontrolled diabetes.
[18] Reversible and irreversible.

►*Cardiovascular:*
Celecoxib – Aggravated hypertension, coronary artery disorder (less than 2%); peripheral gangrene, thrombophlebitis, ventricular fibrillation (less than 0.1%).

Diclofenac – Premature ventricular contractions (less than 1%).

Fenoprofen – Atrial fibrillation, ECG changes, supraventricular tachycardia (less than 1%).

Flurbiprofen – Cerebrovascular ischemia, heart failure, vascular diseases, vasodilation (less than 1%).

Indomethacin – Thrombophlebitis (less than 1%).

Ketoprofen – Peripheral vascular disease, vasodilation (less than 1%).

Meloxicam – Cardiac failure (less than 2%).

Nabumetone – Thrombophlebitis (less than 1%).

Oxaprozin – Blood pressure changes (less than 1%).

Piroxicam – Exacerbation of angina (less than 1%).

Rofecoxib – Atrial fibrillation, bradycardia, hematoma, irregular heartbeat, premature ventricular contraction, venous insufficiency (less than 2%); deep venous thrombosis, transient ischemic attack, unstable angina (less than 0.1%).

Valdecoxib – Aggravated hypertension, aneurysm, bradycardia, cardiomyopathy, cerebrovascular disorder, coronary artery disorder, heart murmur, hemangioma acquired, intermittent claudication, varicose vein (less than 2%); abnormal ECG, aortic stenosis, atrial fibrillation, carotid stenosis, coronary thrombosis, heart block, heart valve disorders, hypertensive encephalopathy, mitral insufficiency, myocardial ischemia, pericarditis, syncope, thrombophlebitis, thrombosis, unstable angina, vasospasm, ventricular fibrillation (less than 0.1%).

►**CNS:**

Celecoxib – Leg cramps, neuralgia, neuropathy (less than 2%); ataxia (less than 0.1%).

Diclofenac – Abnormal coordination, disorientation, irritability, memory disturbance, nightmares, psychotic reaction, tic (less than 1%).

Fenoprofen – Disorientation, personality change, seizures, trigeminal neuralgia (less than 1%).

Flurbiprofen – Ataxia, emotional lability, meningitis, subarachnoid hemorrhage, twitching (less than 1%).

Ibuprofen – Emotional lability, pseudotumor cerebri (less than 1%).

Indomethacin – Aggravation of epilepsy and parkinsonism, coma, depersonalization, dysarthria, peripheral neuropathy, psychic disturbances (including psychotic episodes) (less than 1%).

Ketoprofen – Amnesia, dysphoria, libido disturbances, nightmares, personality disorder (less than 1%).

Ketorolac – Abnormal thinking, euphoria, excessive thirst, extrapyramidal symptoms, hyperkinesis, inability to concentrate, stupor (less than 1%).

Mefenamic acid – Coma, meningitis (less than 1%).

Nabumetone – Agitation, nightmares (less than 1%).

Naproxen – Cognitive dysfunction, inability to concentrate (less than 1%).

Oxaprozin – Sleep disturbance (1% to 3%); weakness (less than 1%).

Piroxicam – Akathisia, coma, meningitis, mood alterations (less than 1%).

Rofecoxib – Median nerve neuropathy, mental acuity decreased, sciatica (less than 2%).

Sulindac – Neuritis, psychic disturbances (including acute psychosis) (less than 1%).

Valdecoxib – Aggravated depression, morbid dreaming, neuralgia, neuropathy, twitching (less than 2%); benign brain neoplasm, manic reaction, psychosis (less than 0.1%).

►**Dermatologic:**

Celecoxib – Cellulitis, contact dermatitis, dermatitis, dry skin, herpes simplex, herpes zoster, injection site reaction, nail disorder, rash erythematous, rash maculopapular, skin disorder, skin nodule (less than 2%).

Diclofenac – Dermatitis (less than 1%).

Etodolac – Cutaneous vasculitis with purpura, hyperpigmentation, maculopapular rash, skin peeling, vesiculobullous rash (less than 1%).

Flurbiprofen – Dry skin, herpes simplex zoster, nail disorder (less than 1%).

Ibuprofen – Photoallergic skin reactions, vesiculobullous eruptions (less than 1%).

Indomethacin – Erythema nodosum, petechiae (less than 1%).

Ketoprofen – Onycholysis, purpuric rash, skin discoloration (less than 1%).

Ketorolac – Pallor (less than 1%).

Meclofenamate – Erythema nodosum (less than 1%).

Mefenamic acid – Toxic epidermal necrosis (less than 1%).

Nabumetone – Acne, pseudoporphyria cutanea tarda (less than 1%).

Naproxen – Epidermal necrolysis, epidermolysis bullosa, photosensitive dermatitis (less than 1%).

Oxaprozin – Pseudoporphyria (less than 1%).

Piroxicam – Bruising, desquamation, erythema, onycholysis, petechial rash, toxic epidermal necrosis, vesiculobullous reaction (less than 1%).

Rofecoxib – Abrasion, atopic dermatitis, basal cell carcinoma, blister, cellulitis, contact dermatitis, herpes simplex, herpes zoster, nail unit disorder, skin erythema, xerosis (less than 2%); severe skin reactions, including Stevens-Johnson syndrome and toxic epidermal necrolysis (less than 0.1%).

Sulindac – Sore or dry mucous membranes (less than 1%).

Valdecoxib – Acne, cellulitis, contact dermatitis, dermatitis, dry skin, herpes simplex, herpes zoster, fungal dermatitis, rash erythematous, rash maculopapular, rash psoriaform, skin hypertrophy, ulceration of skin (less than 2%); basal cell carcinoma, malignant melanoma (less than 0.1%).

►**GI:**

Celecoxib – Diverticulitis, dysphagia, gastroesophageal reflux, hemorrhoids, hepatic function abnormal, hiatal hernia, tenesmus (less than 2%); cholelithiasis, colitis with bleeding, esophageal perforation, ileus, intestinal obstruction, intestinal perforation (less than 0.1%).

Diclofenac – Aphthous stomatitis, bloody diarrhea, cirrhosis, esophageal lesions, hepatic necrosis, hepatorenal syndrome, intestinal perforation (less than 1%).

Etodolac – Cholestatic hepatitis, cholestatic jaundice, duodenitis, intestinal ulceration, liver necrosis, peptic ulcer with or without bleeding and/or perforation, ulcerative stomatitis (less than 1%).

Fenoprofen – Aphthous ulceration of the buccal mucosa, cholestatic hepatitis, metallic taste, peptic ulcer without perforation (less than 1%).

Flurbiprofen – Bloody diarrhea, cholecystitis, cholestatic and noncholestatic jaundice, esophageal disease, exacerbation of inflammatory bowel disease, periodontal abscess, small intestine inflammation with loss of blood and protein (less than 1%).

Ibuprofen – Gastric or duodenal ulcer with bleeding and/or perforation, gingival ulcer (less than 1%).

Indomethacin – Development of ulcerative colitis and regional ileitis, ulcerative stomatitis, toxic hepatitis and jaundice (some fatal cases have been reported), intestinal strictures (diaphragms), GI bleeding without obvious ulcer formation and perforation of pre-existing sigmoid lesions (diverticulum, carcinoma, etc), intestinal ulceration associated with stenosis and obstruction, proctitis, single or multiple ulcerations (including perforation and hemorrhage of the esophagus, stomach, duodenum, or small and large intestines) (less than 1%).

Ketoprofen – Buccal necrosis, cholestatic hepatitis, fecal occult blood, hepatic dysfunction, intestinal ulceration, microvesicular steatosis, GI perforation, salivation, ulcerative colitis (less than 1%).

Meclofenamate – Bleeding and/or perforation with or without obvious ulcer formation, cholestatic jaundice, paralytic ileus (less than 1%).

Meloxicam – Gastroesophageal reflux, intestinal perforation, perforated duodenal ulcer, perforated gastric ulcer, stomatitis ulcerative (less than 2%).

Nabumetone – Duodenitis, dysphagia, gallstones, gingivitis (less than 1%).

Naproxen – GI perforation, nonpeptic GI ulceration, ulcerative stomatitis (less than 1%).

Oxaprozin – Hemorrhoidal bleeding (less than 1%).

Piroxicam – Pain (colic) (less than 1%).

Rofecoxib – Abdominal tenderness, acid reflux, aphthous stomatitis, digestive gas symptoms, duodenal disorder, dysgeusia, gastric disorder, hematochezia, hemorrhoids, infectious gastroenteritis, oral ulcer/lesion/infection (less than 2%); cholecystitis, colitis, colonic malignant neoplasm, duodenal perforation, esophageal ulcer, gastric perforation, intestinal obstruction (less than 0.1%).

Sulindac – Ageusia, bile duct sludging, biliary calculi, cholestasis, GI perforation, intestinal strictures (diaphragm) (less than 1%).

Tolmetin – GI bleeding without evidence of peptic ulcer, perforation (less than 1%).

Valdecoxib – Abnormal stools, diverticulosis, duodenitis, fecal incontinence, gastroesophageal reflux, hematochezia, hemorrhoids, bleeding of hemorrhoids, hepatic function abnormal, hiatal hernia, stool frequency increased, tenesmus (less than 2%); appendicitis, colitis with bleeding, dysphagia, esophageal perforation, ileus, intestinal obstruction, peritonitis, cholelithiasis, gastric carcinoma (less than 0.1%).

►**GU:**

Celecoxib – Breast fibroadenosis, breast neoplasm, breast pain, dysmenorrhea, moniliasis genital, prostatic disorder, urinary incontinence, vaginitis (less than 2%).

Diclofenac – Nocturia (less than 1%).

Etodolac – Leukorrhea, uterine bleeding irregularities (less than 1%).

Fenoprofen – Anuria, mastodynia, nephrosis (less than 1%).

Flurbiprofen – Prostate disease, uterine hemorrhage, vulvovaginitis (less than 1%).

Indomethacin – Breast changes (including enlargement and tenderness, or gynecomastia) (less than 1%).

Ketoprofen – Menometrorrhagia (less than 1%).

Ketorolac – Urinary retention (less than 1%).

Meclofenamate – Nocturia (less than 1%).

Nabumetone – Bilirubinuria, hyperuricemia (less than 1%).

Naproxen – Glomerular nephritis, renal disease (less than 1%).

Oxaprozin – Decreased menstrual flow, increased menstrual flow (less than 1%).

Rofecoxib – Breast mass, menopausal symptoms, nocturia, urinary retention, vaginitis (less than 2%); breast malignant neoplasm, prostatic malignant neoplasm, urolithiasis, worsening of chronic renal failure (less than 0.1%).

Sulindac – Crystalluria, urine discoloration (less than 1%).

Valdecoxib – Amenorrhea, breast neoplasm, dysmenorrhea, glycosuria, leukorrhea, malignant ovarian cyst, mastitis, menorrhagia, menstrual bloating, moniliasis genital, prostatic disorder, pyuria, urinary incontinence (less than 2%); bladder carcinoma, cervical dysplasia, prostate carcinoma, pyelonephritis (less than 0.1%).

▶*Hematologic / Lymphatic:*

Celecoxib – Thrombocythemia (less than 2%).

Diclofenac – Allergic purpura, bruising (less than 1%).

Fenoprofen – Bruising, hemorrhage (less than 1%).

Flurbiprofen – Iron deficiency anemia (less than 1%).

Ibuprofen – Bleeding episodes (less than 1%).

Indomethacin – Anemia secondary to obvious or occult GI bleeding, bone marrow depression, disseminated intravascular coagulation, leukemia, thrombocytopenic purpura (less than 1%).

Ketoprofen – Hemolysis, hypocoagulability (less than 1%).

Meclofenamate – Thrombocytopenic purpura (less than 1%).

Meloxicam – Bilirubinemia (less than 2%).

Nabumetone – Granulocytopenia (less than 1%).

Naproxen – Granulocytopenia (less than 1%).

Rofecoxib – Hypercholesterolemia (less than 2%); lymphoma (less than 0.1%).

Sulindac – Bone marrow depression (including aplastic anemia) (less than 1%).

Tolmetin – Granulocytopenia (less than 1%).

Valdecoxib – Hematoma NOS, leukocytosis, lymphangitis, lymphopenia (less than 2%); embolism, lymphoma-like disorder (less than 0.1%).

▶*Hypersensitivity:*

Ibuprofen – Henoch-Schonlein vasculitis, lupus erythematosus syndrome, syndrome of abdominal pain, fever, chills, nausea and vomiting (less than 1%).

Indomethacin – Acute respiratory distress, angiitis, purpura, rapid fall in blood pressure resembling a shock-like state (less than 1%).

Meclofenamate – Lupus, serum sickness-like syndrome (less than 1%).

Piroxicam – Positive ANA (less than 1%).

Rofecoxib – Hypersensitivity, insect bite reaction (less than 2%); hypersensitivity vasculitis (less than 0.1%).

Sulindac – Hypersensitivity vasculitis, potentially fatal hypersensitivity syndrome (less than 1%).

▶*Metabolic / Nutritional:*

Celecoxib – Diabetes mellitus, hypercholesterolemia, NPN increase (less than 2%); hypoglycemia (less than 0.1%).

Diclofenac – Hypoglycemia, weight loss (less than 1%).

Flurbiprofen – Hyperuricemia (less than 1%).

Ibuprofen – Acidosis, hypoglycemic reactions (less than 1%).

Indomethacin – Glycosuria (less than 1%).

Ketoprofen – Diabetes mellitus (aggravated), hyponatremia (less than 1%).

Meloxicam – Dehydration (less than 2%).

Naproxen – Hypoglycemia (less than 1%).

Piroxicam – Hypoglycemia (less than 1%).

Rofecoxib – Hypercholesterolemia, upper extremity edema (less than 2%); hyponatremia (less than 0.1%).

Valdecoxib – Diabetes mellitus, goiter, hypercholesterolemia, hyperlipemia, hyperuricemia, hypocalcemia (less than 2%); dehydration, hyperparathyroidism (less than 0.1%).

▶*Lab test abnormalities:*

Celecoxib – Alkaline phosphatase increased, CPK increased (less than 2%).

Fenoprofen – Increase in alkaline phosphatase and LDH (less than 1%).

Ibuprofen – Decreased creatinine clearance (less than 1%).

Meloxicam – GGT increased (less than 2%).

Sulindac – Increased prothrombin time (patients taking oral anticoagulants) (less than 1%).

Valdecoxib – Alkaline phosphatase increased, CPK increased, LDH increased (less than 2%).

▶*Musculoskeletal:*

Celecoxib – Arthrosis, bone disorder, fracture accidental, neck stiffness, synovitis, tendinitis (less than 2%).

Flurbiprofen – Myasthenia (less than 1%).

Indomethacin – Involuntary muscle movement (less than 1%).

Rofecoxib – Ankle sprain, arm pain, back strain, bursitis, cartilage trauma, joint swelling, muscular cramp, muscular disorder, muscular spasm, musculoskeletal pain/stiffness, osteoarthritis, tendinitis, traumatic arthropathy, wrist fracture (less than 2%).

Valdecoxib – Fracture accidental, neck stiffness, osteoporosis, synovitis, tendonitis (less than 2%); osteomyelitis, pathological fracture (less than 0.1%).

▶*Respiratory:*

Celecoxib – Bronchospasm aggravated, laryngitis (less than 2%).

Diclofenac – Edema of the pharynx, hyperventilation, laryngeal edema (less than 1%).

Etodolac – Pulmonary infiltration with eosinophilia (less than 1%).

Fenoprofen – Nasopharyngitis (1.2%).

Flurbiprofen – Hyperventilation, laryngitis, pulmonary infarct (less than 1%).

Ketoprofen – Hemoptysis, laryngeal edema (less than 1%).

Mefenamic acid – Respiratory depression (less than 1%).

Nabumetone – Eosinophilic pneumonia, hypersensitivity pneumonitis, idiopathic interstitial pneumonitis (less than 1%).

Naproxen – Eosinophilic pneumonitis (less than 1%).

Oxaprozin – Pulmonary infections (less than 1%).

Piroxicam – Respiratory depression (less than 1%).

Rofecoxib – Allergic rhinitis, laryngitis, nasal congestion, nasal secretion, pulmonary congestion, respiratory infection (less than 2%).

Valdecoxib – Abnormal breath sounds, emphysema, laryngitis, pleurisy (less than 2%); apnea, pleural effusion, pulmonary carcinoma, pulmonary fibrosis, pulmonary hemorrhage, pulmonary infarction, respiratory insufficiency (less than 0.1%).

▶*Special senses:*

Celecoxib – Cataract, deafness, ear abnormality, earache, eye pain, glaucoma, otitis media (less than 2%).

Diclofenac – Amblyopia, night blindness, scotoma, vitreous floaters (less than 1%).

Etodolac – Deafness, photophobia (less than 1%).

Fenoprofen – Burning tongue, optic neuritis (less than 1%).

Flurbiprofen – Corneal opacity, ear disease, glaucoma, parosmia, retinal hemorrhage, retrobulbar neuritis, transient hearing loss (less than 1%).

Ibuprofen – Amblyopia, cataracts, dry eyes, optic neuritis (less than 1%).

Indomethacin – Corneal deposits and retinal disturbances (including those of the macula), deafness (less than 1%).

Ketoprofen – Conjunctivitis sicca, eye pain, retinal hemorrhage and pigmentation change (less than 1%).

Ketorolac – Abnormal taste, abnormal vision (less than 1%).

Meclofenamate – Decreased visual acuity, iritis, macular and perimacular edema, retinal changes including macular fibrosis, reversible loss of color vision, temporary loss of vision (less than 1%).

Meloxicam – Abnormal vision (less than 2%).

Piroxicam – Swollen eyes (less than 1%).

Rofecoxib – Cerumen impaction, dry throat, ophthalmic injection, otic pain, otitis, otitis media, tonsillitis (less than 2%).

Sulindac – Bitter taste, disturbances of retina and vasculature of retina, metallic taste (less than 1%).

Tolmetin – Optic neuropathy, retinal and macular changes (less than 1%).

Valdecoxib – Cataract, conjunctival hemorrhage, ear abnormality, earache, eye pain, halitosis, keratitis, otitis media, periorbital swelling, vision abnormal, xerophthalmia (less than 2%); retinal detachment (less than 0.1%).

▶*Miscellaneous:*

Celecoxib – Allergy aggravated, cyst NOS, hot flushes, infection bacterial/fungal/viral, infection soft tissue, moniliasis, peripheral pain, tooth disorder (less than 2%); sepsis, suicide, sudden death (less than 0.1%).

Diclofenac – Dry mucous membranes, swelling of the lip and tongue (less than 1%).

Ketoprofen – Septicemia, shock (less than 1%).

Ketorolac – Injection site pain (2%).

Mefenamic acid – Death, sepsis (less than 1%).

Meloxicam – Hot flushes (less than 2%).

Piroxicam – Death, sepsis (less than 1%).

Rofecoxib – Abscess, contusion, cyst, dental caries/pain, diaphragmatic hernia, fungal infection, laceration, pelvic pain, postoperative pain, trauma, upper extremity edema, viral syndrome (less than 2%).

Sulindac – Fulminant necrotizing fasciitis (less than 1%).

Valdecoxib – Allergy aggravated, cyst NOS, fungal infection, gout, hot flushes, lipoma, moniliasis, peripheral pain, soft tissue infection, tooth disorder, viral infection (less than 2%); carcinoma, sepsis (less than 0.1%).

Overdosage

➤*Symptoms:* The incidence of acute NSAID overdoses result in minimal or no toxicity. Most reports of toxic signs and symptoms are mild to moderate and include GI distress, nausea, vomiting, lethargy, tinnitus, confusion, headache, and blurred vision. More severe symptoms may include seizures, metabolic acidosis, hypotension, hypothermia, hepatic and renal injury, coma, anaphylactoid reactions, and respiratory depression. Severe poisoning may result in hypertension, acute renal failure, hepatic dysfunction, cardiovascular collapse, and cardiac arrest. Anaphylactoid reactions have been reported with therapeutic ingestion of NSAIDs and may occur following an overdose. Acute overdose studies of **ibuprofen** report ≈ 60% of adults remaining asymptomatic, 30% to 40% suffer mild to moderate symptoms, and < 3% experience severe symptoms. Those at risk for toxicity associated with chronic use include the elderly and those with pre-existing renal, cardiovascular, or hepatic disease. Most organ systems are involved; however, the majority of deaths from chronic use are related to GI effects.

Symptoms may include the following: Drowsiness; dizziness; mental confusion; disorientation; lethargy; paresthesia; numbness; vomiting; gastric irritation; nausea; abdominal pain; intense headache; tinnitus; convulsions; blurred vision; respiratory depression; GI bleeding; hypertension; dyspepsia; ataxia; tremor; hyperpyrexia; epigastric pain; metabolic acidosis; anaphylactoid reactions; heartburn; indigestion; elevations in serum creatinine and BUN; renal impairment, coma, seizures, status epilepticus (**mefenamic acid**); hypotension and tachycardia (acute ingestion of **fenoprofen**); stupor, coma, diminished urine output and hypotension (**sulindac**; deaths have occurred); metabolic acidosis (acute **ibuprofen** overdosage); acute renal failure (**diclofenac** 2 g; **fenoprofen**, **oxaprozin** [rare]).

➤*Treatment:* Treatment of NSAID toxicity is primarily supportive and symptomatic. In addition to supportive measures, the use of oral activated charcoal may help to reduce the absorption and reabsorption of the NSAID. Refer to General Management of Acute Overdosage. Syrup of ipecac and gastric lavage have been recommended, but effectiveness has not been studied in NSAID overdose. Gastric lavage performed > 1 hour after overdosage has little benefit. Take care in administering syrup of ipecac to child ingestions of 100 to 400 mg/kg of **ibuprofen** because ibuprofen at this dose range mimic the symptoms produced by ipecac. Because NSAIDs are rapidly absorbed, decontamination may not benefit > 2- to 4-hour postingestion. Do not give syrup of ipecac to overdose patients at high risk of seizures, especially those who have ingested **mefenamic acid** or high amounts of other NSAIDs.

Because most NSAIDs are highly protein bound, extensively metabolized, and essentially excreted unchanged, elimination enhancement (hemodialysis, forced diuresis, alkalinization of urine, hemoperfusion, and peritoneal dialysis) may be of little value. However, hemodialysis may be necessary in cases of NSAID-induced prolonged or severe renal failure. Multiple doses of activated charcoal for elimination enhancement have been reported in **indomethacin** and **piroxicam** ingestions and therefore, may be applied to **sulindac**, **diclofenac**, **meloxicam**, and **ibuprofen** to interrupt enterohepatic or enteroenteric recirculation. Use this therapy only in severely symptomatic overdoses.

Meclofenamate – Dialysis may be required to correct serious azotemia or electrolyte imbalance.

Meloxicam – In a clinical trial, 4 g oral cholestyramine 3 times daily accelerated meloxicam clearance.

Patient Information

Side effects of NSAIDs can cause discomfort and, rarely, more serious side effects, such as GI bleeding may occur, which may result in hospitalization and even fatalities. NSAIDs are often essential in the management of arthritis and have a major role in treating pain, but they also may be commonly employed for less serious conditions. Apprise patients of potential risks.

Photosensitivity may occur; caution patients to take protective measures (ie, sunscreens, protective clothing) against UV or sunlight until tolerance is determined.

Avoid **aspirin** and alcoholic beverages while taking medication.

Although serious GI tract ulcerations and bleeding can occur without warning symptoms, alert patients for the signs and symptoms of ulcerations and bleeding, and have patients ask for medical advice when observing any indicative sign or symptoms. Apprise patients of the importance of this follow-up.

Inform patients of the warning signs and symptoms of hepatotoxicity (eg, nausea, fatigue, lethargy, pruritus, jaundice, right upper quadrant tenderness, flu-like symptoms). If these occur, instruct patients to stop therapy and seek immediate medical therapy.

Instruct patients to seek immediate emergency help in the case of an anaphylactoid reaction.

Avoid NSAIDs in late pregnancy because it may cause premature closure of the ductus arteriosus.

If GI upset occurs, take with food, milk, or antacids. For GI upset with **tolmetin**, use antacids other than sodium bicarbonate; bioavailability is affected by food and milk. If GI symptoms persist, notify physician.

Advise women who are taking **meclofenamate** for heavy menstrual flow to consult their doctor if they have spotting or bleeding between cycles or worsening of their menstrual blood flow. These symptoms may be signs of the development of a more serious condition that is not appropriately treated with meclofenamate.

Physicians may wish to discuss the potential risks and likely benefits of NSAID treatment with their patients, particularly when the drugs are used for less serious conditions where treatment without NSAIDs may represent an acceptable alternative to both the patient and physician.

Physicians may want to make specific recommendations to patients about when they should take NSAIDs in relation to food and what patients should do if they experience minor GI symptoms associated with them.

May cause drowsiness, vertigo, depression, dizziness, or blurred vision; patients should observe caution while driving or performing other tasks requiring alertness.

Notify physician if skin rash, GI ulceration, bleeding, visual disturbances, weight gain, edema, black stools, or persistent headache occurs.

➤*Mefenamic acid and meclofenamate:* If rash, diarrhea, or other digestive problems occur, discontinue use and consult a physician.

➤*Ibuprofen (otc use):* Do not take for > 3 days for fever, or > 10 days for pain. If symptoms persist, worsen, or if new symptoms develop, contact a physician.

DICLOFENAC

Rx	**Cataflam** (Novartis)	**Tablets:** 50 mg (as potassium)	Sucrose. (CATAFLAM 50). Lt brown. In 100s and UD 100s.
Rx	**Diclofenac Potassium** (Various, eg, Geneva, Mylan, Teva)		In 100s and 500s.
Rx	**Diclofenac Sodium** (Various, eg, Geneva, Roxane, Watson)	**Tablets, delayed-release:** 25 mg (as sodium)	May be enteric-coated. In 60s and 100s.
Rx	**Voltaren** (Novartis)		Enteric-coated. Lactose. (VOLTAREN 25). Yellow, triangular. In 60s, 100s, and UD 100s.
Rx	**Diclofenac Sodium** (Various, eg, Geneva, Martec, Purepac, Roxane, Teva, Watson)	**Tablets, delayed-release:** 50 mg (as sodium)	May be enteric-coated. In 42s, 60s, 100s, 500s, 1000s, and UD 100s.
Rx	**Voltaren** (Novartis)		Enteric-coated. Lactose. (VOLTAREN 50). Lt brown, triangular. In 60s, 100s, 1000s, and UD 100s.
Rx	**Diclofenac Sodium** (Various, eg, Geneva, Martec, Purepac, Roxane, Teva, Watson)	**Tablets, delayed-release:** 75 mg (as sodium)	May be enteric-coated. In 42s, 60s, 100s, 500s, 1000s.
Rx	**Voltaren** (Novartis)		Enteric-coated. Lactose. (VOLTAREN 75). Lt pink, triangular. In 60s, 100s, 1000s, and UD 100s.
Rx	**Diclofenac Sodium** (Various, eg, Geneva, Purepac, Teva)	**Tablets, extended-release:** 100 mg (as sodium)	In 100s.
Rx	**Voltaren-XR** (Novartis)		Sucrose, cetyl alcohol. (Voltaren-XR 100). Lt pink. In 100s and UD 100s.

DICLOFENAC

For complete prescribing information, refer to the NSAIDs group monograph.

Indications

➤*Arthritis:*

Signs and symptoms – For the acute and chronic treatment of signs and symptoms of osteoarthritis (OA) and rheumatoid arthritis (RA) (immediate- or delayed-release tablets).

Chronic therapy – For chronic therapy of OA and RA (extended-release tablets).

➤*Ankylosing spondylitis:* For the treatment of ankylosing spondylitis (immediate- or delayed-release tablets).

➤*Analgesia/Dysmenorrhea:* For the management of pain and primary dysmenorrhea when prompt pain relief is desired (immediate-release tablets).

Administration and Dosage

➤*Approved by the FDA:* July 1988.

➤*OA (immediate- or delayed-release tablets):* 100 to 150 mg/day in divided doses (50 mg twice or 3 times daily or 75 mg twice daily).

Chronic therapy (extended-release tablets) – 100 mg/day. Dosages of 200 mg/day are not recommended for patients with OA. Dosages > 200 mg/day have not been studied.

➤*RA (immediate- or delayed-release tablets):* 100 to 200 mg/day in divided doses (50 mg 3 or 4 times daily or 75 mg twice daily). Dosages > 225 mg/day are not recommended.

Chronic therapy (extended-release tablets) – 100 mg/day. In the rare patient where 100 mg/day is unsatisfactory, the dose may be increased to 100 mg twice daily if the benefits outweigh the clinical risks. Dosages > 225 mg/day are not recommended.

➤*Ankylosing spondylitis:* 100 to 125 mg/day delayed-release tablets as 25 mg 4 times daily, with an extra 25 mg dose at bedtime, if necessary. Dosages > 125 mg/day have not been studied.

➤*Analgesia and primary dysmenorrhea (immediate-release tablets):* Recommended starting dose is 50 mg 3 times daily. In some patients, an initial dose of 100 mg followed by 50 mg doses will provide better relief. After the first day, when the maximum recommended dose may be 200 mg, the total daily dose should generally not exceed 150 mg.

Individualize the diclofenac dosage to the lowest effective dose to minimize adverse effects.

ETODOLAC

Rx	**Etodolac** (Various, eg, Eon, Par, Purepac, Ranbaxy, Taro, Teva, Watson, Zenith Goldline)	**Tablets:** 400 mg	In 100s and 500s.
Rx	**Lodine** (Wyeth-Ayerst)		Lactose. (LODINE 400). Yellow-orange, oval. Film-coated. In 100s and UD 100s.
Rx	**Etodolac** (Various, eg, Eon, Par, Purepac, Ranbaxy, Taro, Teva, Watson, Zenith Goldline)	**Tablets:** 500 mg	In 100s, 500s, and 1000s.
Rx	**Lodine** (Wyeth-Ayerst)		Lactose. (LODINE 500). Blue, oval. Film-coated. In 100s and UD 100s.
Rx	**Etodolac** (Various, eg, ESI Lederle, Purepac, Teva)	**Tablets, extended-release:** 400 mg	In 100s and 500s.
Rx	**Lodine XL** (Wyeth-Ayerst)		Lactose. (LODINE XL 400). Orange-red, capsular-oval shape. Film-coated. In 100s and UD 100s.
Rx	**Etodolac** (Various, eg, ESI Lederle, Teva)	**Tablets, extended-release:** 500 mg	In 100s.
Rx	**Lodine XL** (Wyeth-Ayerst)		Lactose. (LODINE XL 500). Gray-green, capsular-oval shape. Film-coated. In 100s and UD 100s.
Rx	**Etodolac** (Various, eg, ESI Lederle, Teva)	**Tablets, extended-release:** 600 mg	In 100s.
Rx	**Lodine XL** (Wyeth-Ayerst)		Lactose. (LODINE XL 600). Lt. gray, capsular-oval shape. Film-coated. In UD 100s.
Rx	**Etodolac** (Various, eg, Mylan, Par, Taro, Teva, Watson)	**Capsules:** 200 mg	In 100s, 500s, and 1000s.
Rx	**Lodine** (Wyeth-Ayerst)		Lactose. (LODINE 200). Lt. gray and white w/red bands. In 100s and UD 100s.
Rx	**Etodolac** (Various, eg, Mylan, Par, Taro, Teva, Watson)	**Capsules:** 300 mg	In 100s, 500s, and 1000s.
Rx	**Lodine** (Wyeth-Ayerst)		Lactose. (LODINE 300). Lt. gray w/red bands. In 100s and UD 100s.

For complete prescribing information, refer to the NSAIDs group monograph.

Indications

➤*Arthritis:* Acute and long-term use in the management of signs and symptoms of osteoarthritis (OA) and rheumatoid arthritis (RA).

➤*Analgesia:* Management of pain (immediate-release only).

Administration and Dosage

➤*Approved by the FDA:* January 1991.

As with other NSAIDs, use the lowest dose and longest dosing interval for each patient. Therefore, after observing the response to initial therapy with etodolac, adjust the dose and frequency to suit the patient's needs.

Dosage adjustment of etodolac is generally not required in patients with mild to moderate renal impairment. Use etodolac with caution in such patients because, as with other NSAIDs, it may further decrease renal function in some patients with impaired renal function.

➤*Arthritis:*

Immediate-release – The recommended starting dose is 300 mg 2 or 3 times/day, or 400 or 500 mg twice daily. During long-term administration, the dose may be adjusted up or down depending on the clinical response of the patient. A lower dose of 600 mg/day may suffice for long-term administration. In patients who tolerate 1000 mg/day, the dose

may be increased to 1200 mg/day when a higher level of therapeutic activity is required. When treating patients with higher doses, the physician should observe sufficient increased clinical benefit to justify the higher dose. Doses greater than 1000 mg/day have not been adequately evaluated in well-controlled clinical trials.

Extended-release – The recommended starting dose is 400 to 1000 mg given once daily. During long-term administration, the dose may be adjusted up or down, depending on the patient's clinical response, up to a maximum dose of 1200 mg/day. Doses above 1200 mg/day have not been studied, and thus a dose-efficacy relationship at doses beyond 1200 mg/day has not been established.

In chronic conditions, a therapeutic response to therapy with etodolac is sometimes seen within 1 week of therapy, but most often is observed by 2 weeks. After a satisfactory response has been achieved, review and adjust the patient's dose as required.

➤*Analgesia:* Acute pain (immediate-release only) – 200 to 400 mg every 6 to 8 hours. Do not exceed 1200 mg/day. Doses greater than 1000 mg/day have not been adequately evaluated in well controlled clinical trials.

➤*Storage/Stability:* Store at controlled room temperature, 20° to 25°C (68° to 77°F). Dispense immediate-release formulation in light-resistant container. Protect extended-release etodolac from excessive heat and humidity.

FENOPROFEN CALCIUM

Rx	**Fenoprofen** (Various, eg, Geneva, Par, Watson)	**Capsules:** 200 mg	In 100s.
Rx	**Nalfon Pulvules** (Ranbaxy)		(Dista H76 Nalfon 200). White/ocher. In 100s.
Rx	**Fenoprofen** (Various, eg, Geneva, Par, Watson)	**Capsules:** 300 mg	In 100s.
Rx	**Nalfon Pulvules** (Ranbaxy)		(Dista H77 Nalfon). Yellow/ocher. In100s.
Rx	**Fenoprofen** (Various, eg, Watson, Zenith Goldline)	**Tablets:** 600 mg	In 100s, 500s, and 1000s. UD 100s, unit-of-use 30s, 60s, 90s, and 120s.

For complete prescribing information, refer to the NSAIDs group monograph.

Indications

➤*Arthritis:* Relief of the signs and symptoms of rheumatoid arthritis (RA) and osteoarthritis (OA) (in acute flares and exacerbations and long-term management).

➤*Pain:* Relief of mild-to-moderate pain.

Administration and Dosage

Dosage adjustments may be made after initiation of drug therapy or during exacerbations of the disease. Patients with RA generally seem to require larger doses of fenoprofen than those with OA. Employ the smallest dose that yields acceptable control.

Do not exceed 3.2 g/day. If GI upset occurs, take with meals or milk.

➤*RA and OA:* 300 to 600 mg 3 or 4 times daily. Individualize dosage. Improvement may occur in a few days, but 2 to 3 weeks may be required. Dosage adjustments may be made after initiation of drug therapy or during exacerbations of the disease.

➤*Mild-to-moderate pain:* 200 mg every 4 to 6 hours, as needed.

FLURBIPROFEN

Rx	**Flurbiprofen** (Various, eg, Zenith Goldline)	**Tablets:** 50 mg	In 100s.
Rx	**Ansaid** (Pharmacia & Upjohn)		Lactose. (Ansaid 50 mg). White, oval. Film-coated. In 100s, 500s, and 2000s.
Rx	**Flurbiprofen** (Various, eg, Teva, Zenith Goldine)	**Tablets:** 100 mg	In 100s and 500s.
Rx	**Ansaid** (Pharmacia & Upjohn)		Lactose. (Ansaid 100 mg). Blue, oval. Film-coated. In 100s, 500s, 2000s, and UD 100s.

For complete prescribing information, refer to the NSAIDs group monograph.

Indications

➤*Arthritis:* Acute or long-term treatment of the signs and symptoms of rheumatoid arthritis (RA) and osteoarthritis (OA).

Administration and Dosage

➤*Approved by the FDA:* November 1988.

➤*RA and OA:* Initial recommended total daily dose is 200 to 300 mg; administer in divided doses 2, 3, or 4 times daily. Most experience with RA has been with dosage 3 or 4 times/day. The largest recommended single dose in a multiple-dose daily regimen is 100 mg. Tailor the dose to each patient according to the severity of the symptoms and the response to therapy.

Although a few patients have received higher doses, doses > 300 mg/day are not recommended until more clinical experience is obtained.

IBUPROFEN

otc	**Junior Strength Motrin** (McNeil)	**Tablets:** 100 mg	(M 100). Yellow. In 24s.
otc	**Ibuprofen** (Various, eg, Geneva, Goldline, Major, Rugby, Schein, UDL, URL)	**Tablets:** 200 mg	In 24s, 50s, 100s, 250s, 1000s, and UD 100s.
otc	**Advil** (Whitehall-Robins)		Sucrose. (Advil). In 8s, 24s, 50s, 72s, 100s, 165s, and 250s.
otc	**Motrin IB** (McNeil)		**Tablets:** (Motrin IB). In 100s.
			Gelcaps: (Motrin IB). In 8s.
otc	**Haltran** (Lee Pharmaceutical)		In 30s.
otc	**Ibutab** (Zee Medical)		In 24s.
otc	**Midol Maximum Strength Cramp Formula** (Bayer)		(BAYER BAYER BAYER BAYER). In 24s.
otc	**Menadol** (Rugby)		**Captabs:** In 100s.
otc	**Motrin Migraine Pain** (McNeil Consumer)		**Caplets:** (IB). White. In 24s, 50s, and 100s.
Rx	**Ibuprofen** (Various, eg, Geneva, Greenstone Ltd., Major, Schein, UDL, URL, Zenith Goldline)	**Tablets:** 400 mg	In 100s, 360s, 500s, UD 100s, UD 300s, unit-of-use 100s, *Robot ready* 25s, and *Emergi-script* 60s.
Rx	**Motrin** (Pharmacia & Upjohn)		Lactose. (Motrin 400). White. In 100s, 500s, and UD 100s.
Rx	**Ibuprofen** (Various, eg, Geneva, Greenstone Ltd., Major, Schein, UDL, URL, Zenith Goldline)	**Tablets:** 600 mg	In 100s, 270s, 500s, UD 100s, UD 300s, unit-of-use 100s, *Robot ready* 25s, and *Emergi-script* 60s.
Rx	**Motrin** (Pharmacia & Upjohn)		Lactose. (Motrin 600). White, elliptical. In 90s, 100s, 270s, 500s, and UD 100s.
Rx	**Ibuprofen** (Various, eg, Geneva, Greenstone Ltd., Major, Schein, UDL, URL, Zenith Goldline)	**Tablets:** 800 mg	In 100s, 270s, 500s, UD 100s, UD 300s, unit-of-use 100s, *Robot ready* 25s, and *Emergi-script* 60s.
Rx	**Motrin** (Pharmacia & Upjohn)		Lactose. (Motrin 800). White, elliptical. In 100s, 270s, 500s, and UD 100s.
otc	**Children's Advil** (Whitehall-Robins)	**Tablets, chewable:** 50 mg	Aspartame, 2.1 mg phenylalanine. (Advil 50). Fruit and grape flavor. In 24s and 50s.
otc	**Children's Motrin** (McNeil)		Aspartame, 3 mg phenylalanine. Orange flavor. In 24s.
otc	**Motrin, Junior Strength** (McNeil)	**Tablets, chewable:** 100 mg	Aspartame, 6 mg phenylalanine. (MOTRIN 100). Orange flavor. In 24s.
otc	**Junior Strength Advil** (Whitehall-Robins)		Aspartame, 4.2 mg phenylalanine. Grape and fruit flavor. In 24s.
otc	**Advil Liqui-Gels** (Whitehall-Robins)	**Capsules:** 200 mg	Sorbitol. (Advil). Green. In 4s, 20s, 40s, and 80s.
otc	**Advil Migraine** (Whitehall-Robins)		Sorbitol. (Advil). Brown, oval. In 20s.

IBUPROFEN

otc	**Children's Advil** (Wyeth-Ayerst)	**Suspension:** 100 mg/5 ml	Sorbitol, sucrose, EDTA. Fruit flavor. In 119 and 473 ml.
otc	**Children's Motrin** (McNeil-CPC)		Sucrose. Grape, and bubble gum flavor. In 60 and 120 ml.
otc	**Ibuprofen** (Various, eg, Alpharma, Major, Perrigo)		In 118 ml.
otc	**PediaCare Fever** (Pharmacia & Upjohn)		Sucrose. Berry flavor. In 120 ml.
otc	**Pediatric Advil Drops** (Whitehall-Robins)	**Suspension:** 100 mg/2.5 ml	Sorbitol, sucrose, EDTA, glycerin. Grape flavor. In 7.5 ml.
otc	**Ibuprofen** (Perrigo)	**Oral Drops:** 40 mg/ml	In 15 ml.
otc	**Infants' Motrin** (McNeil)		Sorbitol, sucrose. Berry flavor. In 15 ml with dropper.
otc	**PediaCare Fever** (Pharmacia & Upjohn)		Sorbitol, sucrose. Berry flavor. In 15 ml.

For complete prescribing information, refer to the NSAIDs group monograph.

Indications

➤**Arthritis:** Relief of signs and symptoms of rheumatoid arthritis (RA) and osteoarthritis (OA).

➤**Pain:** Relief of mild-to-moderate pain.

➤**Dysmenorrhea:** Treatment of primary dysmenorrhea.

➤**Fever:** Reduction of fever.

Administration and Dosage

➤*Approved by the FDA:* 1974.

The combination of ibuprofen in conjunction with aspirin cannot be recommended.

If the patient consumes ≥ 3 alcoholic drinks every day, taking ibuprofen or other pain relievers/fever reducers may cause stomach bleeding.

➤*Adults:* Do not exceed 3.2 g/day. If GI upset occurs, take with meals or milk.

Arthritis – Individualize dosage. 1.2 to 3.2 g/day (300 mg 4 times daily or 400, 600 or 800 mg 3 or 4 times daily). In chronic conditions, therapeutic response sometimes occurs in a few days to a week, but most often within 2 weeks. RA patients seem to require higher doses than OA patients.

Mild-to-moderate pain – 400 mg every 4 to 6 hours, as necessary.

Primary dysmenorrhea – 400 mg every 4 hours, as necessary.

OTC (minor aches and pains, dysmenorrhea, fever reduction) – 200 mg every 4 to 6 hours while symptoms persist. If pain or fever do not respond to 200 mg, 400 mg may be used. Do not exceed 1.2 g in 24 hours. Do not take for pain for > 10 days or for fever for > 3 days, unless directed by physician. Use the smallest effective dose.

➤*Children:*

Juvenile arthritis – Usual dose is 30 to 40 mg/kg/day in 3 or 4 divided doses; 20 mg/kg/day may be adequate for milder disease. Doses > 50 mg/kg/day are not recommended.

Fever reduction/Pain relief (6 months to 12 years of age) – Adjust dosage on the basis of the initial temperature level. If baseline temperature is ≤ 39.2°C (102.5°F), recommended dose is 5 mg/kg; if baseline temperature is > 39.2°C (102.5°F), recommended dose is 10 mg/kg. Duration of fever reduction is generally 6 to 8 hours. Maximum daily dose is 40 mg/kg.

INDOMETHACIN

Rx	**Indomethacin** (Various, eg, UDL, URL, Zenith Goldline)	**Capsules:** 25 mg	In 50s, 100s, 500s, 1000s, UD 100s, and *Robot* ready 25s.
Rx	**Indocin** (Merck)		Lactose, lecithin. (Indocin/MSD 25). Blue and white. In 100s and 1000s.
Rx	**Indomethacin** (Various, eg, Lederle, UDL, URL, Zenith Goldline)	**Capsules:** 50 mg	In 100s, 500s, 1000s, UD 100s, and *Robot* ready 25s.
Rx	**Indocin** (Merck)		Lactose, lecithin. (Indocin/MSD 50). Blue/white. In 100s.
Rx	**Indomethacin Extended-Release** (Inwood)	**Capsules, sustained-release:** 75 mg	Sucrose, parabens. (IL-3607). Lavender/clear. In 60s and 100s.
Rx	**Indomethacin SR** (Various, eg, Endo, Eon, Inwood, Zenith Goldline)		In 60s, 100s, and 500s.
Rx	**Indocin SR** (Forte Pharma)		(Indocin SR/695). Blue and clear. In unit-of-use 60s.
Rx	**Indocin** (Merck)	**Oral suspension:** 25 mg/5 ml	1% alcohol, sorbitol. Pineapple coconut mint flavor. In 237 ml.
Rx	**Indocin** (Merck)	**Suppositories:** 50 mg	White. In 30s.

For complete prescribing information, refer to the NSAIDs group monograph. For information on parenteral indomethacin, see Agents for Patent Ductus Arteriosus.

Indications

➤**Arthritis:** For active stages of moderate-to-severe rheumatoid arthritis (RA) (including acute flares of chronic disease); moderate-to-severe osteoarthritis (OA); acute gouty arthritis.

➤**Inflammatory conditions:** Moderate-to-severe ankylosing spondylitis; acute painful shoulder (bursitis/tendinitis).

Sustained-release dosage form is not indicated for acute gouty arthritis.

Indomethacin cannot be considered a simple analgesic and should not be used in conditions other than those recommended under Indications.

➤*Unlabeled uses:* Indomethacin has been used for pharmacologic closure of hemodynamically significant patent ductus arteriosus in premature infants weighing between 500 and 1750 g and in whom other supportive measures have been attempted as an alternative to surgical ligation. Standard regimen involves the IV administration of 0.1 to 0.2 mg/kg every 12 hours for 3 doses. See monograph in Agents for Patent Ductus Arteriosus section.

Indomethacin suppresses uterine activity by inhibiting prostaglandin synthesis and has been used to prevent premature labor. Prolonged maternal administration of indomethacin for this purpose could result in prenatal ductus arteriosus closure and increased neonatal morbidity; *avoid this use.*

Topical indomethacin as eye drops in 0.5% and 1% concentrations has been used to treat cystoid macular edema.

Administration and Dosage

Adverse reactions appear to correlate with the dose in most patients. Determine the smallest effective dosage. Always give capsules or oral suspension with food, immediately after meals, or with antacids to reduce gastric irritation.

➤*Moderate-to-severe RA (including acute flares of chronic disease), ankylosing spondylitis, and OA:* 25 mg 2 or 3 times daily. If well tolerated, increase daily dose by 25 or 50 mg (if required by continuing symptoms) at weekly intervals until satisfactory response is obtained or until total daily dose of 150 to 200 mg is reached. Doses above this generally do not increase effectiveness.

In patients who have persistent night pain or morning stiffness, giving a large portion, up to a maximum of 100 mg of the total daily dose at bedtime, either orally or by rectal suppository, may help to relieve pain. The total daily dose should not exceed 200 mg.

In acute flares of chronic RA, it may be necessary to increase dosage by 25 or 50 mg daily. If minor adverse effects develop, reduce dosage rapidly to tolerated dose; observe patient closely. If severe adverse reactions occur, discontinue. After the acute phase of the disease is controlled, attempt to reduce daily dose repeatedly until patient receives smallest effective dose or drug is discontinued.

➤*Acute painful shoulder (bursitis or tendinitis):* 75 to 150 mg daily in 3 or 4 divided doses. Discontinue the drug after inflammation has been controlled for several days. Usual course of therapy is 7 to 14 days.

INDOMETHACIN

➤*Acute gouty arthritis:* 50 mg 3 times daily until pain is tolerable, then rapidly reduce the dose to complete cessation of the drug. Definite relief of pain usually occurs within 2 to 4 hours. Tenderness and heat usually subside in 24 to 36 hours, and swelling gradually disappears in 3 to 5 days. Do not use sustained-release form.

➤*Sustained-release form:* Do not crush. The 75 mg sustained-release capsule can be taken once a day as an alternative to the 25 mg capsule 3 times daily. There will be significant differences between the regimens in indomethacin blood levels, especially after 12 hours. One 75 mg sustained-release capsule twice daily can be substituted for 150 mg/day. Do not use sustained-release form in acute gouty arthritis.

➤*Children:* Effectiveness in children ≤ 14 years of age has not been established.

➤*Storage/Stability:*
Oral suspension and suppositories – Store below 30°C (86°F). Protect oral suspension from freezing.

KETOPROFEN

otc	**Orudis KT** (Whitehall-Robins)	**Tablets:** 12.5 mg	Tartrazine, sugar. (ORUDIS KT). In 24s, 50s, and 100s.
Rx	**Ketoprofen** (Various, eg, Teva)	**Capsules:** 50 mg	In 100s.
Rx	**Ketoprofen** (Various, eg, Qualitest, Teva)	**Capsules:** 75 mg	In 100s and 500s.
Rx	**Ketoprofen** (Andrx)	**Capsules, extended-release:** 100 mg	In 100s and 1000s.
Rx	**Oruvail** (Wyeth-Ayerst)		Sucrose. (Oruvail 100). Pink/dark green. In 100s and *Redipak* 100s.
Rx	**Ketoprofen** (Andrx)	**Capsules, extended-release:** 150 mg	In 100s and 1000s.
Rx	**Oruvail** (Wyeth-Ayerst)		Sucrose. (Oruvail 150). Pink/light green. In 100s and *Redipak* 100s.
Rx	**Ketoprofen** (Andrx)	**Capsules, extended-release:** 200 mg	In 100s and 1000s.
Rx	**Oruvail** (Wyeth-Ayerst)		Sucrose. (Oruvail 200). Pink/White. In 100s and *Redipak* 100s.

For complete prescribing information, refer to the NSAIDs group monograph.

Indications

➤*Capsules:* Acute or long-term treatment of the signs and symptoms of rheumatoid arthritis (RA) and osteoarthritis (OA); mild-to-moderate pain; primary dysmenorrhea.

➤*Capsules, extended-release:* Treatment of the signs and symptoms of RA and OA; not recommended for use in treating acute pain because of its extended-release characteristics.

➤*OTC:* Temporary relief of minor aches and pains associated with common cold, headache, toothache, muscular aches, backache, minor arthritis pain, menstrual cramps, and reduction of fever.

Administration and Dosage

Individualize dosage. May be taken with antacids, food, or milk to minimize adverse GI effects.

➤*RA and OA:* Do not exceed 300 mg/day for the regular-release formulation or 200 mg/day for extended-release capsules.

Starting dose – 75 mg 3 times/day or 50 mg 4 times/day. Reduce initial dose in elderly or debilitated patients or those with impaired renal function.

If minor side effects appear, they may disappear at a lower dose that may still have an adequate therapeutic effect. If well tolerated but not optimally effective, dosage may be increased. Individuals may show better response to 300 mg daily compared with 200 mg, although in well-controlled clinical trials, patients on 300 mg did not show greater mean effectiveness. They did show an increased frequency of upper- and lower-GI distress and headaches. Women had an increased frequency of these adverse effects compared with men. When treating patients with 300 mg/day, observe sufficient increased clinical benefit to offset potential increased risk.

Extended-release – 200 mg once daily.

➤*Mild-to-moderate pain, primary dysmenorrhea:* 25 to 50 mg every 6 to 8 hours as needed. Give smaller doses initially to smaller patients, the elderly, and those with renal or liver disease. Doses > 50 mg may be given, but doses > 75 mg do not display added therapeutic effects. Administer high doses with caution and closely observe patient response. Do not exceed 300 mg/day.

➤*Mild-to-severe renal function impairment:* In patients with mildly impaired renal function, the maximum recommended total daily dose of ketoprofen is 150 mg. In patients with a more severe renal impairment (GFR < 25 ml/min or end-stage renal impairment), the maximum total daily dose should not be > 100 mg.

➤*Hepatic function impairment:* For patients with alcoholic cirrhosis, no significant changes in the kinetic disposition of ketoprofen capsules were observed relative to age-matched normal subjects (see Warnings). It is recommended that for patients with impaired liver function and serum albumin concentration < 3.5 g/dl, the maximum initial total daily dose should be 100 mg.

➤*Hypoalbuminemia/Renal function impairment:* Hypoalbuminemia/reduced renal function increase fraction of free drug (biologically active form); patients with both conditions may be at greater risk of adverse effects. Give lower doses and closely monitor.

➤*Elderly:* In elderly patients, renal function may be reduced with apparently normal serum creatinine or BUN levels. Therefore, it is recommended that the initial dosage of ketoprofen be reduced for patients > 75 years of age.

➤*OTC:*

Adults – 12.5 mg with a full glass of liquid every 4 to 6 hours. If pain or fever persists after 1 hour, follow with 12.5 mg. With experience, some patients may find an initial dose of 25 mg will give better relief. Do not exceed 25 mg in a 4- to 6-hour period or 75 mg in a 24-hour period. Use the smallest effective dose.

Children – Do not give to those < 16 years of age unless directed by a physician.

KETOROLAC TROMETHAMINE

Rx	Ketorolac Tromethamine (Various, eg, Ethex, Teva)	**Tablets**: 10 mg	In 100s and 500s.
Rx	**Toradol** (Roche)		Lactose. (Toradol Roche). White. Film-coated. In 100s.
Rx	Ketorolac Tromethamine (Bedford)	**Injection**: 15 mg/ml	In 1 ml vials.
Rx	**Toradol** (Roche)		In 1 ml *Tubex* syringes and 1 ml fill per 2 ml single-use vial.[1]
Rx	Ketorolac Tromethamine (Bedford)	**Injection**: 30 mg/mL	In 1 and 2 mL single-dose vials and 10 mL multiple-dose vials.
Rx	**Toradol** (Roche)		In 1[2] and 2[3] mL *Tubex* syringes and 1 mL fill per 2 mL and 2 mL fill per 2 mL single-use vials.

[1] With 10% alcohol and 6.68 mg sodium chloride in sterile water.
[2] With 10% alcohol and 4.35 mg sodium chloride in sterile water.

[3] For IM use only. With 10% alcohol and 8.7 mg sodium chloride in sterile water.

For complete prescribing information, refer to the NSAIDs group monograph.

WARNING

Ketorolac is indicated for the short-term (up to 5 days) management of moderately severe acute pain that requires analgesia at the opioid level. It is not indicated for minor or chronic painful conditions. Ketorolac is a potent NSAID analgesic, and its administration carries many risks. The resulting NSAID-related adverse events can be serious in certain patients for whom ketorolac is indicated, especially when the drug is used inappropriately. Increasing the dose beyond the label recommendations will not provide better efficacy but will result in increasing the risk of developing serious adverse events.

GI effects: Ketorolac can cause peptic ulcers, GI bleeding, or perforation. Therefore, it is contraindicated in patients with active peptic ulcer disease, recent GI bleeding or perforation, or a history of peptic ulcer disease or GI bleeding.

Renal effects: Ketorolac is contraindicated in patients with advanced renal impairment and in patients at risk for renal failure because of volume depletion.

Risk of bleeding: Ketorolac inhibits platelet function and is; therefore, contraindicated in patients with suspected or confirmed cerebrovascular bleeding, hemorrhagic diathesis, incomplete hemostasis, and those at high risk of bleeding.

Ketorolac is contraindicated as prophylactic analgesia before any major surgery and is contraindicated intraoperatively when hemostasis is critical because of the increased risk of bleeding.

Hypersensitivity: Hypersensitivity reactions, ranging from bronchospasm to anaphylactic shock, have occurred, and appropriate counteractive measures must be available when administering the first dose of ketorolac. Ketorolac is contraindicated in patients with previously demonstrated hypersensitivity to ketorolac tromethamine or allergic manifestations to aspirin or other NSAIDs.

Intrathecal or epidural administration: Ketorolac is contraindicated for intrathecal or epidural administration because of its alcohol content.

Labor, delivery, and lactation: Use in labor and delivery is contraindicated because ketorolac may adversely affect fetal circulation and inhibit uterine contractions. Use in nursing mothers is contraindicated because of the potential adverse effects of prostaglandin-inhibiting drugs on neonates.

Concomitant use with NSAIDs: Ketorolac is contraindicated in patients currently receiving aspirin or other NSAIDs because of the cumulative risk of inducing serious NSAID-related side effects.

Administration and dosage: Ketorolac (oral) is indicated only as continuation therapy to ketorolac IV/IM; the combined duration of use of IV/IM and oral is not to exceed 5 days because of the increased risk of serious adverse events. The recommended total daily oral dose (maximum, 40 mg) is significantly lower than for IV/IM (maximum, 120 mg; see Administration and Dosage and Transition from IV/IM to oral).

Special populations: Adjust dosage for patients ≥ 65 years of age, for patients < 50 kg (110 lbs) or for body weight (see Administration and Dosage), and for patients with moderately elevated serum creatinine. IV/IM doses are not to exceed 60 mg/day in these patients.

Indications

➤*Moderately severe, acute pain:* Short-term (≤ 5 days) management of moderately severe, acute pain that requires analgesia at the opioid level, usually in a postoperative setting. Initiate therapy with IV/IM, and use oral therapy only as continuation treatment, if necessary. Combined use of IV/IM and oral is not to exceed 5 days of use because of the potential of increasing the frequency and severity of adverse reactions associated with the recommended doses. Switch patients to alternative analgesics as soon as possible. Ketorolac therapy is not to exceed 5 days.

Ketorolac IV/IM has been used concomitantly with morphine and meperidine and has shown an opioid-sparing effect. For breakthrough pain, it is recommended to supplement the lower end of the IV/IM dosage range with low doses of narcotics as needed, unless otherwise contraindicated. Do not administer ketorolac and narcotics in the same syringe (see Administration and Dosage).

Administration and Dosage

➤*Approved by the FDA:* November 1989.

The combined duration of ketorolac IV/IM and oral is not to exceed 5 days. Oral use is only indicated as continuation therapy to IV/IM.

➤*IV/IM:* Ketorolac IV/IM may be used as a single or multiple dose, on a regular or as needed schedule for the management of moderately severe, acute pain that requires analgesia at the opioid level, usually postoperatively. Correct hypovolemia prior to administration. Switch patients to alternative analgesics as soon as possible. Ketorolac therapy is not to exceed 5 days.

When administering IM/IV, the IV bolus must be given ≥ 15 seconds. Give IM administration slowly and deeply into the muscle. The analgesic effect begins in ≈ 30 minutes with maximum effect in 1 to 2 hours after IV or IM dosing. Duration of analgesic effect is usually 4 to 6 hours.

Single-dose treatment – Limit the following regimen to single administration use only:

  IM dosing:
    • < 65 years of age – One 60 mg dose.
    • ≥ 65 years of age, renal impairment, or weight < 50 kg (110 lbs) – One 30 mg dose.
  IV dosing:
    • < 65 years of age – One 30 mg dose.
    • ≥ 65 years of age, renal impairment, or weight < 50 kg (110 lbs) – One 15 mg dose.

Multiple-dose treatment (IV/IM) –
  < 65 years of age: The recommended dose is 30 mg every 6 hours. The maximum daily dose should not exceed 120 mg.
  ≥ 65 years of age, renal impairment (see Warnings), or weight < 50 kg (110 lbs): The recommended dose is 15 mg every 6 hours. The maximum daily dose for these populations should not exceed 60 mg.

For breakthrough pain, do not increase the dose or the frequency of ketorolac. Consider supplementing these regimens with low doses of opioids as needed unless otherwise contraindicated.

Admixture incompatibility – Do not mix IV/IM ketorolac in a small volume (eg, in a syringe) with morphine sulfate, meperidine HCl, promethazine HCl, or hydroxyzine HCl; this will result in precipitation of ketorolac from solution.

➤*Oral:* Indicated only as continuation therapy to ketorolac IV/IM for the management of moderately severe, acute pain that requires analgesia at the opioid level.

Transition from IV/IM to oral – The recommended oral dose is as follows:

  < 65 years of age: 20 mg as a first oral dose for patients who received 60 mg IM single dose, 30 mg IV single dose, or 30 mg multiple dose IV/IM followed by 10 mg every 4 to 6 hours, not to exceed 40 mg/24 hours.

  > 65 years of age, renal impairment, or weight < 50 kg (110 lb): 10 mg as a first oral dose for patients who received a 30 mg IM single dose, 15 mg IV single dose, or 15 mg multiple dose IV/IM followed by 10 mg every 4 to 6 hours, not to exceed 40 mg/24 hours.

Shortening the recommended dosing intervals may result in increased frequency and severity of adverse reactions.

➤*Storage/Stability:*

Injection – Protect from light.

MECLOFENAMATE SODIUM

Rx	Meclofenamate Sodium (Various, eg, Mylan, Schein)	Capsules: 50 mg[1]	In 100s, 500s, and 1000s.
Rx	Meclofenamate Sodium (Various, eg, Mylan, Schein)	Capsules: 100 mg[1]	In 100s, 500s, and 100s.

[1] Meclofenamic acid equivalent, as meclofenamate sodium.

For complete prescribing information, refer to the NSAIDs group monograph.

Indications

➤*Arthritis:* Acute and chronic rheumatoid arthritis (RA) and osteoarthritis (OA).

➤*Pain:* Relief of mild-to-moderate pain.

➤*Dysmenorrhea:* Treatment of primary dysmenorrhea.

➤*Idiopathic heavy menstrual loss:* Treatment of idiopathic heavy menstrual blood loss.

Use requires careful assessment of benefit/risk ratio.

Meclofenamate is not recommended in children because adequate studies to demonstrate safety and efficacy have not been studied.

Administration and Dosage

➤*Approved by the FDA:* 1982.

➤*Mild-to-moderate pain:* 50 mg every 4 to 6 hours. Doses of 100 mg may be required for optimal pain relief. Do not exceed daily dosage of 400 mg.

➤*Excessive menstrual blood loss and primary dysmenorrhea:* 100 mg 3 times daily for up to 6 days, starting at the onset of menstrual flow.

➤*RA and OA:*

Usual dosage – 200 to 400 mg/day in 3 or 4 equal doses.

Initial dosage – Initiate at lower dosage; increase as needed to improve response. Individualize dosage. Do not exceed 400 mg/day. Improvement may occur in a few days; optimum benefit may not occur for 2 to 3 weeks.

Dosage adjustment – After satisfactory response is achieved, adjust as required. A lower dosage may suffice for long-term use. May give with meals or milk. If intolerance occurs, reduce dosage. Discontinue if severe adverse reactions occur.

Functional Class IV – Safety and efficacy are not established in these patients.

➤*Children:* Safety and efficacy in children < 14 years of age have not been established.

MEFENAMIC ACID

Rx	Ponstel (Parke-Davis)	Capsules: 250 mg	Lactose. (FHPC 400). Ivory. In 100s.

For complete prescribing information, refer to the NSAIDs group monograph.

Indications

➤*Pain:* Relief of mild-to-moderate pain in patients ≥ 14 years of age if therapy will be ≤ 1 week.

➤*Dysmenorrhea:* Treatment of primary dysmenorrhea.

Administration and Dosage

As with other NSAIDs, use the lowest dose for each patient. Individualize therapy.

➤*Acute pain:*

Adults (≥ 14 years of age) – 500 mg, then 250 mg every 6 hours as needed, usually not to exceed 1 week. Give with food.

➤*Primary dysmenorrhea:* 500 mg, then 250 mg every 6 hours. Start with onset of bleeding and associated symptoms. Administration should not be necessary for > 2 to 3 days.

➤*Children:* Safety and efficacy in children < 14 years of age have not been established.

MELOXICAM

Rx	Mobic (Boehringer Ingelheim/Abbott)	Tablets: 7.5 mg	Lactose. (M). Yellow, biconvex. In 30s, 100s, and UD 100s.
		15 mg	(15 M). Lactose. Yellow, oblong, biconvex. In 100s.

For complete prescribing information, refer to the NSAIDs group monograph.

Indications

➤*Osteoarthritis:* For relief of the signs and symptoms of osteoarthritis.

Administration and Dosage

➤*Approved by the FDA:* April 14, 2000.

Use the lowest dosage for each patient. For treatment of osteoarthritis, the recommended starting and maintenance dose is 7.5 mg once/day. Some patients may receive additional benefit by increasing the dose to 15 mg once/day. The maximum recommended dose is 15 mg/day. Meloxicam may be taken without regard to meals.

NABUMETONE

Rx	Nabumetone (Various, eg, Eon, Geneva, Teva, UDL)	Tablets: 500 mg	In 100s, 500s, and UD 100s.
Rx	Relafen (SmithKline Beecham)		(Relafen 500). White. Film-coated. Oval. In 100s and UD 100s.
Rx	Nabumetone (Various, eg, Eon, Geneva, Teva)	Tablets: 750 mg	In 100s and 500s.
Rx	Relafen (SmithKline Beecham)		(Relafen 750). Beige. Film-coated. Oval. In 100s and UD 100s.

For complete prescribing information, refer to the NSAIDs group monograph.

Indications

➤*Arthritis:* For acute and chronic treatment of signs and symptoms of osteoarthritis and rheumatoid arthritis.

Administration and Dosage

➤*Approved by the FDA:* December 1991.

Recommended starting dose is 1000 mg as a single dose with or without food. Some patients may obtain more symptomatic relief from 1500 to 2000 mg/day. Nabumetone can be given either once or twice daily. Dosages > 2000 mg/day have not been studied. Use the lowest effective dose for chronic treatment.

NAPROXEN

otc	**Naproxen Sodium** (Various, eg, Goldline)	**Tablets:** 200 mg (220 mg naproxen sodium)	In 24s and 50s.
otc	**Aleve** (Bayer)		**Tablets:** (ALEVE). In 24s, 50s, 100s, and 150s. **Capsules:** In 24s, 50s, 100s, 150s, and 200s. **Gelcaps:** (ALEVE). In 20s, 40s, and 80s.
Rx	**Naproxen Sodium** (Various, eg, Sidmak)	**Tablets:** 250 mg (275 mg naproxen sodium)	In 100s, 500s, 1000s, and UD 100s.
Rx	**Anaprox** (Roche)		(Roche 274). Lt blue, biconvex, oval. In 100s.
Rx	**Naproxen Sodium** (Various, eg, Sidmak)	**Tablets:** 500 mg (550 mg naproxen sodium)	In 100s, 500s, 1000s, and UD 100s.
Rx	**Anaprox DS** (Roche)		(Roche/Anaprox DS). Dark blue, capsule shape. Film-coated. In 100s and 500s.
Rx	**Naproxen** (Various, eg, Lederle, Qualitest, Sidmak, UDL)	**Tablets:** 250 mg	In 30s, 100s, 500s, 1000s, UD 100s, unit-of-use 30s, 60s, 90s, and 120s, and *Robot* ready 25s.
Rx	**Naprosyn** (Roche)		(Roche/Naprosyn 250). Yellow. In 100s and 500s.
Rx	**Naproxen** (Various, eg, Lederle, Qualitest, Sidmak, UDL)	**Tablets:** 375 mg	In 30s, 100s, 500s, 1000s, UD 100s, and unit-of-use 30s, 60s, 90s, and 120s.
Rx	**Naprosyn** (Roche)		(Naprosyn 375). Peach. In 100s and 500s.
Rx	**Naproxen** (Various, eg, Lederle, Qualitest, Sidmak, UDL)	**Tablets:** 500 mg	In 30s, 100s, 500s, 1000s, UD 100s, UD 300s, unit-of- use 30s, 60s, 90s, and 120s, and *Robot* ready 25s.
Rx	**Naprosyn** (Roche)		(Naprosyn 500). Yellow. In 100s and 500s.
Rx	**Naproxen** (Various, eg, Apothecon, Purepac, Roxane, Teva)	**Tablets, delayed-release:** 375 mg	In 100s and 500s.
Rx	**EC-Naprosyn** (Roche)		(EC-Naprosyn 375). White, capsule shape. Enteric- coated. In 100s.
	Naproxen (Various, eg, Apothecon, Purepac, Roxane, Teva)	**Tablets, delayed-release:** 500 mg	In 100s and 500s.
Rx	**EC-Naprosyn** (Roche)		(EC-Naprosyn 500). White, capsule shape. Enteric- coated. In 100s.
Rx	**Naprelan** (Carnrick Laboratories)	**Tablets, controlled-release:** 375 mg (412.5 mg naproxen sodium)	(N375). White, capsule shape. In 100s.
		500 mg (550 mg naproxen sodium)	(N500). White, capsule shape. In 75s.
Rx	**Naprosyn** (Roche)	**Suspension:** 125 mg/5 ml	Sorbitol, sucrose, parabens. Orange-pineapple fla- vor. In 473 ml.
Rx	**Naproxen** (Various, eg, Roxane)		Methylparaben, sorbitol, sucrose. Pineapple-orange flavor. In 15, 20, and 500 ml.

For complete prescribing information, refer to the NSAIDs group monograph.

Indications

➤*Rx:* Relief of mild-to-moderate pain; treatment of primary dysmenorrhea, rheumatoid arthritis (RA), osteoarthritis (OA), ankylosing spondylitis, tendinitis, bursitis, acute gout, juvenile arthritis (**naproxen** only, not **naproxen sodium**).

Delayed-release – Delayed-release naproxen is not recommended for initial treatment of acute pain because absorption is delayed compared with other naproxen formulations.

➤*OTC:* Temporary relief of minor aches and pains associated with the common cold, headache, toothache, muscular aches, backache, minor arthritis pain, pain of menstrual cramps, and reduction of fever.

Administration and Dosage

➤*Rx:* Do not exceed 1.25 g naproxen (1.375 g naproxen sodium) per day.

RA; OA; ankylosing spondylitis; pain; dysmenorrhea; acute tendinitis; bursitis –
Naproxen: 250 to 500 mg twice/day. May increase to 1.5 g/day in patients who tolerate lower doses well for limited periods.
Naproxen suspension: 250 mg (10 ml), 375 mg (15 ml), or 500 mg (20 ml) twice daily.
Delayed-release naproxen (EC-Naprosyn): 375 to 500 mg twice/day. Do not break, crush, or chew tablets.
Controlled-release (Naprelan): 750 mg or 1000 mg once daily. Individualize dosage. Do not exceed 1500 mg/day.

Symptomatic improvement in arthritis usually begins within 1 week; however, treatment for 2 weeks may be required to achieve a therapeutic benefit.
Naproxen sodium: 275 to 550 mg twice daily. May increase to 1.65 g for limited periods.

Morning and evening doses do not have to be equal, and use of the drug more frequently than twice daily is not necessary. Symptomatic arthritis improvement usually begins in 2 weeks; if no improvement is seen, consider a trial for 2 more weeks.

Juvenile arthritis (**naproxen** *only, not* **naproxen sodium**) –
Naproxen: Total daily dose is ≈ 10 mg/kg in 2 divided doses.
• *Suspension* – Use the following as a guide:

Naproxen Suspension: Children's Dose	
Child's weight	Dose
13 kg (29 lb)	2.5 ml (0.5 tsp) bid
25 kg (55 lb)	5 ml (1 tsp) bid
38 kg (84 lb)	7.5 ml (1.5 tsp) bid

Acute gout –
Naproxen: 750 mg, followed by 250 mg every 8 hours until the attack subsides.
Naproxen sodium: 825 mg, then 275 mg every 8 hours until attack subsides.
Controlled-release (Naprelan): 1000 to 1500 mg once daily on the first day followed by 1000 mg once daily until the attack has subsided.

Mild-to-moderate pain; primary dysmenorrhea; acute tendinitis; bursitis –
Naproxen: 500 mg, followed by 500 mg every 12 hours or 250 mg every 6 to 8 hours. Do not exceed a 1.25 g total daily dose. Thereafter, total daily dose should not exceed 1000 mg.
Naproxen sodium: 550 mg, followed by 550 mg every 12 hours or 275 mg every 6 to 8 hours. Do not exceed a 1.375 g total daily dose. Thereafter, total daily dose should not exceed 1100 mg.
Controlled-release (Naprelan): 1000 mg once daily. For patients requiring greater analgesic benefit, 1500 mg/day may be used for a limited period. Thereafter, total daily dose should not exceed 1000 mg.

Children – Safety and efficacy in children < 2 years of age have not been established.

➤*OTC:*

Adults – 200 mg with a full glass of liquid every 8 to 12 hours while symptoms persist. With experience, some patients may find an initial dose of 400 mg followed by 200 mg 12 hours later, if necessary, will give better relief. Do not exceed 600 mg in 24 hours unless otherwise directed. Use the smallest effective dose.

Patients consuming ≥ 3 alcohol-containing drinks per day should consult their doctor for advice on when and how to take naproxen and other pain relievers.

Elderly (> 65 years of age) – Do not take > 200 mg every 12 hours.

Children – Do not give to children < 12 years of age except under the advice and supervision of a physician.

OXAPROZIN

Rx	Oxaprozin (*Eon Labs*)	**Tablets**: 600 mg	(141). White, capsule shape. Film-coated. In 100s, 500s, 1000s, and blister 100s.
Rx	Daypro (Searle)	**Caplets**: 600 mg	(Daypro 1381). White, capsule shape. Scored. Film-coated. In 100s, 500s, and UD 100s.
Rx	Daypro ALTA (Pharmacia)	**Tablets**: 678 oxaprozin potassium (equivalent to 600 mg oxaprozin)	(Searle 1391). Blue, capsule shape. Film-coated. In 100s, 500s, and UD 100s.

For complete prescribing information, refer to the NSAIDs group monograph.

Indications

➤*Arthritis:* Acute and long-term use in the management of signs and symptoms of osteoarthritis (OA) and rheumatoid arthritis (RA).

Administration and Dosage

➤*Approved by the FDA:* October 29, 1992.

➤*RA:* 1200 mg once a day. Smaller and larger doses may be required in individual patients.

➤*OA:* 1200 mg once/day. For patients of low body weight or with milder disease, an initial dosage of 600 mg once/day may be appropriate.

➤*Maximum dose:* 1800 mg/day (or 26 mg/kg, whichever is lower) in divided doses.

Regardless of the indication, individualize the dosage to the lowest effective dose to minimize adverse effects.

PIROXICAM

Rx	Piroxicam (Various, eg, SCS Pharmaceuticals, Teva, UDL, URL, Watson, Zenith Goldline)	**Capsules**: 10 mg	In 100s, 500s, 1000s, and UD 100s.
Rx	Feldene (Pfizer)		Lactose. (Feldene Pfizer 322). Blue/maroon. In 100s.
Rx	Piroxicam (Various, eg, SCS Pharmaceuticals, Teva, UDL, URL, Watson, Zenith Goldline)	**Capsules**: 20 mg	In 100s, 500s, 1000s, and UD 100s.
Rx	Feldene (Pfizer)		Lactose. (Feldene Pfizer 323). Maroon. In 100s, 500s, and UD 100s.

For complete prescribing information, refer to the NSAIDs group monograph.

Indications

➤*Arthritis:* For acute or long-term use in the relief of signs and symptoms of osteoarthritis and rheumatoid arthritis.

Administration and Dosage

➤*Approved by the FDA:* April 1982.

As with other NSAIDs, use the lowest dose for each patient. Individualize therapy.

Initiate and maintain at a single daily dose of 20 mg. May divide daily dose. Although therapeutic effects are evident early in treatment, increase in response progresses over several weeks. Do not assess effect of therapy for 2 weeks. Because of the long half-life of piroxicam, steady-state blood levels are not reached for 7 to 12 days.

➤*Children:* Dosage recommendations and indications for use in children have not been established.

SULINDAC

Rx	Sulindac (Various, eg, Allscripts, Major, Mutual, Mylan, UDL, URL, Warner Chilcott, Watson)	**Tablets**: 150 mg	In 100s, 500s, 1000s, UD 100s.
Rx	Clinoril (Merck)		(MSD 941/Clinoril). Yellow, hexagonal. In 100s.
Rx	Sulindac (Various, eg, Allscripts, Major, Mutual, Mylan, UDL, URL, Warner Chilcott, Watson)	**Tablets**: 200 mg	In 100s, 500s, 1000s, UD 100s.
Rx	Clinoril (Merck)		(MSD 942). Yellow, hexagonal, scored. In 100s.

For complete prescribing information, refer to the NSAIDs group monograph.

Indications

➤*Arthritis:* For acute or long-term use in the relief of signs and symptoms of osteoarthritis (OA) and rheumatoid arthritis (RA); acute gouty arthritis.

➤*Inflammatory conditions:* For acute or long-term use in the relief of signs and symptoms of ankylosing spondylitis; acute painful shoulder (acute subacromial bursitis/supraspinatus tendinitis).

Administration and Dosage

Administer twice a day with food. The usual maximum dosage is 400 mg/day. Dosages > 400 mg/day are not recommended.

➤*OA, RA, and ankylosing spondylitis:* Initial dosage is 150 mg twice a day. Individualize dosage.

Response occurs within 1 week in ≈ 50% of patients with OA, ankylosing spondylitis, and RA. Others may require longer to respond.

➤*Acute painful shoulder (acute subacromial bursitis/supraspinatus tendinitis); acute gouty arthritis:* 200 mg twice/day. After satisfactory response, reduce dosage accordingly.

In acute painful shoulder, therapy for 7 to 14 days is usually adequate. In acute gouty arthritis, therapy for 7 days is usually adequate.

➤*Children:* Safety and efficacy have not been established.

TOLMETIN SODIUM

Rx	Tolmetin Sodium (Various, eg, Mutual, URL)	**Tablets**: 200 mg tolmetin (as sodium)	In 100s.
Rx	Tolectin 200 (McNeil)		18 mg sodium. (McNeil Tolectin 200). White, scored. In 100s.
Rx	Tolmetin Sodium (Various, eg, Mylan, Purepac)	**Tablets**: 600 mg tolmetin (as sodium)	In 100s, 500s, and UD 100s.
Rx	Tolectin 600 (McNeil)		54 mg sodium. (McNeil Tolectin 600). Orange. Film-coated. In 100s and 500s.
Rx	Tolmetin Sodium (Various, eg, Allscripts, Mylan, Purepac, Teva)	**Capsules**: 400 mg tolmetin (as sodium)	In 100s, 500s, 1000s, and UD 100s.
Rx	Tolectin DS (McNeil)		36 mg sodium. (McNeil Tolectin DS). Orange. In 100s, 500s, and UD 100s.

For complete prescribing information, refer to the NSAIDs group monograph.

Indications

➤*Arthritis:* Treatment of acute flares and long-term management of rheumatoid arthritis (RA) and osteoarthritis (OA); treatment of juvenile rheumatoid arthritis.

Safety and efficacy have not been established in children < 2 years of age.

Administration and Dosage

➤*Approved by the FDA:* March 1989.

Expect therapeutic response in a few days to a week. Anticipate progressive improvement during succeeding weeks of therapy. If GI symptoms occur, give with antacids other than sodium bicarbonate; bioavailability is affected by food or milk.

➤*Adults:*

RA and OA – Initially, 400 mg 3 times/day; preferably include dose on arising and at bedtime. To achieve optimal therapeutic effect, adjust the dose according to the patient's response after 1 to 2 weeks. Control is usually achieved at doses of 600 to 1800 mg/day generally in 3 divided doses. Doses > 1800 mg/day have not been studied and are not recommended.

TOLMETIN SODIUM

➤*Children (≥ 2 years of age):* Initially, 20 mg/kg/day in 3 or 4 divided doses. When control is achieved, usual dose ranges from 15 to 30 mg/kg/day. Doses > 30 mg/kg/day have not been studied and are not recommended.

Selective COX-2 Inhibitors

CELECOXIB

Rx	**Celebrex** (Searle)	**Capsules:** 100 mg	Lactose. (7767 100). White. In 100s, 500s, and UD 100s.
		200 mg	Lactose. (7767 200). White. In 100s, 500s, and UD 100s.
		400 mg	(7767 400). White. In 60s and UD 100s.

For complete prescribing information, refer to the NSAIDs group monograph.

Indications

➤*Osteoarthritis (OA):* For relief of the signs and symptoms of OA.

➤*Rheumatoid arthritis (RA):* For relief of signs and symptoms of RA in adults.

➤*Acute pain:* For management of acute pain in adults.

➤*Primary dysmenorrhea:* For treatment of primary dysmenorrhea.

➤*Familial adenomatous polyposis (FAP):* To reduce the number of adenomatous colorectal polyps in FAP, as an adjunct to usual care (eg, endoscopic surveillance, surgery). It is not known whether there is a clinical benefit from a reduction in the number of colorectal polyps in FAP patients, nor whether the effects of celecoxib treatment will persist after the drug is discontinued. The efficacy and safety of celecoxib treatment in patients with FAP beyond 6 months have not been studied.

Administration and Dosage

➤*Approved by the FDA:* December 31, 1998.

Seek the lowest dose of celecoxib for each OA and RA patient. Safety and efficacy in children below 18 years of age have not been evaluated.

➤*OA:* Recommended dosage is 200 mg/day administered as a single dose or as 100 mg twice/day.

➤*RA:* Recommended dosage is 100 to 200 mg twice/day.

➤*Acute pain and primary dysmenorrhea:* Recommended dose is 400 mg initially, followed by an additional 200 mg dose if needed on the first day. On subsequent days, the recommended dose is 200 mg twice daily as needed.

➤*FAP:* Continue usual medical care for FAP patients while on celecoxib. To reduce the number of adenomatous colorectal polyps in patients with FAP, the recommended oral dose is 400 mg (2 × 200 mg capsules) twice daily. Take with food.

➤*Hepatic impairment:* The daily recommended dose of celecoxib in patients with moderate hepatic impairment (Child-Pugh Class II) should be reduced by approximately 50%.

➤*Storage/Stability:* Store at 25°C (77°F); excursions permitted to 15° to 30°C (59° to 86°F).

ROFECOXIB

Rx	**Vioxx** (Merck)	**Tablets:** 12.5 mg	Lactose. (MRK 74 VIOXX). Cream/off-white. In 100s, 1000s, 8000s, unit-of-use 30s, and UD 100s.
		25 mg	Lactose. (MRK 110 VIOXX). Yellow. In 100s, 1000s, 8000s, unit-of-use 30s, and UD 100s.
		50 mg	Lactose. (MRK 114 VIOXX). Orange. In 100s, 500s, 4000s, unit-of-use 30s, and UD 100s.
		Suspension: 12.5 mg/5 mL	Sorbitol, parabens. Strawberry flavor. In 150 mL.
		25 mg/5 mL	Sorbitol, parabens. Strawberry flavor. In 150 mL.

For complete prescribing information, refer to the NSAIDs group monograph.

Indications

➤*Osteoarthritis (OA):* For the relief of the signs and symptoms of OA.

➤*Rheumatoid arthritis (RA):* For the relief of signs and symptoms of RA in adults.

➤*Acute pain:* For the management of acute pain in adults.

➤*Primary dysmenorrhea:* For the treatment of primary dysmenorrhea.

Administration and Dosage

➤*Approved by the FDA:* May 20, 1999.

Use the lowest effective dose for each patient. Tablets may be taken without regards to food.

➤*OA:* The recommended starting dose is 12.5 mg once daily. Some patients may receive additional benefit by increasing the dose to 25 mg once daily. The maximum recommended daily dose is 25 mg.

➤*RA:* Recommended dose is 25 mg once daily. The maximum recommended daily dose is 25 mg.

➤*Acute pain and primary dysmenorrhea:* The recommended dose is 50 mg once daily. The maximum recommended daily dose is 50 mg. Chronic use of 50 mg/day is not recommended. Use of rofecoxib for more than 5 days in the management of pain has not been studied.

➤*Storage/Stability:* Store at 25°C (77°F); excursions permitted to 15° to 30°C (59° to 86°F). Shake suspension before using.

VALDECOXIB

Rx	**Bextra** (Searle)	**Tablets:** 10 mg	Lactose. (10). White, capsule shape. Film-coated. In 100s, 500s, and UD 100s.
		20 mg	Lactose. (20). White, capsule shape. Film-coated. In 100s, 500s, and UD 100s.

For complete prescribing information, refer to the NSAIDs group monograph.

Indications

➤*Osteoarthritis (OA)/Adult rheumatoid arthritis (RA):* For the relief of the signs and symptoms of OA and adult RA.

➤*Primary dysmenorrhea:* Treatment of primary dysmenorrhea.

Administration and Dosage

➤*Approved by the FDA:* November 19, 2001.

➤*OA/Adult RA:* 10 mg once daily.

➤*Primary dysmenorrhea:* 20 mg twice daily, as needed.

➤*Storage/Stability:* Store at 25°C (77°F); excursions permitted to 15° to 30°C (59° to 86°F).

In addition to the agents on the following pages, propranolol and timolol are indicated for migraine prophylaxis (see Beta-Adrenergic Blocking Agents monograph).

Serotonin 5-HT₁ Receptor Agonists

Indications

▶*Migraine treatment:* For the acute treatment of migraine with or without aura in adults.

▶*Cluster headache (sumatriptan injection only):* For the acute treatment of cluster headache episodes.

Actions

▶*Pharmacology:* **Sumatriptan**, **naratriptan**, **zolmitriptan**, **rizatriptan**, **frovatriptan**, **eletriptan**, and **almotriptan** are selective 5-hydroxytryptamine₁ (5-HT₁ or serotonin) receptor agonists.

Drug	High	Weak	None
Almotriptan	5-HT$_{1D}$, 5-HT$_{1B}$, 5-HT$_{1F}$	5-HT$_{1A}$, 5-HT$_7$	5-HT$_{2-4}$, 5-HT$_6$, α-adrenergic, β-adrenergic, adenosine (A$_1$, A$_2$), angiotensin (AT$_1$, AT$_2$), dopaminergic D$_1$ or D$_2$, endothelin (ET$_A$, ET$_B$), tachykinin receptor sites
Eletriptan	5-HT$_{1B}$, 5-HT$_{1D}$, 5-HT$_{1F}$	5-HT$_{1A}$, 5-HT$_{1E}$, 5-HT$_{2B}$, 5-HT$_7$	5-HT$_{2A}$, 5-HT$_{2C}$, 5-HT$_3$, 5-HT$_4$, 5-HT$_{5A}$, 5-HT$_6$, α-adrenergic, and β-adrenergic, dopaminergic D$_1$ or D$_2$, muscarinic, or opioid receptors
Frovatriptan	5-HT$_{1B}$, 5-HT$_{1D}$	none	Benzodiazepine receptor sites
Naratriptan	5-HT$_{1D}$	none	5-HT$_{2-4}$, α-adrenergic, β-adrenergic, dopaminergic, muscarinic, benzodiazepine receptor sites
Rizatriptan	5-HT$_{1B}$, 5-HT$_{1D}$	5-HT$_{1A}$, 5-HT$_{1E}$, 5-HT$_{1F}$, 5-HT$_7$	5-HT$_2$, 5-HT$_3$, α-adrenergic, β-adrenergic, dopaminergic, muscarinic, benzodiazepine receptor sites
Sumatriptan	5-HT$_1$	5-HT$_{1A}$, 5-HT$_{5A}$, 5-HT$_7$	5-HT$_{2-4}$, α-adrenergic, β-adrenergic, dopaminergic, muscarinic, benzodiazepine receptor sites
Zolmitriptan	5-HT$_{1D}$, 5-HT$_{1B}$	5-HT$_{1A}$	5-HT$_{2-4}$, α-adrenergic, β-adrenergic, dopaminergic, muscarinic, histaminic receptor sites

The vascular 5-HT₁ receptor subtype is present on the human basilar artery and in the vasculature of isolated human dura mater. Current theories on the etiology of migraine headaches suggest that symptoms are caused by local cranial vasodilation or the release of vasoactive and proinflammatory peptides from sensory nerve endings in an activated trigeminal system. The therapeutic activity of the serotonin 5-HT₁ receptor agonists in migraine most likely can be attributed to agonist effects at 5-HT$_{1B/1D}$ receptors on the extracerebral, intracranial blood vessels that become dilated during a migraine attack and on nerve terminals in the trigeminal system. Activation of these receptors results in cranial vessel constriction, inhibition of neuropeptide release, and reduced transmission in trigeminal pain pathways.

▶*Pharmacokinetics:*

Pharmacokinetic Parameters of Triptans in Healthy Volunteers and in Patients with Migraine

Drug	Dose and route of administration	T_{max} (h)	C_{max} (mcg/L)	Bioavailability (%)	t½ (h)	AUC (mcg/L•h)	Plasma protein binding (%)
Almotriptan	12.5 mg PO	2.5	49.5	80	3.1	266	≈ 35
	25 mg PO	2.7	64	69	3.6	443	
Eletriptan	20 mg PO	2	–	≈ 50	≈ 4	–	≈ 85
Frovatriptan	2.5 mg PO	3	4.2/7[a]	29.6	25.7	94	≈ 15
	40 mg PO	5	24.7/53.4[a]	17.5	29.7	881	
Naratriptan	2.5 mg PO	2	12.6	74	5.5	98	≈ 28
Rizatriptan	10 mg PO	1, 1.6 to 2.5[b]	19.8	40	2	50	14
Sumatriptan	6 mg SC	0.17	72	96	2	90	14 to 21
	100 mg PO	1.5	54	14	2	158	
	20 mg NAS	1.5	13	15.8	1.8	48	
	25 mg PR	1.5	27	19.2	1.8	78	
Zolmitriptan	2.5 mg PO	1.5, 3[b]	3.3/3.8[a]	39	2.3/2.6[a]	18/21[a]	≈ 25
	5 mg PO	1.5, 3[b]	10	46	3	42	
	5 mg NAS	3	3.93[c]	102[d]	≈ 3	22.4[c]	

[a] Value for men and women, respectively.
[b] Orally-disintegrating tablets.
[c] Values based on 2.5 mg dose.
[d] Compared with oral tablet.

Renal function impairment – Clearance of **zolmitriptan** was reduced by 25% in patients with severe renal impairment (Ccr approximately 5 to 25 mL/min); no significant change was observed in those with moderate renal impairment.

Clearance of **naratriptan** was reduced by 50% in patients with moderate renal impairment (Ccr 18 to 39 mL/min), resulting in an increase in mean half life from 6 hours (healthy) to 11 hours (range, 7 to 20 hours). The mean C_{max} increased by approximately 40%. The effects of severe renal impairment have not been assessed (see Contraindications and Administration and Dosage).

In hemodialysis patients (Ccr less than 2 mL/min/1.73 m²), the AUC for **rizatriptan** was approximately 44% greater than that in patients with normal renal function.

The clearance of **almotriptan** was approximately 65% lower in patients with severe renal impairment (Ccr between 10 and 30 mL/min) and approximately 40% lower in patients with moderate renal impairment (Ccr between 31 and 71 mL/min).

Because less than 10% of **frovatriptan** is excreted in urine after an oral dose, it is unlikely that the exposure to frovatriptan will be affected by renal impairment. The pharmacokinetics of frovatriptan following a single oral dose of 2.5 mg was not different in patients with renal impairment (5 males and 6 females, Ccr 16 to 73 mL/min) vs subjects with normal renal function.

Hepatic function impairment – The liver plays an important role in the presystemic clearance of oral 5-HT₁ agonists. Accordingly, the bioavailability may be markedly increased in patients with liver disease.

Oral: In a small study of hepatically impaired patients, **sumatriptan** AUC and C_{max} increased by approximately 70%, and T_{max} decreased by 40 minutes.

In severely hepatically impaired patients, the mean C_{max}, T_{max}, and AUC of **zolmitriptan** were increased 1.5-, 2-, and 3-fold, respectively. Seven of 27 patients experienced 20 to 80 mm Hg elevations in systolic or diastolic blood pressure after a 10 mg dose. Administer zolmitriptan with caution in patients with liver disease, generally using doses less than 2.5 mg.

Clearance of **naratriptan** was decreased by 30% in patients with moderate hepatic impairment (Child-Pugh grade A or B). This resulted in an approximately 40% increase in the half life (range, 8 to 16 hours). The effects of severe hepatic impairment (Child-Pugh grade C) have not been assessed (see Contraindications).

Following oral administration in patients with hepatic impairment caused by mild to moderate alcoholic cirrhosis of the liver, plasma concentrations of **rizatriptan** were similar in patients with mild hepatic insufficiency compared with a control group of healthy subjects; plasma concentrations of rizatriptan were approximately 30% greater in patients with moderate hepatic insufficiency.

The pharmacokinetics of **almotriptan** have not been assessed in this population. Based on the mechanisms of almotriptan clearance, the maximum decrease expected because of hepatic impairment would be 60%.

The effects of severe hepatic impairment on **eletriptan** metabolism have not been evaluated. Subjects with mild or moderate hepatic impairment demonstrated an increase in AUC (34%) and half life. C_{max} was increased by 18% (see Contraindications).

Elderly – There is a statistically significant increase in **eletriptan** half life (from approximately 4.4 to 5.7 hours) between elderly (65 to 93 years of age) and younger adult subjects (18 to 45 years of age).

Contraindications

Injectable preparations used IV, because of the potential to cause coronary vasospasm; patients with ischemic heart disease (angina pectoris, history of MI, strokes, transient ischemic attacks [TIAs], or documented silent ischemia); Prinzmetal variant angina or other significant underlying cardiovascular disease (see Warnings); patients with signs or symptoms consistent with ischemic heart disease or coronary artery vasospasm; patients with uncontrolled hypertension; concurrent use of (or use within 24 hours of) ergotamine-containing preparations or ergot-type medications such as dihydroergotamine or methysergide; concurrent monoamine oxidase inhibitor (MAOI) therapy (or within 2 weeks of discontinuing an MAOI [except for **eletriptan**]; see Drug Interactions); within 24 hours of another 5-HT₁ agonist; hypersensitivity to the product or any of its ingredients; management of hemiplegic or basilar migraine; ischemic bowel disease.

➤*Naratriptan and sumatriptan:* Cerebrovascular or peripheral vascular syndromes, severe hepatic impairment (Child-Pugh grade C); severe renal impairment (Ccr less than 15 mL/min) (naratriptan only).

➤*Frovatriptan and eletriptan:* Peripheral vascular disease.

➤*Eletriptan:* Severe hepatic impairment.

Warnings

Use 5-HT₁ agonists only when a clear diagnosis of migraine has been established.

➤*Risk of myocardial ischemia or MI and other adverse cardiac events:* Because of the potential of this class of compounds to cause coronary vasospasm, do not give these agents to patients with documented ischemic or vasospastic coronary artery disease (see Contraindications). It is strongly recommended that 5-HT₁ agonists not be given to patients in whom unrecognized coronary artery disease (CAD) is predicted by the presence of risk factors (eg, hypertension, hypercholesterolemia, smoking, obesity, diabetes, strong family history of CAD, female with surgical or physiological menopause, or male older than 40 years of age) unless a cardiovascular evaluation provides satisfactory clinical evidence that the patient is reasonably free of coronary artery and ischemic myocardial disease or other significant underlying cardiovascular disease. The sensitivity of cardiac diagnostic procedures to detect cardiovascular diseases or predisposition to coronary artery vasospasm is modest at best. If, during the cardiovascular evaluation, the patient's medical history, electrocardiogram (ECG), or other investigations reveal findings indicative of, or consistent with, coronary artery vasospasm or myocardial ischemia, do not administer 5-HT₁ agonists (see Contraindications). For patients with risk factors predictive of CAD who are determined to have a satisfactory cardiovascular evaluation, it is strongly recommended that administration of the first dose take place in the setting of a physician's office or similar medically staffed and equipped facility, unless the patient has previously received 5-HT₁ agonists. Because cardiac ischemia can occur in the absence of clinical symptoms, consider obtaining an ECG during the interval immediately following the first use in a patient with risk factors.

It is recommended that patients who are intermittent long-term users of 5-HT₁ agonists who have or acquire risk factors predictive of CAD, as described above, undergo periodic interval cardiovascular evaluation as they continue use.

The systematic approach described above is intended to reduce the likelihood that patients with unrecognized cardiovascular disease will be inadvertently exposed to 5-HT₁ agonists.

Zolmitriptan – There is a report of at least 1 patient experiencing coronary vasospasm without history of cardiac disease and with documented absence of CAD.

Patients with symptomatic Wolff-Parkinson-White syndrome or arrhythmias associated with other cardiac accessory conduction pathway disorders should not receive zolmitriptan.

➤*Cardiac events and fatalities associated with 5-HT₁ agonists:* Serious adverse cardiac events, including acute MI, life-threatening disturbances of cardiac rhythm, and death have been reported within a few hours following the administration of 5-HT₁ agonists. Considering the extent of use of 5-HT₁ agonists in patients with migraine, the incidence of these events is extremely low.

➤*Cerebrovascular events and fatalities with 5-HT₁ agonists:* Cerebral hemorrhage, subarachnoid hemorrhage, stroke, and other cerebrovascular events have been reported in patients treated with 5-HT₁ agonists, and some have resulted in fatalities. In a number of cases, it appears possible that the cerebrovascular events were primary, the agonist having been administered in the incorrect belief that the symptoms experienced were a consequence of migraine, when they were not. It should be noted that patients with migraine may be at increased risk of certain cerebrovascular events (eg, stroke, hemorrhage, TIA).

➤*Other vasospasm-related events:* 5-HT₁ agonists may cause vasospastic reactions other than coronary artery vasospasm. Peripheral vascular ischemia and colonic ischemia with abdominal pain and bloody diarrhea have been reported with 5-HT₁ agonists.

➤*Increases in blood pressure:* Significant elevations in systemic blood pressure, including hypertensive crisis, have been reported on rare occasions in patients with and without a history of hypertension treated with 5-HT₁ agonists. 5-HT₁ agonists are contraindicated in patients with uncontrolled hypertension.

➤*Local irritation:* Approximately 5% of patients noted irritation in the nose and throat after using **sumatriptan** nasal spray. Irritative symptoms such as burning, numbness, paresthesia, discharge, and pain or soreness were noted to be severe in approximately 1% of patients treated. The symptoms were transient and, in approximately 60% of the cases, resolved in less than 2 hours. Limited examinations of the nose and throat did not reveal any clinically noticeable injury in these patients. Adverse events of any kind perceived in the nasopharynx were severe in approximately 1% of patients, and approximately 60% resolved in 1 hour. Nasopharyngeal examinations failed to demonstrate any clinically significant changes with repeated use of sumatriptan nasal spray.

➤*CYP3A4 inhibitors:* In vitro studies have shown that **eletriptan** is metabolized by the CYP3A4 enzyme. A clinical study has shown that coadministration of eletriptan with ketoconazole, erythromycin, verapamil, and fluconazole increased the C_{max} and AUC of eletriptan 3- and 6-fold, 2- and 4-fold, 2- and 3-fold, and 1.4- and 2-fold, respectively. Do not use eletriptan within 72 hours of taking drugs that have demonstrated potent CYP3A4 inhibition.

➤*Hypersensitivity reactions:* Hypersensitivity reactions have occurred on rare occasions, and severe anaphylaxis/anaphylactoid reactions have occurred. Such reactions can be life-threatening or fatal. Refer to Management of Acute Hypersensitivity Reactions.

➤*Renal function impairment:* Use **rizatriptan** and **sumatriptan** with caution in dialysis patients because of a decrease in the clearance (see Pharmacokinetics). After **eletriptan** administration, there was no significant change in clearance observed in subjects with mild, moderate, or severe renal impairment, although blood pressure elevations were observed in this population.

➤*Hepatic function impairment:* Administer with caution to patients with diseases that may alter the absorption, metabolism, or excretion of drugs. The liver plays an important role in the presystemic clearance of oral 5-HT₁ agonists. Accordingly, the bioavailability may be markedly increased in patients with liver disease (see Pharmacokinetics). No dosage adjustment is necessary when **frovatriptan** or **eletriptan** is given to patients with mild to moderate hepatic impairment. Do not use eletriptan in severe hepatic impairment.

➤*Carcinogenesis:* Thyroid follicular cell hyperplasia and thyroid follicular cell adenomas have been observed in rats receiving no more than 400 mg/kg/day **zolmitriptan** for approximately 104 weeks and 90 mg/kg/day **naratriptan** for 13 weeks. An increased incidence of benign c-cell adenomas in the thyroid also was observed in naratriptan animal studies. The lifetime carcinogenic potential of **rizatriptan** was evaluated in a 100-week study in mice and a 106-week study in rats at oral gavage doses up to 125 mg/kg/day. Exposure data were not obtained, but plasma AUCs of parent drug measured in other studies after 5 and 21 weeks of oral dosing in mice and rats, respectively, indicate that the exposures to parent drug at the highest dose level would have been approximately 150 times (mice) and 240 times (rats) the average AUCs measured in humans after three 10 mg doses, the maximum recommended daily dose (MRDD). There was no evidence of an increase in tumor incidence related to rizatriptan in either species.

In a rat study, there was a statistically significant increase in the incidence of pituitary adenomas in males only at 85 mg/kg/day **frovatriptan**, a dose that produced 250 times the exposure achieved at the maximum recommended human dose (MRHD) based on AUC comparisons. In the 26-week transgenic mouse study, there was an increased incidence of subcutaneous sarcomas in females dosed at 200 and 400 mg/kg/day, or 390 and 630 times the human exposure based on AUC comparisons.

In rats, the incidence of testicular interstitial cell adenomas was increased at the high dose of 75 mg/kg/day **eletriptan**. The estimated exposure (AUC) to parent drug at that dose was approximately 6 times that achieved in humans receiving the MRDD of 80 mg. In mice, the incidence of hepatocellular adenomas was increased at the high dose of 400 mg/kg/day eletriptan. The exposure to parent drug (AUC) at that dose was approximately 18 times that achieved in humans receiving the MRDD of 80 mg.

➤*Fertility impairment:* A treatment-related decrease in fertility secondary to a decrease in mating in animals treated with 50 and 500 mg/kg/day **sumatriptan** was observed. A treatment-related decrease in the number of females exhibiting normal estrous cycles at doses of **naratriptan** 170 mg/kg/day or greater and an increase in preimplantation loss at 60 mg/kg/day or greater was observed. Testicular/epididymal atrophy in high-dose male rats accompanied by spermatozoa depletion reduced mating success and may have contributed to the observed preimplantation loss. In a fertility study in rats, altered estrous cyclicity and delays in time to mating were observed in females treated orally with 100 mg/kg/day **rizatriptan**. Plasma drug exposure (AUC) at this dose was approximately 225 times the exposure in humans receiving the MRDD of 30 mg. The no-effect dose was 10 mg/kg/day (approximately 15 times the human exposure at the MRDD). Male and female rats were dosed with **frovatriptan** prior to and during mating and up to implantation at doses of 100, 500, and 1000 mg/kg/day (equivalent to approximately 130, 650, and 1300 times the MRHD on a mg/m² basis). At all dose levels there was an increase in the number of females that mated on the first day of pairing compared with control animals. This occurred in conjunction with a prolongation of the estrous cycle. In addition, females had a decreased mean number of corpora lutea and consequently a lower number of live fetuses per litter, which suggested a partial impairment of ovulation. There were no other fertility-related effects. In a rat fertility and early embryonic development study, there was a prolongation of the estrous cycle at the 200 mg/kg/day **eletriptan** dose because of an increase in duration of estrus. There also were dose-related, statistically significant decreases in mean numbers of corpora lutea per dam at all 3 doses, resulting in decreases in mean numbers of implants and viable fetuses per dam. This suggests a partial inhibition of ovulation by eletriptan. Prolongation of the estrous cycle was observed at a dose of 100 mg/kg/day for **almotriptan**.

➤*Elderly:* Pharmacokinetic disposition of 5-HT₁ agonists in the elderly is similar to that seen in younger adults.

The risk of adverse reactions to **naratriptan** and **sumatriptan** may be greater in elderly patients who have reduced renal function and who are more likely to have decreased hepatic function; they are at higher risk for CAD, and blood pressure increases may be more pronounced. Therefore, the use of naratriptan and sumatriptan in elderly patients is not recommended.

Dose selection of **almotriptan** for an elderly patient should be cautious, usually starting at the low end of the dosing range, reflecting the greater frequency of decreased hepatic, renal, or cardiac function, and of concomitant disease or other drug therapy. The recommended dose for elderly patients with normal renal function for their age is the same as that recommended for younger adults.

Mean blood concentrations of **frovatriptan** in elderly subjects were 1.5 to 2 times higher than those seen in younger adults. Because migraine occurs infrequently in the elderly, clinical experience with frovatriptan is limited to such patients.

Eletriptan has been given to only 50 patients older than 65 years of age. Blood pressure was increased to a greater extent in elderly subjects than in younger subjects. There is no information about the safety and efficacy of zolmitriptan in this population because patients older than 65 years of age were excluded from the controlled clinical trials.

➤*Pregnancy:* Category C. In rats and rabbits, 5-HT₁ agonist administration is associated with embryolethality, fetal abnormalities, and pup mortality. There are no adequate and well-controlled studies in pregnant women. Use during pregnancy only if the potential benefit justifies the potential risk to the fetus.

In reproductive toxicity studies in rats and rabbits, oral administration of **eletriptan** was associated with developmental toxicity (decreased fetal and pup weights and an increased incidence of fetal structural abnormalities). Effects on fetal and pup weights were observed at doses that were 6 to 12 times greater than the clinical MRDD of 80 mg.

When pregnant rats were administered **frovatriptan** during the period of organogenesis at oral doses of 100, 500, and 1000 mg/kg/day (equivalent to 130, 650, and 1300 times the MRHD on a mg/m² basis), there were dose-related increases in incidences of both litters and total numbers of fetuses with dilated ureters, unilateral and bilateral pelvic cavitation, hydronephrosis, and hydroureters.

The manufacturer maintains a **sumatriptan** and **naratriptan** pregnancy registry. Register patients by calling (800) 336-2176.

➤*Lactation:* **Sumatriptan** and **eletriptan** are excreted in human breast milk. In one study of 8 women given a single 80 mg dose of eletriptan, the mean total amount in breast milk over 24 hours was approximately 0.02% of the administered dose. The resulting eletriptan concentration-time profile was similar to that seen in the plasma over 24 hours, with very low concentrations of drug (mean, 1.7 ng/mL) still present in the milk 18 to 24 hours postdose. Lactating rats dosed with **zolmitriptan** had milk levels equivalent to maternal plasma levels at 1 hour and 4 times higher than plasma levels at 4 hours. **Naratriptan**-related material is excreted in the milk of rats. **Rizatriptan** is extensively excreted in rat milk, at a level of 5-fold or greater than maternal plasma levels. Lactating rats dosed with **almotriptan** had milk levels equivalent to maternal plasma levels at 0.5 hours and 7 times higher than plasma levels at 6 hours after dosing. **Frovatriptan** and its metabolites are excreted in the milk of lactating rats with the maximum concentration being 4-fold higher than that seen in blood. Exercise caution when administering to a nursing woman.

➤*Children:* Safety and efficacy have not been established.

Clinical trials have evaluated 25 to 100 mg oral **sumatriptan** in 701 pediatric patients, 0.25 to 2.5 mg **naratriptan** in 300 adolescents 12 to 17 years of age, and 40 mg **eletriptan** in 274 adolescents 11 to 17 years of age. These studies did not establish efficacy. Adverse events observed in these clinical trials were similar in nature to those reported in clinical trials in adults. The frequency of all adverse events in sumatriptan patients appeared to be dose- and age-dependent, with younger patients reporting events more commonly than older adolescents.

The use of 5-HT₁ receptor agonists is not recommended in patients younger than 18 years of age.

Precautions

➤*Chest, jaw, or neck tightness:* Chest, jaw, or neck tightness have occurred after 5-HT₁ agonist administration, and atypical sensations over the precordium (pain, tightness, pressure, heaviness) have occurred, but these rarely have been associated with arrhythmias or ischemic ECG changes. Evaluate patients who experience signs or symptoms suggestive of angina for the presence of CAD or a predisposition to Prinzmetal variant angina before receiving additional doses. Monitor ECG if dosing is resumed and similar symptoms recur.

Similarly, patients who experience other symptoms or signs suggestive of decreased arterial flow, such as ischemic bowel syndrome or Raynaud syndrome, following the use of any 5-HT₁ agonist are candidates for further evaluation.

➤*Seizures:* There have been rare reports of seizures following **sumatriptan** use.

➤*Ophthalmic effects:*
Binding to melanin-containing tissues – Because 5-HT₁ agonists bind to melanin, accumulation in melanin-rich tissues (eg, the eye) could occur over time, raising the possibility of toxicity in these tissues after extended use. Be aware of the possibility of long-term ophthalmologic effects.

Corneal effects – **Sumatriptan**, **naratriptan**, and **almotriptan** cause corneal opacities and defects in dogs; naratriptan also caused transient changes in precorneal tear film. These changes may occur in humans. **Eletriptan** caused transient corneal opacities in dogs receiving 5 mg/kg and above.

➤*Phenylketonurics:* Inform phenylketonuric patients that **rizatriptan** and **zolmitriptan** orally-disintegrating tablets contain phenylalanine (a component of aspartame). Each 5 mg rizatriptan orally-disintegrating tablet contains 1.05 mg phenylalanine, and each 10 mg orally-disintegrating tablet contains 2.1 mg phenylalanine. Each 2.5 mg zolmitriptan orally-disintegrating tablet contains 2.81 mg phenylalanine.

➤*Photosensitivity:* Photosensitization (photoallergy or phototoxicity) may occur; therefore, caution patients to take protective measures (ie, sunscreens, protective clothing) against exposure to sunlight or ultraviolet light (eg, tanning beds) until tolerance is determined.

Drug Interactions

Serotonin 5-HT₁ Receptor Agonist Drug Interactions			
Precipitant drug	Object drug*		Description
Cimetidine	Zolmitriptan	↑	Following coadministration with cimetidine, the half life and AUC of a 5 mg dose of zolmitriptan and its active metabolite were approximately doubled.
Ergot alkaloids (dihydro-ergotamine, methysergide)	5-HT₁ agonists	↑↓	The risk of vasospastic reactions may be increased. Use of 5-HT₁ agonists within 24 hours of treatment with an ergot-containing medication is contraindicated. The AUC and C_max of frovatriptan (2 × 2.5 mg dose) were reduced by ≈ 25% when coadministered with ergotamine tartrate.
Potent CYP3A4 inhibitors (eg, ketoconazole, itraconazole, nefazodone, troleandomycin, clarithromycin, ritonavir, nelfinavir)	Almotriptan Eletriptan	↑	Coadministration of almotriptan and ketoconazole (400 mg/day for 3 days) resulted in an ≈ 60% increase in AUC and maximal plasma concentration of almotriptan. The AUC and C_max of eletriptan are increased with coadministration. Do not use eletriptan within 72 hours of treatment with a potent CYP3A4 inhibitor (see Warnings).

Serotonin 5-HT$_1$ Receptor Agonists

Serotonin 5-HT$_1$ Receptor Agonist Drug Interactions

Precipitant drug	Object drug*		Description
5-HT$_1$ agonists	5-HT$_1$ agonists	↑	The risk of vasospastic reactions may be increased. Coadministration of two 5-HT$_1$ agonists within 24 hours of each other is contraindicated.
MAOIs	Almotriptan Rizatriptan Sumatriptan Zolmitriptan	↑	Use of certain 5-HT$_1$ agonists concomitantly with or within 2 weeks following the discontinuation of an MAOI is contraindicated. If it is necessary to use such agents together, naratriptan, eletriptan, and frovatriptan appear to be less likely to interact with MAOIs.
Oral contraceptives	Frovatriptan	↑	Mean C$_{max}$ and AUC of frovatriptan are 30% higher in those subjects taking oral contraceptives compared with those not taking oral contraceptives.
Propranolol	Zolmitriptan	↔	C$_{max}$ and AUC of zolmitriptan increased 1.5-fold but decreased for the N-desmethyl metabolite by 30% and 15%, respectively. No effects on blood pressure or pulse rate were observed.
	Rizatriptan	↑	In a study of coadministration of 240 mg/day propranolol and a single dose of 10 mg rizatriptan in healthy subjects, mean plasma AUC for rizatriptan was increased by 70% during propranolol administration, and a 4-fold increase was observed in 1 subject.
	Frovatriptan	↑	Propranolol increased the AUC of 2.5 mg frovatriptan in males by 60% and in females by 29%. The C$_{max}$ of frovatriptan was increased 23% in males and 16% in females in the presence of propranolol.
	Eletriptan	↑	C$_{max}$ and AUC of eletriptan were increased by 10% and 33%, respectively, in the presence of propranolol. No interactive increases in blood pressure were observed.
Sibutramine	Naratriptan Rizatriptan Sumatriptan Zolmitriptan	↑	A "serotonin syndrome," including CNS irritability, motor weakness, shivering, myoclonus, and altered consciousness may occur. Coadministration is not recommended. Monitor the patient for adverse effects if concurrent use cannot be avoided.
Almotriptan Frovatriptan Naratriptan Rizatriptan Sumatriptan Zolmitriptan	SSRIs Fluoxetine Fluvoxamine Paroxetine Sertraline	↑	There have been rare reports of weakness, hyperreflexia, and incoordination with combined use of SSRIs. If concomitant treatment is clinically warranted, observe the patient carefully. No interaction was observed when rizatriptan was administered with paroxetine. Fluoxetine had no effect on almotriptan clearance, but C$_{max}$ increased 18%.

* ↑ = Object drug increased. ↓ = Object drug decreased. ↔ = Undetermined clinical effect.

▶*Drug/Food interactions:* Food has no significant effect on oral 5-HT$_1$ agonist bioavailability, but delays **sumatriptan's** T$_{max}$ by approximately 30 minutes and **rizatriptan's** time to reach peak concentration by 1 hour. AUC and C$_{max}$ of **eletriptan** are increased approximately 20% to 30% following oral administration with a high-fat meal.

Adverse Reactions

Serious coronary artery vasospasm, transient myocardial ischemia, ventricular fibrillation/tachycardia, and MI have been associated with 5-HT$_1$ agonists.

Oral – These agents are generally well tolerated. Across all doses, most adverse reactions were mild and transient and did not lead to long-lasting effects. In patients being treated for multiple migraine attacks for 1 year or less with **naratriptan, zolmitriptan, eletriptan,** or **frovatriptan**, 3.6%, 8%, 8.3%, and 5% withdrew from the trial because of adverse experiences, respectively. The most common events were asthenia, dizziness, nausea, paresthesia, fatigue, pain, chest or neck tightness or heaviness, somnolence, warm sensation, dry mouth, headache, flushing, hot or cold sensation, and chest pain.

Frovatriptan: Frovatriptan is generally well tolerated. The incidence of adverse events in clinical trials did not increase when up to 3 doses were used within 24 hours. The majority of adverse events were mild or moderate and transient. The incidence of adverse events in 4 placebo-controlled clinical trials was not affected by gender, age, or concomitant medications commonly used by migraine patients. There were insufficient data to assess the impact of race on the incidence of adverse events.

Oral 5-HT$_1$ Agonist Adverse Reactions (%)[a]

Adverse reaction	Almotriptan 6.25 mg (n=527)	12.5 mg (n=1313)	Eletriptan 20 mg (n=431)	40 mg (n=1774)	80 mg (n=1932)	Frovatriptan 2.5 mg (n=1554)	Naratriptan 1 mg (n=627)	2.5 mg (n=627)	Rizatriptan 5 mg (n=977)	10 mg (n=1167)	Sumatriptan 25 mg (n=417)	50 mg (n=771)	100 mg (n=437)	Zolmitriptan 1 mg (n=163)	2.5 mg (n=498)	5 mg (n=1012)
Atypical sensations																
Hot/Cold sensation	—	—	—	—	—	3	—	—	—	—	—	—	—	—	—	—
Hypesthesia	—	—	—	—	—	—	—	—	—	—	—	—	—	1	1	2
Miscellaneous sensations	—	—	—	—	—	—	2	4	4	5	—	—	—	—	—	—
Paresthesia	1	1	3	3	4	4	1	2	3	4	3	5	3	5	7	9
Warm/Cold sensation	—	—	—	—	—	—	—	—	—	—	3	2	3	—	—	—
Warm/Hot sensation	—	—	2	2	2	—	—	—	—	—	—	—	—	6	5	7
CNS																
Asthenia	—	—	4	5	10	—	—	—	—	—	—	—	—	5	3	9
Dizziness	—	—	3	6	7	8	1	2	4	9	>1	>1	>1	6	8	10
Drowsiness	—	—	—	—	—	—	1	2	—	—	>1	>1	>1	—	—	—
Fatigue	—	—	—	—	—	5	2	2	4	7	2	2	3	—	—	—
Headache	—	—	4	3	4	4	—	—	<2	2	>1	>1	>1	—	—	—
Myasthenia	—	—	—	—	—	—	—	—	—	—	—	—	—	0	1	2
Somnolence	—	—	3	6	7	—	—	—	4	8	—	—	—	5	6	8
Vertigo	—	—	—	—	—	—	—	—	—	—	<1	<1	2	0	0	2
Miscellaneous CNS effects	—	—	—	—	—	—	4	7	—	—	—	—	—	—	—	—
GI																
Abdominal pain/discomfort/stomach pain/cramps/pressure	—	—	1	2	2	—	—	—	—	—	—	—	—	—	—	—
Dry mouth	1	1	2	3	4	3	—	—	3	3	>1	>1	>1	5	3	3
Dyspepsia	—	—	1	2	2	2	—	—	—	—	—	—	—	3	2	1

Serotonin 5-HT₁ Receptor Agonists

Adverse reaction	Almotriptan		Eletriptan			Frovatriptan	Naratriptan		Rizatriptan		Sumatriptan			Zolmitriptan		
Oral 5-HT₁ Agonist Adverse Reactions (%)[a]	6.25 mg (n=527)	12.5 mg (n=1313)	20 mg (n=431)	40 mg (n=1774)	80 mg (n=1932)	2.5 mg (n=1554)	1 mg (n=627)	2.5 mg (n=627)	5 mg (n=977)	10 mg (n=1167)	25 mg (n=417)	50 mg (n=771)	100 mg (n=437)	1 mg (n=163)	2.5 mg (n=498)	5 mg (n=1012)
Dysphagia (including throat tightness/difficulty swallowing)	—	—	1	2	2	—	—	—	—	—	—	—	—	0	0	2
Nausea	4	5	4	6	—	—	—	4	9	6	1	2	—	4	5	8
Pain/Pressure sensations																
Chest tightness pressure, and/or heaviness	—	—	1	2	2	2	—	—	< 2	3	1	2	2	2	3	4
Heaviness	—	—	—	—	—	—	—	—	—	—	< 1	< 1	2	1	2	5
Neck/Throat/Jaw	—	—	—	—	—	—	1	2	< 2	2	< 1	2	3	4	7	10
Pain, location specified/unspecified	—	—	—	—	—	—	—	—	6	9	2	1	1	2	2	3
Pressure	—	—	—	—	—	—	—	—	—	—	< 1	2	2	—	—	—
Regional pain	—	—	—	—	—	—	—	—	< 1	2	—	—	—	—	—	—
Tightness	—	—	—	—	—	—	—	—	—	—	< 1	2	2	—	—	—
Skeletal	—	—	—	—	—	3	—	—	—	—	—	—	—	—	—	—
Other	2	4	3	3	1	1	3	2	2	3	—	—	—	—	—	—
Miscellaneous																
Flushing	—	—	2	2	2	4	—	—	—	—	—	—	—	—	—	—
Myalgia	—	—	—	—	—	—	—	—	—	—	—	—	—	1	1	2
Other	—	—	—	—	—	—	6	7	—	—	—	—	—	—	—	—
Palpitations	—	—	—	—	—	—	—	—	—	—	> 1	> 1	> 1	0	< 1	2
Sweating	—	—	—	—	—	—	—	—	—	—	—	—	—	0	2	3

[a] Data are pooled from separate studies and are not necessarily comparable.

Other adverse reactions include the following:

➤*Almotriptan:*

Cardiovascular – Palpitations, tachycardia, vasodilation (0.1% to 1%); hypertension, syncope (less than 0.1%).

CNS – Dizziness, somnolence (1% or more); anxiety, CNS stimulation, hypesthesia, insomnia, restlessness, shakiness, tremor, vertigo (0.1% to 1%); abnormal coordination, change in dreams, depressive symptoms, euphoria, hyperreflexia, hypertonia, impaired concentration, nervousness, neuropathy, nightmares (less than 0.1%).

Dermatologic – Dermatitis, diaphoresis, erythema, pruritus, rash (0.1% to 1%); photosensitivity reaction (less than 0.1%).

GI – Diarrhea, dyspepsia, vomiting (0.1% to 1%); abdominal cramp or pain, colitis, esophageal reflux, gastritis, gastroenteritis, increased salivation, increased thirst (less than 0.1%).

Metabolic – Hyperglycemia, increased serum CPK (0.1% to 1%); hypercholesterolemia, increased GGT (less than 0.1%).

Musculoskeletal – Muscular weakness, myalgia (0.1% to 1%); arthralgia, arthritis, myopathy (less than 0.1%).

Respiratory – Bronchitis, dyspnea, epistaxis, laryngismus, pharyngitis, rhinitis, sinusitis (0.1% to 1%); hyperventilation, laryngitis, sneezing (less than 0.1%).

Special senses – Conjunctivitis, ear pain, eye irritation, hyperacusis, taste alteration (0.1% to 1%); diplopia, dry eyes, eye pain, nystagmus, otitis media, parosmia, scotoma, tinnitus (less than 0.1%).

Miscellaneous – Headache (1% or more); asthenia, back pain, chest pain, chills, dysmenorrhea, fatigue, neck pain, rigid neck (0.1% to 1%); fever (less than 0.1%).

➤*Eletriptan:*

Cardiovascular – Palpitation (1% or more); hypertension, migraine, peripheral vascular disorder, tachycardia (0.1% to 1%); angina pectoris, arrhythmia, atrial fibrillation, AV block, bradycardia, cerebrovascular disorder, hypotension, syncope, thrombophlebitis, vasospasm, ventricular arrhythmia (less than 0.1%).

CNS – Hypertonia, hypesthesia, vertigo (1% or more); abnormal dreams, agitation, anxiety, apathy, ataxia, confusion, depersonalization, depression, emotional lability, euphoria, hyperesthesia, hyperkinesia, incoordination, insomnia, nervousness, speech disorder, stupor, thinking abnormal, tremor (0.1% to 1%); abnormal gait, amnesia, aphasia, catatonic reaction, dementia, diplopia, dystonia, hallucinations, hemiplegia, hyperalgesia, hypokinesia, hysteria, manic reaction, neuropathy, neurosis, oculogyric crisis, paralysis, psychotic depression, sleep disorder, twitching (less than 0.1%).

Dermatologic – Sweating (1% or more); pruritus, rash, skin disorder (0.1% to 1%); alopecia, dry skin, eczema, exfoliative dermatitis, maculopapular rash, psoriasis, skin discoloration, skin hypertrophy, urticaria (less than 0.1%).

Endocrine – Goiter, thyroid adenoma, thyroiditis (less than 0.1%).

GI – Anorexia, constipation, diarrhea, eructation, esophagitis, flatulence, gastritis, GI disorder, increased salivation, liver function tests abnormal (0.1% to 1%); gingivitis, hematemesis, increased appetite, rectal disorder, stomatitis, tongue disorder, tongue edema, tooth disorder (less than 0.1%).

GU – Impotence, polyuria, urinary frequency, urinary tract disorder (0.1% to 1%); breast pain, kidney pain, leukorrhea, menorrhagia, menstrual disorder, vaginitis (less than 0.1%).

Hematologic/Lymphatic – Anemia, cyanosis, leukopenia, lymphadenopathy, monocytosis, purpura (less than 0.1%).

Metabolic – CPK increased, edema, peripheral edema, thirst (0.1% to 1%); alkaline phosphatase increased, bilirubinemia, hyperglycemia, weight gain, weight loss (less than 0.1%).

Musculoskeletal – Arthralgia, arthritis, arthrosis, bone pain, myalgia, myasthenia (0.1% to 1%); bone neoplasm, joint disorder, myopathy, tenosynovitis (less than 0.1%).

Respiratory – Pharyngitis (1% or more); asthma, dyspnea, respiratory disorder, respiratory tract infection, rhinitis, voice alteration, yawn (0.1% to 1%); bronchitis, choking sensation, cough increased, epistaxis, hiccough, hyperventilation, laryngitis, sinusitis, sputum increased (less than 0.1%).

Special senses – Abnormal vision, conjunctivitis, ear pain, eye pain, lacrimation disorder, photophobia, taste perversion, tinnitus (0.1% to 1%); abnormality of accommodation, dry eyes, ear disorder, eye hemorrhage, otitis media, parosmia, ptosis (less than 0.1%).

Miscellaneous – Back pain, chills, pain (1% or more); face edema, malaise (0.1% to 1%); abdomen enlarged, abscess, accidental injury, allergic reaction, fever, flu syndrome, halitosis, hernia, hypothermia, lab test abnormal, moniliasis, rheumatoid arthritis, shock (less than 0.1%).

➤*Frovatriptan:*

Cardiovascular – Palpitation (1% or more); abnormal ECG, tachycardia (0.1% to 1%); bradycardia (less than 0.1%).

CNS – Anxiety, dysesthesia, hypesthesia, insomnia (1% or more); abnormal gait, agitation, amnesia, asthenia, ataxia, confusion, depersonalization, depression, emotional lability, euphoria, hyperesthesia, impaired concentration, involuntary muscle contractions, migraine aggravated, nervousness, rigors, speech disorder, thinking abnormal, tremor, vertigo (0.1% to 1%); abnormal dreaming, abnormal reflexes, depression aggravated, hypertonia, hypotonia, personality disorder, tongue paralysis (less than 0.1%).

Dermatologic – Sweating increased (1% or more); bullous eruption, pruritus (0.1% to 1%).

GI – Abdominal pain, diarrhea, vomiting (1% or more); anorexia, constipation, dysphagia, esophagospasm, flatulence, saliva increased (0.1% to 1%); change in bowel habits, cheilitis, eructation, gastroesophageal

Serotonin 5-HT₁ Receptor Agonists

reflux, hiccough, peptic ulcer, salivary gland pain, stomatitis, toothache (less than 0.1%).

GU – Micturition frequency, polyuria (0.1% to 1%); abnormal urine, nocturia, renal pain (less than 0.1%).

Hematologic – Epistaxis (0.1% to 1%); purpura (less than 0.1%).

Metabolic / Nutritional – Dehydration, thirst (0.1% to 1%); hypocalcemia, hypoglycemia (less than 0.1%).

Musculoskeletal – Arthralgia, arthrosis, back pain, leg cramps, muscle weakness, myalgia (0.1% to 1%).

Respiratory – Rhinitis, sinusitis (1% or more); pharyngitis, dyspnea, hyperventilation, laryngitis (0.1% to 1%).

Special senses – Tinnitus, vision abnormal (1% or more); abnormal lacrimation, conjunctivitis, earache, eye pain, hyperacusis, taste perversion (0.1% to 1%).

Miscellaneous – Pain (1% or more); fever, hot flushes, malaise, (0.1% to 1%); feeling of relaxation, leg pain, mouth edema, syncope (less than 0.1%).

➤*Naratriptan:*

Atypical sensations – Warm/cold temperature sensations (1% or more); strange feeling and burning/stinging sensation (0.1% to 1%).

Cardiovascular – Abnormal ECG (PR prolongation, QT prolongation, ST/T wave abnormalities, premature ventricular contractions, atrial flutter/fibrillation), increased blood pressure, palpitations, syncope, tachyarrhythmias (0.1% to 1%); bradycardia, heart murmurs, hypotension, varicosities (less than 0.1%).

CNS – Vertigo (1% or more); anxiety, cognitive function disorders, depressive disorders, detachment, equilibrium disorders, sleep disorders, tremors (0.1% to 1%); aggression, agitation, compressed nerve syndromes, confusion, convulsions, coordination disorders, decreased consciousness, dreams, hallucinations, hostility, hyperactivity, hyperesthesia, hypesthesia, motor retardation, muscle twitching/fasciculation, neuralgia, neuritis, panic, paralysis of cranial nerves, psychomotor restlessness, sedation (less than 0.1%).

Dermatologic – Pruritus, skin rashes, sweating, urticaria (0.1% to 1%); acne, allergic skin reactions, dermatitis/dermatosis, folliculitis, hair loss, macular skin/rashes, photodermatitis, photosensitivity, pruritic skin rashes, skin erythema, skin flakiness/dryness (less than 0.1%).

GI – Hyposalivation, vomiting (1% or more); constipation, diarrhea, discomfort/pain, dyspeptic symptoms, gastroenteritis (0.1% to 1%); abnormal bilirubin levels, abnormal liver function tests, altered sense of taste, esophagitis, gastric ulcers, gastritis, hemorrhoids, oral itching and irritation, regurgitation and reflux, salivary gland inflammation (less than 0.1%).

GU – Bladder inflammation, diuresis, polyuria (0.1% to 1%); breast discharge, breast inflammation, decreased libido, endometrium disorders, fallopian tube inflammation, lumps in breast, lumps in female reproductive tract, pyelitis, urinary incontinence, urinary tract hemorrhage, urinary urgency, vaginal inflammation (less than 0.1%).

Hematologic – Increased white cells (0.1% to 1%); anemia, purpura, quantitative red cell or hemoglobin defects, thrombocytopenia (less than 0.1%).

Metabolic / Nutritional – Dehydration, fluid retention, polydipsia, thirst (0.1% to 1%); glycosuria, hypercholesterolemia, hyperglycemia, hyperlipidemia, hypothyroidism, ketonuria, parathyroid neoplasm (less than 0.1%).

Musculoskeletal – Pressure/tightness/heaviness sensations (1% or more); arthralgia, articular rheumatism, joint/muscle stiffness, muscle cramps/spasms, muscle pain, rigidity, tightness (0.1% to 1%); bone/skeletal pain (less than 0.1%).

Respiratory – Bronchitis, cough, pneumonia (0.1% to 1%); airway obstruction/constriction, asthma, pleuritis, tracheitis (less than 0.1%).

Special senses – Photophobia (1% or more); blurred vision (0.1% to 1%); aphasia, difficulty focusing, dry eyes, eye hemorrhage, eye pain/discomfort, scotoma, sensation of eye pressure, (less than 0.1%).

Ear, nose, and throat: Ear, nose, and throat infections (1% or more); phonophobia, sinusitis, tinnitus, upper respiratory tract inflammation (0.1% to 1%); allergic rhinitis, ear/nose/throat hemorrhage, hearing difficulty, labyrinthitis (less than 0.1%).

Miscellaneous – Allergic reactions, allergies, chills, descriptions of odor or taste, edema, fever, swelling (0.1% to 1%); mobility disorders, spasms (less than 0.1%).

Postmarketing reports: These events do not include those already listed in the adverse reactions section above. Because the reports cite events reported spontaneously from worldwide postmarketing experience, frequency of events and the role of naratriptan in their causation cannot be reliably determined.

• *Cardiovascular* – Angina, MI.

• *CNS* – Cerebral vascular accident, including transient ischemic attack, subarachnoid hemorrhage, and cerebral infarction.

• *Miscellaneous* – Dyspnea, hypersensitivity including anaphylaxis/anaphylactoid reactions, in some cases severe (eg, circulatory collapse).

➤*Rizatriptan:*

Cardiovascular – Palpitation (1% or more); arrhythmia, bradycardia, cold extremities, hypertension, tachycardia (0.1% to 1%); angina pectoris (less than 0.1%).

CNS – Euphoria, hypesthesia, mental acuity decreased, tremor (1% or more); agitation, anxiety, ataxia, confusion, depression, disorientation, dream abnormality, dysarthria, gait abnormality, hyperesthesia, insomnia, irritability, memory impairment, nervousness, vertigo (0.1% to 1%); akinesia/bradykinesia, apprehension, depersonalization, dysesthesia, hyperkinesia, hypersomnia, hyporeflexia (less than 0.1%).

Dermatologic – Flushing (1% or more); pruritus, rash, sweating, urticaria (0.1% to 1%); acne, erythema, photosensitivity (less than 0.1%).

GI – Diarrhea, vomiting (1% or more); acid regurgitation, constipation, dyspepsia, dysphagia, flatulence, thirst, tongue edema (0.1% to 1%); anorexia, appetite increased, eructation, gastritis, paralysis (tongue) (less than 0.1%).

GU – Hot flashes (1% or more); menstruation disorder, polyuria, urinary frequency (0.1% to 1%); dysuria (less than 0.1%).

Musculoskeletal – Arthralgia, muscle cramp, muscle spasm, muscle weakness, musculoskeletal pain, myalgia, stiffness (0.1% to 1%).

Respiratory – Dyspnea (1% or more); congestion (nasal), dry nose, dry throat, epistaxis, irritation (nasal), pharyngitis, respiratory congestion (nasal), sinus disorder, upper respiratory tract infection, yawning (0.1% to 1%); cough, hiccough, hoarseness, pharyngeal edema, rhinorrhea, sneezing, tachypnea (less than 0.1%).

Special senses – Blurred vision, burning eye, dry eyes, ear pain, eye irritation, eye pain, tearing, tinnitus (0.1% to 1%); eye swelling, hyperacusis, itching eye, photophobia, photopsia, smell perversion (less than 0.1%).

Miscellaneous – Warm/cold sensations (1% or more); abdominal distention, chills, dehydration, facial edema, hangover effect, heat sensitivity (0.1% to 1%); edema/swelling, fever, orthostatic effects, syncope (less than 0.1%).

Postmarketing reports: The following additional adverse reactions have been reported very rarely and most have been reported in patients with risk factors predictive of CAD: Cerebrovascular accident; MI; myocardial ischemia. The following also have been reported: Dysgeusia; toxic epidermal necrolysis.

➤*Sumatriptan:*

Sumatriptan Adverse Reactions (%)			
Adverse reaction	Tablets	Nasal	Injection
Atypical sensations			
Burning sensation	> 1	0.1 to 1	—
Cold sensation	—	0.1 to 1	—
Dysesthesia	< 0.1	< 0.1	< 0.1
Feeling of heaviness	—	0.1 to 1	—
Feeling strange	—	0.1 to 1	—
Numbness	> 1	0.1 to 1	—
Paresthesia	—	0.1 to 1	0.1 to 1
Pressure sensation	—	0.1 to 1	—
Prickling sensation	—	< 0.1	0.1 to 1
Simultaneous hot/cold sensation	—	—	< 0.1
Stinging sensations	—	—	0.1 to 1
Tickling sensations	—	—	< 0.1
Tight feeling in head	0.1 to 1	0.1 to 1	—
Tingling	—	0.1 to 1	—
Cardiovascular			
Abdominal aortic aneurysm	—	< 0.1	—
Abnormal pulse	—	—	< 0.1
Angina	< 0.1	—	—
Arrhythmia	0.1 to 1	0.1 to 1	0.1 to 1
Atherosclerosis	< 0.1	—	—
Bradycardia	< 0.1	< 0.1	0.1 to 1
Cerebral ischemia	< 0.1	—	—
Cerebrovascular lesion	< 0.1	—	—
ECG changes	0.1 to 1	0.1 to 1	0.1 to 1
Flushing	—	0.1 to 1	—
Heart block	< 0.1	—	—
Hypertension	> 1	0.1 to 1	0.1 to 1
Hypotension	> 1	< 0.1	0.1 to 1
Pallor	0.1 to 1	< 0.1	< 0.1
Palpitations	> 1	0.1 to 1	0.1 to 1
Peripheral cyanosis	< 0.1	—	—
Phlebitis	—	< 0.1	—
Pulsating sensations	0.1 to 1	—	0.1 to 1
Raynaud syndrome	—	—	< 0.1
Syncope	> 1	—	0.1 to 1
Tachycardia	0.1 to 1	0.1 to 1	0.1 to 1

Serotonin 5-HT₁ Receptor Agonists

Sumatriptan Adverse Reactions (%)			
Adverse reaction	Tablets	Nasal	Injection
Thrombosis	< 0.1	—	—
Transient myocardial ischemia	< 0.1	—	—
Vasodilation	< 0.1	—	< 0.1
CNS			
Aggressiveness	< 0.1	—	—
Agitation	< 0.1	0.1 to 1	0.1 to 1
Anxiety	< 0.1	0.1 to 1	—
Apathy	< 0.1	< 0.1	—
Bradylogia	< 0.1	—	—
Chills	—	0.1 to 1	0.1 to 1
Cluster headache	< 0.1	—	—
Confusion	0.1 to 1	0.1 to 1	0.1 to 1
Convulsions	< 0.1	—	—
Depression	0.1 to 1	0.1 to 1	< 0.1
Depressive disorders	< 0.1	—	—
Detachment	< 0.1	—	—
Difficulty concentrating	0.1 to 1	< 0.1	< 0.1
Disturbances of emotion	—	< 0.1	—
Drowsiness/Sedation	—	0.1 to 1	—
Dysarthria	0.1 to 1	< 0.1	< 0.1
Dystonic reaction	< 0.1	—	< 0.1
Euphoria	0.1 to 1	< 0.1	0.1 to 1
Facial pain	0.1 to 1	< 0.1	< 0.1
Facial paralysis	< 0.1	—	—
Globus hystericus	—	—	< 0.1
Hallucinations	< 0.1	—	—
Heat sensitivity	0.1 to 1	—	—
Hunger	< 0.1	< 0.1	—
Hyperesthesia	< 0.1	—	< 0.1
Hysteria	< 0.1	—	< 0.1
Incoordination	0.1 to 1	< 0.1	—
Increased alertness	< 0.1	—	—
Intoxication	—	< 0.1	< 0.1
Memory disturbance	< 0.1	< 0.1	—
Monoplegia	0.1 to 1	< 0.1	< 0.1
Motor dysfunction	< 0.1	—	—
Myoclonia	—	—	< 0.1
Neoplasm of pituitary	—	< 0.1	—
Neuralgia	< 0.1	—	—
Neurotic disorders	< 0.1	—	—
Paralysis	< 0.1	—	—
Personality change	< 0.1	—	—
Phobia	< 0.1	—	—
Phonophobia	> 1	—	—
Photophobia	> 1	—	0.1 to 1
Psychomotor disorders	< 0.1	—	—
Radiculopathy	< 0.1	—	—
Raised intracranial pressure	< 0.1	—	—
Relaxation	—	—	0.1 to 1
Rigidity	< 0.1	—	—
Sensation of lightness	—	0.1 to 1	0.1 to 1
Shivering	0.1 to 1	0.1 to 1	0.1 to 1
Sleep disturbance	0.1 to 1	0.1 to 1	< 0.1
Stress	—	< 0.1	—
Suicide	< 0.1	—	—
Syncope	0.1 to 1	0.1 to 1	—
Transient hemiplegia	—	—	< 0.1
Tremor	0.1 to 1	0.1 to 1	0.1 to 1
Twitching	< 0.1	—	—
Yawning	—	—	< 0.1
Dermatologic			
Dry/Scaly skin	< 0.1	—	—
Eczema	< 0.1	—	—
Erythema	0.1 to 1	0.1 to 1	0.1 to 1
Herpes	—	—	< 0.1
Peeling of skin	—	—	< 0.1
Pruritus	0.1 to 1	0.1 to 1	0.1 to 1
Rash	0.1 to 1	0.1 to 1	0.1 to 1
Seborrheic dermatitis	< 0.1	—	—
Skin nodules	< 0.1	—	—
Skin tenderness	0.1 to 1	—	< 0.1
Sweating	> 1	< 0.1	—
Swelling of face	—	—	< 0.1
Tightness of the skin	< 0.1	—	—
Wrinkling of the skin	< 0.1	—	—

Sumatriptan Adverse Reactions (%)			
Adverse reaction	Tablets	Nasal	Injection
Endocrine/Metabolic			
Dehydration	—	—	< 0.1
Elevated TSH levels	< 0.1	—	—
Endocrine cysts	< 0.1	—	—
Fluid disturbances	< 0.1	—	—
Galactorrhea	< 0.1	< 0.1	—
Hyperglycemia	< 0.1	—	—
Hypoglycemia	< 0.1	< 0.1	—
Hypothyroidism	< 0.1	—	—
Polydipsia	< 0.1	—	< 0.1
Thirst	0.1 to 1	0.1 to 1	0.1 to 1
Weight gain	< 0.1	—	—
Weight loss	< 0.1	< 0.1	—
GI			
Abdominal discomfort	—	0.1 to 1	—
Abdominal distention	< 0.1	—	—
Colitis	—	< 0.1	—
Constipation	0.1 to 1	< 0.1	—
Decreased appetite	< 0.1	< 0.1	< 0.1
Diarrhea	> 1	0.1 to 1	0.1 to 1
Dry mouth	—	< 0.1	—
Dyspeptic symptoms	< 0.1	—	—
Dysphagia	0.1 to 1	0.1 to 1	—
Feelings of GI pressure	< 0.1	—	—
Flatulence/Eructation	—	< 0.1	< 0.1
Gallstones	—	—	< 0.1
Gastritis	< 0.1	—	—
Gastroenteritis	< 0.1	< 0.1	—
GERD	0.1 to 1	0.1 to 1	0.1 to 1
GI bleeding	< 0.1	—	—
GI pain	< 0.1	—	—
GI tract hemorrhage	—	< 0.1	—
Hematemesis	< 0.1	< 0.1	—
Hypersalivation	< 0.1	—	—
Intestinal obstruction	—	< 0.1	—
Melena	< 0.1	< 0.1	—
Oral itching/irritation	< 0.1	—	—
Pancreatitis	—	< 0.1	—
Peptic ulcer	< 0.1	—	< 0.1
Retching	—	—	< 0.1
Salivary gland swelling	< 0.1	—	—
Swallowing disorders	< 0.1	—	—
Taste disturbances	< 0.1	0.1 to 1	0.1 to 1
GU			
Breast cysts	< 0.1	—	—
Breast lumps	< 0.1	—	—
Breast masses	< 0.1	—	—
Breast swelling	< 0.1	—	—
Breast tenderness	0.1 to 1	—	—
Dysuria	—	—	< 0.1
Dysmenorrhea	—	—	< 0.1
Nipple discharge	< 0.1	—	—
Primary malignant breast neoplasm	< 0.1	—	—
Renal calculus	—	—	< 0.1
Urinary frequency	—	—	< 0.1
Musculoskeletal			
Acquired musculoskeletal deformity	< 0.1	—	—
Arthralgia	< 0.1	—	—
Arthritis	—	< 0.1	—
Articular rheumatitis	< 0.1	—	—
Backache	—	< 0.1	< 0.1
Intervertebral disc disorder	—	< 0.1	—
Joint symptoms	—	< 0.1	0.1 to 1
Muscle atrophy	< 0.1	—	—
Muscle cramps	0.1 to 1	< 0.1	—
Muscle stiffness	< 0.1	0.1 to 1	< 0.1
Muscle tightness	< 0.1	—	—
Muscle tiredness	< 0.1	—	< 0.1
Muscle weakness	< 0.1	0.1 to 1	—
Musculoskeletal inflammation	< 0.1	—	—
Myalgia	> 1	0.1 to 1	—
Neck pain/stiffness	—	< 0.1	—
Need to flex calf muscles	—	—	< 0.1
Tetany	< 0.1	< 0.1	—

Serotonin 5-HT₁ Receptor Agonists

Sumatriptan Adverse Reactions (%)			
Adverse reaction	Tablets	Nasal	Injection
Respiratory			
Allergic rhinitis	> 1	—	—
Asthma	0.1 to 1	< 0.1	—
Breathing disorders	< 0.1	—	—
Bronchitis	< 0.1	—	—
Coughing	< 0.1	—	—
Dyspnea	> 1	0.1 to 1	0.1 to 1
Hiccoughs	< 0.1	—	< 0.1
Lower respiratory tract infections	—	0.1 to 1	< 0.1
Sinusitis	> 1	—	—
Upper respiratory tract inflammation	> 1	—	—
Special senses			
Accommodation disorders	< 0.1	—	—
Blindness/Low vision	< 0.1	—	—
Burning/Numbness of tongue	—	< 0.1	—
Conjunctivitis	< 0.1	—	—
Disturbance of smell	0.1 to 1	< 0.1	< 0.1
Ear infection	—	0.1 to 1	—
Ear, nose, throat hemorrhage	> 1	—	—
External ocular disorders	< 0.1	—	—
External otitis	> 1	—	—
Eye edema	< 0.1	—	—
Eye hemorrhage	< 0.1	—	—
Eye irritation	< 0.1	0.1 to 1	0.1 to 1
Eye pain	< 0.1	—	—
Feeling of fullness in ears	< 0.1	—	—
Hearing loss	> 1	0.1 to 1	—
Keratitis	< 0.1	—	—
Lacrimation	0.1 to 1	< 0.1	0.1 to 1
Meniere disease	—	< 0.1	—
Mydriasis	< 0.1	—	—
Nasal inflammation	> 1	—	—
Noise sensitivity	> 1	—	—
Otalgia	0.1 to 1	< 0.1	—
Sclera disorders	< 0.1	—	—
Tinnitus	> 1	—	—
Visual disturbances	< 0.1	< 0.1	—
Miscellaneous			
Anemia	< 0.1	—	—
Chest tightness/discomfort/pressure/heaviness	—	0.1 to 1	—
Dental pain	< 0.1	—	—
Drug abuse	< 0.1	—	—
Fever	—	—	< 0.1
Hypersensitivity	—	—	0.1 to 1
Liver function test disturbance	—	—	0.1 to 1
Serotonin agonist effect	—	—	0.1 to 1

Postmarketing reports (oral, injection): The events enumerated include all except those already listed in the adverse reactions section above or those too general to be informative. Because the reports cite events reported spontaneously from worldwide postmarketing experience, frequency of events and the role of sumatriptan injection in their causation cannot be reliably determined. Systemic reactions following sumatriptan use are likely to be similar regardless of route of administration.

• *Cardiovascular* – Atrial fibrillation, cardiomyopathy, colonic ischemia, Prinzmetal variant angina, pulmonary embolism, shock, thrombophlebitis.

• *CNS* – Cerebrovascular accident, CNS vasculitis, dysphasia, panic disorder, subarachnoid hemorrhage.

• *Dermatologic* – Exacerbation of sunburn, hypersensitivity reactions (allergic vasculitis, erythema, pruritus, rash, shortness of breath, urticaria; in addition, severe anaphylaxis/anaphylactoid reactions have been reported), photosensitivity.

   Injection only: Following SC administration of sumatriptan, contusion, induration, pain, redness, SC bleeding, stinging, swelling, and on rare occasions, lipoatrophy (depression in the skin) or lipohypertrophy (enlargement or thickening of tissue) have been reported.

• *GI* – Ischemic colitis with rectal bleeding, xerostomia.

• *Hematologic* – Hemolytic anemia, pancytopenia, thrombocytopenia.

• *Special senses* – Deafness, ischemic optic neuropathy, loss of vision, retinal artery occlusion, retinal vein thrombosis.

• *Miscellaneous* – Acute renal failure, angioneurotic edema, bronchospasm in patients with and without a history of asthma, cyanosis, death, elevated liver function tests, temporal arteritis.

➤*Zolmitriptan:*

Cardiovascular – Arrhythmias, hypertension, syncope (0.1% to 1%); bradycardia, extrasystoles, postural hypotension, QT prolongation, tachycardia, thrombophlebitis (less than 0.1%).

CNS – Agitation, anxiety, depression, emotional lability, hyperesthesia, insomnia (0.1% to 1%); akathisia, amnesia, apathy, ataxia, cerebral ischemia, dystonia, euphoria, hallucinations, hyperkinesia, hypertonia, hypotonia, irritability (less than 0.1%).

Dermatologic – Pruritus, rash, urticaria (0.1% to 1%).

GI – Esophagitis, gastroenteritis, increased appetite, liver function abnormality, thirst, tongue edema (0.1% to 1%); anorexia, constipation, gastritis, hematemesis, melena, pancreatitis, ulcer (less than 0.1%).

GU – Cystitis, hematuria, polyuria, urinary frequency/urgency (0.1% to 1%); dysmenorrhea, miscarriage (less than 0.1%).

Hematologic – Ecchymosis (0.1% to 1%); cyanosis, eosinophilia, leukopenia, thrombocytopenia (less than 0.1%).

Metabolic – Edema (0.1% to 1%); alkaline phosphatase increased, hyperglycemia (less than 0.1%).

Musculoskeletal – Back pain, leg cramps, tenosynovitis (0.1% to 1%); arthritis, tetany, twitching (less than 0.1%).

Respiratory – Bronchitis, bronchospasm, epistaxis, hiccough, laryngitis, yawn (0.1% to 1%); apnea, voice alteration (less than 0.1%).

Special senses – Dry eye, ear pain, eye pain, hyperacusis, parosmia, tinnitus (0.1% to 1%); diplopia, lacrimation (less than 0.1%).

Miscellaneous – Allergic reaction, chills, facial edema, fever, malaise, photosensitivity (0.1% to 1%).

   Postmarketing reports: The events enumerated include all except those already listed in the adverse reactions section above or those too general to be informative. Because the reports cite events reported spontaneously from worldwide postmarketing experience, frequency of events and the role of zolmitriptan in their causation cannot be reliably determined: Anaphylaxis/anaphylactoid reactions; angina pectoris; coronary artery vasospasm; headache; hypersensitivity reactions including angioedema, ischemic colitis, GI infarction, GI necrosis; MI; transient myocardial ischemia.

Nasal spray –

Zolmitriptan Nasal Spray Adverse Reactions (%)		
Adverse reaction	Zolmitriptan nasal spray 5 mg (n = 236)	Placebo (n = 228)
Atypical sensations		
Hyperesthesia	5	0
Paresthesia	10	6
CNS		
Dizziness	3	4
Somnolence	4	2
GI		
Dry mouth	2	0
Nausea	4	1
Unusual taste	21	3
Pain and pressure sensations		
Pain, location specified	4	1
Pain, throat	4	1
Tightness, throat	2	1
Miscellaneous		
Asthenia	3	1
Disorder/discomfort of nasal cavity	3	2

Other adverse events:

• *Cardiovascular* – Palpitation (1% or more to less than 2%); arrhythmias, hypertension, syncope, tachycardia, thrombophlebitis (0.01%); angina pectoris, atrial fibrillation, bradycardia, MI, vascular disorder, vasodilation (0.001%).

• *CNS* – Headache, insomnia (1% or more to less than 2%); abnormal coordination, abnormal thinking, agitation, amnesia, anxiety, ataxia, circumoral paresthesia, confusion, depersonalization, depression, hypertonia, insomnia, nervousness, speech disorder, tremor, vertigo (0.01%); abnormal dreams, apathy, convulsions, euphoria, hypertonia, irritability, manic reaction, neuropathy, psychosis, tardive dyskinesia (0.001%).

• *Dermatologic* – Pruritus, rash, skin disorder, sweating (0.01%); eczema, erythema, erythema multiforme, hair disorder, neoplasm.

• *Endocrine* – Hyperthyroidism, thyroid edema (0.001%).

• *GI* – Abdominal pain, dysphagia, vomiting (1% or more to less than 2%); diarrhea, dyspepsia, GI disorder, increased saliva, tongue edema, thirst (0.01%); colitis, constipation, eructation, gastritis, GI carcinoma, gingivitis, hepatic neoplasia, increased appetite, intestinal obstruction, jaundice, sialadenitis, stomatitis (0.001%).

- *GU* – Menorrhagia, polyuria (0.01%); breast carcinoma, breast neoplasm, cystitis, dysmenorrhea, enlarged uterine fibroids, fibrocytic breast, kidney pain, metrorrhagia, pyelonephritis, suspicious PAP smear, unintended pregnancy, urinary frequency, urinary tract disorder, urinary tract infection, urine impaired, urogenital neoplasm, uterine disorder, vaginitis (0.001%).
- *Hematologic* – Cyanosis (0.01%); ecchymosis, leukopenia, lymphadenopathy (0.001%).
- *Metabolic/Nutritional* – Dehydration, increased weight, peripheral edema (0.001%).
- *Musculoskeletal* – Arthralgia, joint disorder, myalgia (0.01%); bone pain, osteoporosis, tenosynovitis, twitching (0.001%).
- *Respiratory* – Bronchitis, dyspnea, epistasis, increased cough, laryngeal edema, pharyngitis, rhinitis, sinusitis, throat discomfort, voice alteration (0.01%); hiccough, hyperventilation, increased sputum, laryngitis, yawning (0.001%).
- *Special senses* – Amblyopia, disorder of lacrimation, ear pain, eye pain, parosmia, tinnitus (0.01%); conjunctivitis, dry eye, photophobia, pneumonia, visual field defect (0.001%).
- *Miscellaneous* – Chest tightness, reaction aggravation (1% or more to less than 2%); abnormal laboratory test, allergic reaction, back pain, chest heaviness, chest pain, chest pressure, chills, cyst, edema of the face, flu syndrome, infection, jaw pain, jaw tightening, neck pain, neck tightness, neoplasm, pressure other (0.01%); cellulitis, fever, jaw pressure, neck heaviness (0.001%).

Overdosage

➤*Symptoms:* Based on the pharmacology of serotonin agonists, hypertension and other more serious cardiovascular symptoms can occur. Overdosage in animals has been fatal; possible symptoms include seizure, tremor, inactivity, extremity erythema, reduced respiratory rate, cyanosis, ataxia, mydriasis, injection-site reaction, and paralysis.

➤*Treatment:* There is no specific antidote. Consider GI decontamination (ie, gastric lavage followed by activated charcoal) in patients with suspected overdose. Institute standard supportive care. If chest pain or other symptoms of angina are present, perform ECG monitoring for evidence of ischemia. Based on the elimination half life, continue monitoring patients after overdose for at least 10 hours (**sumatriptan**), 12 hours (**rizatriptan**), 15 hours (**zolmitriptan**), 20 hours (**almotriptan**), 24 hours (**naratriptan**), 48 hours (**frovatriptan**), or 20 hours or more (**eletriptan**).

It is unknown what effect hemodialysis or peritoneal dialysis has on the serum concentrations of these agents.

Patient Information

A patient information leaflet is provided for patients.

➤*Injection (sumatriptan):* Instruct patients who are advised to self-administer sumatriptan in medically unsupervised situations on the proper use of the product prior to doing so for the first time, including loading the auto-injector and discarding the empty syringes.

For adults, the usual dose is a single injection given just below the skin. Administer as soon as migraine symptoms appear, but it may be given at any time during an attack. A second injection may be given if symptoms of migraine return. Do not use more than 2 injections/24 hours, and allow at least 1 hour between each dose.

The patient may experience pain or redness at the site of injection, but this usually lasts less than 1 hour.

➤*Intranasal:* For adults, the usual dose is a single nasal spray into 1 nostril. If headache returns, a second nasal spray may be given 2 hours after the first spray. For any attack where the patient has no response to the first nasal spray, do not use a second nasal spray without first consulting a physician. Do not administer more than 40 mg **sumatriptan** or 10 mg **zolmitriptan** nasal spray in any 24-hour period.

➤*Oral:* Take a single dose with fluids as soon as symptoms of migraine appear; a second dose may be taken if symptoms return, but no sooner than 2 hours (**sumatriptan**, **zolmitriptan**, **eletriptan**) or 4 hours (**naratriptan**) following the first dose. For a given attack, if there is no response to the first dose, do not take a second dose without first consulting a physician. Do not take more than 200 mg sumatriptan, more than 5 mg naratriptan, more than 10 mg zolmitriptan, or more than 80 mg eletriptan in any 24-hour period.

Tell a physician if the patient has risk factors for heart disease (eg, high blood pressure, high cholesterol, obesity, diabetes, smoking, strong family history of heart disease or stroke, a male over 40 years of age, postmenopausal woman).

These agents are intended to relieve migraine but not to prevent or reduce the number of attacks. Use only to treat an actual migraine attack or cluster headache (sumatriptan injection only).

Instruct patients not to use these agents if they are pregnant, think they might be pregnant, are trying to become pregnant, or are not using adequate contraception, unless they have discussed this with a physician. The manufacturer maintains a sumatriptan and naratriptan pregnancy registry. Register patients by calling (800) 336-2176.

If pain, tightness, pressure, or heaviness in the chest, throat, neck, or jaw occurs when using these agents, instruct patients to discuss it with a physician before using more. If the chest pain is severe or does not go away, instruct patients to immediately call a physician.

If sudden or severe abdominal pain occurs following naratriptan or sumatriptan administration, instruct patients to immediately call a physician.

If shortness of breath, wheezing, heart throbbing, swelling of eyelids, face, or lips, skin rash, skin lumps, or hives occur, advise patients to immediately tell a physician. Instruct patients not to take additional doses unless directed by the physician.

If feelings of tingling, heat, flushing (redness of face lasting a short time), heaviness, pressure, drowsiness, dizziness, tiredness, or sickness develop, instruct patients to tell a physician.

Migraine or treatment with **rizatriptan** may cause somnolence in some patients; dizziness also has been reported. Evaluate ability to perform complex tasks during migraine attacks and after administration of rizatriptan.

Instruct patients not to remove the blister from the outer pouch until just prior to dosing zolmitriptan or rizatriptan orally-disintegrating tablets. Instruct patients to peel blister packs open with dry hands and to place the orally-disintegrating tablet on the tongue, where it will dissolve and be swallowed with the saliva.

Inform phenylketonuric patients that rizatriptan and zolmitriptan orally-disintegrating tablets contain phenylalanine (a component of aspartame). Each 5 mg rizatriptan orally-disintegrating tablet contains 1.05 mg phenylalanine and each 10 mg orally-disintegrating tablet contains 2.1 mg phenylalanine. Each 2.5 mg zolmitriptan orally-disintegrating tablet contains 2.81 mg phenylalanine.

Photosensitization (photoallergy or phototoxicity) may occur; therefore, caution patients to take protective measures (ie, sunscreens, protective clothing) against exposure to sunlight or ultraviolet light (eg, tanning beds) until tolerance is determined.

FROVATRIPTAN SUCCINATE

Rx	**Frova** (Elan)	**Tablets:** 2.5 mg (as base)	Lactose. (77). Film-coated. In blister card 9s.

For complete prescribing information, refer to the Serotonin 5-HT₁ Receptor Agonists group monograph.

Indications

➤*Migraine treatment:* For the acute treatment of migraine attacks with or without aura in adults.

Not intended for the prophylactic therapy of migraine or for use in the management of hemiplegic or basilar migraine. The safety and efficacy of frovatriptan have not been established for cluster headache, which is present in an older, predominantly male, population.

Administration and Dosage

➤*Approved by the FDA:* November 9, 2001.

The recommended dosage is a single tablet (2.5 mg) taken orally with fluids.

If the headache recurs after initial relief, a second tablet may be taken, providing there is an interval of at least 2 hours between doses. The total daily dose of frovatriptan should not exceed 3 tablets (3 × 2.5 mg/day).

There is no evidence that a second dose of frovatriptan is effective in patients who do not respond to a first dose of the drug for the same headache.

The safety of treating an average of more than 4 migraine attacks in a 30-day period has not been established.

➤*Storage/Stability:* Store at controlled room temperature, 25°C (77°F); excursions permitted to 15° to 30°C (59° to 86°F). Protect from moisture and light.

Serotonin 5-HT₁ Receptor Agonists

ELETRIPTAN HBr

Rx	Relpax (Pfizer)	**Tablets**: 24.2 mg eletriptan HBr (equivalent to 20 mg base)	Lactose. (REP20 Pfizer). Orange. Film-coated. In blister card 12s.
		48.5 mg eletriptan HBr (equivalent to 40 mg base)	Lactose. (REP40 Pfizer). Orange. Film-coated. In blister card 12s.

For complete prescribing information, refer to the Serotonin 5-HT₁ Receptor Agonists group monograph.

Indications

➤*Migraine:* For acute treatment of migraine with or without aura in adults.

Not intended for the prophylactic therapy of migraine or for use in the management of hemiplegic or basilar migraine. Safety and efficacy of eletriptan have not been established for cluster headache, which is present in an older, predominantly male population.

Administration and Dosage

➤*Approved by the FDA:* December 26, 2002.

Individualize dose. Single doses of 20 and 40 mg were effective for the acute treatment of migraine in adults, with a greater proportion of patients having a response following a 40 mg dose. Individuals may vary in response to doses of eletriptan tablets. An 80 mg dose, although also effective, was associated with an increased incidence of adverse events. Therefore, the maximum recommended single dose is 40 mg.

If, after the initial dose, the headache improves but then returns, a repeat dose may be beneficial. If a second dose is required, it should be taken at least 2 hours after the initial dose. If the initial dose is ineffective, controlled clinical trials have not shown the second dose to be beneficial in treating the same attack. The maximum daily dose should not exceed 80 mg.

The safety of treating an average of more than 3 headaches in a 30-day period has not been established.

➤*CYP3A4 inhibitors:* Eletriptan is metabolized by the CYP3A4 enzyme. Do not use eletriptan within at least 72 hours of treatment with the following potent CYP3A4 inhibitors: Ketoconazole, itraconazole, nefazodone, troleandomycin, clarithromycin, ritonavir, nelfinavir. Do not use eletriptan within 72 hours with drugs that have demonstrated potent CYP3A4 inhibition and have this potent effect described in the Contraindications, Warnings, or Precautions sections of their labeling.

➤*Hepatic impairment:* Do not give eletriptan to patients with severe hepatic impairment because the effect of severe hepatic impairment on eletriptan metabolism was not evaluated. No dose adjustment is necessary in mild to moderate impairment.

➤*Storage/Stability:* Store at 25°C (77°F); excursions permitted to 15° to 30°C (59° to 86°F).

RIZATRIPTAN BENZOATE

Rx	Maxalt (Merck)	**Tablets**: 5 mg (as base)	Lactose. (MRK 266). Pale pink, capsule shape. In unit-of-use carrying case of 6 tablets.
		10 mg (as base)	Lactose. (MAXALT MRK 267). Pale pink, capsule shape. In unit-of-use carrying case of 6 tablets.
Rx	Maxalt-MLT (Merck)	**Tablets, orally disintegrating**: 5 mg (as base)	Lyophilized. 1.05 mg phenylalanine, mannitol, aspartame. White to off-white. Peppermint flavor. In 2 unit-of-use carrying case of 3 tablets (6 tablets total).
		10 mg (as base)	Lyophilized. 2.1 mg phenylalanine, mannitol, aspartame. White to off-white. Peppermint flavor. In 2 unit-of-use carrying case of 3 tablets (6 tablets total).

For complete prescribing information, refer to the Serotonin 5-HT₁ Receptor Agonists group monograph.

Indications

➤*Migraine treatment:* Acute treatment of migraine in adults with or without aura.

Not intended for the prophylactic therapy of migraine or for use in the management of hemiplegic or basilar migraine. Safety and efficacy has not been established for cluster headache, which is present in an older, predominantly male population.

Administration and Dosage

➤*Approved by the FDA:* June 29, 1998.

Single doses of 5 and 10 mg are effective for the acute treatment of migraines in adults. There is little evidence that the 10 mg dose may provide a greater effect than the 5 mg dose. The choice of dose should be made on an individual basis, weighing the possible benefit of the 10 mg dose with the potential risk for increased adverse events.

➤*Redosing:* Doses should be separated by at least 2 hours; no more than 30 mg should be taken in any 24-hour period.

On average, the safety of treating more than 4 headaches in a 30-day period has not been established.

➤*Propranolol patients:* In patients receiving propranolol, use the 5 mg dose of rizatriptan benzoate tablets, up to a maximum of 3 doses in 24 hours.

➤*Orally-disintegrating tablets:* Administration with liquid is not necessary. The orally-disintegrating tablet is packaged in a blister within an outer aluminum pouch. Instruct patients not to remove the blister from the outer pouch until just prior to dosing. The blister pack should then be peeled open with dry hands and the orally-disintegrating tablet placed on the tongue, where it will dissolve and be swallowed with the saliva.

Phenylketonurics – Inform phenylketonuric patients that rizatriptan orally-disintegrating tablets contain phenylalanine (a component of aspartame). Each 5 mg orally-disintegrating tablet contains 1.05 mg phenylalanine, and each 10 mg orally-disintegrating tablet contains 2.1 mg phenylalanine.

➤*Storage/Stability:* Store at room temperature, 15° to 30°C (59° to 86°F). Do not remove the orally-disintegrating tablets from the blister pack until ready to consume.

NARATRIPTAN HCl

Rx	Amerge (GlaxoSmithKline)	**Tablets**: 1 mg (as base)	Lactose. (GX CE3). White, D-shaped. Film-coated. In blister pack 9s.
		2.5 mg (as base)	Lactose. (GX CE5). Green, D-shaped. Film-coated. In blister pack 9s.

For complete prescribing information, refer to the Serotonin 5-HT₁ Receptor Agonists group monograph.

Indications

➤*Migraine treatment:* For the acute treatment of migraine attacks with or without aura in adults.

Naratriptan is not intended for the prophylactic therapy of migraine or for use in the management of hemiplegic or basilar migraine. Safety and efficacy have not been established for cluster headache, which is present in an older, predominantly male population.

Administration and Dosage

Single doses of 1 and 2.5 mg taken with fluid are effective for the acute treatment of migraines in adults. A greater proportion of patients have headache response following a 2.5 mg dose than following a 1 mg dose. Choose the dose on an individual basis, weighing the possible benefit of the 2.5 mg dose with the potential for a greater risk of adverse events. If the headache returns or if the patient has only partial response, the dose may be repeated once after 4 hours, for a maximum dose of 5 mg in a 24-hour period. There is evidence that doses of 5 mg do not provide a greater effect than 2.5 mg.

The safety of treating, on average, more than 4 headaches in a 30-day period has not been established.

➤*Renal/Hepatic function impairment:* The use of naratriptan is contraindicated in patients with severe renal impairment (Ccr less than 15 mL/min) or severe hepatic impairment (Child-Pugh grade C) because of decreased clearance of the drug. In patients with mild to moderate renal or hepatic impairment, do not exceed a maximum daily dose of 2.5 mg over a 24-hour period and consider a lower starting dose.

➤*Storage/Stability:* Store at controlled room temperature, 20° to 25°C (68° to 77°F).

Serotonin 5-HT$_1$ Receptor Agonists

SUMATRIPTAN

Rx	Imitrex (GlaxoSmithKline)	Tablets: 25 mg (as succinate)	(I 25). White, triangular shape. Film-coated. In blister pack 9s.
		50 mg (as succinate)	(IMITREX 50). White, triangular shape. Film-coated. In blister pack 9s.
		100 mg (as succinate)	(IMITREX 100). Pink, triangular shape. Film-coated. In blister pack 9s.
		Injection: 6 mg/0.5 mL (as succinate)	Sodium chloride 7 mg/mL. In 6 mg single-dose vials (0.5 mL in 2 mL) and *STATdose System* (2 prefilled single-dose syringe cartridges, 1 *STATdose Pen*, and instructions for use) injection cartridge pack.[1]
		Spray, nasal: 5 mg	In 100 mcL unit-dose spray device. In 6s.
		20 mg	In 100 mcL unit-dose spray device. In 6s.

[1] Contains 2 prefilled syringe cartridges for refill of *STATdose System* only.

For complete prescribing information, refer to the Serotonin 5-HT$_1$ Receptor Agonists group monograph.

Indications

➤*Migraine treatment:* For the acute treatment of migraine attacks with or without aura in adults.

Tablets and spray are not intended for prophylactic therapy of migraine or for cluster headache, which is present in an older, predominantly male population.

➤*Cluster headache (injection only):* For the acute treatment of cluster headache episodes.

This drug is not for use in the management of hemiplegic or basilar migraine.

Administration and Dosage

➤*Approved by the FDA:* December 28, 1992.

➤*Oral:* Single doses of 25, 50, or 100 mg tablets are effective for the acute treatment of migraine in adults. There is evidence that doses of 50 and 100 mg may provide a greater effect than 25 mg. Doses of 100 mg have not been proven to provide a greater effect than 50 mg. Choose the dose on an individual basis, weighing the possible benefit of a higher dose with the potential for a greater risk of adverse events. If headache returns or the patient has a partial response to the initial dose, the dose may be repeated after 2 hours, not to exceed a total daily dose of 200 mg. If headache returns following an initial treatment with the injection, additional doses of single tablets (up to 100 mg/day) may be given with an interval of at least 2 hours between tablet doses.

Hepatic function impairment – Hepatic function impairment may cause unpredictable elevations in the bioavailability of orally administered sumatriptan. Do not exceed a maximum single dose of 50 mg.

MAOIs – Because of the potential of MAO-A inhibitors to cause unpredictable elevations in the bioavailability of oral sumatriptan, their combined use is contraindicated.

The safety of treating an average of more than 4 headaches in a 30-day period has not been established.

➤*Injection:* The maximum single adult dose is 6 mg injected SC.

Trials failed to show that a clear benefit is associated with the administration of a second 6 mg dose in patients who have failed to respond to a first injection. The maximum recommended dose that may be given in 24 hours is two 6 mg injections separated by at least 1 hour. If side effects are dose-limiting, lower doses may be used. In patients receiving doses lower than 6 mg, use only the single-dose vial dosage form. An auto-injection device is available for use with 6 mg prefilled syringe cartridges to facilitate self-administration in patients in whom this dose is deemed necessary. With this device, the needle penetrates approximately ¼ inch (5 to 6 mm). Because the injection is intended to be given SC, avoid IM or intravascular delivery. Direct patients to use injection sites with an adequate skin and SC thickness to accommodate the length of the needle.

MAO inhibitors – Consider decreased doses of sumatriptan in patients receiving MAOIs.

➤*Intranasal:* Single doses of 5, 10, or 20 mg administered in 1 nostril are effective for the acute treatment of migraine in adults. A greater proportion of patients had headache response following a 20 mg dose than following a 5 to 10 mg dose. Choose the dose on an individual basis, weighing the possible benefit of the 20 mg dose with the potential for a greater risk of adverse events. A 10 mg dose may be achieved by administering a single 5 mg dose in each nostril. There is evidence that doses above 20 mg do not provide a greater effect than 20 mg. If headache returns, the dose may be repeated once after 2 hours, not to exceed a total daily dose of 40 mg.

The safety of treating an average of more than 4 headaches in a 30-day period has not been established.

➤*Storage/Stability:* Store between 2° and 30°C (36° and 86°F). Protect nasal spray and injection from light.

ZOLMITRIPTAN

Rx	Zomig (MedPointe)	Tablets: 2.5 mg	Lactose. (Zomig 2.5). Yellow, scored. Film-coated. In blister pack 6s.
		5 mg	Lactose. (Zomig 5). Pink. Film-coated. In blister pack 3s.
		Spray, nasal: 5 mg	In 100 mcL unit-dose spray device. In 6s.
Rx	Zomig ZMT (MedPointe)	Tablets, orally disintegrating: 2.5 mg	2.81 mg phenylalanine, mannitol, aspartame. (Z). White, bevelled. Orange flavor. In blister pack 6s.

For complete prescribing information, refer to the Serotonin 5-HT$_1$ Receptor Agonists group monograph.

Indications

➤*Migraine treatment:* For the acute treatment of migraine with or without aura in adults.

Zolmitriptan is not intended for prophylactic therapy of migraine or for use in the management of hemiplegic or basilar migraine. Safety and efficacy have not been established for cluster headache, which is present in an older, predominantly male population.

Administration and Dosage

➤*Approved by the FDA:* November 25, 1997.

➤*Tablets:* The initial recommended dose is 2.5 mg or lower (achieved by manually breaking a 2.5 mg tablet in half). If the headache returns, the dose may be repeated after 2 hours, not to exceed 10 mg within a 24-hour period. Response is greater following the 2.5 or 5 mg dose compared with 1 mg. There is little added benefit and increased side effects associated with the 5 mg dose.

➤*Orally-disintegrating tablets:* A single dose of 2.5 mg was effective for the acute treatment of migraines in adults. If the headache returns, the dose may be repeated after 2 hours, not to exceed 10 mg within a 24-hour period. Trials have not adequately established the effectiveness of a second dose if the initial dose is ineffective.

Administration with a liquid is not necessary. The orally-disintegrating tablet is packaged in a blister. Instruct patients not to remove the tab-

let from the blister until just prior to dosing. The blister pack should then be peeled open, and the orally-disintegrating tablet placed on the tongue, where it will dissolve and be swallowed with the saliva. Breaking the orally-disintegrating tablet is not recommended.

On average, the safety of treating more than 3 headaches in a 30-day period has not been established.

➤*Nasal spray:* Administer 1 dose of 5 mg for the treatment of acute migraine. If the headache returns, the dose may be repeated after 2 hours. Do not exceed a maximum daily dose of 10 mg in any 24-hour period. Individuals may vary in response to zolmitriptan. The pharmacokinetics of a 5 mg nasal spray dose is similar to the 5 mg oral formulations. Doses lower than 5 mg can only be achieved through the use of an oral formulation. Therefore, choose the dose and route of administration on an individual basis. The efficacy of a second dose has not been established in placebo-controlled trials.

The safety of treating an average of more than 4 headaches in a 30-day period has not been established.

➤*Hepatic function impairment:* Administer zolmitriptan with caution in patients with liver disease, generally using doses less than 2.5 mg. Patients with moderate to severe hepatic impairment have decreased clearance of zolmitriptan; significant elevation in blood pressure was observed in some patients.

➤*Storage/Stability:* Store at controlled room temperature of 20° to 25°C (68° to 77°F); protect from light and moisture.

Serotonin 5-HT$_1$ Receptor Agonists

ALMOTRIPTAN MALATE

Rx	Axert (Ortho-McNeil)	Tablets: 6.25 mg	Mannitol. (2080). White. In UD 6s.
		12.5 mg	Mannitol. (A). White. In UD 6s.

For complete prescribing information, refer to the Serotonin 5-HT$_1$ Receptor Agonists group monograph.

Indications

➤*Migraine treatment:* For the acute treatment of migraine with or without aura in adults.

Almotriptan is not intended for the prophylactic therapy of migraine or for use in the management of hemiplegic or basilar migraine. Safety and efficacy of almotriptan have not been established for cluster headache, which is present in an older, predominantly male population.

Administration and Dosage

➤*Approved by the FDA:* May 8, 2001.

Doses of 6.25 and 12.5 mg are effective for the acute treatment of migraines in adults, with the 12.5 mg dose tending to be a more effective dose. Individuals may vary in response to doses of almotriptan. Therefore, choose the dose on an individual basis.

If the headache returns, the dose may be repeated after 2 hours, but do not give more than 2 doses within a 24-hour period. Controlled trials have not adequately established the effectiveness of a second dose if the initial dose is ineffective.

The safety of treating an average of more than 4 headaches in a 30-day period has not been established.

➤*Hepatic impairment:* The maximum decrease expected in the clearance of almotriptan because of hepatic impairment is 60%. Therefore, do not exceed a maximum daily dose of 12.5 mg over a 24-hour period, and use a starting dose of 6.25 mg.

➤*Renal impairment:* In patients with severe renal impairment, the clearance of almotriptan was decreased. Therefore, do not exceed a maximum daily dose of 12.5 mg over a 24-hour period, and use a starting dose of 6.25 mg.

➤*Storage/Stability:* Store at 25°C (77°F); excursions permitted to 15° to 30°C (59° to 86°F).

WARNING

Serious and/or life-threatening peripheral ischemia has been associated with the coadministration of dihydroergotamine with potent CYP3A4 inhibitors, including protease inhibitors and macrolide antibiotics. Because CYP3A4 inhibition elevates the serum levels of dihydroergotamine, the risk for vasospasm leading to cerebral ischemia and/or ischemia of the extremities is increased. Hence, concomitant use of these medications is contraindicated.

Indications

➤*Ergotamine:* To abort or prevent vascular headaches such as migraine, migraine variant, and histaminic cephalalgia.

➤*Dihydroergotamine:* For the acute treatment of migraine headaches with or without aura and the acute treatment of cluster headache episodes (injection only). Dihydroergotamine nasal spray is not intended for the prophylactic therapy of migraine or for the management of hemiplegic or basilar migraine.

Administration and Dosage

➤*Ergotamine sublingual:* Initiate therapy as soon as possible after the first symptoms of an attack. Place one 2 mg tablet under the tongue; take another tablet at 30-minute intervals thereafter, if necessary. Do not exceed 3 tablets in any 24-hour period. Do not exceed 5 tablets (10 mg) in any 1 week.

➤*Dihydroergotamine nasal spray:* Start with 1 spray (0.5 mg) in each nostril; repeat in 15 minutes for a total dosage of 4 sprays (2 mg). Studies have shown no additional benefit from acute doses greater than 2 mg for a single migraine administration. The safety of doses greater than 3 mg in a 24-hour period and 4 mg in a 7-day period has not been established. Do not use for chronic daily administration.

➤*Dihydroergotamine injection:* Administer in a dose of 1 mL IV, IM, or SC; may be repeated as needed at 1-hour intervals to a total dose of 3 mL for IM or SC delivery or 2 mL for IV delivery in a 24-hour period. Do not exceed a total weekly dosage of 6 mL. Do not use for chronic daily administration.

Actions

➤*Pharmacology:* Ergotamine has partial agonist or antagonist activity against tryptaminergic, dopaminergic, and alpha-adrenergic receptors, depending upon their site; it is a highly active uterine stimulant. It constricts peripheral and cranial blood vessels and depresses central vasomotor centers.

Ergotamine reduces extracranial blood flow, causes a decline in the amplitude of pulsation in the cranial arteries, and decreases hyperperfusion of the basilar artery territory. It does not reduce cerebral hemispheric blood flow. Small doses increase force and frequency of uterine contractions; larger doses increase resting uterine tone. The gravid uterus is more sensitive to these effects.

Ergotamine is hydrogenated in the 9, 10 position as the mesylate salt. Dihydroergotamine binds with high affinity to $5\text{-HT}_{1D\alpha}$ and $5\text{-HT}_{1D\beta}$ receptors. It also binds with high affinity to serotonin 5-HT_{1A}, 5-HT_{2A}, and 5-HT_{2C} receptors; noradrenaline α_{2A}, α_{2B}, and α_1 receptors; and dopamine D_{2L} and D_3 receptors. The therapeutic activity of dihydroergotamine in migraine generally is attributed to the agonist effect at 5-HT_{1D} receptors. Activation of 5-HT_{1D} receptors located on intracranial blood vessels, including those on arteriovenous anastomoses, leads to vasoconstriction, which correlates with the relief of migraine headache. Dihydroergotamine also possesses oxytocic properties.

➤*Pharmacokinetics:*

Absorption/Distribution – GI and sublingual absorption of ergotamine is poor. Following intranasal administration, however, the mean bioavailability of dihydroergotamine mesylate is 32% relative to the injectable administration. Absorption is variable, probably reflecting intersubject differences of absorption and the technique used for self-administration.

Dihydroergotamine mesylate is 93% plasma protein bound. The apparent steady-state volume of distribution is approximately 800 L.

Metabolism/Excretion – Ergotamine is metabolized by the liver; 90% of the metabolites are excreted in the bile. Unmetabolized drug is erratically secreted in saliva, and only trace amounts of unmetabolized drug are excreted in the feces and urine. Although plasma half-life is about 2 hours, ergotamine has long-lasting effects that may be caused by tissue storage.

Following nasal administration, total metabolites represent only 20% to 30% of plasma AUC. The major metabolite, 8'-β-hydroxydihydroergotamine, exhibits affinity equivalent to its parent for adrenergic and 5-HT receptors and demonstrates equivalent potency in several venoconstrictor activity models. The systemic clearance of dihydroergotamine mesylate following IV and IM administration is 1.5 L/min, which mainly reflects hepatic clearance. After intranasal administration, the urinary recovery of parent drug amounts to about 2% of the administered dose compared with 6% after IM administration. The renal clearance (0.1 L/min) is unaffected by the route of dihydroergotamine

administration. The decline of plasma dihydroergotamine is biphasic with a terminal half-life of about 9 to 10 hours.

Contraindications

Pregnancy, women who may become pregnant (powerful uterine stimulant actions of ergotamine and dihydroergotamine may cause fetal harm; see Warnings); hypersensitivity to ergot alkaloids or any component of the formulation; peripheral vascular disease (eg, thromboangiitis obliterans, luetic arteritis, severe arteriosclerosis, thrombophlebitis, Raynaud's disease); hepatic or renal impairment; severe pruritus; coronary artery disease (CAD); hypertension; sepsis.

There have been reports of serious adverse events associated with the coadministration of dihydroergotamine and potent CYP3A4 inhibitors (eg, protease inhibitors, macrolide antibiotics), resulting in vasospasm that led to cerebral ischemia and/or ischemia of the extremities. The use of potent CYP3A4 inhibitors (ritonavir, nelfinavir, indinavir, erythromycin, clarithromycin, troleandomycin, ketoconazole, itraconazole) with dihydroergotamine is, therefore, contraindicated.

Do not give dihydroergotamine to patients with ischemic heart disease (angina pectoris, history of MI, documented silent ischemia) or to patients who have clinical symptoms or findings consistent with coronary artery vasospasm, including Prinzmetal variant angina.

Dihydroergotamine may increase blood pressure; do not give to patients with uncontrolled hypertension.

Do not use dihydroergotamine, 5-HT_1 agonists (eg, sumatriptan), ergotamine-containing or ergot-type medications, or methysergide within 24 hours of each other.

Do not administer dihydroergotamine to patients with hemiplegic or basilar migraine.

Dihydroergotamine should not be used by nursing mothers.

Do not use dihydroergotamine with peripheral and central vasoconstrictors because the combination may result in additive or synergistic elevation of blood pressure.

Warnings

➤*CYP3A4 inhibitors (eg, macrolide antibiotics, protease inhibitors):* There have been rare reports of serious adverse events in connection with the coadministration of dihydroergotamine and potent CYP3A4 inhibitors, such as protease inhibitors and macrolide antibiotics, resulting in vasospasm that led to cerebral ischemia and/or ischemia of the extremities. Avoid the use of potent CYP3A4 inhibitors with dihydroergotamine. Examples of some of the more potent CYP3A4 inhibitors include: Antifungals ketoconazole and itraconazole, protease inhibitors ritonavir, nelfinavir, and indinavir, and macrolide antibiotics erythromycin, clarithromycin, and troleandomycin. Administer other less potent CYP3A4 inhibitors with caution. Less potent inhibitors include the following: Saquinavir, nefazodone, fluconazole, grapefruit juice, fluoxetine, fluvoxamine, zileuton, clotrimazole. These lists are not exhaustive; consider the effects on CYP3A4 of other agents being considered for concomitant use with dihydroergotamine.

➤*Fibrotic complications:* There have been reports of pleural and retroperitoneal fibrosis in patients following prolonged daily use of injectable dihydroergotamine. Rarely, prolonged daily use of other ergot alkaloid drugs has been associated with cardiac valvular fibrosis. Rare cases also have been reported in association with the use of injectable dihydroergotamine; however, in those cases, patients also received drugs known to be associated with cardiac valvular fibrosis.

➤*Risk of myocardial ischemia and/or MI and other adverse cardiac events:* Do not use dihydroergotamine in patients with documented ischemic or vasospastic coronary artery disease. It is strongly recommended that dihydroergotamine not be given to patients in whom unrecognized CAD is predicted by the presence of risk factors (eg, hypertension, hypercholesterolemia, smoking, obesity, diabetes, strong family history of CAD, females who are surgically or physiologically postmenopausal, or males who are over 40 years of age) unless a cardiovascular evaluation provides satisfactory clinical evidence that the patient is reasonably free of coronary artery and ischemic myocardial disease or other significant underlying cardiovascular disease. The sensitivity of cardiac diagnostic procedures to detect cardiovascular disease or predisposition to coronary artery vasospasm is modest, at best. If during the cardiovascular evaluation, the patient's medical history or electrocardiographic investigations reveal findings indicative of or consistent with coronary artery vasospasm or myocardial ischemia, do not administer dihydroergotamine.

For patients with risk factors predictive of CAD who are shown to have a satisfactory cardiovascular evaluation, it is strongly recommended that administration of the first dose of dihydroergotamine take place in the setting of a physician's office or similar medically staffed and equipped facility unless the patient has previously received dihydroergotamine. Because cardiac ischemia can occur in the absence of clinical symptoms, consider obtaining, on the first occasion of use, an electrocardiogram during the interval immediately following dihydroergotamine in these patients with risk factors.

It is recommended that patients who are intermittent long-term users of dihydroergotamine and who have or acquire risk factors predictive of

CAD, as described above, undergo periodic interval cardiovascular evaluation as they continue to use dihydroergotamine.

The systematic approach described above is currently recommended as a method to identify patients in whom dihydroergotamine may be used to treat migraine headaches with an acceptable margin of cardiovascular safety.

►*Cardiac events and fatalities:* No deaths have been reported in patients using dihydroergotamine. The potential for adverse cardiac events exists. Serious adverse cardiac events, including acute MI, life-threatening disturbances of cardiac rhythm, and death have been reported following the administration of dihydroergotamine. Considering the extent of use of dihydroergotamine in patients with migraine, the incidence of these events is extremely low.

►*Drug-associated cerebrovascular events and fatalities:* Cerebral hemorrhage, subarachnoid hemorrhage, stroke, and other cerebrovascular events have been reported in patients treated with dihydroergotamine; some have resulted in fatalities. It should be noted that patients with migraine may be at increased risk of certain cerebrovascular events (eg, stroke, hemorrhage, transient ischemic attack).

►*Other vasospasm-related events:* Dihydroergotamine, like other ergot alkaloids, may cause vasospastic reactions other than coronary artery vasospasm. Myocardial and peripheral vascular ischemia have been reported with dihydroergotamine.

Dihydroergotamine associated vasospastic phenomena may also cause muscle pains, numbness, coldness, pallor, and cyanosis of the digits. In patients with compromised circulation, persistent vasospasm may result in gangrene or death. Immediately discontinue dihydroergotamine if signs or symptoms of vasoconstriction develop.

►*Increase in blood pressure:* Significant elevation in blood pressure has been reported on rare occasions in patients with and without a history of hypertension treated with dihydroergotamine. Dihydroergotamine is contraindicated in patients with uncontrolled hypertension.

►*Local irritation:* Approximately 30% of patients using dihydroergotamine nasal spray (compared with 9% of placebo patients) have reported irritation in the nose or throat and/or disturbance in taste. Irritative symptoms include congestion, burning sensation, dryness, paresthesia, discharge, epistaxis, pain, or soreness. The symptoms were predominantly mild to moderate in severity and transient. In approximately 70% of the above mentioned cases, the symptoms resolved within 4 hours after dosing with dihydroergotamine.

►*Pregnancy: Category X.* Although no specific teratogenic effects have been found, the fetus suffers if ergotamine is given to the mother. Retarded fetal growth, increased intrauterine death, and resorption occurred in animals, possibly resulting from drug-induced uterine motility and increased vasoconstriction in the placental vascular bed.

Dihydroergotamine possesses oxytocic properties and, therefore, should not be administered during pregnancy. If this drug is used during pregnacy or if the patient becomes pregnant while taking this drug, apprise the patient of the potential hazard to the fetus. There are no adequate studies of dihydroergotamine in human pregnancy, but developmental toxicity has been demonstrated in experimental animals.

►*Lactation:* Ergotamine is secreted into breast milk and has caused symptoms of ergotism (eg, vomiting, diarrhea) in the infant. Exercise caution when administering to a nursing woman. Excessive dosing or prolonged administration may inhibit lactation. It is likely that dihydroergotamine is excreted in human milk, but there are no data on the drug concentration excreted. Because of the potential for these serious adverse events in nursing infants exposed to dihydroergotamine, nursing should not be undertaken while on this medication.

►*Children:* Safety and efficacy for use in children have not been established.

Precautions

►*Coronary artery vasospasm:* Dihydroergotamine may cause coronary artery vasospasm; patients who experience signs or symptoms suggestive of angina following its administration should, therefore, be evaluated for the presence of CAD or a predisposition to variant angina before receiving additional doses. Similarly, patients who experience other symptoms or signs suggestive of decreased arterial flow, such as ischemic bowel syndrome or Raynaud's syndrome following the use of any 5-HT agonist are candidates for further evaluation.

►*Recommended dosage:* Although signs and symptoms of ergotism rarely develop even after long-term intermittent use of ergotamine, exercise care to remain within the limits of recommended dosage.

►*Drug abuse and dependence:* Patients who take ergotamine for extended periods of time may become dependent upon it and require progressively increasing doses for relief of vascular headaches and for prevention of dysphoric effects that follow withdrawal.

Drug Interactions

Ergot Alkaloid Drug Interactions

Precipitant drug	Object drug*		Description
Beta-blockers	Ergot alkaloids	↑	Peripheral ischemia manifested by cold extremities, possible peripheral gangrene may occur.
CYP3A4 inhibitors (eg, protease inhibitors, macrolide antibiotics, ketoconazole, itraconazole, nefazodone, fluconazole, fluoxetine, fluvoxamine, delavirdine, efavirenz)	Ergot alkaloids	↑	The risk of ergot toxicity (ie, peripheral vasospasm/ischemia) may be increased. Coadministration with a potent CYP3A4 inhibitor is contraindicated. Use with caution with less potent CYP3A4 inhibitors (see Warnings and Contraindications).
Nicotine	Ergot alkaloids	↑	Nicotine may provoke vasoconstriction in some patients, predisposing them to a greater ischemic response to ergot therapy.
Sibutramine	Ergot alkaloids	↑	A serotonin syndrome may occur. Coadministration is not recommended. Carefully monitor patients if concurrent use cannot be avoided.
Dihydroergotamine	Nitrates	↓	Functional antagonism between these agents, decreasing the antianginal effects may occur.
Ergot alkaloids	5-HT$_1$ receptor agonists (eg, sumatriptan, frovatriptan, naratriptan, rizatriptan, zolmitriptan)	↑	Risk of vasospastic reactions may be increased. Administration of a 5-HT$_1$ receptor agonist or ergot alkaloid within 24 hours of each other is contraindicated.
Ergot alkaloids	Vasoconstrictors	↑	The pressor effects of concurrent use can combine to cause dangerous hypertension.

* ↑ = Object drug increased.   ↓ = Object drug decreased.

►*Drug/Food interactions:* Administration with grapefruit juice may increase the serum levels of the ergotamine derivative. Use with caution.

Adverse Reactions

►*Ergotamine tartrate:* Nausea and vomiting occur in up to 10% of patients. Numbness and tingling of fingers and toes; muscle pain in the extremities; pulselessness; weakness in the legs; precordial pain; transient tachycardia or bradycardia; localized edema; itching.

►*Dihydroergotamine injection:* Serious cardiac events, including some that have been fatal, have occurred following use of dihydroergotamine injection but are extremely rare. Events reported have included coronary artery vasospasm, transient myocardial ischemia, MI, ventricular tachycardia, and ventricular fibrillation. Fibrotic complications have been reported in association with long-term use of injectable dihydroergotamine.

►*Dihydroergotamine nasal spray:* During clinical studies and the foreign postmarketing experience with dihydroergotamine nasal spray, there have been no fatalities caused by cardiac events.

Dihydroergotamine Nasal Spray Adverse Reactions (%)

Adverse reaction	Dihydroergotamine (N = 597)	Placebo (N = 631)
CNS		
Dizziness	4	2
Somnolence	3	2
Paresthesia	2	2
GI		
Nausea	10	4
Altered sense of taste	8	1
Vomiting	4	1
Diarrhea	2	< 1
Respiratory		
Rhinitis	26	7
Pharyngitis	3	1
Sinusitis	1	1
Miscellaneous		
Application site reaction	6	2
Dry mouth	1	1
Fatigue	1	1
Asthenia	1	0

Ergotamine Derivatives

Dihydroergotamine Nasal Spray Adverse Reactions (%)		
Adverse reaction	Dihydroergotamine (N = 597)	Placebo (N = 631)
Hot flushes	1	< 1
Stiffness	1	< 1

Overdosage

➤*Symptoms:* Some cases of ergotamine poisoning have occurred in patients who have taken less than 5 mg. Usually, however, toxicity is seen at doses in excess of about 15 mg in 24 hours or 40 mg in a few days. Overdosage causes nausea, vomiting, weakness of the legs, pain in limb muscles, numbness and tingling of fingers and toes, precordial pain, tachycardia or bradycardia, hypertension or hypotension, and localized edema and itching with signs and symptoms of ischemia caused by vasoconstriction of peripheral arteries and arterioles. The feet and hands become cold, pale, and numb. Muscle pain occurs while walking and also later at rest. Gangrene may ensue. Confusion, depression, drowsiness, and convulsions are occasional signs of ergotamine toxicity. Overdosage is particularly likely to occur in patients with sepsis or impaired renal or hepatic function. Patients with peripheral vascular disease are especially at risk of developing peripheral ischemia following treatment with ergotamine.

➤*Treatment:* Treatment consists of the withdrawal of the drug followed by symptomatic measures, including attempts to maintain adequate circulation in the affected parts. Anticoagulant drugs, low molecular weight dextran, and potent vasodilators all may be beneficial. IV infusion of sodium nitroprusside has been successful. Vasodilators must be used with special care in the presence of hypotension. Ergotamine is dialyzable.

Patient Information

Once the nasal spray applicator has been prepared, discard it (with any remaining drug) after 8 hours.

Dosage is individualized. Take exactly as prescribed.

Do not exceed the dosing guidelines. Do not use for chronic daily administration.

Do not stop taking or change the dose unless directed by your physician.

Take at the first sign or hint of a migraine attack.

Stop taking the drug and notify your physician if you experience the following: Numbness, tingling, coldness, or paleness in fingers or toes; muscle pain in arms or legs; weakness in legs; chest pain; heart rate changes; sudden worsening of headache; swelling; itching.

DIHYDROERGOTAMINE MESYLATE

Rx	Migranal (Xcel[1])	Spray, nasal: 4 mg/mL[2]	In 1 mL ampuls. Kit: 4 unit dose trays (containing 1 ampul, nasal spray applicator, and breaker cap), patient instruction booklet, patient information sheet, assembly case.
Rx	D.H.E. 45 (Xcel[1])	Injection: 1 mg/mL[3]	In 1 mL amps.
Rx	Dihydroergotamine Mesylate (Various, eg, Bedford, Paddock)		6% alcohol. In 1 mL vials.

[1] Xcel Pharmaceuticals, 6363 Greenwich Drive, Suite 100, San Diego, CA 92122; (858) 202-2700, fax (858) 202-2799.
[2] With 10 mg caffeine and 50 mg dextrose.
[3] With 6.2% alcohol and 15% glycerin.

For complete prescribing information, refer to the Ergotamine Derivatives group monograph.

WARNING

Serious and/or life-threatening peripheral ischemia has been associated with the coadministration of dihydroergotamine with potent CYP3A4 inhibitors, including protease inhibitors and macrolide antibiotics. Because CYP3A4 inhibition elevates the serum levels of dihydroergotamine, the risk for vasospasm leading to cerebral ischemia and/or ischemia of the extremities is increased. Hence, concomitant use of these medications is contraindicated.

Indications

For the acute treatment of migraine headaches with or without aura.

➤*Nasal spray:* Not intended for prophylactic therapy of migraine or management of hemiplegic or basilar migraine.

➤*Injection:* Also indicated for the acute treatment of cluster headache episodes.

Administration and Dosage

Not to be used for chronic daily administration.

➤*Nasal spray:* Not for injection.

Prior to administration, prime the pump by squeezing it 4 times (see patient information sheet or instruction booklet). Once the nasal spray applicator has been prepared, discard any remaining drug in opened ampul after 8 hours.

Administration – One spray (0.5 mg) administered in each nostril. Administer an additional spray (0.5 mg) in each nostril 15 minutes later for a total dosage of 4 sprays (2 mg). Studies have shown no additional benefit from acute doses greater than 2 mg for a single migraine administration. Safety of doses above 3 mg in a 24-hour period and 4 mg in a 7-day period has not been established.

➤*Injection:* Administer in a dose of 1 mL IV, IM, or SC. The dose may be repeated as needed at 1-hour intervals to a total dose of 3 mL for IM or SC delivery or 2 mL for IV delivery in a 24-hour period. Do not exceed a total weekly dosage of 6 mL.

➤*Storage/Stability:* Store below 25°C (77°F). Do not refrigerate or freeze the nasal spray or injection solution.

Injection – Store in light-resistant containers. To assure constant potency, protect the ampuls from light and heat. Administer only if clear and colorless.

ERGOTAMINE TARTRATE

Rx	Ergomar (Lotus Biochemical)	Tablets, sublingual: 2 mg	Lactose, saccharin. (LB 2). Green. In 20s.

For complete prescribing information, refer to the Ergotamine Derivatives group monograph.

Indications

➤*Vascular headache:* As therapy to abort or prevent vascular headache (eg, migraine, migraine variants, so-called histaminic cephalalgia).

Administration and Dosage

Make efforts to initiate therapy as soon as possible after the first symptoms of the attacks are noted because success is proportional to rapidity of treatment and lower dosages will be effective.

Place one 2 mg tablet under the tongue at the first sign of attack or to relieve symptoms after onset of an attack. Take another tablet at half-hour intervals thereafter, if necessary, but do not exceed 3 tablets in any 24-hour period. Limit dosage to not more than 5 tablets (10 mg) in any 1 week.

➤*Storage/Stability:* Protect from light and heat.

ISOMETHEPTENE MUCATE/DICHLORALPHENAZONE/ACETAMINOPHEN

c-iv	Isometheptene/Dichloralphenazone/Acetamino-phen (Various, eg, URL)	Capsules: 65 mg isometheptene mucate, 100 mg dichloralphenazone, 325 mg acetaminophen	In 50s, 100s, 250s, and 500s.
c-iv	Duradrin (Barr)		(DPI 364). Scarlet/White. In 100s, 250s, and 1000s.
c-iv	Midrin (Women First HealthCare)		(MIDRIN). Red. In 50s, 100s, and 250s.
c-iv	Migratine (Major)		Red/White. In 100s and 250s.

Indications

For relief of tension and vascular headaches.

Based on a review of isometheptene mucate by the National Academy of Sciences-National Research Council and/or other information, FDA has classified it as "possibly" effective in the treatment of migraine headache. Final classification of the less-than-effective indication requires further investigation.

Administration and Dosage

➤*Migraine headache:* Usual adult dosage is 2 capsules at once followed by 1 capsule every hour until headache is relieved, up to 5 capsules within a 12-hour period.

➤*Tension headache:* Usual adult dosage is 1 or 2 capsules every 4 hours, up to 8 capsules per day.

➤*Storage/Stability:* Store at controlled room temperature 15° to 30°C (59° to 86°F) in a dry place.

Actions

➤*Pharmacology:* Isometheptene mucate is an unsaturated aliphatic amine with sympathomimetic properties. It acts by constricting dilated cranial and cerebral arterioles, thus reducing the stimuli that lead to vascular headaches.

Dichloralphenazone, a mild sedative, reduces the patient's emotional reaction to the pain of both vascular and tension headaches.

Acetaminophen raises the threshold to painful stimuli, thus exerting an analgesic effect against all types of headaches. Refer to individual monograph.

Contraindications

Glaucoma; severe cases of renal disease; hypertension; organic heart disease; hepatic disease; monoamine oxidase inhibitor (MAOI) therapy (see Drug Interactions).

Warnings

➤*CNS effects:* The capsules contain 100 mg dichloralphenazone. Because of its structural similarity to chloral hydrate, there is a potential for CNS depressant effects. For this reason, caution patients against engaging in hazardous activitoccupations requiring complete mental alertness (eg, operating machinery, driving a motor vehicle) after ingesting the drug. Also, caution patients about possible combined effects with alcohol and other CNS depressant drugs.

➤*Controlled substance:* The capsules are a controlled substance within Schedule IV because of the dichloralphenazone content.

➤*Drug abuse and dependence:* There have been no published reports of withdrawal signs or other signs of abuse associated with the active ingredients contained in the capsules. Because abuse and withdrawal symptoms are possible with chloral hydrate use, they should therefore also be considered possible in those patients taking the capsules in higher doses or for prolonged use. The risk of dependence is increased in patients with a history of alcoholism, drug abuse, or in patients with marked personality disorders. Such dependence-prone individuals should be under careful surveillance when receiving these capsules.

Precautions

➤*Caution:* Observe caution in hypertension and peripheral vascular disease and after recent cardiovascular attacks.

Drug Interactions

➤*MAOIs:* Because isometheptene has sympathomimetic properties, concurrent use may result in severe headache, hypertension, and hyperpyrexia, possibly resulting in hypertensive crisis. Avoid coadministration. If these are used together and hypertension develops, administer phentolamine.

Adverse Reactions

Transient dizziness and skin rash may appear in hypersensitive patients; this usually can be eliminated by reducing the dose.

MIGRAINE COMBINATIONS

	Product & Distributor	Ergotamine tartrate	Caffeine	Other Content	Dosage	How Supplied
Rx	Wigraine Tablets (Organon)	1 mg	100 mg	0.125 mg l-alkaloids of belladonna, 30 mg sodium pentobarbital	2 tablets at first sign of an attack; follow with 1 tablet every hour, if needed. Maximum dose is 6 tablets/attack. Do not exceed 10 tablets/week.	Lactose. (Organon 542). White. In foil strip 20s and 100s.
Rx	Cafergot Supps (Novartis)	2 mg	100 mg	Cocoa butter		(Cafergot Suppository 78-33 Sandoz). In 12s.

For complete information on these ingredients, refer to the individual monographs.

Ingredients

Content given per tablet or suppository.

ERGOTAMINE TARTRATE is used for its specific action against migraine.

CAFFEINE, a cranial vasoconstrictor, is added to ergotamine to enhance vasoconstrictive effects. It may enhance the absorption of ergotamine.

BARBITURATES are used for sedation.

BELLADONNA ALKALOIDS are used for their anticholinergic and antiemetic effects in individuals experiencing excessive nausea and vomiting during attacks.

Indications

	Recommended Uses for Antiemetic/Antivertigo Agents			
Class	Drug	Indications		
		Nausea and Vomiting	Motion Sickness	Vertigo
ANTIDOPAMINERGICS				
Phenothiazines	Chlorpromazine[1]	✔		
	Perphenazine[1]	✔		
	Prochlorperazine	✔		
	Promethazine	✔	✔	
	Thiethylperazine	✔		
Other	Metoclopramide	✔		
ANTICHOLINERGICS				
Antihistamines	Buclizine	✔	✔	
	Cyclizine	✔	✔	
	Dimenhydrinate	✔	✔	✔
	Diphenhydramine		✔	
	Meclizine	✔	✔	✔[2]
Other	Scopolamine		✔	
	Trimethobenzamide	✔		
MISCELLANEOUS				
Miscellaneous	Benzquinamide	✔		
	Cannabinoids	✔		
	Corticosteroids	✔[3]		
	Hydroxyzine HCl	✔[3]		
	Diphenidol	✔		✔
	Phosphorated Carbohydrate Solution	✔		

[1] Also indicated for relief of intractable hiccoughs.
[2] Classified "possibly effective" by the FDA.
[3] This is an *unlabeled* use.

Actions

➤*Pharmacology:* Drug-induced vomiting (eg, drugs, radiation, metabolic disorders) is generally stimulated through the chemoreceptor trigger zone (CTZ), which in turn stimulates the vomiting center (VC) in the brain. Nausea of motion sickness is initiated by stimulation of labyrinthine mechanism of the ear, which sends impulses to CTZ. VC may also be stimulated directly (by GI irritation, motion sickness, vestibular neuritis, etc). Increased activity of central neurotransmitters, dopamine in CTZ or acetylcholine in VC appears to be a major mediator for inducing vomiting.

Patients undergoing cancer chemotherapy often experience nausea and vomiting so intolerable that they may refuse further treatment. Some antineoplastic agents are more emetogenic than others. Prophylaxis with an antiemetic drug before the patient receives chemotherapy and treatment afterward may enable the patient to overcome this unpleasant side effect and continue a potentially curative protocol.

Vertigo is a feeling of whirling or rotation accompanied by involuntary swaying, weakness and lightheadedness. Motion sickness, a functional disorder, is caused by repetitive angular, linear or vertical motion. Both of these conditions are characterized by pallor, sweating, hyperventilation, nausea and vomiting.

The drugs that are effective as antiemetics are the **antidopaminergic** agents (phenothiazines, metoclopramide) which are especially effective for drug-induced emesis. **Anticholinergic agents** (antihistamines, trimethobenzamide, scopolamine) may be more appropriate in motion sickness, labyrinthine disorders, etc. Other agents, whose mechanisms

are not known or that may act differently (eg, hydroxyzine, corticosteroids, cannabinoids), are effective in various types of emesis.

The preceding table indicates manufacturers' recommended uses for agents in this group. Several of these are indicated for uses other than as antiemetic/antivertigo agents. For a full discussion, see individual drug monographs.

Warnings

➤*Children:* Not recommended for uncomplicated vomiting in children; limit use to prolonged vomiting of known etiology for three principal reasons:

1.) Although there is no confirmatory evidence, centrally-acting antiemetics may contribute, in combination with viral illnesses (a possible cause of vomiting in children), to the development of Reye's syndrome, a potentially fatal acute childhood encephalopathy. This syndrome follows a nonspecific febrile illness, and is characterized by an abrupt onset of persistent, severe vomiting, lethargy, irrational behavior, visceral fatty degeneration (especially involving the liver), progressive encephalopathy leading to coma, convulsions and death.

2.) The extrapyramidal symptoms that can occur secondary to some drugs may be confused with the CNS signs of an undiagnosed primary disease responsible for the vomiting, eg, Reye's syndrome or other encephalopathy.

3.) Drugs with hepatotoxic potential may unfavorably alter the course of Reye's syndrome. Avoid such drugs in children whose signs and symptoms (vomiting) could represent Reye's syndrome. It should also be noted that salicylates and acetaminophen are hepatotoxic at large doses. Although it is not known whether at usual doses they would represent a hazard in patients with the underlying hepatic disorder of Reye's syndrome, these drugs, too, should be avoided in children whose signs and symptoms could represent Reye's syndrome, unless alternative methods of controlling fever are not successful.

Children with acute illnesses (eg, chickenpox, CNS infections, measles, gastroenteritis) or dehydration seem to be much more susceptible to neuromuscular reactions, particularly dystonias, than are adults. In such patients, use antiemetics only under close supervision. Do not use dimenhydrinate in children < 2 years of age unless directed by a doctor.

Severe emesis – Severe emesis should not be treated with an antiemetic drug alone; where possible, establish cause of vomiting. Direct primary emphasis toward restoration of body fluids and electrolyte balance, and relief of fever and causative disease process. Avoid overhydration which may result in cerebral edema. Antiemetic effects may impede diagnosis of such conditions as brain tumors, intestinal obstruction and appendicitis, and may obscure signs of toxicity from overdosage of other drugs.

Precautions

➤*Benzyl alcohol:* Some of these products contain benzyl alcohol, which has been associated with a fatal "gasping syndrome" in premature infants.

➤*Tartrazine sensitivity:* Some of these products contain tartrazine, which may cause allergic-type reactions (including bronchial asthma) in susceptible individuals. Although the incidence of sensitivity is low, it is frequently seen in patients who also have aspirin hypersensitivity. Specific products containing tartrazine are identified in the product listings.

➤*Sulfite sensitivity:* Some of these products contain sulfites which may cause allergic-type reactions (eg, hives, itching, wheezing, anaphylaxis) in certain susceptible people. Although the overall prevalence of sulfite sensitivity in the general population is probably low, it is seen more frequently in asthmatics or in atopic nonasthmatic people. Specific products containing sulfites are identified in the product listings.

Patient Information

These agents may cause drowsiness; patients should observe caution while driving or performing other tasks requiring alertness.

Avoid alcohol and other CNS depressants.

Antidopaminergics

CHLORPROMAZINE HCl

Refer to the general discussion of these products in the Antiemetic/Antivertigo Agents group monograph. This is an abbreviated monograph. Complete prescribing information begins in the Antipsychotic Agents group monograph.

Indications

For a complete listing of products, refer to the Antipsychotic Agents monograph.

Control of nausea and vomiting; relief of intractable hiccoughs

Administration and Dosage

Individualize dosage.

➤*Adults:*

Nausea and vomiting –

Oral: 10 to 25 mg every 4 to 6 hours, as needed; increase if necessary.

Rectal: 50 to 100 mg every 6 to 8 hours, as needed.

IM: 25 mg. If no hypotension occurs, give 25 to 50 mg every 3 to 4 hours, as needed, until vomiting stops. Then switch to oral dosage.

Intractable hiccoughs: Orally, 25 to 50 mg 3 or 4 times daily. If symptoms persist for 2 to 3 days, give 25 to 50 mg IM. Should symptoms persist, use slow IV infusion with patient flat in bed. Administer 25 to 50 mg in 500 to 1000 ml of saline. Monitor blood pressure.

Antidopaminergics

CHLORPROMAZINE HCl

➤*Children:*

Nausea and vomiting – Do not use in children < 6 months of age except where potentially lifesaving. Do not use in conditions for which specific children's dosages have not been established. The activity following IM use may last 12 hours.

Oral: 0.25 mg/lb (0.55 mg/kg) every 4 to 6 hours, as needed.
Rectal: 0.5 mg/lb (1.1 mg/kg) every 6 to 8 hours, as needed.
IM: 0.25 mg/lb (0.55 mg/kg) every 6 to 8 hours, as needed.
Maximum IM dosage: Children up to 5 years of age — 40 mg/day.
Children 5 to 12 years of age — 75 mg/day, except in severe cases.

METOCLOPRAMIDE

Rx	Metoclopramide HCl (Quad)	Injection: 5 mg/ml (as monohydrochloride monohydrate)	In 2, 10, 30, 50 and 100 ml vials.
Rx	Reglan (Wyeth-Ayerst)		In 2 and 10 ml amps and 2, 10 and 30 ml vials.
Rx	Reglan (Schwarz Pharma)	Tablets: 5 mg metoclopramide HCl	(AHR Reglan 5). In 100s.
Rx	Metoclopramide (Various)	Tablets: 10 mg (as monohydrochloride mono-hydrate)	In 100s, 500s, 1000s and UD 100s.
Rx	Clopra (Quantum)		(QPL/217). White, scored. In 100s, 500s and 1000s.
Rx	Maxolon (Beecham)		(BMP 192). Blue, scored. In 100s.
Rx	Octamide (Adria)		(Adria 230). In 100s and 500s.
Rx	Reclomide (Major)		In 100s, 500s, 1000s and UD 100s.
Rx	Reglan (Schwarz Pharma)		(Reglan AHR 10). Pink, scored. In 100s, 500s and UD 100s.

Refer to the general discussion of these products beginning in the Antiemetic/Antivertigo monograph. This is an abbreviated monograph. For complete prescribing information refer to the GI Stimulants monograph.

Indications

➤*Parenteral:* Prevention of nausea and vomiting associated with emetogenic cancer chemotherapy.

➤*Unlabeled uses:* Studies have indicated some potential value of metoclopramide (10 mg orally or IV 30 minutes before each meal and at bedtime) in nausea and vomiting of a variety of etiologies (uncontrolled studies report 80% to 90% efficacy), including emesis during pregnancy and labor (5 to 10 mg orally or 5 to 20 mg IV or IM, 3 times/day).

Administration and Dosage

➤*Prevention of chemotherapy-induced emesis:* For doses in excess of 10 mg, dilute injection in 50 ml of a parenteral solution (Dextrose 5% in Water, Sodium Chloride Injection, Dextrose 5% in 0.45% Sodium Chloride, Ringer's or Lactated Ringer's Injection). Infuse slowly IV over not less than 15 minutes, 30 minutes before beginning cancer chemotherapy; repeat every 2 hours for 2 doses, then every 3 hours for 3 doses.

The initial 2 doses should be 2 mg/kg if highly emetogenic drugs such as cisplatin or dacarbazine are used alone or in combination. For less emetogenic regimens, 1 mg/kg/dose may be adequate.

If extrapyramidal symptoms occur, administer 50 mg diphenhydramine IM.

PERPHENAZINE

Rx	Perphenazine (Various, eg, Geneva)	Tablets: 2 mg	In 100s, 1000s, and UD 100s.
Rx	Perphenazine (Various, eg, Geneva)	Tablets: 4 mg	In 100s, 500s, 1000s, and UD 100s.
Rx	Perphenazine (Various, eg, Geneva)	Tablets: 8 mg	In 100s, 500s, 1000s, and UD 100s.
Rx	Perphenazine (Various, eg, Geneva)	Tablets: 16 mg	In 100s, 1000s, and UD 100s.
Rx	Perphenazine (Pharmaceutical Associates)	Oral concentrate: 16 mg/5 mL	Sorbitol, sucrose. Berry flavor. In 118 mL with graduated calibrated dropper.

[1] With sodium bisulfite.

Refer to the general discussion of these products in the Antiemetic/Antivertigo Agents group monograph. This is an abbreviated monograph. For complete prescribing information, refer to the Antipsychotic Agents group monograph.

Indications

Control of severe nausea and vomiting in adults; relief of intractable hiccoughs.

Administration and Dosage

➤*Oral:* 8 to 16 mg daily in divided doses; occasionally, 24 mg may be necessary. Early dosage reduction is desirable.

➤*IM:* Give to seated or recumbent patient; observe patient for a short period afterward.

Adults – 5 mg repeated every 6 hours as necessary. Do not exceed 15 mg in ambulatory or 30 mg in hospitalized patients. For severe conditions, an initial dose of 10 mg may be given. Place patients on oral therapy as soon as possible, usually within 24 hours. In general, reserve higher dosages for hospitalized patients.

Children (> 12 years of age) – The lowest adult dose (5 mg). Pediatric dose not established.

➤*IV:* Use only when necessary to control severe vomiting, intractable hiccoughs or acute conditions such as violent retching during surgery. Limit use to recumbent hospitalized adults in doses not exceeding 5 mg. Give as a diluted solution by either fractional injection or slow drip infusion. In the surgical patient, slow infusion is preferred. When administered in divided doses, dilute 0.5 mg/ml (1 ml mixed with 9 ml saline solution) and give not more than 1 mg/injection at not less than 1 to 2 minute intervals. Discontinue as soon as symptoms are controlled. Do not exceed 5 mg. Hypotensive and extrapyramidal side effects may occur. IV norepinephrine may alleviate hypotension.

➤*Storage/Stability:*

Concentrate – Protect from light. Store between 2° and 30°C (36° and 86°F). Store in carton until contents are used. Shake well.

Injection – Protect from light. Slight yellow discoloration will not alter potency or efficacy; if markedly discolored, discard. Store in carton until used.

PROCHLORPERAZINE

Rx	Prochlorperazine (Various)	Tablets (as maleate): 5 mg	In 12s, 30s, 100s, 1000s and UD 100s.
Rx	Compazine (SmithKline Beecham)		(SKF C66). Yellow-green. In 100s, 1000s and UD 100s.
Rx	Prochlorperazine (Various)	Tablets (as maleate): 10 mg	In 20s, 30s, 100s, 1000s and UD 32s and 100s.
Rx	Compazine (SmithKline Beecham)		(SKF C67). Yellow-green. In 100s, 1000s and UD 100s.
Rx	Prochlorperazine (Various)	Tablets (as maleate): 25 mg	In 100s, 1000s and UD 100s.
Rx	Compazine (SmithKline Beecham)		(SKF C69). Yellow-green. In 100s and 1000s.
Rx	Compazine (SmithKline Beecham)	Spansules (sustained release capsules as maleate): 30 mg	(SKF C47). Black/Clear. In 50s, 500s & UD 100s.
Rx	Compazine (SmithKline Beecham)	Suppositories: 2.5 mg	In 12s.
Rx	Prochlorperazine (Various)		In 12s.
Rx	Compazine (SmithKline Beecham)	5 mg	In 12s.
Rx	Prochlorperazine (Various)		In 12s.
Rx	Compazine (SmithKline Beecham)	25 mg	In 12s.
Rx	Prochlorperazine (Various)		In 12s.
Rx	Compro (Paddock)		In 12s.

Antidopaminergics

PROCHLORPERAZINE

Rx	Compazine (SmithKline Beecham)	Syrup (as edisylate): 5 mg/5 ml	Fruit flavor. In 120 ml.
Rx	Prochlorperazine (Various)	Injection: 5 mg/ml	In 10 ml vials.
Rx	Prochlorperazine (Wyeth-Ayerst)	Injection (as edisylate): 5 mg/ml	In 2 ml amps and 2 and 10 ml vials.
Rx	Compazine (SmithKline Beecham)		In 2 ml amps[1], 2 ml disp. syringes[2] and 10 ml multi-dose vials.[2]

[1] With sodium saccharin and benzyl alcohol.

[2] With sodium sulfite and sodium bisulfite.

Refer to the general discussion of these products in the Antiemetic/Antivertigo Agents group monograph. This is an abbreviated monograph. For complete prescribing information, refer to the Antipsychotic Agents group monograph.

Indications

Control of severe nausea and vomiting.

Administration and Dosage

Do not crush or chew sustained release preparations.

Individualize dosage.

Do not use in pediatric surgery.

➤*Adults:*
Control of severe nausea and vomiting –
Oral: Usually, 5 to 10 mg, 3 or 4 times daily; 15 mg (sustained release) on arising; 10 mg (sustained release) every 12 hours.
Rectal: 25 mg twice daily.
IM: Initially, 5 to 10 mg. If necessary, repeat every 3 or 4 hours. Do not exceed 40 mg/day.
SC: Do not administer SC because of local irritation.

➤*Adult surgery:*
Control of severe nausea and vomiting – Total parenteral dosage should not exceed 40 mg/day. Hypotension may occur if the drug is given IV or by infusion.

IM – 5 to 10 mg, 1 to 2 hours before induction of anesthesia (may repeat once in 30 minutes), or to control acute symptoms during and after surgery (may repeat once).

IV injection – 5 to 10 mg, 15 to 30 minutes before induction of anesthesia, or to control acute symptoms during or after sugery. Repeat once if necessary. Prochlorperazine may be administered either undiluted or diluted in isotonic solution, but do not exceed 10 mg in a single dose of the drug. Do not exceed 5 mg/ml/min. Do not use bolus injection.

IV infusion – 20 mg/L of isotonic solution. Do not dilute in < 1 L of isotonic solution. Add to IV infusion 15 to 30 minutes before induction.

In one study, a dosage of 30 or 40 mg prochlorperazine in 100 ml normal saline was significantly superior to a 10 mg dose in treating cisplatin-induced emesis; toxicity was only moderate.

➤*Children (> 20 pounds or 2 years of age):*
Control of severe nausea and vomiting –
Oral or rectal: More than 1 days' therapy is seldom necessary.
• *20 to 29 lbs (9.1 to 13.2 kg) –* 2.5 mg 1 or 2 times/day (not to exceed 7.5 mg/day).
• *30 to 39 lbs (13.6 to 17.7 kg) –* 2.5 mg 2 or 3 times/day (not to exceed 10 mg/day).
• *40 to 85 lbs (18.2 to 38.6 kg) –* 2.5 mg 3 times/day or 5 mg twice daily (not to exceed 15 mg/day).
IM: 0.06 mg/lb (0.132 mg/kg). Give by deep IM injection. Control is usually obtained with one dose. Duration of action may be 12 hours. Subsequent doses may be given if necessary.

PROMETHAZINE

Refer to the general discussion of these products beginning in the Antiemetic/Antivertigo group monograph. This is an abbreviated monograph. For complete information see Antihistamines.

Indications

For complete listing of promethazine products refer to Antihistamine Product Pages.

➤*Oral or rectal:* Active and prophylactic treatment of motion sickness; prevention and control of nausea and vomiting associated with anesthesia and surgery; antiemetic in postoperative patients.

➤*Parenteral:* Treatment of motion sickness; prevention and control of nausea and vomiting associated with anesthesia and surgery.

Administration and Dosage

➤*Oral and rectal:*

Motion sickness – The average adult dose is 25 mg twice daily. Take the initial dose ½ to 1 hour before travel, and repeat 8 to 12 hours later, if necessary. On succeeding days, administer 25 mg on arising and again before the evening meal. For children, administer 12.5 to 25 mg twice daily.

Nausea and vomiting – The average dose for active therapy in children or adults is 25 mg. Repeat as necessary in doses of 12.5 to 25 mg at 4 to 6 hour intervals.

Children: For nausea and vomiting, the usual dose is 0.5 mg per pound of body weight, and the adjust the dose to the age and weight of the patient and the severity of the condition being treated. For prophylaxis of nausea and vomiting, as during surgery and the postoperative period, the average dose is 25 mg repeated at 4- to 6-hour intervals, as necessary.

➤*Parenteral:* Administer preferably by deep IM injection. Proper IV administration is well tolerated, but hazardous. When used IV, give in a concentration no greater than 25 mg/ml, and at a rate not to exceed 25 mg/min; it is preferable to inject through an appropriate site in tubing of an IV infusion set.

Motion sickness – 12.5 to 25 mg; may repeat as necessary 3 or 4 times a day.

Nausea and vomiting – 12.5 to 25 mg; do not repeat more frequently than every 4 hours. For postoperative nausea and vomiting, administer IM or IV and reduce dosage of analgesics and barbiturates accordingly.

In children < 12 years of age, do not exceed ½ the adult dose. As an adjunct to premedication, use 0.5 mg/lb (1.1 mg/kg) with an equal dose of narcotic or barbiturate and the appropriate dose of an atropine-like drug. Do not use in premature infants or neonates or in vomiting of unknown etiology in children.

Inadvertent intra-arterial injection can result in gangrene of the affected extremity. Subcutaneous injection is contraindicated as it may result in tissue necrosis.

THIETHYLPERAZINE MALEATE

Rx	Torecan (Roxane)	Injection: 5 mg/ml	In 2 ml amps.[1]

[1] With ascorbic acid, sodium metabisulfite and sorbitol.

Refer to the general discussion of these products in the Antiemetic/Antivertigo Agents group monograph. This is an abbreviated monograph. For complete information, see Antipsychotics.

Indications

Relief of nausea and vomiting.

Administration and Dosage

Do not use IV (may cause severe hypotension). Use of this drug has not been studied following intracardiac or intracranial surgery.

When used for nausea or vomiting associated with anesthesia and surgery, administer by deep IM injection at, or shortly before, termination of anesthesia.

➤*Adults:*
Oral and Rectal – 10 to 30 mg daily in divided doses.
IM – 2 ml, 1 to 3 times daily.

➤*Children:* Dosage not determined. Not recommended in children < 12 years of age.

➤*Storage/Stability:* Store suppositories below 25°C (77°F) in a tight container (eg, sealed foil).

Actions

➤*Pharmacology:* Mechanism unknown. Animal experiments suggest a direct action on both the chemoreceptor trigger zone (CTZ) and the vomiting center (VC).

Contraindications

Severe CNS depression; comatose states; hypersensitivity to phenothiazines; IV administration; pregnancy.

Anticholinergics

BUCLIZINE HCl

Rx	Bucladin-S Softabs (Stuart)	Tablets: 50 mg	Tartrazine. (Stuart 864). Yellow, scored. In 100s.

Refer to the general discussion of these products beginning in the Antiemetic/Antivertigo group monograph.

Indications
For the control of nausea, vomiting and dizziness of motion sickness.

Administration and Dosage
Tablets can be taken without swallowing water. Place tablet in mouth and allow to dissolve, or chew or swallow whole.

➤*Adults:* A 50 mg dose usually alleviates nausea. In severe cases, 150 mg/day may be taken. Usual maintenance dose is 50 mg, 2 times daily. In prevention of motion sickness, take 50 mg at least ½ hour before beginning travel. For extended travel, a second 50 mg dose may be taken after 4 to 6 hours.

Actions
➤*Pharmacology:* Acts centrally to suppress nausea and vomiting.

Contraindications
Hypersensitivity to buclizine HCl; pregnancy (see Warnings).

Warnings
➤*Pregnancy:* When administered to the pregnant rat at doses above the human therapeutic range, buclizine induced fetal abnormalities. Clinical data are not adequate to establish safety in early pregnancy.

➤*Children:* Safety and efficacy for use in children have not been established.

Adverse Reactions
Drowsiness, dry mouth, headache and jitteriness.

CYCLIZINE

otc	Marezine (Himmel)	Tablets: 50 mg (as HCl)	(Marezine T4A). Scored. In 12s and 100s.

For complete prescribing information, refer to the Antiemetic/Antivertigo Agents group monograph.

Indications
Prevention and treatment of nausea, vomiting and dizziness of motion sickness.

Administration and Dosage
➤*Oral:*

Adults – 50 mg taken ½ hour before departure; repeat every 4 to 6 hours. Do not exceed 200 mg daily.

Children (6 to 12 years of age) – 25 mg, up to 3 times daily.

➤*Parenteral:* For IM use only.

Adults – 50 mg every 4 to 6 hours, as necessary.

Not recommended for use in children.

Actions
➤*Pharmacology:* Cyclizine has antiemetic, anticholinergic, and antihistaminic properties. It reduces the sensitivity of the labyrinthine apparatus. The action may be mediated through nerve pathways to the vomiting center (VC) from the chemoreceptor trigger zone (CTZ), peripheral nerve pathways, the VC, or other CNS centers.

Cyclizine has an onset of action of 30 to 60 minutes, depending on dosage; the duration of action is 4 to 6 hours and 12 to 24 hours, respectively.

Contraindications
Hypersensitivity to cyclizine.

Warnings
➤*Pregnancy: Category B.* Cyclizine has been teratogenic in rodents, but large scale human studies have not demonstrated adverse fetal effects. Use only when clearly needed and when the potential benefits outweigh the potential hazards to the fetus.

➤*Lactation:* Safety for use in the nursing mother has not been established.

➤*Children:* Safety and efficacy for use in children have not been established. Not recommended for use in children under 12 years of age.

Precautions
➤*Hazardous tasks:* May produce drowsiness; patients should observe caution while driving or performing other tasks requiring alertness.

Because of the anticholinergic action of this agent, use with caution and with appropriate monitoring in patients with glaucoma, obstructive disease of the GI or GU tract and in elderly males with possible prostatic hypertrophy. This drug may have a hypotensive action, which may be confusing or dangerous in postoperative patients.

May have additive effects with alcohol and other CNS depressants (eg, hypnotics, sedatives, tranquilizers, antianxiety agents); use with caution.

Adverse Reactions
➤*Cardiovascular:* Hypotension; palpitations; tachycardia.

➤*CNS:* Drowsiness; restlessness; excitation; nervousness; insomnia; euphoria; blurred vision; diplopia; vertigo; tinnitus; auditory and visual hallucinations (particularly when dosage recommendations are exceeded).

➤*Dermatologic:* Urticaria; rash.

➤*GI:* Dry mouth; anorexia; nausea; vomiting; diarrhea; constipation; cholestatic jaundice.

➤*GU:* Urinary frequency; difficult urination; urinary retention.

➤*Miscellaneous:* Dry nose and throat.

Overdosage
➤*Symptoms:* Moderate overdosage may cause hyperexcitability alternating with drowsiness. Massive overdosage may cause convulsions, hallucinations and respiratory paralysis.

➤*Treatment:* includes appropriate supportive and symptomatic treatment. Refer to General Management of Acute Overdosage. Consider dialysis.

Caution – Do not use morphine or other respiratory depressants.

DIMENHYDRINATE

otc	Dimenhydrinate (Various)	Tablets: 50 mg	In 12s, 100s, 300s, 500s, 1000s and UD 100s.
otc	Calm-X (Republic Drug)		In 16s.
Rx	Dimetabs (Jones Medical)		In 1000s.
otc	Dramamine (Upjohn)		(DRAMAMINE). White, scored. In UD 100s.
otc	Triptone (Commerce)		Long acting. Scored. In 12s.
otc	Dramamine (Upjohn)	Tablets, chewable: 50 mg	(DRAMAMINE).Tartrazine. Aspartame, sorbitol. Orange, scored. Orange flavor. In 8s and 24s.
Rx	Dimenhydrinate (Various)	Injection: 50 mg/ml	In 1 and 10 ml vials and 1 ml amps.
Rx	Dinate (Seatrace)		In 10 ml vials.[1]
Rx	Dramanate (Pasadena)		In 10 ml vials.[1]
Rx	Dymenate (Keene)		In 10 ml vials.[1]
Rx	Hydrate (Hyrex)		In 10 ml vials.[1]
Rx	Dramamine (Upjohn)	Liquid: 15.62 mg/5 ml	In 480 ml.
otc	Dimenhydrinate (Various)	Liquid: 12.5 m/4 ml	In pt and gal.
otc	Dramamine (Upjohn)		5% alcohol. Cherry flavor. In 90 ml.
otc	Children's Dramamine (Upjohn)	Liquid: 12.5 mg per/5 ml	5% alcohol, sucrose. Cherry flavor. In 120 ml.

[1] In benzyl alcohol and propylene glycol.

Anticholinergics

DIMENHYDRINATE

Refer to the general discussion of these products beginning in the Antiemetic/Antivertigo group monograph.

Indications

For the prevention and treatment of nausea, vomiting, dizziness or vertigo of motion sickness.

Administration and Dosage

➤*Adults:*

Oral – 50 to 100 mg every 4 to 6 hours. Do not exceed 400 mg in 24 hours.

IM – 50 mg, as needed.

IV – 50 mg in 10 ml Sodium Chloride Injection given over 2 minutes. Do not inject intra-arterially.

➤*Children:*

Oral (6 to 12 years of age) – 25 to 50 mg every 6 to 8 hours; do not exceed 150 mg in 24 hours.

Oral (2 to 6 years of age) – Up to 12.5 to 25 mg every 6 to 8 hours; do not exceed 75 mg in 24 hours.

IM – 1.25 mg/kg or 37.5 mg/m² 4 times daily; do not exceed 300 mg daily.

➤*Children (< 2 years of age):* Only on advice of a physician.

Actions

➤*Pharmacology:* Dimenhydrinate consists of equimolar proportions of diphenhydramine and chlorotheophylline.

➤*Pharmacokinetics:* Dimenhydrinate has a depressant action on hyperstimulated labyrinthine function. The precise mode of action is not known. The antiemetic effects are believed to be due to the diphenhydramine, an antihistamine also used as an antiemetic agent.

Contraindications

Neonates; patients hypersensitive to dimenhydrinate or its components.

Warnings

➤*Pregnancy: Category B.* Safety for use during pregnancy has not been established. Use only when clearly needed and when the potential benefits outweigh the potential hazards to the fetus.

➤*Lactation:* Small amounts of dimenhydrinate are excreted in breast milk. Because of the potential for adverse reactions in nursing infants, decide whether to discontinue nursing or to discontinue the drug, taking into account the importance of the drug to the mother.

➤*Children:* For infants and children especially, an overdose of antihistamines may cause hallucinations, convulsions or death. Mental alertness may be diminished. In the young child, dimenhydrinate may produce excitation. Do not give to children < 2 years of age unless directed by a physician.

DIPHENHYDRAMINE

Refer to the general discussion of these products beginning in the Antiemetic/Antivertigo group monograph.

Indications

For a complete listing of diphenhydramine HCl products refer to the Antihistamine monograph's product pages.

Treatment and prophylaxis (oral only) of motion sickness.

Administration and Dosage

Individualize dosage.

➤*Oral:* Adults – 25 to 50 mg 3 or 4 times daily.

Precautions

Use with caution in conditions that might be aggravated by anticholinergic therapy (eg, prostatic hypertrophy, stenosing peptic ulcer, pyloroduodenal obstruction, bladder neck obstruction, narrow angle glaucoma, bronchial asthma, cardiac arrhythmias, etc).

➤*Note:* Most IV products contain benzyl alcohol, which has been associated with a fatal "Gasping Syndrome" in premature infants and low birth weight infants.

➤*Benzyl alcohol:* Some of these products contain the preservative benzyl alcohol, which has been associated with a fatal "gasping syndrome" in premature infants.

Drug Interactions

Dimenhydrinate Drug Interactions			
Precipitant drug	Object drug*		Description
Dimenhydrinate	Alcohol, CNS depressants	↑	Concomitant use of alcohol or other CNS depressants with dimenhydrinate may have an additive effect.
Dimenhydrinate	Antibiotics	↑	Use caution when given in conjunction with certain antibiotics that may cause ototoxicity; dimenhydrinate is capable of masking ototoxic symptoms, and irreversible damage may result.

* ↑ = Object drug increased.

Adverse Reactions

➤*Cardiovascular:* Palpitations, hypotension, tachycardia.

➤*CNS:* Drowsiness is most common. Confusion; nervousness; restlessness; headache; insomnia (especially in children); tingling, heaviness and weakness of hands; vertigo; dizziness; lassitude; excitation.

➤*GI:* Nausea; vomiting; diarrhea; epigastric distress; constipation; anorexia.

➤*Ophthalmic:* Blurring of vision; diplopia.

➤*Miscellaneous:* Anaphylaxis; photosensitivity; urticaria; drug rash; hemolytic anemia; difficult or painful urination; nasal stuffiness; tightness of chest; wheezing; thickening of bronchial secretions; dryness of mouth, nose and throat.

Overdosage

➤*Symptoms:* Drowsiness is the usual side effect. Convulsions, coma and respiratory depression may occur with massive overdosage.

➤*Treatment:* No specific antidote is known. If respiratory depression occurs, initiate mechanically assisted respiration and administer oxygen. Treat convulsions with appropriate doses of diazepam. Give phenobarbital (5 to 6 mg/kg) to control convulsions in children. Refer to General Management of Acute Overdosage.

Children > 20 lbs (9.1kg) – 12.5 to 25 mg 3 or 4 times daily (5 mg/kg/24 hrs, or 150 mg/m²/24 hours. Do not exceed 300 mg.

Give first dose 30 minutes before exposure to motion and repeat before meals and upon retiring for the duration of the journey.

➤*Parenteral:* For use only when the oral form is impractical.

Adults – 10 to 50 mg IV or deep IM; 100 mg if required. Maximum daily dosage is 400 mg.

Children – 5 mg/kg/24 hrs or 150 mg/m²/24 hrs, in 4 divided doses, IV or deep IM. Maximum daily dosage is 300 mg.

MECLIZINE

Rx	**Meclizine HCl** (Various)	**Tablets:** 12.5 mg	In 30s, 60s, 100s, 500s, 1000s, and UD 100s.
Rx	**Antivert** (Pfizer US)		(Antivert 210). In 100s, 1000s, and UD 100s.
Rx	**Antrizine** (Major)		In 100s, 500s, and 1000s.
otc/Rx[1]	**Meclizine HCl** (Various)	**Tablets:** 25 mg	In 12s, 20s, 30s, 60s, 100s, 500s, 1000s, and UD 32s and 100s.
Rx	**Antivert/25** (Pfizer US)		(Antivert 211). In 100s, 1000s, and UD 100s.
otc	**Dramamine Less Drowsy Formula** (Pharmacia and Upjohn)		Lactose. In 8s.
otc/Rx[1]	**Meclizine HCl** (Various, eg, Rugby, Goldline)	**Tablets, chewable:** 25 mg	In 20s, 30s, 60s, 100s, 1000s, and UD 100s.
Rx	**Meclizine HCl** (Various)	**Tablets:** 50 mg	In 100s.
Rx	**Antivert/50** (Pfizer US)		(Antivert 214). Scored. In100s.
Rx	**Meni-D** (Seatrace)	**Capsules:** 25 mg	(Meni-D 1-4X Day). Light blue/clear. In 100s.

[1] Products are available *otc* or *Rx*, depending on product labeling.

MECLIZINE

For complete prescribing information, refer to the Antiemetic/Antivertigo Agents group monograph.

Indications

Prevention and treatment of nausea, vomiting, and dizziness of motion sickness.

Meclizine is "possibly effective" for the management of vertigo associated with diseases affecting the vestibular system.

Administration and Dosage

➤*Motion sickness:* Take an initial dose of 25 to 50 mg, 1 hour prior to travel. May repeat dose every 24 hours for the duration of the journey.

➤*Vertigo:* 25 to 100 mg daily in divided doses.

Actions

➤*Pharmacology:* Meclizine has antiemetic, anticholinergic, and antihistaminic properties. It reduces the sensitivity of the labyrinthine apparatus. The action may be mediated through nerve pathways to the vomiting center (VC) from the chemoreceptor trigger zone (CTZ), peripheral nerve pathways, the VC, or other CNS centers.

Meclizine has an onset of action of 30 to 60 minutes, depending on dosage; their duration of action is 4 to 6 hours and 12 to 24 hours, respectively.

Contraindications

Hypersensitivity to meclizine.

Warnings

➤*Pregnancy:* Category B. Meclizine has been teratogenic in rodents, but large scale human studies have not demonstrated adverse fetal effects. Use only when clearly needed and when the potential benefits outweigh the potential hazards to the fetus. It has been suggested that, based on available data, meclizine presents the lowest risk of teratogenicity and is the drug of first choice in treating nausea and vomiting during pregnancy.

➤*Lactation:* Safety for use in the nursing mother has not been established.

➤*Children:* Safety and efficacy for use in children have not been established. Not recommended for use in children < 12 years of age.

Precautions

➤*Hazardous tasks:* May produce drowsiness; patients should observe caution while driving or performing other tasks requiring alertness.

Because of the anticholinergic action of these agents, use with caution and with appropriate monitoring in patients with glaucoma, obstructive disease of the GI or GU tract, and in elderly males with possible prostatic hypertrophy. These drugs may have a hypotensive action, which may be confusing or dangerous in postoperative patients.

May have additive effects with alcohol and other CNS depressants (eg, hypnotics, sedatives, tranquilizers, antianxiety agents); use with caution.

Adverse Reactions

➤*Cardiovascular:* Hypotension; palpitations; tachycardia.

➤*CNS:* Drowsiness; restlessness; excitation; nervousness; insomnia; euphoria; blurred vision; diplopia; vertigo; tinnitus; auditory and visual hallucinations (particularly when dosage recommendations are exceeded).

➤*Dermatologic:* Urticaria; rash.

➤*GI:* Dry mouth; anorexia; nausea; vomiting; diarrhea; constipation; cholestatic jaundice (cyclizine).

➤*GU:* Urinary frequency; difficult urination; urinary retention.

➤*Miscellaneous:* Dry nose and throat.

Overdosage

➤*Symptoms:* Moderate overdosage may cause hyperexcitability alternating with drowsiness. Massive overdosage may cause convulsions, hallucinations, and respiratory paralysis.

➤*Treatment:* Includes appropriate supportive and symptomatic treatment. Refer to General Management of Acute Overdosage. Consider dialysis.

Caution – Do not use morphine or other respiratory depressants.

SCOPOLAMINE, ORAL

Rx	Scopace (Hope Pharm.)	Tablets: 0.4 mg	(HOPE 301). White. In 100s.

Refer to the general discussion of these products beginning in the Antiemetic/Antivertigo group monograph.

Indications

Used as an anticholinergic CNS depressant; in the symptomatic treatment of postencephalitic parkinsonism and paralysis agitans; in spastic states; and locally as a substitute for atropine in ophthalmology.

Scopolamine inhibits excessive motility and hypertonus of the GI tract in irritable colon syndrome, mild dysentery, diverticulitis, pylorospasm, and cardiospasm.

May prevent motion sickness.

Administration and Dosage

The dosage range is 0.4 to 0.8 mg. The dosage may be cautiously increased in parkinsonism and spastic states.

SCOPOLAMINE, TRANSDERMAL

Rx	Transderm-Scop (Novartis Consumer Health, Inc.)	Transdermal Therapeutic System: 1.5 mg scopolamine (delivers ≈ 1 mg scopolamine in vivo over 3 days)	(4345). In 4 unit blister packs.

Refer to the general discussion of these products beginning in the Antiemetic/Antivertigo group monograph.

Indications

In addition to its systemic anticholinergic effects, scopolamine is effective in motion sickness. Refer to the Gastrointestinal Anticholinergic/Antispasmodics monograph.

Prevention of nausea and vomiting associated with motion sickness in adults.

Administration and Dosage

➤*Initiation of therapy:* Apply one system to the postauricular skin (ie, behind the ear) ≥ 4 hours before the antiemetic effect is required. Scopolamine ≈ 1 mg will be delivered over 3 days. Wear only one disc at a time.

➤*Handling:* After applying the disc on dry skin behind the ear, wash hands thoroughly with soap and water, then dry them. Discard the removed disc and wash the hands and application site thoroughly with soap and water to prevent any traces of scopolamine from coming into direct contact with the eyes.

➤*Continuation of therapy:* If the disc is displaced, discard it and place a fresh one on the hairless area behind the other ear. If therapy is required for > 3 days, discard the first disc and place a fresh one on the hairless area behind the other ear.

Actions

➤*Pharmacology:* Scopolamine is a belladonna alkaloid with well-known pharmacological properties. The drug has a long history of oral and parenteral use for central anticholinergic activity, including prophylaxis of motion sickness. The mechanism of action of scopolamine in the CNS is not definitely known but may include anticholinergic effects. The ability of scopolamine to prevent motion-induced nausea is believed to be associated with inhibition of vestibular input to the CNS, which results in inhibition of the vomiting reflex. In addition, scopolamine may have a direct action on the vomiting center within the reticular formation of the brain stem.

➤*Pharmacokinetics:* The transdermal system is a 0.2 mm thick film with 4 layers. It is 2.5 cm^2 in area and contains 1.5 mg scopolamine that is gradually released from an adhesive matrix of mineral oil and polyisobutylene following application to the postauricular skin. An initial priming dose released from the system's adhesive layer saturates the skin binding site for scopolamine and rapidly brings the plasma concentration to the required steady-state level. A continuous controlled release of scopolamine flows from the drug reservoir through the rate controlling membrane to maintain a constant plasma level. Antiemetic protection is produced within several hours following application behind the ear.

➤*Clinical trials:* In clinical studies at sea or in a controlled motion environment, there was a 75% reduction in incidence of motion-induced nausea and vomiting. The system provided significantly greater protection than did oral dimenhydrinate.

Contraindications

Hypersensitivity to scopolamine or any component of the product; glaucoma.

Warnings

Potentially alarming idiosyncratic reactions may occur with therapeutic doses.

SCOPOLAMINE, TRANSDERMAL

➤*Pregnancy: Category C.* Studies in rabbits at plasma levels ≈ 100 times those achieved in humans using a transdermal system revealed a marginal embryotoxic effect. Use in pregnancy only if potential benefits justify potential risk to the fetus.

➤*Lactation:* It is not known whether scopolamine is excreted in breast milk. Exercise caution when administering to a nursing woman.

➤*Children:* Safety and efficacy have not been established. Children are particularly susceptible to the side effects of belladonna alkaloids. Do not use the transdermal system in children.

Precautions

Use with caution in patients with pyloric obstruction, urinary bladder neck obstruction, and in patients suspected of having intestinal obstruction. Use with special caution in the elderly or in individuals with impaired metabolic, liver, or kidney functions because of the increased likelihood of CNS effects.

➤*Potentially hazardous tasks:* May produce drowsiness, disorientation, and confusion. Warn patients against engaging in activities that require mental alertness, such as driving a motor vehicle or operating dangerous machinery.

In patients taking drugs that cause CNS effects, including alcohol, use scopolamine with care.

➤*Drug withdrawal:* Dizziness, nausea, vomiting, headache, and disturbances of equilibrium have been reported in a few patients following discontinuation of the use of the transdermal system. This occurred most often in patients who used the system for > 3 days.

Adverse Reactions

➤*Most common:* Dry mouth (67%); drowsiness (< 17%); transient impairment of eye accommodation including blurred vision and dilation of the pupils. Unilateral fixed and dilated pupil has been reported, apparently from accidentally touching one eye after manipulation of the patch.

➤*Infrequent:* Disorientation; memory disturbances; dizziness; restlessness; hallucinations; confusion; difficulty urinating; rashes or erythema; acute narrow-angle glaucoma; dry, itchy, or red eyes.

Overdosage

➤*Symptoms:* Disorientation, memory disturbances, dizziness, restlessness, hallucinations, or confusion.

➤*Treatment:* Remove the system immediately if these symptoms occur. Initiate appropriate parasympathomimetic therapy if symptoms are severe. Refer to General Management of Acute Overdosage.

For information on overdosage with other dose forms, refer to the GI Anticholinergics/Antispasmodics monograph.

Patient Information

Patient package insert is available with the transdermal product.

Medication may cause dry mouth. May produce drowsiness or blurred vision; patients should observe caution while driving or performing other tasks requiring alertness. If eye pain, blurred vision, dizziness, or rapid pulse occurs, discontinue use and consult physician.

Wash hands thoroughly after handling the transdermal disc. Temporary dilation of the pupils and blurred vision may occur if scopolamine comes in contact with the eyes.

TRIMETHOBENZAMIDE HCl

Rx	**Tigan** (Monarch)	**Capsules**: 300 mg	(Tigan MO79). Purple. In 100s.
Rx	**Trimethobenzamide** (Various)	**Pediatric suppositories**: 100 mg	In 10s.
Rx	**Pediatric Triban** (Great Southern)		In 10s.[1]
Rx	**Tebamide** (G & W Labs)		In 10s.[1]
Rx	**T-Gen** (Goldline)		In 10s.[1]
Rx	**Tigan** (Monarch)		In 10s.[1]
Rx	**Trimazide** (Major)		In 10s.
Rx	**Trimethobenzamide** (Various)	**Adult suppositories**: 200 mg	In 10s and 50s.
Rx	**Tebamide** (G & W Labs)		In 10s[1] and 50s.[1]
Rx	**T-Gen** (Goldline)		In 10s[1] and 50s.[1]
Rx	**Tigan** (Monarch)		In 10s[1] and 50s.[1]
Rx	**Triban** (Great Southern)		In 10s[1] and 50s.[1]
Rx	**Trimazide** (Major)		In 10s.
Rx	**Trimethobenzamide HCl** (Various)	**Injection**: 100 mg/ml	In 2 ml amps and 20 ml vials.
Rx	**Tigan** (Monarch)		In 2 ml amps[3], 20 ml vials,[2] and 2 ml syringe.[4]

[1] With 2% benzocaine.
[2] With phenol.
[3] With methyl- and propylparabens.
[4] With phenol and EDTA.

Refer to the general discussion of these products beginning in the Antiemetic/Antivertigo monograph.

Indications

For the treatment of postoperative nausea and vomiting and for nausea associated with gastroenteritis.

Administration and Dosage

➤*Oral:*

Adults – 300 mg, 3 or 4 times daily.

➤*Rectal:*

Adults – 200 mg, 3 or 4 times daily.

Children (30 to 90 lbs; 13.6 to 40.9 kg) – 100 to 200 mg, 3 or 4 times daily.

(< 30 lbs): 100 mg, 3 or 4 times daily. Do not use in premature or newborn infants.

➤*Injection:* For IM use only.

Adults – 200 mg 3 or 4 times/day. Pain, stinging, burning, redness, and swelling may develop at injection site.

➤*Storage/Stability:* Store at 25°C (77°F). Excursions permitted to 15° to 30°C (59° to 86°F).

Actions

➤*Pharmacokinetics:* Mechanism is obscure, but may be mediated through the chemoreceptor trigger zone; direct impulses to vomiting center are not inhibited.

Contraindications

Hypersensitivity to trimethobenzamide, benzocaine, or similar local anesthetics; parenteral use in children; suppositories in premature infants or neonates.

Warnings

➤*Pregnancy:* Safety for use has not been established. Use only when clearly needed and when the potential benefits outweigh the potential risks to the fetus.

➤*Lactation:* Safety for use in the nursing mother has not been established.

Precautions

Encephalitides, gastroenteritis, dehydration, electrolyte imbalance (especially in children and the elderly or debilitated), and CNS reactions have occurred when used during acute febrile illness.

Exercise caution when giving the drug with alcohol and other CNS-acting agents such as phenothiazines, barbiturates, and belladonna derivatives.

Adverse Reactions

Hypersensitivity reactions; parkinson-like symptoms; hypotension or pain following IM injection; blood dyscrasias; blurred vision; coma; convulsions; depression; disorientation; dizziness; drowsiness; headache; jaundice; muscle cramps; opisthotonos; allergic-type skin reactions. If these occur, discontinue use. While these usually disappear spontaneously, symptomatic treatment may be indicated.

Indications

►*Antiemetic:* Prevention of nausea and vomiting associated with initial and repeat courses of emetogenic cancer therapy, including high-dose cisplatin; prevention of postoperative nausea or vomiting (**ondansetron** and **dolasetron**); prevention of nausea and vomiting associated with radiotherapy in patients receiving either total body irradiation, single high-dose fraction, or daily fractions to the abdomen (oral **ondansetron** and **granisetron**); treatment of postoperative nausea or vomiting (IV **dolasetron**).

►*Unlabeled uses:*

Granisetron – Acute nausea and vomiting following surgery (1 to 3 mg IV).

Dolasetron – Radiotherapy-induced nausea and vomiting (40 mg IV or 0.3 mg/kg IV).

Actions

►*Pharmacology:* Selective 5-hydroxytryptamine₃ (5-HT₃) receptor antagonists are antinauseant and antiemetic agents with little or no affinity for other serotonin receptors, alpha- or beta-adrenergic, dopamine-D_2, histamine-H_1, benzodiazepine, picrotoxin, or opioid receptors.

Serotonin receptors of the 5-HT₃ type are located peripherally on vagal nerve terminals, enteric neurons in the GI tract, and centrally in the chemoreceptor trigger zone. During chemotherapy, mucosal enterochromaffin cells from the small intestine release serotonin, which stimulates the 5-HT₃ receptors. This evokes vagal afferent discharge, inducing vomiting. In IBS, it is presumed the pain, distension, and exaggerated motor response are at least in part caused by stimulation of the 5-HT₃ receptors.

5-HT₃ antagonists have little effect on blood pressure. **Ondansetron** and **granisetron** have little effect on heart rate or ECG. No evidence of an effect on plasma prolactin or aldosterone concentrations has been found. Ondansetron has no effect on esophageal and gastric motility, lower esophageal sphincter pressure or small intestinal transit time, cardiac output, and stroke volume. Multi-day administration of ondansetron and oral granisetron have been shown to slow colonic transit.

►*Pharmacokinetics:*

Distribution – Plasma protein binding is 65% for **granisetron** and 70% to 76% for **ondansetron**. Both drugs distribute into erythrocytes.

5-HT₃ Antagonist Pharmacokinetics	Mean C_{max} (ng/ml)	Mean t½ (hr)	Mean Cl (L/hr/kg)	Mean V_d (L/kg)
IV				
Dolasetron				
Adults (100 mg)	320	7.3	0.564	5.8
Elderly[1] (2 to 4 mcg/kg)	620	6.9	0.498	4.69
Cancer patients				
Adults	505	7.5	0.612	
Adolescents	562	5.5	0.75	
Children	505	4.4	1.152	≈ 5.2
Pediatric surgery	255	4.8	0.786	
Renal function impairment[2]	867	10.9	0.3	
Granisetron (single 40 mcg/kg dose)				
Adults	64	5	0.79	3
Elderly[3]	57	7.5	0.44	4
Cancer patients	84	9	0.38	3
Ondansetron (single 0.15 mg/kg dose)				
Adults	104	4.1	0.35	NA[5]
Elderly[4]	170	5.5	0.262	NA[5]
Cancer/Surgery	NA[5]	3.5	NA[5]	NA[5]
Oral				
Dolasetron				
Adults	556	8.1	0.804	5.8
Elderly[1]	662	7.2	0.57	5.63
Cancer patients				
Adults	NA[5]	7.9	0.774	
Adolescents	374	6.4	1.59	
Children	217	5.5	2.652	
Pediatric surgery	159	5.9	1.248	
Renal function impairment[2]	701	10.7	0.432	
Hepatic function impairment	410	11	0.528	
Granisetron				
Adults (single 1 mg dose)	3.6	6	0.41	4
Cancer patients (1 mg BID × 7 days)	6	NA[5]	0.52	NA[5]

5-HT₃ Antagonist Pharmacokinetics	Mean C_{max} (ng/ml)	Mean t½ (hr)	Mean Cl (L/hr/kg)	Mean V_d (L/kg)
Ondansetron (single 8 mg dose)				
Adults, male (female)	25 (47)	3.6 (4.2)	0.3935 (0.3045)	NA[5]
Elderly,[4] male (female)	37 (46)	4.5 (6)	0.277 (0.249)	NA[5]

[1] 65 to 75 years of age.
[2] Creatinine clearance ≤ 10 ml/min.
[3] ≥ 65 years of age.
[4] ≥ 75 years of age.
[5] NA = not available.

Special populations –

Gender: Plasma concentrations are 30% to 50% lower and less variable in men compared with women given the same oral dose.

►*Clinical trials:*

Granisetron vs dolasetron – In a randomized, double-blind, multicenter study, IV dolasetron was compared with IV granisetron in patients receiving high-dose cisplatin. No statistically significant differences were found between the 2 medications.

Ondansetron vs dolasetron – Three randomized, double-blind, multicenter studies compared ondansetron oral and IV with dolasetron oral and IV. In 2 of the studies, ondansetron and dolasetron were equivalent.

Granisetron vs chlorpromazine – Granisetron injection 40 mcg/kg was compared with the combination of chlorpromazine (50 to 200 mg/24 hrs) and dexamethasone (12 mg) in patients treated with moderately emetogenic chemotherapy, including primarily carboplatin, cisplatin, and cyclophosphamide. Granisetron was superior to the chlorpromazine regimen in preventing nausea and vomiting.

Granisetron vs Chlorpromazine - Prevention of Chemotherapy-Induced Nausea and Vomiting		
Parameter	Granisetron (n = 133)	Chlorpromazine[1] (n = 133)
Response over 24 hours		
Complete response[2]	68%	47%
No vomiting	73%	53%
No more than mild nausea	77%	59%

[1] Patients also received 12 mg dexamethasone.
[2] No vomiting and no moderate or severe nausea.

In other studies of moderately emetogenic chemotherapy, no significant difference in efficacy was found between granisetron doses of 40 and 160 mcg/kg.

Ondansetron vs metoclopramide – Ondansetron injection was compared with metoclopramide in a single-blind trial in 307 patients on cisplatin ≥ 100 mg/m² with or without other chemotherapy agents. Patients received the first dose of ondansetron or metoclopramide 30 minutes before cisplatin. Two additional ondansetron doses were administered 4 and 8 hours later, or five additional metoclopramide doses were administered 2, 4, 7, 10, and 13 hours later. Cisplatin was given over ≤ 3 hours. Episodes of vomiting and retching were tabulated over the 24 hours after cisplatin.

Ondansetron vs Metoclopramide - Prevention of Emesis Induced by Cisplatin (≥ 100 mg/m²) Single-day Therapy[1]		
Parameters	Ondansetron (n = 136) 0.15 mg/kg x 3	Metoclopramide (n = 138) 2 mg/kg x 6
Treatment Response		
0 emetic episodes	40%	30%
1 to 2 emetic episodes	25%	22%
3 to 5 emetic episodes	14%	13%
> 5 emetic episodes/rescued	21%	36%
Median # of emetic episodes	1	2
Median time to first emetic episode (hours)	20.5	4.3
Global satisfaction with control of nausea and vomiting (0-100)[2]	85	63
Acute dystonic reactions	0	8
Akathisia	0	10

[1] In addition to cisplatin, 68% of patients received other chemotherapy agents, including cyclophosphamide, etoposide, and fluorouracil.
[2] Visual analog scale assessment: 0 = not at all satisfied, 100 = totally satisfied.

Dolasetron vs metoclopramide – A randomized, double-blind trial compared single IV doses of dolasetron injection with metoclopramide in 226 (160 men and 66 women) adult cancer patients receiving ≥ 80 mg/m² cisplatin. In this study, dolasetron injection at a dose of 1.8 mg/kg was significantly more effective than metoclopramide in the prevention of chemotherapy-induced nausea and vomiting. In a study

5-HT₃ Receptor Antagonists

of dolasetron in 309 patients (96 men and 213 women) receiving moderately emetogenic chemotherapy such as cyclophosphamide-based regimens, a single 1.8 mg/kg IV dose of dolasetron was equivalent to metoclopramide administered as a 2 mg/kg IV bolus followed by 3 mg/kg IV over 8 hours. Complete response rates were 63% and 52%, respectively.

Contraindications

Hypersensitivity to the drug or components of the product; markedly prolonged QTc or atrioventricular block II to III (**dolasetron**) (see Warnings); patients receiving class I or III antiarrhythmic agents (**dolasetron**) (see Warnings).

Warnings

▶*Postoperatively:* Routine prophylaxis is not recommended for patients in whom there is little expectation that nausea or vomiting will occur postoperatively. In patients in whom nausea or vomiting must be avoided postoperatively, IV **ondansetron** is recommended even when the incidence of postoperative nausea or vomiting is low. For patients who have postoperative nausea or vomiting, ondansetron may be given to prevent further episodes.

▶*Cardiac effects:* Acute, usually reversible, ECG changes (PR and QTc prolongation; QRS widening) caused by **dolasetron** have been observed in healthy volunteers and controlled clinical trials. The active metabolites of dolasetron may block sodium channels, a property unrelated to its ability to block 5-HT₃ receptors. QTc prolongation is primarily caused by QRS widening. Dolasetron appears to prolong both depolarization and, to a lesser extent, repolarization time. The magnitude and frequency of the ECG changes increased with dose (related to peak plasma concentrations of hydrodolasetron but not the parent compound). These ECG interval prolongations usually returned to baseline within 6 to 8 hours, but in some patients were present at 24-hour follow up.

Administer dolasetron with caution in patients who have or may develop prolongation of cardiac conduction intervals, particularly QTc. These include patients with hypokalemia or hypomagnesemia, patients taking diuretics with the potential for inducing electrolyte abnormalities, patients with congenital QT syndrome, patients taking antiarrhythmic drugs or other drugs that lead to QT prolongation, and cumulative high-dose anthracycline therapy.

▶*Peristalsis:* **Ondansetron** does not stimulate gastric or intestinal peristalsis. Do not use instead of nasogastric suction. Use in abdominal surgery may mask a progressive ileus or gastric distension.

▶*Hypersensitivity reactions:* Rare cases of hypersensitivity reactions, sometimes severe (eg, anaphylaxis, bronchospasm, shortness of breath, hypotension, shock, angioedema, urticaria, facial edema) have occurred. Refer to Management of Acute Hypersensitivity Reactions.

▶*Carcinogenesis:* Rats were treated orally with **granisetron** 1, 5, or 50 mg/kg/day (16, 81, and 405 times the recommended human clinical dose). There was a statistically significant increase in the incidence of hepatocellular carcinomas and adenomas. Treatment with granisetron 100 mg/kg/day (1622 times the recommended human dose) produced hepatocellular adenomas in male and female rats.

In a 24-month carcinogenicity study, there was a statistically significant increase in the incidence of combined hepatocellular adenomas and carcinomas in male mice treated with ≥ 150 mg/kg/day (≥ 6.8 times the recommended dose).

Granisetron produced a significant increase in UDS in HeLa cells in vitro and a significantly increased incidence of cells with polyploidy in an in vitro human lymphocyte chromosomal aberration test.

▶*Elderly:* Dosage adjustment is not needed in patients> 65 years of age. Prevention of nausea and vomiting in elderly patients was no different than in younger age groups.

▶*Pregnancy:* Category B. There are no adequate and well-controlled studies in pregnant women. Use during pregnancy only if the potential benefit justifies the potential risk to the fetus.

▶*Lactation:* **Ondansetron** is excreted in the breast milk of rats. It is not known whether 5-HT₃ antagonists are excreted in human breast milk. Exercise caution when 5-HT₃ antagonists are administered to a nursing woman.

▶*Children:*

Granisetron – Safety and efficacy of the injection in children < 2 years of age have not been established. See Administration and Dosage for use in children ≥ 2 years of age. Safety and efficacy of the oral doseform in children have not been established.

Ondansetron – Little information is available about dosage in children ≤ 3 years of age. See Administration and Dosage for use in children 4 to 18 years of age.

Dolasetron – Safety and efficacy in children < 2 years of age have not been established. See Administration and Dosage for use in children ≥ 2 years of age.

Precautions

▶*Benzyl alcohol:* Some of these products contain benzyl alcohol, which has been associated with a fatal "gasping syndrome" in premature infants.

Drug Interactions

Because 5-HT₃ antagonists are metabolized by hepatic cytochrome P450 enzymes, inducers or inhibitors of these enzymes may change the clearance and, hence, the half-life of 5-HT₃ antagonists. However, on the basis of available data, no dosage adjustment is recommended for patients on these drugs.

5-HT₃ Receptor Antagonist Drug Interactions			
Precipitant drug	Object drug*		Description
Atenolol	Dolasetron	↑	Clearance of hydrodolasetron decreased by ≈ 27% when dolasetron was administered IV concomitantly with atenolol.
Cimetidine	Dolasetron	↑	Blood levels of hydrodolasetron increased 24% when dolasetron was coadministered with cimetidine for 7 days.
Rifampin	Dolasetron	↓	Blood levels of hydrodolasetron decreased 28% with coadministration of rifampin for 7 days.
Rifampin	Ondansetron	↓	Plasma concentrations of ondansetron may be reduced, decreasing its antiemetic effect.

* ↑ = Object drug increased. ↓ = Object drug decreased.

▶*Drug/Food interactions:*

Granisetron – When a single dose of oral granisetron 10 mg was administered with food, AUC was decreased by 5% and C$_{max}$ increased by 30% in non-fasting healthy volunteers.

Ondansetron – The extent of absorption of oral ondansetron is significantly increased (≈ 17%) by food but is not believed to be clinically relevant. C$_{max}$ and T$_{max}$ are not significantly affected.

Adverse Reactions

5-HT₃ Receptor Antagonist Adverse Reactions[1] (%)			
Adverse event	Dolasetron	Granisetron	Ondansetron
Cardiovascular			
Hypertension	2.2 to 2.9	2	2.5
Bradycardia	4 to 5.1	-	-
Tachycardia	2.2 to 3	-	-
Hypotension	5.3	-	3 to 5
CNS			
Anxiety/Agitation	-	-	6
Dizziness	2.2 to 4.4	-	7
Drowsiness/Sedation	1.3 to 2.4[2]	-	8
Headache	7 to 24.3[2]	14 to 21	9 to 27[3,4]
Malaise/Fatigue	2.6 to 5.7	-	9 to 13
Chills/Shivering	1.3 to 2.2	5	7
GI			
Abdominal pain	3.2	6	3[3]
Constipation	-	18	6 to 9
Diarrhea	2.1 to 12.4	8	6
Xerostomia	-	-	2
Dyspepsia	2.2 to 3	-	-
Miscellaneous			
Asthenia	-	14	-
Cold sensation	-	-	2
Fever/Pyrexia	3.5 to 4.3	-	2 to 8
Gynecological disorder	-	-	7
Hypoxia	-	-	9
Injection site reaction	-	-	4
Paresthesia	-	-	2
Pruritus	3.1	-	2 to 5
Urinary retention	2[2]	-	5
Weakness	-	-	2[3]
Increase in AST and ALT	3.6	3.4	3.4
Pain	0 to 3.1	2	2
Oliguria	2.6	-	-

[1] Greater than placebo or comparator regardless of route of administration or indication. Data from separate studies; not necessarily comparable.
[2] More common in placebo.
[3] More common with PO tid vs bid dosing.
[4] More common with single high dose IV.

▶*Cardiovascular:*

Ondansetron – Arrhythmias (6%); hypotension (3% to 5%); chest pain (2%); angina, syncope (rare).

Granisetron – Hypertension (2%); angina, arrhythmias, syncope (rare).

Dolasetron – Hypotension; edema, peripheral edema, mobitz I AV block, chest pain, orthostatic hypotension, myocardial ischemia, syncope, severe bradycardia, palpitations, peripheral ischemia, thrombophlebitis/phlebitis (rare); bradycardia; tachycardia; T-wave change; ST-T wave change; sinus arrhythmia; extrasystole (APCs or VPCs); poor R-wave progression; bundle branch block (left and right); nodal arrhythmia; U wave change; atrial flutter/fibrillation. (See Warnings).

➤*CNS:*

Ondansetron – Extrapyramidal syndrome (6%); grand mal seizures (rare).

Granisetron – CNS stimulation; somnolence (3% to 5%); insomnia (< 2% to 3%); extrapyramidal syndrome (rare).

Dolasetron – Flushing; vertigo; paresthesia; tremor; agitation; sleep disorder; depersonalization; ataxia, twitching, confusion, anxiety, abnormal dreaming (rare).

➤*Dermatologic:*

Dolasetron – Rash; increased sweating.

➤*GI:*

Granisetron – Nausea (15%); vomiting (9%); decreased appetite (5%); taste disorder (2%).

Dolasetron – Constipation; dyspepsia; abdominal pain; anorexia; pancreatitis (rare).

➤*GU:*

Dolasetron – Dysuria, polyuria, acute renal failure (rare).

➤*Hematologic:*

Granisetron – Leukopenia (11%); anemia (4%); thrombocytopenia (3%).

Dolasetron – Hematuria, epistaxis, prolonged prothrombin time, PTT increased, anemia, purpura/hematoma, thrombocytopenia (rare).

Ondansetron – Hypokalemia (rare).

➤*Hepatic:*

Dolasetron – Transient increases in AST and ALT (< 1%); hyperbilirubinemia, increased GGT (rare).

➤*Hypersensitivity:*

Dolasetron – Anaphylactic reaction, facial edema, urticaria (rare).

➤*Lab test abnormalities:*

Dolasetron – Transient increases in AST or ALT values have been reported as adverse events in < 1% of adult patients receiving dolasetron in clinical trials. The increases did not appear to be related to

dose or duration of therapy nor associated with symptomatic hepatic disease.

➤*Metabolic/Nutritional:*

Dolasetron – Increased alkaline phosphatase (rare).

➤*Musculoskeletal:*

Ondansetron – Musculoskeletal pain (10%).

Dolasetron – Myalgia, arthralgia (rare).

➤*Respiratory:*

Ondansetron – Bronchospasm (rare).

Dolasetron – Dyspnea, bronchospasm (rare).

➤*Special senses:*

Ondansetron – Transient blurred vision (rare).

Dolasetron – Taste perversion; abnormal vision; tinnitus, photophobia (rare).

➤*Miscellaneous:*

Ondansetron – Wound problem (28%); shivers (7%); postoperative CO_2-related pain (2%); hypersensitivity (rare).

Granisetron – Shivers (5%); alopecia (3%); hypersensitivity (rare).

Overdosage

➤*Symptoms:* A 59-year-old man with metastatic melanoma developed severe hypotension and dizziness 40 minutes after receiving a 15-minute IV infusion of 1000 mg (13 mg/kg) of **dolasetron**.

"Sudden blindness" (amaurosis) of a 2- to 3-minute duration plus severe constipation occurred in one patient who was given a single 72 mg IV dose of **ondansetron**. Hypotension and faintness occurred in a patient who took 48 mg ondansetron orally. Following the infusion of a 32 mg dose of ondansetron over only a 4-minute period, a vasovagal episode with transient second-degree heart block was observed. In all instances, the events completely resolved. Individual doses as large as 145 mg and total daily dosages (3 doses) as large as 252 mg have been administered IV without significant adverse events. Overdosage of up to 38.5 mg **granisetron** injection has been reported without symptoms or with only the occurrence of a slight headache.

➤*Treatment:* Manage patients with appropriate supportive therapy. Following a suspected overdose of **dolasetron** injection, a patient found to have second-degree or higher AV conduction block should undergo cardiac telemetry monitoring. Refer to General Management of Acute Overdosage.

PALONOSETRON HCl

Rx	Aloxi (MGI Pharma)	Injection: 0.25 mg/5 mL (as base)	207.5 mg mannitol. In single-use vials.

For complete prescribing information, refer to the 5-HT₃ Receptor Antagonists group monograph.

Indications

➤*Antiemetic:* For the prevention of acute nausea and vomiting associated with initial and repeat courses of moderately and highly emetogenic cancer chemotherapy; for the prevention of delayed nausea and vomiting associated with initial and repeat courses of moderately emetogenic cancer chemotherapy.

Administration and Dosage

➤*Adults:* The recommended dosage of palonosetron is 0.25 mg administered as a single dose approximately 30 minutes before the start of chemotherapy. Repeated dosing of palonosetron within a 7-day interval is not recommended because the safety and efficacy of frequent (con-

secutive or alternate day) dosing in patients have not been evaluated.

➤*Children:* A recommended IV dosage has not been established for pediatric patients.

➤*Administration:* Infuse IV over 30 seconds. Palonosetron should not be mixed with other drugs. Flush the infusion line with normal saline before and after administration of palonosetron.

➤*Storage/Stability:* Visually inspect parenteral drug products for particulate matter and discoloration before administration whenever solution and container permit.

Store at controlled room temperature 20° to 25°C (68° to 77°F). Excursions permitted to 15° to 30°C (59° to 86°F). Protect from freezing and light.

DOLASETRON MESYLATE

Rx	Anzemet (Aventis)	Tablets: 50 mg	Lactose. (A 50). Pink. Film-coated. In 5s, blister-pack 5s, and UD 10s.
		100 mg	Lactose. (ANZEMET 100). Pink, oval. Film-coated. In 5s, blister-pack 5s, and UD 10s.
		Injection: 20 mg/mL	38.2 mg/mL mannitol. In single-use 0.625 mL amps, 0.625 mL fill in 2 mL *Carpuject*, single-use 5 mL vials, and 25 mL multi-dose vial.

For complete prescribing information, refer to the 5-HT₃ Receptor Antagonists group monograph.

Indications

➤*Antiemetic:* Prevention of nausea and vomiting associated with initial and repeat courses of emetogenic cancer chemotherapy, including high-dose cisplatin (injection only).

Prevention of postoperative nausea and vomiting. As with other antiemetics, routine prophylaxis is not recommended for patients in whom there is little expectation that nausea and/or vomiting will occur postoperatively. In patients where nausea and/or vomiting must be avoided postoperatively, dolasetron injection is recommended even where the incidence of postoperative nausea and/or vomiting is low.

Treatment of postoperative nausea and/or vomiting (injection only).

Administration and Dosage

➤*Approved by the FDA:* September 11, 1997.

Do not exceed the recommended dosage of dolasetron tablets or injection.

➤*Cardiac effects:* Administer dolasetron with caution in patients who have or may develop prolongation of cardiac conduction intervals, particularly QT$_c$. These include patients with hypokalemia or hypomagnesemia, patients taking diuretics with potential for inducing electrolyte abnormalities, patients with congenital QT syndrome, patients taking antiarrhythmic drugs or other drugs that lead to QT prolongation, and cumulative high-dose anthracycline therapy.

➤*Infusion rate:* Dolasetron injection can be infused IV as rapidly as 100 mg/30 seconds or diluted in a compatible IV solution to 50 mL and infused over a period of up to 15 minutes.

DOLASETRON MESYLATE

➤*Prevention of chemotherapy-induced nausea and vomiting:*

Tablets –

Adults: 100 mg within 1 hour before chemotherapy.

Children (2 to 16 years of age): 1.8 mg/kg within 1 hour before chemotherapy, up to a maximum of 100 mg.

IV –

Adults: 1.8 mg/kg as a single dose approximately 30 minutes before chemotherapy. Alternatively, for most patients a fixed dose of 100 mg can be administered over 30 seconds.

Children (2 to 16 years of age): 1.8 mg/kg as a single dose approximately 30 minutes before chemotherapy, up to a maximum of 100 mg.

Extemporaneous oral solution – Dolasetron injection mixed in apple or apple-grape juice may be used for oral dosing in pediatric patients 2 to 16 years of age at 1.8 mg/kg up to a maximum of 100 mg, given within 1 hour before chemotherapy. The diluted product may be kept up to 2 hours at room temperature before use.

➤*Prevention / Treatment of postoperative nausea or vomiting:*

Tablets (prevention only) –

Adults: 100 mg within 2 hours before surgery.

Children (2 to 16 years of age): 1.2 mg/kg within 2 hours before surgery, up to a maximum of 100 mg.

IV (prevention / treatment) –

Adults: 12.5 mg as a single dose approximately 15 minutes before the cessation of anesthesia or as soon as nausea or vomiting presents.

Children (2 to 16 years of age): 0.35 mg/kg as a single dose approximately 15 minutes before the cessation of anesthesia or as soon as nausea or vomiting presents, up to a maximum of 12.5 mg.

Extemporaneous oral solution – Dolasetron injection mixed in apple or apple-grape juice may be used for oral dosing of pediatric patients. When dolasetron injection is administered orally, the recommended oral dosage in pediatric patients 2 to 16 years of age is 1.2 mg/kg up to a maximum 100 mg dose given within 2 hours before surgery. The diluted product may be kept up to 2 hours at room temperature before use.

➤*Admixture compatibility:* Dolasetron is compatible with 0.9% sodium chloride, 5% dextrose, 5% dextrose and 0.45% sodium chloride, 5% dextrose and lactated Ringer's injection, lactated Ringer's injection, and 10% mannitol injection.

Do not mix injection with other drugs. Flush the infusion line before and after administration of dolasetron injection.

➤*Storage / Stability:*

Tablets – Store at 20° to 25°C (68° to 77°F); protect from light.

IV – Store at 20° to 25°C (68° to 77°F) with excursions permitted to 15° to 30°C (59° to 86°F). Protect from light. After dilution, dolasetron injection is stable under normal lighting conditions at room temperature for 24 hours or under refrigeration for 48 hours.

GRANISETRON HCl

Rx	Kytril (Roche)	Tablets: 1 mg (1.12 mg as HCl)	Lactose. (K1). White, triangular. Film-coated. In SUP 20s and unit-of-use 2s.
		Oral solution: 1 mg/5 mL (1.12 mg/5 mL as HCl)	Sorbitol. Orange flavor. In 30 mL.
		Injection: 1 mg/mL (1.12 mg/mL as HCl)	*Single dose:* Preservative-free. 9 mg sodium chloride. In 1 mL vial. *Multidose:* 9 mg sodium chloride, 10 mg benzyl alcohol/1 mL. In 4 mL vial.

For additional information, refer to the 5-HT₃ Receptor Antagonists group monograph.

Indications

➤*Antiemetic:* Prevention of nausea and/or vomiting associated with initial and repeat courses of emetogenic cancer therapy, including high-dose cisplatin.

Nausea and vomiting associated with radiation, including total body irradiation and fractionated abdominal radiation (oral only).

➤*Postoperative nausea and vomiting (injection only):* Prevention and treatment of postoperative nausea and vomiting.

Routine prophylaxis is not recommended in patients in whom there is little expectation that nausea and/or vomiting will occur postoperatively. In patients where nausea and/or vomiting must be avoided during the postoperative period, granisetron injection is recommended even where the incidence of postoperative nausea and/or vomiting is low.

Administration and Dosage

➤*Approved by the FDA:* March 11, 1994 (injection); March 16, 1995 (oral).

➤*Oral:*

Emetogenic chemotherapy – Adult dosage of 2 mg once daily or 1 mg twice daily. In the 2 mg once-daily regimen, two 1 mg tablets or 10 mL of oral solution are given up to 1 hour before chemotherapy. In the 1 mg twice-daily regimen, give the first 1 mg tablet or 1 teaspoonful (5 mL) of oral solution up to 1 hour before chemotherapy and the second tablet or second teaspoonful (5 mL) oral solution 12 hours after the first. Either regimen is administered only on the day(s) chemotherapy is given. Continued treatment while not on chemotherapy has not been found to be useful.

Radiation (total body irradiation or fractionated abdominal radiation) – Adult dose of 2 mg once daily. Two 1 mg tablets or 10 mL of oral solution are taken within 1 hour of radiation.

➤*IV:*

Prevention of chemotherapy-induced nausea and vomiting –

Adults and children 2 years of age or older: 10 mcg/kg administered IV within 30 minutes before initiation of chemotherapy, and only on the day(s) chemotherapy is given.

Infusion preparation: May be administered IV either undiluted over 30 seconds or diluted with 0.9% sodium chloride or 5% dextrose and infused over 5 minutes.

As a general precaution, do not mix solution with other drugs.

Prevention and treatment of postoperative nausea and vomiting –

Adults:

• *Prevention –* 1 mg undiluted granisetron, administered IV over 30 seconds, before induction of anesthesia or immediately before reversal of anesthesia.

• *Treatment –* After surgery, 1 mg undiluted granisetron administered IV over 30 seconds.

➤*Storage / Stability:*

IV – Prepare IV granisetron infusion at the time of administration. However, granisetron is stable for at least 24 hours when diluted in 0.9% sodium chloride or 5% dextrose and stored at room temperature under normal lighting conditions. Once the multidose vial is penetrated, use its contents within 30 days.

Store single-dose and multidose vials at 25°C (77°F); excursions permitted to 15° to 30°C (59° to 86°F). Do not freeze vials. Protect from light.

Oral – Keep tightly closed. Protect from light.

Tablets: Store between 15° to 30°C (59° to 86°F).

Oral solution: Store at 25°C (77°F); excursions permitted to 15° to 30°C (59° to 86°F). Store bottle in an upright position.

5-HT₃ Receptor Antagonists

ONDANSETRON HCl

Rx	Zofran (GlaxoSmithKline)	**Tablets:** 4 mg (as HCl dihydrate)	Lactose. (Zofran 4). White, oval. Film-coated. In 30s, UD 100s, and 1 × 3 daily UD packs.
		8 mg (as HCl dihydrate)	Lactose. (Zofran 8). Yellow, oval. Film-coated. In 30s, UD 100s, and 1 × 3 daily UD packs.
		24 mg (as HCl dihydrate)	Lactose. (GX CF7/24). Pink, oval. Film-coated. In 1 × 1 daily UD packs.
		Solution, oral: 4 mg/5 mL (5 mg as HCl dihydrate)	Sorbitol. Strawberry flavor. In 50 mL bottles.
		Injection: 2 mg/mL (as HCl dihydrate)	Parabens. In 2 mL single-dose vials and 20 mL multidose vials (singles).
		32 mg/50 mL (as HCl dihydrate) (premixed)	Preservative-free. 2500 mg dextrose, 26 mg citric acid, and 11.5 mg sodium citrate/50 mL. In 50 mL single-dose containers.
Rx	Zofran ODT (GlaxoSmithKline)	**Tablets, orally disintegrating:** 4 mg (as base)	< 0.03 mg phenylalanine, aspartame, mannitol, parabens. (Z4). White. Strawberry flavor. In UD 30s.
		8 mg (as base)	< 0.03 mg phenylalanine, aspartame, mannitol, parabens. (Z8). White. Strawberry flavor. In UD 10s and 30s.

For complete prescribing information, refer to the 5-HT₃ Receptor Antagonists group monograph.

Indications

▶*Antiemetic:* Prevention of nausea and vomiting associated with initial and repeat courses of emetogenic cancer chemotherapy, including high-dose cisplatin; prevention of postoperative nausea or vomiting; prevention of nausea and vomiting associated with radiotherapy in patients receiving total body irradiation, single high-dose fraction to the abdomen, or daily fractions to the abdomen (oral); prevention of nausea and vomiting associated with highly emetogenic cancer chemotherapy, including cisplatin ≥ 50 mg/m² (oral).

▶*Unlabeled uses:* Treatment of nausea and vomiting associated with acetaminophen poisoning.

Treatment of acute levodopa-induced psychosis (visual hallucinations).

Nausea and vomiting caused by prostacyclin therapy.

Reduction in bulimic episodes in patients with bulimia nervosa.

Potential benefit in patients with social anxiety disorder.

Treatment of spinal or epidural morphine-induced pruritus.

Administration and Dosage

▶*Approved by the FDA:* December 31, 1992 (oral); January 29, 1999 (orally disintegrating).

▶*Prevention of nausea and vomiting associated with cancer chemotherapy:*

IV – Dilute vial with 50 mL of 5% dextrose or 0.9% NaCl injection before administration. Do not mix with solutions for which compatibility has not been established; in particular, this applies to alkaline solutions because a precipitate may form. Premixed ondansetron in flexible plastic containers does not require dilution.

The recommended IV dosage is three 0.15 mg/kg doses or a single 32 mg dose. With the 3-dose regimen, the first dose is infused over 15 minutes beginning 30 minutes before the start of emetogenic chemotherapy. Subsequent doses are administered 4 and 8 hours after the first dose. The single 32 mg dose is infused over 15 minutes, beginning 30 minutes before the start of emetogenic chemotherapy.

Children: On the basis of the limited available information, the dosage in children 4 to 18 years of age should be three 0.15 mg/kg doses (see above). Little dosing information is available for children ≤ 3 years of age.

Oral (moderately emetogenic cancer chemotherapy) – Recommended dose is 8 mg twice daily. Administer the first dose 30 minutes before the start of emetogenic chemotherapy, with a subsequent dose 8 hours after the first dose. Administer 8 mg twice daily (every 12 hours) for 1 to 2 days after completion of chemotherapy.

Children: For patients ≥ 12 years of age, dosage is the same as for adults; for children 4 to 11 years, give 4 mg 3 times/day. Give the first dose 30 minutes before chemotherapy, with subsequent doses 4 and 8 hours after the first dose. Give 4 mg 3 times/day (every 8 hours) for 1 to 2 days after completion of chemotherapy.

▶*Prevention of nausea and vomiting associated with radiotherapy (oral):* 8 mg 3 times/day.

Total body irradiation – 8 mg 1 to 2 hours before each fraction of radiotherapy administered each day.

Single high-dose fraction radiotherapy to the abdomen – 8 mg 1 to 2 hours before radiotherapy, with subsequent doses every 8 hours after the first dose for 1 to 2 days after completion of radiotherapy.

Daily fractionated radiotherapy to the abdomen – 8 mg 1 to 2 hours before radiotherapy, with subsequent doses every 8 hours after the first dose for each day radiotherapy is given.

Children – There is no experience with tablets or oral solution use in the prevention of radiation-induced nausea and vomiting in children.

▶*Prevention of postoperative nausea or vomiting:*

IV – Ondansetron injection requires no dilution for postoperative nausea and vomiting administration. Immediately before induction of anesthesia, or postoperatively if the patient experiences nausea or vomiting occurring shortly after surgery, administer 4 mg IV undiluted ≥ 30 seconds, preferably over 2 to 5 minutes. Alternatively, 4 mg undiluted may be administered IM as a single injection in adults. In patients who do not achieve adequate control of postoperative nausea and vomiting following a single, prophylactic, preinduction IV dose of ondansetron 4 mg, administration of a second IV dose of 4 mg ondansetron postoperatively does not provide additional control of nausea and vomiting.

Children: Patients 2 to 12 years of age weighing ≤ 40 kg may receive 0.1 mg/kg IV; give a single 4 mg dose for those weighing > 40 kg. Administer over ≥ 30 seconds, preferably over 2 to 5 minutes.

Oral – 16 mg given as a single dose 1 hour before induction of anesthesia.

Children: There is no experience in children with the use of tablets or oral solution in the prevention of postoperative nausea and vomiting.

▶*Prevention of nausea and vomiting associated with highly emetogenic cancer chemotherapy (oral):* The recommended adult oral dosage is 24 mg administered 30 minutes before the start of single-day highly emetogenic chemotherapy, including cisplatin ≥ 50 mg/m². Multi-day, single-dose administration of 24 mg has not been studied. Efficacy of the 32 mg single dose beyond 24 hours in these patients has not been established.

Children – There is no experience with the use of 24 mg tablets.

▶*Rectal suppositories:* Add pulverized ondansetron tablet powder into the melted fatty acid base and mix thoroughly. Pour the melt continuously into the suppository molds until all are filled. Store in light-resistant containers under refrigeration. Stability is reported to be ≥ 30 days. Extemporaneously compounded 16 mg suppositories have been shown to be equivalent to 8 mg tablets; women had higher AUCs.

▶*Solution:* Ondansetron tablets may be compounded extemporaneously with cherry syrup, *Syrpalta, Ora Sweet,* and *Ora Sweet Sugar-Free* to contain ondansetron 0.8 mg/mL (4 mg/5 mL). It is stable for 42 days at 4°C (39°F).

▶*Orally disintegrating tablets:* With dry hands, peel back foil backing from 1 blister, remove tablet, and immediately place on top of the tongue and swallow. Do not push tablet through foil backing. Administration with liquid is not necessary.

▶*Hepatic function impairment:* Do not exceed an 8 mg oral dose. For IV use, a single maximum daily dose of 8 mg infused over 15 minutes beginning 30 minutes before the start of emetogenic chemotherapy is recommended.

▶*Admixture compatibility:* Ondansetron 0.03 and 0.3 mg/mL has been reported to be stable in a total parenteral nutritional admixture (333 mL of 15% amino acids, 500 mL of 70% dextrose, 400 mL of 20% lipids, common therapeutic doses of vitamins and minerals) at 24°C (75°F) for > 48 hours. Ondansetron and dexamethasone sodium phosphate in 5% dextrose injection or 0.9% sodium chloride injection is stable for up to 24 hours when stored at room temperature at 23° to 25°C (73° to 77°F) in PVC bags or glass bottles. Admixtures containing lorazepam, ondansetron, and dexamethasone sodium phosphate in 5% dextrose injection are stable for up to 24 hours at room temperature when stored in glass bottles. Stability of an ondansetron/cisplatin continuous IV infusion combination has been reported to be 7 days when stored under refrigeration at 2° to 8°C (36° to 46°F) for ≥ 24 hours. Admixtures of 0.9% sodium chloride injection, ondansetron 0.1 and 1 mg/mL plus morphine sulfate 1 mg/mL or hydromorphone HCl 0.5 mg/mL are compatible and stable for > 7 days at 32°C (90°F) and for ≥ 31 days at 4° and 22°C (39° and 71°F). Ondansetron 0.05 mg/mL and cyclophosphamide 0.3 mg/mL are stable in 5% dextrose injection or 0.9% sodium chloride injection for 4 days at 23° to 25°C (73° to 77°F) or for 8 days at 4°C (39°F).

In plastic syringes, ondansetron 1.33 mg/mL and **neostigmine, naloxone, midazolam, fentanyl, alfentanil, atropine, morphine,** and **meperidine** are stable for 24 hours at 23° and 4°C (73° and 39°F). Ondansetron 1 mg/mL and **metoclopramide** and **glycopyrrolate** are also stable in plastic syringes for 24 hours at 23° and 4°C (73° and 39°F). Ondansetron 1 mg/mL with **droperidol** 1.25 mg/mL is stable for

ONDANSETRON HCl

≤ 8 hours at ambient temperature. **Propofol** 1 and 5 mg/mL are stable for 4 hours in admixtures with ondansetron 1 mg/mL.

➤*Y-site compatibility:* Ranitidine 0.5 or 2 mg/mL may be administered through a Y-injection port with ondansetron 0.03, 0.1, or 0.3 mg/mL for up to 4 hours. Ondansetron with fluconazole, aztreonam, ceftazidime, or cefazolin are compatible for 4 hours under simulated Y-site conditions.

➤*Storage / Stability:*
Parenteral – Ondansetron IV is stable at room temperature under normal lighting conditions for 48 hours after dilution with the following IV fluids: 0.9% sodium chloride injection; 5% dextrose injection; 5% dextrose and 0.9% sodium chloride injection; 5% dextrose and 0.45% sodium chloride injection; 3% sodium chloride injection.

When stored in polypropylene syringes, ondansetron 2 mg/mL undiluted or concentrations of 0.25, 0.5, or 1 mg/mL is reported to be stable for 3 months at -20°C (-4°F), 14 days at 4°C (39°F), and 48 hours at 22° to 25°C (71° to 77°F).

ALOSETRON HCl

Rx	**Lotronex** (GlaxoSmithKline)	**Tablets:** 0.562 mg (equivalent to 0.5 mg alosetron base)	(GX EX1). White, oval. Film-coated. In 30s.
		1.124 mg (equivalent to 1 mg alosetron base)	Lactose. (GX CT1). Blue, oval. Film-coated. In 30s.

For complete prescribing information refer to the 5-HT$_3$ Receptor Antagonists group monograph.

WARNING

Serious GI adverse events, some fatal, have been reported with the use of alosetron. These events, including ischemic colitis and serious complications of constipation, have resulted in hospitalization, blood transfusion, surgery, and death.

- Only physicians who have enrolled in GlaxoSmithKline's Prescribing Program for *Lotronex*, based on their attestation of qualifications and acceptance of responsibilities, should prescribe alosetron (see Administration and Dosage).
- Alosetron is indicated only for women with severe diarrhea-predominant irritable bowel syndrome (IBS) who have failed to respond to conventional therapy (see Indications). Less than 5% of IBS is considered severe. Before receiving the initial prescription for alosetron, the patient must read and sign the Patient-Physician Agreement.
- Discontinue Alosetron immediately in patients who develop constipation or symptoms of ischemic colitis. Physicians should instruct patients to immediately report constipation or symptoms of ischemic colitis. Do not resume Alosetron in patients who develop ischemic colitis. Physicians should instruct patients who report constipation to immediately contact them if the constipation does not resolve after discontinuation of alosetron. Patients with resolved constipation should resume alosetron only on the advice of their treating physician.

Indications

➤*Irritable bowel syndrome:* Because of serious GI adverse events, some fatal, reported with the use of this drug, alosetron is indicated only for women with severe diarrhea-predominant irritable bowel syndrome (IBS) who have the following:
- Chronic IBS symptoms (generally lasting 6 months or longer),
- had anatomic or biochemical abnormalities of the GI tract excluded, and
- failed to respond to conventional therapy.

Diarrhea-predominant IBS is severe if it includes diarrhea and 1 or more of the following:
- Frequent and severe abdominal pain/discomfort,
- frequent bowel urgency or fecal incontinence,
- disability or restriction of daily activities because of IBS.

Less than 5% of IBS is considered severe.

The safety and efficacy of alosetron HCl in men have not been established.

Administration and Dosage

➤*Approved by the FDA:* February 9, 2000.

For safety reasons, alosetron is approved with marketing restrictions. Only physicians who attest to the following qualifications and accept the following responsibilities, and on that basis enroll in the GlaxoSmithKline Prescribing Program for *Lotronex*, should prescribe alosetron. Physicians must attest that they are able and willing to:
- Diagnose and treat IBS,
- diagnose and manage ischemic colitis,
- diagnose and manage constipation and complications of constipation,
- understand the risks and benefits of treatment with alosetron for severe diarrhea-predominant IBS, including the information in the package insert, Medication Guide, and Patient-Physician Agreement,
- educate patients on the risks and benefits of treatment with alosetron and obtain the patient's signature on the Patient-Physician Agreement form, sign it, place the original signed form in the patient's medical record, and give a copy to the patient,

- report serious adverse events to GlaxoSmithKline at (888) 825-5249 or to the Food and Drug Administration's MedWatch Program at (800) FDA-1088.
- affix program stickers to all prescriptions for alosetron (ie, the original and all subsequent refill prescriptions). Stickers will be provided as part of the GlaxoSmithKline Prescribing Program for *Lotronex*. No telephone, facsimile, or computerized prescriptions are permitted with this program.

To enroll in the Prescribing Program for *Lotronex*, call (888) 825-5249 or visit http://www.lotronex.com.

➤*Usual adult dose:* For safety reasons, start alosetron at a dosage of 1 mg orally once daily for 4 weeks. This dosage may be less constipating than a regimen of 1 mg twice daily. If, after 4 weeks, the 1 mg once daily dosage is well tolerated but does not adequately control IBS symptoms, then the dosage can be increased to 1 mg twice daily. Although the efficacy of the 1 mg once daily dosage in treating diarrhea-predominant IBS has not been evaluated in clinical trials, for safety reasons give consideration to continuing this dosage if well tolerated and IBS symptoms in the individual patient are adequately controlled. Discontinue alosetron in patients who have not had adequate control of IBS symptoms after 4 weeks of treatment with 1 mg twice daily. Alosetron can be taken with or without food.

Discontinue alosetron immediately in patients who develop constipation or signs of ischemic colitis. Do not restart alosetron in patients who develop ischemic colitis.

Clinical trial and postmarketing experience suggest that debilitated patients or patients taking additional medications that decrease GI motility may be at greater risk of serious complications of constipation. Therefore, exercise appropriate caution and follow-up if alosetron is prescribed for these patients (see also Elderly).

➤*Children:* Safety and effectiveness have not been established in pediatric patients.

➤*Elderly:* Postmarketing experience suggests that elderly patients may be at greater risk for complications of constipation; therefore, exercise appropriate caution and follow-up if alosetron is prescribed for these patients.

➤*Renal function impairment:* There are insufficient data available on the biological activity of the metabolites of alosetron. It is unknown if dosage adjustment is needed in patients with renal impairment.

➤*Hepatic function impairment:* No studies have been conducted in patients with hepatic function impairment. Alosetron is extensively metabolized by the liver and increased exposure to alosetron is likely to occur in patients with hepatic impairment. Increased drug exposure may increase the risk of serious adverse events. Use alosetron with caution in patients with hepatic impairment.

➤*Storage / Stability:* Store at 25°C (77°F); excursions permitted to 15° to 30°C (59° to 86°F).

Contraindications

Do not initiate alosetron in patients with constipation. Alosetron is contraindicated in the following patients:
- With a history of chronic or severe constipation or with a history of sequelae from constipation,
- with a history of intestinal obstruction, stricture, toxic megacolon, GI perforation, and/or adhesions,
- with a history of ischemic colitis, impaired intestinal circulation, thrombophlebitis, or hypercoagulable state,
- with current or a history of Crohns disease or ulcerative colitis,
- with active diverticulitis or a history of diverticulitis,
- who are unable to understand or comply with the Patient-Physician Agreement,
- with known hypersensitivity to any component of the product.

Miscellaneous

APREPITANT

Rx	**Emend** (Merck)	**Capsules:** 80 mg	Sucrose. (461 80 mg). White. In 30s and UD[1] 5s.
		125 mg	Sucrose. (462 125 mg). White/Pink. In 30s and UD[1] 5s.

[1] Unit of use tri-fold pack containing one 125 mg capsule and two 80 mg capsules.

Indications

➤*Antiemetic:* Aprepitant, in combination with other antiemetic agents, is indicated for the prevention of acute and delayed nausea and vomiting associated with initial and repeat courses of highly emetogenic cancer chemotherapy, including high-dose cisplatin.

Administration and Dosage

➤*Approved by the FDA:* March 26, 2003.

➤*Dosage regimen:* Aprepitant is given for 3 days as part of a regimen that includes a corticosteroid and a 5-HT$_3$ antagonist. The recommended dose of aprepitant is 125 mg orally 1 hour prior to chemotherapy treatment (day 1) and 80 mg once daily in the morning on days 2 and 3. Aprepitant has not been studied for the treatment of established nausea and vomiting. In clinical studies, the following regimen was used:

Aprepitant Dosage Regimen in Clinical Studies				
	Day 1	Day 2	Day 3	Day 4
Aprepitant[1]	125 mg	80 mg	80 mg	none
Dexamethasone[2]	12 mg orally	8 mg orally	8 mg orally	8 mg orally
Ondansetron[3]	32 mg IV	none	none	none

[1] Aprepitant was administered orally 1 hour prior to chemotherapy treatment on day 1 and in the morning on days 2 and 3.
[2] Dexamethasone was administered 30 minutes prior to chemotherapy treatment on day 1 and in the morning on days 2 through 4. The dose of dexamethasone was chosen to account for drug interactions.
[3] Ondansetron was administered 30 minutes prior to chemotherapy treatment on day 1.

Chronic continuous administration is not recommended. Aprepitant may be taken with or without food.

➤*Concomitant therapy:* The oral dexamethasone doses should be reduced by approximately 50% when coadministered with aprepitant.

The IV methylprednisolone dose should be reduced by approximately 25%, and the oral methylprednisolone dose should be reduced by approximately 50% when coadministered with aprepitant.

➤*Storage/Stability:* Store at 20° to 25° (68° to 77°F).

Actions

➤*Pharmacology:* Aprepitant is a selective high-affinity antagonist of human substance P/neurokinin 1 (NK$_1$) receptors. Aprepitant has little or no affinity for serotonin (5-HT$_3$), dopamine, and corticosteroid receptors, the targets of existing therapies for chemotherapy-induced nausea and vomiting (CINV).

Aprepitant has been shown in animal models to inhibit emesis induced by cytotoxic chemotherapeutic agents such as cisplatin, via central actions. Positron Emission Tomography (PET) studies with aprepitant have shown that it crosses the blood-brain barrier and occupies brain NK$_1$ receptors. Studies show that aprepitant augments the antiemetic activity of the 5-HT$_3$-receptor antagonist ondansetron and the corticosteroid dexamethasone and inhibits both the acute and delayed phases of cisplatin-induced emesis.

➤*Pharmacokinetics:*

Absorption – The mean absolute oral bioavailability of aprepitant is approximately 60% to 65% and the mean peak plasma concentration (C$_{max}$) of aprepitant occurred at approximately 4 hours (T$_{max}$).

The pharmacokinetics of aprepitant are nonlinear across the clinical dose range. In healthy young adults, the increase in AUC$_{0-\infty}$ was 26% greater than dose proportional between 80 and 125 mg single doses administered in the fed state.

Following oral administration of a single 125 mg dose of aprepitant on day 1 and 80 mg once daily on days 2 and 3, the AUC$_{0-24h}$ was approximately 19.6 mcg•h/mL and 21.2 mcg•h/mL on days 1 and 3, respectively. The C$_{max}$ of 1.6 mcg/mL and 1.4 mcg/mL were reached in approximately 4 hours (T$_{max}$) on days 1 and 3, respectively.

Distribution – Aprepitant is greater than 95% bound to plasma proteins. The mean apparent volume of distribution at steady state (Vd$_{ss}$) is approximately 70 L in humans.

Aprepitant crosses the placenta in rats and rabbits and crosses the blood-brain barrier in humans.

Metabolism – Aprepitant undergoes extensive metabolism. In vitro studies using human liver microsomes indicate that aprepitant is metabolized primarily by CYP3A4 with minor metabolism by CYP1A2 and CYP2C19. Metabolism is largely via oxidation at the morpholine ring and its side chains. No metabolism by CYP2D6, CYP2C9, or CYP2E1 was detected. In healthy young adults, aprepitant accounts for approximately 24% of the radioactivity in plasma over 72 hours following a single oral 300 mg dose of [14C]-aprepitant, indicating a substantial presence of metabolites in the plasma. Seven metabolites of

aprepitant, which are only weakly active, have been identified in human plasma.

Excretion – Following administration of a single IV 100 mg dose of [14C]-aprepitant prodrug to healthy subjects, 57% of the radioactivity was recovered in urine and 45% in feces. Aprepitant is eliminated primarily by metabolism; aprepitant is not renally excreted. The apparent plasma clearance of aprepitant ranged from approximately 62 to 90 mL/min. The apparent terminal half-life ranged from approximately 9 to 13 hours.

Special populations –

Gender: The C$_{max}$ for aprepitant is 16% higher in females as compared with males. The half-life of aprepitant is 25% lower in females as compared with males. No dosage adjustment is necessary.

Elderly: Following oral administration of a single 125 mg dose of aprepitant on day 1 and 80 mg once daily on days 2 through 5, the AUC$_{0-24h}$ of aprepitant was 21% higher on day 1 and 36% higher on day 5 in elderly (65 years of age and older) relative to younger adults. The C$_{max}$ was 10% higher on day 1 and 24% higher on day 5 in elderly relative to younger adults. No dosage adjustment is necessary.

Race: Following oral administration of a single 125 mg dose of aprepitant, the AUC$_{0-24h}$ is approximately 25% and 29% higher in Hispanics as compared with whites and blacks, respectively. The C$_{max}$ is 22% and 31% higher in Hispanics as compared with whites and blacks, respectively. No dosage adjustment is necessary.

Hepatic function impairment: Following administration of a single 125 mg dose of aprepitant on day 1 and 80 mg once daily on days 2 and 3 to patients with mild hepatic insufficiency (Child-Pugh score 5 to 6), the AUC$_{0-24h}$ of aprepitant was 11% lower on day 1 and 36% lower on day 3, as compared with healthy subjects given the same regimen. In patients with moderate hepatic insufficiency (Child-Pugh score 7 to 9), the AUC$_{0-24h}$ of aprepitant was 10% higher on day 1 and 18% higher on day 3, as compared with healthy subjects given the same regimen. No dosage adjustment for aprepitant is necessary in patients with mild to moderate hepatic insufficiency.

Renal function impairment: A single 240 mg dose of aprepitant was administered to patients with severe renal insufficiency (Ccr less than 30 mL/min) and to patients with end stage renal disease (ESRD) requiring hemodialysis. In patients with severe renal insufficiency, the AUC$_{0-\infty}$ of total aprepitant (unbound and protein bound) decreased by 21% and C$_{max}$ decreased by 32%, relative to healthy subjects. In patients with ESRD undergoing hemodialysis, the AUC$_{0-\infty}$ of total aprepitant decreased by 42% and C$_{max}$ decreased by 32%. Because of modest decreases in protein binding of aprepitant in patients with renal disease, the AUC of pharmacologically active unbound drug was not significantly affected in patients with renal insufficiency compared with healthy subjects. Hemodialysis conducted 4 or 48 hours after dosing had no significant effect on the pharmacokinetics of aprepitant; less than 0.2% of the dose was recovered in the dialysate. No dosage adjustment is necessary.

Contraindications

Aprepitant is a moderate CYP3A4 inhibitor. Aprepitant should not be used concurrently with pimozide or cisapride. Inhibition of cytochrome P450 isoenzyme 3A4 (CYP3A4) by aprepitant could result in elevated plasma concentrations of these drugs, potentially causing serious or life-threatening reactions. Aprepitant is contraindicated in patients who are hypersensitive to any component of the product.

Warnings

➤*Carcinogenesis:* Treatment with aprepitant at doses of 5 to 125 mg/kg twice per day produced thyroid follicular cell adenomas and carcinomas in male rats. In female rats, it produced increased incidences of hepatocellular adenoma at 25 and 125 mg/kg twice daily, and thyroid follicular adenoma at the 125 mg/kg twice daily dose. Treatment with aprepitant produced skin fibrosarcomas in male mice in 125 and 500 mg/kg/day doses.

➤*Pregnancy:* Category B. There are no adequate and well-controlled studies in pregnant women. Use during pregnancy only if clearly needed.

➤*Lactation:* Aprepitant is excreted in the milk of rats. It is not known whether this drug is excreted in human milk. Because many drugs are excreted in human milk and because of the potential for possible serious adverse reactions in nursing infants from aprepitant and because of the potential for tumorigenicity shown for aprepitant in rodent carcinogenicity studies, a decision should be made whether to discontinue nursing or to discontinue the drug, taking into account the importance of the drug to the mother.

➤*Children:* Safety and efficacy of aprepitant in children have not been established.

Precautions

➤*Long-term therapy:* Chronic continuous use of aprepitant for prevention of nausea and vomiting is not recommended because it has not

APREPITANT

been studied and because the drug interaction profile may change during chronic continuous use.

Drug Interactions

➤*CYP450:* Aprepitant is a substrate, a moderate inhibitor, and an inducer of CYP3A4. Aprepitant is also an inducer of CYP2C9. Use aprepitant with caution in patients receiving concomitant medicinal products, including chemotherapy agents that are primarily metabolized through CYP3A4. Inhibition of CYP3A4 by aprepitant could result in elevated plasma concentrations of these concomitant medicinal products. The effect of aprepitant on the pharmacokinetics of orally administered CYP3A4 substrates is expected to be greater than the effect of aprepitant on the pharmacokinetics of IV administered CYP3A4 substrates.

Chemotherapy agents that are known to be metabolized by CYP3A4 include docetaxel, paclitaxel, etoposide, irinotecan, ifosfamide, imatinib, vinorelbine, vinblastine, and vincristine. In clinical studies, aprepitant was administered commonly with etoposide, vinorelbine, or paclitaxel. The doses of these agents were not adjusted to account for potential drug interactions.

Because of the small number of patients in clinical studies who received the CYP3A4 substrates docetaxel, vinblastine, vincristine, or ifosfamide, particular caution and careful monitoring are advised in patients receiving these agents or other chemotherapy agents metabolized primarily by CYP3A4 that were not studied.

Aprepitant Drug Interactions

Precipitant Drug	Object drug*		Description
CYP3A4 inhibitors (eg, ketoconazole, itraconazole, nefazodone, troleandomycin, clarithromycin, ritonavir, nelfinavir, diltiazem)	Aprepitant	↑	Concurrent use may increase aprepitant plasma concentrations. Use with caution.
CYP3A4 inducers (eg, rifampin, carbamazepine, phenytoin)	Aprepitant	↓	Coadministration may decrease aprepitant plasma concentrations.
Paroxetine	Aprepitant	↓	Concurrent use decreased the AUC by ≈ 25% and C$_{max}$ by ≈ 20% of both aprepitant and paroxetine.
Aprepitant	Paroxetine		
Aprepitant	CYP2C9 substrates (eg, warfarin, tolbutamide, phenytoin)	↓	Aprepitant is a CYP2C9 inducer and has been shown to induce the metabolism of warfarin and tolbutamide, resulting in lower plasma levels. In patients on chronic warfarin therapy, closely monitor the INR in the 2-week period, particularly at 7 to 10 days, following the initiation of aprepitant.
Aprepitant	CYP3A4 substrates (eg, pimozide, cisapride, dexamethasone, methylprednisolone, midazolam, alprazolam, triazolam, docetaxel, paclitaxel, etoposide, irinotecan, ifosfamide, imatinib, vinorelbine, vinblastine, vincristine)	↑	Aprepitant is a moderate inhibitor of CYP3A4 and can increase plasma concentrations of coadministered products that are metabolized through CYP3A4. Aprepitant is contraindicated with pimozide or cisapride (see Contraindications). The dexamethasone dose should be reduced ≈ 50% when given with aprepitant. The dose of IV methylprednisolone should be reduced ≈ 25% and the oral dose reduced ≈ 50% when given with aprepitant.
Aprepitant	Contraceptives, oral	↓	The efficacy of oral contraceptives may be reduced. Alternative or back-up methods of contraception are recommended.

* ↓ = Object drug decreased. ↑ = Object drug increased.

Adverse Reactions

Aprepitant Adverse Reactions in CINV Phase III Studies (Cycle 1) (≥ 3%)

	Aprepitant regimen (N = 544)	Standard therapy (N = 550)
CNS		
Dizziness	6.6	4.4
Headache	8.5	8.7
Insomnia	2.9	3.1

Aprepitant Adverse Reactions in CINV Phase III Studies (Cycle 1) (≥ 3%)

	Aprepitant regimen (N = 544)	Standard therapy (N = 550)
GI		
Abdominal pain	4.6	3.3
Anorexia	10.1	9.5
Constipation	10.3	12.2
Diarrhea	10.3	7.5
Epigastric discomfort	4	3.1
Gastritis	4.2	3.1
Heartburn	5.3	4.9
Nausea	12.7	11.8
Vomiting	7.5	7.6
Lab test abnormalities		
ALT increased	6	4.3
AST increased	3	1.3
Blood urea nitrogen increased	4.7	3.5
Serum creatine increased	3.7	4.3
Proteinuria	6.8	5.3
Miscellaneous		
Asthenia/fatigue	17.8	11.8
Dehydration	5.9	5.1
Fever	2.9	3.5
Hiccups	10.8	5.6
Mucous membrane disorder	2.6	3.1
Neutropenia	3.1	2.9
Tinnitus	3.7	3.8

The following additional clinical adverse experiences (incidence > 0.5% and greater than standard therapy), regardless of causality, were reported in patients treated with aprepitant regimen.

➤*Cardiovascular:* Bradycardia; deep venous thrombosis; hypertension; hypotension; myocardial infarction; pulmonary embolism; tachycardia.

➤*CNS:* Anxiety disorder; confusion; depression; disorientation; peripheral neuropathy; sensory neuropathy.

➤*Dermatologic:* Alopecia; diaphoresis; flushing; rash.

➤*GI:* Acid reflux; deglutition disorder; dysgeusia; dyspepsia; dysphagia; flatulence; obstipation; perforating duodenal ulcer; salivation increased; taste disturbance.

➤*GU:* Dysuria; renal insufficiency.

➤*Hematologic:* Anemia; febrile neutropenia; thrombocytopenia.

➤*Lab test abnormalities:* Alkaline phosphatase increased; hyperglycemia; hyponatremia; leukocytes increased; erythrocyturia; leukocyturia.

The adverse experiences of increased AST and ALT were generally mild and transient.

➤*Metabolic/Nutritional:* Appetite decreased; edema; hypokalemia; weight loss.

➤*Musculoskeletal:* Muscular weakness; musculoskeletal pain; myalgia.

➤*Respiratory:* Cough; dyspnea; lower respiratory infection; nasal secretion; pharyngitis; pneumonitis; respiratory insufficiency; upper respiratory infection.

➤*Miscellaneous:* Diabetes mellitus; malaise; malignant neoplasm; non-small cell lung carcinoma; pelvic pain; septic shock; vocal disturbance.

Stevens-Johnson syndrome was reported in a patient receiving aprepitant with cancer chemotherapy in another CINV study. Angiodema and urticaria were reported in a patient receiving aprepitant in a non-CINV study.

Overdosage

➤*Symptoms:* Single doses up to 600 mg of aprepitant were generally well tolerated in healthy subjects. Aprepitant was generally well tolerated when administered as 375 mg once daily for up to 42 days to patients in non-CINV studies. In 33 cancer patients, administration of a single 375 mg dose of aprepitant on day 1 and 250 mg once daily on days 2 to 5 was generally well tolerated. Drowsiness and headache were reported in one patient who ingested 1440 mg of aprepitant.

➤*Treatment:* In the event of overdose, discontinue use and provide general supportive treatment and monitoring. Because of the antiemetic activity of aprepitant, drug-induced emesis may not be effective.

Aprepitant cannot be removed by hemodialysis.

Miscellaneous

APREPITANT

Patient Information

Instruct patients to take aprepitant only as prescribed. Advise patients to take their first dose (125 mg) of aprepitant 1 hour prior to chemotherapy treatment.

Aprepitant may interact with some drugs including chemotherapy; therefore, advise patients to report to their doctor the use of any prescription, nonprescription medication, or herbal products.

Instruct patients on chronic warfarin therapy to have their clotting status closely monitored in the 2-week period, particularly at 7 to 10 days, following initiation of the 3-day regimen of aprepitant with each chemotherapy cycle.

Administration of aprepitant may reduce the efficacy of oral contraceptives. Advise patients to use alternative or back-up methods of contraception.

DRONABINOL

c-iii	**Marinol** (Unimed)	**Capsules, gelatin:**[1] 2.5 mg	Parabens. (RL). White. In 25s, 60s, and 100s.
		5 mg	Parabens. (RL). Brown. In 25s and 100s.
		10 mg	Parabens. (RL). Orange. In 25s and 60s.

[1] In sesame oil.

Refer to the general discussion of these products beginning in the Antiemetic/Antivertigo Agents monograph.

Indications

➤*Antiemetic:* Treatment of nausea and vomiting associated with cancer chemotherapy in patients not responding adequately to conventional antiemetic treatment.

➤*Appetite stimulation:* Treatment of anorexia associated with weight loss in AIDS patients.

Administration and Dosage

➤*Antiemetic:* Initially, give 5 mg/m^2 1 to 3 hours prior to the administration of chemotherapy, then every 2 to 4 hours after chemotherapy, for a total of 4 to 6 doses/day. If the 5 mg/m^2 dose is ineffective and there are no significant side effects, increase the dose by 2.5 mg/m^2 increments to a maximum of 15 mg/m^2 per dose. Use caution, as the incidence of disturbing psychiatric symptoms increases significantly at this maximum dose. Administration with phenothiazines (eg, prochlorperazine) may improve efficacy (vs either drug alone) without additional toxicity.

➤*Appetite stimulation:* Give 2.5 mg twice daily before lunch and supper. For patients who cannot tolerate 5 mg/day, reduce dosage to 2.5 mg/day as a single evening or bedtime dose. When adverse reactions are absent or minimal and further therapeutic effect is desired, increase to 2.5 mg before lunch and 5 mg before supper (or 5 mg at lunch and 5 mg after supper). Although most patients respond to 2.5 mg twice daily, 10 mg twice daily has been tolerated in ≈ 50% of patients. The dosage may be increased to a maximum of 20 mg/day in divided doses. Use caution in escalating the dosage because of the increased frequency of dose-related adverse reactions at higher dosages.

Actions

➤*Pharmacology:* Dronabinol is the principal psychoactive substance present in *Cannabis sativa* L (marijuana). Nontherapeutic effects of dronabinol are identical to those of marijuana and other centrally active cannabinoids (see Warnings). The mechanism of action is unknown.

Cannabinoids have complex CNS effects, including central sympathomimetic activity. Cannabinoid receptors have been discovered in neural tissues. These receptors may play a role in mediating the effects of dronabinol. Patients may experience mood changes (eg, euphoria, detachment, depression, anxiety, panic, paranoia), decrements in cognitive performance and memory, a decreased ability to control drives and impulses, and alterations of reality (eg, distortions in perception of objects and sense of time, hallucinations). These latter phenomena are more common with larger doses; however, a full-blown picture of psychosis (psychotic organic brain syndrome) may occur in patients receiving doses in the lower portion of the therapeutic range.

Dronabinol, within or slightly above the recommended dose range, increases heart rate and conjunctival injection. Blood pressure effects are inconsistent, but occasional subjects experience orthostatic hypotension or fainting upon standing. In 1 study, a slight but consistent decrease in oral temperature was recorded.

➤*Pharmacokinetics:*

Absorption/Distribution – Following oral administration, dronabinol is almost completely absorbed (90% to 95%). It has a systemic bioavailability of 10% to 20%, an onset of action of ≈ 0.5 to 1 hour, and peak effect at 2 to 4 hours. Duration of psychoactive effects is 4 to 6 hours, but the appetite-stimulant effect may continue for ≥ 24 hours after administration. Dronabinol has a large apparent volume of distribution, ≈ 10 L/kg, because of its lipid solubility. The plasma protein binding of dronabinol and its metabolites is ≈ 97%.

Metabolism/Excretion – Dronabinol undergoes extensive first-pass hepatic metabolism, primarily by microsomal hydroxylation, yielding both active and inactive metabolites. Dronabinol and its principal active metabolite, 11-OH-delta-9-THC, are present in approximately equal concentrations in plasma. Concentrations of both parent drug and metabolite peak at ≈ 2 to 4 hours after oral dosing and decline over several days.

The major route of elimination is biliary excretion. Within 72 hours after oral administration, ≈ 50% of dose is recovered in feces; 10% to 15% appears in urine; < 5% is excreted unchanged in urine. Low levels of dronabinol metabolites have been detected for > 5 weeks in the urine and feces following a single dose. The elimination phase of dronabinol exhibits biphasic kinetics with an alpha half-life of 4 hours and a terminal half-life of 25 to 36 hours. Extended use at recommended doses may cause accumulation of toxic amounts of dronabinol and metabolites.

➤*Clinical trials:*

Appetite stimulation – The initial dosage of dronabinol in all patients was 5 mg/day, given in doses of 2.5 mg 1 hour before lunch and 1 hour before supper. Early morning administration appeared to be associated with an increased frequency of adverse experiences, as compared with dosing later in the day. Side effects (eg, feeling high, dizziness, confusion, somnolence) occurred in 18% of patients at this dosage level; the dosage was reduced to 2.5 mg/day, administered as a single dose at supper or bedtime. Compared with placebo, dronabinol treatment resulted in a statistically significant improvement in appetite as measured by visual analog scale. Trends toward improved body weight and mood and decreases in nausea were also seen. After completing the 6-week study, patients were allowed to continue treatment with dronabinol when there was a sustained improvement in appetite.

Antiemetic – Dronabinol treatment of chemotherapy-induced emesis was evaluated in patients with cancer who received a total of 750 courses of treatment for various malignancies. The antiemetic efficacy was greatest in patients receiving cytotoxic therapy with MOPP for Hodgkin's and non-Hodgkin's lymphomas. Dosages ranged from 2.5 to 40 mg/day, administered in equally divided doses every 4 to 6 hours (4 times daily). Escalating the dose > 7 mg/m^2 increased the frequency of adverse experiences with no additional antiemetic benefit.

Combination antiemetic therapy with dronabinol and a phenothiazine (eg, prochlorperazine) may result in synergistic or additive antiemetic effects and attenuate the toxicities associated with each of the agents.

Contraindications

Hypersensitivity to dronabinol, marijuana, or sesame oil.

Warnings

➤*Tolerance:* Following 12 days of dronabinol, tolerance to the cardiovascular and subjective effects developed at doses up to 210 mg/day. An initial tachycardia induced by dronabinol was replaced successively by normal sinus rhythm and then bradycardia. A fall in supine blood pressure, made worse by standing, was also observed initially. Within days, these effects disappeared, indicating development of tolerance. However, tachyphylaxis and tolerance did not appear to develop to the appetite-stimulant effect. In AIDS patients, the appetite-stimulant effect was sustained for up to 5 months at doses of 2.5 to 20 mg/day.

➤*Patient supervision:* Because of individual variation, clinically determine the period of time the patient needs to be supervised. Closely observe patients within an inpatient setting, if possible. This is especially important during treatment of patients with no prior experience with *Cannabis* or dronabinol. However, even patients experienced with these agents may have serious untoward responses not predicted by prior uneventful exposures. Closely observe any patient who has a psychotic experience with dronabinol until the mental state returns to normal. Do not give additional doses until the patient has been examined and the circumstances evaluated. If the situation warrants, give a lower dose under very close supervision.

➤*Fertility impairment:* In rats, dronabinol doses of 30 to 150 mg/m^2 (0.3 to 1.5 times the maximum recommended human dose in cancer patients and 2 to 10 times that in AIDS patients) reduced ventral prostate, seminal vesicle, and epididymal weights and caused a decrease in seminal fluid volume. Spermatogenesis decreases, developing germ cell numbers, and a number of Leydig cells in the testis were also observed.

➤*Elderly:* Use caution because the elderly are generally more sensitive to the psychoactive effects. In antiemetic studies, no difference in tolerance or efficacy was apparent in patients > 55 years of age.

➤*Pregnancy: Category C.* In mice and rats, dronabinol decreased maternal weight gain and number of viable pups and increased fetal mortality and early resorptions. The dose-dependent effects were less

DRONABINOL

apparent at lower doses. There are no adequate and well-controlled studies in pregnant women. Use during pregnancy only if clearly needed.

➤*Lactation:* Dronabinol is concentrated and excreted in human breast milk, and is absorbed by the nursing baby. Because the effects of chronic exposure to the drug and its metabolites on the infant are unknown, nursing mothers should not use dronabinol.

➤*Children:* Not recommended for AIDS-related anorexia in children because it has not been studied in this population. Dosage for chemotherapy-induced emesis is the same as in adults. Use caution in children because of the psychoactive effects.

Precautions

➤*Hypertension or heart disease:* Use with caution as dronabinol may cause a general increase in central sympathomimetic activity.

➤*Psychiatric patients:* In manic, depressive, or schizophrenic patients, symptoms of these disease states may be exacerbated by the use of cannabinoids.

➤*Drug abuse and dependence:* Dronabinol is highly abusable. Limit prescriptions to the amount necessary for a single cycle of chemotherapy.

It is not known what proportion of individuals exposed chronically to these drugs will develop either psychological or physical dependence. Long-term use of cannabinoids has been associated with disorders of motivation, judgment, and cognition. It is not clear if this is a manifestation of the underlying personalities of chronic users of this class of drugs or if cannabinoids are directly responsible.

A withdrawal syndrome consisting of irritability, insomnia, and restlessness was observed in some subjects within 12 hours following abrupt withdrawal of dronabinol. The syndrome reached its peak intensity at 24 hours when subjects exhibited hot flashes, sweating, rhinorrhea, loose stools, hiccoughs, and anorexia. The syndrome was essentially complete within 96 hours. EEG changes following discontinuation were consistent with a withdrawal syndrome. Several subjects reported impressions of disturbed sleep for several weeks after discontinuing high doses.

➤*Hazardous tasks:* Because of its profound effects on mental status, warn patients not to drive, operate complex machinery, or engage in any activity requiring sound judgment and unimpaired coordination while receiving treatment. Effects may persist for a variable and unpredictable period of time. Dronabinol is highly lipid-soluble, and its metabolites may persist in tissues, including plasma, for days.

Drug Interactions

Some of the following drug interactions occurred following the use of marijuana. Although dronabinol has not been specifically cited in these instances, consider the possibility of a similar interaction.

Cannabinoid Drug Interactions			
Precipitant drug	Object drug*		Description
Dronabinol	Amphetamines Cocaine Sympathomimetics	↑	Additive hypertension, tachycardia, possibly cardiotoxicity, may occur.
Dronabinol	Anticholinergics Antihistamines	↑	Additive or super-additive tachycardia, or drowsiness may occur.
Dronabinol	Antidepressants, tricyclic	↑	Additive tachycardia, hypertension, or drowsiness may occur.
Dronabinol	Alcohol Sedatives Hypnotics Psychomimetics	↑	Additive or synergistic CNS effects may occur. Also, clearance of barbiturates may be decreased, possibly because of inhibition of metabolism.

Cannabinoid Drug Interactions			
Precipitant drug	Object drug*		Description
Cannabinoids	Disulfiram	↑	A reversible hypomanic reaction occurred in a patient who smoked marijuana; confirmed by rechallenge.
Cannabinoids	Fluoxetine	↑	A patient with depression and bulimia became hypomanic after smoking marijuana; symptoms resolved after 4 days.
Cannabinoids	Theophylline	↓	Increased theophylline metabolism was reported with marijuana smoking.

* ↑ = Object drug increased. ↓ = Object drug decreased.

Adverse Reactions

➤*Cardiovascular:* Palpitations, tachycardia, vasodilation (> 1%); conjunctivitis, hypotension (0.3% to 1%).

➤*CNS:* Euphoria (3% to 24%); dizziness, paranoid reaction, somnolence (3% to 10%); asthenia, amnesia, ataxia, confusion, depersonalization, hallucination, abnormal thinking (> 1%); depression, emotional lability, nightmares, speech difficulties, headache, anxiety/nervousness, tremors (< 1%).

➤*Dermatologic:* Flushing (0.3% to 1%); sweating (< 1%).

➤*GI:* Nausea, vomiting (3% to 10%); diarrhea (0.3% to 1%); fecal incontinence, anorexia, hepatic enzyme elevation (< 1%).

➤*Musculoskeletal:* Myalgias (< 1%).

➤*Special senses:* Vision difficulties (> 1%); tinnitus (< 1%).

➤*Respiratory:* Cough, rhinitis, sinusitis (< 1%).

Overdosage

➤*Symptoms:*

Mild intoxication – Drowsiness, euphoria, heightened sensory awareness, altered time perception, reddened conjunctiva, dry mouth, and tachycardia.

Moderate intoxication – Memory impairment, depersonalization, mood alteration, urinary retention, and reduced bowel motility.

Severe intoxication – Decreased motor coordination, lethargy, slurred speech, and postural hypotension.

Apprehensive patients may experience panic reactions, and seizures may occur in patients with existing seizure disorders.

The estimated lethal human dose of IV dronabinol is 30 mg/kg. Significant CNS symptoms in antiemetic studies followed oral doses of 0.4 mg/kg.

➤*Treatment:* Manage potentially serious oral ingestion, if recent, with gut decontamination. In unconscious patients with a secure airway, instill activated charcoal via a nasogastric tube. A saline cathartic or sorbitol may be added to the first dose of activated charcoal. Place patients experiencing depressive, hallucinatory, or psychotic reactions in a quiet area and offer reassurance. Benzodiazepines (5 to 10 mg oral diazepam) may be used for treatment of extreme agitation. Hypotension usually responds to Trendelenburg position and IV fluids. Pressors are rarely required. Refer to General Management of Acute Overdosage.

Patient Information

Avoid alcohol and barbiturates.

May cause dizziness or drowsiness; do not drive or perform hazardous tasks requiring alertness, coordination, or physical dexterity.

Apprise patients of possible changes in mood and other adverse behavioral effects of the drug so they will not panic in the event of such manifestations.

Patients should remain under the supervision of a responsible adult.

Miscellaneous

PHOSPHORATED CARBOHYDRATE SOLUTION

otc	**Emetrol** (Pharmacia & Upjohn)	**Solution:** 1.87 g dextrose, 1.87 g fructose, 21.5 mg phosphoric acid	Methylparaben. Lemon mint or cherry flavor. In 118, 236 and 473 ml.
otc	**Formula EM** (Major)		Methylparaben. Cherry flavor. In 118 ml.
otc	**Nausea Relief** (Zenith Goldline)		Methylparaben. In 118 ml.
otc	**Nausetrol** (Qualitest)	**Solution:** Dextrose, fructose and orthophosphoric acid with controlled hydrogen ion concentration	In 118, 473 and 3785 ml.

Refer to the general discussion beginning in the Antiemetic/Antivertigo Agents monograph.

Indications

➤*Antiemetic:* Relief of nausea caused by upset stomach from intestinal flu, stomach flu and food or drink indiscretions.

➤*Unlabeled uses:* Regurgitation in infants; morning sickness; motion sickness; nausea and vomiting caused by drug therapy or inhalation anesthesia.

Administration and Dosage

Do not dilute. Do not take oral fluids immediately before the dose or for at least 15 minutes after the dose.

➤*Nausea:* Dose may be repeated every 15 minutes until distress subsides. Do not take for > 1 hour or > 5 doses.

Children 2 to 12 years of age – 5 or 10 ml.

Adults – 15 or 30 ml.

➤*Regurgitation in infants:* 5 or 10 ml, 10 to 15 minutes before each feeding; in refractory cases, 10 or 15 ml, 30 minutes before feeding.

➤*Morning sickness:* 15 to 30 ml on arising; repeat every 3 hours or when nausea threatens.

➤*Motion sickness or nausea and vomiting caused by drug therapy or inhalation anesthesia:*

Children – 5 ml doses.

Adults – 15 ml doses.

Actions

➤*Pharmacology:* Hyperosmolar carbohydrate solutions with phosphoric acid relieve nausea and vomiting by a direct local action on the wall of the GI tract that reduces smooth muscle contraction.

Precautions

➤*Nausea:* Nausea may signal a serious condition. If symptoms are not relieved or recur often, consult a physician.

➤*Diabetic patients:* should avoid these preparations because they contain significant amounts of sugar.

➤*Hereditary fructose intolerance:* These preparations contain fructose and should be avoided by individuals with hereditary fructose intolerance.

Adverse Reactions

Large doses of fructose can cause abdominal pain and diarrhea.

Indications

►*Anxiety:* For the management of anxiety disorders or for the short-term relief of the symptoms of anxiety. Anxiety or tension associated with the stress of everyday life usually does not require treatment with an antianxiety agent.

Consult individual drug monographs for specific indications.

In addition to use as antianxiety agents, some benzodiazepines are also useful as hypnotics, anticonvulsants and muscle relaxants. Midazolam, an injectable short-acting benzodiazepine, is used for induction of general anesthesia, preoperative sedation, conscious sedation for diagnostic procedures and to supplement nitrous oxide and oxygen for short surgical procedures (see individual monograph).

►*Unlabeled uses:* Management of irritable bowel syndrome (chlordiazepoxide, diazepam, clorazepate, lorazepam, oxazepam, alprazolam); panic attacks (alprazolam, diazepam); depression (alprazolam); premenstrual syndrome (alprazolam); status epilepticus, chemotherapy-induced nausea and vomiting, acute alcohol withdrawal syndrome, psychogenic catatonia (lorazepam injection); chronic insomnia (lorazepam).

Actions

►*Pharmacology:* Benzodiazepines appear to potentiate the effects of gamma-aminobutyrate (GABA) (ie, they facilitate inhibitory GABA neurotransmission) and other inhibitory transmitters by binding to specific benzodiazepine receptor sites. Recent evidence suggest there are ≥ 2 benzodiazepine receptors, BZ_1 and BZ_2. BZ_1 is thought to be associated with sleep mechanisms; BZ_2 with memory, motor, sensory, and cognitive functions. The activity of the benzodiazepines may involve the following sites: Spinal cord (muscle relaxation); brain stem (anticonvulsant properties); cerebellum (ataxia); limbic and cortical areas (emotional behavior). Anxiolytic effects are distinct from nonspecific consequences of CNS depression (ie, sedation and motor impairment). A distinctive feature of the benzodiazepines is the wide margin of safety between therapeutic and toxic doses. Ataxia and sedation occur only at doses beyond those needed for anxiolytic effects.

Clonazepam suppresses the spike and wave discharge in petit mal seizures and decreases frequency, amplitude, duration and spread of discharge in minor motor seizures.

►*Pharmacokinetics:*

Absorption – The major determinant of the onset and intensity of action of a single oral dose of a benzodiazepine is the rate of absorption from the GI tract. Benzodiazepines are readily absorbed following oral administration.

IM administration of chlordiazepoxide and diazepam results in slow erratic absorption and lower peak plasma levels than oral or IV administration. However, IM administration of diazepam into the deltoid muscle is more likely to be rapid and complete. Lorazepam IM is rapidly and completely absorbed.

Distribution – The highly lipid soluble benzodiazepines are widely distributed in the body tissues and highly bound to plasma proteins (70% to 99%). The duration of action is related to their lipid solubility. Highly lipophilic drugs, like diazepam, are rapidly taken into the brain and then rapidly redistributed throughout the body.

Metabolism – The effect of lipid solubility on duration of action is complicated by hepatic biotransformation to active metabolites. The benzophenone metabolite of alprazolam is inactive, while alpha-hydroxy-alprazolam is $\approx 50\%$ as active as the parent compound; both metabolites have the same half-life as alprazolam. Other benzodiazepines have active metabolites with very long half-lives; cumulative effects occur with chronic administration. Desmethyldiazepam is an active metabolite common to many of these agents (eg, clorazepate, halazepam, diazepam); clorazepate is hydrolyzed in the stomach and absorbed as desmethyldiazepam. Chlordiazepoxide has several active intermediate metabolites. Five metabolites of clonazepam have been identified. Biotransformation of clonazepam is by oxidative hydroxylation and reduction.

Since hepatic biotransformation is the predominant route for benzodiazepine metabolism, the disposition of these drugs may be impaired in patients with chronic liver disease. Oxazepam and lorazepam are metabolized to inactive compounds and therefore have relatively short half-lives and duration of activity. Because of their simple 1-step inactivation, oxazepam or lorazepam may be preferred in patients with liver disease and in the elderly. Sustained clinical effects require multiple daily doses; significant accumulation does not occur. The other agents with prolonged half-lives may be administered as a single daily dose at bedtime. The elimination half-life of diazepam and desmethyldiazepam is prolonged in obese patients; total metabolic clearance does not change.

BENZODIAZEPINE METABOLIC PATHWAYS

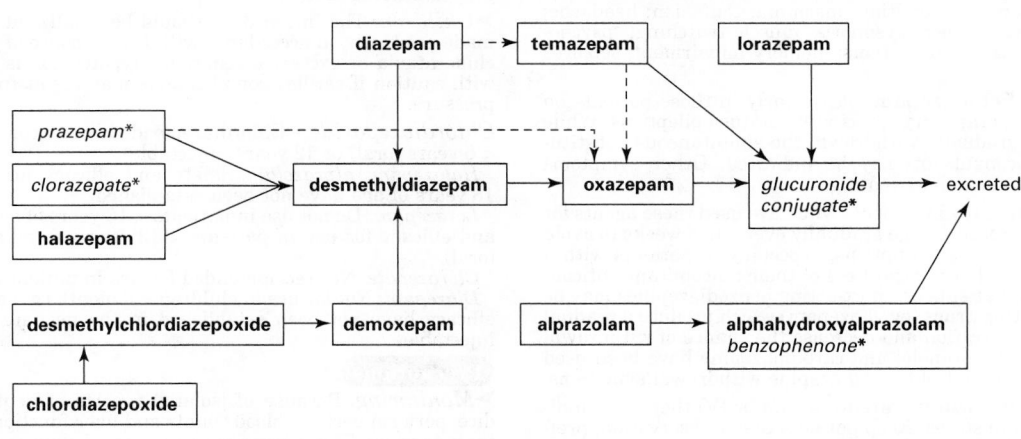

— Major metabolic pathway
- - - Minor metabolic pathway
* Pharmacologically inactive

Excretion – Most of the benzodiazepines are excreted almost entirely in the urine and in the form of oxidized and glucuronide-conjugated metabolites. There is little clinical evidence to suggest that one benzodiazepine is more effective than another. The major differences are reflected in their pharmacokinetic profiles and relative costs. The following table summarizes the major pharmacokinetic variables of these agents:

Benzodiazepine Pharmacokinetics					
Drug	Dosage range (mg/day)[1]	Peak plasma level (hrs)[1]	Elimination t½ (hrs)	Metabolites	Speed of onset[1]	Protein binding
Alprazolam	0.75-4	1-2	6.3-26.9	Alpha-hydroxy-alprazolam; Benzophenone	intermediate	80%
Chlordiazepoxide	15-100	0.5-4	5-30	Desmethylchlordiazepoxide[2]; Demoxepam; Desmethyl-diazepam	intermediate	96%
Clonazepam	1.5-20	1-2	18-50	Inactive 7–amino or 7–acetyl-amino derivatives[2]	intermediate	97%
Clorazepate	15-60	1-2	40-50	Desmethyl-diazepam	fast	97%-98%[3]

Benzodiazepines

Benzodiazepine Pharmacokinetics

Drug	Dosage range (mg/day)[1]	Peak plasma level (hrs)[1]	Elimination t½ (hrs)	Metabolites	Speed of onset[1]	Protein binding
Diazepam	4-40	0.5-2	20-80	Desmethyl-diazepam[2]; nordiazepam	very fast	98%
Halazepam	60-160	1-3	14	Desmethyl-diazepam[2]; 3-hydroxyhalazepam	slow	97%
Lorazepam	2-4	2-4	10-20	Inactive glucuronide conjugate	intermediate	85%
Oxazepam	30-120	2-4	5-20	Inactive glucuronide conjugate	slow	87%

[1] Oral administration.
[2] Major metabolite.

[3] Nordiazepam (active metabolite).

Contraindications

Hypersensitivity to benzodiazepines; psychoses; acute narrow-angle glaucoma (may be used in patients with open-angle glaucoma and appropriate therapy); patients with clinical or biochemical evidence of significant liver disease (clonazepam); intra-arterial use (lorazepam injection); children < 6 months; lactation (diazepam); coadministration with ketoconazole and itraconazole due to inhibition of cytochrome P450 3A (see Warnings).

Warnings

➤*Psychiatric disorders:* These agents are not intended for use in patients with a primary depressive disorder or psychosis, nor in those psychiatric disorders in which anxiety is not a prominent feature.

➤*Long-term use (> 4 months):* Effectiveness has not been assessed by systematic clinical studies. Periodically reassess the usefulness of the drug for the individual patient.

➤*Dependence:* Prolonged use of therapeutic doses can lead to dependence. Withdrawal syndrome has occurred after as little as 4 to 6 weeks treatment. It is more likely if the drug is short-acting (eg, alprazolam), taken regularly for > 3 months and abruptly discontinued.

After rapid decrease of dosage or abrupt discontinuation, withdrawal seizures were reported in **alprazolam** patients.

Onset is within 1 to 10 days; duration of reaction may be 5 days to up to a month depending on agent, dose, etc. Symptoms generally begin with anxiety-like manifestations; the following may occur in ≥ 50% of cases: Increased anxiety; sensory disturbances (paresthesias, hypercusis, photophobia, hypersomnia, metallic taste); concentration difficulties; fatigue; anorexia; dizziness; vomiting; insomnia; confusion; headache; muscle tension/cramps; tremor; dysphoria; muscle twitching; "psychosis"; paranoid delusions; hallucinations; memory impairment; seizures (grand mal).

Abrupt withdrawal of **clonazepam**, particularly in those patients on long-term, high dose therapy, may precipitate status epilepticus. While clonazepam is being gradually withdrawn, the simultaneous substitution of another anticonvulsant may be indicated. Other symptoms include vomiting, diarrhea and sweating.

When discontinuing therapy in patients who have used these agents for prolonged periods, decrease dosage gradually over 4 to 8 weeks to avoid the possibility of withdrawal symptoms, especially in patients with a history of seizures or epilepsy, regardless of their concomitant anticonvulsant drug therapy. Patients on short-acting benzodiazepines may be switched to longer-acting drugs (eg, diazepam) which produce a gradual decrease in drug concentration and decrease the chance of withdrawal symptoms. Clonidine, propranolol and carbamazepine have been used as adjuncts in the treatment of benzodiazepine withdrawal symptoms.

➤*Parenteral administration:* Parenteral (IM or IV) therapy is indicated primarily in acute states. Keep patients under observation, preferably in bed, for ≤ 3 hours.

Do not inject intra-arterially; may produce arteriospasm resulting in gangrene which may require amputation.

Administer parenterally with extreme care (particularly IV) to elderly, very ill and those with limited pulmonary reserve. Because of possible apnea or cardiac arrest, resuscitative facilities should be available. Not recommended for obstetric use. Do not administer to patients in shock, coma or in acute alcohol intoxication.

Hypotension or muscular weakness is possible, particularly when benzodiazepines are used with narcotics, barbiturates or alcohol.

➤*Renal function impairment:* Observe usual precautions in the presence of impaired renal or hepatic function to avoid accumulation of these agents. **Lorazepam** injection is not recommended in these patients. Metabolites of **clonazepam** are excreted by the kidneys; to avoid excess accumulation, exercise caution in patients with impaired renal function. Also, clonazepam is contraindicated in patients with significant liver disease.

➤*Elderly:* The initial dose should be small and dosage increments made gradually, in accordance with the response of the patient, to preclude ataxia or excessive sedation. Hypotension is rare; however, use with caution if cardiac complications may result from a drop in blood pressure.

➤*Pregnancy: Category D* (No category designation for **clonazepam**). Benzodiazepines and their metabolites freely cross the placenta and accumulate in the fetal circulation. An increased risk of congenital malformations associated with the use of minor tranquilizers during the first trimester of pregnancy has been suggested. Malformations reported include cleft lip or palate. Recent studies suggest diazepam use in the first trimester does not cause an increased risk of this. Because use of these drugs is rarely a matter of urgency, avoid them during this period. Consider the possibility that a woman of childbearing potential may be pregnant at the time of institution of therapy. Advise patients that if they become pregnant, or plan to become pregnant, they should discuss the desirability of discontinuing the drug.

Labor and delivery – Benzodiazepines have been found in maternal and cord blood, indicating placental transfer of drug. Therefore, benzodiazepines are not recommended for obstetrical use.

Neonatal withdrawal consisting of severe tremulousness and irritability has been attributed to maternal ingestion of benzodiazepines as well as neonatal flaccidity and respiratory problems. Use during labor has resulted in a "floppy infant" syndrome, manifested by hypotonia, lethargy and sucking difficulties.

Prolonged CNS depression has been observed in neonates, apparently due to inability to biotransform **diazepam** into inactive metabolites.

➤*Lactation:* Benzodiazepines are excreted in breast milk (**lorazepam** not known). Since neonates metabolize benzodiazepines more slowly than adults, accumulation of the drug and its metabolites to toxic levels is possible. Chronic **diazepam** use in nursing mothers reportedly caused infants to become lethargic and to lose weight; do not give to nursing mothers.

➤*Children:* The initial dose should be small and dosage increments made gradually, in accordance with the response of the patient, to preclude ataxia or excessive sedation. Hypotension is rare; however, use with caution if cardiac complications may result from a drop in blood pressure.

Chlordiazepoxide – Chlordiazepoxide is not recommended in children < 6 years (oral) or 12 years (injectable).

Halazepam, alprazolam: Safety and efficacy for use in patients < 18 years of age have not been established.

Lorazepam: Do not use in patients < 18 years of age (injection); safety and efficacy for use in patients < 12 years of age are not established (oral).

Clorazepate: Not recommended for use in patients < 9 years of age.

Diazepam: Not for use in children < 6 months of age (oral); safety and efficacy have not been established in the neonate (≤ 30 days of age; injectable).

Precautions

➤*Monitoring:* Because of isolated reports of neutropenia and jaundice, perform periodic blood counts and liver function tests during long-term therapy. There have been reports of abnormal liver and kidney function tests and of decrease in hematocrit.

➤*Suicide:* In those patients in whom depression accompanies anxiety, suicidal tendencies may be present, and protective measures may be required. Dispense the least amount of drug feasible to the patient.

➤*Paradoxical reactions:* Excitement, stimulation and acute rage have occurred in psychiatric patients and hyperactive aggressive children. These reactions may be secondary to relief of anxiety and usually appear in the first 2 weeks of therapy. Acute hyperexcited states, anxiety, hallucinations, increased muscle spasticity, insomnia and sleep disturbances have also occurred. Should these occur, discontinue the drug. Minor EEG changes, usually low voltage fast activity, have been observed during and after therapy and are of no known significance. Anger, hostility and episodes of mania and hypomania have been reported with **alprazolam**.

➤*Multiple seizure type:* When used in patients in whom several different types of seizure disorders coexist, **clonazepam** may increase the incidence or precipitate the onset of generalized tonic-clonic (grand mal) seizures. This may require the addition of other anticonvulsants or an increase in their dosage.

Diazepam – If use in patients with seizure disorders results in an increase in the frequency or severity of grand mal seizures, there may

Benzodiazepines

be a need to increase the dosage of standard anticonvulsant medication.

➤*Chronic respiratory disease:* **Clonazepam** may produce an increase in salivation. Use with caution in patients if increased salivation causes respiratory difficulty. Due to possibility of respiratory depression, use with caution in such patients.

➤*Benzyl alcohol:* Some of these products contain benzyl alcohol, which has been associated with a fatal "gasping syndrome" in premature infants.

➤*Hazardous tasks:* May produce drowsiness or dizziness; observe caution while driving or performing other tasks requiring alertness.

➤*Tartrazine sensitivity:* Some of these products contain tartrazine, which may cause allergic-type reactions (including bronchial asthma) in susceptible individuals. Although the incidence of tartrazine sensitivity in the general population is low, it is frequently seen in patients who also have aspirin hypersensitivity. Specific products containing tartrazine are identified in the product listings.

Drug Interactions

Benzodiazepine Drug Interactions			
Precipitant drug	Object drug*		Description
Alcohol/CNS depressants (eg, barbiturates, narcotics)	Benzodiazepines	↑	Increased CNS effects (eg, impaired psychomotor function, sedation) may occur.
Benzodiazepines	Alcohol/CNS depressants (eg, barbiturates, narcotics)		
Antacids	Benzodiazepines	↓	Antacids may alter the rate but generally not the extent of GI absorption. Staggering administration times may help avoid possible interaction.
Cimetidine Contraceptives, oral Disulfiram Fluoxetine Isoniazid Ketoconazole Metoprolol Propoxyphene Propranolol Valproic acid	Alprazolam Chlordiazepoxide Clorazepate Diazepam Halazepam	↑	The elimination of benzodiazepines that undergo oxidative hepatic metabolism (alprazolam, chlordiazepoxide, clorazepate, diazepam, halazepam) may be decreased by the following drugs due to inhibition of hepatic metabolism. Pharmacologic effects of these benzodiazepines may be increased and excessive sedation/impaired psychomotor function may occur.
Contraceptives, oral	Lorazepam, Oxazepam	↓	The clearance rate of benzodiazepines that undergo glucuronidation (lorazepam, oxazepam) may be increased.
Probenecid	Benzodiazepines	↑	Probenecid may interfere with benzodiazepine conjugation in the liver, possibly resulting in a more rapid onset or prolonged effect.
Ranitidine	Diazepam	↓	Ranitidine may reduce the GI absorption of diazepam.
Rifampin	Benzodiazepines	↓	The oxidative metabolism of benzodiazepines may be increased due to microsomal enzyme induction. Pharmacologic effects of some benzodiazepines may be decreased.
Scopolamine	Lorazepam	↑	Scopolamine, used concomitantly with parenteral lorazepam, may increase the incidence of sedation, hallucinations and irrational behavior.
Theophyllines	Benzodiazepines	↓	Theophyllines may antagonize the sedative effects of the benzodiazepines.
Benzodiazepines	Digoxin	↑	Digoxin's serum concentrations may be increased. Toxicity characterized by GI and neuropsychiatric symptoms and cardiac arrhythmias may occur. Monitor digoxin serum levels.
Benzodiazepines	Levodopa	↓	Levodopa's antiparkinson efficacy may be decreased by coadministration of benzodiazepines.
Benzodiazepines	Neuromuscular blocking agents	↔	Benzodiazepines may potentiate, counteract or have no effect on the actions of these agents.
Benzodiazepines	Phenytoin	↑	Phenytoin serum concentrations may be increased, resulting in toxicity, but data are conflicting. Phenytoin may increase oxazepam clearance.

* ↑ = Object drug increased. ↓ = Object drug decreased. ↔ = Undetermined clinical effect.

Adverse Reactions

Discontinuation of therapy due to undesirable effects is rare. Transient mild drowsiness is commonly seen in the first few days of therapy. Drowsiness, ataxia and confusion have occurred, especially in the elderly and debilitated. If persistent, reduce dosage. Ataxia is rare with oxazepam and does not appear to be specifically related to dose or age. Other adverse reactions less frequently reported include:

➤*Cardiovascular:* Bradycardia; tachycardia; cardiovascular collapse; hypertension; hypotension; palpitations; edema; phlebitis and thrombosis at IV sites. Decrease in systolic blood pressure has been observed.

➤*CNS:* Sedation and sleepiness; depression; lethargy; apathy; fatigue; hypoactivity; lightheadedness; memory impairment; disorientation; anterograde amnesia; restlessness; confusion; crying; sobbing; delirium; headache; slurred speech; aphonia; dysarthria; stupor; seizures; coma; syncope; rigidity; tremor; dystonia; vertigo; dizziness; euphoria; nervousness; irritability; difficulty in concentration; agitation; inability to perform complex mental functions; akathisia; hemiparesis; hypotonia; unsteadiness; ataxia; incoordination; weakness; vivid dreams; psychomotor retardation; "glassy-eyed" appearance; extrapyramidal symptoms; paradoxical reactions (see Precautions).

➤*Dermatologic:* Urticaria; pruritus; skin rash, including morbilliform, urticarial and maculopapular; dermatitis; hair loss; hirsutism; ankle and facial edema.

➤*GI:* Constipation; diarrhea; dry mouth; coated tongue; sore gums; nausea; anorexia; change in appetite; vomiting; difficulty in swallowing; increased salivation; gastritis.

➤*GU:* Incontinence; changes in libido; urinary retention; menstrual irregularities.

➤*Ophthalmic:* Visual disturbances; diplopia; nystagmus.

➤*Psychiatric:* Behavior problems; hysteria; psychosis; suicidal tendencies.

➤*Miscellaneous:* Depressed hearing; nasal congestion; respiratory disturbances; auditory disturbances; hiccoughs; fever; diaphoresis; paresthesias; muscular disturbance; gynecomastia; galactorrhea; elevations of LDH, alkaline phosphatase, ALT and AST; hepatic dysfunction (including hepatitis and jaundice); leukopenia; blood dyscrasias including agranulocytosis; anemia; thrombocytopenia; eosinophilia; increase or decrease in body weight; dehydration; lymphadenopathy; joint pain; pain, burning and redness following IM injection. Partial airway obstruction has occurred and is believed to be due to excessive sedation at time of procedure (lorazepam injection).

Overdosage

There are no well documented fatal overdoses resulting from oral ingestion of benzodiazepines alone. Most fatalities implicate benzodiazepines only as a component in multiple drug ingestions.

➤*Symptoms:* Mild symptoms include drowsiness, confusion, somnolence, impaired coordination, diminished reflexes and lethargy. These agents rarely cause significant respiratory or circulatory depression, particularly when they are the sole agents ingested. Serious symptoms may include ataxia, hypotonia, hypotension, hypnosis, stages one to three coma, and rarely, death. Consider multiple drug ingestion.

Unlike oral ingestions, IV administration of diazepam is associated with 1.7% incidence of life-threatening reactions, including hypotension and respiratory or cardiac arrest.

➤*Treatment:* Induce vomiting if it has not occurred spontaneously. Employ general supportive measures, along with immediate gastric lavage or ipecac. Follow with activated charcoal administration and a saline cathartic. Monitor respiration, pulse and blood pressure. Administer IV fluids and maintain an adequate airway. Treat hypotension with norepinephrine or metaraminol. With normal kidney function, forced diuresis with osmotic diuretics, IV fluids and electrolytes may accelerate elimination of benzodiazepines. Dialysis is of limited value; however, in more critical situations, renal dialysis and exchange blood transfusions may be indicated. Refer to General Management of Acute Overdosage.

Infusion of 0.5 to 4 mg of physostigmine IV at the rate of 1 mg/minute may reverse symptoms suggestive of central anticholinergic overdose (eg, confusion, memory disturbance, visual disturbances, hallucinations, delirium); however, weigh the hazards associated with the use of physostigmine (eg, induction of seizures) against its possible clinical benefit.

There have been occasional reports of excitation in patients following overdosage with chlordiazepoxide; if this occurs, do not give barbiturates.

Patient Information

May cause drowsiness; avoid driving or other tasks requiring alertness.

Avoid alcohol or other CNS depressants.

May be taken with food or water if stomach upset occurs.

Patients on long-term or high dosage therapy may experience withdrawal symptoms on abrupt cessation of therapy; do not discontinue therapy abruptly or change dosage except on advice of physician.

Concomitant ingestion with antacids may alter the rate of absorption of these drugs (documented with **diazepam** and **chlordiazepoxide**).

▶**Clonazepam, clorazepate** *and* **diazepam**: Patient should carry identification (*Medic Alert*) indicating medication usage and epilepsy.

ALPRAZOLAM

c-iv	**Alprazolam** (Various, eg, Geneva, Mylan, Purepac)	**Tablets**: 0.25 mg	In 100s, 500s, 1000s, and UD 100s.
c-iv	**Xanax** (Pfizer)		Lactose. (Xanax 0.25). White, oval, scored. In 100s, 500s, 1000s, and UD 100s.
c-iv	**Alprazolam** (Various, eg, Geneva, Mylan, Purepac)	**Tablets**: 0.5 mg	In 100s, 500s, 1000s, and UD 100s.
c-iv	**Xanax** (Pfizer)		Lactose. (Xanax 0.5). Peach, oval, scored. In 100s, 500s, 1000s, and UD 100s.
c-iv	**Alprazolam** (Various, eg, Geneva, Mylan, Purepac)	**Tablets**: 1 mg	In 100s, 500s, 1000s, and UD 100s.
c-iv	**Xanax** (Pfizer)		Lactose, FD & C Blue No. 2. (Xanax 1.0). Blue, oval, scored. In 100s, 500s, and 1000s.
c-iv	**Alprazolam** (Various, eg, Mylan, Purepac)	**Tablets**: 2 mg	In 100s and 500s.
c-iv	**Xanax** (Pfizer)		Lactose. (XANAX 2). White, oblong, multi-scored. In 100s and 500s.
c-iv	**Xanax XR** (Pfizer)	**Tablets, extended-release**: 0.5 mg	Lactose. (X 0.5). White, pentagonal. In 60s.
		1 mg	Lactose. (X 1). Yellow, square. In 60s.
		2 mg	Lactose, FD & C Blue No. 2. (X 2). Blue. In 60s.
		3 mg	Lactose, FD & C Blue No. 2. (X 3). Green, triangular. In 60s.
c-iv	**Alprazolam Intensol** (Roxane)	**Oral solution**: 1 mg/mL	Flavorless. In 30 mL with calibrated dropper.

Complete prescribing information begins in the Benzodiazepines monograph.

Indications

▶*Panic disorder (Xanax and Xanax XR):* Treatment of panic disorder, with or without agoraphobia.

▶*Anxiety disorders (immediate-release tablets and intensol):* For the management of anxiety disorders or for the short-term relief of the symptoms of anxiety. Anxiety associated with depression is also responsive.

Alprazolam given sublingually is absorbed as rapidly as after oral administration; completeness of absorption is comparable.

Administration and Dosage

Individualize dosage. Increase cautiously to avoid adverse effects. Reduce gradually when terminating or decreasing daily dose. Decrease no more than 0.5 mg every 3 days.

▶*Anxiety disorders (immediate-release tablets and intensol):* Initial dose is 0.25 to 0.5 mg 3 times/day. Titrate to a maximum total dose of 4 mg/day in divided doses at intervals of 3 to 4 days. If side effects occur with starting dose, decrease dose.

▶*Panic disorder (Xanax and Xanax XR):*

immediate-release tablets – Initial dose is 0.5 mg 3 times/day. Depending on response, increase dose at intervals of 3 to 4 days in increments of no more than 1 mg/day.

Successful treatment has required doses more than 4 mg/day; in controlled studies, doses in the range of 1 to 10 mg/day were used. The mean dosage employed was approximately 5 to 6 mg/day.

Extended-release tablets – Administer once daily, preferably in the morning. Take the tablets intact; do not chew, crush, or break.

Treatment may be initiated with 0.5 to 1 mg once daily. The suggested total daily dose ranges between 3 and 6 mg/day. The suggested total daily dosages will meet the needs of most patients; however, there will be some who require doses greater than 6 mg/day.

Dose maintenance: In controlled trials, a dose range of 1 to 10 mg/day was used. Most patients showed efficacy in the range of 3 to 6 mg/day. Occasionally as much as 10 mg/day was required to achieve successful response.

Immediate/Extended-release tablets –

Dose titration: Depending on response, the dose may be increased at intervals of 3 to 4 days in increments of no more than 1 mg/day. Slower titration to the dose levels may be advisable to allow full expression of the pharmacodynamic effect. Advance dose until an acceptable therapeutic response (ie, a substantial reduction in or total elimination of panic attacks) is achieved, intolerance occurs, or the maximum recommended dose is attained.

Duration: The necessary duration of treatment for responding patients is unknown. However, periodic reassessment is advised. After a period of extended freedom from attacks, a carefully supervised tapered discontinuation may be attempted, but there is evidence that this may often be difficult to accomplish without recurrence of symptoms and/or the manifestations of withdrawal phenomena.

Dose reduction: Because of the danger of withdrawal, avoid abrupt discontinuation. Gradually reduce dosage in all patients when discontinuing therapy or when decreasing the daily dosage. Although there are no systematically collected data to support a specific discontinuation schedule, it is suggested that the daily dosage be decreased by no more than 0.5 mg every 3 days. Some patients may require an even slower dosage reduction. Some patients may prove resistant to all discontinuation regimens.

In any case, reduction of dose must begin under close supervision and must be gradual. If significant withdrawal symptoms develop, reinstitute the previous dosing schedule and attempt a less rapid schedule of discontinuation only after stabilization. In a controlled postmarketing discontinuation study of panic disorder that compared this recommended taper schedule with a slower taper schedule, no difference was observed between groups in the proportion of patients who tapered to zero dose; however, the slower schedule was associated with a reduction in symptoms associated with a withdrawal syndrome.

Switching from immediate-release to extended-release tablets: Patients currently treated with divided doses of immediate-release tablets (eg, 3 to 4 times/day) may be switched to extended-release tablets at the same total daily dose taken once daily. If the therapeutic response after switching is inadequate, dosage may be titrated as outlined above.

▶*Elderly advanced hepatic disease or debilitated patients:*

Immediate-release tablets and intensol – 0.25 mg, given 2 or 3 times/day. Gradually increase if needed and tolerated.

Extended-release tablets – The usual starting dose is 0.5 mg once/day. Gradually increase if needed and tolerated. The elderly may be especially sensitive to the effects of benzodiazepines.

▶*Administration of oral solution:* Alprazolam intensol is a concentrated oral solution. It is recommended that the oral solution be mixed with liquids or semi-solid food such as water, juices, soda or soda-like beverages, applesauce, and puddings. Use only the calibrated dropper provided with this product. Draw into the dropper the amount prescribed for a single dose. Then squeeze the dropper contents into a liquid or semi-solid food. Stir the liquid or food gently for a few seconds. The formulation blends quickly and completely. Consume the entire amount of the mixture of drug and liquid or drug and food immediately. Do not store for future use.

▶*Storage/Stability:* Store at controlled room temperature, 15° to 30°C (59° to 86°F).

CLORAZEPATE DIPOTASSIUM

c-iv	**Clorazepate Dipotassium** (Various, eg, Able, Mylan, Taro, Watson)	**Tablets:** 3.75 mg	In 100s, 500s, 1000s, and UD 100s.
c-iv	**Tranxene T-tab** (Ovation)		FD & C Blue No. 2. (TL). Blue, scored. In 100s, 500s, and UD 100s.
c-iv	**Clorazepate Dipotassium** (Various, eg, Able, Mylan, Taro, Watson)	**Tablets:** 7.5 mg	In 20s, 100s, 500s, 1000s, and UD 100s and 500s.
c-iv	**Tranxene T-tab** (Ovation)		(TM). Peach, scored. In 100s, 500s, and UD 100s.
c-iv	**Clorazepate Dipotassium** (Various, eg, Able, Mylan, Taro, Watson)	**Tablets:** 15 mg	In 100s, 500s, 1000s, and UD 100s.
c-iv	**Tranxene T-tab** (Ovation)		(TN). Lavender, scored. In 100s, 500s, and UD 100s.
c-iv	**Tranxene-SD Half Strength** (Ovation)	**Tablets, extended-release:** 11.25 mg	Lactose. (TX). Blue. In 100s.
c-iv	**Tranxene-SD** (Ovation)	**Tablets, extended-release:** 22.5 mg	Lactose. (TY). Tan. In 100s.

Complete prescribing information begins in the Benzodiazepines monograph. For information on the anticonvulsants use of clorazepate, refer to individual monograph in the Anticonvulsant section.

Indications

►*Anxiety disorders:* For management of anxiety disorders or short-term relief of symptoms of anxiety.

►*Acute alcohol withdrawal:* For the symptomatic relief of acute alcohol withdrawal.

►*Anticonvulsant:* As adjunctive therapy in the management of partial seizures (see Anticonvulsants section).

Administration and Dosage

►*Immediate-release tablets:*

Acute alcohol withdrawal – Day 1: 30 mg initially; followed by 30 to 60 mg in divided doses.

Day 2: 45 to 90 mg in divided doses.

Day 3: 22.5 to 45 mg in divided doses.

Day 4: 15 to 30 mg in divided doses.

Thereafter, gradually reduce the dose to 7.5 to 15 mg/day. Discontinue drug as soon as patient's condition is stable.

The maximum recommended total daily dose is 90 mg. Avoid excessive reductions in the total amount of drug administered on successive days.

►*Anxiety:* 30 mg/day in divided doses. Adjust gradually within the range of 15 to 60 mg/day.

Also may be administered as a single daily dose at bedtime; the initial dose is 15 mg. After the initial dose, the patient may require adjustment of subsequent dosage. Drowsiness may occur at the initiation of treatment and with dosage increments.

►*Elderly or debilitated patients:* Initiate treatment at a dose of 7.5 to 15 mg/day. Lower doses may be indicated.

►*Extended-release tablets:*

Maintenance therapy – Give the 22.5 mg tablet in a single daily dose as an alternate dosage form for patients stabilized on 7.5 mg 3 times/day. Do not use to initiate therapy.

The 11.25 mg tablet may be administered as a single dose every 24 hours as an alternate dosage form for patients stabilized on a dose of 3.75 mg tablets 3 times/day. Not to be used to initiate therapy.

►*Storage/Stability:* Store *Tranxene* below 25°C (77°F). Store clorazepate dipotassium tablets at controlled room temperature, 15° to 30°C (59° to 86°F).

CHLORDIAZEPOXIDE HCl

c-iv	**Chlordiazepoxide HCl** (Various, eg, Barr, Geneva, Major, Watson)	**Capsules:** 5 mg	In 20s, 100s, 500s, 1000s, and UD 100s.
c-iv	**Librium** (ICN Pharmaceuticals)		Lactose, parabens. (LIBRIUM 5). Green and yellow. In 100s.
c-iv	**Chlordiazepoxide HCl** (Various, eg, Barr, Major, UDL, Watson)	**Capsules:** 10 mg	In 20s, 100s, 500s, 1000s, and UD 100s.
c-iv	**Librium** (ICN Pharmaceuticals)		Lactose, parabens. (LIBRIUM 10). Green and black. In 100s.
c-iv	**Chlordiazepoxide HCl** (Various, eg, Barr, Major, UDL, Watson)	**Capsules:** 25 mg	In 20s, 100s, 500s, 1000s, and UD 100s.
c-iv	**Librium** (ICN Pharmaceuticals)		Lactose, parabens. (LIBRIUM 25). Green and white. In 100s.
c-iv	**Librium** (ICN Pharmaceuticals)	**Powder for injection:** 100 mg	In 5 mL amp with 2 mL amp of IM diluent.[1]

[1] With 1.5% benzyl alcohol, polysorbate 80, and 20% propylene glycol.

Complete prescribing information begins in the Benzodiazepines monograph.

Indications

►*Anxiety disorders:* For the management of anxiety disorders or for short-term relief of anxiety symptoms.

►*Acute alcohol withdrawal:* For the symptoms of acute alcohol withdrawal.

►*Preoperative:* For preoperative apprehension and anxiety.

Administration and Dosage

►*Oral:* Individualize dosage.

Mild to moderate anxiety – 5 or 10 mg 3 to 4 times/day.

Severe anxiety – 20 or 25 mg 3 to 4 times/day.

Elderly patients or patients with debilitating disease – 5 mg 2 to 4 times/day.

Preoperative apprehension and anxiety – On days preceding surgery, 5 to 10 mg 3 or 4 times/day.

Acute alcohol withdrawal – 50 to 100 mg; repeat as needed (up to 300 mg). Parenteral form usually used initially. Reduce to maintenance levels.

Children – Initially, 5 mg 2 to 4 times/day. (May be increased in some children to 10 mg 2 or 3 times/day.) Not recommended in children younger than 6 years of age.

►*Parenteral:* Use lower doses (25 to 50 mg) for elderly or debilitated patients and for children 12 years of age or older. Acute symptoms may

be rapidly controlled by parenteral administration; subsequent treatment, if necessary, may be given orally. While 300 mg may be given during a 6-hour period, do not exceed this dose in any 24-hour period. Not recommended in children younger than 12 years of age.

Acute alcohol withdrawal – 50 to 100 mg IM or IV initially; repeat in 2 to 4 hours if necessary.

Acute or severe anxiety – 50 to 100 mg IM or IV initially; then 25 to 50 mg 3 to 4 times/day if necessary.

Preoperative apprehension and anxiety – 50 to 100 mg IM 1 hour prior to surgery.

►*Preparation and administration of injections:* Prepare solution immediately before administration. Discard any unused portion.

IM – Add 2 mL of special IM diluent to contents of 5 mL ampule of chlordiazepoxide sterile powder (100 mg). Avoid excessive pressure when injecting diluent into the ampule containing the powder because bubbles form on the surface of the solution. Agitate gently until completely dissolved. Do not use diluent if it is opalescent or hazy. Do not give solutions made with physiological saline or sterile water for injection IM because of the pain on injection. Give deep IM injection slowly into the upper outer quadrant of the gluteus muscle. Do not give IV solution made with the IM diluent because of the bubbles that form when the IM diluent is added to the chlordiazepoxide powder.

IV – When rapid action is mandatory, administer IV. Add 5 mL of sterile physiological saline or sterile water for injection to contents of amp (100 mg). Agitate gently until thoroughly dissolved. Give injection slowly over 1 minute.

►*Storage/Stability:* Store at 25°C (77°F); excursions permitted to 15° to 30°C (59° to 86°F).

Benzodiazepines

CLONAZEPAM

c-iv	**Clonazepam** (Various, eg, Mylan, PAR, Teva, TorPharm, UDL, Watson)	**Tablets**: 0.5 mg	May contain lactose. In 100s, 500s, 1000s, and UD 100s.
c-iv	**Klonopin** (Roche)		Lactose, FD&C Blue No. 1 and 2. (1/2 KLONOPIN ROCHE). Orange, scored. In 100s.
c-iv	**Clonazepam** (Various, eg, Mylan, PAR, Teva, TorPharm, UDL, Watson)	1 mg	May contain lactose. In 100s, 500s, 1000s, and UD 100s.
c-iv	**Klonopin** (Roche)		Lactose, FD&C Blue No. 1 and 2. (1 KLONOPIN ROCHE). Blue. In 100s.
c-iv	**Clonazepam** (Various, eg, Mylan, PAR, Teva, TorPharm, UDL, Watson)	2 mg	May contain lactose. In 100s, 500s, 1000s, and UD 100s.
c-iv	**Klonopin** (Roche)		Lactose, FD&C Blue No. 1 and 2. (2 KLONOPIN ROCHE). White. In 100s.
c-iv	**Klonopin** (Roche)	**Tablets, orally disintegrating**: 0.125 mg	Mannitol, parabens. (1/8). White. In blister packages of 60.
		0.25 mg	Mannitol, parabens. (1/4). White. In blister packages of 60.
		0.5 mg	Mannitol, parabens. (1/2). White. In blister packages of 60.
		1 mg	Mannitol, parabens. (1). White. In blister packages of 60.
		2 mg	Mannitol, parabens. (2). White. In blister packages of 60.

For additional information, refer to the Benzodiazepines group monograph in the Antianxiety Agents section and to the Anticonvulsants introduction.

Indications

➤*Panic disorder:* For the treatment of panic disorder with or without agoraphobia, as defined by DSM-IV.

➤*Seizure disorder:* Alone or as an adjunct in the treatment of the Lennox-Gastaut syndrome (petit mal variant), akinetic, and myoclonic seizures. May be useful in patients with absence seizures (petit mal) who have failed to respond to succinimides (see Anticonvulsant section).

Administration and Dosage

➤*Panic disorder:* The initial dose for adults is 0.25 mg twice daily. An increase to the target dose for most patients of 1 mg/day may be made after 3 days. Higher doses of 2, 3, and 4 mg/day in a study were less effective than the 1 mg/day dose and were associated with more adverse effects. Nevertheless, it is possible that some individual patients may benefit from doses of up to a maximum dose of 4 mg/day

and, in those instances, the dose may be increased in increments of 0.125 to 0.25 mg twice daily every 3 days until panic disorder is controlled or until side effects make further increases undesired. To reduce the inconvenience of somnolence, administration of one dose at bedtime may be desirable.

➤*Discontinuation:* Discontinue treatment gradually, with a decrease of 0.125 mg twice daily every 3 days until the drug is completely withdrawn. Periodically reevaluate the long-term usefulness of the drug for the individual patient.

➤*Administration:* Administer the tablets with water by swallowing the tablet whole. Administer the orally disintegrating tablet as follows: After opening the pouch, peel back the foil on the blister. Do not push the tablet through foil. Immediately upon opening the blister, using dry hands, remove the tablet and place it in the mouth. Tablet disintegration occurs rapidly in saliva so it can be easily swallowed with or without water.

➤*Storage/Stability:* Store at 25°C (77°F); excursions permitted to 15° to 30°C (59° to 86°F).

DIAZEPAM

c-iv	**Diazepam** (Roxane)	**Oral solution**: 5 mg/5 mL	Sorbitol. Wintergreen-spice flavor. In 500 mL and 5 and 10 mg patient cups.
c-iv	**Diazepam Intensol** (Roxane)	**Oral solution**: 5 mg/mL	19% alcohol. In 30 mL with dropper.
c-iv	**Diazepam** (Various, eg, Barr, Danbury, Ivax, Mylan, Purepac, Zenith)	**Tablets**: 2 mg	May contain lactose. In 100s, 500s, 1000s, and 5000s.
c-iv	**Valium** (Roche)		Lactose. (Roche 2 Valium). White, scored. In 100s and 500s.
c-iv	**Diazepam** (Various, eg, Barr, Danbury, Ivax, Mylan, Purepac, Zenith)	**Tablets**: 5 mg	May contain lactose. In 100s, 500s, 1000s, and 5000s.
c-iv	**Valium** (Roche)		Lactose. (Roche 5 Valium). Yellow, scored. In 100s and 500s.
c-iv	**Diazepam** (Various, eg, Barr, Danbury, Ivax, Mylan, Purepac, Zenith)	**Tablets**: 10 mg	May contain lactose, FD&C Blue No 1. In 100s, 500s, 1000s, and 5000s.
c-iv	**Valium** (Roche)		Lactose, FD&C Blue No 1. (Roche 10 Valium). Blue, scored. In 100s and 500s.
c-iv	**Diazepam** (Various, eg, Abbott)	**Injection**: 5 mg/mL[1]	In 2 mL *Carpuject* cartridges.

[1] With 40% propylene glycol, 10% ethyl alcohol, 5% sodium benzoate, benzoic acid, and 1.5% benzyl alcohol.

Complete prescribing information begins in the Benzodiazepines monograph. Also refer to the Anticonvulsants chapter for further information.

Indications

➤*Anxiety disorders:* For the management of anxiety disorders or for the short-term relief of the symptoms of anxiety.

➤*Acute alcohol withdrawal:* May be useful in symptomatic relief of acute agitation, tremor, impending or acute delirium, tremens, and hallucinosis.

➤*Muscle relaxant:* As an adjunct for the relief of skeletal muscle spasm because of reflex spasm caused by local pathology (eg, inflammation of muscles or joints, secondary to trauma); spasticity caused by upper motor neuron disorders (eg, cerebral palsy, paraplegia); athetosis; stiff-man syndrome. Used parenterally in the treatment of tetanus.

➤*Anticonvulsant:* Parenteral diazepam is a useful adjunct in status epilepticus and severe recurrent convulsive seizures. Oral diazepam may be used adjunctively in convulsive disorders.

➤*Preoperative:* Used parenterally for the relief of anxiety and tension in patients undergoing surgical procedures; IV prior to cardioversion for the relief of anxiety and tension and to diminish patient's recall; as an adjunct prior to endoscopic procedures for apprehension, anxiety, or acute stress reactions and to diminish patient's recall.

Administration and Dosage

➤*Oral:* Individualize dosage. Increase dosage cautiously to avoid adverse effects.

Management of anxiety disorders and relief of symptoms of anxiety (depending upon severity of symptoms) – 2 to 10 mg 2 to 4 times/day.

Acute alcohol withdrawal – 10 mg 3 or 4 times during first 24 hours; reduce to 5 mg 3 or 4 times/day, as needed.

Adjunct in skeletal muscle spasm – 2 to 10 mg 3 or 4 times/day.

Adjunct in convulsive disorders – 2 to 10 mg 2 to 4 times/day.

Elderly patients or in the presence of debilitating disease – 2 to 2.5 mg 1 or 2 times/day initially; increase gradually as needed and tolerated.

Children – 1 to 2.5 mg 3 or 4 times/day initially; increase gradually as needed and tolerated. Not for use in children under 6 months of age. For sedation or muscle relaxation, a dosage of 0.12 to 0.8 mg/kg/24 hours divided 3 to 4 times/day has been recommended.

➤*Oral, solution:* Dosage same as oral tablets.

Intensol – Diazepam intensol is a concentrated oral solution as compared with standard oral liquid medications. It is recommended that the intensol is mixed with liquid or semisolid food such as water, juices,

DIAZEPAM

soda or soda-like beverages, applesauce, and puddings.

Use only the calibrated dropper provided with the product. Draw into the dropper the amount prescribed for a single dose. Then squeeze the dropper contents into a liquid or semi-solid food. Stir the liquid or food gently for a few seconds. Consume the entire amount of the mixture immediately. Do not store for future use.

➤*Parenteral:* Individualize dosage.

Older children and adults – 2 to 20 mg IM or IV, depending on the indication and its severity. In some conditions (eg, tetanus) larger doses may be required. In acute conditions, the injection may be repeated within 1 hour; although, an interval of 3 to 4 hours is usually satisfactory. Use lower doses (2 to 5 mg) and more gradual increases in dosage for elderly and debilitated patients and when other sedatives are administered.

IV – When used IV, observe the following procedures to reduce the possibility of venous thrombosis, phlebitis, local irritation, swelling, and rarely, vascular impairment: Inject slowly, take at least 1 minute per 5 mg (1 mL); do not use small veins (ie, dorsum of hand or wrist); avoid intra-arterial administration or extravasation. Do not mix or dilute with other solutions or drugs in syringe or infusion flask. If not feasible to administer directly IV, inject slowly through infusion tubing as close as possible to the vein insertion. Because of the possibility of precipitation of diazepam in IV fluids and the instability of the drug in plastic (PVC) bags and infusion tubing, IV infusion of diazepam is not recommended. Glass, polypropylene, polyethylene, or polyolefin solution bottles and infusion tubing have been used with negligible loss of diazepam. Once acute symptoms are controlled with injectable diazepam, place patient on oral therapy.

Children – To obtain maximum clinical effect with minimum amount of drug and to reduce the risk of hazardous side effects such as apnea or prolonged periods of somnolence, administer slowly over 3 minutes. Do not exceed 0.25 mg/kg. After an interval of 15 to 30 minutes, the initial dose can be repeated. If relief of symptoms is not obtained after a third dose, appropriate adjunctive therapy is recommended. When IV use is indicated, facilities for respiratory assistance should be readily available.

Moderate anxiety disorders and symptoms of anxiety (adults) – 2 to 5 mg IM or IV. Repeat in 3 to 4 hours if necessary.

Severe anxiety disorders and symptoms of anxiety (adults) – 5 to 10 mg IM or IV. Repeat in 3 to 4 hours if necessary.

Acute alcohol withdrawal (adults) – 10 mg IM or IV initially; then 5 to 10 mg in 3 to 4 hours if necessary.

Endoscopic procedures (adults) –

IV: Titrate dosage to desired sedative response, such as slurring of speech. Administer slowly just prior to procedure. Reduce narcotic dosage by at least one third, and in some cases, they may be omitted; 10 mg or less is usually adequate; up to 20 mg may be used, especially when concomitant narcotics are omitted.

IM: 5 to 10 mg 30 minutes prior to procedure if IV route cannot be used.

Muscle spasm (adults) – 5 to 10 mg IM or IV initially; then 5 to 10 mg in 3 to 4 hours if necessary. Tetanus may require larger doses.

Sedation or muscle relaxation (children) – 0.04 to 0.2 mg/kg/dose every 2 to 4 hours, maximum of 0.6 mg/kg within an 8-hour period.

Tetanus –

Infants (older than 30 days of age): 1 to 2 mg IM or IV slowly, repeated every 3 to 4 hours as necessary.

Children (5 years of age or older): 5 to 10 mg repeated every 3 to 4 hours may be required.

Status epilepticus and severe recurrent convulsive seizures – The IV route is preferred; administer slowly. Use the IM route if IV administration is impossible. Administer 5 to 10 mg initially; repeat if necessary at 10- to 15-minute intervals up to a maximum dose of 30 mg in adults. If necessary, repeat therapy in 2 to 4 hours. Exercise extreme caution in patients with chronic lung disease or unstable cardiovascular status. Although seizures may be controlled promptly, many patients experience a return to seizure activity, presumably because of the short-lived effect of IV diazepam; be prepared to readminister the drug. Diazepam is not recommended for maintenance. Once seizures are controlled, consider other agents for long-term control.

Infants (older than 30 days of age) and children (younger than 5 years of age): Inject 0.2 to 0.5 mg slowly every 2 to 5 minutes up to a maximum of 5 mg.

Children (5 years of age or older): Inject 1 mg every 2 to 5 minutes up to a maximum of 10 mg. Repeat in 2 to 4 hours if necessary. EEG monitoring of seizure may be helpful.

Neonates: 0.3 to 0.75 mg/kg/dose every 15 to 30 minutes for 2 to 3 doses has been suggested.

Preoperative medication (adults) – 10 mg IM before surgery. If atropine, scopolamine, or other premedications are desired, administer in separate syringes.

Cardioversion (adults) – 5 to 15 mg IV, 5 to 10 minutes prior to procedure.

➤*Storage/Stability:* Store at controlled room temperature, 15° to 30°C (59° to 86°F). Protect from light and moisture.

LORAZEPAM

c-iv	**Lorazepam** (Various, eg, Geneva, Major, Mylan, Squibb Mark, UDL)	**Tablets:** 0.5 mg	In 100s, 500s, and 1000s.
		1 mg	In 100s, 500s, and 1000s.
		2 mg	In 100s, 500s, and 1000s.
c-iv	**Lorazepam Intensol** (Roxane)	**Concentrated oral solution:** 2 mg/mL	Alcohol and dye free. In 10 and 30 mL with dropper.
c-iv	**Lorazepam** (Abbott)	**Injection:** 2 mg/mL	In single and 10 mL multidose vials.[a]
c-iv	**Ativan** (Baxter)		In single and 10 mL multidose vials[a], in boxes of 10 *TUBEX*.
c-iv	**Lorazepam** (Abbott)	**Injection:** 4 mg/mL	In single and 10 mL multidose vials.[a]
c-iv	**Ativan** (Baxter)		In single and 10 mL multidose vials[a], in boxes of 10 *TUBEX*.

[a] With PEG 400, propylene glycol, and 2% benzyl alcohol.

Complete prescribing information begins in the Benzodiazepines group monograph. For information on the anticonvulsant use of lorazepam, refer to the individual monograph in the Anticonvulsant section.

Indications

➤*Oral:*

Anxiety disorders – For the management of anxiety disorders or for short-term relief of symptoms of anxiety or anxiety associated with depressive symptoms.

➤*Parenteral:*

Preanesthetic – In adults for preanesthetic medication, producing sedation, relief of anxiety, and a decreased ability to recall events related to surgery.

Status epilepticus – For the treatment of status epilepticus (See Anticonvulsant section).

Administration and Dosage

Individualize dosage. Increase dosage gradually to minimize adverse effects. When higher dosage is indicated, increase the evening dose before the daytime doses.

➤*Oral:* 2 to 6 mg/day (varies from 1 to 10 mg/day) given in divided doses; take the largest dose before bedtime.

Anxiety – Initial dose, 2 to 3 mg/day given 2 or 3 times/day.

Insomnia because of anxiety or transient situational stress – 2 to 4 mg at bedtime.

Elderly or debilitated patients – Initial dose, 1 to 2 mg/day in divided doses; adjust as needed and tolerated.

➤*Parenteral:*

Preanesthetic – Reduce the doses of other CNS depressant drugs.

IM: 0.05 mg/kg up to a maximum of 4 mg. For optimum effect, administer at least 2 hours before operative procedure.

IV: Initial dose is 2 mg total or 0.044 mg/kg (0.02 mg/lb), whichever is smaller. This will sedate most adults; ordinarily, do not exceed in patients over 50 years of age. If a greater lack of recall would be beneficial, doses as high as 0.05 mg/kg up to a total of 4 mg may be given. For optimum effect, give 15 to 20 minutes before the procedure.

➤*Administration:*

IM – Inject undiluted, deep into the muscle mass. Administer narcotic analgesics at their usual preoperative time.

IV – Immediately prior to IV use, dilute with an equal volume of compatible solution (sterile water for injection, sodium chloride injection, or 5% dextrose injection). Do not shake vigorously, as this will result in air entrapment. Inject directly into a vein or into tubing of an existing IV infusion. Do not exceed 2 mg/minute. Have equipment to maintain a patent airway available.

Intensol – Intensol is a concentrated oral solution as compared with standard oral liquid medications. It is recommended that the intensol be mixed with liquid or semi-solid food such as water, juices, soda or soda-like beverage, applesauce, and puddings.

Use only the calibrated dropper provided with this product. Draw into the dropper the amount prescribed for a single dose. Squeeze the drop-

LORAZEPAM

per contents into a liquid or semi-solid food and stir gently for a few seconds. Consume the entire amount of the mixture immediately. Do not store for future use.

►*Concomitant medications:* Reduce the dose of lorazepam by 50% when coadministered with probenecid or valproate. It may be necessary to increase the lorazepam dose in females who are concomitantly taking oral contraceptives.

►*Storage/Stability:*
Injection and oral solution – Refrigerate at 2° to 8°C (36° to 46°F). Protect from light.

Tablets – Store at controlled room temperature, 15° to 30°C (59° to 86°F). Protect from moisture.

OXAZEPAM

c-iv	**Serax** (Alpharma)	**Tablets**: 15 mg	Lactose. (S SERAX 15). Yellow, five-sided. In 100s.
c-iv	**Oxazepam** (Various, eg, Balan, Mark, Moore, Ivax, Squibb)	**Capsules**: 10 mg	In 100s, 500s, and UD 100s.
c-iv	**Serax** (Alpharma)		Lactose. (327 SERAX 10). Pink and white. In 100s.
c-iv	**Oxazepam** (Various, eg, Balan, Mark, Moore, Ivax, Squibb)	**Capsules**: 15 mg	In 100s, 500s, and UD 100s.
c-iv	**Serax** (Alpharma)		Lactose. (328 SERAX 15). Red and white. In 100s.
c-iv	**Oxazepam** (Various, eg, Balan, Mark, Moore, Ivax, Squibb)	**Capsules**: 30 mg	In 100s, 500s, and UD 100s.
c-iv	**Serax** (Alpharma)		Lactose. (329 SERAX 30). Maroon and white. In 100s.

Complete prescribing information begins in the Benzodiazepines group monograph.

Indications

►*Anxiety disorders:* For the management of anxiety disorders or for the short-term relief of the symptoms of anxiety. Anxiety associated with depression also is responsive to oxazepam.

For the management of anxiety, tension, agitation, and irritability in older patients.

Alcoholics with acute tremulousness, inebriation, or with anxiety associated with alcohol withdrawal are responsive to therapy.

Administration and Dosage

Individualize dosage.

►*Mild to moderate anxiety, with associated tension, irritability, agitation, or related symptoms of functional origin or secondary to organic disease:* 10 to 15 mg 3 or 4 times/day.

►*Severe anxiety syndromes, agitation, or anxiety associated with depression:* 15 to 30 mg 3 or 4 times/day.

►*Older patients with anxiety, tension, irritability, and agitation:* Initial dosage is 10 mg 3 times/day. If necessary, increase cautiously to 15 mg 3 or 4 times/day.

►*Alcoholics with acute inebriation, tremulousness, or anxiety on withdrawal:* 15 to 30 mg 3 or 4 times/day.

►*Children (6 to 12 years of age):* Dosage has not been established.

►*Storage/Stability:* Store at controlled room temperature, 15° to 30°C (59° to 86°F).

BUSPIRONE HCl

Rx	**Buspirone HCl** (Various, eg, Amide, Ethex, PAR, Teva, UDL)	**Tablets:** 5 mg (4.6 mg as base)	May contain lactose. In 100s and 500s.
Rx	**BuSpar** (Bristol-Myers Squibb)		Lactose. (MJ 5 mg BuSpar). White, ovoid-rectangular, scored. In 100s and 500s.
Rx	**Buspirone HCl** (Par)	**Tablets:** 7.5 mg (6.85 as base)	May contain lactose. In 100s and 500s.
Rx	**Buspirone HCl** (Various, eg, Amide, Ethex, PAR, Teva, UDL)	**Tablets:** 10 mg (9.1 mg as base)	May contain lactose. In 100s and 500s.
Rx	**BuSpar** (Bristol-Myers Squibb)		Lactose. (MJ 10 mg BuSpar). White, ovoid-rectangular, scored. In 100s and 500s.
Rx	**Buspirone HCl** (Various, eg, Amide, Ethex, PAR, Teva, UDL)	**Tablets:** 15 mg (13.7 mg as base)	May contain lactose. In 100s and 500s.
Rx	**BuSpar** (Bristol-Myers Squibb)		Lactose. (MJ 822/5 5 5). White, ovoid-rectangular, scored. In DIVIDOSE 60s and 180s.
Rx	**Buspirone HCl** (Mylan)	**Tablets:** 30 mg (27.4 mg as base)	Scored. In 60s, 100s, and 180s.
Rx	**BuSpar** (Bristol-Myers Squibb)		Lactose. (824/10 10 10). Pink, scored. In DIVIDOSE 60s.

Indications

➤*Anxiety disorders:* For the management of anxiety disorders or short-term relief of symptoms of anxiety.

Administration and Dosage

➤*Approved by the FDA:* September 29, 1986.

➤*Dosage:* The recommended initial dose is 15 mg daily (7.5 mg 2 times/day). To achieve an optimal therapeutic response, increase the dosage 5 mg/day, at intervals of 2 to 3 days, as needed. Do not exceed 60 mg/day. Divided doses of 20 to 30 mg/day have been commonly used.

The bioavailability of buspirone is increased when given with food as compared with the fasted state. Consequently, patients should take buspirone in a consistent manner with regard to the timing of dosing; either always with or always without food.

➤*Concomitant therapy:* When buspirone is to be given with a potent inhibitor of CYP3A4, the dosage recommendations described in the Drug Interactions section should be followed.

➤*Storage/Stability:* Store at room temperature; protect from temperatures greater than 30°C (86°F). Dispense in a tight, light-resistant container.

Actions

➤*Pharmacology:* Buspirone is an antianxiety agent not chemically or pharmacologically related to the benzodiazepines, barbiturates, or other sedative/anxiolytic drugs. Mechanism of action is unknown. Buspirone differs from benzodiazepines in that it does not exert anticonvulsant or muscle relaxant effects. It also lacks prominent sedative effects associated with more typical anxiolytics. In vitro, buspirone has a high affinity for serotonin ($5\text{-}HT_1A$) receptors; it has no significant affinity for benzodiazepine receptors and does not affect GABA bindings. Buspirone has moderate affinity for brain D_2-dopamine receptors. Some studies suggest that buspirone may have indirect effects on other neurotransmitter systems.

➤*Pharmacokinetics:*

Absorption – Buspirone is rapidly absorbed and undergoes extensive first-pass metabolism. Following oral administration, plasma concentrations of unchanged buspirone are very low and variable between subjects. Peak plasma levels of 1 to 6 ng/mL have been observed 40 to 90 minutes after single oral doses of 20 mg. The single dose bioavailability of unchanged buspirone from a tablet is about 90% of an equivalent dose of solution, but there is large variability.

The effects of food upon the bioavailability of buspirone have been studied in 8 subjects. They were given a 20 mg dose with and without food; the AUC and C_{max} of unchanged buspirone increased by 84% and 116%, respectively, but the total amount of buspirone immunoreactive material did not change. This suggests that food may decrease the extent of presystemic clearance of buspirone (see Administration and Dosage).

A multiple dose study suggests that buspirone has nonlinear pharmacokinetics. Thus, dose increases and repeated dosing may lead to somewhat higher blood levels of unchanged buspirone than predicted from results of single-dose studies.

Distribution – Approximately 86% of buspirone is plasma protein bound. An in vitro study indicated that buspirone did not displace highly protein-bound drugs such as phenytoin, warfarin, and propranolol from plasma protein, and buspirone may displace digoxin.

Metabolism – Buspirone is metabolized primarily by oxidation, which in vitro has been shown to be medicated by cytochrome P450 3A4, producing several hydroxylated derivatives and a pharmacologically active metabolite, 1-pyrimidinyl piperazine (1-PP). Blood samples from humans chronically exposed to buspirone do not exhibit high levels of 1-PP.

Excretion – In a single-dose study, 29% to 63% of the dose was excreted in the urine within 24 hours, primarily as metabolites; fecal excretion accounted for 18% to 38% of the dose. The average elimina-

tion half-life of unchanged buspirone after single doses of 10 to 40 mg is about 2 to 3 hours.

Special populations –

Hepatic function impairment: After multiple-dose administration of buspirone to patients with hepatic impairment, steady-state AUC of buspirone increased 13-fold compared with healthy subjects.

Renal function impairment: After multiple-dose administration of buspirone to renally impaired (Ccr = 10 to 70 mL/min/1.73 m²) patients, steady-state AUC of buspirone increased 4-fold compared with healthy (Ccr at least 80 mL/min/1.73 m²) subjects.

Contraindications

Hypersensitivity to buspirone HCl.

Warnings

Buspirone has no established antipsychotic activity; do not employ in lieu of appropriate antipsychotic treatment.

➤*Physical and psychological dependence:* Buspirone has shown no potential for abuse or diversion and there is no evidence that it causes tolerance or physical or psychological dependence. However, it is difficult to predict from experiments the extent to which a CNS active drug will be misused, diverted, and/or abused once marketed. Consequently, carefully evaluate patients for a history of drug abuse and follow such patients closely, observing them for signs of misuse or abuse (eg, tolerance, drug-seeking behavior).

➤*Renal/Hepatic function impairment:* Since buspirone is metabolized by the liver and excreted by the kidneys, do not use in patients with severe hepatic or renal impairment.

➤*Pregnancy: Category B.* Adequate and well-controlled studies have not been performed in pregnant women. Use during pregnancy only if clearly needed.

➤*Lactation:* The extent of the excretion in breast milk of buspirone or its metabolites is not known. In rats, however, buspirone and its metabolites are excreted in milk. Avoid administration to nursing women, if possible.

➤*Children:* Safety and efficacy of buspirone were evaluated in 2 placebo-controlled 6-week trials involving a total of 559 pediatric patients (ranging from 6 to 17 years of age) with generalized anxiety disorder (GAD). Doses studied were 7.5 to 30 mg twice/day (15 to 60 mg/day). There were no significant differences between buspirone and placebo with regard to the symptoms of GAD.

Precautions

➤*Monitoring:* Effectiveness for more than 3 to 4 weeks has not been demonstrated in controlled trials. However, patients have been treated for a year without ill effect. If used for extended periods, periodically reassess the usefulness of the drug.

➤*Interference with cognitive and motor performance:* Buspirone is less sedating than other anxiolytics and does not produce significant functional impairment. However, its CNS effect may not be predictable. Therefore, caution patients about driving or using complex machinery until they are certain that buspirone does not affect them adversely.

➤*Withdrawal reactions:* Buspirone does not exhibit cross-tolerance with benzodiazepines and other sedative/hypnotic drugs. It will not block the withdrawal syndrome often seen with cessation of therapy with these drugs. Therefore, withdraw patients from their prior treatment gradually before starting buspirone, especially patients who have been using a CNS depressant chronically. Rebound or withdrawal symptoms may occur over varying time periods, depending in part on the type of drug and its effective elimination half-life.

➤*Dopamine receptor binding:* Buspirone can bind to central dopamine receptors; a question has been raised about its potential to cause acute and chronic changes in dopamine-mediated neurological function (eg, dystonia, pseudoparkinsonism, akathisia, tardive dyskinesia). Clinical experience in controlled trials has failed to identify any significant neuroleptic-like activity; however, a syndrome of restlessness has appeared shortly after initiation of treatment in a small fraction of bus-

BUSPIRONE HCl

pirone-treated patients. The syndrome may be explained in several ways. For example, buspirone may increase central noradrenergic activity. Alternatively, the effect may be attributable to dopaminergic effects (ie, may represent akathisia).

Drug Interactions

➤*CYP450 system:* Substances that inhibit CYP3A4, such as ketoconazole or ritonavir, may inhibit buspirone metabolism and increase plasma concentrations of buspirone while substances that induce CYP3A4, such as dexamethasone or certain anticonvulsants (eg, phenytoin, phenobarbital, carbamazepine), may increase the rate of buspirone metabolism. If a patient has been titrated to a stable dosage on buspirone, a dose adjustment of buspirone may be necessary to avoid adverse events attributable to buspirone or diminished anxiolytic activity. Consequently, when administered with a potent inhibitor of CYP3A4, a low dose of buspirone used cautiously is recommended. When used in combination with a potent inducer of CYP3A4 the dosage of buspirone may need adjusting to maintain anxiolytic effect.

Buspirone Drug Interactions			
Precipitant drug	Object drug*		Description
Cimetidine	Buspirone	↑	Coadministration increased buspirone C_{max} (40%) and T_{max} (2-fold), but had minimal effects on AUC.
CYP3A4 inhibitors (eg, itraconazole, ketoconazole, erythromycin, clarithromycin, diltiazem, verapamil, fluvoxamine, ritonavir)	Buspirone	↑	Plasma buspirone concentrations may be elevated because of inhibition of its metabolism (CYP3A4). Adjust buspirone dosage as needed. If given with erythromycin, a low dose of buspirone (eg, 2.5 mg twice/day) is recommended. If given with itraconazole, a low dose of buspirone (eg, 2.5 mg/day) is recommended.
CYP3A4 inducers (eg, rifampin, rifabutin, phenytoin, phenobarbital, carbamazepine, dexamethasone)	Buspirone	↓	Plasma buspirone concentrations may be decreased because of induction of its metabolism (CYP3A4). Adjust the buspirone dose as needed.
Fluoxetine	Buspirone	↓	Effects of buspirone may be decreased. Paradoxical worsening of OCD has occurred.
Nefazodone	Buspirone	↑	Coadministration increased plasma buspirone concentrations (up to 20-fold in C_{max} and up to 50-fold in AUC) and statistically significant decreases (≈ 50%) in plasma concentrations of the buspirone active metabolite. Slight increases (23%) in AUC were observed for nefazodone. If the 2 drugs are to be used in combination, a low dose of buspirone (eg, 2.5 mg/day) is recommended.
Buspirone	Nefazodone		
Buspirone	Diazepam	↑	Although coadministration produced no differences in diazepam kinetic parameters (C_{max}, AUC, and C_{min}), increases (about 15%) in nordiazepam kinetics were seen. Minor effects (dizziness, headache, and nausea) were observed.
Buspirone	Alcohol	↔	Formal studies of the interaction of buspirone with alcohol indicate that buspirone does not increase alcohol-induced impairment in motor and mental performance, but it is prudent to avoid concomitant use.
Buspirone	Haloperidol	↑	Haloperidol and buspirone coadministration may result in increased serum haloperidol concentrations.
Buspirone	MAO inhibitors	↑	There have been reports of elevated blood pressure when buspirone was added to a regimen including an MAOI. Therefore, do not use concomitantly.
Buspirone	Trazodone	↔	One report suggests that concomitant use may have caused 3- to 6-fold elevations of ALT in a few patients. In a similar study attempting to replicate this finding, no interactive effect on hepatic transaminases was identified.

* ↑ = Object drug increased. ↓ = Object drug decreased. ↔ = Undetermined clinical effect.

➤*Drug/Food interactions:* The bioavailability of buspirone is increased when given with food as compared with the fasted state (see Administration and Dosage and Pharmacokinetics).

Grapefruit juice – In a study in healthy volunteers, coadministration of buspirone (10 mg as a single-dose) with grapefruit juice (200 mL double-strength twice/day for 2 days) increased plasma buspirone concentrations (4.3-fold increase in C_{max}; 9.2-fold increase in AUC). Advise patients receiving buspirone to avoid drinking large amounts of grapefruit juice.

Adverse Reactions

Approximately 10% of the 2200 patients in premarketing trials in anxiety disorders lasting 3 to 4 weeks discontinued treatment because of adverse events which included: CNS disturbances (3.4%), primarily dizziness, insomnia, nervousness, drowsiness, and lightheadedness; GI disturbances (1.2%), primarily nausea; miscellaneous disturbances (1.1%), primarily headache and fatigue. In addition, 3.4% of patients had multiple complaints, none of which were primary.

Buspirone Adverse Reactions (%)[a]		
Adverse reaction	Buspirone (n = 477)	Placebo (n = 464)
CNS		
Dizziness	12	3
Drowsiness	10	9
Headache	6	3
Nervousness	5	1
Insomnia	3	3
Lightheadedness	3	< 1
Decreased concentration	2	2
Excitement	2	< 1
Anger/Hostility	2	< 1
Confusion	2	< 1
Numbness	2	< 1
Depression	2	2
Tremor	1	< 1
Incoordination	1	< 1
Paresthesia	1	< 1
GI		
Nausea	8	5
Dry mouth	3	4
Abdominal/Gastric distress	2	2
Diarrhea	2	< 1
Constipation	1	2
Vomiting	1	2
Miscellaneous		
Fatigue	4	4
Weakness	2	< 1
Blurred vision	2	< 1
Tachycardia/Palpitations	1	1
Sweating/Clamminess	1	< 1
Musculoskeletal aches/Pains	1	< 1
Skin rash	1	< 1

[a] Data are pooled from separate studies.

➤*Cardiovascular:* Nonspecific chest pain (at least 1%); syncope, hypotension, hypertension (0.1% to 1%); cerebrovascular accident, CHF, MI, cardiomyopathy, bradycardia (less than 0.1%).

➤*CNS:* Dream disturbances (at least 1%); depersonalization, dysphoria, noise intolerance, euphoria, akathisia, fearfulness, loss of interest, dissociative reaction, hallucinations, involuntary movements, slowed reaction time, suicidal ideation, seizures (0.1% to 1%); feelings of claustrophobia, cold intolerance, stupor, slurred speech, psychosis (less than 0.1%).

➤*Dermatologic:* Edema, pruritus, flushing, easy bruising, hair loss, dry skin, facial edema, blisters (0.1% to 1%); acne and thinning of nails (less than 0.1%).

➤*Endocrine:* Galactorrhea, thyroid abnormality (less than 0.1%).

➤*GI:* Flatulence, anorexia, increased appetite, salivation, irritable colon, rectal bleeding (0.1% to 1%); burning of the tongue (less than 0.1%).

➤*GU:* Decreased or increased libido, urinary frequency, urinary hesitancy, menstrual irregularity and spotting, dysuria (0.1% to 1%); amenorrhea, pelvic inflammatory disease, delayed ejaculation, impotence, enuresis, nocturia (less than 0.1%).

➤*Musculoskeletal:* Muscle cramps, muscle spasms, rigid/stiff muscles, arthralgia (0.1% to 1%); muscle weakness (less than 0.1%).

➤*Respiratory:* Hyperventilation, shortness of breath, chest congestion (0.1% to 1%); epistaxis (less than 0.1%).

➤*Special senses:* Tinnitus, sore throat, nasal congestion (at least 1%); redness and itching of the eyes, altered taste, altered smell, conjunctivitis (0.1% to 1%); inner ear abnormality, eye pain, photophobia, pressure on eyes (less than 0.1%).

BUSPIRONE HCl

➤*Miscellaneous:* Weight gain, fever, roaring sensation in the head, weight loss, malaise (0.1% to 1%); alcohol abuse, bleeding disturbance, loss of voice, hiccoughs (less than 0.1%).

➤*Lab test abnormalities:* Increases in hepatic aminotransferases (AST, ALT) (0.1% to 1%); eosinophilia, leukopenia, thrombocytopenia (less than 0.1%).

Postmarketing – Voluntary reports since introduction have included rare occurrences of allergic reactions (including urticaria), angioedema, cogwheel rigidity, dizziness (rarely reported as vertigo), dystonic reactions, ataxias, extrapyramidal symptoms, dyskinesias (acute and tardive), ecchymosis, emotional lability, serotonin syndrome, transient difficulty with recall, urinary retention, and visual changes (including tunnel vision). Because of the uncontrolled nature of these spontaneous reports, a causal relationship with buspirone treatment has not been determined.

Overdosage

➤*Symptoms:* Doses as high as 375 mg/day were administered to healthy male volunteers. As this dose was approached, the following symptoms were observed: Nausea, vomiting, dizziness, drowsiness, miosis, and gastric distress. No deaths have been reported.

➤*Treatment:* No specific antidote is known. Use general symptomatic and supportive measures along with immediate gastric lavage. Respiration, pulse, and blood pressure should be monitored as in all cases of drug overdosage. Refer to General Management of Acute Overdosage. Dialyzability of buspirone has not been determined.

Patient Information

Take consistently, always with or always without food.

Avoid drinking large amounts of grapefruit juice.

Avoid drinking alcohol and taking other medication (eg, sedatives, tranquilizers) that cause drowsiness.

May cause drowsiness and dizziness. Use caution while driving or performing other tasks requiring alertness. Avoid alcohol and use other CNS depressants with caution.

Inform physician if you are pregnant, become pregnant, or are planning to become pregnant while taking buspirone or if you are breastfeeding.

DOXEPIN HCl

Rx	**Doxepin HCl** (Various, eg, Geneva, Mylan, Par, Schein)	**Capsules:** 10 mg	In 100s, 500s, 1000s and UD 100s.
Rx	**Sinequan** (Roerig)		(Sinequan Roerig 534). In 100s and 1000s.
Rx	**Doxepin HCl** (Various, eg, Geneva, Major, Mylan, Par, Schein)	**Capsules:** 25 mg	In 100s, 500s, 1000s and UD 100s.
Rx	**Sinequan** (Roerig)		(Sinequan Roerig 535). In 100s, 1000s and 5000s.
Rx	**Doxepin HCl** (Various, eg, Major, Mylan, Par, Schein)	**Capsules:** 50 mg	In 100s, 500s, 1000s and UD 100s.
Rx	**Sinequan** (Roerig)		(Sinequan Roerig 536). In 100s, 1000s and 5000s.
Rx	**Doxepin HCl** (Various, eg, Major, Mylan, Par, Schein)	**Capsules:** 75 mg	In 100s, 500s, 1000s and UD 100s.
Rx	**Sinequan** (Roerig)		(Sinequan Roerig 539). In 100s and 1000s.
Rx	**Doxepin HCl** (Various, eg, Mylan, Par, Schein)	**Capsules:** 100 mg	In 100s, 500s, 1000s and UD 100s.
Rx	**Sinequan** (Roerig)		(Sinequan Roerig 538). In 100s and 1000s.
Rx	**Doxepin HCl** (Various, eg, Major, Par)	**Capsules:** 150 mg	In 50s, 100s and 500s.
Rx	**Sinequan** (Roerig)		(Sinequan Roerig 537). In 50s and 500s.
Rx	**Doxepin HCl** (Various, eg, Morton Grove)	**Oral Concentrate:** 10 mg/ml	In 120 ml.
Rx	**Sinequan Concentrate** (Roerig)		Parabens. In 120 ml.

Doxepin is a tricyclic antidepressant that also has antianxiety effects. The following is an abbreviated monograph for doxepin. For complete prescribing information, refer to the Tricyclic Antidepressants monograph.

Indications

➤*Depression/Anxiety:* For the treatment of psychoneurotic patients with depression or anxiety; depression or anxiety associated with alcoholism or organic disease; psychotic depressive disorders with associated anxiety including involutional depression and manic-depressive disorders.

The target symptoms of psychoneurosis that respond to doxepin include anxiety, tension, depression, somatic symptoms and concerns, sleep disturbances, guilt, lack of energy, fear, apprehension and worry.

Administration and Dosage

Individualize dosage.

The total daily dosage may be given on a divided or once-a-day dosage schedule. If the once-a-day schedule is employed, the maximum recommended dose is 150 mg/day, given at bedtime.

Not recommended for use in children < 12 years of age.

➤*Depression/Anxiety:* Start with 75 mg/day. The optimum dose range is 75 to 150 mg/day. May be gradually increased to 300 mg/day for severely ill patients. Additional therapeutic effect is rarely obtained by exceeding a dose of 300 mg/day. Some patients with very mild symptoms or emotional symptoms accompanying organic disease have been controlled on doses as low as 25 to 50 mg/day.

➤*Oral concentrate:* Dilute oral concentrate with ≈ 120 ml of liquid (eg, water; milk; orange, grapefruit, tomato, prune or pineapple juice) just prior to administration; not compatible with a number of carbonated beverages. For patients on methadone maintenance, doxepin concentrate can be mixed with methadone syrup and lemonade, orange juice, water or sugar water. *Do not mix with grape juice.* Preparation and storage of bulk dilutions are not recommended.

HYDROXYZINE

Rx	**Hydroxyzine HCl** (Various, eg, Geneva, Royce, Rugby, Sidmak, Zenith-Goldline)	**Tablets:** 10 mg (as HCl)	In 20s, 30s, 50s, 100s, 250s, 500s, 1000s and UD 32s and 100s.
Rx	**Atarax** (Roerig)		(ATARAX 10). Orange. In 100s, 500s and UD 40s and 100s.
Rx	**Hydroxyzine HCl** (Various, eg, Geneva, Royce, Rugby, Sidmak, Zenith-Goldline)	**Tablets:** 25 mg (as HCl)	In 20s, 30s, 40s, 50s, 60s, 100s, 250s, 500s, 1000s and UD 100s.
Rx	**Atarax** (Roerig)		(ATARAX 25). Green. In 100s, 500s and UD 40s and 100s.
Rx	**Hydroxyzine HCl** (Various, eg, Geneva, Royce, Rugby, Spencer Mead, Zenith-Goldline)	**Tablets:** 50 mg (as HCl)	In 30s and 100s.
Rx	**Atarax** (Roerig)		(ATARAX 50). Yellow. In 100s, 500s and UD 100s.
Rx	**Atarax 100** (Roerig)	**Tablets:** 100 mg (as HCl)	(ATARAX 100). Red. In 100s and UD 100s.
Rx	**Hydroxyzine Pamoate** (Various, eg, Barr, Eon, Geneva, Major, Rugby, Spencer Mead, Zenith-Goldline)	**Capsules:** 25 mg (as pamoate equivalent to HCl)[1]	In 12s, 20s, 50s, 100s, 500s, 1000s and UD 32s and 100s.
Rx	**Vistaril** (Pfizer)		(VISTARIL PFIZER 541). Two-tone green. In 100s, 500s and UD 100s.
Rx	**Hydroxyzine Pamoate** (Various, eg, Barr, Eon, Geneva, Major, Rugby, Spencer Mead, Zenith-Goldline)	**Capsules:** 50 mg (as pamoate equivalent to HCl)[1]	In 12s, 20s, 100s, 500s, 1000s and UD 32s and 100s.
Rx	**Vistaril** (Pfizer)		(VISTARIL PFIZER 542). Green and white. In 100s, 500s and UD 100s.
Rx	**Hydroxyzine Pamoate** (Various, eg, Barr, Rugby, Spencer Mead, Zenith-Goldline)	**Capsules:** 100 mg (as pamoate equivalent to HCl)[1]	In 100s, 500s, 1000s and UD 100s.
Rx	**Vistaril** (Pfizer)		(VISTARIL PFIZER 543). Green/gray. In 100s, 500s, UD 100s.

HYDROXYZINE

Rx	Hydroxyzine HCl (Various, eg, Geneva, Morton Grove, Rugby, UDL, Zenith-Goldline)	Syrup: 10 mg/5 ml (as HCl)	In 16, 120 and 473 ml, gal and UD 5, 12.5 and 25 ml.
Rx	Atarax (Roerig)		Sucrose and menthol. 0.5% alcohol. In 473 ml.
Rx	Vistaril (Pfizer)	Oral Suspension: 25 mg/5 ml (as pamoate equiv. to HCl)[1]	Sorbitol. Lemon flavor. In 120 and 480 ml.
Rx	Hydroxyzine HCl (Various, eg, American Regent, Fujisawa, Schein, Solopak, Steris)	Injection: 25 mg/ml (as HCl)	In 2 ml syringes and 1 and 10 ml vials.
Rx	Vistaril (Roerig)		In 10 ml vials.[2]
Rx	Hydroxyzine HCl (Various, eg, American Pharmaceutical Partners, American Regent)	Injection: 50 mg/ml (as HCl)	In 1 and 10 ml vials.

[1] Hydroxyzine pamoate is administered in doses equivalent to 25, 50 or 100 mg of hydroxyzine HCl.

[2] With benzyl alcohol.

For complete prescribing information, refer to the Antihistamine group monograph and the individual monograph in Antihistamines.

Indications

➤*Anxiety:* Symptomatic relief of anxiety and tension associated with psychoneurosis and as an adjunct in organic disease states in which anxiety is manifest; prior to dental procedures; in acute emotional problems; in alcoholism; allergic conditions with strong emotional overlay (eg, chronic urticaria and pruritus). Hydroxyzine benefits the cardiac patient by its ability to allay the associated anxiety and apprehension attendant to certain types of heart disease.

IM only – For the acutely disturbed or hysterical patient; the acute or chronic alcoholic with anxiety withdrawal symptoms or delirium tremens; as pre- and postoperative and pre- and postpartum adjunctive medication to allay anxiety.

➤*Pruritus:* Management of pruritus caused by allergic conditions such as chronic urticaria, atopic and contact dermatoses, and in histamine-mediated pruritus.

➤*Sedative (oral only):* As a sedative when used as premedication and following general anesthesia.

➤*Antiemetic (parenteral only):* In controlling nausea and vomiting (excluding nausea and vomiting of pregnancy). As pre- and postoperative and pre- and postpartum adjunctive medication to control emesis.

➤*Analgesia, adjunctive therapy (parenteral only):* As pre- and postoperative and pre- and postpartum adjunctive medication to permit reduction in narcotic dosage.

Administration and Dosage

➤*Parenteral:* Hydroxyzine is for deep IM administration only and may be given without further dilution. Avoid IV, SC, or intra-arterial administration (see Warnings). Inject well within the body of a relatively large muscle. In adults, the preferred site is the upper outer quadrant of the buttock or the midlateral thigh. In children, inject into the midlateral muscles of the thigh. In infants and small children, use the periphery of the upper outer quadrant of the gluteal region only when necessary, such as in burn patients, in order to minimize the possibility of sciatic nerve damage.

Use the deltoid area only if well developed, and then only with caution to avoid radial nerve injury. Do not inject into the lower and mid-third of the upper arm.

Start patients on IM therapy when indicated. Maintain on oral therapy whenever practicable. Adjust dosage according to patient's response.

Anxiety –
Adults: 50 to 100 mg 4 times a day.

Pruritus –
Adults: 25 mg 3 or 4 times a day.

Sedative (as premedication and following general anesthesia) –
Adults: 50 to 100 mg.
Children: 0.6 mg/kg.

Antiemetic/Analgesia, adjunctive therapy (parenteral only) –
Adults: 25 to 100 mg IM as pre- and postoperative/pre- and postpartum adjunctive medication to permit reduction of narcotic dosage. Reduce dosage of concomitant CNS depressants by 50%.
Children: 1.1 mg/kg (0.5 mg/lb) IM to control emesis or as pre- and postoperative adjunctive medication to permit reduction of narcotic dosage. Reduce dosage of concomitant CNS depressants by 50%.

➤*Oral:*

Anxiety – The efficacy of hydroxyzine as an antianxiety agent for long-term use (> 4 months) has not been assessed; periodically reevaluate its usefulness.
Adults: 50 to 100 mg 4 times a day.
Children (> 6 years): 50 to 100 mg/day in divided doses.
Children (< 6 years): 50 mg/day in divided doses.

Pruritus –
Adults: 25 mg 3 or 4 times daily.
Children (> 6 years): 50 to 100 mg/day in divided doses.
Children (< 6 years): 50 mg/day in divided doses.

Sedative (as premedication and following general anesthesia) –
Adults: 50 to 100 mg.
Children: 0.6 mg/kg.

Actions

➤*Pharmacology:* Hydroxyzine is a piperazine derivative chemically unrelated to phenothiazine, reserpine, and meprobamate. It is not a cortical depressant but may exert CNS-depressant activity in subcortical areas. Hydroxyzine has demonstrated its clinical efficacy in the management of neuroses and emotional disturbances manifested by anxiety, tension, agitation, apprehension, or confusion. Clinically, it is a rapid-acting true ataraxic (calmative) with a wide margin of safety. It induces a calming effect in anxious, tense, psychoneurotic adults and in anxious, hyperkinetic children without impairing mental alertness.

Primary skeletal muscle relaxation has been demonstrated experimentally. Bronchodilator activity, antihistaminic and analgesic effects have been confirmed clinically. Hydroxyzine has antispasmodic properties, apparently mediated through interference with the mechanism that responds to spasmogenic agents, such as serotonin, acetylcholine, and histamine. An antiemetic effect has also been demonstrated. Hydroxyzine in therapeutic dosage does not increase gastric secretion or acidity and, in most cases, provides mild antisecretory activity.

➤*Pharmacokinetics:* Oral hydroxyzine is rapidly absorbed from the GI tract; clinical effects are usually noted within 15 to 30 minutes after administration. Following a single 100 mg oral dose, peak levels of 82 ng/mL were reached in ≈ 3 hours. Metabolites include cetirizine which has H_1-antagonist activity. Mean elimination half-life is 3 hours but has been reported to be up to 20 hours; half-life may be longer in elderly patients. Hydroxyzine is mainly metabolized by the liver.

Contraindications

Hypersensitivity to hydroxyzine or cetirizine; early pregnancy, lactation (see Warnings); hydroxyzine injection is for IM use only. Do not inject SC, IV, or intra-arterially (see Warnings).

Warnings

➤*Administration:* For deep IM administration only; avoid SC, IV, or intra-arterial injection. Tissue necrosis has been associated with SC or intra-arterial injection; hemolysis has occurred following IV administration. Accidental intra-arterial injection has led to necrosis of the extremity, necessitating amputation of the digits of the affected limb.

➤*Hypersensitivity reactions:* Hypersensitivity reactions have occurred (see Adverse Reactions). Refer to Management of Acute Hypersensitivity Reactions.

➤*Pregnancy:* Clinical data in humans are inadequate to establish safety in early pregnancy. In doses substantially above the human therapeutic range, hydroxyzine has induced fetal abnormalities in animals. Do not use in pregnancy.

➤*Lactation:* It is not known whether this drug is excreted in breast milk; cetirizine, a metabolite of hydroxyzine, has been detected in breast milk. Therefore, do not give hydroxyzine to nursing mothers.

Precautions

➤*ECG changes:* ECG abnormalities, particularly alterations in T-waves similar to those produced by thioridazine and tricyclic antidepressants, have been associated with anxiolytic doses of hydroxyzine HCl.

➤*Porphyria:* Hydroxyzine has been associated with clinical exacerbations of porphyria and is considered unsafe in porphyric patients.

➤*Benzyl alcohol:* Some of the products contain benzyl alcohol, which has been associated with a fatal "gasping syndrome" in premature infants.

HYDROXYZINE

➤*Hazardous tasks:* May produce drowsiness; patients should observe caution while driving or performing other tasks requiring alertness, coordination, or physical dexterity.

Drug Interactions

➤*CNS depressants (eg, narcotics, barbiturates):* Consider the potentiating action when used with hydroxyzine. When CNS depressants are given concomitantly with hydroxyzine, reduce their dosage by 50%. Cardiac arrest has occurred (rare).

Adverse Reactions

Dry mouth; drowsiness is usually transitory and may disappear after a few days of continued therapy or upon dosage reduction; involuntary motor activity, including rare instances of tremor and convulsions, usually with higher than recommended dosage; hypersensitivity reactions have occurred (see Warnings).

Overdosage

➤*Symptoms:* The most common manifestation is oversedation. As in management of any overdosage, consider that multiple agents may have been ingested.

➤*Treatment:* Induce vomiting if it has not occurred spontaneously. Immediate gastric lavage is also recommended. General supportive care is indicated; frequently monitor vital signs and observe the patient closely. Refer to General Management of Acute Overdosage. Control hypotension with IV fluids and levarterenol or metaraminol. Do not use epinephrine; hydroxyzine counteracts its pressor action. There is no specific antidote. It is doubtful that hemodialysis would be of value.

Patient Information

May produce drowsiness; observe caution while driving or performing other tasks requiring alertness, coordination, or physical dexterity. Avoid alcoholic beverages and other CNS depressants; they may intensify this effect.

MEPROBAMATE

c-iv	**Meprobamate** (Various, eg, Watson)	**Tablets:** 200 mg	In 20s, 100s, and 1000s.
c-iv	**Miltown** (Wallace)		Sugar. (Wallace 37 1101). White. In 100s.
c-iv	**Meprobamate** (Various, eg, Watson)	**Tablets:** 400 mg	In 20s, 100s, 500s, 1000s, and UD 100s.
c-iv	**Miltown** (Wallace)		(Wallace 37 1001). White, scored. In 100s, 500s, and 1000s.

Indications

➤*Anxiety:* Management of anxiety disorders or short-term relief of the symptoms of anxiety. Anxiety or tension associated with the stress of everyday life usually does not require treatment with an anxiolytic.

Effectiveness in long-term use (> 4 months) has not been assessed by systematic clinical studies. Periodically reassess usefulness of the drug for the individual patient.

Administration and Dosage

➤*Adults:* 1.2 to 1.6 g/day in 3 to 4 divided doses; do not exceed 2.4 g/day.

➤*Children:* 100 to 200 mg 2 or 3 times daily.

Actions

➤*Pharmacology:* Meprobamate, an antianxiety agent, is a carbamate derivative that has selective effects at multiple sites in the CNS, including the thalamus and limbic system. It also appears to inhibit multineuronal spinal reflexes. Meprobamate is mildly tranquilizing, and has some anticonvulsant and muscle relaxant properties.

➤*Pharmacokinetics:*

Absorption/Distribution – Meprobamate is well absorbed from the GI tract; peak plasma concentrations are reached within 1 to 3 hours. During chronic administration of sedative doses, concentrations in blood range between 5 and 20 mcg/mL. Plasma protein binding is ≈ 15%.

Metabolism/Excretion – The liver metabolizes 80% to 92% of the drug; the remainder is excreted unchanged in the urine. Following a single dose, the plasma half-life ranges from 6 to 17 hours, but during chronic administration, may be as long as 24 to 48 hours. Meprobamate can induce some hepatic microsomal enzymes, but it is not known whether it induces its own metabolism. Excretion is mainly renal (90%), with < 10% appearing in feces.

Contraindications

Acute intermittent porphyria; allergic or idiosyncratic reactions to meprobamate or related compounds (eg, carisoprodol).

Warnings

➤*Drug dependence:* Physical and psychological dependence and abuse may occur. Avoid prolonged use, especially in alcoholics and addiction-prone persons. Consider possibility of suicide attempts. Carefully supervise dose and amounts prescribed; dispense least amount of drug feasible at any one time.

Abrupt discontinuation after prolonged and excessive use may precipitate a recurrence of preexisting symptoms or withdrawal syndrome characterized by anxiety, anorexia, insomnia, vomiting, ataxia, tremors, muscle twitching, confusional states, and hallucinations. Generalized seizures occur in ≈ 10% of cases and are more likely to occur in persons with CNS damage or preexistent or latent convulsive disorders. Onset of withdrawal symptoms usually occurs within 12 to 48 hours after drug discontinuation; symptoms usually cease in the next 12 to 48 hours.

When excessive dosage has continued for weeks or months, reduce gradually over a period of 1 or 2 weeks rather than stopping abruptly. Alternatively, a short-acting barbiturate may be substituted and then gradually withdrawn.

➤*Hypersensitivity reactions:* Usually seen between the first to fourth dose in patients having no previous exposure to the drug. In case of allergic or idiosyncratic reactions, discontinue the drug and initiate appropriate symptomatic therapy, which may include epinephrine, antihistamines and in severe cases, corticosteroids. In evaluating possible allergic reactions, also consider allergy to excipients (see Adverse Reactions). Refer to Management of Acute Hypersensitivity Reactions.

➤*Renal function impairment:* Use with caution to avoid accumulation, since meprobamate is metabolized in the liver and excreted by the kidney.

➤*Elderly:* To avoid oversedation, use lowest effective dose.

➤*Pregnancy:* Meprobamate passes the placental barrier. It is present in umbilical cord blood, at or near maternal plasma levels. An increased risk of congenital malformations is associated with its use during the first trimester of pregnancy. Since few indications exist for this drug in the pregnant woman, use with extreme caution, if at all, during pregnancy. Consider the possibility that a woman of childbearing potential may be pregnant at the time of institution of therapy.

➤*Lactation:* Meprobamate is excreted into breast milk at concentrations 2 to 4 times that of maternal plasma. The effect of this amount of drug on the nursing infant is unknown.

➤*Children:* Do not administer to children < 6 years of age because of a lack of documented evidence of safety and efficacy. The 600 mg tablet is not intended for use in children.

Precautions

➤*Epilepsy:* May precipitate seizures in epileptic patients.

➤*Hazardous tasks:* May produce drowsiness, dizziness, or blurred vision; patients should observe caution while driving or performing other tasks requiring alertness.

Drug Interactions

Meprobamate Drug Interactions			
Precipitant drug	Object drug*		Description
Alcohol	Meprobamate	↑	Acute ingestion may result in a decreased clearance of meprobamate through inhibition of hepatic metabolic systems; enhanced CNS depressant effects may occur. Tolerance may occur with chronic alcohol ingestion, presumably due to enhanced metabolic capacity.
Meprobamate	CNS depressants (eg, barbiturates, narcotics)	↑	Anticipate additive CNS depressant effects.
CNS depressants (eg, barbiturates, narcotics)	Meprobamate		

*↑ = Object drug increased.

Adverse Reactions

➤*Cardiovascular:* Palpitations; tachycardia; various arrhythmias; transient ECG changes; syncope and hypotensive crises (including 1 fatality).

➤*CNS:* Drowsiness; ataxia; dizziness; slurred speech; headache; vertigo; weakness; impairment of visual accommodation; euphoria; overstimulation; paradoxical excitement; fast EEG activity.

➤*GI:* Nausea; vomiting; diarrhea.

➤*Miscellaneous:*

Allergic or idiosyncratic – Usually seen between the first and fourth dose in patients having no previous exposure to the drug.

Milder reactions – Milder reactions are characterized by an itchy, urticarial, or erythematous maculopapular rash which may be generalized or confined to the groin. Other reactions have included the following: Leukopenia; acute nonthrombocytopenic purpura; petechiae; ecchymoses; eosinophilia; peripheral edema; adenopathy; fever; fixed drug eruption with cross reaction to carisoprodol.

More severe reactions – More severe, rare hypersensitivity reactions include the following: Hyperpyrexia; chills; angioneurotic edema; bronchospasm; oliguria; anuria; anaphylaxis; erythema multiforme; exfoliative dermatitis; stomatitis; proctitis. Stevens-Johnson syndrome and bullous dermatitis have also occurred, including 1 fatal case of the latter after administration of meprobamate in combination with prednisolone (see Warnings).

Other – Exacerbation of porphyric symptoms; paresthesias.

➤*Hematologic:* Agranulocytosis and aplastic anemia (rarely fatal) have occurred, but no causal relationship has been established. Rarely, thrombocytopenic purpura.

Overdosage

➤*Symptoms:* Acute intoxication produces drowsiness, lethargy, stupor, ataxia, coma, shock, vasomotor and respiratory collapse and death. Cardiovascular disturbances include arrhythmias, tachycardia, bradycardia and reduced venous return. Profound and persistent hypotension occurs and can appear unexpectedly in mildly comatose patients. Excessive oronasal secretion or relaxation of the pharyngeal wall may cause airway obstruction problems. The following data represent the usual ranges:

Acute simple overdose (meprobamate alone) – Death has occurred with ingestion of as little as 12 g and survival with as much as 40 g.

Blood levels –
0.5 to 3 mg/dl – Therapeutic range.
3 to 10 mg/dl – Mild to moderate overdosage; stupor, light coma.
10 to 20 mg/dl – Deeper coma requiring intensive therapy; some fatalities.
> 20 mg/dl – > 50% fatalities.

MEPROBAMATE

Acute combined overdose – Acute combined overdose with other psychotropic drugs, other CNS depressants or alcohol renders the above values useless as a prognostic indicator.

➤*Treatment:* Because meprobamate is rapidly absorbed, gastric lavage (or emesis in a conscious patient) may be of value only if carried out shortly after ingestion. Ingestion of large amounts may form drug conglomerates in the stomach; continue gastric lavage. Gastroscopy may be indicated. Relapse and death after initial recovery have been attributed to incomplete gastric emptying and delayed absorption. Frequent measurements of vital signs cannot be overemphasized.

Provide symptomatic and supportive treatment. Hypotension may appear rapidly and become persistent unless blood volume is expanded. Avoid fluid overload; fatal pulmonary edema has occurred. Provide respiratory assistance when needed. Exercise care in the treatment of convulsions because of the combined effect of agents on CNS depression. Refer to General Management of Acute Overdosage.

If the patient's condition deteriorates despite assisted respiration, try forced diuresis and pressor agents, then institute hemodialysis. Meprobamate is dialyzable. Hemoperfusion (resin or charcoal) is more effective than hemodialysis. The half-life during hemoperfusion may be reduced more than threefold.

Patient Information

Advise patients that if they become pregnant during therapy or intend to become pregnant, they should consult with their physician about use of the drug.

May cause drowsiness, dizziness or blurred vision; use caution while driving or performing other tasks requiring alertness.

Avoid alcohol and other CNS depressants while taking this drug.

Notify physician if skin rash, sore throat or fever occurs.

Do not crush or chew tablets and sustained release capsules.

Drugs with clinically useful antidepressant effects include the tricyclic antidepressants (TCAs), tetracyclic antidepressants, trazodone, bupropion, venlafaxine, nefazodone, selective serotonin reuptake inhibitors (SSRIs), and the monoamine oxidase inhibitors (MAOIs). The antidepressant agents all appear effective in the treatment of depression. "Major depressive episode" implies a prominent and relatively persistent (nearly every day for ≥ 2 weeks) depressed or dysphoric mood that usually interferes with daily functioning, and includes ≥ 5 of the following 9 symptoms: Depressed mood; markedly diminished interest or pleasure in all, for almost all activities; significant weight loss or gain when not dieting, or decrease or increase in appetite; insomnia or hypersomnia; psychomotor agitation or retardation; fatigue or loss of energy; feelings of worthlessness, or excessive or inappropriate guilt; diminished ability to think or concentrate, or indecisiveness; recurrent thoughts of death, suicidal ideation, or suicide attempt. These symptoms are not because of the direct physiologic effects of a substance or a general medical condition (eg, hypothyroidism). The symptoms are not better accounted for by bereavement (ie, after the loss of a loved one), persist for > 2 months, or are characterized by marked functional impairment, morbid preoccupation with worthlessness, suicidal ideation, psychotic symptoms, or psychomotor retardation.

▶*Mechanism of action:* Effective antidepressant activity has traditionally been associated with the "biogenic amine hypothesis of depression." The theory is that depression is due to reduced functional activity of ≥ 1 of the endogenous monoamines (norepinephrine, serotonin) in the brain. It was believed that certain types of depression were caused by brain neurotransmitter deficiency and that antidepressants relieved depression by inhibiting the reuptake of serotonin and norepinephrine, thereby correcting this deficiency and facilitating neurotransmission. This explanation is now being questioned for several reasons. First, several antidepressant agents lack any apparent effect on neurotransmitter reuptake. More importantly, the blockade of neurotransmitter reuptake occurs within minutes to hours of antidepressant drug initiation, while the antidepressant effects usually take 1 to 4 weeks to manifest.

The emphasis of research has shifted from acute reuptake effects to the slower adaptive changes in norepinephrine and serotonin receptor systems induced by chronic antidepressant therapy. Postsynaptic receptors participate in nerve impulse neurotransmission while the presynaptic receptors regulate neurotransmitter release and reuptake, an important mechanism of neurotransmitter inactivation. Long-term antidepressant treatment produces complex changes in the sensitivities of both presynaptic and postsynaptic receptor sites. The available antidepressant agents may increase the sensitivity of postsynaptic

alpha (α₁) adrenergic and serotonin receptors and may decrease the sensitivity of presynaptic receptor sites. The net effect is the correction (re-regulation) of an abnormal receptor-neurotransmitter relationship. Clinically, this re-regulatory action speeds up the patient's natural recovery process from the depressive episode by normalizing neurotransmission efficacy.

▶*Drug selection:* The non-MAOIs are used more frequently than the MAOIs, mainly because of the perception that MAOIs are less effective than the non-MAOI antidepressants and the risk of hypertensive crisis from ingesting foods containing tyramine or from drug interactions (eg, sympathomimetics) with the MAOIs. However, when MAOIs are used in therapeutic doses, they are probably equally effective to non-MAOIs for the treatment of depression. In general, MAOIs are used for atypical depression.

Base antidepressant drug selection on the patient's history of drug response (if any), the specific drug's side effect profile relative to patient medical conditions and other factors, and clinician familiarity with specific antidepressants. Nortriptyline and desipramine are preferred TCAs in a patient without a history of favorable response to a specific antidepressant because they cause less sedation and have less anticholinergic activity than tertiary TCAs such as amitriptyline and, in the case of nortriptyline, are less likely to cause orthostatic hypotension. Trazodone has less anticholinergic activity than TCAs and causes fewer problems than TCAs when taken in overdose. SSRIs generally lack the adverse reactions (eg, sedation, anticholinergic effects) associated with TCAs, cause few cardiovascular side effects (including orthostasis), are associated with initial weight loss rather than weight gain as is the case with TCAs, and cause fewer problems than TCAs when taken in overdose. Newer information has shown that during long-term use, SSRIs cause similar weight gain as compared with TCAs. However, their use is associated with other side effects such as headache, nervousness, and insomnia. Fluoxetine and paroxetine are recommended to be taken in the morning; sertraline can be taken morning or evening. Use maprotiline, mirtazapine, and bupropion only when other antidepressants have not proven effective. In cases of mild depression, drug therapy and psychotherapy appear to be equally effective.

As a general guideline, continue treatment for 9 months after remission in patients who experience their first episode of depression; following a second episode, continue treatment for 5 years after remission; with a third episode, treat indefinitely.

▶*Actions:* The following table summarizes some of the important pharmacologic and pharmacokinetic data of these agents.

Antidepressant Pharmacologic and Pharmacokinetic Parameters									
0 -none + -slight ++ -moderate +++ -high ++++ -very high +++++ -highest	Major side effects			Amine uptake blocking activity		Half-life (hours)	Therapeutic plasma level (ng/ml)	Time to reach steady state (days)	Dose range (mg/day)
	Anticholinergic	Sedation	Orthostatic hypotension	Norepinephrine	Serotonin				
Tricyclics - Tertiary Amines									
Amitriptyline	++++	++++	++	++	++++	31-46	110-250[1]	4-10	50-300
Clomipramine	+++	+++	++	++	+++++	19-37	80-100	7-14	25-250
Doxepin	++	+++	++	+	++	8-24	100-200[1]	2-8	25-300
Imipramine	++	++	+++	++[2]	++++	11-25	200-350[1]	2-5	30-300
Trimipramine	++	+++	++	+	+	7-30	180[1]	2-6	50-300
Tricyclics - Secondary Amines									
Amoxapine[3]	+++	++	+	+++	++	8[4]	200-500	2-7	50-600
Desipramine	+	+	+	++++	++	12-24	125-300	2-11	25-300
Nortriptyline	++	++	+	++	+++	18-44	50-150	4-19	30-100
Protriptyline	+++	+	+	++++	++	67-89	100-200	14-19	15-60
Tetracyclics									
Maprotiline	++	++	+	+++	0/+	21-25	200-300[1]	6-10	50-225
Mirtazapine	++	+++	++	+++	+++	20-40	-	5	15-45
Triazolopyridine									
Trazodone	+	++++	++	0	+++	4-9	800-1600	3-7	150-600
Aminoketone									
Bupropion[5]	++	++	+	0/+	0/+	8-24	-	1.5-8	200-450
Phenethylamine									
Venlafaxine	0	0	0	+++	+++	5-11[1]	-	3-4	75-375
Phenylpiperazine									
Nefazodone	0/+	++	+	0/+	+++++	2-4	-	4-5	200-600
Selective Serotonin Reuptake Inhibitors									
Citalopram	0/+	0/+	0/+	0/+	++++	33	-	7	20-60
Fluoxetine	0/+	0/+	0/+	0/+	+++++	1-16 days[1]	-	2-4 weeks	20-80

Antidepressant Pharmacologic and Pharmacokinetic Parameters

0 -none + -slight ++ -moderate +++ -high ++++ -very high +++++ -highest	Major side effects			Amine uptake blocking activity		Half-life (hours)	Therapeutic plasma level (ng/ml)	Time to reach steady state (days)	Dose range (mg/day)
	Anticholinergic	Sedation	Orthostatic hypotension	Norepinephrine	Serotonin				
Fluvoxamine	0/+	0/+	0	0/+	+++++	15.6	-	≈ 7	50-300
Paroxetine	0	0/+	0	0/+	+++++	10-24	-	7-14	10-50
Sertraline	0	0/+	0	0/+	+++++	1-4 days[1]	-	7	50-200
Monoamine Oxidase Inhibitors									
Phenelzine	+	+	+	-	-	-	-	-	45-90
Tranylcypromine	+	+	0	-	-	2.4-2.8	-	-	30-60

[1] Parent compound plus active metabolite.
[2] Via desipramine, the major metabolite.
[3] Also blocks dopamine receptors.
[4] 30 hours for major metabolite 8-hydroxyamoxapine.
[5] Inhibits dopamine uptake.

Tricyclic Compounds

Refer to the Antidepressants introduction.

Indications

▶*Depression:* Relief of symptoms of depression (except **clomipramine**). The activating properties of **protriptyline** make it particularly suitable for withdrawn and anergic patients.

Agents with significant sedative action may be useful in depression associated with anxiety and sleep disturbances.

▶*Amoxapine:* Relief of depressive symptoms in patients with neurotic or reactive depressive disorders and endogenous and psychotic depression; depression accompanied by anxiety or agitation.

▶*Doxepin:* Treatment of psychoneurotic patients with depression or anxiety; depression or anxiety associated with alcoholism (not to be taken concomitantly with alcohol); depression or anxiety associated with organic disease (the possibility of drug interaction should be considered if the patient is receiving other drugs concomitantly); psychotic depressive disorders with associated anxiety including involutional depression and manic-depressive disorders. The target symptoms of psychoneurosis that respond particularly well to doxepin include anxiety, tension, depression, somatic symptoms and concerns, sleep disturbances, guilt, lack of energy, fear, apprehension, and worry.

▶*Imipramine:* Treatment of enuresis in children ≥ 6 years of age as temporary adjunctive therapy.

▶*Clomipramine:* Only for treatment of obsessive-compulsive disorder (OCD).

▶*Unlabeled uses:* Analgesic adjuncts for phantom limb pain, chronic pain (migraine, chronic tension headache, diabetic neuropathy, tic douloureux, cancer pain, peripheral neuropathy with pain, postherpetic neuralgia, arthritic pain): Amitriptyline 75 to 300 mg/day; doxepin 30 to 300 mg/day; imipramine 75 to 300 mg/day; nortriptyline 50 to 150 mg/day; desipramine 75 to 300 mg/day; amoxapine 100 to 300 mg/day; protriptyline 15 to 60 mg/day.

Pathologic laughing and weeping secondary to forebrain disease – Amitriptyline 30 to 75 mg/day.

Obstructive sleep apnea – Protriptyline.

Peptic ulcer disease – Trimipramine 25 to 50 mg/day; doxepin 50 to 150 mg/day.

Facilitation of cocaine withdrawal – Desipramine 50 to 200 mg/day; imipramine 150 to 300 mg/day.

Panic disorder – Imipramine; clomipramine; desipramine; nortriptyline. Other antidepressants may also be used.

Eating disorders (effective in bulimia nervosa) – Imipramine; desipramine; amitriptyline.

Premenstrual symptoms – Nortriptyline 50 to 125 mg/day; desipramine 100 to 150 mg/day for depression; clomipramine 25 to 75 mg/day for irritability and dysphoria.

Dermatologic disorders (chronic urticaria and angioedema, nocturnal pruritus in atopic eczema) – Doxepin 10 to 30 mg/day; desipramine 100 to 150 mg/day; nortriptyline 20 to 75 mg/day; amitriptyline 10 to 50 mg/day.

Administration and Dosage

If minor side effects develop, reduce dosage. Discontinue treatment promptly if serious adverse effects or allergic manifestations occur.

▶*Plasma levels:* Determination of plasma levels may be useful in identifying patients who appear to have toxic effects and may have excessively high levels of the drug, or those in whom lack of absorption or noncompliance is suspected. Make adjustments in dosage according to patient's clinical response, not based on plasma levels.

▶*Adolescent, elderly, and outpatients:* Lower dosages are recommended. Initiate therapy at a low dosage and increase gradually, noting the clinical response and any evidence of intolerance. Most antidepressant drugs have a lag period of 10 days to 4 weeks before a therapeutic response is noted. Increasing the dose will not shorten this period but rather increase the incidence of adverse reactions. Following remission, maintenance medication may be required for a longer time at the lowest dose that will maintain remission. Continue maintenance therapy ≥ 3 months to decrease the possibility of relapse.

▶*Single daily dose:* A single daily dose may be used for maintenance therapy. A single daily dose at bedtime is convenient, will minimize daytime side effects (sedation and anticholinergic effects), and the sedative effect at bedtime may be beneficial in patients with sleep disorders. Because of increased risk of cardiovascular and other complications, the elderly may not tolerate single daily doses. **Protriptyline** may have a mild stimulant effect; it is generally not given as a single bedtime dose.

▶*Tricyclic/MAOI combined use:* Tricyclic/MAOI combined use is traditionally contraindicated because of the potential serious adverse reactions (see Drug Interactions). Such combinations may offer significant advantages in patients refractory to more conservative therapy. In conservative dosages, with observance of MAOI dietary restrictions, and under close medical observation, combined therapy has been safe. At least 7 to 10 days should elapse between MAOI discontinuation and TCA institution.

Specific dosage guidelines for individual agents are included in the product listings.

Actions

▶*Pharmacology:* The tricyclic antidepressants (TCAs), structurally related to the phenothiazine antipsychotic agents, possess 3 major pharmacologic actions in varying degrees: Blocking of the amine pump, sedation, and peripheral and central anticholinergic action. In contrast to phenothiazines, which act on dopamine receptors, TCAs inhibit reuptake of norepinephrine or serotonin (5-hydroxytryptamine, 5-HT) at the presynaptic neuron. **Amoxapine**, a metabolite of loxapine, retains some of the postsynaptic dopamine receptor-blocking action of neuroleptics.

Amine uptake inhibition – The amine hypothesis of depression proposes a relationship between depression and levels of CNS bioamines at postsynaptic adrenergic receptors in the brain. TCAs can be characterized by their ability to inhibit presynaptic reuptake of norepinephrine and serotonin (see table in Introduction).

Although amine pump blockade may be immediate, antidepressant response can take days to weeks.

Other pharmacologic effects – Inhibition of histamine and acetylcholine activity. Clinical effects, in addition to antidepressant effects, include sedation, anticholinergic effects, mild peripheral vasodilator effects, and possible "quinidine-like" actions.

▶*Pharmacokinetics:*

Absorption/Distribution – Although the TCAs are well absorbed from the GI tract with peak plasma concentrations occurring in 2 to 4 hours, they undergo a significant first-pass effect. They are highly bound (> 90%) to plasma proteins, lipid soluble, and widely distributed in tissues, including the CNS. Although there is a suggested therapeutic range for many of the TCAs (see table in Introduction), the association between plasma levels and therapeutic effect has not been adequately defined. Wide interpatient variation in steady-state plasma levels at a given dosage is primarily due to differences in the rate of metabolism or first-pass effect. Effective dosage levels vary greatly and must be individualized.

Tricyclic Compounds

Metabolism/Excretion – Metabolism of TCAs occurs in the liver by demethylation, hydroxylation, and glucuronidation, and it varies for each patient. Some intermediate active metabolites include the following:

Amitriptyline ➤ nortriptyline
Amoxapine ➤ 7 hydroxy and 8 hydroxyamoxapine
Clomipramine ➤ desmethylclomipramine
Doxepin ➤ desmethyldoxepin
Imipramine ➤ desipramine

The TCAs are partially secreted into the hepatobiliary circulation and stomach and are reabsorbed and excreted in the urine.

Because of the long half-life, a single daily dose may be given. Up to 2 to 4 weeks may be required to achieve maximal clinical response.

Contraindications

Prior sensitivity to any tricyclic drug. Not recommended for use during the acute recovery phase following MI. Concomitant use of monoamine oxidase inhibitors (MAOIs) is generally contraindicated (see Warnings, Drug Interactions).

➤*Doxepin:* Patients with glaucoma or a tendency to have urinary retention.

Cross-sensitivity may occur among the dibenzazepines (**clomipramine, desipramine, imipramine, nortriptyline,** and **trimipramine**). In addition, dibenzoxepines (**doxepin, amoxapine**) may produce cross-sensitivity. **Amitriptyline** may block the antihypertensive action of guanethidine or similarly active compounds.

Warnings

➤*Tardive dyskinesia:* Tardive dyskinesia, a syndrome consisting of potentially irreversible, involuntary, dyskinetic movements may develop in patients treated with neuroleptics (eg, antipsychotics). **Amoxapine** is not an antipsychotic, but it has substantive neuroleptic activity. Although the syndrome appears most often among the elderly, especially elderly women, it is impossible to determine which patients will develop the syndrome. Whether or not neuroleptic drugs differ in their potential to cause tardive dyskinesia is unknown. For a more complete discussion of tardive dyskinesia, see the Antipsychotic Agents group monograph.

➤*Neuroleptic malignant syndrome (NMS):* NMS is a potentially fatal condition reported in association with antipsychotic drugs and with **amoxapine**. Clinical manifestations of NMS are hyperpyrexia, muscle rigidity, altered mental status, and evidence of autonomic instability (irregular pulse or blood pressure, tachycardia, diaphoresis, and cardiac arrhythmias). The management of NMS should include the following: (1) Immediate discontinuation of antipsychotic drugs, amoxapine, and other drugs not essential to concurrent therapy, (2) intensive symptomatic treatment and medical monitoring, and (3) treatment of any concomitant serious medical problems for which specific treatments are available. There is no general agreement about specific pharmacologic treatment regimens for uncomplicated NMS.

Once the NMS is resolved, use a different antidepressant drug if the patient continues to require antidepressant treatment.

Hyperthermia has occurred with **clomipramine**; most cases occurred when it was used with other drugs (eg, neuroleptics) and may be an example of NMS.

➤*Seizure disorders:* Because TCAs lower the seizure threshold, use with caution in patients with a history of seizures or other predisposing factors (eg, brain damage of varying etiology, alcoholism, concomitant drugs known to lower the seizure threshold). However, seizures have occurred in patients with and without a history of seizure disorders. Seizure was identified as the most significant risk of **clomipramine** use in premarket evaluation.

➤*Anticholinergic effects:* Use with caution in patients with a history of urinary retention, narrow-angle glaucoma, or increased intraocular pressure. In angle-closure glaucoma, even average doses may precipitate an attack. In occasional susceptible patients or in those receiving anticholinergics (including antiparkinson agents), the atropine-like effects may become more pronounced (eg, paralytic ileus). See table in Introduction for relative anticholinergic actions.

➤*Cardiovascular disorders:* Use with extreme caution in patients with cardiovascular disorders because of the possibility of conduction defects, arrhythmias, CHF, sinus tachycardia, MI, strokes, and tachycardia. These patients require cardiac surveillance at all dose levels of the drug. In high doses, TCAs may produce arrhythmias, sinus tachycardia, conduction defects, and prolonged conduction time. Tachycardia and postural hypotension may occur more frequently with **protriptyline**.

➤*Hyperthyroid patients:* Hyperthyroid patients or those receiving thyroid medication require close supervision because of the possibility of cardiovascular toxicity, including arrhythmias.

➤*Psychiatric patients:* Schizophrenic or paranoid patients may exhibit a worsening of psychosis with TCA therapy. In overactive or agitated patients, increased anxiety or agitation may occur. Neuropsychiatric signs and symptoms (eg, delusions, hallucinations, psychotic episodes, confusion, paranoia) have been reported with **clomipramine**

use. Paranoid delusions, with or without associated hostility, may be exaggerated. Reduction of TCA dosage and concomitant antipsychotic therapy (eg, perphenazine) may be necessary.

The possibility of suicide in depressed patients remains during treatment and until significant remission occurs. Patients should not have easy access to large quantities of the drug; advise the physician to prescribe small quantities of TCAs.

➤*Mania/Hypomania:* Hypomanic or manic episodes may occur, particularly in patients with cyclic disorders. Such reactions may necessitate discontinuation of the drug. If needed, **imipramine pamoate** may be resumed in lower doses when these episodes are relieved. Administration of a tranquilizer may be useful in controlling such episodes. Manic-depressive patients may experience a shift to a hypomanic or manic phase, which may necessitate discontinuation and possibly resuming at a lower dose when these episodes are relieved.

➤*MAOIs:* Do not give MAOIs with or immediately following TCAs. Such combinations can produce hyperpyretic crises, severe convulsions, sweating, coma, hyperexcitability, hyperthermia, tachycardia, tachypnea, headache, mydriasis, flushing, confusion, hypotension, disseminated intravascular coagulation, and death. Allow at least 14 days to elapse between MAOI discontinuation and TCA institution. Some TCAs have been used safely and successfully with MAOIs. Initiate TCA cautiously with gradual dosage increase until achieving optimum response. **Furazolidone** may interact similarly with TCAs.

➤*Rash:* Antidepressant drugs can cause skin rashes or "drug fever" in susceptible individuals. These allergic reactions may, in rare cases, be severe. They are more likely to occur during the first few days of treatment but may also occur later. Discontinue if rash or fever develop.

➤*Renal/Hepatic function impairment:* Use with caution and in reduced doses in patients with hepatic impairment; metabolism may be impaired, leading to drug accumulation. **Clomipramine** was occasionally associated with AST and ALT elevations (incidence of ≈ 1% and 3%, respectively) of potential clinical importance (values > 3 times the upper limit of normal) but was not associated with other clinical findings suggestive of hepatic injury. Rare reports of more severe liver injury, some fatal, have been reported. Use caution in treating patients with known liver disease, and periodic monitoring of hepatic enzyme levels is recommended in such patients. Use with caution in patients with significantly impaired renal function.

➤*Elderly:* Be cautious in dose selection for an elderly patient, usually starting at the low end of the dosing range. This reflects the greater frequency of decreased hepatic function, concomitant disease, and other drug therapy in elderly patients. Elderly patients may be sensitive to the anticholinergic side effects of TCAs.

Elderly patients taking **amitriptyline** may be at increased risk for falls; start on low doses of amitriptyline and observe closely.

➤*Pregnancy:* (*Category D* - amitriptyline, imipramine, nortriptyline; *Category C* - amoxapine, clomipramine, desipramine, doxepin, protriptyline, trimipramine). Clinical experience is limited. These agents have demonstrated teratogenicity and embryotoxicity in animals at doses greater than maximum human doses. There have been clinical reports of congenital malformations associated with **imipramine**. Limb reduction anomalies have been reported with **amitriptyline** and **nortriptyline**, and neonatal withdrawal symptoms have been seen with **clomipramine, desipramine,** and **imipramine**. All are isolated reports.

Safety for use during pregnancy has not been established; use only when clearly needed and when the potential benefits outweigh the potential hazards to the fetus.

➤*Lactation:* These agents are excreted into breast milk in low concentrations (approximate milk:plasma ratio of 0.4 to 1.5). Exercise caution when using in a nursing woman.

➤*Children:* Not recommended for patients < 12 years of age. Safety and efficacy have not been established for **amoxapine** in children < 16 years of age, or **clomipramine** in children < 10 years of age. The safety and efficacy of **imipramine** as temporary adjunctive therapy for nocturnal enuresis in pediatric patients < 6 years of age have not been established. The safety of the drug for long-term, chronic use as adjunctive therapy for nocturnal enuresis in pediatric patients ≥ 6 years of age has not been established. Safety and efficacy are not established in the pediatric age group for **trimipramine, nortriptyline, protriptyline,** and **desipramine**.

Do not exceed 2.5 mg/kg/day of **imipramine**. ECG changes of unknown significance have occurred in pediatric patients with doses twice this amount. Effectiveness of imipramine in children for conditions other than nocturnal enuresis has not been established.

Precautions

➤*Monitoring:* Perform baseline and periodic leukocyte and differential counts and liver function studies. Fever or sore throat may signal serious neutrophil depression; discontinue therapy if there is evidence of pathological neutropenia.

Monitor ECG prior to initiation of large doses of TCAs and at appropriate intervals thereafter. Patients with cardiovascular disease require cardiac surveillance at all dosage levels. Elderly patients and patients with cardiac disease or a history of cardiac disease are at special risk of developing cardiac abnormalities with TCAs.

➤*Electroconvulsive therapy:* Electroconvulsive therapy with TCAs may increase the hazards of therapy.

➤*Elective surgery:* Discontinue therapy for as long as possible before elective surgery.

➤*Blood sugar levels:* Elevated and lowered blood sugar levels have occurred.

➤*Sexual dysfunction:* Sexual dysfunction was markedly increased in male patients with OCD taking **clomipramine** (42% ejaculatory failure, 20% impotence) compared with placebo.

➤*Weight changes:* Weight gain has been observed in clinical trials involving all TCAs. Weight gain occurred in 18% of patients receiving **clomipramine**. Some patients had weight gain in excess of 25% of their initial body weight.

➤*Serotonin syndrome:* Some TCAs inhibit neuronal reuptake of serotonin and can increase synaptic serotonin levels (eg, **clomipramine, amitriptyline**). Either therapeutic or excessive doses of these drugs, in combination with other drugs that also increase synaptic serotonin levels (such as MAOIs), can cause a serotonin syndrome consisting of tremor, agitation, delirium, rigidity, myoclonus, hyperthermia, and obtundation.

➤*Benzyl alcohol:* Some of these products contain benzyl alcohol, which has been associated with a fatal "gasping syndrome" in premature infants.

➤*Hazardous tasks:* May impair mental or physical abilities required for the performance of potentially hazardous tasks; have patients observe caution while driving or performing other tasks requiring alertness, coordination, or physical dexterity.

➤*Photosensitivity:* Photosensitization (photoallergy or phototoxicity) may occur; therefore, caution patients to take protective measures (ie, sunscreens, protective clothing) against exposure to ultraviolet light or sunlight until tolerance is determined.

➤*Sulfite sensitivity:* Some of the injectable antidepressant products contain sulfites that may cause allergic-type reactions including anaphylactic symptoms and life-threatening or less-severe asthmatic episodes in certain susceptible people. The overall prevalence of sulfite sensitivity in the general population is unknown but is probably low. Sulfite sensitivity is seen more frequently in asthmatic than in nonasthmatic people. Products containing sulfites are identified in the product listings.

Drug Interactions

➤*P450 system:* Concomitant use of TCAs with other drugs metabolized by cytochrome P450 2D6 may require lower doses than those usually prescribed for either the TCA or the other drug. Therefore, exercise caution in the coadministration of TCAs with other drugs that are metabolized by this isoenzyme, including other antidepressants, phenothiazines, carbamazepine, and type 1C antiarrhythmics (eg, propafenone, flecainide, encainide), or that inhibit this enzyme (eg, quinidine).

Tricyclic Drug Interactions

Precipitant drug	Object drug*		Description
Barbiturates	TCAs	↓	Barbiturates may lower serum levels of TCAs; central and respiratory depressant effects may be additive.
Bupropion	TCAs	↑	Plasma concentrations of TCAs may be elevated, producing an increase in pharmacologic and adverse effects.
Carbamazepine	TCAs	↓	Carbamazepine may decrease TCA levels. Serum carbamazepine levels may be increased resulting in an increase in pharmacologic and toxic effects.
TCAs	Carbamazepine	↑	
Charcoal	TCAs	↓	Charcoal can prevent TCA absorption, thereby reducing their effectiveness or toxicity.
Cimetidine	TCAs	↑	Cimetidine has increased serum TCA concentrations. Anticholinergic symptoms (eg, severe dry mouth, urinary retention, blurred vision) have been associated with elevated TCA serum levels when cimetidine therapy is initiated. Additionally, higher than expected TCA levels have occurred when they are initiated in patients already taking cimetidine. Other H₂ antagonists may be suitable alternatives.
Haloperidol	TCAs	↑	Haloperidol may increase serum concentrations of TCAs; a tonic-clonic seizure occurred in 1 patient.
Histamine H₂ antagonists	TCAs	↑	Increased serum concentrations of the TCAs have occurred; mild symptoms have been noted.
MAO Inhibitors	TCAs	↑	Such combinations can produce hyperpyretic crisis, severe convulsions, sweating, coma, hyperexcitability, hyperthermia, tachycardia, tachypnea, headache, mydriasis, flushing, confusion, hypotension, disseminated intravascular coagulation, and death. However, some MAOIs have been used safely and successfully with TCAs. See Warnings.
Rifamycins	TCAs	↓	TCA levels may be decreased, resulting in a decrease in pharmacologic effects.
Smoking	TCAs	↑	Smoking may increase the metabolic biotransformation of TCAs.
SSRIs	TCAs	↑	SSRIs may increase the pharmacologic and toxic effects of TCAs; symptoms may persist for several weeks after discontinuation of the SSRI. At least 5 weeks may be necessary when switching from fluoxetine to a TCA.
Valproic acid	TCAs	↑	Plasma concentrations and side effects of TCAs may be increased.
Venlafaxine	Desipramine	↑	Desipramine AUC, C_{max}, and C_{min} increased by ≈ 35% in the presence of venlafaxine. The 2-OH-desipramine AUC increased by at least 2.5- to 4.5-fold. The clinical significance of elevated 2-OH-desipramine levels is unknown.
TCAs	Anticholinergics	↑	The anticholinergic effects may be enhanced by the coadministration of certain TCAs. Paralytic ileus may occur.
TCAs	Clonidine	↑	Dangerous elevations in blood pressure and hypertensive crisis have occurred in patients receiving concurrent TCAs. Avoid coadministration.
TCAs	Dicumarol	↑	TCAs may increase the half-life or bioavailability of dicumarol, possibly resulting in increased anticoagulation effects.
TCAs	Guanethidine	↓	TCAs may antagonize guanethidine's antihypertensive action by inhibiting uptake into adrenergic neurons. Avoid this combination when possible; if concurrent therapy is required, monitor blood pressure. At up to 150 mg/day, doxepin may be given with guanethidine without reducing antihypertensive effect.
TCAs	Levodopa	↓	Levodopa absorption may be delayed and its bioavailability decreased by TCAs. Hypertensive episodes have also occurred.
TCAs	Quinolones Grepafloxacin Sparfloxacin	↑	The risk of life-threatening cardiac arrhythmias, including torsades de pointes, may be increased.
TCAs	Sympathomimetics	↓	TCAs potentiate the pressor response of the direct-acting sympathomimetics; dysrhythmias have occurred. The pressor response to the indirect-acting sympathomimetics is decreased by the TCAs.

*↑ = Object drug increased. ↓ = Object drug decreased.

Adverse Reactions

Sedation and anticholinergic effects are reported most frequently. Tolerance to these effects develops, but side effects may be minimized by starting with a low dose and then gradually increasing the dose or reducing dosage.

Anticholinergic – Dry mouth, and rarely, associated sublingual adenitis or gingivitis; blurred vision; disturbance of accommodation; increased intraocular pressure; mydriasis; constipation; paralytic ileus; urinary retention; delayed micturition; urinary tract dilation; hyperpyrexia.

Withdrawal symptoms – Although not indicative of addiction, abrupt cessation after prolonged therapy may produce dizziness, nausea, headache, vomiting, malaise, sleep disturbances, hyperthermia, irritability, or worsening of psychiatric status. Gradual dosage reduction may produce, within 2 weeks, transient symptoms including irritability, restlessness, and dream and sleep disturbance. Rarely mania or hypomania occurred within 2 to 7 days following cessation of chronic therapy.

Enuretic children – Consider adverse reactions reported with adult use. The most common reactions are nervousness, sleep disorders, tiredness, and mild GI disturbances. These usually disappear with continued therapy or dosage reduction. Other reported reactions include the following: Constipation; convulsions; anxiety; emotional instability; syncope; collapse. Do not exceed 2.5 mg/kg/day of **imipramine**.

➤*Cardiovascular:*

General – Arrhythmias; changes in AV conduction; ECG changes (most frequently with toxic doses); flushing; heart block; hot flushes; hypertension; hypotension; orthostatic hypotension; palpitations; precipitation of CHF; premature ventricular contractions; stroke; sudden death; syncope; tachycardia.

Clomipramine – Aneurysm; atrial flutter; bradycardia; bundle branch block; cardiac arrest/failure; cerebral hemorrhage; extrasystoles; MI; myocardial ischemia; pallor; peripheral ischemia; postural hypotension; thrombophlebitis; vasospasm; ventricular fibrillation; ventricular tachycardia.

Desipramine – Hypertensive episodes during surgery. There has been a report of an "acute collapse" and "sudden death" in an 8-year-old (18 kg) male, treated with desipramine for 2 years for hyperactivity. There have been reports of sudden death in children.

➤*CNS:*

General – Agitation; akathisia; alterations in EEG patterns; anxiety; ataxia; coma; confusion (especially in the elderly); disorientation; disturbed concentration; dizziness; drowsiness; dysarthria; exacerbation of psychosis; excitement; excessive appetite; extrapyramidal symptoms including abnormal involuntary movements and tardive dyskinesia; fatigue; hallucinations; delusions; headache; hyperthermia; hypomania; incoordination; insomnia; mania; nervousness; neuroleptic malignant syndrome; nightmares; numbness; panic; paresthesias of extremities; peripheral neuropathy; restlessness; tremors; seizures; tingling; weakness.

Clomipramine – Abnormal dreaming; abnormal gait; abnormal thinking; aggressive reaction; anticholinergic syndrome; apathy; asthenia; aphasia; apraxia; ataxia; catalepsy; cholinergic syndrome; choreoathetosis; coma; convulsions; decrease in memory; delirium; depersonalization; depression; dyskinesia; dysphonia; emotional lability; encephalopathy; euphoria; extrapyramidal disorder; hostility; hemiparesis; hyperkinesia; hyperreflexia; hypertonia; hypnagogic hallucinations; hypoesthesia; hypokinesia; illusion; impaired impulse control; indecisiveness; irritability; leg cramps; manic reaction; migraine; mutism; myoclonus; neuralgia; neuropathy; nystagmus; oculogyric crisis; oculomotor nerve paralysis; panic reaction; paranoia; paresis; phobic disorder; psychosis; psychosomatic disorder; sensory disturbance; schizophrenic reaction; sleep disorder; somnambulism; somnolence; generalized spasm; speech disorder; stimulation; stupor; suicide; suicide attempt; suicidal ideation; teeth-grinding; twitching; vertigo; yawning.

➤*Dermatologic:* **Clomipramine, imipramine** - Acne; alopecia; cellulitis; chloasma; cyst; dermatitis; dry skin; eczema; erythematous rash; folliculitis; genital pruritus; maculopapular rash; photosensitivity reaction; piloerection; psoriasis; pustular rash; seborrhea; skin discoloration; skin hypertrophy; skin ulceration.

➤*GI:*

General – Abdominal pain/cramps; anorexia; aphthous stomatitis; black tongue; constipation; diarrhea; dysphagia; epigastric distress; flatulence; increased pancreatic enzymes; indigestion; GI disorder; nausea and vomiting; parotid swelling; stomatitis; taste disturbance; peculiar taste; ulcerative stomatitis.

Clomipramine – Abnormal hepatic function; blood in stool; cheilitis; chronic enteritis; colitis; discolored feces; duodenitis; dyspepsia; oral/pharyngeal edema; eructation; esophagitis; gastric dilatation; gastric ulcer; gastritis; gastroesophageal reflux; gingival bleeding; gingivitis; glossitis; hemorrhoids; hiccough; increased salivation; intestinal obstruction; irritable bowel syndrome; peptic ulcer; rectal hemorrhage; salivary gland enlargement; tongue ulceration; tooth caries; tooth disorder.

➤*GU:*

General – Gynecomastia and testicular swelling in the male; breast enlargement, menstrual irregularity and galactorrhea in the female; impotence; increased or decreased libido; painful ejaculation; nocturia; testicular swelling; urinary frequency.

Clomipramine – Albuminuria; amenorrhea; anorgasmy; breast engorgement; breast fibroadenosis; breast pain; cervical dysplasia; cystitis; dysmenorrhea; dysuria; endometrial hyperplasia; ejaculation failure; endometriosis; epididymitis; hematuria; lactation (nonpuerperal); leukorrhea; menstrual disorder; micturition disorder/frequency; nocturia; oliguria; ovarian cyst; perineal pain; polyuria; premature ejaculation; prostatic disorder; pyelonephritis; pyuria; renal calculus/cyst/pain; urinary retention; vaginitis; urethral disorder; urinary incontinence; uterine hemorrhage or inflammation; vaginal hemorrhage; vulvar disorder.

➤*Hematologic:*

General – Bone marrow depression including agranulocytosis; aplastic anemia; eosinophilia; leukopenia; purpura; thrombocytopenia.

Clomipramine – Anemia; leukemoid reaction; lymphadenopathy; lymphoma-like disorder.

➤*Hepatic:*

General – Rarely, hepatitis and jaundice (simulating obstructive); elevation in transaminase; changes in alkaline phosphatase; altered liver function.

➤*Hypersensitivity:*

General – Cross-sensitivity with other TCAs; drug fever; edema (general or of face and tongue); itching; petechiae; photosensitization; pruritus; rash; urticaria; vasculitis.

➤*Metabolic / Nutritional:*

General – Change in blood glucose; elevation or depression of blood sugar levels; elevation of prolactin levels; inappropriate ADH secretion.

Clomipramine – Dehydration; diabetes mellitus; fat intolerance; glycosuria; goiter; gout; hypercholesterolemia; hyperglycemia; hyperuricemia; hypokalemia; hypothyroidism; hyperthyroidism.

➤*Musculoskeletal:*

Clomipramine – Arthrosis; bruising; dystonia; exostosis; lupus erythematosus rash; myopathy; myositis; polyarteritis nodosa; torticollis.

➤*Respiratory:*

General – Exacerbation of asthma.

Clomipramine – Bronchitis; bronchospasm; coughing; cyanosis; dyspnea; epistaxis; hemoptysis; hyperventilation; hypoventilation; increased sputum; laryngismus; laryngitis; pharyngitis; pneumonia; rhinitis; sinusitis.

➤*Special senses:*

General – Abnormal lacrimation; tinnitus.

Clomipramine – Abnormal accommodation; abnormal vision; anisocoria; blepharospasm; blepharitis; chromatopsia; conjunctival hemorrhage; conjunctivitis; deafness; diplopia; earache; exophthalmos; eye pain; foreign body sensation; glaucoma; hyperacusis; keratitis; labyrinth disorder; mydriasis; night blindness; ocular allergy; otitis media; parosmia; photophobia; retinal disorder; scleritis; strabismus; taste loss; vestibular disorder; visual field defect.

➤*Miscellaneous:*

General – Alopecia; fever; hyperthermia; hyperpyrexia; local edema; nasal stuffiness; increased perspiration; proneness to falling; weight gain or loss.

Clomipramine – Abnormal skin odor; arthralgia; back pain; chest pain; chills; dependent edema; general edema; fever; halitosis; increased susceptibility to infection; malaise; muscle weakness; myalgia; pain; thirst; withdrawal syndrome.

Overdosage

Children are reportedly more sensitive than adults to acute overdose. Consider any overdose in infants or young children to be serious and potentially fatal. The response of the patient to toxic overdosage of TCAs may vary in severity and is conditioned by factors such as age, amount ingested, amount absorbed, and the interval between ingestion and start of treatment. Deaths may occur from overdosage with this class of drugs. Multiple drug ingestion (including alcohol) is common in deliberate TCA overdose. It is strongly recommended that the physician contact a poison control center for current information on treatment. Signs and symptoms of toxicity develop rapidly after TCA overdose; therefore, hospital monitoring is required as soon as possible.

➤*Symptoms:*

CNS – Early signs include confusion, agitation, hallucinations, drowsiness, and stupor. Seizures are common, especially with **amoxapine**, and may begin within 12 hours after ingestion; status epilepticus may develop. Overdoses with amoxapine are particularly characterized by CNS toxicity, such as coma; acidosis may also occur. Physical examination may reveal clonus, choreoathetosis, hyperactive reflexes, and a positive Babinski's sign.

Anticholinergic – Flushing; dry mouth; mydriasis; dilated pupils; hyperpyrexia; paralytic ileus; urinary retention; decreased GI motility; may not be observed in acute overdose. Anticholinergic effects are not prominent with **amoxapine**.

Cardiovascular – Cardiovascular toxicity is the leading cause of death in overdose. TCAs exert cardiotoxicity because of anticholinergic activity and quinidine-like effect that depresses myocardial contractility, heart rate, and coronary blood flow. Arrhythmias include tachycardia, intraventricular blocks, and complete AV block. Changes in ECG are clinical indicators of TCA toxicity. Any combination of 1) rightward

Tricyclic Compounds

axis of the terminal 40 msec of the QRS complex (a prominent R-wave in lead aVR), 2) QRS duration ≥ 100 msec (≥ 0.1 sec), 3) tachycardia, or 4) QT$_c$ interval ≥ 440 msec suggest serious TCA poisoning. With up to 20 mg/kg, re-entry ventricular arrhythmias, premature ventricular contractions, ventricular tachycardia, or fibrillation may occur. Sudden cardiac arrest has been reported. Pulmonary edema, conduction abnormalities, and hypotension are common. Severe cardiotoxicity usually occurs within 6 hours; however, ECG changes may be noted up to 48 hours postingestion.

Renal – Rhabdomyolysis and renal failure may appear if prolonged seizures or coma occurs. Renal failure may develop 2 to 5 days after toxic overdosage of **amoxapine** in patients who may appear otherwise recovered; acute tubular necrosis with rhabdomyolysis and myoglobinuria is most common. This probably occurs in < 5% of overdose cases, and is typical in those who have experienced multiple seizures.

Other – Respiratory depression, cyanosis, shock, diaphoresis, aspiration, and ARDS may occur in severe overdoses. Hyperthermia and hypothermia have been reported. Polyradiculoneuropathy has been reported with **amitriptyline**. Muscle rigidity, disorders of ocular motility, vomiting, or any other symptoms under adverse events are signs of overdose.

➤*Treatment:* Hospitalize and closely observe with ECG monitoring. Observe for signs of CNS or respiratory depression, hypotension, cardiac dysrhythmias or conduction blocks, and seizures for a minimum of 6 hours even when the amount ingested is thought to be small or the initial degree of intoxication appears slight to moderate. Blood and urine levels are unreliable indicators for clinical management. Closely monitor patients with ECG abnormalities for at least 6 hours and until well after cardiac status returns to normal. A prolonged QRS interval (≥ 100 msec) may indicate the patient is at higher risk for developing seizures, arrhythmias, or hypotension. Relapses may occur after apparent recovery.

Maintain adequate respiratory exchange. Do not use respiratory stimulants. Use normal or half-normal saline to avoid water intoxication, especially in children. Instillation of activated charcoal slurry after large volume gastric lavage may help reduce absorption. Consider gastric lavage in symptomatic patients only after intubation and only if the procedure can be done in the first hour after ingestion. Emesis is contraindicated. Refer to General Management of Acute Overdosage.

Treat cardiovascular effects aggressively. A maximal limb-lead QRS duration of ≥ 0.1 seconds may be an indication of overdose severity. Sodium bicarbonate (hypertonic, 1 M) by IV infusion has effectively treated cardiac dysrhythmias and hypotension. It is usually given 50 mEq (1 mEq/ml) IV bolus, followed by repeated doses to maintain the blood at pH 7.45 to 7.55. If hypotension does not respond to sodium bicarbonate, fluid expansion and vasopressors (eg, norepinephrine 0.1 to 0.2 mcg/kg/min [first choice] or dopamine 10 to 20 mcg/kg/min) may be required. If cardiac dysrhythmias do not respond, lidocaine, bretylium, or phenytoin may be used. Isoproterenol may help control bradyarrhythmias and torsades de pointes ventricular tachycardia while overdrive pacing is being established. Propranolol (0.01 to 0.1 mg/kg/dose over 10 minutes; maximum is 1 mg/dose) is used for life-threatening ventricular arrhythmias in children. The propranolol dose for adults is 1 mg/dose IV administered no faster than 1 mg/min repeated every 2 to 5 minutes until desired response is seen or a maximum of 5 mg has been given. Quinidine, procainamide, and disopyramide are contraindicated for TCA overdose. Serious cardiovascular effects are remarkably rare following **amoxapine** overdosage, and the ECG typically remains within normal limits, except for sinus tachycardia. Hence, prolongation of the QRS interval beyond 100 msec within the first 24 hours is not a useful guide to the severity of overdosage with this drug.

In rare instances, hemoperfusion may be beneficial in acute refractory cardiovascular instability in patients with acute toxicity. Hemodialysis, peritoneal dialysis, exchange transfusions, and forced diuresis have generally been ineffective because of the rapid fixation of TCAs in the tissues.

Treat shock and metabolic acidosis with supportive measures (eg, IV fluids, bicarbonate, oxygen, corticosteroids). Digitalis may increase conduction abnormalities and further irritate an already sensitized myocardium. Exercise care if CHF necessitates rapid digitalization. Closely monitor cardiac function for at least 5 days. Support renal function.

Minimize external stimulation (darken the room) to prevent seizures. Control seizures with benzodiazepines. If these are ineffective, use anticonvulsants (eg, phenytoin, phenobarbital). If phenobarbital and phenytoin are ineffective, consider paralysis or barbiturate coma. Physostigmine is not recommended except to treat life-threatening symptoms that have been unresponsive to other therapies, and then only in consultation with a poison control center. With **amoxapine**, seizures may appear precipitously in otherwise relatively asymptomatic patients. Consider prophylactic anticonvulsants. With other antidepressants, administer diazepam IV bolus (adult: 5 to 10 mg initially that may be repeated every 15 minutes as needed up to 30 mg; child: 0.25 to 0.4 mg/kg dose up to 10 mg/dose) or lorazepam IV bolus (adult: 4 to 8 mg; child: 0.05 to 0.1 mg/kg). Control hyperpyrexia by any available means, including external cooling (ice packs, cooling blankets, sponge baths), benzodiazepines to control agitation and seizures, and paralysis with a neuromuscular blocker, if necessary.

Patient Information

Before using, tell your physician and pharmacist (1) if you have other medical conditions; (2) what other medications you are currently taking (including *otc* and alternative medicines); (3) if you have ever had an unusual or allergic reaction to any TCA; (4) if you are pregnant or may become pregnant; and (5) if you are breastfeeding.

Discontinue drug and get emergency help if any of the following occurs: Seizures; difficult or fast breathing; fever with increased sweating; loss of bladder control; severe muscle stiffness; unusual tiredness or weakness.

Warn patients of the risk of seizure.

Advise patients to complete full course of therapy; may take 4 to 6 weeks to see full benefits.

Warn male patients receiving **clomipramine** of the high incidence of sexual dysfunction.

Given the likelihood that some patients exposed chronically to neuroleptics will develop tardive dyskinesia, it is advised that all patients in whom chronic use is contemplated be given, if possible, full information about this risk. The decision to inform patients or their guardians must obviously take into account the clinical circumstances and the competency of the patient to understand the information provided.

Caution patients against use of alcohol, barbiturates, and other CNS depressants because effects may be exacerbated by TCAs.

Do not discontinue therapy or take other drugs without consent of physician. Abrupt discontinuation of therapy may cause nausea, headache, and malaise.

May cause drowsiness, dizziness, or blurred vision; use caution when driving or performing other tasks requiring alertness, coordination, or physical dexterity. Avoid alcohol and other CNS depressant drugs.

If serious adverse effects occur, dosage should be reduced or treatment should be altered.

Avoid prolonged exposure to sunlight or sunlamps; photosensitivity may occur.

AMITRIPTYLINE HCl

Rx	**Amitriptyline HCl** (Various, eg, Geneva, Mutual, Sidmak, URL, Zenith Goldline)	**Tablets:** 10 mg	In 100s, 1000s, UD 100s, and blister pack 100s and 600s.
Rx	**Amitriptyline HCl** (Various, eg, Geneva, Mutual, Sidmak, UDL, URL, Zenith Goldline)	25 mg	In 100s, 1000s, UD 100s, and blister pack 25s, 100s, and 600s.
Rx	**Amitriptyline HCl** (Various, eg, Geneva, Mutual, Sidmak)	50 mg	In 100s, 1000s, UD 100s, and blister pack 25s, 100s, and 600s.
Rx	**Amitriptyline HCl** (Various, eg, Geneva, Mutual, Sidmak, UDL, Zenith Goldline)	75 mg	In 100s, 500s, 1000s, UD 100s, and blister pack 100s.
Rx	**Amitriptyline HCl** (Various, eg, Geneva, Mutual, Sidmak, UDL, URL, Zenith Goldline)	100 mg	In 100s, 500s, 1000s, UD 100s, and blister pack 100s.
Rx	**Amitriptyline HCl** (Various, eg, Geneva, Mutual, Sidmak, UDL, Zenith Goldline)	150 mg	In 100s, 1000s, and UD 100s.

[1] With dextrose and parabens.

For complete prescribing information, refer to the Tricyclic Compounds group monograph.

Indications

➤*Depression:* For the relief of symptoms of depression. Endogenous depression is more likely to be alleviated than are other depressive states.

Administration and Dosage

➤*Outpatients:* 75 mg/day in divided doses. May gradually increase to 150 mg/day. Make increases preferably in late afternoon or at bedtime. A sedative effect may be apparent before the antidepressant effect is noted. An adequate therapeutic effect may take as long as 30 days to develop.

Alternatively, initiate therapy with 50 to 100 mg at bedtime. Increase by 25 to 50 mg as necessary, to a total of 150 mg/day.

➤*Hospitalized patients:* Hospitalized patients may require 100 mg/

Tricyclic Compounds

AMITRIPTYLINE HCl

day initially. Gradually increase to 200 to 300 mg/day, if necessary.

➤*Adolescent and elderly patients:* 10 mg 3 times/day with 20 mg at bedtime may be satisfactory in adolescent and elderly patients who cannot tolerate higher dosages.

➤*Maintenance:* 40 to 100 mg/day. Total daily dose may be given in a single dose, preferably at bedtime. When patient has satisfactorily improved, reduce dosage to the lowest effective amount. Continue ≥ 3 months to lessen the possibility of relapse.

➤*IM:* Do not administer IV. Initially, 20 to 30 mg IM 4 times/day. The effects may be more rapid with IM than with oral administration. When used for initial therapy in patients unable or unwilling to take tablets, replace the injection with the tablets as soon as possible.

➤*Children:* Not recommended for children < 12 years of age.

AMOXAPINE

Rx	Amoxapine (Various, eg, Geneva, URL, Watson)	**Tablets:** 25 mg	In 30s, 100s, 1000s, and blister pack 100s.
Rx	Amoxapine (Various, eg, Geneva, URL, Watson)	**Tablets:** 50 mg	In 30s, 100s, 500s, 1000s, and blister pack 100s.
Rx	Amoxapine (Various, eg, Geneva, URL, Watson)	**Tablets:** 100 mg	In 30s, 100s, and 1000s.
Rx	Amoxapine (Various, eg, Geneva, URL, Watson)	**Tablets:** 150 mg	In 30s, 100s, and 1000s.

For complete prescribing information, refer to the Tricyclic Compounds group monograph.

Indications

➤*Depression:* For the relief of symptoms of depression in patients with neurotic or reactive depressive disorders as well as endogenous and psychotic depressions. It is indicated for depression accompanied by anxiety or agitation.

Administration and Dosage

Amoxapine is not recommended for patients < 16 years of age.

Usual effective dosage is 200 to 300 mg/day. Three weeks is an adequate trial period providing dosage has reached 300 mg/day (or a lower level of tolerance) for at least 2 weeks. If no response is seen at 300 mg, increase dosage, depending upon tolerance, to 400 mg/day. Hospitalized patients refractory to antidepressant therapy and who have no history of convulsive seizures may have dosage cautiously increased up to 600 mg/day in divided doses.

➤*Adults:* Initially, 50 mg 2 or 3 times daily. Depending upon tolerance, increase dosage to 100 mg 2 or 3 times daily by the end of the first week. Initial dosage of 300 mg/day may cause sedation during the first few days of therapy. Increase above 300 mg/day only if 300 mg/day has been ineffective for at least 2 weeks. Once an effective dosage is established, the drug may be given in a single bedtime dose (not to exceed 300 mg). If the total daily dosage exceeds 300 mg, give in divided doses.

➤*Elderly patients:* Lower dosages are recommended. Initially, 25 mg 2 or 3 times/day. If tolerated, dosage may be increased by the end of the first week to 50 mg 2 or 3 times/day. Although 100 to 150 mg/day may be adequate for many elderly patients, some may require higher dosage; carefully increase up to 300 mg/day. Once an effective dosage is established, give amoxapine in a single bedtime dose, not to exceed 300 mg.

➤*Maintenance:* Maintenance dosage is the lowest dose that will maintain remission. If symptoms reappear, increase dosage to the earlier level until they are controlled. For maintenance therapy at doses of ≤ 300 mg, a single bedtime dose is recommended.

CLOMIPRAMINE HCl

Rx	Clomipramine HCl (Various, eg, Teva, Watson)	**Capsules:** 25 mg	In 100s and 1000s.
Rx	Anafranil (Novartis)		Parabens. (Anafranil 25 mg). Ivory and melon yellow. In 100s and UD 100s.
Rx	Clomipramine HCl (Various, eg, Teva, Watson)	50 mg	In 100s and 1000s.
Rx	Anafranil (Novartis)		Parabens. (Anafranil 50 mg). Ivory and aqua blue. In 100s and UD 100s.
Rx	Clomipramine HCl (Various, eg, Teva, Watson)	75 mg	In 100s and 1000s.
Rx	Anafranil (Novartis)		Parabens. (Anafranil 75 mg). Ivory and yellow. In 100s and UD 100s.

For complete prescribing information, refer to the Tricyclic Compounds group monograph.

Indications

➤*Obsessive-compulsive disorder (OCD):* Treatment of obsessions and compulsions in patients with OCD. The obsessions or compulsions must cause marked distress, be time-consuming, or significantly interfere with social or occupational functioning in order to meet the DSM-IV diagnosis of OCD.

Administration and Dosage

➤*Initial:*

Adults – Initiate at 25 mg daily and gradually increase, as tolerated, to ≈ 100 mg during the first 2 weeks. Administer in divided doses with meals to reduce GI side effects. Thereafter, the dosage may be increased gradually over the next several weeks to a maximum of 250 mg/day. Steady-state plasma levels may not be achieved until 2 to 3 weeks after dosage change. Therefore, after initial titration, it may be appropriate to wait 2 to 3 weeks between further dosage adjustments. After titration, the total daily dose may be given once daily at bedtime to minimize daytime sedation.

Children and adolescents – Initiate at 25 mg daily and gradually increase during the first 2 weeks, as tolerated, to a daily maximum of 3 mg/kg or 100 mg, whichever is smaller. Administer in divided doses with meals to reduce GI side effects. Thereafter, the dosage may be increased to a daily maximum of 3 mg/kg or 200 mg, whichever is smaller. After titration, the total daily dose may be given once daily at bedtime to minimize daytime sedation.

➤*Maintenance:*

Adults, children, and adolescents – The efficacy of clomipramine after 10 weeks has not been documented in controlled trials. However, patients have continued therapy in double-blind studies for up to 1 year without loss of benefit. Adjust the dosage to maintain the patient on the lowest effective dosage and periodically reassess the patient to determine the need for treatment. Give total daily dose once at bedtime.

DESIPRAMINE HCl

Rx	**Desipramine HCl** (Various, eg, Eon, Geneva)	**Tablets:** 10 mg	In 100s and 1000s.
Rx	**Norpramin** (Hoechst Marion Roussel)		(68-7). Blue. Coated. In 100s.[1]
Rx	**Desipramine HCl** (Various, eg, EON, Geneva, Sidmak, URL, Zenith Goldline)	**Tablets:** 25 mg	In 100s, 500s, 1000s, UD 100s, and blister pack 100s and 600s.
Rx	**Norpramin** (Hoechst Marion Roussel)		(NORPRAMIN 25). Yellow. Coated. In 100s and UD 100s.[1]
Rx	**Desipramine HCl** (Various, eg, Eon, Geneva, Sidmak, UDL, URL, Zenith Goldline)	**Tablets:** 50 mg	In 100s, 500s, 1000s, UD 100s, and blister pack 100s and 600s.
Rx	**Norpramin** (Hoechst Marion Roussel)		(NORPRAMIN 50). Green. Coated. In 100s and UD 100s.[1]
Rx	**Desipramine HCl** (Various, eg, Eon, Geneva, Sidmak, UDL, URL)	**Tablets:** 75 mg	In 100s, 500s, 1000s, UD 100s, and blister pack 100s and 600s.
Rx	**Norpramin** (Hoechst Marion Roussel)		(NORPRAMIN 75) Orange. Coated. In 100s.[1]
Rx	**Desipramine HCl** (Various, eg, EON, Geneva, Sidmak)	**Tablets:** 100 mg	In 100s, 500s, and 1000s.
Rx	**Norpramin** (Hoechst Marion Roussel)		(NORPRAMIN 100). Peach. Coated. In 100s.[1]
Rx	**Desipramine HCl** (Various, eg, EON, Geneva, Sidmak)	**Tablets:** 150 mg	In 50s, 100s, and 1000s.
Rx	**Norpramin** (Hoechst Marion Roussel)		(NORPRAMIN 150). White. Coated. In 50s.[1]

[1] With mannitol and sucrose.

For complete prescribing information, refer to the Tricyclic Compounds group monograph.

Indications

➤*Depression:* For the treatment of depression.

Administration and Dosage

Not recommended for use in children < 12 years of age.

Initial therapy may be given in divided doses or as a single daily dose. Maintenance therapy may be administered once daily. Continue a lower maintenance dosage for at least 2 months after a satisfactory response has been achieved.

➤*Adults:* 100 to 200 mg/day. In more severely ill patients, gradually increase to 300 mg/day, if necessary. Do not exceed 300 mg/day. Doses as high as 300 mg should generally be initiated in hospitals. Maintain continued therapy at the optimal dosage level during the active phase of depression. In cases of relapse because of premature drug withdrawal, a prompt response may be obtained by immediate resumption of treatment. Clinical symptoms of intolerance (eg, drowsiness, dizziness, postural hypotension) require dosage reduction.

➤*Elderly and adolescents:* 25 to 100 mg/day. Can be given in divided doses or as a single daily dose. Dosages > 150 mg/day are not recommended.

DOXEPIN HCl

Rx	**Doxepin HCl** (Various, eg, Par, UDL, URL, Watson)	**Capsules :** 10 mg	In 100s, 500s, 1000s, and blister pack 100s.
Rx	**Sinequan** (Roerig)		(Sinequan Roerig 534). In 100s and 1000s.
Rx	**Doxepin HCl** (Various, eg, Par, UDL, Watson)	**Capsules:** 25 mg	In 100s, 500s, 1000s, and blister pack 25s and 100s.
Rx	**Sinequan** (Roerig)		(Sinequan Roerig 535). In 100s, 1000s, and 5000s.
Rx	**Doxepin HCl** (Various, eg, Par, UDL, Watson)	**Capsules:** 50 mg	In 100s, 500s, 1000s, and blister pack 25s and 100s.
Rx	**Sinequan** (Roerig)		(Sinequan Roerig 536). In 100s, 1000s, and 5000s.
Rx	**Doxepin HCl** (Various, eg, Par, UDL)	**Capsules:** 75 mg	In 100s, 500s, 1000s, and blister pack 100s.
Rx	**Sinequan** (Roerig)		(Sinequan Roerig 539). In 100s and 1000s.
Rx	**Doxepin HCl** (Various, eg, Par, UDL, URL)	**Capsules:** 100 mg	In 100s, 500s, 1000s, and blister pack 100s.
Rx	**Sinequan** (Roerig)		(Sinequan Roerig 538). In 100s and 1000s.
Rx	**Doxepin HCl** (Various, eg, Par)	**Capsules:** 150 mg	In 50s, 100s, 500s, and 1000s.
Rx	**Sinequan** (Roerig)		(Sinequan Roerig 537). In 50s and 500s.
Rx	**Doxepin HCl** (Various, eg, Copley, Morton Grove)	**Oral Concentrate:** 10 mg/ml	In 120 ml.
Rx	**Sinequan** (Roerig)		Parabens, peppermint oil, sorbitol. In 118 ml with calibrated dropper.

For complete prescribing information, refer to the Tricyclic Compounds group monograph.

Indications

➤*Depression:* For the treatment of the following:

1.) Psychoneurotic patients with depression or anxiety.
2.) Depression or anxiety associated with alcoholism (not to be taken concomitantly with alcohol).
3.) Depression or anxiety associated with organic disease (the possibility of drug interaction should be considered if the patient is receiving other drugs concomitantly).
4.) Psychotic depressive disorders with associated anxiety including involutional depression and manic-depressive disorders.

The target symptoms of psychoneurosis that respond particularly well to doxepin include anxiety, tension, depression, somatic symptoms and concerns, sleep disturbances, guilt, lack of energy, fear, apprehension, and worry.

Administration and Dosage

Not recommended for use in children < 12 years old.

➤*Mild-to-moderate illness:* Initially, 75 mg/day. Individualize dosage. Usual optimum dosage is 75 to 150 mg/day. Alternatively, the total daily dosage, up to 150 mg, may be given at bedtime. Maximum dose is 150 mg/day.

➤*Mild symptomatology or emotional symptoms accompanying organic disease:* 25 to 50 mg/day is often effective.

➤*More severe anxiety or depression:* Higher doses (eg, 50 mg 3 times/day) may be required; if necessary, gradually increase to 300 mg/day. Additional effectiveness is rarely obtained by exceeding 300 mg/day.

Although optimal antidepressant response may not be evident for 2 to 3 weeks, anti-anxiety activity is rapidly apparent.

➤*Oral concentrate:* Dilute oral concentrate with ≈ 120 ml of water, milk, or fruit juice just prior to administration. The oral concentrate is not physically compatible with a number of carbonated beverages. Do not prepare or store bulk dilutions.

Tricyclic Compounds

IMIPRAMINE HCl

Rx	Imipramine HCl (Various, eg, Geneva, Mutual, Par, URL)	**Tablets:** 10 mg	In 100s, 250s, 500s, and 1000s.
Rx	Tofranil (Novartis)		(Geigy 32). Coral. Sugar-coated. Trianglular. In 100s.
Rx	Imipramine HCl (Various, eg, Geneva, Mutual, Par, URL)	**Tablets:** 25 mg	In 100s, 250s, 500s, and 1000s.
Rx	Tofranil (Novartis)		(Geigy 140). Coral, biconvex. Sugar-coated. In 100s.
Rx	Imipramine HCl (Various, eg, Geneva, Mutual, Par, URL)	**Tablets:** 50 mg	In 50s, 100s, 250s, 500s, 1000s, and UD 20s.
Rx	Tofranil (Novartis)		(Geigy 136). Coral, biconvex. Sugar-coated. In 100s.

For complete prescribing information, refer to the Tricyclic Compounds group monograph.

Indications

►*Depression:* For the relief of symptoms of depression. Endogenous depression is more likely to be alleviated than other depressive states.

►*Childhood enuresis:* May be useful as temporary adjunctive therapy in reducing enuresis in children ≥ 6 years of age.

Administration and Dosage

►*Depression:*

Hospitalized patients – Initially, 100 mg/day orally in divided doses; gradually increase to 200 mg/day, as required. If no response occurs after 2 weeks, increase to 250 to 300 mg/day. Administer once daily, preferably at bedtime.

Outpatients – Initially, 75 mg/day, increased to 150 mg/day. Do not exceed 200 mg/day.

Maintenance: 50 to 150 mg/day or lowest dose that will maintain remission.

Adolescent and geriatric patients – Initially, 30 to 40 mg/day orally; it is generally not necessary to exceed 100 mg/day.

►*Childhood enuresis (≥ 6 years of age):* Initially, 25 mg/day 1 hour before bedtime. If a satisfactory response is not obtained within 1 week, increase up to 50 mg/night if < 12 years of age; up to 75 mg/night if > 12 years of age. A dose > 75 mg/day does not enhance efficacy and increases side effects. Do not exceed 2.5 mg/kg/day. In early night bed-wetters, it may be more effective given earlier and in divided amounts (25 mg midafternoon and at bedtime). Institute a drug-free period after an adequate trial with favorable response. Gradually tapering dosage may reduce tendency to relapse. Children who relapse after discontinuation do not always respond to a subsequent course.

Long-term use efficacy has not been established.

IMIPRAMINE PAMOATE

Rx	Tofranil-PM (Novartis)	**Capsules:**[1] 75 mg	Parabens. (Geigy 20). Coral. In 30s and 100s.
		100 mg	Parabens. (Geigy 40). Dark yellow/coral. In 30s and 100s.
		125 mg	Parabens. (Geigy 45). Ivory/coral. In 30s and 100s.
		150 mg	Parabens. (Geigy 22). Coral. In 30s and 100s.

[1] Strengths are expressed as imipramine HCl equivalent.

For complete prescribing information, refer to the Tricyclic Compounds group monograph.

Indications

►*Depression:* For the relief of symptoms of depression. Endogenous depression is more likely to be alleviated than other depressive states.

Administration and Dosage

►*Hospitalized patients:* Initiate therapy at 100 to 150 mg/day; may be increased to 200 mg/day. If there is no response after 2 weeks, increase dosage to 250 to 300 mg/day.

Dosage higher than 150 mg/day may also be administered on a once-a-day basis after the optimum dosage and tolerance have been determined. The daily dosage may be given at bedtime. In some patients it may be necessary to employ a divided-dose schedule.

As with all tricyclics, the antidepressant effect of imipramine may not be evident for 1 to 3 weeks in some patients.

►*Outpatients:* Initiate therapy at 75 mg/day. Dosage may be increased to 150 mg/day, which is the dose level at which optimum response is usually obtained. If necessary, dosage may be increased to 200 mg/day.

Dosage > 75 mg/day may also be given on a once-a-day basis after the optimum dosage and tolerance have been determined. The daily dose may be given at bedtime. In some patients it may be necessary to employ a divided-dose schedule.

►*Adult maintenance dosage:* Following remission, maintenance medication may be required for a longer period of time at the lowest dose that will maintain remission after which the dosage should gradually be decreased.

The usual maintenance dose is 75 to 150 mg/day. The total daily dose can be administered on a once-a-day basis, preferable at bedtime. In some patients it may be necessary to employ a divided-dose schedule.

In cases of relapse due to premature withdrawal of the drug, reinstitute the effective dosage of imipramine.

►*Adolescent and geriatric patients:* Initiate therapy in these age groups with imipramine HCl at a total daily dosage of 25 to 50 mg because imipramine pamoate does not come in these strengths. Dosage may be increased according to response and tolerance, but it is generally unnecessary to exceed 100 mg/day in these patients. Imipramine pamoate capsules may be used when total daily dosage is established at ≥ 75 mg. The total daily maintenance dosage can be administered on a once-a-day basis, preferably at bedtime.

Tricyclic Compounds

NORTRIPTYLINE HCl

Rx	**Nortriptyline HCl** (Various, eg, Geneva, Teva, UDL)	**Capsules:** 10 mg	In 100s, 500s, 1000s, blister pack 25s, 100s, and 600s, and UD 100s.
Rx	**Pamelor** (Novartis)		(Sandoz PAMELOR 10 mg). In 100s and UD 100s.[1]
Rx	**Nortriptyline HCl** (Various, eg, Geneva, Teva, UDL)	**Capsules:** 25 mg	In 100s, 500s, 1000s, blister pack 25s, 100s, and 600s, and UD 100s.
Rx	**Aventyl HCl Pulvules** (Eli Lilly)		(Lilly H19). White/yellow. In 100s and 500s.
Rx	**Pamelor** (Novartis)		(Sandoz PAMELOR 25 mg). In 100s, 500s, and UD 100s.[1]
Rx	**Nortriptyline HCl** (Various, eg, Geneva, Teva, UDL)	**Capsules:** 50 mg	In 100s, 500s, 1000s, blister pack 25s, 100s, and 600s, and UD 100s.
Rx	**Pamelor** (Novartis)		(Sandoz PAMELOR 50 mg). In 100s and UD 100s.[1]
Rx	**Nortriptyline HCl** (Various, eg, Geneva, Teva)	**Capsules:** 75 mg	In 100s, 500s, 1000s, and blister pack 100s and 600s.
Rx	**Pamelor** (Novartis)		(Sandoz PAMELOR 75 mg). In 100s.[1]
Rx	**Nortriptyline HCl** (Ranbaxy)	**Solution:** 10 mg base/5 ml	In 480 mL.[2]
Rx	**Aventyl HCl** (Eli Lilly)		
Rx	**Pamelor** (Novartis)		In 480 mL.[3]

[1] With benzyl alcohol, EDTA, parabens.
[2] With 4% alcohol, sorbitol.
[3] With 3.4% alcohol.

For complete prescribing information, refer to the Tricyclic Compounds group monograph.

Indications

▶*Depression:* For the relief of symptoms of depression. Endogenous depressions are more likely to be alleviated than are other depressive states.

Administration and Dosage

Not recommended for use in children.

▶*Adults:* 25 mg 3 or 4 times daily; begin at a low level and increase as required. The total daily dose can be given at bedtime. When doses > 100 mg/day are given, plasma levels of nortriptyline should be monitored and maintained in the optimum range of 50 to 150 ng/ml. Doses > 150 mg/day are not recommended. Higher concentrations may be associated with more adverse experiences. Plasma concentrations are difficult to measure, and physicians should consult with the laboratory professional staff.

▶*Elderly and adolescent patients:* 30 to 50 mg daily in divided doses or total daily dose may be given once/day.

PROTRIPTYLINE HCl

Rx	**Protriptyline HCl** (Various, eg, Sidmak)	**Tablets:** 5 mg	In 100s and 1000s.
Rx	**Vivactil** (Merck)		Lactose. (MSD 26). Orange. Oval. Film coated. In 100s.
Rx	**Protriptyline HCl** (Various, eg, Sidmak)	**Tablets:** 10 mg	In 100s and 1000s.
Rx	**Vivactil** (Merck)		Lactose. (MSD 47). Yellow. Oval. Film coated. In 100s and UD 100s.

For complete prescribing information, refer to the Tricyclic Compounds group monograph.

Indications

▶*Depression:* For the treatment of symptoms of mental depression in patients who are under close medical supervision. Its activating properties make it particularly suitable for withdrawn and anergic patients.

Administration and Dosage

Not recommended for use in children.

▶*Adults:* 15 to 40 mg/day divided into 3 or 4 doses. May increase to 60 mg/day. Dosages > 60 mg/day are not recommended. Make any increases in the morning dose.

▶*Adolescent and elderly patients:* Lower dosages are recommended. Initially, 5 mg 3 times/day; increase gradually, if necessary. In elderly, monitor cardiovascular system closely if dose exceeds 20 mg/day.

▶*Maintenance:* When satisfactory improvement has been reached, reduce dosage to the smallest amount that will maintain relief of symptoms.

TRIMIPRAMINE MALEATE

Rx	**Surmontil** (Wyeth)	**Capsules:** 25 mg	Lactose. (Wyeth 4132). Opaque blue/yellow. In 100s.
		50 mg	Lactose. (Wyeth 4133). Opaque blue/orange. In 100s and UD 100s.
		100 mg	Lactose. (Wyeth 4158). Opaque blue/white. In 100s.

For complete prescribing information, refer to the Tricyclic Compounds group monograph.

Indications

▶*Depression:* For the relief of symptoms of depression. Endogenous depression is more likely to be alleviated than other depressive states.

Administration and Dosage

Not recommended for use in children.

▶*Adult outpatients:* Initially, 75 mg/day in divided doses; increase to 150 mg/day. Do not exceed 200 mg/day. The total dosage requirement may be given at bedtime.

▶*Adult hospitalized patients:* Initially, 100 mg/day in divided doses, increase gradually in a few days to 200 mg/day depending upon individual response and tolerance. If improvement does not occur in 2 to 3 weeks, increase to a maximum dose of 250 to 300 mg/day.

▶*Adolescent and elderly patients:* Initially, 50 mg/day, with gradual increments up to 100 mg/day.

▶*Maintenance:* Maintenance medication may be required at the lowest dose that will maintain remission (range, 50 to 150 mg/day). Administer as a single bedtime dose. To minimize relapse, continue maintenance therapy for ≈ 3 months.

Tetracyclic Compounds

Refer to the Antidepressants introduction.

Indications

➤*Depression:* Treatment of depression.

➤*Unlabeled uses:* **Maprotiline** is also effective for the relief of anxiety associated with depression.

Actions

➤*Pharmacology:* The mechanism of action is unknown. Tetracyclics enhance central noradrenergic and serotonergic activity. They do not inhibit monoamine oxidase. Although **maprotiline** and **mirtazapine** are in the same chemical class, they each affect different neurotransmitters and thus have different side effect profiles. Maprotiline primarily acts by blocking reuptake of norepinephrine at nerve endings. This pharmacologic action is thought to be responsible for its antidepressant and anxiolytic effects. They act as antagonists at central presynaptic α_2-adrenergic inhibitory autoreceptors and heteroreceptors, an action that is postulated to result in an increase in central noradrenergic and serotonergic activity.

Mirtazapine is a potent antagonist of $5-HT_2$ and $5-HT_3$ receptors. It does not have significant affinity for the $5-HT_{1A}$ and $5-HT_{1B}$ receptors. It is a potent antagonist of histamine (H_1) receptors, a property that may explain its prominent sedative effects. It is also a moderate antagonist at muscarinic receptors, a property that may explain the relatively low incidence of anticholinergic side effects. Mirtazapine is a moderate peripheral α_1-adrenergic antagonist, a property that may explain the occasional orthostatic hypotension associated with its use.

➤*Pharmacokinetics:*

Maprotiline – The mean time to peak is 12 hours. Steady-state levels measured prior to the morning dose on a 1-dosage regimen demonstrated an average minimum concentration of 238 ng/ml and 95% confidence limits of 181 to 295 ng/ml. Binding to serum proteins is ≈ 88%. Following a 50 mg oral dose of maprotiline in healthy subjects, the peak plasma level occurred between 9 and 16 hours. Range of apparent volume of distribution is 13 to 24 L/kg, and it is more concentrated in the liver, lung, kidney, brain, and heart than in blood. The average elimination half-life in healthy subjects is 43 hours (range, 27 to 58 hours). Maprotiline is metabolized in the liver. After 21 days of IV maprotiline, 57% was found in the urine and 30% in the feces. Maprotiline is excreted via the bile.

Mirtazapine – Mirtazapine is rapidly and completely absorbed following oral administration and has a half–life of ≈ 20 to 40 hours. Peak plasma concentrations are reached within ≈ 2 hours following an oral dose. The presence of food in the stomach has a minimal effect on the rate and extent of absorption and does not require a dosage adjustment. Steady-state plasma levels of mirtazapine are attained within 5 days. Mirtazapine is ≈ 85% bound to plasma protein.

Metabolism/Excretion: Mirtazapine is extensively metabolized after oral administration. Major pathways of biotransformation are demethylation and hydroxylation followed by glucuronide conjugation. In vitro, cytochrome 2D6 and 1A2 are involved in the formation of the 8-hydroxy metabolite of mirtazapine, whereas cytochrome 3A is considered to be responsible for the formation of the N-desmethyl and N-oxide metabolites. Mirtazapine has an absolute bioavailability of ≈ 50%. It is eliminated predominantly via urine (75%) with 15% in feces. Several unconjugated metabolites possess pharmacologic activity but are present in the plasma at very low levels. The (-) enantiomer has an elimination half-life that is approximately twice as long as the (+) enantiomer and, therefore, achieves plasma levels that are ≈ 3 times as high.

Plasma levels are linearly related to dose over a dose range of 15 to 80 mg. The mean elimination half-life of mirtazapine after oral administration ranges from ≈ 20 to 40 hours, with females of all ages exhibiting significantly longer elimination half-lives than males (37 hours vs 26 hours).

Contraindications

Hypersensitivity to maprotiline or mirtazapine; coadministration with monamine oxidase inhibitors (MAOIs; see Warnings).

➤*Maprotiline:* Known or suspected seizure disorders; during acute phase of MI.

Warnings

➤*Agranulocytosis:* In clinical trials, 2 patients treated with **mirtazapine** developed agranulocytosis (absolute neutrophil count [ANC] < 500/mm[3] with associated signs and symptoms [eg, fever, infection]) and a third patient developed severe neutropenia (ANC < 500/mm[3] without any associated symptoms). For these 3 patients, onset of severe neutropenia was detected on days 61, 9, and 14 of treatment, respectively. All 3 patients recovered after mirtazapine was stopped. If a patient develops a sore throat, fever, stomatitis, or other signs of infection, along with a low WBC count, discontinue treatment with the tetracyclic and monitor the patient closely.

➤*Anticholinergic properties:* Administer **maprotiline** with caution in patients with increased intraocular pressure, history of urinary retention, or history of narrow-angle glaucoma because of the drug's anticholinergic properties.

➤*CNS effects:* **Maprotiline** may enhance the response to alcohol, barbiturates, and other CNS depressants, requiring appropriate caution during administration.

➤*Monamine oxidase inhibitors (MAOIs):* Do not give tetracyclics with MAOIs. Allow a minimum of 14 days to elapse after discontinuation of MAOIs before starting a tetracyclic.

➤*Seizures:* Seizures are rare. Most of the seizures have occurred in patients with a history of seizures. In premarketing clinical trials, only 1 seizure was reported among the 2796 patients treated with **mirtazapine**. **Maprotiline** is associated with seizures in overdose and with therapeutic doses. The risk of seizures may be increased when tetracyclics are taken concomitantly with phenothiazines, when the dosage of benzodiazepines is rapidly tapered in patients receiving tetracyclics, or when the recommended dosage of the tetracyclic is exceeded. While a cause-and-effect relationship has not been established, the risk of seizures in patients treated with tetracyclics may be reduced by the following:

• Initiating therapy at a low dosage.
• Maintaining the initial dosage for 2 weeks before raising it gradually in small increments as necessary.
• Keeping the dosage at the minimally effective level during maintenance therapy.

➤*Cardiovascular effects:* Use with caution in patients with a history of MI and angina because of the possibility of conduction defects, arrhythmia, MI, strokes, and tachycardia. Use with caution in patients predisposed to hypotension.

➤*Electroshock therapy:* Avoid concurrent administration of **maprotiline** with electroshock therapy because of the lack of experience in this area.

➤*Renal function impairment:* Following a single 15 mg dose of **mirtazapine**, patients with moderate (glomerular filtration rate [GFR] = 11 to 39 ml/min/1.73 m^2) and severe (GFR < 10 ml/min/1.73 m^2) renal impairment had reductions in mean oral clearance of ≈ 30% and 50%, respectively, compared with healthy subjects.

➤*Hepatic function impairment:* Following a single 15 mg dose of **mirtazapine**, the oral clearance decreased by ≈ 30% in hepatically impaired patients. Use mirtazapine with caution in patients with impaired hepatic function.

➤*Carcinogenesis:* There was an increased incidence of hepatocellular adenoma and carcinoma in male mice at high doses of **mirtazapine** and an increase in thyroid follicular adenoma/cystadenoma and carcinoma in male rats at high doses. Hepatocellular adenoma increased in female rats with mid and high doses of mirtazapine. **Maprotiline** did not show any drug- or dose-related occurrence of carcinogenesis in rats.

➤*Elderly:* Following administration of 20 mg/day **mirtazapine** for 7 days to subjects 25 to 74 years of age, oral clearance was reduced in the elderly subjects compared with the younger subjects. The differences were most striking in males, with a 40% lower clearance in elderly males compared with younger males, while the clearance in elderly females was only 10% lower compared with younger females. Caution is indicated in administering mirtazapine to elderly patients.

➤*Pregnancy:*

Maprotiline – (*Category B*, maprotiline; *Category C*, mirtazapine). There are no adequate and well-controlled studies in pregnant women. Use during pregnancy only if clearly needed.

➤*Lactation:*

Maprotiline – Maprotiline is excreted in breast milk. At steady state, the concentration in milk corresponds closely to the concentrations in whole blood. Exercise caution when maprotiline is administered to a nursing woman.

Mirtazapine – It is not known if mirtazapine is excreted in breast milk. Use caution when mirtazapine is administered to nursing women.

➤*Children:* Safety and efficacy in children (< 18 years of age for **maprotiline**) have not been established.

Precautions

➤*Monitoring:* Discontinue **maprotiline** if there is evidence of pathologic neutrophil depression. Perform leukocyte and differential counts in patients who develop fever and sore throat during therapy.

➤*Somnolence :* Somnolence was reported in 54% of patients treated with **mirtazapine**. Somnolence resulted in discontinuation of treatment in 10.4% of patients. It is unclear whether or not tolerance develops to the somnolent effects. Because mirtazapine has potentially significant effects on performance, caution patients about engaging in activities requiring alertness until they have been able to assess the drug's effect on their psychomotor performance.

➤*Dizziness:* Dizziness was reported in 7% of patients treated with **mirtazapine**. It is unclear whether or not tolerance to the dizziness develops.

➤*Increased appetite/weight gain:* Appetite increase was reported in 17% of patients treated with **mirtazapine**. In some trials, weight gain of ≥ 7% of body weight was reported in 7.5% of patients. Of patients receiving mirtazapine, 8% discontinued because of weight gain.

➤*Cholesterol / Triglycerides:* Nonfasting cholesterol increases to ≥ 20% above the upper limits of normal were observed in 15% of **mirtazapine** patients. In some cases, nonfasting triglyceride increases to ≥ 500 mg/dl were observed in 6% of patients treated with mirtazapine compared with 3% for placebo and 3% for amitriptyline.

➤*Mania / Hypomania:* Mania/Hypomania occurred in ≈ 0.2% of patients receiving **mirtazapine**. Hypomanic or manic episodes have occurred in some patients taking tricyclic antidepressant drugs, particularly in patients with cyclic disorders. Such occurrences have also been noted rarely with **maprotiline**. Although the incidence of mania/hypomania is rare during treatment with tetracyclics, use carefully in patients with a history of mania/hypomania.

➤*Suicide:* Suicidal ideation is inherent in depression and may persist until significant remission occurs. As with any patient receiving antidepressants, closely supervise high-risk patients during initial drug therapy. Physicians should write prescriptions for **mirtazapine** and **maprotiline** for the smallest quantity consistent with good patient management in order to reduce the risk of overdose.

➤*Elective surgery:* Prior to elective surgery, discontinue **maprotiline** for as long as possible, because little is known about the interaction between maprotiline and general anesthetics.

➤*Orthostatic hypotension:* **Mirtazapine** was associated with significant orthostatic hypotension in clinical trials with healthy volunteers. Orthostatic hypotension was infrequently observed in clinical trials with depressed patients.

➤*Lab test abnormalities:* Clinically significant ALT elevations (≥ 3 times the upper limit of the normal range) were observed in 2% of patients exposed to **mirtazapine**. Most of these patients did not develop signs or symptoms associated with compromised liver function. While some patients were discontinued for the ALT increases, in other cases, enzyme levels returned to normal despite continued mirtazapine treatment.

➤*Hazardous tasks:* Caution patients about engaging in hazardous activities until they are reasonably certain that tetracyclics do not adversely affect their ability to engage in such activities; because of their prominent sedative effects, tetracyclics may impair judgement, thinking, and particularly, motor skills.

Drug Interactions

➤*Drugs that are metabolized by or inhibit cytochrome P450 enzymes:* Many drugs are metabolized by or inhibit various cytochrome P450 enzymes (eg, 2D6, 1A2, 3A4). In vitro, **mirtazapine** is a substrate for several of these enzymes, including 2D6, 1A2, and 3A4. While in vitro studies have shown that mirtazapine is not a potent inhibitor of any of these enzymes, an indication that mirtazapine is not likely to have a clinically significant inhibitory effect on the metabolism of other drugs that are substrates for these cytochrome P450 enzymes, the concomitant use of mirtazapine with most other drugs metabolized by these enzymes has not been formally studied. Consequently, it is not possible to make any definitive statements about the risks of coadministration of mirtazapine with such drugs.

Because of the pharmacologic similarity of **maprotiline** to the tricyclic antidepressants, the plasma concentration of maprotiline may be increased when the drug is given concomitantly with hepatic enzyme inhibitors (eg, cimetidine, fluoxetine) and decreased by concomitant administration with hepatic enzyme inducers (eg, barbiturates, phenytoin), as has occurred with tricyclic antidepressants. Adjustment of the dosage of maprotiline may therefore be necessary in such cases.

Tetracyclic Drug Interactions

Precipitant drug	Object drug*		Description
Benzodiazepines	Maprotiline	↑	The risk of seizures may be increased when the dosage of benzodiazepines is rapidly tapered in patients receiving maprotiline (see Warnings).
Phenothiazines	Maprotiline	↑	The risk of seizures may be increased with concomitant use (see Warnings).
Thyroid hormones	Maprotiline	↑	Use caution when administering maprotiline to hyperthyroid patients or those on thyroid medication because of the possibility of enhanced potential for cardiovascular toxicity of maprotiline.
Maprotiline	Anticholinergics, Sympathomimetics	↑	Additive atropine-like effects may occur. Closely supervise and carefully adjust dosage when administering concomitantly.
Maprotiline	Guanethidine	↓	Maprotiline may block the pharmacologic effects of guanethidine or similar drugs.

Tetracyclic Drug Interactions

Precipitant drug	Object drug*		Description
Mirtazapine	Alcohol	↑	Concomitant administration has a minimal effect on plasma levels of mirtazapine. However, the impairment of cognitive and motor skills produced by mirtazapine are additive with those produced by alcohol. Advise patients to avoid alcohol while taking mirtazapine.
Mirtazapine	Diazepam	↑	Concomitant administration has a minimal effect on plasma levels of mirtazapine. However, the impairment of motor skills produced by mirtazapine is additive with those caused by diazepam. Advise patients to avoid diazepam and other similar drugs while taking mirtazapine.

* ↑ = Object drug increased. ↓ = Object drug decreased.

Adverse Reactions

Approximately 16% of the 453 patients who received **mirtazapine** tablets in 6–week controlled US clinical trials discontinued treatment because of an adverse experience, compared with 7% of the 361 placebo-treated patients in those studies. The most common events (≥ 1%) associated with discontinuation and considered to be drug-related (ie, those events associated with dropout at a rate of at least twice that of placebo) included somnolence (10.4%) and nausea (1.5%).

Adverse Reactions: Maprotiline vs Mirtazapine (%)[1]

Adverse reactions	Maprotiline	Mirtazapine
Cardiovascular		
Hypertension	rare	≥ 1
Hypotension	rare	0.1-1
CNS		
Abnormal dreams	-	4
Agitation	2	≥ 1
Anxiety	3	≥ 1
Ataxia	rare	0.1-1
Confusion	rare	2
Dizziness	8	7
Drowsiness	16	-
Extrapyramidal symptoms	rare	0.1-1
Hallucinations	rare	0.1-1
Headache	4	-
Insomnia	2	-
Mania	rare	0.1-1
Nervousness	6	-
Somnolence	-	54
Abnormal thinking	-	3
Tremor	3	2
Weakness and fatigue	4	-
Dermatologic		
Alopecia	rare	< 1
Pruritus	-	≥ 1
Rash	rare	≥ 1
GI		
Dry mouth	22	25
Constipation	6	13
Increased appetite	-	17
Nausea	2	0.1-1
Vomiting	rare	≥ 1
Metabolic/Nutritional		
Edema	rare	1
Peripheral edema	-	2
Weight gain	rare	12
Weight loss	rare	0.1-1
Miscellaneous		
Altered liver function	rare	0.1-1
Asthenia	-	8
Back pain	-	2
Blurred vision	4	-
Dyspnea	-	1
Flu syndrome	-	5
Myalgia	-	2
Urinary frequency	rare	2

[1] Data are pooled from different studies and are not necessarily comparable.

Tetracyclic Compounds

➤*Maprotiline:*

Cardiovascular – Tachycardia, palpitation, arrhythmia, heart block, syncope (rare).

CNS – Disorientation, delusions, restlessness, nightmares, hypomania, exacerbation of psychosis, decrease in memory, feelings of unreality, numbness, tingling, motor hyperactivity, akathisia, seizures, EEG alterations, tinnitus, dysarthria (rare).

Endocrine – Increased or decreased libido, impotence, elevation or depression of blood sugar levels (rare).

GI – Epigastric distress, diarrhea, bitter taste, abdominal cramps, dysphagia (rare).

Hypersensitivity – Skin rash, petechiae, itching, photosensitization, edema, drug fever (rare).

Miscellaneous – Accommodation disturbances, jaundice, mydriasis, urinary retention and delayed micturition, excessive perspiration, flushing, increased salivation, nasal congestion (rare).

Because of maprotiline's pharmacologic similarity to tricyclic antidepressants and isolated reports of the following adverse reactions, consider each reaction when administering maprotiline: Bone marrow depression (including agranulocytosis, eosinophilia, purpura, and thrombocytopenia), MI, stroke, peripheral neuropathy, sublingual adenitis, black tongue, stomatitis, paralytic ileus, gynecomastia in the male, breast enlargement and galactorrhea in the female, and testicular swelling.

Several voluntary reports of interstitial pneumonitis, which were in some cases associated with eosinophilia and increased liver enzymes, have been received since market introduction. However, there is no clear causal relationship.

➤*Mirtazapine:*

Cardiovascular – Vasodilatation (≥ 1%); angina pectoris, MI, bradycardia, ventricular extrasystoles, syncope, migraine (0.1% to 1%); atrial arrhythmia, bigeminy, vascular headache, pulmonary embolus, cerebral ischemia, cardiomegaly, phlebitis, left heart failure (< 0.1%).

CNS – Hypesthesia, apathy, depression, hypokinesia, vertigo, twitching, amnesia, hyperkinesia, paresthesia (≥ 1%); delirium, delusions, depersonalization, dyskinesia, increased libido, abnormal coordination, dysarthria, neurosis, dystonia, hostility, increased reflexes, emotional lability, euphoria, paranoid reaction (0.1% to 1%); aphasia, nystagmus, akathisia, stupor, dementia, diplopia, drug dependence, paralysis, grand mal convulsion, hypotonia, myoclonus, psychotic depression, withdrawal syndrome (< 0.1%).

Dermatologic – Acne, exfoliative dermatitis, dry skin, herpes simplex (0.1% to 1%); urticaria, herpes zoster, skin hypertrophy, seborrhea, skin ulcer (< 0.1%).

Endocrine – Goiter, hypothyroidism (< 0.1%).

GI – Anorexia (≥ 1%); eructation, glossitis, cholecystitis, gum hemorrhage, stomatitis, colitis (0.1% to 1%); tongue discoloration, ulcerative stomatitis, salivary gland enlargement, increased salivation, intestinal obstruction, pancreatitis, aphthous stomatitis, cirrhosis of the liver, gastritis, gastroenteritis, oral moniliasis, tongue edema (< 0.1%).

GU – Urinary tract infection (≥ 1%); kidney calculus, cystitis, dysuria, urinary incontinence, urinary retention, vaginitis, hematuria, breast pain, amenorrhea, dysmenorrhea, leukorrhea, impotence (0.1% to 1%); polyuria, urethritis, metrorrhagia, menorrhagia, abnormal ejaculation, breast engorgement, breast enlargement, urinary urgency (< 0.1%).

Hematologic / Lymphatic – Lymphadenopathy, leukopenia, petechiae, anemia, thrombocytopenia, lymphocytosis, pancytopenia (< 0.1%).

Metabolic / Nutritional – Thirst (≥ 1%); dehydration (0.1% to 1%); gout, AST increased, healing abnormal, acid phosphatase increased, ALT increased, diabetes mellitus (< 0.1%).

Musculoskeletal – Myasthenia, arthralgia (≥ 1%); arthritis, tenosynovitis (0.1% to 1%); pathological fracture, osteoporosis fracture, bone pain, myositis, tendon rupture, arthrosis, bursitis (< 0.1%).

Respiratory – Cough increased, sinusitis (≥ 1%); epistaxis, bronchitis, asthma, pneumonia (0.1% to 1%); asphyxia, laryngitis, pneumothorax, hiccough (< 0.1%).

Special senses – Eye pain, abnormality of accommodation, conjunctivitis, deafness, keratoconjunctivitis, lacrimation disorder, glaucoma, hyperacusis, ear pain (0.1% to 1%); blepharitis, partial transitory deafness, otitis media, taste loss, parosmia (< 0.1%).

Miscellaneous – Malaise, abdominal pain, acute abdominal syndrome (≥ 1%); chills, fever, face edema, ulcer, photosensitivity reaction, neck rigidity, neck pain, enlarged abdomen (0.1% to 1%); cellulitis, substernal chest pain (< 0.1%).

Overdosage

➤*Maprotiline:*

Symptoms – Deaths may occur from overdosage with this class of drugs. Signs and symptoms of maprotiline overdose are similar to those seen with tricyclic overdose. Critical manifestations of overdose include cardiac dysrhythmias, severe hypotension, convulsions, and CNS depression, including coma. Changes in the ECG, particularly in QRS axis or width, are clinically significant indicators of toxicity. Other clinical manifestations include drowsiness, tachycardia, ataxia, vomiting, cyanosis, shock, restlessness, agitation, hyperpyrexia, muscle rigidity, athetoid movements, and mydriasis. Because CHF has been seen with overdosage of tricyclic antidepressants, consider CHF with maprotiline overdosage as well.

Management – Obtain an ECG and immediately initiate cardiac monitoring. Protect the patient's airway, establish an IV line, and initiate gastric decontamination. A minimum of 6 hours of observation with cardiac monitoring and observation for signs of CNS or respiratory depression, hypotension, cardiac dysrhythmias or conduction blocks, and seizures is necessary. If signs of toxicity occur at any time during this period, extended monitoring is required. There are case reports of patients succumbing to fatal dysrhythmias late after tricyclic overdose; these patients had clinical evidence of significant poisoning prior to death and most received inadequate GI decontamination. Monitoring of plasma drug levels should not guide management of the patient.

GI decontamination: All patients suspected of overdose should receive GI decontamination. This should include large volume gastric lavage followed by activated charcoal. Emesis is contraindicated.

Cardiovascular: A maximal limb-lead QRS duration of ≥ 0.1 seconds may be the best indication of the severity of the overdose. Use IV sodium bicarbonate to maintain the serum pH of 7.45 to 7.55. A pH > 7.6 or a Pco_2 < 20 mmHg is undesirable. Dysrhythmias unresponsive to sodium bicarbonate therapy/hyperventilation may respond to lidocaine, bretylium, or phenytoin. Type 1A and 1C antiarrhythmics are generally contraindicated (eg, quinidine, disopyramide, procainamide).

In rare instances, hemoperfusion may be beneficial in acute refractory cardiovascular instability in patients with acute toxicity. However, hemodialysis, peritoneal dialysis, exchange transfusions, and forced diuresis generally have been ineffective.

CNS: In patients with CNS depression, early intubation is advised because of the potential for abrupt deterioration. Control seizures with benzodiazepines, or if these are ineffective, other anticonvulsants (eg, phenobarbital, phenytoin). Physostigmine is not recommended except to treat life-threatening symptoms that have been unresponsive to other therapies and then only in consultation with a poison control center.

➤*Mirtazapine:*

Symptoms – There is very limited experience with mirtazapine overdose. In premarketing clinical studies, there were 8 reports of mirtazapine overdose alone or in combination with other pharmacologic agents. The only drug-overdose death reported while taking mirtazapine was in combination with amitriptyline and chlorprothixene. All other premarketing overdose cases resulted in full recovery. Signs and symptoms reported in association with overdose included disorientation, drowsiness, impaired memory, and tachycardia. There were no reports of ECG abnormalities, coma, or convulsions following overdose with mirtazapine alone.

Management – Employ general measures to manage overdose with any antidepressant. There are no specific antidotes for mirtazapine. If the patient is unconscious, establish and maintain an airway to ensure adequate oxygenation and ventilation. Consider gastric evacuation either by the induction of emesis or lavage or both. Also consider activated charcoal for overdose treatment. Monitoring of cardiac and vital signs is recommended along with general symptomatic and supportive measures.

Consider the possibility of multiple-drug involvement. Consider contacting a poison control center for additional information on the treatment of any overdose.

Patient Information

Warn patients who are to receive **mirtazapine** about the risk of developing agranulocytosis. Instruct patients to contact their physician if they experience any indication of infection such as fever, chills, sore throat, mucous membrane ulceration, or other possible signs of infection. Pay particular attention to any flu-like complaints or other symptoms that might suggest infection.

Caution patients about engaging in hazardous activities until they are reasonably certain that tetracyclics do not adversely affect their ability to engage in such activities; because of their prominent sedative effects, tetracyclics may impair judgement, thinking, and particularly, motor skills.

Advise patients to inform their physician if they are taking or intend to take any prescription, *otc*, or alternative medicinal drugs because there is a potential for tetracyclics to interact with other drugs.

Advise patients to avoid alcohol while taking tetracyclics because of the additive impairment of cognitive and motor skills.

Advise patients to notify their physician if they become pregnant or intend to become pregnant or are breastfeeding during tetracyclic therapy.

Warn patients of the association between seizures and **maprotiline** use. Inform patients that this association is enhanced in patients with a history of seizures and in those taking certain other drugs.

While patients may notice improvement with therapy in 1 to 4 weeks, advise them to continue therapy as directed.

Advise patients to avoid sunlight or sunlamps or wear protective clothing; photosensitivity may occur.

MAPROTILINE HCl

Rx	**Maprotiline HCl** (Various, eg, Mylan)	**Tablets**: 25 mg	In 30s, 100s, and 500s.
Rx	**Maprotiline HCl** (Various, eg, Mylan)	**Tablets**: 50 mg	In 30s, 100s, and 500s.
Rx	**Maprotiline HCl** (Various, eg, Mylan)	**Tablets**: 75 mg	In 30s, 100s, and 500s.

For complete prescribing information, refer to the Tetracyclic Compounds group monograph.

Indications

➤*Depression:* For the treatment of depressive illness in patients with depressive neurosis (dysthymic disorder) and manic-depressive illness, depressed type (major depressive disorder).

Also effective for the relief of anxiety associated with depression.

Administration and Dosage

May be given as a single daily dose or in divided doses. Therapeutic effects are sometimes seen within 3 to 7 days, although 2 to 3 weeks are usually necessary.

➤*Initial adult dosage:* An initial dosage of 75 mg/day is suggested for outpatients with mild-to-moderate depression. In some patients, especially the elderly, an initial dosage of 25 mg/day may be used. Because of the long half-life of maprotiline, maintain the initial dosage for 2 weeks. The dose may then be increased gradually in 25 mg incre-

ments, as required and tolerated. A maximum daily dose of 150 mg/day will result in therapeutic efficacy in most outpatients, but dosages as high as 225 mg/day may be required.

➤*Severe depression:* Give hospitalized patients an initial daily dose of 100 to 150 mg, which may be gradually increased as required and tolerated. Most hospitalized patients with moderate-to-severe depression respond to a daily dose of 150 mg although daily doses as high as 225 mg may be required. Do not exceed 225 mg/day.

➤*Maintenance:* Keep dosage during prolonged maintenance therapy at the lowest effective level. Dosage may be reduced to 75 to 150 mg/day with adjustment depending on therapeutic response.

➤*Elderly:* In general, lower doses are recommended for patients > 60 years of age. Doses of 50 to 75 mg/day are satisfactory as maintenance therapy for elderly patients who do not tolerate higher amounts.

➤*Storage/Stability:* Store at controlled room temperature 15° to 30°C (59° to 86°F). Dispense in a tight, light-resistant container.

MIRTAZAPINE

Rx	**Mirtazapine** (Various, eg, Par, Teva, Watson)	**Tablets**: 15 mg	In 30s, 100s, and 1000s.
Rx	**Remeron** (Organon)		Lactose. (Organon TZ3). Yellow, oval, scored. Film-coated. In 30s, 100s, and UD 100s.
Rx	**Mirtazapine** (Various, eg, Par, Teva, Watson)	**Tablets**: 30 mg	In 30s, 100s, and 1000s.
Rx	**Remeron** (Organon)		Lactose. (Organon TZ5). Red-brown, oval, scored. Film-coated. In 30s and 100s.
Rx	**Mirtazapine** (Various, eg, Par, Teva, Watson)	**Tablets**: 45 mg	In 30s, 100s, and 1000s.
Rx	**Remeron** (Organon)		Lactose. (Organon TZ7). White, oval. Film-coated. In 30s.
Rx	**Remeron SolTab** (Organon)	**Tablets, orally disintegrating**: 15 mg	Aspartame, mannitol, 2.6 mg phenylalanine. (TZ1). In UD 30s and 90s.
		30 mg	Aspartame, mannitol, 5.2 mg phenylalanine. (TZ2). In UD 30s and 90s.
		45 mg	Aspartame, mannitol, 7.8 mg phenylalanine. (TZ4). In UD 30s and 90s.

For complete prescribing information, refer to the Tetracyclic Compounds group monograph.

Indications

➤*Depression:* Treatment of depression.

Administration and Dosage

➤*Approved by the FDA:* June 14, 1996.

➤*Initial treatment:* The recommended starting dosage is 15 mg/day administered in a single dose, preferably in the evening prior to sleep. Patients not responding to the initial 15 mg dose may benefit from dosage increases up to a maximum of 45 mg/day. Do not change dose at intervals of < 1 to 2 weeks.

➤*Maintenance/Extended treatment:* Continue treatment for acute episodes of depression for ≥ 6 months.

➤*Switching to or from a monoamine oxidase inhibitor (MAOI):* At least 14 days should elapse between discontinuation of an MAOI

and initiation of therapy with mirtazapine. In addition, allow ≥ 14 days after stopping mirtazapine before starting an MAOI.

➤*Elderly and renal/hepatic function impairment:* The clearance of mirtazapine is reduced in elderly patients and in patients with moderate-to-severe renal or hepatic impairment. Consequently, plasma mirtazapine levels may be increased in these patient groups compared with levels observed in younger adults without renal or hepatic impairment.

➤*Administration of orally disintegrating tablets:* Open tablet blister pack with dry hands and place tablet on tongue. The tablet will disintegrate rapidly on the tongue and can be swallowed with saliva. Use the tablet immediately after removal from the blister; it cannot be scored. No water is needed. Do not attempt to split the tablet.

➤*Storage/Stability:* Store at 25°C (77°F); excursions permitted to 15° to 30°C (59° to 86°F). Protect from light and moisture. Use orally disintegrating tablets immediately upon opening individual tablet blisters.

TRAZODONE HCl

Rx	**Trazodone HCl** (Various, eg, Barr, Geneva, Ivax, Major, Martec, Mutual, Purepac, Schein, Sidmak, Teva, UDL, URL)	**Tablets**: 50 mg	In 50s, 100s, 500s, 1000s, UD 100s, and *Robot Ready* 25s.
Rx	**Desyrel** (Apothecon)		(Desyrel MJ 775). Orange, scored. Film-coated. In 100s, 1000s, and UD 100s.
Rx	**Trazodone HCl** (Various, eg, Barr, Geneva, Ivax, Major, Mutual, Schein, Sidmak, Teva, UDL, URL)	**Tablets**: 100 mg	In 50s, 100s, 500s, 1000s, UD 100s, and *Robot Ready* 25s.
Rx	**Desyrel** (Apothecon)		(Desyrel MJ 776). White, scored. Film-coated. In 100s, 1000s, and UD 100s.
Rx	**Trazodone HCl** (Various, eg, Barr, Geneva, Major, Martec, Mutual, Sidmak, URL)	**Tablets**: 150 mg	In 100s, 250s, 500s, 1000s, and unit-of-use 30s.
Rx	**Desyrel Dividose** (Apothecon)		(MJ 778 50 50 50). Orange, double-scored. In 100s and 500s.
Rx	**Trazodone HCl** (Barr)	**Tablets**: 300 mg	(barr 733 100 100 100). White, oval, scored. In 100s.
Rx	**Desyrel Dividose** (Apothecon)		(MJ 796 100 100 100). Yellow, double-scored. In 100s.

Indications

➤*Depression:* Treatment of depression.

➤*Unlabeled uses:* Trazodone 50 mg twice daily and tryptophan 500 mg twice daily have been successful in the treatment of aggressive behavior. Dose adjustments were made until therapeutic response was achieved or unacceptable adverse effects developed. Low doses (50 to 100 mg daily) decreased cravings for alcohol, depression, and anxious symptoms in patients with alcoholism. A dosage of 300 mg/day may also be useful for treatment of patients with panic disorder or agoraphobia with panic attacks. Low-dose (25 to 75 mg) trazodone is also used to treat insomnia often in conjunction with a selective serotonin reuptake inhibitor (SSRI) (see Drug Interactions).

Trazodone has been used to treat cocaine withdrawal.

Administration and Dosage

Initiate dosage at a low level and increase gradually. Drowsiness may require the administration of a major portion of the daily dose at bedtime or a reduced dosage. Take shortly after a meal or light snack. Symptomatic relief may be seen during the first week, with optimal effects typically evident within 2 weeks. Of those who respond to therapy, 25% require 2 to 4 weeks of drug administration.

➤*Adults:* An initial dosage is 150 mg/day in divided doses. This may be increased by 50 mg/day every 3 to 4 days. The maximum dosage for outpatients usually should not exceed 400 mg/day in divided doses. Inpatients or more severely depressed subjects may be given up to, but not in excess of, 600 mg/day in divided doses.

➤*Maintenance:* Keep dosage at the lowest effective level when dosing during prolonged maintenance therapy. Once an adequate response has been achieved, dosage may be gradually reduced with subsequent adjustment depending on response.

Although there has been no systematic evaluation of the efficacy of trazodone > 6 weeks, it is recommended that a course of antidepressant drug treatment be continued for several months.

Actions

➤*Pharmacology:* Trazodone is an antidepressant chemically unrelated to tricyclic, tetracyclic, or other known antidepressant agents. The mechanism of antidepressant action is not fully understood. Trazodone is not a monoamine oxidase inhibitor and, unlike amphetamine-type drugs, does not stimulate the CNS. In animals, it selectively inhibits serotonin uptake by brain synaptosomes and potentiates the behavioral changes induced by the serotonin precursor, 5-hydroxy-tryptophan.

➤*Pharmacokinetics:*

Absorption/Distribution – Trazodone is well absorbed after oral administration without selective localization in any tissue. When taken shortly after ingestion of food, there may be an increase in the amount of drug absorbed, a decrease in maximum concentration, and a lengthening in the time to maximum concentration. Peak plasma levels occur in ≈ 1 hour when taken on an empty stomach or in 2 hours when taken with food.

Metabolism/Excretion – Trazodone is extensively metabolized in the liver and is a CYP3A4 substrate; < 1% is excreted unchanged in the urine and feces. Elimination is biphasic, with a half-life of 3 to 6 hours (mean, 4.4) and 5 to 9 hours (mean, 7 to 8) and is unaffected by food. Because the clearance of trazodone from the body is sufficiently variable, in some subjects it may accumulate in the plasma.

Onset of action – For those who responded to trazodone, 33% of the inpatients and 50% of the outpatients had a significant therapeutic response by the end of the first week of treatment. Three-fourths of all responders demonstrated a significant therapeutic effect by the end of the second week. One-fourth of responders required 2 to 4 weeks for a significant therapeutic response.

Contraindications

Hypersensitivity to trazodone; initial recovery phase of MI.

Warnings

➤*Preexisting cardiac disease:* Not recommended for use during the initial recovery phase of MI. Clinical studies and postmarketing reports in patients with preexisting cardiac disease indicate that trazodone may be arrhythmogenic in some patients. Arrhythmias identified include isolated PVCs, ventricular couplets, and short episodes (3 to 4 beats) of ventricular tachycardia. Closely monitor patients with preexisting cardiac disease, particularly for cardiac arrhythmias.

➤*Priapism:* Priapism has been reported in patients receiving trazodone. In patients with prolonged or inappropriate penile erection, discontinue use immediately and consult a physician or go to an emergency room. Injection of alpha-adrenergic stimulants (eg, norepinephrine, epinephrine) may be successful in treating priapism. In many of the cases reported, surgical intervention was required and, in a portion of these cases, permanent impairment of erectile function or impotence resulted. Priapism of the clitoris also has occurred.

➤*Pregnancy: Category C.* Studies in rats and rabbits have revealed increased fetal resorption and congenital anomalies, respectively, when given at 30 to 50 times the maximum human dose and ≈ 15 to 50 times the maximum human dose, respectively. There are no adequate and well-controlled studies in pregnant women. Use during pregnancy only if the potential benefit justifies the potential risk to the fetus.

➤*Lactation:* Trazodone and its metabolites have been found in the milk of rats, suggesting that the drug may be excreted in breast milk. Exercise caution when administering to a nursing mother.

➤*Children:* Safety and efficacy for use in children < 18 years of age have not been established.

Precautions

➤*Suicide:* The possibility of suicide in seriously depressed patients is inherent in the illness and may persist until significant remission occurs. Therefore, prescriptions should be written for the smallest number of tablets consistent with good patient management.

➤*Hypotension:* Hypotension, including orthostatic hypotension and syncope, has occurred. Concomitant administration of antihypertensive therapy with trazodone may require a reduction in the dose of the antihypertensive.

➤*Elective surgery:* There is little known about the interaction between trazodone and general anesthetics; therefore, prior to elective surgery, discontinue trazodone for as long as clinically feasible.

➤*Electroconvulsive therapy:* Avoid concurrent administration with electroconvulsive therapy because of the absence of experience in this area.

➤*Lab test abnormalities:* Occasional low white blood cell and neutrophil counts have been noted, but were not considered clinically significant; however, discontinue the drug in any patient whose white blood cell count or absolute neutrophil count falls below normal levels. White blood cell and differential counts are recommended for patients who develop fever and sore throat (or other signs of infection) during therapy.

➤*Hazardous tasks:* May produce drowsiness, dizziness, or blurred vision; patients should observe caution while driving or performing other tasks requiring alertness, coordination, or physical dexterity.

Drug Interactions

Trazodone Drug Interactions			
Precipitant drug	Object drug*		Description
Trazodone	Alcohol, barbiturates, CNS depressants	↑	Trazodone may enhance the CNS-depressant response to these agents.
Trazodone	Digoxin	↑	Increased serum digoxin levels have been reported to occur in patients receiving concurrent trazodone HCl.

TRAZODONE HCl

Trazodone Drug Interactions			
Precipitant drug	Object drug*		Description
Trazodone	MAOIs	↔	It is not known whether interactions will occur between trazodone and MAOIs. If MAOIs are discontinued shortly before, or are to be given concomitantly with trazodone, initiate therapy cautiously with gradual increase in dosage until optimum response is achieved.
Trazodone	Phenytoin	↑	Phenytoin serum levels were increased with concurrent trazodone therapy.
Trazodone	Warfarin	↑ ↓	There have been reports of increased and decreased prothrombin time occurring in patients taking warfarin and trazodone concurrently.
Carbamazepine	Trazodone	↓	Plasma concentrations of trazodone and its active metabolite may be decreased, producing a decrease in therapeutic effect.
Phenothiazines	Trazodone	↑	Elevated trazodone serum concentrations have occurred, increasing the pharmacologic and toxic effects.
SSRIs Venlafaxine	Trazodone	↑	A "serotonin syndrome," including irritability, increased muscle tone, shivering, myoclonus, and altered consciousness may occur.

* ↑ = Object drug increased. ↓ = Object drug decreased. ↔ = Undetermined clinical effect.

Adverse Reactions

Trazodone Adverse Reactions (%)				
	Inpatients		Outpatients	
Adverse reaction	Trazodone (n = 142)	Placebo (n = 95)	Trazodone (n = 157)	Placebo (n = 158)
Cardiovascular				
Hypertension	2.1	1.1	1.3	< 1
Hypotension	7	1.1	3.8	0
Shortness of breath	< 1	1.1	1.3	0
Syncope	2.8	2.1	4.5	1.3
Tachycardia/Palpitations	0	0	7	7
CNS				
Anger/Hostility	3.5	6.3	1.3	2.5
Confusion	4.9	0	5.7	7.6
Decreased concentration	2.8	2.1	1.3	0
Disorientation	2.1	0	< 1	0
Dizziness/Lightheadedness	19.7	5.3	28	15.2
Drowsiness	23.9	6.3	40.8	19.6
Excitement	1.4	1.1	5.1	5.7
Fatigue	11.3	4.2	5.7	2.5
Headache	9.9	5.3	19.8	15.8
Incoordination	4.9	0	1.9	0
Insomnia	9.9	10.5	6.4	12
Impaired memory	1.4	0	< 1	< 1
Nervousness	14.8	10.5	6.4	8.2
Nightmares/Vivid dreams	< 1	1.1	5.1	5.7
Paresthesia	1.4	0	0	< 1
Tremors	2.8	1.1	5.1	3.8
GI				
Abdominal/Gastric disorder	3.5	4.2	5.7	4.4
Bad taste in mouth	1.4	0	0	0
Constipation	7	4.2	7.6	5.7
Diarrhea	0	1.1	4.5	1.9
Dry mouth	14.8	8.4	33.8	20.3
Nausea/Vomiting	9.9	1.1	12.7	9.5

Trazodone Adverse Reactions (%)				
	Inpatients		Outpatients	
Adverse reaction	Trazodone (n = 142)	Placebo (n = 95)	Trazodone (n = 157)	Placebo (n = 158)
Special senses				
Blurred vision	6.3	4.2	14.7	3.8
Eyes red/tired/itching	2.8	0	0	0
Tinnitus	1.4	0	0	< 1
Miscellaneous				
Allergic skin condition/ edema	2.8	1.1	7	1.3
Aches/Pains	5.6	3.2	5.1	2.5
Decreased appetite	3.5	5.3	0	< 1
Decreased libido	< 1	1.1	1.3	< 1
Head full/heavy	2.8	0	0	0
Malaise	2.8	0	0	0
Nasal/Sinus congestion	2.8	0	5.7	3.2
Sweating/Clamminess	1.4	1.1	< 1	< 1
Weight gain	1.4	0	4.5	1.9
Weight loss	< 1	3.2	5.7	2.5

Other adverse events reported – Occasional sinus bradycardia has occurred in long-term studies; abnormal dreams; agitation; akathisia; allergic reaction; alopecia; anemia; anxiety; aphasia; apnea; arrhythmia; ataxia; atrial fibrillation; breast enlargement or engorgement; cardiac arrest; cardiospasm; cerebrovascular accident; chest pain; chills; cholestasis; clitorism; CHF; conduction block; delayed urine flow; diplopia; early menses; edema; extrapyramidal symptoms; flatulence; grand mal seizures; hallucinations/delusions; hematuria; hemolytic anemia; hirsutism; hyperbilirubinemia; hypersalivation; hypomania; impaired speech; impotence; increased amylase; increased appetite; increased libido; increased salivation; increased urinary frequency; insomnia; leukocytosis; leukonychia; jaundice; lactation; liver enzyme alterations; methemoglobinemia; missed period; muscle twitches; MI; nausea/vomiting (most frequently); numbness; orthostatic hypotension; paresthesia; paranoid reaction; priapism (see Warnings); pruritus; psoriasis; psychosis; rash; retrograde ejaculation; stupor; inappropriate ADH syndrome; tardive dyskinesia; unexplained death; urinary incontinence; urinary retention; urticaria; vasodilation; ventricular ectopic activity (including ventricular tachycardia); vertigo; weakness.

Overdosage

►*Symptoms:* Death from overdose has occurred in patients ingesting trazodone and other drugs concurrently (ie, alcohol, alcohol plus chloral hydrate plus diazepam, amobarbital, chlordiazepoxide, meprobamate).

The most common manifestation of overdose is CNS depression.

The most severe reactions reported with overdose of trazodone alone have been priapism, respiratory arrest, seizures, and ECG changes. Overdosage may cause an increase in incidence or severity of any of the reported adverse reactions.

Clinical manifestations of overdose may include any of those listed in Adverse Reactions, with drowsiness, lethargy, ataxia, nausea, and vomiting reported most frequently. Significant ingestions may produce hypotension, bradycardia, and respiratory depression.

►*Treatment:* There is no specific antidote. Treatment should be symptomatic and supportive for hypotension or excessive sedation. In patients suspected of having an overdose, empty stomach by gastric lavage or administer activated charcoal after control of seizure. Forced diuresis may be useful in elimination of the drug. Refer to General Management of Acute Overdosage.

Patient Information

Take with food. The risk of dizziness/lightheadedness may increase under fasting conditions.

May produce drowsiness or dizziness; advise patients to observe caution while driving or performing other tasks requiring alertness, coordination, or physical dexterity.

Notify physician of dizziness, lightheadedness, or fainting.

Male patients with prolonged, inappropriate, and painful erections should immediately discontinue the drug and consult their physician.

Medication may cause dry mouth, irregular heartbeat, shortness of breath, nausea, and vomiting; notify physician if these become pronounced.

Avoid alcohol and other depressant drugs.

BUPROPION HCl

Rx	**Bupropion HCl** (Various, eg, Geneva, Teva)	**Tablets:** 75 mg	In 100s.
Rx	**Wellbutrin** (GlaxoSmithKline)		(Wellbutrin 75). Yellow-gold. Film-coated. In 100s.
Rx	**Bupropion HCl** (Various, eg, Geneva, Teva)	**Tablets:** 100 mg	In 100s.
Rx	**Wellbutrin** (GlaxoSmithKline)		(Wellbutrin 100). Red. Film-coated. In 100s.
Rx	**Bupropion HCl** (Various, eg, Eon, Watson)	**Tablets, sustained-release (12 hour):** 100 mg	In 60, 100s, and 500s.
Rx	**Budeprion SR** (Impax)		(G 2442). Yellow. Film-coated. In 100s.
Rx	**Wellbutrin SR**[a] (GlaxoSmithKline)		(Wellbutrin SR 100). Blue. Film-coated. In 60s.
Rx	**Bupropion HCl** (Watson)	**Tablets, sustained-release (12 hour):** 150 mg	In 60s and 250s.
Rx	**Wellbutrin SR**[a] (GlaxoSmithKline)		(Wellbutrin SR 150). Purple. Film-coated. In 60s.
Rx	**Wellbutrin SR**[a] (GlaxoSmithKline)	**Tablets, sustained-release (12 hour):** 200 mg	(Wellbutrin SR 200). Lt. pink. Film-coated. In 60s.
Rx	**Wellbutrin XL**[a] (GlaxoSmithKline)	**Tablets, extended-release (24 hour):** 150 mg	(Wellbutrin XL 150). Creamy-white to pale yellow. In 30s.
Rx	**Wellbutrin XL**[a] (GlaxoSmithKline)	**Tablets, extended-release (24 hour):** 300 mg	(Wellbutrin XL 300). Creamy-white to pale yellow. In 30s.

[a] Please note that "SR" refers to the 12-hour tablets and "XL" refers to the 24-hour tablets.

For additional information, refer to the Antidepressants introduction. Bupropion also is used as a smoking deterrent. Refer to the Smoking Deterrents section of this chapter for complete prescribing information.

Indications

➤*Depression:* Treatment of depression.

➤*Unlabeled uses:* Bupropion SR has been shown to be effective in the treatment of neuropathic pain and to enhance weight loss. Bupropion also has been shown to be effective in the treatment of attention deficit hyperactivity disorder.

Administration and Dosage

➤*Approved by the FDA:* December 30, 1985.

➤*General:* It is particularly important to administer bupropion in a manner most likely to minimize the risk of seizure (see Warnings). Do not exceed dose increases of 100 mg/day of the immediate-release formulation in a 3-day period. Gradual escalation of dosage also is important to minimize agitation, motor restlessness, and insomnia often seen during the initial days of treatment. If necessary, these effects may be managed by temporary reduction of dose or the short-term administration of an intermediate- to long-acting sedative-hypnotic. A sedative-hypnotic is not usually required beyond the first week of treatment. Insomnia also may be minimized by avoiding bedtime doses. If distressing, untoward effects supervene, stop dose escalation.

➤*Bupropion immediate-release (IR):* No single dose should exceed 150 mg. Administer 3 times/day, preferably with at least 6 hours between successive doses.

The usual adult dosage is 300 mg/day, given 3 times/day. Begin dosing at 200 mg/day, given as 100 mg twice daily. Based on clinical response, this dosage may be increased to 300 mg/day, given as 100 mg 3 times/day no sooner than 3 days after beginning therapy (see following table).

Bupropion Dosage Regimen					
			Number of tablets		
Treatment day	Total daily dose	Tablet strength	Morning	Midday	Evening
1	200 mg	100 mg	1	0	1
4	300 mg	100 mg	1	1	1

Increasing the dosage above 300 mg/day – As with other antidepressants, the full antidepressant effect of bupropion may not be evident until 4 weeks of treatment or longer. An increase in dosage up to a maximum of 450 mg/day given in divided doses of not more than 150 mg each, may be considered for patients in whom no clinical improvement is noted after several weeks of treatment at 300 mg/day. Dosing above 300 mg/day may be accomplished using the 75 or 100 mg tablets. The 100 mg tablets must be administered 4 times/day with at least 4 hours between successive doses in order not to exceed the limit of 150 mg in a single dose. Discontinue in patients who do not demonstrate an adequate response after an appropriate treatment period at 450 mg/day.

➤*Bupropion SR:* The usual adult target dosage is 300 mg/day given as 150 mg twice daily. Begin dosing with 150 mg/day, given as a single daily dose in the morning. If the 150 mg initial dose is adequately tolerated, increase to 300 mg/day, given as 150 mg twice daily, as early as day 4 of dosing. Allow at least 8 hours between successive doses. Swallow whole; do not crush, divide, or chew.

Increasing the dosage above 300 mg/day – As with other antidepressants, the full antidepressant effect of the SR formula may not be evident until 4 weeks of treatment or longer. Consider an increase in dosage to the maximum of 400 mg/day, given as 200 mg twice daily, for patients in whom no clinical improvement is noted after several weeks at 300 mg/day treatment.

Maintenance – It generally is agreed that acute episodes of depression require several months or longer of sustained pharmacological therapy beyond response to the acute episode. Based on these limited data, it is unknown whether or not the dose of bupropion SR needed for maintenance treatment is identical to the dose needed to achieve an initial response. Periodically reassess patients to determine the need for maintenance treatment and the appropriate dose for such treatment.

➤*Bupropion XL:* The usual adult target dose is 300 mg/day, given once daily in the morning. Dosing should begin at 150 mg/day, given as a single daily dose in the morning. If the 150 mg initial dose is adequately tolerated, an increase to the 300 mg/day target dose, given once daily, may be made as early as day 4 of dosing. There should be an interval of at least 24 hours between successive doses. Swallow whole; do not crush, divide, or chew.

Increasing the dosage above 300 mg/day – As with other antidepressants, the full antidepressant effect of the XL formula may not be evident until 4 weeks of treatment or longer. An increase in dosage to the maximum of 450 mg/day, given as a single dose, may be considered for patients in whom no clinical improvement is noted after several weeks of treatment at 300 mg/day.

Maintenance – It generally is agreed that acute episodes of depression require several months or longer of sustained pharmacological therapy beyond response to the acute episode. Based on these limited data, it is unknown whether or not the dose of bupropion XL needed for maintenance treatment is identical to the dose needed to achieve an initial response. Periodically reassess patients to determine the need for maintenance treatment and the appropriate dose for such treatment.

Switching to Bupropion XL – When switching patients from bupropion tablets to XL tablets or from SR tablets to XL tablets, give the same total daily dose when possible. Patients who are currently being treated with bupropion tablets at 300 mg/day (eg, 100 mg 3 times/day) may be switched to XL tablets 300 mg once daily. Patients who are currently being treated with SR tablets at 300 mg/day (eg, 150 mg twice daily) may be switched to XL tablets 300 mg once daily.

➤*Hepatic function impairment:* Use bupropion with extreme caution in patients with severe hepatic cirrhosis. The dose should not exceed 75 mg once daily (100 mg every day or 150 mg every other day for SR; 150 mg every other day for XL) in these patients. Use bupropion with caution in patients with hepatic impairment (including mild to moderate hepatic cirrhosis) and consider a reduced frequency and/or dose in patients with mild to moderate hepatic cirrhosis.

➤*Renal impairment:* Use bupropion with caution in patients with renal impairment and consider a reduced frequency and/or dose.

➤*Storage/Stability:*

IR – Store at 15° to 25°C (59° to 77°F). Protect from light and moisture.

SR – Store at controlled room temperature, 20° to 25°C (68° to 77°F). Dispense in a tight, light-resistant container.

XL – Store at 25°C (77°F); excursions permitted to 15° to 30°C (59° to 86°F).

Actions

➤*Pharmacology:* Bupropion, an antidepressant of the aminoketone class, is chemically unrelated to other available antidepressant agents. Its structure closely resembles that of diethylpropion; it is related to phenylethylamines. The neurochemical mechanism of the antidepressant effect of bupropion is not known. Bupropion is a relatively weak inhibitor of the neuronal uptake of norepinephrine, serotonin, and dopamine and does not inhibit monoamine oxidase.

Bupropion produces the following dose-related CNS-stimulant effects in animals: Increased locomotor activity, increased rates of responding in various schedule-controlled operant behavior tasks, and, in high doses, induction of mild stereotyped behavior.

➤*Pharmacokinetics:*

Absorption/Distribution – Following oral administration, peak plasma concentrations are usually achieved within 2 hours for bupropion, 3 hours for bupropion SR, and 5 hours for bupropion XL followed by a biphasic decline. The distribution phase has a mean half-life of 3 to 4 hours. Plasma concentrations are dose-proportional following single doses of 100 to 250 mg; however, it is not known if the proportionality between dose and plasma level is maintained in chronic use. Steady-state plasma concentrations of bupropion SR are reached within

BUPROPION HCl

8 days. It appears likely that only a small portion of any oral dose reaches the systemic circulation intact. Bupropion is 84% bound to human albumin at plasma concentrations up to 200 mcg/mL. The extent of protein binding of the hydroxybupropion metabolite is similar to that for bupropion, whereas the extent of protein binding of the threohydrobupropion metabolite is about half that seen with bupropion.

In a study comparing 14-day dosing with 300 mg bupropion XL once daily to the IR formulation of bupropion at 100 mg 3 times/day, equivalence was demonstrated for peak plasma concentration and AUC for bupropion and the 3 metabolites (hydroxybupropion, threohydrobupropion, and erythrohydrobupropion).

In a study comparing chronic dosing with 150 mg bupropion SR twice daily to the IR formulation of bupropion at 100 mg 3 times/day, peak plasma concentrations of bupropion at steady state for bupropion SR were approximately 85% of those achieved with the IR formulation. There was equivalence for bupropion AUCs, as well as equivalence for peak plasma concentration and AUCs for all 3 of the detectable bupropion metabolites. Thus, at steady state, bupropion SR, given twice daily, and the IR formulation of bupropion, given 3 times/day, are essentially bioequivalent for bupropion and the 3 quantitatively important metabolites.

Metabolism/Excretion – The terminal phase has a mean half-life of 14 hours, with a range of 8 to 24 hours. The mean elimination half-life of bupropion after chronic dosing is approximately 21 hours. Following oral administration of 200 mg bupropion, 87% and 10% of the dose were recovered in the urine and feces, respectively; the fraction excreted unchanged was only 0.5%.

Bupropion is extensively metabolized in humans. Three metabolites are active: Hydroxybupropion, which is formed via hydroxylation of the *tert*-butyl group of bupropion, and the amino-alcohol isomers threohydrobupropion and erythrohydrobupropion, which are formed via reduction of the carbonyl group. In vitro findings suggest that CYP2B6 is the principal isoenzyme involved in the formation of hydroxybupropion, while cytochrome P450 isoenzymes are not involved in the formation of threohydrobupropion. Oxidation of the bupropion side chain results in the formation of a glycine conjugate of metachlorobenzoic acid, which is then excreted as the major urinary metabolite. The potency and toxicity of the metabolites relative to bupropion have not been fully characterized. However, it has been demonstrated in an antidepressant screening test in mice that hydroxybupropion is 50% as potent as bupropion, while threohydrobupropion and erythrohydrobupropion are 5-fold less potent than bupropion. This may be of clinical importance because their plasma concentrations are as high or higher than those of bupropion.

Following a single dose in humans, peak plasma concentrations of hydroxybupropion occur approximately 3 hours after administration of bupropion IR, 6 hours after bupropion SR, and 7 hours after bupropion XL. Peak plasma concentrations of hydroxybupropion are approximately 10 times (7 times after bupropion XL administration) the peak level of the parent drug at steady state. The elimination half-life of hydroxybupropion is approximately 20 hours, and its AUC at steady state is about 17 times that of bupropion. The time to peak concentrations for the erythrohydrobupropion and threohydrobupropion metabolites are similar to that of the hydroxybupropion metabolite. However, their elimination half-lives are longer, approximately 33 and 37 hours, respectively, and steady-state AUCs are 1.5 and 7 times that of bupropion, respectively.

Bupropion and its metabolites exhibit linear kinetics following chronic administration of 300 to 450 mg/day.

Special populations –

Hepatic function impairment: The effect of hepatic impairment on the pharmacokinetics of bupropion was characterized in 2 single-dose studies, one in patients with alcoholic liver disease and one in patients with mild to severe cirrhosis. The first study showed that the half-life of hydroxybupropion was significantly longer in 8 patients with alcoholic liver disease than in 8 healthy volunteers (approximately 32 vs approximately 21 hours, respectively).

In the second study, more variability was observed in some of the pharmacokinetic parameters for bupropion (AUC, C_{max}, and T_{max}) and its active metabolites ($t_{\frac{1}{2}}$) in patients with mild to moderate hepatic cirrhosis. In addition, in patients with severe hepatic cirrhosis, the bupropion C_{max} and AUC were substantially increased (mean difference, approximately 70% and 3-fold, respectively) and more variable when compared with values in healthy volunteers; the mean bupropion half-life also was longer (29 hours in patients with severe hepatic cirrhosis vs 19 hours in healthy subjects). For the metabolite hydroxybupropion, the mean C_{max} was approximately 69% lower. For the combined amino-alcohol isomers threohydrobupropion and erythrohydrobupropion, the mean C_{max} was approximately 31% lower. The mean AUC increased by about 1.5-fold for hydroxybupropion and about 2.5-fold for threo/erythrohydrobupropion. The median T_{max} was observed 19 hours later for hydroxybupropion and 31 hours later for threo/erythrohydrobupropion. The mean half-lives for hydroxybupropion and threo/erythrohydrobupropion were increased 5- and 2-fold, respectively, in patients with severe hepatic cirrhosis compared with healthy volunteers.

Hypersensitivity to the drug or its ingredients; seizure disorder; current or prior diagnosis of bulimia or anorexia nervosa; coadministration of a monoamine oxidase inhibitor (MAOI) (see Drug Interactions); in patients being treated with other bupropion products (eg, *Zyban* for smoking cessation); in patients undergoing abrupt discontinuation of alcohol or sedatives (including benzodiazepines).

➤*Other bupropion medications:* Bupropion, bupropion SR, and bupropion XL contain the same active ingredient found in *Zyban*, used as an aid to smoking cessation treatment. Do not use bupropion in combination with *Zyban* or any other medications that contain bupropion.

➤*Anorexia nervosa/bulimia:* Do not give with current or prior diagnosis of bulimia or anorexia nervosa because of a higher incidence of seizures noted in patients treated for bulimia with the IR formulation of bupropion.

➤*Seizures:* Bupropion IR is associated with seizures in approximately 0.4% of patients treated at doses up to 450 mg/day. This incidence of seizures may exceed that of other marketed antidepressants by as much as 4-fold. The estimated seizure incidence increases almost 10-fold between 450 and 600 mg/day. Given the wide variability among individuals and their capacity to metabolize and eliminate drugs, this disproportionate increase in seizure incidence with dose incrementation calls for caution in dosing.

Data for bupropion SR tablets revealed a seizure incidence of approximately 0.1% in patients treated at doses up to 300 mg/day and increases to approximately 0.4% at the maximum recommended dose of 400 mg/day. It is not possible to know if the lower seizure incidence observed in this study involving the SR formulation resulted from the different formulation or the lower dose used. However, the IR and SR formulations are bioequivalent regarding rate and extent of absorption during steady state (the most pertinent condition to estimating seizure incidence) because most observed seizures occur under steady-state conditions. Bupropion XL, while not formally evaluated in clinical trials, may be similar to that presented for the IR and SR formulations of bupropion.

The risk of seizure appears strongly associated with dose. Sudden and large increments in dose may increase risk. While many seizures occurred early in the treatment course, some seizures occurred after several weeks at fixed dose. Discontinue bupropion and do not restart in patients who experience a seizure while on treatment. Predisposing factors that may increase the risk of seizure include history of head trauma or prior seizure, CNS tumor, the presence of severe hepatic cirrhosis, and concomitant medications that lower seizure threshold. Circumstances associated with an increased seizure risk include, among others, excessive use of alcohol or sedatives (including benzodiazepines); addiction to opiates, cocaine, or stimulants; use of OTC stimulants and anorectics; and diabetes treated with oral hypoglycemics or insulin.

Recommendations for reducing seizure risk – (1) The total daily dose does not exceed 450 mg (400 mg SR; 450 mg XL), (2) the daily dose is administered 3 times/day, with each single dose not to exceed 150 mg to avoid high peak concentrations of bupropion and/or its metabolites (twice daily for SR tablets with each single dose not to exceed 200 mg), (3) the rate of incrementation of dose is very gradual.

Use extreme caution when administering to patients with a history of seizure, cranial trauma, or other predisposition toward seizure, or prescribed with other agents (eg, antipsychotics, other antidepressants, theophylline, systemic steroids) that lower seizure threshold.

➤*Hepatotoxicity:* In animals receiving large doses of bupropion chronically, there was an increased incidence of hepatic hyperplastic nodules, hepatocellular hypertrophy, and histologic changes and laboratory tests that suggested mild hepatocellular injury.

➤*Hypersensitivity reactions:* Anaphylactoid/anaphylactic reactions characterized by symptoms such as pruritus, urticaria, angioedema, and dyspnea requiring medical treatment have been reported in clinical trials with bupropion. In addition, there have been rare spontaneous postmarketing reports of erythema multiforme, Stevens-Johnson syndrome, and anaphylactic shock associated with bupropion. Patients should stop taking bupropion and consult a doctor if they experience allergic or anaphylactoid/anaphylactic reactions (eg, skin rash, pruritus, hives, chest pain, edema, shortness of breath) during treatment.

Arthralgia, myalgia, and fever with rash and other symptoms suggestive of delayed hypersensitivity have been reported in association with bupropion. These symptoms may resemble serum sickness.

➤*Renal function impairment:* Use bupropion with caution in patients with renal impairment and consider a reduced frequency and/or dose as bupropion and its metabolites could accumulate in such patients to a greater extent than usual. Closely monitor the patient for adverse effects that could indicate possible high drug or metabolite levels.

➤*Hepatic function impairment:* Use bupropion with extreme caution in patients with severe hepatic cirrhosis. In these patients, a reduced dose and/or frequency is required, as peak bupropion levels are substantially increased and accumulation is likely to occur in such

BUPROPION HCl

patients to a greater extent than usual. Do not exceed 75 mg once a day (100 mg every day or 150 mg every other day for bupropion SR; 150 mg every other day for bupropion XL) in these patients. Use bupropion with caution in patients with hepatic impairment (including mild to moderate hepatic cirrhosis) and consider a reduced frequency and/or dose in patients with mild to moderate hepatic cirrhosis. Closely monitor all patients with hepatic impairment for possible adverse effects that could indicate high drug and metabolite levels.

➤*Carcinogenesis:* In rats, there was an increase in nodular proliferative lesions of the liver at doses of 100 to 300 mg/kg/day.

➤*Mutagenesis:* Bupropion produced a borderline positive response in some strains in the Ames bacterial mutagenicity test. A high oral dose (300 mg/kg, but not 100 or 200 mg/kg) produced a low incidence of chromosomal aberrations in rats. The relevance of these results in human exposure to therapeutic doses is unknown.

➤*Elderly:* Bupropion is extensively metabolized in the liver to active metabolites, which are further metabolized and excreted by the kidneys. The risk of toxic reaction to this drug may be greater in patients with impaired renal function. Because elderly patients are more likely to have decreased renal function, take care in dose selection; it may be useful to monitor renal function.

➤*Pregnancy: Category B.* There are no adequate and well-controlled studies in pregnant women. Use during pregnancy only if clearly needed.

To monitor fetal outcomes of pregnant women exposed to bupropion, GlaxoSmithKline maintains a Bupropion Pregnancy Registry. Health care providers are encouraged to register patients by calling (800) 336-2176.

➤*Lactation:* Bupropion and its metabolites are secreted in breast milk. Because of the potential for serious adverse reactions in nursing infants, decide whether to discontinue nursing or to discontinue the drug, taking into account the importance of the drug to the mother.

➤*Children:* Safety and efficacy in children younger than 18 years of age have not been established.

Precautions

➤*CNS effects:* A substantial proportion of patients experience some degree of increased restlessness, agitation, anxiety, and insomnia, especially shortly after initiation of treatment. Symptoms were sometimes of sufficient magnitude to require treatment with sedative/hypnotic drugs. In approximately 2% of bupropion immediate-release patients, symptoms were sufficiently severe to require discontinuation. Discontinuation was required in 1% and 2.6% of patients treated with 300 and 400 mg/day, respectively, with bupropion SR tablets.

➤*Neuropsychiatric phenomena:* Patients treated with bupropion have shown a variety of neuropsychiatric signs and symptoms including delusions, hallucinations, psychotic episodes, concentration disturbance, confusion, and paranoia. In several cases, neuropsychiatric phenomena abated upon dose reduction and/or withdrawal of treatment.

➤*Psychosis or mania:* Antidepressants can precipitate manic episodes in bipolar manic depressive patients during the depressed phase of their illness and may activate latent psychosis in other susceptible patients.

➤*Altered appetite and weight:* A weight loss of greater than 2.3 kg (5 lbs) occurred in 28% of patients treated with IR bupropion and in at least 14% of patients treated with bupropion SR. This incidence is approximately double that seen in comparable patients treated with tricyclic antidepressants (TCAs) or placebo. Furthermore, 34.5% of patients receiving TCAs gained weight, vs only 9.4% of bupropion IR patients. Consequently, if weight loss is a major presenting sign of a patient's depressive illness, consider the anorectic and/or weight-reducing potential.

➤*Suicide:* The possibility of a suicide attempt is inherent in depression and may persist until significant remission occurs. Accordingly, physicians should write prescriptions for the smallest number of tablets consistent with good patient management.

➤*Cardiac effects:* Hypertension, in some cases severe, requiring acute treatment, has been reported in patients receiving bupropion alone and in combination with nicotine replacement therapy. These events have been observed in patients with and without evidence of pre-existing hypertension. Monitoring of blood pressure is recommended in patients who receive the combination of bupropion and nicotine replacement. There is no clinical experience establishing the safety of bupropion in patients with a recent history of MI or unstable heart disease. Therefore, exercise care if it is used in these groups. Bupropion was associated with a rise in supine blood pressure in the study of patients with CHF, resulting in discontinuation of treatment in 2 patients for exacerbation of baseline hypertension.

➤*Drug abuse and dependence:* Studies in normal volunteers, subjects with a history of multiple-drug abuse, and depressed patients showed some increase in motor activity and agitation/excitement. In individuals experienced with drugs of abuse, a single dose of 400 mg bupropion produced mild amphetamine-like activity as compared with placebo. Studies in rodents and primates have shown that bupropion exhibits some pharmacologic actions common to psychostimulants.

Evidence from single-dose studies suggests that the recommended daily dosage of bupropion when administered in divided doses is not likely to be especially reinforcing to amphetamine or stimulant abusers. However, higher doses, not tested because of seizure risk, may modestly attract those who abuse stimulant drugs.

➤*Photosensitivity:* Photosensitization may occur; therefore, caution patients to take protective measures (ie, sunscreens, protective clothing) against exposure to ultraviolet light or sunlight until tolerance is determined.

Drug Interactions

➤*CYP450:* In vitro studies indicate that bupropion is primarily metabolized to hydroxybupropion by the cytochrome P450 2B6 (CYP2B6) isoenzyme. Therefore, the potential exists for a drug interaction between bupropion and drugs that affect the CYP2B6 metabolism (eg, orphenadrine, cyclophosphamide). While not systemically studied, certain drugs may induce the metabolism of bupropion (eg, carbamazepine, phenobarbital, phenytoin).

Approach with caution coadministration of bupropion with drugs that are metabolized by the cytochrome P450 2D6 (CYP2D6) isoenzyme, including certain antidepressants (eg, nortriptyline, imipramine, desipramine, paroxetine, fluoxetine, sertraline), antipsychotics (eg, haloperidol, risperidone, thioridazine), beta blockers (eg, metoprolol), and type 1C antiarrhythmics (eg, propafenone, flecainide) and initiate coadministration at the lower end of the dose range of the concomitant medication. If bupropion is added to the treatment regimen of a patient already receiving a drug metabolized by CYP2D6, consider the need to decrease the dose of the original medication, particularly for those concomitant medications with a narrow therapeutic index.

➤*Drugs that lower seizure threshold:* Use caution during coadministration of bupropion and agents (eg, antipsychotics, other antidepressants, theophylline, systemic steroids) or treatment regimens (eg, abrupt discontinuation of benzodiazepines) that lower seizure threshold. Use low initial dosing and small gradual dose increases.

Bupropion Drug Interactions			
Precipitant drug	Object drug*		Description
Amantadine Levodopa	Bupropion	↑	There is a higher incidence of adverse experiences with concurrent use of these agents. Use small initial doses and small gradual dose increases of bupropion.
Carbamazepine	Bupropion	↓	Serum concentrations of bupropion may be decreased, decreasing the pharmacologic effects.
MAOIs	Bupropion	↑	Animal data demonstrate bupropion's acute toxicity is enhanced by phenelzine. Coadministration is contraindicated. Allow at least 14 days between discontinuation of an MAOI and initiation of bupropion.
Nicotine replacement	Bupropion	↑	Coadministration may cause hypertension. Monitor blood pressure.
Ritonavir	Bupropion	↑	Large increases in serum bupropion concentrations may occur, increasing the risk of bupropion toxicity. Avoid coadministration.
Bupropion	Alcohol	↑	There have been rare reports of adverse neuropsychiatric events or reduced alcohol tolerance. Minimize or avoid consumption of alcohol during treatment with bupropion.
Bupropion	Drugs metabolized by CYP450 2D6 (eg, SSRIs, many TCAs, beta blockers, type 1C antiarrhythmics, antipsychotics)	↑	Bupropion and hydroxybupropion are inhibitors of the CYP2D6 isoenzyme. If bupropion is added to the treatment regimen of a patient receiving a drug metabolized by CYP2D6, consider a dose reduction in the original medication.
Bupropion	Warfarin	↑	Altered PT or INR are infrequently associated with hemorrhagic or thrombotic complications when bupropion is coadministered with warfarin.

* ↑ = Object drug increased.   ↓ = Object drug decreased.

BUPROPION HCl

Adverse Reactions

Bupropion Adverse Reactions (%)[a]					
Adverse reaction	Bupropion (n = 323)	Placebo (n = 185)	Bupropion SR 300 mg/day (n = 376)	Bupropion SR 400 mg/day (n = 114)	Placebo (n = 385)
Cardiovascular					
Cardiac arrhythmias	5.3	4.3	—	—	—
Flushing	—	—	1	4	< 0.5
Hot flashes	—	—	1	3	1
Hypertension	4.3	1.6	—	—	—
Hypotension	2.5	2.2	—	—	—
Palpitations	3.7	2.2	2	6	2
Syncope	1.2	0.5	—	—	—
Tachycardia	10.8	8.6	—	—	—
CNS					
Agitation	31.9	22.2	3	9	2
Akathisia	1.5	1.1	—	—	—
Akinesia/Bradykinesia	8	8.6	—	—	—
Anxiety	3.1	1.1	5	6	3
CNS stimulation	—	—	2	1	1
Confusion	8.4	4.9	—	—	—
Cutaneous temperature disturbance	1.9	1.6	—	—	—
Decreased libido	3.1	1.6	—	—	—
Delusions	1.2	1.1	—	—	—
Disturbed concentration	3.1	3.8	—	—	—
Dizziness	22.3	16.2	7	11	5
Euphoria	1.2	0.5	—	—	—
Headache/Migraine	25.7	22.2	26/1	25/4	23/1
Hostility	5.6	3.8	—	—	—
Impaired sleep quality	4	1.6	—	—	—
Increased salivary flow	3.4	3.8	—	—	—
Insomnia	18.6	15.7	11	16	6
Irritability	—	—	3	2	2
Memory decreased	—	—	< 0.5	3	1
Nervousness	—	—	5	3	3
Paresthesia	—	—	1	2	1
Pseudoparkinsonism	1.5	1.6	—	—	—
Sedation	19.8	19.5	—	—	—
Sensory disturbance	4	3.2	—	—	—
Somnolence	—	—	2	3	2
Tremor	21.1	7.6	6	3	1
Dermatologic					
Excessive sweating	22.3	14.6	6	5	2
Pruritus	2.2	0	2	4	2
Rash	8	6.5	5	4	1
Urticaria	—	—	2	1	0
GI					
Abdominal pain	—	—	3	9	2
Anorexia	18.3	18.4	5	3	2
Appetite increase	3.7	2.2	—	—	—
Constipation	26	17.3	10	5	7
Diarrhea	6.8	8.6	5	7	6
Dry mouth	27.6	18.4	17	24	7
Dyspepsia	3.1	2.2	—	—	—
Dysphagia	—	—	0	2	0
Nausea/Vomiting	22.9	18.9	13/4	18/2	8/2
GU					
Impotence	3.4	3.1	—	—	—
Menstrual complaints	4.7	1.1	—	—	—
Urinary frequency	2.5	2.2	2	5	2
Urinary retention	1.9	2.2	—	—	—
Urinary tract infection	—	—	1	0	< 0.5
Urinary urgency	—	—	< 0.5	2	0
Vaginal hemorrhage	—	—	0	2	< 0.5
Musculoskeletal					
Arthralgia	—	—	1	4	1
Arthritis	3.1	2.7	0	2	0
Muscle spasms	1.9	3.2	—	—	—
Myalgia	—	—	2	6	3
Twitch	—	—	1	2	< 0.5
Respiratory					
Increased cough	—	—	1	2	1
Pharyngitis	—	—	3	11	2
Sinusitis	—	—	3	1	2
Upper respiratory complaints	5	11.4	—	—	—

BUPROPION HCl

Adverse reaction	Bupropion Adverse Reactions (%)[a]				
	Bupropion (n = 323)	Placebo (n = 185)	Bupropion SR 300 mg/day (n = 376)	Bupropion SR 400 mg/day (n = 114)	Placebo (n = 385)
Special senses					
Amblyopia	—	—	3	2	2
Auditory disturbance	5.3	3.2	—	—	—
Blurred vision	14.6	10.3	—	—	—
Gustatory disturbance	3.1	1.1	—	—	—
Tinnitus	—	—	6	6	2
Taste perversion	—	—	2	4	< 0.5
Miscellaneous					
Asthenia	—	—	2	4	2
Chest pain	—	—	3	4	1
Fatigue	5	8.6	—	—	—
Fever/Chills	1.2	0.5	1	2	< 0.5
Infection	—	—	8	9	6
Pain	—	—	2	3	2
Weight gain	13.6	22.7	—	—	—
Weight loss	23.2	23.2	—	—	—

[a] Data are pooled from separate studies and are not necessarily comparable.

➤*Bupropion XL:* Bupropion XL has not been studied in placebo-controlled trials, although it has been studied in nonplacebo-controlled clinical bioavailability studies.

Discontinuation of treatment –
IR: Adverse reactions caused discontinuation in approximately 10% of patients and volunteers with IR bupropion. The more common events causing discontinuation include the following: Neuropsychiatric disturbances, primarily agitation and abnormalities in mental status (3%); GI disturbances, primarily nausea and vomiting (2.1%); neurological disturbances, primarily seizures, headaches, and sleep disturbances (1.7%); dermatologic problems, primarily rashes (1.4%). Many of these events occurred at doses that exceeded the recommended daily dose.
SR: Adverse reactions caused discontinuation in 9% and 11% of patients treated with 300 and 400 mg/day bupropion SR, respectively. The more common events causing discontinuation include the following: Rash (0.9% to 2.4%); nausea (0.8% to 1.8%); agitation (0.3% to 1.8%); migraine (1.8%).

➤*Other adverse reactions include the following:*
Cardiovascular –
IR: Edema (at least 1%); chest pain, ECG abnormalities (premature beats and nonspecific ST-T changes) (0.1% to 1%); flushing, phlebitis, MI (less than 0.1%).
SR: Postural hypotension, stroke, tachycardia, vasodilation (0.1% to 1%); syncope (less than 0.1%); complete AV block, extrasystoles, hypotension, hypertension (in some cases severe; see Precautions), MI, phlebitis, pulmonary embolism.

CNS –
IR: Ataxia/incoordination, seizure, myoclonus, dyskinesia, dystonia, mania/hypomania, increased libido, hallucinations, decreased sexual function, depression (at least 1%); vertigo, dysarthria, memory impairment, depersonalization, psychosis, dysphoria, mood instability, paranoia, formal thought disorder, frigidity (0.1% to 1%); EEG abnormality, abnormal neurological exam, impaired attention, sciatica, aphasia, suicidal ideation (less than 0.1%).
SR: Abnormal coordination, decreased libido, depersonalization, dysphoria, emotional lability, hostility, hyperkinesia, hypertonia, hypesthesia, suicidal ideation, vertigo (0.1% to 1%); amnesia, ataxia, derealization, hypomania (less than 0.1%); abnormal EEG, akinesia, aphasia, coma, delirium, dysarthria, dyskinesia, dystonia, euphoria, extrapyramidal syndrome, hallucinations, hypokinesia, increased libido, manic reaction, neuralgia, neuropathy, paranoid reaction, unmasking tardive dyskinesia.

Dermatologic –
IR: Nonspecific rashes (at least 1%); alopecia, dry skin (0.1% to 1%); pallor, change in hair color, hirsutism, acne (less than 0.1%).
SR: Maculopapular rash (less than 0.1%); alopecia, angioedema, exfoliative dermatitis, hirsutism.

Endocrine –
IR: Hormone level change (less than 0.1%).
SR: Hyperglycemia, hypoglycemia, syndrome of inappropriate antidiuretic hormone.

GI –
IR: Stomatitis (at least 1%); dysphagia, thirst disturbance, toothache, bruxism, gum irritation, oral edema (0.1% to 1%); rectal complaints, colitis, GI bleeding, intestinal perforation, stomach ulcer, glossitis (less than 0.1%).
SR: Bruxism, gastric reflux, gingivitis, glossitis, increased salivation, mouth ulcers, stomatitis, thirst (0.1% to 1%); tongue edema (less than 0.1%); colitis, esophagitis, GI hemorrhage, gum hemorrhage, intestinal perforation, pancreatitis, stomach ulcer.

GU –
IR: Nocturia (at least 1%); gynecomastia, vaginal irritation, testicular swelling, urinary tract infection, painful erection, retarded ejaculation (0.1% to 1%); glycosuria, dysuria, enuresis, urinary incontinence, menopause, ovarian disorder, pelvic infection, cystitis, dyspareunia, painful ejaculation (less than 0.1%).
SR: Impotence, polyuria, prostate disorder (0.1% to 1%); abnormal ejaculation, cystitis, dyspareunia, dysuria, gynecomastia, menopause, painful erection, salpingitis, urinary incontinence, urinary retention, vaginitis, glycosuria.

Hematologic / Lymphatic –
IR: Lymphadenopathy, anemia, pancytopenia (less than 0.1%).
SR: Ecchymosis (0.1% to 1%); anemia, leukocytosis, leukopenia, lymphadenopathy, pancytopenia, thrombocytopenia. Altered PT and/or INR, infrequently associated with hemorrhagic or thrombotic complications, were observed when bupropion was coadministered with warfarin.

Hepatic –
IR: Liver damage, jaundice (0.1% to 1%).
SR: Abnormal liver function, jaundice (0.1% to 1%); hepatitis, liver damage.

Musculoskeletal –
IR: Musculoskeletal chest pain (less than 0.1%).
SR: Leg cramps, musculoskeletal chest pain (0.1% to 1%); muscle rigidity/fever/rhabdomyolysis, muscle weakness.

Respiratory –
IR: Bronchitis, shortness of breath/dyspnea (0.1% to 1%); epistaxis, rate or rhythm disorder, pneumonia, pulmonary embolism (less than 0.1%).
SR: Bronchospasm (less than 0.1%); pneumonia.

Special senses –
IR: Mydriasis, visual disturbances (0.1% to 1%); diplopia (less than 0.1%).
SR: Accommodation abnormality, dry eye (0.1% to 1%); deafness, diplopia, mydriasis.

Miscellaneous –
IR: Flu-like symptoms (at least 1%); nonspecific pain (0.1% to 1%); body odor, surgically related pain, infection, medication reaction, overdose (less than 0.1%).
SR: Chills, facial edema, edema, peripheral edema, photosensitivity (0.1% to 1%); malaise (less than 0.1%); fever with rash and other symptoms suggestive of delayed hypersensitivity.

➤*Post-marketing:* Voluntary reports of adverse events temporally associated with bupropion IR that have been received since market introduction and which may have no causal relationship with the drug include the following.

Cardiovascular – Hypertension (in some cases severe), orthostatic hypotension, third-degree heart block.

CNS – Coma, delirium, dream abnormalities, paresthesia, unmasking of tardive dyskinesia.

Dermatologic – Stevens-Johnson syndrome, angioedema, exfoliative dermatitis, urticaria.

Endocrine – Syndrome of inappropriate antidiuretic hormone secretion, hyperglycemia, hypoglycemia.

GI – Esophagitis, hepatitis, liver damage.

Hematologic / Lymphatic – Ecchymosis, leukocytosis, leukopenia, thrombocytopenia. Altered PT and/or INR, infrequently associated with hemorrhagic or thrombotic complications, were observed when bupropion was coadministered with warfarin.

Musculoskeletal – Arthralgia, myalgia, muscle rigidity/fever/rhabdomyolysis, muscle weakness.

BUPROPION HCl

Miscellaneous – Fever with rash and other symptoms suggestive of delayed hypersensitivity (these symptoms may resemble serum sickness), tinnitus.

Overdosage

▶*Symptoms:* Thirteen overdoses with bupropion IR occurred during clinical trials; 12 patients ingested 850 to 4200 mg and recovered without significant sequelae. Another patient who ingested 9000 mg bupropion and 300 mg tranylcypromine experienced a grand mal seizure and recovered without further sequelae. Since introduction, overdoses of up to 17,500 mg of the IR formulation have occurred. Seizure was reported in approximately 33% of all cases. Other serious reactions reported with overdoses of the IR formulation of bupropion alone included hallucinations, loss of consciousness, and sinus tachycardia. Fever, muscle rigidity, rhabdomyolysis, hypotension, stupor, coma, and respiratory failure have been reported when bupropion was part of multiple-drug overdoses. Although most patients recovered without sequelae, deaths have been rarely reported with overdoses of the IR formulation of bupropion in patients ingesting massive doses; multiple uncontrolled seizures, bradycardia, cardiac failure, and cardiac arrest prior to death were reported in these patients.

There has been limited experience with overdosage of bupropion SR tablets; 3 cases were reported during clinical trials. One patient ingested 3000 mg of bupropion SR tablets and vomited quickly after the overdose; the patient experienced blurred vision and lightheadedness. A second patient ingested a "handful" of SR tablets and experienced confusion, lethargy, nausea, jitteriness, and seizure. A third patient ingested 3600 mg SR tablets and a bottle of wine; the patient experienced nausea, visual hallucinations, and grogginess. None of the patients experienced further sequelae.

▶*Treatment:* Ensure an adequate airway, oxygenation, and ventilation. Monitor cardiac rhythm and vital signs. EEG monitoring also is recommended for the first 48 hours postingestion. General supportive and symptomatic measures also are recommended. Induction of emesis is not recommended. Gastric lavage with a large-bore orogastric tube with appropriate airway protection, if needed, may be indicated if performed soon after ingestion or in symptomatic patients.

Administer activated charcoal. There is no experience with the use of forced diuresis, dialysis, hemoperfusion, or exchange transfusion in the management of bupropion overdoses. No specific antidotes for bupropion are known.

Because of the dose-related risk of seizures with bupropion, consider hospitalization following suspected overdose. Based on studies in animals, it is recommended that seizures be treated with IV benzodiazepine administration and other supportive measures, as appropriate.

In managing overdosage, consider the possibility of multiple-drug involvement. Consider contacting a poison control center for additional information on the treatment of any overdose.

Patient Information

Advise patients that the bupropion antidepressant (*Wellbutrin*, *Wellbutrin SR*, and *Wellbutrin XL*) contains the same active ingredient as the smoking cessation aid (*Zyban*). Do not use these in combination or with any other medications that contain bupropion.

Advise patients to take bupropion IR in equally divided doses 3 or 4 times/day to minimize the risk of seizure. Take bupropion SR formulation in doses above 150 mg/day in 2 divided doses with at least 8 hours between successive doses to minimize seizure risk. Take bupropion XL once per day, at least 24 hours apart.

Advise patients not to chew, divide, or crush SR or XL tablets.

Advise patients that they may notice something that looks like a tablet in their stool. This is normal. The medication in bupropion XL is contained in a nonabsorbable shell that has been specially designed to slowly release drug in the body. When this process is completed, the empty shell is eliminated from the body.

Advise patients that bupropion may impair ability to perform tasks requiring judgment or motor and cognitive skills. Instruct patients to refrain from driving an automobile or operating complex, hazardous machinery until they are reasonably certain the drug does not adversely affect their performance.

Excessive use or abrupt discontinuation of alcohol or sedatives (including benzodiazepines) may alter the seizure threshold. Some patients have reported lower alcohol tolerance during bupropion treatment. Therefore, instruct patients to minimize the consumption of alcohol and, if possible, avoid completely.

Advise patients to inform their physician or pharmacist if they are taking or plan to take any prescription or OTC drugs or any herbal or natural products.

Advise patients to notify their physician if they become pregnant, intend to become pregnant during therapy, or are breastfeeding.

Tell patients to discontinue bupropion and not restart if they experience a seizure while on treatment.

VENLAFAXINE HCl

Rx	Effexor (Wyeth-Ayerst)	Tablets: 25 mg	Lactose. (25 W 701). Peach, shield shape, scored. In 100s and *Redipak* 100s.
		37.5 mg	Lactose. (37.5 W 781). Peach, shield shape, scored. In 100s and *Redipak* 100s.
		50 mg	Lactose. (50 W 703). Peach, shield shape, scored. In 100s and *Redipak* 100s.
		75 mg	Lactose. (75 W 704). Peach, shield shape, scored. In 100s and *Redipak* 100s.
		100 mg	Lactose. (100 W 705). Peach, shield shape, scored. In 100s and *Redipak* 100s.
Rx	Effexor XR (Wyeth-Ayerst)	Capsules, extended-release: 37.5 mg	(W Effexor XR 37.5). Gray/Peach. In 100s and *Redipak* 100s.
		75 mg	(W Effexor XR 75). Peach. In 100s and *Redipak* 100s.
		150 mg	(W Effexor XR 150). Dk orange. In 100s and *Redipak* 100s.

For additional information, refer to the Antidepressants introduction.

Indications

▶*Depression:* Treatment of major depression.

▶*Anxiety:* Treatment of generalized anxiety disorder (GAD) and social anxiety disorder (SAD) (extended-release [ER] only).

▶*Unlabeled uses:* In some patients, venlafaxine may be beneficial for the treatment of hot flashes; PMDD; PTSD (recommended for use after no response with an SSRI for 8 weeks).

Administration and Dosage

▶*Approved by the FDA:* December 28, 1993.

▶*Venlafaxine immediate-release:*
Depression –

Initial treatment: The recommended starting dosage is 75 mg/day, administered in 2 or 3 divided doses, taken with food. Depending on tolerability and the need for further clinical effect, the dose may be increased to 150 mg/day. If needed, further increase the dosage up to 225 mg/day. When increasing the dose, make increments of up to 75 mg/day at intervals of at least 4 days. In outpatient settings, there was no evidence of usefulness of doses more than 225 mg/day for moderately depressed patients, but more severely depressed inpatients responded to a mean dosage of 350 mg/day. Certain patients, including more severely depressed patients, may respond more to higher doses, up to a maximum of 375 mg/day, generally in 3 divided doses.

Maintenance: It is not known whether the dose needed for maintenance is identical to the dose needed to achieve an initial response. Periodically assess patients to determine the need for maintenance treatment and the appropriate dose for such treatment.

Switching patients from immediate- to extended-release venlafaxine – Depressed patients currently treated at a therapeutic dose with venlafaxine may be switched to venlafaxine ER at the nearest equivalent dose (mg/day; eg, 37.5 mg venlafaxine twice daily to 75 mg venlafaxine ER once daily). However, individual dosage adjustments may be necessary.

Discontinuation – When discontinuing venlafaxine after more than 1 week of therapy, it is generally recommended that the dose be tapered to minimize the risk of discontinuation symptoms. Gradually taper dose over at least a 2-week period in patients who have received venlafaxine.

▶*Venlafaxine ER:*

Depression – Administer venlafaxine ER in a single dose with food either in the morning or in the evening at approximately the same time each day. Swallow each capsule whole with fluid and not divided, crushed, chewed, or placed in water, or it may be administered by carefully opening the capsule and sprinkling the entire contents on a spoonful of applesauce. Swallow this drug/food mixture immediately without chewing, and follow with a glass of water to ensure complete swallowing of the pellets.

Initial treatment: The recommended starting dosage for venlafaxine ER is 75 mg/day administered in a single dose. For some patients, it may be desirable to start at 37.5 mg/day for 4 to 7 days to allow them to adjust to the medication before increasing to 75 mg/day. Patients not responding to the initial 75 mg/day dosage may benefit from dose increases to a maximum of approximately 225 mg/day. Increase dose in increments of up to 75 mg/day as needed, and make at intervals of at least 4 days. In clinical trials establishing efficacy, upward titration was permitted at intervals of at least 2 weeks; the average dosages were approximately 140 to 180 mg/day.

It is not known if higher doses of venlafaxine ER are needed for more severely depressed patients; however, the experience with venlafaxine ER dosages more than 225 mg/day is very limited.

GAD/SAD – The recommended starting dose is 75 mg/day, administered in a single dose. For some patients, it may be desirable to start at 37.5 mg/day for 4 to 7 days to allow them to adjust to the medication before increasing to 75 mg/day. Although a dose-response relationship

VENLAFAXINE HCl

for effectiveness was not clearly established in fixed-dose studies, certain patients not responding to the initial 75 mg/day dose may benefit from dose increases to a maximum of approximately 225 mg/day. Increase dose in increments of up to 75 mg/day, as needed, and make at intervals of not less than 4 days.

Maintenance – It is not known how long a patient with depression, GAD, or SAD should continue to be treated with venlafaxine ER. It is generally agreed that acute episodes of major depression require several months or more of sustained pharmacologic therapy. In patients with SAD, there are no efficacy data beyond 12 weeks of treatment with venlafaxine ER. Periodically reassess the need for continuing medication in patients with GAD or SAD who improve with venlafaxine ER treatment.

Discontinuation of treatment – When discontinuing treatment after at least 1 week of therapy, it is generally recommended that the dose be tapered to minimize the risk of discontinuation symptoms. In clinical trials, tapering was achieved by reducing the daily dose by 75 mg at 1-week intervals. Individualization of tapering may be necessary.

➤*Hepatic function impairment:* Given the decrease in clearance and increase in elimination half-life for both venlafaxine and its active metabolite, O-desmethylvenlafaxine (ODV), observed in patients with hepatic cirrhosis, it is recommended that the total daily dose be reduced 50% in patients with moderate hepatic impairment. Because there was much individual variability in clearance between patients with cirrhosis, it may be necessary to reduce the dose even more than 50%, and individualization of dosing may be desirable in some patients.

➤*Renal function impairment:* Given the decrease in clearance for venlafaxine and the increase in elimination half-life for both venlafaxine and ODV observed in patients with renal impairment (GFR, 10 to 70 mL/min), it is recommended that the total daily dose be reduced 25% to 50% in patients with mild to moderate renal impairment. It is recommended that the total daily dose be reduced 50% and the dose be withheld until the dialysis treatment is completed (4 hours) in patients undergoing hemodialysis. Because there was much individual variability in clearance between patients with renal impairment, individualization of dosing may be desirable in some patients.

➤*Elderly:* No dose adjustment is recommended for elderly patients on the basis of age. However, as with any drug for the treatment of depression or GAD, exercise caution in treating the elderly. When individualizing the dosage, take extra care when increasing the dose.

➤*Switching patients to or from a monoamine oxidase (MAO) inhibitor:* Let at least 14 days elapse between discontinuation of an MAO inhibitor and initiation of therapy with venlafaxine. In addition, allow at least 7 days after stopping venlafaxine before starting an MAO inhibitor.

➤*Storage / Stability:* Store at controlled room temperature, 20° to 25°C (68° to 77°F) in a dry place. Protect from light.

Actions

➤*Pharmacology:* Venlafaxine is chemically unrelated to tricyclic, tetracyclic, or other available antidepressant agents. The mechanism of action is believed to be associated with its potentiation of neurotransmitter activity in the CNS. Venlafaxine and ODV are potent inhibitors of neuronal serotonin and norepinephrine reuptake and weak inhibitors of dopamine reuptake. Venlafaxine and ODV have no significant affinity for muscarinic, histaminergic, or alpha-1 adrenergic receptors in vitro, and they do not possess MAO inhibitory activity.

➤*Pharmacokinetics:* Venlafaxine is well absorbed (at least 92%) and extensively metabolized in the liver. ODV is the only major active metabolite. The absolute bioavailability of venlafaxine is approximately 45%. Approximately 87% of a dose is recovered in the urine within 48 hours as unchanged venlafaxine (5%), unconjugated ODV (29%), conjugated ODV (26%), or other minor inactive metabolites (27%). Renal elimination of venlafaxine and its metabolites is the primary route of excretion. Relative bioavailability from a tablet was 100% when compared with oral solution. Food has no significant effect on the absorption of venlafaxine.

Administration of venlafaxine ER 150 mg every 24 hours generally resulted in lower C_{max} (150 ng/mL for venlafaxine and 260 ng/mL for ODV) and later T_{max} (5.5 hours for venlafaxine and 9 hours for ODV) than for immediate-release venlafaxine tablets (C_{max} for immediate-release venlafaxine 75 mg every 12 hours was 225 ng/mL for venlafaxine and 290 ng/mL for ODV; T_{max} was 2 hours for venlafaxine and 3 hours for ODV). When equal daily doses of venlafaxine were administered as an immediate-release tablet or the ER capsule, the exposure to both venlafaxine and ODV was similar for the 2 treatments, and the fluctuation in plasma concentrations was slightly lower with the ER capsule. Venlafaxine ER, therefore, provides a slower rate of absorption but the same extent of absorption compared with the immediate-release tablet.

The degree of binding of venlafaxine to plasma is approximately 27% at concentrations ranging from 2.5 to 2215 ng/mL. The degree of ODV binding to plasma is approximately 30% at concentrations ranging from 100 to 500 ng/mL. Protein-binding-induced drug interactions with venlafaxine are not expected.

Steady-state concentrations of venlafaxine and ODV in plasma were attained within 3 days of multiple-dose therapy. Plasma clearance, elimination half-life, and steady-state volume of distribution were unaltered after multiple dosing. Mean steady-state plasma clearance of venlafaxine and ODV is approximately 1.3 and 0.4 L/hr/kg, respectively; elimination half-life is approximately 5 and approximately 11 hours, respectively; and steady-state volume of distribution is approximately 7.5 and 5.7 L/kg, respectively. When equal daily doses of venlafaxine were administered as 2 or 3 times/day regimens, the drug exposure (AUC) and fluctuation in plasma levels of venlafaxine and ODV were comparable following both regimens.

Hepatic disease – In 9 patients with hepatic cirrhosis, the pharmacokinetic disposition of both venlafaxine and ODV was significantly altered after oral administration. Venlafaxine and ODV elimination half-life was prolonged approximately 30% and 60%, respectively, and clearance decreased approximately 50% and 30%, respectively, in cirrhotic patients compared with healthy subjects. A large degree of intersubject variability was noted. Three patients with more severe cirrhosis had a more substantial decrease in venlafaxine clearance (approximately 90%) compared with healthy subjects. Dosage adjustment is necessary in these patients (see Administration and Dosage).

Renal disease – Venlafaxine elimination half-life after oral administration was prolonged by approximately 50%, and clearance was reduced approximately 24% in renally impaired patients (GFR, 10 to 70 mL/min) compared with healthy subjects. In dialysis patients, venlafaxine elimination half-life was prolonged approximately 180% and clearance was reduced approximately 57% compared with healthy subjects. Similarly, ODV elimination half-life was prolonged approximately 40% although clearance was unchanged in patients with renal impairment (GFR, 10 to 70 mL/min). In dialysis patients, ODV elimination half-life was prolonged approximately 142% and clearance was reduced approximately 56% compared with healthy subjects. A large degree of intersubject variability was noted. Dosage adjustment is necessary in these patients (see Administration and Dosage).

Contraindications

Hypersensitivity to venlafaxine or any ingredients of the product; concomitant use in patients taking MAO inhibitors.

Warnings

➤*Mutagenesis:* There was a clastogenic response in the in vivo chromosomal aberration assay in rat bone marrow in male rats receiving 200 times on a mg/kg basis, or 50 times on a mg/m² basis, the maximum human daily dose.

➤*MAO inhibitors:* Adverse reactions, some of which were serious, have been reported in patients who have recently been discontinued from an MAO inhibitor and started on venlafaxine, or who have recently had venlafaxine therapy discontinued prior to initiation of an MAO inhibitor. In patients receiving antidepressants with pharmacologic properties similar to venlafaxine in combination with an MAO inhibitor, there have been reports of serious, sometimes fatal, reactions. For a selective serotonin reuptake inhibitor, these reactions have included hyperthermia, rigidity, myoclonus, autonomic instability with possible rapid fluctuations of vital signs, and mental status changes that include extreme agitation progressing to delirium and coma. Some cases presented with features resembling neuroleptic malignant syndrome.

Severe hyperthermia and seizures, sometimes fatal, have been reported in association with the combined use of tricyclic antidepressants and MAO inhibitors. These reactions have also been reported in patients who have recently discontinued these drugs and have been started on an MAO inhibitor. The effects of combined use of venlafaxine and MAO inhibitors have not been evaluated. Therefore, because venlafaxine is an inhibitor of both norepinephrine and serotonin reuptake, it is recommended that venlafaxine not be used in combination with an MAO inhibitor or within 14 days of discontinuing treatment with an MAO inhibitor. Based on the half-life of venlafaxine, allow at least 7 days after stopping venlafaxine before starting an MAO inhibitor.

➤*Sustained hypertension:* Venlafaxine treatment is associated with sustained increases in blood pressure. In a study comparing 3 fixed doses of venlafaxine immediate-release (75, 225, and 375 mg/day) and placebo, a mean increase in supine diastolic blood pressure (SDBP) of 7.2 mm Hg was seen in the 375 mg/day group at week 6 compared with almost no changes in the 75 and 225 mg/day groups and a mean decrease in SDBP of 2.2 mm Hg in the placebo group. There is a dose-dependent increase in the incidence of sustained hypertension for venlafaxine.

Probability of Sustained Elevation in SDBP with Venlafaxine Immediate-Release (%)	
Venlafaxine	Incidence of sustained elevation in SDBP
< 100 mg/day	3
101 to 200 mg/day	5
201 to 300 mg/day	7
> 300 mg/day	13
Placebo	2

VENLAFAXINE HCl

An analysis of patients with sustained hypertension and the 19 venlafaxine immediate-release patients who were discontinued from treatment because of hypertension (less than 1% of total venlafaxine patients) revealed that most of the blood pressure increases were in a modest range (10 to 15 mm Hg, SDBP). Patients treated with venlafaxine ER also experienced increases in SDBP. In various studies in patients treated with 37.5 to 225 mg/day, there were mean increases in SDBP ranging from 0.3 to 1.6 mm Hg. In other premarketing studies, 0.4% to 1.3% of patients discontinued treatment because of elevated blood pressure. Most of the blood pressure increases ranged 12 to 28 mm Hg in SDBP. Nevertheless, sustained increases of this magnitude could have adverse consequences. Therefore, it is recommended that patients receiving venlafaxine have regular monitoring of blood pressure. For patients who experience a sustained increase in blood pressure, consider dose reduction or discontinuation.

➤*Renal/Hepatic function impairment:* Use with caution. In patients with renal impairment (GFR, 10 to 70 mL/min) or cirrhosis of the liver, the clearances of venlafaxine and its active metabolite were decreased thus prolonging the elimination half-lives. A lower dose may be necessary (see Administration and Dosage).

➤*Pregnancy: Category C.* In rats, there was a decrease in pup weight, an increase in stillborn pups, and an increase in pup deaths during the first 5 days of lactation when dosing began during pregnancy and continued until weaning. These effects occurred at 2.5 times (mg/m^2) the maximum human daily dose. There are no adequate and well-controlled studies in pregnant women. Use during pregnancy only if clearly needed.

➤*Lactation:* Venlafaxine and ODV are excreted in breast milk. Because of the potential for serious adverse reactions in nursing infants, decide whether to discontinue breastfeeding or discontinue the drug, taking into account the importance of the drug to the mother.

➤*Children:* Safety and efficacy in patients younger than 18 years of age for immediate-release venlafaxine have not been established.

Safety and efficacy in pediatric patients for venlafaxine ER have not been established.

Precautions

➤*Discontinuation:* Abrupt discontinuation or dose reduction of venlafaxine at various doses has been found to be associated with the appearance of new symptoms, the frequency of which increased with increased dose level and with longer duration of treatment. Reported symptoms include agitation, anorexia, anxiety, confusion, coordination impairment, diarrhea, dizziness, dry mouth, dysphoric mood, fasciculation, fatigue, headache, hypomania, insomnia, nausea, nervousness, nightmares, seizure, sensory disturbance (including shock-like electrical sensations), somnolence, sweating, tremor, vertigo, and vomiting. Therefore, it is recommended that the dosage of venlafaxine ER be tapered gradually and the patient monitored. The period required for tapering may depend on the dose, duration of therapy, and the individual patient. Discontinuation effects are well known to occur with antidepressants.

➤*Anxiety and insomnia:* Anxiety, nervousness, and insomnia were more commonly reported for venlafaxine-treated patients (6%, 13%, and 18%, respectively) vs placebo (3%, 6%, and 10%, respectively), and led to drug discontinuation in 2%, 2%, and 3%, respectively.

In depression trials with the ER form, insomnia was present in 17% of patients vs 11% on placebo, and nervousness in 10% of patients vs 5% placebo. Insomnia and nervousness led to drug discontinuation in 0.9% of patients treated with venlafaxine ER. In GAD trials with the ER form, insomnia was present in 15% of patients vs 10% on placebo, and nervousness in 6% of patients vs 4% on placebo. Insomnia and nervousness led to drug discontinuation in 3% and 2%, respectively, of the patients treated with venlafaxine ER for up to 8 weeks, and 2% and 0.7%, respectively, of the patients treated with venlafaxine ER up to 6 months. In SAD trials with the ER form, insomnia was present in 23% of patients vs 7% on placebo, and nervousness in 11% of patients vs 3% on placebo. Insomnia and nervousness led to drug discontinuation in 3% and 0%, respectively, of the patients treated with venlafaxine ER up to 12 weeks.

➤*Appetite/Weight changes:* Anorexia was more commonly reported for venlafaxine-treated patients (11%) than in placebo-treated patients (2%) during short-term studies. A dose-dependent weight loss was often noted in patients treated for several weeks. Significant weight loss, especially in underweight depressed patients, may be an undesirable result of treatment. A loss of at least 5% of body weight occurred in 6% of patients treated with venlafaxine compared with 1% with placebo and 3% with another antidepressant. However, discontinuation for weight loss associated with venlafaxine was uncommon (0.1%).

With venlafaxine ER, 8% of patients had treatment-emergent anorexia vs 4% on placebo and a loss of at least 5% of body weight occurred in 7% of patients vs 2% with placebo. Discontinuation rates for anorexia and weight loss were 1% and 0.1%, respectively.

In the pool of GAD studies, treatment-emergent anorexia was reported in 8% and 2% of patients receiving venlafaxine ER and placebo for no more than 8 weeks, respectively. A loss of at least 7% of body weight occurred in 3% of the venlafaxine ER-treated and 1% of the placebo-treated patients up to 6 months in these trials. Discontinuation rates for anorexia and weight loss were low for patients receiving venlafaxine ER for up to 8 weeks (0.9% and 0.3%, respectively).

In the pool of SAD studies, treatment-emergent anorexia was reported in 20% and 2% of patients receiving venlafaxine ER and placebo up to 12 weeks, respectively. A loss of 7% or more of body weight occurred in none of the venlafaxine ER-treated or the placebo-treated patients up to 12 weeks in these trials. Discontinuation rates for anorexia and weight loss were low for patients receiving venlafaxine ER up to 12 weeks (0.4% and 0%, respectively).

➤*Mania/Hypomania:* Hypomania or mania occurred in 0.5% of patients treated with venlafaxine and 0.3% of patients on the ER form. Activation of mania/hypomania has also been reported in a small proportion of patients with major affective disorder who were treated with other marketed antidepressants. As with all antidepressants, use venlafaxine cautiously in patients with a history of mania.

➤*Hyponatremia:* Hyponatremia and/or the syndrome of inappropriate antidiuretic hormone secretion (SIADH) may occur with venlafaxine. Take into consideration in patients who are, for example, volume-depleted, elderly, or taking diuretics.

➤*Mydriasis:* Mydriasis has been reported in association with venlafaxine; therefore, monitor patients with raised intraocular pressure or those at risk of acute narrow angle glaucoma.

➤*Seizures:* Seizures were reported in 0.26% of venlafaxine-treated patients; none were reported with venlafaxine ER. Most seizures occurred in patients receiving doses of no more than 150 mg/day. Use venlafaxine cautiously in patients with a history of seizures. Discontinue use in any patient who develops seizures.

➤*Abnormal bleeding:* There have been reports of abnormal bleeding (most commonly ecchymosis) associated with venlafaxine treatment. While a causal relationship to venlafaxine is unclear, impaired platelet aggregation may result from platelet serotonin depletion and contribute to such occurrences.

➤*Suicide:* The possibility of a suicide attempt is inherent in depression and may persist until significant remission occurs. Accompany initial therapy with close supervision of high-risk patients. Write prescriptions for the smallest quantity of tablets consistent with good patient management in order to reduce the risk of overdose.

Observe the same precautions observed when treating patients with depression when treating patients with GAD or SAD.

➤*Concomitant illness:* Caution is advised in administering venlafaxine to patients with diseases or conditions that could affect hemodynamic responses or metabolism. Exercise caution in patients whose underlying medical conditions might be compromised by increases in heart rate (eg, patients with hyperthyroidism, heart failure, or recent MI), particularly when using doses of venlafaxine more than 200 mg/day.

➤*Cardiac patients:* Venlafaxine has not been evaluated in patients with a recent history of MI or unstable heart disease. However, evaluation of the ECGs for patients who received venlafaxine immediate-release in 4- to 6-week double-blind, placebo-controlled trials showed that the incidence of trial-emergent conduction abnormalities did not differ from that with placebo. The mean heart rate in venlafaxine-treated patients was increased relative to baseline by approximately 4 beats/minute.

Evaluation of the ECGs for patients who received venlafaxine ER in 8 to 12 week trials revealed a mean increase from baseline for the QTc interval. The mean change from baseline ranges from 2.8 to 4.7 msec. In these same trials, the mean change from baseline in heart rate for the venlafaxine ER treated patients ranged from 3 to 5 beats per minute.

➤*Drug abuse and dependence:* There was no indication of drug-seeking behavior in the clinical trials. However, it is not possible to predict on the basis of premarketing experience the extent to which a CNS-active drug will be misused, diverted, and/or abused once marketed. Consequently, carefully evaluate patients for history of drug abuse and follow such patients closely, observing them for signs of misuse or abuse of venlafaxine (eg, development of tolerance, incrementation of dose, drug-seeking behavior).

➤*Hazardous tasks:* Caution patients about operating hazardous machinery, including automobiles, until they are reasonably certain that venlafaxine therapy does not adversely affect their ability to engage in such activities.

Drug Interactions

➤*Drugs metabolized by CYP450 isoenzymes:* Venlafaxine is metabolized to its active metabolite, ODV, by cytochrome CYP2D6. Therefore, the potential exists for a drug interaction with drugs that inhibit this CYP2D6-mediated metabolism and venlafaxine. Drugs that reduce the metabolism of venlafaxine to ODV could potentially increase the plasma concentrations of venlafaxine and lower the concentrations of the active metabolite.

In a clinical study involving CYP2D6-poor and -extensive metabolizers, the total concentration of active compounds (venlafaxine plus ODV),

VENLAFAXINE HCl

was similar in the 2 metabolizer groups. Therefore, no dosage adjustment is required when venlafaxine is coadministered with a CYP2D6 inhibitor.

The concomitant use of venlafaxine with a drug treatment that potently inhibits both CYP2D6 and CYP3A4, the primary metabolizing enzymes for venlafaxine, has not been studied. Therefore, use caution if a patient's therapy include venlafaxine and any agents that produce potent simultaneous inhibition of these 2 enzyme systems.

In vitro studies indicate that venlafaxine is a relatively weak inhibitor of CYP2D6. These findings have been confirmed in a clinical drug interaction study comparing the effect of venlafaxine to that of fluoxetine on the CYP2D6-mediated metabolism of dextromethorphan to dextrorphan.

Venlafaxine Drug Interactions

Precipitant drug	Object drug*		Description
Cimetidine	Venlafaxine	↑	Concomitant use resulted in inhibition of first-pass metabolism of venlafaxine in 18 healthy subjects. Oral clearance was reduced by ≈ 43%, and AUC and C_{max} were increased by ≈ 60%. However, cimetidine had no apparent effect on ODV. Consequently, the overall pharmacologic activity is expected to increase only slightly.
MAO inhibitors	Venlafaxine	↑	Serious, sometimes fatal reactions may occur, including hyperthermia, rigidity, myoclonus, autonomic instability with possible rapid fluctuation of vital signs, and mental status changes that include extreme agitation progressing to delirium and coma (see Warnings). Concomitant use is contraindicated.
Venlafaxine	Clozapine	↑	There have been reports of elevated clozapine levels resulting in adverse events including seizures following the addition of venlafaxine.
Venlafaxine	Desipramine	↑	Desipramine AUC, C_{max}, and C_{min} increased ≈ 35% in the presence of venlafaxine. The 2-OH-desipramine AUC increased at least 2.5- to 4.5-fold. The clinical significance of elevated 2-OH-desipramine levels is unknown.
Venlafaxine	Haloperidol	↑	Venlafaxine decreased total oral-dose clearance of a single dose of haloperidol 42%, which resulted in a 70% increase in haloperidol AUC. In addition, the haloperidol C_{max} increased 88%.
Venlafaxine	Indinavir	↓	Venlafaxine resulted in a 28% decrease in the AUC of a single oral dose of indinavir and a 36% decrease in indinavir C_{max}. The clinical significance of this is unknown.
Venlafaxine	Sibutramine Sumatriptan Trazodone	↑	A "serotonin syndrome" including irritability, increased muscle tone, shivering, myoclonus, and altered consciousness may occur.
Venlafaxine	St. John's wort	↑	A "serotonin syndrome," including irritability, increased muscle tone, shivering, myoclonus, and altered consciousness may occur.
Venlafaxine	Warfarin	↑	There have been reports on increases in PT, PTT, or INR when venlafaxine was administered to patients also receiving warfarin.

* ↑ = Object drug increased. ↓ = Object drug decreased.

Adverse Reactions

Common Adverse Events Leading to Discontinuation of Treatment (%)[a,b]

Adverse Reaction	Depression				GAD		SAD	
	IR[c]	Placebo	ER[d]	Placebo	ER[d]	Placebo	ER[d]	Placebo
Cardiovascular								
Hypertension	—	—	1	< 1	—	—	—	—
Vasodilation	—	—	—	—	1	0	—	—
CNS								
Abnormal thinking	—	—	—	—	1	0	—	—
Anxiety	2	1	—	—	—	—	1	< 1
Asthenia	2	< 1	—	—	3	< 1	1	< 1
Dizziness	3	< 1	2	1	4	1	2	0
Headache	3	1	—	—	4	< 1	2	< 1

Common Adverse Events Leading to Discontinuation of Treatment (%)[a,b]

Adverse Reaction	Depression				GAD		SAD	
	IR[c]	Placebo	ER[d]	Placebo	ER[d]	Placebo	ER[d]	Placebo
Insomnia	3	1	1	< 1	3	< 1	3	< 1
Nervousness	2	< 1	—	—	2	< 1	—	—
Paresthesia	—	—	1	0	—	—	—	—
Somnolence	3	1	2	< 1	3	< 1	2	< 1
Tremor	—	—	1	0	1	0	—	—
GI								
Anorexia	—	—	1	< 1	2	< 1	—	—
Diarrhea	—	—	1	0	—	—	—	—
Dry mouth	2	< 1	1	0	2	< 1	—	—
Nausea	6	1	4	< 1	8	< 1	4	0
Vomiting	—	—	—	—	1	< 1	—	—
GU								
Abnormal ejaculation	3	< 1	1	0	—	—	—	—
Decreased libido	—	—	—	—	1	0	—	—
Impotence	—	—	—	—	—	—	3	0
Miscellaneous								
Abnormal vision	—	—	1	0	1	0	—	—
Sweating	2	< 1	—	—	2	< 1	1	0

[a] Two of the major depressive disorder studies with venlafaxine ER were flexible dose, and 1 was fixed dose. Four of the GAD studies with venlafaxine ER were fixed dose, and 1 was flexible dose. Both of the SAD studies with venlafaxine ER were flexible dose.
[b] Data pooled from separate studies and are not necessarily comparable.
[c] IR = Venlafaxine immediate-release.
[d] ER = Venlafaxine extended-release.

Venlafaxine and Venlafaxine ER Adverse Reactions (%)[a]

Adverse reaction	Venlafaxine[b] (n = 1033)	Placebo (n = 609)	Venlafaxine ER[c] (n = 357)	Placebo (n = 285)
Cardiovascular				
Increased blood pressure/ hypertension	2	< 1	4	1
Postural hypotension	1	< 1	—	—
Tachycardia	2	< 1	—	—
Vasodilation	4	3	4[d]	2[d]
CNS				
Abnormal dreams	4	3	7[e]	2[e]
Abnormal thinking	2	1	—	—
Agitation	2	< 1	3	1
Anxiety	6	3	—	—
Asthenia	12	6	8	7
Confusion	2	1	—	—
Decreased libido	2	< 1	3	< 1
Depersonalization	1	< 1	—	—
Depression	1	< 1	3	< 1
Dizziness	19	7	20	9
Headache	25	24	—	—
Hypertonia	3	2	—	—
Insomnia	18	10	17	11
Nervousness	13	6	10	5
Paresthesia	3	2	3	1
Somnolence	23	9	17	8
Tremor	5	1	5	2
Twitching	1	< 1	—	—
Dermatologic				
Pruritus	1	< 1	—	—
Rash	3	2	—	—
GI				
Anorexia	11	2	8	4
Constipation	15	7	8	5
Diarrhea	8	7	—	—
Dry mouth	22	11	12	6
Dyspepsia	5	4	—	—
Flatulence	3	2	4	3
Nausea	37	11	31	12
Vomiting	6	2	4	2
GU				
Abnormal ejaculation/orgasm	12[f]	< 1[f]	16[f,g]	< 1[f,g]
Anorgasmia (female)	—	—	3[h,i]	< 1[h,i]
Impotence	6[f]	< 1[f]	4[f]	< 1[f]
Impaired urination	2	< 1	—	—
Orgasm disturbance	2[g]	< 1[g]	—	—
Urinary frequency	3	2	—	—
Urinary retention	1	< 1	—	—

VENLAFAXINE HCl

Venlafaxine and Venlafaxine ER Adverse Reactions (%)[a]

Adverse reaction	Venlafaxine[b] (n = 1033)	Placebo (n = 609)	Venlafaxine ER[c] (n = 357)	Placebo (n = 285)
Special senses				
Blurred/Abnormal vision	6	2	4[j]	< 1[j]
Mydriasis	2	< 1	—	—
Taste perversion	2	< 1	—	—
Tinnitus	2	< 1	—	—
Miscellaneous				
Chest pain	2	1	—	—
Chills	3	< 1	—	—
Infection	6	5	—	—
Pharyngitis	—	—	7	6
Sweating	12	3	14	3
Trauma	2	1	—	—
Weight loss	1	< 1	3	0
Yawn	3	< 1	3	0

[a] Data pooled from separate studies and are not necessarily comparable.
[b] Events reported by at least 1% of patients treated with venlafaxine immediate-release are included, and are rounded to the nearest %. Events for which the venlafaxine incidence was equal to or less than placebo are not listed in the table, but included the following: Abdominal pain, pain, back pain, flu syndrome, fever, palpitation, increased appetite, myalgia, arthralgia, amnesia, hypesthesia, rhinitis, pharyngitis, sinusitis, cough increased, dysmenorrhea.
[c] Incidence, rounded to the nearest %, for events reported by at least 2% of patients treated with venlafaxine ER, except the following events which had an incidence equal to or less than placebo: Abdominal pain, accidental injury, anxiety, back pain, bronchitis, diarrhea, dysmenorrhea, dyspepsia, flu syndrome, headache, infection, pain, palpitation, rhinitis, and sinusitis.
[d] Mostly "hot flashes."
[e] Mostly "vivid dreams," "nightmares," and "increased dreaming."
[f] Incidence based on number of male patients.
[g] Mostly "delayed ejaculation."
[h] Incidence based on number of female patients.
[i] Mostly "delayed orgasm" or "anorgasmia."
[j] Mostly "blurred vision" and "difficulty focusing eyes."

Venlafaxine Adverse Reactions (%): Dose Comparison

Adverse reaction	Placebo (n = 92)	Venlafaxine 75 mg/day (n = 89)	Venlafaxine 225 mg/day (n = 89)	Venlafaxine 375 mg/day (n = 88)
Cardiovascular				
Hypertension	1.1	1.1	2.2	4.5
Vasodilation	0	4.5	5.6	2.3
GI				
Abdominal pain	3.3	3.4	2.2	8
Anorexia	2.2	14.6	13.5	17
Dyspepsia	2.2	6.7	6.7	4.5
Nausea	14.1	32.6	38.2	58
Vomiting	1.1	7.9	3.4	6.8
CNS				
Agitation	0	1.1	2.2	4.5
Anxiety	4.3	11.2	4.5	2.3
Asthenia	3.3	16.9	14.6	14.8
Dizziness	4.3	19.1	22.5	23.9
Insomnia	9.8	22.5	20.2	13.6
Libido decreased	1.1	2.2	1.1	5.7
Nervousness	4.3	21.3	13.5	12.5
Somnolence	4.3	16.9	18	26.1
Tremor	0	1.1	2.2	10.2
GU				
Abnormal ejaculation/orgasm	0	4.5	2.2	12.5
Impotence	0	5.8	2.1	3.6
(Number of men)	(n = 63)	(n = 52)	(n = 48)	(n = 56)
Miscellaneous				
Abnormality of accommodation	0	9.1	7.9	5.6
Chills	1.1	2.2	5.6	6.8
Infection	2.2	2.2	5.6	2.3
Sweating	5.4	6.7	12.4	19.3
Yawn	0	4.5	5.6	8

Venlafaxine ER Adverse Reactions (%)

Adverse reaction	GAD[a] Venlafaxine ER (n = 1381)	GAD[a] Placebo (n = 555)	SAD[b] Venlafaxine ER (n = 277)	SAD[b] Placebo (n = 274)
Cardiovascular				
Hypertension	—	—	5	4
Palpitation	—	—	3	1
Vasodilatation[c]	4	2	3	1

Venlafaxine ER Adverse Reactions (%)

Adverse reaction	GAD[a] Venlafaxine ER (n = 1381)	GAD[a] Placebo (n = 555)	SAD[b] Venlafaxine ER (n = 277)	SAD[b] Placebo (n = 274)
CNS				
Abnormal dreams[d]	3	2	4	< 1
Agitation	—	—	4	1
Anxiety	—	—	5	3
Asthenia	12	8	17	8
Dizziness	16	11	16	8
Headache	—	—	34	33
Hypertonia	3	2	—	—
Insomnia	15	10	23	7
Libido decreased	4	2	9	< 1
Nervousness	6	4	11	3
Paresthesia	2	1	3	< 1
Somnolence	14	8	16	8
Tremor	4	< 1	4	< 1
Twitching			2	0
GI				
Abdominal pain	—	—	4	3
Anorexia	8	2	20[e]	1[e]
Constipation	10	4	8	4
Diarrhea	—	—	6	5
Dry mouth	16	6	17	4
Nausea	35	12	29	9
Vomiting	5	3	3	2
Weight loss			4	0
GU				
Abnormal ejaculation[f,g,h]	11	< 1	16	1
Eructation	—	—	2	0
Impotence[g,h]	5	< 1	10	1
Orgasmic dysfunction (female)[i,j,k,l]	2	0	8	0
Miscellaneous				
Abnormal vision	5[m]	< 1[m]	6[n]	3[n]
Accidental injury	—	—	5	3
Flu syndrome	—	—	6	5
Sinusitis	—	—	2	1
Sweating	10	3	13	2
Yawn	3	< 1	5	< 1

[a] Adverse events for which the venlafaxine ER reporting rate was less than or equal to the placebo rate are not included. These events are abdominal pain, accidental injury, anxiety, back pain, diarrhea, dysmenorrhea, dyspepsia, flu syndrome, headache, infection, myalgia, pain, palpitation, pharyngitis, rhinitis, tinnitus, and urinary frequency.
[b] Adverse events for which the venlafaxine ER reporting rate was less than or equal to the placebo rate are not included. These events are back pain, depression, dysmenorrhea, dyspepsia, infection, myalgia, pain, pharyngitis, rash, rhinitis, and upper respiratory infection.
[c] Mostly "hot flashes."
[d] Mostly "vivid dreams," "nightmares," and "increased dreaming."
[e] Mostly "decreased appetite" and "loss of appetite."
[f] Includes "delayed ejaculation" and "anorgasmia" in both GAD and SAD patients.
[g] Percentage based on the number of males with GAD (venlafaxine ER = 525, placebo = 220).
[h] Percentage based on the number of males with SAD (venlafaxine ER = 158, placebo = 153).
[i] Includes "delayed orgasm," "abnormal orgasm," and "anorgasmia" in GAD patients.
[j] Percentage based on the number of females with GAD (venlafaxine ER = 856, placebo = 335).
[k] Includes "abnormal orgasm" and "anorgasmia" in SAD patients.
[l] Percentage based on the number of females with SAD (venlafaxine ER = 119, placebo = 121).
[m] Mostly "blurred vision" and "difficulty focusing eyes."
[n] Mostly "blurred vision."

➤*Other ARs observed during premarketing evaluation of immediate- and extended-release venlafaxine:*

Cardiovascular – Angina pectoris, arrhythmia, extrasystoles, hypotension, peripheral vascular disorder (mainly cold feet and/or cold hands), syncope, thrombophlebitis (0.1% to 1%); aortic aneurysm, arteritis, first-degree AV block, bigeminy, bradycardia, bundle branch block, capillary fragility, cerebral ischemia, coronary artery disease, CHF, heart arrest, mitral valve disorder, circulatory disturbance, mucocutaneous hemorrhage, MI, pallor (less than 0.1%).

ER: Postural hypotension tachycardia (at least 1%).

CNS – Migraine, trismus, vertigo (at least 1%); apathy, ataxia, circumoral paresthesia, CNS stimulation, euphoria, hallucinations, hostility, hyperesthesia, hyperkinesia, hypotonia, incoordination, libido increased, manic reaction, myoclonus, neuralgia, neuropathy, psychosis, seizure, abnormal speech, stupor (0.1% to 1%); akinesia, alcohol

VENLAFAXINE HCl

abuse, aphasia, bradykinesia, buccoglossal syndrome, cerebrovascular accident, loss of consciousness, delusions, dementia, dystonia, facial paralysis, abnormal gait, Guillain-Barré syndrome, hypokinesia, neuritis, nystagmus, paresis, psychotic depression, reflexes decreased, reflexes increased, suicidal ideation, torticollis (less than 0.1%).

Immediate-release: Emotional lability (at least 1%); paranoid reaction (0.1% to 1%); akathisia (less than 0.1%).

ER: Amnesia, confusion, depersonalization, hypesthesia, abnormal thinking (at least 1%); emotional lability, akathisia (0.1% to 1%); feeling drunk, hyperchlorhydria, impulse control difficulties, paranoid reaction (less than 0.1%).

Dermatologic – Acne, alopecia, brittle nails, contact dermatitis, dry skin, eczema, skin hypertrophy, maculopapular rash, psoriasis, urticaria (0.1% to 1%); erythema nodosum, exfoliative dermatitis, lichenoid dermatitis, hair discoloration, skin discoloration, furunculosis, hirsutism, leukoderma, pustular rash, vesiculobullous rash, seborrhea, skin atrophy, skin striae (less than 0.1%).

ER: Pruritus (at least 1%); petechial rash (less than 0.1%).

Endocrine – Goiter, hyperthyroidism, hypothyroidism, thyroid nodule, thyroiditis (less than 0.1%).

GI – Bruxism, colitis, dysphagia, tongue edema, esophagitis, gastritis, gastroenteritis, GI ulcer, gingivitis, glossitis, rectal hemorrhage, hemorrhoids, melena, stomatitis, mouth ulceration (0.1% to 1%); cheilitis, cholecystitis, cholelithiasis, hematemesis, GI hemorrhage, gum hemorrhage, hepatitis, ileitis, jaundice, intestinal obstruction, proctitis, increased salivation, soft stools, tongue discoloration (less than 0.1%).

Immediate-release: Eructation (at least 1%); oral moniliasis (less than 0.1%).

ER: Increased appetite (at least 1%); oral moniliasis (0.1% to 1%); esophageal spasm, duodenitis, parotitis, periodontitis (less than 0.1%).

GU – Metrorrhagia, prostatitis, vaginitis (at least 1%); albuminuria, amenorrhea, cystitis, dysuria, hematuria, leukorrhea, menorrhagia, nocturia, bladder pain, breast pain, polyuria, pyuria, urinary incontinence, urinary urgency, vaginal hemorrhage (0.1% to 1%); abortion, anuria, breast discharge, breast engorgement, breast enlargement, endometriosis, fibrocystic breast, calcium crystalluria, cervicitis, ovarian cyst, prolonged erection, gynecomastia (male), hypomenorrhea, kidney calculus, kidney pain, abnormal kidney function, mastitis, menopause, pyelonephritis, oliguria, salpingitis, urolithiasis, uterine hemorrhage, uterine spasm (less than 0.1%).

Immediate-release: Female lactation (0.1% to 1%).

ER: Enlarged prostate, impaired urination (at least 1%); urinary retention (0.1% to 1%); balanitis, female lactation, orchitis, vaginal dryness (less than 0.1%).

Hematologic/Lymphatic – Ecchymosis (at least 1%); anemia, leukocytosis, leukopenia, lymphadenopathy, thrombocythemia, thrombocytopenia (0.1% to 1%); basophilia, increased bleeding time, cyanosis, eosinophilia, lymphocytosis, multiple myeloma, purpura (less than 0.1%).

Lab test abnormalities –

Immediate-release: Patients treated with immediate-release venlafaxine for at least 3 months in placebo-controlled 12-month extension trials had a mean final on-therapy increase in total cholesterol of 9.1 mg/dL. This increase was duration dependent over the 12-month study period and tended to be greater with higher doses. An increase in serum cholesterol from baseline by at least 50 mg/dL and to values at least 261 mg/dL at any time after baseline has been recorded in 5.3% of patients.

ER: Venlafaxine ER capsules treatment for up to 12 weeks in premarketing placebo-controlled trials for major depressive disorder was associated with a mean final on-therapy increase in serum cholesterol concentration of approximately 1.5 mg/dL. Venlafaxine ER treatment for up to 8 weeks and up to 6 months in premarketing placebo-controlled GAD trials was associated with mean final on-therapy increases in serum cholesterol concentration of approximately 1 and 2.3 mg/dL, respectively. Venlafaxine ER treatment for up to 12 weeks in premarketing placebo-controlled SAD trials was associated with mean final on-therapy increases in serum cholesterol concentration of approximately 11.4 mg/dL.

Metabolic/Nutritional – Edema, weight gain (at least 1%); alkaline phosphatase increased, hypercholesterolemia, hyperglycemia, AST increased (0.1% to 1%); alcohol intolerance, bilirubinemia, BUN increased, creatinine increased, diabetes mellitus, gout, abnormal healing, hemochromatosis, hypercalciuria, hyperkalemia, hyperphosphatemia, hyponatremia, hypophosphatemia, hypoproteinemia, uremia (less than 0.1%).

Immediate-release: Glycosuria, hyperuricemia, hypoglycemia, hypokalemia, thirst (0.1% to 1%); dehydration, hyperlipemia, ALT increased (less than 0.1%).

ER: Dehydration, hyperlipemia, hypokalemia, ALT increased, thirst (0.1% to 1%); glycosuria, hyperuricemia, hypocholesteremia, hypoglycemia (less than 0.1%).

Musculoskeletal – Arthritis, arthrosis, bone pain, bone spurs, bursitis, leg cramps, myasthenia, tenosynovitis (0.1% to 1%); pathological fracture, myopathy, osteoporosis, osteosclerosis, rheumatoid arthritis, tendon rupture (less than 0.1%).

ER: Arthralgia (at least 1%); plantar fasciitis (less than 0.1%).

Respiratory – Dyspnea (at least 1%); asthma, chest congestion, epistaxis, hyperventilation, laryngismus, laryngitis, pneumonia, voice alteration (0.1% to 1%); atelectasis, hemoptysis, hypoventilation, hypoxia, larynx edema, pleurisy, pulmonary embolus, sleep apnea (less than 0.1%).

Immediate-release: Bronchitis (at least 1%).

ER: Cough increased (at least 1%).

Special senses – Abnormality of accomodation (at least 1%); cataract, conjunctivitis, corneal lesion, diplopia, dry eyes, eye pain, hyperacusis, otitis media, parosmia, photophobia, taste loss, visual field defect (0.1% to 1%); blepharitis, chromatopsia, conjunctival edema, deafness, glaucoma, retinal hemorrhage, subconjunctival hemorrhage, keratitis, labyrinthitis, miosis, papilledema, decreased pupillary reflex, otitis externa, scleritis, uveitis (less than 0.1%).

Immediate-release: Abnormal vision (at least 1%); exophthalmos (0.1% to 1%).

ER: Mydriasis, taste perversion (at least 1%); exophthalmos (less than 0.1%).

Miscellaneous – Substernal chest pain, neck pain (at least 1%); face edema, intentional injury, malaise, moniliasis, neck rigidity, pelvic pain, photosensitivity reaction, suicide attempt (0.1% to 1%); appendicitis, bacteremia, carcinoma, cellulitis, withdrawal syndrome (less than 0.1%).

Immediate-release: Withdrawal syndrome (less than 0.1%).

ER: Chills, fever (at least 1%).

➤*Adaptation to certain adverse events:* Over a 6-week period, there was evidence of adaptation to some adverse events with continued therapy (eg, dizziness, nausea), but less to other effects (eg, abnormal ejaculation, dry mouth).

➤*Postmarketing:*

Cardiovascular – Deep vein thrombophlebitis; EKG abnormalities such as QT prolongation; cardiac arrhythmias including atrial fibrillation, supraventricular tachycardia, ventricular asystole, ventricular fibrillation (rare), ventricular tachycardia including torsade de pointes (rare).

CNS – Catatonia; delirium; extrapyramidal symptoms including dyskinesia and tardive dyskinesia; neuroleptic malignant syndrome-like events; involuntary movements; serotonin syndrome; shock-like electrical sensations (in some cases, following discontinuation or tapering of the dose); panic.

Dermatologic – Epidermal necrosis/Stevens-Johnson syndrome; erythema multiforme.

Hematologic – Agranulocytosis; aplastic anemia; neutropenia; pancytopenia.

Hepatic -- Hepatic events including GGT elevation, abnormalities of unspecified LFTs, liver damage necrosis, failure, and fatty liver.

Lab test abnormalities – CPK increased; LDH increased.

Miscellaneous – Congenital anomalies; night sweats; pancreatitis; SIADH (usually in the elderly); hemorrhage (including eye and GI bleeding); anaphylaxis; renal failure; rhabdomyolysis; pulmonary eosinophilia; prolactin increased.

Overdosage

➤*Symptoms:* There were 14 premarketing reports of acute overdose with venlafaxine and 2 with venlafaxine ER alone or in combination with other drugs and/or alcohol. The most common symptoms associated with venlafaxine overdose include somnolence, dizziness, nausea, numb hands and feet, and hot-cold spells. All 14 patients recovered without sequelae.

A patient who ingested 2.75 g of venlafaxine was observed to have 2 generalized convulsions and a prolongation of QTc to 500 msec, compared with 405 msec at baseline. Mild sinus tachycardia was reported in 2 of the other patients.

In postmarketing experience, there have been reports of fatalities in patients taking overdoses of venlafaxine, predominantly in combination with alcohol and/or other drugs. ECG changes (eg, prolongation of the QT interval, bundle branch block, QRS prolongation), sinus and ventricular tachycardia, bradycardia, hypotension, altered level of consciousness (ranging from somnolence to coma), seizures, vertigo, and death have been reported.

➤*Treatment:* Treatment should consist of those general supportive and symptomatic measures employed in the management of overdosage with any antidepressant. Ensure an adequate airway, oxygenation, and ventilation. Monitor cardiac rhythm and vital signs. Refer to General Management of Acute Overdosage. Induction of emesis is not recommended. Gastric lavage with a large bore orogastric tube with appropriate airway protection, if needed, may be indicated if performed soon after ingestion or in symptomatic patients. Administer activated charcoal. Because of the large volume of distribution of venlafaxine, forced diuresis, dialysis, hemoperfusion, and exchange transfusion are unlikely to be of benefit. No specific antidotes are known.

In managing overdosage, consider the possibility of multiple drug involvement. Consider contacting a poison control center for additional information on the treatment of any overdose.

VENLAFAXINE HCl

Patient Information

Caution patients about operating hazardous machinery, including automobiles, until they are reasonably certain that venlafaxine therapy does not adversely affect their ability to engage in such activities.

Advise patients to notify their physician if they become pregnant, intend to become pregnant during therapy, or are breastfeeding.

Advise patients to inform their physician or pharmacist if they are taking, or plan to take, any prescription, OTC, or herbal preparations, because there is a potential for interactions.

Advise patients to avoid alcohol while taking venlafaxine.

Advise patients to notify their physician if they develop a rash, hives, or a related allergic phenomenon.

NEFAZODONE HCl

Rx	**Nefazodone HCl** (Various, eg, Eon, Par, Teva)	**Tablets**: 50 mg	In 60s and 100s.
Rx	**Serzone** (Bristol-Myers Squibb)		(BMS 50 mg). Light pink, hexagonal. In 60s.
Rx	**Nefazodone HCl** (Various, eg, Eon, Par, Teva)	**Tablets**: 100 mg	In 60s.
Rx	**Serzone** (Bristol-Myers Squibb)		(BMS 100 mg). White, hexagonal, scored. In 60s.
Rx	**Nefazodone HCl** (Various, eg, Eon, Par, Teva)	**Tablets**: 150 mg	In 60s.
Rx	**Serzone** (Bristol-Myers Squibb)		(BMS 150 mg). Peach, hexagonal, scored. In 60s.
Rx	**Nefazodone HCl** (Various, eg, Eon, Par, Teva)	**Tablets**: 200 mg	In 60s.
Rx	**Serzone** (Bristol-Myers Squibb)		(BMS 200 mg). Light yellow, hexagonal. In 60s.
Rx	**Nefazodone HCl** (Various, eg, Eon, Par, Teva)	**Tablets**: 250 mg	In 60s.
Rx	**Serzone** (Bristol-Myers Squibb)		(BMS 250 mg). White, hexagonal. In 60s.

For additional information, refer to the Antidepressants introduction.

WARNING

Cases of life-threatening hepatic failure have been reported in patients treated with nefazodone. The reported rate in the US is ≈ 1 case of liver failure resulting in death or transplant per 250,000 to 300,000 patient-years of nefazodone treatment. The total patient-years is a summation of each patient's duration of exposure expressed in years. For example, 1 patient-year is equal to 2 patients each treated for 6 months, 3 patients each treated for 4 months, etc (see Warnings).

Ordinarily, do not initiate treatment with nefazodone in individuals with active liver disease or with elevated baseline serum transaminases. There is no evidence that pre-existing liver disease increases the likelihood of developing liver failure, however, baseline abnormalities can complicate patient monitoring.

Advise patients to be alert for signs and symptoms of liver dysfunction (eg, jaundice, anorexia, GI complaints, malaise) and to report them to their doctor immediately if they occur.

Discontinue nefazodone if clinical signs or symptoms suggest liver failure. Patients who develop evidence of hepatocellular injury such as increased serum AST or serum ALT levels ≥ 3 times the upper limit of normal while on nefazodone should be withdrawn from the drug. These patients should be presumed to be at increased risk for liver injury if nefazodone is reintroduced. Accordingly, do not consider such patients for retreatment.

Indications

➤*Depression:* Treatment of depression.

Administration and Dosage

➤*Approved by the FDA:* December 22, 1994 (1S classification).

➤*Initial treatment:* Recommended starting dosage is 200 mg/day, administered in 2 divided doses. In clinical trials, the effective dosage range was generally 300 to 600 mg/day. Consequently, most patients, depending on tolerability and the need for further clinical effect, should have their dose increased. Increase doses in increments of 100 to 200 mg/day, again on a twice-daily schedule, at intervals of ≥ 1 week. Several weeks of treatment may be required to obtain a full antidepressant response.

➤*Elderly/Debilitated patients:* The recommended initial dosage is 100 mg/day on a twice-daily schedule. These patients often have reduced nefazodone clearance or increased sensitivity to the side effects of CNS-active drugs. It also may be appropriate to modify the rate of subsequent dose titration. As steady-state plasma levels do not change with age, the final target dose, based on a careful assessment of the patient's clinical response, may be similar in healthy younger and older patients.

➤*Maintenance/Continuation/Extended treatment:* There is no evidence to indicate how long the depressed patient should be treated with nefazodone. However, it is generally agreed that pharmacologic treatment for acute episodes of depression should continue for ≥ 6 months. Whether the dose of antidepressant needed to induce remission is identical to the dose needed to maintain euthymia is unknown. In clinical trials, > 250 patients were treated for ≥ 1 year.

➤*Switching to or from a monoamine oxidase inhibitor (MAOI):* At least 14 days should elapse between discontinuation of an MAOI and initiation of therapy with nefazodone. In addition, wait ≥ 7 days after stopping nefazodone before starting an MAOI (see Warnings).

➤*Storage/Stability:* Store at room temperature, < 40°C (104°F) and dispense in a tight container.

Actions

➤*Pharmacology:* Nefazodone is an antidepressant with a chemical structure unrelated to selective serotonin reuptake inhibitors, tricyclics, tetracyclics, or MAOIs. The mechanism of action of nefazodone, as with other antidepressants, is unknown. Nefazodone inhibits neuronal uptake of serotonin and norepinephrine.

Nefazodone occupies central 5-HT$_2$ receptors and acts as an antagonist at this receptor. Nefazodone antagonizes alpha$_1$-adrenergic receptors, a property that may be associated with postural hypotension. In vitro, nefazodone had no significant affinity for the following receptors: Alpha$_2$ and beta-adrenergic, 5-HT$_{1A}$, cholinergic, dopaminergic, or benzodiazepine.

➤*Pharmacokinetics:*

Absorption/Distribution – Nefazodone is rapidly and completely absorbed but is subject to extensive metabolism so that its absolute bioavailability is low (≈ 20%) and variable. Food delays absorption of nefazodone and decreases the bioavailability ≈ 20%. Peak plasma concentrations occur at ≈ 1 hour. Half-life is 2 to 4 hours. Nefazodone is widely distributed in body tissues, including the CNS. Volume of distribution ranges from 0.22 to 0.87 L/kg.

Nefazodone and its pharmacologically similar metabolite, hydroxynefazodone, exhibit nonlinear kinetics for dose and time, with AUC and C$_{max}$ increasing more than proportionally with dose increases and more than expected upon multiple dosing over time, compared with single dosing. Data suggest extensive and greater than predicted accumulation of nefazodone and its hydroxy metabolite with multiple dosing. Steady-state plasma nefazodone and metabolite concentrations are attained within 4 to 5 days of initiation of twice-daily dosing or upon dose increase or decrease.

Metabolism/Excretion – Nefazodone is extensively metabolized after oral administration by n-dealkylation and aliphatic and aromatic hydroxylation, and < 1% is excreted unchanged in urine. Three metabolites identified in plasma include hydroxynefazodone (HO-NEF), meta-chlorophenylpiperazine (mCPP), and a triazole-dione metabolite. The AUC (expressed as a multiple of the AUC for nefazodone dosed at 100 mg twice daily) and elimination half-lives (hours), respectively, for these 3 metabolites were as follows: HO-NEF, 0.4 and 1.5 to 4; mCPP, 0.07 and 4 to 8; triazole-dione, 4 and 18.

HO-NEF possesses a pharmacologic profile qualitatively and quantitatively similar to that of nefazodone. mCPP has some similarities to nefazodone but also has agonist activity at some serotonergic receptor subtypes. The pharmacologic profile of the triazole-dione metabolite has not yet been well characterized. In addition to the above compounds, several other metabolites were present in plasma but have not been tested for pharmacologic activity.

The mean half-life of nefazodone ranged between 11 and 24 hours. Approximately 55% was detected in urine and ≈ 20% to 30% in feces. Nefazodone is extensively (> 99%) bound to human plasma proteins in vitro; nefazodone did not alter the in vitro protein binding of chlorpromazine, desipramine, diazepam, diphenylhydantoin, lidocaine, prazosin, propranolol, verapamil, or warfarin. There was a 5% decrease in the protein binding of haloperidol; this is probably of no clinical significance.

Renal function impairment – Renal function impairment (Ccr ranging from 7 to 60 mL/min/1.73 m^2) had no effect on steady-state nefazodone plasma concentrations.

NEFAZODONE HCl

Liver function impairment – In a multiple-dose study of patients with liver cirrhosis, the AUC values for nefazodone and HO-NEF at steady state were ≈ 25% greater than those observed in healthy volunteers.

Age / Gender effects – After single doses of 300 mg, C_{max} and AUC for nefazodone and hydroxynefazodone were up to twice as high in the older patients. However, with multiple doses, differences were much smaller (10% to 20%). A similar result was seen for gender, with a higher C_{max} and AUC in women after single doses but no difference after multiple doses. Initiate treatment with nefazodone at half the usual dose in elderly patients, especially women (see Administration and Dosage); the therapeutic dose range is similar in younger and older patients.

Contraindications

Coadministration with cisapride, pimozide, or carbamazepine (see Warnings and Drug Interactions); patients who were withdrawn from nefazodone because of evidence of liver injury (see Warning box, Warnings); hypersensitivity to nefazodone or other phenylpiperazine antidepressants.

The coadministration of triazolam and nefazodone causes a significant increase in the plasma level of triazolam; a 75% reduction in the initial triazolam dosage is recommended if the 2 drugs are to be given together. Because not all commercially available dosage forms of triazolam permit a sufficient dosage reduction, avoid the coadministration of triazolam and nefazodone for most patients, including the elderly.

Warnings

➤*Hepatotoxicity:* See Warning box. Cases of life-threatening hepatic failure have been reported in patients treated with nefazodone.

The reported rate in the US is ≈ 1 case of liver failure resulting in death or transplant per 250,000 to 300,000 patient-years of use. This represents a rate of ≈ 3 to 4 times the estimated background rate of liver failure. This rate is an underestimate because of under reporting, and the true risk could be considerably greater than this. A large cohort study of antidepressant users found no cases of liver failure leading to death or transplant among nefazodone users in about 30,000 patient-years of exposure. The spontaneous report data and the cohort study results provide estimates of the upper and lower limits of the risk of liver failure in nefazodone-treated patients, but are not capable of providing a precise risk estimate.

The time to liver injury for the reported liver failure cases resulting in death or transplant generally ranged from 2 weeks to 6 months on nefazodone therapy. Although some reports described dark urine and nonspecific prodromal symptoms (eg, anorexia, malaise, GI symptoms), other reports did not describe the onset of clear prodromal symptoms prior to the onset of jaundice.

The physician may consider the value of liver function testing. Periodic serum transaminase testing has not been proven to prevent serious injury, but it is generally believed that early detection of drug-induced hepatic injury along with immediate withdrawal of the suspect drug enhances the likelihood for recovery.

Advise patients to be alert for signs and symptoms of liver dysfunction (eg, jaundice, anorexia, GI complaints, malaise) and to report them to their doctor immediately if they occur. Ongoing clinical assessment of patients should govern physician interventions, including diagnostic evaluations and treatment.

Discontinue nefazodone if clinical signs or symptoms suggest liver failure. Patients who develop evidence of hepatocellular injury such as increased serum AST or serum ALT levels ≥ 3 times the upper limit of normal, while on nefazodone should be withdrawn from the drug. These patients should be presumed to be at increased risk for liver injury if nefazodone is reintroduced. Accordingly, such patients should not be considered for retreatment.

➤*Serious interactions:*

MAO inhibitors – In patients receiving antidepressants with pharmacologic properties similar to nefazodone in combination with an MAOI, there have been reports of serious, sometimes fatal, reactions. For a selective serotonin reuptake inhibitor (SSRI), these reactions have included hyperthermia, rigidity, myoclonus, autonomic instability with possible rapid fluctuations of vital signs, and mental status changes that include extreme agitation progressing to delirium and coma. Some cases presented with features resembling neuroleptic malignant syndrome. Severe hyperthermia and seizures, sometimes fatal, have occurred with the combined use of tricyclic antidepressants and MAOIs. These reactions have also been reported in patients who have recently discontinued these drugs and have been started on an MAOI.

Although the effects of combined use of nefazodone and MAOIs have not been evaluated, because nefazodone is an inhibitor of both serotonin and norepinephrine reuptake, it is recommended that nefazodone not be used in combination with an MAOI, or within 14 days of discontinuing treatment with an MAOI. Allow ≥ 1 week after stopping nefazodone before starting an MAOI.

Triazolobenzodiazepines – Triazolam and alprazolam, metabolized by cytochrome P450 3A4, have revealed substantial and clinically

important increases in plasma concentrations of these compounds when administered concomitantly with nefazodone (see Drug Interactions). If triazolam is coadministered with nefazodone, a 75% reduction in the initial triazolam dosage is recommended. For many patients (eg, the elderly), it is recommended that triazolam not be used in combination with nefazodone. No dosage adjustment is required for nefazodone.

Antihistamines, nonsedating / cisapride / pimozide – Cisapride and pimozide are metabolized by the cytochrome P450 3A4 isozyme; inhibitors of 3A4 can block the metabolism of these drugs, resulting in increased plasma concentrations of the parent drug, which is associated with QT prolongation and with rare cases of serious cardiovascular adverse events, including death, principally because of ventricular tachycardia of the torsades de pointes type. In vitro, nefazodone inhibits 3A4. Consequently, it is recommended that nefazodone not be used in combination with cisapride or pimozide (see Drug Interactions).

➤*Fertility impairment:* A fertility study in rats showed a slight decrease in fertility at 200 mg/kg/day (≈ 3 times the maximum human daily dose).

➤*Elderly:* Initiate treatment at 50% of the usual dose, but titrate upward over the same range as in younger patients (see Administration and Dosage). Observe the usual precautions in elderly patients who have concomitant medical illnesses or who are receiving concomitant drugs.

➤*Pregnancy: Category C.* Increased early pup mortality was seen in rats at a dose ≈ 5 times the maximum human dose, and decreased pup weights were seen at this and lower doses when dosing began during pregnancy and continued until weaning. There are no adequate and well-controlled studies in pregnant women. Use during pregnancy only if the potential benefit justifies the potential risk to the fetus.

➤*Lactation:* It is not known whether nefazodone or its metabolites are excreted in breast milk. Exercise caution when nefazodone is administered to a nursing woman.

➤*Children:* Safety and efficacy in individuals < 18 years of age have not been established.

Precautions

➤*Use in patients with concomitant illness:* Nefazodone has not been evaluated or used to any appreciable extent in patients with a recent history of MI or unstable heart disease. Evaluation of electrocardiograms of 1153 patients who received nefazodone in 6- to 8-week, double-blind, placebo-controlled trials did not indicate that nefazodone is associated with the development of clinically important ECG abnormalities. However, sinus bradycardia, defined as heart rate ≤ 50 bpm and a decrease of ≥ 15 bpm from baseline, was observed in 1.5% of nefazodone-treated patients compared with 0.4% of placebo-treated patients ($P \leq 0.05$). Because patients with a recent history of MI or unstable heart disease were excluded from clinical trials, treat such patients with caution.

➤*Postural hypotension:* Studies revealed that 5.1% of nefazodone patients compared with 2.5% of placebo patients met criteria for a potentially important decrease in blood pressure at some time during treatment (systolic blood pressure ≤ 90 mmHg and a change from baseline of ≥ 20 mmHg). While there was no difference in the proportion of nefazodone and placebo patients having adverse events characterized as syncope (nefazodone, 0.2%; placebo, 0.3%), the rates for adverse events characterized as postural hypotension were as follows: Nefazodone, 2.8%; tricyclic antidepressants, 10.9%; SSRIs, 1.1%; and placebo, 0.8%. Use nefazodone with caution in patients with known cardiovascular or cerebrovascular disease that could be exacerbated by hypotension (eg, history of MI, angina, ischemic stroke) and conditions that would predispose patients to hypotension (eg, dehydration, hypovolemia, treatment with antihypertensive medication).

➤*Mania / Hypomania:* Hypomania or mania occurred in 0.3% of nefazodone-treated unipolar patients, compared with 0.3% of tricyclic- and 0.4% of placebo-treated patients. In patients classified as bipolar, the rate of manic episodes was 1.6% for nefazodone, 5.1% for the combined tricyclic-treated groups, and 0% for placebo-treated patients. Activation of mania/hypomania is a known risk in a small proportion of patients with major affective disorder treated with other marketed antidepressants. As with all antidepressants, use nefazodone cautiously in patients with a history of mania.

➤*Suicide:* The possibility of a suicide attempt is inherent in depression and may persist until significant remission occurs. Closely supervise high-risk patients during initial therapy. Have physicians write prescriptions for the smallest quantity of nefazodone consistent with good patient management to reduce the risk of overdose.

➤*Seizures:* A recurrence of a petit mal seizure was observed in a patient receiving nefazodone who had a history of such seizures. One nonstudy participant reportedly experienced a convulsion (type not documented) following a multiple-drug overdose. Rare occurrences of convulsions (including grand mal seizures) following nefazodone administration have been reported since market introduction. A causal relationship to nefazodone has not been established.

➤*Priapism:* While priapism did not occur during premarketing experience with nefazodone, rare reports of priapism have been received since market introduction. A causal relationship to nefazodone has not been established. If patients present with prolonged or inappropriate

NEFAZODONE HCl

erections, they should discontinue therapy immediately and consult their physicians. If the condition persists for > 24 hours, consult a urologist to determine appropriate management.

➤*Hepatic cirrhosis:* In patients with cirrhosis of the liver, the AUC values of nefazodone and its metabolite HO-NEF were increased by ≈ 25%.

➤*Visual disturbances:* There have been reports of visual disturbances associated with the use of nefazodone, including blurred vision, scotoma, and visual trails. Advise patients to notify their physician if they develop visual disturbances.

➤*Drug abuse and dependence:* Premarketing clinical experience with nefazodone did not reveal any tendency for a withdrawal syndrome or any drug-seeking behavior. However, carefully evaluate patients for a history of drug abuse and follow such patients closely, observing them for signs of misuse or abuse of nefazodone.

➤*Hazardous tasks:* Caution patients about operating hazardous machinery, including automobiles, until they are reasonably certain that nefazodone therapy does not adversely affect their ability to engage in such activities.

➤*Photosensitivity:* Photosensitization (photoallergy or phototoxicity) may occur; therefore, caution patients to take protective measures (ie, sunscreens, protective clothing) against exposure to sunlight or ultra-violet light (eg, tanning beds) until tolerance is determined.

Drug Interactions

➤*Potential interaction with drugs that inhibit or are metabolized by cytochrome P450 (3A4 and 2D6) isozymes:* In vitro, nefazodone is an inhibitor of cytochrome P4503A4. This is consistent with the interaction observed between nefazodone and triazolam and alprazolam, buspirone, atorvastatin, and simvastatin, drugs metabolized by this isozyme. Consequently, caution is indicated in the combined use of nefazodone with any drugs known to be metabolized by the 3A4 isozyme (see Warnings).

Nefazodone and its metabolites in vitro are extremely weak inhibitors of P4502D6. Thus, it is not likely that nefazodone will decrease the metabolic clearance of drugs metabolized by this isozyme.

➤*Drugs highly bound to plasma protein:* Because nefazodone is highly bound to plasma protein, administration to a patient taking another drug that is highly protein bound may cause increased free concentrations of the other drug, potentially resulting in adverse events. Conversely, adverse effects could result from displacement of nefazodone by other highly bound drugs.

Nefazodone Drug Interactions			
Precipitant drug	Object drug*		Description
Anesthetics, general	Nefazodone	↔	Little is known about the potential for interactions between nefazodone and general anesthetics. Prior to elective surgery, discontinue nefazodone for as long as clinically feasible.
Sibutramine	Nefazodone	↑	A "serotonin syndrome," including CNS irritability, motor weakness, shivering, myoclonus, and altered consciousness may occur.
Sumatriptan	Nefazodone	↑	A "serotonin syndrome," including CNS irritability, increased muscle tone, shivering myoclonus, and altered consciousness may occur in some patients. If coadministration cannot be avoided, start with low dosages and closely monitor the patient. Be prepared to provide supportive care, stop the serotonergic agent, and give and antiserotonergic agent (eg, cyproheptadine).
Nefazodone	Alcohol	↔	Although nefazodone did not potentiate the cognitive and psychomotor effects of alcohol in experiments with healthy subjects, the concomitant use of nefazodone and alcohol in depressed patients is not advised.
Nefazodone	Benzodiazepines	↑	Possible increase in CNS-depressant effect. Monitor for increased or decreased CNS effects of benzodiazepines when nefazodone therapy is started or stopped, respectively. An agent that is not eliminated by oxidative metabolism (eg, lorazepam) may be a suitable alternative.
Nefazodone	Buspirone	↑	In healthy volunteers, coadministration resulted in marked increases in plasma buspirone concentrations (increases up to 20-fold in C_{max} and up to 50-fold in AUC) and statistically significant decreases (≈ 50%) in plasma concentrations of the buspirone metabolite 1-pyrimidinylpiperazine. Slight increases in AUC were observed for nefazodone (23%) and its metabolites hydroxynefazodone (17%) and mCPP (9%). Subjects receiving buspirone and nefazodone experienced side effects such as lightheadedness, asthenia, dizziness, and somnolence. If the 2 drugs are to be used in combination, a low dose of buspirone (eg, 2.5 mg twice daily) is recommended. Base subsequent dose adjustment of either drug on clinical assessment.
Buspirone	Nefazodone	↑	
Nefazodone	Carbamazepine	↑	There are reports of elevated serum carbamazepine levels with possible increases in side effects and lower nefazodone levels with possible decreases in efficacy when given concomitantly. Monitor carbamazepine levels and observe the patient for signs and symptoms of carbamazepine side effects or a decrease in therapeutic effect when nefazodone is started or stopped.
Carbamazepine	Nefazodone	↓	
Nefazodone	Cisapride	↑	Increased cisapride plasma concentrations with cardiotoxicity may occur. See Warnings.
Nefazodone	Cyclosporine Tacrolimus	↑	Cyclosporine concentrations and toxicity may be increased. Closely monitor trough cyclosporine whole blood concentrations when nefazodone is started or stopped. Adjust the dose of cyclosporine as needed.
Nefazodone	Digoxin	↑	In 1 study, C_{max}, C_{min}, and AUC of digoxin were increased by 29%, 27%, and 15%, respectively. Plasma level monitoring for digoxin is recommended.
Nefazodone	Haloperidol	↔	Haloperidol apparent clearance decreased by 35% with no significant increase in peak plasma concentrations or time to peak.
Nefazodone	HMG-CoA reductase inhibitors (specifically simvastatin, atorvastatin, lovastatin)	↑	There have been rare reports of rhabdomyolysis when these drugs are given concomitantly. Caution should be used and dosage adjustments are recommended if nefazodone is administered with these specific HMG-CoA reductase inhibitors.
Nefazodone	MAOIs	↑	A "serotonin syndrome" (CNS irritability, shivering, myoclonus, altered consciousness) may occur. Do not coadminister. Allow ≥ 1 week after stopping nefazodone before giving an MAOI. After stopping an MAOI, allow ≥ 2 weeks before giving any serotonin reuptake inhibitor.
Nefazodone	Propranolol	↔	Coadministration resulted in 30% and 14% reductions in C_{max} and AUC of propranolol, respectively, and a 14% reduction in C_{max} for the metabolite, 4-hydroxypropranolol. C_{max}, C_{min}, and AUC of the nefazodone metabolite m-chlorophenylpiperazine were increased by 23%, 54%, and 28%, respectively.
Propranolol	Nefazodone		
Nefazodone	St. John's wort	↑	Increased sedative-hypnotic effects may occur.

* ↑ = Object drug increased. ↓ = Object drug decreased. ↔ = Undetermined clinical effect.

NEFAZODONE HCl

Adverse Reactions

Approximately 16% of the 3496 patients who received nefazodone in worldwide premarketing clinical trials discontinued treatment because of an adverse experience. The more common events in clinical trials associated with discontinuation included: Nausea (3.5%); dizziness (1.9%); insomnia (1.5%); asthenia (1.3%); agitation (1.2%).

Nefazodone Adverse Reactions (%)		
Adverse reaction	Nefazodone (n = 393)	Placebo (n = 394)
Cardiovascular		
Postural hypotension	4	1
Hypotension	2	1
CNS		
Somnolence	25	14
Dizziness	17	5
Insomnia	11	9
Lightheadedness	10	3
Confusion	7	2
Memory impairment	4	2
Paresthesia	4	2
Vasodilation (eg, flushing, feeling warm)	4	2
Abnormal dreams	3	2
Concentration decreased	3	1
Ataxia	2	0
Incoordination	2	1
Psychomotor retardation	2	1
Tremor	2	1
Hypertonia	1	0
Libido decreased	1	< 1
Dermatological		
Pruritus	2	1
Rash	2	1
GI		
Dry mouth	25	13
Nausea	22	12
Constipation	14	8
Dyspepsia	9	7
Diarrhea	8	7
Increased appetite	5	3
Nausea and vomiting	2	1
GU		
Urinary frequency	2	1
Urinary tract infection	2	1
Urinary retention	2	1
Vaginitis (incidence adjusted for gender)	2	1
Breast pain (incidence adjusted for gender)	1	< 1
Metabolic		
Peripheral edema	3	2
Thirst	1	< 1
Respiratory		
Pharyngitis	6	5
Cough increased	3	1
Special senses		
Blurred vision	9	3
Abnormal vision (eg, scotoma, visual trails)	7	1
Tinnitus	2	1
Taste perversion	2	1
Visual field defect	2	0
Miscellaneous		
Headache	36	33
Asthenia	11	5
Infection	8	6
Flu syndrome	3	2
Chills	2	1
Fever	2	1
Neck rigidity	1	0
Arthralgia	1	< 1

Dose Dependency of Nefazodone Adverse Reactions (%)			
Adverse reaction	Nefazodone 300 to 600 mg/day (n = 209)	Nefazodone ≤ 300 mg/day (n = 211)	Placebo (n = 212)
CNS			
Somnolence	28	16	13
Dizziness	22	11	4
Confusion	8	2	1
GI			
Nausea	23	14	12
Constipation	17	10	9
Special senses			
Abnormal vision	10	0	2
Blurred vision	9	3	2
Tinnitus	3	0	1

➤*Cardiovascular:* Sinus bradycardia (1.5%); tachycardia, hypertension, syncope, ventricular extrasystoles, angina pectoris (0.1% to 1%); AV block, CHF, hemorrhage, pallor, varicose vein (< 0.1%).

➤*CNS:* Vertigo, twitching, depersonalization, hallucinations, suicide thoughts/attempt, apathy, euphoria, hostility, abnormal gait, abnormal thinking, attention decreased, derealization, neuralgia, paranoid reaction, dysarthria, increased libido, suicide, myoclonus (0.1% to 1%); hyperkinesia, increased salivation, cerebrovascular accident, hyperesthesia, hypotonia, ptosis, neuroleptic malignant syndrome (< 0.1%).

➤*Dermatologic:* Dry skin, acne, alopecia, urticaria, maculopapular rash, vesiculobullous rash, eczema (0.1% to 1%).

➤*GI:* Gastroenteritis (≥ 1%); eructation, periodontal abscess, abnormal liver function tests, gingivitis, colitis, gastritis, mouth ulceration, stomatitis, esophagitis, peptic ulcer, rectal hemorrhage (0.1% to 1%); glossitis, hepatitis, dysphagia, GI hemorrhage, oral moniliasis, ulcerative colitis (< 0.1%).

➤*GU:* Impotence (≥ 1%); cystitis, urinary urgency, metrorrhagia, amenorrhea, polyuria, vaginal hemorrhage, breast enlargement, menorrhagia, urinary incontinence, abnormal ejaculation, hematuria, nocturia, kidney calculus (0.1% to 1%); uterine fibroids enlarged, uterine hemorrhage, anorgasmia, oliguria (< 0.1%).

➤*Hematologic/Lymphatic:* Ecchymosis, anemia, leukopenia, lymphadenopathy (0.1% to 1%).

➤*Metabolic/Nutritional:* Weight loss, gout, dehydration, lactic dehydrogenase increased, AST and ALT increased (0.1% to 1%); hypercholesterolemia, hypoglycemia (< 0.1%).

➤*Musculoskeletal:* Arthritis, tenosynovitis, muscle stiffness, bursitis (0.1% to 1%); tendinous contracture (< 0.1%).

➤*Respiratory:* Dyspnea, bronchitis (≥ 1%); asthma, pneumonia, laryngitis, voice alteration, epistaxis, hiccough (0.1% to 1%); hyperventilation, yawn (< 0.1%).

➤*Special senses:* Eye pain (≥ 1%); dry eye, ear pain, abnormality of accommodation, diplopia, conjunctivitis, mydriasis, keratoconjunctivitis, hyperacusis, photophobia (0.1% to 1%); deafness, glaucoma, night blindness, taste loss (< 0.1%).

➤*Miscellaneous:* Allergic reaction, malaise, photosensitivity reaction, face edema, hangover effect, abdomen enlarged, hernia, pelvic pain, halitosis (0.1% to 1%); cellulitis (< 0.1%).

Overdosage

➤*Symptoms:* In premarketing clinical studies, there were 7 reports of nefazodone overdose alone or in combination with other pharmacologic agents. The amount of nefazodone ingested ranged from 1000 to 11,200 mg. Commonly reported symptoms included nausea, vomiting, and somnolence. None of the patients died.

In postmarketing experience, overdose with nefazodone alone and in combination with alcohol or other substances has been reported. Commonly reported symptoms were similar to those reported from overdose in premarketing experience. While there have been rare reports of fatalities in patients taking overdoses of nefazodone, predominantly in combination with alcohol or other substances, no causal relationship to nefazodone has been established.

➤*Treatment:* Treatment should consist of those general measures employed in the management of overdosage with any antidepressant. Ensure an adequate airway, oxygenation, and ventilation. Monitor cardiac rhythm and vital signs. General supportive and symptomatic measures are also recommended. Induction of emesis is not recommended. Gastric lavage with a large-bore orogastric tube with appropriate airway protection, if needed, may be indicated if performed soon after ingestion, or in symptomatic patients.

NEFAZODONE HCl

Administer activated charcoal. Because of the wide distribution of nefazodone in body tissues, forced diuresis, dialysis, hemoperfusion, and exchange transfusion are unlikely to be of benefit. No specific antidotes for nefazodone are known.

In managing overdosage, consider the possibility of multiple drug involvement. The physician should consider contacting a poison control center for additional information on the treatment of any overdose.

Patient Information

Instruct patients to continue drug treatment as directed once improvement is noted. It may take several weeks of treatment to obtain the full antidepressant effect.

Inform patients that nefazodone has been associated with liver abnormalities ranging from asymptomatic reversible serum transaminase increases to cases of liver failure resulting in transplant or death. At present, there is no way to predict who is likely to develop liver failure. Ordinarily, patients with active liver disease should not be treated with nefazodone. Patients should be advised to be alert for signs of liver dysfunction (eg, jaundice, anorexia, GI complaints, malaise) and to report them to their doctor immediately if they occur.

Caution patients about operating hazardous machinery, including automobiles, until they are reasonably certain that nefazodone therapy does not adversely affect their ability to engage in such activities.

Avoid alcohol while taking nefazodone.

Advise patients to notify their physician if they become pregnant or intend to become pregnant during therapy or if they are breastfeeding an infant.

Advise patients to inform their physician or pharmacist if they are taking, or plan to take, any prescription, *otc*, or alternative medicinal drugs, because there is a potential for interactions. Significant caution is indicated if nefazodone is to be used in combination with either alprazolam or triazolam, and concomitant use with cisapride or pimozide is contraindicated (see Warnings).

Advise patients to notify their physician if they develop a rash, hives, or a related allergic phenomenon.

Advise patients to notify their physician if they develop visual disturbances.

Advise patients to avoid sunlight and sunlamps or to wear protective clothing; photosensitivity may occur.

Selective Serotonin Reuptake Inhibitors

Refer to the Antidepressants introduction.

Indications

Refer to individual monographs for further information.

SSRIs — Summary of Indications						
Indication ✔ - Labeled X - Unlabeled	Citalopram	Escitalopram	Fluoxetine	Fluvoxamine	Paroxetine	Sertraline
Bulimia nervosa			✔	X		
Depression	✔	✔	✔	X	✔	✔
Generalized anxiety disorder (GAD)	X	✔	X		✔ᵃ	
Obsessive-compulsive disorder (OCD)	X		✔	✔	✔ᵃ	✔
Panic disorder	X	X	✔	X	✔	✔
Premenstrual dysphoric disorder (PMDD)	X		✔ᵇ		✔ᶜ	✔
Posttraumatic stress disorder (PTSD)	X		X		✔ᵃ	✔
Social anxiety disorder				X	✔	✔

ᵃ Immediate-release only.
ᵇ *Sarafem* only.
ᶜ Controlled-release only.

➤*Unlabeled uses:* See the above table.

Fluoxetine – Raynaud phenomenon (20 to 60 mg/day); hot flashes (20 mg/day); second-line prophylaxis of migraines (10 to 40 mg/day).

Paroxetine – Hot flashes (20 mg/day or 12.5 to 25 mg/day controlled-release formulation); diabetic neuropathy.

Actions

➤*Pharmacology:* Selective serotonin reuptake inhibitors (SSRIs) are oral antidepressant agents chemically unrelated to the tricyclic, tetracyclic, or other available antidepressants. The antidepressant action of the SSRIs is presumed to be linked to their inhibition of CNS neuronal uptake of serotonin (5HT). Human and in vitro studies have demonstrated that **fluoxetine** (and its active metabolite S-norfluoxetine), **flu-** **voxamine**, **paroxetine**, **sertraline**, **escitalopram**, and **citalopram** are potent and selective inhibitors of neuronal serotonin reuptake, and they also have a weak effect on norepinephrine and dopamine neuronal reuptake. SSRIs have little affinity for muscarinic, gamma aminobutyric acid (GABA), benzodiazepine, alpha$_1$, alpha$_2$, beta-adrenergic, dopamine (D$_2$), 5-HT$_1$, 5-HT$_2$, and histamine (H$_1$) receptors; antagonism of muscarinic, histaminergic, and alpha$_1$-adrenergic receptors has been associated with various anticholinergic, sedative, and cardiovascular effects for other psychotropic drugs. The chronic administration of sertraline in animals was found to down-regulate brain norepinephrine receptors, as has been observed with other clinically effective antidepressants.

➤*Pharmacokinetics:*

SSRI Pharmacokinetics							
SSRIs	Time to peak plasma concentration (h)	Peak plasma concentration (ng/mL)	Half-life (h)	Protein binding (%)	Time to reach steady state (days)	Primary route of elimination	Bioavailability (%)
Citalopram	≈ 4	nd*	≈ 35	≈ 80	≈ 7	20% renal, fecal	≈ 80
Escitalopram	5	nd*	27 - 32	≈ 56	≈ 7	7% renal	80ᵇ
Fluoxetine	6 - 8	15 - 55	24 - 384ᵃ	≈ 94.5	≈ 28	hepatic	nd*
Fluvoxamine	3 - 8	88 - 546	13.6 - 15.6	≈ 80	≈ 7	≈ 94% renal	53
Paroxetine	5.2	61.7	21	≈ 93-95	≈10	64% renal, 36% fecal	100
Paroxetine CR	6 - 10	30	15 - 20		14		
Sertraline	4.5 - 8.4	nd*	26 - 104ᵃ	98	≈ 7	40% - 45% renal, 40% - 45% fecal	nd*

ᵃ t½ includes the active metabolite.
ᵇ Based on citalopram data.
* nd = No data.

Special populations –
Elderly:
• *Citalopram* – In a single-dose study, citalopram AUC and half-life were increased in the elderly by 30% and 50%, respectively, whereas in a multiple-dose study they were increased by 23% and 30%, respectively.
• *Escitalopram* – Half-life was increased by approximately 50% in elderly subjects, and C$_{max}$ was unchanged.
• *Fluvoxamine* – Mean C$_{max}$ was 40% higher in elderly subjects, and the elimination half-life also increased. The clearance also was reduced by approximately 50%.
• *Paroxetine* – C$_{min}$ concentrations were approximately 70% to 80% higher in elderly patients.
• *Sertraline* – Plasma clearance was approximately 40% lower in elderly patients. Therefore, steady state should be achieved after 2 to 3 weeks in older patients.
Hepatic function impairment:
• *Citalopram* – Oral clearance was reduced by 37% and half-life was doubled in patients with reduced hepatic function.
• *Fluoxetine* – Elimination half-life was prolonged in a study of cirrhotic patients, with a mean of 7.6 days; norfluoxetine elimination also was delayed, with a mean duration of 12 days for cirrhotic patients.
• *Fluvoxamine* – Clearance decreased 30% in patients with hepatic dysfunction.
• *Paroxetine* – Patients with hepatic function impairment had about a 2-fold increase in plasma concentrations (AUC, C$_{max}$).
• *Sertraline* – In patients with mild liver impairment, clearance was reduced, resulting in approximately 3-fold greater exposure.
Renal function impairment:
• *Citalopram* – In patients with mild to moderate renal function impairment, oral clearance was reduced by 17%.

• *Fluoxetine* – In depressed patients on dialysis (N = 12), fluoxetine administered as 20 mg once daily for 2 months produced steady-state fluoxetine and norfluoxetine plasma concentrations comparable with those seen in patients with normal renal function. The possibility exists that renally excreted metabolites of fluoxetine may accumulate to higher levels in patients with severe renal dysfunction.
• *Paroxetine* – The mean plasma concentrations in patients with Ccr less than 30 mL/min were approximately 4 times greater than normal subjects. Patients with Ccr of 30 to 60 mL/min had about a 2-fold increase in plasma concentrations (AUC, C$_{max}$).

Contraindications

Hypersensitivity to SSRIs or any inactive ingredients; in combination with a monoamine oxidase inhibitor (MAOI), or within 14 days of discontinuing an MAOI (see Drug Interactions);administration of thioridazine with **fluoxetine** or within a minimum of 5 weeks after fluoxetine has been discontinued; coadministration of **fluvoxamine** with cisapride, thioridazine or pimozide (see Drug Interactions); concomitant use of thioridazine with **paroxetine**; concomitant use of pimozide with **sertraline**; coadministration of sertraline oral concentrate and disulfiram.

Warnings

➤*Long-term use:* The effectiveness of long-term use of SSRIs for OCD, panic disorder, social anxiety disorder, PMDD, PTSD, GAD, and bulimia has not been systematically evaluated. However, the long-term use of SSRIs for depression has been evaluated and demonstrated to maintain antidepressant response for up to 1 year. Periodically reevaluate the SSRI used for extended periods to determine long-term usefulness of the drug for the individual patient.

➤*MAOIs:* In patients receiving an SSRI in combination with an MAOI, serious, sometimes fatal reactions have occurred, including hyperthermia, rigidity, myoclonus, autonomic instability with possible rapid fluctuations of vital signs, and mental status changes that include confusion, irritability, extreme agitation progressing to delirium, and coma. These reactions also have occurred in patients who have recently discontinued an SSRI and have been started on an MAOI. Some cases presented with features resembling neuroleptic malignant syndrome. While no human data show such an interaction with **paroxetine**, limited animal data suggest that the drugs may act synergistically to elevate blood pressure and evoke behavioral excitation. Therefore, it is recommended that SSRIs not be used in combination with an MAOI or within 14 days of discontinuing treatment with an MAOI. Allow at least 2 weeks after stopping the SSRIs before starting an MAOI; allow at least 5 weeks after stopping **fluoxetine** before starting an MAOI (see Drug Interactions).

➤*Suicide risk:* Patients with major depressive disorder, both adult and pediatric, may experience worsening of their depression and/or the emergence of suicidal ideation and behavior (suicidality), whether or not they are taking antidepressant medications, and this risk may persist until significant remission occurs. Although there has been a long-standing concern that antidepressants may have a role in inducing worsening of depression and the emergence of suicidality in certain patients, a causal role for antidepressants in inducing such behaviors has not been established. Nevertheless, closely observe patients being treated with antidepressants for clinical worsening and suicidality, especially at the beginning of a course of drug therapy or at the time of dose changes, either increases or decreases. Consider changing the therapeutic regimen, including possibly discontinuing the medication, in patients whose depression is persistently worse or whose emergent suicidality is severe, abrupt in onset, or was not part of the patient's presenting symptoms. Write prescriptions for the smallest quantity of tablets or capsules in order to reduce the risk of overdose.

➤*Rash and accompanying events:* Seven percent of patients taking **fluoxetine** have developed a rash and/or urticaria; almost one third were withdrawn from treatment. Clinical findings reported in association with rash include: arthralgias, edema, carpal tunnel syndrome, fever, leukocytosis, lymphadenopathy, mild transaminase elevation, proteinuria, and respiratory distress. Most patients improved promptly with discontinuation of fluoxetine and/or adjunctive treatment with antihistamines or steroids; all patients recovered completely. Two patients treated with fluoxetine developed a serious cutaneous systemic illness. Neither had an unequivocal diagnosis, but one had a leukocytoclastic vasculitis; the other had a severe desquamating syndrome that was considered to be vasculitis or erythema multiforme. Other patients have had systemic syndromes suggestive of serum sickness.

Systemic events, possibly related to vasculitis and including lupus-like syndrome, have developed in patients with rash. Although rare, these events may be serious, involving the lung, kidney, or liver. Death has been associated with the events. Anaphylactoid events, including bronchospasm, angioedema, and urticaria, alone and in combination, have occurred with fluoxetine. Pulmonary events, including inflammatory processes of varying histopathology and/or fibrosis, have occurred rarely. These events have occurred with dyspnea as the only preceding symptom. Whether these systemic events and rash have a common underlying cause or are caused by different etiologies or pathogenic processes is not known. Furthermore, a specific underlying immunologic basis for these events has not been identified. Upon the appearance of rash or of other possibly allergic phenomena for which an alternative etiology cannot be identified, discontinue the SSRI.

➤*Renal function impairment:* In depressed patients on dialysis (N = 12), **fluoxetine** administered as 20 mg once daily for 2 months produced steady-state fluoxetine and norfluoxetine plasma concentrations comparable with those seen in patients with normal renal function. The possibility exists that renally excreted metabolites of fluoxetine may accumulate to higher levels in patients with severe renal dysfunction. Use of a lower or less-frequent dose for renally impaired patients is not routinely necessary (see Administration and Dosage).

Increased plasma concentrations of **paroxetine** occur in subjects with severe renal (Ccr less than 30 mL/min). Reduce the initial dosage of paroxetine in patients with severe renal impairment; if necessary, increase upward titration intervals (see Administration and Dosage).

Because **sertraline** and **escitalopram** are extensively metabolized by the liver, excretion of unchanged drug in the urine is a minor route of elimination. However, use with caution in patients with severe renal impairment.

In patients with mild to moderate renal function impairment, oral clearance of **citalopram** was reduced by 17% compared with healthy subjects. No adjustment of dosage for such patients is recommended. No information is available about pharmacokinetics of citalopram in patients with severely reduced renal function (Ccr less than 20 mL/min). Because citalopram is extensively metabolized, excretion of unchanged drug in urine is a minor route of elimination. Until an adequate number of patients with severe renal impairment have been evaluated during chronic treatment with citalopram, use with caution in such patients.

The mean minimum plasma concentrations in renally impaired patients (Ccr 5 to 45 mL/min) after 4 and 6 weeks of treatment (50 mg twice daily, n = 13) were comparable to each other, suggesting no accumulation of **fluvoxamine** in these patients.

➤*Hepatic function impairment:* SSRIs are extensively metabolized by the liver. Use with caution in patients with severe liver impairment. The elimination half-life of **fluoxetine** was prolonged in a study of cirrhotic patients, with a mean of 7.6 days; norfluoxetine elimination also was delayed, with a mean duration of 12 days. **Fluvoxamine** clearance was decreased by 30%; slowly titrate fluvoxamine during initiation of treatment. Increased plasma concentrations of **paroxetine** occur in patients with severe hepatic impairment. Initial dose should be reduced and upward titration, if necessary, should be at increased intervals. The clearance of **sertraline** is decreased in mild, chronic liver impairment. Give a lower or less-frequent dose in patients with liver impairment; if necessary, increase upward titration intervals.

Citalopram oral clearance was reduced by 37% and half-life was doubled in patients with reduced hepatic function compared with healthy subjects. The recommended dose for most hepatically impaired patients is 20 mg.

In subjects with hepatic impairment, clearance of racemic citalopram was decreased and plasma concentrations were increased. The recommended dose of **escitalopram** in hepatically impaired patients is 10 mg/day.

➤*Carcinogenesis:* In mice and rats given **paroxetine** at 2 to 4 times the maximum recommended human dose (MRHD) on a mg/m² basis, there was a significantly greater number of male rats with reticulum cell sarcomas and a significantly increased linear trend across dose groups for the occurrence of lymphoreticular tumors in male rats. There was a dose-related increase in the incidence of liver adenomas in male mice receiving **sertraline** at 10 to 40 mg/kg (0.25 to 1 times the MRHD on a mg/m² basis). Liver adenomas have a variable rate of spontaneous occurrence in the CD-1 mouse and are of unknown significance to humans. There was an increase in follicular adenomas of the thyroid in female rats receiving sertraline at 40 mg/kg; this was not accompanied by thyroid hyperplasia. While there was an increase in uterine adenocarcinomas in rats receiving sertraline at 10 to 40 mg/kg compared with placebo controls, this effect was not clearly drug-related.

Citalopram was administered in the diet to mice and rats for 18 and 24 months, respectively. There was an increased incidence of small intestine carcinoma in rats receiving 8 or 24 mg/kg/day doses, which are approximately 1.3 and 4 times the MRHD, respectively, on a mg/m² basis. A no-effect dose for this finding was not established. The relevance of these findings to humans is unknown.

➤*Mutagenesis:* **Citalopram** was mutagenic in the in vitro bacterial reverse mutation assay (Ames test) in 2 of 5 bacterial strains (*Salmonella* TA98 and TA1537) in the absence of metabolic activation. It was clastogenic in the in vitro Chinese hamster lung cell assay for chromosomal aberrations in the presence and absence of metabolic activation.

➤*Fertility impairment:* A decrease in fertility was seen with **sertraline** in 1 of 2 rat studies at a dose of 80 mg/kg (4 times the MRHD on a mg/m² basis).

Two fertility studies conducted in rats at doses of up to 7.5 and 12.5 mg/kg/day (approximately 0.9 and 1.5 times the MRHD on a mg/m² basis) indicated that **fluoxetine** had no adverse effects on fertility.

When **citalopram** was administered orally to male and female rats prior to and throughout mating and gestation at doses of 32, 48, and 72 mg/kg/day, mating was decreased at all doses and fertility was decreased at doses of 32 mg/kg/day or more (approximately 5 times the MRHD of 60 mg/day on a body surface area [mg/m²] basis). Gestation duration was increased at 48 mg/kg/day, approximately 8 times the MRHD.

A reduced pregnancy rate was found in reproduction studies in rats at a dose of 15 mg/kg/day **paroxetine**, which is 2.9 times the MRHD for depression or 2.4 times the MRHD for OCD on a mg/m² basis. Irreversible lesions occurred in the reproductive tract of male rats after dosing in toxicity studies for 2 to 52 weeks. These lesions consisted of vacuolation of epididymal tubular epithelium at 50 mg/kg/day and atrophic changes in the seminiferous tubules of the testes with arrested spermatogenesis at 25 mg/kg/day (9.8 and 4.9 times the MRHD for depression; 8.2 and 4.1 times the MRHD for OCD and panic disorder on a mg/m² basis).

➤*Elderly:* The disposition of single doses of **fluoxetine** in healthy elderly subjects (older than 65 years of age) did not differ significantly from that in younger healthy subjects. However, data are insufficient to rule out possible age-related differences during chronic use. Clearance of **fluvoxamine** is decreased by approximately 50% in elderly patients, and greater sensitivity of some older individuals cannot be ruled out. Consequently, slowly titrate fluvoxamine during initiation of therapy. **Paroxetine** pharmacokinetic studies revealed a decreased clearance in the elderly, and a lower starting dose is recommended; there was, however, no overall difference in the adverse event profile between elderly and younger patients, and efficacy was similar. For **sertraline**, the pattern of adverse reactions in the elderly was similar to that in younger patients. However, sertraline plasma clearance may be lower (see Pharmacokinetics). In 2 pharmacokinetic studies, **citalopram** AUC was increased by 23% and 30%, respectively, in elderly subjects as compared with younger subjects, and its half-life was increased by 30% and 50%, respectively. In 2 pharmacokinetic studies, **escitalopram** half-life was increased by approximately 50% in elderly subjects as compared with young subjects and C$_{max}$ was unchanged.

➤*Pregnancy: Category C.* There are no adequate and well-controlled studies in pregnant women. Use during pregnancy only if clearly needed. In a study involving 228 women who had received **fluoxetine** during pregnancy, 5.5% of the women who took fluoxetine in the first trimester delivered infants with major structural anomalies. At doses 0.5 to 4 times the MRHD mg/kg, **sertraline** was associated with delayed ossification in fetuses of rats and rabbits, respectively. The decrease in pup survival was most probably caused by in utero exposure to sertraline. In rats, **fluvoxamine** increased pup mortality at birth and decreased postnatal pup weight and survival. **Paroxetine** reproduction studies in rats revealed no evidence of teratogenic effects. However, in rats, there was an increase in pup deaths during the first 4 days of lactation when dosing occurred during the last trimester of gestation and continued throughout lactation. In 2 rat embryo/fetal development studies, oral administration of **citalopram** (32, 56, or 112 mg/kg/day) to pregnant animals during the period of organogenesis resulted in decreased embryo/fetal growth and survival and an increased incidence of fetal abnormalities (including cardiovascular and skeletal defects) at the high dose, which is approximately 18 times the MRHD. Female rats treated with citalopram from late gestation through weaning increased offspring mortality during the first 4 days after birth, and persistent offspring growth retardation was observed at the highest dose (32 mg/kg/day).

Oral administration of **escitalopram** to pregnant animals during the period of organogenesis resulted in decreased fetal body weight and associated delays in ossification. Maternal toxicity (clinical signs and decreased body weight gain and food consumption) was present at all dose levels. When female rats were treated with escitalopram during pregnancy and through weaning, slightly increased offspring mortality and growth retardation were noted at 48 mg/kg/day. Slight maternal toxicity (clinical signs and decreased body weight gain and food consumption) was seen at this dose.

Neonates exposed to SSRIs or serotonin-norepinephrine reuptake inhibitors (SNRIs) late in the third trimester have developed complications requiring prolonged hospitalization, respiratory support, and tube feeding. Such complications can arise immediately upon delivery. Reported clinical findings have included apnea, constant crying; cyanosis, feeding difficulty, hyperreflexia, hypertonia, hypoglycemia, hypotonia, irritability, jitteriness, respiratory distress, seizures, temperature instability, tremor, vomiting. These features are consistent with either a direct toxic effect of SSRIs and SNRIs or, possibly, a drug discontinuation syndrome. It should be noted that, in some cases, the clinical picture is consistent with serotonin syndrome. When treating a pregnant woman with SSRIs during the third trimester, the physician should carefully consider the potential risks and benefits of treatment.

➤*Lactation:* **Fluoxetine, fluvoxamine, paroxetine, citalopram,** and **escitalopram** are excreted in breast milk. It is not known whether **sertraline** or its metabolites are excreted in breast milk. In one breast milk sample, the concentration of fluoxetine plus norfluoxetine was 70.4 ng/mL; the mother's plasma concentration was 295 ng/mL. No adverse effects were noted in the infant. In another case, an infant nursed by a mother on fluoxetine developed crying, sleep disturbance, vomiting, and watery stools. The infant's plasma drug levels were 340 ng/mL of fluoxetine and 208 ng/mL of norfluoxetine on the second day of feeding. There have been 2 reports of infants experiencing excessive somnolence, decreased feeding, and weight loss in association with breastfeeding from a citalopram-treated mother; in one case, the infant was reported to recover completely upon discontinuation of citalopram by its mother. Exercise caution when SSRIs are administered to a nursing woman. Decide whether to discontinue nursing or discontinue the drug taking into account the importance of the drug to the mother.

➤*Children:* Safety and efficacy in children have not been established.

Regular monitoring of weight and growth is recommended if treatment of a child with an SSRI is to be continued long-term.

The safety and efficacy in pediatric patients younger than 8 years of age in major depressive disorder and younger than 7 years of age in OCD have not been established.

The efficacy of **sertraline** for the treatment of OCD was demonstrated in a 12-week, multicenter, placebo-controlled study with 187 outpatients 6 to 17 years of age. The efficacy of sertraline in pediatric patients with depression, panic disorder, PTSD, PMDD, or social anxiety disorder has not been established.

The efficacy of **fluvoxamine** for the treatment of OCD was demonstrated in a 10-week, multicenter, placebo-controlled study with 120 outpatients 8 to 17 years of age. The adverse event profile was similar to that observed in adult studies. The risks, if any, that may be associated with fluvoxamine's extended use in children and adolescents with OCD have not been systematically assessed. Have the prescriber be mindful that the evidence supporting fluvoxamine use in children

and adolescents derives from relatively short-term clinical studies and from extrapolation of experience gained with adult patients.

> ### Precautions

➤*Monitoring:* In patients receiving SSRIs and suffering from SIADH, displacement syndromes, edematous states, adrenal disease, or conditions of fluid loss, it is recommended that serum electrolytes, especially sodium, as well as BUN and plasma creatinine be monitored regularly. Monitor patients for the emergence of agitation, irritability, and other symptoms, as well as emergence of suicidality, especially at the beginning of drug therapy or at the time of dose changes. Regular monitoring of weight and growth is recommended, especially if treatment of a child with an SSRI is to be continued long-term.

➤*Abnormal bleeding:* Altered platelet function and/or abnormal results from laboratory studies in patients taking **fluoxetine, paroxetine,** or **sertraline** have occurred. There have been reports of abnormal bleeding or purpura in several patients; it is unclear whether the SSRIs had a causative role.

Published case reports have documented the occurrence of bleeding episodes in patients treated with psychotropic drugs that interfere with serotonin reuptake. Subsequent epidemiological studies, both of the case-control and cohort design, have demonstrated an association between the use of psychotropic drugs that interfere with serotonin reuptake and the occurrence of upper GI bleeding. In 2 studies, concurrent use of a nonsteroidal anti-inflammatory drug (NSAID) or aspirin potentiated the risk of bleeding. Although these studies focused on upper GI bleeding, there is reason to believe that bleeding at other sites may be similarly potentiated. Caution patients regarding the risk of bleeding associated with the concomitant use of SSRIs with NSAIDs, aspirin, or other drugs that affect coagulation.

➤*Anxiety, nervousness, and insomnia:* Anxiety, nervousness, and insomnia occurred in 2% to 22% of patients treated with an SSRI. In clinical trials for bulimia nervosa, insomnia occurred in 33% of patients treated with **fluoxetine**.

➤*Altered appetite and weight:* Significant weight loss, especially in underweight depressed or bulimic patients, has occurred. Approximately 3% to 17% of patients treated with an SSRI initially experienced anorexia. Significant weight loss may be an undesirable result of treatment for some patients but on average, patients in controlled trials treated with **paroxetine, citalopram,** or **sertraline** had a minimal 1- to 2-pound weight loss vs smaller changes with placebo. Only rarely have the SSRIs been discontinued because of weight loss or anorexia (see Adverse Reactions); however, after prolonged treatments, patients tend to gain weight. Monitor weight change during therapy.

➤*Activation of mania/hypomania:* Activation of mania/hypomania occurred infrequently in approximately 0.1% to 2.6% of patients taking SSRIs. Activation of mania/hypomania also has occurred in a small proportion of patients with major affective disorder treated with other antidepressants. Use cautiously in patients with a history of mania.

➤*Seizures:* Seizures have occurred with **fluoxetine** (0.1%), **fluvoxamine** (0.2%), **paroxetine** (0.1%), **sertraline** (0.2%), and **citalopram** (0.3%). Sertraline, citalopram, and **escitalopram** have not been evaluated in patients with a seizure disorder. These percentages appear similar to the rate associated with other antidepressants and placebo treatment. Use with care in patients with history of seizures; discontinue therapy if seizures occur.

➤*Cardiac effects:* SSRIs have not been systematically evaluated in patients with a recent history of MI or unstable heart disease. Patients with these diagnoses were generally excluded from clinical studies during the product's premarketing testing. However, the ECGs of patients who received SSRIs in clinical trials were evaluated and the data indicate that they are not associated with the development of clinically significant ECG abnormalities.

➤*Fluoxetine dose changes:* The long elimination half-life of **fluoxetine** and norfluoxetine means that changes in dose will not be fully reflected in plasma for several weeks, affecting titration to final dose and withdrawal from treatment.

➤*Concomitant illness:* Clinical experience is limited. Use caution in patients with diseases or conditions that could affect metabolism or hemodynamic responses.

➤*Glaucoma:* Mydriasis has been reported infrequently in premarketing studies with SSRIs. A few cases of acute angle-closure glaucoma associated with **paroxetine** therapy have been reported in the literature. As mydriasis can cause acute angle closure in patients with narrow-angle glaucoma, use caution when SSRIs are prescribed for patients with narrow-angle glaucoma.

➤*Effects of smoking:* Smokers had a 25% increase in the metabolism of **fluvoxamine** compared with nonsmokers.

➤*Electroconvulsive therapy (ECT):* There are no clinical studies establishing the benefit of the combined use of ECT and SSRIs. Rare prolonged seizure in patients on **fluoxetine** has occurred.

➤*Hyponatremia:* Several cases of **fluoxetine, fluvoxamine, sertraline, paroxetine, escitalopram,** and **citalopram**-induced hyponatremia (some with serum sodium less than 110 mmol/L) have occurred. The hyponatremia appeared to be reversible when fluoxetine, sertraline, paroxetine, citalopram, escitalopram, and fluvoxamine were discontinued. Although these cases were complex with varying possible etiologies, some were possibly because of the syndrome of inappropriate antidiuretic hormone secretion (SIADH). The majority have been in older patients and in patients taking diuretics or who were otherwise volume-depleted.

➤*Diabetes:* **Fluoxetine** may alter glycemic control. Hypoglycemia has occurred during therapy, and hyperglycemia has developed following discontinuation of the drug. The dosage of insulin and/or oral hypoglycemic agents may need to be adjusted when fluoxetine is started or discontinued.

➤*Uricosuric effect:* **Sertraline** is associated with a mean decrease in serum uric acid of approximately 7%. The clinical significance of this weak uricosuric effect is unknown.

➤*Discontinuation of SSRIs:* During marketing of SSRIs and SNRIs, there have been spontaneous reports of adverse events occurring upon discontinuation of these drugs, particularly when abrupt, including the following: agitation, anxiety, confusion, dizziness, dysphoric mood, emotional lability, headache, hypomania, insomnia, irritability, lethargy, and sensory disturbances (eg, paresthesias such as electric shock sensations). While these events are generally self-limiting, there have been reports of serious discontinuation symptoms.

Monitor patients for these symptoms when discontinuing treatment with SSRIs. A gradual reduction in the dose rather than abrupt cessation is recommended whenever possible. If intolerable symptoms occur following a decrease in the dose or upon discontinuation of treatment, then resuming the previously prescribed dose may be considered. Subsequently, the physician may continue decreasing the dose but at a more gradual rate.

➤*Drug abuse and dependence:* Premarketing clinical experience did not reveal any tendency for a withdrawal syndrome or any drug-seeking behavior. It is not possible to predict on the basis of this limited experience the extent to which a CNS-active drug will be misused, diverted, or abused once marketed. Consequently, before starting an SSRI, carefully evaluate patients for history of drug abuse and follow such patients closely, observing them for signs of misuse or abuse.

➤*Hazardous tasks:* Any psychoactive drug may impair judgment, thinking, or motor skills; caution patients about operating hazardous machinery, including automobiles, until they are reasonably certain that the drug treatment does not affect them adversely.

➤*Photosensitivity:* Photosensitization may occur; therefore, caution patients to take protective measures (eg, sunscreens, protective clothing) against exposure to ultraviolet light or sunlight until tolerance is determined.

Drug Interactions

➤*Drugs highly bound to plasma protein:* Because SSRIs are highly bound to plasma protein, administration to a patient taking another drug that is highly protein-bound (eg, warfarin, digoxin) may cause increased free concentrations of the other drug, potentially resulting in adverse events. Conversely, adverse effects could result from displacement of SSRIs by other highly bound drugs.

➤*CYP450 system:* Concomitant use of SSRIs with drugs metabolized by cytochrome P450 2D6 may require lower doses than usually prescribed for either SSRIs or the other drug because SSRIs may significantly inhibit the activity of this isozyme. In most patients (more than 90%), this isozyme is saturated early during dosing. Therefore, coadministration of **paroxetine** with other drugs that are metabolized by this isozyme (eg, certain antidepressants, phenothiazines, risperidone, type IC antiarrhythmics) or drugs that inhibit this enzyme (eg, quinidine) should be approached with caution. **Fluvoxamine** is a relatively weak inhibitor of this isozyme. However, in vitro the drug inhibits the 1A2, 2C9, and 3A4 isozymes, which are involved in the metabolism of warfarin, theophylline, propranolol, and alprazolam. Therapy with medications that are predominantly metabolized by the CYP2D6 system and that have a relatively narrow therapeutic index (eg, flecainide, vinblastine, TCAs) should be initiated at the low end of the dose range if a patient is receiving **fluoxetine** concurrently or has taken it in the previous 5 weeks.

In vitro studies indicate that cytochrome P450 3A4 and 2C19 are the primary enzymes involved in metabolism of **citalopram** and **escitalopram**. Inhibitors of 3A4 (eg, azole antifungals, macrolide antibiotics) and 2C19 (eg, omeprazole) would be expected to increase plasma citalopram levels. Inducers of 3A4 (eg, carbamazepine) would be expected to decrease citalopram and escitalopram levels.

➤*Serotonin syndrome:* The serotonin syndrome is a complication of therapy with serotonergic drugs. It is most commonly observed when 2 drugs that potentiate serotonergic neurotransmission are used concurrently. When this problem occurs with SSRIs, it is most commonly in the setting of other concurrent medications, such as MAOIs, which increase serotonin by different mechanisms. Other such drugs include tryptophan, amphetamines, or other psychostimulants, other antidepressants that increase 5-HT levels, buspirone, lithium, or dopamine agonists (eg, amantadine, bromocriptine). Serotonin syndrome has been reported in 2 patients who were concomitantly receiving linezolid, an antibiotic that is a reversible non-selective MAOI.

➤*Drugs that interfere with hemostasis (eg, NSAIDs, aspirin, warfarin):* Serotonin release by platelets plays an important role in hemostasis. Epidemiological studies of the case-control and cohort design that have demonstrated an association between use of psychotropic drugs that interfere with serotonin reuptake and the occurrence of upper GI bleeding also have shown that concurrent use of an NSAID or aspirin potentiated the risk of bleeding. Thus, caution patients about the use of such drugs concurrently with an SSRI.

SSRI Drug Interactions			
Precipitant drug	Object drug*		Description
Barbiturates	SSRIs Paroxetine	↓	Phenobarbital decreased the AUC and half-life of paroxetine by 25% and 38%, respectively.
Cimetidine	SSRIs	↑	Cimetidine increased steady-state paroxetine concentrations by ≈ 50%. Cimetidine increased sertraline AUC (50%), C_{max} (24%), and half-life (26%). Citalopram and escitalopram AUC (43%) and C_{max} (39%) also increased. Adjust paroxetine dosage as needed.
Cyproheptadine	SSRIs Fluoxetine Paroxetine	↓	The pharmacologic effects of SSRIs may be decreased or reversed.
Linezolid	SSRIs	↑	A serotonin syndrome has been reported to occur after coadministration of linezolid and paroxetine. It may be prudent to allow at least 2 weeks after stopping linezolid before giving an SSRI.
MAO inhibitors	SSRIs	↑	Serious, sometimes fatal, reactions have occurred in patients receiving SSRIs in combination with a MAOI or who have recently discontinued the SSRI and are then started on an MAOI (see Warnings).
Metoclopramide Sibutramine Tramadol	SSRIs	↑	A serotonin syndrome (eg, CNS irritability, shivering, myoclonus, altered consciousness) may occur.
Phenytoin	SSRIs Paroxetine	↓	Phenytoin reduced the AUC and half-life of paroxetine by 50% and 35%, respectively. Also, paroxetine reduced the AUC of phenytoin by 12%, and sertraline, fluoxetine, and fluvoxamine may increase hydantoin levels.
SSRIs Fluoxetine Fluvoxamine Sertraline	Hydantoins	↑↓	
Smoking	SSRIs Fluvoxamine	↓	Smokers had a 25% increase in the metabolism of fluvoxamine.
L-tryptophan	SSRIs	↑	Concurrent use with fluoxetine or paroxetine may produce symptoms related to both central toxicity (eg, headache, sweating, dizziness, agitation, restlessness) and peripheral toxicity (eg, GI distress, nausea, vomiting). Concomitant use is not recommended. Tryptophan may enhance the serotonergic effects of fluvoxamine; use the combination with caution. Severe vomiting has been reported with the coadministration of fluvoxamine and tryptophan.
St. John's wort	SSRIs Paroxetine Sertraline	↑	Increased sedative-hypnotic effects may occur. Avoid concurrent use.

Selective Serotonin Reuptake Inhibitors

SSRI Drug Interactions			
Precipitant drug	Object drug*		Description
SSRIs	Alcohol	↔	Although potentiation of impairment of mental and motor skills caused by alcohol has not occurred, concurrent use is not recommended in patients.
SSRIs	Antidepressants, tricyclic	↑	Plasma TCA levels may be increased; use caution when coadministering. Monitor TCA levels; may need to reduce TCA dose.

SSRIs
  Fluoxetine
  Fluvoxamine
  Sertraline
	Benzodiazepines	↑	Clearance of benzodiazepines metabolized by hepatic oxidation may be decreased; those metabolized by glucuronidation are unlikely to be affected. Coadministration of alprazolam and fluoxetine or fluvoxamine has resulted in increased alprazolam levels and decreased psychomotor performance. Halve the initial alprazolam dose, and titrate to the lowest effective dose. Avoid coadministration of fluvoxamine and diazepam.

SSRIs	Beta blockers	↑	Certain SSRIs may inhibit the metabolism of certain beta blockers. Concurrent use of citalopram or escitalopram and metoprolol produced an increase in metoprolol levels. Fluvoxamine administered with propranolol produced a 5-fold increase in propranolol C_{min}. If propranolol or metoprolol is given with fluvoxamine, reduce the initial beta blocker dose.

SSRIs
  Fluoxetine
  Fluvoxamine
	Buspirone	↓	Effects of buspirone may be decreased; plasma concentrations may be increased with fluvoxamine but clinical response may be decreased. Paradoxical worsening of OCD or serotonin syndrome has occurred.

SSRIs
  Fluoxetine
  Fluvoxamine
	Carbamazepine	↑	Serum carbamazepine levels may be increased with fluoxetine or fluvoxamine, possibly resulting in toxicity. The clearance of citalopram and escitalopram may be increased. The therapeutic effect of sertraline may be decreased.

Carbamazepine	SSRIs
	  Citalopram
	  Escitalopram
	  Sertraline
		↓	

SSRIs
  Fluvoxamine
  Sertraline
	Cisapride	↓	Concurrent use of sertraline and cisapride reduced cisapride AUC and C_{max}. Use with fluvoxamine is contraindicated.

SSRIs
  Citalopram
  Fluoxetine
  Fluvoxamine
  Sertraline
	Clozapine	↑	Elevated serum clozapine levels have occurred. Closely monitor patients on concomitant administration.

SSRIs
  Fluoxetine
  Fluvoxamine
	Cyclosporine	↑	Elevated cyclosporine concentrations were reported in case reports during concomitant administration.

SSRIs Paroxetine	Digoxin	↓	Paroxetine decreased the AUC of digoxin by 15%. The coadministration of paroxetine and digoxin should be undertaken with caution.
SSRIs Fluvoxamine	Diltiazem	↑	Bradycardia has occurred with concurrent use.

SSRIs
  Fluoxetine
  Fluvoxamine
	Haloperidol	↑	Serum concentrations of haloperidol may be increased. Closely monitor patients on concomitant therapy.

SSRIs Citalopram	Ketoconazole	↓	Coadministration decreased ketoconazole C_{max} (21%) and AUC (10%).

SSRIs
  Citalopram
  Escitalopram
  Fluoxetine
  Fluvoxamine
  Sertraline
	Lithium	↑↓	Lithium levels may be increased or decreased by fluoxetine with possible neurotoxicity and increased serotonergic effects. In healthy volunteers, sertraline did not affect lithium levels. It is recommended that plasma lithium levels be monitored following initiation of sertraline, fluoxetine, citalopram, and escitalopram with appropriate adjustments to lithium dose. Concurrent use may enhance serotonergic effects of SSRIs. Use caution when coadministering. Lithium may enhance the serotonergic effects of fluvoxamine. Use with caution in combination; seizures have been reported.

Lithium	SSRIs	↑	
SSRIs Fluvoxamine	Methadone	↑	Significantly increased methadone concentrations have occurred. One patient developed opioid intoxication; another had opioid withdrawal symptoms with fluvoxamine discontinuation.
SSRIs Fluvoxamine	Mexiletine	↑	Mexiletine serum levels may be elevated, increasing the risk of side effects.
SSRIs	NSAIDs	↑	The risk of GI adverse effects may be increased. If possible, avoid concurrent use.

SSRIs
  Fluoxetine
  Fluvoxamine
	Olanzapine	↑	Olanzapine plasma concentrations may be elevated. Observe the patient closely.

SSRIs
  Fluoxetine
  Fluvoxamine
  Paroxetine
	Phenothiazines	↑	Plasma phenothiazine concentrations may be elevated, increasing the pharmacologic and adverse effects, including life-threatening cardiac arrhythmias. Thioridazine is contraindicated with fluvoxamine, fluoxetine, and paroxetine (see Contraindications).

SSRIs
  Fluvoxamine
  Sertraline
	Pimozide	↑	Concurrent use of sertraline and pimozide 2 mg produced a mean increase in pimozide AUC and C_{max} of ≈ 40%, increasing the risk of life-threatening cardiac arrhythmias. Because of pimozide's narrow therapeutic index, administration with sertraline or fluvoxamine is contraindicated.

SSRIs Paroxetine	Procyclidine	↑	Paroxetine increased the AUC, C_{max}, and C_{min} of procyclidine by 35%, 37%, and 67%, respectively. Reduce procyclidine dose if anticholinergic effects occur.
SSRIs Fluoxetine	Propafenone	↑	Coadministration of fluoxetine and propafenone produced elevated propafenone plasma levels. Certain SSRIs may inhibit the metabolism (CYP2D6) of propafenone.
SSRIs Paroxetine	Risperidone	↑	Coadministration may increase risperidone concentrations, increasing the risk of side effects. Serotonin syndrome may occur.
SSRIs Fluoxetine	Ritonavir	↑	The AUC of ritonavir may be increased. Serotonin syndrome may occur.
SSRIs Fluvoxamine	Ropivacaine	↑	Ropivacaine plasma concentrations may be elevated; the pharmacologic effects may be prolonged, increasing the risk of toxicity.

SSRIs
  Fluvoxamine
  Sertraline
	Sulfonylureas
	  Glimepiride
	  Tolbutamide
		↑	Fluvoxamine and sertraline have been shown to decrease the clearance of tolbutamide. Fluvoxamine also has been shown to increase the peak plasma concentration of glimepiride.

SSRIs	Sumatriptan	↑	Weakness, hyperreflexia, and incoordination have occurred with coadministration. Observe patient closely.

Selective Serotonin Reuptake Inhibitors

SSRI Drug Interactions

Precipitant drug	Object drug*		Description
SSRIs	Sympathomimetics	↑	Increased sensitivity to the effect of sympathomimetics and increased risk of serotonin syndrome may occur.
SSRIs Fluvoxamine	Tacrine	↑	Plasma tacrine concentrations may be elevated, increasing the pharmacologic and cholinergic adverse effects.
SSRIs Fluvoxamine Paroxetine	Theophylline	↑	Clearance of theophylline may be decreased by 3-fold when coadministered with fluvoxamine; reduce dosage. Elevated theophylline levels have occurred with paroxetine. It is recommended that theophylline levels be monitored when these drugs are concurrently administered.
SSRIs Fluoxetine Paroxetine	Trazodone	↑	Plasma trazodone levels may be elevated, resulting in increased pharmacologic and toxic effects. If coadministration cannot be avoided, start with a low dose of the SSRI or trazodone.
SSRIs	Warfarin	↑	A pharmacodynamic interaction of altered anticoagulant effects including increased bleeding diathesis with unaltered prothrombin time (PT) may occur with paroxetine or fluoxetine. Coadministration of sertraline and warfarin and citalopram and warfarin has resulted in an 8% and 5% increase in PT, respectively, and delayed PT normalization. Fluvoxamine increased warfarin plasma levels by 98%; PT was prolonged. Monitor PT. Use caution with coadministration and monitor patient.
SSRIs Sertraline	Zolpidem	↑	Coadministration of sertraline and zolpidem produced a shortened onset of action of zolpidem and an increased effect.

* ↑ = Object drug increased. ↓ = Object drug decreased. ↔ = Undetermined clinical effect.

▶ *Drug/Food interactions:* In one study following a single dose of **sertraline** with and without food, sertraline AUC was slightly increased with food and C_{max} was 25% greater. Time to reach peak plasma level decreased from 8 hours post dosing to 5.5 hours. For **paroxetine**, AUC was only slightly increased (6%) when drug was administered with food but the C_{max} was 29% greater, while the time to reach peak plasma concentration decreased from 6.4 hours postdosing to 4.9 hours.

Food does not appear to affect systemic bioavailability of **fluoxetine**, although it may delay absorption by 1 to 2 hours. **Fluvoxamine** and paroxetine CR bioavailability are not affected by food. **Citalopram** and **escitalopram** absorption is not affected by food. Thus, all SSRIs may be given with or without food.

Adverse Reactions

Discontinuation of treatment – In clinical trials, 9.4% to 20% of **paroxetine** patients, 3% to 13% of paroxetine CR patients, 10% to 15% of **sertraline** patients, 22% of **fluvoxamine** patients, 16% of **citalopram** patients, and 6% to 8% of **escitalopram** patients discontinued treatment because of an adverse event.

SSRIs Adverse Reactions (%)[a]

Adverse reaction	Citalopram	Escitalopram	Fluoxetine	Fluvoxamine	Paroxetine IR/CR		Sertraline
Cardiovascular							
Chest pain	—	≥ 1	≥ 1	—	3	1	≥ 1
Hot flushes	0.1 - 1	≥ 1	—	—	—	—	0.1 - 1
Hypertension	0.1 - 1	≥ 1	≥ 1	—	—	2	0.1 - 1
Hypotension (postural)	≥ 1	—	0.1 - 1	≥ 1	≥ 1	0.1 - 1	0.1 - 1
Palpitations	—	≥ 1	1 - 3	3	2 - 3	0.1 - 1	≥ 1
Syncope	0.1 - 1	0.1 - 1	0.1 - 1	≥ 1	≥ 1		0.1 - 1
Tachycardia	≥ 1	0.1 - 1	0.1 - 1	≥ 1	≥ 1	1 - 2	0.1 - 1
Vasodilation	—	—	2 - 3	3	2 - 4	2 - 3	< 0.1
CNS							
Abnormal dreams	—	3	3	—	3 - 4	1	0.1 - 1
Abnormal thinking	—	—	2 - 6	—	0.1 - 1	0.1 - 1	—
Agitation	3	0.1 - 1	≥ 1	2	3 - 6	2 - 3	1 - 6
Amnesia	≥ 1	0.1 - 1	≥ 1	≥ 1	2	0.1 - 1	0.1 - 1
Anxiety	4	—	12 - 13	1 - 5	2 - 6	2 - 5	4
Apathy	≥ 1	0.1 - 1	—	≥ 1	—	—	0.1 - 1
CNS stimulation	—	—	0.1 - 1	2	—	—	—
Concentration, decreased/impaired	≥ 1	≥ 1	—	—	3 - 4	1 - 3	—
Confusion	≥ 1	0.1 - 1	≥ 1	—	1	1	0.1 - 1
Depersonalization	0.1 - 1	0.1 - 1	0.1 - 1	0.1 - 1	3	0.1 - 1	—
Depression	≥ 1	0.1 - 1	—	2	—	2	0.1 - 1
Dizziness	—	4 - 7	2 - 11	2 - 11	6 - 14	6 - 14	6 - 17
Drugged feeling	—	—	—	—	2	—	—
Emotional lability	0.1 - 1	0.1 - 1	≥ 1	0.1 - 1	≥ 1	0.1 - 1	0.1 - 1
Fatigue	5	2-8	—	—	—	—	10 - 16
Headache	—	24	13 - 24	3 - 22	17 - 18	15 - 27	25
Hypertonia	0.1 - 1	—	0.1 - 1	2	0.1 - 1	2 - 3	≥ 1
Hypoesthesia	0.1 - 1	—	0.1 - 1	—	0.1 - 1	0.1 - 1	≥ 1
Hypo-/Hyperkinesia	0.1 - 1	—	—	≥ 1	0.1 - 1	0.1 - 1	0.1 - 1
Insomnia	15	7 - 14	9 - 24	4 - 21	11 - 24	7 - 20	12 - 28
Libido decreased	1 - 4	3 - 7	3 - 9	2	3 - 12	7 - 12	1 - 11
Manic reaction	—	—	—	≥ 1	—	—	1 - 11
Myoclonus/twitching	—	0.1 - 1	0.1 - 1	≥ 1	—	—	0.1 - 1
Nervousness	—	0.1 - 1	3 - 14	2 - 12	2 - 3	1 - 2	—
Paresthesia	≥ 1	2	—	—	3 - 9	2 - 8	5
Psychotic reaction	—	—	—	≥ 1	4	1 - 3	2
Sleep disorder	—	—	≥ 1	0.1-1	—	—	—
Somnolence	18	4 - 13	12 - 13	4 - 22	13 - 24	3 - 22	2 - 15
Tremor	8	0.1 - 1	9 - 12	5	4 - 15	4 - 8	< 1 - 11
Vertigo	0.1 - 1	0.1 - 1	—	0.1 - 1	≥ 1	2	0.1 - 1
Dermatologic							
Acne	0.1 - 1	0.1 - 1	0.1 - 1	0.1 - 1	0.1 - 1	0.1 - 1	0.1 - 1
Pruritus	≥ 1	0.1 - 1	3	—	≥ 1	0.1 - 1	0.1 - 1
Rash	≥ 1	≥ 1	4 - 5	—	2 - 3	≥ 1	3
Sweating, excessive/increased	11	3 - 8	7 - 8	7	1 - 14	6 - 14	3 - 11

Selective Serotonin Reuptake Inhibitors

Adverse reaction	Citalopram	Escitalopram	Fluoxetine	Fluvoxamine	Paroxetine IR/CR		Sertraline
GI							
Abdominal pain	3	2	6	1	4	3-7	2-7
Anorexia	4	—	10 - 11	1 - 6	—		3-11
Constipation	—	3 - 6	5	10	5 - 16	2 - 13	1 - 8
Decreased appetite	—	3			2 - 9	1 - 12	
Diarrhea/loose stools	8	6 - 14	2 - 11	1 - 11	9 - 19	6 - 18	13 - 24
Dry mouth	20	4 - 9	9 - 11	1 - 14	9 - 21	2 - 18	6 - 16
Dyspepsia	5	2 - 6	7 - 8	1 - 10	2 - 5	2 - 13	6 - 13
Dysphagia	0.1 - 1	—	0.1 - 1	2	0.1 - 1	—	0.1 - 1
Flatulence	≥ 1	2	3	4	4	6 - 8	
Gastroenteritis	0.1 - 1	≥ 1	0.1 - 1	0.1 - 1	0.1 - 1	0.1 - 1	0.1 - 1
Increased appetite	≥ 1	≥ 1	≥ 1	—	2 - 4	—	≥ 1
Melena	—	—	0.1 - 1	—	—	—	< 0.1
Nausea	21	15 - 18	9 - 27	9 - 40	15 - 36	17 - 23	13 - 30
Oropharynx disorder	—	—	—	—	2		—
Tooth disorder/caries	—	2	—	3	< 0.1	0.1 - 1	0.1 - 1
Vomiting	4	3	1 - 3	2 - 5	2 - 3	2	4
GU							
Abnormal ejaculation	6	9 - 14	—	8	6 - 28	15 - 27	7 - 19
Female genital disorders	—	—	—	—	2 - 9	2 - 10	—
Male genital disorders, others	—	—	—	—	4 - 10	—	—
Menstrual disorder	—	2	—	—	—	1 - 2	0.1 - 1
Sexual dysfunction/impotence/ anorgasmia	1 - 3	2 - 6	0.1 - 1	2	2 - 13	5 - 10	≥ 1
Urinary frequency	—	≥ 1	2	3	2 - 3	2	0.1 - 1
Urinary tract infection	—	≥ 1	—	0.1 - 1	2	3	—
Urination disorder/retention	0.1 - 1	—	0.1- 1	1	3	2	0.1 - 1
Musculoskeletal							
Arthralgia	2	≥ 1	—	0.1 - 1	≥ 1	2	0.1 - 1
Myalgia	2	≥ 1	—	—	2 - 4	5	≥ 1
Myasthenia	—	—	< 0.1	0.1 - 1	1	< 0.1	—
Myopathy	—	—	< 0.1	< 0.1	2	< 0.1	—
Respiratory							
Bronchitis	0.1 - 1	≥ 1	—	0.1 - 1	0.1 - 1	1 - 2	< 0.1
Cough (increased)	≥ 1	≥ 1	—	≥ 1	≥ 1	1 - 2	0.1 - 1
Dyspnea	0.1 - 1	—	—	2	0.1 - 1	—	0.1 - 1
Pharyngitis	—	—	6 - 10	—	4	8	—
Respiratory disorder	—	—	—	—	7	—	—
Rhinitis	5	5	16 - 23	—	3	4	≥ 1
Sinusitis	3	3	—	≥ 1	4	4 - 8	0.1 - 1
Upper respiratory tract infection	5	—	—	9	—	—	0.1 - 1
Yawn	2	2	3 - 5	2	2 - 5	2 - 5	≥ 1
Special senses							
Amblyopia	—	—	—	3	—	—	—
Taste perversion/change	≥ 1	0.1 - 1	≥ 1	3	2	2	—
Tinnitus	0.1 - 1	≥ 1	≥ 1	—	≥ 1	0.1 - 1	≥ 1
Vision disturbances/blurred vision/ abnormal vision	≥ 1	≥ 1	2 - 3	—	2 - 8	1 - 5	3
Miscellaneous							
Accidental injury/trauma	—	—	1 - 8	≥ 1	3 - 6	3 - 8	—
Allergy/allergic reaction	—	≥ 1	—	0.1 - 1	0.1 - 1	2	< 0.1
Asthenia	—	0.1 - 1	8 - 14	2 - 14	3 - 22	14 - 18	≥ 1
Back pain	—	—	—	—	3	4 - 5	≥ 1
Chills	—	0.1 - 1	≥ 1	2	2	0.1 - 1	—
Edema	0.1 - 1	—	—	≥ 1	0.1 - 1	0.1 - 1	0.1 - 1
Fever	2	≥ 1	2 - 5	—	—	0.1 - 1	0.1 - 1
Flu syndrome	0.1 - 1	5	3 - 12	3	5 - 6	6 - 8	—
Malaise	—	0.1 - 1	0.1 - 1	≥ 1	0.1 - 1	0.1 - 1	< 1 - 10
Pain	—	—	3 - 9	—	—	3	1 - 6
Weight gain	≥ 1	≥ 1	≥ 1	≥ 1	≥ 1	1 - 3	≥ 1
Weight loss	≥ 1	0.1 - 1	2 - 3	≥ 1	0.1 - 1	1	0.1 - 1

[a] Data are pooled from different studies and are not necessarily comparable.

Dose dependency of adverse reactions – A comparison of adverse event rates in a fixed-dose study comparing **paroxetine** 10, 20, 30, and 40 mg/day with placebo revealed a clear dose dependency for some of the more common adverse events associated with paroxetine use.

	Adverse Reactions by Indications of Fluoxetine							
	Depression		OCD		Bulimia		Panic disorder	
Adverse reaction	Fluoxetine (n = 1728)	Placebo (n = 975)	Fluoxetine (n = 266)	Placebo (n = 89)	Fluoxetine (n = 450)	Placebo (n = 267)	Fluoxetine (n = 425)	Placebo (n = 342
CNS								
Abnormal dreams	1	1	5	2	5	3	1	1
Anxiety	12	7	14	7	15	9	6	2
Insomnia	16	9	28	22	33	13	10	7
Libido decreased	3	< 1	11	2	5	1	1	2
Nervousness	14	9	14	15	11	5	8	6

Selective Serotonin Reuptake Inhibitors

Adverse Reactions by Indications of Fluoxetine

Adverse reaction	Depression		OCD		Bulimia		Panic disorder	
	Fluoxetine (n = 1728)	Placebo (n = 975)	Fluoxetine (n = 266)	Placebo (n = 89)	Fluoxetine (n = 450)	Placebo (n = 267)	Fluoxetine (n = 425)	Placebo (n = 342
Somnolence	13	6	17	7	13	5	5	2
Tremor	10	3	9	1	13	1	3	1
Dermatologic								
Rash	4	3	6	3	4	4	2	2
Sweating	8	3	7	< 1	8	3	2	2
GI								
Anorexia	11	2	17	10	8	4	4	1
Diarrhea	12	8	18	13	8	6	9	4
Dry mouth	10	7	12	3	9	6	4	4
Dyspepsia	7	5	10	4	10	6	6	2
Nausea	21	9	26	13	29	11	12	7
GU								
Abnormal ejaculation	< 1	< 1	7	< 1	7	< 1	2	1
Impotence	2	< 1	< 1	< 1	7	< 1	1	< 1
Respiratory								
Pharyngitis	3	3	11	9	10	5	3	3
Sinusitis	1	4	5	2	6	4	2	3
Yawn	< 1	< 1	7	< 1	11	< 1	1	< 1
Miscellaneous								
Asthenia	9	5	15	11	21	9	7	7
Flu syndrome	3	4	10	7	8	3	5	5
Vasodilation	3	2	5	< 1	2	1	1	< 1

Adaptation to certain adverse events – Over a 4- to 6-week period, there was evidence of adaptation to some adverse events with continued therapy (eg, nausea, dizziness), but less to other effects (eg, dry mouth, somnolence, asthenia).

➤*Cardiovascular:*

Citalopram – Angina pectoris, bradycardia, cardiac failure, cerebrovascular accident, extrasystoles, MI, myocardial ischemia (0.1% to 1%); atrial fibrillation, bundle branch block, cardiac arrest, phlebitis, pulmonary embolism, transient ischemic attack (less than 0.1%); chest pain, torsade de pointes, ventricular arrhythmia, QT prolonged (postmarketing).

Escitalopram – Bradycardia, ECG abnormal, varicose vein (0.1% to 1%); atrial fibrillation, hypotension, MI, orthostatic hypotension, pulmonary embolism, QT prolongation, torsade de pointes, ventricular tachycardia (postmarketing).

Fluoxetine – Hemorrhage (at least 1%); angina pectoris, arrhythmia, CHF, hypotension, migraine, myocardial infarct, vascular headache (0.1% to 1%); atrial fibrillation, bradycardia, cerebral embolism, cerebral ischemia, cerebrovascular accident, extrasystoles, heart arrest, heart block, pallor, peripheral vascular disorder, phlebitis, shock, thrombophlebitis, thrombosis, vasospasm, ventricular arrhythmia, ventricular extrasystoles, ventricular fibrillation (less than 0.1%); atrial fibrillation, cerebrovascular accident, heart arrest, pulmonary embolism, pulmonary hypertension, QT prolongation, ventricular tachycardia (including torsade de pointes) (postmarketing).

Fluvoxamine – Angina pectoris, bradycardia, cardiomyopathy, cardiovascular disease, cold extremities, conduction delay, heart failure, MI, pallor, pulse irregular, ST segment changes (0.1% to 1%); AV block, cerebrovascular accident, coronary artery disease, embolus, pericarditis, phlebitis, pulmonary infarction, supraventricular extrasystoles (less than 0.1%); ventricular tachycardia (including torsade de pointes) (postmarketing).

Paroxetine and paroxetine CR – Bradycardia, hematoma, hypotension, supraventricular tachycardia, syncope (0.1% to 1%); angina pectoris, arrhythmia nodal, atrial fibrillation, bundle branch block, cardiospasm, cerebral ischemia, cerebrovascular accident, CHF, heart block, low cardiac output, MI, myocardial ischemia, pallor, phlebitis, pulmonary embolus, supraventricular/ventricular extrasystoles, thrombophlebitis, thrombosis, vascular headache (less than 0.1%); pulmonary hypertension, ventricular fibrillation, ventricular tachycardia (including torsade de pointes) (postmarketing).

Sertraline – Edema (dependent, general, periorbital, peripheral), hypotension, peripheral ischemia, postural dizziness (0.1% to 1%); aggravated hypertension, cerebrovascular disorder, MI, precordial/substernal chest pain (less than 0.1%); atrial arrhythmias, AV block, bradycardia, pulmonary hypertension, QT prolongation, ventricular tachycardia (including torsade de pointes-type arrhythmias) (postmarketing).

➤*CNS:*

Citalopram – Aggravated depression, increased appetite, migraine, suicide attempt (at least 1%); abnormal gait, aggressive reaction, alcohol intolerance, ataxia, delusion, drug dependence, dystonia, euphoria, extrapyramidal disorder, hallucinations, increased libido, involuntary muscle contractions, leg cramps, neuralgia, panic reaction, paranoia, paranoid reaction, psychosis, psychotic depression, rigors (0.1% to 1%); abnormal coordination, catatonic reaction, hyperesthesia, melancholia, ptosis, stupor (less than 0.1%); choreoathetosis; delirium; dyskinesia;

neuroleptic malignant syndrome; serotonin syndrome; withdrawal syndrome; grand mal convulsions (postmarketing).

Escitalopram – Irritability, lethargy, lightheaded feeling, migraine (at least 1%); aggravated depression, aggravated restlessness, anxiety attack, auditory hallucination, bruxism, carbohydrate craving, carpal tunnel syndrome, coordination abnormal, crying abnormal, disorientation, dysequilibrium, excitability, faintness, feeling unreal, forgetfulness, hyperreflexia, jitteriness, panic reaction, restless legs, shaking, sluggishness, suicidal tendency, suicide attempt, tics, tremulousness nervous (0.1% to 1%); abnormal gait, aggression, dystonia, extrapyramidal disorders, grand mal seizures (or convulsions), neuroleptic malignant syndrome, seizures, serotonin syndrome, visual hallucinations (postmarketing).

Fluoxetine – Abnormal gait, acute brain syndrome, akathisia, apathy, ataxia, buccoglossal syndrome, CNS depression, euphoria, hallucinations, hostility, hyperkinesia, incoordination, increased libido, neuralgia, neuropathy, neurosis, paranoid reaction, personality disorder, psychosis, vertigo (0.1% to 1%); abnormal EEG, antisocial reaction, circumoral paresthesia, coma, delusions, dysarthria, dystonia, extrapyramidal syndrome, foot drop, hyperesthesia, neuritis, paralysis, reflexes decreased/increased, stupor, (less than 0.1%); confusion, dyskinesia, movement disorders, neuroleptic malignant syndrome-like events, suicidal ideation, violent behaviors, serotonin syndrome (postmarketing).

Fluvoxamine – Agoraphobia, akathisia, ataxia, CNS depression, convulsion, delirium, delusion, drug dependence, dyskinesia, dystonia, euphoria, extrapyramidal syndrome, gait unsteady, hallucinations, hemiplegia, hostility, hypersomnia, hypochondriasis, hypotonia, hysteria, incoordination, increased salivation, increased libido, neuralgia, paralysis, paranoid reaction, phobia, psychosis, stupor, twitching (0.1% to 1%); akinesia, coma, fibrillations, mutism, obsessions, reflexes decreased, slurred speech, tardive dyskinesia, torticollis, trismus, withdrawal syndrome (less than 0.1%); neuropathy, serotonin syndrome (postmarketing).

Paroxetine and paroxetine CR – Alcohol abuse, ataxia, dyskinesia, dystonia, euphoria, hallucinations, hostility, incoordination, increased libido, lack of emotion, manic reaction, migraine, neuralgia, neurosis, neuropathy, paralysis, paranoid reaction (0.1% to 1%); abnormal gait, akinesia, antisocial reaction, aphasia, choreoathetosis, circumoral paresthesias, coma, convulsion, delirium, delusions, diplopia, drug dependence, dysarthria, extrapyramidal syndrome, fasciculations, grand mal convulsion, hostility, hyperalgesia, hysteria, manic-depressive reaction, meningitis, myelitis, nystagmus, peripheral neuritis, psychosis, psychotic depression, reflexes decreased/increased, stupor, torticollis, trismus, withdrawal syndrome (less than 0.1%); akathisia; irritability; meningitis; myelitis; peripheral neuritis; psychosis; psychotic depression; reflexes decreased; reflexes increased; stupor; extrapyramidal symptoms (which have included akathisia, bradykinesia, cogwheel rigidity, dystonia, and hypertonia), Guillain-Barre syndrome, neuroleptic malignant syndrome-like events, serotonin syndrome associated in some cases with concomitant use of serotonergic drugs and with drugs that may have impaired paroxetine metabolism (symptoms included agitation, confusion, diaphoresis, hallucinations, hyperreflexia, myoclonus, shivering, tachycardia, and tremor), status epilepticus, tremor (postmarketing).

Sertraline – Abnormal coordination, abnormal gait, aggravated depression, aggressive reaction, ataxia, delusion, euphoria, hallucina-

Selective Serotonin Reuptake Inhibitors

tion, hyperesthesia, leg cramps, migraine, nystagmus, paranoid reaction, paroniria (0.1% to 1%); choreoarthrosis, coma, dyskinesia, dysphonia, hyporeflexia, hypotonia, illusion, libido increased, ptosis, somnambulism, suicidal ideation, withdrawal syndrome (less than 0.1%); extrapyramidal symptoms, neuroleptic malignant syndrome-like events, psychosis, serotonin syndrome (postmarketing).

➤*Dermatologic:*

Citalopram – Alopecia, dermatitis, dry skin, eczema, photosensitivity reaction, psoriasis, skin discoloration, urticaria (0.1% to 1%); cellulitis, decreased sweating, hypertrichosis, keratitis, melanosis, pruritus ani (less than 0.1%); angioedema, epidermal necrolysis, erythema multiforme (postmarketing).

Escitalopram – Alopecia, dermatitis, dry lips, dry skin, eczema, folliculitis, furunculosis, lipoma, skin nodule (0.1% to 1%); toxic epidermal necrolysis (postmarketing).

Fluoxetine – Alopecia, contact dermatitis, eczema, maculopapular rash, skin discoloration, skin ulcer, vesiculobullous rash (0.1% to 1%); furunculosis, herpes zoster, hirsutism, petechial rash, photosensitivity, psoriasis, purpuric rash, pustular rash, seborrhea (less than 0.1%); epidermal necrolysis, erythema nodosum, exfoliative dermatitis, Stevens-Johnson syndrome (postmarketing).

Fluvoxamine – Alopecia, dry skin, eczema, exfoliative dermatitis, furunculosis, photosensitivity, seborrhea, skin discoloration, urticaria (0.1% to 1%); bullous eruption, Henoch-Schöenlein purpura, Stevens-Johnson syndrome, toxic epidermal necrolysis, porphyria (postmarketing).

Paroxetine and paroxetine CR – Acne, alopecia, contact dermatitis, dry skin, ecchymosis, eczema, herpes simplex, photosensitivity, urticaria (0.1% to 1%); angioedema, erythema multiforme, erythema nodosum, exfoliative dermatitis, fungal dermatitis, furunculosis, herpes zoster, hirsutism, maculopapular rash, pustular rash, seborrhea, skin discoloration, skin hypertrophy, skin ulcer, vesiculobullous rash, ecchymosis, skin hypertrophy, sweating decreased (less than 0.1%); toxic epidermal necrolysis (postmarketing).

Sertraline – Alopecia, cold clammy skin, dry skin, erythematous rash, maculopapular rash, photosensitivity, urticaria (0.1% to 1%); bullous eruption, contact dermatitis, dermatitis, eczema, hypertrichosis, follicular rash, pustular rash, skin discoloration (less than 0.1%); severe skin reactions that potentially can be fatal, such as Stevens-Johnson syndrome, vasculitis, photosensitivity, and other severe cutaneous disorders (postmarketing).

➤*GI:*

Citalopram – Increased saliva (at least 1%); eructation, esophagitis, gastritis, gingivitis, hemorrhoids, stomatitis, teeth grinding, thirst (0.1% to 1%); cholecystitis, cholelithiasis, colitis, diverticulitis, duodenal ulcer, gastric ulcer, gastroesophageal reflux, glossitis, hiccoughs, jaundice, rectal hemorrhage (less than 0.1%); GI hemorrhage, pancreatitis (postmarketing).

Escitalopram – Abdominal cramp, heartburn (at least 1%); abdominal discomfort, belching, bloating, gagging, gastritis, gastroesophageal reflux, hemorrhoids, increased stool frequency, polyposis gastric, swallowing difficulty (0.1% to 1%); GI hemorrhage, pancreatitis (postmarketing).

Fluoxetine – Abnormal liver function tests, aphthous stomatitis, cholelithiasis, colitis, eructation, esophagitis, gastritis, glossitis, gum hemorrhage, hyperchlorhydria, increased salivation, melena, mouth ulceration, stomach ulcer/hemorrhage, stomatitis, thirst (0.1% to 1%); biliary pain, bloody diarrhea, cholecystitis, duodenal ulcer, enteritis, esophageal ulcer, fecal incontinence, GI hemorrhage, hematemesis, hemorrhage of colon, hepatitis, intestinal obstruction, liver fatty deposit, pancreatitis, peptic ulcer, rectal hemorrhage, salivary gland enlargement, tongue edema (less than 0.1%).

Fluvoxamine – Colitis, eructation, esophagitis, gastritis, GI hemorrhage, GI ulcer, gingivitis, glossitis, hemorrhoids, melena, rectal hemorrhage, stomatitis (0.1% to 1%); biliary pain, cholecystitis, cholelithiasis, fecal incontinence, hematemesis, intestinal obstruction, jaundice (less than 0.1%).

Paroxetine and paroxetine CR – Abnormal liver function tests, bruxism, colitis, dysphagia, eructation, gastritis, gastroesophageal reflux, gingivitis, glossitis, hemorrhoids, increased salivation, pancreatitis, rectal hemorrhage, ulcerative stomatitis (0.1% to 1%); aphthous stomatitis, bloody diarrhea, bulimia, cholelithiasis, duodenitis, enteritis, esophagitis, fecal impaction/incontinence, gum hemorrhage/hyperplasia, hematemesis, hepatitis, hepatosplenomegaly, ileitis, ileus, intestinal obstruction, jaundice, melena, mouth ulceration, peptic ulcer, salivary gland enlargement, stomach ulcer, stomatitis, throat tightness, tongue discoloration, tongue edema, sialadenitis (less than 0.1%).

Sertraline – Eructation, esophagitis, increased saliva, teeth grinding, (0.1% to 1%); aphthous stomatitis, colitis, diverticulitis, fecal incontinence, gastritis, glossitis, gum hyperplasia, hemorrhagic peptic ulcer, hiccough, melena, proctitis, rectal hemorrhage, stomatitis, tenesmus, tongue edema/ulceration, ulcerative stomatitis (less than 0.1%).

➤*GU:*

Citalopram – Dysmenorrhea (3%); amenorrhea, polyuria (at least 1%); breast enlargement, breast pain, dysuria, galactorrhea, micturition frequency, urinary incontinence, vaginal hemorrhage (0.1% to 1%); facial edema, hematuria, oliguria, pyelonephritis, renal calculus, renal pain (less than 0.1%); priapism, spontaneous abortion, acute renal failure (postmarketing).

Escitalopram – Menstrual cramps (at least 1%); blood in urine, breast neoplasm, dysuria, kidney stone, menorrhagia, pelvic inflammation, premenstrual syndrome, spotting between menses, urinary urgency (0.1% to 1%); acute renal failure (postmarketing).

Fluoxetine – Abortion, albuminuria, amenorrhea, breast enlargement, breast pain, cystitis, dysuria, female lactation, fibrocystic breast, hematuria, leukorrhea, menorrhagia, metrorrhagia, nocturia, polyuria, urinary incontinence/urgency, vaginal hemorrhage (0.1% to 1%); breast engorgement, hypomenorrhea, glycosuria, kidney pain, oliguria, priapism, uterine fibroids enlarged, uterine hemorrhage (less than 0.1%); gynecomastia, kidney failure, priapism, vaginal bleeding after drug withdrawal (postmarketing).

Fluvoxamine – Anuria, breast pain, cystitis, delayed menstruation, dysuria, female lactation, hematuria, menopause, menorrhagia, metrorrhagia, nocturia, polyuria, premenstrual syndrome, urinary incontinence/urgency, urination impaired, vaginal hemorrhage, vaginitis (0.1% to 1%); hematospermia, kidney calculus, oliguria (less than 0.1%); priapism (postmarketing).

Paroxetine and paroxetine CR – Dysmenorrhea (at least 1%); albuminuria, amenorrhea, breast pain, cystitis, dysuria, hematuria, menorrhagia, nocturia, polyuria, prostate disorder, prostatitis, pyuria, urinary incontinence/retention/urgency, vaginitis (0.1% to 1%); abortion, breast atrophy/enlargement/neoplasm, ejaculatory disturbance, endometrial disorder; epididymitis, female lactation, fibrocystic breast, kidney calculus, kidney pain, leukorrhea, mastitis, metrorrhagia, nephritis, oliguria, pregnancy and puerperal disorders, salpingitis, urethritis, urinary casts, urolith, uterine fibroids enlarged, uterine spasm, urethritis, vaginal hemorrhage, vaginal moniliasis (less than 0.1%); acute renal failure, priapism (postmarketing).

Sertraline – Amenorrhea, dysmenorrhea, dysuria, intermenstrual bleeding, leukorrhea, nocturia, polyuria, urinary incontinence, vaginal hemorrhage (0.1% to 1%); acute female mastitis, atrophic vaginitis, balanoposthitis, breast enlargement, cystitis, female breast pain, gynecomastia, hematuria, libido increased, menorrhagia, oliguria, priapism, pyelonephritis, renal pain, strangury (less than 0.1%); acute renal failure (postmarketing).

➤*Musculoskeletal:*

Citalopram – Arthritis, muscle weakness, skeletal pain (0.1% to 1%); bursitis, osteoporosis (less than 0.1%).

Escitalopram – Neck/Shoulder pain (3%); arthritis, arthropathy, back discomfort, jaw pain, jaw stiffness, joint stiffness, muscle contractions involuntary, muscle cramp, muscle stiffness, muscle weakness, muscular tone increased (0.1% to 1%).

Fluoxetine – Arthritis, bone pain, bursitis, leg cramps, tenosynovitis (0.1% to 1%); arthrosis, chondrodystrophy, myositis, osteomyelitis, osteoporosis, rheumatoid arthritis (less than 0.1%).

Fluvoxamine – Arthritis, bursitis, generalized muscle spasm, tendinous contracture, tenosynovitis (0.1% to 1%); arthrosis, pathological fracture (less than 0.1%).

Paroxetine and paroxetine CR – Arthritis, arthrosis, tendonitis (0.1% to 1%); bursitis, generalized spasm, myositis, osteoporosis, tenosynovitis, tetany (less than 0.1%).

Sertraline – Arthrosis, dystonia, muscle cramps/weakness (0.1% to 1%).

➤*Respiratory:*

Citalopram – Pneumonia (0.1% to 1%); asthma, bronchospasm, laryngitis, pneumonitis, sputum increased (less than 0.1%).

Escitalopram – Nasal congestion, sinus congestion, sinus headache (at least 1%); asthma, breath shortness, laryngitis, pneumonia, tracheitis (0.1% to 1%).

Fluoxetine – Asthma, epistaxis, hiccoughs, hyperventilation (0.1% to 1%); apnea, atelectasis, cough decreased, emphysema, hemoptysis, hypoventilation, hypoxia, laryngeal edema, lung edema, pneumothorax, stridor (less than 0.1%); eosinophilic pneumonia (postmarketing).

Fluvoxamine – Asthma, epistaxis, hoarseness, hyperventilation (0.1% to 1%); apnea, congestion of upper airway, hemoptysis, hiccoughs, laryngismus, obstructive pulmonary disease, pneumonia (less than 0.1%).

Paroxetine and paroxetine CR – Asthma, epistaxis, hyperventilation, laryngitis, pneumonia, respiratory flu (0.1% to 1%); dysphonia; emphysema, hemoptysis, hiccoughs, lung fibrosis, pulmonary edema, sputum increased, stridor, voice alterations (less than 0.1%).

Sertraline – Bronchospasm, epistaxis (0.1% to 1%); apnea, bradypnea, hemoptysis, hyperventilation, hypoventilation, laryngismus, laryngitis, stridor (less than 0.1%).

Selective Serotonin Reuptake Inhibitors

►*Special senses:*

Citalopram – Conjunctivitis, dry eyes, eye pain (0.1% to 1%); abnormal lacrimation, cataract, diplopia, mydriasis, photophobia, taste loss (less than 0.1%); nystagmus (postmarketing).

Escitalopram – Conjunctivitis, dry eyes, earache, eye infection, eye irritation, metallic taste, pupils dilated, vision abnormal, visual disturbance (0.1% to 1%); diplopia (postmarketing).

Fluoxetine – Ear pain (at least 1%); conjunctivitis, dry eyes, mydriasis, photophobia (0.1% to 1%); blepharitis, deafness, diplopia, exophthalmos, eye hemorrhage, glaucoma, hyperacusis, iritis, parosmia, scleritis, strabismus, taste loss, visual field defect (less than 0.1%); cataract, optic neuritis (postmarketing).

Fluvoxamine – Abnormal accommodation, conjunctivitis, deafness, diplopia, dry eyes, ear pain, eye pain, mydriasis, otitis media, parosmia, photophobia, taste loss, visual field defect (0.1% to 1%); corneal ulcer, retinal detachment (less than 0.1%).

Paroxetine and paroxetine CR – Abnormal accommodation, conjunctivitis, ear ache/pain, eye pain, keratoconjunctivitis, mydriasis, otitis media, (0.1% to 1%); amblyopia, anisocoria, blepharitis, cataract, conjunctival edema, corneal ulcer, deafness, exophthalmos, eye hemorrhage, glaucoma, hyperacusis, night blindness, otitis externa, parosmia, photophobia, ptosis, retinal hemorrhage, taste loss, visual field defect (less than 0.1%).

Sertraline – Abnormal accommodation, conjunctivitis, earache, eye pain, mydriasis (0.1% to 1%); abnormal lacrimation, diplopia, exophthalmos, glaucoma, hyperacusis, labyrinthine disorder, photophobia, scotoma, visual field defect, xerophthalmia (less than 0.1%) blindness, optic neuritis, cataract (postmarketing).

►*Miscellaneous:*

Citalopram – Abnormal glucose tolerance, anemia, epistaxis, increased alkaline phosphatase, increased hepatic enzymes, leukocytosis, leukopenia, lymphadenopathy, purpura (0.1% to 1%); bilirubinemia, coagulation disorder, dehydration, gingival bleeding, goiter, granulocytopenia, gynecomastia, hayfever; hepatitis, hypochromic anemia, hypoglycemia, hypokalemia, hypothyroidism, lymphocytosis, lymphopenia, obesity (less than 0.1%);akathisia, allergic reaction, anaphylaxis, ecchymosis, hemolytic anemia, hepatic necrosis, myoclonus, prolactinemia, prothrombin decreased, rhabdomyolysis, thrombocytopenia, thrombosis (postmarketing).

Escitalopram – Lethargy (3%); pain in limb (at least 1%); anaphylaxis, anemia, bilirubin increased, bruise, edema of extremities, fall, gout, hematoma, hepatic enzymes increased, hypercholesterolemia, hyperglycemia, leg pain, lymphadenopathy cervical, nosebleed, thirst, tightness of chest (0.1% to 1%); angioedema, hepatitis, rhabdomyolysis, SIADH, thrombocytopenia (postmarketing).

Fluoxetine – Anemia, dehydration, ecchymosis, facial edema, generalized edema, gout, hypercholesterolemia, hyperlipemia, hypokalemia, hypothyroidism, intentional overdose, pelvic pain, peripheral edema; suicide attempt (0.1% to 1%); abdominal syndrome acute, alcohol intolerance, alkaline phosphatase increased, ALT increased, blood dyscrasia, BUN increased, creatine phosphokinase increased, diabetic acidosis, diabetes mellitus, hyperkalemia, hyperuricemia, hypocalcemia, hypochromic anemia, hypothermia, intentional injury, iron deficiency anemia, leukopenia, lymphedema, lymphocytosis, neuroleptic malignant syndrome, petechiae, purpura, thrombocythemia, thrombocytopenia (less than 0.1%); aplastic anemia, cholestatic jaundice, hepatic failure/necrosis, hyperprolactinemia, immune-related hemolytic anemia, misuse/abuse, pancreatitis, pancytopenia, sudden unexpected death, thrombocytopenic purpura, hypoglycemia (postmarketing).

Fluvoxamine – Increased liver transaminase (at least 1%); anemia, dehydration, ecchymosis, hypercholesterolemia, hypothyroidism, leukocytosis, lymphadenopathy, neck pain/rigidity, overdose, suicide attempt, thrombocytopenia (0.1% to 1%); cyst, diabetes mellitus, goiter, hyperglycemia, hyperlipidemia, hypoglycemia, hypokalemia, lactate dehydrogenase increased, leukopenia, pelvic pain, purpura, sudden death (less than 0.1%); acute renal failure, agranulocytosis, anaphylactic reaction, aplastic anemia, hepatitis, hyponatremia, ileus, laryngismus, pancreatitis, vasculitis, angioedema (postmarketing).

Paroxetine and paroxetine CR – Trauma (6%); infection (5% to 6%); pain (at least 1%); anemia, AST/ALT increased, facial edema, flu syndrome, leukopenia, lymphadenopathy, moniliasis, neck pain, purpura, peripheral edema, thirst (0.1% to 1%); abnormal erythrocytes, abnormal lymphocytes, abscess, adrenergic syndrome, anisocytosis, anticholinergic syndrome, basophilia, bilirubinemia, bleeding time increased, BUN increased, cellulitis, creatine phosphokinase increased, dehydration, diabetes mellitus, eosinophilia, goiter, gout, hypercalcemia, hypercholesterolemia, hyperglycemia, hyperkalemia, hyperphosphatemia, hyperthyroidism, hypocalcemia, hypochromic anemia, hypoglycemia, hypokalemia, hyponatremia, hypothermia, hypothyroidism, increased alkaline phosphatase, increased lactic dehydrogenase, increased gamma globulins, iron deficiency anemia, ketosis, leukocytosis, lymphedema, lymphocytosis, lymphopenia, microcytic/normocytic anemia, monocytosis, neck rigidity, non-protein nitrogen increased, obesity, pelvic pain, peritonitis, sepsis, thrombocythemia, thrombocytopenia, thyroiditis, ulcer, varicose vein (less than 0.1%); acute pancreatitis,

allergic alveolitis, anaphylaxis, elevated liver function tests (the most severe cases were deaths because of liver necrosis and grossly elevated transaminases associated with severe liver dysfunction), events related to impaired hematopoiesis (including aplastic anemia, pancytopenia, bone marrow aplasia, and agranulocytosis), hemolytic anemia, laryngismus, myopathy, oculogyric crisis which has been associated with concomitant use of pimozide, optic neuritis, porphyria, symptoms suggestive of prolactinemia and galactorrhea, syndrome of inappropriate ADH secretion, vasculitis syndromes (such as Henoch-Schönlein purpura) (postmarketing).

Sertraline – Thirst (0.1% to 1%); abnormal hepatic function, anemia, anterior chamber eye hemorrhage, facial edema, hypoglycemia, pallor, rigors (less than 0.1%); anaphylactoid reaction, angioedema, agranulocytosis, aplastic anemia, galactorrhea, hyperglycemia, hyperprolactinemia, hypothyroidism, increased coagulation time, leukopenia; lupus-like syndrome, oculogyric crisis, pancreatitis, pancytopenia, serum sickness, thrombocytopenia, liver events including elevated enzymes, increased bilirubin, hepatomegaly, hepatitis, jaundice, abdominal pain, vomiting, liver failure, and death (postmarketing).

►*Lab test abnormalities:*

Sertraline – Asymptomatic elevations in serum transaminases (AST or ALT) have occurred infrequently (approximately 0.8%) in association with sertraline administration. These hepatic enzyme elevations usually occurred within the first 1 to 9 weeks of drug treatment and promptly diminished upon drug discontinuation.

Sertraline therapy was associated with small mean increases in total cholesterol (approximately 3%) and triglycerides (approximately 5%) and a small mean decrease in serum uric acid (approximately 7%) of no apparent clinical importance.

Overdosage

►*Symptoms:*

Citalopram – Although there were no reports of fatal citalopram overdose in clinical trials involving overdoses of up to 2,000 mg, postmarketing reports of drug overdoses involving citalopram have included 12 fatalities, 10 in combination with other drugs and/or alcohol, and 2 with citalopram alone (2,800 and 3,920 mg), as well as nonfatal overdoses of up to 6,000 mg. Symptoms most often accompanying citalopram overdose, alone or in combination with other drugs or alcohol, included dizziness, nausea, sinus tachycardia, somnolence, sweating, tremor, and vomiting. In more rare cases, observed symptoms included amnesia, coma, confusion, convulsions, cyanosis, hyperventilation, rhabdomyolysis, and ECG changes (including nodal rhythm, QT_c prolongation, ventricular arrhythmia, and 1 possible case of torsade de pointes).

Escitalopram – There have been reports of escitalopram overdose involving doses of up to 600 mg. All patients recovered and no symptoms associated with the overdoses were reported.

Fluoxetine – Of the 1578 cases of overdose involving fluoxetine, alone or with other drugs, there were 195 deaths. Among 633 adult patients who overdosed on fluoxetine alone, 34 resulted in a fatal outcome, 378 completely recovered, and 15 patients experienced sequelae after overdose, including abnormal accommodation, abnormal gait, confusion, unresponsiveness, nervousness, pulmonary dysfunction, vertigo, tremor, elevated blood pressure, impotence, movement disorder, and hypomania. The remaining 206 patients had an unknown outcome. The most common signs and symptoms associated with nonfatal overdosage were seizures, somnolence, nausea, tachycardia, and vomiting. The largest known ingestion of fluoxetine in adult patients was 8 g in a patient who took fluoxetine alone and who subsequently recovered. However, in an adult patient who took fluoxetine alone, an ingestion as low as 520 mg has been associated with lethal outcome, but causality has not been established.

Among pediatric patients (3 months to 17 years of age), there were 156 cases of overdose involving fluoxetine alone or in combination with other drugs. Six patients died, 127 patients completely recovered, 1 patient experienced renal failure, and 22 patients had an unknown outcome. One of the 6 fatalities was a boy 9 years of age who had a history of OCD, Tourette syndrome with tics, attention deficit disorder, and fetal alcohol syndrome. He had been receiving 100 mg fluoxetine daily for 6 months in addition to clonidine, methylphenidate, and promethazine. Mixed-drug ingestion or other methods of suicide complicated all 6 overdoses in children that resulted in fatalities. The largest ingestion in a pediatric patient was 3 g, which was nonlethal.

Other important adverse events reported with fluoxetine overdose (single or multiple drugs) include coma, delirium, ECG abnormalities (such as QT interval prolongation and ventricular tachycardia, including torsade de pointes-type arrhythmias), hypotension, mania, neuroleptic malignant syndrome-like events, pyrexia, stupor, and syncope.

Fluvoxamine – Of the 462 cases of deliberate or accidental overdose involving fluvoxamine, there were 44 deaths. Of these, 6 were in patients taking fluvoxamine alone and the remaining 38 were in patients taking fluvoxamine along with other drugs. Among nonfatal overdose cases, 373 patients had complete recovery; 4 patients experienced adverse sequelae of overdosage, including persistent mydriasis, unsteady gait, kidney complications (from trauma associated with overdose), and bowel infarction requiring a hemicolectomy. In the remaining 41 patients, the outcome was unknown. The largest known ingestion of fluvoxamine involved 12,000 mg (equivalent of 2 to 3 months' dosage). The patient fully recovered. However, ingestion as low as 1,400 mg have been associated with lethal outcome, indicating considerable prognostic variability.

Commonly (at least 5%) observed adverse events associated with fluvoxamine overdose include coma, hypokalemia, hypotension, nausea, respiratory difficulties, somnolence, tachycardia, and vomiting. Other notable signs and symptoms seen with fluvoxamine overdose (single or multiple drugs) included bradycardia, ECG abnormalities (such as heart arrest, QT interval prolongation, first-degree atrioventricular block, bundle branch block, and junctional rhythm), convulsions, tremor, diarrhea, and increased reflexes.

Paroxetine – Since the introduction of paroxetine in the United States, 342 spontaneous cases of deliberate or accidental overdosage during paroxetine treatment have been reported worldwide. These include overdoses with paroxetine alone and in combination with other substances. Of these, 48 cases were fatal and of the fatalities, 17 appeared to involve paroxetine alone. Eight fatal cases that documented the amount of paroxetine ingested were generally confounded by the ingestion of other drugs or alcohol or the presence of significant comorbid conditions. Of 145 nonfatal cases with known outcome, most recovered without sequelae. The largest known ingestion involved 2,000 mg paroxetine (33 times the maximum recommended daily dose) in a patient who recovered. Commonly reported adverse events associated with paroxetine overdosage include coma, confusion, dizziness, nausea, somnolence, tachycardia, tremor, and vomiting. Other notable signs and symptoms observed with overdoses involving paroxetine (alone or with other substances) include acute renal failure, aggressive reactions, bradycardia, convulsions (including status epilepticus), dystonia, hypertension, hypotension, manic reactions, mydriasis, myoclonus, rhabdomyolysis, serotonin syndrome, stupor, symptoms of hepatic dysfunction (including hepatic failure, hepatic necrosis, jaundice, hepatitis, and hepatic steatosis), syncope, urinary retention, and ventricular dysrhythmias (including torsade de pointes).

Sertraline – Of 1027 cases of overdose involving sertraline worldwide, alone or with other drugs, there were 72 deaths.

Among 634 overdoses in which sertraline was the only drug ingested, 8 resulted in fatal outcome, 75 completely recovered, and 27 patients experienced sequelae after overdosage to include alopecia, decreased libido, diarrhea, ejaculation disorder, fatigue, insomnia, serotonin syndrome, and somnolence. The remaining 524 cases had an unknown outcome. The most common signs and symptoms associated with nonfatal sertraline overdosage were agitation, dizziness, nausea, somnolence, tachycardia, tremor, and vomiting.

The largest known ingestion was 13.5 g in a patient who took sertraline alone and subsequently recovered. However, another patient who took 2.5 g sertraline alone experienced a fatal outcome.

Other important adverse events reported with sertraline overdose (single or multiple drugs) include bradycardia, bundle branch block, coma, convulsions, delirium, hallucinations, hypertension, hypotension, manic reactions, pancreatitis, QT interval prolongation, serotonin syndrome, stupor, and syncope.

➤*Treatment:* There are no specific antidotes. Establish and maintain an airway; ensure adequate oxygenation and ventilation. Activated charcoal, which may be used with sorbitol, may be as or more effective than emesis or lavage.

Monitor cardiac and vital signs along with general symptomatic and supportive measures. SSRI-induced seizures that fail to respond spontaneously may respond to diazepam.

Because of the large volume of distribution of SSRIs, forced diuresis, dialysis, hemoperfusion, and exchange transfusion are unlikely to be of benefit.

Treatment includes usual supportive measures. Refer to General Management of Acute Overdosage.

During overdose management, consider the possibility that multiple medications were ingested. Consider contacting a poison control center for advice.

Patient Information

➤*Hazardous tasks:* Any psychoactive drug may impair judgment, thinking, or motor skills; caution patients about operating hazardous machinery, including automobiles, until they are reasonably certain that the drug treatment does not affect them adversely.

➤*Alcohol:* Although SSRIs have not been shown to increase the impairment of mental and motor skills caused by alcohol, advise patients to avoid alcohol during therapy.

➤*Concomitant medication:* Advise patients to consult their physician or pharmacist before taking concomitant OTC, prescription, or alternative medicinal drugs (see Drug Interactions). Instruct patients to avoid alcohol or other depressant medications.

Caution patients about the concomitant use of SSRIs and NSAIDs, aspirin, or other drugs that affect coagulation because the combined use of psychotropic drugs that interfere with serotonin reuptake and these agents has been associated with an increased risk of bleeding.

➤*Pregnancy or lactation:* Women should notify their physician if they are pregnant, intend to become pregnant, or are breastfeeding.

➤*Rash:* Advise patients to notify their physician if rash, hives, or a related allergic phenomenon develops.

➤*Completing course of therapy:* While patients may notice improvement in 1 to 4 weeks, advise patients to continue therapy as directed.

➤*Photosensitivity:* May cause photosensitivity (sensitivity to sunlight). Instruct patients to avoid prolonged exposure to the sun and other ultraviolet light and to use sunscreens and wear protective clothing until tolerance is determined.

➤*Emergence of adverse reactions:* Encourage patients and their families to be alert to the emergence of akathisia, anxiety, agitation, hostility, hypomania, impulsivity, insomnia, irritability, mania, panic attacks, suicidal ideation, and worsening of depression, especially early during antidepressant treatment. Such symptoms should be reported to the patient's physician, especially if they are severe, abrupt in onset, or were not part of the patient's presenting symptoms.

➤*Controlled-release tablet:* Instruct patients to swallow **paroxetine** CR whole and not to chew or crush.

➤*Citalopram/escitalopram:* Advise patients that **escitalopram** is the active isomer of **citalopram** and that the 2 medications should not be taken concomitantly.

➤*Disulfiram:* Advise patients taking disulfiram not to take concomitant paroxetine oral concentrate because of the alcohol content of the concentrate.

CITALOPRAM HBr

Rx	**Celexa** (Forest)	**Tablets:** 10 mg (as base)	Lactose. (FP 10 mg). Beige, oval. Film-coated. In 100s.
		20 mg (as base)	Lactose. (F P 20 mg). Pink, oval, scored. Film-coated. In 100s and UD 100s.
		40 mg (as base)	Lactose. (F P 40 mg). White, oval, scored. Film-coated. In 100s and UD 100s.
		Solution, oral: 10 mg (as base) per 5 mL	Sorbitol, parabens. Peppermint flavor. In 240 mL.

For complete prescribing information, refer to the SSRIs group monograph.

Indications

➤*Depression:* For the treatment of depression as defined in the DSM-III and DSM-III-R category of major depressive disorder.

➤*Unlabeled uses:* Panic disorder; premenstrual dysphoria (as intermittent administration); posttraumatic stress disorder; generalized anxiety disorder.

Administration and Dosage

➤*Approved by the FDA:* July 24, 1998.

➤*Initial therapy:* 20 mg once daily, generally with an increase to a dose of 40 mg/day. Dose increases usually should occur in increments of 20 mg at intervals of no less than 1 week. Doses greater than 40 mg/day are not ordinarily recommended. Administer once daily in the morning or evening, with or without food. Although certain patients may require a dose of 60 mg/day, the only study pertinent to dose response for effectiveness did not demonstrate an advantage for the 60 mg/day dose over the 40 mg/day dose.

➤*Maintenance therapy:* Antidepressant efficacy was maintained in clinical trials for periods of up to 24 weeks following 6 or 8 weeks of initial treatment (32 weeks total). Periodically re-evaluate the long-term usefulness of the drug for the individual patient if citalopram is used for extended periods.

➤*Elderly/Hepatic function impairment:* 20 mg/day is the recommended dose for most elderly patients and patients with hepatic impairment, with titration to 40 mg/day only for nonresponding patients.

➤*Renal function impairment:* Use with caution in patients with severe renal impairment; however, no dosage adjustment is necessary for patients with mild or moderate renal impairment.

➤*Pregnancy:* Neonates exposed to citalopram and other SSRIs or serotonin-norepinephrine reuptake inhibitors (SNRIs) late in the third trimester have developed complications requiring prolonged hospitalization, respiratory support, and tube feeding. When treating pregnant women with citalopram during the third trimester, the physician should carefully consider the potential risks and benefits of treatment. The physician may consider tapering citalopram in the third trimester.

Selective Serotonin Reuptake Inhibitors

CITALOPRAM HBr

➤*Discontinuation of treatment:* Symptoms associated with discontinuation of citalopram and other SSRIs and SNRIs have been reported. Monitor patients for symptoms (eg, dysphoric mood, irritability, agitation, dizziness, sensory disturbances, anxiety, confusion, headache, lethargy, emotional lability, hypomania) when discontinuing treatment. A gradual reduction in the dose rather than abrupt cessation is recommended whenever possible. If intolerable symptoms occur following a decrease in the dose or upon discontinuation of treatment, then resuming the previously prescribed dose may be considered. Sub-sequently, the physician may continue decreasing the dose but at a more gradual rate.

➤*Switching to or from a monoamine oxidase inhibitor (MAOI):* Allow at least 14 days to elapse between discontinuation of an MAOI and initiation of citalopram. Similarly, allow at least 14 days after stopping citalopram before starting an MAOI.

➤*Storage/Stability:* Store at 25°C (77°F); excursions permitted to 15° to 30°C (59° to 86°F).

ESCITALOPRAM OXALATE

Rx	Lexapro (Forest)	**Tablets:** 5 mg (as base)	Talc. (FL 5). White to off-white. Film-coated. In 100s.
		10 mg (as base)	Talc. (F L 10). White to off-white, scored. Film-coated. In 100s and UD 100s.
		20 mg (as base)	Talc. (F L 20). White to off-white, scored. Film-coated. In 100s and UD 100s.
		Solution, oral: 5 mg (as base) per 5 mL	Sorbitol, parabens. Peppermint flavor. In 240 mL.

For complete prescribing information, refer to the SSRIs group monograph.

Indications

➤*Generalized anxiety disorder (GAD):* For the treatment of GAD.

➤*Major depressive disorder:* For the treatment of major depressive disorder as defined in the DSM-IV.

➤*Unlabeled uses:* Panic disorder.

Administration and Dosage

➤*Approved by the FDA:* August 14, 2002.

Administer once daily in the morning or evening, with or without food.

➤*GAD:*

Initial therapy – 10 mg once daily. If the dose is increased to 20 mg, this should occur after a minimum of 1 week.

Maintenance therapy – GAD is recognized as a chronic condition. The efficacy of escitalopram in the treatment of GAD beyond 8 weeks has not been systematically studied. The physician who elects to use escitalopram for extended periods should periodically reevaluate the long-term usefulness of the drug for the individual patient.

➤*Major depressive disorder:*

Initial therapy – 10 mg once daily. A fixed dose trial of escitalopram demonstrated the effectiveness of 10 and 20 mg but failed to demonstrate a greater benefit of 20 mg over 10 mg. If the dose is increased to 20 mg, this should occur after a minimum of 1 week.

Maintenance therapy – Antidepressant efficacy was maintained on 10 or 20 mg/day in clinical trials for periods of up to 36 weeks following 8 weeks of initial treatment. Periodically reassess to determine the need for maintenance treatment.

➤*Elderly/Hepatic function impairment:* 10 mg/day is the recommended dose for most elderly patients and patients with hepatic impairment.

➤*Renal function impairment:* Use with caution in patients with severe renal impairment; no dosage adjustment is necessary for patients with mild or moderate renal impairment.

➤*Pregnancy:* Neonates exposed to escitalopram and other SSRIs or serotonin-norepinephrine reuptake inhibitors (SNRIs) late in the third trimester have developed complications requiring prolonged hospitalization, respiratory support, and tube feeding. When treating pregnant women with escitalopram during the third trimester, the physician should carefully consider the potential risks and benefits of treatment. The physician may consider tapering escitalopram in the third trimester.

➤*Discontinuation of treatment:* Symptoms associated with discontinuation of escitalopram and other SSRIs and SNRIs have been reported. Monitor patients for these symptoms (eg, dysphoric mood, irritability, agitation, dizziness, sensory disturbances, anxiety, confusion, headache, lethargy, emotional lability, hypomania, insomnia) when discontinuing treatment. A gradual reduction in the dose rather than abrupt cessation is recommended whenever possible. If intolerable symptoms occur following a decrease in the dose or upon discontinuation of treatment, consider resuming the previously prescribed dose. Subsequently, the health care provider may continue decreasing the dose at a more gradual rate.

➤*Switching to or from a monoamine oxidase inhibitor (MAOI):* Allow at least 14 days to elapse between discontinuation of an MAOI and initiation of escitalopram therapy. Similarly, allow at least 14 days after stopping escitalopram before starting an MAOI.

➤*Storage/Stability:* Store at 25°C (77°F); excursions permitted to 15° to 30°C (59° to 86°F).

FLUOXETINE HCl

Rx	Fluoxetine HCl (Various, eg, Geneva, Ivax, Teva)	**Tablets:** 10 mg (as base)	In 30s, 100s, 500s, 1000s, 5000s, and UD 100s.
Rx	Prozac (Eli Lilly/Dista)		(PROZAC 10). Green, elliptical, scored. In 30s and 100s.
Rx	Fluoxetine HCl (Various, eg, Geneva)	**Tablets:** 20 mg (as base)	In 30s, 100s, and 1000s.
Rx	Fluoxetine HCl (Various, eg, Barr, Geneva, Ivax, Par, Teva)	**Capsules:** 10 mg (as base)	May contain parabens, EDTA, or lactose. In 100s, 1000s, 2000s, unit of use 30s, and UD 100s.
Rx	Prozac Pulvules (Eli Lilly/Dista)		(DISTA 3104 Prozac 10 mg). Green. In 100s, 2000s, and blister card 31s.
Rx	Sarafem Pulvules (Warner Chilcott)		(Sarafem 10 mg). Lavender. In blister 28s.
Rx	Fluoxetine HCl (Various, eg, Barr, Geneva, Ivax, Par, Teva)	**Capsules:** 20 mg (as base)	May contain parabens, EDTA, or lactose. In 30s, 100s, 1000s, 2000s, and unit of use 30s.
Rx	Prozac Pulvules (Eli Lilly/Dista)		(DISTA 3105 Prozac 20 mg). Green/Off-white. In 30s, 100s, 2000s, blister card 31s, and UD 100s.
Rx	Sarafem Pulvules (Warner Chilcott)		(Sarafem 20 mg). Pink/Lavender. In blister 28s.
Rx	Fluoxetine HCl (Various, eg, Geneva, Teva)	**Capsules:** 40 mg (as base)	In 30s and 100s.
Rx	Prozac Pulvules (Eli Lilly/Dista)		(DISTA 3107 Prozac 40 mg). Green/Orange. In 30s.
Rx	Prozac Weekly (Eli Lilly/Dista)	**Capsules, delayed-release:** 90 mg (as base)	Sucrose, sugar spheres. (Lilly 3004 90 mg). Green/Clear. Enteric-coated pellets. In blister 4s.
Rx	Fluoxetine HCl (Various, eg, Alpharma, Apotex, Geneva, Teva)	**Solution, oral:** 20 mg per 5 mL (as base)	May contain alcohol, sucrose. In 120 and 473 mL.
Rx	Prozac (Eli Lilly/Dista)		0.23% alcohol, sucrose. Mint flavor. In 120 mL.

For complete prescribing information, refer to the SSRIs group monograph.

Indications

➤*Bulimia nervosa:* For the treatment of binge-eating and vomiting behaviors in patients with moderate to severe bulimia nervosa.

➤*Major depressive disorder:* For the treatment of major depressive disorder as defined in the DSM-IV.

➤*Obsessive-compulsive disorder (OCD):* For the treatment of obsessions and compulsions in patients with OCD, as defined in the DSM-III-R.

➤*Panic disorder:* For the treatment of panic disorder, with or without agoraphobia, as defined in DSM-IV.

➤*Premenstrual dysphoric disorder (PMDD; Sarafem only):* For the treatment of PMDD.

FLUOXETINE HCl

➤*Unlabeled uses:* Posttraumatic stress disorder; Raynaud phenomenon (20 to 60 mg/day); generalized anxiety disorder (20 mg/day); hot flashes (20 mg/day); second-line prophylaxis of migraines (10 to 40 mg/day).

Administration and Dosage

➤*Approved by the FDA:* December 29, 1987.

➤*Bulimia nervosa:*
Initial – 60 mg/day administered in the morning. For some patients, it may be advisable to titrate up to this target dose over several days. Doses above 60 mg/day have not been systematically studied in patients with bulimia.

Maintenance – Patients have been continued on therapy for an additional 52 weeks after an initial 8 weeks of treatment without loss of benefit. Adjust dose to maintain patient on lowest effective dosage. Periodically reassess patients to determine need for continued treatment.

➤*Major depressive disorder:*
Initial –
Adult: 20 mg/day in the morning. Consider a dose increase after several weeks if insufficient clinical improvement is observed. Administer doses above 20 mg/day on a once- (morning) or twice- (eg, morning and noon) daily schedule. Do not exceed a maximum dose of 80 mg/day.
Children (8 to 18 years of age): Initiate treatment with a dose of 10 or 20 mg/day. After 1 week at 10 mg/day, increase the dose to 20 mg/day. However, because of higher plasma levels in lower weight children, the starting and target dose in this group may be 10 mg/day. A dose increase to 20 mg/day may be considered after several weeks if insufficient clinical improvement is observed.

The full antidepressant effect may be delayed until 4 weeks of treatment or longer.

Maintenance – Acute episodes of major depression generally require several months or longer of sustained pharmacologic therapy. Whether the dose of antidepressant needed to induce remission is identical to the dose needed to maintain and/or sustain euthymia is unknown.

Weekly dosing – Initiate *Prozac Weekly* 7 days after the last 20 mg daily dose. If satisfactory response is not maintained, consider re-establishing a daily dosing regimen.

➤*OCD:*
Initial –
Adults: 20 mg/day in the morning. Consider a dose increase after several weeks if insufficient clinical improvement is observed. The full therapeutic effect may be delayed until 5 weeks of treatment or longer. Administer doses above 20 mg/day on a once- (morning) or twice- (morning and noon) daily schedule. A dose range of 20 to 60 mg/day is recommended; however, doses of up to 80 mg/day have been well tolerated. Do not exceed 80 mg/day.
Children (8 to 18 years of age): In adolescents and higher weight children, initiate treatment with a dose of 10 mg/day. After 2 weeks, increase the dose to 20 mg/day. Additional dose increases may be considered after several more weeks if insufficient clinical improvement is observed. A dose range of 20 to 60 mg/day is recommended.

In lower weight children, initiate treatment with a dose of 10 mg/day. Additional dose increases may be considered after several more weeks if insufficient clinical improvement is observed. A dose range of 20 to 30 mg/day is recommended. Experience with daily doses greater than 20 mg is very minimal; there is no experience with doses greater than 60 mg.

Maintenance – OCD is a chronic condition, and it is reasonable to consider continuation for a responding patient. Patients have been continued on therapy for an additional 6 months after an initial 13 weeks of treatment without loss of benefit. Adjust dose to maintain patient on lowest effective dosage. Periodically reassess patient to determine need for continued treatment.

➤*Panic disorder:*
Initial – Initiate treatment with a dose of 10 mg/day. After 1 week, increase the dose to 20 mg/day. The most frequently administered dose in the 2 flexible-dose clinical trials was 20 mg/day. A dose increase may be considered after several weeks if no clinical improvement is observed. Fluoxetine doses above 60 mg/day have not been systematically evaluated in patients with panic disorder.

Maintenance – Panic disorder is a chronic condition and it is reasonable to consider continuation for a responding patient. Nevertheless, periodically reassess patients to determine the need for continued treatment.

➤*PMDD (Sarafem only):*
Initial – 20 mg/day given continuously (every day of the menstrual cycle) or intermittently (defined as starting a daily dose 14 days prior to the anticipated onset of menstruation through the first full day of menses and repeating with each new cycle). The dosing regimen should be determined by the physician based on individual patient characteristics. Do not exceed a maximum dose of 80 mg/day.

Maintenance/Continuation treatment – Systematic evaluation has shown that its efficacy is maintained for periods up to 6 months at a dose of 20 mg/day given continuously and up to 3 months at a dose of 20 mg/day given intermittently. Reassess patients periodically to determine the need for continued treatment.

➤*Hepatic function impairment:* Use lower or less frequent dosing.

➤*Special risk patients:* Consider lower or less frequent dosing for elderly patients, patients with concurrent diseases, or those who are taking multiple medications.

➤*Switching to a tricyclic antidepressant (TCA):* Dosage of TCA may need to be reduced, and plasma TCA concentrations may need to be monitored temporarily when fluoxetine is coadministered or has been recently discontinued.

➤*Switching to or from a monoamine oxidase inhibitor (MAOI):* At least 14 days should elapse between discontinuation of an MAOI and initiation of therapy with fluoxetine. In addition, allow at least 5 weeks, perhaps longer, after stopping fluoxetine before starting an MAOI.

➤*Thioridazine:* Do not administer thioridazine with fluoxetine or within a minimum of 5 weeks after fluoxetine has been discontinued.

➤*Storage/Stability:* Store at controlled room temperature 15° to 30°C (59° to 86°F). Protect from light.

FLUVOXAMINE MALEATE

Rx	Fluvoxamine Maleate (Various, eg, Ivax, Mylan)	Tablets: 25 mg	In 100s and 500s.
Rx	Fluvoxamine Maleate (Various, eg, Ivax, Mylan)	Tablets: 50 mg	In 100s, 500s, and 1000s.
Rx	Fluvoxamine Maleate (Various, eg, Ivax, Mylan)	Tablets: 100 mg	In 100s and 1000s.

For complete prescribing information, refer to the SSRIs group monograph.

Indications

➤*Obsessive-compulsive disorder (OCD):* For the treatment of obsessions and compulsions in patients with OCD, as defined in the DSM-III-R.

➤*Unlabeled uses:* Bulimia nervosa; depression; panic disorder; social phobia.

Administration and Dosage

➤*Approved by the FDA:* December 5, 1994.

➤*Adults:*
Initial – 50 mg as a single daily bedtime dose. In trials, patients were titrated within a range of 100 to 300 mg/day. Increase dose in 50 mg increments every 4 to 7 days, as tolerated, until maximum therapeutic benefit is achieved (not to exceed 300 mg/day). It is advisable to give total daily doses greater than 100 mg in 2 divided doses; if doses are unequal, give larger dose at bedtime.

➤*Children (8 to 17 years of age):*
Initial – 25 mg administered as a single daily dose at bedtime. Physicians should consider age and gender differences when dosing pediatric patients. The maximum dose in children up to 11 years of age should not exceed 200 mg/day. Therapeutic effect in female children may be achieved with lower doses. Dose adjustment in adolescents (up to the adult maximum dose of 300 mg) may be indicated to achieve therapeutic benefit. Increase the dose in 25 mg increments every 4 to 7 days as tolerated, until maximum therapeutic benefit is achieved. Divide total daily doses more than 50 mg into 2 doses. If the 2 divided doses are not equal, give the larger dose at bedtime.

➤*Maintenance:* OCD is a chronic condition, although efficacy has not been documented for beyond 10 weeks in controlled trials; it is reasonable to consider continuation for a responding patient. Adjust dose to maintain patient on lowest effective dosage. Periodically reassess patient to determine need for continued treatment.

➤*Elderly/Hepatic function impairment:* Decreased fluvoxamine clearance has been observed in these patients. It may be appropriate to modify initial dose and subsequent dose titration.

➤*Storage/Stability:* Store at controlled room temperature 15° to 30°C (59° to 86°F). Protect from high humidity and dispense in tight, light-resistant containers.

PAROXETINE HCl

Rx	**Paroxetine HCl** (Various, eg, Apotex, Par, Sandoz)	**Tablets**: 10 mg (as base)	In 30s, 100s, 1000s, and UD 100s.
Rx	**Paxil** (GlaxoSmithKline)		(PAXIL 10). Yellow, oval, scored. Film-coated. In 30s.
Rx	**Pexeva** (Synthon)		(POT 10). White, oval. In 30s.
Rx	**Paroxetine HCl** (Various, eg, Apotex, Par, Sandoz)	**Tablets**: 20 mg (as base)	In 30s, 100s, 1000s, and UD 100s.
Rx	**Paxil** (GlaxoSmithKline)		(PAXIL 20). Pink, oval, scored. Film-coated. In 30s, 100s, and SUP[a] 100s.
Rx	**Pexeva** (Synthon)		(POT 20). Dark orange, oval, scored. In 30s, 100s, and 500s.
Rx	**Paroxetine HCl** (Various, eg, Apotex, Par, Sandoz)	**Tablets**: 30 mg (as base)	In 30s, 100s, 1000s, and UD 100s.
Rx	**Paxil** (GlaxoSmithKline)		(PAXIL 30). Blue, oval. Film-coated. In 30s.
Rx	**Pexeva** (Synthon)		(POT 30). Yellow, oval. In 30s.
Rx	**Paroxetine HCl** (Various, eg, Apotex, Par, Sandoz)	**Tablets**: 40 mg (as base)	In 30s, 100s, 1000s, and UD 100s.
Rx	**Paxil** (GlaxoSmithKline)		(PAXIL 40). Green, oval. Film-coated. In 30s.
Rx	**Pexeva** (Synthon)		(POT 40). Rose, oval. In 30s.
Rx	**Paxil** (GlaxoSmithKline)	**Suspension, oral**: 10 mg (as base) per 5 mL	Parabens, saccharin, sorbitol. Orange flavor. In 250 mL.
Rx	**Paxil CR** (GlaxoSmithKline)	**Tablets, controlled-release**: 12.5 mg (as base)	Lactose. (Paxil CR 12.5). Yellow. Enteric-coated. In 30s and 100s.
		25 mg (as base)	Lactose. (Paxil CR 25). Pink. Enteric-coated. In 30s, 100s, and SUP[a] 100s.
		37.5 mg (as base)	Lactose. (Paxil CR 37.5). Blue. Enteric-coated. In 30s.

[a] SUP = Single unit packages. Intended for institutional use only.

For complete prescribing information, refer to the SSRIs group monograph.

Indications

►*Generalized anxiety disorder (GAD) (immediate-release; except Pexeva):* For the treatment of generalized anxiety disorder, as defined in the DSM-IV.

►*Major depressive disorder (immediate- and controlled-release):* For the treatment of major depressive disorder, as defined in the DSM-III or DSM-IV.

►*Obsessive-compulsive disorder (OCD) (immediate-release):* For the treatment of obsessions and compulsions in patients with OCD, as defined in the DSM-IV.

►*Panic disorder (immediate- and controlled-release):* For the treatment of panic disorder, with or without agoraphobia, as defined in the DSM-IV.

►*Posttraumatic stress disorder (PTSD) (immediate-release; except Pexeva):* For the treatment of PTSD, as defined in the DSM-IV.

►*Premenstrual dysphoric disorder (PMDD) (controlled-release):* For the treatment of PMDD, as defined in the DSM-IV.

►*Social anxiety disorder (immediate- and controlled-release; except Pexeva):* For the treatment of social anxiety disorder, also known as social phobia, as defined in the DSM-IV.

►*Unlabeled uses:* Hot flashes (20 mg/day or 12.5 to 25 mg/day controlled release); diabetic neuropathy.

Administration and Dosage

►*Approved by the FDA:* December 29, 1992.

Swallow controlled-release tablet whole; do not chew or crush.

►*GAD (immediate-release):*

Initial – 20 mg/day. Administer as a single daily dose with or without food, usually in the morning. Usual range is 20 to 50 mg/day. Change doses in 10 mg/day increments and at intervals of at least 1 week. There is not sufficient evidence to suggest a greater benefit to doses higher than 20 mg/day.

Maintenance – Continued therapy for up to 24 weeks has demonstrated a benefit of such maintenance. GAD is recognized as a chronic condition, and it is reasonable to consider continuation of treatment for a responding patient. Make dosage adjustments to maintain the patient on the lowest effective dosage, and periodically reassess patients to determine the need for continued treatment.

►*Major depressive disorder:*

Initial –

Immediate-release: 20 mg/day. Administer as a single daily dose with or without food, usually in the morning. Usual range is 20 to 50 mg/day. As with all drugs for the treatment of major depressive disorder, the full effect may be delayed. Some patients not responding to a 20 mg dose may benefit from dose increases in 10 mg/day increments up to a maximum of 50 mg/day. Change doses at intervals of at least 1 week.

Controlled-release: 25 mg/day. Administer as a single daily dose with or without food, usually in the morning. Usual range is 25 to 62.5 mg/day. As with all drugs for the treatment of major depressive disorder, the full effect may be delayed. Some patients not responding to a 25 mg dose may benefit from dose increases in 12.5 mg/day increments up to a

maximum of 62.5 mg/day. Change doses at intervals of at least 1 week. Swallow controlled-release tablet whole; do not chew or crush.

Maintenance – There is no body of evidence available concerning the duration of paroxetine therapy. It generally is agreed that acute episodes of major depressive disorder require several months or longer of sustained pharmacologic therapy. Whether the dose needed to induce remission is identical to the dose needed to maintain and/or sustain euthymia is unknown. Efficacy of immediate-release paroxetine has been maintained for periods of up to 1 year with doses that averaged approximately 30 mg, which corresponds to a 37.5 mg dose of controlled-release paroxetine based on relative bioavailability considerations.

►*OCD (immediate-release):*

Initial – 20 mg/day. Administer as a single daily dose with or without food, usually in the morning. May be increased in 10 mg/day increments. Change doses at intervals of at least 1 week. The recommended dose is 40 mg/day. Usual range is 20 to 60 mg/day. Do not exceed the maximum dosage of 60 mg/day.

Maintenance – Patients have been continued on therapy for 6 months. However, make dosage adjustments to maintain the patient on the lowest effective dosage, and periodically reassess the patient to determine the need for continued treatment. OCD is a chronic condition, and it is reasonable to consider continuation for a responding patient.

►*Panic disorder:*

Initial –

Immediate-release: 10 mg/day. Administer as a single daily dose with or without food, usually in the morning. May be increased in 10 mg/day increments. The target dose is 40 mg/day. Usual range is 10 to 60 mg/day. Do not exceed the maximum dosage of 60 mg/day. Change doses at intervals of at least 1 week.

Controlled-release: 12.5 mg/day. Administer as a single daily dose with or without food, usually in the morning. Usual range is 12.5 to 75 mg/day. Dose changes should occur in 12.5 mg/day increments. Change doses at intervals of at least 1 week. Do not exceed the maximum dosage of 75 mg/day. Swallow controlled-release tablet whole; do not chew or crush.

Maintenance – Long-term maintenance of efficacy with the immediate-release formulation has been demonstrated in a 3-month relapse prevention trial. In this trial, patients with panic disorder assigned to paroxetine demonstrated a lower relapse rate compared with patients on placebo. Make dosage adjustments to maintain the patient on the lowest effective dosage, and periodically reassess the patient to determine the need for continued treatment. Panic disorder is a chronic condition, and it is reasonable to consider continuation for a responding patient.

►*PMDD (controlled-release):*

Initial – 12.5 mg/day. Administer as a single daily dose with or without food, usually in the morning. Paroxetine CR may be administered either daily throughout the menstrual cycle or limited to the luteal phase of the menstrual cycle, depending on physician assessment. Usual range is 12.5 to 25 mg/day. Change doses at intervals of at least 1 week. Swallow controlled-release tablet whole; do not chew or crush.

Maintenance – The effectiveness for a period exceeding 3 menstrual cycles has not been systematically evaluated in controlled trials. Women commonly report that symptoms worsen with age until relieved by the onset of menopause. It is reasonable to consider continuation of

Selective Serotonin Reuptake Inhibitors

PAROXETINE HCl

treatment for a responding patient; periodically reassess patients to determine the need for continued treatment.

➤*PTSD (immediate-release):*

Initial – 20 mg/day. Administer as a single daily dose with or without food, usually in the morning. Usual range is 20 to 50 mg/day. There is not sufficient evidence to suggest a greater benefit for a dose of 40 mg/day compared with 20 mg/day. Change doses, if indicated, in 10 mg/day increments and at intervals of at least 1 week.

Maintenance – Although the efficacy beyond 12 weeks of dosing has not been demonstrated, PTSD is recognized as a chronic condition, and it is reasonable to consider continuation of treatment for a responding patient. Make dosage adjustments to maintain the patient on the lowest effective dosage, and periodically reassess patients to determine the need for continued treatment.

➤*Social anxiety disorder:*

Initial –

Immediate-release: 20 mg/day. Administer as a single daily dose with or without food, usually in the morning. Usual range is 20 to 60 mg/day. Available information does not suggest any additional benefit for doses above 20 mg/day.

Controlled-release: 12.5 mg/day. Administer as a single daily dose with or without food, usually in the morning. Usual range is 12.5 to 37.5 mg/day. If necessary, increase dose at intervals of at least 1 week, in increments of 12.5 mg/day up to a maximum of 37.5 mg/day. Swallow controlled-release tablets whole; do not chew or crush.

Maintenance – Although the efficacy beyond 12 weeks of dosing has not been demonstrated in controlled clinical trials, social anxiety disorder is recognized as a chronic condition, and it is reasonable to consider continuation of treatment for a responding patient. Make dosage adjustments to maintain the patient on the lowest effective dosage, and periodically reassess the patient to determine the need for continued treatment.

➤*Pregnancy:* Neonates exposed to paroxetine and other SSRIs or selective-norepinephrine reuptake inhibitors (SNRIs) late in the third trimester have developed complications requiring prolonged hospitalization, respiratory support, and tube feeding. When treating pregnant women with paroxetine during the third trimester, the physician should carefully consider the potential risks and benefits of treatment. Consider tapering paroxetine in the third trimester.

➤*Elderly or debilitated or patients with severe renal or hepatic impairment:* The recommended initial dose is 10 mg/day (immediate-release) or 12.5 mg/day (controlled-release). Increases may be made if indicated. Do not exceed 40 mg/day (immediate-release) or 50 mg/day (controlled-release).

➤*Switching patients to or from a monoamine oxidase inhibitor (MAOI):* Allow at least 14 days between discontinuation of an MAOI and initiation of paroxetine therapy. Similarly, allow at least 14 days after stopping paroxetine before starting an MAOI.

➤*Discontinuation of treatment:* Symptoms associated with discontinuation of paroxetine have been reported. When discontinuing treatment, monitor for symptoms such as dizziness, sensory disturbances (eg, paresthesias such as electric shock sensations), agitation, anxiety, nausea, and sweating. A gradual reduction in the dose rather than abrupt cessation is recommended whenever possible. If intolerable symptoms occur following a decrease in the dose or upon discontinuation of treatment, then consider resuming the previously prescribed dose. Subsequently, the physician may continue decreasing the dose but at a more gradual rate.

➤*Administration of suspension:* Shake suspension well before using.

➤*Storage/Stability:*

Tablets – Store immediate-release tablets between 15° and 30°C (59° and 86°F) and controlled-release tablets at or below 25°C (77°F).

Suspension – Store at or below 25°C (77°F).

SERTRALINE HCl

Rx	Zoloft (Pfizer)	**Tablets:** 25 mg (as base)	(ZOLOFT 25 mg). Lt. green, capsule shape, scored. Film-coated. In 50s.
		50 mg (as base)	(ZOLOFT 50 mg). Lt. blue, capsule shape, scored. Film-coated. In 100s, 500s, 5000s, and UD 100s.
		100 mg (as base)	(ZOLOFT 100 mg). Lt. yellow, capsule shape, scored. Film-coated. In 100s, 500s, 5000s, and UD 100s.
		Oral concentrate: 20 mg per mL (as base)	12% alcohol, menthol. In 60 mL.[a]

[a] Dropper dispenser contains dry natural rubber.

For complete prescribing information, refer to the SSRIs group monograph.

Indications

➤*Major depressive disorder:* For the treatment of major depressive disorder as defined in the DSM-III.

➤*Obsessive-compulsive disorder (OCD):* For the treatment of obsessions and compulsions in patients with OCD, as defined in the DSM-III-R.

➤*Panic disorder:* For the treatment of panic disorder with or without agoraphobia, as defined in the DSM-IV.

➤*Posttraumatic stress disorder (PTSD):* For the treatment of PTSD as defined in the DSM-III-R.

➤*Premenstrual dysphoric disorder (PMDD):* For the treatment of PMDD as defined in the DSM-III-R/IV.

➤*Social anxiety disorder:* For the treatment of social anxiety disorder (social phobia) as defined by DSM-IV.

Administration and Dosage

➤*Approved by the FDA:* December 1991.

Administer sertraline once daily in the morning or evening. Given the 24-hour elimination half-life of sertraline, dose changes should not occur at intervals of less than 1 week.

➤*Major depressive disorder:*

Adults, initial treatment – 50 mg once daily.

Maintenance/Continuation/Extended treatment – It is generally agreed that acute episodes of major depressive disorder require several months or longer of sustained pharmacologic therapy. It is not known whether the dose of sertraline needed for maintenance treatment is identical to the dose needed to achieve an initial response. Periodically reassess patients to determine the need for maintenance treatment. Systematic evaluation of sertraline has shown that the antidepressant efficacy is maintained for a period of up to 44 weeks following 8 weeks of initial treatment at doses of 50 to 200 mg/day (mean dose, 70 mg/day).

➤*OCD:*

Adults, initial treatment – 50 mg once daily.

Adults, maintenance/continuation/extended treatment – It is generally agreed that OCD requires several months or longer of sustained pharmacological therapy beyond response to initial treatment.

Systematic evaluation of continuing sertraline for periods of up to 28 weeks in patients with OCD and panic disorder who have responded while taking sertraline during initial treatment phases of 24 to 52 weeks at a dose range of 50 to 200 mg/day has demonstrated a benefit. It is not known whether the dose of sertraline needed for maintenance treatment is identical to the dose needed to achieve an initial response. Nevertheless, periodically reassess patients to determine the need for maintenance treatment.

Children and adolescents – Initiate dosage with 25 mg once daily for children 6 to 12 years of age and 50 mg once daily in adolescents 13 to 17 years of age. While a relationship between dose and effect has not been established for OCD, patients were dosed in a range of 25 to 200 mg/day in trials for children 6 to 17 years of age with OCD. Patients not responding to an initial dose of 25 or 50 mg/day may benefit from dose increases up to a maximum of 200 mg/day. To avoid excess dosing in children with OCD, take into account the generally lower body weights compared with adults when increasing the dose. Given the 24-hour elimination half-life of sertraline, dose changes should not occur at intervals of less than 1 week.

➤*Panic disorder:*

Adults, initial treatment – 25 mg once daily. After 1 week, increase the dose to 50 mg once daily.

Maintenance/Continuation/Extended treatment – It is generally agreed that panic disorder requires several months or longer of sustained pharmacological therapy beyond response to initial treatment. Systematic evaluation of continuing sertraline for periods of up to 28 weeks in patients with OCD and panic disorder who have responded while taking sertraline during initial treatment phases of 24 to 52 weeks at a dose range of 50 to 200 mg/day has demonstrated a benefit. It is not known whether the dose of sertraline needed for maintenance treatment is identical to the dose needed to achieve an initial response. Nevertheless, periodically reassess patients to determine the need for maintenance treatment.

➤*Social anxiety disorder:*

Adults, initial treatment – 25 mg once daily. After 1 week, increase the dose to 50 mg once daily.

Maintenance/Continuation/Extended treatment – Social anxiety disorder is a chronic condition that may require several months or longer of sustained pharmacological therapy beyond response to initial treatment. Systematic evaluation of sertraline has demonstrated that its efficacy in social anxiety disorder is maintained for periods of up to 24 weeks following 20 weeks of treatment at a dose of 50 to 200 mg/day. Make dosage adjustments to maintain patients on the lowest effective

SERTRALINE HCl

dose and periodically reassess patients to determine the need for long-term treatment.

➤*PTSD:*

Adults, initial treatment – 25 mg once daily. After 1 week, increase the dose to 50 mg once daily.

Maintenance/Continuation/Extended treatment – It is generally agreed that PTSD requires several months or longer of sustained pharmacological therapy beyond response to initial treatment. Systematic evaluation of sertraline has demonstrated that its efficacy in PTSD is maintained for periods of up to 28 weeks following 24 weeks of treatment at a dose of 50 to 200 mg/day. It is not known whether the dose of sertraline needed for maintenance treatment is identical to the dose needed to achieve an initial response. Periodically reassess patients to determine the need for maintenance treatment.

➤*PMDD:*

Adults, initial treatment – 50 mg/day, either daily throughout the menstrual cycle or limited to the luteal phase of the menstrual cycle, depending on physician assessment.

While a relationship between dose and effect has not been established for PMDD, patients were dosed in the range of 50 to 150 mg/day with dose increases at the onset of each new menstrual cycle. Patients not responding to a 50 mg/day dose may benefit from dose increases (at 50 mg increments/menstrual cycle) up to 150 mg/day when dosing daily throughout the menstrual cycle, or 100 mg/day when dosing during the luteal phase of the menstrual cycle. If a 100 mg/day dose has been established with luteal phase dosing, utilize a 50 mg/day titration step for 3 days at the beginning of each luteal phase dosing period.

Maintenance/Continuation/Extended treatment – The effectiveness of sertraline in long-term use (ie, for more than 3 menstrual cycles) has not been systematically evaluated in controlled trials. However, as women commonly report that symptoms worsen with age until relieved by the onset of menopause, it is reasonable to consider continuation of a responding patient. Dosage adjustments, which may include changes between dosage regimens (eg, daily throughout the menstrual cycle vs during the luteal phase of the menstrual cycle), may be needed to maintain the patient on the lowest effective dosage. Periodically reassess patients to determine the need for continued treatment.

➤*Hepatic function impairment:* Give a lower or less-frequent dosage in patients with hepatic impairment. Use with caution in these patients.

➤*Switching patients to or from an MAOI:* At least 14 days should elapse between discontinuation of an MAOI and initiation of therapy with sertraline. In addition, allow at least 14 days after stopping sertraline before starting an MAOI.

➤*Oral concentrate:* Dilute prior to use with 4 oz (one-half cup) of water, ginger ale, lemon/lime soda, lemonade, or orange juice only. Do not mix with anything other than the liquids listed. Take the dose immediately after mixing; do not mix in advance. A slight haze may appear after mixing; this is normal. Note: Exercise caution in patients with latex sensitivity as the dropper dispenser contains dry natural rubber.

The oral concentrate is contraindicated with disulfiram because of the alcohol content of the concentrate.

➤*Storage/Stability:* Store at 25°C (77°F); excursions permitted to 15° to 30°C (59° to 86°F).

Monoamine Oxidase Inhibitors

Indications

➤*Depression:* In general, the MAOIs are indicated in patients with atypical (exogenous) depression and in some patients unresponsive to other antidepressive therapy. They are rarely a drug of first choice.

➤*Unlabeled uses:* MAOIs have shown promise in the treatment of bulimia (having characteristics of atypical depression). Phenelzine has been investigated in the treatment of cocaine addiction; careful supervision is required. Anecdotal cases and small studies indicate beneficial effects of phenelzine in patients with night terrors (30 mg twice daily); post-traumatic stress disorder (60 to 75 mg/day); some migraines resistant to other therapies (15 mg 3 times/day); likewise, with tranylcypromine in Binswanger's encephalopathy (40 mg/day), seasonal affective disorder ($\approx$ 30 mg/day), and subjective symptoms in multiple sclerosis patients (10 to 120 mg/day). MAOIs have also been used in the treatment of panic disorder with associated agoraphobia and globus hystericus syndrome.

Actions

➤*Pharmacology:* Monoamine oxidase is a complex enzyme system, widely distributed throughout the body, which is responsible for the metabolic decomposition of biogenic amines (eg, norepinephrine, epinephrine, dopamine, serotonin). Monoamine oxidase inhibitors (MAOIs) inhibit this enzyme system, causing an increase in the concentration of these endogenous amines.

Two types of MAO enzymes have been identified, MAO-A and MAO-B, which exhibit different preferences for substrates and different sensitivities to inhibitors. MAO-A preferentially de-aminates epinephrine, norepinephrine, and serotonin, while MAO-B metabolizes benzylamine and phenylethylamine. Dopamine and tyramine are metabolized by both isozymes. In neural tissues, this enzyme system regulates the metabolic decomposition of catecholamines and serotonin. Hepatic MAO inactivates circulating monoamines or those that are introduced via the GI tract into portal circulation (eg, tyramine).

Except for selegiline, MAOIs currently in use in the US are non-selective. Selegiline, an MAO-B selective agent, is used therapeutically for the treatment of Parkinson's disease. The non-selective agents are used for their antidepressant effects. All of these agents are irreversible inhibitors of MAO, and therefore, may require up to 2 weeks for normal amine metabolism to be restored following drug discontinuation. Studies have also indicated that chronic therapy with MAOIs causes down-regulation in adrenergic and serotonergic receptors.

Drugs that have MAOI activity cause a wide range of clinical effects and have the potential for serious interactions with other substances. Clinicians and patients should be fully aware of the potential hazards associated with their use.

➤*Pharmacokinetics:*

Absorption/Distribution – Limited information is available on MAOI pharmacokinetics. They appear to be well absorbed following oral administration. Peak levels of tranylcypromine and phenelzine are reached in $\approx$ 2 and 3 hours, respectively. However, maximal inhibition of MAO occurs within 5 to 10 days.

Metabolism/Excretion – The hydrazine MAOIs (phenelzine, isocarboxazid) are thought to be metabolized with the release of active metabolites. Inactivation is primarily by acetylation. The clinical effects of phenelzine may continue for up to 2 weeks after discontinuation of therapy. Upon withdrawal of tranylcypromine, MAO activity is recovered in 3 to 5 days (possibly up to 10 days). Phenelzine and isocarboxazid are excreted in the urine mostly as metabolites.

Special populations – "*Slow acetylators*": Slow acetylation of hydrazine MAOIs may yield exaggerated effects after standard dosing.

Contraindications

Hypersensitivity to these agents; pheochromocytoma; CHF; history of liver disease or abnormal liver function tests; severe impairment of renal function; confirmed or suspected cerebrovascular disorders; cardiovascular disease; hypertension; history of headache; coadministration with other MAOIs; dibenzazepine-related agents including tricyclic antidepressants, carbamazepine, and cyclobenzaprine; bupropion; SSRIs; buspirone; sympathomimetics; meperidine; dextromethorphan; anesthetic agents; CNS depressants; antihypertensives; caffeine; cheese or other foods with high tyramine content (see Warnings and Drug Interactions).

Warnings

➤*Hypertensive crises:* The most serious reactions involve changes in blood pressure; it is inadvisable to use these drugs in elderly or debilitated patients or in the presence of hypertension, cardiovascular or cerebrovascular disease, or coadministered with certain drugs or foods (see Warnings and Drug Interactions).

Hypertensive crises have sometimes been fatal. These crises usually occur within several hours after ingestion of a contraindicated substance and are characterized by some or all of the following symptoms: Occipital headache that may radiate frontally; palpitation; neck stiffness/soreness; nausea; vomiting; sweating (sometimes with fever or cold, clammy skin); dilated pupils; photophobia. Either tachycardia or bradycardia may be present and can be associated with constricting chest pain.

Note – Intracranial bleeding (sometimes fatal) has been reported in association with the paradoxical increase in blood pressure. Monitor blood pressure frequently to detect evidence of any pressor response. Do not rely completely on blood pressure readings, but observe patient frequently.

Discontinue therapy immediately if palpitations or frequent headaches occur. These signs may be prodromal of a hypertensive crisis.

Treatment – If a hypertensive crisis occurs, discontinue these drugs immediately and institute therapy to lower blood pressure. Do not use parenteral reserpine. Headaches tend to abate as blood pressure is lowered. Administer alpha-adrenergic blocking agents such as phentolamine 5 mg IV slowly to avoid producing an excessive hypotensive effect. Manage fever by means of external cooling.

Warning to the patient – Warn all patients against eating foods with high tyramine, dopamine, or tryptophan content (see table) during treatment and for 2 weeks after discontinuing MAOIs. Any high-protein food that is aged or undergoes breakdown by putrefaction process to improve flavor is suspect of being able to produce a hypertensive crisis in patients taking MAOIs. Also warn patients against drinking alcoholic beverages and against self-medication with certain proprietary agents such as cold, hay fever, or weight reduction preparations containing sympathomimetic amines while undergoing therapy. Instruct patients not to consume excessive amounts of caffeine in any form and to report promptly the occurrence of headache or other unusual symptoms.

Tyramine-Containing Foods[1]		
Cheese/Dairy Products		
American Blue[2] Boursault[2] Brie	Camembert[2] Cheddar[2] Emmenthaler[2] Gruyere Mozzarella Parmesan	Romano Roquefort Sour cream Stilton[2] Swiss[2] Yogurt
Meat/Fish		
Anchovies Beef or chicken liver,[2] other meats, fish (unrefrigerated, fermented, spoiled, smoked, pickled) Caviar	Fermented sausages (bologna, pepperoni, salami, summer sausage)[2] Dried fish (salted herring) Dry sausage Game meat[2]	Meat extracts Meats prepared with tenderizer Herring, pickled, spoiled[2] Shrimp paste
Alcoholic Beverages (Undistilled)		
Beer (imports, some nonalcoholic)	Red wine (especially Chianti)[2]	Sherry[2] Distilled spirits Liqueurs
Fruit/Vegetables		
Bananas Bean curd Dried fruits (eg, raisins, prunes)	Fruit (eg, avocados, especially overripe) Figs, canned (overripe) Miso soup Raspberries	Sauerkraut[2] Soy sauce Yeast extracts (eg, Marmite)[2]
Foods Containing Other Vasopressors		
Broad beans (eg, fava beans, overripe) – dopa[2]	Caffeine (eg, coffee, tea, colas)	Chocolate – phenylethyl- amine Ginseng

[1] Tyramine contents are not predictable and may vary. The amounts of tyramine are estimated from low to very high.
[2] Contains high to very high amounts of tyramine.

➤*Suicidal risks:* In patients who may be suicidal, no single form of treatment, such as MAOIs, electroconvulsive, or other therapy, should be relied upon as a sole therapeutic measure. Strict supervision and, preferably, hospitalization are advised.

➤*Concomitant antidepressants:* In patients receiving a selective serotonin reuptake inhibitor (SSRI) in combination with an MAOI, there have been reports of serious, sometimes fatal, reactions including hyperthermia, rigidity, myoclonus, autonomic instability with possible rapid fluctuations of vital signs, and mental status changes that include extreme agitation progressing to delirium and coma. These reactions have also occurred in patients who have recently discontinued an SSRI and have been started on a MAOI. Some cases presented with features resembling neuroleptic malignant syndrome. It is recommended that SSRIs not be used in combination with a MAOI, or within 14 days of a MAOI. Allow at least 2 weeks after stopping the SSRI before starting a MAOI (see Drug Interactions). Allow at least 5 weeks after stopping fluoxetine before starting a MAOI.

Do not administer MAOIs with or immediately following tricyclic antidepressants (TCAs). Such combinations can produce seizures, sweating, coma, hyperexcitability, hyperthermia, tachycardia, tachypnea, headache, mydriasis, flushing, confusion, disseminated intravascular coagulation, and death. Allow at least 14 days to elapse between the discontinuation of the MAOIs and the institution of a TCA. Some TCAs have been used safely and successfully in combination with MAOIs.

►*Withdrawal:* Withdrawal may be associated with nausea, vomiting, and malaise. An uncommon withdrawal syndrome following abrupt withdrawal of MAOIs has been infrequently reported. Signs and symptoms of this syndrome generally commence 24 to 72 hours after drug discontinuation and may range from vivid nightmares with agitation to frank psychosis and convulsions. This syndrome generally responds to reinstitution of low-dose MAOI therapy followed by cautious downward titration and discontinuation.

►*Coexisting symptoms:* **Tranylcypromine** and **isocarboxazid** may aggravate coexisting symptoms in depression, such as anxiety and agitation.

►*Renal function impairment:* Observe caution in patients with impaired renal function because there is a possibility of cumulative effects in such patients.

►*Carcinogenesis:* **Phenelzine**, like other hydrazine derivatives, has induced pulmonary and vascular tumors in an uncontrolled lifetime study in mice.

►*Elderly:* Older patients may suffer more morbidity than younger patients during and following an episode of hypertension or malignant hyperthermia with MAOI use. Older patients have less compensatory reserve to cope with any serious adverse reactions. Therefore, use **tranylcypromine** with caution in the elderly.

►*Pregnancy:* Category C. Safety for use during pregnancy has not been established. Use during pregnancy or in women of childbearing age only when clearly needed and when the potential benefits outweigh the potential hazards to the fetus.

Doses of **phenelzine** in pregnant mice well exceeding the maximum recommended human dose have caused a significant decrease in the number of viable offspring per mouse. The growth of dogs and rats has been retarded by doses exceeding the maximum human dose. **Tranylcypromine** passes through the placental barrier of animals into the fetus.

►*Lactation:* Safety for use during lactation has not been established. **Tranylcypromine** is excreted in breast milk. Because of the potential for serious adverse effects in the nursing infant, decide whether to discontinue nursing or the drug, taking into account the importance of the drug to the mother.

►*Children:* Not recommended for patients < 16 years of age.

Precautions

►*Hypotension:* Observe all patients for symptoms of postural hypotension. Hypotensive side effects have occurred in hypertensive as well as healthy and hypotensive patients. Blood pressure usually returns to pretreatment levels rapidly when the drug is discontinued or the dosage is reduced.

At doses > 30 mg/day, postural hypotension is a major side effect and may result in syncope. Make dosage increases more gradually in patients showing a tendency toward hypotension at the beginning of therapy. Postural hypotension may be relieved by the patient lying down until blood pressure returns to normal.

►*Hypomania:* Hypomania has been the most common severe psychiatric side effect reported. This has been largely limited to patients in whom disorders characterized by hyperkinetic symptoms coexist with, but are obscured by, depressive affect; hypomania usually appeared as depression improved. If agitation is present, it may be increased with MAOIs. Hypomania and agitation have also occurred at higher than recommended doses or following long-term therapy.

These drugs may cause excessive stimulation in agitated or schizophrenic patients; in manic-depressive states, it may result in a swing from a depressive to a manic phase.

►*Diabetes:* There is conflicting evidence as to whether MAOIs affect glucose metabolism or potentiate hypoglycemic agents. Consider this if used in diabetics.

►*Epilepsy:* The effect of MAOIs on the convulsive threshold may vary. Do not use with metrizamide; discontinue MAOI ≥ 48 hours prior to myelography and resume ≥ 24 hours postprocedure.

►*Hepatotoxicity:* There is a low incidence of altered liver function or jaundice in patients treated with **isocarboxazid**. In the past, it was difficult to differentiate most cases of drug-induced hepatocellular jaundice from viral hepatitis although this is no longer true. Perform periodic liver chemistry tests during therapy. Discontinue the drug at the first sign of hepatic dysfunction or jaundice.

►*Myocardial ischemia:* MAOIs may suppress anginal pain that would otherwise serve as a warning of myocardial ischemia.

►*Hyperthyroid patients:* Use **tranylcypromine** and **isocarboxazid** cautiously because of increased sensitivity to pressor amines.

►*Switching MAOIs:* In several case reports, hypertensive crisis, cerebral hemorrhage, and death have possibly resulted from switching from one MAOI to another without a waiting period. However, in other patients no adverse reactions occurred. Nevertheless, a waiting period of 10 to 14 days is recommended when switching from one MAOI to another or from a dibenzazepine-related agent (eg, amitriptyline, perphenazine).

►*Drug abuse and dependence:* There have been reports of drug dependency in patients using doses of **tranylcypromine** and **isocarboxazid** significantly in excess of the therapeutic range. Some of these patients had a history of previous substance abuse. The following withdrawal symptoms have been reported: Restlessness; anxiety; depression; confusion; hallucinations; headaches; weakness; diarrhea.

Drug Interactions

MAOI Drug Interactions			
Precipitant drug	Object drug*		Description
Methylphenidate	MAOIs	↑	Coadministration may cause a hypertensive crisis.
Metrizamide	MAOIs	↑	Discontinue MAOIs at least 48 hours before myelography and do not resume for at least 24 hours post-procedure because of the decrease of the seizure threshold.
MAOIs	Anesthetics	↑	Patients taking MAOIs should not undergo elective surgery requiring general anesthesia. Do not give cocaine or local anesthesia containing sympathomimetic vasoconstrictors. Keep in mind the possible combined hypotensive effects of MAOIs and spinal anesthesia. Discontinue the MAOI at least 10 days before elective surgery.
MAOIs	Antidepressants	↑	Do not administer MAOIs together with or immediately following these agents (see Warnings). There have been reports of serious, sometimes fatal, reactions (including hyperthermia, rigidity, myoclonus, autonomic instability with possible fluctuations of vital signs, and mental status changes that include extreme agitation and confusion progressing to delirium and coma). Do not administer MAOIs together or in rapid succession with other MAOIs.
MAOIs	Antidiabetic agents	↑	MAOIs may potentiate the hypoglycemic response to insulin or sulfonylureas and delay recovery from hypoglycemia.
MAOIs	Barbiturates	↑	Give barbiturates at a reduced dose with MAOIs.
MAOIs	Beta blockers	↑	Bradycardia may develop during concurrent use of certain MAOIs and beta blockers.
MAOIs	Bupropion	↑	The concurrent use of an MAOI and bupropion HCl is contraindicated. Allow at least 14 days between discontinuation of an MAOI and initiation of bupropion HCl treatment.
MAOIs	Buspirone	↑	Do not take isocarboxazid in combination with buspirone. Several cases of elevated blood pressure have occurred. Allow at least 10 days between discontinuation of isocarboxazid and institution of buspirone.
MAOIs	Carbamazepine	↑	Hypertensive crises, severe convulsive seizures, coma, or circulatory collapse may occur in patients receiving such combinations.
MAOIs	Cyclobenzaprine	↑	Because cyclobenzaprine is structurally related to the tricyclic antidepressants, use with caution with MAOIs (see MAOIs/Antidepressants).
MAOIs	Dextromethorphan	↑	Hyperpyrexia, abnormal muscle movement, psychosis, bizarre behavior, hypotension, coma, and death have been associated with this combination.
MAOIs	Guanethidine	↓	MAOIs may inhibit the hypotensive effects of guanethidine.
MAOIs	Levodopa	↑	Hypertensive reactions occur if levodopa is given to patients receiving MAOIs.

Monoamine Oxidase Inhibitors

MAOI Drug Interactions

Precipitant drug	Object drug*		Description
MAOIs	Meperidine	↑	Coadministration or use within 2 to 3 weeks of one another may result in agitation, seizures, diaphoresis, and fever, and progress to coma, apnea, and death. Adverse reactions are possible weeks after MAOI withdrawal. Avoid this combination; administer other narcotic analgesics with caution.
MAOIs	Methyldopa	↑	Coadministration may cause loss of blood pressure control or signs of central stimulation (eg, excitation, hallucinations).
MAOIs	Rauwolfia alkaloids	↑	MAOIs inhibit the destruction of serotonin and norepinephrine, which are believed to be released from tissue stores by rauwolfia alkaloids. Exercise caution when rauwolfia is used concomitantly with MAOIs.
MAOIs	Sulfonamide	↑	Coadministration may cause sulfonamide or MAOI toxicity.
Sulfonamide	MAOIs		
MAOIs	Sumatriptan	↑	Systemic exposure to sumatriptan may be increased, producing toxicity.
MAOIs	Sympathomimetics	↑	The MAOIs' potentiation of indirect- or mixed-acting sympathomimetic substances, including anorexiants, may result in severe headache, hypertension, high fever, and hyperpyrexia, possibly resulting in hypertensive crisis; avoid coadministration.
MAOIs	Thiazide diuretics	↑	Exaggerated hypotensive effects may result from concurrent use.
MAOIs	L-Tryptophan	↑	Coadministration may result in hyperreflexia, confusion, disorientation, shivering, myoclonic jerks, agitation, amnesia, delirium, hypomanic signs, ataxia, ocular oscillations, Babinski signs.

* ↑ = Object drug increased. ↓ = Object drug decreased.

➤*Drug/Food interactions:* Warn all patients against eating foods with a high **tyramine** content. Hypertensive crisis may result (see Warnings).

Adverse Reactions

➤*Common:*

Cardiovascular – Orthostatic and postural hypotension; syncope; palpitations; tachycardia.

CNS – Dizziness; headache; hyperreflexia; tremors; muscle twitching; mania; hypomania (see Precautions); confusion; memory impairment; sleep disturbances including hypersomnia and insomnia; weakness; myoclonic movements; fatigue; drowsiness; restlessness; overstimulation including increased anxiety, agitation, and manic symptoms.

GI – Constipation; GI disturbances; nausea; diarrhea; abdominal pain.

Miscellaneous – Edema; dry mouth; elevated serum transaminases; weight gain; sexual disturbances; anorexia; blurred vision; impotence; chills.

➤*Less common:*

CNS – Jitteriness; euphoria; palilalia; paresthesia; chills; myoclonic jerks; anxiety; hyperactivity; lethargy; sedation.

GU – Urinary retention/frequency; impotence.

Hematologic – Hematologic changes including anemia, agranulocytosis and thrombocytopenia; leukopenia.

Ophthalmic – Glaucoma; nystagmus; blurred vision.

Miscellaneous – Sweating; skin rash; hypernatremia; syncope; heavy feeling; palpitations.

➤*Rare:*

CNS – Convulsions; ataxia; shock-like coma; acute anxiety reaction; precipitation of schizophrenia; toxic delirium; manic reaction; headaches without blood pressure elevation; muscle spasm; myoclonic jerks; numbness; confusion; memory loss.

GU – Impaired water excretion compatible with the syndrome of inappropriate secretion of antidiuretic hormone (SIADH).

Hepatic – Reversible jaundice; hepatitis; fatal progressive necrotizing hepatocellular damage.

Metabolic – Hypermetabolic syndrome that may include, but is not limited to, hyperpyrexia, tachycardia, tachypnea, muscular rigidity, elevated CK levels, metabolic acidosis, hypoxia, and coma and may resemble an overdose.

Miscellaneous – Edema of the glottis; transient respiratory and cardiovascular depression following ECT; leukopenia; lupus-like syndrome; fever associated with increased muscle tone; tinnitus; localized scleroderma, cystic acne flare-up, ataxia, akinesia, disorientation, urinary frequency or incontinence, urticaria, fissuring in corner of mouth (tranylcypromine); skin rash; ejaculation problems; tremors.

Overdosage

➤*Symptoms:* Depending on the amount of overdosage, a mixed clinical picture may develop involving signs and symptoms of the CNS, cardiovascular stimulation or depression. Signs and symptoms may be absent or minimal during the initial 12–hour period following ingestion and may develop slowly thereafter, reaching a maximum in 24 to 48 hours. Some symptoms may persist for 8 to 14 days. Immediate hospitalization, with continuous patient monitoring throughout this period, is essential.

Early symptoms of MAOI toxicity include: Irritability; hyperactivity; anxiety; hypotension; vascular collapse; insomnia; restlessness; dizziness; faintness; weakness; drowsiness; hallucinations; trismus; flushing; sweating; tachypnea; tachycardia; movement disorders including grimacing, opisthotonus, rigidity, clonic movements and muscular fasciculation; severe headache. In serious cases, coma, convulsions, hypertension with severe headache, precordial pain, respiratory depression and failure, pyrexia, hyperpyrexia, diaphoresis, cool and clammy skin, cardiorespiratory arrest, incoherence, agitation, mental confusion, extreme dizziness, shock, and death may occur. Rare instances have been reported in which hypertension was accompanied by twitching or myoclonic fibrillation of skeletal muscles with hyperpyrexia, sometimes progressing to generalized rigidity and coma.

➤*Treatment:* Induce emesis or gastric lavage with instillation of charcoal slurry in early poisoning; protect the airway against aspiration. Support respiration by appropriate measures, including management of the airway, use of supplemental oxygen, and mechanical ventilatory assistance, as required. Refer to General Management of Acute Overdosage.

Cardiovascular – Cardiovascular complications include hypertension and hypotension; hence, any cardiovascular agent must be administered cautiously and blood pressure monitored frequently. Severe hypertension may be treated with an alpha-adrenergic blocker (eg, phentolamine, phenoxybenzamine). Beta blocking agents are not necessarily contraindicated and may be useful for tachycardia, tachypnea, and hyperpyrexia; however, more data are needed. Treat hypotension and vascular collapse with IV fluids and, if necessary, titrate blood pressure with an IV infusion of a dilute pressor agent. Administration of pressor amines such as norepinephrine may be of limited value; their effects may be potentiated. Plasma may be of value, as well. Adrenergic agents may produce a markedly increased pressor response.

CNS – CNS stimulation, including convulsions, may be treated with IV diazepam given slowly. Avoid phenothiazine derivatives and CNS stimulants. Monitor body temperature closely. Intensive management of hyperpyrexia may be required. Maintenance of fluid and electrolyte balance is essential.

Hemodialysis, peritoneal dialysis, and charcoal hemoperfusion may be of value in massive overdosage, but sufficient data are not available to recommend their routine use. External cooling is recommended if hyperpyrexia occurs. Barbiturates have been reported to help relieve myoclonic reactions.

The pathophysiologic effects of massive overdosage may persist for several days; recovery from mild overdosage may be expected within 3 to 4 days. Continue treatment for several days until homeostasis is restored. Liver function studies are recommended during the 4 to 6 weeks after recovery. It is not known if tranylcypromine is dialyzable.

Patient Information

Do not discontinue this medication or adjust dosage except on the advice of a physician. Consult physician before taking any other medication, including *otc* items.

Avoid tyramine-containing foods and certain *otc* drug products (see Warnings).

May cause drowsiness or blurred vision; use with caution when driving or performing other tasks requiring alertness, coordination, or physical dexterity.

Dizziness, weakness, or fainting may occur when arising from a sitting position.

Effects may be delayed a few weeks. Take as directed. Avoid alcohol and tryptophan.

Notify physician if severe headache, palpitation, or tachycardia, a sense of constriction in the throat or chest, sweating, dizziness, neck stiffness, nausea or vomiting, or other unusual symptoms occur.

Inform physician and dentist about the use of MAOIs.

PHENELZINE SULFATE

Rx	Nardil (Parke-Davis)	Tablets: 15 mg (as sulfate)	Sucrose, mannitol. (P-D 270). Orange. Biconvex. Sugar coated. In 100s.

For complete prescribing information, refer to the MAOIs group monograph.

Indications

➤*Depression:* Effective in depressed patients clinically characterized as "atypical," "nonendogenous," or "neurotic." These patients often have mixed anxiety and depression and phobic or hypochondriacal features. There is less conclusive evidence of usefulness in severely depressed patients with endogenous features.

Phenelzine sulfate is rarely the first antidepressant drug used. Rather, it is more suitable for use in treatment-resistant patients.

Administration and Dosage

➤*Initial dose:* 15 mg 3 times/day.

➤*Early phase treatment:* Increase dosage to at least 60 mg/day at a fairly rapid pace consistent with patient tolerance. It may be necessary to increase dosage up to 90 mg/day to obtain sufficient MAO inhibition. Many patients do not show a clinical response until treatment at 60 mg has been continued for at least 4 weeks.

➤*Maintenance dose:* After maximum benefit is achieved, reduce dosage slowly over several weeks. Maintenance dose may be as low as 15 mg/day or every other day; continue for as long as required.

TRANYLCYPROMINE SULFATE

Rx	Parnate (SmithKline Beecham)	Tablets: 10 mg (as sulfate)	Lactose. (PARNATE SKF). Rose-red. Film coated. In 100s.

For complete prescribing information, refer to the MAOIs group monograph.

Indications

➤*Depression:* Effective for use with adult outpatients with a Major Depressive Episode without Melancholia according to DSM III diagnosis. Efficacy for use in endogenous depression has not been established.

Administration and Dosage

The usual effective dosage is 30 mg/day in divided doses. Improvement should be seen within 48 hours to 3 weeks after starting therapy. If there is no improvement after 2 weeks, increase dosage in 10 mg/day increments at 1– to 3–week intervals. Dosage range may be extended to a maximum of 60 mg/day from the usual 30 mg/day. Gradually withdraw tranylcypromine when discontinuing therapy.

ISOCARBOXAZID

Rx	Marplan (Oxford)	Tablets: 10 mg	Lactose. Peach. Scored. In 100s.

For complete prescribing information, refer to the MAOIs group monograph.

Indications

➤*Depression:* Treatment of depression. Because of potentially serious side effects, isocarboxazid is not a first-choice antidepressant in the treatment of newly diagnosed depressed patients.

Administration and Dosage

➤*Approved by the FDA:* August 21, 1998.

➤*Initial dosage:* 10 mg twice daily. If tolerated, increase dosage by 10 mg every 2 to 4 days to achieve a dosage of 40 mg by the end of the first week of treatment. Increase dosage by increments of up to 20 mg/ week, if needed and tolerated, to a maximum recommended dosage of 60 mg/day. Daily dosage should be divided into 2 to 4 doses.

➤*Maintenance dosage:* After maximum clinical response is achieved, attempt to reduce the dosage slowly over a period of several weeks without jeopardizing therapeutic response. Beneficial effect may not be seen in some patients for 3 to 6 weeks. If no response is obtained by then, discontinue therapy.

Because of the limited experience with systematically monitored patients receiving isocarboxazid at the higher end of the currently recommended dose range of up to 60 mg/day, caution is indicated in patients for whom a dose of 40 mg/day is exceeded.

WARNING

Clozapine:

Agranulocytosis – Because of a significant risk of agranulocytosis, a potentially life-threatening adverse event, reserve**clozapine** use in 1) the treatment of severely ill patients with schizophrenia who fail to show an acceptable response to adequate courses of standard antipsychotic drug treatment or 2) for reducing the risk of recurrent suicidal behavior in patients with schizophrenia or schizoaffective disorder who are judged to be at risk of re-experiencing suicidal behavior. Patients being treated with clozapine must have a baseline white blood cell (WBC) and differential count before initiation of treatment as well as regular WBC counts during treatment and for 4 weeks after discontinuation of treatment. Clozapine is available only through a distribution system that ensures monitoring of WBC counts according to the schedule described below prior to delivery of the next supply of medication (see Warnings).

Seizures – Seizures have been associated with the use of **clozapine**. Dose appears to be an important seizure predictor, with a greater likelihood at higher clozapine doses. Use caution when administering clozapine to patients having a history of seizures or other predisposing factors. Advise patients not to engage in any activity where sudden loss of consciousness could cause serious risk to themselves or others (see Warnings).

Myocarditis – Analyses of postmarketing safety databases suggest **clozapine** is associated with an increased risk of fatal myocarditis, especially during, but not limited to, the first month of therapy. In patients in whom myocarditis is suspected, discontinue clozapine treatment promptly (see Warnings).

WARNING (cont.)

Other adverse cardiovascular and respiratory effects – Orthostatic hypotension, with or without syncope, can occur with **clozapine** treatment. Rarely, collapse can be profound and be accompanied by respiratory and/or cardiac arrest. Orthostatic hypotension is more likely to occur during initial titration in association with rapid dose escalation. In patients who have had even a brief interval off clozapine (2 or more days since the last dose) start treatment with 12.5 mg once or twice daily (see Warnings). Because collapse, respiratory arrest, and cardiac arrest during initial treatment have occurred in patients who were being administered benzodiazepines or other psychotropic drugs, caution is advised when clozapine is initiated in patients taking a benzodiazepine or any other psychotropic drug (see Warnings).

Mesoridazine, thioridazine: Some antipsychotics have been shown to prolong the QT_c interval in a dose-related manner, and drugs with this potential including **mesoridazine** and **thioridazine** have been associated with a torsade-de-pointes-type arrhythmias and sudden death. Because of its potential for significant, possibly life-threatening, proarrhythmic effects, reserve use of mesoridazine and thioridazine in the treatment of schizophrenic patients who fail to show an acceptable response to adequate courses of treatment with other antipsychotic drugs, either because of insufficient effectiveness or the inability to achieve an effective dose due to intolerable adverse effects from those drugs.

Indications

Antipsychotics — Summary of Indications[a]

Indications ✔ = labeled X = unlabeled	Aripiprazole	Chlorpromazine	Clozapine	Fluphenazine	Haloperidol	Loxapine	Mesoridazine	Molindone	Olanzapine	Perphenazine	Pimozide	Prochlorperazine	Quetiapine	Risperidone	Thioridazine	Thiothixene	Trifluoperazine	Ziprasidone
Psychotic disorders				✔	✔					✔								
Schizophrenia	✔	✔	✔	✔		✔	✔	✔	✔	✔	X	✔	✔	✔	✔	✔	✔	✔
Tourette disorder					✔						✔							
Severe behavioral problems (pediatric patients)		✔			✔									X				
Hyperactivity (pediatric patients)		✔			✔													
Acute manic episodes associated with bipolar disorder	X	✔	X						✔				✔	X				X
Recurrent suicidal behavior			✔															
Nonpsychotic anxiety												✔					✔	
Presurgical apprehension/restlessness		✔																
Nausea/Vomiting		✔		X	X							✔		✔				
Intractable hiccoughs		✔			X													
Tetanus		✔																
Acute intermittent porphyria		✔																
Unlabeled uses																		
Migraines (acute treatment)		X										X						
Psychosis/Agitation in dementia or Alzheimer disease		X			X				X				X	X	X			X
Psychosis in Parkinson disease		X											X	X				
PCP-induced psychosis				X														
Behavioral problems associated with autism														X				
Obsessive-compulsive disorder (refractory to SSRIs)									X					X				

[a] For more detailed information, see the information below and individual drug monographs.

➤*Psychotic disorders:* **Fluphenazine, perphenazine,** and **haloperidol.** For use in the management of the manifestations of psychotic disorders.

➤*Schizophrenia:* **Chlorpromazine, fluphenazine, mesoridazine, perphenazine, prochlorperazine, trifluoperazine, thioridazine, thiothixene, clozapine, loxapine, molindone, aripiprazole, olanzapine, quetiapine, risperidone,** and **ziprasidone.** Clozapine, mesoridazine, and thioridazine should only be used in patients who have failed to respond adequately to other antipsychotic drugs.

➤*Tourette disorder:* **Haloperidol** is indicated for the control of tics and vocal utterances of Tourette disorder in children and adults. **Pimozide** is indicated for the suppression of motor and phonic tics in

patients with Tourette disorder who have failed to respond satisfactorily to standard treatment.

➤*Behavioral problems (pediatric patients):* **Chlorpromazine** and **haloperidol.** For the treatment of severe behavioral problems in children marked by combativeness and/or explosive hyperexcitable behavior (out of proportion to immediate provocations).

➤*Hyperactivity (pediatric patients):* **Chlorpromazine** and **haloperidol.** For the short-term treatment of hyperactive children who show excessive motor activity with accompanying conduct disorders consisting of some or all of the following symptoms: Impulsivity, difficulty sustaining attention, aggressivity, mood lability, poor frustration tolerance.

➤*Acute manic episodes associated with bipolar disorder:* **Chlorpromazine** is indicated to control the manifestations of the manic type of manic-depressive illness. **Olanzapine** is indicated as monotherapy or in combination with lithium or valproate for the short-term treatment of acute manic episodes associated with bipolar I disorder. **Quetiapine** is indicated for the short-term treatment of acute manic episodes associated with bipolar I disorder, as either monotherapy or adjunct therapy to lithium or divalproex.

➤*Recurrent suicidal behavior:* **Clozapine** is indicated for reducing the risk of recurrent suicidal behavior in patients with schizophrenia or schizoaffective disorder who are judged to be at chronic risk for re-experiencing suicidal behavior.

➤*Nonpsychotic anxiety:* **Prochlorperazine** and **trifluoperazine**. For the short-term treatment of generalized nonpsychotic anxiety; however, they are not the first drugs to be used.

➤*Presurgical apprehension/restlessness:* **Chlorpromazine** is indicated for relief of restlessness and apprehension before surgery.

➤*Nausea/Vomiting:* **Chlorpromazine**, **perphenazine**, and **prochlorperazine**. To control severe nausea and vomiting.

➤*Intractable hiccoughs:* **Chlorpromazine**.

➤*Tetanus:* **Chlorpromazine** is indicated as an adjunct in the treatment of tetanus.

➤*Acute intermittent porphyria:* **Chlorpromazine**.

➤*Unlabeled uses:*

Tourette disorder – **Risperidone** has shown efficacy in the treatment of tics in patients with Tourette disorder.

Acute manic episodes associated with bipolar disorder – **Aripiprazole**, **risperidone**, **quetiapine**, or **ziprasidone** may be alternatives when an antipsychotic is needed in the treatment of acute bipolar mania. **Clozapine** may also be an option in the treatment of refractory illness.

Nausea/Vomiting – **Haloperidol** and **fluphenazine** have also been used as antiemetics.

Intractable hiccoughs – **Haloperidol** (2 to 5 mg every 4 to 8 hours) has been used as an alternative agent in the treatment of persistent hiccoughs.

Migraines – **Chlorpromazine** (50 to 100 mg IM) and **prochlorperazine** (10 to 25 mg IM) have been used as abortive treatments of acute migraine attacks in adults.

Psychosis/Agitation in dementia or Alzheimer disease patient – **Haloperidol, olanzapine, risperidone, quetiapine, ziprasidone, clozapine,** and **thioridazine** may be useful in the management of agitation and psychotic events in patients with dementia and Alzheimer disease.

Psychosis in Parkinson disease – In the treatment of psychosis in patients with Parkinson disease, **clozapine** has been shown to be beneficial in alleviating psychosis without compromising motor function. Other alternatives include **quetiapine** and **risperidone**.

PCP psychosis – **Haloperidol** has shown to be effective in improving PCP-induced aggression, combativeness, and schizophreniform symptoms (eg, hallucinations, delusions, disorganized thinking.)

Behavioral problems associated with autism – **Risperidone** was shown to be effective for the treatment of tantrums, aggression, or self-injurious behavior in autistic children.

Behavioral problems (pediatric patients) – **Risperidone** has demonstrated efficacy in reducing aggression in children with a variety of comorbid disorders. Risperidone has also improved severely disruptive behavior in children with subaverage intelligence.

Obsessive-compulsive disorder (refractory to SSRIs) – Patients with OCD refractory to SSRIs may respond to the addition of **risperidone** or **olanzapine**.

Administration and Dosage

See individual product listings for specific dosing.

Individualize dosage. The milligram for milligram potency relationship among all dosage forms has not been precisely established. Increase dosage until symptoms are controlled. Increase dosage gradually in elderly, debilitated or emaciated patients. In continued therapy, gradually reduce dosage to the lowest effective maintenance level after symptoms have been controlled.

Actions

➤*Pharmacology:* The exact mechanism of action of the antipsychotic agents is unknown; however, it is thought to be due to their antagonistic actions on the receptors of several neurotransmitters. The following table provides information on antipsychotic receptor affinity. All produce antagonist effects on the receptors unless otherwise specified.

Antipsychotic Receptor Affinity	
Antipsychotic agent	Receptor affinity
Conventional agents	
Chlorpromazine	**High** — adrenergic **Weak** — peripheral anticholinergic, histaminergic, serotonergic
Fluphenazine	Dopamine D_2, histamine H_1, alpha-adrenergic, serotonin 5-HT_2
Haloperidol	Dopamine D_2, alpha-adrenergic, serotonin 5-HT_2
Loxapine	Dopamine D_2, histamine H_1, alpha-adrenergic, muscarinic M_1
Mesoridazine	Dopamine D_2, histamine H_1, alpha-adrenergic, muscarinic M_1
Molindone	**Low** — dopamine D_2, alpha-adrenergic, serotonin 5-HT_2
Perphenazine	Dopamine D_2, histamine H_1, alpha-adrenergic
Pimozide	Dopamine D_2, alpha-adrenergic, serotonin 5-HT_2
Prochlorperazine	Dopamine D_2, histamine H_1, alpha-D_2adrenergic, serotonin 5-HT_2
Promethazine[a]	Histamine H_1, muscarinic, some serotonin
Thioridazine	Dopamine D_2, histamine H_1, alpha-adrenergic, muscarinic M_1, serotonin 5-HT_2
Thiothixene	**High** — dopamine D_2 **Low** — histamine H_1, alpha-adrenergic
Trifluoperazine	Dopamine D_2, histamine H_1, alpha-adrenergic, muscarinic M_1, serotonin 5-HT_2
Atypical agents	
Aripiprazole	**High** — dopamine D_2[b], D_3, serotonin 5-HT_{1A}[b], 5-HT_{2A} **Moderate** — dopamine D_4, 5-HT_{2C}, 5-HT_7, alpha$_1$-adrenergic, histamine H_1
Clozapine	**High** — dopamine D_4 Other receptors — dopamine D_1, D_2, D_3, D_5, adrenergic, cholinergic, histaminergic, serotonergic
Olanzapine	**High** — serotonin 5-HT_{2A}, 5-HT_{2C}, dopamine D_1, D_2, D_3, D_4, muscarinic M_1, M_2, M_3, M_4, M_5, histamine H_1, alpha$_1$adrenergic **Weak** — $GABA_A$, benzodiazepine receptor, beta-adrenergic
Quetiapine	Serotonin 5-HT_{1A}, 5-HT_2, dopamine D_1, D_2, alpha$_{1 \text{ and } 2}$-adrenergic, histamine H_1
Risperidone	**High** — dopamine D_2 **Low to moderate** — 5-HT_{1C}, 5-HT_{1D}, 5-HT_{1A}, histamine H_1, alpha-adrenergic **Weak** — D_1, haloperidol-sensitive sigma site
Ziprasidone	**High** — dopamine D_2, D_3, 5-HT_{2A}, 5-HT_{2C}, 5-HT_{1A}[1], 5-HT_{1D}, alpha$_1$adrenergic **Moderate** — histamine H_1

[a] Promethazine is classified as a phenothiazine but not indicated as an antipsychotic.
[b] Partial agonist activity.

Conventional (typical) antipsychotics can be grouped into several classes; the phenothiazines, structurally related thioxanthenes, butyrophenones (phenylbutylpiperadines), diphenylbutylpiperadines, and the indolones. As a group, these agents are dopamine receptor antagonists with a higher affinity for D_2 over D_1 receptors. They exhibit varying degrees of selectivity among the cortical dopamine tracts: Nigrostriatal (movement disorders), mesolimbic (relief of hallucinations and delusions), mesocortical (relief of psychosis, worsening of negative symptoms) or tuberoinfundibular (prolactin release). They also bind with varying affinities to nondopaminergic sites, such as cholinergic, alpha$_1$-adrenergic and histaminic receptors, which can partially explain the varied side effect profiles for each agent. Typical antipsychotics are likely to induce extrapyramidal side effects (EPS) and have similar efficacies when used in equipotent doses. Lower-potency agents tend to be more sedating and high-potency agents usually have a higher incidence of acute EPS.

Novel (atypical) antipsychotics were introduced with the development of **clozapine** and can be structurally classified as dibenzepines, benzisoxazoles, or quinolinone. As a group, they have diverse pharmacodynamic profiles differing considerably from the typical antipsychotics but in general have an increased affinity for serotonin 5-HT_2 receptors compared with D_2 receptors. They act upon several neurotransmitter systems including antagonism at one or more types of dopamine receptors (eg, D_1, D_2, D_4, D_5); selectivity for limbic dopamine receptors; antagonism at 1 or more types of serotonin receptors (eg, 5-HT_1, 5-HT_2); antagonism at alpha$_1$ adrenergic receptors; and activity at muscarinic or histamine H_1 receptors. They are considered atypical because of their decreased ability or inability to induce EPS; newer agents also have a decreased propensity to induce agranulocytosis compared with clozapine. Studies indicate that some atypical agents are effective in patients resistant to conventional antipsychotic therapy and may be more effective in relieving negative symptoms than conventional agents.

Pharmacological Parameters of Antipsychotics

Antipsychotic agent	Approx. equiv. dose (mg)	Usual oral daily dose range (mg)	Sedation	EPS	Anticholinergic effects	Orthostatic hypotension	Weight gain
Phenothiazines							
Aliphatic							
Chlorpromazine	100	30-800	+++	++	++	+++	
Piperazine							
Fluphenazine	2	1-40	+	++++	+	+	
Perphenazine	10	12-64	++	++	+	+	
Prochlorperazine		15-150					
Trifluoperazine	5	2-15	+	+++	+	+	
Piperidines							
Mesoridazine	50	100-400	+++	+	+++	++	
Thioridazine	100	150-800	+++	+	+++	+++	
Thioxanthenes							
Thiothixene	4	6-60	+	+++	+	+	
Phenylbutylpiperadines							
Butyrophenone							
Haloperidol	2	1-100	+	++++	+	+	
Diphenylbutylpiperadine							
Pimozide		1-10	+	+++	++	+	
Dihydroindolones							
Molindone	10	15-225	+	++	+	+	
Ziprasidone		40-200	++	++	+	++	+
Dibenzepines							
Dibenzoxazepines							
Loxapine	10	20-250	+	++	+	+	
Dibenzodiazepine							
Clozapine	50	300-900	+++	0	+++	+++	++++
Thienbenzodiazepine							
Olanzapine		5-20	++	+	++	++	++++
Dibenzothiazepine							
Quetiapine		50-800	++	0	0-+	++	+++
Benzisoxazole							
Risperidone		4-16	+	++	0-+	++	+++
Quinolinone							
Aripiprazole		10-30	++	0	0-+	+	+++

++++ = Very high incidence of side effects, +++ = High incidence of side effects, ++ = Moderate incidence of side effects, + = Low incidence of side effects

▶*Pharmacokinetics:*

Metabolism – CYP2D6 is the enzyme responsible for metabolism of many antipsychotics. CYP2D6 is subject to genetic polymorphism and to inhibition by a variety of substrates and some nonsubstrates. Extensive CYP2D6 metabolizers convert drugs rapidly, whereas poor metabolizers convert the drugs much more slowly.

Special populations –

Hepatic function impairment:

• *Aripiprazole* – AUC increased 31% in mild, 8% in moderate, and decreased 20% in severe hepatic impairment.

• *Quetiapine* – Mean oral clearance decreased 30% in patients with hepatic impairment and AUC and C_{max} increased by 3 times. Dosage adjustment may be needed.

• *Ziprasidone* – In patients with clinically significant cirrhosis (Child-Pugh Class A and B), an increase in AUC of 13% and 34% occurred, respectively, and half-life was 7.1 hours compared with 4.8 hours in healthy subjects.

• *Risperidone* – The mean free fraction in plasma was increased by about 35% because of the diminished concentration of albumin and alpha-acid glycoprotein. Reduce dose in hepatic impairment.

Renal function impairment:

• *Aripiprazole* – In patients with severe renal impairment (Ccr less than 30 mL/min), **aripiprazole** and dehydro-aripiprazole C_{max} increased 36% and 53%, respectively. AUC decreased 15% for aripiprazole and increased 7% for dehydro-aripiprazole.

• *Quetiapine* – Patients with severe renal failure (Ccr 10 to 30 mL/min/1.73 m²) had a 25% lower mean oral clearance than normal subjects (Ccr greater than 80 mL/min/1.73m²); however, plasma concentrations were within the same range.

• *Ziprasidone* – Intramuscular **ziprasidone** has not been fully evaluated in renal impairment; however, the cyclodextrin excipient is cleared renally. Therefore, administer IM formulation with caution in these patients.

• *Risperidone* – In patients with moderate to severe renal disease, clearance of the sum of **risperidone** and its active metabolite decreased 60%. Reduce dose in renal disease.

Elderly:

• *Aripiprazole* – Clearance decreased 20% after a single 15 mg dose in patients 65 years of age or older.

• *Quetiapine* – Oral clearance decreased 40% in patients 65 years of age or older. A dosage adjustment may be necessary.

• *Risperidone* – Renal clearance of **risperidone** and its active metabolite were decreased. Modify dose accordingly.

• *Olanzapine* – Mean elimination half-life was about 1.5 times greater in patients 65 years of age or older.

Gender:

• *Aripiprazole* – C_{max} and AUC of **aripiprazole** and dehydro-aripiprazole are 30% to 40% higher in women and correspondingly the oral clearance is lower in women. These differences are largely explained by differences in body weight.

• *Olanzapine* – Clearance is approximately 30% lower in women.

Smoking:

• *Olanzapine* – Clearance is about 40% higher in smokers.

Race:

• *Olanzapine* – Comparisons between study data collected in Japan vs the United States suggest exposure to **olanzapine** could be about 2-fold greater in Japanese patients when equivalent doses are administered.

Antipsychotic Pharmacokinetics

Drug	Bioavailability	Mean C_{max}	T_{max}	Mean Vd	Protein bound (%)	Routes of metabolism	Active metabolite	T½	Routes of excretion
Conventional agents									
Chlorpromazine	20%-40%	25-150 ng/mL	1-4 h	≈ 21 L/kg	92%-97%			24 h	
Fluphenazine	2.7% (oral); 3.4% (SC/IM)	≈ 2.3 ng/mL (oral); 1.3 ng/mL (SC/IM)	≈ 2.8 h (oral); 24-48 h (SC/IM)	20 L/kg				18 h (oral)	
Haloperidol	60%-65% (oral)	≈ 9.2 ng/mL (oral); ≈ 22 ng/mL (IM)	6 days (decanoate)	≈ 18 L/kg	≈ 92%			≈ 18 h (oral); ≈ 3 wk (decanoate)	Feces, urine (≈ 1%)
Loxapine	≈ 100%							8 h	Urine, feces
Mesoridazine								30 h	
Molindone			1.5 h					12 h	Urine, feces
Perphenazine	20%	984 pg/mL	1-3 h	10-34 L/kg		Sulfoxidation, hydroxylation, dealkylation, and glucuronidation by CYP2D6		9-12 h	
Pimozide	> 50%	≈ 10 ng/mL	4 to 12 h	≈ 28 L/kg[a]	99%	N-dealkylation by CYP3A and CYP1A2 to a lesser extent		≈ 55 h	Urine (main route)
Prochlorperazine				20 L/kg				3-5 h (oral); 6.9 h (IV)	

Antipsychotic Pharmacokinetics

Drug	Bioavailability	Mean C$_{max}$	T$_{max}$	Mean Vd	Protein bound (%)	Routes of metabolism	Active metabolite	T$_{1/2}$	Routes of excretion
Promethazine[b]			2-3 h	13 L/kg	76%-80%	N-demethyl-ation and sulfoxidation		5-14 h	Urine, bile
Thioridazine				18 L/kg	99%		mesorida-zine	24 h	
Thiothixene								34 h	
Trifluoperazine								18 h	
Atypical agents									
Aripiprazole	87%		3-5 h	4.9 L/kg[a]	> 99%[c]	Dehydrogena-tion, hydroxylation, and N-dealkylation by CYP3A4 and CYP2D6	Dehydro-aripipra-zole	75[d]-146[e] h	Feces (≈ 55%), urine (≈ 25%)
Clozapine	27%-47%	319 ng/mL[a]	2.5 h	≈ 5.4 L/kg	≈ 97%	Demethylation, hydroxylation, and N-oxidation	Des-methyl metabolite has lim-ited activity	8 h[f]; 12 h[a]	Urine (≈ 50%), feces (≈ 30%)
Olanzapine	≈ 60%	≈ 12.9 ng/mL	≈ 6 h	≈ 1000 L	93% over a concen-tration range of 7-1100 ng/mL	Glucuronida-tion and oxidation by CYP1A2 and CYP2D6		21-54 h	Urine (≈ 57%), feces (≈ 30%)
Quetiapine	≥ 73%	778-1080 mcg/L	1.5 h	≈ 10 L/kg	83%[b]	Sulfoxidation and oxidation by CYP3A4	None	≈ 6 h	Urine (≈ 73%), feces (≈20%)
Risperidone	70%	10 ng/mL	≈ 1 h	1-2 L/kg	90%	Hydroxylation by CYP2D6 and N-dealkylation	9-hy-droxy-risperi-done	3[d]-20[e] h	Urine (≈ 70%), feces (≈ 14%)
Ziprasidone	≈ 60% (oral); 100% (IM)	44.6-139.4 mcg/L	6-8 h (oral); ≈ 60 min (IM)	1.5 L/kg	> 99%	Reduction by aldehyde oxidase, methylation, and oxidation by CYP3A4 and CYP1A2 to a lesser extent		≈ 7 h (oral); 2-5 h (IM)	Feces (≈ 66%), urine (≈ 20%)

[a] At steady-state
[b] Promethazine is classified as a phenothiazine but not indicated as an antipsychotic.
[c] At therapeutic concentrations
[d] Extensive metabolizers
[e] Poor metabolizers
[f] Single dose

Contraindications

Hypersensitivity to drug or any other component of the product (cross-sensitivity between phenothiazines may occur); comatose or greatly depressed states because of CNS depressants or from any other cause (phenothiazines, **clozapine, loxapine, molindone, pimozide, halo-peridol**); coadministration with other drugs that prolong the QT inter-val and in patients with congenital long QT syndrome or history of cardiac arrhythmias (**mesoridazine, thioridazine, pimozide, zipra-sidone**; see Drug Interactions).

►*Phenothiazines:* Suspected or established subcortical brain damage (**fluphenazine**); blood dyscrasias (**perphenazine, trifluoperazine, fluphenazine**); bone marrow depression (**perphenazine, triflu-operazine, fluphenazine**); preexisting liver damage (**perphenazine, trifluoperazine, fluphenazine**); pediatric surgery (**prochlorpera-zine**); hypertensive or hypotensive heart disease of extreme degree (**thioridazine**).

►*Thiothixene:* Circulatory collapse; blood dyscrasias.

►*Haloperidol:* Parkinson disease.

►*Pimozide:* Treatment of simple tics or tics other than those associ-ated with Tourette disorder; in combination with drugs (eg, pemoline, methylphenidate, amphetamines) that may themselves cause motor or phonic tics until it is determined whether or not the drugs, rather than Tourette disorder, are responsible for the tics.

►*Clozapine:* Myeloproliferative disorders; uncontrolled epilepsy; his-tory of **clozapine**-induced agranulocytosis or severe granulocytopenia; should not be used with other agents having a well-known potential to cause agranulocytosis or suppress bone marrow function.

►*Ziprasidone:* Recent acute MI; uncompensated heart failure.

Warnings

►*Tardive dyskinesia (TD):* TD, a syndrome consisting of potentially irreversible, involuntary dyskinetic movements, may develop in patients treated with antipsychotic drugs. Although prevalence of TD appears highest among the elderly, especially women, it is impossible to rely upon prevalence estimates to predict, at the inception of antipsy-chotic treatment, which patients are likely to develop the syndrome. Whether antipsychotic drugs differ in their potential to cause TD is unknown. However, atypical antipsychotics appear to have a lower risk of TD. Both the risk of developing TD and the likelihood that it will become irreversible are increased as duration of treatment and total cumulative dose administered increase. However, the syndrome can develop, although much less commonly, after relatively brief treatment periods at low doses.

There is no known treatment for established cases of TD, although it may remit, partially or completely, if antipsychotics are withdrawn. Antipsychotic treatment itself, however, may suppress (or partially suppress) signs and symptoms of TD, possibly masking the underlying disease process. The effect of symptomatic suppression on the long-term course of the syndrome is unknown.

Given these considerations, prescribe antipsychotics in a manner most likely to minimize the occurrence of tardive dyskinesia. In general, reserve chronic antipsychotic treatment for patients who suffer from a chronic illness that responds to antipsychotic drugs and for whom alter-native, equally effective, but potentially less harmful treatments are not available or appropriate. In patients who require chronic treat-ment, use the smallest dose and the shortest duration of treatment pro-ducing a satisfactory clinical response. Periodically reassess the need for continued treatment.

If signs and symptoms of TD appear, consider drug discontinuation. However, some patients may require treatment despite the presence of the syndrome.

►*Extrapyramidal symptoms (EPS):* Dystonic reactions develop primarily with the use of traditional antipsychotics. EPS has occurred during the administration of **haloperidol** and **pimozide** frequently, often during the first few days of treatment. EPS during the adminis-tration of haloperidol have been reported frequently, often during the first few days of treatment. EPS can be categorized generally as Par-kinson symptoms, akathisia, or dystonia (including opisthotonos and oculogyric crisis). While all can occur at relatively low doses, they occur more frequently and with greater severity at higher doses. The symp-toms may be controlled with dose reductions or administration of anti-parkinson drugs such as benztropine mesylate or trihexyphenidyl HCl. It should be noted that persistent EPS has been reported; the drug may have to be discontinued in such cases.

►*Neuroleptic malignant syndrome (NMS):* A potentially fatal symptom complex sometimes referred to as NMS has been reported in association with administration of antipsychotic drugs. Two possible cases of NMS (2/2387 [0.1%]) have been reported in clinical trials with **quetiapine**. Clinical manifestations of NMS are hyperpyrexia, muscle rigidity, altered mental status, and evidence of autonomic instability (irregular pulse or BP, tachycardia, diaphoresis, cardiac dysrhythmia). Additional signs may include elevated creatine phosphokinase, myoglobinuria (rhabdomyolysis), and acute renal failure. The onset may beafter hours to months of treatment or may occur after discontinuation of therapy. Once started, NMS proceeds rapidly over 24 to 72 hours.

The risk of NMS is higher in patients receiving high-potency, injectable, or depot antipsychotics. NMS may occur with atypical antipsychotics, but the risk is lower. There have been several reported cases of NMS in patients receiving **clozapine** alone or in combination with lithium or other CNS-active agents. The diagnostic evaluation of patients with this syndrome is complicated. In arriving at a diagnosis, it is important to exclude cases where the clinical presentation includes both serious medical illness (eg, pneumonia, systemic infection) and untreated or inadequately treated EPS. Other important considerations in the differential diagnosis include central anticholinergic toxicity, heat stroke, drug fever, and primary CNS pathology.

Include the following in the management of NMS: 1) Immediate discontinuation of antipsychotic drugs and other drugs not essential to concurrent therapy; 2) intensive symptomatic treatment and medical monitoring; and 3) treatment of any concomitant serious medical problems for which specific treatments are available. There is no general agreement about specific pharmacological treatment regimens for NMS.

If a patient requires antipsychotic drug treatment after recovery from NMS, carefully consider the potential reintroduction of drug therapy. Carefully monitor the patient because recurrences of NMS have been reported.

➤*CNS effects:* These agents may impair mental or physical abilities, especially during the first few days. Drowsiness may occur during the first or second week, after which it generally disappears. If troublesome, lower the dosage. Caution patients against activities requiring alertness (eg, operating vehicles or machinery). Use cautiously in depressed patients. Use caution in agitated states with depression, (particularly if a suicidal tendency is recognized). When **haloperidol** is used for mania in cyclic disorders, a rapid mood swing to depression may occur.

Encephalopathic syndrome – An encephalopathic syndrome (characterized by weakness, lethargy, fever, tremulousness and confusion, extrapyramidal symptoms, leukocytosis, elevated serum enzymes, BUN, fasting blood sugar) has occurred in a few patients treated with lithium plus an antipsychotic (**haloperidol**). In some instances, the syndrome was followed by irreversible brain damage. Because of a possible causal relationship between these events and the coadministration of lithium and antipsychotics, closely monitor patients receiving such combined therapy for early evidence of neurologic toxicity and promptly discontinue treatment if such signs appear. This encephalopathic syndrome may be similar to or the same as NMS.

➤*Cardiovascular effects:* Use with caution in patients with cardiovascular disease (history of MI or ischemic heart disease, heart failure, or conduction abnormalities), cerebrovascular disease, conditions that would predispose patients to hypotension (dehydration, hypovolemia, and treatment with antihypertensive medications), or mitral insufficiency. Increased pulse rates occur in most patients. Large doses and parenteral administration should be avoided in patients with impaired cardiovascular systems. To minimize the occurrence of hypotension after injection, keep patient lying down and observe for at least 30 minutes. One result of therapy may be an increase in mental and physical activity. For example, a few patients with angina pectoris have complained of increased pain while taking **trifluoperazine**. Therefore, withdraw the drug from angina patients if an unfavorable response is noted.

ECG changes – A minority of **clozapine** patients experience ECG repolarization changes similar to those seen with other antipsychotic drugs, including S-T segment depression and flattening or inversion of T waves, all of which normalize after discontinuation of clozapine. The clinical significance is unclear. However, several patients have experienced significant cardiac events, including ischemic changes, MI, arrhythmias, and sudden death. In addition there have been postmarketing reports of CHF, pericarditis, and pericardial effusions. Causality assessment was difficult in many of these cases because of serious pre-existing cardiac disease and plausible alternative causes. Rare instances of sudden death have been reported in psychiatric patients, with or without associated antipsychotic drug treatment, and the relationship of these events to antipsychotic drug use is unknown.

Ziprasidone, pimozide, mesoridazine, and **thioridazine** have been shown to prolong the QT interval, and drugs with this potential have been associated with torsade de pointes-type arrhythmias and sudden death. Certain circumstances may increase the risk of torsade de pointes and/or sudden death in association with the used of drugs that prolong the QT interval, including the following: 1) Bradycardia; 2) hypokalemia or hypomagnesemia; 3) concomitant use of other drugs that prolong the QT interval; and 4) presence of congenital prolongation of the QT interval. Perform a baseline ECG and measure serum potassium and magnesium before initiation of treatment and periodically during treatment, especially during a period of dose adjustment. Patients with QT interval over 450 msec should not receive mesoridazine or thioridazine. Ziprasidone should be avoided in patients with histories of significant cardiovascular illness (eg, QT prolongation, recent acute MI, uncompensated heart failure, cardiac arrhythmia). Replete patients with low potassium and/or magnesium with those

electrolytes before proceeding with treatment. Discontinue treatment if the QT interval is over 500 msec. Patients who experience symptoms that may be associated with the occurrence of torsade de pointes (eg, dizziness, palpitations, syncope) may warrant further cardiac evaluation; in particular, consider Holter monitoring. (See Black Box Warning, Contraindications, and Drug Interactions).

Nonspecific ECG changes, usually reversible Q- and T-wave distortions, have been observed in some patients receiving phenothiazines. Nonspecific ECG changes have been observed in some patients receiving **thiothixene**. These changes are usually reversible and frequently disappear on continued thiothixene therapy. The incidence of these changes is lower than that observed with some phenothiazines. The clinical significance of these changes is not known.

Haloperidol has been associated with ECG changes, including QT interval prolongation and ECG pattern changes compatible with the polymorphous configuration of torsade de pointes.

Rare, transient, nonspecific T-wave changes have been reported on ECG in patients taking **molindone**.

Prolongation of the QT interval and torsade de pointes have been reported with risperidone overdoses.

Other drugs that prolong the QT interval have been associated with the occurrence of torsade de pointes. Bradycardia, electrolyte imbalance, concomitant use with other drugs that prolong QT, or the presence of congenital prolongation in QT can increase the risk.

Myocarditis – Postmarketing **clozapine** surveillance data from 4 countries revealed cases of myocarditis, some fatal. The rate of myocarditis in clozapine-treated patients appears to be 17 to 322 times greater than the general population and is associated with an increased risk of fatal myocarditis that is 14 to 161 times greater than the general population. Therefore, consider the possibility of myocarditis in patients receiving clozapine who present with unexplained fatigue, dyspnea, tachypnea, fever, chest pain, palpitations, other signs or symptoms of heart failure, or electrocardiographic findings such as ST-T wave abnormalities or arrhythmias. It is not known whether eosinophilia is a reliable predictor of myocarditis. Tachycardia, which has been associated with clozapine treatment, also has been noted as a presenting sign in patients with myocarditis. Therefore, tachycardia during the first month of therapy warrants close monitoring for other signs of myocarditis. Prompt discontinuation of clozapine treatment is warranted upon suspicion of myocarditis. Patients with clozapine-related myocarditis should not be rechallenged with clozapine.

Cardiomyopathy – Cases of cardiomyopathy have been reported in patients treated with **clozapine**. Approximately 80% of clozapine-treated patients in whom cardiomyopathy was reported were younger than 50 years of age; the duration of treatment with clozapine prior to cardiomyopathy diagnosis varied, but was more than 6 months in 65% of the reports. Dilated cardiomyopathy was most frequently reported. Signs and symptoms suggestive of cardiomyopathy, particularly exertional dyspnea, fatigue, orthopnea, paroxysmal nocturnal dyspnea, and peripheral edema should alert the clinician to perform further investigations. If the diagnosis of cardiomyopathy is confirmed, discontinue clozapine unless the benefit to the patient clearly outweighs the risk.

Pulmonary embolism – Consider the possibility of pulmonary embolism in patients receiving **clozapine** who present with deep vein thrombosis, acute dyspnea, chest pain, or with other respiratory signs and symptoms. Deep vein thrombosis also has been observed in association with clozapine therapy. Whether pulmonary embolus can be attributed to clozapine or some characteristic(s) of its users is not clear, but the occurrence of deep vein thrombosis or respiratory symptomatology should suggest its presence.

Hypotension – Orthostatic hypotension with or without syncope can occur, especially during initial titration in association with rapid dose escalation, and may represent a continuing risk in some patients. In 1 report, initial **clozapine** doses as low as 12.5 mg were associated with collapse and respiratory arrest.

Severe, acute hypotension has occurred with the use of **phenothiazines** and is particularly likely to occur in patients with mitral insufficiency or pheochromocytoma. Rebound hypertension may occur in pheochromocytoma patients.

Carefully watch patients who are undergoing surgery, and who are on large doses of **phenothiazines**, for hypotensive phenomena. It may be necessary to reduce amounts of anesthetics or CNS depressants. The hypotensive effects may occur after the first injection of the antipsychotic, occasionally after subsequent injections, and rarely after the first oral dose. Recovery is usually spontaneous and symptoms disappear within 0.5 to 2 hours. If hypotension occurs, place the patient in a recumbent position. Females have a greater tendency to experience orthostatic hypotension. Patients with hypovolemia have increased sensitivity to the hypotensive effects of these agents. Volume replacement, when needed, should precede use of vasopressors. If a vasopressor is indicated, use phenylephrine or norepinephrine. Avoid using epinephrine in drug-induced hypotension (see Drug Interactions).

Tachycardia – Tachycardia, which may be sustained, also has been observed in approximately 25% of patients taking **clozapine**, with an average increase in pulse rate of 10 to 15 bpm. The sustained tachycardia is not simply a reflex response to hypotension, and is present in all positions monitored. Either tachycardia or hypotension may pose a serious risk for an individual with compromised cardiovascular function. Pulse rates have increased in most patients receiving antipsychotics.

➤*Cerebrovascular effects:* Cerebrovascular adverse events (eg, stroke, transient ischemic attack), including fatalities, were reported in patients (mean age, 85 years; range 73 to 97 years of age) in trials of risperidone in elderly patients with dementia-related psychosis. In placebo-controlled trials, there was a significantly higher incidence of cerebrovascular adverse events in patients treated with risperidone compared to patients treated with placebo. Risperidone is not approved for the treatment of patients with dementia-related psychosis.

➤*Sudden death:* Sudden, unexpected, and unexplained deaths have been reported in psychotic patients receiving phenothiazines. Previous brain damage or seizures may be predisposing factors; avoid high doses in known seizure patients. Several patients have shown sudden flare-ups of psychotic behavior patterns shortly before death. In some cases, death was apparently caused by cardiac arrest; in others, asphyxia was caused by failure of the cough reflex. Autopsy findings usually reveal acute fulminating pneumonia or pneumonitis, aspiration of gastric contents, or intramyocardial lesions. In some patients, cause could not be determined.

Sudden unexpected deaths have occurred in experimental studies of **pimozide** in conditions other than Tourette disorder. These deaths occurred while patients were receiving pimozide dosages in the range of 1 mg/kg. One possible mechanism for such deaths is prolongation of the QT interval predisposing patients to ventricular arrhythmia.

➤*Priapism:* Rare cases of priapism have been associated with **risperidone**, **ziprasidone**, **quetiapine**, **aripiprazole**, and **olanzapine**. While the relationship of the event to these antipsychotics has not been established, other drugs with alpha-adrenergic blocking effects have been reported to induce priapism. Severe priapism may require surgical intervention.

➤*Hyperprolactinemia:* Antipsychotic drugs elevate prolactin levels; the elevation persists during chronic administration. However, in contrast to more typical antipsychotic drugs, **clozapine** therapy produces little or no prolactin elevation. Drugs that antagonize dopamine D_2 receptors elevate prolactin levels. Experiments indicate that approximately 33% of human breast cancers are prolactin-dependent in vitro, a factor of potential importance if the prescription of these drugs is contemplated in a patient with previously detected breast cancer.

Although disturbances such as galactorrhea, amenorrhea, gynecomastia, and impotence have been reported with prolactin-elevating compounds, the clinical significance of elevated serum prolactin levels is unknown for most patients.

Risperidone, **ziprasidone**, and **olanzapine** elevate prolactin levels. As is common with compounds that increase prolactin release, an increase in pituitary gland, mammary gland, and pancreatic islet cell hyperplasia or neoplasia was observed in risperidone carcinogenicity studies conducted in mice and rats. An increase in mammary gland neoplasia was observed in the olanzapine and ziprasidone carcinogenicity studies conducted in mice and in the olanzapine studies in rats.

Elevated prolactin levels were not demonstrated in clinical trials with **quetiapine**. However, increased prolactin levels were observed in rats studied with this compound.

➤*Hyperglycemia and diabetes mellitus:* Severe hyperglycemia, sometimes leading to ketoacidosis, has been reported during **clozapine** treatment in patients with no prior history of hyperglycemia. While a causal relationship to clozapine use has not been definitively established, glucose levels normalized in most patients after discontinuation of clozapine, and a rechallenge in one patient produced a recurrence of hyperglycemia. Consider the possibility of impaired glucose tolerance in patients receiving clozapine who develop symptoms of hyperglycemia, such as polydipsia, polyuria, polyphagia, and weakness. In patients with significant treatment-emergent hyperglycemia, consider discontinuing clozapine.

Hyperglycemia, in some cases extreme and associated with ketoacidosis or hyperosmolar coma or death, has been reported in patients treated with atypical antipsychotics. The relationship between atypical antipsychotic use and hyperglycemia-related adverse events is not completely understood. However, epidemiological studies suggest an increased risk of treatment-emergent hyperglycemia-related adverse events in patients treated with the atypical antipsychotics studied. Precise risk estimates are not available.

Regularly monitor patients with an established diagnosis of diabetes mellitus who are started on atypical antipsychotics for worsening of glucose control. Patients with risk factors for diabetes mellitus (eg, obesity, family history of diabetes) who are starting treatment with atypical antipsychotics should undergo fasting blood glucose testing at baseline and periodically during treatment. Any patient treated with atypical antipsychotics should be monitored for symptoms of hyperglycemia including polydipsia, polyuria, polyphagia, and weakness. Patients who develop symptoms of hyperglycemia during treatment with atypical antipsychotics should undergo fasting blood glucose testing. In some cases, hyperglycemia has resolved when the atypical antipsychotic was discontinued; however, some patients required continuation of antidiabetic treatment despite discontinuation of the suspect drug.

➤*Antiemetic effects:* Drugs with an antiemetic effect can obscure signs of toxicity of other drugs (eg, cancer chemotherapeutic drugs) or mask symptoms of disease (eg, brain tumor, intestinal obstruction, Reye syndrome). They can suppress the cough reflex; aspiration of vomitus is possible.

Risperidone, **thiothixene**, **loxapine**, and **molindone** have an antiemetic effect in animals that may also occur in humans.

➤*Pulmonary:* Cases of bronchopneumonia (some fatal) have followed the use of antipsychotic agents. Lethargy and decreased sensation of thirst caused by central inhibition may lead to dehydration, hemoconcentration, and reduced pulmonary ventilation. If the above signs appear, especially in the elderly, institute remedial therapy promptly.

Use with caution in respiratory impairment caused by acute pulmonary infections or chronic respiratory disorders, such as severe asthma or emphysema. "Silent pneumonias" may develop in patients treated with **phenothiazines**.

➤*Agranulocytosis:* Agranulocytosis, defined as an absolute neutrophil count (ANC) of less than 500/mm³, occurs in association with **clozapine** use at a cumulative incidence at 1 year of approximately 1.3%, based on 15 cases out of 1743 patients exposed to clozapine during clinical testing. All of these cases occurred when the need for close monitoring of WBC counts was already recognized. This reaction could prove fatal if not detected early and therapy interrupted. Of the 149 cases of agranulocytosis reported worldwide in association with clozapine use as of December 31, 1989, 32% were fatal. However, few of these deaths occurred since 1977, when knowledge of clozapine-induced agranulocytosis became more widespread, and close monitoring of WBC counts more widely practiced. In the United States, under a weekly WBC monitoring system with clozapine, there have been 585 cases of agranulocytosis as of August 21, 1997; 19 were fatal. During this period 150,409 patients received clozapine. The incidence rates of agranulocytosis based upon a weekly monitoring schedule, rose steeply during the first 2 months of therapy, peaking in the third month. Among clozapine patients who continued the drug beyond the third month, the weekly incidence of agranulocytosis fell to a substantial degree, so that by the sixth month, the weekly incidence of agranulocytosis was reduced to 3 per 1000 person-years. After 6 months, the weekly incidence of agranulocytosis declined still further, however, never reaching zero.

Patients must have a blood sample drawn for a WBC count before initiation of treatment with **clozapine**, and must have subsequent WBC counts done at least weekly for the first 6 months of treatment, as well as for 4 weeks after discontinuation. The distribution of clozapine is contingent upon performance of the required blood tests (see Administration and Dosage of individual monograph).

Except for evidence of significant bone marrow suppression during initial **clozapine** therapy, there are no established risk factors for the development of agranulocytosis. However, a disproportionate number of the US cases of agranulocytosis occurred in patients of Jewish background compared with the overall proportion of such patients exposed during clozapine's domestic development. Most of the US cases occurred within 4 to 10 weeks of exposure, but neither dose nor duration is a reliable predictor. No patient characteristics have been clearly linked to the development of agranulocytosis in association with clozapine use, but agranulocytosis associated with other antipsychotic drugs occurred with a greater frequency in women, the elderly, and in patients who are cachetic or have serious underlying medical illness; such patients may also be at particular risk with clozapine.

To reduce the risk of agranulocytosis developing undetected, **clozapine** will be dispensed only within the clozapine Patient Management System. For more information, call 1-800-448-5938.

➤*Ophthalmic effects:* As with all drugs that exert anticholinergic effect and/or cause mydriasis, use with caution in patients with a history of glaucoma. During prolonged therapy, ocular changes may occur; these include particle deposition in the cornea and lens, progressing in more severe cases to star-shaped lenticular opacities.

Pigmentary retinopathy – Careful observation should be made for pigmentary retinopathy and lenticular pigmentation (fine lenticular pigmentation has been noted in a small number of patients treated for prolonged periods. Pigmentary retinopathy, which has been observed primarily in patients taking larger than recommended thioridazine doses, is characterized by diminution of visual acuity, brownish coloring of vision, and impairment of night vision; examination of the fundus discloses deposits of pigment.

Cataracts – In dogs receiving **quetiapine** for 6 or 12 months, focal triangular cataracts occurred at the junction of the posterior sutures in the outer cortex of the lens at a dose of 4 times the maximum recommended human dose. The finding may be because of inhibition of cholesterol biosynthesis by quetiapine.

Lens changes have also been observed in patients during long-term treatment, but a causal relationship has not been established. Examination of the lens by methods adequate to detect cataract formation, such as slit-lamp exam, is recommended at initiation of treatment or shortly thereafter, and at 6-month intervals.

➤*Seizure disorders:* Some antipsychotics can lower the convulsive threshold and may precipitate seizures. Grand mal seizures have occurred, particularly in patients with EEG abnormalities or a history of such disorders. Use cautiously in patients with a history of epilepsy or those in a state of alcohol withdrawal. These drugs may be used concomitantly with anticonvulsants; maintain an adequate anticonvulsant dosage (see Drug Interactions).

Seizure has been estimated to occur in association with **clozapine** use at a cumulative incidence at 1 year of approximately 5%, based on the occurrence of 1 or more seizures during its clinical testing prior to domestic marketing. Dose appears to be an important predictor of seizure, with a greater likelihood of seizure at the higher clozapine doses used. Exercise caution in administering clozapine to patients having a history of seizures or other predisposing factors. Because of the substantial risk of seizure associated with clozapine use, advise patients not to engage in any activity where sudden loss of consciousness could cause serious risk to themselves or others.

➤*GI dysmotility:* Esophageal dysmotility and aspiration have been associated with antipsychotic drug use. Aspiration pneumonia is a common cause of morbidity and mortality in elderly patients, in particular those with advanced Alzheimer dementia. Use **quetiapine**, **ziprasidone**, **risperidone**, **olanzapine**, **aripiprazole**, and others cautiously in patients at risk for aspiration pneumonia.

➤*Hypersensitivity reactions:* Patients who have demonstrated a hypersensitivity reaction (eg, blood dyscrasias, jaundice) with a phenothiazine should not be re-exposed to any phenothiazine unless the potential benefits of treatment outweigh the possible hazards.

➤*Renal function impairment:* Administer cautiously to those with diminished renal function. Monitor renal function in long-term therapy; lower the dose or discontinue if BUN becomes abnormal.

➤*Hepatic function impairment:* Jaundice usually occurs between the second and fourth weeks of **phenothiazine** treatment and is regarded as a hypersensitivity reaction. The clinical picture resembles infectious hepatitis with laboratory features of obstructive jaundice. It is usually reversible; however, chronic jaundice has occurred. If fever with flu-like symptoms occurs, perform liver function tests. If tests are abnormal, discontinue treatment. Withhold exploratory laparotomy until extrahepatic obstruction is confirmed. Because of the possibility of liver damage, periodically monitor hepatic function. There is no conclusive evidence that preexisting liver disease makes patients more susceptible to jaundice. Alcoholics with cirrhosis have been successfully treated with **chlorpromazine** without complications. Nevertheless, use cautiously in patients with liver disease. Do not re-expose patients who have experienced jaundice to a **phenothiazine**.

Use with caution in patients with impaired hepatic function. Patients with a history of hepatic encephalopathy caused by cirrhosis have increased sensitivity to the CNS effects of antipsychotic drugs (eg, impaired cerebration and abnormal slowing of the EEG).

Elevations of serum transaminase and alkaline phosphatase, usually transient, have been infrequently observed in some patients. No clinically confirmed cases of jaundice attributable to **thiothixene** have been reported.

Caution is advised in patients using **clozapine** who have concurrent hepatic disease. Hepatitis has been reported in both patients with normal and preexisting liver function abnormalities. Immediately perform liver function tests in patients who develop nausea, vomiting, and/or anorexia during clozapine treatment. If the elevation of these values is clinically relevant or if symptoms of jaundice occur, discontinue clozapine treatment.

Patients with impaired hepatic function may have increases in the free fraction of **risperidone**, possibly resulting in an enhanced effect.

Six percent of **quetiapine** and 2% of **olanzapine** patients had transaminase elevations over 3 times the upper limit of normal. Hepatic enzyme elevations usually occurred within the first 3 weeks of quetiapine treatment and promptly returned to prestudy levels with ongoing treatment. Because quetiapine is extensively metabolized by the liver, higher plasma levels are expected in the hepatically impaired population and dosage adjustment may be needed.

➤*Carcinogenesis:* Antipsychotic drugs elevate prolactin levels, which persist during chronic use. Tissue culture experiments indicate approximately 33% of human breast cancers are prolactin-dependent in vitro, a factor of potential importance if use of these drugs is contemplated in a patient with previously detected breast cancer. Although disturbances such as galactorrhea, amenorrhea, gynecomastia, and impotence have occurred, clinical significance of elevated serum prolactin levels is unknown for most patients. An increase in mammary neoplasia has occurred in rodents after chronic neuroleptic use. Studies, however, have not shown an association between chronic use of these drugs and mammary tumorigenesis.

In mice, **pimozide** causes a dose-related increase in pituitary and mammary tumors.

In female mice at 5 to 20 times the highest initial daily dose of **haloperidol** for chronic or resistant patients, there was a statistically significant increase in mammary gland neoplasia and total tumor incidence; at 20 times the same daily dose there was a statistically significant increase in pituitary gland neoplasia. **Risperidone** administered to rats and mice at doses up to 10 mg/kg for up to 25 months produced statistically significant increases in pituitary gland adenomas, endocrine pancreas adenomas, and mammary gland adenocarcinomas.

The incidence of liver hemangiomas and hemangiosarcomas was significantly increased in 1 mouse study in female mice dosed at 8 mg/kg/day of **olanzapine**. The incidence of mammary gland adenomas and adenocarcinomas also was significantly increased in another study in rodents.

In female mice, the incidences of pituitary gland adenomas and mammary gland adenocarcinomas and adenoacanthomas were increased at dietary doses of 3 to 30 mg/kg/day of **aripiprazole**. The incidence of mammary gland fibroadenomas and adrenocortical carcinomas and combined adrenocortical adenomas/carcinomas also were increased in female rats.

Quetiapine was administered to rats and there were statistically significant increases in thyroid gland follicular adenomas, mammary gland adenomas, and thyroid follicular cell adenomas.

In female mice, there were dose-related increases in the incidences of pituitary gland adenoma and carcinoma, and mammary gland adenocarcinoma at doses of 50, 100, or 200 mg/kg/day of **ziprasidone** tested.

➤*Mutagenesis:* Abnormal sperm and chromosomal aberrations in spermatocytes have occurred in rodents treated with certain antipsychotics.

Aripiprazole and a metabolite were clastogenic in the in vitro chromosomal aberration assay.

Quetiapine produced a reproducible increase in mutations in one *Salmonella typhimurium* tester strain in the presence of metabolic activation.

Ziprasidone produced a reproducible mutagenic response in the Ames assay in 1 strain of *S. typhimurium* in the absence of metabolic activation. Positive results were obtained in both the in vitro mammalian cell gene mutation assay and in the in vitro chromosomal aberration assay in human lymphocytes.

➤*Fertility impairment:* **Quetiapine** decreased mating and fertility in male rats at oral doses of 50 and 150 mg/kg and in female rats at oral doses of 50 mg/kg. An increase in irregular estrus cycles was observed at doses of 10 and 50 mg/kg.

Ziprasidone was shown to increase time to copulation in rats. Fertility rate was reduced at 160 mg/kg/day.

Estrus cycle irregularities and increased corpora lutea were seen at doses of 2, 6, and 20 mg/kg/day of **aripiprazole**. Increased preimplantation loss was seen at 6 and 20 mg/kg, and decreased fetal weight was seen at 20 mg/kg. Male rats had disturbances in spermatogenesis at 60 mg/kg, and prostate atrophy at 40 and 60 mg/kg, but no impairment of fertility was seen.

Risperidone was shown to impair mating, but not fertility, in female rats. In dogs given 0.31 to 5 mg/kg, sperm motility and concentration and serum testosterone were decreased.

Rats treated with **olanzapine** showed impaired male mating performance, but not fertility, at a dose of 22.4 mg/kg/day and female fertility was decreased at a dose of 3 mg/kg/day. Diestrous was prolonged and estrus delayed at 1.1 mg/kg/day; therefore, olanzapine may produce a delay in ovulation.

Female rats administered **pimozide** had prolonged estrus cycles, an effect also produced by other antipsychotics.

➤*Elderly:* Dosages in the lower range are sufficient for most elderly patients. Because these patients appear more susceptible to various cardiovascular, neuromuscular, and anticholinergic reactions, observe patients closely. The prevalence of tardive dyskinesia appears to be highest among the elderly, especially elderly women. Monitor response and adjust dosage accordingly. Increase dosage gradually in elderly patients.

➤*Pregnancy:* Category C; Category B (**clozapine**). Safety for use during pregnancy has not been established. Use only when clearly needed and when potential benefits outweigh potential hazards to the fetus.

There are reported instances of prolonged jaundice, extrapyramidal signs, hyperreflexia or hyporeflexia in newborn infants whose mothers received **phenothiazines**. **Prochlorperazine** is not recommended for use in pregnant patients except in cases of severe nausea and vomiting that are so serious and intractable that drug intervention is required and potential benefits outweigh possible hazards.

Reproductive studies of **chlorpromazine** in rodents have demonstrated potential for embryotoxicity and increased neonatal mortality. Tests in the offspring of the rodent demonstrate decreased performance. The possibility of permanent neurological damage cannot be excluded. It is not recommended that chlorpromazine be given to pregnant patients except when it is essential.

There are reports of cases of limb malformations observed following maternal use of **haloperidol**. Causal relationships were not established in these cases.

Perinatal studies have shown renal papillary abnormalities in offspring of rats treated from mid-pregnancy with **loxapine** doses of 0.6 to 1.8 mg/kg.

In the rat, doses of **pimozide** up to 8 times the maximum human dose resulted in decreased pregnancies and in the retarded development of fetuses. In the rabbit, maternal toxicity, mortality, decreased weight gain, and embryotoxicity including increased resorption were dose-related.

In animal studies, **ziprasidone** and **aripiprazole** demonstrated developmental toxicity, including possible teratogenic effects.

Placental transfer of **risperidone** occurs in rat pups and studies showed a decrease in the number of live pups and an increase in the number of dead pups at birth, and decrease in birth weight in pups. There was one report of a case of agenesis of the corpus callosum in an infant exposed to risperidone in utero. The causal relationship is unknown.

Placental transfer of **olanzapine** occurs in rat pups and studies showed early resorptions and increased numbers of nonviable fetuses.

Animal studies of **quetiapine** showed evidence of embryo/fetal toxicity including delays in skeletal ossification, reduced fetal body weights, increased incidence of a minor soft tissue anomaly, increases in fetal and pup death, and decreases in mean litter weight. Evidence of maternal toxicity was also observed at high doses.

Reproductive studies in animals and clinical experience to date have failed to show a teratogenic effect with **thioridazine**, **thiothixene**, **clozapine**, and **molindone**.

➤*Lactation:* There is evidence that **phenothiazines** are excreted in the breast milk of nursing mothers. Decide whether to discontinue nursing or discontinue the drug, taking into account the importance of the drug to the mother.

Animal studies suggest that **loxapine** (and its metabolites), **risperidone** (and its metabolites), **clozapine**, **olanzapine**, **quetiapine**, and **aripiprazole** may be excreted in breast milk. Risperidone also is excreted in human breast milk. Avoid nursing during loxapine therapy if possible. Women receiving risperidone, clozapine, olanzapine, quetiapine, or aripiprazole should not breastfeed.

Infants should not be nursed during **haloperidol** or **ziprasidone** treatment.

Because of the tumorigenicity and unknown cardiovascular effects in the infant, decide whether to discontinue nursing or discontinue **pimozide**, taking into account the importance of the drug to the mother.

➤*Children:* Children with acute illnesses (eg, chickenpox, CNS infections, measles, gastroenteritis) or dehydration are much more susceptible to neuromuscular reactions, particularly dystonias, than adults. Children seem more prone to develop extrapyramidal reactions, even at moderate doses. Therefore, use the lowest effective dosage.

Extrapyramidal symptoms can occur and be confused with CNS signs of an undiagnosed primary disease responsible for the vomiting (eg, Reye syndrome or other encephalopathy). Avoid antipsychotics and other potential hepatotoxins in children and adolescents whose signs and symptoms suggest Reye syndrome.

Safety and effectiveness of **fluphenazine**, **clozapine**, **haloperidol** (decanoate), **mesoridazine**, **loxapine**, **olanzapine**, **risperidone**, **aripiprazole**, **quetiapine**, and **ziprasidone** in pediatric patients have not been established.

Thiothixene, **perphenazine**, and **molindone** are not recommended in children under 12 years of age. Information on the use and efficacy of **pimozide** in patients less than 12 years of age is limited. **Trifluoperazine** is indicated for the treatment of schizophrenia in children 6 to 12 years of age. When treating children for severe nausea and vomiting, **prochlorperazine** should not to be used in children under 9 kg (20 lb) in weight or 2 years of age. **Chlorpromazine** should not be used in pediatric patients under 6 months of age except where potentially life-saving. Oral **haloperidol** is not intended for children under 3 years of age.

Precautions

➤*Anticholinergic effects:* Use caution in patients with clinically significant prostatic hypertrophy, narrow-angle glaucoma, or a history of paralytic ileus. Anticholinergic effects of **clozapine** are very potent. **Clozapine** use has been associated with varying degrees of impairment of intestinal peristalsis, ranging from constipation to intestinal obstruction, fecal impaction, and paralytic ileus. On rare occasions, these cases have been fatal. Constipation should be initially treated by ensuring adequate hydration, and use of ancillary therapy such as bulk laxatives. **Olanzapine** exhibits in vitro muscarinic receptor affinity and was associated with constipation, dry mouth, and tachycardia. **Thiothixene** and **chlorpromazine** exhibit rather weak anticholinergic properties. **Risperidone**, **aripiprazole**, **ziprasidone**, and **quetiapine** have no affinity for cholinergic muscarinic receptors.

➤*Cholesterol:* **Quetiapine**-treated patients had increases from baseline in cholesterol and triglyceride of 11% and 17%, respectively.

➤*Concomitant conditions:* Use with caution in patients: Exposed to extreme heat or phosphorus insecticides; atropine or related drugs because of additive anticholinergic effects; in a state of alcohol withdrawal; with dermatoses or other allergic reactions to phenothiazine derivatives because of the possibility of cross-sensitivity; who have exhibited idiosyncrasy to other centrally acting drugs. Risperidone has not been evaluated or used to any appreciable extent in patients with a recent history of MI or unstable heart disease; use with caution.

➤*Hematologic:* Various blood dyscrasias have occurred (see Adverse Reactions). In clinical trials, 1% of **clozapine** patients developed eosinophilia, which, in rare cases, can be substantial. If a differential count reveals a total eosinophil count above $4000/mm^3$, clozapine therapy should be interrupted because of the possibility of seizures; do not resume therapy until eosinophil count falls below $3000/mm^3$. If sore throat or other sign of infection occurs, or if white cell and differential counts indicate cellular depression, stop treatment and institute an antibiotic and other suitable therapy. A single case of transient granulocytopenia has been associated with **mesoridazine**. Patients with bone marrow depression with a phenothiazine should not receive any phenothiazines, unless the potential benefits outweigh the possible hazard.

Routine blood counts are advisable during therapy because blood dyscrasias, including leukopenia, agranulocytosis, thrombocytopenic or nonthrombocytopenic purpura, eosinophilia, and pancytopenia have been observed with phenothiazine derivatives.

➤*Myelography:* Discontinue phenothiazines at least 48 hours before myelography because of the possibility of seizures; do not resume therapy for at least 24 hours postprocedure. Do not use phenothiazines to control nausea and vomiting occurring before or after myelography.

➤*Thrombotic thrombocytopenic purpura (TTP):* A single case of TTP was reported in a 28-year-old female patient receiving **risperidone**. She experienced jaundice, fever and bruising, but eventually recovered after receiving plasmapheresis. The relationship to therapy is unknown.

➤*Thyroid:* Severe neurotoxicity (rigidity, inability to walk or talk) may occur in patients with thyrotoxicosis who are also receiving antipsychotics.

Hypothyroidism – **Quetiapine** demonstrated a dose-related decrease in total and free thyroxine (T_4) of approximately 20% at the higher end of the therapeutic dose range that was maximal in the first 2 to 4 weeks of treatment and maintained without adaptation or progression during more chronic therapy. Generally, these changes were of no clinical significance and TSH and TBG were unchanged in most patients, but approximately 0.4% of quetiapine patients did experience TSH increases. Six of the patients with TSH increases needed replacement thyroid treatment.

➤*Hyperpyrexia:* A significant, not otherwise explained rise in body temperature may indicate intolerance to antipsychotics. Discontinue in this case. Disruption of the body's ability to reduce core body temperature has been attributed to antipsychotic agents. Appropriate care is advised for patients who will be experiencing conditions that may contribute to an elevation in core body temperature (eg, exercising strenuously, exposure to extreme heat, receiving concomitant medication with anticholinergic activity, being subject to dehydration). Heat stroke has been reported with **haloperidol** use.

During **clozapine** therapy, patients may experience transient temperature elevations above 100.4°F (38°C), with the peak incidence within the first 3 weeks of treatment. While this fever is generally benign and self-limiting, it may necessitate discontinuing patients from treatment. On occasion, there may be an associated increase or decrease in WBC count. Carefully evaluate patients with fever to rule out the possibility of an underlying infectious process or the development of agranulocytosis. In the presence of high fever, the possibility of NMS must be considered.

➤*Abrupt withdrawal:* These drugs are not known to cause psychic dependence. However, following abrupt withdrawal of high-dose therapy, symptoms such as gastritis, nausea, vomiting, dizziness, headache, restlessness, sweating, increased salivation, and insomnia have occurred. To lessen the likelihood of adverse reactions related to cumulative drug effects, periodically determine whether the maintenance dosage could be lowered or drug therapy discontinued. These symptoms can be reduced by gradual reduction of the dosage or by continuing antiparkinson agents for several weeks after the antipsychotic is withdrawn.

Some patients on **pimozide** or **haloperidol** maintenance treatment experience transient dyskinetic signs after abrupt withdrawal. This may be indistinguishable from the syndrome of persistent tardive dyskinesia except for duration. It is not known whether gradual withdrawal of antipsychotic drugs will reduce the rate of occurrence, but it seems reasonable to gradually withdraw use of the drug.

➤*Suicide:* Suicide remains a possibility in depressed patients during treatment and until significant remission occurs. Do not allow patients of this type to have access to large quantities of the drug.

➤*Cutaneous pigmentation changes:* Rare instances of skin pigmentation have occurred, primarily in females on long-term, high-dose phenothiazine therapy. These changes, restricted to exposed areas of the skin, range from almost imperceptible darkening to a slate gray color, sometimes with a violet hue. Pigmentation may fade following drug discontinuation.

➤*Phenylketonurics:* Inform phenylketonuric patients that some of these products contain phenylalanine.

➤*Benzyl alcohol:* Some of these products contain benzyl alcohol, which has been associated with a fatal "gasping syndrome" in premature infants.

➤*Drug abuse and dependence:* Evaluate patients for history of drug abuse, and observe such patients closely for signs of misuse or abuse (eg, development of tolerance, increases in dose, drug-seeking behavior).

➤*Photosensitivity:* Because photosensitivity has been reported (rarely with **thioridazine**), undue exposure to the sun should be avoided during phenothiazine treatment.

➤*Sulfite sensitivity:* Some of these products contain sulfites that may cause allergic-type reactions, including anaphylactic symptoms and life-threatening or less severe asthmatic episodes in certain susceptible persons. The overall prevalence of sulfite sensitivity in the general population is unknown and probably low. It is seen more frequently in asthmatic or atopic nonasthmatic persons.

Drug Interactions

➤*CYP450:* Several antipsychotics are metabolized by the cytochrome P450 (CYP450) enzyme system. Therefore, several drug interactions may be possible involving drugs that are potent inhibitors or inducers of this enzyme system. Monitor and adjust therapy as needed when these antipsychotics are coadministered with potent inhibitors or inducers of the following isoenzymes.

Antipsychotics and Enzymes Involved with Metabolism	
Antipsychotic agent	Enzyme(s)
Aripiprazole	CYP3A4, 2D6
Clozapine	CYP1A2, 2D6, 3A4
Olanzapine	CYP1A2, 2D6
Perphenazine	CYP2D6
Pimozide	CYP3A, 1A2
Quetiapine	CYP3A4
Risperidone	CYP2D6

Antipsychotics and Enzymes Involved with Metabolism	
Antipsychotic agent	Enzyme(s)
Thioridazine	CYP2D6
Ziprasidone	Aldehyde oxidase, CYP3A4, 1A2

Antipsychotic Contraindications	
Antipsychotic	Contraindicated with
Clozapine	Drugs having a well-known potential to cause agranulocytosis or suppress bone marrow function.
Phenothiazines	Cisapride, sparfloxacin (due to possible additive QT interval prolongation.
Mesoridazine Ziprasidone	Drugs that prolong the QT interval.[a]
Pimozide	Drugs that prolong the QT interval[a]; CYP3A inhibitors (eg, clarithromycin, erythromycin, dirithromycin, troleandomycin, itraconazole, ketoconazole, voriconazole, protease inhibitors, nefazodone, sertraline).
Thioridazine	Drugs that prolong the QT interval[a]; CYP2D6 inhibitors (eg, fluoxetine, paroxetine, fluvoxamine, propranolol, pindolol).

[a] The following drugs may prolong the QT interval and increase the risk of life-threatening cardiac arrhythmias, including torsade de pointes: Antiarrhythmic agents (eg, amiodarone, bretylium, procainamide, sotalol, quinidine, disopyramide, dofetilide), cisapride, gatifloxacin, moxifloxacin, sparfloxacin, pimozide, mesoridazine, thioridazine, ziprasidone, chlorpromazine, droperidol, halofantrine, mefloquine, pentamidine, arsenic trioxide, levomethadyl acetate, dolasetron mesylate, probucol, tacrolimus.

Antipsychotic Drug Interactions			
Precipitant Drug	Object Drug*		Description
Anticholinergic agents	Haloperidol	↓	Decreased serum concentrations of haloperidol, worsening schizophrenic symptoms, and tardive dyskinesia have been reported with coadministration. Coadminister with caution.
Anticholinergic agents	Phenothiazines	↑↓	Therapeutic effects of phenothiazines may be decreased by centrally acting anticholinergics. Coadministration may lead to an increase in anticholinergic effects. Coadminister with caution.
Phenothiazines	Anticholinergic agents		
Antipsychotic agents	Alcohol CNS depressants	↑	Coadministration may lead to enhanced CNS depression, especially impairment of motor skills. Dystonic reactions may be precipitated by alcohol. Avoid concurrent use or use with caution.
Antipsychotic agents	Antihypertensive agents	↑	May enhance the effects of antihypertensive agents. Antipsychotics produce alpha-adrenergic blockage and may potentiate orthostatic hypotension.
Antipsychotic agents	Dopamine Epinephrine	↓	For the treatment of antipsychotic-induced hypotension, do not use epinephrine, dopamine, or other sympathomimetics with beta-agonist activity because beta stimulation may worsen the hypotension caused by the antipsychotic-induced alpha blockade.
Azole antifungal agents	Haloperidol	↑	Haloperidol plasma concentrations may be elevated, increasing risk of side effects with coadministration. Adjust dose of haloperidol as needed.
Beta-blockers (eg, pindolol, propranolol)	Phenothiazines (eg, thioridazine, chlorpromazine)	↑	Coadministration may lead to increased effects from either or both drugs, including increased risk of life-threatening arrhythmias with thioridazine. Thioridazine is contraindicated in patients taking pindolol or propranolol.
Phenothiazines (eg, thioridazine, chlorpromazine)	Beta-blockers (eg, pindolol, propranolol)		
Caffeine	Clozapine	↑	Plasma levels of clozapine may be increased, resulting in increased adverse effects. Avoid caffeine if interaction is suspected.
Carbamazepine	Aripiprazole Olanzapine Risperidone Ziprasidone	↓	The antipsychotic plasma concentrations may be decreased, resulting in decreased therapeutic effect. Adjust antipsychotic dose as needed. When carbamazepine is added to aripiprazole therapy, double the aripiprazole dose.
Carbamazepine	Haloperidol	↓	Therapeutic effects of haloperidol may be decreased. Adjust dose of therapy as needed.
Haloperidol	Carbamazepine	↑	Therapeutic effects of carbamazepine may be increased. Adjust dose of therapy as needed.
Charcoal	Antipsychotics	↓	Charcoal can decrease the absorption of antipsychotics, reducing their effectiveness or toxicity.
Cimetidine	Quetiapine	↑	Cimetidine decreased quetiapine oral clearance 20%.
Citalopram Fluoxetine Fluvoxamine Sertraline	Clozapine	↑	Plasma levels of clozapine may be increased, resulting in increased pharmacologic and toxic effects. Adjust clozapine dose as needed when starting or stopping certain SSRIs.
Clozapine Loxapine	Benzodiazepines	↑	Cases of orthostatic hypotension, collapse, respiratory arrest, and cardiac arrest have been reported with concomitant use of certain benzodiazepines. Coadminister with caution.
Clozapine	Risperidone	↑	Chronic administration of clozapine with risperidone may decrease risperidone clearance.
CYP1A2 inducers (eg, carbamazepine, omeprazole, rifampin)	Clozapine Olanzapine	↓	May decrease clozapine or olanzapine serum concentrations. May need dosage increase for olanzapine. Carbamazepine increased olanzapine clearance 50%.

Antipsychotic Drug Interactions			
Precipitant Drug	Object Drug*		Description
CYP1A2 inhibitors (eg, fluvoxamine)	Clozapine Olanzapine	↑	May increase clozapine or olanzapine serum concentrations. Dose reduction may be needed. Fluvoxamine decreased olanzapine clearance, resulting in a mean increase in C_{max} of 54% in female nonsmokers and 77% in male smokers and AUC increased 52% and 108%, respectively.
CYP3A4 inhibitors (eg, ketoconazole, erythromycin)	Aripiprazole Clozapine Quetiapine Ziprasidone	↑	The plasma concentrations of the antipsychotic may be increased. Reduce aripiprazole dose 50% with coadministration.
Famotidine	Aripiprazole	↓	Coadministration of a single dose of aripiprazole and famotidine resulted in decreased aripiprazole solubility and therefore decreased its rate of absorption, C_{max}, and AUC.
Fluoxetine	Olanzapine	↑	Coadministration resulted in a small (approximately 16%) increase in C_{max} and decrease in olanzapine clearance.
Fluoxetine Paroxetine	Risperidone	↑	Risperidone concentrations may be elevated, increasing the risk of adverse effects. Fluoxetine increased risperidone plasma levels 2.5- to 2.8-fold. Adjust risperidone dose as needed.
Haloperidol	Lithium	↑	Alterations in consciousness, encephalopathy, extrapyramidal effects, fever, leukocytosis, and increased serum enzymes have occurred with coadministration. Monitor coadministration closely and discontinue either drug if interaction is suspected.
Lithium	Haloperidol		
Meperidine	Phenothiazines	↑	Excessive sedation and hypotension may occur with coadministration. Coadministration not recommended.
Phenothiazines	Meperidine		
Olanzapine Quetiapine Risperidone Ziprasidone	Levodopa and dopamine agonists	↓	May antagonize the effects of levodopa and dopamine agonists.
Paroxetine	Phenothiazines	↑	Phenothiazine plasma levels may be increased, increasing the pharmacologic and adverse effects of these agents. Thioridazine is contraindicated. Adjust other phenothiazine doses as needed.
Phenobarbital	Clozapine	↓	Plasma levels of clozapine may be decreased, resulting in decreased pharmacologic effects.
Phenothiazines	Guanethidine	↓	Hypotensive effect of guanethidine is inhibited. Use alternate antihypertensive therapy if BP is uncontrolled.
Phenothiazines	Oral anticoagulants	↓	Phenothiazines may diminish oral anticoagulant effects.
Phenothiazines	Phenytoin	↑↓	Phenothiazines have been reported to increase or decrease phenytoin levels. Monitor phenytoin levels.
Phenothiazines	Thiazide diuretics	↑	Coadministration may potentiate orthostatic hypotension.
Thiazide diuretics	Phenothiazines		
Prochlorperazine	Dofetilide	↑	Elevated dofetilide concentrations may occur with increased risk of ventricular arrhythmia, including torsade de pointes. It is not recommended to use prochlorperazine in patients receiving dofetilide.
Quetiapine	Lorazepam	↑	Lorazepam mean oral clearance was reduced 20% with coadministration.
Quinidine	Aripiprazole	↑	Coadministration increased aripiprazole AUC 112% and decreased the AUC of the active metabolite 35%. Reduce aripiprazole dose 50% with coadministration.
Rifamycins	Haloperidol	↓	Rifamycins may decrease the plasma concentration and therapeutic effects of haloperidol. Adjust haloperidol as needed.
Phenytoin	Quetiapine	↓	Quetiapine plasma levels may be decreased, resulting in decreased pharmacologic effects. Adjust quetiapine dose as needed.
Risperidone	Clozapine	↑	Pharmacologic and adverse effects of clozapine may be increased. Adjust dose as needed.
Risperidone	Valproate	↑	Coadministration resulted in a 20% increase in valproate C_{max}. Adjust therapy as needed.
Ritonavir	Clozapine Perphenazine Risperidone Thioridazine	↑	Increases in serum antipsychotic concentrations may occur, increasing risk of toxicity.
Thioridazine	Quetiapine	↓	Thioridazine increased quetiapine oral clearance 65%.
Valproate	Aripiprazole	↓	Aripiprazole C_{max} and AUC were decreased 25% with coadministration.

↑ = Object drug increased. ↓ = Object drug decreased.

➤*Drug/Lab test interactions:* Phenothiazines may produce false-positive phenylketonuria (PKU) test results. Phenothiazines may cause false-positive pregnancy test results.

➤*Drug/Food interactions:* Grapefruit juice may inhibit the metabolism of **pimozide** via CYP3A. Food slows the absorption of oral **prochlorperazine** and decreases C_{max} 23% and AUC 13%.

Adverse Reactions

Antipsychotic Adverse Reactions[a] (%)

Adverse reactions	Chlorpromazine	Fluphenazine	Haloperidol	Loxapine	Mesoridazine	Molindone	Perphenazine	Pimozide	Prochlorperazine	Thioridazine	Thiothixene	Trifluoperazine	Aripiprazole	Clozapine	Olanzapine	Quetiapine	Risperidone	Ziprasidone, oral (IM)
Cardiovascular																		
Angina pectoris													0.1-1	1		< 0.1	< 0.1	0.1-1
Atrial contractions, premature/ atrial fibrillation/flutter													0.1-1	✔	< 0.1	< 0.1	< 0.1	0.1-1
AV block													0.1-1			< 0.1	0.1-1	< 0.1
Bradycardia						✔							> 1	✔	0.1-1	0.1-1		0.1-1 (≤ 2)
Cardiac arrest	✔						✔		✔	Rare	✔	✔	0.1-1		0.1-1			
Cerebral vascular accident													0.1-1		0.1-1	0.1-1	✔	< 0.1
CHF													0.1-1	✔	0.1-1	< 0.1		
ECG changes	✔	✔	✔	✔	✔	✔	✔	✔	✔	✔	✔	✔		1				✔
Hypertension		✔	✔	✔			✔	✔					> 1	4	2	✔	0.1-1	> 1 (≤ 2)
Hypotension	✔	Rare	✔	✔[b]	✔	Rare	✔	✔[b]	✔[c]	✔	✔	✔[c]	> 1	9	3-5[b]	7[b]	0.1-1	1[b] (≤ 5)
MI													0.1-1	✔			0.1-1	
Palpitation							✔						0.1-1		0.1-1	> 1	0.1-1	
Phlebitis													0.1-1	✔			< 0.1	< 0.1
QTc interval prolongation		✔			✔			✔		✔			0.1-1			0.1-1		✔
Pulmonary embolus													< 0.1	✔	< 0.1		✔	< 0.1
Q- and T-wave distortions	✔							✔				✔						
T-wave flattening					✔			✔		✔						✔	0.1-1	
T-wave inversion					✔			✔		✔						✔	0.1-1	< 0.1
Tachycardia	✔	✔	✔	✔		✔[d]	✔	✔			✔		> 1	25	3	7	3-5	2
Thrombophlebitis, including deep													< 0.1	✔		0.1-1		< 0.1
Twitch													0.1-1	✔		0.1-1		
Vasodilation													0.1-1		0.1-1	0.1-1		(≤ 1)
CNS																		
Accommodation abnormality															0.1-1	< 0.1	0.1-1	
Agitation	✔		✔	✔	✔			✔	✔	✔	✔	✔	✔	4			22-26	> 1 (≤ 2)
Akathisia		✔	✔	Freq	✔	✔	✔	40	✔	✔	✔	✔	10	3	3			8 (≤ 2)
Akinesia			✔	✔	✔			40		✔			< 0.1	4	< 0.1			> 1
Amnesia													0.1-1	✔	0.1-1	0.1-1	0.1-1	> 1
Anxiety			✔										25	1			12-20	(≤ 2)
Apathy													0.1-1			0.1-1	0.1-1	
Asthenia							45						7		10-15	4		5 (≤ 2)
Ataxia					✔		✔						0.1-1	1	0.1-1	0.1-1		> 1
Catatonic-like states	Rare	✔	✔				✔	✔				✔					0.1-1	0.1-1
Confusion		✔	✔	✔			✔[e]			Rare[e]			> 1	3		0.1-1	0.1-1	> 1
Convulsions[f]	✔		✔	✔			✔	✔	✔		Infreq	✔		3				
Delirium													< 0.1	✔	0.1-1	< 0.1	< 0.1	> 1
Depression		✔				✔	10						> 1	1			0.1-1	
Dizziness	✔				✔	✔	✔	✔	✔			✔		19	11-18	10	4-7	8 (3-10)
Dreams, abnormal/ bizarre/increased		✔		✔			3		✔					✔	> 1	0.1-1	≥ 1	
Drowsiness/sedation/ somnolence	✔	✔	✔	✔	✔	✔	✔	25-70	✔	✔	✔	✔	8.7-15.3	39-46	29-35	18	3-8	14 (8-20)
Dysarthria													0.1-1	✔	0.1-1	> 1	0.1-1	> 1
Dyskinesia		✔					✔	✔	✔			✔	0.1-1		≤ 2	0.1-1		> 1
Dystonia	✔	✔	✔	✔	✔		✔	✔	✔	✔	✔	✔	0.1-1		2-3			4
Euphoria		✔				✔							< 0.1		> 1	< 0.1	0.1-1	
Excitement		✔			✔		✔		✔			✔						
Extrapyramidal symptoms	✔	✔	Freq	Freq	✔	✔	✔	Freq	✔	Infreq	✔	✔	✔			✔	17-34	5 (≤ 2)

Antipsychotic Adverse Reactions[a] (%)

Adverse reactions	Conventional Antipsychotics												Atypical Antipsychotics					
	Chlorpromazine	Fluphenazine	Haloperidol	Loxapine	Mesoridazine	Molindone	Perphenazine	Pimozide	Prochlorperazine	Thioridazine	Thiothixene	Trifluoperazine	Aripiprazole	Clozapine	Olanzapine	Quetiapine	Risperidone	Ziprasidone, oral (IM)
CNS																		
Fainting/Faintness	✓			✓	✓		✓	✓										
Fatigue												✓		2			> 1	
Gait abnormal													> 1		6	0.1-1		> 1
Gait, staggering/shuffling	✓				✓					✓		✓						
Hallucinations			✓											✓		0.1-1		
Headache		✓	✓	✓			✓	5-22	✓	Rare		✓	32	7		19	12-14	(3-13)
Hostility													> 1			✓		> 1
Hyperactivity						✓	✓			Rare			0.1-1					
Hyperkinesia								6					0.1-1	1		0.1-1		> 1
Hyperreflexia		✓					✓	✓	✓		✓	✓	0.1-1				< 0.1	< 0.1
Hypesthesia													0.1-1		0.1-1		< 0.1	> 1
Hypokinesia													0.1-1	4	0.1-1			> 1
Incoordination													< 0.1		0.1-1	0.1-1		> 1
Insomnia	✓		✓	✓			✓	10	✓		✓	✓	24	2	12	✓	23-26	< 3
Jitteriness	✓								✓			✓						
Lethargy		✓	✓				✓			Rare				1				
Libido, increased		✓[g]	✓			✓							0.1-1	✓	0.1-1	0.1-1	0.1-1	
Libido decreased/loss of							✓	✓					0.1-1	✓		< 0.1	≥ 5	
Lightheadedness					✓							✓	11					
Malaise													0.1-1		0.1-1	0.1-1	0.1-1	
Migraine															0.1-1	0.1-1	< 0.1	
Motor restlessness (EPS)	✓					✓	✓	✓	✓	✓	✓							
Nervousness													> 1			✓	≥ 1	
Neuroleptic malignant syndrome (NMS)	✓	✓	✓	Freq	✓		✓	✓	✓	✓	✓	✓		✓				
Neuropathy													0.1-1		< 0.1			> 1
Paresthesia			✓										0.1-1		> 1	✓	0.1-1	> 1 (≤ 2)
Pseudoparkinsonism	✓	✓	✓	✓	✓	✓	✓	✓	✓	Infreq	✓	✓		< 1	✓		✓	
Psychosis	Rare	✓	✓		✓		✓		✓	Rare	Infreq	✓	✓	✓		0.1-1		(≤ 1)
Restlessness		✓	✓		✓		✓			Rare	✓			4				
Speech slurred					✓	✓	✓							1				
Suicide attempt/thought													0.1-1/ > 1		> 1	0.1-1		
Stupor													0.1-1			0.1-1	0.1-1	
Syncope					✓						✓			6				
Tardive dyskinesia	✓	✓	✓	✓	✓	✓	✓	✓	✓	✓	✓	✓	0.1-1		0.1-1	0.1-1		> 1
Tardive dystonia	✓		✓							✓								
Tremor	✓		✓		✓	✓	✓		1	✓	✓		✓	2-3	6	4-6	✓	> 1
Trismus	✓				✓		✓			✓	✓		✓					< 0.1
Vertigo			✓										0.1-1	19	0.1-1	0.1-1	0.1-1	> 1
Weakness					✓	✓					✓	✓		1				

Antipsychotic Adverse Reactions[a] (%)

Dermatologic

Adverse reactions	Conventional Antipsychotics												Atypical Antipsychotics					
	Chlorpromazine	Fluphenazine	Haloperidol	Loxapine	Mesoridazine	Molindone	Perphenazine	Pimozide	Prochlorperazine	Thioridazine	Thiothixene	Trifluoperazine	Aripiprazole	Clozapine	Olanzapine	Quetiapine	Risperidone	Ziprasidone, oral (IM)
Acne			✓										0.1-1		0.1-1	0.1-1	0.1-1	
Alopecia			✓	✓									0.1-1		0.1-1		0.1-1	0.1-1
Dermatitis	✓h,i	✓h		✓	✓h,i		✓h,i		✓h	Infreqh,i		✓	< 0.1h	✓	0.1-1	0.1-1	0.1-1	0.1-2h,i,j
Ecchymosis													> 1	✓	5	0.1-1		0.1-1
Eczema		✓					✓		✓			✓	0.1-1	✓	0.1-1	0.1-1	2-4	0.1-1
Erythema		✓			✓		✓		✓	✓		✓				✓		
Maculopapular skin reactions			✓										< 0.1		0.1-1	✓		0.1-1
Pallor							✓			✓					0.1-1		< 0.1	
Photosensitivity	✓	✓	✓				✓		✓	Rare	✓	✓	0.1-1	✓	0.1-1	0.1-1	> 1	> 1
Pruritus		✓			✓	✓	✓			✓	✓	✓	> 1		0.1-1	0.1-1	0.1-1	
Psoriasis													0.1-1			< 0.1	< 0.1	
Purpura, thrombocytopenic	✓	✓					✓		✓			✓						
Rash					✓	✓	✓	8			✓	✓	6	2		4	2-5	4
Rash, vesiculobullous													0.1-1		0.1-1			0.1-1
Seborrhea		✓			✓								0.1-1		0.1-1	0.1-1	≤ 1	
Skin pigmentation changes	✓	✓			✓		✓		✓	✓		✓						
Urticaria		✓					✓		✓	Infreq	✓	✓	< 0.1	✓	< 0.1		< 0.1	0.1-1

Antipsychotic Adverse Reactions[a] (%)

Adverse reactions	Chlorpromazine	Fluphenazine	Haloperidol	Loxapine	Mesoridazine	Molindone	Perphenazine	Pimozide	Prochlorperazine	Thioridazine	Thiothixene	Trifluoperazine	Aripiprazole	Clozapine	Olanzapine	Quetiapine	Risperidone	Ziprasidone, oral (IM)
	Conventional Antipsychotics												Atypical Antipsychotics					
Abdominal discomfort/pain													✓	4		3	1-4	> 1 (≤ 2)
Abdominal distention/enlargement													0.1-1		0.1-1	< 0.1	< 0.1	
Adynamic ileus	✓						✓		✓		✓	✓						
Anorexia		✓	✓		✓		✓	✓		✓	✓	✓	> 1	1		> 1	> 1	2 (≤ 2)
Appetite increased	✓						✓	5	✓		✓	✓	0.1-1	✓	3-6	0.1-1	0.1-1	
Atonic colon	✓								✓			✓						
Constipation	✓	✓	✓	✓	✓	✓	✓	20	✓	✓	Infreq	✓	10	14	9-11	9	7-13	9 (≤ 2)
Diarrhea			✓				✓	5		✓	✓		✓	2		✓	≥ 5	5 (≤ 3)
Diverticulitis																	< 0.1	
Drooling	✓								✓			✓						
Dry mouth	✓	✓	✓	✓	✓	✓	✓	25	✓	✓	Infreq	✓	✓	6	9-22	7	≥ 5	4 (≤ 1)
Dyspepsia			✓										✓	14	7-11	6	5-10	8 (1-3)
Dysphagia	✓						✓	3	✓			✓	0.1-1	✓	0.1-1	0.1-1	0.1-1	0.1-1
Eructation													0.1-1	✓	0.1-1		< 0.1	
Esophageal ulcer/esophagitis													< 0.1		< 0.1		< 0.1	
Fecal impaction		✓					✓						0.1-1	✓	0.1-1			< 0.1
Flatulence													0.1-1		0.1-1	0.1-1	0.1-1	
Gastritis													0.1-1		0.1-1	0.1-1	0.1-1	
Gastroenteritis													0.1-1	✓	0.1-1	0.1-1	< 0.1	
Gastroesophageal reflux													0.1-1	4		0.1-1	< 0.1	
Gingivitis													0.1-1		0.1-1	0.1-1	< 0.1	
Glossitis													< 0.1		< 0.1	< 0.1		
Gum hemorrhage													< 0.1			0.1-1		< 0.1
Hematemesis													< 0.1	✓		< 0.1	< 0.1	< 0.1
Hemorrhoids													0.1-1			0.1-1	0.1-1	
Incontinence, fecal													0.1-1		0.1-1	0.1-1	< 0.1	
Intestinal obstruction													0.1-1	✓	< 0.1	< 0.1	✓	
Melena													< 0.1		0.1-1	0.1-1	0.1-1	< 0.1
Mouth ulceration													0.1-1		0.1-1	0.1-1		
Nausea	✓	✓	✓	✓	✓	✓	✓	✓	✓	✓	✓	✓	14	5	0.1-1	✓	4-6	10 (4-12)
Obstipation	✓					✓	✓			✓	✓	✓						
Paralytic ileus		✓		✓	✓						✓				< 0.1			
Polydipsia				✓				5			✓	✓	0.1-1		> 1	0.1-1	> 1	0.1-1 (≤ 2)
Rectal hemorrhage													0.1-1	✓	0.1-1	0.1-1		< 2
Salivation		✓	✓	✓		✓	✓	14			Infreq		> 1	31	> 1	0.1-1	≤ 2	✓
Stomatitis													0.1-1		0.1-1	0.1-1	0.1-1	0.1-1
Taste altered								5					0.1-1			0.1-1		
Tongue discoloration															< 0.1		< 0.1	
Tongue protrusion	✓	✓					✓		✓			✓						
Tooth caries													0.1-1		0.1-1	0.1-1		
Vomiting			✓	✓	✓		✓	✓		✓	✓	✓	12	3	4	✓	5-7	> 1 (< 3)
Weight gain	✓			✓	✓	✓	✓	✓	✓	✓	✓	✓	8[k]	4	5-6	2	18	10[k]
Weight loss				✓		✓	✓						> 1	✓		0.1-1	0.1-1	

GI

Antipsychotic Adverse Reactions[a] (%)

Conventional Antipsychotics | Atypical Antipsychotics

Category	Adverse reactions	Chlorpromazine	Fluphenazine	Haloperidol	Loxapine	Mesoridazine	Molindone	Perphenazine	Pimozide	Prochlorperazine	Thioridazine	Thiothixene	Trifluoperazine	Aripiprazole	Clozapine	Olanzapine	Quetiapine	Risperidone	Ziprasidone, oral (IM)
GU	Albuminuria													0.1-1		< 0.1			0.1-1
	Amenorrhea	✓			Rare		Infreq	✓		✓	✓	✓	✓	0.1-1		> 1	0.1-1	0.1-1	0.1-1
	Breast engorgement	✓		✓				✓			✓								
	Dysmenorrhea													✓	✓		0.1-1	0.1-1	(≤ 2)
	Ejaculation disorders	✓				✓		✓		✓	✓		✓	0.1-1	1	0.1-1	0.1-1	≥ 5	0.1-1
	Galactorrhea	✓	✓	✓	Rare	✓	Infreq	✓		✓	✓	✓	✓	< 0.1		0.1-1	0.1-1	0.1-1	0.1-1
	Glycosuria	✓						✓		✓		✓	✓	< 0.1		0.1-1	< 0.1		0.1-1
	Gynecomastia	✓	✓	✓	Rare	✓	Infreq	✓		✓	✓	✓	✓	< 0.1		< 0.1	< 0.1	< 0.1	< 0.1
	Hematuria													0.1-1		> 1		0.1-1	0.1-1
	Impotence	✓	✓	✓		✓			15	✓		Infreq	✓	0.1-1	✓	0.1-1	0.1-1	≥ 5	0.1-1
	Incontinence, urinary					✓		✓			✓			> 1		2	0.1-1	0.1-1	
	Mastalgia			✓										< 0.1	✓	0.1-1		0.1-1	
	Menorrhagia						✓							0.1-1		0.1-1		≥ 5	0.1-1
	Menstrual irregularities		✓	✓	Rare			✓			✓	✓	✓						
	Metrorrhagia															> 1	0.1-1		0.1-1
	Nocturia										✓			0.1-1		< 0.1			< 0.1
	Polyuria		✓					✓						0.1-1		0.1-1	< 0.1	> 1	0.1-1
	Priapism	✓		✓		✓	✓			✓	✓		✓	< 0.1	✓	0.1-1			(≤ 1)
	Renal failure, acute		✓											0.1-1			< 0.1		
	Urinary frequency/urgency increased							✓	✓					0.1-1	1	0.1-1	0.1-1		
	Urinary retention	✓		✓	✓	✓	✓	✓			✓	✓		0.1-1	1	0.1-1	0.1-1	> 1	0.1-1
	Vaginal hemorrhage													0.1-1		0.1-1	0.1-1	0.1-1	< 0.1
Hematologic/Lymphatic	Agranulocytosis	✓	✓	Rare	Rare	✓		✓		✓	✓		✓		1				
	Anemia			✓		✓						✓		> 1	✓	0.1-1	0.1-1	0.1-1	0.1-1
	Anemia, aplastic	✓				✓					✓	✓							✓
	Anemia, hemolytic	✓						✓	✓	✓									✓
	Anemia, hypochromic													0.1-1			0.1-1	0.1-1	< 0.1
	Blood dyscrasias		✓					✓		✓			✓						
	Eosinophilia	✓	✓			✓		✓		✓	✓		✓	< 0.1	1	0.1-1			0.1-1
	Hemorrhage													0.1-1		0.1-1		< 0.1	
	Hypercholesterolemia													0.1-1		0.1-1	✓		0.1-1
	Hyperglycemia	✓		✓				✓		✓		✓	✓	0.1-1	✓	0.1-1	0.1-1	✓	0.1-1
	Hyperkalemia													< 0.1		< 0.1			< 0.1
	Hyperlipemia													0.1-1		0.1-1	0.1-1		< 0.1
	Hyperuricemia													< 0.1	✓				< 0.1
	Hypoglycemia	✓		✓				✓		✓		✓	✓	0.1-1		0.1-1	0.1-1	< 0.1	< 0.1
	Hypokalemia													0.1-1		0.1-1	< 0.1	< 0.1	0.1-1
	Hyponatremia			✓					✓					0.1-1	✓	0.1-1		0.1-1	< 0.1
	Hypoproteinemia															< 0.1		< 0.1	< 0.1
	Leukocytosis		✓	✓			Rare						✓	0.1-1	✓	0.1-1	0.1-1	< 0.1	0.1-1
	Leukopenia	✓	✓	✓	Rare	✓	Rare	✓		✓	✓	✓	✓	0.1-1	3	> 1	> 1	< 0.1	0.1-1
	Lymphadenopathy													0.1-1		0.1-1	0.1-1		0.1-1
	Pancytopenia	✓	✓					✓		✓	✓		✓						< 0.1
	Thrombocythemia													< 0.1	✓	0.1-1			< 0.1
	Thrombocytopenia				Rare	✓						✓		0.1-1	✓	0.1-1	< 0.1		< 0.1
Hepatic	ALT/AST elevation			✓								Infreq		0.1-1			✓	0.1-1	0.1-1
	Biliary stasis					✓		✓		✓	✓		✓						
	Cholecystitis													0.1-1				< 0.1	
	Cholelithiasis													0.1-1	✓			< 0.1	
	Hepatitis				Rare									< 0.1	✓	0.1-1		< 0.1	< 0.1
	Jaundice	✓	✓[l]	✓	Rare	✓		✓		✓[l]	✓		✓		✓			✓	< 0.1[l]
	Liver function impaired		✓	✓			Rare	✓		✓			✓		1				

Antipsychotic Adverse Reactions[a] (%)

Category	Adverse reactions	Chlorpromazine	Fluphenazine	Haloperidol	Loxapine	Mesoridazine	Molindone	Perphenazine	Pimozide	Prochlorperazine	Thioridazine	Thiothixene	Trifluoperazine	Aripiprazole	Clozapine	Olanzapine	Quetiapine	Risperidone	Ziprasidone, oral (IM)
Hypersensitivity	Allergic reaction	✓								✓			✓	✓		✓		< 0.1	
	Anaphylactoid reactions	✓	✓					✓		✓		Rare	✓			✓		✓	
Lab Test Abn.	Alkaline phosphatase increased												Infreq	0.1-1		0.1-1	0.1-1		0.1-1
	Cerebrospinal fluid proteins abnormality	✓	✓					✓		✓		✓	✓						
	CPK elevated					✓								> 1	✓				0.1-1
	Creatinine increased													0.1-1			0.1-1	0.1-1	< 0.1
Metabolic/Nutritional	Edema, cerebral	✓	✓				Rare			✓		✓	✓						
	Cyanosis													< 0.1	✓	0.1-1	0.1-1		
	Edema					✓					✓			0.1-1	✓			0.1-1	
	Edema, angioneurotic	✓	✓			✓		✓		✓	✓		✓						
	Edema, facial				✓									0.1-1		0.1-1	0.1-1		> 1
	Edema, laryngeal	✓	✓			✓		✓		✓	✓		✓						
	Edema, peripheral	✓	✓					✓		✓	✓	✓	✓	> 1		3	> 1		0.1-1
	Edema, tongue													0.1-1		0.1-1	0.1-1	< 0.1	0.1-1
Musculoskeletal	Arthralgia/Joint pain													0.1-1	✓	5	0.1-1	2-3	✓
	Arthritis													0.1-1		0.1-1	0.1-1	< 0.1	
	Bone pain													0.1-1		< 0.1	0.1-1		
	Bursitis													0.1-1		0.1-1		< 0.1	
	Muscle rigidity		✓			✓	✓		15		✓	✓		0.1-1	✓				
	Muscle weakness							✓					✓	0.1-1	1		0.1-1		
	Myalgia								3					✓	1		✓	0.1-1	1
	Myoclonus					✓								0.1-1	1		0.1-1		< 0.1
	Myopathy													< 0.1		< 0.1			< 0.1
	Opisthotonos	✓	✓	✓		✓		✓	✓	✓	✓		✓						< 0.1
	Rigidity					✓			10						5			0.1-1	
	Spasm, carpopedal	✓								✓	✓		✓						
	Spasm of neck muscles	✓				✓				✓	✓		✓						
	Torticollis	✓				✓		✓	3	✓	✓		✓					< 0.1	< 0.1
Respiratory	Apnea													< 0.1		0.1-1		✓	
	Asphyxia	✓						✓				✓	✓						
	Aspiration														✓			< 0.1	
	Asthma	✓	✓			✓		✓		✓	✓		✓	0.1-1		0.1-1	0.1-1	< 0.1	
	Cough, increased													3	✓	6	> 1	3	3
	Cough reflex failure	✓						✓		✓		✓	✓						
	Dyspnea					✓								> 1	1	> 1	> 1	≤ 1	> 1
	Epistaxis													0.1-1	✓	0.1-1	0.1-1	0.1-1	0.1-1
	Hemoptysis													< 0.1		0.1-1			< 0.1
	Hyperventilation														✓		< 0.1	0.1-1	
	Nasal congestion	✓	✓			✓	✓	✓		✓	✓	Infreq	✓		1				
	Pharyngitis													✓		4	> 1	2-3	
	Pneumonia													> 1	✓	0.1-1	0.1-1	0.1-1	0.1-1
	Rhinitis													4		7	3	8-10	4 (≤ 1)

Antipsychotic Adverse Reactions[a] (%)

		Conventional Antipsychotics											Atypical Antipsychotics					
Adverse reactions	Chlorpromazine	Fluphenazine	Haloperidol	Loxapine	Mesoridazine	Molindone	Perphenazine	Pimozide	Prochlorperazine	Thioridazine	Thiothixene	Trifluoperazine	Aripiprazole	Clozapine	Olanzapine	Quetiapine	Risperidone	Ziprasidone, oral (IM)
Special senses																		
Blepharitis													0.1-1		0.1-1	0.1-1	< 0.1	0.1-1
Cataracts		✔						✔					0.1-1		0.1-1			0.1-1
Conjunctivitis													> 1	✔	> 1	0.1-1		0.1-1
Diplopia													< 0.1		0.1-1		< 0.1	> 1
Dry eyes													0.1-1		0.1-1	0.1-1		0.1-1
Epithelial keratopathy	✔						✔	✔				✔						
Eye hemorrhage													< 0.1		0.1-1			< 0.1
Glaucoma		✔					✔						✔m	< 0.1	< 0.1			
Lentricular/corneal opacities	✔	✔			✔		✔		✔	✔		✔						
Miosis	✔				✔		✔		✔	✔		✔			< 0.1			
Mydriasis	✔				✔		✔		✔	✔		✔			< 0.1			
Oculogyric crisis	✔	✔	✔	✔			✔	✔	✔			✔	0.1-1					> 1
Parotid swelling							Rare		Rare					✔				
Photophobia		✔					✔						< 0.1				< 0.1	0.1-1
Pigmentary retinopathy	✔						✔		✔									
Tinnitius													0.1-1		0.1-1	0.1-1		0.1-1
Vision abnormal															0.1-1	1-2		3
Vision blurred		✔	✔	✔	✔	✔	✔	✔	✔	✔	Infreq	✔	3					
Visual disturbances		✔												5				
Miscellaneous																		
Accidental injury													✔		12	✔		4
Back pain													✔	1	5	2	≤ 2	(≤ 1)
Chest pain							✔						> 1	1	3	✔	2-3	
Chills													0.1-1	✔	0.1-1	0.1-1		> 1
Choreoathetosis															< 0.1	< 0.1		> 1
Cogwheel rigidity	✔						✔					✔	> 1		0.1-1			> 1 (≤ 1)
Dehydration													0.1-1		0.1-1	0.1-1	< 0.1	0.1-1
Diaphoresis		✔	✔				✔	✔				Infreq	> 1	6	> 1	> 1	0.1-1	(≤ 2)
Fever	✔			✔			✔			✔	✔	✔	2	5	6	2	2-3	> 1
Flu syndrome													> 1		> 1	> 1	0.1-1	> 1 (≤ 1)
Gout													< 0.1		< 0.1	< 0.1		< 0.1
Hyperpyrexia/Hyperthermia	✔	✔	✔	✔	✔		✔	✔	✔	✔	✔	✔						
Hyperthyroidism													< 0.1			< 0.1		< 0.1
Hypertonia													✔		3	> 1		3
Hypothyroidism													0.1-1			0.1-1		< 0.1
Hypotonia													0.1-1		0.1-1		< 0.1	> 1
Mask-like faces	✔						✔					✔						
Moniliasis													< 0.1		0.1-1	0.1-1		
Neck pain/rigidity													> 1	1	0.1-1	0.1-1		
Pain, pelvic													0.1-1		0.1-1	0.1-1		
Pillrolling motion	✔						✔					✔						
Ptosis					✔													
Sudden death	✔	✔	✔		✔		Rare	✔	✔	✔	✔	✔		✔	< 0.1		< 0.1	
Systemic lupus erythematosus-like syndrome	✔	✔			✔		✔		✔	✔		✔						
Thyroiditis															0.1-1		< 0.1	< 0.1
Withdrawal syndrome		✔						✔						1			< 0.1	> 1

✔ = Incidence not reported.
[a] Data are pooled from separate trials and are not necessarily comparable.
[b] Includes orthostatic.
[c] Sometimes fatal.
[d] Especially with sudden marked increase in dosage.
[e] Nocturnal confusion.
[f] Includes petit and grand mal seizures.
[g] In women.
[h] Exfoliative dermatitis included.
[i] Contact dermatitis included.
[j] Fungal dermatitis.
[k] Gained at least 7% body weight.
[l] Includes cholestatic.
[m] Narrow-angle glaucoma.

▶*Other adverse reactions:*

Chlorpromazine: Ocular changes; back muscle rigidity; shock-like reaction.

Fluphenazine: Altered EEG tracings; nonthrombocytopenic purpura; appetite decreased; weight change; local tissue reactions (rare).

Loxapine: Flushed face; numbness; tension.

Mesoridazine: Hypertrophic papillae of tongue; incontinence.

Molindone: Menses resumption; blood glucose alteration; BUN alteration; RBC alteration; thyroid function alteration.

Perphenazine: Pulse-rate change; paranoid reaction; polyphagia; throat tight; ocular changes; inappropriate ADH secretion; limb ache/numbness; shock-like reaction; hypnotic effects; tongue ache; tongue rounding; circulatory collapse (rare).

Pimozide: Adverse behavior effect (5% to 10%); sensitivity of eyes to light (5%); accommodation decrease (4%); speech disorder, stooped posture (2%); gingival hyperplasia, handwriting change (1%); skin irritation; GI distress; tonic spasm; transient dyskinetic signs; periorbital edema; T-wave notching; U-wave appearance.

Thioridazine: Arrhythmias; torsade de pointes-type arrhythmias; autonomic instability; blood glucose alteration; conjunctiva pigmentation; cornea discoloration; altered mental status; paradoxical reaction; irregular pulse; sclera discoloration; altered libido; U-wave appearance; skin eruption (infrequent).

Trifluoperazine: Skin reaction; back muscle rigidity; heat prolongation/intensification.

Haloperidol: BP fluctuations; torsade de pointes-type arrhythmias; hyperammonemia (postmarketing); lymphomonocytosis; RBC count decreased; bronchospasm; laryngospasm; respiration depth increased; retinopathy; heat stroke; local tissue reactions; transient dyskinetic signs.

Atypicals –

Aripiprazole: Ear pain, manic reaction, muscle cramp, dry skin, skin ulcer (at least 1%); deep vein thrombosis, concentration impaired, bloating, periodontal abscess, cystitis, uterine hemorrhage, bilirubinemia, increased BUN, increased lactic dehydrogenase, jaw pain/tightness, depersonalization, diabetes mellitus, iron deficiency anemia, bradykinesia, chest tightness, colitis, dysphoria, dysuria, extrasystoles, eye pain, hiccough, hypersomnia, GI hemorrhage, kidney calculus, laryngitis, leukorrhea, impaired memory, myocardial ischemia, obesity, otitis media, panic attack, peptic ulcer, restless leg, arm rigidity, spasm, thinking slowed, vaginal moniliasis (at least 1%); hyperesthesia, arthrosis (0.1 to 1); cardiomegaly, throat tight, anorgasmia, hepatomegaly, amblyopia, increased lacrimation, tenosynovitis, heat stroke, increased sputum, cerebral ischemia, deafness, macrocytic anemia, aspiration pneumonia, back tightness, increased blinking, blunted affect, cervicitis, cheilitis, decreased consciousness, duodenal ulcer, pulmonary edema, goiter, head heaviness, intracranial hemorrhage, hypernatremia, hypoxia, intestinal perforation, leg rigidity, Mendelson syndrome, dry nasal passages, neck tightness, obsessive thought, otitis externa, pancreatitis, decreased reflexes, respiratory failure, rhabdomyolysis, rheumatoid arthritis, tendonitis, throat pain, urinary burning, urolithiasis, vasovagal reaction buccoglossal syndrome (less than 0.1%).; oral moniliasis; upper respiratory infection; dental pain; QT interval shortened; vaginitis.

Clozapine: Arrhythmias, cardiomyopathy, deep vein thrombosis, ST-depression, aphasia, altered EEG tracings, GI distress, hypothermia, periorbital edema, delusions, amentia, bitter taste, bronchitis, mild cataplexy, chills with fever, cholestasis, poor coordination, ear disorder, epileptiform movements, erythema multiforme, increased ESR, eyelid disorder, bloodshot eyes, gastric ulcer, granulocytopenia, elevated hematocrit, elevated hemoglobin, histrionic movements, hot flashes, acute interstitial nephritis, involuntary movements, irritability, ischemic changes, laryngitis, impaired memory, numbness, overdose, acute pancreatitis, pericardial effusions, pericarditis, petechiae, pleural effusion, pneumonia-like symptoms, premature ventricular contraction, rhabdomyolysis, rhinorrhea, sepsis, shakiness, sneezing, status epilepticus, Stevens-Johnson syndrome, stuttering, abnormal stools, dry throat, throat pain/discomfort, tics, tongue numb/sore, vaginal infections/itch, vasculitis, ventricular fibrillation, wheezing, nightmares, sleep disturbance (4%); neutropenia, WBC decreased (3%); urinary abnormalities (2%); incontinence, cardiac abnormality, leg pain (1%).

Olanzapine: Personality disorder (8%); extremity pain (not joint) (5%); amblyopia (3%); articulation impaired, UTI (2%); angioedema, dental pain, intentional injury (at least 1%); antisocial reaction, CNS stimulation, arthrosis, voice alteration, laryngitis, obsessive compulsive symptoms, phobias, tobacco misuse (0.1% to 1%); normocytic anemia, arteritis, fatty liver deposits, keratoconjunctivitis, nystagmus, ketosis, hangover effect, encephalopathy, hiccough, hyperventilation, hypoxia, lung edema, stridor, breast pain, cystitis, uterine fibroids (less than 0.1%); aphthous stomatitis, enteritis, periodontal abscess, acidosis, bilirubinemia, atelectasis, alcohol misuse, coma (rare).

Quetiapine: UTI, infection, pain, ear pain, dry skin, increased triglycerides (1%); bundle branch block, paranoid reaction, cystitis, vulvovaginitis, leg cramps, increased GGT, alcohol intolerance, bruxism, cerebral ischemia, delusions, depersonalization, diabetes mellitus, dysuria, eye pain, hemiplegia, involuntary movements, leukorrhea, manic reaction, orchitis, pathological fracture, irregular pulse, QRS duration, skin ulcer, abnormal thinking, vaginitis (0.1% to 1%); aphasia, emotional lability, deafness, hand edema, hemolysis, hiccough, neuralgia, neutropenia, skin discoloration, ST abnormality, ST elevated, stuttering, subdural hematoma, T-wave abnormality, water intoxication (less than 0.1%).

Risperidone: Lymphedema (8%); upper respiratory infection (3%); angioedema, cerebral vascular disorder, aggressive reaction (1% to 3%); toothache, sinusitis (2% or less); hyperpigmentation (at least 1%); concentration impaired, hyperkeratosis, nonthrombocytopenic purpura, skin exfoliation, bronchospasm, stridor, xerophthalmia (0.1% to 1%); myocarditis, ST-depression, cholinergic syndrome, emotional lability, nightmares, bullous eruption, furunculosis, hypertrichosis, skin ulceration, verruca, feces discoloration, GI hemorrhage, tongue paralysis, genital pruritus, normocytic anemia, ascites, yawning, eye pain, abnormal lacrimation, photopsia, arthrosis, leg cramps, cachexia, coma, increased sputum, sarcoidosis (less than 0.1%).

Ziprasidone: Injection site pain (7% to 9%); respiratory disorder (8%); personality disorder, speech disorder, furunculosis (2% or less); hypo-

nia, buccoglossal syndrome, accidental fall, hypothermia, motor vehicle accident, flank pain, hypertonia (at least 1%); tooth disorder (less than 1%); cerebral infarct, polycythemia, anorgasmia, male sex dysfunction, tenosynovitis, increased lactic dehydrogenase (0.1% to 1%); bundle branch block, cardiomegaly, myocarditis, keratitis, leukoplakia of the mouth, female sex dysfunction, uterine hemorrhage, basophilia, hypocalcemia, hypochloremia, hypocholesterolemia, lymphedema, lymphocytosis, monocytosis, fatty liver deposits, hepatomegaly, laryngismus, respiratory alkalosis, keratoconjunctivitis, nystagmus, visual field defect, increased BUN, increased GGT, decreased glucose tolerance, ketosis, cerebral infarct, hyperchloremia, oliguria (less than 0.1%).

Overdosage

➤*Symptoms:* CNS depression to the point of somnolence, deep sleep from which patient cannot be aroused, or coma. Hypotension and extrapyramidal symptoms may occur. Other manifestations include: Agitation; restlessness; convulsions; fever; hypothermia; hyperthermia; coma; autonomic reactions; ECG changes; cardiac arrhythmias; tachycardia; hypertension; vomiting; NMS; slurred speech; delirium; respiratory depression or failure; seizures; renal failure (**loxapine**); dry mouth; salivation; ileus; hyperpyrexia; dilated or constricted pupils; cardiac arrest; death.

Other symptoms temporally related to risperidone overdose include torsade de pointes, prolonged QT interval, and cardiopulmonary arrest.

➤*Treatment:* Includes usual supportive measures. Refer to General Management of Acute Overdosage. In case of acute overdosage, establish and maintain an airway and ensure adequate oxygenation and ventilation. Establish IV access and consider gastric lavage (after intubation, if patient is unconscious) and administration of activated charcoal. The possibility of obtundation, seizure, or dystonic reaction of the head and neck following overdose may create a risk of aspiration with induced emesis. Cardiovascular monitoring should commence immediately and include continuous ECG monitoring to detect possible arrhythmias. Treat extrapyramidal symptoms with anticholinergic drugs or diphenhydramine (see Adverse Reactions).

If hypotension occurs, initiate the standard measures for managing circulatory shock, including volume replacement. If a vasoconstrictor is desired, use norepinephrine or phenylephrine. Do not administer epinephrine, dopamine, or other sympathomimetics with beta-agonist activity, because beta stimulation may worsen hypotension of drug-induced alpha blockade (eg, **olanzapine**, **quetiapine**, **risperidone**, **ziprasidone**; see Drug Interactions).

Disopyramide, procainamide, and quinidine carry a theoretical hazard of QT-prolonging effects when administered in patients with acute overdosing. Similarly, it is reasonable to expect that the alpha-adrenergic blocking properties of bretylium might be additive, resulting in problematic hypertension.

Limited experience indicates antipsychotic drugs are not dialyzable.

Because of the long half-life of **pimozide**, patients should be observed for at least 4 days. Additional surveillance after overdosage of **clozapine** and **thioridazine** should be continued for several days because of the risk for delayed effects.

Patient Information

Because some patients exposed chronically to antipsychotics will develop tardive dyskinesia, inform all patients in whom chronic use is contemplated, if possible, about this risk. The decision to inform patients or their guardians must obviously take into account the clinical circumstances and the patient's competence to understand the information (see Warnings).

May cause impaired judgment, thinking, or motor skills; use caution while driving or performing other tasks requiring alertness. Avoid alcohol and other CNS depressants because of possible additive effects and hypotension.

Avoid skin contact with injection and oral concentrates (contact dermatitis may occur). Oral concentrates are most conveniently used when diluted in fruit juices or other liquids. Use immediately after dilution. See individual products for specific guidelines.

Photosensitivity may occur with some antipsychotics. Avoid exposure to ultraviolet light or sunlight. Use sunscreen and protective clothing until tolerance is determined.

Advise patients of the risk of orthostatic hypotension, especially during the period of initial dose titration.

Use caution in hot weather. These drugs may increase susceptibility to heat stroke. Avoid overheating and dehydration.

Notify physician if sore throat, fever, skin rash, impaired vision, tremors, involuntary muscle twitching, muscle stiffness, or jaundice occurs.

Patients should notify their physician if they become pregnant or intend to become pregnant during therapy.

Patients should notify their physician if they are taking, or plan to take, any prescription or over-the-counter drugs or alcohol.

Advise patients not to breastfeed if they are taking **clozapine**, **olanzapine**, **loxapine**, **risperidone**, **aripiprazole**, **ziprasidone**, **haloperidol**, or **quetiapine**. Safety of the typical antipsychotics in the breastfeeding mother has not been established.

False-positive pregnancy tests have occurred with some **phenothiazines** but are less likely to occur when a serum test is used.

Warn patients who are to receive **clozapine** about the significant risk of developing agranulocytosis and that frequent blood tests are required. Patients should report immediately the appearance of lethargy, weakness, fever, sore throat, malaise, mucous membrane ulcer-

ation, or other possible signs of infection. Inform patients of the significant risk of seizures during clozapine treatment. Inform patients that if they stop taking clozapine for more than 2 days, they should not restart their medication at the same dosage, but should contact their physician for dosing instructions.

Phenothiazine Derivatives

CHLORPROMAZINE HCl

Rx	**Chlorpromazine HCl** (Various, eg, Geneva, Major)	**Tablets:** 10 mg	In 100s, 1000s, and UD 100s.
Rx	**Chlorpromazine HCl** (Various, eg, Geneva, Major)	**Tablets:** 25 mg	In 100s, 1000s, and UD 100s.
Rx	**Thorazine** (GlaxoSmithKline)		Lactose, parabens. (SKF T74). Orange. In 100s.
Rx	**Chlorpromazine HCl** (Various, eg, Geneva, Major)	**Tablets:** 50 mg	In 100s, 1000s, and UD 100s.
Rx	**Thorazine** (GlaxoSmithKline)		Lactose, parabens. (SKF T76). Orange. In 100s.
Rx	**Chlorpromazine HCl** (Various, eg, Geneva, Major)	**Tablets:** 100 mg	In 100s, 1000s, and UD 100s.
Rx	**Thorazine** (GlaxoSmithKline)		Lactose, parabens. (SKF T77). Orange. In 100s.
Rx	**Chlorpromazine HCl** (Various, eg, Geneva, Major)	**Tablets:** 200 mg	In 100s, 1000s, and UD 100s.
Rx	**Thorazine** (GlaxoSmithKline)		Lactose, parabens. (SKF T79). Orange. In 100s.
Rx	**Chlorpromazine HCl** (Various, eg, Alpharma)	**Oral concentrate:** 100 mg/mL	May contain parabens, sulfites, sorbitol, and saccharin. In 237 mL with calibrated dropper graduated in 25 mg increments.
Rx	**Thorazine** (GlaxoSmithKline)	**Suppositories (as base):** 100 mg	In 12s.
Rx	**Chlorpromazine HCl** (Various, eg, Elkins-Sinn)	**Injection:** 25 mg/mL	In 1 and 2 mL amps.[a]
Rx	**Thorazine** (GlaxoSmithKline)		In 1 and 2 mL amps.[b]

[a] With sodium metabisulfite and sodium sulfite.

[b] With sodium bisulfite and sodium sulfite.

For complete prescribing information begins in the Antipsychotic Agents group monograph.

Indications

➤*Emesis / Hiccoughs:* For the control of nausea and vomiting and relief of intractable hiccoughs (see Antiemetic/Antivertigo Agents).

➤*Manic-depressive illness:* For the control of manifestations of the manic type of manic-depressive illness.

➤*Porphyria, acute intermittent:* For the treatment of acute intermittent porphyria.

➤*Schizophrenia:* For the treatment of schizophrenia.

➤*Surgery:* For the relief of restlessness and apprehension prior to surgery.

➤*Tetanus:* An adjunct in treatment of tetanus.

➤*Behavioral problems:* For the treatment of severe behavioral problems in children 1 to 12 years of age marked by combativeness and/or explosive hyperexcitable behavior (out of proportion to immediate provocations).

➤*Hyperactivity:* For the short-term treatment of hyperactive children who show excessive motor activity with accompanying conduct disorders consisting of some or all of the following symptoms: Impulsivity, difficulty sustaining attention, aggressivity, mood lability, and poor frustration tolerance.

Administration and Dosage

Individualize dosage based on condition severity. Increase dosage until symptoms are controlled, then gradually reduce dosage to the lowest effective maintenance level. Increase parenteral dosage only if hypotension has not occurred.

➤*Oral concentrate:* Add desired dosage to 60 mL or more of diluent just prior to administration. Suggested vehicles are tomato or fruit juice, milk, simple syrup, orange syrup, carbonated beverages, coffee, tea, or water. Semisolid foods (eg, soups, puddings) may also be used.

➤*Injection:* SC is not advised. Inject IM slowly, deep into upper outer quadrant of buttock. Because of possible hypotensive effects, reserve for bedfast patients or for acute ambulatory cases and keep patient recumbent for at least ½ hour after injection. If irritation is a problem, dilute injection with saline or 2% procaine; do not mix with other agents in the syringe. Avoid injecting undiluted into vein. Use the IV route only for severe hiccoughs, surgery, and tetanus. Slight yellowing will not alter potency. Discard if markedly discolored.

Because of the possibility of contact dermatitis, avoid getting solution on hands or clothing.

➤*Psychotic disorders:* Maximum improvement may not be seen for weeks or even months. Continue optimum dosage for 2 weeks, then gradually reduce to lowest effective maintenance level; 200 mg/day is not unusual. Some patients require higher dosages (eg, 800 mg/day is not uncommon in discharged mental patients).

Hospitalized patients –

Acute schizophrenic or manic states:

• *IM* – 25 mg initially. If necessary, give an additional 25 to 50 mg injection in 1 hour. Increase gradually over several days (up to 400 mg every 4 to 6 hours in exceptionally severe cases) until patient is controlled. Patient usually becomes quiet and cooperative within 24 to 48 hours. Substitute oral dosage and increase until the patient is calm;

500 mg/day is usually sufficient. While gradual increases to 2000 mg or more/day may be necessary, little therapeutic gain is achieved by exceeding 1000 mg/day for extended periods.

Less acutely disturbed:

• *Oral* – 25 mg 3 times/day. Increase gradually until effective dose is reached, usually 400 mg/day.

Outpatients –

Oral: Initial oral dose is 10 mg 3 or 4 times/day or 25 mg 2 or 3 times/day.

More severe cases –

Oral: Give 25 mg 3 times/day. After 1 or 2 days, daily dosage may be increased by 20 to 50 mg at semiweekly intervals until patient becomes calm and cooperative.

Prompt control of severe symptoms –

IM: 25 mg; if necessary, repeat in 1 hour. Give subsequent doses orally, 25 to 50 mg 3 times/day.

➤*Behavioral disorders / Hyperactivity:* Generally, do not use chlorpromazine in children younger than 6 months of age except where potentially lifesaving. It should not be used in conditions for which specific children's dosages have not been established.

Outpatients –

Oral: 0.5 mg/kg (0.25 mg/lb) every 4 to 6 hours, as needed.

Rectal: 1 mg/kg (0.5 mg/lb) every 6 to 8 hours, as needed.

IM: 0.5 mg/kg (0.25 mg/lb) every 6 to 8 hours, as needed.

Hospitalized patients –

Oral: Start with low doses and increase gradually. In severe behavior disorders, 50 to 100 mg/day, or in older children, 200 mg/day or more may be necessary. There is little evidence that improvement in severely disturbed mentally retarded patients is enhanced by doses beyond 500 mg/day.

IM:

• *5 years of age or younger or 50 lbs* – Do not exceed 40 mg/day.

• *5 to 12 years of age or 50 to 100 lbs* – Do not exceed 75 mg/day, except in unmanageable cases.

➤*Surgery:*

Adults –

Preoperative apprehension: 25 to 50 mg orally 2 to 3 hours before surgery or 12.5 to 25 mg IM 1 to 2 hours before surgery.

Intraoperative (to control acute nausea / vomiting):

• *IM* – 12.5 mg. Repeat in ½ hour if necessary and if no hypotension occurs.

• *IV* – 2 mg per fractional injection at 2-minute intervals. Do not exceed 25 mg (dilute 1 mg/mL with saline).

Children –

Preoperative apprehension: 0.5 mg/kg (0.25 mg/lb) orally 2 to 3 hours before operation or 0.5 mg/kg (0.25 mg/lb) IM 1 to 2 hours before operation.

Intraoperative (to control acute nausea / vomiting):

• *IM* – 0.25 mg/kg (0.125 mg/lb); repeat in ½ hour if needed and if no hypotension occurs.

• *IV* – 1 mg per fractional injection at 2-minute intervals; do not exceed IM dosage. Always dilute to 1 mg/mL with saline.

➤*Tetanus:*

Adults – 25 to 50 mg IM 3 or 4 times/day, usually with barbiturates.

CHLORPROMAZINE HCl

For IV use, 25 to 50 mg diluted to at least 1 mg/mL and administered at a rate of 1 mg/min.

Children – 0.5 mg/kg (0.25 mg/lb) IM or IV every 6 to 8 hours. When given IV, dilute to at least 1 mg/mL and administer at a rate of 1 mg per 2 minutes. In children up to 23 kg (50 lbs), do not exceed 40 mg/day; 23 to 45 kg (50 to 100 lbs), do not exceed 75 mg/day, except in severe cases.

➤*Acute intermittent porphyria (adults):* 25 to 50 mg orally 3 or 4 times/day or 25 mg IM 3 or 4 times/day until patient can take oral therapy.

➤*Elderly/Debilitated/Emaciated:* Lower initial doses and more gradual adjustments are recommended.

➤*Storage/Stability:* Store between 15° and 30°C (59° to 86°F). Protect the injection solution from light. The oral concentrate is light sensitive; protect from light and dispense in amber glass bottle. Refrigeration is not required.

FLUPHENAZINE

Rx	**Fluphenazine HCl** (Various, eg, Geneva)	**Tablets:** 1 mg	In 50s, 100s, 500s, 1000s, and UD 100s.
Rx	**Fluphenazine HCl** (Various, eg, Geneva)	**Tablets:** 2.5 mg	In 50s, 100s, 500s, 1000s, and UD 100s.
Rx	**Fluphenazine HCl** (Various, eg, Geneva)	**Tablets:** 5 mg	In 50s, 100s, 500s, 1000s, and UD 100s.
Rx	**Fluphenazine HCl** (Various, eg, Geneva, Par)	**Tablets:** 10 mg	In 50s, 100s, 500s, 1000s, and UD 100s.
Rx	**Fluphenazine HCl** (Various, eg, Pharmaceuticals Associates)	**Elixir:** 2.5 mg/5 mL	May contain 14% alcohol and sucrose. In 60 and 473 mL.
Rx	**Fluphenazine HCl** (American Pharmaceutical Partners)	**Injection:** 2.5 mg/mL	Parabens. In 10 mL vials.
Rx	**Fluphenazine Decanoate** (Various, eg, Bedford Labs, Geneva)	**Injection:** 25 mg/mL	May contain sesame oil and benzyl alcohol. In 5 mL multidose vials.
Rx	**Prolixin Decanoate** (Apothecon)		In sesame oil with benzyl alcohol. In 5 mL multidose vials.

Complete prescribing information begins in the Antipsychotic Agents group monograph.

Indications

➤*Psychotic disorders:* For the management of manifestations of psychotic disorders; esterified formulations (decanoate) are indicated for patients requiring prolonged and parenteral neuroleptic therapy (eg, chronic schizophrenic patients).

Administration and Dosage

Individualize dosage. The oral dose is approximately 2 to 3 times the parenteral dose. Institute treatment with a low initial dosage; increase as necessary. Therapeutic effect is often achieved with doses under 20 mg/day. However, daily doses up to 40 mg may be needed.

➤*Oral:*

Adults – Initially administer 2.5 to 10 mg/day in divided doses at 6 to 8 hour intervals. When symptoms are controlled, reduce dosage gradually to daily maintenance doses of 1 or 5 mg, often given as a single daily dose. Continued treatment is needed to achieve maximum therapeutic benefits; further adjustments in dosage may be necessary during the course of therapy to meet the patient's requirements.

Elderly: Initially, 1 to 2.5 mg/day, adjusted according to response.

For psychotic patients stabilized on a fixed daily dosage of orally administered fluphenazine, conversion from oral therapy to the long-acting injectable fluphenazine decanoate may be indicated.

➤*Injection:*

Hydrochloride formulation – Administer IM. Average starting dose for adult patients is 1.25 mg (0.5 mL) IM. Initial total daily dose may range from 2.5 to 10 mg and should be divided and given at 6- to 8-hour intervals. Use dosages exceeding 10 mg per day with caution. When symptoms are controlled, oral maintenance therapy can generally be instituted often with single daily doses.

Decanoate formulation – Administer IM or SC. Use a dry syringe and needle of at least 21 gauge. A wet needle or syringe may cause the solution to become cloudy. Initiate with 12.5 to 25 mg (0.5 to 1 mL). The onset of action generally appears between 24 and 72 hours after injec-

tion, and the effects of the drug on psychotic symptoms become significant within 48 to 96 hours. Determine subsequent injections and dosage interval in accordance with patient response. When administered as maintenance therapy, a single injection may be effective in controlling schizophrenic symptoms up to 4 weeks or longer. The response to a single dose has been found to last as long as 6 weeks in a few patients on maintenance therapy.

Initially, treat patients who have never taken phenothiazines with a shorter-acting form of the drug before administering the decanoate. This helps to determine the response to fluphenazine and to establish appropriate dosage.

No precise formula can be given to convert to fluphenazine decanoate use. However, in a controlled multicenter study, oral 20 mg/day fluphenazine HCl was equivalent to 25 mg fluphenazine decanoate every 3 weeks. This is an approximate conversion ratio of 0.5 mL (12.5 mg) decanoate every 3 weeks for every 10 mg fluphenazine HCl daily. Do not exceed 100 mg. If doses greater than 50 mg are needed, increase succeeding doses cautiously in 12.5 mg increments.

Once conversion to fluphenazine decanoate is made, careful clinical monitoring of the patient and appropriate dosage adjustment should be made at the time of each injection.

Severely agitated patients: Initially treat with a rapid-acting phenothiazine. When acute symptoms subside, administer 25 mg of the fluphenazine decanoate; adjust subsequent dosage as necessary.

"Poor risk" patients: In "poor risk" patients (known phenothiazine hypersensitivity or with disorders predisposing to undue reactions), cautiously initiate oral or parenteral fluphenazine. When appropriate dosage is established, give equivalent dose of fluphenazine decanoate.

The optimal amount of the drug and the frequency of administration must be determined for each patient because dosage requirements have been found to vary with clinical circumstances as well as with individual response to the drug.

➤*Storage/Stability:* Store tablets, elixir, and injection at room temperature 15° to 30°C (59° to 86°F); avoid excessive heat. Protect from light. Do not freeze elixir or injection.

PERPHENAZINE

Rx	**Perphenazine** (Various, eg, Geneva, Ivax)	**Tablets:** 2 mg	In 100s, 1000s, and UD 100s.
Rx	**Perphenazine** (Various, eg, Geneva, Ivax)	**Tablets:** 4 mg	In 100s, 500s, 1000s, and UD 100s.
Rx	**Perphenazine** (Various, eg, Geneva, Ivax)	**Tablets:** 8 mg	In 100s, 500s, 1000s, and UD 100s.
Rx	**Perphenazine** (Various, eg, Geneva, Ivax)	**Tablets:** 16 mg	In 100s, 1000s, and UD 100s.
Rx	**Perphenazine** (Pharmaceutical Associates)	**Oral concentrate:** 16 mg/5 mL	Sorbitol, sucrose. Berry flavor. In 118 mL with graduated calibrated dropper.

For complete prescribing information refer to the Antipsychotic Agents group monograph.

Indications

➤*Psychotic disorders:* For the treatment of schizophrenia (tablets); management of manifestations of psychotic disorders (oral concentrate).

➤*Emesis:* To control severe nausea and vomiting in adults (see Antiemetic/Antivertigo Agents).

Administration and Dosage

Individualize the dosage and adjust according to the severity of the condition and the response obtained.

➤*Moderately disturbed, nonhospitalized patients with schizophrenia:* 4 to 8 mg 3 times/day initially; reduce as soon as possible to minimum effective dosage.

➤*Hospitalized patients with schizophrenia:* 8 to 16 mg 2 to 4 times/day; avoid dosages greater than 64 mg/day.

Reserve prolonged administration of doses exceeding 24 mg/day for hospitalized patients or patients under continued observation for early detection and management of adverse reactions. An antiparkinsonian agent, such as trihexyphenidyl HCl or benztropine mesylate, is valuable in controlling drug-induced extrapyramidal symptoms.

➤*Oral concentrate:* Dilute perphenazine oral solution (concentrate) only with water, saline, *7-Up*, homogenized milk, carbonated orange drink, and pineapple, apricot, prune, orange, *V-8*, tomato, and grapefruit juices. Do not mix perphenazine oral solution (concentrate) with beverages containing caffeine (eg, coffee, cola), tannics (eg, tea), or pectinates (eg, apple juice) because physical incompatibility may result. Suggested dilution is approximately 2 fluid ounces of diluent for each 5 mL (16 mg) or teaspoonful of perphenazine oral solution (concen-

PERPHENAZINE

trate). A graduated dropper marked to measure 8 mg or 4 mg is supplied with each bottle.

➤*Children:* Not recommended for children younger than 12 years of age.

➤*Elderly:* Geriatric patients are particularly sensitive to the side effects of antipsychotics. Start on lower doses and observe closely.

➤*Storage/Stability:*
Tablets – Store at controlled room temperature 15° to 30°C (59° to 86°F). Dispense in a tight, light-resistant container.

Oral concentrate – Store between 2° and 30°C (36° and 86°F); protect from light. Dispense concentrate in amber bottles; shake well before using.

PROCHLORPERAZINE

Rx	Prochlorperazine (Various, eg, Barr, Geneva, Par, UDL, Ivax)	**Tablets:** 5 mg (as maleate)	In 100s, 500s, 1000s, blister pack 25s, and UD 100s.
Rx	Compazine (GlaxoSmithKline)		Lactose. (SKF C66). Yellow-green. In 100s and UD 100s.
Rx	Prochlorperazine (Various, eg, Barr, Geneva, Par, UDL, Ivax)	**Tablets:** 10 mg (as maleate)	In 100s, 500s, 1000s, blister pack 25s, and UD 100s.
Rx	Compazine (GlaxoSmithKline)		Lactose. (SKF C67). Yellow-green. In 100s and UD 100s.
Rx	Compazine (GlaxoSmithKline)	**Spansules (sustained-release capsules):** 10 mg (as maleate)	Sugar spheres. (10 mg 3344 10 mg SB). Black/Natural. In 50s.
		15 mg (as maleate)	Sugar spheres. (15 mg 3346 15 mg SB). Black/Natural. In 50s.
Rx	Compazine (GlaxoSmithKline)	**Syrup:** 5 mg/5 mL (as edisylate)	Sucrose. Fruit flavor. In 120 mL.
Rx	Prochlorperazine (Various, eg, Abbott)	**Injection:** 5 mg/mL (as edisylate)	In 2 mL vials.
Rx	Compazine (GlaxoSmithKline)		In 2 and 10 mL vials.[a]
Rx	Compazine (GlaxoSmithKline)	**Suppositories:** 2.5 mg	Glycerin and coconut oil. In 12s.
		5 mg	Glycerin and coconut oil. In 12s.
Rx	Prochlorperazine (Various, eg, G & W Labs)	**Suppositories:** 25 mg	In 12s.
Rx	Compazine (GlaxoSmithKline)		Glycerin. In 12s.
Rx	Compro (Paddock)		Glycerin and coconut oil. In 12s.

[a] With sodium saccharin, benzyl alcohol, sodium biphosphate, and sodium tartrate.

For complete prescribing information refer to the Antipsychotic Agents group monograph.

Indications

➤*Schizophrenia:* For the treatment of schizophrenia.

➤*Nonpsychotic anxiety:* For the short-term treatment of generalized nonpsychotic anxiety; however, prochlorperazine is not the first drug of choice for this indication.

➤*Emesis:* To control severe nausea and vomiting (see Antiemetic/Antivertigo Agents). (*Compro* is only indicated for severe nausea and vomiting in adults.)

Administration and Dosage

➤*Adults:* Increase dosage more gradually in debilitated or emaciated patients.

Schizophrenia – Adjust dosage in adult psychiatric disorders to the response of the individual and according to the severity of the condition. Begin with the lowest recommended dose. Although response is ordinarily seen within a day or 2, longer treatment is usually required before maximal improvement is seen.

Oral:
- *Mild conditions* – 5 or 10 mg 3 or 4 times/day.
- *Moderate to severe conditions* – 10 mg 3 or 4 times/day. Gradually increase dosage until symptoms are controlled or side effects become bothersome. When dosage is increased by small increments over 2 or 3 days, side effects either do not occur or are easily controlled. Some patients respond satisfactorily on 50 to 75 mg/day.
- *Severe conditions* – 100 to 150 mg/day.

IM: SC administration is not advisable because of local irritation.

Inject an initial dose of 10 to 20 mg (2 to 4 mL) deeply into the upper outer quadrant of the buttock. Many patients respond shortly after the first injection. Repeat the initial dose every 2 to 4 hours (or, in resistant cases, every hour) to gain control of the patient, if necessary. More than 3 or 4 doses are seldom necessary. After control is achieved, switch patient to an oral form of the drug at the same dosage levels or higher. If, in rare cases, parenteral therapy is needed for a prolonged period, give 10 to 20 mg (2 to 4 mL) every 4 to 6 hours.

Nonpsychotic anxiety in adults –
Oral: 5 mg 3 to 4 times/day; by spansule capsule, usually one 15 mg capsule on arising or one 10 mg capsule every 12 hours. Do not administer in doses of more than 20 mg/day or for longer than 12 weeks.

➤*Children:* Do not use in pediatric patients under 20 lb or younger than 2 years of age. Do not use in conditions for which children's dosages have not been established.

Children seem more prone to develop extrapyramidal reactions, even on moderate doses. Use the lowest effective dose. Occasionally the patients may react to the drug with signs of restlessness and excitement. Do not administer additional doses if this occurs. Take particular precaution in administering the drug to children with acute illnesses or dehydration.

Adjust dosage and frequency of administration according to the severity of the symptoms and the response of the patient. The duration of activity following IM administration may last up to 12 hours. Subsequent doses may be given by the same route if necessary.

Schizophrenia in children –
Oral or rectal: For children 2 to 12 years of age, starting dosage is 2½ mg 2 or 3 times/day. Do not give more than 10 mg on the first day. Then increase dosage according to the patient's response. When writing a prescription for the 2½ mg size suppository, write "2½", not "2.5". This will help avoid confusion with the 25 mg adult size.
- *Children (2 to 5 years of age)* – Usual total daily dose does not exceed 20 mg.
- *Children (6 to 12 years of age)* – Usual total daily dose does not exceed 25 mg.

IM: For ages under 12, calculate the dose on the basis of 0.06 mg/lb of body weight; give by deep IM injection. Control is usually obtained with 1 dose. After control is achieved, switch the patient to an oral form of the drug at the same dosage level or higher.

➤*Elderly:* Dosages in the lower range are sufficient for most elderly patients. Because they appear to be more susceptible to hypotension and neuromuscular reactions, observe such patients closely. Tailor dosage to the individual, carefully monitor response, and adjust dosage accordingly. Increase dosage more gradually in elderly patients.

➤*Compatibility:* Do not mix prochlorperazine injection with other agents in the syringe.

➤*Storage/Stability:* Store injection vials below 30°C (86°F). Do not freeze. Other dose forms can be stored between 15° and 30°C (59° to 86°F). Protect from light.

Phenothiazine Derivatives

TRIFLUOPERAZINE HCl

Rx	Trifluoperazine (Various, eg, Sandoz, UDL)	**Tablets:** 1 mg	In 100s, 500s, 1000s, and UD 100s.
		2 mg	In 100s, 500s, 1000s, and UD 100s.
		5 mg	In 100s, 500s, 1000s, and UD 100s.
		10 mg	In 100s, 500s, 1000s, and UD 100s.

For complete prescribing information refer to the Antipsychotic Agents group monograph.

Indications

➤*Schizophrenia:* For the management of schizophrenia.

➤*Nonpsychotic anxiety:* For the short-term treatment of nonpsychotic anxiety (not the first drug of choice in most patients).

Administration and Dosage

Individualize dosage. Increase dosage more gradually in debilitated or emaciated patients. When maximum response is achieved, reduce dosage gradually to a maintenance level. Use the lowest effective dosage. Patients may be controlled with once- or twice-daily administration.

➤*Schizophrenia:*

Oral –

Adults: 2 to 5 mg orally twice daily. Start small or emaciated patients on the lower dosage. Most patients will show optimum response with 15 or 20 mg/day, although a few may require 40 mg/day or more. Optimum therapeutic dosage levels should be reached within 2 or 3 weeks.

Children (6 to 12 years of age): Adjust dosage to the weight of the child and severity of the symptoms. These dosages are for children 6 to 12 years of age who are hospitalized or under close supervision. Initial dose is 1 mg once or twice daily. Dosage may be increased gradually until symptoms are controlled or until side effects become troublesome. While it is usually not necessary to exceed 15 mg/day, older children with severe symptoms may require higher doses.

➤*Nonpsychotic anxiety:* 1 or 2 mg twice daily. Do not administer more than 6 mg/day or for longer than 12 weeks because trifluoperazine use at higher doses or for longer intervals may cause persistent tardive dyskinesia that may prove irreversible.

➤*Elderly patients:* Usually, lower dosages are sufficient. The elderly appear more susceptible to hypotension and neuromuscular reactions; observe closely and increase dosage gradually.

➤*Storage/Stability:* Store between 15° and 30°C (59° and 86°F).

THIORIDAZINE HCl

Rx	Thioridazine HCl (Various, eg, Geneva, Mylan, URL/Mutual)	**Tablets:** 10 mg	In 60s, 100s, 1000s, and UD 100s.
Rx	Thioridazine HCl (Various, eg, Geneva)	**Tablets:** 15 mg	In 100s, 1000s, and UD 100s.
Rx	Thioridazine HCl (Various, eg, Geneva, Mylan, URL/Mutual)	**Tablets:** 25 mg	In 60s, 100s, 1000s, and UD 100s.
Rx	Thioridazine HCl (Various, eg, Geneva, Mylan, URL/Mutual)	**Tablets:** 50 mg	In 60s, 100s, 1000s, and UD 100s.
Rx	Thioridazine HCl (Various, eg, Geneva, Mylan, URL/Mutual)	**Tablets:** 100 mg	In 60s, 100s, 1000s, and UD 100s.
Rx	Thioridazine HCl (Various, eg, Geneva)	**Tablets:** 150 mg	In 100s and 1000s.
Rx	Thioridazine HCl (Various, eg, Geneva)	**Tablets:** 200 mg	In 100s and 1000s.

For complete prescribing information refer to the Antipsychotic Agents group monograph.

WARNING

Thioridazine has been shown to prolong the QTc interval in a dose-related manner. Drugs with this potential, including thioridazine, have been associated with torsade de pointes-type arrhythmias and sudden death. Because of its potential for significant, possibly life-threatening, proarrhythmic effects, reserve thioridazine use in the treatment of schizophrenic patients who fail to show an acceptable response to adequate courses of treatment with other antipsychotic drugs, either because of insufficient effectiveness or the inability to achieve an effective dose because of intolerable adverse effects from those drugs.

Indications

➤*Schizophrenia:* For the management of schizophrenic patients who fail to respond adequately to treatment with other antipsychotic drugs. Before initiating treatment with thioridazine, it is strongly recommended that a patient be given at least 2 trials, each with a different antipsychotic drug product, at an adequate dose and for an adequate duration (see Warning box).

Administration and Dosage

Dosage must be individualized and the smallest effective dosage should be determined for each patient.

➤*Adults:* Starting dose is 50 to 100 mg 3 times/day with a gradual increment to a maximum of 800 mg/day, if necessary. Once effective control of symptoms has been achieved, the dosage may be reduced gradually to determine the minimum maintenance dose. The total daily dosage ranges from 200 to 800 mg, divided into 2 to 4 doses.

➤*Children:* For patients unresponsive to other agents, the recommended initial dose is 0.5 mg/kg/day given in divided doses. Dosage may be increased gradually until optimum therapeutic effect is obtained or the maximum dose of 3 mg/kg/day has been reached.

➤*Oral concentrate:* Concentrate may be diluted with distilled or acidified tap water or suitable juices. Dilute each dose just prior to administration; preparation and storage of bulk dilutions is not recommended.

➤*Storage/Stability:*

Tablets – Store at controlled room temperature 15° to 30°C (59° to 86°F); dispense in a tight, light-resistant container.

Oral concentrate – Store at controlled room temperature 15° to 30°C (59° to 86°F) in a tight, amber glass bottle.

Thioxanthene Derivatives

THIOTHIXENE

Rx	Thiothixene (Various, eg, Geneva)	Capsules: 1 mg	In 100s, and 1000s.
Rx	Navane (Roerig)		Lactose. In 100s.
Rx	Thiothixene (Various, eg, Geneva)	Capsules: 2 mg	In 100s, 1000s, and UD 100s.
Rx	Navane (Roerig)		Lactose. In 100s.
Rx	Thiothixene (Various, eg, Geneva)	Capsules: 5 mg	In 100s, 1000s, and UD 100s.
Rx	Navane (Roerig)		Lactose. In 100s.
Rx	Thiothixene (Various, eg, Geneva)	Capsules: 10 mg	In 100s, 1000s, and UD 100s.
Rx	Navane (Roerig)		Lactose. In 100s.
Rx	Navane (Roerig)	Capsules: 20 mg	Lactose. In 100s.

For complete prescribing information refer to the Antipsychotic Agents group monograph.

Indications

➤*Schizophrenia:* For the management of schizophrenia.

Administration and Dosage

Individualize dose depending on the chronicity and severity of the symptoms. Use small doses initially and gradually increase to the optimal effective level based on patient response. Some patients have been successfully maintained on once-a-day therapy.

Not recommended for use in children younger than 12 years of age.

➤*Mild conditions:* Initially, 2 mg 3 times/day. If indicated, an increase to 15 mg/day is often effective.

➤*Severe conditions:* Initially, 5 mg twice daily. Optimal is 20 to 30 mg/day. If indicated, 60 mg/day is often effective. Exceeding 60 mg/day rarely increases the beneficial response.

➤*Storage/Stability:* Store at controlled room temperature up to 30°C (86°F).

Phenylbutylpiperadine Derivatives

HALOPERIDOL

Rx	Haloperidol (Various, eg, Geneva, Mylan)	Tablets: 0.5 mg	In 100s, 1000s, and UD 100s.
		1 mg	In 100s, 1000s, and UD 100s.
		2 mg	In 100s, 1000s, and UD 100s.
		5 mg	In 100s, 1000s, and UD 100s.
Rx	Haloperidol (Various, eg, Geneva)	Tablets: 10 mg	In 100s, 1000s, and UD 100s.
		20 mg	In 100s and UD 100s.
Rx	Haloperidol (Various, eg, Ivax, Major)	Oral concentrate: 2 mg (as lactate)/mL	In 15 and 120 mL, and 5 and 10 mL UD 100s.
Rx	Haloperidol (Various, eg, Bedford)	Injection: 5 mg (as lactate)/mL	May contain parabens. In 1 mL vials and 10 mL multidose vials.
Rx	Haldol (McNeil-CPC)		Parabens. In 1 mL amps and 10 mL multidose vials.
Rx	Haloperidol Decanoate (Various, eg, Apotex, Bedford, Gensia Sicor)	Injection: 50 mg (equiv. to 70.5 mg decanoate)/mL	May contain sesame oil and 1.2% benzyl alcohol. In 1 and 5 mL multidose vial.
Rx	Haldol Decanoate 50 (McNeil, Bedford)		In 1 mL amps[a] and 5 mL vials.
Rx	Haloperidol Decanoate (Various, eg, Apotex, Bedford, Gensia Sicor)	Injection: 100 mg (equiv. to 141.04 mg decanoate)/mL	May contain sesame oil and 1.2% benzyl alcohol. In 1 mL and 5 mL multidose vial.
Rx	Haldol Decanoate 100 (McNeil)		In 1 mL amps[a] and 5 mL vials.[a]

[a] In sesame oil with 1.2% benzyl alcohol.

For complete prescribing information refer to the Antipsychotic Agents group monograph.

Indications

➤*Psychotic disorders:* For the treatment of psychotic disorders (eg, schizophrenia). Haloperidol decanoate is for patients who require prolonged parenteral antipsychotic therapy.

➤*Tourette disorder:* For the control of tics and vocal utterances in Tourette disorder.

➤*Behavioral problems:* For the treatment of behavioral problems in children with combative, explosive hyperexcitability that cannot be accounted for by immediate provocation. Reserve for use in these children only after failure to respond to psychotherapy or medications other than antipsychotics.

➤*Hyperactivity:* For short-term treatment of hyperactive children who show excessive motor activity with accompanying conduct disorders consisting of impulsivity, difficulty sustaining attention, aggression, mood lability, or poor frustration tolerance. Reserve for use in these children only after failure to respond to psychotherapy or medications other than antipsychotics.

Administration and Dosage

Individualize dosage. Children, debilitated or geriatric patients, and those with a history of adverse reactions to neuroleptic drugs may require less haloperidol; optimal response is usually obtained with more gradual dosage adjustments and at lower dosage levels. Upon achieving a satisfactory therapeutic response, gradually reduce dosage to the lowest effective maintenance level.

➤*Psychotic disorders:*

Adults: Initial dosage – Moderate symptoms or geriatric or debilitated patients: 0.5 to 2 mg given 2 or 3 times daily; severe symptoms or chronic or resistant patients: 3 to 5 mg 2 or 3 times daily. To achieve prompt control, higher doses may be required.

Patients who remain severely disturbed or inadequately controlled may require dosage adjustment. Daily dosages up to 100 mg may be necessary. Infrequently, doses greater than 100 mg have been used for severely resistant patients; however, safety of prolonged administration of such doses has not been demonstrated.

Children (3 to 12 years of age; weight range 15 to 40 kg) – Do not use in children younger than 3 years of age. Initial dose is 0.5 mg/day (25 to 50 mcg/kg/day). If required, increase in 0.5 mg increments at 5- to 7-day intervals up to 0.15 mg/kg/day or until therapeutic effect is obtained. Total dose may be divided and given 2 or 3 times daily. The dose in this age group has not been well established.

IM administration – 2 to 5 mg haloperidol lactate for prompt control of the acutely agitated schizophrenic patient with moderately severe to very severe symptoms. Depending on response, administer subsequent doses as often as every 60 minutes, although 4- to 8-hour intervals may be satisfactory.

The safety and efficacy of IM administration in children have not been established.

Conversion from IM to oral – Replace the injectable with the oral form as soon as feasible. For an approximation of the total daily dose required, use the parenteral dose administered in the preceding 24 hours; carefully monitor the patient for the first several days. Give the first oral dose within 12 to 24 hours following the last parenteral dose.

➤*Tourette disorder:*

Adults – A starting dose of 0.5 to 1.5 mg 3 times/day by mouth has been suggested; up to about 10 mg/day may be needed. Requirements vary considerably and the dose must be very carefully adjusted to obtain the optimum response.

Children (3 to 12 years of age; 15 to 40 kg) – 0.05 to 0.075 mg/kg/day. Severely disturbed psychotic children may require higher doses.

➤*Behavioral disorders/hyperactivity:*

Children (3 to 12 years of age; 15 to 40 kg) – 0.05 to 0.075 mg/kg/day. Severely disturbed psychotic children may require higher doses.

In severely disturbed, nonpsychotic children or in hyperactive children with conduct disorders, short-term administration may suffice. There is

Phenylbutylpiperadine Derivatives

HALOPERIDOL

little evidence that behavior improvement is further enhanced by dosages greater than 6 mg/day.

▶*Haloperidol decanoate injection:* Individualize dosage and provide close clinical supervision during initiation and stabilization of therapy. The recommended interval between doses is monthly or every 4 weeks. However, variation in patient response may dictate a need for adjustment of the dosing interval as well as the dose. To determine the minimum effective dose, begin with lower initial doses and adjust the dose upward as needed.

Intended for use in chronic psychotic patients who require prolonged parenteral antipsychotic therapy. These patients should be previously stabilized on antipsychotic medication, and should have been treated with, and well tolerated on short-acting haloperidol in order to exclude the possibility of an unexpected adverse sensitivity to haloperidol. Close clinical supervision is required during the initial period of dose adjustment in order to minimize the risk of overdosage or reappearance of psychotic symptoms before the next injection. During dose adjustment or episodes of exacerbation of psychotic symptoms, haloperidol decanoate therapy can be supplemented with short-acting forms of haloperidol.

Haloperidol Decanoate Dosing Recommendations[a]		
Patients	1st Month[b]	Monthly maintenance
Stabilized on low daily oral doses (≤ 10 mg/day)	10 to 15 × daily oral dose	10 to 15 × previous daily oral dose
Elderly or debilitated		
Stabilized on higher doses; risk of relapse	20 × daily oral dose	10 to 15 × previous daily oral dose
Tolerant to oral haloperidol		

[a] Clinical experience with doses greater than 450 mg/month has been limited.
[b] Initial dose should not exceed 100 mg. See below.

Initial dosage – The initial dose should not exceed 100 mg regardless of previous antipsychotic dose requirements. If the conversion requires more than 100 mg of haloperidol decanoate as an initial dose, administer that dose in 2 injections (maximum of 100 mg initially followed by the balance in 3 to 7 days).

Maintenance dosage – Individualize with titration upward or downward based on therapeutic response.

Administration – Administer by deep IM injection. A 21-gauge needle is recommended. The maximum volume per injection site should not exceed 3 mL. Do not administer IV.

▶*Elderly/Debilitated:* Lower initial doses and more gradual adjustments are recommended.

▶*Storage/Stability:*

Tablets – Store at controlled room temperature 15° to 30°C (59° to 86°F). Dispense in tight, light-resistant container.

Injection – Store at controlled room temperature 15° to 30°C (59° to 86°F). Protect from light; do not freeze.

PIMOZIDE

Rx	Orap (Teva)	Tablets: 1 mg	Lactose. (ORAP 1). White, oval, scored. In 100s.
		2 mg	Lactose. (LEMMON ORAP 2). White, oval, scored. In 100s.

For complete prescribing information, refer to the Antipsychotic Agents group monograph.

Indications

▶*Tourette disorder:* For suppression of motor and phonic tics in patients with Tourette disorder who have failed to respond satisfactorily to standard treatment. Pimozide is not intended as a treatment of first choice, nor is it intended for the treatment of tics that are merely annoying or cosmetically troublesome. Reserve pimozide use for Tourette disorder patients whose development and/or daily life function is severely compromised by the presence of motor and phonic tics.

Administration and Dosage

▶*Approved by the FDA:* July 31, 1984.

The suppression of tics by pimozide requires a slow and gradual introduction of the drug. Carefully adjust the patient's dose to a point where the suppression of tics and the relief afforded is balanced against the untoward side effects of the drug. Perform ECG at baseline and periodically thereafter, especially during dosage adjustment.

▶*Tourette:*
Adults –
Initial dose: 1 to 2 mg/day in divided doses. Thereafter, increase dose every other day.

Maintenance dose: Less than 0.2 mg/kg/day or 10 mg/day, whichever is less. Doses greater than 0.2 mg/kg/day or 10 mg/day are not recommended.

Children – Although Tourette disorder most often has its onset between 2 and 15 years of age, information on the use and efficacy of pimozide in patients less than 12 years of age is limited. A 24-week, open-label study in 36 children between 2 and 12 years of age demonstrated that pimozide has a similar safety profile in this age group as in older patients and there were no safety findings that would preclude its use in this age group. Pimozide is not recommended for any childhood condition other than Tourette disorder.

Initiate at a dose of 0.05 mg/kg preferably taken once at bedtime; dose may be increased every third day to a maximum of 0.2 mg/kg, not to exceed 10 mg/day.

Gradual withdrawal – Periodically attempt to reduce dosage to see if tics persist. Increases of tic intensity and frequency may represent a transient, withdrawal-related phenomenon rather than a return of symptoms. Allow 1 or 2 weeks to elapse before concluding that an increase in tic manifestations is due to the underlying disease rather than drug withdrawal. A gradual withdrawal is recommended in any case.

▶*Storage/Stability:* Store at controlled room temperature 15° to 30°C (59° to 86°F) in a tight, light-resistant container.

Dihydroindolone Derivatives

MOLINDONE HCl

Rx	Moban (Endo)	Tablets: 5 mg	Lactose. (Moban 5). Orange. In 100s.
		10 mg	Lactose. (Moban 10). Lavender. In 100s.
		25 mg	Lactose. (Moban 25). Green. In 100s.
		50 mg	Lactose. (Moban 50). Blue. In 100s.

For complete prescribing information refer to the Antipsychotic Agents group monograph.

Indications

▶*Schizophrenia:* For the management of schizophrenia.

Administration and Dosage

Individualize dosage.

▶*Initial dosage:* 50 to 75 mg/day, increase to 100 mg/day in 3 or 4 days. Based on severity of symptomatology, dosage may be titrated up or down depending on individual patient response. An increase to

225 mg/day may be required. Start elderly and debilitated patients on lower dosage.

▶*Maintenance therapy:*

Mild – 5 to 15 mg 3 or 4 times/day.

Moderate – 10 to 25 mg 3 or 4 times/day.

Severe – 225 mg/day may be required.

▶*Storage/Stability:* Store at 25°C (77°F); excursions permitted to 15° to 30°C (59° to 86°F). Dispense in a tight, light-resistant container with child-resistant closure. Keep tightly closed.

CLOZAPINE

Rx	**Clozapine** (Various, eg, Ivax)	**Tablets:** 12.5 mg	In 30s and 100s.
Rx	**Clozapine** (Various, eg, Mylan, UDL, Zenith-Goldline)	**Tablets:** 25 mg	In 100s and 500s.
Rx	**Clozaril** (Novartis)		Lactose, talc. (CLOZARIL 25). Pale yellow, scored. In 100s, 500s, and UD 100s.
Rx	**Clozapine** (Various, eg, Mylan, UDL, Zenith-Goldline)	**Tablets:** 100 mg	In 100s and 500s.
Rx	**Clozaril** (Novartis)		Lactose, talc. (CLOZARIL 100). Pale yellow, scored. In 100s, 500s, and UD 100s.
Rx	**Fazalco** (Alamo)	**Tablets, orally disintegrating:** 25 mg	Aspartame, 1.74 mg phenylalanine. (A01). Yellow, scored. In 48s.
		100 mg	Aspartame, 6.96 mg phenylalanine. (A02). Yellow, scored. In 48s.

For complete prescribing information refer to the Antipsychotic Agents group monograph.

WARNING

Agranulocytosis: Because of a significant risk of agranulocytosis, a potentially life-threatening adverse event, reserve clozapine for use in 1) the treatment of severely ill schizophrenic patients who fail to show an acceptable response to adequate courses of standard antipsychotic drug treatment because of insufficient effectiveness or the inability to achieve an effective dose because of intolerable adverse effects from those drugs, or 2) for reducing the risk of recurrent suicidal behavior in patients with schizophrenia or schizoaffective disorder who are judged to be at risk of re-experiencing suicidal behavior. Consequently, unless the patient is at risk for recurrent suicidal behavior, before initiating treatment with clozapine, it is strongly recommended that a patient be given at least 2 trials, each with a different standard antipsychotic drug product at an adequate dose and for an adequate duration.

Patients who are being treated with clozapine must have a baseline white blood cell (WBC) and differential count before initiation of treatment and regular WBC counts during treatment and for 4 weeks after the discontinuation of clozapine.

Clozapine is available only through a distribution system that ensures monitoring of WBC counts according to the schedule described below prior to delivery of the next supply of medication.

Seizures: Seizures have been associated with the use of clozapine. Dose appears to be an important predictor of seizure, with a greater likelihood at higher clozapine doses. Use caution when administering clozapine to patients who have a history of seizures or other predisposing factors. Advise patients not to engage in any activity where sudden loss of consciousness could cause serious risk to themselves or others.

Myocarditis: Analyses of postmarketing safety databases suggest that clozapine is associated with an increased risk of fatal myocarditis, especially during, but not limited to, the first month of therapy. In patients in whom myocarditis is suspected, promptly discontinue clozapine treatment.

Other adverse cardiovascular and respiratory effects: Orthostatic hypotension, with or without syncope, can occur with clozapine treatment. Rarely, collapse can be profound and be accompanied by respiratory and/or cardiac arrest. Orthostatic hypotension is more likely to occur during initial titration in association with rapid dose escalation. In patients who have had even a brief interval off clozapine (2 or more days since the last dose), start treatment with 12.5 mg once or twice daily (see Administration and Dosage).

Because collapse, respiratory arrest, and cardiac arrest during initial treatment have occurred in patients who were being administered benzodiazepines or other psychotropic drugs, caution is advised when clozapine is initiated in patients taking a benzodiazepine or any other psychotropic drug (see Warnings in Antipsychotic Agents group monograph).

Indications

▶*Schizophrenia:* For the management of severely ill schizophrenic patients who fail to respond adequately to standard drug treatment for schizophrenia.

▶*Recurrent suicidal behavior:* For reducing the risk of recurrent suicidal behavior in patients with schizophrenia or schizoaffective disorder who are judged to be at chronic risk for re-experiencing suicidal behavior, based on history and recent clinical state. Continue clozapine treatment to reduce the risk of suicidal behavior for at least 2 years.

Administration and Dosage

▶*Approved by the FDA:* September 26, 1989.

Clozapine is available only through a distribution system that ensures monitoring of WBC counts according to the schedule described below prior to delivery of the next supply of medication. For more information, call (800) 448-5938. Upon initiation of clozapine therapy, up to a 1 week supply of additional tablets may be provided to the patient to be held for emergencies (eg, weather, holidays).

Drug dispensing should not ordinarily exceed a weekly supply. If a patient is eligible for WBC testing every other week, then a 2-week supply can be dispensed. Dispensing should be contingent on the results of a WBC count.

▶*Monitoring:* Patients must have a blood sample drawn for a WBC count before initiation of treatment with clozapine and must have subsequent WBC counts done at least weekly for the first 6 months of continuous treatment. If WBC counts remain acceptable (WBC at least 3000/mm³, ANC at least 1500/mm³) during this period, WBC counts may be monitored every other week thereafter. After the discontinuation of clozapine, continue weekly WBC counts for an additional 4 weeks.

▶*Initial:* 12.5 mg once or twice daily, and then continue with daily dosage increments of 25 to 50 mg/day, if well tolerated, to achieve a target dose of 300 to 450 mg/day by the end of 2 weeks. Make subsequent dosage increments no more than once or twice weekly, in increments not to exceed 100 mg. Cautious titration and a divided dosage schedule are necessary to minimize the risks of hypotension, seizure, and sedation.

In a multicenter study, patients were titrated during the first 2 weeks up to a maximum dose of 500 mg/day, on a 3 times/day basis. These patients were then dosed in a total daily dose range of 100 to 900 mg/day on a 3 times/day basis thereafter with clinical response and adverse effects as guides to correct dosing.

Clozapine Therapy Guidelines Based on WBC and ANC[a]		
WBC count (mm³)	ANC (mm³)	Guidelines
< 3500, or history of myeloproliferative disorder, or previous clozapine-induced agranulocytosis or granulocytopenia	—	Do not initiate treatment.
< 3500, or > 3500 with a substantial drop[b] from baseline, or presence of immature forms following initiation of treatment	—	Repeat WBC and differential counts. Symptoms of infection include the following: Lethargy, weakness, fever, sore throat.
3000 to 3500 on subsequent counts	> 1500	Perform twice-weekly WBC and differential counts.
< 3000	or < 1500	Interrupt therapy; monitor for flu-like symptoms or other symptoms of infection. Perform WBC count and differential daily. May resume therapy if no signs of infection develop, WBC count > 3000 and ANC > 1500. However, continue twice weekly WBC and differential counts until WBC returns to > 3500, and then monitor WBC weekly for 6 months.
< 2000	or < 1000	Monitor WBC count and differential daily. Consider bone marrow aspiration to ascertain granulopoietic status. If granulopoiesis is deficient, consider protective isolation. If infection develops, perform cultures and institute antibiotics. Do not rechallenge with clozapine because agranulocytosis may develop with a shorter latency.

[a] See manufacturer's product labeling for more specific recommendations.
[b] A substantial drop is defined as a single drop of 3000 or more in the WBC count or a cumulative drop of 3000 or more within 3 weeks.

▶*Dose adjustment:* Continue daily dosing on a divided basis to an effective and tolerable dose level. While many patients may respond adequately at doses between 300 to 600 mg/day, it may be necessary to raise the dose to the 600 to 900 mg/day range. Do not exceed 900 mg/day. The mean and median clozapine doses are approximately 600 mg/day for schizophrenia and 300 mg/day for reducing recurrent suicidal behavior.

Because of the possibility of increased adverse reactions at higher doses, particularly seizures, give patients adequate time to respond to a given dose level before escalation to a higher dose.

Because of the significant risk of agranulocytosis and seizure (events that both present a continuing risk over time), avoid extended treatment of patients failing to show an acceptable level of clinical response.

CLOZAPINE

➤*Maintenance:* Continue clozapine at the lowest level needed to maintain remission. Periodically reassess patients to determine the need for maintenance treatment.

➤*Discontinuation:* In the event of planned termination of clozapine therapy, gradual reduction in dose is recommended over a 1- to 2-week period. However, should a patient's medical condition require abrupt discontinuation (eg, leukopenia), carefully observe the patient for the recurrence of psychotic symptoms and symptoms related to cholinergic rebound (eg, headache, nausea, vomiting, diarrhea). After the discontinuation of clozapine, continue weekly WBC counts for an additional 4 weeks.

➤*Reinitiation of treatment:* When restarting patients who have had even a brief interval off clozapine (ie, 2 days or more since the last dose) it is recommended that treatment be reinitiated with one-half of a 25 mg tablet (12.5 mg) once or twice daily. If that dose is well tolerated, it may be feasible to titrate patients back to a therapeutic dose more quickly than is recommended for initial treatment. However, any patient who has previously experienced respiratory or cardiac arrest with initial dosing, but was then able to be successfully titrated to a therapeutic dose, should be retitrated with extreme caution after even 24 hours of discontinuation.

Monitoring Guidelines for Patients Reinitiated on Clozapine					
Therapy duration	No abnormal blood event and break in therapy is ≤ 1 month	No abnormal blood event and break in therapy is > 1 month	Abnormal blood event and patient is rechallengeable	No abnormal blood event and break in therapy is ≤ 1 year	No abnormal blood event and break in therapy is > 1 year
< 6 months	Continue weekly monitoring left off to complete 6 months	Restart weekly monitoring for 6 months	Restart weekly monitoring for 6 months after recovery from event	—	—
≥ 6 months	—	—		Continue monitoring at every other week intervals	Restart weekly monitoring for 6 months

Certain additional precautions seem prudent. Re-exposure of a patient might enhance the risk of an untoward event's occurrence and increase its severity. Patients discontinued for WBC counts below 2000/mm^3 or an ANC below 1000/mm^3 must not be restarted on clozapine (see Warnings in Antipsychotic Agents group monograph).

➤*Storage/Stability:* Storage temperature should not exceed 30°C (86°F).

Contraindications

Hypersensitivity to clozapine or any other component of the drug; uncontrolled epilepsy; myeloproliferative disorders; history of clozapine-induced agranulocytosis or severe granulocytopenia; simultaneous administration with other agents having a well-known potential to cause agranulocytosis or otherwise suppress bone marrow function; severe CNS depression or comatose states from any cause. Causative factors of agranulocytosis may interact synergistically to increase the risk and/or severity of bone marrow suppression.

Patient Information

Warn patients about the significant risk of developing agranulocytosis. Inform them that weekly blood tests are required to monitor for the occurrence of agranulocytosis and that clozapine tablets will be made available only through a special program designed to ensure the required blood monitoring. Advise patients to report immediately the appearance of lethargy, weakness, fever, sore throat, malaise, mucous membrane ulceration, or other possible signs of infection. Pay particular attention to flu-like complaints or other symptoms that might suggest infection.

Inform patients of the significant risk of seizure during clozapine treatment and advise them to avoid driving and any other potentially hazardous activity while taking clozapine.

Advise patients of the risk of orthostatic hypotension, especially during the period of initial dose titration.

Inform patients that if they stop taking clozapine for more than 2 days, they should not restart their medication at the same dosage but should contact their health care provider for dosing instructions.

Advise women not to breastfeed an infant if they are taking clozapine.

LOXAPINE

Rx	**Loxapine Succinate** (Various, eg, Dixon-Shane, UDL, Watson)	**Capsules:** 5 mg (6.8 mg as loxapine succinate)	In 100s and 1000s.
Rx	**Loxitane** (Watson)		Lactose. (WATSON LOXITANE 5 mg). Dark green. In 100s and 1000s.
Rx	**Loxapine Succinate** (Various, eg, Dixon-Shane, UDL, Watson)	**Capsules:** 10 mg (13.6 mg as loxapine succinate)	In 100s.
Rx	**Loxitane** (Watson)		Lactose. (WATSON LOXITANE 10 mg). Dark green/yellow. In 100s and 1000s.
Rx	**Loxapine Succinate** (Various, eg, Dixon-Shane, UDL, Watson)	**Capsules:** 25 mg (34 mg as loxapine succinate)	In 100s.
Rx	**Loxitane** (Watson)		Lactose. (WATSON LOXITANE 25 mg). Two-tone green. In 100s and 1000s.
Rx	**Loxapine Succinate** (Various, eg, Dixon-Shane, UDL, Watson)	**Capsules:** 50 mg (68.1 mg loxapine succinate)	In 100s.
Rx	**Loxitane** (Watson)		Lactose. (WATSON LOXITANE 50 mg). Dark green/blue. In 100s and 1000s.

For complete prescribing information, refer to the Antipsychotic Agents group monograph.

Indications

➤*Schizophrenia:* For the treatment of schizophrenia.

Administration and Dosage

Individualize dosage. Administer in divided doses, 2 to 4 times/day.

➤*Initial:* 10 mg twice daily. In severely disturbed patients, up to 50 mg/day may be desirable. Increase dosage fairly rapidly over the first 7 to 10 days until symptoms are controlled.

➤*Maintenance:* Reduce dosage to the lowest level compatible with control of symptoms.

Usual therapeutic and maintenance range is 60 to 100 mg/day. Many patients have been maintained satisfactorily at dosages in the range of 20 to 60 mg/day. Dosages higher than 250 mg/day are not recommended.

➤*Storage/Stability:* Store at controlled room temperature, 15° to 30°C (59° to 86°F). Dispense capsules in a tight, child-resistant container.

Dibenzapine Derivatives

OLANZAPINE

Rx	**Zyprexa** (Eli Lilly)	**Tablets:** 2.5 mg	Lactose. (LILLY 4112). White. In 60s, 1000s, and UD 100s.
		5 mg	Lactose. (LILLY 4115). White. In 60s, 1000s, and UD 100s.
		7.5 mg	Lactose. (LILLY 4116). White. In 60s, 1000s, and UD 100s.
		10 mg	Lactose. (LILLY 4117). White. In 60s, 1000s, and UD 100s.
		15 mg	Lactose. (LILLY 4415). Blue, elliptical. In 60s, 1000s, and UD 100s.
		20 mg	Lactose. (LILLY 4420). Pink, elliptical. In 60s, 1000s, and UD 100s.
Rx	**Zyprexa Zydis** (Eli Lilly)	**Tablets, orally disintegrating:** 5 mg	(5). Yellow. In dose pack 30s.[a]
		10 mg	(10). Yellow. In dose pack 30s.[b]
		15 mg	(15). Yellow. In dose pack 30s.[c]
		20 mg	(20). Yellow. In dose pack 30s.[d]
Rx	**Zyprexa IntraMuscular** (Eli Lilly)	**Powder for injection:** 10 mg	In vials.

[a] With aspartame, parabens, mannitol, 0.34 mg phenylalanine.
[b] With aspartame, parabens, mannitol, 0.45 mg phenylalanine.
[c] With aspartame, parabens, mannitol, 0.67 mg phenylalanine.
[d] With aspartame, parabens, mannitol, 0.9 mg phenylalanine.

For complete prescribing information, refer to the Antipsychotic Agents group monograph.

Indications

➤*Bipolar disorder (oral):*

Monotherapy – For the treatment of acute mixed, or manic episodes associated with bipolar I disorder and for the maintenance monotherapy of bipolar disorder.

Combination therapy – In combination with lithium or valproate for the short-term treatment of acute manic episodes associated with bipolar I disorder.

➤*Schizophrenia (oral):* For the treatment of schizophrenia.

➤*Agitation associated with schizophrenia and bipolar I mania (injection):* For the treatment of agitation associated with schizophrenia and bipolar I mania.

Administration and Dosage

➤*Approved by the FDA:* September 30, 1996.

➤*Bipolar disorder (oral):*

Monotherapy – Initial dose is 10 to 15 mg orally once daily without regard to meals. Adjust dosage, if indicated, at 5 mg/day increments or decrements in intervals not less than 24 hours.

Short-term (3 to 4 weeks) antimanic efficacy was demonstrated in a dose range of 5 to 20 mg/day in clinical trials. The safety of doses above 20 mg/day has not been evaluated.

Maintenance monotherapy – The benefit of maintaining bipolar patients on monotherapy with olanzapine at a dose of 5 to 20 mg/day, after achieving a responder status for an average duration of 2 weeks, was demonstrated in a controlled trial. Periodically reevaluate olanzapine use in patients taking the drug for extended periods.

Combination therapy – When coadministered with lithium or valproate, generally begin olanzapine dosing with 10 mg orally once daily without regard to meals.

Short-term (6 weeks) antimanic efficacy was demonstrated in a dose range of 5 to 20 mg/day in clinical trials. The safety of doses above 20 mg/day has not been evaluated in clinical trials.

➤*Schizophrenia (oral):* Initial dose is 5 to 10 mg orally once daily without regard to meals, with a target dose of 10 mg/day within several days of initiation. Adjust dosage, if indicated, at 5 mg/day increments or decrements in intervals not less than 1 week.

Efficacy was demonstrated in a dose range of 10 to 15 mg/day in clinical trials. However, increases in efficacy were not demonstrated in doses above 10 mg/day. Doses above 10 mg/day are recommended only after clinical assessment. The safety of doses above 20 mg/day has not been evaluated in clinical trials.

Maintenance treatment – Periodically reassess patients to determine the need for maintenance treatment.

➤*Administration of orally disintegrating tablets:* Peel back foil on blister; do not push tablet through foil. Using dry hands, remove and place the entire tablet in the mouth. The tablet will disintegrate rapidly in saliva so it can be easily swallowed with or without liquid.

➤*Agitation associated with schizophrenia and bipolar I mania (IM):*

Usual dose – The efficacy of IM olanzapine injection in controlling agitation in these disorders was demonstrated in a dose range of 2.5 to 10 mg. The recommended dose is 10 mg. A lower dose of 5 or 7.5 mg may be considered when clinical factors warrant. If agitation warranting additional IM doses persists following the initial dose, subsequent doses up to 10 mg may be given. However, the efficacy of repeated doses in agitated patients has not be systematically evaluated in controlled clinical trials. Also the safety of total daily doses greater than 30 mg, or 10 mg injections given more frequently than 2 hours after the initial dose, and 4 hours after the second dose have not been evaluated in clinical trials. Maximal dosing of IM olanzapine (eg, three doses of 10 mg given 2 to 4 hours apart) may be associated with a substantial occurrence of significant orthostatic hypotension. Thus, it is recommended that patients requiring subsequent IM injections be assessed for orthostatic hypotension prior to the administration of any subsequent doses of IM olanzapine. The administration of an additional dose to a patient with a clinically significant postural change in systolic blood pressure is not recommended.

If ongoing olanzapine therapy is clinical indicated, oral olanzapine may be initiated in a range of 5 to 20 mg/day as soon as clinically appropriate.

➤*Administration of IM injection:* For IM use only. Do not administer IV or SC. Inject slowly, deep into the muscle mass.

➤*Preparation for administration:* Dissolve the contents of the vial using 2.1 mL sterile water for injection to provide a solution containing approximately 5 mg/mL olanzapine. The resulting solution should appear clear and yellow. Use immediately (within 1 hour) after reconstitution. Discard any unused portion. The following table provides injection volumes for delivering various doses of IM olanzapine for injection.

IM Olanzapine Injection Volume	
Olanzapine dose (mg)	Volume of injection (mL)
10	Withdraw total contents of vial
7.5	1.5
5	1
2.5	0.5

➤*Special populations:*

Oral – The recommended starting dose is 5 mg in patients who are debilitated, who have a predisposition to hypotensive reactions, who otherwise exhibit a combination of factors that may result in slower metabolism of olanzapine (eg, nonsmoking women 65 years of age and older), or who may be more pharmacodynamically sensitive to olanzapine. When indicated, use caution with dose escalation.

Injection – Consider a dose of 5 mg per injection for geriatric patients or when other clinical factors warrant. Consider a lower dose of 2.5 mg per injection for patients who otherwise might be debilitated, be predisposed to hypotensive reactions, or be more pharmacodynamically sensitive to olanzapine.

➤*Storage/Stability:*

Oral – Store at controlled room temperature, 20° to 25°C (68° to 77°F). Protect from light and moisture.

Injection – Protect injection from light; do not freeze. Before reconstitution, store at controlled room temperature, 20° to 25°C (68° to 77°F). Reconstituted injection may be stored at controlled room temperature (20° to 25°C [68° to 77°F]) for up to 1 hour if necessary. Discard any unused portion of reconstituted olanzapine injection.

QUETIAPINE FUMARATE

Rx	Seroquel (AstraZeneca)	Tablets: 25 mg	Lactose. (Seroquel 25). Peach. Film-coated. In 100s and UD 100s.
		100 mg	Lactose. (Seroquel 100). Yellow. Film-coated. In 100s and UD 100s.
		200 mg	Lactose. (Seroquel 200). White. Film-coated. In 100s and UD 100s.
		300 mg	Lactose. (Seroquel 300). White, capsule shape. Film-coated. In 60s and UD 100s.

For complete prescribing information, refer to the Antipsychotic Agents group monograph.

Indications

➤*Schizophrenia:* For the treatment of schizophrenia.

➤*Bipolar mania:* For short-term treatment of acute manic episodes associated with bipolar I disorder, as monotherapy or adjunct therapy to lithium or divalproex.

Administration and Dosage

➤*Approved by the FDA:* September 26, 1997.

➤*Schizophrenia:*

Usual dose – Initial dose of 25 mg twice daily, with increases in increments of 25 to 50 mg 2 or 3 times/day on the second and third day, as tolerated, to a target dose range of 300 to 400 mg/day by the fourth day, given 2 or 3 times/day. Further dosage adjustments, if indicated, should generally occur at intervals of at least 2 days. Dose increments/decrements of 25 to 50 mg twice daily are recommended. Efficacy in schizophrenia was demonstrated in a dose range of 150 to 750 mg/day. The safety of doses greater than 800 mg/day has not been evaluated in clinical trials. The effectiveness of quetiapine for more than 6 weeks has not been systematically evaluated. Periodically re-evaluate the long-term usefulness of the drug for the individual patient.

➤*Bipolar mania:*

Usual dose – When used as monotherapy or adjunct therapy (with lithium or divalproex), initiate quetiapine in twice-daily doses totaling 100 mg/day on day 1, increased to 400 mg/day on day 4 in increments of up to 100 mg/day in twice daily divided doses. Further dosage adjustments up to 800 mg/day by day 6 should be in increments of no more than 200 mg/day. Data indicate that the majority of patients responded between 400 and 800 mg/day. The safety of doses above 800 mg/day has not been evaluated in clinical trials.

➤*Maintenance:* The effectiveness of maintenance treatment is well established for many other antipsychotic drugs. Continue quetiapine in responding patients at the lowest dose needed to maintain remission. Periodically reassess patients.

➤*Hepatic function impairment:* Start patients with hepatic impairment on 25 mg/day. Increase the dose daily in increments of 25 to 50 mg/day to an effective dose, depending on the clinical response and tolerability of the patient.

➤*Special populations:* Consider a slower rate of dose titration and a lower target dose in the elderly, debilitated patients, or those who have a predisposition to hypotensive reactions. Perform dose escalation with caution.

➤*Reinitiation of treatment in patients previously discontinued:* When restarting patients who have had an interval of less than 1 week off of quetiapine, titration of quetiapine is not required; the maintenance dose may be reinitiated. For patients who have been off of quetiapine for more than 1 week, follow the initial titration schedule.

➤*Switching from other antipsychotics:* The period of overlapping antipsychotic administration should be minimized. When switching patients with schizophrenia from depot antipsychotics, if medically appropriate, initiate quetiapine therapy in place of the next scheduled injection. Periodically reevaluate the need for continuing existing EPS medication.

➤*Storage/Stability:* Store at 25°C (77°F); excursions permitted to 15° to 30°C (59° to 86°F).

Benzisoxazole Derivatives

RISPERIDONE

Rx	Risperdal (Janssen)	Tablets: 0.25 mg	Lactose. (JANSSEN Ris 0.25). Dark yellow. In 60s and 500s.
		0.5 mg	Lactose. (JANSSEN Ris 0.5). Red-brown. In 60s and 500s.
		1 mg	Lactose. (JANSSEN R 1). White. In 60s, 500s, and blister pack 100s.
		2 mg	Lactose. (JANSSEN R 2). Orange. In 60s, 500s, and blister pack 100s.
		3 mg	Lactose. (JANSSEN R 3). Yellow. In 60s, 500s, and blister pack 100s.
		4 mg	Lactose. (JANSSEN R 4). Green. In 60s and blister pack 100s.
Rx	Risperdal M-TAB (Janssen)	Tablets, orally disintegrating: 0.5 mg	0.14 mg phenylalanine, mannitol, aspartame, peppermint oil. (R0.5). Light coral. In 7 blister packs of 4 or bingo card of 30.
		1 mg	0.28 mg phenylalanine, mannitol, aspartame, peppermint oil. (R1). Light coral, square. In 7 blister packs of 4 or bingo card of 30.
		2 mg	0.56 mg phenylalanine, mannitol, aspartame, peppermint oil. (R2). Light coral. In 7 blister packs of 4.
Rx	Risperdal (Janssen)	Oral solution: 1 mg/mL	In 30 mL with calibrated pipette.
Rx	Risperdal Consta (Janssen)	Powder for injection: 25 mg	In vials. Dose pack contains prefilled syringe and 2 mL of diluent.
		37.5 mg	
		50 mg	

For complete prescribing information refer to the Antipsychotic Agents group monograph.

Indications

➤*Bipolar mania (oral only):*

Monotherapy – For the short-term treatment of acute manic or mixed episodes associated with bipolar I disorder, as defined in the *DSM-IV*.

Combination therapy – The combination of risperidone with lithium or valproate is indicated for the short-term treatment of acute manic or mixed episodes associated with bipolar I disorder, as defined in the *DSM-IV*.

➤*Schizophrenia:* For the treatment of schizophrenia.

Administration and Dosage

➤*Approved by the FDA:* December 29, 1993.

➤*Oral solution administration:* The oral solution can be mixed with water, coffee, orange juice, or low-fat milk; it is not compatible with cola or tea.

➤*Orally disintegrating tablet administration:* Do not open the blister until ready to administer. For single tablet removal, separate 1 of the 4 blister units by tearing apart at the perforation. Bend the corner where indicated. Peel back foil to expose the tablet. Do not push the tablet through the foil because this could damage the tablet. Using dry hands, remove the tablet from the blister unit, and immediately place the entire tablet on the tongue. Consume the tablet immediately, as the tablet cannot be stored once removed from the blister unit. Tablets disintegrate in the mouth within seconds and can be swallowed subsequently with or without liquid. Advise patients not to split or chew the tablet.

➤*Special populations (oral):* The recommended initial dose is 0.5 mg twice daily in patients who are elderly, debilitated, have severe renal or hepatic impairment, are predisposed to hypotension, or in whom hypotension would pose a risk. Adjust dose at increments of no more than 0.5 mg twice daily. Give increases to dosages above 1.5 mg twice daily at intervals of at least 1 week. In some patients, slower titration may be medically appropriate.

Once-daily dosing in the elderly or debilitated may occur after the patient has been titrated on a twice-daily regimen for 2 to 3 days at the target dose.

➤*Bipolar mania (oral only):*

Usual dose – Administer on a once-daily schedule, starting with 2 to 3 mg/day. If indicated, adjust dosage at intervals of not less than 24 hours and in dosage increments/decrements of 1 mg/day as studied in the short-term, placebo-controlled trials. In these trials, short-term (3 week) antimanic efficacy was demonstrated in a flexible dosage range of 1 to 6 mg/day. Risperidone doses higher than 6 mg/day were not studied.

Maintenance therapy – There is no evidence available from controlled trials to guide a clinician in the longer-term management of a patient who improves during treatment of an acute manic episode with

RISPERIDONE

risperidone. While it is generally agreed that pharmacological treatment beyond an acute response in mania is desirable, both for maintenance of the initial response and for prevention of new manic episodes, there are no systematically obtained data to support the use of risperidone in such longer-term treatment (ie, beyond 3 weeks).

➤*Schizophrenia:*

Oral –

Initial dose: Risperidone can be administered on a twice-daily or once-daily schedule. Initial dose is 1 mg twice daily (day 1), increasing by 1 mg twice daily as tolerated (on days 2 and 3), up to a target dose of 3 mg twice daily (by day 3). Regardless of which regimen is employed, a slower titration may be medically appropriate in some patients. Further dosage adjustments at 1 to 2 mg increments or decrements may be made at intervals of not less than 1 week.

Maximal effect was generally seen in a range of 4 to 8 mg/day. Doses above 6 mg/day for twice-daily dosing were associated with more extrapyramidal symptoms and other adverse effects and generally are not recommended. The safety of doses above 16 mg/day has not been evaluated in clinical trials.

Maintenance therapy: The effectiveness of risperidone 2 to 8 mg/day at delaying relapse was demonstrated in controlled trials in patients who had been clinically stable for at least 4 weeks and then were followed for a period of 1 to 2 years. Periodically, reassess patients to determine the need for maintenance treatment with appropriate dose.

Reinitiation of treatment: When restarting patients who have had an interval off risperidone, follow the initial titration schedule.

Switching from other antipsychotic agents: When switching from other antipsychotic agents to risperidone, immediate discontinuation of the previous antipsychotic treatment may be acceptable for some patients; gradual discontinuation may be more appropriate for other patients. In all cases, minimize the period of overlapping antipsychotic administration. When switching patients from a depot antipsychotic, initiate risperidone therapy in place of the next scheduled injection. Reevaluate the need for continuing existing medications that treat extrapyramidal symptoms.

Injection – For patients who have never taken oral risperidone, establish tolerability with oral risperidone prior to initiating treatment with injectable risperidone.

The recommended dose is 25 mg IM every 2 weeks. Although dose response for effectiveness has not been established for risperidone injection, some patients not responding to 25 mg may benefit from a higher dose of 37.5 or 50 mg. The maximum dose should not exceed 50 mg risperidone injection every 2 weeks.

Give oral risperidone or another antipsychotic medication with the first risperidone injection and continue for 3 weeks (then discontinue) to ensure that adequate therapeutic plasma concentrations are maintained prior to the main release phase of risperidone from the injection site.

Dose adjustments: Do not make upward dosage adjustments more frequently than every 4 weeks. The clinical effects of this dose adjustment should not be anticipated earlier than 3 weeks after the first injection with the higher dose.

Maintenance therapy: Continue responding patients on treatment with risperidone injection at the lowest dose needed. Periodically, reassess patients to determine the need for continued treatment.

Renal/Hepatic impairment: Treat with titrated doses of oral risperidone prior to initiating treatment with risperidone injection. The recommended starting dose is 0.5 mg oral risperidone twice daily during the first week, which can be increased to 1 mg twice daily or 2 mg once daily during the second week. If a dose of at least 2 mg oral risperidone is well tolerated, an injection of 25 mg risperidone can be administered every 2 weeks. Continue oral supplementation for 3 weeks after the first injection until the main release of risperidone from the injection site has begun. In some patients, slower titration may be medically appropriate.

Reinitiation of treatment: When restarting patients who have had an interval off treatment with risperidone injection, supplement with oral risperidone or another antipsychotic medication.

Switching from other antipsychotic agents: Continue previous antipsychotic agents for 3 weeks after the first risperidone injection to ensure that therapeutic concentrations are maintained until the main release phase of risperidone from the injection site has begun. For schizophrenic patients who have never taken oral risperidone, establish tolerability with oral risperidone prior to initiating treatment with risperidone injection. As recommended with other antipsychotic medications, periodically reevaluate the need for continuing existing extrapyramidal symptom medication.

Administration: Administer risperidone injection every 2 weeks by deep IM gluteal injection. A health care professional should administer each injection using the enclosed safety needle. Alternate injections between the 2 buttocks. Do not administer IV.

Do not combine 2 different dosage strengths of risperidone injection in a single administration.

Allow the dose pack from refrigerator to reach room temperature before reconstitution.

It is recommended to use risperidone injection immediately upon suspension in the diluent. It must be used within 6 hours of suspension. Resuspension of risperidone injection is necessary prior to administration because settling occurs over time once the product is in suspension. Keeping the vial upright, shake vigorously back and forth for as long as it takes to resuspend the microspheres.

➤*Storage/Stability:*

Tablets – Store at controlled room temperature (15° to 25°C; 59° to 77°F) away from children. Protect from light and moisture.

Tablets, orally disintegrating – Store at controlled room temperature (15° to 25°C; 59° to 77°F) away from children.

Oral solution – Store at controlled room temperature (15° to 25°C; 59° to 77°F) away from children. Protect from light and freezing.

Injection – Refrigerate the entire dose pack (2° to 8°C; 36° to 46°F) and protect from light. If refrigeration is unavailable, store at temperatures not exceeding 25°C (77°F) for no more than 7 days prior to administration. Once in the suspension, do not expose to temperatures above 25°C (77°F); must be used within 6 hours.

ZIPRASIDONE

Rx	Geodon (Pfizer)	**Capsules:** 20 mg (as HCl)	Lactose. (Pfizer 396). Blue/White. In 60s and UD 80s.
		40 mg (as HCl)	Lactose. (Pfizer 397). Blue/Blue. In 60s and UD 80s.
		60 mg (as HCl)	Lactose. (Pfizer 398). White/White. In 60s and UD 80s.
		80 mg (as HCl)	Lactose. (Pfizer 399). Blue/White. In 60s and UD 80s.
		Powder for Injection: 20 mg (as mesylate)	In single-use vials.

For complete prescribing information refer to the Antipsychotic Agents group monograph.

Indications

➤*Schizophrenia:* For the treatment of schizophrenia.

➤*Acute agitation (injection only):* For the treatment of acute agitation in schizophrenic patients for whom treatment with ziprasidone is appropriate and who need IM antipsychotic medication for rapid control of the agitation.

Administration and Dosage

➤*Approved by the FDA:* February 5, 2001.

When deciding among the alternative treatments available for schizophrenia, consider ziprasidone's greater capacity to prolong the QT/QTc interval compared with other antipsychotic drugs.

➤*Initial treatment:* Administer ziprasidone capsules at an initial daily dose of 20 mg twice daily with food. In some patients, daily dosage subsequently may be adjusted on the basis of individual clinical status up to 80 mg twice daily. If indicated, dosage adjustments generally should occur at intervals of not less than 2 days, as steady state is achieved within 1 to 3 days. In order to ensure use of the lowest effective dose, observe patients for improvement for several weeks before upward dosage adjustment.

Efficacy in schizophrenia was demonstrated in a dose range of 20 to 100 mg twice daily in short-term, placebo-controlled, clinical trials. There were trends toward dose response within the range of 20 to 80 mg twice daily, but results were not consistent. Generally, an increase to a dose greater than 80 mg twice daily is not recommended. The safety of doses above 100 mg twice daily has not been systematically evaluated in clinical trials.

➤*Maintenance treatment:* While there is no body of evidence available to answer the question of how long to treat a patient with ziprasidone, systematic evaluation of ziprasidone has shown that its efficacy in schizophrenia is maintained for periods of up to 52 weeks at a dose of 20 to 80 mg twice daily. No additional benefit was demonstrated for doses above 20 mg twice daily. Periodically reassess patients to determine the need for maintenance treatment.

➤*IM administration:* The recommended dose is 10 to 20 mg administered as required up to a maximum dose of 40 mg/day. Doses of 10 mg may be administered every 2 hours; doses of 20 mg may be administered every 4 hours up to a maximum of 40 mg/day. IM administration of ziprasidone for more than 3 consecutive days has not been studied.

If long-term therapy is indicated, replace IM administration with oral ziprasidone HCl capsules as soon as possible.

Because there is no experience regarding the safety of administering ziprasidone IM to schizophrenic patients already taking oral ziprasidone, coadministration is not recommended.

Benzisoxazole Derivatives

ZIPRASIDONE

➤*Reconstitution:* Administer ziprasidone mesylate by IM injection only. Single-dose vials require reconstitution prior to administration; discard any unused portion.

Add 1.2 mL of sterile water for injection to the vial and shake vigorously until the drug is completely dissolved. Each mL of reconstituted solution contains 20 mg ziprasidone. It must not be mixed with other medicinal products or solvents other than sterile water for injection.

➤*Storage/Stability:*

Capsules – Store at controlled room temperature 15° to 30°C (59° to 86°F).

Injection – Store at controlled room temperature 15° to 30°C (59° to 86°F), in dry form. Protect from light. Following reconstitution, the injection can be stored and protected from light for up to 24 hours at 15° to 30°C (59° to 86°F) or up to 7 days refrigerated at 2° to 8°C (36° to 46°F).

Quinolinone Derivatives

ARIPIPRAZOLE

Rx	Abilify (Bristol-Myers Squibb/Otsuka America)	Tablets: 5 mg	Lactose. (A-007 5). Blue, rectangular. In 30s and blister 100s.
		10 mg	Lactose. (A-008 10). Pink, rectangular. In 30s and blister 100s.
		15 mg	Lactose. (A-009 15). Yellow. In 30s and blister 100s.
		20 mg	Lactose. (A-010 20). White. In 30s and blister 100s.
		30 mg	Lactose. (A-011 30). Pink. In 30s and blister 100s.

For complete prescribing information refer to the Antipsychotic Agents group monograph.

Indications

➤*Schizophrenia:* For the treatment of schizophrenia.

The efficacy of aripiprazole in maintaining stability in patients with schizophrenia who had been symptomatically stable on other antipsychotic medications for periods of 3 months or longer, were discontinued from those other medications, and were then administered aripiprazole 15 mg/day and observed for relapse during a period of up to 26 weeks was demonstrated in a placebo-controlled trial.

Administration and Dosage

➤*Approved by the FDA:* November 15, 2002.

➤*Usual dose:* The recommended starting and target dose is 10 or 15 mg/day administered on a once-daily schedule without regard to meals. Aripiprazole has been systematically evaluated and shown to be effective in a dose range of 10 to 30 mg/day; however, doses higher than 10 or 15 mg/day (the lowest doses in these trials) were not more effective than 10 or 15 mg/day. Dosage increases should not be made before 2 weeks, the time needed to achieve steady state.

➤*Concomitant use with potential CYP3A4 inhibitors:* When coadministration of ketoconazole with aripiprazole occurs, reduce the aripiprazole dose to one-half of the usual dose. When the CYP3A4 inhibitor is withdrawn from combination therapy, increase aripiprazole dose.

➤*Concomitant use with potential CYP2D6 inhibitors:* When coadministration of potential CYP2D6 inhibitors such as quinidine, fluoxetine, or paroxetine with aripiprazole occurs, reduce the aripiprazole dose to at least one-half of its normal dose. When the CYP2D6 inhibitor is withdrawn from combination therapy, increase the aripiprazole dose.

➤*Concomitant use with potential CYP3A4 inducers:* When a potential CYP3A4 inducer such as carbamazepine is added to aripiprazole therapy, double the aripiprazole dose to 20 or 30 mg. Base additional dose increases on clinical evaluation. When carbamazepine is withdrawn from combination therapy, reduce the aripiprazole dose to 10 or 15 mg.

➤*Maintenance therapy:* While there is no body of evidence available to answer the question of how long a patient treated with aripiprazole should remain on it, systematic evaluation of patients with schizophrenia who had been symptomatically stable on other antipsychotic medications for periods of 3 months or longer, were discontinued from those medications, and were then administered aripiprazole 15 mg/day and observed for relapse during a period of up to 26 weeks demonstrated a benefit of such maintenance treatment. Periodically reassess patients to determine the need for maintenance treatment.

➤*Switching from other antipsychotics:* There are no systemically collected data to specifically address switching patients with schizophrenia from other antipsychotics to aripiprazole or concerning coadministration with other antipsychotics. While immediate discontinuation of the previous antipsychotic treatment may be acceptable for some patients with schizophrenia, gradual discontinuation may be more appropriate for others. In all cases, minimize the period of overlapping antipsychotic administration.

➤*Storage/Stability:* Store at 25°C (77°F); excursions permitted to 15° to 30°C (59° to 86°F).

LITHIUM

Rx	Lithium Carbonate (Roxane)	Capsules: 150 mg lithium carbonate (4.06 mEq lithium)	(54 213). White. In 100s, 1000s and UD 100s.
Rx	Lithium Carbonate (Various, eg, Dixon-Shane, Geneva, Goldline, Moore, Roxane)	Capsules: 300 mg lithium carbonate (8.12 mEq lithium)	In 100s, 500s, 1000s and UD 100s.
Rx	Eskalith (SK-Beecham)		(Eskalith SB). Yellow and gray. In 100s.
Rx	Lithium Carbonate (Roxane)	Capsules: 600 mg lithium carbonate (16.24 mEq lithium)	(54 702). White and flesh. In 100s, 1000s and UD 100s.
Rx	Lithium Carbonate (Various, eg, Harber, International Labs, Roxane)	Tablets: 300 mg lithium carbonate (8.12 mEq lithium)	In 100s, 1000s and UD 100s.
Rx	Eskalith (SK-Beecham)		(SKF J09). Gray, scored. In 100s.
Rx	Lithobid (Solvay)	Tablets, slow release: 300 mg lithium carbonate (8.12 mEq lithium)	(Solvay 4492). Peach. Film coated. In 100s, 1000s and UD 100s.
Rx	Lithium Carbonate (Roxane)	Tablets, extended-release: 450 mg lithium carbonate	In 100s.
Rx	Eskalith CR (SK-Beecham)	Tablets, controlled release: 450 mg lithium carbonate (12.18 mEq lithium)	(SKF J10). Buff, scored. In 100s.
Rx	Lithium Citrate (Various, eg, Geneva, Major, PBI, Roxane, Xactdose)	Syrup: 8 mEq lithium (as citrate equivalent to 300 mg lithium carbonate)/5 ml	In 480 and 500 ml and UD 5 and 10 ml.

Complete prescribing information begins in the Antipsychotic Agents group monograph.

WARNING

Toxicity is closely related to serum lithium levels and can occur at therapeutic doses. Facilities for serum lithium determinations are required to monitor therapy.

Indications

➤*Mania:* For the treatment of manic episodes of manic-depressive illness. Maintenance therapy prevents or diminishes the frequency and intensity of subsequent manic episodes in those manic-depressive patients with a history of mania.

➤*Unlabeled uses:* Lithium carbonate (300 to 1000 mg/day) has improved the neutrophil count in patients with cancer chemotherapy-induced neutropenia, in children with chronic neutropenia and in AIDS patients receiving zidovudine.

Lithium has also been used successfully in the prophylaxis of cluster headache; premenstrual tension; bulimia; alcoholism (especially if patient has a concomitant affective disorder such as depression); syndrome of inappropriate secretion of ADH; tardive dyskinesia; hyperthyroidism; postpartum affective psychosis; corticosteroid-induced psychosis.

A topical lithium succinate preparation has been studied in the treatment of seborrheic dermatitis and genital herpes.

Administration and Dosage

Individualize dosage according to both serum levels and clinical response.

LITHIUM

➤*Serum lithium levels:* Draw blood samples immediately prior to the next dose (8 to 12 hours after the previous dose) when lithium concentrations are relatively stable. Do not rely on serum levels alone.

➤*Acute mania:* Optimal patient response is usually established and maintained with 600 mg 3 times daily or 900 mg twice daily for the slow release form. Such doses normally produce an effective serum lithium level ranging between 1 and 1.5 mEq/L.

Determine serum levels twice weekly during the acute phase and until the serum level and clinical condition of the patient have been stabilized.

➤*Long-term use:* The desirable serum levels are 0.6 to 1.2 mEq/L. Dosage will vary, but 300 mg 3 to 4 times daily will usually maintain this level. Monitor serum levels in uncomplicated cases on maintenance therapy during remission every 2 to 3 months.

Actions

➤*Pharmacology:* Lithium is a monovalent cation which competes with calcium, magnesium, potassium and sodium in body tissues and at binding sites. It alters sodium transport in nerve and muscle cells, and effects a shift toward intraneuronal catecholamine metabolism. The specific mechanism of action in mania is unknown, but it does affect the synthesis, storage, release and reuptake of central monoamine neurotransmitters including NE, 5–HT, DA, ACh and GABA. Its antimanic effects may be the result of increases in norepinephrine reuptake and increased serotonin receptor sensitivity.

Lithium also affects distribution of sodium, calcium and magnesium ions. The contribution of these effects to its antimanic qualities is uncertain.

➤*Pharmacokinetics:*

Absorption/Distribution – Lithium is readily absorbed from the GI tract. Absorption is not significantly impaired by food. Peak serum levels occur in 0.5 to 3 hours after administration of conventional tablets and capsules and absorption is complete within 8 hours. Slow-release preparations, however, have a slower and more variable absorption rate with peak levels occurring in 3 to 12 hours. The therapeutic serum level range is from 0.4 to 1 mEq/L. Dose-related adverse effects are not serious at serum levels maintained < 1.5 mEq/L.

Distribution approximates total body water and is complete within ≈ 6 to 10 hours; higher concentrations occur in the bones, the thyroid gland and portions of the brain, than in the serum. Lithium is not protein bound. Although distribution across the blood-brain barrier is slow, the cerebrospinal fluid lithium level is ≈ 40% of the plasma concentration.

Excretion – About 95% of the lithium dose is eliminated by the kidney. Renal clearance is 20% of creatinine clearance (15 to 30 ml/min). It varies with pregnancy, age and renal status of the patient. In the elderly, and in patients with renal impairment, clearance will be low. The average elimination half-life is 24 hours (range, 10 to 50 hours); steady state is reached in 5 to 7 days.

In the kidneys, 80% of lithium is reabsorbed. Lithium and sodium compete for reabsorption in the proximal renal tubule. During periods of sodium depletion (eg, dehydration, diuretic use), the kidney will try to conserve sodium and lithium by reabsorbing > 80% from the proximal tubule. The increased reabsorption causes the lithium serum level to rise, possibly leading to toxicity. Sodium loading will cause increased lithium excretion and the serum levels will decrease.

Warnings

➤*High-risk patients:* The risk of lithium toxicity is very high in patients with significant renal or cardiovascular disease, severe debilitation, dehydration or sodium depletion, or in patients receiving diuretics. Undertake treatment with extreme caution. Daily serum lithium determinations are recommended until the serum level and the clinical condition of the patient are stabilized; hospitalization is necessary.

➤*Encephalopathic syndrome:* Encephalopathic syndrome (characterized by weakness, lethargy, fever, tremulousness, confusion, extrapyramidal symptoms, leukocytosis, elevated serum enzymes, BUN and FBS) has occurred in a few patients given lithium plus a neuroleptic. In some instances, irreversible brain damage occurred. Monitor closely for evidence of neurologic toxicity; discontinue treatment if such signs appear. This syndrome may be similar to or the same as neuroleptic malignant syndrome.

➤*Renal function impairment:* Morphologic changes with glomerular and interstitial fibrosis and nephron atrophy have occurred in patients on chronic lithium therapy (≤ 10% to 20%) and in manic-depressive patients never exposed to lithium. The relationship between such changes and renal function has not been established.

Acquired nephrogenic diabetes insipidus – Acquired nephrogenic diabetes insipidus unresponsive to vasopressin has been associated with chronic lithium administration. Polydipsia and polyuria occur frequently. The mechanism is thought to be the decreased response of the renal tubules to the antidiuretic hormone causing decreased reabsorption of water. Impairment of the concentrating ability of the kidneys is reversed when lithium therapy is discontinued. Management may involve decreasing the dose, discontinuing lithium, or the cautious use of a thiazide diuretic or amiloride. Monitor the patient's renal status.

➤*Elderly:* The decreased rate of excretion in the elderly contributes to a high incidence of toxic effects. Use lower doses and more frequent monitoring.

➤*Pregnancy: Category D.* Lithium crosses the placenta; serum concentration is equal in the mother and fetus. Lithium may cause fetal harm when given to a pregnant woman. Data from lithium birth registries suggest an increase in cardiac and other anomalies, especially Ebstein's anomaly. If the patient becomes pregnant while taking lithium, apprise her of the potential risk to the fetus.

Lithium toxicity in the newborn has included cyanosis, hypotonia, GI bleeding, cardiomegaly, bradycardia, thyroid depression, ECG abnormalities and diabetes insipidus. Most of these are self-limiting. Do not use in pregnancy, especially during the first trimester, unless the potential benefits outweigh potential hazards.

➤*Lactation:* Lithium is excreted in breast milk at about a 50% concentration of maternal serum. Do not nurse during lithium therapy, except in unusual instances where potential benefits to the mother outweigh possible hazards to the infant.

➤*Children:* Safety and efficacy for use in children < 12 years old have not been established. A report of a transient syndrome of acute dystonia and hyperreflexia was reported in a 15 kg child who ingested 300 mg lithium carbonate.

Precautions

➤*Concomitant infection:* Concomitant infection with elevated temperature may necessitate a temporary reduction or cessation of medication.

➤*Tolerance of lithium:* Tolerance of lithium is greater during the acute manic phase and decreases when manic symptoms subside.

➤*Hypothyroidism:* may occur with long-term lithium administration (5% to 15%). Patients may develop enlargement of the thyroid gland and increased thyroid-stimulating hormone (TSH) levels (30%). Lithium-induced hypothyroidism may be treated with thyroid hormone replacement therapy. Hyperthyroidism occurs occasionally.

➤*Sodium depletion:* Lithium decreases renal sodium reabsorption, which could lead to sodium depletion (see Actions). Therefore, the patient must maintain a normal diet (including salt) and an adequate fluid intake (2500 to 3000 ml), at least during the initial stabilization period. Decreased tolerance to lithium may ensue from protracted sweating or diarrhea; if this occurs, administer supplemental fluid and salt.

➤*Parameters to monitor:* Perform the following laboratory tests prior to and periodically during lithium therapy: Serum creatinine; complete blood count (lithium may induce a benign leukocytosis, 10,000 to 18,000 WBC/mm³); urinalysis; sodium and potassium; electrocardiogram; and thyroid function tests. Check lithium serum levels twice weekly until dosage is stabilized. Once steady state has been reached, monitor the level weekly. Once the patient is on maintenance therapy, the level may be checked every 2 to 3 months. Monitor the elderly on maintenance therapy more frequently. Direct physical exams and history toward detection of cardiovascular, renal or organic brain disease.

➤*Hazardous tasks:* Observe caution while driving or performing other tasks requiring alertness.

Drug Interactions

Lithium Drug Interactions			
Precipitant drug	Object drug*		Description
Acetazolamide	Lithium	↓	Increased renal excretion of lithium.
Carbamazepine	Lithium	↑	Increased neurotoxic effects despite therapeutic serum levels and normal dosage range.
Fluoxetine	Lithium	↑	Increased lithium serum levels; mechanism unknown.
Haloperidol	Lithium	↑	Increased neurotoxic effects despite therapeutic serum levels and normal dosage range.
Loop diuretics	Lithium	↑	Increased lithium serum levels; mechanism unknown.
Methyldopa	Lithium	↑	Increased neurotoxic effects with or without increased lithium serum levels.
NSAIDs	Lithium	↑	Decreased renal clearance of lithium possibly caused by inhibition of renal prostaglandin synthesis.
Osmotic diuretics (urea)	Lithium	↓	Increased renal excretion of lithium.
Theophyllines	Lithium	↓	Increased renal excretion of lithium.
Thiazide diuretics	Lithium	↑	Increased lithium serum levels caused by decreased renal lithium clearance.
Urinary alkalinizers	Lithium	↓	Enhanced renal lithium clearance.

LITHIUM

Lithium Drug Interactions			
Precipitant drug	Object drug*		Description
Verapamil	Lithium	↔	Both a reduction in lithium levels and lithium toxicity have occurred.
Lithium	Iodide salts	↑	Synergistic action to more readily produce hypothyroidism.
Lithium	Neuromuscular blocking agents	↑	Neuromuscular blocking effects may be increased; profound and severe respiratory depression may occur.
Lithium	Phenothiazines	↔	Neurotoxicity, decreased phenothiazine concentrations or increased lithium concentrations may occur.
Lithium	Sympatho-mimetics	↓	The pressor sensitivity of the sympathomimetic may be decreased.
Lithium	Tricyclic antide-pressants	↑	Pharmacologic effects of the tricyclic may be increased.

* ↑ = Object drug increased. ↓ = Object drug decreased. ↔ = Undetermined clinical effect.

Adverse Reactions

Adverse reactions are seldom encountered at serum lithium levels < 1.5 mEq/L, except in the occasional patient sensitive to lithium. Mild to moderate toxic reactions may occur at levels from 1.5 to 2.5 mEq/L, and moderate to severe reactions may be seen at levels from 2 to 2.5 mEq/L, depending upon individual response. See Overdosage.

Fine hand tremor, polyuria and mild thirst may occur during initial therapy for the acute manic phase, and may persist throughout treatment. Transient and mild nausea and general discomfort may also appear during the first few days of administration. These side effects usually subside with continued treatment or a temporary reduction or cessation of dosage. If persistent, a cessation of dosage is indicated.

➤*Reactions related to serum levels by organ system (see Overdosage):*

Neurological: Pseudotumor cerebri (increased intracranial pressure and papilledema) has been reported. If undetected, this condition may result in enlargement of the blind spot, constriction of visual fields and eventual blindness caused by optic atrophy. Discontinue lithium, if clinically possible, if this syndrome occurs.

EEG changes: Diffuse slowing; widening of frequency spectrum; potentiation; disorganization of background rhythm.

Neuromuscular: Tremor; muscle hyperirritability (fasciculations, twitching, clonic movements); ataxia; choreo-athetotic movements; hyperactive deep tendon reflexes.

Thyroid: Euthyroid goiter or hypothyroidism (including myxedema) accompanied by lower T_3 and T_4. Iodine 131 uptake may be elevated. (See Precautions.) Paradoxically, rare cases of hyperthyroidism have occurred.

Cardiovascular – Arrhythmia; hypotension; peripheral circulatory collapse; bradycardia; sinus node dysfunction with severe bradycardia (which may result in syncope).

ECG changes: Reversible flattening, isoelectricity or inversion of T-waves.

CNS – Blackout spells; epileptiform seizures; slurred speech; dizziness; vertigo; incontinence of urine or feces; somnolence; psychomotor retardation; restlessness; confusion; stupor; coma; acute dystonia; downbeat nystagmus; blurred vision; startled response; hypertonicity; slowed intellectual functioning; hallucinations; poor memory; tongue movements; tics; tinnitus; cog wheel rigidity.

Dermatologic – Drying and thinning of hair; anesthesia of skin; chronic folliculitis; xerosis cutis; alopecia; exacerbation of psoriasis; acne; angioedema.

GI – Anorexia; nausea; vomiting; diarrhea; dry mouth; gastritis; salivary gland swelling; abdominal pain; excessive salivation; flatulence; indigestion.

GU – Albuminuria; oliguria; polyuria; glycosuria; decreased creatinine clearance; symptoms of nephrogenic diabetes.

Miscellaneous – Fatigue; lethargy; sleepiness; dehydration; weight loss; transient scotomata; impotence/sexual dysfunction; dysgeusia/taste distortion; tightness in chest; hypercalcemia; hyperparathyroidism; salty taste; thirst; swollen lips; swollen, painful joints; fever; polyarthralgia; dental caries.

Reactions unrelated to dosage – Transient EEG and ECG changes; leukocytosis; headache; diffuse nontoxic goiter with or without hypothyroidism; transient hyperglycemia; generalized pruritus with or without rash; cutaneous ulcers; albuminuria; worsening of organic brain syndromes; excessive weight gain; edematous swelling of ankles or wrists; thirst or polyuria, sometimes resembling diabetes insipidus; metallic taste.

The development of painful discoloration of fingers and toes and coldness of the extremities within 1 day of starting lithium treatment has occurred. The mechanism through which these symptoms (resembling Raynaud's syndrome) developed is not known. Recovery followed discontinuation of the drug.

Overdosage

➤*Symptoms:*

Lithium toxicity – Toxic lithium levels are close to therapeutic. The likelihood of toxicity increases with increasing serum lithium levels. Serum lithium levels > 1.5 mEq/L carry a greater risk than lower levels. Do not permit levels to exceed 2 mEq/L during the acute treatment phase. Discontinue the drug if early toxic symptoms occur.

Lithium levels < 2 mEq/L – Diarrhea; vomiting; nausea; drowsiness; muscular weakness; lack of coordination. May be early signs of toxicity.

Lithium levels 2 to 3 mEq/L: Giddiness; ataxia; blurred vision; tinnitus; vertigo; increasing confusion; slurred speech; blackouts; fasciculations; myoclonic twitching or movement of entire limbs; choreoathetoid movements; urinary or fecal incontinence; agitation or manic-like behavior; hyperreflexia; hypertonia; dysarthria.

Lithium levels > 3 mEq/L: Lithium levels > 3 mEq/L may produce a complex clinical picture involving multiple organs and organ systems including: Seizures (generalized and focal); arrhythmias; hypotension; peripheral vascular collapse; stupor; muscle group twitching; spasticity; coma.

➤*Treatment:* Early symptoms of toxicity can usually be treated by dosage reduction or cessation and resumption of the treatment at a lower dose after 24 to 48 hours. In severe cases, first eliminate the ion from the patient. Treatment is essentially the same as that used in barbiturate toxicity: Gastric lavage; correction of fluid and electrolyte imbalance including the use of normal saline; regulation of kidney function. Urea, mannitol and aminophylline all produce significant increases in lithium excretion. Infection prophylaxis, chest x-rays, preservation of respiration and monitoring of thyroid status are essential. Hemodialysis effectively and rapidly lowers serum lithium levels in the severely toxic patient (generally, levels > 3.5 to 4 mEq/L); however, in some circumstances it may be indicated for patients with lower lithium levels. Refer to General Management of Acute Overdosage.

Patient Information

Take immediately after meals or with food or milk to avoid stomach upset.

Stop medication and contact physician if signs of overdose or toxicity occur, such as diarrhea, vomiting, unsteady walking, tremor, drowsiness or muscle weakness.

May impair mental or physical abilities. Use caution while driving or performing other tasks requiring alertness.

Drink 8 to 12 glasses of water or other liquid every day while on this drug. Prolonged exposure to the sun can lead to dehydration. Maintain a regular diet (including salt). Contact physician if fever or diarrhea develops.

Prolonged exposure to the sun can lead to dehydration.

MEMANTINE HCl

Rx	**Namenda** (Forest Laboratories)	**Tablets**: 5 mg	Lactose. (5 FL). Tan, capsule shape. Film-coated. In 60s, UD 100s, and titration paks[1].
		10 mg	Lactose. (10 FL). Gray, capsule shape. Film-coated. In 60s, UD 100s, and titration paks[1].

[1] Titration paks are blister packages containing 49 tablets (28 × 5 mg and 21 × 10 mg).

Indications

➤*Alzheimer disease:* For the treatment of moderate to severe dementia of the Alzheimer type.

➤*Unlabeled uses:* For the treatment of vascular dementia.

Administration and Dosage

➤*Approved by the FDA:* October 17, 2003.

Memantine can be taken with or without food.

➤*Dosage:* The recommended starting dose of memantine is 5 mg once daily. The recommended target dose is 20 mg/day. Increase the dose in 5 mg increments to 10 mg/day (5 mg twice daily), 15 mg/day (5 mg and 10 mg as separate doses), and 20 mg/day (10 mg twice daily). The minimum recommended interval between dose increases is 1 week.

➤*Renal function impairment:* Consider dose reduction in patients with moderate renal impairment. In patients with severe renal impairment, the use of memantine has not been systematically evaluated and is not recommended (see Warnings).

➤*Storage/Stability:* Store at 25°C (77°F); excursions permitted to 15° to 30°C (59° to 86°F).

Actions

➤*Pharmacology:* Persistent activation of CNS N-methyl-D-aspartate (NMDA) receptors by the excitatory amino acid glutamate has been hypothesized to contribute to the symptomatology of Alzheimer disease. Memantine is postulated to exert its therapeutic effect through its action as a low to moderate affinity uncompetitive (open-channel) NMDA receptor antagonist that binds preferentially to the NMDA receptor-operated cation channels. There is no evidence that memantine prevents or slows neurodegeneration in patients with Alzheimer disease.

Memantine showed low to negligible affinity for GABA, benzodiazepine, dopamine, adrenergic, histamine, and glycine receptors and for voltage-dependent Ca^{2+}, Na^+, or K^+ channels. Memantine also showed antagonistic effects at the $5HT_3$ receptor with a potency similar to that for the NMDA receptor and blocked nicotinic acetylcholine receptors with one-sixth to one-tenth the potency.

In vitro studies have shown that memantine does not affect the reversible inhibition of acetylcholinesterase by donepezil, galantamine, or tacrine.

➤*Pharmacokinetics:*

Absorption/Distribution – Following oral administration, memantine is highly absorbed with peak concentrations reached in approximately 3 to 7 hours. Food has no effect on the absorption of memantine. The mean volume of distribution is 9 to 11 L/kg and the plasma protein binding is low (45%). Memantine has linear pharmacokinetics over the therapeutic dose range.

Metabolism/Excretion – Memantine undergoes little metabolism, with the majority (57% to 82%) of an administered dose excreted unchanged in urine; the remainder is converted primarily to 3 polar metabolites: N-gludantan conjugate, 6-hydroxy memantine, and 1-nitroso-deaminated memantine. These metabolites possess minimal NMDA receptor antagonist activity. The hepatic microsomal CYP450 enzyme system does not play a significant role in the metabolism of memantine. Memantine has a terminal elimination half-life of approximately 60 to 80 hours. Renal clearance involves active tubular secretion moderated by pH-dependent tubular reabsorption.

Special populations –

Renal function impairment: Adequate information on the effect of renal impairment on the pharmacokinetics of memantine is not available. Because the major route of elimination is renal, however, it is very likely that subjects with moderate and severe renal impairment will have significantly higher exposure than normal subjects.

Gender: Following multiple-dose administration of memantine 20 mg twice daily, females had approximately 45% higher exposure than males, but there was no difference in exposure when body weight was taken into account.

Contraindications

Known hypersensitivity to memantine or to any excipients used in the formulation.

Warnings

➤*Genitourinary conditions:* Conditions that raise urine pH may decrease the urinary elimination of memantine, resulting in increased plasma levels of memantine. Urine pH is altered by diet, drugs (eg, carbonic anhydrase inhibitors, sodium bicarbonate), and clinical state of the patient (eg, renal tubular acidosis or severe infections of the urinary tract). Use memantine with caution under these conditions.

➤*Renal function impairment:* Inadequate data are available in patients with mild, moderate, and severe renal impairment, but it is likely that patients with moderate renal impairment will have higher exposure than normal subjects. Consider dose reduction in these patients. The use of memantine in patients with severe renal impairment is not recommended.

➤*Pregnancy: Category B.* Slight maternal toxicity, decreased pup weights, and an increased incidence of nonossified cervical vertebrae were seen at an oral dose of 18 mg/kg/day in a study in which rats were given oral memantine beginning premating and continuing through the postpartum period. Slight maternal toxicity and decreased pup weights also were seen at this dose in a study in which rats were treated from day 15 of gestation through the postpartum period. The no-effect dose for these effects was 6 mg/kg, which is 3 times the maximum recommended human dose on a mg/m^2 basis.

There are no adequate and well-controlled studies of memantine in pregnant women. Use during pregnancy only if the potential benefit justifies the potential risk to the fetus.

➤*Lactation:* It is not known whether memantine is excreted in human breast milk. Exercise caution when memantine is administered to a nursing mother.

➤*Children:* There are no adequate and well-controlled trials documenting the safety and efficacy of memantine in any illness occurring in children.

Drug Interactions

➤*NMDA antagonists:* The combined use of memantine with other NMDA antagonists (amantadine, ketamine, and dextromethorphan) has not been systematically evaluated. Approach such use with caution.

➤*Drugs eliminated via renal mechanisms:* Because memantine is eliminated in part by tubular secretion, coadministration of drugs that use the same renal cationic system, including hydrochlorothiazide (HCTZ), triamterene, cimetidine, ranitidine, quinidine, and nicotine, potentially could result in altered plasma levels of both agents. However, coadministration of memantine and HCTZ/triamterene did not affect the bioavailability of either memantine or triamterene, and the bioavailability of HCTZ decreased by 20%.

➤*Drugs that make the urine alkaline:* The clearance of memantine was reduced by approximately 80% under alkaline urine conditions at pH 8. Therefore, alterations of urine pH toward the alkaline condition may lead to an accumulation of the drug with a possible increase in adverse effects. Urine pH is altered by diet, drugs (eg, carbonic anhydrase inhibitors, sodium bicarbonate), and clinical state of the patient (eg, renal tubular acidosis or severe infections of the urinary tract). Use memantine with caution under these conditions.

Adverse Reactions

Memantine Adverse Reactions (%)		
Adverse reaction	Memantine (n = 940)	Placebo (n = 922)
CNS		
Dizziness	7	5
Confusion	6	5
Headache	6	3
Hallucination	3	2
Somnolence	3	2
GI		
Constipation	5	3
Vomiting	3	2
Respiratory system		
Coughing	4	3
Dyspnea	2	1
Miscellaneous		
Hypertension	4	2
Back pain	3	2
Pain	3	1
Fatigue	2	1

Other adverse events occurring with an incidence of at least 2% in memantine-treated patients but at a greater or equal rate on placebo were: Agitation; fall; inflicted injury; urinary incontinence; diarrhea; bronchitis; insomnia; urinary tract infection; influenza-like symptoms; gait abnormal; depression; upper respiratory tract infection; anxiety; peripheral edema; nausea; anorexia; and arthralgia.

Memantine has been administered to approximately 1350 patients with dementia, of whom more than 1200 received the maximum recommended dose of 20 mg/day. Patients received memantine treatment for

MEMANTINE HCl

periods of up to 884 days, with 862 patients receiving at least 24 weeks of treatment and 387 patients receiving 48 weeks or more of treatment.

All adverse events occurring in at least 2 patients are included, except for those already listed in the table above, WHO terms too general to be informative, minor symptoms, or events unlikely to be drug-caused (eg, because they are common in the study population). These adverse events are not necessarily related to memantine treatment and, in most cases, were observed at a similar frequency in placebo-treated patients in the controlled studies.

➤*Cardiovascular:* Syncope, cardiac failure (at least 1%); angina pectoris, bradycardia, myocardial infarction, thrombophlebitis, atrial fibrillation, hypotension, cardiac arrest, postural hypotension, pulmonary embolism, pulmonary edema (0.1% to 1%).

➤*CNS:* Transient ischemic attack, cerebrovascular accident, vertigo, ataxia, hypokinesia, aggressive reaction (at least 1%); paresthesia, convulsions, extrapyramidal disorder, hypertonia, tremor, aphasia, hypesthesia, abnormal coordination, hemiplegia, hyperkinesia, involuntary muscle contractions, stupor, cerebral hemorrhage, neuralgia, ptosis, neuropathy, delusion, personality disorder, emotional lability, nervousness, sleep disorder, libido increased, psychosis, amnesia, apathy, paranoid reaction, thinking abnormal, crying abnormal, appetite increased, paroniria, delirium, depersonalization, neurosis, suicide attempt (0.1% to 1%).

➤*Dermatologic:* Rash (at least 1%); skin ulceration, pruritus, cellulitis, eczema, dermatitis, erythematous rash, alopecia, urticaria (0.1% to 1%).

➤*GI:* Gastroenteritis, diverticulitis, gastrointestinal hemorrhage, melena, esophageal ulceration (0.1% to 1%).

➤*GU:* Frequent micturition (at least 1%); dysuria, hematuria, urinary retention (0.1% to 1%).

➤*Hematologic/Lymphatic:* Anemia (at least 1%); leukopenia (0.1% to 1%).

➤*Metabolic:* Increased alkaline phosphatase, decreased weight (at least 1%); dehydration, hyponatremia, aggravated diabetes mellitus (0.1% to 1%).

➤*Respiratory:* Pneumonia (at least 1%); apnea, asthma, hemoptysis (0.1% to 1%).

➤*Special senses:* Cataract, conjunctivitis (at least 1%); macula lutea degeneration, decreased visual acuity, decreased hearing, tinnitus, blepharitis, blurred vision, corneal opacity, glaucoma, conjunctival hemorrhage, eye pain, retinal hemorrhage, xerophthalmia, diplopia, abnormal lacrimation, myopia, retinal detachment (0.1% to 1%).

➤*Miscellaneous:* Hypothermia, allergic reaction (0.1% to 1%).

Memantine has been commercially available outside the United States since 1982 and has been evaluated in clinical trials including trials in patients with neuropathic pain, Parkinson disease, organic brain syndrome, and spasticity. The following adverse events of possible importance for which there is inadequate data to determine the causal relationship have been reported to be temporally associated with memantine treatment in more than one patient and are not described elsewhere in labeling: Acne; bone fracture; carpal tunnel syndrome; claudication; hyperlipidemia; impotence; otitis media; thrombocytopenia.

Overdosage

➤*Symptoms:* In a documented case of an overdosage with up to 400 mg of memantine, the patient experienced restlessness, psychosis, visual hallucinations, somnolence, stupor, and loss of consciousness. The patient recovered without permanent sequelae.

➤*Treatment:* Because strategies for the management of overdose are continually evolving, contact a poison control center to determine the latest recommendations for the management of an overdose of any drug.

As in any cases of overdosage, utilize general supportive measures and symptomatic treatment. Elimination of memantine can be enhanced by acidification of urine.

Patient Information

Instruct caregivers in the recommended administration (twice daily for doses above 5 mg) and dose escalation (minimum interval of 1 week between dose increases).

TACRINE HCl (Tetrahydroacridinamine; THA)

Rx	Cognex (Parke-Davis)	Capsules: 10 mg	Lactose. (Cognex 10). Yellow/dark green. In 120s and UD 100s.
		20 mg	Lactose. (Cognex 20). Yellow/light blue. In 120s and UD 100s.
		30 mg	Lactose. (Cognex 30). Yellow/orange. In 120s and UD 100s.
		40 mg	Lactose. (Cognex 40). Yellow/lavender. In 120s and UD 100s.

Indications

➤*Alzheimer's disease:* Treatment of mild-to-moderate dementia of the Alzheimer's type.

Administration and Dosage

➤*Approved by the FDA:* September 9, 1993.

The rate of dose escalation may be slowed if a patient is intolerant to the recommended titration schedule. It is not advisable, however, to accelerate the dose incrementation plan. Following initiation of therapy, or any dosage increase, observe patients carefully for adverse effects. Take between meals whenever possible; however, if minor GI upset occurs, take with meals to improve tolerability. Taking tacrine with meals can be expected to reduce plasma levels ≈ 30% to 40%.

➤*Initiation of treatment:* The initial dose of tacrine is 40 mg/day (10 mg 4 times daily). Maintain this dose for ≥ 4 weeks with every other week monitoring of transaminase levels beginning at week 4 of therapy. It is important that the dose not be increased during this period because of the potential for delayed onset of transaminase elevations.

➤*Dose titration:* Following 4 weeks of treatment at 40 mg/day (10 mg 4 times daily), increase the dose to 80 mg/day (20 mg 4 times daily), providing there are no significant transaminase elevations and the patient is tolerating treatment. Titrate patients to higher doses (120 and 160 mg/day in divided doses on a 4 times daily schedule) at 4-week intervals on the basis of tolerance.

➤*Dose adjustment:* Monitor serum transaminase levels (specifically ALT) every other week from at least week 4 to week 16 following initiation of treatment, after which monitoring may be decreased to every 3 months. For patients who develop ALT elevations > 2 times the upper limit of normal, the dose and monitoring regimen should be modified as described in the table below.

A full monitoring and dose titration sequence must be repeated in the event that a patient suspends treatment with tacrine for > 4 weeks.

Recommended Tacrine Dose and Monitoring Regimen Modification in Response to Transaminase Elevations	
Transaminase levels	Treatment and monitoring regimen
≤ 2 × ULN	Continue treatment according to recommended titration and monitoring schedule.
> 2 to ≤ 3 × ULN	Continue treatment according to recommended titration. Monitor transaminase levels weekly until levels return to normal limits.
> 3 to ≤ 5 × ULN	Reduce the daily dose by 40 mg/day. Monitor ALT/SGPT levels weekly. Resume dose titration and every other week monitoring when transaminase levels return to within normal limits.
> 5 × ULN	Stop treatment. Monitor the patient closely for signs and symptoms associated with hepatitis and follow transaminase levels until within normal limits (see Rechallenge).

Experience is limited in patients with ALT > 10 x ULN. The risk of rechallenge must be considered against demonstrated clinical benefit. Patients with clinical jaundice confirmed by a significant elevation in total bilirubin (> 3 mg/dl) or those exhibiting clinical signs or symptoms of hypersensitivity (eg, rash or fever) in association with ALT elevations should immediately and permanently discontinue tacrine and not be rechallenged.

➤*Rechallenge:* Patients who are required to discontinue treatment because of transaminase elevations may be rechallenged once transaminase levels return to within normal limits. Rechallenge of patients exposed to transaminase elevations < 10 x ULN has not resulted in serious liver injury. However, because experience in the rechallenge of patients who had elevations > 10 x ULN is limited, the risks associated with the rechallenge of these patients are not well characterized. Carefully and frequently (weekly) monitor serum ALT when rechallenging such patients. If rechallenged, give patients an initial dose of 40 mg/day (10 mg 4 times daily) and monitor transaminase levels weekly. If, after 6 weeks on 40 mg/day, the patient is tolerating the dosage with no unacceptable elevations in transaminases, recommended dose titration and transaminase monitoring may be resumed.

Continue weekly monitoring of ALT levels for a total of 16 weeks, after which monitoring may be decreased to monthly for 2 months and every 3 months thereafter.

Actions

➤*Pharmacology:* Tacrine is a centrally acting reversible cholinesterase inhibitor, commonly referred to as THA. Although widespread degeneration of multiple CNS neuronal systems eventually occurs, early pathological changes in Alzheimer's disease involve, in a relatively selective manner, cholinergic neuronal pathways that project from the basal forebrain to the cerebral cortex and hippocampus. The resulting deficiency of cortical acetylcholine is believed to account for some of the clinical manifestations of mild to moderate dementia. Tacrine presumably acts by elevating acetylcholine concentrations in the cerebral cortex by slowing the degradation of acetylcholine released by still intact cholinergic neurons. If this theoretical mechanism of action is correct, tacrine's effects may lessen as the disease process advances and fewer cholinergic neurons remain functionally intact. There is no evidence that tacrine alters the course of the underlying dementing process.

➤*Pharmacokinetics:*

Absorption – Tacrine is rapidly absorbed after oral administration. Maximal plasma concentrations occur within 1 to 2 hours. Absolute bioavailability of tacrine is ≈ 17%. Food reduces tacrine bioavailability by ≈ 30% to 40%; however, food has no effect if tacrine is administered at least 1 hour before meals. The effect of achlorhydria on absorption is unknown.

Distribution – Mean volume of distribution of tacrine is ≈ 349 L. Tacrine is ≈ 55% bound to plasma proteins. The extent and degree of distribution within various body compartments has not been systematically studied; however, 336 hours after the administration of a single radiolabeled dose, ≈ 25% was not recovered, suggesting the possibility that tacrine or one or more of its metabolites may be retained.

Metabolism – Tacrine is extensively metabolized by the cytochrome P450 system to multiple metabolites, not all of which have been identified. The vast majority of radiolabeled species present in the plasma following a single dose of radiolabeled tacrine are unidentified (eg, only 5% of radioactivity in plasma has been identified [tacrine and 3-hydroxylated metabolites; 1-, 2- and 4-hydroxytacrine]). Cytochrome P450 IA2 is the principal isozyme involved in metabolism. These findings are consistent with the observation that tacrine or one of its metabolites inhibits the metabolism of theophylline (see Drug Interactions). Following aromatic ring hydroxylation, tacrine metabolites undergo glucuronidation.

Excretion – Tacrine undergoes first-pass metabolism, the extent of which depends on the dose administered. Because the enzyme system involved can be saturated at relatively low doses, a larger fraction of a high dose of tacrine will escape first-pass elimination than a smaller dose. Elimination of tacrine from the plasma is not dose-dependent. The elimination half-life is ≈ 2 to 4 hours. Following initiation of therapy or a change in daily dose, steady-state plasma concentrations will be attained within 24 to 36 hours.

Special populations –

Age: There is no clinically relevant influence of age (50 to 84 years) on tacrine clearance.

Gender: Average tacrine plasma concentrations are ≈ 50% higher in females than in males. This is not explained by differences in body surface area or elimination half-life. The difference is probably because of higher systemic availability after oral dosing and may reflect the known lower activity of cytochrome P450 IA2 in women.

Smoking: Mean plasma tacrine concentrations in current smokers are ≈ ⅓ the concentrations in nonsmokers.

Hepatic function impairment: Although studies in patients with liver disease have not been done, it is likely that functional hepatic impairment will reduce the clearance of tacrine and its metabolites.

Contraindications

Hypersensitivity to tacrine or acridine derivatives; patients previously treated with tacrine who developed treatment-associated jaundice; a serum bilirubin > 3 mg/dl; signs or symptoms of hypersensitivity (eg, rash or fever) in association with ALT/SGPT elevations.

Warnings

➤*Anesthesia:* Tacrine is likely to exaggerate succinylcholine-type muscle relaxation during anesthesia.

➤*Cardiovascular:* Because of its cholinomimetic action, tacrine may have vagotonic effects on heart rate (eg, bradycardia). This action may be particularly important to patients with conduction abnormalities, bradyarrhythmia or "sick sinus syndrome."

➤*GI:* Tacrine is a cholinesterase inhibitor and may be expected to increase gastric acid secretion because of increased cholinergic activity. Therefore, closely monitor patients at increased risk for developing ulcers (eg, history of ulcer disease, concurrent NSAIDs) for symptoms of active or occult GI bleeding. Tacrine can cause nausea, vomiting and loose stools at recommended doses.

➤*Hepatotoxicity:* Prescribe with care in patients with current evidence or history of abnormal liver function indicated by significant abnormalities in serum transaminase (ALT, AST), bilirubin and

TACRINE HCl (Tetrahydroacridinamine; THA)

gamma-glutamyl transpeptidase (GGT) levels. The use of tacrine in patients without a history of liver disease is commonly associated with serum aminotransferase elevations, some to levels ordinarily considered to indicate clinically important hepatic injury. If tacrine is promptly withdrawn following detection of these elevations, clinically evident signs and symptoms of liver injury are rare. Long-term follow-up of patients who experience transaminase elevations, however, is limited; it is, therefore, impossible to exclude with certainty the possibility of chronic sequelae.

One of > 12,000 patients exposed to tacrine in clinical studies and the treatment IND program had documented elevated bilirubin (5.3 x upper limit of normal [ULN]) and jaundice with transaminase levels (AST) nearly 20 x ULN. A dosing regimen employing a more rapid escalation of the daily dose of tacrine may be associated with more serious clinical events.

Cumulative Incidence of ALT Elevations with Tacrine (%)			
Maximum ALT	Males (n = 229)	Females (n = 250)	Total (n = 479)
Within normal limits	53	40	46
> ULN	47	60	54
> 2 x ULN	34	42	38
> 3 x ULN	25	32	29
> 10 x ULN	5	8	6
> 20 x ULN	1	2	2

Experience in 2446 patients who participated in all clinical trials, including the 30-week study, indicates ≈ 50% of patients treated with tacrine can be expected to have at least 1 ALT level above ULN; ≈ 25% of patients are likely to develop elevations > 3 x ULN and ≈ 7% of patients may develop elevations > 10 x ULN. Data collected from the treatment IND program were consistent with those obtained during clinical studies and showed 3% of 5665 patients experiencing an ALT elevation > 10 x ULN. In clinical trials where transaminases were monitored weekly, the median time to onset of the first ALT elevation above ULN was ≈ 6 weeks, with maximum ALT occurring 1 week later, even in instances when treatment was stopped. Under the conditions of forced slow upwards dose titration (increases of 40 mg/day every 6 weeks) employed in clinical studies, 95% of transaminase elevations > 3 x ULN occurred within the first 18 weeks of therapy, and 99% of the 10-fold elevations occurred by the 12th week on ≤ 80 mg. Note, however, that for most patients ALT was monitored weekly and tacrine was stopped when liver enzymes exceeded 3 x ULN. With less frequent monitoring or the less stringent discontinuation criteria, it is possible that marked elevations might be more common. It must also be appreciated that experience with prolonged exposure to the high dose (160 mg/day) is limited. In all cases, transaminase levels returned to within normal limits upon discontinuation of treatment or following dosage reduction, usually within 4 to 6 weeks. This relatively benign experience may be the consequence of careful laboratory monitoring that facilitated the discontinuation of patients early on after the onset of their transaminase elevations. Consequently, frequent monitoring of serum transaminase levels is recommended.

Liver biopsy results in seven patients who received tacrine revealed hepatocellular necrosis in six patients, and granulomatous changes in the seventh. In all cases, liver function tests returned to normal with no evidence of persisting hepatic dysfunction.

Among the 866 patients assigned to tacrine in the 12- and 30-week studies, 212 were withdrawn because they developed transaminase elevations > 3 x ULN. Of these patients, 145 were subsequently rechallenged. During their initial exposure to tacrine, 20 of these 145 had experienced initial elevations > 10 x ULN, while the remainder had experienced elevations between 3 and 10 x ULN. Upon rechallenge with an initial dose of 40 mg/day, only 48 (33%) of the 145 patients developed transaminase elevations > 3 × ULN. Of these patients, 44 had elevations that were between 3 and 10 x ULN and 4 had elevations that were > 10 x ULN. The mean time to onset of elevations occurred earlier on rechallenge than on initial exposure (22 vs 48 days). Of the 145 patients rechallenged, 127 (88%) were able to continue treatment, and 91 of these 127 patients titrated to doses higher than those associated with the initial transaminase elevation.

The incidence of transaminase elevations is higher among females. There are no other known predictors of the risk of hepatocellular injury.

Rechallenge – Patients with clinical jaundice confirmed by a significant elevation in total bilirubin (> 3 mg/dl) or those exhibiting clinical signs or symptoms of hypersensitivity (eg, rash or fever) in association with transaminase elevations should permanently discontinue tacrine and not be rechallenged. Patients who are required to discontinue treatment because of transaminase elevations may be rechallenged once transaminase levels return to within normal limits (see Administration and Dosage). Rechallenge of patients with transaminase elevations < 10 x ULN has not resulted in serious liver injury. However, because experience in the rechallenge of patients who had elevations > 10 x ULN is limited, the risks associated with the rechallenge of

these patients are not well characterized. Use careful, frequent (weekly) monitoring of serum ALT when rechallenging such patients. If rechallenged, give patients an initial dose of 40 mg/day (10 mg 4 times daily) and monitor transaminase levels weekly. If, after 6 weeks on 40 mg/day, the patient is tolerating the dosage with no unacceptable elevations in transaminases, resume recommended dose titration and transaminase monitoring.

Liver biopsy is not indicated in cases of uncomplicated transaminase elevation.

➤*GU:* Cholinomimetics may cause bladder outflow obstruction.

➤*Neurological conditions:*

Seizures – Cholinomimetics are believed to have some potential to cause generalized convulsions; seizure activity may, however, also be a manifestation of Alzheimer's disease.

Worsening of cognitive function – Worsening of cognitive function has been reported following abrupt discontinuation of tacrine or after a large reduction in total daily dose (≥ 80 mg/day).

➤*Pulmonary conditions:* Because of its cholinomimetic action, use tacrine with care in patients with a history of asthma.

Tacrine was mutagenic to bacteria in the Ames test. Unscheduled DNA synthesis was induced in rat and mouse hepatocytes in vitro. Results of cytogenetic (chromosomal aberration) studies were equivocal. Overall, the results of these tests, along with the fact that tacrine belongs to a chemical class (acridines) containing some members that are animal carcinogens, suggest that tacrine may be carcinogenic.

➤*Pregnancy: Category C.* It is not known whether tacrine can cause fetal harm when administered to a pregnant woman or can affect reproductive capacity.

➤*Lactation:* It is not known whether this drug is excreted in breast milk.

➤*Children:* There are no adequate and well controlled trials to document the safety and efficacy of tacrine in any dementing illness occurring in children.

Precautions

➤*Monitoring:* Monitor serum transaminase levels (specifically ALT) every other week from at least week 4 to week 16 following initiation of treatment, after which monitoring may be decreased to every 3 months. Repeat a full monitoring sequence in the event that a patient suspends treatment with tacrine for > 4 weeks. If transaminase elevations occur, modify the dose (see Administration and Dosage).

Continue to monitor ALT levels weekly for a total of 16 weeks, then decrease to monthly for 2 months and to every 3 months thereafter.

➤*Hematology:* An absolute neutrophil count (ANC) < 500/mcl occurred in four patients who received tacrine during the course of clinical trials. Three of the four patients had concurrent medical conditions commonly associated with a low ANC; two of these patients remained on tacrine. The fourth patient, who had a history of hypersensitivity (penicillin allergy), withdrew from the study as a result of a rash and also developed an ANC < 500/mcl, which returned to normal; this patient was not rechallenged, therefore the role played by tacrine in this reaction is unknown. Six patients had an ANC ≤ 1500/mcl, associated with an elevation of ALT. The total clinical experience in > 12,000 patients does not indicate a clear association between tacrine treatment and serious white blood cell abnormalities.

Drug Interactions

➤*P450 system:* Tacrine is primarily eliminated by hepatic metabolism via cytochrome P450 drug metabolizing enzymes. Drug interactions may occur when it is given concurrently with agents such as theophylline, that undergo extensive metabolism via cytochrome P450 IA2.

Tacrine Drug Interactions			
Precipitant drug	Object drug*		Description
Cimetidine	Tacrine	↑	Cimetidine increased the C_{max} and AUC of tacrine by ≈ 54% and 64%, respectively.
Tacrine	Anticholinergics	↓	Because of its mechanism of action, tacrine has the potential to interfere with the activity of anticholinergic medications.
Tacrine	Cholinomimetics/Cholinesterase inhibitors	↑	A synergistic effect is expected when tacrine is given concurrently with succinylcholine, cholinesterase inhibitors or cholinergic agonists (eg, bethanechol).
Tacrine	Theophylline	↑	Coadministration increased theophylline elimination half-life and average plasma levels by ≈ 2-fold; monitor plasma theophylline concentrations and reduce theophylline dose as appropriate.

* ↑ = Object drug increased. ↓ = Object drug decreased.

TACRINE HCl (Tetrahydroacridinamine; THA)

➤*Drug/Food interactions:* Food reduces tacrine bioavailability by ≈ 30% to 40%; however, there is no food effect if tacrine is administered at least 1 hour before meals.

Adverse Reactions

Approximately 17% of 2706 patients who received tacrine withdrew permanently because of adverse events. Transaminase elevations were the most common reason for withdrawals during treatment (8% of all tacrine-treated patients). Apart from withdrawals because of transaminase elevations, 9% withdrew for adverse events. Other adverse events that most frequently led to the withdrawal of tacrine-treated patients in clinical trials were nausea/vomiting (1.5%); agitation (0.9%); rash, anorexia (0.7%); and confusion (0.5%).

The most common adverse events were elevated transaminases, nausea, vomiting, diarrhea, dyspepsia, myalgia, anorexia and ataxia. Of these events, nausea, vomiting, diarrhea, dyspepsia and anorexia appeared to be dose-dependent.

Tacrine Adverse Reactions (%)		
Adverse reaction	Tacrine (n = 634)	Placebo (n = 342)
CNS		
Dizziness	12	11
Confusion	7	7
Ataxia	6	4
Insomnia	6	5
Somnolence	4	3
Tremor	2	< 1
Dermatologic		
Rash	7	5
Facial/Skin flushing	3	< 1
GI		
Nausea/Vomiting	28	9
Diarrhea	16	5
Dyspepsia	9	6
Anorexia	9	3
Abdominal pain	8	7
Flatulence	4	2
Constipation	4	2
GU		
Urination frequency	3	4
Urinary tract infection	3	6
Urinary incontinence	3	3
Psychiatric		
Agitation	7	9
Depression	4	4
Abnormal thinking	3	4
Anxiety	3	2
Hallucination	2	4
Hostility	2	2
Respiratory		
Rhinitis	8	6
Upper respiratory tract infection	3	3
Coughing	3	5
Miscellaneous		
Elevated transaminase	29	2
Headache	11	15
Myalgia	9	5
Fatigue	4	3
Chest pain	4	5
Weight decrease	3	1
Back pain	2	4
Asthenia	2	2
Purpura	2	2

➤*Cardiovascular:* Hypotension, hypertension (≥ 1%); heart failure, myocardial infarction, angina pectoris, cerebrovascular accident, transient ischemic attack, phlebitis, venous insufficiency, abdominal aortic aneurysm, atrial fibrillation or flutter, palpitation, tachycardia, bradycardia, pulmonary embolus, migraine, hypercholesterolemia (0.1% to 1%); heart arrest, premature atrial contractions, A-V block, bundle branch block (< 0.1%).

➤*CNS:* Convulsions, vertigo, syncope, hyperkinesia, paresthesia (≥ 1%); abnormal dreaming, dysarthria, aphasia, amnesia, wandering, twitching, hypesthesia, delirium, paralysis, bradykinesia, movement disorder, cogwheel rigidity, paresis, neuritis, hemiplegia, Parkinson's disease, neuropathy, extrapyramidal syndrome, decreased/absent reflexes (0.1% to 1%); tardive dyskinesia, dysesthesia, dystonia, encephalitis, coma, apraxia, oculogyric crisis, akathisia, oral facial dyskinesia, Bell's palsy, exacerbation of Parkinson's disease (< 0.1%).

➤*Dermatologic:* Increased sweating (≥ 1%); acne, alopecia, dermatitis, eczema, dry skin, herpes zoster, psoriasis, cellulitis, cyst, furuncu-

losis, herpes simplex, hyperkeratosis, basal cell carcinoma, skin cancer (0.1% to 1%); desquamation, seborrhea, squamous cell carcinoma, skin ulcer, skin necrosis, melanoma (< 0.1%).

➤*Endocrine:* Diabetes (0.1% to 1%); hyperthyroid, hypothyroid (< 0.1%).

➤*GI:* Glossitis, gingivitis, dry mouth or throat, stomatitis, increased salivation, dysphagia, esophagitis, gastritis, gastroenteritis, GI hemorrhage, stomach ulcer, hiatal hernia, hemorrhoids, bloody stools, diverticulitis, fecal impaction, fecal incontinence, rectal hemorrhage, cholelithiasis, cholecystitis, increased appetite (0.1% to 1%); duodenal ulcer, bowel obstruction (< 0.1%).

➤*GU:* Hematuria, renal stone, kidney infection, glycosuria, dysuria, polyuria, nocturia, pyuria, cystitis, urinary retention, urination urgency, vaginal hemorrhage, pruritus (genital), breast pain, impotence, prostate cancer (0.1% to 1%); bladder tumor, renal tumor, renal failure, urinary obstruction, breast cancer, ovarian carcinoma, epididymitis (< 0.1%).

➤*Hematologic/Lymphatic:* Anemia, lymphadenopathy (0.1% to 1%); leukopenia, thrombocytopenia, hemolysis, pancytopenia (< 0.1%).

➤*Musculoskeletal:* Fracture, arthralgia, arthritis, hypertonia (≥ 1%); osteoporosis, tendinitis, bursitis, gout (0.1% to 1%); myopathy (< 0.1%).

➤*Psychiatric:* Nervousness (≥ 1%); apathy, increased libido, paranoia, neurosis (0.1% to 1%); suicidal, psychosis, hysteria (< 0.1%).

➤*Respiratory:* Pharyngitis, sinusitis, bronchitis, pneumonia, dyspnea (≥ 1%); epistaxis, chest congestion, asthma, hyperventilation, lower respiratory infection (0.1% to 1%); hemoptysis, lung edema, lung cancer, acute epiglottitis (< 0.1%).

➤*Special senses:* Conjunctivitis (≥ 1%); cataract, dry eyes, eye pain, visual field defect, diplopia, amblyopia, glaucoma, hordeolum, deafness, earache, tinnitus, inner ear infection, otitis media, unusual taste (0.1% to 1%); vision loss, ptosis, blepharitis, labyrinthitis, inner ear disturbance (< 0.1%).

➤*Miscellaneous:* Chill, fever, malaise, peripheral edema (≥ 1%); facial edema, dehydration, weight increase, cachexia, generalized edema, lipoma (0.1% to 1%); heat exhaustion, sepsis, cholinergic crisis, death (< 0.1%).

Overdosage

➤*Symptoms:* Overdosage with cholinesterase inhibitors can cause a cholinergic crisis characterized by severe nausea, vomiting, salivation, sweating, bradycardia, hypotension, collapse and convulsions. Increasing muscle weakness is a possibility and may result in death if respiratory muscles are involved.

The estimated median lethal dose of tacrine following a single oral dose in rats is 40 mg/kg or ≈ 12 times the maximum recommended human dose of 160 mg/day. Dose-related signs of cholinergic stimulation were observed in animals and included vomiting, diarrhea, salivation, lacrimation, ataxia, convulsions, tremor and stereotypic head and body movements.

➤*Treatment:* As in any case of overdose, use general supportive measures. Refer to General Management of Acute Overdosage. Tertiary anticholinergics, such as atropine, may be used as an antidote for tacrine overdosage. IV atropine sulfate titrated to effect is recommended. In adults, the initial atropine dose is 1 to 2 mg IV with subsequent doses based on clinical response. In children, the usual IM or IV dose is 0.05 mg/kg, repeated every 10 to 30 minutes until muscarinic signs and symptoms subside and repeated if they reappear. Atypical increases in blood pressure and heart rate have been reported with other cholinomimetics when coadministered with quaternary anticholinergics such as glycopyrrolate.

It is not known whether tacrine or its metabolites can be eliminated by dialysis (hemodialysis, peritoneal dialysis or hemofiltration).

Patient Information

Advise patients and caregivers that the effect of tacrine therapy is thought to depend on its administration at regular intervals, as directed. Take between meals whenever possible; however, it may be taken with meals to avoid GI upset.

Advise the caregiver about the possibility of adverse effects. Two types should be distinguished: (1) Those occuring in close temporal association with the initiation of treatment or an increase in dose (eg, nausea, vomiting, loose stools, diarrhea); and (2) those with a delayed onset (eg, rash, jaundice, changes in the color of stool [black, very dark or light, eg, acholic]).

Encourage patients and caregivers to inform the physician about the emergence of new events or any increase in the severity of existing adverse clinical events.

Advise caregivers that abrupt discontinuation or a large reduction in total daily dose (≥ 80 mg/day) may cause a decline in cognitive function and behavioral disturbances. Unsupervised increases in the dose of tacrine may also have serious consequences. Changes in dose should not be undertaken in the absence of direct instruction of a physician.

DONEPEZIL HCl

Rx	Aricept (Eisai/Pfizer)	Tablets: 5 mg	White. (ARICEPT 5). In 30s and UD blister pack 100s.
		10 mg	Yellow. (ARICEPT 10). In 30s and UD blister pack 100s.

Indications

➤*Alzheimer's disease:* The treatment of mild-to-moderate dementia of the Alzheimer's type.

Administration and Dosage

The dosages of donepezil are 5 and 10 mg once per day.

The higher dose of 10 mg did not provide a statistically significant clinical benefit greater than that of 5 mg. There is a suggestion, however, based upon order of group mean scores and dose trend analyses of data, that a daily dose of 10 mg donepezil might provide additional benefit for some patients. Do not increase to 10 mg until patients have been on a daily dose of 5 mg for 4 to 6 weeks.

Take donepezil in the evening, just prior to retiring.

Donepezil may be taken with or without food.

➤*Storage / Stability:* Store at controlled room temperature, 15° to 30°C (59° to 86°F).

Actions

➤*Pharmacology:* Donepezil is postulated to exert its therapeutic effect by enhancing cholinergic function. Deficiency of cholinergic neurotransmission may be the cause of Alzheimer's disease. This increase in cholinergic function is accomplished by increasing the concentration of acetylcholine through reversible inhibition of its hydrolysis by acetylcholinesterase (AChE). If this proposed mechanism of action is correct, donepezil's effect may lessen as the disease process advances and fewer cholinergic neurons remain functionally intact. There is no evidence that donepezil alters the course of the underlying dementing process.

➤*Pharmacokinetics:*

Absorption – Donepezil is well absorbed with a relative oral bioavailability of 100% and reaches peak plasma concentrations in 3 to 4 hours. Pharmacokinetics are linear over a dose range of 1 to 10 mg given once daily. Neither food nor time of administration (morning vs evening dose) influences the rate or extent of absorption.

Distribution – Following multiple dose administration, donepezil accumulates in plasma by 4- to 7-fold and steady-state is reached within 15 days. The steady-state volume of distribution is 12 L/kg. Donepezil is ≈ 96% bound to human plasma proteins, mainly to albumins (≈ 75%) and alpha$_1$–acid glycoprotein (≈ 21%) over the concentration range of 2 to 1000 ng/ml.

Metabolism – Donepezil is both excreted in the urine intact and extensively metabolized to four major metabolites, two of which are known to be active and a number of minor metabolites, not all of which have been identified. Donepezil is metabolized by CYP 450 isoenzyme 2D6 and 3A4 and undergoes glucuronidation. Following administration of donepezil, plasma radioactivity was present primarily as intact donepezil (53%) and as 6-O-desmethyl donepezil (11%), which has been reported to inhibit AChE to the same extent as donepezil in vitro and was found in plasma at concentrations equal to ≈ 20% of donepezil.

Excretion – The elimination half-life of donepezil is ≈ 70 hours and the mean apparent plasma clearance is 0.13 L/hr/kg.

Approximately 57% and 15% of the total dose was recovered in urine and feces, respectively, over a period of 10 days, while 28% remained unrecovered, with ≈ 17% of the donepezil dose recovered in the urine as unchanged drug.

Special Populations –

Hepatic function impairment: In a study of 10 patients with stable alcoholic cirrhosis, the clearance of donepezil was decreased by 20% relative to 10 healthy age- and sex-matched subjects.

Renal function impairment: In a study of 4 patients with moderate to severe renal impairment (Cl$_{cr}$ < 22 ml/min/1.72 m^2), the clearance of donepezil did not differ from age- and sex-matched subjects.

Clinical trials:

Thirty-week study – In a 30–week study, 473 patients were randomized to receive single daily doses of placebo or 5 or 10 mg/day of donepezil. The study was divided into a 24–week, double-blind active treatment phase followed by a 6–week single-blind placebo washout period.

Effects on the Alzheimer's Disease Assessment Scale (ADAS cog): After 24 weeks of treatment, the mean differences in the ADAS cog change scores for the donepezil-treated patients compared with the patients on placebo were 2.8 and 3.1 units for the 5 mg/day and 10 mg/day treatments, respectively. These differences were statistically significant.

Following 6 weeks of placebo washout, scores on the ADAS cog for both donepezil treatment groups were indistinguishable from those patients who had received only placebo for 30 weeks. This suggests that the beneficial effects of donepezil abate over 6 weeks following discontinuation

of treatment and do not represent a change in the underlying disease. There is no evidence of a rebound effect 6 weeks after abrupt discontinuation.

Effects on the Clinician's Interview Based Impression of Change (CIBIC-Plus): The mean drug-placebo differences for these groups of patients were 0.35 units and 0.39 units for 5 mg/day and 10 mg/day of donepezil, respectively. These differences were statistically significant. There was no statistically significant difference between the two active treatments.

Fifteen-week study – In a 15–week study, patients were randomized to receive single daily doses of placebo or 5 or 10 mg/day of donepezil for 12 weeks, followed by a 3–week placebo washout period.

Effects on the ADAS cog: After 12 weeks of treatment, the differences in mean ADAS cog change scores were 2.7 and 3 units each, for the 5 and 10 mg/day donepezil treatment groups, respectively. These differences were statistically significant.

Following 3 weeks of placebo washout, scores on the ADAS cog for both donepezil treatment groups increased, indicating that discontinuation of donepezil resulted in a loss of its treatment effect. The duration of this placebo washout period was not sufficient to characterize the rate of loss of the treatment effect, but, the 30–week study demonstrated that treatment effects associated with the use of donepezil abate within 6 weeks of treatment discontinuation.

Effects on the CIBIC-Plus: The differences in mean scores for donepezil-treated patients, compared with the patients on placebo at week 12, were 0.36 units and 0.38 units for the 5 mg/day and 10 mg/day treatment groups, respectively. These differences were statistically significant.

Contraindications

Hypersensitivity to donepezil or to piperidine derivatives.

Warnings

➤*Anesthesia:* Donepezil, as a cholinesterase inhibitor, is likely to exaggerate succinylcholine-type muscle relaxation during anesthesia.

➤*Cardiovascular:* Because of their pharmacological action, cholinesterase inhibitors may have vagotonic effects on heart rate (eg, bradycardia). The potential for this action may be particularly important to patients with "sick sinus syndrome" or other supraventricular cardiac conduction conditions. Syncopal episodes have been reported in association with the use of donepezil.

➤*GI:* Through their primary action, cholinesterase inhibitors may be expected to increase gastric acid secretion because of increased cholinergic activity. Therefore, monitor patients closely for symptoms of active or occult GI bleeding, especially those at increased risk for developing ulcers, eg, those with a history of ulcer disease or those receiving concurrent nonsteroidal anti-inflammatory drugs (NSAIDs). Clinical studies of donepezil have shown no increase, relative to placebo, in the incidence of either peptic ulcer disease or GI bleeding.

Donepezil, as a predictable consequence of its pharmacological properties, has been shown to produce diarrhea, nausea and vomiting. These effects, when they occur, appear more frequently with the 10 mg/day dose than with the 5 mg/day dose. In most cases, these effects have been mild and transient, sometimes lasting 1 to 3 weeks, and have resolved during continued use of donepezil.

➤*GU:* Although not observed in clinical trials, cholinomimetics may cause bladder outflow obstruction.

➤*Seizures:* Cholinomimetics are believed to have some potential to cause generalized convulsions. However, seizure activity also may be a manifestation of Alzheimer's disease.

➤*Pulmonary:* Because of their cholinomimetic actions, prescribe cholinesterase inhibitors with care for patients with a history of asthma or obstructive pulmonary disease.

➤*Pregnancy: Category C.* In a study in which pregnant rats were given up to 10 mg/kg/day from day 17 of gestation through day 20 post partum, there was a slight increase in still births and a slight decrease in pup survival through day 4 post partum at this dose. There are no adequate or well controlled studies in pregnant women. Use donepezil during pregnancy only if the potential benefit justifies the potential risk to the fetus.

➤*Lactation:* It is not known whether donepezil is excreted in breast milk.

➤*Children:* There are no adequate and well controlled trials to document the safety and efficacy of donepezil in any illness occurring in children.

Drug Interactions

Inducers of CYP 2D6 and CYP 3A4 could increase the rate of elimination of donepezil.

DONEPEZIL HCl

Donepezil Drug Interactions

Precipitant drug	Object drug*		Description
Donepezil	Anticholinergics	↓	Because of their mechanism of action, cholinesterase inhibitors have the potential to interfere with the activity of anticholinergic medications.
Donepezil	Cholinomimetics/cholinesterase inhibitors	↑	A synergistic effect may be expected when cholinesterase inhibitors are given concurrently with succinylcholine, similar neuromuscular blocking agents or cholinergic agonists such as bethanechol.
Donepezil	NSAIDs	↑	Donepezil increases gastric acid secretions due to increased cholinergic activity. Therefore, monitor for active or occult GI bleeding.
Donepezil	Furosemide Digoxin Warfarin	↔	Donepezil at concentrations of 0.3 to 10 mcg/ml did not affect the binding of furosemide, digoxin and warfarin to albumin.
Donepezil	Theophylline Cimetidine Warfarin Digoxin	↔	No significant effects on the pharmacokinetics of these drugs have been observed.
Ketoconazole Quinidine	Donepezil	↑	Inhibitors of CYP 450, 3A4 and 2D6, inhibit donepezil metabolism in vitro. Whether there is a clinical effect of these inhibitors is not known.

* ↑ = Object drug increased. ↓ = Object drug decreased. ↔ = Undetermined clinical effect.

Adverse Reactions

Adverse Events Reported for Donepezil (%)

Adverse event	Donepezil (n = 747)	Placebo (n = 355)
CNS		
Insomnia	9	6
Dizziness	8	6
Depression	3	< 1
Abnormal dreams	3	0
Somnolence	2	< 1
GI[1]		
Nausea[2]	11	6
Diarrhea[2]	10	5
Vomiting[3]	5	3
Anorexia	4	2
Musculoskeletal		
Muscle cramps	6	2
Arthritis	2	1
Miscellaneous		
Headache	10	9
Pain, various locations	9	8
Accident	7	6
Fatigue	5	3
Ecchymosis	4	3
Weight decrease	3	1
Frequent urination	2	1
Syncope	2	1

[1] See Warnings.
[2] 1% to 3% discontinued because of adverse reactions.
[3] 1% to 2% discontinued because of adverse reactions.

Other adverse reactions include:

►*Cardiovascular:* Hypertension, vasodilation, atrial fibrillation, hot flashes, hypotension (1%); angina pectoris, postural hypotension, myocardial infarction, AV block (first degree), congestive heart failure, arteritis, bradycardia (see Warnings), peripheral vascular disease, supraventricular tachycardia, deep vein thrombosis (≤ 1%).

►*Dermatologic:* Diaphoresis, urticaria, pruritus (1%); dermatitis, erythema, skin discoloration, hyperkeratosis, alopecia, fungal dermatitis, herpes zoster, nevus, hirsutism, skin striae, night sweats, skin ulcer (≤ 1%).

►*Endocrine:* Diabetes mellitus, goiter (≤ 1%).

►*GI:* Fecal incontinence, GI bleeding (see Warnings), bloating, epigastric pain (1%); eructation, gingivitis, increased appetite, flatulence, periodontal abscess, cholelithiasis, diverticulitis, drooling, dry mouth, fever sore, gastritis, irritable colon, coated tongue, tongue edema, epigastric distress, gastroenteritis, increased transaminases, hemorrhoids, ileus, increased thirst, jaundice, melena, polydypsia, duodenal ulcer, stomach ulcer (≤ 1%).

►*GU:* Urinary incontinence (see Warnings), nocturia (1%); dysuria, hematuria, urinary urgency, metrorrhagia, cystitis, enuresis, prostate hypertrophy, pyelonephritis, inability to empty bladder, breast fibroadenosis, fibrocystic breast, mastitis, pyuria, renal failure, vaginitis (≤ 1%).

►*Hematologic/Lymphatic:* Anemia, thrombocythemia, thrombocytopenia, eosinophilia, erythrocytopenia (≤ 1%).

►*Metabolic/Nutritional:* Dehydration (1%); gout, hypokalemia, increased creatine kinase, hyperglycemia, weight increase, increased lactate dehydrogenase (≤ 1%).

►*Musculoskeletal:* Bone fracture (1%); muscle weakness, muscle fasciculation (≤ 1%).

►*Respiratory:* Dyspnea, sore throat, bronchitis (1%); epistaxis, postnasal drip, pneumonia, hyperventilation, pulmonary congestion, wheezing, hypoxia, pharyngitis, pleurisy, pulmonary collapse, sleep apnea, snoring (≤ 1%).

►*Special senses:* Cataract, eye irritation, vision blurred (1%); dry eyes, glaucoma, earache, tinnitus, blepharitis, decreased hearing, retinal hemorrhage, otitis externa, otitis media, bad taste, conjunctival hemorrhage, ear buzzing, motion sickness, spots before eyes (≤ 1%).

►*Miscellaneous:* Influenza, chest pain, toothache (1%); fever, facial edema, periorbital edema, hernia, hiatal hernia, abscess, cellulitis, chills, generalized coldness, head fullness, head pressure, listlessness (≤ 1%).

Overdosage

►*Symptoms:* Overdosage with cholinesterase inhibitors can result in cholinergic crisis characterized by severe nausea, vomiting, salivation, sweating, bradycardia, hypotension, respiratory depression, collapse and convulsions. Increasing muscle weakness is a possibility and may result in death if respiratory muscles are involved.

►*Treatment:* As in any case of overdose, use general supportive measures. Tertiary anticholinergics such as atropine may be used as an antidote for donepezil overdosage. Intravenous atropine sulfate titrated to effect is recommended: An initial dose of 1 to 2 mg IV with subsequent doses based upon clinical response. Atypical responses in blood pressure and heart rate have been reported with other cholinomimetics when co-administered with quarternary anticholinergics such as glycopyrrolate. It is not known whether donepezil or its metabolites can be removed by dialysis (hemodialysis, peritoneal dialysis or hemofiltration).

RIVASTIGMINE TARTRATE

Rx	**Exelon** (Novartis)	**Capsules:** 1.5 mg (as base)	(Exelon 1.5 mg). Yellow. In 60s, 500s, and UD 100s.
		3 mg (as base)	(Exelon 3 mg). Orange. In 60s, 500s, and UD 100s.
		4.5 mg (as base)	(Exelon 4.5 mg). Red. In 60s, 500s, and UD 100s.
		6 mg (as base)	(Exelon 6 mg). Orange/red. In 60s, 500s, and UD 100s.
		Solution: 2 mg/mL (as base)	In 120 mL bottles.

Indications

➤*Alzheimer's dementia:* For the treatment of mild-to-moderate dementia of the Alzheimer's type.

➤*Unlabeled uses:* Treatment of behavioral effects in Lewy-body dementia.

Administration and Dosage

➤*Approved by the FDA:* April 25, 2000.

The starting dose of rivastigmine is 1.5 mg twice a day. If dose is well tolerated, after a minimum of 2 weeks of treatment, the dose may be increased to 3 mg twice daily. Subsequent increases to 4.5 and 6 mg twice daily should be attempted after a minimum of 2 weeks at the previous dose. If adverse effects (eg, nausea, vomiting, abdominal pain, loss of appetite) cause intolerance during treatment, instruct the patient to discontinue treatment for several doses and then restart at the same or next lower dose level. If treatment is interrupted for longer than several days, reinitiate treatment with the lowest daily dose and titrate as described above. The maximum dose is 6 mg twice daily (12 mg/day).

Take with food in divided doses in the morning and evening.

The dosage of rivastigmine shown to be effective in controlled clinical trials is 6 to 12 mg/day, given as twice daily dosing (daily doses of 3 to 6 mg twice daily). There is evidence from the clinical trials that doses at the higher end of this range may be more beneficial.

Rivastigmine oral solution and capsules may be interchanged at equal doses.

➤*Administration of oral solution:* Instruct caregivers on the correct procedure for administering rivastigmine oral solution (see instruction sheet included with the product).

Remove the oral dosing syringe provided in its protective case and, using the provided syringe, withdraw the prescribed amount of rivastigmine from the container. Each dose of rivastigmine may be swallowed directly from the syringe or first mixed with a small glass of water, cold fruit juice, or soda. Instruct patients to stir and drink the mixture.

➤*Storage/Stability:* Store below 77° F (25° C) in an upright position and protect from freezing.

When rivastigmine oral solution is combined with cold fruit juice or soda, the mixture is stable at room temperature for ≤ 4 hours.

Actions

➤*Pharmacology:* While the precise mechanism of rivastigmine's action is unknown, it is postulated to exert its therapeutic effect by enhancing cholinergic function. This is accomplished by increasing the concentration of acetylcholine through reversible inhibition of its hydrolysis by cholinesterase. If this proposed mechanism is correct, rivastigmine's effect may lessen as the disease process advances and fewer cholinergic neurons remain functionally intact. There is no evidence that rivastigmine alters the course of the underlying dementing process. After a 6 mg dose of rivastigmine, anticholinesterase activity is present in CSF for ≈ 10 hours, with a maximum inhibition of ≈ 60% 5 hours after dosing.

➤*Pharmacokinetics:*

Absorption – Rivastigmine is rapidly and completely absorbed with an absolute bioavailability of ≈ 36% (3 mg dose). It shows linear pharmacokinetics up to 3 mg twice daily but is nonlinear at higher doses. Doubling the dose from 3 to 6 mg twice daily results in a 3-fold increase in AUC. Peak plasma concentrations are reached in ≈ 1 hour. Administration of rivastigmine with food delays absorption (t_{max}) by 90 minutes, lowers C_{max} ≈ 30%, and increases AUC ≈ 30%.

Distribution – Rivastigmine is widely distributed throughout the body with a volume of distribution in the range of 1.8 to 2.7 L/kg. Rivastigmine penetrates the blood-brain barrier, reaching CSF peak concentrations in 1.4 to 2.6 hours. Mean $AUC_{1-12\ hr}$ ratio of CSF/plasma averaged ≈ 40% following 1 to 6 mg twice-daily doses.

Rivastigmine is ≈ 40% bound to plasma proteins at concentrations of 1 to 400 ng/mL, which covers the therapeutic concentration range. Rivastigmine distributes equally between blood and plasma with a blood-to-plasma partition ratio of 0.9 at concentrations ranging from 1 to 400 ng/mL.

Metabolism – Rivastigmine is rapidly and extensively metabolized, primarily via cholinesterase-mediated hydrolysis to the decarbamylated metabolite. Based on evidence from in vitro and animal studies, the major cytochrome P450 isozymes are minimally involved in rivastigmine metabolism. Consistent with these observations is the finding that no drug interactions related to cytochrome P450 have been observed in humans (see Drug Interactions).

Excretion – The elimination half-life is ≈ 1.5 hours, with most elimination as metabolites via the urine. The major pathway of elimination is renal. Following administration of rivastigmine to 6 healthy volunteers, total recovery over 120 hours was 97% in urine and 0.4% in feces. No parent drug was detected in urine. The sulfate conjugate of the decarbamylated metabolite is the major component excreted in urine and represents 40% of the dose. Mean oral clearance of rivastigmine is ≈ 1.8 L/min after 6 mg twice daily.

Special populations –

Nicotine use: Nicotine use increases the oral clearance of rivastigmine by 23%.

Renal function impairment: Following a single 3 mg dose, mean oral clearance of rivastigmine is 64% lower in moderately impaired renal patients. In severely impaired renal patients, mean oral clearance of rivastigmine is 43% higher than in healthy subjects. For unexplained reasons, the severely impaired renal patients had a higher clearance of rivastigmine than moderately impaired patients. However, dosage adjustments may not be necessary in renally impaired patients as the dose of the drug is individually titrated to tolerability.

Hepatic function impairment: Following a single 3 mg dose, mean oral clearance of rivastigmine was 60% lower in hepatically impaired patients than in healthy subjects. After multiple 6 mg twice-daily oral dosing, the mean clearance of rivastigmine was 65% lower in mild and moderate hepatically impaired patients than in healthy subjects. Dosage adjustment is not necessary in hepatically impaired patients as the dose of drug is individually titrated to tolerability.

Elderly: Following a single 2.5 mg oral dose to elderly volunteers (> 60 years of age) and younger volunteers, mean oral clearance of rivastigmine was 30% lower in elderly than in younger subjects.

Contraindications

Hypersensitivity to rivastigmine, carbamate derivatives, or other components of the formulation.

Warnings

➤*GI adverse reactions:* Rivastigmine is associated with significant GI adverse reactions, including nausea and vomiting, anorexia, and weight loss. For this reason, always start patients at a dose of 1.5 mg twice daily and titrate to their maintenance dose. If treatment is interrupted for longer than several days, initiate treatment with the lowest daily dose to reduce the possibility of severe vomiting and its potentially serious sequelae (eg, there has been 1 postmarketing report of severe vomiting with esophageal rupture following inappropriate reinitiation of treatment with a 4.5 mg dose after 8 weeks of treatment interruption).

Nausea and vomiting – In the controlled clinical trials, 47% of the patients treated with a rivastigmine dose in the therapeutic range of 6 to 12 mg/day developed nausea and 31% developed at least 1 episode of vomiting. The rate of vomiting was higher during the titration phase (24% vs 3% for placebo) than in the maintenance phase (14% vs 3% for placebo). The rates were higher in women than men. Five percent of patients discontinued because of vomiting. Vomiting was severe in 2% of rivastigmine-treated patients and was rated as mild or moderate each in 14% of patients. The rate of nausea was higher during the titration phase (43% vs 9% for placebo) than in maintenance phase (17% vs 4% for placebo).

Weight loss – In the controlled trials, ≈ 26% of women on high doses of rivastigmine (> 9 mg/day) had weight loss of ≥ 7% of their baseline weight compared with 6% in the placebo-treated patients. Approximately 18% of the males in the high dose group experienced a similar degree of weight loss compared with 4% in placebo-treated patients. It is not clear how much of the weight loss was associated with anorexia, nausea, vomiting, and diarrhea associated with drug administration.

Anorexia – In the controlled clinical trials, of the patients treated with a rivastigmine dose of 6 to 12 mg/day, 17% developed anorexia compared with 3% of the placebo patients. Neither the time course nor the severity of the anorexia is known.

Peptic ulcers/GI bleeding – Because of their pharmacological action, cholinesterase inhibitors may be expected to increase gastric acid secretion caused by increased cholinergic activity. Therefore, monitor patients closely for symptoms of active or occult GI bleeding, especially those at increased risk for developing ulcers (eg, those with a history of ulcer disease or those receiving concurrent nonsteroidal anti-inflammatory drugs [NSAID]). Clinical studies of rivastigmine have shown no significant increase, relative to placebo, in the incidence of either peptic ulcer disease or GI bleeding.

➤*Anesthesia:* Rivastigmine is likely to exaggerate succinylcholine-type muscle relaxation during anesthesia.

RIVASTIGMINE TARTRATE

►*Cardiovascular effects:* Drugs that increase cholinergic activity may have vagotonic effects on heart rate (eg, bradycardia). The potential for this action may be particularly important in "sick sinus syndrome" or other supraventricular cardiac conduction conditions.

►*Urinary obstruction:* Drugs that increase cholinergic activity may cause urinary obstruction.

►*Seizures:* Drugs that increase cholinergic activity are believed to have some potential for causing seizures. However, seizure activity also may be a manifestation of Alzheimer's disease.

►*Pulmonary effects:* Like other drugs that increase cholinergic activity, use with care in patients with a history of asthma or obstructive pulmonary disease.

►*Mutagenesis:* Rivastigmine was clastogenic in 2 in vitro assays in the presence, but not the absence, of metabolic activation. It caused structural chromosomal aberrations in V79 Chinese hamster lung cells and structural and numerical (polyploidy) chromosomal aberrations in human peripheral blood lymphocytes.

►*Pregnancy: Category B.* Studies in rats showed slightly decreased fetal/pup weights, usually at doses causing some maternal toxicity; decreased weights were seen at doses that were several fold lower than the maximum recommended human dose on a mg/m² basis. There are no adequate or well-controlled studies in pregnant women. Use during pregnancy only if the potential benefit justifies the risk to the fetus.

►*Lactation:* It is not known whether rivastigmine is excreted in breast milk.

Drug Interactions

►*Anticholinergics:* Because of their mechanism of action, cholinesterase inhibitors have the potential to interfere with the activity of anticholinergic medications.

►*Cholinomimetics and other cholinesterase inhibitors:* A synergistic effect may be expected when cholinesterase inhibitors are given concurrently with succinylcholine, similar neuromuscular-blocking agents, or cholinergic agonists such as bethanecol.

Adverse Reactions

The most common adverse events leading to discontinuation, defined as those occurring in ≥ 2% of patients and at twice the incidence seen in placebo patients were nausea, vomiting, anorexia, and dizziness. The most common adverse events (frequency of ≥ 5% and twice the placebo rate) include nausea, vomiting, anorexia, dyspepsia, and asthenia.

Rivastigmine Adverse Reactions (≥ 2%)		
Adverse reaction	Rivastigmine (6 to 12 mg/day) (n = 1189)	Placebo (n = 868)
Patients with any adverse reaction	92	79
CNS		
Dizziness	21	11
Headache	17	12
Insomnia	9	7
Confusion	8	7
Depression	6	4
Anxiety	5	3
Somnolence	5	3
Hallucination	4	3
Tremor	4	1
Syncope	3	2
Aggressive reaction	3	2
GI		
Nausea	47	12
Vomiting	31	6
Diarrhea	19	11
Anorexia	17	3
Abdominal pain	13	6
Dyspepsia	9	4
Constipation	5	4
Flatulence	4	2
Eructation	2	1
Miscellaneous		
Accidental trauma	10	9
Fatigue	9	5
Urinary tract infection	7	6
Asthenia	6	2
Malaise	5	2
Rhinitis	4	3
Increased sweating	4	1
Hypertension	3	2
Influenza-like symptoms	3	2
Weight decrease	3	< 1

In general, adverse reactions were less frequent later in the course of treatment.

Other adverse events observed at a rate of ≥ 2% on rivastigmine 6 to 12 mg/day but at a greater than or equal rate on placebo were chest pain, peripheral edema, vertigo, back pain, arthralgia, pain, bone fracture, agitation, nervousness, delusion, paranoid reaction, upper respiratory tract infections, infection (general), coughing, pharyngitis, bronchitis, rash (general), and urinary incontinence.

►*Cardiovascular:* Hypotension, postural hypotension, cardiac failure, atrial fibrillation, bradycardia, palpitation, angina pectoris, MI (≥ 1%); AV block, bundle branch block, sick sinus syndrome, cardiac arrest, supraventricular tachycardia, peripheral ischemia, pulmonary embolism, thrombosis, deep thrombophlebitis, aneurysm, intracranial hemorrhage, extrasystoles, tachycardia (0.1% to 1%).

►*CNS:* Abnormal gait, ataxia, paresthesia, convulsions, paranoid reaction, confusion (≥ 1%); paresis, apraxia, aphasia, dysphonia, hyperkinesia, hyperreflexia, hypertonia, hypesthesia, hypokinesia, migraine, neuralgia, nystagmus, peripheral neuropathy, abnormal dreaming, amnesia, apathy, delirium, dementia, depersonalization, emotional lability, impaired concentration, decreased libido, personality disorder, suicide attempt, increased libido, neurosis, suicidal ideation, psychosis (0.1% to 1%).

►*Dermatologic:* Rashes of various kinds (eg, maculopapular, eczema, bullous, exfoliative, psoriaform, erythematous) (≥ 1%); alopecia, skin ulceration, urticaria, cold clammy skin, contact dermatitis (0.1% to 1%).

►*Endocrine:* Goiter, hypothyroidism (0.1% to 1%).

►*GI:* Fecal incontinence, gastritis (≥ 1%); dysphagia, esophagitis, gastric ulcer, gastroesophageal reflux, GI hemorrhage, hernia, intestinal obstruction, melena, rectal hemorrhage, gastroenteritis, ulcerative stomatitis, duodenal ulcer, hematemesis, gingivitis, tenesmus, pancreatitis, colitis, dry mouth, increased saliva, glossitis (0.1% to 1%).

►*GU:* Hematuria (≥ 1%); breast pain, impotence, cystitis, atrophic vaginitis, albuminuria, oliguria, acute renal failure, dysuria, micturition urgency, nocturia, polyuria, renal calculus, urinary retention (0.1% to 1%).

►*Hematologic/Lymphatic:* Anemia, epistaxis (≥ 1%); hypochromic anemia, hematoma, thrombocytopenia, purpura, lymphadenopathy, leukocytosis (0.1% to 1%).

►*Hepatic:* Abnormal hepatic function, cholecystitis (0.1% to 1%).

►*Metabolic/Nutritional:* Dehydration, hypokalemia (≥ 1%); diabetes mellitus, gout, hypercholesterolemia, hyperlipemia, hypoglycemia, cachexia, thirst, hyperglycemia, hyponatremia (0.1% to 1%).

►*Musculoskeletal:* Arthritis, leg cramps, myalgia (≥ 1%); cramps, hernia, muscle weakness (0.1% to 1%).

►*Respiratory:* Bronchospasm, laryngitis, apnea (0.1% to 1%).

►*Special senses:* Tinnitus, cataract (≥ 1%); taste perversion, taste loss, conjunctival hemorrhage, blepharitis, diplopia, eye pain, otitis media, glaucoma (0.1% to 1%).

►*Miscellaneous:* Accidental trauma, fever, edema, allergy, hot flushes, rigors (≥ 1%); hemorrhoids, edema periorbital or facial, hypothermia, cold feeling, halitosis, cellulitis, herpes simplex, flushing (0.1% to 1%).

Overdosage

►*Symptoms:* Overdosage with cholinesterase inhibitors can result in cholinergic crisis characterized by severe nausea, vomiting, salivation, sweating, bradycardia, hypotension, respiratory depression, collapse, and convulsions. Increasing muscle weakness is a possibility and may result in death if respiratory muscles are involved.

►*Treatment:* As in any case of overdose, utilize general supportive measures. Refer to General Management of Acute Overdosage. In overdoses accompanied by severe nausea and vomiting, consider the use of antiemetics. In a documented case of a 46 mg overdose with rivastigmine, the patient experienced vomiting, incontinence, hypertension, psychomotor retardation, and loss of consciousness. The patient fully recovered within 24 hours and conservative management was all that was required for treatment.

As rivastigmine has a short plasma half-life of ≈ 1 hour and a moderate duration of acetylcholinesterase inhibition of 8 to 10 hours, do not administer a further dose of rivastigmine for the next 24 hours in cases of asymptomatic overdoses.

Because of the short half-life of rivastigmine, dialysis (hemodialysis, peritoneal dialysis, or hemofiltration) would not be clinically indicated in the event of an overdose.

Patient Information

Advise caregivers of the high incidence of nausea and vomiting associated with the use of the drug along with the possibility of anorexia and weight loss. Encourage caregivers to monitor for these adverse events and inform the physician if they occur. It is critical to inform caregivers that if therapy has been interrupted for more than several days, they should not administer the next dose until discussing it with the physician.

►*Oral solution:* Instruct caregivers in the correct procedure for administering rivastigmine oral solution (see instruction sheet included with the product describing solution administration).

GALANTAMINE HBr

Rx	Reminyl (Janssen)	Tablets: 4 mg (as base)	Lactose. (JANSSEN G 4). Off-white. Film-coated. In 60s.
		8 mg (as base)	Lactose. (JANSSEN G 8). Pink. Film-coated. In 60s.
		12 mg (as base)	Lactose. (JANSSEN G 12). Orange-brown. Film-coated. In 60s.
		Oral solution: 4 mg/mL	Saccharin. In 100 mL w/ calibrated pipette.

Indications

➤*Alzheimer's disease:* Treatment of mild to moderate dementia of the Alzheimer's type.

➤*Unlabeled uses:* Vascular dementia.

Administration and Dosage

➤*Approved by the FDA:* February 28, 2001.

➤*Dosage:* 16 to 32 mg/day given twice daily. As the dose of 32 mg/day is less well tolerated than lower doses and does not provide increased effectiveness, the recommended dose range is 16 to 24 mg/day given twice daily.

Starting dose is 4 mg twice daily (8 mg/day). After a minimum of 4 weeks of treatment, if well tolerated, increase the dose to 8 mg twice daily (16 mg/day). Attempt a further increase to 12 mg twice daily (24 mg/day) only after a minimum of 4 weeks at the previous dose.

Administer galantamine twice daily, preferably with morning and evening meals.

Inform patients and caregivers that if therapy has been interrupted for several days or longer, the patient should be restarted at the lowest dose and the dose escalated to the current dose.

The abrupt withdrawal of galantamine in those patients who had been receiving doses in the effective range was not associated with an increased frequency of adverse events in comparison with those continuing to receive the same doses of that drug. However, the beneficial effects of galantamine are lost when the drug is discontinued.

➤*Hepatic impairment:* Galantamine plasma concentrations may be increased in patients with moderate to severe hepatic impairment. In patients with moderately impaired hepatic function (Child-Pugh 7 to 9), the dose generally should not exceed 16 mg/day. The use of galantamine in patients with severe hepatic impairment (Child-Pugh 10 to 15) is not recommended.

➤*Renal impairment:* For patients with moderate renal impairment, the dose generally should not exceed 16 mg/day. In patients with severe renal impairment (Ccr < 9 mL/min), the use of galantamine is not recommended.

➤*Storage/Stability:* Store galantamine tablets and oral solution at 25°C (77°F); excursions permitted to 15° to 30°C (59° to 86°F).

Actions

➤*Pharmacology:* Galantamine, a tertiary alkaloid, is a competitive and reversible inhibitor of acetylcholinesterase. While the precise mechanism of galantamine's action is unknown, it may exert its therapeutic effect by enhancing cholinergic function. This is accomplished by increasing the concentration of acetylcholine through reversible inhibition of its hydrolysis by cholinesterase. If this mechanism is correct, galantamine's effect may lessen as the disease process advances and fewer cholinergic neurons remain functionally intact. There is no evidence that galantamine alters the course of the underlying dementing process.

➤*Pharmacokinetics:*

Absorption/Distribution – Galantamine is rapidly and completely absorbed with time-to-peak concentration in ≈ 1 hour. Galantamine has an absolute oral bioavailability of ≈ 90%. Bioavailability of the tablet was the same as the bioavailability of an oral solution. Food did not affect the AUC of galantamine but C_{max} decreased by 25% and T_{max} was delayed by 1.5 hours. The mean volume of distribution of galantamine is 175 L.

The plasma protein binding of galantamine is 18% at therapeutically relevant concentrations. In whole blood, galantamine mainly is distributed to blood cells (52.7%). The blood to plasma concentration ratio of galantamine is 1:2.

Metabolism/Excretion – Galantamine is metabolized by hepatic cytochrome P450 enzymes, glucuronidated, and excreted unchanged in the urine. In vitro studies indicated that CYP2D6 and CYP3A4 were the major cytochrome P450 isoenzymes involved in the metabolism of galantamine, and inhibitors of both pathways modestly increase oral bioavailability of galantamine. O-demethylation mediated by CYP2D6 was greater in extensive metabolizers of CYP2D6 than in poor metabolizers. However, in plasma from poor and extensive metabolizers, unchanged galantamine and its glucuronide accounted for much of the sample radioactivity.

Up to 8 hours postdose, unchanged galantamine accounted for 39% to 77% of the total radioactivity in the plasma, and galantamine glucuronide for 14% to 24%. By 7 days, 93% to 99% of the radioactivity had been recovered, with ≈ 95% in urine and ≈ 5% in the feces. Total urinary recovery of unchanged galantamine accounted for ≈ 32% of the dose and that of galantamine glucuronide for ≈ 12%.

After IV or oral administration, ≈ 20% of the dose was excreted as unchanged galantamine in the urine in 24 hours, representing a renal clearance of ≈ 65 mL/min, about 20% to 25% of the total plasma clearance of ≈ 300 mL/min. Galantamine has a terminal elimination half-life of ≈ 7 hours (range, 4.4 to 10) and pharmacokinetics are linear over the range of 8 to 32 mg/day.

The maximum inhibition of anticholinesterase activity of ≈ 40% was achieved in ≈ 1 hour after a single oral dose of 8 mg galantamine in healthy men.

Special populations –

CYP2D6 poor metabolizers: Approximately 7% of the normal population has a genetic variation that leads to reduced levels of activity of the CYP2D6 isozyme. They are referred to as poor metabolizers. After a single oral dose of 4 or 8 mg galantamine, CYP2D6 poor metabolizers demonstrated a similar C_{max} and ≈ 35% AUC increase of unchanged galantamine compared with extensive metabolizers. Dosage adjustment is not necessary in patients identified as poor metabolizers as the dose of drug is individually titrated to tolerability.

Hepatic impairment: Following a single 4 mg dose of galantamine in patients with moderate hepatic impairment, galantamine clearance was decreased by ≈ 25% compared with healthy volunteers. Exposure would be expected to increase further with an increasing degree of hepatic impairment.

Renal impairment: Following a single 8 mg dose of galantamine, AUC increased by 37% and 67% in moderate and severely renal-impaired patients compared with normal volunteers.

Elderly: Data from clinical trials in patients with Alzheimer's disease indicated that galantamine concentrations are 30% to 40% higher than in healthy young subjects.

Gender: No specific pharmacokinetic study was conducted to investigate the effect of gender on the disposition of galantamine, but a population pharmacokinetic analysis indicates that galantamine clearance is ≈ 20% lower in females than in males (explained by lower body weight in females).

Contraindications

Known hypersensitivity to galantamine or to any excipients used in the formulation.

Warnings

➤*Renal function impairment:* In patients with moderately impaired renal function, proceed cautiously with dose titration. In patients with severely impaired renal function (Ccr < 9 mL/min), galantamine is not recommended.

➤*Hepatic function impairment:* In patients with moderately impaired hepatic function, proceed cautiously with dose titration. The use of galantamine in patients with severe hepatic impairment is not recommended.

➤*Pregnancy: Category B.* There are no adequate and well-controlled studies in pregnant women. Use during pregnancy only if the potential benefit justifies the potential risk to the fetus.

➤*Lactation:* It is not known whether galantamine is excreted in breast milk. Galantamine has no indication for use in nursing mothers.

➤*Children:* Safety and efficacy of galantamine in children have not been established. Therefore, the use of galantamine in children is not recommended.

Precautions

➤*Anesthesia:* Galantamine, as a cholinesterase inhibitor, is likely to exaggerate the neuromuscular blockade effects of succinylcholine-type and similar neuromuscular blocking agents during anesthesia.

➤*Cardiovascular conditions:* Because of their pharmacological action, cholinesterase inhibitors have vagotonic effects on the sinoatrial and atrioventricular nodes, leading to bradycardia and AV block. These actions may be particularly important to patients with supraventricular cardiac conduction disorders or to patients taking other drugs concomitantly that significantly slow heart rate. However, postmarketing surveillance of marketed anticholinesterase inhibitors has shown that bradycardia and all types of heart block have been reported in patients with and without known underlying cardiac conduction abnormalities. Therefore, consider all patients to be at risk for adverse effects on cardiac conduction.

In randomized controlled trials, bradycardia was reported more frequently in galantamine-treated patients than in placebo-treated patients, but rarely led to treatment discontinuation. The overall frequency of this event was 2% to 3% for galantamine doses up to 24 mg/day compared with < 1% for placebo. No increased incidence of heart block was observed at the recommended doses.

GALANTAMINE HBr

Patients treated with galantamine ≥ 24 mg/day using the recommended dosing schedule showed a dose-related increase in risk of syncope.

➤*GI conditions:* Cholinomimetics may increase gastric acid secretion because of increased cholinergic activity. Therefore, monitor patients closely for symptoms of active or occult GI bleeding, especially those with an increased risk for developing ulcers (eg, those with a history of ulcer disease or patients using concurrent nonsteroidal anti-inflammatory drugs [NSAIDs]).

Galantamine, as a predictable consequence of its pharmacological properties, has been shown to produce nausea, vomiting, diarrhea, anorexia, and weight loss. In patients who experienced nausea, the median duration was 5 to 7 days.

➤*GU:* Although this was not observed in clinical trials with galantamine, cholinomimetics may cause bladder outflow obstruction.

➤*Neurological conditions:* Cholinesterase inhibitors are believed to have some potential to cause generalized convulsions. However, seizure activity may be a manifestation of Alzheimer's disease.

➤*Pulmonary conditions:* Because of its cholinomimetic action, prescribe galantamine with care to patients with a history of severe asthma or obstructive pulmonary disease.

Drug Interactions

Galantamine Drug Interactions			
Precipitant drug	Object drug*		Description
Cholinesterase inhibitors	Succinylcholine, bethanechol	↑	A synergistic effect is expected when combined.
Succinylcholine, bethanechol	Cholinesterase inhibitors		
Cimetidine	Galantamine	↑	Cimetidine increased the bioavailability of galantamine by ≈ 16%. Ranitidine had no effect.
Ketoconazole	Galantamine	↑	Ketoconazole increased the AUC of galantamine by ≈ 30%.
Paroxetine	Galantamine	↑	Paroxetine increased the oral bioavailability of galantamine by ≈ 40%.
Erythromycin	Galantamine	↑	Erythromycin increased the AUC of galantamine by 10%.

* ↑ = Object drug increased.

Adverse Reactions

In a 5-month trial with escalation of the dose by 8 mg/day every 4 weeks, the overall risk of discontinuation because of an adverse event was 7%, 7%, and 10% for the placebo, 16 mg/day galantamine, and 24 mg/day galantamine groups, respectively, with GI adverse effects the principal reason for discontinuing galantamine. The most frequent adverse events leading to discontinuation in this study are listed in the following table.

Most Frequent Galantamine Adverse Events Leading to Discontinuation[1] (%)			
Adverse reaction	16 mg/day (n = 279)	24 mg/day (n = 273)	Placebo (n = 286)
Nausea	2	4	< 1
Dizziness	2	1	< 1
Vomiting	1	3	0
Anorexia	1	< 1	< 1
Syncope	0	1	0

[1] Placebo-controlled, double-blind trial with 4-week dose escalation schedule.

Adverse Events Occurring in ≥ 5% Galantamine and ≥ 2 Times Placebo[1]			
Adverse event	Galantamine 16 mg/day (n = 279)	Galantamine 24 mg/day (n= 273)	Placebo (n = 286)
Nausea	13	17	5
Diarrhea	12	6	6
Anorexia	7	9	3
Vomiting	6	10	1
Weight decrease	5	5	1

[1] Placebo-controlled trial with 4-week dose escalation schedule.

Galantamine Adverse Events Occurring in ≥ 2% of Patients at a Frequency Greater than Placebo		
Adverse reaction	Galantamine[1] (n = 1040)	Placebo (n = 801)
CNS		
Dizziness	9	6
Headache	8	5
Depression	7	5
Insomnia	5	4
Somnolence	4	3
Tremor	3	2

Galantamine Adverse Events Occurring in ≥ 2% of Patients at a Frequency Greater than Placebo		
Adverse reaction	Galantamine[1] (n = 1040)	Placebo (n = 801)
GI		
Nausea	24	9
Vomiting	13	4
Diarrhea	9	7
Anorexia	9	3
Abdominal pain	5	4
Dyspepsia	5	2
GU		
Urinary tract infection	8	7
Hematuria	3	2
Miscellaneous		
Weight decrease	7	2
Fatigue	5	3
Rhinitis	4	3
Anemia	3	2
Syncope	2	1
Bradycardia	2	1

[1] Adverse events in patients treated with 16 or 24 mg/day of galantamine in 4 placebo-controlled trials are included.

Adverse events occurring with an incidence of ≥ 2% in placebo-treated patients that was either equal to or greater than with galantamine treatment were the following: Constipation, agitation, confusion, anxiety, hallucination, injury, back pain, peripheral edema, asthenia, chest pain, urinary incontinence, upper respiratory tract infection, bronchitis, coughing, hypertension, fall, and purpura.

➤*Other adverse events observed during clinical trials:* These adverse events are not necessarily related to galantamine treatment and in most cases were observed at a similar frequency in placebo-treated patients in the controlled studies.

Cardiovascular – Chest pain (> 1%); postural hypotension, hypotension, dependent edema, cardiac failure, AV block, palpitation, atrial fibrillation, QT prolonged, bundle branch block, supraventricular tachycardia, T-wave inversion, ventricular tachycardia, purpura, epistaxis, thrombocytopenia (0.1% to 1%).

CNS – Vertigo, hypertonia, convulsions, involuntary muscle contractions, paresthesia, ataxia, hypokinesia, hyperkinesia, apraxia, aphasia, apathy, paroniria, paranoid reaction, libido increased, delirium (0.1% to 1%).

GI – Flatulence (> 1%); gastritis, melena, dysphagia, rectal hemorrhage, dry mouth, saliva increased, diverticulitis, gastroenteritis, hiccough (0.1% to 1%); esophageal perforation (< 0.1%).

GU – Incontinence (> 1%); hematuria, micturition frequency, cystitis, urinary retention, nocturia, renal calculi (0.1% to 1%).

Metabolic – Hyperglycemia, alkaline phosphatase increased (0.1% to 1%).

Overdosage

➤*Symptoms:* Signs and symptoms of significant overdosing of galantamine are predicted to be similar to those of overdosing of other cholinomimetics. These effects generally involve the CNS, the parasympathetic nervous system, and the neuromuscular junction. In addition to muscle weakness or fasciculations, some or all of the following signs of cholinergic crisis may develop: Severe nausea, vomiting, GI cramping, salivation, lacrimation, urination, defecation, sweating, bradycardia, hypotension, respiratory depression, collapse, and convulsions. Increasing muscle weakness is a possibility and may result in death if respiratory muscles are involved.

➤*Treatment:* As in any case of overdose, use general supportive measures. Tertiary anticholinergics such as atropine may be used as an antidote for galantamine overdosage. IV atropine sulfate titrated to effect is recommended at an initial dose of 0.5 to 1 mg IV with subsequent doses based on clinical response. Atypical responses in blood pressure and heart rate have been reported with other cholinomimetics when coadministered with quaternary anticholinergics. It is not known whether galantamine or its metabolites can be removed by dialysis (eg, hemodialysis, peritoneal dialysis, hemofiltration).

Patient Information

Instruct caregivers in the recommended administration (twice daily, preferably with morning and evening meal) and dose escalation (dose increases should follow minimum of 4 weeks at prior dose). If therapy has been interrupted for several days or longer, restart the patient at the lowest dose and escalate the dose to the current dose.

Advise patients and caregivers that the most frequent adverse events can be minimized by following the recommended dosage and administration. GI symptoms may be reduced by administering with food or antiemetic medication or ensuring adequate fluid intake.

Instruct caregivers in the correct procedure for administering galantamine oral solution. In addition, inform them of the existence of an instruction sheet (included with the product) describing how the solution is to be administered.

ATOMOXETINE HCl

Rx	Strattera (Eli Lilly)	Capsules: 10 mg (as base)	(LILLY 3227 10 mg). White. In 30s.
		18 mg (as base)	(LILLY 3238 18 mg). Gold/White. In 30s.
		25 mg (as base)	(LILLY 3228 25 mg). Blue/White. In 30s.
		40 mg (as base)	(LILLY 3229 40 mg). Blue. In 30s.
		60 mg (as base)	(LILLY 3239 60 mg). Blue/Gold. In 30s.

Indications

➤*Attention-deficit/hyperactivity disorder (ADHD):* For the treatment of ADHD.

Atomoxetine is indicated as an integral part of a total treatment program for ADHD that may include other measures (psychological, educational, social) for patients with this syndrome. Drug treatment may not be indicated for all patients with this syndrome. Drug treatment is not intended for use in the patient who exhibits symptoms secondary to environmental factors and/or other primary psychiatric disorders, including psychosis. Appropriate educational placement is essential in children and adolescents with this diagnosis; psychosocial intervention is often helpful. When remedial measures alone are insufficient, the decision to prescribe drug treatment medication will depend upon the physician's assessment of the chronicity and severity of the patient's symptoms.

Administration and Dosage

➤*Approved by the FDA:* November 26, 2002.

The safety of single doses over 120 mg and total daily doses above 150 mg have not been systematically evaluated.

➤*Initial treatment:*

Children up to 70 kg – Initiate at a total daily dose of approximately 0.5 mg/kg and increase after a minimum of 3 days to a target total daily dose of approximately 1.2 mg/kg administered as a single daily dose in the morning or as evenly divided doses in the morning and late afternoon/early evening. No additional benefit has been demonstrated for doses higher than 1.2 mg/kg/day. The total daily dose in children and adolescents should not exceed 1.4 mg/kg or 100 mg, whichever is less.

Adults and children over 70 kg – Initiate at a total daily dose of 40 mg and increase after a minimum of 3 days to a target total daily dose of approximately 80 mg administered as a single daily dose in the morning or as evenly divided doses in the morning and late afternoon/early evening. After 2 to 4 additional weeks, the dose may be increased to a maximum of 100 mg in patients who have not achieved an optimal response. There are no data that support increased effectiveness at higher doses. The maximum recommended total daily dose in children over 70 kg and adults is 100 mg.

➤*Maintenance treatment:* There is no evidence available from controlled trials to indicate how long the patient with ADHD should be treated with atomoxetine. However, pharmacological treatment of ADHD may be needed for extended periods. Periodically re-evaluate the long-term usefulness of the drug for the individual patient.

➤*Hepatic function impairment:* For patients with moderate hepatic function impairment (Child-Pugh Class B), reduce initial and target doses to 50% of the normal dose. For patients with severe hepatic function impairment (Child-Pugh Class C), reduce initial and target doses to 25% of normal.

➤*Concomitant use:* In children up to 70 kg body weight administered strong CYP2D6 inhibitors, initiate atomoxetine at 0.5 mg/kg/day and only increase to the usual target dose of 1.2 mg/kg/day if symptoms fail to improve after 4 weeks and the initial dose is well-tolerated.

In children over 70 kg body weight and adults administered strong CYP2D6 inhibitors, initiate atomoxetine at 40 mg/day and only increase to the usual target dose of 80 mg/day if symptoms fail to improve after 4 weeks and the initial dose is well-tolerated.

➤*Discontinuation:* Atomoxetine can be discontinued without being tapered.

➤*Storage/Stability:* Store at 25°C (77°F); excursions permitted to 15° to 30°C (59° to 86°F).

Actions

➤*Pharmacology:* Atomoxetine is a selective norepinephrine reuptake inhibitor. The precise mechanism by which it produces its therapeutic effects in ADHD is unknown, but it is thought to be related to selective inhibition of the presynaptic norepinephrine transporter, as determined in ex vivo uptake and neurotransmitter depletion studies.

➤*Pharmacokinetics:*

Absorption/Distribution – Atomoxetine is well absorbed after oral administration and is minimally affected by food. It is rapidly absorbed after oral administration, with absolute bioavailability of about 63% in extensive metabolizers (EMs) and 94% in poor metabolizers (PMs). Maximal plasma concentrations (C_{max}) are reached approximately 1 to 2 hours after dosing. Administration of atomoxetine with a standard high-fat meal in adults did not affect the extent of oral absorption (AUC) of atomoxetine but did decrease the rate of absorption, resulting in a 37% lower C_{max} and delayed T_{max} by 3 hours. The steady-state volume of distribution after IV administration is 0.85 L/kg. At therapeutic concentrations, 98% of atomoxetine in plasma is bound to protein, primarily albumin.

Metabolism/Excretion – Atomoxetine is metabolized primarily through the CYP2D6 enzymatic pathway. A fraction of the population (about 7% of Caucasians and 2% of African Americans) are PMs of CYP2D6 metabolized drugs. These individuals have reduced activity in this pathway resulting in 10-fold higher AUCs, 5-fold higher peak plasma concentrations, and slower elimination of atomoxetine compared with people with normal activity (EMs).

The major oxidative metabolite formed is 4-hydroxyatomoxetine, which is glucuronidated. 4-Hydroxyatomoxetine is equipotent to atomoxetine as an inhibitor of the norepinephrine transporter but circulates in plasma at much lower concentrations. N-Desmethylatomoxetine is formed by CYP2C19 and other cytochrome P450 enzymes but has substantially less pharmacological activity compared with atomoxetine and circulates in plasma at lower concentrations.

Mean apparent plasma clearance of atomoxetine after oral administration in adult EMs is 0.35 L/h/kg; mean half-life is 5.2 hours. Following oral administration of atomoxetine to PMs, mean apparent plasma clearance is 0.03 L/h/kg; mean half-life is 21.6 hours.

Atomoxetine is excreted primarily as 4-hydroxyatomoxetine-O-glucuronide, mainly in the urine (greater than 80%) and to a lesser extent in the feces (less than 17%). Only a small fraction of the dose is excreted as unchanged atomoxetine (less than 3%).

Special populations –

Hepatic function impairment: Atomoxetine exposure (AUC) is increased, compared with normal subjects, in EM subjects with moderate (Child-Pugh Class B) (2-fold increase) and severe (Child-Pugh Class C) (4-fold increase) hepatic insufficiency. Dosage adjustment is recommended for patients with moderate or severe hepatic insufficiency (see Administration and Dosage).

➤*Clinical trials:* In a randomized, open-label study comparing atomoxetine and methylphenidate treatment in children with ADHD, atomoxetine was found to be associated with therapeutic effects comparable with methylphenidate. Two hundred twenty-eight patients were randomized to atomoxetine (n = 184) or methylphenidate (n = 44). Both drugs were associated with marked improvement in ADHD symptoms as assessed by the parents and investigators. No statistically significant difference between treatment groups on the primary endpoint was observed. Primary endpoint measure was based on an investigator-rated score using the ADHD-IV Rating Scale. Atomoxetine baseline score was approximately 39.4 and endpoint score was approximately 20, vs methylphenidate baseline score of approximately 37.6 and endpoint of approximately 19.8 (P = 0.66). Discontinuations because of adverse events were 5.4% (10/184) in the atomoxetine groups and 11.4% (5/44) for methylphenidate (P = 0.175).

Contraindications

Patients known to be hypersensitive to atomoxetine or other constituents of the product; with a monoamine oxidase inhibitor (MAOI) or within 2 weeks after discontinuing an MAOI; narrow angle glaucoma (see Warnings).

Warnings

➤*Long-term use:* The effectiveness of atomoxetine for long-term use (ie, for more than 9 weeks in child and adolescent patients and 10 weeks in adult patients) has not been systematically evaluated in controlled trials. Therefore, periodically re-evaluate the long-term usefulness of the drug for the individual patient.

➤*MAOIs:* Do not take atomoxetine with an MAOI or within 2 weeks after discontinuing an MAOI. Do not initiate treatment with an MAOI within 2 weeks after discontinuing atomoxetine. With other drugs that affect brain monoamine concentrations, there have been reports of serious, sometimes fatal, reactions (including hyperthermia, rigidity, myoclonus, autonomic instability with possible rapid fluctuations of vital signs, and mental status changes that include extreme agitation progressing to delirium and coma) when taken in combination with an MAOI. Some cases presented with features resembling neuroleptic malignant syndrome. Such reactions may occur when these drugs are given concomitantly or in close proximity.

➤*Narrow angle glaucoma:* In clinical trials, atomoxetine use was associated with an increased risk of mydriasis and therefore its use is not recommended in patients with narrow angle glaucoma.

➤*Growth:* Monitor growth during treatment with atomoxetine. During acute treatment studies (up to 9 weeks), atomoxetine-treated patients lost an average of 0.4 kg, while placebo patients gained an average of 1.5 kg. Weight and height were assessed during open-label studies of 12 and 18 months; mean rates of growth were compared with normal growth curves. Patients treated with atomoxetine for at least

ATOMOXETINE HCl

18 months gained an average of 6.5 kg while mean weight percentile decreased slightly from 68 to 60. For this same group of patients, the average gain in height was 9.3 cm with a slight decrease in mean height percentile from 54 to 50. Whether final adult height or weight is affected by treatment with atomoxetine is unknown. Monitor patients requiring long-term therapy and consider interrupting therapy in patients who are not growing or gaining weight satisfactorily.

►*Hypersensitivity reactions:* Although uncommon, allergic reactions (eg, angioneurotic edema, urticaria, rash) have been reported in patients taking atomoxetine.

►*Pregnancy: Category C.* Pregnant rabbits were treated with up to 100 mg/kg/day (approximately 23 times the maximum human dose on a mg/m² basis) of atomoxetine by gavage throughout the periods of organogenesis. At this dose, in 1 of 3 studies, a decrease in live fetuses and an increase in early resorptions was observed. Slight increases in the incidences of atypical origin of carotid artery and absent subclavian artery were observed. These findings were observed at doses that caused slight maternal toxicity.

Rats were treated with up to approximately 50 mg/kg/day of atomoxetine (approximately 6 times the maximum human dose on a mg/m² basis) in the diet from 2 (females) or 10 (males) weeks prior to mating through the period of organogenesis and lactation. In 1 of 2 studies, decreases in pup weight and pup survival were observed. The decreased pup survival also was seen at 25 mg/kg but not at 13 mg/kg.

No adequate and well-controlled studies have been conducted in pregnant women. Do not use atomoxetine during pregnancy unless the potential benefit justifies the potential risk to the fetus.

►*Lactation:* Atomoxetine and/or its metabolites were excreted in the milk of rats. It is not known if atomoxetine is excreted in human milk. Exercise caution if atomoxetine is administered to a nursing woman.

►*Children:* The safety and efficacy of atomoxetine in pediatric patients less than 6 years of age have not been established. The efficacy of atomoxetine beyond 9 weeks and safety of atomoxetine beyond 1 year of treatment have not been systematically evaluated.

Precautions

►*Cardiac effects:* Use atomoxetine with caution in patients with hypertension, tachycardia, or cardiovascular or cerebrovascular disease because it can increase blood pressure and heart rate. Measure pulse and blood pressure at baseline, following dose increases, and periodically while on therapy.

►*Urinary retention/hesitancy:* In adult ADHD controlled trials, the rates of urinary retention and urinary hesitation (3%, 7/269) were increased among atomoxetine subjects compared with placebo subjects (0%, 0/263). Two adult atomoxetine subjects and no placebo subjects discontinued from controlled clinical trials because of urinary retention. Consider a complaint of urinary retention or urinary hesitancy to be potentially related to atomoxetine.

►*CYP2D6 metabolism:* PMs of CYP2D6 have a 10-fold higher AUC and a 5-fold higher peak concentration to a given dose of atomoxetine compared with EMs. Approximately 7% of the Caucasian population are PMs. The higher blood levels in PMs lead to a higher rate of some adverse events of atomoxetine.

►*Sexual dysfunction:* Atomoxetine appears to impair sexual function in some patients. Changes in sexual desire, performance, and satisfaction are not well assessed in most clinical trials because they need special attention and because patients and physicians may be reluctant to discuss them. Accordingly, estimates of the incidence of untoward sexual experience and performance cited in product labeling are likely to underestimate the actual incidence.

There are no adequate and well-controlled studies examining sexual dysfunction with atomoxetine treatment. While it is difficult to know the precise risk of sexual dysfunction associated with the use of atomoxetine, physicians should routinely inquire about such possible side effects (see Adverse Reactions).

Drug Interactions

Atomoxetine Drug Interactions			
Precipitant drug	Object drug*		Description
Atomoxetine	Albuterol	↑	Administer with caution because the cardiovascular action of albuterol can be potentiated.
CYP2D6 inhibitors	Atomoxetine	↑	Coadministration causes an increase in the AUC and C_max at steady state. Dosage adjustment may be necessary.
MAOIs	Atomoxetine	↑	Coadministration is contraindicated (see Warnings).
Pressor agents	Atomoxetine	↑	Administer with caution because of possible effects on blood pressure.
Atomoxetine	Pressor agents		

* ↑ = Object drug increased.

Adverse Reactions

Atomoxetine was administered to 2067 children or adolescent patients with ADHD and 270 adults with ADHD in clinical studies. During the ADHD clinical trials, 169 patients were treated for longer than 1 year and 526 patients were treated for over 6 months.

►*Children and adolescents:*
Discontinuation of treatment because of adverse events: In acute child and adolescent placebo-controlled trials, 3.5% (15/427) of atomoxetine subjects and 1.4% (4/294) of placebo subjects discontinued for adverse events. For all studies (including open-label and long-term studies), 5% of EMs and 7% of PMs discontinued because of an adverse event. Among atomoxetine-treated patients, aggression, irritability, somnolence, and vomiting (0.5%, n = 2) were the reasons for discontinuation reported by more than 1 patient.

Commonly observed adverse events: The most commonly observed adverse events in patients treated with atomoxetine (incidence of 5% or greater and at least twice the incidence in placebo patients after BID or QD dosing) were the following: Dyspepsia, nausea, vomiting, fatigue, decreased appetite, dizziness, mood swings.

Atomoxetine Common Treatment-Emergent Adverse Reactions in Acute (up to 9 Weeks) Child and Adolescent Trials (%)				
	Percentage of patients reporting from BID trials		Percentage of patients reporting from QD trials	
Adverse reaction	Atomoxetine (N = 340)	Placebo (N = 207)	Atomoxetine (N = 85)	Placebo (N = 85)
CNS				
Headache	27	25	-	-
Irritability	8	5	-	-
Somnolence	7	5	-	-
Dizziness (excluding vertigo)	6	3	-	-
Crying	2	1	-	-
Mood swings	2	0	5	2
GI				
Abdominal pain upper	20	16	16	9
Appetite decreased	14	6	-	-
Vomiting	11	9	15	1
Nausea	7	8	12	2
Dyspepsia	4	2	8	0
Constipation	3	1	0	0
Diarrhea	3	6	4	1
Dry mouth	1	2	4	1
Respiratory				
Cough	11	7	-	-
Rhinorrhea	4	3	-	-
Miscellaneous				
Dermatitis	4	1	-	-
Fatigue	4	5	9	1
Ear infection	3	1	-	-
Influenza	3	1	-	-
Weight decreased	2	0	-	-

The following events were reported by more atomoxetine-treated patients than placebo-treated patients and are possibly related to atomoxetine treatment: Anorexia, blood pressure increased, early morning awakening, flushing, mydriasis, sinus tachycardia, tearfulness. The following events were reported by at least 2% of patients treated with atomoxetine and equal to or less than placebo: Arthralgia, gastroenteritis viral, insomnia, sore throat, nasal congestion, nasopharyngitis, pruritus, sinus congestion, upper respiratory tract infection.

Poor CYP2D6 metabolizers: The following adverse events occurred in at least 2% of PM patients and were twice as frequent or statistically significantly more frequent in PM patients compared with EM patients: Decreased appetite (23% of PMs, 16% of EMs), insomnia (13% of PMs, 7% of EMs), sedation (4% of PMs, 2% of EMs), depression (6% of PMs, 2% of EMs), tremor (4% of PMs, 1% of EMs), early morning awakening (3% of PMs, 1% of EMs), pruritus (2% of PMs, 1% of EMs), mydriasis (2% of PMs, 1% of EMs).

►*Adults:*
Discontinuation of treatment because of adverse events: In the acute adult placebo-controlled trials, 8.5% (23/270) of atomoxetine subjects and 3.4% (9/266) of placebo subjects discontinued for adverse events. Among atomoxetine-treated patients, the reasons for discontinuation reported by more than 1 patient were insomnia (1.1%, n = 3); chest pain, palpitations, urinary retention (0.7%, n = 2).

ATOMOXETINE HCl

Atomoxetine Common Treatment-Emergent Adverse Reactions in Acute (up to 10 Weeks) Adult Trials (%)		
Adverse reaction	Atomoxetine (n = 269)	Placebo (n = 263)
Cardiovascular		
Palpitations	4	1
Hot flushes	3	1
CNS		
Headache	17	17
Insomnia and/or middle insomnia	16	8
Dizziness	6	2
Libido decreased	6	2
Abnormal dreams	4	3
Paresthesia	4	2
Sleep disorder	4	2
Sinus headache	3	1
Dermatologic		
Sweating increased	4	1
Dermatitis	2	1
GI		
Dry mouth	21	6
Nausea	12	5
Appetite decreased	10	3
Constipation	10	4
Dyspepsia	6	4
Flatulence	2	1
GU		
Urinary hesitation and/or urinary retention and/or difficulty in micturition	8	0
Dysmenorrhea[1]	7	3
Erectile disturbance[2]	7	1
Ejaculation failure and/or ejaculation disorder[2]	5	2

Atomoxetine Common Treatment-Emergent Adverse Reactions in Acute (up to 10 Weeks) Adult Trials (%)		
Adverse reaction	Atomoxetine (n = 269)	Placebo (n = 263)
Impotence[2]	3	0
Menstrual disorder[1]	3	2
Prostatitis[2]	3	0
Menses delayed[1]	2	1
Menstruation irregular[1]	2	0
Orgasm abnormal	2	1
Miscellaneous		
Fatigue and/or lethargy	7	4
Sinusitis	6	4
Myalgia	3	2
Pyrexia	3	2
Rigors	3	1
Weight decreased	2	1

[1] Based on total number of females (atomoxetine, n = 95; placebo, n = 91).
[2] Based on total number of males (atomoxetine, n = 174; placebo, n = 172).

The following events were reported by more atomoxetine-treated patients than placebo-treated patients and are possibly related to atomoxetine treatment: Early morning awakening, peripheral coldness, tachycardia. The following events were reported by at least 2% of patients treated with atomoxetine and equal to or less than placebo: Abdominal pain upper, arthralgia, back pain, cough, diarrhea, influenza, irritability, nasopharyngitis, sore throat, upper respiratory tract infection, vomiting.

Overdosage

The effects of overdose greater than twice the maximum recommended daily dose in humans are unknown. Patients who overdose with atomoxetine should be monitored carefully and receive supportive care. Gastric emptying and repeated activated charcoal (with or without cathartics) may prevent systemic absorption.

Psychotherapeutic Combinations

OLANZAPINE AND FLUOXETINE HCl

Rx	**Symbyax** (Eli Lilly)	**Capsules:** 6 mg olanzapine/25 mg fluoxetine	Mustard yellow/Lt. yellow. In 30s, 100s, 1000s, and blister UD 100s.
		6 mg olanzapine/50 mg fluoxetine	Mustard yellow/Lt. grey. In 30s, 100s, 1000s, and blister UD 100s.
		12 mg olanzapine/25 mg fluoxetine	Red/Lt. yellow. In 30s, 100s, 1000s, and blister UD 100s.
		12 mg olanzapine/50 mg fluoxetine	Red/Lt. grey. In 30s, 100s, 1000s, and blister UD 100s.

For additional information, refer to the Selective Serotonin Reuptake Inhibitors and the Antipsychotic Agents group monographs.

Indications

▶*Bipolar disorder:* For the treatment of depressive episodes associated with bipolar disorder.

Administration and Dosage

Administer once daily in the evening, generally beginning with the 6 mg/25 mg capsule. While food has no appreciable effect on the absorption of olanzapine and fluoxetine given individually, the effect of food on the absorption of olanzapine/fluoxetine has not been studied. Dosage adjustments, if indicated, can be made according to efficacy and tolerability. Antidepressant efficacy was demonstrated with olanzapine/fluoxetine in a dose range of olanzapine 6 to 12 mg and fluoxetine 25 to 50 mg. The safety of doses above 18 mg/75 mg has not been evaluated in clinical studies.

▶*Special populations:* Use a starting dose of 6 mg/25 mg for patients with a predisposition to hypotensive reactions, patients with hepatic impairment, or patients who exhibit a combination of factors that may slow the metabolism of olanzapine/fluoxetine (eg, female gender, elderly, nonsmoking status). When indicated, perform dose escalation with caution in these patients. Olanzapine/fluoxetine has not been systemically studied in patients older than 65 years of age or in patients younger than 18 years of age.

▶*Storage/Stability:* Store at 25°C (77°F); excursions permitted to 15° to 30°C (59° to 86°F). Keep tightly closed and protect from moisture.

CHLORDIAZEPOXIDE AND AMITRIPTYLINE

c-iv	**Chlordiazepoxide and Amitriptyline** (Various, eg, Geneva, Lemmon, Par)	**Tablets:** 5 mg chlordiazepoxide and 12.5 mg amitriptyline	In 100s and 500s.
c-iv	**Chlordiazepoxide and Amitriptyline** (Various, eg, Goldline, Lemmon)	**Tablets:** 10 mg chlordiazepoxide and 25 mg amitriptyline	In 100s and 500s.
c-iv	**Limbitrol DS 10-25** (Roche)		(Limbitrol DS). White. Film coated. In 100s, 500s, unit-of-use 50s and UD 100s.

Consider the prescribing information for chlordiazepoxide in the Anti-anxiety Agents monograph and amitriptyline in the Antidepressants monograph.

Indications

Treatment of moderate to severe depression associated with moderate to severe anxiety. The therapeutic response to this combination has occurred earlier and with fewer treatment failures than when either ingredient is used alone. Symptoms likely to respond in the first week of treatment include: Insomnia; feelings of guilt or worthlessness; agitation; psychic and somatic anxiety; suicidal ideation; anorexia.

Administration and Dosage

Initially, administer 10 mg chlordiazepoxide with 25 mg amitriptyline 3 or 4 times daily in divided doses; increase to 6 times daily, as required. Some patients respond to smaller doses and can be maintained on 2 tablets daily.

After a satisfactory response is obtained, reduce dosage to smallest amount needed. The larger portion of the total daily dose may be taken at bedtime. In some patients, a single dose at bedtime may be sufficient. In general, lower dosages are recommended for elderly patients.

CHLORDIAZEPOXIDE AND AMITRIPTYLINE

Contraindications

Hypersensitivity to either benzodiazepines or tricyclic antidepressants; concomitant monoamine oxidase inhibitors (MAOIs; see Drug Interactions); during the acute recovery phase following myocardial infarction.

Drug Interactions

➤*MAOIs:* Hyperpyretic crises, severe convulsions and deaths have occurred in patients receiving a tricyclic antidepressant and an MAOI simultaneously. When it is desired to replace an MAOI with this com-bination, allow a minimum of 14 days to elapse after the former is dis-continued. Cautiously initiate this combination with a gradual increase in dosage until optimum response is achieved.

Patient Information

May cause drowsiness or dizziness; use caution while driving or per-forming other tasks requiring alertness.

Avoid alcohol and other CNS depressants.

Consult a physician before either increasing the dose or abruptly dis-continuing the drug.

PERPHENAZINE AND AMITRIPTYLINE HCl

Rx	**Perphenazine/Amitriptyline** (Various, eg, Bolar, Geneva, Goldline, Lemmon, Par, Rugby, Zenith)	**Tablets:** 2 mg perphenazine and 10 mg ami-triptyline	In 21s, 100s, 500s and 1000s.
Rx	Etrafon 2-10 (Schering)		(Schering ANA or 287). Yellow. In 500s.
Rx	Triavil 2-10 (Lotus Biochemical)		Lactose (LB/2-10). Blue, Triangular, convex-coated. In 100s and 500s.
Rx	**Perphenazine/Amitriptyline** (Various, eg, Bolar, Geneva, Goldline, Lemmon, Par, Rugby, Zenith)	**Tablets:** 2 mg perphenazine and 25 mg ami-triptyline	In 100s, 500s and 1000s.
Rx	Etrafon (Schering)		(Schering ANC or 598). Pink. Sugar coated. In 500s.
Rx	Triavil 2-25 (Lotus Biochemical)		Lactose. (LB/2-25). Lt. orange, triangular, convex-coated. In 100s and 500s.
Rx	**Perphenazine/Amitriptyline** (Various, eg, Bolar, Geneva, Goldline, Lemmon, Par, Rugby, Zenith)	**Tablets:** 4 mg perphenazine and 10 mg ami-triptyline	In 100s, 250s, 500s and 1000s.
Rx	Etrafon-A (Schering)		(Schering ANB or 119). Orange. In 100s, 500s, UD 100s.
Rx	Triavil 4-10 (Lotus Biochemical)		Lactose. (LB/4-10). Beige, triangular, convex-coated. In 100s and 500s.
Rx	**Perphenazine/Amitriptyline** (Various, eg, Bolar, Geneva, Goldline, Lemmon, Par, Rugby, Zenith)	**Tablets:** 4 mg perphenazine and 25 mg ami-triptyline	In 100s, 500s, 800s and 1000s.
Rx	Etrafon-Forte (Schering)		(Schering ANE or 720). Red. Sugar coated. In 500s.
Rx	Triavil 4-25 (Lotus Biochemical)		Lactose. (LB/4-25). Yellow, triangular, convex-coated. In 100s and 500s.
Rx	**Perphenazine/Amitriptyline** (Various, eg, Bolar, Geneva, Goldline, Lemmon, Par, Rugby, Zenith)	**Tablets:** 4 mg perphenazine and 50 mg ami-triptyline	In 100s and 250s.

Consider the prescribing information for perphenazine in the Antipsy-chotic Agents monograph and amitriptyline in the Antidepressants monograph.

Indications

Treatment of moderate to severe anxiety or agitation and depressed mood; patients with depression in whom anxiety or agitation are mod-erate or severe; patients with anxiety and depression associated with chronic physical disease; patients in whom depression and anxiety can-not be clearly differentiated; schizophrenic patients who have associ-ated symptoms of depression.

Many patients presenting symptoms such as agitation, anxiety, insom-nia, psychomotor retardation, functional somatic complaints, tiredness, loss of interest and anorexia have responded well to this combination.

Administration and Dosage

Initially, 2 to 4 mg perphenazine with 10 to 50 mg amitriptyline, 3 or 4 times daily. After a satisfactory response is noted, reduce to smallest amount necessary to obtain relief. Not recommended for use in children.

Patient Information

May cause drowsiness or dizziness, and response to alcohol and other CNS depressants may be enhanced. Use caution while driving or per-forming other tasks requiring alertness.

ERGOLOID MESYLATES (Dihydrogenated Ergot Alkaloids, Dihydroergotoxine)

Rx	**Ergoloid Mesylates** (Various, eg, Ivax, Major, Mutual, URL)	**Tablets, sublingual:** 1 mg	In 100s, 500s, 1000s and UD 100s.
Rx	**Ergoloid Mesylates** (Various, eg, Ivax, Major, Mutual, URL)	**Tablets, oral:** 1 mg	In 60s, 100s, 500s, 1000s and UD 32s, 100s and 1000s.

Indications

➤*Age-related mental capacity decline:* Individuals over 60 years of age who manifest signs and symptoms of an idiopathic decline in men-tal capacity (ie, cognitive and interpersonal skills, mood, self-care, apparent motivation). Patients who respond suffer from some process related to aging or have some underlying dementing condition (ie, pri-mary progressive dementia; Alzheimer's dementia; senile onset; multi-infarct dementia).

Administration and Dosage

The usual starting dose is 1 mg 3 times daily. Alleviation of symptoms is usually gradual; results may not be observed for 3 to 4 weeks. Doses up to 4.5 to 12 mg/day have been used. Up to 6 months of treatment may be necessary to determine efficacy, using doses of at least 6 mg/day.

Actions

➤*Pharmacology:* Ergoloid mesylates contain equal proportions of dihydroergocornine mesylate, dihydroergocristine mesylate and dihy-droergocryptine mesylate.

The mechanism by which ergoloid mesylates produce mental effects is unknown. There is no conclusive evidence they directly affect cerebral arteriosclerosis or cerebrovascular insufficiency. Formerly, it was believed this drug caused cerebral vasodilation by alpha-adrenergic blockade; recent evidence suggests it may act primarily to increase brain metabolism, possibly increasing cerebral blood flow. It does not possess the vasoconstrictor properties of the natural ergot alkaloids.

➤*Pharmacokinetics:* Ergoloid mesylates are rapidly absorbed from the GI tract; peak plasma concentrations are achieved within 0.6 to 3 hours. The drug undergoes rapid first-pass biotransformation in the liver. Sys-temic bioavailability is approximately 6% to 25%. The liquid capsule has a 12% greater bioavailability than the oral tablet. The mean half-life of unchanged ergoloid in plasma is about 2.6 to 5.1 hours.

➤*Clinical trials:* In efficacy studies, modest but statistically signifi-cant changes were observed at the end of 12 weeks in the following parameters: Mental alertness, confusion, recent memory, orientation, emotional lability, self-care, depression, anxiety/fears, cooperation, sociability, appetite, dizziness, fatigue, bothersomeness and an overall impression of clinical status.

Contraindications

Hypersensitivity to ergoloid mesylates.

Acute or chronic psychosis, regardless of etiology.

Precautions

➤*Before prescribing:* Before prescribing ergoloid mesylates, exclude the possibility that the patient's signs and symptoms arise from a potentially reversible and treatable condition. Exclude delirium and dementiform illness secondary to systemic disease, primary neurologi-cal disease or primary disturbance of mood.

➤*Reassess diagnosis:* Periodically reassess the diagnosis and the benefit of current therapy to the patient.

Do not chew or crush sublingual tablets.

Adverse Reactions

Sublingual irritation; transient nausea; GI disturbances.

Patient Information

May cause transient nausea and GI disturbances.

Allow sublingual tablets to completely dissolve under tongue.

The following is a general discussion of nonbarbiturate sedative/hypnotics.

To facilitate comparison, the products are divided into two groups: The miscellaneous nonbarbiturates and the benzodiazepines. Although sedative doses can be given, these agents are primarily intended to be hypnotics (agents that produce drowsiness and facilitate sleep). Agents intended primarily for sedation or tranquilization are discussed in other parts of this chapter.

In the table below, some pharmacokinetic properties of the nonbarbiturate sedative/hypnotics are compared. Do not use this table to predict exact duration of effect, but use as a guide in drug selection.

Nonbarbiturate Sedative/Hypnotics Pharmacokinetic Parameters

| Drug | Adult oral dose | | Onset (min) | Duration of action (hrs) | Half-life (hrs) | Protein binding (%) | Urinary excretion, unchanged (%) |
	Hypnotic	Sedative					
Imidazopyridines							
Zolpidem	10 mg	na*	nd*	nd*	≈ 2.5	92.5	0
Ureides							
Acetylcarbromal	nd*	250-500 mg bid or tid	nd*	nd*	nd*	nd*	nd*
Tertiary Acetylenic Alcohols							
Ethchlorvynol	500 mg	100-200 mg bid or tid	15-60	5	10-20[2]	nd*	40[3]
Piperidine Derivatives							
Glutethimide	250-500 mg	nd*	30	4-8	10-12	50	< 2
Benzodiazepines							
Estazolam	1-2 mg	na*	nd*	nd*	10-24	93	< 5
Flurazepam	15-30 mg	na*	17	7-8	50-100[4]	97	< 1[4]
Quazepam	15 mg	na*	nd*	nd*	25-41	> 95	trace
Temazepam	15-30 mg	na*	nd*	nd*	10-17	98	1.5
Triazolam	0.125-0.5 mg	na*	nd*	nd*	1.5-5.5	90	2
Miscellaneous nonbarbiturates							
Chloral hydrate	0.5-1 g	250 mg tid pc	30	nd*	7-10[1]	35-41	nd*
Paraldehyde	10-30 ml	5-10 ml	10-15	8-12	3.4-9.8	nd*	small
Propiomazine	nd*	10-20 mg	nd*	nd*	nd*	nd*	nd*

* na – Not applicable.   nd = No data.
[1] Trichloroethanol, the principal metabolite.
[2] In acute use, half-life of the distribution phase (1 to 3 hours) is more appropriate.
[3] Free and conjugated forms of the major metabolite, secondary alcohol of ethchlorvynol.
[4] Active metabolite, desalkylflurazepam.

Imidazopyridines

ZOLPIDEM TARTRATE

c-iv	**Ambien** (Sanofi)	**Tablets:** 5 mg	Lactose. (AMB 5 5401). Pink. Film coated. In 100s, 500s and UD 100s.
		10 mg	Lactose. (AMB 10 5421). White. Film coated. In 100s, 500s and UD 100s.

Refer to the general discussion beginning in the Sedatives and Hypnotics, Nonbarbiturate introduction.

Indications

➤*Insomnia:* Short-term treatment.

Administration and Dosage

➤*Adults:* Individualize dosage. Usual dose is 10 mg immediately before bedtime.

Downward dosage adjustment may be necessary when given with agents having known CNS depressant effects because of the potentially additive effects.

➤*Elderly or debilitated patients:* Elderly or debilitated patients may be especially sensitive to the effects of zolpidem. Patients with hepatic insufficiency do not clear the drug as rapidly as healthy individuals. An initial 5 mg dose is recommended in these patients.

➤*Maximum dose:* The total dose should not exceed 10 mg.

Actions

➤*Pharmacology:* Zolpidem is a non-benzodiazepine hypnotic of the imidazopyridine class. Subunit modulation of the GABA receptor chloride channel macromolecular complex is hypothesized to be responsible for sedative, anticonvulsant, anxiolytic and myorelaxant drug properties. The major modulatory site of the GABA receptor complex is located on its alpha subunit and is referred to as the benzodiazepine (BZ) or omega receptor. At least three subtypes of the omega receptor have been identified. While zolpidem is a hypnotic agent with a chemical structure unrelated to benzodiazepines, barbiturates or other drugs with known hypnotic properties, it interacts with a GABA-BZ receptor complex and shares some of the pharmacological properties of the benzodiazepines. In contrast to the benzodiazepines, which non-selectively bind to and activate all three omega receptor subtypes, zolpidem in vitro binds the omega$_1$ receptor preferentially. This selective binding of zolpidem on the omega$_1$ receptor is not absolute, but it may explain the relative absence of myorelaxant and anticonvulsant effects in animal studies as well as the preservation of deep sleep (stage 3 through 4) in human studies of zolpidem at hypnotic doses.

➤*Pharmacokinetics:* The pharmacokinetic profile is characterized by rapid absorption from the GI tract and a short elimination half-life in healthy subjects. In a single-dose crossover study in 45 healthy subjects administered 5 and 10mg, the mean peak concentrations (C_{max}) were 59 (range, 29 to 113) and 121 (range, 58 to 272)ng/ml, respectively, occurring at a mean time (T_{max}) of 1.6 hours for both. The mean elimi-

nation half-life was 2.6 (range, 1.4 to 4.5) and 2.5 (range, 1.4 to 3.8) hours for the 5 and 10mg tablets, respectively. Zolpidem is converted to inactive metabolites that are eliminated primarily by renal excretion. Total protein binding was 92.5% and remained constant, independent of concentration between 40 and 790 ng/ml. Zolpidem did not accumulate in young adults following 20 mg/night for 2 weeks.

The half-life, bioavailability and C_{max} of zolpidem are increased in elderly patients and patients with hepatic function impairment (see Warnings). Food decreases the bioavailability and C_{max} of zolpidem (see Drug Interactions).

In patients with end stage renal failure, zolpidem was not hemodialyzable. No accumulation of unchanged drug appeared after 14 or 21 days. Zolpidem pharmacokinetics were not significantly different in renally impaired patients; therefore, no dosage adjustment is necessary in patients with compromised renal function. However, as a general precaution, closely monitor these patients.

➤*Clinical trials:*

Transient insomnia – Healthy adults experiencing transient insomnia during the first night in a sleep laboratory were evaluated in a double-blind, parallel-group, single-night trial comparing 2 doses of zolpidem (7.5 and 10 mg) and placebo. Both doses were superior to placebo on objective (polysomnographic) measures of sleep latency, sleep duration and number of awakenings.

Chronic insomnia – Adult outpatients with chronic insomnia were evaluated in a double-blind, parallel group, 5 week trial comparing 2 doses of zolpidem tartrate (10 and 15 mg) and placebo. On objective (polysomnographic) measures of sleep latency and sleep efficiency, zolpidem 15 mg was superior to placebo for all 5 weeks; zolpidem 10 mg was superior to placebo on sleep latency for the first 4 weeks and on sleep efficiency for weeks 2 and 4. Zolpidem was comparable to placebo on number of awakenings at both doses studied. Another group was evaluated in a double-blind, parallel-group, 4 week trial comparing 2 doses of zolpidem (10 and 15 mg) and placebo. Zolpidem 10 mg was superior to placebo on a subjective measure of sleep latency for all 4 weeks, and on subjective measures of total sleep time, number of awakenings, and sleep quality for the first treatment week. Zolpidem 15 mg was superior to placebo on a subjective measure of sleep latency for the first 3 weeks, on a subjective measure of total sleep time for the first week, and on number of awakenings and sleep quality for the first 2 weeks.

Next-day residual effects – There was no evidence of residual next-day effects seen with zolpidem in several studies utilizing the Multiple

ZOLPIDEM TARTRATE

Sleep Latency Test (MSLT), the Digit Symbol Substitution Test (DSST) and patient ratings of alertness. In one study involving elderly patients, there was a small but statistically significant decrease in one measure of performance, the DSST, but no impairment was seen in the MSLT.

Rebound effects – There was no objective (polysomnographic) evidence of rebound insomnia at recommended doses in studies evaluating sleep on the nights following discontinuation of zolpidem. There was subjective evidence of impaired sleep in the elderly on the first post-treatment night at doses above the recommended elderly dose of 5 mg.

Memory impairment – Two small studies utilizing objective measures of memory yielded little evidence for memory impairment following zolpidem. There was subjective evidence from adverse event data for anterograde amnesia occurring in association with the administration of zolpidem predominantly at doses > 10 mg.

Effects on sleep stages – In studies that measured the percentage of sleep time spent in each sleep stage, zolpidem generally preserves sleep stages. Sleep time spent in stage 3 to 4 (deep sleep) was found comparable to placebo with only inconsistent, minor changes in REM (paradoxical) sleep at the recommended dose.

Warnings

▶ *Duration of therapy:* Generally limit hypnotics to 7 to 10 days of use; re-evaluate the patient if they are to be taken for > 2 to 3 weeks. Do not prescribe in quantities exceeding a 1 month supply.

▶ *Psychiatric / physical disorder:* Since sleep disturbances may be the presenting manifestation of a physical or psychiatric disorder, initiate symptomatic treatment of insomnia only after a careful evaluation of the patient. The failure of insomnia to remit after 7 to 10 days of treatment may indicate the presence of a primary psychiatric or medical illness which should be evaluated. Worsening of insomnia or the emergence of new thinking or behavior abnormalities may be the consequence of an unrecognized psychiatric or physical disorder. Such findings have emerged during the course of treatment with sedative/hypnotic drugs, including zolpidem. Because some of the important adverse effects of zolpidem appear to be dose-related, it is important to use the smallest possible effective dose, especially in the elderly.

A variety of abnormal thinking and behavior changes have occurred in association with the use of sedative/hypnotics. Some of these changes may be characterized by decreased inhibition (eg, aggressiveness and extroversion that seem out of character), similar to effects produced by alcohol and other CNS depressants. Other reported behavior changes have included bizarre behavior, agitation, hallucinations and depersonalization. Amnesia and other neuropsychiatric symptoms may occur unpredictably. In primarily depressed patients, worsening of depression, including suicidal thinking, has occurred with sedative/hypnotics.

It can rarely be determined with certainty whether a particular instance of the abnormal behaviors listed above are drug-induced, spontaneous in origin, or a result of an underlying psychiatric or physical disorder. Nonetheless, the emergence of any new behavioral sign or symptom of concern requires careful and immediate evaluation.

▶ *Abrupt discontinuation:* Following the rapid dose decrease or abrupt discontinuation of sedative/hypnotics, signs and symptoms similar to those associated with withdrawal from other CNS-depressant drugs have occurred (see Precautions).

▶ *CNS-depressant effects:* Zolpidem, like other sedative/hypnotic drugs, has CNS-depressant effects. Due to the rapid onset of action, only ingest immediately prior to going to bed. Caution patients against engaging in hazardous occupations requiring complete mental alertness, motor coordination or physical dexterity after ingesting the drug (ie, operating machinery or driving a motor vehicle), including potential impairment of the performance of such activities that may occur the day following ingestion of zolpidem. Zolpidem had additive effects when combined with alcohol; therefore, do not take with alcohol. Also caution patients about possible combined effects with other CNS-depressant drugs. Dosage adjustments may be necessary when zolpidem is administered with such agents because of the potentially additive effects.

▶ *Renal function impairment:* Data in end stage renal failure patients repeatedly treated with zolpidem did not demonstrate drug accumulation or alterations in pharmacokinetic parameters. No dosage adjustment in renally impaired patients is required; however, closely monitor these patients (see Pharmacokinetics).

▶ *Hepatic function impairment:* The pharmacokinetics of zolpidem in eight patients with chronic hepatic insufficiency were compared to results in healthy subjects. Following a single 20 mg dose, mean C_{max} and area under the concentration-time curve (AUC) were found to be 2 times (250 vs 499 ng/ml) and 5 times (788 vs 4203 ng•hr/ml) higher, respectively, in the hepatically compromised patients; T_{max} did not change. The mean half-life in cirrhotic patients of 9.9 hrs (range, 4.1 to 25.8 hrs) was greater than that observed in healthy subjects of 2.2 hrs (range, 1.6 to 2.4 hrs). Modify dosing accordingly in patients with hepatic insufficiency (see Administration and Dosage).

▶ *Carcinogenesis:* Zolpidem was administered to rats and mice for 2 years at dosages of 4, 18 and 80 mg/kg/day (26 to 876 times the maxi-

mum recommended human dose on a mg/kg basis). Renal liposarcomas were seen in 4/100 rats (3 males, 1 female) receiving 80 mg/kg/day and a renal lipoma was observed in one male rat at the 18mg/kg/day dose. Incidence rates of lipoma and liposarcoma for zolpidem were comparable to those seen in historical controls and the tumor findings are thought to be a spontaneous occurrence.

▶ *Fertility impairment:* In a rat reproduction study, 100 mg/kg zolpidem resulted in irregular estrus cycles and prolonged precoital intervals, but there was no effect on male or female fertility after daily oral doses of 4 to 100mg.

▶ *Elderly:* Closely monitor these patients. Impaired motor or cognitive performance after repeated exposure or unusual sensitivity to sedative/hypnotic drugs is a concern in the treatment of elderly or debilitated patients. Therefore, the recommended dosage is 5 mg in such patients (see Administration and Dosage) to decrease the possibility of side effects. This recommendation is based on several studies in which the mean C_{max}, half-life and AUC were significantly increased when compared to results in young adults. In one study of eight elderly subjects (> 70 years of age), the means for C_{max}, half-life and AUC significantly increased by 50% (255 vs 384 ng/ml), 32% (2.2 vs 2.9 hrs) and 64% (955 vs 1562 ng•hr/ml), respectively, compared to younger adults (20 to 40 years of age) following a single 20 mg dose. Zolpidem did not accumulate in elderly subjects following nightly oral dosing of 10 mg for 1 week.

▶ *Pregnancy:* Category B. In rats, adverse maternal and fetal effects occurred at 20 and 100 mg/kg and included dose-related maternal lethargy and ataxia, and a dose-related trend to incomplete ossification of fetal skull bones. Underossification of various fetal bones indicates a delay in maturation and is often seen in rats treated with sedative/hypnotic drugs. In rabbits, dose-related maternal sedation and decreased weight gain occurred at all doses tested. At the high dose, 16 mg/kg, there was an increase in postimplantation fetal loss and underossification of sternebrae in viable fetuses. These fetal findings in rabbits are often secondary to reductions in maternal weight gain.

There are no adequate and well controlled studies in pregnant women. Use during pregnancy only if clearly needed. Children born of mothers taking sedative/hypnotic drugs may be at some risk for withdrawal symptoms from the drug during the postnatal period. In addition, neonatal flaccidity has been reported in infants born of mothers who received sedative/hypnotic drugs during pregnancy.

▶ *Lactation:* Studies in lactating mothers indicate that the half-life of zolpidem is similar to that in young healthy volunteers (2.6 hrs). Between 0.004% and 0.019% of the total administered dose is excreted into breast milk, but the effect of zolpidem on the infant is unknown. In a rat study, zolpidem inhibited the secretion of milk. The use of zolpidem in nursing mothers is not recommended.

▶ *Children:* Safety and efficacy in children < 18 years of age have not been established.

Precautions

▶ *Respiratory depression:* Although preliminary studies did not reveal respiratory depressant effects at hypnotic doses in healthy individuals, observe caution if zolpidem is prescribed to patients with compromised respiratory function, since sedative/hypnotics have the capacity to depress respiratory drive.

▶ *Depression:* As with other sedative/hypnotic drugs, administer zolpidem with caution to patients exhibiting signs or symptoms of depression. Suicidal tendencies may be present in such patients and protective measures may be required. Intentional overdosage is more common in this group of patients; therefore, prescribe the least amount of drug that is feasible for the patient at any one time.

▶ *Drug abuse and dependence:* Studies of abuse potential in former drug abusers found that the effects of single doses of zolpidem 40 mg were similar, but not identical, to diazepam 20 mg, while zolpidem 10 mg was difficult to distinguish from placebo.

Sedative/hypnotics have produced withdrawal signs and symptoms following abrupt discontinuation. These reported symptoms range from mild dysphoria and insomnia to a withdrawal syndrome that may include abdominal and muscle cramps, vomiting, sweating, tremors and convulsions. Zolpidem does not reveal any clear evidence for withdrawal syndrome. Nevertheless, the following adverse events included in DSM-III-R criteria for uncomplicated sedative/hypnotic withdrawal were reported during US clinical trials with zolpidem following placebo substitution and occurred within 48 hours following last zolpidem treatment: Fatigue, nausea, flushing, lightheadedness, uncontrolled crying, emesis, stomach cramps, panic attack, nervousness, abdominal discomfort (≤ 1%).

Because individuals with a history of addiction to, or abuse of, drugs or alcohol are at risk of habituation and dependence, they should be under careful surveillance when receiving zolpidem or any other hypnotic.

Drug Interactions

▶ *Drug / Food interactions:* A study of 30 healthy volunteers compared the pharmacokinetics of zolpidem 10 mg when administered while fasting or 20 minutes after a meal. With food, mean AUC and C_{max} were decreased by 15% and 25%, respectively, while mean T_{max}

Imidazopyridines

ZOLPIDEM TARTRATE

was prolonged by 60% (from 1.4 to 2.2 hours). The half-life remained unchanged. For faster sleep onset, do not administer with or immediately after a meal.

Adverse Reactions

Approximately 4% to 6% of patients who received zolpidem at all doses discontinued treatment because of an adverse clinical event. Events most commonly associated with discontinuation were daytime drowsiness (0.5% to 1.6%), amnesia (0.6%), dizziness (0.4% to 0.6%), headache (0.5% to 0.6%), nausea (0.6%) and vomiting (0.5%).

During short-term treatment (up to 10 nights) at doses up to 10 mg, the most commonly observed adverse events were as follows: Drowsiness (2%), dizziness (1%) and diarrhea (1%). During longer term treatment (28 to 35 nights) with doses up to 10 mg, the most commonly observed adverse events were dizziness (5%) and drugged feelings (3%).

Zolpidem Adverse Reactions (Short-Term Trials[1]) (%)		
Adverse reaction	Zolpidem (≤ 10mg) (n = 685)	Placebo (n = 473)
Central and peripheral nervous system		
Headache	7	6
Drowsiness	2	—
Dizziness	1	—
GI		
Nausea	2	3
Diarrhea	1	—
Musculoskeletal		
Myalgia	1	2

[1] From a pool of 11 placebo controlled trials.

Zolpidem Adverse Reactions (Long-Term Trials[1]) (%)		
Adverse reaction	Zolpidem (≤ 10 mg) (n =152)	Placebo (n = 161)
Central and peripheral nervous system		
Headache	19	22
Drowsiness	8	5
Dizziness	5	1
Lethargy	3	1
Drugged feeling	3	—
Lightheaded	2	1
Depression	2	1
Abnormal dreams	1	—
Amnesia	1	—
Anxiety	1	1
Nervousness	1	3
Sleep disorder	1	—
GI		
Nausea	6	6
Dyspepsia	5	6
Diarrhea	3	2
Abdominal pain	2	2
Constipation	2	1
Anorexia	1	1
Vomiting	1	1
Musculoskeletal		
Myalgia	7	7
Arthralgia	4	4
Respiratory		
Upper respiratory tract infection	5	6
Sinusitis	4	2
Pharyngitis	3	1
Rhinitis	1	3
Miscellaneous		
Allergy	4	1
Back pain	3	2
Dry mouth	3	1
Urinary tract infection	2	2
Rash	2	1
Influenza-like symptoms	2	—
Palpitation	2	—
Chest pain	1	—
Fatigue	1	2
Infection	1	1

[1] Treatment of chronic insomnia for 28 to 35 nights.

Other adverse reactions reported with zolpidem are as follows:

➤*Cardiovascular:* Cerebrovascular disorder, hypertension, tachycardia (0.1% to 1%); arrhythmia, arteritis, circulatory failure, extrasystoles, hypertension, aggravated myocardial infarction, phlebitis, pulmonary embolism, pulmonary edema, varicose veins, ventricular tachycardia (< 0.1%).

➤*CNS:* Ataxia, confusion, euphoria, insomnia, vertigo (> 1%); agitation, decreased cognition, detachment, difficulty concentrating, dysarthria, emotional lability, hallucination, hypoesthesia, migraine, paresthesia, sleeping (after daytime dosing), stupor, tremor (0.1% to 1%); abnormal thinking, aggressive reaction, appetite increased, decreased libido, delusion, dementia, depersonalization, dysphasia, feeling strange, hypotonia, hysteria, illusion, intoxicated feeling, leg cramps, manic reaction, neuralgia, neuritis, neuropathy, neurosis, panic attacks, paresis, personality disorder, somnambulism, suicide attempts, tetany, yawning (< 0.1%).

Autonomic nervous system – Increased sweating, pallor, postural hypotension (0.1% to 1%); altered saliva, flushing, glaucoma, hypotension, impotence, syncope, tenesmus (< 0.1%).

➤*Dermatologic:* Acne, bullous eruption, dermatitis, furunculosis, injection-site inflammation, photosensitivity reaction, urticaria (< 0.1%).

➤*GI:* Constipation, dysphagia, flatulence, gastroenteritis, hiccup (0.1% to 1%); enteritis, eructation, esophagospasm, gastritis, hemorrhoids, intestinal obstruction, rectal hemorrhage, tooth caries (< 0.1%).

➤*GU:* Cystitis, urinary incontinence (0.1% to 1%); acute renal failure, dysuria, micturition frequency, polyuria, pyelonephritis, renal pain, urinary retention (< 0.1%).

Reproductive – Menstrual disorder, vaginitis (0.1% to 1%); breast fibroadenosis/neoplasm/pain (< 0.1%).

➤*Hematologic/Lymphatic:* Anemia, hyperhemoglobinemia, leukopenia, lymphadenopathy, macrocytic anemia, purpura (0.1%).

➤*Hepatic:* Increased ALT (0.1% to 1%); abnormal hepatic function, bilirubinemia, increased AST (< 0.1%).

➤*Metabolic/Nutritional:* Hyperglycemia (0.1% to 1%); gout, hypercholesterolemia, hyperlipidemia, increased BUN, periorbital edema, thirst, weight decrease (< 0.1%).

➤*Musculoskeletal:* Arthritis (0.1% to 1%); arthrosis, muscle weakness, sciatica, tendinitis (< 0.1%).

➤*Respiratory:* Bronchitis, coughing, dyspnea (0.1% to 1%); bronchospasm, epistaxis, hypoxia, laryngitis, pneumonia (< 0.1%).

➤*Special senses:* Diplopia, vision abnormal (> 1%); eye irritation/pain, scleritis, taste perversion, tinnitus (0.1% to 1%); corneal ulceration, abnormal lacrimation, photopsia (< 0.1%).

➤*Miscellaneous:* Asthenia, edema, falling, fever, malaise, trauma (0.1% to 1%); allergic reaction, allergy aggravated, abdominal body sensation, anaphylactic shock, face edema, hot flashes, increased ESR, pain, restless legs, rigors, tolerance increased, weight decrease (< 0.1%);menstrual disorder, vaginitis (0.1% to 1%); breast fibroadenosis/neoplasm/pain (< 0.1%).

Immunologic – Abscess, herpes simplex/zoster, otitis externa/media (< 0.1%).

Overdosage

➤*Symptoms:* In reports of overdose with zolpidem alone, impairment of consciousness has ranged from somnolence to light coma. There was one case each of cardiovascular and respiratory compromise. Individuals have fully recovered from zolpidem overdoses up to 400 mg (40 times the maximum recommended dose). Overdose cases involving multiple CNS depressant agents, including zolpidem, have resulted in more severe symptomatology, including fatal outcomes.

➤*Treatment:* Employ general symptomatic and supportive measures along with immediate gastric lavage where appropriate. Administer IV fluids as needed. Refer to General Management of Acute Overdosage. Flumazenil may be useful; in one study it reversed the sedative/hypnotic effects of zolpidem; however, no significant alterations in zolpidem pharmacokinetics were found. Monitor hypotension and CNS depression; treat with appropriate medical intervention. Withhold sedating drugs following overdosage, even if excitation occurs. The value of dialysis in treating overdosage is not determined; hemodialysis studies in patients with renal failure receiving therapeutic doses have demonstrated that zolpidem is not dialyzable.

Patient Information

May cause drowsiness; use caution when performing tasks requiring alertness, coordination or physical dexterity. Avoid alcohol and other CNS depressants while taking this drug.

Ureides

ACETYLCARBROMAL

| Rx | Paxarel (Circle) | Tablets: 250 mg | In 100s. |

Refer to the general discussion beginning in the Sedatives and Hypnotics, Nonbarbiturate introduction.

Indications

Anxiety states; emotional stress; menopausal syndrome; premenstrual tension; insomnia; preoperative or preexamination sedation; fears and psychogenic complications of organic illness; spastic colitis; postoperative and posttraumatic sedation.

Administration and Dosage

➤*Adults:* 250 to 500 mg 2 or 3 times daily.

➤*Children:* Administer proportionately less, according to age and weight.

Actions

➤*Pharmacology:* Acetylcarbromal is a short-acting CNS depressant used as a daytime sedative and as a hypnotic. It releases free bromide which may lead to bromide intoxication. It is metabolized to urea and is readily eliminated. It has generally been replaced by safer, more effective products.

Contraindications

Sensitivity to bromides.

Warnings

➤*Habit formation:* May be habit forming. Should not be used chronically.

➤*Lactation:* Bromides are excreted in breast milk and may cause drowsiness and symptoms of brominism in the nursing infant.

Adverse Reactions

Large doses may cause drowsiness.

Overdosage

➤*Symptoms:* Poisoning with the ureides occurs more often with chronic use than with acute ingestion. Brominism occurs with accumulation of the bromide ion and its displacement of chloride in body fluids. Symptoms related to the CNS, skin, exocrine glands and the GI tract include narcosis, respiratory depression, mental disturbances, impaired thought and memory, dizziness, irritability, dermatitis, conjunctivitis, headache, constipation and gastric distress. Bromide intoxication occurs when serum levels exceed 9 mEq/L.

➤*Treatment:* Treat mild to moderate poisoning by gastric lavage and forced diuresis. Chloride loading with sodium chloride (at least 6 g/day) or ammonium chloride is also useful. Use dialysis when salt loading is contraindicated, when diuresis is not achieved or when serum bromide levels exceed 20 mEq/L. Charcoal hemoperfusion may be effective. Refer also to General Management of Acute Overdosage.

Patient Information

May cause drowsiness; use caution while driving or performing other tasks requiring alertness.

Avoid alcohol and other CNS depressants.

ZALEPLON

c-iv	**Sonata** (King)	**Capsules:** 5 mg	Lactose, tartrazine. (5 mg SONATA). Green/pale green. In 100s.
		10 mg	Lactose, tartrazine. (10 mg SONATA). Green/lt. green. In 100s.

Indications

➤*Insomnia:* Short-term treatment of insomnia.

Administration and Dosage

➤*Approved by the FDA:* August 13, 1999.

The recommended dose of zaleplon for most nonelderly adults is 10 mg. For certain low-weight individuals, 5 mg may be a sufficient dose. Although the risk of certain adverse events associated with zaleplon appears to be dose dependent, the 20 mg dose has been shown to be adequately tolerated and may be considered for the occasional patient who does not benefit from a trial of a lower dose. Doses > 20 mg have not been adequately evaluated and are not recommended. Hypnotics should generally be limited to 7 to 10 days of use, and reevaluation of the patient is recommended if they are to be taken for > 2 to 3 weeks.

Take zaleplon immediately before bedtime or after going to bed and experiencing difficulty falling asleep. Taking it with or immediately after a heavy, high-fat meal results in slower absorption and would be expected to reduce the effect of zaleplon on sleep latency.

➤*Elderly/Debilitated:* Elderly and debilitated patients appear to be more sensitive to the effects of hypnotics; therefore, the recommended dose for these patients is 5 mg. Doses > 10 mg are not recommended.

➤*Hepatic function impairment:* Treat patients with mild-to-moderate hepatic impairment with zaleplon 5 mg because of reduced clearance. Do not use in patients with severe hepatic impairment.

➤*Renal function impairment:* No dose adjustment is necessary in patients with mild-to-moderate renal impairment. It has not been adequately studied in patients with severe renal impairment.

Concomitant cimetidine – Give an initial dose of 5 mg to patients concomitantly taking cimetidine (see Drug Interactions).

Actions

➤*Pharmacology:* Zaleplon is a nonbenzodiazepine hypnotic from the pyrazolopyrimidine class. While zaleplon has a chemical structure unrelated to benzodiazepines, barbiturates, or other drugs with known hypnotic properties, it interacts with the GABA-BZ receptor complex. Subunit modulation of the GABA-BZ receptor chloride channel macromolecular complex is hypothesized to be responsible for some of the pharmacological properties of benzodiazepines, which include sedative, anxiolytic, muscle relaxant, and anticonvulsive effects in animal models.

Zaleplon binds selectively to the brain omega-1 receptor situated on the alpha subunit of the $GABA_A$ receptor complex and potentiates t-butyl-bicyclophosphorothionate (TBPS) binding. Studies of binding of zaleplon to purified $GABA_A$ receptors ($\alpha_1\beta_1\gamma_2$ [omega-1] and $\alpha_2\beta_1\gamma_2$ [omega-2]) have shown that zaleplon has a low affinity for these receptors, with preferential binding to the omega-1 receptor.

➤*Pharmacokinetics:*

Absorption – Zaleplon is rapidly and almost completely absorbed following oral administration. Peak plasma concentrations are attained within ≈ 1 hour after oral administration. Although zaleplon is well absorbed, its absolute bioavailability is ≈ 30% because it undergoes significant presystemic metabolism. A high-fat/heavy meal prolongs the absorption of zaleplon (see Drug Interactions).

Distribution – Zaleplon is a lipophilic compound with a volume of distribution of ≈ 1.4 L/kg following IV administration, indicating substantial distribution into extravascular tissues. The in vitro plasma protein binding is ≈ 60% and is independent of zaleplon concentration over the range of 10 to 1000 ng/ml. Zaleplon is uniformly distributed throughout the blood with no extensive distribution into red blood cells.

Metabolism – After oral administration, zaleplon is extensively metabolized with < 1% of the dose excreted unchanged in urine. Zaleplon is primarily metabolized by aldehyde oxidase to form 5-oxo-zaleplon. Zaleplon is metabolized to a lesser extent by CYP3A4 to form desethylzaleplon, which is quickly converted, presumably by aldehyde oxidase, to 5-oxo-desethylzaleplon. These oxidative metabolites are then converted to glucuronides and eliminated in the urine. All of zaleplon's metabolites are pharmacologically inactive.

Excretion – Following oral or IV administration, zaleplon is rapidly eliminated with a mean half-life of ≈ 1 hour. Assuming normal hepatic blood flow and negligible renal clearance of zaleplon, the estimated hepatic extraction ratio of zaleplon is ≈ 0.7, indicating that zaleplon is subject to high first-pass metabolism.

After administration of zaleplon, 70% of the administered dose is recovered in urine within 48 hours (71% recovered within 6 days), nearly all as zaleplon metabolites and their glucuronides. An additional 17% is recovered in feces within 6 days, most as 5-oxo-zaleplon.

Special populations –

Race: In Japanese subjects, C_{max} and AUC were increased 37% and 64%, respectively. This finding can likely be attributed to differences in body weight or, alternatively, may represent differences in enzyme activities resulting from differences in diet, environment, or other factors.

Contraindications

None known.

Warnings

➤*Duration of therapy:* Because sleep disturbances may be the presenting manifestation of a physical or psychiatric disorder, initiate symptomatic treatment of insomnia only after careful evaluation of the patient. The failure of insomnia to remit after 7 to 10 days of treatment may indicate the need for evaluation of a primary psychiatric or medical illness. Worsening of insomnia or the emergence of new thinking or behavior abnormalities may be the consequence of an unrecognized psychiatric or physical disorder. Such findings have emerged during the course of treatment with sedative/hypnotic drugs, including zaleplon. Because some of the important adverse effects of zaleplon appear to be dose-related, it is important to use the lowest possible effective dose, especially in the elderly (see Administration and Dosage). Do not prescribe zaleplon in quantities exceeding a 1-month supply.

➤*Efficacy:* Zaleplon decreased the time to sleep onset for ≤ 28 days in controlled studies. It has not been shown to increase total sleep time or decrease the number of awakenings.

➤*Abnormal thinking/Behavior changes:* A variety of abnormal thinking and behavior changes have been reported to occur in association with the use of sedatives/hypnotics. Some of these changes may be characterized by decreased inhibition (eg, aggressiveness and extroversion that seem out of character), similar to effects produced by alcohol and other CNS depressants. Other reported behavioral changes have included bizarre behavior, agitation, hallucinations, and depersonalization. Amnesia and other neuropsychiatric symptoms may occur unpredictably. In primarily depressed patients, worsening of depression, including suicidal thinking, has been reported in association with the use of sedatives/hypnotics.

It can rarely be determined with certainty whether a particular instance of the abnormal behaviors listed above are drug-induced, spontaneous in origin, or a result of an underlying psychiatric or physical disorder. Nonetheless, the emergence of any new behavioral sign or symptom of concern requires careful and immediate evaluation.

➤*Rapid dose decrease/Discontinuation:* Following rapid dose decrease or abrupt discontinuation of sedatives/hypnotics, there have been reports of signs and symptoms similar to those associated with withdrawal from other CNS-depressant drugs.

➤*CNS effects:* Zaleplon, like other hypnotics, has CNS-depressant effects. Because of the rapid onset of action, zaleplon should only be ingested immediately prior to going to bed or after the patient has gone to bed and has experienced difficulty falling asleep. Caution patients receiving zaleplon against engaging in hazardous occupations requiring complete mental alertness or motor coordination (eg, operating machinery or driving a motor vehicle) after ingesting the drug, including potential impairment of the performance of such activities that may occur the day following zaleplon ingestion. Zaleplon, as well as other hypnotics, may produce additive CNS-depressant effects when coadministered with other psychotropic medications, anticonvulsants, antihistamines, ethanol, and other drugs that produce CNS depression. Do not take zaleplon with alcohol. Dosage adjustment may be necessary when zaleplon is administered with other CNS-depressant agents because of the potentially additive effects.

➤*Renal function impairment:* Because renal excretion of unchanged zaleplon accounts for < 1% of the administered dose, the pharmacokinetics of zaleplon are not altered in patients with renal insufficiency. No dose adjustment is necessary in patients with mild-to-moderate renal impairment. Zaleplon has not been adequately studied in patients with severe renal impairment.

➤*Hepatic function impairment:* Zaleplon is metabolized primarily by the liver and undergoes significant presystemic metabolism. Consequently, the oral clearance of zaleplon was reduced by 70% and 87% in compensated and decompensated cirrhotic patients, respectively, leading to marked increases in mean C_{max} and AUC (≤ 4-fold and 7-fold in compensated and decompensated patients, respectively) compared with healthy subjects. Reduce the dose of zaleplon to 5 mg in patients with mild-to-moderate hepatic impairment (see Administration and Dosage). Zaleplon is not recommended for use in patients with severe hepatic impairment.

➤*Carcinogenesis:* Mice received doses of 25, 50, 100, and 200 mg/kg/day in the diet for 2 years. These doses are equivalent to 6 to 49 times

ZALEPLON

the maximum recommended human dose (MRHD) of 20 mg on a mg/m² basis. There was a significant increase in the incidence of hepatocellular adenomas in female mice in the high-dose group.

➤*Mutagenesis:* Zaleplon was clastogenic, both in the presence and absence of metabolic activation, causing structural and numerical aberrations (polyploidy and endoreduplication) when tested for chromosomal aberrations in the in vitro Chinese hamster ovary cell assay. In the in vitro human lymphocyte assay, zaleplon caused numerical but not structural aberrations in the presence of metabolic activation at the highest concentrations tested.

➤*Fertility impairment:* In a fertility and reproductive performance study in rats, mortality and decreased fertility were associated with a 100 mg/kg/day oral dose of zaleplon to males and females prior to and during mating. This dose is equivalent to 49 times the maximum recommended human dose (MRHD) of 20 mg on a mg/m² basis. Follow-up studies indicated that impaired fertility was due to an effect on the female.

➤*Elderly:* Impaired motor or cognitive performance after repeated exposure or unusual sensitivity to sedative/hypnotic drugs is a concern in the treatment of elderly or debilitated patients. A dose of 5 mg is recommended for elderly patients to decrease the possibility of side effects (see Administration and Dosage). Closely monitor elderly or debilitated patients.

A total of 628 patients in double-blind, placebo-controlled, parallel-group clinical trials who received zaleplon were ≥ 65 years of age; of these, 311 received 5 mg and 317 received 10 mg. In both sleep laboratory and outpatient studies, elderly patients with insomnia responded to a 5 mg dose with a reduced sleep latency. As a result, 5 mg is the recommended dose in this population. During short-term treatment (14-night studies) of elderly patients with zaleplon, no adverse event with a frequency of ≥ 1% occurred at a significantly higher rate with either 5 or 10 mg zaleplon than with placebo.

➤*Pregnancy:* Category C. In rats, pre- and postnatal growth was reduced in the offspring of dams receiving 100 mg/kg/day. This dose was also maternally toxic, as evidenced by clinical signs and decreased maternal body weight gain during gestation. The no-effect dose for rat offspring growth reduction was 10 mg/kg (a dose equivalent to 5 times the MRHD of 20 mg on a mg/m² basis).

In a pre- and postnatal development study in rats, increased stillbirth and postnatal mortality and decreased growth and physical development were observed in the offspring of female rats treated with doses of ≥ 7 mg/kg/day during the latter part of gestation and throughout lactation. There was no evidence of maternal toxicity at this dose. The no-effect dose for offspring development was 1 mg/kg/day (a dose equivalent to 0.5 times the MRHD of 20 mg on a mg/m² basis). When the adverse effects on offspring viability and growth were examined in a cross-fostering study, they appeared to result from both in utero and lactational exposure to the drug.

There are no studies of zaleplon in pregnant women; therefore, it is not recommended for use in women during pregnancy.

➤*Lactation:* A study in lactating mothers indicated the clearance and half-life of zaleplon is similar to that in young healthy subjects. A small amount of zaleplon is excreted in breast milk with the highest excreted amount occurring during a feeding at ≈ 1 hour after administration. Because the effects of zaleplon on a nursing infant are not known, it is recommended that nursing mothers not take zaleplon.

➤*Children:* The safety and efficacy have not been established.

Precautions

➤*Timing of drug administration:* Take zaleplon immediately before bedtime or after going to bed and experiencing difficulty falling asleep. As with all sedatives/hypnotics, taking zaleplon while ambulatory may result in short-term memory impairment, hallucinations, impaired coordination, dizziness, and lightheadedness.

➤*Concomitant illness:* Clinical experience with zaleplon in patients with concomitant systemic illness is limited. Use with caution in patients with diseases or conditions that could affect metabolism or hemodynamic responses.

➤*Respiratory effects:* Although preliminary studies did not reveal respiratory depressant effects at hypnotic doses of zaleplon in healthy subjects, observe caution if zaleplon is prescribed to patients with compromised respiratory function because sedatives/hypnotics have the capacity to depress respiratory drive. Controlled trials of acute administration of 10 mg in patients with chronic obstructive pulmonary disease or moderate obstructive sleep apnea showed no evidence of alterations in blood gases or apnea/hypopnea index, respectively. However, carefully monitor patients with compromised respiration from preexisting illness.

➤*Depression:* As with other sedative/hypnotic drugs, administer zaleplon with caution to patients exhibiting signs or symptoms of depression. Suicidal tendencies may be present in such patients and protective measures may be required. Intentional overdosage is more common in this group of patients (see Overdosage); therefore, prescribe

the least amount of the drug that is feasible for the patient at any one time.

➤*Drug abuse and dependence:*
Abuse – Two studies assessed the abuse liability of zaleplon at doses of 25, 50, and 75 mg in subjects with known histories of sedative drug abuse. The results of these studies indicate that zaleplon has an abuse potential similar to benzodiazepine and benzodiazepine-like hypnotics.

Dependence – Some patients (mostly those treated with 20 mg) experienced a mild rebound insomnia on the first night following withdrawal that appeared to be resolved by the second night. The use of the Benzodiazepine Withdrawal Symptom Questionnaire and examination for any other withdrawal-emergent events did not detect any other evidence for a withdrawal syndrome following abrupt discontinuation of therapy in premarketing studies.

However, available data cannot provide a reliable estimate of the incidence of dependence during treatment at recommended zaleplon doses. Other sedatives/hypnotics have been associated with various signs and symptoms following abrupt discontinuation, ranging from mild dysphoria and insomnia to a withdrawal syndrome that may include abdominal and muscle cramps, vomiting, sweating, tremors, and convulsions. Seizures have been observed in 2 patients, one of which had a seizure prior to clinical trials with zaleplon. Seizures and death have been seen following the withdrawal of zaleplon from animals at doses many times higher than those proposed for human use. Because individuals with a history of addiction to, or abuse of, drugs or alcohol are at risk of habituation and dependence, they should be under careful surveillance when receiving zaleplon or any other hypnotic.

Tolerance – No development of tolerance to zaleplon was observed for time to sleep onset over 4 weeks.

➤*Tartrazine sensitivity:* Some of these products contain tartrazine (FD&C yellow #5), which may cause allergic-type reactions (including bronchial asthma) in susceptible individuals. Although the incidence of sensitivity is low, it is frequently seen in patients who also have aspirin hypersensitivity. Specific products containing tartrazine are identified in the product listings.

Drug Interactions

➤*Drugs that induce CYP3A4:* CYP3A4 is a minor metabolizing enzyme of zaleplon. Multiple-dose administration of the potent CYP3A4-inducer **rifampin** (600 mg every 24 hours for 14 days); however, reduced zaleplon C_{max} and AUC by ≈ 80%.

➤*Drugs that inhibit CYP3A4:* CYP3A4 is a minor metabolic pathway for the elimination of zaleplon because of the sum of desethylzaleplon (formed via CYP3A4 in vitro) and its metabolites, 5-oxo-desethylzaleplon and 5-oxo-desethylzaleplon glucuronide, account for only 9% urinary recovery of a zaleplon dose. The coadministration of a potent, selective CYP3A4 inhibitor is therefore not expected to produce a clinically important pharmacokinetic interaction with zaleplon; however, there are no clinical studies specifically addressing this question.

➤*Cimetidine:* Cimetidine inhibits both aldehyde oxidase and CYP3A4, the primary and secondary enzymes, respectively, responsible for zaleplon metabolism. Concomitant administration of zaleplon 10 mg and cimetidine 800 mg produced an 85% increase in the mean C_{max} and AUC of zaleplon. Use an initial dose of 5 mg for patients concomitantly treated with cimetidine (see Administration and Dosage).

➤*Drug/Food interactions:* In healthy adults a high-fat/heavy meal prolonged the absorption of zaleplon compared to the fasted state, delaying t_{max} by ≈ 2 hours and reducing C_{max} by ≈ 35%. Zaleplon AUC and elimination half-life were not significantly affected. These results suggest that the effects of zaleplon on sleep onset may be reduced if it is taken with or immediately after a high-fat/heavy meal.

Adverse Reactions

Because some of the important adverse effects of zaleplon appear to be dose-related, it is important to use the lowest possible effective dose, especially in the elderly (see Administration and Dosage).

In clinical trials, 3.1% of 744 patients who received placebo and 3.5% of 2069 patients who received zaleplon discontinued treatment because of an adverse clinical event. This difference was not statistically significant. No event that resulted in discontinuation occurred at a rate of ≥ 1%.

Zaleplon Adverse Reactions (%)			
Adverse reactions	Placebo (n = 277)	Zaleplon 5 or 10 mg (n = 513)	Zaleplon 20 mg (n = 273)
CNS			
Amnesia	1	2	4
Anxiety	2	< 1	3
Depersonalization	< 1	< 1	2
Dizziness	7	7	8
Hallucinations	< 1	< 1	1
Hypesthesia	0	< 1	2
Paresthesia	1	3	3
Somnolence	3	5	5

ZALEPLON

Zaleplon Adverse Reactions (%)			
Adverse reactions	Placebo (n = 277)	Zaleplon 5 or 10 mg (n = 513)	Zaleplon 20 mg (n = 273)
Tremor	1	2	2
Vertigo	< 1	< 1	1
GI			
Anorexia	< 1	< 1	2
Colitis	0	0	1
Dyspepsia	5	4	7
Nausea	7	7	8
Special senses			
Abnormal vision	< 1	< 1	2
Ear pain	0	< 1	1
Eye pain	3	4	4
Hyperacusis	< 1	2	2
Parosmia	1	< 1	2
Miscellaneous			
Abdominal pain	4	5	6
Asthenia	5	5	8
Fever	1	2	2
Headache	31	28	38
Malaise	< 1	< 1	2
Photosensitivity	< 1	< 1	1
Peripheral edema	< 1	< 1	1
Myalgia	4	7	5
Epistaxis	0	< 1	1
Dysmenorrhea	2	2	4

➤*Cardiovascular:* Migraine (≥ 1%); angina pectoris, bundle branch block, hypertension, hypotension, palpitation, syncope, tachycardia, vasodilatation, ventricular extrasystoles (0.1% to < 1%); bigeminy, cerebral ischemia, cyanosis, pericardial effusion, postural hypotension, pulmonary embolus, sinus bradycardia, thrombophlebitis, ventricular tachycardia (< 0.1%).

➤*CNS:* Depression, hypertonia, nervousness, thinking abnormal (mainly difficulty concentrating) (≥ 1%); abnormal gait, agitation, apathy, ataxia, circumoral paresthesia, confusion, emotional lability, euphoria, hyperesthesia, hyperkinesia, hypotonia, incoordination, insomnia, decreased libido, neuralgia, nystagmus (0.1% to < 1%); CNS stimulation, delusions, dysarthria, dystonia, facial paralysis, hostility, hypokinesia, myoclonus, neuropathy, psychomotor retardation, ptosis, decreased/increased reflexes, sleep talking, sleepwalking, slurred speech, stupor, trismus (< 0.1%).

➤*Dermatologic:* Pruritus, rash (≥ 1%); acne, alopecia, contact dermatitis, dry skin, eczema, maculopapular rash, skin hypertrophy, sweating, urticaria, vesiculobullous rash (0.1% to < 1%); melanosis, psoriasis, pustular rash, skin discoloration (< 0.1%).

➤*Endocrine:* Diabetes mellitus, goiter, hypothyroidism (< 0.1%).

➤*GI:* Constipation, dry mouth (≥ 1%); eructation, esophagitis, flatulence, gastritis, gastroenteritis, gingivitis, glossitis, increased appetite, melena, mouth ulceration, rectal hemorrhage, stomatitis (0.1% to < 1%); aphthous stomatitis, biliary pain, bruxism, cardiospasm, cheilitis, cholelithiasis, duodenal ulcer, dysphagia, enteritis, gum hemorrhage, increased salivation, intestinal obstruction, abnormal liver function tests, peptic ulcer, tongue discoloration, tongue edema, ulcerative stomatitis (< 0.1%).

➤*GU:* Bladder pain, breast pain, cystitis, decreased urine stream, dysuria, hematuria, impotence, kidney calculus, kidney pain, menorrhagia, metrorrhagia, urinary frequency, urinary incontinence, urinary urgency, vaginitis (0.1% to < 1%); albuminuria, delayed menstrual period, leukorrhea, menopause, urethritis, urinary retention, vaginal hemorrhage (< 0.1%).

➤*Hematologic/Lymphatic:* Anemia, ecchymosis, lymphadenopathy (0.1% to < 1%); eosinophilia, leukocytosis, lymphocytosis, purpura (< 0.1%).

➤*Metabolic/Nutritional:* Edema, gout, hypercholesteremia, thirst, weight gain (0.1% to < 1%); bilirubinemia, hyperglycemia, hyperuricemia, hypoglycemia, hypoglycemic reaction, ketosis, AST increased, ALT increased, weight loss (< 0.1%).

➤*Musculoskeletal:* Arthritis (≥ 1%); arthrosis, bursitis, joint disorder (mainly swelling, stiffness, and pain), myasthenia, tenosynovitis (0.1% to < 1%); myositis, osteoporosis (< 0.1%).

➤*Respiratory:* Bronchitis (≥ 1%); asthma, dyspnea, laryngitis, pneumonia, snoring, voice alteration (0.1% to < 1%); apnea, hiccough, hyperventilation, pleural effusion, sputum increased (< 0.1%).

➤*Special senses:* Conjunctivitis (≥ 1%); diplopia, dry eyes, photophobia, tinnitus, watery eyes (0.1% to < 1%); abnormality of accommodation, blepharitis, cataract specified, corneal erosion, deafness, eye hemorrhage, glaucoma, labyrinthitis, retinal detachment, taste loss, visual field defect (< 0.1%).

➤*Miscellaneous:* Back pain, chest pain (≥ 1%); substernal chest pain, chills, face edema, generalized edema, hangover effect, neck rigidity (0.1% to < 1%).

Overdosage

There is limited clinical experience with the effects of zaleplon overdosage. Two cases of overdose were reported. One was the accidental ingestion of 20 to 40 mg zaleplon by a 2.5-year-old boy. The second was a 20-year-old man who took 100 mg zaleplon plus 2.25 mg triazolam. Both were treated and recovered uneventfully.

➤*Symptoms:* Expect signs and symptoms of CNS depressant overdose to present as exaggerations of the pharmacological effects noted in preclinical testing. Overdose is usually manifested by degrees of CNS depression ranging from drowsiness to coma. In mild cases, symptoms include drowsiness, mental confusion, and lethargy; in more serious cases, symptoms may include ataxia, hypotonia, hypotension, respiratory depression, rarely coma, and very rarely death.

➤*Treatment:* Use general symptomatic and supportive measures along with immediate gastric lavage when appropriate. Administer IV fluids as needed. Animal studies suggest flumazenil is an antagonist to zaleplon. However, there is no clinical experience with the use of flumazenil as an antidote to a zaleplon overdose. As in all cases of drug overdose, provide general supportive measures and monitor respiration, pulse, blood pressure, and other appropriate signs. Monitor and treat hypotension and CNS depression by appropriate medical intervention. Refer to the General Management of Acute Overdosage.

Patient Information

Take zaleplon immediately before going to bed or after going to bed if there is difficulty falling asleep.

Do not take with or immediately after a high-fat/heavy meal.

Do not use for long periods without talking to a doctor about the risks and benefits of prolonged use.

➤*Side effects:* The most common side effects are drowsiness, dizziness, lightheadedness, and difficulty with coordination.

Zaleplon may cause sleepiness during the day. Daytime drowsiness is best avoided by taking the lowest possible dose.

Hazardous tasks – Patients should use caution while driving or performing other tasks requiring alertness, coordination or physical dexterity.

Do not drink alcohol; it may increase the side effects of zaleplon.

Do not take other medicines without consulting a doctor.

Take exactly as prescribed. Do not change dose without first consulting a doctor.

➤*Memory problems:* Zaleplon may cause amnesia. In most cases, memory problems can be avoided if zaleplon is taken only when the patient is able to get ≥ 4 hours of sleep before being active.

➤*Tolerance:* Development of zaleplon tolerance has not been observed in outpatient clinical studies of ≤ 4 weeks duration; however, it is unknown if the benefits of zaleplon on falling asleep more quickly persist beyond 4 weeks. Use for only a short period of time (eg, 1 or 2 days and generally ≤ 1 or 2 weeks). If sleep problems continue, consult a doctor.

➤*Dependence:* May cause dependence, especially when used regularly for longer than a few weeks or at high doses. Do not discontinue zaleplon abruptly.

➤*Withdrawal:* Withdrawal symptoms may occur if zaleplon is abruptly discontinued after daily use for an extended period of time.

Rebound insomnia (persisting 1 or 2 nights) may occur if zaleplon is stopped.

➤*Changes in behavior and thinking:* Some people have experienced unusual changes in their thinking or behavior that included more outgoing or aggressive behavior than normal, loss of personal identity, confusion, strange behavior, agitation, hallucinations, worsening of depression, and suicidal thoughts.

Store in the original container out of the reach of children.

Refer to the general discussion beginning in the Sedative and Hypnotic, Nonbarbiturate introduction. For information on benzodiazepines used as antianxiety agents, refer to the group monograph in the Antianxiety Agents section.

Indications

➤*Insomnia:* Insomnia characterized by difficulty in falling asleep, frequent nocturnal awakenings or early morning awakening. Can be used for recurring insomnia or poor sleeping habits and in acute or chronic medical situations requiring restful sleep.

Insomnia is often transient and intermittent; therefore, prolonged administration is generally not recommended. Because insomnia may be a symptom of other disorders, consider the possibility that the complaint may be related to a condition for which there is more specific treatment.

Actions

➤*Pharmacology:* Estazolam, flurazepam, quazepam, temazepam and triazolam are benzodiazepine derivatives useful as hypnotics. Benzodiazepines are believed to potentiate gamma aminobutyric acid (GABA) neuronal inhibition. The sedative and anticonvulsant actions involve GABA receptors located in the limbic, neocortical and mesencephalic reticular systems.

At least two benzodiazepine receptor subtypes have been identified in the brain, BZ_1 and BZ_2. BZ_1 is thought to be associated with sleep mechanisms; BZ_2 with memory, motor, sensory and cognitive functions. Quazepam and its active metabolite 2-oxoquazepam have a high affinity for BZ_1 receptors; this selectivity is not seen with estazolam, flurazepam, temazepam and triazolam. It is possible this selectivity of quazepam facilitates GABA transmission; however, further study is needed to determine the clinical significance of this receptor sensitivity.

Benzodiazepines generally decrease sleep latency, the number of awakenings and the time spent in stage 0 (awake stage). Flurazepam, quazepam and temazepam decrease stage 1 (descending drowsiness). Stage 2 (unequivocal sleep) is increased by all benzodiazepines, and most benzodiazepines shorten stages 3 and 4 (slow wave sleep). Temazepam has prolonged stage 3 and shortened stage 4 in neurotic patients or patients with depression. All but flurazepam prolong REM latency. REM sleep is usually shortened, but with temazepam or low-dose flurazepam, this may not be the case. The result of benzodiazepine administration is an increase in total sleep time.

If benzodiazepines are discontinued after 3 or 4 weeks of continued use, the patient may experience REM rebound; however, REM rebound with flurazepam, quazepam and possibly estazolam is slight.

➤*Pharmacokinetics:*

Absorption – These agents are rapidly and completely absorbed within 1 to 3 hours of oral administration. All have high lipid:water distribution coefficients in the non-ionized form. Times to peak plasma concentration range from 0.5 to 2 hours for parent compounds. The major active metabolite of flurazepam reaches peak plasma levels in ≈ 10 hours.

Distribution – Plasma protein binding ranges from 70% to 99% with free-drug concentrations closely approximating CSF levels. IV and rapidly absorbed oral benzodiazepines are rapidly taken into the brain and other highly perfused organs. Redistribution, favoring lipophilic compounds, follows and can greatly influence the duration of CNS effects. They also cross the placenta and are secreted into breast milk.

Metabolism – Benzodiazepines are extensively metabolized in the liver. Biotransformation to active metabolites is an important factor in product selection especially in the elderly or patients with severe liver disease. Flurazepam is biotransformed to an active metabolite, N-desalkylflurazepam, which has a half-life ranging from 47 to 100 hours. Quazepam is extensively metabolized to 2-oxoquazepam, an active metabolite; 2-oxoquazepam is further biotransformed to N-desalkyl-2-oxoquazepam, which is identical to N-desalkylflurazepam and is therefore also active. Temazepam, estazolam and triazolam do not form active long-acting metabolites.

Select Benzodiazepine (Hypnotic) Pharmacokinetic Parameters					
Drug	Usual adult oral dose (mg)	Time to peak plasma levels (hrs)	Half-life (hrs)	Protein binding (%)	Urinary excretion, unchanged (%)
Estazolam	1-2	2	8-28	93	< 5
Flurazepam	15-30	0.5-1 (7.6-13.6)[1]	2-3 (47-100)[1]	97	< 1
Quazepam	7.5-15	2 (1-2)	41 (47-100)[1]	> 95	trace
Temazepam	15-30	1.2-1.6	3.5-18.4 (9-15)	96	0.2
Triazolam	0.125-0.5	1-2	1.5-5.5	78-89	2

[1] N-desalkylflurazepam, active metabolite.

Contraindications

Hypersensitivity to other benzodiazepines; pregnancy (see Warnings); established or suspected sleep apnea (quazepam).

Concurrent use with ketoconazole, itraconazole and nefazodone, medications that significantly impair the oxidative metabolism of **triazolam** mediated by cytochrome P450 3A (CYP3A).

Warnings

➤*Anterograde amnesia:* Anterograde amnesia of varying severity and paradoxical reactions have occurred following therapeutic doses of **triazolam**. Although these effects generally occurred with a 0.5 mg dose, they have also been reported with 0.125 and 0.25 mg doses. These effect may occur with some other benzodiazepines, but data suggest that they may occur at a higher rate with triazolam.

Cases of "traveler's amnesia" have been reported by individuals who have taken **triazolam** to induce sleep while traveling. In some of these cases, insufficient time was allowed for the sleep period prior to awakening and before beginning activity. Also, the concomitant use of alcohol may have been a factor in some cases.

➤*Renal / Hepatic function impairment:* Observe usual precautions under these conditions; the potential for excessive sedation or impaired coordination exists.

Abnormal liver function tests as well as blood dyscrasias have been reported with benzodiazepines.

➤*Elderly:* The risk of developing oversedation, dizziness, confusion or ataxia increases substantially with larger doses of benzodiazepines in elderly and debilitated patients. Initiate with lowest effective dose.

➤*Pregnancy: Category X* (estazolam, quazepam, temazepam, triazolam). Flurazepam is contraindicated in pregnancy.

Teratogenic potential – Benzodiazepines may cause fetal damage when administered during pregnancy. An increased risk of congenital malformations associated with the use of diazepam and chlordiazepoxide during the first trimester of pregnancy has been suggested. Transplacental distribution results in neonatal CNS depression following ingestion of therapeutic doses of a benzodiazepine hypnotic during the last weeks of pregnancy.

Reproduction studies with **temazepam** in animals demonstrated an increased nursling mortality, increased fetal resorptions and increased occurrence of rudimentary ribs. Exencephaly and fusion or asymmetry of the ribs occurred without dose relationship.

Warn the patient of the potential risk to the fetus if there is a likelihood of the patient becoming pregnant while receiving benzodiazepines. Instruct patients to discontinue the drug prior to becoming pregnant. Consider the possibility that a woman of childbearing potential may be pregnant at the time of therapy institution.

Nonteratogenic effects – A child born to a mother taking benzodiazepines may be at some risk of withdrawal symptoms during the postnatal period. Neonatal flaccidity has occurred in an infant whose mother had been receiving benzodiazepines.

A neonate whose mother received 30 mg **flurazepam** nightly for insomnia during the 10 days prior to delivery appeared hypotonic and inactive during the first 4 days of life. Serum levels of N-desalkylflurazepam in the infant indicated transplacental circulation.

➤*Lactation:* Safety for use in the nursing mother has not been established. Benzodiazepines are excreted in breast milk. One study showed only 0.11% of quazepam and its metabolites were excreted in breast milk 48 hours after administration. Animal studies indicate that **triazolam, estazolam** and their metabolites are secreted in milk. Therefore, administration to nursing mothers is not recommended.

➤*Children:*

Flurazepam – Not for use in children < 15 years of age.

Estazolam, quazepam, temazepam, triazolam – Not for use in children < 18 years of age.

Precautions

➤*Monitoring:* When triazolam or estazolam treatment is protracted, obtain periodic blood counts, urinalysis and blood chemistry analyses. Minor EEG changes, usually low-voltage fast activity, are of no known significance.

➤*Depression:* Administer with caution in severely depressed patients or in those in whom there is evidence of latent depression or suicidal tendencies. Signs or symptoms of depression may be intensified by hypnotic drugs. Protective measures may be required. Intentional overdosage is more common in these patients, and the least amount of drug that is feasible should be available to the patient at any one time.

➤*Rebound sleep disorder:* Rebound sleep disorder, which is characterized by recurrence of insomnia to levels worse than before treatment began, may occur following abrupt withdrawal of triazolam, usually during the first 1 to 3 nights. Gradual rather than abrupt discontinuation of the drug may help avoid this syndrome. Rebound insomnia appears to be less likely after withdrawal of agents with intermediate or long half-lives (eg, estazolam, flurazepam, quazepam).

Benzodiazepines

➤*Disturbed nocturnal sleep:* Disturbed nocturnal sleep may occur for the first or second night after discontinuing use.

➤*Early morning insomnia:* Early morning insomnia, or early morning awakenings, appears to be more common with the use of short half-life agents (temazepam, triazolam) than agents with intermediate or long half-lives (estazolam, flurazepam, quazepam). However, daytime sleepiness appears to be more prevalent with the long half-life agents.

➤*Respiratory depression and sleep apnea:* Observe caution. In patients with compromised respiratory function, respiratory depression and sleep apnea have occurred. Estazolam may cause dose-related respiratory depression that is ordinarily not clinically relevant at recommended doses in patients with normal respiratory function. However, patients with compromised respiratory function may be at risk; therefore, monitor appropriately. Benzodiazepines have the capacity to depress respiratory drive, although there are insufficient data to characterize the relative potency of these agents in depressing respiratory drive at clinically recommended doses.

➤*Drug abuse and dependence:* Withdrawal symptoms following abrupt discontinuation of benzodiazepines have occurred in patients receiving excessive doses over extended periods of time. Symptoms are similar to those noted with barbiturates and alcohol following abrupt discontinuance and range from mild dysphoria to abdominal and muscle cramps, vomiting, sweating, tremor and convulsions.

Milder withdrawal symptoms infrequently occur following abrupt discontinuance of higher therapeutic levels of benzodiazepines taken continuously for several months. Exercise caution in administering to individuals known to be addiction-prone or those who may increase the dosage on their own initiative. Limit repeated prescriptions without adequate medical supervision.

Gradual withdrawal is the preferred course for any patient taking benzodiazepines for a prolonged period. Patients with a history of seizures, regardless of their concomitant anti-seizure therapy, should not be withdrawn abruptly from benzodiazepines.

➤*Hazardous tasks:* Observe caution while driving or performing tasks requiring alertness. Be aware of potential impairment of the performance of such activities the day following ingestion.

Amnesia, paradoxical reactions (eg, excitement, agitation) and other adverse behavioral effects may occur unpredictably.

Drug Interactions

Benzodiazepine (Hypnotic) Drug Interactions			
Precipitant drug	Object drug*		Description
Alcohol/CNS depressants	Benzodiazepines	↑	Additive CNS depressant effects. Potential for this interaction continues for several days following flurazepam withdrawal.
Cimetidine	Benzodiazepines (metabolized by oxidation)	↑	The hepatic metabolism of the benzodiazepines may be inhibited, their half-life prolonged and their clearance decreased, possibly resulting in increased pharmacologic and CNS depressant effects. Temazepam, metabolized by glucuronidation, would probably not interact; however, its half-life may be decreased by oral contraceptive agents.
Contraceptives, oral			
Disulfiram			
Isoniazid			
Probenecid	Benzodiazepines	↑	More rapid onset or more prolonged benzodiazepine effect.
Rifampin	Benzodiazepines (metabolized by oxidation)	↓	Increased clearance and decreased half-life of benzodiazepines may occur. Temazepam would probably not interact.
Smoking	Benzodiazepines	↓	Benzodiazepine clearance is increased in cigarette smokers, probably due to enzyme induction.
Theophyllines	Benzodiazepines	↓	Benzodiazepine pharmacologic effects may be antagonized.
Macrolides	Triazolam	↑	Bioavailability of triazolam may be increased.
Benzodiazepines	Digoxin	↑	Digoxin serum levels and toxicity may increase.
Benzodiazepines	Neuromuscular blocking agents (nondepolarizing)	↔	Benzodiazepines may potentiate, counteract or have no effect on these agents.
Benzodiazepines	Phenytoin	↑	Phenytoin serum levels may be increased, resulting in toxicity, but data are conflicting.

* ↑ = Object drug increased. ↓ = Object drug decreased. ↔ = Undetermined clinical effect.

Adverse Reactions

➤*Cardiovascular:* Palpitations; chest pains; tachycardia; hypotension (rare).

➤*CNS:* Headache; nervousness; talkativeness; apprehension; irritability; confusion; euphoria; relaxed feeling; weakness; tremor; lack of concentration; coordination disorders; confusional states/memory impairment; depression; dreaming/nightmares; insomnia; paresthesia; restlessness; tiredness; dysesthesia. Hallucinations, horizontal nystagmus and paradoxical reactions, including excitement, stimulation and hyperactivity were rare. Dizziness, drowsiness, lightheadedness, staggering, ataxia, falling, particularly in elderly or debilitated patients. Severe sedation, lethargy, disorientation and coma are probably indicative of drug intolerance or overdosage.

➤*Dermatologic:* Dermatitis/allergy; sweating, flushes, pruritus, skin rash (rare).

➤*GI:* Heartburn; nausea; vomiting; diarrhea; constipation; GI pain; anorexia; taste alterations; dry mouth; excessive salivation (rare); death from hepatic failure in a patient also receiving diuretics; jaundice; glossitis, stomatitis (triazolam).

➤*Lab test abnormalities:* Elevated AST, ALT, total and direct bilirubin and alkaline phosphatase with **flurazepam**.

➤*Miscellaneous:* Body/joint pain; tinnitus; GU complaints; cramps/pain; congestion. Leukopenia, granulocytopenia, blurred vision, burning eyes, faintness, difficulty in focusing, visual disturbances, shortness of breath, apnea, slurred speech (rare).

➤*Estazolam:* Other adverse reactions reported only for estazolam include the following:

Cardiovascular – Arrhythmia, syncope (< 0.1%).

CNS – Somnolence (42%); asthenia (11%); hypokinesia (8%); hangover (3%); abnormal thinking (2%); anxiety (1%); agitation, amnesia, apathy, emotional lability, hostility, seizure, sleep disorder, stupor, twitch (0.1% to 1%); ataxia, decreased libido, decreased reflexes, neuritis (< 0.1%).

Dermatologic – Urticaria (0.1% to 1%); acne, dry skin, photosensitivity (< 0.1%).

GI – Dyspepsia (2%); decreased/increased appetite, flatulence, gastritis (0.1% to 1%); enterocolitis, melena, mouth ulceration (< 0.1%).

GU – Frequent urination, menstrual cramps, urinary hesitancy/urgency, vaginal discharge/itching (0.1% to 1%); hematuria, nocturia, oliguria, penile discharge, urinary incontinence (< 0.1%).

Respiratory – Cold symptoms (3%); pharyngitis (1%); asthma, cough, dyspnea, rhinitis, sinusitis (0.1% to 1%); epistaxis, hyperventilation, laryngitis (< 0.1%).

Special senses – Ear pain, eye irritation/pain/swelling, photophobia (0.1% to 1%); decreased hearing, diplopia, nystagmus, scotomata (< 0.1%).

Miscellaneous – Lower extremity/back/abdominal pain (1% to 3%); stiffness (1%); allergic reaction, chills, fever, neck/upper extremity pain, thirst, arthritis, muscle spasm, myalgia (0.1% to 1%); edema, jaw pain, swollen breast, thyroid nodule, purpura, swollen lymph nodes, agranulocytosis, increased AST, weight gain/loss, arthralgia (< 0.1%).

Overdosage

➤*Symptoms:* Somnolence; confusion with reduced or absent reflexes; respiratory depression; apnea; hypotension; impaired coordination; slurred speech; seizures; ultimately, coma. Death has occurred with overdoses of benzodiazepines alone and with alcohol.

➤*Treatment:* If excitation occurs, do not use barbiturates. Consider the possibility that multiple agents may have been ingested. Monitor respiration, pulse and blood pressure. Employ general supportive measures. Administer IV fluids and maintain an adequate airway. Perform gastric lavage. Refer to General Management of Acute Overdosage. Hemodialysis and forced diuresis are of little value.

Use of IV pressor agents may be necessary to treat hypotension. Administer IV fluids to encourage diuresis.

Patient Information

Avoid alcohol and other CNS depressants. Do not exceed prescribed dosage.

Do not discontinue medication abruptly after prolonged therapy.

Advise patients that they may experience disturbed nocturnal sleep for the first or second night after discontinuing the drug.

May cause drowsiness or dizziness; observe caution while driving or performing other tasks requiring alertness.

Inform your physician if you are planning to become pregnant, if you are pregnant, or if you become pregnant while taking this medicine.

➤*Triazolam:* Advise patients not to take triazolam in circumstances where a full night's sleep and clearance of the drug from the body are not possible before they would again need to be active and functional.

Benzodiazepines

ESTAZOLAM

Rx	**Estazolam** (Zenith-Goldline)	**Tablets:** 1 mg	In 30s, 100s, 500s and 1000s.
c-iv	**ProSom** (Abbott)		Lactose. (UC). White, scored. In 100s and UD 100s.
Rx	**Estazolam** (Zenith-Goldline)	2 mg	In 30s, 100s, 500s and 1000s.
c-iv	**ProSom** (Abbott)		Lactose. (UD). Coral, scored. In 100s and UD 100s.

For complete prescribing information, refer to the Benzodiazepines group monograph.

Administration and Dosage

➤*Adults:* 1 mg at bedtime; however, some patients may need a 2 mg dose.

➤*Elderly:* If healthy, 1 mg at bedtime; initiate increases with particular care.

➤*Debilitated or small elderly patients:* Consider a starting dose of 0.5 mg, although this is only marginally effective in the overall elderly population.

FLURAZEPAM HCl

c-iv	**Flurazepam** (Various, eg, Goldline, Major, PBI, Warner Chilcott)	**Capsules:** 15 mg	In 100s and 100s.
c-iv	**Dalmane** (Roche)		Orange/ivory. In 100s, 500s, Reverse number pack 100s, UD 100s.
c-iv	**Flurazepam** (Various, eg, Goldline, Major, PBI, Warner Chilcott)	**Capsules:** 30 mg	In 100s and 100s.
c-iv	**Dalmane** (Roche)		(DALMANE 30 ICN). Red/ivory. In 100s, 500s, Reverse number pack 100s, UD 100s.

For complete prescribing information, refer to the Benzodiazepines group monograph.

Administration and Dosage

Individualize dosage.

➤*Adults:* 30 mg before bedtime. In some patients, 15 mg may suffice.

➤*Elderly or debilitated:* Initiate with 15 mg until individual response is determined.

TEMAZEPAM

c-iv	**Restoril** (Sandoz)	**Capsules:** 7.5 mg	Lactose. (Restoril 7.5 mg For Sleep). Blue/pink. In 100s, *ControlPak* 25s, UD 100s.
c-iv	**Temazepam** (Various, eg, Goldline, Lederle, Moore, PBI, Warner Chilcott)	**Capsules:** 15 mg	In 100s, 500s and UD 100s
c-iv	**Restoril** (Sandoz)		(Restoril 15 mg For Sleep). Maroon/pink. In 100s, 500s, *ControlPak* 25s, *Sando Pak* 100s.
c-iv	**Temazepam** (Various, eg, Goldline, PBI, Warner-Chilcott)	**Capsules:** 30 mg	In 100s, 500s and UD 100s.
c-iv	**Restoril** (Sandoz)		(Restoril 30 mg For Sleep). Maroon/blue. In 100s, 500s, *ControlPak* 25s, *Sando Pak* 100s.

For complete prescribing information, refer to the Benzodiazepines group monograph.

Administration and Dosage

➤*Adults:* Individualize dosage. Give 15 to 30 mg before bedtime.

➤*Elderly or debilitated:* Initiate with 15 mg until individual response is determined.

TRIAZOLAM

c-iv	**Triazolam** (Various, eg, Geneva, Goldline, Par, Roxane)	**Tablets:** 0.125 mg	In 10s, 100s, 500s and UD 100s.
c-iv	**Halcion** (Upjohn)		(0.125 Halcion 10). White. In 100s, 500s, UD 100s, *Visipak* 100s.
c-iv	**Triazolam** (Various, eg, Geneva, Goldline, Par, Roxane)	**Tablets:** 0.25 mg	In 10s, 100s, 500s and UD 100s.
c-iv	**Halcion** (Upjohn)		(0.25 Halcion 17). Blue, scored. In 100s, 500s, UD 100s, *Visipak* 100s.

For complete prescribing information, refer to the Benzodiazepines group monograph.

Administration and Dosage

➤*Adults:* 0.125 to 0.5 mg before bedtime.

➤*Elderly or debilitated:* 0.125 to 0.25 mg. Initiate with 0.125 mg until individual response is determined.

QUAZEPAM

c-iv	**Doral** (Wallace)	**Tablets:** 7.5 mg	(7.5 Doral). Light orange w/white speckles. Capsule shaped. In 100s, 500s, UD 100s.
		15 mg	(15 Doral). Light orange w/white speckles. Capsule shaped. In 100s, 500s, UD 100s.

For complete prescribing information, refer to the Benzodiazepines group monograph.

Administration and Dosage

➤*Adults:* Initiate at 15 mg until individual responses are determined; may reduce to 7.5 mg in some patients.

➤*Elderly or debilitated:* Attempt to reduce nightly dosage after the first 1 or 2 nights.

CHLORAL HYDRATE

c-iv	**Chloral Hydrate** (Various, eg, Balan, Dixon-Shane, Goldline, Lannett, URL)	**Capsules:** 500 mg	In 100s, 500s, 1000s and UD100s.
c-iv	**Chloral Hydrate** (Various, eg, Pharmaceutical Assoc., Roxane)	**Syrup:** 250 mg/5 ml	In UD 10 ml (40s and 100s).
c-iv	**Chloral Hydrate** (Various, eg, Balan, Dixon-Shane, Geneva, UDL, URL)	**Syrup:** 500 mg/5 ml	In pt, gal and UD 5 ml (100s) and 10 ml (40s and 100s).
c-iv	**Aquachloral Supprettes** (Polymedica)	**Suppositories:** 324 mg	Tartrazine. In 12s.
c-iv	**Aquachloral Supprettes** (Polymedica)	**Suppositories:** 648 mg	In 12s.

Refer to the general discussion beginning in the Sedative and Hypnotic, Nonbarbiturate introduction.

Indications

Nocturnal sedation; preoperative sedation to lessen anxiety and induce sleep without depressing respiration or cough reflex; in postoperative care and control of pain as an adjunct to opiates and analgesics; preventing or suppressing alcohol withdrawal symptoms (rectal).

Chloral hydrate is effective as a hypnotic only for short-term use; it loses much of its effectiveness for inducing and maintaining sleep after 2 weeks of use.

Administration and Dosage

Take capsules with a full glass of liquid. Administer syrup in ½ glass of water, fruit juice or ginger ale.

➤*Adults:* Single doses or daily dosage should not exceed 2 g.

Hypnotic – 500 mg to 1 g 15 to 30 minutes before bedtime or 30 minutes before surgery.

Sedative – 250 mg 3 times daily after meals.

➤*Children:*

Hypnotic – 50 mg/kg/day, up to 1 g per single dose. May be given in divided doses.

Sedative – 25 mg/kg/day, up to 500 mg per single dose. May be given in divided doses.

Dental sedation – Higher doses than those suggested by the manufacturer are generally used. Doses of 75 mg/kg, supplemented by nitrous oxide may provide better sedation than the lower dose with no change in the vital signs or adverse effects.

Actions

➤*Pharmacology:* The mechanism of action by which the CNS is affected is not known. Hypnotic dosage produces mild cerebral depression and quiet, deep sleep. In therapeutic doses, chloral hydrate has little effect on respiration, blood pressure and reflexes. "Hangover" is less common than with most barbiturates and some benzodiazepines. It has generally been replaced by safer and more effective agents.

➤*Pharmacokinetics:* Chloral hydrate is readily absorbed and metabolized to trichloroethanol, the principal active metabolite. Trichloroethanol has a plasma half-life of 7 to 10 hours; plasma protein binding is 35% to 41%. The drug is converted in the liver and kidney to trichloroacetic acid and excreted in the urine and bile. Although inactive, trichloroacetic acid is 71% to 88% protein bound and can displace other acidic drugs from plasma protein binding sites.

Contraindications

Marked hepatic or renal impairment; severe cardiac disease; gastritis; hypersensitivity or idiosyncrasy to chloral derivatives.

Warnings

➤*Pregnancy: Category C.* Safety for use during pregnancy has not been established. Chloral hydrate crosses the placenta; chronic use during pregnancy may cause withdrawal symptoms in the neonate. Congenital defects have not been reported. Use only when clearly needed and when potential benefits outweigh potential hazards to the fetus.

➤*Lactation:* Chloral hydrate is excreted in breast milk; use by nursing mothers may cause sedation in the infant.

Precautions

➤*Cardiac disease:* Continued use of therapeutic doses does not have a deleterious effect on the heart. However, do not use large doses in patients with severe cardiac disease.

➤*GI conditions:* Avoid use in patients with esophagitis, gastritis or gastric or duodenal ulcers.

➤*Acute intermittent porphyria:* Acute intermittent porphyria attacks may be precipitated by chloral hydrate; use with caution in susceptible patients.

➤*Skin/mucous membrane irritation:* Chloral derivatives irritate the skin and mucous membranes; gastric necrosis has occurred following intoxicating doses.

➤*Drug abuse and dependence:* May be habit forming. Exercise caution in administering to patients prone to addiction. Slurred speech, incoordination, tremulousness and nystagmus should arouse suspicion. Drowsiness, lethargy and hangover are frequently observed from excessive drug intake.

Prolonged use of large doses may result in psychic and physical dependence. Tolerance and psychologic dependence may develop by the second week of continued administration. Chloral hydrate addicts may take huge doses of the drug (up to 12 g nightly). Sudden withdrawal may result in CNS excitation with tremor, anxiety, hallucinations or even delirium, which may be fatal. Gastritis, skin eruptions and parenchymatous renal injury may also occur. Undertake withdrawal in a hospital using supportive therapy similar to that used for barbiturate withdrawal.

➤*Hazardous tasks:* May produce drowsiness; patients should observe caution while driving or performing other tasks requiring alertness.

➤*Tartrazine sensitivity:* Some of these products contain tartrazine, which may cause allergic-type reactions (including bronchial asthma) in susceptible individuals. Although the incidence of tartrazine sensitivity in the general population is low, it is frequently seen in patients who also have aspirin hypersensitivity. Specific products containing tartrazine are identified in the product listings.

Drug Interactions

Chloral Hydrate Drug Interactions			
Precipitant drug	Object drug*		Description
Alcohol	Chloral hydrate	↑	Alcohol may have synergistic effects with chloral hydrate. With alcohol, there is mutual inhibition of metabolism in addition to the combined depressant effect. Disulfiram-like reactions (eg, increased respiration and pulse rate, flushing), although rare, have occurred. Avoid concomitant use.
Chloral hydrate	Alcohol		
Chloral hydrate	Anticoagulants, oral	↑	Hypoprothrombinemic effects may occur by displacement from protein binding sites. However, this effect is usually small and fleeting. Monitor prothrombin levels and adjust coumarin dose accordingly.
Chloral hydrate	CNS depressants	↑	CNS depressants (eg, barbiturates, narcotics) may have additive CNS effects with chloral hydrate coadministration.
CNS depressants	Chloral hydrate		
Furosemide	Chloral hydrate	↑	Administration of chloral hydrate followed by IV furosemide may result in sweating, hot flashes, tachycardia, hypertension, weakness and nausea.
Chloral hydrate	Hydantoins	↓	The elimination of phenytoin may be increased by concurrent chloral hydrate, possibly reducing its effectiveness.

* ↑ = Object drug increased. ↓ = Object drug decreased.

➤*Drug/Lab test interactions:* Chloral hydrate may interfere with the **copper sulfate test** for glycosuria (confirm suspected glycosuria by a glucose oxidase test), **fluorometric tests** for urine catecholamines (do not administer medication for 48 hours preceding the test) or **urinary 17-hydroxycorticosteroid determinations** (when using the Reddy, Jenkins and Thorn procedure).

Adverse Reactions

➤*CNS:* Somnambulism, disorientation, incoherence, paranoid behavior (occasional); excitement, delirium, drowsiness, staggering gait, ataxia, lightheadedness, vertigo, dizziness, nightmares, malaise, mental confusion, headache, hallucinations (rare).

➤*Dermatologic:* Allergic skin rashes including hives, erythema, eczematoid dermatitis, urticaria, scarlatiniform exanthems (occasional).

➤*GI:* Gastric irritation; nausea and vomiting (occasional); flatulence; diarrhea; unpleasant taste to mouth.

➤*Hematologic:* Leukopenia, eosinophilia (occasional).

➤*Miscellaneous:* Hangover, idiosyncratic syndrome, ketonuria (rare).

Overdosage

➤*Symptoms:* Stupor; coma; pinpoint pupils; hypotension; slow or rapid and shallow respiration; hypothermia; areflexia; muscle flaccidity.

Corrosive action – Nausea; vomiting; esophagitis; gastritis; hemorrhagic gastritis; gastric necrosis; enteritis.

CHLORAL HYDRATE

Organ damage – Hepatic damage (jaundice); renal damage (albuminuria); cardiac damage (ventricular and atrial arrhythmias).

Doses > 2 g may produce symptoms of toxicity. The toxic oral dose of chloral hydrate for adults is approximately 5 to 10 g; however, death has occurred following doses of 1.25 and 3 g; some patients have survived after taking 36 g.

➤*Treatment:* Perform gastric lavage or induce vomiting to empty the stomach. Activated charcoal may prevent drug absorption. Treatment includes usual supportive measures. Refer to General Management of Acute Overdosage. Hemoperfusion and hemodialysis are effective, but peritoneal dialysis is not useful. Hemodialysis is reported to promote the clearance of trichloroethanol.

May cause GI upset. Take capsules with a full glass of water or fruit juice; swallow capsules whole – do not chew. Dilute syrup in a half glass of water or fruit juice.

May cause drowsiness; use caution when performing tasks requiring alertness. Avoid alcohol and other CNS depressants.

May be habit forming; do not discontinue the drug abruptly.

PARALDEHYDE

c-iv **Paral** (Forest)	**Liquid (oral, rectal)**	In 30 ml.

Refer to the general discussion beginning in the Sedative and Hypnotic, Nonbarbiturate introduction.

Indications

Sedative and hypnotic. Also used to quiet the patient and to produce sleep in delirium tremens and in other psychiatric states characterized by excitement.

Administration and Dosage

➤*Hypnosis:*

Adults –
  Oral: 4 to 8 ml in milk or iced fruit juice to mask the taste and odor.
  Delirium tremens: 10 to 35 ml may be necessary.
  Rectal: Dissolve in oil as a retention enema. Mix 10 to 20 ml with 1 or 2 parts of olive oil or isotonic sodium chloride solution to avoid rectal irritation.

Children – 0.3 ml/kg orally or rectally.

➤*Sedation:*

Adults – 5 to 10 ml orally or rectally.

Children – 0.15 ml/kg orally or rectally

➤*Storage/Stability:* Upon exposure to light and air, paraldehyde decomposes to acetaldehyde and oxidizes to acetic acid. Do not use if liquid has a brownish color or sharp odor of acetic acid. Keep away from heat, open flame or sparks. Paraldehyde solidifies at approximately 12°C (54°F) and must be liquefied before use. Do not store in direct sunlight or expose to temperatures above 25°C (77°F). Keep product covered in box until use. Discard unused portion. Do not use paraldehyde from a container that has been opened for longer than 24 hours.

Actions

➤*Pharmacology:* Paraldehyde, a polymer of acetaldehyde, is a colorless, bitter tasting liquid with a strong, unpleasant odor; it produces nonspecific, reversible depression of the CNS. With usual therapeutic doses, paraldehyde has little effect on respiration and blood pressure; large doses may cause respiratory depression and hypotension. It has generally been replaced by safer and more effective agents.

➤*Pharmacokinetics:*

Absorption/Distribution – The drug is rapidly absorbed after oral administration. Peak serum concentrations are attained 30 to 60 minutes following oral use. Paraldehyde acts rapidly, producing sleep within 10 to 15 minutes after a therapeutic dose; sleep lasts about 8 to 12 hours.

Metabolism/Excretion – Plasma half-life ranges from 3.4 to 9.8 hours. Approximately 70% to 80% of the drug is metabolized in the liver, 11% to 28% is exhaled unchanged via the lungs and a negligible amount is excreted in the urine. In hepatic disease, elimination rate is decreased and more drug is excreted through the lungs.

Contraindications

Bronchopulmonary disease (excretion of the drug by the lungs); hepatic insufficiency (metabolized by the liver); gastroenteritis (especially if ulceration is present).

Warnings

➤*Mucous membrane irritation:* Paraldehyde is irritating to mucous membranes and must be well diluted. Esophagitis, hemorrhagic gastritis and proctitis have occurred.

➤*Hepatic function impairment:* Patients with liver dysfunction may be more susceptible to effects of paraldehyde.

➤*Pregnancy: Category C.* Paraldehyde crosses the placenta and appears in the fetal circulation. It is not known whether the drug can cause fetal harm. Use during pregnancy only if potential benefits outweigh potential hazards to the fetus.

Labor – Use during labor may cause respiratory depression in the neonate.

➤*Lactation:* Problems in the nursing infant have not been documented; however, consider the risk-benefit.

➤*Children:* Safety and efficacy for use in children have not been established.

Precautions

➤*Strong, unpleasant breath:* Although medically insignificant, paraldehyde has a strong odor that is imparted to the exhaled air for as long as 24 hours after ingestion. The patient is often unaware of the odor.

➤*Habit formation:* May be habit forming; avoid sudden withdrawal after chronic use.

Drug Interactions

➤*Disulfiram:* Disulfiram inhibits acetaldehyde dehydrogenase. Avoid concomitant use.

Adverse Reactions

Prolonged use – Prolonged use may result in addiction resembling alcoholism. Withdrawal may produce delirium tremens and vivid hallucinations. Several cases of metabolic acidosis have occurred in association with paraldehyde addiction, although the etiology is uncertain. Prolonged use may produce yellowing of eyes or skin (hepatitis).

➤*Miscellaneous:* Strong, unpleasant breath may occur (see Precautions).

Overdosage

➤*Symptoms:* Death has occurred following 25 ml orally or 12 ml rectally. The hallmark of toxicity is metabolic acidosis; treat with IV sodium bicarbonate or sodium lactate. Clinical features are: Unconsciousness; coma; rapid, labored respirations; pulmonary hemorrhage; edema; irritation of the throat, stomach and rectum (enema); nausea; vomiting; esophagitis; hemorrhagic gastritis; hepatitis; renal damage; agitation; pseudoketosis; hyperacetaldehydemia; right heart dilation.

➤*Treatment:* Intensive support therapy is paramount. Support respiratory function, treat acidosis and protect the liver. Gastric lavage is inappropriate since the drug is rapidly absorbed after administration. Hemodialysis or peritoneal dialysis may be required to treat acidosis and to support renal function.

May cause GI upset; take with food or mix with milk or iced fruit juice to improve taste.

Avoid alcohol and other sedatives while taking this drug.

May cause drowsiness; use caution while driving or performing tasks requiring alertness.

Do not use paraldehyde in any plastic container; do not dispense with a plastic spoon or syringe.

Discard any unused paraldehyde after opening bottle.

Do not use if liquid has a brownish color or a strong vinegar odor.

DEXMEDETOMIDINE HCl

| *Rx* | **Precedex** (Abbott) | **Injection:** 100 mcg/mL | Preservative-free. 9 mg sodium chloride. In 2 mL vials. |

Indications

➤*Sedation:* For sedation of initially intubated and mechanically ventilated patients during treatment in an intensive care setting.

➤*Unlabeled uses:* To treat shivering; as an adjunct to regional or general anesthesia; as a bridge to ICU sedation and analgesia; as a supplement to regional block in patients undergoing carotid endarterectomy or during awake craniotomy; in selected patients with CHF; to control agitation while receiving noninvasive ventilatory support such as mask continuous or bilevel positive airway pressure; to minimize withdrawal phenomena in critically ill patients who have received long-term benzodiazepines and opioids during their hospitalization.

Administration and Dosage

➤*Approved by the FDA:* December 24, 1999.

Dexmedetomidine should be administered only by people skilled in the management of patients in the intensive care setting. Because of the known pharmacological effects of dexmedetomidine, continuously monitor patients while they receive dexmedetomidine.

➤*Adult:* Loading infusion of 1 mcg/kg over 10 minutes, followed by a maintenance infusion of 0.2 to 0.7 mcg/kg/hr. Adjust the rate of the maintenance infusion to achieve the desired level of sedation. Administer using a controlled infusion device.

Dexmedetomidine is not indicated for infusions lasting > 24 hours.

Dexmedetomidine has been infused continuously in mechanically ventilated patients prior to extubation, during extubation, and postextubation. It is not necessary to discontinue dexmedetomidine prior to extubation provided the infusion does not exceed 24 hours.

➤*Infusion preparation:* Preparation of solutions is the same, whether for the loading dose or maintenance infusion.

To prepare the infusion, withdraw 2 mL of dexmedetomidine and add to 48 mL of 0.9% Sodium Chloride Injection to a total of 50 mL. Shake gently to mix well. Vials are intended for single use only.

Dexmedetomidine must be diluted in 0.9% sodium chloride solution to achieve the required concentrations prior to administration.

Visually inspect parenteral products for particulate matter and discoloration prior to administration. Strict aseptic technique must always be maintained during handling.

➤*Hepatic impairment:* Reduce dosage in patients with impaired hepatic function because of decreased clearance of dexmedetomidine.

➤*Admixture compatibility:* Dexmedetomidine has been shown to be compatible when administered with the following IV fluids and drugs: Lactated Ringers, 5% Dextrose in water, 0.9% Sodium Chloride in water, 20% mannitol, thiopental sodium, etomidate, vecuronium bromide, pancuronium bromide, succinylcholine, atracurium besylate, mivacurium chloride, glycopyrrolate bromide, phenylephrine HCl, atropine sulfate, midazolam, morphine sulfate, fentanyl citrate, and plasma substitute. Compatibility of dexmedetomidine with coadministration of blood, serum, or plasma has not been established.

Compatibility studies have demonstrated the potential for adsorption of dexmedetomidine to some types of natural rubber. Although dexmedetomidine is dosed to effect, it is advisable to use administration components made with synthetic or coated natural rubber gaskets.

➤*Storage / Stability:* Store at controlled room temperature 25°C (77°F).

Actions

➤*Pharmacology:* Dexmedetomidine is a relatively selective α_2-adrenoceptor agonist with sedative properties. α_2-selectivity was observed in animals following slow IV infusion of low and medium doses (10 to 300 mcg/kg). Both α_1 and α_2 activity was observed following slow IV infusion of high doses (≥ 1000 mcg/kg) or with rapid IV administration.

In a study in healthy volunteers (n = 10), respiratory rate and oxygen saturation remained within normal limits. There was no evidence of respiratory depression when dexmedetomidine IV infusion was administered at doses within the recommended dose range (0.2 to 0.7 mcg/kg/hr).

➤*Pharmacokinetics:*

Distribution – Following IV administration, dexmedetomidine exhibits a rapid distribution phase with a half-life of ≈ 6 minutes. The steady-state volume of distribution is ≈ 118 L. Dexmedetomidine protein binding was assessed in the plasma of normal healthy male and female volunteers. The average protein binding was 94%. The fraction of dexmedetomidine bound to plasma proteins was significantly decreased in subjects with hepatic impairment when compared with healthy subjects.

Metabolism – Dexmedetomidine undergoes almost complete biotransformation with very little unchanged dexmedetomidine excreted in the urine and feces. Biotransformation involves both direct glucuronidation as well as cytochrome P450-mediated metabolism. The major metabolic pathways of dexmedetomidine are the following: Direct N-glucuronidation to inactive metabolites; aliphatic hydroxylation (mediated primarily by CYP2A6) of dexmedetomidine to generate 3-hydroxy

dexmedetomidine, the glucuronide of 3-hydroxy dexmedetomidine, and 3-carboxy dexmedetomidine; and N-methylation of dexmedetomidine to generate 3-hydroxy N-methyl dexmedetomidine, 3-carboxy N-methyl dexmedetomidine, and N-methyl O-glucuronide dexmedetomidine.

Excretion – The terminal elimination half-life of dexmedetomidine is ≈ 2 hours, and clearance is estimated to be ≈ 39 L/hr. After 9 days, an average of 95% of the radioactivity following IV administration of radiolabeled dexmedetomidine was recovered in the urine and 4% in the feces. No unchanged dexmedetomidine was detected in the urine. Approximately 85% of the radioactivity recovered in the urine was excreted within 24 hours after the infusion. Fractionation of the radioactivity excreted in the urine demonstrated products of N-glucuronidation accounted for ≈ 34% of the cumulative urinary excretion. In addition, aliphatic hydroxylation of the parent drug to form 3-hydroxy dexmedetomidine, the glucuronide of 3-hydroxy dexmedetomidine, and 3-carboxylic acid dexmedetomidine together represented ≈ 14% of the dose in urine. N-methylation of dexmedetomidine to form 3-hydroxy N-methyl dexmedetomidine, 3-carboxy N-methyl dexmedetomidine, and N-methyl O-glucuronide dexmedetomidine accounted for ≈ 18% of the dose in the urine. The N-methyl metabolite itself was a minor circulating component and was undetected in the urine. Approximately 28% of the urinary metabolites have not been identified.

Renal impairment – Dexmedetomidine pharmacokinetics (C_{max}, T_{max}, AUC, half-life, and volume of distribution) were not significantly different in subjects with severe renal impairment (Ccr < 30 mL/min) compared with healthy subjects. However, the pharmacokinetics of the metabolites of dexmedetomidine have not been evaluated in patients with impaired renal function. Because the majority of metabolites are excreted in the urine, it is possible that the metabolites may accumulate upon long-term infusions in patients with impaired renal function.

Hepatic impairment – In subjects with varying degrees of hepatic impairment (Child-Pugh Class A, B, or C), clearance values for dexmedetomidine were lower than in healthy subjects. The mean clearance values for subjects with mild, moderate, and severe hepatic impairment were 74%, 64%, and 53% of those observed in the healthy subjects, respectively. Mean clearances for free drug were 59%, 51%, and 32% of those observed in healthy subjects, respectively.

Warnings

➤*Cardiac effects:* Clinically significant episodes of bradycardia and sinus arrest have been associated with dexmedetomidine administration in young, healthy volunteers with high vagal tone or with different routes of administration, including rapid IV or bolus administration.

Reports of hypotension and bradycardia have been associated with dexmedetomidine infusion. If medical intervention is required, treatment may include decreasing or stopping the infusion of dexmedetomidine, increasing the rate of IV fluid administration, elevation of the lower extremities, and use of pressor agents. Because dexmedetomidine has the potential to augment bradycardia induced by vagal stimuli, prepare clinicians to intervene. Consider the IV administration of anticholinergic agents (eg, atropine) to modify vagal tone. In clinical trials, atropine or glycopyrrolate were effective in the treatment of most episodes of dexmedetomidine-induced bradycardia. However, in some patients with significant cardiovascular dysfunction, more advanced resuscitative measures were required. Exercise caution when administering dexmedetomidine to patients with advanced heart block.

Transient hypertension has been observed primarily during the loading dose in association with the initial peripheral vasoconstrictive effects of dexmedetomidine. Treatment of the transient hypertension has generally not been necessary, although reduction of the loading infusion rate may be desirable.

➤*Renal function impairment:* Dexmedetomidine is known to be substantially excreted by the kidney and the risk of adverse reactions to this drug may be greater in patients with impaired renal function. Because elderly patients are more likely to have decreased renal function, care should be taken in dose selection in elderly patients, and it may be useful to monitor renal function.

➤*Hepatic function impairment:* Reduce dosage in patients with impaired hepatic function because dexmedetomidine clearance decreases with severity of hepatic impairment.

➤*Mutagenesis:* Dexmedetomidine was clastogenic in the in vitro human lymphocyte chromosome aberration test with, but not without, metabolic activation. Dexmedetomidine was also clastogenic in the in vivo mouse micronucleus test.

➤*Elderly:* In patients > 65 years of age, a higher incidence of bradycardia and hypotension was observed following administration of dexmedetomidine. Consider a dose reduction in patients > 65 years of age.

➤*Pregnancy: Category C.* Fetal toxicity, as evidenced by increased postimplantation losses and reduced number of live pups, was observed in rats at an SC dose of 200 mcg/kg. The no-effect dose was 20 mcg/kg (less than the maximum recommended human IV dose on a mcg/m² basis). Placental transfer of dexmedetomidine was observed when radiolabeled dexmedetomidine was administered SC to pregnant rats.

DEXMEDETOMIDINE HCl

There are no adequate and well-controlled studies in pregnant women. Use during pregnancy only if the potential benefits justify the potential risk to the fetus.

Labor and delivery – Dexmedetomidine is not recommended during labor and delivery, including cesarean section deliveries.

➤*Lactation:* It is not known whether dexmedetomidine is excreted in human breast milk. Radiolabeled dexmedetomidine administered SC to lactating female rats was excreted in milk. Use caution if dexmedetomidine is administered to a nursing woman.

➤*Children:* Dexmedetomidine is not recommended for use in pediatric patients < 18 years of age.

Precautions

➤*Alertness:* Some patients receiving dexmedetomidine have been observed to be arousable and alert when stimulated. This alone should not be considered as evidence of lack of efficacy in the absence of other clinical signs and symptoms.

➤*Advanced heart block and/or severe ventricular dysfunction:* Because dexmedetomidine decreases sympathetic nervous system activity, hypotension or bradycardia may be expected to be more pronounced in hypovolemic patients, in those with diabetes mellitus or chronic hypertension, and in the elderly. In situations where other vasodilators or negative chronotropic agents are administered, coadministration of dexmedetomidine could have an additive pharmacodynamic effect and should be administered with caution.

➤*Withdrawal:* Although not specifically studied, if dexmedetomidine is administered chronically and stopped abruptly, withdrawal symptoms may include nervousness, agitation, and headaches, accompanied or followed by a rapid rise in blood pressure and elevated catecholamine concentrations in the plasma. Do not administer dexmedetomidine for > 24 hours.

➤*Adrenal insufficiency:* Dexmedetomidine had no effect on ACTH-stimulated cortisol release in dogs after a single dose; however, after the SC infusion of dexmedetomidine for 1 week, the cortisol response to ACTH was diminished by ≈ 40%.

➤*Drug abuse and dependence:* Dexmedetomidine is not a controlled substance. The dependence potential of dexmedetomidine has not been studied in humans. However, because studies in rodents and primates have demonstrated that dexmedetomidine exhibits pharmacologic actions similar to those of clonidine, it is possible that dexmedetomidine may produce a clonidine-like withdrawal syndrome upon abrupt discontinuation.

Drug Interactions

➤*CYP450:* In vitro studies in human liver microsomes demonstrated no evidence of cytochrome P450-mediated drug interactions that are likely to be of clinical relevance.

➤*Anesthetics/Sedatives/Hypnotics/Opioids:* Coadministration of dexmedetomidine with anesthetics, sedatives, hypnotics, and opioids is likely to lead to enhanced effects. Specific studies have confirmed these effects with sevoflurane, isoflurane, propofol, alfentanil, and midazolam. No pharmacokinetic interactions between dexmedetomidine and isoflurane, propofol, alfentanil, and midazolam have been demonstrated. However, because of possible pharmacodynamic interactions, when coadministered with dexmedetomidine, a reduction in dosage of dexmedetomidine on the concomitant anesthetic, sedative, hypnotic, or opioid may be required.

In a study of 49 women undergoing hysterectomies, isoflurane minimum alveolar concentration (MAC) was 47% less in combination with dexmedetomidine than when compared with placebo.

Adverse Reactions

Overall, the most frequently observed treatment-emergent adverse events included the following: Hypotension, hypertension, nausea, bradycardia, fever, vomiting, hypoxia, tachycardia, anemia.

Dexmedetomidine Adverse Reactions (> 1%)		
Adverse reaction	Demedetomidine (n = 387)	Placebo (n = 379)
Hypotension	28	13
Hypertension	16	18
Nausea	11	9
Bradycardia	7	3
Fever	5	4
Vomiting	4	6
Atrial fibrillation	4	3
Hypoxia	4	4
Tachycardia	3	5
Hemorrhage	3	4
Anemia	3	2
Dry mouth	3	1
Rigors	2	3
Agitation	2	3
Hyperpyrexia	2	3
Pain	2	2
Hyperglycemia	2	2
Acidosis	2	2
Pleural effusion	2	1
Oliguria	2	< 1
Thirst	2	< 1

The following adverse events were reported in ≤ 1% of patients in the continuous infusion ICU sedation trials.

➤*Cardiovascular:* Blood pressure fluctuation, heart disorder, aggravated hypertension, arrhythmia, ventricular arrhythmia, AV block, cardiac arrest, extrasystoles, atrial fibrillation, heart block, T-wave inversion, tachycardia, supraventricular tachycardia, ventricular tachycardia.

➤*CNS:* Dizziness, headache, neuralgia, neuritis, speech disorder, agitation, confusion, delirium, hallucination, illusion.

➤*GI:* Abdominal pain, diarrhea, vomiting.

➤*Hepatic:* Increased SGGT, increased AST, increased ALT.

➤*Metabolic/Nutritional:* Acidosis, respiratory acidosis, hyperkalemia, increased alkaline phosphatase, thirst.

➤*Respiratory:* Apnea, bronchospasm, dyspnea, hypercapnia, hypoventilation, hypoxia, pulmonary congestion.

➤*Miscellaneous:* Fever, hyperpyrexia, hypovolemia, light anesthesia, pain, rigors, anemia, increased sweating, photopsia, abnormal vision.

Overdosage

The tolerability of dexmedetomidine was noted in 1 study in which healthy subjects were administered doses at and above the recommended dose of 0.2 to 0.7 mcg/kg/hr. The maximum blood concentration achieved in this study was ≈ 13 times the upper boundary of the therapeutic range. The most notable effects observed in 2 subjects who achieved the highest doses were first-degree AV block and second-degree heart block. No hemodynamic compromise was noted with the AV block and the heart block resolved spontaneously within 1 minute.

Five patients received an overdose of dexmedetomidine in the ICU sedation studies. Two of these patients had no symptoms reported; 1 patient received a 2 mcg/kg loading dose over 10 minutes (twice the recommended loading dose) and 1 patient received a maintenance infusion of 0.8 mcg/kg/hr. Two other patients who received a 2 mcg/kg loading dose over 10 minutes experienced bradycardia or hypotension. One patient who received a loading bolus dose of undiluted dexmedetomidine (19.4 mcg/kg) had cardiac arrest from which he was successfully resuscitated.

NONPRESCRIPTION SLEEP AIDS

otc	**Unisom Nighttime Sleep-Aid** (Pfizer)	**Tablets:** 25 mg doxylamine succinate	(Unisom). Blue, scored. Oval. In 8s, 16s, 32s, 48s.
otc	**Dormin** (Randob)	**Tablets:** 25 mg diphenhydramine HCl	In 32s.
otc	**Miles Nervine** (Miles)		(Nervine). In 12s and 30s.
otc	**Nytol** (Block)		Lactose. (N). In 16s, 32s and 72s.
otc	**Simply Sleep** (McNeil)		In 24s and 48s.
otc	**Sleep-eze 3** (Whitehall)		In 12s and 24s.
otc	**Sleepwell 2-nite** (Rugby)		Sucrose. In 72s.
otc	**Sominex** (SmithKline Beecham)		(S). In 16s, 32s and 72s.
otc	**Extra Strength Tylenol PM** (McNeil-CPC)	**Tablets:** 25 mg diphenhydramine, 500 mg acetaminophen	**Tablets:** (Tylenol PM). In 24s, 50s. **Caplets:** (Tylenol PM). In 24s and 50s.
otc	**Exedrine P.M.** (Bristol-Myers Squibb)		Sorbitol. In 20s and 40s.
otc	**Bayer Select Maximum Strength Night Time Pain Relief** (Bayer)		In 24s and 50s.
otc	**Sominex Pain Relief** (SmithKline-Beecham)		In 16s and 32s.
otc	**Tycolene P.M.** (Pfeiffer Pharmaceuticals)		In 50s.
otc	**Extra Strength Doan's P.M.** (Ciba)	**Tablets:** 25 mg diphenhydramine HCl, 500 mg magnesium salicylate	(DOAN'S PM). In 20s.
otc	**Bufferin AF Nite Time** (B-M Squibb)		Parabens. Light blue. In 24s and 50s.
otc	**Unisom with Pain Relief** (Pfizer)	**Tablets:** 50 mg diphenhydramine HCl, 650 mg acetaminophen	In 16s.
otc	**Diphenhydramine HCl** (Rugby)	**Tablets:** 50 mg diphenhydramine HCl	Blue. In 50s.
otc	**Compoz Nighttime Sleep Aid** (Medtech)		Lactose. In 12s and 24s.
otc	**40 Winks** (Roberts Med)		In 30s.
otc	**Maximum Strength Nytol** (Block)		Lactose. (N). In 8s and 16s.
otc	**Snooze Fast** (BDI)		In 36s.
otc	**Midol PM** (Sterling Health)		In 16s.
otc	**Sominex** (SmithKline-Beecham)		(S). In 8s, 16s and 32s.
otc	**Twilite** (Pfeiffer)		Lactose. In 20s.
otc	**Excedrin PM Liquigels** (Bristol-Myers)	**Capsules:** 25 mg diphenhydramine HCl, 500 mg acetaminophen	Sorbitol. In 20s and 40s.
otc	**Extra Strength Tylenol PM Gelcaps** (McNeil-CPC)		EDTA, propylparaben. In 20s and 40s.
otc	**Legatrin PM** (Columbia)	**Tablets:** 50 mg diphenhydramine HCl, 500 mg acetaminophen	In 30s and 50s.
otc	**Melagesic PM** (B.F. Ascher)	**Tablets:** 500 mg acetaminophen, 1.5 mg melatonin.	In 32s.
otc	**Compoz Gel Caps** (Medtech)	**Capsules:** 25 mg diphenhydramine HCl	In 16s.
otc	**Dormin** (Randob)		Lactose. In 32s and 72s.
otc	**Maximum Strength Sleepinal Capsules and Soft Gels** (Thompson)	**Capsules:** 50 mg diphenhydramine HCl	**Capsules:** Lactose. In 16s.
			Soft Gels: Sorbitol. (Sleepinal). In 16s.
otc	**Maximum Strength Unisom SleepGels** (Pfizer)		Sorbitol. (UNISOM). In 8s.
otc	**Nighttime Pamprin** (Chattem)	**Powder:** 50 mg diphenhydramine HCl, 650 mg acetaminophen	Sugar. Apple cinnamon and hot chocolate flavors. In 4s.
otc	**Excedrin P.M.** (B-M Squibb)	**Liquid:** 167 mg acetaminophen, 8.3 mg diphenhydramine HCl/5 ml	10% alcohol, sucrose. Wild berry flavor. In 180 ml.
		Liquid: 1000 mg acetaminophen 50 mg diphenhydramine HCl/30 ml.	10% alcohol, sucrose. Wild berry flavor. In 180 ml.

For complete prescribing information for the antihistamines and for a complete listing of diphenhydramine HCl products, refer to the Antihistamines monograph in the Respiratory Drugs section.

Indications

Aid in the relief of insomnia.

Traditionally, products containing analgesics have been used for relief of insomnia due to minor pain.

Administration and Dosage

Administer 25 mg doxylamine or 50 mg diphenhydramine HCl (76 mg diphenhydramine citrate) before bedtime.

Actions

➤*Pharmacology:* These products contain antihistamines which act on the CNS, producing prominent sedative effects.

Contraindications

Asthma, glaucoma or prostate gland enlargement, except under a physician's advice.

Warnings

➤*Prolonged insomnia:* Not for use > 2 weeks. If insomnia persists for> 2 weeks, consult a physician; it may be a symptom of a serious underlying illness.

➤*Pregnancy:* Consult a physician before using these products. **Doxylamine** should not be taken by pregnant women.

➤*Lactation:* **Doxylamine** should not be taken by a nursing woman.

➤*Children:* Do not use in children < 12 years of age.

Precautions

➤*Hazardous tasks:* May cause drowsiness; observe caution while driving or performing other tasks requiring alertness, coordination or physical dexterity.

Adverse Reactions

Occasional anticholinergic effects may occur with doxylamine.

Overdosage

Antihistamine overdosage reactions may vary from CNS depression to stimulation. See the Antihistamines monograph for a more complete description of reactions.

Patient Information

Avoid alcoholic beverages while taking this product. Do not take this product if you are taking sedatives or tranquilizers without first consulting the physician.

May cause drowsiness; observe caution while driving or performing other tasks requiring alertness, coordination or physical dexterity.

Do not use if you have asthma, glaucoma, emphysema, chronic pulmonary disease, shortness of breath, difficulty in breathing or difficulty in urination due to prostate enlargement unless directed by the physician.

The following general discussion of the barbiturates refers to their use as sedative-hypnotic agents and as anticonvulsants. In addition, barbiturates are discussed under General Anesthetics, Barbiturates.

Indications

The following indications apply to most barbiturates. For specific indications, to the individual monographs.

➤*Sedation:* Although traditionally used as nonspecific CNS depressants for daytime sedation, the barbiturates have generally been replaced by the benzodiazepines.

➤*Hypnotic:* Short-term treatment of insomnia, since barbiturates appear to lose their effectiveness in sleep induction and maintenance after 2 weeks. If insomnia persists, seek alternative therapy (including nondrug) for chronic insomnia.

➤*Preanesthetic:* Used as preanesthetic sedatives.

➤*Anticonvulsant (mephobarbital, phenobarbital):* Treatment of partial and generalized tonic-clonic and cortical focal seizures.

➤*Acute convulsive episodes:* Emergency control of certain acute convulsive episodes (eg, those associated with status epilepticus, cholera, eclampsia, meningitis, tetanus and toxic reactions to strychnine or local anesthetics).

Administration and Dosage

Individualize dosage; consider patient's age, weight and condition. Use parenteral routes only when oral administration is impossible or impractical.

➤*IM injection:* IM injection of the sodium salts should be made deeply into a large muscle. Do not exceed 5 ml at any one site because of possible tissue irritation. Monitor patient's vital signs.

➤*IV:* Restrict to conditions in which other routes are not feasible, either because the patient is unconscious (as in cerebral hemorrhage, eclampsia or status epilepticus), or because the patient resists (as in delirium), or because prompt action is imperative. Slow IV injection is essential; observe patients carefully during administration. Maintain blood pressure, respiration and cardiac function, monitor vital signs and have equipment for resuscitation and artificial ventilation available.

➤*Rectal administration:* Rectally administered barbiturates are absorbed from the colon and are used occasionally in infants for prolonged convulsive states, or when oral or parenteral administration may be undesirable. If the rectal form is not available, the soluble sodium salt may be incorporated in a retention enema.

➤*Elderly/Debilitated:* Reduce dosage because these patients may be more sensitive to barbiturates.

➤*Hepatic/Renal function impairment:* Reduce dosage.

Actions

➤*Pharmacology:* Barbiturates can produce all levels of CNS mood alteration from excitation to mild sedation, hypnosis and deep coma. In sufficiently high therapeutic doses, barbiturates induce anesthesia. Overdosage can produce death.

These agents depress the sensory cortex, decrease motor activity, alter cerebellar function and produce drowsiness, sedation and hypnosis.

Barbiturates have little analgesic action at subanesthetic doses and may increase the reaction to painful stimuli. All barbiturates exhibit anticonvulsant activity in anesthetic doses. However, only phenobarbital and mephobarbital are effective as oral anticonvulsants in subhypnotic doses.

Barbiturates are respiratory depressants; the degree of respiratory depression is dose-dependent. With hypnotic doses, respiratory depression is similar to that which occurs during physiologic sleep and is accompanied by a slight decrease in blood pressure and heart rate.

➤*Pharmacokinetics:*
Absorption – Barbiturates are absorbed in varying degrees following oral, rectal or parenteral administration. The salts are more rapidly absorbed than the acids. The rate of absorption is increased if the sodium salt is ingested as a dilute solution or taken on an empty stomach.

Onset: Onset of action for oral or rectal administration varies from 20 to 60 minutes. For IM administration, onset is slightly faster than the oral route. Following IV administration, onset ranges from almost immediate for pentobarbital sodium and secobarbital to 5 minutes for phenobarbital sodium. Maximal CNS depression may not occur for ≥ 15 minutes after IV administration of phenobarbital sodium.

Duration: Duration of action varies and is related to dose and to the rate at which the barbiturates are redistributed throughout the body. In the following table, the barbiturates are classified according to their duration of action. Do not use this classification to predict the exact duration of effect, but use as a guide in drug selection.

Pharmacokinetics of Sedatives and Hypnotic Barbiturates						
	Half-Life (hrs)		Oral dosage range (mg)		Onset (minutes)	Duration (hours)
Barbiturate	Range	Mean	Sedative[1]	Hypnotic		
Long-Acting Mephobarbital	11 – 67	34	32 – 200	—	30 – ≥ 60	10 – 16
Phenobarbital	53 – 118	79	30 – 120	100 – 320		
Intermediate Amobarbital[2]	16 – 40	25	—	—	45 – 60	6 – 8
Aprobarbital	14 – 34	24	120	40 – 160		
Butabarbital	66 – 140	100	45 – 120	50 – 100		
Short-Acting Pentobarbital	15 – 50	†[3]	40 – 120	100	10 – 15	3 – 4
Secobarbital	15 – 40	28	—	100		

[1] Total daily dose; administered in 2 to 4 divided doses.
[2] Available as injection only.
[3] May follow dose-dependent kinetics. Mean t½ is 50 hrs for 50 mg and 22 hrs for 100 mg.

Distribution – Barbiturates are weak acids that are rapidly distributed to all tissues and fluids with high concentrations in the brain, liver and kidneys. Lipid solubility of the barbiturates is the dominant factor in their distribution. The more lipid soluble the barbiturate, the more rapidly it penetrates body tissue. Barbiturates are bound to plasma and tissue proteins; the degree of binding increases directly as a function of lipid solubility.

Phenobarbital has the lowest lipid solubility, plasma binding and brain protein binding, the longest delay in onset of activity and the longest duration of action. Secobarbital has the highest lipid solubility, plasma protein binding and brain protein binding, the shortest delay in onset of activity and the shortest duration of action.

Excretion – Barbiturates are metabolized primarily by the hepatic microsomal enzyme system, and the metabolic products are excreted in the urine, and less commonly, in the feces. Approximately 25% to 50% of a phenobarbital dose and 13% to 24% of an aprobarbital dose is eliminated unchanged in the urine, whereas the amount of other barbiturates excreted unchanged in the urine is negligible. The excretion of unmetabolized barbiturate is one feature that distinguishes the long-acting agents. The inactive metabolites of the barbiturates are excreted as conjugates of glucuronic acid.

➤*Clinical trials:* Barbiturate-induced sleep reduces the amount of time spent in the rapid eye movement (REM) phase of sleep or dreaming stage. Also, Stages III and IV sleep are decreased. Following abrupt cessation of barbiturates used regularly, patients may experience markedly increased dreaming, nightmares or insomnia.

Secobarbital and pentobarbital lose most of their effectiveness for inducing and maintaining sleep by the end of 2 weeks of continued drug administration, even with the use of multiple doses. Other barbiturates might also be expected to lose their effectiveness for inducing and maintaining sleep after about 2 weeks. However, definitions of tolerance vary; these two barbiturates have been given for weeks to months for chronic sedation with little tolerance developing, although decreased effects on sleep stages occur. In addition, the chronic disruption of the normal sleep pattern may make sleep less satisfying; therefore, dosages may be increased possibly resulting in enhanced tolerance. The short, intermediate and, to a lesser degree, long-acting barbiturates have been widely prescribed for treating insomnia. Although the clinical literature abounds with claims that the short-acting agents are superior for producing sleep, while the intermediate-acting compounds are more effective in maintaining sleep, controlled studies have failed to demonstrate these differential effects.

Mephobarbital has a relatively mild hypnotic effect, but exerts strong sedative effects. When used as a sedative, patients usually become more calm, cheerful and better adjusted to surroundings without clouding of mental faculties. It reportedly produces less sedation than phenobarbital.

Contraindications

Barbiturate sensitivity; manifest or latent porphyria; marked impairment of liver function; severe respiratory disease when dyspnea or obstruction is evident; nephritic patients; patients with respiratory disease where dyspnea or obstruction is present; intra-arterial administration (consequences vary from transient pain to gangrene); SC administration (produces tissue irritation ranging from tenderness and redness to necrosis); previous addiction to the sedative/hypnotic group (ordinary doses may be ineffective and may contribute to further addiction).

Warnings

►*Habit forming:* Tolerance or psychological and physical dependence may occur with continued use (see Drug abuse and dependence in the Precautions section). Administer with caution, if at all, to patients who are mentally depressed, have suicidal tendencies or a history of drug abuse (eg, alcoholics, opiate abusers, other sedative-hypnotic and amphetamine abusers). Limit prescribing and dispensing to the amount required for the interval until the next appointment.

►*IV administration:* Too rapid administration may cause respiratory depression, apnea, laryngospasm or vasodilation with fall in blood pressure. Parenteral solutions of barbiturates are highly alkaline. Therefore, use extreme care to avoid perivascular extravasation or intra-arterial injection. Extravascular injection may cause local tissue damage with subsequent necrosis; consequences of intra-arterial injection may vary from transient pain to gangrene of the limb. Any complaint of pain in the limb warrants stopping the injection.

Phenobarbital sodium may be administered IM or IV as an anticonvulsant for emergency use. When administered IV, it may require ≥ 15 minutes before reaching peak concentrations in the brain. Therefore, injecting phenobarbital sodium until the convulsions stop may cause the brain level to exceed that required to control the convulsions and may lead to severe barbiturate-induced depression.

►*Pain:* Exercise caution when administering to patients with acute or chronic pain, because paradoxical excitement could be induced or important symptoms could be masked. However, the use of barbiturates as sedatives in postoperative surgery and as adjuncts to cancer chemotherapy is well established.

►*Seizure disorders:* Status epilepticus may result from abrupt discontinuation, even when administered in small daily doses in the treatment of epilepsy.

►*Effects on vitamin D:* Barbiturates may increase vitamin D requirements, possibly by increasing the metabolism of vitamin D via enzyme induction. Rickets and osteomalacia have been reported rarely following prolonged use of barbiturates.

►*Renal function impairment:* Barbiturates are excreted either partially or completely unchanged in the urine and are contraindicated in patients with impaired renal function.

►*Hepatic function impairment:* Barbiturates are metabolized primarily by hepatic microsomal enzymes. Administer with caution and initially in reduced doses. Do not use in patients showing premonitory signs of hepatic coma.

►*Elderly:* May produce marked excitement, depression and confusion. In some persons, barbiturates repeatedly produce excitement rather than depression.

►*Pregnancy:* Category D. Barbiturates can cause fetal damage when administered to a pregnant woman. Studies suggest a connection between maternal consumption of barbiturates and a higher incidence of fetal abnormalities. If this drug is used during pregnancy, or if the patient becomes pregnant while taking this drug, apprise her of the potential hazards to the fetus.

Barbiturates readily cross the placental barrier and are distributed throughout fetal tissues. Fetal blood levels approach maternal blood levels following parenteral use.

Withdrawal symptoms occur in infants born to mothers who receive barbiturates throughout the last trimester of pregnancy. Reports include the acute withdrawal syndrome of seizures and hyperirritability from birth to a delayed onset of up to 14 days.

Anticonvulsant use – Because of the strong possibility of precipitating status epilepticus with attendant hypoxia and risk to both mother and unborn child, do not discontinue anticonvulsants when used to prevent major seizures. However, consider discontinuing anticonvulsants prior to and during pregnancy when the nature, frequency and severity of the seizures do not pose a serious threat to the patient. It is not known whether even minor seizures constitute some risk to the embryo or fetus.

Maternal ingestion of anticonvulsants, particularly barbiturates, may be associated with a neonatal coagulation defect that may cause bleeding, usually within 24 hours of birth. The defect is characterized by decreased levels of vitamin K-dependent clotting factors, and prolongation of prothrombin time, partial thromboplastin time or both. Give prophylactic vitamin K to the mother 1 month prior to and during delivery, and to the infant immediately after birth.

Labor and delivery – Hypnotic doses do not appear to significantly impair uterine activity during labor. Full anesthetic doses decrease the force and frequency of uterine contractions. Administration to the mother during labor may result in respiratory depression in the newborn; premature infants are particularly susceptible. If barbiturates are used during labor and delivery, have resuscitation equipment available.

►*Lactation:* Exercise caution when administering to the nursing mother, since small amounts are excreted in breast milk. Drowsiness in the nursing infant has been reported.

►*Children:* In some persons, especially children, barbiturates repeatedly produce excitement rather than depression. Barbiturates may produce irritability, excitability, inappropriate tearfulness and aggression in children. Hyperkinetic states may also be induced and are primarily related to a specific drug sensitivity. Cognitive deficits have been associated with phenobarbital use for complicated febrile seizures in children. Safety and efficacy of amobarbital (children < 6 years of age) and aprobarbital have not been established.

Precautions

►*Monitoring:* During prolonged therapy, perform periodic laboratory evaluation of organ systems, including hematopoietic, renal and hepatic systems.

►*Special risk:* Untoward reactions may occur in the presence of fever, hyperthyroidism, diabetes mellitus and severe anemia. Use with caution.

Use **mephobarbital** with caution in patients with myasthenia gravis and myxedema.

►*Drug abuse and dependence:* Barbiturates may be habit forming. Tolerance, psychological dependence and physical dependence may occur, especially following prolonged use of high doses. Doses in excess of 400 mg/day pentobarbital or secobarbital for ≈ 90 days are likely to produce some degree of physical dependence. A dose of 600 to 800 mg taken for at least 35 days is sufficient to produce withdrawal seizures. The average daily dose for the barbiturate addict is usually about 1.5 g. As tolerance develops, the amount needed to maintain the same level of intoxication increases; tolerance to a fatal dosage, however, does not increase more than two-fold. As this occurs, the margin between an intoxicating dosage and fatal dosage becomes smaller.

Intoxication – Symptoms of acute intoxication include unsteady gait, slurred speech and sustained nystagmus. Mental signs of chronic intoxication include confusion, poor judgment, irritability, insomnia and somatic complaints. If an individual appears to be intoxicated with alcohol to a degree that is radically disproportionate to the amount of alcohol in his/her blood, suspect the use of barbiturates. The lethal dose of a barbiturate is far less if alcohol is also ingested.

Dependence – Symptoms are similar to those of chronic alcoholism and include: A strong desire or need to continue taking the drug; tendency to increase the dose; psychic dependence on the effects of the drug related to subjective and individual appreciation of those effects; and physical dependence on the effects of the drug requiring its presence for maintenance of homeostasis resulting in a definite, characteristic and self-limited abstinence syndrome when the drug is withdrawn.

Withdrawal symptoms – Withdrawal symptoms can be severe and may cause death.

Minor symptoms: These may appear 8 to 12 hours after the last dose of a barbiturate and usually appear in the following order: Anxiety, muscle twitching, tremor of hands and fingers, progressive weakness, dizziness, distortion in visual perception, nausea, vomiting, insomnia and orthostatic hypotension.

Major symptoms: Convulsions and delirium may occur within 16 hours and last up to 5 days after abrupt cessation of these drugs. Intensity of withdrawal symptoms gradually declines in ≈ 15 days.

Treatment of dependence – Treatment of dependence consists of cautious and gradual withdrawal of the drug which takes an extended period of time.

One method involves substituting 30 mg phenobarbital for each 100 to 200 mg dose of barbiturate the patient has been taking. The total daily amount of phenobarbital is administered in 3 to 4 divided doses, not to exceed 600 mg/day. Should signs of withdrawal occur on the first day of treatment, administer an IM loading dose of 100 to 200 mg phenobarbital in addition to the oral dose. After stabilization on phenobarbital, decrease the total daily dose by 30 mg/day as long as withdrawal is proceeding smoothly. A modification of this regimen involves initiating treatment at the patient's regular dosage level and decreasing the daily dosage by 10%, if tolerated. Severely dependent individuals may generally be withdrawn over 2 to 3 weeks.

Infants physically dependent on barbiturates may be given phenobarbital 3 to 10 mg/kg/day. After withdrawal symptoms (eg, hyperactivity, disturbed sleep, tremors, hyperreflexia) are relieved, gradually decrease the dosage of phenobarbital; completely withdraw over 2 weeks.

►*Tartrazine sensitivity:* Some of these products contain tartrazine, which may cause allergic-type reactions (including bronchial asthma) in susceptible individuals. Although the incidence of tartrazine sensitivity in the general population is low, it is frequently seen in patients who also have aspirin hypersensitivity. Specific products containing tartrazine are identified in the product listings.

Drug Interactions

Most reports of clinically significant drug interactions occurring with the barbiturates have involved phenobarbital.

Sedative/Hypnotic Barbiturate Drug Interactions			
Precipitant drug	Object drug*		Description
Alcohol	Barbiturates	↑	Concomitant use may produce additive CNS effects and death.
Charcoal	Barbiturates	↓	Charcoal can reduce the absorption of barbiturates. Depending on the clinical situation, this will reduce their efficacy or toxicity.
Chloramphenicol	Barbiturates	↓	Chloramphenicol may inhibit phenobarbital metabolism. Barbiturates may enhance chloramphenicol metabolism.
Barbiturates	Chloramphenicol	↑	
MAO inhibitors	Barbiturates	↑	MAOIs may enhance the sedative effects of barbiturates.
Rifampin	Barbiturates	↓	Rifampin induces hepatic microsomal enzymes and may decrease the effectiveness of barbiturates.
Valproic acid	Barbiturates	↑	Valproic acid appears to decrease barbiturate metabolism, resulting in an increased effect.
Barbiturates	Anticoagulants	↓	Barbiturates can increase metabolism of anticoagulants resulting in a decreased response. Patients stabilized on anticoagulants may require dosage adjustments if barbiturates are added to or withdrawn from their regimen.
Barbiturates	Beta blockers	↓	Pharmacokinetic parameters of certain β-blockers (metoprolol and propranolol) may be altered by barbiturates. Timolol does not appear to be affected.
Barbiturates	Carbamazepine	↓	Decreased serum carbamazepine levels may occur.
Barbiturates	Clonazepam	↓	Increased clonazepam clearance may occur, which can lead to lower steady-state levels and loss of efficacy.
Barbiturates	Contraceptives, oral	↓	Decreased contraceptive effect may occur due to induction of microsomal enzymes. Menstrual irregularities (spotting, breakthrough bleeding) or pregnancy may occur. An alternate form of birth control is suggested.
Barbiturates	Corticosteroids	↓	Barbiturates may enhance corticosteroid metabolism through the induction of hepatic microsomal enzymes.
Barbiturates	Digitoxin	↓	Barbiturates may increase digitoxin metabolism.
Barbiturates	Doxorubicin	↓	Total doxorubicin plasma clearance may be increased.
Barbiturates	Doxycycline	↓	Phenobarbital decreases doxycycline's half-life and serum levels, which may persist for 2 weeks after barbiturate therapy is discontinued.
Barbiturates	Felodipine	↓	Felodipine plasma levels and bioavailability may be reduced.
Barbiturates	Fenoprofen	↓	Fenoprofen bioavailability may be decreased.
Barbiturates	Griseofulvin	↓	Phenobarbital appears to interfere with the absorption of oral griseofulvin, thus decreasing its blood level; however, the effect on therapeutic response has not been established.
Barbiturates	Hydantoins	↔	The effect of barbiturates on metabolism is unpredictable; monitor hydantoin and barbiturate blood levels frequently if these drugs are given concurrently.
Barbiturates	Methoxyflurane	↑	Enhanced renal toxicity may occur.
Barbiturates	Metronidazole	↓	Barbiturates may decrease the antimicrobial effectiveness of metronidazole.
Barbiturates	Narcotics	↔	Methadone actions may be reduced. CNS depressant effects of meperidine may be prolonged.
Barbiturates	Phenylbutazone	↓	The elimination half-life of phenylbutazone may be reduced.
Barbiturates	Quinidine	↓	Phenobarbital may significantly reduce the serum levels and half-life of quinidine.
Barbiturates	Theophylline	↓	Barbiturates decrease theophylline levels, possibly resulting in decreased effects.
Barbiturates	Verapamil	↓	The clearance of verapamil may be increased and its bioavailability decreased.

* ↓=Object drug decreased.   ↑=Object drug increased.   ↔=Undetermined clinical effect.

Adverse Reactions

The following adverse reactions and their incidence were from observations of hospitalized patients. Because such patients may be less aware of milder adverse effects of barbiturates, the incidence may be higher in fully ambulatory patients.

➤*Cardiovascular:* Bradycardia, hypotension, syncope (< 1%).

➤*CNS:* Somnolence (1% to 3%); agitation, confusion, hyperkinesia, ataxia, CNS depression, nightmares, nervousness, psychiatric disturbance, hallucinations, insomnia, anxiety, dizziness, abnormal thinking, headache, fever (especially with chronic phenobarbital use) (< 1%); vertigo; lethargy; residual sedation (hangover effect); drowsiness.

Emotional disturbances and phobias may be accentuated with phenobarbital use. In some persons, barbiturates repeatedly produce excitement rather than depression; the patient may appear to be inebriated. Irritability and hyperactivity can occur in children.

Barbiturates, when given in the presence of pain, may cause restlessness, excitement and even delirium. Rarely, the use of barbiturates results in localized or diffuse myalgic, neuralgic or arthritic pain, especially in psychoneurotic patients with insomnia. The pain may appear in paroxysms, is most intense in the early morning hours and is most frequently located in the region of the neck, shoulder girdle and upper limbs. Symptoms may last for days after the drug is discontinued.

➤*GI:* Nausea, vomiting, constipation (< 1%); liver damage, particularly with chronic phenobarbital use (< 1%).

➤*Hematologic:* Megaloblastic anemia (rarely, following chronic phenobarbital use).

➤*Hypersensitivity:* Skin rashes, angioedema (particularly following chronic phenobarbital use) (< 1%); exfoliative dermatitis (eg, Stevens-Johnson syndrome and toxic epidermal necrolysis) may be caused by phenobarbital and may be fatal (rare).

Acquired hypersensitivity to barbiturates consists chiefly in allergic reactions that occur especially in persons who tend to have asthma, urticaria, angioedema and similar conditions. Hypersensitivity reactions in this category include localized swelling, particularly of the eyelids, cheeks or lips, and erythematous dermatitis. The skin eruption may be associated with fever, delirium and marked degenerative changes in the liver and other parenchymatous organs.

➤*Local:* Inadvertent intra-arterial injection may produce arterial spasm with resultant thrombosis and gangrene of an extremity. Reactions range from transient pain to severe tissue necrosis and neurological deficit. Injection SC may produce tissue necrosis, pain, tenderness and redness. Injection into or near peripheral nerves may result in permanent neurological deficit. Thrombophlebitis after IV use and pain at IM injection site have been reported.

➤*Respiratory:* Hypoventilation, apnea (< 1%); circulatory collapse; respiratory depression.

Overdosage

The toxic dose of barbiturates varies considerably. In general, an oral dose of 1 g produces serious poisoning in an adult. Death commonly occurs after 2 to 10 g of ingested barbiturate.

➤*Symptoms:* Onset of symptoms may not occur until several hours after ingestion. Acute barbiturate overdosage is manifested by CNS and respiratory depression which may progress to Cheyne-Stokes respiration, areflexia, constriction of the pupils to a slight degree (though in severe poisoning they may show paralytic dilation), nystagmus, ataxia, oliguria, tachycardia, hypotension, lowered body temperature and coma. Typical shock syndrome (eg, apnea, circulatory collapse, respiratory arrest, death) may occur.

In extreme overdose, all electrical activity in the brain may cease, in which case a "flat" EEG normally equated with clinical death cannot be accepted. This effect is fully reversible unless hypoxic damage occurs. Consider the possibility of barbiturate intoxication even in situations that appear to involve trauma.

Complications such as pneumonia, pulmonary edema, cardiac arrhythmias, congestive heart failure and renal failure may occur. Uremia may increase CNS sensitivity to barbiturates if renal function is impaired. Differential diagnosis should include hypoglycemia, head trauma, cerebrovascular accidents, convulsive states and diabetic coma.

➤*Treatment:* Treatment is mainly supportive. Maintain an adequate airway, with assisted respiration and oxygen administration, as necessary. Monitor vital signs and fluid balance. Refer to General Management of Acute Overdosage.

If the patient is conscious and has not lost the gag reflex, emesis may be induced with ipecac. Take care to prevent pulmonary aspiration of vomitus. After completion of vomiting, administer 30 g activated charcoal in a glass of water. Nasogastric administration of multiple doses of activated charcoal has been successful in accelerating the elimination of phenobarbital from the body. If emesis is contraindicated, perform gastric lavage with a cuffed endotracheal tube in place with the patient in the face down position. Activated charcoal may be left in the emptied stomach and a saline cathartic administered.

Administer fluid and other standard treatments for shock, if needed. If renal function is normal, forced diuresis may aid in the elimination of the barbiturate. However, diuresis and peritoneal dialysis are of little value. Alkalinization of the urine increases renal excretion of some barbiturates, especially phenobarbital, aprobarbital and mephobarbital (which is metabolized to phenobarbital).

Hemodialysis and hemoperfusion may be used in severe barbiturate intoxication or if the patient is anuric or in shock. Patient should be rolled from side to side every 30 minutes.

Patient Information

Do not increase the dose of the drug without consulting a physician.

Barbiturates may impair mental or physical abilities required for the performance of potentially hazardous tasks (eg, driving, operating machinery).

Alcohol should not be consumed while taking barbiturates. Concurrent use of barbiturates with other CNS depressants (eg, alcohol, narcotics, tranquilizers and antihistamines) may result in additional CNS depressant effects.

Notify physician if any of the following occurs: Fever; sore throat; mouth sores; easy bruising or bleeding; tiny broken blood vessels under the skin.

Use as an aid to sleep is limited; do not use > 2 weeks.

Long-Acting

PHENOBARBITAL

c-iv	**Phenobarbital** (Various, eg, Harber, Lilly, Major, Moore, PBI, Parmed, Roxane, Rugby, Warner Chilcott)	**Tablets:** 15 mg	In 100s, 1000s, 5000s and UD 100s.
c-iv	**Solfoton** (ECR Pharm.)	**Tablets:** 16 mg	In 100s and 500s.
c-iv	**Phenobarbital** (Various, eg, Goldline, Harber, Lilly, Major, Moore, PBI, Parmed, Roxane, Rugby)	**Tablets:** 30 mg	In 100s, 1000s and 5000s and UD 100s.
c-iv	**Phenobarbital** (Various, eg, Century, Harber, Lilly, Moore, PBI, Parmed, Roxane)	**Tablets:** 60 mg	In 100s, 1000s and UD 100s.
c-iv	**Phenobarbital** (Various, eg, URL)	**Tablets:** 90 mg	In 1000s.
c-iv	**Phenobarbital** (Various, eg, Century, Harber, Lilly, Roxane)	**Tablets:** 100 mg	In 100s and 1000s.
c-iv	**Solfoton** (ECR Pharm.)	**Capsules:** 16 mg	In 100s and 500s.
c-iv	**Phenobarbital** (Pharmaceutical Associates)	**Elixir:** 15 mg/5 ml	13.5% alcohol. Fruit flavor. In pt and UD 5, 10 and 20 ml.
c-iv	**Phenobarbital** (Various, eg, Barre-National, Century, Goldline, Harber, Lilly, Roxane)	**Elixir:** 20 mg/5 ml	Alcohol. In pt, gal, UD 5 ml and UD 7.5 ml.
c-iv	**Phenobarbital Sodium** (Wyeth-Ayerst)	**Injection:** 30 mg/ml	In 1 ml *Tubex.*
c-iv	**Phenobarbital Sodium** (Wyeth-Ayerst)	**Injection:** 60 mg/ml	In 1 ml *Tubex.*
c-iv	**Phenobarbital Sodium** (Wyeth-Ayerst)	**Injection:** 65 mg/ml	In 1 ml vials.
c-iv	**Phenobarbital Sodium** (Various, eg, Elkins-Sinn, Wyeth-Ayerst)	**Injection:** 130 mg/ml	In 1 ml *Tubex* and 1 ml vials.
c-iv	**Luminal Sodium** (Sanofi Winthrop)		In 1 ml amps.[1]

[1] With 10% alcohol and 67.8% propylene glycol.

For complete prescribing information, refer to the Barbiturates group monograph.

Indications

➤*Oral:* Sedative; hypnotic (short-term treatment of insomnia since it appears to lose its effectiveness after 2 weeks); anticonvulsant (treatment of partial and generalized tonic-clonic and cortical focal seizures); emergency control of certain acute convulsive episodes (eg, those associated with status epilepticus, eclampsia, tetanus and toxic reactions to strychnine or local anesthetics).

➤*Parenteral:* Sedative; hypnotic (short-term treatment of insomnia since it appears to lose its effectiveness after 2 weeks); preanesthetic; anticonvulsant (treatment of generalized tonic-clonic and cortical focal seizures); emergency control of acute convulsions (eg, tetanus, eclampsia, status epilepticus).

Administration and Dosage

Individualize dosage. Factors of consideration are age, weight and condition.

➤*Anticonvulsant:* In infants and children, a loading dose of 15 to 20 mg/kg produces blood levels of ≈ 20 mcg/ml shortly after administration. To achieve therapeutic blood levels (10 to 25 mcg/ml), higher dosages per kilogram are generally necessary compared to adults.

➤*Oral:*

Adults –
Sedation: 30 to 120 mg/day in 2 to 3 divided doses. A single dose of 30 to 120 mg may be given at intervals; frequency is determined by response. It is generally considered that no more than 400 mg should be given during a 24 hour period.
Hypnotic: 100 to 200 mg.
Anticonvulsant: 60 to 100 mg/day.

Children –
Anticonvulsant: 3 to 6 mg/kg/day.
Sedation: 8 to 32 mg.
Hypnotic: Determined by age and weight.

➤*Parenteral:* Observe the effect of large doses. Use only when oral use is impossible or impractical.

Adults –
Sedation: 30 to 120 mg/day IM or IV in 2 to 3 divided doses.

Preoperative sedation: 100 to 200 mg, IM only, 60 to 90 min before surgery.
Hypnotic: 100 to 320 mg IM or IV.
Acute convulsions: 200 to 320 mg IM or IV, repeated in 6 hours as necessary.

Children –
Preoperative sedation: 1 to 3 mg/kg IM or IV.
Anticonvulsant: 4 to 6 mg/kg/day for 7 to 10 days to blood level of 10 to 15 mcg/ml, or 10 to 15 mg/kg/day, IV or IM.
Status epilepticus: 15 to 20 mg/kg IV over 10 to 15 minutes. It is imperative to achieve therapeutic levels as rapidly as possible. When given IV, it may require ≥ 15 minutes to attain peak levels in the brain. If injected continuously until convulsions stop, the brain concentration would continue to rise and could exceed that required to control seizures. Since a barbiturate-induced depression may occur, it is important to use the minimal amount required and to wait for the anticonvulsant effect to develop before giving a second dose.

IM – Administer deep IM into one of the large muscles (gluteus maximus, vastus lateralis) or other areas where there is little risk of encountering a nerve trunk or a major artery. Injection into or near peripheral nerves may result in permanent neurological deficit.

IV – Restrict IV use to conditions in which other routes are not feasible, either because the patient is unconscious (as in cerebral hemorrhage, eclampsia or status epilepticus) or because of resistance (as in delirium) or because prompt action is imperative.

No average IV dose reliably produces similar effects in all patients. Possibility of overdose and respiratory depression is remote with slow injection of fractional doses. Observe physical signs closely. Onset of action is usually within 5 minutes of IV use.

In convulsive states, minimize dosage to avoid compounding the depression which may follow convulsions. The injection must be made slowly.

Any vein may be used; administer preferably into a larger vein (to minimize the possibility of thrombosis). Avoid administration into varicose veins, because circulation is retarded. Inadvertent injection into or adjacent to an artery may result in gangrene requiring amputation of an extremity or a portion thereof. Careful technique, including aspiration, is necessary to avoid inadvertent intra-arterial injection.

➤*Elderly/Debilitated:* Reduce dosage; these patients may be more sensitive to the drug.

➤*Hepatic/Renal function impairment:* Reduce dosage.

Long-Acting

MEPHOBARBITAL

c-iv	**Mebaral** (Ovation)	**Tablets:** 32 mg		(M 31). In 250s.
		50 mg		(M 32). In 250s.
		100 mg		(M 33). In 250s.

For complete prescribing information, refer to the Barbiturates group monograph.

Indications

Sedative for the relief of anxiety, tension and apprehension; anticonvulsant for the treatment of grand mal and petit mal epilepsy.

Administration and Dosage

➤*Sedative:*

Adults – 32 to 100 mg 3 or 4 times a day. Optimum dose is 50 mg 3 or 4 times/day.

Children – 16 to 32 mg 3 or 4 times per day.

➤*Epilepsy:*

Adults – Average dose is 400 to 600 mg daily.

Children (< 5 years of age) – 16 to 32 mg 3 or 4 times per day.

Children (> 5 years of age) – 32 to 64 mg 3 or 4 times per day.

Take at bedtime if seizures generally occur at night, and during the day if attacks are diurnal. Start treatment with a small dose and gradually increase over 4 or 5 days until optimum dosage is determined.

➤*Replacement therapy:* Start with a small dose and gradually increase over 4 or 5 days until optimum dose is determined. If the patient has been taking another antiepileptic drug, gradually reduce the dosage of the other drug as the doses of mephobarbital are increased, to guard against the temporary marked attacks that may occur when treatment for epilepsy is changed abruptly. Similarly, when the dose is to be lowered to a maintenance level or to be discontinued, reduce the amount gradually over 4 or 5 days.

➤*Combination drug therapy:* May be used in combination with phenobarbital, in alternating courses or concurrently. When the two are used at the same time, the dose should be about one-half the amount of each used alone. The average daily dose for an adult is from 50 to 100 mg phenobarbital and from 200 to 300 mg mephobarbital. May also be used with phenytoin. When used concurrently, a reduced dose of phenytoin is advisable, but the full dose of mephobarbital may be given. Satisfactory results have been obtained with an average daily dose of 230 mg phenytoin plus about 600 mg mephobarbital.

➤*Elderly/Debilitated:* Reduce dosage since these patients may be more sensitive to the drug.

➤*Hepatic/Renal function impairment:* Reduce dosage.

Intermediate-Acting

AMOBARBITAL SODIUM

c-ii	**Amytal Sodium** (Lilly)	**Powder for Injection**		In 250 and 500 mg vials.

For complete prescribing information, refer to the Barbiturates group monograph.

Indications

Sedation; hypnotic (short-term treatment of insomnia since it appears to lose its effectiveness after 2 weeks); preanesthetic.

Administration and Dosage

Individualize dosage. The maximum single dose for an adult is 1 g.

➤*Sedative:* The usual adult dosage is 30 to 50 mg, 2 or 3 times per day.

➤*Hypnotic:* The usual adult dose is 65 to 200 mg.

➤*IM:* Do not inject a volume > 5 ml IM, regardless of drug concentration, at any one site because of possible tissue irritation. The average IM dose ranges from 65 to 500 mg. Solutions of 20% may be used so that a small volume can contain a large dose. Inject deeply into a large muscle, such as the gluteus maximus. Superficial IM or SC injections may be painful and may produce sterile abscesses or sloughs.

➤*IV:* Restrict IV use to conditions in which other routes are not feasible, either because the patient is unconscious, resists, or because prompt action is imperative. Slow injection is essential. Monitor patients carefully. Do not exceed the rate of 50 mg/min. Ordinarily, 65 to 500 mg may be given to a child 6 to 12 years of age. The final dosage is determined to a great extent by the patient's reaction to the slow administration of the drug.

➤*Preparation of solution:* Add Sterile Water for Injection to the vial and rotate to facilitate solution of the powder. Do not shake the vial.

➤*Elderly/Debilitated:* Reduce dosage since these patients may be more sensitive to the drug.

➤*Hepatic/Renal function impairment:* Reduce dosage.

➤*Storage/Stability:* Do not use a solution which is not absolutely clear after 5 minutes. Amobarbital sodium hydrolyzes in solution or upon exposure to air. No more than 30 minutes should elapse from the time the vial is opened until contents are injected.

BUTABARBITAL SODIUM

c-iii	**Butabarbital Sodium** (Various)	**Tablets:** 15 mg	In 1000s.
c-iii	**Butisol Sodium** (Wallace)		(Butisol Sodium 37 112). Lavender, scored. In 100s and 1000s.
c-iii	**Butabarbital Sodium** (Various)	**Tablets:** 30 mg	In 100s and 1000s.
c-iii	**Butisol Sodium** (Wallace)		Tartrazine. (Butisol Sodium 37 113). Green, scored. In 100s and 1000s.
c-iii	**Butisol Sodium** (Wallace)	**Tablets:** 50 mg	Tartrazine. (Butisol Sodium 37 114). Orange, scored. In 100s.
c-iii	**Butisol Sodium** (Wallace)	**Tablets:** 100 mg	(Butisol Sodium 37 115). Pink, scored. In 100s.
c-iii	**Butabarbital Sodium** (Various, eg, Harber, Major)	**Elixir:** 30 mg/5 ml	In pt.
c-iii	**Butisol Sodium** (Wallace)		7% alcohol, tartrazine, saccharin. In pt and gal.

For complete prescribing information, refer to the Barbiturates group monograph.

Indications

Sedative or hypnotic. Barbiturates appear to lose their effectiveness for sleep induction and maintenance after 2 weeks.

Administration and Dosage

➤*Adults:*

Daytime sedation – 15 to 30 mg, 3 or 4 times daily.

Bedtime hypnotic – 50 to 100 mg.

Preoperative sedation – 50 to 100 mg, 60 to 90 minutes before surgery.

➤*Children:*

Preoperative sedation – 2 to 6 mg/kg; maximum 100 mg.

➤*Elderly/Debilitated:* Reduce dosage; these patients may be more sensitive to the drug.

➤*Hepatic/Renal function impairment:* Reduce dosage.

Short-Acting

SECOBARBITAL SODIUM

c-ii	**Seconal Sodium Pulvules** (Ranbaxy)	**Capsules:** 100 mg	(F40). Orange. In 100s and UD 100s.

For complete prescribing information, refer to the Barbiturates group monograph.

Indications

➤*Oral:* Hypnotic (short-term treatment of insomnia since it appears to lose its effectiveness after 2 weeks); preanesthetic.

Administration and Dosage

➤*Adults:*
Preoperative sedation – 200 to 300 mg 1 to 2 hours before surgery.
Bedtime hypnotic – 100 mg.
➤*Children :*
Preoperative sedation – 2 to 6 mg/kg (max. 100 mg).
➤*Elderly/debilitated:* Reduce dosage; these patients may be more sensitive to the drug.
➤*Hepatic/Renal function impairment:* Reduce dosage.

PENTOBARBITAL SODIUM

c-ii	**Pentobarbital Sodium** (Various)	**Capsules:** 100 mg	In 1000s.
c-ii	**Nembutal** (Ovation)	**Elixir:** Equivalent to 20 mg pentobarbital sodium/5 ml	Saccharin, sucrose, 18% alcohol. In pints.
c-ii	**Pentobarbital Sodium** (Wyeth-Ayerst)	**Injection:** 50 mg/ml	In 2 ml Tubex.[1]

[1] With propylene glycol and 10% alcohol.

For complete prescribing information, refer to the Barbiturates group monograph.

Indications

➤*Oral:* Sedative; hypnotic (short-term treatment of insomnia, since it appears to lose its effectiveness after 2 weeks); preanesthetic.

➤*Rectal:* Sedation (when oral or parenteral administration may be undesirable); hypnotic (short-term treatment of insomnia, since it appears to lose its effectiveness after 2 weeks).

➤*Parenteral:* Sedative; hypnotic (short-term treatment of insomnia since it appears to lose its effectiveness after 2 weeks); preanesthetic; anticonvulsant, in anesthetic doses, for the emergency control of certain acute convulsive episodes (eg, those associated with status epilepticus, eclampsia, meningitis, tetanus and toxic reactions to strychnine or local anesthetics).

Administration and Dosage

➤*Oral:*
Adults –
Sedation: 20 mg 3 or 4 times/day.
Hypnotic: 100 mg at bedtime.
Children –
Sedation: 2 to 6 mg/kg/day, depending on age, weight and degree of sedation desired.
Hypnotic: Base dosage on age and weight.
Preanesthetic: 2 to 6 mg/kg/day (max. 100 mg), depending on age, weight and desired degree of sedation.

➤*Rectal:* Do not divide suppositories.
Adults – 120 to 200 mg.
Children –
12 to 14 years (36.4 to 50 kg; 80 to 110 lbs): 60 or 120 mg.
5 to 12 years (18.2 to 36.4 kg; 40 to 80 lbs): 60 mg.
1 to 4 years (9 to 18.2 kg; 20 to 40 lbs): 30 or 60 mg.
2 months to 1 year (4.5 to 9 kg; 10 to 20 lbs): 30 mg.

➤*Parenteral:* Pentobarbital solutions are highly alkaline. Therefore, exercise extreme care to avoid perivascular extravasation or intra-arterial injection.

IV – Restrict IV use to conditions in which other routes are not feasible, including patient unconsciousness (as in cerebral hemorrhage, eclampsia or status epilepticus), because of resistance (as in delirium), or because prompt action is imperative. Slow IV injection is essential; carefully observe patients during administration. The rate of IV injection should not exceed 50 mg/min. No average IV dose can be relied upon to produce similar effects in different patients. The possibility of overdose and respiratory depression is remote when the drug is injected slowly in fractional doses. The clinical response is the basis for dosage determination, although the patient's weight and age may influence the total amount of the drug required. Watch the physical signs closely to accurately obtain and maintain the desired degree of sedation.

Initially administer 100 mg in the 70 kg adult. Reduce dosage proportionally for pediatric or debilitated patients. At least 1 minute is necessary to determine the full effect. If needed, additional small increments of the drug may be given to a total of 200 to 500 mg for healthy adults.

In convulsive states, keep dosages to a minimum to avoid compounding the depression which may follow convulsions. Inject slowly with regard to the time required for the drug to penetrate the blood-brain barrier.

IM – Inject deeply into a large muscle mass. Do not exceed a volume of 5 ml at any one site because of possible tissue irritation.

Calculate dosage on basis of age, weight and the patient's condition. The usual adult dosage is 150 to 200 mg; children's dosage frequently ranges from 2 to 6 mg/kg as a single IM injection, not to exceed 100 mg.

➤*Elderly/Debilitated:* Reduce dosage; these patients may be more sensitive to the drug.

➤*Hepatic/Renal function impairment:* Reduce dosage.

➤*Storage/Stability:* Do not use if solution is discolored or contains a precipitate.

Oral Combinations

ORAL COMBINATIONS

Combined barbiturate products are promoted to provide a more balanced effect through the combination of those with differing rates of action and dissipation.

c-ii	**Tuinal 100 mg Pulvules** (Lilly)	**Capsules:** 50 mg amobarbital sodium and 50 mg secobarbital sodium	Blue and orange. In 100s.
c-ii	**Tuinal 200 mg Pulvules** (Lilly)	**Capsules:** 100 mg amobarbital sodium and 100 mg secobarbital sodium	Blue and orange. In 100s.

Consider the information given for Barbiturates (see group monograph) when using these products.

Barbiturates

Indications

Induction of anesthesia; supplementation of other anesthetic agents; IV anesthesia for short surgical procedures with minimal painful stimuli; induction of a hypnotic state.

➤*Thiopental (IV):* Control of convulsive states and in neurosurgical patients with increased intracranial pressure if adequate ventilation is provided.

➤*Thiopental (rectal suspension):* Used when preanesthetic sedation or basal narcosis by the rectal route is desired. It may be employed as the sole agent in selected brief, minor procedures where muscular relaxation and analgesia are not required.

Actions

➤*Pharmacology:* The ultrashort-acting barbiturates, thiopental, thiamylal and methohexital, depress the CNS to produce hypnosis and anesthesia without analgesia. Methohexital does not possess muscle relaxant properties. These drugs are frequently used to provide hypnosis during balanced anesthesia with other agents for muscle relaxation and analgesia.

Biotransformation products of thiopental are pharmacologically inactive and mostly excreted in the urine.

➤*Pharmacokinetics:* The rapid onset and brief duration of action of these drugs is a function of their high lipid solubility. They quickly cross the blood-brain barrier, but are rapidly redistributed from the brain to other body tissues, first to highly perfused visceral organs (liver, kidneys, heart) and muscle, and later to fatty tissues.

Administered IV as the sodium salts, these agents produce anesthesia within 1 minute. Recovery after a small dose is rapid, with somnolence and retrograde amnesia. Muscle relaxation occurs at the onset of anesthesia. The duration of anesthetic activity following a single IV dose is 20 to 30 minutes for thiopental and thiamylal, and somewhat shorter for methohexital. Thiopental is readily absorbed by the rectal route when administered as a suspension; onset of action usually occurs within 8 to 10 minutes. Thiopental IV produces hypnosis within 30 to 40 seconds following administration. Repeated doses or continuous infusion of these agents causes accumulation. Slow release of the drug from lipoidal storage sites results in prolonged anesthesia, somnolence and respiratory and circulatory depression. The plasma half-life is 3 to 8 hours.

Contraindications

➤*Absolute:* Latent or manifest porphyria; hypersensitivity to barbiturates; absence of suitable veins for IV administration.

➤*Relative:* Severe cardiovascular disease; hypotension or shock; conditions in which hypnotic effects may be prolonged or potentiated (excessive premedication, Addison's disease, hepatic or renal dysfunction, myxedema, increased blood urea and severe anemia); increased intracranial pressure; asthma; myasthenia gravis; status asthmaticus (thiopental).

If barbiturates are used in conditions involving relative contraindications, reduce dosage and administer slowly.

➤*Rectal suspension:* Patients who are to undergo rectal surgery; presence of inflammatory, ulcerative, bleeding or neoplastic lesions of the lower bowel; patients with acute asthmatic attacks, and variegate or acute intermittent porphyria.

Warnings

➤*Status asthmaticus:* Use **methohexital** and **thiamylal** with extreme caution in patients with status asthmaticus.

➤*Repeated or continuous infusion:* Repeated or continuous infusion may cause cumulative effects resulting in prolonged somnolence and respiratory and circulatory depression. Resuscitative and endotracheal intubation equipment and oxygen should be immediately available. Maintain patency of the airway at all times.

➤*Pregnancy:* Category C (thiopental); Category B (methohexital). Safety for use during pregnancy has not been established. Use only when clearly needed and when the potential benefits outweigh the potential hazards to the fetus.

Thiopental – Thiopental readily crosses the placental barrier.

Methohexital – Methohexital has been used in cesarean section delivery, but because of its solubility and lack of protein binding, it readily and rapidly traverses the placenta.

➤*Lactation:* Small amounts of **thiopental** may appear in breast milk following administration of large doses. Exercise caution when administering barbiturates to a nursing woman.

➤*Children:*
Methohexital – Safety and efficacy in children have not been established.

Precautions

➤*Extravascular injection:* Extravascular injection may cause pain, swelling, ulceration and necrosis. Intra-arterial injection is dangerous and may produce gangrene of an extremity.

➤*Rectal dose:* If evacuation of the instilled rectal dose occurs, assess the effects of any retained portion before administering a repeat dose.

➤*Special risk:* Respiratory depression, apnea or hypotension may occur due to individual variations in tolerance or to the physical status of the patient. Exercise caution in debilitated patients, or those with impaired function of respiratory, circulatory, cardiac, renal, hepatic or endocrine systems.

➤*Drug abuse and dependence:* May be habit-forming.

Drug Interactions

Barbiturate Drug Interactions			
Precipitant Drug	Object Drug*		Description
Narcotics	Barbiturate anesthetics	↑	The barbiturate dose required to induce anesthesia may be reduced. Apnea may be more common with this combination.
Phenothiazines	Barbiturate anesthetics	↑	Preanesthetic use of phenothiazines may raise the frequency and severity of neuromuscular excitation and hypotension in patients who receive barbiturate anesthesia.
Probenecid	Barbiturate anesthetics	↑	The anesthesia produced by the barbiturate may be extended or achieved at lower doses.
Sulfisoxazole	Barbiturate anesthetics	↑	Sulfisoxazole may enhance the anesthetic effects of the barbiturate.

* ↑ = Object drug increased.

➤*Drug/Lab test interactions:* BSP and liver function studies may be influenced by administration of a single dose of barbiturates.

Adverse Reactions

➤*Cardiovascular:* Circulatory depression; thrombophlebitis; hypotension; peripheral vascular collapse; convulsions in association with cardiorespiratory arrest; myocardial depression; cardiac arrhythmias.

➤*CNS:* Emergence delirium; headache; restlessness; anxiety; seizures; prolonged somnolence and recovery.

➤*GI:* Nausea; emesis; abdominal pain. Rectal irritation; diarrhea; cramping; rectal bleeding (rectal administration).

➤*Hypersensitivity:*
Acute allergic reactions – Erythema; pruritus; urticaria; anaphylactic reaction.

➤*Local:* Pain or nerve injury at injection site.

➤*Respiratory:* Respiratory depression including apnea; dyspnea; rhinitis; laryngospasm; bronchospasm; sneezing; coughing.

➤*Miscellaneous:* Salivation; hiccups skin rashes; skeletal muscle hyperactivity; shivering.

Rarely, immune hemolytic anemia with renal failure and radial nerve palsy have occurred.

Overdosage

➤*Symptoms:* Overdosage may occur from too rapid or repeated injections. Too rapid injection may be followed by an alarming fall in blood pressure, even to shock levels. Apnea, occasional laryngospasm, coughing and other respiratory difficulties with excessive or too rapid injections may occur.

➤*Treatment:* In the event of suspected or apparent overdosage, discontinue the drug, maintain or establish a patent airway (intubate if necessary) and administer oxygen with assisted ventilation if necessary. The lethal dose of barbiturates varies and cannot be stated with certainty. Lethal blood levels may be as low as 1 mg/dl for short-acting barbiturates; less if other depressant drugs or alcohol are also present.

THIOPENTAL SODIUM

c-iii	**Thiopental Sodium** (IMS)	**Powder for Injection:** 2% (20 mg/ml)	In 400 mg *Min-I-Mix* vials with *Min-I-Mix* injector.
c-iii	**Pentothal** (Abbott)		In 1, 2.5 and 5 g kits, 400 mg *Ready-to-Mix* syringes and 400 mg *Ready-to-Mix LifeShield* syringes.
c-iii	**Thiopental Sodium** (Various, eg, Gensia, IMS)	**Powder for Injection:** 2.5% (25 mg/ml)	In 250 and 500 mg *Min-I-Mix* vials with *Min-I-Mix* and 500 mg, 1, 2.5, 5 and 10 g kits.
c-iii	**Pentothal** (Abbott)		In 1, 2.5, 5 g and 500 mg kits, 250 and 500 mg *Ready-to-Mix* syringes and 250 and 500 mg *Ready-to-Mix LifeShield* syringes.

For complete prescribing information refer to the Barbiturate Anesthetics group monograph.

Administration and Dosage

➤*Parenteral:* Administer IV only. Individual response is so varied that there can be no fixed dosage. Titrate against patient requirement as governed by age, sex and body weight.

Test dose – Inject a small test dose of 25 to 75 mg to assess tolerance or unusual sensitivity. Observe patient reaction for ≥ 60 seconds.

Anesthesia – Moderately slow induction can be accomplished in the average adult by injection of 50 to 75 mg (2 to 3 ml of a 2.5% solution) at intervals of 20 to 40 seconds, depending on patient response. Once anesthesia is established, additional injections of 25 to 50 mg can be administered whenever the patient moves. Slow injection is recommended to minimize respiratory depression and the possibility of overdosage.

When used for induction in balanced anesthesia with a skeletal muscle relaxant and an inhalation agent, the total dose can be estimated and then injected in two to four fractional doses. With this technique, brief periods of apnea may occur, which may require assisted or controlled pulmonary ventilation. As an initial dose, 210 to 280 mg (3 to 4 mg/kg) is usually required for rapid induction in the average adult (70 kg).

When used as the sole anesthetic agent, the desired level of anesthesia can be maintained by injection of small repeated doses as needed or by using a continuous IV drip in a 0.2% or 0.4% concentration.

Convulsive states following anesthesia (inhalation or local) or other causes – Administer 75 to 125 mg (3 to 5 ml of a 2.5% solution) as soon as possible after the convulsion begins. Convulsions following the use of a local anesthetic may require 125 to 250 mg, given over a 10–minute period.

Neurosurgical patients with increased intracranial pressure – Administer intermittent bolus injections of 1.5 to 3.5 mg/kg to reduce intra-operative elevations of intracranial pressure, if adequate ventilation is provided.

Psychiatric disorders – For narcoanalysis and narcosynthesis, premedication with an anticholinergic agent may precede administration of thiopental. After a test dose, thiopental is injected at a slow rate of 100 mg/min (4 ml/min of a 2.5% solution) with the patient counting backwards from 100.

Alternative thiopental may be administered by rapid IV drip using a 0.2% concentration in 5% Dextrose in Water. The rate of administration should not exceed 50 ml/min.

➤*Preparation of parenteral solution:* Use one of the following diluents: Sterile Water for Injection; 0.9% Sodium Chloride Injection; 5% Dextrose Injection. A 2% or 2.5% solution is most commonly used for intermittent injections, although concentrations vary between 2% and 5%. A 3.4% concentration in Sterile Water for Injection is isotonic. Do not use concentrations < 2% in Sterile Water for Injection because they cause hemolysis.

Use concentrations of 0.2% or 0.4% for continuous IV administration. Prepare them with 5% Dextrose Injection, 0.9% Sodium Chloride Injection or Normosol-R.

➤*Admixture incompatibility:* The most stable solutions are those in water or in isotonic saline, refrigerated and tightly stoppered. Do not mix solutions of succinylcholine, tubocurarine or other drugs that have an acid pH with thiopental solutions.

➤*Storage/Stability:* Freshly prepare parenteral solutions and use promptly; discard unused portions after 24 hours.

METHOHEXITAL SODIUM

c-iv	**Brevital Sodium** (Lilly)	**Powder for Injection:** 2.5 g	In 20 ml vials.

For complete prescribing information, refer to the Barbiturate Anesthetics group monograph.

Administration and Dosage

Pre-anesthetic medication is generally advisable. Any of the recognized pre-anesthetic medications may be used, but the phenothiazines are less satisfactory than the combination of an opiate and a belladonna derivative.

Individualize dosage. Administer IV in a concentration ≤ 1%. Higher concentrations markedly increase the incidence of muscular movements and irregularities in respiration and blood pressure.

➤*Induction:* The dose for induction of anesthesia may range from 50 to 120 mg or more, but averages ≈ 70 mg. Give a 1% solution at ≈ 1 ml/5 seconds. The induction dose usually provides anesthesia for 5 to 7 minutes. Usual dosage in adults ranges from 1 to 1.5 mg/kg.

➤*Maintenance:* Maintenance of anesthesia may be accomplished by intermittent injections of the 1% solution or by continuous IV drip of a 0.2% solution. Intermittent injections of ≈ 20 to 40 mg (2 to 4 ml of a 1% solution) may be given as required, usually every 4 to 7 minutes. For continuous drip, the average rate of administration is ≈ 3 ml of a 0.2% solution/min (1 drop/sec). Individualize the rate of flow for each patient. For longer surgical procedures, gradual reduction in the rate of administration is recommended.

➤*Admixture compatibility/incompatibility:* Do not use bacteriostatic diluents; Sterile Water for Injection is preferred. The 5% Dextrose Injection or 0.9% Sodium Chloride Injection may be used. (Not compatible with Lactated Ringer's Injection). Do not mix methohexital in the same syringe or administer simultaneously during IV infusion through the same needle with acid solutions, such as atropine sulfate, metocurine iodide and succinylcholine chloride (alteration of pH may cause free barbituric acid to be precipitated).

Reconstitution – When the first dilution is made, the solution in the vial will be yellow. When further diluted to make a 1% solution, it must be clear and colorless, or should not be used.

Preparation of 1% Methohexital Solutions	
Vial	Amount diluent (ml)
500 mg	50 ml
2.5 g	250 ml
5.0 g	500 ml

➤*Continuous drip anesthesia:* Prepare a 0.2% solution by adding 500 mg to 250 ml diluent. For this dilution, use 5% Dextrose or Isotonic (0.9%) Sodium Chloride instead of distilled water to avoid extreme hypotonicity.

➤*Storage/Stability:* Reconstituted solutions are chemically stable at room temperature for 24 hours. Store vials at room temperature.

KETAMINE HCl

c-iii	**Ketamine HCl** (Various, eg, Bedford)	**Injection:** 10 mg/ml	In 20 ml vials.[1]
		50 mg/ml	In 10 ml vials.[1]
		100 mg/ml	In 5 ml vials.[1]
c-iii	**Ketalar** (Monarch)	**Injection:** Ketamine base (as HCl): 10 mg/ml	In 20 ml vials (10s).[1]
		50 mg/ml	In 10 ml vials (10s).[1]
		100 mg/ml	In 5 ml vials (10s).[1]

[1] With benzethonium chloride.

WARNING

Emergence reactions: Emergence reactions occur in ≈ 12% of patients. The incidence is least in young (≤ 15 years old) and elderly (> 65 years old) patients. Also less frequent with IM use.

Psychological manifestations – Severity varies between pleasant dream-like states, vivid imagery, hallucinations and emergence delirium sometimes accompanied by confusion, excitement and irrational behavior. The duration is ordinarily a few hours; however, recurrences have been seen up to 24 hours postoperatively. No residual psychological effects are known.

The incidence may be reduced by using lower dosages with IV diazepam. These reactions may be reduced if verbal, tactile and visual patient stimulation is minimized during recovery. This does not preclude monitoring vital signs.

Management – To terminate a severe emergence reaction, a small hypnotic dose of a short-acting or ultrashort-acting barbiturate may be required.

When used on an outpatient basis, do not release patient until recovery from anesthesia is complete. Patients should be accompanied by an adult.

Indications

➤*Diagnostic/Surgical procedures:* Sole anesthetic agent for diagnostic and surgical procedures that do not require skeletal muscle relaxation. Ketamine is best suited for short procedures, but it can be used with additional doses for longer procedures.

➤*Anesthesia:* For induction of anesthesia prior to administration of other general anesthetics.

➤*Supplement:* Used to supplement low-potency agents, such as nitrous oxide.

Administration and Dosage

Individualize dosage.

➤*Induction:*

IV route – Administer over 60 seconds. Initial dose ranges from 1 to 4.5 mg/kg. The average amount to produce 5 to 10 minutes of surgical anesthesia is 2 mg/kg.

Alternatively, in adults, 1 to 2 mg/kg administered at a rate of 0.5 mg/kg/min may be used for induction of anesthesia. In addition, diazepam may be given in 2 to 5 mg doses (total: ≤ 15 mg IV), in a separate syringe over 60 seconds. This may reduce incidence of psychological manifestations during emergence.

Administer slowly (over 60 seconds). More rapid administration may result in respiratory depression and enhanced pressor response.

Note: Do not inject 100 mg/ml concentration IV without proper dilution. Dilute with equal volume Sterile Water for Injection, Normal Saline or 5% Dextrose in Water.

IM route – Initial dose ranges from 6.5 to 13 mg/kg. A dose of 10 mg/kg will usually produce 12 to 25 minutes of surgical anesthesia.

➤*Maintenance:* Increments of one-half to the full induction dose may be repeated as needed for maintenance of anesthesia. The larger the total dose administered, the longer the time to complete recovery.

Adults induced with ketamine augmented with IV diazepam may be maintained on ketamine given by slow microdrip infusion at 0.1 to 0.5 mg/minute, augmented with 2 to 5 mg IV diazepam, given as needed. Often, ≤ 20 mg of IV diazepam total for combined induction and maintenance will suffice. The incidence of psychological manifestations during emergence may be reduced.

Dilution – To prepare a dilute solution containing 1 mg/ml, transfer 10 ml (50 mg/ml vial) or 5 ml (100 mg/ml vial) to 500 ml of 5% Dextrose Injection or Sodium Chloride (0.9%) Injection and mix well.

Vials of 10 mg/ml are not recommended for dilution.

If fluid restriction is required, add ketamine to a 250 ml infusion, as described above, to provide a 2 mg/ml concentration.

Admixture incompatibility – Barbiturates and ketamine are incompatible (precipitate); do not inject from same syringe. Do not mix ketamine and diazepam in syringe or infusion flask.

Ketamine is clinically compatible with the commonly used general and local anesthetic agents when an adequate respiratory exchange is maintained.

➤*Storage/Stability:* Store between 15° to 30°C (59° to 86°F). Protect from light.

Actions

➤*Pharmacology:* Ketamine is a rapid-acting general anesthetic producing an anesthetic state characterized by profound analgesia, normal pharyngeal-laryngeal reflexes, normal or slightly enhanced skeletal muscle tone, cardiovascular and respiratory stimulation and occasionally, a transient and minimal respiratory depression. A patent airway is maintained partly by virtue of unimpaired pharyngeal and laryngeal reflexes.

The anesthetic state produced by ketamine has been termed "dissociative anesthesia" in that it appears to selectively interrupt association pathways of the brain before producing somatesthetic sensory blockade. It may selectively depress the thalamoneocortical system before significantly obtunding the more ancient cerebral centers and pathways (reticular-activating and limbic systems).

➤*Pharmacokinetics:* Following IV administration, the ketamine concentration has an initial slope (α-phase) lasting ≈ 45 minutes with a half-life of 10 to 15 minutes, corresponding to anesthetic effect. Anesthetic action is terminated by redistribution from CNS and by hepatic biotransformation. The major metabolite is ≈ ⅓ as active as ketamine. The β-phase half-life of ketamine is 2.5 hours.

Elevation of blood pressure begins shortly after injection, reaches a maximum in minutes and returns to pre-anesthetic values within 15 minutes. The systolic and diastolic blood pressure peaks from 10% to 50% above pre-anesthetic levels.

An IV dose of 2 mg/kg usually produces surgical anesthesia within 30 seconds after injection, lasting 5 to 10 minutes. Additional increments can be administered IV or IM to maintain anesthesia without significant cumulative effects.

IM doses of 9 to 13 mg/kg usually produce surgical anesthesia within 3 to 4 minutes and last ≈ 12 to 25 minutes.

Contraindications

Patients in whom a significant elevation of blood pressure would be a serious hazard; hypersensitivity to the drug.

Warnings

➤*Cardiac effects:* Monitor cardiac function continuously during the procedure in patients with hypertension or cardiac decompensation.

➤*Respiratory effects:* Respiratory depression may occur with overdosage or too rapid a rate of administration, in which case employ supportive ventilation. Mechanical support of respiration is preferred to administration of analeptics.

➤*Tonic-clonic movements:* Purposeless and tonic-clonic movements of extremities may occur during the course of anesthesia. These movements do not imply a light plane and are not indicative of the need for additional doses of the anesthetic.

➤*Emergence reactions and psychological manifestation:* See Warning Box.

➤*Pregnancy: Category C.* Safety for use during pregnancy, including obstetrics, has not been established; use is not recommended.

Precautions

➤*Respiratory surgery/diagnostic procedures:* Do not use in surgery or diagnostic procedures of the pharynx, larynx or bronchial tree. Do not administer ketamine alone because pharyngeal and laryngeal reflexes are usually active. Muscle relaxants, with proper attention to respiration, may be required.

➤*Vomiting:* Vomiting has been reported following administration. Laryngeal-pharyngeal reflexes may offer some airway protection, however the possibility of aspiration must be considered because protective reflexes may also be diminished by supplementary anesthetics and muscle relaxants.

➤*Visceral pain:* In surgical procedures involving visceral pain pathways, supplement with an agent that obtunds visceral pain.

➤*Preoperative preparation:* Give atropine, scopolamine or another drying agent at an appropriate interval prior to induction.

➤*Alcohol:* Use with caution in chronic alcoholics and acutely alcohol intoxicated patients.

➤*Resuscitative:* Resuscitative equipment should be ready for use.

➤*Cerebrospinal fluid pressure:* Cerebrospinal fluid pressure increase has been reported following administration.

KETAMINE HCl

➤*Hazardous tasks:* Warn patients not to drive, operate hazardous machinery or engage in hazardous activities for 24 hours or more after anesthesia.

Drug Interactions

Ketamine Drug Interactions			
Precipitant drug	Object drug*		Description
Ketamine	Nondepolarizing muscle relaxants	↑	Ketamine may increase the neuromuscular effects resulting in prolonged respiratory depression.
Ketamine	Thiopental	↓	The hypnotic effect of thiopental may be antagonized.
Barbiturates/Narcotics	Ketamine	↑	Prolonged recovery time may occur if used with ketamine.
Halothane	Ketamine	↓	Cardiac output, blood pressure and pulse rate may be decreased. Halothane blocks the cardiovascular stimulatory effects of ketamine. Closely monitor cardiac function if ketamine and halothane are used together.
Theophyllines	Ketamine	↔	Unpredictable extensor-type seizures have been reported with coadministration.
Thyroid hormones	Ketamine	↑	Concurrent use may produce hypertension and tachycardia.

* ↑ = Object drug increased. ↓ = Object drug decreased. ↔ = Undetermined effect.

Adverse Reactions

➤*Cardiovascular:* Elevated blood pressure and pulse rate (frequent); hypotension; bradycardia; arrhythmia.

➤*CNS:* Enhanced skeletal muscle tone manifested by tonic and clonic movements, sometimes resembling seizures.

➤*GI:* Anorexia; nausea; vomiting.

➤*Ophthalmic:* Diplopia; nystagmus; slight elevation in intraocular pressure.

➤*Psychiatric:* (See Warning Box).

➤*Respiratory:* Although respiration is frequently stimulated, severe depression of respiration or apnea may occur following rapid IV administration of high doses. Laryngospasm and other forms of airway obstruction have occurred.

➤*Miscellaneous:* Local pain and exanthema at the injection site (infrequent); transient erythema or morbilliform rash.

Overdosage

Respiratory depression may occur with overdosage or too rapid administration rate; employ supportive ventilation. Mechanical support of respiration is preferred to analeptic use.

ETOMIDATE

Rx	Amidate (Abbott)	Injection: 2 mg/ml	In 10, 20 ml amps, 20 ml *Abboject*.

Indications

➤*Anesthesia:* Induction of general anesthesia.

➤*Supplementation:* Supplementation of subpotent anesthetic agents, such as nitrous oxide in oxygen, during maintenance of anesthesia for short operative procedures.

➤*Unlabeled uses:* Etomidate has been used for prolonged sedation of critically ill patients or ventilator-dependent patients; however, this use has been associated with increased risks, including acute adrenal insufficiency and increased mortality.

Administration and Dosage

➤*Induction of anesthesia:* For IV use only. Adults and children > 10 years of age, 0.2 to 0.6 mg/kg. Usual dose is 0.3 mg/kg, injected over 30 to 60 seconds.

Concomitant anesthesia – Smaller increments may be given to adults during short operative procedures to supplement subpotent anesthetic agents. Compatible with commonly used preanesthetic medication.

Actions

➤*Pharmacology:* Etomidate, a nonbarbiturate hypnotic without analgesic activity, has fewer cardiovascular depressant effects than thiopental sodium. Up to 0.6 mg/kg in patients with severe cardiovascular disease has little or no effect on myocardial metabolism, cardiac output, peripheral circulation or pulmonary circulation. Hemodynamic effects are qualitatively similar to those of thiopental sodium. Etomidate lowers cerebral blood flow and cerebral oxygen consumption. It will usually lower intracranial pressure slightly and intraocular pressure moderately.

➤*Pharmacokinetics:* Injection IV produces hypnosis rapidly, usually within 1 minute. Duration is usually 3 to 5 minutes. Immediate recovery period will usually be shortened in adults by ≈ 0.1 mg IV fentanyl, 1 or 2 min before induction of anesthesia, probably because less etomidate is generally required. Protein binding, primarily to albumin, is ≈ 76%. Etomidate is rapidly metabolized in the liver. Plasma levels of unchanged drug decrease rapidly up to 30 minutes following injection and thereafter more slowly with a half-life of ≈ 75 minutes. Approximately 75% of the dose is excreted in the urine, mostly as metabolite (80%).

Contraindications

Hypersensitivity to etomidate.

Warnings

➤*Corticosteroid replacement:* Although no changes in vital signs or increased mortality have been reported with etomidate-induced reduced plasma cortisol levels, consider exogenous corticosteroid replacement in patients undergoing severe stress.

➤*Myoclonus:* Prior IV narcotic or benzodiazepine administration may reduce the incidence of these involuntary muscle movements.

➤*Renal/Hepatic function impairment:* Limited pharmacokinetic data in patients with cirrhosis and esophageal varices suggest that the volume of distribution and elimination half-life of etomidate are approximately double that seen in healthy subjects.

➤*Pregnancy: Category C.* Etomidate has embryocidal effects in rats when given in doses 1 and 4 times the human dose and has caused maternal toxicity in rats and rabbits. Use only when clearly needed and when the potential benefits outweigh the unknown potential hazards to the fetus. Use in labor and delivery is not recommended.

➤*Lactation:* Some etomidate is excreted in breast milk. Use caution when administering to a nursing mother.

➤*Children:* Safety and efficacy for use in children < 10 years of age have not been established. Use is not recommended.

Drug Interactions

➤*Verapamil:* The anesthetic effect of etomidate may be increased with prolonged respiratory depression and apnea.

Adverse Reactions

Most frequent – Transient skeletal muscle movements (32%) classified as myoclonic in the majority of cases (74%; see Warnings); transient venous pain (20%); tonic movements (10%); eye movements (9%); averting movements (7%).

➤*Cardiovascular:* Hypertension; hypotension; tachycardia; bradycardia; arrhythmias.

➤*Miscellaneous:* Hyperventilation; hypoventilation; apnea of short duration (5 to 90 seconds with spontaneous recovery); laryngospasm; hiccoughs; snoring; postoperative nausea or vomiting following induction of anesthesia.

MIDAZOLAM HCl

c-iv	Versed (Roche)	Syrup: 2 mg/ml	Sorbitol. Cherry flavor. In 118 ml of syrup, with press-in bottle adapter, 4 single-use, graduated, oral dispensers, and 4 tip caps.
c-iv	Midazolam HCl (Various, eg, Abbott, Bedford)	Injection: 1 mg (as HCl)/ml	In 2 and 5 ml vials and *Carpuject* vials and 10 ml vials.
c-iv	Versed (Roche)		In 2, 5 and 10 ml vials.[1]
c-iv	Midazolam HCl (Various, eg, Abbott, Bedford)	5 mg (as HCl)/ml	In 1, 2, and 5 ml vials and *Carpuject* vials, 10 ml vials, and 2 ml syringes.
c-iv	Versed (Roche)		In 1, 2, 5 and 10 ml vials, 2 ml *Tel-E-Ject* syringes.[1]

[1] With 1% benzyl alcohol and EDTA.

Benzodiazepine compounds used as antianxiety agents appear under the Antianxiety Agents monograph.

MIDAZOLAM HCl

WARNING

Midazolam IV has been associated with respiratory depression and respiratory arrest. In some cases, where this was not recognized promptly and treated effectively, death or hypoxic encephalopathy resulted. Use midazolam IV only in hospital or ambulatory care settings, including physicians' offices, that provide for continuous monitoring of respiratory and cardiac function. Assure immediate availability of resuscitative drugs and equipment and personnel trained in their use. (See Warnings.)

The initial IV dose for conscious sedation may be as little as 1 mg, but should not exceed 2.5 mg in a normal healthy adult. Lower doses are necessary for older (> 60 years) or debilitated patients and in patients receiving concomitant narcotics or other CNS depressants. Never give the initial dose and all subsequent doses as a bolus; administer over at least 2 minutes and allow an additional 2 or more minutes to fully evaluate sedative effect. Use of 1 mg/ml formulation or dilution of 1 mg/ml or 5 mg/ml formulation is recommended to facilitate slower injection. See Administration and Dosage for complete dosing information.

Indications

▶*Preoperative sedation (IV and IM):* Preoperative sedation, anxiolysis and amnesia.

▶*Sedation/Anesthesia (IV):* Sedation, anxiolysis and amnesia prior to or during short diagnostic, therapeutic or endoscopic procedures, either alone or with other CNS depressants; for induction of general anesthesia before administration of other anesthetic agents; to supplement nitrous oxide and oxygen (balanced anesthesia); infusion for sedation of intubated and mechanically ventilated patients as a component of anesthesia or during treatment in a critical care setting.

▶*Unlabeled uses:* Treatment of epileptic seizures (10 to 15 mg); alternative for the termination of refractory status epilepticus.

Administration and Dosage

Administer IV or IM only.

Individualize dosage. Midazolam is a potent sedative agent which requires slow administration. Midazolam is 3 to 4 times as potent per mg as diazepam. Because serious and life-threatening cardiorespiratory events have been reported, make provisions for monitoring, detection and correction of these reactions for every patient, regardless of age or health status. Excessive doses or rapid or single bolus IV doses may result in respiratory depression or arrest. (See Warnings.)

▶*Elderly or debilitated patients:* In general, lower doses are required. Adjust the IV dosage according to the type and amount of premedication used.

▶*Preoperative sedation anxiolysis and amnesia (IM):* Inject deep in a large muscle mass. 0.07 to 0.08 mg/kg (≈ 5 mg for an average adult) up to 1 hour before surgery. For patients > 60 years of age, debilitated, chronically ill or receiving concomitant CNS depressants, the dose must be individualized and reduced. Onset is in 15 minutes, peaking at 30 to 60 minutes. Atropine or scopolamine and reduced narcotic doses may be coadministered.

▶*Sedation, anxiolysis or amnesia for procedures (IV):* Use midazolam either alone or with a narcotic. For peroral procedures, use an appropriate topical anesthetic. For bronchoscopic procedures, use narcotic premedication.

Use 1 mg/ml to facilitate slower injection. Dilute the 1 and 5 mg/ml formulations with 0.9% sodium chloride or 5% dextrose in water. Individualize dosage. Do not give by rapid or single bolus IV. Response will vary with age, physical status and concomitant medications, but may also vary independent of these factors. (See Warnings.)

Healthy adults < 60 years of age – Titrate slowly to the desired effect (eg, the initiation of slurred speech). Some patients may respond to as little as 1 mg. Give no more than 2.5 mg over at least 2 minutes. Wait an additional 2 or more minutes to fully evaluate the sedative effect. If further titration is necessary, use small increments to the appropriate level of sedation. Wait an additional 2 or more minutes after each increment to fully evaluate sedative effect. A total dose> 5 mg is usually not necessary.

If narcotic premedication or other CNS depressants are used, patients will require ≈ 30% less midazolam than unpremedicated patients.

Patients ≥ 60 years of age, debilitated/chronically ill patients – The danger of underventilation or apnea is greater and the peak effect may take longer in these patients; reduce increments and slow the rate of injection.

Titrate slowly to desired effect (eg, initiation of slurred speech). Some patients may respond to as little as 1 mg. Give ≤ 1.5 mg over ≥ 2 minutes. Wait an additional 2 or more minutes to fully evaluate sedative effect. If additional titration is needed, give at a rate of no more than 1 mg over 2 minutes, waiting an additional 2 or more minutes each time to fully evaluate sedative effect. Total doses > 3.5 mg are not usually necessary.

If CNS depressant premedications are used in these patients, they will require at least 50% less midazolam than healthy young unpremedicated patients.

Maintenance – Give in increments of 25% of the dose used to first reach the sedative endpoint, only by slow titration, especially in the elderly/chronically ill/debilitated. Give only if thorough evaluation clearly indicates need for additional sedation.

▶*Induction of general anesthesia, before use of other anesthetics (IV):* Individual response is variable, particularly when a narcotic premedication is not used. Titrate dosage to desired clinical effect according to patient's age and clinical status. When midazolam is used before other IV agents for induction of anesthesia, the initial dose of each agent may be significantly reduced, at times as low as 25% of the usual initial dose of the individual agents.

Unpremedicated patients – An average adult < 55 years of age will initially require 0.3 to 0.35 mg/kg over 20 to 30 seconds, allowing 2 minutes for effect. If needed to complete induction, use increments of ≈ 25% of initial dose; may complete induction with volatile liquid inhalational anesthetics. Up to 0.6 mg/kg total dose may be used, but may prolong recovery.

Unpremedicated patients > 55 years of age or with severe systemic disease or other debilitation may require less midazolam. For patients > 55 years of age, an initial dose is 0.3 mg/kg. For patients with severe systemic disease or other debilitation, an initial dose of 0.2 to 0.25 mg/kg will usually suffice; in some cases, as little as 0.15 mg/kg.

Premedicated patients – Give 0.15 to 0.35 mg/kg. In average adults < 55 years of age, give 0.25 mg/kg over 20 to 30 seconds and allow 2 minutes for effect. Use 0.2 mg/kg for good risk (ASA I & II) surgical patients> 55 years of age. In patients with severe systemic disease or debilitation, 0.15 mg/kg may suffice.

Narcotic premedication used during clinical trials included fentanyl (1.5 to 2 mcg/kg IV, given 5 minutes before induction), morphine (individualized, up to 0.15 mg/kg IM) or meperidine (individualized, up to 1 mg/kg IM). Sedative premedications were hydroxyzine pamoate (100 mg orally) and sodium secobarbital (200 mg orally). Except for IV fentanyl, give all other premedications ≈ 1 hr before midazolam.

▶*Maintenance of anesthesia (IV):* Maintenance of anesthesia (IV) for short surgical procedures, as a component of balanced anesthesia. Give incremental injections of ≈ 25% of the induction dose in response to signs of lightening of anesthesia and repeat as necessary.

▶*Continuous infusion:* Dilute 5 mg/ml to a concentration of 0.5 mg/ml with 0.9% Sodium Chloride or 5% Dextrose in Water.

Usual adult dose – If a loading dose is necessary to rapidly initiate sedation, 0.01 to 0.05 mg/kg (≈ 0.5 to 4 mg for a typical adult) may be given slowly or infused over several minutes. This dose may be repeated at 10 to 15 minute intervals until adequate sedation is achieved. For maintenance of sedation, the usual initial infusion rate is 0.02 to 0.1 mg/kg/hr (1 to 7 mg/hr). Higher loading or maintenance infusion rates may occasionally be required in some patients. Use the lowest recommended doses in patients with residual effects from anesthetic drugs or in those concurrently receiving other sedatives or opioids.

Individual response to midazolam is variable. Titrate the infusion rate to the desired level of sedation. Perform assessment of sedation at regular intervals and adjust the midazolam infusion rate up or down by 25% to 50% of the initial infusion rate to assure adequate titration of sedation level. Larger adjustments or even a small incremental dose may be necessary if rapid changes in the level of sedation are indicated. In addition, decrease the infusion rate by 10% to 25% every few hours to find the minimum effective infusion rate. Finding the minimum effective infusion rate decreases the potential accumulation of midazolam and provides for the most rapid recovery once the infusion is terminated. Patients who exhibit agitation, hypertension or tachycardia in response to noxious stimulation, but who are otherwise adequately sedated, may benefit from concurrent administration of an opioid analgesic. Addition of an opioid will generally reduce the minimum effective midazolam infusion rate.

Pediatric (non-neonatal): To initiate sedation, an IV loading dose of 0.05 to 0.2 mg/kg administered over at least 2 to 3 minutes can be used to establish the desired clinical effect in patients whose trachea is intubated. This loading dose may be followed by a continuous IV infusion to maintain the effect. Assisted ventilation is recommended for pediatric patients who are receiving other CNS depressant medications such as pioids. Initiate continuous IV infusions of midazolam at a rate of 0.06 to 0.12 mg/kg/hr (1 to 2 mcg/kg/min). The rate of infusion can be increased or decreased (generally by 25% of the initial or subsequent infusion rate) as required, or supplemental IV doses of midazolam can be administered to increase or maintain the desired effect. Frequent assessment at regular intervals using standard pain/sedation scale is recommended.

• *Hemodynamically compromised patients* – When initiating an infusion with midazolam in hemodynamically compromised patients, titrate the usual loading dose of midazolam in small increments and monitor the patient for hemodynamic instability (eg, hypotension). Monitor respiratory rate and oxygen saturation carefully.

Neonatal: In intubated preterm and term neonates, initiate continuous IV infusions of midazolam at a rate of 0.03 mg/kg/hr (0.5 mcg/kg/

MIDAZOLAM HCl

min) in neonates < 32 weeks of age and 0.06 mg/kg/hr (1 mcg/kg/min) in neonates > 32 weeks of age. Do not use IV loading doses in neonates; rather the infusion may be run more rapidly for the first several hours to establish therapeutic plasma levels. Frequently reassess the rate of infusion, particularly after the first 24 hours, so as to administer the lowest possible effective dose and reduce the potential for drug accumulation. This is particularly important because of the potential for adverse effects related to metabolism of the benzyl alcohol.

▶*Children:*

Sedation, anxiolysis or amnesia (IM) – Sedation after IM midazolam is age- and dose-dependent; higher doses may result in deeper and more prolonged sedation. Doses of 0.1 to 0.15 mg/kg are usually effective and do not prolong emergence from general anesthesia. For more anxious patients, doses up to 0.5 mg/kg have been used. Although not systemically studied, the total dose usually does not exceed 10 mg. If midazolam is given with an opioid, the initial dose of each must be reduced.

Sedation, anxiolysis or amnesia (IV) – Administer the initial dose of midazolam over 2 to 3 minutes. Because midazolam is water soluble, it takes approximately three times longer than diazepam to achieve peak EEG effects; therefore one must wait an additional 2 to 3 minutes to fully evaluate the sedative effect before initiating a procedure or repeating a dose. If further sedation is necessary, continue to titrate with small increments until the appropriate level of sedation is achieved. If other medications capable of depressing the CNS are coadministered, consider the peak effect of those concomitant medications and adjust the dose of midazolam.

< 6 months old – Pediatric patients < 6 months old are particularly vulnerable to airway obstruction and hypoventilation; therefore titration with small increments to clinical effect and careful monitoring are essential.

6 months to 5 years of age – Initial dose 0.05 to 0.1 mg/kg. A total dose up to 0.6 mg/kg may be necessary to reach the desired endpoint but usually does not exceed 6 mg. Prolonged sedation and risk of hypoventilation may occur with higher doses.

6 to 12 years of age – Initial dose 0.025 to 0.05 mg/kg; total dose up to 0.4 mg/kg may be needed to reach the desired endpoint but usually does not exceed 10 mg. Prolonged sedation and risk of hypoventilation may be associated with higher doses.

12 to 16 years of age – Dose as adults.

▶*Compatibility:* May be mixed in same syringe with: Morphine; meperidine; atropine; scopolamine. Midazolam, at a concentration of 0.5 mg/ml, is compatible with 5% Dextrose in Water and 0.9% Sodium Chloride for up to 24 hours and Lactated Ringer's solution for up to 4 hours.

▶*Storage/Stability:* Store at 15° to 30°C (59° to 86°F).

Actions

▶*Pharmacology:* Midazolam is a short-acting benzodiazepine CNS depressant.

In patients without intracranial lesions, induction is associated with a moderate decrease in cerebrospinal fluid pressure, similar to thiopental. Preliminary data in intracranial surgical patients with normal intracranial pressure but decreased compliance show comparable elevations of intracranial pressure with midazolam and with thiopental during intubation.

Induction doses depress the ventilatory response to carbon dioxide stimulation for 15 minutes or more beyond the duration of ventilatory depression following administration of thiopental. Impairment of ventilatory response is more marked in patients with chronic obstructive pulmonary disease (COPD). Sedation with IV midazolam does not adversely affect the mechanics of respiration; total lung capacity and peak expiratory flow decrease significantly, but static compliance and maximum expiratory flow at 50% of awake total lung capacity (V_{max}) increase.

Induction is associated with a slight to moderate decrease in mean arterial pressure, cardiac output, stroke volume and systemic vascular resistance. Slow heart rates (less than 65/minute), particularly in patients taking propranolol for angina, tend to rise slightly; faster heart rates (eg, 85/minute) tend to slow slightly.

▶*Pharmacokinetics:*

Absorption/Distribution – The mean absolute bioavailability following IM use is > 90% with mean peak plasma concentrations (C_{max}) of 90 ng/ml occuring within 30 minutes. C_{max} and time to peak (T_{max}) for the 1–hydroxy metabolite following the IM dose were 8 ng/ml and 1 hour, respectively. Midazolam has a large volume of distribution (Vd) of 1 to 3.1 L/kg. Peak concentrations of midazolam as well as 1-hydroxymethyl midazolam after IM administration are about one-half of those achieved after equivalent IV doses. The concentration of midazolam is 10- to 30-fold greater than that of 1–hydroxymethyl midazolam after single IV administration. Midazolam can accumulate in peripheral tissues with continuous infusion. Maintain the lowest effective midazolam infusion rate to reduce effects of accumulation.

Midazolam is ≈ 97% plasma protein bound, primarily to albumin. It crosses the placenta and enters fetal circulation.

Metabolism/Excretion – Elimination of the parent drug takes place via hepatic metabolism of midazolam to hydroxylated metabolites that are conjugated and excreted in the urine. Midazolam IV has an elimination half-life of 1.8 to 6.4 hours and a plasma clearance (Cl) of 0.25 to 0.54 L/hr/kg; < 0.5% of the dose is excreted in the urine intact. The biotransformation of midazolam is mediated by cytochrome P450 3A4. 1–hydroxy-midazolam accounts for 60% to 70% of biotransformation while 4–hydroxy-midazolam constitutes ≤ 5%. 1–hydroxy-midazolam is at least as potent as the parent compound and may contribute to the net pharmacologic activity of midazolam. The affinities of 1– and 4–hydroxy-midazolam for the benzodiazepine receptor are ≈ 20% and 7%, respectively, relative to midazolam. Midazolam follows linear kinetics at IV doses of 0.15 to 0.3 mg/kg but clearance is successively reduced by ≈ 30% at doses of 0.45 to 0.6 mg/kg indicating non-linear kinetics in this dose range.

Onset/Duration – Onset of IM sedation in adults is 15 minutes; peak sedation, 30 to 60 minutes. Sedative effects in the pediatric population begin within 5 minutes and peak at 15 to 30 minutes depending upon the dose administered.

Sedation after IV injection was achieved within 3 to 5 minutes. The time of onset is affected by total dose administered and the concurrent administration of narcotic premedication. In endoscopy patients, 71% had no recall of introduction of the endoscope; 82% had no recall of endoscope withdrawal.

When given IV, anesthesia induction occurs in ≈1.5 minutes when narcotic premedication is given and in 2 to 2.5 minutes without narcotic or with sedative premedication. Some memory impairment was noted in 90% of patients. Midazolam does not delay awakening from general anesthesia, which usually occurs within 2 hours but may take up to 6 hours.

Plasma concentration-effect relationship – At plasma concentrations > 100 ng/ml there is ≥ 50% probability that patients will be sedated but respond to verbal commands (sedation score = 3). At 200 ng/ml there is ≥ 50% probability that patients will be asleep but respond to glabellar tap (sedation score = 4).

Congestive heart failure (CHF) – Patients with CHF have a 2–fold increase in the elimination half-life, a 25% decrease in the plasma clearance and a 40% increase in volume of distribution.

Renal function impairment – There was a 2-fold increase in clearance and volume of distribution in patients with chronic renal failure. Midazolam clearance may be reduced (1.9 vs 2.8 ml/min/kg) and the half-life prolonged (7.6 vs 13 hr) in acute renal failure (ARF) patients. The renal clearance of the 1–hydroxy-midazolam glucuronide was prolonged in the ARF patients (4 vs 136 ml/min) and the half-life was prolonged (12 hr vs > 25 hr). Plasma levels accumulated to ≈ 10 times that of the parent drug.

Hepatic function impairment – The mean half-life of midazolam is increased 2.5–fold in alcoholic patients. Clearance is reduced by 50% and the Vd increased by 20%.

Pediatrics – In pediatric patients, weight-normalized clearance is similar or higher (0.19 to 0.8 L/hr/kg) than in adults and the terminal elimination half-life (0.78 to 3.3 hours) is similar to or shorter than in adults. In seriously ill neonates, the terminal elimination half-life of midazolam is substantially prolonged (6.5 to 12 hours) and the clearance reduced (0.07 to 0.12 L/hr/kg).

Obesity – The mean half-life is greater in obese patients (5.9 vs 2.3 hours) because of an increase of ≈ 50% in the Vd, corrected for total body weight. Clearance is not significantly affected.

Elderly – Plasma half-life is ≈ 2–fold higher in the elderly. The mean Vd based on total body weight increases consistently between 15% to 100% and mean Cl is decreased ≈ 25%.

Contraindications

Hypersensitivity to benzodiazepines; acute narrow-angle glaucoma (use in open-angle glaucoma only if patients are receiving appropriate therapy).

Warnings

▶*Respiratory depression:* Prior to IV administration in any dose, ensure the immediate availability of oxygen, resuscitative equipment and skilled personnel for the maintenance of a patent airway and support of ventilation. Continuously monitor patients for early signs of underventilation or apnea, which can lead to hypoxia/cardiac arrest. Continue to monitor vital signs during recovery period. Because midazolam IV depresses respiration and because opioid agonists and other sedatives can add to this depression, administer midazolam as an induction agent only by a person trained in general anesthesia. The immediate availability of specific reversal agents (eg, flumazenil) is highly recommended. Use in conscious sedation only when a person skilled in early detection of underventilation, maintaining a patent airway and supporting ventilation is present. Titrate slowly when used for sedation, anxiolysis and amnesia, do not administer midazolam by rapid or single bolus IV administration.

▶*Serious cardiorespiratory adverse events:* Serious cardiorespiratory adverse events have occurred, including respiratory depression, airway obstruction, desaturation, apnea, respiratory arrest or cardiac arrest, sometimes resulting in death or permanent neurologic injury.

MIDAZOLAM HCl

There have been rare reports of hypotensive episodes requiring treatment during or after diagnostic or surgical manipulations in patients who received midazolam. Hypotension may occur more frequently in conscious sedation patients premedicated with a narcotic. Adverse hemodynamic events have been reported in pediatric patients with cardiovascular instability.

▶*Improper dosing:* Reactions such as agitation, involuntary movements (including tonic/clonic movements and muscle tremor), hyperactivity and combativeness have been reported. These reactions may be caused by inadequate or excessive dosing or improper administration of midazolam; however, consider cerebral hypoxia or true paradoxical reactions. Should such reactions occur, evaluate response to each dose of midazolam and all other drugs, including local anesthetics, before proceeding.

Neonates – Reversal of such responses with flumazenil has been reported in pediatric patients. Avoid rapid injection in the neonatal population. IV injection (< 2 minutes) has been associated with severe hypotension in neonates, particularly when the patient has also received fentanyl. Severe hypotension has also been observed in neonates receiving a continuous infusion of midazolam who then receive a rapid IV injection of fentanyl. Seizures have been reported in several neonates following rapid IV administration. The neonate has reduced or immature organ function and is also vulnerable to profound or prolonged respiratory effects of midazolam.

▶*Ophthalmic:* Measurements of intraocular pressure in patients without eye disease show a moderate lowering following induction with midazolam.

▶*Do not administer:* Do not administer to patients in shock or coma, or in acute alcohol intoxication with depression of vital signs. Exercise particular care in use of midazolam IV in patients with uncompensated acute illnesses, such as severe fluid or electrolyte disturbances.

▶*Intra-arterial injection:* Intra-arterial injection hazards are unknown; therefore, take extreme precautions against unintended intra-arterial injection. Avoid extravasation.

▶*Abrupt withdrawal:* Withdrawal symptoms (convulsions, hallucinations, tremor, abdominal and muscle cramps, vomiting and sweating) may occur following abrupt discontinuation of benzodiazepines, including midazolam. Abdominal distension, nausea, vomiting and tachycardia are prominent symptoms of withdrawal in infants. Severe withdrawal symptoms are usually limited to patients receiving excessive doses over an extended period of time. Milder withdrawal symptoms (eg, dysphoria and insomnia) generally follow abrupt discontinuance of benzodiazepines taken therapeutically for several months. After extended therapy, avoid abrupt discontinuation and gradually taper dosage.

▶*Higher risk:* Higher risk surgical patients, elderly or debilitated patients require lower dosages for induction of anesthesia, whether premedicated or not. Patients with COPD are unusually sensitive to the respiratory depressant effect of midazolam. Patients with chronic renal failure and patients with CHF eliminate midazolam more slowly. Because elderly patients frequently have inefficient function of one or more organ systems, and because dosage requirements decrease with age, reduce initial dosage of midazolam and consider possibility of profound or prolonged effect.

With concomitant CNS depressant medication, decrease IV doses by 50% for elderly and debilitated patients. These patients will probably take longer to recover completely after induction of anesthesia.

▶*Renal function impairment:* Patients with renal impairment may have longer elimination half-lives for midazolam and its metabolites, which may result in slower recovery.

▶*Carcinogenesis:* In mice given 80 mg/kg/day of midazolam for 2 years, there was a marked increase in the incidence of hepatic tumors in female mice, and a small but statistically significant increase in benign thyroid follicular cell tumors in male mice.

▶*Pregnancy: Category D.* An increased risk of congenital malformations is associated with the use of benzodiazepine drugs. If this drug is used during pregnancy, apprise the patient of the potential hazard to the fetus.

Labor and delivery – Following IM administration of 0.05 mg/kg, both venous and umbilical arterial serum concentrations were lower than maternal concentrations.

Because midazolam is transferred transplacentally and because other benzodiazepines given in the last weeks of pregnancy have resulted in neonatal CNS depression, midazolam is not recommended for obstetrical use.

▶*Lactation:* Midazolam is excreted in breast milk. Exercise caution when administering to a nursing mother.

▶*Children:* As a group, pediatric patients generally require higher dosages of midazolam (mg/kg) than do adults. Younger (< 6 years old) pediatric patients may require higher dosages (mg/kg) than older pediatric patients and may require closer monitoring. In obese pediatric patients, calculate the dose based on ideal body weight. The neonate has reduced or immature organ function and is also vulnerable to profound or prolonged respiratory effects of midazolam.

Precautions

▶*Intracranial pressure/circulatory side effects:* Midazolam does not protect against the increase in intracranial pressure or circulatory effects associated with endotracheal intubation under light general anesthesia.

▶*Benzyl alcohol:* The midazolam injection contains benzyl alcohol, which has been associated with a fatal "gasping syndrome" in premature infants.

▶*Hazardous tasks:* No patient should operate hazardous machinery or a motor vehicle until the effects of the drug, such as drowsiness, have subsided or until the day after anesthesia and surgery, whichever is longer.

Drug Interactions

Caution is advised when midazolam is administered concomitantly with drugs that are known to inhibit the P450 3A4 enzyme system such as cimetidine, erythromycin, diltiazem, verapamil, ketaconazole and itraconazole. These drug interactions may result in prolonged sedation caused by a decrease in plasma clearance of midazolam.

Midazolam Drug Interactions			
Precipitant drug	Object drug*		Description
Midazolam	Anesthetics, inhalation	↑	Inhalation anesthetics may need to be reduced if midazolam is used as an induction agent. IV administration decreases minimum alveolar concentration (MAC) of halothane required for general anesthesia. This correlates with midazolam dosage.
Midazolam	CNS depressants	↑	Barbiturates, alcohol or other CNS depressants may increase risk of hypoventilation, airway obstruction, desaturation or apnea and contribute to prolonged effect with midazolam. Narcotic premedication also depresses ventilatory response to carbon dioxide stimulation.
Midazolam	Narcotic analgesics	↑	Narcotics, secobarbital and droperidol used as premedications accentuate midazolam's hypnotic effect. Adjust midazolam dosage according to the premedication used. Hypotension occurs more frequently with IV midazolam and meperidine in conscious sedation. Severe hypotension has been reported with concomitant administration of fentanyl.
Midazolam	Propofol	↑	The pharmacologic effects of propofol may be increased.
Midazolam	Thiopental	↑	A moderate reduction in induction dosage requirements (≈ 15%) has been noted following use of IM midazolam for premedication.
Azole antifungal agents	Midazolam	↑	Serum concentrations of certain benzodiazepines may be increased and prolonged, producing enhanced CNS depression and prolonged effects.
Cimetidine	Midazolam	↑	Serum levels of some benzodiazepines may be increased. Certain actions, especially sedation, may be enhanced.
Contraceptives, oral	Midazolam	↑	Coadministration of combination oral contraceptives and benzodiazepines that undergo oxidation may result in a prolongation of benzodiazepine half-life.
Ethanol	Midazolam	↑	Increased CNS effects with acute ethanol ingestion. Tolerance may occur with chronic ethanol use.
Fluvoxamine	Midazolam	↑	Reduced clearance, prolonged half-life, and increased serum concentrations of certain benzodiazepines may occur. Sedation or ataxia may be increased.
Indinavir	Midazolam	↑	Possibly prolonged sedation and respiratory depression.
Rifamycins	Midazolam	↓	The pharmacokinetic parameters of benzodiazepines may be altered (eg, increase in drug and metabolite clearance and decrease in elimination half-life).
Ritonavir	Midazolam	↑	Possibly severe sedation and respiratory depression.
Theophyllines	Midazolam	↓	The sedative effects of benzodiazepines may be antagonized by theophyllines.

MIDAZOLAM HCl

Midazolam Drug Interactions			
Precipitant drug	Object drug*		Description
Valproic acid	Midazolam	↑	Pharmacokinetic parameters of benzodiazepines may be increased. Liver metabolism of some benzodiazepines may be decreased.
Verapamil	Midazolam	↑	Effects of certain benzodiazepines may be increased, producing increased CNS depression and prolonged effects.

* ↑ = Object drug increased.   ↓ = Object drug decreased.

Adverse Reactions

See Warnings concerning serious cardiorespiratory events and paradoxical reactions.

Fluctuations in vital signs are most frequent and include decreased tidal volume or respiratory rate decrease (IV – 23.3%; IM – 10.8%); apnea (IV – 15.4%); variations in blood pressure and pulse rate.

IM – Headache (1.3%); pain at injection site (3.7%); induration and redness (0.5%), muscle stiffness (0.3%).

IV – The following were observed mainly following IV administration:
Respiratory: Coughing (1.3%); laryngospasm, bronchospasm, dyspnea, hyperventilation, wheezing, shallow respirations, airway obstruction, tachypnea (< 1%).
Cardiovascular: Bigeminy, premature ventricular contractions, vasovagal episode, bradycardia, tachycardia, nodal rhythm (< 1%).
➤*CNS:* Oversedation (1.6%); headache (1.5%); drowsiness (1.2%); retrograde amnesia, euphoria, confusion, argumentativeness, nervousness, agitation, anxiety, grogginess, restlessness, emergence delirium, prolonged emergence from anesthesia, dreaming during emergence, insomnia, nightmares, tonic/clonic movements, involuntary or athetoid movements, ataxia, dizziness, dysphoria, slurred speech, dysphonia, paresthesia (< 1%).
➤*Dermatologic:* Hives, hive-like elevation at injection site, swelling or feeling of burning, warmth, or coldness at injection site, rash, pruritus (< 1%).
➤*GI:* Hiccoughs (3.9%); nausea (2.8%); vomiting (2.6%); acid taste, excessive salivation, retching (< 1%).
➤*Special senses:* Blurred vision, diplopia, nystagmus, pinpoint pupils, cyclic eyelid movements, visual disturbance, difficulty focusing, blocked ears, loss of balance (< 1%).
➤*Miscellaneous:* Tenderness at injection site (5.6%); pain during injection (5%); redness (2.6%); induration (1.7%); phlebitis (0.4%); yawning, lethargy, chills, weakness, toothache, faint feeling, hematoma (< 1%).

Children – Desaturation (4.6%); apnea (2.8%); hypotension (2.7%); paradoxical reactions (2%); hiccough (1.2%); seizure-like activity (1.1%); nystagmus (1.1%).

Overdosage

➤*Symptoms:* Symptoms are similar to other benzodiazepines; sedation, somnolence, confusion, impaired coordination and reflexes, coma, and untoward effects on vital signs.

➤*Treatment:* Monitor respiration, pulse rate, and blood pressure and employ supportive measures. Maintain a patent airway and support ventilation. Start an IV infusion. Treat hypotension with IV fluid therapy, repositioning, judicious use of vasopressors, and other appropriate measures. The value of peritoneal dialysis, forced diuresis, or hemodialysis is unknown.

Flumazenil, a specific benzodiazepine-receptor antagonist, is indicated for the complete or partial reversal of the sedative effects of benzodiazepines and may be used in situations when an overdose with a benzodiazepine is known or suspected (see the Flumazenil monograph in the Antidotes section). Flumazenil is intended as an adjunct to, not as a substitute for, proper management of benzodiazepine overdose. Monitor patients treated with flumazenil for resedation, respiratory depression, and other residual benzodiazepine effects for an appropriate period after treatment. Flumazenil will only reverse benzodiazepine-induced effects but will not reverse the effects of other concomitant medications. Refer to General Management of Acute Overdosage.

Patient Information

Inform physician about any alcohol consumption and other medicine being taken, especially blood pressure medication and antibiotics, including nonprescription drugs. Alcohol has an increased effect when consumed with benzodiazepines; therefore, exercise caution regarding simultaneous ingestion of alcohol during benzodiazepine treatment.

Inform the physician if pregnant, planning to become pregnant, or breastfeeding.

Patients receiving continuous infusion of midazolam in critical care settings over an extended period of time may experience symptoms of withdrawal following abrupt discontinuation.

PROPOFOL

Rx	**Propofol** (Baxter)	Injectable emulsion: 10 mg/mL	In 20 mL single-use vials and 50 and 100 mL single-use infusion vials.[1]
Rx	**Diprivan** (AstraZeneca)		In 20 mL single-use amps, 50 and 100 mL single-use infusion vials, and 50 mL prefilled single-use syringes.[2]

[1] With 100 mg/mL soybean oil, 22.5 mg/mL glycerol, 12 mg/mL egg yolk phospholipid, and 0.25 mg/mL sodium metabisulfite. pH = 4.5 to 6.4.

[2] With 100 mg/mL soybean oil, 22.5 mg/mL glycerol, 12 mg/mL egg lecithin, and 0.005% EDTA. pH = 7 to 8.5.

Indications

➤*Anesthesia:* Induction or maintenance of anesthesia as part of a balanced anesthetic technique for inpatient and outpatient surgery in adults and children ≥ 3 years of age. Can also be used for maintenance of anesthesia as part of a balanced anesthetic technique for inpatient and outpatient surgery in adult patients and pediatric patients > 2 months of age. Propofol is not recommended for induction of anesthesia in patients < 3 years of age or for maintenance of anesthesia in patients < 2 months of age because safety and efficacy have not been established in those populations.

➤*Monitored anesthesia care (MAC) sedation:* Propofol can be used to initiate and maintain MAC sedation during diagnostic procedures in adults, and it may also be used for MAC sedation in conjunction with local/regional anesthesia in patients undergoing surgical procedures.

➤*Intensive care unit (ICU) sedation:* Continuous sedation and control of stress responses in intubated or respiratory-controlled adult patients in ICUs. Not indicated in pediatric ICU sedation because safety and efficacy have not been established.

Administration and Dosage

➤*Approved by the FDA:* October 1989.

➤*Administration:* Individualize dosage and rate of administration and titrate to the desired effect, according to clinically relevant factors, including preinduction and concomitant medications, age, American Society of Anesthesiologists (ASA) physical classification, and level of debilitation of the patient.

In the elderly, debilitated, and ASA III/IV patients, do not use rapid bolus doses as this will increase cardiorespiratory effects including hypotension, apnea, airway obstruction, or oxygen desaturation.

Propofol blood concentrations at steady state are generally proportional to infusion rates, especially within an individual patient. Undesirable effects such as cardiorespiratory depression are likely to occur at higher blood levels which result from bolus dosing or rapid increase in the infusion rate. An adequate interval (3 to 5 minutes) must be allowed between clinical dosage adjustments in order to assess drug effects.

When administering propofol by infusion, syringe pumps or volumetric pumps are recommended to provide controlled infusion rates. When infusing propofol to patients undergoing magnetic resonance imaging, metered control devices may be used if mechanical pumps are impractical.

Changes in vital signs (increases in pulse rate, blood pressure, sweating, and/or tearing) that indicate a response to surgical stimulation or lightening of anesthesia may be controlled by the administration of 25 to 50 mg (2.5 to 5 mL) incremental boluses and/or by increasing the infusion rate.

For minor surgical procedures (ie, body surface), 60% to 70% nitrous oxide can be combined with a variable rate infusion to provide satisfactory anesthesia. With more stimulating surgical procedures (eg, intra-abdominal), or if supplementation with nitrous oxide is not provided, increase administration rate(s) of propofol or opioids in order to provide adequate anesthesia.

Always titrate infusion rates downward in the absence of clinical signs of light anesthesia until a mild response to surgical stimulation can be perceived in order to avoid the administration of propofol at rates higher than are clinically necessary. Generally, achieve infusion rates of 50 to 100 mcg/kg/min in adults during maintenance in order to optimize recovery times.

Other drugs that cause CNS depression (eg, hypnotics/sedatives, inhalational anesthetics, opioids) can increase CNS depression induced by

PROPOFOL

propofol. Morphine premedication (0.15 mg/kg) with nitrous oxide 67% in oxygen decreases the necessary propofol injection maintenance infusion rate and therapeutic blood concentrations when compared to non-narcotic (eg, lorazepam) premedication.

►*Induction of general anesthesia:*

Adults – Most adult patients < 55 years of age and classified ASA I/II require 2 to 2.5 mg/kg of propofol for induction when unpremedicated or when premedicated with oral benzodiazepines or IM opioids. For induction, titrate propofol (≈ 40 mg every 10 seconds) against the response of the patient until the clinical signs show the onset of anesthesia.

Elderly, debilitated, or ASA III/IV patients – Because of the reduced clearance and higher blood concentrations, most elderly, debilitated, or ASA III/IV patients require ≈ 1 to 1.5 mg/kg (≈ 20 mg every 10 seconds) of propofol for induction of anesthesia according to their condition and responses. Do not use a rapid bolus, as this will increase the likelihood of undesirable cardiorespiratory depression, including hypotension, apnea, airway obstruction, and/or oxygen desaturation.

Children – Most patients 3 through 16 years of age and classified ASA I/II require 2.5 to 3.5 mg/kg for induction when unpremedicated or when lightly premedicated with oral benzodiazepines or IM opioids. Within this dosage range, younger pediatric patients may require higher induction doses than older pediatric patients. A lower dosage is recommended for pediatric patients classified as ASA III/IV. Attempt to minimize pain on injection when administering propofol to pediatric patients. Boluses of propofol may be administered via small veins if pretreated with lidocaine or via antecubital or larger veins.

Neurosurgical patients – Slower induction is recommended using boluses of 20 mg every 10 seconds. Slower boluses or infusions of propofol for induction of anesthesia, titrated to clinical responses, will generally result in reduced induction dosage requirements (1 to 2 mg/kg).

Cardiac anesthesia – Morphine premedication (0.15 mg/kg) with nitrous oxide 67% in oxygen has been shown to decrease the necessary propofol maintenance infusion rates and therapeutic blood concentrations when compared to nonnarcotic (lorazepam) premedication. Determine the rate of propofol administration based on the patient's premedication and adjust according to clinical responses.

Avoid rapid bolus injection. Use a slow rate of ≈ 20 mg every 10 seconds until induction onset (0.5 to 1.5 mg/kg). In order to assure adequate anesthesia, when propofol is used as the primary agent, maintenance infusion rates should not be < 100 mcg/kg/min and should be supplemented with analgesic levels of continuous opioid administration. When an opioid is used as the primary agent, propofol maintenance rates should be < 50 mcg/kg/min and care should be taken to ensure amnesia with concomitant benzodiazepines. Higher doses of propofol will reduce the opioid requirements (see table below). When propofol is used as the primary anesthetic, it should not be administered with the high-dose opioid technique, as this may increase the likelihood of hypotension.

Propofol Cardiac Anesthesia Techniques		
Primary agent	Rate	Secondary agent/rate (following induction with primary agent)
Propofol		Opioid[1] 0.05 to 0.075 mcg/kg/min (no bolus)
Preinduction anxiolysis	25 mcg/kg/min	
Induction	0.5 to 1.5 mcg/kg over 60 sec	
Maintenance (titrated to clinical response)	100 to 150 mcg/kg/min	
Opioid[2]		Propofol 50 to 100 mcg/kg/min (no bolus)
Induction	25 to 50 mcg/kg	
Maintenance	0.2 to 0.3 mcg/kg/min	

[1] Opioid is defined in terms of fentanyl equivalents, ie, 1 mcg fentanyl = 5 mcg alfentanil (for bolus), 10 mcg alfentanil (for maintenance), or 0.1 mcg sufentanil.
[2] Take care to ensure amnesia with concomitant benzodiazepine therapy.

►*Maintenance of general anesthesia:*

Adults – In adults, anesthesia can be maintained by administering propofol by infusion or intermittent IV bolus injection. The patient's clinical response will determine the infusion rate or the amount and frequency of incremental injections.

Continuous infusion: Propofol 100 to 200 mcg/kg/min administered in a variable rate infusion with 60% to 70% nitrous oxide and oxygen provides anesthesia for patients undergoing general surgery. Maintenance by infusion should immediately follow the induction dose in order to provide satisfactory or continuous anesthesia during the induction phase. During this initial period following the induction dose, higher rates of infusion are generally required (150 to 200 mcg/kg/min) for the first 10 to 15 minutes. Subsequently decrease infusion rates 30% to 50% during the first half hour of maintenance. Generally, rates of 50 to 100 mcg/kg/min in adults should be achieved during maintenance in order to optimize recovery times.

Intermittent bolus: Increments of propofol 25 to 50 mg (2.5 to 5 mL) may be administered with nitrous oxide in adult patients undergoing general surgery. The incremental boluses should be administered when changes in vital signs indicate a response to surgical stimulation or light anesthesia.

Children – Propofol administered as a variable rate infusion supplemented with nitrous oxide 60% to 70% provides satisfactory anesthesia for most children ≥ 2 months of age, ASA class I or II, undergoing general anesthesia.

In general, for the pediatric population, maintenance by infusion of propofol at a rate of 200 to 300 mcg/kg/min should immediately follow the induction dose. Following the first half hour of maintenance, infusion rates of 125 to 150 mcg/kg/min are typically needed. Titrate propofol to achieve the desired clinical effect. Younger children may require higher maintenance infusion rates than older children.

►*Initiation of MAC sedation:*

Adults – Either an infusion or a slow injection method may be used while closely monitoring cardiorespiratory function. With the infusion method, sedation may be initiated by infusing propofol at 100 to 150 mcg/kg/min (6 to 9 mg/kg/hr) for a period of 3 to 5 minutes and titrating to the desired clinical effect while closely monitoring respiratory function. With the slow injection method for initiation, patients will require ≈ 0.5 mg/kg administered over 3 to 5 minutes and titrated to clinical responses. When propofol is administered slowly over 3 to 5 minutes, most patients will be adequately sedated, and the peak drug effect can be achieved while minimizing undesirable cardiorespiratory effects occurring at high plasma levels.

Elderly, debilitated, or ASA III/IV patients – Do not use rapid (single or repeated) bolus dose administration for MAC sedation. The rate of administration should be over 3 to 5 minutes and the dosage of propofol should be reduced to ≈ 80% of the usual adult dosage in these patients according to their condition, responses, and changes in vital signs.

Can be the sole agent for maintenance of MAC sedation during surgical/diagnostic procedures, supplemented with opioids or benzodiazepines, which increase sedative and respiratory effects and may also result in a slower recovery profile.

►*Maintenance of MAC sedation:* Propofol can be administered as the sole agent for maintenance as MAC sedation during surgical/diagnostic procedures.

Adults – A variable rate infusion method is preferable over an intermittent bolus dose method. With the variable rate infusion method, patients will generally require maintenance rates of 25 to 75 mcg/kg/min (1.5 to 4.5 mg/kg/hr) during the first 10 to 15 minutes of sedation maintenance. Subsequently decrease infusion rates over time to 25 to 50 mcg/kg/min and adjust to clinical response. In titrating to clinical effect, allow ≈ 2 minutes for onset of peak drug effect.

Always titrate downward in the absence of clinical signs of light sedation until mild responses to stimulation are obtained in order to avoid sedative administration at rates higher than are clinically necessary.

If intermittent bolus method is used, 10 or 20 mg (1 or 2 mL) increments can be given and titrated to desired level of sedation. With the intermittent bolus method of sedation maintenance, there is the potential for respiratory depression, transient increases in sedation depth, or prolongation of recovery.

Elderly, debilitated, or ASA III/IV patients – Do not use rapid (single or repeated) bolus dose administration for MAC sedation. Reduce the rate of administration and the dosage to ≈ 80% of the usual adult dosage in these patients according to their condition, responses, and changes in vital signs.

►*ICU sedation:*

Adults – For intubated, mechanically ventilated adult patients, initiate slowly with a continuous infusion to titrate to desired clinical effect and minimize hypotension.

In clinical studies, the mean infusion maintenance rate for all patients was ≈ 27 mcg/kg/min. The maintenance infusion rates required to maintain adequate sedation ranged from 2.8 to 130 mcg/kg/min. The infusion rate was lower in patients > 55 years of age (≈ 20 mcg/kg/min) compared to patients < 55 years of age (≈ 38 mcg/kg/min). In these studies, morphine or fentanyl was used as needed for analgesia.

Most adult ICU patients recovering from the effects of general anesthesia or deep sedation will require maintenance rates of 5 to 50 mcg/kg/min (0.3 to 3 mg/kg/hr) individualized and titrated to clinical response. With medical ICU patients or patients who have recovered from the effect of general anesthesia or deep sedation, the rate of administration of ≥ 50 mcg/kg/min may be required to achieve adequate sedation. These higher rates may increase the likelihood of hypotension.

Although there are reports of reduced analgesic requirements, most patients received opioids for analgesia during maintenance of ICU sedation. Some patients also received benzodiazepines or neuromuscular blocking agents. During long-term maintenance of sedation, some ICU patients were awakened once or twice every 24 hours for assessment of neurologic or respiratory function.

PROPOFOL

In post-coronary artery bypass graft (CABG) patients, the maintenance rate of propofol administration was usually low (median, 11 mcg/kg/min) because of the intraoperative adminstration of high opioid doses.

Avoid discontinuation prior to weaning or for daily evaluation of sedation levels. This may result in rapid awakening with associated anxiety, agitation, and resistance to mechanical ventilation. Adjust infusions to maintain light sedation through these processes.

Propofol Dosage Guidelines[1]		
Indication	Induction/Initiation	Maintenance
General anesthesia (outpt/inpt):		
Healthy < 55 years	2 to 2.5 mg/kg (40 mg every 10 sec until onset)	100 to 200 mcg/kg/min intermittent bolus; increments of 20 to 50 mg as needed
Elderly, debilitated, ASA III/IV	1 to 1.5 mg/kg (20 mg every 10 sec until onset)	50 to 100 mcg/kg/min
General anesthesia (pediatric): > 3 years	2.5 to 3.5 mg/kg over 20 to 30 sec	200 to 300 mcg/kg/min (1st 30 min) 125 to 150 mcg/kg/min (remainder)
General anesthesia (cardiac):	0.5 to 1.5 mg/kg (a slow rate of ≈ 20 mg every 10 sec until onset); avoid rapid bolus induction	Primary propofol injection with secondary opioid: 100 to 150 mcg/kg/min Low-dose propofol injection w/ primary opioids: 50 to 100 mcg/kg/min (no bolus)
General anesthesia (neuro):	1 to 2 mg/kg (20 mg every 10 sec until onset	100 to 200 mcg/kg/min
MAC sedation:		
Healthy < 55 years:		
Slow infusion/ variable rate	100 to 150 mcg/kg/min for 3 to 5 min	25 to 75 mcg/kg/min for 10 to 15 min; decreased to 25 to 50 mcg/kg/min
Slow injection/ intermittent bolus	0.5 mg/kg over 3 to 5 min	Incremental bolus doses of 10 to 20 mg
Elderly, debilitated, ASA III/IV patients:		
Slow infusion/ variable rate	Usually same as healthy adult, but avoid rapid bolus dose	80% of adult dose; do not use rapid bolus dose
Slow injection/ intermittent bolus	Usually same as healthy adult, but avoid rapid bolus dose	80% of adult dose; do not use rapid bolus dose
ICU sedation:	Initial infusion: 5 mcg/kg/min for ≥ 5 min Subsequent increments of 5 to 10 mcg/kg/min over 5 to 10 min intervals until desired sedation level is achieved	Infusion rates of 5 to 50 mcg/kg/min or higher may be required

[1] Following the first half hour of maintenance, if clinical signs of light anesthesia are not present, decrease the infusion rate.

►*Handling:* Always maintain strict aseptic technique during handling. Propofol injectable emulsion is a single-use parenteral product that contains sodium metabisulfite (0.25 mg/mL) or 0.005% EDTA to retard the rate of growth of microorganisms in the event of accidental extrinsic contamination. However, propofol injectable emulsion can still support the growth of microorganisms as it is not an antimicrobially preserved product under USP standards. Do not use if contamination is suspected.

►*Admixture compatibility and stability:* Although propofol appears to be compatible with other therapeutic agents for a very limited amount of time, the manufacturers do not recommend mixing it with other agents prior to administration.

►*Dilution prior to administration:* Propofol is provided as a ready-to-use formulation. However, should dilution be necessary, only dilute with 5% Dextrose Injection and do not dilute to a concentration < 2 mg/mL because it is an emulsion. In diluted form it is more stable when in contact with glass than with plastic (95% potency after 2 hours of running infusion in plastic).

►*Administration with other fluids:* Compatibility of propofol with the coadministration of blood/serum/plasma has not been established (see Warnings). Propofol is compatible with the following IV fluids when administered using a y-type infusion set: 5% Dextrose Injection; Lactated Ringer's Injection; Lactated Ringer's and 5% Dextrose Injection; 5% Dextrose and 0.45% Sodium Chloride Injection; 5% Dextrose and 0.2% Sodium Chloride Injection.

►*Storage/Stability:* Do not use if there is evidence of separation of the phases of the emulsion.

Discard any unused portions of propofol or solutions containing propofol at the end of the anesthetic procedure or at 6 hours, whichever occurs sooner; for ICU sedation, discard after 12 hours (if administered directly from the vial or prefilled syringe) or 6 hours (if transferred to a syringe or other container).

Store at 4° to 22°C (40° to 72°F). Do not freeze. Protect from light. Shake well before use.

Propofol undergoes oxidative degradation in the presence of oxygen, and is therefore packaged under nitrogen to eliminate this degradation path.

Actions

►*Pharmacology:* Propofol is an IV hypnotic/sedative agent for induction and maintenance of anesthesia or sedation. IV injection of a therapeutic dose produces hypnosis rapidly and smoothly with minimal excitation, usually within 40 seconds from the start of an injection. As with other rapidly acting IV anesthetic agents, the half-time of blood-brain equilibration is ≈ 1 to 3 minutes, and this accounts for the rapid induction of anesthesia.

Pharmacodynamic properties of propofol depend on the therapeutic blood propofol concentrations. Steady-state concentrations are generally proportional to infusion rates, especially within an individual patient. Undesirable side effects such as cardiorespiratory depression are likely to occur at higher blood levels that result from bolus dosing or rapid increase in infusion rate. Allow an adequate interval (3 to 5 minutes) between clinical dosage adjustments in order to assess drug effects.

The hemodynamic effects of propofol injection during induction of anesthesia vary. If spontaneous ventilation is maintained, major cardiovascular effects are arterial hypotension (sometimes > 30% decrease) with little or no change in heart rate and no appreciable decrease in cardiac output. If ventilation is assisted or controlled (positive pressure ventilation), degree and incidence of decrease in cardiac output are accentuated. Addition of a potent opioid (eg, fentanyl) as a premedication further decreases cardiac output and respiratory drive.

If anesthesia is continued by infusion of propofol, endotracheal intubation and surgical stimulation may return arterial pressure towards normal. However, cardiac output may remain depressed. In comparative clinical studies, hemodynamic effects of propofol during induction are generally more pronounced than with traditional IV induction agents.

Induction of anesthesia with propofol is frequently associated with apnea. In 1573 adult patients given propofol (2 to 2.5 mg/kg), apnea lasted 0 to 30 sec in 7%, 30 to 60 seconds in 24%, and > 60 seconds in 12% of patients. In 218 children from birth to 16 years of age assessable for apnea who received bolus doses of propofol 1 to 3.6 mg/kg, the values were 12%, 10%, and 5%, respectively. During maintenance, propofol causes a decrease in ventilation usually associated with an increase in carbon dioxide tension which may be marked depending on the rate of administration and other concurrent agents (eg, opioids, sedatives).

In humans and animals, propofol does not suppress the adrenal response to ACTH. Preliminary findings in patients with normal intraocular pressure indicate that propofol anesthesia produces a decrease in intraocular pressure, which may be associated with a concomitant decrease in systemic vascular resistance. Animal studies and limited experience in susceptible patients have not indicated any propensity of propofol to induce malignant hyperthermia. Propofol is rarely associated with elevation of plasma histamine levels and does not cause signs of histamine release.

►*Pharmacokinetics:* Following an IV bolus dose, plasma levels initially decline rapidly due to both high metabolic clearance and rapid drug distribution into tissues. Distribution accounts for about half of this decline following a bolus of propofol.

However, distribution is not constant over time, but decreases as body tissues equilibrate with plasma and become saturated. The rate at which equilibration occurs is a function of the rate and duration of the infusion. When equilibration occurs, there is no longer a net transfer of propofol between tissues and plasma.

Discontinuation of the recommended doses of propofol after the maintenance of anesthesia for ≈ 1 hour, or for sedation in the ICU for 1 day, results in a prompt decrease in blood propofol concentrations and rapid awakening. Longer infusions (10 days of ICU sedation) result in accumulation of significant tissue stores of propofol, such that the reduction in circulating propofol is slowed and the time to awakening is increased.

By daily titration of propofol dosage to achieve only the minimum effective therapeutic concentration, rapid awakening within 10 to 15 minutes will occur even after long-term administration. However, if higher than necessary infusion levels have been maintained for a long time, propofol will be redistributed from fat and muscle to the plasma, and this return of propofol from peripheral tissues will slow recovery.

The large contribution of distribution (≈ 50%) to the fall of propofol plasma levels following brief infusions means that after very long infusions (at steady state), about half the initial rate will maintain the same plasma levels. Thus, titration to clinical response and daily evaluation of sedation levels are important during use of propofol infusion for ICU sedation, especially infusions of long duration.

PROPOFOL

Special populations –

Adults: Clearance ranges from 23 to 50 mL/kg/min. It is chiefly eliminated by hepatic conjugation to inactive metabolites that are excreted by the kidneys. A glucuronide conjugate accounts for ≈ 50% of dose. Steady-state volume of distribution approaches 60 L/kg. Terminal half-life after a 10-day infusion is 1 to 3 days.

Elderly: With increasing age, the dose needed to achieve a defined anesthetic endpoint (dose requirement) decreases. This does not appear to be an age-related change. With increasing age, higher peak plasma levels occur, which can explain the decreased dose requirement. These higher levels can predispose patients to cardiorespiratory effects, including hypotension, apnea, airway obstruction, or oxygen desaturation. Lower doses are, therefore, recommended in the elderly.

Children: The pharmacokinetics of propofol were studied in 53 children between 3 and 12 years of age who received propofol for periods of ≈ 1 to 2 hours. The observed distribution and clearance of propofol in these children were similar to adults.

Hepatic/Renal function impairment: Propofol pharmacokinetics do not appear to be different in patients with chronic hepatic cirrhosis or chronic renal impairment compared to adults with normal hepatic and renal function.

Contraindications

When general anesthesia or sedation are contraindicated; hypersensitivity to propofol or components of the product.

Warnings

➤*Administration:* Only people trained in the administration of general anesthesia and not involved in the conduct of the surgical/diagnostic procedure should administer propofol. Continuously monitor patients. Facilities for maintenance of a patent airway, artificial ventilation, and oxygen enrichment and circulatory resuscitation must be immediately available. For sedation of intubated, mechanically ventilated patients in the ICU, administer only by people skilled in the management of critically ill patients and trained in cardiovascular resuscitation and airway management.

In elderly, debilitated, or ASA III/IV patients, do not use rapid (single or repeated) bolus administration during general anesthesia or MAC sedation in order to minimize undesirable cardiorespiratory depression, including hypotension, apnea, airway obstruction, or oxygen desaturation.

➤*Blood/Plasma coadministration:* Do not coadminister through the same IV catheter with blood or plasma because compatibility has not been established. In vitro, aggregates of the globular component of the emulsion vehicle have occurred with blood/plasma/serum from humans and animals.

➤*Aseptic technique:* Always maintain strict aseptic techniques during handling because propofol is a single-use parenteral product and contains no antimicrobial preservatives. The vehicle is capable of supporting growth of micro-organisms. Failure to follow aseptic handling procedures may result in microbial contamination causing fever, infection/sepsis, life-threatening illnesses, or death.

➤*Anaphylaxis:* Rarely, features of anaphylaxis, which may include angioedema, bronchospasm, erythema, and hypotension, have occurred after the administration of propofol, although the use of other drugs in most instances makes the relationship to propofol unclear.

➤*Elderly:* Use a lower induction dose and a slower maintenance rate of administration (see Precautions).

➤*Pregnancy: Category B.* Reproduction studies have been performed in rats and rabbits at IV doses of 15 mg/kg/day (approximately equivalent to the recommended human induction dose on a mg/m² basis) and have revealed no evidence of impaired fertility or harm to the fetus caused by propofol. However, propofol has been shown to cause maternal deaths in rats and rabbits and decreased pup survival during the lactating period in dams treated with 15 mg/kg/day. The pharmacological activity (anesthesia) of the drug on the mother is probably responsible for the adverse effects seen in the offspring. However, there are no adequate and well-controlled studies in pregnant women. Use during pregnancy only if clearly needed.

Labor and delivery – Not recommended for obstetrics, including cesarean section deliveries. Propofol crosses the placenta and may be associated with neonatal depression.

➤*Lactation:* Not recommended for use in nursing mothers because propofol is excreted in breast milk and the effects of oral absorption of small amounts of propofol are not known.

➤*Children:* Safety and efficacy of propofol have been established for induction of anesthesia in children ≥ 3 years of age and for the maintenance of anesthesia in children ≥ 2 months of age. Not recommended for the induction of anesthesia in children < 3 years of age, in the maintenance of anesthesia in children < 2 months of age, or for ICU or MAC sedation in children because safety and efficacy have not been established. In pediatric patients, administration of fentanyl concomitantly with propofol may result in serious bradycardia. Although no causal relationship has been established, serious adverse events (including fatalities) have been reported in children with respiratory tract infections given propofol for ICU sedation. In pediatric patients, abrupt discontinuation following prolonged infusion may result in flushing of the hands and feet, agitation, tremulousness, and hyperirritability. Increased incidences of bradycardia (5%), agitation (4%), and jitteriness (9%) also have been reported.

Precautions

➤*Monitoring:* MAC sedation patients should be continuously monitored by people not involved in the conduct of the surgical or diagnostic procedure; oxygen supplementation should be immediately available and provided where clinically indicated. Monitor oxygen saturation in all patients. Continuously monitor patients for early signs of hypotension, apnea, airway obstruction, or oxygen desaturation. These cardiorespiratory effects are more likely to occur following rapid initiation (loading) boluses or during supplemental maintenance boluses, especially in the elderly, debilitated, or ASA III/IV patients.

➤*Special risk patients:* Use a lower induction dose and a slower maintenance rate of administration in elderly, debilitated, and ASA III/IV patients (see Administration and Dosage). Continuously monitor patients for early signs of significant hypotension or bradycardia. Treatment may include increasing the rate of IV fluid administration, elevation of lower extremities, use of pressor agents, or administration of atropine. Apnea often occurs during induction and may persist for > 60 seconds. Ventilatory support may be required. Because propofol is an emulsion, use caution in patients with lipid metabolism disorders (eg, primary hyperlipoproteinemia, diabetic hyperlipidemia, pancreatitis).

➤*Discharge of patient:* Satisfy the clinical criteria for discharge from the recovery/day surgery area established for each institution before discharge of the patient from the care of the anesthesiologist.

➤*Epilepsy:* When administered to an epileptic patient, there may be a risk of seizure during the recovery phase.

➤*Transient local pain:* Transient local pain may occur during IV injection, which may be reduced if the larger veins of the forearm or antecubital fossa are used or by prior injection of IV lidocaine (1 mL of a 1% solution). Venous sequelae (phlebitis or thrombosis) have occurred rarely (< 1%). In 2 well-controlled clinical studies using dedicated IV catheters, no instances of venous sequelae were reported up to 14 days following induction. Intentional injection into SC or perivascular tissues of animals caused minimal tissue reaction. Intra-arterial injection in animals did not induce local tissue effects. Accidental intra-arterial injections have been reported in patients, and other than pain, there were no major sequelae.

➤*Perioperative myoclonia:* Perioperative myoclonia, rarely including convulsions and opisthotonus, has occurred.

➤*Pulmonary edema:* Pulmonary edema has been reported rarely with propofol use, although a causal relationship is not known.

➤*Cardiovascular effects:* Propofol has no vagolytic activity and has been associated with reports of bradycardia, asystole, and, rarely, cardiac arrest. Consider the IV administration of anticholinergic agents (eg, atropine, glycopyrrolate) to modify potential increases in vagal tone caused by concomitant agents (eg, succinylcholine) or surgical stimuli. There have been rare reports of cardiac arrest. Monitor patients for early signs of significant hypotension or cardiovascular depression, which may be profound. These effects are responsive to discontinuation of propofol, IV fluid administration, or vasopressor therapy.

➤*Hyperlipidemia:* Because propofol is formulated in an oil-in-water emulsion, elevations in serum triglycerides may occur when it is administered for extended periods of time. Monitor patients at risk of hyperlipidemia for increases in serum triglycerides or serum turbidity. Adjust if fat is being inadequately cleared from the body. A reduction in the quantity of concurrently administered lipids is indicated to compensate for the amount of lipid infused as part of the formulation; 1 mL of propofol contains ≈ 0.1 g of fat (1.1 kcal).

➤*Neurosurgical anesthesia:* When propofol is used in patients with increased intracranial pressure (ICP) or impaired cerebral circulation, avoid significant decreases in mean arterial pressure because of the resultant decreases in cerebral perfusion pressure. To avoid significant hypotension and decreases in cerebral perfusion pressure, use an infusion or slow bolus of ≈ 20 mg every 10 seconds instead of rapid, more frequent, and larger boluses. Slower induction titrated to clinical responses generally will result in reduced induction dosage requirements (1 to 2 mg/kg). When increased ICP is suspected, hyperventilation and hypocarbia should accompany use of propofol.

➤*Cardiac anesthesia:* Use slower rates of administration in premedicated patients, geriatric patients, patients with recent fluid shifts, or patients who are hemodynamically unstable. Correct any fluid deficits prior to administration. In those patients where additional fluid therapy may be contraindicated, other measures (eg, elevation of lower extremities, use of pressor agents) may be useful to offset the hypotension that is associated with the induction of anesthesia with propofol.

➤*Additives:*

Sodium metabisulfite – Propofol formulations that contain sodium metabisulfite, a sulfite, may cause allergic-type reactions including anaphylactic symptoms and life-threatening or less severe asthmatic episodes in certain susceptible people. The overall prevalence of sulfite sensitivity in the general population is unknown and probably low. Sulfite sensitivity is seen more frequently in asthmatic than nonasthmatic people.

PROPOFOL

EDTA – EDTA is a strong chelator of trace metals, including zinc. Although with propofol there are no reports of decreased zinc levels or zinc deficiency-related adverse events, do not infuse propofol for > 5 days without providing a drug holiday to safely replace estimated or measured urine zinc losses.

In clinical trials, mean urinary zinc loss was ≈ 2.5 to 3 mg/day in adult patients and 1.5 to 2 mg/day in pediatric patients.

In patients who are predisposed to zinc deficiency, such as those with burns, diarrhea, or major sepsis, consider the need for supplemental zinc during prolonged therapy.

At high doses (2 to 3 g/day) EDTA has been reported, on rare occasions, to be toxic to the renal tubules. Studies to date in patients with normal or impaired renal function, have not shown any alterations in renal function with propofol injectable emulsion containing 0.005% EDTA. In patients at risk for renal impairment, check urinalysis and urine sediment before initiation of sedation and then monitor on alternate days during sedation.

➤*Drug abuse and dependence:* Rare cases of self-administration of propofol by health care professionals have been reported. Manage propofol to prevent the risk of diversion.

Drug Interactions

➤*CNS depressants:* CNS depressants (eg, hypnotics/sedatives, inhalational anesthetics, opioids) can increase the CNS depression induced by propofol. Morphine premedication with nitrous oxide decreases the necessary propofol maintenance infusion rate and therapeutic blood concentrations when compared to nonnarcotic (eg, lorazepam) premedication (see Administration and Dosage). In addition, the induction dose requirements of propofol may be reduced in patients with IM or IV premedication, particularly with narcotics alone or in combination with sedatives. These agents may increase the anesthetic or sedative effects of propofol and may also result in more pronounced decreases in systolic, diastolic, and mean arterial pressures and cardiac output.

Adverse Reactions

➤*Anesthesia/MAC sedation:*

Cardiovascular – Hypotension (3% to 10%); arrhythmia, tachycardia, bradycardia (1% to 3%); hemorrhage/bleeding, premature atrial contractions, syncope, atrial fibrillation, atrial arrhythmia, AV heartblock, bigeminy, bundle branch block, cardiac arrest, abnormal ECG, edema, extrasystole, heart block, hypertension, MI, myocardial ischemia, PVCs, ST segment depression, supraventricular tachycardia, ventricular fibrillation (< 1%).

CNS – Movement (3% to 10%); hypertonia/dystonia, paresthesia, abnormal dreams, agitation, anxiety, bucking/jerking/thrashing, chills/shivering, clonic/myoclonic movement, combativeness, confusion, delirium, depression, dizziness, emotional lability, euphoria, fatigue, headache, hysteria, insomnia, moaning, rigidity, seizures, somnolence, tremor, twitching, amorous behavior, hypotonia, hallucinations, neuropathy, opisthotonos (< 1%).

Dermatologic – Rash, pruritus (1% to 3%); flushing, diaphoresis, urticaria (< 1%).

GI – Hypersalivation, cramping, diarrhea, dry mouth, enlarged parotid, nausea, swallowing, vomiting (< 1%).

GU – Cloudy urine, oliguria, urine retention (< 1%).

Local – Burning/stinging or pain (17.6%); hives/itching, phlebitis, redness/discoloration (< 1%).

Respiratory – Apnea (1% to 3%); bronchospasm, burning in throat, wheezing, cough, dyspnea, hiccough, hypoventilation, hyperventilation, hypoxia, laryngospasm, pharyngitis, sneezing, tachypnea, upper airway obstruction, decreased lung function (< 1%).

Special senses – Amblyopia, diplopia, ear pain, eye pain, taste perversion, tinnitus, conjunctival hyperemia, nystagmus, abnormal vision (< 1%).

Miscellaneous – Awareness, extremity pain, fever, increased drug effect, neck rigidity/stiffness, chest/trunk pain, myalgia, coagulation disorder, leukocytosis, hyperkalemia, asthenia, hyperlipidemia, anaphylaxis/anaphylactoid reaction, perinatal disorder, anticholinergic syndrome, hypomagnesemia (< 1%).

➤*ICU sedation:*

Cardiovascular – Hypotension (26%); bradycardia, decreased cardiac output (1% to 3%); arrhythmia, atrial fibrillation, bigeminy, cardiac arrest, extrasystole, ventricular tachycardia, right heart failure (< 1%).

CNS – Agitation, chills/shivering, intracranial hypertension, seizures, somnolence, abnormal thinking (< 1%).

Metabolic/Nutritional – Hyperlipidemia (3% to 10%); increased BUN, creatinine, and osmolality, dehydration, hyperglycemia, metabolic acidosis (< 1%).

Respiratory – Respiratory acidosis during weaning (3% to 10%); hypoxia (< 1%).

Miscellaneous – Fever, sepsis, trunk pain, weakness, rash, ileus, abnormal liver function, green urine, kidney failure (< 1%).

➤*Children:* Generally, the adverse reaction profile in children 6 days to 16 years of age is similar to adults. The following reactions have occurred: Hypotension, movement (17%); burning/stinging or pain (10%); hypertension (8%); rash (5%); pruritus (2%); nodal tachycardia (1.6%); arrhythmia (1.2%); apnea.

Overdosage

If accidental overdosage occurs, discontinue propofol immediately. Overdosage is likely to cause cardiorespiratory depression. Treat respiratory depression by artificial ventilation with oxygen. Cardiovascular depression may require raising the patient's legs, increasing the flow rate of IV fluids, and administering pressor agents or anticholinergic agents. Refer to General Management of Acute Overdosage.

Patient Information

Performance of activities requiring mental alertness, coordination, or physical dexterity may be impaired for some time after general anesthesia or sedation.

DROPERIDOL

Rx	**Droperidol** (Various, eg, Abbott Hospital, American Regent)	**Injection:** 2.5 mg/mL	In 2 mL vials.
Rx	**Inapsine** (Akorn)		In 1 and 2 mL amps or vials.

WARNING

Cases of QT prolongation or torsade de pointes have been reported in patients receiving droperidol at doses at or below recommended doses. Some cases have occurred in patients with no known risk factors for QT prolongation and some cases have been fatal.

Because of its potential for serious proarrhythmic effects and death, reserve droperidol for use in the treatment of patients who fail to show an acceptable response to other adequate treatments, because of insufficient effectiveness or the inability to achieve an effective dose due to intolerable adverse effects from those drugs.

Cases of QT prolongation and serious arrhythmias (eg, torsade de pointes) have been reported in patients treated with droperidol. Based on these reports, all patients should undergo a 12-lead ECG prior to administration of droperidol to determine if a prolonged QT interval (ie, QTc > 440 msec for males or 450 msec for females) is present. If there is a prolonged QT interval, do not administer droperidol. For patients in whom the potential benefit of droperidol treatment is felt to outweigh the risks of potentially serious arrhythmias, perform ECG monitoring prior to treatment and continue for 2 to 3 hours after completing treatment to monitor for arrhythmias.

Droperidol is contraindicated in patients with known or suspected QT prolongation, including patients with congenital long QT syndrome.

Administer droperidol with extreme caution to patients who may be at risk for development of prolonged QT syndrome (eg, CHF, bradycardia, use of a diuretic, cardiac hypertrophy, hypokalemia, hypomagnesemia, or administration of other drugs known to increase the QT interval). Other risk factors may include age > 65 years, alcohol abuse, and use of agents such as benzodiazepines, volatile anesthetics, and IV opiates. Initiate droperidol at a low dose and adjust upward, with caution, as needed to achieve the desired effect.

Indications

➤ *Neuroleptic/Antiemetic:* To reduce the incidence of nausea and vomiting in surgical and diagnostic procedures.

➤ *Unlabeled uses:* Breakthrough chemotherapy-induced nausea and vomiting (0.5 to 2 mg IV or IM every 3 to 4 hours as needed); acute treatment of chemotherapy-induced nausea and vomiting (0.5 to 2 mg IV or IM before chemotherapy).

Administration and Dosage

Individualize dosage. Some of the factors to be considered in determining the dose are age, body weight, physical status, underlying pathological condition, use of other drugs, type of anesthesia to be used, and surgical procedure involved.

Administer additional doses with caution and only if the potential benefit outweighs the potential risk.

Monitor vital signs and ECG routinely.

➤ *Adults:* The maximum recommended initial dose of droperidol is 2.5 mg IM or slow IV. Additional 1.25 mg doses may be administered to achieve the desired effect.

➤ *Children (2 to 12 years of age):* The maximum recommended initial dose is 0.1 mg/kg, taking into account the patient's age and other clinical factors.

➤ *Admixture compatibilities:* Droperidol in a concentration of 2.5 mg/mL is physically compatible for at least 15 minutes with the following admixed in a syringe: Atropine sulfate, butorphanol tartrate, chlorpromazine HCl, cimetidine HCl (stable for 4 hours), dimenhydrinate, diphenhydramine HCl, fentanyl citrate, glycopyrrolate (stable for 48 hours), hydroxyzine HCl, meperidine HCl, metoclopramide HCl, midazolam HCl (stable for 4 hours under fluorescent light), morphine sulfate, nalbuphine HCl (stable for 36 to 48 hours), ondansetron HCl (stable for 8 hours at 23°C [73°F]), pentazocine lactate, perphenazine, prochlorperazine edisylate, promazine HCl, promethazine HCl, scopolamine HBr. Precipitation occurs if mixed with barbiturates.

Visually inspect parenteral drug products for particulate matter and discoloration prior to administration, whenever solution and container permit. If such abnormalities are observed, do not administer the drug.

➤ *Storage/Stability:* Store at room temperature 15° to 25°C (59° to 77°F). Protect from light.

Actions

➤ *Pharmacology:* Droperidol produces marked tranquilization and sedation. It allays apprehension and provides a state of mental detachment and indifference while maintaining a state of reflex alertness. Droperidol produces an antiemetic effect as evidenced by the antagonism of apomorphine in dogs. It lowers the incidence of nausea and vomiting during surgical procedures and provides antiemetic protection in the postoperative period. It also produces mild alpha-adrenergic

blockade, peripheral vascular dilatation, and reduction of the pressor effect of epinephrine, resulting in hypotension and decreased peripheral vascular resistance. Droperidol may decrease pulmonary arterial pressure (particularly if it is abnormally high). It may reduce the incidence of epinephrine-induced arrhythmias, but it does not prevent other cardiac arrhythmias.

➤ *Pharmacokinetics:* The onset of action occurs in 3 to 10 minutes following IV or IM administration. The peak effect may not be apparent for 30 minutes. The duration of the sedative and tranquilizing effect is generally 2 to 4 hours. Alteration of alertness may persist as long as 12 hours.

Contraindications

Known or suspected QT prolongation (ie, QTc interval > 440 msec for males or 450 msec for females); includes patients with congenital long QT syndrome.

Hypersensitivity to droperidol.

Droperidol is not recommended for any use other than for the treatment of perioperative nausea and vomiting in patients for whom other treatments are ineffective or inappropriate (see Warnings).

Warnings

Fluids and other countermeasures to manage hypotension should be readily available.

As with other CNS depressant drugs, patients who have received droperidol should have appropriate surveillance.

➤ *Risks for prolonged QT syndrome:* Administer with extreme caution in the presence of risk factors for development of prolonged QT syndrome such as the following:
1.) Clinically significant bradycardia (< 50 bpm),
2.) any clinically significant cardiac disease,
3.) treatment with Class I and Class III antiarrhythmics,
4.) treatment with monoamine oxidase inhibitors (MAOIs),
5.) concomitant treatment with other drug products known to prolong the QT interval, and
6.) electrolyte imbalance, in particular hypokalemia and hypomagnesemia, or concomitant treatment with drugs (eg, diuretics) that may cause electrolyte imbalance.

➤ *Cardiac conduction:* Cases of QT prolongation and serious arrhythmias (eg, torsade de pointes, ventricular arrythmias, cardiac arrest, and death) have been observed during postmarketing treatment with droperidol. Some cases have occurred in patients with no known risk factors and at doses at or below recommended doses. There has been at least 1 case of nonfatal torsade de pointes confirmed by rechallenge.

Based on these reports, all patients should undergo a 12-lead ECG prior to administration of droperidol to determine if prolonged QT interval (ie, QTc > 440 msec for males or 450 msec for females) is present. If there is a prolonged QT interval, do not administer droperidol. For patients in whom the potential benefit of droperidol treatment is felt to outweigh the risks of potentially serious arrhythmias, perform ECG monitoring prior to treatment and continue for 2 to 3 hours after completing treatment to monitor for arrhythmias.

➤ *Concomitant narcotic analgesic therapy:* It is recommended that opioids, when required, initially be used in reduced doses.

➤ *Neuroleptic malignant syndrome:* As with other neuroleptic agents, very rare reports of neuroleptic malignant syndrome (altered consciousness, muscle rigidity, and autonomic instability) have occurred in patients who have received droperidol. Since it may be difficult to distinguish neuroleptic malignant syndrome from malignant hyperpyrexia in the perioperative period, consider prompt treatment with dantrolene if increases in temperature, heart rate, or carbon dioxide production occur.

➤ *Special risk patients:* Reduce the initial dose of droperidol in the elderly, debilitated, and other poor-risk patients. Consider the effect of the initial dose in determining incremental doses.

➤ *Renal/Hepatic function impairment:* Administer with caution because of the importance of these organs in the metabolism and excretion of drugs.

➤ *Pregnancy: Category C.* There are no adequate and well-controlled studies in pregnant women. Use only when the potential benefit justifies the potential risk to the fetus. Droperidol administered IV has caused a slight increase in newborn rat mortality at 4.4 times the upper human dose. Following IM administration, increased mortality of the offspring at 1.8 times the upper human dose is attributed to CNS depression in the dams.

Labor and delivery – There are insufficient data to support the use of droperidol in labor and delivery. Therefore, such use is not recommended.

➤ *Lactation:* It is not known whether droperidol is excreted in breast milk. Exercise caution when administering to a nursing mother.

DROPERIDOL

➤*Children:* Safety for use in children < 2 years of age have not been established.

Precautions

➤*Hypotension:* If hypotension occurs, consider the possibility of hypovolemia and manage with appropriate parenteral fluid therapy. Reposition patient to improve venous return to the heart when operative conditions permit. In spinal and peridural anesthesia, tilting the patient into a head-down position may result in a higher level of anesthesia than desired and impair venous return to the heart. Exercise care in moving and positioning patients because of the possibility of orthostatic hypotension. If volume expansion with fluids plus other countermeasures do not correct the hypotension, consider using pressor agents other than epinephrine. Epinephrine may paradoxically decrease the blood pressure in patients treated with droperidol because of the alpha-adrenergic blocking action of droperidol.

➤*Decreased pulmonary artery pressure:* Droperidol also may decrease pulmonary arterial pressure; this fact should be considered by those who conduct diagnostic or surgical procedures where interpretation of pulmonary arterial pressure measurements might determine final management of the patient.

➤*EEG:* When the EEG is used for postoperative monitoring, the EEG pattern may slowly return to normal.

➤*Pheochromocytoma:* In patients with diagnosed/suspected pheochromocytoma, severe hypertension and tachycardia have been observed after the administration of droperidol.

Drug Interactions

Any drug known to have the potential to prolong the QT interval should not be used together with droperidol. Possible pharmacodynamic interactions can occur between droperidol and potentially arrhythmogenic agents such as class I or III antiarrhythmics, antihistamines that prolong the QT interval, antimalarials, calcium channel blockers, neuroleptics that prolong the QT interval, and antidepressants.

Use caution when patients are taking concomitant drugs known to induce hypokalemia or hypomagnesemia as they may precipitate QT prolongation and interact with droperidol. These would include diuretics, laxatives, and supraphysiological use of steroid hormones with mineralocorticoid potential.

Droperidol Drug Interactions			
Precipitant drug	Object drug*		Description
Droperidol	Anesthesia	↑	Certain forms of conduction anesthesia (eg, spinal anesthesia, some peridural anesthetics) can cause peripheral vasodilation and hypotension because of sympathetic blockade. Droperidol can alter circulation through other mechanisms.
CNS depressants (eg, barbiturates, tranquilizers, opioids, general anesthetics)	Droperidol	↑	CNS depressants have additive or potentiating CNS effects with droperidol; thus, droperidol dose will be less than usual. Likewise, following the droperidol, reduce the dose of other CNS depressants.
Droperidol	CNS depressants (eg, barbiturates, tranquilizers, opioids, general anesthetics)		

Droperidol Drug Interactions			
Precipitant drug	Object drug*		Description
Epinephrine	Droperidol	↑	Epinephrine may paradoxically enhance droperidol-induced hypotension because of the alpha-adrenergic blocking action of droperidol. Epinephrine is not recommended as treatment of droperidol-induced hypotension.
Parenteral analgesics (eg, fentanyl)	Droperidol	↑	Hypertension has been reported following coadministration of droperidol and fentanyl or other parenteral analgesics and may be due to unexplained alterations in sympathetic activity following large doses.

* ↑ = Object drug increased.

Adverse Reactions

➤*Cardiovascular:* QT interval prolongation, torsade de pointes, cardiac arrest, and ventricular tachycardia have been reported. Some of these cases were associated with death. Some cases occurred in patients with no known risk factors, and some were associated with droperidol doses at or below recommended doses.

Physicians should be alert to palpitations, syncope, or other symptoms suggestive of episodes of irregular cardiac rhythm in patients taking droperidol and promptly evaluate such cases (see Warnings).

Most common are mild to moderate hypotension and tachycardia, which usually subside without treatment. If hypotension occurs and is severe or persists, the possibility of hypovolemia should be considered and managed with appropriate parenteral fluid therapy. Hypertension, with or without pre-existing hypertension, has been reported following administration of droperidol combined with fentanyl or other parenteral analgesics. This may be due to unexplained alterations in sympathetic activity following large doses; however, it also is frequently attributed to anesthetic or surgical stimulation during light anesthesia. QT prolongation has been reported, and there is ≥ 1 case of nonfatal torsade de pointes confirmed by rechallenge.

➤*CNS:* Most common include dysphoria, postoperative drowsiness, restlessness, hyperactivity, and anxiety that can be the result of inadequate dosage (lack of adequate treatment effect) or of an adverse drug reaction (part of the symptom complex of akathisia). Extrapyramidal signs and symptoms (dystonia, akathisia, oculogyric crisis) may develop and usually can be controlled with anticholinergic agents. Postoperative hallucinatory episodes (sometimes associated with transient periods of mental depression) also have been reported.

➤*Miscellaneous:* Other less common reported adverse reactions include anaphylaxis, dizziness, chills or shivering, laryngospasm, and bronchospasm. Neuroleptic malignant syndrome (altered consciousness, muscle rigidity, and autonomic instability) very rarely has occurred.

Overdosage

➤*Symptoms:* Manifestations of overdosage are extension of pharmacologic actions and may include QT prolongation and serious arrhythmias (eg, torsade de pointes).

➤*Treatment:* In the presence of hypoventilation or apnea, administer oxygen and assist or control respiration as indicated. Maintain a patent airway; an oropharyngeal airway or endotracheal tube might be indicated. Observe the patient for 24 hours; maintain body warmth and fluid intake. If hypotension occurs and is severe or persists, consider hypovolemia and manage with appropriate parenteral fluid therapy. If significant extrapyramidal reactions occur in the context of an overdose, administer an anticholinergic. Refer to General Management of Acute Overdosage.

CYCLOPROPANE

Administration and Dosage

The information on General Anesthetic Gases is not intended to supply complete information on actions, uses, cautions and contraindications. Recommended uses and product availability are given. Consult detailed literature before using. These agents should be administered only by those with appropriate training and experience.

Supplied in orange cylinders.

Actions

➤*Pharmacology:* An anesthetic gas with a rapid onset of action. May be used for analgesia and induction and maintenance of anesthesia. Produces skeletal muscle relaxation in full anesthetic doses. Adminis-

ter in a closed system with oxygen. Disadvantages include difficulty in detection of planes of anesthesia, occasional laryngospasm and cardiac arrhythmia. Postanesthetic nausea, vomiting and headache are frequent.

Precautions

➤*Malignant hyperthermia:* Malignant hyperthermia may be triggered by most of the potent, fat-soluble, inhalational anesthetics and by many skeletal muscle relaxants, especially when used as prophylaxis and treatment.

➤*Caution:* Cyclopropane/oxygen mixtures are flammable and EXPLOSIVE. Due to this undesirable property, cyclopropane is rarely used.

ETHYLENE

Administration and Dosage

The information on General Anesthetic Gases is not intended to supply complete information on actions, uses, cautions and contraindications. Recommended uses and product availability are given. Consult detailed literature before using. These agents should be administered only by those with appropriate training and experience.

Supplied in red cylinders.

Actions

➤*Pharmacology:* An anesthetic gas with rapid onset and recovery. Provides adequate analgesia but has poor muscle relaxation properties. Must be administered in high (80%) concentrations with oxygen (20%). Advantages include minimal bronchospasm and laryngospasm and minimal postanesthetic vomiting. Ethylene is nontoxic; hypoxia is the primary complication.

Precautions

➤*Caution:* Ethylene/oxygen mixtures are flammable and EXPLOSIVE. Due to this undesirable property, ethylene is rarely used.

NITROUS OXIDE (N₂O)

Administration and Dosage

The information on General Anesthetic Gases is not intended to supply complete information on actions, uses, cautions and contraindications. Recommended uses and product availability are given. Consult detailed literature before using. These agents should be administered only by those with appropriate training and experience.

Supplied in blue cylinders.

Actions

➤*Pharmacology:* The most commonly used anesthetic gas, nitrous oxide is a weak anesthetic usually used in combination with other anesthetics. It does not cause skeletal muscle relaxation. The chief danger in the use of nitrous oxide is hypoxia; at least 20% oxygen should be used. An increased risk of renal and hepatic diseases and peripheral neuropathy has been reported in dental personnel who work in areas where nitrous oxide is used.

The gas can diffuse into air-containing cavities faster than nitrogen can leave, causing potentially dangerous pressure accumulation (eg, middle

ear abnormalities, bowel obstruction, pneumothorax). Nitrous oxide also oxidizes and inactivates vitamin B_{12}, thus affecting some enzymes. This action may be linked to observations of adversely affected hematological, immune, neurological and reproductive systems.

Precautions

➤*Adverse effects:* In high concentrations, nitrous oxide may cause vomiting, respiratory depression and death. A primary advantage of nitrous oxide is that it is nonexplosive.

➤*Malignant hyperthermia:* Malignant hyperthermia may be triggered by most of the potent, fat-soluble, inhalational anesthetics and by many skeletal muscle relaxants, especially when used as prophylaxis and treatment.

➤*Drug abuse and dependence:* Abuse and dependence have been documented, with speculation that interaction with the endogeneous opioid system may be involved.

HALOTHANE

Rx	Halothane (Abbott)	In 250 ml.[1]

[1] With 0.01% thymol.

[2] With 0.01% thymol and up to 0.00025% ammonia.

Indications

Induction and maintenance of general anesthesia.

Administration and Dosage

The information on General Anesthetic Volatile Liquids is not intended to supply complete information on actions, uses, cautions and contraindications. Recommended uses and product availability are given. Consult detailed literature before using. Should be administered only by those with appropriate training and experience.

Halothane may be administered by the nonrebreathing technique, partial rebreathing or closed technique. The induction dose varies. The maintenance concentration varies from 0.5% to 1.5%. May be administered with either oxygen or a mixture of oxygen and nitrous oxide.

Actions

➤*Pharmacology:* An inhalation anesthetic. Induction and recovery are rapid and depth of anesthesia can be rapidly altered. Halothane is not an irritant to the respiratory tract, and no increase in salivary or bronchial secretions ordinarily occurs. Pharyngeal and laryngeal reflexes are rapidly obtunded. It causes bronchodilation. Hypoxia, aci-

dosis or apnea may develop during deep anesthesia. It sensitizes the myocardium to the action of epinephrine and norepinephrine; the combination may cause serious cardiac arrhythmias. Halothane produces moderate muscular relaxation. Muscle relaxants are used as adjuncts to maintain lighter levels of anesthesia.

Warnings

➤*Hepatic function impairment:* Halothane administration has been associated with hepatic dysfunction. There may be two types: One characterized by increased serum enzyme levels (20% to 25% of patients) and the other, fulminant hepatic failure (1 in 7000 to 1 in 30,000). Patients at particular risk appear to be middle-aged obese females with previous closely spaced halothane administration.

Precautions

➤*Malignant hyperthermia:* Malignant hyperthermia may be triggered by most of the potent, fat-soluble, inhalational anesthetics and by many skeletal muscle relaxants, especially when used concurrently. Monitor the patient closely; dantrolene (see individual monograph) has been used as prophylaxis and treatment.

METHOXYFLURANE

Rx	Penthrane (Abbott)	In 15 and 125 ml.[1]

[1] With 0.01% butylated hydroxytoluene.

Indications

Usually used in combination with oxygen and nitrous oxide, to provide anesthesia for surgical procedures in which the total duration of administration is anticipated to be ≤ 4 hours, and in which methoxyflurane is not to be used in concentrations that will provide skeletal muscle relaxation.

May be used alone or in combination with oxygen and nitrous oxide for analgesia in obstetrics and in minor surgical procedures.

Administration and Dosage

The information on General Anesthetic Volatile Liquids is not intended to supply complete information on actions, uses, cautions and contraindications. Recommended uses and product availability are given. Consult detailed literature before using. Should be administered only by those with appropriate training and experience.

➤*Analgesia and anesthesia:* 0.3% to 0.8%.

➤*Induction:* Up to 2%.

➤*Maintenance:* 0.1% to 2% is adequate for maintenance when administered in a carrier gas flow of oxygen and at least 50% nitrous oxide.

Actions

➤*Pharmacology:* Provides anesthesia or analgesia. After surgical anesthesia, analgesia and drowsiness may persist after consciousness has returned. This may reduce the need for narcotics in the immediate postoperative period.

When used alone in safe concentration, it will not produce appreciable skeletal muscle relaxation; use a muscle relaxant as an adjunct. Bronchiolar constriction or laryngeal spasm is not ordinarily provoked.

Warnings

➤*Renal function impairment:* May cause renal failure or damage due to release of the fluoride ion.

Precautions

➤*Malignant hyperthermia:* Malignant hyperthermia may be triggered by most of the potent, fat-soluble, inhalational anesthetics and by many skeletal muscle relaxants, especially when used concurrently. Monitor the patient closely; dantrolene (see individual monograph) has been used as prophylaxis and treatment.

ENFLURANE

Rx	Enflurane (Abbott)	In 125 and 250 mL.
Rx	Ethrane (Ohmeda)	In 125 and 250 mL.
Rx	Compound 347 (Minrad)	In 250 mL.

Indications

Induction and maintenance of general anesthesia. Provides analgesia for vaginal delivery. Also used to supplement other general anesthetic agents during delivery by cesarean section.

Administration and Dosage

The information on General Anesthetic Volatile Liquids is not intended to supply complete information on actions, uses, cautions and contraindications. Recommended uses and product availability are given. Consult detailed literature before using. Should be administered only by those with appropriate training and experience.

➤*Induction:* 2% to 4.5% produces anesthesia in 7 to 10 minutes.

➤*Maintenance:* Surgical levels of anesthesia may be maintained with 0.5% to 3% concentrations. Maintenance concentration should not exceed 3%.

Actions

➤*Pharmacokinetics:* An inhalation anesthetic. Induction and recovery from anesthesia are rapid. There is mild stimulus to salivation or tracheobronchial secretions. Pharyngeal and laryngeal reflexes are readily obtunded. The level of anesthesia changes rapidly. Reduces ven-

tilation as depth of anesthesia increases. High $PaCO_2$ levels can be obtained at deeper levels of anesthesia if ventilation is not supported. Provokes a sigh response reminiscent of that seen with diethyl ether.

Progressive increases in depth of anesthesia produce increasing hypotension. Heart rate remains relatively constant without significant bradycardia; cardiac rhythm remains stable and is unaffected by carbon dioxide elevation in arterial blood.

Muscle relaxation – Muscle relaxation may be adequate for intra-abdominal operations at normal levels of anesthesia. If greater relaxation is necessary, muscle relaxants may be used.

Warnings

➤*Renal function impairment:* May cause renal failure or may damage already impaired kidneys due to release of fluoride ion.

Precautions

➤*Malignant hyperthermia:* Malignant hyperthermia may be triggered by most of the potent, fat-soluble, inhalational anesthetics and by many skeletal muscle relaxants, especially when used concurrently. Monitor the patient closely; dantrolene (see individual monograph) has been used as prophylaxis and treatment.

ISOFLURANE

Rx	**Isoflurane** (Abbott)	In 100 mL.
Rx	**Forane** (Anaquest)	In 100 mL.
Rx	**Terrell** (Minrad)	In 100 and 250 mL.

Indications

Induction and maintenance of general anesthesia.

Administration and Dosage

The information on General Anesthetic Volatile Liquids is not intended to supply complete information on actions, uses, cautions and contraindications. Recommended uses and product availability are given. Consult detailed literature before using. Should be administered only by those with appropriate training and experience.

➤*Induction:* Inspired concentrations of 1.5% to 3% isoflurane usually produce surgical anesthesia in 7 to 10 minutes.

➤*Maintenance:* Surgical levels of anesthesia may be sustained with a 1% to 2.5% concentration when nitrous oxide is used concomitantly.

Actions

➤*Pharmacokinetics:* Induction and recovery from isoflurane anesthesia are rapid. Its mild pungency limits the rate of induction, although excessive salivation or tracheobronchial secretions do not appear to be stimulated. Pharyngeal and laryngeal reflexes are readily obtunded. The level of anesthesia changes rapidly; it is a profound respiratory depressant. Monitor respiration closely and support when necessary. As the dose is increased, tidal volume decreases and respiratory rate is unchanged. This depression is partially reversed by surgical stimulation.

Blood pressure – Blood pressure decreases with induction of anesthesia, progresses with increasing depth, but returns toward normal with surgical stimulation. Progressive increases in depth of anesthesia produce decreases in blood pressure. Nitrous oxide diminishes the concentration of isoflurane required and may reduce the arterial hypotension seen with isoflurane alone. With controlled ventilation and normal $PaCO_2$, cardiac output is maintained through an increase in heart rate which compensates for a reduction in stroke volume. The hypercapnia attending isoflurane anesthesia further increases heart rate and raises cardiac output above awake levels. Isoflurane does not sensitize the myocardium to exogenously administered epinephrine.

Muscle relaxation – Muscle relaxation is adequate for intra-abdominal operations at normal levels of anesthesia. Complete muscle paralysis is attained with small doses of muscle relaxants.

Precautions

➤*Malignant hyperthermia:* Malignant hyperthermia may be triggered by most of the potent, fat-soluble, inhalational anesthetics and by many skeletal muscle relaxants, especially when used concurrently. Monitor the patient closely; dantrolene (see individual monograph) has been used as prophylaxis and treatment.

DESFLURANE

Rx	**Suprane** (Ohmeda)	In 240 ml.

Indications

➤*Anesthesia:* An inhalation agent for induction or maintenance of anesthesia for inpatient and outpatient surgery in adults.

Administration and Dosage

➤*Approved by the FDA:* September 18, 1992.

The information on General Anesthetic Volatile Liquids is not intended to supply complete information on actions, uses, cautions and contraindications. Recommended uses and product availability are given. Consult detailed literature before using. Should be administered only by those with appropriate training and experience.

Deliver desflurane from a vaporizer specifically designed and designated for use with desflurane. The administration of general anesthesia must be individualized based on the patient's response.

➤*Preanesthetic medication:* Issues such as whether or not to premedicate and the choice of premedicant(s) must be individualized. In clinical studies, patients scheduled to be anesthetized with desflurane frequently received IV preanesthetic medication, such as opioids or benzodiazepines.

➤*Induction:* In adults, a frequent starting concentration was 3%, increased in 0.5% to 1% increments every 2 to 3 breaths. End-tidal concentrations of 4% to 11% desflurane, with and without N_2O, produced anesthesia within 2 to 4 minutes.

After induction in adults with an IV drug such as thiopental or propofol, desflurane can be started at approximately 0.5 to 1 MAC, whether the carrier gas is O_2 or N_2O/O_2.

➤*Maintenance:* Surgical levels of anesthesia in adults may be maintained with concentrations of 2.5% to 8.5% with or without the concomitant use of nitrous oxide. In children, surgical levels of anesthesia may be maintained with concentrations of 5.2% to 10% with or without the concomitant use of nitrous oxide.

During the maintenance of anesthesia, increasing concentrations produce dose-dependent decreases in blood pressure. Excessive decreases in blood pressure may be due to depth of anesthesia and in such instances may be corrected by decreasing the inspired concentration of desflurane.

Concentrations of desflurane exceeding 1 MAC may increase heart rate. Thus, with this drug an increased heart rate may not serve reliably as a sign of inadequate anesthesia. The use of desflurane decreases the required doses of neuromuscular blocking agents.

Actions

➤*Pharmacology:* Desflurane is a volatile liquid inhalation anesthetic minimally biotransformed in the liver. Less than 0.02% of the desflurane absorbed can be recovered as urinary metabolites (compared to 0.2% for isoflurane). Minimum alveolar concentration (MAC) of desflurane in oxygen for a 25-year-old adult is 7.3%. The MAC of desflurane decreases with increasing age and with addition of depressants such as opioids or benzodiazepines. Changes in the clinical effects of desflurane rapidly follow changes in the inspired concentration.

Although desflurane can be used in adults for the inhalation induction of anesthesia via mask, it produces a high incidence of respiratory irritation (coughing, breathholding, apnea, increased secretions, laryngospasm).

Do not use desflurane as the sole agent for anesthetic induction in patients with coronary artery disease or any patients where increases in heart rate or blood pressure are undesirable. If desflurane is to be used in patients with coronary artery disease, use in combination with other medications for induction of anesthesia, preferably IV opioids and hypnotics.

Desflurane is not recommended for induction of general anesthesia in infants or children because of a high incidence of moderate to severe laryngospasm, coughing, breathholding and secretions.

Warnings

➤*Children:* Desflurane is not recommended for induction of anesthesia in children because of a high incidence of moderate to severe upper airway adverse events. After induction of anesthesia with agents other than desflurane, and tracheal intubation, desflurane is indicated for maintenance of anesthesia in infants and children.

Precautions

➤*Malignant hyperthermia:* Malignant hyperthermia may be triggered by most of the potent, fat-soluble, inhalational anesthetics and by many skeletal muscle relaxants, especially when used concurrently. Monitor the patient closely; dantrolene (see individual monograph) has been used as prophylaxis and treatment.

SEVOFLURANE

| *Rx* | **Ultane** (Abbott) | | In 250 mL. |

Indications

➤*Anesthesia:* Induction and maintenance of general anesthesia in adult and pediatric patients for inpatient and outpatient surgery.

Administration and Dosage

➤*Approved by the FDA:* June 7, 1995.

The information on General Anesthetic Volatile Liquids is not intended to supply complete information on actions, uses, precautions, and contraindications. Recommended uses and product availability are given. Consult detailed literature before using. Sevoflurane should be administered only by those with appropriate training and experience.

The concentration of sevoflurane being delivered from a vaporizer should be known. This may be accomplished by using a vaporizer calibrated specifically for sevoflurane. Administration of general anesthesia must be individualized based on patient response.

➤*Replacement of CO_2 absorbents:* Before administration of sevoflurane, replace the CO_2 absorbent if it is desiccated. The exothermic reaction that occurs with sevoflurane and CO_2 absorbents is increased when the CO_2 absorbent becomes desiccated, such as after an extended period of dry gas flow through the CO_2 absorbent canisters. Extremely rare cases of spontaneous fire in the respiratory circuit of the anesthesia machine have been reported during sevoflurane use in conjunction with the use of a desiccated CO_2 absorbent. Rapid changes in the color of some CO_2 absorbents or an unusually delayed rise in the delivered (inspired) gas concentration of sevoflurane compared with the vaporizer setting may indicate excessive heating of the CO_2 absorbent canister and chemical breakdown of sevoflurane.

➤*Preanesthetic medication:* No specific premedication is either indicated or contraindicated. The decision as to whether or not to premedicate and choice of premedication is left to the discretion of the anesthesiologist.

➤*Induction:* Sevoflurane has a nonpungent odor and does not cause respiratory irritation; it is suitable for mask induction in children and adults.

➤*Maintenance:* Surgical levels of anesthesia can usually be obtained with concentrations of 0.5% to 3% with or without the concomitant use of nitrous oxide. Sevoflurane can be administered with any type of anesthesia circuit.

➤*Storage / Stability:* Store at controlled room temperature (15° to 30°C; 59° to 86°F).

Actions

➤*Pharmacology:* Sevoflurane is an inhalational anesthetic. Minimum alveolar concentration (MAC) of sevoflurane in oxygen for an adult 40 years of age is 2.1%. The MAC of sevoflurane decreases with age.

Alveolar concentration/inspired concentration (F_A/F_I) of sevoflurane was compared with F_A/F_I data of other halogenated anesthetics in healthy volunteers. When all data were normalized to isoflurane, the uptake and distribution of sevoflurane was faster than isoflurane and halothane but slower than desflurane. Sevoflurane is a dose-related cardiac depressant. It does not produce increases in heart rate at doses less than 2 MAC.

➤*Pharmacokinetics:*

Metabolism / Excretion – Sevoflurane is metabolized by cytochrome P450 2E1 to hexafluoroisopropanol (HFIP) with release of inorganic fluoride and CO_2. Once formed HFIP is rapidly conjugated with glucuronic acid and eliminated as a urinary metabolite. No other metabolic pathways for sevoflurane have been identified. In vivo metabolism studies suggest that approximately 5% of the sevoflurane dose may be metabolized.

The low solubility of sevoflurane facilitates rapid elimination via the lungs. In healthy volunteers, rate of elimination was similar compared with desflurane, but faster compared with halothane or isoflurane. Up to 3.5% of the sevoflurane dose appears in the urine as inorganic fluoride. Studies on fluoride indicate that up to 50% of fluoride clearance is nonrenal (via fluoride being taken up into bone).

Contraindications

Sevoflurane can cause malignant hyperthermia. Do not use in patients with known sensitivity to sevoflurane or to other halogenated agents nor in patients with known or suspected susceptibility to malignant hyperthermia.

Precautions

➤*Malignant hyperthermia:* Malignant hyperthermia may be triggered by most of the potent inhalational anesthetics. Treatment of malignant hyperthermia includes discontinuation of triggering agents, administration of IV dantrolene sodium and supportive therapy. Sevoflurane may present an increased risk in patients with known sensitivity to volatile halogenated anesthetic agents (see Contraindications).

This information on local anesthetics is not intended to be comprehensive. Consult standard textbooks for further discussion of techniques and applications.

WARNING

Obstetrical anesthesia: The 0.75% concentration of **bupivacaine** is not recommended for obstetrical anesthesia. Cardiac arrest with difficult resuscitation or death has occurred during use for epidural anesthesia in obstetrical patients. Resuscitation has been difficult or impossible despite adequate preparation and appropriate management. Cardiac arrest has occurred after convulsions resulting from systemic toxicity, presumably following unintentional intravascular injection. Reserve the 0.75% concentration for surgical procedures where a high degree of muscle relaxation and prolonged effect are necessary.

Historically, pregnant patients were reported to have a high risk for cardiac arrhythmias, cardiac/circulatory arrest, and death when bupivacaine was inadvertently rapidly injected IV. Avoid 0.75% levobupivacaine in obstetrical patients. The concentration is indicated only for nonobstetrical surgery requiring profound muscle relaxation and long duration. For Cesarean section, the 5 mg/mL (0.5%) levobupivacaine solution in doses up to 150 mg is recommended.

Have resuscitative equipment and drugs immediately available when any local anesthetic is used.

Do not use preparations containing preservatives for caudal epidural anesthesia. When using preparations without preservatives, discard any unused drug remaining in vial.

Indications

Refer to individual product listings.

Administration and Dosage

The dose of local anesthetic administered varies with the procedure, vascularity of the tissues, depth of anesthesia, degree of required muscle relaxation, duration of anesthesia desired, and the physical condition of the patient. Reduce dosages for children, the elderly, debilitated patients, and patients with cardiac or liver disease.

➤*Infiltration or regional block anesthesia:* Always inject slowly, with frequent aspirations, to prevent intravascular injection.

For detailed Administration and Dosage, refer to individual product listings and specific manufacturers' labeling.

Actions

➤*Pharmacology:* These agents prevent generation and conduction of nerve impulses by inhibiting ionic fluxes, increasing electrical excitation threshold, slowing nerve impulse propagation, and reducing rate of rise of action potential. Progression of anesthesia is related to the diameter, myelination, and conduction velocity of affected nerve fibers. The order of loss of nerve function is: Pain, temperature, touch, proprioception, and skeletal muscle tone.

Systemic absorption of local anesthetics affects the cardiovascular system and CNS. At blood concentrations achieved with normal therapeutic doses, changes in cardiac conduction, excitability, refractoriness, contractility, and peripheral vascular resistance are minimal. However, toxic blood concentrations depress cardiac conduction and excitability, which may lead to atrioventricular block and ultimately to cardiac arrest. In addition, with toxic blood concentrations, myocardial contractility may be depressed and peripheral vasodilation may occur, leading to decreased cardiac output and arterial blood pressure.

Following systemic absorption, toxic blood concentrations can produce CNS stimulation, depression, or both. Apparent central stimulation may manifest as restlessness, tremors, and shivering, which may progress to convulsions. Depression and coma may occur, possibly progressing ultimately to respiratory arrest. Local anesthetics have a primary depressant effect on the medulla and on higher centers. The depressed stage may occur without a prior stage of CNS stimulation.

The use of vasoconstrictors (eg, epinephrine) with local anesthetics promotes local hemostasis, decreases systemic absorption and prolongs duration of action.

➤*Pharmacokinetics:* Various pharmacokinetic parameters can be significantly altered by the presence of hepatic or renal disease, addition of epinephrine, factors affecting urinary pH, renal blood flow, administration route and age of patient, and the presence or absence of epinephrine in the anesthetic solution.

Injectable Local Anesthetics Pharmacokinetics

Anesthetic	Onset (minutes)	Duration (hours)	Equivalent anesthetic concentration (%)	pKa	Partition coefficient	Systemic protein binding (%)
Esters						
Procaine[1]	2-5	0.25-1	2	9.1	0.02[3]	5.8[4]
(w/epinephrine)	nd	0.5-1.5				
(Epidural)[2]	15-25	0.5-1.5				
Chloroprocaine[1]	6-12	0.5	2	9	0.14[3]	nd
(w/epinephrine)	nd	0.5-1.5				
(Epidural)[2]	5-15	0.5-1.5				
Tetracaine[1]	≤ 15	2-3	0.25	8.5	4.1[3]	75.6[5]
(Epidural)[2]	20-30	3-5				
(Spinal)	nd	1.25-3				
Amides						
Lidocaine[1]	< 2	0.5-1	1	7.9	2.9[3]	64.3
(w/epinephrine)	< 2	2-6				
(Epidural)[2]	5-15	1-3				
(Spinal)	nd	0.5-1.5				
Prilocaine[1]	< 2	≥ 1	1	7.9	0.9[3]	55
(w/epinephrine)	< 2	2.25				
(Epidural)[2]	5-15	1-3				
Mepivacaine[1]	3-5	0.75-1.5	1	7.8	0.8[3]	77.5[5]
(w/epinephrine)	nd	2-6				
(Epidural)[2]	5-15	1-3				
(Spinal)	nd	0.5-1.5				
Bupivacaine[1]	5	2-4	0.25	8.2	27.5[3]/1565[6]	95.6[5]
(w/epinephrine)	nd	3-7				
(Epidural)[2]	10-20	3-5				
(Spinal)	nd	1.25-2.5				
Levobupivacaine	—	—	—	8.09	1624[6]	> 97[5]
(Epidural)[7]	≈ 10	≈ 8	nd			
Articaine	—	—	nd	7.8	17[8]	60-80
(w/epinephrine)	1-6	1				
Ropivacaine	—	—	nd	8.07	2.9[9]	94
(Epidural)	10-30	0.5-6				

[1] Values in this line are for infiltrative anesthesia. nd – No data.
[2] With epinephrine 1:200,000.
[3] n-Heptane/Buffer, pH 7.4.
[4] Nerve homogenate binding.
[5] Plasma protein binding.
[6] Oleyl alcohol/water buffer.
[7] Administration in Cesarean section.
[8] n-octanol/Soerensen buffer, pH 7.35.
[9] n-heptane buffer.

Rate of systemic absorption depends on total dose and concentration of drug, vascularity of administration site, and presence of vasoconstrictors. Depending on route, local anesthetics are distributed to some extent to all body tissues. High concentrations are found in highly perfused organs (eg, liver, lungs, heart, brain). Rate and extent of placental diffusion are determined by plasma protein binding, ionization, and lipid solubility. Fetal/maternal ratios are inversely related to degree of protein binding. Only free, unbound drug is available for placental transfer. Drugs with the highest protein binding capacity may have the lowest fetal/maternal ratios. Lipid soluble, nonionized drugs readily enter fetal blood from maternal circulation.

The onset of local anesthesia is dependent on the dissociation constant (pKa), lipid solubility, pH at the injection site, protein binding and molecular size. In general, local anesthetics with high lipid solubility or low pKa have a faster onset.

Local anesthetics are divided into 2 groups: Esters, which are derivatives of para-aminobenzoic acid, and amides, which are derivatives of aniline. The "ester" local anesthetics are metabolized by hydrolysis of the ester linkage by plasma esterase, probably plasma cholinesterase. The "amide" local anesthetics are metabolized primarily in the liver, then excreted primarily in the urine as metabolites, with a small fraction of unchanged drug.

Contraindications

Hypersensitivity to local anesthetics or any components of the products, para-aminobenzoic acid (esters only) or parabens; congenital or idiopathic methemoglobinemia (**prilocaine**); spinal and caudal anesthesia in septicemia, existing neurologic disease, spinal deformities, and severe hypertension, hemorrhage, shock, or heart block; subarachnoid administration (**chloroprocaine**).

➤*Bupivacaine/Levobupivacaine:* Obstetrical paracervical block anesthesia (such use has resulted in fetal bradycardia and death); IV regional anesthesia (Bier block; cardiac arrest and death have occurred) (see Warnings).

Warnings

➤*Head and neck area:* Small doses of local anesthetics injected into the head and neck area, including retrobulbar, dental, and stellate ganglion blocks, may produce adverse reactions similar to systemic toxicity seen with unintentional intravascular injections of larger doses. The injection procedures require the utmost care. Confusion, convulsions, respiratory depression or arrest, and cardiovascular stimulation or depression have been reported. These reactions may be caused by intraarterial injection of the local anesthetic with retrograde flow to cerebral circulation. They also may be caused by puncture of the dural sheath of the optic nerve during retrobulbar block with diffusion of any local anesthetic along the subdural space to the midbrain. Observe patient carefully. Monitor respiration and circulation. Do not exceed dosage recommendations.

Ophthalmic surgery – When local anesthetic solutions are used for retrobulbar block, complete corneal anesthesia usually precedes onset of clinically acceptable external ocular muscle akinesia. Therefore, presence of akinesia rather than anesthesia alone should determine readiness of the patient for surgery. Clinicians who perform retrobulbar blocks should be aware that there have been reports of respiratory arrest following local anesthetic injection.

Dentistry – Because of the long duration of anesthesia of **bupivacaine with epinephrine**, caution patients about the possibility of inadvertent trauma to tongue, lips, and buccal mucosa and advise against chewing solid foods or testing anesthetized area by biting or probing.

Cardiovascular reactions – Cardiovascular reactions are depressant. They may be the result of direct drug effect, the result of vasovagal reaction, particularly if the patient is in the sitting position. Failure to recognize premonitory signs such as sweating, feeling of faintness, changes in pulse, or sensorium may result in progressive cerebral hypoxia and seizure, or serious cardiovascular catastrophe. Place patient in recumbent position and administer oxygen.

➤*Intravascular or subarachnoid administration:* It is essential that aspiration for blood or cerebrospinal fluid (where applicable) be done prior to injecting any local anesthetic, both the original dose and all subsequent doses, to avoid intravascular or subarachnoid injection. However, a negative aspiration does not ensure against an intravascular or subarachnoid injection.

In performing **ropivacaine** blocks, unintended intravascular injection is possible and may result in cardiac arrhythmia or cardiac arrest. The potential for successful resuscitation has not been studied in humans. Administer ropivacaine in incremental doses. It is not recommended for emergency situations where a fast onset of surgical anesthesia is necessary. Historically, pregnant patients were reported to have a high risk for cardiac arrhythmias, cardiac/circulatory arrest, and death when 0.75% **bupivacaine** was inadvertently rapidly injected IV.

➤*Spinal anesthesia:* The following conditions may preclude the use of spinal anesthesia, depending upon the physician's evaluation of the situation and ability to deal with the following complications or complaints that may occur:
• Pre-existing diseases of the CNS, such as those attributable to pernicious anemia, poliomyelitis, syphilis, or tumor.
• Hematological disorders predisposing to coagulopathies or patients on anticoagulant therapy. Trauma to a blood vessel during the conduct of spinal anesthesia may, in some instances, result in uncontrollable CNS hemorrhage or soft tissue hemorrhage.
• Chronic backache and preoperative headache.
• Hypotension and hypertension.
• Technical problems (persistent paresthesias, persistent bloody tap).
• Arthritis or spinal deformity.
• Extremes of age.
• Psychosis or other causes of poor cooperation by the patient.

➤*Hypersensitivity reactions:* These include anaphylaxis and may occur in a small segment of the population allergic to para-aminobenzoic acid derivatives (eg, procaine, tetracaine, benzocaine). The amide-type local anesthetics have not shown cross-sensitivity with the esters.

Reactions resulting in fatality have occurred on rare occasions with the use of local anesthetics, even in the absence of a history of hypersensitivity.

Administer ester-type local anesthetics cautiously to patients with abnormal or reduced levels of plasma esterases.

➤*Renal function impairment:* Use **mepivacaine** with caution in patients with renal disease.

➤*Hepatic function impairment:* Because amide-type local anesthetics are metabolized primarily in the liver and ester-type local anesthetics are hydrolyzed by plasma cholinesterase produced by the liver, patients with hepatic disease, especially severe hepatic disease, may be more susceptible to potential toxicity. Use cautiously in such patients.

➤*Elderly:* Repeated doses may cause accumulation of the drug or its metabolites or slow metabolic degradation; give reduced doses.

➤*Pregnancy:* Category B (**levobupivacaine, lidocaine, prilocaine, ropivacaine**). *Category C* (**articaine, bupivacaine, chloroprocaine, mepivacaine, procaine, tetracaine**). Safety for use in pregnant women, other than those in labor, has not been established. Local anesthetics rapidly cross the placenta. When used for epidural, caudal, paracervical, or pudendal block, they can cause varying degrees of maternal, fetal, and neonatal toxicity involving alterations of the CNS, peripheral vascular tone, and cardiac function. The incidence and degree of toxicity depend upon the procedure, type and amount of drug used, and technique of administration.

Labor, delivery, and abortion – Fetal bradycardia and fetal acidosis may occur in patients receiving anesthetics for paracervical block. Always monitor fetal heart rate prior to and during paracervical anesthesia. Added risk appears to be present in prematurity, toxemia of pregnancy, and fetal distress. Weigh the possible advantages against dangers when considering paracervical block in these conditions. The use of some local anesthetics during labor and delivery may be followed by diminished muscle strength and tone for the infant's first day or 2 of life.

Careful adherence to recommended dosage is extremely important. Failure to achieve adequate analgesia via intended paracervical or pudendal block or both with these doses may indicate intravascular or fetal intracranial injection. Babies so affected present with unexplained neonatal depression at birth and usually manifest seizures within 6 hours. Prompt use of supportive measures and forced urinary excretion of the local anesthetic have been used successfully.

Maternal hypotension – Maternal hypotension has resulted from regional anesthesia. Local anesthetics produce vasodilation by blocking sympathetic nerves. Elevating the patient's legs and positioning her on her left side will help prevent decreases in blood pressure. Continuously monitor fetal heart rate; electronic monitoring is advisable. It is extremely important to avoid aortacaval compression by the gravid uterus during administration of regional block.

Epidural, caudal, paracervical, or pudendal anesthesia – These may alter the forces of parturition through changes in uterine contractility or maternal expulsive efforts. Epidural anesthesia has been reported to prolong the second stage of labor by removing the parturient's reflex urge to bear down or by interfering with motor function. The use of obstetrical anesthesia may increase the need for forceps assistance.

Maternal convulsions and cardiovascular collapse following use of some local anesthetics for paracervical block in early pregnancy (as anesthesia for elective abortion) suggest that systemic absorption may be rapid. Therefore, do not exceed the recommended maximum dose. Inject slowly, with frequent aspirations. Allow a 5-minute interval between sides.

➤*Lactation:* Safety for use in the nursing mother has not been established. **Bupivacaine** has been reported to be excreted in breast milk. However, it is not known whether local anesthetic drugs are excreted in breast milk.

➤*Children:* Because of lack of clinical experience, the administration of **bupivacaine** to children < 12 years of age and bupivacaine 0.75% in dextrose to children < 18 years of age is not recommended.

Safety and efficacy of **tetracaine, levobupivacaine,** and **ropivacaine** in children have not been established.

Lidocaine 0.5% to 2% with or without epinephrine (except for dentistry indications) is not indicated in children ≤ 3 years of age. Lidocaine 5% in dextrose is not indicated in children < 16 years of age. Lidocaine 1.5% in dextrose is not indicated in children.

Articaine is not indicated in children < 4 years of age. **Chloroprocaine** is not indicated in children < 3 years of age.

Reduce dosages in children, commensurate with age, body weight, and physical condition.

Precautions

➤*Dosage:* Use the lowest dosage that results in effective anesthesia to avoid high plasma levels and serious adverse effects. Inject slowly, with frequent aspirations before and during the injection, to avoid intravascular injection. Perform syringe aspirations before and during each supplemental injection in continuous (intermittent) catheter techniques. During the administration of epidural anesthesia, it is recommended that a test dose be administered initially and that the patient be monitored for CNS toxicity and cardiovascular toxicity, as well as for signs of unintended intrathecal administration, before proceeding.

➤*Inflammation or sepsis:* Use local anesthetic procedures with caution when there is inflammation or sepsis in the region of proposed injection.

➤*CNS toxicity:* Monitor cardiovascular and respiratory vital signs and state of consciousness after each injection. Restlessness, anxiety, incoherent speech, lightheadedness, numbness, and tingling of the mouth and lips, metallic taste, tinnitus, dizziness, blurred vision, tremors, twitching, depression, or drowsiness may be early signs of CNS toxicity.

➤*Malignant hyperthermia:* Many drugs used during anesthesia are considered potential triggering agents for familial malignant hyperthermia. It is not known whether local anesthetics may trigger this reaction and the need for supplemental general anesthesia cannot be predicted in advance; therefore, have a standard protocol for management available.

➤*Vasoconstrictors:* Use solutions containing a vasoconstrictor with caution and in carefully circumscribed quantities in areas of the body supplied by end arteries or having otherwise compromised blood supply (eg, digits, nose, external ear, penis). Use with extreme caution in patients whose medical history and physical evaluation suggest the existence of hypertension, peripheral vascular disease, arteriosclerotic heart disease, cerebral vascular insufficiency, or heart block; these individuals may exhibit exaggerated vasoconstrictor response.

Serious dose-related cardiac arrhythmias may occur if preparations containing a vasoconstrictor such as epinephrine are employed in patients during or following the administration of potent inhalation agents.

➤*IV regional anesthesia:* Cardiac arrest and death are reported with the use of **bupivacaine** for IV regional anesthesia (Bier block). Bupivacaine is not recommended for this technique.

➤*Special risk:*

Debilitated patients/acutely ill patients/the elderly/children – Repeated doses may cause accumulation of the drug or its metabolites or slow metabolic degradation. Give reduced doses. Use anesthetics with caution in patients with severe disturbances of cardiac rhythm, hypotension, shock, or heart block. Also use local anesthetics with caution in patients with impaired cardiovascular function because they may be less able to compensate for functional changes associated with the prolongation of A-V conduction produced by these drugs.

➤*Sulfite sensitivity:* Some of these products contain sulfites. Sulfites may cause allergic-type reactions (eg, hives, itching, wheezing, anaphylaxis) in certain susceptible people. Although the overall prevalence of sulfite sensitivity in the general population is probably low, it is seen more frequently in asthmatics or in atopic nonasthmatic people.

Drug Interactions

➤*Intercurrent use:* Mixtures of local anesthetics are sometimes employed to compensate for the slower onset of one drug and the shorter duration of action of the second drug. Toxicity is probably additive with mixtures of local anesthetics, but some experiments suggest synergisms. Exercise caution regarding toxic equivalence when mixtures of local anesthetics are employed.

Some preparations contain vasoconstrictors. Keep this in mind when using concurrently with other drugs that may interact with vasoconstrictors (refer to the Vasopressors Used in Shock monographs).

➤*CYP450:* The metabolism of **levobupivacaine** may be affected by the known CYP3A4 inducers (eg, phenytoin, phenobarbital, rifampin), CYP3A4 inhibitors (azole antimycotics, eg, ketoconazole; certain protease inhibitors, eg, ritonavir; macrolide antibiotics, eg, erythromycin; and calcium channel antagonists, eg, verapamil), CYP1A2 inducers (omeprazole), and CYP1A2 inhibitors (furafylline and clarithromycin). Dosage adjustment may be warranted when levobupivacaine is concurrently administered with CYP3A4 inhibitors and CYP1A2 inhibitors as systemic levobupivacaine levels may rise, resulting in toxicity.

The plasma concentration of **ropivacaine** was reduced 70% during coadministration of fluvoxamine (25 mg twice daily for 2 days), a selective and potent CYP1A2 inhibitor. Thus strong inhibitors of cytochrome P4501A2 such as fluvoxamine, given concomitantly during administration of ropivacaine, can interact with ropivacaine, leading to increased ropivacaine plasma levels. Exercise caution when CYP1A2 inhibitors are coadministered. Possible interactions with drugs known to be metabolized by CYP1A2 via competitive inhibition (eg, theophylline, imipramine) may also occur. Coadministration of a selective and potent inhibitor of CYP3A4, ketoconazole (100 mg bid for 2 days with ropivacaine infusion administered 1 hour after ketoconazole) caused a 15% reduction in in vivo plasma clearance of ropivacaine.

Injectable Local Anesthetic Drug Interactions			
Precipitant drug	Object drug*		Description
Local anesthetics	Sedatives	↑	If employed to reduce patient apprehension during dental procedures, use reduced doses, since local anesthetics used in combination with CNS depressants may have additive effects. Give young children minimal doses of each agent.
Local anesthetics	Sulfonamides	↓	The para-aminobenzoic acid metabolite of procaine, chloroprocaine, and tetracaine inhibits the action of sulfonamides. Therefore, do not use procaine, chloroprocaine, or tetracaine in any condition in which a sulfonamide drug is employed.

* ↑ = Object drug increased.   ↓ = Object drug decreased.

Adverse Reactions

The most common acute adverse reactions are related to the CNS and cardiovascular systems. These are generally dose-related and may result from overdosage, rapid absorption from the injection site, diminished tolerance, or unintentional intravascular injection.

➤*Cardiovascular:* Myocardial depression, hypotension (with spinal anesthesia caused by vasomotor paralysis and pooling of blood in the venous bed), hypertension, decreased cardiac output, heart block, bradycardia, ventricular arrhythmias (including tachycardia and fibrillation), cardiac arrest, and fetal bradycardia (see Warnings).

➤*CNS:* Restlessness, anxiety, dizziness, tinnitus, blurred vision, chills, pupil constriction or tremors may occur, possibly proceeding to convulsions ($\approx$ 0.1% of local anesthetic epidural administrations). Excitement may be transient or absent, with depression being the first manifestation. This may quickly be followed by drowsiness merging into unconsciousness and respiratory arrest.

Postspinal headache, meningismus, arachnoiditis, palsies, apprehension, double vision, euphoria, sensation of heat, cold, numbness, and spinal nerve paralysis (spinal anesthesia) have also occurred.

➤*GI:* Nausea, vomiting.

➤*Hypersensitivity:* Cutaneous lesions, urticaria, pruritus, erythema, angioneurotic edema (including laryngeal edema), sneezing, syncope, excessive sweating, elevated temperature, and anaphylactoid symptoms (including severe hypotension). Skin testing is of limited value.

➤*Respiratory:* Respiratory impairment or paralysis caused by level of anesthesia (spinal) extending to upper thoracic and cervical segments (see Warnings).

➤*Miscellaneous:* Occasional unintentional penetration of the subarachnoid space by the catheter may occur. Subsequent adverse effects may depend partially on amount of drug administered intrathecally. These may include the following: High or total spinal block; hypotension secondary to spinal block; urinary retention; fecal or urinary incontinence; loss of perineal sensation and sexual function; persistent anesthesia; paresthesia, weakness, and paralysis of the lower extremities and loss of sphincter control; headache and backache; septic meningitis; meningismus; slowing of labor and increased incidence of forceps delivery; cranial nerve palsies caused by traction on nerves from loss of cerebrospinal fluid; arachnoiditis; persistent motor, sensory, or autonomic deficit of some lower spinal segments with slow (several months), incomplete, or no recovery.

Methemoglobinemia – **Prilocaine** may produce dose-dependent methemoglobinemia. While methemoglobin values of < 20% do not generally produce any clinical symptoms, evalute the appearance of cyanosis at 2 to 4 hours following administration in terms of the patient's status.

➤*Articaine:*

Articaine Adverse Reactions (≥ 1%)	
Adverse reaction	Articaine (n = 882)
Pain	13
Headache	4
Face edema	1
Gingivitis	1
Infection	1
Paresthesia	1

The following list includes adverse and intercurrent events that were recorded in ≥ 1 patients, but occurred at an overall rate of < 1% and were considered clinically relevant.

Cardiovascular – Hemorrhage; migraine; syncope; tachycardia.

CNS – Dizziness; dry mouth; facial paralysis; hyperesthesia; increased salivation; nervousness; neuropathy; paresthesia; somnolence.

Dermatologic – Pruritus; skin disorder.

GI – Abdominal pain; constipation; diarrhea; dyspepsia; glossitis; gum hemorrhage; mouth ulceration; nausea; stomatitis; tongue edema; tooth disorder; vomiting.

Hematologic/Lymphatic – Ecchymosis; lymphadenopathy.

Metabolic/Nutritional – Edema; thirst.

Musculoskeletal – Arthralgia; myalgia; osteomyelitis.

Respiratory – Pharyngitis; rhinitis.

Special senses – Ear pain; taste perversion.

Miscellaneous – Accidental injury; asthenia; back pain; dysmenorrhea; injection site pain; malaise; neck pain.

➤*Levobupivacaine:*

Levobupivacaine Adverse Reactions (≥ 1%)	
Adverse reaction	Levobupivacaine (n = 509)
Cardiovascular	
Hypotension	19.6
ECG abnormal	3.1
Bradycardia	2.2
Tachycardia	1.8
Hypertension	1
CNS	
Fetal distress	9.6
Delivery delayed	6.3
Dizziness	5.1
Headache	4.5
Hypoesthesia	2.6
Paresthesia	1.8
Somnolence	1.2
Anxiety	1
Dermatologic	
Pruritus	3.7
Purpura	1.4

Levobupivacaine Adverse Reactions (≥ 1%)	
Adverse reaction	Levobupivacaine (n = 509)
GI	
Nausea	11.6
Vomiting	8.3
Abdomen enlarged	2.9
Constipation	2.8
Flatulence	2.4
Abdominal pain	2.2
Dyspepsia	2
Diarrhea	1
GU	
Albuminuria	2.9
Hematuria	2
Urine abnormal	1.8
Urinary incontinence	1.2
Breast pain (female)	1
Urine flow decreased	1
Urinary tract infection	1
Miscellaneous	
Anemia	9.6
Postoperative pain	7.3
Fever	6.5
Back pain	5.7
Pain	3.5
Rigors	2.9
Diplopia	2.6
Hypothermia	2.2
Hemorrhage in pregnancy	1.8
Wound drainage increased	1.4
Coughing	1.2
Leukocytosis	1.2
Anesthesia, local	1

The following adverse events were reported at an overall rate of < 1% and were considered clinically relevant.

Cardiovascular – Postural hypotension; arrhythmia; extrasystoles; atrial fibrillation; cardiac arrest.

CNS – Hypokinesia; involuntary muscle contraction; spasm (generalized); tremor; syncope; confusion.

Dermatologic – Increased sweating; skin discoloration.

Respiratory – Apnea; bronchospasm; dyspnea; pulmonary edema; respiratory insufficiency.

Miscellaneous – Asthenia; edema; elevated bilirubin; ileus.

➤*Ropivacaine:* For the indications of epidural administration in surgery, Cesarean section, postoperative pain management, peripheral nerve block, and local infiltration, the following treatment-emergent adverse events were reported with an incidence of ≥ 5% in all clinical studies (n = 3988): Hypotension (37%); nausea (24.8%); vomiting (11.6%); bradycardia (9.3%); fever (9.2%); pain (8%); postoperative complications (7.1%); anemia (6.1%); paresthesia (5.6%); headache, pruritus (5.1%); back pain (5%).

Urinary retention, dizziness, rigors, hypertension, tachycardia, anxiety, oliguria, hypesthesia, chest pain, hypokalemia, dyspnea, cramps, and urinary tract infection occurred with an incidence of 1% to 5%.

Ropivacaine Adverse Events (≥ 1%) in Adult Patients Receiving Regional or Local Anesthesia[1]		
Adverse reaction	Ropivacaine (n = 1661)	Bupivacaine (n =1433)
Cardiovascular		
Hypotension	32.3	28.5
Bradycardia	5.8	5.1
CNS		
Headache	5.1	4.7
Paresthesia	4.9	4
Dizziness	2.5	1.6
Anxiety	1.3	0.8
GI		
Nausea	17	14.4
Vomiting	7	6.1
GU		
Urinary retention	1.4	1.4
Breast disorder, breast feeding	1.3	0.8

Ropivacaine Adverse Events (≥ 1%) in Adult Patients Receiving Regional or Local Anesthesia[1]		
Adverse reaction	Ropivacaine (n = 1661)	Bupivacaine (n =1433)
Miscellaneous		
Back pain	4.4	5.2
Pain	4.3	5
Pruritus	3.8	2.8
Fever	3.7	2.6
Rigors (chills)	2.5	1.7
Postoperative complications	2.5	3.1
Hypesthesia	1.6	1.7
Progression of labor poor/failed	1.4	1.5
Rhinitis	1.1	0.9

[1] Surgery, labor, Cesarean section, postoperative pain management, peripheral nerve block, local infiltration.

The following adverse events were reported during the clinical program in > 1 patient (n = 3988), occurred at an overall incidence of < 1%, and were considered relevant.

Cardiovascular – Vasovagal reaction; syncope; postural hypotension; nonspecific ECG abnormalities; extrasystoles; nonspecific arrhythmias; atrial fibrillation; ST segment changes; MI; deep vein thrombosis; phlebitis; pulmonary embolism.

CNS – Tremor; Horner's syndrome; paresis; dyskinesia; neuropathy; vertigo; coma; convulsion; hypokinesia; hypotonia; ptosis; stupor; agitation; confusion; somnolence; nervousness; amnesia; hallucination; emotional lability; insomnia; nightmares.

Dermatologic – Rash; urticaria.

GI – Fecal incontinence; tenesmus; neonatal vomiting.

GU – Poor progression of labor; uterine atony; urinary incontinence; micturition disorder.

Special senses – Tinnitus; hearing abnormalities; vision abnormalities.

Respiratory – Bronchospasm; coughing.

Miscellaneous – Injection site pain; hypothermia; malaise; asthenia; accident or injury; jaundice; hypomagnesemia; myalgia.

For the indication of epidural anesthesia for surgery, the 15 most common adverse events were compared between different concentrations of **ropivacaine** and **bupivacaine**. The following table is based on data from trials in the US and other countries where ropivacaine was administered as an epidural anesthetic for surgery.

Ropivacaine Common Adverse Events (Epidural Administration) (%)					
	Ropivacaine			Bupivacaine	
Adverse reaction	5 mg/mL (n = 256)	7.5 mg/mL (n = 297)	10 mg/mL (n = 207)	5 mg/mL (n = 236)	7.5 mg/mL (n = 174)
Hypotension	38.7	49.2	54.6	38.6	51.1
Nausea	13.3	22.9	—	17.4	20.7
Bradycardia	11.3	19.5	19.3	13.6	14.4
Back pain	7	7.7	16.4	8.9	13.2
Vomiting	7	11.1	11.1	8.1	8
Headache	4.7	6.7	7.7	5.5	5.2
Fever	3.1	1.7	8.7	4.7	—
Chills	2.3	2.4	2.9	1.7	1.7
Urinary retention	2	2.7	4.8	4.2	—
Paresthesia	2	3.4	2.4	3	—
Pruritus	—	4.7	1.4	—	4

Overdosage

Acute emergencies from local anesthetics are generally related to high plasma levels encountered during therapeutic use or to unintended subarachnoid injection.

➤*Management:* The first consideration is prevention.

Convulsions – Convulsions, as well as underventilation or apnea, are caused by unintentional subarachnoid injection; maintain patent airway and assist or control ventilation with oxygen and a delivery system capable of permitting immediate positive airway pressure by mask. Evaluate circulation. If convulsions persist despite respiratory support, and if the status of the circulation permits, give small increments of an ultra short-acting barbiturate (eg, thiopental) or a benzodiazepine (eg, diazepam) IV. Circulatory depression may require administration of IV fluids and a vasopressor.

If not treated immediately, convulsions and cardiovascular depression can result in hypoxia, acidosis, bradycardia, arrhythmias, and cardiac arrest. Underventilation or apnea may produce these same signs and also lead to cardiac arrest if ventilatory support is not instituted. If cardiac arrest occurs, institute standard cardiopulmonary resuscitative measures.

Endotracheal intubation may be indicated.

The supine position is dangerous in pregnant women at term because of aortacaval compression by the gravid uterus. Therefore, during treatment of systemic toxicity, maternal hypotension or fetal bradycardia following regional block, maintain the parturient in the left lateral decubitus position if possible, or accomplish manual displacement of the uterus off the great vessels. Resuscitation of obstetrical patients may take longer than resuscitation of nonpregnant patients and closed-chest cardiac compression may be ineffective. Rapid delivery of the fetus may improve the response to resuscitation efforts.

Patient Information

When appropriate, inform patients in advance that they may experience temporary loss of sensation and motor activity, usually in the lower half of the body, following proper administration of caudal or epidural anesthesia.

Advise the patient to exert caution to avoid inadvertent trauma to the lips, tongue, cheek, mucosae, or soft palate when these structures are anesthetized. The ingestion of food should therefore be postponed until normal function returns.

Advise the patient to consult the dentist if anesthesia persists or a rash develops.

Amide Local Anesthetics

ARTICAINE HCl

Rx	Septocaine (Septodont)	Injection: 4% with 1:100,000 epinephrine	In 1.7 mL cartridges in boxes and cans of 50.[1]

[1] With 1.6 mg/mL sodium chloride and 0.5 mg/mL sodium metabisulfite.

For complete prescribing information, refer to the Injectable Local Anesthetics group monograph.

Indications

For local, infiltrative, or conductive anesthesia in simple and complex dental and periodontal procedures.

Administration and Dosage

➤*Approved by the FDA:* April 3, 2000.

Articaine HCl Recommended Dosages[1]		
Procedure	Volume (mL)	Total dose of articaine HCl (mg)
Infiltration	0.5 to 2.5	20 to 100
Nerve block	0.5 to 3.4	20 to 136
Oral surgery	1 to 5.1	40 to 204

[1] The above suggested volumes serve only as a guide. Other volumes may be used provided the total maximum recommended dose is not exceeded.

➤*Maximum recommended dosages:*

Adults – For healthy adults, the maximum dose of articaine administered by submucosal infiltration and nerve block should not exceed 7 mg/kg (0.175 mL/kg) or 3.2 mg/lb (0.0795 mL/lb) of body weight.

Children – Use in pediatric patients < 4 years of age is not recommended. Determine the quantity to be injected by the age and weight of the child and the magnitude of the operation. Do not exceed the equivalent of 7 mg/kg (0.175 mL/kg) or 3.2 mg/lb (0.0795 mL/lb) of body weight.

BUPIVACAINE HCl

Rx	Bupivacaine HCl (Abbott)	Injection: 0.25%	In 20, 30, and 50 mL amps, 10 and 30 mL vials, 50 mL multidose vials,[1] and 50 mL *Abboject*.
Rx	Marcaine (Abbott)		In 50 mL single-dose amps, 10 and 30 mL single-dose vials, 50 mL multidose vials.[1]
Rx	Sensorcaine (AstraZeneca)		In 50[1] mL multidose vials.
Rx	Sensorcaine MPF (AstraZeneca)		In 30 mL single-dose amps and 10 and 30 mL single-dose vials.
Rx	Bupivacaine HCl (Abbott)	Injection: 0.5%	In 10 and 30 mL vials, 20 and 30 mL amps, 30 mL *Abboject*, and 50 mL multidose vials.[1]
Rx	Marcaine (Abbott)		In 10 and 30 mL single-dose vials, 30 mL single-dose amps, and 50 mL multidose vials.[1]
Rx	Sensorcaine (AstraZeneca)		In 50[1] mL multidose vials.
Rx	Sensorcaine MPF (AstraZeneca)		In 10 and 30 mL single-dose vials.
Rx	Bupivacaine HCl (Abbott)	Injection: 0.75%	In 20 and 30 mL amps and 10 and 30 mL vials.
Rx	Marcaine (Abbott)		In 30 mL single-dose amps and 10 and 30 mL single-dose vials.
Rx	Sensorcaine MPF (AstraZeneca)		In 30 mL single-dose amps and 10 and 30 mL single-dose vials.
Rx	Bupivacaine HCl with Epinephrine 1:200,000 (Abbott)	Injection: 0.25% with 1:200,000 epinephrine	In 50 mL amps, 10 and 30 mL vials, and 50 mL flip-top multidose vials.[1]
Rx	Marcaine (Abbott)		In 50 mL amps[2] and 10,[2] 30,[2] and 50[1],[2] mL vials.
Rx	Sensorcaine (AstraZeneca)		In 50 mL multidose vials.[1]
Rx	Sensorcaine MPF (AstraZeneca)		In 10 and 30 mL single-dose vials.[3]
Rx	Bupivacaine HCl with Epinephrine 1:200,000 (Abbott)	Injection: 0.5% with 1:200,000 epinephrine	In 30 mL amps, 10 and 30 mL vials, and 50 mL flip-top multidose vials.[1]
Rx	Marcaine (Abbott)		In 3 and 30 mL single-dose amps[2] and 10 and 30 mL single-dose vials.[2]
Rx	Sensorcaine (AstraZeneca)		In 50 mL multidose vials.[1]
Rx	Sensorcaine MPF (AstraZeneca)		In 5 mL single-dose amps and 10 and 30 mL single-dose vials.[3]
Rx	Marcaine (Eastman-Kodak)		In 1.8 mL dental cartridges.[2]
Rx	Bupivacaine HCl with Epinephrine 1:200,000 (Abbott)	Injection: 0.75% with 1:200,000 epinephrine	In 30 mL amps.
Rx	Marcaine (Abbott)		In 30 mL amps.[2]
Rx	Sensorcaine-MPF Spinal (AstraZeneca)	Injection: 0.75% in 8.25% dextrose	In 2 mL amps.
Rx	Bupivacaine Spinal (Abbott)		Preservative-free. In 2 mL amps.

[1] With 1 mg methylparaben per mL.
[2] With 0.5 mg sodium metabisulfite and 0.1 mg EDTA per mL.
[3] With 0.5 mg sodium metabisulfite per mL.

For complete prescribing information, refer to the Injectable Local Anesthetics group monograph.

Amide Local Anesthetics

BUPIVACAINE HCl

Indications

➤*Local infiltration and sympathetic block:* 0.25% solution.

➤*Lumbar epidural:* 0.25%, 0.5%, and 0.75% solutions (0.75% nonobstetrical).

➤*Subarachnoid block:* 0.75% solution in 8.25% dextrose.

➤*Caudal block:* 0.25% and 0.5% solutions.

➤*Peripheral nerve block:* 0.25% and 0.5% solutions.

➤*Retrobulbar block:* 0.75% solution.

➤*Dental block and epidural test dose:* 0.5% solution with epinephrine.

Administration and Dosage

Avoid the rapid injection of a large volume of a local anesthetic solution and use fractional (incremental) doses. Administer the smallest dose and concentration required to produce the desired result.

The duration of anesthesia is such that for most indications, a single dose is sufficient.

➤*Maximum dosage:* Maximum dosage limit must be individualized. Most experience is with single doses up to 225 mg with epinephrine 1:200,000 and 175 mg without epinephrine. These doses may be repeated up to once every 3 hours. The duration of anesthetic effect may be prolonged by the addition of epinephrine.

➤*Epidural anesthesia:* During epidural administration of bupivacaine, administer 0.5% and 0.75% solutions in incremental doses of 3 to 5 mL with sufficient time between doses to detect toxic manifestations of unintentional intravascular or intrathecal injection. In obstetrics, use only the 0.5% and 0.25% concentrations; incremental doses of 3 to 5 mL of the 0.5% solution not exceeding 50 to 100 mg at any dosing interval are recommended. Repeat doses should be preceded by a test dose containing epinephrine if not contraindicated. Use only the single-dose amps and single-dose vials for caudal or epidural anesthesia; the multidose vials contain a preservative and, therefore, should not be used for these procedures.

➤*Test dose for caudal and lumbar epidural blocks:* The test dose of bupivacaine (0.5% with 1:200,000 epinephrine in a 3 mL amp) is recommended for use as a test dose when clinical conditions permit prior to caudal and lumbar epidural blocks. Carefully monitor pulse rate and other signs immediately following each test dose administration to detect possible intravascular injection, and allot adequate time for onset of spinal block to detect possible intrathecal injection. An intravascular or subarachnoid injection is still possible even if results of the test dose are negative. The test dose itself may produce a systemic toxic reaction, high spinal or cardiovascular effects from the epinephrine.

➤*Obstetrical use (0.75% in 8.25% dextrose only):* Doses as low as 6 mg have been used for vaginal delivery under spinal anesthesia. The dose range of 7.5 to 10.5 mg (1 to 1.4 mL) has been used for Cesarean section under spinal anesthesia. In recommended doses, bupivacaine produces complete motor and sensory block. A dose of 7.5 mg (1 mL) generally has proven satisfactory for spinal anesthesia for lower extremity and perineal procedures including transurethral resection of the prostate (TURP) and vaginal hysterectomy. A dose of 12 mg (1.6 mL) has been used for lower abdominal procedures such as abdominal hysterectomy, tubal ligation, and appendectomy. These doses are recommended as a guide for use in the average adult and may be reduced for the elderly or debilitated patients.

➤*Use in dentistry (0.5% with epinephrine only):* For infiltration and block injection in the maxillary and mandibular area when a longer duration of local anesthetic action is desired, such as for oral surgical procedures generally associated with significant postoperative pain, an average dose of 1.8 mL (9 mg) per injection site usually will suffice; an occasional second dose of 1.8 mL (9 mg) may be used if necessary to produce adequate anesthesia after making allowance for a 2- to 10-minute onset time. The total dose for all injection sites spread out over a single dental sitting usually should not exceed 90 mg for a healthy adult patient (ten 1.8 mL injections). Inject slowly and with frequent aspirations.

➤*Recommended dosages in various procedures:*

Bupivacaine Recommended Concentrations and Doses

Type of block	Concentration	Each dose (mL)	Each dose (mg)	Motor block[1]
Local infiltration	0.25%[2]	up to max.	up to max.	—
Epidural	0.75%[2,3]	10 to 20	75 to 150	complete
	0.5%[2]	10 to 20	50 to 100	moderate to complete
	0.25%[2]	10 to 20	25 to 50	partial to moderate
Caudal	0.5%[2]	15 to 30	75 to 150	moderate to complete
	0.25%[2]	15 to 30	37.5 to 75	moderate
Peripheral nerves	0.5%[2]	5 to max.	25 to max.	moderate to complete
	0.25%[2]	5 to max.	12.5 to max.	moderate to complete
Retrobulbar	0.75%[2]	2 to 4	15 to 30	complete
Sympathetic	0.25%	20 to 50	50 to 125	—
Epidural test dose	0.5% w/epinephrine	2 to 3	10 to 15 (10 to 15 mcg epinephrine)	—

[1] With continuous (intermittent) techniques, repeat doses increase the degree of motor block. The first repeat dose of 0.5% may produce complete motor block. Intercostal nerve block with 0.25% may also produce complete motor block for intra-abdominal surgery.
[2] Solutions with or without epinephrine.
[3] For single-dose use, not for intermittent epidural technique. Not for obstetrical anesthesia.

➤*Storage/Stability:* Store at controlled room temperature, 15° to 30°C (59° to 86°F).

LEVOBUPIVACAINE HCl

Rx	Chirocaine (Purdue Frederick)	Injection: 2.5 mg/mL (as base)	Preservative-free. In 10 and 30 mL single-dose vials.[1]
		5 mg/mL (as base)	Preservative-free. In 10 and 30 mL single-dose vials.[1]
		7.5 mg/mL (as base)	Preservative-free. In 10 and 30 mL single-dose vials.[1]

[1] With sodium chloride.

For complete prescribing information, refer to the Injectable Local Anesthetics group monograph.

Indications

Production of local or regional anesthesia for surgery and obstetrics and for postoperative pain management.

➤*Surgical anesthesia:* Epidural, peripheral nerve blockade, or local infiltration.

➤*Pain management:* Continuous epidural infusion or intermittent epidural neural blockade; continuous or intermittent peripheral neural blockade or local infiltration.

For continuous epidural analgesia, levobupivacaine may be administered in combination with epidural fentanyl or clonidine.

Administration and Dosage

➤*Approved by the FDA:* August 5, 1999.

Avoid the rapid injection of a large volume of a local anesthetic solution; always use fractional doses. Administer the smallest dose and concentration required to produce the desired result.

Use an adequate test dose (3 to 5 mL) of a short-acting local anesthetic solution containing epinephrine prior to induction of complete nerve block. Repeat this test dose if the patient is moved in such a fashion as to have displaced the epidural catheter. It is recommended that adequate time be allowed for the onset of anesthesia following administration of each test dose.

Levobupivacaine Dosage Recommendations

Indication	Concentration	Dose (mL)	Dose (mg)
Surgical anesthesia			
Epidural for surgery	0.5% to 0.75%	10 to 20	50 to 150
Epidural for Cesarean section	0.5%	20 to 30	100 to 150
Peripheral nerve	0.25% to 0.5%	30	75 to 150
Ophthalmic	0.75%	0.4 mL/kg 5 to 15	1 to 2 mg/kg 37.5 to 112.5
Local infiltration	0.25%	60	150
Pain management[1]			
Labor analgesia (epidural bolus)	0.25%	10 to 20	25 to 50
Postoperative pain (epidural infusion)	0.125% to 0.25%[2]	4 to 10 mL/hr	5 to 25 mg/hr

[1] In pain management, levobupivacaine can be used epidurally with fentanyl or clonidine.
[2] Make dilutions of levobupivacaine standard solutions with preservative-free 0.9% saline according to standard hospital procedures for sterility.

Epidural doses of up to 375 mg have been administered incrementally to patients during a surgical procedure.

LEVOBUPIVACAINE HCl

The maximum dose in 24 hours for intraoperative block and postoperative pain management was 695 mg.

The maximum dose administered as a postoperative epidural infusion over 24 hours was 570 mg.

The maximum dose administered to patients as a single fractionated injection was 300 mg for brachial plexus block.

LIDOCAINE HCl

Rx	**Lidocaine HCl** (Various, eg, Abbott)	**Injection:** 0.5%	In 50 mL single-dose vials and 50 mL multidose vials.[1]
			In 50 mL multidose vials.[2]
Rx	**Xylocaine** (AstraZeneca)		In 50 mL single-dose vials.
Rx	**Xylocaine MPF** (AstraZeneca)		
Rx	**Lidocaine HCl** (Various, eg, Abbott, American Regent, Elkins-Sinn)	**Injection:** 1%	In 2 and 5 mL amps, 5 mL vials,[3] 30 mL single-dose vials, 20,[1] 30,[1] and 50 mL[1] multidose vials, 5 mL syringes, and cartridges.
Rx	**Xylocaine** (AstraZeneca)		In 10, 20, and 50 mL multidose vials.[2]
Rx	**Xylocaine MPF** (AstraZeneca)		In 2, 5 and 30 mL amps, 10 and 20 mL *PolyAmp DuoFit*, and 2, 5, 10, and 30 mL single-dose vials.
Rx	**Lidocaine HCl** (Various, eg, Abbott)	**Injection:** 1.5%	In 20 mL amps.
Rx	**Xylocaine MPF** (AstraZeneca)		In 20 mL amps, 10 and 20 mL *PolyAmp DuoFit*, and 5 and 10 mL single-dose vials.
Rx	**Lidocaine HCl** (Various, eg, Abbott, American Regent, Elkins-Sinn)	**Injection:** 2%	In 2 and 10 mL amps, 5 mL vials,[3] 10 mL single-dose vials, 20[1] and 50 mL[1] multidose vials, and 5 mL syringes.
Rx	**Xylocaine** (AstraZeneca)		In 10, 20, and 50 mL multidose vials[2] and 1.8 mL cartridges.
Rx	**Xylocaine MPF** (AstraZeneca)		In 2 and 10 mL amps, 10 mL *PolyAmp DuoFit*, and 2, 5, and 10 mL single-dose vials.
Rx	**Lidocaine HCl** (Abbott)	**Injection:** 4%	In 5 mL single-dose amps.
Rx	**Xylocaine MPF** (AstraZeneca)		In 5 mL amps and 5 mL syringe with laryngotracheal cannula.
Rx	**Lidocaine and Epinephrine** (Abbott)	**Injection:** 0.5% with 1:200,000 epinephrine	In 50 mL multidose vials.[4]
Rx	**Xylocaine** (AstraZeneca)		In 50 mL multidose vials.[2]
Rx	**Lidocaine and Epinephrine** (Abbott)	**Injection:** 1% with 1:100,000 epinephrine	In 20, 30, and 50 mL multidose vials.[4]
Rx	**Xylocaine** (AstraZeneca)		In 10, 20, and 50 mL multidose vials.[2]
Rx	**Lidocaine and Epinephrine** (Abbott)	**Injection:** 1% with 1:200,000 epinephrine	In 30 mL single-dose amps.[5]
Rx	**Xylocaine MPF** (AstraZeneca)		In 30 mL amps and 5, 10, and 30 mL single-dose vials.[5]
Rx	**Lidocaine HCl** (Abbott)	**Injection:** 1.5% with 1:200,000 epinephrine	In 5 and 30 mL amps and 30 mL single-dose vials.[5]
Rx	**Lidocaine and Epinephrine** (Abbott)		In 5 and 30 mL single-dose amps and 30 mL single-dose vials.[5]
Rx	**Xylocaine MPF** (AstraZeneca)		In 5 and 30 mL amps and 5, 10, and 30 mL single-dose vials.[5]
Rx	**Octocaine** (Septodont)	**Injection:** 2% with 1:50,000 epinephrine	In 1.8 mL cartridges.[6]
Rx	**Xylocaine** (AstraZeneca)		In 1.8 mL dental cartridges.[5]
Rx	**Lidocaine HCl and Epinephrine** (Eastman Kodak)		In 1.8 mL dental cartridges.[5]
Rx	**Lidocaine and Epinephrine** (Various, eg, Abbott, Eastman Kodak)	**Injection:** 2% with 1:100,000 epinephrine	In 1.8 mL cartridges and 20, 30, and 50 mL multidose vials.[7]
Rx	**Octocaine** (Septodont)		In 1.8 mL cartridges.[6]
Rx	**Xylocaine** (AstraZeneca)		In 10,[4] 20[4] and 50 mL[4] multidose vials and 1.8 mL cartridges.[5]
Rx	**Lidocaine and Epinephrine** (Abbott)	**Injection:** 2% with 1:200,000 epinephrine	In 20 mL single-dose vials.[5]
Rx	**Xylocaine MPF** (AstraZeneca)		In 20 mL amps and 5, 10, and 20 mL single-dose vials.[5]
Rx	**Lidocaine HCl** (Abbott)	**Injection:** 1.5% with 7.5% dextrose	In 2 mL amps.
Rx	**Xylocaine** (AstraZeneca)		In 2 mL amps.
Rx	**Xylocaine-MPF** (AstraZeneca)		In 2 mL amps.
Rx	**Lidocaine HCl** (Abbott)	**Injection:** 5% with 7.5% dextrose	In 2 mL single-dose amps.
Rx	**Xylocaine MPF** (AstraZeneca)		In 2 mL amps.

[1] May contain methylparaben.
[2] With methylparaben.
[3] Preservative-free.
[4] With methylparaben and sodium metabisulfite.
[5] With sodium metabisulfite.
[6] With sodium bisulfite.
[7] May contain sodium metabisulfite and methylparaben.

For complete prescribing information, refer to the Injectable Local Anesthetics group monograph.

Indications

▶*Infiltration:*
Percutaneous – 0.5% or 1% solution.

IV regional – 0.5% solution.

▶*Peripheral nerve block:*
Brachial – 1.5% solution.

Dental – 2% solution.

Intercostal or paravertebral – 1% solution.

Pudendal or paracervical obstetrical (each side) – 1% solution.

▶*Sympathetic nerve blocks:*
Cervical (stellate ganglion) or lumbar – 1% solution.

▶*Central neural blocks:*
Epidural –
  Thoracic: 1% solution.
  Lumbar:
  • *Analgesia* – 1% solution.
  • *Anesthesia* – 1.5% or 2% solution.

▶*Caudal:*
Obstetrical analgesia – 1% solution.
Surgical anesthesia – 1.5% solution.

LIDOCAINE HCl

➤*Spinal anesthesia:* 5% solution with dextrose.

➤*Low spinal or saddle block anesthesia:* 1.5% solution with dextrose.

➤*Retrobulbar or transtracheal injection:* 4% solution.

➤*Epidural test dose:* 1.5% with 1:200,000 epinephrine.

➤*Epidural anesthesia:* 1%, 1.5%, or 2% with 1:200,000 epinephrine.

➤*Dental procedures:* 2% with 1:100,000 or 1:50,000 epinephrine.

Administration and Dosage

Avoid the rapid injection of a large volume of local anesthetic solution and use fractional (incremental) doses. Administer the smallest dose and concentration required to produce the desired result.

➤*Maximum dosage:* For normal healthy adults, the individual maximum recommended dose of lidocaine with epinephrine should not exceed 7 mg/kg (3.5 mg/lb) of body weight and, in general, it is recommended that the maximum total dose not exceed 500 mg. When used without epinephrine, the maximum individual dose should not exceed 4.5 mg/kg (2 mg/lb) of body weight, and in general, it is recommended that the maximum total dose does not exceed 300 mg. For continuous epidural or caudal anesthesia, do not administer the maximum recommended dosage at intervals of < 90 minutes. When continuous lumbar or caudal epidural anesthesia is used for nonobstetrical procedures, more drug may be administered if required to produce adequate anesthesia.

The maximum recommended dose per 90 minute period of lidocaine for paracervical block in obstetrical patients and nonobstetrical patients is 200 mg total. One half of the dose is usually administered to each side. Inject slowly 5 minutes between sides.

➤*Test dose for caudal and lumbar epidural block:* As a precaution against the adverse experiences sometimes observed following unintentional penetration of the subarachnoid space, administer a test dose such as 2 to 3 mL of 1.5% lidocaine at least 5 minutes prior to injecting the total volume required for a caudal or lumbar epidural block. Repeat the test dose if the patient is moved in a manner that may have displaced the catheter. Epinephrine, if contained in the test dose (10 to 15 mcg have been suggested) may serve as a warning of unintentional intravascular injection. If injected into a blood vessel, this amount of epinephrine is likely to produce a transient "epinephrine response" within 45 seconds, consisting of an increase in heart rate and systolic blood pressure, circumoral pallor, palpitations, and nervousness in the unsedated patient. Avoid the rapid injection of a large volume of lidocaine injection through the catheter, and when feasible, administer fractional doses.

➤*Epidural anesthesia:* The dosage varies with the number of dermatomes to be anesthetized (generally, 2 to 3 mL of the indicated concentration per dermatome).

➤*Surgical anesthesia:* The dosage recommended for abdominal anesthesia is 1.5 to 2 mL (75 to 100 mg).

➤*Low spinal or saddle block anesthesia:* The dosage recommended for normal vaginal delivery is ≈ 1 mL (50 mg). For Cesarean section and those deliveries requiring intrauterine manipulation, 1.5 mL (75 mg) is usually adequate.

➤*Retrobulbar injection:* The suggested dose for a 70 kg person is 3 to 5 mL (120 to 200 mg), ie, 1.7 to 3 mg/kg or 0.9 to 1.5 mg/lb of body weight. A portion of this is injected retrobulbarly and the rest may be used to block the facial nerve.

➤*Transtracheal injection:* For local anesthesia by the transtracheal route, inject 2 to 3 mL through a large enough needle so that the injection can be made rapidly. By injecting during inspiration, some of the drug will be carried into the bronchi and the resulting cough will distribute the rest of the drug over the vocal cords and the epiglottis.

Occasionally, it may be necessary to spray the pharynx by oropharyngeal spray to achieve complete analgesia. For the combination of the injection and spray, it should rarely be necessary to use > 5 mL (200 mg), ie, 3 mg/kg or 1.5 mg/lb of body weight.

➤*Dental procedures:* In oral infiltration and mandibular block, initial dosages of 1 to 5 mL (½ to 2½ cartridges) of lidocaine 2% with epinephrine 1:50,000 or 1:100,000 usually are effective. In children < 10 years of age, it is rarely necessary to administer > ½ cartridge (0.9 to 1 mL or 18 to 20 mg) per procedure.

➤*Recommended dosages in various procedures:*

Recommended Dosages of Lidocaine Injection for Various Anesthetic Procedures in Healthy Adults			
	Lidocaine injection (without epinephrine)		
Procedure	Concentration (%)	Volume (mL)	Total dose (mg)
Infiltration			
Percutaneous	0.5 or 1	1 to 60	5 to 300
IV regional	0.5	10 to 60	50 to 300
Peripheral nerve blocks			
Brachial	1.5	15 to 20	225 to 300
Dental	2	1 to 5	20 to 100
Intercostal	1	3	30
Paravertebral	1	3 to 5	30 to 50
Pudendal (each side)	1	10	100
Paracervical obstetrical analgesia (each side)	1	10	100
Sympathetic nerve blocks			
Cervical (stellate ganglion)	1	5	50
Lumbar	1	5 to 10	50 to 100
Central neural blocks			
Epidural[1]			
Thoracic	1	20 to 30	200 to 300
Lumbar			
Analgesia	1	25 to 30	250 to 300
Anesthesia	1.5	15 to 20	225 to 300
	2	10 to 15	200 to 300
Caudal			
Obstetrical analgesia	1	20 to 30	200 to 300
Surgical anesthesia	1.5	15 to 20	225 to 300

[1] Dose determined by number of dermatomes to be anesthetized (2 to 3 mL/dermatome).

➤*Storage/Stability:* Store at 15° to 30°C (59° to 86°F).

MEPIVACAINE HCl

Rx	**Carbocaine** (Abbott)	**Injection:** 1%	In 30 mL single-dose vials and 50 mL[1] multidose vials.
Rx	**Polocaine** (AstraZeneca)		In 50 mL multidose vials.[1]
Rx	**Polocaine MPF** (AstraZeneca)		In 30 mL single-dose vials.[1]
Rx	**Carbocaine** (Abbott)	**Injection:** 1.5%	In 30 mL single-dose vials.
Rx	**Polocaine MPF** (AstraZeneca)		In 30 mL single-dose vials.
Rx	**Carbocaine** (Abbott)	**Injection:** 2%	In 20 mL single-dose vials and 50 mL[1] multidose vials.
Rx	**Polocaine** (AstraZeneca)		In 50 mL multidose vials.[1]
Rx	**Polocaine MPF** (AstraZeneca)		In 20 mL single-dose vials.
Rx	**Mepivacaine HCl** (Septodont)	**Injection:** 3%	In 1.8 mL dental cartridge.
Rx	**Carbocaine** (Eastman-Kodak)		In 1.8 mL dental cartridge.[2]
Rx	**Polocaine** (AstraZeneca)		In 1.8 mL dental cartridge.[3]
Rx	**Carbocaine with Neo-Cobefrin** (Eastman-Kodak)	**Injection:** 2% with 1:20,000 levonordefrin	In 1.8 mL dental cartridge.[2]
Rx	**Mepivacaine HCl and Levonordefrin** (Septodont)		In 1.8 mL dental cartridge.[3]
Rx	**Polocaine with Levonordefrin** (AstraZeneca)		In 1.8 mL dental cartridge.[4]

[1] With methylparaben.
[2] With acetone sodium bisulfite.

[3] With sodium bisulfite.
[4] With sodium metabisulfite.

For complete prescribing information, refer to the Injectable Local Anesthetics group monograph.

Indications

➤*Peripheral nerve block (eg, cervical, brachial, intercostal, pudendal):* 1% or 2% solution.

➤*Transvaginal block (paracervical plus pudendal):* 1% solution.

➤*Paracervical block in obstetrics:* 1% solution.

➤*Caudal and epidural block:* 1%, 1.5%, or 2% solution.

➤*Infiltration:* 0.5% (via dilution) or 1% solution

➤*Therapeutic block (pain management):* 1% or 2% solution.

➤*Dental procedures (infiltration or nerve block):* 3% solution or 2% solution with levonordefrin.

Amide Local Anesthetics

MEPIVACAINE HCl

Administration and Dosage

Avoid the rapid injection of a large volume of a local anesthetic solution and use fractional (incremental) doses. Administer the smallest dose and concentration required to produce the desired result.

➤*Maximum dosage:* The recommended single adult dose (or the total of a series of doses given in 1 procedure) for unsedated, healthy, normal-sized individuals should not usually exceed 400 mg. The total dose for any 24-hour period should not exceed 1000 mg. Carefully measure the pediatric dose as a percentage of the total adult dose, based on weight, and do not exceed 5 to 6 mg/kg (2.5 to 3 mg/lb) in pediatric patients, especially those weighing < 30 lb. In pediatric patients < 3 years of age or weighing < 30 lb, use concentrations < 2% (eg, 0.5% to 1.5%).

➤*Dental procedures (infiltration or nerve block):* In the upper or lower jaw, the average dose of 1 cartridge usually will suffice. Five cartridges (180 mg of the 2% solution or 270 mg of the 3% solution) usually are adequate to effect anesthesia of the entire oral cavity.

➤*Recommended dosages in various procedures:*

Mepivacaine HCl Recommended Concentrations and Doses				
Procedure	Conc. (%)	Total dose mL	Total dose mg	Comments
Cervical, brachial, intercostal, pudendal nerve block	1	5 to 40	50 to 400	Pudendal block: one half of total dose injected each side.
	2	5 to 20	100 to 400	
Transvaginal block (paracervical plus pudendal)	1	up to 30 (both sides)	up to 300 (both sides)	One-half of total dose injected each side.

Mepivacaine HCl Recommended Concentrations and Doses				
Procedure	Conc. (%)	Total dose mL	Total dose mg	Comments
Paracervical block	1	up to 20 (both sides)	up to 200 (both sides)	One half of total dose injected each side. This is maximum recommended dose per 90-minute period in obstetrical and nonobstetrical patients. Inject slowly, 5 minutes between sides.
Caudal and epidural block	1	15 to 30	150 to 300	Use only single-dose vials that do not contain a preservative.
	1.5	10 to 25	150 to 375	
	2	10 to 20	200 to 400	
Infiltration	1	up to 40	up to 400	An equivalent amount of a 0.5% solution (prepared by diluting the 1% solution with Sodium Chloride Injection) may be used for large areas.
Therapeutic block (pain management)	1	1 to 5	10 to 50	—
	2	1 to 5	20 to 100	

➤*Storage/Stability:* Store at 15° to 30°C (59° to 86°F).

PRILOCAINE HCl

Rx	Citanest Plain (AstraZeneca)	Injection: 4%	In 1.8 mL cartridge.
Rx	Citanest Forte (AstraZeneca)	Injection: 4% with 1:200,000 epinephrine	In 1.8 mL cartridge.[1]

[1] With sodium metabisulfite.

For complete prescribing information, refer to the Injectable Local Anesthetics group monograph.

Indications

➤*For local anesthesia by nerve block or infiltration in dental procedures:* 4% solution.

Administration and Dosage

Administer the least volume of injection required.

➤*Maximum dosage:* In patients weighing < 150 lbs (70 kg), administer no more than 4 mg/lb (8 mg/kg). In patients weighing ≥ 150 lbs, administer no more than 600 mg (8 cartridges) as a single injection. In children < 10 years of age, it is rarely necessary to administer more than one-half cartridge (40 mg).

➤*Inferior alveolar block:* There are no practical clinical differences between prilocaine with and without epinephrine when used for inferior alveolar blocks.

➤*Maxillary infiltration:* Prilocaine without epinephrine is recommended for use in maxillary infiltration anesthesia for procedures in which the painful aspects can be completed within 15 minutes after the injection. For long procedures, or those involving maxillary posterior teeth where soft tissue numbness is not troublesome to the patient, prilocaine with epinephrine is recommended.

For most routine procedures, initial dosages of 1 to 2 mL of prilocaine with or without epinephrine usually will provide adequate infiltration or major nerve block anesthesia.

➤*Storage/Stability:* Store at ≈ 25°C (77°F).

ROPIVACAINE HCl

Rx	Naropin (AstraZeneca)	Injection: 0.2%	Preservative-free. In 10 and 20 mL *PolyAmp DuoFit*, 20 mL single-dose vials, and 100 and 200 mL single-dose infusion bottles.
		0.5%	Preservative-free. In 10 and 20 mL *PolyAmp DuoFit* and 30 mL single-dose vials.
		0.75%	Preservative-free. In 10 and 20 mL *PolyAmp DuoFit*.
		1%	Preservative free. In 10 and 20 mL *PolyAmp DuoFit* and 10 and 20 mL single-dose vials.

For complete prescribing information, refer to the Injectable Local Anesthetics group monograph.

Indications

For the production of local or regional anesthesia for surgery, postoperative pain management, and obstetrical procedures.

Administration and Dosage

➤*Approved by the FDA:* September 24, 1996.

Avoid the rapid administration of a large volume of local anesthetic solution and use fractional (incremental) doses. Administer the smallest dose and concentration required to produce the desired result.

Use an adequate test dose (3 to 5 mL of a short-acting local anesthetic containing epinephrine) prior to induction of complete block. Repeat this test dose if patient movement potentiates epidural catheter displacement. Ropivacaine epidural infusions can be used for up to 24 hours.

Ropivacaine Dosage Recommendations					
Procedures	Concentration (mg/mL)	Volume (mL)	Dose (mg)	Onset (min)	Duration (hours)
Surgical anesthesia					
Lumbar epidural administration	5 (0.5%)	15 to 30	75 to 150	15 to 30	2 to 4
Surgery	7.5 (0.75%)	15 to 25	113 to 188	10 to 20	3 to 5
	10 (1%)	15 to 20	150 to 200	10 to 20	4 to 6
Lumbar epidural administration	5 (0.5%)	20 to 30	100 to 150	15 to 25	2 to 4
Cesarean section	7.5 (0.75%)	15 to 20	113 to 150	10 to 20	3 to 5
Thoracic epidural administration	5 (0.5%)	5 to 15	25 to 75	10 to 20	na
Surgery	7.5 (0.75%)	5 to 15	38 to 113	10 to 20	na
Major nerve block	5 (0.5%)	35 to 50	175 to 250	15 to 30	5 to 8
(eg, brachial plexus block)	7.5 (0.75%)	10 to 40	75 to 300	10 to 25	6 to 10
Field block (eg, minor nerve blocks and infiltration)	5 (0.5%)	1 to 40	5 to 200	1 to 15	2 to 6

Amide Local Anesthetics

ROPIVACAINE HCl

Ropivacaine Dosage Recommendations

Procedures	Concentration (mg/mL)	Volume (mL)	Dose (mg)	Onset (min)	Duration (hours)
Labor pain management					
Lumbar epidural administration					
Initial dose	2 (0.2%)	10 to 20	20 to 40	10 to 15	0.5 to 1.5
Continuous infusion[1]	2 (0.2%)	6 to 14 mL/hr	12 to 28 mg/hr	na	na
Incremental injections (top-up)[1]	2 (0.2%)	10 to 15 mL/hr	20 to 30 mg/hr	na	na
Postoperative pain management					
Lumbar epidural administration					
Continuous infusion[2]	2 (0.2%)	6 to 14 mL/hr	12 to 28 mg/hr	na	na
Thoracic epidural administration					
Continuous infusion[2]	2 (0.2%)	6 to 14 mL/hr	12 to 28 mg/hr	na	na
Infiltration	2 (0.2%)	1 to 100	2 to 200	1 to 5	2 to 6
(eg, minor nerve block)	5 (0.5%)	1 to 40	5 to 200	1 to 5	2 to 6

[1] Median dose of 21 mg/hour was administered by continuous infusion or incremental injections (top-ups) over a median delivery time of 5.5 hours.
[2] Cumulative doses up to 770 mg of ropivacaine over 24 hours (intraoperative block plus postoperative infusion): Continuous epidural infusion at rates up to 28 mg/hr for 72 hours have been well tolerated in adults, ie, 2016 mg plus surgical dose of ≈ 100 to 150 mg as top-up.

➤*Storage/Stability:* Store at controlled room temperature, 20° to 25°C (68° to 77°F).

Ester Local Anesthetics

CHLOROPROCAINE HCl

Rx	**Nesacaine** (AstraZeneca)	Injection: 1%	In 30 mL multidose vials.[1]
Rx	**Chloroprocaine HCl** (Bedford)	Injection: 2%	In 20 mL single-dose vials.[2]
Rx	**Nesacaine** (AstraZeneca)		In 30 mL multidose vials.[1]
Rx	**Nesacaine-MPF** (AstraZeneca)		In 20 mL single-dose vials.[2]
Rx	**Chloroprocaine HCl** (Bedford)	Injection: 3%	In 20 mL single-dose vials.[2]
Rx	**Nesacaine-MPF** (AstraZeneca)		In 20 mL single-dose vials.[2]

[1] With methylparaben and EDTA.
[2] Preservative-free.

For complete prescribing information, refer to the Injectable Local Anesthetics group monograph.

Indications

➤*Infiltration and peripheral nerve block:* 1% to 2% solution. 1% and 2% solutions with preservatives are not to be used for lumbar or caudal epidural administration.

Mandibular – 2% solution.

Infraorbital – 2% solution.

Brachial plexus – 2% solution.

Digital (without epinephrine) – 1% solution.

Pudendal block – 2% solution.

Paracervical block – 1% solution.

➤*Infiltration, peripheral and central nerve block, including lumbar and caudal epidural block:* 2% or 3% solution (without preservatives).

Administration and Dosage

Chloroprocaine may be administered as a single injection or continuously through an indwelling catheter.

Avoid the rapid injection of a large volume of a local anesthetic solution and use fractional (incremental) doses. Administer the smallest dose and concentration required to produce the desired result.

➤*Maximum dosage:* The maximum single recommended doses of chloroprocaine in adults are: Without epinephrine, 11 mg/kg, not to exceed a maximum total dose of 800 mg; with epinephrine (1:200,000), 14 mg/kg, not to exceed a maximum total dose of 1000 mg.

➤*Test dose for caudal and lumbar epidural block:* In order to guard against adverse experiences sometimes noted following unintended penetration of the subarachnoid space, the following procedure modification is recommended: Use an adequate test dose (3 mL of chloroprocaine 3% injection or 5 mL of chloroprocaine 2% injection) prior to induction of complete block. This test dose should be repeated if the patient is moved in such a fashion as to have displaced the epidural catheter. Allow adequate time for onset of anesthesia following administration of each test dose.

➤*Caudal and lumbar epidural block:* For caudal anesthesia, the initial dose is 15 to 25 mL of a 2% or 3% solution. Repeated doses may be given at 40- to 60-minute intervals.

For lumbar epidural anesthesia, 2 to 2.5 mL per segment of a 2% or 3% solution can be used. The usual total volume of chloroprocaine injection is from 15 to 25 mL. Repeated doses 2 to 6 mL less than the original dose may be given at 40- to 50-minute intervals.

➤*Infiltration and peripheral nerve block:*

Suggested Chloroprocaine Doses for Infiltration and Peripheral Nerve Block

Anesthetic procedure	Concentration (%)	Volume (mL)	Total dose (mg)
Mandibular	2	2 to 3	40 to 60
Infraorbital	2	0.5 to 1	10 to 20
Brachial plexus	2	30 to 40	600 to 800
Digital (without epinephrine)	1	3 to 4	30 to 40
Pudendal	2	10 each side	400
Paracervical	1	3 per each of 4 sites	up to 120

➤*Pediatric dosage:* The maximum dose is determined by the child's age and weight and should not exceed 11 mg/kg (5 mg/lb). Concentrations of 0.5% to 1% are suggested for infiltration and 1% to 1.5% for nerve block. Some of the lower concentrations for use in infants and smaller children are not available in prepackaged containers; it will be necessary to dilute available concentrations with the amount of 0.9% sodium chloride injection necessary to obtain the required final concentration.

➤*Preparation of epinephrine injections:* To prepare a 1:200,000 epinephrine-chloroprocaine injection, add 0.1 mL of a 1:1000 epinephrine injection to 20 mL of chloroprocaine injection.

➤*Storage/Stability:* Keep from freezing. Protect from light. Store at controlled room temperature, 15° to 30°C (59° to 86°F).

Ester Local Anesthetics

PROCAINE HCl

Rx	Procaine HCl (Various, eg, Abbott)	Injection: 1%	In 30 mL multidose vials.[1]
Rx	Novocain (Abbott)		In 2 mL *Uni-Amps*, 6 mL single-dose amps,[2] and 30 mL multidose vials.[3]
Rx	Procaine HCl (Various, eg, Abbott, IDE)	Injection: 2%	In 30 mL multidose vials.[1]
Rx	Novocain (Abbott)		In 30 mL multidose vials.[3]
Rx	Novocain (Abbott)	Injection: 10%	In 2 mL *Uni-Amps*.[2]

[1] May contain sodium metabisulfite.
[2] With acetone sodium bisulfite.
[3] With acetone sodium bisulfite and chlorobutanol.

For complete prescribing information, refer to the Injectable Local Anesthetics group monograph.

Indications

➤*Infiltration anesthesia:* 0.25% to 0.5% (via dilution) solution.

➤*Peripheral nerve block:* 0.5% (via dilution), 1% and 2% solution.

➤*Spinal anesthesia:* 10% solution.

Administration and Dosage

Avoid the rapid injection of a large volume of a local anesthetic solution and use fractional (incremental) doses. Administer the smallest dose and concentration required to produce the desired result.

➤*Maximum dosage:* The usual total dose during 1 treatment should not exceed 1000 mg. In pediatric patients, 15 mg/kg of a 0.5% solution for local infiltration is the maximum recommended dose.

➤*Dilution instructions:* To prepare 60 mL of a 0.5% solution (5 mg/mL), dilute 30 mL of the 1% solution with 30 mL 0.9% sodium chloride injection. To prepare 60 mL of a 0.25% solution (2.5 mg/mL), dilute 15 mL of the 1% solution with 45 mL 0.9% sodium chloride injection. Add 0.5 to 1 mL of epinephrine 1:1000 per 100 mL anesthetic solution for vasoconstrictive effect (1:200,000 to 1:100,000).

➤*Infiltration anesthesia:* For infiltration anesthesia, 350 to 600 mg of a 0.25% to 0.5% solution generally is considered to be a single safe total dose.

➤*Peripheral nerve block:* For peripheral nerve block, 0.5% solution (up to 200 mL), 1% solution (up to 100 mL), or 2% solution (up to 50 mL). The use of the 2% solution usually should be limited to cases requiring a small volume of anesthetic solution (10 to 25 mL). An anesthetic solution of 0.5 to 1 mL of epinephrine 1:1000 per 100 mL may be added for vasoconstrictive effect (1:200,000 or 1:100,000).

➤*Spinal anesthesia:*

Recommended Procaine Dosage for Spinal Anesthesia				
	Procaine 10% solution			
Extent of anesthesia	Volume of 10% solution (mL)	Volume of diluent (mL)	Total dose (mg)	Site of injection (lumbar interspace)
Perineum	0.5	0.5	50	4th
Perineum and lower extremities	1	1	100	3rd or 4th
Up to costal margin	2	1	200	2nd, 3rd, or 4th

The diluent may be sterile normal saline, sterile distilled water, spinal fluid, and for hyperbaric technique, sterile dextrose solution.

The usual rate of injection is 1 mL/5 seconds. Full anesthesia and fixation usually occur in 5 minutes.

➤*Storage/Stability:* Store at controlled room temperature, 15° to 30°C (59° to 86°F).

TETRACAINE HCl

Rx	Pontocaine HCl (Abbott)	Injection: 1%	In 2 mL amps.[1]
		0.2% in 6% dextrose	In 2 mL amps.
		0.3% in 6% dextrose	In 5 mL amps.
		Powder for reconstitution: 20 mg	In *Niphanoid* (instantly soluble) amps.

[1] With acetone sodium bisulfite.

For complete prescribing information, refer to the Injectable Local Anesthetics group monograph.

Indications

➤*Spinal anesthesia (saddle block):* 0.2% solution in dextrose.

➤*Spinal anesthesia (high, median, and low):* 0.3% solution in dextrose.

➤*Spinal anesthesia, prolonged (2 to 3 hours):* 1% solution.

Administration and Dosage

Administer the lowest dosage needed to provide effective anesthesia.

➤*Reconstitution:* If the *Niphanoid* is preferred, it is first dissolved in 10% dextrose solution in a ratio of 1 mL dextrose to 10 mg of the anesthetic. Further dilution is made with an equal volume of spinal fluid. The resulting solution now contains 5% dextrose with 5 mg of anesthetic agent/mL.

➤*Spinal anesthesia (high, median, low, and saddle block):*

Suggested Tetracaine Dosage for Spinal Anesthesia (High, Median, Low, and Saddle Block)			
Extent of anesthesia	Dose of tetracaine (mg)	Volume of solution (mL)	Site of injection (lumbar interspace)
Saddle block for obstetrics	2 to 4	1 to 2 of 0.2%	4th
Low spinal for perineal operations	3 to 6	1 to 2 of 0.3%	4th
Median spinal for operations on lower abdomen	9 to 12	3 to 4 of 0.3%	3rd or 4th

Suggested Tetracaine Dosage for Spinal Anesthesia (High, Median, Low, and Saddle Block)			
Extent of anesthesia	Dose of tetracaine (mg)	Volume of solution (mL)	Site of injection (lumbar interspace)
High spinal for operations on upper abdomen	15[1]	5 of 0.3%	2nd, 3rd, or 4th

[1] Doses exceeding 15 mg are rarely required and should be used only in exceptional cases.

➤*Spinal anesthesia (prolonged):*

Suggested Tetracaine Doses for Prolonged Spinal Anesthesia					
	Using *Niphanoid*		Using 1% solution		
Extent of anesthesia	Dose of *Niphanoid* (mg)	Volume of spinal fluid (mL)	Dose of solution (mL)	Volume of spinal fluid (mL)	Site of injection (lumbar interspace)
Perineum	5[1]	1	0.5 (= 5 mg)[1]	0.5	4th
Perineum and lower extremities	10	2	1 (= 10 mg)	1	3rd or 4th
Up to costal margin	15 to 20[2]	3	1.5 to 2 (= 15 to 20 mg)[2]	1.5 to 2	2nd, 3rd, or 4th

[1] For vaginal delivery (saddle block), from 2 to 5 mg in dextrose.
[2] Doses exceeding 15 mg are rarely required and should be used only in exceptional cases. Inject solution at rate of ≈ 1 mL/5 seconds.

➤*Storage/Stability:* Store under refrigeration, 2° to 8°C (36° to 46°F).

COMBINATION LOCAL ANESTHETICS

Rx	Duocaine (Amphastar)	Injection: 10 mg/mL lidocaine HCl/ 3.75 mg/mL bupivacaine HCl	Preservative-free. In 10 mL single-dose vials. In cartons of 25.

For complete prescribing information, refer to the Injectable Local Anesthetics group monograph.

Indications

➤*Surgical anesthesia:* For the production of local or regional anesthesia for ophthalmologic surgery by peripheral nerve block techniques such as parabulbar, retrobulbar, and facial blocks. May be used with or without epinephrine and/or hyaluronidase.

Administration and Dosage

➤*Approved by the FDA:* May 23, 2003.

➤*Peribulbar nerve block:* 6 to 12 mL lidocaine/bupivacaine solution (60 to 120 mg lidocaine and 22 to 45 mg bupivacaine). This technique produces akinesia of the superior oblique muscles, the eyelids, and the orbicularis oculi muscle.

➤*Retrobulbar and facial nerve block:* 2 to 5 mL lidocaine/bupivacaine solution (20 to 50 mg lidocaine and 7 to 18 mg bupivacaine). A portion of the dose is injected retrobulbarly, and the remainder may be used to block the facial nerve.

➤*Maximum dosage:* Individualize maximum dosage limit in each case after evaluating the size and physical status of the patient, as well as the usual rate of systemic absorption from a particular injection site.

For healthy adults, the individual maximum recommended dose of lidocaine/bupivacaine without epinephrine should not exceed 0.18 mL/kg (0.08 mL/lb) of body weight, and, in general, it is recommended that the maximum total dose not exceed 12 mL (120 mg lidocaine and 45 mg bupivacaine). When used with epinephrine, the maximum individual dose should not exceed 0.28 mL/kg (0.14 mL/lb) of body weight, and, in general, it is recommended that the maximum total dose not exceed 20 mL (200 mg lidocaine and 75 mg bupivacaine).

➤*Storage/Stability:* Store at 15° to 25°C (59° to 77°F). Discard unused portion after initial use.

Anticonvulsant drugs include a variety of agents, all possessing the ability to depress abnormal neuronal discharges in the CNS, thus inhibiting seizure activity. Because of differences in pharmacology, therapeutic use, and adverse reaction potential, these agents are discussed in groups as follows:

- Barbiturates
- Hydantoins
- Succinimides
- Oxazolidinediones
- Benzodiazepines
- Adjuvants to anticonvulsants

➤*Warnings:*

Pregnancy – Reports suggest an association between use of anticonvulsant drugs by women with epilepsy and an elevated incidence of birth defects in children born to these women. Data are more extensive with respect to phenytoin and phenobarbital; other reports indicate a possible similar association with other anticonvulsants. Other factors (eg, genetics or the seizure disorder per se) may also contribute to the higher incidence of birth defects. The great majority of mothers receiving anticonvulsant medication deliver healthy infants.

Do not discontinue anticonvulsant drugs in patients in whom the drug is administered to prevent major seizures because of the strong possibility of precipitating status epilepticus with attendant hypoxia and risk to both the mother and the unborn child. Consider discontinuation of anticonvulsants prior to and during pregnancy when the nature, frequency, and severity of the seizures do not pose a serious threat to the patient. It is not known whether even minor seizures constitute some risk to the developing embryo or fetus.

An increase in seizure frequency during pregnancy occurs in a high proportion of patients because of altered phenytoin absorption or metabolism. Periodic measurement of serum phenytoin levels is particularly valuable in the management of pregnant epileptic patients as a guide to an appropriate adjustment of dosage. However, postpartum restoration of the original dosage will probably be indicated.

Reports suggest that maternal ingestion of anticonvulsant drugs, particularly barbiturates and hydantoins, is associated with a neonatal coagulation defect that may cause bleeding during the early (usually within 24 hours of birth) neonatal period. The defect is characterized by decreased levels of vitamin K-dependent clotting factors, and prolongation of either the prothrombin time or the partial thromboplastin time, or both. It has been suggested that prophylactic vitamin K be given to the mother 1 month prior to and during delivery, and to the infant immediately after birth.

In addition to the reports of increased incidence of congenital malformations, such as cleft lip/palate and heart malformations in children of women receiving phenytoin and other antiepileptic drugs, there have been more recent reports of a fetal hydantoin syndrome. This consists of prenatal growth deficiency, microcephaly, and mental deficiency in children born to mothers who have received phenytoin, barbiturates, alcohol, or trimethadione. However, these features are all interrelated and are frequently associated with intrauterine growth retardation from other causes.

There have been isolated reports of malignancies, including neuroblastoma, in children whose mothers received phenytoin during pregnancy.

Seizures – Seizures may be classified based on their clinical form. The following is based on the International Classification of Epileptic Seizures:[†]

1.) Partial seizures (generally involve 1 hemisphere of the brain at onset)
    a.) Simple (consciousness not impaired)
    b.) With motor symptoms (Jacksonian, adversive)
    c.) With somatosensory or other special sensory symptoms
    d.) With autonomic symptoms
    e.) With psychic symptoms
    f.) Complex (consciousness impaired)
    g.) Simple partial onset followed by impaired consciousness
    h.) Impaired consciousness at onset
    i.) Secondarily generalized
    j.) Simple partial seizures evolving to generalized tonic-clonic seizures
    k.) Complex partial seizures evolving to generalized tonic-clonic seizures
    l.) Simple partial seizures evolving to complex partial seizures, then to generalized tonic-clonic seizures.
2.) Generalized seizures (involve both hemispheres of the brain at onset, consciousness usually impaired)
    a.) Absence
    b.) Typical
    c.) Atypical
    d.) Myoclonic
    e.) Clonic
    f.) Tonic
    g.) Tonic-clonic
    h.) Atonic
3.) Localization-related (focal)
    a.) Idiopathic
    b.) Benign focal epilepsy of childhood
    c.) Symptomatic
    d.) Chronic progressive epilepsia partialis continua
    e.) Temporal-lobe
    f.) Extratemporal
4.) Generalized epilepsy
    a.) Idiopathic
    b.) Benign neonatal convulsions
    c.) Childhood absence
    d.) Juvenile myoclonic
    e.) Other
    f.) Cryptogenic or symptomatic
    g.) West syndrome (infantile spasms)
    h.) Early myoclonic encephalopathy
    i.) Lennox-Gastaut syndrome
    j.) Progressive myoclonic epilepsy
5.) Special syndromes
    a.) Febrile seizures
6.) Unclassified

Withdrawal of anticonvulsants – A long-term prospective study suggests that epileptic adults may remain seizure-free if their anticonvulsant is withdrawn following at least 2 years of a single therapy regimen. Approximately one-third of patients relapsed following withdrawal of the anticonvulsants.

Predictors of relapse include the following: Seizure type (highest relapse rates occurred with complex partial seizures with secondary generalization and generalized seizures).

Number of seizures (higher risk with > 100 seizures before control).

Number of drugs (highest rate with patients taking 2 or 3 drugs).

Treatment duration (longer duration of drug treatment resulted in higher relapse rate).

EEG classification (lower relapse rate with less severe EEG abnormalities).

Type of drug (higher relapse rate following withdrawal of valproic acid).

	**Anticonvulsants: Indications and Pharmacokinetics**
	Drug	Labeled indications	Protein binding (%)	Metabolism/ Excretion	t½ (hrs)	Therapeutic serum levels (mcg/mL)
Barbiturates	Phenobarbital[1] (PB)	Status epilepticus Cortical focal Tonic-clonic	40-60	Liver; 25% eliminated unchanged in urine	53-140	20-40
Hydantoins	Ethotoin	Tonic-clonic Psychomotor	nd	Liver; renal excretion of metabolites	3-9[3]	15-50
Hydantoins	Mephenytoin	Tonic-clonic Psychomotor Focal Jacksonian	nd	Liver	95 (active metabolite)	nd
Hydantoins	Phenytoin	Tonic-clonic Psychomotor Status epilepticus	≈ 90	Liver; renal excretion. < 5% excreted unchanged	Dose-dependent[2]	10-20

† Commission on Classification and Terminology of the International League Against Epilepsy. *Epilepsia.* 1981;22:489-501 and 1989;30:389-99.

Anticonvulsants: Indications and Pharmacokinetics

	Drug	Labeled indications	Protein binding (%)	Metabolism/ Excretion	t½ (hrs)	Therapeutic serum levels (mcg/mL)
Succinimides	Ethosuximide	Absence	0	Liver; 25% excreted unchanged in urine	30 (children 7-9 yrs) 40-60 (adults)	40-100
Succinimides	Methsuximide	Absence	nd	Liver; < 1% excreted unchanged in urine	< 2 (40, active metabolite)	nd
Succinimides	Phensuximide	Absence	nd	Urine, bile	8 (active metabolite)	nd
Oxazolidinediones	Trimethadione	Absence	0	Demethylated to dimethadione; 3% excreted unchanged	6-13 days (dimetha-dione)	≥ 700 (dimethadione)
Benzodiazepines	Clonazepam	Absence Myoclonic Akinetic	50-85	5 metabolites identi-fied; urine is major excre-tion route	18-60	20-80 ng/ml
Benzodiazepines	Clorazepate	Partial[4]	97	Hydrolyzed in stom-ach to desmethyldiaz-epam (active); metabolized in liver, renally excreted	30-100	nd
Benzodiazepines	Diazepam	Status epilepticus[4] Convulsive disor-ders, all forms[4]	97-99	Liver, active metabo-lites	20-50	nd
Adjuncts to anticonvulsants	Lamotrigine	Partial (adults)	≈ 55	Glucuronic acid con-jugation to inactive metabolites; 94% excreted in urine, 2% in feces.	≈ 33[5]	nd
Adjuncts to anticonvulsants	Carbamazepine	Tonic-clonic Mixed Psychomotor	≈ 75	Liver to active 10, 11–epoxide. 72% excreted in urine, 28% in feces	18-54 (initial) 10-20[5] ≈ 6 (10, 11- epoxide)	4-12
Adjuncts to anticonvulsants	Felbamate[6]	Partial (adults) Partial/general-ized assoc. with Lennox-Gastaut syndrome (chil-dren)	22-25	40% to 50% unchanged in urine, 40% as uniden-tified metabolites and conjugates	20-23	nd[7]
Adjuncts to anticonvulsants	Gabapentin	Partial (adults) with and without secondary gener-alization	< 3	Not appreciably metabo-lized; excreted in urine unchanged	5-7	nd
Adjuncts to anticonvulsants	Primidone	Tonic-clonic Psychomotor Focal	20-25	Metabolized to PB and PEMA, both active	5-15 (primidone) 10-18 (PEMA) 53-140 (PB)	5-12 (primidone) 15-40 (PB)
Adjuncts to anticonvulsants	Valproic acid	Absence	80-94	Liver; excreted in urine	5-20	50-150

[1] Other barbiturates are also used as anticonvulsants. See Sedatives/Hypnotics section.
[2] Exhibits dose-dependent, nonlinear pharmacokinetics.
[3] Below 8 mcg/ml; > 8 mcg/ml, t½ not defined due to dose-dependent, nonlinear phar-macokinetics.
[4] Recommended for adjunctive use.
[5] Following multiple administrations (150 mg twice daily) to normal volunteers taking no other medications, lamotrigine induced its own metabolism, resulting in a 25% decrease in half-life compared to values obtained in the same volunteers following a single dose. Evidence gathered from other sources suggests that self-induction may not occur when lamotrigine is given as adjunctive therapy in patients receiving enzyme-inducing antiepileptic drugs (EIAEDs).
[6] Because of cases of aplastic anemia, it has been recommended that the use of this drug be discontinued unless, in the judgment of the physician, continued therapy is war-ranted. Refer to the specific monograph.
[7] Value of monitoring blood levels not established.

Hydantoins

Refer to the general discussion beginning in the Anticonvulsants intro-duction.

Indications

Control of grand mal and psychomotor seizures.

▶*Phenytoin:* To prevent and treat seizures occurring during or follow-ing neurosurgery.

Parenteral – For the control of status epilepticus of the grand mal type.

▶*Unlabeled uses:* Phenytoin is useful as an antiarrhythmic agent, particularly in cardiac glycoside-induced arrhythmias. (Oral loading dose = 14 mg/kg; oral maintenance = 200 to 400 mg/day. IV loading dose = 50 mg every 5 minutes to total dose of 1 g; IV maintenance dose = 200 to 400 mg/day.) Pharmacokinetic, electrophysiologic and ECG effects of phenytoin are summarized in the Antiarrhythmic Agents monograph.

Phenytoin has been used as an alternative to magnesium sulfate for severe preeclampsia (15 mg/kg IV, given as 10 mg/kg initially and 5 mg/kg 2 hours later).

Phenytoin has been used in the treatment of trigeminal neuralgia (tic douloureux), recessive dystrophic epidermolysis bullosa and junctional epidermolysis bullosa.

Actions

▶*Pharmacology:* The primary site of action of the hydantoins appears to be the motor cortex, where the spread of seizure activity is inhibited. Possibly by promoting sodium efflux from neurons, hydan-toins tend to stabilize the threshold against hyperexcitability caused by excessive stimulation or environmental changes capable of reducing membrane sodium gradient. This includes the reduction of post-tetanic potentiation at synapses. Loss of posttetanic potentiation prevents cor-tical seizure foci from detonating adjacent cortical areas. Hydantoins reduce the maximal activity of brain stem centers responsible for the tonic phase of grand mal seizures.

Phenytoin is available as phenytoin acid (chewable tablets, suspension) or phenytoin sodium (capsules, injection); phenytoin sodium contains 92% phenytoin.

▶*Pharmacokinetics:*

Absorption/Distribution – Phenytoin is slowly absorbed from the small intestine. Rate and extent of absorption varies and is dependent on the product formulation. Bioavailability may differ among products of different manufacturers. Oral phenytoin sodium extended reaches peak plasma levels in 12 hours; phenytoin sodium prompt peaks within 1.5 to 3 hours. Administration IM results in precipitation of phenytoin at the injection site, resulting in slow and erratic absorption, which may continue for up to 5 days or more; 50% to 75% of an IM dose is absorbed within 24 hours. Plasma levels vary and are significantly lower than those achieved with an equal oral dose. Plasma protein binding is 87% to 93% and is lower in uremic patients and neonates. Volume of distribution averages 0.6 L/kg.

Phenytoin's therapeutic plasma concentration is 10 to 20 mcg/ml, although many patients achieve complete seizure control at lower serum concentrations. At plasma concentrations > 20 mcg/ml, far-lateral nystagmus may occur and at concentrations > 30 and 40 mcg/ml, ataxia and gross mental changes are usually seen.

Metabolism/Excretion – Phenytoin is metabolized in the liver to inactive hydroxylated metabolites and excreted in the urine by tubular secretion. The metabolism of phenytoin is capacity-limited and shows saturability. The major metabolite is 5–(p–hydroxyphenyl)-5–phenylhydantoin (p–HPPH); 1% to 5% is excreted unchanged. Because the elimination of p–HPPH glucuronide is rate-limited by its formation from phenytoin, measurement of the metabolite in urine can be used to assess the rate of phenytoin metabolism, patient compliance or bioavailability. Elimination is exponential (first-order) at plasma concentrations < 10 mcg/ml, and plasma half-life ranges from 6 to 24 hours. Dose-dependent elimination is apparent at higher concentrations, and half-life increases; values of 20 to 60 hours may be found at therapeutic levels. A genetically determined limitation in ability to metabolize phenytoin has occurred. Good correlation is generally seen between total phenytoin plasma concentration and therapeutic effects. Serum level monitoring is essential.

Contraindications

Hypersensitivity to hydantoins.

➤*Phenytoin:* Because of its effect on ventricular automaticity, do not use phenytoin in sinus bradycardia, sino-atrial block, second and third degree AV block or in patients with Adams-Stokes syndrome.

Warnings

➤*Abrupt withdrawal:* Abrupt withdrawal in epileptic patients may precipitate status epilepticus. Reduce dosage, discontinue or substitute other anticonvulsant medication gradually.

➤*Other seizures:* Hydantoins are not indicated in seizures due to hypoglycemia or other metabolic causes. Perform appropriate diagnostic procedures.

➤*Phenytoin:* Use with caution in hypotension and severe myocardial insufficiency.

➤*Hypersensitivity reactions:* In the event of an allergic or hypersensitivity reaction, rapid substitution of alternative therapy may be necessary. Alternative therapy should be an anticonvulsant not belonging to the hydantoin chemical class. Phenytoin hypersensitivity reactions are not typical; they may present as one of many different syndromes (eg, lymphoma, hepatitis, Stevens-Johnson syndrome) and may include such symptoms as fever, rash, arthralgias or lymphadenopathy.

➤*Hepatic function impairment:* Biotransformation of hydantoins occurs in the liver; elderly patients or those with impaired liver function or severe illness may show early signs of toxicity. Discontinue drug if hepatic dysfunction occurs.

Induced abnormalities – Phenytoin-induced hepatitis is one of the more commonly reported hypersensitivity syndromes.

➤*Pregnancy:* Refer to information for use during pregnancy in the Anticonvulsants introduction. If megaloblastic anemia occurs during gestation, consider folic acid therapy.

➤*Lactation:* These drugs are excreted in breast milk. Because of the potential for serious adverse reactions in nursing infants, decide whether to discontinue nursing or to discontinue the drug.

Precautions

➤*Hematologic effects:* Perform blood counts and urinalyses when therapy is begun and at monthly intervals for several months thereafter. Blood dyscrasias have occurred. Avoid use in combination with other drugs known to adversely affect the hematopoietic system. Be alert for general malaise, sore throat, fever, mucous membrane bleeding, glandular swelling, petechiae, easy bruising, epistaxis, cutaneous reactions and other symptoms indicative of blood dyscrasias. Signs of marked depression of the blood count indicate the need for drug withdrawal.

Some evidence suggests that hydantoins may interfere with folic acid metabolism, precipitating megaloblastic anemia.

➤*Dermatologic effects:* Discontinue these drugs if a skin rash appears. If the rash is exfoliative, purpuric or bullous, do not resume use. If the rash is milder (measles-like or scarlatiniform), resume therapy after the rash has completely disappeared. If rash recurs upon reinstitution of therapy, further medication is contraindicated.

➤*Lymph node hyperplasia:* Lymph node hyperplasia has been associated with hydantoins, and may represent a hypersensitivity reaction. Rarely, this may progress to frank malignant lymphoma. If lymph node enlargement occurs, attempt to substitute another anticonvulsant drug or drug combination.

Differentiate lymphadenopathy from other lymph gland pathology. Lymphadenopathy which simulates Hodgkin's disease has been observed. If a lymphoma-like syndrome develops, withdraw the drug and observe the patient closely for regression of signs and symptoms before resuming treatment.

Monoclonal gammopathy and multiple myeloma have occurred during prolonged phenytoin therapy.

➤*Hyperglycemia:* Hyperglycemia, resulting from the drug's inhibitory effect on insulin release, has occurred. Hydantoins may also raise blood sugar levels in hyperglycemic persons.

➤*Cardiovascular:* Death from cardiac arrest has occurred after too-rapid IV administration, sometimes preceded by marked QRS widening. Observe the patient closely when the drug is administered IV when possible SA node depression exists. Administer cautiously in the presence of advanced AV block. Do not exceed an IV infusion rate of 50 mg/minute.

➤*Grand mal and petit mal seizures:* Drugs that control grand mal seizures are not effective for petit mal seizures. Therefore, if both conditions are present, combined drug therapy is needed.

➤*Slow metabolism:* A small percentage of individuals treated with hydantoins metabolize the drug slowly. Slow metabolism may be due to limited enzyme availability and lack of induction. It appears to be genetically determined. Metabolism of phenytoin is dose-dependent.

➤*Osteomalacia:* Osteomalacia has been associated with phenytoin therapy.

➤*Acute intermittent porphyria:* Administer hydantoins cautiously to patients with acute intermittent porphyria.

Drug Interactions

The following drug interactions have occurred with the use of phenytoin; however, they may occur when using any of the hydantoins.

➤*Increased pharmacologic effects:* Increased pharmacologic effects of hydantoins may occur when the following drugs are administered concurrently. Mechanisms of these interactions may include:

Hydantoin Drug Interactions: Increased Hydantoin Effects			
Inhibit metabolism		Displace anticonvulsant	Unknown
Allopurinol	Metronidazole	Salicylates[1]	Chlorpheniramine
Amiodarone	Miconazole	Tricyclic antidepressants	Ibuprofen
Benzodiazepines	Omeprazole	Valproic acid[2]	Phenothiazines
Chloramphenicol	Phenacemide		
Cimetidine	Phenylbutazone		
Disulfiram	Succinimides		
Ethanol	Sulfonamides		
(acute ingestion)	Trimethoprim		
Fluconazole	Valproic acid[2]		
Isoniazid			

[1] **Salicylates** displace phenytoin from its plasma protein binding sites in a dose-dependent manner; no significant change occurs in the free phenytoin level.
[2] **Valproic acid** affects phenytoin disposition in different ways. Displacement of phenytoin from plasma proteins increases the free fraction and decreases total phenytoin levels; the concentration of unbound phenytoin is not significantly altered. Increased levels may result from inhibition of phenytoin metabolism. Conversely, phenytoin increases metabolism of valproic acid.

➤*Decreased pharmacologic effects:* Decreased pharmacologic effects of hydantoins may occur when the following drugs are administered concurrently. Mechanisms of these interactions may include:

Hydantoin Drug Interactions: Decreased Hydantoin Effects		
Increase metabolism	Decrease absorption	Unknown
Barbiturates[1]	Antacids	Antineoplastics
Carbamazepine[2]	Charcoal	Folic acid[3]
Diazoxide	Sucralfate	Influenza virus vaccine[4]
Ethanol		Loxapine
(chronic ingestion)		Nitrofurantoin
Rifampin		Pyridoxine
Theophylline		

[1] **Barbiturates'** effect on phenytoin is variable and unpredictable. Addition of phenytoin generally increases phenobarbital serum concentrations. Individual monitoring is needed, especially when starting or stopping either drug.
[2] **Carbamazepine's** effect on phenytoin is variable. Carbamazepine serum levels may also be decreased.
[3] See also Drug/Food interactions.
[4] **Influenza virus vaccine** may increase, decrease, or have no effect on total serum phenytoin concentrations.

➤*Phenytoin:* Phenytoin may decrease the pharmacologic effects of the following drugs:

Hydantoin Drug Interactions: Decreased Effects of Other Drugs

Increased metabolism by phenytoin		Other
Acetaminophen[1]	Haloperidol	Cyclosporine
Amiodarone	Methadone	Dopamine
Carbamazepine	Metyrapone[2]	Furosemide
Cardiac glycosides	Mexiletine	Levodopa
Corticosteroids	Oral contraceptives	Levonorgestrel
Dicumarol	Quinidine	Mebendazole
Disopyramide	Theophylline	Nondepolarizing muscle relaxants
Doxycycline	Valproic acid	Phenothiazines
Estrogens		Sulfonylureas

[1] **Acetaminophen** Although the therapeutic effects of acetaminophen may be reduced by concomitant phenytoin use, the potential hepatotoxicity of acetaminophen may be increased, especially with chronic phenytoin use.
[2] See also Drug/Lab test interactions.

Hydantoin Drug Interactions

Precipitant drug	Object drug*		Descriptions
Clonazepam	Phenytoin	↓↑	Plasma levels of clonazepam or phenytoin may be decreased with concomitant use, or phenytoin toxicity may occur.
Phenytoin	Clonazepam	↓	
Corticosteroid	Phenytoin	↓	Corticosteroid use may mask systemic manifestations of phenytoin hypersensitivity reactions.
Phenytoin	Dopamine	↓	Five critically ill patients requiring dopamine to maintain blood pressure developed severe hypotension when IV phenytoin was administered.
Phenytoin	Lithium	↑	Lithium toxicity may be increased by coadministration of phenytoin. Marked neurologic symptoms were reported despite normal serum levels of lithium.
Phenytoin	Meperidine	↑	Meperidine's analgesic effectiveness may be decreased, while the toxic effects could be increased by phenytoin. The hepatic metabolism of meperidine is increased, but the formation of normeperidine, a potentially toxic metabolite, is increased.
Phenytoin	Primidone	↑	Primidone's pharmacologic effects may be increased by phenytoin administration; toxicity has occurred. The metabolic conversion of primidone to phenobarbital and phenylethylmalonamide (PEMA) may also be increased. Monitor serum concentrations of primidone and primidone metabolites following alterations in hydantoin therapy.
Phenytoin	Warfarin	↑	Warfarin may be displaced by phenytoin; in one report, a patient died of bleeding complications.
Phenytoin Carbamazepine	Cisatracurium Besylate	↓	Resistance to the neuromuscular blocking action of nondepolarizing agents has been demonstrated in patients chronically administered phenytoin or carbamazepine. Slightly shorter durations of neuromuscular block may be anticipated and infusion rate requirements may be higher.

* ↑ = Object drug increased. ↓ = Object drug decreased.

➤*Drug/Lab test interactions:* Phenytoin may interfere with the **metyrapone** and the 1 mg **dexamethasone** tests. Discontinuing hydantoins prior to metyrapone testing would be ideal, but not practical; consider doubling the oral metyrapone dose.

➤*Drug/Food interactions:* Several case reports and single-dose studies suggest that enteral nutritional therapy may decrease phenytoin concentrations; however, this has not been substantiated. Monitor phenytoin concentrations. Consider giving phenytoin 2 hours before and after the enteral feeding, or stopping the enteral therapy for 2 hours before and after phenytoin administration.

Long-term phenytoin therapy may result in folate deficiency, possibly progressing to megaloblastic anemia (rare).

Adverse Reactions

➤*Cardiovascular:*

Phenytoin IV – Cardiovascular collapse; CNS depression; hypotension (when the drug is administered rapidly IV). Rate of administration is very important; do not exceed 50 mg/minute. Severe cardiotoxic reactions and fatalities have occurred with atrial and ventricular conduction depression and ventricular fibrillation, most commonly in elderly or gravely ill patients.

➤*CNS:*

Most common – Nystagmus; ataxia; dysarthria; slurred speech; mental confusion; dizziness; insomnia; transient nervousness; motor twitchings; diplopia; fatigue; irritability; drowsiness; depression; numbness; tremor; headache. These side effects may disappear by reducing dosage. Psychotic disturbances and increased seizures have occurred, but a definite causal relationship is uncertain. Choreoathetosis following IV phenytoin infusion has occurred.

➤*Dermatologic:* Manifestations sometimes accompanied by fever have included scarlatiniform, morbilliform, maculopapular, urticarial and nonspecific rashes; a morbilliform rash is the most common. Rashes are more frequent in children and young adults. Serious forms which may be fatal include bullous, exfoliative or purpuric dermatitis, lupus erythematosus syndrome, Stevens-Johnson syndrome and toxic epidermal necrolysis. Hirsutism and alopecia have occurred.

➤*Endocrine:* Diabetes insipidus; hyperglycemia.

➤*GI:* Nausea; vomiting; diarrhea; constipation. Administration of the drug with or immediately after meals may help prevent GI discomfort.

Gingival hyperplasia – Gingival hyperplasia occurs frequently with phenytoin; incidence may be reduced by good oral hygiene, including gum massage, frequent brushing and appropriate dental care.

➤*Hepatic:* Toxic hepatitis and liver damage may occur and rarely can be fatal. Hypersensitivity reactions with hepatic involvement include hepatocellular degeneration and fatal hepatocellular necrosis. Hepatitis, jaundice and nephrosis have been reported, but a definite cause and effect relationship has not been established. See Warnings.

➤*Hematologic:* Hematopoietic complications, some fatal, include thrombocytopenia, leukopenia, granulocytopenia, agranulocytosis and pancytopenia. Macrocytosis and megaloblastic anemia usually respond to folic acid therapy. Eosinophilia; monocytosis; leukocytosis; simple anemia; hemolytic anemia; aplastic anemia; ecchymosis.

➤*Lab test abnormalities:* Phenytoin may decrease serum thyroxine and free thyroxine concentrations. Although these decreases are generally not associated with clinical hypothyroidism, some patients may develop goiter or hypothyroidism.

➤*Respiratory:* Pneumonia; pharyngitis; sinusitis; hyperventilation; rhinitis; apnea; aspiration pneumonia; asthma; dyspnea; atelectasis; increased cough/sputum; epistaxis; hypoxia; pneumothorax; hemoptysis; bronchitis; chest pain; pulmonary fibrosis.

➤*Special senses:* Tinnitus; diplopia; taste perversion; amblyopia; deafness; visual field defect; eye pain; conjunctivitis; photophobia; hyperacusis; mydriasis; parosmia; ear pain; tast loss.

➤*Miscellaneous:* Polyarthropathy; hyperglycemia; weight gain; chest pain; edema; IgA depression; fever; photophobia; conjunctivitis; gynecomastia; periarteritis nodosa; pulmonary fibrosis; soft tissue injury at the injection site with and without extravasation of IV phenytoin; lymph node hyperplasia (see Precautions).

Connective tissue system – Coarsening of the facial features; enlargement of the lips; Peyronie's disease.

Overdosage

➤*Symptoms:* The lethal dose in adults is estimated to be 2 to 5 g. Initial symptoms are nystagmus, ataxia and dysarthria; the patient may then become comatose and hypotensive, with pupils unresponsive. At plasma concentrations > 20 mcg/ml, far-lateral nystagmus may occur and at concentrations > 30 mcg/ml, ataxia is usually seen. Significantly diminished mental capacity occurs at levels > 40 mcg/ml. Death is due to respiratory and circulatory depression.

➤*Treatment:* Treatment is nonspecific; there is no known antidote. Refer to General Management of Acute Overdosage. Consider hemodialysis, since phenytoin is not completely bound to plasma proteins. Total exchange transfusion has been utilized in the treatment of severe intoxication in children.

Patient Information

Take medication with food to reduce GI upset.

Phenytoin suspension must be thoroughly shaken immediately prior to use.

Do not discontinue medication abruptly or change dosage, except on advice of physician.

Maintain good oral hygiene (regular brushing and flossing) while taking phenytoin. Inform dentist of medication usage.

Patients should carry identification (*Medic Alert*) indicating medication usage and epilepsy.

May cause drowsiness, dizziness or blurred vision; alcohol may intensify these effects. Observe caution while driving or performing other tasks requiring alertness, coordination or physical dexterity. Notify physician if drowsiness, slurred speech or impaired coordination (ataxia) occurs.

Do not use capsules which are discolored.

Hydantoins

►*Diabetic patients:* Monitor urine sugar regularly and report any abnormalities to physician.

Notify physician if any of the following occurs: Skin rash; severe nausea or vomiting; swollen glands; bleeding, swollen or tender gums; yellow- ish discoloration of the skin or eyes; joint pain; unexplained fever; sore throat; unusual bleeding or bruising; persistent headache; malaise; any indication of an infection or bleeding tendency; pregnancy.

ETHOTOIN

Rx	Peganone (Ovation)	Tablets: 250 mg	Lactose. White, scored. In 100s.

For complete prescribing information, refer to the Hydantoins group monograph.

Administration and Dosage

Administer in 4 to 6 divided doses daily. Take after food; space doses as evenly as practicable. Initial dosage should be conservative.

►*Adults:* The initial daily dose should be ≤ 1 g, with subsequent gradual dosage increases over several days. The usual adult maintenance dose is 2 to 3 g/day; < 2 g/day is ineffective in most adults.

►*Pediatric:* Dosage depends upon the age and weight of the patient. Initial dose should not exceed 750 mg/day. The usual maintenance dose in children ranges from 500 mg to 1 g/day, although occasionally 2 g or rarely 3 g daily may be necessary.

►*Replacement therapy:* Reduce the dosage of the other drug gradually as that of ethotoin is increased. Ethotoin may eventually replace the other drug, or the optimal dosage of both anticonvulsants may be established.

►*Concomitant anticonvulsant therapy:* Ethotoin is compatible with all commonly employed anticonvulsant medications with the possible exception of phenacemide. In grand mal seizures, concomitant use with phenobarbital may be beneficial. It may be used in combination with drugs such as trimethadione or paramethadione, as an adjunct in those patients with petit mal associated with grand mal seizures.

FOSPHENYTOIN SODIUM

Rx	Cerebyx (Parke-Davis)	Injection: 150 mg (100 mg phenytoin sodium)	In 2 ml vials.
		750 mg (500 mg phenytoin sodium)	In 10 ml vials.

For complete prescribing information, refer to the Hydantoins group monograph.

Administration and Dosage

The dose, concentration in dosing solutions and infusion rate of IV fosphenytoin is expressed as phenytoin sodium equivalents (PE) to avoid the need to perform molecular weight-based adjustments when converting between fosphenytoin and phenytoin sodium doses. Prescribe and dispense fosphenytoin in phenytoin sodium equivalent units (PE). Fosphenytoin has important differences in administration from those for parenteral phenytoin sodium.

Dilute fosphenytoin in 5% Dextrose or 0.9% Saline Solution for Injection to a concentration ranging from 1.5 to 25 mg PE/ml.

►*Status epilepticus:* The loading dose 15 to 20 mg PE/kg administered at 100 to 150 mg PE/min.

Because the full antiepileptic effect of phenytoin, whether given as fosphenytoin or parenteral phenytoin, is not immediate, other measures, including concomitant administration of an IV benzodiazepine, will usually be necessary for control of status epilepticus.

►*Nonemergent and maintenance dosing:*
Loading dose – 10 to 20 mg PE/kg given IV or IM.

Maintenance dose – 4 to 6 mg PE/kg/day.

Because of the risk of hypotension, administer at a rate of ≤ 150 mg PE/min.

Continuously monitor the electrocardiogram, blood pressure and respiratory function and observe the patient throughout the period of maximal serum phenytoin concentrations, ≈ 10 to 20 min after the end of the infusion.

►*Renal / Hepatic function impairment:* Due to an increased fraction of unbound phenytoin in patients with renal or hepatic disease, or in those with hypoalbuminemia, interpret total phenytoin plasma concentrations with caution. Unbound phenytoin concentrations may be more useful in these patients. After IV administration, fosphenytoin clearance to phenytoin may be increased without a similar increase in phenytoin clearance. This has the potential to increase the frequency and severity of adverse events.

►*Elderly:* Age does not have a significant impact on the pharmacokinetics of fosphenytoin following administration. Phenytoin clearance is decreased slightly in elderly patients and lower or less frequent dosing may be required.

►*Storage / Stability:* Refrigerate at 2° to 8°C (36° to 46°F). Do not store at room temperature for more than 48 hours.

PHENYTOIN SODIUM, PARENTERAL

Rx	Phenytoin Sodium (Elkins-Sinn)	Injection: 50 mg/ml (46 mg phenytoin)[1]	In 2 and 5 ml Dosette amps, 2 ml Dosette vials and 5 ml vials.

[1] With propylene glycol and alcohol.

For complete prescribing information, refer to the Hydantoins group monograph.

Administration and Dosage

Phenytoin sodium contains 92% phenytoin.

►*IV administration:* The addition of phenytoin solution to an IV infusion is not recommended due to lack of solubility and resultant precipitation.

Inject parenteral phenytoin slowly and directly into a large vein through a large-gauge needle or IV catheter.

Do not exceed an IV infusion rate of 50 mg/minute in adults or 1 to 3 mg/kg/minute in neonates. There is a relatively small margin between full therapeutic effect and minimally toxic doses. Monitor ECG and blood pressure continuously. In status epilepticus, the IV route is preferred because of the delay in absorption with IM administration.

Follow each IV injection with an injection of sterile saline through the same needle or IV catheter to avoid local venous irritation due to alkalinity of the solution. Avoid continuous infusion.

Soft tissue irritation and injury, with and without extravasation of IV phenytoin, have occurred at the injection site.

Although not recommended, some studies indicate that an IV infusion of phenytoin may be feasible if proper precautions are observed, such as a suitable vehicle (eg, Sodium Chloride 0.9% or Lactated Ringer's injection), appropriate concentration, preparing the infusion shortly before administration and using an inline filter.

►*IM administration:* Avoid the IM route due to erratic absorption of phenytoin and pain and muscle damage at the injection site. When IM administration is required for a patient previously stabilized orally, compensating dosage adjustments are necessary to maintain therapeutic plasma levels; an IM dose 50% greater than the oral dose is necessary. When returned to oral administration, reduce the dose by 50% of the original oral dose for 1 week to prevent excessive plasma levels due to sustained release from IM tissue sites. Determine serum drug levels when possible drug interactions are suspected.

If the patient requires > 1 week of IM therapy, consider alternative routes (eg, gastric intubation), using oral preparations. For periods < 1 week, the patient shifted back from IM administration should receive ½ the original oral dose for the same period of time the patient received IM therapy. Monitor plasma levels.

►*Status epilepticus:* In adults, administer loading dose of 10 to 15 mg/kg slowly. Follow by maintenance doses of 100 mg orally or IV every 6 to 8 hours. For neonates and children, oral absorption of phenytoin is unreliable; IV loading dose is 15 to 20 mg/kg in divided doses of 5 to 10 mg/kg. If administration does not terminate the seizure, consider the use of other anticonvulsants, IV barbiturates, general anesthesia or other measures.

►*Neurosurgery (prophylactic dosage):* 100 to 200 mg IM at ≈ 4 hour intervals during surgery and the postoperative period.

►*Storage / Stability:* The solution is suitable for use as long as it remains free of haziness and precipitate. Upon refrigeration or freezing, a precipitate might form; this will dissolve again after the solution is allowed to stand at room temperature. The solution is still suitable for use. Use only a clear solution. A faint yellow color may develop, but has no effect on the potency of the solution.

PHENYTOIN and PHENYTOIN SODIUM, ORAL

For complete prescribing information, refer to the Hydantoins group monograph.

Administration and Dosage

Phenytoin sodium contains 92% phenytoin.

Individualize dosage. Determine serum levels for optimal dosage adjustments; the clinically effective serum level is usually in the range of 10 to 20 mcg/ml.

Monitor serum concentrations and exercise care when switching a patient from the sodium salt to the free acid form or vice versa. The free acid form of phenytoin is used in the *Dilantin Infatabs* and *Dilantin-125* suspension, as opposed to the sodium salt in the other products. Because there is an ≈ 8% increase in drug content with the free acid form, dosage adjustment and serum monitoring may be necessary.

➤*Loading dose:* Some authorities have advocated use of an oral loading dose of phenytoin in adults who require rapid steady-state serum levels and where IV administration is not desirable. Reserve this dosing regimen for patients in a clinic or hospital setting where phenytoin serum levels can be monitored. Patients with a history of renal or liver disease should not receive the oral loading regimen.

Initially, 1 g of phenytoin capsules is divided into 3 doses (400 mg, 300 mg, 300 mg) and administered at intervals of 2 hours. Normal maintenance dosage is then instituted 24 hours after the loading dose, with frequent serum level determinations.

➤*Adults:* Adults who have received no previous treatment may be started on 100 mg capsule/tablet or 125 mg suspension 3 times daily; individualize dosage. Satisfactory maintenance dosage - 300 to 400 mg/day. An increase to 600 mg/day (625 mg/day suspension) may be necessary.

➤*Pediatric:* Initially, 5 mg/kg/day in 2 or 3 equally divided doses with subsequent dosage individualized to a maximum of 300 mg/day. Daily maintenance dosage - 4 to 8 mg/kg. Children over 6 years may require the minimum adult dose (300 mg/day). If the daily dosage cannot be divided equally, the larger dose should be given before retiring.

➤*Single daily dosage:* In adults, if seizure control is established with divided doses of three 100 mg extended phenytoin sodium capsules daily, once-a-day dosage with 300 mg may be considered. Once-a-day dosage offers convenience to the patient or to nursing personnel for institutionalized patients; it may improve compliance and it is intended to be used only for patients requiring this amount of drug daily. Caution patients not to miss a dose. Only extended phenytoin sodium capsules are recommended once-a-day.

➤*Bioavailability:* Because of potential bioavailability differences between products, brand interchange is not recommended. Dosage adjustments may be required when switching from the extended to the prompt products.

PHENYTOIN

Rx	**Dilantin Infatab** (Parke-Davis)	**Tablets, chewable:** 50 mg	(P-D 007). Saccharin, sucrose. Yellow, scored. Triangular. In 100s and UD 100s.
Rx	**Phenytoin** (Alpharma)	**Suspension, oral:** 125 mg/5 ml	≤ 0.6% alcohol, sucrose. In 240 ml.
Rx	**Dilantin-125** (Parke-Davis)		≤ 0.6% alcohol, sucrose. Orange-vanilla flavor. In 240 ml.

For complete prescribing information, refer to the Hydantoins group monograph.

Administration and Dosage

Not for once-a-day dosing.

PHENYTOIN SODIUM, PROMPT

Rx	**Phenytoin Sodium** (Various, eg, Major, Parmed, Zenith)	**Capsules:** 100 mg (92 mg phenytoin)	In 100s, 1000s and UD 100s.

For complete prescribing information, refer to the Hydantoins group monograph.

Administration and Dosage

Not for once-a-day dosing.

➤*Dissolution rate:* Not < 85% in 30 minutes.

PHENYTOIN SODIUM, EXTENDED

Rx	**Dilantin Kapseals** (Parke-Davis)	**Capsules:** 30 mg (27.6 mg phenytoin)	Lactose, sucrose. (P-D 365). Transparent w/pink band. In 100s.
Rx	**Phenytoin Sodium** (Various, eg, Goldline, Major)	**Capsules:** 100 mg (92 mg phenytoin)	Clear. In 100s and 1000s.
Rx	**Dilantin Kapseals** (Parke-Davis)		Lactose, sucrose. (DILANTIN 100 mg). Transparent w/orange band. In 100s, 1000s and UD 100s.
Rx	**Phenytek** (Bertek)	**Capsules:** 200 mg	(BERTEK 670). Blue. In 30s and 100s.
Rx	**Phenytek** (Bertek)	**Capsules:** 300 mg	(BERTEK 750). Blue. In 30s and 100s.

For complete prescribing information, refer to the Hydantoins group monograph.

Administration and Dosage

May be used for once-a-day dosing.

Refer to the general discussion beginning in the Anticonvulsants introduction.

Indications

Control of absence (petit mal) seizures.

➤*Methsuximide:* For petit mal seizures when refractory to other drugs.

Actions

➤*Pharmacology:* Succinimides suppress the paroxysmal three cycle per second spike and wave activity associated with lapses of consciousness common in absence (petit mal) seizures. The frequency of epileptiform attacks is reduced, apparently by motor cortex depression and elevation of the threshold of the CNS to convulsive stimuli.

➤*Pharmacokinetics:*

Absorption / Distribution – These agents are readily absorbed from the GI tract. Peak serum levels of ethosuximide are achieved in 3 to 7 hours; peak levels of methsuximide and phensuximide are reached in 1 to 4 hours. Therapeutic serum concentrations of ethosuximide range from 40 to 100 mcg/ml.

Metabolism / Excretion – Ethosuximide is extensively metabolized to inactive metabolites; ≈ 20% is excreted unchanged via the kidneys. The plasma half-life is 30 hours in children and 60 hours in adults. Less than 1% of a dose of methsuximide is recovered unchanged in urine; plasma half-lives range from 2.6 to 4 hours. Phensuximide is excreted in urine and in bile; half-life is ≈ 4 hours.

Contraindications

Hypersensitivity to succinimides.

Warnings

➤*Hematologic effects:* Blood dyscrasias, some fatal, have occurred; therefore, perform periodic blood counts. Should signs or symptoms of infection (eg, sore throat, fever) develop, consider blood counts at that point.

➤*Lupus:* Cases of systemic lupus erythematosus have occurred.

➤*Renal / Hepatic function impairment:* Succinimides have produced morphological and functional changes in animal liver. Abnormal liver and renal function have been reported in humans. For this reason, administer with extreme caution to patients with known liver or renal disease. Perform periodic urinalyses and liver function studies for all patients receiving these drugs.

➤*Pregnancy:* Refer to information for use during pregnancy in the Anticonvulsant introduction.

Precautions

➤*Grand mal seizures:* Succinimides, when used alone in mixed types of epilepsy, may increase the frequency of grand mal seizures in some patients.

➤*Dosage changes / other medication:* It is important to proceed slowly when increasing or decreasing dosage, and when adding or eliminating other medication. Abrupt withdrawal of anticonvulsant medication may precipitate absence (petit mal) status.

➤*Acute intermittent porphyria:* Use phensuximide with caution.

Drug Interactions

Succinimide Drug Interactions			
Precipitant drug	Object drug*		Description
Succinimides	Hydantoins	↑	Serum hydantoin levels may be increased.
Succinimides	Primidone	↓	Lower primidone and phenobarbital levels may occur.
Valproic acid	Succinimides	↔	Both increases and decreases in succinimide levels have occurred.

* ↑ = Object drug increased. ↓ = Object drug decreased. ↔ = Undetermined clinical effect.

Adverse Reactions

The following have been reported with one or more of the succinimides:

➤*CNS:* Drowsiness; ataxia; dizziness; irritability; nervousness; headache; blurred vision; myopia; photophobia; hiccoughs; euphoria; dreamlike state; lethargy; hyperactivity; fatigue; insomnia. Drowsiness, ataxia and dizziness are the most frequent **methsuximide** side effects.

➤*Dermatologic:* Pruritus; urticaria; Stevens-Johnson syndrome; pruritic erythematous rashes; skin eruptions; erythema multiforme; systemic lupus erythematosus; alopecia; hirsutism.

➤*GI:* (frequent): Nausea; vomiting; vague gastric upset; cramps; anorexia; diarrhea; weight loss; epigastric and abdominal pain; constipation.

➤*GU:* Urinary frequency, renal damage, hematuria (**phensuximide**); vaginal bleeding; microscopic hematuria.

➤*Hematologic:* Eosinophilia; granulocytopenia; leukopenia; agranulocytosis; monocytosis; pancytopenia, with or without bone marrow suppression.

➤*Psychiatric:* Confusion; instability; mental slowness; depression; hypochondriacal behavior; sleep disturbances; night terrors; aggressiveness; inability to concentrate. These effects may be noted particularly in patients who have previously exhibited psychological abnormalities. There have been rare reports of paranoid psychosis, suicidal behavior, auditory hallucinations, increased libido and increased state of depression.

➤*Miscellaneous:* Periorbital edema; hyperemia; muscle weakness; swelling of the tongue; gum hypertrophy.

Overdosage

The therapeutic range of ethosuximide serum levels is 40 to 100 mcg/ml, although levels as high as 150 mcg/ml have occurred without signs of toxicity. Methsuximide levels > 40 mcg/ml have caused toxicity; coma has been seen at levels of 150 mcg/ml.

➤*Symptoms:*

Acute overdosage – Confusion; sleepiness; unsteadiness; flaccid muscles; coma with slow, shallow respiration; hypotension; cyanosis; hypo- or hyperthermia; absent reflexes; nausea; vomiting; CNS depression including coma with respiratory depression.

Chronic overdosage – Skin rash; confusion; ataxia; dizziness; drowsiness; hangover; depression; irritability; poor judgment; periorbital edema; proteinuria; hepatic dysfunction; fatal bone marrow aplasia; delayed onset of coma; nausea; vomiting; muscular weakness; hematuria; casts; nephrosis.

➤*Treatment:* Treatment includes usual supportive measures. Refer to General Management of Acute Overdosage. Charcoal hemoperfusion may be indicated. Hemodialysis may be useful for ethosuximide. Forced diuresis and exchange transfusions are ineffective.

Patient Information

If GI upset occurs, take with food or milk.

Do not discontinue medication abruptly or change dosage, except on advice of physician.

Patients should carry identification (Medic Alert) indicating medication usage and epilepsy.

May cause drowsiness, dizziness or blurred vision; alcohol may exacerbate these effects. Use caution while driving or performing other tasks requiring alertness, coordination or physical dexterity.

Notify physician if any of the following occurs: Skin rash, joint pain, unexplained fever, sore throat, unusual bleeding or bruising, drowsiness, dizziness, blurred vision or pregnancy.

➤*Phensuximide:* Phensuximide may discolor the urine pink, red or red-brown. This is not harmful.

ETHOSUXIMIDE

Rx	**Ethosuximide** (Sidmak)	**Capsules:** 250 mg	In 100s.
Rx	**Zarontin** (Parke-Davis)		Sorbitol. (PD 237). In 100s.
Rx	**Ethosuximide** (Copley)	**Syrup:** 250 mg/5 ml	Saccharin, sucrose. Raspberry flavor. In 483 ml.
Rx	**Zarontin** (Parke-Davis)		Raspberry flavor. Saccharin, sucrose. In pt.

For complete prescribing information, refer to the Succinimides group monograph.

Administration and Dosage

➤*Children (3 to 6 years of age):* Initial dose – 250 mg/day.

➤*Children and adults (≥ 6 years of age):* 500 mg/day.

➤*Maintenance therapy:* Individualize dosage. Increase by small increments. One method is to increase the daily dose by 250 mg every 4 to 7 days until control is achieved with minimal side effects. Administer dosages exceeding 1.5 g/day in divided doses only under strict supervision. The optimal dose for most children is 20 mg/kg/day.

➤*Concomitant therapy:* May be administered in combination with other anticonvulsants when other forms of epilepsy coexist with absence (petit mal) seizures.

METHSUXIMIDE

Rx	**Celontin** (Parke-Davis)	**Capsules:** 150 mg	In 100s.
		300 mg	In 100s.

For complete prescribing information, refer to the Succinimides group monograph.

Indications

▶*Seizures:* For the control of absence (petit mal) seizures that are refractory to other drugs.

Administration and Dosage

Individualize therapy according to patient response. A suggested schedule is 300 mg/day for the first week. If required, increase at weekly intervals by 300 mg/day for 3 weeks, up to a dosage of 1200 mg/day.

Optimal dosage is the amount of methsuximide that is barely sufficient to control seizures so that side effects may be kept to a minimum. The 150 mg capsule facilitates pediatric administration.

▶*Concomitant therapy:* May be administered in combination with other anticonvulsants when other forms of epilepsy coexist with absence (petit mal) seizures.

▶*Storage/Stability:* Store at 25°C (77°F); excursions permitted to 15° to 30°C (59° to 86°F). Protect from light, moisture, and excessive heat (40°C; 104°F).

ZONISAMIDE

Rx	**Zonegran** (Elan)	**Capsules:** 25 mg	(ZONEGRAN 25). White. In 100s.
		50 mg	(ZONEGRAN 50). White/Gray. In 100s.
		100 mg	(ZONEGRAN 100). White/Red. In 100s.

Indications

➤*Epilepsy:* Adjunctive therapy in the treatment of partial seizures in adults with epilepsy.

Administration and Dosage

➤*Approved by the FDA:* March 27, 2000.

➤*Adults:* The initial dose is 100 mg/day. After 2 weeks, the dose may be increased to 200 mg/day for at least 2 weeks. It can be increased to 300 and 400 mg/day, with the dose stable for at least 2 weeks, to achieve steady state at each level. Because of the long half-life of zonisamide, up to 2 weeks may be required to achieve steady-state levels upon reaching a stable dose or following dosage adjustment. Administer zonisamide once or twice daily. Zonisamide may be taken with or without food. Swallow the capsules whole.

Although the regimen described is one that has been shown to be tolerated, the prescriber may wish to prolong the duration of treatment at lower doses to fully assess the effects of zonisamide at steady state, noting that many of the side effects of zonisamide are more frequent at doses of 300 mg/day and above. Although there is some evidence of greater response at doses above 100 to 200 mg/day, the increase appears small, and formal dose-response studies have not been conducted. Evidence from controlled trials suggest that zonisamide doses of 100 to 600 mg/day are effective, but there is no suggestion of increasing response above 400 mg/day. There is little experience with doses greater than 600 mg/day.

➤*Discontinuation of therapy:* Abrupt withdrawal of zonisamide in patients with epilepsy may precipitate increased seizure frequency or status epilepticus. Gradually reduce dose of zonisamide.

➤*Storage/Stability:* Store at 25°C (77°F); excursions permitted to 15° to 30°C (59° to 86°F) in a dry place; protect from light.

Actions

➤*Pharmacology:* The precise mechanism(s) of action is unknown. Zonisamide demonstrated anticonvulsant activity in several experimental models. In animals, zonisamide was effective against tonic extension seizures induced by maximal electroshock but ineffective against clonic seizures induced by SC pentylenetetrazol. Zonisamide raised the threshold for generalized seizures in the kindled rat model and reduced the duration of cortical focal seizures induced by electrical stimulation of the visual cortex in cats. Furthermore, it suppressed interictal spikes and the secondary generalized seizures produced by cortical application of tungstic acid gel in rats or by cortical freezing in cats. The relevance of these models to human epilepsy is unknown.

Zonisamide may produce these effects through action at sodium and calcium channels. In vitro pharmacological studies suggest that zonisamide blocks sodium channels and reduces voltage-dependent, transient inward currents (T-type Ca^{2+} currents), consequently stabilizing neuronal membranes and suppressing neuronal hypersynchronization. In vitro binding studies have demonstrated that zonisamide binds to the GABA/benzodiazepine receptor ionophore complex in an allosteric fashion, which does not produce changes in chloride flux. Other in vitro studies have demonstrated that zonisamide (10 to 30 mcg/mL) suppresses synaptically driven electrical activity without affecting postsynaptic GABA or glutamate responses (cultured mouse spinal cord neurons) or neuronal or glial uptake of [³H]-GABA (rat hippocampal slices). Thus, zonisamide does not appear to potentiate the synaptic activity of GABA. In vivo microdialysis studies demonstrated that zonisamide facilitates dopaminergic and serotonergic neurotransmission. It also has weak carbonic anhydrase inhibiting activity, but this pharmacologic effect is not thought to be a major contributing factor in the antiseizure activity of zonisamide.

➤*Pharmacokinetics:*

Absorption – Following a 200 to 400 mg oral zonisamide dose, peak plasma concentrations (range, 2 to 5 mcg/mL) in healthy volunteers occur within 2 to 6 hours. In the presence of food, the time to maximum concentration is delayed, occurring at 4 to 6 hours, but food has no effect on the bioavailability of zonisamide.

Distribution – The apparent volume of distribution of zonisamide is about 1.45 L/kg following a 400 mg oral dose. At concentrations of 1 to 7 mcg/mL, it is approximately 40% bound to human plasma proteins. Zonisamide extensively binds to erythrocytes, resulting in an 8-fold higher concentration of zonisamide in red blood cells (RBCs) than in plasma.

Metabolism/Excretion – The elimination half-life of zonisamide in plasma is about 63 hours. The elimination half-life in RBCs is approximately 105 hours. Zonisamide is excreted primarily in urine as parent drug and as the glucuronide of a metabolite. Following multiple dosing, 62% was recovered in the urine, with 3% in the feces by day 10. Zonisamide undergoes acetylation to form N-acetyl zonisamide and reduc-

tion to form the open ring metabolite, 2-sulfamoylacetyl phenol (SMAP). Of the excreted dose, 35% was recovered as zonisamide, 15% as N-acetyl zonisamide, and 50% as the glucuronide of SMAP. Reduction of zonisamide to SMAP is mediated by cytochrome P450 isozyme 3A4 (CYP3A4). Zonisamide does not induce its own metabolism. Plasma clearance of zonisamide is approximately 0.3 to 0.35 mL/min/kg in patients not receiving enzyme-inducing antiepilepsy drugs (AEDs). The clearance of zonisamide is increased to 0.5 mL/min/kg in patients concurrently on enzyme-inducing AEDs.

Renal clearance is about 3.5 mL/min. The clearance of an oral dose of zonisamide from RBCs is 2 mL/min.

Special populations –

Renal function impairment: Single 300 mg zonisamide doses were administered to 3 groups of volunteers. Group 1 was a healthy group with a creatinine clearance (Ccr) ranging from 70 to 152 mL/min. Groups 2 and 3 had Ccr ranging from 14.5 to 59 mL/min and 10 to 20 mL/min, respectively. Zonisamide renal clearance decreased with decreasing renal function (3.42, 2.5, and 2.23 mL/min, respectively). Marked renal impairment (Ccr less than 20 mL/min) was associated with an increase in zonisamide AUC of 35%.

Contraindications

Hypersensitivity to sulfonamides or zonisamide.

Warnings

➤*Oligohydrosis and hyperthermia in pediatric patients:* Oligohydrosis, sometimes resulting in heat stroke and hospitalization, is seen in association with zonisamide in pediatric patients.

During the preapproval development program in Japan, 1 case of oligohydrosis was reported in 403 pediatric patients, an incidence of 1 case per 285 patient-years of exposure. While there were no cases reported in the US or European development programs, less than 100 pediatric patients participated in these trials.

In the first 11 years of marketing in Japan, 38 cases were reported, an estimated reporting rate of about 1 case per 10,000 patient-years of exposure. In the first year of marketing in the United States, 2 cases were reported, an estimated reporting rate of about 12 cases per 10,000 patient-years of exposure. These rates are underestimates of the true incidence because of under-reporting. There has been 1 report of heat stroke in an 18-year-old patient in the United States.

Decreased sweating and an elevation in body temperature above normal characterized these cases. Many cases were reported after exposure to elevated environmental temperatures. Heat stroke, requiring hospitalization, was diagnosed in some cases. There have been no reported deaths.

Pediatric patients appear to be at an increased risk for zonisamide-associated oligohydrosis and hyperthermia. Closely monitor patients, especially pediatric patients, treated with zonisamide for evidence of decreased sweating and increased body temperature, particularly in warm or hot weather. Use caution when zonisamide is prescribed with other drugs that predispose patients to heat-related disorders; these drugs include, but are not limited to, carbonic anhydrase inhibitors and drugs with anticholinergic activity.

The safety and efficacy of zonisamide in pediatric patients have not been established. Zonisamide is not approved for use in pediatric patients.

➤*Cognitive/Neuropsychiatric adverse events:* Use of zonisamide was frequently associated with CNS-related adverse events. The most significant of these can be classified into the following 3 general categories: 1) Psychiatric symptoms, including depression and psychosis; 2) psychomotor slowing, difficulty with concentration, and speech or language problems, in particular, word-finding difficulties; and 3) somnolence or fatigue.

Psychomotor slowing and difficulty with concentration occurred in the first month of treatment and were associated with doses above 300 mg/day. Speech and language problems tended to occur after 6 to 10 weeks of treatment and at doses above 300 mg/day. Although in most cases these events were of mild to moderate severity, they at times led to withdrawal from treatment.

Somnolence and fatigue were frequently reported CNS adverse events during clinical trials with zonisamide. Although in most cases these events were of mild to moderate severity, they led to withdrawal from treatment in 0.2% of the patients enrolled in controlled trials. Somnolence and fatigue tended to occur within the first month of treatment. Somnolence and fatigue occurred most frequently at doses of 300 to 500 mg/day. Caution patients about this possibility and take special care if they drive, operate machinery, or perform any hazardous task.

ZONISAMIDE

Among all epilepsy patients treated with zonisamide in clinical trials, 0.89% were discontinued and 1.4% were hospitalized because of reported psychosis or related symptoms.

➤*Potentially fatal reactions to sulfonamides:* Fatalities have occurred, although rarely, as a result of severe reactions to sulfonamides (zonisamide is a sulfonamide) including Stevens-Johnson syndrome (SJS), toxic epidermal necrolysis (TEN), fulminant hepatic necrosis, agranulocytosis, aplastic anemia, and other blood dyscrasias. Such reactions may occur when a sulfonamide is readministered, regardless of the route of administration. If signs of hypersensitivity or other serious reactions occur, discontinue zonisamide immediately. Refer to Management of Acute Hypersensitivity Reactions.

➤*Serious skin reactions:* Discontinue zonisamide in patients who develop an otherwise unexplained rash or observe them frequently. Seven deaths from severe rash (SJS and TEN) were reported in the first 11 years of marketing in Japan. All of the patients were receiving other drugs in addition to zonisamide. In postmarketing experience from Japan, a total of 49 cases of SJS or TEN have been reported, a reporting rate of 46 per million patient-years of exposure. Although this rate is greater than background, it is probably an underestimate of the true incidence because of underreporting. There were no confirmed cases of SJS or TEN in the US, European, or Japanese development programs.

➤*Serious hematological events:* Two confirmed cases of aplastic anemia and 1 confirmed case of agranulocytosis were reported in the first 11 years of marketing in Japan, rates greater than generally accepted background rates. There were no cases of aplastic anemia and 2 confirmed cases of agranulocytosis in the US, European, or Japanese development programs. There is inadequate information to assess the relationship, if any, between dose and duration of treatment and these events.

➤*Abrupt withdrawal:* Abrupt withdrawal of zonisamide in patients with epilepsy may precipitate increased seizure frequency or status epilepticus. Reduce or discontinue dose gradually.

➤*Renal function impairment:* In several clinical studies, zonisamide was associated with a statistically significant 8% mean increase from the baseline of serum creatinine and blood urea nitrogen (BUN) compared with essentially no change in the placebo patients. The increase appeared to persist over time but was not progressive; this has been interpreted as an effect on glomerular filtration rate (GFR). There were no episodes of unexplained acute renal failure in clinical development. The decrease in GFR appeared within the first 4 weeks of treatment. In a 30-day study, the GFR returned to baseline within 2 to 3 weeks of drug discontinuation. There is no information about reversibility, after drug discontinuation, of the effects of GFR after long-term use. Discontinue zonisamide in patients who develop acute renal failure or a clinically significant, sustained increase in the creatinine/BUN concentration. Do not use zonisamide in patients with renal failure (estimated GFR less than 50 mL/min) as there has been insufficient experience concerning drug dosing and toxicity.

➤*Fertility impairment:* Rats treated with zonisamide (20, 60, or 200 mg/kg) before mating and during the initial gestation phase showed signs of reproductive toxicity (decreased corpora lutea, implantations, and live fetuses) at all doses. The low dose in this study is approximately 0.5 times the maximum recommended human dose (MRHD) on a mg/m² basis. The effect of zonisamide on human fertility is unknown.

➤*Elderly:* Single dose pharmacokinetic parameters are similar in elderly and young healthy volunteers. In general, use caution in selecting a dose for an elderly patient, usually starting at the low end of the dosing range because of their greater frequency of decreased hepatic, renal, or cardiac function, and of concomitant disease or other drug therapy.

➤*Pregnancy:* Category C. Zonisamide was teratogenic in mice, rats, and dogs and embryolethal in monkeys when administered during the period of organogenesis. Fetal abnormalities or embryo-fetal deaths occurred in these species at zonisamide dosage and maternal plasma levels similar to or lower than therapeutic levels in humans, indicating that use of this drug in pregnancy entails a significant risk to the fetus. A variety of external, visceral, and skeletal malformations was produced in animals by prenatal exposure to zonisamide. Cardiovascular defects were prominent in both rats and dogs. There are no adequate studies in pregnant women. Use zonisamide during pregnancy only if the potential benefit outweighs the potential risk to the fetus.

Advise women of childbearing potential who are given zonisamide to use effective contraception.

➤*Lactation:* It is not known whether zonisamide is excreted in breast milk. Because of potentially serious adverse reactions in nursing infants from zonisamide, decide whether to discontinue nursing or discontinue the drug, taking into account the importance of the drug to the mother. Use in nursing mothers only if the benefits outweigh the risks.

➤*Children:* Cases of oligohydrosis and hyperpyrexia have been reported (see Warnings). Safety and efficacy of zonisamide in pediatric patients younger than 16 years of age have not been established.

Precautions

➤*Lab test abnormalities:* In several clinical studies, zonisamide was associated with a mean increase in the concentration of serum creatinine and blood urea nitrogen (BUN) of approximately 8% over the baseline measurement. Consider monitoring renal function periodically.

Zonisamide was associated with an increase in serum alkaline phosphatase. In the randomized, controlled trials, a mean increase of approximately 7% over the baseline was associated with zonisamide compared with a 3% mean increase in placebo-treated patients. These changes were not statistically significant. The clinical relevance of these changes is unknown.

➤*Hazardous tasks:* Zonisamide may produce drowsiness, especially at higher doses. Advise patients not to drive a car or operate other complex machinery until they have gained experience on zonisamide sufficient to determine whether it affects performance.

Drug Interactions

➤*CYP 450:* Drugs that induce liver enzymes increase the metabolism and clearance of zonisamide and decrease its half-life. The half-life of zonisamide following a 400 mg dose in patients concurrently on enzyme-inducing AEDs such as phenytoin, carbamazepine, or phenobarbital was between 27 to 38 hours; the half-life of zonisamide in patients concurrently on the nonenzyme-inducing AED, valproate, was 46 hours. Concurrent medication with drugs that induce or inhibit CYP3A4 would be expected to alter serum concentrations of zonisamide. Zonisamide is not expected to interfere with the metabolism of other drugs that are metabolized by cytochrome P450 isozymes.

➤*Drug/Food interactions:* The time to maximum concentration of zonisamide is delayed in the presence of food, but no effect on bioavailability occurs.

Adverse Reactions

The most commonly observed adverse events associated with the use of zonisamide in controlled clinical trials that were not seen at an equivalent frequency among placebo-treated patients were the following: Somnolence, anorexia, dizziness, headache, nausea, agitation/irritability.

In controlled clinical trials, 12% of patients receiving zonisamide as adjunctive therapy discontinued because of an adverse event compared with 6% receiving placebo. Approximately 21% of the 1336 patients with epilepsy who received zonisamide in clinical studies discontinued treatment because of an adverse event. The adverse events most commonly associated with discontinuation were the following: Somnolence, fatigue, or ataxia (6%); anorexia (3%); difficulty concentrating (2%); difficulty with memory, mental slowing, nausea/vomiting (2%); weight loss (1%). Many of these adverse events were dose-related.

Zonisamide Adverse Reactions Occurring in at Least 2% of Zonisamide-Treated Patients		
Adverse reaction	Zonisamide (n = 269)	Placebo (n = 230)
CNS		
Agitation/Irritability	9	4
Anxiety	3	2
Ataxia	6	1
Confusion	6	3
Depression	6	3
Difficulty concentrating	6	2
Difficulty with memory	6	2
Dizziness	13	7
Fatigue	8	6
Headache	10	8
Insomnia	6	3
Mental slowing	4	2
Nervousness	2	1
Nystagmus	4	2
Paresthesia	4	1
Schizophrenic/ Schizophreniform behavior	2	0
Somnolence	17	7
Tiredness	7	5
GI		
Abdominal pain	6	3
Anorexia	13	6
Constipation	2	1
Diarrhea	5	2
Dyspepsia	3	1
Nausea	9	6
Special senses		
Difficulties in verbal expression	2	< 1
Diplopia	6	3

ZONISAMIDE

Zonisamide Adverse Reactions Occurring in at Least 2% of Zonisamide-Treated Patients		
Adverse reaction	Zonisamide (n = 269)	Placebo (n = 230)
Speech abnormalities	5	2
Taste perversion	2	0
Miscellaneous		
Dry mouth	2	1
Ecchymosis	2	1
Flu syndrome	4	3
Rash	3	2
Rhinitis	2	1
Weight loss	3	2

➤*Cardiovascular:* Bradycardia, hypertension, hypotension, palpitation, syncope, tachycardia, thrombophlebitis, vascular insufficiency (0.1% to 1%); atrial fibrillation, heart failure, pulmonary embolus, ventricular extrasystoles (less than 0.1%).

➤*CNS:* Abnormal gait, convulsion, hyperesthesia, incoordination, tremor (at least 1%); abnormal dreams, cerebrovascular accident, decreased libido, dysarthria, euphoria, hyperkinesia, hypertonia, increased reflexes, movement disorder, neuropathy, paresthesia, peripheral neuritis, twitching, vertigo (0.1% to 1%); circumoral paresthesia, dyskinesia, dystonia, encephalopathy, facial paralysis, hypokinesia, myoclonus, oculogyric crisis (less than 0.1%).

➤*Dermatologic:* Pruritus (at least 1%); acne, alopecia, dry skin, eczema, hirsutism, maculopapular rash, pustular rash, sweating, urticaria, vesiculobullous rash (0.1% to 1%).

➤*GI:* Vomiting (at least 1%); cholelithiasis, dysphagia, flatulence, gastritis, gastro-duodenal ulcer, gastroenteritis, gingivitis, glossitis, gum hemorrhage, gum hyperplasia, melena, rectal hemorrhage, stomatitis, ulcerative stomatitis (0.1% to 1%); cholangitis, cholecystitis, cholestatic jaundice, colitis, duodenitis, esophagitis, fecal incontinence, hematemesis, mouth ulceration (less than 0.1%).

➤*GU:* Amenorrhea, dysuria, hematuria, impotence, nocturia, polyuria, urinary frequency, urinary incontinence, urinary retention, urinary urgency (0.1% to 1%); albuminuria, bladder calculus, bladder pain, enuresis, gynecomastia, mastitis, menorrhagia (less than 0.1%).

➤*Hematologic/Lymphatic:* Anemia, immunodeficiency, leukopenia, lymphadenopathy (0.1% to 1%); microcytic anemia, petechia, thrombocytopenia (less than 0.1%).

➤*Metabolic/Nutritional:* Dehydration, edema, peripheral edema, thirst, weight gain (0.1% to 1%); hypoglycemia, hyponatremia, increased ALT/AST, increased LDH (less than 0.1%).

➤*Musculoskeletal:* Arthralgia, arthritis, leg cramps, myalgia, myasthenia (0.1% to 1%).

➤*Respiratory:* Increased cough, pharyngitis (at least 1%); dyspnea (0.1% to 1%); apnea, hemoptysis (less than 0.1%).

➤*Special senses:* Amblyopia, tinnitus (at least 1%); conjunctivitis, deafness, glaucoma, parosmia, visual field defect (0.1% to 1%); iritis, photophobia (less than 0.1%).

➤*Miscellaneous:* Accidental injury, asthenia (at least 1%); allergic reaction, chest pain, face edema, flank pain, malaise, neck rigidity (0.1% to 1%); lupus erythematosus (less than 0.1%).

Status epilepticus – Among patients treated with zonisamide across all epilepsy studies (controlled and uncontrolled), 1% of patients had an event reported as status epilepticus.

Sudden unexplained death in epilepsy – During the development of zonisamide, 9 sudden unexplained deaths occurred among 991 patients with epilepsy receiving zonisamide for whom accurate exposure data are available. Some of the deaths could represent seizure-related deaths in which the seizure was not observed.

Kidney stones – Among 991 patients treated during the development of zonisamide, 40 patients (4%) with epilepsy receiving zonisamide developed clinically possible or confirmed kidney stones (eg, clinical symptomatology, sonography), a rate of 34 per 1000 patient-years of exposure (40 patients with 1168 years of exposure). The analyzed stones were composed of calcium or urate salts. In general, increasing fluid intake and urine output can help reduce the risk of stone formation, particularly in those with predisposing factors. It is unknown; however, whether these measures will reduce the risk of stone formation in patients treated with zonisamide.

Overdosage

➤*Symptoms:* Experience with zonisamide daily doses over 800 mg/day is limited. During zonisamide clinical development, 3 patients ingested unknown amounts of zonisamide as suicide attempts, and all 3 were hospitalized with CNS symptoms. One patient became comatose and developed bradycardia, hypotension, and respiratory depression; the zonisamide plasma level was 100.1 mcg/mL measured 31 hours postingestion. Plasma levels fell with a half-life of 57 hours, and the patient became alert 5 days later.

➤*Treatment:* No specific antidotes for zonisamide overdosage are available. Following a suspected recent overdose, induce emesis or perform gastric lavage with the usual precautions to protect the airway. General supportive care is indicated, including frequent monitoring of vital signs and close observation. Zonisamide has a long half-life. Because of the low protein binding of zonisamide (40%), renal dialysis may not be effective. Refer to General Management of Acute Overdosage.

Patient Information

Zonisamide may produce drowsiness, especially at higher doses. Advise patients not to drive a car or operate other complex machinery until they have gained experience on zonisamide sufficient to determine whether it affects performance.

Advise patients to contact the physician immediately if a rash develops or seizures worsen.

Advise patients to contact the physician immediately if they develop signs or symptoms, such as sudden back pain, abdominal pain, or blood in the urine that could indicate a kidney stone. Increasing fluid intake and urine output may reduce the risk of stone formation, particularly in those with predisposing risk factors for stones.

Contact the physician immediately if a child has been taking zonisamide and is not sweating as usual with or without fever.

Because zonisamide can cause hematological complications, advise patients to contact the physician immediately if they develop a fever, sore throat, oral ulcers, or easy bruising.

As with other AEDs, inform patients to contact the physician if they intend to become pregnant or are pregnant during zonisamide therapy. Notify a physician if intending to breastfeed or are breastfeeding.

Benzodiazepines

CLONAZEPAM

c-iv	**Clonazepam** (Various, eg, Major, Mylan, PAR, Teva, TorPharm, UDL, Watson)	**Tablets:** 0.5 mg	May contain lactose. In 100s, 500s, 1000s, and UD 100s.
c-iv	**Klonopin** (Roche)		Lactose. (1/2 Klonopin/Roche). Orange, scored. In 100s.
c-iv	**Clonazepam** (Various, eg, Major, Mylan, PAR, Teva, TorPharm, UDL, Watson)	**Tablets:** 1 mg	May contain lactose. In 100s, 500s, 1000s, and UD 100s.
c-iv	**Klonopin** (Roche)		Lactose. (1 Klonopin/Roche). Blue. In 100s.
c-iv	**Clonazepam** (Various, eg, Major, Mylan, PAR, Teva, TorPharm, UDL, Watson)	**Tablets:** 2 mg	May contain lactose. In 100s, 500s, and UD 100s.
c-iv	**Klonopin** (Roche)		Lactose. (2 Klonopin/Roche). White. In 100s.
c-iv	**Klonopin Wafers** (Roche)	**Tablets, orally disintegrating:** 0.125 mg	Mannitol, parabens. (⅛). White. In blister pack 60s.
		0.25 mg	Mannitol, parabens. (¼). White. In blister pack 60s.
		0.5 mg	Mannitol, parabens. (½). White. In blister pack 60s.
		1 mg	Mannitol, parabens. (1). White. In blister pack 60s.
		2 mg	Mannitol, parabens. (2). White. In blister pack 60s.

Refer to the general discussion beginning in the Anticonvulsants introduction. For complete prescribing information, refer to the Benzodiazepine monograph in the Antianxiety Agents section.

Indications

➤*Seizure disorders:* Used alone or as adjunctive treatment of Lennox-Gastaut syndrome (petit mal variant), akinetic, and myoclonic seizures. May be useful in patients with absence (petit mal) seizures who have failed to respond to succinimides.

➤*Panic disorders:* For the treatment of panic disorder, with or without agoraphobia, as defined in DSM-IV (see Antianxiety Agents section).

Administration and Dosage

➤*Seizure disorders:*

Adults – Do not exceed initial dose of 1.5 mg/day in 3 divided doses. Increase in increments of 0.5 to 1 mg every 3 days until seizures are adequately controlled or until side effects preclude any further increase. Individualize maintenance dosage. Maximum recommended dosage is 20 mg/day.

Up to 30% of patients have shown a loss of anticonvulsant activity, often within 3 months of administration; dosage adjustment may re-establish efficacy.

Infants and children (up to 10 years of age or 30 kg) – To minimize drowsiness, the initial dose must be between 0.01 and 0.03 mg/kg/day, not to exceed 0.05 mg/kg/day, given in 2 or 3 divided doses. Increase dosage by no more than 0.25 to 0.5 mg every third day until a daily maintenance dose of 0.1 to 0.2 mg/kg has been reached, unless seizures are controlled or side effects preclude further increase. When possible, divide the daily dose into 3 equal doses. If doses are not equally divided, give the largest dose at bedtime.

➤*Administration:* Swallow tablet whole with water. Administer the orally disintegrating tablet as follows: After opening the pouch, peel back the foil on the blister. Do not push the tablet through foil. Immediately upon opening the blister, using dry hands, remove the tablet and place it in the mouth. Tablet disintegration occurs rapidly in saliva so it can be easily swallowed with or with out water.

➤*Storage/Stability:* Store at 25°C (77°F); excursions permitted to 15° to 30° (59° to 86°F).

CLORAZEPATE DIPOTASSIUM

c-iv	**Clorazepate** (Various, eg, Able, Mylan, Taro, UDL, Watson)	**Tablets:** 3.75 mg	In 100s, 500s, 1000s, and UD 100s.
c-iv	**Tranxene T-Tab** (Ovation)		FD&C Blue No. 2. (TL). Blue, six-sided, scored. In 100s, 500s, and UD 100s.
c-iv	**Clorazepate** (Various, eg, Able, Mylan, Taro, UDL, Watson)	**Tablets:** 7.5 mg	In 100s, 500s, 1000s, and UD 100s.
c-iv	**Tranxene T-Tab** (Ovation)		(TM). Peach, six-sided, scored. In 100s, 500s, and UD 100s.
c-iv	**Clorazepate** (Various, eg, Able, Mylan, Taro, UDL, Watson)	**Tablets:** 15 mg	In 100s, 500s, 1000s, and UD 100s.
c-iv	**Tranxene T-Tab** (Ovation)		(TN). Lavender, six-sided, scored. In 100s, 500s, and UD 100s.
c-iv	**Tranxene-SD Half Strength** (Abbott)	**Tablets, extended-release:** 11.25 mg	FD&C Blue No. 2, lactose. (TX). Blue. In 100s.
c-iv	**Tranxene-SD** (Abbott)	**Tablets, extended-release:** 22.5 mg	Lactose. (TY). Tan. In 100s.

Refer to the general discussion beginning in the Anticonvulsants introduction. For complete prescribing information, refer to the Benzodiazepine monograph in the Antianxiety Agents section.

Indications

➤*Alcohol withdrawal:* For the symptomatic relief of acute alcohol withdrawal (see monograph in the Antianxiety Agents section).

➤*Anxiety:* For the management of anxiety disorders or for the short-term relief of the symptoms of anxiety (see monograph in the Antianxiety Agents section).

➤*Partial seizures:* Used as adjunctive therapy in the management of partial seizures.

Administration and Dosage

To minimize drowsiness, do not exceed recommended initial dosages and increments.

➤*Partial seizures:*

Adults and children (older than 12 years of age) – Maximum initial dose is 7.5 mg orally 3 times/day. Increase by no more than 7.5 mg/week and do not exceed 90 mg/day.

Children (9 to 12 years of age) – Maximum initial dose is 7.5 mg orally 2 times/day. Increase by no more than 7.5 mg/week; do not exceed 60 mg/day. Not recommended in patients younger than 9 years of age.

➤*Extended-release (ER) tablets:* A 22.5 mg ER tablet may be administered as a single dose once daily as an alternate dosage form for patients stabilized on a dose of 7.5 mg 3 times/day; do not use to initiate therapy.

The 11.25 mg ER tablets may be administered as a single dose once daily as an alternate dosage form for patients stabilized on a dose of 3.75 mg 3 times/day; do not use to initiate therapy.

➤*Storage/Stability:* Store below 25°C (77°F).

DIAZEPAM

c-iv	**Diazepam** (Various, eg, Barr, Danbury, Ivax, Mylan, Purepac, UDL)	**Tablets:** 2 mg	In 100s, 500s, 1000s, 5000s, and UD 100s.
c-iv	**Valium** (Roche)		Lactose. (Roche 2 Valium). White, scored. Round with cut out V. In 100s and 500s.
c-iv	**Diazepam** (Various, eg, Barr, Danbury, Ivax, Mylan, Purepac, UDL)	**Tablets:** 5 mg	In 100s, 500s, 1000s, 5000s, and UD 100s.
c-iv	**Valium** (Roche)		Lactose. (Roche 5 Valium). Yellow, scored. Round with cut out V. In 100s and 500s.

DIAZEPAM

c-iv	**Diazepam** (Various, eg, Barr, Danbury, Ivax, Mylan, Purepac, UDL)	**Tablets:** 10 mg	In 100s, 500s, 1000s, 5000s, and UD 100s.
c-iv	**Valium** (Roche)		FD&C Blue No. 1, lactose. (Roche 10 Valium). Blue, scored. Round with cut out V. In 100s and 500s.
c-iv	**Diazepam** (Roxane)	**Solution:** 1 mg/mL	Sorbitol. Orange. Wintergreen-spice flavor. In 500 mL and UD 5 and 10 mL.
c-iv	**Diazepam Intensol** (Roxane)	**Solution, concentrate (Intensol):** 5 mg/mL	Alcohol. In 30 mL w/dropper.
c-iv	**Diazepam** (Various, eg, Abbott, Steris, Zenith Goldline)	**Injection:** 5 mg/mL	1.5% benzyl alcohol, 10% alcohol. In 2 mL cartridges.
c-iv	**Diastat** (Xcel)	**Gel, rectal:** 2.5 mg (pediatric)	1.5% benzyl alcohol, 10% ethyl alcohol. In twin packs. Includes lubricating jelly and plastic applicator with flexible, molded tip in 2 lengths.
		5 mg (pediatric)	1.5% benzyl alcohol, 10% ethyl alcohol. In twin packs. Includes lubricating jelly and plastic applicator with flexible, molded tip in 2 lengths.
		10 mg	1.5% benzyl alcohol, 10% ethyl alcohol. In twin packs. Includes lubricating jelly and plastic applicator with flexible, molded tip in 2 lengths.
		15 mg (adult)	1.5% benzyl alcohol, 10% ethyl alcohol. In twin packs. Includes lubricating jelly and plastic applicator with flexible, molded tip in 2 lengths.
		20 mg (adult)	1.5% benzyl alcohol, 10% ethyl alcohol. In twin packs. Includes lubricating jelly and plastic applicator with flexible, molded tip in 2 lengths.

Refer to the general discussion beginning in the Anticonvulsants introduction. For complete prescribing information, refer to the Benzodiazepine monograph in the Antianxiety Agents section.

Indications

➤*Acute alcohol withdrawal (except rectal gel):* Useful in the symptomatic relief of acute agitation, tremor, impending or acute delirium tremens, and hallucinosis (see Antianxiety Agents section).

➤*Antianxiety disorders (except rectal gel):* For the management of anxiety disorders or for the short-term relief of the symptoms of anxiety (see Antianxiety Agents section).

➤*Convulsive disorders:*

Oral – Adjunctive therapy in convulsive disorders. Effectiveness as sole therapy has not been proven.

Rectal – For the management of selected, refractory patients with epilepsy on stable regimens of anti-epileptic agents who require intermittent use of diazepam to control bouts of increased seizure activity.

➤*Muscle spasm (except rectal gel):* Adjunct for the relief of skeletal muscle spasm caused by reflex spasm to local pathology (eg, inflammation of the muscle or joints or secondary to trauma); spasticity caused by upper motor neuron disorders (eg, cerebral palsy, paraplegia); athetosis; stiff-man syndrome; tetanus (parenteral only) (see Skeletal Muscle Relaxants section).

➤*Status epilepticus/severe recurrent convulsive seizures (parenteral only):* Adjunctive therapy in status epilepticus and severe recurrent convulsive seizures.

➤*Surgical procedures (except rectal gel):* As an adjunct prior to endoscopic and surgical procedures if apprehension, anxiety, or acute stress reactions are present and to diminish patients recall of the procedures. Intravenously, prior to cardioversion, for the relief of anxiety and tension (see Antianxiety Agents section).

Administration and Dosage

➤*Convulsive disorders:* Individualize dosage. Some patients may require higher doses than those given below. In such cases, increase dosage cautiously to avoid adverse effects. Use lower doses and slowly increase the dose in elderly or debilitated patients and when other sedative drugs are administered.

➤*Convulsive disorders (tablets, oral solution, Intensol):*

Adults – 2 to 10 mg 2 to 4 times/day.

Elderly or debilitated patients – 2 to 2.5 mg once or twice daily initially. Increase gradually as needed and tolerated. Limit dosage to the smallest effective amount to preclude the development of ataxia or oversedation.

Children at least 6 months of age – Not for use in children younger than 6 months of age. Give 1 to 2.5 mg 3 or 4 times/day initially; increase gradually as needed and tolerated.

➤*Intensol preparation:* Intensol is a concentrated oral solution and must be mixed with liquid or semi-solid food (eg, water, juices, soda or soda-like beverages), applesauce, puddings). Consume the entire amount immediately. Do not store.

➤*Rectal:* 0.2 to 0.5 mg/kg, depending on age. Calculate the recommended dose by rounding upward to the next available unit dose. A second dose, when required, may be given 4 to 12 hours after the first dose. Do not treat more than 5 episodes/month or more than 1 episode every 5 days.

Children 2 to 5 years of age – 0.5 mg/kg.

Children 6 to 11 years of age – 0.3 mg/kg.

Adults and children older than 12 years of age – 0.2 mg/kg.

The following table provides acceptable weight ranges for each dose:

Diazepam Rectal Dosing Based on Age and Weight			
2 to 5 years of age weight (kg)	6 to 11 years of age weight (kg)	≥ 12 years of age weight (kg)	Dose (mg)
6 to 11	10 to 18	14 to 27	5
12 to 22	19 to 37	28 to 50	10
23 to 33	38 to 55	51 to 75	15
34 to 44	56 to 74	76 to 111	20

A 2.5 mg supplemental dose may be given for patients requiring more precise dose titration or as a partial replacement dose for patients who may expel a portion of the first dose.

Elderly and/or debilitated patients – Adjust dosage downward to reduce ataxia or oversedation.

➤*Status epilepticus/severe recurrent convulsive seizures (parenteral only):*

Administration – The IV route is preferred in the convulsing patient. However, if IV administration is impossible, the IM route may be used. Inject deeply into the muscle. Inject IV slowly (at least 1 minute for each 5 mg). Do not use small veins (eg, dorsum of hand or wrist); avoid intra-arterial use and extravasation.

Adults – 5 to 10 mg initially. May be repeated at 10- to 15-minute intervals up to a maximum dose of 30 mg if necessary. Therapy may be repeated in 2 to 4 hours; however, residual active metabolites may persist. Exercise extreme caution in individuals with chronic lung disease or unstable cardiovascular status.

Children at least 5 years of age – 1 mg every 2 to 5 minutes up to a maximum of 10 mg. Repeat in 2 to 4 hours if necessary. EEG monitoring of the seizure may be helpful.

Infants older than 30 days of age and children younger than 5 years of age – 0.2 to 0.5 mg slowly every 2 to 5 minutes up to a maximum of 5 mg. Repeat in 2 to 4 hours if necessary. EEG monitoring of the seizure may be helpful.

Although seizures may be brought under control promptly, a significant proportion of patients experience a return to seizure activity because of the short-lived effect of IV diazepam. Be prepared to readminister. Not recommended for maintenance; once seizures are controlled, administer agents indicated for long-term seizure control.

➤*Admixture incompatibility:* Do not mix or dilute with other solutions or drugs in syringe or infusion flask. If it is not feasible to administer directly IV, it may be slowly injected through the infusion tubing as close as possible to the vein insertion.

➤*Tonic status epilepticus:* Tonic status epilepticus has been precipitated in patients treated with IV diazepam for petit mal status or petit mal variant status.

➤*Special-risk patients:* Use extreme care in administering IV diazepam to the elderly, to very ill patients, and to those with limited pulmonary reserve; apnea or cardiac arrest may occur.

➤*Storage/Stability:*

Injection – Protect from light. Store at room temperature, 15° to 30°C (59° to 86°F). Do not use if solution is darker than slightly yellow or contains a precipitate.

Tablets, Intensol, rectal gel – Store at controlled room temperature 15° to 30°C (59° to 86°F). Protect from moisture.

Benzodiazepines

LORAZEPAM

c-iv	**Lorazepam** (Abbott)	**Injection:** 2 mg/mL	In single and 10 mL multidose vials.[1]
c-iv	**Ativan** (Baxter)		In single and 10 mL multidose vials.[1]
c-iv	**Lorazepam** (Abbott)	**Injection:** 4 mg/mL	In single and 10 mL multidose vials.[1]
c-iv	**Ativan** (Baxter)		In single and 10 mL multidose vials.[1]

[1] With PEG 400, propylene glycol, and 2% benzyl alcohol.

Complete prescribing information begins in the Benzodiazepines group monograph. For information on the antianxiety use of lorazepam, refer to the individual monograph in the Antianxiety section.

Indications

➤*Preanesthetic:* Used in adults for preanesthetic medication to produce sedation, relieve anxiety, and decrease the ability to recall events related to surgery (see Antianxiety monograph).

➤*Status epilepticus:* For the treatment of status epilepticus.

Administration and Dosage

Individualize dosage. Increase dosage gradually to minimize adverse effects. When higher dosage is indicated, increase the evening dose before the daytime doses.

➤*Status epilepticus:* 4 mg IV given slowly (2 mg/min). If seizures continue or recur after a 10- to 15-minute observation period, an additional 4 mg IV dose may be slowly administered.

IM – IM administration is not preferred in the treatment of status epilepticus because therapeutic lorazepam levels may not be reached as quickly as with IV administration. However, when an IV port is not available, the IM route may prove useful.

➤*Administration:*

IV – Immediately prior to IV use, dilute with an equal volume of compatible solution (sterile water for injection, sodium chloride injection, or 5% dextrose injection). Do not shake vigorously, as this will result in air entrapment. Inject directly into a vein or into tubing of an existing IV infusion. Do not exceed 2 mg/min. Have equipment available to maintain a patent airway.

IM – Inject undiluted deep into the muscle mass.

➤*Concomitant medications:* Reduce the dose of lorazepam by 50% when coadministered with probenecid or valproate. It may be necessary to increase the lorazepam dose in females who are concomitantly taking oral contraceptives.

➤*Storage/Stability:* Refrigerate at 2° to 8°C (36° to 46°F). Protect from light.

CARBAMAZEPINE

Rx	**Carbamazepine** (Various, eg, Ivax, Shire, Taro, Teva, UDL)	**Tablets, chewable:** 100 mg	May contain corn starch, sorbitol, sucrose. In 100s, 500s, and UD 50s and 100s.
Rx	**Tegretol** (Novartis)		Sucrose. (Tegretol 52 52). Pink, red-speckled, scored. In 100s and UD 100s.
Rx	**Carbamazepine** (Various, eg, Ivax, Taro, Teva, Tor-Pharm, UDL)	**Tablets:** 200 mg	May contain corn starch, lactose. In 100s, 500s, 1000s, and UD 100s and 300s.
Rx	**Epitol** (Teva)		Lactose. (Epitol 93-93). White, scored. In 100s.
Rx	**Tegretol** (Novartis)		(Tegretol 27 27). Pink, scored. Capsule shape. In 100s, 1000s, and UD 100s.
Rx	**Tegretol-XR** (Novartis)	**Tablets, extended-release:** 100 mg	Mannitol. (T 100 mg). Yellow. In 100s.
		200 mg	Mannitol. (T 200 mg). Pink. In 100s.
		400 mg	Mannitol. (T 400 mg). Brown. In 100s.
Rx	**Carbatrol** (Shire)	**Capsules, extended-release:** 100 mg	Lactose. (Shire). Bluish green. In 14s and 120s.
		200 mg	Lactose. (Shire). Lt. gray and bluish green. In 30s and 120s.
		300 mg	Lactose. (Shire). Black and bluish green. In 30s and 120s.
Rx	**Carbamazepine** (Various, eg, Alpharma, Taro)	**Suspension:** 100 mg/5 mL	May contain saccharin, sorbitol, sucrose, parabens. In 450 mL and UD 10 mL.
Rx	**Tegretol** (Novartis)		Sorbitol, sucrose. Citrus/vanilla flavor. In 450 mL.
Rx	**Carbamazepine** (Alpharma)	200 mg/10 mL	Sorbitol, sucrose. Citrus/vanilla flavor. In 10 mL dose cups.

Refer to the general discussion beginning in the Anticonvulsants introduction.

WARNING

Aplastic anemia and agranulocytosis have been reported in association with carbamazepine therapy. The risk of developing these reactions is 5 to 8 times greater than in the general population; however, the overall risk of these reactions in the untreated general population is low (approximately 6 and 2 patients per 1 million per year for agranulocytosis and aplastic anemia, respectively). Although reports of transient or persistent decreased platelet or white blood cell counts are not uncommon in association with the use of carbamazepine, data are not available to estimate accurately their incidence or outcome; however, the vast majority of the cases of leukopenia have not progressed to the more serious conditions of aplastic anemia or agranulocytosis. Because of the very low incidence of agranulocytosis and aplastic anemia, the vast majority of minor hematologic changes observed in monitoring of patients on carbamazepine are unlikely to signal the occurrence of either abnormality. Nonetheless, obtain complete pretreatment hematological testing as a baseline. If a patient exhibits low or decreased white blood cell or platelet counts during the course of treatment, monitor the patient closely. Consider discontinuation of the drug if any evidence of significant bone marrow depression develops.

Indications

►*Epilepsy:* For the treatment of partial seizures with complex symptoms (psychomotor, temporal lobe); patients with these seizures appear to show greatest improvement. For generalized tonic-clonic seizures (grand mal), mixed seizure patterns, or other partial or generalized seizures.

►*Trigeminal neuralgia:* For the treatment of pain associated with true trigeminal neuralgia. Beneficial results also have been reported in glossopharyngeal neuralgia.

►*Unlabeled uses:* For the treatment of restless leg syndrome; alternative/adjunctive treatment for certain symptoms associated with borderline personality disorder; alternative to benzodiazepines for managing alcohol withdrawal; adjunctive therapy for schizophrenia.

Alternative or adjunctive treatment for manic or mixed episodes of bipolar disorder – Initial dose of 200 to 600 mg/day in 2 to 4 divided doses. Usual maintenance dose of 1000 mg/day; maximum dose of 1600 mg/day.

Treatment of postherpetic neuralgia – Initial dose of 100 mg at bedtime; increase by 100 mg every 3 days until dosage is 200 mg 2 times/day, response is adequate, or blood drug level is 6 to 12 mcg/mL.

Administration and Dosage

Individualize dosage. A low initial daily dosage with gradual increase is advised. As soon as adequate control is achieved, reduce dosage gradually to the minimum effective level. Take with meals.

Because a given dose of carbamazepine suspension will produce higher peak levels than the same dose given as the tablet, start with low doses (children 6 to 12 years of age, ½ teaspoon 4 times/day) and increase slowly to avoid unwanted side effects.

Do not administer carbamazepine suspension simultaneously with other liquid medications or diluents.

►*Capsules, extended-release:* Extended-release capsules may be opened and the beads sprinkled over food such as a teaspoon of applesauce or other similar food products if this method of administration is preferred. Do not crush or chew the capsules or their contents. Extended-release capsules can be taken with or without meals.

►*Conversion from tablets to suspension:* Convert by administering the same number of milligrams per day in smaller, more frequent doses (eg, twice daily tablets to 3 times/day suspension).

►*Conversion from conventional tablets to extended-release tablets:* Extended-release carbamazepine is for twice daily administration. Administer the same total daily milligram dose of extended-release carbamazepine. Swallow extended-release carbamazepine tablets whole, and never crush or chew. Inspect extended-release carbamazepine tablets for chips or cracks; do not consume damaged tablets. Extended-release carbamazepine tablet coating is not absorbed and is excreted in the feces; these coatings may be noticeable in the stool.

►*Combination therapy:* When adding to existing anticonvulsant therapy, add the drug gradually while the other anticonvulsants are maintained or gradually decreased, except phenytoin, which may have to be increased.

Carbamazepine Dosages								
Indication		Initial dose			Titration		Maintenance	Maximum daily dose
Epilepsy	Tablets[a]	Extended-release formulations	Suspension	Tablets	Extended-release formulations	Suspension	All formulations	All formulations
Adults and children over 12 years of age	200 mg twice daily	200 mg twice daily	100 mg 4 times/day	Increase at weekly intervals of no more than 200 mg/day using a 3- or 4-times/day regimen	Increase at weekly intervals of no more than 200 mg/day using a 2 times/day regimen	Increase at weekly intervals of no more than 200 mg/day using a 3- or 4-times/day regimen	Adjust to minimum effective level, usually 800 to 1200 mg/day	12 to 15 years of age: 1000 mg/day 16 years of age and older: 1200 mg/day Adults, rare instances: 1600 mg/day

CARBAMAZEPINE

		Carbamazepine Dosages						
Indication	Initial dose			Titration			Maintenance	Maximum daily dose
Epilepsy	Tablets[a]	Extended-release formulations	Suspension	Tablets	Extended-release formulations	Suspension	All formulations	All formulations
Children 6 to 12 years of age	100 mg twice daily	Tablets: 100 mg twice daily Capsules: N/A[b]	50 mg 4 times/day	Increase at weekly intervals of no more than 100 mg/day using a 3- or 4-times/day regimen	Increase at weekly intervals of no more than 100 mg/day using a 2 times/day regimen	Increase at weekly intervals of no more than 100 mg/day using a 3- or 4-times/day regimen	Adjust to minimum effective level, usually 400 to 800 mg/day	Tablets/suspension: 1000 mg/day. Capsules: 35 mg/kg/day
Children younger than 6 years of	10 to 20 mg/kg/day 2 or 3 times/day	N/A[b]	10 to 20 mg/kg/day 4 times/day	Increase weekly to achieve optimal clinical response administered 3- or 4-times/day	N/A	Increase weekly to achieve optimal clinical response administered 3- or 4-times/day	Ordinarily, optimal responses are achieved at daily doses less than 35 mg/kg	35 mg/kg/day
Trigeminal neuralgia	100 mg twice daily	Tablets: 100 mg twice daily Capsules: 200 mg once daily	50 mg 4 times/day	May increase by up to 200 mg/day using 100 mg increments every 12 hr as needed	May increase by up to 200 mg/day using 100 mg increments every 12 hours as needed	May increase by 50 mg/day 4 times/day as needed	Usually 400 to 800 mg/day; attempt to reduce the dosage or discontinue the drug at least once every 3 months	1200 mg/day

[a] Dosing applies to conventional tablets and chewable tablets.

[b] Children receiving total daily dosages of 400 mg immediate-release carbamazepine or greater may be converted to the same total daily dosage of the extended-release capsules using a twice daily regimen.

➤*Storage/Stability:* Shake suspension well before using. Do not store above 30°C (86°F); protect from moisture and light.

Actions

➤*Pharmacology:* Carbamazepine is an anticonvulsant effective in the treatment of psychomotor and grand mal seizures, as well as trigeminal neuralgia.It is an iminostilbene derivative chemically related to the tricyclic antidepressants and unrelated to other anticonvulsants or agents used to control the pain of trigeminal neuralgia. Its mechanism of action is unknown. It appears to act by reducing polysynaptic responses and blocking post-tetanic potentiation.

➤*Pharmacokinetics:*

Absorption/Distribution – The suspension, conventional tablet, and extended-release tablet deliver equivalent amounts of drug to the systemic circulation; however, the suspension is absorbed somewhat faster (T_{max} 1.5 hours) and the extended-release tablet/capsule slightly slower (T_{max} 3 to 19 hours) than the conventional tablet (T_{max} 4 to 5 hours). The bioavailability of the extended-release tablet was 89% compared with suspension. Following a twice-daily dosage regimen, the suspension has higher peak levels and lower trough levels than those obtained from the tablet formulation for the same dosage regimen. However, the suspension given 3 times/day affords steady-state plasma levels comparable with the tablets given twice daily when administered at the same total daily dose. Following a twice-daily dosage regimen, extended-release tablets afford steady-state plasma levels comparable with conventional tablets given 4 times/day when administered at the same total daily dose. Plasma levels are variable and may range from 0.5 to 25 mcg/mL, with no apparent relationship to the daily intake of the drug. Usual adult therapeutic levels are between 4 and 12 mcg/mL. Carbamazepine is 76% bound to plasma proteins. The CSF/serum ratio is 0.22, similar to 24% unbound carbamazepine in serum. Transplacental passage of carbamazepine is rapid (30 to 60 minutes); the drug accumulates in fetal tissues, with higher levels found in the liver and kidney than in the brain and lungs.

Metabolism/Excretion – Carbamazepine is metabolized in the liver by the P450 3A4 isozyme to the 10,11–epoxide, which also has anticonvulsant activity. Because it can induce its own metabolism, the half-life is variable. Initial half-life ranges from 25 to 65 hours and decreases to 12 to 17 hours with repeated doses. The half-life of the metabolite is somewhat shorter than that of the parent drug. After administration, 72% is found in urine and 28% in feces. Urinary products are composed largely of hydroxylated and conjugated metabolites, with only 3% unchanged carbamazepine.

Children – There is a poor correlation between plasma concentrations of carbamazepine and the *Tegretol* dose in children. Carbamazepine is more rapidly metabolized to carbamazepine-10,11-epoxide in the younger age group than in adults. In children below the age of 15, there is an inverse relationship between CBZ-E/CBZ ratio and increasing age.

Contraindications

History of bone marrow depression; hypersensitivity to carbamazepine and tricyclic compounds; concomitant use of monoamine oxidase (MAO) inhibitors. Discontinue MAO inhibitors for at least 14 days before carbamazepine administration (see Drug Interactions).

Warnings

➤*Minor pain:* This drug is not a simple analgesic. Do not use for the relief of minor aches or pains.

➤*Dermatologic:* Severe dermatologic reactions, including toxic epidermal necrolysis (Lyell syndrome) and Stevens-Johnson syndrome, have been reported with carbamazepine. These reactions have been extremely rare; however, a few fatalities have been reported.

➤*Hematologic:* Patients with a history of adverse hematologic reaction to any drug may be particularly at risk.

➤*Anticholinergic effects:* Carbamazepine has shown mild anticholinergic activity; therefore, use with caution in patients with increased intraocular pressure.

➤*CNS effects:* Because of the drug's relationship to other tricyclic compounds, the possibility of activating latent psychosis and confusion or agitation in elderly patients exists.

➤*Hypersensitivity reactions:* Hypersensitivity reactions to carbamazepine have been reported in patients who previously experienced this reaction to anticonvulsants, including phenytoin and phenobarbital. Obtain a history of hypersensitivity reactions for the patient and the immediate family members. If positive, use caution in prescribing carbamazepine. Multi-organ hypersensitivity reactions occurring days to weeks or months after initiating treatment have been reported in rare cases (see Adverse Reactions). Consider discontinuation of carbamazepine if any evidence of hypersensitivity develops.

➤*Carcinogenesis:* Carbamazepine administered to rats for 2 years at doses of 25 to 250 mg/kg/day resulted in a dose-related increase in the incidence of hepatocellular tumors in females and benign interstitial cell adenomas in the testes of males.

➤*Pregnancy: Category D.* Carbamazepine can cause fetal harm when administered to a pregnant woman. Epidemiological data suggest that there may be an association between the use of carbamazepine during pregnancy and congenital malformations, including spina bifida. Compared with monotherapy, there may be a higher prevalence of teratogenic effects associated with the use of anticonvulsants in combination therapy. Therefore, if therapy is to be continued, monotherapy may be preferable for pregnant women.

Use only when clearly needed and when the potential benefits outweigh the potential hazards to the fetus. For information on use during pregnancy, refer to the Anticonvulsants introduction.

➤*Lactation:* Carbamazepine and its epoxide metabolite are transferred in to breast milk. The ratio of the concentration in breast milk to that in maternal plasma is about 0.4 for carbamazepine and about 0.5 for the epoxide. The estimated doses given to the newborn during breastfeeding are in the range of 2 to 5 mg/day for carbamazepine and 1 to 2 mg/day for the epoxide. Because of the potential for serious adverse reactions, decide whether to discontinue nursing or to discontinue the drug, taking into account the importance of the drug to the mother.

➤*Children:* Carbamazepine's effectiveness for use in the management of pediatric patients with epilepsy is derived from clinical investiga-

CARBAMAZEPINE

tions performed in adults and in vitro systems. The generally accepted therapeutic range of total carbamazepine in plasma (ie, 4 to 12 mcg/mL) is the same in children and adults. The safety of carbamazepine in pediatric patients has been systematically studied up to 6 months of age.

Precautions

➤*Monitoring:* Obtain complete pretreatment blood counts, including platelets and possibly reticulocytes and serum iron, as a baseline. If, in the course of treatment, a patient exhibits low or decreased white blood cell or platelet counts, monitor the patient closely. Consider discontinuation of the drug if any evidence of significant bone marrow depression develops.

Perform baseline liver function tests and periodic evaluations. Discontinue drug immediately if liver dysfunction occurs. Obtain baseline and periodic eye examinations (eg, slit lamp, funduscopy, tonometry), urinalysis, and BUN determinations.

Monitoring of blood levels may be particularly useful in cases of dramatic increase in seizure frequency, for verification of compliance and in determining the cause of toxicity when more than 1 medication is being used.

➤*Hepatic effects:* Hepatic effects, ranging from slight elevations in liver enzymes to rare cases of hepatic failure have been reported. In some cases, hepatic effects may progress despite discontinuation of the drug.

➤*Hyponatremia:* Hyponatremia has been reported in association with carbamazepine use either alone or in combination with other drugs.

➤*Absence seizures:* Absence seizures (petit mal) do not appear to be controlled by carbamazepine. Use with caution in patients with a mixed seizure disorder that includes atypical absence seizures because carbamazepine has been associated with increased frequency of generalized convulsions in these patients.

➤*Special risk:* Prescribe carbamazepine only after benefit-to-risk appraisal in patients with a history of the following: Cardiac, hepatic, or renal damage; adverse hematologic reaction to other drugs; interrupted courses of therapy with the drug.

➤*Hazardous tasks:* May produce drowsiness, dizziness, or blurred vision; inform patients to observe caution while driving or performing other tasks requiring alertness, coordination, or physical dexterity.

Drug Interactions

➤*P450 3A4:* Inhibitors of the 3A4 isozyme that have been shown or would be expected to increase plasma carbamazepine levels include cimetidine, clarithromycin, danazol, diltiazem, erythromycin, fluoxetine, isoniazid, itraconazole, ketoconazole, loratadine, niacinamide, nicotinamide, propoxyphene, troleandomycin, valproate, and verapamil.

Inducers of the 3A4 isozyme that have been shown or that would be expected to decrease plasma carbamazepine levels include cisplatin, doxorubicin, felbamate, phenobarbital, phenytoin, primidone, rifampin, and theophylline.

Carbamazepine Drug Interactions			
Precipitant drug	Object drug*		Description
Azole antifungal agents	Carbamazepine	↑	Plasma concentrations of carbamazepine may be elevated, increasing clinical and adverse effects. Closely monitor carbamazepine levels when an azole antifungal agent is started or stopped.
Barbiturates	Carbamazepine	↓	Decreased plasma carbamazepine concentrations may occur, resulting in possible loss of effectiveness. Closely monitor carbamazepine levels and consider discontinuing the barbiturate or adjusting the dose of carbamazepine as needed.
Charcoal	Carbamazepine	↓	Charcoal may decrease the GI absorption of carbamazepine (see Overdosage).
Cimetidine	Carbamazepine	↑	Carbamazepine plasma levels may increase; carbamazepine toxicity may result. Interaction appears to be of greater clinical importance when cimetidine is added to carbamazepine during the first 4 weeks of therapy.
Danazol	Carbamazepine	↑	Carbamazepine levels increased 38% to 123% within 30 days of danazol administration. Avoid concomitant administration if possible.
Diltiazem	Carbamazepine	↑	Serum carbamazepine concentrations may be increased; carbamazepine toxicity may result. Monitor serum carbamazepine levels and observe the patient.
Felbamate	Carbamazepine	↓	Serum levels of either agent may be decreased resulting in a loss of effectiveness. An average decrease of 25% in carbamazepine levels has been reported.
Carbamazepine	Felbamate	↓	
Hydantoins	Carbamazepine	↓	Both increased and decreased hydantoin plasma levels as well as decreased carbamazepine plasma levels have occurred during coadministration. Monitor serum concentrations of both drugs, particularly when starting or stopping one drug.
Carbamazepine	Hydantoins	↔	
Isoniazid	Carbamazepine	↑	Carbamazepine toxicity, isoniazid hepatotoxicity, or both may result. Isoniazid is suspected to inhibit carbamazepine metabolism and carbamazepine may increase isoniazid degradation to hepatotoxic metabolites.
Carbamazepine	Isoniazid		
Lamotrigine	Carbamazepine	↑	Lamotrigine levels may be reduced by 40%; carbamazepine half-life was reported to be reduced 1.7 hours per 100 mg. Also, serum levels of the active epoxide carbamazepine metabolite may be elevated.
Carbamazepine	Lamotrigine	↓	
Macrolide antibiotics (eg, clarithromycin, erythromycin, troleandomycin)	Carbamazepine	↑	Carbamazepine toxicity has occurred shortly after initiation of erythromycin; adding 8 to 33 mg/kg/day troleandomycin caused acute toxicity within 24 to 48 hours; addition of 250 mg clarithromycintwice daily for 10 days increased carbamazepine levels 60% despite a 22% reduction in carbamazepine dose.
MAO inhibitors	Carbamazepine	↑	Coadministration is contraindicated. Discontinue MAOI at least 14 days prior to administration of carbamazepine.
Carbamazepine	MAO inhibitors		
Nefazodone	Carbamazepine	↑	Elevated serum carbamazepine levels and lower nefazodone levels may result. Coadministration is contraindicated.
Carbamazepine	Nefazodone	↓	
Propoxyphene	Carbamazepine	↑	Increases in carbamazepine levels between 45% and 77% have been reported. Decreased carbamazepine clearance as a result of propoxyphene inhibition of hepatic metabolism has been proposed.
Protease inhibitors	Carbamazepine	↑	Carbamazepine levels may be elevated, increasing risk of toxicity, while the protease inhibitor levels may be decreased, resulting in antiretroviral treatment failure.
Carbamazepine	Protease inhibitors	↓	
SSRIs Fluoxetine Fluvoxamine	Carbamazepine	↑	Carbamazepine levels may be increased, producing possible toxicity.
Tricyclic antidepressants	Carbamazepine	↑	Carbamazepine toxicity was reported in 1 patient on concomitant desipramine. Lower imipramine, desipramine, amitriptyline, and doxepin levels have been reported with coadministration. A 60% reduction in nortriptyline levels requiring a doubling of the nortriptyline dose to achieve therapeutic levels also was reported after addition of carbamazepine.
Carbamazepine	Tricyclic antidepressants	↓	
Valproic acid	Carbamazepine	↔	Decreased valproic acid levels with possible loss of seizure control may occur. Variable changes in carbamazepine levels may occur. Monitor serum levels and observe for ≥ 1 month after starting or stopping either drug.
Carbamazepine	Valproic acid	↓	
Verapamil	Carbamazepine	↑	Concomitant therapy has resulted in symptoms of carbamazepine toxicity within 36 to 96 hours. Mean increases in total and free plasma carbamazepine levels were 46% and 33%, respectively.
Carbamazepine	Acetaminophen	↓	Carbamazepine may increase the metabolism of acetaminophen, increasing the risk of acetaminophen-induced hepatotoxicity and/or decreasing its effectiveness. Risk appears greatest during acetaminophen overdosage.

CARBAMAZEPINE

Carbamazepine Drug Interactions			
Precipitant drug	Object drug*		Description
Carbamazepine	Anticoagulants	↓	Carbamazepine may increase the metabolism of these agents due to induction of hepatic microsomal enzyme induction. Hypoprothrombinemic effect of the anticoagulants may be decreased. Monitor prothrombin times when starting or stopping carbamazepine therapy.
Carbamazepine	Benzodiazepines	↓	The pharmacological effects of benzodiazepines may be reduced. Adjust benzodiazepine dose as needed.
Carbamazepine	Bupropion	↓	Carbamazepine increases the hepatic P450 3A4 metabolism of bupropion and has been reported to decrease bupropion peaks by 87% and AUC by 90%.
Carbamazepine	Clozapine	↓	The pharmacological effects of clozapine may be reduced. Adjust the dose of clozapine as needed.
Carbamazepine	Contraceptives, oral and levonorgestrel subdermal implant contraceptives	↓	A decrease in contraceptive effectiveness, possibly leading to unintended breakthrough bleeding and/or pregnancy may occur. The AUC for an ethinyl estradiol/levonorgestrel oral contraceptives was reduced. Alternative contraceptive methods are recommended if coadministered.
Carbamazepine	Cyclosporine	↓	Cyclosporine levels may be decreased. Carbamazepine may induce the hepatic metabolism of cyclosporine. Monitor cyclosporine levels and observe the patient for signs of rejection or toxicity if carbamazepine is added or discontinued, respectively.
Carbamazepine	Doxycycline	↓	Doxycycline half-life and serum levels may be reduced. Consider the use of another tetracycline.
Carbamazepine	Felodipine	↓	The pharmacological effects of felodipine may be decreased. Patients receiving long-term concomitant therapy may require higher doses of felodipine to achieve therapeutic plasma levels.
Carbamazepine	Haloperidol	↓	Haloperidol serum levels and efficacy may be decreased by carbamazepine. A 60% decrease in levels has been reported.
Carbamazepine	Lithium	↑	Increased CNS toxicity may occur during concomitant therapy.
Carbamazepine	Nondepolarizing neuromuscular blockers	↓	Nondepolarizing muscle relaxants may have shorter than expected duration or be less effective. Reported pancuronium and atracurium postoperative recovery times were 42% to 70% faster.
Carbamazepine	Olanzapine	↓	Olanzapine plasma concentrations may be reduced. Adjust olanzapine dose as needed.
Carbamazepine	Primidone	↑↓	Primidone levels may be increased or decreased and carbamazepine levels may be decreased. Monitor serum levels of both and adjust dosages as needed.
Primidone	Carbamazepine		
Carbamazepine	Succinimides (eg, ethosuximide, methsuximide, phensuximide)	↓	Succinimide levels may be decreased.
Carbamazepine	Theophyllines	↑↓	Theophylline levels may be increased or decreased and carbamazepine levels may be decreased. Adjust doses accordingly as needed.
Theophyllines	Carbamazepine	↓	
Carbamazepine	Tiagabine	↓	Tiagabine levels may be reduced.
Carbamazepine	Topiramate	↓	Carbamazepine may decrease topiramate plasma levels. Monitor topiramate levels and adjust dose accordingly.
Carbamazepine	Voriconazole	↓	Voriconazole levels may be reduced. Coadministration is contraindicated.
Carbamazepine	Ziprasidone	↓	Ziprasidone plasma concentrations may be reduced. Monitor the clinical response to ziprasidone and adjust dose as needed.

* ↑ = Object drug increased.   ↓ = Object drug decreased.   ⟷ = Undetermined clinical effect.

➤*Drug/Lab test interactions:*
Thyroid function – Thyroid function tests show decreased values with carbamazepine.

Pregnancy tests – Interference with some pregnancy tests has been reported.

➤*Drug/Food interactions:*
Grapefruit juice – Serum carbamazepine levels may be elevated. Avoid coadministration of carbamazepine with grapefruit products.

Adverse Reactions

If adverse reactions are so severe that the drug must be discontinued, abrupt discontinuation in a responsive epileptic patient may lead to seizures or status epilepticus.

Most frequent – Dizziness; drowsiness; nausea; unsteadiness; vomiting. To minimize such reactions, initiate therapy at low doses.

➤*Cardiovascular:* Aggravation of coronary artery disease; aggravation of hypertension; arrhythmias; AV block; CHF; hypotension; syncope and collapse; thromboembolism; thrombophlebitis. Some cardiovascular complications have resulted in fatalities.

➤*CNS:* Abnormal involuntary movements; confusion; depression with agitation; disturbances of coordination; dizziness; drowsiness; fatigue; headache; hyperacusis; paralysis and other symptoms of cerebral arterial insufficiency; peripheral neuritis and paresthesias; speech disturbances; talkativeness; visual hallucinations.

➤*Dermatologic:* Aggravation of disseminated lupus erythematosus and toxic epidermal necrolysis (Lyell syndrome); alopecia; alterations in pigmentation; diaphoresis; erythema multiforme and nodosum; exfoliative dermatitis; photosensitivity reactions; pruritic and erythematous rashes; purpura; Stevens-Johnson syndrome; urticaria. Discontinuation of therapy may be necessary.

➤*GI:* Abdominal pain; anorexia; constipation; diarrhea; dryness of mouth and pharynx; gastric distress; glossitis and stomatitis; nausea; vomiting.

➤*GU:* Acute urinary retention; albuminuria; azotemia; elevated BUN; glycosuria; impotence; microscopic deposits in urine; oliguria with hypertension; renal failure; urinary frequency.

➤*Hematologic:* Acute intermittent porphyria; agranulocytosis; aplastic anemia; bone marrow depression; eosinophilia; leukocytosis; leukopenia; pancytopenia; thrombocytopenia (see Warning Box).

➤*Hepatic:* Abnormal liver function tests; cholestatic/hepatocellular jaundice; hepatic failure (rare); hepatitis.

➤*Hypersensitivity:* Multi-organ hypersensitivity reactions occurring days to weeks or months after initiating treatment have been reported in rare cases. Signs or symptoms may include, but are not limited to, abnormal liver function tests, arthralgia, disorders mimicking lymphoma, eosinophilia, fever, hepatosplenomegaly, leukopenia, lymphadenopathy, skin rashes, and vasculitis. These signs and symptoms may occur in various combinations and not necessarily concurrently. Signs and symptoms may initially be mild. Various organs, including but not limited to, colon, immune system, kidneys, liver, lungs, myocardium, pancreas, and skin may be affected (see Precautions).

➤*Lymphatic:* Adenopathy or lymphadenopathy.

➤*Metabolic:* Decreased plasma calcium levels; fever and chills; frank water intoxication, with decreased serum sodium (hyponatremia) and confusion; inappropriate antidiuretic hormone (ADH) secretion syndrome.

➤*Musculoskeletal:* Aching joints and muscles; leg cramps.

➤*Ophthalmic:* Blurred vision; conjunctivitis; nystagmus; transient diplopia and oculomotor disturbances; scattered, punctate cortical lens opacities.

➤*Pulmonary:* Pulmonary hypersensitivity characterized by dyspnea, fever, pneumonitis, or pneumonia.

➤*Miscellaneous:* Aseptic meningitis accompanied by myoclonus and peripheral eosinophilia; edema; pancreatitis; isolated cases of lupus erythematosus-like syndrome; tinnitus.

Overdosage

➤*Toxic doses:*
Lowest known lethal dose –
Adults: 3.2 g (a woman 24 years of age died from cardiac arrest and a man 24 years of age died of pneumonia and hypoxic encephalopathy).
Children: 4 g (a girl 14 years of age died from cardiac arrest).
Small children: 1.6 g (a girl 3 years of age died of aspiration pneumonia).

CARBAMAZEPINE

▶*Symptoms:* Signs and symptoms first appear after 1 to 3 hours of ingestion. Neuromuscular disturbances are the most prominent. Cardiovascular disorders are generally mild, and severe cardiac complications occur only when very high doses (greater than 60 g) have been ingested.

Respiration – Irregular breathing; respiratory depression.

Cardiovascular – Conduction disorders; EEG may show dysrhythmias; hypotension or hypertension; shock; tachycardia.

CNS – Impaired consciousness ranging to adiadochokinesia; ataxia; athetoid movements; ballism; convulsions, especially in small children; deep coma; dizziness; drowsiness; dysmetria; initial hyperreflexia followed by hyporeflexia; motor restlessness; muscular twitching; mydriasis; nystagmus; opisthotonos; psychomotor disturbances; tremor.

GI / GU – Anuria or oliguria; nausea; urinary retention; vomiting.

Laboratory findings – Isolated instances of overdosage have included acetonuria, glycosuria, leukocytosis, and reduced leukocyte count.

▶*Treatment:* The prognosis in cases of severe poisoning is dependent upon prompt elimination of the drug. Even when more than 4 hours have elapsed following ingestion of the drug, irrigate the stomach repeatedly, especially if the patient also has consumed alcohol. There is no specific antidote. Refer to General Management of Acute Overdosage. Charcoal administration is effective in increasing the total body clearance of carbamazepine. The recommended dosage is 50 to 100 g initially followed by a rate of at least 12.5 g/hour, preferably via a nasogastric tube; continue until the patient is symptom free.

Dialysis is indicated only in severe poisoning associated with renal failure. Replacement transfusion is indicated in severe poisoning in small children.

In treating convulsions, diazepam or barbiturates may aggravate respiratory depression (especially in children), cause hypotension, and coma. Do not use barbiturates if MAO inhibitors also have been taken by the patient either in overdosage or in recent therapy (within 1 week).

Monitor – Monitor respiration, ECG, blood pressure, body temperature, pupillary reflexes, and kidney and bladder function for several days.

Treatment of blood count abnormalities – If evidence of significant bone marrow depression develops: Discontinue drug; perform daily CBC, platelet and reticulocyte counts; perform bone marrow aspiration and trephine biopsy immediately, and repeat with sufficient frequency to monitor recovery. Fully developed aplastic anemia requires intensive monitoring and therapy; seek specialized consultation.

Special periodic studies might be helpful as follows: White cell and platelet antibodies; [59]Fe – ferrokinetic studies; peripheral blood cell typing; cytogenetic studies on marrow and peripheral blood; bone marrow cultures for colony-forming units; hemoglobin electrophoresis for A_2 and F hemoglobin; serum folic acid; B_{12} levels.

Patient Information

Advise patients that carbamazepine may produce drowsiness, dizziness, or blurred vision; advise patients to observe caution while driving or performing other tasks requiring alertness, coordination, or physical dexterity.

Advise patients to notify physician if any of the following occurs: Unusual bleeding or bruising, fever, sore throat, rash or ulcers in the mouth, lymphadenopathy, and petechial or purpuric hemorrhage, and in the case of liver reactions, anorexia, nausea/vomiting, or jaundice.

Advise patients to take with food; however, the extended-release capsules can be taken with or without food.

Inform patients that the extended-release tablet coating is not absorbed and is excreted in the feces; these coatings may be noticeable in the stool.

Inform patients not to administer carbamazepine suspension simultaneously with other liquid medications.

Advise patients taking the suspension to shake well before administering.

Inform patients that the capsule formulation may be opened and the beads sprinkled over food such as applesauce or other similar foods. Do not crush or chew the capsule contents.

MAGNESIUM SULFATE

Rx	Magnesium Sulfate[1] (Abbott)	Injection: 4%[2] (0.325 mEq/mL)	In 100, 500, and 1000 mL single-dose flexible containers.
		8%[2] (0.65 mEq/mL)	In 50 mL single-dose flexible containers.
Rx	Magnesium Sulfate[1] (Various, eg, Abbott)	Injection: 12.5% (1 mEq/mL)	Preservative-free. In 8 mL single-dose vials.
Rx	Magnesium Sulfate[1] (Various, eg, Abbott, American Pharmaceutical Partners, American Regent)	Injection: 50% (4 mEq/mL)	Preservative-free. In 2 and 10 mL single-dose amps, 2, 10, and 20 mL single-dose vials, 50 mL multi-dose vials, and 5 and 10 mL syringes.

[1] As heptahydrate.

[2] In water for injection.

For further information refer to the general discussion beginning in the Anticonvulsants introduction. Refer to monographs in the Mineral and IV Nutritional Therapy sections.

Indications

▶*Acute nephritis in children:* To control hypertension, encephalopathy, and convulsions associated with acute nephritis in children.

▶*Hypomagnesemia:* For replacement therapy in magnesium deficiency, especially in acute hypomagnesemia accompanied by signs of tetany similar to those observed in hypocalcemia. When added to total parenteral nutrition therapy, to correct or prevent hypomagnesemia that may arise during the course of therapy (see the monograph in the IV Nutritional Therapy section).

▶*Seizures associated with eclampsia:* For seizure prevention and control in severe pre-eclampsia or eclampsia without producing deleterious CNS depression in the mother or infant.

▶*Unlabeled uses:* Magnesium sulfate is commonly used as a tocolytic agent in the management of preterm labor.

Magnesium sulfate (2 g IV over 1 to 2 minutes for adults) has been shown to prevent recurrences of torsades de pointes by suppressing early-after depolarizations.

In patients with severe acute asthma, the IV administration of magnesium sulfate may improve pulmonary function when given as an adjunct to standard therapy.

Administration and Dosage

Individualize dosage. Monitor the patient's clinical status to avoid toxicity. Discontinue as soon as the desired effect is obtained. Repeat doses are dependent on the continuing presence of the patellar reflex and adequate respiratory function.

▶*Acute nephritis in children:* For nephritic seizures, the dose for children is 20 to 40 mg/kg IM as needed to control seizures. Dilute the 50% concentration to a 20% solution and give 0.1 to 0.2 mL/kg of the 20% solution.

▶*Seizures associated with eclampsia:* Initial dose is 10 to 14 g magnesium sulfate. To initiate therapy, 4 g magnesium sulfate in water for injection (premixed) or 4 to 5 g in 250 mL of 5% dextrose injection or 0.9% sodium chloride injection may be administered IV. Simultaneously, 4 to 5 g magnesium sulfate may be administered IM into each buttock using undiluted 50% magnesium sulfate.

Alternatively, the initial IV dose of 4 g may be given by diluting the 50% solution to a 10% or 20% concentration; the diluted fluid (40 mL of a 10% solution or 20 mL of a 20% solution) may then be injected IV over a period of 3 to 4 minutes.

After the initial IV dose, some clinicians administer 1 to 2 g/hr by constant IV infusion. Subsequent IM doses of 4 to 5 g magnesium sulfate may be injected into alternate buttocks every 4 hours, depending on the presence of the patellar reflex, adequate respiratory function, and absence of signs of magnesium toxicity. Continue therapy until paroxysms cease.

A serum magnesium level of 3 to 6 mg/dL (2.5 to 5 mEq/L) is considered optimal for control of seizures. Do not exceed a total daily dose of 30 to 40 g magnesium sulfate.

▶*Renal function impairment:* Obtain serum magnesium concentrations frequently. Maximum dose is 20 g/48 hours.

▶*IV administration:* Solutions for IV infusion must be diluted to a concentration of 20% or less prior to administration. Generally, do not exceed 1.5 mL of a 10% concentration (or its equivalent) per minute (150 mg/min) as the rate of IV injection, except in severe eclampsia with seizures.

▶*IM administration:* For adults, deep IM injection of the undiluted (50%) solution is appropriate. For children, dilute to a 20% or less concentration prior to injection.

▶*Compatibility:* The diluents commonly used are 5% dextrose injection and 0.9% sodium chloride injection.

▶*Incompatibility:* Magnesium sulfate in solution may result in a precipitate when mixed with solutions containing the following: Alcohol (in high concentrations), alkali carbonates and bicarbonates, alkali hydroxides, arsenates, barium, calcium, clindamycin phosphate, heavy metals, hydrocortisone sodium succinate, phosphates, polymyxin B sulfate, procaine HCl, salicylates, strontium, and tartrates.

The potential incompatibility will often be influenced by the changes in the concentration of reactants and the pH of the solutions.

Magnesium may reduce the antibiotic activity of streptomycin, tetracycline, and tobramycin when given together.

▶*Storage / Stability:* Store at controlled room temperature 15° to 30°C (59° to 86°F).

MAGNESIUM SULFATE

Actions

▶*Pharmacology:* Magnesium prevents or controls convulsions by blocking neuromuscular transmission and decreasing the amount of acetylcholine liberated at the end plate by the motor nerve impulse. Magnesium has a CNS depressant effect, but it does not adversely affect the mother, fetus, or neonate when used as directed in eclampsia or pre-eclampsia. Normal plasma magnesium levels range from 1.5 to 2.5 mEq/L. Effective anticonvulsant serum levels range from 2.5 or 3 to 7.5 mEq/L.

One gram magnesium sulfate (heptahydrate) provides 8.12 mEq (4.1 mmol) magnesium.

▶*Pharmacokinetics:*

Absorption/Distribution – Approximately 1% to 2% of total body magnesium is located in the extracellular fluid space. Magnesium is 30% bound to albumin.

With IV use, the onset of anticonvulsant action is immediate and lasts approximately 30 minutes. With IM use, onset occurs in 1 hour and persists for 3 to 4 hours.

Metabolism/Excretion – Magnesium is not metabolized. It is excreted solely by the kidney at a rate proportional to the serum concentration and glomerular filtration rate.

Contraindications

Heart block or myocardial damage; do not give in toxemia of pregnancy during the 2 hours preceding delivery.

Warnings

▶*Aluminum toxicity:* Some products may contain aluminum. See individual product labeling for ingredients.

If kidney function is impaired aluminum may reach toxic levels with prolonged parenteral administration. Premature neonates are particularly at risk because their kidneys are immature, and they require large amounts of calcium and phosphate solutions, which contain aluminum.

Research indicates that patients with impaired kidney function, including premature neonates, who receive parenteral levels of aluminum at greater than 4 to 5 mcg/kg/day accumulate aluminum at levels associated with CNS and bone toxicity. Tissue loading may occur at lower rates of administration.

▶*IV use:* IV use in eclampsia is reserved for immediate control of life-threatening convulsions. Administer slowly to avoid producing hypermagnesemia.

▶*Renal function impairment:* Because magnesium is excreted by the kidneys, parenteral use in the presence of renal insufficiency may lead to magnesium intoxication. Use with caution (see Administration and Dosage).

▶*Elderly:* Elderly patients often require reduced dosage because of impaired renal function.

▶*Pregnancy: Category A.* Magnesium sulfate has not been shown to increase the risk of fetal abnormalities if administered during all trimesters. The possibility of fetal harm appears remote; however, use only if clearly needed.

▶*Lactation:* Because magnesium is distributed into milk, exercise caution when administering to a nursing mother. The American Academy of Pediatrics considers magnesium sulfate compatible with breastfeeding.

▶*Children:* When administered by continuous IV infusion (especially for more than 24 hours preceding delivery) to control convulsions in toxemic mothers, the newborn may show signs of magnesium toxicity, including neuromuscular or respiratory depression. Hypermagnesemia in the newborn may require resuscitation and assisted ventilation via endotracheal intubation or intermittent positive pressure ventilation as well as IV calcium.

Elevated magnesium levels in the newborn may persist for up to 7 days; elimination half-life is approximately 43.2 hours.

Precautions

▶*Monitoring:* Monitor serum magnesium levels and clinical status to avoid overdosage. See Overdosage for serum level/toxicity relationships. Clinical indications of a safe dosage regimen include the presence of the patellar reflex (knee jerk) and absence of respiratory depression (approximately 16 breaths or more/minute).

▶*Urine output:* Maintain at a level of 100 mL every 4 hours.

Drug Interactions

▶*CNS depressants:* When barbiturates, narcotics, other hypnotics (or systemic anesthetics), or other CNS depressants are to be given in conjunction with magnesium, adjust their dosage with caution because of additive CNS depressant effects of magnesium.

▶*Neuromuscular blockers:* Magnesium sulfate potentiates the neuromuscular blockade produced by neuromuscular blocking agents.

Adverse Reactions

▶*Miscellaneous:*

Hypocalcemia – Hypocalcemia with signs of tetany secondary to magnesium sulfate therapy for eclampsia has occurred.

Magnesium intoxication – Magnesium intoxication is the usual cause of adverse effects that include the following: Cardiac and CNS depression preceeding respiratory paralysis, circulatory collapse, depressed reflexes, flaccid paralysis, flushing, hypotension, hypothermia, sweating.

Overdosage

▶*Symptoms:* Sharp drop in blood pressure and respiratory paralysis. Disappearance of the patellar reflex is a useful clinical sign to detect the onset of magnesium intoxication. ECG changes reported include increased PR interval, increased QRS complex, and prolonged QT interval. Heart block and asystole may occur.

An approximate correlation of magnesium toxicity vs serum level is presented in the table.

Effects of Magnesium Toxicity vs Serum Level	
Serum level (mEq/L)	Effect
1.5 to 3	Normal serum concentration
> 3	Nausea, vomiting, weakness, flushing
> 5	ECG changes (including prolonged PR, QRS, QT intervals)
7 to 10	Hypotension, loss of deep tendon reflexes, sedation
> 10	Arrhythmias, muscle paralysis, respiratory arrest, hypotension
> 14	Respiratory arrest, asystole, death

▶*Treatment:* Provide artificial ventilation until a calcium salt can be injected IV to antagonize the effects of magnesium. A dose of 5 to 10 mEq of 10% calcium gluconate usually will reverse the respiratory depression and heart block. Peritoneal dialysis or hemodialysis may be required in extreme cases.

ACETAZOLAMIDE

Rx	**Acetazolamide** (Various, eg, Mutual, Taro, URL)	**Tablets:** 125 mg	May contain lactose. In 50s, 100s, 250s, 500s, and 1000s.
Rx	**Acetazolamide** (Various, eg, Lannett, Mutual, Taro, Watson)	**Tablets:** 250 mg	May contain lactose. In 50s, 100s, 250s, 500s, and 1000s.
Rx	**Acetazolamide** (Bedford Labs)	**Powder for injection, lyophilized:** 500 mg	Preservative-free. In vials.

Refer to the general discussion beginning in the Anticonvulsants introduction. For complete prescribing information, refer to the Carbonic Anhydrase Inhibitors group monograph in the Renal and Genitourinary Agents.

Indications

▶*Centrencephalic epilepsies (petit mal, unlocalized seizures):* The best results have been in petit mal seizures in children. Good results, however, have been seen in children and adults with other seizure disorders.

▶*Edema:* For the adjunctive treatment of edema caused by CHF and drug-induced edema (see Carbonic Anhydrase Inhibitors in the Diuretics section).

▶*Glaucoma:* For the adjunctive treatment of open-angle glaucoma, secondary glaucoma, and preoperatively in acute angle-closure glaucoma where delay of surgery is desired to lower intraocular pressure (see Carbonic Anhydrase Inhibitors in the Diuretics section).

▶*High altitude sickness (tablets only):* For the prevention or amelioration of symptoms associated with acute altitude (mountain) sickness in climbers attempting rapid ascent and in those who are very susceptible despite gradual ascent (see Carbonic Anhydrase Inhibitors in the Diuretics section).

Administration and Dosage

▶*Epilepsy:* 8 to 30 mg/kg/day in divided doses. Optimum range is 375 to 1000 mg/day.

▶*Concomitant anticonvulsant therapy:* When given in combination with other anticonvulsants, the starting dose is 250 mg/day. Increase to levels as indicated above.

▶*Replacement therapy:* Change from other medication to acetazolamide gradually.

▶*Administration of parenteral solution:* Direct IV administration is preferred. IM administration is painful because of the alkaline pH of the solution.

ACETAZOLAMIDE

➤*Reconstitution of parenteral solution:* Reconstitute each 500 mg vial with at least 5 mL sterile water for injection. Use within 12 hours of reconstitution. Discard any unused portion.

➤*Oral suspension:* A 25 mg/mL suspension compounded from 250 mg tablets with 70% sorbitol in a suspension vehicle of magnesium aluminum silicate, carboxymethylcellulose sodium, sweeteners, flavoring, preservatives, humectants, and pH adjusters was stable for at least 79 days at 5°, 22°, and 30°C (41°, 72°, and 86°F). Store in amber glass bottles at pH 4 to 5.

Preparation – Pulverize twelve 250 mg tablets to a fine powder in a mortar. Add approximately 20 mL of vehicle in geometric proportions and mix to uniform paste. Transfer contents of mortar to an amber glass bottle and add enough of the vehicle to bring the final volume to 120 mL. Label the bottle "Shake well before using" and "Protect from light" with an expiration date of 60 days.

➤*Storage / Stability:* Store at controlled room temperature, 15° to 30° C (59° to 86°F).

Refrigerate reconstituted solution at 2° to 8°C (36° to 46°F). Use within 12 hours of reconstitution; contains no preservative.

OXCARBAZEPINE

Rx	Trileptal (Novartis)	**Tablets:** 150 mg	(T/D C/G). Yellow, oval, scored. Film-coated. In 100s, 1000s, and UD 100s.
		300 mg	(TE/TE CG/CG). Yellow, oval, scored. Film-coated. In 100s, 1000s, and UD 100s.
		600 mg	(TF/TF CG/CG). Yellow, oval, scored. Film-coated. In 100s, 1000s, and UD 100s.
		Suspension: 300 mg/5 mL	Saccharin, sorbitol, ethanol. In 250 mL with dosing syringe and adapter.

Indications

➤*Epilepsy:* For use as monotherapy or adjunctive therapy in the treatment of partial seizures in adults and children 4 to 16 years of age with epilepsy.

➤*Unlabeled uses:* Alternative treatment for bipolar disorder.

Administration and Dosage

➤*Approved by the FDA:* January 17, 2000.

Give all dosing in a twice-daily regimen. Oxcarbazepine may be taken with or without food.

➤*Adults:*

Adjunctive therapy – Initiate treatment with a dose of 600 mg/day, given in a twice-daily regimen. If clinically indicated, the dose may be increased by a maximum of 600 mg/day at approximately weekly intervals; the recommended daily dose is 1200 mg/day. Daily doses more than 1200 mg/day show somewhat greater effectiveness in controlled trials, but most patients were not able to tolerate the 2400 mg/day dose, primarily because of CNS effects. Closely observe and monitor the plasma levels of the concomitant antiepileptic drugs (AEDs) during the period of oxcarbazepine titration, as these plasma levels may be altered, especially at oxcarbazepine doses greater than 1200 mg/day.

Conversion to monotherapy – Patients receiving concomitant AEDs may be converted to monotherapy by initiating treatment with oxcarbazepine at 300 mg twice daily while simultaneously initiating the reduction of the concomitant AEDs' dose. Withdraw the concomitant AEDs over 3 to 6 weeks, while reaching the maximum dose of oxcarbazepine in approximately 2 to 4 weeks. Oxcarbazepine may be increased as clinically indicated by a maximum increment of 600 mg/day at approximate weekly intervals to achieve the recommended daily dose of 2400 mg/day. A daily dose of 1200 mg/day has been shown in 1 study to be effective in patients in whom monotherapy has been initiated with oxcarbazepine.

Initiation of monotherapy – Initiate at a dose of 600 mg/day (given in a twice-daily regimen). Increase by 300 mg/day every third day to a dose of 1200 mg/day. Controlled trials in these patients examined the effectiveness of a 1200 mg/day dose; a dose of 2400 mg/day has been shown to be effective in patients converted from other AEDs to oxcarbazepine monotherapy.

➤*Pediatric patients 4 to 16 years of age:*

Adjunctive therapy – Initiate at a daily dose of 8 to 10 mg/kg not to exceed 300 mg twice daily. Achieve the target maintenance dose of oxcarbazepine over 2 weeks, according to patient weight, using the following table.

Weight (kg)	Target maintenance dose (mg/day)
20 to 29	900
29.1 to 39	1200
> 39	1800

In the clinical trial in which the intention was to reach these target doses, the median daily dose was 31 mg/kg with a range of 6 to 51 mg/kg.

Conversion to monotherapy – Patients receiving concomitant AEDs may be converted to monotherapy by initiating treatment at approximately 8 to 10 mg/kg/day given in a twice-daily regimen, while simultaneously initiating the reduction of the dose of the concomitant AEDs. The concomitant AEDs can be completely withdrawn over 3 to 6 weeks, while oxcarbazepine may be increased as clinically indicated by a maximum increment of 10 mg/kg/day at approximately weekly intervals to achieve the recommended daily dose.

Initiation of monotherapy – Patients not currently being treated with antiepileptic drugs may have monotherapy initiated with oxcarbazepine. Initiate at a dose of 8 to 10 mg/kg/day given in a twice-daily regimen. Increase the dose by 5 mg/kg/day every third day to the recommended daily dose shown in the table below.

Maintenance Doses of Oxcarbazine for Children During Monotherapy	
Weight (kg)	Dose (mg/day)
20	600 to 900
25	900 to 1200
30	900 to 1200
35	900 to 1500
40	900 to 1500
45	1200 to 1500
50	1200 to 1800
55	1200 to 1800
60	1200 to 2100
65	1200 to 2100
70	1500 to 2100

➤*Renal function impairment (Ccr less than 30 mL/min):* Initiate therapy at one-half the usual starting dose (300 mg/day), and increase slowly to achieve the desired clinical response.

➤*Storage / Stability:* Store at 25°C (77°F); excursions permitted to 15° to 30°C (59° to 86°F). Dispense in tight container.

Store oral suspension in the original container. Shake well before using. Use within 7 weeks of first opening the bottle.

Actions

➤*Pharmacology:* Oxcarbazepine activity is primarily exerted through the 10-monohydroxy metabolite (MHD) of oxcarbazepine. The precise mechanism by which oxcarbazepine and MHD exert their antiseizure effect is unknown; however, in vitro electrophysiological studies indicate that they produce blockade of voltage-sensitive sodium channels, resulting in stabilization of hyperexcited neural membranes, inhibition of repetitive neuronal firing, and diminution of propagation of synaptic impulses. These actions are thought to be important in the prevention of seizure spread in the intact brain. In addition, increased potassium conductance and modulation of high-voltage activated calcium channels may contribute to the anticonvulsant effects of the drug. No significant interactions of oxcarbazepine or MHD with brain neurotransmitters or modulator receptor sites have been demonstrated.

➤*Pharmacokinetics:*

Absorption – Following oral administration of oxcarbazepine, it is completely absorbed and extensively metabolized to its pharmacologically active MHD metabolite. After single dose administration of the tablets and suspension to healthy male volunteers under fasted conditions, the median T_{max} was 4.5 (range, 3 to 13 hours and 6 hours, respectively). Food does not effect the rate or extent of oxcarbazepine absorption.

Steady-state plasma concentrations of MHD are reached within 2 to 3 days in patients when oxcarbazine is given twice a day. At steady state, the pharmacokinetics of MHD are linear and show dose proportionality over the dose range of 300 to 2400 mg/day.

Distribution – The apparent volume of distribution of MHD is 49 L. Approximately 40% of MHD is bound to serum proteins, predominantly to albumin. Binding is independent of the serum concentration within the therapeutically relevant range. Oxcarbazepine and MHD do not bind to alpha-1-acid glycoprotein.

Metabolism – Oxcarbazepine is rapidly reduced by cytosolic enzymes in the liver to its MHD, which is primarily responsible for the pharmacological effect of oxcarbazepine. MHD is metabolized further by conjugation with glucuronic acid. Minor amounts (ie, 4% of the dose) are oxidized to the pharmacologically inactive 10,11-dihydroxy metabolite (DHD).

Excretion – The half-life of the parent drug is approximately 2 hours, while the half-life of MHD is approximately 9 hours. Oxcarbazepine is excreted from the body mostly in the form of metabolites, predominantly by the kidneys. More than 95% of the dose appears in the urine, with less than 1% as unchanged oxcarbazepine. Fecal excretion accounts for less than 4% of the administered dose. Approximately 80%

OXCARBAZEPINE

of the dose is excreted in the urine either as glucuronides of MHD (49%) or as unchanged MHD (27%); the inactive DHD accounts for approximately 3%, and conjugates of MHD and oxcarbazepine account for 13% of the dose.

Special populations –

Renal function impairment: When oxcarbazepine is administered as a single 300 mg dose in renally impaired patients (Ccr less than 30 mL/min), the elimination half-life of MHD is prolonged to 19 hours, with a 2-fold increase in AUC.

Elderly: Following administration of single (300 mg) and multiple (600 mg/day) doses of oxcarbazine to elderly volunteers (60 to 82 years of age), the maximum plasma concentrations and AUC values of MHD were 30% to 60% higher than in younger volunteers (18 to 32 years of age). Comparisons of Ccr in young and elderly volunteers indicate that the difference was caused by age-related reductions in Ccr.

Children: After a single-dose administration of 5 to 15 mg/kg of oxcarbazepine, the dose-adjusted AUC values of MHD were 30% to 40% lower in children younger than 8 years of age than in children older than 8 years of age. The clearance in children older than 8 years of age approaches that of adults.

Contraindications

Known hypersensitivity to oxcarbazepine or any of its components.

Warnings

➤*Hyponatremia:* Clinically significant hyponatremia (sodium less than 125 mmol/L) generally occurred during the first 3 months of treatment with oxcarbazepine, although there were patients who first developed a serum sodium less than 125 mmol/L more than 1 year after initiation of therapy. Most patients who developed hyponatremia were asymptomatic, but patients in the clinical trials were frequently monitored. Some had their oxcarbazepine dose reduced or discontinued or had their fluid intake restricted for hyponatremia. Whether or not these maneuvers prevented the occurrence of more severe events is unknown. Cases of symptomatic hyponatremia have been reported during postmarketing use. In clinical trials, patients whose treatment with oxcarbazepine was discontinued because of hyponatremia generally experienced normalization of serum sodium within a few days without additional treatment.

Measure serum sodium levels for patients during maintenance treatment with oxcarbazepine, particularly if the patient is receiving other medications known to decrease serum sodium levels (eg, drugs associated with inappropriate ADH secretion) or if symptoms possibly indicating hyponatremia develop (eg, nausea, malaise, headache, lethargy, confusion, obtundation, or increase in seizure frequency or severity).

➤*History of hypersensitivity reaction to carbamazepine:* Approximately 25% to 30% of patients who have had hypersensitivity reactions to carbamazepine will experience a hypersensitivity reaction with oxcarbazepine. Treat with oxcarbazepine only if the potential benefit justifies the potential risk.

➤*Renal function impairment:* There is a linear correlation between Ccr and the renal clearance of MHD (see Administration and Dosage).

➤*Carcinogenesis:* In mice, a dose-related increase in the incidence of hepatocellular adenomas was observed at oxcarbazepine doses of at least 70 mg/kg/day or approximately 0.1 times the maximum recommended human dose (MRHD) on a mg/m² basis. In rats, the incidence of hepatocellular carcinomas was increased in females treated with oxcarbazepine at doses at least 25 mg/kg/day (0.1 times the MRHD on a mg/m² basis), and incidences of hepatocellular adenomas or carcinomas were increased in males and females treated with MHD at doses of 600 mg/kg/day (2.4 times the MRHD on a mg/m² basis) and at least 250 mg/kg/day (equivalent to the MRHD on a mg/m² basis), respectively. There was an increase in the incidence of benign testicular interstitial cell tumors in rats at 250 mg oxcarbazepine/kg/day and at least 250 mg MHD/kg/day, and an increase in the incidence of granular cell tumors in the cervix and vagina in rats at 600 mg MHD/kg/day.

➤*Mutagenesis:* Oxcarbazepine increased mutation frequencies in the Ames test in vitro in the absence of metabolic activation in 1 of 5 bacterial strains. Oxcarbazepine and MHD produced increases in chromosomal aberrations and polyploidy in the Chinese hamster ovary assay in vitro in the absence of metabolic activation.

➤*Fertility impairment:* In a fertility study in which rats were administered MHD (50, 150, or 450 mg/kg) orally prior to and during mating and early gestation, estrous cyclicity was disrupted and numbers of corpora lutea, implantations, and live embryos were reduced in females receiving the highest dose (approximately 2 times the MRHD on a mg/m² basis).

➤*Elderly:* Following administration of single (300 mg) and multiple (600 mg/day) doses of oxcarbazepine to elderly volunteers (60 to 82 years of age), the maximum plasma concentrations and AUC values of MHD were 30% to 60% higher than in younger volunteers (18 to 32 years of age). Comparisons of Ccr in young and elderly volunteers indicate that the difference was caused by age-related reductions in Ccr.

➤*Pregnancy: Category C.* Increased incidences of fetal structural abnormalities and other manifestations of developmental toxicity (embryolethality, growth retardation) were observed in the offspring of animals treated with either oxcarbazepine or MHD during pregnancy at doses similar to the MRHD.

When pregnant rats were given oxcarbazepine (30, 300, or 1000 mg/kg) orally throughout the period of organogenesis, increased incidences of fetal malformations (craniofacial, cardiovascular, and skeletal) and variations were observed at the intermediate and high doses (approximately 1.2 to 4 times, respectively, the MRHD on a mg/m² basis). Increased embryofetal death and decreased fetal body weights were seen at the high dose. Doses of at least 300 mg/kg were also maternally toxic (decreased body weight gain, clinical signs), but there is no evidence to suggest that teratogenicity was secondary to the maternal effects.

In a study in which pregnant rabbits were orally administered MHD (20, 100, or 200 mg/kg) during organogenesis, embryofetal mortality was increased at the highest dose (1.5 times the MRHD on a mg/m² basis). This dose produced only minimal maternal toxicity.

In a study in which female rats were dosed orally with oxcarbazepine (25, 50, or 150 mg/kg) during the latter part of gestation and throughout the lactation period, a persistent reduction in body weights and altered behavior (decreased activity) were observed in offspring exposed to the highest dose (0.6 times the MRHD on a mg/m² basis). Oral administration of MHD (25, 75, or 250 mg/kg) to rats during gestation and lactation resulted in a persistent reduction in offspring weights at the highest dose (equivalent to the MRHD on a mg/m² basis).

Oxcarbazepine and its metabolite are transferred through the placenta.

There are no adequate and well-controlled clinical studies of oxcarbazepine in pregnant women; however, it is closely related structurally to carbamazepine, which is considered to be teratogenic in humans. Therefore, it is likely that oxcarbazepine is a human teratogen. Use during pregnancy only if the potential benefit justifies the potential risk to the fetus.

➤*Lactation:* Oxcarbazepine and its active metabolite MHD are excreted in human breast milk. A milk-to-plasma concentration ratio of 0:5 was found for both. Because of the potential for serious adverse reactions, decide whether to discontinue nursing or to discontinue the drug in nursing women, taking into account the importance of the drug to the mother.

➤*Children:* Oxcarbazepine has been shown to be effective as adjunctive therapy or monotherapy for partial seizures in patients 4 to 16 years of age.

Precautions

➤*CNS effects:* Oxcarbazepine has been associated with cognitive symptoms including psychomotor slowing, difficulty with concentration, and speech or language problems; somnolence or fatigue; and coordination abnormalities, including ataxia and gait disturbances.

➤*Withdrawal of AEDs:* Withdraw gradually to minimize the potential of increased seizure frequency.

➤*Lab test abnormalities:* Serum sodium levels less than 125 mmol/L have been observed in patients treated with oxcarbazepine. Experience from clinical trials indicates that serum sodium levels return toward normal when the oxcarbazepine dosage is reduced or discontinued or when the patient is treated conservatively (eg, fluid restriction).

Laboratory data from clinical trials suggest that oxcarbazepine use was associated with decreases in T_4, without changes in T_3 or TSH.

Drug Interactions

➤*Cytochrome P450:* Oxcarbazepine inhibits CYP2C19 and induces CYP3A4/5 with potentially important effects on plasma concentrations of other drugs. In addition, several AEDs that are cytochrome P450 inducers can decrease plasma concentrations of oxcarbazepine and MHD.

Oxcarbazepine and its pharmacologically active MHD have little or no capacity to function as inhibitors for most of the human cytochrome P450 enzymes evaluated (CYP1A2, CYP2A6, CYP2C9, CYP2D6, CYP2E1, CYP4A9, and CYP4A11), with the exception of CYP2C19 and CYP3A4/5. Although inhibition of CYP3A4/5 by oxcarbazepine and MHD did occur at high concentrations, it is not likely to be of clinical significance. However, the inhibition of CYP2C19 by oxcarbazepine and MHD is clinically relevant.

In vitro, the UDP-glucuronyl transferase level was increased, indicating induction of this enzyme. Increases of 22% with MHD and 47% with oxcarbazepine were observed. As MHD, the predominant plasma substrate, is only a weak inducer of UDP-glucuronyl transferase, it is unlikely to have an effect on drugs that are mainly eliminated by conjugation through UDP-glucuronyl transferase (eg, valproic acid).

In addition, oxcarbazepine and MHD induce a subgroup of the cytochrome P450 3A family (CYP3A4 and CYP3A5) responsible for the metabolism of dihydropyridine calcium antagonists and oral contraceptives, resulting in a lower plasma concentration of these drugs.

As binding of MHD to plasma proteins is low (40%), clinically significant interactions with other drugs through competition for protein-binding sites are unlikely.

OXCARBAZEPINE

Strong inducers of CYP450 enzymes (ie, carbamazepine, phenytoin, phenobarbital) have been shown to decrease the plasma levels of MHD.

Oxcarbazepine Drug Interactions			
Precipitant drug	Object drug*		Description
Carbamazepine	Oxcarbazepine	↓	Concurrent use of carbamazepine and oxcarbazepine decreased MHD[1] concentration by ≈ 40%.
Phenobarbital	Oxcarbazepine	↓	Administration of phenobarbital with oxcarbazepine decreased MHD[1] concentrations ≈ 25% while phenobarbital concentrations increased ≈ 14%.
Oxcarbazepine	Phenobarbital	↑	
Phenytoin	Oxcarbazepine	↓	Coadministration of phenytoin with oxcarbazepine (600 to 1800 mg/day) caused a 30% decrease in MHD[1] AUC. Higher doses of oxcarbazepine (> 1200 to 2400 mg/day) increased phenytoin concentrations up to 40%. A decrease in phenytoin dose may be required when given with oxcarbazepine in doses > 1200 mg/day.
Oxcarbazepine	Phenytoin	↑	
Oxcarbazepine	Felodipine	↓	The AUC of felodipine decreased by 28% when repeatedly administered in combination with oxcarbazepine.

Oxcarbazepine Drug Interactions			
Precipitant drug	Object drug*		Description
Oxcarbazepine	Oral contraceptives	↓	The mean AUC of ethinyl estradiol decreased by 48% to 52% and the mean AUC of levonorgestrel decreased by 32% to 52% when administered in combination with oxcarbazepine.
Valproic acid	Oxcarbazepine	↓	Concurrent use of valproic acid and oxcarbazepine decreased MHD[1] concentrations ≈ 18%.
Oxcarbazepine	Lamotrigine	↓	Oxcarbazepine administration reduced serum concentrations of lamotrigine 29%. Adjust the dose of lamotrigine as needed.
Verapamil	Oxcarbazepine	↓	Verapamil administration resulted in a 20% decrease of oxcarbazepine (MHD)[1] plasma levels.

* ↑ = Object drug increased. ↓ = Object drug decreased.
[1] MHD = pharmacologically active 10-monohydroxy metabolite of oxcarbazepine.

Adverse Reactions

Oxcarbazepine (OXC) Adverse Reactions in Adults (%)								
	Patients on Adjunctive Therapy Treated with Oxcarbazepine (mg/day)				Patients on Monotherapy Previously Treated with Other AEDs (mg/day)		Patients on Monotherapy Not Previously Treated with Other AEDs (mg/day)	
Adverse reactions	OXC 600 (n = 163)	OXC 1200 (n = 171)	OXC 2400 (n = 126)	Placebo (n = 166)	OXC 2400 (n = 86)	OXC 300 (n = 86)	OXC (n = 55)	Placebo (n = 49)
CNS								
Headache	32	28	26	23	31	15	13	10
Dizziness	26	32	49	13	28	8	22	6
Somnolence	20	28	36	12	19	5		
Anxiety					7	5		
Ataxia	9	17	31	5	7	1	5	0
Vertigo	6	12	15	2	3	0		
Abnormal gait	5	10	17	1				
Insomnia	4	2	3	1	6	3		
Tremor	3	8	16	5	6	3	4	0
Amnesia					5	1	4	2
Convulsions aggravated					5	2		
Emotional lability					3	2		
Hypoesthesia					3	1		
Nervousness	2	4	2	1	7	0	5	2
Agitation	1	1	2	1				
Abnormal coordination	1	3	2	1	2	1	4	2
Abnormal EEG	0	0	2	0				
Speech disorder	1	1	3	0	2	0		
Confusion	1	1	2	1	7	0		
Cranial injury nos[1]	1	0	2	1				
Dysmetria	1	2	3	0				
Abnormal thinking	0	2	4	0				
Dermatologic								
Acne	1	2	2	0				
Hot flushes					2	1		
Purpura					2	0		
Rash							4	2
GI								
Nausea	15	25	29	10	22	7	16	12
Vomiting	13	25	36	5	15	5	7	6
Abdominal pain	10	13	11	5	5	3		
Anorexia					5	3		
Dry mouth					3	0		
Rectum hemorrhage					2	0		
Toothache					2	1		
Diarrhea	5	6	7	6	7	5	7	2
Dyspepsia	5	5	6	2	6	1	5	4
Constipation	2	2	6	4			5	0

OXCARBAZEPINE

Oxcarbazepine (OXC) Adverse Reactions in Adults (%)							
Adverse reactions	Patients on Adjunctive Therapy Treated with Oxcarbazepine (mg/day)				Patients on Monotherapy Previously Treated with Other AEDs (mg/day)		Patients on Monotherapy Not Previously Treated with Other AEDs (mg/day)	
	OXC 600 (n = 163)	OXC 1200 (n = 171)	OXC 2400 (n = 126)	Placebo (n = 166)	OXC 2400 (n = 86)	OXC 300 (n = 86)	OXC (n = 55)	Placebo (n = 49)
Gastritis	2	1	2	1				
GU								
Urinary tract infection					5	1		
Micturition frequency					2	1		
Vaginitis					2	0		
Metabolic/Nutritional								
Hyponatremia	3	1	2	1	5	0		
Thirst					2	0		
Musculoskeletal								
Muscle weakness	1	2	2	0				
Back pain							4	2
Sprains/Strains	0	2	2	1				
Respiratory								
Rhinitis	2	4	5	4				
Upper respiratory tract infection					10	5	7	0
Coughing					5	0		
Bronchitis					3	0		
Pharyngitis					3	0		
Epistaxis							4	0
Chest infection							4	0
Sinusitis							4	2
Special senses								
Diplopia	14	30	40	5	12	1		
Nystagmus	7	20	26	5	2	0		
Taste perversion					5	0		
Earache					2	1		
Ear infection nos[1]					2	0		
Abnormal vision	6	14	13	4	14	2	4	0
Abnormal accommodation	0	0	2	0				
Miscellaneous								
Fatigue	15	12	15	7	21	5		
Fever					3	0		
Allergy					2	0		
Generalized edema					2	1		
Chest pain					2	0		
Asthenia	6	3	6	5				
Edema, legs	2	1	2	1				
Weight increase	1	2	2	1				
Abnormal feeling	0	1	2	0				
Falling down nos[1]							4	0
Lymphadenopathy					2	0		
Hypotension	0	1	2	0				
Infection viral					7	5		
Infection					2	0		

[1] nos = not otherwise specified

Adjunctive therapy/monotherapy in adults previously treated with other AEDs – The most commonly observed (at least 5%) adverse experiences seen in association with oxcarbazepine and substantially more frequent than in placebo-treated patients were the following: Dizziness, somnolence, diplopia, fatigue, nausea, vomiting, ataxia, abnormal vision, abdominal pain, tremor, dyspepsia, abnormal gait.

Approximately 23% of 1537 adult patients discontinued treatment because of an adverse experience. The adverse experiences most commonly associated with discontinuation were the following: Dizziness (6.4%), diplopia (5.9%), ataxia (5.2%), vomiting (5.1%), nausea (4.9%), somnolence (3.8%), headache (2.9%), fatigue (2.1%), abnormal vision (2.1%), tremor (1.8%), abnormal gait (1.7%), rash (1.4%), hyponatremia (1%).

Monotherapy in adults not previously treated with other AEDs – Approximately 9% of 295 adult patients discontinued treatment because of an adverse experience. The adverse experiences most commonly associated with discontinuation were the following: Dizziness, nausea, rash (1.7%); headache (1.4%).

Pediatric Patients on Adjunctive/Monotherapy Previously Treated with Other AEDs (≥ 2%)		
Adverse reactions	OXC (n = 171)	Placebo (n = 139)
CNS		
Headache	31	19
Somnolence	31	13
Dizziness	28	8
Ataxia	13	4
Emotional lability	8	4
Abnormal gait	8	3
Tremor	6	4
Speech disorder	3	1
Impaired concentration	2	1
Convulsions	2	1
Involuntary muscle contractions	2	1
Vertigo	2	0

OXCARBAZEPINE

Pediatric Patients on Adjunctive/Monotherapy Previously Treated with Other AEDs (≥ 2%)		
Adverse reactions	OXC (n = 171)	Placebo (n = 139)
Dermatologic		
Bruising	4	2
Increased sweating	3	0
GI		
Vomiting	33	14
Nausea	19	5
Constipation	4	1
Dyspepsia	2	0
Respiratory		
Rhinitis	10	9
Pneumonia	2	1
Special senses		
Diplopia	17	1
Abnormal vision	13	1
Nystagmus	9	1
Miscellaneous		
Fatigue	13	9
Allergy	2	0
Asthenia	2	1

Adjunctive therapy/monotherapy in pediatric patients previously treated with other AEDs – The most commonly observed (at least 5%) adverse experiences seen in association with oxcarbazepine in pediatric patients were similar to those seen in adults.

Approximately 11% of the 456 pediatric patients discontinued treatment because of an adverse experience. The adverse experiences most commonly associated with discontinuation were the following: Somnolence (2.4%); vomiting (2%); ataxia (1.8%); diplopia, dizziness (1.3%); fatigue, nystagmus (1.1%).

Monotherapy in pediatric patients not previously treated with other AEDs – Approximately 9.2% of 152 pediatric patients discontinued treatment because of an adverse experience. The adverse experiences most commonly associated (at least 1%) with discontinuation were rash (5.3%) and maculopapular rash (1.3%).

➤*Cardiovascular:* Bradycardia; cardiac failure; cerebral hemorrhage; hypertension; postural hypotension; palpitation; syncope; tachycardia.

➤*CNS:* Aggressive reaction; amnesia; anguish; anxiety; apathy; aphasia; aura; aggravated convulsions; delirium; delusion; depressed level of consciousness; dysphonia; dystonia; emotional lability; euphoria; extrapyramidal disorder; feeling drunk; hemiplegia; hyperkinesia; hyperreflexia; hypoesthesia; hypokinesia; hyporeflexia; hypotonia; hysteria; decreased/increased libido; manic reaction; migraine; involuntary muscle contractions; nervousness; neuralgia; oculogyric crisis; panic disorder; paralysis; paroniria; personality disorder; psychosis; ptosis; stupor; tetany.

➤*Dermatologic:* Acne; alopecia; angioedema; bruising; contact dermatitis; eczema; facial rash; flushing; folliculitis; heat rash; hot flushes; photosensitivity reaction; genital pruritus; psoriasis; purpura; erythematous rash; maculopapular rash; vitiligo; urticaria.

➤*GI:* Increased appetite; blood in stool; cholelithiasis; colitis; duodenal ulcer; dysphagia; enteritis; eructation; esophagitis; flatulence; gastric ulcer; gingival bleeding; gum hyperplasia; hematemesis; rectum hemorrhage; hemorrhoids; hiccough; dry mouth; biliary pain; hypochondrium pain right; retching; sialoadenitis; stomatitis; ulcerative stomatitis.

➤*GU:* Dysuria; hematuria; intermenstrual bleeding; leukorrhea; menorrhagia; micturition frequency; renal pain; urinary tract pain; polyuria; priapism; renal calculus.

➤*Hematologic:* Leukopenia; thrombocytopenia.

➤*Lab test abnormalities:* Increased gamma-GT; hyperglycemia; hypocalcemia; hypoglycemia; hypokalemia; elevated liver enzymes; increased serum transaminase.

➤*Respiratory:* Asthma; dyspnea; epistaxis; laryngismus; pleurisy.

➤*Special senses:* Abnormal accommodation; cataract; conjunctival hemorrhage; eye edema; hemianopia; mydriasis; otitis externa; photophobia; scotoma; taste perversion; tinnitus; xerophthalmia.

➤*Miscellaneous:* Fever; malaise; precordial chest pain; rigors; weight decrease; hypertonia muscle; procedure dental oral; procedure female reproductive; procedure musculoskeletal; procedure skin; systemic lupus erythematosus.

Postmarketing – The following adverse events not seen in controlled clinical trials have been observed in named patient programs or postmarketing experience.

➤*Dermatologic:* Erythema multiforme; Stevens-Johnson syndrome; toxic epidermal necrolysis.

➤*Miscellaneous:* Multiorgan hypersensitivity disorders characterized by features such as rash, fever, lymphadenopathy, abnormal liver function tests, eosinophilia, and arthralgia.

Overdosage

Isolated cases of overdose with oxcarbazepine have been reported. The maximum dose taken was approximately 24,000 mg. All patients recovered with symptomatic treatment.

➤*Treatment:* There is no specific antidote. Administer symptomatic and supportive treatment as appropriate. Consider removal of the drug by gastric lavage and/or inactivation by administering activated charcoal.

Patient Information

Inform patients that approximately 25% to 30% of patients who have exhibited hypersensitivity reactions to carbamazepine may experience hypersensitivity reactions to oxcarbazepine.

Additional nonhormonal forms of contraception are recommended when using oxcarbazepine because of a reduction in hormonal contraceptive efficacy.

Advise patients to exercise caution if alcohol is taken in combination with oxcarbazepine therapy because of a possible additive sedative effect.

Oxcarbazepine may cause dizziness and somnolence. Accordingly, advise patients not to drive or operate machinery until they have gained sufficient experience on oxcarbazepine to gauge whether it adversely affects their ability to drive or operate machinery.

FELBAMATE

Rx	Felbatol[1] (Wallace Labs)	Tablets: 400 mg	Lactose. (Wallace 0430). Yellow, scored. Capsule shape. In 100s and UD 100s.
		600 mg	Lactose. (Wallace 0431). Peach, scored. Capsule shape. In 100s and UD 100s.
		Suspension: 600 mg/5 ml	Sorbitol, parabens, saccharin. In 240 and 960 ml.

[1] It has been recommended that use of this drug be discontinued if aplastic anemia or hepatic failure occurs unless, in the judgment of the physician, continued therapy is warranted. See Warning box. For further information contact Wallace Labs at 800–526–3840.

Refer to the general discussion beginning in the Anticonvulsants introduction.

WARNING

Aplastic anemia: The use of felbamate is associated with a marked increase in the incidence of aplastic anemia. Accordingly, use only in patients whose epilepsy is so severe that the risk of aplastic anemia is deemed acceptable in light of the benefits conferred by its use (see Indications). Ordinarily, a patient should not be placed on or continued on felbamate without consideration of appropriate expert hematologic consultation.

Among felbamate-treated patients, aplastic anemia (pancytopenia in the presence of bone marrow largely depleted of hematopoietic precursors) occurs at an incidence that may be > 100-fold greater than that seen in the untreated population (eg, two to five million people per year). The risk of death in patients with aplastic anemia generally varies as a function of its severity and etiology. Current estimates of the overall case-fatality rate are in the range of 20% to 30%, but rates as high as 70% have been reported in the past.

A reliable estimate cannot be made of the syndrome's incidence or its case-fatality rate or to identify the factors, if any, that might conceivably be used to predict who is at greater or lesser risk.

The clinical manifestations of aplastic anemia may not be seen until after a patient has been on felbamate for several months (eg, 5 to 30 weeks); however, the injury to bone marrow stem cells may occur weeks to months earlier, placing patients at risk for developing anemia for a variable and unknown period after drug discontinuation.

It is not known whether or not the risk of developing aplastic anemia changes with duration of exposure, dose or concomitant use of antiepileptic drugs or other drugs.

Aplastic anemia typically develops without premonitory clinical or laboratory signs. The full-blown syndrome presents with signs of infection, bleeding or anemia. Accordingly, routine blood testing cannot be reliably used to reduce the incidence of aplastic anemia, but it will, in some cases, allow the detection of the hematologic changes before the syndrome declares itself clinically. Discontinue felbamate if any evidence of bone marrow depression occurs.

Hepatic failure: Hepatic failure resulting in fatalities has been reported with a marked increase in frequency in patients receiving felbamate. Accordingly, only use felbamate in patients whose epilepsy is so severe that the potential benefits of seizure control outweigh the risk of liver failure.

Although full information is not yet available, the number of cases reported greatly exceeds the number that is expected based on the annual incidence of acute liver failure in the US (eg, ≈ 2000 cases/year).

Reliable estimates cannot be made of the incidence of hepatic failure or to identify the factors, if any, that might be used to predict which patient is at greater or lesser risk.

It is not known whether the risk of developing hepatic failure changes with duration of exposure, dosage or concomitant use of other antiepileptic drugs or other drugs.

Avoid use in patients with a history of hepatic dysfunction.

Patients prescribed felbamate should have liver function tests (AST, ALT, bilirubin) performed before initiating felbamate and at 1- to 2-week intervals while treatment continues. A patient who develops abnormal liver function tests should be immediately withdrawn from felbamate treatment.

Indications

Felbamate is not indicated as a first-line antiepileptic treatment (see Warnings). Felbamate is recommended for use only in those patients who respond inadequately to alternative treatments and whose epilepsy is so severe that a substantial risk of aplastic anemia or liver failure is deemed acceptable in light of the benefits conferred by its use.

➤*Partial seizures:* Monotherapy or adjunctive therapy in the treatment of partial seizures with and without generalization in adults with epilepsy.

➤*Lennox-Gastaut syndrome:* Adjunctive therapy in the treatment of partial and generalized seizures associated with Lennox-Gastaut syndrome in children.

Administration and Dosage

➤*Approved by the FDA:* July 29, 1993.

➤*Discontinuation of therapy:* Because of reports of aplastic anemia and hepatic failure in association with felbamate, it has been recommended to discontinue use of the drug if these conditions develop unless the physician decides that withdrawal would pose an even greater risk to the patient (see Warning Box).

Patients should not discontinue the drug on their own. If the decision is made to discontinue therapy, felbamate may be discontinued by reducing the dosage by one-third increments every 4 to 5 days. As with any antiepileptic, abrupt discontinuation may result in an increase in seizure frequency; however, if it is necessary to discontinue felbamate abruptly, it may be stopped without tapering as long as the patient is covered by adequate dosages of other antiepileptics.

The following prescribing information is applicable to those physicians who opt to continue the use of felbamate in select patients.

Felbamate is used as monotherapy and adjunctive therapy in adults and as adjunctive therapy in children. When the drug is added to or substituted for existing antiepileptic drugs (AEDs), it is necessary to reduce the dosage of those AEDs in the range of 20% to 33% to minimize side effects.

➤*Adults (≥ 14 years of age):* Most of the patients received 3600 mg/day in clinical trials.

Monotherapy (initial therapy) – Felbamate has not been systematically evaluated as initial monotherapy. Initiate at 1200 mg/day in divided doses 3 or 4 times daily. Titrate previously untreated patients under close clinical supervision, increasing the dosage in 600 mg increments every 2 weeks to 2400 mg/day based on clinical response and thereafter to 3600 mg/day if clinically indicated.

Conversion to monotherapy – Initiate at 1200 mg/day in divided doses 3 or 4 times daily. Reduce the dosage of concomitant AEDs by one-third at initiation of felbamate therapy. At week 2, increase the felbamate dosage to 2400 mg/day while reducing the dosage of other AEDs up to an additional one-third of their original dosage. At week 3, increase the felbamate dosage up to 3600 mg/day and continue to reduce the dosage of other AEDs as clinically indicated.

Adjunctive therapy – Add felbamate at 1200 mg/day in divided doses 3 or 4 times daily while reducing present AEDs by 20% to control plasma concentrations of concurrent phenytoin, valproic acid, phenobarbital and carbamazepine (and its metabolites). Further reductions of the concomitant AED dosage may be necessary to minimize side effects caused by drug interactions. Increase the felbamate dosage by 1200 mg/day increments at weekly intervals to 3600 mg/day. Most side effects during adjunctive therapy resolve as the dosage of concomitant AEDs is decreased.

Felbamate/Concomitant AED Dosage (Adults): Adjunctive Therapy			
Drugs	Week 1	Week 2	Week 3
Dosage reduction of concomitant AEDs	Reduce original dose by 20% to 33%[1]	Reduce original dose by up to an additional 33%[1]	Reduce as clinically indicated
Felbamate dosage	1200 mg/day initial dose	2400 mg/day therapeutic dosage range	3600 mg/day therapeutic dosage range

[1] See Adjunctive Therapy and Conversion to Monotherapy sections.

While the previous conversion guidelines may result in a felbamate 3600 mg/day dose within 3 weeks, in some patients, titration to 3600 mg/day has been achieved in as little as 3 days with appropriate adjustment of other AEDs.

➤*Children with Lennox-Gastaut syndrome (ages 2 to 14 years):* *Adjunctive therapy –* Add felbamate at 15 mg/kg/day in divided doses 3 or 4 times daily while reducing present AEDs by 20% to control plasma levels of concurrent phenytoin, valproic acid, phenobarbital and carbamazepine (and its metabolites). Further reductions of the concomitant AED dosage may be necessary to minimize side effects caused by drug interactions. Increase the felbamate dosage by 15 mg/kg/day increments at weekly intervals to 45 mg/kg/day. Most side effects during adjunctive therapy resolve as the dosage of concomitant AEDs is decreased.

➤*Storage / Stability:*
Suspension – Shake well before using. Store at room temperature.

Actions

➤*Pharmacology:* Felbamate is an oral antiepileptic agent. The mechanism by which it exerts its anticonvulsant activity is unknown, but in animals, felbamate has properties in common with other anticonvulsants. Felbamate is effective in mice and rats in the maximal electroshock test, the SC pentylenetetrazol seizure test and the SC pic-

FELBAMATE

rotoxin seizure test. Felbamate also exhibits anticonvulsant activity against seizures induced by intracerebroventricular administration of glutamate in rats and N-methyl-D,L-aspartic acid in mice. Protection against maximal electroshock-induced seizures suggests that felbamate may reduce seizure spread, an effect possibly predictive of efficacy in generalized tonic-clonic or partial seizures. Protection against pentylenetetrazol-induced seizures suggests that felbamate may increase seizure threshold, an effect considered to be predictive of potential efficacy in absence seizures.

Receptor-binding studies in vitro indicate that felbamate has weak inhibitory effects on GABA-receptor binding and benzodiazepine receptor binding and is devoid of activity at the MK-801 receptor binding site of the NMDA receptor-ionophore complex. However, felbamate interacts as an antagonist at the strychnine-insensitive glycine recognition site of the NMDA receptor-ionophore complex.

There was a mean decrease in respiratory rate of ≈ 1 respiration/min during adjunctive therapy in children. In adults, statistically significant mean reductions in body weight were observed during monotherapy and adjunctive therapy. In children, there were mean decreases in body weight during adjunctive therapy and monotherapy; however, these mean changes were not statistically significant. These mean reductions in adults and children were $\approx 5\%$ of the mean weights at baseline.

➤*Pharmacokinetics:*

Absorption/Distribution – Felbamate is well absorbed after oral administration. Over 90% of the dose is recovered in the urine. Pharmacokinetic parameters of the tablet and suspension are similar.

The apparent volume of distribution was 756 ± 82 ml/kg after a 1200 mg dose. Felbamate C_{max}, C_{min} and AUC are proportionate to dose. Multiple daily doses of 1200, 2400 and 3600 mg gave C_{min} values of 30 ± 5, 55 ± 8 and 83 ± 21 mcg/ml, respectively (n = 10). Felbamate gave dose-proportional steady-state peak plasma concentrations in children ages 4 to 12 over a range of 15, 30 and 45 mg/kg/day with peak concentrations of 17, 32 and 49 mcg/ml, respectively.

Metabolism/Excretion – Following oral administration, felbamate is the predominant plasma species ($\approx 90\%$). About 40% to 50% of absorbed dose appears unchanged in urine, and an additional 40% is present as unidentified metabolites and conjugates. About 15% is present as parahydroxyfelbamate, 2-hydroxyfelbamate and felbamate monocarbamate, none of which have significant anticonvulsant activity. Binding to plasma protein was independent of concentrations between 10 and 310 mcg/ml. Binding ranged from 22% to 25%, mostly to albumin.

Felbamate is excreted with a terminal half-life of 20 to 23 hours, which is unaltered after multiple doses. Clearance after a single 1200 mg dose is 26 ± 3 ml/hr/kg; after multiple daily doses of 3600 mg, it is 30 ± 8 ml/hr/kg.

Contraindications

Hypersensitivity to felbamate or ingredients of the product; hypersensitivity reactions to other carbamates; history of any blood dyscrasia or hepatic dysfunction.

Warnings

➤*Aplastic anemia:* There have been cases of aplastic anemia, some fatal, in association with the use of felbamate (see Warning Box).

➤*Hepatic failure:* There have been cases of acute liver failure, some fatal, in association with the use of felbamate (see Warning Box).

➤*Discontinuation:* Antiepileptic drugs should not be suddenly discontinued because of the possibility of increasing seizure frequency (see Administration and Dosage).

➤*Carcinogenesis:* There was a statistically significant increase in hepatic cell adenomas in high-dose male and female mice (1200 mg/kg) and in high-dose female rats (100 mg/kg). Hepatic hypertrophy was significantly increased in a dose-related manner in mice. There was a statistically significant increase in benign interstitial cell tumors of the testes in male rats receiving high-dose felbamate.

As a result of the synthesis process, felbamate could contain small amounts of two known animal carcinogens, the genotoxic compound ethyl carbamate (urethane) and the nongenotoxic compound methyl carbamate. It is theoretically possible that a 50 kg patient receiving 3600 mg of felbamate could be exposed to ≤ 0.72 mcg urethane and 1800 mcg methyl carbamate. These daily doses are $\approx 1/35,000$ (urethane) and 1/5500 (methyl carbamate) on a mg/kg basis of the dose levels carcinogenic in rodents. Any presence of these two compounds in felbamate used in the lifetime carcinogenicity studies was inadequate to cause tumors.

➤*Elderly:* Clinical experience has not identified differences in responses between the elderly and younger patients. In general, dosage selection for an elderly patient should be cautious, usually starting at the low end of the dosing range, reflecting the greater frequency of decreased hepatic, renal or cardiac function and of concomitant disease or other drug therapy.

➤*Pregnancy: Category C.* Placental transfer of felbamate occurs in rat pups. The no-effect dose for rat pup mortality was 6.9 times the human dose on a mg/kg basis. There are no studies in pregnant women. Use during pregnancy only if clearly needed.

➤*Lactation:* Felbamate has been detected in breast milk. The effect on the nursing infant is unknown. In rats, there was a decrease in pup weight and an increase in pup deaths during lactation.

➤*Children:* Safety and efficacy in children, other than those with Lennox-Gastaut syndrome, have not been established.

Precautions

➤*Monitoring:* Perform full hematologic evaluations before, during and for a significant period of time after discontinuation of felbamate therapy. While it might appear prudent to perform frequent CBCs in patients while continuing therapy, there is no evidence that such monitoring will provide early detection of marrow suppression before aplastic anemia occurs. Obtain complete pretreatment blood counts, including platelets and reticulocytes, at baseline. Consult a hematologist if any hematologic abnormalities are detected during the course of treatment. Discontinue if any evidence of bone marrow depression occurs.

Perform liver function testing (AST, ALT, bilirubin) before felbamate is started and at 1- to 2-week intervals during therapy. Discontinue immediately if any liver abnormalities are detected during the course of treament.

➤*Photosensitivity:* Photosensitization (photoallergy or phototoxicity) may occur; therefore, caution patients to take protective measures against exposure to ultraviolet light or sunlight (eg, sunscreens, protective clothing) until tolerance is determined.

Drug Interactions

Felbamate Drug Interactions		
Precipitant drug	Object drug*	Description
Felbamate	Phenytoin ↑	Felbamate causes an increase in steady-state phenytoin levels. To maintain phenytoin levels and achieve felbamate dosages of 3600 mg/day, an ≈ 40% dose reduction of phenytoin was necessary in some patients. In contrast, phenytoin causes an approximate doubling of felbamate clearance, resulting in an ≈ 45% decrease in steady-state levels.
Phenytoin	Felbamate ↓	
Felbamate	Phenobarbital ↑	Coadministration causes an increase in phenobarbital plasma concentrations. Phenobarbital may reduce plasma felbamate levels. Steady-state plasma felbamate concentrations were 29% lower than the mean concentrations of a group of newly diagnosed subjects with epilepsy also receiving 2400 mg felbamate a day.
Phenobarbital	Felbamate ↓	
Felbamate	Carbamazepine ↓	Felbamate causes a decrease in steady-state carbamazepine levels and an increase in steady-state carbamazepine epoxide (metabolite) levels. In addition, carbamazepine causes an ≈ 50% increase in felbamate clearance, resulting in an ≈ 40% decrease in steady-state trough levels.
Carbamazepine	Felbamate ↓	
Felbamate	Methsuximide ↑	Increased normethsuximide levels requiring methsuximide dose reduction was reported in three patients.
Felbamate	Valproic acid ↑	Felbamate causes an increase in steady-state valproic acid levels. Valproic acid does not appear to affect felbamate levels.

*↑= Object drug increased. ↓ = Object drug decreased.

FELBAMATE

Adverse Reactions

Felbamate Adverse Reactions (%)						
	Adults				Children	
	Monotherapy		Adjunctive therapy		Lennox-Gastaut	
Adverse reaction	Felbamate (n = 58)	Valproate (n = 50)	Felbamate (n = 114)	Placebo (n = 43)	Felbamate (n = 31)	Placebo (n = 27)
CNS						
Insomnia	8.6	4	17.5	7	16.1	14.8
Headache	6.9	18	36.8	9.3	6.5	18.5
Anxiety	5.2	2	5.3	4.7	—	—
Somnolence	—	—	19.3	7	48.4	11.1
Dizziness	—	—	18.4	14	—	—
Nervousness	—	—	7	2.3	16.1	18.5
Tremor	—	—	6.1	2.3	—	—
Abnormal gait	—	—	5.3	0	9.7	0
Depression	—	—	5.3	0	—	—
Paresthesia	—	—	3.5	2.3	—	—
Ataxia	—	—	3.5	0	6.5	3.7
Dry mouth	—	—	2.6	0	—	—
Stupor	—	—	2.6	0	—	—
Abnormal thinking	—	—	—	—	6.5	3.7
Emotional lability	—	—	—	—	6.5	0
Miosis	—	—	—	—	6.5	0
Dermatologic						
Acne	3.4	0	—	—	—	—
Rash	3.4	0	3.5	4.7	9.7	7.4
GI						
Dyspepsia	8.6	2	12.3	7	6.5	3.7
Vomiting	8.6	2	16.7	4.7	38.7	14.8
Constipation	6.9	2	11.4	2.3	12.9	0
Diarrhea	5.2	0	5.3	2.3	—	—
ALT increased	5.2	2	3.5	0	—	—
Nausea	—	—	34.2	2.3	6.5	0
Anorexia	—	—	19.3	2.3	54.8	14.8
Abdominal pain	—	—	5.3	0	—	—
Hiccups	—	—	—	—	9.7	3.7
GU						
Urinary incontinence	—	—	—	—	6.5	7.4
Intramenstrual bleeding	3.4	0	—	—	—	—
UTI	3.4	2	—	—	—	—
Hematologic						
Purpura	—	—	—	—	12.9	7.4
Leukopenia	—	—	—	—	6.5	0
Respiratory						
Upper respiratory tract infection	8.6	4	5.3	7	45.2	25.9
Rhinitis	6.9	0	—	—	—	—
Sinusitis	—	—	3.5	0	—	—
Pharyngitis	—	—	2.6	0	9.7	3.7
Coughing	—	—	—	—	6.5	0
Special senses						
Diplopia	3.4	4	6.1	0	—	—
Otitis media	3.4	0	—	—	9.7	0
Taste perversion	—	—	6.1	0	—	—
Abnormal vision	—	—	5.3	2.3	—	—
Miscellaneous						
Hypophosphatemia	3.4	0	—	—	—	—
Myalgia	—	—	2.6	0	—	—
Fatigue	6.9	4	16.8	7	9.7	3.7
Weight decrease	3.4	0	—	—	6.5	0
Facial edema	3.4	0	—	—	—	—
Fever	—	—	2.6	4.7	22.6	11.1
Chest pain	—	—	2.6	0	—	—
Pain	—	—	—	—	6.5	0

➤*Cardiovascular:* Palpitation, tachycardia (≥ 1%); supraventricular tachycardia (< 0.1%).

➤*CNS:* Agitation, psychological disturbance, aggressive reaction (≥ 1%); hallucination, euphoria, suicide attempt, migraine (0.1% to 1%).

➤*Dermatologic:* Pruritus (≥ 1%); urticaria, bullous eruption (0.1% to 1%); buccal mucous membrane swelling, Stevens-Johnson syndrome (< 0.1%).

➤*GI:* AST increased (≥ 1%); esophagitis, appetite increased (0.1% to 1%); GGT elevated (< 0.1%).

➤*Hematologic:* Lymphadenopathy, leukopenia, leukocytosis, thrombocytopenia, granulocytopenia (0.1% to 1%); positive antinuclear factor test, qualitative platelet disorder, agranulocytosis (< 0.1%).

➤*Metabolic/Nutritional:* Hypokalemia, hyponatremia, LDH increased, alkaline phosphatase increased, hypophosphatemia (0.1% to 1%); CPK increased (< 0.1%).

➤*Miscellaneous:* Weight increase, asthenia, malaise, influenza-like symptoms (≥ 1%); dystonia (0.1% to 1%); anaphylactoid reaction, substernal chest pain, photosensitivity allergic reaction (< 0.1%).

Overdosage

➤*Symptoms:* Four subjects inadvertently received felbamate as adjunctive therapy in dosages ranging from 5400 to 7200 mg/day for 6 to 51 days. One subject who received 5400 mg/day as monotherapy for 1 week reported no adverse experiences. Another subject attempted suicide by ingesting 12,000 mg in a 12-hour period. The only adverse experiences reported were mild gastric distress and a resting heart rate of 100 bpm. No serious adverse reactions have been reported.

FELBAMATE

▶*Treatment:* Employ general supportive measures if overdosage occurs. Refer to General Management of Acute Overdosage. It is not known if felbamate is dialyzable.

Patient Information

Inform patients that the use of felbamate is associated with aplastic anemia and hepatic failure, potentially fatal conditions acutely or over a long period of time.

Instruct patients to take felbamate only as prescribed.

Avoid prolonged exposure to sunlight or sunlamps; may cause photosensitivity.

Advise patients to immediately report any signs of infection, bleeding, easy bruising, or signs of anemia (eg, fatigue, weakness, lassitude) to the physician.

Advise patients to follow their physician's directives for liver function testing before starting and at frequent intervals while taking felbamate.

GABAPENTIN

Rx	Neurontin (Pfizer)	**Capsules:** 100 mg	Lactose, talc. (PD Neurontin/100 mg). White. In 100s and UD 50s.
		300 mg	Lactose, talc. (PD Neurontin/300 mg). Yellow. In 100s and UD 50s.
		400 mg	Lactose, talc. (PD Neurontin/400 mg). Orange. In 100s and UD 50s.
		Tablets: 600 mg	Talc. (Neurontin 600). White, elliptical. Film-coated. In 100s, 500s, and UD 50s.
		800 mg	Talc. (Neurontin 800). White, elliptical. Film-coated. In 100s, 500s, and UD 50s.
		Solution, oral: 250 mg/5 mL	Xylitol. Cool strawberry anise flavor. In 470 mL.

Refer to the general discussion beginning in the Anticonvulsants introduction.

Indications

▶*Epilepsy:* Adjunctive therapy in the treatment of partial seizures with and without secondary generalization in patients over 12 years of age with epilepsy. Also indicated as adjunctive therapy for partial seizures in children 3 to 12 years of age.

▶*Postherpetic neuralgia:* For management of postherpetic neuralgia in adults.

▶*Unlabeled uses:* Tremors associated with multiple sclerosis; neuropathic pain; bipolar disorder; migraine prophylaxis.

Administration and Dosage

▶*Approved by the FDA:* December 30, 1993.

Can be taken with or without food.

▶*Postherpetic neuralgia:* In adults with postherpetic neuralgia, gabapentin therapy may be initiated as a single 300 mg dose on day 1, 600 mg/day on day 2 (divided twice daily), and 900 mg/day on day 3 (divided 3 times daily). The dose can subsequently be titrated up as needed for pain relief to a daily dose of 1800 mg (divided 3 times daily). In clinical studies, efficacy was demonstrated over a range of doses from 1800 mg/day to 3600 mg/day with comparable effects across the dose range. Additional benefit of using doses greater than 1800 mg/day was not demonstrated.

▶*Epilepsy:* Recommended for add-on therapy in patients 3 years of age and older.

Patients older than 12 years of age – The effective dose is 900 to 1800 mg/day in divided doses (3 times/day) using 300 or 400 mg capsules, or 600 or 800 mg tablets. The starting dose is 300 mg 3 times/day. If necessary, the dose may be increased using 300 or 400 mg capsules, or 600 or 800 mg tablets 3 times/day up to 1800 mg/day. Dosages up to 2400 mg/day have been well tolerated in long-term clinical studies. Doses of 3600 mg/day have also been administered to a small number of patients for a relatively short duration, and have been well tolerated. The maximum time between doses in the 3 times daily schedule should not exceed 12 hours.

Pediatric patients 3 to 12 years of age – The starting dose should range from 10 to 15 mg/kg/day in 3 divided doses, and the effective dose reached by upward titration over a period of approximately 3 days. The effective dose of gabapentin in patients 5 years of age and older is 25 to 35 mg/kg/day and given in divided doses (3 times/day). The effective dose in pediatric patients 3 and 4 years of age is 40 mg/kg/day and given in divided doses (3 times/day). Gabapentin may be administered as the oral solution, capsule, tablet, or using combinations of these formulations. Dosages up to 50 mg/kg/day have been well tolerated in a long-term clinical study. The maximum time interval between doses should not exceed 12 hours.

It is not necessary to monitor gabapentin plasma concentrations to optimize therapy. Further, because there are no significant pharmacokinetic interactions with other commonly used antiepileptic drugs, the addition of gabapentin does not alter the plasma levels of these drugs appreciably.

If gabapentin is discontinued or an alternate anticonvulsant medication is added to the therapy, this should be done gradually over a minimum of 1 week.

▶*Renal function impairment:*

Gabapentin Dosage Based on Renal Function in Patients ≥ 12 Years of Age

Creatinine clearance (mL/min)	Total daily dose range (mg/day)	Dose regimen (mg)				
≥ 60	900 to 3600	300 tid	400 tid	600 tid	800 tid	1200 tid
> 30 to 59	400 to 1400	200 bid	300 bid	400 bid	500 bid	700 bid
> 15 to 29	200 to 700	200 qd	300 qd	400 qd	500 qd	700 qd

Gabapentin Dosage Based on Renal Function in Patients ≥ 12 Years of Age

Creatinine clearance (mL/min)	Total daily dose range (mg/day)	Dose regimen (mg)				
15[a]	100 to 300	100 qd	125 qd	150 qd	200 qd	300 qd
Posthemodialysis supplemental dose (mg)[b]						
Hemodialysis		125[b]	150[b]	200[b]	250[b]	350[b]

[a] For patients with creatinine clearance (Ccr) < 15 mL/min, reduce daily dose in proportion to Ccr (eg, patients with a Ccr of 7.5 mL/min should receive one-half the daily dose that patients with a Ccr of 15 mL/min receive.

[b] Patients on hemodialysis should receive maintenance doses based on estimates of Ccr as indicated in the upper portion of the table and a supplemental posthemodialysis dose administered after each 4 hours of hemodialysis as indicated in the lower portion of the table.

Ccr is difficult to measure in outpatients. In patients with stable renal function, Ccr can be reasonably well estimated using the equation of Cockcroft and Gault:

$$\text{Males:} \quad \frac{\text{Weight (kg)} \times (140 - \text{age})}{72 \times \text{serum creatinine (mg/dL)}} = \text{Ccr}$$

Females: $0.85 \times$ above value

Use of gabapentin in patients under 12 years of age with compromised renal function has not been studied.

▶*Storage / Stability:*

Capsules and tablets – Store at 25°C (77°F); excursions permitted to 15° to 30°C (59° to 86°F).

Oral solution – Store refrigerated (2° to 8°C; 36° to 46°F).

Actions

▶*Pharmacology:* The mechanism by which gabapentin exerts its anticonvulsant action is unknown, but in animals it has properties in common with other anticonvulsants. Gabapentin exhibits antiseizure activity in mice and rats in the maximal electroshock and pentylenetetrazole seizure models and other preclinical models (eg, strains with genetic epilepsy). The relevance of these models to human epilepsy is not known.

The mechanism by which gabapentin exerts its analgesic action is unknown, but in animal models of analgesia, gabapentin prevents allodynia and hyperalgesia. In particular, gabapentin prevents pain-related responses in several models of neuropathic pain in rats or mice (eg, spinal nerve ligation models, streptozocin-induced diabetes model, spinal cord injury model, acute herpes zoster infection model). Gabapentin also decreases pain-related responses after peripheral inflammation (carrageenan footpad test, late phase of formalin test). Gabapentin did not alter immediate pain-related behaviors (rat tail flick test, formalin footpad acute phase, acetic acid abdominal constriction test, footpad heat irradiation test). The relevance of these models to human pain is not known.

Gabapentin is structurally related to the neurotransmitter gamma-aminobutyric acid (GABA) but it does not interact with GABA receptors, it is not converted metabolically into GABA or a GABA agonist. Gabapentin is not an inhibitor of GABA uptake or degradation. Gabapentin does not exhibit affinity for a number of other common receptor sites. In vitro studies have revealed a gabapentin binding site in areas of rat brain including neocortex and hippocampus.

All pharmacological actions following gabapentin administration are due to the activity of the parent compound; gabapentin is not appreciably metabolized.

▶*Pharmacokinetics:*

Absorption – Gabapentin bioavailability is not dose-proportional (ie, as dose is increased, bioavailability decreases). Bioavailability of gabapentin is approximately 60%, 47%, 34%, 33%, and 27% following 900, 1200, 2400, 3600, and 4800 mg/day given in 3 divided doses, respectively. Food has only a slight effect on the rate and extent of absorption.

GABAPENTIN

Distribution – Gabapentin circulates largely unbound (less than 3%) to plasma protein. The apparent volume of distribution after 150 mg IV administration is approximately 58 L. In patients with epilepsy, steady-state predose (C_{min}) concentrations of gabapentin in cerebrospinal fluid (CSF) were approximately 20% of the corresponding plasma concentrations.

Metabolism / Excretion – Gabapentin is eliminated from the systemic circulation by renal excretion as unchanged drug; it is not appreciably metabolized.

Gabapentin elimination half-life is 5 to 7 hours and is unaltered by dose or following multiple dosing. Elimination rate constant, plasma clearance, and renal clearance are directly proportional to Ccr (see Warnings and Special Populations). In elderly patients and in patients with impaired renal function, gabapentin plasma clearance is reduced. Gabapentin can be removed from plasma by hemodialysis.

Special populations:

• *Renal insufficiency* – Subjects with renal insufficiency were administered single 400 mg oral doses. The mean half-life ranged from about 6.5 (patients with Ccr greater than 60 mL/min) to 52 hours (Ccr less than 30 mL/min) and renal clearance from about 90 mL/min (greater than 60 mL/min group) to about 10 mL/min (less than 30 mL/min). Mean plasma clearance decreased from approximately 190 to 20 mL/min. Dosage adjustment in patients with compromised renal function is necessary (see Administration and Dosage).

• *Children* – Gabapentin pharmacokinetics were determined in 48 pediatric subjects between the ages of 1 month and 12 years following a dose of approximately 10 mg/kg. Peak plasma concentrations were similar across the entire age group and occurred 2 to 3 hours postdose. In general, pediatric subjects between 1 month and less than 5 years of age achieved approximately 30% lower exposure (AUC) than that observed in those 5 years of age and older. Accordingly, oral clearance normalized per body weight was higher in the younger children. Apparent oral clearance of gabapentin was directly proportional to Ccr. Gabapentin elimination half-life averaged 4.7 hours and was similar across the age groups studied.

A population pharmacokinetic analysis was performed in 253 pediatric subjects between 1 month and 13 years of age. Patients received 10 to 65 mg/kg/day given 3 times/day. Apparent oral clearance (CL/F) was directly proportional to Ccr and this relationship was similar following a single dose and at steady state. Higher oral clearance values were observed in children under 5 years of age compared with those observed in children 5 years of age and older, when normalized per body weight. The clearance was highly variable in infants under 1 year of age. The normalized CL/F values observed in pediatric patients 5 years of age and older were consistent with values observed in adults after a single dose. The oral volume of distribution normalized per body weight was constant across the age range.

These pharmacokinetic data indicate that the effective daily dose in pediatric patients with epilepsy 3 and 4 years of age should be 40 mg/kg/day to achieve average plasma concentrations similar to those achieved in patients 5 years of age and older receiving gabapentin at 30 mg/kg/day (see Administration and Dosage).

Hemodialysis – In a study in anuric subjects (n = 11), the apparent elimination half-life of gabapentin on nondialysis days was about 132 hours; during dialysis, the apparent half-life of gabapentin was reduced to 3.8 hours. Hemodialysis thus has a significant effect on gabapentin elimination in anuric subjects. Dosage adjustment in patients undergoing hemodialysis is necessary (see Administration and Dosage).

Age – The effect of age was studied in subjects 20 to 80 years of age. Apparent oral clearance of gabapentin decreased as age increased, from about 225 mL/min in those under 30 years of age to about 125 mL/min in those over 70 years of age. Renal clearance also declined with age; however, the decline in the renal clearance of gabapentin with age can largely be explained by the decline in renal function. Reduction of gabapentin dose may be required in patients who have age-related compromised renal function (see Administration and Dosage).

Contraindications

Hypersensitivity to the drug or its ingredients.

Warnings

➤*Neuropsychiatric adverse events (3 to 12 years of age):* Gabapentin use in pediatric patients with epilepsy 3 to 12 years of age is associated with the occurrence of CNS-related adverse events. The most significant of these can be classified into the following categories:

1.) emotional lability (primarily behavioral problems),
2.) hostility, including aggressive behaviors,
3.) thought disorder, including concentration problems and change in school performance, and
4.) hyperkinesia (primarily restlessness and hyperactivity).

Among the gabapentin-treated patients, most of the events were mild to moderate in intensity.

In controlled trials in pediatric patients 3 to 12 years of age, the incidence of these adverse events was the following: Emotional lability, 6% (gabapentin-treated patients) vs 1.3% (placebo-treated patients); hostility, 5.2% vs 1.3%; hyperkinesia, 4.7% vs 2.9%; and thought disorder,

1.7% vs 0. One of these events, a report of hostility, was considered serious. Discontinuation of gabapentin treatment occurred in 1.3% of patients reporting emotional lability and hyperkinesia and 0.9% of gabapentin-treated patients reporting hostility and thought disorder. One placebo-treated patient withdrew as a result of emotional lability.

➤*Withdrawal-precipitated seizure:* Do not abruptly discontinue antiepileptic drugs because of the possibility of increasing seizure frequency.

➤*Status epilepticus:* In the placebo-controlled studies in patients older than 12 years of age, the incidence of status epilepticus in patients receiving gabapentin was 0.6% vs 0.5% with placebo. Among the patients treated with gabapentin, 31 (1.5%) had status epilepticus. Of these, 14 patients had no prior history of status epilepticus either before treatment or while on other medications. Because adequate historical data are not available, it is impossible to say whether or not treatment with gabapentin is associated with a higher or lower rate of status epilepticus than would be expected to occur in a similar population not treated with gabapentin.

➤*Sudden and unexplained deaths in patients with epilepsy:* During the course of premarketing development of gabapentin, 8 sudden and unexplained deaths were recorded among 2203 patients. Some of these could represent seizure-related deaths where the seizure was not observed (eg, at night). This represents an incidence of 0.0038 deaths per patient-year. Although this rate exceeds that expected in a healthy population matched for age and sex, it is within the range of estimates for the incidence of sudden unexplained deaths in patients with epilepsy not receiving gabapentin.

➤*Carcinogenesis:* An unexpectedly high incidence of pancreatic acinar adenocarcinomas was identified in male, but not female, rats. The clinical significance of this finding is unknown. In clinical studies comprising 2085 patient-years of exposure, new tumors were reported in 10 patients, and pre-existing tumors worsened in 11 patients during or up to 2 years following discontinuation of gabapentin.

➤*Elderly:* Clinical studies of gabapentin in epilepsy did not include sufficient numbers of subjects 65 years of age and older to determine whether they responded differently from younger subjects. Other reported clinical experience has not identified differences in responses between the elderly and younger patients. In general, dose selection for an elderly patient should be cautious, usually starting at the low end of the dosing range, reflecting the greater frequency of decreased hepatic, renal, or cardiac function, and of concomitant disease or other drug therapy.

This drug is known to be substantially excreted by the kidney, and the risk of toxic reactions to this drug may be greater in patients with impaired renal function. Because elderly patients are more likely to have decreased renal function, care should be taken in dose selection and dose should be adjusted based on Ccr values in these patients (see Pharmacology, Adverse Reactions, and Administration and Dosage).

➤*Pregnancy: Category C.* Gabapentin is fetotoxic in rodents, causing delayed ossification of several bones in the skull, vertebrae, forelimbs, and hindlimbs. These effects occurred when pregnant mice received oral doses of 1000 or 3000 mg/kg/day during the period of organogenesis, or approximately 1 to 4 times the maximum dose of 3600 mg/day.

When rats were dosed prior to and during mating and throughout gestation, pups from all dose groups (500, 1000, and 2000 mg/kg/day) were affected. These doses are equivalent to approximately 1 to 5 times the maximum human dose. There was an increased incidence of hydroureter or hydronephrosis in rats. The doses at which the effects occurred are approximately 1 to 5 times the maximum human dose of 3600 mg/day.

In rabbits, an increased incidence of postimplantation fetal loss occurred in dams exposed to 60, 300, and 1500 mg/kg/day, or less than approximately ¼ to 8 times the maximum human dose.

There are no adequate and well-controlled studies in pregnant women. Use during pregnancy only if the potential benefit justifies the potential risk to the fetus.

➤*Lactation:* Gabapentin is secreted in breast milk. A nursed infant could be exposed to a maximum dose of approximately 1 mg/kg/day of gabapentin. Because the effect on the nursing infant is unknown, use gabapentin in women who are nursing only if the benefits clearly outweigh the risks.

➤*Children:*

Postherpetic neuralgia – Safety and effectiveness of gabapentin in the management of postherpetic neuralgia in pediatric patients have not been established.

Epilepsy – Effectiveness as adjunctive therapy in the treatment of partial seizures in pediatric patients below 3 years of age has not been established.

Precautions

➤*Monitoring:* Clinical trial data do not indicate that routine monitoring of clinical laboratory parameters is necessary for the safe use of gabapentin. The value of monitoring blood concentrations has not been established. Gabapentin may be used in combination with other antiepileptic drugs without concern for alteration of the blood concentrations of gabapentin or of other antiepileptic drugs.

GABAPENTIN

Drug Interactions

Gabapentin is not appreciably metabolized nor does it interfere with the metabolism of commonly coadministered antiepileptic drugs.

Gabapentin Drug Interactions			
Precipitant drug	Object drug*		Description
Antacids	Gabapentin	↓	Antacids reduced the bioavailability of gabapentin by about 20%. This decrease in bioavailability was about 5% when gabapentin was given 2 hours after the antacid. It is recommended that gabapentin be taken at least 2 hours following antacid administration.
Cimetidine	Gabapentin	↑	The mean apparent oral clearance of gabapentin fell by 14% and Ccr fell by 10% with concurrent cimetidine. Thus, cimetidine seemed to alter the renal excretion of gabapentin and creatinine. This small decrease in gabapentin excretion is not expected to be of clinical importance.
Hydrocodone	Gabapentin	↑	Coadministration increases gabapentin AUC values by 14%. Coadministration decreases hydrocodone C_{max} and AUC values in a dose-dependent manner. C_{max} and AUC values were 3% and 4% lower, respectively, after administration of 125 mg gabapentin and 21% to 22% lower, respectively after administration of 500 mg gabapentin. The mechanism for this interaction and the magnitude of interaction at other doses is unknown.
Gabapentin	Hydrocodone	↓	
Morphine	Gabapentin	↑	Coadministration of 60 mg morphine 2 hours prior to administration of 600 mg gabapentin resulted in an increase in gabapentin AUC by 44%. The magnitude of interaction at other doses is unknown.
Gabapentin	Contraceptives, oral	↑	The C_{max} of norethindrone was 13% higher when coadministered with gabapentin; this interaction is not expected to be of clinical importance.

* ↑ = Object drug increased. ↓ = Object drug decreased.

▶*Drug/Lab test interactions:* Because false positive readings were reported with the *Ames N-Multistix SG* dipstick test for urinary protein when gabapentin was added to other antiepileptic drugs, the more specific sulfosalicylic acid precipitation procedure is recommended to determine the presence of urine protein.

Adverse Reactions

▶*Postherpetic neuralgia:* The most commonly observed adverse events associated with the use of gabapentin in adults, not seen at an equivalent frequency among placebo-treated patients, were dizziness, somnolence, and peripheral edema.

In the 2 controlled studies in postherpetic neuralgia, 16% of the 336 patients who received gabapentin and 9% of the 227 patient who received placebo discontinued treatment because of an adverse event. The adverse events that most frequently led to withdrawal in gabapentin-treated patients were dizziness, somnolence, and nausea.

Gabapentin Adverse Reactions in Postherpetic Neuralgia (%)		
Adverse reaction	Gabapentin (N = 336)	Placebo (N = 227)
CNS		
Dizziness	28	7.5
Somnolence	21.4	5.3
Asthenia	5.7	4.8
Ataxia	3.3	0
Abnormal thinking	2.7	0
Abnormal gait	1.5	0
Incoordination	1.5	0
Amnesia	1.2	0.9
Hypesthesia	1.2	0.9
Headache	3.3	3.1
Metabolic/Nutritional		
Peripheral edema	8.3	2.2
Weight gain	1.8	0
Hyperglycemia	1.2	0.4

Gabapentin Adverse Reactions in Postherpetic Neuralgia (%)		
Adverse reaction	Gabapentin (N = 336)	Placebo (N = 227)
GI		
Diarrhea	5.7	3.1
Dry mouth	4.8	1.3
Constipation	3.9	1.8
Nausea	3.9	3.1
Vomiting	3.3	1.8
Abdominal pain	2.7	2.6
Flatulence	2.1	1.8
Special senses		
Amblyopia[a]	2.7	0.9
Conjunctivitis	1.2	0
Diplopia	1.2	0
Otitis media	1.2	0
Miscellaneous		
Infection	5.1	3.5
Accidental injury	3.3	1.3
Rash	1.2	0.9
Pharyngitis	1.2	0.4

[a] Reported as blurred vision.

Other events in more than 1% of patients but equally or more frequent in the placebo group included pain, tremor, neuralgia, back pain, dyspepsia, dyspnea, and flu syndrome.

There were no clinically important differences between men and women in the types and incidence of adverse events. Because there were few patients whose race was reported as other than white, there are insufficient data to support a statement regarding the distribution of adverse events by race.

▶*Epilepsy:* The most commonly observed adverse events associated with the use of gabapentin in combination with other antiepileptic drugs in patients older than 12 years of age, not seen at an equivalent frequency among placebo-treated patients, were somnolence, dizziness, ataxia, fatigue, and nystagmus. The most commonly observed adverse events reported with the use of gabapentin in combination with other antiepileptic drugs in pediatric patients 3 to 12 years of age, not seen at an equal frequency among placebo-treated patients, were viral infection, fever, nausea/vomiting, somnolence, and hostility.

Approximately 7% of the 2074 individuals over 12 years of age and approximately 7% of the 449 pediatric patients 3 to 12 years of age who received gabapentin in premarketing clinical trials discontinued treatment because of an adverse events. The adverse events most commonly associated with withdrawal in patients over 12 years of age were somnolence (1.2%); ataxia (0.8%); fatigue, nausea, vomiting, dizziness (0.6%). The adverse events most commonly associated with withdrawal in pediatric patients were emotional lability (1.6%); hostility (1.3%); and hyperkinesia (1.1%).

Gabapentin Adverse Reactions in Epilepsy Treatment (%)		
Adverse reaction	Gabapentin[a] (> 12 years of age) (N = 543)	Gabapentin[a] (3 to 12 years of age) (N = 119)
CNS		
Somnolence	19.3	8.4
Dizziness	19.3	2.5
Ataxia	12.5	—
Nystagmus	8.3	—
Hostility	—	7.6
Tremor	6.8	—
Emotional lability	> 1	4.2
Hyperkinesia	—	2.5
Nervousness	2.4	—
Dysarthria	2.4	—
Amnesia	2.2	—
Depression	1.8	—
Abnormal thinking	1.7	—
Twitching	1.3	—
Abnormal coordination	1.1	—
Headache	> 1	> 2
Convulsions	> 1	> 2
Confusion	> 1	—
Insomnia	> 1	—
Dermatologic		
Pruritus	1.3	—
Abrasion	1.3	—
Rash	> 1	—
Acne	> 1	—

GABAPENTIN

Gabapentin Adverse Reactions in Epilepsy Treatment (%)		
Adverse reaction	Gabapentin[a] (> 12 years of age) (N = 543)	Gabapentin[a] (3 to 12 years of age) (N = 119)
GI		
Nausea/Vomiting	> 1	8.4
Dyspepsia	2.2	—
Dryness of mouth/throat	1.7	—
Constipation	1.5	—
Dental abnormalities	1.5	—
Increased appetite	1.1	—
Abdominal pain	> 1	—
Diarrhea	> 1	> 2
Anorexia	—	> 2
Musculoskeletal		
Myalgia	2	—
Fracture	1.1	—
Respiratory		
Rhinitis	4.1	> 2
Bronchitis	—	3.4
Pharyngitis	2.8	> 2
Respiratory infection	—	2.5
Coughing	1.8	> 2
Upper respiratory infection	—	> 2
Special senses		
Diplopia	5.9	—
Amblyopia[b]	4.2	—
Otitis media	—	> 2
Miscellaneous		
Fatigue	11	3.4
Viral infection	> 1	10.9
Fever	> 1	10.1
Weight increase	2.9	3.4
Back pain	1.8	—
Peripheral edema	1.7	—
Impotence	1.5	—
Leukopenia	1.1	—
WBC decreased	1.1	—
Vasodilation	1.1	—

[a] Plus background antiepileptic drug therapy.
[b] Amblyopia often was described as blurred vision.

Among the treatment-emergent adverse events occurring at an incidence of at least 10% of gabapentin-treated patients, somnolence and ataxia appeared to exhibit a positive dose-response relationship.

Adult patients older than 12 years of age –

Cardiovascular: Hypertension (at least 1%); angina pectoris, hypotension, intracranial hemorrhage, murmur, palpitations, peripheral vascular disorder, tachycardia (0.1% to 1%); atrial fibrillation, bradycardia, cerebrovascular accident, deep thrombophlebitis, heart block, heart failure, hypercholesterolemia, hyperlipidemia, MI, pericardial effusion, pericardial rub, pericarditis, premature atrial contraction, pulmonary embolus, pulmonary thrombosis, thrombophlebitis, ventricular extrasystoles (fewer than 0.1%).

CNS: Anxiety, decreased/absent/increased reflexes, hostility, hyperkinesia, paresthesia, vertigo (at least 1%); abnormal dreaming, agitation, apathy, aphasia, cerebellar dysfunction, CNS tumors, decrease or loss of libido, decreased position sense, depersonalization, dysesthesia, doped-up sensation, dystonia, euphoria, facial paralysis, feeling high, hallucination, hemiplegia, hypesthesia, hypotonia, migraine, paranoia, paresis, positive Babinski sign, psychosis, stupor, subdural hematoma, suicidal, syncope (0.1% to 1%); antisocial reaction, apraxia, choreoathetosis, encephalopathy, fine motor control disorder, hyperesthesia, hypokinesia, hysteria, increased libido, local myoclonus, mania, meningismus, nerve palsy, neurosis, orofacial dyskinesia, personality disorder, subdued temperament, suicide gesture (fewer than 0.1%).

Dermatologic: Alopecia, cyst, dry skin, eczema, herpes simplex, hirsutism, increased sweating, seborrhea, urticaria (0.1% to 1%); desquamation, herpes zoster, leg ulcer, local swelling, maceration, melanosis, photosensitivity reaction, psoriasis, scalp seborrhea, skin discoloration, skin necrosis, skin nodules, skin papules, subcutaneous nodule (fewer than 0.1%).

Endocrine: Cushingoid appearance, goiter, hyperthyroid, hypoestrogen, hypothyroid (fewer than 0.1%).

GI: Anorexia, flatulence, gingivitis (at least 1%); bloody stools, fecal incontinence, gastroenteritis, glossitis, gum hemorrhage, hemorrhoids, hepatomegaly, increased salivation, stomatitis, thirst (0.1% to 1%); blisters in mouth, colitis, dysphagia, eructation, esophageal spasm, esophagitis, hematemesis, hiatal hernia, irritable bowel syndrome, lip hemorrhage, pancreatitis, peptic ulcer, perleche, proctitis, rectal hemorrhage, salivary gland enlarged, tooth discoloration (fewer than 0.1%).

GU: Abnormal ejaculation, amenorrhea, breast cancer, cystitis, dys-

menorrhea, dysuria, hematuria, inability to climax, menorrhagia, urinary retention/incontinence, urination frequency, vaginal hemorrhage (0.1% to 1%); acute renal failure, anuria, breast pain, epididymitis, genital pruritus, glycosuria, kidney pain, leukorrhea, nephrosis, nocturia, ovarian failure, pyuria, renal stone, swollen testicle, testicle pain, urination urgency, vaginal pain (fewer than 0.1%).

Hematologic/Lymphatic: Purpura (at least 1%; most often described as bruises resulting from physical trauma); anemia, lymphadenopathy, thrombocytopenia (0.1% to 1%); bleeding time increased, lymphocytosis, non-Hodgkin's lymphoma, WBC count increased (fewer than 0.1%).

Musculoskeletal: Arthralgia (at least 1%); arthritis, joint stiffness/swelling, positive Romberg test, tendinitis (0.1% to 1%); bursitis, contracture, costochondritis, osteoporosis (fewer than 0.1%).

Respiratory: Pneumonia (at least 1%); apnea, dyspnea, epistaxis (0.1% to 1%); aspiration pneumonia, bronchospasm, hyperventilation, hiccup, hypoventilation, laryngitis, lung edema, mucositis, nasal obstruction, snoring (fewer than 0.1%).

Special senses: Abnormal vision (at least 1%); bilateral or unilateral ptosis, cataract, conjunctivitis, dry eyes, ear fullness, earache, eye hemorrhage, eye pain, eye twitching, hearing loss, hordeolum, inner ear infection, otitis, photophobia, taste loss, tinnitus, unusual taste, visual field defect (0.1% to 1%); abnormal accommodation, blindness, chorioretinitis, corneal disorders, degenerative eye changes, eustachian tube dysfunction, eye focusing problem, eye itching, glaucoma, iritis, labyrinthitis, lacrimal dysfunction, miosis, odd smells, otitis externa, perforated ear drum, retinal degeneration, retinopathy, sensitivity to noise, strabismus, watery eyes (fewer than 0.1%).

Miscellaneous: Asthenia, facial edema, malaise (at least 1%); allergy, chill, generalized edema, weight decrease (0.1% to 1%); alcohol intolerance, hangover effect, lassitude, strange feelings (fewer than 0.1%).

Pediatric patients 3 to 12 years of age –

CNS: Aura disappeared; occipital neuralgia.

Respiratory: Hoarseness, pseudocroup.

Miscellaneous: Coagulation defect; dehydration; infectious mononucleosis; hepatitis; sleep walking.

▶*Clinical trials in adults with neuropathic pain of various etiology:*

Cardiovascular – Cardiovascular disorder, cerebrovascular accident, CHF, hypertension, hypotension, MI, migraine, palpitation, peripheral vascular disorder, syncope, vasodilation (0.1% to 1%); angina pectoris, heart failure, increased capillary fragility, phlebitis, thrombophlebitis, varicose vein (fewer than 0.1%).

CNS – Confusion, depression (at least 1%); abnormal dreams, anxiety, circumoral paresthesia, depersonalization, dysarthria, emotional lability, euphoria, hyperesthesia, hypokinesia, insomnia, libido decreased, nervousness, neuropathy, nystagmus, paresthesia, reflexes decreased, speech disorder, stupor, vertigo (0.1% to 1%); agitation, hypertonia, libido increased, movement disorder, myoclonus, vestibular disorder (fewer than 0.1%).

Dermatologic – Dry skin, fungal dermatitis, furunculosis, herpes simplex, herpes zoster, pruritus, psoriasis, skin disorder, skin ulcer, sweating, urticaria, vesiculobullous rash (0.1% to 1%); acne, hair disorder, maculopapular rash, nail disorder, skin carcinoma, skin discoloration, skin hypertrophy (fewer than 0.1%).

GI – Abnormal stools, anorexia, gastritis, gastroenteritis, GI disorder, increased appetite, liver function tests abnormal, oral moniliasis, periodontal abscess, thirst, tongue disorder, tooth disorder (0.1% to 1%); cholecystitis, cholelithiasis, duodenal ulcer, fecal incontinence, gamma glutamyl transpeptidase increased, gingivitis, intestinal obstruction, intestinal ulcer, melena, mouth ulceration, rectal disorder, rectal hemorrhage, stomatitis (fewer than 0.1%).

GU – Breast pain, dysuria, impotence, menstrual disorder, polyuria, urinary incontinence, urinary retention, urinary tract infection, vaginal moniliasis (0.1% to 1%); cystitis, ejaculation abnormal, gynecomastia, nocturia, pyelonephritis, swollen penis, swollen scrotum, urinary frequency, urinary urgency, urine abnormality (fewer than 0.1%).

Hematologic/Lymphatic – Anemia, ecchymosis, (0.1% to 1%); lymphadenopathy, lymphoma-like reaction, prothrombin decreased (fewer than 0.1%).

Metabolic/Nutritional – Edema, gout, hypoglycemia, weight loss (0.1% to 1%); alkaline phosphatase increased, diabetic ketoacidosis, lactic dehydrogenase increased (fewer than 0.1%).

Musculoskeletal – Arthralgia, arthritis, arthrosis, leg cramps, myalgia, myasthenia (0.1% to 1%); joint disorder, shin bone pain, tendon disorder (fewer than 0.1%).

Respiratory – Asthma, bronchitis, cough increased, epistaxis, lung disorder, pneumonia, rhinitis, sinusitis (0.1% to 1%); hemoptysis, voice alteration (fewer than 0.1%).

Special senses – Abnormal vision, deafness, ear pain, eye disorder, taste perversion (0.1% to 1%); conjunctival hyperemia, diabetic retinopathy, eye pain, fundi with microhemorrhage, retinal vein thrombosis, taste loss (fewer than 0.1%).

Miscellaneous – Abscess, allergic reaction, cellulitis, chest pain, chills, chills and fever, diabetes mellitus, face edema, malaise, neck pain, mucous membrane disorder (0.1% to 1%); abnormal BUN value, body odor, cyst, fever, hernia, lump in neck, pelvic pain, sepsis, viral

GABAPENTIN

infection (fewer than 0.1%).

►*Postmarketing experiences:*

Miscellaneous – Angioedema; blood glucose fluctuation; erythema multiforme; elevated liver function tests; fever; hyponatremia; jaundice; Stevens-Johnson syndrome.

Overdosage

►*Symptoms:* Signs of acute toxicity in animals included ataxia, labored breathing, ptosis, sedation, hypoactivity, or excitation. Acute oral overdoses of gabapentin up to 49 g have been reported. In these cases, double vision, slurred speech, drowsiness, lethargy, and diarrhea were observed. All patients recovered with supportive care.

►*Treatment:* Gabapentin can be removed by hemodialysis. Although hemodialysis has not been performed in the few overdose cases reported, it may be indicated by the patient's clinical state or in patients with significant renal impairment.

Patient Information

Instruct patients to take gabapentin only as prescribed.

Advise patients that gabapentin may cause dizziness, somnolence, and other symptoms and signs of CNS depression. Accordingly, advise them to neither drive a car nor operate other complex machinery until they have gained sufficient experience on gabapentin to gauge whether or not it affects their mental or motor performance adversely.

LAMOTRIGINE

Rx	Lamictal (GlaxoSmithKline)	**Tablets:** 25 mg	Lactose. (Lamictal 25). White, shield shape, scored. In 100s.
		100 mg	Lactose. (Lamictal 100). Peach, shield shape, scored. In 100s.
		150 mg	Lactose. (Lamictal 150). Cream, shield shape, scored. In 60s.
		200 mg	Lactose. (Lamictal 200). Blue, shield shape, scored. In 60s.
Rx	Lamictal Chewable Dispersible (GlaxoSmithKline)	**Tablets, chewable:** 2 mg	Saccharin. (LTG 2). White to off-white. Black currant flavor. In 30s.
		5 mg	Saccharin. (GX CL2). White to off-white, caplet shape. Black currant flavor. In 100s.
		25 mg	Saccharin. (GX CL5). White, elliptical. Black currant flavor. In 100s.

Refer to the general discussion beginning in the Anticonvulsants introduction.

WARNING

Serious rashes requiring hospitalization and discontinuation of treatment have been reported in association with lamotrigine use. The incidence of these rashes, which include Stevens-Johnson syndrome, is approximately 0.8% in pediatric patients (less than 16 years of age) and 0.3% in adults receiving lamotrigine as adjunctive therapy.

In clinical trials of bipolar and other mood disorders, the rate of serious rash was 0.08% (0.8 per 1000) in adult patients receiving lamotrigine as initial monotherapy and 0.13% (1.3 per 1000) in adult patients receiving lamotrigine as adjunctive therapy.

In a prospectively followed cohort of 1983 pediatric patients taking adjunctive lamotrigine for epilepsy, there was 1 rash-related death. Rare cases of toxic epidermal necrolysis and/or rash-related death have occurred, but their numbers are too few to permit a precise estimate of the rate.

Because the rate of serious rash is greater in pediatric patients than in adults, it bears emphasis that lamotrigine is approved only for use in pediatric patients younger than 16 years of age who have seizures associated with the Lennox-Gastaut syndrome or in patients with partial seizures (see Indications).

Other than age, no factors have been identified that are known to predict the risk of occurrence or the severity of rash associated with lamotrigine. It is suggested, yet to be proven, that the risk of rash also may be increased by 1) coadministration of lamotrigine with valproic acid, 2) exceeding the recommended initial dose of lamotrigine, or 3) exceeding the recommended dose escalation for lamotrigine. However, cases have been reported in the absence of these factors.

Nearly all cases of life-threatening rashes associated with lamotrigine have occurred within 2 to 8 weeks of treatment initiation. However, isolated cases have been reported after prolonged treatment (eg, 6 months). Accordingly, duration of therapy cannot be relied upon as a means to predict the potential risk heralded by the first appearance of a rash.

Although benign rashes also occur with lamotrigine, it is not possible to predict reliably which rashes will prove to be serious or life-threatening. Accordingly, discontinue lamotrigine at the first sign of rash, unless the rash is clearly not drug-related. Discontinuation of treatment may not prevent a rash from becoming life-threatening or permanently disabling or disfiguring.

Indications

►*Epilepsy, adjunctive therapy:* Adjunctive therapy in the treatment of partial seizures and as adjunctive therapy in the generalized seizures of Lennox-Gastaut syndrome in pediatric (at least 2 years of age) and adult patients.

►*Epilepsy, monotherapy:* Conversion to monotherapy in adults with partial seizures who are receiving treatment with a single enzyme-inducing antiepileptic drug (EIAED) (eg, carbamazepine, phenytoin, phenobarbital).

Safety and efficacy have not been established as initial monotherapy, for conversion to monotherapy from a non-enzyme-inducing antiepileptic drug (AED) (eg, valproate), or for simultaneous conversion to monotherapy from 2 or more concomitant AEDs.

Safety and efficacy in patients younger than 16 years of age, other than those with partial seizures and the generalized seizures of Lennox-Gastaut syndrome, have not been established (see Warning Box).

►*Bipolar disorder:* For the maintenance treatment of bipolar I disorder to delay the time to occurrence of mood episodes (eg, depression, mania, hypomania, mixed episodes) in patients treated for acute mood episodes with standard therapy.

►*Unlabeled uses:* Lamotrigine may be useful in adults with generalized tonic-clonic (GTC), absence seizures, myoclonic seizures, and drug-resistant seizures in epilepsy syndromes with multiple seizures type.

Administration and Dosage

►*Approved by the FDA:* December 27, 1994.

►*General dosing considerations:* The risk of nonserious rash is increased when exceeding the recommended initial dose and/or the rate of dose escalation of lamotrigine. Therefore, closely follow the dosing recommendations.

It is recommended that lamotrigine not be restarted in patients who discontinued because of rash associated with prior treatment with lamotrigine, unless the potential benefits clearly outweigh the risks. If the decision is made to restart a patient who has discontinued lamotrigine, then assess the need to restart with the initial dosing recommendations. It is recommended that, the greater the interval of time since the previous dose, the greater consideration be given to restarting with the initial dosing recommendations. If a patient has discontinued lamotrigine for a period of more than 5 half-lives, it is recommended that initial dosing recommendations and guidelines be followed.

►*Epilepsy, adjunctive therapy:* For dosing guidelines below, EIAEDs include phenytoin, carbamazepine, phenobarbital, and primidone.

Lamotrigine added to AEDs other than EIAEDs and valproic acid – The effect of AEDs other than EIAEDs and valproic acid on the metabolism of lamotrigine is not currently known. Therefore, no specific dosing guidelines can be provided in that situation. Exercise conservative starting doses and dose escalations (as with concomitant valproic acid). Maintenance dosing would be expected to fall between the maintenance dose with valproic acid and the maintenance dose when added to EIAEDs without valproic acid.

►*Patients 2 to 12 years of age with epilepsy:*

Lamotrigine Added to an AED Regimen Containing Valproic Acid in Patients 2 to 12 Years of Age			
Weeks 1 and 2	0.15 mg/kg/day in 1 or 2 divided doses, rounded down to the nearest whole tablet.		
Weeks 3 and 4	0.3 mg/kg/day in 1 or 2 divided doses, rounded down to the nearest whole tablet.		
Weight-based dosing can be achieved by using the following guide:			
If the patient's weight is:		Give this daily dose using the most appropriate combination of 2 and 5 mg lamotrigine tablets	
Greater than	And less than	Weeks 1 and 2	Weeks 3 and 4
6.7 kg	14 kg	2 mg every other day	2 mg every day
14.1 kg	27 kg	2 mg every day	4 mg every day
27.1 kg	34 kg	4 mg every day	8 mg every day
34.1 kg	40 kg	5 mg every day	10 mg every day

LAMOTRIGINE

Lamotrigine Added to an AED Regimen Containing Valproic Acid in Patients 2 to 12 Years of Age
Usual maintenance dose: 1 to 5 mg/kg/day (maximum, 200 mg/day in 1 or 2 divided doses). To achieve the usual maintenance dose, increase subsequent doses every 1 to 2 weeks as follows: Calculate 0.3 mg/kg/day, round this amount down to the nearest whole tablet, and add this amount to the previously administered daily dose. The usual maintenance dose in patients adding lamotrigine to valproic acid alone ranges from 1 to 3 mg/kg/day. Maintenance doses in patients weighing less than 30 kg may need to be increased by as much as 50%, based on clinical response.

The smallest available strength of lamotrigine chewable dispersible tablets is 2 mg. Administer only whole tablets. If the calculated dose cannot be achieved using whole tablets, round down to the nearest whole tablet.

Lamotrigine Added to EIAEDs (Without Valproic Acid) in Patients 2 to 12 Years of Age	
Weeks 1 and 2	0.6 mg/kg/day in 2 divided doses, rounded down to the nearest whole tablet.
Weeks 3 and 4	1.2 mg/kg/day in 2 divided doses, rounded down to the nearest whole tablet.
Usual maintenance dose: 5 to 15 mg/kg/day (maximum, 400 mg/day in 2 divided doses). To achieve the usual maintenance dose, increase subsequent doses every 1 to 2 weeks as follows: Calculate 1.2 mg/kg/day, round this amount down to the nearest whole tablet, and add this amount to the previously administered daily dose. Maintenance doses in patients weighing less than 30 kg may need to be increased by as much as 50%, based on clinical response.	

➤*Patients older than 12 years of age with epilepsy:* Recommended dosing guidelines for lamotrigine added to valproic acid, and guidelines for lamotrigine added to EIAEDs are summarized in the following tables.

Lamotrigine Added to AED Regimen Containing Valproic Acid in Patients > 12 Years of Age	
Weeks 1 and 2	25 mg every other day
Weeks 3 and 4	25 mg every day
Usual maintenance dose: 100 to 400 mg/day (1 or 2 divided doses). To achieve maintenance, doses may be increased by 25 to 50 mg/day every 1 to 2 weeks. The usual maintenance dose in patients adding lamotrigine to valproic acid alone ranges from 100 to 200 mg/day.	

Lamotrigine Added to EIAEDs (Without Valproic Acid) in Patients > 12 Years of Age	
Weeks 1 and 2	50 mg/day
Weeks 3 and 4	100 mg/day in 2 divided doses
Usual maintenance dose: 300 to 500 mg/day (in 2 divided doses). To achieve maintenance, increase doses by 100 mg/day every 1 to 2 weeks.	

➤*Conversion from a single EIAED to monotherapy with lamotrigine in patients 16 years of age and older with epilepsy:* The goal of the transition regimen is to effect the conversion to monotherapy with lamotrigine under conditions that ensure adequate seizure control while mitigating the risk of serious rash associated with the rapid titration of lamotrigine.

The conversion regimen involves first titrating lamotrigine to the target dose (500 mg/day in 2 divided doses) while maintaining the dose of the EIAED at a fixed level. Secondly, withdraw concomitant EIAED by 20% decrements each week over a 4-week period.

The recommended maintenance dose of lamotrigine as monotherapy is 500 mg/day given in 2 divided doses. Because of an increased risk of rash, do not exceed the recommended initial dose and subsequent dose escalations (see Warning Box).

➤*Usual epilepsy maintenance dose:* In patients receiving multidrug regimens employing EIAEDs without valproic acid, maintenance doses of adjunctive lamotrigine as high as 700 mg/day have been used. In patients receiving valproic acid alone, maintenance doses of adjunctive lamotrigine as high as 200 mg/day have been used.

➤*Renal function impairment:* Base initial doses on the patient's AED regimen (see above); reduced maintenance doses may be effective for patients with significant renal function impairment. Use with caution in these patients.

➤*Hepatic function impairment:* Generally, reduce initial, escalation, and maintenance doses by approximately 50% in patients with moderate (Child-Pugh Grade B) and 75% in patients with severe (Child-Pugh Grade C) hepatic impairment. Adjust escalation and maintenance doses according to clinical response.

➤*Dosage regimen for bipolar disorder:* The target dose of lamotrigine is 200 mg/day (100 mg/day in combination with valproate and 400 mg/day in combination with carbamazepine or other enzyme-inducing drugs). Doses above 200 mg/day are not recommended. Treatment with lamotrigine is introduced, based on concurrent medications, according to the regimen outlined in the following table.

Escalation Regimen for Lamotrigine for Patients with Bipolar Disorder	For patients not taking carbamazepine (or other enzyme-inducing drugs) or valproic acid	For patients taking valproic acid	For patients taking carbamazepine (or other enzyme-inducing drugs) and not taking valproic acid
Weeks 1 and 2	25 mg daily	25 mg every other day	50 mg daily
Weeks 3 and 4	50 mg daily	25 mg daily	100 mg daily, in divided doses
Week 5	100 mg daily	50 mg daily	200 mg daily, in divided doses
Week 6	200 mg daily	100 mg daily	300 mg daily, in divided doses
Week 7	200 mg daily	100 mg daily	up to 400 mg daily, in divided doses

➤*Dosage adjustment for bipolar disorder:* If other psychotropic medications are withdrawn following stabilization, the dose of lamotrigine should be adjusted. For patients discontinuing valproate, the dose of lamotrigine should be doubled over a 2-week period in equal weekly increments (see following table). For patients discontinuing carbamazepine or other enzyme inducing agents, the dose of lamotrigine should remain constant for the first week and then should be decreased by half over a 2-week period in equal weekly decrements. The dose of lamotrigine may then be further adjusted to the target dose (200 mg) as clinically indicated.

If other drugs are subsequently introduced, the dose of lamotrigine may need to be adjusted. In particular, the introduction of valproate requires reduction in the dose of lamotrigine.

Adjustments to Lamotrigine Dosing for Patients with Bipolar Disorder Following Discontinuation of Psychotropic Medications	Discontinuation of psychotropic drugs excluding valproic acid, carbamazepine, or other enzyme-inducing drugs	After discontinuation of valproic acid	After discontinuation of carbamazepine or other enzyme-inducing drugs
		Current lamotrigine dose (mg/day) 100	Current lamotrigine dose (mg/day) 400
Week 1	Maintain current lamotrigine dose	150	400
Week 2	Maintain current lamotrigine dose	200	300
Week 3 onward	Maintain current lamotrigine dose	200	200

➤*Discontinuation:* For patients receiving lamotrigine in combination with other AEDs, consider a re-evaluation for all AEDs in the regimen if a change in seizure control or an appearance or worsening of adverse experiences is observed.

If a decision is made to discontinue therapy with lamotrigine, a stepwise reduction of dose over 2 weeks or more (approximately 50% per week) is recommended unless safety concerns require a more rapid withdrawal.

Discontinuing an EIAED prolongs the half-life of lamotrigine; discontinuing valproic acid shortens the half-life of lamotrigine.

➤*Target plasma levels:* A therapeutic plasma concentration range has not been established for lamotrigine. Base dosing of lamotrigine on therapeutic response.

➤*Administration of chewable dispersible tablets:* Swallow lamotrigine chewable dispersible tablets whole, chewed, or dispersed in water or diluted fruit juice. If chewed, consume a small amount of water or diluted fruit juice to aid in swallowing.

To disperse chewable dispersible tablets, add the tablets to a small amount of liquid (1 teaspoon or enough to cover the medication). Approximately 1 minute later, when the tablets are completely dispersed, swirl the solution and consume the entire quantity immediately. Do not attempt to administer partial quantities of the dispersed tablets.

➤*Storage/Stability:* Store at 25°C (77°F); excursions permitted to 15 to 30°C (59 to 86°F). Store in a dry place.

Actions

➤*Pharmacology:* Lamotrigine, an AED of the phenyltriazine class, is chemically unrelated to existing AEDs. The precise mechanism(s) by which lamotrigine exerts its anticonvulsant action is unknown. In animals, lamotrigine prevented seizure spread in the maximum electroshock and pentylenetetrazol tests and prevented seizures in the visually and electrically evoked after-discharge tests for antiepileptic activity. One proposed mechanism involves an effect on sodium channels. In vitro studies suggest that it inhibits voltage-sensitive sodium

LAMOTRIGINE

channels, thereby stabilizing neuronal membranes and consequently modulating presynaptic transmitter release of excitatory amino acids (eg, glutamate, aspartate).

Lamotrigine has a weak inhibitory effect on the serotonin 5-HT$_3$ receptor. It does not exhibit high-affinity binding to the following neurotransmitter receptors: Adenosine A$_1$ and A$_2$; adrenergic α_1, α_2, and β; dopamine D$_1$ and D$_2$; γ-aminobutyric acid (GABA) A and B; histamine H$_1$; kappa opioid; muscarinic acetylcholine; serotonin 5-HT$_2$. Studies have failed to detect an effect of lamotrigine on dihydropyridine-sensitive calcium channels. It had weak effects at sigma opioid receptors. It did not inhibit the uptake of norepinephrine, dopamine, or serotonin.

Animal studies demonstrated that the 2-N-methyl metabolite causes dose-dependent prolongations of the PR interval, widening of the QRS complex, and at higher doses, complete AV conduction block. Similar cardiovascular effects are not anticipated in humans because only trace amounts of the 2-N-methyl metabolite (less than 0.6% of the dose) have been found in human urine. However, plasma concentrations of this metabolite could be increased in patients with a reduced capacity to glucuronidate lamotrigine (eg, liver disease).

In vitro, lamotrigine inhibits dihydrofolate reductase, the enzyme that catalyzes reduction of dihydrofolate to tetrahydrofolate. Inhibition of this enzyme may interfere with biosynthesis of nucleic acids and proteins. When lamotrigine was given to pregnant rats during organogenesis, fetal, placental, and maternal folate concentrations were reduced. Significantly reduced concentrations of folate are associated with teratogenesis (see Pregnancy). Folate concentrations were reduced in male rats given repeated oral doses of lamotrigine. Reduced concentrations were partially returned to normal when supplemented with folinic acid.

▶ Pharmacokinetics:

Absorption / Distribution – Lamotrigine is rapidly and completely absorbed after oral administration with negligible first-pass metabolism (absolute bioavailability is 98%). The bioavailability is not affected by food. Peak plasma concentrations occur from 1.4 to 4.8 hours following drug administration.

In healthy volunteers not receiving other medications and given single doses, the plasma concentrations of lamotrigine increased in direct proportion to the dose administered over the range of 50 to 400 mg.

The lamotrigine chewable/dispersible tablets were found to be equivalent, whether they were administered as dispersed in water, chewed and swallowed, or swallowed as whole, to the lamotrigine compressed tablets in terms of rate and extent of absorption.

Estimates of the mean apparent volume of distribution (Vd/F) of lamotrigine following oral administration ranged from 0.9 to 1.3 L/kg. Vd/F is independent of dose and is similar following single and multiple doses in patients with epilepsy and in healthy volunteers.

Lamotrigine is approximately 55% protein-bound and does not displace other AEDs (eg, carbamazepine, phenobarbital, phenytoin) from protein-binding sites.

Mean Lamotrigine Pharmacokinetic Parameters in Adult Patients with Epilepsy or Healthy Volunteers[a]			
Adult study population	T$_{max}$ (h)	t½ (h)	Cl/F (mL/min/kg)
Patients taking EIAEDs:[b]			
Single dose (n = 24)	2.3	14.4	1.1
Multiple dose (n = 17)	2	12.6	1.21
Patients taking EIAEDs + valproic acid:			
Single dose (n = 25)	3.8	27.2	0.53
Patients taking valproic acid only:			
Single dose (n = 4)	4.8	58.8	0.28
Healthy volunteers taking valproic acid:			
Single dose (n = 6)	1.8	48.3	0.3
Multiple dose (n = 18)	1.9	70.3	0.18
Healthy volunteers taking no other medications:			
Single dose (n = 179)	2.2	32.8	0.44
Multiple dose (n = 36)	1.7	25.4	0.58

[a] The majority of parameter means determined in each study had coefficients of variation between 20% and 40% for half-life and Cl/F, and between 30% and 70% for T$_{max}$. The overall mean values were calculated from individual study means that were weighted based on the number of volunteers/patients in each study.
[b] Examples of EIAEDs are carbamazepine, phenobarbital, phenytoin, and primidone.

Metabolism / Excretion – Lamotrigine is metabolized predominantly by glucuronic acid conjugation; the major metabolite is an inactive 2-N-glucuronic acid conjugate. Lamotrigine was recovered in the urine (94%) and in the feces (2%). The urine contained unchanged lamotrigine (10%) and the 2-N-glucuronide (76%). Other identified metabolites include a 5-N-glucuronide (10%) and a 2-N-methyl metabolite (0.14%). The urine contained unidentified minor metabolites (4%).

Following multiple administrations (150 mg twice daily) to healthy volunteers taking no other medications, lamotrigine induced its own metabolism resulting in a 25% decrease in half-life and a 37% increase in plasma clearance at steady state compared with values obtained in the same volunteers following a single dose. Evidence suggests that self-induction by lamotrigine may not occur when given as adjunctive therapy in patients receiving EIAEDs.

The clearance of lamotrigine is affected by the coadministration of antiepileptic drugs. Lamotrigine is eliminated more rapidly in patients who have been taking hepatic EIAEDs, including carbamazepine, phenytoin, phenobarbital, and primidone. However, valproic acid actually decreases the clearance of lamotrigine (eg, more than doubles the elimination half-life of lamotrigine). If lamotrigine is administered to a patient receiving valproic acid, give lamotrigine at reduced dosage, less than 50% of the dose used in patients not receiving valproic acid (see Drug Interactions and Administration and Dosage).

Special populations –

Renal function impairment: Twelve volunteers with chronic renal failure (mean Ccr = 13 mL/min; range, 6 to 23) and another 6 undergoing hemodialysis were each given 100 mg lamotrigine. The mean plasma half-lives determined in the study were 42.9 hours (chronic renal failure), 13 hours (during hemodialysis), and 57.4 hours (between hemodialysis) compared with 26.2 hours in healthy volunteers. On average, approximately 20% (range, 5.6 to 35.1) lamotrigine present was eliminated by hemodialysis during a 4-hour session.

Hepatic function impairment: The pharmacokinetics of lamotrigine following a single 100 mg dose of lamotrigine were evaluated in 24 subjects with moderate to severe hepatic dysfunction and compared with 12 subjects without hepatic impairment. The median apparent clearance of lamotrigine was 0.31, 0.24, or 0.1 mL/kg/min in patients with Grade A, B, or C (Child-Pugh Classification) hepatic impairment, respectively, compared with 0.34 mL/kg/min in the healthy controls. Median half-life of lamotrigine was 36, 60, or 110 hours in patients with Grade A, B, or C hepatic impairment, respectively, vs 32 hours in healthy controls.

Elderly: The pharmacokinetics of lamotrigine following a single 150 mg dose of lamotrigine were evaluated in 12 elderly volunteers between 65 and 76 years of age (mean Ccr = 61 mL/min; range, 33 to 108 mL/min). The mean half-life of lamotrigine in these subjects was 31.2 hours (range, 24.5 to 43.4 hours) and the mean clearance was 0.4 mL/min/kg (range, 0.26 to 0.48 mL/min/kg).

Children: The pharmacokinetics of lamotrigine following a single 2 mg/kg dose were evaluated in 2 studies of pediatric patients with epilepsy. All patients were receiving concomitant therapy with other AEDs.

Population pharmacokinetic analyses involving patients 2 to 18 years of age demonstrated that lamotrigine clearance was influenced predominantly by total body weight and concurrent AED therapy. The oral clearance of lamotrigine was higher, on a body weight basis, in pediatric patients than in adults. Weight-normalized lamotrigine clearance was higher in those subjects weighing less than 30 kg, compared with those weighing greater than 30 kg. Accordingly, patients weighing less than 30 kg may need an increase of as much as 50% in maintenance doses, based on clinical response, as compared with subjects weighing more than 30 kg being administered the same AEDs (see Administration and Dosage). These analyses also revealed that, after accounting for body weight, lamotrigine clearance was not significantly influenced by age. Thus, administer the same weight-adjusted doses to children irrespective of differences in age. Concomitant AEDs that influence lamotrigine clearance in adults were found to have similar effects in children.

Mean Pharmacokinetic Parameters in Pediatric Patients with Epilepsy			
Pediatric study population	T$_{max}$ (h)	t½. (h)	Cl/F (mL/min/kg)
10 months to 5.3 years of age			
Patients taking EIAEDs (n = 10)	3	7.7	3.62
Patients taking AEDs with no known effect on drug-metabolizing enzymes (n = 7)	5.2	19	1.2
Patients taking valproic acid only (n = 8)	2.9	44.9	0.47
5 to 11 years of age			
Patients taking EIAEDs (n = 7)	1.6	7	2.54
Patients taking EIAEDs plus valproic acid (n = 8)	3.3	19.1	0.89
Patients taking valproic acid only[a] (n = 3)	4.5	65.8	0.24
13 to 18 years of age			
Patients taking EIAEDs (n = 11)	*	*	1.3
Patients taking EIAEDs plus valproic acid (n = 8)	*	*	0.5
Patients taking valproic acid only (n = 4)	*	*	0.3

[a] Two subjects were included in the calculation for mean T$_{max}$.
* Parameter not estimated.

Race: The oral clearance of lamotrigine was 25% lower in nonwhites than whites.

▶ Clinical trials:

Monotherapy with lamotrigine in adults with partial seizures already receiving treatment with a single EIAED – The effectiveness of monotherapy with lamotrigine was established in a multicenter,

LAMOTRIGINE

double-blind clinical trial enrolling 156 adult outpatients with partial seizures. The patients experienced 4 or more simple partial, complex partial, and/or secondarily generalized seizures during each of 2 consecutive 4-week periods while receiving carbamazepine or phenytoin monotherapy during baseline. Lamotrigine (target dose of 500 mg/day) or valproic acid (1000 mg/day) was added to either carbamazepine or phenytoin monotherapy over a 4-week period. Patients were then converted to monotherapy with lamotrigine or valproic acid during the next 4 weeks, then continued on monotherapy for an additional 12-week period.

Study endpoints were completion of all weeks of study treatment or meeting an escape criterion. Criteria for escape relative to baseline were the following:

1.) Doubling of average monthly seizure count,
2.) doubling of highest consecutive 2-day seizure frequency,
3.) emergence of a new seizure type (defined as a seizure that did not occur during the 8-week baseline) that is more severe than seizure types that occur during study treatment, or
4.) clinically significant prolongation of GTC seizures. The primary efficacy variable was the proportion of patients in each treatment group who met escape criteria.

The percentage of patients who met escape criteria was 42% in the lamotrigine group and 69% in the valproic acid group. The difference in the percentage of patients meeting escape criteria was statistically significant ($P = 0.0012$) in favor of lamotrigine.

Patients in the control group were intentionally treated with a relatively low dose of valproate; as such, the sole objective of this study was to demonstrate the effectiveness and safety of monotherapy with lamotrigine and cannot be interpreted to imply the superiority of lamotrigine to an adequate dose of valproate.

Contraindications

Hypersensitivity to the drug or its components.

Warnings

➤*Dermatologic effects or serious rash:* See Warning Box regarding the risk of serious rashes requiring hospitalization and discontinuation of lamotrigine. Use caution, especially in pediatric patients.

Serious rashes associated with hospitalization and discontinuation of lamotrigine have been reported. Rare deaths have been reported, but their numbers are too few to permit a precise estimate of the rate. There are suggestions, yet to be proven, that the risk of rash also may be increased by 1) coadministration of lamotrigine with valproic acid, 2) exceeding the recommended initial dose of lamotrigine, or 3) exceeding the recommended dose escalation for lamotrigine. However, cases have been reported in the absence of these factors.

In epilepsy clinical trials, approximately 10% of all patients exposed to lamotrigine developed a rash. In the Bipolar Disorder clinical trials, 14% of patients exposed to lamotrigine developed a rash. Typically, rash occurs in the first 2 to 8 weeks of treatment initiation. Lamotrigine-associated rashes do not appear to have unique identifying features. However, isolated cases have been reported after prolonged treatment (eg, 6 months). Accordingly, duration of therapy cannot be relied upon as a means to predict the potential risk heralded by the first appearance of a rash.

Although benign rashes also occur with lamotrigine, it is not possible to predict reliably which rashes will prove to be serious or life threatening. Accordingly, discontinue lamotrigine at the first sign of rash, unless the rash is clearly not drug-related. Discontinuation of treatment may not prevent a rash from becoming life-threatening or permanently disabling or disfiguring.

It is recommended that lamotrigine not be restarted in patients who discontinued use due to rash associated with prior treatment with lamotrigine unless the potential benefits clearly outweigh the risks. If the decision is made to restart a patient who has discontinued lamotrigine, assess the need to restart with the initial dosing recommendations (See Administration and Dosage).

Children – The incidence of serious rash associated with hospitalization and discontinuation of lamotrigine in a prospectively followed cohort of pediatric patients receiving adjunctive therapy was approximately 0.8% of 1983 patients. When 14 of these cases were reviewed by 3 expert dermatologists, there was considerable disagreement as to their proper classification. There was 1 rash-related death in this 1983-patient cohort. Additionally, there have been rare cases of toxic epidermal necrolysis with and without permanent sequelae and/or death in US and foreign postmarketing experience. It bears emphasis, accordingly, that lamotrigine is only approved for use in those patients less than 16 years of age who have partial seizures or generalized seizures associated with the Lennox-Gastaut syndrome.

There is evidence that the inclusion of valproic acid in a multidrug regimen increases the risk of serious, potentially life-threatening rash in pediatric patients. In pediatric patients who used valproic acid concomitantly, 1.2% of 482 experienced a serious rash compared with 0.6% of 952 patients not taking valproic acid.

Adults – Serious rash, resulting in hospitalization and discontinuation, occurred in 0.3% of the 3348 subjects who participated in premar-

keting clinical trials of epilepsy. In the bipolar and other mood disorders clinical trials, the rate of serious rash was 0.08% of 1233 of adult patients who received lamotrigine as initial monotherapy and 0.13% of 1538 of adult patients who received lamotrigine as adjunctive therapy. No fatalities occurred among these individuals, but rare cases of rash have been associated with a fatal outcome in reports from postmarketing experience. Among the rashes leading to hospitalization were Stevens-Johnson syndrome, toxic epidermal necrolysis, angioedema, and a rash associated with a number of the following systemic manifestations: Fever, lymphadenopathy, facial swelling, hematologic and hepatologic abnormalities.

There is evidence that the inclusion of valproic acid in a multidrug regimen increases the risk of serious, potentially life-threatening rash in adults. Of 584 patients administered lamotrigine with valproic acid in clinical trials, 1% were hospitalized in association with rash. In contrast, 0.16% of 2398 patients given lamotrigine without valproic acid were hospitalized.

Other examples of serious and potentially life-threatening rash that did not lead to hospitalization also occurred in premarketing development. Among these, 1 case was reported to be Stevens-Johnson-like.

➤*Withdrawal seizures:* As with other AEDs, do not abruptly discontinue lamotrigine because of the possibility of increasing seizure frequency. Unless safety concerns require a more rapid withdrawal, taper the dose of lamotrigine over a period of 2 weeks or more (see Administration and Dosage).

➤*Addition of lamotrigine to a multidrug regimen that includes valproic acid:* Because valproic acid reduces the clearance of lamotrigine, the dosage of lamotrigine in the presence of valproic acid is less than half of that required in its absence (see Administration and Dosage).

➤*Acute multiorgan failure:* Multiorgan failure, which in some cases has been fatal or irreversible, has been observed in patients receiving lamotrigine. Fatalities associated with multiorgan failure and various degrees of hepatic failure have been reported in 2 of 3796 adult patients and 4 of 2435 pediatric patients who received lamotrigine in clinical trials. No such fatalities have been reported in bipolar patients in clinical trials. Rare fatalities from multiorgan failure have also been reported in compassionate plea and postmarketing use. The majority of these deaths occurred in association with other serious events, including status epilepticus and overwhelming sepsis, and hantavirus making it difficult to identify the initiating cause.

Additionally, 3 patients developed multiorgan dysfunction and disseminated intravascular coagulation 9 to 14 days after lamotrigine was added to their AED regimens. Rash and elevated transaminases were also present in all patients and rhabdomyolysis was noted in 2 patients. Both pediatric patients were receiving concomitant therapy with valproic acid, while the adult patient was being treated with carbamazepine and clonazepam. All patients subsequently recovered with supportive care after treatment with lamotrigine was discontinued.

➤*Blood dyscrasias:* There have been reports of blood dyscrasias that may or may not be associated with the hypersensitivity syndrome. These have included neutropenia, leukopenia, anemia, thrombocytopenia, pancytopenia, and, rarely, aplastic anemia, and pure red cell aplasia.

➤*Hypersensitivity reactions:* Hypersensitivity reactions, some fatal or life-threatening, have occurred. Some of these reactions have included clinical features of multiorgan failure/dysfunction such as hepatic abnormalities and evidence of disseminated intravascular coagulation. It is important to note that early manifestations of hypersensitivity (eg, fever, lymphadenopathy) may be present even though a rash is not evident. If such symptoms are present, evaluate the patient immediately. Discontinue lamotrigine if an alternative etiology for the signs or symptoms cannot be established.

Prior to initiation of treatment, instruct patients that a rash or other signs or symptoms of hypersensitivity (eg, fever, lymphadenopathy) may occur and that it may indicate a serious medical event. Should it occur, report promptly to physician.

➤*Elderly:* In general, exercise caution in dose selection for elderly patients, usually starting at the low end of the dosing range, reflecting the greater frequency of decreased hepatic, renal, or cardiac function and the greater frequency of concomitant diseases or other drug therapy.

➤*Pregnancy: Category C.* Maternal toxicity and secondary fetal toxicity producing reduced fetal weight or delayed ossification were seen in mice, rats, but not in rabbits at doses up to 1.2, 0.5, and 1.1 times, respectively, on a mg/m^2 basis, the highest usual human maintenance dose (ie, 500 mg/day). In rat dams administered an IV dose at 0.6 times the highest usual human maintenance dose, the incidence of intrauterine death without signs of teratogenicity was increased.

When pregnant rats were orally dosed at 0.1, 0.14, or 0.3 times the highest human maintenance dose (on a mg/m^2 basis) during the latter part of gestation (days 15 to 20), maternal toxicity and fetal death were seen. In dams, food consumption and weight gain were reduced, and the gestation period was slightly prolonged (22.6 vs 22 days in the control group). Stillborn pups were found in all 3 drug-treated groups with the highest number in the high-dose group. Postnatal death was also seen, but only in the 2 highest doses, and occurred between days 1 and

LAMOTRIGINE

20. Some of these deaths appear to be drug-related and not secondary to the maternal toxicity. A no-observed-effect level could not be determined for this study.

Although lamotrigine was not found to be teratogenic, it decreases fetal folate concentrations in rats, an effect associated with teratogenesis in animals and humans. There are no adequate and well-controlled studies in pregnant women. Use during pregnancy only if the potential benefit justifies the potential risk to the fetus. Refer to Warnings in the Anticonvulsants introduction.

Pregnancy exposure registry – To facilitate the monitoring of fetal outcomes in pregnant women exposed to lamotrigine prior to known fetal outcomes, the manufacturer maintains a Lamotrigine Pregnancy Registry. Physicians can register patients by calling (800) 336-2176. Patients can enroll themselves in the North American Antiepileptic Drug Pregnancy Registry by calling (888) 233-2334.

➤*Lactation:* Preliminary data indicate that lamotrigine passes into breast milk. Because the effects on the infant exposed to lamotrigine by this route are unknown, breastfeeding is not recommended.

➤*Children:* Lamotrigine is indicated as adjunctive therapy for partial seizures in patients above 2 years of age and for the generalized seizures of Lennox-Gastaut syndrome. Safety and efficacy for other uses in patients younger than 16 years of age have not been established. Safety and efficacy in patients below the age of 18 years with bipolar disorder have not been established.

Precautions

➤*Monitoring:* The value of monitoring plasma concentrations of lamotrigine has not been established. Because of the possible pharmacokinetic interactions between lamotrigine and other AEDs being taken concomitantly (see Drug Interactions), monitoring of the plasma levels of lamotrigine and concomitant AEDs may be indicated, particularly during dosage adjustments. In general, exercise clinical judgment regarding monitoring of plasma levels of lamotrigine and other AEDs.

➤*Sudden unexplained death in epilepsy (SUDEP):* During premarketing development, 20 sudden and unexplained deaths were recorded among 4700 patients with epilepsy (5747 patient-years of exposure). Some of these could represent seizure-related deaths in which the seizure was not observed (eg, at night). This represents an incidence of 0.0035 deaths per patient-year. Although this rate exceeds that expected in a healthy population matched for age and sex, it is within the range of estimates for the incidence of SUDEP in patients not receiving lamotrigine. It is reassuring that the similarity of estimated SUDEP rates in patients receiving lamotrigine and those receiving another antiepileptic drug that underwent clinical testing in a similar population at about the same time; importantly, that drug is chemically unrelated to lamotrigine. This evidence suggests, although it does not prove, that the high SUDEP rates reflect population rates, not a drug effect.

➤*Status epilepticus:* Valid estimates of the incidence of treatment-emergent status epilepticus among lamotrigine-treated patients are difficult to obtain. At a minimum, 7 of 2343 adult patients had episodes that could unequivocally be described as status epilepticus. In addition, variably defined episodes of seizure exacerbation (eg, seizure clusters, seizure flurries) were reported.

➤*Suicide:* The possibility of a suicide attempt is inherent in Bipolar Disorder, and close supervision of high-risk patients should accompany drug therapy. Write prescriptions for lamotrigine for the smallest quantity of tablets consistent with good patient management, in order to reduce the risk of overdose. Overdoses have been reported for lamotrigine, some of which have been fatal (see Overdosage).

➤*Melanin-containing tissues:* Because lamotrigine binds to eye and other melanin-containing tissues, it could accumulate in melanin-rich tissues over time. This raises the possibility that lamotrigine may cause toxicity in these tissues after extended use. Although there are no specific recommendations for periodic ophthalmological monitoring, be aware of the possibility of long-term effects.

➤*Special risk:* Caution is advised when using lamotrigine in patients with diseases or conditions that could affect metabolism or elimination of the drug, such as renal, hepatic, or cardiac functional impairment.

Hepatic metabolism to the glucuronide followed by renal excretion is the principal route of elimination of lamotrigine. The use of lamotrigine in patients with impaired liver function may be associated with risks (see Actions and Administration and Dosage).

A study in individuals with severe chronic renal failure (mean Ccr = 13 mL/min) not receiving other AEDs indicated that the elimination half-life of unchanged lamotrigine is prolonged relative to individuals with normal renal function. Until adequate numbers of patients with severe renal impairment have been evaluated during chronic treatment with lamotrigine, use with caution in these patients, generally using a reduced maintenance dose for patients with significant impairment.

Drug Interactions

➤*Folate inhibitors:* Lamotrigine is an inhibitor of dihydrofolate reductase. Be aware of this action when administering other medications that inhibit folate metabolism.

Lamotrigine Drug Interactions

Precipitant drug	Object drug[*]		Description
Acetaminophen	Lamotrigine	↓	Serum lamotrigine concentrations may be reduced, producing a decrease in therapeutic effects. With chronic administration of acetaminophen, if an interaction is suspected, it may be necessary to adjust the dose of lamotrigine.
Carbamazepine	Lamotrigine	↓	Lamotrigine concentration is decreased by ≈ 40%. Carbamazepine-epoxide levels may be increased.
Lamotrigine	Carbamazepine	↑	
Contraceptives, oral Progestins	Lamotrigine	↓	Lamotrigine plasma concentrations may be reduced. Adjust the dose of lamotrigine as needed.
Oxcarbazepine	Lamotrigine	↓	Oxcarbazepine administration reduced serum concentrations of lamotrigine 29%. Adjust the dose of lamotrigine as needed.
Primidone Phenobarbital	Lamotrigine	↓	Lamotrigine concentration is decreased ≈ 40%.
Phenytoin	Lamotrigine	↓	Lamotrigine concentration is decreased ≈ 40%.
Rifamycins	Lamotrigine	↓	Lamotrigine plasma levels may be reduced. Adjust the dose of lamotrigine as needed.
Succinimides (eg, ethosuximide)	Lamotrigine	↓	Lamotrigine serum concentrations may be reduced, decreasing the therapeutic effects. Adjust the dose of lamotrigine as needed.
Valproic acid	Lamotrigine	↑	The addition of valproic acid increased lamotrigine steady-state concentration > 2-fold. Trough steady-state valproic acid concentration decreased by ≈ 25% when lamotrigine was added in 1 study. Another study showed no change in valproic acid concentrations.
Lamotrigine	Valproic acid	↓	

[*] ↑ = Object drug increased. ↓ = Object drug decreased.

Adverse Reactions

Adjunctive therapy in adults with epilepsy – The most commonly observed (5% or more) adverse experiences associated with the use of lamotrigine in combination with other antiepileptic drugs were the following: Dizziness, diplopia, ataxia, blurred vision, nausea and vomiting (dose-related), somnolence, headache, and rash. Dizziness, diplopia, ataxia, and blurred vision occurred more commonly in patients receiving carbamazepine with lamotrigine than in patients receiving other EIAEDs with lamotrigine. Clinical data suggest a higher incidence of rash, including serious rash, in patients receiving concomitant valproic acid than in patients not receiving valproic acid (see Warnings).

Approximately 11% of the 3378 adult patients who received lamotrigine as adjunctive therapy in premarketing clinical trials discontinued treatment because of an adverse experience. The adverse events most commonly associated with discontinuation were rash (3%), dizziness (2.8%), and headache (2.5%).

Lamotrigine Adverse Reactions in Placebo-Controlled Adjunctive Trials[a] (≥ 2%)

Adverse reaction	Lamotrigine (n = 711)	Placebo (n = 419)
CNS		
Dizziness	38	13
Headache	29	19
Ataxia	22	6
Somnolence	14	7
Incoordination	6	2
Insomnia	6	2
Tremor	4	1
Depression	4	3
Anxiety	4	3
Convulsion	3	1
Irritability	3	2
Speech disorder	3	0
Concentration disturbance	2	1
Seizure exacerbation	2	1
Dermatologic		
Rash	10	5
Pruritus	3	2

LAMOTRIGINE

Lamotrigine Adverse Reactions in Placebo-Controlled Adjunctive Trials[a] (≥ 2%)

Adverse reaction	Lamotrigine (n = 711)	Placebo (n = 419)
GI		
Nausea	19	10
Vomiting	9	4
Diarrhea	6	4
Abdominal pain	5	4
Dyspepsia	5	2
Constipation	4	3
Tooth disorder	3	2
Anorexia	2	1
GU (female patients only)	(n = 365)	(n = 207)
Dysmenorrhea	7	6
Vaginitis	4	1
Amenorrhea	2	1
Respiratory		
Rhinitis	14	9
Pharyngitis	10	9
Cough increased	8	6
Special senses		
Diplopia	28	7
Blurred vision	16	5
Vision abnormality	3	1
Miscellaneous		
Flu syndrome	7	6
Fever	6	4
Neck pain	2	1
Arthralgia	2	0

[a] Patients in these adjunctive studies were receiving 1 to 3 concomitant EIAEDs in addition to lamotrigine or placebo. Patients may have reported multiple adverse experiences during the study or at discontinuation; thus, patients may be included in more than 1 category.

Monotherapy in adults with epilepsy – The most commonly observed (5% or more) adverse experiences during the monotherapy phase of the controlled trial in adults not seen at an equivalent rate in the control group were vomiting, coordination abnormality, dyspepsia, nausea, dizziness, rhinitis, anxiety, insomnia, infection, pain, weight decrease, chest pain, and dysmenorrhea. The most commonly observed (5% or more) adverse experiences associated with the use of lamotrigine during the conversion to monotherapy (add-on) period were the following: dizziness, headache, nausea, asthenia, coordination abnormality, vomiting, rash, somnolence, diplopia, ataxia, accidental injury, tremor, blurred vision, insomnia, nystagmus, diarrhea, lymphadenopathy, pruritus, and sinusitis. Approximately 10% of patients who received lamotrigine as monotherapy in premarketing clinical trials discontinued treatment because of an adverse experience. The adverse events most commonly associated with discontinuation were rash (4.5%), headache (3.1%), and asthenia (2.4%).

Dose-Related Adverse Events from a Randomized, Placebo-Controlled Trial in Adults (%)

Adverse reaction	Lamotrigine 300 mg (n = 71)	Lamotrigine 500 mg (n = 72)	Placebo (n = 73)
Ataxia	10	28	10
Blurred vision	11	25	10
Diplopia	24	49	8
Dizziness	31	54	27
Nausea	18	25	11
Vomiting	11	18	4

Other events that occurred in more than 1% of patients, but equally or more frequently in the placebo group included the following: Asthenia; back pain; chest pain; flatulence; menstrual disorder; myalgia; paresthesia; respiratory disorder; urinary tract infection.

Adverse Events in Adults with Partial Seizures in a Controlled Monotherapy Trial[a] (≥ 2%)

Adverse reaction	Lamotrigine[b] (n = 43)	Low-dose valproic acid[c] (n = 44)
CNS		
Coordination abnormality	7	0
Dizziness	7	0
Anxiety	5	0
Insomnia	5	2
GI		
Vomiting	9	0
Dyspepsia	7	2
Nausea	7	2
GU (female patients only)	(n = 21)	(n = 28)
Dysmenorrhea	5	0

Adverse Events in Adults with Partial Seizures in a Controlled Monotherapy Trial[a] (≥ 2%)

Adverse reaction	Lamotrigine[b] (n = 43)	Low-dose valproic acid[c] (n = 44)
Miscellaneous		
Rhinitis	7	2
Chest pain	5	2
Infection	5	2
Weight decrease	5	2
Pain	5	0

[a] Patients were converted to lamotrigine or valproic acid monotherapy from adjunctive therapy with carbamazepine or phenytoin. Patients may have reported multiple adverse experiences during the study; thus, patients may be included in more than 1 category.
[b] Up to 500 mg/day.
[c] 1000 mg/day.

Adjunctive therapy in pediatric patients with epilepsy – The most commonly observed (5% or more) adverse experiences seen with lamotrigine use as adjunctive treatment in pediatric patients were infection, vomiting, rash, fever, somnolence, accidental injury, dizziness, diarrhea, abdominal pain, nausea, ataxia, tremor, asthenia, bronchitis, flu syndrome, and diplopia.

In 339 patients 2 to 16 years of age, 4.2% of patients on lamotrigine and 2.9% of patients on placebo discontinued due to adverse experiences. The most commonly reported adverse experiences that led to discontinuation were rash for patients treated with lamotrigine and deterioration of seizure control for patients treated with placebo.

Approximately 11.5% of the 1081 pediatric patients who received lamotrigine as adjunctive therapy in premarketing clinical trials discontinued treatment because of an adverse experience. The adverse events most commonly associated with discontinuation were rash (4.4%), reaction aggravated (1.7%), and ataxia (0.6%).

Adverse Events in Placebo-Controlled Adjunctive Trials in Pediatric Patients (≥ 2%)

Adverse reaction	Lamotrigine[a] (n = 168)	Placebo (n = 171)
CNS		
Somnolence	17	15
Dizziness	14	4
Ataxia	11	3
Tremor	10	1
Emotional lability	4	2
Gait abnormality	4	2
Thinking abnormality	3	2
Convulsions	2	1
Nervousness	2	1
Vertigo	2	1
Dermatologic		
Rash	14	12
Eczema	2	1
Pruritus	2	1
GI		
Abdominal pain	10	5
Vomiting	20	16
Diarrhea	11	9
Nausea	10	2
Constipation	4	2
Dyspepsia	2	1
Tooth disorder	2	1
GU		
Male and female patients		
Urinary tract infection	3	0
Male patients only	(n = 93)	(n = 92)
Penis disorder	2	0
Respiratory		
Pharyngitis	14	11
Bronchitis	7	5
Increased cough	7	6
Sinusitis	2	1
Bronchospasm	2	1
Special senses		
Diplopia	5	1
Blurred vision	4	1
Ear disorder	2	1
Visual abnormality	2	0

LAMOTRIGINE

Adverse Events in Placebo-Controlled Adjunctive Trials in Pediatric Patients (≥ 2%)		
Adverse reaction	Lamotrigine[a] (n = 168)	Placebo (n = 171)
Miscellaneous		
Fever	15	14
Accidental injury	14	12
Asthenia	8	4
Flu syndrome	7	6
Pain	5	4
Facial edema	2	1
Photosensitivity	2	0
Hemorrhage	2	1
Lymphaden-opathy	2	1
Edema	2	0

[a] Dose up to 15 mg/kg/day or a maximum of 750 mg/day.

Bipolar disorder – Adverse events that occurred in at least 5% of patients and were numerically more common during the dose escalation phase of lamotrigine in these trials (when patients may have been receiving concomitant medications) compared with the monotherapy phase were the following: Headache (25%), rash (11%), dizziness (10%), diarrhea (8%), dream abnormality (6%), and pruritus (6%).

During the monotherapy phase of the double-blind, placebo-controlled trials of 18 months' duration, 13% of 227 patients who received lamotrigine (100 to 400 mg/day), 16% of 190 patients who received placebo, and 23% of 166 patients who received lithium discontinued therapy because of an adverse experience. The adverse events which most commonly led to discontinuation of lamotrigine were rash (3%) and mania/hypomania/mixed mood adverse events (2%). Approximately 16% of 2401 patients who received lamotrigine (50 to 500 mg/day) for bipolar disorder in premarketing trials discontinued therapy because of an adverse experience; most commonly due to rash (5%) and mania/hypomania/mixed mood adverse events (2%).

Adverse Events in 2 Placebo-Controlled Trials in Adults with Bipolar I Disorder[a] (≥ 5%)		
Adverse reaction	Lamotrigine (n = 227)	Placebo (n = 190)
CNS		
Insomnia	10	6
Somnolence	9	7
GI		
Nausea	14	11
Xerostemia (dry mouth)	6	4
Abdominal pain	6	3
Constipation	5	2
Vomiting	5	2
Respiratory		
Rhinitis	7	4
Pharyngitis	5	4
Exacerbation of cough	5	3
Miscellaneous		
Back pain	8	6
Fatigue	8	5
Rash (non serious)[b]	7	5

[a] Patients in these studies were converted to lamotrigine (100 to 400 mg/day) or placebo monotherapy from add-on therapy with other psychotropic medications. Patients may have reported multiple adverse experiences during the study; thus, patients may be included in more than 1 category.
[b] In the overall bipolar and other mood disorders clinical trials, the rate of serious rash was 0.08% of 1233 of adult patients who received lamotrigine as initial monotherapy and 0.13% of 1538 of adult patients who received lamotrigine as adjunctive therapy (see Warnings).

These adverse events were usually mild to moderate in intensity. Other events that occurred in 5% or more patients but equally or more frequently in the placebo group included the following: Dizziness, mania, headache, infection, influenza, pain, accidental injury, diarrhea, and dyspepsia. Adverse events that occurred with a frequency of less than 5% and greater than 1% of patients receiving lamotrigine and numerically more frequent than placebo were the following:

➤*CNS:* Amnesia, depression, agitation, emotional lability, dyspraxia, abnormal thoughts, dream abnormality, hypoesthesia, and migraine.

➤*Metabolic/Nutritional:* Weight gain, edema.

➤*Musculoskeletal:* Arthralgia, myalgia.

➤*Miscellaneous:* Fever, neck pain, flatulence, sinusitis, urinary frequency. Two patients experienced seizures shortly after abrupt withdrawal of lamotrigine. However, there were confounding factors that may have contributed to the occurrence of seizures in these bipolar patients.

➤*Other adverse events observed for adult and pediatric patients:*
Cardiovascular – Flushing, hot flashes, hypertension, palpitations, postural hypotension, syncope, tachycardia, vasodilation (0.1% to 1%); angina pectoris, atrial fibrillation, deep thrombophlebitis, ECG abnormality, MI (less than 0.1%).

CNS – Confusion, paresthesia (1% or more); akathisia, apathy, aphasia, CNS depression, depersonalization, dysarthria, dyskinesia, euphoria, hallucinations, hostility, hyperkinesia, hypertonia, libido decreased, memory decrease, mind racing, movement disorder, myoclonus, panic attack, paranoid reaction, personality disorder, psychosis, sleep disorder, stupor, suicidal ideation (0.1% to 1%); cerebellar syndrome, cerebrovascular accident, cerebral sinus thrombosis, choreoathetosis, CNS stimulation, delirium, delusions, dysphoria, dystonia, extrapyramidal syndrome, faintness, grand mal convulsions, hemiplegia, hyperalgesia, hyperesthesia, hypokinesia, hypotonia, manic depression reaction, neuralgia, neurosis, paralysis, peripheral neuritis (less than 0.1%).

Dermatologic – Acne, alopecia, hirsutism, maculopapular rash, skin discoloration, urticaria, (0.1% to 1%); angioedema, erythema, erythema multiforme, exfoliative dermatitis, fungal dermatitis, herpes zoster, leukoderma, petechial rash, pustular rash, seborrhea, Stevens-Johnson syndrome, vesiculobullous rash (less than 0.1%).

Endocrine – Goiter, hypothyroidism (less than 0.1%).

GI – Dysphagia, eructation, gastritis, gingivitis, increased appetite, increased salivation, mouth ulceration (0.1% to 1%); GI hemorrhage, glossitis, gum hemorrhage, gum hyperplasia, hematemesis, hemorrhagic colitis, hepatitis, melena, stomach ulcer, stomatitis, thirst, tongue edema (less than 0.1%).

GU – Abnormal ejaculation, breast pain, hematuria, impotence, menorrhagia, polyuria, urinary incontinence, urine abnormality (0.1% to 1%); acute kidney failure, anorgasmia, breast abscess, breast neoplasm, creatinine increase, cystitis, dysuria, epididymitis, female lactation, kidney pain/failure, nocturia, urinary retention, urinary urgency, vaginal moniliasis (less than 0.1%).

Hematologic/Lymphatic – Ecchymosis, leukopenia (0.1% to 1%); anemia, eosinophilia, fibrin decrease, fibrinogen decrease, iron deficiency anemia, leukocytosis, lymphocytosis, macrocytic anemia, petechia, thrombocytopenia (less than 0.1%).

Metabolic – Abnormal liver function tests, AST increase (0.1% to 1%); alcohol intolerance, alkaline phosphatase increase, ALT increase, bilirubinemia, general edema, GGT increase, hyperglycemia (less than 0.1%).

Musculoskeletal – Arthritis, leg cramps, myasthenia, twitching (0.1% to 1%); bursitis, joint disorder, muscle atrophy, muscle spasm, pathological fracture, tendinous contracture (less than 0.1%).

Respiratory – Yawn (0.1% to 1%); hiccough, hyperventilation (less than 0.1%).

Special senses – Amblyopia (more than 1%); abnormality of accommodation, conjunctivitis, dry eyes, ear pain, photophobia, taste perversion, tinnitus (0.1% to 1%); deafness, lacrimation disorder, oscillopsia, parosmia, ptosis, strabismus, taste loss, uveitis, visual field defect (less than 0.1%).

Miscellaneous – Allergic reaction, chills, halitosis, malaise (0.1% to 1%); abdomen enlarged, abscess, suicide attempt (less than 0.1%).

➤*Postmarketing reports:* These adverse experiences have not been listed above, and data are insufficient to support an estimate of their incidence or to establish causation.

Hematologic/Lymphatic – Agranulocytosis, aplastic anemia, disseminated intravascular coagulation, hemolytic anemia, neutropenia, pancytopenia, red cell aplasia.

Miscellaneous – Esophagitis, pancreatitis, lupus-like reaction, vasculitis, apnea, hypersensitivity reaction, multiorgan failure, progressive immunosuppression, tics. Rhabdomyolysis has been observed in patients experiencing hypersensitivity reactions. Exacerbation of parkinsonian symptoms in patients with pre-existing Parkinson disease have been reported.

Overdosage

➤*Symptoms:* Overdoses involving quantities up to 15 g have been reported for lamotrigine, some of which have been fatal. Overdose has resulted in ataxia, nystagmus, increased seizures, decreased level of consciousness, coma, and intraventricular conduction delay.

➤*Treatment:* There are no specific antidotes for lamotrigine. Following a suspected overdose, hospitalization is advised. General supportive care is indicated, including frequent monitoring of vital signs and close observation of the patient (refer to General Management of Acute Overdosage). If indicated, perform gastric lavage and give activated charcoal. Observe usual precautions to protect the airway. Keep in mind that lamotrigine is rapidly absorbed. It is uncertain whether hemodialysis is an effective means of removing lamotrigine from the blood. In 6 renal failure patients, approximately 20% of the amount of lamotrigine in the body was removed during 4 hours of hemodialysis. Contact a poison control center for information on the management of lamotrigine overdosage.

LAMOTRIGINE

Patient Information

Advise patients to notify physician immediately if they develop a rash or other signs of hypersensitivity (eg, fever, lymphadenopathy), or if they acutely develop any worsening of seizure control.

Advise patients that lamotrigine may cause dizziness, somnolence, and other symptoms and signs of CNS depression. Advise patients to neither drive a car nor to operate other complex machinery until they have gained sufficient experience on lamotrigine to gauge whether or not it adversely affects their mental and/or motor performance.

Advise patients that other adverse reactions may include headache, blurred or double vision, lack of coordination, sleepiness, nausea, vomiting, and insomnia.

Advise patients to notify their physician if they become pregnant, intend to become pregnant, if they intend to breastfeed, or are breastfeeding.

Although most patients who develop rash while receiving lamotrigine have mild to moderate symptoms, some may develop a serious skin reaction that requires hospitalization. Rarely, deaths have been reported. These serious skin reactions are most likely to happen within the first 2 to 8 weeks of treatment. Serious skin reactions occur more often in children than in adults.

It is not possible to predict whether a mild rash will develop into a more serious reaction. Therefore, advise patients to notify their physician if they experience a skin rash, hives, fever, swollen lymph glands, painful sores in the mouth or around the eyes, or swelling of lips or tongue. These symptoms may be the first signs of a serious reaction.

Swallow tablets whole. Chewing the tablets may leave a bitter taste.

Lamotrigine chewable dispersible tablets may be swallowed whole, chewed, or mixed in water or diluted fruit juice. If the tablets are chewed, consume a small amount of water or diluted fruit juice to aid in swallowing.

To disperse lamotrigine chewable dispersible tablets, add the tablets to a small amount of liquid (1 teaspoon or enough to cover the medication) in a glass or spoon. Approximately 1 minute later, when the tablets are completely dispersed, mix the solution and take the entire amount immediately.

LEVETIRACETAM

Rx	**Keppra** (UCB Pharma)	**Tablets:** 250 mg	(ucb 250). Blue, oblong, scored. Film-coated. In 120s.
		500 mg	(ucb 500). Yellow, oblong, scored. Film-coated. In 120s.
		750 mg	(ucb 750). Orange, oblong, scored. Film-coated. In 120s.
		Oral solution: 100 mg/mL	Dye free. Parabens. Grape flavor. In 480 mL.

Refer to the general discussion beginning in the Anticonvulsants introduction.

Indications

➤*Epilepsy:* Adjunctive therapy in the treatment of partial onset seizures in adults with epilepsy.

Administration and Dosage

➤*Approved by the FDA:* November 30, 1999.

➤*Dosage:* Initiate treatment with 1000 mg/day given as twice daily dosing (500 mg twice/day). Additional dosing increments may be given (1000 mg/day additional every 2 weeks) to a maximum recommended daily dose of 3000 mg. Doses greater than 3000 mg/day have been used in open-label studies for 6 months and longer. There is no evidence that doses of more than 3000 mg/day confer additional benefit.

Give orally with or without food.

➤*Withdrawal seizure:* Withdraw levetiracetam gradually to minimize the potential of increased seizure frequency.

➤*Renal function impairment:* Individualize dosing according to the patient's renal function status. Recommended doses and adjustment for dose are shown in the following table.

Levetiracetam Dosing Adjustment Regimen for Patients with Impaired Renal Function			
Group	Creatinine clearance (mL/min)	Dosage (mg)	Frequency
Normal	> 80	500 to 1500	every 12 h
Mild	50 to 80	500 to 1000	every 12 h
Moderate	30 to 50	250 to 750	every 12 h
Severe	< 30	250 to 500	every 12 h
ESRD patients using dialysis	—	500 to 1000[a]	every 24 h

[a] Following dialysis, a 250 to 500 mg supplemental dose is recommended.

➤*Storage/Stability:* Store at 25°C (77°F); excursions permitted to 15° to 30°C (59° to 86°F).

Actions

➤*Pharmacology:* Levetiracetam is chemically unrelated to other antiepileptic drugs. The precise mechanism by which levetiracetam exerts its antiepileptic effect is unknown. The antiepileptic activity of levetiracetam was assessed in a number of animal models of epileptic seizures. Levetiracetam did not inhibit single seizures induced by maximal stimulation with electrical current or different chemoconvulsants and showed only minimal activity in submaximal stimulation and in threshold tests. However, protection was observed against secondarily generalized activity from focal seizures induced by pilocarpine and kainic acid, 2 chemoconvulsants that induce seizures that mimic some features of human complex partial seizures with secondary generalization. Levetiracetam also displayed inhibitory properties in the kindling model in rats, another model of human complex partial seizures, during kindling development and in the fully kindled state. The predictive value of these animal models for specific types of human epilepsy is uncertain.

In vitro and in vivo recordings of epileptiform activity from the hippocampus have shown that levetiracetam inhibits burst firing without affecting normal neuronal excitability, suggesting that levetiracetam may selectively prevent hypersynchronization of epileptiform burst firing and propagation of seizure activity.

Levetiracetam at concentrations of up to 10 mcM did not demonstrate binding affinity for a variety of known receptors such as those associated with benzodiazepines, gamma-aminobutyric acid (GABA), glycine, N-methyl-D-aspartate (NMDA), re-uptake sites, and second messenger systems. Furthermore, in vitro studies have failed to find an effect of levetiracetam on neuronal voltage-gated sodium or T-type calcium currents. Levetiracetam does not appear to directly facilitate GABAergic neurotransmission, but has been shown to oppose the activity of negative modulators of GABA- and glycine-gated currents in neuronal cell culture.

➤*Pharmacokinetics:*

Absorption/Distribution – Levetiracetam is rapidly and almost completely absorbed, with peak plasma concentrations occurring approximately 1 hour following oral administration in fasted subjects. The oral bioavailability of levetiracetam tablets is 100%, and the tablets and oral solution are bioequivalent in rate and extent of absorption. Food does not affect the extent of absorption of levetiracetam but it decreases C_{max} by 20% and delays T_{max} by 1.5 hours.

The pharmacokinetics of levetiracetam are linear over the dose range of 500 to 5000 mg. Steady state is achieved after 2 days of multiple twice daily dosing. Levetiracetam and its major metabolite are less than 10% bound to plasma proteins.

Metabolism – Levetiracetam is not extensively metabolized. The major metabolic pathway is the enzymatic hydrolysis of the acetamide group, which produces the carboxylic acid metabolite, ucb L057 (24%) and is not dependent on any liver cytochrome P450 isoenzymes. The major metabolite is inactive in animal seizure models. Two minor metabolites were identified as the product of hydroxylation of the 2-oxo-pyrrolidine ring (2% of dose) and opening of the 2-oxo-pyrrolidine ring in position 5 (1% of dose). There is no enantiomeric interconversion of levetiracetam or its major metabolite.

Excretion – Levetiracetam plasma half-life in adults is about 7 hours and is unaffected by either dose or repeated administration. Levetiracetam is eliminated from the systemic circulation by renal excretion as unchanged drug, which represents 66% of administered dose. The total body clearance is 0.96 mL/min/kg and the renal clearance is 0.6 mL/min/kg. The mechanism of excretion is glomerular filtration with subsequent partial tubular reabsorption. The metabolite ucb L057 is excreted by glomerular filtration and active tubular secretion with a renal clearance of 4 mL/min/kg. Levetiracetam elimination is correlated to creatinine clearance (Ccr); clearance is reduced in patients with impaired renal function.

Special populations –

Gender: Levetiracetam C_{max} and AUC were 20% higher in women compared to men. However, clearances adjusted for body weight were comparable.

Elderly: Pharmacokinetics of levetiracetam were evaluated in 16 elderly subjects (61 to 88 years of age) with Ccr ranging from 30 to 74 mL/min. Following oral administration of twice daily dosing for 10 days, total body clearance decreased by 38% and the half-life was 2.5 hours longer in the elderly compared with healthy adults. This is most likely because of the decrease in renal function in these subjects (see Warnings).

Children: Pharmacokinetics of levetiracetam were evaluated in 24 pediatric patients (6 to 12 years of age) after single dose (20 mg/kg). The apparent clearance of levetiracetam was approximately 40% higher than in adults.

LEVETIRACETAM

Renal function impairment: The disposition of levetiracetam was studied in subjects with varying degrees of renal function. Total body clearance of levetiracetam is reduced in patients with impaired renal function by 40% in the mild renal impairment group (Ccr = 50 to 80 mL/min), 50% in the moderate group (Ccr = 30 to 50 mL/min), and 60% in the severe group (Ccr less than 30 mL/min).

In anuric (end-stage renal disease) patients, the total body clearance decreased 70% compared with healthy subjects (Ccr greater than 80 mL/min). Approximately 50% of the pool of levetiracetam in the body is removed during a standard 4-hour hemodialysis procedure (see Warnings, Administration and Dosage).

Hepatic function impairment: In subjects with mild (Child-Pugh A) to moderate (Child-Pugh B) hepatic impairment, the pharmacokinetics of levetiracetam were unchanged. In patients with severe hepatic impairment (Child-Pugh C), total body clearance was 50% that of healthy subjects, but decreased renal clearance accounted for most of the decrease. No dose adjustment is needed for patients with hepatic impairment.

Contraindications

Hypersensitivity to the drug or any of its ingredients.

Warnings

➤*CNS effects:*

Somnolence – In controlled trials of patients with epilepsy, 14.8% of levetiracetam-treated patients reported somnolence compared with 8.4% of placebo patients. There was no clear dose response up to 3000 mg/day. In a study where there was no titration, approximately 45% of patients receiving 4000 mg/day reported somnolence. The somnolence was considered serious in 0.3% of the levetiracetam-treated patients compared with 0% in the placebo group. About 3% of levetiracetam-treated patients discontinued treatment because of somnolence vs 0.7% with placebo. In 1.4% of levetiracetam-treated patients and in 0.9% of placebo patients the dose was reduced, while 0.3% of the levetiracetam-treated patients were hospitalized because of somnolence.

Asthenia – In controlled trials of patients with epilepsy, 14.7% of levetiracetam-treated patients reported asthenia vs 9.1% with placebo. Treatment was discontinued in 0.8% of levetiracetam-treated patients vs 0.5% with placebo. In 0.5% of levetiracetam-treated patients and in 0.2% of placebo patients the dose was reduced.

Coordination difficulties – A total of 3.4% of levetiracetam-treated patients experienced coordination difficulties (reported as either ataxia, abnormal gait, or incoordination) vs 1.6% with placebo. A total of 0.4% of levetiracetam-treated patients in controlled trials discontinued treatment because of ataxia vs 0% with placebo. In 0.7% of levetiracetam-treated patients and in 0.2% of placebo patients the dose was reduced because of coordination difficulties, while one of the levetiracetam-treated patients was hospitalized because of worsening of preexisting ataxia.

Somnolence, asthenia, and coordination difficulties occurred most frequently within the first 4 weeks of treatment.

Psychotic symptoms – In controlled trials of patients with epilepsy, 5 (0.7%) of levetiracetam-treated patients experienced psychotic symptoms compared with 1 (0.2%) placebo patient. Two (0.3%) levetiracetam-treated patients were hospitalized and their treatment was discontinued. Both events, reported as psychosis, developed within the first week of treatment and resolved within 1 to 2 weeks following treatment discontinuation. Two other events, reported as hallucinations, occurred after 1 to 5 months and resolved within 2 to 7 days while the patients remained on treatment. In 1 patient experiencing psychotic depression occurring within a month, symptoms resolved within 45 days while the patient continued treatment. A total of 13.3% of levetiracetam patients experienced other behavioral symptoms (eg, aggression, anger, irritability, agitation, hostility, anxiety, apathy, emotional lability, depersonalization, depression) compared with 6.2% of placebo patients. Approximately half of these patients reported these events within the first 4 weeks. A total of 1.7% of levetiracetam-treated patients discontinued treatment because of these events vs 0.2% with placebo. The treatment dose was reduced in 0.8% of levetiracetam-treated patients and in 0.5% of placebo patients. A total of 0.8% of levetiracetam-treated patients had a serious behavioral event (vs 0.2% with placebo) and were hospitalized.

In addition, 4 (0.5%) levetiracetam-treated patients attempted suicide vs 0% with placebo. One of these patients successfully committed suicide. In the other 3 patients, the events did not lead to discontinuation or dose reduction. The events occurred after patients had been treated for 1 to 6 months.

➤*Withdrawal seizure:* Withdraw antiepileptic drugs, including levetiracetam, gradually to minimize the potential of increased seizure frequency.

➤*Renal function impairment:* Clearance of levetiracetam is decreased in patients with renal function impairment and is correlated with Ccr. Take caution in dosing patients with moderate and severe renal impairment and patients undergoing hemodialysis. Reduce dosage in patients with impaired renal function receiving levetiracetam and give supplemental doses to patients after dialysis (see Actions, Administration and Dosage).

➤*Elderly:* No overall differences in safety were observed between subjects 65 years of age and older and younger subjects. There were insufficient numbers of elderly subjects in controlled trials of epilepsy to adequately assess the effectiveness of levetiracetam in these patients.

Levetiracetam is known to be substantially excreted by the kidney, and the risk of adverse reactions to this drug may be greater in patients with impaired renal function. Because elderly patients are more likely to have decreased renal function, take care in dose selection; it may be useful to monitor renal function.

➤*Pregnancy:* Category C. In animal studies, levetiracetam produced evidence of developmental toxicity at doses similar to or greater than human therapeutic doses.

Administration to female rats throughout pregnancy and lactation was associated with increased incidences of minor fetal skeletal abnormalities and retarded offspring growth pre- and/or postnatally at doses of 350 mg/kg/day or greater (approximately equivalent to the maximum recommended human dose [MRHD] of 3000 mg on a mg/m² basis) and with increased pup mortality and offspring behavioral alterations at a dose of 1800 mg/kg/day (6 times the MRHD).

Treatment of pregnant rabbits during the period of organogenesis resulted in increased embryofetal mortality and increased incidences of minor fetal skeletal abnormalities at doses of 600 mg/kg/day and greater (approximately 4 times MRHD) and in decreased fetal weights and increased incidences of fetal malformations at a dose of 1800 mg/kg/day (12 times the MRHD). Maternal toxicity was also observed at 1800 mg/kg/day.

When pregnant rats were treated during the period of organogenesis, fetal weights were decreased and the incidence of fetal skeletal variations was increased at a dose of 3600 mg/kg/day (12 times the MRHD).

There are no adequate and well-controlled studies in pregnant women. Use levetiracetam during pregnancy only if the potential benefit justifies the potential risk to the fetus.

Pregnancy exposure registry – To facilitate monitoring fetal outcomes of pregnant women exposed to levetiracetam, physicians should encourage patients to register before fetal outcome is known (eg, ultrasound, results of amniocentesis) in the Antiepileptic Drug Pregnancy Registry by calling (888) 233-2334.

➤*Lactation:* Levetiracetam is excreted in breast milk. Because of the potential for serious adverse reactions in nursing infants from levetiracetam, a decision should be made whether to discontinue nursing or discontinue the drug, taking into account the importance of the drug to the mother.

➤*Children:* Safety and efficacy in patients younger than 16 years of age have not been established.

Precautions

➤*Hematologic effects:* Minor but statistically significant decreases compared with placebo in total mean RBC count (0.03×10^6/mm²), mean hemoglobin (0.09 g/dL), and mean hematocrit (0.38%), were seen in levetiracetam-treated patients in controlled trials.

A total of 3.2% of treated and 1.8% of placebo patients had at least 1 possibly significant (2.8×10^9/L or less) decreased WBC, and 2.4% of treated and 1.4% of placebo patients had at least 1 possibly significant (1×10^9/L or less) decreased neutrophil count. Of the treated patients with a low neutrophil count, all but 1 rose toward or to baseline with continued treatment. No patient was discontinued secondary to low neutrophil counts.

➤*Hazardous tasks:* Patients should use caution while driving or performing other tasks requiring alertness, coordination or physical dexterity.

Drug Interactions

➤*Drug/Food interactions:* Food does not affect the extent of absorption of levetiracetam, but it decreases C_{max} by 20% and delays T_{max} by 1.5 hours.

Adverse Reactions

The most frequently reported adverse events associated with the use of levetiracetam in combination with other antiepileptic drugs (AEDs) were somnolence, asthenia, infection, and dizziness. Asthenia, somnolence, and dizziness appeared to occur predominantly during the first 4 weeks of treatment with levetiracetam.

Treatment-Emergent Adverse Reactions in Placebo-Controlled Add-On Studies of Levetiracetam-Treated Patients (≥ 1%)		
Adverse reaction	Levetiracetam (n = 769)	Placebo (n = 439)
CNS		
Somnolence	15	8
Headache	14	13
Dizziness	9	4
Depression	4	2
Nervousness	4	2
Ataxia	3	1
Vertigo	3	1
Amnesia	2	1

LEVETIRACETAM

Treatment-Emergent Adverse Reactions in Placebo-Controlled Add-On Studies of Levetiracetam-Treated Patients (≥ 1%)		
Adverse reaction	Levetiracetam (n = 769)	Placebo (n = 439)
Anxiety	2	1
Hostility	2	1
Paresthesia	2	1
Emotional lability	2	0
Respiratory		
Pharyngitis	6	4
Rhinitis	4	3
Increased cough	2	1
Sinusitis	2	1
Miscellaneous		
Asthenia	15	9
Infection	13	8
Pain	7	6
Anorexia	3	2
Diplopia	2	1

Other events reported by 1% or more of patients treated with levetiracetam but as or more frequent in the placebo group were the following: Abdominal pain; accidental injury; amblyopia; arthralgia; back pain; bronchitis; chest pain; confusion; constipation; convulsion; diarrhea; increased drug level; dyspepsia; ecchymosis; fever; flu syndrome; gastroenteritis; gingivitis; grand mal convulsion; fungal infection; insomnia; nausea; otitis media; rash; abnormal thinking; tremor; urinary tract infection; vomiting; weight gain.

In well-controlled clinical studies, 15% of patients receiving levetiracetam and 11.6% receiving placebo either discontinued or had a dose reduction as a result of an adverse event.

Adverse Reactions Most Commonly Associated with Discontinuation or Dose Reduction of Levetiracetam in Patients with Epilepsy (%)		
Adverse reaction	Levetiracetam (n = 769)	Placebo (n = 439)
Somnolence	4.4	1.6
Convulsion	3	3.4
Dizziness	1.4	0
Asthenia	1.3	0.7
Rash	0	1.1

➤*Lab test abnormalities:* Although most laboratory tests are not systematically altered with levetiracetam treatment, there have been relatively infrequent abnormalities seen in hematologic parameters and liver function tests.

➤*Postmarketing:* Leukopenia; neutropenia; pancytopenia; thrombocytopenia.

Overdosage

➤*Symptoms:* The highest known dose of levetiracetam received in the clinical development program was 6000 mg/day. Other than drowsiness, there were no adverse events in the few known cases of overdose. Cases of somnolence, agitation, aggression, depressed level of consciousness, respiratory depression, and coma were observed with levetiracetam overdoses in postmarketing use.

➤*Treatment:* There is no specific antidote for overdose with levetiracetam. If indicated, attempt elimination of unabsorbed drug by emesis or gastric lavage; observe usual precautions to maintain airway. General supportive care of the patient is indicated, including monitoring of vital signs and observation of the clinical status of patient. Refer to the General Management of Acute Overdosage. Contact a Certified Poison Control Center for up-to-date information on the management of overdose with levetiracetam.

Standard hemodialysis procedures result in significant clearance of levetiracetam (approximately 50% in 4 hours); consider in cases of overdose. Although hemodialysis has not been performed in the few known cases of overdose, it may be indicated by the patient's clinical state or in patients with significant renal impairment.

Patient Information

Advise patients to notify their physician if they become pregnant or intend to become pregnant during therapy.

Advise patients that levetiracetam may cause dizziness and somnolence. Accordingly, advise patients not to drive or operate machinery or engage in other hazardous activities until they have gained sufficient experience on levetiracetam to gauge whether it adversely affects their performance of these activities.

Advise patients to swallow the tablets whole. Patients should not chew or crush tablets. Oral solution should be used if the patient cannot swallow the tablets. A medicine dropper or medicine cup should be used to measure the oral solution. A teaspoon should not be used. Their pharmacist can provide a medicine dropper or medicine cup to help them measure.

Advise patients to call their health care provider right away if any of the following symptoms appear: Extreme sleepiness, tiredness, and weakness; problems with muscle coordination (problems walking and moving); mood and behavior changes (eg, aggression, anger, anxiety, apathy, depression, hostility, irritability, hallucinations, thoughts of suicide).

Advise patients that the most common side effects are sleepiness, weakness, dizziness, infection. These side effects could happen at any time, but happen most often within the first 4 weeks of treatment, except infection.

PRIMIDONE

Rx	**Primidone** (Lannett)	**Tablets:** 50 mg	In 100s, 500s, and 1000s.
Rx	**Mysoline** (Xcel Pharm.)		Lactose. (Mysoline 50 M). White, scored. Square. In 100s and 500s.
Rx	**Primidone** (Various, eg, Danbury, Lannett, Major)	**Tablets:** 250 mg	In 100s, 500s, and 1000s.
Rx	**Mysoline** (Xcel Pharm)		Lactose. (Mysoline 250 M). Yellow, scored. Square. In 100s, 1000s, and UD 100s.

Refer to the general discussion beginning in the Anticonvulsants introduction.

Indications

➤*Epilepsy:* For the control of grand mal, psychomotor, or focal epileptic seizures, either alone or with other anticonvulsants. It may control grand mal seizures refractory to other anticonvulsants.

➤*Unlabeled uses:*

Essential tremor – Primidone at doses of 50 to 750 mg/day has demonstrated effectiveness in the treatment of essential tremor.

Administration and Dosage

Individualize dosage. The therapeutic efficacy of a dosage regimen takes several weeks before it can be assessed.

In some cases, serum blood level determinations of primidone may be necessary for optimal dosage adjustment. The clinically effective serum level for primidone is between 5 to 12 mcg/mL.

➤*Adults and children (8 years of age and older):* Patients who have received no previous treatment may be started on primidone according to the following regimen:
- *Days 1 to 3* – 100 to 125 mg at bedtime.
- *Days 4 to 6* – 100 to 125 mg twice daily.
- *Days 7 to 9* – 100 to 125 mg 3 times/day.
- *Day 10 to maintenance* - 250 mg 3 to 4 times/day. If required, increase dose to 250 mg 5 to 6 times/day, but do not exceed doses of 500 mg 4 times/day (2 g/day).

➤*Children (younger than 8 years of age):* The following regimen may be used to initiate therapy:
- *Days 1 to 3* – 50 mg at bedtime.

- *Days 4 to 6* – 50 mg twice daily.
- *Days 7 to 9* – 100 mg twice daily.
- *Day 10 to maintenance* - 125 to 250 mg 3 times/day or 10 to 25 mg/kg/day in divided doses.

➤*Patients already receiving other anticonvulsants:* Start primidone at 100 to 125 mg at bedtime and gradually increase to maintenance level as the other drug is gradually decreased. Continue this regimen until satisfactory dosage level is achieved for the combination or the other drug is completely withdrawn. When therapy with primidone alone is the objective, do not complete the transition in less than 2 weeks.

➤*Storage/Stability:* Store at room temperature, approximately 25°C (77°F). Dispense in tight, light-resistant container.

Actions

➤*Pharmacology:* Primidone raises electroshock or chemoshock seizure thresholds or alters seizure patterns in animals. Mechanism of antiepileptic action is unknown.

Primidone and its 2 metabolites, phenobarbital and phenylethylmalonamide (PEMA), have anticonvulsant activity. In addition, PEMA potentiates the activity of phenobarbital in animals.

➤*Pharmacokinetics:*

Absorption/Distribution – Primidone is rapidly and almost completely absorbed after oral administration, although individual variability exists. Peak concentrations are usually observed approximately 3 hours after ingestion. Primidone and PEMA are bound to plasma proteins to only a small extent.

Metabolism/Excretion – Primidone is converted to 2 active metabolites, phenobarbital and PEMA. The plasma half-life ranges between 5

PRIMIDONE

to 15 hours. The half-life of PEMA is approximately 16 hours. Both metabolites accumulate during long-term therapy. The appearance of phenobarbital in plasma may be delayed several days upon primidone initiation. Approximately 40% of the drug is excreted unchanged in the urine.

Contraindications

Porphyria; hypersensitivity to phenobarbital.

Warnings

➤*Status epilepticus:* Abrupt withdrawal of antiepileptic medication may precipitate *status epilepticus.*

➤*Therapeutic efficacy:* Therapeutic efficacy of a dosage regimen takes several weeks to assess.

➤*Pregnancy: Category D.* The effects of primidone in pregnancy are unknown.

Neonatal hemorrhage, with a coagulation defect resembling vitamin K deficiency, has been described in newborns whose mothers were taking primidone and other anticonvulsants. Pregnant women taking anticonvulsant therapy should receive prophylactic vitamin K therapy for 1 month prior to and during delivery. (See Warnings in the Anticonvulsants Introduction.)

➤*Lactation:* Primidone appears in breast milk in substantial quantities. It is suggested that undue somnolence and drowsiness in nursing newborns of primidone-treated mothers be taken as an indication to discontinue nursing.

Precautions

➤*Monitoring:* Because therapy generally extends over prolonged periods, perform complete blood counts and a sequential multiple analysis test every 6 months.

➤*Hazardous tasks:* Patients should use caution while driving or performing other tasks requiring alertness, coordination or physical dexterity.

Drug Interactions

Primidone Drug Interactions			
Precipitant drug	Object drug*		Description
Carbamazepine	Primidone	↓	Concomitant primidone and carbamazepine may result in decreased primidone, its metabolite phenobarbital, and carbamazepine serum concentrations.
Primidone	Carbamazepine		
Hydantoins (eg, phenytoin)	Primidone	↑	Hydantoins may increase serum primidone and its metabolites. Patients on concomitant treatment with hydantoins and primidone should be monitored closely following any alteration in hydantoin therapy.
Succinimides (eg, ethosuximide, methsuximide)	Primidone	↓	Coadministration of primidone and a succinimide may result in lower primidone and phenobarbital serum concentrations.
Valproic Acid	Primidone	↑	Plasma primidone concentrations may be elevated, increasing the pharmacologic and adverse effects. Primidone dosage may need to be decreased in some patients.
Primidone	Anticoagulants (eg, warfarin sodium)	↓	Primidone reduces the effect of anticoagulants. Monitor anticoagulation dose and tailor doses as needed.
Primidone	Beta-blockers (eg, propranolol)	↓	Pharmacokinetic effects of certain beta-blockers may be reduced. Consider a higher beta-blocker dose during coadministration of primidone.
Primidone	Corticosteroids (eg, prednisone)	↓	Decreased effect of corticosteroid may be observed. If possible, avoid this combination.
Primidone	Doxycycline	↓	Coadministration may decrease doxycycline half-life and serum levels, possibly resulting in a decreased therapeutic effect. These effects may persist for weeks following primidone discontinuation. Consider an alternate tetracycline.

Primidone Drug Interactions			
Precipitant drug	Object drug*		Description
Primidone	Estrogens Oral contraceptives	↓	AUC of estrogen may be decreased. Contraceptive failure has been reported. Alternate contraception methods are recommended.
Primidone	Ethanol	↑	Impaired hand-eye coordination, additive CNS effects, and death have been noted upon acute ingestion. Chronic ethanol ingestion may manifest as drug tolerance. Avoid concomitant use.
Primidone	Felodipine	↓	Pharmacologic effects of felodipine may be decreased. Patients receiving long-term treatment with both drugs may require higher doses of felodipine.
Primidone	Methadone	↓	The actions of methadone may be reduced. Patients receiving chronic methadone treatment may experience opiate withdrawal symptoms. A higher dose of methadone may be required during coadministration with primidone.
Primidone	Metronidazole	↓	Therapeutic failure of metronidazole has been observed. May need to use higher initial metronidazole doses in patients also receiving primidone.
Primidone	Nifedipine	↓	Decreased serum nifedipine concentrations, possibly reducing efficacy have been observed. Titrate dose according to response. A larger nifedipine dose may be needed.
Primidone	Quinidine	↓	Primidone appears to produce decreased quinidine serum concentrations and a decreased quinidine elimination half-life.
Primidone	Theophyllines	↓	Decreased theophylline levels, possibly resulting in reduced therapeutic effects have been observed. Increased theophylline dosages may be required with use of primidone.

* ↑ = Object drug increased.   ↓ = Object drug decreased.

Adverse Reactions

➤*CNS:* Ataxia, vertigo (these tend to disappear with continued therapy or with reduction of initial dosage); drowsiness; emotional disturbances; fatigue; hyperirritability.

➤*GI:* Anorexia, nausea, vomiting.

➤*Hematologic:* Megaloblastic anemia may occur as a rare idiosyncrasy and responds to folic acid without necessity of discontinuing medication. Granulocytopenia, agranulocytosis, and red-cell hypoplasia and aplasia have been reported rarely.

➤*Special senses:* Diplopia, nystagmus.

➤*Miscellaneous:* Impotence; morbilliform skin eruptions.

Patient Information

Drowsiness, dizziness, or muscular incoordination may occur initially, but these symptoms usually disappear with continued therapy. Observe caution while driving or performing other tasks requiring alertness, coordination, or physical dexterity.

Do not discontinue medication abruptly or change dosage, except on advice of a health care provider.

Notify health care provider if skin rash or fever occurs or if patient becomes pregnant.

Have patients carry identification (*Medic Alert*) indicating medication usage and epilepsy.

TIAGABINE HCl

Rx	Gabitril Filmtabs (Cephalon)	Tablets: 2 mg	Lactose. (FJ). Peach. Film coated. In 100s.
		4 mg	Lactose. (FK). Yellow. Film coated. In 100s, 500s and *Abbo-Pac* 100s.
		12 mg	Lactose. (FL). Green. Ovaloid. Film coated. In 100s, 500s and *Abbo-Pac* 100s.
		16 mg	Lactose. (FM). Blue. Ovaloid. Film coated. In 100s, 500s and *Abbo-Pac* 100s.

Refer to the general discussion beginning in the Anticonvulsants introduction.

Indications

➤*Partial seizures:* Adjunctive therapy for treatment of partial seizures.

Administration and Dosage

➤*Approved by the FDA:* September 30, 1997.

Tiagabine is given orally and should be taken with food.

➤*Children (12 to 18 years):* Initiate tiagabine at 4 mg once daily. Modification of concomitant antiepilepsy drugs is not necessary, unless clinically indicated. The total daily dose of tiagabine may be increased by 4 mg at the beginning of week 2. Thereafter, the total daily dose of may be increased by 4 to 8 mg at weekly intervals until clinical response is achieved or up to 32 mg/day. Give the total daily dose in two to four divided doses. Doses > 32 mg/day have been tolerated in a small number of adolescent patients for a relatively short duration.

➤*Adults and children > 18 years:* Initiate tiagabine at 4 mg once daily. Modification of concomitant antiepilepsy drugs is not necessary, unless clinically indicated. The total daily dose of tiagabine may be increased by 4 to 8 mg at weekly intervals until clinical response is achieved or up to 56 mg/day. Give the total daily dose in two to four divided doses. Doses > 56 mg/day have not been systematically evaluated in adequate well controlled trials.

Experience is limited in patients taking total daily doses > 32 mg/day using twice-daily dosing. A typical dosing titration regimen for patients taking enzyme-inducing antiepilepsy drugs (AEDs) is provided.

Typical Dosing Titration Regimen of Tiagabine for Patients Taking Enzyme-Inducing AEDs		
Week	Initiation and titration schedule	Total daily dose
Week 1	Initiate at 4 mg once daily	4 mg/day
Week 2	Increase total daily dose by 4 mg	8 mg/day (in 2 divided doses)
Week 3	Increase total daily dose by 4 mg	12 mg/day (in 3 divided doses)
Week 4	Increase total daily dose by 4 mg	16 mg/day (in 2 to 4 divided doses)
Week 5	Increase total daily dose by 4 to 8 mg	20 to 24 mg/day (in 2 to 4 divided doses)
Week 6	Increase total daily dose by 4 to 8 mg	24 to 32 mg/day (in 2 to 4 divided doses)
Usual adult maintenance dose	32 to 56 mg/day in 2 to 4 divided doses	

Actions

➤*Pharmacology:* The precise mechanism by which tiagabine exerts its antiseizure effect is unknown, although it is believed to be related to its ability (in vitro) to enhance the activity of gamma aminobutyric acid (GABA), the major inhibitory neurotransmitter in the CNS. These experiments have shown that tiagabine binds to recognition sites associated with the GABA uptake carrier. It is thought that, by this action, tiagabine blocks GABA uptake into presynaptic neurons, permitting more GABA to be available for receptor binding on the surfaces of postsynaptic cells. This suggests that tiagabine prevents the propagation of neural impulses that contribute to seizures by a GABA-ergic action.

Based on in vitro binding studies, tiagabine does not significantly inhibit the uptake of dopamine, norepinephrine, serotonin, glutamate, or choline and shows little or no binding to dopamine D_1 and D_2, muscarinic, serotonin $5HT_{1A}$, $5HT_2$, and $5HT_3$, beta-1 and 2 adrenergic, alpha-1 and alpha-2 adrenergic, histamine H_2 and H_3, adenosine A_1 and A_2, opiate µ, K_1, NMDA glutamate and GABA receptors. It also lacks significant affinity for sodium or calcium channels. Tiagabine binds to histamine H_1, serotonin $5HT_{1B}$, benzodiazepine, and chloride channel receptors at concentrations 20 to 400 times those inhibiting the uptake of GABA.

➤*Pharmacokinetics:*

Absorption/Distribution – Absorption of tiagabine is rapid and nearly complete (> 95%), with an absolute oral bioavailability of ≈ 90%. Peak plasma concentrations occur at ≈ 45 minutes in the fasting state.

A high fat meal decreases the rate (mean T_{max} is prolonged to 2.5 hours, and mean C_{max} is reduced by ≈ 40%), but not the extent (AUC) of tiagabine absorption.

The pharmacokinetics of tiagabine are linear over the single dose range of 2 to 24 mg. Following multiple dosing, steady state is achieved within 2 days. Tiagabine is 96% bound to plasma proteins, mainly to albumin and α1–acid glycoprotein. While the relationship between tiagabine plasma concentrations and clinical response is not currently understood, trough plasma concentrations from < 1 to 234 ng/ml were observed in controlled clinical trials at doses of 30 to 56 mg/day.

Metabolism/Excretion – The metabolism of tiagabine has not been fully elucidated; at least two metabolic pathways have been identified in humans: 1) thiophene ring oxidation leading to the formation of 5–oxo-tiagabine; and 2) glucuronidation. The 5–oxo-tiagabine metabolite does not contribute to the pharmacologic activity of tiagabine.

Tiagabine is likely to be metabolized primarily by the P450 3A (CYP3A) isoform, although contributions to the metabolism of tiagabine from CYP1A2, CYP2D6 or CYP2C19 have not been excluded. Mean systemic plasma clearance is 109 ml/min and the average elimination half-life for tiagabine in healthy subjects ranged from 7 to 9 hours. The elimination half-life decreased by 50% to 65% in hepatic enzyme-induced patients with epilepsy compared to uninduced patients with epilepsy.

Elimination half-life is only 4 to 7 hours in patients receiving hepatic enzyme-inducing drugs (carbamazepine, phenytoin, primidone and phenobarbital).

Approximately 2% of an oral dose of tiagabine is excreted unchanged, with 25% and 63% of the remaining dose excreted into the urine and feces, respectively, primarily as metabolites.

Diurnal effect: A diurnal effect on the pharmacokinetics of tiagabine was observed. Mean-steady state C_{min} values were 40% lower in the evening than in the morning. Tiagabine steady-state AUC values were also found to be 15% lower following the evening dose compared with the morning dose.

Special populations –

Hepatic function impairment: In patients with moderate hepatic impairment (Child-Pugh Class B), clearance of unbound tiagabine was reduced by ≈ 60%.

Children: The apparent clearence and volume of distribution of tiagabine per unit body surface area or per kg were fairly similar in 25 children (age 3 to 10 years) and in adults taking enzyme-inducing antiepilepsy drugs ([AEDs] eg, carbamazepine or phenytoin). In children who were taking a non-inducing AED (eg, valproate), the clearance of tiagabine based upon body weight and body surface area was 2 and 1.5–fold higher, respectively, than in uninduced adults with epilepsy.

➤*Clinical trials:* Two placebo controlled trials examined the effectiveness of tiagabine. Both trials included an open screening phase during which patients were titrated to an optimal dose and then treated with this dose for an additional 4 weeks. After this open phase, patients were randomized to one of two blinded treatment sequences (tiagabine followed by placebo or placebo followed by tiagabine), each lasting 7 weeks (with a 3 week washout). The reductions in seizure rates were statistically significant in both studies.

Contraindications

Hypersensitivity to the drug or its ingredients.

Warnings

➤*Withdrawal seizures:* Do not abruptly discontinue antiepilepsy drugs because of the possibility of increasing seizure frequency. Withdraw tiagabine gradually to minimize the potential for increased seizure frequency, unless safety concerns require a more rapid withdrawl.

➤*Cognitive/neuropsychiatric adverse events:* Adverse events most often associated with the use of tiagabine were related to the CNS. The most significant of these can be classified into two general catagories: 1) Impaired concentration, speech or language problems, and confusion (effects on thought processes); and 2) somnolence and fatigue (effects on level of consciousness). The majority of these events were mild to moderate. In controlled clinical trials, these events led to discontinuation of treatment with tiagabine in 6% of patients compared to 2% of the placebo-treated patients. A total of 1.6% of the tiagabine-treated patients in the controlled trials were hospitalized secondary to the occurrence of these events compared to 0% of the placebo-treated patients. Some of these events were dose-related and usually began during initial titration.

➤*EEG abnormalities:* Patients with a history of spike and wave discharges on EEG have been reported to have exacerbations of their EEG abnormalities associated with these cognitive/neuropsychiatric events. This raises the possibility that these clinical events may, in some cases, be a manifestation of underlying seizure activity. In the documented

TIAGABINE HCl

cases of spike and wave discharges on EEG with cognitive/neuropsychiatric events, patients usually continued tiagabine, but required dosage adjustment.

➤*Status epilepticus:* In the three double-blind, placebo-controlled, parallel-group studies, the incidence of any type of status epilepticus (simple, complex, or generalized tonic-clonic) in patients receiving tiagabine was 0.8% vs 0.7% receiving placebo. Among the patients treated with tiagabine across all epilepsy studies (controlled and uncontrolled), 5% had some form of status epilepticus. Of the 5%, 57% of patients experienced complex partial status epilepticus. A critical risk factor for status epilepticus was the presence of the condition history; 33% of patients with a history of status epilepticus had recurrence during tiagabine treatment. Because adequate information about the incidence of status epilepticus in a similar population of patients with epilepsy who have not received treatment with tiagabine is not available, it is impossible to state whether or not treatment with tiagabine is associated with a higher or lower rate of status epilepticus than would be expected to occur in a similar population not treated with tiagabine.

➤*Sudden unexpected death in epilepsy (SUDEP):* There have been as many as 10 cases of SUDEP during the clinical development of tiagabine among 2531 patients with epilepsy (3831 patient-years of exposure).

This represents an estimated incidence of 0.0026 deaths per patient-year. This rate is within the range of estimates for the incidence of SUDEP not receiving tiagabine (ranging from 0.0005 for the general population with epilepsy, 0.003 to 0.004 for clinical trial populations similar to that in the clinical development program for tiagabine, to 0.005 for patients with refractory epilepsy). The estimated SUDEP rates in patients receiving tiagabine are also similar to those observed in patients receiving other antiepilepsy drugs, chemically unrelated to tiagabine, that underwent clinical testing in similar populations at about the same time. This evidence suggests that the SUDEP rates reflect population rates, not a drug effect.

➤*Hepatic function impairment:* Because the clearance of tiagabine is reduced in patients with liver disease, dosage reduction or longer dosing intervals may be necessary in these patients.

➤*Carcinogenesis:* In rats, a study of the potential carcinogenicity associated with tiagabine administration showed that 200 mg/kg/day for 2 years resulted in small, but statistically significant increases in the incidences of hepatocellular adenomas in females and Leydig cell tumors of the testes in males.

➤*Mutagenesis:* Tiagabine produced an increase in structural chromosome aberration frequency in human lymphocytes in vitro in the absence of metabolic activation.

➤*Pregnancy: Catagory C.* Tiagabine has adverse effects on embryo-fetal development, including teratogenic effects, when administered to pregnant rats and rabbits at doses greater than in the human therapeutic dose. There are no adequate and well controlled studies in pregnant women. Use tiagabine during pregnancy only if clearly needed.

➤*Lactation:* Tiagabine or its metabolites are excreted in the milk of rats. Use in women who are nursing only if the benefits clearly outweigh the risks.

➤*Children:* Safety and efficacy in children < 12 years old have not been established.

Precautions

➤*Concomitant enzyme-inducing antiepilepsy drug (AED):* Virtually all experience with tiagabine has been obtained in patients receiving at least one concomitant enzyme-inducing AED. Use in non-induced patients (eg, patients receiving valproate monotherapy) may require lower doses or a slower dose titration of tiagabine for clinical response. Patients taking a combination of inducing and non-inducing drugs (eg, carbamazepine and valproate) should be considered to be induced.

➤*Generalized weakness:* Moderately severe to incapacitating generalized weakness has been reported following administration of tiagabine in 28 of 2531 (≈1%) patients with epilepsy. The weakness resolved in all cases after a reduction in dose or discontinuation of tiagabine.

➤*Ophthalmic effects:* There is evidence in animal studies of residual binding in the retina and uvea after 3 weeks (the latest time point measured). Although not directly measured, melanin binding is suggested. The ability of available tests to detect potentially adverse consequences, if any, of the binding of tiagabine to melanin-containing tissue is unknown and there was no systematic monitoring for relevant ophthalmological changes during the clinical development of tiagabine. However, long-term (up to 1 year) toxicological studies of tiagabine in dogs showed no treatment-related ophthalmoscopic changes and macro- and microscopic examinations of the eye were unremarkable. Accordingly, although no specific recommendations for periodic ophthalmologic monitoring exists, be aware of the possibility of long-term ophthalmologic effects.

➤*Rash:* Four patients treated with tiagabine during the product's pre-marketing clinical testing developed what were considered to be serious rashes. In two patients, the rash was described as maculopapular; in one it was described as vesiculobullous; and in the fourth case, a diagnosis of Stevens-Johnson syndrome was made. In none of the 4 cases is it certain that tiagabine was the primary, or even a contributory, cause of the rash. Nevertheless, drug associated rash can, if extensive and serious, cause irreversible morbidity, even death.

➤*Therapeutic drug monitoring:* A therapeutic range for tiagabine plasma concentrations has not been established. In controlled trials, trough plasma concentrations observed among patients randomized to doses of tiagabine that were statistically significantly more effective than placebo ranged from < 1 to 234 ng/ml. Because of the potential for pharmacokinetic interactions between tiagabine and drugs that induce or inhibit hepatic metabolizing enzymes, it may be useful to obtain plasma levels of tiagabine before and after changes are made in the therapeutic regimen.

Drug Interactions

Tiagabine Drug Interactions			
Precipitant drug	Object drug*		Description
Tiagabine	Valproate	↔	Tiagabine causes a slight decrease (≈ 10%) in steady-state valproate concentrations. Valproate significantly decreased tiagabine binding in vitro from 96.3% to 94.8%, which resulted in an increase of ≈ 40% in the free tiagabine concentration. The clinical relevance of this in vitro finding is unknown.
Valproate	Tiagabine	↔	Tiagabine clearance is 60% greater in patients taking carbamazepine, phenobarbital or phenytoin with or without other enzyme-inducing antiepilepsy drugs (AEDs).
Carbamazepine	Tiagabine	↔	
Phenytoin			
Phenobarbital			

* ↔ = Undetermined clinical effect.

➤*Drug/Food interactions:* A high-fat meal decreases the rate (mean T_{max} is prolonged to 2.5 hours, and mean C_{max} is reduced by ≈ 40%), but not the extent (AUC) of tiagabine absorption.

Adverse Reactions

Approximately 21% of patients who received tiagabine in clinical trials of epilepsy discontinued treatment because of an adverse event. The adverse events most commonly associated with discontinuation were dizziness (1.7%), somnolence (1.6%), depression (1.3%), confusion (1.1%) and asthenia (1.1%).

The most commonly observed adverse events associated with the use of tiagabine in combination with other antiepilepsy drugs greater than those in placebo-treated patients were dizziness/lightheadedness, asthenia/lack of energy, somnolence, nausea, nervousness/irritability, tremor, abdominal pain and abnormal thinking/difficulty with concentration or attention.

Tiagabine Adverse Reactions (%)[1]		
Adverse reaction	Tiagabine (n = 494)	Placebo (n = 275)
CNS		
Dizziness	27	15
Asthenia	20	14
Somnolence	18	15
Nervousness	10	3
Tremor	9	3
Insomnia	6	4
Difficulty with concentration/attention	6	2
Ataxia	5	3
Confusion	5	3
Speech disorder	4	2
Difficulty with memory	4	3
Parasthesia	4	2
Depression	3	1
Emotional lability	3	2
Abnormal gait	3	2
Hostility	2	1
Nystagmus	2	1
Language problems	2	0
Agitation	1	0
GI		
Nausea	11	9
Diarrhea	7	3
Vomiting	7	4
Increased appetite	2	0
Mouth ulceration	1	0
Respiratory		
Pharyngitis	7	4
Cough increased	4	3
Skin		
Rash	5	4
Pruritus	2	0

TIAGABINE HCl

Tiagabine Adverse Reactions (%)[1]		
Adverse reaction	Tiagabine (n = 494)	Placebo (n = 275)
Miscellaneous		
Abdominal pain	7	3
Pain (unspecified)	5	3
Vasodilation	2	1
Myasthenia	1	0

[1] Patients in these add-on studies were receiving 1 to 3 concomitant enzyme-inducing antiepilepsy drugs in addition to tiagabine or placebo. Patients may have reported multiple adverse experiences; thus, patients may be included in > 1 catagory.

Overdosage

►*Symptoms:* Experience of acute overdose with tiagabine is limited. Eleven patients in clinical trials took single doses of tiagabine up to 800 mg. All patients fully recovered, usually within 1 day. The most common symptoms reported after overdose included somnolence, impaired consciousness, agitation, confusion, speech difficulty, hostility, depression, weakness, and myoclonus. One patient who ingested a single dose of 400 mg experienced generalized tonic-clonic status epilepticus, which responded to IV phenobarbital.

Eleven individuals (including 5 children < 7 years of age) not in tiagabine clinical trials accidentally ingested tiagabine in a single dose up to 20 mg. These individuals were asymptomatic in 6 cases. Symptoms exhibited in ≥ 1 of the other 5 individuals included ataxia, confusion, somnolence, impaired consciousness, impaired speech, agitation, lethargy, drowsiness, and myoclonus. One individual experienced a tonic-clonic seizure but was taking other agents which may be associated with seizures. All individuals recovered, usually within 1 day.

►*Treatment:* There is no specific antidote for overdose. If indicated, achieve elimination of unabsorbed drug by emesis or gastric lavage; observe usual precautions to maintain the airway. General supportive care of the patient is indicated including monitoring of vital signs and observation of clinical status of the patient. Because tiagabine is mostly metabolized by the liver and is highly protein bound, dialysis is unlikely to be beneficial. Refer to General Management of Acute Overdosage.

Patient Information

Instruct patients to take tiagabine with food.

Advise patients that tiagabine may cause dizziness, somnolence, and other symptoms and signs of CNS depression. Accordingly, advise them neither to drive nor to operate other complex machinery until they have gained sufficient experience on tiagabine to gauge whether or not it affects their mental or motor performance adversely. Because of the possible additive depressive effects, also use caution when patients are taking other CNS depressents in combination with tiagabine.

Because teratogenic effects were seen in the offspring of rats exposed to maternally toxic doses of tiagabine and experience in humans is limited, advise patients to notify their physician if they become pregnant or intend to become pregnant during therapy.

Because of the possibility that tiagabine may be excreated in breast milk, advise patients to notify their physician if they intend to breastfeed or are breastfeeding an infant.

TOPIRAMATE

Rx	**Topamax** (Ortho-McNeil)	**Tablets:** 25 mg	Lactose. (TOP 25). White. In 60s.
		50 mg	Lactose. (TOPAMAX 50). Light-yellow. In 60s.
		100 mg	Lactose. (TOPAMAX 100). Yellow. In 60s.
		200 mg	Lactose. (TOPAMAX 200). Salmon. In 60s.
		Capsules, sprinkle: 15 mg	Sucrose. (TOP 15 mg). White/clear. In 60s.
		25 mg	Sucrose. (TOP 25 mg). White/clear. In 60s.

Refer to the general discussion beginning in the Anticonvulsants introduction.

Indications

►*Partial onset seizures:* As adjunctive therapy for partial onset seizures in adults and children 2 to 16 years of age.

►*Tonic-clonic seizures:* As adjunctive therapy for primary generalized tonic-clonic seizures in adults and children 2 to 16 years of age.

►*Seizures associated with Lennox-Gastaut syndrome:* As adjunctive therapy in patients 2 years of age and older with seizures associated with Lennox-Gastaut syndrome.

►*Unlabeled uses:* Alcohol dependence, binge eating disorder, bulimia nervosa, cluster headaches, infantile spasms, migraine prevention, and weight loss in obesity.

Administration and Dosage

►*Approved by the FDA:* December 24, 1996.

It is not necessary to monitor topiramate plasma concentrations to optimize therapy.

Because of the bitter taste, do not break tablets.

Topiramate can be taken without regard to meals.

►*Adults (17 years of age and older):* The recommended total daily dose as adjunctive therapy in adults with partial seizures is 200 to 400 mg/day in 2 divided doses, and 400 mg/day in 2 divided doses as adjunctive treatment in adults with primary generalized tonic-clonic seizures. It is recommended that therapy be initiated at 25 to 50 mg/day followed by titration to an effective dose in increments of 25 to 50 mg/week. Titrating in increments of 25 mg/week may delay the time to reach an effective dose.

Doses greater than 400 mg/day (600, 800, and 1000 mg/day) have not been shown to improve responses. Doses more than 1600 mg/day have not been studied.

In the study of primary generalized tonic-clonic seizures, the initial titration rate was slower than in previous studies; the assigned dose was reached at the end of 8 weeks.

►*Children (2 to 16 years of age):* The recommended total daily dose as adjunctive therapy is approximately 5 to 9 mg/kg/day in 2 divided doses. Begin titration at no more than 25 mg (based on a range of 1 to 3 mg/kg/day) nightly for the first week. Then increase the dosage at 1- or 2-week intervals by increments of 1 to 3 mg/kg/day (administered in 2 divided doses) to achieve optimal clinical response. Guide dose titration by clinical outcome.

In the study of primary generalized tonic-clonic seizures the initial titration rate was slower than in previous studies; the assigned dose of 6 mg/kg/day was reached at the end of 8 weeks.

►*Concomitant therapy:* On occasion, the addition of topiramate to phenytoin may require an adjustment of the phenytoin dose to achieve optimal clinical outcome. The addition or withdrawal of phenytoin and/or carbamazepine during adjunctive therapy with topiramate may require adjustment of the topiramate dose.

►*Sprinkle capsules:* Swallow whole or administer by carefully opening the capsule and sprinkling the entire contents on a small amount (teaspoon) of soft food such as applesauce, custard, ice cream, oatmeal, pudding, or yogurt. Swallow this drug/food mixture immediately; do not chew. Do not store for future use.

►*Withdrawal:* Withdraw anti-epileptic drugs, including topiramate, gradually to minimize the potential of increased seizure frequency.

►*Hepatic function impairment:* In hepatically impaired patients, topiramate plasma concentrations may be increased. Administer with caution.

►*Renal function impairment:* In renally impaired subjects (Ccr less than 70 mL/min/1.73 m²), 50% of the usual adult dose is recommended. Such patients will require a longer time to reach steady state at each dose.

►*Hemodialysis:* Topiramate is cleared by hemodialysis at a rate 4 to 6 times greater than a healthy individual; a prolonged period of dialysis may cause topiramate levels to fall below that required to maintain an antiseizure effect. To avoid rapid drops in topiramate plasma concentration during hemodialysis, a supplemental dose of topiramate may be required. The actual adjustment will take into account the following: 1) The duration of the dialysis period, 2) the clearance rate of the dialysis system being used, and 3) the effective renal clearance of topiramate in the patient being dialyzed.

►*Storage/Stability:* Store tablets in a tightly closed container at room temperature 15° to 30°C (59° to 86°F). Store sprinkle capsules in a tightly closed container at 25°C (77°F) or less. Protect tablets and capsules from moisture.

Actions

►*Pharmacology:* Topiramate is a sulfamate-substituted monosaccharide with a broad spectrum of anti-epileptic activity. The precise mechanism by which topiramate exerts its antiseizure effect is unknown; however, preclinical studies have revealed 4 properties that may contribute to topiramate's anti-epileptic efficacy. Electrophysiological and biochemical evidence suggests that topiramate, at pharmacologically relevant concentrations, blocks voltage-dependent sodium channels, augments the activity of the neurotransmitter gamma-aminobutyrate at some subtypes of the GABA-A receptor, antagonizes the kainate subtype of the glutamate receptor, and inhibits the carbonic anhydrase enzyme, particularly isozymes 2 and 4.

►*Pharmacokinetics:*

Absorption/Distribution – Absorption of topiramate is rapid, with peak plasma concentrations occurring at approximately 2 hours follow-

TOPIRAMATE

ing a 400 mg oral dose. The relative bioavailability of topiramate from the tablet formulation is approximately 80% compared with a solution. The bioavailability of topiramate is not affected by food.

Pharmacokinetics of topiramate are linear with dose proportional increases in plasma concentration over dose range studies (200 to 800 mg/day). Steady state is reached in approximately 4 days in patients with normal renal function. Topiramate is 13% to 17% bound to human plasma proteins over the concentration range of 1 to 250 mcg/mL.

Metabolism/Excretion – Topiramate is not extensively metabolized and is primarily eliminated unchanged in the urine (approximately 70% of an administered dose). Six metabolites have been identified in humans, none of which constitutes more than 5% of an administered dose. The metabolites are formed via hydroxylation, hydrolysis, and glucuronidation. There is evidence of renal tubular reabsorption of topiramate. The mean plasma elimination half-life is 21 hours after single or multiple doses. Overall, plasma clearance is approximately 20 to 30 mL/min following oral administration.

Bioequivalency – The sprinkle capsule formulation is bioequivalent to the immediate-release tablet formulation and, therefore, may be substituted as therapeutically equivalent.

Special populations –

Hemodialysis: Topiramate is cleared by hemodialysis. Using a high efficiency, counterflow, single pass-dialysate hemodialysis procedure, topiramate dialysis clearance was 120 mL/min with blood flow through the dialyzer at 400 mL/min. This high clearance (compared with 20 to 30 mL/min total oral clearance in healthy adults) will remove a clinically significant amount of topiramate from the patient over the hemodialysis treatment period. Therefore, a supplemental dose may be required (see Administration and Dosage).

Renal function impairment: The clearance of topiramate was reduced 42% in moderately renally impaired subjects (Ccr 30 to 69 mL/min/1.73 m^2) and 54% in severely renally impaired subjects (Ccr less than 30 mL/min/1.73 m^2) compared with normal renal function subjects (Ccr greater than 70 mL/min/1.73 m^2). Because topiramate is presumed to undergo significant tubular reabsorption, it is uncertain whether this experience can be generalized to all situations of renal impairment. It is conceivable that some forms of renal disease could differentially affect glomerular filtration rate and tubular reabsorption, resulting in a clearance of topiramate not predicted by creatinine clearance. However, 50% of the usual starting and maintenance dose is recommended in patients with moderate or severe renal impairment.

Hepatic function impairment: In hepatically impaired subjects, topiramate clearance may be decreased; the underlying mechanism is not well understood.

Children: Pharmacokinetics of topiramate were evaluated in patients 4 to 17 years of age receiving 1 or 2 other anti-epileptic drugs. Clearance was independent of dose. Pediatric patients have a 50% higher clearance and consequently shorter elimination half-life than adults. Consequently, the plasma concentration for the same mg/kg dose may be lower in pediatric patients compared with adults. As in adults, hepatic enzyme-inducing anti-epileptic drugs decrease the steady-state plasma concentrations of topiramate.

Contraindications

History of hypersensitivity to any component of this product.

Warnings

➤*Acute myopia and secondary angle-closure glaucoma:* A syndrome consisting of acute myopia associated with secondary angle-closure glaucoma has been reported in patients receiving topiramate. Symptoms include acute onset of decreased visual acuity and/or ocular pain. Ophthalmologic findings can include myopia, anterior chamber shallowing, ocular hyperemia (redness), and increased intraocular pressure. Mydriasis may or may not be present. This syndrome may be associated with supraciliary effusion resulting in anterior displacement of the lens and iris with secondary angle-closure glaucoma. Symptoms typically occur within 1 month of initiating topiramate therapy. In contrast to primary narrow-angle glaucoma, which is rare before 40 years of age, secondary angle-closure glaucoma associated with topiramate has been reported in pediatric patients as well as adults. The primary treatment to reverse symptoms is discontinuation of topiramate as rapidly as possible, according to the judgment of the treating physician. Other measures, in conjunction with discontinuation of topiramate, may be helpful.

Elevated intraocular pressure of any etiology, if left untreated, can lead to serious sequelae including permanent vision loss.

➤*Metabolic acidosis:* Hyperchloremic, non-anion gap, metabolic acidosis (ie, decreased serum bicarbonate below the normal reference range in the absence of chronic respiratory alkalosis) is associated with topiramate treatment. This metabolic acidosis is caused by renal bicarbonate loss because of the inhibitory effect of topiramate on carbonic anhydrase. Such electrolyte imbalance has been observed with the use of topiramate in placebo-controlled clinical trials and in the postmarketing period. Generally, topiramate-induced metabolic acidosis occurs early in treatment, although cases can occur at any time during treatment. Bicarbonate decrements usually are mild to moderate (average decrease of 4 mEq/L at daily doses of 400 mg in adults and at

approximately 6 mg/kg/day in pediatric patients); rarely, patients can experience severe decrements to values below 10 mEq/L. Conditions or therapies that predispose to acidosis (eg, renal disease, severe respiratory disorders, status epilepticus, diarrhea, surgery, ketogenic diet, drugs) may be additive to the bicarbonate lowering effects of topiramate.

Some manifestations of acute or chronic metabolic acidosis may include hyperventilation, nonspecific symptoms such as fatigue and anorexia, or more severe sequelae including cardiac arrhythmias or stupor. Chronic, untreated metabolic acidosis may increase the risk for nephrolithiasis or nephrocalcinosis, and also may result in osteomalacia (referred to as rickets in pediatric patients) and/or osteoporosis with an increased risk for fractures. Chronic metabolic acidosis in pediatric patients also may reduce growth rates. A reduction in growth rate eventually may decrease the maximal height achieved. The effect of topiramate on growth and bone-related sequelae has not been systematically investigated.

Measurement of baseline and periodic serum bicarbonate during topiramate treatment is recommended. If metabolic acidosis develops and persists, consider reducing the dose or discontinuing topiramate (using dose tapering). If the decision is made to continue patients on topiramate in the face of persistent acidosis, consider alkali treatment.

Adults – In adults, the incidence of persistent treatment-emergent decreases in serum bicarbonate (levels of less than 20 mEq/L at 2 consecutive visits or at the final visit) in controlled clinical trials for adjunctive treatment of epilepsy was 32% for 400 mg/day, and 1% for placebo. Metabolic acidosis has been observed at doses as low as 50 mg/day. The incidence of a markedly abnormally low serum bicarbonate (ie, absolute value less than 17 mEq/L and greater than 5 mEq/L decrease from pretreatment) in these trials was 3% for 400 mg/day, and 0% for placebo. Serum bicarbonate levels have not been systematically evaluated at daily doses greater than 400 mg/day.

Children – In pediatric patients (younger than 16 years of age), the incidence of persistent treatment-emergent decreases in serum bicarbonate in placebo-controlled trials for adjunctive treatment of Lennox-Gastaut syndrome or refractory partial onset seizures was 67% for topiramate (at approximately 6 mg/kg/day), and 10% for placebo. The incidence of a markedly abnormally low serum bicarbonate (ie, absolute value less than 17 mEq/L and greater than 5 mEq/L decrease from pretreatment) in these trials was 11% for topiramate and 0% for placebo. Cases of moderately severe metabolic acidosis have been reported in patients as young as 5 months of age, especially at daily doses above 5 mg/kg/day.

➤*Oligohidrosis and hyperthermia:* Oligohidrosis (decreased sweating), infrequently resulting in hospitalization, has been reported in association with topiramate use. Decreased sweating and an elevation in body temperature above normal characterized these cases. Some of the cases were reported after exposure to elevated environmental temperatures.

The majority of the reports have been in children. Closely monitor patients, especially pediatric patients, treated with topiramate for evidence of decreased sweating and increased body temperature, especially in hot weather. Use caution when topiramate is prescribed with other drugs that predispose patients to heat-related disorders; these drugs include, but are not limited to, other carbonic anhydrase inhibitors and drugs with anticholinergic activity.

➤*Withdrawal:* Withdraw anti-epileptic drugs, including topiramate, gradually to minimize the potential of increased seizure frequency.

➤*CNS adverse events:*

Adults – Adverse events most often associated with the use of topiramate were CNS-related. The most significant of these can be classified into 2 general categories: 1) Psychomotor slowing, difficulty with concentration, and speech or language problems, in particular, word-finding difficulties and 2) somnolence or fatigue. Additional nonspecific CNS effects occasionally observed with topiramate as add-on therapy include dizziness or imbalance, confusion, memory problems, and exacerbation of mood disturbances (eg, irritability, depression).

Reports of psychomotor slowing, speech and language problems, and difficulty with concentration and attention were common. Although in some cases these events were mild to moderate, at times they led to withdrawal from treatment. The incidence of psychomotor slowing is only marginally dose-related, but language problems and difficulty with concentration or attention clearly increased in frequency with increasing dosage.

Somnolence and fatigue were the most frequently reported adverse events during clinical trials with topiramate. These events generally were mild to moderate and occurred early in therapy. While the incidence of somnolence does not appear to be dose-related, fatigue increases at dosages more than 400 mg/day.

Children – In double-blind clinical studies, the incidences of cognitive/neuropsychiatric adverse events in pediatric patients generally were lower than previously observed in adults. These events included psychomotor slowing, difficulty with concentration/attention, speech disorders/related speech problems, and language problems. The most frequently reported neuropsychiatric events in this population were somnolence and fatigue. No patients discontinued treatment because of adverse events in double-blind trials.

TOPIRAMATE

➤*Sudden unexplained death in epilepsy:* During the course of pre-marketing development of topiramate tablets, 10 sudden and unexplained deaths were recorded among a cohort of treated patients (2796 subject years of exposure). This represents an incidence of 0.0035 deaths per patient year. Although this rate exceeds that expected in a healthy population matched for age and sex, it is within the range of estimates for the incidence of sudden unexplained deaths in patients with epilepsy not receiving topiramate (ranging from 0.0005 for the general population of patients with epilepsy, to 0.003 for a clinical trial population similar to that in the topiramate program, to 0.005 for patients with refractory epilepsy).

➤*Renal function impairment:* The major route of elimination of unchanged topiramate and its metabolites is via the kidney. Dosage adjustment may be required (see Administration and Dosage and Pharmacokinetics).

➤*Hepatic function impairment:* In hepatically impaired patients, administer topiramate with caution because clearance may be decreased.

➤*Carcinogenesis:* An increase in urinary bladder tumors was observed in mice given topiramate (20, 75, and 300 mg/kg) for 21 months. The elevated bladder tumor incidence, which was statistically significant in males and females receiving 300 mg/kg, was primarily because of the increased occurrence of a smooth muscle tumor considered histomorphologically unique to mice. Plasma exposures in mice receiving 300 mg/kg were approximately 0.5 to 1 times steady-state exposures measured in patients receiving topiramate monotherapy at the recommended human dose (RHD) of 400 mg, and 1.5 to 2 times steady-state topiramate exposures in patients receiving 400 mg of topiramate plus phenytoin. The relevance of this finding to human carcinogenic risk is uncertain.

➤*Pregnancy: Category C.* Topiramate has demonstrated selective developmental toxicity, including teratogenicity, in animal studies. When oral doses of 20, 100, or 500 mg/kg were administered to pregnant mice during the period of organogenesis, the incidence of fetal malformations (primarily craniofacial defects) was increased at all doses. The low dose is approximately 0.2 times the RHD of 400 mg/day on a mg/m^2 basis. Fetal body weights and skeletal ossification were reduced at 500 mg/kg in conjunction with decreased maternal body weight gain.

In rat studies (oral doses of 20, 100, and 500 mg/kg or 0.2, 2.5, 30, and 400 mg/kg), the frequency of limb malformations (eg, ectrodactyly, micromelia, amelia) was increased among the offspring of dams treated with 400 mg/kg (10 times the RHD on a mg/m^2 basis) or greater during the organogenesis period of pregnancy. Embryotoxicity (eg, reduced fetal body weights, increased incidence of structural variations) was observed at doses as low as 20 mg/kg (0.5 times the RHD on a mg/m^2 basis). Clinical signs of maternal toxicity were seen at 400 mg/kg or more, and maternal body weight gain was reduced during treatment with 100 mg/kg or more.

In rabbit studies (20, 60, and 180 mg/kg or 10, 35, and 120 mg/kg orally during organogenesis), embryo/fetal mortality was increased at 35 mg/kg or more (2 times the RHD on a mg/m^2 basis), and teratogenic effects (primarily rib and vertebral malformations) were observed at 120 mg/kg (6 times the RHD on a mg/m^2 basis). Evidence of maternal toxicity (eg, decreased body weight gain, clinical signs, mortality) was seen at 35 mg/kg or more.

When female rats were treated during the latter part of gestation and throughout lactation (0.2, 4, 20, and 100 mg/kg or 2, 20, and 200 mg/kg), offspring exhibited decreased viability and delayed physical development at 200 mg/kg (5 times the RHD on a mg/m^2 basis) and reductions in pre- and/or postweaning body weight gain at 2 mg/kg or more (0.05 times the RHD on a mg/m^2 basis). Maternal toxicity (eg, decreased body weight gain, clinical signs) was evident at 100 mg/kg or more.

In a rat embryo/fetal development study with a postnatal component (0.2, 2.5, 30, or 400 mg/kg during organogenesis; noted above), pups exhibited delayed physical development at 400 mg/kg (10 times the RHD on a mg/m^2 basis) and persistent reductions in body weight gain at 30 mg/kg or more (1 time the RHD on a mg/m^2 basis).

There are no studies using topiramate in pregnant women. Use topiramate during pregnancy only if the potential benefit outweighs the potential risk to the fetus.

In postmarketing experience, cases of hypospadias have been reported in male infants exposed in utero to topiramate, with or without other anticonvulsants; however, a causal relationship with topiramate has not been established.

➤*Lactation:* Topiramate is excreted in the milk of lactating rats. Limited observations in patients suggest an extensive secretion of topiramate into breast milk. Weigh the potential benefit to the mother against the potential risk to the infant.

➤*Children:* Safety and efficacy in children younger than 2 years of age have not been established. Topiramate is associated with metabolic acidosis; chronic untreated metabolic acidosis in pediatric patients may cause osteomalacia (rickets) and may reduce growth rates. A reduction in growth rate may eventually decrease the maximal height achieved.

The effect of topiramate on growth and bone-related sequelae has not been systematically investigated (see Warnings).

Precautions

➤*Monitoring:* Measurement of baseline and periodic serum bicarbonate during topiramate treatment is recommended. Closely monitor patients, especially pediatric patients, for evidence of decreased sweating and increased body temperature, especially in hot weather.

➤*Kidney stones:* A total of 1.5% of 2086 patients exposed to topiramate during its development reported the occurrence of kidney stones, an incidence approximately 2 to 4 times greater than that expected in a similar, untreated population. As in the general population, the incidence of stone formation among topiramate-treated patients was higher in men. Kidney stones also have been reported in pediatric patients.

An explanation for the association of topiramate and kidney stones may lie in the fact that topiramate is a weak carbonic anhydrase inhibitor. Carbonic anhydrase inhibitors (eg, acetazolamide, dichlorphenamide) promote stone formation by reducing urinary citrate excretion and by increasing urinary pH. The concomitant use of topiramate with other carbonic anhydrase inhibitors or potentially in patients on a ketogenic diet may create a physiological environment that increases the risk of kidney stone formation and should be avoided.

Increased fluid intake increases urinary output, lowering substance concentration involved in stone formation. Hydration is recommended to reduce new stone formation.

➤*Paresthesia:* Paresthesia, an effect associated with the use of other carbonic anhydrase inhibitors, appears to be a common effect of topiramate.

➤*Photosensitivity:* Photosensitization (photoallergy or phototoxicity) may occur; therefore, caution patients to take protective measures (ie, sunscreens, protective clothing) against exposure to sunlight or ultraviolet light (eg, tanning beds) until tolerance is determined.

Drug Interactions

Topiramate Drug Interactions			
Precipitant drug	Object drug*		Description
Carbamazepine	Topiramate	↓	Carbamazepine may increase the metabolism of topiramate causing a 40% decrease in serum concentrations. Adjust the dose if needed.
Hydantoins (eg, phenytoin)	Topiramate	↓	Hydantoins may increase the metabolism of topiramate causing a 48% decrease in serum concentration. Topiramate may decrease the metabolism of hydantoins causing a 25% increase in serum concentrations in some patients. Adjust the dose if needed.
Topiramate	Hydantoins (eg, phenytoin)	↑	
Metformin	Topiramate	↑	Coadministration caused decreased topiramate plasma clearance. Metformin C$_{max}$ and AUC increased by 18% and 25%, respectively, and clearance decreased by 20%. The clinical significance of these effects are not known.
Topiramate	Metformin		
Valproic acid	Topiramate	↓	Coadministration caused a 14% decrease in topiramate serum concentrations and an 11% decrease in valproic acid serum concentrations.
Topiramate	Valproic acid		
Topiramate	Alcohol; CNS depressants	↑	Use topiramate with extreme caution because of the potential to cause CNS depression, as well as other cognitive or neuropsychiatric adverse events.
Topiramate	Carbonic anhydrase inhibitors (eg, acetazolamide)	↑	Concomitant use may increase the risk of renal stone formation and should be avoided (see Precautions).
Topiramate	Contraceptives; oral Estrogens	↓	Topiramate reduced the ethinyl estradiol AUC by 18% to 30% and plasma concentrations by 15% to 25%. Oral contraceptive efficacy may be reduced and breakthrough bleeding may occur. Consider an alternate method of contraception or increasing the estrogen dose.
Topiramate	Digoxin	↓	Serum digoxin AUC is decreased by 12% with concomitant topiramate administration. The clinical relevance of this observation has not been established.

* ↑ = Object drug increased. ↓ = Object drug decreased.

TOPIRAMATE

Adverse Reactions

Approximately 28% of adult epilepsy patients who received topiramate dosages of 200 to 1600 mg/day in clinical studies discontinued treatment because of the following: Anorexia (2.7%); ataxia (2.1%); confusion (3.1%); depression (2.6%); difficulty with concentration/attention (2.9%); fatigue, memory difficulties, somnolence (3.2%); dizziness, weight decrease (2.5%); nervousness (2.3%); paresthesia (2%); psychomotor slowing (4%). Approximately 11% of pediatric patients who received topiramate at dosages up to 30 mg/kg/day discontinued treatment because of the following: Aggravated convulsions (2.3%); difficulty with concentration/attention (1.6%); language problems, personality disorder, somnolence (1.3%).

Topiramate Adverse Reactions in Placebo-Controlled Add-On Trials (%)[a],[b]

Adverse reaction	Pediatric topiramate dosage 5 to 9 mg/kg/day (n = 98)	Adult topiramate dosage 200 to 400 mg/day (n = 183)	Adult topiramate dosage 600 to 1000 mg/day (n = 414)
Cardiovascular			
Bradycardia	1	—	—
Hypertension	1	—	—
CNS			
Aggressive reaction	9	3	3
Agitation	—	3	3
Apathy	—	1	3
Appetite increased	1	—	—
Asthenia	—	6	3
Ataxia	6	16	14
Cognitive problems	—	3	3
Confusion	4	11	14
Convulsions, grand mal	1	—	—
Coordination abnormal	—	4	4
Depersonalization	—	1	2
Depression	—	5	13
Difficulty with concentration/attention	10	6	14
Difficulty with memory	5	12	14
Dizziness	4	25	32
Emotional lability	—	3	3
Fatigue	16	15	30
Gait abnormal	8	3	2
Hyperkinesia	5	—	—
Hypesthesia	—	2	1
Hyporeflexia	2	—	—
Insomnia	8	—	—
Language problems	—	6	10
Libido decreased	—	2	< 1
Mood problems	—	4	9
Muscle contractions, involuntary	—	2	2
Nervousness	14	16	19
Neurosis	1	—	—
Nystagmus	—	10	11
Paresthesia	1	11	19
Personality disorder (behavior problems)	11	—	—
Psychomotor slowing	3	13	21
Somnolence	26	29	28
Speech disorders/Related speech problems	4	13	11
Stupor	—	2	1
Tremor	—	9	9
Vertigo	—	1	2
Dermatologic			
Alopecia	2	—	—
Dermatitis	2	—	—
Eczema	1	—	—
Hypertrichosis	2	—	—
Increased sweating	—	1	< 1
Pallor	1	—	—
Rash, erythematous	2	1	< 1
Seborrhea	1	—	—
Skin discoloration	1	—	—
Skin disorder	3	2	1
GI			
Abdominal pain	—	6	7
Anorexia	24	10	12
Constipation	5	4	3
Dry mouth	—	2	4

Topiramate Adverse Reactions in Placebo-Controlled Add-On Trials (%)[a],[b]

Adverse reaction	Pediatric topiramate dosage 5 to 9 mg/kg/day (n = 98)	Adult topiramate dosage 200 to 400 mg/day (n = 183)	Adult topiramate dosage 600 to 1000 mg/day (n = 414)
Dyspepsia	—	7	6
Dysphagia	1	—	—
Fecal incontinence	1	—	—
Flatulence	1	—	—
Gastroenteritis	3	2	1
Gastroesophageal reflux	1	—	—
GI disorder	—	1	0
Gingivitis	—	1	1
Glossitis	1	—	—
Gum hyperplasia	1	—	—
Nausea	6	10	12
Saliva increased	6	—	—
GU			
Amenorrhea	—	2	2
Breast pain	—	4	0
Hematuria	—	2	< 1
Leukorrhea	2	—	—
Menorrhagia	—	2	1
Menstrual disorder	—	2	1
Micturition frequency	—	1	2
Nocturia	1	—	—
Prostatic disorder	—	2	0
Urinary incontinence	4	2	1
Urinary tract infection	—	2	3
Urine abnormal	—	1	< 1
Hematologic			
Hematoma	1	—	—
Leukopenia	2	2	1
Prothrombin increased	1	—	—
Purpura	8	—	—
Thrombocytopenia	1	—	—
Metabolic/Nutritional			
Edema	—	2	1
Hypoglycemia	1	—	—
Thirst	2	—	—
Weight decrease	9	9	13
Weight increase	1	—	—
Respiratory			
Dyspnea	—	1	2
Epistaxis	4	2	1
Pharyngitis	—	6	3
Pneumonia	5	—	—
Respiratory disorder	1	—	—
Rhinitis	—	7	6
Sinusitis	—	5	6
Special senses			
Diplopia	1	10	10
Eye abnormality	2	—	—
Hearing decreased	—	2	1
Lacrimation abnormal	1	—	—
Myopia	1	—	—
Taste perversion	—	2	4
Vision abnormal	2	13	10
Miscellaneous			
Allergy	2	2	3
Back pain	1	5	3
Body odor	—	1	0
Chest pain	—	4	2
Hot flushes	—	2	1
Infection	—	2	1
Infection, viral	7	2	< 1
Influenza-like symptoms	—	3	4
Injury	14	—	—
Leg pain	—	2	4
Moniliasis	—	1	0
Myalgia	—	2	2
Rigors	—	1	< 1
Skeletal pain	—	1	0

[a] Patients in these add-on trials were receiving 1 to 2 concomitant anti-epileptic drugs in addition to topiramate or placebo.
[b] Data are pooled from separate studies and are not necessarily comparable.

TOPIRAMATE

Incidence of Dose-Related Adverse Events From Placebo-Controlled, Add-On Trials in Adults with Partial Onset Seizures (%)			
	Topiramate dosage (mg/day)		
Adverse reaction	200 (n = 45)	400 (n = 68)	600 to 1000 (n = 414)
Anorexia	4	6	12
Anxiety	2	3	10
Confusion	9	10	14
Depression	9	7	13
Fatigue	11	12	30
Difficulty with concentration/attention	7	9	14
Language problems	2	9	10
Mood problems	0	6	9
Nervousness	13	18	19
Weight decrease	4	9	13

➤*Other adverse events:* Other adverse events that occurred in more than 1% of adults treated with 200 to 400 mg of topiramate in placebo-controlled trials but with equal or greater frequency in the placebo group were the following: Aggravated convulsions, anxiety, coughing, diarrhea, dysmenorrhea, eye pain, fever, headache, injury, insomnia, muscle weakness, pain, personality disorder, rash, upper respiratory tract infection, and vomiting.

➤*Cardiovascular:* Hypertension (1% or more); angina pectoris, AV block, DVT, hypotension, postural hypotension, syncope, vasodilation (0.1% to 1%); pulmonary embolism, vasospasm (less than 0.1%).

➤*CNS:* Euphoria, hallucination, hypertonia, insomnia, psychosis, suicide attempt (1% or more); abnormal dreaming, apraxia, delirium, delusion, dyskinesia, dysphonia, dystonia, EEG abnormal, encephalopathy, hyperesthesia, neuropathy, neurosis, paranoia, paranoid reaction (0.1% to 1%); cerebellar syndrome, libido increased, manic reaction, tongue paralysis, upper motor neuron lesion (less than 0.1%).

➤*Dermatologic:* Acne (1% or more); abnormal hair texture, decreased sweating, flushing, photosensitivity reaction, urticaria (0.1% to 1%); chloasma (less than 0.1%).

➤*GI:* Diarrhea, vomiting (1% or more); enlarged abdomen, esophagitis, gastritis, gingival bleeding, melena, hemorrhoids, stomatitis, tongue edema (0.1% to 1%).

➤*GU:* Dysuria, impotence, renal calculus (1% or more); albuminuria, breast discharge, ejaculation disorder, oliguria, polyuria, renal pain, urinary retention (0.1% to 1%).

➤*Hematologic/Lymphatic:* Anemia (1% or more); eosinophilia, granulocytopenia, lymphadenopathy, lymphopenia, thrombocythemia (0.1% to 1%); lymphocytosis, marrow depression, pancytopenia, polycythemia (less than 0.1%).

➤*Hepatic:* ALT, AST, gamma-GT increased (0.1% to 1%).

➤*Metabolic/Nutritional:* Dehydration (1% or more); acidosis, facial edema, hyperglycemia, hyperlipidemia, hypocalcemia, hypokalemia, increased alkaline phosphatase (0.1% to 1%); creatinine increased, diabetes mellitus, hyperchloremia, hypernatremia, hypocholesterolemia, hyponatremia, hypophosphatemia (less than 0.1%).

➤*Musculoskeletal:* Arthralgia (1% or more); arthrosis (0.1% to 1%).

➤*Special senses:* Conjunctivitis, tinnitus (1% or more); abnormal accommodation, parosmia, photophobia, ptosis, scotoma, strabismus, taste loss, visual field defect, xerophthalmia (0.1% to 1%); iritis, mydriasis (less than 0.1%).

➤*Miscellaneous:* Phlebitis (0.1% to 1%); alcohol intolerance (less than 0.1%).

➤*Postmarketing:* Bullous skin reactions (including erythema multiforme, Stevens-Johnson syndrome, toxic epidermal necrolysis), hepatic failure (including fatalities), hepatitis, pancreatitis, pemphigus, renal tubular acidosis.

Overdosage

➤*Symptoms:* Signs and symptoms of overdosage include the following: Abdominal pain, abnormal coordination, agitation, blurred vision, convulsions, depression, diplopia, dizziness, drowsiness, hypotension, lethargy, mentation impaired, metabolic acidosis, speech disturbance, and stupor. The clinical consequences were not severe in most cases, but deaths have been reported after poly-drug overdoses involving topiramate.

➤*Treatment:* If the ingestion is recent in acute topiramate overdose, immediately empty the stomach by lavage. Activated charcoal has been shown to adsorb topiramate in vitro. Ensure appropriately supportive treatment. Hemodialysis is an effective means of removing topiramate from the body.

A patient who ingested a dose between 96 and 110 g topiramate was admitted to the hospital with coma lasting 20 to 24 hours followed by full recovery after 3 to 4 days.

Patient Information

Instruct patients to seek immediate medical attention if they experience blurred vision or periorbital pain.

Closely monitor patients, especially pediatric patients, for evidence of decreased sweating and increased body temperature, especially in hot weather.

Instruct patients, particularly those with predisposing factors, to maintain an adequate fluid intake in order to minimize the risk of renal stone formation.

Warn patients about the potential for somnolence, dizziness, confusion, and difficulty concentrating and advise them not to drive or operate machinery until they have gained sufficient experience with topiramate to gauge whether it adversely affects their mental or motor performance.

Advise patients that topiramate may decrease the effectiveness of oral contraceptives. Advise patients to report any change in their menstrual cycle and to consider an alternate method of contraception.

Topiramate may cause photosensitivity (sensitivity to sunlight). Instruct patients to avoid prolonged exposure to the sun and other ultraviolet light. Instruct patients to use sunscreens and wear protective clothing until tolerance is determined.

Advise patients to consider additional food intake if weight loss occurs on this medication.

Inform the patient that sprinkle capsules may be sprinkled on a small amount (teaspoon) of soft food, such as applesauce, custard, ice cream, oatmeal, pudding, or yogurt. Advise the patient to swallow the entire spoonful of the sprinkle/food mixture immediately. Do not chew. Instruct the patient to drink fluids immediately in order to make sure all of the mixture is swallowed. Do not store sprinkle/food mixture for use at a later time.

VALPROIC ACID and DERIVATIVES

Rx	Valproic Acid (Various, eg, Qualitest, Sidmak, UDL, Upsher Smith, Vangard, Watson)	Capsules: 250 mg (as valproic acid)	In 10s, 30s, 31s, and 100s.
Rx	Depakene (Abbott)		Parabens, corn oil. (Depakene). Orange. In 100s.
Rx	Depakote (Abbott)	Tablets, delayed-release (enteric-coated): 125 mg (as divalproex sodium)	Talc. Salmon pink. In 100s and *Abbo-Pac* UD 100s.
		250 mg (as divalproex sodium)	Talc. Peach. In 100s, 500s, and *Abbo-Pac* UD 100s.
		500 mg (as divalproex sodium)	Talc. Lavender. In 100s, 500s, and *Abbo-Pac* UD 100s.
Rx	Depakote ER (Abbott)	Tablets, extended-release: 250 mg (as divalproex sodium)	Lactose. (a HF). White, oval. In 60s, 100s, 500s, and *Abbo-Pac* UD 100s.
		500 mg (as divalproex sodium)	Lactose, polydextrose. (a HC). Gray, oval. In 100s, 500s, and *Abbo-Pac* UD 100s.
Rx	Depakote (Abbott)	Capsules, sprinkle: 125 mg (as divalproex sodium)	White/Blue. In 100s and *Abbo-Pac* UD 100s.
Rx	Valproic Acid (Various, eg, Alpharma, Hi-Tech, Major, Morton Grove, Pharmaceutical Associates, Qualitest, Teva, Xactdose)	Syrup: 250 mg (as sodium valproate)/5 mL	In 473 mL.
Rx	Depakene (Abbott)		Parabens, sorbitol, sucrose. In 473 mL.
Rx	Valproate Sodium (Bedford)	Injection: 100 mg/mL (as valproate sodium)	Preservative free. In 5 mL single-dose vials.
Rx	Depacon (Abbott)		EDTA. Preservative free. In 5 mL single-dose vials.

Refer to the general discussion beginning in the Anticonvulsants introduction.

WARNING

Hepatotoxicity: Hepatic failure resulting in fatalities has occurred in patients receiving valproic acid and its derivatives. Children under 2 years of age are at a considerably increased risk of developing fatal hepatotoxicity, especially those on multiple anticonvulsants, those with congenital metabolic disorders, those with severe seizure disorders accompanied by mental retardation, and those with organic brain disease. In this patient group, use with extreme caution and as a sole agent. Weigh benefits of therapy against risks. Above this age group, the incidence of fatal hepatotoxicity decreases considerably in progressively older patient groups. These incidents usually have occurred during the first 6 months of treatment. Serious or fatal hepatotoxicity may be preceded by nonspecific symptoms such as loss of seizure control in epileptic patients, malaise, weakness, lethargy, facial edema, anorexia, and vomiting. Monitor patients closely for appearance of these symptoms. Perform liver function tests prior to therapy and at frequent intervals thereafter, especially during the first 6 months.

Teratogenicity: Valproate can produce teratogenic effects such as neural tube defects (eg, spina bifida). Accordingly, the use of valproate products in women of childbearing potential requires that the benefits of its use be weighed against the risk of injury to the fetus. This is especially important when the treatment of a spontaneously reversible condition not ordinarily associated with permanent injury or risk of death (eg, migraine) is contemplated (see Warnings). An information sheet describing the teratogenic potential of valproate is available for patients.

Pancreatitis: Cases of life-threatening pancreatitis have been reported in children and adults receiving valproate. Some of the cases have been described as hemorrhagic with a rapid progression from initial symptoms to death. Cases have been reported shortly after initial use as well as after several years of use. Warn patients and guardians that abdominal pain, nausea, vomiting, and/or anorexia can be symptoms of pancreatitis that require prompt medical evaluation. If pancreatitis is diagnosed, discontinue valproate. Initiate alternative treatment for the underlying medical condition as clinically indicated.

Indications

➤*Epilepsy:* For use as sole and adjunctive therapy in the treatment of simple and complex absence seizures and adjunctively in patients with multiple seizure types that include absence seizures; as monotherapy and adjunctive therapy in the treatment of patients with complex partial seizures that occur in isolation or in association with other types of seizures.

Valproate sodium injection is indicated as an IV alternative in patients for whom oral administration of valproate products is temporarily not feasible.

➤*Mania (divalproex sodium delayed-release tablets):* Treatment of manic episodes associated with bipolar disorder.

➤*Migraine (divalproex sodium delayed-release and extended-release [ER] tablets):* As prophylaxis of migraine headaches.

➤*Unlabeled uses:* May be a useful adjunct in schizophrenic patients with EEG abnormalities suggestive of seizure activity, or in those patients with agitated or violent behavior.

Administration and Dosage

➤*Oral products:* Bedtime administration may minimize effects of CNS depression. GI irritation may be minimized by taking with food or by slowly increasing the dose. Delayed-release divalproex sodium (espe-

cially initiating therapy with a lower dose) may reduce the incidence of irritative GI effects. Swallow the extended-release tablets whole; do not crush or chew. Swallow the valproic acid capsules without chewing to avoid local irritation of the mouth and throat.

➤*Sprinkle capsules:* May be swallowed whole or the capsules may be opened and the entire contents may be sprinkled on a small amount (teaspoonful) of soft food such as applesauce or pudding. Swallow drug/food mixture immediately; do not chew. Do not store for future use.

➤*Valproic acid syrup or capsule dosing:* The following table is a guide for the initial daily dose of valproic acid (15 mg/kg/day) syrup and capsules.

Valproic Acid Syrup and Capsule Initial Dosing Guide

Weight		Total daily dose (mg)	Number of capsules or teaspoonfuls of syrup		
kg	lb		Dose 1	Dose 2	Dose 3
10 to 24.9	22 to 54.9	250	0	0	1
25 to 39.9	55 to 87.9	500	1	0	1
40 to 59.9	88 to 131.9	750	1	1	1
60 to 74.9	132 to 164.9	1000	1	1	2
75 to 89.9	165 to 197.9	1250	2	1	2

➤*Injection:* For IV use only. Administer as a 60-minute infusion (but not more than 20 mg/min) with the same frequency as the oral products. Use of valproate sodium injection for periods of more than 14 days has not been studied. Switch patients to oral valproate products as soon as it is clinically feasible.

Rapid infusion of IV valproate sodium has been associated with an increase in adverse events. Infusion times of less than 60 minutes or rates of infusion more than 20 mg/min have limited experience in patients with epilepsy (see Adverse Reactions). Administer IV as a 60-minute infusion, as noted above. Dilute with at least 50 mL of a compatible diluent. Discard any unused portion of the vial contents.

Compatibility and stability – Valproate sodium injection was found to be physically compatible and chemically stable in dextrose (5%) injection, sodium chloride (0.9%) injection, and lactated ringer's injection for at least 24 hours when stored in glass or polyvinyl chloride (PVC) bags at controlled room temperature (15° to 30°C; 59° to 86°F).

➤*Conversion from oral products to injection:* When switching from oral products, the total daily dose of valproate sodium injection should be equivalent to the total daily dose of the oral product and administered at the same frequency. Closely monitor patients receiving doses near the maximum recommended daily dose of 60 mg/kg/day, particularly those not receiving enzyme-inducing drugs. If the total daily dose exceeds 250 mg, give in a divided regimen. The equivalence between injectable and oral valproate products at steady state was only evaluated in an every-6-hour regimen. If given less frequently (ie, 2 or 3 times a day), trough levels might fall below those of an oral dosage form given via the same regimen; closely monitor trough plasma levels.

➤*Younger children:* Younger children, especially those receiving enzyme-inducing drugs, will require larger maintenance doses to attain targeted valproic acid concentrations.

➤*Elderly:* Reduce the starting dose because of a decrease in unbound clearance of valproate; base therapeutic dose on clinical response. Starting doses lower than 250 mg can only be achieved in the elderly by the use of divalproex sodium delayed-release tablets. Dosage should be increased more slowly and with regular monitoring for fluid and nutritional intake, dehydration, somnolence, and other adverse events.

➤*Dose-related adverse reactions:* Because the frequency of adverse effects (particularly elevated liver enzymes and thrombocytopenia) may be dose-related, weigh the benefit of improved therapeutic effect with higher doses against the possibility of a greater incidence of adverse reactions. The probability of thrombocytopenia appears to increase sig-

VALPROIC ACID and DERIVATIVES

nificantly at total valproate concentrations of 110 mcg/mL or more (females) or 135 mcg/mL or more (males) (see Warnings).

➤ *Complex partial seizures:* Adults and children 10 years of age and older.

Monotherapy – Initiate therapy at 10 to 15 mg/kg/day; increase by 5 to 10 mg/kg/week to achieve optimal clinical response. Ordinarily, optimal clinical response is achieved at daily doses below 60 mg/kg/day. If satisfactory clinical response has not been achieved, plasma levels should be measured to determine whether or not they are in the usually accepted therapeutic range (50 to 100 mcg/mL). No recommendation can be made regarding the safety of valproate for use at doses above 60 mg/kg/day.

The probability of thrombocytopenia increases significantly at total trough valproate plasma concentrations above 110 mcg/mL in females and 135 mcg/mL in males. Weigh the benefit of improved seizure control with higher doses against the possibility of a greater incidence of adverse reactions.

Conversion to monotherapy: Initiate therapy at 10 to 15 mg/kg/day. Increase the dosage by 5 to 10 mg/kg/week to achieve optimal clinical response. Ordinarily, optimal clinical response is achieved at daily doses below 60 mg/kg/day. If satisfactory clinical response has not been achieved, measure plasma levels to determine whether or not they are in the usually accepted therapeutic range (50 to 100 mcg/mL). Concomitant antiepilepsy drug (AED) dosage ordinarily can be reduced by approximately 25% every 2 weeks. This reduction may be started at initiation of therapy or delayed by 1 to 2 weeks if there is a concern that seizures are likely to occur with a reduction. The speed and duration of withdrawal of the concomitant AED can be highly variable; monitor patients closely during this period for increased seizure frequency.

Adjunctive therapy – Divalproex sodium or valproic acid may be added to the patient's regimen at a dosage of 10 to 15 mg/kg/day. The dosage may be increased by 5 to 10 mg/kg/week to achieve optimal clinical response. Ordinarily, optimal clinical response is achieved at daily doses below 60 mg/kg/day. If satisfactory clinical response has not been achieved, measure plasma levels to determine whether or not they are in the usually accepted therapeutic range (50 to 100 mcg/mL). No recommendation can be made regarding the safety of valproate for use at doses above 60 mg/kg/day. If the total daily dose exceeds 250 mg, administer in divided doses.

➤ *Simple and complex absence seizures:* The recommended initial dose is 15 mg/kg/day, increasing at 1-week intervals by 5 to 10 mg/kg/day until seizures are controlled or side effects preclude further increases. The maximum recommended dosage is 60 mg/kg/day. If the total daily dose exceeds 250 mg, give in divided doses.

In epileptic patients previously receiving valproic acid therapy, initiate divalproex sodium at the same daily dose and dosing schedule. After the patient is stabilized on divalproex tablets, a dosing schedule of 2 or 3 times a day may be elected in selected patients.

Divalproex sodium ER is only approved in adults and children 10 years of age and older for this medication.

➤ *Conversion from Depakote to Depakote ER:* In adult and pediatric patients 10 years of age and older, patients with epilepsy previously receiving *Depakote*, *Depakote ER* should be administered once daily using a dose 8% to 20% higher than the total daily dose of *Depakote*. For patients whose *Depakote* total daily dose cannot be directly converted to *Depakote ER*, consideration may be given at the clinician's discretion to increase the patient's *Depakote* total daily dose to the next higher dosage before converting to the appropriate total daily dose of *Depakote ER*.

Dose Conversion from *Depakote* to *Depakote ER*	
Depakote total daily dose (mg)	*Depakote ER* (mg)
500ᵃ to 625	750
750ᵃ to 875	1000
1000ᵃ to 1125	1250
1250 to 1375	1500
1500 to 1625	1750
1750	2000
1875 to 2000	2250
2125 to 2250	2500
2375	2750
2500 to 2750	3000
2875	3250
3000 to 3125	3500

ᵃ These total daily doses of *Depakote* cannot be directly converted to an 8% to 20% higher total daily dose of *Depakote ER* because the required dosing strengths of *Depakote ER* are not available. Consideration may be given at the clinician's discretion to increase the patient's *Depakote* total daily dose to the next higher dosage before converting to the appropriate total daily dose of *Depakote ER*.

There are insufficient data to allow a conversion factor recommendation for patients with *Depakote* doses above 3125 mg/day.

Plasma valproate C_{min} concentrations for *Depakote ER* on average are equivalent to *Depakote*, but may vary across patients after conversion.

➤ *Mania (divalproex sodium delayed-release tablets):* Initial dose is 750 mg daily in divided doses; increase as rapidly as possible to achieve the lowest therapeutic dose that produces the desired clinical effect or the desired range of plasma concentrations. In acute mania trials, patients were dosed to a clinical response with a trough plasma concentration between 50 and 125 mcg/mL. Maximum concentrations generally were achieved within 14 days. Maximum recommended dosage is 60 mg/kg/day.

➤ *Migraine:*

Divalproex sodium delayed-release tablets – Starting dose is 250 mg orally twice daily. Some patients may benefit from doses up to 1000 mg/day. There is no evidence that higher doses lead to greater efficacy.

Divalproex sodium ER tablets – The recommended starting dose is 500 mg once daily for 1 week, thereafter increasing to 1000 mg once daily. Although doses other than 1000 mg once daily have not been evaluated in patients with migraines, the effective dose range of delayed-released tablets in these patients is 500 to 1000 mg/day. As with other valproate products, individualize doses of the ER tablets and adjust the dose as necessary. When ER tablets are given in doses 8% to 20% higher than the total daily dose of the delayed-release tablets, the two formulations are bioequivalent. If a patient requires smaller dose adjustments than that available with the ER tablets, use the delayed-release tablets instead.

➤ *Therapeutic serum levels:* Therapeutic serum levels for most patients with seizures will range from 50 to 100 mcg/mL; however, a good correlation has not been established between daily dose, serum level and therapeutic effect.

➤ *Storage/Stability:* Store divalproex sodium delayed-release tablets and syrup below 30°C (86°F). Store sprinkle capsules below 25°C (77°F). Store capsules at 15° to 25°C (59° to 77°F). Store ER tablets at 25°C (77°F); excursions permitted to 15° to 30°C (59° to 86°F). Store vials at controlled room temperature 15° to 30°C (59° to 86°F). Discard unused portion of vial.

Actions

➤ *Pharmacology:* This group includes valproic acid, sodium valproate (the sodium salt), and divalproex sodium, a stable coordination compound containing equal proportions of valproic acid and sodium valproate. Regardless of form, dosage is expressed as valproic acid equivalents.

Although the mechanism of action is not established, its activity may be related to increased brain levels of gamma-aminobutyric acid (GABA).

➤ *Pharmacokinetics:*

Absorption – Following oral administration, valproate sodium is rapidly converted to valproic acid in the stomach. Valproic acid is rapidly absorbed from the GI tract. Absorption of the drug is delayed slightly but not decreased by administration with meals; administration of the drug with milk products does not affect the rate or degree of absorption. Following oral administration of divalproex sodium, divalproex sodium dissociates into valproic acid in the GI tract.

The absolute bioavailability of divalproex ER tablets administered as a single dose after a meal was approximately 90% relative to IV infusion. When given in equal total daily doses, the bioavailability of ER tablets is less than that of the delayed-release tablets. The ER tablet given once daily produced an average bioavailability of 89% relative to divalproex delayed-release tablets given 2, 3, or 4 times daily. Maximum valproate plasma concentrations in these studies were achieved on average 4 to 17 hours after the ER dose intake. After multiple dosing, the ER tablet given once daily has been shown to produce a percent fluctuation that is 10% to 20% lower than that of regular delayed-release tablets given 2, 3, or 4 times daily.

The relationship between plasma concentration and clinical response is not well documented. One contributing factor is the nonlinear, concentration-dependent protein binding of valproate, which affects the clearance of the drug. Thus, monitoring of total serum valproate cannot provide a reliable index of the bioactive valproate species.

Equivalent doses of IV and oral products deliver equivalent quantities of valproate ion systemically. Although the rate of valproate ion absorption may vary with the formulation administered (liquid, solid, or sprinkle), conditions of use (eg, fasting or postprandial), and the method of administration (eg, whether the contents of the capsule are sprinkled on food or the capsule is taken intact), these differences should be of minor clinical importance under the steady state conditions achieved with chronic use in the treatment of epilepsy. Whether or not rate of absorption influences the efficacy of valproate as an antimanic or antimigraine agent is unknown. However, it is possible that differences among the various valproate products in T_{max} and C_{max} could be important upon initiation of treatment but in chronic use is unlikely to be affected.

Distribution – Valproic acid is rapidly distributed. Volume of distribution of total or free valproic acid is 11 or 92 L/1.73 m², respectively. Valproic acid has been detected in CSF (approximately 10% of total concentrations) and milk (about 1% to 10% of serum concentrations).

VALPROIC ACID and DERIVATIVES

Therapeutic range is commonly considered to be 50 to 100 mcg/mL of total valproate, although some patients may be controlled with lower or higher plasma concentrations.

The plasma protein binding of valproate is concentration-dependent and the free fraction increases from approximately 10% at 40 mcg/mL to 18.5% at 130 mcg/mL. Protein binding of valproate is reduced in the elderly, in patients with chronic hepatic diseases, in patients with renal impairment, and in the presence of other drugs (eg, aspirin). Conversely, valproate may displace certain protein-bound drugs (eg, phenytoin, carbamazepine, warfarin, tolbutamide).

Metabolism / Excretion – Primarily metabolized in liver; 30% to 50% of an administered dose is excreted as glucuronide conjugate in the urine. Mitochondrial β-oxidation is the other major metabolic pathway, typically accounting for over 40% of the dose. Usually, less than 15% to 20% is eliminated by other oxidative mechanisms. Less than 3% of an administered dose is excreted unchanged in urine.

Mean plasma clearance for total and free valproate is 0.56 and 4.6 L/h/1.73 m², respectively. Mean terminal half-life for valproate monotherapy ranges from 9 to 16 hours. The estimates cited apply primarily to patients who are not taking drugs that affect hepatic metabolizing enzyme systems. For example, patients taking enzyme-inducing antiepileptic drugs (carbamazepine, phenytoin, and phenobarbital) will clear valproate more rapidly. Because of these changes in valproate clearance, monitoring of antiepileptic concentrations should be intensified whenever concomitant antiepileptics are introduced or withdrawn.

Special populations –

Children: Children within the first 2 months of life have a markedly decreased ability to eliminate valproate compared to older children and adults. This is a result of reduced clearance as well as increased volume of distribution (in part due to decreased plasma protein binding). For example, in one study, the half-life in children under 10 days ranged from 10 to 67 hours compared to a range of 7 to 13 hours in children older than 2 months. Pediatric patients (ie, between 3 months and 10 years of age) have 50% higher clearances expressed on weight than do adults. Over 10 years of age, children have pharmacokinetic parameters that approximate those of adults.

Elderly: The capacity of elderly patients (range, 68 to 89 years of age) to eliminate valproate has been shown to be reduced compared to younger adults (age range, 22 to 26). Intrinsic clearance is reduced by 39%; the free fraction is increased by 44%. Accordingly, the initial dosage should be reduced in the elderly.

Hepatic function impairment: In one study, the clearance of free valproate was decreased by 50% in 7 patients with cirrhosis and by 16% in 4 patients with acute hepatitis, compared with 6 healthy subjects. In that study, the half-life of valproate was increased from 12 to 18 hours. Liver disease is also associated with decreased albumin concentrations and larger unbound fractions (2 to 2.6 fold increase) of valproate.

Renal function impairment: A slight reduction (27%) in the unbound clearance of valproate has been reported in patients with renal failure (Ccr less than 10 mL/min); however, hemodialysis typically reduces valproate concentrations by about 20%. Protein binding in these patients is substantially reduced; thus, monitoring total concentrations may be misleading.

Contraindications

Hepatic disease/significant hepatic dysfunction (see Warnings); hypersensitivity to the drug; known urea cycle disorders (see Warnings).

Warnings

➤*Pancreatitis:* Cases of life-threatening pancreatitis have been reported in children and adults receiving valproate. Some of the cases have been described as hemorrhagic with rapid progression from initial symptoms to death. Some cases have occurred shortly after initial use as well as after several years of use. The rate based upon the reported cases exceeds that expected in the general population, and there have been cases in which pancreatitis recurred after rechallenge with valproate. In clinical trials, there were 2 cases of pancreatitis without alternative etiology in 2416 patients, representing 1044 patient-years experience. Warn patients and guardians that abdominal pain, nausea, vomiting, and/or anorexia can be symptoms of pancreatitis that require prompt medical evaluation. If pancreatitis is diagnosed, discontinue valproate. Initiate alternative treatment for the underlying medical condition as clinically indicated.

➤*Urea cycle disorders (UCDs):* Hyperammonemic encephalopathy, sometimes fatal, has been reported following initiation of valproate therapy in patients with UCDs, a group of uncommon genetic abnormalities, particularly ornithine transcarbamylase deficiency. Prior to the initiation of valproate therapy, consider evaluation for UCD in the following patients: 1) those with a history of unexplained encephalopathy or coma, encephalopathy associated with a protein load, pregnancy-related or postpartum encephalopathy, unexplained mental retardation, or history of elevated plasma ammonia or glutamine; 2) those with cyclical vomiting and lethargy, episodic extreme irritability, ataxia, low BUN, or protein avoidance; 3) those with a family history of UCD or a family history of unexplained infant deaths (particularly males); 4) those with other signs or symptoms of UCD. Patients who develop symptoms of unexplained hyperammonemic encephalopathy while receiving valproate therapy should receive prompt treatment

(including discontinuation of valproate therapy) and be evaluated for underlying urea cycle disorders.

➤*Thrombocytopenia:* The frequency of adverse effects (particularly elevated liver enzymes and thrombocytopenia) may be dose-related. In a clinical trial of divalproex sodium as monotherapy in patients with epilepsy, 27% receiving approximately 50 mg/kg/day on average, had at least 1 value of platelets less than or equal to 75×10^9/L. Approximately half of these patients had treatment discontinued, with return of platelet counts to normal. In the remaining patients, platelet counts normalized with continued treatment. The probability of thrombocytopenia appears to increase significantly at total valproate plasma concentrations at least 110 mcg/mL in females or at least 135 mcg/mL in males. The therapeutic benefit, which may accompany the higher doses, should therefore be weighed against the possibility of a greater incidence of adverse effects.

➤*Acute head injuries:* A study evaluating the effect of IV valproate in the prevention of posttraumatic seizures in patients with acute head injuries found a higher incidence of death in valproate treatment groups compared with the IV phenytoin treatment group (13% vs 8.5%, respectively). Until further information is available, it seems prudent not to use valproate sodium injection in patients with acute head trauma for the prophylaxis of posttraumatic seizures.

➤*Hepatotoxicity:* See Warning Box. Use caution in patients who have a history of hepatic disease. These incidents usually have occurred during the first 6 months of treatment. Serious or fatal hepatotoxicity may be preceded by nonspecific symptoms such as malaise, weakness, lethargy, facial edema, anorexia, and vomiting. Closely monitor patients for these symptoms. Perform liver function tests prior to therapy and at frequent intervals thereafter, especially during the first 6 months. Physicians should not rely totally on serum biochemistry because these tests may not be abnormal in all instances, but should also consider the results of careful interim medical history and physical examination.

Patients on multiple anticonvulsants, children, those with congenital metabolic disorders, those with severe seizure disorders accompanied by mental retardation, and those with organic brain disease may be at particular risk. Experience has indicated that children under 2 years of age are at considerably increased risk of developing fatal hepatotoxicity, especially those with the aforementioned conditions. When valproate products are used in this patient group, they should be used with extreme caution and as a sole agent. Weigh the benefits of therapy against the risks. Use of valproate sodium injection has not been studied in children below 2 years of age. Above this age group, experience has indicated that the incidence of fatal hepatotoxicity decreases considerably in progressively older patient groups.

Discontinue immediately in the presence of significant hepatic dysfunction, suspected or apparent. In some cases, hepatic dysfunction has progressed in spite of drug discontinuation. The frequency of adverse effects (particularly elevated liver enzymes and thrombocytopenia) may be dose-related.

➤*Long-term use in mania:* Safety and effectiveness for long-term use in mania (more than 3 weeks) have not been systematically evaluated in clinical trials. Continually re-evaluate the drug's usefulness if it is used for extended periods.

➤*Discontinuation:* Do not abruptly discontinue in patients in whom the drug is administered to prevent major seizures because of the strong possibility of precipitating status epilepticus with attendant hypoxia and threat to life.

➤*Carcinogenesis:* Increased incidences of subcutaneous fibrosarcomas and benign pulmonary adenomas have occurred in male rodents given 10% to 50% the human dose for 2 years. The significance of these findings for humans is unknown.

➤*Fertility impairment:* Chronic toxicity studies in animals demonstrated reduced spermatogenesis and testicular atrophy. The effect of valproate on testicular development and on sperm production and fertility in humans is unknown.

➤*Elderly:* In a double-blind, multicenter trial of valproate in elderly patients with dementia (mean age, 83 years), doses were increased by 125 mg/day to a target dose of 20 mg/kg/day. A significantly higher proportion of valproate patients had somnolence compared with placebo, and although not statistically significant, there was a higher proportion of patients with dehydration. Discontinuations for somnolence were also significantly higher than with placebo. In some patients with somnolence (approximately 50%), there was associated reduced nutritional intake and weight loss. There was a trend for the patients who experienced these events to have a lower baseline albumin concentration, lower valproate clearance, and a higher BUN. In elderly patients, increase dosage more slowly and with regular monitoring for fluid and nutritional intake, dehydration, somnolence, and other adverse events. Consider dose reductions or discontinuation of valproate in patients with decreased food or fluid intake and in patients with excessive somnolence (see Administration and Dosage).

A reduced starting dose is recommended (see Administration and Dosage).

➤*Pregnancy:* Category D. The incidence of neural tube defects in the fetus may be increased in mothers receiving valproic acid during the first trimester. The CDC estimates the risk of valproic acid-exposed women having children with spina bifida to be approximately 1% to 2%.

VALPROIC ACID and DERIVATIVES

According to published and unpublished reports, valproic acid may produce teratogenic effects in the offspring of human females receiving the drug during pregnancy. Other congenital anomalies (eg, craniofacial defects, cardiovascular malformations, and anomalies involving various body systems), compatible and incompatible with life, have been reported.

There are multiple reports in the clinical literature that indicate that the use of antiepileptic drugs during pregnancy results in an increased incidence of birth defects in the offspring. Although data are more extensive with respect to trimethadione, paramethadione, phenytoin, and phenobarbital, reports indicate a possible similar association with the use of other antiepileptic drugs. Therefore, administer antiepileptic drugs to women of childbearing potential only if they are clearly shown to be essential in the management of their seizures. Do not abruptly discontinue antiepileptic drugs administered to prevent major seizures because of the strong possibility of precipitating status epilepticus with attendant hypoxia and threat to life. Consider tests to detect neural tube and other defects using current accepted procedures a part of routine prenatal care in childbearing women receiving valproate.

Patients taking valproate may develop clotting abnormalities. A patient who had low fibrinogen when taking multiple anticonvulsants, including valproate, gave birth to an infant with afibrinogenemia who subsequently died of hemorrhage. If valproate is used in pregnancy, carefully monitor the clotting parameters. Hepatic failure, resulting in the death of a newborn and of an infant, have been reported following the use of valproate during pregnancy.

➤*Lactation:* Concentrations of valproic acid in breast milk are 1% to 10% of serum concentrations. It is not known what effect this would have on a nursing infant. Consider discontinuing nursing when valproate products are administered to a nursing woman.

➤*Children:* See Warning Box. Experience has indicated that pediatric patients under 2 years of age are at a considerably increased risk of developing fatal hepatotoxicity, especially those with the aforementioned conditions (see Warning Box). When valproate products are used in this patient group, they should be used with extreme caution and as a sole agent. Weigh the benefits of therapy against the risks. Above 2 years of age, experience in epilepsy has indicated that the incidence of fatal hepatoxicity decreases considerably in progressively older patient groups.

Younger children, especially those receiving enzyme-inducing drugs, will require larger maintenance doses to attain targeted total and unbound valproic acid concentrations. The variability in free fraction limits the clinical usefulness of monitoring total serum valproic acid concentrations. Interpretation of valproic acid concentrations in children should include consideration of factors that affect hepatic metabolism and protein binding.

The safety and efficacy of divalproex sodium ER tablets for the prophylaxis of migraine headaches in pediatric patients has not been established. The safety and efficacy of divalproex ER for the treatment of complex partial seizures, simple and complex absence seizures, and multiple seizure types that include absence seizures has not been established in pediatric patients younger than 10 years of age.

Use of valproate sodium injection has not been studied in children below 2 years of age.

The safety and efficacy of divalproex sodium for the treatment of acute mania has not been studied in individuals under 18 years of age. The safety and efficacy of divalproex sodium for the prophylaxis of migraines has not been studied in individuals below 16 years of age.

Precautions

➤*Hematologic effects:* Thrombocytopenia, inhibition of the secondary phase of platelet aggregation and abnormal coagulation parameters (eg, low fibrinogen) have occurred. The probability of thrombocytopenia appears to increase significantly at total valproate plasma concentrations of at least 110 mcg/mL in females and/or at least 135 mcg/mL in males. Determine platelet counts and coagulation tests before initiating therapy, at periodic intervals and prior to surgery. Hemorrhage, bruising, or a hemostasis/coagulation disorder are indications for reduction of dosage or withdrawal of therapy.

➤*Hyperammonemia:* Hyperammonemia has been reported in association with valproate therapy and may be present despite normal liver function tests. In patients who develop unexplained lethargy and vomiting or changes in mental status, hyperammonemic encephalopathy should be considered and an ammonia level should be measured. If ammonia is increased, discontinue valproate therapy. Initiate appropriate interventions for treatment of hyperammonemia; such patients should undergo investigation for underlying urea cycle disorders (see Warnings).

Asymptomatic elevations of ammonia are more common and when present, require close monitoring of plasma ammonia levels. If the elevation persists, consider discontinuation of valproate therapy.

➤*Suicidal ideation:* Suicidal ideation may be a manifestation of certain psychiatric disorders and may persist until a significant remission of symptoms occurs. Closely supervise high-risk patients during initial drug therapy.

➤*Hazardous tasks:* Patients should use caution while driving or performing other tasks requiring alertness, coordination or physical dexterity.

Drug Interactions

Valproic Acid Drug Interactions			
Precipitant drug	Object drug*		Description
Charcoal	Valproic acid	↓	Valproic acid absorption is decreased.
Chlorpromazine	Valproic acid	↑	Valproate t½ and trough levels may increase, clearance may decrease.
Cholestyramine	Valproic acid	↓	Serum concentrations and bioavailability of valproic acid may be reduced, resulting in a decrease in therapeutic effects. Administer valproic acid at least 3 hours before, but not within 3 hours following cholestyramine.
Cimetidine	Valproic acid	↑	Small but potentially significant decrease in valproate clearance and increase in t½.
Erythromycin	Valproic acid	↑	Erythromycin may increase serum valproic acid concentrations, producing valproic acid toxicity.
Felbamate	Valproic acid	↑	Coadministration revealed a 35% increase in mean peak valproate levels.
Rifampin	Valproic acid	↓	In 1 study, rifampin increased the oral clearance of valproate by 40%.
Salicylates (eg, aspirin)	Valproic acid	↑	Salicylates may displace valproic acid from protein binding sites and may also alter the metabolic pathways. Monitor serum concentrations.
Valproic acid	Tricyclic antidepressants	↑	Plasma concentrations and side effects of the tricyclic antidepressant may be increased. Coadministration resulted in a 21% decrease in the plasma clearance of amitriptyline and a 34% decrease in the net clearance of nortriptyline.
Valproic acid	Carbamazepine	↑	Variable changes in carbamazepine concentrations with increased levels of the active metabolite; decreased valproic acid levels with possible loss of seizure control may occur.
Carbamazepine	Valproic acid	↓	
Valproic acid	Clonazepam	↔	Concomitant use may induce absence status in patients with a history of absence type seizures.
Valproic acid	Diazepam	↑	Valproate displaces diazepam from its plasma albumin binding sites and inhibits its metabolism.
Valproic acid	Ethosuximide	↑↓	Increases and decreases in ethosuximide blood levels and decreases in valproic acid levels have been reported. Valproic acid appears to inhibit the metabolism of ethosuximide.
Ethosuximide	Valproic acid	↓	
Valproic acid	Lamotrigine	↑	Serum valproic acid concentrations may be decreased while lamotrigine levels increase. In one study, coadministration increased the half-life of lamotrigine from 26 to 70 hours. Lamotrigine dose should be reduced.
Lamotrigine	Valproic acid	↓	
Valproic acid	Barbiturates	↑	Valproic acid may decrease hepatic metabolism of barbiturates. Barbiturate dosage may need to be decreased in some patients.
Valproic acid	Hydantoins (eg, phenytoin)	↑	Increased action of phenytoin, even at therapeutic levels; increased metabolism of valproic acid with decreased pharmacologic effects may occur.
Hydantoins (eg, phenytoin)	Valproic acid	↓	
Valproic acid	Tolbutamide	↔	The unbound fraction of tolbutamide may be increased from 20% to 50%. The clinical relevance of this displacement is unknown.
Valproic acid	Warfarin	↑	The potential exists for valproate to displace warfarin from protein binding sites. Monitor coagulation tests.
Valproic acid	Zidovudine	↑	Zidovudine clearance was decreased by 38% in 6 HIV-seropositive patients.

* ↑ = Object drug increased.   ↓ = Object drug decreased.   ↔ = Undetermined clinical effect.

VALPROIC ACID and DERIVATIVES

▶*Drug/Lab test interactions:* Valproic acid is partially eliminated in the urine as a keto-metabolite, which may lead to a false interpretation of the urine ketone test. There have been reports of altered thyroid function tests associated with valproic acid. The clinical significance is unknown.

Adverse Reactions

Adverse reaction	Tablets Migraine	Mania	Epilepsy Adjunctive therapy for complex partial seizures	High-dose[b]	Low-dose[b]	Extended-release Migraine	Injection
CNS							
Asthenia	20	10	27	21	10	-	-
Somnolence	17	19	27	30	18	7	1.7
Dizziness	12	12	25	18	13	1-5	5.2
Tremor	9	-	25	57	19	1-5	0.6
Ataxia	-	1-5	8	-	-	-	-
Emotional lability	1-5	-	6	-	-	-	-
Abnormal thinking	1-5	1-5	6	-	-	-	-
Amnesia	-	-	5	7	4	-	0.9
Euphoria	-	-	-	-	-	-	-
Headache	-	-	31	≥5	≥5	-	4.3
Hypesthesia	-	-	-	-	-	-	0.6
Nervousness	-	-	-	11	7	1-5	0.9
Paresthesia	1-5	1-5	-	-	-	-	0.9
Insomnia	1-5	1-5	-	15	9	1-5	-
Depression	1-5	1-5	-	5	4	-	-
GI							
Nausea	31	22	48	34	26	15	3.2
Dyspepsia	13	9	8	11	10	7	-
Diarrhea	12	-	13	23	19	7	0.9
Vomiting	11	12	27	23	15	7	1.3
Abdominal pain	9	9	23	12	9	7	1.1
Increased appetite	6	-	-	-	-	1-5	-
Constipation	1-5	-	5	-	-	-	-
Anorexia	1-5	1-5	12	11	4	-	-
Hematologic/ Lymphatic							
Thrombocyto-penia	-	-	-	24	1	-	-
Ecchymosis	1-5	1-5	-	5	4	-	-
Respiratory							
Flu syndrome	-	-	12	-	-	-	-
Infection	-	-	12	20	13	-	-
Bronchitis	-	-	5	-	-	-	-
Rhinitis	1-5	1-5	5	-	-	1-5	-
Pharyngitis	-	-	-	8	2	1-5	0.6
Dyspnea	1-5	1-5	-	5	1	-	-
Special senses							
Nystagmus	-	-	8	7	1	-	-
Diplopia	-	1-5	16	-	-	-	-
Amblyopia/ Blurred vision	-	1-5	12	8	4	-	-
Taste perversion	1-5	-	-	-	-	-	1.9
Tinnitus	1-5	1-5	-	7	1	1-5	-
Miscella-neous							
Weight gain	8	-	-	9	4	1-5	-
Back pain	8	-	-	-	-	-	-
Alopecia	7	1-5	6	24	13	-	-
Fever	1-5	1-5	6	-	-	-	-
Weight loss	-	-	6	-	-	-	-
Chest pain	1-5	1-5	-	-	-	-	1.7
Injection site inflammation	-	-	-	-	-	-	0.6
Injection site pain	-	-	-	-	-	-	2.6
Injection site reaction	-	-	-	-	-	-	2.4

Adverse reaction	Tablets Migraine	Mania	Epilepsy Adjunctive therapy for complex partial seizures	High-dose[b]	Low-dose[b]	Extended-release Migraine	Injection
Pain (unspecified)	-	-	-	-	-	-	1.3
Vasodilation	1-5	1-5	-	-	-	-	0.9
Sweating	-	-	-	-	-	-	0.9
Peripheral edema	1-5	1-5	-	8	3	-	-
Infection	-	-	-	-	-	15	-
Rash	1-5	6	-	-	-	1-5	-

[a] Data are pooled from separate trials and are not necessarily comparable.
[b] Monotherapy for complex partial seizures. Since patients were being titrated off another antiepilepsy drug during the first portion of the trial, it is not possible, in many cases, to determine whether the following adverse events can be ascribed to divalproex sodium alone, or the combination of divalproex sodium and other antiepilepsy drugs.

▶*Valproate sodium injection:* The adverse events that can result from valproate sodium injection use include all of those associated with oral forms of valproate. The following describes experience specifically with valproate sodium injection. Valproate sodium injection has been generally well tolerated in clinical trials involving 111 healthy adult male volunteers and 352 patients with epilepsy given at doses of 125 to 6000 mg (total daily dose). A total of 2% of patients discontinued treatment with valproate sodium injection because of adverse events. The most common adverse events leading to discontinuation were 2 cases each of nausea/vomiting and elevated amylase. Other adverse events leading to discontinuation were hallucinations, pneumonia, headache, injection site reaction, and abnormal gait. Dizziness and injection site pain were observed more frequently at 100 mg/min infusion rate than at rates up to 33 mg/min. At a 200 mg/min rate, dizziness and taste perversion occurred more frequently than at a 100 mg/min rate. The maximum rate of infusion studied was 200 mg/min.

In a separate clinical safety trial, 112 patients with epilepsy were given infusions of valproate sodium (up to 15 mg/kg) over 5 to 10 minutes (1.5 to 3 mg/kg/min). The common adverse events (greater than 2%) were somnolence (10.7%); dizziness, paresthesia, asthenia (7.1%); nausea (6.3%), and headache (2.7%). While the incidence of these adverse events was generally higher than in the table above (experience encompassing the standard, much slower infusion rates), eg, somnolence (1.7%), dizziness (5.2%), paresthesia (0.9%), asthenia (0%), nausea (3.2%), and headache (4.3%), a direct comparison between the incidence of adverse events in the 2 cohorts cannot be made because of differences in patient populations and study designs.

Ammonia levels have not been systematically studied after IV valproate, so that an estimate of the incidence of hyperammonemia after IV valproate sodium cannot be provided. Hyperammonemia with encephalopathy has been reported in 2 patients after infusions of valproate sodium.

▶*Complex partial seizures:*

Cardiovascular – Hypertension, palpitation, tachycardia, bradycardia (more than 1% to less than 5%).

CNS – Sedation has occurred (alone and in combination) and usually disappears upon reduction of other anticonvulsant medication. Anxiety, confusion, abnormal gait, paresthesia, hypertonia, incoordination, abnormal dreams, personality disorder (more than 1% to less than 5%); bradycardia; emotional upset; depression; psychosis; aggression; hyperactivity; behavioral deterioration; hostility; tremor (may be dose-related); hallucinations; ataxia; headache; nystagmus; diplopia; asterixis; "spots before eyes;" dysarthria; dizziness; hypesthesia; vertigo; incoordination; parkinsonism; coma (rare, alone or in conjunction with phenobarbital); encephalopathy with and without fever (rare, developed shortly after introduction of valproate monotherapy without evidence of hepatic dysfunction or inappropriately high plasma levels); reversible cerebral atrophy and dementia (several reports). Although recovery has been described following drug withdrawal, there have been fatalities in patients with hyperammonemic encephalopathy, particularly in patients with underlying urea cycle disorders (see Warnings and Precautions).

Dermatologic – Dry skin, rash, pruritus, petechiae (more than 1% to less than 5%); transient hair loss; skin rash; erythema multiforme; photosensitivity; generalized pruritus; Stevens-Johnson syndrome. Rare cases of toxic epidermal necrolysis have been reported including a fatal case in a 6-month-old infant taking valproate and several other concomitant medications. An additional case of toxic epidermal necrosis resulting in death was reported in a 35-year-old AIDS patient taking several concomitant medications and with a history of multiple cutaneous drug reactions.

Endocrine – Abnormal thyroid function tests; parotid gland swelling.

GI – Flatulence, hematemesis, eructation, periodontal abscess (more than 1% to less than 5%); indigestion; constipation; anorexia with

VALPROIC ACID and DERIVATIVES

weight loss; increased appetite with weight gain. Use of delayed-release divalproex sodium may reduce GI side effects in some patients.

GU – Amenorrhea, dysmenorrhea, urinary frequency, urinary incontinence, vaginitis (more than 1% to less than 5%). Irregular menses; secondary amenorrhea; breast enlargement; galactorrhea; polycystic ovary disease (rare); enuresis; urinary tract infection.

Hematologic – Valproic acid inhibits the secondary phase of platelet aggregation; this may be reflected in altered bleeding time. Thrombocytopenia; bruising; hematoma formation; epistaxis; frank hemorrhage; relative lymphocytosis; macrocytosis; hypofibrinogenemia; leukopenia; eosinophilia; anemia (including macrocytic with or without folate deficiency); bone marrow suppression; pancytopenia; aplastic anemia; acute intermittent porphyria.

Hepatic – Minor elevations of AST, ALT, and LDH (frequent, dose-related); increases in serum bilirubin and abnormal changes in other liver function tests (occasionally). These results may reflect potentially serious hepatotoxicity. (See Warning Box and Warnings).

Metabolic – Hyperammonemia (see Precautions); hyponatremia; inappropriate ADH secretion; Fanconi syndrome (rare and seen primarily in children); hyperglycinemia associated with a fatal outcome in a patient with pre-existent nonketotic hyperglycinemia; decreased carnitine concentrations.

Musculoskeletal – Arthralgia, leg cramps, myalgia, myasthenia, twitching (more than 1% to less than 5%).

Respiratory – Epistaxis, pneumonia, sinusitis, cough increased (more than 1% to less than 5%).

Special senses – Abnormal vision, deafness, taste perversion, otitis media (more than 1% to less than 5%). Hearing loss, ear pain.

Miscellaneous – Back pain, malaise (more than 1% to less than 5%); extremity edema; weakness; acute pancreatitis (including fatal cases); lupus erythematosus; fever; bone pain; cutaneous vasculitis; anaphylaxis.

➤*Mania:* The following additional adverse events were reported in greater than 1% to 5% of patients.

Cardiovascular – Hypertension, hypotension, palpitations, postural hypotension, tachycardia.

CNS – Abnormal dreams, abnormal gait, agitation, catatonic reaction, confusion, dysarthria, hallucinations, hypertonia, hypokinesia, reflexes increased, tardive dyskinesia, vertigo.

Dermatologic – Discoid lupus erythematosus, dry skin, furunculosis, maculopapular rash, seborrhea.

GI – Fecal incontinence, flatulence, gastroenteritis, glossitis, periodontal abscess.

GU – Dysmenorrhea, dysuria, urinary incontinence.

Metabolic/Nutritional – Edema.

Musculoskeletal – Arthralgia, arthrosis, leg cramps, twitching.

Special senses – Conjunctivitis, deafness, dry eyes, ear pain, eye pain.

Miscellaneous – Chills, chills and fever, neck pain, neck rigidity.

➤*Migraine:* The following adverse events were reported (greater than 1% to 5%):

CNS – Abnormal dreams, abnormal gait, confusion, hypertonia, speech disorder, vertigo.

Dermatologic – Pruritus.

GI – Dry mouth, flatulence, GI disorder (unspecified), stomatitis, tooth disorder.

GU – Cystitis, metrorrhagia, vaginal hemorrhage.

Metabolic/Nutritional – AST increase, ALT increase.

Musculoskeletal – Leg cramps, myalgia.

Respiratory – Cough increased, sinusitis.

Special senses – Conjunctivitis, ear disorder.

Miscellaneous – Accidental injury, chills, face edema, malaise, viral infection.

Overdosage

➤*Symptoms:* Overdosage may result in somnolence, heart block, and deep coma. Patients have recovered with a valproate serum concentration as high as 2120 mcg/mL. Fatalities have been reported.

➤*Treatment:* Use general supportive measures and carefully maintain adequate urinary output. The fraction of drug not bound to protein is high and hemodialysis plus hemoperfusion may result in significant removal of drug. Naloxone has reversed CNS depressant effects. It theoretically could reverse anticonvulsant effects; use caution in patients with epilepsy. See General Management of Acute Overdosage.

Patient Information

If GI upset occurs, take with food.

Do not chew capsules; swallow whole to avoid irritation of mouth and throat.

Because divalproex sodium may produce CNS depression, especially when combined with another CNS depressant (eg, alcohol), advise patients against engaging in hazardous activities, such as driving an automobile or operating dangerous machinery, until it is known that they do not become drowsy from the drug.

Sprinkle capsules may be swallowed whole or may be administered by carefully opening the capsule and sprinkling the entire contents on a small amount (teaspoonful) of soft food such as applesauce or pudding. The drug/food mixture should be swallowed immediately (avoid chewing) and not stored for future use.

Warn patients and guardians that abdominal pain, nausea, vomiting, and/or anorexia can be symptoms of pancreatitis and require further medical evaluation promptly.

Because divalproex sodium has been associated with certain types of birth defects, advise female patients of childbearing age considering the use of divalproex sodium for the prevention of migraine to read the patient information leaflet.

Do not crush or chew ER tablets; swallow whole.

The specially coated particles in the sprinkle capsules have been observed in the stool, but this occurrence has not been associated with clinically significant effects.

Inform patients of the signs and symptoms associated with hyperammonemic encephalopathy and tell them to inform the prescriber if any of these symptoms occur.

➤*Diabetic patients:* Medication may interfere with urine tests for ketones.

ATRACURIUM BESYLATE

Rx	Tracrium (GlaxoWellcome)	Injection: 10 mg/ml[1]	In 5 ml single-use and 10 ml multi-dose vials.[2]

[1] With benzenesulfonic acid.

[2] With 0.9% benzyl alcohol.

> ## WARNING
>
> Atracurium should be used only by those skilled in airway management and respiratory support. Equipment and personnel must be immediately available for endotracheal intubation and support of ventilation, including use of positive pressure oxygen. Adequacy of respiration must be assured through assisted or controlled ventilation. Have anticholinesterase reversal agents immediately available.

Indications

As an adjunct to general anesthesia to facilitate endotracheal intubation; to relax skeletal muscle during surgery or mechanical ventilation.

Administration and Dosage

To avoid patient distress, do not administer before unconsciousness has been induced.

Administer IV. IM use may result in tissue irritation.

Use a peripheral nerve stimulator to monitor twitch suppression and recovery.

Adjust the rate of administration according to patient response as determined by peripheral nerve stimulation.

➤Bolus doses for intubation and maintenance of neuromuscular blockade:

Initial adult dose – 0.4 to 0.5 mg/kg (1.7 to 2.2 times ED_{95}) IV bolus. Expect good conditions for nonemergency intubation in 2 to 2.5 minutes in most patients; maximum neuromuscular blockade is achieved ≈ 3 to 5 minutes after injection.

Maintaining neuromuscular blockade during prolonged surgical procedures – 0.08 to 0.1 mg/kg. The first maintenance dose is generally required 20 to 45 minutes after initial injection. Give maintenance doses at regular intervals, every 15 to 25 minutes under balanced anesthesia, slightly longer under isoflurane or enflurane. Higher doses (up to 0.2 mg/kg) permit maintenance dosing at longer intervals.

Histamine release – Initially, 0.3 to 0.4 mg/kg given slowly or in divided doses over 1 minute (see Precautions).

Neuromuscular disease, severe electrolyte disorders or carcinomatosis – Consider dosage reductions in which potentiation of neuromuscular blockade or difficulties with reversal have been demonstrated. There has been no clinical experience in these patients and no specific dosage adjustments. No dosage adjustments are required for patients with renal diseases.

Following use of succinylcholine for intubation under balanced anesthesia – Initially, 0.3 to 0.4 mg/kg. Further reductions may be desirable with the use of potent inhalational anesthetics. Permit the patient to recover from the effects of succinylcholine prior to atracurium administration. Data are insufficient to recommend specific initial doses following administration of succinylcholine in infants and children.

Pediatrics – No dosage adjustments required for patients ≥ 2 years old. An initial dose of 0.3 to 0.4 mg/kg is recommended for infants (1 month to 2 years old) under halothane anesthesia. More frequent maintenance doses may be required.

➤Use by infusion: After administration of an initial bolus dose of 0.3 to 0.5 mg/kg, give a diluted solution by continuous infusion for maintenance of neuromuscular blockade during extended surgical procedures. Long-term use in the ICU has not been studied sufficiently to support dosage recommendations. Accuracy is best achieved using a precision infusion device.

Initiate infusion only after early evidence of spontaneous recovery from the bolus dose. An initial infusion rate of 9 to 10 mcg/kg/min may be required to rapidly counteract the spontaneous recovery of neuromuscular function. Thereafter, a rate of 5 to 9 mcg/kg/min should maintain continuous neuromuscular blockade in the range of 89% to 99% in most patients under balanced anesthesia.

In patients undergoing cardiopulmonary bypass with induced hypothermia, the rate of infusion required to maintain adequate surgical relaxation during hypothermia (25° to 28°C) is approximately half the rate required during normothermia.

Atracuruim Infusion Rates Concentrations for 0.2 and 0.5 mg/ml		
Drug delivery rate (mcg/kg/min)	Infusion delivery rate (ml/kg/min)	
	0.2 mg/ml[1]	0.5 mg/ml[2]
5	0.025	0.01
6	0.03	0.012
7	0.035	0.014

Atracuruim Infusion Rates Concentrations for 0.2 and 0.5 mg/ml		
Drug delivery rate (mcg/kg/min)	Infusion delivery rate (ml/kg/min)	
	0.2 mg/ml[1]	0.5 mg/ml[2]
8	0.04	0.016
9	0.045	0.018
10	0.05	0.02

[1] 2 ml of 1% (10 mg/ml) added to 98 ml diluent.
[2] 5 ml of 1% (10 mg/ml) added to 95 ml diluent.

➤Admixture compatibility: Prepare infusion solutions by admixing atracurium with an appropriate diluent: 5% Dextrose Injection, 0.9% Sodium Chloride Injection or 5% Dextrose and 0.9% Sodium Chloride Injection. Do not use Lactated Ringer's Injection. The amount of infusion solution required per minute will depend upon the concentration and dose desired (see table). Use infusion solutions within 24 hours of preparation. Discard unused solutions.

Atracurium has an acid pH; do not mix with alkaline solutions (eg, barbiturates) in the same syringe or administer simultaneously during IV infusion through the same needle. The drug may be inactivated and precipitated.

➤Storage / Stability: Atracurium loses potency at the rate of 6% per year under refrigeration (5°C; 41°F). Rate of loss in potency increases to ≈ 5% per month at 25°C (77°F). Refrigerate at 2° to 8°C (36° to 46°F) to preserve potency. Do not freeze. Upon removal from refrigeration, use atracurium within 14 days even if refrigerated.

Store solutions containing 0.2 or 0.5 mg/ml either under refrigeration or at room temperature for 24 hours without significant loss of potency.

Actions

➤Pharmacology: Atracurium, a nondepolarizing skeletal muscle relaxant, antagonizes the neurotransmitter action of acetylcholine by binding competitively with cholinergic receptor sites on the motor endplate.

Atracurium is a less potent histamine releaser than d-tubocurarine or metocurine. Histamine release is minimal with initial doses up to 0.5 mg/kg, and hemodynamic changes are minimal within the recommended dose range. A moderate histamine release and significant fall in blood pressure have occurred following 0.6 mg/kg. The effects were generally short-lived and manageable.

➤Pharmacokinetics: Essentially linear within the range of 0.3 to 0.6 mg/kg.

Onset, peak and duration of action – The time to onset of paralysis decreases and the duration of maximum effect increases with increasing doses. The duration of neuromuscular blockade is ≈ ⅓ to ½ that of d-tubocurarine, metocurine and pancuronium at initially equipotent doses.

The ED_{95} (dose required to produce 95% suppression of the muscle twitch response with balanced anesthesia) has averaged 0.23 mg/kg (0.11 to 0.26 mg/kg). An initial dose of 0.4 to 0.5 mg/kg generally produces maximum neuromuscular blockade within 3 to 5 minutes of injection, with good or excellent intubation conditions within 2 to 2.5 minutes in most patients. Recovery from neuromuscular blockade (under balanced anesthesia) begins ≈ 20 to 35 minutes after injection; recovery to 25% of control is achieved ≈ 35 to 45 minutes after injection, and recovery is usually 95% complete ≈ 60 to 70 minutes after injection.

Repeated administration of maintenance doses has no cumulative effect on the duration of neuromuscular blockade if recovery is allowed to begin prior to repeat dosing. After the initial dose, the first maintenance dose (0.08 to 0.1 mg/kg) is generally required within 20 to 45 minutes, and subsequent doses are required at ≈ 15 to 25 minute intervals.

Recovery – Recovery proceeds more rapidly than recovery from d-tubocurarine, metocurine and pancuronium. Regardless of dose, the time from start of recovery to complete (95%) recovery is ≈ 30 minutes under balanced anesthesia and ≈ 40 minutes under halothane, enflurane or isoflurane anesthesia. Repeated doses have no cumulative effect on recovery time.

Excretion – The elimination half-life is ≈ 20 minutes. The duration of neuromuscular blockade does not correlate with plasma pseudocholinesterase levels and is not altered by the absence of renal function. Atracurium is inactivated in plasma via two nonoxidative pathways. Some placental transfer occurs.

Contraindications

Hypersensitivity to atracurium besylate.

ATRACURIUM BESYLATE

Warnings

►*Anesthesia:* Atracurium has no known effect on consciousness, pain threshold or cerebration. Use only with adequate anesthesia.

►*Elderly:* No differences have been identified in effectiveness, safety or dosage requirements.

►*Pregnancy: Category C.* There are no adequate and well controlled studies in pregnant women. Use during pregnancy only if the potential benefits outweigh the potential hazards to the fetus.

Labor and delivery – Atracurium (0.3 mg/kg) has been administered to 26 pregnant women during delivery by cesarean section. No harmful effects occurred in any of the newborn infants, although small amounts crossed the placental barrier. Consider the possibility of respiratory depression in the newborn.

It is not known whether muscle relaxants given during vaginal delivery have immediate or delayed adverse effects on the fetus or increase the likelihood that resuscitation of the newborn will be necessary. The possibility of forceps delivery may increase.

►*Lactation:* It is not known whether this drug is excreted in breast milk. Safety for use in the nursing mother has not been established.

►*Children:* Safety and efficacy for children < 1 month old are not established.

Precautions

►*Histamine release:* Exercise caution, especially when substantial histamine release would be hazardous (eg, patients with clinically significant cardiovascular disease, severe anaphylactoid reactions or asthma). The recommended initial dose is lower (0.3 to 0.4 mg/kg); administer slowly or in divided doses over 1 minute.

►*Benzyl alcohol:* This product contains benzyl alcohol, which has been associated with a fatal "gasping syndrome" in premature infants.

►*Bradycardia:* Bradycardia during anesthesia may be more common with atracurium than with other muscle relaxants because atracurium has no clinically significant effects on heart rate. It will not counteract bradycardia or vagal stimulation.

►*Neuromuscular diseases:* Usage in neuromuscular diseases in which potentiation of nondepolarizing agents has been noted (eg, myasthenia gravis, Eaton-Lambert syndrome) may cause profound effects. The use of a peripheral nerve stimulator is especially important for assessing neuromuscular blockade in these patients. Take similar precautions in patients with severe electrolyte disorders or carcinomatosis.

►*Malignant hyperthermia (MH):* Halogenated anesthetic agents and succinylcholine are recognized as the principal pharmacologic triggering agents in MH-susceptible patients; however, because MH can develop in the absence of established triggering agents, the clinician should be prepared to recognize and treat MH in any patient scheduled for general anesthesia. Reports of MH have been rare in cases in which atracurium has been used.

►*Long-term use:* Average infusion rates of 11 to 13 mcg/kg/min (range: 4.5 to 29.5) were required to achieve adequate neuromuscular block. These data suggest that there is wide interpatient variability in dosage requirements. Dosage requirements may decrease or increase with time. Following discontinuation of infusion of atracurium, spontaneous recovery of four twitches in a train-of-four occurred in an average of ≈ 30 minutes (range: 15 to 75 min) and spontaneous recovery to a train-of-four ratio > 75% (the ratio of the height of the fourth to the first twitch in a train-of-four) occurred in an average of ≈ 60 minutes (range: 32 to 108 min).

When atracurium is used in the ICU, it is recommended that neuromuscular transmission be monitored continuously during administration with the help of a nerve stimulator. Do not give additional doses of atracurium or any other neuromuscular blocking agent before there is a definite response to T_1 (first twitch). If no response is elicited, discontinue infusion administration until a response returns.

Drug Interactions

Atracurium Drug Interactions			
Precipitant drug	Object drug*		Description
Diuretics	Atracurium	↑	The neuromuscular blocking effects of atracurium may be increased by thiazide diuretics. Hypokalemia enhances the neuromuscular blockade, possibly by hyperpolarizing the end-plate membrane, increasing resistance to depolarization.

Atracurium Drug Interactions			
Precipitant drug	Object drug*		Description
General anesthetics (enflurane, isoflurane, halothane) Antibiotics (eg, aminoglycosides, polypeptide antibiotics) Lithium Verapamil Procainamide Quinidine	Atracurium	↑	These medications may enhance the neuromuscular blocking action of atracurium. Neuromuscular blockade was prolonged 20% by halothane and 35% by enflurane and isoflurane.
Magnesium sulfate	Atracurium	↑	When administered for the management of toxemia of pregnancy, may enhance neuromuscular blockade of pancuronium. However, in one patient, reversal of neuromuscular blockade was not affected by magnesium sulfate.
Other muscle relaxants	Atracurium	↔	If administered during the same procedure, consider the possibility of a synergistic or antagonist effect.
Phenytoin Theophylline	Atracurium	↓	Phenytoin and theophylline may cause resistance to, or reversal of, the neuromuscular blocking action of atracurium.
Succinylcholine	Atracurium	↑	Succinylcholine does not enhance duration, but quickens onset and may increase depth of atracurium-induced neuromuscular blockade.
Acetylcholinesterase inhibitors (eg, neostigmine, edrophonium and pyridostigmine	Atracurium	↓	Antagonism is inhibited and neuromuscular block is reversed by acetylcholinesterase inhibitors.
Corticosteroids	Atracurium	↑	Prolonged weakness may occur.

* ↑ = Object drug increased. ↓ = Object drug decreased. ↔ = Undetermined effect.

Adverse Reactions

The following adverse reactions are among those reported most frequently, but data are insufficient to estimate incidence.

►*Cardiovascular:* Hypotension, vasodilatation (flushing), tachycardia, bradycardia.

►*Dermatologic:* Rash, urticaria, reaction at injection site.

►*Hypersensitivity:* Allergic reactions (anaphylactic or anaphylactoid responses), rarely severe.

►*Musculoskeletal:* Inadequate block, prolonged block.

►*Respiratory:* Dyspnea, bronchospasm, laryngospasm.

Atracurium Adverse Reactions				
	Initial dose (mg/kg)			
Adverse reaction	0 - 0.3 (n = 485)	0.31 - 0.5[1] (n = 366)	≥ 0.6 (n = 24)	Total (n = 875)
Skin flush	1%	8.7%	9.2%	5%
Erythema	0.6%	0.5%	0%	0.6%
Itching	0.4%	0%	0%	0.2%
Wheezing/Bronchial secretions	0.2%	0.3%	0%	0.2%
Hives	0.2%	0%	0%	0.1%
Vital sign change[2] (≥ 30%)	(n = 365)	(n = 144)	(n = 21)	(n = 530)
Mean arterial pressure				
Increase	1.9%	2.8%	0%	2.1%
Decrease	1.1%	2.1%	14.3%	1.9%
Heart rate				
Increase	1.6%	2.8%	4.8%	2.1%
Decrease	0.8%	0%	0%	0.6%

[1] Recommended range for most patients.
[2] Clinical trials (n = 530) patients without cardiovascular disease.

Overdosage

Excessive doses produce enhanced pharmacological effects. Overdosage may increase risk of histamine release and cardiovascular effects, especially hypotension. Provide cardiovascular support as needed. Ensure airway and ventilation. Longer neuromuscular blockade may occur. Use an anticholinesterase reversing agent (eg, neostigmine, edrophonium, pyridostigmine) with an anticholinergic such as atropine or glycopyrrolate.

CISATRACURIUM BESYLATE

| Rx | Nimbex (GlaxoWellcome) | **Injection:** 2 mg/ml | In 5 and 10[1] ml vials. |
| | | 10 mg/ml | In 20 ml vials. |

[1] Contains 0.9% benzyl alcohol as a preservative.

Indications

▶*Neuromuscular blocker:* An intermediate-onset/intermediate-duration neuromuscular blocking agent for inpatients and outpatients as an adjunct to general anesthesia, to facilitate tracheal intubation and to provide skeletal muscle relaxation during surgery or mechanical ventilation in the ICU.

Administration and Dosage

Administer IV only. The dosage information provided below is intended as a guide only. The use of a peripheral nerve stimulator will permit the most advantageous use of cisatracurium, minimize the possibility of overdosage or underdosage and assist in the evaluation of recovery.

▶*Adults:*

Initial doses – One of two intubating doses of cisatracurium may be chosen, based on the desired time to intubation and the anticipated length of surgery. Doses of 0.15 and 0.2 mg/kg, as components of a propofol/nitrous oxide/oxygen induction-intubation technique, may produce generally good or excellent conditions for tracheal intubation in 2 and 1.5 minutes, respectively, with clinically effective durations of action during propofol anesthesia of 55 and 61 minutes, respectively. Lower doses may result in a longer time for the development of satisfactory conditions.

▶*Elderly/Renal function impairment:* Because slower times to onset of complete neuromuscular block were observed in elderly and renal dysfunction patients, extending the interval between administration of cisatracurium and the intubation attempt for these patients may be required to achieve adequate intubation conditions.

A dose of 0.03 mg/kg is recommended for maintenance of neuromuscular block during prolonged surgery, which sustains neuromuscular block for ≈ 20 minutes. Maintenance dosing is generally required 40 to 50 minutes following an initial dose of 0.15 mg/kg and 50 to 60 minutes following an initial dose of 0.2 mg/kg; the need for maintenance doses should be determined by clinical criteria.

▶*Children (2 to 12 years of age):* The recommended dose is 0.1 mg/kg over 5 to 10 seconds during either halothane or opioid anesthesia. When given during stable opioid/nitrous oxide/oxygen anesthesia, 0.1 mg/kg produces maximum neuromuscular block in an average of 2.8 minutes and clinically effective block for 28 minutes.

▶*Continuous infusion:*

Infusion in the OR – After an initial bolus dose, a diluted solution can be given by continuous infusion to adults and children ≥ 2 years of age for maintenance of neuromuscular block during extended surgery. Adjust the rate of administration according to the patient's response as determined by peripheral nerve stimulation.

Initiate the infusion only after early evidence of spontaneous recovery from the initial bolus dose. An initial infusion rate of 3 mcg/kg/min may be required to rapidly counteract the spontaneous recovery of neuromuscular function. Thereafter, a rate of 1 to 2 mcg/kg/min should be adequate to maintain continuous neuromuscular block in the range of 89% to 99% in most pediatric and adult patients. Consider reduction of the infusion rate by up to 30% to 40% when administered during stable isoflurane or enflurane anesthesia.

The rate of infusion of atracurium required to maintain adequate surgical relaxation in patients undergoing coronary artery bypass surgery with induced hypothermia (25° to 28°C; 77° to 82°F) is approximately half the rate required during normothermia. Based on the structural similarity between cisatracurium and atracurium, a similar effect on the infusion rate of cisatracurium may be expected.

Spontaneous recovery from neuromuscular block following discontinuation of infusion of cisatraurium may be expected to proceed at a rate comparable to that following administration of a single bolus dose.

▶*Infusion in the ICU:* The principles for infusion of cisatracurium, in the OR are also applicable to use in the ICU. An infusion rate of ≈ 3 mcg/kg/min should provide adequate neuromuscular block in adult patients in the ICU. Following recovery from neuromuscular block, readministration of a bolus dose may be necessary to quickly re-establish neuromuscular block prior to reinstitution of the infusion.

▶*Infusion rate tables:* The amount of infusion solution/min will depend on the concentration in the infusion solution, the desired dose and the patient's weight.

Infusion Rates of Cisatracurium for Maintenance of Neuromuscular Block During Opioid/ NitrousOxide/Oxygen Anesthesia

Patient weight (kg)	Drug delivery rate (mcg/kg/min)					Drug delivery rate (mcg/kg/min)				
	1	1.5	2	3	5	1	1.5	2	3	5
	Infusion delivery rate (ml/hr) for a concentration of 0.1 mg/ml					Infusion delivery rate (ml/hr) for a concentration of 0.4 mg/ml				
10	6	9	12	18	30	1.5	2.3	3	4.5	7.5
45	27	41	54	81	135	6.8	10.1	13.5	20.3	33.8
70	42	63	84	126	210	10.5	15.8	21	31.5	52.5
100	60	90	120	180	300	15	22.5	30	45	75

▶*Admixture compatibility/incompatibility:* Cisatracurium injection is acidic (pH = 3.25 to 3.65) and may not be compatible with alkaline solutions having a pH > 8.5 (eg, barbiturate solutions). Cisatracurium is compatible with: 5% Dextrose Injection; 0.9% Sodium Chloride Injection; 5% Dextrose and 0.9% Sodium Chloride Injection; sufentanil; alfentanil HCl; fentanyl; midazolam HCl; droperidol. Cisatracurium is not compatible with propofol or ketorolac for Y-site administration.

▶*Storage/Stability:* Refrigerate vials at 2° to 8°C (36° to 46°F) in the carton. Protect from light. Do NOT freeze. Upon removal from refrigeration to room temperature (25°C; 77°F), use within 21 days even if rerefrigerated. Cisatracurium diluted in 5% Dextrose Injection, 0.9% NaCl Injection or 5% Dextrose and 0.9% NaCl Injection to 0.1 mg/ml may be refrigerated or stored at room temperature for 24 hours without significant loss of potency. Dilutions to 0.1 or 0.2 mg/ml in 5% Dextrose and Lactated Ringer's Injection may be refrigerated for 24 hours. Cisatracurium should not be diluted in Lactated Ringer's Injection due to chemical instability.

Actions

▶*Pharmacology:* Cisatracurium is a nondepolarizing skeletal muscle relaxant. Compared with other neuromuscular blocking agents, it is intermediate in its onset and duration of action. Cisatracurium is one of 10 isomers of atracurium besylate and constitutes ≈ 15% of the mixture. Cisatracurium binds competitively to cholinergic receptors on the motor end-plate to antagonize the action of acetylcholine, resulting in block of neuromuscular transmission. This action is antagonized by acetylcholinesterase inhibitors such as neostigmine.

The neuromuscular blocking potency of cisatracurium is ≈ 3–fold that of atracurium. The time to maximum block is up to 2 minutes longer for equipotent doses of cisatracurium vs atracurium. The clinically effective duration and rate of spontaneous recovery from equipotent doses are similar.

Repeat maintenance doses or a continuous infusion for up to 3 hours is not associated with development of tachyphylaxis or cumulative neuromuscular blocking effects. The time needed to recover from successive maintenance doses does not change with the number of doses administered as long as partial recovery is allowed to occur between doses. Maintenance doses can therefore be administered at relatively regular intervals with predictable results. The rate of spontaneous recovery of neuromuscular function after infusion is independent of the duration of infusion end comparable to the rate of recovery following initial doses.

Long-term infusion (up to 6 days) during mechanical ventilation in the ICU has been evaluated. Patients treated with cisatracurium recovered neuromuscular function following termination of infusion in ≈ 55 minutes vs 178 minutes with vecuronium. In a study comparing cisatracurium and atracurium, patients recovered neuromuscular function in ≈ 50 minutes for both drugs.

In children, cisatracurium has a lower ED_{95} than in adults. At 0.1 mg/kg during opioid anesthesia, cisatracurium had a faster onset and shorter duration of action in children. Recovery following reversal is faster in children.

▶*Pharmacokinetics:*

Metabolism/Excretion – The neuromuscular blocking activity is due to parent drug. The degradation of cisatracurium is largely independent of liver metabolism. Cisatracurium undergoes Hofmann elimination (a pH and temperature dependent chemical process) to form laudanosine and the monoquaternary acrylate metabolite, neither of which has any neuromuscular blocking activity.

CISATRACURIUM BESYLATE

The liver and kidney play a minor role in the elimination of cisatracurium but are primarily pathways for the elimination of metabolites. Therefore, the half-life of metabolites (including laudanosine) are longer in patients with kidney or liver dysfunction and metabolite concentrations may be higher after long-term use. Most importantly, C_{max} values of laudanosine are significantly lower in healthy surgical patients receiving infusions of cisatracurium than in patients receiving infusions of atracurium (mean C_{max}: 60 and 342 ng/ml, respectively). Because cisatracurium is three times more potent than atracurium and lower doses are required, the corresponding laudanosine concentrations following cisatracurium are one-third those that would be expected following an equipotent dose of atracurium.

Approximately 80% of the CL is accounted for by Hofmann elimination and the remaining 20% by renal and hepatic elimination. Following administration to 6 healthy male patients, 95% of the dose was recovered in the urine (mostly as conjugated metabolites) and 4% in the feces; < 10% of the dose was excreted as unchanged parent drug in the urine.

In the studies of healthy surgical patients, mean half-life values ranged from 22 to 29 minutes. The mean half-life values of laudanosine were 3.1 and 3.3 hours in healthy surgical patients receiving cisatracurium or atracurium, respectively. During IV infusions of cisatracurium, C_{max} of laudanosine and the MQA metabolite are ≈ 6% and 11% of the parent compound, respectively.

Special populations:
• *Elderly patients (≥ 65 years of age)* – Volumes of distribution were slightly larger in elderly patients than in young patients resulting in slightly longer half-life values. The rate of equilibration between plasma cisatracurium concentrations and neuromuscular block was slower in elderly patients than in young patients.

• *Hepatic disease* – In 13 patients with end-stage liver disease undergoing liver transplantation and 11 healthy adult patients undergoing elective surgery, the slightly larger volumes of distribution in liver transplant patients were associated with slightly higher plasma clearances of cisatracurium. The times to maximum block were ≈ 1 minute faster in liver transplant patients than in healthy adult patients. The half-life of metabolites are longer in patients with hepatic disease and concentrations may be higher after long-term administration.

• *Renal dysfunction* – In 13 healthy adult patients and 15 patients with endstage renal disease (ESRD) undergoing elective surgery, the times to 90% block were ≈ 1 minute slower in ESRD patients following 0.1 mg/kg. There were no differences in the durations or rates of recovery of cisatracurium between ESRD and healthy adult patients. The half-life of the metabolites is longer in patients with renal failure and concentrations may be higher after long-term administration.

• *ICU patients* – The pharmacokinetics of cisatracurium, atracurium and their metabolites were determined in 12 ICU patients. The plasma clearances of cisatracurium and atracurium are similar. The volume of distribution was larger and the half-life was longer for cisatracurium. The minor differences in pharmacokinetics were not associated with any differences in the recovery profiles.

• *Other patient factors* – Gender and obesity were associated with statistically significant effects on the pharmacokinetics or pharmacodynamics of cisatracurium; these factors were not associated with clinically significant alterations in the predicted onset or recovery profile.

Contraindications

Hypersensitivity to cisatracurium or other bis-benzylisoquinolinium agents; hypersensitivity to benzyl alcohol (10 ml vials only).

Warnings

➤*Administration:* Administer in carefully adjusted dosage by or under the supervision of experienced clinicians who are familiar with the drug's actions and the possible complications of its use. The drug should not be administered unless personnel and facilities for resuscitation and life support (tracheal intubation, artificial ventilation, oxygen therapy) and an antagonist of cisatracurium are immediately available. It is recommended that a peripheral nerve stimulator be used to measure neuromuscular function during administration in order to monitor drug effect, determine the need for additional doses and confirm recovery from neuromuscular block.

➤*Patient distress:* Cisatracurium has no known effect on consciousness, pain threshold or cerebration. To avoid distress to the patient, neuromuscular block should not be induced before unconsciousness.

➤*Benzyl alcohol:* The 10 ml multiple dose vials contain benzyl alcohol. In neonates, benzyl alcohol has been associated with neurological and other complications which are sometimes fatal. Single use vials (5 and 20 ml) do not contain benzyl alcohol.

➤*Renal/Hepatic function impairment:* The onset time was ≈ 1 minute faster in patients with end-stage liver disease and ≈ 1 minute slower in patients with renal dysfunction vs healthy adult control patients. Recovery profile was not altered.

➤*Elderly:* Cisatracurium was safely administered during clinical trials to 145 elderly patients (> 65 years of age) with significant cardiovascular disease. The time to maximum block is ≈ 1 minute slower in elderly patients.

➤*Pregnancy: Category B.* There are no adequate and well controlled studies in pregnant women. Use during pregnancy only if clearly needed.

➤*Lactation:* It is not known whether cisatracurium is excreted in breast milk. Exercise caution following administration to a nursing woman.

➤*Children:* Cisatracurium has not been studied in patients < 2 years of age.

Precautions

➤*Endotracheal intubation:* Because of its intermediate onset of action, cisatraturium is not recommended for rapid sequence endotracheal intubation.

➤*Neuromuscular diseases:* Neuromuscular blocking agents may have a profound effect in patients with neuromuscular diseases (eg, myasthenia gravis and the myasthenic syndrome). In these and other conditions in which prolonged neuromuscular block is a possibility (eg, carcinomatosis), the use of a peripheral nerve stimulator and a dose of ≤ 0.02 mg/kg is recommended to assess the level of neuromuscular block and to monitor dosage requirements.

➤*Burns:* Patients with burns have developed resistance to nondepolarizing neuromuscular blocking agents, including atracurium. The extent of altered response depends on the size of the burn and the time elapsed since the burn injury. Based on structural similarity to atracurium, consider the possibility of increased dosing requirements and shortened duration if cisatracurium is administered to burn patients.

➤*Hemiparesis/Paraparesis:* Patients with hemiparesis or paraparesis may demonstrate resistance to nondepolarizing muscle relaxants in the affected limb. To avoid inaccurate dosing, preform neuromuscular monitoring on a non-paretic limb.

➤*Electrolyte disturbance:* Acid-base or serum electrolyte abnormalities may potentiate or antagonize the action of neuromuscular blocking agents.

➤*Malignant hyperthermia (MH):* Because MH can develop in the absence of established triggering agents, the clinician should be prepared to recognize and treat MH in any patient undergoing general anesthesia.

➤*Long-term use in the ICU:* Long-term infusion (up to 6 days) during mechanical ventilation in the ICU has been safely used. Laudanosine, a major, biologically active metabolite of atracurium and cisatracurium without neuromuscular blocking activity, produces transient hypotension and, in higher doses, cerebral excitatory effects (generalized muscle twitching and seizures) when administered to animals. There have been rare spontaneous reports of seizures in ICU patients who have received atracurium or other agents; these patients usually had predisposing causes. There are insufficient data to determine whether or not laudanosine contributes to seizures in ICU patients. Consistent with the decreased infusion rate requirements for cisatracurium, laudanosine concentrations were lower in patients receiving cisatracurium than in patients receiving atracurium for up to 48 hours.

Drug Interactions

Cisatracurium Besylate Drug Interactions			
Precipitant drug	Object drug*		Description
Antibiotics (eg, aminoglycosides, tetracyclines, bacitracin, polymyxins, lincomycin, clindamycin, colistin, sodium colistimethate) Magnesium salts Lithium Local anesthetics Procainamide Quinidine	Neuromuscular blocking agents (cisatracurium besylate)	↑	Agents that may enhance the neuromuscular blocking action of agents such as cisatracurium.

CISATRACURIUM BESYLATE

Cisatracurium Besylate Drug Interactions			
Precipitant drug	Object drug*		Description
Nitrous oxide/oxygen with either isoflurane or enflurane	Cisatracurium besylate	↑	Isoflurane or enflurane administered with nitrous oxide/oxygen may prolong the clinically effective duration of action of initial and maintenance doses of cisatracurium and decrease the required infusion rate. In long surgical procedures during enflurane and isoflurane anesthesia, less frequent maintenance dosing, lower maintenance doses or reduced infusion rates of cisatracurium may be necessary. The average infusion rate requirement may be decreased by as much as 30% to 40%.
Phenytoin Carbamazepine	Cisatracurium besylate	↓	Resistance to the neuromuscular blocking action of nondepolarizing agents has been demonstrated in patients chronically administered phenytoin or carbamazepine. Slightly shorter durations of neuromuscular block may be anticipated and infusion rate requirements may be higher.
Succinylcholine	Cisatracurium besylate	↑	The time to onset of maximum block following cisatracurium is ≈ 2 minutes faster with prior administration of succinylcholine.

* ↑ = Object drug increased.   ↓ = Object drug decreased.

Adverse Reactions

Bradycardia (0.4%); hypotension, flushing, bronchospasm (0.2%); rash (0.1%).

Overdosage

Overdosage with neuromuscular blocking agents may result in neuromuscular block beyond the time needed for surgery and anesthesia. The primary treatment if maintenance of a patent airway and controlled ventilation until recovery of normal neuromuscular function is assured. Once recovery from neuromuscular block begins, further recovery may be facilitated by use of an anticholinesterase agent (eg, neostigmine, edrophonium) in conjunction with an anticholinergic agent.

▶*Antagonism of neuromuscular block:* Antagonists (such as neostigmine and edrophonium) should not be administered when complete neuromuscular block is evident or suspected. The use of a peripheral nerve stimulator to evaluate recovery and antagonism of neuromuscular block is recommended.

Evaluate patients administered antagonists for evidence of adequate clinical recovery. Ventilation must be supported until no longer required.

DOXACURIUM CHLORIDE

Rx Nuromax (GlaxoWellcome)	Injection: 1 mg/ml	In 5 ml multiple-dose vials.[1]

[1] With 0.9% benzyl alcohol.

WARNING

Administer in carefully adjusted doses by or under the supervision of experienced clinicians who are familiar with the drug's actions and the possible complications of its use. Do not administer unless facilities for intubation, artificial respiration, oxygen therapy and an antagonist are immediately available. Employ a peripheral nerve stimulator to monitor drug response, need for additional relaxants and adequacy of spontaneous recovery or antagonism.

Doxacurium has no known effect on consciousness, pain threshold or cerebration; to avoid patient distress, do not induce neuromuscular blockade before unconsciousness.

Indications

Adjunct to general anesthesia, to provide skeletal muscle relaxation during surgery; to provide skeletal muscle relaxation for endotracheal intubation or to facilitate mechanical ventilation.

Administration and Dosage

▶*Approved by the FDA:* March 1991.

For IV use only.

▶*Individualization of dosages:*

Elderly/renal function impairment – The potential for a prolongation of block may be reduced by decreasing the initial dose and titrating the dose.

Obese patients (≥ 30% more than ideal body weight [IBW] for height) – Determine the dose using the patient's IBW, according to the following formulae:

Men: IBW (kg) = (106 + [6 × inches in height above 5 feet])/2.2

Women: IBW (kg) = (100 + [5 × inches in height above 5 feet])/2.2

Severe liver disease – Dosage requirements are variable; some patients may require a higher than normal initial dose to achieve clinically effective block. Once adequate block is established, the clinical duration of block may be prolonged in such patients relative to patients with normal liver function.

Other conditions – As with other nondepolarizing neuromuscular blocking agents, a reduction of doxacurium dose must be considered in cachectic or debilitated patients, in patients with neuromuscular diseases, severe electrolyte abnormalities, or carcinomatosis, and in other patients in whom potentiation of neuromuscular block or difficulty with reversal is anticipated. Increased doses of doxacurium may be required in burn patients (see Precautions).

▶*Adults:*

Initial doses – When administered as a component of a thiopental/narcotic induction-intubation paradigm as well as for production of long-duration neuromuscular block during surgery, 0.05 mg/kg (2 × ED$_{95}$) produces good-to-excellent conditions for tracheal intubation in 5 minutes in ≈ 90% of patients. Lower doses may result in a longer time for development of satisfactory intubation conditions. Clinically effective neuromuscular block may be expected to last ≈ 100 minutes on average (range, 39 to 232) following 0.05 mg/kg administered to patients receiving balanced anesthesia.

Reserve an initial dose of 0.08 mg/kg (3 × ED$_{95}$) for instances in which a need for very prolonged neuromuscular block is anticipated. In ≈ 90% of patients, good-to-excellent intubation conditions may be expected in 4 minutes after this dose; however, clinically effective block may be expected to persist ≥ 160 minutes (range, 110 to 338).

If doxacurium is administered during steady-state isoflurane, enflurane or halothane anesthesia, consider reduction of the dose by one-third.

When succinylcholine is administered to facilitate tracheal intubation in patients receiving balanced anesthesia, an initial dose of 0.025 mg/kg (ED$_{95}$) doxacurium provides ≈ 60 minutes (range, 9 to 145) of clinically effective neuromuscular block for surgery. For a longer duration of action, a larger initial dose may be administered.

Maintenance doses – Maintenance dosing will generally be required ≈ 60 minutes after an initial dose of 0.025 mg/kg or 100 minutes after an initial dose of 0.05 mg/kg during balanced anesthesia. Repeated maintenance doses administered at 25% T$_1$ recovery may be expected to be required at relatively regular intervals in each patient. The interval may vary considerably between patients. Maintenance doses of 0.005 and 0.01 mg/kg each provide an average 30 minutes (range, 9 to 57) and 45 minutes (range, 14 to 108), respectively, of additional clinically effective neuromuscular block. For shorter or longer desired durations, smaller or larger maintenance doses may be administered.

▶*Children:* When administering during halothane anesthesia, an initial dose of 0.03 mg/kg (ED$_{95}$) produces maximum neuromuscular block in ≈ 7 minutes (range, 5 to 11) and clinically effective block for an average of 30 minutes (range, 12 to 54). Under halothane anesthesia, 0.05 mg/kg produces maximum block in ≈ 4 minutes (range, 2 to 10) and clinically effective block for 45 minutes (range, 30 to 80). Maintenance doses are generally required more frequently in children than in adults. Because of the potentiating effect of halothane seen in adults, a higher dose of doxacurium may be required in children receiving balanced anesthesia than in children receiving halothane anesthesia to achieve a comparable onset and duration of neuromuscular block. Doxacurium has not been studied in children < 2 years of age.

▶*Admixture incompatibility:*

Y-site administration – Doxacurium injection may not be compatible with alkaline solutions with a pH > 8.5 (eg, barbiturate solutions).

▶*Admixture compatibility:* 5% Dextrose Injection; 0.9% Sodium Chloride Injection; 5% Dextrose and 0.9% Sodium Chloride Injection; Lactated Ringer's Injection; 5% Dextrose/Lactated Ringer's Injection; sufentanil citrate; alfentanil HCl; fentanyl citrate.

▶*Storage/Stability:* Store at room temperature of 15° to 25°C (59° to 77°F). Do not freeze.

Doxacurium diluted up to 1:10 in 5% Dextrose Injection or 0.9% Sodium Chloride Injection is physically and chemically stable when stored in polypropylene syringes at 5° to 25° C (41° to 77° F), for up to 24 hours. Immediate use of the diluted product is preferred; discard any unused portion of diluted doxacurium after 8 hours.

Actions

▶*Pharmacology:* Doxacurium chloride is a long-acting, nondepolarizing skeletal muscle relaxant for IV administration. It binds competi-

Nondepolarizing Neuromuscular Blockers

DOXACURIUM CHLORIDE

tively to cholinergic receptors on the motor end-plate to antagonize the action of acetylcholine, resulting in a block of neuromuscular transmission. This action is antagonized by acetylcholinesterase inhibitors, such as neostigmine.

Doxacurium is $\approx$ 2.5 to 3 times more potent than pancuronium and 10 to 12 times more potent than metocurine. Doxacurium in doses of 1.5 to 2 x ED_{95} has a clinical duration of action similar to that of equipotent doses of pancuronium and metocurine. The average ED_{95} (dose required to produce 95% suppression of the adductor pollicis muscle twitch response to ulnar nerve stimulation) is 0.025 mg/kg (range, 0.02 to 0.033) in adults receiving balanced anesthesia.

The onset and clinically effective duration (time from injection to 25% recovery) of doxacurium administered alone or after succinylcholine during stable balanced anesthesia are shown in the following table:

Pharmacodynamic Dose Response to Doxacurium During Balanced Anesthesia[1]			
	Initial doxacurium dose (mg/kg)		
Parameter	0.025[2] (n = 34)	0.05 (n = 27)	0.08 (n = 9)
Time to maximum block (min)	9.3 (5.4 - 16)	5.2 (2.5 - 13)	3.5 (2.4 - 5)
Clinical duration (min; time to 25% recovery)	55 (9 - 145)	100 (39 - 232)	160 (110 - 338)

[1] Values shown are means (range).
[2] Doxacurium administered after 10% to 100% recovery from an intubating dose of succinylcholine.

Initial doses of 0.05 mg/kg (2 x ED_{95}) and 0.08 mg/kg (3 x ED_{95}) given during thiopental-narcotic anesthesia induction produce good-to-excellent conditions for tracheal intubation in 5 and 4 minutes (which are before maximum block), respectively.

The mean time for spontaneous T_1 (first twitch) recovery from 25% to 50% of control following initial doses of doxacurium is $\approx$ 26 minutes (range, 7 to 104) during balanced anesthesia. The mean time for spontaneous T_1 recovery from 25% to 75% is 54 minutes (range, 14 to 184).

Most patients required pharmacologic reversal prior to full spontaneous recovery from neuromuscular block. As with other long-acting neuromuscular blocking agents, doxacurium may be associated with prolonged times to full spontaneous recovery. Following an initial dose of 0.025 mg/kg, some patients may require as long as 4 hours to exhibit full spontaneous recovery.

Cumulative neuromuscular blocking effects are not associated with repeated administration of maintenance doses of doxacurium at 25% T_1 recovery. As with initial doses, however, the duration of action following maintenance doses may vary considerably among patients.

The doxacurium ED_{95} for children 2 to 12 years of age receiving halothane anesthesia is $\approx$ 0.03 mg/kg. Children require higher doses on a mg/kg basis than adults to achieve comparable levels of block. The onset, time and duration of block are shorter in children than adults. During halothane anesthesia, doses of 0.03 and 0.05 mg/kg produce maximum block in $\approx$ 7 and 4 minutes, respectively. The duration of clinically effective block is $\approx$ 30 minutes after an initial dose of 0.03 mg/kg and $\approx$ 45 minutes after 0.05 mg/kg.

The neuromuscular block produced by doxacurium may be antagonized by anticholinesterase agents. The more profound the neuromuscular block at reversal, the longer the time and the greater the dose of anticholinesterase required for recovery of neuromuscular function.

Hematologic – In healthy adult patients, children (2 to 12 years of age) and patients with serious cardiovascular disease undergoing coronary artery bypass grafting, cardiac valvular repair or vascular repair, doxacurium produced no dose-related effects on mean arterial blood pressure or heart rate.

Doses of 0.03 to 0.08 mg/kg (1.2 to 3 x ED_{95}) were not associated with dose-dependent changes in mean plasma histamine concentration. Adverse experiences typically associated with histamine release (eg, bronchospasm, hypotension, tachycardia, cutaneous flushing, urticaria) are very rare.

➤*Pharmacokinetics:* The pharmacokinetics are linear. The pharmacokinetics are similar in healthy young adult and elderly patients. The time to maximum block is longer in elderly patients than in young adult patients (11.2 vs 7.7 minutes at 0.025 mg/kg). In addition, the clinically effective durations of block are more variable and tend to be longer in healthy elderly patients.

A longer half-life can be expected in patients with end-stage kidney disease; in addition, these patients may be more sensitive to the neuromuscular blocking effects of doxacurium. The time to maximum block was slightly longer and the clinically effective duration of block was prolonged in patients with end-stage kidney disease.

Sensitivity to the neuromuscular blocking effects of doxacurium was highly variable in patients undergoing liver transplantation. Three of seven patients developed $\leq$ 50% block, indicating that a reduced sensitivity to doxacurium may occur in such patients. In those patients who developed > 50% neuromuscular block, the time to maximum block and the clinically effective duration tended to be longer than in healthy young adult patients.

Pharmacokinetic and Pharmacodynamic Parameters of Doxacurium[1]							
	Healthy young adult patients (22 to 49 years)				Kidney transplant patients	Liver transplant patients	Healthy elderly patients (67 to 72 yrs)
	Dose (mg/kg)				Dose (mg/kg)	Dose (mg/kg)	Dose (mg/kg)
Parameter	0.015 (n = 9)	0.025 (n = 8)	0.05 (n = 8)	0.08 (n = 8)	0.015 (n = 8)	0.015 (n = 7)	0.025 (n = 8)
Elimination half-life (min)	99 (48 - 193)	86 (25 - 171)	123 (61 - 163)	98 (47 - 163)	221 (84 - 592)	115 (69 - 148)	96 (50 - 114)
Volume of distribution at steady state (L/kg)	0.22 (0.11- 0.43)	0.15 (0.1-0.21)	0.24 (0.13-0.3)	0.22 (0.16-0.33)	0.27 (0.17-0.55)	0.29 (0.17-0.35)	0.22 (0.14-0.4)
Plasma clearance (ml/min/kg)	2.66 (1.35-6.66)	2.22 (1.02-3.95)	2.62 (1.21-5.7)	2.53 (1.88-3.38)	1.23 (0.48-2.4)	2.3 (1.96-3.05)	2.47 (1.58-3.6)
Maximum block (%)	86 (59-100)	97 (88-100)	100	100	98 (95-100)	70 (0-100)	96 (90-100)
Clinically effective duration of block[2] (min)	36 (19-80)	68 (35-90)	91 (47-132)	177 (74-268)	80 (29-133)	52 (20-91)	97 (36-179)

[1] Values shown are means (range).

[2] Time from injection to 25% recovery of the control twitch height.

Consecutively administered maintenance doses of 0.005 mg/kg, each given at 25% T_1 recovery following the preceding dose, do not result in a progressive increase in the plasma concentration of doxacurium or a progressive increase in the depth or duration of block produced by each dose.

Doxacurium is not metabolized; the major elimination pathway is excretion of unchanged drug in urine and bile. In studies of healthy adult patients, 24% to 38% of an administered dose was recovered as parent drug in urine over 6 to 12 hours after dosing. High bile concentrations (relative to plasma) have been found 35 to 90 minutes after administration. The overall extent of biliary excretion is unknown.

Plasma protein binding is $\approx$ 30%.

Contraindications

Hypersensitivity to the drug.

Warnings

➤*Antagonism of neuromuscular block:* Antagonists (such as neostigmine) should not be administered prior to the demonstration of some spontaneous recovery from neuromuscular block. The time for recovery of neuromuscular function following administration of neostigmine is dependent upon the level of residual neuromuscular block at the time of attempted reversal; longer recovery times may be anticipated when neostigmine is administered at more profound levels of block (eg, at < 25% T_1 recovery).

➤*Benzyl alcohol:* Doxacurium injection contains benzyl alcohol. In newborn infants, benzyl alcohol has been associated with an increased incidence of neurological and other complications that are sometimes fatal.

➤*Renal / Hepatic function impairment:* Consider the possibility of prolonged neuromuscular block in patients undergoing renal transplantation and the possibility of a variable onset and duration of neu-

DOXACURIUM CHLORIDE

romuscular block in patients undergoing liver transplantation when doxacurium is used.

►*Elderly:* In elderly patients, the onset of maximum block is slower and the duration of neuromuscular block is more variable and may be longer than in young patients.

►*Pregnancy: Category C.* There are no adequate or well controlled studies in pregnant women. Use during pregnancy only if the potential benefit justifies the risk to the fetus.

Obstetrics (cesarean section) – Because the duration of action of doxacurium exceeds the usual duration of operative obstetrics (cesarean section), doxacurium is not recommended for use in patients undergoing cesarean section.

►*Lactation:* It is not known whether doxacurium is excreted in breast milk. Exercise caution following administration to a nursing woman.

►*Children:* Doxacurium has not been studied in children < 2 years of age. See Actions and Administration and Dosage for use in children 2 to 12 years of age.

Precautions

►*Neuromuscular diseases:* Neuromuscular blocking agents may have a profound effect in patients with neuromuscular diseases (eg, myasthenia gravis and the myasthenic syndrome). In these and other conditions in which prolonged neuromuscular block is a possibility (eg, carcinomatosis), use a peripheral nerve stimulator and a small test dose of doxacurium to assess the level of neuromuscular block and to monitor dosage requirements. Shorter acting muscle relaxants may be more suitable.

►*Burn victims:* Resistance to nondepolarizing neuromuscular blocking agents may develop in patients with burns depending upon the time elapsed since the injury and the size of the burn.

►*Acid-base or serum electrolyte abnormalities:* Acid-base or serum electrolyte abnormalities may potentiate or antagonize the action of neuromuscular blocking agents. Their action may be enhanced by magnesium salts administered for the management of eclampsia or preeclampsia.

►*Obesity:* Administration of doxacurium on the basis of actual body weight is associated with a prolonged duration of action in obese patients (see Actions). Base the dose upon ideal body weight in obese patients (see Administration and Dosage).

►*Malignant hyperthermia (MH):* Doxacurium has not been studied in MH-susceptible patients. Because MH can develop in the absence of established triggering agents, be prepared to recognize and treat MH in any patient receiving general anesthesia.

►*Long-term use:* Information on the use of doxacurium in the ICU is limited. No evidence of tachyphylaxis, accumulation or prolonged recovery has been observed.

When doxacurium is used in the ICU, monitor neuromuscular transmission continuously during administration with the help of a nerve stimulator. Do not give additional doses of doxacurium or any other neuromuscular blocking agent before there is a definite response to T_1 or to the first twitch. If no response is elicited, bolus administration should be delayed until a response returns.

►*Benzyl alcohol:* This product contains the preservative benzyl alcohol, which has been associated with a fatal "gasping syndrome" in premature infants.

Drug Interactions

Doxacurium Chloride Drug Interactions			
Precipitant drug	Object drug*		Description
Antibiotics (eg, aminoglycosides, tetracyclines, bacitracin, polymyxins, lincomycin, clindamycin, colistin and sodium colistimethate)	Doxacurium	↑	May enhance the neuromuscular blocking action of nondepolarizing agents.
Carbamazepine Phenytoin	Doxacurium	↓	Carbamazepine and phenytoin lengthen the time of onset of neuromuscular block induced by doxacurium and shorten the duration of block.
Inhalational anesthetics	Doxacurium	↑	Isoflurane, enflurane, and halothane decrease the ED_{50} of doxacurium by 30% to 45% and may also prolong the duration of action by up to 25%.
Lithium Local anesthetics Magnesium salts Procainamide Quinidine	Doxacurium	↑	May enhance the neuromuscular blocking action of nondepolarizing agents.

* ↑ = Object drug increased. ↓ = Object drug decreased.

Adverse Reactions

The most frequent adverse effect of nondepolarizing blocking agents is an extension of the pharmacological action beyond the time needed for surgery and anesthesia. This effect may vary from skeletal muscle weakness to profound and prolonged skeletal muscle paralysis resulting in respiratory insufficiency and apnea that require manual or mechanical ventilation until recovery (see Overdosage). Inadequate reversal of neuromuscular block from doxacurium is possible.

►*Cardiovascular:* Hypotension, flushing (0.3%); ventricular fibrillation, myocardial infarction (< 0.1%).

►*Dermatologic:* Urticaria, injection site reaction (< 0.1%).

►*Respiratory:* Bronchospasm, wheezing (< 0.1%).

►*Special senses:* Diplopia (< 0.1%).

►*Miscellaneous:* Difficult neuromuscular block reversal, prolonged drug effect, fever (< 0.1%).

Overdosage

Overdosage with neuromuscular blocking agents may result in neuromuscular block beyond the time needed for surgery and anesthesia. The primary treatment is maintenance of a patent airway and controlled ventilation until recovery of normal neuromuscular function. Once evidence of recovery is observed, further recovery may be facilitated by administration of an anticholinesterase agent (eg, neostigmine, edrophonium) in conjunction with an appropriate anticholinergic agent.

MIVACURIUM CHLORIDE

Rx	**Mivacron** (Abbott Hospital)	**Injection:** 2 mg/ml	In 5 and 10 ml single use vials in Water for Injection.

Indications

As an adjunct to general anesthesia, to facilitate tracheal intubation and to provide skeletal muscle relaxation during surgery or mechanical ventilation.

Administration and Dosage

►*Approved by the FDA:* January 22, 1992.

Administer IV only. Individualize doses. Factors that may warrant dosage adjustment include but may not be limited to: The presence of significant kidney, liver or cardiovascular disease, obesity (patients weighing ≥ 30% more than ideal body weight for height), asthma, reduction in plasma cholinesterase activity and the presence of inhalational anesthetic agents. The use of a peripheral nerve stimulator will permit the most advantageous use of mivacurium, minimize the possibility of overdosage or underdosage, and assist in the evaluation of recovery.

►*Renal or hepatic impairment:* 0.15 mg/kg for facilitation of tracheal intubation. However, the clinically effective duration of block produced by this dose is about 1.5 times longer in patients with end-stage kidney disease and about 3 times longer in patients with end-stage liver disease. Decrease infusion rates by as much as 50% in these patients depending on the degree of renal or hepatic impairment.

►*Reduced plasma cholinesterase activity:* Use with great caution, if at all, in patients known or suspected of being homozygous for the atypical plasma cholinesterase gene (see Warnings). Doses of 0.03 mg/kg produced complete neuromuscular block for 26 to 128 minutes in three such patients; thus initial doses > 0.03 mg/kg are not recommended in homozygous patients. Infusions of mivacurium are not recommended in homozygous patients.

Mivacurium has been used safely in patients heterozygous for the atypical plasma cholinesterase gene and in genotypically normal patients with reduced plasma cholinesterase activity. After recommended intubating doses, the clinically effective duration of block in heterozygous patients may be approximately 10 minutes longer. Use lower infusion rates in these patients.

►*Drugs or conditions causing potentiation of or resistance to neuromuscular block:* Cachectic or debilitated patients, patients with neuromuscular diseases or carcinomatosis. In these or other patients in whom potentiation of neuromuscular block or difficulty with reversal may be anticipated, decrease initial dose. A test dose of ≤ 0.015 to 0.02 mg/kg (lower end of the dose-response curve) is recommended.

The neuromuscular blocking action of mivacurium is potentiated by isoflurane or enflurane anesthesia. The initial dose of 0.15 mg/kg may be used for intubation prior to the administration of these agents. If mivacurium is first administered after establishment of stable-state isoflurane or enflurane anesthesia, reduce the initial dose by as much

MIVACURIUM CHLORIDE

as 25%, and reduce the infusion rate by as much as 35% to 40%. A greater potentiation of the neuromuscular blocking action may be expected with higher concentrations of enflurane or isoflurane. The use of halothane requires no adjustment of the initial dose of mivacurium but may prolong the duration of action and decrease the average infusion rate by as much as 20%.

When mivacurium is administered to patients receiving certain antibiotics, magnesium salts, lithium, local anesthetics, procainamide and quinidine, longer durations of neuromuscular block may be expected and infusion requirements may be lower.

➤*Burns:* While patients with burns develop resistance to nondepolarizing neuromuscular blocking agents, they may also have reduced plasma cholinesterase activity. Consequently a test dose of not more than 0.015 to 0.02 mg/kg is recommended, followed by additional dosing guided by the use of a neuromuscular block monitor.

➤*Cardiovascular disease:* In patients with clinically significant cardiovascular disease, use an initial dose of ≤ 0.15 mg/kg, administered over 60 seconds.

➤*Obesity (patients weighing ≥ 30% more than their ideal body weight [IBW]):* Determine the initial dose using the patient's IBW, according to the following formulas:

Men: IBW in kg = (106 + [6 x inches in height above 5 feet])/2.2

Women: IBW in kg = (100 + [5 x inches in height above 5 feet])/2.2

➤*Allergy and sensitivity:* In patients with any history suggestive of a greater sensitivity to the release of histamine or related mediators (eg, asthma), use an initial dose of ≤ 0.15 mg/kg, administered over 60 seconds.

➤*Adults:*

Initial doses – 0.15 mg/kg administered over 5 to 15 seconds for facilitation of tracheal intubation for most patients. When administered as a component of a thiopental/opioid/nitrous oxide/oxygen induction-intubation technique, 0.15 mg/kg (2 x ED_{95}) produces generally good-to-excellent conditions for tracheal intubation in 2.5 minutes. Lower doses may result in a longer time for development of satisfactory intubation conditions. Administration of doses ≥ 0.2 mg/kg is associated with the development of transient decreases in blood pressure in some patients.

Clinically effective neuromuscular block may last for 15 to 20 minutes (range, 9 to 38) and spontaneous recovery may be 95% complete in 25 to 30 minutes (range, 16 to 41) following 0.15 mg/kg administered to patients receiving opioid/nitrous oxide/oxygen anesthesia. Maintenance dosing is generally required approximately 15 minutes after an initial dose of 0.15 mg/kg during opioid/nitrous oxide/oxygen anesthesia. Maintenance doses of 0.1 mg/kg each provide approximately 15 minutes of additional clinically effective block. For shorter or longer durations of action, smaller or larger maintenance doses may be administered.

Continuous infusion – Continuous infusion may be used to maintain neuromuscular block. Upon early evidence of spontaneous recovery from an initial dose, an initial infusion rate of 9 to 10 mcg/kg/min is recommended. If continuous infusion is initiated simultaneously with the administration of an initial dose, use a lower initial infusion rate (eg, 4 mcg/kg/min). In either case, adjust the initial infusion rate according to the response to peripheral nerve stimulation and to clinical criteria. On average, an infusion rate of 6 to 7 mcg/kg/min (range, 1 to 15) will maintain neuromuscular block within the range of 89% to 99% for extended periods in adults receiving opioid/nitrous oxide/oxygen anesthesia. Consider reduction of the infusion rate by up to 35% to 40% when mivacurium is administered during stable-state conditions of isoflurane or enflurane anesthesia.

➤*Children:*

Initial doses – Dosage requirements on a mg/kg basis are higher in children, and onset and recovery of neuromuscular block occur more rapidly. The recommended dose for facilitating tracheal intubation in children 2 to 12 years of age is 0.2 mg/kg administered over 5 to 15 seconds. When administered during stable opioid/nitrous oxide/oxygen anesthesia, 0.2 mg/kg produces maximum neuromuscular block in an average of 1.9 minutes (range, 1.3 to 3.3) and clinically effective block for 10 minutes (range, 6 to 15). Maintenance doses are generally required more frequently in children than in adults. Administration of mivacurium doses above the recommended range (> 0.2 mg/kg) is associated with transient decreases in MAP in some children.

Continuous infusion – Children require higher mivacurium infusion rates. During opioid/nitrous oxide/oxygen anesthesia, the infusion rate required to maintain 89% to 99% neuromuscular block averages 14 mcg/kg/min (range, 5 to 31). The principles for infusion in adults are also applicable to children (see above).

➤*Infusion rate tables:* For adults and children, the amount of infusion solution required per hour depends upon the clinical requirements of the patient, the concentration of mivacurium in the infusion solution and the patient's weight. Consider the contribution of the infusion solution to the fluid requirements of the patient. The following tables provide guidelines for delivery in ml/hr (equivalent to microdrops/min when 60 microdrops = 1 ml) of mivacurium premixed infusion (0.5 mg/ml) and of mivacurium injection (2 mg/ml).

Infusion Rates for Maintenance of Neuromuscular Block During Opioid/Nitrous Oxide/Oxygen Anesthesia Using Mivacurium Premixed Infusion (0.5 mg/ml)										
Patient weight (kg)	Drug delivery rate (mcg/kg/min)									
	4	5	6	7	8	10	14	16	18	20
	Infusion delivery rate (ml/hr)									
10	5	6	7	8	10	12	17	19	22	24
15	7	9	11	13	14	18	25	29	32	36
20	10	12	15	17	19	24	34	38	43	48
25	12	15	18	21	24	30	42	48	54	60
35	17	21	26	29	34	42	59	67	76	84
50	24	30	36	42	48	60	84	96	108	120
60	29	36	43	50	58	72	101	115	130	144
70	34	42	50	59	67	84	118	134	151	168
80	39	48	58	67	77	96	134	154	173	192
90	44	54	65	76	86	108	151	173	194	216
100	48	60	72	84	96	120	168	192	216	240

Infusion Rates for Maintenance of Neuromuscular Block During Opioid/Nitrous Oxide/Oxygen Anesthesia Using Mivacurium Injection (2 mg/ml)										
Patient weight (kg)	Drug delivery rate (mcg/kg/min)									
	4	5	6	7	8	10	14	16	18	20
	Infusion delivery rate (ml/hr)									
10	1.2	1.5	1.8	2.1	2.4	3	4.2	4.8	5.4	6
15	1.8	2.3	2.7	3.2	3.6	4.5	6.3	7.2	8.1	9
20	2.4	3	3.6	4.2	4.8	6	8.4	9.6	10.8	12
25	3	3.8	4.5	5.3	6	7.5	10.5	12	13.5	15
35	4.2	5.3	6.3	7.4	8.4	10.5	14.7	16.8	18.9	21
50	6	7.5	9	10.5	12	15	21	24	27	30
60	7.2	9	10.8	12.6	14.4	18	25.2	28.8	32.4	36
70	8.4	10.5	12.6	14.7	16.8	21	29.4	33.6	37.8	42
80	9.6	12	14.4	16.8	19.2	24	33.6	38.4	43.2	48
90	10.8	13.5	16.2	18.9	21.6	27	37.8	43.2	48.6	54
100	12	15	18	21	24	30	42	48	54	60

➤*Mivacurium premixed infusion in flexible plastic containers:*
Caution – Do not introduce additives into this solution. Do not administer unless solution is clear and container is undamaged. Mivacurium premixed infusion is intended for single patient use only. Discard the unused portion.

Warning – Do not use flexible plastic container in series connections.

➤*Mivacurium injection compatibility and admixtures:*
Y-site administration – Mivacurium may not be compatible with alkaline solutions having a pH> 8.5 (eg, barbiturate solutions).

Mivacurium is compatible with: 5% Dextrose Injection, USP; 0.9% Sodium Chloride Injection, USP; 5% Dextrose and 0.9% Sodium Chloride Injection, USP; Lactated Ringer's Injection, USP; 5% Dextrose in Lactated Ringer's Injection; sufentanil; alfentanil; fentanyl; midazolam; droperidol.

➤*Dilution stability:* Mivacurium diluted to 0.5 mg/ml in 5% Dextrose Injection, USP, 5% Dextrose and 0.9% Sodium Chloride Injection, USP, 0.9% Sodium Chloride Injection, USP, Lactated Ringer's Injection, USP or 5% Dextrose in Lactated Ringer's Injection is physically and chemically stable when stored in PVC (polyvinyl chloride) bags at 5° to 25°C (41° to 77°F) for up to 24 hours. Prepare admixtures of mivacurium for single patient use only and use within 24 hours of preparation. Discard the unused portion of diluted mivacurium after each use.

➤*Storage/Stability:* Store injection and premixed infusion at room temperature of 15° to 25°C (59° to 77°F). Avoid exposure to direct ultraviolet light. Do not freeze. Avoid excessive heat.

Actions

➤*Pharmacology:* Mivacurium is a short-acting, nondepolarizing skeletal muscle relaxant for IV administration. Mivacurium binds competitively to cholinergic receptors on the motor end-plate to antagonize the action of acetylcholine, resulting in a block of neuromuscular transmission. This action is antagonized by acetylcholinesterase inhibitors, such as neostigmine.

Pharmacodynamics – The time to maximum neuromuscular block is similar to intermediate-acting agents (eg, atracurium). The clinically effective duration of action of the stereoisomers in mivacurium is one-

MIVACURIUM CHLORIDE

third to one-half that of intermediate-acting agents and 2 to 2.5 times that of succinylcholine.

The average ED_{95} (dose required to produce 95% suppression of the adductor pollicis muscle twitch response to ulnar nerve stimulation) of mivacurium is 0.07mg/kg (range, 0.06 to 0.09) in adults receiving opioid/nitrous oxide/oxygen anesthesia. The pharmacodynamics of doses of mivacurium $\geq ED_{95}$ administered over 5 to 15 seconds during opioid/nitrous oxide/oxygen anesthesia are summarized in the following table. The mean time for spontaneous recovery of the twitch response from 25% to 75% of control amplitude is about 6 minutes (range, 3 to 9) following an initial dose of 0.15mg/kg, and 7 to 8 minutes (range, 4 to 24) following initial doses of 0.2 or 0.25 mg/kg.

Pharmacodynamic Dose Response to Mivacurium During Opioid/Nitrous Oxide/Oxygen Anesthesia[1]					
		Time to Spontaneous Recovery			
Initial dose (mg/kg)	Time to maximum block (min)	5% recovery (min)	25% recovery[2] (min)	95% recovery[3] (min)	T_4/T_1 ratio $\geq 75\%$[3] (min)
Adults					
0.07 to 0.1 (n = 47)	4.9 (2-7.6)	11 (7-19)	13 (8-24)	21 (10-36)	21 (10-36)
0.15 (n = 50)	3.3 (1.5-8.8)	13 (6-31)	16 (9-38)	26 (16-41)	26 (15-45)
0.2 (n = 50)	2.5 (1.2-6)	16 (10-29)	20 (10-36)	31 (15-51)	34 (19-56)
0.25 (n = 48)	2.3 (1-4.8)	19 (11-29)	23 (14-38)	34 (22-64)	43 (26-75)
Children 2 to 12 years					
0.11 to 0.12 (n = 17)	2.8 (1.2-4.6)	5 (3-9)	7 (4-10)	—	—
0.2 (n = 18)	1.9 (1.3-3.3)	7 (3-12)	10 (6-15)	19 (14-26)	16 (12-23)
0.25 (n = 9)	1.6 (1-2.2)	7 (4-9)	9 (5-12)	—	—

[1] Values shown are medians of means (range).
[2] Clinically effective duration of neuromuscular block.
[3] Data available for as few as 40% of adults in specific dose groups and for 22% of children in the 0.2 mg/kg dose group due to administration of reversal agents or additional doses of mivacurium prior to 95% recovery or T_4/T_1 ratio recovery to $\geq 75\%$.

Volatile anesthetics may decrease the dosing requirement for mivacurium and prolong the duration of action; the magnitude of these effects may be increased as the concentration of the volatile agent is increased. Isoflurane and enflurane may decrease the effective dose of mivacurium by as much as 25%, and may prolong the clinically effective duration of action and decrease the average infusion requirement by as much as 35% to 40%. Halothane has little or no effect on the ED_{50} of mivacurium, but may prolong the duration of action and decrease the average infusion requirement by as much as 20% (see Administration and Dosage).

Administration over 60 seconds does not alter the time to maximum neuromuscular block or the duration of action. The duration of action of the stereoisomers of mivacurium may be prolonged in patients with reduced plasma cholinesterase (pseudocholinesterase) activity (see Precautions and Administration and Dosage).

Interpatient variability in duration of action occurs. However, analysis of data from 224 diverse patients in clinical studies indicated that approximately 90% of the patients had clinically effective durations of block within 8 minutes of the median duration predicted from the dose-response data. Variations in plasma cholinesterase activity were not associated with clinically significant effects or duration. The variability in duration, however, was greater in patients with plasma cholinesterase activity at or slightly below the lower limit of the normal range.

A dose of 0.15 mg/kg (2 x ED_{95}) administered during the induction of anesthesia produced generally good-to-excellent conditions for tracheal intubation in 2.5 minutes. Doses of 0.2 and 0.25 mg/kg (3 and 3.5 x ED_{95}) yielded similar conditions in 2 minutes.

Repeated administration of maintenance doses or continuous infusion for up to 2.5 hours is not associated with development of tachyphylaxis or cumulative neuromuscular blocking effects in ASA Physical Status I-II patients. Spontaneous recovery of neuromuscular function after infusion is independent of the duration of infusion and comparable to recovery reported for single doses.

The neuromuscular block produced by the stereoisomers in mivacurium is readily antagonized by anticholinesterase agents. The more profound the neuromuscular block at the time of reversal, the longer the time and the greater the dose of anticholinesterase agent required for recovery of neuromuscular function.

Children: In children 2 to 12 years, mivacurium has a higher ED_{95} (0.1mg/kg), faster onset, and shorter duration of action than in adults. The mean time for spontaneous recovery of the twitch response from 25% to 75% of control amplitude is about 5 minutes (n = 4) following an

initial dose of 0.2 mg/kg. Recovery following reversal is faster in children than in adults.

Hematologic – Administration of doses up to and including 0.15 mg/kg (2 x ED_{95}) over 5 to 15 seconds to ASA Physical Status I-II patients during opioid/nitrous oxide/oxygen anesthesia is associated with minimal change in mean arterial blood pressure (MAP) or heart rate.

Higher doses of ≥ 0.2 mg/kg (≥ 3 x ED_{95}) may be associated with transient decreases in MAP and increases in heart rate in some patients. These decreases in MAP are usually maximal within 1 to 3 minutes following the dose, typically resolved without treatment in an additional 1 to 3 minutes, and are usually associated with increases in plasma histamine concentration. Decreases in MAP can be minimized by administering mivacurium over 30 or 60 seconds.

Analysis of 426 patients in clinical studies receiving initial doses ≤ 0.3 mg/kg (2 times the recommended intubating dose) during anesthesia showed that high initial doses and a rapid rate of injection contributed to a greater probability of experiencing a decrease of $\geq 30\%$ in MAP after administration. Obese patients also had a greater probability of experiencing a decrease of $\geq 30\%$ in MAP when dosed on the basis of actual body weight, thereby receiving a larger dose than if dosed on the basis of ideal body weight.

Children experience minimal changes in MAP or heart rate after doses ≤ 0.2 mg/kg over 5 to 15 seconds, but higher doses (≥ 0.25 mg/kg) may be associated with transient decreases in MAP.

➤*Pharmacokinetics:*

Metabolism / Excretion – Enzymatic hydrolysis by plasma cholinesterase is the primary mechanism for inactivation of mivacurium and yields a quaternary alcohol and a quaternary monoester metabolite. Renal and biliary excretion of unchanged mivacurium are minor elimination pathways; urine and bile are important elimination pathways for the two metabolites. Each metabolite is unlikely to produce clinically significant neuromuscular, autonomic or cardiovascular effects. The following table describes the results from a study of 9 adult patients receiving an infusion of mivacurium at 5 mcg/kg/min for 60 minutes followed by 10 mcg/kg/min for 60 minutes. Mivacurium is a mixture of isomers which do not interconvert in vivo. The two more potent isomers, *cis-trans* (36% of the mixture) and *trans-trans* (57% of the mixture), have very high clearances that exceed cardiac output reflecting the extensive metabolism by plasma cholinesterase. The volume of distribution is relatively small, reflecting limited tissue distribution secondary to the polarity and large molecular weight of mivacurium. The combination of high metabolic clearance and low distribution volume results in the short elimination half-life of approximately 2 minutes for the two active isomers. The pharmacokinetics of the *cis-trans* and *trans-trans* isomers are dose-proportional. The *cis-cis* isomer (6% of the mixture) has approximately one-tenth the neuromuscular blocking potency of the *trans-trans* and *cis-trans* isomers in cats and data suggest that it produces minimal (< 5%) neuromuscular block during a 2 hour infusion.

Stereoisomer Pharmacokinetic Parameters of Mivacurium in ASA Physical Status I-II Adult Patients (n = 9)[1]			
Parameter	*trans-trans* isomer	*cis-trans* isomer	*cis-cis* isomer
Elimination half-life (min)	2.3 (1.4-3.6)	2.1 (0.8-4.8)	55 (32-102)
Volume of distribution (L/kg)	0.15 (0.06-0.24)	0.27 (0.08-0.56)	0.31 (0.18-0.46)
Plasma clearance (ml/min/kg)	53 (32-105)	99 (52-230)	4.2 (2.4-5.4)

[1] Values shown are mean (range).

Special populations – Preliminary evidence indicates that reduced clearance of one or more isomers is responsible for the longer duration of action of mivacurium seen in patients with end-stage kidney or liver disease. The data did not provide a pharmacokinetic explanation for the 15% to 20% longer duration of block seen in the elderly.

Contraindications

Allergic hypersensitivity to mivacurium or other benzylisoquinolinium agents, as manifested by reactions such as urticaria, severe respiratory distress or hypotension; use of multi-dose vials in patients with allergy to benzyl alcohol.

Warnings

➤*Administration:* Administer in carefully adjusted dosage by or under the supervision of experienced clinicians who are familiar with the drug's actions and the possible complications of its use. The drug should not be administered unless personnel and facilities for resuscitation and life support (tracheal intubation, artificial ventilation, oxygen therapy), and an antagonist of mivacurium are immediately available. Use a peripheral nerve stimulator to measure neuromuscular function during administration in order to monitor drug effect.

➤*Conscious patients:* Mivacurium has no known effect on consciousness, pain threshold, or cerebration. To avoid distress to the patient, neuromuscular block should not be induced before unconsciousness.

MIVACURIUM CHLORIDE

➤*Renal function impairment:* The clinically effective duration of action of 0.15 mg/kg mivacurium was about 1.5 times longer in patients with end-stage kidney disease, presumably due to reduced clearance of one or more isomers.

➤*Hepatic function impairment:* The clinically effective duration of action of 0.15 mg/kg mivacurium was 3 times longer in patients with end-stage liver disease than in healthy patients and is likely related to the markedly decreased plasma cholinesterase activity (30% of healthy patient values) which could decrease the clearance of one or more isomers.

➤*Elderly:* Mivacurium was safely administered during clinical trials to 64 elderly patients ($\geq$ 65 years of age), including 31 patients with significant cardiovascular disease. The duration of neuromuscular block may be slightly longer in elderly patients than in young adult patients.

➤*Pregnancy: Category C.* There are no adequate and well controlled studies in pregnant women. Use during pregnancy only if the potential benefit justifies the potential risk to the fetus.

➤*Lactation:* It is not known whether mivacurium or any of the stereoisomers are excreted in breast milk. Exercise caution following administration to a nursing woman.

➤*Children:* Mivacurium has not been studied in children < 2 years of age (see Administration and Dosage for use in children 2 to 12 years of age). In children 2 to 12 years of age, mivacurium has a faster onset, a shorter duration, and recovery following reversal is faster compared to adults (see Pharmacodynamics).

Precautions

➤*Histamine release:* Although mivacurium is not a potent histamine releaser, the possibility of substantial histamine release must be considered. Release of histamine is related to the dose and speed of injection.

Exercise caution in administering mivacurium to patients with clinically significant cardiovascular disease and patients with any history suggesting a greater sensitivity to the release of histamine or related mediators (eg, asthma). In such patients, use an initial dose of $\leq$ 0.15 mg/kg, administered over 60 seconds; maintain adequate hydration and carefully monitor hemodynamic status.

➤*Obese patients:* Obese patients may be more likely to experience clinically significant transient decreases in MAP than non-obese patients when the dose is based on actual rather than ideal body weight. Determine the initial dose using the patient's ideal body weight.

➤*Bradycardia:* Recommended doses have no clinically significant effects on heart rate; therefore, mivacurium will not counteract the bradycardia produced by many anesthetic agents or by vagal stimulation.

➤*Neuromuscular diseases:* Neuromuscular blocking agents may have a profound effect in patients with neuromuscular diseases (eg, myasthenia gravis and the myasthenic syndrome). In these and other conditions in which prolonged neuromuscular block is a possibility (eg, carcinomatosis), the use of a peripheral nerve stimulator and a dose of $\leq$ 0.015 to 0.02 mg/kg is recommended.

➤*Burn patients:* Mivacurium has not been studied, but resistance to nondepolarizing neuromuscular blocking agents may develop in patients with burns depending upon the time elapsed since the injury and the size of the burn. Patients with burns may have reduced plasma cholinesterase activity which may offset this resistance.

➤*Acid-base or serum electrolyte abnormalities:* Acid-base or serum electrolyte abnormalities may potentiate or antagonize the action of neuromuscular blocking agents; their action may be enhanced by magnesium salts administered for the management of toxemia of pregnancy.

➤*Reduced plasma cholinesterase activity:* Mivacurium is metabolized by plasma cholinesterase. Prolonged neuromuscular block following administration of mivacurium must be considered in patients with reduced plasma cholinesterase (pseudocholinesterase) activity. Plasma cholinesterase activity may be diminished in the presence of genetic abnormalities of plasma cholinesterase (eg, patients heterozygous or homozygous for the atypical plasma cholinesterase gene), pregnancy, liver or kidney disease, malignant tumors, infections, burns, anemia, decompensated heart disease, peptic ulcer or myxedema. Plasma cholinesterase activity may also be diminished by chronic administration of oral contraceptives, glucocorticoids, or certain MAO inhibitors and by irreversible inhibitors of plasma cholinesterase (eg, organophosphate insecticides, echothiophate, certain antineoplastic drugs).

Mivacurium has been used safely in patients heterozygous for the atypical plasma cholinesterase gene. At doses of 0.1 to 0.2 mg/kg, the clinically effective duration of action was 8 to 11 minutes longer in patients heterozygous for the atypical gene than in genotypically normal patients.

As with succinylcholine, patients homozygous for the atypical plasma cholinesterase gene (1 in 2500 patients) are extremely sensitive to the neuromuscular blocking effect of mivacurium. In three such adult patients, a small dose of 0.03 mg/kg (approximately the $ED_{10\ -20}$ in genotypically normal patients) produced complete neuromuscular block for 26 to 128 minutes. Once spontaneous recovery had begun, neuromuscular block in these patients was antagonized with conventional doses of neostigmine. One adult patient, who was homozygous for the atypical plasma cholinesterase gene, received a dose of 0.18 mg/kg and exhibited complete neuromuscular block for about 4 hours. The patient was extubated after 8 hours; reversal was not attempted. Use with great caution, if at all, in patients known to be or suspected of being homozygous for the atypical plasma cholinesterase gene.

Drug Interactions

Mivacurium can be expected to interact similarly to other nondepolarizing neuromuscular blockers. Refer to the Nondepolarizing Neuromuscular Blockers – Curare Preparations group monograph.

Adverse Reactions

Prolonged neuromuscular block was reported in 3 of 2074 patients. The most common adverse experience was transient, dose-dependent cutaneous flushing about the face, neck or chest, most frequently after the initial dose in about 20% of adult patients who received 0.15 mg/kg over 5 to 15 seconds. Flushing typically began within 1 to 2 minutes after the dose and lasted for 3 to 5 minutes. Of 60 patients who experienced flushing after 0.15 mg/kg, one patient also experienced mild hypotension that was not treated, and one patient experienced moderate wheezing that was successfully treated.

➤*Cardiovascular:* Flushing (15%); tachycardia, bradycardia, cardiac arrhythmia, phlebitis (<1%).

➤*Dermatologic:* Rash, urticaria, erythema, injection site reaction (< 1%).

➤*Respiratory:* Bronchospasm, wheezing, hypoxemia (< 1%).

➤*Miscellaneous:*

Hypotension – 1% to 2% of healthy adults given $\geq$ 0.2 mg/kg over 5 to 15 seconds and 2% to 4% of cardiac surgery patients given $\geq$ 0.2 mg/kg over 60 seconds were treated for decreases in blood pressure associated with the administration of mivacurium.

Other – Prolonged drug effect, dizziness, muscle spasms (< 1%).

Overdosage

Overdosage with neuromuscular blocking agents may result in neuromuscular block beyond the time needed for surgery and anesthesia. The primary treatment is maintenance of a patent airway and controlled ventilation until recovery of normal neuromuscular function is ensured. Once evidence of recovery from neuromuscular block is observed, further recovery may be facilitated by administration of an anticholinesterase agent (eg, neostigmine, edrophonium) in conjunction with an appropriate anticholinergic agent. Overdosage may increase the risk of hemodynamic side effects, especially decreases in blood pressure. If needed, cardiovascular support may be provided by proper positioning of the patient, fluid administration, or vasopressor agent administration.

➤*Antagonism of neuromuscular block:* Antagonists (such as neostigmine) should not be administered when complete neuromuscular block is evident or suspected. Use a peripheral nerve stimulator to evaluate recovery and antagonism of neuromuscular block. Administration of 0.03 to 0.064 mg/kg neostigmine or 0.5 mg/kg edrophonium at $\approx$ 10% recovery from neuromuscular block produced 95% recovery of the muscle twitch response and a T_4/T_1 ratio $\geq$ 75% in about 10 minutes. The times from 25% recovery of the muscle twitch response to T_4/T_1 ratio $\geq$ 75% following these doses of antagonists averaged about 7 to 9 minutes. In comparison, average times for spontaneous recovery from 25% to $T_4/T_1 \geq$ 75% were 12 to 13 minutes. Evaluate patients receiving antagonists for adequate clinical evidence of antagonism (eg, 5 second head lift and grip strength). Ventilation must be supported until no longer required.

Antagonism may be delayed in the presence of debilitation, carcinomatosis, and the concomitant use of certain broad-spectrum antibiotics, anesthetic agents and other drugs which enhance neuromuscular block or cause respiratory depression. Management is the same as that of prolonged neuromuscular block.

Nondepolarizing Neuromuscular Blockers

ROCURONIUM BROMIDE

Rx	**Zemuron** (Organon)	**Injection:** 10 mg/mL	In 5 mL and 10 mL multi-dose vials.

> ### WARNING
>
> This drug should be administered by adequately trained individuals familiar with its actions, characteristics, and hazards (see Warnings).

Indications

For inpatients and outpatients as an adjunct to general anesthesia to facilitate both rapid sequence and routine tracheal intubation, and to provide skeletal muscle relaxation during surgery or mechanical ventilation.

Administration and Dosage

➤*Approved by the FDA:* March 17, 1994.

For IV use only. Consider individualization of dosage in each case.

The following dosage information is intended to serve as an initial guide to clinicians familiar with other neuromuscular blocking agents to acquire experience with rocuronium. The monitoring of twitch response is recommended to evaluate recovery from rocuronium and decrease the hazards of overdosage if additional doses are administered.

➤*Rapid sequence intubation:* In appropriately premedicated and adequately anesthetized patients, 0.6 to 1.2 mg/kg will provide excellent or good intubating conditions in most patients in less than 2 minutes.

➤*Dose for tracheal intubation:* The recommended initial dose regardless of anesthetic technique is 0.6 mg/kg. Neuromuscular block sufficient for intubation (at least 80% block) is attained in a median time of 1 minute (range, 0.4 to 6) and most patients have intubation completed within 2 minutes. Maximum blockade is achieved in most patients in less than 3 minutes. This dose may be expected to provide 31 minutes (range, 15 to 85) of clinical relaxation under opioid/nitrous oxide/oxygen anesthesia. Under halothane, isoflurane, and enflurane anesthesia, expect some extension of the period of clinical relaxation.

A lower dose (0.45 mg/kg) may be used. Neuromuscular block sufficient for intubation (at least 80% block) is attained in a median time of 1.3 minutes (range, 0.8 to 6.2) and most patients have intubation completed within 2 minutes. Maximum blockade is achieved in most patients in less than 4 minutes. This dose may be expected to provide 22 minutes (range, 12 to 31) of clinical relaxation under opioid/nitrous oxide/oxygen anesthesia. Patients receiving this low dose of 0.45 mg/kg who achieve less than 90% block (about 16% of these patients) may have a more rapid time to 25% recovery (12 to 15 minutes).

Should there be reason for the selection of a larger bolus dose in individual patients, initial doses of 0.9 or 1.2 mg/kg can be given during surgery under opioid/nitrous oxide/oxygen anesthesia without adverse effects to the cardiovascular system. These doses will provide at least 80% block in most patients in less than 2 minutes, with maximum blockade occurring in most patients in less than 3 minutes. Doses of 0.9 and 1.2 mg/kg may be expected to provide 58 (range, 27 to 111) and 67 minutes (range, 38 to 160), respectively, of clinical relaxation under opioid/nitrous oxide/oxygen anesthesia.

➤*Maintenance:* Maintenance doses of 0.1, 0.15, and 0.2 mg/kg, administered at 25% recovery of control T_1 (defined as 3 twitches of train-of-four), provide a median of 12 (range, 2 to 31), 17 (range, 6 to 50), and 24 minutes (range, 7 to 69) of clinical duration under opioid/nitrous oxide/oxygen anesthesia. In all cases, guide dosing based on the clinical duration following initial dose or prior maintenance dose, and do not administer until recovery of neuromuscular function is evident. A clinically insignificant cumulation of effect with repetitive maintenance dosing has been observed.

➤*Continuous infusion:* Initiate infusion at an initial rate of 10 to 12 mcg/kg/min only after early evidence of spontaneous recovery from an intubating dose. Because of the rapid redistribution and the associated rapid spontaneous recovery, initiation of the infusion after substantial return of neuromuscular function (more than 10% of control T_1) may necessitate additional bolus doses to maintain adequate block for surgery.

Upon reaching the desired level of neuromuscular block, the infusion must be individualized for each patient. Adjust the rate of administration according to the patient's twitch response as monitored with the use of a peripheral nerve stimulator. In clinical trials, infusion rates have ranged from 4 to 16 mcg/kg/min.

Inhalation anesthetics, particularly enflurane and isoflurane, may enhance the neuromuscular blocking action of nondepolarizing muscle relaxants. In the presence of steady-state concentrations of enflurane or isoflurane, it may be necessary to reduce the rate of infusion by 30% to 50% at 45 to 60 min after the intubating dose.

Spontaneous recovery and reversal of neuromuscular blockade following discontinuation of rocuronium may be expected to proceed at rates comparable to that following comparable total doses administered by repetitive bolus injections (See Pharmacology).

Infusion solutions can be prepared by mixing rocuronium with an appropriate infusion solution such as 5% glucose in water or lactated Ringer's (see Admixture compatibility). Discard unused portions of infusion solutions.

➤*Children:* Initial doses of 0.6 mg/kg in children under halothane anesthesia produce excellent to good intubating conditions within 1 minute. The median time to maximum block was 1 minute (range, 0.5 to 3.3). This dose will provide a median time of clinical relaxation of 41 minutes (range, 24 to 68) in children 3 months to 1 year of age and 27 minutes (range, 17 to 41) in children 1 to 12 year of age. Maintenance doses of 0.075 to 0.125 mg/kg, administered upon return of T_1 to 25% of control, provide clinical relaxation for 7 to 10 minutes.

Spontaneous recovery proceeds at approximately the same rate in children 3 months to 1 year of age as in adults, but is more rapid in children 1 to 12 years of age than adults. A continuous infusion initiated at a rate of 12 mcg/kg/min upon return of T_1 to 10% of control (one twitch present in the train-of-four), may also be used to maintain neuromuscular blockade in children. The infusion must be individualized for each patient. Adjust the rate of administration according to the patient's twitch response as monitored with the use of a peripheral nerve stimulator. Spontaneous recovery and reversal of neuromuscular blockade following discontinuation of rocuronium may be expected to proceed at rates comparable to that following similar total exposure to single bolus doses.

➤*Obesity:* In obese patients, base the initial dose of rocuronium 0.6 mg/kg on the patient's actual body weight.

➤*Elderly:* Geriatric patients (65 years of age and older) exhibited a slightly prolonged median clinical duration of 46 (range, 22 to 73), 62 (range, 49 to 75), and 94 minutes (range, 64 to 138) under opioid/nitrous oxide/oxygen anesthesia following doses of 0.6, 0.9 and 1.2 mg/kg, respectively. Maintenance doses of 0.1 and 0.15 mg/kg administered at 25% recovery of T_1 provide approximately 13 and 33 minutes of clinical duration under opioid/nitrous oxide/oxygen anesthesia. The median rate of spontaneous recovery of T_1 from 25% to 75% in geriatric patients is 17 min (range, 7 to 56), which is not different from that in other adults.

➤*Admixture compatibility:* Rocuronium is compatible in solution with 0.9% NaCl solution, sterile water for injection, 5% glucose in water, lactated Ringer's, and 5% glucose in saline. Use within 24 hours of mixing with these solutions.

➤*Admixture incompatibility:* Rocuronium, which has an acid pH, should not be mixed with alkaline solutions (eg, barbiturates) in the same syringe or administered simultaneously during IV infusion through the same needle.

➤*Storage/Stability:* Store under refrigeration, 2° to 8°C (36° to 46°F). Do not freeze. Upon removal from refrigeration to room temperature storage conditions (25°C; 77°F), use within 60 days. Use opened vials within 30 days.

Actions

➤*Pharmacology:* Rocuronium injection is a nondepolarizing neuromuscular blocking agent with a rapid to intermediate onset (depending on dose) and intermediate duration. It acts by competing for cholinergic receptors at the motor end-plate. This action is antagonized by acetylcholinesterase inhibitors such as neostigmine and edrophonium.

The ED_{95} (dose required to produce 95% suppression of the first [T_1] mechanomyographic [MMG] response of the adductor pollicis muscle [thumb] to indirect supramaximal train-of-four stimulation of the ulnar nerve) during opioid/nitrous oxide/oxygen anesthesia is approximately 0.3 mg/kg. Patient variability around the ED_{95} dose suggests that 50% of patients will exhibit T_1 depression of 91% to 97%.

Intubating Conditions in Patients with Intubations Initiated at 60 to 70 seconds		
Rocuronium dose (mg/kg; administered over 5 sec)	Patients with excellent or good intubating conditions[1]	Time to completion of intubation (min; median)
Adults[2] 18 to 64 y		
0.45 (n = 43)	86%	1.6
0.6 (n = 51)	96%	1.6
Pediatric 1 to 12 y		
0.6 (n = 12)	100%	1
Pediatric 3 mo to 1 y		
0.6 (n = 18)	100%	1

[1] Excellent intubating conditions = jaw relaxed, vocal cords apart and immobile, no diaphragmatic movement; good intubating conditions = same as excellent but with some diaphragmatic movement.
[2] Excludes patients undergoing cesarean section.

ROCURONIUM BROMIDE

Time to Onset and Clinical Duration[a] Following Initial (Intubating) Dose (Median)

Rocuronium dose (mg/kg; administered over 5 sec)	Time to ≥ 80% block (min)	Time to maximum block (min)	Clinical duration[a] (min)
Adults 18 to 64 y[b]			
0.45 (n = 50)	1.3	3	22
0.6 (n = 142)	1	1.8	31
0.9 (n = 20)	1.1	1.4	58
1.2 (n = 18)	0.7	1	67
Elderly ≥ 65 y[b]			
0.6 (n = 31)	2.3	3.7	46
0.9 (n = 5)	2	2.5	62
1.2 (n = 7)	1	1.3	94
Pediatric 3 mo to 1 y[c]			
0.6 (n = 17)	-	0.8	41
0.8 (n = 9)	-	0.7	40
Pediatric 1 to 12 y[c]			
0.6 (n = 27)	0.8	1	26
0.8 (n = 18)	-	0.5	30

[a] Clinical duration = time until return to 25% of control T_1. Patients receiving doses of 0.45 mg/kg who achieved less than 90% block (16% of these patients had approximately 12 to 15 minutes to 25% recovery).
[b] Under opioid/nitrous oxide/oxygen anesthesia.
[c] Under halothane anesthesia.

There were no reports of less than satisfactory clinical recovery of neuromuscular function.

The neuromuscular blocking action of rocuronium may be enhanced in the presence of potent inhalation anesthetics.

Hemodynamics – There were no dose-related effects on the incidence of changes from baseline (at least 30%) in mean arterial blood pressure (MAP) or heart rate associated with rocuronium over the dose range of 0.12 to 1.2 mg/kg within 5 minutes after rocuronium administration and prior to intubation. Increases or decreases in MAP were observed in 2% to 5% of geriatric and other adult patients and in about 1% of pediatric patients. Heart rate changes (at least 30%) occurred in 2% or less of geriatric and other adult patients. Tachycardia (at least 30%) occurred in 12 of 127 children. Laryngoscopy and tracheal intubation following rocuronium administration were accompanied by transient tachycardia (at least 30% increases) in about 33% of adult patients under opioid/nitrous oxide/oxygen anesthesia. Animal studies have indicated that the ratio of vagal:neuromuscular block following rocuronium administration is less than vecuronium but greater than pancuronium. The tachycardia observed in some patients may result from this vagal blocking activity.

Histamine release – Clinically significant concentrations of plasma histamine occurred in 1 of 88 patients. Clinical signs of histamine release (eg, flushing, rash, bronchospasm) associated with the administration of rocuronium were reported in 9 of 1137 (0.8%) patients.

►*Pharmacokinetics:*

Absorption/Distribution – Following IV administration, rocuronium plasma levels follow a 3 compartment open model. The rapid distribution half-life is 1 to 2 minutes and the slower distribution half-life is 14 to 18 minutes. Rocuronium is approximately 30% bound to plasma proteins. In geriatric and other adult surgical patients undergoing either opioid/nitrous oxide/oxygen or inhalational anesthesia, the observed pharmacokinetic profile was essentially unchanged.

Tissue redistribution accounts for most (about 80%) of the initial amount of rocuronium administered. As tissue compartments fill with continued dosing (4 to 8 hours), less drug is redistributed away from the site of action and, for an infusion-only dose, the rate to maintain neuromuscular blockade falls to about 20% of the initial infusion rate. The use of a loading dose and a smaller infusion rate reduces the need for adjustment of dose.

Mean Rocuronium Pharmacokinetic Parameters

Parameters	Adults (n = 22; ages 27 to 58 y)	Elderly (n = 20; ≥ 65 y)	Normal renal/hepatic function (n = 10)	Renal transplant patients (n = 10)	Hepatic dysfunction patients (n = 9)
Clearance (L/kg/h)	0.25	0.21	0.16	0.13	0.13
Volume of distribution at steady state (L/kg)	0.25	0.22	0.26	0.34	0.53
Half-life β elimination (h)	1.4	1.5	2.4	2.4	4.3

Metabolism/Excretion – In animals, rocuronium is eliminated primarily by the liver. The rocuronium analog 17-desacetyl-rocuronium, a metabolite, has been rarely observed in the plasma or urine of humans administered single doses of 0.5 to 1 mg/kg with or without a subsequent infusion (for up to 12 hours). In the cat, 17-desacetyl-rocuronium has approximately one-twentieth the neuromuscular blocking potency of rocuronium. In general, patients undergoing cadaver kidney transplant have a small reduction in clearance, which is offset pharmacokinetically by a corresponding increase in volume, such that the net effect is an unchanged plasma half life.

Special populations –

Renal function impairment: Subjects with renal failure have clinical durations that are similar to but somewhat more variable than the duration that one would expect in subjects with normal renal function.

Hepatic function impairment: Patients with demonstrated liver cirrhosis have a marked increase in their volume of distribution resulting in a plasma half life approximately twice that of patients with normal hepatic function. Hepatically impaired patients, because of the large increase in volume, may demonstrate clinical durations approaching 1.5 times that of subjects with normal hepatic function. Individualize the dose to the needs of the patient.

Children –

Mean Rocuronium Pharmacokinetics in Children

Parameters	Patient age range		
	3 to < 12 mo (n = 6)	1 to < 3 y (n = 5)	3 to < 8 y (n = 7)
Clearance (L/kg/h)	0.35	0.32	0.44
Volume of distribution at steady state (L/kg)	0.3	0.26	0.21
Half-life β elimination (h)	1.3	1.1	0.8

Contraindications

Hypersensitivity to rocuronium.

Warnings

►*Administration:* Administer in carefully adjusted dosages by or under the supervision of experienced clinicians familiar with the drug's actions and the possible complications of its use. The drug should not be administered unless facilities for intubation, artificial respiration, oxygen therapy, and an antagonist are immediately available. It is recommended that clinicians administering neuromuscular blocking agents such as rocuronium use a peripheral nerve stimulator to monitor drug response, need for additional relaxant, and adequacy of spontaneous recovery or antagonism.

►*CNS effects:* Rocuronium has no known effect on consciousness, pain threshold, or cerebration. Therefore, its administration must be accompanied by adequate anesthesia or sedation.

►*Myasthenia gravis:* In patients with myasthenia gravis or myasthenic (Eaton-Lambert) syndrome, small doses of nondepolarizing neuromuscular blocking agents may have profound effects. In such patients, a peripheral nerve stimulator and use of a small test dose may be of value in monitoring the response to administration of muscle relaxants.

►*Pulmonary hypertension:* Rocuronium may be associated with increased pulmonary vascular resistance; therefore, caution is appropriate in patients with pulmonary hypertension or valvular heart disease.

►*Burns:* Patients with burns are known to develop resistance to nondepolarizing neuromuscular blocking agents, probably because of up-regulation of postsynaptic skeletal muscle cholinergic receptors.

►*Hypersensitivity reactions:* Although rare, severe anaphylactic reactions to neuromuscular blocking agents have been reported. These reactions have, in some cases, been life threatening. Because of the potential severity of these reactions, take the necessary precautions, such as making appropriate emergency treatment immediately available. Take special precautions in patients who have had previous anaphylactic reactions to other neuromuscular blocking agents, since allergic crossreactivity has been reported in this class of drugs.

►*Renal function impairment:* Because of the limited role of the kidney in the excretion of rocuronium, usual dosing guidelines should be adequate. Rocuronium 0.6 mg/kg has been evaluated in 3 trials (n = 30) in patients undergoing renal transplant surgery, or shunt procedures in preparation for dialysis. The mean clinical duration of 54 ± 22 minutes min was not considered prolonged compared to 46 ± 12 minutes in normal patients; however, there was substantial variation (range, 22 to 90 minutes).

►*Hepatic function impairment:* Since rocuronium is primarily excreted by the liver, use with caution in patients with clinically significant hepatic disease. After 0.6 mg/kg rocuronium, the median clinical duration of 60 minutes (range, 35 to 166) was moderately prolonged in patients with significant hepatic disease compared with 42 minutes in patients with normal hepatic function. The median recovery time of 53 minutes was also prolonged in patients with cirrhosis compared with 20 minutes in patients with normal hepatic function. Four of

ROCURONIUM BROMIDE

8 patients with cirrhosis did not achieve complete block. These findings are consistent with the increase in volume of distribution at steady state observed in patients with significant hepatic disease. If used for rapid sequence induction in patients with ascites, an increased initial dosage may be necessary to assure complete block. Duration will be prolonged in these cases. The use of doses higher than 0.6 mg/kg has not been studied.

➤*Pregnancy:* Category C. There are no adequate and well-controlled studies in pregnant women. Use during pregnancy only if the potential benefit justifies the potential risk to the fetus. Rocuronium is not recommended for rapid sequence induction in cesarean section patients.

➤*Children:* The use of rocuronium in children younger than 3 months of age and older than 14 years of age has not been studied (See Administration and Dosage).

Precautions

➤*Special populations:* Resistance to nondepolarizing agents consistent with up-regulation of skeletal muscle acetylcholine receptors is associated with burns, disuse atrophy, denervation, and direct muscle trauma. Receptor up-regulation also may contribute to the resistance to nondepolarizing muscle relaxants, which sometimes develops in patients with cerebral palsy, patients chronically receiving anticonvulsant agents such as carbamazepine or phenytoin or with chronic exposure to nondepolarizing agents.

Other nondepolarizing neuromuscular blocking agents have been found to exhibit profound neuromuscular blocking effects in cachectic or debilitated patients, patients with neuromuscular diseases, and patients with carcinomatosis. In these or other patients in whom potentiation of neuromuscular block or difficulty with reversal may be anticipated, consider a decrease from the recommended initial dose.

➤*Tolerance:* As with other nondepolarizing neuromuscular blocking drugs, apparent tolerance to rocuronium may develop rarely during chronic administration in the ICU. While the mechanism for development of this resistance is not known, receptor up-regulation may be a contributing factor. It is strongly recommended that neuromuscular transmission be monitored continuously during administration and recovery with the help of a nerve stimulator. Do not give additional doses of rocuronium or any other neuromuscular blocking agent until there is a definite response (one twitch of the train-of-four) to nerve stimulation. Prolonged paralysis and/or skeletal muscle weakness may be noted during initial attempts to wean patients from the ventilator who have chronically received neuromuscular blocking drugs in the ICU. Therefore, only use in this setting if the specific advantages of the drug outweigh the risk.

➤*Malignant hyperthermia (MH):* Because rocuronium is always used with other agents, and the occurrence of MH during anesthesia is possible even in the absence of known triggering agents, be familiar with early signs, confirmatory diagnosis and treatment of MH prior to the start of any anesthetic.

➤*Altered circulation time:* Conditions associated with slower circulation time (eg, cardiovascular disease, advanced age) may be associated with a delay in onset time. Because higher doses of rocuronium produce a longer duration of action, do not increase the initial dosage in these patients to reduce onset time; instead, when feasible, allow more time for the drug to achieve onset of effect.

➤*Electrolyte and acid-base imbalance:* Rocuronium-induced neuromuscular blockade was modified by alkalosis and acidosis in animals. Both respiratory and metabolic acidosis prolonged the recovery time. The potency of rocuronium was significantly enhanced in metabolic acidosis and alkalosis, but was reduced in respiratory alkalosis. In addition, experience with other drugs has suggested that acute (eg, diarrhea) or chronic (eg, adrenocortical insufficiency) electrolyte imbalance may alter neuromuscular blockade. Since electrolyte imbalance and acid-base imbalance are usually mixed, either enhancement or inhibition may occur.

➤*Extravasation:* In animals, rocuronium was well tolerated following IV, intra-arterial, and perivenous administration with only a slight irritation of surrounding tissues observed after perivenous administration. In humans, if extravasation occurs it may be associated with signs or symptoms of local irritation; terminate the injection or infusion immediately and restart in another vein.

Drug Interactions

Rocuronium Drug Interactions			
Precipitant drug	Object drug*		Description
Antibiotics (eg, aminoglycosides, vancomycin, tetracyclines, bacitracin, polymyxin, colistin, sodium colistimethate)	Rocuronium	↑	Coadministration may enhance the neuromuscular blocking action of rocuronium.

Rocuronium Drug Interactions			
Precipitant drug	Object drug*		Description
Azathioprine	Rocuronium	↓	Azathioprine has caused reversal of neuromuscular blocking effects when coadministered with other nondepolarizing muscle relaxants. Consider this possibility for rocuronium.
Carbamazepine	Rocuronium	↓	Rocuronium may have shorter than expected duration or be less effective when given with carbamazepine.
Diuretics	Rocuronium	↔	Diuretics may lead to electrolyte imbalances, which in turn, may modify neuromuscular blockade (see Precautions).
Inhalational anesthetics (eg, halothane, enflurane, isoflurane)	Rocuronium	↑	The use of these drugs with rocuronium will enhance neuromuscular blockade. Potentiation is most prominent with enflurane followed by isoflurane.
Ketamine	Rocuronium	↑	Ketamine has enhanced the actions of other nondepolarizing muscle relaxants, contributing to profound and severe respiratory depression. Consider this possibility for rocuronium.
Magnesium sulfate	Rocuronium	↑	Magnesium sulfate, administered for toxemia of pregnancy, may potentiate the actions of rocuronium.
Phenytoin	Rocuronium	↓	Rocuronium may have shorter than expected duration or be less effective when given with phenytoin.
Quinidine	Rocuronium	↑	The use of quinidine during recovery from use of other muscle relaxants suggests that recurrent paralysis may occur. Consider this possibility for rocuronium.
Succinylcholine	Rocuronium	↑	Prior administration enhances the neuromuscular blocking effect of rocuronium and its duration of action. If succinylcholine is used before rocuronium, delay administration of rocuronium until recovery from succinylcholine has been observed.
Theophyllines	Rocuronium	↓	Theophyllines have produced a dose-dependent reversal of neuromuscular blocking effects with other nondepolarizing muscle relaxants. Consider this possibility for rocuronium.
Verapamil	Rocuronium	↑	Verapamil has caused enhanced effects of other nondepolarizing muscle relaxants. Respiratory depression may be prolonged. Consider this possibility for rocuronium.

* ↑ = Object drug increased. ↓ = Object drug decreased. ↔ = Undetermined clinical effect.

Adverse Reactions

➤*Cardiovascular:* Abnormal ECG, arrhythmia, hypertension, tachycardia, and transient hypotension (less than 1%).

➤*Dermatologic:* Injection site edema, pruritus, and rash (less than 1%).

➤*GI:* Nausea and vomiting (less than 1%).

➤*Respiratory:* Asthma (bronchospasm, rhonchi, wheezing) and hiccup (less than 1%).

➤*Miscellaneous:* There have been reports of severe allergic reactions (anaphylactic and anaphylactoid reactions and shock) with rocuronium, including some that have been life-threatening and rarely fatal (see Warnings).

Overdosage

No cases of significant accidental or intentional overdose with rocuronium have been reported. Overdosage with neuromuscular blocking agents may result in neuromuscular block beyond the time needed for surgery and anesthesia. The primary treatment is maintenance of a patent airway and controlled ventilation until recovery of normal neuromuscular function is assured. Once evidence of recovery from neuromuscular block is observed, further recovery may be facilitated by administration of an anticholinesterase agent (eg, neostigmine, edrophonium) in conjunction with an appropriate anticholinergic agent.

ROCURONIUM BROMIDE

➤*Management of prolonged neuromuscular blockade:* Do not administer antagonists (such as neostigmine) prior to the demonstration of some spontaneous recovery from neuromuscular blockade. The use of a nerve stimulator to document recovery and antagonism of neuromuscular blockade is recommended.

Evaluate patients for adequate clinical evidence of antagonism (eg, 5 sec head lift, adequate phonation, ventilation, upper airway maintenance). Ventilation must be supported until no longer required.

Antagonism may be delayed in the presence of debilitation, carcinomatosis, and concomitant use of certain broad spectrum antibiotics, anesthetic agents or other drugs that enhance neuromuscular blockade or separately cause respiratory depression. Under such circumstances the management is the same as that of prolonged neuromuscular blockade.

PANCURONIUM BROMIDE

Rx	Pancuronium Bromide (Various, eg, Elkins-Sinn, Gensia Sicor)	Injection: 1 mg/mL	In 10 mL vials.[1]
		2 mg/mL	In 2 and 5 mL vials, amps.[1]

[1] With benzyl alcohol.

> **WARNING**
>
> This drug should be administered by adequately trained individuals familiar with its actions, characteristics, and hazards (see Warnings).

Indications

Adjunct to general anesthesia to facilitate tracheal intubation and to provide skeletal muscle relaxation during surgery or mechanical ventilation.

Administration and Dosage

For IV use only. Individualize dosage.

➤*Concomitant therapy:* Because potent inhalation agents or prior administration of succinylcholine enhance the intensity and duration of pancuronium, the lower end of the recommended initial dosage range may suffice when pancuronium bromide is first used after intubation with succinylcholine and/or after maintenance doses of volatile liquid inhalational anesthetics are started.

➤*Adults:* In adults under balanced anesthesia, the initial IV dosage is 0.04 to 0.1 mg/kg. Later, use incremental doses starting at 0.01 mg/kg. These increments slightly increase the magnitude of the blockade and significantly increase the duration of blockade because a significant number of myoneural junctions are still blocked when there is clinical need for more drug.

Skeletal muscle relaxation for endotracheal intubation – Bolus dose of 0.06 to 0.1 mg/kg. Conditions satisfactory for intubation usually occur in 2 to 3 min.

Cesarean section – The dosage to provide relaxation for intubation and operation and the dosage to provide relaxation following use of succinylcholine for intubation (see Drug Interactions) are the same as for general surgical procedures.

➤*Children:* With the exception of neonates, dosage requirements are the same as for adults. Neonates are especially sensitive to this drug class during the first month of life. Give a test dose of 0.02 mg/kg to assess responsiveness.

➤*Admixture compatibility:* Pancuronium is compatible in solution with 0.9% sodium chloride injection, 5% dextrose injection, 5% dextrose and sodium chloride, and lactated Ringer's injection.

➤*Storage/Stability:* Refrigerate at 2° to 8°C (36° to 46°F) to maintain potency for 2 years. If stored at 18° to 22°C (65° to 72°F), potency is maintained for 6 months.

Mixed with compatible solutions in glass or plastic containers, pancuronium will remain stable for 48 hours with no alteration in potency or pH.

Actions

➤*Pharmacology:* Pancuronium, a nondepolarizing neuromuscular blocking agent, possesses all of the characteristic pharmacological actions of this class of drugs (curariform). It acts by competing for cholinergic receptors at the motor end-plate. The antagonism to acetylcholine is inhibited, and neuromuscular block is reversed by anticholinesterase agents such as pyridostigmine, neostigmine, and edrophonium. It is approximately 5 times as potent as d-tubocurarine chloride and approximately one-third less potent than vecuronium.

The most characteristic circulatory effects of pancuronium studied under halothane anesthesia are a moderate rise in heart rate, mean arterial pressure, and cardiac output; systemic vascular resistance is not changed significantly and central venous pressure may fall slightly. The heart rate rise is related inversely to the rate immediately before administration of pancuronium, blocked by prior administration of atropine, and appears unrelated to the concentration of halothane or dose of pancuronium. Histamine release rarely occurs.

The ED_{95} (dose required to produce 95% suppression of the muscle twitch response) is approximately 0.05 mg/kg under balanced anesthesia and 0.03 mg/kg under halothane anesthesia. These doses produce effective skeletal muscle relaxation (as judged by time from maximum effect to 25% recovery of control twitch height) for approximately 22 minutes. The duration from injection to 90% recovery of control

twitch height usually occurs in approximately 65 minutes. The intubating dose of 0.1 mg/kg (balanced anesthesia) will effectively abolish twitch response within approximately 4 minutes; time from injection to 25% recovery from this dose is approximately 100 minutes. Supplemental doses slightly increase the magnitude of blockade and significantly increase the duration of blockade.

➤*Pharmacokinetics:*

Absorption/Distribution – Pancuronium exhibits strong binding to gamma globulin and moderate binding to albumin. Approximately 87% is bound to plasma protein. The volume of distribution ranges from 241 to 280 mL/kg.

Metabolism/Excretion – The elimination half-life of pancuronium ranges between 89 to 161 minutes. Plasma clearance is approximately 1.1 to 1.9 mL/min/kg. Approximately 40% of the total dose of pancuronium has been recovered in urine as unchanged pancuronium and its metabolites, and approximately 11% has been recovered in bile. As much as 25% of an injected dose may be recovered as 3-hydroxy metabolite, which is half as potent a blocking agent as pancuronium. Less than 5% of the injected dose is recovered as 17-hydroxy metabolite and 3.17-dihydroxy metabolite, which have been judged to be approximately 50 times less potent than pancuronium.

Special populations –

Renal function impairment: In patients with renal failure, the elimination half-life is doubled and the plasma clearance is reduced by approximately 60%. The volume of distribution is variable and, in some cases, elevated. The rate of recovery of neuromuscular blockade, as determined by peripheral nerve stimulation is variable and sometimes much slower than normal.

Hepatic function impairment: In patients with cirrhosis, the volume of distribution is increased by approximately 50%, the plasma clearance is decreased by approximately 22%, and the elimination half-life is doubled. Similar results were noted in patients with biliary obstruction, except that plasma clearance was less than half the normal rate. The initial dose to achieve adequate relaxation may thus be high in patients with hepatic and/or biliary tract dysfunction, while the duration of action is greater than usual.

Contraindications

Hypersensitivity to pancuronium.

Warnings

➤*Administration:* Pancuronium bromide injection should be administered in carefully adjusted doses by or under the supervision of experienced clinicians who are familiar with its actions and the possible complications that might occur following its use. Do not administer the drug unless facilities for intubation, artificial respiration, oxygen therapy, and reversal agents are immediately available. The clinician must be prepared to assist or control respiration.

➤*CNS effects:* Pancuronium has no known effect on consciousness, the pain threshold, or cerebration. Accompany administration by adequate anesthesia and sedation.

➤*Myasthenia gravis:* In patients with myasthenia gravis or the myasthenic (Eaton-Lambert) syndrome, small doses of pancuronium may have profound effects. In such patients, a peripheral nerve stimulator and use of a small test dose may be of value in monitoring the response to administration of muscle relaxants.

➤*Renal/Hepatic/Pulmonary function impairment:* Although it has been used successfully in preexisting pulmonary, hepatic, or renal disease, exercise caution in these situations, especially in renal disease, because a major portion of pancuronium is excreted unchanged in the urine. The elimination half-life is doubled, and the plasma clearance is reduced in patients with renal failure; at the same time, the rate of recovery of neuromuscular blockade is variable and sometimes much slower than normal (see Pharmacokinetics).

➤*Pregnancy: Category C.* It is not known whether pancuronium bromide can cause fetal harm when administered to a pregnant woman or if it can affect reproduction capacity. Give pancuronium bromide to a pregnant woman only if the administering clinician decides that the benefits outweigh the risks.

May be used in cesarean section, but reversal of pancuronium may be unsatisfactory in patients receiving magnesium sulfate for toxemia of pregnancy because magnesium salts enhance neuromuscular blockade.

PANCURONIUM BROMIDE

Usually, reduce dosage. Interval between use of pancuronium and delivery should be reasonably short to avoid clinically significant placental transfer.

►*Children:* Dose response studies in children indicate that, with the exception of neonates, dosage requirements are the same as for adults. Neonates are especially sensitive to nondepolarizing neuromuscular blocking agents, such as pancuronium bromide, during the first month of life. It is recommended that a test dose of 0.02 mg/kg be given first in this group to measure responsiveness (see Administration and Dosage).

The prolonged use in neonates undergoing mechanical ventilation has been associated in rare cases with severe skeletal muscle weakness that may be first noted during attempts to wean such patients from the ventilator; these patients usually receive other drugs such as antibiotics which may enhance neuromuscular blockade. Microscopic changes consistent with disuse atrophy have been noted at autopsy. Although a cause-and-effect relationship has not been established, the benefit-to-risk ratio must be considered when there is a need for neuromuscular blockade to facilitate long-term mechanical ventilation of neonates.

Rare cases of unexplained, clinically significant methemoglobinemia have been reported in premature neonates undergoing emergency anesthesia and surgery that included combined use of pancuronium, fentanyl and atropine. A direct cause-and-effect relationship has not been established.

Precautions

►*Monitoring:* Use of a peripheral nerve stimulator will usually be of value for monitoring of neuromuscular blocking effect, avoiding overdosage and assisting in evaluation of recovery.

►*Altered circulation time:* Conditions associated with slower circulation time (cardiovascular disease, old age and edematous states resulting in increased volume of distribution) may contribute to a delay in onset time; do not increase dosage.

►*Hepatic or biliary tract disease:* The doubled elimination half-life and reduced plasma clearance determined in patients with hepatic and/or biliary tract disease, as well as limited data showing that recovery time is prolonged an average of 65% in patients with biliary tract obstruction, suggest that prolongation of neuromuscular blockade may occur. At the same time, these conditions are characterized by an approximately 50% increase in volume of distribution of pancuronium, suggesting that the total initial dose to achieve adequate relaxation may be high in some cases. The possibility of slower onset, higher total dosage, and prolongation of neuromuscular blockage must be considered when pancuronium is used in these patients.

►*Long-term use:* In rare cases, long-term use of neuromuscular blocking drugs to facilitate mechanical ventilation may be associated with prolonged paralysis and/or skeletal muscle weakness that may first be noted during attempts to wean such patients from the ventilator. Typically, such patients receive other drugs such as broad spectrum antibiotics, narcotics and/or steroids and may have electrolyte imbalance and diseases that lead to electrolyte imbalance, hypoxic episodes of varying duration, acid-base imbalance and extreme debilitation, any of which may enhance the actions of a neuromuscular blocking agent. Additionally, patients immobilized for extended periods frequently develop symptoms consistent with disuse muscle atrophy. Therefore, when there is a need for long-term mechanical ventilation, the benefits-to-risk ratio of neuromuscular blockade must be considered.

►*Severe obesity or neuromuscular disease:* Patients with severe obesity or neuromuscular disease may pose airway and/or ventilatory problems requiring special care before, during, and after the use of neuromuscular blocking agents such as pancuronium.

►*Electrolyte imbalance:* Electrolyte imbalance and diseases that lead to electrolyte imbalance, such as adrenal cortical insufficiency, alter neuromuscular blockade. Depending on the nature of the imbalance, either enhancement or inhibition may be expected.

►*Benzyl alcohol:* Benzyl alcohol, contained in some of these products as a preservative, has been associated with a fatal "gasping syndrome" in premature infants.

Drug Interactions

Pancuronium Bromide Drug Interactions			
Precipitant drug	Object drug*		Description
Antibiotics (eg, aminoglycosides, tetracyclines, bacitracin, polymyxin B, capreomycin, vancomycin, clindamycin, lincomycin, colistin, and sodium colistimethate)	Pancuronium	↑	Parenteral/intraperitoneal administration of high doses of certain antibiotics may intensify or produce neuromuscular block on its own. If these agents are used preoperatively or in conjunction with pancuronium during surgery, unexpected prolongation of neuromuscular block is a possibility.
Azathioprine	Pancuronium	↓	Azathioprine may cause reversal of neuromuscular blocking effects of pancuronium.
Carbamazepine	Pancuronium	↓	Pancuronium may have shorter than expected duration or be less effective when given with carbamazepine.
Diuretics	Pancuronium	↔	Diuretics may lead to electrolyte imbalances, which in turn may modify neuromuscular blockade (See Precautions).
Inhalational anesthetics (eg, halothane, enflurane, isoflurane)	Pancuronium	↑	Use of these drugs with pancuronium will enhance neuromuscular blockade. Potentiation is most prominent with use of enflurane and isoflurane.
Ketamine	Pancuronium	↑	Ketamine may enhance the actions of pancuronium, possibly contributing to profound and severe respiratory depression.
Magnesium sulfate	Pancuronium	↑	Magnesium sulfate, administered for toxemia of pregnancy, may potentiate the actions of pancuronium, possibly resulting in profound and severe respiratory depression.
Metocurine/Tubocurarine	Pancuronium	↑	The combination of pancuronium and either metocurine or tubocurarine appears to be synergistic; however, the duration of blockade is not prolonged.
Phenytoin	Pancuronium	↓	Pancuronium may have shorter than expected duration or be less effective when given with phenytoin.
Quinidine, quinine	Pancuronium	↑	Pancuronium effects may be enhanced.
Succinylcholine	Pancuronium	↑	Prior administration enhances the neuromuscular blocking effect of pancuronium and its duration of action. If succinylcholine is used before pancuronium, delay administration of pancuronium until the effects of succinylcholine begin to subside. If a small dose of pancuronium is given at least 3 minutes prior to the administration of succinylcholine to reduce the incidence of and intensity of succinylcholine-induced fasciculations, this dose may induce a degree of neuromuscular block sufficient to cause respiratory depression in some patients.
Theophyllines	Pancuronium	↓	Theophyllines may produce a dose-dependent reversal of neuromuscular blocking effects of pancuronium.
Verapamil	Pancuronium	↑	Nondepolarizing muscle relaxant effects may be enhanced. Respiratory depression may be prolonged. Avoid concurrent use if possible.
Pancuronium	Halothane/Tricyclic antidepressants	↑	Patients receiving chronic tricyclic antidepressant therapy who are anesthetized with halothane should have pancuronium administered with caution because severe ventricular arrhythmias may result from the combination. The severity of arrhythmias appears, in part, related to the dose of pancuronium.

* ↑ = Object drug increased.   ↓ = Object drug decreased.   ↔ = Undetermined clinical effect.

PANCURONIUM BROMIDE

Adverse Reactions

Hypersensitivity reactions – Hypersensitivity reactions (rare), eg, bronchospasm, flushing, redness, hypotension, tachycardia, and other reactions are possibly mediated by histamine release.

Neuromuscular – The most frequent reactions are an extension of pharmacological actions beyond the time period needed. This varies from skeletal muscle weakness to profound and prolonged skeletal muscle paralysis, resulting in respiratory insufficiency or apnea. Inadequate reversal of the neuromuscular blockade is possible. Manage adverse reactions by manual or mechanical ventilation until there is adequate recovery. Prolonged paralysis and/or skeletal muscle weakness have been reported after long-term use to support mechanical ventilation in the intensive care unit.

➤*Cardiovascular:* Arterial pressure, cardiac output, and increase in heart rate; decrease in central venous pressure (see Actions).

➤*Dermatologic:* Transient rash (occasional).

➤*GI:* Salivation during light anesthesia, especially with no anticholinergic premedication.

Overdosage

Residual neuromuscular blockade beyond the time needed may occur, manifested by skeletal muscle weakness, decreased respiratory reserve, low tidal volume, or apnea. May use peripheral nerve stimulator to assess degree of residual neuromuscular blockade.

➤*Management of prolonged neuromuscular blockade:* Pyridostigmine bromide, neostigmine, or edrophonium, in conjunction with atropine or glycopyrrolate, will usually antagonize the action of pancuronium. Judge satisfactory reversal by adequacy of skeletal muscle tone and respiration. Failure of prompt reversal (within 30 minutes) may occur in the presence of extreme debilitation and carcinomatosis and with concomitant use of certain broad spectrum antibiotics or anesthetic agents and other drugs that enhance neuromuscular blockade or cause respiratory depression of their own. Under such circumstances, the management is the same as that of prolonged neuromuscular blockade; support ventilation by artificial means until the patient has resumed respiratory control.

PIPECURONIUM BROMIDE

Rx	**Arduan** (Organon)	**Powder for Injection (lyophilized)**[1]: 10 mg	In 10 ml vials.

[1] Freeze-dried cake with 380 mg mannitol.

WARNING

Administer pipecuronium in carefully adjusted dosage by or under the supervision of experienced clinicians familiar with the drug's actions and the possible complications of its use. Do not administer unless facilities for intubation, artificial respiration, oxygen therapy and an antagonist are within immediate reach. Clinicians administering long-acting neuromuscular blocking agents should employ a peripheral nerve stimulator to monitor drug response, need for additional relaxant and adequacy of spontaneous recovery or antagonism.

Indications

As an adjunct to general anesthesia; to provide skeletal muscle relaxation during surgery; to provide skeletal muscle relaxation for endotracheal intubation.

Pipecuronium is only recommended for procedures anticipated to last ≥ 90 minutes.

Administration and Dosage

For IV use only. Administer by or under the supervision of experienced clinicians familiar with the use of neuromuscular blocking agents. Individualize dosage.

The dosage information that follows serves as an initial guide to clinicians familiar with other neuromuscular block to acquire experience with pipecuronium. The monitoring of twitch response is recommended to evaluate recovery from pipecuronium and decrease the hazards of overdosage if additional doses are administered.

Clinicians administering long-acting neuromuscular blocking agents such as pipecuronium should employ a peripheral nerve stimulator to monitor drug response, need for additional relaxant and adequacy of spontaneous recovery or antagonism.

➤*Individualize dosage:* The table below is to assist those physicians who wish to adjust dosage based on ideal body weight and renal function.

For small patients with decreased renal function, the initial dose is < 70 to 85 mcg/kg, ie, < 2 times the average ED$_{95}$ dose, which is generally the recommended intubating dose for neuromuscular blocking agents. Use extra care during intubation of any patient in whom, in order to decrease the possibility of prolonged clinical duration, < 70 mcg/kg is used for intubation. Dosing in accordance with the following table may reduce the variability in clinical duration to bring ≈ 20% more patients to within ± 30 minutes of the duration predicted by the dose adjusted by ideal body weight and calculated creatinine clearance.

Calculated Dose of Pipecuronium (mg)[1]							
Creatinine clearance (ml/min)[3]	Ideal body weight (kg)[2]						Dose in mcg/kg
	50	60	70	80	90	100	
≤ 40	2.5[4]	3[4]	3.5[4]	4[4]	4.5[4]	5[4]	50[4]
60	2.5[4]	3[4]	3.8	4.9	6.2	7.7	55
80	2.6	3.7	5	6.5	8.3	10[5]	70
≥ 100	3.2	4.6	6.3	8.2	9[5]	10[5]	85 to 100[5]

[1] Based on ideal body weight (IBW) in kg and estimated creatinine clearance; mg = ml if 10 mg vial is reconstituted with 10 ml.
[2] IBW (kg): Men = (106 + [6 lbs/inch in height > 5 ft])/2.2. Women = (100 + [5 lbs/inch in height > 5 ft])/2.2. Use actual body weight in the calculation if it is < IBW.
[3] Estimated Ccr = [{(140 - age in years) × IBW (kg)} ÷ 72 x serum creatinine (mg/dl)}] × 0.85 (for females only).
[4] Minimum calculated dose for intubation; anticipate prolonged clinical blockade.
[5] Maximum calculated dose for intubation; anticipate use of maintenance doses.

➤*Endotracheal intubation:* The recommended initial dose under balanced anesthesia, halothane, isoflurane or enflurane anesthesia in patients with normal renal function who are not obese is 0.07 to 0.085 mg/kg (70 to 85 mcg/kg). Good to excellent intubating conditions are generally provided within 2.5 to 3 minutes. Maximum blockade, usually > 95%, is achieved in ≈ 5 minutes. Doses in this range provide ≈1 to 2 hours of clinical relaxation under balanced anesthesia (range, 47 to 124 minutes). Under halothane, isoflurane and enflurane anesthesia, expect extension of the period of clinical relaxation.

For obese patients (≥ 30% above ideal body weight for height), it is particularly important to consider dosage adjustment according to ideal body weight.

➤*Use following succinylcholine:* If succinylcholine is used to facilitate endotracheal intubation, pipecuronium may be administered after recovery from succinylcholine paralysis. In patients with normal renal function who are not obese, starting doses of 0.05 mg/kg of pipecuronium are recommended and will provide ≈ 45 minutes of clinical relaxation. In nonobese patients with normal renal function, higher pipecuronium doses of 0.07 to 0.085 mg/kg, if administered after recovery from succinylcholine, are associated with approximately the same clinical duration as pipecuronium without prior succinylcholine administration.

➤*Maintenance dosing:* Maintenance doses of 0.01 to 0.015 mg/kg (10 to 15 mcg/kg) administered at 25% recovery of control T_1, provide ≈ 50 minutes (range, 17 to 175 minutes) clinical duration under balanced anesthesia. Consider a lower dose in patients receiving inhalation anesthetics. In all cases, guide dosing based on the clinical duration following initial dose or prior maintenance dose, and do not administer until signs of neuromuscular function are evident.

➤*Children:* Infants (3 months to 1 year) under balanced anesthesia or halothane anesthesia manifest similar dose response to pipecuronium as do adults on a mcg/kg basis. Children (1 to 14 years) under balanced anesthesia or halothane anesthesia may be less sensitive than adults. The clinical duration of doses averaging 0.04 mg/kg (40 mcg/kg) in infants and 0.057 mg/kg (57 mcg/kg) in children, ranged from 10 to 44 minutes and from 18 to 52 minutes, respectively. These doses were ≈ 1.2 times ED$_{95}$.

➤*IV compatibility:* 0.9% NaCl solution; 5% Dextrose in Saline; 5% Dextrose in Water; Lactated Ringer's; Sterile Water for Injection; Bacteriostatic Water for Injection.

Pipecuronium is not recommended for dilution into or administration from large volume IV solutions.

➤*Storage/Stability:* Store at 2° to 30°C (35° to 86°F). Protect from light.

When reconstituted with Bacteriostatic Water for Injection – Contains benzyl alcohol. Use within 5 days. May be stored at room temperature or refrigerated.

When reconstituted with compatible IV solutions – Refrigerate vial. Use within 24 hours. Single use only. Discard unused portion.

Actions

➤*Pharmacology:* Pipecuronium bromide, a long-acting nondepolarizing neuromuscular blocker, possesses the characteristic pharmacological actions of this drug class (curariform). It competes for cholinergic receptors at the motor end-plate. This action is antagonized by acetylcholinesterase inhibitors, such as neostigmine.

➤*Pharmacokinetics:* The individual cumulative ED$_{95}$ (dose required to produce 95% suppression of T_1 [first twitch] of the train-of-four or 95% suppression of single-twitch response) during balanced anesthesia has averaged 41 mcg/kg (range, 20 to 91 mcg/kg). Maximum blockade is

PIPECURONIUM BROMIDE

achieved in ≈ 5 minutes following single doses of 70 to 85 mcg/kg. Under balanced anesthesia, following single doses of 70 mcg/kg, time to recovery to 25% of control (clinical duration) ranged from 30 to 175 minutes. Clinical duration following 80 to 85 mcg/kg single doses varied between 40 to 211 minutes. Pipecuronium has an onset time and clinical duration similar to those of pancuronium bromide at comparable doses.

No significant differences were observed in mean clinical duration of single 100 mcg/kg doses compared with doses of 80 to 85 mcg/kg. Doses >100 mcg/kg are not recommended because of the possibility of even longer duration of action.

The mean time for spontaneous recovery from 25% to 50% of control T_1 is ≈ 24 minutes (range, 8 to 131 minutes).

Pipecuronium can be administered following recovery from succinylcholine when the latter is used to facilitate endotracheal intubation. Preliminary data suggest that, if a single dose of 50 mcg/kg is administered under these conditions, prolongation in clinical duration may be noted (range, 23 to 95 minutes following succinylcholine vs 8 to 50 minutes without it). Initial doses of 70 to 85 mcg/kg used without succinylcholine have produced good to excellent intubation conditions within 2.5 to 3 minutes of injection, which is before maximum blockade.

Mean clinical duration of first maintenance doses of 10 to 15 mcg/kg given at 25% recovery of control T_1 is ≈ 50 minutes (range, 17 to 175 minutes).

Obesity – Clinical durations > 120 minutes for the dose of 70 mcg/kg or > 150 minutes for doses of ≥ 80 mcg/kg occurred in ≈ 8% of cases. In ≈ ⅓ of such cases, dosage was administered to obese patients (defined as ≥ 30% above ideal body weight for height) based on actual body weight. Prolonged clinical duration was ≈ 2 times more common in obese patients.

Renal function impairment – There is an inverse relationship between renal function and clinical duration; the mean clinical duration more than doubles when the calculated creatinine clearance decreases from 100 to 40 ml/min.

Preliminary Pharmacokinetic Parameters of Pipecuronium[1]		
	Mean (range)[2]	
Parameter	Normal renal and hepatic function (n = 4)	Renal transplant (n = 7)
Clearance (L/hr/kg)	0.12 (0.1 - 0.14)	0.08 (0.02 - 0.12)
Volume of distribution at steady state (L/kg)	0.25 (0.12 - 0.37)	0.37 (0.28 - 0.51)
Half-life distribution (min)	6.22 (1.34 - 10.66)	4.33 (1.69 - 6.17)
Half-life elimination (hr)	1.7 (0.9 - 2.7)	4 (2 - 8.2)

[1] Due to the small number of subjects and the interpatient variation, this information is a general guide only. Definitive concentration-effect and pharmacokinetic relationships have not yet been established.

[2] Determined after rapid administration of a single bolus dose of 70 mcg/kg.

The 3–deacetyl metabolite has been detected in the urine of humans undergoing coronary artery bypass surgery. Fifty-six percent of the administered dose was recovered in the urine, of which 41% was unchanged drug, and the remaining 15% was the 3–deacetyl metabolite. No metabolites were found in the plasma.

Warnings

▶*Antagonism of neuromuscular blockade:* Antagonists (such as neostigmine) should not be administered prior to the demonstration of some spontaneous recovery from neuromuscular blockade. The use of a nerve stimulator to document recovery and antagonism of neuromuscular blockade is recommended.

Evaluate patients for adequate clinical evidence of antagonism (eg, 5–second head lift, adequate phonation, ventilation and upper airway maintenance). As with other neuromuscular blocking agents, physicians should be alert to the possibility that the action of the drugs used to antagonize neuromuscular blockade may wear off before plasma levels of pipecuronium have declined sufficiently.

Antagonism may be delayed in the presence of debilitation, carcinomatosis, and concomitant use of certain broad-spectrum antibiotics or

anesthetic agents and other drugs that enhance neuromuscular blockade or separately cause respiratory depression. Management is same as that of prolonged neuromuscular blockade.

Edrophonium doses of 0.5 mg/kg are not as effective as neostigmine doses of 0.04 mg/kg in antagonizing pipecuronium-induced neuromuscular block and is often inadequate. Therefore, the use of edrophonium 0.5 mg/kg is not recommended to antagonize pipecuronium-induced neuromuscular blockade. The use of greater (1 mg/kg) doses of edrophonium or of pyridostigmine has not been investigated.

▶*Hemodynamics:* Clinically significant bradycardia, hypotension and hypertension have occurred. The most common observations, comparing vital signs immediately prior to initial dosage with pipecuronium and 2 minutes after injection, are a slight decrease in heart rate and systolic and diastolic blood pressure.

▶*Myasthenia gravis or myasthenic (Eaton-Lambert) syndrome:* Small doses of nondepolarizing neuromuscular blocking agents may have profound effects. Shorter acting muscle relaxants may be more suitable for these patients.

▶*Long-term use:* Pipecuronium is not recommended for use in patients requiring prolonged mechanical ventilation in the ICU or prior to or following other nondepolarizing neuromuscular blocking agents.

▶*Renal function impairment:* Because it is primarily excreted by the kidney, and because some shorter acting drugs (vecuronium and atracurium) have a more predictable duration of action in patients with renal dysfunction, use with extra caution in patients with renal failure (see Administration and Dosage; Actions).

▶*Pregnancy: Category C.* There are no adequate and well controlled studies in pregnant women. Use during pregnancy only if the potential benefit justifies the potential risk to the fetus.

Obstetrics (cesarean section) – There are insufficient data on placental transfer of pipecuronium and possible related effect(s) upon the neonate following cesarean section delivery. In addition, the duration of action of pipecuronium exceeds the duration of operative obstetrics (cesarean section). Therefore, pipecuronium is not recommended for use in patients undergoing cesarean section.

▶*Children:* Infants (3 months to 1 year of age) under balanced anesthesia or halothane anesthesia manifest similar dose response to pipecuronium as do adults on a mcg/kg basis. Children (1 to 14 years of age) under balanced anesthesia or halothane anesthesia, may be less sensitive than adults. Infants appear to be more sensitive to pipecuronium, but the duration of action is shorter in infants. There are no data on either onset time or clinical duration of larger doses in infants or children. There are no data on maintenance dosing in infants and children.

Precautions

▶*Bradycardia:* Pipecuronium has little or no effect on the heart rate, and it will not counteract the bradycardia produced by many opioid anesthetics or vagal stimulation.

▶*Increased volume of distribution:* Conditions associated with an increased volume of distribution (eg, slower circulation time in cardiovascular disease, old age, edematous states) may be associated with a delay in onset time. Because higher doses may produce a longer duration of action, the initial dosage should not usually be increased to enhance onset time.

▶*Obesity:* The most common patient condition associated with prolonged clinical duration is obesity, defined as ≥ 30% over ideal body weight. Base dose on ideal body weight for height in obese patients (see Administration and Dosage).

▶*Malignant hyperthermia (MH):* Human MH has not been reported with the administration of pipecuronium. Because pipecuronium is never used alone, and because the occurrence of MH during anesthesia is possible even in the absence of known triggering agents, clinicians should be familiar with early signs, confirmatory diagnosis and treatment of MH prior to the start of any anesthetic.

▶*CNS:* Pipecuronium has no known effect on consciousness, pain threshold or cerebration. Therefore administration must be accompanied by adequate anesthesia.

▶*Fluid/Electrolyte imbalance:* Experience with other drugs has suggested that acute (eg, diarrhea) or chronic (eg, adrenocortical insufficiency) electrolyte imbalance may alter neuromuscular blockade. Because electrolyte imbalance and acid-base imbalance are usually mixed, either enhancement or inhibition may occur.

PIPECURONIUM BROMIDE

Drug Interactions

Pipecuronium Bromide Drug Interactions

Precipitant drug	Object drug*		Description
Anesthetics, inhalational	Pipecuronium	↑	Use of volatile inhalation anesthetics enhances the activity of other neuromuscular blocking agents on the order of enflurane> isoflurane > halothane. Minimal effects are generally observed on onset time and peak effect. In routine use of neuromuscular blocking agents, only clinical duration is generally affected (prolonged). Use of isoflurane has resulted in an increase in mean clinical duration of 12%. In 25 patients first anesthetized with enflurane for ≥ 5 minutes, the mean clinical duration was increased by 50%. Therefore, anticipate a prolonged clinical duration following initial or maintenance doses and prolonged recovery from the neuromuscular blocking effect of pipecuronium.
Antibiotics (eg, aminoglycosides; tetracyclines; bacitracin; polymyxin B; colistin; sodium colistimethate)	Pipecuronium	↑	Parenteral/intraperitoneal administration of high doses of certain antibiotics may intensify or produce neuromuscular block on their own. If these antibiotics are used in conjunction with pipecuronium during surgery, consider prolongation of neuromuscular block a possibility.
Magnesium salts	Pipecuronium	↑	Administration for the management of toxemia of pregnancy may enhance neuromuscular blockade.
Quinidine	Pipecuronium	↑	Experience concerning injection of quinidine during recovery from use of other muscle relaxants suggests that recurrent paralysis may occur. This possibility must also be considered for pipecuronium.
Succinylcholine	Pipecuronium	↑	Pipecuronium can be administered following recovery from succinylcholine when the latter is used to facilitate endotracheal intubation. The use of pipecuronium before succinylcholine, in order to attenuate some of the side effects of succinylcholine, is not recommended. (See Pharmacokinetics.)

* ↑ = Object drug increased.

Adverse Reactions

The most frequent side effect of nondepolarizing blocking agents is an extension of the drug's pharmacological action beyond the time period needed for surgery and anesthesia. Clinical signs may vary from skeletal muscle weakness to skeletal muscle paralysis resulting in respiratory insufficiency or apnea. This may be due to the drug's effect or inadequate antagonism.

➤*Cardiovascular:* Hypotension (2.5%); bradycardia (1.4%); hypertension, myocardial ischemia, cerebrovascular accident, thrombosis, atrial fibrillation, ventricular extrasystole (< 1%).

➤*Metabolic/Nutritional:* Hypoglycemia, hyperkalemia, increased creatinine (< 1%).

➤*Musculoskeletal:* Muscle atrophy, difficult intubation (< 1%).

➤*Respiratory:* Dyspnea, respiratory depression, laryngismus, atelectasis (< 1%).

➤*Miscellaneous:* Hypesthesia, CNS depression, anuria, rash, urticaria (< 1%).

Overdosage

➤*Treatment:* Support ventilation by artificial means until no longer required. Intensified monitoring of vital organ function is required for the period of paralysis and during an extended period postrecovery.

VECURONIUM BROMIDE

Rx	**Vecuronium Bromide** (Various, eg, Abbott, Baxter, Bedford)	**Powder for Injection:** 10 mg[1]	In 10 mL vials.
Rx	**Norcuron** (Organon)		In 10 mL vials with and without diluent.[2]
Rx	**Vecuronium Bromide** (Various, eg, Abbott, Baxter, Bedford)	**Powder for Injection:** 20 mg[1]	In 20 mL vials.
Rx	**Norcuron** (Organon)		In 20 mL vials without diluent.

[1] May contain mannitol.
[2] Contains 0.9% benzyl alcohol.

WARNING

Do not administer unless facilities for intubation, artificial respiration, oxygen therapy and reversal agents are immediately available. Be prepared to assist or control respiration.

Indications

To use as an adjunct to general anesthesia, to facilitate endotracheal intubation and to provide skeletal muscle relaxation during surgery or mechanical ventilation.

Administration and Dosage

For IV use only. Individualize dosage.

Vecuronium has no known effect on consciousness, pain threshold or cerebration. Administration must be accompanied by adequate anesthesia.

➤*Initial adult dose:* 0.08 to 0.1 mg/kg (1.4 to 1.75 times the ED_{90}) as an IV bolus injection to produce good or excellent nonemergency intubation conditions in 2.5 to 3 minutes. Under balanced anesthesia, clinically required neuromuscular blockade lasts ≈ 25 to 30 minutes, with recovery to 25% of control achieved in ≈ 25 to 40 minutes and recovery to 95% of control in 25 to 40 minutes. In the presence of potent inhalation anesthetics, vecuronium's neuromuscular blocking effect is enhanced. If vecuronium is first administered > 5 minutes after the start of inhalation agents or when steady state has been achieved, the initial dose may be reduced by ≈ 15%.

Prior administration of succinylcholine may enhance vecuronium's neuromuscular blocking effect and duration of action. If intubation is performed using succinylcholine, a reduction of initial dose of vecuronium to 0.04 to 0.06 mg/kg with inhalation anesthesia and 0.05 to 0.06 mg/kg with balanced anesthesia may be required.

➤*Maintenance dosage:* During prolonged surgical procedures, 0.01 to 0.015 mg/kg is recommended. The first maintenance dose is generally required within 25 to 40 minutes. Use clinical criteria to determine the need for maintenance doses. Because the drug lacks cumulative effects, subsequent maintenance doses may be administered at ≈ 12 to 15 minute intervals under balanced anesthesia, and slightly longer under inhalation agents. (If less frequent administration is desired, administer higher maintenance doses.)

If larger doses are necessary, initial doses ranging from 0.15 mg/kg up to 0.28 mg/kg have been given with proper ventilation during surgery under halothane without cardiovascular effects.

After an intubating dose of 0.08 to 0.1 mg/kg, a continuous infusion of 0.001 mg/kg/min can be initiated ≈ 20 to 40 minutes later. Infusion of vecuronium should be initiated only after early evidence of spontaneous recovery from the bolus dose.

➤*Children (10 to 17 years):* Administer adult dosage.

➤*Admixture compatibility:* 0.9% Sodium Chloride, 5% Dextrose in Saline or Water, Lactated Ringer's Solution and Sterile Water for Injection.

➤*Storage/Stability:* Store at 15° to 30°C (59° to 86°F). Protect from light. May be stored at room temperature or refrigerated. When reconstituted with supplied bacteriostatic water for injection, use within 5 days.

When reconstituted with sterile water for injection or other compatible IV solutions, refrigerate vial. Use within 24 hours. Single use only. Discard unused portion.

Actions

➤*Pharmacology:* Vecuronium bromide, a nondepolarizing neuromuscular blocking agent of intermediate duration, possesses the pharmacologic actions of the curariform class. It competes for cholinergic receptors at the motor end-plate, and its effects are reversed by acetylcholinesterase inhibitors. Vecuronium is about ⅓ more potent than pancuronium, but its duration of activity is shorter at initially equipotent doses. The time to onset of paralysis decreases and the duration of maximum effect increases with increasing doses.

VECURONIUM BROMIDE

▶*Pharmacokinetics:*

Onset, peak and duration of action – The ED_{90} (dose required to produce 90% suppression of the muscle twitch response with balanced anesthesia) averages 0.057 mg/kg (0.049 to 0.062 mg/kg). Following an initial IV dose of 0.08 to 0.1 mg/kg, vecuronium produces the first depression of twitch in 1 minute, good intubation conditions within 2.5 to 3 minutes and maximum neuromuscular blockade within 3 to 5 minutes. Under balanced anesthesia, the recovery time to 25% of control is ≈ 25 to 40 minutes after injection; recovery is usually 95% complete in 45 to 65 minutes.

Repeated maintenance doses have little or no cumulative effect on duration of blockade. The first maintenance dose is generally required in 25 to 40 minutes, and subsequent doses are required at 12 to 15 minute intervals.

Recovery index (time from 25% to 75% recovery) is ≈ 15 to 25 minutes under balanced or halothane anesthesia, more rapid than recovery from pancuronium.

Absorption/Distribution – Following a single IV dose, the distribution half-life is ≈ 4 minutes. Plasma protein binding is 60% to 80%.

Metabolism/Excretion – Only unchanged vecuronium bromide has been detected in human plasma. One metabolite, 3-deacetyl vecuronium, has been identified in urine and in bile at concentrations of 10% and 25%, respectively, of the injected dose. Elimination half-life is 65 to 75 minutes in healthy surgical patients and in renal failure patients. A shortened half-life of ≈ 35 to 40 minutes has been reported in late pregnancy. The volume of distribution at steady state is ≈ 300 to 400 ml/kg; systemic rate of clearance is ≈ 3 to 4.5 ml/min/kg.

In patients with cirrhosis or cholestasis, recovery time may be doubled. Renal failure does not appear to significantly affect recovery times.

Urine recovery of vecuronium bromide varies from 3% to 35% in 24 hours. Approximately 25% to 50% may be excreted in bile within 42 hours.

Contraindications

Hypersensitivity to vecuronium.

Warnings

▶*Myasthenia gravis:* In patients who have myasthenia gravis or myasthenic (Eaton-Lambert) syndrome, small doses of vecuronium may have profound effects. In such patients, a peripheral nerve stimulator and use of a small test dose may be of value in monitoring the response to muscle relaxants.

▶*Long-term use:* Long-term IV infusion to support mechanical ventilation in ICU has not been studied sufficiently to support dosage recommendations.

Whenever the use of vecuronium or any neuromuscular blocking agent is contemplated in the ICU, it is recommended that neuromuscular transmission be monitored continuously during administration and recovery with the help of a nerve stimulator. Use of a peripheral nerve stimulator for adequate monitoring of neuromuscular blocking effect will preclude inadvertent excess dosing. Additional doses of vecuronium, or any other neuromuscular blocking agent, should not be given before there is a definite response to T_1 (first twitch). If no response is elicited, infusion administration should be discontinued until a response returns.

▶*Renal/Hepatic function impairment:* Vecuronium is well tolerated without significant prolongation of neuromuscular blocking effect in patients with renal failure who have been optimally prepared for surgery by dialysis. If anephric patients cannot be prepared for non-elective surgery, prolongation of neuromuscular blockade may occur; therefore, consider a lower initial dose of the drug.

Patients with cirrhosis or cholestasis have prolonged recovery times. Current data do not permit dosage recommendations in patients with impaired liver function.

▶*Pregnancy: Category C.* Safety for use during pregnancy has not been established. Use only when clearly needed and when the potential benefits outweigh the unknown potential hazards to the fetus.

▶*Children:* Infants < 1 year of age but > 7 weeks, also tested under halothane anesthesia, are moderately more sensitive to vecuronium on a mg/kg basis than adults and take ≈ 1½ times as long to recover. Available information does not permit recommendations for usage in neonates.

Precautions

▶*Altered circulation time:* Conditions associated with slower circulation time (cardiovascular disease, old age and edematous states resulting in increased volume of distribution) may contribute to a delay in onset time; therefore, do not increase dosage.

▶*Severe obesity or neuromuscular disease:* Severe obesity or neuromuscular disease may pose airway or ventilatory problems requiring special care before, during and after the use of vecuronium.

▶*Malignant hyperthermia (MH):* Many drugs used in anesthetic practice are suspected of being capable of triggering MH. Data are insufficient to establish whether vecuronium is capable of triggering MH.

▶*Electrolyte imbalance:* Electrolyte imbalance and diseases which lead to electrolyte imbalance, such as adrenal cortical insufficiency, have altered neuromuscular blockade. Depending on the nature of the imbalance, either enhancement or inhibition may be expected.

▶*Benzyl alcohol:* Benzyl alcohol, contained in some of these products as a preservative, has been associated with a fatal "gasping syndrome" in premature infants.

Drug Interactions

Vecuronium Bromide Drug Interactions			
Precipitant drug	Object drug*		Description
Antibiotics (eg, aminoglycosides, tetracyclines, bacitracin, polymyxin B, colistin and sodium colistimethate)	Vecuronium	↑	Parenteral/intraperitoneal administration of high doses of certain antibiotics may intensify or produce neuromuscular blockade on their own. If these or other newly introduced antibiotics are used with vecuronium during surgery, consider the possibility of unexpected prolongation of neuromuscular block.
Inhalational anesthetics (eg, enflurane, isoflurane and halothane)	Vecuronium	↑	Inhalational anesthetics given with vecuronium will enhance neuromuscular blockade. Potentiation is most prominent with use of enflurane and isoflurane. With the above agents, the initial dose of vecuronium may be the same as with balanced anesthesia unless the inhalational anesthetic has been administered for a sufficient time at a sufficient dose to have reached clinical equilibrium. If vecuronium is first administered > 5 minutes after the start of the inhalation of enflurane, isoflurane or halothane, or when steady state has been achieved, the intubating dose of vecuronium may be decreased by ≈ 15%.
Magnesium salts	Vecuronium	↑	Magnesium salts, administered for the management of toxemia of pregnancy, may enhance the neuromuscular blockade of vecuronium.
Quinidine	Vecuronium	↑	Recurrent paralysis may occur with injection of quinidine during recovery from use of other muscle relaxants. Consider this possibility with vecuronium.
Succinylcholine	Vecuronium	↑	Prior administration of succinylcholine may enhance vecuronium's neuromuscular blocking effect and its duration of action. If succinylcholine is used first, delay the administration of vecuronium until the succinylcholine effect shows signs of wearing off.

* ↑ = Object drug increased.

Adverse Reactions

The most frequent adverse reaction to nondepolarizing blocking agents as a class is an extension of the drug's pharmacological action. This may vary from skeletal muscle weakness to profound and prolonged skeletal muscle paralysis resulting in respiratory insufficiency or apnea.

Vecuronium in doses up to 3 times those needed for clinical relaxation did not produce clinically significant changes in systolic, diastolic or mean arterial pressure.

Inadequate reversal of the neuromuscular blockade is possible. Manage these adverse reactions by manual or mechanical ventilation until recovery. Little or no increase in intensity of blockade or duration of action of vecuronium is noted from the use of thiobarbiturates, narcotic analgesics, nitrous oxide or droperidol. (See Overdosage.)

▶*Hypersensitivity:* Hypersensitivity reactions such as bronchospasm, flushing, redness, hypotension, tachycardia and other reactions commonly associated with histamine release are unlikely to occur.

Overdosage

Excessive doses can produce enhanced pharmacological effects. This may be manifested by skeletal muscle weakness, decreased respiratory reserve, low tidal volume or apnea. Use a peripheral nerve stimulator to assess the degree of residual neuromuscular blockade and to differentiate residual neuromuscular blockade from other causes of decreased respiratory reserve.

SUCCINYLCHOLINE CHLORIDE

Rx	**Anectine** (GlaxoWellcome)	**Injection:** 20 mg/ml	In 10 ml vials.[1]
Rx	**Quelicin** (Abbott)		In 5 ml *Abboject* (single-dose) syringeand 10 ml vials.[2]
Rx	**Succinylcholine Chloride** (Organon)		In 10 ml vials.[3]
Rx	**Quelicin** (Abbott)	**Injection:** 50 mg/ml	In 10 ml amps.
Rx	**Anectine Flo-Pack** (GlaxoWellcome)	**Powder for infusion:** 500 mg	In vials.
		Powder for infusion: 1 g	In vials.

[1] With methylparaben.
[2] With methyl- and propylparabens.

[3] With benzyl alcohol.

WARNING

Use succinylcholine only if skilled in the management of artificial respiration and when facilities are instantly available for tracheal intubation and for providing adequate ventilation of the patient, including the administration of oxygen under positive pressure and the elimination of carbon dioxide. The clinician must be prepared to assist or control respiration.

Indications

►*Anesthesia:* Adjunct to general anesthesia to facilitate endotracheal intubation, and to induce skeletal muscle relaxation during surgery or mechanical ventilation.

Administration and Dosage

Individualize dosage.

To avoid patient distress, administer after unconsciousness has been induced.

►*Short surgical procedures:* The average dose required to induce muscle relaxation of short duration is 0.6 mg/kg IV. The optimum dose varies among individuals and may range from 0.3 to 1.1 mg/kg. Maximum paralysis may persist for ≈ 2 minutes. Recovery takes place within 4 to 6 minutes.

Following an injection of an effective dose of succinylcholine, relaxation sufficient for endotracheal intubation generally occurs in ≈ 1 minute. Administer more succinylcholine at appropriate intervals if relaxation is not complete.

►*Long surgical procedures:* Dosage depends on duration of procedure and the need for muscle relaxation. Average rate for an adult ranges between 2.5 and 4.3 mg/min. Solutions containing 0.1% to 0.2% (1 to 2 mg/ml) are commonly used for continuous IV drip. The more dilute solution is probably preferable for ease of control of the administration rate of relaxation. Give this 1 mg/ml IV drip solution at 0.5 to 10 mg/minute to obtain required amount of relaxation. The 0.2% solution may be useful when it is desirable to avoid overburdening circulation with a large volume of fluid.

►*Prolonged muscular relaxation:* Prolonged muscular relaxation may be achieved with intermittent IV injections. Give an initial dose of 0.3 to 1.1 mg/kg then give 0.04 to 0.07 mg/kg at appropriate intervals to maintain the required degree of relaxation.

►*Children:*

IV – For infants and small children, 2 mg/kg; for older children and adolescents, 1 mg/kg. IV bolus use may result in profound bradycardia or, rarely, asystole. As in adults, the incidence of bradycardia is higher after a second dose. Reduce occurrence of bradyarrhythmias by pre-treatment with atropine.

IM – In the absence of a suitable vein for IV administration, a dose of 3 to 4 mg/kg (not exceeding a total dose of 150 mg) is suggested. The onset of effect is usually observed in ≈ 2 to 3 minutes.

►*Preparation of solution:* Use only freshly prepared solutions. Succinylcholine is incompatible with alkaline solutions and will precipitate if mixed or administered together. Discard unused solutions within 24 hours. Inject separately; do not mix in the same syringe or administer simultaneously through the same needle with solutions of short-acting barbiturates, such as sodium thiopental or other drugs with an alkaline pH.

►*Storage/Stability:* Refrigerate at 2° to 8°C (36° to 46°F). Multi-dose vials are stable for ≤ 14 days at room temperature without significant loss of potency.

Powder for infusion does not require refrigeration.

Actions

►*Pharmacology:* Succinylcholine is an ultrashort-acting depolarizing skeletal muscle relaxant. Like acetylcholine, it combines with cholinergic receptors of the motor endplate to produce depolarization observed as fasciculations. Neuromuscular transmission is then inhibited so long as an adequate concentration of succinylcholine remains at the receptor site; the neuromuscular block produces a flaccid paralysis.

Paralysis usually appears in the following muscles consecutively: Levator muscles of the eyelids, mastication muscles, limb muscles, abdominal muscles, glottis muscles, the intercostals, the diaphragm and all other skeletal muscles.

Succinylcholine has no effect on consciousness, pain threshold or cerebration; use only with adequate anesthesia. While it has no direct effect upon the myocardium, changes in rhythm may result from vagal stimulation, such as may result from surgical procedures (particularly in children) or from potassium-mediated alterations in electrical conductivity. These effects are enhanced by cyclopropane and halogenated anesthetics. Succinylcholine slightly increases intraocular pressure, which may persist after the onset of complete paralysis. Tachyphylaxis occurs with repeated doses. It has no direct effect on the uterus or other smooth muscles. Because the drug is highly ionized and has a low lipid solubility, it does not readily cross the placenta.

When succinylcholine is given over a prolonged period of time, the characteristic depolarizing neuromuscular block (Phase I block) may change to a block that superficially resembles a nondepolarizing block (Phase II block). This may be associated with prolonged respiratory depression or apnea in patients who manifest the transition to Phase II block. After confirmation by peripheral nerve stimulation, reverse with anticholinesterase drugs such as neostigmine (see Precautions).

►*Pharmacokinetics:*

Onset and duration – Following IV injection, complete muscular relaxation occurs within 30 to 60 seconds and with single administration, lasts ≈ 4 to 6 minutes. Following IM injection, onset of action may vary from 2 to 3 minutes. Muscular relaxation of longer duration can be achieved by repeated injections at appropriate intervals or by continuous IV infusion.

Metabolism – The drug is rapidly hydrolyzed by plasma cholinesterase to succinylmonocholine (a nondepolarizing muscle relaxant), then more slowly to succinic acid and choline. Succinylmonocholine can accumulate and cause prolonged paralysis due to its slower rate of hydrolysis. Correlation has been found between pseudocholinesterase levels and duration of action. About 10% is excreted unchanged in the urine.

Contraindications

Hypersensitivity to succinylcholine or any components of these products; patients with genetically determined disorders of plasma pseudocholinesterase; personal or familial history of malignant hyperthermia; myopathies associated with elevated creatine phosphokinase (CPK) values; acute narrow-angle glaucoma; penetrating eye injuries.

Warnings

►*Malignant hyperthermia (MH):* The abrupt onset of MH, a rare hypermetabolic process of skeletal muscle, may be triggered by succinylcholine. Early premonitory signs include: Muscle rigidity, particularly involving jaw muscles; tachycardia and tachypnea unresponsive to increased depth of anesthesia; evidence of increased oxygen requirement and carbon dioxide production (change in color of the CO_2 absorber); rising temperature; metabolic acidosis. Considerations important to the management of this problem are: Early recognition of premonitory signs; immediate discontinuation of anesthesia and succinylcholine (either agent may induce the syndrome); implementation of supportive measures including administration of oxygen and sodium bicarbonate, lowering body temperature, restoration of fluid and electrolyte balance, maintenance of adequate urinary output and administration of IV dantrolene (see the dantrolene monograph). Establish a standard protocol to implement when the syndrome becomes apparent.

►*Controlling respiration:* Use succinylcholine only when facilities for endotracheal intubation, artificial respiration and oxygen administration are instantly available. Be prepared to assist or control respiration.

►*Myasthenia gravis:* Myasthenia gravis patients have shown resistance to succinylcholine.

►*Myalgia:* Succinylcholine may cause myalgia. Aspirin 600 mg 1 hour before anesthesia has been shown to reduce myalgia.

►*Pregnancy: Category C.* Safety for use during pregnancy has not been established. It is not known whether the drug can cause fetal harm when administered to a pregnant woman or can affect reproduction capacity. Use in pregnant women only when clearly needed and when potential benefits outweigh potential hazards.

SUCCINYLCHOLINE CHLORIDE

Pseudocholinesterase levels are decreased by $\approx 24\%$ during pregnancy and for several days postpartum. Therefore, pregnant patients may be expected to show greater sensitivity (prolonged apnea) to succinylcholine than nonpregnant patients.

Labor and delivery – Succinylcholine is commonly used to provide muscle relaxation during cesarean section. While small amounts cross the placenta, the amount that enters fetal circulation after a single 1 mg/kg dose to the mother should not endanger the fetus. However, because the amount of drug that crosses the placenta depends on the concentration gradient between the maternal and fetal circulations, residual neuromuscular blockade (apnea and flaccidity) may occur in the neonate after repeated high doses to the mother or in the presence of atypical pseudocholinesterase in the mother.

➤*Lactation:* It is not known whether this drug is excreted in breast milk. Exercise caution when succinylcholine is administered to a nursing woman.

➤*Children:* There are rare reports of ventricular dysrhythmias and cardiac arrest secondary to acute rhabdomyolysis with hyperkalemia in healthy children. Many of these children were subsequently found to have a skeletal muscle myopathy, such as Duchenne's muscular dystrophy, which had clinical signs that were not obvious. The syndrome often presents as sudden cardiac arrest within minutes after the administration of succinylcholine. These children are usually, but not exclusively, males and most frequently ≤ 8 years of age. There have also been reports in adolescents. There may be no signs or symptoms to alert the practitioner to which patients are at risk. A careful history and physical may identify developmental delays suggestive of a myopathy. A preoperative creatine kinase could identify some but not all patients at risk. Because of the abrupt onset of this symptom, routine resuscitative measures are likely to be unsuccessful. Careful monitoring of the electrocardiogram may alert the practitioner to peaked T-waves (an early sign). Administration of IV calcium, bicarbonate and glucose with insulin, with hyperventilation have resulted in successful resuscitation in some of the reported cases. Extraordinary and prolonged resuscitative efforts have been effective in some cases. As in adults, the incidence of bradycardia in children is higher following the second succinylcholine dose.

Precautions

➤*Use with caution:* Use with caution in cardiovascular, hepatic, pulmonary, metabolic or renal disorders. Administer with great caution to patients with severe burns, electrolyte imbalance, hyperkalemia, those receiving quinidine and those who are digitalized or recovering from severe trauma, as serious cardiac arrhythmias or cardiac arrest may result. Observe caution in patients with preexisting hyperkalemia or those who are paraplegic, who have suffered spinal cord injury or have degenerative or dystrophic neuromuscular disease, because such patients tend to become severely hyperkalemic when succinylcholine is given.

➤*Prolonged blockade:* Prolonged blockade may occur in patients with hypokalemia, hypocalcemia, hepatic disorders, cardiovascular and pulmonary disorders.

➤*Low plasma pseudocholinesterase:* Low plasma pseudocholinesterase may be associated with a prolonged paralysis of respiration following succinylcholine. Low levels are often found in patients with severe liver disease or cirrhosis, anemia, burns, malnutrition, dehydration, cancer, collagen diseases, abnormal body temperatures, myxedema, pregnancy, exposure to neurotoxic insecticides; in those receiving antimalarial drugs, anticancer drugs, irradiation, MAO inhibitors, oral contraceptives, pancuronium, chlorpromazine, echothiophate iodide or neostigmine; or in those with a recessive hereditary trait. Administer minimal doses with extreme care to such patients. If low plasma pseudocholinesterase activity is suspected, administer a test dose of 5 to 10 mg or produce relaxation by the cautious administration of a 0.1% IV drip.

➤*Nondepolarizing blockade:* During repeated or prolonged administration of succinylcholine, the characteristic Phase I block may convert to a Phase II block. Prolonged respiratory depression or apnea may be observed in patients manifesting this transition. The transition from Phase I to Phase II block was reported in seven of seven patients studied under halothane anesthesia after an accumulated dose of 2 to 4 mg/kg succinylcholine (administered in repeated, divided doses). The onset of Phase II block coincided with the onset of tachyphylaxis and prolongation of spontaneous recovery. In another study, using balanced anesthesia (N_2O/O_2/narcotic-thiopental) and succinylcholine infusion, the transition was less abrupt with great variability in the dose required to produce Phase II block. Of 32 patients studied, 24 developed Phase II block. Tachyphylaxis was not associated with the transition, and 50% of the patients who developed Phase II block experienced prolonged recovery.

When Phase II block is suspected, base the decision to reverse the block with an anticholinesterase drug upon a positive diagnosis using a peripheral nerve stimulator, because an anticholinesterase agent will potentiate a succinylcholine-induced Phase I block. Phase II block is indicated by fade of responses to successive stimuli (preferably "train of four"). Accompany anticholinesterase drugs to reverse Phase II block by appropriate doses of atropine to prevent cardiac arrhythmias. After adequate reversal of Phase II block with an anticholinesterase agent, observe the patient for at least 1 hour for signs of return of muscle relaxation. Do not attempt reversal unless: (1) A peripheral nerve stimulator is used to determine the presence of Phase II block, and (2) spontaneous recovery of muscle twitch has occurred for at least 20 minutes and has reached a plateau with further recovery proceeding slowly; this delay ensures complete hydrolysis of succinylcholine by pseudocholinesterase prior to administration of the anticholinesterase agent.

Concurrent use of a depolarizing and a nondepolarizing (competitive) muscle relaxant is not recommended because a prolonged mixed block may occur. In this instance, determine the dominant feature of the block by the use of a nerve stimulator and treat accordingly.

➤*Ophthalmic:* Succinylcholine causes a slight, transient increase in intraocular pressure immediately after its injection and during the fasciculation phase; slight increases may persist after onset of complete paralysis. Use with caution, if at all, during intraocular surgery and in patients with glaucoma.

➤*Patients with fractures or muscle spasm:* Patients with fractures or muscle spasm require caution because the muscle fasciculations may cause additional trauma.

Reduce muscle fasciculations and hyperkalemia by administering a small dose of a nondepolarizing relaxant prior to succinylcholine. If other relaxants are to be used during the procedure, consider the possibility of a synergistic or antagonistic effect.

➤*Intracranial pressure:* Succinylcholine may cause a transient increase in intracranial pressure; however, adequate anesthetic induction prior to administration of succinylcholine will minimize this effect.

➤*Intragastric pressure:* Succinylcholine may increase intragastric pressure, which could result in regurgitation and possible aspiration of stomach contents.

➤*Benzyl alcohol:* Some of these products contain the preservative benzyl alcohol, which has been associated with a fatal "gasping syndrome" in premature infants.

SUCCINYLCHOLINE CHLORIDE

Drug Interactions

Succinylcholine Drug Interactions			
Precipitant drug	Object drug*		Description
Amphotericin B Thiazide diuretics	Succinylcholine	↑	Amphotericin B and thiazide diuretics may increase effects of succinylcholine secondary to induced electrolyte imbalance. Patients with hypocalcemia and hypokalemia usually require reduced succinylcholine doses.
Cimetidine	Succinylcholine	↑	Cimetidine inhibits pseudocholinesterase.
Cyclophosphamide	Succinylcholine	↑	Cyclophosphamide decreases plasma pseudocholinesterase.
Diazepam	Succinylcholine	↓	Diazepam may reduce the duration of neuromuscular blockade produced by succinylcholine.
Inhalation anesthetics (eg, cyclopropane, diethyl ether, halothane, nitrous oxide)	Succinylcholine	↑	Coadministration with succinylcholine may increase incidence of bradycardia, arrhythmias, sinus arrest, and apnea, as well as the occurrence of malignant hyperthermia in susceptible individuals.
IV procaine	Succinylcholine	↑	IV procaine competes for the enzyme and may prolong the effect of succinylcholine.
Narcotic analgesics	Succinylcholine	↑	Narcotic analgesics may increase the incidence of bradycardia and sinus arrest.
Nondepolarizing muscle relaxants	Succinylcholine	↑↓	Consider the possibility of a synergistic or antagonistic effect with succinylcholine.
Phenelzine, promazine, oxytocin, certain nonpenicillin antibiotics, quinidine, beta-adrenergic blocking agents, procainamide, lidocaine, trimethaphan, lithium carbonate, furosemide, magnesium sulfate, quinine, chloroquine, and isoflurane	Succinylcholine	↑	All of these drugs may enhance the neuromuscular blocking action of succinylcholine.
Succinylcholine	Digitalis glycosides	↑	Succinylcholine may cause a sudden potassium extrusion from muscle cells, possibly causing arrhythmias or ventricular fibrillation in digitalized patients. Toxicity (cardiac arrhythmias) of both drugs may be increased.

* ↑ = Object drug increased. ↓ = Object drug decreased.

Adverse Reactions

As with other neuromuscular blockers, the potential for releasing histamine is present following succinylcholine use. However, serious histamine-mediated flushing, hypotension, and bronchoconstriction are uncommon in normal clinical usage.

Adverse reactions consist primarily of an extension of the drug's pharmacological actions. Profound and prolonged muscle relaxation may occur, resulting in respiratory depression to the point of apnea. Hypersensitivity and anaphylactic reactions have been reported rarely. The following reactions have been reported:

➤*Cardiovascular:* Bradycardia (frequently noted after a second IV injection of a 2% solution in children); tachycardia; hypertension; hypotension; cardiac arrest; arrhythmias.

➤*Respiratory:* Respiratory depression or apnea.

➤*Miscellaneous:* Malignant hyperthermia (see Warnings); increased intraocular pressure (see Precautions); muscle fasciculation; postoperative muscle pain; excessive salivation; hyperkalemia; rash; myoglobinemia; myoglobinuria; perioperative dreams (children); myalgia; jaw rigidity; rhabdomyolysis with possible myoglobinuric acute renal failure.

Overdosage

Overdosage with succinylcholine may result in neuromuscular block beyond the time needed for surgery and anesthesia. This may be manifested by skeletal muscle weakness, decreased respiratory reserve, low tidal volume, or apnea. The primary treatment is maintenance of a patent airway and respiratory support until recovery of normal respiration is assured. Depending on the dose and duration of succinylcholine administration, the characteristic depolarizing neuromuscular block (Phase I) may change to a block with characteristics superficially resembling a nondepolarizing block (Phase II).

Centrally Acting

BACLOFEN

Rx	Baclofen (Various, eg, Ivax, Watson)	**Tablets:** 10 mg	In 30s, 100s, 250s, 500s, and 1000s.
Rx	Lioresal (Novartis)		(Lioresal 1010). White, scored, oval. In 100s and UD 100s.
Rx	Baclofen (Various, eg, Ivax, Watson)	**Tablets:** 20 mg	In 30s, 100s, 250s, 500s, and 1000s.
Rx	Lioresal (Novartis)		(Lioresal 2020). White, scored, capsule shape. In 100s and UD 100s.
Rx	Kemstro (Schwarz)	**Tablets, orally disintegrating:** 10 mg	Mannitol, aspartame, 3.9 mg phenylalanine. (10 SP 351). Scored. Orange flavor. In 100s.
Rx	Kemstro (Schwarz)	20 mg	Mannitol, aspartame, 7.9 mg phenylalanine. (20 SP 352). Scored. Orange flavor. In 100s.
Rx	Lioresal Intrathecal (Medtronic)	**Intrathecal:** 0.05 mg/mL (50 mcg/mL)	Preservative-free. In single-use amps.
		10 mg/20 mL (500 mcg/mL)	Preservative-free. In single-use amps (1 amp refill kit).
		10 mg/5 mL (2000 mcg/mL)	Preservative-free. In single-use amps (2 or 4 amp refill kits).

WARNING

Abrupt discontinuation of intrathecal baclofen, regardless of the cause, has resulted in sequelae that include high fever, altered mental status, exaggerated rebound spasticity, and muscle rigidity, which in rare cases has advanced to rhabdomyolysis, multiple organ-system failure, and death.

Prevention of abrupt discontinuation of intrathecal baclofen requires careful attention to programming and monitoring of the infusion system, refill scheduling and procedures, and pump alarms. Advise patients and caregivers of the importance of keeping scheduled refill visits and educate them on the early symptoms of baclofen withdrawal. Give special attention to patients at apparent risk (eg, spinal cord injuries at T-6 or above, communication difficulties, history of withdrawal symptoms from oral or intrathecal baclofen). Consult the technical manual of the implantable infusion system for additional postimplant clinician and patient information (see Warnings).

Indications

➤*Oral:* For the alleviation of signs and symptoms of spasticity resulting from multiple sclerosis, particularly for the relief of flexor spasms, concomitant pain, clonus, and muscular rigidity. Patients should have reversible spasticity so that treatment will aid in restoring residual function.

May be of some value in patients with spinal cord injuries and other spinal cord diseases.

Baclofen is not indicated in the treatment of skeletal muscle spasm resulting from rheumatic disorders, stroke, cerebral palsy, and Parkinson's disease (because efficacy has not been established).

➤*Intrathecal:* Management of severe spasticity. For spasticity of spinal cord origin, reserve chronic infusion of intrathecal baclofen via an implantable pump for patients who are unresponsive to oral baclofen therapy or who experience intolerable CNS side effects at effective doses. Patients with spasticity caused by traumatic brain injury should wait at least 1 year after injury before considering long-term intrathecal baclofen therapy. Intended for use by the intrathecal route in single bolus test doses (via spinal catheter or lumbar puncture) and, for chronic use, only in implantable pumps approved by the FDA specifically for baclofen administration into the intrathecal space.

Intrathecal therapy may be considered an alternative to destructive neurosurgical procedures. Prior to implantation of a device for chronic intrathecal infusion, patients must show a response in a screening trial (see Administration and Dosage).

➤*Unlabeled uses:*

Oral – Treatment of trigeminal neuralgia (tic douloureux); intractable hiccoughs; to reduce choreiform movements in patients with Huntington's chorea; to reduce rigidity in patients with parkinsonism syndrome; to reduce spasticity in patients with cerebral lesions, cerebral palsy, or rheumatic disorders; to reduce spasticity in patients with cerebrovascular stroke; acquired periodic alternating nystagmus; acquired pendular nystagmus; to reduce the number of gastroesophageal reflux episodes (single 40 mg dose); Tourette syndrome in children (20 mg 3 times daily); prophylactic treatment of migraine; neuropathic pain.

Intrathecal – Generalized dystonia associated with cerebral palsy.

Administration and Dosage

➤*Oral:* Individualize dosage. Start at a low dosage and increase gradually until the optimum effect is achieved (usually 40 to 80 mg daily).

The following dosage titration schedule is suggested: 5 mg 3 times daily for 3 days; 10 mg 3 times daily for 3 days; 15 mg 3 times daily for 3 days; 20 mg 3 times daily for 3 days. Thereafter, additional increases may be necessary, but the total daily dose should not exceed 80 mg daily (20 mg 4 times daily).

The lowest effective dose is recommended. If benefits are not evident after a reasonable trial period, withdraw the drug slowly.

➤*Intrathecal:* Refer to the manufacturer's manual for the implantable intrathecal infusion pump for specific instructions and precautions for programming the pump or refilling the reservoir.

Screening phase – Prior to pump implantation and initiation of chronic infusion of baclofen, patients must demonstrate a positive clinical response to a bolus dose administered intrathecally in a screening trial. The screening trial employs baclofen at a concentration of 50 mcg/mL. The screening procedure is as follows: Administer an initial bolus containing 50 mcg/mL into the intrathecal space by barbotage over a period of not less than 1 minute. Observe the patient over the ensuing 4 to 8 hours. A positive response consists of a significant decrease in muscle tone or frequency or severity of spasm. If the initial response is less than desired, a second bolus injection may be administered 24 hours after the first. This second screening bolus dose consists of 75 mcg/1.5 mL. Again, observe the patient for an interval of 4 to 8 hours. If the response is still inadequate, a final bolus screening dose of 100 mcg/2 mL may be administered 24 hours later.

Do not consider patients who do not respond to a 100 mcg intrathecal bolus as candidates for an implanted pump for chronic infusion.

Children – The starting screening dose for pediatric patients is the same as in adult patients (ie, 50 mcg). However, for very small patients, a screening dose of 25 mcg may be tried first.

Postimplant dose titration period – To determine the initial total daily dose of baclofen following implant, double the screening dose that gave a positive effect, and administer over a 24-hour period, unless the efficacy of the bolus dose was maintained for more than 8 hours, in which case the starting daily dose should be the screening dose delivered over a 24-hour period. Do not increase the dose in the first 24 hours (ie, until the steady state is achieved).

Spasticity of spinal cord origin (adults) – For adult patients, after the first 24 hours, increase the daily dose slowly by 10% to 30% increments and only once every 24 hours until the desired clinical effect is achieved. If there is not a substantive clinical response to increases in the daily dose, check for proper pump function and catheter patency.

Monitor patients closely in a fully equipped and staffed environment during the screening phase and dose-titration period immediately following implant. Resuscitative equipment should be immediately available for use in case of life-threatening or intolerable side effects.

Spasticity of cerebral origin (adults) – After the first 24 hours, increase the daily dose slowly by 5% to 15% once every 24 hours until the desired clinical effect is achieved.

Children – After the first 24 hours, increase the daily dose slowly by 5% to 15% only once every 24 hours until the desired effect is achieved.

Maintenance therapy –

Spasticity of spinal cord origin: The clinical goal is to maintain muscle tone as close to normal as possible and to minimize the frequency and severity of spasms to the extent possible without inducing intolerable side effects. Very often, the maintenance dose needs to be adjusted during the first few months of therapy while patients adjust to changes in lifestyle because of the alleviation of spasticity. During periodic refills of the pump, the daily dose may be increased by 10% to 40%, but no more than 40%, to maintain adequate symptom control. The daily dose may be reduced by 10% to 20% if patients experience side effects. Most patients require gradual increases in dose over time to maintain optimal response during chronic therapy. A sudden large requirement for dose escalation suggests a catheter complication (eg, catheter kink or dislodgement).

Maintenance dosage for long-term continuous infusion ranged from 12 to 2003 mcg/day, with most patients adequately maintained on 300 to 800 mcg/day. There is limited experience with daily doses greater than 1000 mcg/day. Determination of the optimal dose requires individual titration. Use the lowest dose with an optimal response.

Spasticity of cerebral origin: During periodic refills of the pump, the daily dose may be increased by 5% to 20% but no more than 20% to

BACLOFEN

maintain adequate symptom control. The daily dose may be reduced by 10% to 20% if patients experience side effects.

Maintenance dosage for long-term continuous infusion of baclofen ranged from 22 to 1400 mcg/day, with most patients adequately maintained on 90 to 703 mcg/day. In clinical trials, only 3 of 150 patients required daily doses greater than 1000 mcg/day.

Children: Use same dosing recommendations for patients with spasticity of cerebral origin. Pediatric patients under 12 years of age seemed to require a lower daily dose in clinical trials. Average daily dose for patients under 12 years of age was 274 mcg/day, with a range of 24 to 1199 mcg/day. Dosage requirement for pediatric patients over 12 years of age does not seem to be different from that of adult patients. Determination of the optimal baclofen dose requires individual titration. Use the lowest dose with an optimal response.

Potential need for dose adjustments in chronic use – During long-term treatment, approximately 5% of patients become refractory to increasing doses. There is not sufficient experience to make firm recommendations for tolerance treatment; however, this tolerance has been treated on occasion in the hospital by a drug holiday consisting of the gradual reduction of baclofen intrathecal over a 2- to 4-week period and switching to alternative methods of spasticity management. After the drug holiday, baclofen intrathecal may be restarted at the initial continuous infusion dose.

Additional considerations pertaining to dose adjustments – It may be important to titrate the dose to maintain some degree of muscle tone and allow occasional spasms to help support circulatory function, to possibly prevent the formation of deep vein thrombosis, and to optimize activities of daily living and ease of care.

Except in overdose-related emergencies, the dose ordinarily should be reduced slowly if the drug is discontinued for any reason.

Attempt to discontinue concomitant oral antispasticity medication to avoid possible overdose or adverse drug interactions prior to screening or following implant and initiation of chronic intrathecal baclofen infusion. Reduction and discontinuation of oral antispasmodics should be done slowly and with careful monitoring by the physician. Avoid abrupt reduction or discontinuation of concomitant antispastics.

Pump dose adjustment and titration – In most patients, it will be necessary to increase the dose gradually over time to maintain effectiveness; a sudden requirement for substantial dose escalation typically indicates a catheter complication.

Reservoir refilling must be performed by fully trained and qualified personnel following the directions provided by the pump manufacturer. Carefully calculate refill intervals to prevent depletion of the reservoir, as this would result in the return of severe spasticity.

Use extreme caution when filling an FDA-approved implantable pump equipped with an injection port that allows direct access to the intrathecal catheter. Direct injection into the catheter through the access port may cause a life-threatening overdose.

Dilution instructions – Dilute with sterile preservative-free Sodium Chloride for Injection. For patients who require concentrations other than 500 or 2000 mcg/mL, intrathecal baclofen must be diluted.

Delivery regimen – Baclofen intrathecal is most often administered in a continuous infusion mode immediately following implant. For those patients implanted with programmable pumps who have achieved relatively satisfactory control on continuous infusion, further benefit may be attained using more complex schedules of delivery. For example, patients who have increased spasms at night may require a 20% increase in their hourly infusion rate. Program changes in flow rate to start 2 hours before the time of desired clinical effect.

➤*Storage / Stability:*

Oral – Do not store above 30°C (86°F).

Intrathecal – Does not require refrigeration. Do not store above 30°C (86°F). Do not freeze. Do not heat sterilize.

Actions

➤*Pharmacology:* The precise mechanism of action is unknown. Baclofen can inhibit both monosynaptic and polysynaptic reflexes at the spinal level, possibly by hyperpolarization of afferent terminals, although actions at supraspinal sites may also contribute to its clinical effect. It is a structural analog of the inhibitory neurotransmitter gamma-aminobutyric acid (GABA) and may exert its effects by stimulation of the GABA$_B$ receptor subtype. Baclofen has CNS depressant properties as indicated by production of sedation with tolerance, somnolence, ataxia, and respiratory and cardiovascular depression.

When introduced directly into the intrathecal space, effective cerebrospinal fluid (CSF) concentrations are achieved with resultant plasma concentrations 100 times less than those occurring with oral administration.

➤*Pharmacokinetics:*

Oral – Baclofen is rapidly and extensively absorbed and eliminated. Absorption may be dose-dependent, reduced with increasing doses. It is excreted primarily by the kidney in unchanged form and there is relatively large intersubject variation in absorption or elimination.

Intrathecal –

Bolus: The onset of action is generally 0.5 to 1 hour after an intrathecal bolus dose. Peak spasmolytic effect is seen at approximately 4 hours after dosing and effects may last 4 to 8 hours. Onset, peak response, and duration of action may vary with individual patients depending on the dose and severity of symptoms. After a bolus lumbar injection of 50 or 100 mcg in 7 patients, the average CSF elimination half-life was 1.51 hours over the first 4 hours, and the average CSF clearance was approximately 30 mL/hour.

Continuous infusion: The antispastic action is first seen at 6 to 8 hours after initiation of continuous infusion. Maximum activity is observed in 24 to 48 hours. The mean CSF clearance was approximately 30 mL/hour in 10 patients on continuous intrathecal infusion.

The pharmacokinetics of CSF clearance of baclofen calculated from intrathecal bolus or continuous infusion studies approximates CSF turnover, suggesting elimination is by bulk-flow removal of CSF.

Concurrent plasma concentrations during intrathecal administration are expected to be low (0 to 5 ng/mL). Limited data suggest that a lumbar-cisternal concentration gradient of approximately 4:1 is established along the neuroaxis during baclofen infusion.

Contraindications

Hypersensitivity to baclofen.

➤*Intrathecal:* IV, IM, SC, or epidural administration.

Warnings

➤*Intrathecal administration:* Because of the possibility of potentially life-threatening CNS depression, cardiovascular collapse, or respiratory failure, physicians must be adequately trained and educated in chronic intrathecal infusion therapy.

Do not implant the pump system until the patient's response to bolus injection is adequately evaluated. Evaluation (consisting of a screening procedure; see Administration and Dosage) requires that baclofen be administered into the intrathecal space via catheter or lumbar puncture. Because of the risks associated with the screening procedure and dosage adjustment following pump implantation, conduct these phases in a medically supervised and adequately equipped environment following the instructions outlined in Administration and Dosage.

➤*Fatalities:* There were 16 deaths among the 576 patients treated with baclofen intrathecal for spasticity of spinal cord origin in premarketing and postmarketing studies. Because these patients were treated in uncontrolled clinical settings, it is impossible to determine definitively what role, if any, baclofen played in their deaths.

➤*Infection:* Patients should be infection-free prior to the screening trial with baclofen intrathecal because a systemic infection may interfere with an assessment of the patient's response.

Patients should be infection-free prior to pump implantation because an infection may increase the risk of surgical complications. Moreover, a systemic infection may complicate dosing.

➤*Abrupt drug withdrawal:*

Oral – Hallucinations and seizures have occurred on abrupt withdrawal. Except in cases of serious adverse reactions, reduce dose slowly when drug is discontinued.

Intrathecal – Abrupt withdrawal of intrathecal baclofen has resulted in high fever, altered mental status, exaggerated rebound spasticity, and muscle rigidity that in rare cases progressed to rhabdomyolysis, multiple-organ system failure, and death. In most cases, symptoms of withdrawal appeared within hours to a few days following interruption of baclofen therapy. Common reasons for abrupt interruption of intrathecal baclofen therapy included malfunction of the catheter (especially disconnection), low volume in the pump reservoir, end of pump battery life, and human error.

Early symptoms of baclofen withdrawal may include return of baseline spasticity, pruritus, hypotension, and paresthesias. Some clinical characteristics of the advanced intrathecal baclofen withdrawal syndrome may resemble autonomic dysreflexia, infection (sepsis), malignant hyperthermia, neuroleptic-malignant syndrome, or other conditions associated with a hypermetabolic state or widespread rhabdomyolysis.

The suggested treatment for intrathecal baclofen withdrawal is the restoration of intrathecal baclofen at or near the same dosage as before therapy was interrupted.

➤*Pump implantation (intrathecal):* Following surgical implantation of the pump, particularly during the initial phases of pump use, and on each occasion that the dosing rate of the pump or the concentration of intrathecal baclofen in the reservoir is adjusted, close medical monitoring is required until it is certain that the patient's response to the infusion is acceptable and reasonably stable.

Use extreme caution when filling an FDA approved implantable pump. Such pumps should only be refilled through the reservoir refill septum. However, some pumps also are equipped with a catheter access port that allows direct access to the intrathecal catheter. Direct injection into the catheter access port may cause a life-threatening overdose.

➤*Stroke (oral):* Baclofen has not significantly benefitted patients with stroke; they also have poor drug tolerance.

BACLOFEN

➤*Renal function impairment:* Because baclofen is primarily excreted unchanged through the kidneys, administer with caution to patients with impaired renal function. Dosage reduction may be necessary.

➤*Pregnancy: Category C.* Oral baclofen increases the incidence of omphaloceles (ventral hernias) in rat fetuses given approximately 13 times the maximum oral dose recommended for human use; this dose also caused reductions in food intake and weight gain in dams. There are no studies in pregnant women. Use only when clearly needed and when potential benefits outweigh potential hazards to the fetus.

➤*Lactation:* In mothers treated with oral baclofen in therapeutic doses, the active substance passes into the breast milk. It is not known whether detectable levels of drug are present in the breast milk of nursing mothers receiving intrathecal baclofen. As a general rule, undertake nursing while a patient is receiving intrathecal baclofen only if the potential benefit justifies the potential risk to the infant.

➤*Children:*

Oral – Safety for use in children under 12 years of age has not been established.

Intrathecal – Safety in children under 4 years of age has not been established.

Precautions

➤*Epilepsy:* Monitor the clinical state and EEG at regular intervals, as deterioration in seizure control and EEG changes have occurred in patients taking this drug.

Seizures have been reported during overdose and withdrawal from intrathecal baclofen as well as in patients maintained on therapeutic doses of intrathecal baclofen.

➤*Spasticity:* Titrate dose with caution where spasticity is utilized to sustain upright posture and balance in locomotion or whenever spasticity is utilized to obtain increased function.

➤*Ovarian cysts (oral):* Ovarian cysts have been found by palpation in about 4% of multiple sclerosis patients treated with baclofen for up to 1 year. In most cases, these cysts disappeared spontaneously while patients continued to receive the drug. Ovarian cysts are estimated to occur spontaneously in about 1% to 5% of the normal female population.

➤*Psychotic disorders:* Cautiously treat patients suffering from psychotic disorders, schizophrenia, or confusional states, and keep under careful surveillance because exacerbations of these conditions have been observed with oral administration.

➤*Autonomic dysreflexia (intrathecal):* Use intrathecal baclofen with caution in patients with a history of autonomic dysreflexia. The presence of nociceptive stimuli or abrupt withdrawal may cause an autonomic dysreflexic episode.

➤*Drowsiness:* Because of the possibility of sedation, patients should observe caution while driving or performing other tasks requiring alertness, coordination, or physical dexterity.

Adverse Reactions

➤*Intrathecal:*

	Baclofen Adverse Events (≥ 1%)					
	Spasticity of spinal origin			Spasticity of cerebral origin		
Adverse reaction	Screening[1] (N = 576)	Titration[2] (N = 474)	Mainten-ance[3] (N = 430)	Screening[1] (N = 211)	Titration[2] (N = 153)	Mainten-ance[3] (N = 150)
Cardiovascular						
Hypertension	0.2	0.6	0.5	-	-	-
Hypotension	1	0.2	1.9	1.9	0.7	2
CNS						
Agitation	-	-	-	0.5	0	1.3
Anxiety	0.2	0.4	0.9	-	-	-
Asthenia	0.7	1.3	1.4	0	0	2
Convulsion	0.5	1.3	4.7	0.9	3.3	10
Confusion	0.5	0.6	2.3	-	-	-
Depression	0	0	1.6	-	-	-
Dizziness	1.7	1.9	7.9	2.4	2.6	8
Hallucinations	0.3	0.4	0.5	-	-	-
Headache	1.6	2.5	5.1	6.6	7.8	10.7
Insomnia	0	0.4	1.6	-	-	-
Paresthesia	2.4	2.1	6.7	1.9	0.7	3.3
Somnolence	5.7	5.9	20.9	7.6	10.5	18.7
Thinking abnormal	-	-	-	0.5	1.3	0.7
Dermatologic						
Pruritus	-	-	-	0	0	4
Urticaria	0.2	0.2	1.2	-	-	-

	Baclofen Adverse Events (≥ 1%)					
	Spasticity of spinal origin			Spasticity of cerebral origin		
Adverse reaction	Screening[1] (N = 576)	Titration[2] (N = 474)	Mainten-ance[3] (N = 430)	Screening[1] (N = 211)	Titration[2] (N = 153)	Mainten-ance[3] (N = 150)
GI						
Anorexia	0	0.4	0.9	-	-	-
Constipation	0.2	1.5	5.1	0.5	1.3	2
Diarrhea	0	0.8	2.3	0.5	0.7	2
Dry mouth	0.2	0.4	3.3	0.5	0	1.3
Nausea	-	-	-	1.4	3.3	7.3
Nausea/ Vomiting	1.6	2.3	5.6	6.6	10.5	4
Vomiting	-	-	-	6.2	8.5	4
GU						
Impotence	0.2	0.4	1.6	-	-	-
Urinary frequency	0	0.6	0.9	-	-	-
Urination impaired	-	-	-	0	0	2
Urinary incontinence	0	0.8	1.4	0	0	2
Urinary retention	0.7	1.7	1.9	0.9	6.5	8
Musculoskeletal						
Back pain	-	-	-	0.9	0.7	2
Hypertonia	-	-	-	0	0.7	6
Hypotonia	5.4	13.5	25.3	2.4	14.4	34.7
Respiratory						
Dyspnea	0.3	0	1.2	-	-	-
Hypoventilation	0.2	0.8	2.1	1.4	1.3	4
Pneumonia	0.2	0.2	1.2	0	0	2
Special senses						
Amblyopia	0.5	0.2	2.3	-	-	-
Diplopia	0	0.4	0.9	-	-	-
Miscellaneous						
Accidental injury	-	0.2	3.5	-	-	-
Chills	-	-	-	0.5	0	1.3
Coma	0	1.5	0.9	0.5	0	1.3
Death	0.2	0.4	3	-	-	-
Dysautonomia	0.2	0.2	0.9	-	-	-
Fever	0.5	0.2	0.7	-	-	-
Increased salivation	-	-	-	0	2.6	2.7
Pain	0	0.6	3	0	0	4
Peripheral edema	0	0	2.3	0	0	3.3
Speech disorder	0	0.2	3.5	0.5	0.7	0.7
Tremor	-	-	-	0.5	0	1.3

[1] Following administration of test bolus.
[2] Two-month period following implant.
[3] Beyond 2 months following implant.

Spasticity of spinal origin: The most commonly observed adverse events with spasticity of spinal origin that were not seen at an equivalent incidence among placebo-treated patients were the following: Somnolence, dizziness, nausea, hypotension, headache, convulsions, hypotonia.

Adverse events most commonly associated with discontinuation included the following: Pump pocket infections, meningitis, wound dehiscence, gynecological fibroids, pump overpressurization.

Spasticity of cerebral origin:

• *Commonly observed* – In premarketing clinical trials, the most commonly observed adverse events associated with use of intrathecal baclofen that were not seen in equivalent incidence among placebo-treated patients included the following: Agitation, constipation, somnolence, chills, urinary retention, hypotonia, and leukocytosis.

• *Associated with discontinuation of treatment* – The 9 adverse events leading to discontinuation of treatment were the following: Infection (3), CSF leaks (2), meningitis (2), drainage (1), and unmanageable trunk control (1).

• *Incidence in controlled trials* – The following events occurred among the 62 patients receiving intrathecal baclofen in 2 randomized, placebo-controlled trials involving cerebral palsy and head injury patients, respectively: Leukocytosis, nystagmus, agitation, constipation, somnolence, nausea, vomiting, chills, urinary retention, hypotonia.

Fatalities: See Warnings.

In addition, the following adverse events were reported in pre- and postmarketing studies and foreign studies and are arranged in decreasing order of frequency:

BACLOFEN

Cardiovascular –
 Spasticity of spinal origin: Postural hypotension; bradycardia; palpitations; syncope; ventricular arrhythmia; deep thrombophlebitis; pallor; tachycardia.
 Spasticity of cerebral origin: Bradycardia.

CNS –
 Spasticity of spinal origin: Abnormal gait; abnormal thinking; tremor; amnesia; twitching; vasodilation; cerebrovascular accident; nystagmus; personality disorder; psychotic depression; cerebral ischemia; emotional lability; euphoria; hypertonia; ileus; drug dependence; incoordination; paranoid reaction; ptosis.
 Spasticity of cerebral origin: Akathisia; ataxia; confusion; depression; opisthotonos; amnesia; anxiety; hallucinations; hysteria; insomnia; nystagmus; personality disorder; reflexes decreased; vasodilation.

Dermatologic –
 Spasticity of spinal origin: Alopecia; sweating.
 Spasticity of cerebral origin: Rash; sweating; alopecia; contact dermatitis; skin ulcer.

GI –
 Spasticity of spinal origin: Flatulence; dysphagia; dyspepsia; gastroenteritis.
 Spasticity of cerebral origin: Dysphagia; fecal incontinence; GI hemorrhage; tongue disorder.

GU –
 Spasticity of spinal origin: Hematuria; kidney failure.
 Spasticity of cerebral origin: Abnormal ejaculation; kidney calculus; oliguria; vaginitis.

Hematologic / Lymphatic –
 Spasticity of spinal origin: Anemia.
 Spasticity of cerebral origin: Leukocytosis; petechial rash.

Metabolic / Nutritional –
 Spasticity of spinal origin: Weight loss; albuminuria; dehydration; hyperglycemia.

Respiratory –
 Spasticity of spinal origin: Respiratory disorder; aspiration pneumonia; hyperventilation; pulmonary embolus; rhinitis.
 Spasticity of cerebral origin: Apnea; dyspnea; hyperventilation.

Special senses –
 Spasticity of spinal origin: Abnormal vision; abnormality of accommodation; photophobia; taste loss; tinnitus.
 Spasticity of cerebral origin: Abnormality of accommodation.

Miscellaneous –
 Spasticity of spinal origin: Suicide; lack of drug effect; abdominal pain; hypothermia; neck rigidity; chest pain; chills; face edema; flu syndrome; overdose.
 Spasticity of cerebral origin: Death; fever; abdominal pain; carcinoma; malaise; hypothermia.

➤*Oral:*

Cardiovascular – Hypotension (≤ 9%); palpitations; chest pain; syncope (rare).

CNS – Drowsiness (10% to 63%); dizziness (5% to 15%); headache (4% to 8%); insomnia (2% to 7%); fatigue (2% to 4%); confusion (1% to 11%); euphoria; excitement; depression; hallucinations; paresthesia; muscle pain; tinnitus; coordination disorder; tremor; rigidity; dystonia; ataxia; nystagmus; strabismus; miosis; mydriasis; diplopia; dysarthria; slurred speech, blurred vision, epileptic seizures (rare).

Dermatologic – Rash; pruritus; excessive perspiration.

GI – Nausea (4% to 12%); constipation (2% to 6%); dry mouth; anorexia; taste disorder; coma; respiratory depression; seizures. abdominal pain; vomiting; diarrhea; positive test for occult blood in stool (rare).

GU – Urinary frequency (2% to 6%); enuresis; urinary retention; dysuria; impotence; inability to ejaculate; nocturia; hematuria (rare).

Lab test abnormalities – Increased AST; elevated alkaline phosphatase; elevation of blood sugar.

Respiratory – Dyspnea (rare); nasal congestion.

Miscellaneous – Weakness (5% to 15%); ankle edema; weight gain.

Overdosage

➤*Oral:*

Symptoms – Vomiting; muscular hypotonia; drowsiness; accommodation disorders; coma; respiratory depression; seizures.

Treatment – In the alert patient, administer activated charcoal, followed by lavage. In the obtunded patient, secure the airway with a cuffed endotracheal tube before beginning lavage (do not induce emesis). Maintain adequate respiratory exchange; do not use respiratory stimulants.

➤*Intrathecal:*

Symptoms – Pay special attention to recognizing the signs and symptoms of overdosage, especially during the initial screening and dose-titration phase of treatment, but also during re-introduction of intrathecal baclofen after a period of interruption in therapy. Symptoms may include: Drowsiness; lightheadedness; dizziness; somnolence; respiratory depression; seizures; rostral progression of hypotonia; loss of consciousness progressing to coma of up to 72 hours duration. In most cases reported, coma was reversible without sequelae after drug was discontinued. Symptoms of overdose were reported in a sensitive adult patient after receiving a 25 mcg intrathecal bolus.

Treatment – There is no specific antidote; however, the following steps should ordinarily be undertaken: (1) Remove residual solution from the pump as soon as possible; (2) intubate patients with respiratory depression, if necessary, until the drug is eliminated.

Anecdotal reports suggest that IV physostigmine may reverse central side effects, notably drowsiness and respiratory depression. Use caution in administering physostigmine IV, however, because its use has been associated with the induction of seizures and bradycardia.

 Physostigmine doses for adult patients: Administer 2 mg of physostigmine IM or IV at a slow, controlled rate of no more than 1 mg/min. Dosage may be repeated if life-threatening signs, such as arrhythmia, convulsions, or coma occur.

 Physostigmine doses for pediatric patients: Administer 0.02 mg/kg physostigmine IM or IV; do not give more than 0.5 mg/min. The dosage may be repeated at 5 to 10 minute intervals until a therapeutic effect is obtained or a maximum dose of 2 mg is attained.

Physostigmine may not be effective in reversing large overdoses, and patients may need to be maintained with respiratory support.

If lumbar puncture is not contraindicated, consider withdrawing 30 to 40 mL of CSF to reduce CSF baclofen concentration.

Patient Information

May cause drowsiness, dizziness, and fatigue. Patients should observe caution while driving or performing other tasks requiring alertness, coordination, or physical dexterity.

Avoid alcohol and other CNS depressants.

Do not discontinue therapy except on advice of physician. Abrupt withdrawal may result in hallucinations.

May cause frequent urge to urinate or painful urination, constipation, nausea, headache, insomnia, or confusion. Notify physician if these effects persist.

CARISOPRODOL

Rx	**Carisoprodol** (Various, eg, Major, Mutual, Parmed, Schein)	**Tablets:** 350 mg	In 30s, 60s, 100s, 500s, 1000s, and UD 100s.
Rx	**Soma** (Wallace)		(Soma 37 Wallace 2001). White. In 100s, 500s, and UD 500s.

Indications

➤*Musculoskeletal conditions:* As an adjunct to rest, physical therapy, and other measures for the relief of discomfort associated with acute, painful musculoskeletal conditions.

Administration and Dosage

➤*Adults:* 350 mg 3 or 4 times daily; take the last dose at bedtime.

Actions

➤*Pharmacology:* Carisoprodol is a congener of meprobamate. The mode of action of carisoprodol has not been clearly identified but may be related to its sedative properties. Carisoprodol does not directly relax tense skeletal muscles in man. In animals, the drug produces muscle relaxation by blocking interneuronal activity in the descending reticular formation and spinal cord.

➤*Pharmacokinetics:* The onset of action is rapid (30 minutes) and the duration is 4 to 6 hours. It is metabolized in the liver and excreted in the urine.

Contraindications

Acute intermittent porphyria; allergic or idiosyncratic reactions to carisoprodol or related compounds such as meprobamate.

Warnings

➤*Idiosyncratic reactions:* Idiosyncratic reactions may appear rarely within minutes or hours of the first dose of carisoprodol. Symptoms include the following: Extreme weakness, transient quadriplegia, dizziness, ataxia, temporary loss of vision, diplopia, mydriasis, dysarthria, agitation, euphoria, confusion, and disorientation. Symptoms usually subside over the next several hours. Supportive and symptomatic therapy, including hospitalization, may be necessary.

➤*Drug dependence:* In 1 study, abrupt cessation of 100 mg/kg/day (about 5 times the recommended daily adult dosage) was followed in

CARISOPRODOL

some patients by mild withdrawal symptoms such as abdominal cramps, insomnia, chills, headache, and nausea. Delirium and convulsions did not occur. In clinical use, psychological dependence and abuse have been rare, and there have been no reports of significant abstinence signs. Nevertheless, use the drug with caution in addiction-prone individuals.

➤*Renal / Hepatic function impairment:* Exercise caution in administration to patients with compromised liver or kidney function.

➤*Pregnancy:* Safety for use during pregnancy has not been established. Use during pregnancy or in women of childbearing potential only when clearly needed and when the potential benefits outweigh the potential hazards to the fetus.

➤*Lactation:* Carisoprodol is excreted in breast milk at concentrations 2 to 4 times that of maternal plasma. Consider this factor when use of the drug is contemplated in lactating patients.

➤*Children:* Not recommended for use in children under 12 years of age.

Precautions

➤*Hazardous tasks:* May impair the mental or physical abilities required for the performance of potentially hazardous tasks; patients should observe caution while driving or performing other tasks requiring alertness, coordination or physical dexterity.

Adverse Reactions

➤*Cardiovascular:* Tachycardia; postural hypotension; facial flushing.

➤*CNS:* Dizziness; drowsiness; vertigo; ataxia; tremor; agitation; irritability; headache; depressive reactions; syncope; insomnia.

➤*GI:* Nausea; vomiting; hiccoughs; epigastric distress.

➤*Miscellaneous:*
Allergic or idiosyncratic (occasional) – Usually seen within the first to fourth doses in patients having had no previous contact with the drug. Skin rash, erythema multiforme, pruritus, eosinophilia and fixed drug eruption with cross-reaction to meprobamate have been reported. Severe reactions are manifested by asthmatic episodes, fever, weakness, dizziness, angioneurotic edema, smarting eyes, hypotension and anaphylactoid shock.

If such reactions occur, discontinue carisoprodol and initiate appropriate symptomatic therapy. Refer to Management of Acute Hypersensitivity Reactions.

Overdosage

➤*Symptoms:* Stupor, coma, shock, respiratory depression and, very rarely, death. The effects of an overdosage of carisoprodol and alcohol or other CNS depressants or psychotropic agents can be additive even when one of the drugs has been taken in the usual recommended dosage.

➤*Treatment:* Includes usual supportive measures. Refer to General Management of Acute Overdosage.

Although carisoprodol overdosage experience is limited, the following treatments have been successful with the related drug, meprobamate: Diuresis, osmotic (mannitol) diuresis, peritoneal dialysis and hemodialysis (carisoprodol is dialyzable).

Monitor urine output and avoid overhydration. Observe for possible relapse due to incomplete gastric emptying and delayed absorption. Carisoprodol can be measured in biological fluids by gas chromatography.

Patient Information

May take with food or meals if GI upset occurs.

May cause drowsiness or dizziness. Patients should observe caution while driving or performing other tasks requiring alertness, coordination or physical dexterity. Avoid alcohol and other CNS depressants.

If dizziness (postural hypotension) occurs, avoid sudden changes in posture; use caution when climbing stairs, etc.

CHLORPHENESIN CARBAMATE

Rx	Maolate (Upjohn)	Tablets: 400 mg	Tartrazine. (Maolate). Tan, scored. In 50s and 500s.

Indications

➤*Musculoskeletal conditions:* As an adjunct to rest, physical therapy and other measures for relief of discomfort associated with acute, painful musculoskeletal conditions.

Administration and Dosage

➤*Initial:* 800 mg 3 times daily until the desired effect is obtained.

➤*Maintenance:* May reduce to 400 mg 4 times daily, or less, as required.

Safe use for periods exceeding 8 weeks has not been established.

Actions

➤*Pharmacology:* Chlorphenesin is chemically related to mephenesin. Its mode of action has not been identified, but may be related to its sedative properties. It has no direct action on striated muscle, the motor endplate or the nerve fiber. It does not directly relax tense skeletal muscles.

➤*Pharmacokinetics:* The drug is readily absorbed from the GI tract. Peak plasma concentrations of chlorphenesin are reached 1 or 3 hours after administration and half-life is approximately 3.5 hours.

Contraindications

Hypersensitivity to chlorphenesin carbamate.

Warnings

➤*Hypersensitivity reactions:* Occasionally, anaphylactoid reactions and drug fever occur. Such reactions indicate discontinuing the drug. Refer to Management of Acute Hypersensitivity Reactions.

➤*Hepatic function impairment:* Use with caution in patients with preexisting liver disease or impaired hepatic function.

➤*Pregnancy:* Safety for use has not been established. Use during pregnancy and in women of childbearing potential only if clearly needed and when the potential benefits outweigh the potential hazards.

➤*Lactation:* Safety for use has not been established. Use in the nursing mother only when clearly needed and when the potential benefits outweigh the potential hazards.

➤*Children:* Safety and efficacy are not established. Use is not recommended.

Precautions

➤*Duration:* Safe use for periods exceeding 8 weeks has not been established.

➤*Hazardous tasks:* May impair mental or physical abilities required for the performance of potentially hazardous tasks; patients should observe caution while driving or performing other tasks requiring alertness, coordination or physical dexterity.

➤*Tartrazine sensitivity:* This product contains tartrazine, which may cause allergic-type reactions (including bronchial asthma) in susceptible individuals. Although the incidence of tartrazine sensitivity in the general population is low, it is frequently seen in patients who also have aspirin hypersensitivity.

Adverse Reactions

➤*CNS:* Drowsiness; dizziness; confusion; paradoxical stimulation; insomnia; increased nervousness; headache. Dose reduction will usually control these symptoms.

➤*GI:* Nausea; epigastric distress; GI bleeding (two cases, not established as drug-related).

➤*Hematologic:* Leukopenia, thrombocytopenia, agranulocytosis, pancytopenia (rare).

➤*Hypersensitivity:* Anaphylactoid reactions and drug fever (see Warnings).

Overdosage

➤*Symptoms:* One patient who attempted suicide by ingesting 12 g was slightly nauseated and drowsy for about 6 hrs, but recovered with routine supportive therapy.

➤*Treatment:* Includes usual supportive measures. Refer to General Management of Acute Overdosage.

Patient Information

May cause drowsiness or dizziness. Patients should observe caution while driving or performing other tasks requiring alertness, coordination or physical dexterity. Avoid alcohol and other CNS depressants.

CHLORZOXAZONE

Rx	Chlorzoxazone (Various, eg, Goldline)	Tablets: 250 mg	In 100s and 1000s.
Rx	Paraflex (McNeil Pharm.)	Caplets: 250 mg	(Paraflex). Peach. In 100s.
Rx	Remular-S (Inter. Ethical)	Tablets: 250 mg	In 100s.
Rx	Chlorzoxazone (Various, eg, Goldline, IDE, Royce, Rugby, Schein)	Tablets: 500 mg	In 100s, 500s and 1000s.
Rx	Parafon Forte DSC (McNeil Pharm.)	Caplets: 500 mg	(McNeil Parafon Forte DSC). Lt. green, scored. In 100s, 500s and UD 100s.

Indications

➤*Musculoskeletal conditions:* As an adjunct to rest, physical therapy and other measures for the relief of discomfort associated with acute, painful musculoskeletal conditions.

Administration and Dosage

➤*Adults:*

Usual dosage – 250 mg 3 or 4 times daily. Initial dosage for painful musculoskeletal conditions is 500 mg 3 or 4 times daily. If response is inadequate, increase to 750 mg 3 or 4 times daily. As improvement occurs, dosage can usually be reduced.

Actions

➤*Pharmacology:* Mode of action is not identified, but may be related to its sedative properties. Acts primarily at the spinal cord level and subcortical areas of the brain, inhibiting multisynaptic reflex arcs involved in producing and maintaining skeletal muscle spasm of varied etiology. This results in reduced skeletal muscle spasm, relief of pain and increased mobility of involved muscles. It does not directly relax tense skeletal muscles.

➤*Pharmacokinetics:* Serum levels can be detected in the first 30 minutes after administration and peak in 1 to 2 hours. Onset of action is 1 hour; effects last 3 to 4 hours. The drug is rapidly metabolized and excreted in urine, primarily as a glucuronide conjugate. Half-life is ≈ 60 minutes; < 1% of a dose is excreted unchanged in urine in 24 hours.

Contraindications

Intolerance to chlorzoxazone.

Warnings

➤*Hypersensitivity reactions:* Use with caution in patients with known allergies or a history of allergic drug reactions. If a sensitivity reaction occurs such as urticaria, redness or itching, discontinue use. Refer to Management of Acute Hypersensitivity Reactions.

➤*Hepatic function impairment:* If signs or symptoms of liver dysfunction are observed, discontinue use.

➤*Pregnancy:* Safety for use has not been established. Use only when clearly needed and when the potential benefits outweigh the potential hazards.

Precautions

➤*Hazardous tasks:* May produce drowsiness or dizziness; patients should observe caution while driving or performing other tasks requiring alertness, coordination or physical dexterity.

Adverse Reactions

The drug is well tolerated and seldom produces undesirable adverse reactions.

➤*CNS:* Drowsiness; dizziness; lightheadedness; malaise; overstimulation.

➤*Dermatologic:* Allergic-type skin rashes, petechiae, ecchymoses (rare).

➤*GI:* GI disturbances; GI bleeding (rare).

➤*Hypersensitivity:* Angioneurotic edema, anaphylaxis (very rare). See Warnings.

➤*Hepatic:* Chlorzoxazone was suspected of causing liver damage in some patients. The clinical picture was compatible with either a viral or drug-induced hepatitis. In most cases the patients recovered when the drug was stopped.

➤*Miscellaneous:* Urine discoloration.

Overdosage

➤*Symptoms:* Initially, nausea, vomiting or diarrhea together with drowsiness, dizziness, lightheadedness or headache may occur. Early in the course, there may be malaise or sluggishness followed by marked loss of muscle tone, making voluntary movement impossible. Deep tendon reflexes may be decreased or absent. The sensorium remains intact, and there is no peripheral loss of sensation. Respiratory depression may occur with rapid, irregular respiration and intercostal and substernal retraction. Blood pressure is lowered, but shock has not been observed.

➤*Treatment:* Treatment is supportive. Cholinergic drugs or analeptic drugs are of no value and should not be used. Refer to General Management of Acute Overdosage.

Patient Information

Take with food or water if GI upset occurs. Notify physician of skin rash or itching.

May cause drowsiness, dizziness or lightheadedness. Observe caution while driving or performing other tasks requiring alertness, coordination or physical dexterity. Avoid alcohol and other CNS depressants.

Medication may discolor urine orange or purple-red.

CYCLOBENZAPRINE HCl

Rx	Flexeril (McNeil)	Tablets: 5 mg	Lactose. (FLEXERIL). Yellow-orange, 5 sided D-shape. Film-coated.
Rx	Cyclobenzaprine HCl (Various, eg, Goldline, Major, Moore, Parmed, Rugby, Schein)	Tablets: 10 mg	In 30s, 100s and 1000.
Rx	Flexeril (McNeil)		Lactose. Yellow. Film-coated.

Indications

➤*Musculoskeletal conditions:* Adjunct to rest and physical therapy for relief of muscle spasm associated with acute painful musculoskeletal conditions.

➤*Unlabeled uses:* Cyclobenzaprine (10 to 40 mg/day) appears to be a useful adjunct in the management of the fibrositis syndrome.

Administration and Dosage

Give 10 mg 3 times daily (range, 20 to 40 mg daily in divided doses). Do not exceed 60 mg/day. Do not use longer than 2 or 3 weeks.

Actions

➤*Pharmacology:* Cyclobenzaprine, structurally related to the tricyclic antidepressants (TCAs), relieves skeletal muscle spasm of local origin without interfering with muscle function. It is ineffective in muscle spasm due to CNS disease. In animals, the drug reduces or abolishes muscle hyperactivity, does not act at the neuromuscular junction or directly on skeletal muscle, and acts primarily within the CNS at the brain stem as opposed to spinal cord levels; however, its action on the latter may contribute to its overall skeletal muscle relaxant activity. The net effect is a reduction of tonic somatic motor activity, influencing both gamma and alpha motor systems.

Animal studies also show a similarity between the effects of cyclobenzaprine and TCAs, including reserpine antagonism, norepinephrine potentiation, potent peripheral and central anticholinergic effects and sedation. In animals, cyclobenzaprine causes a slight to moderate increase in heart rate.

➤*Pharmacokinetics:* Cyclobenzaprine is well absorbed after oral administration, but there is a large intersubject variation in plasma levels. Peak plasma levels are reached in 4 to 6 hours. The onset of action occurs in 1 hour with a duration of 12 to 24 hours. It is highly bound to plasma proteins, extensively metabolized primarily to glucuronide-like conjugates and excreted primarily via the kidneys. Elimination half-life is 1 to 3 days.

➤*Clinical trials:* Cyclobenzaprine significantly improves the signs and symptoms of skeletal muscle spasm as compared with placebo. Clinical responses include improvement in muscle spasm, local pain and tenderness, increased range of motion and less restriction in activities of daily living. Clinical improvement was observed as early as the first day of therapy. In controlled trials comparing cyclobenzaprine, diazepam and placebo, cyclobenzaprine demonstrated comparable or greater improvement in muscle spasm when compared with diazepam. Side effects were comparable.

CYCLOBENZAPRINE HCl

Contraindications

Hypersensitivity to cyclobenzaprine; concomitant use of monoamine oxidase (MAO) inhibitors or within 14 days after their discontinuation (see Drug Interactions); acute recovery phase of myocardial infarction (MI) and in patients with arrhythmias, heart block or conduction disturbances, or congestive heart failure (CHF); hyperthyroidism.

Warnings

➤*Spasticity:* Cyclobenzaprine is not effective in the treatment of spasticity associated with cerebral or spinal cord disease, or in children with cerebral palsy.

➤*Duration:* Use only for short periods (up to 2 or 3 weeks); effectiveness for more prolonged use is not proven. Muscle spasm associated with acute, painful musculoskeletal conditions is generally of short duration; specific therapy for longer periods is seldom warranted.

➤*Similarity to TCAs:* Cyclobenzaprine is closely related to the TCAs. In short-term studies for indications other than muscle spasm associated with acute musculoskeletal conditions, and usually at doses greater than those recommended, some of the more serious CNS reactions noted with the TCAs have occurred. Because of pharmacologic similarities to tricyclic drugs, consider certain withdrawal symptoms with cyclobenzaprine, although they have not been reported. Abrupt cessation of treatment after prolonged administration may produce nausea, headache and malaise; these do not indicate addiction.

➤*Pregnancy: Category B.* Use only when clearly needed and when the potential benefits outweigh the unknown potential hazards to the fetus.

➤*Lactation:* It is not known whether cyclobenzaprine is excreted in breast milk. Some of the TCAs are excreted in breast milk. Exercise caution when administering cyclobenzaprine to a nursing woman.

➤*Children:* Safety and efficacy in children < 15 years of age have not been established.

Precautions

➤*Anticholinergic effects:* Because of its anticholinergic action, use with caution in patients with a history of urinary retention, angle-closure glaucoma and increased intraocular pressure.

➤*Hazardous tasks:* May impair mental or physical abilities required for performance of hazardous tasks; patients should observe caution while driving or performing other tasks requiring alertness, coordination and physical dexterity.

Drug Interactions

Because of similarities to the TCAs, consider all interactions listed in the Tricyclic Antidepressants monograph.

➤*MAO inhibitors:* Hyperpyretic crisis, severe convulsions and death have occurred in patients receiving TCAs and MAO inhibitors. Cyclobenzaprine may interact similarly.

Adverse Reactions

Because of the similarities to TCAs, consider all reactions listed in the Adverse Reaction section in the Tricyclic Antidepressants monograph.

➤*Cardiovascular:* Tachycardia, syncope, arrhythmias, vasodilation, palpitations, hypotension (< 1%); chest pain; edema; hypertension; myocardial infarction; heart block; stroke.

➤*CNS:* Drowsiness (39%); dizziness (11%); fatigue, tiredness, asthenia, blurred vision, headache, nervousness (1% to 3%); convulsions, ataxia, vertigo, dysarthria, paresthesia, tremors, hypertonia, malaise, tinnitus, diplopia (< 1%); decreased or increased libido; abnormal gait; delusions; peripheral neuropathy; Bell's palsy; alteration in EEG patterns; extrapyramidal symptoms.

➤*Dermatologic:* Sweating, skin rash, urticaria, pruritus (< 1%); photosensitization; alopecia.

➤*GI:* Dry mouth (27%); nausea, constipation, dyspepsia, unpleasant taste (1% to 3%); vomiting, anorexia, diarrhea, GI pain, gastritis, thirst, flatulence, ageusia (< 1%); paralytic ileus; tongue discoloration; stomatitis; parotid swelling.

➤*GU:* Urinary frequency or retention (< 1%); impaired urination; dilation of urinary tract; impotence; testicular swelling; gynecomastia; breast enlargement; galactorrhea.

➤*Hematologic/Lymphatic:* Purpura; bone marrow depression; leukopenia; eosinophilia; thrombocytopenia.

➤*Hepatic:* Abnormal liver function, hepatitis, jaundice, cholestasis (< 1%).

➤*Metabolic/Nutritional:* Elevation and lowering of blood sugar levels; weight gain or loss.

➤*Musculoskeletal:* Muscle twitching, local weakness (< 1%); myalgia.

➤*Psychiatric:* Confusion (1% to 3%); disorientation, insomnia, depressed mood, abnormal sensations, anxiety, agitation, abnormal thinking and dreaming, hallucinations, excitement (< 1%).

➤*Miscellaneous:* Edema of face and tongue (< 1%); inappropriate ADH syndrome; dyspnea.

Overdosage

➤*Symptoms:* High doses may cause temporary confusion, disturbed concentration, transient visual hallucinations, agitation, hyperactive reflexes, muscle rigidity, vomiting or hyperpyrexia, in addition to the effects listed under adverse reactions. Overdosage may cause drowsiness, hypothermia, tachycardia and other cardiac arrhythmias such as bundle branch block, ECG evidence of impaired conduction and CHF, dilated pupils, convulsions, severe hypotension, stupor and coma. Paradoxical diaphoresis has been reported.

➤*Treatment:* Treatment includes usual supportive measures. Refer to General Management of Acute Overdosage. Obtain an ECG and closely monitor cardiac function if there is any evidence of dysrhythmia.

Physostigmine, 1 to 3 mg IV, has been used to reverse anticholinergic effects. However, profound bradycardia and asystole may occur as a result. The role of physostigmine is not clear; avoid its use if other therapeutic agents are successful in reversing cardiac dysrhythmias.

Dialysis is probably of no value because of low plasma concentrations of the drug.

Patient Information

May cause drowsiness, dizziness or blurred vision. Patients should observe caution while driving or performing other tasks requiring alertness, coordination or physical dexterity.

Avoid alcohol and other CNS depressants.

May cause dry mouth.

DIAZEPAM

c-iv	**Diazepam** (Various, eg, Barr, Major, Mylan, Parmed, Zenith)	**Tablets:** 2 mg	In 100s, 500s, 1000s and 5000s.
c-iv	**Valium** (Roche)		(2 Valium/ Roche). White, scored. In 100s, 500s and Tel-E-Dose 100s.
c-iv	**Diazepam** (Various, eg, Barr, Major, Mylan, Zenith)	**Tablets:** 5 mg	In 100s, 500s, 1000s, 2500s and 5000s.
c-iv	**Valium** (Roche)		(5 Valium / Roche). Yellow, scored. In 100s, 500s and Tel-E-Dose 100s.
c-iv	**Diazepam** (Various, eg, Barr, Major, Mylan, Zenith)	**Tablets:** 10 mg	In 100s, 500s, 1000s, 2500s and 5000s.
c-iv	**Valium** (Roche)		(10 Valium / Roche). Blue, scored. In 100s, 500s and Tel-E-Dose 100s.
c-iv	**Diazepam** (Roxane)	**Oral Solution:** 5 mg/5 ml	Wintergreen-spice flavor. In UD 5 and 10 ml.
c-iv	**Diazepam Intensol** (Roxane)	**Concentrated Oral Solution:** 5 mg/ml	In 30 ml with calibrated dropper.
c-iv	**Diazepam** (Various, eg, Winthrop)	**Injection:** 5 mg/ml	In 2 ml amps, 1, 2, 5 and 10 ml vials and 1 and 2 ml syringes.

[1] With 40% propylene glycol, 10% ethyl alcohol, 5% sodium benzoate and 1.5% benzyl alcohol.

The following is an abbreviated monograph. For complete prescribing information, refer to the Benzodiazepines monograph in the Antianxiety Agents section.

Indications

An adjunct for the relief of skeletal muscle spasm due to reflex spasm to local pathology (such as inflammation of the muscles or joints, or secondary to trauma); spasticity caused by upper motor neuron disorders (eg, cerebral palsy and paraplegia); athetosis; stiff-man syndrome. Injectable diazepam may also be used as an adjunct in tetanus.

Also used as an antianxiety agent (see Benzodiazepines monograph in the Antianxiety Agents section) and an anticonvulsant (see the Diazepam monograph in the Anticonvulsants section).

Administration and Dosage

➤*Oral:* Individualize dosage for maximum beneficial effect.

Adults – 2 to 10 mg 3 or 4 times daily.

Geriatric or debilitated patients – 2 to 2.5 mg 1 or 2 times daily initially, increasing as needed and tolerated.

Children – 1 to 2.5 mg 3 or 4 times daily initially, increasing as needed and tolerated (not for use in children under 6 months of age).

Intensol – Dosages are same as those listed above. Mix with liquid or semi-solid food such as water, juices, soda or soda-like beverages, applesauce and puddings. Stir in gently. Consume the entire mixture immediately. Do not store for future use.

DIAZEPAM

Sustained release – 15 to 30 mg once daily.

➤*Parenteral:* Use lower doses (2 to 5 mg) and slow dosage increases for elderly or debilitated patients and when other sedatives are given. When acute symptoms are controlled with the injectable form, administer oral therapy if further treatment is required.

Neonates (≤ 30 days of age) – Safety and efficacy have not been established. Prolonged CNS depression has been observed in neonates, apparently due to inability to biotransform diazepam into inactive metabolites.

Children – Give slowly over 3 minutes in a dosage not to exceed 0.25 mg/kg. After a 15 to 30 minute interval, the initial dosage can be safely repeated. If relief is not obtained after a third administration, begin adjunctive therapy appropriate to the condition being treated.

➤*IM:* Inject deeply into the muscle.

➤*IV:* Inject slowly, taking at least 1 minute for each 5 mg (1 ml). Do not use small veins (ie, dorsum of hand or wrist). Avoid intra-arterial administration or extravasation. Do not mix or dilute with other solutions or drugs.

Adults – 5 to 10 mg, IM or IV initially, then 5 to 10 mg in 3 to 4 hours, if necessary. For tetanus, larger doses may be required.

Children – For tetanus in infants > 30 days of age, 1 to 2 mg IM or IV slowly; repeat every 3 to 4 hours as necessary. In children ≥ 5 years of age, 5 to 10 mg. Repeat every 3 to 4 hours if necessary to control tetanus spasms. Have respiratory assistance available.

Actions

➤*Pharmacology:* In animals, diazepam acts on the thalamus and hypothalamus, inducing calming effects. Diazepam has no demonstrable peripheral autonomic blocking action, nor does it produce extrapyramidal side effects; however, animals treated with diazepam do have a transient ataxia at higher doses.

Major muscle relaxant actions occur in two proposed sites: At the spinal level resulting in enhancement of GABA-mediated presynaptic inhibition, and at supraspinal sites, probably in the brain stem reticular formation.

METAXALONE

Rx	Skelaxin (King)	Tablets: 400 mg	(C 8662). Pale rose, scored. In 100s and 500s.
		800 mg	(8667 S). Pink, oval, scored. In 100s and 500s.

Indications

➤*Musculoskeletal conditions:* As an adjunct to rest, physical therapy and other measures for the relief of discomfort associated with acute, painful musculoskeletal conditions.

Administration and Dosage

➤*Adults and children (> 12 years):* 800 mg 3 to 4 times daily.

Actions

➤*Pharmacology:* The mechanism of action of metaxalone has not been established, but it may be caused by general CNS depression. The drug has no direct action on the contractile mechanism of striated muscle, the motor endplate or the nerve fiber. Metaxalone does not directly relax tense skeletal muscles.

➤*Pharmacokinetics:* Onset of action is 1 hour and duration of action is 4 to 6 hours. Peak plasma levels of ≈ 300 mcg/ml occur 2 hours after administration of 800 mg metaxalone. The half-life is 2 to 3 hours; metabolites are excreted in the urine.

Contraindications

Hypersensitivity to metaxalone; known tendency to drug-induced hemolytic or other anemias; significantly impaired renal or hepatic function.

Warnings

➤*Hepatic function impairment:* Administer with great care to patients with preexisting liver damage and perform serial liver function studies as required. Elevations in cephalin flocculation tests without concurrent changes in other liver function parameters have been noted.

➤*Pregnancy:* Human experience has not revealed evidence of fetal injury, but the possibility of infrequent or subtle damage to the human fetus cannot be excluded. Do not use during pregnancy, especially during early pregnancy, or in women who may become pregnant, unless the potential benefits outweigh the potential hazards to the fetus.

➤*Lactation:* It is not known whether this drug is excreted in breast milk. Safety for use in the nursing mother has not been established.

➤*Children:* Safety and efficacy for use in children ≤ 12 years of age have not been established.

Drug Interactions

➤*Drug/Lab test interactions:* False-positive Benedict's tests, caused by an unknown reducing substance, have been noted. A glucose-specific test will differentiate findings.

Adverse Reactions

➤*CNS:* Drowsiness; dizziness; headache; nervousness; irritability.

➤*GI:* Nausea; vomiting; GI upset.

➤*Miscellaneous:* Hypersensitivity reaction (light rash with or without pruritus); leukopenia; hemolytic anemia; jaundice.

Overdosage

Employ gastric lavage and supportive therapy as indicated. No documented case of major toxicity has been reported. Refer to General Management of Acute Overdosage.

Patient Information

May cause drowsiness or dizziness. Patients should observe caution while driving or performing other tasks requiring alertness, coordination or physical dexterity.

Avoid alcohol and other CNS depressants.

Notify physician if skin rash or yellowish discoloration of the skin or eyes occurs.

METHOCARBAMOL

Rx	Methocarbamol (Various, eg, Geneva, Lederle, Major, Schein, UDL, Zenith-Goldline)	Tablets: 500 mg	In 100s, 500s and UD 100s.
Rx	Robaxin (Schwarz Pharma)		Saccharin. (Robaxin AHR). Light orange. In 100s, 500s, *Disco-Pak* 100s.
Rx	Methocarbamol (Various, eg, Geneva, Lederle, Major, Schein, UDL, Zenith-Goldline)	Tablets: 750 mg	In 60s, 100s, 500s and UD 100s.
Rx	Robaxin-750 (Schwarz Pharma)		Saccharin. (AHR Robaxin-750). Orange. Capsule-shaped. In 100s, 500s and *Disco-Pak* 100s.
Rx	Methocarbamol (Various, eg, Schein)	Injection: 100 mg/ml	In 10 ml vials.
Rx	Robaxin (Wyeth-Ayerst)		In 10 ml vials.[1]

[1] In solution of polyethylene glycol 300. After mixing with IV infusion fluids, do not refrigerate.

Indications

➤*Musculoskeletal conditions:* Adjunctive therapy to rest, physical therapy, and other measures for the relief of discomfort associated with acute, painful musculoskeletal conditions.

➤*Tetanus:* May have a beneficial effect in the control of neuromuscular manifestations of tetanus.

Administration and Dosage

➤*Parenteral:* For IV and IM use only. Not recommended for SC administration. Do not exceed total adult dosage of 3 g for > 3 consecutive days except in the treatment of tetanus. Repeat this course after a lapse of 48 hours if the condition persists. Base dosage and frequency on severity of the condition and the therapeutic response.

For the relief of symptoms of moderate degree, 1 g may be adequate. Injection need not be repeated, as tablets will sustain the relief. For severe cases or in postoperative conditions in which oral use is not feasible, 2 to 3 g may be required.

IV – Administer undiluted directly IV at a maximum rate of 3 ml/minute. May also be added to an IV drip of Sodium Chloride Injection or 5% Dextrose Injection; do not dilute one vial given as a single dose to > 250 ml for IV infusion. Avoid vascular extravasation which may result in thrombophlebitis. The patient should be recumbent during and for at least 10 to 15 minutes following injection.

IM – Do not inject > 5 ml into each gluteal region; repeat at 8 hour intervals, if needed. As symptoms are relieved, change to tablets.

METHOCARBAMOL

Tetanus – Methocarbamol does not replace the usual procedure of debridement, tetanus antitoxin, penicillin, tracheotomy, attention to fluid balance and supportive care. Add methocarbamol injection to the regimen as soon as possible.

Adults: Inject 1 or 2 g directly into the IV tubing. An additional 1 or 2 g may be added to the infusion bottle so that a total of ≤ 3 g is given as the initial dose. Repeat procedure every 6 hours until conditions allow for the insertion of a nasogastric tube. Crushed methocarbamol tablets suspended in water or saline may then be given through the nasogastric tube. Total daily oral doses ≤ 24 g may be required.

Children: A minimum initial dose of 15 mg/kg is recommended. Give by injection into the tubing or by IV infusion with an appropriate quantity of fluid. Repeat every 6 hours as indicated.

➤*Oral (Adults):*

Initial – 1.5 g 4 times daily.

Maintenance – 1 g 4 times daily; 750 mg every 4 hours; or 1.5 g 3 times daily.

For the first 48 to 72 hours, 6 g/day are recommended. (For severe conditions 8 g daily may be administered.) Thereafter, reduce to ≈ 4 g daily.

Actions

➤*Pharmacology:* Mechanism of action has not been established, but may be caused by general CNS depression. The drug has no direct action on the contractile mechanism of striated muscle, motor endplate or nerve fiber. It does not directly relax tense skeletal muscles.

➤*Pharmacokinetics:* Methocarbamol has an onset of action of 30 minutes. Peak plasma levels occur ≈ 2 hours after administration of 2 g. The half-life is from 1 to 2 hours; inactive metabolites are excreted in the urine and small amounts in the feces.

Contraindications

Hypersensitivity to methocarbamol or any ingredient of the product.

➤*Parenteral:* Because of the presence of polyethylene glycol 300 in the vehicle, do not administer parenteral methocarbamol to patients with known or suspected renal pathology.

Warnings

➤*Pregnancy:* Safe use of methocarbamol has not been established with regard to possible adverse effects upon fetal development. Therefore, do not use the drug in women who are or who may become pregnant, particularly during early pregnancy unless, in the judgment of the physician, the potential benefits outweigh the possible hazards.

➤*Lactation:* It is not known whether methocarbamol is excreted in breast milk. Exercise caution when administering to a nursing woman. The American Academy of Pediatrics classifies methocarbamol as compatible with breastfeeding.

➤*Children:* Safety and efficacy in children < 12 years old are not established, except in tetanus. See directions for use in tetanus under Administration and Dosage.

Precautions

➤*Rate of injection:* Rate of injection should not exceed 3 ml/minute. Since solution is hypertonic, avoid vascular extravasation. A recumbent position reduces likelihood of adverse reactions.

➤*Total parenteral dosage:* Total parenteral dosage should not exceed 3 g per day for > 3 consecutive days, except in the treatment of tetanus.

➤*Epilepsy:* Use the injectable form cautiously in suspected or known epileptics.

Drug Interactions

➤*Drug/Lab test interactions:* Methocarbamol may cause a color interference in certain screening tests for **5-hydroxyindoleacetic acid (5-HIAA)** and **vanillylmandelic acid (VMA)**.

Adverse Reactions

➤*Parenteral:* Certain reactions may have been caused by an overly rapid rate of IV injection.

Cardiovascular – Syncope; hypotension; bradycardia. In most cases of syncope, there was spontaneous recovery. In others, epinephrine, injectable steroids or injectable antihistamines were employed to hasten recovery.

CNS – Dizziness; lightheadedness; vertigo; headache; drowsiness; fainting; mild muscular incoordination. Reports of convulsive seizures during IV use include instances in epileptics. Psychic trauma of the procedure may be a contributing factor. Several observers have reported success in terminating epileptiform seizures with methocarbamol, but its use in patients with epilepsy is not recommended.

Dermatologic – Urticaria; pruritus; rash; flushing.

Ophthalmic – Blurred vision; conjunctivitis with nasal congestion; nystagmus; diplopia.

Miscellaneous – GI upset; metallic taste; sloughing or pain at the injection site; thrombophlebitis; anaphylactic reaction; fever.

➤*Oral:* Lightheadedness; dizziness; drowsiness; nausea; urticaria; pruritus; rash; conjunctivitis with nasal congestion; blurred vision; headache; fever.

Overdosage

➤*Symptoms:* Overdose, often in conjunction with alcohol or other CNS depressants, is marked by coma and other signs of CNS depression.

➤*Treatment:* Supportive. Refer to General Management of Acute Overdosage.

Patient Information

May cause drowsiness, dizziness or lightheadedness. Patients should observe caution while driving or performing other tasks requiring alertness, coordination or physical dexterity. Avoid alcohol and other CNS depressants.

Urine may darken to brown, black or green.

Notify physician if skin rash, itching, fever or nasal congestion occurs.

ORPHENADRINE CITRATE

Rx	**Orphenadrine Citrate** (Various)	**Tablets:** 100 mg	In 30s, 100s, 500s and 1000s.
Rx	**Orphenadrine Citrate** (Apothecon)	**Tablets, sustained release:** 100 mg	Lactose. (INV 336). White. In 100s and 500s.
Rx	**Norflex** (3M Pharm)		(3M 221). White. In 100s and 500s.
Rx	**Orphenadrine Citrate** (Various, eg, Rugby)	**Injection:** 30 mg per ml	In 2 ml amps and 10 ml vials.
Rx	**Banflex** (Forest Pharm.)		In 10 ml vials.
Rx	**Flexon** (Various, eg, Keene)		In 10 ml vials.
Rx	**Norflex** (3M Pharm)		In 2 ml amps.[1]

[1] With sodium bisulfite.

Indications

➤*Musculoskeletal conditions:* As an adjunct to rest, physical therapy and other measures for relief of discomfort associated with acute, painful musculoskeletal conditions.

➤*Unlabeled uses:* Orphenadrine 100 mg at bedtime may be beneficial in the treatment of quinine-resistant leg cramps.

Administration and Dosage

➤*Oral:* 100 mg each morning and evening. Do not crush or chew sustained release preparations.

➤*Parenteral:* 60 mg IV or IM. May repeat every 12 hours.

Actions

➤*Pharmacology:* The mode of action of orphenadrine has not been identified, but may be related to its analgesic properties. It acts centrally at the brain stem; it does not directly relax tense skeletal muscles. It possesses anticholinergic actions.

➤*Pharmacokinetics:* Peak plasma levels occur 2 hours after administration of 100 mg orphenadrine; duration of action is 4 to 6 hours. The half-life is approximately 14 hours for the parent drug, and 2 to 25 hours for metabolites. Excretion is via urine and feces. Most of orphenadrine is degraded to eight known metabolites.

Contraindications

Glaucoma; pyloric or duodenal obstruction; stenosing peptic ulcers; prostatic hypertrophy; obstruction of the bladder neck; cardiospasm (megaesophagus) and myasthenia gravis; hypersensitivity to orphenadrine.

Warnings

➤*Hypersensitivity reactions:* Hypersensitivity reactions may occur. Refer to Management of Acute Hypersensitivity Reactions.

➤*Pregnancy: Category C.* It is not known whether orphenadrine can cause fetal harm or affect reproduction capacity. Use in pregnancy only when clearly neded.

➤*Lactation:* It is not known whether orphenadrine is excreted in breast milk.

➤*Children:* Safety and efficacy for use in children have not been established. Not recommended for use in the pediatric age group.

ORPHENADRINE CITRATE

Precautions

➤*Cardiac disease:* Use with caution in patients with cardiac decompensation, coronary insufficiency, cardiac arrhythmias or tachycardia.

➤*Long-term therapy:* Safety of continuous long-term therapy has not been established; periodically monitor blood, urine and liver function values.

➤*Hazardous tasks:* May cause transient episodes of lightheadedness, dizziness or syncope. Patients should observe caution while driving or performing other tasks requiring alertness, coordination or physical dexterity.

➤*Sulfite sensitivity:* Some of these products contain sulfites which may cause allergic-type reactions (eg, hives, itching, wheezing, anaphylaxis) in certain susceptible persons. Although the overall prevalence of sulfite sensitivity in the general population is probably low, it is seen more frequently in asthmatics or in atopic nonasthmatic persons. Specific products containing sulfites are identified in the product listings.

Drug Interactions

Orphenadrine Drug Interactions			
Precipitant drug	Object drug[*]		Description
Amantadine	Orphenadrine	↑	Anticholinergic effects may be increased.
Orphenadrine	Haloperidol	↔	Worsening of schizophrenic symptoms, decreased haloperidol levels and development of tardive dyskinesia may occur.
Orphenadrine	Phenothiazines	↓	Therapeutic effects of phenothiazines may be decreased.

[*] ↑ = Object drug increased. ↓ = Object drug decreased. ↔ = Undetermined effect.

Adverse Reactions

Adverse effects are mainly due to the anticholinergic effects of orphenadrine and are usually associated with higher doses.

Dry mouth is the first side effect to appear. When daily dose is increased, possible effects include:

➤*Cardiovascular:* Tachycardia, palpitation, transient syncope.

➤*CNS:* Weakness, headache, dizziness, lightheadedness, confusion (in elderly patients), hallucinations, agitation, tremor, drowsiness.

➤*GI:* Vomiting, nausea, constipation, gastric irritation.

➤*GU:* Urinary hesitancy and retention.

➤*Hematologic:* Rarely, aplastic anemia; a causal relationship has not been established.

➤*Hypersensitivity:* Urticaria and other dermatoses (sometimes pruritic). Rarely, anaphylactic reaction following IM injection (rare). See Warnings.

➤*Ophthalmic:* Blurred vision, pupil dilation, increased ocular tension.

Overdosage

➤*Symptoms:* The lethal dose of orphenadrine in adults is 2 to 3 g. Intoxication is very rapid and death can occur within 3 to 5 hours preceded by deep coma, seizures and shock. Serious cardiac rhythm disturbances are common.

➤*Treatment:* Prevent further absorption by gastric lavage. Hemodialysis may not be helpful.

Patient Information

May cause drowsiness, dizziness, blurred vision or fainting. Observe caution while driving or performing tasks requiring alertness, coordination or physical dexterity.

Avoid alcohol and other CNS depressants.

May cause dry mouth, difficult urination, constipation, headache and GI upset. Notify physician if these effects persist, or if skin rash or itching, rapid heart rate, palpitations or mental confusion occurs.

TIZANIDINE HCl

Rx	Tizanidine HCl (Various, eg, Par, Teva)	Tablets: 2 mg (as base)	In 150s and 300s.
Rx	Zanaflex (Athena Neurosciences)		Lactose. (592). White, scored. In 150s.
Rx	Tizanidine HCl (Various, eg, Eon, Par, Teva)	Tablets: 4 mg (as base)	In 150s, 300s, and 1000s.
Rx	Zanaflex (Athena Neurosciences)		Lactose. (594). White, scored. In 150s.

Indications

➤*Muscle spasticity:* For the acute and intermittent management of increased muscle tone associated with spasticity.

Administration and Dosage

➤*Approved by the FDA:* November 27, 1996.

A single oral dose of 8 mg tizanidine reduces muscle tone in patients with spasticity for a period of several hours. The effect peaks at ≈ 1 to 2 hours and dissipates between 3 to 6 hours. Effects are dose-related.

Although single doses of < 8 mg have not been demonstrated to be effective in controlled clinical studies, the dose-related nature of tizanidine's common adverse events make it prudent to begin therapy with single oral doses of 4 mg. Increase the dose gradually (2 to 4 mg steps) to optimum effect (satisfactory reduction of muscle tone at a tolerated dose).

The dose can be repeated at 6– to 8–hour intervals, as needed, to a maximum of three doses in 24 hours. Do not exceed 36 mg/day.

Experience with single doses exceeding 8 mg and daily doses exceeding 24 mg is limited. There is essentially no experience with repeated, single, daytime doses > 12 mg or total daily doses > 36 mg.

Actions

➤*Pharmacology:* Tizanidine is a centrally acting α_2-adrenergic agonist. It presumably reduces spasticity by increasing presynaptic inhibition of motor neurons. In animal models, tizanidine has no direct effect on skeletal muscle fibers or the neuromuscular junction, and no major effect on monosynaptic spinal reflexes. The effects of tizanidine are greatest on polysynaptic pathways. The overall effect of these actions is thought to reduce facilitation of spinal motor neurons.

The imidazole chemical structure of tizanidine is related to that of the antihypertensive drug clonidine and other α_2-adrenergic agonists. Pharmacologic studies in animals show similarities between the two compounds, but tizanidine was found to have one-tenth to one-fiftieth of the potency of clonidine in lowering blood pressure.

➤*Pharmacokinetics:*

Absorption/Distribution – Following oral administration, tizanidine is essentially completely absorbed. Peak effect occurs 1 to 2 hours after dosing, and the effect dissipates between 3 to 6 hours. The absolute oral bioavailability is ≈ 40% because of extensive first-pass metabolism in the liver. Peak plasma concentrations occur at 1.5 hours. Tizanidine is widely distributed throughout the body; mean steady-state volume of distribution is 204 L/kg following IV administration in healthy adult volunteers. It is ≈ 30% bound to plasma proteins.

Food: Food increases C_{max} by ≈ 33% and shortens time-to-peak concentration by ≈ 40 minutes, but the extent of tizanidine absorption is not affected.

Metabolism/Excretion – Tizanidine has extensive first-pass metabolism in the liver, ≈ 95% of the administered dose is metabolized. Tizanidine has a half-life of ≈ 2.5 hours. Metabolites are not known to be active; their half-lives range from 20 to 40 hours. Following single and multiple oral dosing of tizanidine, an average of 60% and 20% of total drug is recovered in the urine and feces, respectively.

Elderly: Following single dose administration of 6 mg, younger subjects cleared the drug four times faster than the elderly subjects.

➤*Clinical trials:* In one study, patients with multiple sclerosis were randomized to receive single oral doses of drug or placebo. A statistically significant reduction of the Ashworth score for tizanidine compared with placebo was detected at 1, 2 and 3 hours after treatment. The greatest reduction in muscle tone was 1 to 2 hours after treatment. By 6 hours after treatment, muscle tone in the 8 and 16 mg tizanidine groups was indistinguishable from muscle tone in placebo-treated patients. Although 16 mg produced a larger effect, adverse events including hypotension were more common and more severe than in the 8 mg group.

In a multiple-dose study, 118 patients with spasticity secondary to spinal cord injury were randomized to either placebo or tizanidine. Patients were titrated over 3 weeks up to a maximum tolerated dose of 36 mg daily given in three unequal doses (eg, 10 mg given in the morning and afternoon and 16 mg given at night). Patients were then maintained on their maximally tolerated dose for 4 additional weeks (eg, maintenance phase). At endpoint, there was a statistically significant reduction in muscle tone in the tizanidine-treated group compared with placebo. The reduction in muscle tone was not associated with a reduction in muscle strength (a desirable outcome) but also did not lead to any consistent advantage of tizanidine-treated patients on measures of activities of daily living.

Contraindications

Hypersensitivity to tizanidine or any components of the drug.

Warnings

➤*Chronic and multiple dosing:* Clinical experience with long-term use of tizanidine at doses of 8 to 16 mg single doses or total daily doses

Centrally Acting

TIZANIDINE HCl

of 24 to 36 mg is limited. Approximately 75 patients have been exposed to individual doses of ≥ 12 mg for 1 year or more and ≈ 80 patients have been exposed to total daily doses of 30 to 36 mg/day for ≥ 1 year.

➤*Hypotension:* Tizanidine is an α_2-adrenergic agonist (like clonidine) and can produce hypotension. In a single dose study, 66% of patients treated with 8 mg had a 20% reduction in either diastolic or systolic blood pressure. The reduction was seen within 1 hour after dosing, peaked 2 to 3 hours after dosing and was associated, at times, with bradycardia, orthostatic hypotension, lightheadedness/dizziness and rarely syncope. The hypotensive effect is dose-related and has been measured following single doses of ≥ 2 mg.

The chance of significant hypotension may possibly be minimized by titration of the dose and by focusing attention on signs and symptoms of hypotension prior to dose advancement. In addition, patients moving from a supine to a fixed upright position may be at increased risk for hypotension and orthostatic effects.

➤*Hepatotoxicity:* Tizanidine occasionally causes liver injury, most often hepatocellular in type. In controlled clinical studies, ≈ 5% of patients treated with tizanidine had elevations of liver function tests (ALT, AST) to > 3 times the upper limit of normal (or 2 times if baseline levels were elevated) compared with 0.4% in the control patients. Most cases resolved rapidly upon drug withdrawal with no reported residual problems. In occasional symptomatic cases, nausea, vomiting, anorexia and jaundice have been reported. In postmarketing experience, three deaths associated with liver failure have occurred in patients treated with tizanidine. In one case, a 49-year-old male developed jaundice and liver enlargement following 2 months of tizanidine treatment, primarily at 6 mg three times a day. A liver biopsy showed multilobular necrosis without eosinophilic infiltration. Another patient, treated with tizanidine at a dose of 4 mg/day, was also on carbamazepine when he developed cholestatic jaundice after 2 months of treatment; this patient died with pneumonia ≈ 20 days later. Another patient, treated with tizanidine for 11 days, was also treated with dantrolene for ≈ 2 weeks prior to developing fatal fulminant hepatic failure.

Monitoring of aminotransferase levels is recommended during the first 6 months of treatment (eg, baseline, 1, 3 and 6 months) and periodically thereafter, based on clinical status.

➤*Sedation:* In the multiple dose, controlled clinical studies, 48% of patients receiving any dose of tizanidine reported sedation as an adverse event. In 10% of these cases, the sedation was rated as severe compared with < 1% in the placebo-treated patients. Sedation may interfere with everyday activity.

Patients began noting this effect 30 minutes following dosing. The effect peaked 1.5 hours following dosing. Of the patients who received a single dose of 16 mg, 51% continued to report drowsiness 6 hours following dosing compared with 13% in the patients receiving placebo or 8 mg tizanidine.

In the multiple dose studies, the prevalence of patients with sedation peaked following the first week of titration, and then remained stable for the duration of the maintenance phase of the study.

➤*Hallucinations/Psychotic-like symptoms:* Tizanidine use has been associated with hallucinations. Formed, visual hallucinations or delusions have been reported in 5 of 170 patients (3%). These 5 cases occurred within the first 6 weeks. Most of the patients were aware that the events were unreal. One patient developed psychoses in association with the hallucinations. One patient among these five continued to have problems for ≥ 2 weeks following discontinuation of tizanidine.

➤*Renal function impairment:* Use tizanidine with caution in patients with renal insufficiency (creatinine clearance < 25 ml/min), as clearance is reduced by > 50%. In these patients, during titration, reduce the individual doses. If higher doses are required, increase individual doses rather than dosing frequency. Monitor these patients closely for the onset or increase in severity of the common adverse events (dry mouth, somnolence, asthenia and dizziness) as indicators of potential overdose.

➤*Hepatic function impairment:* Because of the potential toxic hepatic effect of tizanidine, use the drug only with extreme caution in patients with impaired hepatic function.

➤*Elderly:* Use tizanidine with caution in elderly patients because clearance is decreased 4–fold.

➤*Pregnancy:* Category C. Tizanidine has not been studied in pregnant women. Use in pregnant women only if clearly needed.

➤*Lactation:* It is not known whether tizanidine is excreted in breast milk, although as a lipid soluble drug, it might be expected to pass into breast milk.

➤*Children:* There are no adequate and well controlled studies to document the safety and efficacy of tizanidine in children.

Precautions

➤*Monitoring:* Monitoring of aminotransferase levels is recommended during the first 6 months of treatment (eg, baseline, 1, 3 and 6 months) and periodically thereafter, based on clinical status (see Warnings).

➤*Cardiovascular:* Prolongation of the QT interval and bradycardia were noted in chronic toxicity studies in dogs at doses equal to the maximum human dose on a mg/m^2 basis. ECG evaluation was not performed in the controlled clinical studies. Reduction in pulse rate has been noted in association with decreases in blood pressure in the single dose controlled study.

➤*Ophthalmic:* Dose-related retinal degeneration and corneal opacities have been found in animal studies at doses equivalent to approximately the maximum recommended dose on a mg/m^2 basis. There have been no reports of corneal opacities or retinal degeneration in the clinical studies.

Drug Interactions

Tizanidine Drug Interactions			
Precipitant Drug	Object Drug*'		Description
Alcohol	Tizanidine	↑	Alcohol increased the AUC of tizanidine by ≈ 20% while also increasing its C$_{max}$ by ≈ 15%. This was associated with an increase in side effects of tizanidine. The CNS depressant effects of tizanidine and alcohol are additive.
Contraceptives, Oral	Tizanidine	↑	Use with caution in women taking oral contraceptives, as clearance of tizanidine is reduced by ≈ 50% in such patients. In these patients, during titration, reduce the individual doses.
Tizanidine	Acetaminophen	↓	Tizanidine delayed the T$_{max}$ of acetaminophen by 16 minutes. Acetaminophen did not affect the pharmacokinetics of tizanidine.
Tizanidine	Antihypertensives	↑	Caution is advised when tizanidine is to be used in patients receiving concurrent antihypertensive therapy. Do not use with other α_2-adrenergic agonists.

* ↑ = Object drug increased. ↓ = Object drug decreased.

➤*Drug/Food interactions:* Food increases tizanidine C$_{max}$ by ≈ 33% and shortens time-to-peak concentration by ≈ 40 minutes, but extent of absorption is not affected.

Adverse Reactions

Common adverse events leading to discontinuation – The adverse events most frequently leading to withdrawal of tizanidine-treated patients in the controlled clinical studies were asthenia, somnolence, dry mouth (3%); increased spasm or tone, dizziness (2%).

Most frequent adverse events – The most frequent adverse events were dry mouth, somnolence/sedation, asthenia and dizziness; 75% of the patients rated the events as mild to moderate and 25% of the patients rated the events as being severe. These events appeared to be dose-related.

Tizanidine Adverse Reactions (Incidence Greater Than Placebo, %)		
Adverse reaction	Placebo (n = 261)	Tizanidine (n = 264)
CNS		
Asthenia (tiredness)	16	41
Dizziness	4	16
Dyskinesia	0	3
Nervousness	< 1	3
Somnolence	10	48
GI		
Constipation	1	4
Dry mouth	10	49
Pharyngitis	1	3
Vomiting	0	3
GU		
Urinary frequency	2	3
UTI	7	10
Lab test abnormalities		
ALT increased	< 1	3
Liver function tests	< 1	3
Miscellaneous		
Amblyopia	< 1	3
Flu syndrome	2	3
Infection	5	6
Rhinitis	2	3
Speech disorder	0	3

TIZANIDINE HCl

➤*Cardiovascular:* Vasodilation, postural hypotension, syncope, migraine, arrhythmia (0.1% to 1%); angina pectoris, coronary artery disorder, heart failure, myocardial infarct, phlebitis, pulmonary embolus, ventricular extrasystoles, ventricular tachycardia (rare).

➤*CNS:* Depression, anxiety, paresthesia (1%); tremor, emotional lability, convulsion, paralysis, thinking abnormal, vertigo, abnormal dreams, agitation, depersonalization, euphoria, migraine, stupor, dysautonomia, neuralgia (0.1% to 1%); dementia, hemiplegia, neuropathy (rare).

➤*Dermatologic:* Rash, sweating, skin ulcer (1%); pruritus, dry skin, acne, alopecia, urticaria (0.1% to 1%); exfoliative dermatitis, herpes simplex, herpes zoster, skin carcinoma (rare).

➤*GI:* Abdominal pain, diarrhea, dyspepsia (1%); dysphasia, cholelithiasis, fecal impaction, flatulence, GI hemorrhage, hepatitis, melena (0.1% to 1%); gastroenteritis, hematemesis, hepatoma, intestinal obstruction, liver damage (rare).

➤*GU:* Urinary urgency, cystitis, menorrhagia, pyelonephritis, urinary retention, kidney calculus, uterine fibroids enlarged, vaginal moniliasis, vaginitis (0.1% to 1%); albuminuria, glycosuria, hematuria, metrorrhagia (rare).

➤*Hematologic/Lymphatic:* Ecchymosis, hypercholesterolemia, anemia, hyperlipemia, leukopenia, leukocytosis, sepsis (0.1% to 1%); petechia, purpura, thrombocythemia, thrombocytopenia (rare).

➤*Metabolic/Nutritional:* Edema, hypothyroidism, weight loss (0.1% to 1%); adrenal cortex insufficiency, hyperglycemia, hypokalemia, hyponatremia, hypoproteinemia, respiratory acidosis (rare).

➤*Musculoskeletal:* Myasthenia, back pain (1%); pathological fracture, arthralgia, arthritis, bursitis (0.1% to 1%).

➤*Respiratory:* Sinusitis, pneumonia, bronchitis (0.1% to 1%); asthma (rare).

➤*Special senses:* Ear pain, tinnitus, deafness, glaucoma, conjunctivitis, eye pain, optic neuritis, otitis media, retinal hemorrhage, visual field defect (0.1% to 1%); iritis, keratitis, optic atrophy (rare).

➤*Miscellaneous:* Fever (1%); allergic reaction, moniliasis, malaise, abscess, neck pain, sepsis, cellulitis, death, overdose (0.1% to 1%); carcinoma, congenital anomaly, suicide attempt (rare).

Overdosage

One significant overdosage of tizanidine has been reported. Attempted suicide by a 46-year-old male with multiple sclerosis resulted in coma very shortly after ingestion of 100 tizanidine tablets. Pupils were not dilated and nystagmus was not present. The patient had marked respiratory depression with Cheyne-Stokes respiration. Gastric lavage and forced diuresis with furosemide and mannitol were instituted. The patient recovered several hours later without sequelae. Laboratory findings were normal.

➤*Treatment:* Should overdosage occur, undertake basic steps to ensure the adequacy of an airway and the monitoring of cardiovascular and respiratory systems. Refer to General Management of Acute Overdosage.

Patient Information

Advise patients of the limited clinical experience with tizanidine both in regard to duration of use and the higher doses required to reduce muscle tone.

Because of the possibility of tizanidine lowering blood pressure, warn patients about the risk of clinically significant orthostatic hypotension.

Because of the possibility of sedation, warn patients about performing activities requiring alertness, such as driving a vehicle or operating machinery. Instruct patients that the sedation may be additive when tizanidine is taken in conjunction with other drugs or substances (eg, alcohol) that act as CNS depressants.

DANTROLENE SODIUM

Rx	**Dantrium** (Procter & Gamble Pharm.)	**Capsules:** 25 mg	(Dantrium 25 mg 0149 0030). Lactose. Orange and light brown. In 100s, 500s and UD 100s.
		50 mg	(Dantrium 50 mg 0149 0031). Lactose. Orange and dark brown. In 100s.
		100 mg	(Dantrium 100 mg 0149 0033). Lactose. Orange and light brown. In 100s and UD 100s.
Rx	**Dantrium Intravenous** (Procter & Gamble Pharm.)	**Powder for Injection:** 20 mg/vial. ($\approx$ 0.32 mg/ml after reconstitution)	With 3 g mannitol per vial. In 70 ml vials.

WARNING

Dantrolene has a potential for hepatotoxicity. Do not use in conditions other than those recommended. The incidence of symptomatic hepatitis (fatal and nonfatal) reported in patients taking up to 400 mg/day is much lower than in those taking $\geq$ 800 mg/day. Even sporadic short courses of these higher dose levels within a treatment regimen markedly increased the risk of serious hepatic injury. Liver dysfunction, as evidenced by liver enzyme elevations, has been observed in patients exposed to the drug for varying periods of time. Overt hepatitis has been most frequently observed between the third and twelfth months of therapy. Risk of hepatic injury appears to be greater in females, in patients > 35 years of age and in patients taking other medications in addition to dantrolene.

Monitor hepatic function, including frequent determinations of AST or ALT. If no observable benefit is derived from therapy after 45 days, discontinue use.

Use the lowest possible effective dose for each patient.

Indications

▶*Spasticity:*

Oral – For the control of clinical spasticity resulting from upper motor neuron disorders such as spinal cord injury, stroke, cerebral palsy or multiple sclerosis. It is of particular benefit to the patient whose functional rehabilitation has been retarded by the sequelae of spasticity. Such patients must have presumably reversible spasticity where relief of spasticity will aid in restoring residual function.

▶*Malignant hyperthermia:*

IV – Management of the fulminant hypermetabolism of skeletal muscle characteristic of malignant hyperthermia crisis, along with appropriate supportive measures.

Preoperatively, and sometimes postoperatively, to prevent or attenuate the development of clinical and laboratory signs of malignant hyperthermia in individuals judged to be susceptible to malignant hyperthermia.

Oral – Preoperatively to prevent or attenuate the development of signs of malignant hyperthermia in susceptible patients who require anesthesia or surgery. Currently accepted clinical practices in the management of such patients must still be adhered to (careful monitoring for early signs of malignant hyperthermia, minimizing exposure to triggering mechanisms and prompt use of IV dantrolene and indicated supportive measures if signs of malignant hyperthermia appear).

Following a malignant hyperthermia crisis to prevent recurrence of malignant hyperthermia.

▶*Unlabeled uses:* Exercise-induced muscle pain; neuroleptic malignant syndrome; heat stroke.

Administration and Dosage

▶*Chronic spasticity:* Prior to administration, consider the potential response to treatment. Decreased spasticity sufficient to allow a daily function not otherwise attainable should be the therapeutic goal. Establish a therapeutic goal (regain and maintain a specific function such as therapeutic exercise program, utilization of braces, transfer maneuvers, etc) before beginning therapy. Increase dosage until the maximum performance compatible with the dysfunction due to underlying disease is achieved. No further increase in dosage is then indicated.

Titrate and individualize dosage. In view of the potential for liver damage in long-term use, discontinue therapy if benefits are not evident within 45 days.

Adults – Begin with 25 mg once daily; increase to 25 mg, 2 to 4 times daily; then by increments of 25 mg up to as high as 100 mg, 2 to 4 times daily if necessary. Most patients will respond to 400 mg/day or less; higher doses are rarely needed. (See Warning Box.) Maintain each dosage level for 4 to 7 days to determine response. Adjust dosage to achieve maximal benefit without adverse effects.

Children – Use a similar approach. Start with 0.5 mg/kg twice daily; increase to 0.5 mg/kg, 3 or 4 times daily; then by increments of 0.5 mg/kg, up to 3 mg/kg, 2 to 4 times daily if necessary. Do not exceed doses higher than 100 mg 4 times daily.

▶*Malignant hyperthermia:*

Preoperative prophylaxis (MH) – Dantrolene may be given orally or IV to patients judged susceptible to malignant hyperthermia as part of the overall patient management to prevent or attenuate development of clinical and laboratory signs of MH.

Oral – Give 4 to 8 mg/kg/day orally in 3 or 4 divided doses for 1 or 2 days prior to surgery, with last dose given $\approx$ 3 or 4 hours before scheduled surgery with a minimum of water. This dosage will usually be associated with skeletal muscle weakness and sedation (sleepiness or drowsiness) or excessive GI irritation (nausea or vomiting); adjust within the recommended dosage range to avoid incapacitation or excessive GI irritation.

IV – 2.5 mg/kg $\approx$ 1 hour before anesthesia and infused over $\approx$ 1 hour. Additional dantrolene IV may be indicated during anesthesia and surgery by malignant hyperthermia signs or prolonged surgery. Individualize additional doses.

Treatment – As soon as the malignant hyperthermia reaction is recognized, discontinue all anesthetic agents. Use of 100% oxygen is recommended. Administer dantrolene by continuous rapid IV push beginning at a minimum dose of 1 mg/kg, and continuing until symptoms subside or a maximum cumulative dose of 10 mg/kg has been reached. If the physiologic and metabolic abnormalities reappear, repeat the regimen. NOTE: Administration should be continuous until symptoms subside. The effective dose to reverse the crisis depends upon the degree of susceptibility to malignant hyperthermia, the amount and time of exposure to the triggering agent and the time elapsed between onset of the crisis and initiation of treatment.

Children – Dose is the same as for adults.

Post-crisis follow-up – Following a malignant hyperthermia crisis, give 4 to 8 mg/kg/day orally, in 4 divided doses for 1 to 3 days to prevent recurrence. IV dantrolene may be used when oral administration is not practical. The IV dose must be individualized, starting with 1 mg/kg or more as the clinical situation dictates.

▶*Preparation of solution:* Add 60 ml of Sterile Water for Injection, USP (without a bacteriostatic agent) to each vial, and shake until solution is clear. Protect from direct light, and use within 6 hours. Store reconstituted solutions at controlled room temperature (15° to 30°C or 59° to 86°F). Avoid prolonged exposure to light.

Actions

▶*Pharmacology:* In isolated nerve-muscle preparation, dantrolene produced relaxation by affecting contractile response of the skeletal muscle at a site beyond the myoneural junction and directly on the muscle itself. In skeletal muscle, the drug dissociates the excitation-contraction coupling, probably by interfering with the release of calcium from the sarcoplasmic reticulum. This effect appears more pronounced in fast muscle fibers than in slow ones, but generally affects both. A CNS effect occurs, with drowsiness, dizziness and generalized weakness occasionally present. Although dantrolene does not appear to directly affect the CNS, the extent of its indirect effect is unknown. The administration of IV dantrolene is also associated with loss of grip strength and weakness in the legs.

Malignant hyperthermia – In anesthetic-induced malignant hyperthermia syndrome, evidence points to an intrinsic abnormality of muscle tissue. In affected humans, "triggering agents" may induce a sudden rise in myoplasmic calcium by accelerating its release from sarcoplasmic reticulum. This rise in myoplasmic calcium activates acute catabolic processes common to the malignant hyperthermia crisis.

Dantrolene may prevent such changes within the muscle cell by interfering with calcium release from the sarcoplasmic reticulum to the myoplasm. Thus, physiologic, metabolic and biochemical changes associated with the crisis may be reversed or attenuated. Administration of IV dantrolene, combined with supportive measures, is effective in reversing the hypermetabolic process of malignant hyperthermia. Oral dantrolene will also attenuate or prevent the development of signs of malignant hyperthermia, provided that currently accepted practices in the management of such patients are adhered to; IV dantrolene should also be available for use should the signs of malignant hyperthermia appear.

▶*Pharmacokinetics:*

Absorption/Distribution – Absorption after oral administration is incomplete and slow but consistent, and dose-related blood levels are obtained.

Slightly greater amounts of dantrolene are associated with red blood cells than with the plasma fraction of blood. Significant amounts are reversibly bound to plasma proteins, mostly albumin; this binding is readily reversible. Its plasma protein binding is affected by some drugs (see Drug Interactions).

DANTROLENE SODIUM

Metabolism – Metabolic patterns are similar in adults and children. Dantrolene is found in measurable amounts in blood and urine; the major metabolites noted are the 5-hydroxy analog and the acetamido analog. Mean half-life in adults is 9 hours after a 100 mg oral dose and 4 to 8 hours after IV administration. Since it is probably metabolized by hepatic microsomal enzymes, metabolism enhancement by other drugs is possible. However, neither phenobarbital nor diazepam appears to affect metabolism.

Contraindications

➤*Oral:* Active hepatic disease, such as hepatitis and cirrhosis; where spasticity is utilized to sustain upright posture and balance in locomotion or to obtain or maintain increased function; treatment of skeletal muscle spasm resulting from rheumatic disorders.

Warnings

➤*Hepatic effects:* Fatal and nonfatal liver disorders of an idiosyncratic or hypersensitivity type may occur. At the start of therapy, perform baseline liver function studies (AST, ALT, alkaline phosphatase, total bilirubin). If abnormalities exist, the potential for hepatotoxicity could be enhanced.

Perform liver function studies at appropriate intervals during therapy. If such studies reveal abnormal values, generally discontinue therapy. Consider reinitiation or continuation only when drug benefits have been of major importance. Some laboratory values may return to normal with continued therapy; others may not.

If symptoms of hepatitis accompanied by liver function test abnormalities or jaundice appear, discontinue therapy. If caused by dantrolene and detected early, abnormalities may revert to normal when the drug is discontinued.

Therapy has been reinstituted in a few patients who have developed clinical or laboratory evidence of hepatocellular injury. Attempt reinstitution only in patients who clearly need dantrolene, after previous symptoms and laboratory abnormalities have cleared. Hospitalize the patient and restart the drug in very small and gradually increasing doses. Monitor laboratory values frequently, and withdraw the drug immediately if there is any indication of recurrent liver involvement. Some patients have reacted with liver abnormality upon administration of a challenge dose, while others have not.

Use with caution in females and in patients > 35 years of age; there is a greater likelihood of drug-induced, potentially fatal hepatocellular disease in these populations.

➤*Long-term use:* Safety and efficacy have not been established. Chronic studies in animals at dosages > 30 mg/kg/day showed growth or weight depression, signs of hepatopathy and possible occlusion nephropathy; all were reversible upon cessation of treatment.

Continued long-term administration is justified if use of the drug: Significantly reduces painful or disabling spasticity such as clonus; significantly reduces the intensity or degree of nursing care required; rids the patient of any annoying manifestation of spasticity considered important by the patient.

Brief withdrawal for 2 to 4 days will frequently demonstrate exacerbation of the manifestations of spasticity and may serve to confirm a clinical impression.

In view of the potential for liver damage in long-term use, discontinue therapy if benefits are not evident within 45 days.

➤*Malignant hyperthermia (MH):* IV use is not a substitute for previously known supportive measures. These measures include discontinuing the suspected triggering agents, attending to increased oxygen requirements, managing the metabolic acidosis, instituting cooling when necessary, attending to urinary output and monitoring electrolyte imbalance.

There have been occasional reports of death following malignant hyperthermia crisis even when treated with IV dantrolene; incidence figures are not available. Most of these deaths can be accounted for by late recognition, delayed treatment, inadequate dosage, lack of supportive therapy, intercurrent disease or the development of delayed complications such as renal failure or disseminated intravascular coagulopathy. In some cases, there are insufficient data to completely rule out therapeutic failure of dantrolene.

Rare reports of fatality in MH crisis, despite initial satisfactory response to IV dantrolene, involve patients who could not be weaned from dantrolene after initial treatment.

➤*Hepatic function impairment:* Use with caution in patients with a history of previous liver disease or dysfunction.

➤*Carcinogenesis:* An increased incidence of benign and malignant mammary tumors and hepatic lymphangiomas and hepatic angiosarcomas has occurred in animals. Carcinogenicity in humans cannot be fully excluded; weigh this possible risk of chronic administration against the benefits of the drug for the individual patient.

➤*Pregnancy: Category C* (parenteral). Dantrolene is embryocidal in the rabbit and decreases pup survival in the rat when given at doses seven times the human oral dose. There are no adequate and well controlled studies in pregnant women. Use only when clearly needed and when the potential benefits outweigh the potential hazards to the fetus.

➤*Labor and delivery* – In one uncontrolled study, 100 mg/day of prophylactic oral dantrolene was administered to term pregnant patients awaiting labor and delivery. Dantrolene readily crossed the placenta, with maternal and fetal whole blood levels approximately equal at delivery; neonatal levels then fell ≈ 50%/day for 2 days before declining sharply. No neonatal respiratory and neuromuscular side effects were detected at low dose. More data, at higher doses, are needed before definitive conclusions can be made.

One patient developed postpartum uterine atony following dantrolene administration after a cesarean section.

➤*Lactation:* Do not use in nursing women.

➤*Children:* Safety for use in children < 5 years of age has not been established. Because of the possibility that adverse effects could become apparent only after many years, a benefit-risk consideration of long-term use is particularly important.

Precautions

➤*Extravasation:* Because of the high pH of the IV formulation, prevent extravasation into the surrounding tissues.

➤*Special risk:* Use with caution in patients with impaired pulmonary function, particularly those with obstructive pulmonary disease; severely impaired cardiac function due to myocardial disease; a history of previous liver disease or dysfunction.

➤*Hazardous tasks:* Patients should use caution while driving or performing other tasks requiring alertness, coordination or physical dexterity.

➤*Photosensitivity:* Photosensitization may occur; therefore, caution patients to take protective measures (eg, sunscreens, protective clothing) against exposure to ultraviolet light or sunlight until tolerance is determined.

Drug Interactions

Dantrolene Drug Interactions			
Precipitant drug	Object drug*		Description
Clofibrate	Dantrolene	↓	Plasma protein binding of dantrolene may be reduced.
Dantrolene	Verapamil	↑	Hyperkalemia and myocardial depression occurred in one patient during concurrent use.
Estrogens	Dantrolene	↑	Although a definite drug interaction is not established, hepatotoxicity occurred more often in women > 35 years old receiving these agents concurrently.
Warfarin	Dantrolene	↓	Plasma protein binding of dantrolene may be reduced.

* ↑ = Object drug increased. ↓ = Object drug decreased.

Adverse Reactions

➤*Oral:* Most frequent – Drowsiness; dizziness; weakness; general malaise; fatigue; diarrhea. These effects are generally transient, occur early in treatment and can often be obviated by beginning with a low dose and increasing gradually until an optimal regimen is established. Diarrhea may be severe and may necessitate temporary withdrawal of therapy. If diarrhea recurs upon readministration, discontinue use.

Cardiovascular – Tachycardia; erratic blood pressure; phlebitis.

CNS – Speech disturbance; seizure; headache; lightheadedness; visual disturbance; diplopia; alteration of taste; insomnia; mental depression/confusion; increased nervousness.

Dermatologic – Abnormal hair growth; acne-like rash; pruritus; urticaria; eczematoid eruption; sweating.

GI – Constipation; GI bleeding; anorexia; dysphagia; gastric irritation; abdominal cramps; hepatitis (see Warnings).

GU – Increased urinary frequency; hematuria; crystalluria; difficult erection; urinary incontinence; nocturia; dysuria; urinary retention.

Musculoskeletal – Myalgia; backache.

Miscellaneous – Chills; fever; feeling of suffocation; excessive tearing; pleural effusion with pericarditis.

➤*Parenteral:* The following adverse reactions are in approximate order of severity: Pulmonary edema developing during treatment of MH crisis (diluent volume and mannitol needed to deliver IV dantrolene possibly contributed); thrombophlebitis following IV dantrolene (actual incidence figures not available); urticaria and erythema (possibly associated with IV dantrolene); death (see Warnings).

None of the serious reactions occasionally reported with long-term oral dantrolene use, such as hepatitis, seizures, and pleural effusion with pericarditis, have been reasonably associated with short-term dantrolene IV therapy.

DANTROLENE SODIUM

Overdosage

There is no known antidote. Employ general supportive measures along with immediate gastric lavage. Administer IV fluids in fairly large quantities to avert the possibility of crystalluria. Maintain an adequate airway; have artificial resuscitation equipment available. Monitor ECG; observe patient carefully. No experience has been reported with dialysis.

Patient Information

May cause drowsiness, dizziness or lightheadedness. Patients should exercise caution while driving or performing other tasks requiring alertness, coordination or physical dexterity.

Avoid alcohol and other CNS depressants.

Avoid prolonged exposure to sunlight; photosensitivity may occur.

May cause weakness, malaise, fatigue, nausea and diarrhea. Notify physician if these effects persist.

Notify physician if skin rash, itching, bloody or black tarry stools or yellowish discoloration of the skin or eyes occurs.

Dantrolene IV may decrease grip strength and increase weakness of leg muscles, especially walking down stairs.

Exercise caution at meals on the day of administration because difficulty swallowing and choking has been reported.

SKELETAL MUSCLE RELAXANT COMBINATIONS

Rx	**Methocarbamol w/ASA** (Various, eg, Moore, Par)	**Tablets:** 400 mg methocarbamol and 325 mg aspirin. *Dose: 2 tablets 4 times daily*	In 15s, 30s, 40s, 100s, 500s and 1000s.
Rx	**Carisoprodol Compound** (Various, eg, Moore, Rugby)	**Tablets:** 200 mg carisoprodol and 325 mg aspirin. *Dose: 1 or 2 tablets 4 times daily*	In 15s, 30s, 40s, 100s, 500s and 1000s.
Rx	**Sodol Compound** (Major)		In 100s and 500s.
Rx	**Soma Compound** (Wallace)		(Soma C Wallace-2103). White and orange. In 100s, 500s and UD500s.
c-iii	**Soma Compound w/Codeine** (Wallace)	**Tablets:** 200 mg carisoprodol, 325 mg aspirin and 16 mg codeine phosphate. *Dose: 1 or 2 tablets 4 times daily*	(Soma CC Wallace-2403). White and yellow. In 100s.[1]
Rx	**Flexaphen** (Trimen)	**Capsules:** 250 mg chlorzoxazone and 300 mg acetaminophen. *Dose: 2 capsules 4 times daily*	Tan. In 100s.
Rx	**Lobac** (Seatrace)	**Capsules:** 200 mg salicylamide, 20 mg phenyltoloxamine and 300 mg acetaminophen. *Dose: 2 capsules 4 times daily*	(Seatrace). Eggshell. In 24s and 100s.
Rx	**Norgesic** (3M Pharm)	**Tablets:** 25 mg orphenadrine citrate, 385 mg aspirin and 30 mg caffeine. *Dose: 1 or 2 tablets 3 or 4 times daily*	(NORGESIC 3M). Green, white and yellow. In 100s, 500s and UD 100s.
Rx	**Orphengesic** (Par)		Lactose. (Par 472). Bilayered white/green. In 100s and 500s.
Rx	**Orphengesic Forte** (Par)	**Tablets:** 50 mg orphenadrine citrate, 770 mg aspirin and 60 mg caffeine. *Dose: ½ or 1 tablet 3 or 4 times daily*	Lactose. (Par 473). Bilayered white/green, capsule shape, scored. In 100s and 500s.

[1] With sodium metabisulfite.

Indications

➤*Uses:* The methocarbamol and aspirin combinations and the carisoprodol and aspirin (with or without codeine) combinations are indicated as adjuncts to rest, physical therapy and other measures for relief of discomfort associated with acute, painful musculoskeletal conditions. The other combinations are classified as *"probably effective"* for this indication. Components of these combinations include:

MUSCLE RELAXANTS – Methocarbamol; Chlorzoxazone; Carisoprodol; Orphenadrine Citrate; (see individual monographs).

ANALGESICS – Acetaminophen; Aspirin; Codeine; (see individual monographs).

CAFFEINE – Caffeine (see individual monograph), used as a CNS stimulant, also has minor analgesic activity.

Precautions

➤*Sulfite sensitivity:* Some of these products contain sulfites, which may cause allergic-type reactions (eg, hives, itching, wheezing, anaphylaxis) in certain susceptible people. Although the overall prevalence of sulfite sensitivity in the general population is probably low, it is seen more frequently in asthmatics or in atopic nonasthmatic people. Specific products containing sulfites are identified in the product listings.

▶*Parkinsons's Disease:* Parkinsonism is a neurological disease with a variety of origins characterized by tremor, rigidity, akinesia, and disorders of posture and equilibrium. The onset is slow and progressive with symptoms advancing over months to years.

Although the biochemical basis of parkinsonism is complex, the primary defect appears to be an imbalance of neurotransmitters (ie, a relative excess of acetylcholine and a deficiency/absence of dopamine in the basal ganglia). Other central neurotransmitters may have some modifying influence on these primary substances. This defect may be part of a more generalized, structural, and enzymatic defect.

Currently, therapy for Parkinson's disease is palliative, as there is no cure for this disease. The goal of therapy is to provide maximum relief from the symptoms and to attempt to maintain the independence and mobility of the patient.

Drug therapy of Parkinson's disease is aimed at correcting or modifying these neurotransmitter defects by inhibiting the effects of acetylcholine or enhancing the effects of dopamine.

▶*Anticholinergic agents:* Centrally-acting anticholinergics tend to diminish the characteristic tremor. Patients with minimal involvement who are functioning relatively well may not require medication. However, as the disease progresses, the anticholinergics may be considered.

▶*Dopaminergic agents:* Dopamine deficiency appears to be the central feature of the pathogenesis of parkinsonism. **Levodopa**, the immediate precursor of dopamine, directly increases dopamine content in the brain; it is currently the most effective treatment for parkinsonism. Other drugs are available that also affect the dopamine content of the brain: **Bromocriptine** and **pergolide** directly stimulate dopamine receptors. Pergolide is 10 to 1000 times more potent than bromocriptine on a milligram per milligram basis; **amantadine** may increase dopamine at the receptor either by releasing intact striatal dopamine stores or by blocking neuronal dopamine reuptake; **selegiline** increases dopaminergic activity through inhibition of monoamine oxidase type B; however, other mechanisms may exist such as interference of dopamine reuptake at the synapse.

Levodopa is used for symptomatic patients with moderate disabilities; therapy is usually initiated with a combination of levodopa and carbidopa (a dopa decarboxylase inhibitor that prevents peripheral metabolism of levodopa). Unfortunately, the response to levodopa gradually diminishes after 2 to 5 years in most patients, at which time the dopaminergic agonists, bromocriptine or pergolide, selegiline, or amantadine may be added to the drug regimen. Amantadine may also be used in patients with minimal involvement when the patients cannot tolerate an anticholinergic drug.

The table below summarizes the drug therapy available for parkinsonism:

Drug Therapy for Parkinsonism						
	Indications					
Drugs	Postencephalitic	Arteriosclerotic	Idiopathic	Drug/chemical induced	Adjunct to Levodopa/Carbidopa	Usual daily dose range (mg)
Anticholinergics						
Benztropine	✔	✔	✔	✔		0.5-6.5
Biperiden	✔	✔	✔	✔		2-8
Diphenhydramine	✔	✔	✔	✔		10-400
Ethopropazine	✔	✔	✔	✔		50-600
Procyclidine	✔	✔	✔	✔		7.5-20
Trihexyphenidyl	✔	✔	✔	✔	✔	1-15
Dopaminergic Agents						
Amantadine	✔	✔	✔	✔		200-400
Bromocriptine	✔		✔			12.5-100
Carbidopa/Levodopa	✔		✔	✔[1]		10/100-200/2000
Levodopa	✔	✔	✔	✔[1]		500-8000
Pergolide					✔	1-5
Selegiline					✔	10

[1] Not effective in drug-induced extrapyramidal symptoms.

Anticholinergics

Indications

Adjunctive therapy in all forms of parkinsonism (postencephalitic, arteriosclerotic and idiopathic) and in the control of drug-induced extrapyramidal disorders. Refer to individual drug monographs for specific indications of individual agents.

Administration and Dosage

Dosage depends upon the age of the patient, etiology of the disease, and individual responsiveness. The dosage required for treatment of drug-induced extrapyramidal symptoms will depend on the severity of the side effects. Maintain flexible dosage to permit individualized dosing. In general, younger and postencephalitic patients require and tolerate somewhat higher doses than older patients and those with arteriosclerotic or idiopathic-type parkinsonism.

Give before or after meals, as determined by patient's reaction. Postencephalitic patients (more prone to excessive salivation) may prefer to take it after meals and may, in addition, require small amounts of atropine. If the mouth dries excessively, take before meals, unless it causes nausea. If taken after meals, thirst can be allayed by mint candies, chewing gum, or water.

Actions

▶*Pharmacology:* The anticholinergic agents, although generally less effective than levodopa, are useful in the treatment of all forms of parkinsonism: Postencephalitic, arteriosclerotic, idiopathic, and drug-induced extrapyramidal symptoms. They reduce the incidence and severity of akinesia, rigidity, and tremor by ≈ 20%; secondary symptoms such as drooling are also reduced. In addition to suppressing central cholinergic activity, these agents may also inhibit the reuptake and storage of dopamine at central dopamine receptors, thereby prolonging the action of dopamine.

The naturally occurring belladonna alkaloids (atropine, scopolamine, hyoscyamine) are active anticholinergic agents; however, they have largely been replaced by synthetic agents (eg, benztropine, trihexyphenidyl) with a more selective CNS activity. Peripheral anticholinergic side effects (eg, urinary retention, tachycardia, constipation) frequently limit the size of dosages utilized.

Antihistamines (eg, diphenhydramine) with central anticholinergic effects are also used; they may have a lower incidence of peripheral side effects than the belladonna alkaloids or synthetic derivatives. These agents are generally better tolerated by elderly patients. Some antihistamines provide mild antiparkinson effects, and are useful for initiating therapy in patients with minimal symptoms. Because of their sedative effects, the antihistamines may be useful in certain patients with insomnia.

In spite of limited efficacy, anticholinergics are useful in mild cases of Parkinson's disease where risks and demands of levodopa therapy are not warranted.

▶*Pharmacokinetics:* Little pharmacokinetic data are available for these agents. The following table lists some of the available parameters.

Various Antiparkinson Anticholinergic Pharmacokinetic Parameters				
Anticholinergic	Time to peak concentration (hrs)	Peak concentration (mcg/L)	Half-life (hrs)	Oral bioavailability (%)
Benztropine[1]				
Biperiden	1-1.5	4-5	18.4-24.3	29
Diphenhydramine	2-4	65-90	4-15	50-72
Procyclidine	1.1-2	80	11.5-12.6	52-97
Trihexyphenidyl	1-1.3	87.2	5.6-10.2	≈ 100

[1] No data available.

Contraindications

Hypersensitivity to any component; glaucoma, particularly angle-closure glaucoma (simple type glaucomas do not appear to be adversely affected); pyloric or duodenal obstruction; stenosing peptic ulcers; prostatic hypertrophy or bladder neck obstructions; achalasia (megaesophagus); myasthenia gravis; megacolon.

▶*Benztropine:* Children < 3 years of age; use with caution in older children.

Warnings

➤*Ophthalmic:* Incipient narrow-angle glaucoma may be precipitated by these drugs. Perform gonioscopy and closely monitor intraocular pressures at regular intervals.

➤*Elderly:* Geriatric patients, particularly > 60 years of age, frequently develop increased sensitivity to anticholinergic drugs and require strict dosage regulation. Occasionally, mental confusion and disorientation may occur; agitation, hallucinations, and psychotic-like symptoms may develop.

➤*Pregnancy:* Category C. Safety for use during pregnancy has not been established. Use only when clearly needed and when the potential benefits outweigh the potential hazards to the fetus.

➤*Lactation:* Safety for use in the nursing mother has not been established. An inhibitory effect on lactation may occur. Although infants are particularly sensitive to anticholinergic agents, no adverse effects have been reported in nursing infants whose mothers were taking atropine.

➤*Children:* Safety and efficacy for use in children have not been established.

Precautions

➤*Concomitant conditions:* Use caution in patients with tachycardia, cardiac arrhythmias, hypertension, hypotension, prostatic hypertrophy (particularly in the elderly), or any tendency toward urinary retention, liver or kidney disorders, and obstructive disease of the GI or GU tract.

➤*CNS:* When used to treat extrapyramidal reactions resulting from phenothiazines in psychiatric patients, antiparkinson agents may exacerbate mental symptoms and precipitate a toxic psychosis. The possibility of antiparkinson agents masking the development of persistent extrapyramidal symptoms with prolonged phenothiazine therapy has not been investigated. Whether to administer prophylactic anticholinergics to prevent drug-induced extrapyramidal effects is controversial.

In addition, 19% to 30% of patients given anticholinergics develop depression, confusion, delusions, or hallucinations. Also, **benztropine** given in large doses or to susceptible patients may cause weakness and inability to move particular muscle groups. Dosage may have to be adjusted.

Tardive dyskinesia – Tardive dyskinesia may appear in some patients on long-term therapy with phenothiazines and related agents, or may occur after therapy has been discontinued. Antiparkinson agents do not alleviate the symptoms of tardive dyskinesia and, in some instances, may aggravate such symptoms.

➤*Heat illness:* Give with caution during hot weather, especially when given concomitantly with other atropine-like drugs to the elderly, the chronically ill, alcoholics, those who have CNS disease, and those who work in a hot environment. Anhidrosis may occur more readily when some disturbance of sweating already exists. Decrease dosage so that the ability to maintain body heat equilibrium by perspiration is not impaired. Severe anhidrosis and fatal hyperthermia have occurred.

➤*Dry mouth:* If dry mouth is so severe that there is difficulty in swallowing or speaking, or if loss of appetite and weight occurs, reduce dosage or discontinue the drug temporarily.

➤*Abuse potential:* Some patients may use these agents for mood elevations or psychedelic experiences. Cannabinoids, barbiturates, opiates, and alcohol may have additive effects with anticholinergics. It is important to be aware of this potential abuse situation.

➤*Hazardous tasks:* May impair mental or physical abilities; patients should observe caution while driving or performing other tasks requiring alertness.

Drug Interactions

Anticholinergic Drug Interactions			
Precipitant drug	Object drug*		Description
Amantadine	Anticholinergics	↑	Amantadine and anticholinergic coadministration may result in an increased incidence of anticholinergic side effects. These effects disappear when the anticholinergic dose is reduced.
Anticholinergics	Digoxin	↑	Digoxin serum levels may be increased by anticholinergics when digoxin is administered as a slow dissolution oral tablet.
Anticholinergics	Haloperidol	↓	Haloperidol and anticholinergic coadministration may result in worsening of schizophrenic symptoms, decreased haloperidol serum concentrations, and development of tardive dyskinesia.

Anticholinergic Drug Interactions			
Precipitant drug	Object drug*		Description
Anticholinergics	Levodopa	↓	Anticholinergics may decrease gastric motility resulting in increased gastric deactivation of levodopa and decreased intestinal absorption, possibly leading to a reduction in levodopa's efficacy. Other reports refute these findings.
Anticholinergics	Phenothiazines	↓	The pharmacologic/therapeutic actions of phenothiazines may be reduced by concurrent anticholinergics. An increase in the incidence of anticholinergic side effects has occurred.
Phenothiazines	Anticholinergics	↑	

↑ = Object drug increased. ↓ = Object drug decreased.

Adverse Reactions

➤*Cardiovascular:* Tachycardia; palpitations; hypotension; postural hypotension; mild bradycardia.

➤*CNS:* Disorientation; confusion; memory loss; hallucinations; psychoses; agitation; nervousness; delusions; delirium; paranoia; euphoria; excitement; lightheadedness; dizziness; headache; listlessness; depression; drowsiness; weakness; giddiness; paresthesia; heaviness of the limbs.

➤*GI:* Dry mouth; acute suppurative parotitis; nausea; vomiting; epigastric distress; constipation; dilation of the colon; paralytic ileus; development of duodenal ulcer.

➤*Hypersensitivity:* Skin rash; urticaria; other dermatoses.

➤*Musculoskeletal:* Muscular weakness; muscular cramping.

➤*Ophthalmic:* Blurred vision; mydriasis; diplopia; increased intraocular tension; angle-closure glaucoma; dilation of pupils.

➤*Renal:* Urinary retention; urinary hesitancy; dysuria.

➤*Miscellaneous:* Elevated temperature; flushing; numbness of fingers; decreased sweating, hyperthermia, heat stroke (see Precautions); difficulty in achieving or maintaining an erection.

Overdosage

➤*Symptoms:* Characterized by the adverse reactions and may also include the following: Circulatory collapse; cardiac arrest; respiratory depression or arrest; CNS depression preceded or followed by stimulation; intensification of mental symptoms or toxic psychosis in mentally ill patients treated with neuroleptic drugs (eg, phenothiazines); shock; coma; stupor; seizures; convulsions; ataxia; anxiety; incoherence; hyperactivity; combativeness; anhidrosis; hyperpyrexia; fever; hot, dry, flushed skin; dry mucous membranes; dysphagia; foul-smelling breath; decreased bowel sounds; dilated and sluggish pupils.

➤*Treatment:* Immediately following acute ingestion, remove remaining drug from stomach by inducing emesis or by gastric lavage (contraindicated in precomatose, convulsive or psychotic states). Activated charcoal is an effective adsorbent.

Treatment of overdosage is symptomatic. To relieve the peripheral effects, 5 mg of pilocarpine may be given orally at repeated intervals.

Artificial respiration and oxygen therapy may be needed for respiratory depression. A short-acting barbiturate or diazepam may be used for CNS excitement or convulsions; use with caution to avoid subsequent depression; institute supportive care for depression. Urinary retention may require catheterization. Hyperpyrexia is best treated with alcohol sponges, ice bags, or other cold applications. To counteract mydriasis and cycloplegia, a local miotic may be used. Darken room for photophobia. Treat circulatory collapse with fluids and vasopressors. The relapse intervals lengthen as the anticholinergic agent is metabolized; observe patient for 8 to 12 hours after last relapse.

Physostigmine salicylate reverses most cardiovascular and CNS effects of overdosage. In *adults*, 1 to 2 mg IM or IV given slowly (no more than 1 mg/min) is effective. In *children*, start with 0.02 mg/kg IM or by slow IV injection (no more than 0.5 mg/min). If necessary, repeat at 5- to 10-minute intervals until a therapeutic effect or a maximum dose of 2 mg is attained. Avoid rapid injection to reduce the possibility of physostigmine-induced convulsions. Give physostigmine cautiously. It can precipitate seizures, cholinergic crisis, bradyarrhythmias, and asystole. Use in a setting where advanced life support is available.

Patient Information

If GI upset occurs, may be taken with food.

May cause drowsiness, dizziness, or blurred vision; observe caution while driving or performing other tasks requiring alertness until response to drug is known.

Avoid alcohol and other CNS depressants.

May cause dry mouth; sucking hard candy, adequate fluid intake, or good oral hygiene may relieve this symptom. Difficult urination or con-

Anticholinergics

stipation may occur; constipation may be relieved by use of stool softeners. Notify physician if effects persist.

Notify physician if rapid or pounding heartbeat, confusion, eye pain or rash occurs.

Use caution in hot weather. This medication may increase susceptibility to heat stroke.

BELLADONNA ALKALOIDS

Refer to the general discussion in the Antiparkinson Agents introduction. Complete prescribing information begins in the Antiparkinson Agent Anticholinergics group monograph.

scribing information on the belladonna alkaloids (atropine, scopolamine HBr, hyoscyamine sulfate and levorotatory alkaloids of belladonna) see Gastrointestinal Anticholinergics/Antispasmodics monograph.

Indications

Belladonna alkaloids may be used in symptomatic treatment of parkinsonism, in addition to their use as antispasmodics. For complete pre-

BENZTROPINE MESYLATE

Rx	Benztropine Mesylate (Various, eg, Harber, Moore, Par, Parmed, Rugby)	Tablets: 0.5 mg	In 100s and UD 100s.
Rx	Cogentin (MSD)		(MSD 21). White, scored. In 100s.
Rx	Benztropine Mesylate (Various, eg, Goldline, Moore, Purepac, Rugby, Vangard)	Tablets: 1 mg	In 100s, 1000s and UD 100s.
Rx	Benztropine Mesylate (Various, eg, Goldline, Moore, Purepac, Rugby, Vangard)	Tablets: 2 mg	In 100s, 1000s and UD 100s.
Rx	Cogentin (MSD)	Injection: 1 mg/ml	In 2 ml amps.

Refer to the general discussion in the Antiparkinson Agents introduction. Complete prescribing information begins in the Antiparkinson Agent Anticholinergics group monograph.

Indications

For use as an adjunct in the therapy of all forms of parkinsonism. May also be used in the control of extrapyramidal disorders (except tardive dyskinesia) due to neuroleptic drugs (eg, phenothiazines).

Administration and Dosage

➤ *Injection:* Injection is useful for psychotic patients with acute dystonic reactions or other reactions which make oral medication difficult or impossible, or when a more rapid response is desired.

Since there is no significant difference in onset of action after IV or IM injection, there is usually no need to use the IV route. Improvement is sometimes noticeable a few minutes after injection. In emergency situations, when the condition of the patient is alarming, 1 to 2 ml will normally provide quick relief. If the parkinsonian effect begins to return, repeat the dose.

➤ *Dosage titration:* Because of cumulative action, initiate therapy with a low dose, increase in increments of 0.5 mg gradually at 5 or 6 day intervals to the smallest amount necessary for optimal relief. Maximum daily dose is 6 mg.

Generally, older patients and thin patients cannot tolerate large doses.

➤ *Dosage intervals:* Some patients experience greatest relief by taking the entire dose at bedtime; others react more favorably to divided doses, 2 to 4 times a day. The drug's long duration of action makes it

particularly suitable for bedtime medication; its effects may last throughout the night, enabling patients to turn in bed during the night more easily, and to rise in the morning.

➤ *Parkinsonism:* 1 to 2 mg/day, with a range of 0.5 to 6 mg/day, orally or parenterally.

Idiopathic parkinsonism – Start with 0.5 to 1 mg at bedtime; 4 to 6 mg per day may be required.

Postencephalitic parkinsonism – 2 mg per day in one or more doses. In highly sensitive patients, begin therapy with 0.5 mg at bedtime; increase as necessary.

➤ *Concomitant therapy:* If other antiparkinson agents are to be reduced or discontinued, do so gradually. Many patients obtain greatest relief with combination therapy.

➤ *Drug-induced extrapyramidal disorders:* Administer 1 to 4 mg once or twice daily.

Acute dystonic reactions – 1 to 2 ml IM or IV usually relieves the condition quickly. After that, 1 to 2 mg orally 2 times daily usually prevents recurrence.

Extrapyramidal disorders which develop soon after initiating treatment with neuroleptic drugs are likely to be transient. A dosage of 1 to 2 mg orally 2 or 3 times a day usually provides relief within 1 or 2 days. After 1 or 2 weeks, withdraw drug to determine its continued need. If such disorders recur, reinstitute benztropine.

Certain drug-induced extrapyramidal disorders which develop slowly may not respond to benztropine.

BIPERIDEN

Rx	Akineton (Par)	Tablets: 2 mg (as HCl)	(11). White, scored. In 100s and 1000s.

Refer to the general discussion in the Antiparkinson Agents introduction. Complete prescribing information begins in the Antiparkinson Agent Anticholinergics group monograph.

Indications

Adjunct in the therapy of all forms of parkinsonism (postencephalitic, arteriosclerotic and idiopathic). Useful in the control of extrapyramidal disorders secondary to neuroleptic drug therapy (eg, phenothiazines).

Administration and Dosage

➤ *Parkinsonism:* 2 mg 3 or 4 times daily, orally. Individualize dosage with dosing titrated to a maximum of 16 mg/24 hours.

➤ *Drug-induced extrapyramidal disorders:* 2 mg 1 to 3 times daily.

DIPHENHYDRAMINE

For complete prescribing information and product availability, see Antihistamines group monograph. Also refer to the general discussion in the Antiparkinson Agents introduction and the Antiparkinson Agent Anticholinergics group monograph.

Indications

For parkinsonism and drug-induced extrapyramidal reactions in the elderly unable to tolerate more potent agents; mild cases of parkinsonism (including drug-induced) in other age groups; in other cases of parkinsonism (including drug-induced) in combination with centrally-acting anticholinergic agents.

Administration and Dosage

➤ *Oral:* Adults – 25 to 50 mg 3 to 4 times daily.

Children > 20 lbs (9 kg) – 12.5 to 25 mg 3 or 4 times daily or 5 mg/kg/day. Do not exceed 300 mg/day or 150 mg/m²/day.

➤ *Parenteral:* Administer IV or deeply IM.

Adults – 10 to 50 mg; 100 mg if required. Maximum daily dosage is 400 mg.

Children – 5 mg/kg/day or 150 mg/m²/day, divided into 4 doses. Maximum daily dosage is 300 mg.

Anticholinergics

PROCYCLIDINE

Rx	Kemadrin (Glaxo Wellcome)	Tablets: 5 mg	(Kemadrin S3A). White, scored. In 100s.

Refer to the general discussion in the Antiparkinson Agents introduction. Complete prescribing information begins in the Antiparkinson Agent Anticholinergics group monograph.

Indications

➤*Parkinsonism:* Treatment of parkinsonism, including the postencephalitic, arteriosclerotic and idiopathic types. Partial control of the parkinsonism symptoms is the usual therapeutic accomplishment. Procyclidine is usually more efficacious in the relief of rigidity than tremor; but tremor, fatigue, weakness and sluggishness are frequently improved. It can be substituted for all previous medications in mild and moderate cases. For the control of more severe cases, add other drugs to procyclidine therapy, as warranted.

➤*Drug-induced extrapyramidal symptoms:* Procyclidine relieves the symptoms of extrapyramidal dysfunction which accompany phenothiazine and rauwolfia therapy. It also controls sialorrhea resulting from neuroleptic medication.

Administration and Dosage

➤*Parkinsonism (for patients who have received no other therapy):* Initially, 2.5 mg 3 times daily after meals. If well tolerated, gradually increase dose to 5 mg; administer 3 times daily, and occasionally before retiring, if necessary. In some cases, smaller doses may be effective.

Transferring patients from other therapy – Substitute 2.5 mg 3 times daily for all or part of the original drug. Procyclidine is then increased as required; the other drug is correspondingly omitted or decreased until complete replacement is achieved. Individualize dosage.

➤*For drug-induced extrapyramidal symptoms:* Begin with 2.5 mg 3 times daily; increase by 2.5 mg daily increments until the patient obtains relief of symptoms. Individualize dosage. In most cases, results will be obtained with 10 to 20 mg daily.

TRIHEXYPHENIDYL HCl

Rx	Trihexyphenidyl HCl (Various, eg, Balan, Bolar, Danbury, Moore, Raway, Schein)	Tablets: 2 mg	In 30s, 100s, 250s, 1000s and UD 100s.
Rx	Trihexy-2 (Geneva)		White. In 100s and 1000s.
Rx	Trihexyphenidyl HCl (Various, eg, Balan, Bolar, Danbury, Lannett, Moore, Schein)	Tablets: 5 mg	In 100s, 250s, 1000s and UD 100s.
Rx	Trihexy-5 (Geneva)		White. In 100s and 1000s.

Refer to the general discussion in the Antiparkinson Agents introduction. Complete prescribing information begins in the Antiparkinson Agent Anticholinergics group monograph.

Indications

Adjunct in the treatment of all forms of parkinsonism (postencephalitic, arteriosclerotic and idiopathic); adjuvant therapy with levodopa; for the control of drug-induced extrapyramidal disorders. The sustained release dosage form is indicated for maintenance therapy after patients have been stabilized on tablets or elixir.

Administration and Dosage

➤*Parkinsonism:* Initially, administer 1 to 2 mg the first day; increase by 2 mg increments at intervals of 3 to 5 days, until a total of 6 to 10 mg is given daily. Many patients derive maximum benefit from a total daily dose of 6 to 10 mg; however, postencephalitic patients may require a total daily dose of 12 to 15 mg. Trihexyphenidyl is tolerated best if divided into 3 doses and taken at mealtimes. High doses may be divided into 4 parts, administered at mealtimes and at bedtime.

Concomitant use with levodopa – The usual dose of each may need to be reduced. Conversely, trihexyphenidyl decreases the total bioavailability of levodopa. Careful adjustment is necessary, depending on side effects and degree of symptom control. Trihexyphenidyl 3 to 6 mg/day in divided doses is usually adequate.

➤*Concomitant use with other anticholinergics:* May be substituted, in whole or in part, for other anticholinergics. The usual procedure is partial substitution initially, with progressive reduction in the other medication as the dose of trihexyphenidyl is increased.

➤*Drug-induced extrapyramidal disorders:* Size and frequency of dose are determined empirically. Start with a single 1 mg dose. Daily dosage usually ranges between 5 to 15 mg, although reactions have been controlled on as little as 1 mg/day. If reactions are not controlled in a few hours, progressively increase subsequent doses until control is achieved. Control may be more rapidly achieved by temporarily reducing tranquilizer dose when instituting trihexyphenidyl; then adjust both drugs until desired ataractic effect is retained without onset of extrapyramidal reactions.

It is sometimes possible to maintain the patient on reduced dosage after the reactions have remained under control for several days. These reactions have remained in remission for long periods after discontinuing therapy.

➤*Sustained release:* Because of the relatively high dosage in sustained release capsules, do not use for initial therapy. Once patients are stabilized on conventional dosage forms, they may be switched to sustained release capsules on a milligram per milligram of total daily dose basis. Administer as a single dose after breakfast or in 2 divided doses 12 hours apart. Most patients will be adequately maintained on the sustained release form, but some may develop an exacerbation of parkinsonism and may require treatment with tablets or elixir.

AMANTADINE HCl

Rx	Amantadine HCl (Various)	Capsules: 100 mg	In 100s.
Rx	Amantadine HCl (Various, eg, Barre-National, Copley)	Syrup: 50 mg/5 ml	In pt.
Rx	Symmetrel (Du Pont)		Parabens, sorbitol. In pt.

This is an abbreviated monograph. For full prescribing information, refer to the Antiviral Agents monograph. Also refer to the general discussion in the Antiparkinson Agents introduction.

Indications

➤*Parkinson's disease/syndrome and drug-induced extrapyramidal reactions:* Idiopathic Parkinson's disease (paralysis agitans); postencephalitic parkinsonism; arteriosclerotic parkinsonism; drug-induced extrapyramidal reactions; symptomatic parkinsonism following injury to the nervous system by carbon monoxide intoxication.

Administration and Dosage

➤*Parkinson's disease:* 100 mg twice/day when used alone. Onset of action is usually within 48 hrs. Initial dose is 100 mg/day for patients with serious associated medical illnesses or those receiving high doses of other antiparkinson drugs. After one to several weeks at 100 mg once/day, increase to 100 mg twice/day, if necessary. Patients whose responses are not optimal at 200 mg/day may occasionally benefit from an increase up to 400 mg/day in divided doses; supervise closely. Patients initially benefiting from amantadine often experience decreased efficacy after a few months. Benefit may be regained by increasing to 300 mg/day, or by temporary discontinuation for several weeks. Other antiparkinson drugs may be necessary.

Concomitant therapy – Some patients who do not respond to anticholinergic antiparkinson drugs may respond to amantadine. When each is used with marginal benefit, concomitant use may produce additional benefit.

When amantadine and levodopa are initiated concurrently, the patient can exhibit rapid therapeutic benefits. Maintain the dose at 100 mg/day or twice/day, while levodopa is gradually increased to optimal benefit. When amantadine is added to optimal, well tolerated doses of levodopa, additional benefit may result; this includes minimizing the fluctuations in improvement which sometimes occur on levodopa alone. Patients who require a reduction in their usual dose of levodopa because of side effects may regain lost benefit with addition of amantadine.

➤*Renal function impairment:* The following table is designed to yield steady-state plasma concentrations of 0.7 to 1 mcg/ml.

Suggested Dosage Guidelines for Amantadine in Impaired Renal Function		
Creatinine clearance (ml/min/1.73 m^2)	Estimated half-life (hours)	Suggested maintenance regimen[a]
100	11	100 mg twice a day or 200 mg daily
80	14	100 mg twice a day
60	19	200 mg alternated with 100 mg daily
50	23	100 mg daily
40	29	100 mg daily
30	40	200 mg twice weekly
20	66	100 mg 3 times weekly
10	178	200 mg alternated with 100 mg every 7 days
Three times weekly chronic hemodialysis	199	200 mg alternated with 100 mg every 7 days

[a] Loading dose on first day of 200 mg. Reproduced with permission from Horadam VW, Sharp JG, Smilack JD, McAnalley BH, Garriott JC, Stephens MK, et al. Pharmacokinetics of amantadine HCl in subjects with normal and impaired renal function. *Ann Intern Med.* 1981;94(Pt 1):454-458.

➤*Drug-induced extrapyramidal reactions:* 100 mg twice/day. Patients with suboptimal responses may benefit from 300 mg/day in divided doses.

Actions

➤*Pharmacology:* The exact mechanism of action is unknown, but amantadine is thought to release dopamine from intact dopaminergic terminals that remain in the substantia nigra of parkinson patients. Dopamine release may also occur from other central sites.

Amantadine is less effective than levodopa in the treatment of Parkinson's disease, but slightly more effective than anticholinergic agents. Although anticholinergic-type side effects have been noted with amantadine when used in patients with drug-induced extrapyramidal reactions, there is a lower incidence of these side effects than with anticholinergic antiparkinson drugs.

BROMOCRIPTINE MESYLATE

Rx	Parlodel SnapTabs (Sandoz)	Tablets: 2.5 mg (as mesylate)	(Parlodel 2½). White, scored. In 30s and 100s.
Rx	Parlodel (Sandoz)	Capsules: 5 mg (as mesylate)	(Parlodel 5 mg). Caramel/white. In 30s & 100s.

This is an abbreviated monograph. Bromocriptine is also used in the treatment of amenorrhea/galactorrhea, female infertility, acromegaly and prevention of physiological lactation. For full prescribing information, refer to the monograph in the Endocrine/Metabolic chapter. Also refer to the general discussion in the Antiparkinson Agents introduction.

Indications

➤*Parkinson's disease:* In the treatment of idiopathic or postencephalitic Parkinson's disease.

Administration and Dosage

➤*Parkinson's disease:* Initiate treatment at a low dosage and individualize; increase the daily dosage slowly until a maximum therapeutic response is achieved. If possible, maintain the dosage of levodopa during this introductory period.

Initially, use 1.25 mg (one-half of a 2.5 mg tablet) twice daily with meals. Assess dosage titrations every 2 weeks to ensure that the lowest dosage producing an optimal therapeutic response is not exceeded. If necessary, increase the dosage every 2 to 4 weeks by 2.5 mg/day with meals. If it is necessary to reduce the dose because of adverse reactions, reduce dose gradually in 2.5 mg increments. Usual range is 10 to 40 mg/day.

The safety of bromocriptine has not been demonstrated in dosages exceeding 100 mg/day.

Actions

➤*Pharmacology:* Bromocriptine, a dopamine agonist, may relieve akinesia, rigidity and tremor in patients with Parkinson's disease. It produces its therapeutic effect by directly stimulating the dopamine receptors in the corpus striatum. Experiments in rodents suggest a direct action of bromocriptine on striatal dopamine receptors.

As adjunctive treatment to levodopa (alone or with a peripheral decarboxylase inhibitor), bromocriptine therapy may provide additional therapeutic benefits in those patients who are currently maintained on optimal dosages of levodopa, those who are beginning to develop tolerance to levodopa therapy, and those who are experiencing levodopa "end of dose failure." Bromocriptine may permit reducing the maintenance dose of levodopa and thus, may ameliorate the occurrence or severity of adverse reactions associated with long-term levodopa therapy such as abnormal involuntary movements (eg, dyskinesias) and the marked swings in motor function ("on-off" phenomenon). Continued efficacy of bromocriptine during treatment of > 2 years has not been established.

Data are insufficient to evaluate benefit from treating newly diagnosed Parkinson's disease with bromocriptine. Studies show more adverse reactions (notably nausea, hallucinations, confusion and hypotension) in bromocriptine-treated patients than in levodopa/carbidopa-treated patients. Patients unresponsive to levodopa are poor candidates for bromocriptine.

CARBIDOPA

Rx	**Lodosyn**[1] (Bristol-Myers Squibb Primary Care)	**Tablets:** 25 mg carbidopa		(MSD 129). Orange, scored. In 100s.

[1] Most patients may be maintained on carbidopa/levodopa combination products. *Lodosyn* is available to physicians for use in patients requiring individual titration of carbidopa and levodopa.

Carbidopa is used only with levodopa. See levodopa monograph. Also refer to the general discussion in the Antiparkinson Agents introduction.

WARNING

When carbidopa is to be given to patients being treated with levodopa, give the two drugs at the same time, starting with no more than 20% to 25% of the previous daily dosage of levodopa. At least 8 hours should elapse between the last dose of levodopa and initiation of therapy with carbidopa and levodopa.

Indications

Carbidopa has no effect when given alone. It is indicated only for use with levodopa.

For use with levodopa in the treatment of the symptoms of idiopathic Parkinson's disease, postencephalitic parkinsonism and symptomatic parkinsonism which may follow injury to the nervous system by carbon monoxide intoxication and manganese intoxication.

Carbidopa permits administration of lower doses of levodopa, more rapid dosage titration and a somewhat smoother response. However, patients with markedly irregular ("on-off") response to levodopa do not benefit from the addition of carbidopa. Carbidopa is effective in patients who do not have adequate reduction in nausea and vomiting when the carbidopa/levodopa combination provides < 70 mg/day of carbidopa. Carbidopa is used with levodopa in the occasional patient whose dosage requirement of carbidopa and levodopa necessitates separate titration of each entity.

➤*Unlabeled uses:* Carbidopa is also used to reduce the peripheral metabolism of L-5-hydroxytryptophan (L-5HTP) when used to treat post-anoxic intention myoclonus (see the L-5HTP monograph in the Keeping Up section).

Administration and Dosage

Carbidopa/levodopa combinations are the preferred method of administration (see Levodopa/Carbidopa monograph) but occasionally a patient may require individual titration of these drugs.

Determine optimal daily dosage by careful titration. Peripheral dopa decarboxylase is saturated by carbidopa at ≈ 70 to 100 mg/day. Patients who require only low doses of levodopa (eg, < 700 mg when given as carbidopa/levodopa 1:10) will receive doses of carbidopa which theoretically do not saturate peripheral dopa decarboxylase.

➤*Maximum daily dose:* Do not exceed 200 mg. If the patient is taking carbidopa/levodopa, calculate the total amount of additional carbidopa to be administered each day.

➤*Patients receiving carbidopa/levodopa who require additional carbidopa:* Some patients may not have adequate reduction in nausea and vomiting when the dosage of carbidopa is < 70 mg a day, and the dosage of levodopa is < 700 mg a day. When these patients are taking 10 mg carbidopa/100 mg levodopa, 25 mg carbidopa may be given with the first dose each day. Additional doses of 12.5 mg or 25 mg may be given during the day with each dose. When patients are taking 25 mg carbidopa/250 mg levodopa, 25 mg carbidopa may be given with any dose, as required, for optimum therapeutic response.

➤*Dosage adjustment:* Add or omit to 1 tablet per day. Because therapeutic and adverse responses occur more rapidly with combined therapy than with levodopa alone, closely monitor patients. Dyskinesias may require dosage reduction. Blepharospasm may be a useful early sign of excess dosage.

Other standard antiparkinson agents may be continued while carbidopa and levodopa are administered; the dosage of such drugs may require adjustment.

If general anesthesia is required, continue therapy as long as patient is allowed to take oral fluids and medication. When therapy is temporarily interrupted, resume usual daily dosage as soon as patient is able to take oral medication.

Actions

➤*Pharmacology:* Carbidopa inhibits decarboxylation of peripheral levodopa. It does not cross blood-brain barrier and does not affect levodopa metabolism within the CNS.

Since its decarboxylase inhibiting activity is limited to extracerebral tissues, administration of carbidopa with levodopa makes more levodopa available for transport to the brain. Carbidopa does not have any overt pharmacodynamic actions in the recommended doses. Normally, pyridoxine HCl (vitamin B_6), in oral doses of 10 to 25 mg, may reverse the effects of levodopa by increasing the rate of aromatic amino acid decarboxylation. Carbidopa inhibits this action of pyridoxine HCl.

Since levodopa competes with certain amino acids, levodopa absorption may be impaired in some patients on a high protein diet.

➤*Clinical trials:* Carbidopa reduces the amount of levodopa required by ≈ 70% to 75%. When administered with levodopa, carbidopa increases plasma levels and plasma half-life of levodopa, and decreases plasma and urinary dopamine and homovanillic acid. Coadministration produces greater urinary excretion of levodopa in proportion to excretion of dopamine than separate administration. Reduced formation of dopamine in extracerebral tissues, such as the heart, may protect against dopamine-induced cardiac arrhythmias.

Contraindications

Patients hypersensitive to carbidopa or levodopa.

Warnings

➤*Neuroleptic malignant-like syndrome:* Neuroleptic malignant-like syndrome including muscular rigidity, elevated body temperature, mental changes and increased serum creatine phosphokinase has been reported when antiparkinsonian agents were withdrawn abruptly. Therefore, carefully observe patients when the dosage of levodopa is reduced abruptly or discontinued, especially if the patient is receiving neuroleptics.

➤*Discontinue levodopa:* Discontinue levodopa at least 8 hours before concomitant therapy with carbidopa/levodopa is started. When combination therapy is initiated, reduce levodopa to 20% to 25% of the previous levodopa dosage (see Administration and Dosage).

Carbidopa does not decrease adverse reactions due to central effects of levodopa.

➤*Dyskinesias:* Carbidopa permits more levodopa to reach the brain and more dopamine to be formed. Dyskinesias may occur sooner and at lower dosages with coadministration than with levodopa alone, and may require dosage reduction.

➤*Elderly:* Elderly patients may require less carbidopa/levodopa due to an age related decrease in peripheral dopa decarboxylase.

➤*Pregnancy:* Although effects in pregnancy are unknown, both levodopa and carbidopa/levodopa have caused visceral and skeletal malformations in rabbits. Use only when clearly needed and when potential benefits outweigh potential hazards to the fetus.

➤*Lactation:* Do not administer to the nursing mother.

➤*Children:* Safety for use in children < 18 years old is not established.

Drug Interactions

➤*Tricyclic antidepressants:* Concomitant use has, in rare reports, caused adverse reactions, including hypertension and dyskinesia.

Adverse Reactions

Carbidopa has not been demonstrated to have any overt pharmacodynamic actions in the recommended doses. The only adverse reactions reported have been with concomitant use of carbidopa and levodopa. (See levodopa monograph.)

Levels of BUN, creatinine and uric acid are lower during concomitant administration of carbidopa and levodopa than with levodopa alone.

LEVODOPA

Rx	**Larodopa** (Roche)	**Tablets:** 100 mg		(LARODOPA 100). Pink, scored. In 100s.
Rx	**Larodopa** (Roche)	**Tablets:** 500 mg		Pink, scored. In100s.

Refer to the general discussion in the Antiparkinson Agents introduction.

Indications

Treatment of idiopathic, postencephalitic and symptomatic parkinsonism which may follow injury to the nervous system by carbon monoxide and manganese intoxication, and in elderly patients with parkinsonism associated with cerebral arteriosclerosis.

➤*Concomitant therapy:* Levodopa is often used in combination with carbidopa, which inhibits decarboxylation of levodopa and makes more

levodopa available for transport to the brain (see Levodopa/Carbidopa monograph).

Selegiline and pergolide are each used as adjuncts in the management of parkinsonian patients being treated with levodopa/carbidopa; the dose of the levodopa/carbidopa may be decreased with concomitant therapy (see individual monographs).

➤*Unlabeled uses:* Levodopa has been used with some benefit to relieve herpes zoster (shingles) pain and restless legs syndrome.

LEVODOPA

Administration and Dosage

In order to reduce the high incidence of adverse reactions, individualize therapy and gradually increase dosage to the desired therapeutic level.

Determine the optimal daily dose for maximal improvement with tolerated side effects and titrate for each patient.

▶Initial: Administer 0.5 to 1g daily, divided into 2 or more doses; give with food.

Increase gradually in increments not exceeding 0.75 g/day every 3 to 7 days, as tolerated. Do not exceed 8 g/day, except for exceptional patients. A significant therapeutic response may not be obtained for 6 months.

In the event general anesthesia is required, therapy may be continued as long as the patient is able to take oral fluids and medication. If therapy is temporarily interrupted, the usual daily dosage may be administered as soon as the patient is able to take oral medication. Whenever therapy has been interrupted for longer periods, adjust dosage gradually; however, in many cases, the patient can be rapidly titrated to his previous therapeutic dosage.

Actions

▶Pharmacology: The symptoms of Parkinson's disease are related to depletion of striatal dopamine. Dopamine does not cross the blood-brain barrier; however, levodopa, the metabolic precursor of dopamine, does cross the blood-brain barrier. It is decarboxylated into dopamine in the basal ganglia and in the periphery. Hence, blood dopamine is markedly increased, accounting for many of levodopa's pharmacologic and adverse effects.

▶Pharmacokinetics:

Absorption/Distribution – Levodopa is absorbed from the small bowel; peak plasma levels occur in 0.5 to 2 hours, and may be delayed in the presence of food. The rate of absorption is dependent upon the rate of gastric emptying, pH of gastric juice, and the length of time the drug is exposed to degradative enzymes of gastric mucosa and intestinal flora.

Metabolism/Excretion – The drug is extensively metabolized (> 95%) in the periphery and by the liver; < 1% of unchanged drug penetrates the CNS. Plasma half-life ranges from 1 to 3 hours. It is excreted primarily in the urine. The major urinary metabolites of levodopa appear to be dihydroxyphenylacetic acid (DOPAC) and homovanillic acid (HVA). In 24 hour urine samples, HVA accounts for 13% to 42% of the ingested dose of levodopa.

Contraindications

Hypersensitivity to the drug; narrow-angle glaucoma; patients on MAOI therapy (does not apply to MAOI-type B agents such as selegiline). Discontinue MAOIs 2 weeks prior to initiating levodopa therapy.

Because levodopa may activate a malignant melanoma, do not use in patients with suspicious, undiagnosed skin lesions or history of melanoma.

Warnings

▶Concomitant conditions: Administer cautiously to patients with severe cardiovascular or pulmonary disease, bronchial asthma, occlusive cerebrovascular disease, renal, hepatic or endocrine disease, affective disorders, major psychoses and cardiac arrhythmias. Periodically evaluate hepatic, hematopoietic, cardiovascular and renal functions during extended therapy in all patients.

▶Myocardial infarction: Administer cautiously to patients with a history of myocardial infarction who have residual atrial, nodal or ventricular arrhythmias. Use in a facility with a coronary or intensive care unit.

▶Upper GI hemorrhage: Upper GI hemorrhage may occur in those patients with a history of peptic ulcer.

▶Psychiatric patients: Observe all patients for the development of depression with suicidal tendencies. Treat psychotic patients with caution.

▶Pregnancy: Safety for use during pregnancy has not been established. Use only when clearly needed and when potential benefits outweigh potential hazards to the fetus. At dosages in excess of 200mg/kg/day, levodopa has an adverse effect in rodents on fetal and postnatal growth and viability.

▶Lactation: Do not use in nursing mothers.

▶Children: Safety for use in children < 12 years has not been established.

Precautions

▶Wide-angle glaucoma: Patients with chronic wide-angle glaucoma may be treated cautiously with levodopa, if the intraocular pressure is well controlled and the patient is carefully monitored for changes in intraocular pressure during therapy.

▶"On-off" phenomenon: Some patients who initially respond to levodopa therapy may develop the "on-off" phenomenon, a condition where patients suddenly oscillate between improved clinical status and loss of therapeutic effect (abrupt onset of akinesia). This effect may occur

within minutes or hours and is associated with long-term levodopa treatment. Approximately 15% to 40% of patients develop this phenomenon after 2 to 3 years of treatment; this frequency increases after 5 years. In other patients, a deteriorating response to levodopa occurs ("wearing-off" effect).

Suggestions to alleviate these conditions include keeping the dose low, reserving the drug for severe cases, or the use of a "drug holiday" which includes complete withdrawal of levodopa for a period of time (5 to 14 days) followed by a slow reintroduction of the drug at a lower dose. A protein-restricted diet and adjunctive therapy (eg, pergolide, selegiline), allowing for a decreased levodopa dose, may also be beneficial. Further study is needed.

▶Tartrazine sensitivity: Some of these products contain tartrazine, which may cause allergic-type reactions (including bronchial asthma) in certain susceptible individuals. Although the overall incidence of tartrazine sensitivity is low, it is frequently seen in patients who also have aspirin hypersensitivity. Specific products containing tartrazine are identified in the product listings.

Drug Interactions

Levodopa Drug Interactions			
Precipitant drug	Object drug*		Description
Antacids	Levodopa	↑	Levodopa bioavailability may be increased, possibly increasing its efficacy.
Anticholinergics	Levodopa	↓	Increased gastric deactivation and decreased intestinal absorption of levodopa may occur.
Benzodiazepines	Levodopa	↓	Levodopa's therapeutic value may be attenuated.
Hydantoins	Levodopa	↓	Levodopa's effectiveness may be reduced.
Methionine	Levodopa	↓	Levodopa's effectiveness may be reduced.
Metoclopramide	Levodopa	↔	Levodopa's bioavailability may be increased; levodopa may decrease the effects of metoclopramide on gastric emptying and lower esophageal pressure.
MAO inhibitors	Levodopa	↑	Hypertensive reactions occur with levodopa and MAOI coadministration. Avoid concurrent use. The MAO-type B inhibitor selegiline is used with levodopa and is not associated with such a reaction.
Papaverine	Levodopa	↓	Levodopa's effectiveness may be reduced.
Pyridoxine	Levodopa	↓	Levodopa's effectiveness is reduced.
Tricyclic antidepressants	Levodopa	↓	Delayed absorption and decreased bioavailability of levodopa may occur. Hypertensive episodes have occurred.

* ↑ = Object drug increased ↓ = Object drug decreased ↔ = Undetermined effect

▶Drug/Lab test interactions: The Coombs test has occasionally become positive during extended therapy. Elevations of uric acid have occurred with the colorimetric method, but not with the uricase method.

▶Drug/Food interactions: In six of nine patients, meals reduced the peak plasma concentrations of levodopa by 29%; the peak was delayed by 34 minutes. A protein-restricted diet may also help minimize the "fluctuations" (decreased response to levodopa at the end of each day or at various times of day) that occur in some patients.

Adverse Reactions

Elevations of BUN, AST, ALT, LDH, bilirubin, alkaline phosphatase, or protein-bound iodine have been reported; the significance of these findings is not known. Occasional reduction in WBC, hemoglobin and hematocrit have occurred.

Leukopenia has occurred; it required temporary cessation of levodopa therapy.

Frequent – Adventitious movements, such as choreiform or dystonic movements (10% to 90%); anorexia (50%); nausea and vomiting (80%) with or without abdominal pain and distress; dry mouth; dysphagia; dysgeusia (4.5% to 22%); sialorrhea; ataxia; increased hand tremor; headache; dizziness; numbness; weakness and faintness; bruxism; confusion; insomnia; nightmares; hallucinations and delusions; agitation and anxiety; malaise; fatigue; euphoria.

Less frequent – Cardiac irregularities or palpitations; orthostatic hypotension (symptomatic 5%); bradykinesia (the "on-off" phenomenon; see Precautions); mental changes, including paranoid ideation, psychotic episodes, depression with or without suicidal tendencies, and dementia; urinary retention; muscle twitching and blepharospasm (may be taken as an early sign of overdosage; consider dosage reduction); trismus; burning sensation of the tongue; bitter taste; diarrhea;

LEVODOPA

constipation; flatulence; flushing; skin rash; increased sweating; bizarre breathing patterns; urinary incontinence; diplopia; blurred vision; dilated pupils; hot flashes; weight gain or loss; dark sweat or urine.

Rare – GI bleeding; duodenal ulcer; hypertension; phlebitis; hemolytic anemia; agranulocytosis; oculogyric crises; sense of stimulation; hiccoughs; edema; loss of hair; hoarseness; priapism; activation of latent Horner's syndrome.

Overdosage

➤*Treatment:* For acute overdosage, employ general supportive measures, along with immediate gastric lavage. Administer IV fluids judiciously and maintain an adequate airway. Refer to General Management of Acute Overdosage.

Monitor ECG and carefully observe the patient for the possible development of arrhythmias; if required, give appropriate antiarrhythmic therapy. Consider the possibility of multiple drug ingestion.

Patient Information

Effects may be delayed from several weeks to a few months.

May cause GI upset; take with food.

Avoid vitamin products containing vitamin B_6 (pyridoxine HCl). See Drug Interactions.

Observe caution while driving or performing other tasks requiring alertness.

If fainting, lightheadedness or dizziness (orthostatic hypotension) occurs, avoid sudden changes in posture; notify physician of this effect.

Medication may cause darkening of the urine or sweat. This effect is not harmful.

➤*Diabetic patients:* Medication may interfere with urine tests for sugar or ketones. Report any abnormal results to physician before adjusting dosage of antidiabetic medications.

Notify physician if any of the following occur: Uncontrollable movements of the face, eyelids, mouth, tongue, neck, arms, hands or legs; mood or mental changes; irregular heartbeats or palpitations; difficult urination; severe or persistent nausea and vomiting.

LEVODOPA AND CARBIDOPA

Rx	Carbidopa & Levodopa (Lemmon)	Tablets: 10 mg carbidopa and 100 mg levodopa	(93 292). Blue, mottled, scored. In 100s and 1000s.
Rx	Sinemet-10/100 (Bristol-Myers Squibb Primary Care)		(SINEMET 647). Dark blue, scored. Oval. In 100s and UD 100s.
Rx	Carbidopa & Levodopa (Lemmon)	Tablets: 25 mg carbidopa and 100 mg levodopa	(93 293). Yellow, mottled, scored. In 100s and 1000s.
Rx	Sinemet-25/100 (Bristol-Myers Squibb Primary Care)		(SINEMET650). Yellow, scored. Oval. In 100s and UD 100s.
Rx	Carbidopa & Levodopa (Lemmon)	Tablets: 25 mg carbidopa and 250 mg levodopa	(93 294). Blue, mottled, scored. In 100s and 1000s.
Rx	Sinemet-25/250 (Bristol-Myers Squibb Primary Care)		(SINEMET 654). Light blue, scored. Oval. In 100s and UD 100s.
Rx	Sinemet CR (Bristol-Myers Squibb Primary Care)	Tablets, sustained release: 25 mg carbidopa, 100 mg levodopa	(SINEMET CR 601). Pink. Biconvex. Oval. In 100s and UD 100s.
		50 mg carbidopa and 200 mg levodopa	(SINEMET CR 521). Peach, scored. Oval, biconvex. In 100s and UD 100s.
Rx	Carbidopa and Levodopa (Mylan)	Tablets, extended-release: 25 mg carbidopa and 100 mg levodopa	(MYLAN/88). Purple, oval, unscored, biconvex. In 100s and 500s.
		50 mg carbidopa and 200 mg levodopa	(MYLAN/94). Purple, oval, scored, biconvex. In 100s and 500s.

These agents are used in combination because carbidopa inhibits decarboxylation of levodopa and makes more levodopa available for transport to the brain. For complete information on each of the components refer to the individual monographs. Also refer to the general discussion in the Antiparkinson Agents introduction.

Indications

Treatment of symptoms of idiopathic Parkinson's disease (paralysis agitans), postencephalitic parkinsonism and symptomatic parkinsonism which may follow injury to the nervous system by carbon monoxide and manganese intoxication.

Administration and Dosage

The optimum daily dose must be determined by careful titration in each patient.

➤*Patients not receiving levodopa:*

Sinemet – 1 tablet of 25 mg carbidopa/100 mg levodopa 3 times daily or 10 mg carbidopa/100 mg levodopa 3 or 4 times daily. Dosage may be increased by 1 tablet every day or every other day, as necessary, until a dosage of 8 tablets a day is reached.

Tablets of the two ratios (eg, 1:4, 25/100 or 1:10, 10/100 and 25/250) may be given separately or combined as needed to provide the optimum dosage.

Provide at least 70 to 100 mg carbidopa per day. When more carbidopa is required, substitute one 25/100 tablet for each 10/100 tablet. When more levodopa is required, substitute the 25/250 tablet for the 25/100 or 10/100 tablet.

Sinemet CR – 1 tablet twice daily at intervals of not less than 6 hours. Doses and dosing intervals may be increased or decreased based on response. Most patients have been adequately treated with 2 to 8 tablets per day (divided doses) at intervals of 4 to 8 hours while awake. Higher doses (≥ 12 tablets per day) and intervals < 4 hours have been used but are not usually recommended. If an interval of < 4 hours is used or if the divided doses are not equal, give the smaller doses at the end of the day. Allow at least a 3 day interval between dosage adjustments.

Sinemet CR may be administered as whole or half tablets which should not be crushed or chewed.

➤*Patients currently treated with levodopa:* Levodopa must be discontinued at least 8 hours before therapy with levodopa/carbidopa. Substitute the combination drug at a dosage that will provide approximately 25% of the previous levodopa dosage.

Sinemet – Suggested starting dosage is 1 tablet of 25 mg carbidopa/250 mg levodopa 3 or 4 times a day for patients taking > 1500 mg levodopa or 25 mg carbidopa/100 mg levodopa for patients taking < 1500 mg levodopa.

Sinemet CR – Usually 1 tablet twice daily.

➤*Patients currently treated with conventional carbidopa/levodopa preparations:* Substitute dosage with *Sinemet CR* at an amount that provides ≈ 10% more levodopa per day, although this may need to be increased to a dosage that provides up to 30% more levodopa per day. Use intervals of 4 to 8 hours while awake.

Guidelines for Initial Conversion from *Sinemet* to *Sinemet CR* (50/100 mg tablets)	
Sinemet Total daily levodopa dose (mg)	*Sinemet CR* (50/100 mg tablets) Suggested dosage regimen
300 to 400	1 tablet twice daily
500 to 600	1½ tablets twice daily or 1 tablet 3 times daily
700 to 800	Total of 4 tablets in ≥ 3 divided doses (eg, 1½ tablets am, 1½ tablets early pm, 1 tablet later pm)
900 to 1000	Total of 5 tablets in ≥ 3 divided doses (eg, 2 tablets am, 2 tablets early pm, 1 tablet later pm)

➤*Combination therapy:* Other antiparkinson drugs can be given concurrently; dosage adjustment may be necessary.

Sinemet – Sinemet (25/100 or 10/100) can be added to the dosage regimen of *Sinemet CR* in selected patients with advanced disease who need additional levodopa.

Actions

➤*Pharmacology:* The sustained release formulation is designed to release the ingredients over a 4 to 6 hour period. There is less variation in plasma levodopa levels than with the conventional formulation. However, the sustained release form is less systemically bioavailable (70% to 75%) and may require increased daily doses to achieve the same level of symptomatic relief.

➤*Pharmacokinetics:* The half-life of levodopa may be prolonged following the sustained release form because of continuous absorption. In elderly subjects, the mean time to peak levodopa concentration was 2 hours for sustained release vs 0.5 hours for conventional. The maximum levodopa concentration of levodopa following the sustained release form was ≈ 35% of the conventional form.

➤*Clinical trials:* In clinical trials, patients receiving the sustained release form did not experience quantitatively significant reductions in "off" time (motor fluctuations) compared to the conventional form; however, global ratings of improvement were better.

LEVODOPA AND CARBIDOPA

Warnings

➤*CNS effects:* Certain adverse CNS effects (eg, dyskinesias) will occur at lower dosages and sooner during therapy with the sustained release form.

Drug Interactions

➤*Drug/Food interactions:* Administration of a single dose of the sustained release form with food increased the extent of levodopa availability by 50% and increased peak levodopa concentrations by 25%.

Adverse Reactions

In clinical trials, the adverse reaction profile of the sustained release form did not differ substantially from that of the conventional form.

ENTACAPONE

Rx	Comtan (Novartis)	**Tablets:** 200 mg	Mannitol, sucrose. (COMTAN). Film-coated. Oval, brownish-orange. In 10s, 100s, and 500s.

Indications

➤*Parkinson's disease:* As an adjunct to levodopa/carbidopa to treat patients with idiopathic Parkinson's disease who experience the signs and symptoms of end-of-dose "wearing-off." The effectiveness of entacapone has not been systematically evaluated in patients with idiopathic Parkinson's disease who do not experience end-of-dose "wearing-off."

Administration and Dosage

➤*Approved by the FDA:* October 22, 1999.

The recommended dose of entacapone is one 200 mg tablet administered concomitantly with each levodopa/carbidopa dose to a maximum of 8 times daily (200 mg x 8 = 1600 mg/day). Clinical experience with daily doses > 1600 mg is limited.

Always administer entacapone in combination with levodopa/carbidopa. Entacapone has no antiparkinsonian effect of its own.

In clinical trials, the majority of patients required a decrease in daily levodopa dose if their daily dose of levodopa had been ≥ 800 mg, or if they had moderate or severe dyskinesias prior to treatment with entacapone.

Reducing the daily levodopa dose or extending the interval between doses may be necessary to optimize patient reponse. In clinical trials, the average reduction in the daily levodopa dose was ≈ 25% in those patients requiring a levodopa dose reduction. (More than 58% of patients with levodopa doses > 800 mg daily required such a reduction.)

Entacapone can be combined with the immediate- and sustained-release formulations of levodopa/carbidopa.

Entacapone may be taken with or without food.

➤*Withdrawing patients from entacapone:* Rapid withdrawal or abrupt reduction in the entacapone dose could lead to emergence of signs and symptoms of Parkinson's disease, and may lead to hyperpyrexia and confusion, a symptom complex resembling neuroleptic malignant syndrome (see Precautions). Consider this syndrome in the differential diagnosis for any patient who develops a high fever or severe rigidity. If a decision is made to discontinue treatment with entacapone, monitor patients closely and adjust other dopaminergic agents as needed. Although tapering entacapone has not been evaluated, it seems reasonable to withdraw patients slowly if the decision to discontinue treatment is made.

Actions

➤*Pharmacology:* Entacapone is a selective and reversible inhibitor of catechol-*O*-methyltransferase (COMT).

In mammals, COMT is distributed throughout various organs with the highest activity in the liver and kidney. COMT is also present in the heart, lung, smooth and skeletal muscles, intestinal tract, reproductive organs, various glands, adipose tissue, skin, blood cells, and neuronal tissues, especially the glial cells. COMT catalyzes the transfer of the methyl group of S-adenosyl-L-methionine to the phenolic group of substrates that contain a catechol structure. Physiological substrates of COMT include dopa, catecholamines (dopamine, norepinephrine, and epinephrine), and their hydroxylated metabolites. COMT eliminates biologically active catechols and other hydroxylated metabolites. In the presence of a decarboxylase inhibitor, COMT becomes the major metabolizing enzyme for levodopa, catalyzing the metabolism to 3-methoxy-4-hydroxy-L-phenylalanine (3-OMD) in the brain and periphery.

Entacapone is believed to act by inhibiting COMT and altering the plasma pharmacokinetics of levodopa. When entacapone is given in conjunction with levodopa and an aromatic amino acid decarboxylase inhibitor (such as carbidopa), plasma levels of levodopa are greater and more sustained than after administration of levodopa and an aromatic amino acid decarboxylase inhibitor alone. It is believed that these more sustained plasma levels of levodopa result in more constant dopaminergic stimulation in the brain, leading to alleviation of the signs and symptoms of Parkinson's disease. The higher levodopa levels also lead to increased levodopa adverse effects, sometimes requiring a decrease in the levodopa dose.

In animals, while entacapone enters the CNS to a minimal extent, it has been shown to inhibit central COMT activity. In humans, entacapone inhibits COMT in peripheral tissues. The effects of entacapone on central COMT activity in humans have not been studied.

COMT activity in erythrocytes – In healthy volunteers, entacapone reversibly inhibits human erythrocyte COMT activity after oral administration. There is a linear correlation between entacapone dose and erythrocyte COMT inhibition, the maximum inhibition being 82% following an 800 mg single dose. With a 200 mg single dose of entacapone, maximum inhibition of erythrocyte COMT activity is on average 65% with a return to baseline level within 8 hours.

Effect on pharmacokinetics of levodopa and its metabolites – When 200 mg entacapone is administered together with levodopa/carbidopa, entacapone increases the area under the curve (AUC) of levodopa by ≈ 35% and the elimination half-life of levodopa is prolonged from 1.3 to 2.4 hours. In general, the average peak levodopa plasma concentration and the time of its occurrence (T_{max} of 1 hour) are unaffected. The onset of effect occurs after the first dose and is maintained during long-term treatment. Studies in patients with Parkinson's disease suggest that the maximal effect occurs with 200 mg entacapone. Plasma levels of 3-OMD are markedly and dose-dependently decreased by entacapone when administered with levodopa/carbidopa.

➤*Pharmacokinetics:*

Absorption – Entacapone is rapidly absorbed, with a T_{max} of ≈ 1 hour. The absolute bioavailability following oral administration is 35%. Food does not affect the pharmacokinetics of entacapone.

Distribution – The volume of distribution of entacapone at steady-state after IV injection is small (20 L). Entacapone does not distribute widely into tissues because of its high plasma protein binding. Based on in vitro studies, the plasma protein binding of entacapone is 98% over the concentration range of 0.4 to 50 mcg/ml. Entacapone mainly binds to serum albumin.

Metabolism/Excretion – Entacapone is almost completely metabolized prior to excretion, with only a small amount (0.2% of dose) excreted unchanged in the urine. The main metabolic pathway is isomerization to the *cis*-isomer followed by direct glucuronidation of the parent and *cis*-isomer; the glucuronide conjugate is inactive. After oral administration, 10% of the parent and metabolite are excreted in the urine and 90% in the feces.

Special populations:

Hepatic function impairment: A single 200 mg dose of entacapone, without levodopa/dopa decarboxylase inhibitor coadministration, showed ≈ 2-fold higher AUC and C_{max} values in patients with a history of alcoholism and hepatic impairment (n = 10) compared with healthy subjects (n = 10). All patients had biopsy-proven liver cirrhosis caused by alcohol. According to Child-Pugh grading, 7 patients with liver disease had mild hepatic impairment and 3 patients had moderate hepatic impairment. Biliary excretion appears to be the major route of excretion; only ≈ 10% of the entacapone dose is excreted in urine as parent compound and conjugated glucuronide. Consequently, administer entacapone with care to patients with biliary obstruction.

Renal function impairment: The pharmacokinetics of entacapone have been investigated after a single 200 mg entacapone dose, without levodopa/dopa decarboxylase inhibitor coadministration, in a renal impairment study. There were 3 groups: Healthy subjects (n = 7; Ccr > 1.12 ml/sec/1.73 m²), moderate impairment (n = 10; Ccr ranging from 0.6 to 0.89 ml/sec/1.73 m²), and severe impairment (n = 7; Ccr ranging from 0.2 to 0.44 ml/sec/1.73 m²). No important effects of renal function on entacapone pharmacokinetics were found.

Entacapone pharmacokinetics are linear over the dose range of 5 to 800 mg and are independent of levodopa/carbidopa coadministration. The elimination of entacapone is biphasic, with an elimination half-life of 0.4 to 0.7 hours based on the β-phase and 2.4 hours based on the γ-phase. The γ-phase accounts for ≈ 10% of the total AUC. The total body clearance after IV administration is 850 ml/min. After a single 200 mg dose of entacapone, the C_{max} is ≈ 1.2 mcg/ml.

Contraindications

Hypersensitivity to the drug or its ingredients.

Warnings

➤*Monoamine oxidase (MAO) inhibitors:* MAO and COMT are the 2 major enzyme systems involved in the metabolism of catecholamines. Therefore, it is theoretically possible that the combination of entacapone and a non-selective MAO inhibitor (eg, phenelzine, tranylcypromine) would result in inhibition of the majority of pathways responsible for normal catecholamine metabolism. For this reason, do not treat patients concomitantly with entacapone and a non-selective MAO inhibitor.

ENTACAPONE

Entacapone can be taken concomitantly with a selective MAO-B inhibitor (eg, selegiline).

➤*Drugs metabolized by COMT:* When a single 400 mg dose of entacapone was given together with IV isoproterenol and epinephrine without a levodopa/dopa decarboxylase inhibitor, the overall mean maximal changes in heart rate during infusion were ≈ 50% and 80% higher than with placebo for isoprenaline and epinephrine, respectively.

Therefore, adminster drugs known to be metabolized by COMT (ie, isoproterenol, epinephrine, norepinephrine, dopamine, dobutamine, methyldopa, apomorphine, isoetherine, bitolterol) with caution in patients receiving entacapone regardless of the route of administration (including inhalation), as their interaction may result in increased heart rates, arrhythmias, and excessive changes in blood pressure.

Ventricular tachycardia was noted in one 32-year-old healthy male volunteer in an interaction study after epinephrine infusion and oral entacapone administration. Treatment with propranolol was required. A causal relationship to entacapone administration appears probable but cannot be attributed with certainty.

➤*Hepatic function impairment:* Treat patients with hepatic impairment with caution. The AUC and C_{max} of entacapone approximately doubled in patients with documented liver disease compared with controls (see Pharmacokinetics and Administration and Dosage).

➤*Carcinogenesis:* Rats were treated orally once daily with entacapone doses of 20, 90, or 400 mg/kg. An increased incidence of renal tubular adenomas and carcinomas was found in male rats treated with the highest dose of entacapone. Plasma exposures (AUC) associated with this dose were ≈ 20 times higher than estimated plasma exposures of humans receiving the maximum recommended daily dose (MRDD) of entacapone (MRDD = 1600 mg). Although no treatment related tumors were observed in animals receiving the lower doses, the carcinogenic potential of entacapone has not been fully evaluated. The carcinogenic potential of entacapone administered in combination with levodopa/carbidopa has not been evaluated.

➤*Mutagenesis:* Entacapone was mutagenic and clastogenic in the in vitro mouse lymphoma/thymidine kinase assay in the presence and absence of metabolic activation, and was clastogenic in cultured human lymphocytes in the presence of metabolic activation.

➤*Pregnancy:* Category C. In embryofetal development studies, entacapone was administered to pregnant animals throughout organogenesis at doses of up to 1000 mg/kg/day in rats and 300 mg/kg/day in rabbits. Increased incidences of fetal variations were evident in rats treated with the highest dose in the absence of overt signs of maternal toxicity. The maternal plasma drug exposure (AUC) associated with this dose was ≈ 34 times the estimated plasma exposure in humans receiving the MRDD of 1600 mg. Increased frequencies of abortions and late/total resorptions and decreased fetal weights were observed in the litters of rabbits treated with maternotoxic doses of ≥ 100 mg/kg/day (plasma AUCs 0.4 times those in humans receiving the MRDD). There was no evidence of teratogenicity in these studies.

However, when entacapone was administered to female rats prior to mating and during early gestation, an increased incidence of fetal eye anomalies (macrophthalmia, microphthalmia, anophthalmia) was observed in the litters of dams treated with doses of 160 mg/kg/day (plasma AUCs 7 times those in humans receiving the MRDD) or greater, in the absence of maternotoxicity.

Entacapone is given concomitantly with levodopa/carbidopa, which is known to cause visceral and skeletal malformations in rabbits. The teratogenic potential of entacapone in combination with levodopa/carbidopa was not assessed in animals.

There is no experience from clinical studies regarding the use of entacapone in pregnant women. Therefore, use during pregnancy only if the potential benefit justifies the potential risk to the fetus.

➤*Lactation:* In animal studies, entacapone was excreted into maternal rat milk. It is not known whether entacapone is excreted in human breast milk. Exercise caution when entacapone is administered to a nursing woman.

➤*Children:* There is no identified potential use of entacapone in pediatric patients.

Precautions

➤*Hypotension/Syncope:* Dopaminergic therapy in patients with Parkinson's disease has been associated with orthostatic hypotension. Entacapone enhances levodopa bioavailability and, therefore, might be expected to increase the occurrence of orthostatic hypotension. However, in entacapone clinical trials, no differences from placebo were seen for measured orthostasis or symptoms of orthostasis. Orthostatic hypotension was documented at least once in 2.7% and 3% of the patients treated with 200 mg entacapone and placebo, respectively. A total of 4.3% and 4% of the patients treated with 200 mg entacapone and placebo, respectively, reported orthostatic symptoms at some time during their treatment and also had ≥ 1 documented episode of orthostatic hypotension. However, the episode of orthostatic symptoms was not accompanied by vital sign measurements. Neither baseline treatment with dopamine agonists or selegiline, nor the presence of ortho-

stasis at baseline, increased the risk of orthostatic hypotension in patients treated with entacapone compared with patients on placebo.

In the large controlled trials, ≈ 1.2% and 0.8% of 200 mg entacapone and placebo patients, respectively, reported ≥ 1 episode of syncope. Reports of syncope were generally more frequent in patients in both treatment groups who had an episode of documented hypotension (although the episodes of syncope, obtained by history, were themselves not documented with vital sign measurement).

➤*Diarrhea:* In clinical trials, diarrhea devloped in 10% and 4% of patients treated with 200 mg entacapone and placebo, respectively. In patients treated with entacapone, diarrhea was generally mild-to-moderate in severity (8.6%) but was regarded as severe in 1.3% of patients. Diarrhea resulted in drug withdrawal in 1.7% of patients, 1.2% with mild and moderate diarrhea, and 0.5% with severe diarrhea. Diarrhea generally resolved after discontinuation of entacapone. Two patients with diarrhea were hopitalized. Typically, diarrhea presents within 4 to 12 weeks after entacapone is started, but it may appear as early as the first week and as late as many months after treatment initiation.

➤*Hallucinations:* Dopaminergic therapy in Parkinson's disease patients has been associated with hallucinations. In clinical trials, hallucinations developed in ≈ 4% of patients treated with 200 mg entacapone or placebo. Hallucinations led to drug discontinuation and premature withdrawal from clinical trials in 0.8% and 0% of patients treated with 200 mg entacapone and placebo, respectively. Hallucinations led to hospitalization in 1% and 0.3% of patients in the 200 mg entacapone and placebo groups, respectively.

➤*Dyskinesia:* Entacapone may potentiate the dopaminergic side effects of levodopa and may cause or exacerbate preexisting dyskinesia. Although decreasing the dose of levodopa may ameliorate this side effect, many patients in controlled trials continued to experience frequent dyskinesias, despite a reduction in their levodopa dose. The rates of withdrawal for dyskinesia were 1.5% and 0.8% for 200 mg entacapone and placebo, respectively.

➤*Dopaminergic therapy reactions:* The events listed below are rare events known to be associated with the use of drugs that increase dopaminergic activity, although, they are most often associated with the use of direct dopamine agonists:

Rhabdomyolysis – Cases of severe rhabdomyolysis have been reported with entacapone use. The complicated nature of these cases makes it impossible to determine what role, if any, entacapone played in their pathogenesis. Severe prolonged motor activity including dyskinesia may account for rhabdomyolysis. However, one case included fever and alteration of consciousness. Therefore, it is possible that the rhabdomyolysis may be a result of the syndrome described in the Hyperpyrexia and confusion section.

Hyperpyrexia and confusion –
Tapering of dose: Cases of a symptom complex resembling neuroleptic malignant syndrome characterized by elevated temperature, muscular rigidity, altered consciousness, and elevated creatine phosphokinase (CPK) have been reported in association with the rapid dose reduction or withdrawal of other dopaminergic drugs. Several cases with similar signs and symptoms have been reported in association with entacapone therapy, although no information about dose manipulation is available. The complicated nature of these cases makes it difficult to determine what role, if any, entacapone may have played in their pathogenesis. No cases have been reported following the abrupt withdrawal or dose reduction of entacapone treatment during clinical studies.

Prescribers should exercise caution when discontinuing entacapone treatment. When considered necessary, withdrawal should proceed slowly. If a decision is made to discontinue treatment with entacapone, recommendations include monitoring the patient closely and adjusting other dopaminergic treatments as needed. Consider this syndrome in the differential diagnosis for any patient who develops a high fever or severe rigidity. Tapering entacapone has not been systematically evaluated.

Fibrotic complications – Cases of retroperitoneal fibrosis, pulmonary infiltrates, pleural effusion, and pleural thickening have been reported in some patients treated with ergot-derived dopaminergic agents. These complications may resolve when the drug is discontinued, but complete resolution does not always occur. Although these adverse events are believed to be related to the ergoline structure of these compounds, whether other nonergot-derived drugs (eg, entacapone) that increase dopaminergic activity can cause them is unknown. It should be noted that the expected incidence of fibrotic complications is so low that even if entacapone caused these complications at rates similar to those attributable to other dopaminergic therapies, it is unlikely that it would have been detected in a cohort of the size exposed to entacapone. Four cases of pulmonary fibrosis were reported during clinical development of entacapone; 3 of these patients were also treated with pergolide and 1 with bromocriptine. Treatment duration with entacapone ranged from 7 to 17 months.

➤*Renal toxicity:* In a 1-year toxicity study, entacapone (plasma exposure 20 times that in humans receiving the MRDD of 1600 mg) caused an increased incidence of nephrotoxicity in male rats characterized by regenerative tubules, thickening of basement membranes, infiltration of mononuclear cells, and tubular protein casts. These effects were not associated with changes in clinical chemistry parameters, and there is

ENTACAPONE

no established method to monitor for the possible occurrence of these lesions in humans. Although possible, there is currently no evidence that this toxicity could represent a species-specific effect.

➤*Biliary excretion:* As most entacapone excretion is via the bile, exercise caution when drugs known to interfere with biliary excretion, glucuronidation, and intestinal beta-glucuronidase are given concurrently with entacapone. These include probenecid, cholestyramine, and some antibiotics (eg, erythromycin, rifamipicin, ampicillin, chloramphenicol).

➤*Lab test abnormalities:* Entacapone is an iron chelator. The impact of entacapone on the body's iron stores is unknown; however, a tendency towards decreasing serum iron concentrations was noted in clinical trials. In a controlled clinical study, serum ferritin levels (as a marker of iron deficiency and subclinical anemia) were not changed with entacapone compared with placebo after 1 year of treatment and there was no difference in rates of anemia or decreased hemoglobin levels.

Drug Interactions

In vitro studies of human cytochrome P450 (CYP) enzymes showed that entacapone inhibited the CYP isoenzymes 1A2, 2A6, 2C9, 2C19, 2D6, 2E1, and 3A only at very high concentrations (IC50 from 200 to > 1000 mcM; an oral 200 mg dose achieves a highest level of ≈ 5 mcM in people); therefore, these enzymes would not be expected to be inhibited in clinical use.

Entacapone Drug Interactions

Precipitant drug	Object drug*		Description
MAO inhibitors	Entacapone	↑	MAO and COMT are the 2 major enzyme systems involved in catecholamine metabolism. Therefore, it is theoretically possible that the combination of entacapone and a non-selective MAO inhibitor (eg, phenelzine, tranylcypromine) would result in inhibition of the majority of the pathways responsible for normal catecholamine metabolism. For this reason, patients should ordinarily not be treated concomitantly with entacapone and a non-selective MAO inhibitor (see Warnings). Entacapone may be taken concomitantly with a selective MAO-B inhibitor (eg, selegiline).
Probenecid Cholestyramine Erythromycin Rifamipicin Ampicillin Chloramphenicol	Entacapone	↑	As most entacapone excretion is via the bile, exercise caution when drugs known to interfere with biliary excretion, glucuronidation, and intestinal beta-glucuronidase are given concurrently with entacapone.
Entacapone	Isoproterenol Epinephrine Norepinephrine Dopamine Dobutamine Methyldopa Apomorphine Isoetherine Bitolterol	↑	Administer drugs known to be metabolized by COMT (ie, isoproterenol, epinephrine, norepinephrine, dopamine, dobutamine, methyldopa, apomorphine, isoetherine, bitolterol) with caution in patients receiving entacapone regardless of the route of administration (including inhalation), as their interaction may result in increased heart rates, possibly arrhythmias, and excessive changes in blood pressure (see Warnings).

* ↑ = Object drug increased.

Adverse Reactions

The most commonly observed adverse events (> 5%) in the double-blind, placebo-controlled trials (n = 1003) associated with the use of entacapone and not seen at an equivalent frequency among the placebo-treated patients were: Dyskinesia/hyperkinesia, nausea, urine discoloration, diarrhea, and abdominal pain.

Approximately 14% of the 603 patients given entacapone in the double-blind, placebo-controlled trials discontinued treatment because of adverse events compared with 9% of the 400 patients who received placebo. The most frequent causes of discontinuation (for entacapone and placebo, respectively) in decreasing order are: Psychiatric reasons (2% vs 1%), diarrhea (2% vs 0%), dyskinesia/hyperkinesia (2% vs 1%), nausea (2% vs 1%), abdominal pain (1% vs 0%), and aggravation of Parkinson's disease symptoms (1% vs 1%).

Entacapone Adverse Reactions (≥1%)

Adverse reaction	Entacapone (n = 603)	Placebo (n = 400)
CNS		
Dyskinesia	25	15
Hyperkinesia	10	5
Hypokinesia	9	8
Dizziness	8	6
Anxiety	2	1
Somnolence	2	0
Agitation	1	0
GI		
Nausea	14	8
Diarrhea	10	4
Abdominal pain	8	4
Constipation	6	4
Vomiting	4	1
Dry mouth	3	0
Dyspepsia	2	1
Flatulence	2	0
Gastritis	1	0
GI disorders	1	0
Miscellaneous		
Sweating increased	2	1
Back pain	2	1
Taste perversion	1	0
Dyspnea	3	1
Purpura	2	1
Urine discoloration	10	0
Back pain	4	2
Fatigue	6	4
Asthenia	2	1
Infection, bacterial	1	0

Overdosage

➤*Symptoms:* There have been no reports of accidental or intentional overdose with entacapone. However, COMT inhibition by entacapone treatment is dose-dependent. A massive overdose of entacapone may theoretically produce a 100% inhibition of the COMT enzyme, thereby preventing the metabolism of endogenous and exogenous catechols.

The highest single dose of entacapone administered to humans was 800 mg, resulting in a plasma concentration of 14.1 mcg/ml. The highest daily dose given to humans was 2400 mg, administered in 1 study as 400 mg 6 times daily with levodopa/carbidopa for 14 days in 15 Parkinson's disease patients, and in another study as 800 mg 3 times daily for 7 days in 8 healthy volunteers. At this daily dose, the peak plasma concentrations of entacapone averaged 2 mcg/ml (at 45 min, compared with 1 and 1.2 mcg/ml with 200 mg entacapone at 45 min). Abdominal pain and loose stools were the most commonly observed adverse events. Daily doses as high as 2000 mg entacapone have been administered as 200 mg 10 times daily with levodopa/carbidopa or levodopa/benserazide for ≥ 1 year in 10 patients, for ≥ 2 years by 8 patients, and for ≥ 3 years in 7 patients. However, overall clinical experience with daily doses > 1600 mg is limited.

Range of lethal entacapone plasma concentrations based on animal data was 80 to 130 mcg/ml in mice. Respiratory difficulties, ataxia, hypoactivity, and convulsions were observed in mice after high oral doses.

➤*Treatment:* Management of entacapone overdose is symptomatic; there is no known antidote. Hospitalization is advised, and general supportive care is indicated. There is no experience with hemodialysis or hemoperfusion, but these procedures are unlikely to be of benefit because entacapone is highly bound to plasma proteins. An immediate gastric lavage and repeated doses of charcoal over time may hasten the elimination of entacapone by decreasing its absorption/reabsorption from the GI tract. Carefully monitor the adequacy of the respiratory and circulatory systems and employ appropriate supportive measures. Review for the possibility of drug interactions, especially with catechol-structured drugs. Refer to General Management of Acute Overdosage.

Patient Information

Instruct patients to take entacapone only as prescribed.

Inform patients that hallucinations can occur.

Advise patients that they may develop postural (orthostatic) hypotension with or without symptoms such as dizziness, nausea, syncope, and sweating. Hypotension may occur more frequently during initial therapy. Accordingly, caution patients against rising rapidly after sitting or lying down, especially after prolonged periods, and especially at the initiation of entacapone treatment.

Advise patients that they should neither drive a car nor operate other complex machinery until they have gained sufficient experience on entacapone to gauge whether or not it affects their mental or motor per-

ENTACAPONE

formance adversely. Because of the possible additive sedative effects, use caution when patients are taking other CNS depressants in combination with entacapone.

Inform patients that nausea may occur, especially at the initiation of treatment with entacapone.

Advise patients of the possibility of an increase in dyskinesia.

Advise patients that treatment with entacapone may cause a change in urine color (a brownish-orange discoloration) that is not clinically relevant. In controlled trials, 10% of patients treated with entacapone reported urine discoloration compared with 0% of placebo patients.

Although entacapone has not been shown to be teratogenic in animals, it is always given in conjunction with levodopa/carbidopa, which is known to cause visceral and skeletal malformations in the rabbit. Accordingly, advise patients to notify their physicians if they become pregnant or intend to become pregnant during therapy (see Warnings).

Entacapone is excreted into maternal milk in rats. Because of the possibility that entacapone may be excreted into human maternal milk, advise patients to notify their physicians if they intend to breastfeed or are breastfeeding an infant.

CARBIDOPA, LEVODOPA, AND ENTACAPONE

Rx	Stalevo 50 (Novartis)	**Tablets:** 12.5 mg carbidopa, 50 mg levodopa, and 200 mg entacapone	Mannitol, sucrose. (LCE 50). Film-coated. Round, bi-convex, brownish- or greyish-red. In 100s and 250s.
Rx	Stalevo 100 (Novartis)	25 mg carbidopa, 100 mg levodopa, and 200 mg entacapone	Mannitol, sucrose. (LCE 100). Film-coated. Oval, brownish- or greyish-red. In 100s and 250s.
Rx	Stalevo 150 (Novartis)	37.5 mg carbidopa, 150 mg levodopa, and 200 mg entacapone	Mannitol, sucrose. (LCE 150). Film-coated. Ellipse shape, brownish- or greyish-red. In 100s and 250s.

For complete prescribing information on each of the components refer to the individual monographs. Also refer to the general discussion in the Antiparkinson Agents introduction.

Indications

➤*Parkinson disease:* To treat patients with idiopathic Parkinson disease; to substitute (with equivalent strength of each of the 3 components) for immediate release carbidopa/levodopa and entacapone previously administered as individual products; to replace immediate release carbidopa/levodopa therapy (without entacapone) when patients experience the signs and symptoms of end-of-dose "wearing-off" (only for patients taking a total daily dose of levodopa of 600 mg or less and not experiencing dyskinesias).

Administration and Dosage

➤*Approved by the FDA:* June 13, 2003.

Do not fractionate individual tablets and administer only 1 tablet at each dosing interval. Individualize therapy and adjust according to the desired therapeutic response.

Use carbidopa, levodopa, and entacapone combination as a substitute for patients already stabilized on equivalent doses of carbidopa/levodopa and entacapone. Some patients who have been stabilized on a given dose of carbidopa/levodopa may be treated with carbidopa, levodopa, and entacapone combination if a decision has been made to add entacapone.

The optimum daily dosage of carbidopa, levodopa, and entacapone combination must be determined by careful titration in each patient. Carbidopa, levodopa, and entacapone combination tablets are available in 3 strengths, each in a 1:4 ratio of carbidopa to levodopa and combined with 200 mg of entacapone in a standard release formulation.

Studies show that peripheral dopa decarboxylase is saturated by carbidopa at approximately 70 to 100 mg/day. Patients receiving less than this amount of carbidopa are more likely to experience nausea and vomiting. Experience with total daily dosages of carbidopa greater than 200 mg is limited.

Clinical experience with daily doses above 1600 mg of entacapone is limited. It is recommended that no more than 1 carbidopa, levodopa, and entacapone combination tablet be taken at each dosing administration. Thus, the maximum recommended daily dose of carbidopa, levodopa, and entacapone combination is 8 tablets/day.

➤*Transferring patients currently treated with carbidopa/levodopa and entacapone to carbidopa, levodopa, and entacapone combination tablet:*

Carbidopa/levodopa – There is no experience in transferring patients currently treated with formulation of carbidopa/levodopa other than immediate release carbidopa/levodopa with a 1:4 ratio (controlled release formulations, or standard release presentations with a 1:10 ratio of carbidopa/levodopa) and entacapone to carbidopa, levodopa, and entacapone combination.

Entacapone – Patients who are currently treated with entacapone 200 mg tablet with each dose of standard release carbidopa/levodopa, can be directly switched to the corresponding strength of carbidopa, levodopa, and entacapone combination containing the same amounts of levodopa and carbidopa. For example, patients receiving 1 tablet of standard release carbidopa/levodopa 25/100 mg and 1 tablet of entacapone 200 mg at each administration can be switched to a single *Stalevo 100* tablet (containing 25 mg of carbidopa, 100 mg of levodopa, and 200 mg of entacapone).

➤*Transferring patients not currently treated with entacapone tablets from carbidopa/levodopa to carbidopa, levodopa, and entacapone combination tablets:* In patients with Parkinson disease who experience the signs and symptoms of end-of-dose "wearing-off" on their current standard release carbidopa/levodopa treatment, clinical experience shows that patients with a history of moderate or severe dyskinesias or taking more than 600 mg/day of levodopa are likely to require a reduction in daily levodopa dose when entacapone is added to their treatment. Since dose adjustment of the individual components is impossible with fixed dose products, it is recommended that patients first be titrated individually with a carbidopa/levodopa product (ratio 1:4) and an entacapone product, and then transferred to a corresponding dose of carbidopa, levodopa, and entacapone combination once the patient's status has stabilized.

In patients who take a total daily levodopa dose up to 600 mg and who do not have dyskinesias, an attempt can be made to transfer to the corresponding daily dose of carbidopa, levodopa, and entacapone combination. However, even in these patients, a reduction of carbidopa/levodopa or entacapone may be necessary, and the provider is reminded that this may not be possible with carbidopa, levodopa, and entacapone combination. Because entacapone prolongs and enhances the effects of levodopa, individualize therapy and adjust if necessary according to the desired therapeutic response.

➤*Maintenance therapy:* Individualize therapy and adjust for each patient according to the desired therapeutic response.

When less levodopa is required, reduce the total daily dosage of carbidopa/levodopa by decreasing the strength of carbidopa, levodopa, and entacapone combination at each administration or by decreasing the frequency of administration by extending the time between doses.

When more levodopa is required, take the next higher strength of carbidopa, levodopa, and entacapone combination and/or increase the frequency of doses, up to a maximum of 8 times daily and not to exceed the maximum daily dose recommendations as outlined above.

➤*Addition of other antiparkinsonian medications:* Standard drugs for Parkinson disease may be used concomitantly while carbidopa, levodopa, and entacapone combination is being administered, although dosage adjustments may be required.

➤*Interruption of therapy:* Sporadic cases of a symptom complex resembling Neuroleptic Malignant Syndrome (NMS) have been associated with dose reductions and withdrawal of levodopa preparations. Observe patients carefully if abrupt reduction or discontinuation of carbidopa, levodopa, and entacapone combination is required, especially if the patient is receiving neuroleptics.

If general anesthesia is required, carbidopa, levodopa, and entacapone combination may be continued as long as the patient is permitted to take fluids and medication by mouth. If therapy is interrupted temporarily, observe the patient for symptoms resembling NMS, and the usual daily dosage may be administered as soon as the patient is able to take oral medication.

➤*Hepatic function impairment:* Treat patients with hepatic impairment with caution. The AUC and C_{max} of entacapone approximately doubled in patients with documented liver disease, compared with controls. However, these studies were conducted with single-dose entacapone without levodopa/dopa decarboxylase inhibitor coadministration, and therefore the effects of liver disease on the kinetics of chronically administered entacapone have not been evaluated.

➤*Storage/Stability:* Store at 25°C (77°F); excursions permitted to 15° to 30°C (59° to 86°F).

PERGOLIDE MESYLATE

Rx	Pergolide Mesylate (Teva)	Tablets: 0.05 mg	Lactose. (7160). Ivory, capsule shape, scored. In 100s.
Rx	Permax (Amarin)		Lactose. (A024). Ivory, rectanglar, scored. In 30s.
Rx	Pergolide Mesylate (Teva)	Tablets: 0.25 mg	Lactose. (7159). Mottled green, capsule shape, scored. In 100s.
Rx	Permax (Amarin)		Lactose. (A025). Green, rectanglar, scored. In 100s.
Rx	Pergolide Mesylate (Teva)	Tablets: 1 mg	Lactose. (7161). Mottled pink, capsule shape, scored. In 100s.
Rx	Permax (Amarin)		Lactose. (A026). Pink, rectanglar, scored. In 100s.

Refer to the general discussion in the Antiparkinson Agents introduction.

Indications

➤*Parkinson disease:* Adjunctive treatment to levodopa/carbidopa in the management of the signs and symptoms of Parkinson disease.

➤*Unlabeled uses:* Restless legs syndrome.

Administration and Dosage

➤*Approved by the FDA:* December 30, 1988.

Initiate with a daily dose of 0.05 mg for the first 2 days. Gradually increase the dosage by 0.1 or 0.15 mg/day every third day over the next 12 days of therapy. The dosage then may be increased by 0.25 mg/day every third day until an optimal therapeutic dosage is achieved.

Pergolide is usually administered in divided doses 3 times/day. During dosage titration, the dosage of concurrent levodopa/carbidopa may be cautiously decreased.

In clinical studies, the mean therapeutic daily dosage of pergolide was 3 mg/day. The average concurrent daily dosage of levodopa/carbidopa (expressed as levodopa) was approximately 650 mg/day. The efficacy of pergolide at doses above 5 mg/day has not been systematically evaluated.

Actions

➤*Pharmacology:* Pergolide mesylate is a potent dopamine receptor agonist at D_1 and D_2 receptor sites. It is 10 to 1000 times more potent than bromocriptine on a milligram per milligram basis. Pergolide inhibits the secretion of prolactin; it causes a transient rise in serum concentrations of growth hormone and a decrease in serum concentrations of luteinizing hormone. In Parkinson disease, pergolide is believed to exert its therapeutic effect by directly stimulating postsynaptic dopamine receptors in the nigrostriatal system.

➤*Pharmacokinetics:*

Absorption/Distribution – Following oral administration, approximately 55% of the dose can be recovered from the urine and 5% from expired CO_2, suggesting that a significant fraction is absorbed. Pergolide is approximately 90% bound to plasma proteins.

Metabolism/Excretion – At least 10 metabolites have been detected, including N-despropylpergolide, pergolide sulfoxide, and pergolide sulfone. Pergolide sulfoxide and sulfone are dopamine agonists in animals. It is not known whether any other metabolites are active. The major route of excretion is via the kidney.

➤*Clinical trials:* In a multicenter study of patients with mild to moderate Parkinson disease who were intolerant to levodopa/carbidopa, pergolide use permitted a 5% to 30% reduction in daily levodopa dose. Patients on pergolide maintained an equivalent or better clinical status than exhibited at baseline. These patients had been on levodopa/carbidopa for 3.9 years (range, 2 days to 16.8 years).

Contraindications

Hypersensitivity to pergolide or other ergot derivatives.

Warnings

➤*Symptomatic hypotension:* In clinical trials, approximately 10% of patients taking pergolide with levodopa vs 7% taking placebo with levodopa experienced symptomatic orthostatic and/or sustained hypotension, especially during initial treatment. With gradual dosage titration, tolerance to the hypotension usually develops. Warn patients of the risk, begin therapy with low doses, and increase the dosage in carefully adjusted increments over a period of 3 to 4 weeks (see Administration and Dosage).

➤*Hallucinosis:* In controlled trials, pergolide with levodopa caused hallucinosis in approximately 14% of patients as opposed to 3% taking placebo with levodopa. It caused discontinuation of treatment in approximately 3% of those enrolled; tolerance was not observed.

➤*Fatalities:* In 1 trial, 2 of 187 patients on placebo died vs 1 of 189 patients on pergolide. Of the 2299 patients on pergolide in premarketing studies, 143 died while on the drug or shortly after discontinuing it. The study patients were elderly, ill, and at high risk for death. It seems unlikely that pergolide played any role in these deaths, but the possibility that pergolide shortens patient survival cannot be excluded.

➤*Carcinogenesis:* A 2-year carcinogenicity study was conducted in mice and rats; the highest doses tested were approximately 340 and 12 times the maximum human oral dose. A low incidence of uterine neoplasms occurred in rats and mice. Endometrial adenomas and carcinomas were observed in rats. Endometrial sarcomas were observed in mice. The occurrence of these neoplasms is probably attributable to the high estrogen/progesterone ratio that would occur in rodents as a result of the prolactin-inhibiting action of pergolide. The endocrine mechanisms believed to be involved in the rodents are not present in humans.

➤*Fertility impairment:* In male and female mice, fertility was maintained at 0.6 and 1.7 mg/kg/day but decreased at 5.6 mg/kg/day. Prolactin may be involved in stimulating and maintaining progesterone levels required for implantation in mice; therefore, the impaired fertility at high dose may occur because of depressed prolactin levels.

➤*Elderly:* There was an increased incidence of confusion, somnolence, and peripheral edema in patients 65 years of age and over. This drug is known to be substantially excreted by the kidney and the risk of toxic reactions to this drug may be greater in patients with impaired renal function. Elderly patients are more likely to have decreased renal function; therefore take care in dose selection and consider monitoring renal function.

➤*Pregnancy: Category B.* There are no adequate and well-controlled studies in pregnant women. Among women who received pergolide for endocrine disorders, there were 33 pregnancies that resulted in healthy babies and 6 pregnancies that resulted in congenital abnormalities (3 major, 3 minor); a causal relationship has not been established. Use during pregnancy only if clearly needed.

➤*Lactation:* It is not known whether this drug is excreted in breast milk. Pergolide may interfere with lactation. Because many drugs are excreted in human milk and because of the potential for serious adverse reactions to nursing infants, decide whether to discontinue nursing or to discontinue the drug, taking into account the importance of the drug to the mother.

➤*Children:* Safety and efficacy have not been established.

Precautions

➤*Monitoring:* There have been rare reports of pleuritis, pleural effusion, pleural fibrosis, pericarditis, pericardial effusion, cardiac valvulopathy involving 1 or more valves, or retroperitoneal fibrosis in patients taking pergolide. In some cases, symptoms or manifestations of cardiac valvulopathy improved after discontinuation of pergolide. Use caution when using pergolide in patients with a history of these conditions, particularly those patients who experienced the events while taking ergot derivatives. Carefully monitor, clinically and with appropriate radiographic and laboratory studies, those patients with a history of such events while taking pergolide.

➤*Cardiac dysrhythmias:* Exercise caution in patients prone to cardiac dysrhythmias. In a study comparing pergolide and placebo, patients on pergolide had significantly more episodes of atrial premature contractions and sinus tachycardia.

The use of pergolide in patients on levodopa may cause and/or exacerbate pre-existing states of confusion and hallucinations (see Warnings) or pre-existing dyskinesia.

➤*Discontinuation of therapy:* Abrupt discontinuation of pergolide in patients receiving it chronically as an adjunct to levodopa may precipitate the onset of hallucinations and confusion; these may occur within a span of several days. Discontinue pergolide gradually whenever possible, even if the patient is to remain on levodopa.

➤*Neuroleptic malignant syndrome (NMS):* A symptom complex resembling the NMS (characterized by elevated temperature, muscular rigidity, altered consciousness, and autonomic instability), with no other obvious etiology, has been reported in association with rapid dose reduction, withdrawal of, or changes in antiparkinsonian therapy, including pergolide.

Drug Interactions

➤*Dopamine antagonists:* Dopamine antagonists (eg, neuroleptics: phenothiazines, butyrophenones, thioxanthines) or metoclopramide may diminish the effectiveness of pergolide, a dopamine agonist.

➤*Protein binding:* Because pergolide mesylate is approximately 90% bound to plasma proteins, exercise caution if pergolide is coadministered with other drugs known to affect protein binding.

PERGOLIDE MESYLATE

Adverse Reactions

Pergolide Adverse Reactions (%)		
Adverse reaction	Pergolide (N = 189)	Placebo (N = 187)
Cardiovascular		
Postural hypotension	9	7
Vasodilation	3.2	< 1
Palpitation	2.1	< 1
Hypotension	2.1	< 1
Syncope	2.1	1.1
Hypertension	1.6	1.1
Arrhythmia	1.1	< 1
MI	1.1	< 1
CNS		
Dyskinesia	62.4	24.6
Dizziness	19.1	13.9
Hallucinations	13.8	3.2
Dystonia	11.6	8
Confusion	11.1	9.6
Somnolence	10.1	3.7
Insomnia	7.9	3.2
Anxiety	6.4	4.3
Tremor	4.2	7.5
Depression	3.2	5.4
Abnormal dreams	2.7	4.3
Personality disorder	2.1	< 1
Psychosis	2.1	0
Abnormal gait	1.6	1.6
Akathisia	1.6	0
Extrapyramidal syndrome	1.6	1.1
Incoordination	1.6	< 1
Paresthesia	1.6	3.2
Akinesia	1.1	1.1
Hypertonia	1.1	0
Neuralgia	1.1	< 1
Speech disorder	1.1	1.6
Dermatologic		
Rash	3.2	2.1
Sweating	2.1	2.7
GI		
Nausea	24.3	12.8
Constipation	10.6	5.9
Diarrhea	6.4	2.7
Dyspepsia	6.4	2.1
Anorexia	4.8	2.7
Dry mouth	3.7	< 1
Vomiting	2.7	1.6
GU		
Urinary frequency	2.7	6.4
Urinary tract infection	2.7	3.7
Hematuria	1.1	< 1
Musculoskeletal		
Arthralgia	1.6	2.1
Bursitis	1.6	< 1
Myalgia	1.1	< 1
Twitching	1.1	0
Respiratory		
Rhinitis	12.2	5.4
Dyspnea	4.8	1.1
Epistaxis	1.6	< 1
Hiccough	1.1	0
Special senses		
Abnormal vision	5.8	5.4
Diplopia	2.1	0
Taste perversion	1.6	0
Eye disorder	1.1	0
Miscellaneous		
Peripheral edema	7.4	4.3
Pain	7	2.1
Abdominal pain	5.8	2.1
Injury, accident	5.8	7
Headache	5.3	6.4
Asthenia	4.2	4.8
Chest pain	3.7	2.1
Flu syndrome	3.2	2.1
Neck pain	2.7	1.6
Back pain	1.6	2.1
Surgical procedure	1.6	< 1

Pergolide Adverse Reactions (%)		
Adverse reaction	Pergolide (N = 189)	Placebo (N = 187)
Edema	1.6	0
Weight gain	1.6	0
Anemia	1.1	< 1
Chills	1.1	0
Facial edema	1.1	0
Infection	1.1	0

➤*Most common:*

CNS – Dyskinesia; hallucinations; somnolence; insomnia.

GI – Nausea; constipation; diarrhea; dyspepsia.

Respiratory – Rhinitis.

➤*Discontinuation:* Of approximately 1200 patients receiving pergolide treatment, 27% discontinued treatment because of adverse events; most commonly these were related to the nervous system (15.5%), primarily hallucinations (7.8%), and confusion (1.8%).

➤*Fatalities:* See Warnings.

➤*Additional adverse reactions that occurred in 1% or less of approximately 1800 patients:*

Cardiovascular – Postural hypotension, syncope, hypertension, palpitations, vasodilations, CHF (1%); MI, tachycardia, heart arrest, abnormal ECG, angina pectoris, thrombophlebitis, bradycardia, ventricular extrasystoles, cerebrovascular accident, ventricular tachycardia, cerebral ischemia, atrial fibrillation, varicose veins, pulmonary embolus, AV block, shock (0.1% to 1%); vasculitis, pulmonary hypertension, pericarditis, migraine, heart block, cerebral hemorrhage (less than 0.1%).

CNS – Dyskinesia, dizziness, hallucinations, confusion, somnolence, insomnia, dystonia, paresthesia, depression, anxiety, tremor, akinesia, extrapyramidal syndrome, abnormal gait, abnormal dreams, incoordination, psychosis, personality disorder, nervousness, choreoathetosis, amnesia, paranoid reaction, abnormal thinking, headache (1%); akathisia, neuropathy, neuralgia, hypertonia, delusions, convulsion, increased or decreased libido, euphoria, emotional lability, vertigo, myoclonus, coma, apathy, paralysis, neurosis, hyperkinesia, ataxia, acute brain syndrome, torticollis, meningitis, manic reaction, hypokinesia, hostility, agitation, hypotonia (0.1% to 1%); stupor, neuritis, intracranial hypertension, hemiplegia, facial paralysis, brain edema, myelitis (fewer than 0.1%).

Dermatologic – Sweating, rash (1%); skin discoloration, pruritus, acne, skin ulcer, alopecia, dry skin, skin carcinoma, seborrhea, hirsutism, herpes simplex, eczema, fungal dermatitis, herpes zoster (0.1% to 1%); vesiculobullous rash, subcutaneous nodule, skin nodule, benign skin neoplasm, lichenoid dermatitis (fewer than 0.1%).

Endocrine – Hypothyroidism, adenoma, diabetes mellitus, inappropriate ADH (0.1% to 1%); endocrine disorder, thyroid adenoma (less than 0.1%).

GI – Nausea, vomiting, dyspepsia, diarrhea, constipation, dry mouth, dysphagia (1%); flatulence, abnormal liver function tests, increased appetite, salivary gland enlargement, thirst, gastroenteritis, gastritis, periodontal abscess, intestinal obstruction, nausea and vomiting, gingivitis, esophagitis, cholelithiasis, tooth caries, hepatitis, stomach ulcer, melena, hepatomegaly, hematemesis, eructation (0.1% to 1%); sialadenitis, peptic ulcer, pancreatitis, jaundice, glossitis, fecal incontinence, duodenitis, colitis, cholecystitis, aphthous stomatitis, esophageal ulcer (less than 0.1%).

GU – Urinary tract infection, urinary frequency, urinary incontinence, hematuria, dysmenorrhea (1%); dysuria, breast pain, menorrhagia, impotence, cystitis, urinary retention, abortion, vaginal hemorrhage, vaginitis, priapism, kidney calculus, fibrocystic breast, lactation, uterine hemorrhage, urolithiasis, salpingitis, pyuria, metrorrhagia, menopause, kidney failure, breast carcinoma, cervical carcinoma (0.1% to 1%); amenorrhea, bladder carcinoma, breast engorgement, epididymitis, hypogonadism, leukorrhea, nephrosis, pyelonephritis, urethral pain, uricaciduria, withdrawal bleeding (fewer than 0.1%).

Hematologic / Lymphatic – Anemia (1%); leukopenia, lymphadenopathy, leukocytosis, thrombocytopenia, petechia, megaloblastic anemia, cyanosis (0.1% to 1%); purpura, lymphocytosis, eosinophilia, thrombocythemia, acute lymphoblastic leukemia, polycythemia, splenomegaly (less than 0.1%).

Metabolic / Nutritional – Peripheral edema, weight loss, weight gain (1%); dehydration, hypokalemia, hypoglycemia, iron deficiency anemia, hyperglycemia, gout, hypercholesterolemia (0.1% to 1%); electrolyte imbalance, cachexia, acidosis, hyperuricemia (less than 0.1%).

Musculoskeletal – Twitching, myalgia, arthralgia (1%); bone pain, tenosynovitis, myositis, bone sarcoma, arthritis (0.1% to 1%); osteoporosis, muscle atrophy, osteomyelitis (less than 0.1%).

Respiratory – Rhinitis, dyspnea, pneumonia, pharyngitis, increased cough (1%); epistaxis, hiccough, sinusitis, bronchitis, voice alteration, hemoptysis, asthma, lung edema, pleural effusion, laryngitis, emphysema, apnea, hyperventilation (0.1% to 1%); pneumothorax, lung fibrosis, larynx edema, hypoxia, hypoventilation, hemothorax, lung carcinoma (less than 0.1%).

PERGOLIDE MESYLATE

Special senses – Abnormal vision, diplopia (1%); otitis media, conjunctivitis, tinnitus, deafness, taste perversion, ear or eye pain, glaucoma, eye hemorrhage, photophobia, visual field defect (0.1% to 1%); blindness, cataract, retinal detachment, retinal vascular disorder (less than 0.1%).

Miscellaneous – Asthenia, accidental injury, pain, abdominal pain, chest pain, back pain, flu syndrome, neck pain, fever (1%); facial edema, chills, enlarged abdomen, malaise, neoplasm, hernia, pelvic pain, sepsis, cellulitis, moniliasis, abscess, jaw pain, hypothermia (0.1% to 1%); acute abdominal syndrome, lupus-erythematosus syndrome (less than 0.1%).

Postmarketing – Neuroleptic malignant syndrome.

Overdosage

➤*Symptoms:* There is no clinical experience with massive overdosage. The largest overdose involved a young hospitalized adult patient who intentionally took 60 mg of pergolide. He experienced vomiting, hypotension, and agitation. Another patient receiving a daily dosage of 7 mg pergolide unintentionally took 19 mg/day for 3 days, after which his vital signs were normal but he experienced severe hallucinations. Within 36 hours of resuming the prescribed dose, the hallucinations stopped. One patient unintentionally took 14 mg/day for 23 days instead of her prescribed 1.4 mg/day dosage. She experienced severe involuntary movements and tingling in her arms and legs. Another patient who inadvertently received 7 mg instead of the prescribed 0.7 mg experienced palpitations, hypotension, and ventricular extrasystoles. The highest total daily dose (prescribed for several patients with refractory Parkinson disease) has exceeded 30 mg.

Animal studies indicate that the manifestations of overdosage in humans may include nausea, vomiting, convulsions, decreased blood pressure, and CNS stimulation.

➤*Treatment:* Management of overdosage may require supportive measures to maintain arterial blood pressure. Monitor cardiac function; an antiarrhythmic agent may be necessary. If signs of CNS stimulation are present, a phenothiazine or other butyrophenone neuroleptic agent may be indicated; the efficacy of such drugs in reversing the effects of overdose has not been assessed.

Protect the patient's airway and support ventilation and perfusion. Meticulously monitor and maintain within acceptable limits the patient's vital signs, blood gases, and serum electrolytes. Absorption of drugs from the GI tract may be decreased by giving activated charcoal, which, in many cases, is more effective than emesis or lavage. Consider charcoal instead of, or in addition to, gastric emptying. Repeated doses of charcoal over time may hasten elimination of some drugs that have been absorbed. Safeguard the patient's airway when employing gastric emptying or charcoal.

There is no experience with dialysis or hemoperfusion, and these procedures are unlikely to be of benefit.

Patient Information

Inform patients and their families of the common adverse consequences of the use of pergolide (see Adverse Reactions) and the risk of hypotension (see Warnings).

Because pergolide may cause somnolence, caution patients about operating hazardous machinery, including automobiles, until they are reasonably certain that pergolide therapy does not affect them adversely. Because of the possible additive sedative effects, caution patients who are taking other CNS depressants in combination with pergolide.

Advise patients to notify a physician if they become or intend to become pregnant during therapy or are breast-feeding.

SELEGILINE HCl (L-Deprenyl)

Rx	**Selegiline HCl** (Various, eg, Endo Labs)	**Tablets:** 5 mg	In 60s and 500s.
Rx	**Carbex** (Du Pont Pharma)		Lactose. (E620). White, oval. In 60s.
Rx	**Eldepryl** (Somerset)	**Capsules:** 5 mg	Lactose. (Eldepryl 5mg). Aqua blue. In 60s and 300s.

Refer to the general discussion in the Antiparkinson Agents introduction.

Indications

➤*Parkinson's disease:* Adjunct in the management of Parkinsonian patients being treated with levodopa/carbidopa who exhibit deterioration in the quality of their response to this therapy.

Administration and Dosage

➤*Parkinsonian patients receiving levodopa/carbidopa therapy who demonstrate a deteriorating response to this treatment:* 10 mg/day administered as divided doses of 5 mg each taken at breakfast and lunch. There is no evidence that additional benefit will be obtained from the administration of higher doses. In general, avoid higher doses because of the increased risk of side effects.

After 2 to 3 days of treatment, attempt to reduce the dose of levodopa/carbidopa. A reduction of 10% to 30% appears typical. Further reductions of levodopa/carbidopa may be possible during continued selegiline therapy.

Actions

➤*Pharmacology:* Selegiline hydrochloride is a levorotatory acetylenic derivative of phenethylamine. The mechanism of action in the adjunctive treatment of Parkinson's disease is not fully understood. Inhibition of monoamine oxidase (MAO) type B activity is of primary importance; selegiline may act through other mechanisms to increase dopaminergic activity.

Selegiline is an irreversible inhibitor of MAO by acting as a "suicide" substrate for the enzyme; ie, it is converted by MAO to an active moiety that combines irreversibly with the active site or the enzyme's essential FAD cofactor. Because selegiline has greater affinity for type B than for type A active sites, it can serve as a selective inhibitor of MAO type B at the recommended dose.

MAOs are widely distributed throughout the body; their concentration is especially high in liver, kidney, stomach, intestinal wall and brain. MAOs are currently subclassified into two types, A and B, which differ in their substrate specificity and tissue distribution in humans. Intestinal MAO is predominantly type A, while most of that in the brain is type B. In CNS neurons, MAO plays an important role in the catabolism of catecholamines (dopamine, norepinephrine and epinephrine) and serotonin. MAOs are also important in the catabolism of various exogenous amines found in a variety of food and drugs. MAO in the GI tract and liver (primarily type A) provides vital protection from exogenous amines (eg, tyramine) that have the capacity, if absorbed intact, to cause a hypertensive crisis.

Selegiline may have pharmacological effects unrelated to MAO type B inhibition. There is some evidence that it may increase dopaminergic activity by other mechanisms, including interfering with dopamine reuptake at the synapse. Effects resulting from selegiline administration may also be mediated through its metabolites. Two of its three principal metabolites, amphetamine and methamphetamine, have pharmacological actions of their own; they interfere with neuronal uptake and enhance release of several neurotransmitters (eg, norepinephrine, dopamine, serotonin). However, the extent to which these metabolites contribute to the effects of selegiline are unknown.

➤*Pharmacokinetics:*

Absorption/Distribution – Selegiline is rapidly absorbed; ≈ 73% of a dose is absorbed; maximum plasma concentration occurs 0.5 to 2 hours following administration. Following use of a single oral 10 mg dose in 12 healthy subjects, serum levels of intact selegiline were below the limit of detection (< 10 ng/ml).

Metabolism/Excretion – The drug is rapidly metabolized. Three metabolites, N-desmethyldeprenyl (the major metabolite; mean half-life 2 hours), amphetamine (mean half-life 17.7 hours), and methamphetamine (mean half-life 20.5 hours), were found in serum and urine. Over 48 hours, 45% of the dose appeared in the urine as these 3 metabolites. Unchanged selegiline is not detected in urine. The rate of MAO-B regeneration following discontinuation of treatment has not been quantitated. It is this rate, dependent upon de novo protein synthesis, that seems likely to determine how fast normal MAO-B activity can be restored.

➤*Clinical trials:* Selegiline's benefit in Parkinson's disease has only been documented as an adjunct to levodopa/carbidopa. Its effectiveness as a sole treatment is unknown, but attempts to treat Parkinson's disease with nonselective MAO inhibitor monotherapy have been unsuccessful.

Contraindications

Hypersensitivity to the drug; use with meperidine (this contraindication is often extended to other opioids; see Drug Interactions).

Warnings

➤*Maximum dose:* Do not use at daily doses exceeding those recommended (10 mg/day) because of the risks associated with nonselective inhibition of MAO.

The selectivity of selegiline for MAO-B may not be absolute even at the recommended daily dose of 10 mg/day and selectivity is further diminished with increasing daily doses. The precise dose at which selegiline becomes a nonselective inhibitor of all MAOs is unknown, but may be in the range of 30 to 40 mg/day.

➤*Pregnancy: Category C.* It is not known whether selegiline can cause fetal harm when administered to a pregnant woman or can affect reproduction capacity. Use during pregnancy only if clearly needed.

➤*Lactation:* It is not known whether selegiline is excreted in breast milk.

➤*Children:* The effects of selegiline in children have not been evaluated.

SELEGILINE HCl (L-Deprenyl)

Precautions

➤*Hypertensive crisis:* In theory, because MAO-A of the gut is not inhibited, patients treated with selegiline at a dose of 10 mg/day can take medications containing pharmacologically active amines and consume tyramine-containing foods without risk of uncontrolled hypertension. Clinical experience appears to confirm this prediction. The pathophysiology of the tyramine reaction is complicated and, in addition to its ability to inhibit MAO-B selectively, selegiline's apparent freedom from this reaction has been attributed to an ability to prevent tyramine and other indirect acting sympathomimetics from displacing norepinephrine from adrenergic neurons.

It seems prudent to assume that selegiline can only be used safely without dietary restrictions at doses where it presumably selectively inhibits MAO-B (eg, 10 mg/day). Attention to the dose-dependent nature of selegiline's selectivity is critical if it is to be used without elaborate restrictions placed on diet and concomitant drug use.

➤*Levodopa side effects:* Some patients given selegiline may experience an exacerbation of levodopa-associated side effects, presumably due to the increased amounts of dopamine reacting with supersensitive post-synaptic receptors. These effects may be mitigated by reducing the dose of levodopa/carbidopa by ≈10% to 30%.

Drug Interactions

Selegine Drug Interactions			
Precipitant drug	Object drug *		Description
Selegiline	Fluoxetine	↑	Death has occurred following initiation of nonselective MAOIs shortly after discontinuation of fluoxetine. To date, this has not been reported with selegiline; however, in general, avoid this combination. At least 5 weeks should elapse between discontinuation of fluoxetine and initiation of an MAOI; at least 14 days between discontinuation of an MAOI and initation of fluoxetine.
Selegiline	Meperidine	↑	Because of reports of fatal interactions, MAOIs are ordinarily contraindicated for use with meperidine. This warning is often extended to other opioids. In general, avoid this combination. Stupor, muscular rigidity, severe agitation and elevated temperature have been reported in a man receiving selegiline and meperidine. This is typical of the interaction of meperidine and MAOIs. Other serious reactions (eg, severe agitation, hallucinations, death) have occurred.

* ↑ = Object drug increased

Adverse Reactions

The following events led to discontinuation of treatment with selegiline (in decreasing order of frequency): Nausea; hallucinations; confusion; depression; loss of balance; insomnia; orthostatic hypotension; increased akinetic involuntary movements; agitation; arrhythmias; bradykinesia; chorea; delusions; hypertension; new or increased angina pectoris; syncope.

Selegiline Adverse Reactions (%)		
Adverse reactions	Selegiline (n = 49)	Placebo (n = 50)
Nausea	10	3
Dizziness/lightheaded/fainting	7	1
Abdominal pain	4	2
Confusion	3	0
Hallucinations	3	1
Dry mouth	3	1
Vivid dreams	2	0
Dyskinesias	2	5
Headache	2	1
Ache, generalized	1	0

Selegiline Adverse Reactions (%)		
Adverse reactions	Selegiline (n = 49)	Placebo (n = 50)
Anxiety/tension	1	1
Diarrhea	1	0
Insomnia	1	1
Lethargy	1	0
Leg pain	1	0
Low back pain	1	0
Palpitations	1	0
Urinary retention	1	0
Weight loss	1	0

The following adverse reactions were reported in prospectively monitored clinical trials (n = 920).

➤*Cardiovascular:* Orthostatic hypotension; hypertension; arrhythmia; palpitations; new/ increased angina pectoris; hypotension; tachycardia; peripheral edema; sinus bradycardia; syncope.

➤*CNS:*

Motor/Coordination/Extrapyramidal – Increased tremor; chorea; loss of balance; restlessness; blepharospasm; increased bradykinesia; facial grimace; falling down; heavy leg; stiff neck; tardive dyskinesia; dystonic symptoms; dyskinesia; involuntary movements; freezing; festination; increased apraxia; muscle cramps.

Mental status/behavioral/psychiatric – Hallucinations; dizziness; confusion; anxiety; depression; drowsiness; behavior/mood changes; dreams/nightmares; tiredness; delusions; disorientation; lightheadedness; lethargy; malaise; apathy; overstimulation; vertigo; personality change; sleep disturbance; restlessness; weakness; transient irritability.

Pain/Altered sensation – Headache; back/leg pain; tinnitus; migraine; supraorbital pain; throat burning; generalized ache; chills; numbness of fingers/toes; taste disturbance.

➤*Dermatologic:* Increased sweating; diaphoresis; facial hair; hair loss; hematoma; rash; photosensitivity.

➤*GI:* Nausea; vomiting; constipation; weight loss; anorexia; poor appetite; dysphagia; diarrhea; heartburn; rectal bleeding, GI bleeding (exacerbation of preexisting ulcer disease).

➤*GU:* Slow urination; transient nocturia; prostatic hypertrophy; urinary hesitancy/retention/frequency; sexual dysfunction.

➤*Miscellaneous:* Asthma; diplopia; shortness of breath; speech affected; dry mouth; blurred vision.

Adverse reactions reported at doses > 10 mg/day include – Muscle twitch; myoclonic jerks; impaired memory; increased energy; transient euphoria; bruxism; transient anorgasmia; decreased penile sensation.

Overdosage

➤*Symptoms:* Some individuals exposed to doses of 600 mg of dl-selegiline suffered hypotension and psychomotor agitation.

Since the selective inhibition of MAO-B is achieved only at doses in the range recommended for the treatment of Parkinson's disease (eg, 10 mg/day), overdoses are likely to cause significant inhibition of both MAO-A and B. Consequently, the signs and symptoms of overdose may resemble those observed with nonselective MAO inhibitors. Refer to the MAOI monograph in the Antidepressants section.

➤*Treatment:* The following is based on the assumption that selegiline overdose may be modeled by nonselective MAO inhibitor poisoning. Treat hypotension and vascular collapse with IV fluids and, if necessary, blood pressure titration with an IV infusion of a dilute pressor agent. Adrenergic agents may produce a markedly increased pressor response. Refer to General Management of Acute Overdosage.

Patient Information

Advise patients of possible need to reduce levodopa dosage after therapy initiation.

Advise patients not to exceed the daily recommended dose of 10 mg. Explain the risk of using higher daily doses of selegiline, and provide a brief description of the tyramine reaction. It may be useful to inform patients (or their families) about the signs and symptoms associated with MAO inhibitor-induced hypertensive reactions. In particular, urge patients to immediately report any severe headache, other atypical or unusual symptoms not previously experienced.

TOLCAPONE

Rx	Tasmar (Roche)	**Tablets:** 100 mg	Lactose. (Tasmar 100 Roche). Beige, hexagonal, biconvex. Film coated. In 90s.
		200 mg	Lactose. (Tasmar 200 Roche). Reddish brown, hexagonal, biconvex. Film coated. In 90s.

Refer to the general discussion in the Antiparkinson Agents introduction.

WARNING

Because of the risk of potentially fatal, acute fulminant liver failure, use tolcapone in patients with Parkinson's disease on levodopa/carbidopa who are experiencing symptom fluctuations and are not responding satisfactorily to, or are not appropriate candidates for other adjunctive therapies.

Because of the risk of liver injury, withdraw patients from tolcapone who fail to show substantial clinical benefit within 3 weeks of initiation of treatment.

Do not initiate therapy if the patient exhibits clinical evidence of liver disease or 2 ALT or AST values greater than the upper limit of normal. Treat patients with severe dyskinesia or dystonia with caution.

Patients who develop evidence of hepatocellular injury and are withdrawn from the drug for any reason may be at increased risk for liver injury if tolcapone is reintroduced. Accordingly, do not consider such patients for retreatment.

Cases of severe hepatocellular injury, including fulminant liver failure resulting in death, have been reported in postmarketing use. Three cases of fatal fulminant hepatic failure have been reported from ≈ 60,000 patients providing ≈ 40,000 patient-years of worldwide use. This incidence may be 10- to 100-fold higher than the background incidence in the general population. Underreporting of cases may lead to significant underestimation of the increased risk associated with tolcapone.

Advise a prescriber who elects to use tolcapone in face of the increased risk of liver injury to monitor patients for evidence of emergent liver injury. Instruct patients about the need for self-monitoring for classical signs of liver disease (eg, clay-colored stools, jaundice) and nonspecific ones (eg, fatigue, appetite loss, lethargy).

Although frequent laboratory monitoring for evidence of hepatocellular injury is essential, it is not clear that baseline and periodic monitoring of liver enzymes will prevent fulminant liver failure. However, it is generally believed that early detection of drug-induced hepatic injury along with immediate withdrawal of the suspect drug enhances the likelihood for recovery. It is also widely held, without a robust body of evidence, that patients with preexisting hepatic disease are more vulnerable to hepatotoxins. Accordingly, the following liver monitoring program is recommended.

Conduct appropriate tests to exclude the presence of liver disease before starting treatment with tolcapone. Determine baseline levels of ALT and AST and every 2 weeks for the first year of therapy, every 4 weeks for the next 6 months, and every 8 weeks thereafter. Monitor liver enzymes before increasing the dose to 200 mg 3 times daily, and reinitiate at the frequency above.

Discontinue tolcapone if ALT or AST exceeds the upper limit of normal or if clinical signs and symptoms suggest the onset of hepatic failure (persistent nausea, fatigue, lethargy, anorexia, jaundice, dark urine, pruritus, and right upper quandrant tenderness).

Indications

➤*Parkinson's disease:* As an adjunct to levodopa and carbidopa for the treatment of signs and symptoms of idiopathic Parkinson's disease.

Administration and Dosage

➤*Approved by the FDA:* January 30, 1998.

Because of the risk of potentially fatal, acute fulminant liver failure, use tolcapone in patients with Parkinson's disease on levodopa/carbidopa who are experiencing symptom fluctuations and are not responding satisfactorily to, or are not appropriate candidates for other adjunctive therapies.

Because of the risk of liver injury, withdraw patients from tolcapone who fail to show substantial clinical benefit within 3 weeks of initiation of treatment.

Do not initiate therapy if the patient exhibits clincal evidence of liver disease or 2 ALT or AST values greater than the upper limit of normal. Treat patients with severe dyskinesia or dystonia with caution.

Patients who develop evidence of hepatocellular injury while on tolcapone and are withdrawn from the drug for any reason may be at increased risk for liver injury if tolcapone is reintroduced. Accordingly, do not consider such patients for retreatment.

Therapy with tolcapone may be initiated with 100 mg 3 times daily, with or without food always as an adjunct to levodopa/carbidopa therapy. The recommended daily dose is also 100 mg 3 times daily. In clinical trials, elevations in ALT occurred more frequently at the dose of 200 mg 3 times daily. While it is unknown whether the risk of acute fulminant liver failure is increased at the 200 mg dose, it would be pru-

dent to use 200 mg only if the anticipated incremental clinical benefit is justified. If a patient fails to show the expected incremental benefit on the 200 mg dose after 3 weeks of treatment (regardless of dose), discontinue tolcapone.

In clinical trials, the first tolcapone dose of the day was always taken with the first levodopa/carbidopa dose of the day, and the subsequent tolcapone doses were given ≈ 6 to 12 hours later.

To optimize an individual patient's response, reductions in daily levodopa dose may be necessary. In clinical trials, the average reduction in daily levodopa dose was ≈ 30% in those patients requiring a levodopa dose reduction (> 70% of patients with levodopa doses > 600 mg/day required such a reduction). Patients with moderate or severe dyskinesias before beginning treatment also required levodopa dosage reductions.

Tolcapone can be combined with the immediate and sustained release formulation of levodopa/carbidopa.

➤*Renal/Hepatic function impairment:* Do not initiate therapy in any patient with liver disease or 2 ALT or AST values greater than the upper limit of normal.

No dosage adjustment of tolcapone is recommended for patients with mild-to-moderate renal impairment. The safety of tolcapone has not been examined in subjects who had creatinine clearance < 25 ml/min.

➤*Withdrawing patients from tolcapone:* If a decision is made to discontinue treatment with tolcapone, then it is recommended to closely monitor the patient and adjust other dopaminergic treatments as needed. Tapering tolcapone has not been systemically evaluated. As the duration of COMT inhibition with tolcapone is generally 5 to 6 hours on average, decreasing the frequency of dosage to twice or once a day may not in itself prevent withdrawal effects.

Actions

➤*Pharmacology:* Tolcapone is a selective and reversible inhibitor of catechol-O-methyltransferase (COMT), used in the treatment of Parkinson's disease as an adjunct to levodopa/carbidopa therapy.

COMT is distributed throughout various organs. The highest activities are in the liver and kidney. COMT catalyses the transfer of the methyl group of S-adenosyl-L-methionine to the phenolic group of substrates that contain a catechol structure. Physiological substrates of COMT include dopa, catecholamines (dopamine, norepinephrine, epinephrine), and their hydroxylated metabolites. The function of COMT is the elimination of biologically active catechols and some other hydroxylated metabolites. In the presence of a decarboxylase inhibitor, COMT becomes the major metabolizing enzyme for levodopa catalyzing the metabolism to 3-methoxy-4-hydroxy-L-phenylalanine (3-OMD) in the brain and periphery.

The precise mechanism of action of tolcapone is unknown, but it is believed to be related to its ability to inhibit COMT and alter the plasma pharmacokinetics of levodopa. When tolcapone is given in conjunction with levodopa and an aromatic amino acid decarboxylase inhibitor, such as carbidopa, plasma levels of levodopa are more sustained than after administration of levodopa and an aromatic amino acid decarboxylase inhibitor alone. It is believed that these sustained plasma levels of levodopa result in more constant dopaminergic stimulation in the brain, leading to greater effects on the signs and symptoms of Parkinson's disease in patients, as well as increased levodopa adverse effects, sometimes requiring a decrease in the dose of levodopa. Tolcapone enters the CNS to a minimal extent but has been shown to inhibit central COMT activity in animals.

In healthy volunteers, oral tolcapone reversibly inhibits human erythrocyte COMT activity. The inhibition is closely related to plasma tolcapone concentrations.

➤*Pharmacokinetics:*

Absorption/Distribution – Tolcapone is rapidly absorbed with a T_{max} of ≈ 2 hours. The absolute bioavailability following oral administration is ≈ 65%. Food given within 1 hour before and 2 hours after dosing decreases the relative bioavailability by 10% to 20%. Pharmacokinetics are linear over the dose range of 50 to 400 mg, independent of levodopa/carbidopa coadministration. With 3 times daily dosing of 100 or 200 mg, C_{max} is ≈ 3 and 6 mcg/ml, respectively.

The steady-state volume of distribution is small (9 L). Tolcapone does not distribute widely into tissues because of its high plasma protein binding, which is > 99.9%. Tolcapone binds mainly to serum albumin.

Metabolism/Excretion – Tolcapone is almost completely metabolized prior to excretion, with only a very small amount (0.5% of dose) found unchanged in urine. The elimination half-life is 2 to 3 hours, and no significant accumulation occurs. The main metabolic pathway of tolcapone is glucuronidation; the glucuronide conjugate is inactive. In addition, the compound is methylated by COMT to 3-O-methyl-tolcapone. Tolcapone is metabolized to a primary alcohol (hydroxylation of the methyl group), that is subsequently oxidized to the carboxylic acid. In vitro experiments suggest that the oxidation may be catalyzed by cyto-

TOLCAPONE

chrome P450 3A4 and 2A6. The reduction to an amine and subsequent N-acetylation occur to a minor extent. After oral administration, 60% is excreted in urine and 40% in feces.

Special populations –

Hepatic function impairment: Moderate non-cirrhotic liver disease had no impact on the pharmacokinetics of tolcapone. However, in patients with moderate cirrhotic liver disease (Child-Pugh Class B), clearance and volume of distribution of unbound tolcapone was reduced by almost 50%. This reduction may increase the average concentration of unbound drug by 2-fold.

Contraindications

Hypersensitivity to the drug or its ingredients; patients with liver disease; patients who were withdrawn from tolcapone because of evidence of tolcapone-induced hepatocellular injury; patients with a history of nontraumatic rhabdomyolysis or hyperpyrexia and confusion possibly related to medication.

Warnings

➤*Hepatic failure:* See Warning Box.

➤*MAO inhibitors:* Monoamine oxidase (MAO) and COMT are the 2 major enzyme systems involved in the metabolism of catecholamines. It is theoretically possible, therefore, that the combination of tolcapone and a non-selective MAO inhibitor (eg, phenelzine, tranylcypromine) would result in inhibition of the majority of the pathways responsible for normal catecholamine metabolism. For this reason, patients should ordinarily not be treated concomitantly with tolcapone and a non-selective MAO inhibitor. Tolcapone can be taken concomitantly with a selective MAO-B inhibitor (eg, selegiline).

➤*Hepatic enzyme abnormalities:* In controlled trials, increases to > 3 times the upper limit of normal (ULN) in ALT or AST occurred in ≈ 1% of patients at 100 mg 3 times daily and 3% of patients at 200 mg 3 times daily. Females were more likely than males to have an increase in hepatic enzymes (≈ 5% vs 2%). Approximately > 33% of patients with elevated enzymes had diarrhea. Increases to > 8 × ULN in hepatic enzymes occurred in 0.3% of patients treated with 100 mg 3 times daily and 0.7% at 200 mg 3 times daily. Elevated enzymes led to discontinuation in 0.3% and 1.7% of patients treated with 100 and 200 mg 3 times daily, respectively. Elevations usually occurred within 6 weeks to 6 months of starting treatment. In about half the cases, enzyme levels returned to baseline within 1 to 3 months while patients continued tolcapone treatment. When treatment was discontinued, enzymes generally declined within 2 to 3 weeks but in some cases took as long as 1 to 2 months to return to normal.

One patient, a 55-year-old woman treated with tolcapone 200 mg 3 times daily for 53 days, had diarrhea followed 4 days later by yellowing of the skin and eyes. She died 7 days after the onset of diarrhea. No liver function tests were performed after the onset of symptoms. Monitor liver function tests (see Precautions).

➤*Renal function impairment:* No dosage adjustment is needed in patients with mild-to-moderate renal impairment; however, patients with severe renal impairment should be treated with caution (see Administration and Dosage).

➤*Hepatic function impairment:* Because of the risk of liver injury, do not initiate tolcapone therapy in patients with liver disease. For similar reasons, do not initiate treatment in patients who have 2 ALT or AST values greater than the upper limit of normal (see Warning Box) or any other evidence of hepatocellular dysfunction.

➤*Carcinogenesis:* An increased incidence of uterine adenocarcinomas in female rats occurred at exposure equivalent to 26.4 times the human exposure. Renal tubular injury and renal tubular tumor formation was evident in rats. A low incidence of renal tubular cell adenomas occurred in middle- and high-dose female rats; tubular cell carcinomas occurred in middle- and high-dose male and high-dose female rats, with a statistically significant increase in high-dose males.

Minimal-to-marked damage to the renal tubules, consisting of proximal tubule cell degeneration, single-cell necrosis, hyperplasia, and karyocytomegaly, occurred at the doses associated with renal tumors. Renal tubule damage, characterized by proximal tubule cell degeneration and the presence of atypical nuclei, and 1 adenocarcinoma in a high-dose male, were observed in a 1-year study in rats receiving doses of tolcapone of 150 and 450 mg/kg/day. These histopathological changes suggest the possibility that renal tumor formation might be secondary to chronic cell damage and sustained repair, but this relationship has not been established. The relevance of these findings to humans is not known.

➤*Pregnancy:* Category C. In rabbits, an increased rate of abortion occurred at a dose of ≥ 100 mg/kg/day (3.7 times the daily clinical dose on a mg/m² basis). Evidence of maternal toxicity (decreased weight gain, death) was observed at 300 mg/kg in rats and 400 mg/kg in rabbits. When tolcapone was administered to female rats during the last part of gestation and throughout lactation, decreased litter size and impaired growth and learning performance in female pups were observed at a dose of 250/150 mg/kg/day (dose reduced from 250 to 150 mg/kg/day) during late gestation caused by high rate of maternal mortality.

Tolcapone is always given concomitantly with levodopa/carbidopa, which is known to cause visceral and skeletal malformations in rabbits. The combination of tolcapone (100 mg/kg/day) with levodopa/carbidopa (80/20 mg/kg/day) produced an increased incidence of fetal malformations (primarily external and skeletal digit defects) compared with levodopa/carbidopa alone when pregnant rabbits were treated throughout organogenesis.

In a combination embryo-fetal development study in rats, fetal body weights were reduced by the combination of tolcapone (10, 30, and 50 mg/kg/day) and levodopa/carbidopa (120/30 mg/kg/day) and by levodopa/carbidopa alone.

There is no experience from clinical studies regarding the use of tolcapone in pregnant women. Therefore, use during pregnancy only if the potential benefit justifies the potential risk to the fetus.

➤*Lactation:* In animal studies, tolcapone was excreted in maternal rat milk. It is not known whether tolcapone is excreted in human breast milk. Exercise caution when tolcapone is administered to a nursing woman.

➤*Children:* There is no identified potential use of tolcapone in pediatric patients.

Precautions

➤*Monitoring:* Although frequent laboratory monitoring for evidence of hepatocellular injury is essential, it is not clear that baseline and periodic monitoring of liver enzymes will prevent fulminant liver failure. However, it is generally believed that early detection of drug-induced hepatic injury along with immediate withdrawal of the suspect drug enhances the likelihood for recovery. It is also widely held, without a robust body of evidence, that patients with preexisting hepatic disease are more vulnerable to hepatotoxins. Accordingly, the following liver monitoring program is recommended:

Before starting treatment, the physician should conduct appropriate tests to exclude the presence of liver disease. In patients determined to be appropriate candidates for treatment with tolcapone, serum glutamic-pyruvic transaminase (ALT) and serum glutamic-oxaloacetic transaminase (AST) levels should be determined at baseline and then every 2 weeks for the first year of therapy, every 4 weeks for the next 6 months, and every 8 weeks thereafter.

If the dose is increased to 200 mg 3 times daily, liver enzyme monitoring should take place before increasing the dose and be reinitiated at the frequency above.

Discontinue tolcapone if ALT or AST exceeds the upper limit of normal or if clinical signs and symptoms suggest the onset of hepatic failure (persistent nausea, fatigue, lethargy, anorexia, jaundice, dark urine, pruritus, and right upper quandrant tenderness).

➤*Special populations:* Do not initiate therapy if the patient exhibits clinical evidence of active liver disease or 2 ALT or AST values greater than the upper limit of normal. Treat patients with severe dyskinesia, dystonia, or severe renal impairment with caution.

➤*Hypertension/Syncope:* Dopaminergic therapy in Parkinson's disease patients has been associated with orthostatic hypotension. Tolcapone enhances levodopa bioavailability and, therefore, may increase the occurrence of orthostatic hypotension. In tolcapone clinical trials, orthostatic hypotension was documented at least once in 8%, 14%, and 13% of the patients treated with placebo, 100, and 200 mg tolcapone 3 times daily, respectively. A total of 2%, 5%, and 4% of the patients treated with placebo, 100, and 200 mg tolcapone 3 times daily, respectively, reported orthostatic symptoms at some time during their treatment and also had ≥ 1 episode of orthostatic hypotension documented; however, the episode of orthostatic symptoms itself was invariably not accompanied by vital sign measurements. Patients with orthostasis at baseline were more likely than patients without symptoms to have orthostatic hypotension during the study, regardless of treatment group. In addition, the effect was greater in tolcapone-treated patients than in placebo-treated patients. Baseline treatment with dopamine agonists or selegiline did not appear to increase the likelihood of experiencing orthostatic hypotension when treated with tolcapone. Approximately 0.7% of the patients treated with tolcapone (5% of patients who were documented to have had ≥ 1 episode of orthostatic hypotension) eventually withdrew from treatment because of adverse events presumably related to hypotension.

➤*Diarrhea:* In clinical trials, patients treated with placebo, 100, and 200 mg tolcapone 3 times daily developed diarrhea at an incidence of ≈ 8%, 16%, and 18%, respectively, that most commonly led to discontinuation, and led to hospitalization in 0.3%, 0.7%, and 1.7% of patients, respectively. Generally, diarrhea resolved after discontinuation of tolcapone.

Typically, diarrhea presents 6 to 12 weeks after tolcapone is started, but it may appear as early as 2 weeks and as late as many months after the initiation of treatment. Clinical trial data suggested that diarrhea associated with tolcapone use may sometimes be associated with anorexia (decreased appetite).

Follow all cases of persistent diarrhea with an appropriate work-up (including occult blood samples).

➤*Hallucinations:* In clinical trials, patients treated with placebo, 100, and 200 mg tolcapone 3 times daily developed hallucinations at an

TOLCAPONE

incidence of ≈ 5%, 8%, and 10%, respectively, which led to drug discontinuation and premature withdrawal from clinical trials in 0.3%, 1.4%, and 1% of patients and required hospitalization in 0%, 1.7%, and 0% of patients, respectively.

In general, hallucinations present shortly after the initiation of therapy with tolcapone (typically within the first 2 weeks). Data suggest that hallucinations associated with tolcapone use may be responsive to levodopa dose reduction. Patients whose hallucinations resolved had a mean levodopa dose reduction of 175 to 200 mg (20% to 25%). Hallucinations were commonly accompanied by confusion and, to a lesser extent, sleep disorder (insomnia), and excessive dreaming.

➤*Dyskinesia:* Tolcapone may potentiate the dopaminergic side effects of levodopa and may cause or exacerbate preexisting dyskinesia. Although decreasing the dose of levodopa may ameliorate this side effect, many patients in controlled trials continued to experience frequent dyskinesias despite a reduction in their doses of levodopa. The rates of withdrawal for dyskinesia were 0%, 0.3%, and 1% for placebo, 100, and 200 mg tolcapone 3 times daily, respectively.

➤*Rhabdomyolysis:* Cases of severe rhabdomyolysis, with 1 case of multiorgan system failure rapidly progressing to death, have been reported. The complicated nature of these cases makes it impossible to determine what role, if any, tolcapone played in their pathogenesis. Severe prolonged motor activity including dyskinesia may account for rhabdomyolysis. However, some cases included fever, alteration of consciousness, and muscular rigidity. Therefore, it is possible that the rhabdomyolysis may be a result of the syndrome described in Withdrawal emergent hyperpyrexia and confusion section.

➤*Hematuria:* The rates of hematuria in placebo controlled trials were ≈ 2%, 4%, and 5% with placebo, 100, and 200 mg tolcapone 3 times daily, respectively. The etiology of the increase with tolcapone has not always been explained (for example, by urinary tract infection or coumadin therapy).

➤*Events reported with dopaminergic therapy:* The events listed below are known to be associated with the use of drugs that increase dopaminergic activity, although they are most often associated with the use of direct dopamine agonists. While cases of withdrawal-emergent hyperpyrexia and confusion have been reported in association with tolcapone withdrawal (see below), the expected incidence of fibrotic complications is so low that, even if tolcapone caused these complications at rates similar to those attributable to other dopaminergic therapies, it is unlikely that even a single example would have been detected in a cohort of the size exposed to tolcapone.

Withdrawal-emergent hyperpyrexia and confusion – Four cases of a symptom complex, resembling the neuroleptic malignant syndrome (characterized by elevated temperature, muscular rigidity, and altered consciousness), similar to that reported in association with the rapid dose reduction or withdrawal of other dopaminergic drugs, have been reported in association with the abrupt withdrawal or lowering of the tolcapone dose. In 3 of these cases, CPK was elevated. One patient died, and the other 3 patients recovered over periods of ≈ 2, 4, and 6 weeks.

Fibrotic complications – Cases of retroperitoneal fibrosis, pulmonary infiltrates, pleural effusion, and pleural thickening have been reported in some patients treated with ergot-derived dopaminergic agents. While these complications may resolve when the drug is discontinued, complete resolution does not always occur. Although these adverse events are believed to be related to the ergoline structure of these compounds, whether other, nonergot-derived drugs (eg, tolcapone) that increase dopaminergic activity can cause them is unknown.

Three cases of pleural effusion, 1 with pulmonary fibrosis, occurred during clinical trials. These patients were also on concomitant dopamine agonists (pergolide or bromocriptine) and had a history of cardiac disease or pulmonary path-ology (nonmalignant lung lesion).

Drug Interactions

➤*Cytochrome P450:* Because of its affinity to cytochrome P450 2C9 in vitro, tolcapone may interfere with drugs whose clearance is dependent on this metabolic pathway, such as tolbutamide and warfarin. However, in an in vivo interaction study, tolcapone did not change the pharmacokinetics of tolbutamide. Therefore, clinically relevant interactions involving cytochrome P450 2C9 appear unlikely. Because clinical information is limited regarding the combination of warfarin and tolcapone, monitor coagulation parameters when these 2 drugs are coadministered.

➤*Protein binding:* Although tolcapone is highly protein-bound, tolcapone in vitro did not displace other highly protein-bound drugs from their binding sites at therapeutic concentrations.

➤*Drugs metabolized by COMT:* Tolcapone may influence the pharmacokinetics of drugs metabolized by COMT. However, no effects were seen on pharmacokinetics of the COMT substrate carbidopa. The effect of tolcapone on the pharmacokinetics of other drugs of this class such as α-methyldopa, dobutamine, apomorphine, and isoproterenol has not been evaluated. Consider a dose reduction of such compounds when they are coadministered with tolcapone.

➤*Levodopa:* When tolcapone is administered with levodopa/carbidopa, it increases the relative bioavailability (AUC) of levodopa by ≈ 2-fold. This is caused by a decrease in levodopa clearance resulting in

a prolongation of the terminal elimination half-life of levodopa (from ≈ 2 to 3.5 hours). In general, the average peak levodopa plasma concentration (C_{max}) and the T_{max} are unaffected.

➤*Drug / Food interactions:* Food given within 1 hour before or 2 hours after tolcapone decreases relative bioavailability by 10% to 20%.

Adverse Reactions

Cases of severe hepatocellular injury, including fulminant liver failure resulting in death, have been reported in postmarketing use. Three cases of fatal fulminant hepatic failure have been reported from ≈ 60,000 patients providing ≈ 40,000 patient-years of worldwide use. This incidence may be 10- to 100-fold higher than the background incidence in the general population.

Approximately 16% of the 592 patients who participated in the double-blind, placebo controlled trials discontinued treatment because of adverse events compared with 10% of the 298 patients who received placebo. Diarrhea was the most frequent cause of discontinuation (≈ 6% in tolcapone patients vs 1% on placebo).

Tolcapone Adverse Reactions (≥ 1%)		
	Placebo	Tolcapone (3 times daily)
Adverse reaction	(n=298)	100 mg (n=296)	200 mg (n=298)
Cardiovascular			
Orthostatic complaints	14	17	17
Chest pain	1	3	1
Hypotension	1	2	2
Chest discomfort	1	1	2
CNS			
Dyskinesia	20	42	51
Sleep disorder	18	24	25
Dystonia	17	19	22
Excessive dreaming	17	21	16
Somnolence	13	18	14
Confusion	9	11	10
Dizziness	10	13	6
Headache	7	10	11
Hallucination	5	8	10
Syncope	3	4	5
Balance loss	2	3	2
Hyperkinesia	1	3	2
Paresthesia	2	3	1
Hypokinesia	1	1	3
Agitation	0	1	1
Irritability	0	1	1
Mental deficiency	0	1	1
Hyperactivity	0	1	1
Panic reaction	0	1	0
Euphoria	0	1	0
Hypertonia	0	0	1
Dermatologic			
Sweating increased	2	4	7
Dermal bleeding	0	1	1
Skin tumor	0	1	0
Alopecia	0	1	0
GI			
Nausea	18	30	35
Anorexia	13	19	23
Diarrhea	8	16	18
Vomiting	4	8	10
Constipation	5	6	8
Xerostomia	2	5	6
Abdominal pain	3	5	6
Dyspepsia	2	4	3
Flatulence	2	2	4
GU			
Urinary tract infection	4	5	5
Urine discoloration	1	2	7
Micturition disorder	1	2	1
Uterine tumor	1	1	0
Musculoskeletal			
Muscle cramps	17	17	18
Stiffness	1	2	2
Arthritis	1	2	1
Neck pain	1	2	2
Respiratory			
Upper respiratory tract infection	3	5	7
Dyspnea	2	3	3
Sinus congestion	0	2	1
Ophthalmic			
Cataract	0	1	0
Eye inflammation	0	1	1

TOLCAPONE

Tolcapone Adverse Reactions (≥ 1%)			
	Placebo	Tolcapone (3 times daily)	
Adverse reaction	(n=298)	100 mg (n=296)	200 mg (n=298)
Miscellaneous			
Falling	4	4	6
Fatigue	6	7	3
Influenza	2	3	4
Burning	0	2	1
Malaise	0	1	0
Fever	0	0	1

Other events reported by ≥ 1% of patients treated with tolcapone that were equally or more frequent in the placebo group were arthralgia, limb pain, anxiety, micturition frequency, fractures, blurred vision, pneumonia, paresis, lethargy, asthenia, peripheral edema, abnormal gait, taste alteration, weight decrease, and sinusitis.

Effects of gender and age on adverse reactions – Experience in clinical trials have suggested that patients > 75 years of age may be more likely to develop hallucinations while these same patients may be less likely to develop dystonia. Females may be more likely to develop somnolence than males.

Overdosage

►*Symptoms:* The highest dose of tolcapone administered to humans was 800 mg 3 times daily, with and without levodopa/carbidopa coadministration. This was in a 1-week study in elderly, healthy volunteers. The peak plasma concentrations of tolcapone at this dose were 30 mcg/ml on average (compared with 3 and 6 mcg/ml with 100 and 200 mg tolcapone, respectively). Nausea, vomiting, and dizziness were observed, particularly in combination with levodopa/carbidopa.

The threshold for the lethal plasma concentration for tolcapone based on animal data is > 100 mcg/ml. Respiratory difficulties were observed in rats at high oral (gavage) and IV doses and in dogs with rapidly injected IV doses.

►*Treatment:* Hospitalization is advised. General supportive care is indicated. Refer to General Management of Acute Overdosage. Given the very high protein binding of tolcapone, hemodialysis is unlikely to be of benefit.

Patient Information

Do not use tolcapone until there has been a complete discussion of the risks and the patient has provided written informed consent.

Inform patients of the clinical signs and symptoms that suggest the onset of hepatic injury (persistent nausea, fatigue, lethargy, anorexia, jaundice, dark urine, pruritus, and right upper quandrant tenderness). Advise patients to contact physician immediately if symptoms of hepatic failure occur. Inform patients of the need to have regular blood tests to monitor liver enzymes.

Inform patients that hallucinations can occur.

Inform patients that they may develop postural (orthostatic) hypotension with or without symptoms such as dizziness, nausea, syncope, and sometimes sweating. Hypotension may occur more frequently during initial therapy. Accordingly, caution patients against rising rapidly after sitting or lying down, especially if they have been doing so for prolonged periods and especially at the initiation of tolcapone treatment.

Advise patients not to drive cars or operate other complex machinery until they have gained sufficient experience with tolcapone to gauge whether or not it affects their mental or motor performance adversely. Because of the possible additive sedative effects, use caution when patients are taking other CNS depressants in combination with tolcapone.

Inform patients that nausea may occur, especially at initiation of tolcapone treatment.

Advise patients of the possibility of an increase in dyskinesia or dystonia.

Although tolcapone has not been teratogenic in animals, it is always given in conjunction with levodopa/carbidopa, which is known to cause visceral and skeletal malformations in the rabbit. Accordingly, advise patients to notify their physicians if they become pregnant or intend to become pregnant during therapy (see Warnings).

Tolcapone is excreted into maternal milk in rats. Because of the possibility that tolcapone may be excreted into human breast milk, advise patients to notify their physicians if they intend to breastfeed or are breastfeeding an infant.

DOPAMINE RECEPTOR AGONISTS, NON-ERGOT

For additional information, refer to the Antiparkinson Agents introduction.

Indications

➤*Parkinson's disease:* For the treatment of the signs and symptoms of idiopathic Parkinson's disease.

Actions

➤*Pharmacology:* **Pramipexole** and **ropinirole**, non-ergot dopamine agonists for Parkinson's disease, have high relative in vitro specificity and full intrinsic activity at the D_2 subfamily of dopamine receptors, binding with higher affinity to D_3 than to D_2 or D_4 receptor subtypes. The relevance of D_3 receptor binding in Parkinson's disease is unknown. Ropinirole also has moderate in vitro affinity for opioid receptors, and its metabolites have negligible in vitro affinity for dopamine D_1, $5HT_1$, $5HT_2$, benzodiazepine, GABA, muscarinic, alpha$_1$-, alpha$_2$- and beta-adrenoreceptors.

The precise mechanism of action as a treatment for Parkinson's disease is unknown, although it is believed to be related to stimulation of dopamine receptors in the striatum.

➤*Pharmacokinetics:* Non-ergot dopamine agonists are rapidly absorbed, reaching peak concentrations in ≈ 1 to 2 hours. They are extensively distributed throughout the body with a volume of distribution of ≈ 500 L. **Pramipexole** also distributes into red blood cells with an erythrocyte-to-plasma ratio of ≈ 2. Steady-state concentrations of non-ergot dopamine agonists are achieved within 2 days after dosing. Urinary excretion is the major route of elimination with > 88% of the dose recovered in the urine.

Select Pharmacokinetic Parameters of Non-Ergot Dopamine Receptor Agonists

	Absolute bioavailability (%)	Protein binding (%)	Half-life (hrs)[1]	Clearance (ml/min)	P450 metabolism
Pramipexole	> 90	15	8 (12)	400	None; ≈ 90% excreted unchanged
Ropinirole	55	30 to 40	6	783	Extensive (CYP1A2); 1 to 2% excreted unchanged

[1] In elderly patients > 65 years of age.

Food – Food does not affect the extent of absorption but increases the time to achieve maximum plasma levels by 1 hour for pramipexole and 2.5 hours for ropinirole.

Special populations – Adjustment of initial doses based on gender, weight or age is not necessary because therapy is initiated at subtherapeutic doses and gradually titrated for optimal therapeutic effect.

Smoking – Cigarette smoking is expected to increase the clearance of ropinirole since CYP1A2 is known to be induced by smoking.

Renal impairment – The clearance of **pramipexole** was decreased ≈ 75% in patients with severe renal impairment (CCl ≈ 20 ml/min) and was 60% lower in patients with moderate renal impairment (CCl ≈ 40 ml/min). Use a lower initial and maintenance dose of pramipexole in these patients.

No dosage adjustment for **ropinirole** is necessary for patients with moderate renal impairment (CCl 30 to 50 ml/min). The effects of severe renal impairment have not been studied.

Hepatic impairment – Plasma levels of **ropinirole** may increase and clearance may decrease; titrate ropinirole with caution in patients with impaired hepatic function.

➤*Clinical trials:* In all studies, one or more of the Unified Parkinson's Disease Rating Scale (UPDRS) subparts served as the primary outcome assessment measure. This is a four-part, multi-item rating scale intended to evaluate mentation (part I), activities of daily living (part II), motor performance (part III) and complications of therapy (part IV).

Early Parkinson's disease (without levodopa) – In a study involving 335 patients, the group treated with 0.375 mg **pramipexole** titrated over 7 weeks up to a maximum of 4.5 mg/day and maintained over 6 months achieved statistically significant improvements over placebo in mean baseline USDRS part II (1.9 vs -0.4, respectively) and part III (5 vs -0.8, respectively) scores. Statistically significant differences were seen by week 2 for activities of daily living (part II) and by week 3 for motor performance (part III).

In another study of 63 patients, the treatment group titrated for 10 weeks on **ropinirole** 0.5 mg twice daily to a maximum of 5 mg twice daily and then maintained through week 12 achieved a statistically significant mean percentage improvement over placebo in USDRS part III scores (43% vs 21%). At the end of 12 weeks, 71% of ropinirole-treated patients (vs 41% placebo) were considered "responders" by experiencing a ≥ 30% reduction in their baseline score. Statistically significant dif-

ferences were seen by week 2 for motor performance (part III) and after week 8 for percentage of responders.

Advanced Parkinson's disease (with levodopa) – In the following trials, patients had a mean disease duration of 9 years and had been exposed to levodopa for ≈ 7 to 8 years. Primary assessments were USDRS part II or part III, reduction in levodopa and amount of "off" time. Patients were treated with levodopa and could also be on concomitant selegiline, anticholinergics or amantadine; the non-ergot dopamine agonist was titrated to a maximal tolerable dose and then maintained throughout the remainder of the 6 month trial period.

Patients in a **pramipexole** study (n=360) were initiated on 0.375 mg/day and titrated to ≤ 4.5 mg/day in 3 divided doses. The pramipexole group achieved statistically significant mean improvements from baseline over the placebo group in USDRS part II scores at 2 weeks and in part III scores at 3 weeks. Levodopa dosage reduction occurred in 76% of pramipexole patients vs 54% of placebo patients; the average reduction in dose was 27%. The mean number of "off" hours decreased in the treatment group only by 2 hours.

A **ropinirole** study involving 148 patients initiated patients at 0.25 mg three times daily and titrated upward to a minimum of 2.5 mg/day but ≤ 8 mg/day. At 6 months, 28% of patients treated with ropinirole vs 11% in the placebo group had achieved a ≥ 20% reduction in both their levodopa dose and in the proportion of awake time in the "off" condition. Mean reduction in levodopa dosage was achieved in 19.4% of ropinirole patients and in 3% of placebo; the average levodopa dose reduction in the ropinirole group was 31%. The mean number of "off" hours decreased from 6.4 to 4.9 hours/day for the ropinirole group and from 7.3 to 6.4 hours/day for the placebo group.

Contraindications

Hypersensitivity to the product or any of its components.

Warnings

➤*Symptomatic hypotension:* Dopamine agonists appear to impair the systemic regulation of blood pressure, with resulting orthostatic hypotension especially during dose escalation. Parkinson's disease patients appear to have impaired capacity to respond to an orthostatic challenge. Therefore, these patients require careful monitoring for signs and symptoms of orthostatic hypotension while being treated with dopaminergic agonists, especially during dose escalation.

➤*Syncope:* Syncope, sometimes associated with bradycardia, was observed in association with **ropinirole** therapy. In patients with early Parkinson's disease treated with ropinirole (without levodopa), 11.5% had syncope compared with 1.4% on placebo. Most of these cases occurred > 4 weeks after initiation of therapy of ropinirole and were usually associated with a recent increase in dose.

Of 208 patients being treated with both **levodopa** and **ropinirole** in advanced Parkinson's disease trials, syncope was reported in 2.9% vs 1.7% with placebo.

➤*Hallucinations:* Hallucinations were observed in a greater number of patients receiving dopaminergics than placebo. In early Parkinson's disease, hallucinations were observed in ≈ 5% to 9% of treated patients vs ≈ 1.5% to 2.5% for the placebo group. In patients with advanced Parkinson's disease receiving concomitant levodopa, hallucinations were observed in ≈ 10% to 16.5% of patients receiving dopaminergics vs ≈ 4% receiving placebo.

Elderly – Age appears to increase the risk of hallucinations attributable to dopaminergics. Elderly patients (> 65 years of age) with early and advanced Parkinson's disease have experienced hallucinations ≈ 7 and ≈ 5 times more often, respectively, than their younger counterparts when treated with dopaminergics.

➤*Renal function impairment:* Reduce initial and maintenance doses of **pramipexole** for patients with moderate to severe renal impairment (see Administration and Dosage).

➤*Fertility impairment:* A significant increase in testicular Leydig cell adenomas was observed in male rats treated with **ropinirole** at all doses tested (eg, ≥ 1.5 mg/kg [0.6 times the maximum recommended human dose on a mg/m^2 basis]). The relevance of this occurrence to humans is of questionable significance. An increase in benign uterine endometrial polyps at a dose of 50 mg/kg/day (10 times the maximum recommended human dose on a mg/m^2 basis) was observed in female mice treated with ropinirole.

➤*Elderly:* The incidence of hallucinations appears to increase with age (see Hallucinations in Warnings).

➤*Pregnancy: Category C.* There are no adequate and well-controlled studies in pregnant women. In animals, **ropinirole** has been shown to have adverse effects on embryo-fetal development, including teratogenic effects, decreased fetal body weight, increased fetal death and digital malformation. Use during pregnancy only if the potential benefit outweighs the potential risk to the fetus.

➤*Lactation:* Treatment with these agents has resulted in an inhibition of prolactin secretion in humans. It is not known whether these drugs are excreted in breast milk. Decide whether to discontinue nursing or the drug, taking into account the importance of the drug to the mother.

DOPAMINE RECEPTOR AGONISTS, NON-ERGOT

➤*Children:* Safety and efficacy have not been established.

Precautions

➤*Monitoring:* Monitor for signs and symptoms of orthostatic hypotension (see Warnings).

➤*Dyskinesia:* Dopamine receptor agonists may potentiate the dopaminergic side effects of levodopa and may cause or exacerbate preexisting dyskinesia. Decreasing the dose of levodopa may ameliorate this side effect.

➤*Retinal pathology:* Pathologic changes (degeneration and loss of photoreceptor cells) were observed in the retinas of albino rats receiving dopamine receptor agonists in a 2-year study. The potential significance of this effect in humans has not been established, but cannot be disregarded because disruption of a mechanism that is universally present in vertebrates (eg, disk shedding) may be involved.

➤*Withdrawal-emergent hyperpyrexia and confusion:* Although not reported with these specific agents, a symptom complex resembling the neuroleptic malignant syndrome (characterized by elevated temperature, muscular rigidity, altered consciousness and autonomic instability) with no other obvious etiology, has occurred in association with rapid dose reduction, withdrawal of or changes in antiparkinsonian dopaminergic therapy.

➤*Fibrotic complication:* Cases of retroperitoneal fibrosis, pulmonary infiltrates, pleural effusion and pleural thickening have occurred in some patients treated with ergot-derived dopaminergic agents. While these complications may resolve when the drug is discontinued, complete resolution does not always occur.

Although these adverse events are believed to be related to the ergoline structure of these compounds, whether non-ergot-derived dopamine agonists can cause these reactions is unknown.

➤*CNS effects:* Use concomitant CNS depressants with caution because of the possible additive sedative effects.

➤*Rhabdomyolysis:* A single case of rhabdomyolysis occurred in a 49-year-old male with advanced Parkinson's disease treated with **pramipexole**. The patient was hospitalized with an elevated CPK (10,631 IU/L). The symptoms resolved with discontinuation of the medication.

➤*Binding to melanin:* **Ropinirole** binds to melanin-containing tissues (eg, eyes, skin) in pigmentated rats. After a single dose, long-term retention of the drug was demonstrated with a half-life in the eye of 20 days. It is not known if ropinirole accumulates in these tissues over time.

Drug Interactions

Non-Ergot Dopamine Receptor Agonist Drug Interactions			
Precipitant drug	Object drug*		Description
Non-ergot dopamine agonists	Levodopa	↑	Concomitant administration increased levodopa C_{max} (20% to 40%); pramipexole C_{max} decreased from 2.5 to 0.5 hours.
Cimetidine	Pramipexole	↑	Cimetidine caused a 50% increase in pramipexole AUC and a 40% increase in its half-life.
Estrogen	Ropinirole	↑	Estrogens (mainly ethinyl estradiol, 0.6 to 3 mg over a 4-month to 23-year period) reduced the oral clearance of ropinirole by 36% in 16 patients. Dosage adjustment may not be needed because ropinirole is titrated to effect. However, dose adjustment may be required if estrogen therapy is stopped or started during treatment with ropinirole.
Ciprofloxacin	Ropinirole	↑	Coadministration with ciprofloxacin, an inhibitor of CYP1A2, increased ropinirole AUC by 84% on average and C_{max} by 60%.
Drugs eliminated via renal secretion (eg, cimetidine, ranitidine, diltiazem, triamterene, verapamil, quinidine, quinine)	Pramipexole	↑	Coadministration of drugs that are secreted by the cationic transport system may decrease the oral clearance of pramipexole by ≈ 20%.
Inhibitors of CYP1A2 (eg, cimetidine, ciprofloxacin, diltiazem, enoxacin, erythromycin, fluvoxamine, mexiletine, norfloxacin, tacrine)	Ropinirole	↑	Potential exists for substrates or inhibitors of CYP1A2 to alter ropinirole's clearance. If therapy with a potent CYP1A2 inhibitor is stopped or started during ropinirole treatment, dose adjustment may be required.
Dopamine antagonists (eg, phenothiazines, butyrophenones, thioxanthenes, metoclopramide)	Nonergot dopamine agonists	↓	Because these agents are dopamine agonists, it is possible that dopamine antagonists, such as the neuroleptics, may diminish their effectiveness.

* ↑ = Object drug increased.   ↓ = Object drug decreased.

➤*Drug/Food interactions:* **Pramipexole** and **ropinirole** T_{max} are increased by ≈ 1 and 2.5 hours, respectively, when taken with food, although the extent of absorption is not affected.

Adverse Reactions

➤*Early Parkinson's disease (without levodopa):* The most commonly observed adverse events (> 5%) shared by the non-ergot dopamine receptor agonists were nausea, dizziness, somnolence, dyspepsia, constipation, asthenia and hallucinations.

Approximately 24% of **ropinirole**-treated patients discontinued treatment because of adverse events vs 13% for placebo. The most common adverse events for discontinuing therapy were nausea (6.4%); dizziness (3.8%); aggravated Parkinson's disease, hallucinations, somnolence, vomiting, headache (1.3%). In **pramipexole** studies, ≈ 12% of treated patients vs 11% in the placebo group discontinued therapy because of adverse events. Hallucinations (3.1%); dizziness, nausea (2.1%); somnolence, extrapyramidal syndrome (1.6%); headache and confusion (1.3%) were the most common reason for discontinuation.

Non-Ergot Dopamine Receptor Agonist Adverse Reactions in Early Parkinson's Disease (without Levodopa)[1] (%)		
Adverse reaction	Pramipexole (n = 388)	Ropinirole (n = 157)
Autonomic nervous system		
Increased sweating	-	6
Dry mouth	-	5
Flushing	-	3
Cardiovascular		
Syncope	-	12
Orthostatic symptoms	-	6
Hypertension	-	5
Palpitations	-	3

Non-Ergot Dopamine Receptor Agonist Adverse Reactions in Early Parkinson's Disease (without Levodopa)[1] (%)		
Adverse reaction	Pramipexole (n = 388)	Ropinirole (n = 157)
Atrial fibrillation	-	2
Extrasystoles	-	2
Hypotension	-	2
Tachycardia	-	2
CNS		
Dizziness	25	40
Somnolence	22	40
Insomnia	17	-
Hallucinations[2]	9	5
Confusion	4	5
Amnesia	4	3
Hypesthesia	3	4
Yawning	-	3
Dystonia	2	-
Akathisia	2	-
Thinking abnormalities	2	-
Hyperkinesia	-	2
Impaired concentration	-	2
Vertigo	-	2
Decreased libido	1	-
Myoclonus	1	-
GI		
Nausea	28	60
Constipation	14	-
Vomiting	-	12
Dyspepsia	-	10

DOPAMINE RECEPTOR AGONISTS, NON-ERGOT

Non-Ergot Dopamine Receptor Agonist Adverse Reactions in Early Parkinson's Disease (without Levodopa)[1] (%)		
Adverse reaction	Pramipexole (n = 388)	Ropinirole (n = 157)
Abdominal pain	-	6
Anorexia	4	4
Flatulence	-	3
Dysphagia	2	-
Metabolic/Nutritional		
Peripheral edema	5	4
Decreased weight	2	0
Respiratory		
Pharyngitis	-	6
Rhinitis	-	4
Sinusitis	-	4
Bronchitis	-	3
Dyspnea	-	3
Special senses		
Abnormal vision	3	6
Eye abnormality	-	3
Xerophthalmia	-	2
Miscellaneous		
Asthenia	14	6
Fatigue	-	11
Viral infection	-	11
Pain	-	8
Edema	5	7
Urinary tract infection	-	5
Chest pain	-	4
Malaise	2	3
Fever	1	-
Impotence	2	3
Peripheral ischemia	-	3
Increased alkaline phosphatase	-	3

[1] Data pooled from separate studies; not necessarily comparable.
[2] See Warnings.

▶*Advanced Parkinson's disease (with levodopa):* The most commonly observed adverse events (> 5%) shared by the non-ergot dopamine receptor agonists were dyskinesia, dizziness, extrapyramidal syndrome/aggravated Parkinsonism, somnolence, insomnia, injury, hallucinations, confusion, urinary frequency/infection, constipation and dry mouth.

Approximately 24% of patients treated with **ropinirole** and levodopa discontinued therapy because of adverse events vs 18% of patients given placebo and levodopa. The most common adverse events causing discontinuation of treatment were dizziness (2.9%); dyskinesia, vomiting, confusion (2.4%); nausea, hallucinations, anxiety (1.9%) and increased sweating (1.4%). In patients treated with **pramipexole** and levodopa, ≈ 12% discontinued therapy as a result of adverse reactions vs 16% in the placebo group. Therapy was discontinued most often because of hallucinations (2.7%); orthostatic hypotension (2.3%); dyskinesia (1.9%); extrapyramidal syndrome (1.5%); dizziness and confusion (1.2%).

Non-Ergot Dopamine Receptor Agonist Adverse Reactions in Advanced Parkinson's Disease (with Levodopa)[1] (%)		
Adverse reaction	Pramipexole (n=260)	Ropinirole (n=208)
Cardiovascular		
Postural hypotension	53	2
Syncope	-	3
CNS		
Dyskinesia	47	34
Extrapyramidal syndrome	28	-
Insomnia	27	-
Dizziness	26	26
Somnolence	9	20
Hallucinations	17	10
Headache	-	17
Dream abnormalities	11	3
Confusion	10	9
Falls	-	10
Dystonia	8	-
Gait abnormalities/ hypokinesia	7	5
Hypertonia	7	-
Amnesia	6	5
Tremor/twitching	2	6
Nervousness	-	5

Non-Ergot Dopamine Receptor Agonist Adverse Reactions in Advanced Parkinson's Disease (with Levodopa)[1] (%)		
Adverse reaction	Pramipexole (n=260)	Ropinirole (n=208)
Paresthesia	-	5
Akathisia	3	-
Thinking abnormalities	3	-
Paresis	-	3
Paranoid reaction	2	-
Delusions	1	-
Sleep disorders	1	-
GI		
Nausea	-	30
Constipation	10	6
Abdominal pain	-	9
Vomiting	-	7
Diarrhea	-	5
Dysphagia	-	2
Flatulence	-	2
Increased saliva	-	2
GU		
Urinary frequency	6	-
Urinary tract infection	4	6
Urinary incontinence	2	2
Pyuria	-	2
Metabolic/Nutritional		
Peripheral edema	2	-
Increased creatine PK	1	-
Musculoskeletal		
Arthritis	3	3
Twitching	2	6
Bursitis	2	-
Myasthenia	1	-
Respiratory		
Pneumonia	2	9
Dyspnea	4	3
Rhinitis	3	-
Special senses		
Accommodation abnormalities	4	-
Vision abnormalities	3	-
Diplopia	1	-
Miscellaneous		
Accidental injury	17	-
Asthenia	10	-
Dry mouth	7	5
Increased sweating	-	7
Increased drug level	3	-
Pain	-	-
General edema	4	-
Chest pain	3	-
Malaise	3	-
Skin disorders	2	-
Anemia	-	2
Weight decrease	-	2

[1] Data pooled from separate studies; not necessarily comparable.

Overdosage

There is no clinical experience with massive overdosage. One patient with a 10-year history of schizophrenia took **pramipexole** 11 mg/day for 2 days (two to three times the recommended daily dose). No adverse events were reported related to the increased dose. Blood pressure remained stable, although pulse rate increased to between 100 and 120 beats/minute. Of ten patients ingesting > 24 mg/day, one experienced mild oro-facial dyskinesia, another experienced intermittent nausea. Other symptoms reported with accidental overdoses were: Agitation, increased dyskinesia, grogginess, sedation, orthostatic hypotension, chest pain, confusion, vomiting and nausea. The largest overdose reported was 435 mg taken over a 7-day period (62.1 mg/day).

▶*Treatment:* There is no known antidote for overdosage of a dopamine agonist. If signs of CNS stimulation are present, a phenothiazine or other butyrophenone neuroleptic agent may be indicated; the efficacy of such drugs in reversing the effects of overdosage has not been assessed. Management of overdose may require general supportive measures along with gastric lavage, IV fluids and ECG monitoring. A negligible amount of **pramipexole** is removed by dialysis. Refer to General Management of Acute Overdosage.

Patient Information

Inform patients that hallucinations can occur and that the elderly are at a higher risk than younger patients with Parkinson's disease.

DOPAMINE RECEPTOR AGONISTS, NON-ERGOT

Patients may develop postural hypotension with or without symptoms such as dizziness, nausea, fainting or blackouts and sometimes sweating. Hypotension may occur more frequently during initial therapy. Accordingly, caution patients against rising rapidly after sitting or lying down, especially if they have been doing so for prolonged periods and at the initiation of treatment with pramipexole.

Advise patients that they may experience somnolence and that they should neither drive a car nor operate other complex machinery until they have gained sufficient experience with the drug to gauge whether or not it affects their mental or motor performance adversely. Inform patients of the possible additive sedative effects when taken in combination with other CNS depressants.

Because **ropinirole** has been shown to have adverse effects on embryo-fetal development, advise patients to notify their physician if they become pregnant or intend to become pregnant during therapy.

Advise patients to notify their physicians if they intend to breastfeed or are breastfeeding an infant.

If patients develop nausea, advise them that taking this medication with food may reduce the occurrence of nausea.

PRAMIPEXOLE

Rx	Mirapex (Boehringer Ingelheim)	Tablets: 0.125 mg	(U 2). White. In 63s.
		0.25 mg	(UU 44). White, scored. Oval. In 90s.
		0.5 mg	Mannitol. (UU 88). White, scored. Oval. In 90s and UD 100s.
		1 mg	(UU 66). White, scored. In 90s.
		1.5 mg	(UU 3737). White, scored. In 90s.

For complete prescribing information, refer to the Dopamine Receptor Agonists, Non-Ergot group monograph.

Indications

➤*Parkinson's disease:* For the treatment of the signs and symptoms of idiopathic Parkinson's disease.

Administration and Dosage

➤*Approved by the FDA:* July 2, 1997.

Titrate pramipexole gradually in all patients. Increase the dosage to achieve a maximum therapeutic effect balanced against the principal side effects of dyskinesia, hallucinations, somnolence and dry mouth.

May be taken with food to reduce the occurrence of nausea.

➤*Initial treatment:* Increase dosages gradually from a starting dose of 0.375 mg/day given in three divided doses and do not increase more frequently than every 5 to 7 days. A suggested ascending dosage schedule used in clinical studies is shown in the following table:

Ascending Dosage Schedule of Pramipexole		
Week	Dosage (mg)	Total daily dose (mg)
1	0.125 three times/day	0.375
2	0.25 three times/day	0.75
3	0.5 three times/day	1.5
4	0.75 three times/day	2.25
5	1 three times/day	3
6	1.25 three times/day	3.75
7	1.5 three times/day	4.5

➤*Maintenance treatment:* Pramipexole is effective and well tolerated over a dosage range of 1.5 to 4.5 mg/day administered in equally divided doses 3 times per day with or without concomitant levodopa ($\approx$ 800 mg/day).

In a fixed-dose study in early Parkinson's disease patients, doses of 3, 4.5 and 6 mg/day did not provide any significant benefit beyond that achieved at a daily dose of 1.5 mg/day.

When pramipexole is used in combination with levodopa, consider a reduction of the levodopa dosage. In a controlled study in advanced Parkinson's disease, the dosage of levodopa was reduced by an average of 27% from baseline.

➤*Renal function impairment:*

Pramipexole Dosage with Renal Function Impairment		
Creatinine clearance (ml/min)	Starting dose (mg)	Maximum dose (mg)
> 60	0.125 three times/day	1.5 three times daily
35-59	0.125 two times/day	1.5 twice daily
15-34	0.125 one time/day	1.5 once daily
< 15 or hemodialysis patients	The use of pramipexole has not been adequately studied in this group of patients.	

➤*Discontinuation of treatment:* It is recommended that pramipexole be discontinued over a period of 1 week; in some studies, however, abrupt discontinuation was uneventful.

ROPINIROLE HCl

Rx	Requip[1] (SmithKline Beecham)	Tablets: 0.25 mg	(SB4890). White, pentagonal, film-coated *Tiltab* with beveled edges. In 30s and 100s.
		0.5 mg	(SB4891). Yellow, pentagonal, film-coated *Tiltab* with beveled edges. In 30s and 100s.
		1 mg	(SB4892). Pale green, pentagonal, film-coated *Tiltab* with beveled edges. In 30s and 100s.
		2 mg	(SB4893). Pale yellowish pink, pentagonal, film-coated *Tiltab* with beveled edges. In 30s and 100s.
		5 mg	(SB4894). Pale blue, pentagonal, film-coated *Tiltab* with beveled edges. In 30s and 100s.

[1] Contains lactose.

For complete prescribing information, refer to the Dopamine Receptor Agonists, Non-Ergot group monograph.

Indications

➤*Parkinson's disease:* For the treatment of the signs and symptoms of idiopathic Parkinson's disease.

Administration and Dosage

➤*Approved by the FDA:* September 23, 1997.

Take 3 times daily. Ropinirole can be taken with or without food. Advise patients that taking ropinirole with food may reduce the occurrence of nausea.

The recommended starting dose is 0.25 mg 3 times daily. Based on individual patient response, dosage should then be titrated in weekly increments as described in the table below. After week 4, if necessary, daily dosage may be increased by 1.5 mg/day on a weekly basis up to a dose of 9 mg/day, and then by ≤ 3 mg/day weekly to a total dose of 24 mg/day.

Ascending-Dose Schedule of Ropinirole		
Week	Dosage	Total daily dose
1	0.25 mg 3 times/day	0.75 mg
2	0.5 mg 3 times/day	1.5 mg
3	0.75 mg 3 times/day	2.25 mg
4	1 mg 3 times/day	3 mg

When ropinirole is administered as adjunct therapy to levodopa, the concurrent dose of levodopa may be decreased gradually as tolerated.

Discontinue ropinirole gradually over a 7-day period. Decrease the frequency of administration from three times daily to twice daily for 4 days. For the remaining 3 days, decrease the frequency to once daily prior to complete withdrawal of ropinirole.

APOMORPHINE HYDROCHLORIDE

Rx   **Apokyn** (Mylan Bertek)   **Injection:** 10 mg/mL   Sodium metabisulfite. 2 mL glass ampules and 3 mL cartridges.

For complete prescribing information, refer to the Dopamine Receptor Agonists, Non-Ergot group monograph.

Indications

➤*Parkinson disease:* For the acute, intermittent treatment of hypomobility, "off" episodes ("end-of-dose wearing off" and unpredictable "on/off" episodes) associated with advanced Parkinson disease. Apomorphine has been studied as an adjunct to other medications.

Administration and Dosage

➤*Approved by the FDA:* April 20, 2004.

Always express the prescribed dose of apomorphine in mL to avoid confusion, and doses greater than 0.6 mL (6 mg) are not recommended. Patients and caregivers must receive detailed instructions in the preparation and injection of doses, with particular attention paid to the correct use of the dosing pen.

For subcutaneous administration only.

➤*Concomitant medication:* Do not initiate apomorphine without the use of a concomitant antiemetic. Most antiemetic experience is with trimethobenzamide and this should generally be used. Start trimethobenzamide (300 mg 3 times daily orally) 3 days prior to the initial dose of apomorphine and continue during at least the first 2 months of therapy.

Based on reports of profound hypotension and loss of consciousness when apomorphine was administered with ondansetron, the concomitant use of drugs of the 5HT₃ antagonist class is contraindicated.

➤*Dosage:* Titrate the dose of apomorphine on the basis of effectiveness and tolerance, starting at 0.2 mL (2 mg) and up to a maximum recommended dose of 0.6 mL (6 mg) as follows:

Give patients in an "off" state a 0.2 mL (2 mg) test dose in a setting where blood pressure can be closely monitored by medical personnel. Check supine and standing blood pressure predose and at 20, 40, and 60 minutes postdose. Do not consider patients who develop clinically significant orthostatic hypotension in response to this test dose of apomorphine candidates for treatment. If the patient tolerates the 0.2 mL (2 mg) dose and responds, use the starting dose of 0.2 mL (2 mg) on an as-needed basis to treat existing "off" episodes. If needed, the dose can be increased in 0.1 mL (1 mg) increments every few days on an outpatient basis.

The general principle guiding dosing (described in detail below) is to determine a dose (0.3 or 0.4 mL) that the patient will tolerate as a test dose under monitored conditions, and then begin an outpatient dosing trial (periodically assessing both efficacy and tolerability) using a dose 0.1 mL (1 mg) lower than the tolerated test dose.

For patients who tolerate the test dose of 0.2 mL (2 mg) but achieve no response, a dose of 0.4 mL (4 mg) may be administered at the next observed "off" period, but no sooner than 2 hours after the initial test dose of 0.2 mL (2 mg). Check supine and standing blood pressure predose and at 20, 40, and 60 minutes postdose. If the patient tolerates a test dose of 0.4 mL (4 mg), the starting dose should be 0.3 mL (3 mg) used on an as-needed basis to treat existing "off" episodes. If needed, the dose can be increased in 0.1 mL (1 mg) increments every few days on an outpatient basis. If a patient does not tolerate a test dose of 0.4 mL (4 mg), a test dose of 0.3 mL (3 mg) may be administered during a separate "off" period, no sooner than 2 hours after the test dose of 0.4 mL (4 mg). Check supine and standing blood pressure predose and at 20, 40, and 60 minutes postdose. If the patient tolerates the 0.3 mL (3 mg) test dose, the starting dose should be 0.2 mL (2 mg) used on an as-needed basis to treat existing "off" episodes. If needed, and the 0.2 mL (2 mg) dose is tolerated, the dose can be increased to 0.3 mL (3 mg) after a few days. In such a patient, the dose should ordinarily not be increased to 0.4 mL (4 mg) on an outpatient basis.

Most patients studied in the apomorphine development program responded to 0.3 to 0.6 mL (3 to 6 mg). There is no evidence from controlled trials that doses greater than 0.6 mL (6 mg) give an increased effect, and these doses are not recommended. The average frequency of dosing was 3 times per day in the development program, and there is limited experience with single doses greater than 0.6 mL (6 mg), dosing more than 5 times per day, and with total daily doses greater than 2 mL (20 mg).

If a single dose of apomorphine is ineffective for a particular "off" period, do not give a second dose for that "off" episode. The efficacy of a second dose for a single "off" episode has not been systematically studied and the safety of redosing has not been characterized.

➤*Interruption of therapy:* Patients who have a significant interruption in therapy (more than a week) should be restarted on a 0.2 mL (2 mg) dose and gradually titrated to effect.

➤*Hepatic function impairment:* For patients with mild and moderate hepatic function impairment, exercise caution because of the increased C_{max} and AUC in these patients.

➤*Renal function impairment:* For patients with mild and moderate renal function impairment, reduce the testing dose and subsequent starting dose to 0.1 mL (1 mg).

➤*Storage/Stability:* Store at 25°C (77°F). Excursions permitted to 15° to 30°C (59° to 86°F).

ADENOSINE PHOSPHATE

Rx	**Adenosine Phosphate** (Various, eg, Pasadena)	**Injection:** 25 mg/ml in an aqueous solution	In 10 and 30 ml vials.[1]

[1] May contain benzyl alcohol.

Indications

➤*Varicose veins:* Symptomatic relief of complications with stasis dermatitis.

➤*Unlabeled uses:* Adenosine monophosphate has been used to treat herpes infections.

Adenosine is currently being investigated for use in increasing blood flow to brain tumors and in porphyria cutanea tarda.

Administration and Dosage

Administer IM only. Not for IV use.

➤*Initial:* Administer 25 to 50 mg once or twice daily until symptoms subside.

➤*Maintenance:* 25 mg 2 or 3 times weekly.

➤*Storage / Stability:* Store at room temperature 15° to 30°C (59° to 86°F).

Actions

➤*Pharmacology:* Adenosine is converted to adenosin monophosphate (A_5MP) which is associated with many normal biochemical processes. The mechanism of action is not understood. Clinical benefits may result from correction of underlying biochemical imbalances or deficiences at the cellular level. The drug may also be a neurotransmitter.

Contraindications

History of myocardial infarction; cerebral hemorrhage.

Warnings

➤*Anaphylactoid reactions:* If a patient complains of dyspnea and chest tightness following an injection, do not administer further injections. Immediately institute treatment for allergic reactions. Refer to Management of Acute Hypersensitivity Reactions.

➤*Pregnancy: Category C.* Safe use has not been established with respect to adverse effects upon fetal development. Do not use in women of childbearing potential or during early pregnancy unless the benefits outweigh the potential hazards.

➤*Children:* Not recommended for use in children. Clinical experience has been insufficient to establish safety or a suitable dosage regimen.

Precautions

➤*Benzyl alcohol:* This product contains the preservative benzyl alcohol, which has been associated with a fatal "gasping syndrome" in premature infants.

Adverse Reactions

Flushing, dizziness, palpitations, hypotension, dyspnea, epigastric discomfort, nausea, occasional local rash and diureses, increase in symptoms of bursitis and tendinitis.

Anticholinesterase Muscle Stimulants

Indications

►*Myasthenia gravis:* Treatment of myasthenia gravis.

►*Urinary retention:* The prevention and treatment of postoperative distention and urinary retention after mechanical obstruction has been excluded.

►*Reversal of nondepolarizing muscle relaxants:* Reversal of nondepolarizing muscle relaxants (**pyridostigmine** and **neostigmine**).

►*Unlabeled uses:* Diagnosis of myasthenia gravis (0.022 mg/kg/dose IM × 1).

Actions

►*Pharmacology:* These drugs facilitate transmission of impulses across the myoneural junction by inhibiting the destruction of acetylcholine by cholinesterase. They differ in duration of action and in adverse effects. Equivalent doses, onset and duration of action are summarized below.

Drug	Route	Equivalent Dosage (mg)	Onset (min)	Duration (hours)	Indications
Ambenonium	PO	5-10	20-30	3-8	Myasthenia gravis
Edrophonium	IM	10	2-10	0.17-0.67	Diagnosis myasthenia gravis
	IV	10	< 1	0.08-0.33	Diagnosis myasthenia gravis;[1] Nondepolarizing muscle relaxant antagonist
Neostigmine	PO	15	45-75	2-4	Myasthenia gravis
	IM	1.5	20-30	2-4	Myasthenia gravis
	IV	0.5	4-8	2-4	Diagnosis myasthenia gravis; Nondepolarizing muscle relaxant antagonist
Pyridostigmine	PO	60	20-30	3-6	Myasthenia gravis
	IM	2	< 15	2-4	Myasthenia gravis
	IV	2	2-5	2-4	Myasthenia gravis; Nondepolarizing muscle relaxant antagonist

[1] Also used to evaluate treatment requirements in myasthenia gravis.

Contraindications

Hypersensitivity to anticholinesterases; mechanical intestinal and urinary obstructions; peritonitis (**neostigmine**); history of reaction to bromides (**neostigmine** and **pyridostigmine**).

Warnings

►*Use with caution:* Use with caution in patients with bronchial asthma, epilepsy, bradycardia, recent coronary occlusion, vagotonia, hyperthyroidism, cardiac arrhythmias or peptic ulcer. Treat transient bradycardia with atropine sulfate. Isolated instances of cardiac and respiratory arrest, believed to be vagotonic effects, have occurred. When large doses are given, prior or simultaneous injection of atropine sulfate may be advisable. Use separate syringes.

►*Cholinergic/Masthenic crisis:* Overdosage may result in cholinergic crisis, characterized by increasing muscle weakness that, through involvement of the respiratory muscles, may lead to death. Myasthenic crisis because of an increase in disease severity is also accompanied by extreme muscle weakness and may be difficult to distinguish from cholinergic crisis. Differentiation is extremely important; use **edrophonium** and clinical judgment.

Treatment of the two conditions differs radically: Myasthenic crisis requires more intensive anticholinesterase therapy; cholinergic crisis calls for withdrawal of all drugs of this type and immediate use of atropine. Have a syringe containing 1 mg of atropine sulfate immediately available to be given IV to counteract severe cholinergic reactions. Use atropine to abolish or blunt GI side effects or other muscarinic reactions; however, such use may lead to inadvertent induction of cholinergic crisis by masking signs of overdosage.

►*Used as antagonists to nondepolarizing muscle relaxants:* Obtain adequate recovery of voluntary respiration and neuromuscular transmission prior to discontinuing respiratory assistance. Observe continuously. If there is doubt concerning adequacy of recovery from the nondepolarizing muscle relaxant, continue artificial ventilation.

►*Supervision:* Great care and supervision are required with **ambenonium**. Because ambenonium has a more prolonged action than other antimyasthenic drugs, simultaneous use with other cholinergics is contraindicated except under strict supervision. Therefore, when a patient is to be given the drug, suspend use of all other cholinergics until the patient has been stabilized.

►*Hypersensitivity reactions:* Because of possible hypersensitivity in an occasional patient, have atropine and epinephrine readily available when using parenteral therapy.

►*Pregnancy:* (*Category C* – neostigmine.) Safety for use during pregnancy has not been established. Transient muscular weakness occurred in ≈ 20% of infants born to mothers treated with these drugs during pregnancy. Use only when clearly needed and when the potential benefits outweigh the potential hazards to the fetus.

Anticholinesterase drugs may cause uterine irritability and induce premature labor when given IV to pregnant women near term.

►*Lactation:* **Pyridostigmine** is excreted in breast milk. Because they are ionized at physiologic pH, **ambenonium** and **neostigmine** would not be expected to be excreted in breast milk.

►*Children:* Safety and efficacy for use of **neostigmine** in children are not established.

Precautions

►*Anticholinesterase insensitivity:* Anticholinesterase insensitivity may develop for brief or prolonged periods. Carefully monitor the patient; respiratory assistance may be needed. Reduce or withhold dosages until the patient again becomes sensitive.

Drug Interactions

Anticholinesterase Muscle Stimulants Drug Interactions			
Precipitant drug	Object drug*		Description
Anticholinesterase muscle stimulants	Anticholinesterase drugs	↑	Exercise caution in patients with myasthenic symptoms who are receiving other anticholinesterase muscle stimulants. Because symptoms of anticholinesterase overdose (cholinergic crisis) may mimic underdosage (myasthenic weakness), the condition may be worsened.
Anticholinesterase muscle stimulants	Succinylcholine	↑	Neuromuscular blocking effects may be increased. Prolonged respiratory depression with extended periods of apnea may occur. Provide respiratory support as needed.
Aminoglycoside antibiotics (eg, neomycin, streptomycin, kenamycin)	Anticholinesterase muscle stimulants	↑	Aminoglycoside antibiotics have a mild but definite nondepolarizing blocking action which may accentuate neuromuscular block.
Local and general anesthetics Antiarrhythmics	Anticholinesterase muscle stimulants	↓	Use cautiously, if at all, in patients with myasthenia gravis. The neostigmine dose may have to be increased accordingly.
Atropine Belladonna derivatives	Anticholinesterase muscle stimulants	↑	Routine administration of these agents may suppress the parasympathomimetic (muscarinic) symptoms of excessive GI stimulation leaving only the more serious symptoms of fasciculation and paralysis of voluntary muscles as signs of overdosage.
Corticosteroids	Anticholinesterase muscle stimulants	↓	May decrease the anticholinesterase effects of these agents. Conversely, anticholinesterase effects may increase after stopping corticosteroids. Provide respiratory support as needed.
Depolarizing muscle relaxants (eg, succinylcholine, decamethonium)	Anticholinesterase muscle stimulants	↑	Neostigmine may prolong the Phase I block of these drugs. Use these drugs in myasthenic patients only when definitely indicated. Carefully adjust the anticholinesterase dosage.
Magnesium	Anticholinesterase muscle stimulants	↓	Magnesium has a direct depressant effect on skeletal muscle, and it may antagonize the beneficial effects of anticholinesterase therapy.
Mecamylamine	Anticholinesterase muscle stimulants	↑	Do not administer to patients receiving this ganglionic blocking agent.
Methocarbamol	Anticholinesterase muscle stimulants	↓	A single case report indicates this drug may have impaired the effect of **pyridostigmine** in a patient with myasthenia gravis.

* ↑ = Object drug increased. ↓ = Object drug decreased.

Adverse Reactions

►*Cardiovascular:* Arrhythmias (especially bradycardia); fall in cardiac output leading to hypotension; tachycardia; AV block; nodal rhythm; nonspecific EKG changes; cardiac arrest; syncope.

►*CNS:* Convulsions; dysarthria; dysphonia; dizziness; loss of consciousness; drowsiness; headache.

►*Dermatologic:* Skin rash (**pyridostigmine** and **neostigmine**; subsides upon discontinuance); thrombophlebitis (IV).

➤*GI:* Increased salivary, gastric and intestinal secretions; nausea; vomiting; dysphagia; increased peristalsis; diarrhea; abdominal cramps; flatulence.

➤*Hypersensitivity:* Allergic reactions and anaphylaxis.

➤*Musculoskeletal:* Weakness; fasciculations; muscle cramps and spasms; arthralgia.

➤*Respiratory:* Increased tracheobronchial secretions; laryngospasm; bronchiolar constriction; respiratory muscle paralysis; central respiratory paralysis; dyspnea; respiratory depression; respiratory arrest; bronchospasm.

➤*Miscellaneous:* Urinary frequency and incontinence; urinary urgency; diaphoresis; rash; urticaria; flushing; alopecia (**pyridostigmine**).

Overdosage

➤*Symptoms:* When the drug produces overstimulation, the clinical picture is one of increasing parasympathomimetic action that is more or less characteristic when not masked by the use of atropine. Signs and symptoms of overdosage, including cholinergic crises, vary considerably. They are usually manifested by increasing GI stimulation with epigastric distress, abdominal cramps, diarrhea and vomiting, excessive salivation, pallor, cold sweating, urinary urgency, blurring of vision and eventually fasciculation and paralysis of voluntary muscles, including those of the tongue (thick tongue and difficulty in swallowing), shoulder, neck and arms. Miosis, increase in blood pressure with or without bradycardia and subjective sensations of internal trembling, and often severe anxiety and panic may complete the picture. A cholinergic crisis is usually differentiated from the weakness and paralysis of myasthenia gravis insufficiently treated by cholinergic drugs by the fact that myasthenic weakness is not accompanied by any of the above signs and symptoms, except the last two subjective ones (anxiety and panic).

➤*Treatment:* Because the warning of overdosage is minimal, the existence of a narrow margin between the first appearance of side effects and serious toxic effects must be borne in mind constantly. If signs of overdosage occur (excessive GI stimulation, excessive salivation, miosis and more serious fasciculations of voluntary muscles), discontinue temporarily all cholinergic medication and administer from 0.5 to 1 mg (1/120 to 1/60 grain) of atropine IV. A total atropine dose of 5 to 10 mg or more may be required. Give other supportive treatment as indicated (artificial respiration, tracheotomy, oxygen, etc).

Patient Information

Notify physician if nausea, vomiting, diarrhea, sweating, increased salivary secretions, irregular heartbeat, muscle weakness, severe abdominal pain or difficulty in breathing occurs.

AMBENONIUM CHLORIDE

Rx	**Mytelase** (Sanofi Winthrop)	**Tablets:** 10 mg	Scored. In 100s.

For complete prescribing information, refer to the Anticholinesterase Muscle Stimulants group monograph.

Indications

➤*Myasthenia gravis:* Treatment of myasthenia gravis.

Administration and Dosage

Individualize dosage. The amount of medication necessary to control symptoms may fluctuate in each patient. Because maximum therapeutic effectiveness (optimal muscle strength and no GI disturbances) is highly critical, closely supervise.

Ambenonium has a longer duration of action than other agents and requires administration only every 3 or 4 hours, depending on clinical response. Medication is usually not required throughout the night.

➤*Moderately severe myasthenia:* 5 to 25 mg 3 or 4 times daily (range, 5 mg to 75 mg/dose). Start with 5 mg and increase gradually to determine optimum dose. Adjust at 1 to 2 day intervals to avoid drug accumulation and overdosage.

A few patients require greater doses for adequate control, but increasing dosage > 200 mg daily requires exacting supervision to avoid overdosage.

Edrophonium may be used to evaluate adequacy of maintenance dose. See the edrophonium monograph.

EDROPHONIUM CHLORIDE

Rx	**Enlon** (Ohmeda)	**Injection:** 10 mg/ml	In 15 ml vials.[1]
Rx	**Reversol** (Organon)		In 10 ml vials (25s).[1]
Rx	**Tensilon** (ICN)		In 1 ml amps,[2] 10 ml vials.[1]

[1] With 0.45% phenol and 0.2% sodium sulfite.

[2] With 0.2% sodium sulfite.

Complete prescribing information for these products begins in the Anticholinesterase Muscle Stimulants group monograph.

Indications

Differential diagnosis of myasthenia gravis; adjunct in evaluating treatment requirements in myasthenia gravis; evaluate emergency treatment in myasthenic crises. Because of its brief duration of action, it is not useful in maintenance therapy.

Curare antagonist to reverse neuromuscular block produced by curare, tubocurarine or gallamine; adjunct in treating respiratory depression caused by curare overdose.

Administration and Dosage

➤*Differential diagnosis of myasthenia gravis:*

Adults, IV – Prepare tuberculin syringe of 10 mg edrophonium with IV needle. Inject 2 mg IV in 15 to 30 sec. Leave needle in situ. If no reaction occurs after 45 sec, inject remaining 8 mg. If cholinergic reaction (muscarinic side effects, skeletal muscle fasciculations, increased muscle weakness) occurs after 2 mg injection, discontinue test; give atropine sulfate 0.4 to 0.5 mg IV. After 30 min, test may be repeated.

Adults, IM – In adults with inaccessible veins, inject 10 mg IM. Retest subjects who demonstrate hyperreactivity (cholinergic reaction) after 30 minutes with 2 mg IM to rule out false-negative reactions.

Children, IV – Up to 34 kg (75 lbs), 1 mg; > 34 kg (> 75 lbs), 2 mg. If no response after 45 seconds, may titrate up to 5 mg in children < 34 kg (< 75 lbs), and up to 10 mg in heavier children, given in 1 mg increments every 30 to 45 seconds. In infants, give 0.5 mg. Alternatively, the following schedule is recommended: Total dose is 0.2 mg/kg. Give 0.04 mg/kg initially as a test dose, then in 1 mg increments if no reaction occurs within 1 minute. Maximum dose is 10 mg total.

Children, IM – Up to 34 kg (75 lbs), 2 mg; > 34 kg (> 75 lbs), 5 mg. There is a 2 to 10 minute delay in reaction.

➤*Evaluation of treatment requirements in myasthenia gravis:* 1 to 2 mg IV 1 hour after oral intake of the treatment drug. Responses are summarized below:

Response to Edrophonium Test in Myasthenia Gravis			
Response to edrophonium test	Myasthenic[1]	Adequate[2]	Cholinergic[3]
Muscle strength (ptosis, diplopia, dysphonia, dysphagia, dysarthria, respiration, limb strength)	Increased	No change	Decreased
Fasciculations (orbicularis oculi, facial muscles, limb muscles)	Absent	Present or absent	Present or absent
Side effects (lacrimation, diaphoresis, salivation, abdominal cramps, nausea, vomiting, diarrhea)	Absent	Minimal	Severe

[1] *Myasthenic response:* Occurs in untreated myasthenics and may establish diagnosis; in patients under treatment, it indicates inadequate therapy.

[2] *Adequate response:* Observed in stabilized patients; a typical response in normal individuals. In addition, forced lid closure is often observed in psychoneurotics.

[3] *Cholinergic response:* Seen in myasthenics overtreated with anticholinesterases.

➤*Edrophonium test in crisis:* When a patient is apneic, secure controlled ventilation immediately. Do not test with edrophonium until respiration is adequate. If patient is *cholinergic,* edrophonium will increase oropharyngeal secretions and further weaken respiratory muscles. If crisis is *myasthenic,* the test clearly improves respiration and the patient can receive a longer acting IV anticholinesterase. Do not have > 2 mg in syringe. Give 1 mg IV initially; carefully observe cardiac response. If, after 1 min, this dose does not further impair the patient, inject the remaining 1 mg. If no clear improvement of respiration occurs after 2 mg, discontinue all anticholinesterase therapy and control ventilation by tracheostomy and assisted respiration.

Anticholinesterase Muscle Stimulants

EDROPHONIUM CHLORIDE

➤*Curare antagonist:* Give 10 mg slowly IV over 30 to 45 seconds to detect onset of cholinergic reaction. Repeat when necessary. Maximal dose is 40 mg. Do not give before use of curare, tubocurarine or gallamine triethiodide; use when needed. When given to counteract curare overdosage, carefully observe the effect of each dose on respiration before repeating, and employ assisted ventilation.

Precautions

➤*Sulfite sensitivity:* Some of these products contain sulfites, which may cause allergic-type reactions (eg, hives, itching, wheezing, anaphylaxis) in certain susceptible people. Although the overall prevalence of sulfite sensitivity in the general population is probably low, it is seen more frequently in asthmatics or in atopic nonasthmatic people. Specific products containing sulfites are identified in the product listings.

EDROPHONIUM CHLORIDE/ATROPINE SULFATE

Rx	Enlon-Plus (Ohmeda)	Injection: 10 mg edrophonium chloride and 0.14 mg atropine sulfate	In 5 ml amps[1] and 15 ml multidose vials.[2]

[1] With 2 mg sodium sulfite.
[2] With 2 mg sodium sulfite and 4.5 mg phenol.

Complete prescribing information for these products begins in the Anticholinesterase Muscle Stimulants monograph.

Indications

As a reversal agent or antagonist of nondepolarizing neuromuscular blocking agents.

Adjunctively in the treatment of respiratory depression caused by curare overdosage.

Not effective against depolarizing neuromuscular blocking agents. Not recommended for use in the differential diagnosis of myasthenia gravis.

Administration and Dosage

➤*Approved by the FDA:* November 6, 1991.

Dosages of edrophonium and atropine injection range from 0.05 to 0.1 ml/kg given slowly over 45 seconds to 1 minute at a point of at least 5% recovery of twitch response to neuromuscular stimulation (95% block). The dosage delivered is 0.5 to 1 mg/kg edrophonium and 0.007 to 0.014 mg/kg atropine. A total dosage of 1 mg/kg edrophonium should rarely be exceeded. Monitor response carefully and secure assisted or controlled ventilation. Satisfactory reversal permits adequate voluntary respiration and neuromuscular transmission (as tested with a peripheral nerve stimulator). Recurarization has not been reported after satisfactory reversal has been attained.

➤*Storage/Stability:* Store between 15° to 26°C (59° to 78°F).

Actions

➤*Pharmacology:* Atropine is added to edrophonium to counteract the unavoidable muscarinic side effects (eg, bradycardia, bronchoconstriction, increased secretions) of edrophonium.

Precautions

➤*Sulfite sensitivity:* This product contains sulfites, which may cause allergic-type reactions (eg, hives, itching, wheezing, anaphylaxis) in certain susceptible people. Although the overall prevalence of sulfite sensitivity in the general population is probably low, it is seen more frequently in asthmatics or in atopic nonasthmatic people. Specific products containing sulfites are identified in the product listings.

NEOSTIGMINE

Rx	Neostigmine Methylsulfate (Various)	Injection: 1:1000	In 10 ml vials.
Rx	Prostigmin (ICN)		In 10 ml vials.[1]
Rx	Neostigmine Methylsulfate (Various)	Injection: 1:2000	In 1 ml amps and 10 ml vials.
Rx	Prostigmin (ICN)		In 1 ml amps[2] and 10 ml vials.[1]
Rx	Neostigmine Methylsulfate (Various)	Injection: 1:4000	In 1 ml amps.
Rx	Prostigmin (ICN)		In 1 ml amps.[2]

[1] With 0.45% phenol.
[2] With 0.2% methyl- and propylparabens.

For complete prescribing information, refer to the Anticholinesterase Muscle Stimulants group monograph.

Indications

➤*Symptomatic control of myasthenia gravis:* In acute myasthenic crisis where difficulty in breathing and swallowing is present, use the parenteral form.

➤*Antidote for nondepolarizing neuromuscular blocking agents:* Antidote for nondepolarizing neuromuscular blocking agents (eg, tubocurarine, metocurine, gallamine or pancuronium) after surgery.

➤*Urinary retention:* Prevention and treatment of postoperative distention and urinary retention after mechanical obstruction has been excluded.

For additional indications refer to Neostigmine Methylsulfate monograph.

Administration and Dosage

➤*Symptomatic control of myasthenia gravis:*

Oral – 15 to 375 mg/day. Consider possibility of cholinergic crisis before exceeding dosage. The average dosage is 150 mg given over 24 hours; for children, 2 mg/kg/day orally divided every 3 to 4 hours. The interval between doses is of paramount importance; it must be individualized. Frequently, therapy is required day and night. Larger portions of the total daily dose may be given at times of greater fatigue (afternoon, mealtimes, etc).

Parenteral – Inject 1 ml of the 1:2000 solution (0.5 mg) SC or IM. Individualize subsequent doses. For children, 0.01 to 0.04 mg/kg/dose IM, IV or SC every 2 to 3 hours as needed.

➤*Antidote for nondepolarizing neuromuscular blocking agents:* When administered IV, also give atropine sulfate (0.6 to 1.2 mg) IV several minutes before the neostigmine. Give 0.5 to 2 mg neostigmine by slow IV injection and repeat as required; however, only in exceptional cases should total dose exceed 5 mg.

Infants – 0.025 to 0.1 mg/kg/dose (doses at low end of range probably are adequate), with atropine (0.01 to 0.04 mg/kg; 0.4 mg for each mg of neostigmine) or glycopyrrolate (0.004 to 0.02 mg/kg; 0.2 mg for each mg of neostigmine).

Children – 0.025 to 0.08 mg/kg/dose, with atropine (0.01 to 0.03 mg/kg; 0.4 mg for each mg of neostigmine) or glycopyrrolate (0.004 to 0.015 mg/kg; 0.2 mg for each mg of neostigmine).

Keep the patient well ventilated and maintain a patent airway until complete recovery. Administer drug when patient is being hyperventilated and the carbon dioxide level of blood is low.

Never administer in the presence of high concentrations of halothane or cyclopropane. In cardiac cases and severely ill patients, titrate the exact dose of neostigmine required using a peripheral nerve stimulator. With bradycardia, increase pulse rate to ≈ 80/minute with atropine before administering neostigmine.

➤*Prevention of postoperative distention and urinary retention:* One ml of the 1:4000 solution (0.25 mg) SC or IM as soon as possible after operation; repeat every 4 to 6 hours for 2 or 3 days.

➤*Treatment of postoperative distention:* One ml of the 1:2000 solution (0.5 mg) SC or IM as required.

➤*Treatment of urinary retention:* One ml of the 1:2000 solution (0.5 mg) SC or IM. If urination does not occur within an hour, catheterize. After the patient has voided, or the bladder has been emptied, continue the 0.5 mg injections every 3 hours for at least 5 injections.

PYRIDOSTIGMINE BROMIDE

Rx	Pyridostigmine Bromide (Various, eg, Geneva, Watson)	Tablets: 60 mg	Scored. In 100s and 500s.
Rx	Mestinon (ICN)		Lactose. (MESTINON 60 ICN). Scored. In 100s and 500s.
Rx	Mestinon (ICN)	Tablets, extended-release: 180 mg	(ICN-M180). Scored. In 30s.
Rx	Mestinon (ICN)	Syrup: 60 mg/5mL	Sucrose, sorbitol, 5% alcohol. Raspberry flavor. In 480 mL.
Rx	Mestinon (ICN)	Injection: 5 mg/mL[1]	In 2 mL amps.

[1] With 0.2% parabens and 0.02% sodium citrate.

For complete prescribing information, refer to the Anticholinesterase Muscle Stimulants group monograph.

Indications

➤*Myasthenia gravis:* Treatment of myasthenia gravis.

➤*Reversal of nondepolarizing muscle relaxants (IV only):* Reversal of nondepolarizing muscle relaxants such as curariform drugs and gallamine triethiodide.

➤*Unlabeled uses:*

Treatment of myasthenia gravis in children – 7 mg/kg/24 hours orally divided into 5 or 6 doses; 0.05 to 0.15 mg/kg/dose IM or IV every 4 to 6 hours.

Administration and Dosage

➤*Myasthenia gravis:*

Oral – Individualize dosage.

Adults: 600 mg/day (range, 60 to 1500 mg), spaced to provide maximum relief.

Extended-release tablets: 180 to 540 mg once or twice daily. Individual needs vary markedly. Use dosage intervals of at least 6 hours. Do not crush or chew. For optimum control, rapidly acting regular tablets or syrup also may be needed.

Parenteral – To supplement oral dosage preoperatively and postoperatively, during labor and postpartum, during myasthenic crisis or when oral therapy is impractical, give approximately 1/30 the oral dose, either IM or very slowly IV. Observe patient closely for cholinergic reactions, particularly if the IV route is used.

Neonates of myasthenic mothers may have transient difficulty in swallowing, sucking, and breathing. Injectable pyridostigmine may be indicated (by symptoms and use of the edrophonium test) until syrup can be taken. Dosage requirements range from 0.05 to 0.15 mg/kg IM. It is important to differentiate between cholinergic and myasthenic crises in neonates.

Pyridostigmine, given parenterally 1 hour before second stage labor is complete, enables patients to have adequate strength during labor and provides protection to infants in the immediate postnatal state.

➤*Reversal of nondepolarizing muscle relaxants:*

Parenteral – Give atropine sulfate (0.6 to 1.2 mg) IV immediately prior to pyridostigmine to minimize side effects. Pyridostigmine 10 or 20 mg IV is usually sufficient. Full recovery usually occurs in no more than 15 minutes, but at least 30 minutes may be required. Satisfactory reversal is evident by adequate voluntary respiration, respiratory measurements, and use of a peripheral nerve stimulator device. Keep patient well ventilated and maintain a patent airway until complete recovery of normal respiration.

Once satisfactory reversal has been attained, recurarization has not been reported. Failure of pyridostigmine injection to provide prompt (30 minutes or less) reversal may occur (eg, extreme debilitation, carcinomatosis, or with concomitant use of certain broad-spectrum antibiotics or anesthetic agents, notably ether).

➤*Storage/Stability:* Store at controlled room temperature 15° to 30°C (59° to 86°F).

GUANIDINE HCl

Rx	Guanidine HCl (Key)	Tablets: 125 mg	Mannitol. (KEY 74). In 100s.

Indications

➤*Myasthenic syndrome of Eaton-Lambert:* To reduce symptoms of muscle weakness and easy fatigability associated with myasthenic syndrome of Eaton-Lambert. Not indicated for myasthenia gravis.

➤*Unlabeled uses:* Guanidine has been used in the treatment of botulism.

Administration and Dosage

Initial dosage is 10 to 15 mg/kg/day in 3 or 4 divided doses; gradually increase to 35 mg/kg/day or up to the development of side effects. As individual tolerance is highly variable, the dosage must be carefully titrated. Continue the tolerable dose. Occasionally, removal of the primary neoplastic lesion may result in improvement of symptoms, permitting drug discontinuation.

➤*Storage/Stability:* Store between 15° and 30°C (59° and 86°F).

Actions

➤*Pharmacology:* Guanidine enhances the release of acetylcholine following a nerve impulse. It appears to slow the rates of depolarization and repolarization of muscle cell membranes.

Contraindications

Intolerance or allergy to guanidine.

Warnings

➤*Fatal bone marrow suppression:* Fatal bone marrow suppression, apparently dose-related, can occur. Follow baseline blood studies by frequent complete blood cell count (CBC) and differential counts. Discontinue use if bone marrow suppression occurs. Avoid concurrent therapy with other drugs that may cause bone marrow suppression.

➤*Pregnancy:* Safety for use during pregnancy has not been established. Use only when clearly needed and when potential benefits outweigh potential hazards to the fetus.

➤*Lactation:* Guanidine is excreted in breast milk; discontinue breast-feeding.

➤*Children:* Safety for use in children has not been established.

Precautions

➤*Renal effects:* Renal function may be affected in some patients. Perform regular urine examinations and serum creatinine determinations.

Adverse Reactions

➤*Cardiovascular:* Palpitations; tachycardia; atrial fibrillation; hypotension.

➤*CNS:* Paresthesia of lips, face, hands, feet; cold sensations in hands, feet; nervousness; lightheadedness; increased irritability; jitteriness; tremor; trembling sensations; ataxia; emotional lability; psychotic state; confusion; mood changes; hallucinations.

➤*Dermatologic:* Rash; flushing or pink complexion; folliculitis; petechiae; purpura; ecchymoses; sweating; skin eruptions; dryness and scaling of the skin.

➤*GI:* Dry mouth; anorexia; gastric irritation; nausea; diarrhea; abdominal cramping. GI side effects may preclude use.

➤*Hematologic:* Bone marrow depression with anemia, leukopenia, and thrombocytopenia (see Warnings).

➤*Hepatic:* Abnormal LFTs.

➤*Renal:* Creatinine elevation; uremia; chronic interstitial nephritis; renal tubular necrosis; acute interstitial nephritis.

➤*Miscellaneous:* Sore throat; fever.

Overdosage

➤*Symptoms:* Mild GI disorders (eg, anorexia, increased peristalsis, diarrhea) are early warnings that tolerance is being exceeded. These symptoms may be relieved by atropine, but consider dosage reduction. Slight numbness and/or tingling of the lips and fingertips has occurred shortly after taking a guanidine dose; this is not an indication to discontinue treatment or reduce dosage.

Severe intoxication is characterized by nervous hyperirritability, fibrillary tremors and convulsive contractions of muscle, salivation, vomiting, diarrhea, hypoglycemia, and circulatory disturbances.

➤*Treatment:* Calcium gluconate IV may control the neuromuscular and convulsive symptoms and relieve other toxic manifestations. Atropine is more effective than calcium in relieving the GI symptoms, circulatory disturbances, and changes in blood sugar.

Patient Information

Notify physician if sore throat, fever, skin rash, flushing, GI upset (eg, nausea, diarrhea), nervousness, or tremor occurs.

DISULFIRAM

Rx　　**Antabuse** (Odyssey)　　　　　　　**Tablets:** 250 mg　　　　　　Lactose. (OP 706). In 100s.

<table>
<tr><td colspan="2" align="center">**WARNING**</td></tr>
<tr><td colspan="2">Never give to a patient in a state of alcohol intoxication or without the patient's full knowledge. Instruct the patient's relatives accordingly.</td></tr>
</table>

Indications

An aid in the management of selected chronic alcoholics who want to remain in a state of enforced sobriety so that supportive and psychotherapeutic treatment may be applied to best advantage.

Administration and Dosage

➤*Approved by the FDA:* December 8, 1983.

Do NOT administer until the patient has abstained from alcohol for at least 12 hours.

➤*Initial dosage schedule:* Administer a maximum of 500 mg/day in a single dose for 1 to 2 weeks. Although usually taken in the morning, if a sedative effect is experienced, take at bedtime or decrease dosage.

➤*Maintenance regimen:* The average maintenance dose is 250 mg/day (range, 125 to 500 mg), not to exceed 500 mg/day. NOTE: Occasional disulfiram patients report that they are able to drink alcoholic beverages with impunity and without any symptomatology. Such patients must be presumed to be disposing of their tablets without actually taking them. Until such patients are observed reliably taking their daily tablets (preferably crushed and well-mixed with liquid), do not assume that disulfiram is ineffective.

➤*Duration of therapy:* Continue use until the patient is fully recovered socially, and a basis for permanent self-control is established. Maintenance therapy may be required for months or even years.

➤*Trial with alcohol:* The test reaction has been largely abandoned. Do not administer a test reaction to a patient older than 50 years of age. A clear, detailed, and convincing description of the reaction is felt to be sufficient in most cases.

Where a test reaction is deemed necessary, the suggested procedure is: After the first 1 to 2 weeks of therapy with 500 mg/day, a drink of 15 mL of 100 proof whiskey or equivalent is taken slowly. This test dose may be repeated once only so that total dose does not exceed 30 mL whiskey. Once a reaction develops, stop alcohol consumption. Only perform such tests when the patient is hospitalized and facilities, including oxygen, are available.

➤*Management of disulfiram-alcohol reaction:* In severe reactions, institute supportive measures to restore blood pressure and treat shock. Other recommendations include: Oxygen or carbogen (95% oxygen and 5% carbon dioxide), vitamin C IV in massive doses (1 g), and ephedrine sulfate. Antihistamines have also been used IV. Monitor potassium levels, particularly in patients on digitalis, since hypokalemia has been reported.

➤*Storage/Stability:* Store at controlled room temperature at 15° to 30°C (59° to 86°F)

Actions

➤*Pharmacology:* Disulfiram produces a sensitivity to alcohol which results in a highly unpleasant reaction when the patient under treatment ingests even small amounts of alcohol. Disulfiram blocks oxidation of alcohol at the acetaldehyde stage by inhibiting aldehyde dehydrogenase. The concentration of acetaldehyde in the blood may be 5 to 10 times higher than that achieved during normal alcohol metabolism. Accumulation of acetaldehyde produces the disulfiram-alcohol reaction (see Warnings). This reaction, which is proportional to the dosage of both disulfiram and alcohol, persists as long as alcohol is being metabolized. Disulfiram does not influence alcohol elimination. Prolonged administration of disulfiram does not produce tolerance; the longer a patient remains on therapy, the more sensitive the patient becomes to alcohol.

➤*Pharmacokinetics:*

Absorption – Disulfiram is slowly absorbed from the GI tract. The average time to reach maximum plasma concentrations were 8 to 10 hours for disulfiram and its metabolites.

Metabolism/Excretion – Disulfiram is rapidly metabolized to diethyldithiocarbamate which is then metabolized in the liver to its glucoronide and methyl ester and to diethylamine, carbon disulfide, and sulfate ions. Disulfiram is slowly eliminated from the body. The metabolites are primarily excreted in the urine and carbon disulfide is exhaled in the breath. Ingestion of alcohol may produce unpleasant symptoms for 1 to 2 weeks after the last dose of disulfiram.

Contraindications

Severe myocardial disease or coronary occlusion; psychoses; hypersensitivity to disulfiram or to other thiuram derivatives used in pesticides and rubber vulcanization; patients receiving or who have recently received metronidazole, paraldehyde, alcohol, or alcohol-containing preparations (eg, cough syrups, tonics).

Warnings

➤*Hepatic Toxicity:* Hepatic toxicity including hepatic failure resulting in transplantation or death has been reported. Severe and sometimes fatal hepatitis associated with disulfiram therapy may develop even after many months of therapy. Hepatic toxicity has occurred in patients with or without prior history of abnormal liver function. Advise patients to immediately notify their physician of any early symptoms of hepatitis (eg, fatigue, weakness, malaise, anorexia, nausea, vomiting, jaundice, dark urine).

➤*Administration:* Never administer to an intoxicated patient or without the patient's knowledge (see Warning Box). The patient must be fully informed of the disulfiram-alcohol reaction. The patient must be strongly cautioned against surreptitious drinking while taking the drug, and fully aware of the possible consequences. Warn patient to avoid alcohol in disguised forms (eg, in sauces, vinegars, cough mixtures, aftershave lotions, back rubs). Also, warn that reactions may occur with alcohol up to 14-days after ingesting disulfiram.

➤*Disulfiram-alcohol reaction:* Disulfiram plus alcohol, even small amounts, produces flushing, throbbing in head and neck, throbbing headaches, respiratory difficulty, nausea, copious vomiting, sweating, thirst, chest pain, palpitations, dyspnea, hyperventilation, tachycardia, hypotension, syncope, marked uneasiness, weakness, vertigo, blurred vision, and confusion. In severe reactions there may be respiratory depression, cardiovascular collapse, arrhythmias, myocardial infarction, acute congestive heart failure, unconsciousness, convulsions, and death. The intensity of the reaction is proportional to the amounts of disulfiram and alcohol ingested. Mild reactions may occur in the sensitive individual when the blood alcohol concentration is as low as 5 to 10 mg/dL. Symptoms are fully developed at 50 mg/dL, and unconsciousness usually results at 125 to 150 mg/dL. The duration of the reaction varies from 30 to 60 minutes to several hours.

➤*Concomitant conditions:* Because of the possibility of an accidental disulfiram-alcohol reaction, use with caution in patients with diabetes mellitus, hypothyroidism, epilepsy, cerebral damage, chronic and acute nephritis, or hepatic cirrhosis or insufficiency.

➤*Carcinogenesis:* In rats, simultaneous ingestion of disulfiram and nitrate in the diet for 78 weeks has been reported to cause tumors, and it has been suggested that disulfiram may react with nitrites in the rat stomach to form a nitrosamine, which is tumorigenic. Disulfiram alone in the rats diet did not lead to such tumors. The relevance of this finding to humans is not known at this time.

➤*Hypersensitivity reactions:* Evaluate patients with a history of rubber contact dermatitis for hypersensitivity to thiuram derivatives before administering disulfiram. Refer to General Management of Acute Hypersensitivity Reactions.

➤*Pregnancy: Category C.* Safety for use during pregnancy has not been established.

➤*Lactation:* It is not known whether this drug is excreted in human milk. Do not give disulfiram to breastfeeding mothers.

➤*Children:* Safety and efficacy in pediatric patients have not been established.

Precautions

➤*Monitoring:* Perform baseline and follow-up LFTs (10 to 14 days) to detect hepatic dysfunction resulting from therapy. Perform a CBC and serum chemistries.

➤*Dependence and addiction:* Alcoholism may accompany or be followed by dependence on narcotics or sedatives. Barbiturates have been coadministered with disulfiram without untoward effects, but consider the possibility of initiating a new abuse.

➤*Ethylene dibromide:* Do not expose patients to ethylene dibromide or its vapors. This precaution is based on preliminary results of animal research which suggest a toxic interaction between inhaled ethylene dibromide and ingested disulfiram results in a higher incidence of tumors and mortality in rats.

Drug Interactions

Disulfiram Drug Interactions			
Precipitant drug	Object drug*		Description
Isoniazid	Disulfiram	↑	Observe patients receiving isoniazid and disulfiram for the appearance of unsteady gait or marked changes in behavior; discontinue disulfiram or reduce the dose if such signs appear.
Metronidazole	Disulfiram	↑	Patients may exhibit acute toxic psychosis or confusional state when taking metronidazole in combination with disulfiram, requiring discontinuation of 1 or both of the agents.

DISULFIRAM

Disulfiram Drug Interactions			
Precipitant drug	Object drug*		Description
Disulfiram	Alcohol	↑	Disulfiram causes a severe alcohol-intolerance reaction (eg, flushing and increased respiration, pulse rate, and cardiac output). Death has been reported. Avoid alcohol in all forms. See Warnings.
Disulfiram	Benzodiazepines	↑	Disulfiram decreases the plasma clearance of benzodiazepines metabolized by oxidation, possibly resulting in increased CNS depressant actions. When benzodiazepine therapy is indicated, use oxazepam, temazepam, or lorazepam since they are metabolized by glucuronidation.
Disulfiram	Caffeine	↑	Cardiovascular and CNS stimulation effects of caffeine may be increased by disulfiram.
Disulfiram	Chlorzoxazone	↑	Disulfiram inhibits the hepatic metabolism of chlorzoxazone. Derease the dose of chlorzoxazone if increased CNS depression occur.
Disulfiram	Cocaine	↑	Cardiovascular side effects of cocaine may be increased when used concurrently with disulfiram.
Disulfiram	Hydantoins (eg, phenytoin)	↑	Serum hydantoin levels may be increased by disulfiram, resulting in an increase in the pharmacologic and toxic effects. Monitor hydantoin levels and adjust the dosage as needed.
Disulfiram	Theophyllines	↑	Disulfiram may inhibit the metabolism of the theophylline, thus increasing its effects. Monitor the theophylline level and adjust dose accordingly.
Disulfiram	Tricyclic antidepressants	↑	Tricyclic antidepressants and disulfiram coadministration may result in acute organic brain syndrome. The bioavailability of the antidepressant may also be increased.

Disulfiram Drug Interactions			
Precipitant drug	Object drug*		Description
Disulfiram	Warfarin	↑	Disulfiram may increase the anticoagulant effect of warfarin. Monitor prothrombin time and adjust the warfarin dosage as necessary.

* ↑ = Object drug increased.

Adverse Reactions

➤*CNS:* Drowsiness; fatigue; headache. Psychotic reactions have been noted, often attributable to high dosage, combined toxicity (metronidazole or isoniazid), or to the unmasking of underlying psychoses.

Neurologic – Peripheral neuropathy; peripheral neuritis; polyneuritis; optic neuritis.

➤*Dermatologic:* Occasional skin eruptions are, as a rule, readily controlled by antihistamines; acneform eruptions; allergic dermatitis.

➤*GI:* Metallic or garlic-like aftertaste, usually during the first 2 weeks of therapy.

➤*Hepatic:* Multiple cases of cholestatic and fulminant hepatitis as well as hepatic failure resulting in transplantation or death have been associated with disulfiram use.

➤*Miscellaneous:* Impotence.

Patient Information

Never use in intoxicated individuals or without an individual's knowledge.

Do not take for at least 12 hours after drinking alcohol. A reaction may occur for up to 2 weeks after disulfiram has been stopped.

Avoid alcohol in all forms. This includes the following: Alcoholic beverages, vinegars, many liquid medications (including prescription and nonprescription products), some sauces, aftershave lotions, colognes, liniments, and others.

Always read product labels or ask your pharmacist about alcohol content of all liquid medications before choosing one.

May cause drowsiness. Use caution while driving or performing other tasks requiring alertness.

The alcohol-disulfiram reaction can have serious effects on the heart and respiratory systems.

Always carry identification indicating you are taking disulfiram. Include the phone numbers of your doctor or the medical facility that should be contacted in case of reaction.

Indications

As an aid to smoking cessation for the relief of nicotine withdrawal symptoms. Use as part of a comprehensive behavioral smoking-cessation program.

▶*Unlabeled uses:* In 2 children, use of nicotine polacrilex gum and haloperidol improved symptoms (eg, tics) of Tourette's syndrome. Further study is needed.

Administration and Dosage

Withdrawal from nicotine in addicted individuals is characterized by craving, nervousness, restlessness, irritability, mood lability, anxiety, drowsiness, sleep disturbances, impaired concentration, increased appetite, minor somatic complaints (headache, myalgia, constipation, fatigue), and weight gain. Nicotine toxicity is characterized by nausea, abdominal pain, vomiting, diarrhea, diaphoresis, flushing, dizziness, disturbed hearing/vision, confusion, weakness, palpitations, altered respiration, and hypotension.

The following table includes dosing, duration of therapy, and availability information for nicotine replacement therapy products.

Nicotine Replacement Pharmacotherapy			
Type of therapy	Dosage	Duration	Availability
Gum	< 24 cigarettes/day: 2 mg gum up to 24 pieces/day	up to 12 weeks	*otc*
	> 25 cigarettes/day: 4 mg gum up to 24 pieces/day		
Inhaler	6 to 16 cartridges/day	up to 6 months	*Rx only*
Transdermal patch	21 mg/24 hr 14 mg/24 hr 7 mg/24 hr	4 to 6 weeks then 2 weeks then 2 weeks	*otc*
	15 mg/16 hr	6 weeks	
Nasal spray	8 to 40 doses/day	3 to 6 months	*Rx only*

Actions

▶*Pharmacology:* Nicotine, the chief alkaloid in tobacco products, binds stereoselectively to acetylcholine receptors at the autonomic ganglia, in the adrenal medulla, at neuromuscular junctions, and in the brain. Two types of CNS effects are believed to be the basis of nicotine's positively reinforcing properties. A stimulating effect, exerted mainly in the cortex via the locus ceruleus, produces increased alertness and cognitive performance. A "reward" effect via the "pleasure system" in the brain is exerted in the limbic system. At low doses the stimulant effects predominate, while at high doses the reward effects predominate. Intermittent IV administration of nicotine activates neurohormonal pathways, releasing acetylcholine, norepinephrine, dopamine, serotonin, vasopressin, beta-endorphin, growth hormone, and adrenocorticotropic hormone (ACTH).

The cardiovascular effects of nicotine include peripheral vasoconstriction, tachycardia, and elevated blood pressure. Acute and chronic tolerance to nicotine develops from smoking tobacco or ingesting nicotine preparations. Acute tolerance (a reduction in response for a given dose) develops rapidly (< 1 hour), but at distinct rates for different physiologic effects (eg, skin temperature, heart rate, subjective effects). Withdrawal symptoms, such as cigarette craving, can be reduced in some individuals by plasma nicotine levels lower than those for smoking.

Nicotine polacrilex contains nicotine bound to an ion exchange resin in a chewing gum base. The **nicotine transdermal system** is a multilayered unit containing nicotine as the active agent that provides systemic delivery of nicotine for up to 24 hours (*Nicotrol*, up to 16 hours) following its application to intact skin.

▶*Pharmacokinetics:*

Absorption/Distribution –

Nicotine: Nicotine as tobacco smoke is absorbed rapidly through the lungs. Nicotine is a weak base; absorption through mucous membranes depends on pH. Nicotine gum is buffered at an alkaline pH to increase absorption through the buccal mucosa. The volume of distribution of IV nicotine is ≈ 2 to 3 L/kg. Plasma protein binding is < 5%.

Gum: The nicotine is bound to an ion exchange resin and is released only during chewing; nicotine will not be released in significant amounts if the gum is swallowed. The blood level of nicotine will depend upon the vigor and duration of chewing. The trough level of nicotine obtained by smoking 1 cigarette/hour is ≈ 2 times that of chewing one 2 mg piece of gum.

Transdermal: Following application, ≈ 68% of the nicotine released from the system enters the systemic circulation. The remainder of the nicotine released from the system is lost via evaporation from the edge. All systems are labeled by the actual amount of nicotine absorbed by the patient.

After application, plasma concentrations rise rapidly, plateau within 2 to 12 hours, and then slowly decline until the system is removed, after which they decline more rapidly. Following the second daily application, steady-state plasma nicotine concentrations are achieved and are on average 25% to 30% higher compared with single-dose applications.

Plasma nicotine concentrations are proportional to dose and are similar for all sites of application on the upper body and upper outer arm.

Half-hourly smoking of cigarettes produces average plasma nicotine concentrations of ≈ 44 ng/mL. Average plasma nicotine concentrations from transdermal nicotine are ≈ 5 to 17 ng/mL.

Inhaler: Most of the nicotine released from the inhaler is deposited in the mouth with only a fraction of the dose released (< 5%) reaching the lower respiratory tract. Eight deep inhalations over 20 minutes releases on average 4 mg of nicotine content from each cartridge, of which 2 mg is systemically absorbed. Peak plasma concentrations are typically reached within 15 minutes after inhalation ends. Absorption of nicotine through the buccal mucosa is relatively slow. Nicotine arterial plasma concentration peaks and declines seen with cigarette smoking are not achieved with the inhaler. After use of a single inhaler, the arterial nicotine concentration rises slowly to an average of 6 ng/mL in contrast to those of a cigarette, which increase rapidly and reach a mean C_{max} of ≈ 49 ng/mL within 5 minutes.

Intermittent use of the nicotine inhaler typically produces nicotine plasma levels of 6 to 8 ng/mL, corresponding to ≈ 33% of those achieved with cigarette smoking.

Nasal spray: Following administration of 2 sprays of nicotine nasal spray (1 mg), ≈ 53% enters the systemic circulation. Plasma concentrations of nicotine rise rapidly, reaching maximum venous concentrations of 12 ng/mL in 15 minutes. The apparent absorption half-life of nicotine is ≈ 3 minutes. There is a wide variation among subjects in the plasma nicotine concentrations for the spray. Peak nicotine concentrations similar to whose seen after smoking 1 cigarette (17 ng/mL) were seen in 20% of subjects after a 1 mg dose of spray.

Metabolism/Excretion –

Nicotine: Nicotine is rapidly and extensively metabolized by the liver. More than 20 metabolites have been identified, all of which are believed to be less active than the parent compound. The primary plasma metabolite, cotinine, has a half-life of 15 to 20 hours, and concentrations that exceed nicotine by 10-fold. About 10% of the nicotine absorbed is excreted unchanged in the urine. This may be increased up to 30% with high urinary flow rates and urine pH < 5. The half-life of nicotine averages 1 to 2 hours. Nicotine accumulates in the body over 6 to 9 hours of regular smoking. Thus, smoking results in a nicotine exposure that lasts 24 hours a day. Persistence of nicotine in the brain results in changes in nicotinic receptors in the brain. Changes in receptor numbers or function are presumably the substrate for nicotine withdrawal syndrome.

Transdermal: Following removal of transdermal nicotine, plasma nicotine concentrations decline exponentially with an apparent mean half-life of 3 to 4 hours due to continued absorption from the skin depot. Most nonsmoking patients will have nondetectable nicotine concentrations in 10 to 12 hours.

Nicotine Pharmacokinetics					
Parameter	Smoking	Gum	Transdermal	Nasal spray	Inhaler
Time to peak levels (hours)	ND[1]	0.25 to 0.5	2 to 12	0.25	0.25
Peak plasma level (ng/mL)	44	5 to 10	5 to 17	12	6
Half-life (hours)	15 to 20[2]	3 to 4	3 to 4	1 to 2	ND

[1] No data.
[2] Refers to cotinine, the primary plasma metabolite of nicotine.

▶*Clinical trials:*

Nicotine replacement therapy – In a randomized, comparative trial of smokers averaging ≥ 10 cigarettes/day, who received nicotine replacement therapy in the form of 2 or 4 mg **gum**, a 15 mg **transdermal patch**, a **nasal spray**, or an **inhaler**, compliance was 38%, 82%, 15%, and 11%, respectively. The patch was easiest to use, with the inhaler, followed by the spray as the most embarrassing to use. There were no significant differences between products with regard to their effect on withdrawal symptoms, difficulty not smoking, urges to smoke at week 1, or body weight gain at week 12. At week 12, abstinence rates for the gum, patch, nasal spray, and inhaler were 20%, 21%, 24%, and 24%, respectively.

In an analysis of the results of 40 trials comparing 2 mg of gum, 4 mg of gum, and transdermal patch, efficacy was highly significant for both gum and patches. Nicotine gum (2 mg) had an overall efficacy of 6%, greater in self-referred than in invited subjects (11% vs 3%). Efficacy in "high dependence" smokers (as assessed by a questionnaire) was 16% (range, 7% to 25%), but in "low dependence" smokers there was no significant effect. The 4 mg gum was effective in ≈ 33% of "high dependence" smokers. The efficacy of the transdermal patch (9% overall) was less strongly related to nicotine dependence, perhaps because the patch cannot deliver a bolus of nicotine to satisfy craving.

In a review of trials that directly compared 4 vs 2 mg of gum in highly dependent smokers, the odds ratio of abstinence found a significant benefit in favor of 4 mg gum (odds ratio 2.67, 95% confidence interval 1.69 to 4.22).

Contraindications

Hypersensitivity to nicotine or any components of the products, including menthol.

Warnings

➤*Nicotine risks:* Nicotine from any source can be toxic and addictive. Smoking causes lung disease, cancer, and heart disease, and may adversely affect pregnant women or the fetus. For any smoker, with or without concomitant disease or pregnancy, the risk of nicotine replacement in a smoking cessation program should be weighed against the hazard of continued smoking, and the likelihood of achieving cessation of smoking without nicotine replacement.

➤*Renal/Hepatic function impairment:* Because nicotine is extensively metabolized and its total system clearance is dependent on liver blood flow, anticipate some influence of hepatic impairment on drug kinetics (reduced clearance). Only severe renal impairment should affect clearance of nicotine or its metabolites from circulation.

➤*Carcinogenesis:* Nicotine does not apear to be a carcinogen in laboratory animals. Nicotine and its metabolites increased the incidences of tumors in the cheek pouches of hamsters and forestomach of rats, respectively, when given in combination with tumor-initiators. One study, which could not be replicated, suggested that cotinine, the primary metabolite of nicotine, may cause lymphoreticular sarcoma in the large intestine of rats.

➤*Fertility impairment:* In rats and rabbits, implantation can be delayed or inhibited by a reduction in DNA synthesis that appears to be caused by nicotine. Studies have shown a decrease in litter size in rats treated with nicotine during gestation.

➤*Elderly:* Nicotine **inhaler** and **nasal spray** therapy appeared to be as effective in elderly patients ≥ 60 years of age as in younger smokers.

➤*Pregnancy:* Category *D* (**inhaler, spray, transdermal patch**); Category *C* (**gum**). Tobacco smoke contains nicotine, hydrogen cyanide, and carbon monoxide. The harmful effects of cigarette smoking on maternal and fetal health are clearly established. These include low birth weight (21% to 39% of all infants), an increased risk of spontaneous abortion, increased perinatal mortality, and decreased placental perfusion. Smoking causes a decrease in the oxygen-carrying capacity of hemoglobin when carbon monoxide passes through the placenta. Nicotine causes vasoconstriction and decreased placenta blood flow. Smoking interferes with the body's ability to process essential vitamins and minerals, resulting in decreased intestinal synthesis of vitamin B_{12}, calcium loss from bones, and decreased usage of vitamin C. In general, smokers have a nutrient-poor diet. Smoking during pregnancy increases the risk of ectopic pregnancy, spontaneous abortion, preterm birth, premature rupture of membranes, placenta previa, abruptio placenta, and chorioamnionitis.

No association has been found between maternal smoking and congenital anomalies; however, nicotine and cotinine are found in higher concentrations in infants whose mothers smoke.

Second-hand smoking is an increasing concern for its potential effects on infants and siblings. There is an association between maternal smoking and sudden infant death syndrome, but it is unclear whether it is from in utero exposure or postnatal passive exposure, or both.

Nicotine was shown to produce skeletal abnormalities in the offspring of mice when toxic doses were given to the dams.

A nicotine bolus (up to 2 mg/kg) to pregnant rhesus monkeys caused acidosis, hypercarbia, and hypotension (fetal and maternal concentrations were ≈ 20 times those achieved after smoking 1 cigarette in 5 minutes). Fetal breathing movements were reduced in the fetal lamb after IV injection of 0.25 mg/kg nicotine to the ewe (equivalent to smoking 1 cigarette every 20 seconds for 5 minutes). Uterine blood flow was reduced ≈ 30% after infusion of 0.1 mcg/kg/min nicotine to pregnant rhesus monkeys (equivalent to smoking ≈ 6 cigarettes every minute for 20 minutes).

The inhaler and nasal spray do not deliver hydrogen cyanide and carbon monoxide. However, because they do deliver nicotine, it is presumed that the inhaler and the nasal spray can cause fetal harm when administered to a pregnant woman. The effect of nicotine delivered by the inhaler and nasal spray has not been examined in pregnancy and the specific effects of nicotine inhaler and nasal spray therapy on fetal development are unknown. Spontaneous abortion during nicotine replacement therapy has been reported; as with smoking, nicotine as a contributing factor cannot be excluded. Pregnant smokers should be encouraged to attempt cessation using education and behavioral interventions before using pharmacological approaches. If the inhaler or nasal spray are used during pregnancy, or if the patient becomes pregnant while using it, the patient should be apprised of the potential hazard to the fetus. Inhaler and spray therapy should be used during pregnancy only if the likelihood of smoking cessation justifies the potential risk of using it by the pregnant patient who might continue to smoke.

➤*Lactation:* Nicotine and cotinine pass freely into breast milk up to 2 hours after maternal smoking; the milk to plasma ratio averages 2.9. Nicotine is absorbed orally. An infant has the ability to clear nicotine by hepatic first-pass clearance; however, the efficiency of removal is probably lowest at birth. Nicotine concentrations in milk can be expected to be lower with **inhaler** and **nasal spray** nicotine therapy when used as directed than with cigarette smoking, as maternal plasma nicotine concentrations are generally reduced with nicotine replacement. Decide whether to discontinue nursing or to discontinue the drug, weighing the risk of exposure of the infant to nicotine from replacement therapy against the risks associated with the infant's exposure to nicotine from continued smoking by the mother and from nicotine therapy alone or in combination with continued smoking.

➤*Children:* Safety and efficacy in children/adolescents < 18 years of age who smoke have not been evaluated.

Cigarette smoke contains many compounds including carbon monoxide, dioxin, cyanide, and cadmium. Studies have shown residual effects beyond the neonatal period, including growth deficits, and deficiencies in intellectual, emotional, and behavioral development. These manifest as poor auditory responsiveness, fine motor tremors, hypertonicity, and decreases in verbal comprehension.

The amounts of nicotine that are tolerated by adult smokers can produce symptoms of poisoning and could prove fatal if inhaled, ingested, or bucally absorbed by children or pets. An inhaler or nasal spray cartridge container contains ≈ 60% (6 mg) of its initial drug content when discarded. Therefore, caution patients to keep the used and unused systems out of the reach of children and pets.

Precautions

➤*General:* Urge the patient to stop smoking completely when initiating nicotine replacement therapy. Inform patients that if they continue to smoke while using the product, they may experience adverse effects due to peak nicotine levels higher than those experienced from smoking alone. If there is a clinically significant increase in cardiovascular or other effects attributable to nicotine, the treatment should be discontinued. Physicians should anticipate that concomitant medications may need dosage adjustment (see Drug Interactions). Sustained use (> 6 months) of inhaler or nasal spray by patients who stop smoking has not been studied and is not recommended (see Drug Abuse and Dependence).

➤*Bronchospastic disease:* The **inhaler** has not been specifically studied in asthma or chronic pulmonary disease. Nicotine is an airway irritant and might cause bronchospasm. The inhaler should be used with caution in patients with bronchospastic disease. Other forms of nicotine replacement might be preferable in patients with severe bronchospastic airway disease.

Asthma, bronchospasm, and reactive airway disease exacerbation of bronchospasm in patients with pre-existing asthma has been reported. Use of the **nasal spray** in patients with severe reactive airway disease is not recommended.

➤*Nasal disorders:* Use of the **nasal spray** is not recommended in patients with known chronic nasal disorders (eg, allergy, rhinitis, nasal polyps, sinusitis) because such use has not been adequately studied. The effect of the nasal spray on the nasal mucosa topical application of either nicotine or tobacco products is irritating to the nasal mucosa and physicians should consider both the risks and benefits to the patient before initiating or continuing nasal spray therapy. The effect of the nasal spray on the nasal mucosa was studied in 39 cigarette smokers who used the nasal spray for 1 month. When compared with baseline, random biopsies taken after 4 weeks of treatment revealed 1 patient with persistence of pre-existing dysplasia and 1 patient with a newly found dysplasia. In both, dysplasia was not seen after a recovery period of 8 weeks. Forty-two patients who used the nasal spray for > 6 months underwent follow-up ear, nose, and throat examinations 1 to 3 months after discontinuing the use of the spray. Many reported local irritant effects of the spray during spray use, but none showed persistent mucosal injury that the examining physician could attribute to use of the product. The clinical significance of these findings is not known, but extended use of the product > 6 months is not recommended.

➤*Cardiovascular:* Weigh the benefits against the risks of nicotine in patients with certain cardiovascular and peripheral vascular diseases. Specifically, screen and evaluate patients with coronary heart disease (history of MI or angina pectoris), serious cardiac arrhythmias, or vasospastic diseases (Buerger's disease, Prinzmetal variant angina, Raynaud's phenomena) before nicotine is prescribed. There have been occasional reports of tachycardia and palpitations associated with nicotine replacement therapy; therefore, if cardiovascular symptoms occur, discontinue the drug. Generally, do not use during the immediate post-MI period, nor in patients with serious arrhythmias or with severe or worsening angina pectoris.

Accelerated hypertension – Nicotine therapy constitutes a risk factor for development of malignant hypertension in patients with accelerated hypertension. **Inhaler** therapy should be used with caution in these patients and only when the benefits of including nicotine replacement in a smoking cessation program outweigh the risks.

➤*Endocrine:* Because of the action of nicotine on the adrenal medulla (release of catecholamines), use with caution in patients with hyperthyroidism, pheochromocytoma, or insulin-dependent diabetes.

➤*Oral/GI:* Because nicotine delays healing in peptic ulcer disease, use in patients with active or inactive peptic ulcer only when benefits of including nicotine in a smoking cessation program outweigh risks.

➤*Dental:* When used over an extended time, nicotine **gum** may cause severe occlusal stress due to its heavier viscosity than ordinary chewing gum. Nicotine gum may cause loosening of inlays or fillings, can stick to dentures, and cause damage to oral mucosa and natural teeth. Hard, sugarless candy between doses of gum is recommended to help provide oral stimulation required by some patients. Temporol mandibular joint dysfunction and pain have also been reported with excessive chewing.

➤*Drug abuse and dependence:*

Inhaler – The nicotine inhaler is likely to have a low abuse potential based on slower absorption, smaller fluctuations, and lower blood levels of nicotine when compared with cigarettes. However, nicotine withdrawal symptoms were noted in clinical trials during tapering and discontinuation of the nicotine inhaler. Dependence can occur from transference of tobacco-related nicotine dependence to the inhaler. The use of the inhaler for > 6 months is not recommended. Encourage patients to withdraw gradually from therapy after 3 months of usage to minimize the risk of dependence. If necessary, dose reduction can be gradually achieved over a 6- to 12-week period.

Nasal spray – Nicotine nasal spray has a dependence potential intermediate between other nicotine-based therapies and cigarettes. The nasal spray is distinct from other nicotine-based smoking cessation therapies in its greater speed of onset, greater capacity of self-titration of dose, and frequent, rapid fluctuations of plasma nicotine concentration. Dependence on nicotine nasal spray occurred during clinical trials. Feelings of dependency were reported by 32% of active spray users and 13% of placebo spray users. Such dependence may represent transference of tobacco-related nicotine dependence to the nasal spray. Some patients (15% to 20%) used the active spray for longer than recommended (6 to 12 months) and 5% used a higher dose than recommended. Some patients experienced anxiety after discontinuing the spray and some reported craving the spray rather than cigarettes.

Drug Interactions

Smoking cessation, with or without nicotine substitutes, may alter response to concomitant medication in ex-smokers.

Cigarette smoking is an inducer of CYP1A2 enzymes, the primary mechanism for drug interactions. For drugs whose metabolism is stimulated by enzyme inducers, the dose may need to be increased upon initiation of inducer (smoking) therapy and decreased when the inducer (smoking) is discontinued.

Smoking Drug Interactions			
Precipitant drug	Object drug*		Description
Smoking	Alcohol	↓	May decrease the rate of absorption and peak serum concentration.
Smoking	Benzodiazepines (diazepam, chlordiazepoxide)	↓	Smoking may decrease sedation and drowsiness probably by CNS stimulation.
Smoking	Beta adrenergic blockers	↓	Sympathetic activation by nicotine may decrease end-organ responsiveness. Beta blockers may be less effective for blood pressure and heart rate control in smokers.
Smoking	Caffeine Clozapine Fluvoxamine Olanzapine Tacrine Theophylline	↓	Smoking is an inducer of CYP1A2 enzymes. It can increase clearance and decrease AUC, mean plasma concentration, half-life, and volume of distribution.
Smoking	Clorazepate Lidocaine (oral)	↓	Smoking can decrease AUC.
Smoking	Estradiol	↓	Smoking can increase 2-hydroxylation with possible antiestrogenic effects.
Smoking	Flecanide Imipramine	↓	Can increase clearance and decrease serum concentrations.
Smoking	Heparin	↓	Smoking can increase clearance and decrease half-life. The smoker may require higher doses of heparin.
Smoking	Insulin	↓	Smoking can cause decreased SC absorption resulting in higher insulin requirements for smokers.
Smoking	Mexiletine	↓	Smoking may increase oral clearance and decrease half-life.
Smoking	Opioids (dextropropoxyphene, pentazocine)	↓	Smoking can decrease the analgesic effect; therefore, smokers may require higher doses for analgesia.

Smoking Drug Interactions			
Precipitant drug	Object drug*		Description
Smoking	Propranolol	↓	Smoking can increase oral clearance.
Smoking Nicotine	Catecholamines Cortisol	↑	Smoking and nicotine can increase circulating cortisol and catecholamines. Therapy with adrenergic agonists or adrenergic blockers may need to be adjusted upon changes in nicotine therapy or smoking status.

* ↑ = Object drug increased. ↓ = Object drug decreased.

➤*Nasal spray:* The extent of absorption and peak plasma concentration is slightly reduced in patients with the common cold/rhinitis. In addition, the time to peak concentration is prolonged. The use of a nasal vasoconstrictor such as xylometazoline in patients with rhinitis will further prolong the time to peak.

Adverse Reactions

Assessment of adverse events in patients who participated in controlled clinical trials is complicated by the occurrence of signs and symptoms of nicotine withdrawal in some patients and nicotine excess in others. The incidence of adverse events is compounded by the many minor complaints that smokers commonly have, continued smoking by many patients, and the local irritation from the active drug and placebo.

➤*Inhaler:*

Nicotine Inhaler Adverse Reactions (%)		
Adverse reaction	Drug	Placebo
Local irritation (mouth, throat)	40	18
Coughing	32	12
Rhinitis	23	16
Dyspepsia	18	9
Headache	26	15

Local – Taste complaints, pain in jaw and neck, tooth disorders, sinusitis (≥ 3%).

Miscellaneous – Influenza-like symptoms, pain, back pain, allergy, paresthesias, flatulence, fever (≥ 3%).

   Withdrawal: Dizziness, anxiety, sleep disorder, depression, withdrawal syndrome, drug dependence, fatigue, myalgia (≥ 3%).

   Nicotine-related: Nausea, diarrhea, hiccough (≥ 3%).

   Smoking-related: Chest discomfort, bronchitis, hypertension (≥ 3%).

➤*Nasal spray:*

   Common smoker complaints: Chest tightness, dyspepsia, paresthesias in limbs, constipation, and stomatitis.

   Withdrawal symptoms: Anxiety, irritability, restlessness, cravings, dizziness, impaired concentration, weight increase, emotional lability, somnolence, fatigue, increased sweating, insomnia (≥ 5%); confusion, depression, apathy, tremor, increased appetite, incoordination, increased dreaming (< 5%).

   Local irritation: Moderate-to-severe in 94% of patients during the first 2 days of treatment, declining to 81% after 3 weeks of treatment (rated moderate-to-mild); runny nose; throat irritation; watering eyes; sneezing; cough; nasal congestion; subjective comments related to the taste or usage of the dosage form; sinus irritation; transient epistaxis; eye irritation; transient changes in sense of smell; pharyngitis; paresthesias of the nose, mouth, or head; numbness of the nose or mouth; burning of the nose or eyes; earache; facial flushing; transient changes in sense of taste; hoarseness; nasal ulcer or blister.

   Dependence: Feelings of dependence and calming were reported by more patients on active spray than placebo.

   Others (not attributable to intercurrent illness):

Nicotine Nasal Spray Adverse Reactions (> 1%)		
Adverse reaction	Drug	Placebo
Headache	18	15
Back pain	6	4
Dyspnea	5	6
Nausea	5	5
Arthralgia	5	1
Menstrual disorder	4	4
Palpitation	4	4
Flatulence	4	3
Tooth disorder	4	1
Gum disorder	4	1
Myalgia	3	4
Abdominal pain	3	3
Confusion	3	3

Nicotine Nasal Spray Adverse Reactions (> 1%)		
Adverse reaction	Drug	Placebo
Acne	3	1
Dysmenorrhea	3	0
Pruritus	2	3

CNS – Aphasia, amnesia, migraine, numbness (< 1%).

GI – Dry mouth, hiccough, diarrhea (< 1%).

Respiratory – Bronchitis, bronchospasm, increased sputum (< 1%).

Miscellaneous – Peripheral edema, pain, allergy, purpura, rash, abnormal vision (< 1%).

➤*Gum:*

Miscellaneous – Injury to mouth, teeth, or dental work; belching; increased salivation; mild jaw muscle ache; sore mouth or throat.

➤*Transdermal:*

Miscellaneous – Erythema, pruritus, and/or burning at the application site.

Overdosage

➤*Symptoms:* Signs and symptoms of acute nicotine poisoning include the following: Pallor, cold sweat, nausea, salivation, vomiting, abdominal pain, diarrhea, headache, dizziness, disturbed hearing and vision, tremor, mental confusion, weakness. Prostration, hypotension, and respiratory failure may ensue with large overdoses. Lethal doses produce convulsions quickly; death follows as a result of peripheral or central respiratory paralysis or, less frequently, cardiac failure. The oral minumum acute lethal dose for nicotine in adult humans is reported to be 40 to 60 mg.

➤*Treatment:* Large oral nicotine ingestions cause vomiting, and the consequences of an overdose will vary. Institute gastric lavage and/or activated charcoal (with protected airway) when appropriate. Avoid syrup of ipecac.

Other supportive measures include diazepam or barbiturates for seizures, atropine for excessive bronchial secretions or diarrhea, respiratory support for respiratory failure, and vigorous fluid support for hypotension and cardiovascular collapse.

Nasal spray – A full bottle of nicotine nasal spray contains 100 mg of nicotine and would be expected to be irritating if sprayed in the eyes, mouth, or ears. Treat eye exposure with copious water irrigation for 20 minutes.

Inhaler – One cartridge of nicotine inhaler contains 10 mg of nicotine, of which, ≈ 4 mg is delivered nicotine. It is unlikely that an excessive nicotine overdose will occur via inhalation, but should such an overdose occur, the patient should contact a physician immediately. Refer patients ingesting nicotine inhaler cartridges to a health care facility for management. Administer repeated doses of activated charcoal as long as the cartridge remains in the GI tract because the cartridge will continue to release nicotine for many hours. The cartridge can be identified with a radiogram.

Transdermal – Remove the patch, flush the skin with water, and dry. Do not use soap, which may increase nicotine absorption. If the patch has been ingested, administer activated charcoal. In an unconscious patient, secure an airway before administering activated charcoal via a nasogastric tube. As long as the patch remains in the GI tract, administer repeated doses of charcoal because the patch will continue to release nicotine. A saline cathartic or sorbitol may be added to the first dose of activated charcoal to enhance passage of the patch.

NICOTINE TRANSDERMAL SYSTEM

	Product/Distributor	Dose absorbed in 24 hours (mg/day)	How supplied
otc	**Nicotine Transdermal System Step 1** (Various, eg, Novartis, Watson)	21	In 7 and 30 systems per box.
otc	**Nicotine Transdermal System Step 2** (Various, eg, Novartis, Watson)	14	In 7 and 30 systems per box.
otc	**Nicotine Transdermal System Step 3** (Various, eg, Novartis, Watson)	7	In 7 and 30 systems per box.
otc	**Nicoderm CQ Step 1** (GlaxoSmithKline Consumer)	21	In 7 and 14 systems per box; original and clear patches.
otc	**Nicoderm CQ Step 2** (GlaxoSmithKline Consumer)	14	In 14 systems per box; original and clear patches.
otc	**Nicoderm CQ Step 3** (GlaxoSmithKline Consumer)	7	In 14 systems per box; original and clear patches.
otc	**Nicotrol Step 1** (Pharmacia)	15[1]	In 7s and 14s.
otc	**Nicotrol Step 2** (Pharmacia)	10[1]	In 7s and 14s.
otc	**Nicotrol Step 3** (Pharmacia)	5[1]	In 7s and 14s.

[1] Dose absorbed in 16 hours.

For complete prescribing information, refer to the Nicotine group monograph.

Indications

➤*Smoking cessation:* To reduce withdrawal symptoms, including nicotine craving, associated with quitting smoking.

Administration and Dosage

➤*Approved by the FDA:* November 1991.

Advise patients to ask their doctor before using the patch if less than 18 years of age, are pregnant or nursing, have heart disease, have had a recent heart attack or irregular heartbeat, have high blood pressure not controlled with medication, take prescription medicine for depression or asthma, are allergic to adhesive tape, or have skin problems.

Advise patients not to use the patch if they use snuff, nicotine gum, or other nicotine-containing products; continue to smoke; or chew tobacco. Instruct patients not to smoke even if not wearing the patch. Nicotine in skin will be entering the bloodstream for several hours after the patch is removed. Advise patients to stop using the patch and see their doctor if skin redness caused by the patch does not go away after 4 days or if their skin swells or a rash develops. Also, have patients stop if they develop irregular heartbeats or palpitations or symptoms of nicotine overdose (eg, nausea, vomiting, dizziness, weakness, rapid heartbeat).

Recommended Dosing Schedule of Transdermal Nicotine for Healthy Patients		
	Duration	
Dose	Per strength of patch	Entire course of therapy
Nicoderm[1] 21 mg/day 14 mg/day 7 mg/day	First 6 weeks Next 2 weeks Last 2 weeks	8 to 10 weeks

Recommended Dosing Schedule of Transdermal Nicotine for Healthy Patients		
	Duration	
Dose	Per strength of patch	Entire course of therapy
Nicotrol 15 mg/16 hours 10 mg/16 hours 5 mg/16 hours	First 6 weeks Next 2 weeks Last 2 weeks	10 weeks

[1] Start with 14 mg/day for 6 weeks for patients who smoke less than 10 cigarettes/day. Decrease dose to 7 mg/day for the final 2 weeks.

➤*Application of system:* Apply the system promptly upon its removal from the protective pouch and removal of backing. Apply only once a day to a hairless, clean, dry skin site on upper arm or hip. Hold for 10 seconds. Wash hands thoroughly after application. Do not wear more than 1 patch at a time. Do not cut patch in half or into smaller pieces.

Nicoderm – The patch may be worn for 16 to 24 hours. If the patient craves a cigarette when he/she wakes up, advise the patient to wear the patch for 24 hours. After 16 or 24 hours, remove the used system and apply a new system to an alternate skin site. Do not leave patch on for more than 24 hours because it may irritate your skin and loses strength after 24 hours. Apply at the same time each day. Do not use patch for more than 8 to 10 weeks. If patients have vivid dreams or other sleep disturbances, they may remove the patch at bedtime and apply a new one in the morning.

Nicotrol – Each day, apply a new system upon waking and remove at bedtime. If the patient forgets to remove the patch at bedtime, that person may have vivid dreams or other sleep disruptions. Do not wear patch for more than 16 hours.

➤*Disposal:* When the used system is removed from the skin, fold it over and place in the protective pouch that contained the new system or in the disposal tray, if provided. Wash hands. Immediately dispose of the used system in such a way to prevent its access by children or pets.

➤*Storage/Stability:* Store at 20° to 25°C (68° to 77°F).

NICOTINE POLACRILEX (Nicotine resin complex)

otc	**Commit** (GlaxoSmithKline Consumer)	**Lozenge:** 2 mg nicotine (as polacrilex) per lozenge	Aspartame[1] and mannitol. In 72s.
		4 mg nicotine (as polacrilex) per lozenge	Aspartame[1] and mannitol. In 72s.
otc	**Nicotine Gum** (Various, eg, Rugby)	**Chewing gum:** 2 mg nicotine (as polacrilex) per square	In 48s and 108s.
otc	**Nicorette** (GlaxoSmithKline Consumer)		In orange, mint, and original flavors. In 48s, 108s, and 168s.
otc	**Nicotine Gum** (Various, eg, Rugby)	**Chewing gum:** 4 mg nicotine (as polacrilex) per square.	In 48s and 108s.
otc	**Nicorette** (GlaxoSmithKline Consumer)		In orange, mint, and original flavors. In 48s, 108s, and 168s.

[1] Contains 3.4 mg phenylalanine.

For complete prescribing information, refer to the Nicotine group monograph.

Indications

➤*Smoking cessation:* To reduce withdrawal symptoms, including nicotine craving, associated with quitting smoking.

Administration and Dosage

➤*Approved by the FDA:* January 1984.

Advise patient to stop smoking completely when beginning to use the gum or lozenge.

➤*Gum:* If the patient smokes less than 25 cigarettes/day, start with the 2 mg nicotine gum. If the patient smokes 25 or more cigarettes/day, start with the 4 mg nicotine gum. Refer to the dosing schedule in the table below.

Instruct patient to chew the gum slowly until it tingles, then park it between the cheek and gum. When the tingle is gone, instruct patient to begin chewing again until the tingle returns. Repeat the process until most of the tingle is gone (about 30 minutes).

Advise patient not to eat or drink for 15 minutes before chewing the nicotine gum or while chewing a piece. To improve the chances of quitting, chew at least 9 pieces/day for the first 6 weeks. If there are strong and frequent cravings, use a second piece within the hour. However, do not continuously use 1 piece after another because this may cause hiccoughs, heartburn, nausea, or other side effects.

Advise the patient not use more than 24 pieces/day and to stop using the nicotine gum at the end of 12 weeks. If there is still a need to use the nicotine gum, have the patient contact a physician.

➤*Lozenge:* If the patient smokes his/her first cigarette more than 30 minutes after waking up, start with the 2 mg nicotine lozenge. If the patient smokes their first cigarette within 30 minutes of waking up, start with the 4 mg nicotine lozenge. Refer to the dosing schedule in the table below.

Instruct the patient to place the lozenge in the mouth and allow it to slowly dissolve (about 20 to 30 minutes). Minimize swallowing. Advise the patient not to chew or swallow the lozenge. The patient may feel a warm or tingling sensation. Advise the patient to occasionally move the lozenge from one side of the mouth to the other until completely dissolved.

Advise the patient not to eat or drink 15 minutes before using or while the lozenge is in the mouth. To improve the chances of quitting, use at least 9 lozenges/day for the first 6 weeks. Do not use more than one lozenge at a time or continuously use one lozenge after another because this may cause hiccoughs, heartburn, nausea, or other side effects.

Advise the patient not to use more than 5 lozenges in 6 hours or more than 20 lozenges/day and to stop using the nicotine lozenge at the end of 12 weeks. If there is still a need to use the nicotine lozenge, have the patient contact a physician.

Nicotine Polacrilex Dosing Schedule		
Weeks 1 to 6	Weeks 7 to 9	Weeks 10 to 12
1 piece of gum or lozenge every 1 to 2 hours	1 piece of gum or lozenge every 2 to 4 hours	1 piece of gum or lozenge every 4 to 8 hours

➤*Disposal:*

Gum – Place used chewing pieces in a wrapper and dispose of in such a way to prevent its access by children or pets. Pieces of nicotine gum may have enough nicotine to make children or pets sick. In case of overdose, contact a medical professional or Poison Control Center.

Lozenge – Nicotine lozenges may have enough nicotine to make children or pets sick. If you need to remove the lozenge, wrap it in paper and throw away in the trash. In case of overdose, contact a medical professional or Poison Control Center.

➤*Storage/Stability:* Store at 20° to 25°C (68° to 77°F). Protect from light.

NICOTINE INHALATION SYSTEM

Rx	**Nicotrol Inhaler** (Pharmacia)	**Inhaler:** 4 mg delivered (10 mg/cartridge)	Kit contains mouthpiece, storage trays each containing 6 cartridges, plastic storage case, and patient information leaflet. In 42s and 168s.

For complete prescribing information, refer to the Nicotine group monograph.

Indications

➤*Smoking cessation:* As an aid in smoking cessation for the relief of nicotine withdrawal symptoms. Inhaler therapy is recommended for use as part of a comprehensive behavioral smoking cessation program.

Administration and Dosage

➤*Approved by the FDA:* May 2, 1997.

Patients must desire to stop smoking and should be instructed to stop smoking completely as they begin using the inhaler.

➤*Initial dosage:* The initial dosage of the nicotine inhaler is individualized. Patients may self-titrate to the level of nicotine they require. Most successful patients in the clinical trials used between 6 and 16 cartridges per day. Best effect was achieved by frequent continuous puffing (20 minutes). The recommended duration of treatment is 3 months, after which patients may be weaned from the inhaler by gradual reduction of the daily dose over the following 6 to 12 weeks.

Encourage patients to use at least 6 cartridges/day at least for the first 3 to 6 weeks of treatment. In clinical trials, the average daily dose was more than 6 (range, 3 to 18) cartridges for patients who successfully quit smoking. Additional doses may be needed to control the urge to smoke with a maximum of 16 cartridges daily for up to 12 weeks. Regular use of the inhaler during the first week of treatment may help patients adapt to the irritant effects of the product. Some patients may exhibit signs or symptoms of nicotine withdrawal or excess that will require an adjustment of the dosage.

➤*Gradual reduction of dose (up to 12 weeks):* Most patients will need to gradually discontinue the use of the inhaler after the initial treatment period. Gradual reduction of dose may begin after 12 weeks of initial treatment and may last for up to 12 weeks. Recommended strategies for discontinuing use include suggesting to patients that they use the product less frequently, keep a tally of daily usage, try to meet a steadily reducing target, or set a planned "quit date" for stopping use of the product.

➤*Individualization of dosage:* The goal of the inhaler therapy is complete abstinence. If a patient is unable to stop smoking by the fourth week of therapy, discontinue treatment.

Treat patients who are successfully abstinent on the inhaler at the selected dosage for up to 12 weeks, then gradually reduce use of the inhaler over the next 6 to 12 weeks. Some patients may not require gradual reduction of dosage and may abruptly stop treatment successfully. The safe use of this product for more than 6 months has not been established.

Controlled clinical trials of nicotine products suggest that palpitations, nausea, and sweating are more often symptoms of nicotine excess, whereas anxiety, nervousness, and irritability are more often symptoms of nicotine withdrawal.

➤*Safety and handling:* See patient information sheet for instructions on handling and disposal. After using the inhaler, carefully separate the mouthpiece, remove the used cartridge, and throw it away, out of the reach of children and pets. Store the mouthpiece in the plastic storage case for further use. The mouthpiece is reusable and should be cleaned regularly with soap and water.

➤*Storage/Stability:* Store at room temperature not to exceed 25°C (77°F). Protect cartridges from light.

NICOTINE NASAL SPRAY

Rx	Nicotrol NS (Pharmacia)	Spray pump: 0.5 mg nicotine/actuation (10 mg/mL)	Parabens, EDTA. Each unit has a glass container mounted with metered spray pump (delivers ≈ 200 applications). In 10 mL bottles.

For complete prescribing information, refer to the Nicotine group monograph.

Indications

►*Smoking cessation:* As an aid to smoking cessation for the relief of nicotine withdrawal symptoms. The nasal spray should be used as a part of a comprehensive behavioral smoking cessation program.

Safety and efficacy of continued use of nicotine nasal spray for periods longer than 6 months have not been adequately studied and such use is not recommended.

Administration and Dosage

►*Approved by the FDA:* March 22, 1996.

Instruct patients to stop smoking completely when they begin using the product. Instruct them not to sniff, swallow, or inhale through the nose as the spray is being administered. They should also be advised to administer the spray with the head tilted back slightly.

►*Dosage:* Each actuation of the nasal spray delivers a metered 50 mcL spray containing 0.5 mg nicotine. One dose is 1 mg of nicotine (2 sprays, 1 in each nostril). Start patients with 1 or 2 doses per hour, which may be increased up to a maximum recommended dose of 40 mg (80 sprays, somewhat less than ½ of the bottle) per day. For best results, encourage patients to use at least the recommended minimum of 8 doses/day, as less is unlikely to be effective. In clinical trials, the patients who successfully quit smoking used the product heavily when nicotine withdrawal was at its peak, sometimes up to the recommended maximum of 40 doses/day (in heavier smokers).

Nicotine Nasal Spray Dosing Recommendations			
Maximum recommended duration of treatment	Recommended doses/hr	Maximum doses/hr	Maximum doses/day
3 months	1 to 2[1]	5	40

[1] One dose = 2 sprays (1 in each nostril). One dose delivers 1 mg of nicotine to the nasal mucosa.

►*Discontinuation:* No tapering strategy has been shown to be optimal in clinical studies. Many patients simply stopped using the spray at their last clinic visit. Recommended strategies for discontinuation of use include suggesting the following to patients: Use only ½ a dose (1 spray) at a time, use the spray less frequently, keep a tally of daily usage, try to meet a steadily reducing usage target, skip a dose by not medicating every hour, or set a planned "quit date" for stopping use of the spray.

►*Individualization of dosage:* The goal of the nasal spray therapy is complete abstinence. If a patient is unable to stop smoking by the fourth week of therapy, discontinue treatment. Regular use of the spray during the first week of treatment may help patients adapt to the irritant effects of the spray. Patients who are successfully abstinent on the nasal spray should be treated at the selected dosage for up to 8 weeks, following which use of the spray should be discontinued over the next 4 to 6 weeks. Some patients may not require gradual reduction of dosage and may abruptly stop treatment successfully. Treatment with the nasal spray for longer periods has not been shown to improve outcome, and the safety of use for periods longer than 6 months has not been established.

Controlled clinical trials of nicotine products suggest that palpitations, nausea, and sweating are more often symptoms of nicotine excess; whereas anxiety, nervousness, and irritability are more often symptoms of nicotine withdrawal.

►*Safety and handling:* Take care in handling the nasal spray during periods of opening and closing the container. It may break if dropped. If this occurs, the spill should be cleaned up immediately with an absorbent cloth/paper towel. Take care to avoid contact of the solution with the skin and wash the area several times. Should even a small amount of the nasal spray come in contact with the skin, lips, mouth, eyes, or ears, immediately rinse the affected areas with water. Dispose of used bottles with the child-resistant cap in place. Used bottles should be disposed of in such a way as to prevent access by children or pets.

►*Storage/Stability:* Store at room temperature not to exceed 30°C (86°F).

BUPROPION HCl

Rx	Zyban (GlaxoSmithKline)	Tablets, sustained-release: 150 mg	(ZYBAN 150). Purple. Film-coated. In 60s.

Bupropion is also used as an antidepressant. Refer to the Antidepressants section for complete prescribing information.

Indications

►*Smoking cessation:* An aid to smoking cessation treatment.

►*Unlabeled uses:* Bupropion SR has been shown to be effective in the treatment of neuropathic pain and to enhance weight loss. Bupropion also has been shown to be effective in the treatment of attention deficit hyperactivity disorder.

Administration and Dosage

►*Approved by the FDA:* May 14, 1997.

►*Usual dose:* The recommended and maximum dose of bupropion is 300 mg/day, given as 150 mg twice daily. Begin dosing at 150 mg/day given every day for the first 3 days, followed by a dose increase for most patients to the usual recommended dose of 300 mg/day. There should be an interval of at least 8 hours between successive doses. Do not give doses above 300 mg/day (see Warnings). Swallow whole; do not crush, divide, or chew.

Initiate treatment with bupropion while the patient is still smoking because about 1 week of treatment is required to achieve steady-state blood levels of bupropion. Patients should set a "target quit date" within the first 2 weeks of treatment with bupropion, generally in the second week. Continue treatment for 7 to 12 weeks; base duration of treatment on the relative benefits and risks for individual patients. If a patient has not made significant progress towards abstinence by week 7 of therapy with bupropion, it is unlikely that he or she will quit during that attempt; discontinue treatment. Dose tapering of bupropion is not required when discontinuing treatment. It is important that patients continue to receive counseling and support throughout treatment with bupropion and for a period of time thereafter.

►*Maintenance:* Nicotine dependence is a chronic condition. Some patients may need continuous treatment. Systematic evaluation of bupropion 300 mg/day for maintenance therapy demonstrated that treatment for up to 6 months was effective. Whether to continue treatment with bupropion for periods longer than 12 weeks for smoking cessation must be determined for individual patients.

►*Combination treatment:* Combination treatment with bupropion and nicotine transdermal system (NTS) may be prescribed for smoking cessation. Monitoring for treatment-emergent hypertension in patients treated with the combination of bupropion and NTS is recommended.

►*Hepatic function impairment:* Use extreme caution in patients with severe hepatic cirrhosis. The dose should not exceed 150 mg every other day in these patients. Use bupropion with caution in patients with hepatic impairment (including mild to moderate hepatic cirrhosis) and consider a reduced frequency of dosing in patients with mild to moderate hepatic cirrhosis (see Warnings).

►*Renal function impairment:* Use caution in patients with renal impairment and consider a reduced frequency of dosing (see Warnings).

►*Storage/Stability:* Store at controlled room temperature, 20° to 25°C (68° to 77°F). Dispense in tight, light-resistant containers.

Actions

►*Pharmacology:* Bupropion is a non-nicotine aid to smoking cessation. It is a relatively weak inhibitor of the neuronal uptake of norepinephrine, serotonin, and dopamine, and does not inhibit monoamine oxidase. The mechanism by which bupropion enhances the ability of patients to abstain from smoking is unknown. However, it is presumed that this action is mediated by noradrenergic or dopaminergic mechanisms.

►*Pharmacokinetics:*

Absorption – Bupropion is a racemic mixture that follows biphasic pharmacokinetics best described by a 2-compartment model.

Following oral administration of bupropion to healthy volunteers, peak plasma concentrations of 91 and 143 ng/mL were achieved within 3 hours. At steady state, the mean C_{max} was 136 ng/mL following a 150 mg dose every 12 hours.

Food: Food increased bupropion C_{max} by 11%, and the extent of absorption (AUC) by 17%. The T_{max} was prolonged by 1 hour, but these were of no clinical significance.

Distribution – Bupropion is 84% plasma protein bound in vitro. The extent of protein binding of the hydroxybupropion metabolite is similar to that for bupropion, whereas the protein binding of threohydrobupropion metabolite is about 50% of that seen with bupropion. The volume of distribution estimated from a single 150 mg dose is 1950 L. The distribution phase has a mean half-life of 3 to 4 hours.

Metabolism – Bupropion is extensively metabolized in humans to 3 active metabolites: Hydroxybupropion, threohydrobupropion, and erythrohydrobupropion. In mice, the potency of hydroxybupropion is comparable to bupropion, while the other metabolites are ⅒ to ½ as potent. Plasma concentrations of the metabolites are higher than those of bupropion. In vitro findings suggest that CYP2B6 is the principal isoenzyme involved in the formation of hydroxybupropion, while cyto-

BUPROPION HCl

chrome P450 isoenzymes are not involved in the formation of threohydrobupropion. There is potential for drug interactions when bupropion is coadministered with drugs metabolized by the CYP2B6 isoenzyme (see Drug Interactions).

Peak plasma concentrations of hydroxybupropion occur approximately 6 hours after administration of a single dose, and are approximately 10 times the peak level of the parent drug at steady state. The AUC at steady state is about 17 times that of bupropion. The times to peak concentrations for erythrohydrobupropion and threohydrobupropion are similar to that of the hydroxybupropion metabolite, and steady-state AUCs are 1.5 and 7 times that of bupropion, respectively.

Excretion – Bupropion and its metabolites follow linear kinetics with chronic administration of 150 to 300 mg/day. Following chronic dosing of bupropion 150 mg every 12 hours for 14 days, the mean clearance at steady state was 160 L/hr. The mean elimination half-life of bupropion is approximately 21 hours. The estimated half-lives of the metabolites, from a multiple-dose study, were the following: 20 hours for hydroxybupropion, 37 hours for threohydrobupropion, and 33 hours for erythrohydrobupropion. Steady-state plasma concentrations of bupropion and its metabolites are reached within 5 to 8 days, respectively.

Following oral administration of 200 mg ^{14}C-bupropion, 87% and 10% of the dose was recovered in the urine and feces, respectively. The fraction of the oral dose of bupropion excreted unchanged was 0.5%.

Special populations –

Hepatic function impairment: The half-life of hydroxybupropion was significantly prolonged in subjects with alcoholic liver disease (approximately 32 hours vs approximately 21 hours). The differences in half-life for bupropion and the other metabolites were minimal.

➤*Clinical trials:* In a comparative study, 4 treatments were evaluated: Bupropion 300 mg/day, NTS 21 mg/day, combination of bupropion 300 mg/day plus NTS 21 mg/day, and placebo. Patients were treated for 9 weeks.

Patients treated with either bupropion or NTS or combination achieved greater 4-week abstinence rates than patients treated with placebo. Although the treatment combination of bupropion and NTS displayed the highest rates of continuous abstinence throughout the study, the quit rates for the combination were not significantly higher than for bupropion alone.

Contraindications

Coadministration with a monoamine oxidase (MAO) inhibitor (see Drug Interactions), *Wellbutrin*, *Wellbutrin SR*, or any medications that contain bupropion; current or prior diagnosis of bulimia or anorexia nervosa, seizure disorders (see Warnings); patients who have shown an allergic response to bupropion or other ingredients in the formulation; patients undergoing abrupt discontinuation of alcohol or sedatives (including benzodiazepines).

Warnings

➤*Other bupropion medications:* Bupropion is the active ingredient found in *Wellbutrin* and *Wellbutrin SR*, used to treat depression. Do not use this product in combination with *Wellbutrin*, *Wellbutrin SR*, or any other medications that contain bupropion.

➤*Anorexia nervosa/bulimia:* Do not give with current or prior diagnosis of bulimia or anorexia nervosa because of a higher incidence of seizures noted in patients treated for bulimia with the immediate-release formulation of bupropion.

➤*Seizures:* Because the use of bupropion is associated with a dose-dependent risk of seizures, do not prescribe doses over 300 mg/day for smoking cessation. The seizure rate associated with doses of sustained-release bupropion up to 300 mg/day is approximately 0.1%. Data for the immediate-release formulation of bupropion revealed a seizure incidence of approximately 0.4% in depressed patients treated at doses in a range of 300 to 450 mg/day. In addition, the estimated seizure incidence increases almost 10-fold between 450 and 600 mg/day.

Predisposing factors that may increase the risk of seizure with bupropion use include history of head trauma or prior seizure, CNS tumor, the presence of severe hepatic cirrhosis, and concomitant medications that lower seizure threshold.

Circumstances associated with an increased seizure risk include the following, among others: Excessive use of alcohol or sedatives (including benzodiazepines); abrupt withdrawal from alcohol or other sedatives; addiction to opiates, cocaine, or stimulants; use of OTC stimulants and anorectics; diabetes treated with oral hypoglycemics or insulin.

Concomitant medications – Many medications (eg, antipsychotics, antidepressants, theophylline, systemic steroids) and treatment regimens (eg, abrupt discontinuation of benzodiazepines) are known to lower seizure threshold.

Reducing the risk of seizures – Retrospective analysis suggests that the risk of seizures may be minimized if patients adhere to the following:

• The total daily dose of bupropion does not exceed 300 mg (the maximum recommended dose for smoking cessation),

• the recommended dose for most patients (300 mg/day) is administered in divided doses (150 mg twice daily),

• and no single dose exceeds 150 mg.

Administer with extreme caution to patients with a history of seizures, cranial trauma, or other predisposition(s) toward seizures or patients treated with other agents (eg, antipsychotics, antidepressants, theophylline, systemic steroids) or treatment regimens (eg, abrupt discontinuation of a benzodiazepine) that lower seizure threshold.

➤*Hepatotoxicity:* An increase in incidence of hepatic hyperplastic nodules, hepatocellular hypertrophy, and various histologic changes suggesting mild hepatocellular injury were noted in animals receiving chronic, large doses of bupropion.

➤*Hypersensitivity reactions:* Anaphylactoid/anaphylactic reactions characterized by symptoms such as pruritus, urticaria, angioedema, and dyspnea requiring medical treatment have been reported at a rate of about 1 to 3 per 1000 in clinical trials of bupropion. In addition, there have been rare postmarketing reports of erythema multiforme, Stevens-Johnson syndrome, and anaphylactic shock associated with bupropion.

Advise patients to stop taking bupropion and consult their doctor if they experience allergic or anaphylactoid/anaphylactic reactions (eg, rash, pruritus, hives, chest pain, edema, shortness of breath) during treatment.

Arthralgia, myalgia, and fever with rash and other symptoms suggestive of delayed hypersensitivity have been reported in association with bupropion. These symptoms may resemble serum sickness.

➤*Renal function impairment:* No studies have been conducted in patients with renal impairment. Bupropion is extensively metabolized in the liver to active metabolites, which are further metabolized and excreted by the kidneys. Use bupropion with caution in patients with renal impairment and consider a reduced frequency of dosing as bupropion and its metabolites may accumulate in such patients to a greater extent than usual. Closely monitor the patient for possible adverse effects that could indicate high drug or metabolite levels.

➤*Hepatic function impairment:* The half-life of hydroxybupropion was significantly prolonged in subjects with alcoholic liver disease (approximately 32 hours vs approximately 21 hours). The differences in half-life for bupropion and the other metabolites were minimal.

Use with extreme caution in patients with severe hepatic cirrhosis. In these patients, a reduced frequency of dosing is required. The dose should not exceed 150 mg every other day.

Use with caution in patients with hepatic impairment (including mild to moderate hepatic cirrhosis) and reduced frequency of dosing should be considered in patients with mild to moderate hepatic cirrhosis. Closely monitor all patients with hepatic impairment for possible adverse effects that could indicate high drug and metabolite levels.

➤*Carcinogenesis:* In rats, there was an increase in nodular proliferative lesions of the liver at doses of 100 to 300 mg/kg/day (approximately 3 to 10 times the maximum recommended human dose [MRHD] on a mg/m^2 basis).

➤*Elderly:* A pharmacokinetic study, single and multiple dose, suggested that the elderly are at increased risk for accumulation of bupropion and its metabolites. Because elderly patients are more likely to have decreased renal function, take care in dose selection. It may be useful to monitor renal function.

➤*Pregnancy: Category B.* Teratology studies have been performed in rats and rabbits. There is no evidence of impaired fertility or harm to the fetus caused by bupropion. There are no adequate and well-controlled studies in pregnant women. Use during pregnancy only if clearly needed. Encourage pregnant smokers to attempt cessation using educational and behavioral interventions before pharmacological approaches are used.

To monitor fetal outcomes of pregnant women exposed to bupropion, the manufacturer maintains a bupropion pregnancy registry. Health care providers are encouraged to register patients by calling (800) 336-2176.

➤*Lactation:* Bupropion and its metabolites are secreted in breast milk. Because of the potential for serious adverse reactions in breastfeeding infants from bupropion, decide whether to discontinue breastfeeding or discontinue the drug, taking into account the importance of the drug to the mother.

➤*Children:* Clinical trials with bupropion did not include individuals under 18 years of age. Therefore, the safety and efficacy in a pediatric smoking population have not been established.

Precautions

➤*Insomnia:* In 1 trial, 29% of patients treated with 150 mg/day and 35% of patients treated with 300 mg/day experienced insomnia vs 21% with placebo. Symptoms were sufficiently severe to require discontinuation of treatment in 0.6% of patients treated with bupropion and none of the placebo patients.

In another trial, 40% of the patients treated with 300 mg/day of bupropion, 28% of the patients treated with 21 mg/day NTS, and 45% of the patients treated with the combination of bupropion and NTS experienced insomnia vs 18% with placebo. Symptoms were sufficiently severe to require discontinuation of treatment in 0.8% of patients treated with bupropion and 0% of the patients in the other 3 treatment groups.

BUPROPION HCl

Insomnia may be minimized by avoiding bedtime doses and, if necessary, reduction in dose.

➤*Neuropsychiatric phenomena:* The incidence of neuropsychiatric side effects was generally comparable with placebo. Depressed patients treated with bupropion show a variety of neuropsychiatric signs and symptoms including delusions, hallucinations, psychosis, concentration disturbance, paranoia, and confusion. In some cases, these symptoms abated upon dose reduction or withdrawal of treatment.

➤*Psychosis or mania:* Antidepressants can precipitate manic episodes in bipolar disorder patients during the depressed phase of their illness and may activate latent psychosis in other susceptible individuals. The sustained-release formulation of bupropion is expected to pose similar risks. There were no reports of activation of psychosis or mania in clinical trials conducted in nondepressed smokers.

➤*Cardiac effects:* Hypertension, in some cases severe, requiring acute treatment, has been reported in patients receiving bupropion alone and in combination with nicotine replacement therapy. These events have been observed in patients with and without evidence of pre-existing hypertension.

Data from a comparative study of bupropion, NTS, the combination of sustained-release bupropion plus NTS, and placebo as an aid to smoking cessation suggest a higher incidence of treatment-emergent hypertension in patients treated with the combination of bupropion and NTS. In this study, 6.1% of patients treated with the combination of bupropion and NTS had treatment-emergent hypertension compared with 2.5%, 1.6%, and 3.1% of patients treated with bupropion, NTS, and placebo, respectively. The majority of these patients had evidence of pre-existing hypertension. Monitoring of blood pressure is recommended in patients who receive the combination of bupropion and nicotine replacement.

Use caution in patients with a recent history of MI or unstable heart disease. Bupropion was well-tolerated in depressed patients who had previously developed orthostatic hypotension while receiving tricyclic antidepressants and was generally well tolerated in depressed patients with stable CHF. Bupropion was associated with a rise in supine blood pressure in the study of patients with CHF, resulting in discontinuation of treatment in 2 patients for exacerbation of baseline hypertension.

➤*Drug abuse and dependence:* Bupropion is likely to have a low abuse potential. There have been a few reported cases of drug dependence and withdrawal symptoms associated with the immediate-release formulation of bupropion. In studies of abuse liability, individuals experienced with drugs of abuse reported that bupropion produced a feeling of euphoria and desirability. In these subjects, a single dose of 400 mg (1.33 times the recommended daily dose) of bupropion produced mild, amphetamine-like effects compared with placebo.

Keep in mind that bupropion may induce dependence when evaluating the desirability of including the drug in smoking cessation programs of individual patients.

Drug Interactions

➤*CYP450:* In vitro studies indicate that bupropion is primarily metabolized to hydroxybupropion by the CYP2B6 isoenzyme. Therefore, the potential exists for a drug interaction between bupropion and drugs that affect the CYP2B6 isoenzyme (eg, orphenadrine, cyclophosphamide). The threohydrobupropion metabolite does not appear to be produced by the cytochrome P450 isoenzymes.

Because bupropion is extensively metabolized, the coadministration of other drugs may affect its clinical activity. In particular, certain drugs may induce the metabolism of bupropion (eg, carbamazepine, phenobarbital, phenytoin) while other drugs may inhibit the metabolism of bupropion (eg, cimetidine).

Physiological changes resulting from smoking cessation itself, with or without treatment with bupropion, may alter the pharmacokinetics of some concomitant medications, which may require dosage adjustment.

Bupropion Drug Interactions

Precipitant drug	Object drug*		Description
Carbamazepine	Bupropion	↓	Serum concentrations of bupropion may be decreased.
Amantadine Levodopa	Bupropion	↑	A higher incidence of adverse experiences may occur during coadministration. Use small initial doses and gradual dose increases of bupropion.
MAO inhibitors	Bupropion	↑	In animals, the acute toxicity of bupropion is enhanced by the MAO inhibitor phenelzine. Coadministration is contraindicated. Allow at least 14 days between discontinuing an MAO inhibitor and starting bupropion.
Nicotine replacement	Bupropion	↑	Coadministration may cause hypertension. Monitor blood pressure.

Bupropion Drug Interactions

Precipitant drug	Object drug*		Description
Ritonavir	Bupropion	↑	Large increases in serum bupropion concentrations may occur, increasing the risk of bupropion toxicity. Avoid coadministration.
Bupropion	Alcohol	↑	There have been rare reports of adverse neuropsychiatric events or reduced alcohol tolerance. Minimize or avoid consumption of alcohol during treatment with bupropion.
Bupropion	Antidepressants (eg, nortriptyline, imipramine, desipramine, paroxetine, fluoxetine, sertraline) Antipsychotics (eg, haloperidol, risperidone, thioridazine) Beta-blockers (eg, metoprolol) Type 1C antiarrhythmics (eg, propafenone, flecainide)	↑	Bupropion and hydroxybupropion are inhibitors of the CYP2D6 isoenzyme. If bupropion is added to the treatment regimen of a patient receiving a drug metabolized by CYP2D6, consider a dose reduction in the original medication.

* ↑ = Object drug increased. ↓ = Object drug decreased.

➤*Drugs that lower seizure threshold:* Coadministration of bupropion and agents (eg, antipsychotics, antidepressants, theophylline, systemic steroids) or treatment regimens (eg, abrupt discontinuation of benzodiazepines) that lower seizure threshold should be undertaken only with extreme caution (see Contraindications).

Adverse Reactions

Bupropion Adverse Reactions[1]

Adverse reaction	Bupropion 100 to 300 mg/day (n = 461)	Bupropion 300 mg/day (n = 243)	NTS 21 mg/day (n = 243)	Bupropion and NTS (n = 244)
Cardiovascular				
Hot flashes	1	-	-	-
Hypertension	1	1	< 1	2
Palpitations	-	2	0	1
CNS				
Anxiety	-	8	6	9
Disturbed concentration	-	9	3	9
Dizziness	8	10	2	8
Dream abnormality	-	5	18	13
Dysphoria	-	< 1	1	2
Insomnia	31	40	28	45
Nervousness	-	4	< 1	2
Somnolence	2	-	-	-
Thinking abnormality	1	-	-	-
Tremor	2	1	< 1	2
Dermatologic				
Application site reaction	-	11[2]	17[2]	15[2]
Dry skin	2	-	-	-
Pruritus	3	3	1	5
Rash	3	4	3	3
Urticaria	1	2	0	2
GI				
Abdominal pain	-	3	4	1
Anorexia	1	3	1	5
Constipation	-	8	4	9
Diarrhea	-	4	4	3
Dry mouth	11	10	4	9
Increased appetite	2	-	-	-
Mouth ulcer	-	2	1	1
Nausea	-	9	7	11
Thirst	-	< 1	< 1	2
Musculoskeletal				
Arthralgia	4	5	3	3
Myalgia	2	4	3	5
Respiratory				
Bronchitis	2	-	-	-
Dyspnea	-	1	0	2
Epistaxis	-	2	1	1
Increased cough	-	3	5	< 1

BUPROPION HCl

Bupropion Adverse Reactions[1]				
Adverse reaction	Bupropion 100 to 300 mg/day (n = 461)	Bupropion 300 mg/day (n = 243)	NTS 21 mg/day (n = 243)	Bupropion and NTS (n = 244)
Pharyngitis	-	3	2	3
Rhinitis	-	12	11	9
Sinusitis	-	2	2	2
Special senses				
Taste perversion	2	3	1	3
Tinnitus	-	1	0	< 1
Miscellaneous				
Accidental injury	-	2	2	1
Allergic reaction	1	-	-	-
Chest pain	-	< 1	1	3
Facial edema	-	< 1	0	1
Neck pain	2	2	1	< 1

[1] Data are pooled from separate studies and are not necessarily comparable.
[2] Patients randomized to bupropion or placebo received placebo patches.

Other adverse reactions with both the sustained-release and immediate-release formulations:

➤*Cardiovascular:* Flushing, migraine, postural hypotension, stroke, tachycardia, vasodilation (0.1% to 1%); syncope (fewer than 0.1%); cardiovascular disorder; complete AV block; extrasystoles; hypotension; hypertension; MI; phlebitis; pulmonary embolism.

➤*CNS:* Agitation, depression, irritability, headache (at least 1%); abnormal coordination, CNS stimulation, confusion, decreased libido, decreased memory, depersonalization, emotional lability, hostility, hyperkinesia, hypertonia, hypesthesia, paresthesia, suicidal ideation, vertigo (0.1% to 1%); amnesia, ataxia, derealization, hypomania (fewer than 0.1%); abnormal electroencephalogram (EEG); akinesia; aphasia; coma; delirium; delusions; dysarthria; dyskinesia; dystonia; euphoria; extrapyramidal syndrome; hallucinations; hypokinesia; increased libido; manic reaction; neuralgia; neuropathy; paranoid reaction; unmasking tardive dyskinesia.

➤*Dermatologic:* Sweating (at least 1%); acne, dry skin (0.1% to 1%); maculopapular rash (fewer than 0.1%); angioedema; alopecia; exfoliative dermatitis; hirsutism.

➤*Endocrine:* Hyperglycemia; hypoglycemia; syndrome of inappropriate antidiuretic hormone.

➤*GI:* Dyspepsia, flatulence, vomiting (at least 1%); abnormal liver function, bruxism, dysphagia, gastric reflux, gingivitis, glossitis, jaundice, stomatitis (0.1% to 1%); edema of the tongue (fewer than 0.1%); colitis; esophagitis; GI hemorrhage; gum hemorrhage; hepatitis; increased salivation; intestinal perforation; liver damage; pancreatitis; stomach ulcer; stool abnormality.

Dry mouth – The incidence of dry mouth may be related to the dose of bupropion. May be minimized by reducing dose.

➤*GU:* Urinary frequency (at least 1%); impotence, polyuria, urinary urgency (0.1% to 1%); abnormal ejaculation; cystitis; dyspareunia; dysuria; gynecomastia; menopause; painful erection; prostate disorder; salpingitis; urinary incontinence; urinary retention; urinary tract disorder; vaginitis.

➤*Hematologic/Lymphatic:* Ecchymosis (0.1% to 1%); anemia; leukocytosis; leukopenia; lymphadenopathy; pancytopenia; thrombocytopenia.

➤*Metabolic/Nutritional:* Edema, increased weight, peripheral edema (0.1% to 1%); glycosuria.

➤*Musculoskeletal:* Leg cramps, twitching, musculoskeletal chest pain (0.1% to 1%); arthritis; muscle rigidity/fever/rhabdomyolysis; muscle weakness.

➤*Special senses:* Amblyopia (at least 1%); accommodation abnormality, dry eye (0.1% to 1%); deafness; diplopia; mydriasis.

➤*Miscellaneous:* Asthenia, fever, headache (at least 1%); back pain, chills, inguinal hernia, pain, photosensitivity (0.1% to 1%); bronchospasm; malaise (fewer than 0.1%); pneumonia.

Arthralgia, myalgia, fever with rash, and other symptoms suggestive of delayed hypersensitivity may resemble serum sickness.

Discontinuation of treatment – Adverse events were sufficiently troublesome to cause discontinuation of treatment in 8% of the 706 patients treated with bupropion and 5% of the 313 patients treated with placebo. The more common events leading to discontinuation of treatment with bupropion included nervous system disturbances (3.4%), primarily tremors, and skin disorders (2.4%), primarily rashes.

Overdosage

➤*Symptoms:* There has been limited experience with overdosage of the sustained-release formulation of bupropion; 3 such cases were reported during clinical trials in depressed patients. One patient ingested 3000 mg of bupropion sustained-release tablets and vomited quickly after the overdose; the patient experienced blurred vision and lightheadedness. A second patient ingested a "handful" of bupropion sustained-release tablets and experienced confusion, lethargy, nausea, jitteriness, and seizure. A third patient ingested 3600 mg of bupropion sustained-release tablets and a bottle of wine; the patient experienced nausea, visual hallucinations, and "grogginess." None of the patients experienced further sequelae.

There has been extensive experience with overdosages of the immediate-release formulation of bupropion. Thirteen overdoses occurred during clinical trials in depressed patients. Twelve patients ingested 850 to 4200 mg and recovered without significant sequelae. Another patient who ingested 9000 mg of the immediate-release formulation of bupropion and 300 mg of tranylcypromine experienced a grand mal seizure and recovered without further sequelae.

Since its introduction, overdoses of up to 17,500 mg of the immediate-release formulation of bupropion have been reported. Seizure was reported in approximately 1/3 of all cases. Other serious reactions reported with the immediate-release formulation of bupropion alone included hallucinations, loss of consciousness, and sinus tachycardia. Fever, muscle rigidity, rhabdomyolysis, hypotension, stupor, coma, and respiratory failure have been reported when the immediate-release formulation of bupropion was part of multiple-drug overdoses.

Although most patients recovered without sequelae, deaths associated with overdoses of the immediate-release formulation of bupropion alone have been reported rarely in patients ingesting massive doses of the drug. Multiple uncontrolled seizures, bradycardia, cardiac failure, and cardiac arrest prior to death were reported in these patients.

➤*Treatment:* Ensure adequate airway, oxygenation, and ventilation. Monitor cardiac rhythm and vital signs. EEG monitoring is also recommended for the first 48 hours postingestion. General supportive and symptomatic measures are also recommended. Induction of emesis is not recommended. Gastric lavage with a large-bore orogastric tube with appropriate airway protection, if needed, may be indicated if performed soon after ingestion or in symptomatic patients. Administer activated charcoal. There is no experience with the use of forced diuresis, dialysis, hemoperfusion, or exchange transfusion in the management of bupropion overdoses. No specific antidotes for bupropion are known.

Because of the dose-related risk of seizures with bupropion, hospitalization following suspected overdose should be considered. Based on studies in animals, it is recommended that seizures be treated with IV benzodiazepine administration and other supportive measures, as appropriate.

In managing overdosage, consider the possibiltiy of multiple drug involvement. The physician should consider contacting a poison control center for additional information on the treatment of any overdose.

Refer to Management of Acute Overdosage.

Patient Information

Read all the patient information provided on a separate leaflet for patients. Physicians are advised to review the leaflet with their patients.

Advise patients to stop taking bupropion and consult a doctor if they experience allergic or anaphylactoid/anaphylactic reactions (eg, skin rash, pruritus, hives, chest pain, edema, shortness of breath) during treatment.

Zyban contains the same active ingredient found in *Wellbutrin* and *Wellbutrin SR* used to treat depression. Bupropion products should not be used in conjunction with other products that contain bupropion.

Advise patients not to chew, divide, or crush SR tablets.

Rx **Rilutek** (Rhone-Poulenc Rorer) **Tablets:** 50 mg (RPR 202). White. Capsule shape. Film coated. In 60s.

Indications

➤*Amyotrophic lateral sclerosis (ALS):* Treatment of patients with ALS. Riluzole extends survival or time to tracheostomy.

Administration and Dosage

➤*Approved by the FDA:* December 12, 1995.

The recommended dose is 50 mg every 12 hours. No increased benefit can be expected from higher daily doses, but adverse events are increased.

Take at least 1 hour before or 2 hours after a meal to avoid decreased bioavailability.

➤*Storage/Stability:* Protect from bright light.

Actions

➤*Pharmacology:* The etiology and pathogenesis of amyotrophic lateral sclerosis (ALS; Lou Gehrig's disease) are not known, although a number of hypotheses have been advanced. One hypothesis is that motor neurons, made vulnerable through either genetic predisposition or environmental factors, are injured by glutamate. In some cases of familial ALS the enzyme superoxide dismutase has been defective.

The mode of action of riluzole, a benzathiazole, is unknown. Its pharmacological properties include the following, some of which may be related to its effect: 1) an inhibitory effect on glutamate release; 2) inactivation of voltage-dependent sodium channels; and 3) ability to interfere with intracellular events that follow transmitter binding at excitatory amino acid receptors.

In a single study, riluzole delayed median time to death in a transgenic mouse model of ALS. These mice express human superoxide dismutase bearing one of the mutations found in one of the familial forms of human ALS.

It is also neuroprotective in in vivo models of neuronal injury involving excitotoxic mechanisms. It protected cultured rat motor neurons from the excitotoxic effects of glutamic acid and prevented death of cortical neurons induced by anoxia.

Because of its blockade of glutamatergic neurotransmission, riluzole also exhibits myorelaxant and sedative properties in animals at doses of 30 mg/kg (about 20 times the recommended human daily dose), and anticonvulsant properties at 2.5 mg/kg.

➤*Pharmacokinetics:*

Absorption/Distribution – Riluzole is well absorbed ($\approx$ 90%), with average absolute oral bioavailability of $\approx$ 50%. Pharmacokinetics are linear over a dose range of 25 to 100 mg every 12 hours. A high fat meal decreases absorption, reducing AUC $\approx$ 20% and peak blood levels by $\approx$ 45%. The mean elimination half-life of riluzole is 12 hours after repeated doses. With multiple dose administration, riluzole accumulates in plasma by about 2–fold, and steady-state is reached in < 5 days. Riluzole is 96% bound to plasma proteins, mainly to albumin and lipoproteins.

Metabolism/Excretion – Riluzole is extensively metabolized to six major and a number of minor metabolites, not all of which have been identified. Some metabolites appear pharmacologically active in vitro. The metabolism is mostly hepatic and consists of cytochrome P450 dependent hydroxylation and glucuronidation.

There is marked inter-individual variability in the clearance of riluzole, probably attributable to variability of CYP1A2 activity, the principal isozyme involved in N-hydroxylation.

In vitro studies using liver microsomes show that hydroxylation of the primary amine group producing N-hydroxyriluzole is the main metabolic pathway. Cytochrome P450 1A2 is the principal isozyme involved in N-hydroxylation. Whereas direct glucuroconjugation of riluzole (involving the glucurotransferase isoform UGT-HP4) is very slow in human liver microsomes, N-hydroxyriluozoe is readily conjugated at the hydroxylamine group resulting in the formation of O- (> 90%) and N-glucuronides.

Following a single 150 mg dose to six healthy males, 90% and 5% was recovered in the urine and feces, respectively, over 7 days. Glucuronides accounted for > 85% of the metabolites in urine. Only 2% was recovered in the urine as unchanged drug.

Special populations –

Hepatic/Renal disease: Because riluzole is extensively metabolized and subsequently excreted in the urine, it is likely that functional hepatic and renal impairment will reduce the clearance of riluzole and its metabolites and lead to higher plasma levels (see Warning).

Elderly: Age related decreased reanl function would be expected to give higher plasma levels of riluzole and metabolites. However, in controlled clinical trials, in which $\approx$ 30% of patients were > 65 years of age., there were no differences in adverse events between younger and older patients (see Warnings).

Gender: CYP 1A2 activity has been reported to be lower in women than in men. Therefore, a gender effect may result in higher blood concentrations of riluzole and its metabolites in women (see Precautions).

No gender effect on favorable or adverse events of riluzole was seen in controlled trials, however.

Smoking: Cigarette smoking is known to induce CYP 1A2. Patients who smoke cigarettes would be expected to eliminate riluzole faster. However, there is no information on the effect of, or need for, dosage adjustment in these patients.

Race: Clearance of riluzole in Japanese subjects native to Japan was found to be 50% lower compared with whites after normalizing for body weight. Although it is not clear if this differenc is due to genetic or environmental factors (eg, smoking, alcohol, coffee, dietary preferences), it is possible that Japanese subjects may possess a lower capacity (oxidative or conjugative) for metabolizing riluzole (see Precautions).

➤*Clinical trials:* The efficacy of riluzole as a treatment of ALS was established in two trials in which the time to tracheostomy or death was longer for patients randomized to riluzole than for those randomized to placebo. These studies admitted patients with either familial or sporadic ALS, a disease duration of < 5 years and a baseline forced vital capacity $\geq$ 60%. Although riluzole improved early survival in both studies, measures of muscle strength and neurological function did not show a benefit. Among the patients in whom treatment failed during the study (tracheostomy or death) there was a difference between the treatment groups in median survival of $\approx$ 60 to 90 days. There was no statistically significant difference in mortality at the end of the studies.

Contraindications

Severe hypersensitivity reacts to riluzole or any of the tablet components.

Warnings

➤*Neutropenia:* Among $\approx$ 4000 patients given riluzole for ALS, there were three cases of marked neutropenia (absolute neutrophil < 500/mm^3), all seen within the first 2 months of treatment. In one case, neutrophil counts rose on continued treatment. In a second case, counts rose after therapy was stopped. A third case was more complex, with marked anemia as well as neutropenia and the etiology of both is uncertain. Warn patients to report any febrile illness to the physicians. The report of febrile illness should promt the checking of white blood cell counts.

➤*Renal function impairment:* Use with caution in patients with concomitant renal insufficiency.

➤*Hepatic function impairment:* Use with care in patients with current evidence or history of abnormal liver function indicated by significant abnormalities in serum transaminase (SGPT, SGOT), bilirubin or gamma-glutamate transferase (GGT) levels. Baseline elevations of several LFTs (especially elevated bilirubin) should preclude the use of riluzole.

Riluzole, even in patients without a prior history of liver disease. causes serum aminotransferase elevations. Experience in almost 800 ALS patients indicates that $\approx$ 50% of riluzole-treated patients will experience at least one SGPT level above the upper limit of normaul (ULN), $\approx$ 8% will hve elevations> 3 $\times$ ULN and $\approx$ 2% will have elevations > 5 $\times$ ULN. A single non-ALS patient with epilepsy treated with concomitant carbamazepine and phenobarbital experienced marked, rapid elevations of liver enzymes with jaundice for four months after starting riluzole; these returned to normal 7 weeks after treatment discontinuation.

Maximum increases in serum SGPT usually occurred within 3 months after the start of therapy and were usually transient when < 5 $\times$ ULN. In trials, if SGPT levels were < 5 $\times$ ULN, treatment continued and SGPT levels usually returned to below 2 $\times$ ULN within 2 to 6 monhts. However, treatment in studies was discontinued if SGPT levels exceeded 5 $\times$ ULN, so that there is no experience with continued treatmetn of ALS patiens once GSPT values exceed 5 $\times$ ULN. There were rare instances of jaundice.

Monitor liver chemistries (see Precautions).

➤*Fertility impairment:* Riluzole imipaired fertility when administered to male and female rats prior to and during mating at an oral dose of 15 mg/kg or 1.5 times the maximum daily dose (see Pregnancy).

➤*Elderly:* Age-related compromised renal and hepatic function may cause a decrease in clearance of riluzole. In controlled clinical trials, $\approx$ 30% of patients were > 65 years old. There were no differences in adverse effects between younger and older patients.

➤*Pregnancy:* Category C. Administration of riluzole to pregnant animals during the period of organogenesis caused embryotoxicity in rats and rabbits at doses of 27 and 60 mg/kg, respectively, or 2.6 and 11.5 times, respectively, the recommended maximum human daily dose. Evidence of maternal toxicity was also observed at these doses. When administered to rats prior to and during mating (males and females) and throughout gestation and lactation (females), riluzole produced adverse effects on pregnancy (decreased implantations, increased intrauterine death) and offspring viability and growth at an oral dose of 15 mg/kg.

RILUZOLE

There are no adequate and well controlled studies in pregnant women. Use during pregnancy only if the potential benefit justifies the potential risk to the fetus.

➤*Lactation:* In rat studies, riluzole was detected in maternal milk. It is not known whether riluzole is excreted in breast milk. Because the potential for serious adverse reactions in nursing infants from riluzole is unknown, advise women not to breastfeed during treatment with riluzole.

➤*Children:* The safety and efficacy in children have not been established.

Precautions

➤*Monitoring:* Measure serum aminotransferases including SGPT levels before and during therapy. Evaluate serum SGPT levels every month during the first 3 months of treatment, every 3 months during the remainder of the first year and periodically thereafter. Evaluate serum SGPT levels more frequently in patients who develop elevations (see Warnings).

As noted in the Warnings section, there is no experience with continued treatment of patients once SGPT exceeds 5 × ULN. If a decision is made to continue to treat these patients, frequent monitoring (at least weekly) of complete liver function is recommended. Discontinue treatment if SGPT exceeds 10 × ULN or if clinical jaundice develops. Because there is no experience with rechallenge of patients who have had riluzole discontinued for SGPT > 5 × ULN, no recommendations about restarting riluzole can be made.

In the two controlled trials in patients with ALS, the frequency with which values for hemoglobin, hematocrit and erythrocyte counts fell below the lower limit of normal was greater in riluzole-treated patients than in placebo-treated patients; however, these changes were mild and transient. The proportions of patients observed with abnoramlly low values for these parameters showed a dose-response relationship. Only one patient was discontinued from treatment because of severe anemia. The significance of this finding is unknown.

➤*Special populations:* Females and Japanese patients may possess a lower metabolic capacity to eliminate riluzole compared with male and white subjects, respectively.

Drug Interactions

➤*Effect of other drugs on riluzole metabolism:* In vitro studies using human liver microsomal preparations suggest that CYP1A2 is the principal isozyme involved in the initial oxidative metabolism of riluzole and therefore potential interactions may occur when riluzole is given concurrently with agents that affect CYP1A2 activity. Potential inhibitors of CYP1A2 (eg, caffeine, theophylline, amitriptyline, quinolones) could decrease the rate of riluzole elimination, while inducers of CYP1A2 (eg, cigarette smoke, charcoal-broiled food, rifampin, omeprazole) could increase the rate of riluzole elimination.

➤*Drug/Food interactions:* A high fat meal decreases absorption of riluzole, reducing AUC by ≈ 20% and peak blood levels by ≈ 45%.

Adverse Reactions

The most commonly observed adverse reactions associated with the use of riluzole were: Asthenia, nausea, dizziness, diarrhea, anorexia, vertigo, somnolence, circumoral paresthesia (dose-related); decreased lung function; abdominal pain; pneumonia; vomiting.

Approximately 14% of patients with ALS who received riluzole in premarketing clinical trials discontinued treatment because of an adverse experience. Of those patients who discontinued due to adverse events, the most commonly reported were: Nausea, abdominal pain, constipation and SGPT elevations.

Riluzole Adverse Reactions (%)				
	Riluzole			Placebo (n = 320)
Adverse Reaction	50 mg/day (n = 237)	100 mg/day (n = 313)	200 mg/day (n = 244)	
Cardiovascular				
Hypertension	6.8	5.1	3.3	4.1
Tachycardia	1.3	2.6	2	13
Phlebitis	0.4	1	0.8	0.3
Palpitation	0.4	0.6	1.2	0.9
Postural hypotension	0.8	0	1.6	0.6
CNS				
Hypertonia	5.9	6.1	5.3	5.9
Depression	4.2	4.5	6.1	5
Dizziness	5.1	3.8	12.7	2.5
Dry mouth	3	3.5	2	3.4
Insomnia	2.1	3.5	2.9	3.4
Somnolence	0.8	1.9	4.1	1.3
Vertigo	2.5	1.9	4.5	0.9
Circumoral paresthesia	1.3	1.6	3.3	0

Riluzole Adverse Reactions (%)				
	Riluzole			Placebo (n = 320)
Adverse Reaction	50 mg/day (n = 237)	100 mg/day (n = 313)	200 mg/day (n = 244)	
Dermatologic				
Pruritus	3.8	3.8	2.5	3.1
Eczema	0.8	1.6	1.6	0.6
Alopecia	0	1	1.2	0.6
Exfoliative dermatitis	0	0.6	1.2	0
GI				
Nausea	12.2	16.3	20.5	10.6
Vomiting	4.2	4.2	4.5	1.6
Dyspepsia	2.5	3.8	6.1	5
Anorexia	3.8	3.2	8.6	3.8
Diarrhea	5.5	2.9	9	3.1
Flatulence	2.5	2.6	2	1.9
Stomatitis	0.8	1	1.2	0
Tooth disorder	0	1	1.2	0.3
Oral moniliasis	0.4	0.6	1.2	0.3
GU				
Urinary tract infection	2.5	2.6	4.5	2.2
Dysuria	0	1	1.2	0.3
Metabolic/Nutritional				
Weight loss	4.6	4.8	3.7	4.7
Peripheral edema	4.2	2.9	3.3	2.2
Respiratory				
Decreased lung function	13.1	10.2	16	9.4
Rhinitis	8.9	6.4	7.8	6.3
Increased cough	2.1	2.6	3.7	1.6
Sinusitis	0.4	1	1.6	0.9
Miscellaneous				
Asthenia	14.8	19.2	20.1	12.2
Headache	8	7.3	7	6.6
Abdominal pain	6.8	5.1	7.8	3.8
Arthralgia	5.1	3.5	1.6	3.4
Back pain	1.7	3.2	4.1	2.5
Aggravation reaction	0.4	1.3	2	0.9
Malaise	0.4	0.6	1.2	0

➤*Cardiovascular:* Syncope, hypotension, heart failure, migraine, peripheral vascular disease, angina pectoris, myocardial infarction, ventricular extrasystoles, cerebral hemorrhage, atrial fibrillation, bundle branch block, congestive heart failure, pericarditis, lower extremity embolus, myocardial ischemia, shock (0.1% to 1%); bradycardia, cerebral ischemia, hemorrhage, mesenteric artery occlusion, subarachnoid hemorrhage, supraventricular tachycardia, thrombosis, ventricular fibrillation, ventricular tachycardia (≤ 0.1%).

➤*CNS:* Agitation, tremor (≥ 1%); hallucinations, personality disorders, abnormal thinking, coma, paranoid reaction, manic reaction, ataxia, extrapyrimidal syndrome, hypokinesis, urinary retention, emotional ability, delusions, apathy, hypesthesia, incoordination, confusion, convulsion, leg cramps, amnesia, dysarthria, increased libido, stupor, subdural hematoma, abnormal gait, delirium, depersonalization, facial paralysis, hemiplegia, decreased libido, myoclonus (0.1% to 1%); abnormal dreams, acute brain syndrome, CNS depression, dementia, cerebral embolism, euphoria, hypotonia, ileus, peripheral neurities, psychosis, psychotic depression, schizophrenic reaction, trismus, wristdrop (≤ 0.1%).

➤*Dermatologic:* Skin ulceration, urticaria, psoriasis, seborrhea, skin disorder, fungal dermatitis (0.1% to 1%); engioedema, contact dermatitis, erythema multiforme, furunculosis, skin moniliasis, skin granuloma, skin nodule (≤ 0.1%).

➤*Endocrine:* Diabetes mellitus, thyroid neoplasia (0.1% to 1%); diabetes insipidus, parathyroid disorder (≤ 0.1%).

➤*GI:* Increased appetite, intestinal obstruction, fecal impaction, GI hemorrhage, GI ulceration, gastritis, fecal incontinence, jaundice, hepatitis, glossitis, gum hemorrhage, pancreatitis, tenesmus, esophageal stenosis (0.1% to 1%); cheilitis, cholecystitis, hematemesis, melena, biliary pain, proctitis, pseudomembranous enterocolitis, enlarged salivary gland, tongue discoloration, tooth caries (≤ 0.1%).

➤*GU:* Urinary urgency, urine abnormality, urinary incontinence, kidney calculus, hematuria, impotence, prostate carcinoma, kidney pain, metorrhagia, priapism (0.1% to 1%); amenorrhea, breast abscess, breast pain, nephritis, nocturia, pyelonephritis, enlarged uterine fibroids, uterine hemorrhage, vaginal moniliasis (≤ 0.1%).

RILUZOLE

➤*Hematologic/Lymphatic:* Anemia, leukocytosis, leukopenia, ecchymosis (0.1% to 1%); neutropenia, aplastic anemia, cyanosis, hypochromic anemia, iron deficiency anemia, lymphadenopathy, petechiae, purpura (≤ 0.1%).

➤*Musculoskeletal:* Athrosis, myasthenia, bone neoplasm (0.1% to 1%); bone necrosis, osteoporosis, tetany (≤ 0.1%).

➤*Respiratory:* Hiccough, pleural disorder, asthma, epistaxis, hemoptysis, yawn, hyperventilation, lung edema, hypoventilation, lung carcinoma, hypoxia, laryngitis, pleural effusion, pneumothorax, respiratory monoliasis, stridor (0.1% to 1%).

➤*Special senses:* Amblyopia, ophthalmitis (0.1% to 1%); blepharitis, cataract, deafness, diplopia, ear pain, glaucoma, hyperacusis, photophobia, taste loss, vestibular disorder (≤ 0.1%).

➤*Metabolic/Nutritional:* Gout, respiratory acidosis, edema, thirst, hypokalemia, hyponatremia, weight gain (0.1% to 1%); generalized edema, hypercalcemia, hypercholesteremia (≤ 0.1%).

➤*Miscellaneous:* Adverse events that occurred in > 2% of patients treated with 100 mg/day but equally or more frequently in the placebo group included: Accidental injury; apnea; bronchitis; constipation; death; dysphagia; dyspnea; flu syndrome; heart arrest; increased sputum; pneumonia; respiratory disorder. Dizziness did occur more commonly in females (11%) than in males (4%).

Hostility (≥ 1); abscess, sespsis, photosensitivity reaction, cellulitis, face edema, hernia, peritonitis, attempted suicide, injection site reaction, chills, flu syndrome, intentional injury, enlarged abdomen, neoplasm (0.1% to 1%); acrodynia, hypothermia, moniliasis, rheumatoid arthritis (≤ 0.1%).

➤*Lab test abnormalities:* Increased gamma glutamyl transferase, abnormal liver function/tests, increased alkaline phosphatase, positive direct Coombs test, increased gamma globulins (0.1% to 1%); increased lactic dehydrogenase (≤ 0.1%).

Overdosage

No specific antidote or treatment information is available. In the event of overdose, discontinue therapy immediately. Treatment should be supportive and directed toward alleviating symptoms.

Patient Information

Advise patients to report any febrile illness to their physicians.

Advise patients to take riluzole at the same time of day (eg, in the morning and evening) each day. If a dose is missed, take the next tablet as originally planned.

Warn patients about the potential for dizziness, vertigo or somnolence and advise them not to drive or operate machinery until they have gained sufficient experience on riluzole to gauge whether or not it affects their mental or motor performance adversely.

Whether alcohol increases risk of serious hepatotoxicity with riluzole is unknown; discourage riluzole-treated patients from drinking alcohol in excess.

HYALURONIC ACID DERIVATIVES

Rx	**Hyalgan** (Sanofi-Synthe-labo)	**Solution:** 20 mg sodium hyaluronate/2 mL[1]	2 mL vials and prefilled syringes.
Rx	**Supartz** (Smith & Nephew)	**Solution:** 25 mg sodium hyaluronate/2.5 mL[2]	2.5 mL prefilled syringe.
Rx	**Synvisc** (Wyeth)	**Solution:** 16 mg hylan polymers (hylan G-F 20)/2 mL[3]	2 mL glass syringe with 3 disposable syringes.
Rx	**Orthovisc** (Ortho Biotech)	**Injection:** 30 mg hyaluronan,[4] 18 mg sodium chloride.	In 2 mL single use vials.

[1] Molecular weight is 500,000 to 730,000 daltons.
[2] Molecular weight is 620,000 to 1,170,000 daltons.
[3] Molecular weight is 6,000,000 daltons on average.
[4] Molecular weight is 1,000,000 to 2,900,000 daltons.

Sodium hyaluronate is also used as an ophthalmic agent. For complete prescribing information, refer to the individual monograph in the Ophthalmics section.

Indications

➤*Osteoarthritis symptoms:* For the treatment of pain in osteoarthritis of the knee in patients who have failed to respond adequately to conservative nonpharmacologic therapy and simple analgesics (eg, acetaminophen).

Administration and Dosage

➤*Approved by the FDA:* May 28, 1997.

Administer 2 mL (2.5 mL for *Supartz*) by intra-articular injection in affected knee once weekly for the recommended number of injections per treatment cycle. If treatment is bilateral, use a separate 2 mL (2.5 mL for *Supartz*) vial/syringe for each knee. Do not prepare injection site with skin disinfectants containing quarternary ammonium salts; precipitation of drug can occur. Do not give other intra-articular injectables concomitantly (see Warnings).

➤*Treatment cycle:*

Hyalgan – Give a total of 5 injections/treatment cycle using a 20 gauge needle. Inject local anesthetic (eg, lidocaine) SC prior to administration. Studies with a follow-up period of 60 days have shown that patients may experience benefit with 3 injections given at weakly intervals.

Supartz – Give a total of 5 injections/treatment cycle using a 22 to 23 gauge needle. Injection of a local anesthetic (eg, lidocaine) SC prior to administration may be recommended.

Synvisc – Give a total of 3 injections/treatment cycle using an 18 to 22 gauge needle. Remove synovial fluid or effusion before each injection.

Orthovisc – Inject into the knee joint in a series of intra-articular injections 1 week apart for 3 or 4 injections.

➤*Joint effusion:* If present, remove effusion before administering therapy. Do not use the same syringe for removing fluid and injecting hyaluronic acid derivatives. However, use the same needle for injecting **hylan G-F 20**.

➤*Storage / Stability:*

Hyalgan and Supartz – Products are intended for single use; use immediately once opened and discard any unused portion. Store in original package below 25°C (less than 77°F); do not freeze.

Synvisc – Products are intended for single use; use immediately once opened and discard any unused portion. Store in original package below 30°C (less than 86°F); protect from light; do not freeze.

Actions

➤*Pharmacology:* Hyaluronic acid is a naturally occurring polysaccharide of the glycosaminoglycan family containing repeating disaccharide units of sodium-glucuronate-N-acetylgucosamine. Certain disease states can affect the integrity and rheology of synovial fluid and in the case of osteoarthritis (OA), decrease its viscosity and elasticity. This results from both a decrease in the molecular size and concentration of hyaluronan within the synovial fluid. Intra-articular viscosupplementation with hyaluronic acid, high molecular weight fractions of purified natural sodium hyaluronate, and cross-linked polymers of hyaluronan known as hylans are aimed at improving the elasticity and viscosity of synovial fluid for the treatment of OA. Exact mechanism(s) of action of hyaluronic acid derivatives is/are unknown.

➤*Pharmacokinetics:* The molecular weight of the agent may have an effect on its half-life. The higher the molecular weight, the longer the half-life may be. Higher molecular weights also appear to lead to increased elasticity of the synovial fluid.

➤*Clinical trials:* Patients with OA of the knee with moderate to severe pain were randomized to receive *Hyalgan* or placebo intra-articular injections once weekly for 5 weeks or naproxen 500 mg twice daily for 26 weeks. A greater percentage of sodium hyaluronate patients (56%) than placebo (41%) or naproxen (45%) achieved a predefined improvement in a 50 foot walk by week 5 and maintained this improvement through week 26.

Contraindications

Hypersensitivity to hyaluronan or any components of the product; infections or skin diseases in the area of the injection site; concomitant skin disinfectants containing quarternary ammonium salts (see Warnings).

Warnings

➤*Quarternary ammonium salts:* Avoid concomitant use of disinfectants for skin preparation containing quarternary ammonium salts; precipitation of drug may occur.

➤*Intra-articular administration:* Administer by intra-articular injection only. Avoid intravascular, extra-articular, synovial tissue and capsule administration; rare systemic adverse events have been reported with **hylan G-F 20**. Safety and efficacy of intra-articular administration in locations other than the knee and for conditions other than osteoarthritis have not been established. Use **hylan G-F 20** with caution when evidence of lymphatic or venous stasis exists in treatment leg. The safety and efficacy of **hylan G-F 20** in severely inflamed knee joints have not been established.

Do not coadminister with other intra-articular injectables. Safety and efficacy have not been established and may be altered by dilutional effects.

➤*Inflammatory arthritis:* Transient increases in inflammation in the injected knee following injections with **sodium hyaluronate** have been reported in some patients with inflammatory arthritis (eg, rheumatoid or gouty arthritis).

➤*Hypersensitivity reactions:* Anaphylactoid reactions have occurred with **sodium hyaluronate**. The incidents resolved with favorable outcomes upon discontinuation of therapy. Five allergic reactions were reported in the **sodium hyaluronate** group. All 5 events were classified as mild to moderate. These were: Hayfever, reaction on face and neck, cutaneous reaction on forearms and knees, and an undefined mild allergy reaction. No anaphylactic reactions were observed.

➤*Pregnancy:* Safety and efficacy have not been established in pregnant women. Give to a pregnant woman only if potential benefits outweigh the potential risks.

➤*Lactation:* It is not known if hyaluronic acid derivatives are excreted in breast milk. Safety and efficacy have not been established in lactating women. Exercise caution when administering to a breast-feeding woman.

➤*Children:* Safety and efficacy have not been established.

Precautions

➤*Avian allergies:* These products are extracted from chicken/rooster combs. Use caution in patients allergic to avian proteins, feathers, and egg products.

➤*Joint effusion:* Remove joint effusion before using hyaluronic acid derivatives.

➤*Latex sensitivity:* Administer **hylan G-F 20** with caution to patients with a possible history of latex sensitivity, because the packaging contains dry natural rubber.

➤*Treatment cycle:* The efficacy of a single treatment cycle of less than the recommended number of injections has not been established; 5 injections of *Hyalgan*, 5 injections of *Supartz*, 3 injections of *Synvisc*. Safety and efficacy of repeat cycles have not been established.

Adverse Reactions

➤*Hyalgan:*

CNS – Headache (18%).

GI – GI complaints (29%, severe in 2.4%).

Local – Injection site pain (23%); skin reaction, including ecchymosis and rash (14%); joint pain and swelling (13%, severe in 1.2%); pruritus (7%); positive bacterial cultures of aspirated effusion from the treated knee (1.2%).

➤*Supartz:*

CNS – Headache (4.4%); dizziness (1% to 4%).

GI – Abdominal pain, diarrhea, dyspepsia, nausea (1% to 4%).

Local – Injection site reaction, including application/injection site reaction, injection site inflammation, and purpura (5.7%); injection site pain (4.2%).

Musculoskeletal – Arthralgia (17.8%); arthropathy/arthrosis/arthritis (11%).

Respiratory – Upper respiratory infection, sinusitis, bronchitis, rhinitis (1% to 4%).

Miscellaneous – Back pain (6.5%); pain, non-specific (6%); flu-like symptoms, UTI, inflicted injury, leg pain, discomfort in legs, fall (1% to 4%).

HYALURONIC ACID DERIVATIVES

▶*Synvisc:*

Dermatologic – Rash, thorax and back (2%); pruritus (2%).

Musculoskeletal – Calf cramps, muscle pain.

Local – Knee pain or swelling (2.2% of injections, 7.2% of patients).

Miscellaneous – Ankle edema, tonsillitis with nausea, low back sprain, hemorrhoid problems, tachyarrhythmia, phlebitis with varicosities.

▶*Postmarketing:*

Hyalgan –

Fever: Seven cases of fever were reported, in which 3 were associated with local reactions; pyogenic arthritis was ruled out for all 3 cases. All fever patients discontinued treatment and all resolved.

Shock: One patient reported incident of shock (hypotensive crisis). The incident resolved and treatment was continued.

Synvisc –

CNS: Headache, dizziness, chills, paresthesia, malaise (rare).

Dermatological: Rash; itching; hives (rare).

Local: The most common adverse events reported have been pain, swelling, and/or effusion in the injected knee. In some cases the effusion was considerable and caused pronounced pain. In some instances, patients have presented with knees that were tender, warm, and red. It is important to rule out infection or cystalline arthopathies in such cases. Synovial fluid aspirates of varying volumes have revealed a range of cell counts, from very few to over 50,000 cells/mm^3. Reported treatments included symptomatic therapy (eg, rest, ice, heat, elevation, simple analgesics, NSAIDs) and/or arthrocentesis. Intra-articular corticosteroids have been used when infection was excluded. Rarely, arthroscopy has been performed. The occurrence of post-injection effusion may be associated with patient history of effusion, advanced stage of disease, and/or the number of injections a patient receives. Reactions generally abate within a few days. Clinical benefit from the treatment may still occur after such reactions.

Miscellaneous: Nausea, fever, muscle cramps, peripheral edema, flushing facial edema, intra-articular infections, respiratory difficulties, thrombocytopenia (rare).

Patient Information

Provide patients with a copy of Patient Information sheet prior to use.

Inform patients that transient pain/swelling of the treated joint may occur.

Advise patients to avoid strenuous or prolonged (more than 1 hour) weight-bearing activities (eg, jogging, tennis) within 48 hours following treatment.

Advise patients receiving **hylan G-F 20** that transient effusion may occur. In some cases the effusion may be considerable and cause pronounced pain; advise patients to consult with physician if swelling is extensive.

HYALURONIC ACID

| Rx | Restylane (Medicis Aesthetics) | Gel for injection: 20 mg/mL | In single-use prefilled syringes. |

Indications

▶*Facial wrinkles and folds:* For mid to deep dermal implantation for the correction of moderate to severe facial wrinkles and folds, such as nasolabial folds.

The safety and efficacy of hyaluronic acid for the treatment of anatomic regions other than nasolabial folds have not been established.

Administration and Dosage

▶*Approved by the FDA:* December 12, 2003.

▶*Injection:* Before injecting, press the rod carefully until a small droplet is visible at the tip of the needle. Inject, applying even pressure on the plunger rod while slowly pulling the needle backwards. The wrinkle should be lifted and eliminated by the end of the injection. It is important that the injection is stopped just before the needle is pulled out of the skin to prevent material from leaking out or ending up too superficially in the skin. Typical usage for each treatment session is less than 2 mL per treatment site; however, based on clinical studies, limit patients to 1.5 mL per treatment site.

Only correct to 100% of the dermal volume effect. Do not overcorrect. With cutaneous contour deformities, the best results are obtained if the defect can be manually stretched to the point where it is eliminated. The degree and duration of the correction depend on the character of the defect treated, the tissue stress at the implant site, the depth of the implant in the tissue, and the injection technique. Markedly indurated defects may be difficult to correct.

▶*Postinjection:* When the injection is completed, gently massage the treated site so that it conforms to the contour of the surrounding tissue. If an overcorrection has occurred, massage the area firmly between the fingers or against an underlying superficial bone to obtain optimal results.

▶*Administration:* The injection technique may vary with regard to the depth of injection and the administered quantity. The linear threading technique, serial puncture injections, or a combination of the 2 have been used with success.

The correct injection technique is crucial for the final result of the treatment.

Administer using a thin gauge needle (30 g × ½″). The needle is inserted at an approximate angle of 30° parallel to the length of the wrinkle or fold. The bevel of the needle should face upwards and the substance should be injected into the middle of the dermis. For mid-dermis placement, the contour of the needle should be visible but not the color of it. If the product is injected too deep or IM, the duration of the effect will be shorter. If the product is injected too superficially, this may result in visible lumps and/or grayish discoloration.

▶*Administration precautions:* If so called blanching is observed (ie, the overlying skin turns a whitish color), stop the injection immediately and massage the area until it returns to a normal color.

▶*Retreatment:* If the wrinkle needs further treatment, repeat the same procedure with several punctures of the skin until a satisfactory result is obtained. Additional treatment may be necessary to achieve the desired correction. With patients who have localized swelling, the degree of correction is sometimes difficult to judge at the time of treatment. In these cases, it is better to invite the patient to a touch-up session after 1 to 2 weeks.

▶*Admixture incompatibilities:* Do not mix hyaluronic acid with other products prior to injection. Hyaluronic acid is supplied in a syringe ready for use. Never mix with other products prior to injection of the device.

▶*Storage/Stability:* Hyaluronic acid must be used prior to the expiration date. Store at a temperature up to 25°C (77°F). Do not freeze and protect from sunlight. Refrigeration is not needed.

Do not resterilize hyaluronic acid because this may damage or alter the product. Hyaluronic acid is packaged for single-patient use.

Hyaluronic acid is a clear, colorless gel without particulates. In the event that the content of a syringe shows signs of separation and/or appears cloudy, do not use the syringe.

Actions

▶*Pharmacology:* Hyaluronic acid is generated by *Streptococcus* species of bacteria, chemically crosslinked with BDDE, stabilized, and suspended in a physiologic buffer.

▶*Clinical trials:* A randomized, controlled trial evaluated the safety and effectiveness of hyaluronic acid for the treatment of facial wrinkles and folds compared with *Zyplast*, a cross-linked collagen dermal implant. Using hyaluronic acid on randomized nasal labial folds and the control treatment on the opposite nasal folds, effectiveness of treatment was evaluated at 6 months and safety evaluated at 12 months. The primary endpoint was the difference in effect of hyaluronic acid and *Zyplast* on the visual severity of the nasolabial folds 6 months after baseline. The primary evaluation was the 5-point wrinkle severity rating scale (SRS) score. Baseline was defined to begin at the follow-up, demonstrating that optimal correction had been maintained for 2 weeks. Optimal correction was defined to be the best cosmetic result obtainable as determined by the evaluating physician. A specific, objective score or goal for correction was not defined and 2 injectable implant sessions were expected. Hyaluronic acid was shown to be safe and effective when compared with *Zyplast* as to duration of the augmentation of nasolabial folds at 6 months follow-up. Based on the per patient evaluation by the evaluating investigator, the SRS scores at 6 months demonstrated that SRS for hyaluronic acid was lower (better) than control in 78 patients; hyaluronic acid was equal to control in 46 patients; and hyaluronic acid was higher (worse) than control in 13 patients.

Contraindications

Severe allergies manifested by history of anaphylaxis or history or presence of multiple severe allergies.

Hyaluronic acid contains trace amounts of gram-positive bacterial proteins and is contraindicated for patients with a history of allergies to such material.

Use in breast augmentation and for implantation into bone, tendon, ligament, or muscle.

Hyaluronic acid must not be implanted into blood vessels. Implantation into dermal vessels may cause vascular occlusion, infarction, or embolic phenomena.

Warnings

▶*Skin eruptions:* Defer the use of hyaluronic acid at specific sites in which an active inflammatory process (skin eruptions such as cysts, pimples, rashes, or hives) or infection is present until the inflammatory process has been controlled.

▶*Injection-site reactions:* Injection-site reactions to hyaluronic acid have been observed as consisting mainly of short-term inflammatory symptoms starting early after treatment and with less than 7 days duration.

HYALURONIC ACID

➤*Superficial necrosis:* Localized superficial necrosis may occur after injection in the glabellar area. This may be the result of injury, obstruction, or compromise of the blood vessels.

➤*Long-term use:* Long-term safety and effectiveness of use beyond 1 year have not been investigated in clinical trials.

➤*Infection:* As with all transcutaneous procedures, hyaluronic acid implantation carries a risk of infection.

➤*Keloid formation or hypertrophic scarring:* The safety of hyaluronic acid in patients with increased susceptibility to keloid formation and hypertrophic scarring has not been studied. Do not use hyaluronic acid in patients with known susceptibility to keloid formation or hypertrophic scarring.

➤*Hypersensitivity reactions:* Hypersensitivity as an inflammatory reaction to hyaluronic acid has been observed with swelling, redness, tenderness, induration, and rarely acneiform papules at the injection site (see Adverse Reactions).

➤*Pregnancy:* Safety and efficacy have not been established in pregnant women. Give to a pregnant woman only if potential benefits outweigh the potential risks.

➤*Lactation:* It is not known if hyaluronic acid derivatives are excreted in breast milk. Safety and efficacy have not been established in lactating women.

➤*Children:* Safety and efficacy of hyaluronic acid in children have not been established.

Precautions

➤*Inflammatory reaction:* If laser treatment, chemical peeling, or any other procedure based on active dermal response is considered after treatment with hyaluronic acid, there is a possible risk of an inflammatory reaction at the implant site. This also applies if hyaluronic acid is administered before the skin has healed completely after such a procedure.

➤*Blanching:* If so called blanching is observed (ie, the overlying skin turns a whitish color), stop the injection immediately and massage the area until it returns to a normal color.

➤*Photosensitivity/Cold weather:* Minimize exposure of the treated area to excessive sun, UV lamp exposure, and extreme cold weather until any initial swelling and redness has resolved.

➤*Special risk:* Use with caution in patients on immunosuppressive therapy. Patients who are using substances that reduce coagulation, such as aspirin and NSAIDs, may experience increased bruising or bleeding at injection sites.

Adverse Reactions

In a study of 138 patients at 6 centers, adverse events reported in hyaluronic acid patient diaries during 14 days after treatment are reported in the following table. Patients in the study received hyaluronic acid injections in 1 side of the face, and a bovine collagen dermal filler (*Zyplast*) in the other side of the face.

Maximum Intensity of Symptoms After Initial Treatment (%)					
	Hyaluronic acid side			*Zyplast* side		
	Mild	Moderate	Severe	Mild	Moderate	Severe
Bruising	23.2	25.4	3.6	31.2	16.7	0.7
Itching	22.5	8	0	19.6	4.4	0
Pain	29	24.6	3.6	33.3	7.2	1.4
Redness	40.6	39.1	5.1	52.2	26.8	5.8
Swelling	39.1	44.2	3.6	47.1	25.4	1.4
Tenderness	43.5	31.2	2.9	50.7	12.3	1.4
Other	10.1	10.9	3.6	14.5	7.2	2.2

Duration of Adverse Events After Initial Treatment (%)							
	Hyaluronic acid side				*Zyplast* side		
	Number of days				Number of days		
	1	2 to 7	8 to 13	≥ 14	1	2 to 7	8 to 13	≥ 14
Bruising	5.1	40.6	4.4	2.2	5.1	38.4	3.6	1.4
Itching	8	18.1	4.4	0	5.8	15.9	2.2	0
Pain	21	34.8	1.4	0	22.5	18.1	0.7	0.7
Redness	13.8	49.3	13	8.7	13.8	51.4	10.9	8.7
Swelling	11.6	60.9	11.6	2.9	10.1	50.7	11.6	1.4
Tenderness	15.2	56.5	4.4	1.4	19.6	39.1	4.4	1.4
Other	5.1	16.7	2.2	0.7	7.2	10.9	4.4	1.4

Other Adverse Events[a] (%)	
Adverse event	Incidence (N = 138)
CNS	
Depression	2.2
Depression aggravated	2.2
Headache	1.4
Migraine	1.4
Dermatologic	
Acne	3.6
Contact dermatitis	1.4
Respiratory	
Bronchitis	1.4
Pneumonia	1.4
Sinusitis	5
Upper respiratory tract infection	4.3
Miscellaneous	
Allergic reaction[b]	1.4
Arthralgia	1.4
Back pain	2.2
Herpes simplex	1.4
Hypercholesterolemia	1.4
Inflicted injury	5.8
Osteoporosis	1.4
Tooth disorder	2.9
Urinary incontinence	1.4

[a] From physician case report forms.
[b] One case of seasonal allergy and one reaction to make-up in the periorbital area.

➤*Postmarketing:*

Dermatologic – Inflammatory reaction has been observed with swelling, redness, tenderness, induration, and rarely acneiform papules at the injection site with onset at 1 to several weeks after initial treatment in previously unexposed individuals, and in less than 7 days following treatment in patients known to have been previously exposed. Average duration of this effect is 2 weeks.

Miscellaneous – Allergic reaction, bacterial infection, necrosis.

Adverse reactions should be reported to Medicis Aesthetics at (866) 222-1480.

Patient Information

Counsel the patient and discuss the appropriate indications, risks, benefits, and expected response to the hyaluronic acid treatment.

If the treated area is swollen directly after the injection, an ice pack can be applied on the site for a short period.

Patients may have mild to moderate injection-site reactions, which typically resolve in a few days.

Minimize exposure of the treated area to excessive sun and UV lamp exposure and extreme cold weather until any initial swelling and redness has resolved.

BOTULINUM TOXIN TYPE A

Rx	**Botox** (Allergan)	**Powder for Injection (vacuum dried):** 100 units of vacuum-dried *Clostridium botulinum* toxin type A neurotoxin complex[1]	Preservative-free. 0.5 mg albumin (human), 0.9 mg sodium chloride. In single-use vials.
Rx	**Botox Cosmetic** (Allergan)		Preservative-free. 0.5 mg albumin (human), 0.9 mg sodium chloride. In single-use vials.

[1] One unit corresponds to the calculated median lethal intraperitoneal dose (LD$_{50}$) in mice.

For more information, refer to Botulinum Toxin Type A monograph in the Ophthalmic and Otic Agents chapter.

Indications

➤*Cervical dystonia (CD) (Botox only):* For the treatment of CD in adults to decrease the severity of abnormal head position and neck pain associated with CD.

➤*Glabellar lines (Botox Cosmetic only):* For the temporary improvement in the appearance of moderate to severe glabellar lines associated with corrugator or procerus muscle activity in adult patients 65 years of age or younger.

➤*Unlabeled uses:* Treatment of hemifacial spasms, spasmodic torticollis (ie, clonic twisting of the head), oromandibular dystonia, spasmodic dysphonia (laryngeal dystonia) and for other dystonias (eg, writer's cramp, focal task-specific dystonias). Botulinum toxin is being assessed in the treatment of head and neck tremor unresponsive to pharmacologic therapy. Designated an orphan drug for the treatment of dynamic muscle contracture in pediatric cerebral palsy patients.

Other reported uses of botulinum toxin type A include the following: Acquired nystagmus, oscillopsia, tremor, tics, detrusor sphincter dyssynergia, achalasia, anismus/vaginismus, cosmesis, hyperhidrosis, myofacial pain, temporomandibular joint dysfunction, cervicogenic headache, and spasticity.

Administration and Dosage

➤*Approved by the FDA:* December 1989.

➤*CD (Botox only):*

Patients with known history of tolerance – The mean dose administered to patients in the phase 3 study was 236 U (25% to 75%; range, 198 U to 300 U). The dose was divided among the affected muscles. Tailor dosing in initial and sequential treatment sessions to the individual patient based on the patient's head and neck position, localization of pain, muscle hypertrophy, patient response, and adverse event history.

Patients without prior use – The initial dose for a patient without prior use of botulinum toxin type A should be at a lower dose, with subsequent dosing adjusted based on individual response. Limiting the total dose injected into the sternocleidomastoid muscles to 100 U or less may decrease the occurrence of dysphagia.

A 25, 27, or 30-gauge needle may be used for superficial muscles, and a longer 22-gauge needle may be used for deeper musculature. Localization of the involved muscles with electromyographic guidance may be useful.

Clinical improvement generally begins within the first 2 weeks after injection with maximum clinical benefit at approximately 6 weeks postinjection. In the phase 3 study, most subjects were observed to have returned to pretreatment status by 3 months posttreatment.

Dilution technique – To reconstitute vacuum-dried botulinum toxin type A, use sterile normal saline without a preservative; 0.9% Sodium Chloride Injection is the recommended diluent. Draw up the proper amount of diluent in the appropriate size syringe, and slowly inject the diluent into the vial. Because botulinum toxin type A is denatured by bubbling or similar violent agitation, inject the diluent into the vial gently. Discard the vial if a vacuum does not pull the diluent into the vial. Gently mix botulinum toxin type A with the saline by rotating the vial. Record the date and time of reconstitution on the space on the label. Administer within 4 hours after reconstitution.

The use of 1 vial for more than 1 patient is not recommended because the product and diluent do not contain a preservative.

Botulinum Toxin Type A Dilution	
Diluent added (0.9% Sodium Chloride Injection)	Resulting dose (U/0.1 mL)
1 mL	10 U
2 mL	5 U
4 mL	2.5 U
8 mL	1.25 U

Note – These dilutions are calculated for an injection volume of 0.1 mL. A decrease or increase in the botulinum toxin type A dose is also possible by administering a smaller or larger injection volume – from 0.05 mL (50% decrease in dose) to 0.15 mL (50% increase in dose).

The method for performing the potency assay is specific to Allergan's botulinum toxin type A. Because of specific details of this assay such as the vehicle, dilution scheme, and laboratory protocols for the various potency assays, units of biological activity of botulinum toxin type A cannot be compared with nor converted into units of any other botulinum toxin or any toxin assessed with any other specific assay method.

Preparation – An injection of botulinum toxin type A is prepared by drawing into an appropriately sized sterile syringe an amount of the properly diluted toxin (see Dilution Table) slightly greater than the intended dose. Air bubbles in the syringe barrel are expelled and the syringe is attached to an appropriate injection needle. Confirm patency of the needle. Injection volume in excess of the intended dose is expelled through the needle into an appropriate waste container to assure patency of the needle and to confirm that there is no syringe-needle leakage. Use a new sterile needle and syringe to enter the vial on each occasion for dilution or removal of botulinum toxin type A.

➤*Glabellar lines (Botox Cosmetic only):* Inject IM only.

Reconstitute with 0.9% sterile, nonpreserved saline (100 units in 2.5 mL saline) prior to IM injection. The resulting formulation will be 4 U/0.1 mL and a total treatment dose of 20 U in 0.5 mL. The duration of activity of botulinum toxin type A for glabellar lines is approximately 3 to 4 months. Injection intervals should be no more frequent than every 3 months and should be performed using the lowest effective dose. The safety and efficacy of more frequent dosing have not been clinically evaluated; more frequent dosing is not recommended.

Dilution technique – Using a 21-gauge, 2.5-inch length needle and an appropriately sized syringe, draw up a total of 2.5 mL of 0.9% sterile saline. Insert the needle at a 45° angle and slowly inject into the vial. Discard the vial if a vacuum does not pull the diluent into the vial. Gently rotate the vial and record the date and time of reconstitution on the space on the label.

Draw at least 0.5 mL of the properly reconstituted toxin into the sterile syringe, preferably a tuberculin syringe, and expel any air bubbles in the syringe barrel. Remove the needle used to reconstitute the product and attach a 30-gauge needle. Confirm the patency of the needle.

➤*Storage/Stability:* Store unopened vials in a refrigerator (2° to 8°C; 36° to 46°F) for up to 24 months. Do not use after the expiration date on the vial. Administer within 4 hours after reconstitution. During these 4 hours, store reconstituted botulinum toxin type A in a refrigerator (2° to 8°C; 36° to 46°F). Reconstituted botulinum toxin type A should be clear, colorless, and free of particulate matter.

Actions

➤*Pharmacology:* Botulinum toxin neurotoxin complex is a sterile, vacuum-dried form of purified botulinum toxin type A, produced from a fermentation of the Hall strain of *Clostridium botulinum* type A grown in a medium-containing casein hydrolysate and yeast extract. Botulinum toxin type A blocks neuromuscular conduction by binding to receptor sites on motor nerve terminals, entering the nerve terminals, and inhibiting the release of acetylcholine. This inhibition occurs as the neurotoxin cleaves SNAP-25, a protein integral to the successful docking and release of acetylcholine from vesicles situated within nerve endings. When injected IM at therapeutic doses, botulinum toxin type A produces a partial chemical denervation of the muscle, resulting in a localized reduction in muscle activity. In addition, the muscle may atrophy, axonal sprouting may occur, and extrajunctional acetylcholine receptors may develop; thus, slowly reversing muscle denervation produced by botulinum toxin type A.

Contraindications

Presence of infection at the proposed injection site(s); hypersensitivity to any ingredient in the formulation.

Warnings

➤*Neuropathic disorders:* Individuals with peripheral motor neuropathic diseases (eg, amyotrophic lateral sclerosis, motor neuropathy) or neuromuscular junctional disorders (eg, myasthenia gravis, Lambert-Eaton syndrome) should only receive botulinum toxin type A with caution. Patients with neuromuscular disorders may be at increased risk of clinically significant systemic effects including severe dysphagia and respiratory compromise from typical doses of botulinum toxin type A. Published medical literature has reported rare cases of administration of a botulinum toxin to patients with known or unrecognized neuromuscular disorders where the patients have shown extreme sensitivity to the systemic effects of typical clinical doses. In some of these cases, dysphagia has lasted several months and required placement of a gastric feeding tube.

➤*Dysphagia:* Dysphagia is a commonly reported adverse event following treatment of CD patients with all botulinum toxins. In these patients, there are reports of rare cases of dysphagia severe enough to warrant the insertion of a gastric feeding tube. There are also rare case reports where subsequent to the finding of dysphagia, a patient developed aspiration pneumonia and died.

➤*Albumin:* This product contains albumin, a derivative of human blood. Based on effective donor screening and product manufacturing processes, it carries an extremely remote risk for transmission of viral diseases. A theoretical risk for transmission of Creutzfeldt-Jakob disease (CJD) also is considered extremely remote. No cases of transmission of viral diseases or CJD have ever been identified for albumin.

BOTULINUM TOXIN TYPE A

➤*Dosage, systemic toxicity:* Do not exceed the recommended dosages and frequencies of administration. Risks resulting from administration at higher dosages are not known. Should accidental injection or oral ingestion occur, medically supervise the person for several days on an outpatient basis for signs or symptoms of systemic weakness or muscle paralysis.

➤*Cardiovascular events:* There have been rare reports following administration of botulinum toxin type A for other indications of adverse events involving the cardiovascular system, including arrhythmia and MI, some with fatal outcomes. Some of these patients had risk factors including pre-existing cardiovascular disease.

➤*Hypersensitivity reactions:* As with all biologic products, have epinephrine and other precautions available if anaphylactic reaction occurs. Refer to General Management of Acute Hypersensitivity Reactions.

➤*Elderly:* In general, be cautious in dose selection for an elderly patient, usually starting at the low end of the dosing range, reflecting the greater frequency of decreased hepatic, renal, or cardiac function, and of concomitant disease or other drug therapy.

➤*Pregnancy: Category C.* When pregnant mice and rats were injected IM during the period of organogenesis, the developmental no observed effect level (NOEL) of botulinum toxin type A was 4 U/kg. Higher doses (8 or 16 U/kg) were associated with reductions in fetal body weights or delayed ossification, which may be reversible.

In a range-finding study in rabbits, daily injection of 0.125 U/kg/day (days 6 to 18 of gestation) and 2 U/kg (days 6 and 13 of gestation) produced severe maternal toxicity, abortions, or fetal malformations. Higher doses resulted in death of the dams. The rabbit appears to be a very sensitive species to botulinum toxin type A.

There are no adequate and well-controlled studies of botulinum toxin type A in pregnant women. Because animal reproductive studies are not always predictive of human response, administer this product during pregnancy only if the potential benefit justifies the potential risk to the fetus. If this drug is used during pregnancy, or if the patient becomes pregnant while taking this drug, apprise the patient of the potential risks, including abortion or fetal malformations, which have been observed in rabbits.

Administration of *Botox Cosmetic* is not recommended during pregnancy.

➤*Lactation:* It is not known whether this drug is excreted in breast milk. Exercise caution when botulinum toxin type A is administered to a nursing woman.

➤*Children:* Safety and efficacy in children less than 16 years of age have not been established for CD.

Use for glabellar lines is not recommended in children.

Precautions

➤*Safe and effective use:* Safe and effective use of botulinum toxin type A depends upon proper storage of the product, selection of the correct dose, and proper reconstitution and administration techniques. Physicians administering botulinum toxin type A must understand the relevant neuromuscular and orbital anatomy and any alterations to the anatomy caused by prior surgical procedures, and standard electromyographic techniques.

➤*CD:* Patients with smaller neck muscle mass and patients who require bilateral injections into the sternocleidomastoid muscle have been reported to be at greater risk for dysphagia. Limiting the dose injected into the sternocleidomastoid muscle may reduce the occurrence of dysphagia. Injections into the levator scapulae may be associated with an increased risk of upper respiratory tract infection and dysphagia.

➤*Injection site:* Use caution when botulinum toxin type A treatment is used in the presence of inflammation at the proposed injection site(s) or when excessive weakness or atrophy is present in the target muscle(s).

➤*Immunogenicity:* Treatment with botulinum toxin type A may result in the formation of antibodies that may reduce the effectiveness of subsequent treatments with botulinum toxin type A for glabellar lines or other indications. Formation of neutralizing antibodies to botulinum toxin type A may reduce the effectiveness of botulinum toxin type A treatment of the appearance of glabellar lines or other clinical indications such as CD, blepharospasm, and strabismus by inactivating the biological activity of the toxin. The rate of formation of neutralizing antibodies in patients receiving botulinum toxin type A has not been well studied.

The observed incidence of neutralizing activity in an assay may be influenced by several factors including sample handling, concomitant medications, and underlying disease. For these reasons, comparison of the incidence of neutralizing activity to botulinum toxin type A with the incidence reported to other products may be misleading.

The results from some studies suggest that botulinum toxin type A injections at more frequent intervals or at higher doses may lead to greater incidence of antibody formation. The potential for antibody for-

mation may be minimized by injecting with the lowest effective dose given at the longest feasible intervals between injections.

➤*Ophthalmic:* Reduced blinking from injection of the orbicularis muscle can lead to corneal exposure, persistent epithelial defect, and corneal ulceration, especially in patients with VII nerve disorders. In the use of botulinum toxin type A for the treatment of blepharospasm, 1 case of corneal perforation in an aphakic eye requiring corneal grafting occurred because of this effect. Employ careful testing of corneal sensation in eyes previously operated upon, avoidance of injection into the lower lid area to avoid ectropion, and vigorous treatment of any epithelial defect. This may require protective drops, ointment, therapeutic soft contact lenses, or closure of the eye by patching or other means.

Inducing paralysis in 1 or more extraocular muscles may produce spatial disorientation, double vision, or past pointing. Covering the affected eye may alleviate these symptoms.

➤*Dermatologic:* Use caution when botulinum toxin type A treatment is used in patients who have an inflammatory skin problem at the injection site, marked facial asymmetry, ptosis, excessive dermatochalasis, deep dermal scarring, thick sebaceous skin, or the inability to substantially lessen glabellar lines by physically spreading them apart, as these patients were excluded from the Phase 3 safety and efficacy trials.

Drug Interactions

➤*Aminoglycosides:* The effect of botulinum toxin may be potentiated by aminoglycoside antibiotics or any other drug that interferes with neuromuscular transmission. Exercise caution when botulinum toxin type A is used in patients taking these drugs.

The effect of administering different botulinum neurotoxin serotypes at the same time or within several months of each other is unknown. Excessive neuromuscular weakness may be exacerbated by administration of another botulinum toxin prior to the resolution of the effects of a previously administered botulinum toxin.

Adverse Reactions

In general, adverse events occur within the first week following injection of botulinum toxin type A and while generally transient, may have a duration of several months.

A report of acute angle closure glaucoma 1 day after receiving an injection of botulinum toxin for blepharospasm was received, with recovery 4 months later after laser iridotomy and trabeculectomy. Focal facial paralysis, syncope, and exacerbation of myasthenia gravis also have been reported after treatment of blepharospasm.

➤*CD:* In CD patients evaluated for safety in double-blind and open-label studies following injection of botulinum toxin type A, the most frequently reported adverse reactions were dysphagia (19%), upper respiratory tract infection (12%), neck pain (11%), and headache (11%).

Other events reported in 2% to 10% of patients in any 1 study in decreasing order of incidence include the following: Increased cough, flu syndrome, back pain, rhinitis, dizziness, hypertonia, soreness at injection site, asthenia, oral dryness, speech disorder, fever, nausea, and drowsiness. Stiffness, numbness, diplopia, ptosis, and dyspnea have been reported rarely.

Dysphagia and symptomatic general weakness may be attributable to an extension of the pharmacology of botulinum toxin type A resulting from the spread of the toxin outside the injected muscles.

The most common severe adverse event associated with the use of botulinum toxin type A injection in patients with CD is dysphagia with about 20% of these cases also reporting dyspnea (see Warnings). Most dysphagia is reported as mild or moderate in severity. However, it may rarely be associated with more severe signs and symptoms (see Warnings).

Additionally, reports in the literature include a case of a female patient who developed brachial plexopathy 2 days after injection of 120 U for the treatment of CD and reports of dysphonia in patients who have been treated for CD.

Cardiovascular – There have been rare reports of adverse events involving the cardiovascular system, including arrhythmia and MI, some with fatal outcomes. Some of these patients had risk factors including cardiovascular disease. The exact relationship of these events to the botulinum toxin injection has not been established.

Local – Localized pain, tenderness, or bruising may be associated with the injection. Local weakness of the injected muscle(s) represents the expected pharmacological action of botulinum toxin. However, weakness of adjacent muscles also may occur because of spreading of the toxin.

Miscellaneous – There have been rare spontaneous reports of death, sometimes associated with dysphagia, pneumonia, or other significant debility after treatment with botulinum toxin.

Postmarketing: The following events have been reported since the drug has been marketed and a causal relationship to the botulinum toxin injection is unknown: Skin rash (including erythema multiforme, urticaria, and psoriasiform eruption), pruritus, and allergic reaction.

➤*Glabellar lines:* In clinical trials, the most frequently reported adverse events following injection of botulinum toxin type A were headache, respiratory infection, flu syndrome, blepharoptosis, and nausea.

BOTULINUM TOXIN TYPE A

Less frequently occurring (less than 3%) adverse reactions included pain in the face, erythema at the injection site, and muscle weakness. While local weakness of the injected muscle(s) is representative of the expected pharmacological action of botulinum toxin, weakness of adjacent muscles may occur as a result of the spread of toxin. These events are thought to be associated with the injection and occurred within the first week. The events generally were transient but may last several months.

Botox Cosmetic Adverse Reactions (%)		
Adverse reaction	Botulinum toxin type A (n = 405)	Placebo (n = 130)
Overall	43.7	41.5
CNS		
Headache	13.3	17.7
Dizziness	1.2	1.5
Paresthesia	1	0.8
Anxiety	0.7	0
Twitch	0.7	0
Dermatologic		
Erythema	1.7	1.5
Skin tightness	1	0
Skin irritation	0.7	0
GI		
Nausea	3	2.3
Dyspepsia	1	0
Tooth disorder	1	0
Liver function abnormal	0.7	1.5
Respiratory		
Infection	3.5	3.8
Bronchitis	1.5	0.8
Sinusitis	1.5	0.8
Pharyngitis	1.2	1.5
Dyspnea	0.7	0
Sinus infection	0.7	1.5
Laryngitis	0.7	0
Rhinitis	0.7	1.5
Miscellaneous		
Blepharoptosis	3.2	0
Pain in face	2.2	0.8
Flu syndrome	2	1.5
Muscle weakness	2	0
Ecchymosis	1.7	2.3
Pain at injection site	1.7	0.8

Botox Cosmetic Adverse Reactions (%)		
Adverse reaction	Botulinum toxin type A (n = 405)	Placebo (n = 130)
Edema at injection site	1.5	2.3
Pain in back	1	2.3
Urinary tract infection	1	0.8
Hypertension	1	0
Accidental injury	0.7	0.8

In published literature of the use of botulinum toxin type A for facial lines, there has been a single reported incident of diplopia, which resolved completely in 3 weeks. Transient ptosis, the most frequently reported complication, has been reported in the literature in approximately 5% of patients.

Between January 1, 1990, and August 31, 2000, there have been 7 spontaneous reports of serious adverse events documented as being related to the reported cosmetic use of botulinum toxin type A, including anaphylactic reaction, myasthenia gravis, decreased hearing, ear noise and localized numbness, blurred vision and retinal vein occlusion, glaucoma, and vertigo with nystagmus.

Overdosage

▶*Symptoms:* Signs and symptoms of overdose are not apparent immediately postinjection. Should accidental injection or oral ingestion occur, medically supervise the patient for up to several weeks for signs or symptoms of systemic weakness or muscle paralysis.

▶*Treatment:* An antitoxin is available in the event of immediate knowledge of an overdose or misinjection. In the event of overdosage or injection into the wrong muscle, additional information may be obtained by contacting Allergan Pharmaceuticals at (800) 433-8871 from 8 am to 4 pm Pacific Time, or at (714) 246-5954 for a recorded message at other times. The antitoxin will not reverse any botulinum toxin-induced muscle weakness effects already apparent by the time of antitoxin administration.

Patient Information

As with any treatment with the potential to allow previously sedentary patients to resume activities, caution these patients to resume activity slowly and carefully following administration.

Advise patients or caregivers to seek immediate medical attention if swallowing, speech, or respiratory disorders arise.

Inform patients with CD of the possibility of experiencing dysphagia, which is typically mild to moderate, but could be severe. Rare consequences of severe dysphagia include aspiration, dyspnea, pneumonia, and the need to reestablish an airway.

BOTULINUM TOXIN TYPE B

Rx	**Myobloc** (Elan Pharm)	**Solution, injectable:**[1] 5000 U/mL	Preservative free. In 3.5 mL single-use vials.[2]

[1] One unit corresponds to the calculated median lethal intraperitoneal dose (LD$_{50}$) in mice.

[2] With 0.05% human serum albumin, 0.01 M sodium succinate, 0.1 M sodium chloride.

Indications

▶*Cervical dystonia (CD):* For the treatment of patients with CD to reduce the severity of abnormal head position and neck pain associated with CD.

Administration and Dosage

▶*Approved by the FDA:* December 11, 2000.

▶*Cervical dystonia:* The recommended initial dose of botulinum toxin type B for patients with a history of tolerating botulinum toxin injections is 2500 to 5000 U divided among affected muscles. Give patients without a history of tolerating botulinum toxin injections a lower initial dose. Optimize subsequent dosing according to the patient's individual response. The duration of effect in patients responding to botulinum toxin type B treatment has been observed in studies to be between 12 and 16 weeks at doses of 5000 U or 10,000 U. Botulinum toxin type B should be administered by physicians familiar and experienced in the assessment and management of patients with CD. Units of biological activity of botulinum toxin type B cannot be compared with or converted into units of any other botulinum toxin.

▶*Storage/Stability:* Store under refrigeration at 2° to 8°C (36° to 46°F) for up to 21 months. Do not freeze. Do not shake. After dilution with normal saline, the product must be used within 4 hours as the formulation does not contain a preservative.

Actions

▶*Pharmacology:* Botulinum toxin type B injectable solution is a sterile liquid formulation of a purified neurotoxin that acts at the neuromuscular junction to produce flaccid paralysis. The neurotoxin is produced by fermentation of the bacterium *Clostridium botulinum* type B (Bean strain).

The 7 serologically distinct botulinum neurotoxins, designated A through G, share a common structural organization consisting of 1 heavy chain and 1 light chain polypeptide linked by a single disulfide bond. These toxins inhibit acetylcholine release at the neuromuscular junction via a 3-stage process: 1) Heavy chain mediated neurospecific binding of the toxin, 2) internalization of the toxin by receptor-mediated endocytosis, and 3) ATP and pH dependent translocation of the light chain to the neuronal cytosol where it acts as a zinc-dependent endoprotease cleaving polypeptides essential for neurotransmitter release. Botulinum toxin type B specifically has been demonstrated to cleave synaptic vesicle associated membrane protein (VAMP, also known as synaptobrevin), which is a component of the protein complex responsible for docking and fusion of the synaptic vesicle to the presynaptic membrane, a necessary step for neurotransmitter release.

Contraindications

Known hypersensitivity to any ingredient in the formulation.

Warnings

▶*Neuropathic disorders:* Exercise caution when administering botulinum toxin type B to individuals with peripheral motor neuropathic diseases (eg, amyotrophic lateral sclerosis, motor neuropathy) or neuromuscular junctional disorders (eg, myasthenia gravis, Lambert-Eaton syndrome). Patients with neuromuscular disorders may be at increased risk of clinically significant systemic effects including severe dysphagia and respiratory compromise from typical doses of botulinum toxin type B. Published medical literature has reported rare cases of administration of a botulinum toxin to patients with known or unrecognized neuromuscular disorders where the patients have shown extreme sensitivity to the systemic effects of typical clinical doses. In some cases, dysphagia has lasted months and required placement of a gastric feeding tube.

▶*Botulism:* There were no documented cases of botulism resulting from the IM injection of botulinum toxin type B in patients with CD treated in clinical trials. However, if botulism is clinically suspected, hospitalization for the monitoring of systemic weakness or paralysis

BOTULINUM TOXIN TYPE B

and respiratory function (incipient respiratory failure) may be required.

➤*Dysphagia:* Dysphagia is a commonly reported adverse event following treatment with all botulinum toxins in cervical dystonia patients. In the medical literature, there are reports of rare cases of dysphagia severe enough to warrant the insertion of a gastric feeding tube. There are also rare case reports where subsequent to the finding of dysphagia, a patient developed aspiration pneumonia and died.

➤*Viral diseases:* This product contains albumin, a derivative of human blood. Based on effective donor screening and product manufacturing processes, it carries an extremely remote risk for transmission of viral diseases. A theoretical risk for transmission of Creutzfeldt-Jakob disease (CJD) also is considered extremely remote. No cases of transmission of viral diseases or CJD have ever been identified with albumin.

➤*Pregnancy: Category C.* Animal reproduction studies have not been conducted with botulinum toxin type B. It is also not known whether it can cause fetal harm when administered to a pregnant woman or can affect reproduction capacity. Give botulinum toxin type B to a pregnant woman only if clearly needed.

➤*Lactation:* It is not known if this drug is excreted in human milk. Exercise caution when botulinum toxin type B is administered to a nursing woman.

➤*Children:* Safety and efficacy in pediatric patients have not been established.

Precautions

Only 9 subjects without a history of tolerating injections of type A botulinum toxin have been studied. Initiate treatment of botulinum toxin naive patients at lower doses (see Adverse Reactions). During repeated treatment studies, 446 subjects were followed with periodic ELISAbased evaluations for development of antibody responses against botulinum toxin type B. Of these patients, 12% had positive ELISAassays at baseline. Patients began to develop new ELISAresponses after a single treatment session with botulinum toxin type B. By 6 months after initiating treatment, estimates for ELISApositive rate were 20%, which continued to rise to 36% at 1 year and 50% positive ELISA status at 18 months. Serum neutralizing activity was primarily not seen in patients until after 6 months. Estimated rates of development were 10% at 1 year and 18% at 18 months in the overall group of patients, based on analysis of samples from ELISApositive individuals. The clinical significance of development of antibodies has not been determined.

Drug Interactions

Coadminister botulinum toxin type B and aminoglycosides or other agents interfering with neuromuscular transmission (eg, curare-like compounds) with caution as the effect of the toxin may be potentiated.

The effect of administering different botulinum neurotoxin serotypes at the same time or within < 4 months of each other is unknown. However, neuromuscular paralysis may be potentiated by coadministration or overlapping administration of different botulinum toxin serotypes.

Adverse Reactions

The most commonly reported adverse events associated with botulinum toxin type B treatment in all studies were dry mouth, dysphagia, dyspepsia, and injection site pain. Dry mouth and dysphagia were the adverse reactions most frequently resulting in discontinuation of treatment. There was an increased incidence of dysphagia with increased dose in the sternocleidomastoid muscle. The incidence of dry mouth showed some dose-related increase with doses injected into the splenius capitis, trapezius, and sternocleidomastoid muscles.

Only 9 subjects without a history of tolerating injections of type A botulinum toxin have been studied. Adverse event rates have not been adequately evaluated in these patients.

Botulinum Toxin Type B Adverse Reactions Following Single Treatment Session (%)

Adverse reaction	Dosing groups			
	2500 U (n = 31)	5000 U (n = 67)	10,000 U (n = 106)	Placebo (n = 104)
CNS				
Dizziness	3	3	6	2
Neck pain related to CD	0	16	17	16
Headache	10	16	11	8
Torticollis	0	4	8	7
Pain related to CD/Torticollis	10	4	7	4
GI				
Dry mouth	3	12	34	3
Dysphagia	16	10	25	3
Dyspepsia	3	0	10	5
Nausea	10	3	8	5
Miscellaneous				
Injection site pain	16	12	15	9
Infection	13	19	15	15
Pain	6	6	13	10
Flu syndrome	6	9	8	4
Arthralgia	0	1	7	5
Back pain	3	4	7	3
Cough increased	3	6	7	3
Myasthenia	3	4	6	3
Asthenia	3	0	6	4
Accidental injury	0	4	5	4
Rhinitis	3	1	5	6

The following additional adverse events were reported in ≥ 2% of patients:

➤*CNS:* Headache related to injection; migraine; anxiety; tremor; hyperesthesia; somnolence; confusion; pain related to CD/torticollis; vertigo.

➤*Dermatologic:* Pruritus; ecchymosis

➤*GI:* GI disorder; vomiting; glossitis; stomatitis; tooth disorder.

➤*GU:* Urinary tract infection; cystitis; vaginal moniliasis.

➤*Metabolic/Nutritional:* Peripheral edema; edema; hypercholesterolemia.

➤*Musculoskeletal:* Arthritis; joint disorder.

➤*Respiratory:* Dyspnea; lung disorder; pneumonia.

➤*Special senses:* Amblyopia; otitis media; abnormal vision; taste perversion; tinnitus.

➤*Miscellaneous:* Allergic reaction; fever; chest pain; chills; hernia; malaise; abscess; cyst; neoplasm; viral infection; vasodilation.

Overdosage

➤*Symptoms:* Symptoms of overdose are not likely to present immediately following injection(s). Should a patient ingest the product or be accidently overdosed, monitor the patient for up to several weeks for signs and symptoms of systemic weakness or paralysis.

➤*Treatment:* In the event of an overdose, an antitoxin may be administered. Contact Elan Pharmaceuticals (888) 638-7605 for additional information and your State Health Department to process a request for antitoxin through the Centers for Disease Control and Prevention in Atlanta, GA. The antitoxin will not reverse any botulinum toxin induced muscle weakness effects already apparent by the time of antitoxin administration.

The agents in this section are used in combination with other products in the treatment of *H. pylori.* No agents are used alone. For additional information, refer to the *H. pylori* Treatment Guidelines in the Appendix or the individual monographs. In addition, combination packages are available for the treatment of *H. pylori.* Generally, these packages contain several individual drug products that are specifically packaged for the convenience of the patient. Refer to prescribing information for each individual agent.

AMOXICILLIN

Indications

➤*Eradication of H. pylori:* In combination with lansoprazole and clarithromycin or lansoprazole alone for the eradication of *H. pylori* in patients with duodenal ulcers.

Administration and Dosage

1 g twice daily for 14 days (triple therapy) or 1 g 3 times daily (double therapy).

BISMUTH

Indications

➤*Eradication of H. pylori:* In combination with other products for the eradication of *H. pylori.*

Administration and Dosage

525 mg 4 times a day in combination with other products.

CLARITHROMYCIN

Indications

➤*Eradication of H.pylori:* In combination with omeprazole or lansoprazole for the treatment of patients with an active duodenal ulcer associated with *H. pylori* infection.

Administration and Dosage

500 mg 3 times a day for days 1 to 14.

LANSOPRAZOLE

Indications

➤*Duodenal ulcer:* In combination with clarithromycin and/or amoxicillin for the eradication of *H. pylori* infection in patients with active or recurrent duodenal ulcers.

Administration and Dosage

30 mg twice daily for for 14 days (triple therapy) or 30 mg 3 times daily for 14 days (double therapy).

METRONIDAZOLE

Indications

➤*Eradication of H. pylori:* In combination with other products for the eradication of *H. pylori.*

Administration and Dosage

250 mg 4 times a day in combination with other products.

OMEPRAZOLE

Indications

➤*Eradication of H. pylori:* In combination with clarithromycin for treatment of patients with an active duodenal ulcer associated with *H. pylori* infection.

Administration and Dosage

40 mg once daily for days 1 to 14 and 20 mg once daily for days 15 to 28.

TETRACYCLINE

Indications

➤*Eradication of H. pylori:* In combination with other products for the eradication of *H. pylori.*

Administration and Dosage

500 mg 4 times a day in combination with other products.

BISMUTH SUBSALICYLATE, METRONIDAZOLE AND TETRACYCLINE HCl COMBINATION

Rx	Helidac (Procter & Gamble)	Tablets: 262.4 mg bismuth subsalicylate	(PG 11). Pink, chewable. In 8s.
		250 mg metronidazole	(PG 10). White. In 4s.
		Capsules: 500 mg tetracycline	(PG 12). Pale orange and white. In 4s.

For more information, refer to the *H. pylori* agents and individual monographs.

Administration and Dosage

➤*Adults:* Take 525 mg bismuth subsalicylate, 250 mg metronidazole and 500 mg tetracycline plus an H₂ antagonist 4 times daily at meals and at bedtime for 14 days. Chew and swallow the bismuth subsalicylate tablets. Swallow the metronidazole tablet and tetracycline capsule whole with a full glass of water (8 ounces). Take concomitantly prescribed H₂ antagonist therapy as directed.

Ingestion of adequate amounts of fluid, particularly with the bedtime dose of tetracycline HCl, is recommended to reduce the risk of esophageal irritation and ulceration.

Missed doses can be made up by continuing the normal dosing schedule until the medication is gone. Do not take double doses. If more than four doses are missed, contact the physician.

LANSOPRAZOLE, AMOXICILLIN, AND CLARITHROMYCIN COMBINATION

Rx	Prevpac (TAP Pharmaceuticals)	Daily administration pack: Two 30 mg *Prevacid* (lansoprazole) capsules, four 500 mg *Trimox* (amoxicillin) capsules, and two 500 mg *Biaxin* (clarithromycin) tablets.

Indications

➤*Eradication of H. pylori:* Eradication of *H. pylori* to reduce risk of duodenal ulcer recurrence.

Administration and Dosage

➤*Adults:* 30 mg lansoprazole, 1 g amoxicillin, and 500 mg clarithromycin administered together twice daily (morning and evening) for 14 days.

Do not use in patients with creatinine clearance < 30 mL/min.

Indications

▶*Duodenal ulcer:*

Short-term treatment – Most patients heal within 4 weeks; there is rarely reason to use full dosage for > 6 to 8 weeks.

Maintenance therapy – Reduced dosages after healing of active ulcer. Patients have been maintained on continued **cimetidine** (400 mg at bedtime) for up to 5 years.

▶*Gastric ulcer:*

Treatment (benign, active) – Short-term treatment. Most patients heal in 6 wks.

Maintenance (ranitidine) – Reduced dosage after healing of acute ulcer.

▶*Gastroesophageal reflux disease (GERD), including endoscopically diagnosed erosive esophagitis:* **Ranitidine** and **nizatidine** are also indicated for symptomatic relief of associated heartburn.

▶*Erosive esophagitis (ranitidine):* Maintenance treatment for erosive esophagitis.

▶*Pathological hypersecretory conditions (cimetidine, famotidine, ranitidine):* eg, Zollinger-Ellison syndrome, systemic mastocytosis, multiple endocrine adenomas.

▶*Upper GI bleeding (cimetidine):* Prevention in critically ill patients.

▶*Heartburn, acid indigestion and sour stomach:*

Cimetidine (otc only) – Relief of these symptoms.

Famotidine (otc only) – Relief of these symptoms and prevention of these symptoms brought on by consuming food and beverages.

▶*Unlabeled uses:*

Histamine H$_2$ antagonists – As part of a multi-drug regimen to eradicate *Helicobacter pylori* in the treatment of peptic ulcer.

Cimetidine – Oral 400 to 600 mg or IV 300 mg, 60 to 90 minutes before anesthesia to prevent aspiration pneumonitis.

Doses of 1 g/day have been used with variable success to treat primary hyperparathyroidism and to control secondary hyperparathyroidism in chronic hemodialysis patients.

Treatment of chronic viral warts in children (25 to 40 mg/kg/day in divided doses).

The combination of H$_1$ and H$_2$ antagonists may be useful in chronic idiopathic urticaria not responding to H$_1$ antagonists alone. It may also be useful for itching and flushing in anaphylaxis, pruritus, urticaria and contact dermatitis (IV).

Cimetidine IV may be useful in acetaminophen overdose by reducing formation of the toxic intermediate via the cytochrome P450 oxidase system, thereby protecting against hepatotoxicity.

Cimetidine has been used for dyspepsia (400 mg twice/day); however, other studies do not confirm its effectiveness.

Cimetidine may improve overall survival in patients with colorectal cancer.

Other potential uses include: Prophylaxis of stress-induced ulcers; tinea capitis; herpes virus infection; hirsute women.

Ranitidine – Ranitidine has shown some value in protection against aspiration of acid during anesthesia. In one study, oral ranitidine 2 to 3.5 mg/kg was effective in decreasing gastric acidity in children before anesthesia induction.

Ranitidine 150 mg twice daily may be effective in preventing gastroduodenal mucosal damage that may be associated with long-term NSAIDs, including aspirin.

Ranitidine controls acute upper GI bleeding (150 mg IV or 300 mg/day orally).

Effective in preventing stress ulcers IV (0.125 to 0.25 mg/kg/hr) or orally.

Famotidine – Famotidine may be effective in upper GI bleeding (20 mg twice daily).

Prevention of stress ulcers (40 mg/day).

During and before anesthesia to prevent pulmonary aspiration of gastric acid (40 mg IM or orally).

Histamine H$_2$ Antagonists: Summary of Indications

✔ – Labeled x – Unlabeled	Cimetidine	Famotidine	Nizatidine	Ranitidine
Duodenal ulcer				
Treatment	✔	✔	✔	✔
Maintenance	✔	✔	✔	✔
GERD (including erosive esophagitis)	✔	✔	✔	✔
Gastric ulcer				
Treatment	✔	✔	✔	✔
Maintenance				✔

Histamine H$_2$ Antagonists: Summary of Indications

✔ – Labeled x – Unlabeled	Cimetidine	Famotidine	Nizatidine	Ranitidine
Pathological hypersecretory conditions	✔	✔		✔
Heartburn/acid indigestion/ sour stomach	✔[1,2]	✔[1,3]		
Erosive esophagitis, maintenance				✔
Prevent upper GI bleeding	✔	x		x
Peptic ulcer[4]	x	x	x	x
Prevent aspiration pneumonitis	x	x		x
Prophylaxis of stress ulcers	x	x		x
Prevent gastric NSAID damage				x
Hyperparathyroidism	x			
Secondary hyperparathyroidism in hemodialysis	x			
Tinea capitis	x			
Herpes virus infection	x			
Hirsute women	x			
Chronic idiopathic urticaria	x			
Anaphylaxis (dermatological)	x			
Acetaminophen overdose	x			
Dyspepsia	x			
Warts	x			
Colorectal cancer	x			

[1] *otc* use only.
[2] Relief of symptoms only.
[3] Relief and prevention of symptoms.
[4] As part of a multi-drug regimen to eradicate *Helicobacter pylori*.

Actions

▶*Pharmacology:* Histamine H$_2$ antagonists are reversible competitive blockers of histamine at the H$_2$ receptors, particularly those in the gastric parietal cells. The H$_2$ antagonists are highly selective, do not affect the H$_1$ receptors, and are not anticholinergic agents. Potent inhibitors of all phases of gastric acid secretion, they inhibit secretions caused by histamine, muscarinic agonists and gastrin. They also inhibit fasting and nocturnal secretions, and secretions stimulated by food, insulin, caffeine, pentagastrin and betazole. In addition, the volume and the hydrogen ion concentration of gastric juice are reduced. **Cimetidine**, **ranitidine** and **famotidine** have no effect on gastric emptying, and cimetidine and famotidine have no effect on lower esophageal sphincter pressure. Ranitidine, **nizatidine** and famotidine have little or no effect on fasting or postprandial serum gastrin. Ranitidine is 5 to 12 times more potent and famotidine is 30 to 60 times more potent than cimetidine on a molar basis in controlling gastric acid hypersecretion, although there is no indication that the greater potency offers any advantage.

The histamine H$_2$ antagonists are effective in alleviating symptoms and in preventing complications of peptic ulcer disease. The drugs have similar adverse reaction profiles. Cimetidine appears to have the greatest degree of antiandrogenic (eg, gynecomastia, impotence) and CNS (eg, mental confusion) effects. Cimetidine inhibits the cytochrome P450 oxidase system that affects other drugs (eg, warfarin, theophylline). Ranitidine also affects the microsomal enzyme system, but its influence on elimination of other drugs is not significant. Famotidine and nizatidine do not affect the cytochrome P450 enzyme system.

Treatment failures – Treatment failures have been documented with all of the H$_2$ antagonists. Because all of the drugs act to inhibit gastric acid secretion, it is doubtful that ulcers "resistant" to one drug will heal with another.

Cimetidine –

  Antisecretory activity:

  • *Nocturnal* – Cimetidine 800 mg at bedtime reduces mean hourly hydrogen ion (H$^+$) activity by > 85% over 8 hours in duodenal ulcer patients, with no effect on daytime acid secretion. The 1600 mg bedtime dose produces 100% inhibition of mean hourly H$^+$ activity over an 8 hour period in ulcer patients, but also reduces H$^+$ activity by 35% for an additional 5 hours the next morning. Both the 400 mg twice daily and 300 mg 4 times daily doses decrease nocturnal acid secretion in a dose-related manner, 47% to 83% over 6 to 8 hours and 54% over 9 hours, respectively.

By the first hour after a standard meal, 300 mg inhibited gastric acid secretion in ulcer patients by at least 50% and during the next 2 hours by at least 75%. A 300 mg breakfast dose continued for at least 4 hours, with partial suppression of the rise in gastric acid secretion following lunch in duodenal ulcer patients.

Total pepsin output is also reduced as a result of the decrease in volume of gastric juice. Cimetidine 300 mg inhibited the rise in intrinsic factor concentration produced by betazole, but some intrinsic factor was secreted at all times.

Ranitidine – Basal, nocturnal, and betazole-stimulated secretion are most sensitive to inhibition by ranitidine, responding almost completely to doses of ≤ 100 mg. Ranitidine does not affect pepsin secretion or pentagastrin-stimulated intrinsic factor secretion. Other pharmacological actions include an increase in gastric nitrate-reducing organisms; small, transient, dose-related increases in serum prolactin after IV bolus injections of ≥ 100 mg and possible impairment of vasopressin release. No effect on prolactin levels has been noted with recommended oral or IV doses.

Famotidine – The acid concentration and volume of gastric secretion are suppressed, while changes in pepsin secretion are proportional to volume output. Exocrine pancreatic function is not affected. After oral use, the onset of antisecretory effect occurred within 1 hour; the maximum effect was dose-dependent, occurring within 1 to 3 hours. Duration of secretion inhibition by doses of 20 and 40 mg was 10 and 12 hours, respectively.

After IV administration, the maximum effect was achieved within 30 minutes. Single IV doses of 10 and 20 mg inhibited nocturnal secretion for 10 and 12 hours, respectively.

There is no cumulative effect with repeated doses. The nocturnal intragastric pH was raised by evening doses of 20 and 40 mg to mean values of 5 and 6.4, respectively. When famotidine was given after breakfast, the basal daytime interdigestive pH at 3 and 8 hours after 20 or 40 mg was raised to about 5.

Nizatidine – Nizatidine's effect on gastric acid secretion is presented in the following table:

Effect of Oral Nizatidine on Gastric Acid Secretion

Method	Time after dose (hrs)	% Inhibition of gastric acid output by dose (mg)				
		20-50	75	100	150	300
Basal	up to 8	45-57	–	72	–	–
Nocturnal	up to 10	57	–	73	–	90
Betazole	up to 3	–	93	–	100	99
Pentagastrin	up to 6	–	25	–	64	67
Meal	up to 4	41	64	–	98	97
Caffeine	up to 3	–	73	–	85	96

Total pepsin output was reduced in proportion to the reduced volume of gastric secretions. Oral administration of 75 to 300 mg nizatidine increased betazole-stimulated secretion of intrinsic factor. There was no effect on hormone levels, including androgens.

➤*Pharmacokinetics:*

Pharmacokinetic Properties of Histamine H₂ Antagonists

H₂ receptor antagonist	Bioavailability (%)	Time to peak plasma concentration (hrs)	Peak plasma concentration[1] (mcg/mL)	Half-life (hrs)	Protein binding (%)	Volume of distribution (L/kg)	Elimination (%)		
							Urine, unchanged		Metabolized
							Oral	IV	
Cimetidine	60-70	0.75-1.5	0.7-3.2 (300 mg dose) (3.5-7.5 IV)	≈ 2[2]	13-25	0.8-1.2	48	75	30-40
Famotidine	40-45	1-3	0.076-0.1 (40 mg dose)	2.5-3.5[3]	15-20	1.1-1.4	25-30	65-70	30-35
Nizatidine	> 90	0.5-3	0.7-1.8/ 1.4-3.6 (150/300 mg dose)	1-2[3]	≈ 35	0.8-1.5	60	na[4]	< 18
Ranitidine	50-60 (90-100 IM)	1-3 (0.25 IM)	0.44-0.55 (0.58 IM)	2-3[3]	15	1.2-1.9	30-35	68-79	< 10

[1] Dose-dependent.
[2] Increased in renal and hepatic impairment and in the elderly.
[3] Increased in renal impairment.
[4] na = not applicable.

Additional pharmacokinetic data for these agents are discussed individually.

Cimetidine – Absorption may be decreased by antacids, but is unaffected by food. Both oral and parenteral administration provide comparable serum levels. Plasma concentrations of 0.5 to 1 mcg/mL are required to suppress basal or gastric acid secretion; however, plasma concentrations of cimetidine have not correlated with duodenal ulcer healing. Blood concentrations remain above those required to provide 80% inhibition of basal gastric acid secretion for 4 to 5 hours following a 300 mg dose. Cimetidine is widely distributed. Following oral administration, ≈ 30% to 40% is metabolized in the liver, the sulfoxide being the major metabolite. Cimetidine is not significantly removed by hemodialysis or peritoneal dialysis.

Ranitidine – Absorption of oral ranitidine is not significantly impaired by the administration of food. Coadministration of antacids may reduce its absorption. Hepatic metabolism results in 3 metabolites. Maintenance of serum concentrations necessary to inhibit 50% of

stimulated gastric acid secretion (36 to 94 ng/mL) is 12 hours orally and 6 to 8 hours IV. However, blood levels bear no consistent relationship to dose or degree of acid inhibition.

Famotidine – Plasma levels after multiple doses of famotidine are similar to those after single doses. Famotidine is eliminated by renal (65% to 70%) and metabolic (30% to 35%) routes. The only metabolite identified is the S-oxide.

Nizatidine – A concentration of 1000 mcg/L is equivalent to 3 mcmol/L; a dose of 300 mg is equivalent to 905 mcmol. Plasma concentrations 12 hours after administration are < 10 mcg/L. Plasma clearance is 40 to 60 L/hour. Because of the short half-life and rapid clearance, drug accumulation would not be expected in individuals with normal renal function who take either 300 mg at bedtime or 150 mg twice daily. Nizatidine exhibits dose proportionality over the recommended dose range.

Antacids consisting of aluminum and magnesium hydroxides with simethicone decrease nizatidine absorption by ≈ 10%. With food, AUC and maximum concentration increase by ≈ 10%.

In humans, < 7% of an oral dose is metabolized as N2-monodesmethylnizatidine, an H₂-receptor antagonist. Other likely metabolites are the N2-oxide (< 5% of the dose) and the S-oxide (< 6% of the dose). More than 90% of an oral dose of nizatidine is excreted in the urine within 12 hours. Renal clearance is ≈ 500 mL/min, which indicates excretion by active tubular secretion. Less than 6% is eliminated in the feces.

➤*Clinical trials:*
Comparative studies –

Duodenal Ulcer Healing Rates – Comparison of H₂ Antagonists[1]			
Drug	Dose (mg/day)	Healing rate	
		4 week	8 week
Cimetidine	1000	60% to 84%	82% to 95%
Famotidine	40	67% to 77%	
Nizatidine	300	73% to 81%	
Ranitidine	300	63% to 77%	

[1] Combined results. Studies did not compare all drugs simultaneously.

In the treatment of gastric ulcers, healing rates after 6 weeks of therapy with ranitidine 150 mg twice daily or cimetidine 300 mg 4 times daily were 65% to 70%; after 8 weeks of treatment, the rates increased to 75% to 85%.

Studies evaluating an evening meal or bedtime dose of ranitidine 150 mg or cimetidine 400 mg for duodenal ulcer maintenance therapy indicated the relapse rate was lower in ranitidine patients. However, these doses are not equipotent in reducing gastric acid secretion. A 1-year multicenter study indicated that nizatidine 150 mg at night is similar in efficacy to ranitidine in preventing ulcer recurrence.

Contraindications

Hypersensitivity to individual agents or to other H₂-receptor antagonists.

Warnings

➤*Benzyl alcohol:* Benzyl alcohol contained in some of these products as a preservative, has been associated with a fatal "gasping syndrome" in premature infants.

➤*Hypersensitivity reactions:* Rare cases of anaphylaxis have occurred, as well as rare episodes of hypersensitivity (eg, bronchospasm, laryngeal edema, rash, eosinophilia). Refer to Management of Acute Hypersensitivity Reactions.

➤*Renal function impairment:* Because these agents are excreted primarily via the kidneys, decreased clearance may occur; reduced dosage may be necessary (see Administration and Dosage).

➤*Hepatic function impairment:* Observe caution. Decreased clearance may occur; these agents are partly metabolized in the liver. In normal renal function with uncomplicated hepatic dysfunction, **nizatidine** disposition is similar to that in healthy individuals.

➤*Elderly:* Safety and efficacy appear similar to those of younger patients; however, the elderly may have reduced renal function. Ulcer healing rates, adverse events, and laboratory abnormalities in patients 65 to 82 years of age on **ranitidine** were no different from younger patients. Decreased **cimetidine** clearance may be more common.

➤*Pregnancy:* (*Category B* – **cimetidine**, **famotidine**, **ranitidine**, **nizatidine**). Cimetidine crosses the placenta. There are no adequate and well controlled studies with these agents in pregnant women. Use only when clearly needed and when the potential benefits outweigh the potential hazards to the fetus.

➤*Lactation:*
Cimetidine – Cimetidine is excreted in breast milk with milk:plasma ratios of ≈ 5:1 to 12:1. Potential daily infant ingestion is ≈ 6 mg. Do not nurse.

Ranitidine – Ranitidine is excreted in breast milk with milk:plasma ratios of 1:1 to 6.7:1. Exercise caution when administering to a nursing mother.

Nizatidine – Nizatidine is excreted in breast milk in a concentration of 0.1% of the oral dose in proportion to plasma concentrations. Decide whether to discontinue nursing or discontinue the drug, taking into account the importance of the drug to the mother.

Famotidine – Famotidine is excreted in the breast milk of rats. It is not known whether it is excreted in human breast milk. Decide whether to discontinue nursing or to discontinue the drug, taking into account the importance of the drug to the mother.

➤*Children:* Safety and efficacy are not established. **Cimetidine** is not recommended for children < 16 years of age, unless anticipated benefits outweigh potential risks. In very limited experience, cimetidine 20 to 40 mg/kg/day has been used. *OTC* use is not recommended in children < 12 years of age.

Precautions

➤*Gastric malignancy:* Symptomatic response to these agents does not preclude gastric malignancy. Rare transient healing of gastric ulcers has occurred with **cimetidine** despite subsequently documented malignancy. Follow gastric ulcer patients closely.

➤*Reversible CNS effects:* Reversible CNS effects (eg, mental confusion, agitation, psychosis, depression, anxiety, hallucinations, disorientation) have occurred with **cimetidine**, predominantly in severely ill patients. These confusional states usually develop within 2 to 3 days after initiation of therapy and clear within 3 to 4 days following discontinuation. Advancing age (≥ 50 years) and preexisting liver or renal disease appear to be contributing factors. In several cases, the mental confusion has been associated with elevated trough serum concentrations (> 1.25 mcg/mL).

➤*Hepatocellular injury:* Hepatocellular injury may occur with **nizatidine** as evidenced by elevated liver enzymes (AST, ALT, or alkaline phosphatase). In some cases, there was a marked elevation of AST, ALT enzymes (> 500 IU/L) and, in a single instance, ALT was > 2000 IU/L. However, the overall occurrence of elevated liver enzymes and elevations to 3 times the upper limit of normal did not significantly differ from placebo-treated patients. All abnormalities were reversible after discontinuation of nizatidine.

Occasionally, reversible hepatitis, hepatocellular or hepatocanalicular or mixed, with or without jaundice has occurred with oral **ranitidine**. ALT values have increased to at least twice pretreatment levels with IV ranitidine administered for ≥ 5 days.

Laboratory test monitoring – Laboratory test monitoring for liver abnormalities is appropriate.

➤*Rapid IV administration:* Rapid IV administration of **cimetidine** has been followed by rare instances of cardiac arrhythmias and hypotension. Bradycardia, tachycardia, and premature ventricular beats in association with rapid administration of IV **ranitidine** may occur rarely, usually in patients predisposed to cardiac rhythm disturbances.

➤*Antiandrogenic effect:* **Cimetidine** has a weak antiandrogenic effect in animals. Gynecomastia in patients treated for ≥ 1 month may occur. In patients with pathological hypersecretory states, this occurred in ≈ 4% of cases; in all others, the incidence was ≈ 0.3% to 1%. No evidence of endocrine dysfunction was found; the condition remained unchanged or returned to normal with continuing treatment.

➤*Immunocompromised patients:* Decreased gastric acidity, including that produced by acid-suppressing agents such as H₂ antagonists, may increase the possibility of strongyloidiasis.

Drug Interactions

➤*Cimetidine:* Cimetidine reduces the hepatic metabolism of drugs metabolized via the cytochrome P450 pathway, delaying elimination and increasing serum levels. Drugs metabolized by hepatic microsomal enzymes, particularly those of low therapeutic ratio or in patients with renal or hepatic impairment, may require dosage adjustment. Concomitant cimetidine with any of the following drugs may result in their increased pharmacologic effects or toxicity.

Cimetidine Drug Interactions (Decreased Hepatic Metabolism)		
Benzodiazepines[1]	Metronidazole	Sulfonylureas
Caffeine	Moricizine	Tacrine
Calcium channel blockers	Pentoxifylline	Theophyllines[2]
Carbamazepine	Phenytoin	Triamterene
Chloroquine	Propafenone	Tricyclic antidepressants
Labetalol	Propranolol	Valproic acid
Lidocaine	Quinidine	Warfarin
Metoprolol	Quinine	

[1] Does not include agents metabolized by glucuronidation (lorazepam, oxazepam, temazepam).
[2] Does not include dyphylline.

➤*Cytochrome P450:* **Ranitidine** (which weakly binds to cytochrome P450 in vitro), **famotidine**, and **nizatidine** do not inhibit the cytochrome P450-linked oxygenase enzyme system in the liver. Drug interactions with these agents mediated by inhibition of hepatic metabolism are not expected. However, some interactions may occur with these agents (see table).

Following are additional interactions that may occur with cimetidine as well as potential interactions with the other H₂ antagonists:

Histamine H₂ Antagonist Drug Interactions			
Precipitant drug	Object drug*		Description
Antacids Anticholinergics Metoclopramide	H₂ antagonists	↓	These agents may decrease the absorption of cimetidine. However, 1 study suggested cimetidine absorption is unaffected by concomitant multiple-dose antacid administration. Ranitidine absorption may be decreased by concurrent antacids; data conflict. Avoid simultaneous administration. Bioavailability of famotidine and nizatidine may be slightly decreased; no special precautions are necessary.
Cigarette smoking	Cimetidine	↓	Cigarette smoking reverses cimetidine-induced inhibition of nocturnal gastric secretion, hindering ulcer healing. Cigarette use is closely related to ulcer recurrence.
Cimetidine	Ferrous salts Indomethacin Ketoconazole Tetracyclines	↓	Pharmacologic effects of these agents may be decreased by cimetidine due to decreased absorption.
Cimetidine	Carmustine	↑	Bone marrow suppression (toxicity) of carmustine may be enhanced by cimetidine, possibly due to additive effect or inhibition of carmustine metabolism.
Cimetidine	Digoxin	↓	Serum digoxin concentrations may decrease during coadministration.
Cimetidine	Flecainide	↑	Pharmacologic effects of flecainide may be increased.
Cimetidine	Fluconazole	↓	Fluconazole plasma levels may be reduced, possibly due to decreased absorption.
Cimetidine	Fluorouracil	↑	Fluorouracil serum concentrations may be increased following chronic cimetidine use.
Cimetidine	Narcotic analgesics	↑	Toxic effects (eg, respiratory depression) may be increased.
Cimetidine Ranitidine	Procainamide	↑	Cimetidine may increase plasma levels of procainamide and its cardioactive metabolite n-acetyl-procainamide (NAPA) by decreasing renal tubular secretion. Ranitidine may decrease the renal clearance and increase AUC of procainamide. One study reported no effect of ranitidine on procainamide or NAPA elimination.
Cimetidine	Succinylcholine	↑	The neuromuscular blocking effects may be increased by cimetidine. Prolonged respiratory depression with extended periods of apnea may occur.
Cimetidine	Tocainide	↓	Cimetidine may decrease the pharmacologic effects of tocainide.
Nizatidine	Salicylates	↑	Increased serum salicylate levels occurred when nizatidine was administered to patients receiving very high doses of aspirin (3.9 g/day).
Ranitidine	Diazepam	↓	Diazepam's pharmacologic effects may be decreased due to decreased GI absorption by ranitidine. Staggering administration times may avoid this interaction.
Ranitidine	Sulfonylureas	↑	Ranitidine may increase the hypoglycemic effect of glipizide; 1 glyburide patient developed severe hypoglycemia after ranitidine. This did not occur in 2 studies with glyburide or tolbutamide. Glipizide dosage adjustment may be needed.
Ranitidine	Theophyllines	↔	Case reports indicate theophylline plasma levels may be increased by ranitidine, possibly increasing pharmacologic and toxic effects. However, controlled studies indicate an interaction does not occur. If this interaction occurs, it is rare.
Ranitidine	Warfarin	↑	Ranitidine may interfere with warfarin clearance (data conflict; significance not established). Hypoprothrombinemic effects may increase; may need adjustment.
H₂ antagonists	Ethanol	↑	Concurrent use may increase plasma ethanol levels and AUC. This interaction may have minimal clinical importance.

* ↑ = Object drug increased.   ↓ = Object drug decreased.   ↔ = Undetermined clinical effect.

➤*Drug/Lab test interactions:* False-positive tests for urobilinogen may occur during **nizatidine** therapy. False-positive tests for urine protein with *Multistix* may occur during **ranitidine** therapy; testing with sulfosalicylic acid is recommended.

➤*Drug/Food interactions:* Food may increase bioavailability of **famotidine** and **nizatidine**; this is of no clinical consequence. **Cimetidine** and **ranitidine** are not affected.

Adverse Reactions

Histamine H₂ Antagonist Adverse Reactions				
Adverse reaction	Cimetidine	Famotidine	Nizatidine	Ranitidine
CNS Headache	1%[1]	4.7%	†	†
Somnolence/Fatigue	1%	†	2.4%	rare
Dizziness	1%	1.3%	†	rare
Confusional states[2]	1%	†	rare	rare
Hallucinations	1%	†		rare
Agitation/Anxiety		†		†
Depression		†		rare
Insomnia		†	†	rare
Dermatologic Exfoliative dermatitis/erythroderma	†		†	
Alopecia	rare[2]	†		rare
Rash	†	†	†	†
Erythema multiforme	rare			rare
Pruritus/Urticaria		†	0.5%	
GI Nausea		†	†	†
Vomiting		†	†	†
Abdominal discomfort		†	†	†
Diarrhea	1%	1.7%	†	†
Constipation		1.2%	†	†
Pancreatitis	rare[2]			rare
Cholestatic/Hepatocellular effects	rare to 1%[2]		rare	†
Hematologic Agranulocytosis	rare			rare
Granulocytopenia	rare			†[2]
Thrombocytopenia	rare	†	†	†[2]
Autoimmune hemolytic/aplastic anemia	rare			rare
Miscellaneous Cardiac arrhythmias[3]/Arrest	rare		rare	rare
Gynecomastia	0.3%-4%		rare	†
Impotence	1%[2]	†	†	†
Loss of libido		†	†	†
Arthralgia	rare[2]	†		rare
Bronchospasm	†	†		
Hypersensitivity reactions	rare[2]			rare
Transient pain at injection site	†[4]	†	na[5]	†

† Occurs, no incidence reported or not well established.
[1] May be severe.
[2] Reversible.
[3] With rapid IV administration.
[4] IM.
[5] na – Not applicable.

In addition to the adverse effects listed in the table, the following have been reported:

Cimetidine – Reversible exacerbation of joint symptoms with preexisting arthritis, including gouty arthritis (1%); peripheral neuropathy; delirium; cutaneous vasculitis; phytobezoar formation; galactorrhea; neutropenia (including agranulocytosis) in patients with serious concomitant illnesses receiving drugs or treatment known to produce neutropenia.

Rare: Reversible interstitial nephritis and urinary retention; myalgia; polymyositis; epidermal necrolysis; strongyloidiasis hyperinfection in immunocompromised patients (extremely rare; see Precautions).

Impotence: Reversible impotence in patients with pathological hypersecretory disorders (eg, Zollinger-Ellison syndrome) receiving cimetidine, particularly in high doses, for 12 to 79 months (mean, 38 months). However, in large scale surveillance studies at regular dosages, the incidence has not exceeded that of the general population.

Ranitidine – Vertigo, reversible blurred vision (suggestive of a change in accommodation), malaise, reversible leukopenia, pancytopenia (sometimes with marrow hypoplasia), anaphylaxis, angioneurotic edema (rare). Transient local burning or itching may occur with IV administration.

Famotidine – Anorexia; dry mouth; musculoskeletal pain; paresthesias; grand mal seizure (one report); acne; dry skin; flushing; tinnitus; taste disorder; fever; asthenia; palpitations; orbital edema; conjunctival injection.

Nizatidine – Sweating (1%); asymptomatic ventricular tachycardia; hyperuricemia unassociated with gout or nephrolithiasis; eosinophilia; fever.

➤*Lab test abnormalities:* Small increases in serum creatinine and elevated ALT levels (at least twice pretreatment levels) occurred with **ranitidine**. Small possibly dose-related increases in plasma creatinine and serum transaminase occurred with **cimetidine**; these are not common and do not signify deteriorating renal function. Elevated AST, ALT and alkaline phosphatase levels occur with **nizatidine** (see Precautions).

Overdosage

➤*Symptoms:* There is no experience with deliberate overdosage. Toxic doses in animals are associated with rapid respiration or respiratory failure, tachycardia, muscular tremors, vomiting, restlessness, pallor of mucous membranes or redness of mouth and ears, hypotension, collapse and cholinergic-type effects including lacrimation, salivation, emesis, miosis and diarrhea.

Reported ingestions of up to 20 g **cimetidine** have been associated with transient adverse effects similar to those encountered in normal clinical experience. Two deaths have occurred in adults who reportedly ingested > 40 g on a single occasion.

Famotidine doses of up to 640 mg/day have been given to patients with pathological hypersecretory conditions with no serious adverse effects.

➤*Treatment:* Symptomatic and supportive. Remove unabsorbed material from the GI tract, monitor the patient and employ supportive therapy. Refer to General Management of Acute Overdosage.

With **nizatidine**, renal dialysis for 4 to 6 hours increased plasma clearance by ≈ 84%.

Physostigmine has been reported to arouse obtunded patients with evidence of **cimetidine**-induced CNS toxicity; data are insufficient to recommend this use.

Patient Information

Inform physician or pharmacist of any concomitant drug therapy, especially when taking **cimetidine**.

Stagger doses of antacids and **cimetidine** or **ranitidine**.

These agents may be taken without regard to meals.

➤*OTC:* Do not take maximum daily dosage for > 2 weeks continuously except under the advice and supervision of a physician.

CIMETIDINE

otc	**Cimetidine** (Zenith Goldline)	**Tablets:** 200 mg	In 30s and 50s.
otc	**Tagamet HB 200** (SmithKline Beecham)		In 30s and 50s.
Rx	**Cimetidine** (Various, eg, Endo, Major, Mylan, Novopharm, Penn Labs, Schein)	**Tablets:** 200 mg	In 100s, 500s and 1000s.
Rx	**Cimetidine** (Various, eg, Goldline, Major, Mylan, Novopharm, Penn Labs, Schein)	**Tablets:** 300 mg	In 100s, 500s and 1000s.
Rx	**Tagamet** (SK-Beecham)		(Tagamet 300 SB). Light green. In 100s.
Rx	**Cimetidine** (Various, eg, Endo, Goldline, Major, Mylan, Novopharm, Penn Labs, Schein)	**Tablets:** 400 mg	In 100s, 500s, and 1000s.
Rx	**Tagamet** (SK-Beecham)		(Tagamet 400 SB). Light green. Capsule shape. In 60s.
Rx	**Cimetidine** (Various, eg, Endo, Goldline, Major, Mylan, Penn Labs, Schein)	**Tablets:** 800 mg	In 100s, 500s and 1000s.
Rx	**Tagamet** (SK-Beecham)		(Tagamet 800 SB). Light green. Oval. In 30s.
Rx	**Cimetidine Oral Solution** (Barre-National)	**Liquid:** 300 mg (as HCl) per 5 mL	2.8% alcohol, parabens, saccharin, sorbitol. Mint-peach flavor. In 240 and 470 mL.
Rx	**Cimetidine** (Endo)	**Injection:** 150 mg (as HCl) per mL	5 mg phenol per mL. In 2 mL vials and 8 mL multi-dose vials.

For complete prescribing information, refer to the Histamine H₂ Antagonists group monograph.

Indications

➤*Duodenal ulcer:* Short-term treatment and maintenance therapy.

➤*Benign gastric ulcer:* Short-term treatment.

➤*Gastroesophageal reflux disease (GERD), erosive:* Treatment of erosive GERD

➤*Pathological hypersecretory conditions:* Treatment of pathological hypersecretory conditions.

➤*GI bleeding:* Prevention of upper GI bleeding in critically ill patients.

➤*Heartburn, acid indigestion and sour stomach (otc only):* Relief of these symptoms.

Administration and Dosage

➤*Approved by the FDA:* 1977.

➤*Oral:*

Duodenal ulcer –

Short-term treatment of active duodenal ulcer: 800 mg at bedtime. Alternate regimens are 300 mg 4 times a day with meals and at bedtime, or 400 mg twice a day. Give antacids as needed for pain relief. While healing often occurs during the first few weeks, continue treatment for 4 to 6 weeks unless healing is demonstrated by endoscopy.

Maintenance therapy: 400 mg at bedtime.

Active benign gastric ulcer – For short-term treatment, 800 mg at bedtime or 300 mg 4 times a day with meals and at bedtime. The preferred regimen is 800 mg at bedtime based on convenience and lowered potential for drug interaction. There is no information concerning usefulness of treatment periods longer than 8 weeks.

Erosive gastroesophageal reflux disease (GERD) –

Adults: 1600 mg daily in divided doses (800 mg twice daily or 400 mg 4 times a day) for 12 weeks. Use beyond 12 weeks has not been established.

Pathological hypersecretory conditions – 300 mg 4 times a day with meals and at bedtime. If necessary, give 300 mg doses more often. Individualize dosage. Do not exceed 2400 mg/day; continue as long as clinically indicated.

Heartburn, acid indigestion and sour stomach (otc only) – 200 mg (2 tablets) with water as symptoms occur or as directed, up to twice daily (up to 4 tablets in 24 hrs). Do not take maximum dose for > 2 weeks continuously unless otherwise directed by a physician.

Children: Do not give to children < 12 years of age unless otherwise directed.

➤*Parenteral:* For hospitalized patients with pathological hypersecretory conditions or intractable ulcers, or patients unable to take oral medication. The usual dose is 300 mg IM or IV every 6 to 8 hours. If it is necessary to increase dosage, do so by more frequent administration of a 300 mg dose, not to exceed 2400 mg/day.

Prevention of upper GI bleeding – Continuous IV infusion of 50 mg/ hour. Patients with creatinine clearance < 30 mL/min should receive half the recommended dose. Treatment beyond 7 days has not been studied.

GERD – The doses and regimen for parenteral administration in patients with GERD have not been established.

➤*IM:* Administer undiluted.

➤*IV:* Dilute in 0.9% Sodium Chloride Injection or other compatible IV solution to a total volume of 20 mL; inject ≥ 2 minutes.

➤*Intermittent IV infusion:* Dilute 300 mg in at least 50 mL of 5% Dextrose Injection or other compatible IV solution; infuse over 15 to 20 minutes.

➤*Continuous IV infusion:* 37.5 mg/hour (900 mg/day). For patients requiring a more rapid elevation of gastric pH, continuous infusion may be preceded by a 150 mg loading dose administered by IV infusion as described above. Dilute 900 mg cimetidine injection in a compatible IV fluid (see Stability) for a constant rate infusion over a 24 hour period.

Note: Cimetidine may be diluted in 100 to 1000 mL; however, a volumetric pump is recommended if the volume for 24 hour infusion is < 250 mL.

➤*Plastic containers:* Do not add drugs to the solution in these containers or introduce any additives.

➤*Admixture incompatibility:* Incompatible with aminophylline and barbiturates in IV solutions. Incompatible in the same syringe with pentobarbital sodium and a pentobarbital sodium/atropine sulfate combination. In one study, cimetidine and aminophylline were chemically stable and physically compatible for 48 hours at room temperature when admixed in 5% Dextrose in Water.

➤*Severely impaired renal function:* Accumulation may occur. Use the lowest dose; 300 mg every 12 hours orally or IV has been recommended. According to the patient's condition, dosage frequency may be increased to every 8 hours or even further with caution. Whether hemodialysis reduces the level of circulating cimetidine is controversial. Give the dose at the end of hemodialysis. When liver impairment is also present, further dosage reductions may be necessary.

➤*Storage/Stability:* Stable for 48 hours at room temperature when added to commonly used IV solutions (eg, 0.9% Sodium Chloride Injection, 5% or 10% Dextrose Injection, Lactated Ringer's Solution, 5% Sodium Bicarbonate Injection) or when added to a total parenteral nutrition admixture containing amino acids, dextrose, fat emulsion, electrolytes and vitamins. When diluted to a concentration of 15 mg/mL in sterile water for injection and stored in glass vials, cimetidine was stable for 14 days at 22°C (71°F) and for 42 days at 4°C (39.2°F).

Premixed, single-dose – Avoid exposure of the premixed product to excessive heat. The product should be stored at controlled room temperature (15° to 30°C; 59° to 86°F). Brief exposure up to 40°C does not adversely affect premixed product.

RANITIDINE HCl

otc	**Ranitidine** (Various, eg, Goldline)	**Tablets:** 75 mg (as base)	In 30s.
otc	**Zantac 75** (Warner-Lambert)		(Z 75). In 4s, 10s, 20s, 30s, 60s, and 80s.
Rx	**Ranitidine** (Various, eg, Apotex, Geneva, Mylan, Ranbaxy, Teva, UDL, Watson)	**Tablets:** 150 mg (as base)	In 60s, 100s, 500s, 1000s, 5000s, and UD 100s.
Rx	**Zantac** (GlaxoSmithKline)		(Zantac 150 Glaxo). Peach, 5-sided. Film-coated. In 60s, 180s, 500s, 1000s, and UD 100s.
Rx	**Ranitidine** (Various, eg, Apotex, Geneva, Mylan, Ranbaxy, Teva, Watson)	**Tablets:** 300 mg (as base)	In 30s, 100s, 250s, 500s, 1000s, 2500s, and UD 100s.
Rx	**Zantac** (GlaxoSmithKline)		(Zantac 300 Glaxo). Yellow, capsule shape. Film-coated. In 30s, 250s and UD 100s.
Rx	**Zantac EFFERdose** (GlaxoSmithKline)	**Tablets, effervescent:** 25 mg (as base)	(GS 25C). White/pale yellow. In 60s.[a]
		150 mg (as base)	(Zantac 150 427). White/pale yellow. In 60s.[b]
Rx	**Ranitidine HCl** (Various, eg, Alpharma)	**Syrup:** 15 mg (as base) per mL	May contain alcohol. In UD 10 mL.
Rx	**Zantac** (GlaxoSmithKline)		7.5% alcohol, saccharin, sorbitol, parabens. Peppermint flavor. In 480 mL.
Rx	**Zantac** (GlaxoSmithKline)	**Injection:** 1 mg (as base) per mL	Preservative free. In premixed 50 mL single-dose plastic containers.[c]
		25 mg (as base) per mL	In 2 and 6 mL vials.[d]

[a] With aspartame; 2.81 mg phenylalanine and 30.52 mg sodium/tablet.
[b] With aspartame; 16.84 mg phenylalanine and 183.12 mg sodium/tablet

[c] Premixed in 0.45% sodium chloride.
[d] With phenol.

For complete prescribing information, refer to the Histamine H₂ Antagonists group monograph.

Indications

➤*Duodenal ulcer:* Short-term treatment of active ulcer and maintenance therapy after healing of acute ulcers.

➤*Gastric ulcer:* Short-term treatment of active, benign ulcer and maintenance therapy after healing of acute ulcer.

➤*Pathological hypersecretory conditions:* Treatment of pathological hypersecretory conditions (eg, Zollinger-Ellison syndrome, systemic mastocytosis).

➤*Gastroesophageal reflux disease (GERD):* Treatment of GERD.

➤*Erosive esophagitis:*

Treatment – Treatment of endoscopically diagnosed erosive esophagitis, and for symptomatic relief of associated heartburn.

Maintenance – Maintenance of healing erosive esophagitis.

➤*IV:* Indicated in some hospitalized patients with pathological hypersecretory conditions or intractable duodenal ulcers, or as an alternative to the oral dosage form for short-term use in patients who are unable to take oral medication.

➤*Heartburn (otc only):* Relieves heartburn associated with acid indigestion and sour stomach. Prevents heartburn associated with acid indigestion and sour stomach brought on by certain foods and beverages.

Administration and Dosage

➤*Approved by the FDA:* June 1983.

➤*Oral:*

Adults –

Duodenal ulcer:
• *Treatment* – 150 mg orally twice daily. An alternate dosage of 300 mg once daily after the evening meal or at bedtime can be used for patients in whom dosing convenience is important; 100 mg twice daily is as effective as the 150 mg dose in inhibiting gastric acid secretion.
• *Maintenance* – 150 mg at bedtime.
Pathological hypersecretory conditions: 150 mg orally twice a day. More frequent doses may be necessary. Individualize dosage and continue as long as indicated. Doses up to 6 g/day have been used.
Gastric ulcer:
• *Treatment* – 150 mg twice daily.
• *Maintenance* – 150 mg at bedtime.
GERD: 150 mg twice daily.
Erosive esophagitis:
• *Treatment* – 150 mg 4 times daily.
• *Maintenance* – 150 mg twice daily.
Heartburn (otc only):
• *Treatment* – For relief of symptoms, swallow 1 tablet with a glass of water.
• *Prevention* – To prevent symptoms, swallow 1 tablet with a glass of water 30 to 60 minutes before eating food or drinking beverages that cause heartburn.
• *Maintenance* – Can be used up to twice daily (up to 2 tablets in 24 hours).

Children – The safety and effectiveness of ranitidine have been established in children from 1 month to 16 years of age. There is insufficient information about the pharmacokinetics of ranitidine in neonatal patients < 1 month of age to make dosing recommendations. Do not give *otc* ranitidine to children < 12 years of age unless directed by physician.

Active duodenal and gastric ulcers:
• *Treatment* – 2 to 4 mg/kg/day twice daily to a maximum of 300 mg/day.
• *Maintenance* – 2 to 4 mg/kg once daily to a maximum of 150 mg/day.
GERD and erosive esophagitis: Although limited data exist for these conditions in pediatric patients, published literature supports a dosage of 5 to 10 mg/kg/day, usually given as 2 divided doses.

Preparation –
Zantac 25 EFFERdose tablets: Dissolve 1 tablet in no less than 5 mL (1 teaspoonful) of water in an appropriate measuring cup. Wait until the tablet is completely dissolved before administering the solution to the infant/child. The solution may be administered by medicine dropper for infants.
Zantac 150 EFFERdose tablets: Dissolve each dose in ≈ 6 to 8 oz. of water before drinking.

➤*Parenteral:*
IM – 50 mg (2 mL) every 6 to 8 hours. (No dilution necessary.)
Intermittent bolus – 50 mg (2 mL) every 6 to 8 hours. Dilute 50 mg in 0.9% Sodium Chloride or other compatible IV solution to a concentration no greater than 2.5 mg/mL (20 mL). Inject at a rate no greater than 4 mL/min (5 minutes).
Intermittent IV infusion – 50 mg (2 mL) every 6 to 8 hours. Dilute 50 mg in 5% Dextrose Injection or other compatible IV solution to a concentration no greater than 0.5 mg/mL (100 mL) and infuse at a rate no greater than 5 to 7 mL/minute, or use 50 mL of 1 mg/mL premixed solution and infuse over 15 to 20 minutes; do not exceed 400 mg/day.

Premixed injection – Requires no dilution and should be infused over 15 to 20 minutes. Administer by slow IV drip infusion only. Do not introduce additives into the solution. If used with a primary IV fluid system, discontinue primary solution during premixed infusion.

Continuous IV infusion – Add ranitidine injection to 5% Dextrose Injection or other compatible IV solution (see Storage/Stability). Deliver at a rate of 6.25 mg/hr (eg, 150 mg [6 mL] ranitidine injection in 250 mL of 5% Dextrose Injection at 10.7 mL/hr).

For Zollinger-Ellison patients, dilute ranitidine injection in 5% Dextrose Injection or other compatible IV solution (see Storage/Stability) to a concentration ≤ 2.5 mg/mL. Start the infusion at a rate of 1 mg/kg/hr. If after 4 hours either the measured gastric acid output is > 10 mEq/hr or the patient becomes symptomatic, adjust the dose upwards in 0.5 mg/kg/hr increments and remeasure the acid output. Doses up to 2.5 mg/kg/hr and infusion rates as high as 220 mg/hr have been used.

➤*Children:* The recommended IV dose in pediatric patients is for a total daily dose of 2 to 4 mg/kg, to be divided and administered every 6 to 8 hours up to a maximum of 50 mg given every 6 to 8 hours. Limited data in neonatal patients (< 1 month of age) receiving ECMO have shown that a dose of 2 mg/kg is usually sufficient to increase gastric pH to > 4 for at least 15 hours. Therefore, consider doses of 2 mg/kg given every 12 to 24 hours or as a continuous infusion.

➤*Renal impairment (Ccr < 50 mL/min):* 150 mg orally every 24 hours or 50 mg parenterally every 18 to 24 hours. The frequency of dosing may be increased to every 12 hours or further with caution. Hemodialysis reduces the level of circulating ranitidine. Adjust dosage timing so that a scheduled dose coincides with the end of hemodialysis.

➤*Elderly:* Elderly patients are more likely to have decreased renal function; therefore, exercise caution in dose selection. It also may be useful to monitor renal function.

➤*Storage/Stability:*
Tablets – Store between 15° and 30°C (59° and 86°F) in a dry place. Protect from light. Replace cap securely after each opening.

RANITIDINE HCl

Effervescent tablets – Store between 2° and 30°C (36° and 86°F).

Syrup – Store between 4° and 25°C (39° and 77°F). Dispense in tight, light-resistant containers.

Parenteral – Undiluted ranitidine injection tends to exhibit a yellow color that may intensify over time without adversely affecting potency.

Ranitidine injection is stable for 48 hours at room temperature when added to or diluted with most commonly used IV solutions (eg, 0.9% Sodium Chloride Injection, 5% or 10% Dextrose Injection, Lactated Ringer's injection, 5% Sodium Bicarbonate Injection).

Store the premixed injection between 2° and 25°C (36° and 77°F) and the injection between 4° and 30°C (39° and 86°F). Protect from light.

NIZATIDINE

otc	**Axid AR** (Whitehall-Robins)	**Tablets:** 75 mg	(AXID AR). In 12s and 30s.
Rx	**Nizatidine** (Various, eg, Eon, Ivax, Mylan, Par)	**Capsules:** 150 mg	In 60s, 100s, 500s, 1000s, and UD 100s.
Rx	**Axid Pulvules** (Lilly)		(Lilly 3144/Axid 150 mg). Yellow. In 60s, 500s, and *Identi-Dose* 100s and 620s.
Rx	**Nizatidine** (Various, eg, Eon, Ivax, Mylan, Par)	**Capsules:** 300 mg	In 30s, 100s, and 500s.
Rx	**Axid Pulvules** (Lilly)		(Lilly 3145/Axid 300 mg). Yellow/brown. In 30s.

For complete prescribing information, refer to the Histamine H₂ Antagonists group monograph.

Indications

➤*Duodenal ulcer:* Treatment of active ulcer for up to 8 weeks and maintenance therapy after healing of active ulcer.

➤*Benign gastric ulcer:* Treatment of active benign ulcer for up to 8 weeks.

➤*Gastroesophageal reflux disease (GERD):* For endoscopically diagnosed esophagitis, including erosive and ulcerative esophagitis, and associated heartburn due to GERD.

➤*Heartburn (otc only):* Relief of heartburn, acid indigestion, and sour stomach and prevention of these symptoms brought on by consuming food and beverages.

Administration and Dosage

➤*Approved by the FDA:* April 1988.

For adult use only (≥ 12 years of age for *otc*).

➤*Duodenal ulcer:*

Acute therapy – 300 mg once daily at bedtime. An alternative dosage regimen is 150 mg twice daily. Most heal in 4 weeks.

Maintenance therapy – 150 mg once daily at bedtime.

➤*GERD:* 150 mg twice daily.

➤*Benign gastric ulcer:* 300 mg given either as 150 mg twice daily or 300 mg once daily at bedtime.

➤*Heartburn, acid indigestion, and sour stomach (otc only):* Can be used up to twice daily (up to 2 tablets in 24 hours).

Relief – For relief of symptoms, take 1 tablet with a full glass of water.

Prevention – For prevention of symptoms, take 1 tablet with a full glass of water right before eating or up to 60 minutes before consuming food and beverages that cause heartburn.

➤*Moderate-to-severe renal insufficiency:*

Nizatidine Dosage in Renal Insufficiency		
	Dosage	
Creatinine clearance	Active duodenal ulcer, GERD, benign gastric ulcer	Maintenance therapy
20 to 50 mL/min	150 mg/day	150 mg every other day
< 20 mL/min	150 mg every other day	150 mg every 3 days

FAMOTIDINE

otc	**Famotidine** (Ivax)	**Tablets:** 10 mg	In 18s, 30s, 50s, and 70s.
otc	**Pepcid AC** (J & J Merck)		(Pepcid AC). In 2s, 6s, 18s, 30s, 60s, and 90s.
Rx	**Famotidine** (Various, eg, Geneva, Ivax, Teva, UDL, Watson, Zenith Goldline)	**Tablets:** 20 mg	May contain lactose. In 30s, 100s, 500s, 1000s, UD 100s, and *Robot-Ready* 25s.
Rx	**Pepcid** (Merck)		(MSD 963 PEPCID). Beige, U-shape. Film-coated. In 1000s, 10,000s, unit-of-use 30s, 90s, and 100s, UD 100s, and *Uniblister* 31s.
otc	**Pepcid AC Maximum Strength** (J & J Merck)		In 25s.
Rx	**Famotidine** (Various, eg, Geneva, Ivax, Teva, Watson, Zenith Goldline)	**Tablets:** 40 mg	May contain lactose. In 30s, 100s, 500s, 1000s, and UD 100s.
Rx	**Pepcid** (Merck)		(MSD 964 PEPCID). Lt. brownish orange, U-shape. Film-coated. In 1000s, 10,000s, unit-of-use 30s, 90s, and 100s, UD 100s, and *Uniblister* 31s.
otc	**Pepcid AC** (J & J Merck)	**Gelcaps:** 10 mg	(PEPCID AC). In 30s, 50s, 60s, and 90s.
otc	**Pepcid AC** (J & J Merck)	**Tablets, chewable:** 10 mg	Aspartame, lactose, mannitol, 1.4 mg phenylalanine. (PEPCID AC). In 6s, 18s, 30s, 50s, 60s, and 68s.
Rx	**Pepcid RPD** (Merck)	**Tablets, orally disintegrating:** 20 mg	Aspartame, mannitol, 1.05 mg phenylalanine. Mint flavor. Pale rose, hexagonal. In UD 30s and 100s.
		40 mg	Aspartame, mannitol, 2.1 mg phenylalanine. Mint flavor. Pale rose, hexagonal. In UD 30s and 100s.
Rx	**Pepcid** (Merck)	**Powder for oral suspension:** 40 mg/5 mL when reconstituted	Parabens, sucrose. Cherry-banana-mint flavor. In bottles of 400 mg.
Rx	**Famotidine** (Various, eg, American Pharma, Baxter, Bedford, Wyeth-Ayerst)	**Injection:** 10 mg/mL	May contain mannitol or benzyl alcohol. In 1 and 2 mL single-dose vials and 4, 20, and 50 mL multiple-dose vials.
Rx	**Pepcid** (Merck)		Mannitol. In 2 mL single-dose vials[a] and 4 and 20 mL multi-dose vials.[b]
Rx	**Pepcid** (Merck)	**Injection (premixed):** 20 mg/50 mL	Preservative-free. In 50 mL single-dose *Galaxy* containers.

[a] Preservative free.

[b] With 0.9% benzyl alcohol.

For complete prescribing information, refer to the Histamine H₂ Antagonists group monograph.

Indications

➤*Duodenal ulcer:* Short-term treatment of active ulcer and maintenance therapy after healing of active ulcer.

➤*Benign gastric ulcer:* Short-term treatment of active benign ulcer.

➤*Pathological hypersecretory conditions:* Treatment of pathological hypersecretory conditions (eg, Zollinger-Ellison syndrome).

➤*Gastroesophageal reflux disease (GERD):* Short-term treatment of GERD. Also for short-term treatment of esophagitis due to GERD, including erosive or ulcerative disease diagnosed by endoscopy (short-term treatment).

➤*IV:* Indicated in some hospitalized patients with pathological hypersecretory conditions or intractable ulcers, or as an alternative to the oral dosage forms for short-term use in patients who are unable to take oral medication.

➤*Heartburn, acid indigestion, and sour stomach (otc only):* Relieves heartburn associated with acid indigestion and sour stomach and prevents heartburn associated with acid indigestion and sour stomach brought on by eating or drinking certain food and beverages.

FAMOTIDINE

Administration and Dosage

➤*Approved by the FDA:* October 1986.

➤*Oral:*

Duodenal ulcer –

  Acute therapy: 40 mg/day at bedtime. Most heal in 4 weeks; there is rarely reason to use full dosage for more than 6 to 8 weeks. 20 mg twice daily is also effective.

  Maintenance therapy: 20 mg once a day at bedtime.

Benign gastric ulcer –

  Acute therapy: 40 mg once a day at bedtime.

Pathological hypersecretory conditions – Individualize dosage. The adult starting dose is 20 mg every 6 hours; some patients may require a higher starting dose. Continue as long as clinically indicated. Doses up to 160 mg every 6 hours have been administered to some patients with severe Zollinger-Ellison syndrome.

GERD – 20 mg twice daily for up to 6 weeks. For esophagitis including erosions and ulcerations and accompanying symptoms due to GERD, 20 or 40 mg twice daily for up to 12 weeks.

Children – Studies suggest the following starting doses in pediatric patients 1 to 16 years of age.

  Peptic ulcer: 0.5 mg/kg/day orally at bedtime or divided twice daily up to 40 mg/day.

  GERD with or without esophagitis including erosions and ulcerations: 1 mg/kg/day orally divided twice daily up to 40 mg twice daily.

While published uncontrolled studies suggest effectiveness of famotidine in the treatment of GERD and peptic ulcer, data in pediatric patients are insufficient to establish percent response with dose and duration of therapy. Therefore, individualize treatment duration (initially based on adult duration recommendations) and dose based on clinical response or pH determination (gastric or esophageal) and endoscopy. Published uncontrolled clinical studies in pediatric patients have employed doses up to 1 mg/kg/day for peptic ulcer and 2 mg/kg/day for GERD with or without esophagitis including erosions and ulcerations. No pharmacokinetic or pharmacodynamic data are available on pediatric patients younger than 1 year of age.

Heartburn, acid indigestion, and sour stomach (otc only) –

  Acute therapy: 1 tablet with water.,

  Prevention: 1 tablet 10 to 60 minutes before eating food or drinking a beverage that is expected to cause symptoms.,

  Use: Can be used up to twice daily (up to 2 tablets in 24 hours). Do not take maximum dose for more than 2 weeks continuously unless otherwise directed by a physician.

  Children: Do not give to children under 12 years of age unless otherwise directed.

➤*Parenteral:*

IV – In some hospitalized patients with pathological hypersecretory conditions or intractable ulcers, or in patients unable to take oral medication, give famotidine IV 20 mg every 12 hours. Doses and regimen for GERD are not established.

Children – Individualize dosage. Starting dose in pediatric patients 1 to 16 years of age is 0.25 mg/kg IV (injected over a period of at least 2 minutes or as a 15-minute infusion) every 12 hours up to 40 mg/day.

Preparation of IV solutions – Dilute 2 mL famotidine IV (solution containing 10 mg/mL) with 0.9% sodium chloride injection or other compatible IV solution to a total volume of either 5 or 10 mL and inject over not less than 2 minutes.

Preparation of IV infusion solutions – Famotidine IV may also be administered as an infusion, 2 mL diluted with 100 mL of 5% dextrose or other compatible solution, and infused over 15 to 30 minutes. A premixed solution is also available containing famotidine premixed with 0.9% sodium chloride.

➤*Renal function impairment:* To avoid excess accumulation of the drug in patients with moderate (Ccr less than 50 mL/min) or severe renal insufficiency (Ccr less than 10 mL/min) the dose may be reduced to half the dose or the dosing interval may be prolonged to 36 to 48 hours, as indicated.

➤*Storage/Stability:*

Tablets/Orally disintegrating tablets/oral suspension dry powder and suspension – Store at 25°C (77°F); excursions permitted to 15° to 30°C (59° to 86°F). Protect suspension from freezing. Discard unused suspension after 30 days.

Pepcid AC Maximum Strength – Store at 20° to 30°C (68° to 86°F).

Injection – Solution is stable for 7 days at room temperature when added to or diluted with most commonly used IV solutions (eg, water for injection, 0.9% sodium chloride injection, 5% or 10% dextrose injection, lactated Ringer's injection, 5% sodium bicarbonate injection). When added to or diluted with 5% sodium bicarbonate injection, a precipitate may form at higher concentrations of famotidine injection (more than 0.2 mg/mL). Although diluted famotidine injection has been shown to be stable for 7 days at room temperature, there are no data on the maintenance of sterility after dilution. Therefore, it is recommended that if not used immediately after preparation, diluted solutions of famotidine injection should be refrigerated and used within 48 hours.

Store injection (non-premixed) at 2° to 8°C (36° to 46°F). Store premixed injection at room temperature (25°C; 77°F). Avoid exposure of the premixed product to excessive heat; brief exposure to temperatures up to 35°C (95°F) does not adversely affect the product. One study showed stability of famotidine admixed in dextrose or saline in polyvinyl chloride minibags and polypropylene syringes for 15 days at room temperature.

HISTAMINE H$_2$ ANTAGONIST COMBINATIONS

otc	**Pepcid Complete** (J & J Merck)	**Tablets, chewable:** 10 mg famotidine, 800 mg calcium carbonate, 165 mg magnesium hydroxide	Lactose, sugar. (P). Mint flavor. In 5s, 15s, 25s, and 50s.

For complete prescribing information, refer to the Histamine H$_2$ Antagonists group monograph.

Indications

➤*Heartburn:* Relieves heartburn associated with acid indigestion and sour stomach.

Administration and Dosage

➤≥ *12 years of age:* To relieve symptoms, chew 1 tablet before swallowing. Do not use > 2 tablets in 24 hours. Do not swallow tablet whole; chew completely.

➤*Storage/Stability:* Store at 25° to 30°C (77° to 86°F).

Indications

▶*Gastric ulcers:* For treatment or symptomatic relief of various gastric disorders including gastric and duodenal ulcers, gastroesophageal reflux disease (GERD), or pathological hypersecretory conditions. Refer to individual monographs for specific indications.

▶*Unlabeled uses:* Posterior laryngitis (**omeprazole** 40 mg at bedtime for 6 to 24 weeks); efficacy of pancreatin enhanced for treatment of steatorrhea in cystic fibrosis patients.

Actions

▶*Pharmacology:* **Omeprazole**, **lansoprazole**, **rabeprazole**, and **pantoprazole** belong to a class of antisecretory compounds, the substituted benzimidazoles, that do not exhibit anticholinergic or histamine H_2 antagonistic properties, but that suppress gastric acid secretion by specific inhibition of the H^+/K^+ ATPase enzyme system at the secretory surface of the gastric parietal cell. Because this enzyme system is the "acid (proton) pump" within the gastric mucosa, these agents have been characterized as gastric acid pump inhibitors; they block the final step of acid production. This effect is dose-related and inhibits both basal and stimulated acid secretion regardless of the stimulus.

Because of the normal physiologic effect caused by the inhibition of gastric acid secretion, blood flow in the antrum, pylorus, and duodenal bulb decreases. These agents increase serum pepsinogen levels and decrease pepsin activity. As with other agents that elevate intragastric pH, increases in gastric pH are associated with increases in nitrate-reducing bacteria and elevation of nitrate concentration in gastric juice in patients with gastric ulcer.

Serum gastrin levels increase parallel with inhibition of acid secretion. No further increase in serum gastrin occurs with continued treatment. Gastrin values usually returned to pretreatment levels within 1 to 2 weeks (omeprazole), 4 weeks (lansoprazole), or 3 months (pantoprazole) after discontinuation of therapy.

▶*Pharmacokinetics:*

Absorption / Distribution – **Omeprazole**, **lansoprazole**, **rabeprazole**, and **pantoprazole** are acid-labile. Omeprazole and lansoprazole are formulated as enteric-coated granules, while rabeprazole and pantoprazole are formulated as enteric-coated tablets. Absorption is rapid and begins after the granules leave the stomach. Peak plasma concentrations and AUC are approximately proportional, but because of a saturable first-pass effect, a greater than linear response in peak plasma concentration and AUC occurs with omeprazole at doses > 40 mg.

Metabolism / Excretion – These agents are extensively metabolized by the liver. Several metabolites have been identified. These metabolites have very little or no antisecretory activity. The plasma elimination half-life of proton pump inhibitors does not reflect duration of suppression of gastric acid secretion. Thus, the plasma elimination half-life is < 2 hours while the acid inhibitory effect lasts > 24 hours, apparently because of prolonged binding to the parietal H^+/K^+ ATPase enzyme. When the drug is discontinued, secretory activity returns over 3 to 5 days.

Little unchanged drug is excreted in urine. Approximately 33% of **lansoprazole** and the majority of **omeprazole** ($\approx$ 77%), **rabeprazole** ($\approx$ 90%), and **pantoprazole** ($\approx$ 71%) is eliminated in urine. The remainder of the dose is excreted in feces. This implies a significant biliary excretion of the metabolites of omeprazole and lansoprazole.

Select Pharmacokinetics of Proton Pump Inhibitors

Drug	Absolute bioavailability (%)	T_{max} (hours)	t½ (hours)	Duration of action (hours)	Clearance (mL/min)	Protein binding (%)
Omeprazole	$\approx$ 30 to 40[1]	0.5 to 3.5	0.5 to 1	$\leq$ 72	500 to 600	$\approx$ 95
Lansoprazole	> 80	$\approx$ 1.7	1.5	> 24	—	97
Rabeprazole	52	2 to 5	1 to 2	> 24	301 to 588	96.3
Pantoprazole	$\approx$ 77	2.4	$\approx$ 1	> 24	127 to 233	$\approx$ 98

[1] The bioavailability of omeprazole increases slightly upon repeat administration.

Special populations:

• *Hepatic function impairment –* In patients with chronic hepatic disease, the bioavailability of **omeprazole** increased to $\approx$ 100%, reflecting decreased first-pass effect; plasma half-life increased to nearly 3 hours. Plasma clearance averaged 70 mL/min, compared with 500 to 600 mL/min in healthy subjects. However, no dosage adjustment is necessary.

In patients with various degrees of chronic hepatic disease, the mean plasma half-life of **lansoprazole** was prolonged from 1.5 hours to 3.2 to 7.2 hours. An increase in mean AUC of up to 500% was observed at steady state in hepatically impaired patients compared with healthy subjects. Consider dose reduction in patients with severe hepatic disease.

In patients with chronic, mild-to-moderate hepatic disease, the AUC of **rabeprazole** doubled, the elimination half-life increased 2- to 3-fold, and the total body clearance decreased to less than half compared with healthy patients after a 20 mg oral dose. No dosage adjustment is required for patients with mild-to-moderate impairment. No information exists on rabeprazole disposition in patients with severe hepatic impairment.

In patients with mild-to-moderate hepatic impairment, maximum **pantoprazole** concentrations increased 1.5-fold, serum half-life increased 7 to 9 hours, and AUC increased 5- to 7-fold compared with healthy subjects; however, these values were no greater than those observed in slow CYP2C19 metabolizers. No dosage adjustment is required for patients with mild-to-moderate impairment. The pharmacokinetics have not been well characterized in patients with severe hepatic impairment.

• *Renal function impairment –* In patients with chronic renal impairment (creatinine clearance, 10 to 62 mL/min/1.73 m^2), the disposition of **omeprazole** was similar to that in healthy volunteers but with a slight increase in bioavailability. Because urinary excretion is a primary route of elimination of omeprazole metabolites, their elimination slowed in proportion to the decreased creatinine clearance. However, no dosage adjustment is necessary.

In patients with severe renal insufficiency, plasma protein binding decreased by 1% to 1.5% after administration of 60 mg of **lansoprazole**. Patients with renal insufficiency had a shortened elimination half-life and decreased total AUC (free and bound). However, AUC for free lansoprazole in plasma was not related to the degree of renal impairment, and C_{max} and T_{max} were not different from subjects with healthy kidneys. No dosage adjustment is necessary.

In patients with stable end-stage renal impairment requiring maintenance hemodialysis with creatinine clearance $\leq$ 5 mL/min, no difference in **rabeprazole** pharmacokinetics compared with healthy subjects was observed after a 20 mg dose. No dosage adjustment is necessary.

In patients with severe renal impairment, the pharmacokinetics of **pantoprazole** were similar to that of healthy subjects. No dosage adjustment is necessary.

• *Elderly –* In the elderly, the elimination rate of **omeprazole** was somewhat decreased and bioavailability was increased. Omeprazole was 76% bioavailable with a 40 mg oral dose in elderly volunteers vs 58% in young volunteers. Nearly 70% of the dose was recovered in urine as metabolites; no unchanged drug was detected. The plasma clearance of omeprazole was 250 mL/min and its plasma half-life averaged 1 hour. However, no dosage adjustment is necessary.

The clearance of **lansoprazole** is decreased in the elderly, with elimination half-life increased by $\approx$ 50% to 100%. Because the mean half-life in the elderly remains between 1.9 to 2.9 hours, repeated once-daily dosing does not result in accumulation of lansoprazole. Peak plasma levels were not increased in the elderly. No dosage adjustment is necessary.

In healthy elderly subjects receiving **rabeprazole** 20 mg once daily for 7 days, AUC values doubled and C_{max} increased by 60% compared with a younger control group. No dosage adjustment is necessary.

In elderly subjects receiving **pantoprazole**, the AUC increased by 43% and the C_{max} increased by 26% compared with younger subjects. However, no dosage adjustment is necessary.

• *Race –* An increase in AUC of **omeprazole** of $\approx$ 4-fold was noted in Asian subjects compared with white subjects. Consider dose adjustment for Asian subjects, particularly where maintenance of healing of erosive esophagitis is indicated.

In healthy Japanese men, the AUC was $\approx$ 50% to 60% greater than values derived from pooled data from healthy men in the US.

▶*Clinical trials:*

Duodenal and Gastric Ulcer Healing Rates with Omeprazole and Lansoprazole vs Ranitidine (%)[1]

Ulcer	Omeprazole		Ranitidine	Lansoprazole			Ranitidine
	20 mg	40 mg	150 mg bid	15 mg	30 mg	60 mg	300 mg hs
Duodenal ulcer							
Week 2	83	83	53	35	44.2	39.1	30.5
Week 4	97	100	82	92.3	80.3	89.9	70.5
Week 8	100	100	94	—	—	—	—
Gastric ulcer							
Week 4	63.5	78.1	56.3	64.6	58.1	53.3	—
Week 8	81.5	91.4	78.4	92.2	96.8	93.2	—

[1] Data pooled from separate studies. Not comparable.

An international randomized, double-blind, active-controlled trial was conducted in 205 patients comparing 20 mg rabeprazole once daily with 20 mg omeprazole once daily. Rabeprazole and omeprazole were comparable in healing duodenal ulcers. The percentages of patients with endoscopic healing at 2 and 4 weeks are presented below.

Healing of Duodenal Ulcers: Rabeprazole vs Omeprazole (% Patients Healed)

Week	Rabeprazole 20 mg (n = 102)	Omeprazole 20 mg (n = 103)
2	69	61
4	98	93

	Erosive Esophagitis Healing Rates with Proton Pump Inhibitors (%)										
	Omeprazole		Lansoprazole			Rabeprazole			Pantoprazole		
Week	20 mg (n = 83)	40 mg (n = 87)	15 mg (n = 69)	30 mg (n = 65)	60 mg (n = 72)	10 mg (n = 27)	20 mg (n = 25)	40 mg (n = 26)	10 mg (n = 153)	20 mg (n = 158)	40 mg (n = 162)
4	39	45	67.6	81.3	80.6	63	56	54	45.6	58.4	75
6	—	—	87.7	95.4	94.3	—	—	—	—	—	—
8	74	75	90.9	95.4	94.4	93	84	85	66	83.5	92.6

H. pylori – In 2 multicenter US studies (n = 498), the following regimens were studied for treatment of *H. pylori*: **Omeprazole** 40 mg/day plus clarithromycin 500 mg 3 times daily for 14 days followed by omeprazole 20 mg/day for 14 days or omeprazole 40 mg/day for 14 days. In 2 foreign studies (n = 369), the dose regimen was the same as that used in the US studies except for 1 study, where omeprazole 40 mg/day was used throughout the 28-day treatment period. Clinical studies in the US evaluated the efficacy of **lansoprazole** in combination with amoxicillin capsules and clarithromycin tablets as triple 14-day therapy or in combination with amoxicillin capsules as dual 14-day therapy for the eradication of *H. pylori*. Triple therapy: Lansoprazole 30 mg twice daily/amoxicillin 1 g twice daily/clarithromycin 500 mg twice daily. Dual therapy: Lansoprazole 30 mg 3 times daily/amoxicillin 1 g 3 times daily.

	H. pylori Healing Rates[1] with Proton Pump Inhibitors		
	Dual therapy		Triple therapy
Study	Omeprazole	Lansoprazole	Lansoprazole
US	64 to 74	—	—
Non-US	74 to 83		
1	—	70	86
2	—	61	83

[1] Data pooled from several different studies. Not comparable.

Contraindications

Hypersensitivity to any component of the formulation; substituted benzimidazoles (**rabeprazole**).

Warnings

►*Atrophic gastritis:* Atrophic gastritis has been noted occasionally in gastric corpus biopsies from patients treated long-term with **omeprazole**.

►*Hepatic function impairment:* In patients with various degrees of chronic hepatic disease, the mean plasma half-life of **lansoprazole** was prolonged ≈ 2 to 6 hours, and an increase in the mean AUC of ≤ 500% was observed at steady state. Consider dose reduction in severe hepatic disease (see Administration and Dosage).

►*Carcinogenesis:* In two 24-month carcinogenicity studies in rats, **omeprazole** at daily doses ≈ 4 to 352 times the human dose produced gastric enterochromaffin-like (ECL) cell carcinoids in a dose-related manner in male and female rats; the incidence was markedly higher in female rats that had higher blood levels of omeprazole. In addition, ECL cell hyperplasia was present in all treated groups of both sexes.

Gastric biopsy specimens from the body of the stomach from ≈ 150 patients treated continuously with **lansoprazole** for ≥ 1 year have not shown evidence of gastric ECL cell effects similar to those seen in rat studies. Longer-term data are needed to rule out the possibility of an increased risk of development of gastric tumors in patients receiving long-term lansoprazole therapy.

In a study with rats, **rabeprazole** produced gastric ECL cell hyperplasia in male and female rats and ECL cell carcinoid tumors in female rats at all test doses (lowest dose was 0.1 times the human exposure at the recommended dose for GERD). In a study with CD-1 mice, no tumors were observed at doses up to 1.6 times the human exposure at the recommended dose for GERD. In > 400 patients treated with rabeprazole 10 or 20 mg/day for up to 1 year, the incidence of ECL hyperplasia increased with time and dose. No patient developed the adenomatoid, dysplastic, or neoplastic changes of ECL cells in the gastric mucosa, and no patient developed the carcinoid tumors observed in rats.

In a 24-month study with rats treated with 0.1 to 40 times the human exposure of a 50 kg person dosed at 40 mg/day on a body surface basis, dose-related ECL cell hyperplasia and benign and malignant neuroendocrine cell tumors were observed. Other GI tumors, as well as tumors of the liver and thyroid gland, were also observed. Other studies in rats and mice have produced similar findings. In 39 patients treated with **pantoprazole** 40 to 240 mg/day for up to 5 years, a moderate increase in ECL cell density was observed starting after the first year of use. The effect appeared to plateau after 4 years.

►*Elderly:* Bioavailability of **omeprazole** may be increased (see Pharmacokinetics).

The clearance of **lansoprazole** is decreased in the elderly, with an ≈ 50% to 100% increase of elimination half-life (see Pharmacokinetics).

AUC values and C_{max} of **rabeprazole** and **pantoprazole** were increased in elderly subjects compared with healthy controls (see Pharmacokinetics), but no dosage adjustment is recommended.

►*Pregnancy:* Category C (**omeprazole**); Category B (**lansoprazole, rabeprazole, pantoprazole**). In rabbits, doses 17 to 172 times the human dose of omeprazole produced dose-related increases in embryolethality, fetal resorptions, and pregnancy disruptions. In rats, dose-related embryo/fetal toxicity and postnatal developmental toxicity were observed in offspring of parents treated with 35 to 345 times the human dose. In pregnant rats and rabbits, no evidence of impaired fertility or harm to the fetus was observed with lansoprazole, rabeprazole, and pantoprazole. However, there are no adequate and well-controlled studies in pregnant women. Use during pregnancy only if the potential benefit justifies the risk to the fetus.

►*Lactation:* It is not known whether these agents are excreted in breast milk. **Lansoprazole** and **pantoprazole** and their metabolites are excreted in the milk of rats. In rats, **omeprazole** administration during late gestation and lactation at doses of 35 to 345 times the human dose resulted in decreased weight gain in pups. Decreased body weight of rat pups was observed when rabeprazole was administered to rats in late gestation and during lactation at doses 195 times the human dose for body surface area. Because of the potential for serious adverse reactions in nursing infants, and because of the potential for tumorigenicity shown in rat carcinogenicity studies, decide whether to discontinue nursing or to discontinue the drug, taking into account the importance of the drug to the mother.

►*Children:* Safety and efficacy in children have not been established.

Precautions

►*Gastric malignancy:* Symptomatic response to therapy with proton pump inhibitors does not preclude gastric malignancy.

Drug Interactions

Proton pump inhibitors cause a profound and long-lasting inhibition of gastric acid secretion; therefore, it is theoretically possible that **lansoprazole, omeprazole, pantoprazole,** and **rabeprazole** may interfere with the absorption of drugs where gastric pH is an important determinant of bioavailability (eg, ketoconazole, ampicillin, iron salts, digoxin, cyanocobalamin).

►*P450 system:* **Omeprazole** may interact with other drugs also metabolized via the cytochrome P450 system. There are clinical reports of interaction with other drugs metabolized via the cytochrome P450 (CYP450) system (eg, cyclosporine, disulfiram, benzodiazepines). **Lansoprazole** is metabolized through the CYP450 system via CYP3A and CYP2C19 isoenzymes; however, lansoprazole does not have clinically significant interactions with other drugs metabolized by the CYP450 system. **Rabeprazole** is metabolized by the CYP450 drug metabolizing enzyme system. **Pantoprazole** is metabolized through the CYP450 system primarily through the CYPC19 and CYP3A4 isoenzymes; however, clinically relevant interactions of pantoprazole with other drugs with the same metabolic pathways are not expected. In clinical trials, antacids were used concomitantly with these agents.

Proton Pump Inhibitor Drug Interactions			
Precipitant drug	Object drug*		Description
Clarithromycin	Omeprazole	↑	Coadministration of omeprazole and clarithromycin may result in increases in plasma levels of omeprazole, clarithromycin, and 14-hydroxy-clarithromycin.
Omeprazole	Clarithromycin		
Sucralfate	Lansoprazole Omeprazole	↓	Coadministration delayed absorption and reduced proton pump inhibitor bioavailability by ≈ 17%. Therefore, take these agents ≥ 30 minutes prior to sucralfate.
Omeprazole	Benzodiazepines Diazepam Flurazepam Triazolam	↑	Omeprazole produced a 130% increase in the half-life of diazepam, probably caused by inhibition of oxidative metabolism. Plasma levels were also increased and total clearance of diazepam was decreased.
Omeprazole	Phenytoin	↑	Omeprazole reduced the plasma clearance of phenytoin by 15% and increased its half-life by 27%, probably caused by inhibition of oxidative metabolism.

Proton Pump Inhibitor Drug Interactions			
Precipitant drug	Object drug*		Description
Lansoprazole	Theophylline	↓	A 10% increase in theophylline clearance occurred. Additional titration of theophylline dosage may be required.
Omeprazole	Warfarin	↑	Omeprazole may prolong the elimination of warfarin via inhibition of oxidative metabolism.

* ↑ = Object drug increased. ↓ = Object drug decreased.

➤*Drug/Food interactions:* Both C_{max} and AUC are diminished by ≈ 50% if **lansoprazole** is given 30 minutes after food as opposed to in the fasting condition. There is no significant food effect if given before meals.

Adverse Reactions

Omeprazole is generally well tolerated. In clinical trials of 3096 patients (including duodenal ulcer, Zollinger-Ellison syndrome and resistant ulcer patients), the following adverse experiences occurred in ≥ 1% of patients:

Selected Adverse Reactions (%): Omeprazole vs Ranitidine			
Adverse reaction	Omeprazole (n = 465)	Ranitidine (n = 195)	Placebo (n = 64)
CNS			
Headache	6.9	7.7	6.3
Dizziness	1.5	2.6	0
Asthenia	1.1	1.5	1.6
GI			
Diarrhea	3	2.1	3.1
Abdominal pain	2.4	2.1	3.1
Nausea	2.2	4.1	3.1
Vomiting	1.5	1.5	4.7
Constipation	1.1	0	0
Miscellaneous			
Upper respiratory tract infection	1.9	2.6	1.6
Rash	1.5	0	0
Cough	1.1	1.5	0
Back pain	1.1	0.5	0

In general, **lansoprazole** treatment has been well tolerated in both short-term and long-term trials. The following adverse events were reported in ≥ 1% of patients: Diarrhea (3.6%); abdominal pain (1.8%); nausea (1.4%). Headache occurred at > 1% incidence but was more common with placebo. The incidence of diarrhea is similar between placebo and lansoprazole 15 and 30 mg patients (2.9%, 1.4% and 4.2%, respectively), but higher with lansoprazole 60 mg (7.4%). The most commonly reported adverse event during maintenance therapy was diarrhea. The most frequently reported adverse events for dual- and triple-therapy regimens were diarrhea (8%) and headache (7%). Taste disturbance (5%) also occurred with triple therapy.

In clinical trials with **rabeprazole**, the only adverse event occurring in > 1% of patients and appearing with greater frequency than placebo was headache (2.4% vs placebo 1.6%). The following adverse events occurred in ≥ 1% of patients treated with **pantoprazole** in short-term domestic trials and were considered by the investigators to be possibly, probably, or definitely related to the drug: Headache; diarrhea; flatulence; abdominal pain; rash; eructation; insomnia; hyperglycemia.

The following adverse reactions occurred in < 1% of patients:

➤*Cardiovascular:* Chest pain/angina; palpitation; hypertension; tachycardia.

Omeprazole – Bradycardia; peripheral edema; elevated blood pressure.

Lansoprazole – Cerebrovascular accident; hypotension; MI; shock (circulatory failure); vasodilation.

Rabeprazole – MI; abnormal electrocardiogram; migraine; syncope; bundle branch block; sinus bradycardia; bradycardia, pulmonary embolus, supraventricular tachycardia, thrombophlebitis, vasodilation, QTc prolongation, ventricular tachycardia (rare).

Pantoprazole – Arrhythmia; cardiovascular disorder; chest pain substernal; CHF; abnormal electrocardiogram; hemorrhage; hypotension; myocardial ischemia; retinal vascular disorder; syncope; tachycardia; thrombophlebitis; thrombosis; vasodilation.

➤*CNS:* Anxiety; apathy; confusion; depression; hallucinations; aggravated hostility; nervousness; paresthesia.

Omeprazole – Vertigo; insomnia; tremors; somnolence; dream abnormalities; hemifacial dysesthesia; aggression.

Lansoprazole – Agitation; amnesia; dizziness/syncope; hemiplegia; decreased libido; abnormal thinking.

Rabeprazole – Insomnia; dizziness; somnolence; hypertonia; neuralgia; vertigo; convulsion; abnormal dreams; decreased libido; neuropathy; tremor; agitation, amnesia, confusion, extrapyramidal syndrome, hyperkinesia (rare).

Pantoprazole – Abnormal dreams; convulsion; dry mouth; dysarthria; emotional lability; hyperkinesia; hypesthesia; decreased libido; neuralgia; neuritis; decreased reflexes; sleep disorder; somnolence; abnormal thinking; tremor; vertigo.

➤*Dermatologic:* Rash; urticaria; pruritus; alopecia.

Omeprazole – Severe, generalized skin reactions, including toxic epidermal necrolysis (rare, some fatal); Stevens-Johnson syndrome; erythema multiforme (some severe); skin inflammation; angioedema; dry skin; hyperhidrosis; purpura; petechiae.

Lansoprazole – Acne.

Rabeprazole – Bullous and other drug eruptions of the skin; sweating; dry skin, herpes zoster, psoriasis, skin discoloration (rare).

Pantoprazole – Acne; contact dermatitis; dry skin; eczema; fungal dermatitis; hemorrhage; herpes simplex; herpes zoster; lichenoid dermatitis; maculopapular rash; pain; skin disorder; skin ulcer; sweating; severe dermatologic reactions, including erythema multiforme, Stevens-Johnson syndrome, and toxic epidermal necrolysis (some fatal).

➤*GI:* Anorexia; fecal discoloration; dry mouth; flatulence; gastric fundic gland polyps.

Omeprazole – Pancreatitis (some fatal); irritable colon; esophageal candidiasis; mucosal atrophy of the tongue.

Gastroduodenal carcinoids have been reported in patients with Zollinger-Ellison syndrome on long-term treatment with **omeprazole**. This finding is believed to be a manifestation of the underlying condition, which is known to be associated with such tumors.

During treatment with omeprazole, gastric fundic gland polyps have been noted rarely. These polyps are benign and appear to be reversible when treatment is discontinued.

Lansoprazole – Melena; bezoar; cardiospasm; cholecystitis; cholelithiasis; cholelithiasis; constipation; thirst; dyspepsia; dysphagia; eructation; esophageal stenosis; esophageal ulcer; esophagitis; gastroenteritis; GI hemorrhage; hematemesis; increased appetite; increased salivation; rectal hemorrhage; stomatitis; tenesmus; ulcerative colitis; vomiting.

Rabeprazole – Diarrhea; nausea; abdominal pain; vomiting; dyspepsia; constipation; eructation; gastroenteritis; rectal hemorrhage; melena; cholelithiasis; mouth ulceration; stomatitis; dysphagia; gingivitis; cholecystitis; increased appetite; abnormal stools; colitis; esophagitis; glossitis; pancreatitis; proctitis; bloody diarrhea, cholangitis, duodenitis, GI hemorrhage, salivary gland enlargment, thirst (rare).

Pantoprazole – Aphthous stomatitis; cardiospasm; colitis; cholecystitis; cholelithiasis; duodenitis; dysphagia; enteritis; esophageal hemorrhage; esophagitis; GI carcinoma; GI hemorrhage; GI moniliasis; gingivitis; glossitis; halitosis; hematemesis; increased appetite; melena; mouth ulceration; oral moniliasis; pancreatitis; periodontal abscess; periodontitis; rectal hemorrhage; stomach ulcer; stomatitis; abnormal stools; tongue discoloration; ulcerative colitis.

➤*GU:* Hematuria; glycosuria; gynecomastia.

Omeprazole – Acute interstitial nephritis (some with positive rechallenge); urinary tract infection; microscopic pyuria; urinary frequency; proteinuria; testicular pain; elevated serum creatinine; hematuria; glycosuria.

Lansoprazole – Abnormal menses; albuminuria; breast tenderness; impotence; kidney calculus; urinary retention; breast enlargement/gynecomastia.

Rabeprazole – Cystitis; urinary frequency; dysmenorrhea; dysuria; kidney calculus; metrorrhagia; polyuria; breast enlargement, impotence, leukorrhea, menorrhagia, orchitis, urinary incontinence (rare).

Pantoprazole – Albuminuria; balanitis; breast pain; cystitis; dysmenorrhea; dysuria; epididymitis; impotence; kidney calculus; kidney pain; nocturia; prostatic disorder; pylenoephritis; scrotal edema; urethral pain; urethritis; urinary tract disorder; impaired urination; vaginitis.

➤*Hematologic:* Anemia; hemolysis.

Omeprazole – Pancytopenia (rare); agranulocytosis (some fatal); thrombocytopenia; neutropenia; anemia; leukocytosis; hemolytic anemia.

Lansoprazole – Agranulocytosis; aplastic anemia; hemolytic anemia; leukopenia; neutropenia; pancytopenia; thrombocytopenia; thrombotic thrombocytopenic purpura.

Rabeprazole – Ecchymosis; leukopenia; lymphadenopathy; hypochromic anemia; pancytopenia; thrombocytopenia.

Pantoprazole – Ecchymosis; eosinophilia; hypochromic anemia; iron deficiency anemia; leukocytosis; leukopenia; thrombocytopenia.

➤*Hepatic:* Elevated AST, ALT, alkaline phosphatase, and bilirubin.

Lansoprazole – Increased γ-glutamyl transpeptidase.

Omeprazole – Elevated γ-glutamyl transpeptidase; overt liver disease, including hepatocellular, cholestatic, or mixed hepatitis; liver necrosis (some fatal); hepatic failure (some fatal); hepatic encephalopathy.

Pantoprazole – Biliary pain; bilirubinemia; cholestatic jaundice; hepatitis; increased γ-glutamyl transpeptidase.

Rabeprazole – Jaundice; hepatic encephalopathy, hepatitis, hepatoma, liver fatty deposit (rare).

➤*Lab test abnormalities:*

Lansoprazole – Abnormal liver function tests; increased globulins; increased glucocorticoids; increased LDH; increased gastrin levels; abnormal AG ratio; increased/decreased/abnormal WBC and platelets; abnormal RBC; eosinophilia; hyperlipemia; increased/decreased electrolytes; increased/decreased cholesterol; increased AST; increased ALT; increased creatinine; increased alkaline phosphatase; bilirubinemia.

Rabeprazole – Abnormal platelets; albuminuria; increased creatine phosphokinase; abnormal erythrocytes; hypercholesterolemia; hyperglycemia; hyperlipemia; hypokalemia; hyponatremia; leukorrhea; abnormal liver function tests; prostatic specific antigen increase; increased ALT; urine abnormality; abnormal WBC.

Pantoprazole – Increased creatinine; hypercholesterolemia; hyperuricemia.

➤*Metabolic:* Gout; weight gain; hypoglycemia.

Omeprazole – Hyponatremia.

Lansoprazole – Diabetes mellitus; edema; goiter; hyperglycemia; weight loss.

Rabeprazole – Peripheral edema; edema; dehydration; weight loss.

Pantoprazole – Diabetes mellitus; goiter; dehydration; edema; gout; peripheral edema; thirst; weight loss.

➤*Musculoskeletal:* Arthralgia; myalgia.

Omeprazole – Muscle cramps; muscle weakness; leg pain; joint pain.

Lansoprazole – Arthritis; musculoskeletal pain.

Rabeprazole – Arthritis; leg cramps; bone pain; arthrosis; bursitis; twitching (rare).

Pantoprazole – Arthritis; arthrosis; bone disorder; bone pain; bursitis; joint disorder; leg cramps; neck rigidity; tenosynovitis.

➤*Respiratory:* Epistaxis.

Omeprazole – Pharyngeal pain.

Lansoprazole – Asthma; bronchitis; increased cough; dyspnea; hemoptysis; hiccough; pneumonia; upper respiratory tract infection/inflammation.

Rabeprazole – Dyspnea; asthma; laryngitis; hiccough; hyperventilation; apnea, hypoventilation (rare).

Pantoprazole – Asthma; hiccough; laryngitis; lung disorder; pneumonia; voice alteration.

➤*Special senses:* Taste perversion; tinnitus.

Lansoprazole – Deafness; eye pain; visual field defect; otitis media; blurred vision; speech disorder.

Rabeprazole – Cataract; amblyopia; glaucoma; dry eyes; abnormal vision; otitis media; corneal opacity, blurry vision, diplopia, deafness, eye pain, retinal degeneration, strabismus (rare).

Pantoprazole – Abnormal vision; amblyopia; cataract specified; deafness; diplopia; ear pain; extraocular palsy; glaucoma; otitis externa.

➤*Miscellaneous:* Fever; malaise.

Omeprazole – Pain; fatigue; abdominal swelling; allergic reactions, including, rarely, anaphylaxis.

Lansoprazole – Asthenia; candidiasis; chest pain (not otherwise specified); flu syndrome; halitosis; infection (not otherwise specified); anaphylactoid-like reaction.

Rabeprazole – Asthenia; allergic reaction; chills; chest pain substernal; neck rigidity; photosensitivity reaction; hyperthyroidism; hypothyroidism; abdomen enlarged, face edema, hangover effect (rare); sudden death; coma and hyperammonemia; rhabdomyolysis; disorientation and delirium; interstitial pneumonia; TSH elevations; agranulocytosis; hemolytic anemia.

Pantoprazole – Abscess; allergic reaction; chills; cyst; face edema; generalized edema; heat stroke; hernia; abnormal laboratory test; moniliasis; neoplasm; nonspecified drug reaction; anaphylaxis; angioedema (Quincke's edema); anterior ischemic optic neuropathy.

Combination therapy with clarithromycin – Adverse experiences observed in controlled clinical trials using combination therapy with **omeprazole** and clarithromycin that differed from those previously described for omeprazole alone were the following: Taste perversion (15%); tongue discoloration, rhinitis (2%); pharyngitis, flu syndrome (1%).

Overdosage

➤*Symptoms:* Overdosage with **omeprazole** has been reported rarely. Doses ranged from 320 to 900 mg (16 to 45 times the usual recommended dose). Symptoms were transient and included confusion, drowsiness, blurred vision, tachycardia, nausea, diaphoresis, flushing, headache, and dry mouth. No serious clinical outcome has been reported. No specific antidote for omeprazole overdosage is known.

In 1 overdose case, a patient consumed 600 mg of **lansoprazole** with no adverse reaction.

There has been no experience with large overdoses of **rabeprazole**. The maximum reported overdose was 80 mg. There were no signs or symptoms associated with any overdose. Patients with Zollinger-Ellison syndrome have been treated with up to 120 mg daily.

Two reports of overdose with 400 and 600 mg of **pantoprazole** have been reported with no adverse effects observed. There has been 1 report of suicide involving an overdose of 560 mg pantoprazole; however, the death was more reasonably attributed to other drugs ingested.

➤*Treatment:* **Omeprazole**, **lansoprazole**, **pantoprazole**, and **rabeprazole** are extensively protein bound and are not readily dialyzable. Treatment should be symptomatic and supportive. Refer to General Management of Acute Overdosage.

Patient Information

Take before eating. Take **pantoprazole** with or without food.

Swallow capsules or tablets whole; do not open, chew, split, or crush.

For patients who have problems swallowing capsules, **lansoprazole** can be opened and the intact granules within can be sprinkled on 1 tablespoon of either applesauce, *Ensure* pudding, cottage cheese, yogurt, or strained pears, and swallowed immediately. Do not chew or crush the granules.

Lansoprazole capsules may be emptied into a small volume of either orange juice or tomato juice (60 mL; ≈ 2 oz), mixed briefly and swallowed immediately. To ensure complete delivery of the dose, rinse the glass with ≥ 2 volumes of juice and swallow the contents immediately. The granules have also been shown in vitro to remain intact when exposed to apple, cranberry, grape, orange, pineapple, prune, tomato, and *V-8* vegetable juice and stored for up to 30 minutes.

Antacids may be used while taking these drugs.

OMEPRAZOLE

otc	**Prilosec OTC**[1] (AstraZeneca)	**Tablets, delayed-release:** 20 mg	Lactose, mannitol. (742 PRILOSEC 20). Amethyst. In 1000s, unit-of-use 30s, and UD 100s.
Rx	**Omeprazole** (Various, eg, Kremers-Urban, Mylan)	**Capsules, delayed-release:** 10 mg	In 30s and 100s.
Rx	**Prilosec** (AstraZeneca)		Lactose, mannitol. (606 PRILOSEC 10). Apricot and amethyst. In 1000s and unit-of-use 30s.
Rx	**Omeprazole** (Various, eg, Allscripts, H.J. Harkins, Kremers-Urban, Lek, Mylan)	**Capsules, delayed-release:** 20 mg	In 30s and 100s.
Rx	**Prilosec** (AstraZeneca)	**Capsules, delayed-release:** 40 mg	Lactose, mannitol. (743 PRILOSEC 40). Apricot and amethyst. In 100s, 1000s, and unit-of-use 30s.
Rx	**Zegerid** (Santarus)	**Powder for oral suspension:** 20 mg	Sucrose, sucralose, sodium bicarbonate (460 mg sodium/dose), xanthan gum. In 30 unit-dose packets.

[1] As omeprazole magnesium.

For complete prescribing information, refer to the Proton Pump Inhibitors group monograph.

Indications

➤*Duodenal ulcer:* For short-term treatment of active duodenal ulcer.

➤*Duodenal ulcer associated with H. pylori (except Zegerid):* In combination with clarithromycin to eradicate *H. pylori*. In patients with a 1-year history of duodenal ulcers or active duodenal ulcers, use in combination with clarithromycin and amoxicillin to eradicate *H. pylori*.

➤*Gastric ulcer (except Zegerid):* For short-term treatment (4 to 8 weeks) of active benign gastric ulcer.

➤*Erosive esophagitis:* For short-term treatment (4 to 8 weeks) of erosive esophagitis diagnosed by endoscopy; to maintain healing of erosive esophagitis.

➤*Gastroesophageal reflux disease (GERD):* For the treatment of heartburn and other symptoms associated with GERD.

➤*Hypersecretory conditions (except Zegerid):* For long-term treatment of hypersecretory conditions (eg, Zollinger-Ellison syndrome, multiple endocrine adenomas, systemic mastocytosis).

OMEPRAZOLE

▶*Unlabeled uses:* Posterior laryngitis (omeprazole 40 mg at bedtime, 6 to 24 weeks); enhanced efficacy of pancreatin (for treatment of steatorrhea in cystic fibrosis patients).

Administration and Dosage

Take before eating. Do not open, crush, or chew the capsule; swallow whole. In clinical trials, antacids were used concomitantly with omeprazole.

▶*Duodenal ulcer:*

Treatment – 20 mg daily for 4 to 8 weeks; most patients heal within 4 weeks, although some may require an additional 4 weeks of therapy.

Associated with H. pylori –

Triple therapy (omeprazole/clarithromycin/amoxicillin): Omeprazole 20 mg plus clarithromycin 500 mg plus amoxicillin 1000 mg each given twice daily for 10 days. If an ulcer is present at the initiation of therapy, continue omeprazole 20 mg for an additional 18 days.

Dual therapy (omeprazole/clarithromycin): Omeprazole 40 mg once daily plus clarithromycin 500 mg 3 times daily for 14 days. If an ulcer is present at the initiation of therapy, continue omeprazole 20 mg for an additional 14 days.

For additional prescribing information for clarithromycin or amoxicillin, refer to the Clarithromycin monograph or the Amoxicillin monograph.

▶*Gastric ulcer, treatment:* 40 mg once a day for 4 to 8 weeks.

▶*Erosive esophagitis:*

Treatment – 20 mg daily for 4 to 8 weeks (see Indications).

Maintenance – 20 mg daily.

▶*GERD:*

GERD without esophageal lesions – 20 mg daily for 4 weeks.

GERD with erosive esophagitis – 20 mg daily for 4 to 8 weeks.

The efficacy of omeprazole used for > 8 weeks has not been established. In the rare patient not responding to 8 weeks of treatment, an additional 4 weeks of treatment may help. If there is recurrence of erosive esophagitis or GERD, an additional 4- to 8-week course of omeprazole may be considered.

▶*Preparation and administration of oral suspension:* Take on an empty stomach 1 hour before a meal. The powder for oral suspension is supplied as unit dose packets containing an immediate-release formulation of 20 mg omeprazole.

Directions for use – Empty packet contents into a small cup containing 2 tablespoons of water. Do not use other liquids or foods. Stir well and drink immediately. Refill cup with water and drink.

▶*Pathological hypersecretory conditions:* Individualize dosage. Initial adult dose is 60 mg/day. Doses up to 120 mg 3 times daily have been administered. Administer daily dosages > 80 mg in divided doses. Some patients with Zollinger-Ellison syndrome have been treated continuously for > 5 years.

▶*Storage/Stability:* Store tablets at 20° to 25°C (68° to 77°F). Store capsules at 15° to 30°C (59° to 86°F) in a tight container protected from light and moisture. Store powder for oral suspension packets at 25°C (69° to 77°F); excursions permitted to 15° to 30°C (59° to 86°F).

ESOMEPRAZOLE MAGNESIUM

Rx	Nexium (AstraZeneca)	Capsules, delayed-release: 20 mg	Sugar spheres, talc. (NEXIUM 20 mg). Amethyst. In 90s, 1000s, unit-of-use 30s, and UD 100s.
		40 mg	Sugar spheres, talc. (NEXIUM 40 mg). Amethyst. In 90s, 1000s, unit-of-use 30s, and UD 100s.

For complete prescribing information, refer to the Proton Pump Inhibitors group monograph. Refer to the Penicillins and Macrolides group monographs for complete prescribing information for amoxicillin and clarithromycin.

Indications

▶*Erosive esophagitis:* For the short-term treatment (4 to 8 weeks) in the healing and symptomatic resolution of diagnostically confirmed erosive esophagitis; to maintain symptom resolution and healing of erosive esophagitis.

▶*Gastroesophageal reflux disease (GERD):* For the treatment of heartburn and other symptoms associated with GERD.

▶*Helicobacter pylori eradication to reduce the risk of duodenal ulcer recurrence:*

Triple therapy – In combination with amoxicillin and clarithromycin for the treatment of *H. pylori* infection and duodenal ulcer disease (active or history of within the past 5 years) to eradicate *H. pylori*. Eradication of *H. pylori* has been shown to reduce the risk of duodenal ulcer recurrence.

Perform susceptibility testing in patients who fail therapy. If resistance to clarithromycin is demonstrated or susceptibility testing is not possible, institute alternative antimicrobial therapy.

Administration and Dosage

▶*Approved by the FDA:* February 20, 2001.

Swallow whole and take at least 1 hour before eating.

Esomeprazole Recommended Adult Dosage Schedule		
Indication	Dose (mg)	Frequency
GERD		
Healing of erosive esophagitis	20 or 40	Once daily for 4 to 8 weeks[a]
Maintenance of healing of erosive esophagitis	20	Once daily[b]
Symptomatic GERD	20	Once daily for 4 weeks[c]

Esomeprazole Recommended Adult Dosage Schedule		
Indication	Dose (mg)	Frequency
H. pylori eradication to reduce the risk of duodenal ulcer recurrence (triple therapy)		
Esomeprazole	40	Once daily for 10 days
Amoxicillin	1000	Twice daily for 10 days
Clarithromycin	500	Twice daily for 10 days

[a] The majority of patients are healed within 4 to 8 weeks. For patients who do not heal after 4 to 8 weeks, consider an additional 4 to 8 weeks of treatment.
[b] Controlled studies did not extend beyond 6 months.
[c] If symptoms do not resolve completely after 4 weeks, consider an additional 4 weeks of treatment.

▶*Difficulty swallowing:* For patients who have difficulty swallowing capsules, add 1 tablespoon of applesauce to an empty bowl, open the esomeprazole capsule, and carefully empty the pellets onto the applesauce. Mix the pellets with the applesauce and swallow immediately. Do not heat or chew the applesauce. Do not chew or crush the pellets. Do not store the pellet/applesauce mixture for future use.

▶*Administration per nasogastric tube:* For patients who have a nasogastric tube in place, open the esomeprazole capsules and empty the intact granules into a 60 mL syringe. Mix with 50 mL of water. Replace the plunger and shake the syringe vigorously for 15 seconds. Hold the syringe with the tip up and check for granules remaining in the tip. Attach the syringe to a nasogastric tube, and deliver the contents of the syringe through the nasogastric tube into the stomach. After administering the granules, flush the nasogastric tube with additional water. Do no administer the pellets if they have dissolved or disintegrated.

The suspension must be used immediately after preparation.

▶*Hepatic function impairment:* For patients with severe liver impairment (Child Pugh class C), do not exceed a dose of 20 mg.

▶*Storage/Stability:* Store at 25°C (77°F); excursions permitted to 15° to 30°C (59° to 86°F). Keep tightly closed.

LANSOPRAZOLE

Rx	Prevacid (TAP Pharm)	Tablets, orally disintegrating, delayed-release[1]: 15 mg	Mannitol, lactose, aspartame, 2.5 mg phenylalanine. White to yellowish-white with orange to dark brown speckles. Strawberry flavor. In UD 30s.
		30 mg	Mannitol, lactose, aspartame, 5.1 mg phenylalanine. White to yellowish-white with orange to dark brown speckles. Strawberry flavor. In UD 30s.
		Capsules, delayed-release[1]: 15 mg	(PREVACID 15). Sugar spheres, sucrose. Pink/Green. In 1000s, unit-of-use 30s, and UD 30s.
		30 mg	(PREVACID 30). Sugar spheres, sucrose. Pink/Black. In 100s, 1000s, and UD 100s.
		Granules for oral suspension, delayed-release[1]: 15 mg	Sugar, mannitol, docusate sodium. Strawberry flavor. In UD 30s.
		30 mg	Sugar, mannitol, docusate sodium. Strawberry flavor. In UD 30s.
Rx	Prevacid IV (TAP Pharm)	Powder for injection, lyophilized: 30 mg/vial	60 mg mannitol, 10 mg meglumine. In single-dose vials with in-line filters.

[1] Contains enteric-coated granules.

LANSOPRAZOLE

For complete prescribing information, refer to the Proton Pump Inhibitors group monograph.

Indications

➤*Duodenal ulcer (oral only):* For short-term treatment (up to 4 weeks) for healing and symptomatic relief of active duodenal ulcer; to maintain healing of duodenal ulcers.

➤*Duodenal ulcer associated with Helicobacter pylori (oral only):* In combination with amoxicillin with or without clarithromycin for the eradication of *H. pylori* infection in patients with active or recurrent duodenal ulcers. Eradication has been shown to reduce the risk of duodenal ulcer recurrence.

Triple therapy – In combination with amoxicillin plus clarithromycin for the treatment of *H. pylori* infection and duodenal ulcer disease (active or 1-year history of a duodenal ulcer) to eradicate *H. pylori*.

Dual therapy – In combination with amoxicillin for treatment in patients with *H. pylori* infection and duodenal ulcer disease (active or 1-year history of duodenal ulcer) who are allergic or intolerant to clarithromycin or in whom resistance to clarithromycin is known or suspected.

➤*Gastric ulcer (oral only):* For short-term treatment (up to 8 weeks) for healing and symptomatic relief of active benign gastric ulcer; treatment of NSAID-associated gastric ulcer in patients who continue NSAID use; for reducing the risk of NSAID-associated gastric ulcer in patients with a history of a documented gastric ulcer who require the use of an NSAID.

➤*Gastroesophageal reflux disease (GERD) (oral only):* For short-term treatment of heartburn and other symptoms associated with GERD.

➤*Erosive esophagitis:* For short-term treatment (up to 8 weeks) for healing and symptomatic relief of all grades of erosive esophagitis; to maintain healing of erosive esophagitis.

IV formulation – When patients are unable to take the oral formulations, the IV formulation is indicated as an alternative for the short-term treatment (up to 7 days) of all grades of erosive esophagitis. The safety and efficacy of the IV formulation as an initial treatment of erosive esophagitis have not been demonstrated.

➤*Pathological hypersecretory conditions, including Zollinger-Ellison syndrome (oral only):* For long-term treatment of pathological hypersecretory conditions, including Zollinger-Ellison syndrome.

Administration and Dosage

➤*Approved by the FDA:* May 10, 1995.

Take before meals.

Do not be crush or chew lansoprazole products.

➤*Duodenal ulcer:*

Treatment – 15 mg once daily for 4 weeks.

Maintenance – 15 mg once daily to maintain healing of duodenal ulcers.

Associated with H. pylori –

Triple therapy: 30 mg lansoprazole plus 500 mg clarithromycin and 1 g amoxicillin twice daily (every 12 hours) for 10 or 14 days.

Dual therapy: 30 mg lansoprazole plus 1 g amoxicillin 3 times/day (every 8 hours) for 14 days for patients intolerant or resistant to clarithromycin.

➤*Gastric ulcer:*

Treatment – 30 mg once daily for up to 8 weeks.

Associated with NSAIDs –

Healing: 30 mg once daily for up to 8 weeks. Controlled studies did not extend beyond indicated duration.

Risk reduction: 15 mg once daily for up to 12 weeks. Controlled studies did not extend beyond indicated duration.

➤*GERD:*

Adults – 15 mg once daily for up to 8 weeks.

Children 1 to 11 years of age (short-term treatment) –

30 kg or less: 15 mg/day for up to 12 weeks. The lansoprazole dose was increased (up to 30 mg twice daily) in some pediatric patients after 2 or more weeks of treatment if they remained symptomatic. For pediatric patients unable to swallow an intact capsule, see Difficulty swallowing.

Over 30 kg: 30 mg/day for up to 12 weeks. The lansoprazole dose was increased (up to 30 mg twice daily) in some pediatric patients after 2 or more weeks of treatment if they remained symptomatic. For pediatric patients unable to swallow an intact capsule, see Difficulty swallowing.

➤*Erosive esophagitis:*

Adults –

Treatment: 30 mg once daily for up to 8 weeks. For patients who do not heal within 8 weeks (5% to 10%), it may be helpful to give an additional 8 weeks of treatment. If there is a recurrence of erosive esophagitis, consider an additional 8-week course.

Maintenance: 15 mg once daily to maintain healing of erosive esophagitis.

IV formulation: In patients unable to take oral therapy, 30 mg/day administered by IV infusion over 30 minutes for up to 7 days. Once the patient is able to take medications orally, therapy can be switched to an oral lansoprazole formulation for a total of 6 to 8 weeks.

Children 1 to 11 years of age (short-term treatment) –

30 kg or less: 15 mg/day for up to 12 weeks. The lansoprazole dose was increased (up to 30 mg twice daily) in some pediatric patients after 2 or more weeks of treatment if they remained symptomatic. For pediatric patients unable to swallow an intact capsule, see Difficulty swallowing.

Over 30 kg: 30 mg/day for up to 12 weeks. The lansoprazole dose was increased (up to 30 mg twice daily) in some pediatric patients after 2 or more weeks of treatment if they remained symptomatic. For pediatric patients unable to swallow an intact capsule, see Difficulty swallowing.

➤*Hypersecretory conditions, including Zollinger-Ellison syndrome:* Individualize dosage. Recommended starting dose is 60 mg once daily. Dosages up to 90 mg twice daily have been administered. Administer daily dosages of greater than 120 mg in divided doses. Some patients with Zollinger-Ellison syndrome have been treated with lansoprazole for longer than 4 years.

➤*Hepatic function impairment:* Consider dosage adjustment in patients with severe liver disease.

➤*Nasogastric (NG) tube (capsules):* For patients who have an NG tube in place, lansoprazole can be opened and the intact granules mixed in 40 mL of apple juice. Do not use other liquids. Inject through the NG tube into the stomach. After administering the granules, flush the NG tube with additional apple juice to clear the tube.

➤*Difficulty swallowing:*

Capsules – For patients who have difficulty swallowing capsules, lansoprazole can be opened and the intact granules contained within can be sprinkled on 1 tablespoon of applesauce, *Ensure* pudding, cottage cheese, yogurt, or strained pears and swallowed immediately. Alternatively, the delayed-release capsules may be emptied into a small volume of apple, orange, or tomato juice (60 mL; approximately 2 oz), mixed briefly, and swallowed immediately. To ensure complete delivery of the dose, rinse the glass with 2 or more volumes of juice and swallow the contents immediately. Use in other foods and liquids has not been studied clinically and, therefore, is not recommended.

Oral suspension – Empty packet contents into 2 tablespoons of water. Do not use other liquids or foods. Stir well and drink immediately. If any material remains after drinking, add more water, stir, and drink immediately. Do not give through enteral administration tubes.

Orally disintegrating tablets – Place the tablet on the tongue. Allow it to disintegrate with or without water until the particles can be swallowed. The tablet typically disintegrates in less than 1 minute. *SoluTabs* are not designed to be swallowed intact or chewed.

IV formulation – Dilute with 5 mL sterile water for injection. Administer using in-line filter provided. The filter must be used to remove precipitate that may form when the reconstituted drug product is mixed with IV solutions.

• Inject 5 mL of sterile water for injection into a 30 mg vial of lansoprazole. The resulting solution will contain 6 mg/mL lansoprazole.

• Mix gently until the powder is dissolved.

• Dilute the reconstituted solution in either 50 mL of 0.9% sodium chloride injection, lactated Ringer's injection, or 5% dextrose in water.

Administration: An in-line filter must be used. Administer over 30 minutes. A dedicated line is not required; however, the IV line should be flushed before and after administration with 0.9% sodium chloride injection, lactated Ringer's injection, or 5% dextrose injection. Do not administer with other drugs or diluents as this may cause incompatibilities.

➤*Storage/Stability:*

Oral – Store at 25°C (77°F); excursions permitted to 15° to 30°C (59° to 86°F).

IV – Store powder for injection at 25°C (77°F); excursions permitted to 15° to 30°C (59° to 86°F). Protect from light. The reconstituted solution can be held for 1 hour when stored at 25°C (77°F) prior to further dilution. Store the admixture at 25°C (77°F). Administer within the designated time period listed in the table below. No refrigeration is required.

IV Lansoprazole Stability		
Diluent	pH	Administer within (hours)
0.9% sodium chloride injection	≈ 10.2	24
Lactated Ringer's injection	≈ 10	24
5% dextrose injection	≈ 9.5	12

RABEPRAZOLE SODIUM

Rx	**Aciphex** (Eisai)	**Tablets, delayed-release:** 20 mg	Mannitol. (ACIPHEX 20). Lt. yellow. Enteric-coated. In 30s, 90s, and UD 100s.

For complete prescribing information, refer to the Proton Pump Inhibitors group monograph.

Indications

➤*Duodenal ulcers:* Short-term (up to 4 weeks) treatment in the healing and symptomatic relief of duodenal ulcers. Most patients heal within 4 weeks.

➤*Erosive/Ulcerative gastroesophageal reflux disease (GERD):* For short-term (4 to 8 weeks) treatment in the healing and symptomatic relief of erosive or ulcerative GERD. For those patients who have not healed after 8 weeks of treatment, consider an additional 8-week course.

➤*Maintenance of healing of erosive or ulcerative GERD:* For maintaining healing and reduction in relapse rates of heartburn symptoms in patients with erosive or ulcerative GERD.

➤*GERD:* For treatment of daytime and nighttime heartburn and other symptoms associated with GERD.

➤*Hypersecretory conditions:* For the long-term treatment of pathological hypersecretory conditions, including Zollinger-Ellison syndrome.

➤*Helicobacter pylori eradication to reduce risk of duodenal ulcer recurrence:* Rabeprazole in combination with amoxicillin and clarithromycin as a 3-drug regimen is indicated for treatment of *H. pylori* infection and duodenal ulcer disease (active or history within the past 5 years) to eradicate *H. pylori*. Eradication of *H. pylori* has been shown to reduce the risk of duodenal ulcer recurrence.

Administration and Dosage

➤*Approved by the FDA:* August 19, 1999.

Swallow tablets whole. Do not chew, crush, or split.

➤*Duodenal ulcers:* 20 mg once daily after the morning meal for a period of up to 4 weeks. Most patients with duodenal ulcers heal within 4 weeks. A few patients may require additional therapy to achieve healing.

➤*Erosive or ulcerative GERD:*

Treatment – 20 mg once daily for 4 to 8 weeks. For those patients who have not healed after 8 weeks of treatment, consider an additional 8-week course.

Maintenance – 20 mg once daily.

➤*GERD:* 20 mg once daily for 4 weeks. If symptoms do not resolve completely after 4 weeks, an additional course of treatment may be considered.

➤*Hypersecretory conditions, including Zollinger-Ellison syndrome:* The dosage of rabeprazole in patients with pathological hypersecretory conditions varies with the individual patient. The recommended adult oral starting dose is 60 mg once daily. Adjust doses to individual patient needs and continue for as long as clinically indicated. Some patients may require divided doses. Doses up to 100 mg/day and 60 mg twice daily have been administered. Some patients with Zollinger-Ellison syndrome have been treated continuously with rabeprazole for up to 1 year.

➤*H. pylori eradication to reduce risk of duodenal ulcer recurrence:* The 3-drug regimen is as follows: Rabeprazole 20 mg twice daily for 7 days, amoxicillin 1000 mg twice daily for 7 days, and clarithromycin 500 mg twice daily for 7 days. All 3 medications should be taken twice daily with the morning and evening meals. It is important that patients comply with the full 7-day regimen.

Perform susceptibility testing in patients who fail therapy. If resistance to clarithromycin is demonstrated or susceptibility testing is not possible, institute alternative antimicrobial therapy.

➤*Hepatic impairment:* Administration of rabeprazole to patients with mild to moderate liver impairment resulted in increased exposure and decreased elimination. Because of the lack of clinical data on rabeprazole in patients with severe hepatic impairment, use caution in these patients.

➤*Storage/Stability:* Store at 25°C (77°F); excursions permitted to 15° to 30°C (59° to 86°F). Protect from moisture.

PANTOPRAZOLE SODIUM

Rx	**Protonix** (Wyeth-Ayerst)	**Tablets, delayed-release:** 20 mg	Mannitol. (P20). Yellow, oval. In 90s.
		40 mg	Mannitol. (PROTONIX). Yellow, oval. In 90s, 100s, 1000s, and *Redipak* blister strips of 10 (10s).
Rx	**Protonix I.V.** (Wyeth-Ayerst)	**Powder for injection, freeze-dried:** 40 mg/vial	EDTA. In vials.

For complete prescribing information, refer to the Proton Pump Inhibitors group monograph.

Indications

➤*Oral:*

Treatment of erosive esophagitis associated with gastroesophageal reflux disease (GERD) – Short-term treatment (up to 8 weeks) in the healing and symptomatic relief of erosive esophagitis associated with GERD. For those patients who have not healed after 8 weeks of treatment, an additional 8-week course of pantoprazole may be considered.

Maintenance of healing of erosive esophagitis – Maintenance of healing of erosive esophagitis and reduction in relapse rates of day- and nighttime heartburn symptoms in patients with GERD. Controlled studies did not extend beyond 12 months.

Pathological hypersecretory conditions including Zollinger-Ellison syndrome – For long-term treatment of pathological hypersecretory conditions including Zollinger-Ellison syndrome.

➤*IV:*

GERD associated with a history of erosive esophagitis – Short-term treatment (7 to 10 days) of GERD with a history of erosive esophagitis, as an alternative to oral therapy in patients who are unable to continue taking oral pantoprazole. Safety and efficacy of IV pantoprazole as initial treatment for GERD with a history of erosive esophagitis have not been demonstrated.

Pathological hypersecretion associated with Zollinger-Ellison syndrome – Treatment of pathological hypersecretory conditions associated with Zollinger-Ellison syndrome or other neoplastic conditions.

Administration and Dosage

➤*Approved by the FDA:* February 2, 2000.

➤*Oral:* Swallow tablets whole, with or without food in the stomach. Concomitant administration of antacids does not affect the absorption of pantoprazole. Do not split, chew, or crush tablets. If patients are unable to swallow a 40 mg tablet, two 20 mg tablets may be taken.

Erosive esophagitis associated with GERD – 40 mg once daily for up to 8 weeks. For patients who have not healed after 8 weeks of treatment, an additional 8-week course of pantoprazole may be considered.

Maintenance of healing of erosive esophagitis – 40 mg daily.

Pathological hypersecretory conditions including Zollinger-Ellison syndrome – The dosage in patients with pathological hypersecretory conditions varies with the individual patient. The recommended adult starting dose is 40 mg twice daily. Adjust dosage regimens to individual patient needs and continue for as long as clinically indicated. Doses up to 240 mg/day have been administered. Some patients have been treated continuously for more than 2 years.

➤*IV:* Administer through a dedicated line or through a Y site. Flush the IV line before and after administration of IV pantoprazole with 5% Dextrose Injection, 0.9% Sodium Chloride Injection, or Lactated Ringer's Injection. Do not simultaneously administer IV pantoprazole through the same line with other IV solutions.

Discontinue treatment with IV pantoprazole as soon as the patient is able to resume treatment with pantoprazole delayed-release tablets.

Parenteral routes of administration other than IV are not recommended.

Treatment of GERD associated with a history of erosive esophagitis – As an alternative to continued oral therapy, 40 mg pantoprazole once daily by infusion for 7 to 10 days. Safety and efficacy of IV pantoprazole as a treatment for GERD in patients with a history of erosive esophagitis for more than 10 days have not been demonstrated.

Reconstitution:
• *15-minute infusion* – Reconstitute IV pantoprazole with 10 mL of 0.9% Sodium Chloride Injection, and further dilute (admix) with 100 mL of 5% Dextrose Injection, 0.9% Sodium Chloride Injection, or Lactated Ringer's Injection to a final concentration of approximately 0.4 mg/mL.
• *2-minute infusion* – Reconstitute IV pantoprazole with 10 mL of 0.9% sodium chloride injection to a final concentration of approximately 4 mg/mL.

Administration:
• *15-minute infusion* – Administer IV pantoprazole admixtures over a period of approximately 15 minutes at a rate of approximately 7 mL/min.
• *2-minute infusion* – The total volume from vial should be administered over at least 2 minutes.

Pathological hypersecretion associated with Zollinger-Ellison syndrome – The dosage of IV pantoprazole in patients with pathological hypersecretory conditions associated with Zollinger-Ellison syndrome or other neoplastic conditions varies with individual patients. The recommended adult dosage is 80 mg every 12 hours. The frequency

PANTOPRAZOLE SODIUM

of dosing can be adjusted to individual patient needs based on acid output measurements. In those patients who need a higher dosage, 80 mg every 8 hours is expected to maintain acid output below 10 mEq/h. Daily doses higher than 240 mg or administered for more than 6 days have not been studied. Perform transition from oral to IV and from IV to oral formulations of gastric acid inhibitors in such a manner to ensure continuity of effect of suppression of acid secretion. Patients with Zollinger-Ellison syndrome may be vulnerable to serious clinical complications of increased acid production even after a short period of loss of effective inhibition.

Reconstitution:

• *15-minute infusion* – Reconstitute each vial with 10 mL of 0.9% Sodium Chloride Injection. The contents of the 2 vials should be combined and further diluted (admixed) with 80 mL of 5% Dextrose Injection, 0.9% Sodium Chloride Injection, or Lactated Ringer's Injection to a total volume of 100 mL with a final concentration of approximately 0.8 mg/mL.

• *2-minute infusion* – Reconstitute with 10 mL of 0.9% sodium chloride injection per vial to a final concentration of approximately 4 mg/mL.

Administration:

• *15-minute infusion* – Administer IV over a period of approximately 15 minutes at a rate of approximately 7 mL/min.

• *2-minute infusion* – The total volume from both vials should be administered IV over a period of at least 2 minutes.

►*Storage / Stability:*

Oral – Store delayed-release tablets at 20° to 25°C (68° to 77°F). Excursions permitted to 15° to 30°C (59° to 86°F).

IV – Store IV pantoprazole at 2° to 8°C (36° to 46°F). Protect from light. Do not freeze reconstituted product.

The reconstituted solution may be stored for up to 2 hours at room temperature prior to further dilution; the admixed solution may be stored for up to 22 hours at room temperature prior to IV infusion. Neither the reconstituted solution nor the admixed solution need to be protected from light.

Incompatibilities – Midazolam has been shown to be incompatible with Y-site administration of pantoprazole injection and pantoprazole may not be compatible with products containing zinc. Immediately stop use if precipitation or discoloration occurs.

SUCRALFATE

Rx	**Sucralfate** (Various, eg, Eon Labs, Major, Martec, Teva)	**Tablets:** 1 g	In 100s and 500s.
Rx	**Carafate** (Axcan Scandipharm)		(Carafate 1712). Light pink, oblong, scored. In 100s, 120s, and 500s.
Rx	**Sucralfate** (Precision Dose)	**Suspension:** 1 g/10 mL	Methylparaben, sorbitol. In 10 mL unit dose cups.
Rx	**Carafate** (Axcan Scandipharm)		Sorbitol, methylparaben. In 415 mL.

Indications

➤*Duodenal ulcer:* Short-term treatment (up to 8 weeks) of active duodenal ulcer.

➤*Maintenance therapy (tablets only):* Duodenal ulcer patients at reduced dosage after healing of acute ulcers.

➤*Unlabeled uses:* Sucralfate has been used in the following conditions: Accelerating healing of gastric ulcers; long-term treatment of gastric ulcers; treatment of reflux and peptic esophagitis; treatment of NSAID- and aspirin-induced GI symptoms and mucosal damage; prevention of stress ulcers and GI bleeding in critically ill patients. Because increased gastric pH may be implicated in causing nosocomial infections in critically ill patients, sucralfate may offer an advantage over antacids and histamine H_2 antagonists in stress ulcer prophylaxis.

Sucralfate in suspension has also been used in treatment of oral and esophageal ulcers caused by radiation, chemotherapy, and sclerotherapy.

Administration and Dosage

➤*Active duodenal ulcer:*

Adults – 1 g 4 times daily on an empty stomach (at least 1 hour before meals and at bedtime).

Take antacids as needed for pain relief, but not within ½ hour before or after sucralfate.

While healing with sucralfate may occur within the first 2 weeks, continue treatment for 4 to 8 weeks unless healing is demonstrated by x-ray or endoscopic examination.

➤*Maintenance therapy (tablets only):*

Adults – 1 g twice daily.

➤*Storage/Stability:*

Suspension – Store at controlled room temperature, 20° to 25°C (68° to 77°F).

Actions

➤*Pharmacology:* The exact mechanism(s) of action of sucralfate in peptic ulcer disease is unclear, but the therapeutic effects result from local (ie, at the ulcer site) rather than systemic activity.

Sucralfate does not appreciably affect gastric acid output or concentration. Following an oral dose, sucralfate rapidly reacts with hydrochloric acid in the stomach to form a highly condensed, viscous, adhesive, paste-like substance with the capacity to buffer acid and binds to the surface of gastric and duodenal ulcers.

A major portion of a dose of sucralfate binds electrostatically to positively charged protein molecules in the damaged mucosa of the GI tract to form insoluble, stable complexes. Only a small amount actually dissipates in the GI contents. The insoluble complexes form an adherent, protective barrier at the ulcer site.

The barrier formed at the ulcer site protects the ulcer from the potential ulcerogenic properties of pepsin, acid, and bile, thus allowing the ulcer to heal.

➤*Pharmacokinetics:*

Absorption – Sucralfate is minimally absorbed from the GI tract following an oral dose. Poor absorption may result from the high polarity and low solubility of the drug in the GI tract. The duration of action depends on the time that the drug is in contact with this site because sucralfate exerts its effects directly at the site of the ulcer. The drug's viscous adhesiveness, slow reaction with acid, and high affinity for damaged mucosa contribute to its prolonged action. Following oral administration, binding to the ulcer site has been shown for up to 6 hours, and 30% of the dose is retained within the GI tract for at least 3 hours.

Distribution – Distribution into human tissues and fluids following systemic absorption has not been identified. Approximately 95% of the dose remains in the GI tract, with only minute amounts being distributed into liver, kidneys, skeletal muscle, adipose tissue, and skin.

Excretion – Following reaction of sucralfate with hydrochloric acid, nonmetabolized sucrose sulfate is formed in the GI tract.

Warnings

➤*Chronic renal failure/dialysis:* During sucralfate administration, small amounts of aluminum are absorbed from the GI tract. Concomitant use with other aluminum-containing products (eg, antacids) may increase the total body burden of aluminum. Patients with normal renal function receiving these agents concomitantly adequately excrete aluminum in the urine. However, patients with chronic renal failure or receiving dialysis have impaired excretion of absorbed aluminum, and sucralfate does not cross dialysis membranes. Aluminum accumulation

and toxicity (eg, aluminum osteodystrophy, osteomalacia, encephalopathy) have occurred. Use with caution in these patients.

➤*Pregnancy: Category B.* There are no adequate and well-controlled studies in pregnant women. Use this drug during pregnancy only if clearly needed.

➤*Lactation:* It is not known whether this drug is excreted in breast milk. Exercise caution when sucralfate is administered to a nursing mother.

➤*Children:* Safety and efficacy in children have not been established.

Precautions

➤*Ulcer recurrence:* Duodenal ulcer is a chronic recurrent disease. While short-term treatment can completely heal the ulcer, do not expect a successful course to alter posthealing frequency or severity of duodenal ulceration.

Drug Interactions

Sucralfate Drug Interactions			
Precipitant drug	Object drug*		Description
Sucralfate	Antacids, aluminum-containing	↑	The total body burden of aluminum may be increased with sucralfate coadministration. See Warnings.
Sucralfate	Anticoagulants	↓	A decrease in the hypoprothrombinemic effect of warfarin may occur.
Sucralfate	Diclofenac	↓	The pharmacologic effects of diclofenac may be decreased.
Sucralfate	Digoxin	↓	Serum digoxin levels may be reduced, decreasing the therapeutic effects.
Sucralfate	Histamine H_2 antagonists Cimetidine Ranitidine	↓	Bioavailability of the histamine H_2 antagonists may be decreased. Administering the histamine H_2 antagonist ≥ 2 hours before sucralfate may eliminate the interaction.
Sucralfate	Hydantoins	↓	Phenytoin absorption may be decreased.
Sucralfate	Ketoconazole	↓	Ketoconazole bioavailability may be decreased.
Sucralfate	Levothyroxine	↓	The effects of levothyroxine may be decreased.
Sucralfate	Penicillamine	↓	Penicillamine's effectiveness may be lessened or negated.
Sucralfate	Quinidine	↓	Serum quinidine levels may be reduced, decreasing the therapeutic effects.
Sucralfate	Quinolones	↓	Bioavailability of the quinolones may be decreased. Administering the quinolone ≥ 2 hours before sucralfate may eliminate the interaction.
Sucralfate	Tetracycline	↓	Tetracycline bioavailability may be decreased.
Sucralfate	Theophylline	↓	Theophylline bioavailability may be decreased.

* ↑ = Object drug increased. ↓ = Object drug decreased.

Adverse Reactions

Adverse reactions in clinical trials were minor and rarely led to drug discontinuation.

Constipation was the most frequent complaint (2%). Other adverse effects include: Diarrhea, nausea, vomiting, gastric discomfort, indigestion, flatulence, dry mouth, rash, pruritus, back pain, headache, dizziness, insomnia, sleepiness, vertigo (less than 0.5%). There have been postmarketing reports of hypersensitivity reactions (including urticaria, angioedema, respiratory difficulty, rhinitis, laryngospasm, and facial swelling).

Overdosage

Risks associated with overdosage appear minimal.

Patient Information

Take on an empty stomach at least 1 hour before meals and at bedtime.

Do not take antacids ½ hour before or after taking sucralfate.

MISOPROSTOL

Rx	**Misoprostol** (Various, eg, Greenstone)	**Tablets:** 100 mcg	(G 5007). White. In unit-of-use 60s and 120s.
Rx	**Cytotec** (Pfizer)		(SEARLE 1451). White. In UD 100s and unit-of-use 60s and 120s.
Rx	**Misoprostol** (Various, eg, Greenstone)	**Tablets:** 200 mcg	(G 5008). White, hexagonal. In unit-of-use 60s and 100s.
Rx	**Cytotec** (Pfizer)		(SEARLE 1461). White, hexagonal. In UD 100s and unit-of-use 60s and 100s.

WARNING

Misoprostol administration in pregnant women can cause abortion, premature birth, or birth defects. Uterine rupture has been reported when misoprostol was administered in pregnant women to induce labor or to induce abortion beyond the eighth week of pregnancy (see Precautions). Pregnant women should not take misoprostol to reduce the risk of ulcers induced by nonsteroidal anti-inflammatory drugs (NSAIDs) (see Contraindications, Warnings, and Precautions).

Advise patients of the abortifacient property and warn them not to give the drug to others.

Do not use misoprostol for reducing the risk of NSAID-induced ulcers in women of childbearing potential unless the patient is at high risk of developing complications from gastric ulcers associated with use of the NSAIDs or at high risk of developing gastric ulceration. In such patients, misoprostol may be prescribed if the patient:

- has had a negative serum pregnancy test within 2 weeks prior to beginning therapy;
- is capable of complying with effective contraceptive measures;
- has received oral and written warnings of the hazards of misoprostol, the risk of possible contraception failure, and the danger to other women of childbearing potential should the drug be taken by mistake; and
- will begin misoprostol only on the second or third day of the next normal menstrual period.

Indications

➤*Gastric ulcer:* To reduce the risk of NSAID (including aspirin)-induced gastric ulcers in patients at high risk of complications from a gastric ulcer (eg, the elderly and patients with concomitant debilitating disease), as well as patients at high risk of developing gastric ulceration (eg, patients with a history of ulcer). Misoprostol should be taken for the duration of NSAID therapy. It had no effect, compared with placebo, on GI pain or discomfort associated with NSAIDs.

➤*Unlabeled uses:*

Cervical ripening and labor induction – Vaginal misoprostol has been proven safe and effective for cervical ripening and labor induction. However, vaginal misoprostol is associated with a higher frequency of excessive uterine contractility and intervention (see Warnings).

Pregnancy termination – Misoprostol has been used in combination with mifepristone for pregnancy termination. Patients taking mifepristone must take 400 mcg misoprostol orally 2 days after taking mifepristone unless a complete abortion has already been confirmed before that time.

Postpartum hemorrhage – Vaginal administration of misoprostol for the treatment of serious postpartum hemorrhage in the presence of uterine atony (see Warnings).

Chronic, idiopathic constipation – Short-term trials have shown an acceleration of intestinal transit in healthy individuals and in those with chronic constipation. Improvement in stool frequency in patients with chronic constipation has been seen with treatment doses of 200 mcg 2 to 4 times/day.

Administration and Dosage

➤*Approved by the FDA:* 1988.

➤*Adults:* 200 mcg 4 times/day with food. If this dose cannot be tolerated, 100 mcg can be used. Take misoprostol for the duration of NSAID therapy as prescribed. Take with meals, and take the last dose of the day at bedtime.

➤*Renal impairment/Elderly:* Dosage adjustment is not routinely needed, but dosage can be reduced if the 200 mcg dose is not tolerated.

➤*Storage/Stability:* Store at or below 25°C (77°F) in a dry area.

Actions

➤*Pharmacology:* Misoprostol, a synthetic prostaglandin E_1 analog, has antisecretory (inhibiting gastric acid secretion) and mucosal (in animals) protective properties. NSAIDs inhibit prostaglandin synthesis; a deficiency of prostaglandins within the gastric mucosa may lead to diminishing bicarbonate and mucus secretion and may contribute to the mucosal damage caused by these agents. Misoprostol can increase bicarbonate and mucus production.

Prostaglandin receptor binding is saturable, reversible, and stereospecific. The sites have a high affinity for misoprostol, for its acid metabolite, and for other E type prostaglandins, but not for F or I prostaglandins and unrelated compounds, such as histamine or cimeti-

dine. It is likely that these specific receptors allow misoprostol taken with food to be effective topically, despite the lower serum concentrations attained.

Misoprostol produces a moderate decrease in pepsin concentration during basal conditions but not during histamine stimulation. It has no significant effect on fasting or postprandial gastrin nor on intrinsic factor output.

Effects on gastric acid secretion – Misoprostol over the range of 50 to 200 mcg inhibits basal and nocturnal gastric acid secretion, and acid secretion in response to a variety of stimuli, including meals, histamine, pentagastrin, and coffee. Activity is apparent 30 minutes after oral administration and persists for at least 3 hours. Only the 200 mcg dose had substantial effects on nocturnal secretion or on histamine and meal-stimulated secretion.

Uterine effects – Misoprostol produces uterine contractions that may endanger pregnancy (see Warning Box).

➤*Pharmacokinetics:*

Absorption/Distribution – Misoprostol is extensively absorbed and undergoes rapid de-esterification to its free acid, which is responsible for its clinical activity and, unlike the parent compound, is detectable in plasma. In healthy volunteers, misoprostol is rapidly absorbed after oral administration with a time to reach peak concentration of misoprostol acid of approximately 12 minutes.

Mean plasma levels after single doses show a linear relationship with doses over the range of 200 to 400 mcg. No accumulation was noted in multiple-dose studies; plasma steady state was achieved within 2 days.

The serum protein binding of misoprostol acid is less than 90% and is concentration-independent in the therapeutic range.

Metabolism/Excretion – Misoprostol does not affect the hepatic mixed function oxidase (cytochrome P-450) enzyme system in animals. Misoprostol has a terminal half-life of 20 to 40 minutes. After oral administration of radiolabeled misoprostol, about 80% of detected radioactivity appears in urine.

Special populations –

Renal function impairment: Patients with varying degrees of renal impairment showed an approximate doubling of half-life, C_{max}, and AUC compared with healthy individuals, but there was no clear correlation between the degree of impairment and AUC.

Elderly: In subjects over 64 years of age, the AUC for misoprostol acid is increased.

Contraindications

History of allergy to prostaglandins; pregnant women to reduce the risk of ulcers induced by NSAIDs.

Warnings

➤*Cardiovascular:* Use caution when administering misoprostol to patients with pre-existing cardiovascular disease.

➤*Duodenal ulcers:* Misoprostol does not reduce the risk of duodenal ulcers in patients on NSAIDs.

➤*Renal function impairment:* Pharmacokinetic studies in patients with varying degrees of renal impairment showed an approximate doubling of half-life, maximum concentration, and AUC, but no clear correlation between degree of impairment and AUC was shown. No routine dosage adjustment is recommended, but dosage may need to be reduced if the usual dose is not tolerated.

➤*Fertility impairment:* Misoprostol, when administered to breeding male and female rats at doses 6.25 to 625 times the maximum recommended human therapeutic dose, produced dose-related pre- and postimplantation losses and a significant decrease in the number of live pups born at the highest dose. These findings suggest the possibility of a general adverse effect on fertility in males and females.

➤*Elderly:* In subjects over 64 years of age, the AUC for misoprostol acid is increased; however, no routine dosage adjustment is recommended. Reduce the dose if the usual dose is not tolerated.

➤*Pregnancy: Category X.* Misoprostol may endanger pregnancy (may cause abortion) and thereby cause harm to the fetus when administered to a pregnant woman. Misoprostol may produce uterine contractions, uterine bleeding, and expulsion of the products of conception. Abortions caused by misoprostol may be incomplete. If a woman is or becomes pregnant while taking this drug to reduce the risk of NSAID-induced ulcers, discontinue the drug and apprise the patient of potential hazards to the fetus.

Congenital anomalies sometimes associated with fetal death have been reported subsequent to the unsuccessful use of misoprostol as an abortifacient, but the drug's teratogenic mechanism has not been demonstrated. Several reports in the literature associate the use of

MISOPROSTOL

misoprostol during the first trimester of pregnancy with skull defects, cranial nerve palsies, facial malformations, and limb defects.

Labor and delivery – Misoprostol can induce or augment uterine contractions. Vaginal administration of misoprostol, outside of its approved indication, has been used as a cervical ripening agent, for the induction of labor, and for treatment of serious postpartum hemorrhage in the presence of uterine atony. A major adverse effect of the obstetrical use of misoprostol is hyperstimulation of the uterus, which may progress to uterine tetany with marked impairment of uteroplacental blood flow, uterine rupture (requiring surgical repair, hysterectomy, and/or salpingo-oophorectomy), or amniotic fluid embolism. Pelvic pain, retained placenta, severe genital bleeding, shock, fetal bradycardia, and fetal and maternal death have been reported.

There may be an increased risk of uterine tachysystole, uterine rupture, meconium passage, meconium staining of amniotic fluid, and Cesarean delivery due to uterine hyperstimulation with the use of higher doses of misoprostol, including the manufactured 100 mcg tablet. The risk of uterine rupture increases with advancing gestational ages and with prior uterine surgery, including Cesarean delivery. Grand multiparity also appears to be a risk factor for uterine rupture.

When misoprostol is used for cervical ripening or induction of labor, the effect of misoprostol on the later growth, development, and functional maturation of the child have not been established. Information on misoprostol's effect on the need for forceps delivery or other intervention is unknown.

➤*Lactation:* It is unlikely that misoprostol is excreted in breast milk because it is rapidly metabolized. However, it is not known if the active metabolite (misoprostol acid) is excreted in breast milk. Therefore, do not administer to nursing mothers because the potential excretion of misoprostol acid could cause significant diarrhea in nursing infants.

➤*Children:* Safety and efficacy in children have not been established.

Precautions

➤*Women of childbearing potential:* Advise women of childbearing potential that they must not be pregnant when misoprostol therapy is initiated and that they must use an effective contraception method while taking misoprostol (see Warning Box).

➤*Diarrhea:* Diarrhea is dose-related and usually develops early in the course of therapy (after 13 days), usually is self-limiting (often resolving after 8 days), but sometimes requires discontinuation of misoprostol. Rare instances of profound diarrhea, leading to severe dehydration, have been reported. If misoprostol is prescribed, carefully monitor patients with an underlying condition such as inflammatory bowel disease, or those in whom dehydration, were it to occur, would be dangerous. The incidence of diarrhea can be minimized by administering after meals and at bedtime and by avoiding coadministration of misoprostol with magnesium-containing antacids.

Drug Interactions

➤*Antacids:* Antacids reduce the total availability of misoprostol acid, but this does not appear clinically important.

➤*Drug/Food interactions:* Maximum plasma concentrations of misoprostol acid are diminished when taken with food.

Adverse Reactions

Misoprostol Adverse Reactions (%)[1]	
Adverse reaction	Incidence
GI	
Diarrhea	13 to 40
Abdominal pain	7 to 20
Nausea[2]	3.2
Flatulence[2]	2.9
Headache[2]	2.4
Dyspepsia[2]	2
Vomiting[2]	1.3
Constipation[2]	1.1
GU	
Spotting	0.7
Cramps	0.6
Hypermenorrhea	0.5
Menstrual disorder	0.3
Dysmenorrhea	0.1

[1] Data are pooled from different trials and are not necessarily comparable.
[2] No significant difference in incidence compared with placebo.

➤*Infrequent adverse reactions:* The following adverse events were infrequently reported. Causal relationships have not been established but cannot be excluded.

Cardiovascular – Chest pain; edema; diaphoresis; hypotension; hypertension; arrhythmia; phlebitis; increased cardiac; enzymes; syncope; MI (some fatal); thromboembolic events (eg, pulmonary embolism, arterial thrombosis, cardiovascular accident).

CNS – Anxiety; change in appetite; depression; drowsiness; dizziness; thirst; impotence; loss of libido; sweating increase; neuropathy; neurosis; confusion.

Dermatologic – Rash; dermatitis; alopecia; pallor; breast pain.

GI – GI bleeding; GI inflammation/infection; rectal disorder; abnormal hepatobiliary function; gingivitis; reflux; dysphagia; amylase increase.

GU – Polyuria; dysuria; hematuria; UTI.

Hematologic – Anemia; abnormal differential; thrombocytopenia; purpura; ESR increased.

Metabolic/Nutritional – Glycosuria; gout; increased nitrogen; increased alkaline phosphatase.

Musculoskeletal – Arthralgia; myalgia; muscle cramps; stiffness; back pain.

Respiratory – Upper respiratory tract infection; bronchitis; bronchospasm; dyspnea; pneumonia; epistaxis.

Special senses – Abnormal taste; abnormal vision; conjunctivitis; deafness; tinnitus; earache.

Miscellaneous – Aches/pains; anaphylaxis; asthenia; fatigue; fever; rigors; weight changes.

Overdosage

➤*Symptoms:* The toxic dose in humans has not been determined. Cumulative total daily doses of 1600 mcg have been tolerated with only symptoms of GI discomfort. In animals, the acute toxic effects are the following: diarrhea; GI lesions; focal cardiac, hepatic, and renal tubular necrosis; testicular atrophy; respiratory difficulties; CNS depression. Clinical signs that may indicate an overdose are sedation, tremor, convulsions, dyspnea, abdominal pain, diarrhea, fever, palpitations, hypotension, or bradycardia.

➤*Treatment:* Treat with supportive therapy; refer to Management of Acute Overdosage.

It is not known if misoprostol acid is dialyzable. However, because misoprostol is metabolized like a fatty acid, it is unlikely that dialysis would be appropriate treatment for overdosage.

Patient Information

Advise patients to read the patient information leaflet.

Advise patients not to take misoprostol to reduce the risk of NSAID-induced ulcers if pregnant (see Warning Box). Misoprostol can cause abortion (sometimes incomplete, which could lead to dangerous bleeding and require hospitalization or surgery), premature birth, or birth defects. Advise patients it is important to avoid pregnancy by using an effective contraception method while taking this medication and for at least 1 month or through 1 menstrual cycle after the medication is stopped. Misoprostol has been reported to cause the uterus to rupture (tear) when given after the eighth week of pregnancy. Rupture (tearing) of the uterus can result in severe bleeding, hysterectomy, or maternal or fetal death.

If patient becomes pregnant during misoprostol therapy, advise patient to stop taking misoprostol and contact health care provider immediately. Remind patients that even if they are on a means of birth control, it is still possible to become pregnant.

Advise patient that misoprostol may cause diarrhea, abdominal cramping, or nausea in some people. In most cases, these problems develop during the first few weeks of therapy and stop after about a week. The patient can minimize possible diarrhea by taking misoprostol with food.

Because side effects usually are mild to moderate and usually go away in a matter of days, most patients can continue to take misoprostol. Advise patients to call their doctor if they experience prolonged difficulty (more than 8 days), severe diarrhea, cramping, or nausea.

Advise patients to take misoprostol only according to the directions given by the health care provider.

Advise patients not to give misoprostol to anyone else.

Indications

Hyperacidity: Symptomatic relief of upset stomach associated with hyperacidity (heartburn, gastroesophageal reflux, acid indigestion, and sour stomach); hyperacidity associated with peptic ulcer and gastric hyperacidity.

Aluminum carbonate: Treatment, control, or management of hyperphosphatemia or for use with a low phosphate diet to prevent formation of phosphate urinary stones.

Calcium carbonate: Treating calcium deficiency states (ie, post-menopausal/senile osteoporosis). See Calcium monograph in Minerals and Electrolytes, Oral section.

Magnesium oxide: Treatment of magnesium deficiencies or magnesium depletion from malnutrition, restricted diet, alcoholism, or magnesium-depleting drugs.

Unlabeled uses: Antacids with aluminum and magnesium hydroxides or aluminum hydroxide alone effectively prevent significant stress ulcer bleeding. Antacids are also effective in treatment and maintenance of duodenal ulcer and may be effective in treating gastric ulcer. Antacids are also recommended, initially, for gastroesophageal reflux disease.

Aluminum hydroxide has been used to reduce phosphate absorption in hyperphosphatemia in patients with chronic renal failure.

Calcium carbonate may also be used to bind phosphate.

Administration and Dosage

Administration and dosage depends on the condition being treated and the agent being used. See individual products for specific information.

Liquid doseforms are usually preferred because of their rapid action and greater activity; however, tablets may be more acceptable and convenient, particularly when patients are away from home or where the liquid would be inconvenient to carry. Other doseforms are available but do not appear to offer any significant advantage.

Actions

Pharmacology: Antacids neutralize gastric acidity, resulting in an increase in the pH of the stomach and duodenal bulb. Additionally, by increasing the gastric pH above 4, they inhibit the proteolytic activity of pepsin. Antacids do not "coat" the mucosal lining, but may have a local astringent effect. Antacids also increase the lower esophageal sphincter tone. Aluminum ions inhibit smooth muscle contraction, thus inhibiting gastric emptying. Use aluminum-containing products with caution in patients with gastric outlet obstruction.

A systemic antacid (eg, sodium bicarbonate) is readily absorbed and capable of producing systemic electrolyte disturbances and alkalosis. A nonsystemic antacid forms compounds that are not absorbed to a significant extent and thus does not exert an appreciable systemic effect unless use is chronic, high-dose, or the patient has confounding pathology. However, nonsystemic antacids may alter urinary pH in some patients.

Acid neutralizing capacity (ANC) – ANC is a consideration in selecting an antacid. It varies for commercial antacid preparations and is expressed as mEq/mL. Milliequivalents of ANC is defined by the mEq of HCl required to keep an antacid suspension at pH 3.5 for 10 minutes in vitro. An antacid must neutralize ≥ 5 mEq/dose. Also, any ingredient must contribute ≥ 25% of the total ANC of a given product to be considered an antacid. Antacids with high ANC are usually more effective in vivo. Sodium bicarbonate and calcium carbonate have the greatest neutralizing capacity but are not suitable for chronic therapy because of systemic effects. Suspensions have greater neutralizing capacity than powders or tablets. For maximum effectiveness, chew tablets thoroughly. If ingested in the fasting state, antacids reduce acidity for approximately 20 to 40 minutes because of rapid gastric emptying. If ingested 1 hour after meals, they reduce gastric acidity for at least 3 hours.

Alginic acid – Alginic acid, an ingredient found with sodium bicarbonate in some antacid products, is not an antacid; however, in the presence of saliva, it reacts with sodium bicarbonate to form sodium alginate. Its protective effect is due to its foaming, viscous, and floating properties.

Phosphate binding – Aluminum-containing antacids bind with phosphate ions in the intestine to form insoluble aluminum phosphate, which is excreted in the feces. This is of value in treating hyperphosphatemia of chronic renal failure. Calcium carbonate can also suppress phosphate concentrations. The aluminum salt with useful phosphate binding capacity is aluminum hydroxide.

Warnings

Sodium content: Sodium content of antacids may be significant. Patients with hypertension, CHF, marked renal failure, or those on restricted or low-sodium diets should use a low-sodium preparation. The sodium content of most commercial antacid preparations is found in the product listings.

"Acid rebound": Antacids may cause dose-related rebound hyperacidity because they may increase gastric secretion or serum gastrin levels. Early data implicated calcium carbonate as the only agent that caused "acid rebound;" however, it is now clear that most antacids may

result in this effect. In addition, the effect may not be clinically significant because the "acid rebound" may be compensated for by buffers in the antacid.

Milk-alkali syndrome: Milk-alkali syndrome, an acute illness with symptoms of headache, nausea, irritability, and weakness, or a chronic illness with alkalosis, hypercalcemia, and possibly, renal impairment, has occurred following the concurrent use of high-dose calcium carbonate and sodium bicarbonate.

Hypophosphatemia: Prolonged use of aluminum-containing antacids may result in hypophosphatemia in normophosphatemic patients if phosphate intake is not adequate. In its more severe forms, hypophosphatemia can lead to anorexia, malaise, muscle weakness, and osteomalacia.

Renal function impairment: Use magnesium-containing products with caution, particularly when > 50 mEq magnesium is given daily. Hypermagnesemia and toxicity may occur because of decreased clearance of the magnesium ion. Approximately 5% to 20% of orally administered magnesium salts can be systemically absorbed.

Prolonged use of aluminum-containing antacids in patients with renal failure may result in or worsen dialysis osteomalacia. Elevated tissue aluminum levels contribute to the development of the dialysis encephalopathy and osteomalacia syndromes. Small amounts of aluminum are absorbed from the GI tract and renal excretion of aluminum is impaired in renal failure. Aluminum is not well removed by dialysis because it is bound to albumin and transferrin, which do not cross dialysis membranes. As a result, aluminum is deposited in bone, and dialysis osteomalacia may develop when large amounts of aluminum are ingested orally by patients with impaired renal function.

Pregnancy: A pregnant woman should consult a physician before using an antacid.

Precautions

GI hemorrhage: Use aluminum hydroxide with care in patients who have recently suffered massive upper GI hemorrhage.

Lipid effects: In 1 study, administration of an aluminum hydroxide-containing antacid reduced LDL cholesterol by 18.5% after 4 months in hypercholesterolemic patients. Although HDL was also reduced (to a lesser extent), the HDL/LDL ratio increased by 13%. Similar results were noted in a smaller pilot study. In another study, calcium carbonate reduced LDL by 4.4% and increased HDL by 4.1%. Further studies are needed to determine the role of antacids in hypercholesterolemia.

Buffered aspirin solutions: Caution against use of these antacid/analgesic combinations in chronic pain syndromes. Alkalinization of urine accelerates aspirin excretion, and systemic alkalosis and increased sodium load may occur.

Drug Interactions

	Antacid Drug Interactions				
	Antacid[1]				
Drug	Aluminum salts	Calcium salts	Magnesium salts	Sodium bicarbonate	Magnesium-aluminum combinations
Allopurinol	↓				
Amphetamines				↑	
Benzodiazepines	↑		↓	↓	↓
Captopril					↓
Chloroquine	↓		↓		
Corticosteroids	↓		↓		
Dicumarol			↑		
Diflunisal	↓				
Digoxin	↓		↓		
Ethambutol	↓				
Flecainide				↑	
Fluoroquinolones		↓			↓
Histamine H₂ antagonists	↓		↓		↓
Hydantoins		↓	↓		↓
Iron salts	↓	↓	↓	↓	↓
Isoniazid	↓				
Ketoconazole				↓	↓
Levodopa					↑
Lithium				↓	
Methenamine				↓	
Methotrexate				↓	
Nitrofurantoin			↓		
Penicillamine	↓		↓		↓
Phenothiazines	↓		↓		↓
Quinidine		↑	↑	↑	↑

Antacid Drug Interactions					
	Antacid[1]				
Drug	Aluminum salts	Calcium salts	Magnesium salts	Sodium bicarbonate	Magnesium-aluminum combinations
Salicylates		↓		↓	↓
Sodium poly-styrene sulfonate					‡[2]
Sulfonylureas			↑	↓	↑
Sympatho-mimetics				↑	
Tetracyclines	↓	↓	↓	↓	↓
Thyroid hor-mones	↓				
Ticlopidine	↓		↓		↓
Valproic acid					↑

[1] Pharmacologic effect increased (↑) or decreased (↓) by antacids.
[2] Concomitant use may cause metabolic alkalosis in patients with renal impairment.

Antacids may interfere with drugs by:

1.) Increasing the gastric pH altering disintegration, dissolution, solubility, ionization and gastric emptying time. Absorption of weakly acidic drugs is decreased, possibly resulting in decreased drug effect (eg, digoxin, phenytoin, chlorpromazine, isoniazid). Weakly basic drug absorption is increased possibly resulting in toxicity or adverse reactions (eg, pseudoephedrine, levodopa).
2.) Adsorbing or binding drugs to their surface resulting in decreased bioavailability (eg, tetracycline). Magnesium trisilicate and magnesium hydroxide have the greatest ability to adsorb drugs; calcium carbonate and aluminum hydroxide have an intermediate ability to adsorb drugs.
3.) Increasing urinary pH affecting the rate of drug elimination. The effect is inhibition of the excretion of basic drugs (eg, quinidine, amphetamines) and enhanced excretion of acidic drugs (eg, salicylates). Sodium bicarbonate has the most pronounced effect on urinary pH.

Staggering the administration times of the interacting drug and the antacid by ≥ 2 hours will often help avoid undesirable drug interactions. Refer to individual product monographs for information.

Adverse Reactions

Magnesium-containing antacids – Laxative effect as saline cathartic may cause diarrhea; hypermagnesemia in renal failure patients (see Warnings).

Aluminum-containing antacids – Constipation (may lead to intestinal obstruction); aluminum-intoxication, osteomalacia and hypophosphatemia (see Precautions); accumulation of aluminum in serum, bone and the CNS (aluminum accumulation may be neurotoxic); encephalopathy.

Antacids – Dose-dependent rebound hyperacidity and milk-alkali syndrome (see Warnings).

Patient Information

►*Chewable tablets:* Thoroughly chew before swallowing. Follow with a glass of water.

►*Effervescent tablets:* Allow to completely dissolve in water. Allow most of the bubbling to stop before drinking.

►*Drug interaction precaution:* Antacids may interact with certain prescription drugs. If you are presently taking a prescription drug, do not take an antacid without checking with your physician or pharmacist.

Magnesium-containing products may act as a saline cathartic in larger doses and produce a laxative effect and may cause diarrhea; aluminum and calcium-containing products may cause constipation. Magnesium/aluminum antacid mixtures are used to avoid bowel function changes.

Notify physician if relief is not obtained or if there are any symptoms that suggest bleeding, such as black tarry stools or "coffee ground" vomitus.

Taking too much of these products can cause the stomach to secrete excess stomach acid. Consult your physician or pharmacist about the appropriate dose. Do not use the maximum dosage of antacids for > 2 weeks, except under the supervision of a physician.

MAGNESIA (Magnesium Hydroxide)

otc	**Phillips' Chewable** (Sterling Health)	**Tablets, chewable:** 311 mg	Sucrose. (Phillips). Mint flavor. In 100s and 200s.
otc	**Milk of Magnesia** (Various, eg, Geneva, Goldline, Rugby, UDL)	**Liquid:** 400 mg/5 mL	In 360 mL, pt and gal, UD 15 and 30 mL.
otc	**Phillips' Milk of Magnesia** (Sterling Health)		Original, mint and cherry flavors. In 120, 360 and 780 mL.
otc	**Concentrated Phillips' Milk of Magnesia** (Sterling Health)	**Liquid:** 800 mg/5 mL	Sorbitol, sugar. Strawberry flavor. In 240 mL.

For complete prescribing information, refer to the Antacids group monograph.

Administration and Dosage

►*Antacid dose, adults and children > 12 years of age:*
Liquid – 5 to 15 mL up to 4 times daily with water.

Liquid, concentrated – 2.5 to 7.5 mL up to 4 times daily with water.
Tablets – 622 mg to 1244 mg up to 4 times daily.
Laxative dose – See product listing in Laxative monograph.

ALUMINUM HYDROXIDE GEL

				Sodium[1] (mg)	ANC[1] (mEq)
otc	**Amphojel** (Wyeth-Ayerst)	**Tablets:** 600 mg	(Wyeth). Saccharin. In 100s.		
otc	**Alu-Cap** (3M Pharm)	**Capsules:** 400 mg	Red/green. In 100s.		8.5
otc	**Dialume** (RPR)	**Capsules:** 500 mg	In 500s.	≤ 1.2	
otc	**Aluminum Hydroxide Gel** (Various, eg, Goldline, Pharm Assoc, Rugby, UDL)	**Suspension:** 320 mg per 5 mL	In 360 and 480 mL, UD 15 and 30 mL.		
otc	**Concentrated Aluminum Hydroxide Gel** (Roxane)	**Suspension:** 450 mg per 5 mL	Peppermint flavor. In 500 mL and UD 30 mL.	1-2	
		675 mg per 5 mL	Creamsicle flavor. In 180 and 500 mL, UD 20 and 30 mL.		
otc	**Concentrated Aluminum Hydroxide Gel** (Various, eg, Pharm Assoc, Roxane)	**Liquid:** 600 mg per 5 mL	In 30, 180 and 480 mL.		
otc	**AlternaGEL** (J & J-Merck)		In 150 and 360 mL.		

[1] Acid neutralizing capacity and sodium content per capsule, tablet or 5 mL.

For complete prescribing information, refer to the Antacids group monograph.

Administration and Dosage

►*Tablets/Capsules:* 500 to 1500 mg 3 to 6 times daily, between meals and at bedtime.

►*Suspension:* 5 to 30 mL as needed between meals and at bedtime or as directed.

CALCIUM CARBONATE

				Sodium[1] (mg)	ANC[1] (mEq)
otc	**Amitone** (Menley & James)	**Tablets, chewable:** 350 mg	Sucrose. Peppermint flavor. In 100s.	< 2	
otc sf	**Mallamint** (Roberts)	**Tablets, chewable:** 420 mg	Mint flavor. In 1000s, Sani-Pak 1000s and 4 dose boxes.	< 0.1	
otc	**Trial Antacid** (Zee Medical)		Sorbitol. Spearmint flavor. In 24s.		
otc	**Antacid Tablets** (Goldline)	**Tablets, chewable:** 500 mg	Sucrose. Assorted flavors. In 150s.	≤ 2	
otc	**Dicarbosil** (BIRA)		Peppermint flavor. White. In rolls of 12.	< 2	10
otc	**Equilet** (Mission)		In 150s.	< 0.35	
otc	**Tums** (SK-Beecham)		Sucrose. (TUMS). Peppermint, assort. flavors. In 36s, 75s, 150s and 400s.	≤ 2	
otc	**Maalox Antacid/Calcium Supplement** (Novartis)	**Tablets, chewable:** 600 mg	Aspartame, 0.5 mg phenylalanine, dextrose, mannitol. Lemon flavor. In 85s.	1	
otc	**Maalox Quick Dissolve** (Novartis)		Aspartame, 0.5 mg phenylalanine, dextrose, mannitol. (Maalox QD). Lemon, wild berry, and wintergreen flavors. In 30s, 45s, and 85s.		
otc	**Extra Strength Alkets Antacid** (Roberts Pharm)	**Tablets, chewable:** 750 mg	Peppermint. In 96s.		
otc	**Extra Strength Antacid** (Various, eg, Goldline, Major)		In 96s.		
otc	**Extra Strength Tums E-X** (SK-Beecham)		Sucrose. (TUMS). Assorted flavors. In 24s, 48s and 96s.	≤ 2	
otc	**Tums Smooth Dissolve** (GlaxoSmithKline)		Sorbitol, dextrose, sucrose (2 g sugar). In peppermint and assorted fruit flavors. In 45s.		
otc	**Alka-Mints** (Bayer)	**Tablets, chewable:** 850 mg	Sorbitol, sugar. (Alka-Mints). Assorted flavors and spearmint. In 75s.	< 5	
otc	**Maalox Maximum Strength Quick Dissolve** (Novartis)	**Tablets, chewable:** 1000 mg	Aspartame, 0.9 mg phenylalanine, dextrose, mannitol. (MS Maalox QD+). Wild berry and wintergreen flavors. In 35s and 65s.	2	
otc	**Calcium Carbonate** (Various, eg, Medirex, Vangard)	**Tablets:** 500 mg	In 100s, 120s and UD 100s.		
otc	**Calcium Carbonate** (Various, eg, Major, Moore)	**Tablets:** 600 mg	In 60s, 72s, 150s and UD 100s.		
otc	**Calcium Carbonate** (Various, eg, Lilly, Rugby)	**Tablets:** 650 mg	In 100s and 1000s.		
otc	**Calcium Carbonate** (Roxane)	**Tablets:** 1250 mg	In 100s and UD 100s.		
otc	**Chooz** (Schering-P)	**Gum tablets:** 500 mg	Sucrose, glucose. Mint flavor. In 16s.		
otc	**Surpass** (Wrigley)	**Gum:** 300 mg	Aspartame, sorbitol. 3.9 mg phenylalanine. Wintergreen flavor. In 10s.		
otc	**Surpass Extra Strength** (Wrigley)	**Gum:** 450 mg	Aspartame, sorbitol. 3.9 mg phenylalanine. Fruit flavor. In 10s.		
otc	**Calcium Carbonate** (Roxane)	**Suspension:** 1250 mg per 5 mL	Sorbitol. Mint flavor. In 500 mL, UD 5 mL.		

[1] Acid-neutralizing capacity and sodium content per tablet, lozenge or 5 mL.

For complete prescribing information, refer to the Antacids group monograph.

➤*Dosage:* 0.5 to 1.5 g as needed.

▮ Administration and Dosage ▮
Contains 40% calcium; 20 mEq calcium/g.

MAGNESIUM OXIDE

				ANC[1] (mEq)
otc	**Mag-Ox 400** (Blaine)	**Tablets:** 400 mg	In 100s, 1000s and UD 100s.	
otc	**Maox 420** (Manne Co)	**Tablets:** 420 mg	Tartrazine. In 250s and 1000s.	21
otc	**Magnesium Oxide** (Various, eg, Major)	**Tablets:** 500 mg	In 100s.	
otc	**Uro-Mag** (Blaine)	**Capsules:** 140 mg	In 100s and 1000s.	

[1] Acid neutralizing capacity per capsule or tablet.

For complete prescribing information, refer to the Antacids group monograph.

➤*Tablets:* 400 to 800 mg/day.

▮ Administration and Dosage ▮
➤*Capsules:* 140 mg 3 to 4 times daily.

MAGALDRATE (Aluminum Magnesium Hydroxide Sulfate)

otc	**Riopan** (Whitehall)	**Suspension:** 540 mg per 5 mL	Saccharin, sorbitol. Mint flavor. In 360 mL.
otc	**Magaldrate** (Various, eg, Moore)	**Liquid:** 540 mg per 5 mL	In 355 mL.
otc	**Iosopan** (Goldline)		In 355 mL.

For complete prescribing information, refer to the Antacids group monograph.

➤*Dosage:* 5 to 10 mL between meals and at bedtime.

▮ Administration and Dosage ▮
Magaldrate is a chemical entity of aluminum and magnesium hydroxides (not a physical mixture). It contains the equivalent of 29% to 40% magnesium oxide and 18% to 26% aluminum oxide.

SODIUM BICARBONATE

| otc | **Sodium Bicarbonate** (Various, eg, Rugby) | **Tablets:** 325 mg | In 1000s. |
| otc | **Sodium Bicarbonate** (Various, eg, Rugby) | **Tablets:** 650 mg | In 1000s. |

[1] Sodium content per tablet.

For complete prescribing information, refer to the Antacids group monograph.

Administration and Dosage

Contains 27% sodium.

►*Dosage:* 0.3 to 2 g 1 to 4 times daily.

SODIUM CITRATE

				Sodium[1] (mg)
otc	**Citra pH** (ValMed)	**Solution:** 450 mg	Sucrose. Clear. In 30 mL.	105.67

[1] Sodium content per 5 mL.

For complete prescribing information, refer to the Antacids group monograph.

Administration and Dosage

30 mL daily.

ANTACIDS

Antacid Combinations

CAPSULES AND TABLETS
Content given in mg per tablet or gelcap. 23 mg sodium = 1 mEq.

	Product & distributor	Aluminum Hydroxide	Magnesium Hydroxide	Calcium Carbonate	Other Content	Sodium (mg)	How supplied
otc	Rolaids Tablets (Pfizer Consumer)		110	550	Dextrose, sucrose		Chewable. Peppermint, spearmint, and cherry flavors. In 12s, 36s, 150s, 250s, and 300s.
otc	Rolaids Extra Strength Tablets (Pfizer Consumer)		135	675	Dextrose, sucrose		Chewable. Cool strawberry, freshmint, fruit, and tropical punch flavors. In 10s, 30s, and 100s.
otc	Rolaids Multi-Symptom Tablets (Pfizer Consumer)		135	675	60 mg simethicone, dextrose, sucrose		Chewable. Cool mint and berry flavors. In 10s, 30s, and 60s.
otc	Mintox Tablets (Major)	200	200		Saccharin		Chewable. Mint flavor. In 100s.
otc	RuLox #1 Tablets (Rugby)		200				Chewable. Mint flavor. In 100s and 1000s.
otc	RuLox #2 Tablets (Rugby)	400	400		Sorbitol		Chewable. Mint flavor. In 100s and 1000s.
otc sf	Titralac Extra Strength Tablets (3M Pharm.)			750	Saccharin	0.6	Chewable. Spearmint flavor. In 100s.
otc	Mylanta Gelcaps (J&J Merck)			311	232 mg magnesium carbonate, parabens, EDTA		In 24s and 50s.
otc	Mylagen Gelcaps (Goldline)				232 mg magnesium carbonate		In 24s.
otc	Gas-Ban (Roberts Med)			300	40 mg simethicone		In UD 8s and 1000s.
otc sf	Calglycine Antacid (Rugby)			420	150 mg glycine.		In 250s and 1000s.
otc sf	Titralac Tablets (3M Pharm.)				Saccharin	0.3	Chewable. Spearmint flavor. In 40s, 100s and 1000s.
otc	Titralac Plus Tablets (3M Pharm.)				21 mg simethicone, saccharin	1.1	Chewable. (TITRALAC PLUS). Spearmint flavor. In 100s.
otc	Foamicon Tablets (Invamed)	80			Alginic acid, sodium bicarbonate, 20 mg magnesium trisilicate, calcium stearate, sugar, sucrose	18.4	Chewable. White. In 100s.
otc	Gaviscon Tablets (SK-Beecham)				Alginic acid, sodium bicarbonate, 20 mg magnesium trisilicate, sucrose, calcium stearate	18.4	Chewable. (GAVISCON 1175). In 30s and 100s.
otc	Double Strength Gaviscon-2 Tablets (SK-Beecham)	160			Alginic acid, sodium bicarbonate, 40 mg magnesium trisilicate, sucrose	36.8	Chewable. In 48s.
otc	Gaviscon Extra Strength Relief Formula Tablets (SK-Beecham)				105 mg magnesium carbonate, alginic acid, sodium bicarbonate, sucrose, calcium stearate	29.9	Chewable. In 30s and 100s.
otc	Extra Strength Alenic Alka Tablets (Rugby)				105 mg magnesium carbonate	29.9	Chewable. Butterscotch flavor. In 100s.
otc	Extra Strength Genaton Tablets (Goldline)				105 mg magnesium carbonate, alginic acid, sodium bicarbonate, sucrose, calcium stearate	29.9	Chewable. In 100s.

ANTACIDS

Antacid Combinations

CAPSULES AND TABLETS

	Product & distributor	Aluminum Hydroxide	Magnesium Hydroxide	Calcium Carbonate	Other Content	Sodium (mg)	How supplied
otc	Almacone Tablets (Rugby)	200	200		20 mg simethicone		Chewable. Yellow/white. Peppermint flavor. In 100s and 1000s.
otc	Trial AG Tablets (Zee Medical)				25 mg simethicone, sucrose, mannitol		Lemon flavor. In 20s.
otc	Gelusil Tablets (Parke-Davis)				25 mg simethicone, sorbitol, sugar	< 5	Chewable. (P-D GELUSIL 034). Peppermint flavor. In 100s.
otc	Mintox Plus Tablets (Major)				25 mg simethicone, saccharin, sucrose		Chewable. In 100s.
otc	Mylanta Double Strength Tablets (J&J-Merck)	400	400		40 mg simethicone, saccharin, sorbitol		Chewable. (MYLANTA DS). Mint and cherry flavors. In 24s and 60s.
otc	Calcium Rich Rolaids Tablets (Warner-Lambert)		80	412		0.4	Chewable. Original, cherry, spearmint and assorted fruit flavors. In 12s, 36s, 75s and 150s.
otc	Advanced Formula Di-Gel Tablets (Schering-Plough)		128	280	20 mg simethicone, sucrose		Chewable. Mint and lemon-orange flavors. In 30s, 60s. and 90s.
otc	Riopan Plus Tablets (Whitehall)				480 mg magaldrate, 20 mg simethicone, sorbitol, sucrose		Chewable. Cool mint flavor. In 50s and 100s.
otc	Riopan Plus Double Strength Tablets (Whitehall)				1080 mg magaldrate, 20 mg simethicone, saccharin, sorbitol, sucrose		Chewable. Cool mint flavor. In 60s.

Refer to the general discussion of these products in the Antacids group monograph.

LIQUIDS

Content given in mg per 5 mL. 23 mg sodium = 1 mEq.

	Product & Distributor	Aluminum Hydroxide	Magnesium Hydroxide	Calcium Carbonate	Other Content	Sodium (mg)	How Supplied
otc	Mylanta Regular Strength Liquid (J&J Merck)	200	200		20 mg simethicone, parabens, saccharin, sorbitol		In original, cherry, and mint flavors. In 150 mL (original), 360 mL (all flavors), and 720 mL (original and cherry).
otc	Alamag Suspension (Goldline)	225	200		Sorbitol, sucrose, parabens	< 1.25	Mint flavor. In 355 mL.
otc	Maalox Suspension (Rhone-Poulenc Rorer)				Saccharin, sorbitol, parabens		Mint creme and cherry creme flavors. In 148, 355 and 769 mL.
otc	Alamag Plus Suspension (Goldline)				25 mg simethicone, parabens, saccharin, sorbitol		Lemon flavor. In 355 mL.
otc	Mintox Suspension (Major)				Parabens, saccharin, sorbitol	1.4	Mint flavor. In 355 and 780 mL.
otc	RuLox Suspension (Rugby)				Simethicone, saccharin, sorbitol, parabens		Mint flavor. In 360 and 769 mL and gal.
otc	Aludrox Suspension (Wyeth-Ayerst)	307	103		Simethicone, saccharin, sorbitol, parabens		In 355 mL.
otc	Mylanta Maximum Strength Liquid (J&J Merck)	400	400		40 mg simethicone, parabens, saccharin, sorbitol		Original, cherry, and mint flavors. In 360 mL (all flavors) and 720 mL (original flavor).
otc	Extra Strength Maalox Suspension (Rhone-Poulenc Rorer)	500	450		40 mg simethicone, parabens, saccharin, sorbitol		Cherry creme, lemon creme and mint creme flavors. In 148, 355 and 769 mL.
otc	Maalox TC Suspension (Novartis)	600	300		Parabens, sorbitol		Mint flavor. In 355 mL.
otc	Maalox Anti-Gas Extra Strength (Novartis)	500	450		40 mg simethicone, calcium saccharin, sorbitol, parabens.		In cherry and mint flavors. In 769 mL.
otc	Extra Strength Mintox Plus Liquid (Major)	500	450		40 mg simethicone, parabens, saccharin, sorbitol		Lemon Swiss creme flavor. In 355 mL.
otc	Simaal Gel 2 Liquid (Schein)	500	400		40 mg simethicone		In 360 mL.
otc	Gaviscon Extra Strength Relief Formula Liquid (SK-Beecham)	254			237.5 mg magnesium carbonate, parabens, EDTA, saccharin, sorbitol, simethicone, sodium alginate		Cool mint flavor. In 355 mL.

ANTACIDS

Antacid Combinations

LIQUIDS

	Product & Distributor	Aluminum Hydroxide	Magnesium Hydroxide	Calcium Carbonate	Other Content	Sodium (mg)	How Supplied
otc	**Alenic Alka Liquid** (Rugby)	31.7			137.3 mg magnesium carbonate, sodium alginate, EDTA, saccharin, sorbitol, parabens	13	Spearmint flavor. In 355 mL.
otc	**Gaviscon Liquid** (SK-Beecham)				119.3 mg magnesium carbonate, sodium alginate, EDTA, saccharin, sorbitol, parabens	13	Cool mint flavor. In 177 and 355 mL.
otc	**Marblen Liquid** (Fleming)			520	400 mg magnesium carbonate		Peach/Apricot flavor. In 473 mL.
sf	**Titralac Plus Liquid** (3M Personal Health Care)			500	20 mg simethicone, parabens, saccharin, sorbitol	0.15	Mint flavor. In 360 mL.
otc	**Almacone Liquid** (Rugby)	200	200		20 mg simethicone		In 360 mL and gal.
otc	**Di-Gel Liquid** (Schering-Plough)				20 mg simethicone, saccharin, sorbitol, parabens		Mint and lemon-orange flavors. In 180 and 360 mL.
otc	**Mi-Acid Liquid** (Major)				20 mg simethicone, parabens, sorbitol		In 355 and 780 mL.
otc	**Mylagen Liquid** (Goldline)				20 mg simethicone, parabens, sorbitol, sucrose		In 355 mL.
otc	**Mygel Suspension** (Geneva)				20 mg simethicone	< 1.25	In 355 mL.
otc	**Mylanta** (J&J-Merck)				20 mg simethicone		In 360 mL.
otc	**Alumina, Magnesia, and Simethicone Suspension** (Roxane)	213	200		20 mg simethicone, sorbitol, parabens, saccharin (lemon, mint, cherry only)		Original, lemon, mint, and cherry flavors. In 150 (original), 355 (original, cherry, lemon, mint), and 720 (original, cherry) mL.
otc	**Gas Ban DS Liquid** (Roberts)	400	400		20 mg simethicone, parabens, sorbitol		In UD 15 and 30 mL.
otc	**Mygel II Suspension** (Geneva)				40 mg simethicone		In 150 mL.
otc	**Almacone II Double Strength Liquid** (Rugby)				40 mg simethicone		In 360 mL.
otc	**Mylagen II Liquid** (Goldline)				40 mg simethicone, saccharin, sorbitol		In 360 mL and gal.
otc	**Mi-Acid II Liquid** (Major)				40 mg simethicone, parabens, sorbitol, sucrose	< 1.25	In 355 mL.
otc	**Mylanta Double Strength Liquid** (J&J-Merck)				40 mg simethicone, parabens, sorbitol		In 355 mL.
otc	**RuLox Plus Suspension** (Rugby)	500	450		40 mg simethicone, sorbitol, parabens		Cherry and cool mint creme flavors. In 150 and 360 mL.
otc	**Iosopan Plus Liquid** (Goldline)				40 mg simethicone, saccharin, sorbitol, parabens		Lemon creme flavor. In 355 mL.
otc	**Magaldrate Plus Suspension** (Various, eg, Moore)				540 mg magaldrate, 40 mg simethicone		In 355 mL.
otc	**Mylanta Supreme** (Johnson & Johnson/Merck)		135	400	540 mg magaldrate, 40 mg simethicone		In 360 mL.
					Saccharin, sorbitol.		Mint, lemon, and cherry flavors. In 355 mL.

Refer to the general discussion of these products in the Antacids group monograph.

ANTACIDS

Antacid Combinations

POWDERS AND EFFERVESCENT TABLETS

Content given per dose or tablet.

	Product and Distributor	Sodium Bicarbonate (mg)	Other Content	Sodium (mg)	How Supplied
otc	**Bromo Seltzer Effervescent Granules** (Warner-Lambert)	2781	325 mg acetaminophen, 2224 mg citric acid (when dissolved, forms 2848 mg sodium citrate), sugar	761	In 127.5 g.
otc	**Sparkles Effervescent Granules** (Lafayette)	2000	1500 mg citric acid, simethicone		In UD 50s.
otc	**Gold Alka-Seltzer Effervescent Tablets** (Bayer)	958[1]	832 mg citric acid, 312 mg potassium bicarbonate	311	In 20s and 36s.
otc	**Original Alka-Seltzer Effervescent Tablets** (Bayer)	1700	325 mg aspirin, 1000 mg citric acid, 9 mg phenylalanine	506	Aspartame. Lemon-lime flavor. In 24s.
otc	**Zee-Seltzer Effervescent Tablets** (Zee Medical)	1916	325 mg aspirin, 1000 mg citric acid	524	In 12s.
otc	**Original Alka-Seltzer Effervescent Tablets** (Bayer)	1916[1]	325 mg aspirin, 1000 mg citric acid	567	In 36s.
otc	**Extra Strength Alka-Seltzer Effervescent Tablets** (Bayer)	1985[1]	500 mg aspirin, 1000 mg citric acid	588	In 12s and 24s.

[1] Heat-treated.

Refer to the general discussion of these products in the Antacids group monograph.

Indications

The general uses for these agents are listed below. Refer to the individual product listings for specific indications.

➤*Peptic ulcer:* Adjunctive therapy for peptic ulcer. These agents suppress gastric acid secretion. There is no conclusive evidence they aid in the healing of a peptic ulcer, decrease the rate of recurrence or prevent complications. Anticholinergics are used much less frequently in modern ulcer management.

➤*Other GI conditions:* Functional GI disorders (diarrhea, pylorospasm, hypermotility, neurogenic colon), irritable bowel syndrome (spastic colon, mucous colitis), acute enterocolitis, ulcerative colitis, diverticulitis, mild dysenteries, pancreatitis, splenic flexure syndrome and infant colic.

➤*Biliary tract:* For spastic disorders of the biliary tract. Given in conjunction with a narcotic analgesic.

➤*Urogenital tract:* Uninhibited hypertonic neurogenic bladder.

➤*Bradycardia:* Atropine is used in the suppression of vagally mediated bradycardias.

➤*Preoperative medication:* Atropine, scopolamine, hyoscyamine and glycopyrrolate are used as preanesthetic medication to control bronchial, nasal, pharyngeal, and salivary secretions; and to block cardiac vagal inhibitory reflexes during induction of anesthesia and intubation. Scopolamine is used for preanesthetic sedation and for obstetric amnesia.

➤*Antidotes for poisoning by cholinergic drugs:* Atropine is used for poisoning by organophosphorous insecticides, chemical warfare nerve gases and as an antidote for mushroom poisoning due to muscarine in certain species such as *Amanita muscaria* (see Pralidoxime Chloride monograph).

➤*Miscellaneous uses:* Calming delirium; motion sickness (scopolamine), see Antiemetic/Antivertigo Agents group monograph; parkinsonism, see Antiparkinson Agents group monograph.

➤*Unlabeled uses:*
Bronchial asthma – Atropine and related agents are effective in some patients with cholinergic-mediated bronchospasm. Use in chronic lung disease is not generally recommended; these agents reduce bronchial secretions resulting in decreased fluidity and thickening of residual secretion.

Glycopyrrolate may be effective in the treatment of bronchial asthma; doses of 1 mg (nebulization) and 1.3 mg (solution) have been used.

Actions

➤*Pharmacology:* Anticholinergics are also known as antimuscarinic drugs. In addition to the Anticholinergics/Antispasmodics discussed below, related drugs include: Anticholinergic Antiparkinson Agents, Cycloplegic Mydriatics and Urinary Anticholinergics. See specific monographs.

GI anticholinergics are used primarily to decrease motility (smooth muscle tone) in GI, biliary and urinary tracts and for antisecretory effects. Antispasmodics, related compounds, decrease GI motility by acting on smooth muscle.

Gastrointestinal Anticholinergic/Antispasmodic Dosage		
	Adult Dosage	
Drug	Oral	Parenteral
Anticholinergics Atropine	0.4-0.6 mg	0.4-0.6 mg
Scopolamine		0.32-0.65 mg
L-hyoscyamine	0.125-0.25 mg tid-qid (0.375 to 0.7 mg q 12 hrs – sustained release)	0.25-0.5 mg q 4 h
L-alkaloids of belladonna	0.25-0.5 mg tid	
Belladonna alkaloids	0.18-0.3 mg tid-qid	
Quaternary Anticholinergics Methscopolamine bromide	2.5 mg ac; 2.5-5 mg hs	
Clidinium bromide	2.5-5 mg tid-qid	
Glycopyrrolate	1-2 mg bid-tid	0.1-0.2 mg tid-qid
Mepenzolate bromide	25-50 mg qid	
Methantheline bromide	50-100 mg q 4-6 hrs	
Propantheline bromide	7.5-15 mg tid; 30 mg hs	
Tridihexethyl chloride	25-50 mg tid-qid	
Antispasmodics Dicyclomine HCl	20-40 mg qid	20 mg qid

These agents inhibit the muscarinic actions of acetylcholine at postganglionic parasympathetic neuroeffector sites including smooth muscle, secretory glands and CNS sites. Large doses may block nicotinic receptors at the autonomic ganglia and at the neuromuscular junction.

Specific anticholinergic responses are dose-related. Small doses inhibit salivary and bronchial secretions and sweating; moderate doses dilate the pupil, inhibit accommodation and increase heart rate (vagolytic effect); larger doses decrease motility of GI and urinary tracts; very large doses inhibit gastric acid secretion.

➤*Pharmacokinetics:*
Absorption/Distribution –
Belladonna alkaloids: Belladonna alkaloids are rapidly absorbed after oral use. They readily cross blood-brain barrier, and affect the CNS. The major difference between these agents is that atropine at usual therapeutic doses is a stimulant, whereas scopolamine is a CNS depressant. Undesirable peripheral and central effects occur at doses sufficient to control GI motility and gastric acid secretion.

Atropine has a half-life of about 2.5 hours; 94% of a dose is eliminated through the urine in 24 hours.

Quaternary anticholinergics: Synthetic or semisynthetic derivatives structurally related to the belladonna alkaloids, they are poorly and unreliably absorbed orally. Because they do not cross the blood-brain barrier, CNS effects are negligible. They are also less likely to affect the pupil or ciliary muscle of the eye. Duration of action is more prolonged than alkaloids. In addition, they may cause some degree of ganglionic blockade; neuromuscular blockade may occur at toxic doses.

Antispasmodics: The tertiary ammonium compounds have little or no antimuscarinic activity, and therefore, no significant effect on gastric acid secretion. They exhibit a nonspecific direct relaxant effect on smooth muscle.

Contraindications

➤*Hypersensitivity:* Hypersensitivity to anticholinergic drugs; patients hypersensitive to belladonna or to barbiturates may be hypersensitive to **scopolamine**.

➤*Ocular:* Narrow-angle glaucoma; adhesions (synechiae) between the iris and lens.

➤*Cardiovascular:* Tachycardia; unstable cardiovascular status in acute hemorrhage; myocardial ischemia.

➤*GI:* Obstructive disease (eg, achalasia, pyloroduodenal stenosis or pyloric obstruction, cardiospasm); paralytic ileus; intestinal atony of the elderly or debilitated; severe ulcerative colitis; toxic megacolon complicating ulcerative colitis; hepatic disease.

➤*GU:* Obstructive uropathy (eg, bladder neck obstruction due to prostatic hypertrophy); renal disease.

➤*Musculoskeletal:* Myasthenia gravis.

➤*Asthma:* **Atropine** is contraindicated in asthma patients.

➤**Dicyclomine**: Infants < 6 months of age (see Warnings).

Warnings

➤*Heat prostration:* Heat prostration can occur with anticholinergic drug use (fever and heat stroke due to decreased sweating) in the presence of a high environmental temperature.

➤*Diarrhea:* Diarrhea may be an early symptom of incomplete intestinal obstruction, especially in patients with ileostomy or colostomy. Treatment of diarrhea with these drugs is inappropriate and possibly harmful.

➤*Parkinsonism:* Vomiting, malaise, sweating and salivation may occur in patients with parkinsonism upon sudden withdrawal of large doses of **scopolamine**.

➤*Anticholinergic psychosis:* Anticholinergic psychosis has been reported in sensitive individuals given anticholinergic drugs. CNS signs and symptoms include confusion, disorientation, short-term memory loss, hallucinations, dysarthria, ataxia, coma, euphoria, decreased anxiety, fatigue, insomnia, agitation and mannerisms, and inappropriate affect. These CNS signs and symptoms usually resolve 12 to 24 hours after drug discontinuation.

➤*Gastric ulcer:* Gastric ulcer may produce a delay in gastric emptying time and may complicate therapy (antral stasis).

➤*Elderly:* Elderly patients may react with excitement, agitation, drowsiness and other untoward manifestations to even small doses of anticholinergic drugs.

➤*Pregnancy:* Category B (**glycopyrrolate**, parenteral); Category C (**hyoscyamine, atropine, scopolamine, isopropamide, propantheline, methantheline**). Hyoscyamine crosses the placenta; atropine and scopolamine cross the placenta rapidly after IV use. Effects on the fetus depend on maturity of its parasympathetic nervous system. In neonates, scopolamine may depress respiration and contribute to neonatal hemorrhage due to reduction in vitamin K-dependent clotting factors.

Safety for use during pregnancy has not been established. Use only when clearly needed and when the potential benefits outweigh the potential hazards to the fetus.

Labor and delivery – **Scopolamine** does not affect uterine contractions during labor or increase duration of labor. It crosses the placenta but has not been reported to affect the fetus adversely.

➤*Lactation:* **Hyoscyamine** is excreted in breast milk; other anticholinergics (especially **atropine**) may be excreted in milk, causing infant toxicity, and may reduce milk production. Documentation is lacking or conflicting. Generally, do not use in nursing women.

➤*Children:* Safety and efficacy are not established. **Hyoscyamine** has been used in infant colic. Safety and efficacy of **glycopyrrolate** in children < 12 are not established for peptic ulcer.

There are reports of infants in the first 3 months of life, administered **dicyclomine** syrup, who experienced respiratory distress, seizures, syncope, asphyxia, pulse rate fluctuations, muscular hypotonia, and coma. These symptoms occurred within minutes of ingestion and lasted 20 to 30 minutes; this suggests that they were a consequence of local irritation or aspiration rather than a pharmacologic effect. A few deaths have been reported in infants ≤ 3 months of age. Two of these were associated with excessively high dicyclomine blood levels. Dicyclomine is contraindicated in infants < 6 months of age.

Precautions

➤*Use with caution in the following:*

Cardiovascular – Coronary heart disease; CHF; cardiac arrhythmias; tachycardia; hypertension.

GI – Hepatic disease; early evidence of ileus, as in peritonitis; ulcerative colitis (large doses may suppress intestinal motility and precipitate or aggravate toxic megacolon); hiatal hernia associated with reflux esophagitis (anticholinergics may aggravate it).

GU – Renal disease; prostatic hypertrophy. Patients with prostatism can have dysuria and may require catheterization.

Ocular – Glaucoma; light irides. If there is mydriasis and photophobia, wear dark glasses. Use caution in the elderly because of increased incidence of glaucoma.

Pulmonary – Debilitated patients with chronic lung disease; reduction in bronchial secretions can lead to inspissation and formation of bronchial plugs. Use cautiously in patients with asthma or allergies.

Miscellaneous – Autonomic neuropathy; hyperthyroidism.

In pain or severe anxiety, scopolamine is usually given with analgesics or sedatives to avoid behavioral disturbances. Risk of hyperpyrexia is increased in patients with fever. In elderly patients, confusional states are more common.

➤*Special risk:* Use cautiously in infants, small children, and people with Down's syndrome, brain damage, or spastic paralysis.

➤*Hazardous tasks:* Patients should use caution while driving or performing other tasks requiring alertness, coordination or physical dexterity.

➤*Tartrazine sensitivity:* Some of these products contain tartrazine (FD&C yellow #5), which may cause allergic-type reactions (including bronchial asthma) in susceptible individuals. Although the incidence of sensitivity is low, it is frequently seen in patients who also have aspirin hypersensitivity. Specific products containing tartrazine are identified in the product listings.

➤*Sulfite sensitivity:* Some of these products contain sulfites that may cause allergic-type reactions (including anaphylactic symptoms and life-threatening or less severe asthmatic episodes) in certain susceptible persons. The overall prevalence of sulfite sensitivity in the general population is unknown and probably low. It is seen more frequently in asthmatic or atopic nonasthmatic persons.

Drug Interactions

➤*Amantadine:* Coadministration of anticholinergics may result in an increase in anticholinergic side effects. Consider decreasing the anticholinergic dose.

➤*Atenolol:* The pharmacologic effects may be increased by concurrent anticholinergic administration. **Metoprolol** and **propranolol** were not affected in 2 studies.

➤*Digoxin:* Pharmacologic effects may be increased by anticholinergic coadministration. This may be product specific, (ie, slow-dissolving digoxin tablets interact whereas digoxin capsules and elixir are not affected). However, because USP standards require a minimum dissolution rate, tablets available in the US are not likely to be affected.

➤*Phenothiazines:* The antipsychotic effectiveness may be decreased by anticholinergic coadministration. Anticholinergic side effects may also be increased by concurrent therapy. Adjust the phenothiazine dose as necessary.

➤*Tricyclic antidepressants:* Anticholinergic coadministration may increase anticholinergic side effects (eg, dry mouth, constipation, urinary retention) because of an additive effect. A tricyclic antidepressant with less anticholinergic activity may be beneficial.

Adverse Reactions

➤*Cardiovascular:* Palpitations; bradycardia (following low doses of **atropine**); tachycardia (after higher doses).

➤*CNS:* Headache; flushing; nervousness; drowsiness; weakness; dizziness; confusion; insomnia; fever (especially in children); mental confusion or excitement especially in elderly patients with even small doses. Large doses may produce CNS stimulation (restlessness, tremor). In the presence of pain, **scopolamine** may produce excitement, restlessness, hallucinations, or delirium. Parenteral **dicyclomine** may cause temporary lightheadedness.

➤*Dermatologic:* Severe allergic reactions including anaphylaxis, urticaria, and other dermal manifestations. Local irritation may occur with parenteral **dicyclomine.**

➤*GI:* Xerostomia; altered taste perception; nausea; vomiting; dysphagia; heartburn; constipation; bloated feeling; paralytic ileus.

➤*GU:* Urinary hesitancy and retention; impotence.

➤*Ophthalmic:* Blurred vision; mydriasis; photophobia; cycloplegia; increased intraocular pressure; dilated pupils.

➤*Miscellaneous:* Suppression of lactation; nasal congestion; decreased sweating.

Overdosage

➤*Symptoms:*

GI – Dry mouth; thirst; vomiting; nausea; abdominal distention; difficulty swallowing.

CNS – Theoretically, a curare-like action may occur (ie, neuromuscular blockade leading to muscular weakness and paralysis); CNS stimulation; delirium; drowsiness; restlessness; anxiety; stupor; fever; disorientation; dizziness; headache; seizures; hallucinations; ataxia; convulsions; coma; psychotic behavior; other signs of an acute organic psychosis.

Cardiovascular – Circulatory failure; rapid pulse and respiration; vasodilation; tachycardia with weak pulse; hypertension; hypotension; respiratory depression; palpitations.

GU – Urinary urgency with difficulty in micturition.

Ocular – Blurred vision; photophobia; dilated pupils.

Miscellaneous – Leukocytosis; flushed hot dry skin; rash; respiratory failure.

Children – Children, especially those with Down's syndrome, spastic paralysis, or brain damage, are more sensitive than adults to toxic effects.

➤*Treatment:* Induce emesis or perform gastric lavage, then administer activated charcoal slurry, and supportive and symptomatic therapy, as indicated. See also General Management of Acute Overdosage.

Physostigmine by slow IV injection of 0.2 to 4 mg has been used to reverse anticholinergic effects. Because physostigmine is rapidly metabolized, the patient may relapse into coma after 1 to 2 hours; repeat doses as necessary to a total of 6 mg (2 mg in children). However, profound bradycardia, asystole, and seizures may occur (see Antidotes monograph). The role of physostigmine is not clear; avoid it if other therapeutic agents successfully reverse cardiac dysrhythmias.

Neostigmine methylsulfate 0.25 to 2.5 mg IV, repeated as needed, may be given.

Diazepam, short-acting barbiturates, IV sodium thiopental (2% solution), or chloral hydrate (100 to 200 mL of a 2% solution) by rectal infusion may control excitement. **Hyoscyamine** is dialyzable, but hemodialysis is ineffective for atropine poisoning. Treat hyperpyrexia with physical cooling measures.

If the curare-like effect progresses to paralysis of respiratory muscles, institute artificial respiration and maintain until effective respiratory action returns.

Patient Information

Usually taken 30 to 60 minutes before a meal.

May cause drowsiness, dizziness, or blurred vision; patients should observe caution while driving or performing other tasks requiring alertness.

Notify physician if rash, flushing, or eye pain occurs.

May cause dry mouth, difficulty in urination, constipation or increased sensitivity to light; notify physician if these effects persist or become severe.

Belladonna Alkaloids

L-HYOSCYAMINE SULFATE

Rx	**Anaspaz** (Ascher)	**Tablets:** 0.125 mg	(225/295). In 100s and 500s.
Rx	**ED-SPAZ** (Edwards)		White, scored. In 100s.
Rx	**Levsin** (Schwarz Pharma)		(SCHWARZ 531). White, scored. In 100s and 500s.
Rx	**Cystospaz** (PolyMedica)	**Tablets:** 0.15 mg	(W 2225). Blue. In 100s.
Rx	**A-Spas S/L** (Hyrex)	**Tablets, sublingual:** 0.125 mg	White. In 100s.
Rx	**Levsin/SL** (Schwarz Pharma)		(Schwarz 532). Blue-green, scored. Octagonal. Peppermint flavor. In 100s and 500s.
Rx	**Symax-SL** (Capellon)		(SL 125). Green. In 100s.
Rx	**Hyoscyamine Sulfate** (Various, eg, Econolab, Ethex, Global, Goldline)	**Tablets, extended release:** 0.375 mg	In 100s and 1000s.
Rx	**Levbid** (Schwarz Pharma)		(SP538). Orange, scored. Capsule shape. In 100s.
Rx	**Symax-SR** (Capellon)	**Tablets, sustained release:** 0.375 mg	(SR 375). Green, scored, capsule shape. In 100s.
Rx	**Neosol** (Breckenridge)	**Tablets, orally disintegrating:** 0.125 mg	Mint flavor. White. In 100s.
Rx	**NuLev** (Schwarz Pharma)		Aspartame, mannitol. 1.7 mg phenylalanine. (SP 111). White. Mint flavor. In 100s.
Rx	**Hyoscyamine Sulfate** (Ethex)	**Capsules, extended release:** 0.375 mg	In 100s.
Rx	**Hyoscyamine Sulfate** (Various, eg, Econolab, Ethex)	**Capsules, timed release:** 0.375 mg	In 100s.
Rx	**Levsinex Timecaps** (Schwarz Pharma)		(SCHWARZ 537). Brown/clear. In 100s and 500s.
Rx	**Hyoscyamine Sulfate** (Goldline)	**Solution:** 0.125 mg/mL	5% alcohol. In 15 mL w/dropper.
Rx	**Levsin Drops** (Schwarz Pharma)		5% alcohol. Sorbitol. Orange flavor. In 15 mL.
Rx	**Levsin** (Schwarz Pharma)	**Elixir:** 0.125 mg/5 mL	20% alcohol. Sorbitol. Orange flavor. In pt.
Rx	**Levsin** (Schwarz Pharma)	**Injection:** 0.5 mg/mL	In 1 mL amps and 10 mL[1] vials.
Rx	**IB-Stat** (InKine)	**Oral spray:** 0.125 mg/mL (0.125 mg/spray)	5.3% alcohol, liquid sugar, methylparaben, sorbitol. In 30 mL.

[1] With 1.5% benzyl alcohol and 0.1% sodium metabisulfite.

For complete prescribing information, refer to the Gastrointestinal Anticholinergics/Antispasmodics group monograph.

Indications

➤*GI:* To aid in the control of gastric secretion, visceral spasm, hypermotility in spastic colitis, spastic bladder, pylorospasm, and associated abdominal cramps. To relieve symptoms in functional intestinal disorders (eg, mild dysenteries and diverticulitis), infant colic, biliary, and renal colic. As adjunctive therapy in peptic ulcer; irritable bowel syndrome (irritable colon, spastic colon, mucous colitis, acute enterocolitis, functional GI disorders); neurogenic bowel disturbances including splenic flexure syndrome and neurogenic colon; to reduce pain and hypersecretion in pancreatitis.

➤*Respiratory tract:* As a "drying agent" in the relief of symptoms of acute rhinitis.

➤*CNS:* In parkinsonism to reduce rigidity and tremors and to control associated sialorrhea and hyperhidrosis. May be used for poisoning by anticholinesterase agents.

➤*GU:* Cystitis; renal colic.

➤*Cardiovascular:* Certain cases of partial heart block associated with vagal activity.

➤*Parenteral:* Reduces duodenal motility to facilitate the diagnostic radiologic procedure, hypotonic duodenography. May also improve radiologic visibility of the kidneys.

➤*Preoperative medication:* Parenteral hyoscyamine is indicated as a preoperative antimuscarinic to reduce salivary, tracheobronchial, and pharyngeal secretions; to reduce volume and acidity of gastric secretions; to block cardiac vagal inhibitory reflexes during induction of anesthesia and intubation. Hyoscyamine protects against peripheral muscarinic effects such as bradycardia and excessive secretions produced by halogenated hydrocarbons and cholinergic agents such as physostigmine, neostigmine, and pyridostigmine given to reverse actions of curariform agents.

Administration and Dosage

➤*Oral:*

Adults – 0.125 to 0.25 mg, 3 or 4 times/day orally or sublingually; or 0.375 to 0.75 mg in sustained-release form every 12 hours.

Children – Individualize dosage according to weight.

➤*Parenteral:* 0.25 to 0.5 mg SC, IM, or IV, 2 to 4 times daily, as needed.

ATROPINE SULFATE

Rx	**Sal-Tropine** (Hope)	**Tablets:** 0.4 mg	In 100s.
Rx	**Atropine Sulfate** (Abbott)	**Injection:** 0.05 mg/mL	In 5 mL Abboject syringes.
Rx	**Atropine Sulfate** (Abbott)	**Injection:** 0.1 mg/mL	In 5 and 10 mL Abboject syringes.
Rx	**Atropine Sulfate** (Various, eg, Elkins-Sinn, GlaxoWellcome, Loch, Moore, Rugby, Schein, Vortech)	**Injection:** 0.3 mg/mL	In 1 and 30 mL vials.
		0.4 mg/mL	In 1 mL amps and 1, 20, and 30 mL vials.
		0.5 mg/mL	In 1 and 30 mL vials and 5 mL syringes.
		0.8 mg/mL	In 0.5 and 1 mL amps and 0.5 mL syringes.
		1 mg/mL	In 1 mL amps and vials and 10 mL syringes.
Rx	**AtroPen** (Meridian Medical Technologies)	**Injection:** 0.5 mg	Glycerin, phenol. In pre-filled auto-injectors.
		1 mg	Glycerin, phenol. In pre-filled auto-injectors.
		2 mg	Glycerin, phenol. In pre-filled auto-injectors.

For complete prescribing information, refer to the Gastrointestinal Anticholinergics/Antispasmodics group monograph. For information on the Atropine Sulfate Ophthalmic preparations, refer to the individual monograph.

Indications

Antisialogogue for preanesthetic medication to prevent or reduce secretions of the respiratory tract.

Treatment of parkinsonism. Rigidity and tremor are relieved by the apparently selective depressant action.

Restore cardiac rate and arterial pressure during anesthesia when vagal stimulation produced by intra-abdominal surgical traction causes a sudden decrease in pulse rate and cardiac action.

Lessen the degree of atrioventricular heart block when increased vagal tone is a major factor in the conduction defect as in some cases due to digitalis.

Overcome severe bradycardia and syncope due to a hyperactive carotid sinus reflex.

Antidote (with external cardiac massage) for cardiovascular collapse from the injudicious use of a choline ester (cholinergic) drug, pilocarpine, physostigmine, or isofluorophate.

Relieve pylorospasm, hypertonicity of small intestine, and hypermotility of colon.

Relax the spasm of biliary and ureteral colic and bronchial spasm.

Relaxation of the upper GI tract and colon during hypertonic radiography.

ATROPINE SULFATE

Diminish the tone of the detrusor muscle of the urinary bladder in the treatment of urinary tract disorders.

Control the crying and laughing episodes in patients with brain lesions.

In cases of closed head injuries that cause acetylcholine to be released or to be present in cerebrospinal fluid, which in turn causes abnormal EEG patterns, stupor, and neurological signs.

Relieve hypertonicity of the uterine muscle.

Management of peptic ulcer.

Control rhinorrhea of acute rhinitis or hay fever.

➤*Poisoning:* Treatment of anticholinesterase poisoning from organophosphorous insecticides; as an antidote for mushroom poisoning due to muscarine, in certain species such as *Amanita muscaria.*

For the treatment of poisoning by susceptible organophosphorous nerve agents having cholinesterase activity as well as organophosphorous or carbamate insecticides. Also intended as initial treatment of the muscarinic symptoms of insecticide or nerve agent poisonings (generally breathing difficulties due to increased secretions). Pralidoxime chloride may serve as an important adjunct to atropine therapy.

Administration and Dosage

➤*Adults:* 0.4 to 0.6 mg.

➤*Children:*

Atropine Dosage Recommendations in Children		
Weight		Dose
lb	kg	mg
7 to 16	3.2 to 7.3	0.1
16 to 24	7.3 to 10.9	0.15
24 to 40	10.9 to 18.1	0.2
40 to 65	18.1 to 29.5	0.3
65 to 90	29.5 to 40.8	0.4
> 90	40.8	0.4 to 0.6

➤*Hypotonic radiography:* 1 mg IM.

➤*Surgery:* Give SC, IM or IV. The average adult dose is 0.5 mg (range 0.4 to 0.6 mg). As an antisialogogue, it is usually injected IM prior to induction of anesthesia. In children, it has been suggested to use a dose of 0.01 mg/kg to a maximum of 0.4 mg, repeated every 4 to 6 hours as needed. A recommended infant dose is 0.04 mg/kg (infants < 5 kg) or 0.03 mg/kg (infants > 5 kg), repeated every 4 to 6 hours as needed. During surgery, the drug is given IV when reduction in pulse rate and cessation of cardiac action are due to increased vagal activity. However, if the anesthetic is cyclopropane, use doses less than 0.4 mg and give slowly to avoid production of ventricular arrhythmia. Usual doses reduce severe bradycardia and syncope associated with hyperactive carotid sinus reflex.

➤*Bradyarrhythmias:* The usual IV adult dosage ranges from 0.4 to 1 mg every 1 to 2 hours as needed; larger doses, up to a maximum of 2 mg, may be required. In children, IV dosage ranges from 0.01 to 0.03 mg/kg. Atropine is also a specific antidote for cardiovascular collapse resulting from injudicious administration of choline ester. When cardiac arrest has occurred, external cardiac massage or other method of resuscitation is required to distribute the drug after IV injection.

➤*Poisoning:* In anticholinesterase poisoning from exposure to insecticides, give large doses of ≥ 2 to 3 mg parenterally; repeat until signs of atropine intoxication appear. In "rapid" type of mushroom poisoning, give in doses sufficient to control parasympathomimetic signs before coma and cardiovascular collapse supervene.

AtroPen – Primary protection against exposure to chemical nerve agent and insecticide poisoning is the wearing of protective garments including masks, designed specifically for this use. Individuals should not rely solely upon the availability of antidotes such as atropine and pralidoxime to provide complete protection from chemical nerve agent and insecticide poisoning. Immediate evacuation from the contaminated environment is essential. Decontamination of the poisoned individual should occur as soon as possible. If dermal exposure has occurred, clothing should be removed and the hair and skin washed thoroughly with sodium bicarbonate or alcohol as soon as possible.

The *AtroPen* Auto-injector should be administered as soon as symptoms of organophosphorous. or carbamate poisoning appear (eg, usually tearing, excessive oral secretions, wheezing, muscle fasciculations). In moderate to severe poisoning, the administration of more than 1 *AtroPen* may be required until atropinization is achieved (flushing, mydriasis, tachycardia, dryness of the mouth and nose).

No more than 3 *AtroPen* injections should be used unless the patient is under the supervision of a trained medical provider. Different dose strengths of the *AtroPen* are available depending on the recipient's age and weight.

AtroPen Dosing	
Patient group	Dose strength
Adults and children weighing more than 90 lbs (generally over 10 years of age)	2 mg
Children weighing 40 to 90 lbs (generally 4 to 10 years of age)	1 mg
Children weighing 15 to 40 lbs (generally 6 months to 4 years of age)*	0.5 mg

* Children weighing less than 15 lbs (generally younger than 6 months of age) should ordinarily not be treated with the *AtroPen* auto-injector. Atropine doses for these children should be individualized at doses of 0.05 mg/kg.

Concomitant therapy: In severe poisonings, it may also be desirable to concurrently administer an anticonvulsant if seizure is suspected in the unconscious individual since the classic tonic-clonic jerking may not be apparent due to the effects of the poison. In poisonings due to organophosphorous nerve agents and insecticides, it also may be helpful to concurrently administer a cholinesterase reactivator such as pralidoxime chloride.

Pralidoxime (if used) is most effective if administered immediately or soon after the poisoning. Generally, little is accomplished if pralidoxime is given more than 36 hours after termination of exposure unless the poison is known to age slowly or re-exposure is possible, such as in delayed continuing GI absorption of ingested poisons. Fatal relapses, thought to be due to delayed absorption, have been reported after initial improvement. Continued administration for several days may be useful in such patients.

An anticonvulsant such as diazepam may be administered to treat convulsions if suspected in the unconscious individual. The effects of nerve agents and some insecticides can mask the motor signs of a seizure.

Mild symptoms: One *AtroPen* is recommended if 2 or more of the following mild symptoms of nerve agent (nerve gas) or insecticide exposure appear in situations where exposure is known or suspected:
• Blurred vision, miosis
• Excessive unexplained teary eyes
• Excessive unexplained runny nose
• Increased salivation such as sudden unexplained excessive drooling
• Chest tightness or difficulty breathing
• Tremors throughout the body or muscular twitching
• Nausea and/or vomiting
• Unexplained wheezing or coughing
• Acute onset of stomach cramps
• Tachycardia or bradycardia

Severe symptoms: Two additional *AtroPen* injections given in rapid succession are recommended 10 minutes after receiving the first *AtroPen* injection if the victim develops any of the following severe symptoms. If possible, a person other than the victim should administer the second and third *AtroPen* injections. If a victim is encountered who is either unconscious or has any of the severe symptoms, immediately administer 3 *AtroPen* injections into the victim's mid-lateral thigh in rapid succession using the appropriate weight-based *AtroPen* dose.
• Strange or confused behavior
• Severe difficulty breathing or severe secretions from the lungs/airway
• Severe muscular twitching and general weakness
• Involuntary urination and defecation (feces)
• Convulsions
• Unconsciousness

Emergency care of the severely poisoned individual should include removal of oral and bronchial secretions, maintenance of a patent airway, supplemental oxygen and, if necessary, artificial ventilation. In general, atropine should not be used until cyanosis has been overcome since atropine may produce ventricular fibrillation and possible seizures in the presence of hypoxia.

Close supervision of all moderately to severely poisoned patients is indicated for at least 48 to 72 hours.

Administration:
1.) Snap the grooved end of the plastic sleeve down and over the yellow safety cap. Remove the *AtroPen* from the plastic sleeve. Do not place fingers on the green tip.
2.) Firmly grasp the *AtroPen* with the green tip pointed down.
3.) Pull off the yellow safety cap with your other hand.
4.) Aim and firmly jab the green tip straight down (a 90° angle) against the outer thigh. The *AtroPen* device will then activate and deliver the medicine. It is okay to inject through clothing, but make sure pockets at the injection site are empty. Very thin people and small children also should be injected in the thigh, but before giving the *AtroPen*, bunch up the thigh to provide a thicker area for injection.
5.) Hold the auto-injector firmly in place for at least 10 seconds to allow the injection to finish.
6.) Remove the *AtroPen* and massage the injection site for several seconds. If the needle is not visible, check to be sure the yellow safety cap has been removed, and repeat steps 3 and 5, but press harder.

Belladonna Alkaloids

ATROPINE SULFATE

▶*Storage/Stability:*

AtroPen – Store at 25°C (77°F); excursions permitted to 15° to 30°C (59° to 86°F). Keep from freezing; protect from light.

SCOPOLAMINE HBr (Hyoscine HBr)

Rx	**Scopace** (Hope Pharm)	**Tablets, soluble:** 0.4 mg	(Hope 301). White. In 100s.
Rx	**Scopolamine HBr** (Various, eg, Loch)	**Injection:** 0.3 mg/mL	In 1 mL vials.
Rx	**Scopolamine HBr** (Various, eg, GlaxoWellcome)	**Injection:** 0.4 mg/mL	In 0.5 mL amps and 1 mL vials.
Rx	**Scopolamine HBr** (GlaxoWellcome)	**Injection:** 0.86 mg/mL	In 0.5 mL amps.[1]
Rx	**Scopolamine HBr** (Various, eg, Loch)	**Injection:** 1 mg/mL	In 1 mL vials.

[1] With alcohol and mannitol.

For complete prescribing information, refer to the Gastrointestinal Anticholinergics/Antispasmodics group monograph.

Indications

▶*Tablets:* Inhibits excessive motility and hypertonus of the GI tract in such conditions as the irritable colon syndrome, mild dysentery, diverticulitis, pylorospasm, and cardiospasm; may also prevent motion sickness.

▶*Injection:* Preanesthetic sedation and obstetric amnesia in conjunction with analgesics; also used for calming delirium.

Motion sickness (see Antiemetic/Antivertigo Agents monograph).

Administration and Dosage

▶*Tablets:* 0.4 to 0.8 mg. Dosage may be cautiously increased in parkinsonism and spastic states.

▶*Injection:* Give SC or IM; may give IV after dilution with Sterile Water for Injection.

Adults – 0.32 to 0.65 mg.

Children – 0.006 mg/kg (0.003 mg/lb). Maximum dosage, 0.3 mg.

BELLADONNA

Rx	**Belladonna Tincture** (Various, eg, Lannett, Life, Lilly, Rugby, Texas Drug)	**Liquid:** 27 to 33 mg belladonna alkaloids/ 100 mL	65% to 70% alcohol. In 120 mL, pt and gal.

For complete prescribing information, refer to the Gastrointestinal Anticholinergics/Antispasmodics group monograph.

Indications

▶*GI:* As adjunctive therapy in the treatment of peptic ulcer, functional digestive disorders (including spastic, mucous and ulcerative colitis), diarrhea, diverticulitis, pancreatitis.

▶*GU:* Dysmenorrhea, nocturnal enuresis.

▶*CNS:* Parkinsonism (idiopathic and postencephalitic). Large doses may provide some symptomatic relief; tremor, rigidity, sialorrhea and oculogyric crises are reduced; posture, gait and speech are improved.

▶*Other:* Motion sickness; nausea and vomiting of pregnancy.

Administration and Dosage

▶*Belladonna tincture:* Adults - 0.6 to 1 mL, 3 to 4 times daily.

Children – 0.03 mL/kg (0.8 mL/m^2) 3 times daily.

Actions

▶*Pharmacology:* Belladonna, a crude botanical preparation, contains the anticholinergic alkaloids hyoscyamine (which racemizes to atropine on extraction), scopolamine (hyoscine) and other minor alkaloids. Belladonna leaf contains approximately 0.35% alkaloids. Pharmaceutical preparations of belladonna include belladonna tincture, which contains 27 to 33 mg alkaloids/100 mL.

Quaternary Anticholinergics

METHSCOPOLAMINE BROMIDE

Rx	**Pamine** (Kenwood/Bradley)	**Tablets:** 2.5 mg	White. In 100s and 500s.
Rx	**Pamine Forte** (Kenwood Therapeutics)	**Tablets:** 5 mg	(PAMINE 5). White, oval. In 60s.

For complete prescribing information, refer to the Gastrointestinal Anticholinergics/Antispasmodics group monograph.

Indications

Adjunctive therapy in the treatment of peptic ulcer.

Administration and Dosage

2.5 mg 30 minutes before meals and 2.5 to 5 mg at bedtime.

GLYCOPYRROLATE

Rx	**Robinul** (Horizon)	**Tablets:** 1 mg	Lactose. (HPC 200). White, scored. In 100s and 500s.
Rx	**Robinul Forte** (Horizon)	**Tablets:** 2 mg	Lactose. (Horizon 205). White, scored. In 100s.
Rx	**Glycopyrrolate** (Various, eg, American Regent, Quad, Schein, Texas Drug, VHA)	**Injection:** 0.2 mg per mL	In 1, 2, 5 and 20 mL vials.
Rx	**Robinul** (Robins)		In 1, 2, 5 and 20 mL vials.[1]

[1] With 0.9% benzyl alcohol.

For complete prescribing information, refer to the Gastrointestinal Anticholinergics/Antispasmodics group monograph.

Indications

▶*Oral:* Adjunctive therapy in the treatment of peptic ulcer.

▶*Parenteral:* Used preoperatively to reduce salivary, tracheobronchial and pharyngeal secretions; to reduce the volume and free acidity of gastric secretions; to block cardiac vagal inhibitory reflexes during induction of anesthesia and intubation. May be used intraoperatively to counteract drug-induced or vagal traction reflexes with the associated arrhythmias. Glycopyrrolate protects against the peripheral muscarinic effects (eg, bradycardia and excessive secretions) of cholinergic agents such as neostigmine and pyridostigmine given to reverse the neuromuscular blockade due to nondepolarizing muscle relaxants.

Administration and Dosage

Not recommended for children under age 12 for the management of peptic ulcer.

▶*Oral:* 1 mg 3 times daily or 2 mg 2 to 3 times daily.

Maintenance – 1 mg 2 times daily.

▶*Parenteral:*

Peptic ulcer – 0.1 to 0.2 mg IM or IV 3 or 4 times daily.

Preanesthetic medication – 0.002 mg/lb (0.004 mg/kg) IM, 30 minutes to 1 hour prior to anesthesia. Children less than 2 years of age may require up to 0.004 mg/lb. Children under 12, give 0.002 to 0.004 mg/lb IM.

Intraoperative medication – Adults, 0.1 mg IV. Repeat as needed at 2 to 3 minute intervals. Children, give 0.002 mg/lb (0.004 mg/kg) IV, not to exceed 0.1 mg in a single dose; may be repeated at 2 to 3 minute intervals.

Reversal of neuromuscular blockade – Adults and children, 0.2 mg for each 1 mg neostigmine or 5 mg pyridostigmine. Administer IV simultaneously.

Quaternary Anticholinergics

MEPENZOLATE BROMIDE

Rx	Cantil (Hoechst Marion Roussel)	**Tablets:** 25 mg	Tartrazine. (Merrell 37). Yellow. In 100s.

For complete prescribing information, refer to the Gastrointestinal Anticholinergics/Antispasmodics group monograph.

Indications

Adjunctive therapy in the treatment of peptic ulcer.

Administration and Dosage

➤*Adults:* 25 to 50 mg 4 times daily with meals and at bedtime.

➤*Children:* Safety and efficacy have not been established.

PROPANTHELINE BROMIDE

Rx	Pro-Banthine (Schiapparelli Searle)	**Tablets:** 7.5 mg	(RPC 073). White, sugar coated. In 100s.
Rx	Propantheline Bromide (Various, eg, Goldline, Harber, Moore, Par, Richlyn, Roxane, Rugby)	**Tablets:** 15 mg	In 100s, 500s, 1000s, and UD 100s.
Rx	Pro-Banthine (Schiapparelli Searle)		(Searle 601) Peach, sugar coated. In 100s, 500s, and UD 100s.

For complete prescribing information, refer to the Gastorintestinal anticholinergics/Antispasmodics group monograph.

Indications

Adjunctive therapy in the treatment of peptic ulcer.

➤*Unlabeled uses:* Propantheline has been used for its antisecretory and antispasmodic effects.

Administration and Dosage

➤*Adults:* 15 mg 30 minutes before meals and 30 mg at bedtime. For patients with mild manifestations, geriatric patients or those of small stature, take 7.5 mg, 3 times daily.

➤*Children:*

Peptic ulcer – Safety and efficacy have not been established.

Antisecretory – 1.5 mg/kg/day divided 3 to 4 times daily.

Antispasmodic – 2 to 3 mg/kg/day divided every 4 to 6 hours and at bedtime.

Antispasmodics

DICYCLOMINE HCl

Rx	Dicyclomine HCl (Various, eg, Bolar, Goldline, Lederle, Major, Rugby)	**Capsules:** 10 mg	In 30s, 100s, 120s, 1000s, and UD 100s.
Rx	Bentyl (Axcan Scandipharm)		(Bentyl 10). In 100s, 500s, and UD 100s.
Rx	Byclomine (Major)		In 100s, 250s, 1000s, and UD 100s.
Rx	Di-Spaz (Vortech)		In 1000s.
Rx	Dicyclomine HCl (Various, eg, Bolar, Goldline, Lederle, Major, Rugby)	**Tablets:** 20 mg	In 15s, 20s, 30s, 100s, 120s, 250s, 1000s, and UD 100s.
Rx	Bentyl (Axcan Scandipharm)		(Bentyl 20) In 100s, 500s, 1000s, and UD 100s.
Rx	Byclomine (Major)		In 100s, 250s, 1000s, and UD 100s.
Rx	Dicyclomine HCl (Various, eg, Moore, Ritchie)	**Capsules :** 20 mg	In 100s, and 1000s.
Rx	Dicyclomine HCl (Various, eg, Gen-King, Goldline, Harber, Moore, Qualitest, Rugby)	**Syrup:** 10 mg/5 mL	In 118 mL, pt, and gal.
Rx	Bentyl (Axcan Scandipharm)		Saccharin in pt.
Rx	Dicyclomine HCl (Various, eg, Baxter, Goldline, Major, Moore, Ritchie, Rugby, Steris)	**Injection:** 10 mg/mL	In 2 and 10 mL vials.
Rx	Bentyl (Axcan Scandipharm)		In 2 mL amps and 10 mL vials.
Rx	Dibent (Hauck)		In 10 mL vials.
Rx	Dilomine (Kay Drug)		In 10 mL vials.
Rx	Di-Spaz (Vortech)		In 10 mL vials.
Rx	Or-Tyl (Ortega)		In 10 mL vials.

For complete prescribing information, refer to the Gastrointestinal Anticholinergics/Antispasmodics group monograph.

Indications

Treatment of functional bowel/irritable bowel syndrome (irritable colon, spastic colon, mucous colitis).

Administration and Dosage

➤*Oral:*

Adults – The only oral dose shown to be effective is 160 mg/day in 4 equally divided doses. However, because of side effects, begin with 80 mg/day (in 4 equally divided doses). Increase dose to 160 mg/day unless side effects limit dosage.

➤*Parenteral:* IM only. Not for IV use.

Adults – 80 mg/day in 4 divided doses.

GASTROINTESTINAL ANTICHOLINERGICS/ANTISPASMODICS

Refer to the general discussion of these products in the GI Anticholinergics/Antispasmodics group monograph.

Actions

▶ *Pharmacology:* Combination anticholinergic preparations may include the following components:

Sedatives and antianxiety agents – See: Barbiturates, Prochlorperazine, Hydroxyzine, Meprobamate, Chlordiazepoxide.

Ergotamine tartrate – Ergotamine tartrate provides inhibition of the sympathetic nervous system.

GI ANTICHOLINERGIC COMBINATIONS, CAPSULES AND TABLETS

Content given per tablet or capsule.

	Product and Distributor	Anticholinergic	Sedative, Antianxiety Agent or Other	Daily Dose (Tablets)	How Supplied
Rx	**Barbidonna No. 2 Tablets** (Wallace)	0.025 mg atropine sulfate, 0.0074 mg scopolamine HBr, 0.1286 mg hyoscyamine sulfate	32 mg phenobarbital	3	Lactose. (Wallace 311). Lt. brown, scored. In 100s.
Rx	**Barbidonna Tablets** (Wallace)	0.025 mg atropine sulfate, 0.0074 mg scopolamine HBr, 0.1286 mg hyoscyamine sulfate	16 mg phenobarbital	3 to 6	Lactose. (Wallace 301). White, scored. In 100s and 500s.
Rx	**Belladonna Alkaloids w/Phenobarbital Tablets** (Various, eg, Goldline, Major, Westward)	0.0194 mg atropine sulfate, 0.0065 mg scopolamine HBr, 0.1037 mg hyoscyamine HBr or sulfate	16.2 mg phenobarbital	3 to 8	In 50s, 100s, 1000s and UD 100s.
Rx	**Hyosophen Tablets** (Rugby)				(Rugby 3920). White, scored. In 100s and 1000s.
Rx	**Spasmolin Tablets** (Various, eg, Global)				In 100s and 1000s.
Rx	**Butibel Tablets** (Wallace)	15 mg belladonna extract	15 mg butabarbital sodium	4 to 8	(Butibel 37/046). Red. In 100s.
Rx	**Chlordiazepoxide w/Clidinium Bromide Capsules** (Various, eg, Chelsea Labs, Eon, Goldline, Major, Moore, Schein)	2.5 mg clidinium	5 mg chlordiazepoxide HCl	3 to 8	In 100s, 500s, 1000s and UD 100s.
Rx	**Librax Capsules** (Roche)				Parabens, lactose. Green. In 100s, 500s and Tel-E-Dose 100s.
Rx	**Bellamine Tablets** (Major)	0.2 mg levorotatory alkaloids of belladonna	40 mg phenobarbital, 0.6 mg ergotamine tartrate	1 in morning and night	In 100s.

Refer to the general discussion of these products in the GI Anticholinergics/Antispasmodics group monograph.

GI ANTICHOLINERGIC COMBINATIONS, TABLETS, SUSTAINED RELEASE

Content given per tablet.

	Product and Distributor	Anticholinergic	Sedative or Antianxiety Agent	Other Content	Daily Dose (Tablets)	How Supplied
Rx	**Bel-Phen-Ergot SR Tablets** (Goldline)	0.2 mg l-alkaloids of belladonna	40 mg phenobarbital, 0.6 mg ergotamine tartrate	Lactose	2	In 100s.

Refer to the general discussion of these products in the GI Anticholinergics/Antispasmodics group monograph.

GI ANTICHOLINERGIC COMBINATIONS, LIQUIDS

Content given per 5 mL liquid and 1 mL drops.

	Product and Distributor	Anticholinergic	Sedative	Other Content	Daily Dose	How Supplied
Rx	**Hyosophen Elixir** (Rugby)	0.0194 mg atropine sulfate, 0.0065 mg scopolamine HBr, 0.1037 mg hyoscyamine HBr or sulfate	16.2 mg phenobarbital	23% alcohol, sugar, sorbitol	15 to 40 mL	In 120 mL, pt and gal.
Rx	**Antispasmodic Elixir**[1] (Various, eg, Goldline, Qualitest, RID, UDL)				*Children:* 4.5 kg to 45.4 kg - 0.5 to 5 mL q4h or 0.75 to 7.5 mL q6h, respectively	In 120 mL, pt, and gal.
Rx	**Butibel Elixir** (Wallace)	15 mg belladonna extract	15 mg butabarbital sodium	7% alcohol, sucrose, saccharin	20 to 40 mL. *Children* ≥ 6 - 10 mL; *Children* < 6 - 5 to 10 mL	Orange flavor. In pt.
Rx sf	**Antrocol Elixir** (ECR)	0.195 mg atropine sulfate	16 mg phenobarbital	20% alcohol	15 to 40 mL. *Children* - 0.5 mL per 15 lbs every 4 to 6 hours	In pt.

[1] May contain alcohol.

Refer to the general discussion of these products at the beginning of the GI Anticholinergics/Antispasmodics group monograph.

MESALAMINE (5-aminosalicylic acid, 5-ASA)

Rx	Asacol (Procter & Gamble)	Tablets, delayed release: 400 mg	Lactose. (Asacol NE). Red-brown. Capsule shape. In 100s.
Rx	Pentasa (Hoechst Marion Roussel)	Capsules, controlled release: 250 mg	Sugar. (2010 Pentasa 250 mg). Green/blue. In 240s and UD 80s.
Rx	Canasa (Axcan Scandipharm)	Suppositories: 500 mg	Hard fat base. Light tan. In 30s.
Rx	FIV-ASA (Paddock)		In 30s.

Indications

➤*Chronic inflammatory bowel disease:*

Oral – Remission and treatment of mildly to moderately active ulcerative colitis.

Rectal – Treatment of active mild to moderate distal ulcerative colitis, proctosigmoiditis or proctitis.

Administration and Dosage

➤*Oral:*

Tablets – 800 mg 3 times daily for a total dose of 2.4 g/day for 6 weeks.

Capsules – 1 g 4 times daily for a total dose of 4 g for up to 8 weeks.

➤*Suppository:* One suppository (500 mg) 2 times daily. Retain the suppository in the rectum for 1 to 3 hours or more if possible to achieve maximum benefit. While the effect may be seen within 3 to 21 days, the usual course of therapy is 3 to 6 weeks depending on symptoms and sigmoidoscopic findings. Studies have not assessed whether the suppositories will modify relapse rates after the 6 week short-term treatment.

Actions

➤*Pharmacology:* Sulfasalazine is split by bacterial action in the colon into sulfapyridine (SP) and mesalamine (5-ASA). It is thought that the mesalamine component is therapeutically active in ulcerative colitis. The usual oral dose of sulfasalazine for active ulcerative colitis in adults is 3 to 4 g per day in divided doses, which provides 1.6 g free mesalamine to the colon. Each suspension enema delivers up to 4 g mesalamine to the left side of the colon; each suppository delivers 500 mg to the rectum.

The mechanism of action of mesalamine (and sulfasalazine) is unknown, but appears to be topical rather than systemic. Mucosal production of arachidonic acid (AA) metabolites, both through cyclooxygenase pathways (ie, prostanoids) and through lipoxygenase pathways (ie, leukotrienes [LTs] and hydroxyeicosatetraenoic acids [HETEs]) is increased in patients with chronic inflammatory bowel disease, and it is possible that mesalamine diminishes inflammation by blocking cyclooxygenase and inhibiting prostaglandin (PG) production in the colon.

➤*Pharmacokinetics:*

Absorption/Distribution –

Rectal: Mesalamine administered rectally as a suspension enema is poorly absorbed from the colon and is excreted principally in the feces during subsequent bowel movements. The extent of absorption is dependent upon the retention time of the drug product, and there is considerable individual variation. At steady state, approximately 10% to 30% of the daily 4 g dose can be recovered in cumulative 24 hour urine collections. Other than the kidneys, the organ distribution and other bioavailability characteristics of absorbed mesalamine are not known. The compound undergoes acetylation, but whether this process takes place at colonic or systemic sites has not been elucidated.

Oral:

• *Tablets* – Mesalamine tablets are coated with an acrylic-based resin that delays release of mesalamine until it reaches the terminal ileum and beyond. Approximately 28% is absorbed after oral ingestion, leaving the remainder available for topical action and excretion in the feces. Absorption is similar with or without food. Mesalamine from oral mesalamine tablets appears to be more extensively absorbed than that released from sulfasalazine. Maximum plasma levels of mesalamine and N-acetyl-5-ASA following multiple doses are ≈ 1.5 to 2 times higher than those following an equivalent dose of sulfasalazine; combined parent drug and metabolite areas under the concentration-time curve and urine drug dose recoveries are also ≈ 1.3 to 1.5 times higher. The time to reach maximum plasma concentration for mesalamine and its metabolite is usually delayed (because of the delayed release formulation) and ranges from 4 to 12 hours.

• *Capsules* – Mesalamine capsules are ethylcellulose-coated, controlled release formulations designed to release therapeutic quantities of the drug throughout the GI tract; 20% to 30% of mesalamine is absorbed. In contrast, when mesalamine is administered orally as an unformulated 1 g aqueous suspension, mesalamine is ≈ 80% absorbed. Plasma mesalamine concentration peaked at ≈ 1 mcg/mL 3 hours after administration of a 1 g dose and declined in a biphasic manner. Mean terminal half-life was 42 minutes after IV administration. N-acetyl-5-ASA peaked at ≈ 3 hours at 1.8 mcg/mL, and its concentration followed a biphasic decline.

Metabolism/Excretion –

Rectal: Whatever the metabolic site, most absorbed mesalamine is excreted in urine as the N-acetyl-5-ASA metabolite. Patients demonstrated plasma levels of 2 mcg/mL 10 to 12 hours after administration; about 66% of this was the N-acetyl metabolite. While the elimination half-life of mesalamine is short (0.5 to 1.5 hr), the acetylated metabolite exhibits a half-life of 5 to 10 hours. In addition, steady-state plasma levels demonstrated a lack of accumulation of either free or metabolized drug during repeated daily administrations.

Oral:

• *Tablets* – Following oral administration, the absorbed mesalamine is rapidly acetylated in the gut mucosal wall and by the liver. It is excreted mainly by the kidneys as N-acetyl-5-ASA. The half-lives of elimination for mesalamine and the metabolite are usually about 12 hours, but are variable ranging from 2 to 15 hours. There is large intersubject variability in plasma concentrations of mesalamine and N-acetyl-5-ASA and in their elimination half-lives following use of the tablets.

• *Capsules* – Elimination of free mesalamine and salicylates in feces increased proportionally with the dose. N-acetyl-5-ASA was the primary compound excreted in the urine (19% to 30%).

Contraindications

Hypersensitivity to mesalamine, salicylates or any component of the formulation.

Warnings

➤*Intolerance/Colitis exacerbation:* Mesalamine has been implicated in the production of an acute intolerance syndrome or exacerbation of colitis (≈ 3% of patients) characterized by cramping, acute abdominal pain and bloody diarrhea, and occasionally fever, headache, malaise, pruritus, conjunctivitis and rash. Symptoms usually abate when mesalamine is discontinued. Reevaluate the patient's history of sulfasalazine intolerance, if any. If a rechallenge is performed to validate the hypersensitivity, do it under close supervision and only if clearly needed, giving consideration to reduced dosage. One patient previously sensitive to sulfasalazine was rechallenged with 400 mg oral mesalamine; within 8 hours she experienced headache, fever, intensive abdominal colic and profuse diarrhea and was readmitted as an emergency. She responded poorly to steroids; 2 weeks later, a pancolectomy was required.

➤*Pancolitis:* While using mesalamine some patients have developed pancolitis. However, extension of upper disease boundary or flare-ups occurred less often in mesalamine patients than in placebo patients.

➤*Hypersensitivity reactions:* In a clinical trial, most patients who were hypersensitive to sulfasalazine were able to take mesalamine enemas without evidence of any allergic reaction. Nevertheless, exercise caution when mesalamine is initially used in patients known to be allergic to sulfasalazine. Instruct these patients to discontinue therapy if signs of rash or fever become apparent.

➤*Renal function impairment:* Renal impairment, including minimal change nephropathy, and acute and chronic interstitial nephritis, has occurred. In animals, the kidney is the principal target organ for toxicity; at doses ≈ 15 to 20 times the recommended human dose, mesalamine causes renal papillary necrosis. Exercise caution when using mesalamine in patients with renal dysfunction or a history of renal disease. Evaluate renal function of all patients prior to therapy and periodically during therapy.

The possibility of increased absorption of mesalamine and concomitant renal tubular damage as noted in preclinical studies must be kept in mind. Carefully monitor patients who receive concurrent oral products which liberate mesalamine and those with preexisting renal disease with urinalysis, BUN and creatinine studies.

➤*Pregnancy: Category B.* There are no adequate and well controlled studies in pregnant women for either sulfasalazine or 5-ASA. Use during pregnancy only if clearly needed. Mesalamine is known to cross the placental barrier.

➤*Lactation:* Low concentrations of mesalamine and higher concentrations of N-acetyl-5-ASA have been detected in breast milk. Clinical significance has not been determined. However, exercise caution when administering to a nursing woman.

➤*Children:* Safety and efficacy for use in children have not been established.

Precautions

➤*Pericarditis:* Pericarditis has occurred rarely with mesalamine-containing products including sulfasalazine. Cases of pericarditis have also occurred as manifestations of inflammatory bowel disease. In cases reported with mesalamine rectal suspension, there have been positive rechallenges. In one of these cases, however, a second rechallenge with sulfasalazine was negative throughout a 2 month follow-up. Investigate chest pain or dyspnea in mesalamine-treated patients with this in mind. Discontinuation of the drug may be warranted in some patients, but rechallenge can be performed under careful clinical observation.

➤*Sulfite sensitivity:* Some of these products contain sulfites that may cause allergic-type reactions (including anaphylactic symptoms and life-threatening or less severe asthmatic episodes) in certain susceptible persons. The overall prevalence of sulfite sensitivity in the general

MESALAMINE (5-aminosalicylic acid, 5-ASA)

population is unknown and probably low. It is seen more frequently in asthmatic or atopic nonasthmatic persons.

Epinephrine is the preferred treatment for serious allergic or emergency situations even though epinephrine injection contains sodium or potassium metabisulfite. The alternatives to using epinephrine in a life-threatening situation may not be satisfactory. The presence of a sulfite(s) in epinephrine injection should not deter the administration of the drug for treatment of serious allergic or other emergency situations.

Adverse Reactions

Mesalamine is usually well tolerated. Most adverse effects have been mild and transient.

Mesalamine Adverse Reactions (%)[1]

Adverse reaction	Oral Tablets (n = 152)	Oral Capsules (n = 451)	Rectal Suppository (n = 168)
CNS			
Asthenia	7	—	1.2
Chills	3	—	—
Dizziness	8	< 1	3
Fever	7	0.9	1.2
Headache	35	2.2	6.5
Insomnia	✔[2]	< 1	—
Malaise/Fatigue/Weakness	1-2	< 1	—
Sweating	3	< 1	—
Dermatologic			
Acne	1-2	0.2	1.2
Itching	—	—	—
Pruritus	3	< 1	—
Rash/Spots	6	1.3	1.2
GI			
Abdominal pain/cramps/discomfort	18	1.1	3
Bloating	—	—	—
Colitis exacerbation	3	0.4	1.2
Constipation	5	< 1	—
Diarrhea	7	3.5	3
Dyspepsia	6	—	—
Eructation	16	< 1	—
Flatulence/Gas	3	—	3.6
Hemorrhoids	—	—	—
Nausea	13	3.1	1.2
Pain on insertion of enema	—	—	—
Rectal pain/soreness/burning	—	—	1.8
Vomiting	5	1.1	—
Musculoskeletal			
Arthralgia	5	< 1	—
Arthritis	1-2	—	—
Back pain	7	—	—
Hypertonia	5	—	—
Leg/Joint pain	✔[2]	< 1	—
Myalgia	3	< 1	—
Respiratory			
Cold/Sore throat	—	—	1.8
Cough increased	1-2	—	—
Pharyngitis	11	—	—
Rhinitis	5	—	—
Miscellaneous			
Chest pain	3	—	—
Conjunctivitis	1-2	< 1	—
Dysmenorrhea	3	—	—
Edema	3	< 1	1.2
Flu syndrome	3	—	—
Hair loss[3]	✔[2]	< 1	—
Pain	14	—	—
UTI/Urinary burning	✔[2]	—	—

[1] Data are pooled from separate studies and are not necessarily comparable.
[2] ✔ = Occurred, no incidence reported.
[3] Mild hair loss characterized by "more hair in the comb." There are at least six additional cases in the literature of mild hair loss with mesalamine or sulfasalazine. Retreatment is not always associated with repeated hair loss.

Other adverse reactions reported with oral mesalamine include the following:

►*Cardiovascular:* Pericarditis (see Precautions); myocarditis; vasodilation; migraine; palpitations; pericarditis; fatal myocarditis; chest pain; T-wave abnormalities.

►*CNS:* Anxiety; depression; somnolence; emotional lability; hyperesthesia; vertigo; nervousness; confusion; paresthesia; tremor; peripheral neuropathy; transverse myelitis; Guillain-Barré syndrome.

►*GI:* Anorexia; pancreatitis (also for rectal); gastroenteritis; gastritis; increased appetite; cholecystitis; dry mouth; oral ulcers; perforated peptic ulcer; bloody diarrhea; tenesmus; duodenal ulcer, dysphagia; esophageal ulcer; fecal incontinence; GI bleeding; oral moniliasis; rectal bleeding; stool abnormalities (color/texture change).

►*GU:* Interstitial nephritis, nephropathy (see Warnings); dysuria; urinary urgency; hematuria; epididymitis; menorrhagia; amenorrhea; metrorrhagia; hypomenorrhea; nephrotic syndrome; urinary frequency; albuminuria; nephrotoxicity.

►*Dermatologic:* Psoriasis; pyoderma gangrenosum; dry skin; erythema nodosum; urticaria; eczema; nail disorder; photosensitivity; lichen planus.

►*Hematologic:* Agranulocytosis; thrombocytopenia; eosinophilia; leukopenia; anemia; lymphadenopathy; ecchymosis; thrombocythemia.

►*Respiratory:* Sinusitis; interstitial pneumonitis; asthma exacerbation; pulmonary infiltrates; fibrosing alveolitis.

►*Special senses:* Ear/Eye pain; taste perversion; blurred vision; tinnitus.

►*Miscellaneous:* Neck pain; abdominal enlargement; facial edema; gout; hypersensitivity pneumonitis; asthenia; breast pain; Kawasaki-like syndrome.

►*Lab test abnormalities:* Elevated AST, ALT, alkaline phosphatase, serum creatinine, BUN, amylase, lipase, GGTP and LDH. Hepatitis occurs rarely. More commonly, asymptomatic elevations of liver enzymes have occurred which usually resolve during continued use or with discontinuation of the drug.

Overdosage

►*Symptoms:* Mesalamine is an aminosalicylate, and symptoms of salicylate toxicity may be possible, such as tinnitus, vertigo, headache, confusion, drowsiness, sweating, hyperventilation, vomiting and diarrhea. Severe intoxication with salicylates can lead to disruption of electrolyte balance and blood pH, hyperthermia and dehydration.

One case of overdosage has been reported. A 3-year-old male ingested 2 g of mesalamine tablets. He was treated with ipecac and charcoal, and no adverse events occurred. Oral doses in mice and rats of ≈ 5000 mg/kg cause significant lethality.

►*Treatment:* Conventional therapy for salicylate toxicity may be beneficial in the event of acute overdosage. This includes prevention of further GI tract absorption by emesis and, if necessary, by gastric lavage. Correct fluid and electrolyte imbalance by the administration of appropriate IV therapy. Maintain adequate renal function.

Patient Information

►*Tablets:* Swallow tablets whole; do not break the outer coating, which is designed to remain intact to protect the active ingredient. In 2% to 3% of patients, intact or partially intact tablets are found in the stool. If this occurs repeatedly, notify the physician.

►*Suppository:* Remove the foil wrapper. Avoid excessive handling of the suppository which is designed to melt at body temperature. Insert completely into rectum with gentle pressure, pointed end first.

OLSALAZINE SODIUM

Rx	**Dipentum** (Celltech)	**Capsules:** 250 mg	(Dipentum 250 mg). Beige. In 100s and 500s.

Indications

Maintenance of remission of ulcerative colitis in patients intolerant of sulfasalazine.

Administration and Dosage

1 g per day in 2 divided doses.

Actions

➤*Pharmacology:* Olsalazine sodium is a sodium salt of a salicylate compound that is effectively bioconverted to 5–aminosalicylic acid (mesalamine; 5–ASA), which has anti-inflammatory activity in ulcerative colitis. Approximately 98% to 99% of an oral dose will reach the colon where each molecule is rapidly converted into two molecules of 5-ASA by colonic bacteria and the low prevailing redox potential found in this environment. More than 0.9 g mesalamine would usually be made available in the colon from 1 g olsalazine. The liberated 5-ASA is absorbed slowly, resulting in very high local concentrations in the colon.

The mechanism of action of mesalamine is unknown, but appears topical rather than systemic. It possibly diminishes colonic inflammation by blocking cyclooxygenase and inhibiting colon prostaglandin production in bowel mucosa.

In rats the kidney is the major target organ of olsalazine toxicity. At an oral daily dose of ≥ 400 mg/kg, olsalazine treatment produced nephritis and tubular necrosis in a 4 week study, interstitial nephritis and tubular calcinosis in a 6 month study and renal fibrosis, mineralization and transitional cell hyperplasia in a 1 year study.

➤*Pharmacokinetics:* After oral administration, ≈ 2.4% of a single 1 g oral dose is absorbed. Maximum serum concentrations appear after approximately 1 hour, and are low (eg, 1.6 to 6.2 mcmol/L) even after a 1 g single dose. Olsalazine has a very short serum half-life of ≈ 0.9 hours and is > 99% bound to plasma proteins. Urinary recovery is < 1%. Total oral olsalazine recovery ranges from 90% to 97%.

About 0.1% of an oral dose is metabolized in liver to olsalazine-O-sulfate (olsalazine-S), which has a half-life of 7 days and accumulates to steady state in 2 to 3 weeks. Patients on daily 1 g doses for 2 to 4 yrs show a stable plasma concentration of olsalazine-S (3.3 to 12.4 mcmol/L). Olsalazine-S is> 99% plasma protein bound. Its long half-life is mainly due to slow dissociation from the protein binding site. Less than 1% of olsalazine and olsalazine-S appears undissociated in plasma.

Serum concentrations of 5-ASA are detected after 4 to 8 hours. The peak levels of 5–ASA after an oral dose of 1 g olsalazine are low (0 to 4.3 mcmol/L). Of the total urinary 5-ASA, > 90% is in the form of N-acetyl-5-ASA (Ac-5-ASA).

Ac-5-ASA is acetylated (deactivated) in ≥ 2 sites, colonic epithelium and liver. Ac-5-ASA is found in serum, with peak values of 1.7 to 8.7 mcmol/L after a single 1 g dose. In urine, ≈ 20% of total 5-ASA is found almost exclusively as Ac-5-ASA. Remaining 5-ASA is partially acetylated and excreted in feces. After dosing, the concentration of 5-ASA in the colon has been calculated to be 18 to 49 mmol/L. No accumulation of 5-ASA or Ac-5-ASA in plasma has been detected. 5–ASA and Ac-5-ASA are 74% and 81% bound to plasma proteins, respectively.

➤*Clinical trials:* In 1 controlled study, ulcerative colitis patients in remission were randomized to olsalazine 500 mg 3 times daily or placebo; relapse rates at 6 months were compared. For the 52 olsalazine patients, 12 relapses occurred; for the 49 placebo patients, 22 relapses occurred. This difference in relapse rates was significant.

In a second controlled study, 164 ulcerative colitis patients in remission were randomized to olsalazine 500 mg twice a day or sulfasalazine 1 g twice a day and relapse rates were compared after 6 months. The relapse rate for olsalazine was 19.5% while that for sulfasalazine was 12.2%; the difference was not significant.

Contraindications

Hypersensitivity to salicylates.

Warnings

➤*Carcinogenesis:* In animals, olsalazine was tested at daily doses of 200 to 2000 mg/kg/day (approximately 10 to 100 times the human maintenance dose). Urinary bladder transitional cell carcinomas were found in three male rats (6%); liver hemangiosarcomata were found in two male mice (4%).

➤*Pregnancy: Category C.* Olsalazine produces fetal developmental toxicity (ie, reduced fetal weights, retarded ossifications and immaturity of visceral organs) when given during organogenesis to pregnant rats in doses 5 to 20 times the human dose (100 to 400 mg/kg). There are no adequate and well controlled studies in pregnant women. Use during pregnancy only if potential benefit justifies potential risk to the fetus.

➤*Lactation:* Oral olsalazine given to lactating rats in doses 5 to 20 times the human dose produced growth retardation in their pups. It is not known whether this drug is excreted in human milk. Exercise caution when administering to a nursing woman.

➤*Children:* Safety and efficacy in children have not been established.

Precautions

➤*Diarrhea:* About 17%, resulting in drug withdrawal in 6%; appears dose-related, but may be difficult to distinguish from underlying disease symptoms.

➤*Exacerbation of the symptoms of colitis:* Exacerbation of the symptoms of colitis, thought to have been caused by mesalamine or sulfasalazine, has been noted.

➤*Renal abnormalities:* Renal abnormalities were not reported in clinical trials with olsalazine; however, the possibility of renal tubular damage due to absorbed mesalamine or its n-acetylated metabolite must be kept in mind, particularly for patients with preexisting renal disease. In these patients, monitor urinalysis, BUN and creatinine determination.

Adverse Reactions

Overall, 10.4% of patients discontinued olsalazine because of an adverse experience compared with 6.7% of placebo patients.

Osalazine Adverse Reactions		
Adverse Reactions	Olsalazine (n = 441)	Placebo (n = 208)
CNS		
Headache	5%	4.8%
Fatigue/Drowsiness/Lethargy	1.8%	2.9%
Depression	1.5%	—
Vertigo/Dizziness	1%	—
Insomnia	—	2.4%
Dermatologic		
Rash	2.3%	1.4%
Itching	1.3%	—
GI		
Diarrhea	11.1%	6.7%
Pain/Cramps	10.1%	7.2%
Nausea	5%	3.9%
Dyspepsia	4%	4.3%
Bloating	1.5%	1.4%
Anorexia	1.3%	1.9%
Vomiting	1%	—
Stomatitis	1%	—
Blood in stool	—	3.4%
Miscellaneous		
Arthralgia	4%	2.9%
Upper respiratory tract infection	1.5%	—
Withdrawal from therapy (No. Patients)		
Diarrhea	26	10
Nausea	3	2
Abdominal pain	5	0
Rash/Itching	5	0
Headache	3	0
Heartburn	2	0
Rectal bleeding	1	0
Insomnia	1	0
Dizziness	1	0
Anorexia	1	0
Lightheadedness	1	0
Depression	1	0
Miscellaneous	4	3

A causal relationship to the drug has not been demonstrated for the following:

➤*Cardiovascular:* Pericarditis; second degree heart block; hypertension; orthostatic hypotension; peripheral edema; chest pains; tachycardia; palpitations; bronchospasm; shortness of breath.

➤*CNS:* Paresthesia; tremors; mood swings; irritability; fever; chills.

➤*Dermatologic:* Erythema nodosum; photosensitivity; erythema; hot flashes; alopecia.

OLSALAZINE SODIUM

➤*GI:* Pancreatitis; rectal bleeding; flare in symptoms; rectal discomfort; epigastric discomfort; flatulence; granulomatous hepatitis and nonspecific, reactive hepatitis. A patient developed mild cholestatic hepatitis with sulfasalazine and when changed to olsalazine 2 weeks later. Withdrawal of olsalazine led to complete recovery.

➤*GU:* Urinary frequency; dysuria; hematuria; proteinuria; impotence; menorrhagia.

➤*Hematologic:* Leukopenia; neutropenia; lymphopenia; eosinophilia; thrombocytopenia; anemia; reticulocytosis.

➤*Lab test abnormalities:* Elevated ALT or AST.

➤*Musculoskeletal:* Muscle cramps.

➤*Special senses:* Dry mouth; dry eyes; watery eyes; blurred vision.

Overdosage

Symptoms of acute toxicity were decreased motor activity and diarrhea in all species tested and, in addition, vomiting in dogs.

Patient Information

Take with food. Take in evenly divided doses.

Contact your physician if diarrhea occurs (reported in $\approx$ 17% of subjects in clinical studies).

BALSALAZIDE DISODIUM

Rx	Colazal (Salix)	Capsules: 750 mg	≈ 86 mg sodium. (CZ). Beige. In 280s.

Indications

➤*Active ulcerative colitis:* Treatment of mildly to moderately active ulcerative colitis.

Administration and Dosage

➤*Approved by the FDA:* July 18, 2000.

➤*Ulcerative colitis:* Take three 750 mg capsules 3 times a day for a total daily dose of 6.75 g for a duration of 8 weeks. Some patients in clinical trials required treatment for ≤ 12 weeks. Safety and efficacy of balsalazide disodium beyond 12 weeks have not been established.

Actions

➤*Pharmacology:* Balsalazide is delivered intact to the colon where it is cleaved by bacterial azoreduction to release equimolar quantities of mesalamine, which is the therapeutically active portion of the molecule and 4-aminobenzoyl-β-alanine. The recommended dose of 6.75 g/day for the treatment of active disease provides 2.4 g of free 5-aminosalicylic acid to the colon.

The 4-aminobenzoyl-β-alanine carrier moiety released when balsalazide is cleaved is only minimally absorbed and is largely inert. The mechanism of action of 5-aminosalicylic acid is unknown but appears to be topical rather than systemic. Mucosal production of arachidonic acid metabolites, both through the cyclooxygenase pathways (eg, prostanoids) and through the lipoxygenase pathways (eg, leukotrienes, hydroxyeicosatetraenoic acids) is increased in patients with chronic inflammatory bowel disease, and it is possible that 5-aminosalicylic acid diminishes inflammation by blocking production of arachidonic acid metabolites in the colon.

➤*Pharmacokinetics:*

Absorption – In healthy individuals, the systemic absorption of intact balsalazide was very low and variable. The mean C_{max} occurs ≈ 1 to 2 hours after single oral doses of 1.5 or 2.25 g. In a study of ulcerative colitis patients receiving balsalazide 1.5 g twice daily for > 1 year, systemic drug exposure, based on mean AUC values, was ≤ 60 times greater (8 to 480 ng•hr/mL) after equivalent multiple doses of 1.5 g twice daily when compared with healthy subjects who received the same dose. There was a large intersubject variability in the plasma concentration of balsalazide vs time profiles in all studies, thus its half-life could not be determined.

Distribution – The binding of balsalazide to human plasma proteins was ≥ 99%.

Metabolism – The products of the azoreduction of this compound, 5-aminosalicylic acid and 4-aminobenzoyl-β-alanine, and their N-acetylated metabolites have been identified in plasma, urine, and feces.

Excretion – Less than 1% of an oral dose was recovered as parent compound, 5-aminosalicylic acid, or 4-aminobenzoyl-β-alanine in the urine of healthy subjects after single and multiple doses of balsalazide while ≤ 25% of the dose was recovered as the N-acetylated metabolites. In a study with 10 healthy volunteers, 65% of a single 2.25 g dose of balsalazide was recovered as 5-aminosalicylic acid, 4-aminobenzoyl-β-alanine, and the N-acetylated metabolites in feces, while < 1% of the dose was recovered as parent compound.

Less than 1% of an oral dose was recovered as intact balsalazide in the urine. Less than 4% of the dose was recovered as 5-aminosalicylic acid, while virtually no 4-aminobenzoyl-β-alanine was detected in urine. The urinary recovery of the N-acetylated metabolites comprised 20% to 25% of the balsalazide dose.

Contraindications

Hypersensitivity to salicylates or any of the components of balsalazide capsules or balsalazide metabolites.

Warnings

➤*Renal function impairment:* There have been no reported incidents of renal impairment in patients taking balsalazide. Renal toxicity has been observed in patients given other mesalamine products. Therefore, exercise caution when administering balsalazide to patients with known renal dysfunction or a history of renal disease.

➤*Pregnancy: Category B.* There are no adequate and well-controlled studies in pregnant women. Use during pregnancy only if the potential benefit justifies the potential risk to the fetus.

➤*Lactation:* It is not known whether balsalazide is excreted in breast milk. Exercise caution when administering to a nursing woman.

➤*Children:* Safety and efficacy of balsalazide in pediatric patients have not been established.

Precautions

➤*Exacerbation of symptoms:* Of the 259 patients treated with 6.75 g/day of balsalazide, exacerbation of the symptoms of colitis, possibly related to drug use, has been reported in 3 patients.

➤*Pyloric stenosis:* Patients with pyloric stenosis may have prolonged gastric retention of balsalazide capsules.

Adverse Reactions

More than 1000 patients received treatment in clinical trials. In 4 controlled trials, patients receiving a balsalazide dose of 6.75 g/day most frequently reported (≥ 3%) the following reactions: Headache (8%); abdominal pain (6%); diarrhea and nausea (5%); vomiting, respiratory infection, and arthralgia (4%). Withdrawal from therapy because of adverse reactions was comparable among patients on balsalazide and placebo.

Balsalazide Adverse Events (≥ 1%)	
Adverse reaction	Balsalazide 6.75 g/day (n = 259)
Headache	8
Abdominal pain	6
Nausea	5
Diarrhea	5
Vomiting	4
Respiratory	4
Arthralgia	4
Rhinitis	2
Insomnia	2
Fatigue	2
Rectal bleeding	2
Flatulence	2
Fever	2
Dyspepsia	2
Pharyngitis	2
Pain	2
Coughing	2
Back pain	2
Anorexia	2
Urinary tract	1
Sinusitis	1
Myalgia	1
Frequent stools	1
Flu-like disorder	1
Dry mouth	1
Dizziness	1
Cramps	1
Constipation	1

Some adverse events, such as abdominal pain, fatigue, and nausea, were reported more frequently in women than in men. Abdominal pain, rectal bleeding, and anemia can be part of the clinical presentation of ulcerative colitis.

The following adverse events have been infrequently reported by patients taking balsalazide during clinical trials (n = 513) for the treatment of active acute ulcerative colitis or from foreign post-marketing reports. In most cases, no relationship to balsalazide has been established.

➤*Cardiovascular:* Bradycardia; deep venous thrombosis; hypertension; leg ulcer; palpitations; pericarditis.

➤*CNS:* Aphasia; dysphonia; abnormal gait; hypertonia; hypoesthesia; paresis; generalized spasm; tremor; anxiety; depression; nervousness; somnolence.

➤*Dermatologic:* Alopecia; angioedema; dermatitis; dry skin; erythema nodosum; erythematous rash; pruritus; pruritus ani; psoriasis; skin ulceration.

➤*GI:* Increased amylase; bowel irregularity; aggravated ulcerative colitis; diarrhea with blood; diverticulosis; epigastric pain; eructation; fecal incontinence; abnormal feces; gastroenteritis; giardiasis; glossitis; hemorrhoids; melena; benign neoplasm; pancreatitis; ulcerative stomatitis; frequent stools; tenesmus; tongue discoloration.

➤*Hematologic:* Anemia; epistaxis; increased plasma fibrinogen; hemorrhage; decreased prothrombin; increased prothrombin; thrombocythemia.

BALSALAZIDE DISODIUM

➤*Hepatic:* Increased bilirubin; abnormal hepatic function; increased AST; increased ALT.

➤*GU:* Menstrual disorder; hematuria; interstitial nephritis; micturition frequency; polyuria; pyuria.

➤*Immunologic:* Abscess; decreased immunoglobins; infection; moniliasis; viral infection.

➤*Lymphatic:* Eosinophilia; granulocytopenia; leukocytosis; leukopenia; lymphadenopathy; lymphoma-like disorder; lymphopenia.

➤*Metabolic/Nutritional:* Increased creatine phosphokinase; hypocalcemia; hypokalemia; hypoproteinemia; increased LDH; weight decrease; weight increase.

➤*Musculoskeletal:* Arthritis; arthropathy; stiffness in legs.

➤*Respiratory:* Bronchospasm; dyspnea; hemoptysis.

➤*Special senses:* Conjunctivitis; earache; ear infection; iritis; parosmia; taste perversion; tinnitus; abnormal vision.

➤*Miscellaneous:* Enlarged abdomen; asthenia; chest pain; chills; edema; hot flushes; malaise.

➤*Postmarketing:* The following events have been identified during post-approval use in clinical practice. Because they are reported voluntarily from a population of unknown size, estimates of frequency cannot be made. These events have been chosen for inclusion because of a combination of seriousness, frequency of reporting, or potential causal connection to mesalamine.

GI – Reports of hepatotoxicity, including elevated liver function tests (AST, ALT, GGT, LDH, alkaline phosphatase, bilirubin), jaundice, cholestatic jaundice, cirrhosis, hepatocellular damage including liver necrosis and liver failure. Some of these cases were fatal; however, no fatalities associated with these events were reported in balsalazide clinical trials. One case of Kawasaki-like syndrome, which included hepatic function changes, was also reported; however, this event was not reported in balsalazide clinical trials.

Overdosage

If an overdose occurs with balsalazide use, treatment should be supportive with particular attention to the correction of electrolyte abnormalities. Refer to General Management of Acute Overdosage.

SULFASALAZINE

Rx	**Sulfasalazine** (Various, eg, Mutual Pharm, Watson)	**Tablets:** 500 mg	In 50s, 100s, 500s and 1000s.
Rx	**Azulfidine** (Pharmacia & Upjohn)		(101 KPh). Gold, scored. In 100s, 300s and UD 100s.
Rx	**Azulfidine EN-tabs** (Pharmacia & Upjohn)	**Tablets, delayed-release:** 500 mg	(102 KPh). Gold, elliptical. Enteric coated. In 100s and 300s.

Sulfasalazine is also indicated for use in rheumatoid arthritis. Refer to the monograph in the Biologic and Immunologic Agents chapter.

Indications

➤*Ulcerative colitis:* In the treatment of mild-to-moderate ulcerative colitis, and as adjunctive therapy in severe ulcerative colitis; for the prolongation of the remission period between acute attacks of ulcerative colitis.

➤*Rheumatoid arthritis (RA; enteric-coated tablets):* For complete prescribing information, refer to the monograph in the Biologic and Immunologic Agents chapter. In the treatment of patients with RA who have responded inadequately to salicylates or other nonsteroidal anti-inflammatory drugs (NSAIDs).

➤*Juvenile rheumatoid arthritis (JRA; enteric-coated tablets):* For complete prescribing information, refer to the monograph in the Biologic and Immunologic Agents chapter. In the treatment of pediatric patients ≥ 6 years of age with polyarticular-course JRA who have responded inadequately to salicylates or other NSAIDs.

➤*Unlabeled uses:* Ankylosing spondylitis; Crohn's disease; psoriatic arthritis (2 g/day).

Administration and Dosage

Individualize dosage. Give the drug in evenly divided doses over each 24-hour period; intervals between nighttime doses should not exceed 8 hours, with administration after meals recommended when feasible. Swallow tablets whole; do not crush or chew. Experience suggests that with daily dosages of ≥ 4 g, the incidence of adverse effects tends to increase. Instruct patients receiving these dosages about the appearance of adverse effects, and carefully observe patients for these effects.

Some patients may be sensitive to treatment with sulfasalazine. Various desensitization-like regimens have been reported to be effective. These regimens suggest starting with a total daily dose of 50 to 250 mg initially, and doubling it every 4 to 7 days until the desired therapeutic level is achieved. If the symptoms of sensitivity recur, discontinue sulfasalazine. Do not attempt desensitization in patients who have a history of agranulocytosis, or who have experienced an anaphylactoid reaction while previously receiving sulfasalazine.

➤*Ulcerative colitis:*
Initial therapy –
   Adults: 3 to 4 g daily in evenly divided doses. It may be advisable to initiate therapy with a lower dosage (eg, 1 to 2 g daily), to reduce possible GI intolerance.
   Children ≥ 2 years of age: 40 to 60 mg/kg body weight in each 24-hour period, divided into 3 to 6 doses.

Maintenance therapy –
   Adults: 2 g daily.
   Children ≥ 2 years of age: 30 mg/kg body weight in each 24-hour period, divided into 4 doses.

It is often necessary to continue medication even when clinical symptoms, including diarrhea, have been controlled. When endoscopic examination confirms satisfactory improvement, reduce dosage to a maintenance level. If diarrhea recurs, increase dosage to previously effective levels.

Actions

➤*Pharmacology:* The mode of action of sulfasalazine or its metabolites, 5-aminosalicyclic acid (5-ASA) and sulfapyridine (SP), is still under investigation, but may be related to the anti-inflammatory or immunomodulatory properties that have been observed in animals and in vitro, to its affinity for connective tissue, or to the relatively high concentration it reaches in serous fluids, the liver, and intestinal walls. In ulcerative colitis, clinical studies utilizing rectal administration of sulfasalazine, SP, and 5-ASA have indicated the major therapeutic action may reside in the 5-ASA moiety. The relative contribution of the parent drug and the major metabolites in RA is unknown.

➤*Pharmacokinetics:*
Absorption – The absolute bioavailability of orally administered sulfasalazine is < 15% for parent drug. In the intestine, sulfasalazine is metabolized by intestinal bacteria to SP and 5-ASA. Of the two, SP is relatively well absorbed from the colon and highly metabolized with an estimated bioavailability of 60%. 5-ASA is much less well absorbed with an estimated bioavailability of 10% to 30%. Detectable serum concentrations of sulfasalazine have been found in healthy subjects within 90 minutes after the dose. In comparison, peak plasma levels of both SP and 5-ASA occur ≈ 10 hours after dosing.

Distribution – Following IV injection, the calculated volume of distribution (Vd_{ss}) for sulfasalazine was ≈ 7.5 L. Sulfasalazine is highly bound to albumin (> 99.3%), while SP is only ≈ 70% bound to albumin. Acetylsulfapyridine (AcSP), the principal metabolite of SP, is ≈ 90% bound to plasma proteins.

Metabolism – The observed plasma half-life for IV sulfasalazine is 7.6 hours. The primary route of metabolism of SP is via acetylation to form AcSP. The rate of metabolism of SP to AcSP is dependent on acetylator phenotype. In fast acetylators, the mean plasma half-life of SP is 10.4 hours, while in slow acetylators it is 14.8 hours. SP can also be metabolized to 5-hydroxy-sulfapyridine (SPOH) and N-acetyl-5-hydroxy-sulfapyridine. 5-ASA is primarily metabolized in both the liver and intestine to N-acetyl-5-aminosalicylic acid via a non-acetylation-phenotype-dependent route. Because of low plasma levels produced by 5-ASA after oral administration, reliable estimates of plasma half-life are not possible.

Excretion – Absorbed SP and 5-ASA and their metabolites are primarily eliminated in the urine either as free metabolites or as glucuronide conjugates. The majority of 5-ASA stays within the colonic lumen and is excreted as 5-ASA and acetyl-5-ASA with the feces. The calculated clearance of sulfasalazine following IV administration was 1 L/hour. Renal clearance was estimated to account for 37% of total clearance.

Elderly – Elderly patients with RA showed a prolonged plasma half-life for sulfasalazine, SP, and their metabolites.

Fast / Slow acetylators – The metabolism of SP to AcSP is mediated by polymorphic enzymes such that two distinct populations of slow and fast metabolizers exist. Approximately 60% of the white population can be classified as belonging to the slow acetylator phenotype. These subjects will display a prolonged plasma half-life for SP (14.8 vs 10.4 hours) and an accumulation of higher plasma levels of SP than fast acetylators. Subjects who were slow acetylators of SP showed a higher incidence of adverse events.

Contraindications

Pediatric patients < 2 years of age; intestinal or urinary obstruction; porphyria; hypersensitivity to sulfasalazine, its metabolites, salicylates, or sulfonamides.

Warnings

➤*Porphyria:* Do not administer sulfonamides to patients with porphyria as these drugs have been reported to precipitate an acute attack.

➤*GI intolerance:* Sulfasalazine enteric-coated tablets are particularly indicated in patients with ulcerative colitis who cannot take uncoated sulfasalazine tablets because of GI intolerance, and in whom there is evidence that this intolerance is not primarily the result of high blood levels of sulfapyridine and its metabolites (eg, patients experiencing nausea and vomiting with the first few doses of the drug, or patients in whom a reduction in dosage does not alleviate the adverse GI effects).

➤*Special risk patients:* The presence of clinical signs such as sore throat, fever, pallor, purpura, or jaundice may be indications of serious blood disorders. Use with caution in patients with severe allergy or bronchial asthma.

➤*Deaths:* Deaths associated with the administration of sulfasalazine have been reported from hypersensitivity reactions, agranulocytosis, aplastic anemia, other blood dyscrasias, renal and liver damage, irreversible neuromuscular and CNS changes, and fibrosing alveolitis. If toxic or hypersensitivity reactions occur, discontinue sulfasalazine immediately.

➤*Renal / Hepatic function impairment:* Only after critical appraisal should sulfasalazine be given to patients with hepatic or renal damage or blood dyscrasias.

➤*Carcinogenesis:* Sulfasalazine was tested at 84, 168 and 337.5 mg/kg/day doses in rats. A statistically significant increase in the incidence of urinary bladder transitional cell papillomas was observed in male rats. In female rats, two (4%) of the 337.5 mg/kg rats had transitional cell papilloma of the kidney. The increased incidence of neoplasms in the urinary bladder and kidney of rats was also associated with an increase in the renal calculi formation and hyperplasia of transitional cell epithelium. For the mouse study, sulfasalazine was tested at 675, 1350 and 2700 mg/kg/day. The incidence of hepatocellular adenoma or carcinoma in male and female mice was significantly greater than the control at all doses tested.

➤*Fertility impairment:* Oligospermia and infertility have been observed in men treated with sulfasalazine. Withdrawal of the drug appears to reverse these effects.

➤*Pregnancy: Category B.* There are no adequate and well-controlled studies in pregnant women. Use during pregnancy only if clearly needed.

A national survey evaluated the outcome of pregnancies associated with inflammatory bowel disease (IBD). In 186 pregnancies in women treated with sulfasalazine alone or sulfasalazine and concomitant steroid therapy, the incidence of fetal morbidity and mortality was compa-

SULFASALAZINE

rable both to that of 245 untreated IBD pregnancies and to pregnancies in the general population.

A study of 1455 pregnancies associated with exposure to sulfonamides, including sulfasalazine, indicated that the group of drugs was not associated with fetal malformation. A review of the medical literature covering 1155 pregnancies in women with ulcerative colitis suggested that the outcome was similar to that expected in the general population.

Sulfasalazine and sulfapyridine pass the placental barrier. Although sulfapyridine has been shown to have poor bilirubin-displacing capacity, there is potential for kernicterus.

➤*Lactation:* Sulfonamides are excreted in breast milk. In newborns, they compete with bilirubin for binding sites on the plasma proteins and may cause kernicterus. Insignificant amounts of uncleaved sulfasalazine have been found in breast milk, whereas the sulfapyridine levels in breast milk are ≈ 30% to 60% of those in the maternal serum. Sulfapyridine has been shown to have a poor bilirubin-displacing capacity. Exercise caution.

➤*Children:* The safety and efficacy of sulfasalazine in pediatric patients < 2 years of age with ulcerative colitis have not been established. It has been reported that the frequency of adverse events in patients with systemic-course juvenile arthritis is high.

Precautions

➤*Monitoring:* Perform complete blood counts, including differential white cell count, and liver function tests before starting sulfasalazine and every second week during the first 3 months of therapy. During the second 3 months, perform the same tests monthly and, thereafter, once every 3 months and as clinically indicated. Also perform urinalysis and an assessment of renal function periodically during treatment.

The determination of serum sulfapyridine levels may be useful because concentrations > 50 mcg/mL appear to be associated with an increased incidence of adverse reactions.

➤*Ulcerative colitis relapse:* Inform patients with this condition that ulcerative colitis rarely remits completely, and that the risk of relapse can be substantially reduced by continued administration of sulfasalazine at a maintenance dosage.

➤*Glucose-6-phosphate dehydrogenase deficiency:* Observe patients with glucose-6-phosphate dehydrogenase deficiency closely for signs of hemolytic anemia. This reaction is frequently dose-related.

➤*Undisintegrated tablets:* Isolated instances have occurred where sulfasalazine enteric-coated tablets have passed undisintegrated. If this is observed, discontinue the administration of the drug immediately.

➤*Adequate fluid intake:* Maintain adequate fluid intake in order to prevent crystalluria and stone formation.

Drug Interactions

Sulfasalazine Drug Interactions			
Precipitant drug	Object drug*		Description
Sulfasalazine	Digoxin	↓	Reduced absorption of digoxin has been reported when coadministered with sulfasalazine.
Sulfasalazine	Folic acid	↓	Reduced GI absorption of folic acid has been reported when coadministered with sulfasalazine. Periodically monitor patients taking sulfasalazine. If folate deficiency is noted, potential treatment measures include increasing dietary folate, giving sulfasalazine between meals, and administering additional folic acid or folinic acid.
Sulfonamides (eg, sulfasalazine)	Sulfonylureas (eg, glipizide)	↑	Sulfonamides may impair hepatic metabolism of sulfonylureas or alter plasma protein binding. Monitor blood glucose and decrease the sulfonylurea dose as necessary.

* ↑ = Object drug increased.   ↓ = Object drug decreased.

Adverse Reactions

The most common adverse reactions associated with sulfasalazine in ulcerative colitis are anorexia, headache, nausea, vomiting, gastric distress, and reversible oligospermia. These occur in ≈ 33% of patients. Less frequent adverse reactions are skin rash, pruritus, urticaria, fever, Heinz body anemia, hemolytic anemia, and cyanosis, which may occur at a frequency of ≤ 1 in 30 patients.

Similar adverse reactions are associated with use in adult RA, although there was a greater incidence of some reactions. In RA studies, the following common adverse reactions were noted: Nausea (19%); dyspepsia, rash (13%); headache (9%); abdominal pain, vomiting (8%); fever (5%); dizziness, stomatitis, pruritus, abnormal liver function tests (4%); leukopenia (3%); thrombocytopenia (1%). One report showed a 10% rate of immunoglobulin suppression, which was slowly reversible and rarely accompanied by clinical findings.

The following adverse reactions occur rarely (≈ ≤ 1 in 1000 patients).

➤*CNS:* Transverse myelitis; convulsions; meningitis; transient lesions of the posterior spinal column; cauda equina syndrome; Guillain-Barré syndrome; peripheral neuropathy; mental depression; vertigo; hearing loss; insomnia; ataxia; hallucinations; tinnitus; drowsiness.

➤*GI:* Hepatitis; pancreatitis; bloody diarrhea; impaired folic acid absorption; impaired digoxin absorption; stomatitis; diarrhea; abdominal pains; neutropenic enterocolitis.

➤*Hematologic:* Aplastic anemia; agranulocytosis; leukopenia; megaloblastic (macrocytic) anemia; purpura; thrombocytopenia; hypoprothrombinemia; methemoglobinemia; congenital neutropenia; myelodysplastic syndrome.

➤*Hypersensitivity:* Erythema multiforme (Stevens-Johnson syndrome); exfoliative dermatitis; epidermal necrolysis (Lyell's syndrome) with corneal damage; anaphylaxis; serum sickness syndrome; pneumonitis with or without eosinophilia; vasculitis; fibrosing alveolitis; pleuritis; pericarditis with or without tamponade; allergic myocarditis; polyarteritis nodosa; lupus erythematosus-like syndrome; hepatitis and hepatic necrosis with or without immune complexes; fulminant hepatitis, sometimes leading to liver transplantation; parapsoriasis variformis acuta (Mucha-Haberman syndrome); rhabdomyolysis; photosensitization; arthralgia; periorbital edema; conjunctival and scleral injection; alopecia.

➤*Renal:* Toxic nephrosis with oliguria and anuria; nephritis; nephrotic syndrome; hematuria; crystalluria; proteinuria; hemolytic-uremic syndrome.

➤*Miscellaneous:* Urine discoloration; skin discoloration.

Children – In general, the adverse reactions in JRA patients are similar to those seen in patients with adult RA except for a high frequency of serum sickness-like syndrome in systemic-course JRA.

Overdosage

➤*Symptoms:* Symptoms of overdosage may include nausea, vomiting, gastric distress, and abdominal pains. In more advanced cases, CNS symptoms (eg, drowsiness, convulsions) may be observed. Serum sulfapyridine concentrations may be used to monitor the progress of recovery from overdosage. Doses of regular sulfasalazine tablets of 16 g/day have been given to patients without mortality.

➤*Treatment:* Gastric lavage or emesis plus catharsis as indicated. Alkalinize urine. If kidney function is normal, force fluids. If anuria is present, restrict fluids and salt, and treat appropriately. Catheterization of the ureters may be indicated for complete renal blockage by crystals. The low molecular weight of sulfasalazine and its metabolites may facilitate their removal by dialysis. For agranulocytosis, discontinue the drug immediately, hospitalize the patient, and institute appropriate therapy.

Patient Information

If sore throat, fever, pallor, purpura, or jaundice occur, have patients contact their physician.

Instruct patients to take sulfasalazine in evenly divided doses, preferably after meals, and to swallow the tablets whole.

Advise patients that sulfasalazine may produce an orange-yellow discoloration of the urine or skin.

Instruct patients to drink plenty of water.

CELECOXIB

Rx	**Celebrex** (Searle)	**Capsules:** 100 mg	Lactose, gelatin. (7767 100). White and blue. In 100s, 500s, and UD 100s.
		200 mg	Lactose, gelatin. (7767 200). White and gold. In 100s, 500s, and UD 100s.
		400 mg	(7767 400). White. In 60s and UD 100s.

For complete prescribing information, refer to the celecoxib monograph in the Central Nervous System chapter.

Indications

➤*Familial adenomatous polyposis (FAP):* To reduce the number of adenomatous colorectal polyps in FAP as an adjunct to usual care (eg, endoscopic surveillance, surgery). It is not known whether there is a clinical benefit from a reduction in the number of colorectal polyps in FAP patients. It is also not known whether the effects of celecoxib treatment will persist after celecoxib is discontinued. The efficacy and safety of celecoxib treatment in patients with FAP > 6 months have not been studied.

Administration and Dosage

➤*FAP:* To reduce the number of adenomatous colorectal polyps in patients with FAP, the recommended oral dose is 400 mg twice daily taken with food. Celecoxib treatment in FAP has not been shown to reduce the risk of GI cancer or the need for prophylactic colectomy or other FAP-related surgeries. Therefore, do not alter the usual care of FAP patients because of the concurrent administration of celecoxib. In particular, do not decrease the frequency of routine endoscopic surveillance and prophylactic colectomy and do not delay other FAP-related surgeries.

➤*Hepatic insufficiency:* Reduce the daily recommended dose of celecoxib capsules in patients with moderate hepatic impairment (Child-Pugh Class II) by ≈ 50%.

Actions

➤*Clinical trials:*

FAP – Celecoxib was evaluated to reduce the number of adenomatous colorectal polyps. A randomized, double-blind, placebo-controlled study was conducted in 83 patients with FAP. The study population included 58 patients with a prior subtotal or total colectomy and 25 patients with an intact colon. Thirteen patients had the attenuated FAP phenotype.

One area in the rectum and up to 4 areas in the colon were identified at baseline for specific follow-up, and polyps were counted at baseline and following 6 months of treatment. The mean reduction in the number of colorectal polyps was 28% for celecoxib 400 mg twice daily, 12% for celecoxib 100 mg twice daily, and 5% for placebo. The reduction in polyps observed with celecoxib 400 mg twice daily was statistically superior to placebo at the 6-month timepoint (p = 0.003).

INFLIXIMAB

| Rx | **Remicade** (Centocor) | **Powder for injection, lyophilized:** 100 mg | 500 mg sucrose. Preservative-free. In 20 mL single-use vials. |

Indications

➤*Rheumatoid arthritis (RA):* In combination with methotrexate for reducing the signs and symptoms and inhibiting the progression of structural damage and improving physical function in patients with moderately to severely active RA who have had an inadequate response to methotrexate.

➤*Crohn disease, moderate to severe:* For reducing signs and symptoms and inducing and maintaining clinical remission in patients with moderately to severely active Crohn disease who have had an inadequate response to conventional therapy.

➤*Crohn disease, fistulizing:* For reducing the number of draining enterocutaneous and rectovaginal fistulas and maintaining fistula closure. The safety and efficacy of therapy continued beyond 3 doses have not been established.

➤*Unlabeled uses:* For possible treatment of plaque psoriasis, ankylosing spondylitis, ulcerative colitis, psoriatic arthritis, psoriasis, Behcet syndrome, uveitis, and juvenile arthritis.

Administration and Dosage

➤*Approved by the FDA:* August 24, 1998.

➤*RA:* 3 mg/kg given as an IV infusion followed with additional similar doses at 2 and 6 weeks after the first infusion, then every 8 weeks thereafter. Give infliximab in combination with methotrexate. For patients who have an incomplete response, consider adjusting the dose up to 10 mg/kg or treating as often as every 4 weeks.

➤*Crohn disease or fistulizing Crohn disease:* 5 mg/kg given as an induction regimen at 0, 2, and 6 weeks followed by a maintenance regimen of 5 mg/kg every 8 weeks thereafter. For patients who respond and then lose their response, consider treatment with 10 mg/kg. Patients who do not respond by week 14 are unlikely to respond with continued dosing; consider discontinuing infliximab in these patients.

➤*Preparation and administration instructions:* Infliximab vials do not contain antibacterial preservatives. Therefore, use the vials immediately after reconstitution. Do not re-enter or store. Reconstitute with 10 mL sterile water for injection. Further dilute the total dose to 250 mL with 0.9% sodium chloride injection. The infusion concentration should range between 0.4 and 4 mg/mL. Begin infusion within 3 hours of preparation.

1.) Calculate the dose and the number of vials needed (each vial contains 100 mg of infliximab). Calculate the total volume of reconstituted solution required.
2.) Reconstitute each infliximab vial with 10 mL sterile water for injection using a syringe equipped with a 21-gauge or smaller needle. Remove the flip top from the vial and wipe the top with an alcohol swab. Insert the syringe needle into the vial through the center of the rubber stopper and direct the stream of sterile water for injection to the glass wall of the vial. Do not use the vial if the vacuum is not present. Gently swirl the solution by rotating the vial to dissolve the lyophilized powder. Avoid prolonged or vigorous agitation. Do not shake. Foaming of the solution on reconstitution is not unusual. Allow the reconstituted solution to stand for 5 minutes. The solution should be colorless to light yellow and opalescent. It may develop a few translucent particles as infliximab is a protein. Do not use if opaque particles, discoloration, or other foreign particles are present.
3.) Dilute the total volume of the reconstituted infliximab solution dose to 250 mL with 0.9% sodium chloride injection (withdraw a volume of 0.9% sodium chloride injection equal to the volume of reconstituted infliximab from the 0.9% sodium chloride injection 250 mL bottle or bag). Slowly add the total volume of reconstituted infliximab solution to the 250 mL infusion bottle or bag. Gently mix.
4.) Administer the infusion solution over a period of not less than 2 hours; an infusion set with an in-line, sterile, nonpyrogenic, low-protein-binding filter (pore size of 1.2 mcm or less) must be used. Do not store or reuse any unused portion of the infusion solution.
5.) No physical biochemical compatibility studies have been conducted to evaluate the coadministration of infliximab with other agents. Do not infuse infliximab concomitantly in the same IV line with other agents.
6.) Inspect parenteral drug products visually for particulate matter and discoloration prior to administration whenever solution and container permit. If visibly opaque particles, discoloration, or other foreign particulates are observed, do not use the solution.

➤*Storage/Stability:* Store the lyophilized product under refrigeration at 2° to 8°C (36° to 46°F). Do not freeze. Do not use beyond the expiration date. This product contains no preservative.

Actions

➤*Pharmacology:* Infliximab is a chimeric IgG1κ monoclonal antibody. It is produced by a recombinant cell line cultured by continuous perfusion and is purified by a series of steps that includes measures to inactivate and remove viruses.

Infliximab neutralizes the biological activity of tumor necrosis factor alpha (TNFα) by high-affinity binding to its soluble and transmembrane forms and inhibits TNFα receptor binding. Infliximab does not neutralize TNFβ (lymphotoxin α), a related cytokine that uses the same receptors as TNFα. Biological activities attributed to TNFα include the following: Induction of proinflammatory cytokines (eg, IL-1, IL-6), leukocyte migration enhancement by increasing endothelial layer permeability and expression of adhesion molecules by endothelial cells and leukocytes, activation of neutrophil and eosinophil functional activity, and induction of acute phase reactants and other liver proteins, as well as tissue-degrading enzymes produced by synoviocytes and/or chondrocytes. Cells expressing transmembrane TNFα bound by infliximab can be lysed in vitro or in vivo. Infliximab inhibits the functional activity of TNFα in a wide variety of in vitro bioassays using human fibroblasts, endothelial cells, neutrophils, B- and T-lymphocytes, and epithelial cells. Anti-TNFα antibodies reduce disease activity in the cotton-top tamarin colitis model and decrease synovitis and joint erosions in a murine model of collagen-induced arthritis. Infliximab prevents disease in transgenic mice that develop polyarthritis as a result of constitutive expression of human TNFα, and, when administered after disease onset, allows eroded joints to heal.

Elevated concentrations of TNFα have been found in the joints of RA patients and the stools of Crohn disease patients and correlate with elevated disease activity. In Crohn disease, infliximab reduces infiltration of inflammatory cells and TNFα production in inflamed areas of the intestine and reduces the proportion of mononuclear cells from the lamina propria able to express TNFα and interferon. In RA, treatment with infliximab reduced infiltration of inflammatory cells into inflamed areas of the joint as well as expression of molecules mediating cellular adhesion and vascular cell adhesion molecule-1, chemoattraction, and tissue degradation. After treatment with infliximab, patients with Crohn disease or RA have decreased levels of serum IL-6 and C-reactive protein compared with baseline. However, peripheral blood lymphocytes from infliximab-treated patients showed no significant decrease in number or in proliferative responses to in vitro mitogenic stimulation when compared with cells from untreated patients.

➤*Pharmacokinetics:* A study of single IV infusions of 3 to 20 mg/kg in Crohn disease or RA patients showed a linear relationship between the dose and the maximum serum concentration. The volume of distribution at steady state was independent of dose and indicated that infliximab was distributed primarily within the vascular compartment. The median terminal half-life of infliximab ranged between 8 to almost 10 days.

No systemic accumulation of infliximab occurred upon continued repeated administration at 4- or 8-week intervals following the initial 0, 2, and 6 week induction regimen.

Contraindications

In patients with moderate or severe (NYHA Class III/IV) CHF (see Warnings).

Hypersensitivity to any murine proteins or other components of the product.

Warnings

➤*CHF:* Do not administer doses greater than 5 mg/kg to patients with CHF. Use infliximab with caution in patients with mild heart failure (NYHA Class I/II). Monitor patients closely; infliximab must not be continued in patients who develop new or worsening symptoms of heart failure.

In a study evaluating infliximab in NYHA Class III/IV CHF patients (left ventricular ejection fraction 35% or less), higher incidences of mortality and hospitalization because of worsening heart failure were seen in infliximab-treated patients, especially those treated with 10 mg/kg. One hundred and fifty patients were treated with 3 infusions of infliximab 5 or 10 mg/kg or placebo over 6 weeks. At 28 weeks, 4 of 101 patients treated with infliximab (1 at 5 mg/kg and 3 at 10 mg/kg) died, compared with no deaths among the 49 placebo-treated patients. In follow-up at 38 weeks, 9 patients treated with infliximab (2 at 5 mg/kg and 7 at 10 mg/kg) died, compared with 1 death among the placebo-treated patients. At 28 weeks, 14 of 101 patients treated with infliximab (3 at 5 mg/kg and 11 at 10 mg/kg) were hospitalized for worsening CHF compared with 5 of the 49 placebo-treated patients.

➤*Risk of infections:* Serious infections, including sepsis, have been reported in patients receiving TNF-blocking agents. Some of these infections have been fatal. Many of the serious infections in patients treated with infliximab occurred in patients on concomitant immuno-

INFLIXIMAB

suppressive therapy that, in addition to their Crohn disease or RA, could predispose them to infections. Do not give infliximab to patients with a clinically important active infection. Exercise caution when considering the use of infliximab in patients with a chronic infection or a history of recurrent infections. Monitor patients for signs and symptoms of infection while on or after treatment with infliximab. Closely monitor new infections. If a patient develops a serious infection, discontinue infliximab therapy (see Warning Box, Adverse Reactions).

Cases of histoplasmosis, coccidioidomycosis, listeriosis, pneumocystosis, tuberculosis, other bacterial, mycobacterial, and fungal infections have been observed in patients receiving infliximab. For patients who have resided in regions where histoplasmosis or coccidioidomycosis is endemic, carefully consider the benefits and risks of infliximab treatment before initiation of infliximab therapy.

➤*Autoimmunity:* Treatment with infliximab therapy may result in the formation of autoantibodies and, rarely, in the development of a lupus-like syndrome. Discontinue treatment if a patient develops symptoms suggestive of a lupus-like syndrome following treatment with infliximab.

➤*Neurologic events:* Infliximab and other agents that inhibit TNF have been associated in rare cases with optic neuritis, seizure, and new onset or exacerbation of clinical symptoms and/or radiographic evidence of CNS demyelinating disorders, including multiple sclerosis. Exercise caution in considering the use of infliximab in patients with pre-existing or recent-onset CNS demyelinating or seizure disorders.

➤*Hypersensitivity reactions:* Infliximab has been associated with hypersensitivity reactions that vary in their time of onset. Urticaria, dyspnea, and hypotension have occurred during or within 2 hours of infliximab infusion. However, in some cases, serum sickness-like reactions have been observed in Crohn disease patients 3 to 12 days after infliximab therapy was reinstituted following an extended period without infliximab treatment. Symptoms associated with these reactions include the following: Fever, rash, headache, sore throat, myalgias, polyarthralgias, hand and facial edema, dysphagia. These reactions were associated with a marked increase in antibodies to infliximab, loss of detectable serum concentrations of infliximab, and possible loss of drug efficacy. Discontinue infliximab for severe reactions. Have medications for the treatment of hypersensitivity reactions (eg, acetaminophen, antihistamines, corticosteroids, epinephrine) available for immediate use in the event of a reaction. Refer to Management of Acute Hypersensitivity Reactions.

➤*Elderly:* Because there is a higher incidence of infections in the elderly population in general, use caution when treating the elderly.

➤*Pregnancy: Category B.* No evidence of maternal toxicity, embryotoxicity, or teratogenicity was observed in a developmental toxicity study conducted in mice. Doses up to 40 mg/kg were shown to produce no adverse effects in animal reproduction studies. It is not known whether infliximab can cause fetal harm when administered to a pregnant woman or can affect reproduction capacity. Give to a pregnant woman only if clearly needed.

➤*Lactation:* It is not known whether infliximab is excreted in human breast milk or absorbed systemically after ingestion. Because of the potential for adverse reactions in nursing infants from infliximab, decide whether to discontinue nursing or discontinue the drug, taking into account the importance of the drug to the mother.

➤*Children:* Safety and efficacy have not been established.

Precautions

➤*Malignancy:* Patients with a long duration of Crohn disease or RA and chronic exposure to immunosuppressant therapies are more prone to develop lymphomas (see Adverse Reactions). The impact of infliximab treatment on these phenomena is unknown.

➤*Immunogenicity:* Treatment with infliximab can be associated with the development of antibodies to infliximab. The incidence of antibodies to infliximab in patients given a 3-dose induction regimen followed by maintenance dosing was approximately 10%. A higher incidence of antibodies to infliximab was observed in Crohn disease patients receiving infliximab after drug-free intervals of more than 16 weeks. The majority of antibody-positive patients had low titers. Patients who were antibody-positive were more likely to experience an infusion reaction. Antibody development was lower among Crohn disease and RA patients receiving immunosuppressant therapies such as 6-mercaptopurine, azathioprine, and methotrexate.

➤*Vaccinations:* No data are available on the response to vaccination or on the secondary transmission of infection by live vaccines in patients receiving anti-TNF therapy. Do not coadminister live vaccines.

Adverse Reactions

The most common reasons for discontinuation of treatment were infusion-related reactions (eg, dyspnea, flushing, headache, rash). Adverse events have been reported in a higher proportion of RA patients receiving the 10 mg/kg dose than the 3 mg/kg dose; however, no differences were observed in the frequency of adverse events between the 5 and 10 mg/kg doses in patients with Crohn disease.

Infusion-related reactions –

Acute infusion reactions: An infusion reaction was defined as any adverse event occurring during the infusion or within 1 to 2 hours after the infusion. In all clinical trials, approximately 20% of infliximab-treated patients experienced an infusion reaction compared with 10% of placebo-treated patients. Among all infliximab infusions, 3% were accompanied by nonspecific symptoms such as fever or chills; 1% were accompanied by cardiopulmonary reactions (eg, primarily chest pain, hypotension, hypertension, dyspnea); and less than 1% were accompanied by pruritus, urticaria, or the combined symptoms of pruritus/urticaria and cardiopulmonary reactions. Serious infusion reactions occurred in less than 1% of patients and included anaphylaxis, convulsions, erythematous rash, and hypotension. Approximately 3% of patients discontinued infliximab because of infusion reactions, and all patients recovered with treatment and/or discontinuation of infusion. Infliximab infusions beyond the initial infusion were not associated with a higher incidence of reactions.

Patients who became positive for antibodies to infliximab were more likely (approximately 2- to 3-fold) to develop infusion reactions than those who were negative. Use of concomitant immunosuppressant agents appeared to reduce the frequency of antibodies to infliximab and infusion reactions.

Reactions following readministration: In a study in which 37 of 41 patients with Crohn disease retreated with infliximab following a 2- to 4-year period without infliximab treatment, 10 patients experienced adverse events manifesting 3 to 12 days following infusion, of which 6 were considered serious. Signs and symptoms included myalgia and/or arthralgia with fever and/or rash; some patients also experienced pruritus, facial, hand, or lip edema, dysphagia, urticaria, sore throat, and headache. Patients experiencing these adverse events had not experienced infusion-related adverse events associated with their initial infliximab therapy. Of these patients, adverse events occurred in 9 of 23 (39%) who had received the liquid formulation, which is no longer in use, and 1 of 14 (7%) who received the lyophilized formulation. The clinical data are not adequate to determine if occurrence of these reactions is due to differences in formulation. Patients' signs and symptoms improved substantially or resolved with treatment in all cases. There are insufficient data on the incidence of these events after drug-free intervals of 1 to 2 years. However, these events have been observed infrequently in clinical trials and postmarketing surveillance at intervals of up to 1 year.

Infections – In infliximab clinical trials, treated infections were reported by 35% of infliximab-treated patients (average of 53 weeks of follow-up) and by 26% of placebo-treated patients (average of 41 weeks of follow-up). When longer observation of patients on infliximab was accounted for, the event rate was similar for both groups. The infections most frequently reported were respiratory tract infections (eg, sinusitis, pharyngitis, bronchitis) and urinary tract infections. No increased risk of serious infections or sepsis has been observed with infliximab compared with placebo. Among infliximab-treated patients, these serious infections included pneumonia, abscess, skin ulceration, bacterial infection, cellulitis, and sepsis. Three opportunistic infections were reported; coccidioidomycosis (which resulted in death), nocardiosis, and cytomegalovirus. Tuberculosis was reported in 2 patients, 1 of whom died due to miliary tuberculosis. Other cases of tuberculosis, including disseminated tuberculosis, also have been reported postmarketing. Most of the cases of tuberculosis occurred within the first 2 months after initiation of therapy with infliximab and may reflect recrudescence of latent disease. Fifteen percent of patients with fistulizing Crohn's disease developed a new fistula-related abscess during a 54-week trial.

Auto-antibodies/lupus-like syndrome – Approximately 52% of infliximab-treated patients in clinical trials who were antinuclear antibody (ANA) negative at baseline developed a positive ANA during the trial compared with approximately 19% of placebo-treated patients. Anti-dsDNA antibodies were newly detected in approximately 17% of infliximab-treated patients compared with 0% of placebo-treated patients. Reports of lupus and lupus-like syndromes, however, remain uncommon.

In clinical studies, 6 patients were diagnosed with a possible lupus-like syndrome, 3 with RA and 3 with Crohn's disease. All 6 patients improved following discontinuation of therapy and appropriate medical treatment. No patients had CNS or renal involvement. No cases of lupus-like reactions have been observed in up to 3 years of long-term follow-up.

Malignancies/Lymphoproliferative disease – In completed clinical studies of infliximab for up to 102 weeks, 18 of 1678 patients developed 19 new or recurrent malignancies. These were non-Hodgkin B-cell lymphoma, breast cancer, melanoma, squamous, rectal adenocarcinoma, and basal cell carcinoma. There are insufficient data to determine whether infliximab contributed to the development of these malignancies. The observed rates and incidences were similar to those expected for the populations studied (see Precautions).

Other adverse reactions – Safety data are available from 1678 infliximab-treated patients, including 555 with RA, 1106 with Crohn disease, and 17 with conditions other than RA or Crohn disease. Adverse events reported in 5% or more of all patients with RA receiving 4 or more infusions are in the following table. The types and frequencies of adverse reactions observed were similar in infliximab-treated

INFLIXIMAB

RA and Crohn disease patients except for abdominal pain which occurred in 26% of infliximab-treated patients with Crohn disease. In the Crohn disease studies, there were insufficient numbers and duration of follow-up for patients who never received infliximab to provide meaningful comparisons.

Infliximab Adverse Reactions Occurring in Patients Receiving ≥ 4 Infusions for RA (≥ 5%)		
Adverse reaction	Infliximab (n = 430)	Placebo (n = 81)
CNS		
Headache	29	21
Fatigue	13	9
Insomnia	6	4
Depression	8	2
Dermatologic		
Rash	18	7
Pruritus	9	2
GI		
Nausea	24	23
Diarrhea	19	19
Abdominal pain	17	12
Dyspepsia	10	9
Musculoskeletal		
Arthralgia	13	7
Back pain	13	5
Myalgia	6	6
Respiratory		
Upper respiratory tract infection	40	35
Pharyngitis	17	12
Sinusitis	20	7
Coughing	18	9
Dyspnea	6	2
Rhinitis	14	14
Miscellaneous		
Urinary tract infection	14	12
Fever	13	11
Chest pain	7	6
Moniliasis	8	2
Hypertension	10	6
Abscess	6	5

The most common serious adverse events observed in clinical trials were infections. Other serious adverse events occurring in 0.2% or more or clinically significant adverse events by body system were as follows:

➤*Cardiovascular:* MI; circulatory failure; hypotension; syncope; arrhythmia; bradycardia; cardiac arrest; tachycardia; pulmonary edema; brain infarction; thrombophlebitis.

➤*CNS:* Meningitis; neuritis; peripheral neuropathy; confusion; dizziness; suicide attempt.

➤*Dermatologic:* Increased sweating; ulceration.

➤*GI:* Constipation; ileus; GI hemorrhage; intestinal obstruction; intestinal perforation; intestinal stenosis; pancreatitis; peritonitis; proctalgia.

➤*Hematologic:* Hemolytic anemia; anemia; thrombocytopenia; leukopenia; pancytopenia.

➤*Hepatic:* Cholelithiasis; hepatitis; cholecystitis; biliary pain.

➤*Musculoskeletal:* Intervertebral disk herniation; tendon disorder.

➤*Respiratory:* Lower respiratory tract infection; adult respiratory distress syndrome; pleural effusion; pleurisy; respiratory insufficiency; pulmonary embolism.

➤*Miscellaneous:* Allergic reaction; surgical/procedural sequelae; serum sickness; menstrual irregularity; renal failure; dehydration; diaphragmatic hernia; edema; basal cell and breast neoplasms; lymphoma; cellulitis; sepsis; lymphadenopathy; renal calculus.

A greater proportion of patients in an RA trial who received infliximab plus methotrexate experienced transient mild (less than 2 times the upper limit of normal) or moderate (greater than or equal to 2 but less than 3 times the upper limit of normal) elevations in AST or ALT (49% and 47%, respectively) compared with patients treated with placebo plus methotrexate (27% and 35%, respectively). Six (1.8%) patients treated with infliximab and methotrexate experienced more prolonged elevations in their ALT.

➤*Postmarketing:* In postmarketing experience, infections have been observed with various pathogens including viral, bacterial, fungal, and protozoal organisms. Infections have been noted in all organ systems and have been reported in patients receiving infliximab alone or in combination with immunosuppressive agents.

Additional adverse events reported from postmarketing experience with infliximab include demyelinating disorders (eg, multiple sclerosis, optic neuritis), Guillain-Barré syndrome, interstitial pneumonitis/fibrosis, neuropathies, hemolytic anemia, idiopathic thrombocytic purpura, thrombotic thrombocytopenic purpura, and transverse myelitis.

In postmarketing experience, cases of anaphylactic-like reactions, including laryngeal/pharyngeal edema and severe bronchospasm, and seizure have been associated with infliximab administration.

Overdosage

Single doses up to 20 mg/kg have been administered without any direct toxic effect. In case of overdosage, it is recommended that the patient be monitored for any signs or symptoms of adverse reactions or effects and appropriate symptomatic treatment instituted immediately.

Patient Information

Tuberculosis, invasive fungal infections, and other serious infections that can be fatal may occur in patients who take this medicine. Patients receiving this medicine should be tested for hidden tuberculosis infection with a skin test. Tuberculosis should be treated before starting this medicine.

Do not use this medication if you are allergic to any ingredient in this medicine including mouse-derived proteins.

Contact your doctor at once if severe rash, hives, difficulty breathing, fainting, or other signs of an allergic reaction occur.

Update immunizations before starting this medicine.

Avoid vaccinations with live virus vaccines (eg, measles, mumps, oral polio) while you are taking this medicine. Vaccinations may be less effective.

This medicine may cause dizziness. Use caution while driving or performing other tasks requiring alertness, coordination, or physical dexterity.

TEGASEROD MALEATE

Rx **Zelnorm** (Novartis)	**Tablet:** 2 mg	Lactose. (NVR DL). In UD 60s.
	6 mg	Lactose. (NVR EH). In UD 60s.

Indications

➤*Irritable bowel syndrome (IBS):* For the short-term treatment of women with IBS whose primary bowel symptom is constipation.

The safety and efficacy of tegaserod in men have not been established.

Administration and Dosage

➤*Approved by the FDA:* July 24, 2002.

➤*Dose:* The recommended dose is 6 mg taken twice daily orally before meals for 4 to 6 weeks. For those patients who respond to therapy at 4 to 6 weeks, an additional 4- to 6-week course may be considered.

The efficacy of tegaserod beyond 12 weeks has not been studied.

➤*Storage/Stability:* Store at 25°C (77°F); excursions permitted to 15° to 30°C (59° to 86°F). Protect from moisture.

Actions

➤*Pharmacology:* Tegaserod is a 5-HT$_4$ receptor partial agonist that binds with high affinity at human 5-HT$_4$ receptors, whereas it has no appreciable affinity for 5-HT$_3$ or dopamine receptors. It has moderate affinity for 5-HT$_1$ receptors. Tegaserod, by acting as an agonist at neuronal 5-HT$_4$ receptors, triggers the release of further neurotransmitters such as calcitonin gene-related peptide from sensory neurons. The activation of 5-HT$_4$ receptors in the GI tract stimulates the peristaltic reflex and intestinal secretion, as well as inhibits visceral sensitivity. In vivo studies showed that tegaserod enhanced basal motor activity and normalized impaired motility throughout the GI tract. In addition, studies demonstrated that tegaserod moderated visceral sensitivity during colorectal distention in animals.

➤*Pharmacokinetics:*

Absorption – Peak plasma concentrations are reached approximately 1 hour after oral dosing. The absolute bioavailability of tegaserod when administered to fasting subjects is approximately 10%. The pharmacokinetics are dose-proportional over the 2 to 12 mg range given twice daily for 5 days. There was no clinically relevant accumulation of tegaserod in plasma when a 6 mg twice-daily dose was given for 5 days.

Distribution – Tegaserod is approximately 98% bound to plasma proteins, predominantly alpha-1-acid glycoprotein. Tegaserod exhibits pronounced distribution into tissues following IV dosing with a volume of distribution at steady state of approximately 368 L.

Metabolism – Tegaserod is metabolized mainly via 2 pathways. The first is a presystemic acid catalyzed hydrolysis in the stomach followed by oxidation and conjugation that produces the main metabolite of tegaserod, 5-methoxyindole-3-carboxylic acid glucuronide. The main metabolite has negligible affinity for 5-HT$_4$ receptors in vitro. In humans, systemic exposure to tegaserod was not altered at neutral gastric pH values. The second metabolic pathway of tegaserod is direct glucuronidation that leads to generation of 3 isomeric N-glucuronides.

Excretion – The plasma clearance of tegaserod is approximately 77 L/h with an estimated terminal half-life (t$_{1/2}$) of approximately 11 hours following IV dosing. Approximately two thirds of the orally administered dose of tegaserod is excreted unchanged in the feces, with the remaining one third excreted in the urine, primarily as the main metabolite.

Special populations –

  Renal function impairment: In subjects with severe renal impairment requiring dialysis (Ccr 15 mL/min/1.73 m^2 or less), C$_{max}$ and AUC of the main pharmacologically inactive metabolite of tegaserod increased 2- and 10-fold, respectively, in subjects with severe renal impairment compared with healthy controls. No dosage adjustment is required in patients with mild to moderate renal impairment. Tegaserod is not recommended in patients with severe renal impairment.

  Hepatic function impairment: In subjects with mild hepatic impairment, mean AUC was 31% higher and C$_{max}$ 16% higher compared with subjects with normal hepatic function. No dosage adjustment is required in patients with mild impairment; however, caution is recommended when using tegaserod in this patient population. Tegaserod has not been studied adequately in patients with moderate and severe hepatic impairment and, therefore, is not recommended in these patients.

Contraindications

Severe renal impairment; moderate or severe hepatic impairment; history of bowel obstruction, symptomatic gallbladder disease, suspected sphincter of Oddi dysfunction, or abdominal adhesions; known hypersensitivity to the drug or any of its excipients.

Warnings

➤*Carcinogenesis:* In mice, dietary administration of tegaserod for 104 weeks produced mucosal hyperplasia and adenocarcinoma of the small intestine at 600 mg/kg/day. There was no evidence of carcinogenicity at a lower dose of 200 or 60 mg/kg/day.

➤*Pregnancy:* Category B. Reproduction studies have been performed in rats at oral doses of up to 100 mg/kg/day (approximately 15 times the human exposure at 6 mg twice daily based on plasma AUC$_{0-24h}$) and rabbits at oral doses of up to 120 mg/kg/day (approximately 51 times the human exposure at 6 mg twice daily based on plasma AUC$_{0-24h}$) and have revealed no evidence of impaired fertility or harm to the fetus caused by tegaserod. Because animal reproduction studies are not always predictive of human response, use this drug during pregnancy only if clearly needed.

➤*Lactation:* Tegaserod and its metabolites are excreted in the milk of lactating rats with a high milk-to-plasma ratio. It is not known whether tegaserod is excreted in human milk. Many drugs that are excreted in human milk have potential for serious adverse reactions in nursing infants. Based on the potential for tumorigenicity shown for tegaserod in the mouse carcinogenicity study, decide whether to discontinue nursing or discontinue the drug, taking into account the importance of the drug to the mother.

➤*Children:* Safety and efficacy have not been established in children under 18 years of age.

Precautions

➤*Diarrhea:* Do not initiate tegaserod in patients who are currently experiencing or frequently experience diarrhea. Discontinue tegaserod immediately in patients with new or sudden worsening of abdominal pain. The majority of tegaserod patients reporting diarrhea had a single episode. In most cases, diarrhea occurred within the first week of treatment. Typically, diarrhea resolved with continued therapy. Patients should consult their physician if they experience severe diarrhea or if the diarrhea is accompanied by severe cramping, abdominal pain, or dizziness.

In the Phase 3 clinical studies, 8.8% of patients receiving tegaserod reported diarrhea as an adverse experience compared with 3.8% of patients receiving placebo. Overall, the discontinuation rate from the studies because of diarrhea was 1.6% among the tegaserod-treated patients.

In 2 clinical studies of 4 to 8 weeks duration designed to assess the safety and tolerability of tegaserod in IBS patients with diarrhea as a predominant symptom (N = 162), no serious adverse events were observed; 6% of tegaserod-treated patients discontinued treatment because of diarrhea or abdominal pain.

➤*Abdominal surgeries:* An increase in abdominal surgeries was observed on tegaserod (0.3%) vs placebo (0.2%) in the Phase 3 clinical studies. The increase was primarily because of a numerical imbalance in cholecystectomies reported in patients treated with tegaserod (0.17%) vs placebo (0.06%). A causal relationship between abdominal surgeries and tegaserod has not been established.

Drug Interactions

Tegaserod Drug Interactions

Precipitant drug	Object drug*		Description
Tegaserod	Digoxin	↓	Coadministration reduces peak plasma concentrations and exposure of digoxin ≈ 15%. This reduction of bioavailability is not considered clinically relevant and, therefore, a dose adjustment is unlikely to be required.
Tegaserod	Oral contraceptives	↓	Coadministration reduced peak concentrations and exposure of levonorgestrel 8%. This is not expected to alter the risk of ovulation and, therefore, no alteration in contraceptive therapy is necessary.

↓ = Object drug decreased.

➤*Drug/Food interactions:* When the drug is administered with food, the bioavailability of tegaserod is reduced 40% to 65% and C$_{max}$ by approximately 20% to 40%. Similar reductions in plasma concentration occur when tegaserod is administered to subjects within 30 minutes prior to a meal or 2.5 hours after a meal. T$_{max}$ of tegaserod is prolonged from approximately 1 hour to 2 hours when taken following a meal, but decreased to 0.7 hours when taken 30 minutes prior to a meal.

Adverse Reactions

Tegaserod Adverse Reactions Occurring in ≥ 1% of IBS Patients vs Placebo

Adverse reaction	Tegaserod 6 mg twice daily (n = 1327)	Placebo (n = 1305)
CNS		
Headache	15	12
Dizziness	4	3
Migraine	2	1

TEGASEROD MALEATE

Tegaserod Adverse Reactions Occurring in ≥ 1% of IBS Patients vs Placebo		
Adverse reaction	Tegaserod 6 mg twice daily (n = 1327)	Placebo (n = 1305)
GI		
Abdominal pain	12	11
Diarrhea	9	4
Nausea	8	7
Flatulence	6	5
Musculoskeletal		
Back pain	5	4
Arthropathy	2	1
Miscellaneous		
Accidental trauma	3	2
Leg pain	1	< 1

The following adverse events also occurred during treatment with tegaserod:

➤*Cardiovascular:* Hypotension, angina pectoris, syncope, arrhythmia, bundle branch block, supraventricular tachycardia.

➤*CNS:* Attempted suicide, impaired concentration, emotional lability, increased appetite, sleep disorder, depression, vertigo.

➤*Dermatologic:* Pruritus, increased sweating, flushing.

➤*GI:* Irritable colon, fecal incontinence, tenesmus, increased appetite, eructation, increased AST, increased ALT, bilirubinemia, cholecystitis, appendicitis, subileus.

➤*GU:* Ovarian cyst, miscarriage, menorrhagia, albuminuria, frequent micturition, polyuria, renal pain.

➤*Musculoskeletal:* Back pain, cramps.

➤*Miscellaneous:* Pain, facial edema, increased creatine phosphokinase, breast carcinoma, asthma.

➤*Postmarketing:*
GI – Suspected sphincter of Oddi spasm, bile duct stone, and cholecystitis with elevated transaminases.

Overdosage

There have been no reports of human overdosage with tegaserod. Single oral doses of 120 mg of tegaserod were administered to 3 healthy volunteers in 1 study. All 3 subjects developed diarrhea and headache. Two of these subjects also reported intermittent abdominal pain, and 1 developed orthostatic hypotension. In 28 healthy subjects exposed to doses of tegaserod from 90 to 180 mg/day for several days, adverse events were diarrhea (100%), headache (57%), abdominal pain (18%), flatulence (18%), nausea (7%), and vomiting (7%).

Based on the large distribution volume and high protein binding of tegaserod, it is unlikely that tegaserod could be removed by dialysis. In cases of overdosage, treat symptomatically and institute supportive measures as appropriate.

Patient Information

Advise patients to take tegaserod before a meal.

Indications

➤*Constipation:* Treatment of constipation.

➤*Rectal/Bowel examinations:* Certain stimulant, lubricant, and saline laxatives are used to evacuate the colon for rectal and bowel examinations.

➤*Prophylaxis:* Laxatives, generally **fecal softeners** or **mineral oil**, are useful prophylactically in patients who should not strain during defecation (ie, following anorectal surgery, MI).

➤*Psyllium:* Useful in patients with irritable bowel syndrome and diverticular disease.

➤*Polycarbophil:* For constipation or diarrhea associated with conditions such as irritable bowel syndrome and diverticulosis; acute non-specific diarrhea.

➤*Mineral oil (enema):* Relief of fecal impaction.

➤*Docusate sodium:* Prevention of dry, hard stools.

➤*Unlabeled uses:* **Psyllium** appears to be useful in the reduction of cholesterol levels as an adjunct to a dietary program.

Actions

➤*Pharmacology:* Laxatives function by promoting active electrolyte secretion, decreasing water and electrolyte absorption, increasing intraluminal osmolarity, or increasing hydrostatic pressure in the gut.

	Laxatives	Onset of action (hr)	Site of action	Mechanism of action	Comments
Saline	Dibasic sodium phosphate[1,2] Magnesium citrate Magnesium hydroxide Magnesium sulfate Monobasic sodium phosphate[1,2] Sodium biphosphate[1]	0.5-3	Small and large intestine	Attract/Retain water in intestinal lumen, increasing intraluminal pressure; cholecystokinin release.	May alter fluid and electrolyte balance. Sulfate salts are considered the most potent.
Stimulant/Irritant	Cascara	6-8	Colon	Direct action on intestinal mucosa or nerve plexus; alters water and electrolyte secretion.	May prefer castor oil when more complete evacuation is required.
	Bisacodyl tablets Casanthranol Senna	6-10			
	Bisacodyl suppository	0.25-1			
Bulk-producing	Methylcellulose Polycarbophil Psyllium	12-72	Small and large intestine	Holds water in stool to increase bulk-stimulating peristalsis; forms emollient gel.	Safe; minimal side effects. Take with plenty of water (240 mL/dose).
Emollient	Mineral oil	6-8	Colon	Retards colonic absorption of fecal water; softens stool.	May decrease absorption of fat-soluble vitamins.
Fecal softeners/ Surfactants	Docusate[3]	12-72	Small and large intestine	Facilitates admixture of fat and water to soften stool.	Beneficial in anorectal conditions in which passage of a firm stool is painful.
Hyperosmotic	Glycerin suppository	0.25-1	Colon	Local irritation; hyperosmotic action.	Sodium stearate in preparation causes local irritation.
	Lactulose	24-48	Colon	Osmotic effect retains fluid in the colon, lowering the pH and increasing colonic peristalsis.	Also indicated in portal-systemic encephalopathy.
Miscellaneous	Castor oil	2-6	Small intestine	Direct action on intestinal mucosa or nerve plexus; alters water and electrolyte secretion.	Castor oil is converted to ricinoleic acid (active component) in the gut.

Table heading: Pharmacologic Actions of Laxatives

[1] Onset of action for rectal preparations is 2 to 15 minutes.
[2] Colon is site of action for rectal preparations.

[3] Site of action for potassium salt is in the colon.

Calcium polycarbophil is a hydrophilic agent. As a bulk laxative, it retains free water within the intestinal lumen and indirectly opposes dehydrating forces of the bowel, promoting well-formed stools. In diarrhea, when the intestinal mucosa is incapable of absorbing water at normal rates, it absorbs free fecal water, forming a gel and producing formed stools. Thus, in diarrhea and constipation, it works by restoring a more normal moisture level and providing bulk.

Lactulose, a synthetic disaccharide analog of lactose containing galactose and fructose, decreases blood ammonia concentrations and reduces the degree of portal-systemic encephalopathy.

The human GI tissue does not have an enzyme capable of hydrolysis of this disaccharide; as a result, oral doses pass to the colon virtually unchanged. After reaching the colon, lactulose is metabolized by bacteria resulting in the formation of lactic acid, formic acid, acetic acid, and carbon dioxide. These products produce an increased osmotic pressure and slightly acidify the colonic contents, resulting in an increase in stool water content and stool softening. Because the colonic contents are more acidic than the blood, ammonia can migrate from the blood into the colon. The acid colonic contents convert NH_3 to the ammonium ion $[NH_4]^+$, trapping it and preventing its absorption. The laxative action of the lactulose metabolites then expels the trapped ammonium ion from the colon.

➤*Pharmacokinetics:* **Lactulose** is poorly absorbed. When given orally, only small amounts reach the blood. Urinary excretion is ≤ 3% and is essentially complete within 24 hours. Lactulose does not exert its effect until it reaches the colon. Transit time through the colon may be slow; therefore, 24 to 48 hours may be required to produce a normal bowel movement.

Contraindications

Hypersensitivity to any ingredient; nausea, vomiting, or other symptoms of appendicitis; fecal impaction; intestinal obstruction; undiagnosed abdominal pain; patients who require a low galactose diet (**lactulose**).

Do not give **docusate sodium** if **mineral oil** is being given.

Warnings

➤*Constipation:* Prior to using laxatives, consider living habits affecting bowel function, including disease state and drug history. Treatment and prevention of constipation include the following: Adequate fluid intake (4 to 6 glasses [8 oz] of water daily), proper dietary habits including increasing fiber intake, responding to the urge to defecate, and daily exercise. Restrict self-medication to short-term therapy of constipation; chronic use of laxatives (particularly stimulants) may lead to dependence.

Agents That May Cause Constipation	
Prostaglandin synthesis inhibitors	Non-potassium sparing diuretics
Anticholinergics	Ganglionic blockers
Antihistamines	Iron preparations
Phenothiazines	Barium sulfate
Tricyclic antidepressants	Clonidine
Benztropine	Polystyrene sodium sulfonate
Trihexyphenidyl	Antacids containing either calcium
Opiates	carbonate or aluminum hydroxide

➤*Fluid and electrolyte balance:* Excessive laxative use may lead to significant fluid and electrolyte imbalance. Monitor patients periodically.

Preparations containing sodium should be used cautiously by individuals on a sodium-restricted diet, and in the presence of edema, CHF, renal failure, or borderline hypertension.

Megacolon, bowel obstruction, imperforate anus, or CHF – Do not use **sodium phosphate** and **sodium biphosphate** in these patients; hypernatremic dehydration may occur.

Abuse/Dependency – Chronic use of laxatives may result in fluid and electrolyte imbalances, steatorrhea, osteomalacia, diarrhea, cathartic colon, and liver disease. Also known as laxative abuse syndrome (LAS), it is difficult to diagnose. It is often seen in women with depression, personality disorders, or anorexia nervosa. Many agents can be detected in urine or stool samples; however, it is important to follow up negative test results if LAS is suspected, because patients may be intermittent abusers or change laxative products frequently.

Cathartic colon – Cathartic colon, a poorly functioning colon, results from the chronic abuse of stimulant cathartics.

➤*Melanosis coli:* Melanosis coli is a darkened pigmentation of the colonic mucosa resulting from chronic use of anthraquinone derivatives (**casanthrol, cascara sagrada, senna**).

➤*Lipid pneumonitis:* Lipid pneumonitis may result from oral ingestion and aspiration of **mineral oil**, especially when patient reclines. The young, elderly, and debilitated are at greatest risk.

➤*Electrocautery procedures:* A theoretical hazard may exist for patients being treated with **lactulose** who may undergo electrocautery procedures during proctoscopy or colonoscopy. Accumulation of H_2 gas in significant concentration in the presence of an electrical spark may result in an explosion. Although this complication has not been reported with lactulose, patients should have a thorough bowel cleansing with a nonfermentable solution. Insufflation of CO_2 as an additional safeguard may be pursued, but is considered a redundant measure.

➤*Renal function impairment:* Up to 20% of the magnesium in magnesium salts may be absorbed. Use caution with products containing phosphate, sodium, magnesium, or potassium salts in the presence of renal dysfunction. Use **sodium phosphate** and **sodium biphosphate** with caution in these patients; hyperphosphatemia, hypernatremia, acidosis, and hypocalcemia may occur.

➤*Pregnancy:* Category B. (**Lactulose, magnesium sulfate**). Category C. (**Casanthranol, cascara sagrada, danthron, docusate sodium, docusate calcium, docusate potassium, mineral oil, senna**). Do not use **castor oil** during pregnancy; its irritant effect may induce premature labor. Mineral oil may decrease absorption of fat-soluble vitamins. Improper use of saline cathartics can lead to dangerous electrolyte imbalance. If needed, limit use to bulk-forming or surfactant laxatives.

➤*Lactation:* Anthraquinone derivatives (eg, **casanthranol, cascara sagrada, danthron**) are excreted in breast milk resulting in a potential increased incidence of diarrhea in the nursing infant. Magnesium emulsions administered orally did not affect the stools of nursing infants, although magnesium content in breast milk was slightly elevated compared with untreated patients. Sennosides A and B (eg, **senna**) are not excreted in breast milk. It is not known whether **docusate calcium, docusate potassium, docusate sodium, lactulose**, and **mineral oil** are excreted in breast milk.

➤*Children:* Administer with caution. Dosage is product specific. Do not administer enemas to children < 2 years of age. Infants receiving **lactulose** may develop hyponatremia and dehydration.

Precautions

➤*Monitoring:* In the overall management of portal-systemic encephalopathy, there is serious underlying liver disease with complications such as electrolyte disturbance (eg, hypokalemia, hypernatremia), which may require other specific therapy. Elderly, debilitated patients who receive **lactulose** for > 6 months should have serum electrolytes (potassium, chloride) and carbon dioxide measured periodically.

➤*Diabetic patients:* **Lactulose** syrup contains galactose (< 1.6 g/15 mL) and lactose (< 1.2 g/15 mL). Use with caution in these individuals.

➤*Concomitant laxative use:* Do not use other laxatives, especially during the initial phase of therapy for portal-systemic encephalopathy; the resulting loose stools may falsely suggest adequate lactulose dosage.

➤*Rectal bleeding or failure to respond:* Rectal bleeding or failure to respond to therapy may indicate a serious condition, which may require further medical attention.

➤*Urine discoloration:* Discoloration of acidic urine to yellow-brown or black may occur with **cascara sagrada** or **senna**. Pink-red, red-violet, or red-brown discoloration of alkaline urine may occur with cascara sagrada or senna.

➤*Impaction or obstruction:* Impaction or obstruction may be caused by bulk-forming agents if temporarily arrested in their passage through the alimentary canal (eg, patients with esophageal strictures). Administer bulk-forming agents with plenty of fluid (240 mL/dose).

➤*Melanosis coli:* Anthraquinone derivatives (**casanthrol, cascara sagrada**, and **senna**) may cause melanosis coli, a harmless discoloring of colonic mucosa, persisting ≤ 6 months following discontinuation.

➤*Tartrazine sensitivity:* Some of these products contain tartrazine, which may cause allergic-type reactions (including bronchial asthma) in susceptible individuals. Although the incidence of tartrazine sensitivity in the general population is low, it is frequently seen in patients who also have aspirin hypersensitivity. Specific products containing tartrazine are identified in the product listings.

Drug Interactions

Laxative Drug Interactions			
Precipitant drug	Object drug*		Description
Surfactants (eg, docusate)	Mineral oil	↑	When concomitantly administered, surfactants (eg, docusate) may increase mineral oil absorption.
Milk Antacids H_2 antagonists Protein pump inhibitors	Bisacodyl	↑	Avoid administration 1 to 2 hours before bisacodyl tablets; concomitant administration may cause the enteric coating to dissolve, resulting in gastric lining irritation or dyspepsia.
Mineral oil	Lipid-soluble vitamins	↓	Absorption of lipid-soluble vitamins may decrease during prolonged mineral oil administration.
Neomycin and other anti-infectives	Lactulose	↔	Reports conflict about concomitant use of lactulose syrup. The elimination of certain colonic bacteria may interfere with desired degradation of lactulose and prevent acidification of colonic contents. Monitor patient if concomitant oral anti-infectives are given.
Antacids	Lactulose	↓	Nonabsorbable antacids given concurrently with lactulose may inhibit the desired lactulose-induced drop in colonic pH.

* ↑ = Object drug increased. ↓ = Object drug decreased. ↔ = Undetermined clinical effect.

Adverse Reactions

Diarrhea; nausea; vomiting; perianal irritation; fainting; bloating; flatulence; cramps.

Obstruction of the esophagus, stomach, small intestine, and colon has occurred when bulk-forming laxatives are administered without adequate fluids or in patients with intestinal stenosis.

Large doses of **mineral oil** may cause anal seepage, resulting in itching (pruritus ani), rectal inflammation, and perianal discomfort.

Lactulose – Gaseous distention with flatulence, belching, abdominal discomfort such as cramping (≈ 20%); nausea; vomiting. Excessive dosage can lead to diarrhea.

Overdosage

There have been no reports of accidental **lactulose** overdose. It is expected that diarrhea and abdominal cramps would be the major symptoms; discontinue the drug.

Patient Information

Direct attention to proper dietary fiber intake, adequate fluids, and regular exercise.

Do not use in the presence of abdominal pain, nausea, or vomiting.

Laxative use is only a temporary measure; do not use > than 1 week. When regularity returns, discontinue use. Prolonged, frequent, or excessive use may result in dependence or electrolyte imbalance.

Notify physician if unrelieved constipation, rectal bleeding, or symptoms of electrolyte imbalance (eg, muscle cramps or pain, weakness, dizziness) occur.

Pink-red, red-violet, red-brown, yellow-brown, or black discoloration of urine may occur with **cascara sagrada** or **senna**.

Refrigerate **magnesium citrate** solutions to improve taste.

Take with a full glass of water or juice.

➤*Mineral oil:* Preferably administered on an empty stomach.

➤*Bisacodyl tablets:* Swallow whole; do not take within 1 to 2 hours of antacids, prescription or *otc* H_2 antagonists, proton pump inhibitors, or milk.

➤*Lactulose:* May be mixed with fruit juice, water, or milk to increase palatability.

May cause belching, flatulence, or abdominal cramps; notify physician if these effects become bothersome or if diarrhea occurs.

Do not take other laxatives while on lactulose therapy.

In the event that unusual diarrheal condition occurs, contact your physician.

SALINE LAXATIVES

otc	**Epsom Salt** (Various, eg, Humco)	**Granules:** Magnesium sulfate. *Dose:* Adults ≥ 12 years - 5 to 10 mL in ½ glass of water. Children 6 to 12 years - 2.5 to 5 mL in ½ glass of water.	In 120 g and 1 and 4 lbs.
otc	**Milk of Magnesia – Concentrated** (Roxane)	**Suspension:** Equiv. to 30 mL milk of magnesia *Dose:* 10 to 20 mL.	In 100 and 400 mL and UD 10 mL.
otc	**Phillips' Milk of Magnesia, Concentrated** (Bayer)	**Suspension:** Magnesium hydroxide 800 mg/5 mL *Dose:* Adults and children ≥ 12 years – 15 to 30 mL. Children 6 to 11 years - 7.5 to 15 mL Children 2 to 5 years - 2.5 to 7.5 mL	Sorbitol, sugar. Strawberry creme flavor. In 240 mL.
otc	**Milk of Magnesia** (Various, eg, Geneva, Goldline, Humco, Roxane, Rugby, URL)	**Suspension:** Magnesium hydroxide 400 mg/5 mL *Dose:* Adults and children ≥ 12 years - 30 to 60 mL/day, taken with liquid. Children 6 to 11 years - 15 to 30 mL/day Children 2 to 5 years - 5 to 15 mL/day	In 180, 360, 480 mL and UD 30 mL, gallon
otc	**Phillips' Milk of Magnesia** (Bayer)		Saccharin (mint); sorbitol, sugar (cherry). Mint, cherry, and regular flavors. In 120, 360, and 780 mL.
otc sf	**Magnesium Citrate Solution** (Humco)	**Solution:** 1.75 g magnesium citrate/30 mL *Dose:* Adults and children ≥ 12 years - ½ to 1 bottle Children 6 to 12 years - ⅓ to ½ bottle	Saccharin. Cherry and lemon flavors. In 296 mL.
otc sf	**Fleet Phospho-soda** (Fleet)	**Solution:** 2.4 g monobasic sodium phosphate and 0.9 g dibasic sodium phosphate/5 mL *Dose:* Adults and children ≥ 12 years - 20 to 45 mL/day Children 10 to 11 years - 10 to 20 mL/day Children 5 to 9 years - 5 to 10 mL/day	556 mg sodium/5 mL. Saccharin. Regular and ginger-lemon flavors. In 45, 90, and 240 mL.

For complete prescribing information, refer to the Laxatives group monograph.

Irritant or Stimulant Laxatives

CASCARA SAGRADA

otc	**Cascara Sagrada** (Various, eg, Rugby)	**Tablets:** 325 mg *Dose:* Adults and children ≥ 12 years - 1 tablet/day	In 100s and 1000s.
otc	**Aromatic Cascara Fluidextract** (Various, eg, Goldline, Hi-Tech Pharmacal Co., Inc., Rugby)	**Liquid:** *Dose:* Adults and children ≥ 12 years - 2 to 6 mL single daily dose	19% alcohol. In 473 mL.
otc	**Cascara Aromatic** (Humco)	**Liquid:** *Dose:* Adults and children ≥ 12 years - 2.5 to 5 mL in a single daily dose Children 2 to < 12 years - ⅙ to ½ teaspoonful	18% alcohol. In 120 and 473 mL.

For complete prescribing information, refer to the Laxatives group monograph.

SENNOSIDES

otc	**Senexon** (Rugby)	**Tablets:** 8.6 mg sennosides *Dose:* Adults and children ≥ 12 years - 2 tablets once or twice daily Children 6 to < 12 years - 1 tablet once or twice/day	Lactose. In 100s and 1000s.
otc	**ex•lax** (Novartis Consumer)	**Tablets:** 15 mg sennosides *Dose:* Adults and children ≥ 12 years - 2 tablets once or twice daily w/ water Children 6 to < 12 years - 1 tablet once or twice daily w/ water	Sucrose. (ex-lax 1). In 8s, 30s, and 60s.
otc	**ex•lax chocolated** (Novartis Consumer)	**Tablets:** 15 mg sennosides *Dose:* Adults and children ≥ 12 years - 2 tablets once or twice daily w/ water Children 6 to < 12 years - 1 tablet once or twice daily w/ water	Sugar, oil, dry milk. Chocolated. In 6s, 18s, and 48s.
otc	**Lax-Pills** (G & W Labs)	**Tablets:** 15 mg sennosides *Dose:* Adults and children ≥ 12 years - 2 tablets once or twice daily w/ water Children 6 to < 12 years - 1 tablet once or twice daily w/ water	In blister pack 30s and 60s.
otc	**Lax-Pills** (G & W Labs)	**Tablets:** 25 mg sennosides *Dose:* Adults and children ≥ 12 years - 2 tablets once or twice daily w/ water Children 6 to < 12 years - 1 tablet once or twice daily w/ water	In blister pack 24s and 48s.
otc	**Maximum Relief ex•lax** (Novartis Consumer)	**Tablets:** 25 mg sennosides *Dose:* Adults and children ≥ 12 years - 2 tablets once or twice daily w/ water Children 6 to < 12 years - 1 tablet once or twice daily w/ water	Sucrose. (ex-lax 1). In 24s and 48s.
otc	**Senokot** (Purdue Frederick)	**Tablets:** 8.6 mg sennosides *Dose:* Adults and children ≥ 12 years - Start w/ 2 tablets/day not to exceed 4 tablets twice/day Children 6 to < 12 years - Start w/ 1 tablet/day not to exceed 2 tablets twice/day Children 2 to < 6 years - ½ tablet/day not to exceed 1 tablet twice/day	Lactose. In 10s, 20s, 50s, 100s, 1000s, and UD 100s.
		Granules: 15 mg/5 mL sennosides *Dose:* Adults and children ≥ 12 years - Start w/ 1 tsp/day not to exceed 2 tsp twice/day Children 6 to < 12 years - ½ tsp/day not to exceed 1 tsp twice/day Children 2 to < 6 years - ¼ tsp/day not to exceed ½ tsp twice/day	Sucrose. In 56, 170, and 340 g.
		Syrup: 8.8 mg/5 mL sennosides *Dose:* Adults and children ≥ 12 years - 2 to 3 tsp/day not to exceed 3 tsp twice/day Children 6 to < 12 years - 1 to 1½ tsp/day not to exceed 1½ tsp twice/day Children 2 to < 6 years - ½ to ¾ tsp/day not to exceed ¾ tsp twice/day	Alcohol free. Parabens, sucrose. In 59 and 237 mL.
otc	**Senna-Gen** (Zenith-Goldline)	**Tablets:** 8.6 mg sennosides. *Dose:* Adults and children ≥ 12 years - 2 to 4 tablets once or twice daily Children 6 to < 12 years - 1 to 2 tablets once or twice daily Children 2 to < 6 years - ½ to 1 tablet once or twice daily	Lactose. In 100s and 1000s.
otc	**SenokotXTRA** (Purdue Fredrick)	**Tablets:** 17 mg sennosides *Dose:* Adults and children ≥ 12 years - Start w/ 1 tablet/day not to exceed 2 tablets twice/day Children 6 to < 12 years - Start w/ ½ tablet/day not to exceed 1 tablet twice/day	Lactose. In 12s and 36s.

Irritant or Stimulant Laxatives

SENNOSIDES

otc	**Black-Draught** (Monticello Drug Co.)	**Tablets:** 6 mg sennosides *Dose:* Adults and children ≥ 12 years - 2 tablets once or twice/day Children 6 to < 12 years - 1 tablet once or twice/day	Sucrose. In 30s.
		Granules: 20 mg sennosides/5 mL *Dose:* Adults and children ≥ 12 years - As a tea: ¼ to ½ cup	Tartrazine, sucrose. In 22.5 g.
otc	**Fletcher's Castoria** (Mentholatum)	**Liquid:** 33.3 mg/mL senna concentrate *Dose:* Children 6 to 15 years – 10 to 15 mL ≤ 2 times/day Children 2 to 5 years – 5 to 10 mL ≤ 2 times/day	Alcohol free, sucrose, parabens. In 74 and 150 mL.

For complete prescribing information, refer to the Laxatives group monograph.

BISACODYL

otc	**Gentlax** (Purdue Frederick)	**Tablets:** 5 mg	Sugar, sucrose. In 20s and 100s.
otc	**Bisacodyl** (Various, eg, Global Source, Major, UDL, URL)	**Tablets, enteric-coated:** 5 mg	In 25s, 50s, 100s, 1000s and UD 100s.
otc	**Alophen** (Numark)		Sugar. In 100s.
otc	**Bisa-Lax** (Bergen Brunswig)		In 25s and 50s.
otc	**Dulcolax** (Ciba Consumer)		Lactose, sucrose, parabens. (BI 12). In 10s, 25s, 50s, and 100s.
otc	**Fleet Laxative** (Fleet)		Sucrose. In 25s and 100s.
otc	**Modane** (Savage Labs.)		Lactose. In 100s.
otc	**Bisac-Evac** (G & W Labs)		In 25s.
otc	**Caroid** (Mentholatum Co.)		Sugar. In 100s.
otc	**Correctol** (Schering-Plough)		Talc, lactose, sugar. (Correctol). In 30s, 60s, and 90s.
otc	**Feen-a-mint** (Schering-Plough)		Talc, lactose, sugar. (Feen-a-mint). In 30s.
otc	**Doxidan** (Pharmacia)	**Tablets, delayed release:** 10 mg	In 10s, 30s, and 90s.
otc	**Bisacodyl** (Various, eg, Global Source, URL)	**Suppositories:** 10 mg	In 12s, 16s, and 100s.
otc	**Bisacodyl Uniserts** (Upsher-Smith)		In 12s.
otc	**Bisa-Lax** (Bergen Brunswig)		Hydrogenated vegetable oil. In 50s.
otc	**Dulcolax** (Novartis Consumer Health)		In 4s, 8s, 16s, and 50s.
otc	**Bisac-Evac** (G & W Labs.)		In 8s, 12s, 50s, 100s, 500s, and 1000s.
otc	**Fleet Laxative** (Fleet)		In 4s, 12s, 50s, and 100s.

For complete prescribing information, refer to the Laxatives group monograph.

> ### Administration and Dosage

➤**Tablets:** Swallow whole; do not chew. Do not take within 1 hour of antacids or milk.

Adults and children ≥ 12 years – 10 to 15 mg (usually 10) as a single dose once daily.

Children 6 to < 12 years – 5 mg once daily.

➤**Suppositories:**
Adults – 10 mg once daily to stimulate bowel movement.
Children 6 to < 12 years – 5 mg once daily.

Bulk-Producing Laxatives

PSYLLIUM

otc	**Metamucil** (Procter & Gamble)	**Capsules:** 0.52 g psyllium husk *Dose:* Adults 12 years of age and older - 2 to 6 capsules for increasing daily fiber intake; 6 capsules for cholesterol-lowering use. Take with 8 oz liquid (swallow 1 capsule at a time) up to tid.	In 100s and 160s.
otc sf	**Fiberall Tropical Fruit Flavor** (Heritage Consumer)	**Powder:** 3.5 g psyllium hydrophilic mucilloid per dose *Dose:* 1 rounded tsp (5 to 5.9 g) in 6 oz cool water or juice once daily followed immediately by ½ glass of water. After 1 week, may take ≤ 3 servings/day.	Aspartame. In 454 g and UD 10 g packets.
otc	**Fiberall Orange Flavor** (Heritage Consumer)		Aspartame. In 480 g.
otc	**Genfiber** (Goldline Consumer)	**Powder:** 3.4 g psyllium hydrophilic mucilloid fiber and 14 calories per dose. *Dose:* Adults - 1 rounded tsp in 8 oz liquid 1 to 3 times/day. Children 6 to 12 years - ½ rounded tsp in 8 oz liquid 1 to 3 times/day.	Dextrose. In 595 g.
otc	**Genfiber, Orange Flavor** (Goldline Consumer)	**Powder:** 3.4 g psyllium hydrophilic mucilloid per dose. *Dose:* Adults - 1 rounded tablespoon in 8 oz liquid 1 to 3 times/day. Children 6 to 12 years - ½ rounded tablespoon in 8 oz liquid 1 to 3 times/day.	Sucrose. Orange flavor. In 397 g.
otc sf	**Hydrocil Instant** (Numark)	**Powder:** 3.5 g psyllium hydrophilic mucilloid/dose *Dose:* 1 level scoopful (3.7 g) in liquid	In 250 g.
otc sf	**Konsyl** (Konsyl Pharm.)	**Powder:** 6 g psyllium. *Dose:* 1 packet or rounded tsp (6 g) in liquid	In 300 and 450 g and UD 6 g packets.
otc sf	**Konsyl Easy Mix Formula** (Konsyl Pharm.)	**Powder:** 6 g psyllium, 4.4 mg Na, 48 mg Ca, 4 mg P, 0.06 mg Zn, 42 mg K, 0.35 g carbohydrates, 4 calories/5 mL *Dose:* 1 teaspoon (5 mL) or 6.3 g packet	In 200 g and packets.
otc	**Metamucil Orange Flavor, Smooth Texture** (Procter & Gamble)	**Powder:** ≈ 3.4 g psyllium husk, 5 mg sodium, 12 g carbohydrates, and 45 calories per dose *Dose:* Adults and children ≥ 12 years - 1 rounded tablespoon in liquid, 1 to 3 times a day. Children 6 to 12 years - ½ adult dose	Sucrose. In 420, 630, and 1368 g, and 100 UD single-dose packs (100s).
otc sf	**Metamucil, Sugar Free, Smooth Texture** (Procter & Gamble)	**Powder:** ≈ 3.4 g psyllium husk, 5 g carbohydrates, 4 mg sodium, and 20 calories per dose *Dose:* Adults and children ≥ 12 years - 1 rounded tsp in liquid, 1 to 3 times a day. Children 6 to 12 years - ½ adult dose	In 425 g and packets of 30s or 100s.
otc sf	**Metamucil, Sugar Free, Orange Flavor, Smooth Texture** (Procter & Gamble)	**Powder:** ≈ 3.4 mg psyllium husk, 5 g carbohydrates, 5 mg sodium, 20 calories per dose. *Dose:* Adults and children ≥ 12 years - 1 rounded tsp in liquid 1 to 3 times a day. Children 6 to 12 years - ½ adult dose	Aspartame, 25 mg phenylalanine per dose. In 210, 420, 630, and 660 g.
otc	**Metamucil Orange Flavor, Original Texture** (Procter & Gamble)	**Powder:** ≈ 3.4 g psyllium husk, 10 g carbohydrates, 5 mg sodium, 40 calories/dose *Dose:* Adults and children ≥ 12 years - 1 rounded tablespoon in 8 oz. liquid ≤ 3 times/day Children 6 to 12 years - ½ adult dose	Sucrose. In 210, 420, 538, and 630 g.

Bulk-Producing Laxatives

PSYLLIUM

otc	**Metamucil Original Texture** (Procter & Gamble)	**Powder:** ≈ 3.4 g psyllium husk, 6 g carbohydrates, 3 mg sodium, 25 calories/dose *Dose:* Adults and children ≥ 12 years - 1 rounded tsp in 8 oz. liquid ≤ 3 times/day Children 6 to 12 years - ½ adult dose	Sucrose. In 822 g and packets of 30.
otc	**Reguloid, Orange** (Rugby)	**Powder:** ≈ 3.4 g psyllium mucilloid/tbsp *Dose:* Adults ≥ children 12 years - 1 rounded tbsp, 1 to 3 times daily in 8 oz. liquid. Children 6 to 12 years - ½ adult dose	Sucrose. Orange flavor. In 369 and 540 g.
otc sf	**Reguloid, Sugar Free Orange** (Rugby)	**Powder:** ≈ 3.4 g psyllium hydrophilic mucilloid per rounded tsp *Dose:* Adults and children ≥ 12 years - 1 rounded tsp in 8 oz liquid, 1 to 3 times/day. Children 6 to 12 years - ½ adult dose in 8 oz liquid 1 to 3 times/day	Aspartame, 30 mg phenyl-alanine per dose. In 284 and 426 g
otc sf	**Reguloid, Sugar Free Regular** (Rugby)	**Powder:** ≈ 3.4 g psyllium hydrophilic mucilloid per dose *Dose:* Adults and children ≥ 12 years - 1 rounded tsp in 8 oz liquid, 1 to 3 times/day. Children 6 to 12 years - ½ adult dose in 8 oz liquid 1 to 3 times a day.	Aspartame, 6 mg phenyl-alanine per dose. In 284 and 426 g.
otc	**Natural Fiber Laxative** (Apothecary)	**Powder:** ≈ 3.4 g psyllium hydrophillic mucilloid/7 g dose. 14 calories/dose. *Dose:* Adults and children ≥ 12 years - 7 g 1 to 3 times/day Children 6 to 12 years - ½ adult dose	Sodium free. In 390 g.
otc	**Syllact** (Wallace)	**Powder:** 3.3 g psyllium seed husks and ≈ 14 calories per rounded tsp *Dose:* Adults and children ≥ 12 years - 1 rounded tsp in 8 oz liquid, 1 to 3 times daily. Children 6 to < 12 years – ½ to 1 rounded tsp. in 8 oz liquid 1 to 3 times/day	Dextrose, saccharin, para-bens. Fruit flavor. In 284 g.
otc	**Konsyl-D** (Konsyl Pharm.)	**Powder:** 3.4 g psyllium, 14 calories per rounded tsp *Dose:* Adults and children ≥ 12 years - 1 tsp 1 to 3 times/day Children 6 to < 12 years - ½ tsp 1 to 3 times/day	Dextrose. In 325 and 500 g and UD 6.5 g.
otc	**Reguloid** (Rugby)		Dextrose. 14 calories per rounded tsp. In 369 and 540 g.
otc	**Perdiem Fiber Therapy** (Novartis Consumer Health)	**Granules:** 4.03 g psyllium, 1.8 mg sodium, 36.1 mg potassium and 4 calories/rounded tsp (6 g) *Dose:* Adults - 1 to 2 rounded tsp with 8 oz liquid, once or twice daily. Do not chew. Children 7 to 11 years - 1 rounded tsp with 8 oz liquid once or twice daily	Sucrose. Dye free. Mint flavor. In 100 and 250 g.
otc	**Serutan** (Menley & James)	**Granules:** 2.5 g psyllium and < 0.03 g sodium per heaping tsp *Dose:* Adults - 1 to 3 heaping tsp on cereal or other food, 1 to 3 times daily. Children 6 to 12 years - ½ to 1½ heaping tsp with 8 oz liquid.	Saccharin, sugar. In 170 and 540 g.
otc	**Metamucil** (Procter & Gamble)	**Wafers:** ≈ 3.4 g psyllium husk/dose, 17 g carbohydrates, 20 mg sodium, 5 g fat, 120 calories/dose *Dose:* Adults and children ≥ 12 years - 2 wafers w/ 8 oz. liquid ≤ 3 times/day Children 6 to 12 years - 1 wafer w/ 8 oz. liquid ≤ 3 times/day	Sugar, fructose, molasses, sucrose. Cinnamon spice and apple crisp flavors. In 24s.

For complete prescribing information, refer to the Laxatives group monograph.

POLYCARBOPHIL

otc	**Equalactin** (Numark)	**Tablets, chewable:** 625 mg calcium polycarbophil (equivalent to 500 mg polycarbophil)	Citrus flavor. In 24s and 48s.
otc	**Konsyl Fiber** (Konsyl)	**Tablets:** 500 mg polycarbophil	In 90s.
otc	**Fiber-Lax** (Rugby)	**Tablets:** 625 mg calcium polycarbophil (equivalent to 500 mg polycarbophil)	In 60s, 90s, and 500s.
otc	**Bulk Forming Fiber Laxative** (Goldline Consumer)		Film-coated. In 60s.
otc	**FiberCon** (Lederle)		Calcium carbonate. (LL F66). In 36s, 60s, 90s, and 150s.

For complete prescribing information, refer to the Laxatives group monograph.

Indications

►*Constipation/Diarrhea:* Treatment of constipation or diarrhea associated with conditions such as irritable bowel syndrome and diverticulosis; acute nonspecific diarrhea.

Administration and Dosage

►*Adults and children ≥ 12 years of age:* 1 g 1 to 4 times daily or as needed. Do not exceed 4 g in 24 hours.

►*Children 6 to < 12 years of age:* 500 mg ≤ 4 times daily or as needed. Do not exceed 2 g/day.

►*Children < 6 years of age:* Products vary. Consult product labeling for specific guidelines.

For severe diarrhea, repeat dose every 30 min; do not exceed maximum daily dose.

When using as a laxative, drink 8 oz water or other liquid with each dose.

MISCELLANEOUS BULK-PRODUCING LAXATIVES

otc	**Citrucel** (GlaxoSmithKline)	**Powder:** 2 g methylcellulose per heaping tbsp	Sucrose. Orange flavor. In 480 and 846 g.
otc sf	**Citrucel Sugar Free** (GlaxoSmithKline)	**Powder:** 2 g methylcellulose, 52 mg phenylalanine per leveled scoop	Aspartame. Orange flavor. In 245 and 480 g.
otc	**Citrucel** (GlaxoSmithKline)	**Tablets:** 500 g methylcellulose	Maltodextrin. (CIT). Capsule shape. In 164s.
otc	**Unifiber** (Niche)	**Powder:** Powdered cellulose	In 150, 270, and 480 g.
otc	**Maltsupex** (Wallace)	**Tablets, coated:** 750 mg malt soup extract	Parabens. In 100s.
		Powder: 8 g malt soup extract per level scoop	In 227 and 454 g.
		Liquid: 16 g malt soup extract per tbsp	In 237 and 473 mL.

For complete prescribing information, refer to the Laxatives group monograph.

Administration and Dosage

Take with a full glass of water; encourage additional fluid intake.

►*Citrucel:*

Adults and children ≥ 12 years of age – 1 heaping tbsp (19 g) in 8 oz cold water, 1 to 3 times daily.

Children 6 to < 12 years of age – ½ the adult dose in 8 oz cold water, once daily.

►*Unifiber:* Dose is 1 tbsp into a glass with 3 or 4 oz. of fruit juice, milk, or water, or mix with soft foods such as applesauce, mashed potatoes, or pudding. Can be taken up to 3 times daily if needed or as recommended by a doctor.

►*Maltsupex:*

Tablets – Adults, 12 to 36 g/day. Initially, 4 tablets 4 times daily (at meals and bedtime).

Powder – Adults, up to 32 g twice daily for 3 or 4 days, then 16 to 32 g at bedtime. Children 6 to 12 years, up to 16 g twice daily for 3 or 4 days; 2 to 6 years, 8 g twice daily for 3 or 4 days. For infants < 2 years, con-

Bulk-Producing Laxatives

MISCELLANEOUS BULK-PRODUCING LAXATIVES

sult a doctor.

Liquid – Adults, 2 tbsp twice daily for 3 or 4 days, then 1 to 2 tbsp at bedtime. Children 6 to 12 years, 1 tbsp twice daily for 3 or 4 days; 2 to 6 years, ½ tbsp twice daily for 3 or 4 days. For infants < 2 years, consult a doctor.

Emollients

MINERAL OIL

otc	Mineral Oil (Various, eg, Fleet, Paddock)	**Liquid**: Mineral oil	In 180 and 473 mL.
otc	Kondremul Plain (Heritage Consumer Prod.)	**Emulsion**: Mineral oil	Irish moss, acacia, glycerin. In 480 mL.

For complete prescribing information, refer to the Laxatives group monograph.

Administration and Dosage

▶*Dose:*

Adults and children ≥ 12 years of age – 15 to 45 mL, take at bedtime; *Kondremul,* 30 to 75 mL.

Children 6 to < 12 years of age – 5 to 15 mL; *Kondremul,* 10 to 25 mL.

Fecal Softeners/Surfactants

DOCUSATE SODIUM (Dioctyl Sodium Sulfosuccinate; DSS)

otc	ex-lax Stool Softener (Novartis Consumer Health)	**Tablets**: 100 mg *Dose:* Adults and children ≥ 12 years - 100 to 300 mg/day Children 2 to < 12 years - 100 mg/day	Methylparabens. Caplet shape. In 40s.
otc	Colace (Purdue)	**Capsules**: 50 mg *Dose:* Adults and children ≥ 12 years - 50 to 300 mg/day Children 6 to 12 years - 50 to 150 mg/day	(RPC 052). In 30s, 60s, and UD 100s.
otc	Colace (Purdue)	**Capsules**: 100 mg *Dose:* Adults and children ≥ 12 years - 100 to 300 mg/day Children 6 to 12 years - 100 mg/day Children 2 to 6 years - Products vary. Consult product labeling for specific guidelines.	In 30s, 60s, 250s, 1000s, and UD 100s.
otc	D-S-S (Magno-Humphries)		In 100s.
otc	Non-Habit Forming Stool Softener (Rugby)		Sorbitol, parabens. In 100s and 1000s.
otc	Stool Softener (Rugby)		Lactose, tartrazine. In 1000s.
otc	Regulax SS (Republic)		In 60s, 100s, and 1000s.
otc	Docusate Sodium (Various, eg, Geneva, UDL, URL)	**Capsules**: 250 mg *Dose:* Adults and children ≥ 12 years - 250 mg/day	In 100s and 1000s, and UD 100s.
otc	Stool Softener (Rugby)		Lactose. In 1000s.
otc	Docusate Sodium (UDL)	**Capsules, soft gel**: 50 mg *Dose:* Adults and children ≥ 12 years - 50 to 300 mg/day Children 2 to < 12 years - 50 mg/day	In 100s and UD 100s.
otc	Docusate Sodium (Various, eg, Goldline Consumer, UDL, URL)	**Capsules, soft gel**: 100 mg *Dose:* Adults and children ≥ 12 years - 100 to 300 mg/day Children 6 to < 12 years - 100 mg/day Children 2 to 6 years - Products vary. Consult product labeling for specific guidelines.	In 100s, 1000s, and UD 100s and 300s.
otc	D.O.S. (Goldline Consumer)		Parabens. In 100s and 1000s.
otc	Genasoft (Goldline Consumer)		Methylparaben. In 60s.
otc	Phillips' Liqui-Gels (Bayer Consumer)		Parabens, sorbitol. (Phillips). In 10s, 30s, and 50s.
otc	Sof-lax (Fleet)		5 mg sodium/gelcap. In 60s.
otc	Docusate Sodium (Various, eg, Schein)	**Capsules, soft gel**: 250 mg *Dose:* Adults and children ≥ 12 years - 250 mg/day	In 100s.
otc	Stool Softener (Rugby)		Sorbitol, parabens. In 100s and 1000s.
otc	D.O.S. (Goldline Consumer)		Oblong. Red-orange. In 100s and 500s.
otc	Docusate Sodium (Roxane)	**Syrup**: 50 mg per 15 mL *Dose:* Adults and children ≥ 12 years - 50 to 100 mg Children 6 to 12 years - 50 mg Children 3 to 5 years - 33 mg	Saccharin, sucrose, parabens. In UD 15 and 30 mL (100s).
otc	Docu (Hi-Tech Pharmacal Co.)	**Syrup**: 20 mg per 5 mL *Dose:* Adults and children ≥ 12 years - 60 to 180 mg/day Children 6 to 12 years - 40 mg 1 to 3 times/day Children 3 to 6 years - 20 to 60 mg/day	5% alcohol. In 480 mL.
otc	Diocto (Various, eg, Alpharma)	**Syrup**: 60 mg per 15 mL	In 480 mL. *Dose:* Adults and children ≥ 12 years - 60 to 360 mg/day Children 2 to 12 years - Dosage varies. Consult product labeling for specific guidelines. Generally, 40 to 150 mg/day.
otc	Colace (Purdue)		≤ 1% alcohol. Menthol, parabens, sucrose. In 237 and 473 mL. *Dose:* Adults and children ≥ 12 years - 60 to 300 mg/day Children 6 to 12 years - 40 to 120 mg/day Children 3 to 6 years - 20 to 60 mg/day Children < 3 years - 10 to 40 mg/day
otc	Silace (Silarx)		≤ 1% alcohol. In 473 mL. *Dose:* Adults and children ≥ 12 years - 60 to 180 mg/day Children 6 to 12 years - 40 mg 1 to 3 times/day
otc	Docusate Sodium (Roxane)	**Syrup**: 100 mg/30 mL *Dose:* Adults and children ≥ 12 years - 50 to 100 mg Children 6 to 12 years - 50 mg Children 3 to 5 years - 33 mg	Saccharin, sucrose, parabens. In UD 15 and 30 mL (100s).

Fecal Softeners/Surfactants

DOCUSATE SODIUM (Dioctyl Sodium Sulfosuccinate; DSS)

otc	**Diocto** (Various, eg, Goldline Consumer, Rugby)	**Liquid:** 150 mg per 15 mL	In 480 mL. *Dose:* Adults and children ≥ 12 years - 50 to 350 mg/day Children 2 to < 12 years - Dosage varies. Consult product labeling for specific guidelines. Generally, 20 to 150 mg/day.
otc	**Colace** (Purdue)		Parabens. In 30 and 480 mL. *Dose:* Children 3 to 6 years - 20 mg 1 to 3 times/day
otc	**Docu** (Hi-Tech Pharmacal Co.)		In 480 mL. *Dose:* Adults and children > 12 years - 50 to 200 mg/day Children 6 to 12 years - 40 to 120 mg/day Children 3 to 6 years - 20 to 60 mg/day

For complete prescribing information, refer to the Laxatives group monograph.

Administration and Dosage

➤*Liquid:* Give in milk, fruit juice, or infant formula to mask taste. In enemas, add 50 to 100 mg (5 to 10 mL liquid) to a retention or flushing enema.

DOCUSATE CALCIUM (Dioctyl Calcium Sulfosuccinate)

otc	**Docusate Calcium** (Various)	**Capsules:** 240 mg	In 100s, 500s, and UD 100s and 300s.
otc	**Stool Softener** (Apothecary)		In 50s.
otc	**Stool Softener DC** (Rugby)		Sorbitol, parabens. In 100s, 500s, and 1000s.
otc	**Surfak Liquigels** (Pharmacia & Upjohn)	**Capsules, soft gel:** 240 mg	Sorbitol, parabens. Red. In 10s, 30s, 100s, 500s, and UD 100s.
otc	**DC Softgels** (Goldline)		In 100s and 500s.

For complete prescribing information, refer to the Laxatives group monograph.

Administration and Dosage

➤*Adults and children ≥ 12 years of age:* 240 mg daily until bowel movements are normal.

Hyperosmotic Agents

GLYCERIN

otc	**Glycerin** (Various, eg, Apothecary)	**Suppositories:** Glycerin	**Adults:** In 10s, 12s, 25s, 50s, and 100s.
			Pediatric: In 10s, 12s, and 25s.
otc	**Sani-Supp** (G & W Labs)		**Adults:** In 10s, 25s, and 50s.
			Pediatric: In 10s and 25s.
otc	**Colace** (Purdue)		**Adults:** In 12s, 24s, 48s, and 100s.
otc	**Colace Infant/Child** (Purdue)		**Pediatric:** In 12s and 24s.
otc	**Fleet Babylax** (Fleet)	**Liquid:** 4 mL per applicator	In 6 applicators.

For complete prescribing information, refer to the Laxatives group monograph.

Administration and Dosage

➤*Suppositories:* Insert 1 suppository high in the rectum and retain 15 to 30 minutes; it need not melt to produce laxative action.

➤*Rectal liquid:* With gentle, steady pressure, insert stem with tip pointing towards navel. Squeeze unit until nearly all the liquid is expelled, then remove. A small amount of liquid will remain in unit.

LACTULOSE

Rx	**Lactulose** (Various, eg, Zenith Goldline)	**Solution:** 10 g lactulose per 15 mL. (< 1.6 g galactose, < 1.2 g lactose and ≤ 1.2 g of other sugars).	In 237, 473, 960, and 1893 mL.
Rx	**Cephulac** (Hoechst-Marion Roussel)		In 473 mL, 1.9 L, and UD 30 mL.
Rx	**Cholac** (Alra)		In 30, 240, 480, 960, 1920, and 3785 mL.
Rx	**Constulose** (Alpharma)		In 237 and 946 mL.
Rx	**Enulose** (Alpharma)		In 473 mL and 1.89 L.
Rx	**Kristalose** (Bertek)	**Crystals for reconstitution:** Lactulose (< 0.3 g galactose and lactose/10 g).	In 10 g (30s) and 20 g (30s).

For complete prescribing information, refer to the Laxatives group monograph.

Indications

➤*Chronulac, Duphalac, Constulose:* Treatment of constipation.

➤*Cephulac, Cholac, Enulose:* Prevention and treatment of portal-systemic encephalopathy, including hepatic pre-coma and coma. Lactulose reduces blood ammonia levels by 25% to 50%; this generally parallels improved mental state and EEG patterns.

Clinical response has been observed in ≈ 75% of patients. An increase in protein tolerance is also frequent. In chronic portal-systemic encephalopathy, lactulose has been given for > 2 years in controlled studies.

Administration and Dosage

➤*Chronulac, Duphalac, Constulose:*

Treatment of constipation – 15 to 30 mL (10 to 20 g lactulose) daily, increased to 60 mL/day, if necessary.

➤*Cephulac, Cholac, Enulose:* Prevent and treat portal-systemic encephalopathy

Oral –

Adults: 30 to 45 mL, 3 or 4 times/day. Adjust dosage every day or two to produce 2 or 3 soft stools daily. Hourly doses of 30 to 45 mL may be used to induce rapid laxation in the initial phase of therapy. When the laxative effect has been achieved, reduce dosage to recommended daily dose. Improvement may occur within 24 hours, but may not begin before 48 hours or later. Continuous long-term therapy is indicated to lessen severity and prevent recurrence of portal-systemic encephalopathy.

Children: There is little information on use in children and adolescents. The goal is to produce 2 or 3 soft stools daily. Recommended initial daily oral dose in infants is 2.5 to 10 mL in divided doses. For older children and adolescents, the total daily dose is 40 to 90 mL. If the initial dose causes diarrhea, reduce immediately. If diarrhea persists, discontinue use.

Rectal – Administer to adults during impending coma or coma stage of portal-systemic encephalopathy when the danger of aspiration exists or when endoscopic or intubation procedures interfere with oral administration. The goal of treatment is reversal of the coma stage so the patient can take oral medication. Reversal of coma may occur within 2 hours of the first enema. Start recommended oral doses before enema is stopped entirely.

Lactulose may be given as a retention enema via a rectal balloon catheter. Do not use cleansing enemas containing soap suds or other alkaline agents.

Mix 300 mL lactulose with 700 mL water or physiologic saline and retain for 30 to 60 minutes. The enema may be repeated every 4 to

Hyperosmotic Agents

LACTULOSE

6 hours. If the enema is inadvertently evacuated too promptly, it may be repeated immediately.

May be more palatable when mixed with fruit juice, water, or milk.

➤*Storage/Stability:* Store below 86°F (30°C); do not freeze.

Enemas

MISCELLANEOUS ENEMAS

otc	**Fleet** (Fleet)	**Disposable enema:** 7 g dibasic sodium phosphate and 19 g monobasic sodium phosphate per 118 mL delivered dose (4.4 g sodium per dose) *Dose:* Adults – 118 mL. Children 2 to < 12 years – 59 mL.	In squeeze bottles. **Pediatric:** In 66 mL.
otc	**Fleet Bisacodyl** (Fleet)	**Disposable enema:** 10 mg bisacodyl per 30 mL delivered dose *Dose:* Adults and children ≥ 12 years – 30 mL.	**Adult:** In 133 mL. In 37 mL squeeze bottles.
otc	**Fleet Mineral Oil** (Fleet)	**Disposable enema:** Mineral oil *Dose:* Adults and children ≥ 12 years – 118 mL. Children 2 to < 12 years – 59 mL.	In 133 mL plastic squeeze bottles.
otc	**Therevac-SB** (Jones Medical)	**Disposable enema:** 283 mg docusate sodium in a base of soft soap, polyethylene glycol, and 275 mg glycerin per 4 mL ampule *Dose:* 4 mL.	In UD 30s.
otc	**Therevac-Plus** (Jones Medical)	**Disposable enema:** 283 mg docusate sodium, 275 mg glycerin, and 20 mg benzocaine in a base of soft soap, polyethylene glycol per 4 mL ampule *Dose:* 4 mL.	In 50s and UD 30s.

For complete prescribing information, refer to the Laxatives group monograph.

CO₂-RELEASING SUPPOSITORIES

otc	**Ceo-Two** (Beutlich)	**Suppositories:** Sodium bicarbonate and potassium bitartrate in a water-soluble polyethylene glycol base. Before inserting, moisten suppository with warm water.	In 10s.

For complete prescribing information, refer to the Laxatives group monograph.

Bowel Evacuants

POLYETHYLENE GLYCOL-ELECTROLYTE SOLUTION (PEG-ES)

Rx	**CoLyte** (Schwarz Pharma)	**Powder for Oral Solution:** 1 gal: 227.1 g PEG 3350, 21.5 g sodium sulfate, 6.36 g sodium bicarb, 5.53 g NaCl, 2.82 g KCl.	Regular and pineapple flavors. In bottles.
		4 L: 240 g PEG 3350, 22.72 g sodium sulfate, 6.72 g sodium bicarb, 5.84 g NaCl, 2.98 g KCl.	Citrus berry, lemon lime, cherry, and pineapple flavors. In bottles.
Rx	**GoLYTELY** (Braintree Labs.)	**Powder for Oral Solution:** 236 g PEG 3350, 22.74 g sodium sulfate, 6.74 g sodium bicarb, 5.86 g NaCl, 2.97 g KCl.	In disposable jugs.
		227.1 g PEG 3350, 21.5 g sodium sulfate, 6.36 g sodium bicarb, 5.53 g NaCl, 2.82 g KCl.	In packets.
Rx	**NuLytely** (Braintree Labs.)	**Powder for Reconstitution:** 420 g PEG 3350, 5.72 g sodium bicarb, 11.2 g NaCl, 1.48 g KCl.	Cherry, lemon-lime, and orange flavors. In 4 L disposable jugs.
Rx	**OCL** (Abbott)	**Oral Solution:** 146 mg NaCl, 168 mg sodium bicarb, 1.29 g sodium sulfate decahydrate, 75 mg KCl, 6 g PEG 3350, 30 mg polysorbate 80/100 mL.	In 1500 mL (3 pack).

For complete prescribing information, refer to the Laxatives group monograph.

Indications

For bowel cleansing prior to GI examination.

➤*Unlabeled uses:* PEG electrolyte solutions are useful in the management of acute iron overdose in children. In a 33-month-old, 2953 mL/kg was administered over 5 days.

Administration and Dosage

The patient should fast 3 to 4 hours prior to ingestion of the solution; do not give solid foods < 2 hours before solution is administered.

One method is to schedule patients for midmorning exam, allowing 3 hours for drinking and 1 hour to complete bowel evacuation. Another method is to give the solution the evening before the exam, particularly if the patient is to have a barium enema. No foods, except clear liquids, are permitted after solution administration.

➤*Adults:* Dosage is 4 L of oral solution prior to GI exam. May be given via a nasogastric tube to patients unwilling or unable to drink the preparation. Drink 240 mL every 10 minutes until 4 L are consumed or until the rectal effluent is clear. Rapid drinking of each portion is preferred to drinking small amounts continuously. Nasogastric tube administration is at the rate of 20 to 30 mL/min (1.2 to 1.8 L/hour). The first bowel movement should occur in ≈ 1 hour.

➤*Preparation of solution:* Tap water may be used to reconstitute the solution. Shake container vigorously several times to ensure that the powder is completely dissolved.

After reconstitution to 4 L volume with water, the solution contains PEG 3350 17.6 mmol/L, sodium 125 mmol/L, sulfate 40 mmol/L (*Colyte*80 mmol/L), chloride 35 mmol/L, bicarbonate 20 mmol/L, and potassium 10 mmol/L.

➤*Storage/Stability:* Refrigerate reconstituted solution (chilling before administration improves palatability); use within 48 hours.

Actions

➤*Pharmacology:* Oral solution induces diarrhea, which rapidly cleanses the bowel, usually within 4 hours. Polyethylene glycol 3350 (PEG 3350) and the electrolyte concentration result in virtually no net absorption or excretion of ions or water. Large volumes may be given without significant changes in water or electrolyte balance.

Contraindications

GI obstruction; gastric retention; bowel perforation; toxic colitis, megacolon, or ileus.

Warnings

Do not add flavorings or additional ingredients to solution before use.

➤*Pregnancy: Category C.* Safety has not been established. Use only when clearly needed and when the benefits outweigh the potential hazards to the fetus.

➤*Children:* Safety and efficacy for use in children have not been established.

Several studies in infants and children from 3 to 14 years of age showed PEG-electrolyte solutions are safe and effective in bowel evacuation.

Precautions

➤*Regurgitation/Aspiration:* Observe unconscious or semiconscious patients with impaired gag reflex and those who are otherwise prone to regurgitation or aspiration during use, especially if given via a nasogastric tube. If GI obstruction or perforation is suspected, rule out these contraindications before administration.

If a patient experiences severe bloating, distention, or abdominal pain, slow or temporarily discontinue administration until symptoms abate.

➤*Severe ulcerative colitis:* Use with caution.

Drug Interactions

Oral medication given within 1 hour of start of therapy may be flushed from the GI tract and not absorbed.

Adverse Reactions

Nausea, abdominal fullness, and bloating are the most common adverse reactions (occurring in up to 50% of patients). Abdominal cramps, vomiting, and anal irritation occur less frequently. These adverse reactions are transient. Isolated cases of urticaria, rhinorrhea, and dermatitis have been reported, which may represent allergic reactions.

Bowel Evacuants

POLYETHYLENE GLYCOL (PEG) SOLUTION

| *Rx* | **MiraLax** (Braintree Labs.) | **Powder for Oral Solution:** 255 g PEG 3350 | In 14 oz. |
| | | 527 g PEG 3350 | In 26 oz. |

For complete prescribing information, refer to the Laxatives group monograph.

Indications

For the treatment of occasional constipation. Do not use for > 2 weeks.

Administration and Dosage

The usual dose is 17 g of powder/day in 8 ounces of water. Each bottle is supplied with a measuring cap marked to contain 17 g of laxative powder when filled to the indicated line.

Two to 4 days (48 to 96 hours) may be required to produce a bowel movement.

MISCELLANEOUS BOWEL EVACUANTS

otc	**X-Prep Liquid** (Gray)	Senna extract, parabens, 50 g sugar. Alcohol free. In 74 mL.	
otc	**Tridrate Bowel Cleansing System** (Lafayette)	19 g magnesium citrate. 3 bisacodyl tablets (5 mg each). 1 bisacodyl suppository (10 mg).	
otc	**X-Prep Bowel Evacuant Kit-1** (Gray)	74 mL **X-Prep** liquid: Extract of senna concentrate, 50 g sugar, sucrose, parabens. Alcohol-free. 2 **Senokot-S** tablets: Standardized senna concentrate and 50 mg docusate sodium per tablet, lactose. 1 **Rectolax** suppository: 10 mg bisacodyl.	
otc	**Fleet Prep Kit 1** (Fleet)	45 mL **Phospho-soda** (21.6 g monobasic sodium phosphate and 8.1 g dibasic sodium phosphate). 4 bisacodyl tablets (5 mg each). Enteric-coated. 1 bisacodyl suppository (10 mg).	
otc	**Fleet Prep Kit 2** (Fleet)	45 mL **Phospho-soda** (21.6 g monobasic sodium phosphate and 8.1 g dibasic sodium phosphate). 4 bisacodyl tablets (5 mg each). Enteric-coated. 1 bagenema.	
otc	**Fleet Prep Kit 3** (Fleet)	45 mL **Phospho-soda** (21.6 g monobasic sodium phosphate and 8.1 g dibasic sodium phosphate). 4 bisacodyl tablets (5 mg each). Enteric-coated. One 30 mL bisacodyl enema (10 mg).	
Rx	**Visicol** (InKine Pharmaceutical)	**Tablets:** 1.102 g sodium phosphate monobasic monohydrate, 0.398 g sodium phospahte dibasic anhydrous (total of 1.5 g sodium phosphate). In 40s.	

For complete prescribing information, refer to the Laxatives group monograph.

Miscellaneous Laxatives

CASTOR OIL

otc	**Castor Oil** (Various, eg, Humco, Paddock)	**Liquid:** *Dose:* Adults and children ≥ 12 years - 15 to 60 mL/day. Children 2 to < 12 years - 5 to 15 mL/day.	In 60, 120, and 480 mL.
otc	**Purge** (Fleming)	**Liquid:** 95% castor oil. *Dose:* Adults - 30 to 60 mL Children - Adjust between infant and adult dosage. Infants - 2.5 to 7.5 mL	Lemon flavor. In 30 and 60 mL.
otc	**Emulsoil** (Paddock)	**Emulsion:** 95% castor oil with emulsifying agents. *Dose:* Adults and children ≥ 12 years - 15 to 60 mL/day mixed with ½ to 1 glass liquid. Children 2 to < 12 years - 5 to 15 mL mixed with ½ to 1 glass liquid.	Butylparaben. In 63 mL.
otc *sf*	**Neoloid** (Kenwood)	**Emulsion:** 36.4% castor oil with 0.1% sodium benzoate, 0.2% potassium sorbate. *Dose:* Adults and children ≥ 12 years - 45 to 60 mL/day. Children 2 to < 12 years - 15 to 30 mL/day	Mint flavor. In 118 mL.

For complete prescribing information, refer to the Laxatives group monograph.

Laxative Combinations

LAXATIVE COMBINATIONS, CAPSULES AND TABLETS

		Docusate (mg)	Senna Concentrate (mg)	Casanthranol (mg)	Cascara Sagrada (mg)	Other Content and How Supplied
otc	**Senokot-S Tablets** (Purdue Frederick)	50[1]	8.6[2]			Lactose. In 10s, 30s, 60s, 1000s, and UD 100s.
otc	**PeriColace Tablets** (Purdue)	50[1]	8.6[2]			In 10s, 30s, and 60s.
otc	**ex-lax Gentle Strength Caplets** (Novartis)	65[1]	10[2]			Lactose, methylparaben, polydextrose. (ex-lax). In 24s.
otc	**Docusate w/ Casanthranol Caps** (Various, eg, Paddock, Schein, URL)	100[1]		30		In 100s, 1000s, and UD 100s, 300s, and 600s.
otc	**DSS 100 Plus Capsules** (Magno-Humphries)					In 60s.
otc	**Laxative & Stool Softener** (Rugby)					Parabens, sorbitol. In 100s.
otc	**Peri-Colace Capsules** (Roberts)					Sorbitol, parabens. In 30s, 60s, 250s, 1000s, and UD 100s.
otc	**Peri-Dos Softgels (Capsules)** (Goldline)					Sorbitol, parabens. Maroon. In 100s and 1000s.
otc	**Nature's Remedy Tablets** (Block Drug)				150	100 mg aloe, lactose. In 15s, 30s, and 60s.

[1] As sodium.   [2] As sennosides.

LAXATIVE COMBINATIONS, CAPSULES AND TABLETS

For complete prescribing information, refer to the Laxatives group monograph.

Administration and Dosage

➤*Adults:* 1 to 4 capsules/tablets per day. Products vary. Consult product labeling for specific guidelines.

➤*Children < 12 years of age:* Products vary. Consult product labeling for specific guidelines.

Ingredients

In addition to the laxatives listed on the previous pages, these combinations include casanthranol as a stimulant laxative.

LAXATIVE COMBINATIONS, LIQUIDS

otc	**Diocto C** (Various, eg, Alpharma, Rugby)	**Syrup:** 60 mg docusate sodium and 30 mg casanthranol per 15 mL	In 480 mL.
otc	**Peri-Colace** (Roberts)		10% alcohol. Sorbitol, sucrose, parabens. In 240 and 480 mL.
otc sf	**Liqui-Doss** (Ferndale)	**Emulsion:** Mineral oil in an emulsifying base	Alcohol free. In 60 and 480 mL.
otc	**Haley's M-O** (Bayer)	**Liquid:** ≈ 900 mg magnesium hydroxide and 3.75 mL mineral oil per 15 mL	Saccharin (vanilla creme only). Regular or vanilla creme. In 360 (both) and 780 mL (vanilla creme only).
otc	**Black-Draught** (Monticello)	**Syrup:** 90 mg per 15 mL casanthranol with senna extract, rhubarb, methyl salicylate, and menthol	5% alcohol. Tartrazine, parabens, sucrose, saccharin. In 60 and 150 mL.
otc	**Silace-C** (Silarx)	**Syrup:** 30 mg casanthranol, 60 mg docusate sodium per 15 mL	10% alcohol. In 473 mL.
otc sf	**Concentrated Milk of Magnesia-Cascara** (Roxane)	**Suspension:** 15 mL equiv. to 30 mL milk of magnesia, USP, and 5 mL aromatic cascara fluid extract, USP	7% alcohol. In UD 15 mL.

For complete prescribing information, refer to the Laxatives group monograph.

Administration and Dosage

➤*Dose:*

Adults – 5 to 60 mL. Products vary. Consult product labeling for specific guidelines.

Children < 12 years of age – Products vary. Consult product labeling for specific guidelines.

LAXATIVE COMBINATIONS, GRANULES

otc	**Perdiem Overnight Relief** (Novartis Consumer Health)	**Granules:** 3.25 g psyllium, 0.74 g senna, 1.8 mg sodium, 35.5 mg potassium, and 4 calories per rounded teaspoonful	Dye free. Sucrose. Mint flavor. In 100, 250, and 400 g.

For complete prescribing information, refer to the Laxatives group monograph.

Administration and Dosage

➤*Dose:*

Adults and children ≥ 12 years of age – 1 or 2 rounded tsp, 1 to 2 times daily, with ≥ 8 oz cool liquid. Do not chew.

Children 7 to 11 years of age – 1 rounded tsp 1 to 2 times daily with ≥ 8 oz cool liquid. Do not chew.

For severe constipation – May take ≤ 2 rounded tsp every 6 hours, not to exceed 5 tsp/24 hours.

DIFENOXIN HCl WITH ATROPINE SULFATE

c-iv	**Motofen** (Carnrick)	**Tablets:** 1 mg difenoxin (as HCl) and 0.025 mg atropine sulfate	Dye free. (C 8674). White, scored. Five-sided. In 50s and 100s.

Indications

Adjunctive therapy in management of acute nonspecific diarrhea and acute exacerbations of chronic functional diarrhea.

Administration and Dosage

➤*Adults:* Recommended starting dose: 2 tablets, then 1 tablet after each loose stool; 1 tablet every 3 to 4 hours as needed. The total dosage during any 24 hour treatment period should not exceed 8 tablets. For diarrhea in which clinical improvement is not observed in 48 hours, continued administration is not recommended. For acute diarrhea and acute exacerbations of functional diarrhea, treatment beyond 48 hours is usually not necessary.

➤*Children:* Studies in children < 12 years old are inadequate to evaluate safety and efficacy. Contraindicated in children < 2 years old.

Actions

➤*Pharmacology:* Difenoxin is an antidiarrheal agent chemically related to meperidine. Atropine sulfate is present to discourage deliberate overdosage.

Animal studies have shown that difenoxin manifests its antidiarrheal effect by slowing intestinal motility. The mechanism of action is by a local effect on the gastrointestinal wall.

Difenoxin is the principal active metabolite of diphenoxylate and is effective at one-fifth the dosage of diphenoxylate.

➤*Pharmacokinetics:* Difenoxin is rapidly and extensively absorbed orally. Mean peak plasma levels of 160 ng/mL occur within 40 to 60 minutes in most patients following a 2 mg dose. Plasma levels decline to less than 10% of their peak values within 24 hours and to less than 1% of their peak values within 72 hours. This decline parallels the appearance of difenoxin and its metabolites in the urine. Difenoxin is metabolized to an inactive hydroxylated metabolite. Both the drug and its metabolites are excreted, mainly as conjugates, in urine and feces.

Contraindications

Diarrhea associated with organisms that penetrate the intestinal mucosa (eg, toxigenic *E. coli*, *Salmonella* sp, *Shigella*;) and pseudomembranous colitis associated with broad-spectrum antibiotics. Antiperistaltic agents may prolong or worsen diarrhea.

Children < 2 years of age because of the decreased margin of safety of drugs in this class in younger age groups.

Hypersensitivity to difenoxin, atropine or any of the inactive ingredients; jaundice.

Warnings

Difenoxin HCl with atropine sulfate is not innocuous; strictly adhere to dosage recommendations. It is not recommended for children < 2 years of age. Overdosage may result in severe respiratory depression and coma, possibly leading to permanent brain damage or death (see Overdosage).

➤*Fluid and electrolyte balance:* The use of this drug does not preclude the administration of appropriate fluid and electrolyte therapy. Dehydration, particularly in children, may further influence the variability of response and may predispose to delayed difenoxin intoxication. Drug-induced inhibition of peristalsis may result in fluid retention in the colon, and this may further aggravate dehydration and electrolyte imbalance. If severe dehydration or electrolyte imbalance is manifested, withhold the drug until appropriate corrective therapy has been initiated.

➤*Ulcerative colitis:* Agents which inhibit intestinal motility or delay intestinal transit time have induced toxic megacolon. Consequently, carefully observe patients with acute ulcerative colitis. Discontinue promptly if abdominal distention occurs or if other untoward symptoms develop.

➤*Liver and kidney disease:* Use with extreme caution in patients with advanced hepato-renal disease and in all patients with abnormal liver function tests since hepatic coma may be precipitated.

➤*Atropine:* A subtherapeutic dose of atropine has been added to difenoxin to discourage deliberate overdosage. A recommended dose is not likely to cause prominent anticholinergic side effects, but avoid in patients in whom anticholinergic drugs are contraindicated. Observe the warnings and precautions for use of anticholinergic agents. In children, signs of atropinism may occur even with recommended doses, particularly in patients with Down's syndrome.

➤*Pregnancy: Category C.* Reproduction studies in rats and rabbits with doses up to 75 times the human therapeutic dose demonstrated no evidence of teratogenesis. Pregnant rats receiving oral doses 20 times the maximum human dose had an increase in delivery time as well as a significant increase in the percent of stillbirths. Neonatal survival in rats was also reduced with most deaths occurring within 4 days of delivery. There are no well controlled studies in pregnant women. Use during pregnancy only if the potential benefit justifies the potential risk to the fetus.

➤*Lactation:* Because of the potential for serious adverse reactions in nursing infants, decide whether to discontinue nursing or to discontinue the drug, taking into account the importance of the drug to the mother.

➤*Children:* Contraindicated in children under 2 years of age. Safety and efficacy in children below the age of 12 have not been established. See Overdosage section for information on hazards from accidental poisoning in children.

Precautions

➤*Drug abuse and dependence:* Addiction to (dependence on) difenoxin is theoretically possible at high dosage. Therefore, do not exceed recommended dosage. Because of the structural and pharmacological similarities of difenoxin to drugs with definite addiction potential, administer with caution to patients receiving addicting drugs, to addiction-prone individuals, or to those whose histories suggest they may increase the dosage on their own initiative.

Drug Interactions

Difenoxin Drug Interactions			
Precipitant drug	Object drug*		Description
Difenoxin	Barbiturates, tranquilizers, narcotics, and alcohol	↑	Barbiturates, tranquilizers, narcotics, and alcohol may be potentiated by coadministration of difenoxin. Closely monitor patients.
Difenoxin	MAOIs	↑	Because the chemical structure of difenoxin is similar to meperidine, concurrent use with MAOIs may, in theory, precipitate a hypertensive crisis.

*↑ = Object drug increased.

Adverse Reactions

Anticholinergic – In view of the small amount of atropine present (0.025 mg/tablet), effects such as dryness of the skin and mucous membranes, flushing, hyperthermia, tachycardia and urinary retention are very unlikely to occur, except perhaps in children.

Many adverse effects reported during clinical investigation are difficult to distinguish from symptoms of diarrheal syndrome. However, the following events have occurred:

➤*CNS:* Dizziness, lightheadedness (5%); drowsiness (4%); headache (2.5%); tiredness, nervousness, insomnia, confusion (< 1%).

➤*GI:* Nausea (7%), vomiting, dry mouth (3%); epigastric distress, constipation (≤ 1%).

➤*Ophthalmic:* Burning eyes, blurred vision (infrequent).

Overdosage

➤*Symptoms:* Initial signs may include dryness of the skin and mucous membranes, flushing, hyperthermia and tachycardia followed by lethargy or coma, hypotonic reflexes, nystagmus, pinpoint pupils and respiratory depression.

➤*Treatment:* Gastric lavage, establishment of a patent airway and, possibly, mechanically assisted respiration are advised. Refer to General Management of Acute Overdosage.

Naloxone may be used in the treatment of respiratory depression. When administered IV, the onset is generally apparent within 2 minutes. Naloxone may also be administered SC or IM providing a slightly less rapid onset but a more prolonged effect.

Because the duration of action of difenoxin is longer than that of naloxone, improvement of respiration following administration may be followed by recurrent respiratory depression. Continuous observation is necessary until the effect of difenoxin on respiration (which may persist for many hours) has passed. Supplemental IM naloxone doses may be used to produce a longer lasting effect. Treat all possible overdosages as serious; observe for at least 48 hours, preferably under continuous hospital care.

Although signs of overdosage and respiratory depression may not be evident soon after ingestion of difenoxin, respiratory depression may occur 12 to 30 hours later.

Patient Information

Adhere strictly to recommended dosage schedules. Keep out of reach of children since accidental overdosage may result in severe, even fatal, respiratory depression.

May cause dizziness or drowsiness; use caution while driving or performing other tasks requiring alertness, coordination or physical dexterity.

DIPHENOXYLATE HCl WITH ATROPINE SULFATE

C-V	**Diphenoxylate HCl w/Atropine Sulfate** (Various, eg, Mylan, Purepac, Rugby, Schein)	**Tablets:** 2.5 mg diphenoxylate HCl and 0.025 mg atropine sulfate	In 100s, 500s, 1000s, 2500s and UD 100s.
C-V	**Logen** (Goldline)		White. In 100s, 500s & 1000s.
C-V	**Lomotil** (Searle)		Sorbitol, sucrose. (Searle 61). White. In 100s, 500s, 1000s, 2500s, UD 100s.
C-V	**Lonox** (Geneva)		White. In 100s, 500s, 1000s & UD 100s.
C-V	**Diphenoxylate HCl w/ Atropine Sulfate** (Various, eg, Goldline, Roxane, Rugby)	**Liquid:** 2.5 mg diphenoxylate HCl and 0.025 mg atropine sulfate per 5 mL	In 60 mL, UD 4 and 10 mL.
C-V	**Lomanate** (Qualitest)		In 60 mL.
C-V	**Lomotil** (Searle)		15% alcohol. Sorbitol. Cherry flavor. In 60 mL w/dropper.

Indications

Adjunctive therapy in the management of diarrhea.

Administration and Dosage

➤*Adults:* Individualize dosage. Initial dose is 5 mg 4 times a day.

➤*Children:* See Warnings. In children 2 to 12 years of age, use liquid form only. The recommended initial dosage is 0.3 to 0.4 mg/kg daily, in 4 divided doses.

Diphenoxylate w/Atropine Pediatric Dosage			
	Approximate weight		Dosage (mL)
Age (years)	kg	lb	(4 times daily)
2	11-14	24-31	1.5-3
3	12-16	26-35	2-3
4	14-20	31-44	2-4
5	16-23	35-51	2.5-4.5
6-8	17-32	38-71	2.5-5
9-12	23-55	51-121	3.5-5

This pediatric schedule is the best approximation of an average dose recommendation which may be adjusted downwards according to the overall nutritional status and degree of dehydration encountered in the sick child.

➤*Reduce dosage:* Reduce dosage as soon as initial control of symptoms is achieved. Maintenance dosage may be as low as ¼ of the initial daily dosage. Do not exceed recommended dosage. Clinical improvement of acute diarrhea is usually observed within 48 hours. If clinical improvement of chronic diarrhea is not seen within 10 days after a maximum daily dose of 20 mg, symptoms are unlikely to be controlled by further use.

Actions

➤*Pharmacology:* Diphenoxylate, a constipating meperidine congener, lacks analgesic activity. High doses (40 to 60 mg) cause opioid activity, (eg, euphoria, suppression of morphine abstinence syndrome, physical dependence after chronic use).

➤*Pharmacokinetics:* Bioavailability of tablet vs liquid is ≈ 90%. Diphenoxylate is rapidly, extensively metabolized to diphenoxylic acid (difenoxine), the active major metabolite. Elimination half-life is ≈ 12 to 14 hrs. An average of 14% of drug and metabolites are excreted over 4 days in urine, 49% in feces. Urinary excretion of unmetabolized drug is < 1%; difenoxine plus its glucuronide conjugate constitutes ≈ 6%.

Contraindications

Children < 2 years old due to greater variability of response; hypersensitivity to diphenoxylate or atropine; obstructive jaundice; diarrhea associated with pseudomembranous enterocolitis or enterotoxin-producing bacteria (see Warnings).

Warnings

➤*Diarrhea:* Diphenoxylate may prolong or aggravate diarrhea associated with organisms that penetrate intestinal mucosa (ie, toxigenic *Escherichia coli, Salmonella, Shigella*) or in pseudomembranous enterocolitis associated with broad-spectrum antibiotics. Do not use diphenoxylate in these conditions. In some patients with acute ulcerative colitis, diphenoxylate may induce toxic megacolon. Discontinue therapy if abdominal distention or other untoward symptoms develop.

➤*Fluid / electrolyte balance:* Dehydration, particularly in younger children, may influence variability of response and may predispose to delayed diphenoxylate intoxication. Inhibition of peristalsis may result in fluid retention in the intestine, which may further aggravate dehydration and electrolyte imbalance. If severe dehydration or electrolyte imbalance occurs, withhold the drug until initiating corrective therapy.

➤*Hepatic function impairment:* Use with extreme caution in patients with advanced hepato-renal disease or abnormal liver function; hepatic coma may be precipitated.

➤*Pregnancy: Category C.* There are no adequate and well controlled studies in pregnant women. Use in women of childbearing potential only when clearly needed and when the potential benefits outweigh the potential hazards to the fetus.

➤*Lactation:* Exercise caution when administering to a nursing mother. Diphenoxylic acid may be excreted in breast milk and atropine is excreted in breast milk.

➤*Children:* Use with caution; signs of atropinism may occur with recommended doses, particularly in Down's syndrome patients. Use with caution in young children due to variable response. Not recommended in children < 2 years old.

Precautions

➤*Drug abuse and dependence:* In recommended doses, diphenoxylate has not produced addiction and is devoid of morphine-like subjective effects. At high doses, it exhibits codeine-like subjective effects; therefore, addiction to diphenoxylate is possible. A subtherapeutic dose of atropine may discourage deliberate abuse.

➤*Hazardous tasks:* Patients should use caution while driving or performing other tasks requiring alertness, coordination or physical dexterity.

Drug Interactions

Diphenoxylate Drug Interactions			
Precipitant drug	Object drug*		Description
Diphenoxylate	MAOIs	↑	Since the chemical structure of diphenoxylate is similar to meperidine, concurrent use may precipitate hypertensive crises.
Diphenoxylate	Barbiturates, tranquilizers, and alcohol	↑	Diphenoxylate may potentiate the depressant action. Closely observe the patient when these medications are used concomitantly.

* ↑ = Object drug increased.

Adverse Reactions

Atropine effects – Dry skin and mucous membranes, flushing, hyperthermia, tachycardia, urinary retention, especially in children.

➤*CNS:* Dizziness; drowsiness; sedation; headache; malaise; lethargy; restlessness; euphoria; depression; numbness of extremities; confusion.

➤*GI:* Anorexia; nausea; vomiting; abdominal discomfort; paralytic ileus; toxic megacolon; pancreatitis.

➤*Hypersensitivity:* Pruritus; gum swelling; angioneurotic edema; urticaria; anaphylaxis.

Overdosage

➤*Symptoms:* Initial signs include dry skin and mucous membranes, mydriasis, restlessness, flushing, hyperthermia and tachycardia followed by lethargy or coma, hypotonic reflexes, nystagmus and pinpoint pupils. Severe, even fatal, respiratory depression may result. Signs of overdosage and respiratory depression may not be evident soon after ingestion; respiratory depression may occur 12 to 30 hours later.

➤*Treatment:* includes usual supportive measures. Refer to General Management of Acute Overdosage. Gastric lavage, induction of emesis, establishment of a patent airway, and, possibly, mechanically assisted respiration are advised. Use naloxone for respiratory depression (see individual monograph). Diphenoxylate's duration of action is longer than that of naloxone; improved respiration after administration may be followed by recurrent respiratory depression. Consequently, continuous observation for at least 48 hours is necessary until diphenoxylate's effect on respiration has passed. Activated charcoal may significantly decrease bioavailability of diphenoxylate. In non-comatose patients, 100 g activated charcoal slurry can be given immediately after induction of vomiting or gastric lavage.

Patient Information

Do not exceed prescribed dosage. Avoid alcohol and other CNS depressants.

May cause drowsiness or dizziness; use caution while driving or performing other tasks requiring alertness, coordination or physical dexterity.

May cause dry mouth.

Notify physician if diarrhea persists or if fever, palpitations or abnormal distention occur.

LOPERAMIDE HCl

otc	**Diar-aid Caplets** (Thompson)	**Tablets:** 2 mg	In 12s.
otc	**Imodium A-D Caplets** (McNeil-CPC)		Lactose. (Imodium Janssen). In 6s and 12s.
otc	**K-Pek II** (Rugby)		Lactose. (122). Capsule shape. In 12s.
Rx	**Loperamide** (Various, eg, Mylan, Novopharm)	**Capsules:** 2 mg	In 100s, 500s and 1000s.
otc	**Neo-Diaral** (Roberts)		In UD 8s and 250s.
otc	**Loperamide** (Various, eg, Barre-National, Roxane)	**Liquid:** 1 mg/5 mL	In 60 and 118 mL.
otc	**Imodium A-D** (McNeil-CPC)		5.25% alcohol. Cherry/licorice flavor. In 60, 90 and 120 mL.
otc	**Pepto Diarrhea Control** (Procter & Gamble)	**Liquid:** 1 mg/mL	5.25% alcohol, parabens. Cherry flavor. In 60 and 120 mL.

Indications

➤*Rx:* Control and symptomatic relief of acute nonspecific diarrhea and of chronic diarrhea associated with inflammatory bowel disease.

For reducing the volume of discharge from ileostomies.

➤*OTC:* Control of symptoms of diarrhea, including traveler's diarrhea.

➤*Unlabeled uses:* In one study, the combination of loperamide (4 mg loading dose, 2 mg after each loose stool) plus trimethoprim-sulfamethoxazole for 3 days resulted in more rapid relief from traveler's diarrhea than either agent alone.

Administration and Dosage

➤*Rx: Acute diarrhea:* Adults: 4 mg followed by 2 mg after each unformed stool. Do not exceed 16 mg/day. Clinical improvement is usually observed within 48 hours.

➤*Children:* First day doses:

Loperamide Pediatric Dosage (First Day Schedule)

Age (years)	Weight (kg)	Doseform	Amount
2-5	13-20	liquid	1 mg tid
6-8	20-30	liquid or capsule	2 mg bid
8-12	> 30	liquid or capsule	2 mg tid

This dosage may be adjusted downwards according to the overall nutritional status and degree of dehydration encountered in the sick child.

Subsequent doses – Administer 1 mg/10 kg only after a loose stool. Total daily dosage should not exceed recommended dosages for the first day.

➤*Chronic diarrhea:*

Adults – 4 mg followed by 2 mg after each unformed stool until diarrhea is controlled; then, individualize dosage. When optimal daily dosage (average, 4 to 8 mg) has been established, administer as a single dose or in divided doses.

If clinical improvement is not observed after treatment with 16 mg/day for at least 10 days, symptoms are unlikely to be controlled by further use. Continue administration if diarrhea cannot be adequately controlled with diet or specific treatment.

➤*Children:* Dose has not been established.

➤*OTC: Acute diarrhea, including traveler's diarrhea:*

Adults – 4 mg after first loose bowel movement followed by 2 mg after each subsequent loose bowel movement but no more than 8 mg/day for no more than 2 days.

Children –

9 to 11 years old (60 to 95 lbs): 2 mg after first loose bowel movement followed by 1 mg after each subsequent loose bowel movement but no more than 6 mg/day for no more than 2 days.

6 to 8 years old (48 to 59 lbs): 1 mg after first loose bowel movement followed by 1 mg after each subsequent loose bowel movement but no more than 4 mg/day for no more than 2 days.

• *< 6 years old (up to 47 lbs)* – Consult physician (not for use in children < 6 years of age).

Actions

➤*Pharmacology:* Loperamide slows intestinal motility and affects water and electrolyte movement through the bowel. It inhibits peristalsis by a direct effect on the circular and longitudinal muscles of the intestinal wall. It reduces daily fecal volume, increases viscosity and bulk density and diminishes the loss of fluid and electrolytes. Tolerance to the antidiarrheal effect has not been observed.

In morphine-dependent monkeys, loperamide at higher than recommended doses prevented signs of morphine withdrawal. However, in humans, opiate-like effects have not been demonstrated after > 2 years of therapeutic use of loperamide.

➤*Pharmacokinetics:*

Absorption/Distribution – Loperamide is 40% absorbed after oral administration and does not penetrate well into the brain. Peak plasma levels occur approximately 5 hours after capsule administration, 2.5 hours after liquid administration and are similar for both formulations.

Metabolism/Excretion – The apparent elimination half-life is 10.8 hrs (range, 9.1 to 14.4 hrs). Of a 4 mg oral dose, 25% is excreted unchanged in the feces, and 1.3% is excreted in the urine as free drug and glucuronic acid conjugate within 3 days.

Contraindications

Hypersensitivity to the drug and in patients who must avoid constipation.

➤*OTC use:* Bloody diarrhea; body temperature > 101°F.

Warnings

➤*Diarrhea:* Do not use loperamide in acute diarrhea associated with organisms that penetrate the intestinal mucosa (enteroinvasive *Escherichia coli*, *Salmonella* and *Shigella*) or in pseudomembranous colitis associated with broad-spectrum antibiotics.

➤*Acute ulcerative colitis:* In some patients with acute ulcerative colitis, agents which inhibit intestinal motility or delay intestinal transit time may induce toxic megacolon. Discontinue therapy promptly if abdominal distention occurs or if other untoward symptoms develop in patients with acute ulcerative colitis.

➤*Fluid/electrolyte depletion:* Fluid/electrolyte depletion may occur in patients who have diarrhea. Loperamide use does not preclude administration of appropriate fluid and electrolyte therapy.

➤*Pregnancy: Category B.* There are no adequate and well controlled studies in pregnant women. Safety for use during pregnancy is not established. Use only when clearly needed and when potential benefits outweigh potential hazards to fetus.

➤*Lactation:* It is not known whether loperamide is excreted in breast milk. Safety for use in the nursing mother has not been established.

➤*Children:* Not recommended for use in children < 2 years old. Use special caution in young children because of the greater variability of response in this age group. Dehydration may further influence variability of response. Dosage has not been established for children in treatment of chronic diarrhea.

Precautions

➤*Acute diarrhea:* If clinical improvement is not observed in 48 hours, discontinue use.

➤*Hepatic dysfunction:* Monitor patients with hepatic dysfunction closely for signs of CNS toxicity because of the apparent large first-pass biotransformation.

➤*Drug abuse and dependence:* Physical dependence in humans has not been observed.

Adverse Reactions

Adverse experiences are generally minor and self-limiting; they are more commonly observed during the treatment of chronic diarrhea: Abdominal pain, distention or discomfort; constipation; dry mouth; nausea; vomiting; tiredness; drowsiness or dizziness; hypersensitivity reactions (including skin rash).

Overdosage

➤*Symptoms:* Constipation, CNS depression and GI irritation. In clinical trials, nausea and vomiting occurred in an adult who took 60 mg within 24 hours. Ingestion of up to 60 mg loperamide in a single dose caused no significant adverse effects in healthy subjects. A 15-month-old, 8 kg child developed opioid toxicity (eg, pale skin, increased pulse rate, respiratory depression) following a 1 g dose of loperamide.

➤*Treatment:* Activated charcoal administered promptly after loperamide ingestion can reduce the amount of drug absorbed into systemic circulation by up to ninefold.

LOPERAMIDE HCl

Monitor for CNS depression for at least 24 hrs; if it occurs, give naloxone. Children may be more sensitive to CNS effects. If responsive to naloxone, monitor vital signs for symptom recurrence for at least 24 hrs after the last naloxone dose. In view of loperamide's prolonged action and naloxone's short duration (1 to 3 hrs) (see individual monograph), monitor closely; repeat naloxone as indicated.

May cause drowsiness or dizziness; patients should observe caution while driving or performing other tasks requiring alertness, coordination or physical dexterity.

May cause dry mouth. Drink plenty of clear fluids to help prevent dehydration, which may accompany diarrhea.

Notify physician if diarrhea does not stop after a few days or if abdominal pain or distention or fever occurs. Do not exceed prescribed dosage.

BISMUTH SUBSALICYLATE (BSS)

otc	**Bismatrol** (Major)	**Tablets, chewable:** 262 mg	Saccharin. In 240 mL.
otc	**Peptic Relief** (Rugby)		Dextrose, sorbitol. In 30s.
otc sf	**Pepto-Bismol** (Procter & Gamble)		< 2 mg sodium/tablet. Saccharin, mannitol. (Pepto-Bismol). Pink. Original and cherry flavors. In 30s, 42s (cherry). In 24s, 42s (original).
otc	**Kaopectate Children's** (Pharmacia)	**Liquid:** 87 mg/5 mL	Sucrose. Cherry flavor. In 236 mL.
otc	**Pink Bismuth** (Various, eg, Goldline)	**Liquid:** 130 mg/15 mL	In 240 mL.
otc	**Pink Bismuth** (Various, eg, Goldline)	**Liquid:** 262 mg/15 mL	In 240 mL.
otc	**Kaopectate** (Pharmacia)		Sucrose. In 236 and 355 mL (regular flavor) and 236 and 355 mL (peppermint flavor).
otc	**Peptic Relief** (Rugby)		Saccharin, sorbitol. In 237 mL.
otc sf	**Pepto-Bismol** (Procter & Gamble)		5 mg sodium/15 mL. Saccharin. In 120, 240, 360 & 480 mL.
otc sf	**Pepto-Bismol Maximum Strength** (P & G)	**Liquid:** 524 mg/15 mL	< 5 mg sodium/15 mL. Saccharin. In 120, 240 and 360 mL.
otc	**Kaopectate Extra Strength** (Pharmacia)	**Liquid:** 525 mg/15 mL	Sucrose. Peppermint flavor. In 236 mL.

Indications

For indigestion without causing constipation; nausea; control of diarrhea, including traveler's diarrhea, within 24 hours. Also relieves abdominal cramps.

➤*Unlabeled uses:* Bismuth subsalicylate (BSS) has been used to prevent traveler's diarrhea (enterotoxigenic *Escherichia coli*), in doses of 2.1 g/day (2 tablets 4 times daily before meals and at bedtime) for up to 3 weeks during brief periods of high risk. The suspension has also been used (4.2 g/day). BSS has been effective in up to 65% of patients.

BSS has also been used for chronic infantile diarrhea (2.5 mL every 4 hours for children 2 to 24 months old; 5 mL for those 24 to 48 months old; 10 mL for those 48 to 70 months old) and for symptoms of Norwalk virus-induced gastroenteritis.

Administration and Dosage

➤*Adults:* 2 tablets or 30 mL.

➤*Children:*

9 to 12 years of age – 1 tablet or 15 mL.

6 to 9 years of age – ⅔ tablet or 10 mL.

3 to 6 years of age – ⅓ tablet or 5 mL.

< 3 years of age – Consult physician.

Repeat dosage every 30 minutes to 1 hour, as needed, up to 8 doses in 24 hours.

Actions

➤*Pharmacology:* BSS appears to have antisecretory and antimicrobial effects in vitro and may have some anti-inflammatory effects. The salicylate moiety provides the antisecretory effect, while the bismuth moiety may exert direct antimicrobial effects against bacterial and viral enteropathogens.

➤*Pharmacokinetics:* BSS undergoes chemical dissociation in the GI tract. Two BSS tablets yield 204 mg salicylate. Following ingestion, salicylate is absorbed, with> 90% recovered in the urine; plasma levels are similar to levels achieved after a comparable dose of aspirin. Absorption of bismuth is negligible.

Precautions

➤*Impaction:* Impaction may occur in infants and debilitated patients.

➤*Radiologic examinations:* May interfere with radiologic examinations of GI tract. Bismuth is radiopaque.

Drug Interactions

Bismuth Subsalicylate (BSS) Drug Interactions			
Precipitant drug	Object drug*		Description
BSS	Aspirin	↑	BSS contains salicylate. If taken with aspirin and ringing of the ears occurs, discontinue use.
BSS	Tetracyclines	↓	BSS may decrease GI absorption and bioavailability of tetracyclines, reducing their efficacy.

* ↑ = Object drug increased.   ↓ = Object drug decreased.

Shake liquid well before using. Chew tablets or allow to dissolve in mouth.

Stool may temporarily appear gray-black.

If diarrhea is accompanied by high fever or continues for > 2 days, consult physician.

ANTIDIARRHEAL COMBINATION PRODUCTS

otc	**Kaolin w/Pectin** (Various, eg, Roxane, Wyeth-Ayerst)	**Suspension:** 90 g kaolin, 2 g pectin/30 mL. *Dose:* After each bowel movement. *Adults* - 60 to 120 mL/dose.	In 180 mL, pt and UD 30 mL.
otc	**Kapectolin** (Various, eg, Goldline, Major)	*Children - 6 to 12 years:* 30 to 60 mL/dose. *3 to 6 years:* 15 to 30 mL/dose.	In 360 mL.
otc	**Parepectolin** (Rhone-Poulenc Rorer)	**Concentrated liquid:** 600 mg attapulgite/15 mL. *Dose:* After each bowel movement up to 7 doses/day. *Adults* – 30 mL/dose. *Children - 6 to 12 years:* 15 mL/dose. *3 to < 6 years:* 7.5 mL/dose.	Sucrose. In 240 mL.
otc	**K-Pek** (Rugby)	**Suspension:** 750 mg attapulgite/15 mL. *Dose:* After each bowel movement up to 6 doses/day. *≥ 12* – 30 mL. *Children - 6 to < 12 years:* 15 mL/dose. *3 to < 6 years:* 7.5 mL/dose.	EDTA, methylparaben. sucrose. In 237 and 473 mL.
otc	**Kaodene Non-Narcotic** (Pfeiffer)	**Liquid:** 3.9 g kaolin, 194.4 mg pectin/30 mL, bismuth subsalicylate. *Dose:* 1 to 3 doses/day or after each loose stool. *Adults* – 45 mL/dose. *Children - 6 to 12 years:* 22.5 mL/dose. *3 to 6 years:* 15 mL/dose.	Alcohol free. Sucrose. In 120 mL.
otc	**Diasorb** (Columbia)	**Tablets:** 750 mg activated attapulgite. *Dose:* After each bowel movement up to 3 doses/day. *Adults* - 4/dose. *Children – 6 to 12 years:* 2/dose. *3 to 6 years:* 1/dose.	Sorbitol. In 24s.
		Liquid: 750 mg activated attapulgite/5 mL. *Dose:* After each bowel movement up to 3 doses/day. *Adults* – 20 mL/dose. *Children - 6 to 12 years:* 10 mL/dose. *3 to 6 years:* 5 mL/dose.	Sugar free. Sorbitol, saccharin. Cola flavor. In 120 mL.
otc	**Kaopectate Maximum Strength** (Upjohn)	**Caplets:** 750 mg attapulgite. *Dose:* After each bowel movement up to 6 doses/day. *Adults* - 2/dose. *Children - 6 to 12 years:* 1/dose.	Sucrose. In 12s and 20s.

Indications

For the symptomatic treatment of diarrhea by reducing intestinal motility or adsorbing fluid.

Warnings

►*Diarrhea from other causes:* Do not use antiperistaltic agents for diarrhea associated with pseudomembranous enterocolitis or in diarrhea caused by toxigenic bacteria.

►*Salicylate absorption:* Salicylate absorption may occur from bismuth subsalicylate; therefore, observe caution in patients with bleeding disorders or salicylate sensitivity and in children.

►*Ingredients:* The use of the ingredients in combination in the following products as nonspecific antidiarrheal agents has, to a large extent, been empiric. Adequate controlled clinical studies demonstrating the efficacy of these antidiarrheal combinations are lacking. The FDA has determined that the following ingredients are *not* generally recognized as safe and effective and are misbranded when present in *otc* antidiarrheal preparations: Aluminum hydroxide, atropine sulfate, calcium carbonate, carboxymethylcellulose, glycine, homatropine methylbromide, hyoscyamine sulfate, *Lactobacillus acidophilus* and *bulgaricus*, opium (powdered and tincture), paregoric, phenyl salicylate, scopolamine hydrobromide and zinc phenolsulfonate.

In 1986, in the tentative final monograph for these agents, the FDA considered attapulgite a Category I agent (safe and effective) and placed kaolin and pectin in Category III (insufficient data to permit classification). Recently, however, an FDA advisory committee recommended that the FDA reverse the classifications, making attapulgite Category III and kaolin and pectin Category I. Further studies are pending.

Activated attapulgite, kaolin and **pectin** are used for their adsorbent and protectant actions.

Bismuth salts have antacid and adsorbent properties.

SIMETHICONE

otc	**Simethicone** (Various)	**Drops:** 40 mg per 0.6 mL	In 30 mL w/calibrated oral syringe.
otc	**Flatulex** (Dayton)		In 30 mL w/calibrated dropper.
otc	**Genasyme Drops** (Goldline)		Hydroxypropyl methylcellulose, saccharin calcium, sodium benzoate, sodium citrate. In 30 mL.
otc	**Mylicon** (J&J-Merck)		In 30 mL dropper bottle.
otc	**Degas** (Invamed)	**Tablets, chewable:** 80 mg	Sucrose. In 100s.
otc	**Gas Relief** (Rugby)		In 100s.
otc	**Gax-X** (Sandoz)		(Gas-X). White, scored. In 12s, 30s.
otc	**Genasyme** (Goldline)		Chewable. In 100s.
otc	**Maalox Anti-Gas** (R-P Rorer)		Sucrose. Lemon flavor. In 12s.
otc	**Extra Strength Gas-X** (Sandoz)	**Tablets, chewable:** 125 mg	(Gas-X). Yellow, scored. In 18s.
otc	**Gas Relief** (Rugby)		Dextrose, sugar, sorbitol. In 60s and 100s.
otc	**Maximum Strength Mylanta Gas** (J&J-Merck)		Sorbitol. White, scored. In 12s and 60s.
otc	**Maalox Extra Strength Anti-Gas** (Novartis)	**Tablets, chewable:** 150 mg	Mannitol, sucrose. Lemon and peppermint flavors. In 10s.
otc	**Phazyme** (Reed & Carnrick)	**Tablets:** 60 mg	Enteric coated inner core. In 50s, 100s and 1000s.
otc	**Phazyme 95** (Reed & Carnrick)	**Tablets:** 95 mg	Enteric coated inner core. In 50s, 100s, 500s and Consumer Pak 10s.
otc	**Phazyme 125** (Reed & Carnrick)	**Capsules:** 125 mg	(Phazyme 125). Red. In 50s.
otc	**Gas-X Extra Strength** (Sandoz)	**Capsules, softgel:** 125 mg	Sorbitol. In 10s and 30s.

Indications

For relief of the painful symptoms of excess gas in the digestive tract. Used as an adjunct in the treatment of many conditions in which gas retention may be a problem, such as: Postoperative gaseous distention, air swallowing, functional dyspepsia, peptic ulcer, spastic or irritable colon, or diverticulosis.

➤*Unlabeled uses:* Simethicone has been used for treating the symptoms of infant colic. It is generally administered with meals.

Administration and Dosage

➤*Capsules:* 125 mg, 4 times daily after each meal and at bedtime.

➤*Tablets:* 40 to 125 mg, 4 times daily after each meal and at bedtime. Chew thoroughly.

➤*Drops:* Take after meals and at bedtime. Shake well before using.

Children < 2 years of age – 20 mg 4 times daily up to 240 mg/day. For ease of administration, dosage can be mixed with 30 mL cool water, infant formula or other suitable liquids.

Children 2 to 12 years of age – 40 mg 4 times daily.

Adults – 40 to 80 mg 4 times daily up to 500 mg/day.

Actions

➤*Pharmacology:* The defoaming action relieves flatulence by dispersing and preventing the formation of mucus-surrounded gas pockets in the GI tract. It acts in the stomach and intestines to change the surface tension of gas bubbles, enabling them to coalesce; thus, gas is freed and eliminated more easily by belching or passing flatus.

CHARCOAL

otc	**Charcoal Plus DS** (Kramer)	**Tablets:** 250 mg	Sorbitol. In 120s.
otc	**Charcoal** (Various, eg, Nature's Bounty, Rugby)	**Capsules:** 260 mg	In 50s and 100s.
otc	**CharcoCaps** (Requa)		In 8s, 36s and 100s.

Indications

For relief of intestinal gas, diarrhea and GI distress associated with indigestion and accompanying cramps or odor.

For the prevention of nonspecific pruritus associated with kidney dialysis treatment.

For use as an antidote in poisonings, see individual monograph in the Endocrine/Metabolic chapter.

Administration and Dosage

Usual adult dosage is 500 to 520 mg after meals or at first sign of discomfort. Repeat as needed, up to 5 g daily.

Actions

➤*Pharmacology:* Charcoal is an adsorbent, detoxicant and soothing agent. It reduces the volume of intestinal gas and relieves related discomfort.

Warnings

➤*Diarrhea:* If diarrhea persists for > 2 days or is accompanied by fever, consult physician.

➤*High dosage or prolonged use:* High dosage or prolonged use does not cause side effects or harm the patient's nutritional state.

➤*Children:* Do not use in children < 3 years of age.

Drug Interactions

Activated charcoal can adsorb drugs while they are in the GI tract. Therefore, take charcoal 2 hours before, or 1 hour after other medication.

Charcoal Drug Interactions				
Precipitant drug	Object drug*			Description
Charcoal	Acetaminophen Barbiturates Carbamazepine Digitoxin Digoxin Furosemide Glutethimide Hydantoins Methotrexate Nizatidine Phenothiazines	Phenylbutazones Propoxyphene Salicylates Sulfones Sulfonylureas Tetracyclines Theophyllines Tricyclic antidepressants Valproic acid	↓	Charcoal can reduce absorption of these drugs and actually remove them from the systemic circulation which may reduce the effectiveness of a given agent. Charcoal is also used as an antidote for drug overdoses (refer to the individual monograph in the Endocrine/Metabolic chapter).

* ↓ = Object drug decreased.

CHARCOAL AND SIMETHICONE

otc	**Flatulex** (Dayton)	**Tablets:** 250 mg activated charcoal and 80 mg simethicone	Green. In 100s.

Indications

For the relief of gas pain and associated symptoms.

Administration and Dosage

1 tablet 3 times daily and at bedtime.

Actions

➤*Pharmacology:* Charcoal reduces the volume of gas. Simethicone disperses and prevents the formation of mucus-surrounded gas pockets, and allows for their elimination. For further information on simethicone, refer to the individual monograph.

ORLISTAT

Rx	Xenical (Roche)	Capsules: 120 mg	(Roche XENICAL 120). Dark blue. In 90s.

Indications

►*Obesity management:* For management of obesity including weight loss and weight maintenance when used in conjunction with a reduced-calorie diet. Orlistat is also indicated to reduce the risk for weight regain after prior weight loss. Orlistat is indicated for obese patients with an initial body mass index (BMI) ≥ 30 kg/m², or ≥ 27 kg/m² in the presence of other risk factors (eg, hypertension, diabetes, dyslipidemia).

The following table illustrates body mass index (BMI) according to a variety of weights and heights. The BMI is calculated by dividing weight in kilograms by height in meters squared. For example, a person who weighs 180 lbs and is 5'5'' would have a BMI of 30.

Body Mass Index (BMI), kg/m²*																					
Height (ft/in)	Weight (lb)																				
	120	130	140	150	160	170	180	190	200	210	220	230	240	250	260	270	280	290	300	310	320
4'10''	25	27	29	31	34	36	38	40	42	44	46	48	50	52	54	57	59	61	63	65	67
4'11''	24	26	28	30	32	34	36	38	40	43	45	47	49	51	53	55	57	59	61	63	65
5'0''	23	25	27	29	31	33	35	37	39	41	43	45	47	49	51	53	55	57	59	61	63
5'1''	23	25	27	28	30	32	34	36	38	40	42	44	45	47	49	51	53	55	57	59	61
5'2''	22	24	26	27	29	31	33	35	37	38	40	42	44	46	48	49	51	53	55	57	59
5'3''	21	23	25	27	28	30	32	34	36	37	39	41	43	44	46	48	49	51	53	55	57
5'4''	21	22	24	26	28	29	31	33	34	36	38	40	41	43	45	46	48	50	51	53	55
5'5''	20	22	23	25	27	28	30	32	33	35	37	38	40	42	43	45	47	48	50	52	53
5'6''	19	21	23	24	26	27	29	31	32	34	36	37	39	40	42	44	45	47	48	50	52
5'7''	19	20	22	24	25	27	28	30	31	33	35	36	38	39	41	42	44	46	47	49	50
5'8''	18	20	21	23	24	26	27	29	30	32	34	35	37	38	40	41	43	44	46	47	49
5'9''	18	19	21	22	24	25	27	28	30	31	33	34	36	37	38	40	41	43	44	46	47
5'10''	17	19	20	22	23	24	26	27	29	30	32	33	35	36	37	39	40	42	43	45	46
5'11''	17	18	20	21	22	24	25	27	28	29	31	32	34	35	36	38	39	41	42	43	45
6'0''	16	18	19	20	22	23	24	26	27	29	30	31	33	34	35	37	38	39	41	42	43
6'1''	16	17	19	20	21	22	24	25	26	28	29	30	32	33	34	36	37	38	40	41	42
6'2''	15	17	18	19	21	22	23	24	26	27	28	30	31	32	33	35	36	37	39	40	41

* Conversion factors: Weight in lbs ÷ 2.2 = weight in kilograms (kg)Height in inches × 0.0254 = height in meters (m)1 foot = 12 inches.

Administration and Dosage

►*Approved by the FDA:* April 26, 1999.

The recommended dose of orlistat is one 120 mg capsule 3 times a day with each main meal containing fat (during or up to 1 hour after the meal).

Place the patient on a nutritionally balanced, reduced-calorie diet that contains ≈ 30% of calories from fat. Distribute the daily intake of fat, carbohydrate, and protein over 3 main meals. If a meal is occasionally missed or contains no fat, the dose of orlistat can be omitted.

Because orlistat reduces the absorption of some fat-soluble vitamins and beta-carotene, counsel patients to take a multivitamin containing fat-soluble vitamins to ensure adequate nutrition. Instruct the patient to take the supplement once a day, ≥ 2 hours before or after the administration of orlistat, such as at bedtime.

Doses > 120 mg 3 times a day have not been shown to provide additional benefit.

Based on fecal fat measurements, the effect of orlistat is seen as soon as 24 to 48 hours after dosing. Upon discontinuation of therapy, fecal fat content usually returns to pretreatment levels within 48 to 72 hours.

Safety and effectiveness beyond 2 years have not been determined at this time.

Actions

►*Pharmacology:* Orlistat is a reversible lipase inhibitor for obesity management that acts by inhibiting the absorption of dietary fats. It exerts its therapeutic activity in the lumen of the stomach and small intestine by forming a covalent bond with the active serine residue site of gastric and pancreatic lipases. Consequently, the inactivated enzymes are unavailable to hydrolyze dietary fat in the form of triglycerides into absorbable free fatty acids and monoglycerides. Undigested triglycerides are not absorbed, resulting in a caloric deficit that may have a positive effect on weight control. Therefore, systemic absorption of the drug is not needed for activity. At the recommended therapeutic dose of 120 mg 3 times a day, orlistat inhibits dietary fat absorption by ≈ 30%.

In several studies of up to 6 weeks duration, the effects of therapeutic doses of orlistat on GI and systemic physiological processes were assessed in healthy-weight and obese subjects. Post-prandial cholecystokinin plasma concentrations were lowered after multiple doses of orlistat in 2 studies but not significantly different from placebo in 2 other experiments. There were no clinically significant changes observed in gallbladder motility, bile composition or lithogenicity, or colonic cell proliferation rate, and no clinically significant reduction of gastric emptying time or gastric acidity. In addition, no effects on plasma triglyceride levels or systemic lipases were observed with the administration of orlistat in these studies. In a 3-week study of 28 healthy male volunteers, orlistat (120 mg 3 times a day) did not significantly affect the balance of calcium, magnesium, phosphorus, zinc, copper, and iron.

A simple maximum effect (E_{max}) model was used to define the dose-response curve of the relationship between orlistat daily dose and fecal fat excretion as representative of GI lipase inhibition. The dose-response curve demonstrated a steep portion for doses up to ≈ 400 mg daily, followed by a plateau for higher doses. At doses > 120 mg 3 times a day, the percentage increase in effect was minimal.

►*Pharmacokinetics:*

Absorption – Systemic exposure to orlistat is minimal. Peak plasma concentrations occurred at ≈ 8 hours following oral dosing with 360 mg orlistat; plasma concentrations of intact orlistat were near the limits of detection (< 5 ng/mL). In therapeutic studies involving monitoring of plasma samples, detection of intact orlistat in plasma was sporadic and concentrations were low (< 10 ng/mL or 0.02 mcm), without evidence of accumulation, and consistent with minimal absorption.

The average absolute bioavailablity of intact orlistat was assessed in studies with male rats at oral doses of 150 and 1000 mg/kg/day and in male dogs at oral doses of 100 and 1000 mg/kg/day and found to be 0.12% and 0.59% in rats and 0.7% and 1.9% in dogs, respectively.

Distribution – In vitro orlistat was > 99% bound to plasma proteins (lipoproteins and albumin were major binding proteins). Orlistat minimally partitioned into erythrocytes.

Metabolism – Based on animal data, it is likely that the metabolism of orlistat occurs mainly within the GI wall. In obese patients, 2 metabolites, M1 (4-member lactone ring hydrolyzed) and M3 (M1 with N-formyl leucine moiety cleaved), accounted for ≈ 42% in plasma. M1 and M3 have an open beta-lactone ring and extremely weak lipase inhibitory activity (1000- and 2500-fold less than orlistat, respectively). In view of this low inhibitory activity and the low plasma levels at the therapeutic dose (average of 26 and 108 ng/mL for M1 and M3, respectively, 2 to 4 hours after a dose), these metabolites are considered pharmacologically inconsequential. The primary metabolite M1 had a short half-life (≈ 3 hours) whereas the secondary metabolite M3 disappeared at a slower rate (half-life, ≈ 13.5 hours). In obese patients, steady-state plasma levels of M1, but not M3, increased in proportion to orlistat doses.

Excretion – Fecal excretion was the major route of elimination following a single oral dose of 360 mg orlistat in healthy and obese subjects. Orlistat and its M1 and M3 metabolites also underwent biliary excretion. Approximately 97% was excreted in feces; 83% of that was found to be unchanged orlistat. The cumulative renal excretion was < 2%. The time to reach complete excretion (fecal plus urinary) was 3 to 5 days. The disposition of orlistat appeared to be similar between healthy-weight and obese subjects. Based on limited data, the half-life of the absorbed drug is in the range of 1 to 2 hours.

►*Clinical trials:* Observational epidemiologic studies have established a relationship between obesity and visceral fat and the risks for cardiovascular disease, type 2 diabetes, certain forms of cancer, gallstones, certain respiratory disorders, and an increase in overall mortality. These studies suggest that weight loss, if maintained, may produce health benefits for obese patients who have or are at risk of developing weight-related comorbidities. The long-term effects of orlistat on mor-

ORLISTAT

bidity and mortality associated with obesity have not been established.

One-year results – Weight loss was observed within 2 weeks of initiation of therapy and continued for 6 to 12 months. Pooled data from 5 clinical trials indicated that the overall mean weight loss from randomization to the end of 6 months and 1 year of treatment in the intent-to-treat population were 12.4 lbs and 13.4 lbs in the patients treated with orlistat and 6.2 lbs and 5.8 lbs in the placebo-treated patients, respectively. During the 4-week placebo lead-in period of the studies, an additional 5 to 6 lb weight loss was also observed in the same patients. Of the patients who completed 1 year of treatment, 57% of the patients treated with orlistat (120 mg 3 times a day) and 31% of the placebo-treated patients lost ≥ 5% of their baseline body weight.

Population as a whole – The changes in metabolic, cardiovascular, and anthropometric risk factors associated with obesity based on pooled data for 5 clinical studies, regardless of the patient's risk factor status at randomization, are presented in the following table. One year of therapy with orlistat resulted in relative improvement in several risk factors.

Mean Change in Risk Factors from Randomization Following 1-year Treatment[1]		
Risk factor	Orlistat 120 mg[2]	Placebo[2]
Anthropometric		
Waist circumference, cm	−6.45	−4.04
Hip circumference, cm	−5.31	−2.96
Cardiovascular		
Systolic blood pressure, mmHg	−1.01	+0.58
Diastolic blood pressure, mmHg	−1.19	+0.46
Metabolic		
Total cholesterol	−2%	+5%
LDL cholesterol	−4%	+5%
HDL cholesterol	+9.3%	+12.8%
LDL/HDL	−0.37	−0.2
Triglycerides	+1.34%	+2.9%
Fasting glucose, mmol/L	−0.04	0
Fasting insulin, pmol/L	−6.7	+5.2

[1] Treatment designates 120 mg orlistat 3 times a day plus diet or placebo plus diet.
[2] Intent-to-treat population at week 52, observed data based on pooled data from 5 studies.

Population with abnormal risk factors – The changes from randomization following 1-year treatment in the population with abnormal lipid levels (LDL ≥ 130 mg/dL, LDL/HDL ≥ 3.5, HDL < 35 mg/dL) were greater for orlistat compared with placebo with respect to LDL cholesterol (−7.83% vs +1.14%) and the LDL/HDL ratio (−0.64 vs −0.46). HDL increased in the placebo group by 20.1% and in the orlistat group by 18.8%. In the population with abnormal blood pressure at baseline (systolic BP ≥ 140 mmHg), the change in systolic BP from randomization to 1 year was greater for orlistat (−10.89 mmHg) than placebo (−5.07 mmHg). For patients with a diastolic blood pressure ≥ 90 mmHg, orlistat patients decreased by −7.9 mmHg while the placebo patients decreased by −5.5 mmHg. Fasting insulin decreased more for orlistat than placebo (−39 vs −16 pmol/L) from randomization to 1 year in the population with abnormal baseline values (≥ 120 pmol/L). A greater reduction in waist circumference for orlistat vs placebo (−7.29 vs −4.53 cm) was observed in the population with abnormal baseline values (≥ 100 cm).

Effect on weight regain – Three studies were designed to evaluate the effects of orlistat compared with placebo in reducing weight regain after a previous weight loss achieved following either diet alone or prior treatment with orlistat. The diet used during the 1-year weight regain portion of the studies was a weight-maintenance diet, rather than a weight-loss diet, and patients received less nutritional counseling than patients in weight-loss studies. In one study, patients treated with placebo regained 52% of the weight they had previously lost while the patients treated with orlistat regained 26% of the weight they had previously lost. In a second study, patients treated with placebo regained 63% of the weight they had previously lost while the patients treated with orlistat regained 35% of the weight they had lost. In another study, patients treated with placebo regained 53% of the weight they had previously lost while the patients treated with orlistat regained 32% of the weight that they had lost.

Two-year results – The treatment effects of orlistat were examined for 2 years in four of the five 1-year weight management clinical studies previously discussed. At the end of year 1, the patients' diets were reviewed and changed where necessary. The diet prescribed in the second year was designed to maintain patients' current weight. Orlistat was shown to be more effective than placebo in long-term weight control in 4 large, multicenter, 2-year, double-blind, placebo-controlled studies. Pooled data from 4 clinical studies indicate that 40% of all patients treated with orlistat 120 mg 3 times a day and 24% of patients treated with placebo who completed 2 years of the same therapy had ≥ 5% loss of body weight from randomization. Pooled data from 4 clinical studies indicate that the relative weight loss advantage between

orlistat 120 mg 3 times a day and placebo treatment groups was the same after 2 years as for 1 year, indicating that the pharmacologic advantage of orlistat was maintained over 2 years.

Population as a whole – The relative differences in risk factors between treatment with orlistat and placebo were similar to the results following 1 year of therapy for total cholesterol, LDL cholesterol, LDL/HDL ratio, triglycerides, fasting glucose, fasting insulin, diastolic blood pressure, waist circumference, and hip circumference. The relative differences between treatment groups for HDL cholesterol and systolic blood pressure were less than that observed in the year 1 results.

Population with abnormal risk factors – The relative differences in risk factors between treatment with orlistat and placebo were similar to the results following 1 year of therapy for LDL and HDL cholesterol, triglycerides, fasting insulin, diastolic blood pressure, and waist circumference. The relative differences between treatment groups for LDL/HDL ratio and isolated systolic blood pressure were less than that observed in the year 1 results.

Patients with type 2 diabetes – A 1-year, double-blind, placebo-controlled study in type 2 diabetic patients (n = 321) stabilized on sulfonylureas was conducted. Of patients treated with orlistat, 30% achieved a ≥ 5% reduction in body weight from randomization compared with 13% of the placebo-treated patients. The following table describes the changes over 1 year of treatment with orlistat compared with placebo in sulfonylurea usage and dose reduction as well as in hemoglobin HbA1c, fasting glucose, and insulin.

Mean Changes in Body Weight and Glycemic Control Following 1-year Treatment with Orlistat in Patients with Type 2 Diabetes		
Parameter	Orlistat 120 mg (n = 162)	Placebo (n = 159)
% patients who discontinued dose of oral sulfonylurea	11.7%	7.5%
% patients who decreased dose of oral sulfonylurea	31.5%	21.4%
Average reduction in sulfonylurea medication dose	−22.8%	−9.1%
Body weight change (lbs)	−8.9	−4.2
HbA1c	−0.18%	+0.28%
Fasting glucose, mmol/L	−0.02	+0.54
Fasting insulin, pmol/L	−19.68	−18.02

In addition, orlistat (n = 162) compared to placebo (n = 159) was associated with significant lowering for total cholesterol (−1% vs +9%), LDL cholesterol (−3% vs +10%), LDL/HDL ratio (−0.26 vs −0.02), and triglycerides (+2.54% vs +16.2%), respectively. For HDL cholesterol, there was a +6.49% increase on orlistat and +8.6% increase on placebo. Systolic blood pressure increased by +0.61 mmHg on orlistat and increased by +4.33 mmHg on placebo. Diastolic blood pressure decreased by −0.47 mmHg for orlistat and by −0.5 mmHg for placebo.

Glucose tolerance in obese patients – Two-year studies that included oral glucose tolerance tests were conducted in obese patients not previously diagnosed or treated for type 2 diabetes and whose baseline oral glucose tolerance test (OGTT) status at randomization was either normal, impaired, or diabetic.

The progression from a normal OGTT at randomization to a diabetic or impaired OGTT following 2 years of treatment with orlistat (n = 251) or placebo (n = 207) were compared. Following treatment with orlistat, 0% and 7.2% of the patients progressed from normal to diabetic and normal to impaired, respectively, compared with 1.9% and 12.6% of the placebo treatment group, respectively.

In patients found to have an impaired OGTT at randomization, the percent of patients improving to normal or deteriorating to diabetic status following 1 and 2 years of treatment with orlistat compared with placebo are presented. After 1 year of treatment, 45.8% of the placebo patients and 73% of the orlistat patients had a normal OGTT while 10.4% of the placebo patients and 2.6% of the orlistat patients became diabetic. After 2 years of treatment, 50% of the placebo patients and 71.7% of the orlistat patients had a normal OGTT while 7.5% of placebo patients were found to be diabetic and 1.7% of orlistat patients were found to be diabetic after treatment.

Contraindications

Chronic malabsorption syndrome or cholestasis; hypersensitivity to orlistat or to any component of this product.

Warnings

➤*Causes of obesity:* Organic causes of obesity (eg, hypothyroidism) should be excluded before prescribing orlistat.

➤*Pregnancy: Category B.* There are no adequate and well-controlled studies of orlistat in pregnant women. Orlistat is not recommended for use during pregnancy.

➤*Lactation:* It is not known if orlistat is secreted in breast milk. Therefore, orlistat should not be taken by nursing women.

➤*Children:* Safety and efficacy in pediatric patients have not been established.

ORLISTAT

Precautions

➤*Diet:* Advise patients to adhere to dietary guidelines (see Administration and Dosage). GI events (see Adverse Reactions) may increase when orlistat is taken with a diet high in fat (> 30% total daily calories from fat). The daily intake of fat should be distributed over 3 main meals. If orlistat is taken with any one meal very high in fat, the possibility of GI effects increases.

➤*Vitamin supplement:* Counsel patients to take a multivitamin supplement that contains fat-soluble vitamins to ensure adequate nutrition because orlistat reduces the absorption of some fat-soluble vitamins and beta-carotene. In addition, the levels of vitamin D and beta-carotene may be low in obese patients compared with non-obese people. Instruct the patient to take the supplement once a day ≥ 2 hours before or after the administration of orlistat, such as at bedtime.

The following table illustrates the percentage of patients who developed a low vitamin level on ≥ 2 consecutive visits during 1 and 2 years of therapy in studies in which patients were not previously receiving vitamin supplementation.

Incidence of Low Vitamin Values in Nonsupplemented Patients with Normal Baseline Values Receiving Orlistat		
Vitamin	Placebo	Orlistat
Vitamin A	1%	2.2%
Vitamin D	6.6%	12%
Vitamin E	1%	5.8%
Beta-carotene	1.7%	6.1%

➤*Urinary oxalate:* Some patients may develop increased levels of urinary oxalate following treatment. Exercise caution when prescribing orlistat to patients with a history of hyperoxaluria or calcium oxalate nephrolithiasis.

➤*Diabetic patients:* Weight-loss induction by orlistat may be accompanied by improved metabolic control in diabetic patients, which might require a reduction in dose of oral hypoglycemic medication (eg, sulfonylureas, metformin) or insulin.

➤*Misuse potential:* As with any weight-loss agent, the potential exists for misuse of orlistat in inappropriate patient populations (eg, patients with anorexia nervosa or bulimia). See Indications for recommended prescribing guidelines.

Drug Interactions

Orlistat Drug Interactions			
Precipitant drug	Object drug*		Description
Orlistat	Cyclosporine	↔	Because changes in cyclosporine absorption have been reported with variations in dietary intake, caution is advised in the concomitant use of orlistat plus diet in patients receiving cyclosporine therapy.
Orlistat	Fat-soluble vitamins	↓	A pharmacokinetic interaction study showed a 30% reduction in beta-carotene supplement absorption when concomitantly administered with orlistat. Orlistat inhibited absorption of a vitamin E acetate supplement by ≈ 60%. The effect on the absorption of supplemental vitamin D, vitamin A, and nutritionally derived vitamin K is not known at this time.
Orlistat	Pravastatin	↑	In 24 healthy-weight, mildly hypercholesterolemic subjects receiving orlistat 120 mg 3 times a day for 10 days, the effect was additive to the lipid-lowering effect of pravastatin. Modest increases (≈ 30%) in pravastatin plasma concentrations were observed during coadministration with orlistat.
Orlistat	Warfarin	↔	In 12 healthy-weight subjects, administration of orlistat 120 mg 3 times a day for 16 days did not result in any change in either warfarin pharmacokinetics or pharmacodynamics. Although undercarboxylated osteocalcin, a marker of vitamin K nutritional status, was unaltered with orlistat administration, vitamin K levels tended to decline in subjects taking orlistat. Therefore, as vitamin K absorption may be decreased with orlistat, monitor patients on chronic stable doses of warfarin who are prescribed orlistat closely for changes in coagulation parameters.

* ↓ = Object drug decreased. ↑ = Object drug increased. ↔ = Undetermined clinical effect.

Adverse Reactions

GI symptoms were the most commonly observed (≥ 5%, at least twice that of placebo) treatment-emergent adverse events associated with the use of orlistat and are primarily a manifestation of the mechanism of action. These and other commonly observed adverse reactions were generally mild and transient, and they decreased during the second year of treatment. In general, the first occurrence of these events was within 3 months of starting therapy. Overall, ≈ 50% of all episodes of GI adverse events associated with orlistat treatment lasted for < 1 week, and a majority lasted for ≤ 4 weeks. However, GI adverse events may occur in some individuals over a period of ≥ 6 months.

Commonly Observed Adverse Reactions with Orlistat (%)				
	Year 1		Year 2	
Adverse reaction	Orlistat (n = 1913)	Placebo (n = 1466)	Orlistat (n = 613)	Placebo (n = 524)
Oily spotting	26.6	1.3	4.4	0.2
Flatus with discharge	23.9	1.4	2.1	0.2
Fecal urgency	22.1	6.7	2.8	1.7
Fatty/Oily stool	20	2.9	5.5	0.6
Oily evacuation	11.9	0.8	2.3	0.2
Increased defecation	10.8	4.1	2.6	0.8
Fecal incontinence	7.7	0.9	1.8	0.2

Discontinuation of treatment – In controlled clinical trials, 8.8% of patients treated with orlistat discontinued treatment because of adverse events, compared with 5% of placebo-treated patients. The most common adverse events resulting in discontinuation of treatment were gastrointestinal.

The following table lists other treatment-emergent adverse events from 7 multicenter, double-blind, placebo-controlled clinical trials that occurred at a frequency of ≥ 2% among patients treated with orlistat 120 mg 3 times a day and with an incidence that was greater than placebo during year 1 and year 2:

Other Orlistat Treatment-Emergent Adverse Reactions (%)				
	Year 1		Year 2	
Adverse reaction	Orlistat (n = 1913)	Placebo (n = 1466)	Orlistat (n = 613)	Placebo (n = 524)
CNS				
Anxiety	4.7	2.9	2.8	2.1
Depression	—[1]	—	3.4	2.5
Dizziness	5.2	5	—	—
Headache	30.6	27.6	—	—
Dermatologic				
Dry skin	2.1	1.4	-	-
Rash	4.3	4	-	-
GI				
Abdominal pain/discomfort	25.5	21.4	-	-
Gingival disorder	4.1	2.9	2	1.5
Infectious diarrhea	5.3	4.4	—	—
Nausea	8.1	7.3	3.6	2.7
Rectal pain/discomfort	5.2	4	3.3	1.9
Tooth disorder	4.3	3.1	2.9	2.3
Vomiting	3.8	3.5		
Musculoskeletal				
Arthritis	5.4	4.8	—	—
Back pain	13.9	12.1	—	—
Joint disorder	2.3	2.2	—	—
Myalgia	4.2	3.3	—	—
Pain lower extremities	—	—	10.8	10.3
Tendinitis	—	—	2	1.9
Reproductive, female				
Menstrual irregularity	9.8	7.5	—	—
Vaginitis	3.8	3.6	2.6	1.9
Respiratory				
Ear, nose, and throat symptoms	2	1.6	—	—
Influenza	39.7	36.2	—	—
Lower respiratory tract infection	7.8	6.6	—	—
Upper respiratory tract infection	38.1	32.8	26.1	25.8
Miscellaneous				
Fatigue	7.2	6.4	3.1	1.7
Otitis	4.3	3.4	2.9	2.5
Pedal edema	—	—	2.8	1.9
Sleep disorder	3.9	3.3	—	—
Urinary tract infection	7.5	7.3	5.9	4.8

[1] — = None reported at a frequency ≥ 2% and greater than placebo.

ORLISTAT

Overdosage

Single doses of 800 mg orlistat and multiple doses of up to 400 mg 3 times a day for 15 days have been studied in healthy-weight and obese subjects without significant adverse findings. Should a significant overdose occur, observe the patient for 24 hours. Systemic effects attributable to the lipase-inhibiting properties of orlistat should be rapidly reversible.

Patient Information

Instruct patients to read the Patient Information before starting treatment with orlistat and each time their prescription is renewed.

METOCLOPRAMIDE

Rx	Metoclopramide HCl (Various, eg, Goldline, Invamed, Major)	**Tablets:** 5 mg as (monohydrochloride monohydrate)	In 100s, 500s and 1000s.
Rx	Reglan (Schwarz Pharma)		Lactose. (Reglan 5 AHR). Green. Elliptical. In 100s and *Dis-Co* UD 100s.
Rx	Metoclopramide HCl (Various, eg, Geneva, Goldline, Invamed, Major, Martec, Parmed, Rugby, Schein, Warner-C)	**Tablets:** 10 mg (as monohydrochloride monohydrate)	In 100s, 500s, 1000s, 2500s and UD 100s.
Rx	Maxolon (SK-Beecham)		Lactose. (BMP 192). Blue, scored. In 100s.
Rx	Reglan (Schwarz Pharma)		(Reglan AHR 10). Pink, scored. Capsule shape. In 100s, 500s and *Dis-Co* UD 100s.
Rx	Metoclopramide HCl (Various, eg, Goldline, Major, Roxane, Rugby, Warner-C)	**Syrup:** 5 mg/5 mL (as monohydrochloride monohydrate)	In 480 mL and UD 10 mL.
Rx	Metoclopramide HCl (Various, eg, DuPont, Smith & Nephew SoloPak)	**Injection:** 5 mg/mL (as monohydrochloride monohydrate)	In 2, 10, 20 and 30 mL vials and 2 mL amps.
Rx	Octamide PFS (Adria)		Preservative free. In 2, 10 and 30 mL single-dose vials.
Rx	Reglan (Wyeth-Ayerst)		Preservative free. In 2 and 10 mL amps and 2, 10 and 30 mL vials.

Indications

➤*Diabetic gastroparesis:* Relief of symptoms associated with acute and recurrent diabetic gastroparesis (diabetic gastric stasis). Usual manifestations of delayed gastric emptying (ie, nausea, vomiting, heartburn, persistent fullness after meals, anorexia) respond within different time intervals. Significant relief of nausea occurs early and improves over 3 weeks. Relief of vomiting and anorexia may precede the relief of abdominal fullness by ≥ 1 week.

➤*Oral:*

Symptomatic gastroesophageal reflux – Short-term (4 to 12 weeks) therapy for adults with symptomatic documented gastroesophageal reflux who fail to respond to conventional therapy.

➤*Parenteral:* For prevention of nausea and vomiting associated with emetogenic cancer chemotherapy.

Prophylaxis of postoperative nausea and vomiting when nasogastric suction is undesirable.

Single doses may facilitate small bowel intubation when the tube does not pass the pylorus with conventional maneuvers.

Stimulates gastric emptying and intestinal transit of barium in cases where delayed emptying interferes with radiological examination of the stomach or small intestine.

➤*Unlabeled uses:* Used to improve lactation. Doses of 30 to 45 mg/day have increased milk secretion, possibly by elevating serum prolactin levels. (See Warnings.)

Studies have indicated some potential value of metoclopramide in the following conditions: Nausea and vomiting of a variety of etiologies (uncontrolled studies report 80% to 90% efficacy), including emesis during pregnancy and labor (see Warnings); gastric ulcer; anorexia nervosa (due to GI stimulation); to improve patient response to ergotamine, analgesics and sedatives in migraine, perhaps by enhancing absorption of the other medications; treatment of postoperative gastric bezoars (10 mg 3 or 4 times daily); diabetic cystoparesis (atonic bladder); esophageal variceal bleeding.

Administration and Dosage

➤*Diabetic gastroparesis:* 10 mg 30 minutes before each meal and at bedtime for 2 to 8 weeks.

Determine initial route of administration by the severity of symptoms. With only the earliest manifestations of diabetic gastric stasis, initiate oral administration. If symptoms are severe, begin with parenteral therapy. Administer 10 mg IV over 1 to 2 minutes. Parenteral administration up to 10 days may be required before symptoms subside, then oral administration may be instituted. Reinstitute therapy at the earliest manifestation.

➤*Symptomatic gastroesophageal reflux:* 10 to 15 mg orally up to 4 times daily 30 minutes before each meal and at bedtime. If symptoms occur only intermittently or at specific times of the day, single doses up to 20 mg prior to the provoking situation may be preferred rather than continuous treatment. Occasionally, patients who are more sensitive to the therapeutic or adverse effects of metoclopramide (eg, elderly) will require only 5 mg per dose. Guide therapy directed at esophageal lesions by endoscopy. Therapy > 12 weeks has not been evaluated and cannot be recommended.

➤*Prevention of postoperative nausea and vomiting:* Inject IM near the end of surgery. The usual adult dose is 10 mg; however, doses of 20 mg may be used.

➤*Prevention of chemotherapy-induced emesis:* Infuse slowly IV over ≥ 15 minutes, 30 minutes before beginning cancer chemotherapy; repeat every 2 hours for 2 doses, then every 3 hours for 3 doses.

The initial 2 doses should be 2 mg/kg if highly emetogenic drugs such as cisplatin or dacarbazine are used alone or in combination. For less emetogenic regimens, 1 mg/kg/dose may be adequate.

If extrapyramidal symptoms occur, administer 50 mg diphenhydramine IM.

➤*IV admixture:* When diluted in a parenteral solution, administer IV slowly over a period of not less than 15 minutes.

Preparation/Storage of solution – For doses > 10 mg, dilute injection in 50 mL of a parenteral solution. The preferred parenteral solution is Sodium Chloride Injection, which when combined with metoclopramide, can be stored frozen for up to 4 weeks. Metoclopramide is degraded when admixed and frozen with Dextrose 5% in Water. Metoclopramide diluted in Sodium Chloride Injection, Dextrose 5% in Water, Dextrose 5% in 0.45% Sodium Chloride, Ringer's Injection or Lactated Ringer's Injection may be stored up to 48 hours (without freezing) after preparation if protected from light. All dilutions may be stored unprotected from light under normal light conditions up to 24 hours after preparation.

➤*Direct IV injection:* Inject undiluted metoclopramide slowly IV allowing 1 to 2 minutes for 10 mg, since a transient but intense feeling of anxiety and restlessness, followed by drowsiness, may occur with rapid administration.

Facilitation of small bowel intubation – If the tube has not passed the pylorus with conventional maneuvers in 10 minutes, administer a single undiluted dose slowly IV over 1 to 2 minutes.

Recommended single dose –
Adults: 10 mg (2 mL).
Children (6 to 14 years): 2.5 to 5 mg (0.5 to 1 mL).
Children (< 6 years): 0.1 mg/kg.

Radiological examinations – In patients where delayed gastric emptying interferes with radiological examination of the stomach or small intestine, a single dose may be administered slowly IV over 1 to 2 minutes.

➤*Rectal administration:* For outpatient treatment when oral dosing is not possible, suppositories containing 25 mg metoclopramide have been extemporaneously compounded (5 pulverized oral tablets in polyethylene glycol). Administer 1 suppository 30 to 60 minutes before each meal and at bedtime.

➤*Renal/Hepatic function impairment:* Because metoclopramide is excreted principally through the kidneys, in those patients whose creatinine clearance is < 40 mL/min, initiate therapy at approximately one-half the recommended dosage. Depending on clinical efficacy and safety considerations, the dosage may be increased or decreased as appropriate.

See Overdosage section for information regarding dialysis.

Metoclopramide undergoes minimal hepatic metabolism, except for simple conjugation. Its safe use has been described in patients with advanced liver disease whose renal function was normal.

➤*Admixture compatibilities/incompatibilities:*
Physically and chemically compatible up to 48 hours – Cimetidine; mannitol; potassium acetate; potassium chloride; potassium phosphate.

Physically compatible up to 48 hours – Ascorbic acid; benztropine; cytarabine; dexamethasone sodium phosphate; diphenhydramine; doxorubicin; heparin sodium; hydrocortisone sodium phosphate; lidocaine; magnesium sulfate; multivitamin infusion (must be refrigerated) vitamin B complex with ascorbic acid.

Incompatible – Cephalothin; chloramphenicol; sodium bicarbonate.

Actions

➤*Pharmacology:* Metoclopramide stimulates motility of the upper GI tract without stimulating gastric, biliary or pancreatic secretions. Its mode of action is unclear, but it appears to sensitize tissues to the action of acetylcholine. The effect on motility does not depend on intact vagal innervation, but it can be abolished by anticholinergic drugs.

METOCLOPRAMIDE

Metoclopramide increases the tone and amplitude of gastric (especially antral) contractions, relaxes the pyloric sphincter and the duodenal bulb, and increases peristalsis of the duodenum and jejunum, resulting in accelerated gastric emptying and intestinal transit. It increases the resting tone of the lower esophageal sphincter. It has little, if any, effect on colon or gallbladder motility. In patients with gastroesophageal reflux and reduced lower esophageal sphincter pressure (LESP), single oral doses produce dose-related increases in LESP. Effects on LESP begin at about 5 mg and increase through 20 mg. The increase in LESP from a 5 mg dose lasts about 45 minutes and that of 20 mg lasts between 2 and 3 hours. Increased rate of stomach emptying has been observed with single oral doses of 10 mg.

Like the phenothiazines and related dopamine antagonists, metoclopramide produces sedation and, rarely, may produce extrapyramidal reactions. It also induces release of prolactin and transiently increases circulating aldosterone levels.

The antiemetic properties of metoclopramide appear to be a result of its antagonism of central and peripheral dopamine receptors. Dopamine produces nausea and vomiting by stimulation of the medullary chemoreceptor trigger zone (CTZ), and metoclopramide blocks stimulation of the CTZ by agents like levodopa or apomorphine which are known to increase dopamine levels or to possess dopamine-like effects. Metoclopramide also inhibits the central and peripheral effects of apomorphine and abolishes the slowing of gastric emptying caused by apomorphine.

In gastroesophageal reflux, the principal effect of metoclopramide is on symptoms of postprandial and daytime heartburn with less observed effect on nocturnal symptoms. If symptoms are confined to particular situations, such as following the evening meal, consider use of metoclopramide as single doses prior to the provocative situation, rather than using the drug throughout the day. In one study, patients with episodes of evening or nocturnal heartburn had significant improvement in the incidence and symptoms of heartburn following treatment with a single 10 mg dose either before or after the evening meal or at bedtime for 1 to 3 months. Healing of esophageal ulcers and erosions has been endoscopically demonstrated at the end of a 12 week trial using doses of 15 mg 4 times daily. As there is no documented correlation between symptoms and healing of esophageal lesions, endoscopically monitor patients with documented lesions.

➤*Pharmacokinetics:*

Absorption/Distribution – Metoclopramide is rapidly and well absorbed. Onset of action is 1 to 3 minutes following an IV dose, 10 to 15 minutes following IM administration, and 30 to 60 minutes following an oral dose. Effects persist for 1 to 2 hours.

Relative to an IV dose of 20 mg, the absolute oral bioavailability of metoclopramide is 80% ± 15.5%. Peak plasma concentrations occur at about 1 to 2 hours after a single oral dose. Similar time to peak is observed after individual doses at steady state. The area under the drug concentration-time curve increases linearly with doses from 20 to 100 mg; peak concentrations also increase linearly with dose. The whole body volume of distribution is high (about 3.5 L/kg) which suggests extensive distribution of drug to the tissues.

Metabolism/Excretion – Approximately 85% of an orally administered dose appears in the urine within 72 hours. Of the 85% eliminated in the urine, about one-half is present as free or conjugated metoclopramide. The average elimination half-life in individuals with normal renal function is 5 to 6 hours. The drug is not extensively bound to plasma proteins (about 30%).

Renal impairment affects the clearance of metoclopramide. In a study of patients with varying degrees of renal impairment, a reduction in creatinine clearance was correlated with a reduction in plasma clearance, renal clearance, non-renal clearance, and increase in elimination half-life. Decrease the dose in renal function impairment to avoid drug accumulation (see Administration and Dosage).

Contraindications

When stimulation of GI motility might be dangerous (eg, in the presence of GI hemorrhage, mechanical obstruction or perforation); pheochromocytoma (the drug may cause a hypertensive crisis, probably due to release of catecholamines from the tumor; control such crises with phentolamine); sensitivity or intolerance to metoclopramide; epileptics or patients receiving drugs likely to cause extrapyramidal reactions (the frequency and severity of seizures or extrapyramidal reactions may be increased).

Warnings

➤*Depression:* Depression has occurred in patients with and without a history of depression. Symptoms have ranged from mild to severe and have included suicidal ideation and suicide. Give metoclopramide to patients with a history of depression only if the expected benefits outweigh the potential risks.

➤*Extrapyramidal symptoms:* Extrapyramidal symptoms, manifested primarily as acute dystonic reactions, occur in ≈ 0.2% to 1% of patients treated with the usual adult dosages of 30 to 40 mg/day. These usually are seen during the first 24 to 48 hours of treatment, occur more frequently in children and young adults, and are even more frequent at the higher doses used in prophylaxis of vomiting due to cancer

chemotherapy. These symptoms may include involuntary movements of limbs and facial grimacing, torticollis, oculogyric crisis, rhythmic protrusion of tongue, bulbar type of speech, trismus or dystonic reactions resembling tetanus. Rarely, dystonic reactions may present as stridor and dyspnea, possibly due to laryngospasm. If symptoms occur, they usually subside following 50 mg diphenhydramine IM. Benztropine 1 to 2 mg IM may also be used to reverse these reactions.

➤*Parkinson-like symptoms:* Parkinson-like symptoms have occurred, more commonly within the first 6 months after beginning treatment with metoclopramide, but occasionally after longer periods. These symptoms generally subside within 2 to 3 months following discontinuance of metoclopramide. Give metoclopramide cautiously, if at all, to patients with preexisting Parkinson's disease, since such patients may experience exacerbation of parkinsonian symptoms when taking metoclopramide.

➤*Tardive dyskinesia:* Tardive dyskinesia, a syndrome consisting of potentially irreversible, involuntary, dyskinetic movements, may develop in patients treated with metoclopramide. Although prevalence of the syndrome appears to be highest among the elderly, especially elderly women, it is impossible to predict which patients are likely to develop the syndrome. Both the risk of developing the syndrome and the likelihood that it will become irreversible are believed to increase with the duration of treatment and the total cumulative dose. Less commonly, the syndrome can develop after relatively brief treatment periods at low doses; in these cases, symptoms appear more likely to be reversible.

There is no known treatment for established cases of tardive dyskinesia although the syndrome may remit, partially or completely, within several weeks to months after metoclopramide is withdrawn. Metoclopramide itself, however, may suppress (or partially suppress) the signs of tardive dyskinesia, thereby masking the underlying disease process. The effect of this symptomatic suppression upon the long-term course of the syndrome is unknown. Therefore, the use of metoclopramide for the symptomatic control of tardive dyskinesia is not recommended.

➤*Hypertension:* In one study of hypertensive patients, IV metoclopramide released catecholamines. Use caution in hypertensive patients.

➤*Anastomosis or closure of the gut:* Giving a promotility drug such as metoclopramide could theoretically put increased pressure on suture lines following a gut anastomosis or closure. Although adverse events related to this possibility have not been reported to date, consider the possibility when deciding whether to use metoclopramide or nasogastric suction in the prevention of postoperative nausea and vomiting.

➤*Carcinogenesis:* Elevated prolactin levels persist during chronic administration. Approximately one-third of human breast cancers are prolactin-dependent in vitro; use caution if metoclopramide is contemplated in a patient with previously detected breast cancer. Although galactorrhea, amenorrhea, gynecomastia and impotence have occurred with prolactin-elevating drugs, the clinical significance of elevated serum prolactin levels is unknown. An increase in mammary neoplasms has been found in rodents after chronic administration of prolactin-stimulating neuroleptic drugs; however, studies have not shown an association and evidence is not conclusive.

➤*Pregnancy:* Category B. Metoclopramide crosses the placenta. However, there are no adequate and well controlled studies in pregnant women. In several case reports, no effects on the fetus occurred following the use of metoclopramide during pregnancy for nausea and vomiting and reflux esophagitis. Use only when clearly needed and when the potential benefits outweigh the potential hazards to the fetus.

➤*Lactation:* Metoclopramide is excreted into breast milk and may concentrate at about twice the plasma level at 2 hours postdose. In a mother receiving 30 mg/day, the amount to the infant would be < 45 mcg/kg/day, which is much less than the maximum daily recommended dose in infants. Therefore, there appears to be no risk to the nursing infant with maternal doses ≤ 45 mg/day. However, exercise caution when administering to a nursing mother.

➤*Children:* Infants and children (ages 21 days to 3.3 years) with symptomatic gastroesophageal reflux have been treated with metoclopramide at a dosage of 0.5 mg/kg/day; symptoms improved, the duration of the disease was shortened, and surgery was avoided. One infant with GI manifestations of congenital myotonic dystrophy was successfully treated with metoclopramide (0.3 mg/kg/day).

Methemoglobinemia has occurred in premature and full term neonates given metoclopramide orally, IV or IM, 1 to 4 mg/kg/day for 1 to ≥ 3 days; this did not occur at 0.5 mg/kg/day. Reverse methemoglobinemia by IV administration of methylene blue.

Precautions

➤*Hypoglycemia:* Gastroparesis (gastric stasis) may be responsible for poor diabetic control. Exogenously administered insulins may act before food has left the stomach, leading to hypoglycemia.

➤*Hazardous tasks:* Patients should use caution while driving or performing other tasks requiring alertness, coordination or physical dexterity.

METOCLOPRAMIDE

Drug Interactions

Metoclopramide Drug Interactions			
Precipitant drug	Object drug*		Description
Metoclopramide	Alcohol	↑	Metoclopramide increases the rate of absorption of alcohol by decreasing the time it takes alcohol to reach the small intestine where it is rapidly absorbed.
Metoclopramide	Cimetidine	↓	Bioavailability of cimetidine may be reduced due to decreased absorption as a result of faster gastric transit time.
Metoclopramide	Cyclosporine	↑	A faster gastric emptying time may allow for an increase in cyclosporine absorption, possibly increasing its immunosuppressive and toxic effects.
Metoclopramide	Digoxin	↓	Digoxin absorption, plasma levels and therapeutic effects may be decreased. The capsule, elixir and tablets with a high dissolution rate are least affected.
Metoclopramide	Levodopa	↑	These agents have opposite effects on dopamine receptors. The bioavailability of levodopa may be increased, and levodopa may decrease the effects of metoclopramide on gastric emptying and lower esophageal pressure. Metoclopramide is relatively contraindicated in Parkinson's disease patients.
Levodopa	Metoclopramide	↓	
Metoclopramide	MAO inhibitors	↑	Since metoclopramide releases catecholamines in patients with essential hypertension, use cautiously, if at all, in patients receiving MAO inhibitors.
Metoclopramide	Succinylcholine	↑	By inhibiting plasma cholinesterase, metoclopramide may increase the neuromuscular blocking effects of succinylcholine.
Anticholinergics Narcotic analgesics	Metoclopramide	↓	The effects of metoclopramide on GI motility are antagonized by these agents.

* ↑ = Object drug increased.   ↓ = Object drug decreased.

Adverse Reactions

Approximately 20% to 30% of patients experience side effects that are usually mild, transient and reversible upon drug withdrawal. Incidence also correlates with dose and duration of metoclopramide use. Doses of 2 mg/kg for control of cisplatin-induced vomiting have produced CNS and GI side effects with an incidence of 81% and 43%, respectively.

Extrapyramidal symptoms (EPS; 1% to 9%) – Acute dystonic reactions, the most common type of EPS associated with metoclopramide, occur in approximately 0.2% of patients treated with 30 to 40 mg/day. In cancer chemotherapy patients receiving 1 to 2 mg/kg/dose, the incidence is 2% in patients ≥ 30 years of age and ≥ 25% in children and young adults who have not had prophylactic administration of diphenhydramine. Symptoms include involuntary movements of limbs, facial grimacing, torticollis, oculogyric crisis, rhythmic protrusion of tongue, bulbar type of speech, trismus, opisthotonus (tetanus-like reactions) and rarely, stridor and dyspnea possibly due to laryngospasm; ordinarily these symptoms are readily reversed by diphenhydramine (see Warnings).

Parkinson-like symptoms may include bradykinesia, tremor, cogwheel rigidity, mask-like facies (see Warnings).

Tardive dyskinesia most frequently is characterized by involuntary movements of the tongue, face, mouth or jaw, and sometimes by involuntary movements of the trunk or extremities; movements may be choreoathetotic in appearance (see Warnings).

Motor restlessness (akathisia) may consist of feelings of anxiety, agitation, jitteriness, and insomnia, as well as inability to sit still, pacing and foot-tapping. These symptoms may disappear spontaneously or respond to a reduction in dosage.

➤*Cardiovascular:* Hypotension; hypertension (see Warnings); supraventricular tachycardia; bradycardia.

➤*CNS:*

12% to 24% – Restlessness, drowsiness, fatigue, lassitude (≈ 10%); akathisia (1% to 8%); dizziness (3%; ≈ 70% in cancer chemotherapy patients treated with 1 to 22 mg/kg doses); anxiety; dystonia; insomnia; headache; myoclonus; confusion; mental depression with suicidal ideation (see Warnings); convulsive seizures; hallucinations.

➤*Endocrine:* Galactorrhea, amenorrhea, gynecomastia, impotence secondary to hyperprolactinemia (see Warnings); fluid retention secondary to transient elevation of aldosterone. Elevated serum prolactin levels may cause galactorrhea, reversible amenorrhea, nipple tenderness and gynecomastia in males.

➤*GI:* Nausea and bowel disturbances, primarily diarrhea (2% to 9%).

➤*Hematologic:* Neutropenia; leukopenia; agranulocytosis; methemoglobinemia (especially with overdosage in neonates). (See Overdosage.)

➤*Hypersensitivity:* A few cases of rash, urticaria or bronchospasm, especially in patients with a history of asthma. Rarely, angioneurotic edema, including glossal or laryngeal edema.

➤*Miscellaneous:* Urinary frequency; incontinence; visual disturbances; porphyria; neuroleptic malignant syndrome (NMS), potentially fatal, is comprised of the symptom complex of hyperthermia, altered consciousness, muscular rigidity and autonomic dysfunction; transient flushing of the face and upper body, without alterations in vital signs, following high IV doses; cases of hepatotoxicity, characterized by such findings as jaundice and altered liver function tests, when metoclopramide was administered with other drugs with known hepatotoxic potential.

Overdosage

➤*Symptoms:* Drowsiness, disorientation and extrapyramidal reactions which are self-limiting and usually disappear within 24 hours. Muscle hypertonia, irritability and agitation are common.

➤*Treatment:* Anticholinergic or antiparkinson drugs or antihistamines with anticholinergic properties may help control extrapyramidal reactions. Hemodialysis appears ineffective in removing metoclopramide, probably because of the small amount of the drug in blood relative to tissues. Similarly, continuous ambulatory peritoneal dialysis does not remove significant amounts of drug. It is unlikely that dosage would need to be adjusted to compensate for losses through dialysis.

Methemoglobinemia has occurred in premature and full-term neonates who were given overdoses of metoclopramide (1 to 4 mg/kg/day orally, IM or IV for 1 to ≥ 3 days). Methemoglobinemia has not been reported in neonates treated with 0.5 mg/kg/day in divided doses. Methemoglobinemia can be reversed by the IV administration of methylene blue. Also see General Management of Acute Overdosage.

Patient Information

May produce drowsiness and dizziness; observe caution while driving or performing other tasks requiring alertness, coordination or physical dexterity.

Notify physician if involuntary movement of eyes, face or limbs occurs.

Take medication 30 minutes before each meal.

DEXPANTHENOL (Dextro-Pantothenyl Alcohol)

Rx	**Dexpanthenol** (Various)	Injection: 250 mg per mL	In 10 mL and 2 mL vials.
Rx	**Ilopan** (Adria)		In UD *Stat-Pak* 2 mL disp. syringes.[1]

[1] Syringes contain no more than 0.5% chlorobutanol.

Indications

Prophylactic use immediately after major abdominal surgery to minimize the possibility of paralytic ileus; intestinal atony causing abdominal distention; postoperative or postpartum retention of flatus; postoperative delay in resumption of intestinal motility; paralytic ileus.

Administration and Dosage

➤*Prevention of postoperative adynamic ileus:* 250 or 500 mg IM. Repeat in 2 hours, followed by doses every 6 hours until danger of adynamic ileus has passed.

➤*Treatment of adynamic ileus:* 500 mg IM. Repeat in 2 hours, followed by doses every 6 hours, as needed.

➤*IV administration:* Not for direct IV administration. The 500 mg dose has been mixed with IV bulk solutions such as glucose or Lactated Ringer's and infused slowly IV.

Actions

➤*Pharmacology:* Dexpanthenol is the alcohol analog of D-pantothenic acid. Pantothenic acid is a precursor of coenzyme A, which is a cofactor for enzyme-catalyzed reactions involving transfer of acetyl groups. The final step in acetylcholine synthesis is the choline acetylase transfer of an acetyl group from acetylcoenzyme A to choline. Acetylcholine, the neurohumoral transmitter in the parasympathetic system, maintains normal intestinal functions. Decreased acetylcholine content results in decreased peristalsis and, in extreme cases, adynamic ileus. Dexpanthenol's mechanism of action is unknown.

Choline – Choline, in addition to being the precursor for acetylcholine, is essential for normal transport of fat, as a constituent of the phospholipid lecithin, and as an intermediary methyl donor in intermediary metabolism. Choline has the same pharmacological actions as acetylcholine but is less active; single oral 10 g doses produce no obvious pharmacodynamic response.

DEXPANTHENOL (Dextro-Pantothenyl Alcohol)

In 1 study, urinary concentrations of pantothenic acid increased 10- to 50-fold above baseline during a 4-hour period following 100 mg dexpanthenol. Within 24 hours, urinary levels were only slightly above baseline.

Contraindications

Hemophilia; ileus caused by mechanical obstruction.

Warnings

➤*Hypersensitivity reactions:* If signs of a hypersensitivity reaction appear, discontinue the drug. Refer to Management of Acute Hypersensitivity Reactions.

➤*Pregnancy: Category C.* It is not known whether dexpanthenol can cause fetal harm when administered to a pregnant woman or can affect reproduction capacity. Give to a pregnant woman only when clearly needed.

➤*Lactation:* It is not known whether this drug is excreted in breast milk. Exercise caution when administering the drug to a nursing woman.

➤*Children:* Safety and efficacy for use in children have not been established.

Precautions

➤*Mechanical obstruction:* If ileus is secondary to mechanical obstruction, direct primary attention to the obstruction. Management of adynamic ileus includes the following: Correction of any fluid and electrolyte imbalance (especially hypokalemia), anemia, and hypoproteinemia; treatment of infection; avoidance of drugs that decrease GI motility; GI tract decompression when considerably distended by nasogastric suction or by use of a long intestinal tube.

Drug Interactions

Dexpanthenol Drug Interactions			
Precipitant drug	Object drug*		Description
Dexpanthenol	Antibiotics, barbiturates, or narcotics	↑	Allergic reactions have occurred rarely during concomitant use of dexpanthenol.
Dexpanthenol	Succinylcholine	↑	Temporary respiratory difficulty occurred following dexpanthenol administration 5 minutes after succinylcholine was discontinued. Succinylcholine's effects appeared to have been prolonged. Do not administer within 1 hour of succinylcholine.

* ↑ = Object drug increased.

Adverse Reactions

Itching; tingling; difficulty breathing; red patches of skin; generalized dermatitis; urticaria; slight drop in blood pressure; intestinal colic (30 minutes after administration); vomiting; diarrhea (10 days postsurgery); agitation in an elderly patient.

DIGESTIVE ENZYMES

Content given per capsule, tablet, or 0.7 g powder.

	Product and Distributor[a]	Lipase (USP units)	Protease (USP units)	Amylase (USP units)	How Supplied
	PANCREATIN				
Rx	**Ku-Zyme Capsules**[b] (Schwarz Pharma)	1200	15,000	15,000	(SCHWARZ 4122). Yellow/White. In 100s.
Rx	**Kutrase Capsules**[b] (Schwarz Pharma)	2400	30,000	30,000	(SCHWARZ 4175). Green/White. In 100s.
	PANCRELIPASE				
Rx	**Pancrease MT 4 Capsules**[b] (McNeil)	4000	12,000	12,000	(McNEIL PANCREASE MT 4). Yellow/Clear. Enteric-coated microtablets. In 100s.
Rx	**Pancrecarb MS-4 Delayed-Release Capsules**[b] (Digestive Care)	4000	25,000	25,000	(DCI PANCRECARB MS-4). Clear. Enteric-coated microspheres. In 100s.
Rx	**Pancrelipase Capsules**[b] (Various, eg, Global)	4500	25,000	20,000	Enteric-coated microspheres. In 100s and 250s.
Rx	**Lipram 4500 Delayed-Release Capsules**[b] (Global)				(0115 7035). White. Enteric-coated microspheres. In 100s and 250s.
Rx	**Pancrease Capsules**[b] (McNeil)				Sucrose. Dye free. (McNEIL Pancrease). White/Clear. Enteric-coated microspheres. In 100s and 250s.
Rx	**Ultrase Capsules**[b] (Axcan Scandipharm)				Sugar. (ULTRASE). White. Enteric-coated microspheres. In 100s.
Rx	**Creon 5 Delayed-Release Capsules**[b] (Solvay)	5000	18,750	16,600	(SOLVAY 1205). Orange/Blue. Enteric-coated *Minimicrospheres.* In 100s and 250s.
Rx	**Lipram-CR5 Delayed-Release Capsules**[b] (Global)				(0115 7057). Natural/White. Enteric-coated microspheres. In 100s and 250s.
Rx	**Pancrelipase Tablets**[b] (Various, eg, Contract Pharmacal)	8000	30,000	30,000	May contain lactose. In 100s and 500s.
Rx	**Ku-Zyme HP Capsules**[b] (Schwarz Pharma)				Lactose. (SCHWARZ 525). White. In 100s.
Rx	**Panokase Tablets**[b] (Breckenridge)				Lactose. In 100s and 500s.
Rx	**Plaretase 8000 Tablets**[b] (Ethex)				(ETH 416). Tan. In 100s and 500s.
Rx	**Viokase 8 Tablets**[b] (Axcan Scandipharm)				Lactose. (VIOKASE 9111). Tan. In 100s and 500s.
Rx	**Pancrecarb MS-8 Delayed-Release Capsules**[b] (Digestive Care)	8000	45,000	40,000	(DCI PANCRECARB MS-8). Clear. Enteric-coated microspheres. In 100s and 250s.
otc	**PAN-2400 Capsules** (Bio-Tech)	9,816	60,214	75,900	In 100s.
Rx	**Lipram-PN10 Delayed-Release Capsules**[b] (Global)	10,000	30,000	30,000	(0115 7040). Natural/Brown. Enteric-coated microspheres. In 100s.
Rx	**Pancrease MT 10 Capsules**[b] (McNeil)				(McNEIL PANCREASE MT 10). Pink/Clear. Enteric-coated microtablets. In 100s.
Rx	**Creon 10 Delayed-Release Capsules**[b] (Solvay)	10,000	37,500	33,200	(SOLVAY 1210). Brown/Natural. Enteric-coated *Minimicrospheres.* In 100s and 250s.
Rx	**Lipram-CR10 Delayed-Release Capsules**[b] (Global)				(0115 7036). Brown/Flesh. Enteric-coated microspheres. In 100s and 250s.
Rx	**Lipram-UL12 Delayed-Release Capsules**[b] (Global)	12,000	39,000	39,000	(0115 7042). Natural/White. Enteric-coated microspheres. In 100s.
Rx	**Ultrase MT 12 Capsules**[b] (Axcan Scandipharm)				(ULTRASE MT12). White/Yellow. Enteric-coated minitablets. In 100s.
Rx	**Pancrelipase Capsules**[b] (Various, eg, Mutual)	16,000	48,000	48,000	Enteric-coated microspheres. In 100s and 250s.
Rx	**Lipram-PN16 Delayed-Release Capsules**[b] (Global)				(0115 7023). Flesh. Enteric-coated microspheres. In 100s.
Rx	**Pancrease MT 16 Capsules**[b] (McNeil)				(McNEIL PANCREASE MT 16). Salmon/Clear. Enteric-coated microtablets. In 100s.
Rx	**Pancrelipase Tablets**[b] (Various, eg, Contract Pharmacal)	16,000	60,000	60,000	May contain lactose. In 100s and 500s.
Rx	**Viokase 16 Tablets**[b] (Axcan Scandipharm)				Lactose. (V[16] 9116). Tan, oval. In 100s and 500s.
Rx	**Viokase Powder**[b,c] (Axcan Scandipharm)	16,800	70,000	70,000	Lactose. In 227 g.
Rx	**Lipram-UL18 Delayed-Release Capsules**[b] (Global)	18,000	58,500	58,500	(0115 7041). Flesh/White. Enteric-coated microspheres. In 100s.
Rx	**Ultrase MT 18 Capsules**[b] (Axcan Scandipharm)				(ULTRASE MT18). Gray/White. Enteric-coated minitablets. In 100s.
Rx	**Lipram-PN20 Delayed-Release Capsules**[b] (Global)	20,000	44,000	56,000	(0115 7055). Flesh/Natural. Enteric-coated microspheres. In 100s.
Rx	**Pancrease MT 20 Capsules**[b] (McNeil)				(McNEIL/PANCREASE MT 20). White. Enteric-coated microtablets. In 100s.
Rx	**Lipram-UL20 Delayed-Release Capsules**[b] (Global)	20,000	65,000	65,000	(0115 7043). Brown. Enteric-coated microspheres. In 100s and 500s.
Rx	**Ultrase MT 20 Capsules**[b] (Axcan Scandipharm)				(ULTRASE MT20). Light gray/yellow. Enteric-coated minitablets. In 100s and 500s.
Rx	**Creon 20 Delayed-release Capsules**[b] (Solvay)	20,000	75,000	66,400	(SOLVAY 1220). Orange/Natural. Enteric-coated *Minimicrospheres.* In 100s and 250s.
Rx	**Lipram-CR20 Delayed-Release Capsules**[b] (Global)				(0115 7024). Brown/White. Enteric-coated microspheres. In 100s and 250s.

[a] Product tables do not imply bioequivalence (see page xi). Also refer to Bioequivalency (in Administration and Dosage).

[b] Porcine-derived enzymes.
[c] Amount in ¼ teaspoon.

Indications

Enzyme replacement therapy in patients with deficient exocrine pancreatic secretions, such as in cystic fibrosis, chronic pancreatitis, post-pancreatectomy, ductal obstructions caused by cancer of the pancreas or common bile duct, pancreatic insufficiency, and for steatorrhea of malabsorption syndrome and postgastrectomy (Billroth II and Total) or post-GI surgery (eg, Billroth II gastroenterostomy).

Presumptive test for pancreatic function, especially in pancreatic insufficiency caused by chronic pancreatitis.

Administration and Dosage

➤*Bioequivalency:* These products are not bioequivalent and cannot be interchanged without physician supervision. Variability not only occurs at the product level, but may also be clinically significant from one batch of product to the next.

Pancrelipase capsules and tablets are required to contain between 90% and 150% of the labeled lipase activity. Pancrelipase delayed-release capsules are required to contain between 90% and 165% of the labeled lipase activity, and not less than 90% of amylase and protease labeled activities. No USP standards have currently been identified for pancreatin capsules.

DIGESTIVE ENZYMES

➤*Enzyme supplementation:* Take capsules or tablets with meals or snacks. Adjust dosage based on severity of the exocrine pancreatic enzyme deficiency. The number of tablets, capsules, or dosage given with meals or snacks should be estimated by assessing which dose minimizes steatorrhea and maintains good nutritional status. Dose increases, if required, should be made slowly, with careful monitoring of response and symptomatology.

To protect enteric coating, do not crush or chew the microspheres or microtablets. Where swallowing of capsules is difficult, they may be opened and shaken onto a small quantity of soft non-hot food (eg, applesauce, gelatin) that does not require chewing. Swallow immediately without chewing as the proteolytic action may cause irritation of the mucosa. Follow with a glass of juice or water to ensure complete swallowing of the microspheres/microtablets. Microsphere contact with foods having a pH greater than 5.5 can dissolve the enteric coating.

➤*Ku-Zyme, Pancrecarb, Ultrase, Ultrase MT:* Initiate with 1 or 2 capsules with each meal or snack.

➤*Kutrase:* Take 1 capsule with each meal or snack.

➤*Ku-Zyme HP:* Take 1 to 3 capsules with each meal or snack. In severe deficiencies, increase the dose to 8 capsules with meals or increase the frequency to hourly intervals if nausea, cramps, or diarrhea do not occur.

➤*Pancrease, Pancrease MT 4:*

Infants (up to 12 months) – 2000 to 4000 lipase units/120 mL of formula or breast milk.

Under 4 years of age – Initiate with 1000 lipase units/kg/meal up to a maximum of 2500 lipase units/kg/meal.

Over 4 years of age – Initiate with 400 lipase units/kg/meal up to a maximum of 2500 lipase units/kg/meal.

The total daily dose reflects approximately 3 meals and 2 to 3 snacks/day. If doses greater than 2500 lipase units/kg/meal are required, then further investigation is warranted to rule out other causes of malabsorption. Doses greater than 2500 lipase units/kg/meal should be used with caution and only if they are documented to be effective by 3-day fecal fat measures. It is unknown if doses this high are safe.

➤*Pancrelipase, Lipram:*

Children 6 months to less than 1 year of age – 2000 lipase units/meal.

Children 1 to 6 years of age – 4000 to 8000 lipase units with each meal and 4000 units with snacks.

Children 7 to 12 years of age – 4000 to 12,000 lipase units with each meal and with snacks.

Adults – 4000 to 20,000 lipase units with each meal and with snacks.

➤*Creon 5:*

Adults and children over 6 years of age – Usual starting dose is 2 to 4 capsules/meal or snack.

Children under 6 years of age – The exact dosage should be selected based on clinical experience with this age group. Initiate with 1 to 2 capsules/meal or snack.

Cystic fibrosis patients – Usual doses are 1500 to 3000 lipase units/kg/meal. Doses in excess of 6000 lipase units/kg/meal are not recommended.

➤*Creon 10:*

Adults and children over 6 years of age – Usual starting dose is 1 to 2 capsules/meal or snack.

Children under 6 years of age – Usual starting dose is up to 1 capsule per meal or snack.

Cystic fibrosis patients – Usual doses are 1500 to 3000 lipase units/kg/meal. Doses in excess of 6000 lipase units/kg/meal are not recommended.

➤*Creon 20:*

Adults and children over 6 years of age – Typical starting dose is 1 capsule/meal or snack.

Children under 6 years of age – Select the exact dosage based on clinical experience for this age group.

Cystic fibrosis patients – Usual doses are 1500 to 3000 lipase units/kg/meal. Doses in excess of 6000 lipase units/kg/meal are not recommended.

➤*Panokase, Plaretase, Viokase (tablets):*

Cystic fibrosis and chronic pancreatitis patients – Dose ranges from 8000 to 32,000 lipase units (1 to 4 tablets [*Plaretase, Panokase, Viokase 8*] or 1 to 2 tablets [*Viokase 16*]). Take with meals.

Pancreatectomy or obstruction of pancreatic ducts – Take 1 to 2 tablets (*Plaretase, Panokase, Viokase 8*) or 1 tablet (*Viokase 16*) every 2 hours.

➤*Viokase (powder):*

Cystic fibrosis – Take 0.7 g (¼ tsp) with meals.

➤*Storage/Stability:*

Creon, Ku-Zyme, Kutrase, Ultrase, Ultrase MT – Store at controlled room temperature 15° to 25°C (59° to 86°F) in a dry place. Protect from high humidity. Do not refrigerate.

Ku-Zyme HP, Lipram, Pancrease, Pancrease MT, Pancrecarb, Pancrelipase, Panokase, Plaretase, Viokase – Store at room temperature not exceeding 25°C (77°F) in a dry place. Protect from high humidity. Store in tight containers. Do not refrigerate.

Actions

➤*Pharmacology:* Digestive enzymes (pancreatic enzymes) hydrolyze fats to glycerol and fatty acids, change proteins into peptides and amino acids, and starch into dextrins and maltose. These agents exert their primary actions in the duodenum and upper jejunum. Once the digestive enzymes accomplish their catalytic function to hydrolyze food, the digestive enzymes may be inactivated by anti-enzymes, excreted by intestinal mucosa, or by protease digestion. The digested enzyme fragments may be absorbed from the intestine and subsequently excreted in the urine. The inactivated enzymes are excreted in the feces. Fat malabsorption (steatorrhea) and protein maldigestion occur when the pancreas loses more than 90% of its ability to produce digestive enzymes. The resultant diarrhea and malabsorption can be reasonably managed if 30,000 lipase units are delivered to the duodenum during a 4-hour period with and after a meal, representing approximately 10% of the normal pancreatic output.

The USP defines standards for 2 pancreatic enzyme preparations, pancreatin and pancrelipase. Pancreatin (a substance containing principally amylase, lipase, and protease) contains not less than 2 USP units of lipase activity, and not less than 25 USP units of amylase as well as protease activity. Pancrelipase (a substance containing principally lipase, and also containing amylase and protease) contains not less than 24 USP units of lipase activity, and not less than 100 USP units of amylase as well as protease activity.

Contraindications

Hypersensitivity to pork protein or enzymes; acute pancreatitis; acute exacerbations of chronic pancreatic diseases.

Warnings

➤*Colonic strictures:* Cases of fibrotic strictures in the colon have been reported primarily in cystic fibrosis patients with the use of enzyme supplements, generally at dosages above the recommended range. Some cases required surgery, including resection of the bowel. If symptoms suggestive of GI obstruction occur, consider the possibility of bowel strictures.

➤*Treatment failure:* Treatment failures have been reported in cystic fibrosis patients when brand name products were replaced by a generic substitution. Use care and monitor closely when switching patients from one product to another.

➤*Replacement therapy:* Pancreatic exocrine replacement therapy should not delay or supplant treatment of the primary disorder.

➤*Pregnancy:* Category B (*Pancrease, Pancrease MT*). Reproduction studies have been conducted in rats and rabbits at doses 0.44 and 0.35 times the maximum daily human dose, respectively, and have revealed no evidence of impaired fertility or harm to the fetus caused by *Pancrease MT*. However, there are no adequate and well-controlled studies in pregnant women. Use during pregnancy only if clearly needed.

Category C (*Creon, Ku-Zyme, Ku-Zyme HP, Kutrase, Lipram, Pancrelipase, Panokase, Plaretase, Ultrase, Ultrase MT, Viokase*). It is not known whether the drug can cause fetal harm when administered to a pregnant woman or can affect reproduction capacity. Give to a pregnant woman only if clearly needed. The enteric coating component, diethyl phthalate, has been teratogenic in rats with high intraperitoneal dosing.

➤*Lactation:* It is not known whether pancreatin is excreted in breast milk. Exercise caution when administering to a nursing mother.

➤*Children:* Colonic strictures, particularly in children with cystic fibrosis, have been associated with doses generally above the recommended dosing range (see Warnings). Patients currently receiving doses above 2500 lipase units/kg/meal or 4000 lipase units/g fat/day should be re-evaluated and the dosage either immediately decreased or titrated downward to the lowest effective clinical dose as assessed by 3-day fecal fat excretion.

Precautions

➤*Excessive doses:* Excessive doses may cause nausea, abdominal cramps, or diarrhea. Extremely high doses have been associated with hyperuricosuria and hyperuricemia.

➤*Pork sensitivity:* Use pork products with caution in patients sensitive to pork. Discontinue use if symptoms of sensitivity appear and initiate symptomatic and supportive treatment if necessary. Individuals previously sensitized to trypsin, pancreatin, or pancrelipase may have allergic reactions.

DIGESTIVE ENZYMES

➤*Irritation of skin/mucous membranes:* Do not spill powder on hands because it may irritate skin. The dust of finely powdered concentrates irritates the nasal mucosa and the respiratory tract. Inhalation of airborne powder can precipitate an asthma attack. Asthma also can occur in patients sensitized to pancreatic enzyme concentrates.

Drug Interactions

Digestive Enzymes Drug Interactions			
Precipitant drug	Object drug*		Description
Antacids	Digestive enzymes	↓	Calcium carbonate or magnesium hydroxide may negate the beneficial effect of the enzymes.
Digestive enzymes	Folic acid	↓	Impaired folic acid absorption by oral pancreatic enzymes may lead to folic acid deficiency.
Digestive enzymes	Iron	↓	The serum iron response to oral iron may be decreased by concomitant pancreatic extracts.

* ↓ = Object drug decreased.

Adverse Reactions

The most frequently reported adverse reactions are GI in nature. Less frequently, allergic-type reactions also have been observed. Other adverse reactions reported include the following: Colonic structures; diarrhea; abdominal pain; intestinal obstruction; vomiting; intestinal stenosis; constipation; dermatitis; flatulence; nausea; melena; weight decrease; pain; bloating; cramping. Perianal irritation and, rarely, inflammation with large doses may occur with pancreatin. Extremely high doses have been associated with hyperuricemia and hyperuricosuria.

Overdosage

Overdosage may cause diarrhea or transient intestinal upset. No acute toxic reactions have been reported.

Patient Information

Take before or with meals. Take with plenty of fluids.

Do not inhale powder dosage form or powder from capsules because it may irritate skin or mucous membranes.

To protect enteric coating, do not crush or chew the microspheres/tablets in the enteric-coated capsule formulations.

Do not switch products without consulting your physician.

Actions

➤*Pharmacology:* Gastric acidifiers counterbalance a deficiency of hydrochloric acid in the gastric juice and destroy or inhibit growth of putrefactive microorganisms in ingested food. A deficiency of hydrochloric acid is often associated with pernicious anemia, allergies, gastric carcinoma and congenital achlorhydria.

Contraindications

Gastric hyperacidity or peptic ulcer.

GLUTAMIC ACID HCl

otc	**Glutamic Acid HCl** (Various)	**Capsules**: 340 mg	In 100s.

For complete prescribing information, refer to the Gastric Acidifiers group monograph.

340 mg contains approximately 1.8 mEq hydrochloric acid.

Administration and Dosage

1 to 3 capsules 3 times daily before meals.

DEHYDROCHOLIC ACID

Rx	**Dehydrocholic Acid** (Various, eg, Goldline)	**Tablets:** 250 mg	In 100s.
otc	**Cholan-HMB** (Ciba Consumer)		Lactose. Dye free. (Cholan HMB). In 100s.
otc	**Decholin** (Miles Pharm.)		Lactose. In 100s.

Indications

Temporary relief of constipation.

Adjunctive therapy of biliary stasis, without complete mechanical obstruction of the common or hepatic bile ducts, where hydrocholeresis is desired.

Administration and Dosage

250 to 500 mg 3 times daily after meals. Thereafter, titrate dosage to individual patient's needs. Do not exceed 1.5 g in 24 hours.

When used as a laxative, a bowel movement is generally produced in 6 to 12 hours.

Actions

➤*Pharmacology:* Dehydrocholic acid is an oxidation product of cholic acid (a natural bile acid). At recommended dosage levels, dehydrocholic acid exerts laxative and hydrocholeretic (increased volume and water content of bile) actions. The mechanisms of action are unknown. Unlike the natural bile acids and their conjugates, dehydrocholic acid does not readily form micelles (small aggregates of bile acids, fats and phospholipids necessary for normal fat absorption).

Contraindications

Significant cholelithiasis; presence of jaundice; marked hepatic insufficiency; complete obstruction of the common or hepatic bile ducts or of the GI or GU tracts; hypersensitivity to bile acids or their conjugates; use as a diuretic or adjunct.

Warnings

➤*Rectal bleeding:* Rectal bleeding or failure to have a bowel movement after use as a laxative may indicate a serious condition. Discontinue use and consult a physician.

➤*Duration:* Do not use as a laxative for > 1 week unless directed otherwise.

➤*GI effects:* Do not use as a laxative if abdominal pain, nausea or vomiting are present unless directed otherwise.

➤*Elderly:* Use with caution. If promotion of true bile flow is desired, use a cholagogue.

➤*Children:* No data supporting a recommended pediatric dose are available. Therefore, do not use in children < 12 years of age.

Adverse Reactions

Hypersensitivity (pruritus, dermatitis).

URSODIOL (Ursodeoxycholic acid)

Rx	Ursodiol (Watson)	**Capsules:** 300 mg	(Watson 3159). White. In 100s.
Rx	Actigall (Watson)		(ACTIGALL 300 mg). White and pink. In 100s.

WARNING

Gallbladder stone dissolution with ursodiol treatment requires months of therapy. Complete dissolution does not occur in all patients and recurrence of stones within 5 years has been observed in up to 50% of patients who do dissolve their stones on bile acid therapy. Carefully select patients for therapy with ursodiol, and consider alternative therapies.

Indications

►*Gallstone disolution:* Dissolution of gallstones in patients with radiolucent, noncalcified, gallbladder stones < 20 mm in greatest diameter in whom elective cholecystectomy would be undertaken except for the presence of increased surgical risk due to systemic disease, advanced age, idiosyncratic reaction to general anesthesia, or for those patients who refuse surgery.

Administration and Dosage

►*Radiolucent gallbladder stones:* 8 to 10 mg/kg/day given in 2 or 3 divided doses.

Obtain ultrasound images of the gallbladder at 6 month intervals for the first year of therapy to monitor gallstone response. If gallstones appear to have dissolved, continue therapy and confirm dissolution on a repeat ultrasound within 1 to 3 months. Most patients who eventually achieve complete stone dissolution will show partial or complete dissolution at the first on-treatment reevaluation. If partial stone dissolution is not seen by 12 months, likelihood of success is greatly reduced.

►*Storage / Stability:* Do not store above 30°C (86°F).

Actions

►*Pharmacology:* Ursodiol, intended for dissolution of radiolucent gallstones, is a naturally occurring bile acid found in small quantities in normal human bile and in larger quantities in the biles of certain species of bears. Ursodiol suppresses hepatic synthesis and cholesterol secretion, and also inhibits intestinal absorption of cholesterol. It has little inhibitory effect on synthesis and secretion into bile of endogenous bile acids, and does not appear to affect phospholipid secretion into bile.

With repeated dosing, bile ursodeoxycholic acid concentrations reach steady state in about 3 weeks. Although insoluble in aqueous media, cholesterol can be solubilized in at least two ways in the presence of dihydroxy bile acids. In addition to solubilizing cholesterol in micelles, ursodiol acts by an apparently unique mechanism to cause dispersion of cholesterol as liquid crystals in aqueous media. Thus, even though administration of high doses (eg, 15 to 18 mg/kg/day) does not result in a concentration of ursodiol higher than 60% of the total bile acid pool, ursodiol-rich bile solubilizes cholesterol. The overall effect of ursodiol is to increase the concentration level at which saturation of cholesterol occurs. The various actions of ursodiol combine to change the bile of patients with gallstones from cholesterol-precipitating to cholesterol-solubilizing.

After ursodiol dosing is stopped, its concentration in bile falls exponentially, declining to about 5% to 10% of its steady-state level in about 1 week.

►*Pharmacokinetics:* About 90% of a therapeutic dose of ursodiol is absorbed in the small bowel after oral administration. After absorption, ursodiol enters the portal vein and undergoes extraction from portal blood by the liver (ie, "first-pass" effect) where it is conjugated with either glycine or taurine and is then secreted into the hepatic bile ducts. Ursodiol in bile is concentrated in the gallbladder and expelled into the duodenum in gallbladder bile via the cystic and common ducts by gallbladder contractions provoked by physiologic responses to eating.

Small quantities of ursodiol appear in the systemic circulation and very small amounts are excreted into urine. A small portion of orally administered drug undergoes bacterial degradation with each cycle of enterohepatic circulation. Ursodiol can be both oxidized and reduced, yielding either 7-keto-lithocholic acid or lithocholic acid, respectively. Free ursodiol, 7-keto-lithocholic acid and lithocholic acid are relatively insoluble in aqueous media and larger proportions of these compounds are excreted via the feces. Reabsorbed free ursodiol is reconjugated by the liver. Eighty percent of lithocholic acid formed in the small bowel is excreted in the feces, but the 20% that is absorbed is sulfated in the liver to relatively insoluble lithocholyl conjugates which are excreted into bile and lost in feces. Absorbed 7-keto-lithocholic acid is stereospecifically reduced in the liver to chenodiol.

►*Clinical trials:* Based on clinical trials in 868 patients with radiolucent gallstones treated for 6 to 78 months with ursodiol doses ranging from about 5 to 20 mg/kg/day, a dose of about 8 to 10 mg/kg/day appeared to be best. Complete stone dissolution occurs in about 30% of unselected patients with uncalcified gallstones < 20 mm in maximal diameter treated for up to 2 years. Patients with calcified gallstones prior to treatment, or patients who develop stone calcification or gallbladder nonvisualization on treatment, and patients with stones larger

than 20 mm in maximal diameter rarely dissolve their stones. The chance of gallstone dissolution is increased up to 50% in patients with floating or floatable stones (ie, those with high cholesterol content), and is inversely related to stone size for those < 20 mm in maximal diameter. Complete dissolution was observed in 81% of patients with stones up to 5 mm in diameter. Age, sex, weight, degree of obesity and serum cholesterol level are not related to the chance of stone dissolution with ursodiol.

Partial stone dissolution occurring within 6 months of beginning therapy with ursodiol appears to be associated with a > 70% chance of eventual complete stone dissolution with further treatment; partial dissolution observed within 1 year of starting therapy indicates a 40% probability of complete dissolution.

Stone recurrence after dissolution with ursodiol therapy was seen within 2 years in 30% of patients. Stone recurrence occurs in up to 50% of patients within 5 years of complete stone dissolution with ursodiol therapy. Obtain serial ultrasonographic examinations to monitor for recurrence of stones; establish radiolucency of the stones before instituting another course of ursodiol. A prophylactic dose of ursodiol has not been established.

Alternative therapies – Watchful waiting has the advantage that no therapy may ever be required. For patients with silent or minimally symptomatic stones, the rate of development of moderate to severe symptoms or gallstone complications is between 2% and 6% per year; 7% to 27% in 5 years. Presumably the rate is higher for patients already having symptoms.

Surgery (cholecystectomy) offers the advantage of immediate and permanent stone removal, but carries a high risk in some patients. About 5% of cholecystectomized patients have residual symptoms of retained common duct stones. The spectrum of surgical risk varies as a function of age and the presence of disease other than cholelithiasis.

Contraindications

Presence of calcified cholesterol stones, radiopaque stones or radiolucent bile pigment stones (ursodiol will not dissolve these stones; hence, patients with such stones are not candidates for ursodiol); patients with compelling reasons for cholecystectomy including unremitting acute cholecystitis, cholangitis, biliary obstruction, gallstone pancreatitis or biliary-gastrointestinal fistula; allergy to bile acids; chronic liver disease.

Warnings

►*Length of therapy:* Safety of use of ursodiol beyond 24 months is not established.

►*Gallbladder nonvisualization:* Nonvisualizing gallbladder by oral cholecystogram prior to the initiation of therapy is not a contraindication to ursodiol therapy. However, gallbladder nonvisualization developing during ursodiol treatment predicts failure of complete stone dissolution and therapy should be discontinued.

►*Carcinogenesis:* Bile acids might be involved in the pathogenesis of human colon cancer in patients who have undergone a cholecystectomy; direct evidence is lacking.

►*Pregnancy: Category B.* There have been no adequate and well controlled studies in pregnant women, but inadvertent exposure of four women to therapeutic doses of the drug in the first trimester of pregnancy during the ursodiol trials led to no evidence of effects on the fetus or newborn baby. The possibility that ursodiol can cause fetal harm cannot be ruled out; hence, do not use the drug during pregnancy.

►*Lactation:* It is not known whether ursodiol is excreted in breast milk. Exercise caution when ursodiol is administered to a nursing mother.

►*Children:* Safety and efficacy for use in children have not been established.

Precautions

►*Hepatic effects:* Ursodiol therapy has not been associated with liver damage. Lithocholic acid, a naturally occurring bile acid and metabolite of ursodiol, is known to be a liver-toxic metabolite. This bile acid is formed in the gut from ursodiol less efficiently and in smaller amounts than that seen from chenodiol. Lithocholic acid is detoxified in the liver by sulfation and although man appears to be an efficient sulfater, it is possible that some patients may have a congenital or acquired deficiency in sulfation, thereby predisposing them to lithocholate-induced liver damage. Therefore, measure AST and ALT at the initiation of therapy, after 1 and 3 months of therapy, and every 6 months thereafter.

Patients with significant abnormalities in liver tests at any point should be monitored frequently; evaluate carefully for worsening gallstone disease which, in the controlled clinical trials, has been the only identified cause of significant liver test abnormality. Discontinue therapy with ursodiol if increased levels persist.

URSODIOL (Ursodeoxycholic acid)

Drug Interactions

Ursodiol Drug Interactions			
Precipitant drug	Object drug*		Description
Antacids	Ursodiol	↓	Aluminum-based antacids adsorb bile acids in vitro and interfere with the action of ursodiol by reducing its absorption.
Bile acid sequestrants	Ursodiol	↓	Cholestyramine and colestipol may interfere with the action of ursodiol by reducing its absorption.
Clofibrate Estrogens Oral Contraceptives	Ursodiol	↓	These agents (and perhaps other lipid-lowering drugs) increase hepatic cholesterol secretion, and encourage cholesterol gallstone formation and hence may counteract the effectiveness of ursodiol.

* ↓ = Object drug decreased.

Adverse Reactions

➤*Dermatologic:* Pruritus; rash; urticaria; dry skin; sweating; hair thinning. One patient with preexisting psoriasis apparently developed exacerbation of itching which remitted on withdrawal of the drug.

➤*GI:* Nausea; vomiting; dyspepsia; metallic taste; abdominal pain; biliary pain; cholecystitis; constipation; stomatitis; flatulence. Doses of 8 to 10 mg/kg/day rarely cause diarrhea (< 1%); in one study, incidence of mild, transient diarrhea was 6%.

➤*Miscellaneous:* Headache; fatigue; anxiety; depression; sleep disorder; arthralgia; myalgia; back pain; cough; rhinitis.

Overdosage

The most likely manifestation of severe overdose with ursodiol would probably be diarrhea; treat symptomatically. Treatment includes usual supportive measures. Refer to General Management of Acute Overdosage.

MONOCTANOIN

Rx	Moctanin (Ethitek)	Infusion: Glyceryl-l-mono-octanoate (80-85%), glyceryl-l-mono-decanoate (10-15%), glyceryl-l-2-di-octanoate (10-15%), free glycerol (2.5% maximum)	In 120 mL ready-for-use bottles with disposable bottle hangers.

Indications

➤*Gallstone dissolution:* A solubilizing agent for cholesterol (radiolucent) gallstones retained in the biliary tract following cholecystectomy, via perfusion of the common bile duct, when other means of removing cholesterol stones retained in the common bile duct have failed or cannot be undertaken.

Administration and Dosage

Determine the value of monoctanoin therapy. Gallstones must be radiolucent and readily accessible to the perfusate. If recently removed stones are available, analyze them for composition or incubate in monoctanoin at body temperature with stirring. If analysis shows the stone to be other than cholesterol or if no dissolution is observed after 72 hours of incubation, do not institute or discontinue therapy.

Do not administer IV or IM. Perfuse into the biliary tract either directly via catheter inserted through the T-tube or a catheter inserted through the mature sinus tract through a nasobiliary tube placed endoscopically. The gravity feed method is recommended if a positive pressure infusion pump is not available. The tip of the catheter must be placed as close to the stone(s) as possible (preferably within 1 cm) to ensure stone contact and complete bathing. Monoctanoin is effective only when in direct contact with the stone.

Add 13 mL of Sterile Water for Injection to each 120 mL vial to reduce the viscosity and enhance the bathing of the stone(s). This dilution reduces the viscosity by nearly 50%. The drug should enter the body at 37°C (98.6°F) and be maintained at this temperature during administration.

Continuously perfuse on a 24 hour basis at a rate of 3 to 5 mL/hr. Continuous perfusion usually requires 2 to 10 days for elimination or size reduction of stones. If, after 10 days, cholangiography shows neither elimination nor reduction in size or density of stones, perform endoscopy to determine advisability of additional perfusion based on friability, softness or reduction of stone density.

If abdominal pain, nausea, diarrhea or emesis occurs and is not tolerated, stop perfusion for 1 hour, aspirate duct, then restart; if symptoms persist, stop perfusion for 1 hour, aspirate duct, then restart at a reduced rate of 3 mL/hr; if symptoms still persist, temporarily discontinue perfusion during meals.

➤*Storage/Stability:* When stored at temperatures below 15°C (59°F), the drug may form a semisolid. To reliquify, heat to 21° to 27°C (70° to 80°F). Store at room temperature 15° to 30°C (59° to 86°F).

Actions

➤*Pharmacology:* Monoctanoin is a semisynthetic esterified glycerol intended for cholesterol stone dissolution via perfusion of the common bile duct. The mixed mono-di-glyceride has the following approximate composition: Glyceryl-l-mono-octanoate (80% to 85%); glyceryl-l-mono-decanoate and glyceryl-l-2-di-octanoate (10% to 15%); and free glycerol (maximum 2.5%).

Monoctanoin is readily hydrolyzed by pancreatic and other digestive lipases. The liberated fatty acids are excreted or absorbed and metabolized in a normal fashion.

Treatment results in complete stone dissolution about 33% of the time and in reduction in stone size in approximately 33% of patients. When reduced in size, these stones may pass spontaneously or may be more susceptible to simple physical extraction. Complete dissolution is much more likely when there is a single stone (almost 50%) than when there are multiple stones (about 20%). Complete dissolution is lower in diabetic patients (about 10%).

Contraindications

Impaired hepatic function; significant biliary tract infection; history of recent duodenal ulcer or jejunitis; porto-systemic shunting (such that there is saturation of the hepatic uptake and metabolism of material absorbed from the gut lumen); acute pancreatitis, or any active life-threatening problems that would be complicated by perfusion into the biliary tract.

Warnings

➤*Rate of administration:* Intended for biliary tract perfusion only; not for parenteral use. Monoctanoin is irritating to GI and biliary tracts. The irritation seems closely related to biliary tract pressure and rate of perfusion; monitor both closely. Such irritation is reversible and disappears 2 to 7 days after therapy. (See Adverse Reactions.)

➤*Ascending cholangitis:* Ascending cholangitis has occurred, possibly related to obstruction in the common bile duct. If fever, anorexia, chills, leukocytosis, severe right upper quadrant abdominal pain or increasing jaundice occurs, discontinue treatment.

➤*GI effects:* Biopsies from the gastric antrum, duodenum and bile ducts have shown diffuse erythema in the antral and duodenal mucosa. Duodenal erosion and inflammatory cell infiltration have occurred. Multiple duodenal ulcerations adjacent to the infusion catheter were observed in one patient. No mucosal abnormalities were seen 1 month after therapy was discontinued.

➤*Pregnancy:* Category C. It is not known whether monoctanoin can cause fetal harm when administered to a pregnant woman or if it can affect reproduction capacity. Use during pregnancy only when clearly needed and when potential benefits outweigh potential hazards to the fetus.

➤*Lactation:* It is not known whether monoctanoin is excreted in breast milk. Exercise caution when administering to a nursing woman.

➤*Children:* Safety and efficacy for use in children have not been established.

Precautions

➤*Hepatic function:* Monitor liver function tests in all patients. Use caution in patients with obstructive jaundice due to stones.

Adverse Reactions

The incidences of adverse reactions are based on 326 patients. Overall, most adverse reactions were mild GI symptoms related to perfusion rate and biliary pressure. Some were tolerated; some abated with reduced perfusion rate and discontinuation during meals.

➤*GI:* Abdominal pain/discomfort (50.3%); nausea (32%); vomiting (20%); diarrhea (19%); anorexia (3%); loose stool (1.5%); indigestion (1.2%); increased serum amylase, burning epigastrium, increased fistula drainage, bile shock (< 1%).

➤*Miscellaneous:* Fever (6.3%); leukopenia, pruritus, fatigue/lethargy, intolerance, chills, depression, diaphoresis, headache, hypokalemia, allergic reaction (< 1%). One patient developed lupus erythematosus, which abated when the drug was discontinued. Five deaths have been attributed to cholangitis, gallbladder perforation and biliary peritonitis, pulmonary embolism, preexisting jaundice and pancreatitis and sepsis, CHF and renal failure, respectively.

NYSTATIN

Rx	**Nystatin** (Various, eg, Geneva, Major, NMC, Parmed)	**Oral suspension:** 100,000 units/mL	In 5, 60 and 480 mL.
Rx	**Nilstat** (Lederle)		Cherry flavor. In 60 and 473 mL.
Rx	**Mycostatin Pastilles** (Bristol-Myers Oncology)	**Troches:** 200,000 units	In 30s.
Rx	**Nystatin** (Paddock)	**Bulk Powder:** 50 million units	
Rx	**Nilstat** (Lederle)	**Bulk Powder:** 150 million units	
Rx	**Nystatin** (Paddock)		
Rx	**Nystatin** (Paddock)	**Bulk Powder:** 500 million units	
Rx	**Nilstat** (Lederle)	**Bulk Powder:** 1 billion units	
Rx	**Nystatin** (Paddock)		
Rx	**Nilstat** (Lederle)	**Bulk Powder:** 2 billion units	
Rx	**Nystatin** (Paddock)		
Rx	**Nystatin** (Paddock)	**Bulk Powder:** 5 billion units	

Indications

➤*Candidiasis:* Treatment of oral candidiasis.

For information on nystatin for treatment of intestinal candidiasis, refer to the monograph in the Antifungals Agents section.

Administration and Dosage

➤*Oral suspension:*

Adults and children – 400,000 to 600,000 units 4 times daily (one half of dose in each side of mouth, retaining the drug as long as possible before swallowing).

Infants – 200,000 units 4 times daily (100,000 units in each side of mouth).

Premature and low birth weight infants – Limited clinical studies indicate that 100,000 units 4 times daily is effective.

➤*Troches (pastilles):*

Adults and children – 200,000 to 400,000 units 4 or 5 times daily, for as long as 14 days, if necessary. Do not chew or swallow whole. To achieve maximum effect from the medication, the troches must be allowed to dissolve slowly in the mouth; therefore, patients, including children and the elderly, must be competent to utilize the dosage form as intended. Discontinue dosage if symptoms persist after the initial 14 day treatment period.

➤*Powder for extemporaneous compounding:*

Adults and children – Add ⅛ tsp (≈ 500,000 units) to ≈ ½ cup of water and stir well. Administer 4 times daily. Use immediately after mixing; do not store.

Continue local treatment at least 48 hours after perioral signs and symptoms have disappeared and cultures have returned to normal.

To improve oral retention of the drug, nystatin (250,000 units) has been administered for oral candidiasis in the form of flavored frozen popsicles.

Actions

➤*Pharmacology:* Nystatin, an antifungal antibiotic, is both fungistatic and fungicidal in vitro against a wide variety of yeasts and yeast-like fungi. It is a polyene antibiotic of undetermined structural formula that is obtained from *Streptomyces noursei*. It binds to sterols in the cell membrane of the fungus with a resultant change in membrane permeability.

Pharmacokinetics: Following oral administration, nystatin is sparingly absorbed with no detectable blood levels. Most of the orally administered drug is passed unchanged in the stool.

Contraindications

Hypersensitivity to nystatin.

Warnings

➤*Systemic mycoses:* Nystatin is not indicated for the treatment of systemic mycoses.

➤*Pregnancy: Category C.* Safety for use during pregnancy has not been established. Use only if clearly needed and when the potential benefits outweigh the potential hazards to the fetus.

Adverse Reactions

➤*GI:* Nausea, vomiting, GI distress and diarrhea occur occasionally with large doses.

Overdosage

Oral doses of nystatin > 5,000,000 units/day have caused nausea and GI upset.

Patient Information

Retain the drug in the mouth as long as possible.

Continue use at least 2 days after symptoms have subsided.

TANNIC ACID

otc	**Zilactin Medicated** (Zila Pharm.)	**Gel:** 7% suspended in 80% alcohol	In 7.5 g.

Indications

For temporary relief of pain, burning and itching caused by cold sores, fever blisters and canker sores.

Administration and Dosage

At first symptoms, apply every 4 hours for the first three days and then as needed. Wipe affected areas dry before applying.

Actions

➤*Pharmacology:* These products form a thin pliable film over sores or blisters within 60 seconds of application. This protective film, if used in the mouth, normally withstands eating and drinking.

Precautions

➤*Do not use in or around eyes:* If contact occurs, flush immediately and continuously with clear water for 10 minutes. Consult physician immediately if pain or irritation persists.

➤*Stinging sensation:* A slight, temporary stinging sensation may occur when the drug is applied to an open sore or blister.

➤*Infection:* If infection persists beyond 10 days, discontinue use and consult a physician.

CLOTRIMAZOLE

Rx	**Mycelex** (Bayer)	**Troches:** 10 mg	(MYCELEX 10). White. In 70s and 140s.

For information on topical and vaginal clotrimazole, refer to individual monographs.

Indications

➤*Treatment:* Local treatment of oropharyngeal candidiasis.

➤*Prophylaxis:* To reduce the incidence of oropharyngeal candidiasis in patients immunocompromised by conditions that include chemotherapy, radiotherapy or steroid therapy utilized in the treatment of leukemia, solid tumors or renal transplantation.

Administration and Dosage

Dissolve troche slowly in mouth in order to achieve maximum effect.

➤*Treatment:* Adminster 1 troche 5 times a day for 14 consecutive days. Only limited data are available on safety and efficacy after pro-

longed administration; therefore, limit therapy to short-term use if possible.

➤*Prophylaxis:* Administer 1 troche 3 times daily for the duration of chemotherapy or until steroids are reduced to maintenance levels.

➤*Storage/Stability:* Store below 30°C (56°F); avoid freezing.

Actions

➤*Pharmacology:* A broad spectrum antifungal agent that inhibits yeast growth by altering cell membrane permeability. It is fungicidal in vitro against *Candida albicans* and other *Candida* sp.

➤*Pharmacokinetics:* Following oral administration, long-term concentration in saliva appears related to the slow release of drug from the oral mucosa to which clotrimazole is apparently bound. Dosing every 3 hours maintains effective salivary levels for most strains of *Candida*.

CLOTRIMAZOLE

Contraindications

Hypersensitivity to clotrimazole.

Warnings

➤*Systemic mycoses:* Clotrimazole is not indicated for the treatment of systemic mycoses.

➤*Prophylactic use:* There are no data to establish safety and efficacy for prophylactic use in patients immunocompromised by etiologies other than those listed in indications.

➤*Pregnancy: Category C.* Clotrimazole is embryotoxic in rats and mice given doses 100 times the adult human dose, possibly secondary to maternal toxicity. Doses of 120 times the human dose in mice from 9 weeks before mating through weaning was associated with impairment of mating, decreased number of viable young and decreased survival to weaning. There are no adequate and well controlled studies in pregnant women. Use only when clearly needed and when the potential benefits outweigh the potential hazards to the fetus.

➤*Children:* Safety and efficacy for use in children under 3 years of age have not been established; therefore, use in these patients is not recommended. Safety and efficacy of the prophylactic use of clotrimazole troches in children have not been established.

Precautions

➤*Abnormal liver function tests:* AST levels were minimally elevated in ≈ 15% of patients in clinical trials. It was often impossible to distinguish effects of clotrimazole from other therapy and the underlying disease (malignancy in most cases). Assess hepatic function periodically, particularly in patients with preexisting hepatic impairment.

Because patients must allow the troche to dissolve slowly in the mouth to achieve maximum effect, they must be of such an age or physical/mental condition to comprehend such instructions.

Adverse Reactions

Abnormal liver function test; elevated AST levels were reported in ≈ 15% of patients in clinical trials (see Precautions).

Nausea; vomiting; unpleasant mouth sensations; pruritus.

Patient Information

To achieve maximum effect, allow troche to dissolve slowly in the mouth.

CHLORHEXIDINE GLUCONATE

Rx	PerioChip (Astra)	Chip: 2.5 mg	Glycerin, hydrolyzed gelatin. Orange-brown, rectangular (rounded at 1 end). In 10s.
Rx	Peridex (Procter & Gamble)	Oral Rinse: 0.12%	In 480 mL.[1]
Rx	PerioGard (Colgate Oral)		In 473 mL with 15 mL dose cup.[1]

[1] With 11.6% alcohol, saccharin.

Indications

➤*Gingivitis (rinse only):* For the treatment of gingivitis as characterized by gingival redness and swelling, including bleeding upon probing.

➤*Scaling and root planing, as adjunct (chip only):* As an adjunct to scaling and root planing procedures for reduction of pocket depth in patients with adult periodontitis. May be used as a part of a periodontal maintenance program, which includes good oral hygiene and scaling and root planing.

Administration and Dosage

➤*Rinse:* Initiate therapy directly following dental prophylaxis. Reevaluate and give a thorough prophylaxis every 6 months.

Use twice daily as an oral rinse for 30 seconds, morning and evening after brushing teeth. Usual dosage is 15 mL (marked in cap) of undiluted drug. Not intended for ingestion; expectorate after rinsing.

➤*Chip:* Insert 1 chip into a periodontal pocket with probing pocket depth (PD) ≥ 5 mm. Up to 8 chips may be inserted in a single visit. Treatment is recommended to be administered once every 3 months in pockets with PD remaining ≥ 5 mm.

Isolate the periodontal pocket and dry the surrounding area prior to chip insertion. Grasp the chip using forceps (such that the rounded end points away from the forceps), and insert it into the periodontal pocket to its maximum depth. If necessary, the chip can be further maneuvered into position using the tips of the forceps or a flat instrument. The chip does not need to be removed because it biodegrades completely.

In the unlikely event of chip dislodgement (in the 2 pivotal clinical trials, only 8 chips were reported lost), several actions are recommended, depending on the day of chip loss. If dislodgement occurs ≥ 7 days after placement, the dentist should consider the subject to have received a full course of treatment. If dislodgement occurs within 48 hours after placement, insert a new chip. If dislodgement occurs > 48 hours after placement, the dentist should not replace the chip but reevaluate the patient at 3 months and insert a new chip if the pocket depth has not been reduced to < 5 mm.

➤*Storage/Stability:* Do not freeze the rinse. Refrigerate the chip at 2° to 8°C (36° to 46°F).

Actions

➤*Pharmacology:* Chlorhexidine provides microbicidal activity during oral rinsing. The clinical significance is not clear. Microbiological sampling of plaque has shown a reduction of aerobic and anaerobic bacteria, ranging from 54% to 97% through 6 months of use.

In a 6-month clinical study, there were no significant changes in bacterial resistance, overgrowth of potentially opportunistic organisms or other adverse changes in the oral microbial ecosystem. The number and resistance of bacteria in plaque had returned to baseline levels 3 months after use was discontinued.

➤*Pharmacokinetics:* Approximately 30% of chlorhexidine is retained in the oral cavity following rinsing and is slowly released into the oral fluids. Chlorhexidine is poorly absorbed from the GI tract. The mean peak plasma level of 0.206 mcg/g was reached 30 minutes after ingestion of 300 mg. Detectable levels were not present in the plasma 12 hours after administration. Excretion occurred primarily through the feces (≈ 90%); < 1% was excreted in the urine.

Contraindications

Hypersensitivity to chlorhexidine gluconate.

Warnings

➤*Necrotizing ulcerative gingivitis:* Chlorhexidine gluconate has not been tested in acute nectrotizing ulcerative gingivitis.

➤*Calculus deposits:* An increase in supragingival calculus was noted in clinical testing in chlorhexidine users. It is not known if use results in an increase in subgingival calculus. Remove calculus deposits by dental prophylaxis at 6 month intervals.

➤*Hypersensitivity reactions:* Hypersensitivity and generalized allergic reactions have been reported rarely. Have epinephrine 1:1000 immediately available. Refer to Management of Acute Hypersensitivity Reactions.

➤*Pregnancy: Category B.* Safety for use during pregnancy has not been established. Use only if clearly needed and when the potential benefits outweigh the potential hazards to the fetus.

➤*Lactation:* It is not known whether this drug is excreted in breast milk. Exercise caution when administering to a nursing mother.

➤*Children:* Efficacy has not been established in children < 18 years of age.

Precautions

➤*Gingivitis and periodontitis:* The presence or absence of gingival inflammation following treatment should not be used as a major indicator of underlying periodontitis.

➤*Staining:* Staining of oral surfaces, such as tooth surfaces, restorations, and the dorsum of the tongue may occur. In clinical testing, 56% of users exhibited a measurable increase in facial anterior stain, compared with 35% of control users after 6 months. Stain will be more pronounced in patients who have heavier accumulations of unremoved plaque.

Stain resulting from use does not adversely affect health of the gingivae or other oral tissues. Stain can be removed from most tooth surfaces by conventional professional prophylactic techniques. Use discretion when prescribing to patients with anterior facial restorations with rough surfaces or margins. If natural stain cannot be removed from these surfaces by dental prophylaxis, exclude patients from treatment if permanent discoloration is unacceptable. Stain in these areas may be difficult to remove and rarely may necessitate replacement of restorations.

➤*Taste perception alteration:* Taste perception alteration may occur while undergoing treatment. Most patients accommodate with continued use. Permanent taste alterations have not been reported.

Adverse Reactions

➤*Miscellaneous:*

Most common – Increase in staining of teeth and other oral surfaces, increase in calculus formation, altered taste perception (see Warnings and Precautions).

➤*Local:* Minor irritation and superficial desquamation of the oral mucosa, particularly among children. Transient parotitis has occurred.

Overdosage

Ingestion of 30 to 60 mL by a small child (≈ 10 kg body weight) might result in gastric distress, including nausea, or signs of alcohol intoxication. Seek medical attention if a small child ingests 120 mL or if signs of alcohol intoxication develop.

CARBAMIDE PEROXIDE (Urea Peroxide)

otc	**Cankaid Liquid** (Dickinson)	**Solution:** 10% in anhydrous glycerol	EDTA. In 22.5 mL.
otc	**Gly-Oxide Liquid** (GlaxoSmithKline)	**Solution:** 10%	In 15 and 60 mL.
otc	**Orajel Perioseptic** (Del)	**Liquid:** 15%	Saccharin, sorbitol, EDTA, methylparaben, ethyl alcohol. In 240 mL.

Indications

➤*Oral care:* For relief of minor oral inflammation such as canker sores, denture irritation, postdental procedure irritation, and irritation related to inflamed gums. Used to aid oral hygiene when normal cleansing measures are inadequate or when patient wears orthodontic or dental appliances.

Administration and Dosage

➤*Solution:* Apply undiluted up to 4 times daily after meals and at bedtime, or as directed. Place several drops onto affected area and expectorate after 2 to 3 minutes. To treat widespread inflammation or hard to reach areas, place 10 drops on tongue, mix with saliva, swish for several minutes, and expectorate. For everyday use, apply product to toothbrush, cover with toothpaste, brush normally, and expectorate.

➤*Liquid:* Swish around in the mouth over the affected area for at least 1 minute and then expectorate. Use up to 4 times daily after meals and at bedtime or as directed by a doctor.

➤*Storage/Stability:* Protect from excessive heat and direct sunlight.

Actions

➤*Pharmacology:* Releases oxygen to help gently remove unhealthy tissue, then cleanse and soothe canker sores and minor wounds and inflammations. Also inhibits odor-forming bacteria.

Warnings

➤*Irritation:* If sore mouth symptoms do not improve in 7 days, or if irritation, pain, or redness persists or worsens, or if swelling, rash, or fever develops, discontinue use of product and see a dentist or doctor promptly.

➤*Children:* Do not use in children under 2 years of age unless otherwise directed.

Patient Information

Severe or persistent oral inflammation, denture irritation, or gingivitis may be serious. If these or unexpected side effects occur, consult physician or dentist promptly.

Discontinue use if condition persists or worsens.

Do not use in children under 2 years of age unless directed by physician or dentist.

PILOCARPINE HCl

Rx	**Salagen** (MGI Pharma)	**Tablets:** 5 mg	(MGI 705). White. Film-coated. In 100s.
		7.5 mg	(SAL 7.5). Blue. Film-coated. In 100s.

For information on the ophthalmic use of pilocarpine, refer to the individual monograph in the Ophthalmics chapter.

Indications

➤*Dry mouth:* Treatment of symptoms of dry mouth from salivary gland hypofunction caused by radiotherapy for cancer of the head and neck; treatment of symptoms of dry mouth in patients with Sjogren's syndrome.

Administration and Dosage

➤*Approved by the FDA:* March 22, 1994.

➤*Head and neck cancer patients:* The recommended dose for the initiation of treatment is 5 mg 3 times/day. Adjust dosage according to therapeutic response and tolerability. The usual dosage range is 3 to 6 tablets or 15 to 30 mg/day (not to exceed 2 tablets/dose). Although early improvement may be realized, at least 12 weeks of uninterrupted therapy may be necessary to assess whether a beneficial response will be achieved. The incidence of the most common adverse events increases with dose. Use the lowest dose that is tolerated and effective for maintenance.

➤*Sjogren's syndrome:* The recommended dose is 5 mg taken 4 times/day. Efficacy was established by 6 weeks of use.

➤*Hepatic function impairment:* Regardless of the indication, the starting dose in patients with moderate hepatic impairment should be 5 mg twice daily, followed by adjustment based on therapeutic response and tolerability. Patients with mild hepatic insufficiency do not require dosage reductions. The use of pilocarpine in patients with severe hepatic insufficiency is not recommended.

➤*Storage/Stability:* Store at controlled room temperature (15° to 30°C; 59° to 86°F).

Actions

➤*Pharmacology:* Pilocarpine is a cholinergic parasympathomimetic agent exerting a broad spectrum of pharmacologic effects with predominant muscarinic action. Pilocarpine in appropriate dosage can increase secretion by the exocrine glands. The sweat, salivary, lacrimal, gastric, pancreatic, intestinal glands, and the mucous cells of the respiratory tract may be stimulated. Dose-related smooth muscle stimulation of the intestinal tract may cause increased tone, increased motility, spasm, and tenesmus. Bronchial smooth muscle tone may increase. The tone and motility of urinary tract, gallbladder, and biliary duct smooth muscle may be enhanced. Pilocarpine may have paradoxical effects on the cardiovascular system. The expected effect of a muscarinic agonist is vasodepression, but administration of pilocarpine may produce hypertension after a brief episode of hypotension. Bradycardia and tachycardia have been reported with use of pilocarpine.

➤*Pharmacokinetics:* In a study in 12 healthy male volunteers, there was a dose-related increase in unstimulated salivary flow following single 5 and 10 mg oral doses. The stimulatory effect was time-related with an onset at 20 minutes and peak at 1 hour with a duration of 3 to 5 hours.

In a multiple-dose pharmacokinetic study in male volunteers following 2 days of 5 or 10 mg oral pilocarpine given at 8 am, noon, and 6 pm, the mean elimination half-life was 0.76 and 1.35 hours for the 5 and 10 mg doses, respectively. T_{max} was 1.25 and 0.85 hours and C_{max} was 15 and 41 ng/mL, respectively. The AUC was 33 and 108 ng•h/mL, respectively, following the last 6-hour dose.

Inactivation of pilocarpine is thought to occur at neuronal synapses and probably in plasma. Pilocarpine and its minimally active or inactive degradation products, including pilocarpic acid, are excreted in the urine.

When taken with a high-fat meal, there was a decrease in the rate of absorption of pilocarpine. Mean T_{max} was 1.47 and 0.87 hours and mean C_{max} was 51.8 and 59.2 ng/mL for fed and fasted states, respectively.

Special populations –

Elderly: In 5 healthy elderly female volunteers, the mean C_{max} and AUC were approximately twice that of elderly males and young healthy male volunteers.

Hepatic function impairment: In patients with mild to moderate hepatic impairment (n = 12), administration of a single 5 mg dose resulted in a 30% decrease in total plasma clearance and a doubling of exposure (as measured by AUC). Peak plasma levels also were increased by about 30% and half-life was increased to 2.1 hours.

Contraindications

Uncontrolled asthma; hypersensitivity to pilocarpine; when miosis is undesirable (eg, in acute iritis and in narrow-angle [angle closure] glaucoma).

Warnings

➤*Cardiovascular disease:* Patients with significant cardiovascular disease may be unable to compensate for transient changes in hemodynamics or rhythm induced by pilocarpine. Pulmonary edema has been reported as a complication of pilocarpine toxicity from high ocular doses given for acute angle-closure glaucoma. Administer pilocarpine with caution and under close medical supervision in patients with significant cardiovascular disease.

The dose-related cardiovascular effects of pilocarpine include hypotension, hypertension, bradycardia, and tachycardia.

➤*Ocular effects:* Ocular formulations of pilocarpine have caused visual blurring, which may result in decreased visual acuity, especially at night and in patients with central lens changes, and impairment of depth perception. Advise caution while driving at night or performing hazardous activities in reduced lighting.

➤*Pulmonary disease:* Pilocarpine increases airway resistance, bronchial smooth muscle tone, and bronchial secretions. Administer with caution and under close medical supervision in patients with controlled asthma, chronic bronchitis, or chronic obstructive pulmonary disease requiring pharmacologic therapy.

➤*Hepatic function impairment:* Based on decreased plasma clearance observed in patients with moderate hepatic impairment, the starting dose in these patients should be 5 mg twice daily, followed by adjustment based on therapeutic response and tolerability. Patients with mild hepatic insufficiency (Child-Pugh score of 5 to 6) do not require dosage reductions. To date, pharmacokinetic studies in subjects with severe hepatic impairment (Child-Pugh score of 10 to 15) have not been carried out. The use of pilocarpine in these patients is not recommended.

PILOCARPINE HCl

►*Carcinogenesis:* In rats, a dosage of 18 mg/kg/day, which yielded a systemic exposure approximately 100 times larger than the maximum systemic exposure observed clinically, resulted in a statistically significant increase in the incidence of benign pheochromocytomas in both males and females and a statistically significant increase in the incidence of hepatocellular adenomas in female rats.

►*Fertility impairment:* Oral administration of pilocarpine to male and female rats at a dosage of 18 mg/kg/day, which yielded a systemic exposure approximately 100 times larger than the maximum systemic exposure observed clinically, resulted in impaired reproductive function, including reduced fertility, decreases sperm motility, and morphologic evidence of abnormal sperm. It is unclear whether the reduction in fertility was due to effects on male animals, female animals, or males and females. In dogs, exposure to pilocarpine at a dosage of 3 mg/kg/day (approximately 3 times the maximum recommended human dose when compared on the basis of body surface area (mg/m^2) estimates) for 6 months resulted in evidence of impaired spermatogenesis. The data obtained in these studies suggest that pilocarpine may impair the fertility of male and female humans. Administer pilocarpine tablets to individuals who are attempting to conceive a child only if the potential benefit justifies potential fertility impairment.

►*Elderly:* In placebo-controlled trials in Sjogren's syndrome patients, the mean age of patients was approximately 55 years of age (range, 21 to 85 years of age). The adverse events reported by those over 65 years of age and those 65 years of age and younger were comparable except for notable trends for urinary frequency, diarrhea, and dizziness.

►*Pregnancy:* Category C. Pilocarpine was associated with a reduction in mean fetal body weight and an increase in the incidence of skeletal variations when given to pregnant rats at a dosage of 90 mg/kg/day (approximately 26 times the maximum recommended dose for a 50 kg human). These effects may have been secondary to maternal toxicity. In another study, oral administration of pilocarpine to female rats during gestation and lactation at a dosage of 36 mg/kg/day (approximately 10 times the maximum recommended dose for a 50 kg human when compared on the basis of body surface area (mg/m^2) estimates) resulted in an increased incidence of stillbirths; decreased neonatal survival and reduced mean body weight of pups were observed at dosages of 18 mg/kg/day (approximately 5 times the maximum recommended dose for a 50 kg human when compared on the basis of body surface area (mg/m^2) estimates) and above. There are no adequate and well-controlled studies in pregnant women. Use during pregnancy only if the potential benefit justifies the potential risk to the fetus.

►*Lactation:* It is not known whether this drug is excreted in breast milk. Because of the potential for serious adverse reactions in nursing infants, decide whether to discontinue nursing or to discontinue the drug, taking into account the importance of the drug to the mother.

►*Children:* Safety and efficacy in children have not been established.

Precautions

►*Toxicity:* Pilocarpine toxicity is characterized by an exaggeration of its parasympathomimetic effects. These may include the following: Headache; visual disturbance; lacrimation; sweating; respiratory distress; GI spasm; nausea; vomiting; diarrhea; AV block; tachycardia; bradycardia; hypotension; hypertension; shock; mental confusion; cardiac arrhythmia; tremors.

►*Biliary tract:* Administer with caution to patients with known or suspected cholelithiasis or biliary tract disease. Contractions of the gallbladder or biliary smooth muscle could precipitate complications including cholecystitis, cholangitis, and biliary obstruction.

►*Renal colic:* Pilocarpine may increase ureteral smooth muscle tone and could theoretically precipitate renal colic (or ureteral reflux), particularly in patients with nephrolithiasis.

►*Psychiatric disorder:* Cholinergic agonists may have dose-related CNS effects. Consider this when treating patients with underlying cognitive or psychiatric disturbances.

Drug Interactions

Pilocarpine (Oral) Drug Interactions			
Precipitant drug	Object drug*		Description
Pilocarpine	Anticholinergics	↓	Pilocarpine may antagonize the anticholinergic effects of drugs used concomitantly. Consider these effects when anticholinergic properties may be contributing to the therapeutic effect of concomitant medication (eg, atropine, inhaled ipratropium).
Pilocarpine	Beta blockers	↑	Use coadministration with caution because of possible conduction disturbances.

* ↑ = Object drug increased. ↓ = Object drug decreased.

►*Drug/Food interactions:* The rate of absorption of pilocarpine is decreased when taken with a high-fat meal. Maximum concentration is decreased and time to reach maximum concentration is increased.

Adverse Reactions

►*Head and neck cancer patients:* The most frequent adverse experiences associated with pilocarpine were a consequence of the expected pharmacologic effects.

Pilocarpine Adverse Reactions (%)				
		Pilocarpine		
Adverse reaction	Placebo (n = 152)	5 mg tid (n = 141)	10 mg tid (n = 121)	5 or 10 mg tid (n = 212)
Sweating	9	29	68	-
Nausea	4	6	15	-
Rhinitis	7	5	14	-
Diarrhea	5	4	7	-
Chills	< 1	3	15	-
Flushing	3	8	13	-
Urinary frequency	7	9	12	-
Dizziness	4	5	12	-
Asthenia	3	6	12	-
Headache	8	-	-	11
Dyspepsia	5	-	-	7
Lacrimation	8	-	-	6
Edema	4	-	-	5
Abdominal pain	4	-	-	4
Amblyopia	2	-	-	4
Vomiting	1	-	-	4
Pharyngitis	8	-	-	3
Hypertension	1	-	-	3

The following events were reported at dosages of 7.5 to 30 mg/day (1% to 2%) – Abnormal vision, conjunctivitis, dysphagia, epistaxis, myalgias, pruritus, rash, sinusitis, tachycardia, taste perversion, tremor, voice alteration.

The following events also were reported (less than 1%). Causal relation is unknown. –
Cardiovascular: Bradycardia; ECG abnormality; palpitations; syncope.
CNS: Anxiety; confusion; depression; abnormal dreams; hyperkinesia; hypesthesia; nervousness; paresthesias; speech disorder; twitching.
GI: Anorexia; increased appetite; esophagitis; GI disorder; tongue disorder.
GU: Dysuria; metrorrhagia; urinary impairment.
Hematologic: Leukopenia; lymphadenopathy.
Respiratory: Increased sputum; stridor; yawning.
Special senses: Deafness; eye pain; glaucoma.
Miscellaneous: Body odor; hypothermia; mucous membrane abnormality; seborrhea. In long-term treatment of 2 patients with underlying cardiovascular disease, 1 experienced an MI and the other an episode of syncope.

►*Sjogren's syndrome patients:* The adverse events reported by those over 65 years of age and those 65 years of age and younger were comparable except for notable trends for urinary frequency, diarrhea, and dizziness. The incidences of urinary frequency and diarrhea in the elderly were about double those in the nonelderly. The incidence of dizziness was about 3 times as high in the elderly as in the nonelderly. These adverse experiences were not considered to be serious. In the 2 placebo-controlled studies, the most common adverse events related to drug use were sweating, urinary frequency, chills, and vasodilation (flushing). The most commonly reported reason for patient discontinuation of treatment was sweating. Expected pharmacologic effects of pilocarpine include the following adverse experiences.

Pilocarpine Adverse Experiences (%)		
Adverse event	5 mg qid (20 mg/day) (n = 255)	Placebo qid (n = 253)
Sweating	40	7
Urinary frequency	10	4
Nausea	9	9
Flushing	9	2
Rhinitis	7	8
Diarrhea	6	7
Chills	4	2
Increased salivation	3	0
Asthenia	2	2
Headache	13	19
Flu syndrome	9	9
Dyspepsia	7	7
Dizziness	6	7
Pain	4	2
Sinusitis	4	5
Abdominal pain	3	4
Vomiting	3	1
Pharyngitis	2	5
Rash	2	3
Infection	2	6

PILOCARPINE HCl

The following events were reported in Sjogren's syndrome patients at incidences of 1% to 2% at dosing of 20 mg/day: Accidental injury; allergic reaction; back pain; blurred vision; constipation; increased cough; edema; epistaxis; face edema; fever; flatulence; glossitis; lab test abnormalities, including chemistry, hematology, and urinalysis; myalgia; palpitation; pruritus; somnolence; stomatitis; tachycardia; tinnitus; urinary incontinence, urinary tract infection; vaginitis.

The following events were reported rarely in Sjogren's syndrome patients (fewer than 1%) at dosing of 10 to 30 mg/day. Causal relation is unknown.

Cardiovascular: Angina pectoris, arrhythmia, ECG abnormality, hypotension, hypertension, intracranial hemorrhage, migraine, MI.

CNS: Abnormal dreams, abnormal thinking, aphasia, confusion, depression, emotional lability, hyperkinesia, hypesthesia, insomnia, leg cramps, nervousness, paresthesias, tremor.

Dermatologic: Alopecia, contact dermatitis, dry skin, eczema, erythema nodosum, exfoliative dermatitis, herpes simplex, skin ulcer, vesiculobullous rash.

GI: Abnormal liver function tests, anorexia, bilirubinemia, cholelithiasis, colitis, dry mouth, eructation, gastritis, gastroenteritis, GI disorder, gingivitis, hepatitis, increased sputum, melena, nausea and vomiting, pancreatitis, parotid gland enlargement, salivary gland enlargement, taste loss, tongue disorder, tooth disorder.

GU: Breast pain, dysuria, mastitis, menorrhagia, metrorrhagia, ovarian disorder, pyuria, salpingitis, urethral pain, urinary urgency, vaginal hemorrhage, vaginal moniliasis.

Hematologic: Abnormal WBC, abnormal platelets, hematuria, lymphadenopathy, thrombocythemia, thrombocytopenia, thrombosis.

Metabolic/Nutritional: Hypoglycemia, peripheral edema.

Musculoskeletal: Arthralgia, arthritis, bone disorder, myasthenia, pathological fracture, spontaneous bone fracture, tendon disorder, tenosynovitis.

Respiratory: Bronchitis, dyspnea, hiccough, laryngismus, laryngitis, pneumonia, viral infection, voice alteration.

Special senses: Abnormal vision, cataract, conjunctivitis, dry eyes, ear disorder, ear pain, eye disorder, eye hemorrhage, glaucoma, lacrimation disorder, retinal disorder, taste perversion.

Miscellaneous: Chest pain, cyst, death, moniliasis, neck pain, neck rigidity, photosensitivity reaction.

The following adverse experiences have been reported rarely with ocular pilocarpine: AV block, agitation, ciliary congestion, confusion, delusion, depression, dermatitis, eyelid twitching, iris cysts, macular hole, malignant glaucoma, middle ear disturbance, shock, and visual hallucination.

Overdosage

Pilocarpine fatal overdosage resulting from poisoning has been reported at doses presumed to be greater than 100 mg in 2 hospitalized patients; 100 mg is considered potentially fatal. Treat overdosage with atropine titration (0.5 to 1 mg SC or IV) and use supportive measures to maintain respiration and circulation. Epinephrine (0.3 to 1 mg SC or IM) also may be of value in the presence of severe cardiovascular depression or bronchoconstriction. Refer to General Management of Acute Overdosage. It is not known if pilocarpine is dialyzable.

Patient Information

Inform patients that pilocarpine may cause visual disturbances, especially at night, that could impair their ability to drive safely.

If a patient sweats excessively while taking pilocarpine and cannot drink enough liquid, have the patient consult a physician. Dehydration may develop.

CEVIMELINE HCl

Rx **Evoxac** (Daiichi Pharm.)	**Capsules:** 30 mg	Lactose. White. In 100s and 500s.

Indications

➤*Sjögren's Syndrome:* For the treatment of dry mouth symptoms in patients with Sjögren's Syndrome.

Administration and Dosage

➤*Approved by the FDA:* January 11, 2000.

The recommended dose of cevimeline is 30 mg taken 3 times/day. There is insufficient safety information to support doses > 30 mg 3 times/day. There is also insufficient evidence for additional efficacy of cevimeline at doses > 30 mg 3 times/day.

Actions

➤*Pharmacology:* Cevimeline is a cholinergic agonist that binds to muscarinic receptors. Muscarinic agonists in sufficient dosage can increase secretion of exocrine glands, such as salivary and sweat glands, and increase tone of the smooth muscle in the GI and urinary tracts.

➤*Pharmacokinetics:*

Absorption – After administration of a single 30 mg dose, cevimeline was rapidly absorbed with a mean time to peak concentration of 1.5 to 2 hours. No accumulation of active drug or its metabolites was observed following multiple dose administration. When administered with food, absorption decreases, with a fasting T_{max} of 1.53 hours, a T_{max} of 2.86 hours, and a 17.3% reduction in peak concentration.

Distribution – Cevimeline has a volume of distribution of ≈ 6 L/kg and is < 20% bound to human plasma proteins.

Metabolism – Isozymes CYP2D6 and CYP3A3/4 are responsible for the metabolism of cevimeline. After 24 hours, 86.7% of the dose was recovered (16% unchanged, 44.5% as *cis* and trans-sulfoxide, 22.3% of the dose as glucuronic acid conjugate, and 4% of the dose as N-oxide of cevimeline). Approximately 8% of the trans-sulfoxide metabolite is then converted into the corresponding glucuronic acid conjugate and eliminated. Cevimeline did not inhibit cytochrome P450 isozymes 1A2, 2A6, 2C9, 2C19, 2D6, 2E1, and 3A4.

Excretion – The mean half-life of cevimeline is ≈ 5 hours. After 24 hours, 84% of a 30 mg dose of cevimeline was excreted in urine. After 7 days, 97% of the dose was recovered in the urine and 0.5% was recovered in the feces.

Contraindications

Uncontrolled asthma; known hypersensitivity to cevimeline; when miosis is undesirable (eg, acute iritis, narrow-angle [angle-closure] glaucoma).

Warnings

➤*Cardiovascular:* Cevimeline can potentially alter cardiac conduction or heart rate. Patients with significant cardiovascular disease may potentially be unable to compensate for transient changes in hemodynamics or rhythm induced by cevimeline. Use cevimeline with caution and under close medical supervision in patients with a history of cardiovascular disease evidenced by angina pectoris or MI.

➤*Pulmonary:* Cevimeline can potentially increase airway resistance, bronchial smooth muscle tone, and bronchial secretions. Administer cevimeline with caution and under close medical supervision to patients with asthma, chronic bronchitis, or chronic obstructive pulmonary disease.

➤*Ocular:* Ophthalmic formulations of muscarinic agonists have been reported to cause visual blurring that may result in decreased visual acuity (especially at night and in patients with central lens changes) and impairment of depth perception. Advise caution while driving at night or performing hazardous activities in reduced lighting.

➤*Carcinogenesis:* Lifetime carcinogenicity studies were conducted in CD-1 mice and F-344 rats. A statistically significant increase in the incidence of adenocarcinomas of the uterus in female rats that received cevimeline at a dosage of 100 mg/kg/day (≈ 8 times the maximum human exposure based on comparison of AUC data).

➤*Fertility impairment:* Female rats that were treated with cevimeline at dosages ≤ 45 mg/kg/day from 14 days prior to mating through day 7 of gestation exhibited a statistically significantly smaller number of implantations than did control animals.

➤*Elderly:* Although clinical studies of cevimeline included subjects > 65 years of age, the numbers were not sufficient to determine whether they respond differently from younger subjects. Exercise special care when cevimeline treatment is initiated in an elderly patient, considering the greater frequency of decreased hepatic, renal, or cardiac function, and of concomitant disease or other drug therapy in the elderly.

➤*Pregnancy:* Category C. Cevimeline was associated with a reduction in the mean number of implantations when given to pregnant Sprague-Dawley rats from 14 days prior to mating through day 7 of gestation at a dosage of 45 mg/kg/day (≈ 5 times the maximum recommended dose for a 60 kg human when compared on the basis of body surface area estimates). This effect may have been secondary to maternal toxicity. There are no adequate and well-controlled studies in pregnant women. Use cevimeline during pregnancy only if the potential benefit justifies the potential risk to the fetus.

➤*Lactation:* It is not known whether this drug is secreted in breast milk. Because of the potential for serious adverse reactions in nursing infants from cevimeline, decide whether to discontinue nursing or discontinue the drug, taking into account the importance of the drug to the mother.

➤*Children:* Safety and efficacy have not been established.

Precautions

➤*Toxicity:* Cevimeline toxicity is characterized by an exaggeration of its parasympathomimetic effects. These may include the following: Headache, visual disturbance, lacrimation, sweating, respiratory distress, GI spasm, nausea, vomiting, diarrhea, atrioventricular block,

CEVIMELINE HCl

tachycardia, bradycardia, hypotension, hypertension, shock, mental confusion, cardiac arrhythmia, and tremors.

➤*Biliary tract:* Administer with caution to patients with a history of cholelithiasis. Contractions of the gallbladder or biliary smooth muscle could precipitate complications such as cholecystitis, cholangitis, and biliary obstruction.

➤*Renal colic:* Administer with caution to patients with a history of nephrolithiasis. An increase in the ureteral smooth muscle tone could theoretically precipitate renal colic or ureteral reflux in patients with nephrolithiasis.

Drug Interactions

Cevimeline Drug Interactions			
Precipitant drug	Object drug*		Description
Cevimeline	Beta blockers	↑	Administer cevimeline with caution to patients taking beta adrenergic antagonists because of the possibility of conduction disturbances.
Cevimeline	Parasympathomimetics	↑	Drugs with parasympathomimetic effects administered concurrently with cevimeline may be expected to have additive effects.
Cevimeline	Antimuscarinics	↓	Cevimeline might interfere with desirable antimuscarinic effects of drugs used concomitantly.

* ↑ = Object drug increased. ↓ = Object drug decreased.

➤*CYP450 system:* Drugs that inhibit CYP2D6 and CYP3A3/4 also inhibit the metabolism of cevimeline. Use with caution in individuals known or suspected to be deficient of CYP2D6 activity, based on previous experience, as they may be at a higher risk of adverse events. In an in vitro study, cytochrome P450 isozymes 1A2, 2A6, 2C9, 2C19, 2D6, 2E1, and 3A4 were not inhibited by exposure to cevimeline.

➤*Drug/Food interactions:* When cevimeline is administered with food, absorption decreases, with a fasting T_{max} of 1.53 hours, a T_{max} of 2.86 hours, and a 17.3% reduction in peak concentration.

Adverse Reactions

In clinical trials, 11.1% of patients discontinued treatment with cevimeline because of adverse events.

Cevimeline Adverse Reactions (%)		
Adverse reaction	Cevimeline 30 mg 3 times/day (n = 533)	Placebo (n = 164)
Excessive sweating	18.7	2.4
Headache	14.4	20.1
Nausea	13.8	7.9
Sinusitis	12.3	10.9
Upper respiratory tract infection	11.4	9.1
Rhinitis	11.2	5.4
Diarrhea	10.3	10.3
Dyspepsia	7.8	8.5
Abdominal pain	7.6	6.7
Urinary tract infection	6.1	3
Coughing	6.1	3
Pharyngitis	5.2	5.4
Vomiting	4.6	2.4
Injury	4.5	2.4
Back pain	4.5	4.2
Rash	4.3	6
Conjunctivitis	4.3	3.6
Dizziness	4.1	7.3
Bronchitis	4.1	1.2
Arthralgia	3.7	1.8
Surgical intervention	3.3	3
Fatigue	3.3	1.2
Pain	3.3	3
Skeletal pain	2.8	1.8
Insomnia	2.4	1.2
Hot flushes	2.4	0
Excessive salivation	2.2	0.6
Rigors	1.3	1.2
Anxiety	1.3	1.2
Urinary frequency	0.9	1.8

Cevimeline Adverse Reactions (%)		
Adverse reaction	Cevimeline 30 mg 3 times/day (n = 533)	Placebo (n = 164)
Asthenia	0.5	0
Flushing	0.3	0.6
Polyuria	0.1	0.6

The following events were reported in Sjögren's patients at incidences < 3% and ≥ 1%: Constipation, tremor, abnormal vision, hypertonia, peripheral edema, chest pain, myalgia, fever, anorexia, eye pain, earache, dry mouth, vertigo, salivary gland pain, pruritus, influenza-like symptoms, eye infection, postoperative pain, vaginitis, skin disorder, depression, hiccough, hyporeflexia, infection, fungal infection, sialoadenitis, otitis media, erythematous rash, pneumonia, edema, salivary gland enlargement, allergy, gastroesophageal reflux, eye abnormality, migraine, tooth disorder, epistaxis, flatulence, toothache, ulcerative stomatitis, anemia, hypoesthesia, cystitis, leg cramps, abscess, eructation, moniliasis, palpitation, increased amylase, xerophthalmia, allergic reaction.

The following events were reported rarely in treated Sjögren's patients (< 1%); causal relationship is unknown:

➤*Cardiovascular:* Abnormal ECG, heart disorder, heart murmur, aggravated hypertension, hypotension, arrhythmia, extrasystoles, T-wave inversion, tachycardia, supraventricular tachycardia, angina pectoris, MI, pericarditis, pulmonary embolism, peripheral ischemia, superficial phlebitis, purpura, deep thrombophlebitis, vascular disorder, vasculitis hypertension.

➤*CNS:* Carpal tunnel syndrome, coma, abnormal coordination, dysesthesia, dyskinesia, dysphonia, aggravated multiple sclerosis, involuntary muscle contractions, neuralgia, neuropathy, paresthesia, speech disorder, agitation, confusion, depersonalization, aggravated depression, abnormal dreaming, emotional lability, manic reaction, paroniria, somnolence, abnormal thinking, hyperkinesia, hallucination.

➤*Dermatologic:* Acne, alopecia, burn, dermatitis, contact dermatitis, lichenoid dermatitis, eczema, furunculosis, hyperkeratosis, lichen planus, nail discoloration, nail disorder, onychia, onychomycosis, paronychia, photosensitivity reaction, rosacea, scleroderma, seborrhea, skin discoloration, dry skin, skin exfoliation, skin hypertrophy, skin ulceration, urticaria, verruca, bullous eruption, cold clammy skin.

➤*Endocrine:* Increased glucocorticoids, goiter, hypothyroidism.

➤*GI:* Appendicitis, increased appetite, ulcerative colitis, diverticulitis, duodenitis, dysphagia, enterocolitis, gastric ulcer, gastritis, gastroenteritis, GI hemorrhage, gingivitis, glossitis, rectum hemorrhage, hemorrhoids, ileus, irritable bowel syndrome, melena, mucositis, esophageal stricture, esophagitis, oral hemorrhage, peptic ulcer, periodontal destruction, rectal disorder, stomatitis, tenesmus, tongue discoloration, tongue disorder, geographic tongue, tongue ulceration, dental caries.

➤*GU:* Epididymitis, prostatic disorder, abnormal sexual function, amenorrhea, female breast neoplasm, malignant female breast neoplasm, female breast pain, positive cervical smear test, dysmenorrhea, endometrial disorder, intermenstrual bleeding, leukorrhea, menorrhagia, menstrual disorder, ovarian cyst, ovarian disorder, genital pruritus, uterine hemorrhage, vaginal hemorrhage, atrophic vaginitis, albuminuria, bladder discomfort, increased blood urea nitrogen, dysuria, hematuria, micturition disorder, nephrosis, nocturia, increased nonprotein nitrogen, pyelonephritis, renal calculus, abnormal renal function, renal pain, strangury, urethral disorder, abnormal urine, urinary incontinence, decreased urine flow, pyuria.

➤*Hematologic:* Thrombocytopenic purpura, thrombocythemia, thrombocytopenia, hypochromic anemia, eosinophilia, granulocytopenia, leucopenia, leukocytosis, cervical lymphadenopathy, lymphadenopathy.

➤*Hepatic:* Cholelithiasis, increased gamma-glutamyl transferase, increased hepatic enzymes, abnormal hepatic function, viral hepatitis, increased AST/ALT.

➤*Metabolic/Nutritional:* Dehydration, diabetes mellitus, hypercalcemia, hypercholesterolemia, hyperglycemia, hyperlipemia, hypertriglyceridemia, hyperuricemia, hypoglycemia, hypokalemia, hyponatremia, thirst.

➤*Musculoskeletal:* Arthritis, aggravated arthritis, arthropathy, femoral head avascular necrosis, bone disorder, bursitis, costochondritis, planta fascilitis, muscle weakness, osteomyelitis, osteoporosis, synovitis, tendinitis, tenosynovitis.

➤*Respiratory:* Asthma, bronchospasm, chronic obstructive airway disease, dyspnea, hemoptysis, laryngitis, nasal ulcer, pleural effusion, pleurisy, pulmonary congestion, pulmonary fibrosis, respiratory disorder.

➤*Special senses:* Deafness, decreased hearing, motion sickness, parosmia, taste perversion, blepharitis, cataract, corneal opacity, corneal ulceration, diplopia, glaucoma, anterior chamber eye hemorrhage, keratitis, keratoconjunctivitis, mydriasis, myopia, photopsia, retinal deposits, retinal disorder, scleritis, vitreous detachment, tinnitus.

CEVIMELINE HCl

➤*Miscellaneous:* Aggravated allergy, precordial chest pain, abnormal crying, hematoma, leg pain, edema, periorbital edema, activated pain trauma, pallor, changed sensation temperature, weight decrease/increase, choking, mouth edema, syncope, malaise, face edema, substernal chest pain, basal cell carcinoma, squamous carcinoma, fall, food poisoning, heat stroke, joint dislocation, postoperative hemorrhage, cellulitis, herpes simplex, herpes zoster, bacterial infection, viral infection, genital moniliasis, sepsis, aggravated rheumatoid arthritis, lupus erythematosus rash, lupus erythematosus syndrome.

In 1 subject with lupus erythematosis receiving concomitant multiple therapy, a highly elevated ALT level was noted after the fourth week of cevimeline therapy. In 2 other subjects receiving cevimeline in the clinical trials, very high AST levels were noted. The significance of these findings is unknown.

Overdosage

➤*Treatment:* Manage signs and symptoms of acute overdosage in a manner consistent with that indicated for other muscarinic agonists; institute general supportive measures. Refer to General Management of Acute Overdosage. If medically indicated, atropine may be of value as an antidote for emergency use in patients who have had an overdose of cevimeline. If medically indicated, epinephrine may also be of value in the presence of severe cardiovascular depression or bronchoconstriction. It is not known if cevimeline is dialyzable.

Patient Information

Inform patients that cevimeline may cause visual disturbances, especially at night, that could impair their ability to drive safely.

If a patient sweats excessively while taking cevimeline, consult a health care provider and advise the patient to drink extra water as dehydration may develop.

SALIVA SUBSTITUTES

otc	**Saliva Substitute** (Roxane)	**Solution:** Sorbitol, sodium carboxymethylcellulose, methylparaben	In 120 mL bottle.
otc	**Moi-Stir** (Kingswood)	**Solution:** Dibasic sodium phosphate, magnesium, calcium chloride, sodium chloride, and potassium chlorides, sorbitol, sodium carboxymethylcellulose, parabens	In 120 mL spray.
otc	**Moi-Stir Swabsticks** (Kingswood)	**Swabsticks:** Dibasic sodium phosphate, magnesium, calcium chloride, sodium chloride, and potassium chlorides, sorbitol, sodium carboxymethylcellulose, parabens	In packets (3s).
otc	**Entertainer's Secret** (KLI Corp)	**Solution:** Sodium carboxymethylcellulose, potassium chloride, dibasic sodium phosphate, parabens, aloe vera gel, glycerin	In 60 mL spray.
otc	**Salivart** (Gebauer)	**Solution:** Sodium carboxymethylcellulose, sorbitol, sodium chloride, potassium chloride, calcium chloride, magnesium chloride, dibasic potassium phosphate, nitrogen (as propellant)	Preservative-free. In 75 mL aerosol spray cans.
otc	**MouthKote** (Parnell)	**Solution:** Xylitol, sorbitol, yerba santa, citric acid, ascorbic acid, sodium benzoate, saccharin	Lemon-lime flavor. In 60 and 240 mL spray.

Indications

These products are used as saliva substitutes to relieve dry mouth and throat in xerostomia, which may be caused by the following: Surgery or radiation near the salivary glands; chemotherapy; Sjogren syndrome; Bell palsy; HIV/AIDS; lupus; diabetes; aging; emotional factors; dry throat; scratchy, hoarse voice; medications (eg, antidepressants, antihistamines, antihypertensives); infection or dysfunction of the salivary glands.

Administration and Dosage

Refer to specific product labeling for additional dosage guidelines.

➤*Spray:* Hold close to mouth and spray for one-half second or less to relieve dryness. May be used as often as needed to moisten and lubricate; may swallow or expectorate.

➤*Swabsticks:* Swab and cleanse all intraoral surfaces for 2 to 3 minutes using all 3 disposable swabsticks. Repeat procedure every 3 to 4 hours while awake or more frequently if needed.

➤*Storage/Stability:* Store at controlled room temperature, 15° to 30°C (59° to 86°F). Contents under pressure. Protect from direct sunlight and heat above 38°C (100°F).

DOXYCYCLINE

Rx	**Periostat** (CollaGenex)	**Tablets:** 20 mg (as hyclate)	Lactose. (PS 20). White. In 60s, 100s, and 1000s.
Rx	**Atridox** (CollaGenex)	**Injection:** 42.5 mg (as hyclate, 10%)	In 2 syringe mixing system[1] and blunt cannula.

[1] Syringe A contains 450 mg *Atrigel* Delivery System. Syringe B contains 50 mg doxycycline hyclate equivalent to 42.5 mg doxycycline.

For information on the anti-infective use of doxycycline, refer to individual monograph in the Anti-Infectives, Systemic chapter.

Indications

➤*Periodontitis:*

Tablet – As an adjunct to scaling and root planing to promote attachment level gain and to reduce pocket depth in patients with adult periodontitis.

Injection – For chronic adult periodontitis for a gain in clinical attachment, reduction in probing depth, and reduction in bleeding on probing.

Administration and Dosage

➤*Approved by the FDA:* September 30, 1998.

➤*Tablets:* The dosage of doxycycline for periodontitis differs from that of doxycycline used to treat infections. Exceeding the recommended dosage may result in an increased incidence of side effects including the development of resistant microorganisms.

Doxycycline 20 mg twice daily as an adjunct following scaling and root planing (SRP) may be administered for up to 9 months. Take twice daily at 12 hour intervals, usually in the morning and evening. It is recommended that if doxycycline is taken close to meal times, allow at least 2 hours before or after meals. Safety beyond 12 months and efficacy beyond 9 months have not been established.

Administration of adequate amounts of fluid is recommended to wash down the drug and reduce the risk of esophageal irritation and ulceration.

➤*Injection:* Doxycycline injection is a variable-dose product dependent on the size, shape, and number of pockets being treated.

Preparation for use –
1.) Remove the pouched product from refrigeration at least 15 minutes prior to mixing.
2.) Couple Syringe A (liquid delivery system) and Syringe B (drug powder).
3.) Inject the liquid contents of Syringe A (indicated by purple stripe) into Syringe B (doxycycline powder) and then push the contents back into syringe A. This entire operation is 1 mixing cycle.
4.) Complete 100 mixing cycles at a pace of 1 cycle per second using

brisk strokes. *If immediate use is desired, skip to step 7.*
5.) If necessary, the coupled syringes can be stored in the resealable pouch at room temperature for a maximum of 3 days.
6.) After storage, perform an additional 10 mixing cycles just prior to use. *Continue with immediate use instructions.*
7.) The contents will be in Syringe A (indicated by purple stripe). Hold the coupled syringes vertically with Syringe A at the bottom. Pull back on the Syringe A plunger and allow the contents to flow down the barrel for several seconds.
8.) Uncouple the 2 syringes and attach the blunt cannula to Syringe A. *The product is now ready for application.*

Administration – Doxycycline does not require local anesthesia for placement.

Bend the cannula to resemble a periodontal probe and explore the periodontal pocket in a manner similar to periodontal probing. Keeping the cannula tip near the base of the pocket, express the product into the pocket until the formulation reaches the top of the gingival margin. Withdraw the cannula tip from the pocket. In order to separate the tip from the formulation, turn the tip of the cannula towards the tooth, press the tip against the tooth surface, and pinch the string of formulation from the tip of the cannula. Variations on this technique may be needed to achieve separation between doxycycline and cannula.

If desired, using an appropriate dental instrument, doxycycline may be packed into the pocket. Dipping the edge of the instrument in water before packing will help keep doxycycline from sticking to the instrument and will help speed coagulation of doxycycline. To aid coagulation, put a few drops of water onto the surface of doxycycline once in the pocket. If necessary, add more doxycycline as described above and pack it into the pocket until the pocket is full.

Cover the pockets containing doxycycline with either *Coe-Pak* periodontal dressing or *Octyldent* dental adhesive.

Application of doxycycline may be repeated 4 months after initial treatment.

➤*Storage/Stability:*

Tablets – Store at controlled room temperature (15° to 30°C; 59° to 86°F) and dispense in tight, light-resistant containers.

Injection – Store at 2° to 8°C (36° to 46°F).

DOXYCYCLINE

Actions

▶*Pharmacology:* Doxycycline is a broad-spectrum semisynthetic tetracycline. Doxycycline is bacteriostatic, inhibiting bacterial protein synthesis due to disruption of transfer RNA and messenger RNA at ribosomal sites. In vitro testing has shown that *Porphyromonas gingivalis*, *Prevotella intermedia*, *Campylobacter rectus*, and *Fusobacterium nucleatum*, which are associated with periodontal disease, are susceptible to doxycycline at concentrations less than or equal to 6 mcg/mL.

Doxycycline has been shown to inhibit collagenase activity in vitro. Additional studies have shown that doxycycline reduces the elevated collagenase activity in the gingival crevicular fluid of patients with adult periodontitis. The clinical significance of these findings is not known.

The dosage of doxycycline achieved with doxycycline tablets during administration is well below the concentration required to inhibit microorganisms commonly associated with adult periodontitis. Do not use this product for reducing the numbers of or eliminating those microorganisms associated with periodontitis.

▶*Pharmacokinetics:*

Absorption –

Tablets: After oral administration, doxycycline hyclate is rapidly and nearly completely absorbed from the GI tract. Doxycycline is eliminated with a half-life of approximately 18 hours by renal and fecal excretion of the unchanged drug. In a single-dose study in healthy volunteers, concomitant administration of doxycycline with a 1000 calorie, high-fat, high-protein meal that included dairy products resulted in a decrease in the rate and extent of absorption and delay in the time to maximum concentrations.

Injection: Doxycycline levels in gingival crevicular fluid (GCF) peaked (-1500 mcg/mL and -2000 mcg/mL for *Coe-Pak* and *Octyldent* groups, respectively) 2 hours following treatment with doxycycline injection. These levels remained above 1000 mcg/mL through 18 hours, at which time the levels began to decline gradually. However, local levels of doxycycline remained well above the minimum inhibitory concentration (MIC90) for periodontal pathogens (6 mcg/mL or below) through day 7. In contrast, subjects receiving oral doxycycline had peak GCF levels of -2.5 mcg/mL at 12 hours following the initial oral dosing with levels declining to -0.2 mcg/mL by day 7. High variability was observed for doxycycline levels in GCF for oral and injection treatment groups.

The maximum concentration of doxycycline in saliva was achieved at 2 hours after both treatments with doxycycline injection, with means of 4.05 and 8.788 mcg/mL and decreased to 0.36 and 0.23 mcg/mL at day 7 for the *Coe-Pak* and *Octyldent* groups, respectively.

The concentration of doxycycline in serum following treatment of doxycycline injection never exceeded 0.1 mcg/mL.

Distribution – Doxycycline is greater than 90% bound to plasma proteins. Its apparent volume of distribution is between 52.6 and 134 L.

Metabolism – Major metabolites of doxycycline have not been identified. However, enzyme inducers such as barbiturates, carbamazepine, and phenytoin decrease the half-life of doxycycline.

Excretion – Doxycycline is eliminated unchanged in the urine and feces. Half-life averaged approximately 18 hours in subjects receiving a single 20 mg doxycycline dose. It is variously reported that between 29% and 55.4% of an administered dose can be accounted for in the urine by 72 hours.

Pharmacokinetic Parameters for Doxycycline					
	n	C_{max} (ng/mL)	T_{max} (h)	Cl/F (L/h)	$t_{1/2}$ (h)
Single dose 20 mg (tablet)	20	≈ 362	1.4 (1 to 2.5)	≈ 3.85	≈ 18.1
Steady-state 20 mg BID (tablet)[1]	30	≈ 790	2 (0.98 to 12)	≈ 3.76	Not determined

[1] Steady-state data were obtained from normal volunteers administered a bioequivalent formulation.

Special populations –

Gender: Doxycycline pharmacokinetics were compared in 9 men and 11 women under fed and fasted conditions. While female subjects had a higher rate (C_{max}) and extent of absorption (AUC), these differences are thought to be caused by differences in body weight/lean body mass. Differences in other pharmacokinetic parameters were not significant.

▶*Clinical trials:*

Injection – In 2 well-controlled, multi-center, parallel-design, 9-month clinical trials, 831 patients with chronic adult periodontitis characterized by a mean probing depth of 5.9 to 6 mm were enrolled. Subjects received 1 of the following 4 treatments: 1) Doxycycline injection, 2) SRP, 3) vehicle control, or 4) oral hygiene. All subjects received a second administration of the initially randomized treatment 4 months after their baseline treatment. Changes in the efficacy parameters, attachment level, pocket depth, and bleeding on probing, between baseline and month 9 showed the following: 1) Doxycycline injection was superior to vehicle control and oral hygiene, and 2) doxycycline met the decision rule of being at least 75% as good as SRP (the standard of at least 75% as good as SRP is required for any product approved as a

stand alone therapy for periodontitis). Additional research would be necessary to establish long-term comparability to SRP.

A third clinical trial was conducted to determine whether the product can be left in the pocket to bioabsorb or be expelled naturally and achieve comparable clinical results. In this study, the product was retained with *Octyldent* dental adhesive rather than *Coe-Pak* periodontal dressing as in the previously mentioned studies. This was a 3-arm, randomized, controlled, parallel group, single-blind trial that enrolled 605 subjects. Subjects received 1 of the following 3 treatments: 1) Doxycycline injection with *Coe-Pak* removed after 7 days as in the pivotal trials, 2) doxycycline injection retained with *Octyldent* and left to bioabsorb or be expelled naturally, or 3) vehicle control with *Octyldent* left to bioabsorb or be expelled naturally.

The results support the use of doxycycline injection retained with *Octyldent* and left to bioabsorb or be expelled naturally.

Contraindications

Use in nursing mothers; hypersensitivity to any of the tetracyclines. Use of *Periostat* is contraindicated in infancy and childhood.

Warnings

▶*Tooth discoloration:* Use of the tetracycline class during tooth development (last half of pregnancy, infancy, and childhood to 8 years of age) may cause permanent discoloration of the teeth (yellow-gray-brown). This adverse reaction is more common during long-term use of the drugs but has been observed following repeated short-term courses. Enamel hypoplasia has also been reported. Therefore, do not use tetracycline drugs in this age group or in pregnant or nursing mothers unless the potential benefits outweigh the potential risks.

▶*Bone growth:* All tetracyclines form a stable calcium complex in any bone-forming tissue. A decrease in fibula growth rate has been observed in premature infants given oral tetracyclines in doses of 25 mg/kg every 6 hours. This reaction was shown to be reversible when the drug was discontinued.

▶*Photosensitivity:* Photosensitivity manifested by an exaggerated sunburn reaction has been observed in some individuals taking tetracyclines. Advise patients apt to be exposed to direct sunlight or ultraviolet light that this reaction can occur with tetracycline drugs, and to discontinue treatment at the first evidence of skin erythema.

▶*Renal function impairment:* The catabolic action of the tetracyclines may cause an increase in BUN. Studies to date indicate that this does not occur with the use of doxycycline in patients with impaired renal function.

▶*Mutagenesis:* Data from an in vitro assay with Chinese hamster ovary cells for potential to cause chromosomal aberrations suggest that doxycycline hyclate is a weak clastogen.

▶*Fertility impairment:* Oral administration of doxycycline hyclate to male and female Sprague-Dawley rats adversely affected fertility and reproductive performance, as evidenced by increased time for mating to occur; reduced sperm motility, velocity, and concentration; abnormal sperm morphology; and increased pre- and postimplantation losses. Doxycycline hyclate induced reproductive toxicity at all dosages that were examined in this study, as even the lowest dosage tested (50 mg/kg/day) induced a statistically significant reduction in sperm velocity. Note that 50 mg/kg/day is approximately 10 times the amount of doxycycline hyclate contained in the recommended daily dose of doxycycline for a 60 kg human when compared on the basis of body surface area estimates (mg/m^2). Although doxycycline impairs the fertility of rats when administered at sufficient dosage, the effect on human fertility is not known.

▶*Pregnancy:* Category D. Doxycycline can cause fetal harm when administered to a pregnant woman. Results of animal studies indicate that tetracyclines cross the placenta, are found in fetal tissues, and can have toxic effects on the developing fetus (often related to retardation of skeletal development). Evidence of embryotoxicity has also been noted in animals treated early in pregnancy. If any tetracyclines are used during pregnancy or if the patient becomes pregnant while taking this drug, inform the patient of the potential hazard to the fetus.

Doxycycline injection has not been clinically tested in pregnant women.

▶*Lactation:* Tetracyclines are excreted in human milk. Because of the potential for serious adverse reactions in nursing infants from doxycycline, use in nursing mothers is contraindicated.

It is not known if doxycycline is excreted in human milk following use of doxycycline injection.

▶*Children:* The use of doxycycline in infancy and childhood is contraindicated.

The safety and efficacy of doxycycline injection in pediatric patients have not been established.

Precautions

▶*Monitoring:* In long-term therapy, perform periodic laboratory evaluations of organ systems, including hematopoietic, renal, and hepatic studies.

▶*Opportunistic microorganism overgrowth:* While no overgrowth by opportunistic microorganisms such as yeast was noted during clinical studies, as with other antimicrobials, doxycycline therapy may

DOXYCYCLINE

result in overgrowth of nonsusceptible microorganisms, including fungi.

The use of tetracyclines may increase the incidence of vaginal candidiasis.

Use doxycycline with caution in patients with a history or predisposition to oral candidiasis. The safety and efficacy of doxycycline have not been established for the treatment of periodontitis in patients with coexistent oral candidiasis.

Take appropriate measures if superinfection is suspected.

➤*Dental implants:* Doxycycline injection has not been clinically tested for use in the regeneration of alveolar bone, either in preparation for or in conjunction with the placement of endosseous (dental) implants or in the treatment of failing implants.

➤*Extremely severe periodontal defects:* Doxycycline injection has not been clinically evaluated in patients with conditions involving extremely severe periodontal defects with very little remaining periodontium.

➤*Immunocompromised patients:* Doxycycline injection has not been clinically tested in immunocompromised patients (eg, patients with immunocompromised diabetes, chemotherapy, radiation therapy, or infections with HIV).

Drug Interactions

Doxycycline Drug Interactions			
Precipitant	Object drug*		Description
Doxycycline	Anticoagulants	↑	Patients who are on anticoagulant therapy may require downward adjustment of their anticoagulant dosage.
Doxycycline	Beta-lactam antibiotics (eg, penicillins)	↓	Pharmacologic and therapeutic action of penicillins may be reduced. Avoid this combination if possible.
Doxycycline	Digoxin	↑	Doxycycline may result in increased serum digoxin levels in a small subset of patients (≈ 10%). Monitor patients for increased digoxin levels.
Doxycycline	Contraceptives, oral	↓	Concurrent use of tetracyclines may render oral contraceptives less effective.
Doxycycline	Isotretinoin	↑	Risk of pseudotumor cerebri (benign intracranial hypertension) may be increased. Concomitant use of isotretinoin and a tetracycline is not recommended.
Doxycycline	Theophyllines	↑	The incidence of adverse reactions to theophyllines may be increased. Monitor theophylline levels and adjust dose as needed.
Antacids	Doxycycline	↓	Absorption of doxycycline is impaired by antacids containing aluminum, calcium, or magnesium. Absorption is also impaired by bismuth subsalicylate.
Barbiturates Carbamazepine Phenytoin	Doxycycline	↓	Barbiturates, carbamazepine, and phenytoin decrease the half-life of doxycycline.
Cholestyramine Colestipol	Doxycycline	↓	Coadministration may decrease or delay the absorption of doxycycline, therefore decreasing the serum concentrations. Adjust the doxycycline dose, if needed.
Iron-containing products	Doxycycline	↓	Absorption of tetracyclines is impaired by iron-containing products. Avoid coadministration. Minimize interaction by separating administration by 3 to 4 h or by using an enteric-coated or sustained-release formulation of the iron salt.
Methoxyflurane	Doxycycline	↑	The concurrent use of tetracycline and methoxyflurane has been reported to result in fatal renal toxicity.
Doxycycline	Methoxyflurane		
Rifamycins (eg, rifampin)	Doxycycline	↓	Rifampin may decrease the serum concentration and half-life of doxycycline. Monitor the patient's clinical response.
Urinary alkalinizers	Doxycycline	↓	Coadministration of doxycycline and urinary alkalinizers may result in increased excretion of doxycycline. Separate use of these agents by 3 to 4 hours.

* ↑ = Object drug increased.   ↓ = Object drug decreased.

➤*Drug/Lab test interactions:* False elevations of urinary catecholamine levels may occur because of interference with the fluorescence test.

➤*Drug/Food interactions:* In a single-dose study in healthy volunteers, concomitant administration of doxycycline with a 1000 calorie, high-fat, high-protein meal that included dairy products resulted in a decrease in the rate and extent of absorption and delay in the time to maximum concentrations.

Adverse Reactions

The most frequent adverse reactions occurring in studies involving treatment with doxycycline or placebo are listed in the following table.

Incidence of Adverse Reactions in Oral Doxycycline Clinical Trials (%)		
Adverse reaction	Doxycycline 20 mg BID (n = 213)	Placebo (n = 215)
GI		
Nausea	8	6
Toothache	7	13
Tooth disorder	6	9
Diarrhea	6	4
Dyspepsia	6	2
Sore throat	5	6
Periodontal abscess	4	10
Acid indigestion	4	3
Respiratory		
Sinus congestion	5	5
Coughing	4	5
Sinus headache	4	4
Sinusitis	3	8
Bronchitis	3	2
Gum pain	< 1	3
Miscellaneous		
Headache	26	26
Common cold	22	21
Flu symptoms	11	19
Joint pain	6	4
Injury	5	8
Rash	4	3
Menstrual cramp	4	2
Pain	4	2
Back pain	3	4
Backache	2	4
Infection	2	3
Muscle pain	1	3

The following table lists the incidence of treatment-emergent adverse events from all causalities, across all treatment groups, occurring in at least 1% of the entire study population in doxycycline injection clinical trials.

Incidence of Adverse Reactions in Doxycycline Injection Clinical Trials (%)		
Adverse reaction	Doxycycline (n = 609)	Placebo (n = 413)
GI		
Gum discomfort, pain, or soreness; loss of attachment; increased pocket depth	18.1	23
Toothache, pressure sensitivity	14.3	14.3
Peridontal abscess, exudate, infection, drainage, extreme mobility, suppuration	9.9	10.9
Thermal tooth sensitivity	7.7	8.5
Soft tissue erythema, sore mouth, unspecified pain	4.3	5.3
Gum inflammation, swelling, sensitivity	4.1	5.8
Indigestion, upset stomach, stomachache	3.6	4.1
Diarrhea	3.3	2.4
Tooth mobility, bone loss	2	0.7
Nausea and vomiting	1.8	0.7
Periapical abscess, lesion	1.5	1.9
Endodontic abscess, pulpitis	1.5	1.5
Jaw pain	1.1	0.5
Bleeding gums	1	0.7
Fistula	0.8	1.5
Tooth loss	0.8	1.5
Aphthous ulcer, canker sores	0.7	1.7
Musculoskeletal		
Muscle aches	6.4	4.6
Backache	3.6	5.3
Lower back pain	1.6	1.7
Pain in arms or legs	1.5	2.2
Neck pain	1.3	1.7
Shoulder pain	1	1

DOXYCYCLINE

Incidence of Adverse Reactions in Doxycycline Injection Clinical Trials (%)		
Adverse reaction	Doxycycline (n = 609)	Placebo (n = 413)
Respiratory		
Common cold	25.5	25.2
Flu, respiratory	6.1	9
Sore throat	5.7	6.5
Stuffy head, postnasal drip, congestion	5.6	7.7
Sinus infection	5.3	2.7
Cough	3.6	6.1
Flu	2.8	2.9
Bronchitis	2.3	1.9
Allergies	1	1
Miscellaneous		
Headache	27.3	28.1
Broken tooth	5.1	4.1
Premenstrual tension syndrome	4.4	3.1
Sleeplessness	3.4	1.5
Tension headache	1.8	0.7
Ear infection	1.6	1.9
Body aches, soreness	1.6	1.2
High blood pressure	1.6	0.2
Skin infection or inflammation	1.3	1
Fever	1	1.9

The following adverse reactions have been observed in patients receiving tetracyclines:

➤*GI:* Anorexia, nausea, vomiting, diarrhea, glossitis, dysphagia, enterocolitis, and inflammatory lesions (with vaginal candidiasis) in the anogenital region. Hepatotoxicity has been reported rarely. Rare instances of esophagitis and esophageal ulcerations have been reported in patients receiving the capsule forms of the drugs in the tetracycline class. Most of these patients took medications immediately before going to bed.

➤*Dermatologic:* Maculopapular and erythematous rashes. Exfoliative dermatitis has been reported but is uncommon. Photosensitivity (see Warnings).

➤*Renal:* Rise in BUN has been reported and is apparently dose-related (see Warnings).

➤*Hypersensitivity:* Urticaria, angioneurotic edema, anaphylaxis, anaphylactoid purpura, serum sickness, pericarditis, and exacerbation of systemic lupus erythematosus.

➤*Hematologic:* Hemolytic anemia, thrombocytopenia, neutropenia, and eosinophilia have been reported.

Overdosage

➤*Treatment:* In case of overdosage, discontinue medication, treat symptomatically, and institute supportive measures. Dialysis does not alter serum half-life and thus would not be of benefit in treating cases of overdose.

Patient Information

➤*Tablets:* Avoid taking at the same time with antacids, dairy products (eg, milk, cheese, ice cream), or iron-containing products. If any of these products must be taken, take them at least 2 hours before or after taking this medicine.

May cause permanent change in color of teeth. Do not take this medicine during the last half of pregnancy or give to children 8 years of age and younger to avoid possible color change in teeth.

May cause sensitivity to sunlight. Avoid prolonged exposure to the sun and other ultraviolet light. Use sunscreens and wear protective clothing until tolerance is determined.

➤*Injection:* Avoid mechanical oral hygiene procedures (ie, tooth brushing, flossing) on any treated areas for 7 days or after injection treatment.

Avoid excessive sunlight or artificial ultraviolet light while receiving doxycycline injection.

Doxycycline may decrease the effectiveness of birth control pills.

MINOCYCLINE HCl

Rx	**Arestin** (Cord Logistics)	Microspheres, sustained-release: 1 mg	In UD 12s.

For information on the anti-infective (systemic) use of minocycline, refer to tetracyclines in the Anti-infective chapter.

Indications

➤*Adult periodontitis:* As an adjunct to scaling and root planing procedures for reduction of pocket depth in patients with adult periodontitis; may be used as part of a periodontal maintenance program that includes good oral hygiene and scaling and root planing.

Administration and Dosage

➤*Approved by the FDA:* February 16, 2001.

Minocycline microspheres are provided as a dry powder and packaged in a unit-dose cartridge, which is inserted into a cartridge handle to administer the product. The oral health care professional removes the disposable cartridge from its pouch and connects the cartridge to the handle mechanism. Minocycline is a variable dose product, dependent on the size, shape, and number of pockets being treated. In US clinical trials, up to 121 unit-dose cartridges were used in a single visit and up to 3 treatments, at 3-month intervals, were administered in pockets with a pocket depth of 5 mm or greater.

Minocycline microspheres administration does not require local anesthesia. Professional subgingival administration is accomplished by inserting the unit-dose cartridge into the base of the periodontal pocket and then pressing the thumb ring in the handle mechanism to expel the powder, while gradually withdrawing the tip from the base of the pocket. The handle mechanism should be sterilized between patients. Minocycline microspheres do not have to be removed, as they are bioresorbable; an adhesive or dressing is not required.

➤*Storage/Stability:* Store at 20° to 25°C (68° to 77°F)/60% relative humidity. Excursions permitted to 15° to 30°C (59° to 86°F). Avoid exposure to excessive heat.

Actions

➤*Pharmacokinetics:*

Absorption/Distribution – In a pharmacokinetic study, 18 patients (10 men and 8 women) with moderate to advanced chronic periodontitis were treated with a mean dose of 46.2 mg (25 to 112 unit doses) of minocycline microspheres. After fasting for at least 10 hours, patients received subgingival application of minocycline microspheres (1 mg/ treatment site) following scaling and root planing at a minimum of 30 sites on at least 8 teeth. Investigational drug was administered to all eligible sites at least 5 mm in probing depth. Mean dose normalized saliva AUC and C_{max} were found to be approximately 125 and 1000 times higher than those of serum parameters, respectively.

➤*Microbiology:* Minocycline, a member of the tetracycline class of antibiotics, has a broad spectrum of activity. It is bacteriostatic and exerts its antimicrobial activity by inhibiting protein synthesis. In vitro susceptibility testing has shown that the organisms *Porphyromonas gingivalis, Prevotella intermedia, Fusobacterium nucleatum, Eikenella corrodens,* and *Actinobacillus actinomycetemcomitans,* which are associated with periodontal disease, are susceptible to minocycline at concentrations of up to 8 mcg/mL.

The emergence of minocycline-resistant bacteria in single-site plaque samples was studied in subjects before and after treatment with minocycline microspheres at 2 centers. There was a slight increase in the numbers of minocycline-resistant bacteria at the end of the 9-month study period; however, the number of subjects studied was small and the clinical significance of these findings is unknown.

➤*Clinical trials:* In 2 well-controlled, multicenter, investigator-blind, vehicle-controlled, parallel-design studies, 748 patients with generalized moderate to advanced adult periodontitis characterized by a mean probing depth of 5.9 and 5.81 mm, respectively, were enrolled. Subjects received 1 of 3 treatments:

1.) Scaling and root planing;
2.) scaling and root planing plus vehicle (bioresorbable polymer, PGLA); and
3.) scaling and root planing plus minocycline microspheres.

MINOCYCLINE HCl

To qualify for the study, patients were required to have 4 teeth with periodontal pockets of 6 to 9 mm that bled on probing. Treatment was administered to all sites with mean probing depths of 5 mm or greater. Retreatment occurred at 3 and 6 months after initial treatment, and any new site with pocket depth 5 mm or greater also received treatment. Patients treated with minocycline microspheres were found to have statistically significantly reduced probing pocket depth compared with those treated with scaling and root planing alone or scaling and root planing plus vehicle at 9 months after initial treatment.

Probing Pocket Depth at Baseline and Change in Pocket Depth at 9 Months from 2 Multicenter US Clinical Trials						
	Study OPI-103A (N = 368)			Study OPI-103B (N = 380)		
Time	SRP[1] alone (n = 124)	SRP[1] + vehicle (n = 123)	SRP[1] + minocycline microspheres (n = 121)	SRP[1] alone (n = 126)	SRP[1] + vehicle (n = 126)	SRP[1] + minocycline microspheres (n = 128)
PD[2] (mm) at baseline, mean	≈ 5.88	≈ 5.91	≈ 5.88	≈ 5.79	≈ 5.82	≈ 5.81
PD[2] (mm) change from baseline at 9 months, mean	≈ -1.04	≈ -0.9	≈ -1.2[3,4]	≈ -1.32	≈ -1.3	≈ -1.63[4,5]

[1] SRP = Scaling and root planing.
[2] PD = Pocket depth.
[3] Significantly different from SRP ($P \le 0.05$).
[4] Significantly different from SRP + vehicle ($P \le 0.001$).
[5] Significantly different from SRP ($P \le 0.001$).

When these studies are combined, the mean pocket depth change at 9 months was -1.18 mm, -1.1 mm, and -1.42 mm for SRP alone, SRP + vehicle, and SRP + minocycline microspheres, respectively.

Contraindications

Known sensitivity to minocycline or tetracyclines.

Warnings

➤*Tooth discoloration:* The use of drugs of the tetracycline class during tooth development (last half of pregnancy, infancy, and childhood to 8 years of age) may cause permanent discoloration of the teeth (yellow-gray-brown). This adverse reaction is more common during the long-term use of the drugs but has been observed following repeated short-term courses. Enamel hypoplasia also has been reported. Therefore, do not use tetracyclines in this age group, or in pregnant or nursing women, unless the potential benefits outweigh the potential risks.

➤*Photosensitivity:* Photosensitivity manifested by an exaggerated sunburn reaction has been observed in some individuals taking tetracyclines. Advise patients apt to be exposed to direct sunlight or ultraviolet light that this reaction may occur with tetracycline drugs, and discontinue treatment at the first evidence of skin erythema.

➤*Carcinogenesis:* Dietary administration of minocycline in long-term tumorigenicity studies in rats resulted in evidence of thyroid tumor production. Minocycline also has been found to produce thyroid hyperplasia in rats and dogs. In addition, there has been evidence of oncogenic activity in rats in studies with a related antibiotic, oxytetracycline (ie, adrenal and pituitary tumors).

➤*Fertility impairment:* Fertility and general reproduction studies have provided evidence that minocycline impairs fertility in male rats.

➤*Pregnancy: Category D.* Minocycline microspheres have not been clinically tested in pregnant women. Results of animal studies indicate that tetracyclines cross the placenta, are found in fetal tissues, and can have toxic effects on the developing fetus (often related to retardation of skeletal development). If any tetracyclines are used during pregnancy, or if the patient becomes pregnant while taking the drug, apprise the patient of the potential hazard to the fetus.

➤*Lactation:* Tetracyclines are excreted in human milk. Because of the potential for serious adverse reactions in nursing infants from the tetracyclines, a decision should be made whether to discontinue nursing or discontinue the drug, taking into account the importance of the drug to the mother.

➤*Children:* Because adult periodontitis does not affect children, safety and efficacy of minocycline microspheres in pediatric patients cannot be established.

Precautions

➤*Acutely abscessed periodontal pocket:* The use of minocycline microspheres in acutely abscessed periodontal pocket has not been studied and is not recommended.

➤*Other dental procedures:* Minocycline microspheres have not been clinically tested for use in the regeneration of alveolar bone, either in preparation for or in conjunction with the placement of endosseous (dental) implants or in the treatment of failing implants.

➤*Nonsusceptible microorganism overgrowth:* Use of minocycline microspheres may result in overgrowth of nonsusceptible microorganisms, including fungi. The effect of treatment for longer than 6 months has not been studied.

➤*Candidiasis:* Use minocycline microspheres with caution in patients with a history of predisposition to oral candidiasis. The safety and efficacy of minocycline microspheres has not been established for the treatment of periodontitis in patients with coexistent oral candidiasis.

➤*Immunocompromise:* Minocycline microspheres have not been clinically tested in immunocompromised patients (such as those immunocompromised by diabetes, chemotherapy, radiation therapy, or HIV infection).

➤*Superinfection:* If superinfection is suspected, take appropriate measures.

Adverse Reactions

The most frequently reported nondental, treatment-emergent adverse events in the 3 multicenter US trials were headache, infection, flu syndrome, and pain.

Minocycline Adverse Reactions (≥ 3%)			
Adverse reaction	SRP[1] alone (N = 250)	SRP[1] + vehicle (N = 249)	SRP[1] + minocycline microspheres (N = 423)
Percent of patients with treatment-emergent adverse reactions	62.4	71.9	68.1
Total number of adverse reactions	543	589	987
Periodontitis	25.6	28.1	16.3
Tooth disorder	12	13.7	12.3
Tooth caries	9.2	11.2	9.9
Dental pain	8.8	8.8	9.9
Stomatitis	8.4	6.8	6.4
Infection	8	9.6	7.6
Headache	7.2	11.6	9
Gingivitis	7.2	8.8	9.2
Flu syndrome	3.2	6.4	5
Pharyngitis	3.2	1.6	4.3
Infection, dental	4	3.6	3.8
Pain	4	1.2	4.3
Mucous membrane disorder	2.4	0.8	3.3
Dyspepsia	2	0	4
Mouth ulceration	1.6	3.2	5

[1] SRP = Scaling and root planing.

Patient Information

After treatment, avoid eating hard, crunchy, or sticky foods for 1 week and postpone brushing for a 12-hour period. Avoid touching treated areas. Postpone the use of interproximal cleaning devices for 10 days after administration of minocycline microspheres. Advise patients that although some mild to moderate sensitivity is expected during the first week after scaling and root planing and administration of minocycline microspheres, they should notify the dentist promptly if pain, swelling, or other problems occur.

AMLEXANOX

| *Rx* | **Aphthasol** (Access) | **Paste:** 5% | Benzyl alcohol, mineral oil, petrolatum. In 5 g. |

Indications

➤*Aphthous ulcers:* Aphthous ulcer treatment in people with healthy immune systems.

Administration and Dosage

➤*Approved by the FDA:* December 17, 1996.

Apply as soon as possible after noticing symptoms of an aphthous ulcer and use 4 times daily, preferably following oral hygiene after breakfast, lunch, dinner, and at bedtime. Squeeze a dab of paste (approximately 0.25 inch [0.5 cm]) onto a fingertip. With gentle pressure, dab paste onto each ulcer in mouth. Use medication until ulcer heals. If significant healing or pain reduction has not occurred in 10 days, advise the patient to consult a dentist or physician.

➤*Storage / Stability:* Store at controlled room temperature (15° to 30°C [59° to 86°F]).

Actions

➤*Pharmacology:* The mechanism of action by which amlexanox accelerates healing of aphthous ulcers is unknown. In vitro, amlexanox is a potent inhibitor of the formation or release of inflammatory mediators (histamine and leukotrienes) from mast cells, neutrophils, and mononuclear cells. Given orally to animals, amlexanox has demonstrated antiallergic and anti-inflammatory activities and suppresses both immediate and delayed-type hypersensitivity reactions. The relevance of these activities of amlexanox to its effects on aphthous ulcers has not been established.

➤*Pharmacokinetics:*

Absorption – After a single oral application of 100 mg of paste (5 mg amlexanox), maximal serum levels of approximately 120 ng/mL are observed at 2.4 hours. Most of the systemic absorption of amlexanox is via the GI tract, and the amount absorbed directly through the active ulcer is not a significant portion of the applied dose.

Distribution – With multiple applications 4 times daily, steady-state levels were reached within 1 week and no accumulation was observed within 4 weeks.

Metabolism / Excretion – The elimination half-life is 3.5 hours in healthy individuals. Approximately 17% of the dose is eliminated into the urine as unchanged amlexanox, a hydroxylated metabolite, and their conjugates.

➤*Clinical trials:* The safety of amlexanox oral paste 5% was established in a study in which 100 patients with aphthous ulcers applied the medication 4 times daily for 28 days with no significant topical or systemic adverse effects. The effectiveness was demonstrated in 3 controlled clinical studies of patients with mild to moderate aphthous ulcers. Amlexanox oral paste 5% accelerated healing of aphthous ulcers in a statistically significant manner as compared with vehicle and no treatment.

Contraindications

Hypersensitivity to amlexanox or other ingredients in the formulation.

Warnings

➤*Pregnancy:* Category B. There are no adequate and well-controlled studies in pregnant women. Use during pregnancy only if clearly needed.

➤*Lactation:* Amlexanox was found in the milk of rats; therefore, exercise caution when administering amlexanox oral paste to a nursing woman.

➤*Children:* Safety and efficacy in pediatric patients have not been established.

Precautions

➤*Local irritation:* In the event that rash or contact mucositis occurs, discontinue use.

Adverse Reactions

Transient pain, stinging, or burning at the site of application (1% to 2%); contact mucositis, nausea, diarrhea (< 1%).

Overdosage

None reported. However, ingestion of a full tube of 5 g of paste would result in systemic exposure well below the maximum nontoxic dose of amlexanox in animals. GI upset such as diarrhea and vomiting could result from an overdose.

Patient Information

Apply the paste as soon as possible after noticing the symptoms of an aphthous ulcer. Continue to use the paste 4 times daily, preferably following oral hygiene after breakfast, lunch, dinner, and at bedtime.

Squeeze a dab of paste (approximately 0.25 inch [0.5 cm]) onto a fingertip. Dab the paste onto each ulcer in the mouth using gentle pressure.

Wash hands immediately after applying amlexanox oral paste.

Wash eyes promptly if they should come in contact with the paste.

Use the paste until the ulcer heals. If significant healing or pain reduction has not occurred in 10 days, consult your dentist or physician.

SULFURIC ACID/SULFONATED PHENOLICS

| *Rx* | **Debacterol** (Henry Schein/Sullivan-Schein Dental) | **Liquid:** 30% sulfuric acid and 22% sulfonated phenolics | In 1 mL prefilled, single-use applicator.[1] |

[1] Swab applicator contains 0.2 mL of product.

Indications

➤*Ulcerating lesions:* Topical treatment of ulcerating lesions of the oral cavity, such as recurrent aphthous stomatitis (canker sores). Provides relief from pain and discomfort of oral mucosal ulcers and helps decrease the risk of infection of the ulcerated tissue.

Not intended for the treatment of vesicular lesions, such as cold sores or fever blisters.

Administration and Dosage

Immediately before applying, thoroughly dry the ulcerated area of oral mucosa that is to be treated using a sterile cotton-tipped applicator or some similar method. After drying the lesion, hold swab with the colored ring end up. Bend the colored ring tip gently to the side until it snaps to release the liquid inside. Liquid flows down into the white tip applicator. Then apply the coated applicator directly to the dried ulcer bed. A very brief stinging sensation is experienced immediately upon application of the liquid to the ulcer. Hold the cotton-tipped applicator in contact with the ulcer for at least 5 seconds while using a rolling motion to thoroughly coat the entire ulcer bed, the ulcer rim, and the surrounding halo of normal mucosa. Do not hold the applicator on the ulcer for more than 10 seconds. The sulfuric acid/sulfonated phenolics liquid will not harm the normal oral mucosa when used as directed. Then thoroughly rinse out the mouth with water and spit out the rinse water. The stinging sensation and ulcer pain will subside almost immediately after the water rinse.

One application per ulcer treatment is usually sufficient. However, if the ulcer pain returns shortly after rinsing with water, it is an indication that some part of the ulcer was not covered with the sulfuric acid/sulfonated phenolics liquid. A second application should then be applied to the ulcer immediately during the same treatment session until it remains pain-free after rinsing. It is not recommended that more than 1 treatment session be performed on any individual mucosal ulcer. Do not reapply the product to the same lesion after it is free of pain.

➤*Storage / Stability:* Store at room temperature, 15° to 30°C (59° to 86°F).

Actions

➤*Pharmacology:* The liquid contains sulfonated phenolics, which are antiseptic agents with topical analgesic properties, and sulfuric acid, which is a tissue denaturant and sterilizing agent, in an aqueous solution.

Contraindications

Known allergy to sulfonated phenolics.

Warnings

Keep out of the reach of children. Do not use if allergic to sulfonated phenolics.

➤*Prolonged use:* Because of its nature, prolonged use on normal tissue should be avoided. The sulfuric acid/sulfonated phenolics liquid will eventually necrotize and slough all tissue to which it is applied in sufficient volume; apply carefully.

➤*Pregnancy:* Category C.

➤*Children:* Safety and efficacy in children under 12 years of age have not been established.

Precautions

➤*External use only:* Avoid eye contact.

Adverse Reactions

May cause local irritation upon administration. If excess irritation occurs during use, a rinse with sodium bicarbonate (baking soda) solution will neutralize the reaction (use 2.5 mL in 120 mL of water).

Mouth and Throat Products

Indications

These products are indicated in minor sore throat and in minor irritation of the throat or mouth.

Administration and Dosage

Do not use for > 2 days or in children < 2 years of age, unless directed by physician. For dosage guidelines, refer to the specific package labeling.

Actions

➤*Pharmacology:*

Benzocaine and dyclonine – Benzocaine and dyclonine are local anesthetics.

Cetylpyridinium chloride, eucalyptus oil, thymol and hexylresorcinol – Cetylpyridinium chloride, eucalyptus oil, thymol, and hexylresorcinol have antiseptic activity.

Menthol, camphor, capsicum, dyclonine and phenol – Menthol, camphor, capsicum, dyclonine, and phenol are used for their antipruritic, local anesthetic and counterirritant activities.

Hydrocortisone and triamcinolone (corticosteroids) – Hydrocortisone and triamcinolone (corticosteroids) are used for their anti-inflammatory activities.

Warnings

➤*Severe/Persistent sore throat:* Severe and persistent sore throat or sore throat accompanied by high fever, headache, nausea and vomiting may be serious. Consult physician promptly.

Precautions

➤*Tartrazine sensitivity:* Some of these products contain tartrazine (FD&C yellow #5), which may cause allergic-type reactions (including bronchial asthma) in susceptible individuals. Although the incidence of sensitivity is low, it is frequently seen in patients who also have aspirin hypersensitivity. Specific products containing tartrazine are identified in the product listings.

LOZENGES AND TROCHES

otc sf	**Cylex** (Pharmakon)	**Lozenges:** 15 mg benzocaine, 5 mg cetylpyridinium chloride	Sorbitol. Cherry flavor. In 12s.
otc sf	**Mycinettes** (Pfeiffer)	**Lozenges:** 15 mg benzocaine	Sorbitol, saccharin, menthol. Cherry flavor. In 12s.
otc	**Spec-T** (Apothecon)	**Lozenges:** 10 mg benzocaine	Sucrose. In 10s.
otc sf	**Cepacol Maximum Strength** (J.B. Williams)		Menthol. Cherry and cool mint flavors. In 16s.
otc	**Vicks Chloraseptic Sore Throat** (Richardson-Vicks)	**Lozenges:** 6 mg benzocaine, 10 mg menthol	Cool mint, cherry, menthol flavors. In 18s.
otc	**Vicks Children's Chloraseptic** (Richardson-Vicks)	**Lozenges:** 5 mg benzocaine	Corn syrup, sucrose. Grape flavor. In 18s.
otc	**Sucrets Children's Sore Throat** (SK-Beecham)	**Lozenges:** 1.2 mg dyclonine HCl	Corn syrup, sucrose. Cherry flavor. In 24s.
otc	**Cēpacol Throat** (J.B. Williams)	**Lozenges:** 0.07% cetylpyridinium chloride, 0.3% benzyl alcohol	Tartrazine. In 27s and 40s.
otc	**Kof-Eze** (Roberts Med)	**Lozenges:** 6 mg menthol	In 4s and 500s.
otc	**Sucrets Maximum Strength** (SK-Beecham)	**Lozenges:** 3 mg dyclonine HCl, menthol	Corn syrup, sucrose. Wintergreen and vapor black cherry flavors. In 24s, 48s and 55s.
otc	**Vapor Lemon Sucrets** (SK-Beecham)	**Lozenges:** 2 mg dyclonine HCl	Sucrose, corn syrup. In 18s.
otc	**Sucrets Sore Throat** (SK-Beecham)	**Lozenges:** 2.4 mg hexylresorcinol	In regular and mentholated flavors. In 24s.
otc sf	**Cēpastat Extra Strength** (Heritage Consumer Prod.)	**Lozenges:** 29 mg phenol, menthol, eucalyptus oil	Sorbitol. In 18s.
otc sf	**Cēpastat Cherry** (Heritage Consumer Prod.)	**Lozenges:** 14.5 mg phenol, menthol	Saccharin, sorbitol. Cherry flavor. In 18s.
otc sf	**N'ice 'n Clear** (SK-Beecham)	**Lozenges:** 5 mg menthol	Sorbitol. Cool peppermint, cherry eucalyptus and menthol eucalyptus flavors. In 16s.
otc	**Robitussin Honey Cough** (Whitehall-Robins)	**Lozenges:** 5 mg menthol	Herbal with natural honey center. Corn syrup, sorbitol, sucrose. In 20s. Honey lemon tea flavor: Corn syrup, sucrose. In 25s.
otc	**Vicks Menthol Cough Drops** (Richardson-Vicks)	**Lozenges:** Menthol, thymol, eucalyptus oil, camphor, tolu balsam	Benzyl alcohol. Menthol flavor. In 14s and 40s.
otc	**Maximum Strength Halls-Plus** (Warner-Lambert)	**Lozenges:** 10 mg menthol	Corn syrup, sucrose. In regular, cherry, mentholyptus and honey-lemon flavors. In 10s and 25s.
otc	**Extra Strength Vicks Cough Drops** (Richardson-Vicks)	**Lozenges:** 8.4 mg menthol	Corn syrup, sucrose. Menthol flavor. In 9s and 30s.
otc	**Extra Strength Vicks Cough Drops** (Richardson-Vicks)	**Lozenges:** 10 mg menthol	Corn syrup, sucrose. Cherry and honey lemon flavors. In 9s and 30s.
otc	**Robitussin Cough Drops** (Robins)	**Lozenges:** 7.4 mg menthol, eucalyptus oil.	Sucrose, corn syrup. (R). In cherry and menthol eucalyptus flavors. In 9s and 25s.
		10 mg menthol, eucalyptus oil.	Sucrose, corn syrup. (R). Honey-lemon flavor. In 9s and 25s.
otc	**Get Better Bear Sore Throat Pops** (Whitehall)	**Lozenge on a stick:** 19 mg pectin	Corn syrup, sucrose, parabens. Cherry and grape flavored. In 10s.
otc	**Cēpacol Anesthetic** (J.B. Williams)	**Troches:** 10 mg benzocaine, 0.07% cetylpyridinium chloride	Tartrazine. In 18s and 24s.
otc sf	**Hall's Sugar Free Mentho-Lyptus** (Warner-Lambert)	**Tablets:** 6 mg menthol, 2.8 mg eucalyptus oil	Mountain menthol flavor. In 25s.
		Tablets: 5 mg menthol, 2.8 mg eucalyptus oil	Citrus blend and black cherry flavors. In 25s.

MOUTHWASHES AND SPRAYS

	Product	Composition	Other Ingredients
otc	**TiSol** (Parnell)	**Solution:** 1% benzyl alcohol, 0.04% menthol, 0.9% isotonic NaCl	EDTA, sorbitol. In 237 mL.
otc	**Listerine, Natural Citrus** (Pfizer Consumer)	**Mouthwash:** 0.064% thymol, 0.092% eucalyptol, 0.06% methyl salicylate, 0.042% menthol, 21.6% alcohol	Sorbitol, sucralose. In 250 and 500 mL and 1 and 1.5 L.
otc	**Listerine, Tartar Control** (Pfizer Consumer)	**Mouthwash:** 0.064% thymol, 0.092% eucalyptol, 0.06% methyl salicylate, 0.042% menthol, 21.6% alcohol	Sorbitol, sucrose. Wintermint flavor. In 250 and 500 mL and 1 and 1.5 L.
otc	**FreshBurst Listerine** (GlaxoWellcome)	**Rinse:** 0.064% thymol, 0.092% eucalyptol, 0.06% methyl salicylate, 0.042% menthol, 21.6% alcohol	Sorbitol, saccharin. In 250 mL.
otc	**Scope** (Procter & Gamble)	**Rinse:** Cetylpyridinium chloride, 67.9% SD alcohol 38-F	Tartrazine, saccharin. Original mint and wintergreen flavors. In 90, 180, 360, 720, 1080 and 1440 mL.
otc sf	**Sucrets** (SK-Beecham)	**Throat Spray:** 0.1% dyclonine HCl, 10% alcohol	Sorbitol. Mint and cherry flavors. In 90 and 180 mL.
otc sf	**Sore Throat Spray** (Major)	**Throat Spray:** 1.4% phenol	Alcohol free. Saccharin. Cherry and menthol flavors. In 177 mL.
otc sf	**Phenaseptic** (Rugby)	**Throat Spray:** 1.4% phenol	Saccharin. Cherry flavor. In 177 mL.
otc sf	**Green Throat Spray** (Clay-Park Labs)	**Throat Spray:** 1.4% phenol	Alcohol free. Glycerin, saccharin. In 473 mL.
otc sf	**Red Throat Spray** (Clay-Park Labs)	**Throat Spray:** 1.4% phenol	Alcohol free. Glycerin, saccharin. In 177 mL.
otc	**Cheracol Sore Throat** (Roberts)	**Throat Spray:** 1.4% phenol, 12.5% alcohol	Sorbitol, saccharin. Cherry flavor. In 180 mL.
otc sf	**Mycinette** (Pfeiffer)	**Throat Spray:** 1.4% phenol, 0.3% alum (aluminum ammonium sulfate)	Alcohol free. Regular, cherry, mint and cool blue menthol flavors. In 180 mL.
otc	**Throto-Ceptic** (S.S.S. Company)	**Spray/Gargle:** 1.4% phenol, 0.5% alum (aluminum ammonium sulfate)	Mint, cherry, cool blue menthol, or regular flavors. In 171 mL.
otc	**N'ice** (SK-Beecham)	**Throat Spray:** 0.12% menthol, 25% glycerin, 23% alcohol	Glucose, saccharin, sorbitol. Peppermint flavor. In 180 mL.
otc	**Children's Vicks Chloraseptic** (Procter & Gamble)	**Throat Spray:** 0.5% phenol	Alcohol free. Saccharin, sorbitol. Grape flavor. In 177 mL.
otc	**Listermint Arctic Mint** (GlaxoWellcome)	**Mouthwash:** Glycerin, poloxamer 335, PEG 600, sodium lauryl sulfate, sodium benzoate, benzoic acid, zinc chloride	Saccharin. In 946 mL.
otc	**Cepacol** (J.B. Williams)	**Mouthwash:** 0.05% cetylpyridinium chloride, 14% alcohol	Tartrazine, saccharin. In 360, 540, 720, 960 mL.
otc	**Advanced Formula Plax** (Pfizer)	**Mouthwash:** Tetrasodium pyrophosphate, alcohol	Saccharin. Original, peppermint and softmint flavors. In 120, 240, 473, 720 and 1740 mL.
otc	**Listerine** (GlaxoWellcome)	**Mouthwash:** 0.06% thymol, 0.09% eucalyptol, 0.06% methyl salicylate, 0.04% menthol, 26.9% alcohol (regular flavor), 21.6% alcohol (cool mint flavor)	Sorbitol, saccharin (Cool Mint). Regular, cool mint flavors. In 90, 180, 360, 540, 720, 960, 1440 mL.
otc	**Phylorinol** (Schaffer)	**Mouthwash:** 0.6% phenol, methyl salicylate	Alcohol free. Sorbitol. In 240 mL.
otc sf	**Vicks Chloraseptic** (Procter & Gamble)	**Mouthrinse/gargle:** 1.4% phenol	Alcohol free. Saccharin. Menthol flavor. In 355 mL.

MISCELLANEOUS MOUTH AND THROAT PREPARATIONS

otc	**Dent's Extra Strength Toothache Gum** (C.S. Dent)	**Gum:** Benzocaine	In 1 g.
otc	**Maximum Strength Orajel** (Del Pharm)	**Liquid:** 20% benzocaine, 44.2% ethyl alcohol, phenol	Tartrazine, saccharin. In 13.3 mL.
otc *sf*	**Orajel Mouth-Aid** (Del Pharm)	**Liquid:** 20% benzocaine, 0.1% cetylpyridinium chloride, 70% ethyl alcohol, povidone	Tartrazine, saccharin. In 13.3 mL.
otc	**Orajel P.M. Nighttime Formula Toothache Pain Relief** (Del Pharm)	**Cream:** 20% benzocaine, menthol, methyl salicylate, saccharin	In 5.4 g.
otc	**Tanac** (Del Pharm)	**Liquid:** 10% benzocaine, 0.12% benzalkonium chloride	Saccharin. In 13 mL.
otc	**Anbesol** (Whitehall)	**Liquid:** 6.3% benzocaine, 0.5% phenol, 70% alcohol, menthol, camphor, povidone-iodine	In 9 and 22 mL.
otc	**Orasol** (Goldline)	**Liquid:** 6.3% benzocaine, 0.5% phenol, 70% alcohol, povidone-iodine	In 14.79 mL.
otc *sf*	**Tanac Roll-On** (Del Pharm)	**Liquid:** 5% benzocaine, 0.12% benzalkonium chloride	Saccharin. In 8.8 mL.
otc	**Dent's Maximum Strength Toothache Drops** (C.S. Dent)	**Liquid:** Benzocaine, 74% alcohol, 0.09% chlorobutanol anhydrous	In 3.7 mL.
otc	**Double-Action Toothache Kit** (C.S. Dent)	**Liquid:** Benzocaine, 74% alcohol, 0.09% chlorobutanol anhydrous	Also contains *Maranox Pain Relief Tablets* containing 325 mg acetaminophen. In 8 tablets with 3.7 mL drops.
otc	**Orasept** (Pharmakon Labs)	**Liquid:** 12.16% tannic acid, 1.53% methylbenzethonium Cl, 53.31% denatured ethyl alcohol, camphor, menthol, benzyl alcohol, spearmint oil and oil of Cassia	In 15 mL.
otc	**Phylorinol** (Schaffer)	**Liquid:** 0.6% phenol, boric acid, strong iodine solution, sodium copper chlorophyll	Sorbitol. In 240 mL.
otc	**Maximum Strength Anbesol** (Whitehall)	**Liquid:** 20% benzocaine, 60% alcohol, polyethylene glycol	Saccharin. In 9 mL.
otc	**Red Cross Toothache** (Mentholatum)	**Liquid:** 85% eugenol, sesame oil	In 3.7 mL with cotton pellets and tweezers.
otc *sf*	**Ulcerease** (Med-Derm)	**Liquid:** 0.6% liquefied phenol, glycerin, sodium bicarbonate, sodium borate	Alcohol free. In 180 mL.
otc	**Curasore** (S.S.S. Company)	**Liquid:** 1% pramoxine HCl	Ethyl alcohol, ethyl ether. In 15 mL.
otc	**Benzodent** (P & G)	**Ointment:** 20% benzocaine	In 30 g.
otc	**Blistex** (Blistex)	**Ointment:** 0.5% camphor, 0.5% phenol, 1% allantoin, lanolin	Mineral oil base. In 4.2 and 10.5 g.
otc	**Lip Medex** (Blistex)	**Ointment:** Petrolatum, 1% camphor, 0.54% phenol, cocoa butter, lanolin	In 210 g.
otc	**Abreva** (SmithKline Beecham Consumer)	**Cream:** 10% docosanol, benzyl alcohol, light mineral oil	In 2 g.
otc	**Numzit Teething** (Goody's)	**Lotion:** 0.2% benzocaine, 12.1% alcohol, 0.02% saccharin, 2% glycerin, 0.5% kelgin MU	Methylparaben, saccharin. In 15 mL.
otc *sf*	**Babee Teething** (Pfeiffer)	**Lotion:** 2.5% benzocaine, 0.02% cetalkonium chloride, camphor, eucalyptol, menthol	Dye free. Alcohol. In 15 mL.
otc	**Pfeiffer's Cold Sore** (Pfeiffer)	**Lotion:** 7% gum benzoin, camphor, menthol, eucalyptol, 85% alcohol	In 15 mL.
otc	**Banadyne-3** (Norstar)	**Solution:** 4% lidocaine, menthol 1%, 45% alcohol	In 7.5 mL.
otc	**Peroxyl Dental Rinse** (Colgate)	**Solution:** 1.5% hydrogen peroxide, 6% alcohol	Mint flavor. In 240 mL and pint.
otc	**Amosan** (Oral-B)	**Powder:** Sodium peroxyborate monohydrate (derived from sodium perborate)	Saccharin. Peppermint, menthol and vanilla flavors. In 1.7 g UD packets (20s and 40s).
otc	**Maximum Strength Orajel** (Del Pharm)	**Gel:** 20% benzocaine	Saccharin. In 9.45 g.
otc	**Maximum Strength Anbesol** (Whitehall)	**Gel:** 20% benzocaine, 60% alcohol, carbomer 934P, polyethylene glycol	Saccharin. In 7.2 g.
otc *sf*	**Orajel Brace-aid** (Del Pharm)	**Gel:** 20% benzocaine	Saccharin. In 14.1 g.
otc *sf*	**Orajel Mouth-Aid** (Del Pharm)	**Gel:** 20% benzocaine, 0.02% benzalkonium chloride, 0.1% zinc chloride	Saccharin. In 9.45 g.
otc	**SensoGARD** (Block)	**Gel:** 20% benzocaine	Parabens. In 0.5 g.
otc	**Numzident** (Goody's)	**Gel:** 10% benzocaine, 47.86% PEG 400 N.F., 10% PEG 3350 NF	Saccharin. Cherry-vanilla flavor. In 15 g.
otc	**Zilactin-B Medicated** (Zila)	**Gel:** 10% benzocaine, 76% alcohol	In 7.5 g.
otc *sf*	**Orajel/d** (Del Pharm)	**Gel:** 10% benzocaine	Saccharin. In 9.45 g.
otc	**Baby Anbesol** (Whitehall)	**Gel:** 7.5% benzocaine	EDTA, saccharin. In 7.2 g.
otc	**Baby Orajel Nighttime** (Del Pharm)	**Gel:** 10% benzocaine	Alcohol free. Saccharin, sorbitol. Cherry flavor. In 6 g.
otc	**Baby Orajel Tooth & Gum Cleanser** (Del Pharm)	**Gel:** 2% poloxamer 407, 0.12% simethicone	Parabens, saccharin, sorbitol. In 14.2 g.
otc	**Numzit Teething** (Goody's)	**Gel:** 7.5% benzocaine, 0.018% peppermint oil, 0.09% clove leaf oil, 66.2% PEG-400, 26.1% PEG-3350	0.036% saccharin. In 14.1 g.
otc	**hda Toothache Gel** (S.S.S. Company)	**Gel:** 6.5% benzocaine	Benzyl alcohol, glycerin. In 15 mL bottle with applicator.
otc *sf*	**Anbesol** (Whitehall)	**Gel:** 6.3% benzocaine, 0.5% phenol, 70% alcohol, camphor	In 7.5 g.

MISCELLANEOUS MOUTH AND THROAT PREPARATIONS

otc	**Toothache Gel** (Roberts Med)	**Gel:** Benzocaine, oil of cloves, benzyl alcohol, propylene glycol	In 15 g.
otc	**Probax** (Fischer)	**Gel:** 2% propolis, petrolatum, mineral oil, lanolin	In 3.5 g.
otc	**Tanac** (Del Pharm)	**Gel:** 1% dyclonine HCl, 0.5% allantoin, petrolatum, lanolin	In 9.45 g.
otc	**Rembrandt Canker Pain Relief Kit** (Den-Mat Corp.)	**Gel:** 5% benzocaine **Rinse:** Methylparaben, saccharin **Paste:** 0.15% fluoride ion from sodium monofluorophosphate w/v ½.	In 28 g. In 37 mL. In 34 g.
otc	**Orabase-B** (Colgate)	**Paste:** 20% benzocaine, mineral oil	In 5 and 15 g.
Rx	**Orabase HCA** (Colgate)	**Paste:** 0.5% hydrocortisone acetate, 5% polyethylene, mineral oil	In 5 g.
Rx	**Kenalog in Orabase** (Apothecon)	**Paste:** 0.1% triamcinolone acetonide	In 5 g.
Rx	**Oralone Dental** (Thames)	**Paste:** 0.1% triamcinolone acetonide	In 5 g.
otc	**Orabase-Plain** (Colgate)	**Paste:** Plasticized hydrocarbon gel	In 5 and 15 g.
otc	**Tanac Dual Core** (Del Pharm)	**Stick:** 7.5% benzocaine, 6% tannic acid, 0.75% octyl dimethyl PABA, 0.2% allantoin, 0.12% benzalkonium chloride	Cetyl alcohol, butylparaben. In 2.84 g stick.
otc	**Blistex** (Blistex)	**Lip Balm:** SPF 10. 0.5% camphor, 0.5% phenol, 1% allantoin, 2% dimethicone, 6.6% padimate O, 2.5% oxybenzone, petrolatum	Parabens. In 4.5 g.
otc	**Herpecin-L** (Campbell Labs)	**Lip Balm:** Allantoin, padimate O	In 2.8 g.
otc	**Blistex** (Blistex)	**Lip Balm:** 1% camphor, 1% menthol, 0.5% phenol, petrolatum, cocoa butter, lanolin, mixed waxes, oil of cloves	In 0.25 and 0.38 oz.
otc	**Chap Stick Medicated Lip Balm** (Robins)	**Lip Balm:** 1% camphor, 0.6% menthol, 0.5% phenol, petrolatum, mineral oil, cocoa butter, lanolin	Parabens. In jars (7 g), squeezable tubes (10 g) and sticks (4.2 g).
otc	**3 in 1 Toothache Relief** (C.S. Dent)	**Gum, Liquid, Lotion/Gel:** Benzocaine	In family first-aid packs.
otc	**Kank-a** (Blistex)	**Liquid/Film:** 20% benzocaine, benzoin compound tincture, SD alcohol 38b, benzyl alcohol, castor oil	Saccharin. In 9.9 mL.
otc	**Ulcerease** (Med-Derm)	**Liquid:** 0.6% liquified phenol, glycerin, sodium borate	In 180 mL.
otc	**Dent's Lotion-Jel** (C.S. Dent)	**Lotion/Gel:** Benzocaine	In 6 g.

PREPARATIONS FOR SENSITIVE TEETH

otc	**Denquel Sensitive Teeth** (Procter & Gamble)	**Toothpaste:** 5% potassium nitrate	Mint flavor. In 48, 90 and 135 g.
otc	**Sensodyne Cool Gel** (Block)	**Toothpaste:** Potassium nitrate, sodium fluoride	Saccharin, sorbitol, parabens. In 28.3 g.
otc	**Sensodyne-F** (Block)	**Toothpaste:** Potassium nitrate, sodium monofluorophosphate	Saccharin, sorbitol. In 72 and 138 g.
otc	**Sensodyne-SC** (Block)	**Toothpaste:** 10% strontium Cl hexa-hydrate	Saccharin, sorbitol, parabens. In 26 g.
otc	**Sensitivity Protection Crest** (Procter & Gamble)	**Toothpaste:** Sodium fluoride, potassium nitrate	Mint flavor. In 175 g.
otc	**Sensodyne Fresh Mint** (Block)	**Toothpaste:** Potassium nitrate, sodium monofluorophosphate	Sorbitol, saccharin. In 26 g.
Rx	**Triamcinolone Acetonide Dental 0.1%** (Various, eg, Qualitest, Taro)	**Paste:** 0.1% triamcinolone acetonide	In 5 g.

▶ Administration and Dosage

These toothpastes are specially formulated to replace regular toothpaste for people with sensitive teeth. Use daily as in regular dental care.

CHLOROPHYLL DERIVATIVES (Chlorophyllin)

otc *sf*	**Chlorophyll** (Freeda)	**Tablets:** 20 mg chlorophyll	In 100s, 250s and 500s.
otc	**PALS** (Palisades)	**Tablets:** 100 mg chlorophyllin copper complex	In 100s.
otc	**Chloresium** (Rystan)	**Tablets:** 14 mg chlorophyllin copper complex	In 100s and 1000s.
otc	**Chloresium** (Rystan)	**Solution:** 0.2% chlorophyllin copper complex in an isotonic saline solution	In 240 mL and qt.
otc	**Chloresium** (Rystan)	**Ointment:** 0.5% water-soluble chlorophyllin copper complex in a hydrophilic base	In 30 and 120 g and lb.

Indications

➤*Oral:* To control fecal odors in colostomy, ileostomy or incontinence; also for certain breath and body odors.

➤*Topical:* To promote normal healing, relieve pain and inflammation, and reduce malodors in wounds, burns, surface ulcers, cuts, abrasions and skin irritations.

Administration and Dosage

➤*Topical:*

Ointment – Apply generously and cover with gauze, linen or other appropriate dressing. Change no more often than every 48 to 72 hours.

Solution – Apply full strength as continuous wet dressing.

➤*Oral:*

Adults and children (> 12 years of age) – 1 to 2 tablets/day; may be increased to 3 tablets/day.

Children (< 12 years of age) – Consult physician.

➤*Ostomies:* In ostomies, take tablets orally or place in the appliance.

Warnings

➤*Diarrhea:* If cramping or diarrhea occur, reduce the dosage.

Adverse Reactions

Oral – No toxic effects have been reported. A temporary mild laxative effect may occur; the stool is commonly stained dark green.

Topical – Sensitivity reactions are extremely rare; only a few instances of slight itching or irritation have been reported.

BISMUTH SUBGALLATE

otc	**Devrom** (Parthenon)	**Tablets:** 200 mg	Lactose, sugar. Chewable. In 100s.

Indications

To control fecal odors in colostomy, ileostomy or incontinence.

Administration and Dosage

Take 1 or 2 tablets 3 times daily with meals. Chew or swallow whole.

Adverse Reactions

A temporary darkening of the tongue or stool may occur.

The anorectal preparations are used primarily for the symptomatic relief of the discomfort associated with hemorrhoids and perianal itching or irritation. In addition to the products specifically listed in this section, many of the Topical Local Anesthetics and Topical Corticosteroids may also be used locally in anorectal therapy (see specific monographs in the Dermatologics chapter).

Ingredients

The various components of these products are briefly discussed below. For complete information on specific indications, contraindications, precautions and adverse effects of ingredients, refer to the appropriate monographs as indicated.

➤*Hydrocortisone:* Hydrocortisone (see additional monographs in the Endocrine/Metabolic and Dermatologics chapters) reduces inflammation, itching and swelling.

➤*Local anesthetics:* Local anesthetics (benzocaine, pramoxine) temporarily relieve pain, itching and irritation. The most frequent adverse effects of topical local anesthetic use are allergic reactions (eg, burning, itching). Their safety and efficacy when used intrarectally require further evaluation (see additional monographs in the Dermatologics chapter).

➤*Vasoconstrictors:* Vasoconstrictors (ephedrine, phenylephrine) reduce swelling and congestion of anorectal tissues. They relieve local itching by a slight anesthetic effect. These agents are not effective in stopping bleeding from venous tissues.

➤*Astringents:* Astringents (witch hazel, zinc oxide) coagulate the protein in skin cells, protecting the underlying tissue and decreasing the cell volume. They lessen mucus and other secretions, and relieve anorectal irritation and inflammation.

➤*Antiseptics:* Antiseptics (benzalkonium chloride, phenylmercuric nitrate) are not of therapeutic value when applied to the anorectal area. There is no convincing evidence that they prevent infection in the anorectal area. Many are present as preservatives.

➤*Emollients / protectants:* Emollients (glycerin, lanolin, mineral oil, petrolatum, zinc oxide, cocoa butter, shark liver oil, bismuth salts) form a physical barrier on the skin and lubricate tissues, preventing irritation of the anorectal area and water loss from the stratum corneum. Many of these substances are used as bases and carriers of pharmacologically active compounds.

➤*Counterirritants:* Counterirritants (camphor) evoke a feeling of comfort, cooling, tingling or warmth and distract the perception of pain and itching.

➤*Keratolytics:* Keratolytics (resorcinol) cause desquamation and sloughing of epidermal surface cells and may help to expose underlying tissue to therapeutic agents.

➤*Wound-healing agents:* Wound-healing agents (balsam peru, skin respiratory factor or srf, yeast cell derivative) are claimed to promote wound healing or tissue repair. Effectiveness of these compounds has not been conclusively demonstrated.

➤*Anticholinergic agents:* Anticholinergic agents inhibit the action of acetylcholine. Because these agents produce their action systemically, they are not effective in ameliorating local symptoms of anorectal disease.

Patient Information

Maintain normal bowel function by proper diet, adequate fluid intake and regular exercise.

Products for external use only are not to be used intrarectally. Apply external products sparingly after, rather than before, a bowel movement. If possible, wash, rinse and dry the area before use.

Avoid excessive laxative use.

Stool softeners or bulk laxatives may be useful adjunctive therapy.

In general, patients with conditions such as diabetes, hypertension, hyperthyroidism or cardiovascular disease should not use products containing vasoconstrictors.

Products containing resorcinol should not be used on open wounds.

If anorectal symptoms do not improve in 7 days, or if bleeding, protrusion, seepage or pain occurs, consult a physician.

STEROID-CONTAINING PRODUCTS

Rx	**Proctocort** (Monarch Pharmaceuticals)	**Cream:** 1% hydrocortisone	Stearyl and benzyl alcohols. In 30 g with applicator.
Rx	**Dermol HC** (Dermol)		Mineral oil, lanolin and cetyl alcohols, parabens. In 30 g.
Rx	**Analpram-HC** (Ferndale)	**Cream:** 1% hydrocortisone acetate, 1% pramoxine HCl	Cetyl alcohol, 0.1% potassium sorbate, 0.1% sorbic acid. In 30 g.
Rx	**ProctoCream-HC** (Schwarz Pharma)		In 30 g.
Rx	**Analpram-HC** (Ferndale)	**Cream:** 2.5% hydrocortisone acetate, 1% pramoxine HCl	0.1% potassium sorbate, 0.1 % sorbic acid, cetyl alcohol. In 30 g.
Rx	**Anusol-HC** (Monarch)	**Cream:** 2.5% hydrocortisone	Petrolatum, EDTA, benzyl and stearyl alcohols. In 30 g.
Rx	**ProctoCream-HC** (Schwarz Pharma)	**Cream:** 2.5% hydrocortisone	Glycerin, stearyl alcohol, benzyl alcohol. In 30 g.
Rx	**Dermol HC** (Dermol)	**Cream:** 2.5% hydrocortisone	Mineral oil, lanolin and cetyl alcohols, parabens. In 30 g.
Rx	**Dermol HC** (Dermol)	**Ointment:** 1% hydrocortisone	Mineral oil, white petrolatum. In 30 g.
Rx	**Cortifoam** (Schwarz Pharma)	**Aerosol Foam:** 10% hydrocortisone acetate	Parabens. 90 mg/applicatorful. In 14 applications.
Rx	**Proctofoam-HC** (Schwarz Pharma)	**Aerosol Foam:** 1% hydrocortisone acetate, 1% pramoxine HCl	Parabens, cetyl alcohol, stearyl alcohol. In 10 g (≥ 14 applications) w/applicator.
Rx	**Pramoxine HC** (Rugby)		Parabens, cetyl alcohol. In 10 g with applicator.
Rx	**Proctocort** (Monarch Pharmaceuticals)	**Suppositories:** 30 mg hydrocortisone acetate	In 12s.
Rx	**Hydrocortisone Acetate** (Various, eg, Able, Clay-Park, Cypress, Major, Paddock)	**Suppositories:** 25 mg hydrocortisone acetate	In 12s and 24s.
Rx	**Anucort-HC** (G & W)		Vegetable oil. In 12, 24s and 100s.
Rx	**Anusol-HC** (Parke-Davis)		In 12s and 24s.
Rx	**Cort-Dome High Potency** (Bayer)		In 12s.
Rx	**Hemril-HC Uniserts** (Upsher-Smith)		Vegetable oil. In 12s.
Rx	**Hemorrhoidal HC** (Various, eg, Schein, Geneva, Goldline)		In 12s, 24s, 50s, 100s & UD 12s.

Refer to the general discussion of these products in the Anorectal Preparations Introduction.

LOCAL ANESTHETIC-CONTAINING PRODUCTS

otc	Tronolane (Ross)	**Cream:** 1% pramoxine HCl	Zinc oxide, parabens. In 30 and 60 g
otc	Americaine (Novartis Consumer)	**Ointment:** 20% benzocaine	In 22.5 g
otc	Medicone (EE Dickinson)	**Ointment:** 20% benzocaine	Mineral oil, white petrolatum. In 30 g
otc	Anusol (Parke-Davis)	**Ointment:** 1% pramoxine HCl	12.5% zinc oxide, mineral oil and cocoa butter. In 30 g with applicator.
otc	ProctoFoam NS (Schwarz Pharma)	**Aerosol Foam:** 1% pramoxine HCl	In 15 g with applicator.
otc	Fleet Pain Relief (Fleet)	**Pads:** 1% pramoxine HCl, 12% glycerin	In 100s.

Refer to the general discussion of these products in the Anorectal Preparations Introduction.

PERIANAL HYGIENE PRODUCTS

otc	Balneol Perianal Cleansing (Solvay)	**Lotion:** Mineral oil, lanolin oil	Methylparaben. In 120 mL.
otc	Tucks Clear (Warner Wellcome)	**Gel:** 50% hamamelis water, 10% glycerin	Benzyl alcohol, EDTA. In 19.8 g.
otc	Sensi-Care Perineal Skin Cleanser Solution (ConvaTec)	**Solution:** Sodium C_{12-14} olefin sulfonate, disodium cocoamphodiacetate.	Aloe vera. In 120 and 240 mL.
otc	Preparation H Cleansing (Whitehall)	**Tissues:** Propylene glycol, phenoxyethanol	Alcohol free. Parabens, citric acid. In 15s and 40s.
otc	Tucks (Parke-Davis)	**Pads:** 50% witch hazel and 10% glycerin with 0.003% benzalkonium Cl	In 40s & 100s.
otc	Tucks Take-Alongs (Parke-Davis)		In 12s.
otc	Fleet Medicated Wipes (Fleet)	**Pads:** 50% hamamelis water, 7% alcohol, 10% glycerin, benzalkonium chloride and methylparaben	In 100s.

Refer to the general discussion of these products in the Anorectal Preparations Introduction.

MISCELLANEOUS ANORECTAL COMBINATION PRODUCTS

otc	Preparation H Cooling Gel (Whitehall-Robins)	**Gel:** 50% witch hazel, 0.25% phenylephrine HCl. 7.5% alcohol, EDTA, parabens.	In 51 g.
otc	Preparation H (Whitehall-Robins)	**Cream:** 18% petrolatum, 12% glycerin, 3% shark liver oil, 0.25% phenylephrine HCl, cetyl alcohol, stearyl alcohol, EDTA, lanolin, parabens	In 27 and 54 g.
		Ointment: 71.9% petrolatum, 14% mineral oil, 3% shark liver oil, 0.25% phenylephrine HCl, corn oil, glycerin, lanolin, lanolin alcohol, parabens, tocopherol	In 30 and 60 g.
otc	Formulation R (G & W)	**Cream:** 18% petrolatum, 12% glycerin, 0.25% phenylephrine HCl.	In 52 g.
		Ointment: 71.9% petrolatum, 14% mineral oil, 0.25% phenylephrine HCl	Parabens. In 28.4 and 56.8 g.
otc	Hem-Prep (G & W)	**Ointment:** 0.025% phenylephrine HCl, 11% zinc oxide, white petrolatum	In 42.5 g
otc	Preparation H (Whitehall)	**Suppositories:** 3% shark liver oil, 79% cocoa butter, corn oil, EDTA, parabens and tocopherol	In 12s, 24s, 36s and 48s.
otc	Wyanoids Relief Factor (Wyeth)	**Suppositories:** 79% cocoa butter, 3% shark liver oil, corn oil, EDTA, parabens and tocopherol	In 12s.
otc	Nupercainal (Ciba Consumer)	**Suppositories:** 2.1 g cocoa butter, 0.25 g zinc oxide and sodium bisulfite	In 12s and 24s.
otc	Anusol (GlaxoWellcome)	**Suppositories:** 51% topical starch, benzyl alcohol, soy bean oil, tocopheryl acetate	In 12s.
otc	Hemril Uniserts (Upsher-Smith)	**Suppositories:** 2.25% bismuth subgallate, 1.75% bismuth resorcin compound, 1.2% benzyl benzoate, 11% zinc oxide, 1.8% balsam peru in hydrolyzed vegetable oil base	In 12s and 50s.
otc	Rectagene (Pfeiffer)	**Suppositories:** Live yeast cell derivative supplying 2000 units Skin Respiratory Factor per ounce and shark liver oil in a cocoa butter base	In 12s.
otc	Rectagene II (Pfeiffer)	**Suppositories:** 2.25% bismuth subgallate, 1.75% bismuth resorcin compound, 1.2% benzyl benzoate, 1.8% peruvian balsam, 11% zinc oxide, bismuth subiodide, calcium phosphate in a hydrogenated vegetable oil base	In 12s.
otc	Pazo Hemorrhoid (Bristol-Myers)	**Suppositories:** 3.8 mg ephedrine sulfate, 96.5 mg zinc oxide, vegetable oil	In 12s and 24s.
otc	Hem-Prep (G & W)	**Suppositories:** 0.25% phenylephrine HCl, 11% zinc oxide	In 12s.
otc	Tronolane (Ross)	**Suppositories:** 11% zinc oxide and 95% hard fat	In 10s and 20s.
otc	Hemorid For Women (Thompson Medical)	**Cream:** 30% white petrolatum, 20% mineral oil, 1% pramoxine HCl, 0.25% phenylephrine HCl, aloe vera gel, parabens, cetyl and stearyl alcohols	In 28.3 g.

Refer to the general discussion of these products in the Anorectal Preparations Introduction.

Indications

▶*Oral:* Penicillins are generally indicated in the treatment of mildly to moderately severe infections caused by penicillin-sensitive microorganisms.

▶*Penicillinase-resistant penicillins:* The percentage of staphylococcal isolates resistant to penicillin G outside the hospital is increasing, approximating the high percentage found in the hospital. Therefore, use a penicillinase-resistant penicillin as initial therapy for any suspected staphylococcal infection until culture and sensitivity results are known.

When treatment is initiated before definitive culture and sensitivity results are known, consider that these agents are only effective in the treatment of infections caused by pneumococci, group A beta-hemolytic streptococci and penicillin G-resistant and penicillin G-sensitive staphylococci.

▶*Parenteral:* In patients with severe infection or when there is nausea, vomiting, gastric dilatation, cardiospasm or intestinal hypermotility. Parenteral aqueous penicillin G (eg, potassium, sodium) is the dosage form of choice in severe infections caused by penicillin-sensitive microorganisms when rapid and high penicillin serum levels are required.

For specific labeled indications, refer to individual drug monographs.

Administration and Dosage

Therapy may be initiated prior to obtaining results of bacteriologic studies when there is reason to believe the causative organisms may be susceptible. Once results are known, adjust therapy.

Dosage for any individual patient must take into consideration the severity of infection, the susceptibility of the organisms causing the infection and the status of the patient's host defense mechanism. Duration of therapy depends on the severity of the infection.

Continue treatment of all infections for a minimum of 48 to 72 hours beyond the time that the patient becomes asymptomatic or evidence of bacterial eradication has been obtained, unless single-dose therapy is employed. A minimum of 10 days treatment is recommended for any infection caused by group A beta-hemolytic streptococci to prevent the occurrence of acute rheumatic fever or acute glomerulonephritis.

Patients with a history of rheumatic fever or chorea and receiving continuous prophylaxis may harbor increased numbers of penicillin-resistant organisms.

Actions

▶*Pharmacology:* Penicillins are bactericidal antibiotics that include natural and semisynthetic derivatives. These agents contain the 6-β-aminopenicillanic acid nucleus and have a similar mechanism of action. All penicillins share cross-allergenicity. Significant differences among agents include: Resistance to gastric acid inactivation; resistance to inactivation by penicillinase; spectrum of antimicrobial activity. In addition to the prototype penicillin G, this class includes an acid-stable penicillin G derivative (penicillin V), penicillinase-resistant penicillins, the aminopenicillins and the extended spectrum derivatives. Bacampicillin is hydrolyzed in vivo to ampicillin; amoxicillin is closely related to ampicillin. Several of these penicillins are also available in combination with agents that inactivate β-lactamase enzymes (eg, clavulanic acid, sulbactam), thereby extending the antibiotic spectrum to include many bacteria normally resistant to it and to other β-lactam antibiotics (see Pharmacokinetics). The available combinations include ampicillin/sulbactam; amoxicillin/potassium clavulanate; ticarcillin/potassium clavulanate and piperacillin/tazobactam sodium.

Penicillins					
	Routes of administration	Penicillinase-resistant	Acid stable	% Protein bound	May be taken with meals
Natural					
Penicillin G	IM-IV	no	no	60	†¹
Penicillin V	Oral	no	no	80	yes
Penicillinase-Resistant					
Cloxacillin	Oral	yes	yes	95	no
Dicloxacillin	Oral	yes	yes	98	no
Nafcillin	IM-IV-Oral	yes	yes	87 to 90	no
Oxacillin	IM-IV-Oral	yes	yes	94	no
Aminopenicillins					
Amoxicillin	Oral	no	yes	20	yes
Amoxicillin/potassium clavulanate	Oral	yes	yes	18/25	yes
Ampicillin	IM-IV-Oral	no	yes	20	no
Ampicillin/sulbactam	IM-IV	yes	†¹	28/38	†¹
Bacampicillin	Oral	no	yes	20	yes
Extended-Spectrum					
Carbenicillin	Oral	no	yes	50	no
Mezlocillin	IM-IV	no	†¹	16 to 42	†¹
Piperacillin	IM-IV	no	†¹	16	†¹
Piperacillin/tazobactam sodium	IV	yes	†¹	30/30	†¹
Ticarcillin	IM-IV	no	†¹	45	†¹
Ticarcillin/potassium clavulanate	IV	yes	†¹	45/9	†¹

¹ Available only for IM or IV use.

Mechanism – Penicillins inhibit the biosynthesis of cell wall mucopeptide. They are bactericidal against sensitive organisms when adequate concentrations are reached, and they are most effective during the stage of active multiplication. Inadequate concentrations may produce only bacteriostatic effects.

▶*Pharmacokinetics:*

Absorption – Because gastric acidity, stomach emptying time and other factors affecting absorption may vary considerably, serum levels may be reduced to nontherapeutic levels in certain individuals. Penicillin V shows less individual variation than penicillin G and has become the only natural penicillin available for oral administration. Nafcillin's oral absorption is inferior to oxacillin, cloxacillin and dicloxacillin. Ampicillin and carbenicillin indanyl have good GI absorption, but amoxicillin and bacampicillin are more completely absorbed.

Absorption of most penicillins is affected by food; these medications are best taken on an empty stomach, 1 hour before or 2 hours after meals. Penicillin V may be given with meals; however blood levels may be slightly higher when given on an empty stomach. Amoxicillin, bacampicillin tablets and amoxicillin/potassium clavulanate may be given without regard to meals.

Peak serum levels occur ≈ 1 hour after oral use. After a 500 mg oral dose, peak serum concentrations for oxacillin, cloxacillin and dicloxacillin range from 5 to 7, 7.5 to 14.4 and 10 to 17 mcg/mL, respectively. One hour after a 1 g oral nafcillin dose, average serum concentration was 1.19 mcg/mL (range, 0 to 3.12). IM injections of 1 g nafcillin, 560 mg oxacillin and 1 g methicillin produced peak serum levels in 0.5 to 1 hour of 7.61, 15 and 17 mcg/mL, respectively.

Parenteral penicillin G (sodium and potassium) gives rapid and high but transient blood levels; derivatives provide prolonged penicillin blood levels with IM use. Procaine penicillin G, an equimolecular suspension of procaine and penicillin G, must be given IM; it dissolves slowly at the injection site and plateaus in about 4 hours; levels decline gradually over 15 to 20 hours. Benzathine penicillin G IM also must be given IM only; is absorbed very slowly from the injection site and is hydrolyzed to penicillin G; hence, serum levels are much lower but more prolonged, sustaining serum levels for up to 4 weeks.

Distribution – Penicillins are bound to plasma proteins, primarily albumin, in varying degrees (see table in Pharmacology section). They diffuse readily into most body tissues and fluids, including kidneys, liver, lungs, heart, skin, synovial fluid, intestines, bile, peritoneal fluid, bronchial and wound secretions, bone, prostate, pericardial and ascitic fluids, spleen and other tissues. Penetration into cerebrospinal fluid (CSF), the brain and the eye occurs only with inflammation. CSF levels usually do not exceed 5% of penicillin G's peak serum concentration. Penicillins cross the placenta and appear in amniotic fluid and cord serum.

Excretion – Penicillins are excreted largely unchanged in the urine by glomerular filtration and active tubular secretion. Nonrenal elimination includes hepatic inactivation and excretion in bile; this is only a minor route for all penicillins except nafcillin and oxacillin. Excretion by renal tubular secretion can be delayed by coadministration of probenecid. Excretion is delayed in neonates and infants. Elimination half-life of most penicillins is short (≤ 1.4 hr). Impaired renal function prolongs the serum half-life of penicillins eliminated primarily by renal excretion. The half-life is not greatly affected for nafcillin, oxacillin, cloxacillin and dicloxacillin because of increased biotransformation and biliary excretion. Because piperacillin is excreted by biliary and renal routes, it can be used safely in appropriate dosage in patients with severe renal impairment and in the treatment of hepatobiliary infections.

β-lactamase inhibitors: (Clavulanic acid, sulbactam and tazobactam). These have weak antimicrobial activity but irreversibly inactivate bacterial β-lactamase enzymes. Used with β-lactam antibiotics, they protect antibiotics from inactivation by β-lactamase-producing organisms.

Clavulanic acid – Used in combination with amoxicillin and ticarcillin, it inhibits plasmid-mediated β-lactamases (eg, *Haemophilus influenzae, Neisseria gonorrheae, Escherichia coli, Salmonella, Shigella,* staphylococci) and chromosomal-mediated β-lactamases (eg, *Klebsiella, Bacteroides fragilis* and *Legionella*). It does not inhibit β-lactamases produced by *Enterobacter, Serratia, Morganella, Citrobacter, Pseudomonas* or *Acinetobacter* species.

Clavulanic acid is well absorbed orally and widely distributed to many body tissues. Half-life is ≈ 1 hour; 35% to 45% is excreted unchanged in the urine during the first 6 hours after administration. Probenecid does not alter renal excretion of clavulanic acid.

Sulbactam – Another β-lactamase inhibitor, this extends the bacterial spectrum of ampicillin to include such β-lactamase-producing organisms as *S. aureus, H. influenzae, B. fragilis* and most strains of *E. coli*.

Tazobactam – This is a penicillanic acid sulfone β-lactamase inhibitor and has poor activity against chromosomal β-lactamases of Enterobacteriaceae but has good activity against many of the plasmid β-lactamases. Tazobactam extends the spectrum but does not increase the activity of piperacillin against *Pseudomonas aeruginosa.* The currently recommended piperacillin dose in piperacillin/tazobactam is less than the recommended dose of piperacillin when used alone for serious infections and may prove ineffective in the treatment of some *P. aeruginosa* infections. The manufacturer recommends concomitant aminoglycoside therapy when treating *P. aeruginosa* nosocomial pneumonia.

▶*Microbiology:* The following table indicates the organisms that are generally susceptible to the penicillins in vitro:

Organisms Generally Susceptible to Penicillins

✓ = generally susceptible

Organisms	Natural penicillins — Penicillin G	Penicillin V	Penicillinase-resistant — Cloxacillin	Dicloxacillin	Nafcillin	Oxacillin	Aminopenicillins — Amoxicillin	Ampicillin	Bacampicillin	Amoxicillin/potassium clavulanate	Ampicillin/sulbactam	Extended spectrum — Carbenicillin	Mezlocillin	Piperacillin	Ticarcillin	Ticarcillin/potassium clavulanate	Piperacillin/tazobactam sodium
Gram-positive																	
Staphylococci	✓[1]	✓[1]	✓	✓	✓	✓	✓[1]	✓[1]	✓[1]	✓	✓	✓[1]		✓[1]	✓[1]		
Staphylococcus aureus	✓[1]	✓[1]	✓	✓	✓	✓				✓	✓	✓[1]	✓[1]	✓[1]	✓[1]	✓	✓[5]
Staphyloccus epidermidis																	✓[5]
Streptococci	✓	✓					✓				✓						
Streptococcus pneumoniae	✓	✓	✓	✓	✓	✓	✓	✓	✓	✓	✓	✓	✓	✓	✓	✓	✓[2]
Beta-hemolytic streptococci	✓	✓			✓		✓	✓	✓	✓	✓	✓	✓	✓	✓	✓	✓
Enterococcus (Streptococcus) faecalis	✓[4]	✓					✓	✓	✓	✓	✓	✓	✓	✓	✓	✓	✓
Streptococcus viridans	✓	✓			✓		✓	✓	✓	✓	✓	✓		✓			✓
Corynebacterium diphtheriae	✓	✓															
Bacillus anthracis	✓	✓						✓									
Streptococcus agalactiae															✓		
Streptococcus pyogenes																	✓
Erysipelothrix rhusiopathiae	✓																
Listeria monocytogenes	✓	✓					✓	✓			✓						
Gram-negative																	
Escherichia coli	✓						✓	✓	✓	✓	✓	✓	✓	✓	✓	✓	✓
Haemophilus influenzae							✓	✓	✓	✓	✓	✓	✓	✓[2]	✓	✓	✓
Haemophilus parainfluenzae													✓				
Eikenella corrodens											✓						
Bacteroides melaninogenicus																	✓
Pseudomonas sp.															✓		
Klebsiella sp.								✓	✓	✓	✓		✓	✓		✓	✓
Neisseria gonorrhoeae	✓[1]	✓					✓	✓	✓	✓	✓	✓	✓	✓	✓	✓	
Neisseria meningitidis	✓							✓		✓	✓						✓[2]
Proteus mirabilis	✓						✓	✓	✓	✓	✓	✓	✓	✓	✓	✓	✓
Salmonella sp.	✓							✓									
Shigella sp.	✓							✓									
Morganella morganii											✓	✓	✓	✓	✓	✓	✓
Proteus vulgaris													✓	✓		✓	✓
Providencia rettgeri													✓	✓		✓	✓
Providencia stuartii													✓	✓			
Enterobacter sp.	✓											✓	✓	✓	✓	✓	✓
Citrobacter sp.												✓	✓	✓	✓	✓	✓
Pseudomonas aeruginosa												✓	✓	✓	✓	✓	✓
Serratia sp.												✓	✓	✓	✓	✓	✓
Acinetobacter sp.												✓	✓	✓	✓		
Streptobacillus moniliformis	✓	✓															
Moraxella (Branhamella) catarrhalis										✓	✓			✓		✓	✓
Anaerobic																	
Clostridium sp.	✓	✓					✓	✓		✓	✓	✓	✓	✓	✓	✓	✓
Peptococcus sp.	✓	✓					✓	✓		✓	✓	✓	✓	✓	✓	✓	✓
Peptostreptococcus sp.	✓	✓						✓		✓	✓	✓	✓	✓	✓	✓	✓
Bacteroides sp.	✓[3]									✓	✓		✓	✓		✓	✓
Fusobacterium sp.	✓									✓	✓		✓	✓		✓	✓
Eubacterium sp.	✓												✓	✓	✓		
Treponema pallidum	✓	✓															
Actinomyces bovis	✓	✓												✓			
Veillonella sp.													✓	✓	✓	✓	

[1] Non-penicillinase-producing.
[2] Non-beta-lactamase-producing.
[3] Many strains of *B. fragilis* are resistant.
[4] Bacteriostatic effect.
[5] Non-methicillin/oxacillin-resistant strains.

Contraindications

History of hypersensitivity to penicillins, cephalosporins, imipenem, or β-lactamase inhibitors (piperacillin/tazobactam).

Do not treat severe pneumonia, empyema, bacteremia, pericarditis, meningitis and purulent or septic arthritis with an oral penicillin during the acute stage.

History of amoxicillin/clavulanate potassium-associated cholestatic jaundice/hepatic dysfunction (amoxicillin/clavulanate potassium only).

Warnings

►*Bleeding abnormalities:* **Ticarcillin, mezlocillin or piperacillin** may induce hemorrhagic manifestations associated with abnormalities of coagulation tests (eg, bleeding time, prothrombin time, platelet aggregation). Upon withdrawal of the drug, bleeding should cease and coagulation abnormalities revert to normal. Observe patients with renal impairment, in whom excretion of these drugs is delayed, for prolonged bleeding manifestations.

►*Cystic fibrosis:* These patients have a higher incidence of side effects (eg, fever, rash) when treated with extended spectrum penicillins (eg, piperacillin, carbenicillin). This may be caused by the higher IgE, IgG and eosinophil levels in this population.

►*Hypersensitivity reactions:* Serious and occasionally fatal immediate hypersensitivity reactions have occurred. The incidence of anaphylactic shock is between 0.015% and 0.04%. Anaphylactic shock resulting in death has occurred in ≈ 0.002% of the patients treated. Although anaphylaxis is more frequent following parenteral therapy, it may occur with oral use. Accelerated reactions (including urticaria and laryngeal edema) and delayed reactions (serum sickness-like reactions) may also occur. These reactions are likely to be immediate and severe in penicillin-sensitive individuals with a history of atopic conditions (see Adverse Reactions).

Hypersensitivity myocarditis – This is not dose-dependent and may occur at any time during treatment. The initial reaction involves rash, fever and eosinophilia. The second stage reflects cardiac involvement: Sinus tachycardia, ST-T changes, slight increase in cardiac enzymes (creatine phosphokinase) and cardiomegaly.

An urticarial rash, not representing a true penicillin allergy, occasionally occurs with **ampicillin** (9%). This reaction is more frequent in patients on allopurinol (14% to 22.4%), patients with lymphatic leukemia (90%) and in those with infectious mononucleosis (43% to 100%). Typically, the rash appears 7 to 10 days after the start of oral ampicillin therapy and remains for a few days to a week after drug discontinuance. In most cases, the rash is maculopapular, pruritic and generalized.

Before therapy, inquire about previous hypersensitivity reactions to penicillins, cephalosporins and other allergens. Skin testing with benzylpenicilloyl-polylysine may be used to evaluate penicillin hypersensitivity (see individual monograph in In Vivo Diagnostic Aids section).

Desensitization: Patients with a positive skin test to one of the penicillin determinants can be desensitized, which is a relatively safe procedure. This is recommended in instances when penicillin must be given (eg, neurosyphilis, congenital syphilis, syphilis in pregnancy) where no proven alternatives exist. This can be done orally, IV or SC; however, oral is thought to be safest and easiest. Various protocols are described, but each protocol utilizes the same principles, which involve gradually increasing doses of penicillin, increasing each dose every 15 to 20 minutes. For example, one oral protocol using penicillin V uses 14 total doses, each dose given 15 minutes apart. The units per dose are doubled at each interval (eg, 100, 200, 400, 800) for a total cumulative dose of 1.3 million units over 4 hours. After desensitization, maintain patients on penicillin for the duration of therapy.

Cross-allergenicity with cephalosporins: Individuals with a history of penicillin hypersensitivity have experienced severe reactions when treated with a cephalosporin. The incidence of cross-allergenicity between penicillins and cephalosporins is estimated to range from 5% to 16%; however, it is possible the incidence is much lower, possibly 3% to 7%.

Urticaria, other skin rashes and serum sickness-like reactions may be controlled by antihistamines and, if necessary, corticosteroids. Discontinue use unless the condition being treated is life-threatening and amenable only to penicillin therapy. Serious anaphylactoid reactions require emergency measures. See Management of Acute Hypersensitivity Reactions.

►*Renal function impairment:* Because carbenicillin is primarily excreted by the kidney, patients with severe renal impairment (creatinine clearance, < 10 mL/min) will not achieve the therapeutic urine levels of carbenicillin.

In patients with creatinine clearance 10 to 20 mL/min, it may be necessary to adjust dosage to prevent accumulation of the drug.

The dosage of penicillin G should be reduced in patients with severe renal impairment, with additional modifications when hepatic disease accompanies the renal impairment.

►*Pregnancy:* Category B. There are no adequate or well controlled studies in pregnant women. Penicillins cross the placenta.

Use during pregnancy only if clearly needed.

Labor and delivery – Oral aminopenicillins are poorly absorbed during labor. It is not known whether use has immediate or delayed adverse effects on the fetus or alters normal labor.

►*Lactation:* Penicillins are excreted in breast milk in low concentrations; use may cause diarrhea, candidiasis or allergic response in the nursing infant. Ampicillin use by nursing mothers may lead to sensitization of infants; therefore make a decision to discontinue nursing or to discontinue ampicillin, taking into account the importance of the drug to the mother.

►*Children:* Safety and efficacy of carbenicillin, piperacillin and the β-lactamase inhibitor/penicillin combinations have not been established in infants and children < 12 years old. Penicillins are excreted largely unchanged by the kidney. Because of incompletely developed renal function in infants, the rate of elimination will be slow. Penicillinase-resistant penicillins (especially methicillin) may not be completely excreted, with abnormally high blood levels resulting. Oral aminopenicillins are not absorbed as well in neonates as in adults. Use caution in administering to newborns and evaluate organ system function frequently. Frequent blood levels are advisable, with dosage adjustments when necessary. Monitor all newborns closely for clinical and laboratory evidence of toxic or adverse effects.

Precautions

►*Monitoring:* Perform bacteriologic studies to determine causative organisms and their susceptibility so that appropriate therapy is administered.

Obtain blood cultures, white blood cell and differential cell counts prior to initiation of therapy and at least weekly during therapy with penicillinase-resistant penicillins. Measure AST and ALT during therapy to monitor for liver function abnormalities.

Perform periodic urinalysis, BUN and creatinine determinations during therapy with penicillinase-resistant penicillins, and consider dosage alterations if these values become elevated. If renal impairment is known or suspected, reduce the total dosage and monitor blood levels to avoid possible neurotoxic reactions.

Monitoring is particularly important in newborns, infants and when high dosages are used.

►*Streptococcal infections:* Therapy must be sufficient to eliminate the organism (a minimum of 10 days); otherwise, sequelae (eg, endocarditis, rheumatic fever) may occur. Take cultures after treatment to confirm that streptococci have been eradicated.

►*Sexually transmitted diseases:* When treating gonococcal infections in which primary and secondary syphilis are suspected, perform proper diagnostic procedures, including darkfield examinations and monthly serological tests for at least 4 months. All cases of penicillin-treated syphilis should receive clinical and serological examinations every 6 months for 2 to 3 years. Test all syphilis patients for HIV infection.

►*Resistance:* The number of strains of staphylococci resistant to penicillinase-resistant penicillins has been increasing; widespread use of penicillinase-resistant penicillins may result in an increasing number of resistant staphylococcal strains. Interpret resistance to any penicillinase-resistant penicillin as evidence of clinical resistance to all. Cross-resistance with cephalosporin derivatives also occurs frequently.

►*Pseudomembranous colitis:* This has occurred with the use of broad spectrum antibiotics because of overgrowth of *Clostridia* sp; therefore, it is important to consider its diagnosis in patients who develop diarrhea in association with antibiotic use. Mild cases may respond to drug discontinuation alone. Manage moderate-to-severe cases with fluid, electrolyte and protein supplementation. If it is not relieved by drug withdrawal, or when it is severe, oral vancomycin is the treatment of choice.

►*Procaine sensitivity:* If sensitivity to the procaine in **penicillin G procaine** is suspected, inject 0.1 mL of a 1% to 2% procaine solution intradermally. Development of erythema, wheal, flare or eruption indicates procaine sensitivity; treat by the usual methods. Do not use procaine penicillin preparations.

►*Parenteral administration:* Inadvertent intravascular administration, including direct intra-arterial injection or injection immediately adjacent to arteries, has resulted in severe neurovascular damage, including transverse myelitis with permanent paralysis, gangrene requiring amputation of digits and more proximal portions of extremities, and necrosis and sloughing at and surrounding the injection site. Such severe effects have occurred following injections into the buttock, thigh and deltoid areas. Other serious complications include immediate pallor, mottling or cyanosis of the extremity, both distal and proximal to the injection site, followed by bleb formation; severe edema requiring anterior or posterior compartment fasciotomy in the lower extremity. These severe effects have most often occurred in infants and small children. Promptly consult a specialist if any evidence of a compromise of the blood supply occurs at, proximal to, or distal to the site of injection.

Quadriceps femoris fibrosis and atrophy have occurred following repeated IM injections of penicillin preparations into the anterolateral thigh.

Take particular care with IV administration because of the possibility of thrombophlebitis. Higher than recommended IV doses of most of the penicillins may cause neuromuscular excitability or convulsions.

Avoid SC and fat layer injections; pain and induration may occur. If these occur, apply an ice pack.

►*Electrolyte imbalance:* Administer **aqueous penicillin G** IV in high doses (> 10 million units) slowly because of electrolyte imbalance from either the potassium or sodium content. When sodium restriction is necessary (eg, cardiac patients), make periodic electrolyte determinations and monitor cardiac status.

Patients given continuous IV therapy with **potassium penicillin G** in high dosage (> 10 million units daily) may suffer severe or even fatal potassium poisoning, particularly if renal insufficiency is present. Hyperreflexia, convulsions, coma, cardiac arrhythmias and cardiac arrest may be indicative of this syndrome. High dosage of **sodium salts of penicillins** may result in or aggravate CHF because of high sodium intake. Individuals with liver disease or those receiving cytotoxic therapy or diuretics rarely demonstrated a decrease in serum potassium concentrations with high doses of **piperacillin**.

Sodium penicillin G contains 2 mEq sodium per million units, **potassium penicillin G** contains 1.7 mEq potassium and 0.3 mEq sodium per million units. The sodium content of other IV penicillin derivatives is listed below:

Sodium Content of IV Penicillins			
Penicillin	Maximum recommended daily dose (g)	Sodium content (mEq/g)[1]	Sodium (mEq/day)[1],[2]
Ampicillin sodium	14	2.9 to 3.1	40.6 to 43.4
Mezlocillin sodium	24	1.85	44.4
Nafcillin sodium	6	2.9	17.4
Oxacillin sodium	6	2.5 to 3.1	15 to 18.6
Piperacillin sodium	24	1.85	44.4
Piperacillin/tazobactam sodium	12	2.35	28.2
Ticarcillin disodium	18	5.2 to 6.5	93.6 to 117

[1] 1 mEq sodium equals 23 mg.
[2] Based on maximum daily dose.

Hypokalemia – This has occurred in a few patients receiving **mezlocillin, ticarcillin** and **piperacillin**. It may also occur in patients with low potassium reserves and in patients receiving cytotoxic therapy or diuretics. Monitor serum potassium and supplement when necessary.

►*Superinfection:* Use of antibiotics (especially prolonged or repeated therapy) may result in bacterial or fungal overgrowth of nonsusceptible organisms. Such overgrowth may lead to a secondary infection. Take appropriate measures if this occurs.

Indwelling IV catheters encourage superinfections.

►*Tartrazine sensitivity:* Some of these products contain tartrazine, which may cause allergic-type reactions (including bronchial asthma) in susceptible individuals. Although the incidence of tartrazine sensitivity in the general population is low, it is frequently seen in patients who also have aspirin hypersensitivity. Specific products containing tartrazine are identified in the product listings.

►*Sulfite sensitivity:* Some of these products contain sodium formaldehyde sulfoxylate, a sulfite that may cause allergic-type reactions including anaphylactic symptoms and life-threatening or less severe asthmatic episodes in certain susceptible people. The overall prevalence of sulfite sensitivity in the general population is unknown and probably low. Sulfite sensitivity is seen more frequently in asthmatic than in nonasthmatic people.

Drug Interactions

Penicillin Drug Interactions			
Precipitant drug	Object drug*		Description
Penicillins, parenteral	Aminoglycosides, parenteral	↔	Although these agents are often used together to achieve a synergistic action, certain penicillins may inactivate certain aminoglycosides in vitro. Do not mix in the same IV solution. Also, oral neomycin may reduce the serum concentrations of oral penicillin.
Penicillins, parenteral	Anticoagulants	↑	Large IV doses of penicillins can increase bleeding risks of anticoagulants by prolonging bleeding time. Conversely, nafcillin and dicloxacillin have been associated with warfarin resistance.
Penicillins, oral	Beta blockers	↔	Ampicillin may reduce the bioavailability of atenolol. Case reports indicated that beta blockers may potentiate anaphylactic reactions of penicillin.

Penicillin Drug Interactions			
Precipitant drug	Object drug*		Description
Penicillins	Contraceptives, oral	↓	The efficacy of oral contraceptives may be reduced and increased breakthrough bleeding may occur. Although infrequently reported, contraceptive failure is possible; the use of an additional form of contraception during penicillin therapy is advisable.
Penicillins, parenteral	Heparin	↑	An increased risk of bleeding may occur, possibly because of additive effects.
Allopurinol	Ampicillin	↑	The rate of ampicillin-induced skin rash appears much higher when coadministered with allopurinol than with either drug by itself (see Warnings).
Chloramphenicol	Penicillins	↔	Synergistic effects may develop, but antagonism has been reported in animal studies.
Erythromycin	Penicillins	↔	In vitro tests and clinical studies have demonstrated both antagonism and synergism with coadministration.
Tetracyclines	Penicillins	↓	The bacteriostatic action of tetracycline derivatives may impair the bactericidal effects of penicillins.
Nafcillin	Cyclosporine	↓	Administered concomitantly subtherapeutic cyclosporine levels have been reported. When used concomitantly in organ transplant patients, the cyclosporine levels should be monitored.
Mezlocillin, Piperacillin	Vecuronium	↑	Mezlocillin, along with other ureidopenicillins, has been reported in one study to prolong neuromuscular blockage of vecuronium. Caution is indicated when mexlocillin is used perioperatively. Piperacillin when used concomitantly with vecuronium has been implicated in the prolongation of the neuromuscular blockade of vecuronium. It is expected that the neuromuscular blockade produced by any of the non-depolarizing muscle relaxants could be prolonged in the presence of piperacillin.
Aspirin, phenylbutazone, sulfonamides, indomethacin, thiazide diuretics, furosemide, ethacrynic acid	Penicillin G	↑	These drugs may compete with penicillin G for renal tubular secretion and thus prolong the serum half-life of penicillin.
Probenecid	Penicillins (renally excreted)	↑	Probenecid administered concomitantly with piperacillin/tazobactam prolongs the half-life of piperacillin by 21% and tazobactam by 71%. Carbenicillin indanyl sodium blood levels may be increased and prolonged by concurrent administration of probenecid.

* ↑ = Object drug increased.   ↓ = Object drug decreased.   ↔ = Undetermined clinical effect.

►*Drug/Lab test interactions:* False-positive **urine glucose** reactions may occur with penicillin therapy if Clinitest, Benedict's Solution or Fehling's Solution are used. It is recommended that enzymatic glucose oxidase tests (such as *Clinistix* or *Tes-Tape*) be used. Positive **Coombs' tests** have occurred. Positive direct antiglobulin tests (DAT) have been reported after large IV doses of **piperacillin; clavulanic acid** has also been reported to cause a positive DAT. High urine concentrations of some penicillins may produce false-positive protein reactions (pseudoproteinuria) with the following methods: Sulfosalicylic acid and boiling test, acetic acid test, biuret reaction and nitric acid test. The bromphenol blue (*Multi-Stix*) reagent strip test has been reported to be reliable.

►*Drug/Food interactions:* Absorption of most penicillins is affected by food; these medications are best taken on an empty stomach, 1 hour before or 2 hours after meals. **Penicillin V** may be given with meals; however, blood levels may be slightly higher when taken on an empty stomach. **Amoxicillin, amoxicillin/potassium clavulanate** and **bacampicillin** tablets may be given without regard to meals.

Adverse Reactions

►*Cardiovascular:* Cardiac arrest; tachycardia; palpitations; pulmonary hypertension; pulmonary embolism; syncope; vasovagal reaction; cerebrovascular accident; hypotension; vasodilation.

►*CNS:* Penicillins have caused neurotoxicity (manifested as lethargy, neuromuscular hyperirritability, hallucinations, convulsions and seizures) when given in large IV doses, especially in patients with renal failure. Mental disturbances including anxiety, confusion, agitation, depression, hallucinations, weakness, seizures, combativeness and expressed "fear of impending death" have been reported in individuals following single-dose therapy for gonorrhea with **penicillin G procaine**, which may have been a reaction to procaine. Reactions have been transient, lasting from 15 to 30 minutes. Dizziness, fatigue, insomnia, reversible hyperactivity and prolonged muscle relaxation have occurred.

►*GI:* Glossitis; stomatitis; gastritis; sore mouth or tongue; dry mouth; furry tongue; black "hairy" tongue; abnormal taste sensation; nausea; vomiting; abdominal pain or cramp; epigastric distress; diarrhea or bloody diarrhea; rectal bleeding; flatulence; enterocolitis; pseudomembranous colitis; intestinal necrosis (see Precautions). Incidence of symptoms, particularly diarrhea, is less with amoxicillin and bacampicillin than with ampicillin.

►*GU:* Vaginitis; neurogenic bladder; hematuria; proteinuria; renal failure; impotence; priapism.

►*Hematologic/Lymphatic:*

Bleeding abnormalities – Hemorrhagic manifestations associated with abnormalities of coagulation tests such as clotting and prothrombin time have occurred and are more likely to occur in patients with renal failure (see Warnings).

Anemia; hemolytic anemia; thrombocytopenia; thrombocytopenic purpura; eosinophilia; leukopenia; granulocytopenia; neutropenia; bone marrow depression; agranulocytosis; lymphadenopathy; a reduction of hemoglobin or hematocrit; prolongation of bleeding and prothrombin time; decrease in WBC and lymphocyte counts; increase in lymphocytes, monocytes, basophils and platelets. These reactions are usually reversible on discontinuation of therapy, and are believed to be hypersensitivity phenomena. A slight thrombocytosis occurred in < 1% of patients treated with amoxicillin and clavulanate potassium. Atypical lymphocytosis has been observed in one pediatric patient receiving ampicillin/sulbactam sodium.

►*Hypersensitivity:* Adverse reactions (estimated incidence, 0.7% to 10%) are more likely to occur in individuals with previously demonstrated hypersensitivity. In penicillin-sensitive individuals with a history of allergy, asthma or hay fever, the reactions may be immediate and severe (see Warnings).

Allergic symptoms include urticaria; angioneurotic edema; laryngospasm; bronchospasm; hypotension; vascular collapse; death; maculopapular to exfoliative dermatitis; vesicular eruptions; erythema multiforme (rarely, Stevens-Johnson syndrome); reactions resembling serum sickness (chills, fever, edema, arthralgia, arthritis, malaise); laryngeal edema; skin rashes; prostration; allergic vasculitis; pruritus; asthenia; pain, headache.

►*Local:* Pain (accompanied by induration) at the site of injection; ecchymosis; deep vein thrombosis; hematomas; atrophy; skin ulcer; neurovascular reactions including warmth, vasospasm, pallor, mottling, gangrene, numbness of the extremities, cyanosis of the extremities and neurovascular damage. Vein irritation and phlebitis can occur, particularly when undiluted solution is injected directly into the vein. Tissue necrosis due to extravasated **nafcillin** has been successfully modified with hyaluronidase.

►*Renal:* Interstitial nephritis (eg, oliguria, proteinuria, hematuria, hyaline casts, pyuria) and nephropathy are infrequent and usually associated with high doses of parenteral penicillins; however, this has occurred with all of the penicillins. Such reactions are hypersensitivity responses and are usually associated with fever, skin rash and eosinophilia. Elevations of creatinine or BUN may occur.

►*Miscellaneous:* Anorexia; joint disorder; periostitis; myoglobinuria; rhabdomyolysis; exacerbation of arthritis; hypoxia; apnea; dyspnea; diaphoresis; blurred vision; blindness; hyperthermia; itchy eyes, transient hepatitis and cholestatic jaundice (rare); sciatic neuritis caused by IM injection of penicillin. The Jarisch-Herxheimer reaction has been reported in the treatment of syphilis.

►*Lab test abnormalities:* Elevations of AST, ALT, bilirubin and LDH have been noted in patients receiving semisynthetic penicillins (particularly **oxacillin** and **cloxacillin**); such reactions are more common in infants. Elevations of serum alkaline phosphatase and hypernatremia, and reduction in serum potassium, albumin, total proteins and uric acid may occur. Decreased hemoglobin, hematocrit, RBC, WBC, neutrophils, lymphocytes, platelets and increased lymphocytes, monocytes, basophils, eosinophils and platelets; increased BUN and creatinine; presence of RBCs and hyaline casts in urine (**ampicillin sodium and sulbactam sodium**). Evidence indicates glutamic oxaloacetic transaminase (GOT) is released at the site of IM injection of **ampicillin**. Increased amounts of this enzyme in the blood do not necessarily indicate liver involvement.

Hemorrhagic manifestations associated with abnormalities of coagulation tests such as clotting and prothrombin time have occurred and are more likely to occur in patients with renal failure (see Warnings).

Overdosage

Penicillin overdosage can result in neuromuscular hyperexcitability or convulsive seizures. Dose-related toxicity may arise with the use of massive doses of IV penicillins (40 to 100 million units/day), particularly in patients with severe renal impairment. Manifestations may include agitation, confusion, asterixis, hallucinations, stupor, coma, multifocal myoclonus, seizures and encephalopathy. Hyperkalemia is also possible.

In case of overdosage, discontinue penicillin, treat symptomatically and institute supportive measures as required. Refer to General Management of Acute Overdosage. If necessary, hemodialysis may be used to reduce blood levels of **penicillin**, although the degree of effectiveness of this procedure is questionable. Hemodialysis does not accelerate the rate of clearance of **nafcillin** from the blood. The metabolic by-products of **carbenicillin indanyl sodium**, **indanyl sulfate** and **glucuronide**, as well as free **carbenicillin**, are dialyzable. In renal function impairment, aminopenicillins can be removed by hemodialysis, but not peritoneal dialysis. The molecular weight, degree of protein binding and pharmacokinetic profile of **sulbactam** and **clavulanic acid** suggest these compounds may also be removed by hemodialysis.

Patient Information

Complete full course of therapy.

Take on an empty stomach 1 hour before or 2 hours after meals. Absorption of penicillin V, amoxicillin, bacampicillin tablets and amoxicillin/potassium clavulanate is not significantly affected by food.

Take each oral cloxacillin dose with a full glass of water. Do not take with fruit juice or a carbonated beverage.

Take at even intervals, preferably around the clock.

Notify physician if skin rash, itching, hives, severe diarrhea, shortness of breath, wheezing, black tongue, sore thoat, nausea, vomiting, fever, swollen joints or any unusual bleeding or bruising occurs.

Discard any liquid forms of **penicillin** after 7 days if stored at room temperature or after 14 days if refrigerated.

Natural Penicillins

PENICILLIN G (AQUEOUS)

Rx	**Penicillin G Potassium** (Baxter)	**Injection, premixed, frozen:** 1,000,000 units	In 50 mL Galaxy containers.
		2,000,000 units	In 50 mL Galaxy containers.
		3,000,000 units	In 50 mL Galaxy containers.
Rx	**Pfizerpen** (Pfizer)	**Powder for Injection:** 1,000,000 units	≈ 6.8 mg sodium (0.3 mEq), 65.6 mg potassium (1.68 mEq)/million units. In vials.
		Powder for Injection: 5,000,000 units	≈ 6.8 mg sodium (0.3 mEq), 65.6 mg potassium (1.68 mEq)/million units. In vials.
		Powder for Injection: 20,000,000 units per vial	≈ 6.8 mg sodium (0.3 mEq), 65.6 mg potassium (1.68 mEq)/million units. In vials.

For complete prescribing information, refer to the Penicillins group monograph.

Administration and Dosage

►*Infants:* Preferably administered IV as 15- to 30-minute infusions.

>*7 days old* – 75,000 units/kg/day in divided doses every 8 hours (meningitis – 200,000 to 300,000 units/kg/day every 6 hours).

< *7 days old* – 50,000 units/kg/day in divided doses every 12 hours; group B streptococcus – 100,000 units/kg/day; meningitis – 100,000 to 150,000 units/kg/day).

Streptococci in groups A, C, G, H, L and M are very sensitive to penicillin G. Some group D organisms are sensitive to the high serum levels obtained with aqueous penicillin G.

Penicillin G injection should be administered by IV infusion.

Natural Penicillins

PENICILLIN G (AQUEOUS)

Parenteral Penicillin G Use and Dosages in Adults	
Indications	Adult dosage
Labeled uses:	
Meningococcal meningitis/septicemia:	24 million units/day; 1 to 2 million units IM every 2 hours; or 20 to 30 million units/day continuous IV drip for 14 days or until afebrile for 7 days; or 200,000 to 300,000 units/kg/day every 2 to 4 hours in divided doses for a total of 24 doses
Actinomycosis:	
For cervicofacial cases	1 to 6 million units/day
For thoracic and abdominal disease	10 to 20 million units/day IV every 4 to 6 hours for 6 weeks. May be followed by oral penicillin V, 500 mg 4 times daily for 2 to 3 months
Clostridial infections: Botulism (adjunctive therapy to antitoxin), gas gangrene and tetanus (adjunctive therapy to human tetanus immune globulin)	20 million units/day every 4 to 6 hours as adjunct to antitoxin
Fusospirochetal infections: Severe infections of oropharynx, lower respiratory tract and genital area	5 to 10 million units/day every 4 to 6 hours
Rat-bite fever (Spirillum minus, Streptobacillus moniliformis), Haverhill fever:	12 to 20 million units/day every 4 to 6 hours for 3 to 4 weeks
Listeria infections (Listeria monocytogenes):	
Meningitis (adults)	15 to 20 million units/day every 4 to 6 hours for 2 weeks
Endocarditis (adults)	15 to 20 million units/day every 4 to 6 hours for 4 weeks
Pasteurella infections (Pasteurella multocida): Bacteremia and meningitis	4 to 6 million units/day every 4 to 6 hours for 2 weeks
Erysipeloid (Erysipelothrix rhusiopathiae): Endocarditis	12 to 20 million units/day every 4 to 6 hours for 4 to 6 weeks
Diphtheria: Adjunct to antitoxin to prevent carrier state	2 to 3 million units/day in divided doses every 4 to 6 hours for 10 to 12 days
Anthrax: (B. anthracis is often resistant)	Minimum 5 million units/day; 12 to 20 million units/day have been used
Serious streptococcal infections (S. pneumoniae): Empyema, pneumonia, pericarditis, endocarditis, meningitis	5 to 24 million units/day in divided doses every 4 to 6 hours
Syphilis:[1] Neurosyphilis[1]	18 to 24 million units/day IV (3 to 4 million units every 4 hours) for 10 to 14 days. Many recommend benzathine penicillin G 2.4 million units IM weekly for 3 weeks following the completion of this regimen
Disseminated gonococcal infections: (eg, meningitis, endocarditis, arthritis)	10 million units/day every 4 to 6 hours, with the exception of meningococcal meningitis/septicemia, ie, every 2 hours
Unlabeled uses:	
Lyme disease (Borrelia burgdorferi):	
Erythema chronicum migrans	Use oral penicillin V
Neurologic complications (eg, meningitis, encephalitis)	200,000 to 300,000 units/kg/day (up to 20 million units) IV for 10 to 14 days
Carditis	200,000 to 300,000 units/kg/day (up to 20 million units) IV for 10 days with cardiac monitoring and a temporary pacemaker for complete heart block
Arthritis	200,000 to 300,000 units/kg/day (up to 20 million units) IV for 10 to 20 days

[1] CDC 1998 Sexually Transmitted Diseases Treatment Guidelines. *Morbidity and Mortality Weekly Report* 1997 Jan 23;47 (No. RR-1):1-118.

Parenteral Penicillin G Use and Dosages in Children	
Indications	Pediatric dosage
Serious streptococcal infections, such as pneumonia and endocarditis (*S. pneumoniae*) and meningococcus:	150,000 units/kg/day divided in equal doses every 4 to 6 hours; duration depends on infecting organism and type of infection
Meningitis caused by susceptible strains of pneumococcus and meningococcus:	250,000 units/kg/day divided in equal doses every 4 hours for 7 to 14 days depending on the infecting organism (maximum dose of 12 to 20 million units/day)
Disseminated gonococcal infections (penicillin-susceptible strains):	*Weight < 45 kg:*
Arthritis	100,000 units/kg/day in 4 equally divided doses for 7 to 10 days
Meningitis	250,000 units/kg/day in equal doses every 4 hours for 10 to 14 days
Endocarditis	250,000 units/kg/day in equal doses every 4 hours for 4 weeks
	Weight ≥ 45 kg:
Arthritis, meningitis, endocarditis	10 million units/day in 4 equally divided doses with the duration of therapy depending on the type of infection
Syphilis (congenital and neurosyphilis) after the newborn period:	200,000 to 300,000 units/kg/day (administered as 50,000 units/kg every 4 to 6 hours) for 10 to 14 days
Congenital syphilis:[1] Symptomatic or asymptomatic infants	*Infants:* 50,000 units/kg/dose IV every 12 hours the first 7 days, thereafter every 8 hours for total of 10 days. *Children:* 50,000 units/kg every 4 to 6 hours for 10 days.
Diphtheria (adjunctive therapy to antitoxin and for prevention of carrier state):	150,000 to 250,000 units/kg/day in equal doses every 6 hours for 7 to 10 days
Rat-bite fever; Haverhill fever (with endocarditis caused by S. moniliformis):	150,000 to 250,000 units/kg/day in equal doses every 4 hours for 4 weeks

[1] CDC 1998 Sexually Transmitted Diseases Treatment Guidelines. *Morbidity and Mortality Weekly Report* 1997 Jan 23;47 (No. RR-1):1-118.

▶*Renal impairment:* Penicillin G is relatively nontoxic and dosage adjustments are generally required only in cases of severe renal impairment. The recommended dosage regimen is as follows:

Creatinine clearance < 10 mL/min; administer a full loading dose followed by one-half of the loading dose every 8 to 10 hours.

Uremic patients with a creatinine clearance > 10 mL/min; administer a full loading dose followed by one-half of the loading dose every 4 to 5 hours.

Since alpha-hemolytic streptococci resistant to penicillin may be found when patients are receiving continuous oral penicillin for secondary

Natural Penicillins

PENICILLIN G (AQUEOUS)

prevention of rheumatic fever, prophylactic agents other than penicillin may be prescribed in addition to their continuous rheumatic fever prophylactic regimen.

Penicillin G potassium contains 1.7 mEq potassium and 0.3 mEq sodium per million units; penicillin G sodium contains 2 mEq sodium per million units.

Give recommended daily dosage IM or by continuous IV infusion.

➤*IM:* Keep total volume of injection small. The IM route is the preferred route of administration. Solutions containing ≤ 100,000 units/mL may be used with a minimum of discomfort. Use greater concentrations as required.

➤*Continuous IV infusion:* When larger doses are required, administer aqueous solutions by means of continuous IV infusion. Determine volume and rate of fluid administration required by the patient in a 24-hour period. Add appropriate daily dosage to this fluid.

➤*Intrapleural or other local infusion:* If fluid is aspirated, give infusion in a volume equal to one fourth or one half the amount of fluid aspirated; otherwise, prepare as for the IM injection.

➤*Intrathecal use:* Must be highly individualized. Use only with full consideration of the possible irritating effects of penicillin when used by this route. The preferred route of therapy in bacterial meningitis is IV, supplemented by IM injection. It has been suggested that intrathecal use has no place in therapy.

➤*Preparation of solutions:* Depending on the route of administration, use sterile water for injection, isotonic sodium chloride injection, or dextrose injection. Penicillins are rapidly inactivated in the presence of carbohydrate solutions at alkaline pH.

➤*Storage/Stability:* The dry powder is stable and does not require refrigeration. Sterile solutions may be kept in the refrigerator for 1 week without loss of potency. Solutions prepared for IV infusion are stable at room temperature for ≥ 24 hours.

Premixed, frozen solution – Thaw frozen container at room temperature (25°C; 77°F) or in a refrigerator (5°C; 41°F). Do not force thaw by immersion in water baths or by microwave irradiation.

The thawed solution is stable for 24 hours at room temperature or for 14 days under refrigeration. Do not refreeze thawed antibiotics.

PENICILLIN G PROCAINE, INJECTABLE

| *Rx* | **Penicillin G Procaine** (Monarch) | Injection: 600,000 units/vial | In 1 mL *Tubex.*[1] |
| | | Injection: 1,200,000 units/vial | In 2 mL *Tubex.*[1] |

[1] With parabens and povidone.

For complete prescribing information, refer to the Penicillins group monograph.

Indications

A long-acting parenteral penicillin (IM only) indicated in the treatment of moderately severe infections caused by penicillin G-sensitive microorganisms that are sensitive to low and persistent serum levels achievable with this dosage form. Therapy should be guided by bacteriological studies (including susceptibility tests) and by clinical response. When high sustained serum levels are required, use aqueous penicillin G (see individual monograph).

➤*Note:* This drug is no longer indicated in the treatment of gonorrhea.

Administration and Dosage

Administer by deep IM injection only into the upper outer quadrant of the buttock. In neonates, infants, and small children, the midlateral

aspect of the thigh may be preferable. When doses are repeated, rotate the injection site. Do not inject into or near an artery or nerve. Penicillin G procaine must never be used IV.

Streptococci in groups A, C, G, H, L, and M are very sensitive to penicillin G. Other groups, including group D (enterococci), are resistant. Use aqueous penicillin for streptococcal infections with bacteremia.

An increasing number of strains of staphylococci are resistant to penicillin G, emphasizing the need for culture and sensitivity studies.

➤*Newborns:* Avoid use in these patients because sterile abscesses and procaine toxicity are of much greater concern in newborns than in older children.

Severe pneumonia, empyema, bacteremia, pericarditis, meningitis, peritonitis, and arthritis of pneumococcal etiology are better treated with aqueous penicillin G during the acute stage.

Penicillin G Procaine Uses and Dosages	
Organisms/Infections	Dosage
Pneumococcal infections: Moderately severe upper respiratory tract infections	*Adults:* 600,000 to 1 million units/day IM *Children (< 60 lbs, 27 kg):* 300,000 units/day IM
Streptococcal infections (group A): Moderately severe to severe tonsillitis, erysipelas, scarlet fever, upper respiratory tract, and skin and soft tissue infections	*Adults:* 600,000 to 1 million units/day IM for a minimum of 10 days *Children (< 60 lbs, 27 kg):* 300,000 units/day IM
Bacterial endocarditis – Only in extremely sensitive infections (Group A streptococci)	600,000 to 1 million units/day IM
Staphylococcal infections: Moderately severe infections of the skin and soft tissue	*Adults:* 600,000 to 1 million units/day IM *Children (< 60 lbs, 27 kg):* 300,000 units/day
Diphtheria: Adjunctive therapy with antitoxin	300,000 to 600,000 units/day IM for 14 days.
Carrier state	300,000 units/day IM for 10 days
Anthrax: Cutaneous	600,000 to 1 million units/day IM. Continue prophylaxis until exposure to *Bacillus anthracis* has been excluded. If exposure is confirmed and vaccine is available, continue prophylaxis for 4 weeks and until 3 doses of vaccine have been administered, or for 30 to 60 days if vaccine is not available.
Vincent's gingivitis and pharyngitis (fusospirochetosis)	600,000 to 1 million units/day IM. Obtain necessary dental care in infections involving gum tissue.
Erysipeloid	600,000 to 1 million units/day IM
Rat-bite fever (Streptobacillus moniliformis and Spirillum minus)	600,000 to 1 million units/day IM
Syphilis: Primary, secondary, and latent with a negative spinal fluid (adults and children > 12 years of age)	600,000 units/day IM for 8 days; total, 4.8 million units
Late (tertiary, neurosyphilis, and latent syphilis with positive spinal fluid examination or no spinal fluid examination)	600,000 units/day IM for 10 to 15 days; total, 6 to 9 million units
Neurosyphilis[1] (as an alternative to the recommended regimen of penicillin G aqueous)	2.4 million units/day IM plus probenecid 500 mg orally 4 times/day, both for 10 to 14 days; many recommend benzathine penicillin G 2.4 million/units IM following the completion of this regimen
Congenital syphilis[1]	*Children < 70 lb (32 kg):* 50,000 units/kg/day (administered as a single IM dose) for 10 to 14 days.
Yaws, bejel, and pinta	Treat same as syphilis in corresponding stage of disease

[1] CDC 2002 Sexually Transmitted Diseases Treatment Guidelines. *MMWR Morbid Mortal Wkly Rept.* 2002;51(RR-6):1-82.

Inspect parenteral drug products visually for particulate matter and discoloration prior to administration whenever solution and container permit.

➤*Storage/Stability:* Store in the refrigerator (2° to 8°C; 36° to 46°F). Keep from freezing.

Natural Penicillins

PENICILLIN G BENZATHINE, INTRAMUSCULAR

Rx	**Bicillin L-A** (Monarch)	Injection: 600,000 units/dose	In 1 mL *Tubex.*[1]
		1,200,000 units/dose	In 2 mL *Tubex.*[1]
		2,400,000 units/dose	In 4 mL prefilled syringe.[1]
Rx	**Permapen** (Roerig)	Injection: 1,200,000 units/dose	In 2 mL *Isoject.*[2]

[1] With povidone and parabens.

[2] With polyvinylpyrrolidone and parabens.

For complete prescribing information, refer to the Penicillins group monograph.

Indications

Treatment of infections caused by penicillin-G-sensitive microorganisms that are susceptible to the low and very prolonged serum levels common to this particular dosage form.

When high sustained serum levels are required, use injectable penicillin G, either IM or IV.

➤*Upper respiratory tract infection (mild to moderate):* Caused by susceptible streptococci.

➤*Venereal diseases:* Syphilis, yaws, bejel, and pinta.

➤*Prophylaxis of rheumatic fever or chorea:* Use of penicillin G benzathine has proven effective in preventing recurrence of these conditions. It also has been used as follow-up prophylactic therapy for rheumatic heart disease and acute glomerulonephritis.

Administration and Dosage

Shake well before using.

➤*For IM use only:* Do not administer IV.

➤*Administer by deep IM injection:* Administer in the upper outer quadrant of the buttock. Do not inject into or near an artery or nerve. Because of the high concentration of suspended material in this product, the needle may be blocked if the injection is not made at a slow, steady rate. In neonates, infants, and small children, the midlateral aspect of the thigh may be preferable. When doses are repeated, rotate the injection site. Do not administer IV.

Penicillin G Benzathine Uses and Dosages	
Organisms/Infections	Dosage
Streptococcal (group A): Upper respiratory tract infections	*Adults:* 1.2 million units IM as a single injection *Older children:* 900,000 units IM as a single injection *Infants and children (< 60 lbs; 27 kg):* 300,000 to 600,000 units
Syphilis:[1] 　*Early syphilis* - Primary, secondary, or latent syphilis	*Adults:* 2.4 million units IM in single dose *Children:* 50,000 units/kg IM, up to adult dosage
Gummas and cardiovascular syphilis[1] - Latent	*Adults:* 2.4 million units IM once weekly for 3 weeks *Children:* 50,000 units/kg IM, up to adult dosage
Neurosyphilis[1]	Aqueous penicillin G, 18 to 24 million units/day IV (3 to 4 million units every 4 hours) for 10 to 14 days. Many recommend benzathine penicillin G, 2.4 million IM units once/week for up to 3 weeks following completion of this regimen. or Procaine penicillin G, 2.4 million units/day IM *plus* probenecid 500 mg orally 4 times daily, both for 10 to 14 days. Many recommend benzathine penicillin G, 2.4 million units IM once/week for up to 3 weeks following completion of this regimen.
Syphilis in pregnancy[1]	Dosage schedule appropriate for stage of syphilis recommended for nonpregnant patients.
Congenital syphilis	*Children < 2 years of age:* 50,000 units/kg/body weight *Children 2 to 12 years of age:* Adjust dosage based on adult dosage schedule.
Yaws, bejel, and pinta	1.2 million units IM in a single dose
Prophylaxis for rheumatic fever and glomerulonephritis	Following an acute attack, may be given IM in doses of 1.2 million units once a month or 600,000 units every 2 weeks

[1] CDC 2002 Sexually Transmitted Diseases Treatment Guidelines. *MMWR Morbid Mortal Wkly Rept.* 2002;51(RR-6):1-82.

➤*Storage/Stability* Refrigerate at 2° to 8°C (36° to 46°F); avoid freezing.

PENICILLIN G BENZATHINE AND PROCAINE COMBINED, INTRAMUSCULAR

Rx	**Bicillin C-R** (Monarch)	600,000 units/dose (300,000 units each penicillin G benzathine and penicillin G procaine)	In 1 mL *Tubex.*[1]
		1,200,000 units/dose (600,000 units each penicillin G benzathine and penicillin G procaine)	In 2 mL *Tubex.*[1]
		2,400,000 units/dose (1,200,000 units each penicillin G benzathine and penicillin G procaine)	In 4 mL syringe.[1]
Rx	**Bicillin C-R 900/300** (Monarch)	Injection: 1,200,000 units/dose (900,000 units penicillin G benzathine and 300,000 units penicillin G procaine)	In 2 mL *Tubex.*[1]

[1] With parabens, lecithin and povidone.

For complete prescribing information, refer to the Penicillins group monograph.

Indications

Treatment of moderately severe infections caused by microorganisms that are susceptible to the serum levels of penicillin G achievable with this dosage form. Guide therapy by bacteriological studies and clinical response. When high, sustained serum levels are required, use IV or IM aqueous penicillin G (potassium or sodium). Do not use this drug in the treatment of venereal diseases, including syphilis and gonorrhea or yaws, bejel, and pinta. The following infections usually will respond to adequate doses of this drug:

➤*Streptococcal infections:* Moderately severe to severe infections of the upper respiratory tract, skin and soft tissue infections, scarlet fever, and erysipelas.

➤*Pneumococcal infections:* Moderately severe pneumonia and otitis media.

Administration and Dosage

For IM injection only. Do not inject into or near an artery or nerve, or IV, or admix with other IV solutions.

➤*Administer by deep IM injection:* Administer in the upper outer quadrant of the buttock. In infants, neonates, and small children, the midlateral aspect of the thigh may be preferable. When doses are repeated, rotate the injection site. Discontinue delivery of the dose if the subject complains of severe immediate pain at the injection site. Because of the high concentration of suspended material in this product, the needle may be blocked if the injection is not made at a slow, steady state. Do not administer IV.

➤*Streptococcal infections:* Streptococci in groups A, C, G, H, L, and M are very sensitive to penicillin G. Other groups, including group D (enterococci), are resistant. Penicillin G sodium or potassium is recommended for streptococcal infections with bacteremia.

Treatment with the recommended dosage is usually given in a single session using multiple IM sites when indicated. An alternative dosage schedule may be used, giving half the total dose on day 1 and half on day 3. This will also ensure adequate serum levels over a 10-day period; however, use only when the patient's cooperation can be ensured.

Adults and children (more than 60 lbs; 27 kg) – 2.4 million units IM.

Children (30 to 60 lbs; 14 to 27 kg) – 900,000 to 1.2 million units IM.

Infants and children (less than 30 lbs; 14 kg) – 600,000 units IM.

Natural Penicillins

PENICILLIN G BENZATHINE AND PROCAINE COMBINED, INTRAMUSCULAR

➤*Pneumococcal infections (except pneumococcal meningitis):* Repeat every 2 or 3 days until the patient has been afebrile for 48 hours. Severe pneumonia, empyema, bacteremia, pericarditis, meningitis, peritonitis, and arthritis of pneumococcal etiology are better treated with aqueous penicillin G during the acute stage.

Children – 600,000 units IM.

Adults – 1.2 million units IM.

➤*Storage/Stability:* Refrigerate at 2° to 8°C (36° to 46°F). Protect from freezing.

PENICILLIN V (Phenoxymethyl Penicillin)

Rx	Penicillin VK (Various, eg, Teva)	Tablets: 250 mg	In 100s, and 1000s.
Rx	Veetids (Geneva)		Lactose. (BL V1). White. Film-coated. In 100s and 1000s.
Rx	Penicillin VK (Various, eg, Teva)	Tablets: 500 mg	In 100s and 500s.
Rx	Veetids (Geneva)		Lactose. (BL V2). White. Film-coated. In 100s and 1000s.
Rx	Penicillin VK (Various, eg, Teva)	Powder for Oral Solution: 125 mg/5 mL when reconstituted	In 100 and 200 mL.
Rx	Veetids (Geneva)		DL-menthol, saccharin, sucrose. In 100 and 200 mL.
Rx	Penicillin VK (Various, eg, Teva)	Powder for Oral Solution: 250 mg/5 mL when reconstituted	In 100 and 200 mL.
Rx	Veetids (Geneva)		DL-menthol, saccharin, sucrose. In 100 and 200 mL.

For complete prescribing information, refer to the Penicillins group monograph.

Indications

Treatment of infections caused by susceptible strains of the designated organisms in the conditions listed below:

➤*Streptococcal infections (mild to moderately severe):* Those of the upper respiratory tract, including scarlet fever and mild erysipelas.

➤*Pneumococcal infections (mild to moderately severe):* Those of the respiratory tract, including otitis media.

➤*Staphylococcal infections (mild):* Those of skin and soft tissue.

➤*Fusospirochetosis (Vincent's gingivitis and pharyngitis; mild to moderately severe):* Those of the oropharynx.

➤*For prevention:* To prevent recurrence following rheumatic fever or chorea.

Administration and Dosage

250 mg = 400,000 units.

Do not treat severe pneumonia, empyema, bacteremia, pericarditis, meningitis, and arthritis with oral penicillin V during the acute stage.

Streptococci in groups A, C, G, H, L and M are very sensitive to penicillin. Other groups, including group D (enterococci), are resistant.

An increasing number of strains of staphylococci are resistant to penicillin, emphasizing the need for culture and susceptibility studies.

Penicillin V Uses and Dosages for Adults and Children > 12 Years of Age	
Organisms/Infections	Dosage
Labeled uses:	
Streptococcal infections: Mild to moderately severe infections of the upper respiratory tract, including scarlet fever and mild erysipelas	125 to 250 mg orally every 6 to 8 hours for 10 days
Pharyngitis in children	25 to 50 mg/kg/day divided every 6 hours for 10 days
Pneumococcal infections: Mild to moderately severe respiratory tract infections including otitis media	250 to 500 mg orally every 6 hours until afebrile at least 2 days
Staphylococcal infections: Mild infections of skin and soft tissue	250 to 500 mg orally every 6 to 8 hours
Fusospirochetosis (Vincent's infection) of the oropharynx: Mild to moderately severe infections	250 to 500 mg orally every 6 to 8 hours
For prevention of recurrence following rheumatic fever or chorea	125 to 250 mg orally 2 times/day on a continuing basis
Unlabeled uses:	
Prophylactic treatment of children with sickle cell anemia or splenectomy: To reduce the incidence of S. pneumoniae septicemia	3 months to 5 years of age: 125 mg orally 2 times/day > 5 years of age: 250 mg BID
Actinomycosis	Penicillin G 10 to 20 mg/day IV for 4 to 6 week, then Penicillin V 2 to 4 g/day for 6 to 12 months
Early Lyme disease (Borrelia burgdorferi): Erythema migrans	500 mg orally 4 times a day for 10 to 20 days
Anthrax: Postexposure prophylaxis - Confirmed or suspected exposure to Bacillus anthracis	Adults: 7.5 mg/kg orally 4 times/day Children < 9 years of age: 50 mg/kg/day orally divided 4 times/day Continue prophylaxis until exposure to B. anthracis has been excluded. If exposure is confirmed and vaccine is available, continue prophylaxis for 4 weeks and until 3 doses of vaccine have been administered or for 30 to 60 days if vaccine if not available.

➤*Mixing oral solutions:* Prepare solution at time of dispensing as follows: Tap bottle until all powder flows freely. Add about one half of the total amount of water for reconstitution and shake well to wet powder. Add the remainder of the water and shake well again.

➤*Storage/Stability:* Reconstituted oral solution must be stored in refrigerator. Discard unused portion after 14 days.

Penicillinase-Resistant Penicillins

NAFCILLIN SODIUM

Rx	Nafcillin Injection (Baxter)	Injection: 1 g (as base)	In 50 mL single-dose *Galaxy* bags.
		2 g (as base)	In 100 mL in single-dose *Galaxy* bags.

For complete prescribing information, refer to the Penicillins group monograph.

Indications

Treatment of infections caused by penicillinase-producing staphylococci that have demonstrated susceptibility to the drug.

May be used to initiate therapy in suspected cases of resistant staphylococcal infections prior to the availability of susceptibility test results. Do not use in infections caused by organisms susceptible to penicillin G. If the susceptibility tests indicate that the infection is due to an organism other than a resistant *Staphylococcus*, do not continue therapy.

Nafcillin-probenecid therapy is generally limited to those infections where very high serum levels of nafcillin are necessary.

Administration and Dosage

➤*Dose:* The usual IV dosage for adults is 500 mg every 4 hours. For severe infections, 1 g every 4 hours is recommended.

➤*Administration:* Administer slowly over at least 30 to 60 minutes to minimize the risk of vein irritation and extravasation.

➤*Duration:* Duration of therapy varies with the type and severity of infection as well as the overall condition of the patient; therefore, determine duration by the clinical and bacteriological response of the patient. In severe staphylococcal infections, continue nafcillin therapy for at least 14 days. Continue therapy for at least 48 hours after the patient has become afebrile, and asymptomatic and cultures are negative. The treatment of endocarditis and osteomyelitis may require a longer duration of therapy.

NAFCILLIN SODIUM

▶*Solution:* Thaw frozen container at room temperature (25°C or 77°F) or under refrigeration (5°C or 41°F). Do not force thaw by immersion in water baths or by microwave irradiation.

Components of the solution may precipitate in the frozen state and will dissolve upon reaching room temperature with little or no agitation. Agitate after solution has reached room temperature. If after visual inspection the solution remains cloudy or if an insoluble precipitate is noted or if any seals or outlet ports are not intact, discard the container.

▶*Caution:* Do not use plastic containers in series connections. Such use could result in air embolism because of residual air being drawn

from the primary container before administration of the fluid from the secondary container is complete.

▶*Hepatic/Renal function impairment:* For patients with hepatic insufficiency and renal failure, measure nafcillin serum levels and adjust dosage accordingly.

▶*Elderly:* With IV administration, particularly in elderly patients, take care because of the possibility of thrombophlebitis.

▶*Other medication:* Do not add supplementary medication to nafcillin injection.

▶*Storage/Stability:* Store at or below −20°C (−4°F). The thawed 1 and 2 g solutions are stable for 21 days under refrigeration (5°C or 41°F) or 72 hours at room temperature (25°C or 77°F). Do not refreeze.

OXACILLIN SODIUM

Rx	Oxacillin Sodium (Various, eg, Geneva)	**Powder for Oral Solution:** 250 mg/5 mL when reconstituted	In 100 mL.
		Powder for Injection: 500 mg	In vials.
		Powder for Injection: 1 g	In vials, *ADD-Vantage* vials, and piggyback vials.
		Powder for Injection: 2 g	In vials, *ADD-Vantage* vials, and piggyback vials.
		Powder for Injection: 10 g	In bulk vials.

For complete prescribing information, refer to the Penicillins group monograph.

Indications

Treatment of infections caused by penicillinase-producing staphylococci. May be used to initiate therapy when a staphylococcal infection is suspected. (See Indications in the group monograph concerning use of penicillinase-resistant penicillins.)

Administration and Dosage

Treat serious or life-threatening infections, such as staphylococcal septicemia or other deep-seated severe infection, initially with parenteral

treatment; oral oxacillin may be given for follow-up therapy. Duration of therapy varies with the type and severity of infection as well as the overall condition of the patient. Therefore, it should be determined by the clinical and bacteriological response of the patient. In severe staphylococcal infections, continue therapy with penicillinase-resistant penicillins for at least 14 days. Continue therapy for at least 48 hours after the patient has become afebrile and asymptomatic and cultures are negative. The treatment of endocarditis and osteomyelitis may require a longer term of therapy.

Oxacillin Dosage		
	Adults	Children (< 40 kg)
Oral		
Mild to moderate infection	500 mg every 4 to 6 hours	50 mg/kg/day in equally divided doses every 6 hours
Severe infection	1 g every 4 to 6 hours (following parenteral therapy)	100 mg/kg/day in equally divided doses every 4 to 6 hours (following parenteral therapy)
Parenteral (IM or IV)		
Mild to moderate infection	250 to 500 mg IM or IV every 4 to 6 hours	50 mg/kg/day IM or IV in equally divided doses every 6 hours
Severe infection	1 g IM or IV every 4 to 6 hours	100 mg/kg/day IM or IV in equally divided doses every 4 to 6 hours. **Premature/neonates:** 25 mg/kg/day IM or IV

Inject slowly IV over a period of approximately 10 minutes.

▶*Preparation of solution:*

IM use – Use sterile water for injection. Add 1.4 mL to the 250 mg vial, 2.7 mL to the 500 mg vial, 5.7 mL to the 1 g vial, 11.5 mL to the 2 g vial, and 23 mL to the 4 g vial. Shake well until a clear solution is obtained. After reconstitution, vials will contain 250 mg of active drug per 1.5 mL of solution. The reconstituted solution is stable for 3 days at 21°C (70°F) or for 1 week under refrigeration (4°C; 40°F).

Direct IV use – Use sterile water for injection or sodium chloride for injection. Add 5 mL to the 250 mg and 500 mg vials, 10 mL to the 1 g vial, 20 mL to the 2 g vial, and 40 mL to the 4 g vial. Withdraw the

entire contents and administer slowly over a period of approximately 10 minutes.

IV drip – Reconstitute as directed above (for direct IV use) prior to diluting with IV solution.

Admixture incompatibility – If another agent is used in conjunction with oxacillin therapy, do not physically mix it with oxacillin; administer it separately.

▶*Storage/Stability:* The reconstituted oral solution is stable for 3 days at room temperature or 14 days under refrigeration.

Stability Periods for Oxacillin Sodium for Injection									
	Concentrations at room temperature (25°C)			Concentrations under refrigeration (4°C)		Concentrations frozen (−15°C)			
Solution	10 to 100 mg/mL	10 to 30 mg/mL	0.5 to 2 mg/mL	10 to 100 mg/mL	10 to 30 mg/mL	50 to 100 mg/mL	250 mg/ 1.5 mL	100 mg/mL	10 to 100 mg/mL
Sterile water for injection	4 days			7 days		30 days	30 days		
Isotonic NaCl	4 days			7 days				30 days	
M/6 molar sodium lactate solution		24 hr			4 days				30 days
5% dextrose in water			6 hr		4 days				30 days
5% dextrose in 0.45% NaCl		24 hr			4 days				30 days
10% invert sugar			6 hr		4 days				30 days
Lactated Ringer's solution			6 hr		4 days				30 days

Penicillinase-Resistant Penicillins

DICLOXACILLIN SODIUM

Rx	Dicloxacillin Sodium (Various, eg, Teva)	**Capsules:** 250 mg	In 40s, 100s, 500s, and UD 100s.
		500 mg	In 30s, 40s, 50s, 100s, 500s, and UD 100s.

For complete prescribing information, refer to the Penicillins group monograph.

Indications

Treatment of infections caused by penicillinase-producing staphylococci. May be used to initiate therapy when a staphylococcal infection is suspected (see Indications in the group monograph concerning use of penicillinase-resistant penicillins).

Administration and Dosage

Dicloxacillin sodium is best absorbed when taken on an empty stomach, preferably 1 to 2 hours before meals.

Recommended Dosages for Dicloxacillin in Mild to Moderate and Severe Infections			
Adults		Children	
Mild to moderate	Severe	Mild to moderate	Severe
125 mg every 6 hours	250 mg every 6 hours	12.5 mg/kg/day[1] in equally divided doses every 6 hours	25 mg/kg/day[1] in equally divided doses every 6 hours.

[1] Patients weighing less than 40 kg (88 lbs).

In severe staphylococcal infections, continue therapy with penicillinase-resistant penicillins for at least 14 days. Continue therapy for at least 48 hours after the patient has become afebrile and asymptomatic and cultures are negative. The treatment of endocarditis and osteomyelitis may require a longer term of therapy.

Treat infections caused by Group A beta-hemolytic streptococci for at least 10 days to help prevent the occurrence of acute rheumatic fever or acute glomerulonephritis.

Penicillin-probenecid therapy generally is limited to those infections where very high serum levels of penicillin are necessary. Do not use oral preparations of the penicillinase-resistant penicillins as initial therapy in serious, life-threatening infections.

Aminopenicillins

AMPICILLIN

Rx	Ampicillin (Various, eg, Teva)	**Capsules:** 250 mg (as trihydrate)	In 100s and 500s.
Rx	Principen (Geneva)		Lactose. (BRISTOL 7992). Lt. gray/scarlet. In 100s, 500s, and UD 100s.
Rx	Ampicillin (Various, eg, Teva)	**Capsules:** 500 mg (as trihydrate)	In 100s and 500s.
Rx	Principen (Geneva)		Lactose. (BRISTOL 7993). Lt. gray/scarlet. In 100s, 500s, and UD 100s.
Rx	Principen (Geneva)	**Powder for Oral Suspension:** 125 mg/5 mL (as trihydrate) when reconstituted	Sucrose. Fruit flavor. In 100, 150, and 200 mL.
Rx	Principen (Geneva)	**Powder for Oral Suspension:** 250 mg/5 mL (as trihydrate) when reconstituted	Sucrose. Fruit flavor. In 100 and 200 mL.
Rx	Ampicillin Sodium (Various, eg, APP, Geneva)	**Powder for Injection:**[1] 250 mg	In vials.
Rx	Ampicillin Sodium (Various, eg, APP, Geneva)	**Powder for Injection:**[1] 500 mg	In vials.
Rx	Ampicillin Sodium (Various, eg, APP)	**Powder for Injection:**[1] 1 g	In vials.
Rx	Ampicillin Sodium (Various, eg, APP)	**Powder for Injection:**[1] 2 g	In vials.

[1] Contains approximately 2.9 mEq of sodium/g.

For complete prescribing information, refer to the Penicillins group monograph.

Indications

Ampicillin is indicated in the treatment of infections caused by susceptible strains of the designated organisms listed below:

➤*Respiratory tract:* For infections caused by nonpenicillinase-producing *Haemophilus influenzae*, penicillinase (injection only) and non-penicillinase-producing staphylococci, and streptococci including *Streptococcus pneumoniae*.

➤*GI tract:* For infections caused by *Shigella*, *Salmonella typhosa* and other *Salmonella*, *Escherichia coli*, *Proteus mirabilis*, and enterococci.

➤*GU tract:* For infections caused by *E. coli*, *P. mirabilis*, enterococci, *Shigella*, *S. typhosa* and other *Salmonella*, and nonpenicillinase-producing *Neisseria gonorrhoeae*.

➤*Bacterial meningitis (injection only):* For infections caused by *Neisseria meningitides*, *E. coli*, Group B streptococci, and *Listeria monocytogenes*. Note: The addition of an aminoglycoside with ampicillin may increase its effectiveness against gram-negative bacteria.

➤*Septicemia and endocarditis (injection only):* For infections caused by *Streptococcus* sp., penicillin G susceptible staphylococci, enterococci, *E. coli*, *P. mirabilis*, and *Salmonella* sp. Note: The addition of an aminoglycoside may enhance the effectiveness of ampicillin when treating streptococcal endocarditis.

Administration and Dosage

Reserve parenteral form (IM or IV) for moderately severe and severe infections and for patients unable to take oral medication. Change to oral therapy as soon as appropriate. Take capsules and oral solution 30 minutes before or 2 hours after meals to maximize absorption.

Larger doses may be required for severe or chronic infections. Except for the single dose regimen for gonorrhea, continue therapy for a minimum of 48 to 72 hours after the patient becomes asymptomatic or evidence of bacterial eradication has been obtained. In infections caused by hemolytic strains of streptococci, a minimum of 10 days of treatment is recommended to guard against the risk of rheumatic fever or glomerulonephritis. In the treatment of chronic urinary or GI infections, frequent bacteriologic and clinical appraisal is necessary during therapy and may be necessary for several months afterwards. Stubborn infections may require treatment for several weeks. Smaller doses than those indicated should not be used.

In the treatment of complications of gonorrheal urethritis, such as prostatitis and epididymitis, prolonged and intensive therapy is recommended. Cases of gonorrhea with a suspected primary lesion of syphilis should have dark-field examinations before receiving treatment. In all other cases where concomitant syphilis is suspected, perform monthly serologic tests for a minimum of 4 months.

➤*Renal function impairment:* Increase dosing interval to 6 to 12 hours in moderate renal impairment (Ccr 10 to 50 mL/min) and 12 to 24 hours in severe renal impairment (Ccr less than 10 mL/min).

Ampicillin Uses and Dosages	
Organisms/Infections	Dosage
Labeled uses:	
Enterococcal endocarditis	12 g/day IV either continuously or in equally divided doses every 4 hours plus 1 mg/kg IM or IV gentamicin every 8 hours for 4 to 6 weeks.
Respiratory tract and soft tissue infections	*Parenteral:* Patients ≥ 40 kg – 250 to 500 mg every 6 hours; < 40 kg – 25 to 50 mg/kg/day in equally divided doses at 6- to 8-hour intervals
	Oral: Patients> 20 kg – 250 mg every 6 hours; ≤ 20 kg – 50 mg/kg/day in equally divided doses at 6- to 8-hour intervals
Bacterial meningitis	Adults/Children: 150 to 200 mg/kg/day in equally divided doses every 3 to 4 hours. Initial treatment is usually by IV, followed by IM injections.

Aminopenicillins

AMPICILLIN

Ampicillin Uses and Dosages	
Organisms/Infections	Dosage
Septicemia:	Adults/Children: 150 to 200 mg/kg/day. Give IV at least 3 days; continue IM every 3 to 4 hours.
GI and GU infections: Other than *N. gonorrhoeae*[1]	*Oral:* Adults/Children> 20 kg - 500 mg orally every 6 hours. Use larger doses for severe or chronic infections, if needed. Children ≤ 20 kg - 100 mg/kg/day every 6 hours
N. gonorrhoeae	*Oral:* Single dose of 3.5 g administered simultaneously with 1 g probenecid *Parenteral:* Adults/children ≥ 40 kg - 500 mg IV or IM every 6 hours Children < 40 kg - 50 mg/kg/day IV or IM in equally divided doses at 6- to 8-hour intervals
Urethritis caused by *N. gonorrhoeae* in males	*Parenteral:* Adult males - Two 500 mg doses, IV or IM, at an interval of 8 to 12 hours. Treatment may be repeated if necessary or extended if required. In complicated gonorrheal urethritis (eg, prostatitis, epididymitis), prolonged and intensive therapy is recommended.
Unlabeled uses: *Prevention of bacterial endocarditis:*[2] For dental, oral or upper respiratory tract procedures in patients unable to take oral medications	2 g (50 mg/kg for children), both IM or IV 30 minutes prior to procedure
For GU/GI (excluding esophageal) procedures: High-risk	*Adults:* 2 g ampicillin IM/IV plus 1.5 mg/kg gentamicin 30 minutes prior to procedure; 6 hours later, ampicillin 1 g IM/IV or amoxicillin 1 g orally *Children:* Ampicillin 50 mg/kg (not to exceed 2 g) IM/IV plus gentamicin 1.5 mg/kg 30 minutes prior to procedure; 6 hours later, ampicillin 25 mg/kg IM/IV or amoxicillin 25 mg/kg orally
Moderate risk	*Adults:* Amoxicillin 2 g orally 1 hour before procedure, or ampicillin 2 g IM/IV within 30 minutes of starting the procedure. *Children:* Amoxicillin 50 mg/kg orally 1 hour before procedure, or ampicillin 50 mg/kg IM/IV within 30 minutes of starting the procedure.
Prophylaxis for neonatal Group B streptococcal disease: If culture positive or risk factors are present[2]	*During labor:* Give 2 g IV (load), then 1 g IV every 4 hour until delivery
Preterm, premature rupture of the membranes in Group B negative women	2 g IV every 6 hours plus erythromycin 250 mg IV every 8 hours for 48 hours; followed by amoxicillin 250 mg plus erythromycin base 333 mg every 8 hours orally for 5 days.

[1] Ampicillin is not included in the current (2002) CDC recommendations for the treatment of gonorrhea.

[2] Gilbert DN, Moellering Jr. RC, Sande MA. *The Sanford Guide to Antimicrobial Therapy.* 31 ed., 2001.

➤*Preparation of solutions:* Use only freshly prepared solutions. Administer IM and IV injections within 1 hour after preparation because the potency may decrease significantly after this period. Reconstitute with sterile or bacteriostatic water for injection.

For IM use – Dissolve contents of a vial with the amount of sterile water for injection or bacteriostatic water for injection listed in the table below:

Preparation of Ampicillin IM Solutions			
Vial strength	Diluent (mL)	Withdrawable volume (mL)	Concentration (mg/mL)
250 mg	0.9	1	250
500 mg	1.7	2	250
1 g	3.4	4	250
2 g	6.8	8	250

Direct IV administration – Add 5 mL sterile water for injection or bacteriostatic water for injection to the 250 and 500 mg vials and administer slowly over a 3 to 5 minute period. Ampicillin for injection 1 or 2 g also may be given by direct IV administration. Dissolve in 7.4 or 14.8 mL sterile water for injection or bacteriostatic water for injection, respectively. Administer slowly over at least 10 to 15 minutes.

Caution: More rapid administration may result in convulsive seizures.

IV drip – Dilute as above for direct IV use prior to further dilution with compatible IV solutions.

➤*Storage/Stability:*
Parenteral –

Stability of Ampicillin Infusion Solutions at Room Temperature (25°C; 77°F)		
IV solution	Concentrations up to (mg/mL)	Stability (h)
0.9% sodium chloride	30	8
5% dextrose in water	2	4
5% dextrose in water	10 to 20	2

Stability of Ampicillin Infusion Solutions at Room Temperature (25°C; 77°F)		
IV solution	Concentrations up to (mg/mL)	Stability (h)
5% dextrose in 0.45% sodium chloride solution	2	4
10% invert sugar in water	2	4
M/6 sodium lactate solution	30	8
Lactated Ringer's solution	30	8
Sterile water for injection	30	8

Stability of Ampicillin Infusion Solutions Refrigerated (4°C; 39°F)		
IV solution	Concentrations up to (mg/mL)	Stability (h)
Sterile water for injection	30	48
Sterile water for injection	20	72
0.9% sodium chloride	30	48
0.9% sodium chloride	20	72
Lactated Ringer's solution	30	24
M/6 sodium lactate solution	30	8
5% dextrose in water	20	4
5% dextrose in 0.45% NaCl	10	4
10% invert sugar	20	3

Stability studies on ampicillin sodium in various IV solutions indicate that the drug will lose less than 10% activity at the temperatures noted for the time periods and concentrations stated. tore powder for injection at controlled room temperature 15° to 30°C (59° to 80°F).

Oral – Store capsules at room temperature. Avoid excessive heat. Reconstituted oral solution is stable for 7 days at room temperature (not exceeding 25°C; 77°F) or 14 days refrigerated. Keep tightly closed.

AMPICILLIN SODIUM AND SULBACTAM SODIUM

Rx	**Ampicillin and Sulbactam** (ESI Lederle)	**Powder for injection:** 1.5 g (1 g ampicillin sodium/ 0.5 g sulbactam sodium)	In vials.
Rx	**Unasyn** (Roerig)		
Rx	**Ampicillin and Sulbactam** (ESI Lederle)	3 g (2 g ampicillin sodium/1 g sulbactam sodium)	In vials, bottles, and *ADD-Vantage* vials.
Rx	**Unasyn** (Roerig)		In vials.
Rx	**Unasyn** (Roerig)	15 g (10 g ampicillin sodium/5 g sulbactam sodium)	In vials, bottles, and *ADD-Vantage* vials.
			In bulk package.

For complete prescribing information, refer to the Penicillins group monograph.

Indications

For the treatment of infections caused by susceptible strains of the microorganisms in the conditions listed below.

➤*Skin and skin structure infections:* Those caused by β-lactamase-producing strains of *Staphylococcus aureus*, *Escherichia coli*†, *Klebsiella*† sp. (including *K. pneumoniae*†), *Proteus mirabilis*†, *Bacteroides fragilis*†, *Enterobacter*† sp. and *Acinetobacter calcoaceticus*†.

➤*Intra-abdominal infections:* Those caused by β-lactamase-producing strains of *E. coli*, *Klebsiella* sp. (including *K. pneumoniae*†), *Bacteroides* sp. (including *B. fragilis*), *Enterobacter*† sp.

➤*Gynecological infections:* Those caused by β-lactamase-producing strains of *E. coli*† and *Bacteroides* sp.† (including *B. fragilis*†).

While this combination is indicated only for the conditions listed above, infections caused by ampicillin-susceptible organisms also are amenable to treatment because of the ampicillin content. Therefore, mixed infections caused by ampicillin-susceptible organisms and β-lactamase-producing organisms susceptible to this combination should not require the addition of another antibiotic.

Administration and Dosage

Give IV or IM.

➤*Adult:* 1.5 g (1 g ampicillin + 0.5 g sulbactam) to 3 g (2 g ampicillin + 1 g sulbactam) every 6 hours. Do not exceed 4 g/day sulbactam.

➤*Children:* Do not routinely exceed 14 days of IV therapy. Safety and efficacy of IM administration have not been established.

Children 1 year of age or older – 300 mg/kg/day IV (200 mg ampicillin/100 mg sulbactam) in divided doses every 6 hours.

Children 40 kg or more – Dose according to adult recommendations; total sulbactam dose should not exceed 4 g/day.

The safety and efficacy of ampicillin/sulbactam sodium have been established for pediatric patients 1 year of age or older for skin and skin structure infections as approved in adults but have not been established for pediatric patients for intra-abdominal infections.

➤*Renal function impairment:* The elimination kinetics of ampicillin and sulbactam are similarly affected; hence, the ratio of one to the other will remain constant despite the renal function. In patients with renal impairment, administer as follows:

Ampicillin/Sulbactam Dosage Guide For Patients With Renal Impairment		
Ccr (mL/min/1.73 m^2)	Half-life (hours)	Recommended dosage
≥ 30	1	1.5 to 3 g q 6 to 8 h
15-29	5	1.5 to 3 g q 12 h
5-14	9	1.5 to 3 g q 24 h

➤*Preparation for IV use:* Reconstitute powder for IV and IM use with any of the compatible diluents described below. Allow solutions to stand after dissolution so that any foaming will dissipate. This permits visual inspection for complete solubilization.

1.5 and 3 g bottles – Reconstitute to desired concentrations (3 to 45 mg/mL) with any of the following diluents. Discard unused solutions after indicated times.

Preparation of Ampicillin/Sulbactam for IV Use		
Diluent	Maximum concentration (mg/mL)	Stability
Sterile water for injection	45 (30/15)	8h @ 25°C
	45 (30/15)	48 h @ 4°C
	30 (20/10)	72 h @ 4°C
0.9% sodium chloride injection	45 (30/15)	8h @ 25°C
	45 (30/15)	48 h @ 4°C
	30 (20/10)	72 h @ 4°C
5% dextrose injection	30 (20/10)	2h @ 25°C
	30 (20/10)	4 h @ 4°C
	3 (2/1)	4h @ 25°C
Lactated Ringer's injection	45 (30/15)	8 h @ 25°C
	45 (30/15)	24 h @ 4°C
M/6 sodium lactate injection	45 (30/15)	8 h @ 25°C
	45 (30/15)	8 h @ 4°C
5% dextrose in 0.45% saline	3 (2/1)	4 h @ 25°C
	15 (10/5)	4 h @ 4°C
10% invert sugar	3 (2/1)	4 h @ 25°C
	30 (20/10)	3 h @ 4°C

If piggyback bottles are unavailable, use standard vials of sterile powder. Initially, reconstitute with sterile water for injection to yield 375 mg/mL (250 mg ampicillin/125 mg sulbactam/mL). Then immediately dilute to yield 3 to 45 mg/mL (2 to 30 mg ampicillin/1 to 15 mg sulbactam/mL). Inject slowly over at least 10 to 15 minutes or infuse in greater dilutions with 50 to 100 mL diluent over 15 to 30 minutes.

The *ADD-Vantage* system is intended as single-dose for IV administration after dilution with the *ADD-Vantage Flexible Diluent Container* containing 50 mL (1.5 g vial only), 100 mL or 250 mL of 0.9% sodium chloride injection only. Once diluted, the solution is stable at a maximum concentration of 30 (20/10) mg/mL for 8 hours at 25°C, 77°F. Therefore, the final diluted soution should be completely administered within 8 hours to assure proper potency.

➤*Preparation for IM injection:* Reconstitute with sterile water for injection or 0.5% or 2% lidocaine HCl injection. Consult the following table for recommended volumes needed to obtain 375 mg/mL solutions (250 mg ampicillin/125 mg sulbactam/mL). Use only freshly prepared solutions; give within 1 hour after preparation.

Preparation of Ampicillin/Sulbactam for IM Use		
Vial size	Diluent to be added	Withdrawal volume
1.5 g	3.2 mL	4 mL
3 g	6.4 mL	8 mL

➤*Admixture incompatibility:* When concomitant aminoglycosides are indicated, reconstitute and administer this product and aminoglycosides separately; aminopenicillins inactivate aminoglycosides in vitro.

➤*Storage/Stability:* Store at or below 30°C (86°F) prior to reconstitution.

AMOXICILLIN

Rx	**Amoxicillin** (Various, eg, Ranbaxy, Teva)	**Tablets, chewable:** 125 mg (as trihydrate)	In 100s.
Rx	**Trimox** (Apothecon)		Mannitol, sucrose. (BMS37). Pink, flat-faced. In 60s.
Rx	**Amoxicillin** (Ranbaxy)	**Tablets, chewable:** 200 mg (as trihydrate)	In 20s.
Rx	**Amoxil** (GlaxoSmithKline)		Aspartame, 1.82 mg phenylalanine. (AMOXIL 200). Pale pink. Cherry-banana-peppermint flavor. In 20s and 100s.
Rx	**Amoxicillin** (Various, eg, Ranbaxy, Teva)	**Tablets, chewable:** 250 mg (as trihydrate)	In 100s, 250s, and 500s.
Rx	**Trimox** (Apothecon)		Mannitol, sucrose. (BMS 38). Pink, flat-faced. In 100s and 500s.
Rx	**Amoxicillin** (Ranbaxy)	**Tablets, chewable:** 400 mg (as trihydrate)	In 20s and 100s.
Rx	**Amoxil** (GlaxoSmithKline)		Aspartame, 3.64 mg phenylalanine. (AMOXIL 400). Pale pink. Cherry-banana-peppermint flavor. In 20s and 100s.

† Efficacy for these organisms in this organ system was studied in fewer than 10 infections.

AMOXICILLIN

Rx	**Amoxicillin** (Various, eg, Ranbaxy, Teva)	**Tablets:** 500 mg (as trihydrate)	In 20s and 100s.
Rx	**Amoxil** (GlaxoSmithKline)		(Amoxil 500). Pink, capsule shape. Film-coated. In 20s, 100s, and 500s.
Rx	**Amoxicillin** (Various, eg, Ranbaxy, Teva)	**Tablets:** 875 mg (as trihydrate)	In 20s, 100s, and 500s.
Rx	**Amoxil** (GlaxoSmithKline)		(Amoxil 875). Pink, capsule shape, scored. Film-coated. In 20s, 100s, 500s.
Rx	**Amoxicillin** (Various, eg, Ranbaxy, Teva)	**Capsules:** 250 mg (as trihydrate)	In 100s, 500s, and 1000s.
Rx	**Amoxil** (GlaxoSmithKline)		(Amoxil 250). Blue/Pink. In 500s.
Rx	**Trimox** (Apothecon)		(Bristol 7278). Flesh/Maroon. In 30s, 100s, 500s, and UD 100s.
Rx	**Amoxicillin** (Various, eg, Ranbaxy, Teva)	**Capsules:** 500 mg (as trihydrate)	In 50s, 100s, and 500s.
Rx	**Amoxil** (GlaxoSmithKline)		(Amoxil 500). Blue/Pink. In 500s.
Rx	**Trimox** (Apothecon)		(Bristol 7279). Flesh/Maroon. In 30s, 100s, 500s, and UD 100s.
Rx	**Amoxil Pediatric Drops** (GlaxoSmithKline)	**Powder for oral suspension:** 50 mg/mL (as trihydrate) when reconstituted	Sucrose. Bubble-gum flavor. In 15 and 30 mL.
Rx	**Amoxicillin** (Various, eg, Teva)	**Powder for oral suspension:** 125 mg/5 mL (as trihydrate) when reconstituted	In 80, 100, and 150 mL.
Rx	**Amoxil** (GlaxoSmithKline)		Sucrose. Strawberry flavor. In 80 and 150 mL.
Rx	**Trimox** (Apothecon)		Sucrose. In 80, 100, and 150 mL.
Rx	**Amoxicillin** (Ranbaxy)	**Powder for oral suspension:** 200 mg/5 mL (as trihydrate) when reconstituted	Fruit flavor. In 50, 75, and 100 mL.
Rx	**Amoxil** (GlaxoSmithKline)		Sucrose. Bubble-gum flavor. In 50, 75, and 100 mL.
Rx	**Amoxicillin** (Various, eg, Teva)	**Powder for oral suspension:** 250 mg/5 mL (as trihydrate) when reconstituted	In 80, 100, and 150 mL.
Rx	**Amoxil** (GlaxoSmithKline)		Sucrose. Bubble-gum flavor. In 100 and 150 mL.
Rx	**Trimox** (Apothecon)		Sucrose. In 80, 100, and 150 mL.
Rx	**Amoxicillin** (Ranbaxy)	**Powder for oral suspension:** 400 mg/5 mL (as trihydrate) when reconstituted	Fruit flavor. In 50, 75, and 100 mL.
Rx	**Amoxil** (GlaxoSmithKline)		Sucrose. Bubble-gum flavor. In 50, 75, and 100 mL.
Rx	**DisperMox** (Ranbaxy)	**Tablets for oral suspension:** 200 mg	Aspartame, 5.6 mg phenylalanine. (RX565). Lt. pink, mottled. Strawberry flavor. In 20s, 60s, 1000s, and UD 100s.
		400 mg	Aspartame, 5.6 mg phenylalanine. (RX567). Lt. pink, mottled. Strawberry flavor. In 20s, 60s, 500s, and UD 100s.

For complete prescribing information, refer to the Penicillins group monograph. For information on amoxicillin therapy in *Helicobacter pylori* infection, refer to the *H. pylori* Agents monograph in the GI chapter.

Indications

Amoxicillin is indicated in the treatment of infections due to susceptible (only β-lactamase-negative) strains of the designated microorganisms in the conditions listed below:

➤*Ear, nose, and throat:* Infections caused by *Streptococcus* sp. (α- and β-hemolytic strains only), *S. pneumoniae*, *Staphylococcus* sp., or *Haemophilus influenzae*.

➤*GU tract:* Infections caused by *Escherichia coli*, *Proteus mirabilis*, or *Enterococcus faecalis*.

➤*Skin and skin structure:* Infections caused by *Streptococcus* sp. (α- and β-hemolytic strains only), *Staphylococcus* sp., or *E. coli*.

➤*Lower respiratory tract:* Infections caused by *Streptococcus* sp. (α- and β-hemolytic strains only), *S. pneumoniae*, *Staphylococcus* sp., or *H. influenzae*.

➤*Gonorrhea, acute uncomplicated (anogenital and urethral infections):* Infections caused by *Neisseria gonorrhoeae* (males and females).

Administration and Dosage

Amoxicillin capsules, chewable tablets, and oral suspensions may be given without regard to meals. The 400 mg suspension, 400 mg chewable tablet, and 875 mg tablet have been studied only when administered at the start of a light meal. However, food effect studies have not been performed with the 200 and 500 mg formulations.

➤*Neonates and infants 12 weeks (3 months) of age and younger*: Because of incompletely developed renal function affecting elimination of amoxicillin in this age group, the recommended upper dose of amoxicillin is 30 mg/kg/day divided every 12 hours.

Amoxicillin Uses and Dosages	
Organisms/Infections	Dosage
Labeled uses:	
Ear/Nose/Throat/Skin/Skin structure/GU tract	*Mild/Moderate:*
	Adults and children ≥ 40 kg: 500 mg every 12 hours or 250 mg every 8 hours
	Children > 3 months and < 40 kg: 25 mg/kg/day in divided doses every 12 hours or 20 mg/kg/day in divided doses every 8 hours
	Severe:
	Adults and children ≥ 40 kg: 875 mg every 12 hours or 500 mg every 8 hours
	Children > 3 mos and < 40 kg: 45 mg/kg/day in divided doses every 12 hours or 40 mg/kg/day in divided doses every 8 hours
Lower respiratory tract	*Adults and children ≥ 40 kg:* 875 mg every 12 hours or 500 mg every 8 hours
	Children > 3 months and < 40 kg: 45 mg/kg/day in divided doses every 12 hours or 40 mg/kg/day in divided doses every 8 hours
Gonorrhea:[1] Acute, uncomplicated anogenital and urethral infections in males and females	*Adults:* 3 g as single oral dose
	Prepubertal children (> 2 yrs): 50 mg/kg amoxicillin combined with 25 mg/kg probenecid as a single dose
Unlabeled uses:	
Prophylaxis for bacterial endocarditis: For dental, oral, respiratory tract, or esophageal; and for moderate-risk patients undergoing GU/GI procedures	*Adults:* 2 g orally 1 hour prior to procedure
	Children: 50 mg/kg orally 1 hour prior to procedure

AMOXICILLIN

Amoxicillin Uses and Dosages	
Organisms/Infections	Dosage
Early Lyme disease: Localized or disseminated associated with erythema migrans without neurological involvement or third-degree AV heart block	500 mg 3 times/day for 14 to 21 days
Anthrax: Postexposure prophylaxis following confirmed or suspected exposure to *Bacillus anthracis*.	*Adults:* 500 mg orallly 3 times/day
	Children < 9 years of age: 80 mg/kg/day orally divided into 2 to 3 doses.
	Continue prophylaxis until exposure has been excluded. If exposure is confirmed and vaccine is available, continue prophylaxis for 4 weeks and until 3 doses of vaccine have been administered or for 30 to 60 days if vaccine is unavailable.

[1] All patients with gonorrhea should be evaluated for syphilis (see Precautions in the group monograph).

The spectrum of amoxicillin is essentially identical to ampicillin, except that ampicillin is more effective against *Shigella* sp. Amoxicillin has the advantage of more complete absorption than ampicillin, a 3-times/day regimen for most infections, and less diarrhea than ampicillin.

Larger doses may be required for persistent or severe infections. Dosing for infections caused by less susceptible organisms should follow the recommendations for severe infections.

The children's dose is intended for individuals whose weight will not cause the calculated dosage to be greater than that recommended for adults; the children's dose should not exceed the maximum adult dose.

It should be recognized that in the treatment of chronic urinary tract infections, frequent bacteriological and clinical appraisals are necessary. Smaller doses than those recommended above should not be used. Even higher doses may be needed at times. In stubborn infections, therapy may be required for several weeks. It may be necessary to continue clinical or bacteriological follow-up for several months after cessation of therapy. Except for gonorrhea, continue treatment for a minimum of 48 to 72 hours beyond the time that the patient becomes asymptomatic or evidence of bacterial eradication has been obtained. It is recommended that there be at least 10 days of treatment for any infection caused by *Streptococcus pyogenes* to prevent the occurrence of acute rheumatic fever.

➤*Renal function impairment:* Patients with impaired renal function do not generally require a reduction in dose unless the impairment is severe. Severely impaired patients with a glomerular filtration rate of less than 30 mL/min should not receive the 875 mg tablet. Patients with a glomerular filtration rate of 10 to 30 mL/min should receive 500 or 250 mg every 12 hours, depending on the severity of the infection. Patients with a less than 10 mL/min glomerular filtration rate should receive 500 or 250 mg every 24 hours, depending on severity of the infection.

Hemodialysis patients should receive 500 or 250 mg every 24 hours, depending on severity of the infection. They should receive an additional dose both during and at the end of dialysis.

There are currently no dosing recommendations for pediatric patients with impaired renal function.

➤*Mixing oral suspension:* Prepare suspension at time of dispensing as follows: Tap bottle until all powder flows freely. Add approximately one third of the total amount of water for reconstitution and shake vigorously to wet powder. Add remainder of the water and again shake vigorously. Shake well before using.

Administration – Place required amount of suspension directly on the child's tongue for swallowing. Alternate means: Add required amount of suspension to formula, milk, fruit juice, water, ginger ale, or cold drinks; take immediately and consume in its entirety.

➤*Mixing pediatric drops:* Prepare pediatric drops at time of dispensing as follows: Add the required amount of water to the bottle and shake vigorously. Each milliliter of suspension will then contain amoxicillin trihydrate equivalent to 50 mg amoxicillin. Shake well before using.

➤*Mixing tablets for oral suspension:* Mix 1 tablet in approximately 10 mL of water. Drink entire mixture, rinse with small amount of water, and drink the contents to ensure entire dose is taken. Do not chew or swallow tablets. The tablets will not rapidly dissolve in mouth.

The tablet is not recommended to be mixed with any liquid other than water, as studies have only been conducted using water.

➤*Storage / Stability:* Store *Amoxil* capsules and 125 and 250 mg unreconstituted powder at or below 20°C (68°F); store 200 and 400 mg unreconstituted powder, chewable tablets, and tablets at or below 25°C (77°F). Store *Trimox* capsules and unreconstituted powder at or below 20°C (68°F); store chewable tablets at controlled room temperature (15° to 30°C; 59° to 86°F). Dispense in tight containers.

Any unused portion of the reconstituted suspension must be discarded after 14 days. Refrigeration is preferable, but not required.

AMOXICILLIN AND POTASSIUM CLAVULANATE (Co-amoxiclav)

Rx	**Augmentin** (GlaxoSmithKline)	**Tablets:** 250 mg amoxicillin (as trihydrate) and 125 mg clavulanic acid[1]	0.63 mEq potassium. (Augmentin 250/125). White, oval. Film-coated. In 30s and UD 100s.
Rx	**Amoxicillin, Clavulanate Potassium** (Various, eg, Geneva, Ranbaxy, Teva)	**Tablets:** 500 mg amoxicillin (as trihydrate) and 125 mg clavulanic acid[1]	In 20s.
Rx	**Augmentin** (GlaxoSmithKline)		0.63 mEq potassium. (Augmentin 500/125). White, oval. Film-coated. In 20s and UD 100s.
Rx	**Amoxicillin, Clavulanate Potassium** (Various, eg, Geneva, Lek, Ranbaxy, Teva)	**Tablets:** 875 mg amoxicillin (as trihydrate) and 125 mg clavulanic acid[1]	In 20s.
Rx	**Augmentin** (GlaxoSmithKline)		0.63 mEq potassium. (Augmentin 875). White, capsule shape, scored. In 20s and UD 100s.
Rx	**Augmentin XR** (GlaxoSmithKline)	**Tablets, extended-release:** 1000 mg amoxicillin and 62.5 mg clavulanic acid	**Unscored tablets:** 0.32 mEq potassium, 1.27 mEq sodium. (AC 1000/62.5). White, oval. Film-coated. In 28s (7 day XR pack) and 40s (10 day XR pack). **Scored tablets:** 0.32 mEq potassium, 1.27 mEq sodium. (AUGMENTIN XR). White, oval. Film-coated. In 28s (7 day XR pack) and 40s (10 day XR pack).
Rx	**Augmentin** (GlaxoSmithKline)	**Tablets, chewable:** 125 mg amoxicillin (as trihydrate) and 31.25 mg clavulanic acid[1]	0.16 mEq potassium, saccharin, mannitol. (BMP 189). Yellow, mottled. Lemon-lime flavor. In 30s.
Rx	**Amoxicillin, Clavulanate Potassium** (Geneva)	**Tablets, chewable:** 200 mg amoxicillin (as trihydrate) and 28.5 mg clavulanic acid[1]	In UD 20s.
Rx	**Augmentin** (GlaxoSmithKline)		0.14 mEq potassium, saccharin, mannitol, aspartame.[2] (AUGMENTIN 200). Pink, mottled. Cherry-banana flavor. In 20s.
Rx	**Augmentin** (GlaxoSmithKline)	**Tablets, chewable:** 250 mg amoxicillin (as trihydrate) and 62.5 mg clavulanic acid[1]	0.32 mEq potassium, saccharin, mannitol. (BMP 190). Yellow, mottled. Lemon-lime flavor. In 30s.
Rx	**Amoxicillin, Clavulanate Potassium** (Geneva)	**Tablets, chewable:** 400 mg amoxicillin (as trihydrate) and 57 mg clavulanic acid[1]	In UD 20s.
Rx	**Augmentin** (GlaxoSmithKline)		0.29 mEq potassium, saccharin, mannitol, aspartame.[3] (AUGMENTIN 400). Pink, mottled. Cherry-banana flavor. In 20s.

Aminopenicillins

AMOXICILLIN AND POTASSIUM CLAVULANATE (Co-amoxiclav)

Rx	**Augmentin** (GlaxoSmithKline)	**Powder for oral suspension**: 125 mg amoxicillin and 31.25 mg clavulanic acid[1] per 5 mL	0.16 mEq potassium/5 mL, saccharin, mannitol. Banana flavor. In 75, 100, and 150 mL.
Rx	**Amoxicillin, Clavulanate Potassium** (Geneva)	**Powder for oral suspension**: 200 mg amoxicillin and 28.5 mg clavulanic acid[1] per 5 mL	In 100 mL.
Rx	**Augmentin** (GlaxoSmithKline)		0.14 mEq potassium/5 mL, saccharin, mannitol, aspartame.[4] Orange-raspberry flavor. In 50, 75, and 100 mL.
Rx	**Augmentin** (GlaxoSmithKline)	**Powder for oral suspension**: 250 mg amoxicillin and 62.5 mg clavulanic acid[1] per 5 mL	0.32 mEq potassium/5 mL, saccharin, mannitol. Orange flavor. In 75, 100, and 150 mL.
Rx	**Amoxicillin, Clavulanate Potassium** (Geneva)	**Powder for oral suspension**: 400 mg amoxicillin and 57 mg clavulanic acid[1] per 5 mL	In 100 mL.
Rx	**Augmentin** (GlaxoSmithKline)		0.29 mEq potassium/5 mL, saccharin, mannitol, aspartame.[4] Orange-raspberry flavor. In 50, 75, and 100 mL.
Rx	**Augmentin ES-600** (GlaxoSmithKline)	**Powder for oral suspension**: 600 mg amoxicillin (as trihydrate) and 42.9 mg clavulanic acid per 5 mL[1]	0.23 mEq potassium/5 mL, aspartame.[4] Orange-raspberry flavor. In 75 mL.

[1] As the potassium salt.
[2] Contains 2.1 mg phenylalanine.

[3] Contains 4.2 mg phenylalanine.
[4] Contains 7 mg phenylalanine/5 mL.

For complete prescribing information, refer to the Penicillins group monograph.

Indications

▶*Lower respiratory infections:* Those caused by β-lactamase-producing strains of *Haemophilus influenzae* and *Moraxella catarrhalis.*

▶*Otitis media and sinusitis:* Those caused by β-lactamase-producing strains of *H. influenzae* and *M. (Branhamella) catarrhalis.*

▶*Skin and skin structure infections:* Those caused by β-lactamase-producing strains of *Staphylococcus aureus, Escherichia coli,* and *Klebsiella* sp.

▶*Urinary tract infections:* Those caused by β-lactamase-producing strains of *Escherichia coli, Klebsiella* sp., and *Enterobacter* sp.

▶*Augmentin ES 600:*

Acute otitis media (Augmentin ES-600) – For the treatment of pediatric patients with recurrent or persistent acute otitis media due to *Streptococcus pneumoniae* (penicillin MICs less than or equal to 2 mcg/mL), *H. influenzae* (including β-lactamase-producing strains), *M. catarrhalis* (including β-lactamase-producing strains) characterized by the following risk factors: Antibiotic exposure for acute otitis media within the preceding 3 months, and either of the following:
• Age of 2 years or younger, or
• daycare attendance.

Note: Acute otitis media due to *S. pneumoniae* alone can be treated with amoxicillin. *Augmentin ES-600* is not indicated for the treatment of acute otitis media due to *S. pneumoniae* with penicillin MIC at least 4 mcg/mL.

▶*Augmentin XR:*

Community-acquired pneumonia (Augmentin XR) – For the treatment of patients with community-acquired pneumonia or acute bacterial sinusitis due to confirmed or suspected β-lactamase-producing pathogens (ie, *H. influenzae, M. catarrhalis, H. parainfluenzae, K. pneumoniae,* or methicillin-susceptible *S. aureus*) and *S. pneumoniae* with reduced susceptibility to penicillin (ie, penicillin MICs equal to 2 mcg/mL). *Augmentin XR* is not indicated for the treatment of infections due to *S. pneumoniae* with penicillin MICs 4 mcg/mL or more. Data are limited with regard to infections due to *S. pneumoniae* with penicillin MICs 4 mcg/mL or more.

Note – Acute bacterial sinusitis or community-acquired pneumonia due to a penicillin-susceptible strain of *S. pneumoniae* plus a β-lactamase-producing pathogen can be treated with another *Augmentin* product containing lower daily doses of amoxicillin. Acute bacterial sinusitis or community-acquired pneumonia due to *S. pneumoniae* alone can be treated with amoxicillin.

While amoxicillin/potassium clavulanate is indicated only for the conditions listed above, infections caused by ampicillin-susceptible organisms are also amenable to this drug because of its amoxicillin content. Therefore, mixed infections caused by ampicillin-susceptible organisms and β-lactamase-producing organisms susceptible to amoxicillin/potassium clavulanate should not require an additional antibiotic. Therapy may be instituted prior to obtaining the results from bacteriologic and susceptibility studies when there is reason to believe the infection may involve any of the β-lactamase-producing organisms listed above. Once the results are known, adjust therapy.

Administration and Dosage

▶*Augmentin:* May be administered without regard to meals; however, absorption of clavulanate potassium is enhanced when taken at the start of a meal. To minimize the potential for GI intolerance, give the drug at the start of a meal.

Contraindicated in patients with a history of amoxicillin/clavulanate potassium-associated cholestatic jaundice/hepatic dysfunction. Use with caution in patients with evidence of hepatic dysfunction.

Tablet interchangeability – Because the 250 and 500 mg tablets contain the same amount of clavulanic acid (125 mg as potassium salt), two 250 mg tablets are not equivalent to one 500 mg tablet. The 875 mg tablet also contains 125 mg potassium clavulanate. In addition, the 250 mg tablet and 250 mg chewable tablet do not contain the same amount of potassium clavulanate and should not be substituted for each other, as they are not interchangeable.

Adults – One 500 mg tablet every 12 hours or one 250 mg tablet every 8 hours.

Suspension: Adults who have difficulty swallowing may be given the 125 mg/5 mL or 250 mg/5 mL suspension in place of the 500 mg tablet or give 200 mg/5 mL or 400 mg/5 mL suspension in place of the 875 mg tablet.

Severe infections and respiratory tract infections: One 875 mg tablet every 12 hours or one 500 mg tablet every 8 hours.

Renal function impairment: This does not generally require a dose reduction unless impairment is severe. Severely impaired patients with a glomerular filtration rate (GFR) of less than 30 mL/min should not receive the 875 mg tablet. Give patients with a GFR of 10 to 30 mL/min 500 or 250 mg every 12 hours, depending on the severity of infection. Give patients with a GFR less than 10 mL/min 500 or 250 mg every 24 hours, depending on severity of infection. Give hemodialysis patients 500 or 250 mg every 24 hours, and an additional dose both during and at the end of dialysis.

Hepatic function impairment: Dose with caution and monitor hepatic function.

Children –

Less than 3 months of age: 30 mg/kg/day divided every 12 hours, based on the amoxicillin component. Use of the 125 mg/5 mL oral suspension is recommended.

3 months of age or older: Children's dose is based on amoxicillin content. Refer to the following table. Because of the different amoxicillin to clavulanic acid ratios in the 250 mg tablets (250/125) vs the 250 mg chewable tablets (250/62.5), do not use the 250 mg tablet until the child weighs 40 kg or more.

40 kg or more: Dose according to adult recommendations.

Amoxicillin/Potassium Clavulanate Dosing in Children ≥ 3 Months of Age		
	Dosing regimen	
Infections	200 mg/5 mL or 400 mg/5 mL (q 12 hr)[1,2]	125 mg/5 mL or 250 mg/5 mL (q 8 hr)[2]
Otitis media,[3] sinusitis, lower respiratory tract infections, severe infections	45 mg/kg/day	40 mg/kg/day
Less severe infections	25 mg/kg/day	20 mg/kg/day

[1] The every-12-hour regimen is associated with significantly less diarrhea; however, the 200 and 400 mg formulations (suspension and chewable tablets) contain aspartame and should not be used by phenylketonurics.

[2] Each strength of the suspension is available as a chewable tablet for use by older children.
[3] Recommended duration is 10 days.

▶*Augmentin ES-600: Augmentin ES-600,* 600 mg/5 mL, does not contain the same amount of clavulanic acid (as the potassium salt) as any of the other *Augmentin* suspensions. *Augmentin ES-600* contains 42.9 mg clavulanic acid per 5 mL whereas *Augmentin* 200 mg/5 mL suspension contains 28.5 mg clavulanic acid per 5 mL and the 400 mg/5 mL suspension contains 57 mg clavulanic acid per 5 mL. Therefore, *Augmentin* 200 mg/5 mL and 400 mg/5 mL suspensions should not be substituted for *Augmentin ES-600,* as they are not interchangeable.

AMOXICILLIN AND POTASSIUM CLAVULANATE (Co-amoxiclav)

Dosage –

Pediatric patients 3 months and older: Based on the amoxicillin component (600 mg/5 mL), the recommended dose of *Augmentin ES-600* is 90 mg/kg/day divided every 12 hours, administered for 10 days (see table below).

Recommended Dose of *Augmentin ES-600*	
Body weight (kg)	Volume of *Augmentin ES-600* providing 90 mg/kg/day
8	3 mL twice daily
12	4.5 mL twice daily
16	6 mL twice daily
20	7.5 mL twice daily
24	9 mL twice daily
28	10.5 mL twice daily
32	12 mL twice daily
36	13.5 mL twice daily

Pediatric patients weighing 40 kg or more: Experience with *Augmentin ES-600* in this group is not available.

Adults: Experience with *Augmentin ES-600* in adults is not available and adults who have difficulty swallowing should not be given *Augmentin ES-600* in place of the *Augmentin* 500 mg or 875 mg tablet.

Hepatic impairment: Dose hepatically impaired patients with caution and monitor hepatic function at regular intervals.

Mixing oral suspension – Prepare a suspension at time of dispensing as follows: Tap bottle until all the powder flows freely. Add approximately two thirds of the total amount of water for reconstitution and shake vigorously to suspend powder. Add remainder of the water and again shake vigorously.

Administration – To minimize the potential for GI intolerance, take at the start of a meal. Absorption of clavulanate potassium may be enhanced when the drug is administered at the start of a meal.

➤*Augmentin XR:* Take at the start of a meal to enhance the absorption of amoxicillin and minimize the potential for GI intolerance. Absorption of the amoxicillin component is decreased when *Augmentin XR* is taken on an empty stomach.

The recommended dose is 4000 mg/250 mg daily according to the following table.

Augmentin XR Dosing		
Indication	Dose	Duration
Acute bacterial sinusitis	2 tablets q 12 h	10 days
Community-acquired pneumonia	2 tablets q 12 h	7 to 10 days

Augmentin tablets (250 or 500 mg) cannot be used to provide the same dosages as *Augmentin XR* extended-release tablets. This is because *Augmentin XR* contains 62.5 mg clavulanic acid, while the *Augmentin* 250 and 500 mg tablets each contain 125 mg clavulanic acid. In addition, the extended-release tablet provides an extended time course of plasma amoxicillin concentrations compared with immediate-release tablets. Thus, 2 *Augmentin* 500 mg tablets are not equivalent to 1 *Augmentin XR* tablet.

The scored *Augmentin XR* tablets are available for greater convenience for adult patients who have difficulty swallowing. The scored *Augmentin XR* tablet may be broken in half at score line. The scored tablet is not intended to reduce the dosage of medication taken; as stated in the table above, the recommended dose of *Augmentin XR* is 2 tablets twice daily every 12 hours.

Renally impaired patients – The pharmacokinetics of *Augmentin XR* have not been studied in patients with renal impairment. *Augmentin XR* is contraindicated in severely impaired patients with a creatinine clearance of less than 30 mL/min and in hemodialysis patients.

Hepatically impaired patients – Dose hepatically impaired patients with caution and monitor hepatic function at regular intervals.

Children – Safety and efficacy in pediatric patients below 16 years of age have not been established.

➤*Storage/Stability:* Refrigerate reconstituted suspension and discard after 10 days. Shake well before using. Store tablets and dry powder at or below 25°C (77°F); dispense in the original container.

Extended-Spectrum Penicillins

TICARCILLIN DISODIUM

Rx	Ticar (GlaxoSmithKline)	Powder for Injection: 3 g	In 3 g vials.

For complete prescribing information, refer to the Penicillins group monograph.

Indications

For treatment of the following: Bacterial septicemia, skin/soft tissue infections, acute and chronic respiratory tract infections caused by susceptible strains of *Pseudomonas aeruginosa*, *Proteus* sp. (both indole-positive and indole-negative), and *Escherichia coli*. Although clinical improvement has been shown, bacteriological cures cannot be expected in patients with chronic respiratory disease or cystic fibrosis.

➤*GU tract infections:* Complicated and uncomplicated infections caused by susceptible strains of *P. aeruginosa*, *Proteus* sp. (both indole-positive and indole-negative), *E. coli*, *Enterobacter*, and *Streptococcus faecalis* (enterococcus).

➤*Infections caused by susceptible anaerobic bacteria:* Bacterial septicemia; lower respiratory tract infections such as empyema, anaerobic pneumonitis, and lung abscess; intra-abdominal infections such as peritonitis and intra-abdominal abscess (typically resulting from anaerobic organisms resident in the normal GI tract); infections of the female pelvis and genital tract such as endometritis, pelvic inflammatory disease, pelvic abscess, and salpingitis; skin and soft tissue infections.

Although ticarcillin is primarily indicated in gram-negative infections, consider its in vitro activity against gram-positive organisms in infections caused by both gram-negative and gram-positive organisms.

Based on the in vitro synergism between ticarcillin and gentamicin, amikacin, or tobramycin against certain strains of *P. aeruginosa*, combined therapy has been successful using full therapeutic dosages.

Administration and Dosage

Use IV therapy in higher doses in serious urinary tract and systemic infections. IM injections should not exceed 2 g/injection. Seriously ill patients should receive higher doses.

Ticarcillin Uses and Dosages	
Organisms/Infections	Dosage
Bacterial septicemia, respiratory tract infections, skin and soft tissue infections, intra-abdominal infections and infections of the female pelvis and genital tract	*Adults:* 200 to 300 mg/kg/day by IV infusion in divided doses every 4 or 6 hours (3 g every 4 hour or 4 g every 6 hours), depending on weight of patient and severity of infection *Children (< 40 kg):* 200 to 300 mg/kg/day by IV infusion in divided doses every 4 or 6 hours[1]
Urinary tract infections: Complicated infections	*Adults and children:* 150 to 200 mg/kg/day IV infusion in divided doses every 4 or 6 hours. Usual dose for average adult (70 kg) is 3 g 4 times/day
Uncomplicated infections	*Adults:* 1 g IM or direct IV every 6 hr. *Children (< 40 kg):* 50 to 100 mg/kg/day IM or direct IV in divided doses every 6 or 8 hours
Neonates: Severe infections (sepsis) caused by susceptible strains of *Pseudomonas* sp., *Proteus* sp., and *E. coli*	Give IM or by 10- to 20-min IV infusions
< 2 kg	*Age < 7 days* – 75 mg/kg/12 h (150 mg/kg/day) *Age > 7 days* – 75 mg/kg/8 h (225 mg/kg/day)
≥ 2 kg	*Age < 7 days* – 75 mg/kg/8 h (225 mg/kg/day) *Age > 7 days* – 100 mg/kg/8 h (300 mg/kg/day)

[1] Daily dose for children should not exceed adult dosage.

TICARCILLIN DISODIUM

➤*Renal function impairment:*

Dosage Adjustments of Ticarcillin in Renal Insufficiency	
Organisms/Infections	Dosage
Dosage in renal insufficiency[1]	Initial loading dose of 3 g IV, then base IV doses on Ccr and type of dialysis
Ccr (mL/min) –	
> 60	3 g every 4 h
30 to 60	2 g every 4 h
10 to 30	2 g every 8 h
< 10	2 g every 12 hr or 1 g IM every 6 h
< 10 with hepatic dysfunction	2 g every 24 h or 1 g IM every 12 h
Patients on peritoneal dialysis	3 g every 12 h
Patients on hemodialysis	2 g every 12 h and 3 g after each dialysis

[1] Half-life in patients with renal failure is approximately 13 hours.

Children weighing more than 40 kg (88 lbs) should receive adult dose. In children less than 40 kg, data are insufficient to recommend an optimum dose.

➤*IM:* Inject well into a relatively large muscle. For initial reconstitution, use sterile water for injection, sodium chloride Injection, or 1% lidocaine HCl solution (without epinephrine). Do not use more than 1 g of reconstituted ticarcillin in a single IM injection.

Reconstitute each gram of ticarcillin with 2 mL sterile water for injection, sodium chloride Injection, or 1% lidocaine HCl solution (without epinephrine) to obtain a concentration of approximately 385 mg/mL. Each 2.6 mL of the resulting solution will contain 1 g of ticarcillin.

➤*IV:* For initial reconstitution, use sodium chloride injection, 5% dextrose injection, or Lactated Ringer's injection.

Reconstitute each g of ticarcillin with 4 mL of compatible IV solution to obtain approximately 200 mg/mL concentration. When dissolved, dilute further if desired. When injecting solution directly, administer as slowly as possible to avoid vein irritation.

For IV infusions, administer by continuous or intermittent IV drip. Administer intermittent infusion over a 30-minute to 2-hour period in equally divided doses. Concentrations of approximately 50 mg/mL or more will reduce the incidence of vein irritation.

➤*Admixture incompatibilities:* Do NOT mix ticarcillin together with gentamicin, amikacin, or tobramycin in the same IV solution, because of the gradual inactivation of gentamicin, amikacin, or tobramycin under these circumstances. The therapeutic effect of these drugs remains unimpaired when administered separately.

Stability and Storage of Ticarcillin IV Solutions			
		Stability (loss of potency < 10%)	
Concentration	Compatible diluents	Controlled room temperature (21° to 24°C; 70° to 75°F)	Refrigeration (4°C; 40°F)
10 mg/mL and 100 mg/mL	Sodium chloride injection	72 h	14 days
	5% dextrose injection	72 h	14 days
	Lactated Ringer's injection	48 h	14 days

➤*Storage/Stability:* Do not use refrigerated solutions stored longer than 72 hours for multidose purposes. Discard unused solutions after the time periods mentioned in the above table. After reconstitution and dilution to a concentration of 10 to 100 mg/mL, this solution can be frozen at −18°C (0°F) and stored for up to 30 days. The thawed solution must be used within 24 hours. Store dry powder at room temperature or below.

TICARCILLIN AND CLAVULANATE POTASSIUM

Rx	Timentin (GlaxoSmithKline)	**Powder for Injection:** 3 g ticarcillin (as disodium) and 0.1 g clavulanic acid (as potassium)[1]	In 3.1 g vials, piggyback bottles, *ADD-Vantage* vials and 31 g pharmacy bulk packages.[2]
		Injection, solution: 3 g ticarcillin (as disodium) and 0.1 g clavulanic acid (as potassium)/100 mL[3]	In 100 mL premixed, frozen *Galaxy* plastic containers.

[1] Contains 4.75 mEq sodium and 0.15 mEq potassium/g.
[2] Pharmacy bulk package contains 30 g ticarcillin (as disodium) and 1 g clavulanic acid.
[3] Contains 18.7 mEq sodium and 0.5 mEq potassium/100 mL.

For complete prescribing information, refer to the Penicillins group monograph.

Indications

Treatment of infections caused by susceptible strains of these designated organisms:

➤*Septicemia:* This includes bacteremia caused by β-lactamase-producing strains of *Klebsiella* sp., *Escherichia coli*, *Staphylococcus aureus*, and *Pseudomonas aeruginosa* (and other *Pseudomonas* species).

➤*Lower respiratory tract infections:* Those caused by β-lactamase-producing strains of *S. aureus*, *Haemophilus influenzae*, and *Klebsiella* sp.

➤*Bone and joint infections:* Those caused by β-lactamase-producing strains of *S. aureus*.

➤*Skin and skin structure infections:* Those caused by β-lactamase-producing strains of *S. aureus*, *Klebsiella* sp., and *E. coli*.

➤*Urinary tract infections:* Complicated and uncomplicated infections caused by β-lactamase-producing strains of *E. coli*, *Klebsiella* sp., *P. aeruginosa* (and other *Pseudomonas* species), *Citrobacter* sp., *Enterobacter cloacae*, *Serratia marcescens*, *S. aureus*.

➤*Gynecologic infections:* Endometritis caused by β-lactamase-producing strains of *Bacteroides melaninogenicus*, *Enterobacter* sp. (including *E. cloacae*), *E. coli*, *K. pneumoniae*, *S. aureus*, and *Staphylococcus epidermidis*.

➤*Intra-abdominal infections:* Peritonitis caused by β-lactamase-producing strains of *E. coli*, *K. pneumoniae*, and *Bacteroides fragilis* group.

While this combination is indicated only for the conditions listed above, infections caused by ticarcillin-susceptible organisms also are amenable to this combination treatment caused by its ticarcillin content.

Treatment of mixed infections and for presumptive therapy prior to the identification of the causative organisms.

Based on the in vitro synergism between this drug and aminoglycosides against certain strains of *P. aeruginosa*, combined therapy has been successful, especially in patients with impaired host defenses. Use drugs in full therapeutic doses. When results of culture and susceptibility tests become available, adjust antimicrobial therapy.

Administration and Dosage

➤*Approved by the FDA:* December 17, 1997.

Administer by IV infusion over 30 minutes.

Generally, continue treatment for at least 2 days after signs and symptoms of infection have disappeared. The usual duration is 10 to 14 days; however, difficult and complicated infections may require more prolonged therapy.

Frequent bacteriologic and clinical appraisal is necessary during therapy of chronic urinary tract infections and may be required for several months after therapy has been completed; persistent infections may require treatment for several weeks; do not use doses smaller than those indicated.

In certain infections involving abscess formation, perform appropriate surgical drainage in conjunction with antimicrobial therapy.

When administering in combination with another antimicrobial (eg, an aminoglycoside), administer each drug separately.

➤*Adults:*

Ticarcillin/Clavulanate Potassium Administration in Adults			
	Systemic and urinary tract infections	Gynecological infections	
		Moderate	Severe
Adults ≥ 60 kg	3.1 g every 4 to 6 h	200 mg/kg/day every 6 h	300 mg/kg/day every 4 h
Adults < 60 kg	200 to 300 mg/kg/day every 4 to 6 h		

There are no sufficient data to support the use of this product in pediatric patients younger than 3 months of age or for the treatment of septicemia or infections in the pediatric population where the suspected or proven pathogen is *H. influenzae* type b.

➤*Children:*

Dosage Guidelines for Ticarcillin/Clavulanate Potassium in Children ≥ 3 Months of Age		
	Mild to moderate infections	Severe infections
Children ≥ 60 kg	3.1 g every 6 h	3.1 g every 4 h
Children < 60 kg (dosed at 50 mg/kg/dose)	200 mg/kg/day every 6 h	300 mg/kg/day every 4 h

➤*Renal function impairment:*

Dosage of Ticarcillin/Clavulanate Potassium in Renal Insufficiency[1]	
Ccr (mL/min)	Dosage
> 60	3.1 g every 4 h
30 to 60	2 g every 4 h
10 to 30	2 g every 8 h
< 10	2 g every 12 h
< 10 with hepatic dysfunction	2 g every 24 h

TICARCILLIN AND CLAVULANATE POTASSIUM

Dosage of Ticarcillin/Clavulanate Potassium in Renal Insufficiency[1]	
Ccr (mL/min)	Dosage
Patients on peritoneal dialysis	3.1 g every 12 h
Patients on hemodialysis	2 g every 12 h supplemented with 3.1 g after each dialysis

[1] Initial loading dose is 3.1 g. Follow with doses based on Ccr and type of dialysis.

➤*Preparation of infusion solution:* Reconstitute by adding ≈ 13 mL of Sterile Water for Injection or NaCl Injection. Shake well. The resulting ticarcillin concentration is ≈ 200 mg/mL and 6.7 mg/mL clavulanic acid for the 3.1 g dose. Conversely, each 5 mL of the 3.1 g dose reconstituted with ≈ 13 mL of diluent will contain ≈ 1 g ticarcillin and 33 mg clavulanic acid.

Further dilute the solution with sodium chloride injection, 5% dextrose injection or Lactated Ringer's injection to a concentration between 10 to 100 mg/mL. Administer over 30 minutes by direct infusion or through a Y-type IV infusion set already in place. If this method or the piggyback method is used, temporarily discontinue administering any other solutions during the infusion of ticarcillin and clavulanate potassium.

➤*Admixture incompatibility:* Incompatible with sodium bicarbonate.

➤*Storage / Stability:* The concentrated stock solution (200 mg/mL) is stable for up to 6 hours at room temperature (21° to 23°C; 70° to 75°F) or up to 72 hours under refrigeration (4°C; 40°F); if further diluted to a concentration between 10 and 100 mg/mL with any of the recommended diluents, the following stability periods apply:

Stability and Storage for IV Solution of Ticarcillin/Clavulanate Potassium				
		Stability		
Concentration	Compatible diluents	Controlled room temp	Refrigerated	Frozen
10 mg/mL to 100 mg/mL	Sodium chloride injection	24 h	7 days	30 days
	5% dextrose injection	24 h	3 days	7 days
	Lactated Ringer's injection	24 h	7 days	30 days

Unused solutions must be discarded after the time period stated above. Use all thawed solutions within 8 hours. Do not refreeze thawed solutions.

Premixed, frozen solutions – Store at ≤ –20°C (– 4°F). Thaw at room temperature 22°C (72°F) or in a refrigerator 4°C (39°F). Do not force thaw by immersion in water baths or by microwave irradiation. Thawed solution is stable for 7 days if stored under refrigeration or for 24 hours at room temperature. Do not refreeze.

Actions

➤*Pharmacology:* The formulation of ticarcillin with clavulanic acid protects ticarcillin from degradation by β-lactamase enzymes (see group monograph).

PIPERACILLIN SODIUM

Rx	**Piperacillin Sodium** (American Pharmaceutical Partners)	**Powder for injection**: Contains 1.85 mEq (42.5 mg) sodium/g 2 g	In vials.
Rx	**Pipracil** (Lederle)		In vials and *ADD-Vantage* vials.
Rx	**Piperacillin Sodium** (American Pharmaceutical Partners)	**Powder for injection**: Contains 1.85 mEq (42.5 mg) sodium/g 3 g	In vials.
Rx	**Pipracil** (Lederle)		In vials, infusion bottles.
Rx	**Piperacillin Sodium** (American Pharmaceutical Partners)	**Powder for injection**: Contains 1.85 mEq (42.5 mg) sodium/g 40 g	In vials.
Rx	**Pipracil** (Lederle)		In pharmacy bulk vials.

For complete prescribing information, refer to the Penicillins group monograph.

Indications

Treatment of mixed infections and presumptive therapy prior to the identification of the causative organisms. Also, it may be used as single-drug therapy in some situations where two antibiotics are normally used.

➤*Intra-abdominal infections (including hepatobiliary and surgical infections):* Those caused by *Escherichia coli*; *Pseudomonas aeruginosa*; enterococci; *Clostridium* sp.; anaerobic cocci; *Bacteroides* sp., including *B. fragilis*.

➤*Urinary tract infections (UTIs):* Those caused by *E. coli, Klebsiella* sp., *P. aeruginosa, Proteus* sp., including *P. mirabilis* and enterococci.

➤*Gynecologic infections (including endometritis, pelvic inflammatory disease, pelvic cellulitis):* Those caused by *Bacteroides* sp., including *B. fragilis*; anaerobic cocci; *Neisseria gonorrhoeae*; enterococci (*Streptococcus faecalis*).

➤*Septicemia (including bacteremia):* Due to *E. coli, Klebsiella* sp., *Enterobacter* sp., *Serratia* sp., *P. mirabilis, S. pneumoniae*, enterococci, *P. aeruginosa, Bacteroides* sp. and anaerobic cocci.

➤*Lower respiratory tract infections:* Those caused by *E. coli, Klebsiella* sp., *Enterobacter* sp., *P. aeruginosa, Serratia* sp., *Haemophilus influenzae, Bacteroides* sp. and anaerobic cocci. Although improvement has been noted in cystic fibrosis patients, long-term bacterial eradication may not be achieved.

➤*Skin and skin structure infections:* Those caused by *E. coli; Klebsiella* sp.; *Serratia* sp.; *Acinetobacter* sp.; *Enterobacter* sp.; *P. aeruginosa*; indole-positive *Proteus* sp.; *P. mirabilis; Bacteroides* sp., including *B. fragilis*; anaerobic cocci; enterococci.

➤*Bone and joint infections:* Those caused by *P. aeruginosa*, enterococci, *Bacteroides* sp. and anaerobic cocci.

➤*Gonococcal infections:* Treatment of uncomplicated gonococcal urethritis.

➤*Streptococcal infections:* Infections caused by streptococcus species including group A β-hemolytic streptococci and *S. pneumoniae*; however, these infections are ordinarily treated with more narrow spectrum penicillins.

➤*Prophylaxis:* For prophylactic use in surgery including intra-abdominal (GI and biliary) procedures, vaginal and abdominal hysterectomy and cesarean section. Effective prophylaxis depends on the time of administration; give ½ to 1 hour before the operation so that effective levels can be achieved in the wound prior to the procedure.

Stop the prophylactic use of piperacillin within 24 hours. Continuing administration of any antibiotic increases the possibility of adverse reactions, but in the majority of surgical procedures does not reduce the incidence of subsequent infections. If there are signs of infection, obtain specimens for culture so that appropriate therapy can begin.

Administration and Dosage

Administer IM or IV. The *ADD-Vantage* vial is NOT for IM use. For serious infections, give 3 to 4 g every 4 to 6 hours as a 20-to 30-minute IV infusion. Maximum daily dose is 24 g/day, although higher doses have been used. Limit IM injections to 2 g/site. The average duration of treatment is 7 to 10 days, except in the treatment of gynecologic infections, in which it is from 3 to 10 days; the duration should be guided by the patient's clinical and bacteriological progress. Continue for at least 48 to 72 hours after the patient becomes asymptomatic. Antibiotic therapy for group A β-hemolytic streptococcal infections should be maintained for at least 10 days to reduce the risk of rheumatic fever or glomerulonephritis.

➤*Hemodialysis:* Maximum dose is 6 g/day (2 g every 8 hours). Hemodialysis removes 30% to 50% of piperacillin in 4 hours; administer an additional 1 g after each dialysis.

➤*Renal failure and hepatic insufficiency:* Measure serum levels to provide additional guidance for adjusting dosage; however, this may not be practical.

➤*Infants and children < 12 years of age:* Dosages have not been established; however, the following dosages have been suggested:

Neonates –
Less than 36 weeks old: 75 mg/kg IV every 12 hours in the first week of life, then every 8 hours in the second week.
Full-term: 75 mg/kg IV every 8 hours the first week of life, then every 6 hours thereafter.

Children – Other conditions, 200 to 300 mg/kg/day, up to a maximum of 24 g/day divided every 4 to 6 hours.

➤*Concomitant therapy:* Use with aminoglycosides has been successful, especially in patients with impaired host defenses. Use both drugs in full therapeutic doses.

Piperacillin Uses and Dosages	
Organisms/Infections	Dosage
Serious infections: Septicemia, nosocomial pneumonia, intra-abdominal infections, aerobic and anaerobic gynecologic infections and skin and soft tissue infections:	12 to 18 g/day IV (200 to 300 mg/kg/day) in divided doses every 4 to 6 hrs
Renal impairment –	
Creatinine clearance 20 to 40 mL/min	12 g/day; 4 g every 8 hrs
< 20 mL/min	8 g/day; 4 g every 12 hrs

Extended-Spectrum Penicillins

PIPERACILLIN SODIUM

Piperacillin Uses and Dosages

Organisms/Infections	Dosage
Urinary tract infections: Complicated (normal renal function)	8 to 16 g/day IV (125 to 200 mg/kg/day) in divided doses every 6 to 8 hrs
Renal impairment	
Creatinine clearance 20 to 40 mL/min	9 g/day; 3 g every 8 hrs
< 20 mL/min	6 g/day; 3 g every 12 hrs
Uncomplicated UTI and most community-acquired pneumonia (normal renal function)	6 to 8 g/day IM or IV (100 to 125 mg/kg/day) in divided doses every 6 to 12 hrs
Uncomplicated UTI with renal impairment –	
Creatinine clearance < 20 mL/min	6 g/day; 3 g every 12 hrs
Uncomplicated gonorrhea infections:	2 g IM in a single dose with 1 g probenecid ½ hr prior to injection
Prophylaxis: Intra-abdominal surgery	2 g IV just prior to anesthesia; 2 g during surgery; 2 g every 6 hrs post-op for no more than 24 hrs

Piperacillin Uses and Dosages

Organisms/Infections	Dosage
Vaginal hysterectomy	2 g IV just prior to anesthesia; 2 g 6 hrs after initial dose; 2 g 12 hrs after first dose
Cesarean section	2 g IV after cord is clamped; 2 g 4 hrs after initial dose; 2 g 8 hrs after first dose
Abdominal hysterectomy	2 g IV just prior to anesthesia; 2 g on return to recovery room; 2 g after 6 hrs

Diluents for Reconstitution of Piperacillin

Sterile Water for Injection	Bacteriostatic[1] Sodium Chloride Injection
Bacteriostatic Water[1] for Injection	Dextrose 5% in Water
Sodium Chloride Injection	Dextrose 5% and 0.9% Sodium Chloride
	Lidocaine HCl 0.5% to 1% (w/o epinephrine)[2]

[1] Either parabens or benzyl alcohol.
[2] For IM use only. Lidocaine is contraindicated in patients with a known history of hypersensitivity to local anesthetics of the amide type.

Piperacillin Solutions

IV Solutions	IV Admixtures	*ADD-Vantage* vials
Dextrose 5% in Water	0.9% Sodium Chloride [+ KCl 40 mEq]	Dextrose 5% in Water
0.9% Sodium Chloride	5% Dextrose in Water [+ KCl 40 mEq]	0.9% Sodium Chloride
Dextrose 5% and 0.9% Sodium Chloride	5% Dextrose/0.99% Sodium Chloride [+ KCl 40 mEq]	
Lactated Ringer's Injection[1]	Ringer's Injection [+ KCl 40 mEq]	
Dextran 6% in 0.9% Sodium Chloride	Lactated Ringer's Injection[1] [+ KCl 40 mEq]	

[1] When piperacillin is further diluted with Lactated Ringer's Injection, the diluted solution must be administered within 2 hours.

➤*IV administration:*
Reconstitution directions – Reconstitute each g piperacillin with at least 5 mL of a suitable diluent (except lidocaine HCl 0.5% to 1% without epinephrine) listed above. Shake well until dissolved. Reconstituted solution may be further diluted to the desired volume (eg, 50 or 100 mL) in the above listed IV solutions and admixtures.

Reconstitution directions for bulk vial – Reconstitute the 40 g vial with 172 mL of a suitable diluent (except lidocaine HCl 0.5% to 1% without epinephrine) listed above to achieve a concentration of 1 g per 5 mL.

➤*Directions for administration:*
Intermittent IV infusion – Infuse diluted solution over a period of about 30 minutes. During infusion it is desirable to discontinue the primary IV solution.

IV injection (bolus) – Reconstituted solution should be injected slowly over a 3- to 5-minute period to help avoid vein irritation.

➤*IM administration:*
Reconstitution directions – Reconstitute each g of piperacillin with 2 mL of a suitable diluent listed in the previous table to achieve a concentration of 1 g per 2.5 mL. Shake well until dissolved.

Directions for administration – When indicated by clinical and bacteriological findings, IM administration of 6 to 8 g daily, in divided doses, may be used for initiation of therapy. In addition, consider IM administration of the drug for maintenance therapy after clinical and bacteriologic improvement has been obtained with IV piperacillin sodium treatment. Administration IM should not exceed 2 g per injection at any one site. The preferred site is the upper outer quadrant of the buttock (ie, gluteus maximus). Use the deltoid area only if well developed, and then only with caution to avoid radial nerve injury. Injections IM should not be made into the lower or mid-third of the upper arm.

➤*Storage/Stability:* Stable in both glass and plastic containers when reconstituted with recommended diluents and when diluted with the IV solutions and IV admixtures indicated above.

Extensive stability studies have demonstrated chemical stability (potency, pH and clarity) through 24 hours at room temperature, up to 1 week refrigerated, and up to 1 month frozen (–10° to –20°C; 14° to –4°F). (*Note:* The 40 g bulk vial should not be frozen after reconstitution.) However, appropriate consideration of aseptic technique and individual hospital policy may recommend discarding unused portions after storage for 48 hours under refrigeration and recommend discarding after 24 hours storage at room temperature.

CARBENICILLIN INDANYL SODIUM

Rx	Geocillin (Roerig)	**Tablets:** 382 mg carbenicillin (118 mg indanyl sodium ester)	Yellow. Film coated. Capsule shape. In 100s and UD 100s.

For complete prescribing information, refer to the Penicillins group monograph.

Indications

➤*Acute and chronic infections of the upper and lower urinary tract and in asymptomatic bacteriuria:* Those caused by susceptible strains of *Escherichia coli, Proteus mirabilis, Morganella morganii, Providencia rettgeri, P. vulgaris, Pseudomonas* sp., *Enterobacter* sp. and enterococci. Also indicated in the treatment of prostatitis caused by susceptible strains of *E. coli,* enterococcus (*S. faecalis*), *P. mirabilis* and *Enterobacter* species.

Administration and Dosage

➤*Urinary tract infections:*
E. coli, Proteus sp. and *Enterobacter sp.* – 382 to 764 mg carbenicillin 4 times daily.

Pseudomonas sp. and enterococci – 764 mg carbenicillin 4 times daily.

➤*Prostatitis caused by E. coli, P. mirabilis, Enterobacter sp. and enterococcus (S. faecalis):* 764 mg carbenicillin 4 times daily.

Carbenicillin indanyl sodium blood levels may be increased and prolonged by concurrent administration of probenecid.

PIPERACILLIN SODIUM AND TAZOBACTAM SODIUM

Rx	**Zosyn** (Wyeth)	**Powder for Injection, lyophilized:** 2.25 g (2 g piperacillin/0.25 g tazobactam)	4.69 mEq sodium. Preservative-free. In vials and *ADD-Vantage* vials.
		3.375 g (3 g piperacillin/0.375 g tazobactam)	7.04 mEq sodium. Preservative-free. In vials and *ADD-Vantage* vials.
		4.5 g (4 g piperacillin/0.5 g tazobactam)	9.39 mEq sodium. Preservative-free. In vials and *ADD-Vantage* vials.
		40.5 g (36 g piperacillin/4.5 g tazobactam)	84.5 mEq sodium. Preservative-free. In bulk vials.
		Injection:[1] 2.25 g/50 mL (2 g piperacillin/0.25 g tazobactam)	5.7 mEq sodium. In *Galaxy* containers.
		3.375 g/50 mL (3 g piperacillin/0.375 g tazobactam)	8.6 mEq sodium. In *Galaxy* containers.
		4.5 g/100 mL (4 g piperacillin/0.5 g tazobactam)	11.4 mEq sodium. In *Galaxy* containers.

[1] Supplied as frozen, iso-osmotic solution in single-dose plastic containers.

For complete prescribing information, refer to the Penicillins group monograph.

Indications

For the treatment of patients with moderate to severe infections caused by piperacillin-resistant, piperacillin/tazobactam susceptible, β-lactamase-producing strains of the microorganisms in the conditions listed below.

➤*Appendicitis (complicated by rupture or abscess) and peritonitis:* Caused by piperacillin-resistant, β-lactamase-producing strains of *Escherichia coli* or these members of the *Bacteroides* group: *B. fragilis, B. ovatus, B. thetaiotaomicron* or *B. vulgatus.*

➤*Uncomplicated and complicated skin and skin structure infections:* Those including cellulitis, cutaneous abscesses and ischemic/diabetic foot infections caused by piperacillin-resistant, β-lactamase-producing strains of *Staphylococcus aureus.*

➤*Postpartum endometritis or pelvic inflammatory disease:* Caused by piperacillin-resistant, β-lactamase-producing strains of *E. coli.*

➤*Community-acquired pneumonia (moderate severity only):* Caused by piperacillin-resistant, β-lactamase-producing strains of *Haemophilus influenzae.*

➤*Nosocomial pneumonia (moderate to severe):* Caused by piperacillin-resistant, β-lactamase-producing strains of *S. aureus* and by piperacillin/tazobactam-susceptible *Acinetobacter baumanii, H. influenzae, Klebsiella pneumoniae,* and *Pseudomonas aeruginosa* in combination with an aminoglycoside.

Piperacillin/tazobactam is indicated only for the specified conditions listed above. However, infections caused by piperacillin-susceptible organisms for which piperacillin is effective are also amenable to piperacillin/tazobactam treatment because of its piperacillin content. The treatment of mixed infections caused by piperacillin-susceptible organisms and piperacillin-resistant, β-lactamase-producing organisms susceptible to piperacillin/tazobactam should not require adding another antibiotic. An exception is in the treatment of *P. aeruginosa* in nosocomial pneumonia, which should be treated in combination with an aminoglycoside.

Administration and Dosage

➤*Approved by the FDA:* October 22, 1993.

Administer by IV infusion over 30 minutes. The usual total daily dose for adults is 3.375 g every 6 hours totaling 13.5 g (12 g piperacillin/1.5 g tazobactam) for 7 to 10 days.

➤*Nosocomial pneumonia:* Start with 4.5 g every 6 hours plus an aminoglycoside. The recommended total daily dose is 18 g (16 g piperacillin/2 g tazobactam) for 7 to 14 days. Continue the aminoglycoside in patients from whom *P. aeruginosa* is isolated. If it is not isolated, the aminoglycoside may be discontinued at the discretion of the treating physician as guided by the severity of the infection and the patient's clinical and bacteriological progress.

➤*Renal function impairment:* In patients with renal insufficiency (Ccr 40 mL/min or less), adjust the IV dose to the degree of actual renal function impairment. In patients with nosocomial pneumonia receiving concomitant aminoglycoside therapy, adjust the aminoglycoside dosage according to the manufacturer's recommendations.

Piperacillin Sodium and Tazobactam Sodium Dosage Recommendations[1]

Creatinine clearance (mL/min)	All indications (except nosocomial pneumonia)	Nosocomial pneumonia
> 40	3.375 g every 6 hours	4.5 g every 6 hours
20-40[2]	2.25 g every 6 hours	3.375 g every 6 hours
< 20[2]	2.25 g every 8 hours	2.25 g every 6 hours
Hemodialysis[3]	2.25 g every 12 hours	2.25 g every 8 hours
CAPD	2.25 g every 12 hours	2.25 g every 8 hours

[1] Dosage provided is "total" combined piperacillin/tazobactam.
[2] Creatinine clearance for patients not receiving hemodialysis.
[3] Administer 0.75 g following each hemodialysis session on hemodialysis days.

➤*Hemodialysis:* The maximum dose is 2.25 g every 12 hours for all indications other than nosocomial pneumonia and 2.25 g every 8 hours for nosocomial pneumonia. In addition, because hemodialysis removes 30% to 40% of a dose, give one additional 0.75 g dose following each dialysis period. Peritoneal dialysis removes approximately 6% and 21% of the piperacillin and tazobactam doses, respectively. No additional dosage of piperacillin/tazobactam is necessary for continuous ambulatory peritoneal dialysis (CAPD) patients.

➤*Reconstitution:* Reconstitute conventional vials with 5 mL of compatible diluent per gram of piperacillin. Shake well until dissolved. Dilute to at least 50 mL to 150 mL. Administer over a period of at least 30 minutes.

➤*Compatible reconstituted diluents:* These include 0.9% sodium chloride for injection, sterile water for injection (maximum recommended volume is 50 mL), 5% dextrose, bacteriostatic saline/parabens, bacteriostatic water/parabens, bacteriostatic saline/benzyl alcohol, and bacteriostatic water/benzyl alcohol. Lactated Ringer's solution is not compatible.

➤*Compatible IV diluent solutions:* These include 0.9% sodium chloride for injection, sterile water for injection (maximum recommended volume per dose is 50 mL), 5% dextrose, and 6% dextran in saline.

➤*ADD-Vantage system admixtures:* These include 5% dextrose in water (50 or 100 mL) and 0.9% sodium chloride (50 or 100 mL).

➤*Coadministration infusion:* During the infusion it is desirable to discontinue the primary infusion solution. When cotherapy with aminoglycosides is indicated, reconstitute piperacillin/tazobactam and the aminoglycoside, and administer separately (because of the in vitro inactivation of the aminoglycoside by the penicillin).

➤*Storage/Stability:* Store piperacillin/tazobactam vials and *ADD-Vantage* vials at controlled room temperature (20° to 25°C [68° to 77°F]) prior to reconstitution. Use single-dose vials immediately after reconstitution. Discard any unused portion after 24 hours if stored at room temperature or after 48 hours if stored at refrigerated temperature (2° to 8°C [36° to 46°F]). Do not freeze vials after reconstitution. Stability in the IV bags has been demonstrated for up to 24 hours at room temperature and up to 1 week at refrigerated temperature. Stability in an ambulatory IV infusion pump has been demonstrated for a period of 12 hours at room temperature. Stability with the admixed *ADD-Vantage* system has been demonstrated through 24 hours at room temperature. Do not refrigerate or freeze the admixed *ADD-Vantage* after reconstitution.

Indications

For specific approved indications, refer to individual drug monographs.

Administration and Dosage

►*Duration of therapy:* Continue administration for a minimum of 48 to 72 hours after fever abates or after evidence of bacterial eradication has been obtained. A minimum of 10 days treatment is recommended for group A β-hemolytic streptococci infections to guard against the risk of rheumatic fever or glomerulonephritis.

►*Perioperative prophylaxis:* Discontinue prophylactic use within 24 hours after the surgical procedure. In surgery where infection may be particularly devastating (eg, open heart surgery, prosthetic arthroplasty), may continue prophylactic use for 3 to 5 days following surgery completion. If there are signs of infection, obtain cultures and perform sensitivity tests so appropriate therapy may be instituted.

Actions

►*Pharmacology:* Cephalosporins are structurally and pharmacologically related to penicillins. **Cefoxitin** and **cefotetan** (cephamycins) and **loracarbef** (a carbacephem) are included because of their similarity.

Most cephalosporins and related compounds are divided into first, second and third generation agents (see table). Within each group, differentiation is primarily by pharmacokinetics; groups are divided by antibacterial spectrum. In general, progression from first to third generation reveals broadening gram-negative spectrum, loss of efficacy against gram-positive organisms, greater efficacy against resistant organisms and increased cost. However, this classification scheme is becoming less clearly defined as newer agents enter the market. The decision to use a specific agent in the clinical setting should be primarily based on bacterial spectrum, route of administration, side effect profile and indications.

Mechanism – Cephalosporins inhibit mucopeptide synthesis in the bacterial cell wall, making it defective and osmotically unstable. The drugs are usually bactericidal, depending on organism susceptibility, dose, tissue concentrations and the rate at which organisms are multiplying. They are more effective against rapidly growing organisms forming cell walls.

►*Pharmacokinetics:*

Pharmacokinetic Parameters of Cephalosporins									
	Drug	Routes	Half-Life			Protein bound (%)	Recovered unchanged in urine (%)	Peak serum level 1 g IV dose (mcg/ml)	Sodium (mEq/g)
			Normal renal function (minutes)	ESRD[1] (hours)	Hemodialysis (hours)				
First	Cefadroxil	Oral	78-96	20-25	3-4	20	> 90	—	—
	Cefazolin	IM-IV	90–120	3-7	9-14	80-86	60-80	185	2-2.1
	Cephalexin	Oral	50-80	19-22	4-6	10	> 90	—	—
	Cephapirin	IM-IV	36	1.8-4	1.8	44-50	70	73	2.4
	Cephradine	Oral/IM-IV	48-80	8-15	—	8-17	> 90	86	6[2]
Second	Cefaclor	Oral	35-54	2-3	1.6-2.1	25	60-85	—	—
	Cefmetazole	IM-IV	72-90	—	—	65	85	—	2
	Cefonicid	IM-IV	270	11	—	90	99	221.3	3.7
	Cefotetan	IM-IV	180-276	13-35	5	88-90	51-81	158	3.5
	Cefoxitin	IV	40-60	20	4	73	85	110	2.3
	Cefprozil	Oral	78	5.2-5.9	decreased	36	60	—	—
	Cefuroxime	Oral/IM-IV	80	16-22[3]	3.5	50	66-100	100[4]	2.4[3]
	Loracarbef	Oral	60	32	4	25	> 90	—	—
Third	Cefdinir	Oral	100	16	3.2	60-70	12-18	—	—
	Cefepime	IM-IV	102-138	17-21	11-16	20	85	79	—
	Cefixime	Oral	180-240	11.5	—	65	50	—	—
	Cefoperazone	IM-IV	120	1.3-2.9	2	82-93	20-30	73-153	1.5
	Cefotaxime	IM-IV	60	3-11	2.5	30-40	60	42-102	2.2
	Cefpodoxime[5]	Oral	120-180	9.8	—	21-29	29-33	—	—
	Ceftazidime	IM-IV	114-120	14-30	—	< 10	80-90	69-90	2.3
	Ceftibuten	Oral	144	13.4-22.3	2-4	65	56	—	—
	Ceftizoxime	IM-IV	102	25-30	6	30	80	60-87	2.6
	Ceftriaxone	IM-IV	348-522	15.7	14.7	85-95	33-67	151	3.6

[1] ESRD = End stage renal disease (Ccr < 10 ml/min/1.73 m^2).
[2] Also available in sodium-free form.
[3] Injection only.
[4] Following 1.5 g IV dose.
[5] Extended-spectrum agent.

CEPHALOSPORINS AND RELATED ANTIBIOTICS

Organisms Generally Susceptible to Cephalosporins

✓ = generally susceptible
++ = demonstrated in vitro activity

Organisms	First Generation					Second Generation									Cefepime[1]	Cefixime	Third Generation						
	Cefadroxil	Cefazolin	Cephalexin	Cephapirin	Cephradine	Cefaclor	Cefonicid	Cefoxitin	Cefuroxime	Cefmetazole	Cefotetan	Cefprozil	Loracarbef	Cefdinir			Cefoperazone	Cefotaxime	Cefpodoxime[2]	Ceftazidime	Ceftibuten	Cefizoxime	Ceftriaxone
Gram-positive																							
Staphylococci[3]	✓	✓	✓[4]	✓	✓	✓[4]	✓[4]	✓	✓	✓	✓	✓	✓	✓[5]	✓[6]		✓	✓[5]	✓[4]	✓		✓	✓
Staphylococcus aureus														✓[5]									
Staphylococcus epidermidis									++					✓[5]									
Staphylococcus saprophyticus							++	++	++				++	++[6]									
Streptococci, beta-hemolytic	✓	✓	✓	✓	✓	✓	✓	✓	✓	✓	✓	✓	✓	++	++	✓	✓	✓	✓	✓		✓	✓
Streptococcus agalactiae						++			++				++										
Streptococcus bovis	✓	✓	✓	✓	✓	✓	✓	✓	✓	✓		✓	✓			✓							
Streptococcus pneumoniae	✓	✓	✓	✓	✓	✓	✓	✓	✓	✓	✓	✓	✓	✓[7]	✓	✓	✓	✓	✓	✓	✓[7]	✓	✓
Streptococcus pyogenes	✓			✓		✓	✓	✓	✓	✓	✓	✓	✓	✓	✓[8]	✓	✓	✓	✓	✓	✓	✓	✓
Streptococcus viridans						++			++		++		++	++	++	✓			++	++			
Gram-negative																							
Acinetobacter sp.															++		✓[4]	✓		++		✓	++
Citrobacter sp.		++[4]				++	++		✓[4]	++	++	++	++	++	++	++	✓	✓	++	✓		++	++
Enterobacter sp.		✓				++	++		✓[4]	++	✓	++	++	++	++	++	✓	✓	++	✓		✓	✓
Escherichia coli	✓	✓	✓	✓	✓	✓	✓	✓	✓	✓	✓	✓	✓	✓	✓	✓	✓	✓	✓	✓	✓	✓	✓
Haemophilus influenzae				✓		✓[5]	✓[5]	✓[5]	✓[5]	✓[5]	✓[5]	✓[5]	✓[5]	✓[5]	++[5]	✓[5]	✓[5]	✓[5]	✓[5]	✓[5]	✓[5]	✓[5]	✓[5]
Haemophilus parainfluenzae					++	++	✓[5]		++	✓[5]	✓[5]		++	✓[5]	++	✓[5]	✓	✓	++	++		✓	✓
Hafnia alvei														++	++	++[5]			++	++			
Klebsiella sp.	✓	✓	✓	✓	✓	✓	✓	✓	✓	✓	✓	✓	✓	✓	✓	✓	✓	✓	✓	✓		✓	✓
Klebsiella pneumoniae		++	++			++	++			++		++		++	++	++				++			
Moraxella (Branhamella) catarrhalis	++					✓[5]		✓	✓	++	++	✓[5]	✓[5]	✓[5]	✓[5]	✓[5]	✓		✓		✓[5]		
Morganella (Proteus) morganii								✓		++	++		++		++			✓		✓	✓[5]		✓
Neisseria catarrhalis			✓	✓			✓	✓	✓[4]									✓		✓		✓	✓
Neisseria gonorrhoeae						++	++	✓	✓	✓	++				✓	++		✓		✓		✓	✓
Neisseria meningitidis								✓	✓	✓	✓		+[3]			++	✓[5]	✓	✓[4]	++			✓
Pasteurella multocida							++			++	++				++	++	++			++		++	++
Proteus inconstans	✓												++										
Proteus mirabilis	✓	✓	✓	✓	✓	✓	✓	✓	✓	✓	✓	✓	✓	✓	✓	✓	✓	✓	✓	✓		✓	✓
Proteus vulgaris								✓		++	✓			++	++	++	✓	✓	++	✓		✓	✓
Providencia sp.						✓	✓	✓		++					++	++	✓	++	++	++		++	++
Providencia rettgeri						++		✓		++	++					++	✓	++	++	++		✓[4]	✓[4]
Pseudomonas aeruginosa				✓							++		+[3]		++		✓[5]	✓[4]	✓[4]	✓		✓[4]	✓[4]
Salmonella sp.											++				++		++	✓	++	✓		✓	✓
Salmonella typhi	✓	✓	✓	✓	✓	✓	✓	✓	✓	✓	✓	✓	✓	++		++	✓	✓	✓	✓		✓[4]	✓[4]
Serratia sp.											++					✓		++	++	✓		++	++
Shigella sp.	✓						✓		✓	++	++	++	++	++		++	✓	++	++	✓		✓	✓
Yersinia enterocolitica										✓	✓		++	++		++	++	++	++	++		++	++

CEPHALOSPORINS AND RELATED ANTIBIOTICS

✓ = generally susceptible
+ = demonstrated in vitro activity

Organisms Generally Susceptible to Cephalosporins

Organisms	First Generation					Second Generation									Third Generation								
	Cefadroxil	Cefazolin	Cephalexin	Cephapirin	Cephradine	Cefaclor	Cefonicid	Cefoxitin	Cefuroxime	Cefmetazole	Cefotetan	Cefprozil	Loracarbef	Cefdinir	Cefepime[1]	Cefixime	Cefoperazone	Cefotaxime	Cefpodoxime[2]	Ceftazidime	Ceftibuten	Ceftizoxime	Ceftriaxone
Anaerobes																							
Bacteroides sp.						✓		✓	✓	✓	✓[4]	+					✓	✓		✓[4]		+	✓
Bacteroides fragilis								✓	✓	✓	✓						✓	✓				✓	+
Clostridium sp.							+	✓	✓	✓	✓	+					✓	✓		+		+	+
Clostridium difficile											+	+	+				+						
Eubacterium sp.							+						+				+			+			+
Fusobacterium sp.							+	✓	✓	✓	✓	+	+				+	✓				+	+
Peptococcus sp.						+	+	✓	✓	+	✓	+	+				✓	✓		+		✓	+
Peptococcus niger						+	+						+										
Peptostreptococcus sp.						+	+	✓	✓	+	✓	+	+				✓	✓	+	+		✓	+
Porphyromonas asaccharolytica											✓												
Prevotella bivia											✓												
Prevotella digiens											✓												
Prevotella melaninogenica											+												
Prevotella oralis											+												
Propionibacterium acnes						+					+		+										
Propionibacterium sp.											+												
Veillonella sp.																							
Other																							
Borrelia burgdorferi									✓														

[1] Including some β-lactamase-producing strains.
[2] Extended-spectrum agent.
[3] Methicillin-susceptible strains only.
[4] Some strains are resistant.
[5] Penicillin-susceptible strains only.
[6] Lancefield's group A streptococci.
[7] Some other references consider this fourth generation.
[8] Coagulase-positive, coagulase-negative, and penicillinase-producing.

Absorption – **Cephalexin, cephradine, cefaclor, cefixime, cefprozil, cefadroxil, ceftibuten** and **loracarbef** are well absorbed from the GI tract; absorption of these agents (except cefadroxil and cefprozil) may be delayed by food, but the amount absorbed is not affected. Peak plasma levels of loracarbef (capsules) are decreased by food and occur later. After oral administration, **cefuroxime axetil** is absorbed from the GI tract and rapidly hydrolyzed in the intestinal mucosa and blood to cefuroxime. **Cefpodoxime proxetil** is a pro-drug that is absorbed from the GI tract and de-esterified to its active metabolite, cefpodoxime. The absorption of oral cefuroxime and cefpodoxime is increased when given with food. **Cefdinir** may be taken without regard to meals.

Distribution – Cephalosporins are widely distributed to most tissues and fluids. First and second generation agents do not readily enter cerebrospinal fluid (CSF), except **cefuroxime**, even when meninges are inflamed. Third generation compounds (little data for **cefixime**) and cefuroxime readily diffuse into the CSF of patients with inflamed meninges. However, CSF levels of **cefoperazone** are relatively low. No data are available for **cefdinir** human CSF penetration. Therapeutic levels are reached in bone after usual doses of most agents. **Cefazolin** penetrates acutely inflamed bone at higher concentrations than in normal bone.

High concentrations of **ceftriaxone** and **cefoperazone** are attained in bile. Therapeutic levels of **ceftizoxime, cefuroxime, cefotetan, ceftazidime, cefoxitin** and **cefonicid** are attained in bile. Bile levels of **cefazolin** can reach or exceed serum levels by up to five times in patients without obstructive biliary disease.

Metabolism / Excretion – **Cefuroxime axetil** is metabolized to free cefuroxime plus acetaldehyde and acetic acid. **Cephapirin** is metabolized to less active compounds; however, desacetylcephapirin contributes to the drug's antibacterial activity. Desacetylcefotaxime, a major metabolite of **cefotaxime**, contributes to the bactericidal activity and increases the spectrum to include anaerobes, specifically *Bacteroides* sp; the synergy with the parent drug appears to extend the dosing interval to 8 to 12 hours because of the prolonged metabolite half-life. **Cefpodoxime proxetil** is a pro-drug that is de-esterified to its active metabolite, cefpodoxime. **Cefdinir** is not appreciably metabolized and is primarily excreted renally. Most cephalosporins and metabolites are primarily excreted renally. **Cefoperazone** is excreted mainly in the bile; peak serum levels and serum half-lives are unchanged, even in patients with severe renal insufficiency. In hepatic dysfunction, serum half-life and urinary excretion are increased.

➤*Microbiology:* Refer to the previous tables for organisms generally susceptible to cephalosporins.

β*-lactamase resistance* – First generation cephalosporins are generally inactivated by β-lactamase-producing organisms. Newer agents are distinguished by an increasing resistance to β-lactamase inactivation. **Cefonicid, cefdinir, loracarbef** and **cefixime** have a high degree of stability to some β–lactamases. **Cefoxitin, cefuroxime, ceftriaxone, cefotaxime, ceftizoxime, cefmetazole** and **cefotetan** have a high degree of stability in the presence of both penicillinases and cephalosporinases produced by gram-negative and gram-positive bacteria. **Cefoperazone, cefpodoxime** and **ceftazidime** are highly stable in the presence of β-lactamases produced by most gram-negative pathogens and are active against some organisms that are resistant to other β-lactam antibiotics because of β-lactamase production. **Cefepime** has a broad spectrum of activity against gram-positive and gram-negative bacteria but has a low affinity for chromosomally encoded beta-lactamases. **Cefaclor** is stable in the presence of some β-lactamases. **Cefprozil** has in vitro activity against a broad range of gram-positive and gram-negative bacteria.

Contraindications

Hypersensitivity to cephalosporins or related antibiotics (see Warnings).

Warnings

➤*Cross-allergenicity with penicillin:* Administer cautiously to penicillin-sensitive patients. There is evidence of partial cross-allergenicity; cephalosporins cannot be assumed to be an absolutely safe alternative to penicillin in the penicillin-allergic patient. The estimated incidence of cross-sensitivity is 5% to 16%; however, it is possibly as low as 3% to 7%.

➤*Serum sickness-like reactions:* Erythema multiforme or skin rashes accompanied by polyarthritis, arthralgia and, frequently, fever have been reported; these reactions usually occurred following a second course of therapy. Signs and symptoms occur after a few days of therapy and resolve a few days after drug discontinuation with no serious sequelae. Antihistamines and corticosteroids may be of benefit in managing symptoms.

➤*Seizures:* Several cephalosporins have been implicated in triggering seizures, particularly in patients with renal impairment when the dosage was not reduced. If seizures associated with drug therapy occur, discontinue the drug. Anticonvulsant therapy can be given if clinically indicated.

➤*Coagulation abnormalities:* **Cefmetazole, cefoperazone, cefotetan** and **ceftriaxone** may be associated with a fall in prothrombin activity. Those at risk include patients with renal impairment, cancer, impaired vitamin K synthesis or low vitamin K stores (eg, chronic hepatic disease or malnutrition), as well as patients receiving a protracted course of antimicrobial therapy. Monitor prothrombin time for patients at risk and administer exogenous vitamin K as indicated. Vitamin K administration may be necessary if the prothrombin time is prolonged before therapy.

➤*Pseudomembranous colitis:* This occurs with cephalosporins (and other broad spectrum antibiotics); consider this diagnosis in patients who develop diarrhea with antibiotic use. Colitis may range in severity from mild to life-threatening. Treatment alters normal flora of the colon and may permit overgrowth of *Clostridia* species. A toxin produced by *C. difficile* is a primary cause of antibiotic-associated colitis. Cholestyramine and colestipol resins bind the toxin in vitro.

Mild cases of colitis may respond to drug discontinuation alone. Manage moderate-to-severe cases by sigmoidoscopy, bacteriologic studies and with fluid, electrolyte and protein supplementation, as indicated. When the colitis is not relieved by drug discontinuation, or when it is severe, oral vancomycin (see individual monograph) is treatment of choice. Rule out other causes of colitis.

Prescribe broad-spectrum antibiotics with caution in individuals with a history of GI disease, especially colitis.

➤*Immune hemolytic anemia:* This has been observed in patients receiving cephalosporin class antibiotics. Rare cases of severe hemolytic anemia, including fatalities, have been reported in association with cephalosporins. If a patient develops anemia any time within 2 to 3 weeks subsequent to the start of therapy, the diagnosis of cephalosporin-associated anemia should be considered and the drug stopped until the etiology is determined with certainty. Blood transfusions may be administered as needed. Patients who receive prolonged courses of cephalosporins for treatment of infections should have periodic monitoring for signs and symptoms of hemolytic anemia, including a measurement of hematological parameters where appropriate.

➤*Renal function impairment:* Cephalosporins may be nephrotoxic; use with caution in the presence of markedly impaired renal function (creatinine clearance [Ccr] rate of < 50 ml/min/1.73 m²). In the elderly and in patients with known or suspected renal impairment, monitor carefully prior to and during therapy.

Reduce total daily antibiotic dosage in patients with transient or persistent reduction of urinary output caused by renal insufficiency; high and prolonged serum concentrations can occur in such patients from usual doses. See individual product monographs for information on dosage adjustments in impaired renal function.

➤*Hepatic function impairment:* **Cefoperazone** is extensively excreted in bile. Serum half-life increases 2-fold to 4-fold in patients with hepatic disease or biliary obstruction. If higher dosages are used (> 4 g), monitor serum concentrations.

➤*Elderly:* In elderly patients, dosage adjustments based on decreased renal function may be necessary.

➤*Pregnancy: Category B.* Safety for use during pregnancy is not established. Use only when potential benefits outweigh potential hazards to the fetus. Cephalosporins appear safe for pregnant patients, but relatively few controlled studies exist.

These agents cross the placenta; peak umbilical cord concentrations for the various agents range from 3 to 29 mcg/ml following doses of 0.5 to 2 g. These data yielded a maternal:fetal serum ratio range of 0.16 to 1. Drug levels in cord blood after administration of **cefazolin** are ≈ ¼ to ⅓ maternal drug levels. **Cefotetan** reaches therapeutic levels in cord blood.

In addition, the pharmacokinetic parameters of these drugs appear to change in the pregnant woman; tendencies are toward shorter half-lives, lower serum levels, larger volumes of distribution and increased clearance.

➤*Lactation:* Most of these agents are excreted in breast milk in small quantities. Levels range from 0.16 to 4 mcg/ml, or a breast milk:maternal serum ratio of 0.01 to 0.5 following 0.5 to 2 g doses. **Cefdinir** was not detected in breast milk following single 600 mg doses. However, consider these problems for the nursing infant: Modification/alteration of bowel flora; pharmacological effects; interference with interpretation of culture results if a fever/infection workup is needed. **Ceftibuten** has not been studied.

➤*Children:* When using cephalosporins in infants, consider the relative benefit to risk. In neonates, accumulation of cephalosporin antibiotics, with resulting prolongation of drug half-life, has occurred.

In children ≥ 3 months of age, higher doses of **cefoxitin** have been associated with an increased incidence of eosinophilia and elevated AST.

In children ≥ 6 months of age, **ceftizoxime** has been associated with transient elevated levels of eosinophils, AST, ALT and CPK.

Safety and efficacy in children < 1 month (**cefazolin** and **cefaclor** capsule and suspension),< 3 months (**cefuroxime, cephapirin** and **cefoxitin**), < 5 months (**cefpodoxime**), < 6 months (**cefdinir, loracarbef, cefixime, ceftozoxime** and **cefprozil**), < 9 months (**oral cephradine**) and < 1 year (**cefepime** and **parenteral cephradine**) have not been established.

Safety and efficacy of **cefaclor** extended release tablets in children < 16 years of age have not been established.

Safety and efficacy of **cefonicid, cefmetazole, cefoperazone, cephalexin** and **cefotetan** in children have not been established.

Precautions

➤*Parenteral use:* Inject IM preparations deep into musculature; properly dilute IV preparations and administer over an appropriate time interval. See individual product monographs. Prolonged or high dosage IV use may be associated with thrombophlebitis; use small IV needles, larger veins and alternate infusion sites.

➤*Gonorrhea:* In the treatment of gonorrhea, all patients should have a serologic test for syphilis. Patients with incubating syphilis (seronegative without clinical signs of syphilis) are likely to be cured by the regimens used for gonorrhea.

➤*Benzyl alcohol:* Some cephalosporin products contain benzyl alcohol. In neonates, benzyl alcohol has been associated with neurological and other complications which are sometimes fatal. Benzyl alcohol-containing cephalosporin products should not be used in neonates.

➤*Superinfection:* Use of antibiotics (especially prolonged or repeated therapy) may result in bacterial or fungal overgrowth of nonsusceptible organisms. Such overgrowth may lead to a secondary infection. Take appropriate measures if this occurs.

Drug Interactions

Cephalosporin Drug Interactions			
Precipitant drug	Object drug*		Description
Cephalosporins Cefazolin Cetmetazole Cefoperazone Cefotetan	Ethanol	↑	Alcoholic beverages consumed concurrently with or ≤ 72 hours after cefoperazone, cefazolin, cefmetazole or cefotetan may produce acute alcohol intolerance (disulfiram-like reaction). These antibiotics possess a methyltetrazolethiol side chain that may inhibit aldehyde dehydrogenase. The reaction begins within 30 minutes after alcohol ingestion and may subside 30 minutes to several hours afterwards; the reaction may occur ≤ 3 days after the last dose of the antibiotic.
Cephalosporins	Aminoglycosides	↑	Aminoglycoside nephrotoxicity may be potentiated by concurrent use of some cephalosporins, specifically cephalothin. Monitor renal function closely.
Cephalosporins Cefazolin Cefmetazole Cefoperazone Cefotetan	Anticoagulants	↑	Hypoprothrombinemic effects of anticoagulants may be increased by cephalosporins with the methyltetrazolethiol side chain (cefazolin, cefmetazole, cefoperazone, cefotetan). Bleeding complications may occur (see Warnings). Bleeding disorders have occurred with some of the other cephalosporins; therefore, the risk might be increased in anticoagulated patients. The concurrent use of heparin may also theoretically increase the risk of bleeding.
Cephalosporins Cephalothin	Polypeptide antibiotics	↑	The nephrotoxic effects of colistimethate may be increased by cephalothin. Monitor renal function.
Probenecid	Cephalosporins	↑	Probenecid may increase and prolong cephalosporin plasma levels by competitively inhibiting renal tubular secretion. This is most significant for cephalosporins eliminated primarily by tubular secretion.
Antacids	Cephalosporins Cefaclor Cefdinir Cefpodoxime	↓	Plasma concentrations of cefaclor extended release tablets, cefdinir and cefpodoxime may be reduced by coadministration of antacids. If antacids are required during administration of these antibiotics, the cephalosporin should be taken 2 hours before or after the antacid. Cefprozil and ceftibuten do not appear to be affected by coadministration of antacids.
H₂ antagonists	Cephalosporins Cefpodoxime Cefuroxime	↓	Plasma concentrations of cefpodoxime and cefuroxime may be reduced by coadministration of H₂ antagonists, decreasing the antibiotic effect. Cefaclor extended release tablets do not appear to be affected by coadministration of H₂ antagonists.

Cephalosporin Drug Interactions			
Precipitant drug	Object drug*		Description
Iron supplements	Cephalosporins Cefdinir	↓	Iron supplements and foods fortified with iron reduce the absorption of cefdinir by 80% and 30%, respectively. If iron supplements are needed during cefdinir therapy, cefdinir should be taken 2 hours before or after the supplement. Iron-fortified infant formula (2.2 mg elemental iron/6 oz) has no effect on cefdinir absorption.
Loop diuretics	Cephalosporins	↑	Use cephalosporins with caution in patients receiving potent diuretics (eg, loop diuretics). The risk of nephrotoxicity may be increased. Monitor renal function.

* ↑ = Object drug increased. ↓ = Object drug decreased.

➤*Drug/Lab test interactions:* A false-positive reaction for **urine glucose** may occur with Benedict's solution, Fehling's solution or with *Clinitest* tablets, but not with enzyme-based tests such as *Clinistix* and *Tes-Tape*.

Cephradine may cause false-positive reactions in urinary protein tests that use sulfosalicylic acid.

Cefuroxime may cause a false-negative reaction in the ferricyanide test for **blood glucose**.

Cefdinir may cause a false-positive reaction for ketones in urine when measured using nitroprusside but not nitroferricynide.

A false-positive direct **Coombs' test** has occurred in some patients receiving cephalosporins, particularly those with azotemia, in hematologic studies, in transfusion cross-matching procedures when **antiglobulin tests** are performed on the minor side or in Coombs' testing of newborns of mothers receiving cephalosporins before parturition. This reaction is nonimmunological.

Cephalosporins may falsely elevate **urinary 17-ketosteroid** values.

High concentrations of **cephalothin** or **cefoxitin** (> 100 mcg/ml) may interfere with measurement of creatinine levels by the Jaffe reaction and produce false results. Serum samples from patients on cefoxitin should not be analyzed for creatinine if obtained within 2 hours of drug use. **Cefotetan** may affect these measurements.

➤*Drug/Food interactions:* Food increases absorption of **cefpodoxime** and oral **cefuroxime**.

Adverse Reactions

➤*Cardiovascular:* Hypotension; palpitations; chest pain; vasodilation; syncope.

➤*CNS:* Headache; dizziness; vertigo; lethargy; fatigue; paresthesia; confusion; anxiety; hyperactivity; nervousness; insomnia; hypertonia; somnolence. Generalized tonic-clonic seizures, mild hemiparesis and extreme confusion after large doses in renal failure (**cefazolin**).

➤*Dermatologic:* Urticaria; diaphoresis; flushing; cutaneous moniliasis.

➤*GI:* Nausea; vomiting; diarrhea; constipation; anorexia; thirst; glossitis; oral candidiasis and moniliasis; abdominal pain; flatulence; heartburn; gastritis; stomach cramps; eructation; melena; bleeding peptic ulcer; ileus; gall bladder sludge; dyspepsia; colitis, including pseudomembranous colitis, can appear during or after treatment (see Warnings); adverse GI effects after parenteral use of some cephalosporins.

➤*GU:* Transitory elevations in BUN with and without elevated serum creatinine; pyuria; dysuria; vaginitis; vaginal discharge; genito-anal pruritus; genital candidiasis and moniliasis; reversible interstitial nephritis; hematuria; toxic nephropathy; acute renal failure (rare); casts in urine (**ceftriaxone**).

➤*Hematologic:* Eosinophilia; transient neutropenia; lymphocytosis; leukocytosis; leukopenia; thrombocythemia; thrombocytopenia; agranulocytosis; granulocytopenia; hemolytic anemia; bone marrow depression; pancytopenia; decreased platelet function; bleeding in association with hypoprothrombinemia; anemia; aplastic anemia; hemorrhage; transient thrombocytosis; neutropenia caused by an immunologic reaction and characterized by rapid destruction of peripheral neutrophils may require drug discontinuation; transient fluctuations in leukocyte counts, predominantly lymphocytosis; slight decreases in neutrophil count; decreased hemoglobin or hematocrit; disturbances in vitamin K-dependent clotting function (increased PT); increased platelet and increased bleeding. Lymphopenia, monocytosis, basophilia (ceftriaxone, rare and may be accompanied by jaundice, glycosuria, bronchospasm, palpitations and epistaxis).

➤*Hepatic:* Elevated AST, ALT, total bilirubin, alkaline phosphatase, LDH; hepatomegaly; hepatitis; jaundice; cholestasis; cholestatic jaundice; hepatic failure.

➤*Hypersensitivity:* Anaphylaxis; angioedema; Stevens-Johnson syndrome; erythema multiforme; toxic epidermal necrolysis; renal dysfunction; toxic nephropathy; hepatic dysfunction (including cholestasis); aplastic anemia; hemolytic anemia; hemorrhage; erythema; maculopapular rash; urticaria; pruritus.

➤*Local:* Pain; induration; temperature elevation and tenderness from IM injection; sterile abscesses from accidental SC injection; local swelling; inflammation; burning, cellulitis, paresthesia, phlebitis and thrombophlebitis following IV or IM administration.

➤*Musculoskeletal:* Myalgia; arthralgia; rhabdomyolysis; exacerbation of myasthenia gravis (**cefoxitin**).

➤*Respiratory:* Asthma; laryngeal edema; dyspnea; interstitial pneumonitis; bronchitis; bronchospasm; pneumonia; respiratory failure; epistaxis (**ceftriaxone**, rare); rhinitis (**loracarbef**).

➤*Miscellaneous:* Facial edema; swollen tongue; fever; chills; malaise; asthenia; dysgeusia; glucosuria; encephalopathy in renally impaired patients receiving unadjusted dosage regiment (**cefepime**); Jarisch-Herxheimer reaction (**cefuroxime**); muscle cramps, stiffness, spasms of neck, pain/tightness in chest, pain/bleeding in urethra, kidney pain, tachycardia, lockjaw-type reaction (**cefuroxime**, single dose for gonorrhea); elevated CPK (IM **ceftizoxime** or **cefaclor** extended release tablets); mild-to-moderate hearing loss reported in some pediatric patients (**cefuroxime**).

Overdosage

➤*Parenteral cephalosporins:* Inappropriately large doses may cause seizures, particularly in renal impairment. Reduce dosage when renal function is impaired. If seizures occur, promptly discontinue drug; administer anticonvulsants if clinically indicated; consider hemodialysis in cases of overwhelming overdosage.

Patient Information

➤*For oral preparations:* Complete full course of therapy.

May cause GI upset; may take with food or milk. Take **cefpodoxime** and **cefuroxime** with food to increase absorption.

A false-positive reaction for urine glucose may occur with the nonspecific urine tests. Use an enzyme-based test.

➤*Cephradine:*

Diabetics – Notify physician before changing diet or dosage of medication.

➤*Phenylketonurics:* **Cefprozil** oral suspension contains phenylalanine 28 mg/5 ml.

➤*Antacids:* Those containing magnesium or aluminum interfere with the absorption of cefdinir. If this type of antacid is required during **cefdinir** therapy, take cefdinir 2 hours before or after the antacid.

CEFPODOXIME PROXETIL

Rx	Vantin (Pharmacia & Upjohn)	**Tablets:** 100 mg	Lactose. (U3617). Orange. Film coated. In 20s, 100s and UD 100s.
		200 mg	Lactose. (U3618). Coral red. Film coated. In 20s, 100s and UD 100s.
		Granules for suspension: 50 mg/5 ml	Lactose, sucrose. Lemon creme flavor. In 50, 75 and 100 ml bottles.
		100 mg/5 ml	Lactose, sucrose. Lemon creme flavor. In 50 and 100 ml bottles.

For complete prescribing information, refer to the Cephalosporins group monograph.

Indications

➤*Lower respiratory tract:*

Acute, community-acquired pneumonia – Due to *Streptococcus pneumoniae* or *Haemophilus influenzae* (including beta-lactamase-producing strains).

Chronic bronchitis – Acute bacterial exacerbation caused by *S. pneumoniae*, *H. influenzae* (non-beta-lactamase-producing strains only) or *M. catarrhalis*.

Data are insufficient to establish efficacy in patients with acute bacterial exacerbations of chronic bronchitis caused by β-lactamase-producing *H. influenzae*.

➤*Upper respiratory tract:*

Acute otitis media – Due to *S. pneumoniae*, *H. influenzae* (including β-lactamase-producing strains) or *Moraxella (Branhamella) catarrhalis*.

Pharyngitis/tonsillitis – Due to *S. pyogenes*.

Only IM penicillin is effective in prophylaxis of rheumatic fever. Cefpodoxime is generally effective in eradication of streptococci from the oropharynx. However, efficacy for prophylaxis of subsequent rheumatic fever is not established.

➤*Sexually transmitted diseases:*

Acute, uncomplicated urethral and cervical gonorrhea – Due to *Neisseria gonorrhoeae* (including penicillinase-producing strains).

Acute, uncomplicated ano-rectal infections in women – Due to *N. gonorrhoeae* (including penicillinase-producing strains).

Efficacy of cefpodoxime in males with rectal infections caused by *N. gonorrhoeae* is not established. Data do not support the use of cefpodoxime in treatment of pharyngeal infections caused by *N. gonorrhoeae* in men or women.

➤*Skin and skin structures:*

Uncomplicated infections – Those caused by *Staphylococcus aureus* (including penicillinase-producing strains) or *S. pyogenes*. Surgically drain abscesses as clinically indicated.

In clinical trials, successful treatment of uncomplicated skin and skin structure infections was dose-related. The effective therapeutic dose for skin infections was higher than those used in other recommended indications.

➤*Urinary tract:*

Uncomplicated infections (cystitis) – Due to *Escherichia coli*, *Klebsiella pneumoniae*, *Proteus mirabilis* or *S. saprophyticus*.

In considering the use of cefpodoxime in the treatment of cystitis, weigh cefpodoxime's lower bacterial eradication rates against the increased eradication rates and different safety profiles of some other classes of approved agents.

Administration and Dosage

➤*Approved by the FDA:* August 7, 1992.

Administer tablets with food to enhance absorption. Administer oral suspension without regard to food.

Dosage/Duration of Cefpodoxime			
Type of infection	Total daily dose	Dose frequency	Duration
Adults ≥ 13 years of age			
Acute community-acquired pneumonia	400 mg	200 mg every 12 hrs	14 days
Acute bacterial exacerbations of chronic bronchitis (tablets)	400 mg	200 mg every 12 hrs	10 days
Uncomplicated gonorrhea (men and women) and rectal gonococcal infections (women)	200 mg	single dose	
Skin and skin structure	800 mg	400 mg every 12 hrs	7 to 14 days
Pharyngitis/tonsillitis	200 mg	100 mg every 12 hrs	5 to 10 days
Uncomplicated urinary tract infection	200 mg	100 mg every 12 hrs	7 days
Children (age 5 months through 12 years):[1]			
Acute otitis media	10 mg/kg/day (max 400 mg/day)	10 mg/kg every 24 hrs (max 400 mg/dose) or 5 mg/kg every 12 hrs (max 200 mg/dose)	10 days
Pharyngitis/tonsillitis	10 mg/kg/day (max 200 mg/day)	5 mg/kg every 12 hours (max 100 mg/dose)	5 to 10 days

[1] Do not exceed adult recommended doses.

➤*Renal function impairment:* For patients with severe renal impairment (creatinine clearance [Ccr] < 30 ml/min), increase the dosing intervals to every 24 hours. Hemodialysis patients use a dose frequency of three times a week after hemodialysis.

When only the serum creatinine level is available, the following calculation may be used to estimate Ccr (ml/min). For this estimate to be valid, the serum creatinine level should represent a steady state of renal function.

CEFPODOXIME PROXETIL

Males: $\dfrac{\text{Weight (kg)} \times (140 - \text{age})}{72 \times \text{serum creatinine (mg/dL)}} = \text{Ccr}$

Females: $0.85 \times \text{above value}$

➤*Cirrhosis:* Cefpodoxime pharmacokinetics in cirrhotic patients (with or without ascites) are similar to those in healthy subjects. Dose adjustment is not necessary.

➤*Storage/Stability:* Store the suspension in a refrigerator at 2° to 8°C (36° to 46°F). Discard unused portion after 14 days.

CEFACLOR

Rx	**Cefaclor** (Various, eg, Apothecon, Mylan, Rugby, URL)	**Capsules:** 250 mg	In 30s, 100s, 500s and 1000s.
Rx	**Ceclor Pulvules** (Eli Lilly)		(3061). White and purple. In 15s, 100s and UD 100s.
Rx	**Cefaclor** (Various, eg, Apothecon, Mylan, Rugby, URL)	**Capsules:** 500 mg	In 15s, 100s and 500s.
Rx	**Cefaclor** (Zenith Goldline)	**Tablets, extended release:** 375 mg	(X 4194 500). Blue, oval. In 100s.
		500 mg	
Rx	**Cefaclor** (Various, eg, Apothecon, Mylan, Rugby, URL, Zenith Goldline)	**Powder for oral suspension:** 125 mg/5 ml	In 75 and 150 ml.
	Ceclor (Eli Lilly)		Sucrose. Strawberry flavor. In 75 and 150 ml.
Rx	**Cefaclor** (Various, eg, Apothecon, Mylan, Rugby, URL, Zenith Goldline)	**Powder for oral suspension:** 187 mg/5 ml	In 50 and 100 ml.
	Ceclor (Eli Lilly)		Sucrose. Strawberry flavor. In 50 and 100 ml.
Rx	**Cefaclor** (Various, eg, Apothecon, Mylan, Rugby, URL, Zenith Goldline)	**Powder for oral suspension:** 250 mg/5 ml	In 75 and 150 ml.
	Ceclor (Eli Lilly)		Sucrose. Strawberry flavor. In 75 and 150 ml.
Rx	**Cefaclor** (Various, eg, Apothecon, Mylan, Rugby, URL, Zenith Goldline)	**Powder for oral suspension:** 375 mg/5 ml	In 50 and 100 ml.
	Ceclor (Eli Lilly)		Sucrose. Strawberry flavor. In 50 and 100 ml.

For complete prescribing information, refer to the Cephalosporins group monograph.

Indications

➤*Lower respiratory tract infections:* These include pneumonia caused by *Streptococcus pneumoniae*, *H. influenzae* and *S. pyogenes* (group A β-hemolytic streptococci).

➤*Upper respiratory tract infections:* These include pharyngitis and tonsillitis caused by *S. pyogenes* (group A β-hemolytic streptococci).

➤*Otitis media:* Due to *S. pneumoniae*, *H. influenzae*, staphylococci and *S. pyogenes* (group A β-hemolytic streptococci).

➤*Skin and skin structure infections:* Those caused by *Staphylococcus aureus* and *S. pyogenes* (group A β-hemolytic streptococci).

➤*Urinary tract infections:* These include pyelonephritis and cystitis caused by *Escherichia coli*, *Proteus mirabilis*, *Klebsiella* sp. and coagulase-negative staphylococci.

➤*Tablets, extended release:*

Acute bacterial exacerbations of chronic bronchitis – Due to *H. influenzae* (non-β-lactamase-producing strains only), *M. catarrhalis* (including β-lactamase-producing strains) or *S. pneumoniae*.

Secondary bacterial infections of acute bronchitis – Due to *H. influenzae* (non-β-lactamase-producing strains only), *M. catarrhalis* (including β-lactamase-producing strains) or *S. pneumoniae*.

Pharyngitis and tonsillitis – Due to *S. pyogenes*.

Uncomplicated skin/skin structure infections – Those caused by *S. aureus* (methicillin-susceptible).

Administration and Dosage

➤*Adults:* Usual dosage is 250 mg every 8 hours. In severe infections or those caused by less susceptible organisms, dosage may be doubled.

Capsules – Food does not affect the extent of absorption.

Tablets, extended release – Administer with food to enhance absorption. Do not cut, crush or chew.

Equivalence: Until data are available, the extended release tablet should not be assumed to be equivalent to the tablet or suspension formulations.

Acute bacterial exacerbations of chronic bronchitis – 500 mg every 12 hours for 7 days.

The effectiveness of the extended release tablets against β-lactamase producing *H. influenzae* has not been established.

Secondary bacterial infection of acute bronchitis – 500 mg every 12 hours for 7 days.

The effectiveness of the extended release tablets against β-lactamase producing *H. influenzae* has not been established.

Pharyngitis or tonsillitis – 375 mg every 12 hours for 10 days.

Uncomplicated skin and skin structure infections – 375 mg every 12 hours for 7 to 10 days.

The effectiveness of the extended release tablets against *S. pyogenes* has not been established.

➤*Children:* Give 20 mg/kg/day in divided doses every 8 hours. In more serious infections, such as otitis media and infections caused by less susceptible organisms, administer 40 mg/kg/day, with a maximum dosage of 1 g/day. Do not exceed adult recommended doses.

Twice daily treatment option – For otitis media and pharyngitis, the total daily dosage may be divided and administered every 12 hours.

➤*Storage/Stability:* Refrigerate suspension after reconstitution; discard after 14 days.

CEPHALEXIN

Rx	**Cephalexin** (Various, eg, Geneva, Lederle, Rugby)	**Capsules:** 250 mg	In 100s, 500s, 1000s, UD 20s and 100s.
Rx	**Keflex** (Dista)		(Dista H69/Keflex 250). White/light green. In 20s, 100s and UD 100s.
Rx	**Cephalexin** (Various, eg, Geneva, Lederle, Major, Rugby)	500 mg	In 100s, 250s, 500s, 1000s, UD 20s and 100s.
Rx	**Biocef** (Inter. Ethical Labs)		In 100s.
Rx	**Keflex** (Dista)		(Dista H71/Keflex 500). Two-tone green. In 20s and UD 100s.
Rx	**Cephalexin** (Various, eg, Barr, Lederle, Zenith-Goldline)	**Tablets:** 250 mg	In 20s, 100s and 500s.
Rx	**Cephalexin** (Various, eg, Barr, Lederle, Schein, Zenith-Goldline)	500 mg	In 20s, 100s and 500s.
Rx	**Cephalexin** (Various, eg, Geneva, Lederle, Zenith-Goldline)	**Powder for oral suspension:** 125 mg/5 ml	In 100 and 200 ml.
Rx	**Cephalexin** (Various, eg, Barr, Geneva, Lederle, Zenith-Goldline)	250 mg/5 ml	In 100 and 200 ml.
Rx	**Biocef** (Inter. Ethical Labs)		In 100 ml.
Rx	**Keflex** (Dista)		In 100, 200 and UD 100 ml.

For complete prescribing information, refer to the Cephalosporins group monograph.

CEPHALEXIN

Indications

▶*Respiratory tract infections:* Those caused by *Streptococcus pneumoniae* and group A β-hemolytic streptococci.

▶*Otitis media:* Due to *S. pneumoniae, Haemophilus influenzae,* staphylococci, streptococci and *M. catarrhalis.*

▶*Skin and skin structure infections:* Those caused by staphylococci or streptococci.

▶*Bone infections:* Those caused by staphylococci or *Proteus mirabilis.*

▶*GU infections:* These include acute prostatitis caused by *Escherichia coli, P. mirabilis* and *Klebsiella* sp.

Administration and Dosage

▶*Adults:* 1 to 4 g/day in divided doses. Usual dose – 250 mg every 6 hours. Streptococcal pharyngitis, skin and skin structure infections, uncomplicated cystitis in patients > 15 years – 500 mg every 12 hours. May need larger doses for more severe infections or less susceptible organisms. If dose is > 4 g/day, use parenteral drugs.

▶*Children:* Do not exceed adult recommended doses.

Monohydrate – 25 to 50 mg/kg/day in divided doses. For streptococcal pharyngitis in patients > 1 year and for skin and skin structure infections, divide total daily dose and give every 12 hours. In severe infections, double the dose.

Otitis media: 75 to 100 mg/kg/day in 4 divided doses.

β-hemolytic streptococcal infections: Continue treatment for at least 10 days.

▶*Storage / Stability:* Refrigerate reconstituted suspension; discard after 14 days.

CEPHALEXIN HCl MONOHYDRATE

Rx	**Keftab** (Biovail)	**Tablets:** 500 mg	(4143). Dark green. In 100s.

Actions

▶*Pharmacokinetics:*

Absorption – Cephalexin HCl monohydrate does not require conversion in the stomach before absorption.

CEFADROXIL

Rx	**Cefadroxil** (Various, eg, Major)	**Capsules:** 500 mg[1]	In 100s.
Rx	**Duricef** (Bristol-Myers Squibb)		(PPP 784). In 20s, 50s, 100s and UD 100s.
Rx	**Cefadroxil** (Various, eg, Major)	**Tablets:** 1 g[1]	In 24s, 50s, 100s and 500s.
Rx	**Duricef** (Bristol-Myers Squibb)		(PPP 785). In 50s, 100s, UD 40s and 100s.
Rx	**Duricef** (Bristol-Myers Squibb)	**Powder for oral suspension:** 125 mg/5 ml	Orange-pineapple flavor. In 50 and 100 ml.
		250 mg/5 ml	Sucrose. Orange-pineapple flavor. In 50 and 100 ml.
		500 mg/5 ml	Sucrose. Orange-pineapple flavor. In 75 and 100 ml.

[1] As monohydrate.

For complete prescribing information, refer to the Cephalosporins group monograph.

Indications

▶*Urinary tract infections:* Those caused by *Escherichia coli, Proteus mirabilis* and *Klebsiella* sp.

▶*Skin and skin structure infections:* Those caused by staphylococci or streptococci.

▶*Pharyngitis and tonsillitis:* Due to group A β-hemolytic streptococci.

Administration and Dosage

Can be given without regard to meals. Shake suspension well before using.

▶*Urinary tract infections:* For uncomplicated lower urinary tract infection (ie, cystitis), the usual dosage is 1 or 2 g/day in single or 2 divided doses. For all other urinary tract infections, the usual dosage is 2 g/day in 2 divided doses.

▶*Skin and skin structure infections:* 1 g/day in single or 2 divided doses.

▶*Pharyngitis and tonsillitis:*

Group A β-hemolytic streptococci – 1 g/day in single or 2 divided doses for 10 days.

▶*Children:* Do not exceed adult recommended doses.

Urinary tract infections, skin and skin structure infections – 30 mg/kg/day in divided doses every 12 hours.

Pharyngitis, tonsillitis – 30 mg/kg/day in single or 2 divided doses. For β-hemolytic streptococcal infections, continue treatment for ≥ 10 days.

▶*Renal function impairment:* Adjust dosage according to creatinine clearance rates to prevent drug accumulation.

Initial adult dose – 1 g; the maintenance dose (based on creatinine clearance rate, ml/min/1.73 m²) is 500 mg at the intervals below:

Cefadroxil Dosage in Renal Impairment	
Creatinine clearance (ml/min)	Dosage interval (hours)
0-10	36
10-25	24
25-50	12
> 50	No adjustment

▶*Storage / Stability:* Refrigerate reconstituted suspension; discard after 14 days.

CEPHRADINE

Rx	**Cephradine** (Various, eg, Baxter, Biocraft, Geneva, Lederle, Lemmon, Major, Parmed, Teva, Zenith)	**Capsules:** 250 mg	In 24s, 40s, 100s, 500s and UD 100s.
Rx	**Velosef** (Bristol-Myers Squibb)		Lactose. (113S601). In 12s.
Rx	**Cephradine** (Various, eg, Baxter, Biocraft, Geneva, Lederle, Lemmon, Major, Parmed, Zenith)	**Capsules:** 500 mg	In 24s, 40s, 100s, 500s and UD 100s.
Rx	**Velosef** (Bristol-Myers Squibb)		Lactose. (114S601). In 12s.
Rx	**Cephradine** (Various, eg, Biocraft, Geneva, Parmed, Teva)	**Powder for oral suspension:** 125 mg/5 ml when reconstituted	In 100 and 200 ml.
Rx	**Velosef** (Bristol-Myers Squibb)		Sucrose. Fruit flavor. In 100 ml.
Rx	**Cephradine** (Various, eg, Biocraft, Teva)	**Powder for oral suspension:** 250 mg/5 ml when reconstituted	In 100 and 200 ml.
Rx	**Velosef** (Bristol-Myers Squibb)		Sucrose. Fruit flavor. In 100 ml.

For complete prescribing information, refer to the Cephalosporins group monograph.

Indications

▶*Respiratory tract infections:* For example, tonsillitis, pharyngitis and lobar pneumonia, caused by group A β-hemolytic streptococci and *Streptococcus pneumoniae.*

▶*Otitis media:* Due to group A β-hemolytic streptococci, *S. pneumoniae, Haemophilus influenzae* and staphylococci.

▶*Skin and skin structure infections:* Those caused by staphylococci (penicillinase/nonpenicillinase-producing) and β-hemolytic streptococci.

▶*Urinary tract infections:* Those (including prostatitis) caused by *Escherichia coli, Proteus mirabilis* and *Klebsiella* species.

Cephradine may be used in the treatment of some enterococcal (*S. faecalis*) infections confined to the urinary tract. The high concentrations of cephradine achieved in the urinary tract will be effective against many strains of enterococci for which disc susceptibility studies indicate relative resistance. Ampicillin is the drug of choice for enterococcal urinary tract (*S. faecalis*) infections.

CEPHRADINE

Administration and Dosage

May be given without regard to meals.

➤*Adults:*

Skin, skin structures and respiratory tract infections (other than lobar pneumonia) – Usual dose is 250 mg every 6 hours or 500 mg every 12 hours.

For lobar pneumonia – 500 mg every 6 hours or 1 g every 12 hours.

For uncomplicated urinary tract infections – The usual dose is 500 mg every 12 hours. In more serious infections and prostatitis, 500 mg every 6 hours or 1 g every 12 hours. Severe or chronic infections may require larger doses (≤ 1 g every 6 hours).

➤*Children:* No adequate information is available on the efficacy of twice daily regimens in children < 9 months of age. For children ≥ 9 months, the usual dose is 25 to 50 mg/kg/day, in equally divided doses every 6 or 12 hours. For otitis media caused by *H. influenzae*, 75 to 100 mg/kg/day in equally divided doses every 6 or 12 hours is recommended; do not exceed 4 g/day.

➤*All patients, regardless of age and weight:* Larger doses (≤ 1 g four times/day) may be given for severe or chronic infections.

➤*Renal function impairment:*

Patients not on dialysis – Use the following initial dosage schedule as a guideline based on creatinine clearance. Further modification in the dosage schedule may be required because of individual variations in absorption.

Cephradine Dosage in Renal Impairment		
Ccr (ml/min)	Dose (mg)	Time Interval (hours)
> 20	500	6
5 to 20	250	6
< 5	250	12

Patients on chronic, intermittent hemodialysis – 250 mg initially; repeat at 12 hours and after 36 to 48 hours. Children may require dosage modification proportional to their weight and severity of infection.

➤*Storage/Stability:* Do not store above 30°C (86°F) prior to reconstitution. After reconstitution, suspensions retain their potency for 7 days at room temperature and 14 days if refrigerated.

LORACARBEF

Rx	Lorabid (Monarch)	**Pulvules (capsules):** 200 mg	(3170). Blue/gray. In 30s.
		400 mg	(3171). Blue/pink. In 30s.
		Powder for oral suspension: 100 mg/5 ml	Parabens, sucrose. Strawberry bubble gum flavor. In 50, 75 and 100 ml.
		200 mg/5 ml	Parabens, sucrose. Strawberry bubble gum flavor. In 50, 75 and 100 ml.

For complete prescribing information, refer to the Cephalosporins group monograph.

Indications

➤*Lower respiratory tract:*

Secondary bacterial infection of acute bronchitis – Also, acute bacterial exacerbations of chronic bronchitis caused by *S. pneumoniae*, *H. influenzae* or *M. catarrhalis* (both including β-lactamase-producing strains).

Pneumonia – Due to *S. pneumoniae* or *H. influenzae* (non-β-lactamase-producing strains only).

➤*Upper respiratory tract:*

Otitis media – Due to *S. pneumoniae*, *H. influenzae* (including β-lactamase-producing strains), *M. catarrhalis* (including β-lactamase-producing strains), *S. pyogenes*.

In a patient population with significant numbers of β-lactamase-producing organisms, loracarbef's clinical cure and bacteriological eradication rates were somewhat less than those observed with a product containing a β-lactamase inhibitor. Take into account loracarbef's decreased potential for toxicity vs products containing β-lactamase inhibitors along with susceptibility patterns of common microbes.

Acute maxillary sinusitis – Due to *S. pneumoniae*, *H. influenzae* (non-β-lactamase-producing strains only) or *M. catarrhalis* (including β-lactamase-producing strains).

In a patient population with significant numbers of β-lactamase-producing organisms, loracarbef's clinical cure and bacteriological eradication rates were somewhat less than those observed with a product containing a β-lactamase inhibitor. Take into account loracarbef's decreased potential for toxicity vs products containing β-lactamase inhibitors along with susceptibility patterns of common microbes.

Pharyngitis and tonsillitis – Due to *S. pyogenes*. Usual drug of choice in treatment and prevention of streptococcal infections, including prophylaxis of rheumatic fever, is IM penicillin. Loracarbef is generally effective in eradicating *S. pyogenes* from the nasopharynx; however, data establishing efficacy of loracarbef in subsequent prevention of rheumatic fever are not available at present.

➤*Skin and skin structure:*

Uncomplicated skin and skin structure infections – Those caused by *S. aureus* (including penicillinase-producing) or *S. pyogenes*. Surgically drain abscesses as indicated.

➤*Urinary tract:*

Uncomplicated UTIs (cystitis) – Due to *E. coli* or *S. saprophyticus*.

In considering the use of loracarbef in the treatment of cystitis, weigh its lower bacterial eradication rates and lower potential for toxicity against the increased eradication rates and increased potential for toxicity demonstrated by some other classes.

Uncomplicated pyelonephritis – Due to *E. coli*.

Administration and Dosage

➤*Approved by the FDA:* December 31, 1991.

Administer ≥ 1 hour before or 2 hours after a meal.

Dosage/Duration of Loracarbef		
Population/Infection	Dosage (mg)	Duration (days)
Adults ≥ 13 years of age		
Lower respiratory tract		
Secondary bacterial infection of acute bronchitis	200-400 q 12 hrs	7
Acute bacterial exacerbation of chronic bronchitis	400 q 12 hrs	7
Pneumonia	400 q 12 hrs	14
Upper respiratory tract		
Pharyngitis/Tonsillitis	200 q 12 hrs	10[1]
Sinusitis	400 q 12 hrs	10
Skin and skin structure		
Uncomplicated	200 q 12 hrs	7
Urinary tract		
Uncomplicated cystitis	200 q 24 hrs	7
Uncomplicated pyelonephritis	400 q 12 hrs	14
Infants and children (6 months to 12 years)[2]		
Upper respiratory tract		
Acute otitis media[3]	30 mg/kg/day in divided doses q 12 hrs	10
Acute maxillary sinusitis	15 mg/kg/day in divided doses q 12 hrs	10[1]
Pharyngitis/Tonsillitis		
Skin and skin structure		
Impetigo	15 mg/kg/day in divided doses q 12 hrs	7

[1] In treatment of infections caused by *S. pyogenes*, administer for ≥ 10 days.
[2] Do not exceed adult recommended doses.
[3] Use suspension; it is more rapidly absorbed than capsules, resulting in higher peak plasma concentrations when given at the same dose.

Loracarbef Pediatric Suspension Dosage									
	Daily dose 15 mg/kg/day				Daily dose 30 mg/kg/day				
Weight	100 mg/5 ml twice daily		200 mg/5 ml twice daily		100 mg/5 ml twice daily		200 mg/5 ml twice daily		
lb	kg	ml	tsp	ml	tsp	ml	tsp	ml	tsp
15	7	2.6	0.5	—	—	5.2	1	2.6	0.5
29	13	4.9	1	2.5	0.5	9.8	2	4.9	1
44	20	7.5	1.5	3.8	0.75	—	—	7.5	1.5
57	26	9.8	2	4.9	1	—	—	9.8	2

➤*Renal function impairment:* Use usual dose and schedule in patients with creatinine clearance (Ccr) levels ≥ 50 ml/min. Patients with Ccr between 10 and 49 ml/min may be given half the recommended dose at the usual dosage interval. Patients with Ccr levels < 10 ml/min may receive recommended dose given every 3 to 5 days; patients on hemodialysis should receive another dose following dialysis.

When only serum creatinine is available, the following formula may be used to convert this value into Ccr. The equation assumes the patient's renal function is stable.

$$\text{Males:} \quad \frac{\text{Weight (kg)} \times (140 - \text{age})}{72 \times \text{serum creatinine (mg/dL)}} = \text{Ccr}$$

Females: 0.85 × above value

LORACARBEF

Reconstitution of oral suspension – Add 30, 45 or 60 ml water in two portions to the dry mixture in the 50, 75 or 100 ml bottle, respectively.

➤*Storage/Stability:* After mixing, the suspension may be kept at room temperature, 15° to 30°C (59° to 86°F), for 14 days without significant loss of potency. Keep tightly closed. Discard unused portion after 14 days.

CEFPROZIL

Rx	Cefzil (Bristol-Myers Squibb)	Tablets: 250 mg (as anhydrous)	(7720 250). Light orange. Film coated. In 100s and UD 100s.
		500 mg (as anhydrous)	(7721 500). White. Film coated. In 50s, 100s and UD 100s.
		Powder for oral suspension:[1] 125 mg/5 ml (as anhydrous)	Bubble gum flavor. In 50, 75 and 100 ml.
		250 mg/5 ml (as anhydrous)	Bubble gum flavor. In 50, 75 and 100 ml.

[1] Contains sucrose, aspartame and phenylalanine (28 mg/5 ml).

For complete prescribing information, refer to the Cephalosporins group monograph.

Indications

➤*Pharyngitis/tonsillitis:* Due to *Streptococcus pyogenes*.

Note: Usual drug of choice in treatment and prevention of streptococcal infections, including rheumatic fever prophylaxis, is IM penicillin. Cefprozil is generally effective in eradicating *S. pyogenes* from nasopharynx; however, substantial data establishing efficacy in subsequent prevention of rheumatic fever are not available.

➤*Otitis media:* Due to *S. pneumoniae, Haemophilus influenzae* and *Moraxella catarrhalis*.

Note: In the treatment of otitis media caused by β-lactamase producing organisms, cefprozil had bacteriologic eradication rates somewhat lower than those observed with a product containing a specific β-lactamase inhibitor. In considering the use of cefprozil, balance lower overall eradication rates against the susceptibility patterns of the common microbes in a given geographic area and the increased potential for toxicity with products containing β-lactamase inhibitors.

➤*Acute sinusitis:* Due to *S. pneumoniae, H. influenzae* (including β-lactamase-producing strains) and *M. catarrhalis* (including β-lactamase-producing strains).

➤*Secondary bacterial infection of acute bronchitis and acute bacterial exacerbation of chronic bronchitis:* Due to *S. pneumoniae, H. influenzae* (including β-lactamase-producing strains) and *Moraxella catarrhalis* (including β-lactamase-producing strains).

➤*Uncomplicated skin and skin structure infections:* Due to *Staphylococcus aureus* (including penicillinase-producing strains) and *S. pyogenes*.

Administration and Dosage

➤*Approved by the FDA:* December 1991.

Cefprozil Dosage and Duration		
Population/Infection	Dosage (mg)	Duration (days)
Adults (≥ 13 years of age)		
Pharyngitis/Tonsillitis	500 q 24 hrs	10[1]
Acute sinusitis (use higher dose for moderate-to-severe infections)	250 q 12 hrs or 500 q 12 hrs	10
Secondary bacterial infection of acute bronchitis and acute bacterial exacerbation of chronic bronchitis	500 q 12 hrs	10
Uncomplicated skin and skin structure infections	250 q 12 hrs, 500 q 24 hrs or 500 q 12 hrs	10
Children (2 to 12 years)[2]		
Pharyngitis/Tonsillitis	7.5 mg/kg q 12 hrs	10[1]
Uncomplicated skin and skin structure infections	20 mg/kg q 24 hrs	10
Infants and children (6 months to 12 years)[2]		
Otitis media	15 mg/kg q 12 hrs	10
Acute sinusitis (use higher dose for moderate-to-severe infections)	7.5 mg/kg q 12 hrs or 15 mg/kg q 12 hrs	10

[1] For infections caused by *S. pyogenes*, administer for ≥ 10 days.
[2] Not to exceed adult recommended doses.

➤*Renal function impairment:* For creatinine clearance (Ccr) of 30 to 120 ml/min, use standard dosage and dosing interval. For Ccr < 30 ml/min, use a dosage 50% of standard at the standard dosing interval.

Cefprozil is in part removed by hemodialysis; therefore, administer after the completion of hemodialysis.

➤*Storage/Stability:*

Suspension – Refrigerate after reconstitution; discard after 14 days.

CEFTIBUTEN

| Rx | Cedax (Schering-Plough) | Capsules: 400 mg | Parabens. (Cedax 400). White. In 20s and UD 40s. |
| | | Powder for oral suspension: 90 mg/5 ml | Sucrose. Cherry flavor. In 30, 60, 90 and 120 ml. |

For complete prescribing information, refer to the Cephalosporins group monograph.

Indications

➤*Acute bacterial exacerbations of chronic bronchitis:* Caused by *Haemophilus influenzae* (including β-lactamase-producing strains), *Moraxella catarrhalis* (including β-lactamase-producing strains) and *Streptococcus pneumoniae* (penicillin-susceptible strains only).

In acute bacterial exacerbations of chronic bronchitis clinical trials where *Moraxella catarrhalis* was isolated from infected sputum at baseline, ceftibuten clinical efficacy was 22% less than control.

➤*Acute bacterial otitis media:* Caused by *H. influenzae* (including β-lactamase-producing strains), *M. catarrhalis* (including β-lactamase-producing strains) or *S. pyogenes*.

Although ceftibuten used empirically was equivalent to comparators in the treatment of clinically or microbiologically documented acute otitis media, the efficacy against *S. pneumoniae* was 23% less than control. Therefore, give ceftibuten empirically only when adequate antimicrobial coverage against *S. pneumoniae* has been previously administered.

➤*Pharyngitis and tonsillitis:* Caused by *S. pyogenes*.

Only penicillin by the IM route has been shown to be effective in the prophylaxis of rheumatic fever. Ceftibuten is generally effective in the eradication of *S. pyogenes* from the oropharynx; however, data establishing efficacy for prophylaxis of subsequent rheumatic fever are not available.

Administration and Dosage

➤*Approved by the FDA:* December 20, 1995.

Ceftibuten suspension must be administered ≥ 2 hours before or 1 hour after a meal.

Ceftibuten Dosage and Duration			
Type of infection	Daily maximum dose	Dose and frequency	Duration
Adults ≥ 12 years of age Acute bacterial exacerbations of chronic bronchitis caused by *H. influenzae, M. catarrhalis* or *Streptococcus pneumoniae* Pharyngitis and tonsillitis caused by *S. pyogenes* Acute bacterial otitis media caused by *H. influenzae, M. catarrhalis* or *S. pyogenes*	400 mg	400 mg qd	10 days
Children[1] Pharyngitis and tonsillitis caused by *S. pyogenes* Acute bacterial otitis media caused by *H. influenzae, M. catarrhalis* or *S. pyogenes*	400 mg	9 mg/kg qd	10 days

[1] Do not exceed adult recommended doses.

CEFTIBUTEN

Ceftibuten Oral Suspension Pediatric Dosage Chart[1]			
Weight		90 mg/5 ml	180 mg/5 ml
kg	lb		
10	22	5 ml (1 tsp) qd	2.5 ml (½ tsp) qd
20	44	10 ml (2 tsp) qd	5 ml (1 tsp) qd
40	88	20 ml (4 tsp) qd	10 ml (2 tsp) qd

[1] Children > 45 kg should receive the maximum daily dose of 400 mg

➤*Renal function impairment:* Ceftibuten may be administered at normal doses in the presence of impaired renal function with creatinine clearance of ≥ 50 ml/min. The recommendations for dosing in patients with varying degrees of renal insufficiency are presented in the following table.

Ceftibuten Dosage in Renal Impairment	
Creatinine clearance (ml/min)	Recommended dosing schedule
> 50	9 mg/kg or 400 mg q 24 h (normal dosing schedule)
30-49	4.5 mg/kg or 200 mg q 24 h
5-29	2.25 mg/kg or 100 mg q 24 h

➤*Hemodialysis patients:* In patients undergoing hemodialysis two or three times weekly, a single 400 mg dose of ceftibuten capsules or a single dose of 9 mg/kg (maximum of 400 mg) oral suspension may be administered at the end of each hemodialysis session.

Directions for Mixing Ceftibuten Suspension			
Final concentration	Bottle size	Amount of water	Directions
90 mg/5 ml	30 ml	Suspend in 28 ml	First, tap bottle to loosen powder. Then, add water in two portions, shaking well after each aliquot.
	60 ml	Suspend in 53 ml	
	90 ml	Suspend in 78 ml	
	120 ml	Suspend in 103 ml	
180 mg/5 ml	30 ml	Suspend in 28 ml	
	60 ml	Suspend in 53 ml	
	120 ml	Suspend in 103 ml	

➤*Storage / Stability:*
Suspension – After mixing, the suspension may be kept for 14 days and must be stored in the refrigerator. Keep tightly closed. Shake well before each use. Discard any unused portion after 14 days.

CEFDINIR

Rx	**Omnicef** (Abbott)	**Capsules:** 300 mg	(OMNICEF). Lavender and turquoise. In 60s.
		Oral suspension: 125 mg/5 ml	Sucrose. Cream-colored. Strawberry-flavored. In 60 and 100 ml.

For complete prescribing information, refer to the Cephalosporins group monograph.

⬤ Indications

➤*Adults and adolescents:*
Community-acquired pneumonia – Caused by *Haemophilus influenzae* (including β-lactamase-producing strains), *H. parainfluenzae* (including β-lactamase-producing strains), *Streptococcus pneumoniae* (penicillin-susceptible strains only) and *Moraxella catarrhalis* (including β-lactamase-producing strains).

Acute exacerbations of chronic bronchitis – Caused by *H. influenzae* (including β-lactamase producing strains), *H. parainfluenzae* (including β-lactamase-producing strains), *S. pneumoniae* (penicillin-susceptible strains only) and *M. catarrhalis* (including β-lactamase-producing strains).

Acute maxillary sinusitis – Caused by *H. influenzae* (including β-lactamase-producing strains), *S. pneumoniae* (penicillin-susceptible strains only) and *M. catarrhalis* (including β-lactamase-producing strains).

Pharyngitis / Tonsillitis – Caused by *S. pyogenes.*

Uncomplicated skin and skin structure infections – Caused by *Staphylococcus aureus* (including β-lactamase-producing strains) and *S. pyogenes.*

➤*Children:*
Acute bacterial otitis media – Caused by *H. influenzae* (including β-lactamase-producing strains), *S. pneumoniae* (penicillin-susceptible strains only) and *M. catarrhalis* (including β-lactamase-producing strains).

Pharyngitis / Tonsillitis – Caused by *S. pyogenes.*

Uncomplicated skin and skin structure infections – Caused by *S. aureus* (including β-lactamase-producing strains) and *S. pyogenes.*

➤*NOTE:* Cefdinir is effective in the eradication of *S. pyogenes* from the oropharynx. Cefdinir has not, however, been studied for the prevention of rheumatic fever following *S. pyogenes* pharyngitis/tonsillitis. Only IM penicillin has been demonstrated to be effective for the prevention of rheumatic fever.

⬤ Administration and Dosage

➤*Approved by the FDA:* December 4, 1997.

➤*Adults / Adolescents:* The recommended dosage and duration of treatment for infections in adults and adolescents are described in the following chart; the total daily dose for all infections is 600 mg. Once-daily dosing for 10 days is as effective as twice-daily dosing. Once-daily dosing has not been studied in pneumonia or skin infections; therefore, administer twice daily in these infections. Capsules may be taken without regard to meals.

Cefdinir Dosage in Adults and Adolescents (≥ 13 years of age)		
Type of infection	Dosage	Duration
Community-acquired pneumonia	300 mg q 12 hrs	10 days
Acute exacerbations of chronic bronchitis	300 mg q 12 hrs or	10 days
	600 mg q 24 hrs	10 days
Acute maxillary sinusitis	300 mg q 12 hrs or	10 days
	600 mg q 24 hrs	10 days
Pharyngitis/Tonsillitis	300 mg q 12 hrs or	5 to 10 days
	600 mg q 24 hrs	10 days
Uncomplicated skin and skin structure infections	300 mg q 12 hrs	10 days

➤*Children (6 months through 12 years of age):* The recommended dosage and duration of treatment for infections in pediatric patients are described in the following chart; the total daily dose for all infections is 14 mg/kg, up to a maximum dose of 600 mg/day. Once-daily dosing for 10 days is as effective as twice-daily dosing. Once-daily dosing has not been studied in skin infections; therefore, administer twice daily in this infection. Oral suspension may be administered without regard to meals.

Cefdinir Dosage in Pediatric Patients (Age 6 Months Through 12 years)		
Type of infection	Dosage	Duration
Acute bacterial otitis media	7 mg/kg q 12 h or	10 days
	14 mg/kg q 24 h	10 days
Acute maxillary sinusitis	7 mg/kg q 12 h or	10 days
	14 mg/kg q 24 h	10 days
Pharyngitis/Tonsillitis	7 mg/kg q 12 h or	5 to 10 days
	14 mg/kg q 24 h	10 days
Uncomplicated skin and skin structure infections	7 mg/kg q 12 h	10 days

Cefdinir for Oral Suspension Pediatric Dosage Chart		
Weight		125 mg/5 ml
kg	lb	
9	20	2.5 ml (½ tsp) q 12 h or 5 ml (1 tsp) q 24 h
18	40	5 ml (1 tsp) q 12 h or 10 ml (2 tsp) q 24 h

CEFDINIR

Cefdinir for Oral Suspension Pediatric Dosage Chart		
Weight		
kg	lb	125 mg/5 ml
27	60	7.5 ml (1½ tsp) q 12 h or 15 ml (3 tsp) q 24 h
36	80	10 ml (2 tsp) q 12 h or 20 ml (4 tsp) q 24 h
≥ 43[1]	95	12 ml (2½ tsp) q 12 h or 24 ml (5 tsp) q 24 h

[1] Pediatric patients who weigh ≥ 43 kg should receive the maximum daily dose of 600 mg.

➤*Renal function impairment:* For adult patients with creatinine clearance < 30 ml/min, the dose of cefdinir should be 300 mg given once daily.

Creatinine clearance is difficult to measure in outpatients. However, the following formula may be used to estimate creatinine clearance (Ccr) in adult patients. For estimates to be valid, serum creatinine levels should reflect steady-state levels of renal function.

$$\text{Males:} \quad \frac{\text{Weight (kg)} \times (140 - \text{age})}{72 \times \text{serum creatinine (mg/dL)}} = \text{Ccr}$$

Females: $0.85 \times$ above value

The following formula may be used to estimate creatinine clearance in pediatric patients.

$$\text{Ccr (mL/min/1.73 m}^2\text{)} = K \times \frac{\text{body length or height (cm)}}{\text{serum creatinine (mg/dL)}}$$

where K=0.55 for pediatric patients > 1 year of age and 0.45 for infants (≤ 1 year).

For pediatric patients with a creatinine clearance of < 30 ml/min/1.73 m², the dose of cefdinir should be 7 mg/kg (≤ 300 mg) given once daily.

➤*Hemodialysis:* Hemodialysis removes cefdinir from the body. In patients maintained on chronic hemodialysis, the recommended initial dosage regimen is a 300 mg or 7 mg/kg dose every other day. At the conclusion of each hemodialysis session, 300 mg (or 7 mg/kg) should be given. Subsequent doses (300 mg or 7 mg/kg) are then administered every other day.

➤*Reconstitution of oral suspension:* For the 60 ml bottle, add 39 ml water; for the 120 ml bottle, add 65 ml water. Shake well before each use.

➤*Storage/Stability:* After mixing, the suspension can be stored at room temperature (25°C; 77°F). The container should be kept tightly closed, and the suspension should be shaken well before each administration. The suspension may be used for 10 days, after which any unused portion must be discarded.

CEFAZOLIN SODIUM

Rx	Cefazolin Sodium (Apothecon)	Powder for Injection:[1] 500 mg	In vials and piggyback vials.
Rx	Ancef (SmithKline Beecham)		In vials and piggyback vials.
Rx	Cefazolin Sodium (Apothecon)	Powder for Injection:[1] 1 g	In vials and piggyback vials.
Rx	Ancef (SmithKline Beecham)		In vials and piggyback vials.
Rx	Zolicef (Apothecon)		In 10 ml vials.
Rx	Cefazolin Sodium (Apothecon)	Powder for Injection:[1] 5 g	In vials and piggyback vials.
Rx	Ancef (SmithKline Beecham)		In bulk vials.
Rx	Cefazolin Sodium (Apothecon)	Powder for Injection:[1] 10 g	In pharmacy bulk packages.
Rx	Ancef (SmithKline Beecham)		In bulk vials.
Rx	Cefazolin Sodium (Apothecon)	Powder for Injection:[1] 20 g	In pharmacy bulk packages.
Rx	Ancef (SmithKline Beecham)	Injection:[1] 500 mg	Dextrose. Premixed, frozen. In 50 ml plastic containers.
Rx	Ancef (SmithKline Beecham)	Injection:[1] 1 g	Dextrose. Premixed, frozen. In 50 ml plastic containers.

[1] Contains 2.1 mEq sodium/g.

For complete prescribing information, refer to the Cephalosporins group monograph.

Indications

➤*Respiratory tract infections:* Caused by *Streptococcus pneumoniae*, *Klebsiella* species, *Haemophilus influenzae*, *Staphylococcus aureus* (penicillinase/non-penicillinase-producing) and group A β-hemolytic streptococci.

➤*Genitourinary tract infections (eg, prostatitis, epididymitis):* Caused by *Escherichia coli*, *Proteus mirabilis*, *Klebsiella* species and some strains of *Enterobacter* and enterococci.

➤*Skin and skin structure infections:* Caused by *S. aureus* (penicillinase/non-penicillinase-producing), group A β-hemolytic streptococci and other strains of streptococci.

➤*Biliary tract infections:* Caused by *E. coli*, various strains of streptococci, *P. mirabilis*, *Klebsiella* species and *S. aureus*.

➤*Bone and joint infections:* Caused by *S. aureus*.

➤*Septicemia:* Caused by *S. pneumoniae*, *S. aureus* (penicillinase/non-penicillinase-producing), *P. mirabilis*, *E. coli* and *Klebsiella* species.

➤*Endocarditis:* Caused by *S. aureus* (penicillinase/non-penicillinase-producing) and group A β-hemolytic streptococci.

➤*Perioperative prophylaxis:* May reduce the incidence of certain postoperative infections in patients undergoing contaminated or potentially contaminated surgical procedures (eg, vaginal hysterectomy and cholecystectomy in high risk patients such as those> 70 years of age, with acute cholecystitis, obstructive jaundice or common duct bile stones).

May also be effective in surgical patients in whom infection at the operative site would present a serious risk (eg, open heart surgery and prosthetic arthroplasty).

Administration and Dosage

Total daily dosages are the same for IV and IM administration.

➤*Mild infections caused by susceptible gram-positive cocci:* 250 to 500 mg every 8 hours.

➤*Moderate-to-severe infections:* 500 mg to 1 g every 6 to 8 hours.

➤*Pneumococcal pneumonia:* 500 mg every 12 hours.

➤*Severe, life-threatening infections (eg, endocarditis, septicemia):* 1 to 1.5 g every 6 hours. Rarely, 12 g/day have been used.

➤*Acute uncomplicated urinary tract infections:* 1 g every 12 hours.

➤*Perioperative prophylaxis:*

Preoperative – 1 g IV or IM, 0.5 to 1 hour prior to surgery.

Intraoperative (≥ 2 hours) – 0.5 to 1 g IV or IM during surgery at appropriate intervals.

Postoperative – 0.5 to 1 g IV or IM every 6 to 8 hours for 24 hours after surgery. Prophylactic administration may be continued for 3 to 5 days, especially where the occurrence of infection may be particularly devastating (eg, open heart surgery, prosthetic arthroplasty).

➤*Renal function impairment:* All reduced dosage recommendations apply after an initial loading dose appropriate to the severity of the infection.

Cefazolin Dosage in Renal Impairment				
		Dose		
Serum creatinine (mg/dl)	Ccr (ml/min)	Mild-to-moderate infection (mg)	Moderate-to-severe infection (mg)	Dosage interval (hrs)
≤ 1.5	≥ 55	250 to 500	500 to 1000	6-8
1.6-3	35-54	250 to 500	500 to 1000	≥ 8
3.1-4.5	11-34	125 to 250	250 to 500	12
≥ 4.6	≤ 10	125 to 250	250 to 500	18-24

➤*Children:* Do not exceed adult recommended doses.

Mild-to-moderately severe infections – A total daily dosage of 25 to 50 mg/kg (≈ 10 to 20 mg/lb) in three or four equal doses.

Severe infections – Total daily dosage may be increased to 100 mg/kg (45 mg/lb).

Pediatric Dosage of Cefazolin[1]									
		25 mg/kg/day				50 mg/kg/day			
		Approx. single dose		Volume needed 125 mg/ml		Approx. single dose		Volume needed 225 mg/ml	
Weight									
lbs	kg	mg q 8 hrs	mg q 6 hrs	mg q 8 hrs	mg q 6 hrs	mg q 8 hrs	mg q 6 hrs	mg q 8 hrs	mg q 6 hrs
10	4.5	40	30	0.35 ml	0.25 ml	75	55	0.35 ml	0.25 ml
20	9	75	55	0.6 ml	0.45 ml	150	110	0.7 ml	0.5 ml
30	13.6	115	85	0.9 ml	0.7 ml	225	170	1 ml	0.75 ml

CEFAZOLIN SODIUM

Pediatric Dosage of Cefazolin[1]								
		25 mg/kg/day			50 mg/kg/day			
Weight		Approx. single dose	Volume needed 125 mg/ml		Approx. single dose	Volume needed 225 mg/ml		
lbs	kg	mg q 8 hrs	mg q 6 hrs	mg q 8 hrs	mg q 6 hrs	mg q 8 hrs	mg q 6 hrs	mg q 8 hrs	mg q 6 hrs
40	18.1	150	115	1.2 ml	0.9 ml	300	225	1.35 ml	1 ml
50	22.7	190	140	1.5 ml	1.1 ml	375	285	1.7 ml	1.25 ml

[1] Infants (premature and < 1 month): Safety not established; use is not recommended. Do not exceed adult recommended doses.

Renal function impairment – Recommendations apply after an initial loading dose.

Ccr 40 to 70 ml/min, 60% of normal daily dose every 12 hrs; Ccr 20 to 40 ml/min, 25% of normal daily dose every 12 hrs; Ccr 5 to 20 ml/min, 10% of normal daily dose every 24 hrs.

➤*IM administration:* Inject into a large muscle mass. Pain on injection is infrequent.

➤*Intermittent IV infusion:* Administer in a volume control set or in a separate, secondary IV container. Reconstituted 500 mg or 1 g may be diluted in 50 to 100 ml of: 0.9% NaCl Injection; 5% or 10% Dextrose Injection; 5% Dextrose in Lactated Ringer's Injection; 5% Dextrose and 0.2%, 0.45% or 0.9% NaCl; Lactated Ringer's Injection; 5% or 10% Invert Sugar in Sterile Water for Injection; 5% Sodium Bicarbonate (*Ancef*); Ringer's Injection; *Normosol-M* in D5-W; *Ionosol B* w/Dextrose 5%; *Plasma-Lyte* with 5% Dextrose.

➤*Direct IV injection:* Dilute reconstituted 500 mg or 1 g in minimum of 5 ml Sterile Water for Injection. Inject slowly into vein or through IV tubing over 3 to 5 min.

➤*Preparation of solution: IM:* Reconstitute with Sterile Water, Bacteriostatic Water or 0.9% Sodium Chloride Injections. Shake well until dissolved.

➤*IV:* Dilute as required.

➤*Storage/Stability:* Reconstituted cefazolin is stable for 24 hours at room temperature, 96 hours refrigerated (5°C; 41°F).

Frozen solution – Store at -20°C (-4°F). Do not force thaw by immersion in water baths or by microwave irradiation. The thawed solution maintains satisfactory potency for 48 hours at 25°C (77°F) and for 30 days under refrigeration (5°C; 41°F).

CEFMETAZOLE SODIUM

Rx	Zefazone (Pharmacia & Upjohn)	Injection:[1] 1 g/50 ml	Frozen, iso-osmotic, premixed solution in single dose plastic container.
		2 g/50 ml	Frozen, iso-osmotic, premixed solution in a single dose plastic container.

[1] 2.7 mEq sodium/g.

Complete prescribing information for these products begins in the Cephalosporins.

Indications

➤*Urinary tract infections (complicated or uncomplicated):* Caused by *E. coli*.

➤*Lower respiratory tract infections:* Pneumonia and bronchitis caused by *S. pneumoniae*, *S. aureus* (penicillinase-and non-penicillinase-producing strains), *E. coli*, *H. influenzae* (non-penicillinase-producing strains).

➤*Skin and structure infections:* *S. aureus* (penicillinase- and non-penicillinase-producing strains), *S. epidermidis*, *S. pyogenes*, *S. agalactiae*, *E. coli*, *P. mirabilis*, *P. vulgaris*, *M. morganii*, *P. stuartii*, *K. pneumoniae*, *K. oxytoca*, *B. fragilis*, *B. melaninogenicus*.

➤*Intra-abdominal infections:* *E. coli*, *K. pneumoniae*, *K. oxytoca*, *B. fragilis*, *C. perfringens*.

➤*Prophylaxis:* Preoperative administration may reduce the incidence of certain postoperative infections in patients who undergo cesarean section, abdominal or vaginal hysterectomy, cholecystectomy (high-risk patients) and colorectal surgery.

Administration and Dosage

➤*Adults:*

General guidelines – 2 g IV every 6 to 12 hours for 5 to 14 days.

➤*Prophylaxis:*

Cefmetazole Dosing Regimen for Surgical Prophylaxis	
Surgery	Dosing Regimen
Vaginal hysterectomy	2 g single dose 30 to 90 min before surgery or 1 g doses 30 to 90 min before surgery and repeated 8 and 16 hours later.
Abdominal hysterectomy	1 g doses 30 to 90 min before surgery and repeated 8 and 16 hours later.
Cesarean section	2 g single dose after clamping cord or 1 g doses after clamping cord; repeated at 8 and 16 hours.

Cefmetazole Dosing Regimen for Surgical Prophylaxis	
Surgery	Dosing Regimen
Colorectal surgery[1]	2 g single dose 30 to 90 minutes before surgery or 2 g doses 30 to 90 minutes before surgery and repeated 8 and 16 hours later.
Cholecystectomy (high risk)	1 g doses 30 to 90 minutes before surgery and repeated 8 and 16 hours later.

[1] All patients studied received preoperative bowel preparation with mechanical cleansing, oral neomycin or kanamycin and oral erythromycin.

➤*Renal function impairment:*

Cefmetazole Dosage Guidelines in Renal Function Impairment			
Renal function	Creatinine clearance (ml/min/1.73 m^2)	Dose (g)	Frequency (hrs)
Mild impairment	50-90	1 to 2	q 12
Moderate impairment	30-49	1 to 2	q 16
Severe impairment	10-29	1 to 2	q 24
Essentially no function	< 10	1 to 2	q 48[1]

[1] Administered after hemodialysis.

➤*Reconstitution:* Reconstitute with Sterile Water for Injection, Bacteriostatic Water for Injection or 0.9% Sodium Chloride Injection.

➤*Storage/Stability:* Following reconstitution, cefmetazole maintains satisfactory potency for 24 hours at room temperature (25°C; 77°F), for 7 days under refrigeration (8°C; 46°F) and for 6 weeks in the frozen state (≤ -20°C; -4°F).

Primary solutions may be further diluted to concentrations of 1 to 20 mg/ml in 0.9% Sodium Chloride Injection, 5% Dextrose Injection, Lactated Ringer's Injection or 1% Lidocaine solution without Epinephrine and maintain potency for 24 hours at room temperature (25°C; 77°F), for 7 days under refrigeration (8°C; 46°F) and for 6 weeks in the frozen state (≤ -20°C; -4°F).

Do not refreeze thawed solutions. Discard unused solutions or frozen material.

CEFOXITIN SODIUM

Rx	Cefoxitin (American Pharmaceutical Partners)	Powder for Injection: 1 g	In vials and infusion bottles.
Rx	Mefoxin (Merck)		In vials and infusion bottles.[1]
Rx	Cefoxitin (American Pharmaceutical Partners)	Powder for Injection: 2 g	In vials and infusion bottles.
Rx	Mefoxin (Merck)		In vials and infusion bottles.[1]
Rx	Cefoxitin (American Pharmaceutical Partners)	Powder for Injection: 10 g	In pharmacy bulk packages.
Rx	Mefoxin (Merck)		In bulk bottles.[1]
Rx	Mefoxin (Merck)	Injection: 1 g	Dextrose. Premixed, frozen. In 50 ml plastic containers.
		2 g	Dextrose. Premixed, frozen. In 50 ml plastic containers.

[1] Contains 2.3 mEq sodium/g.

For complete prescribing information, refer to the Cephalosporins group monograph.

Indications

Cefoxitin and cephalothin were comparable for management of infections caused by susceptible gram-positive cocci and gram-negative rods.

Many infections caused by gram-negative bacteria resistant to some cephalosporins and penicillins respond to cefoxitin.

➤*Lower respiratory tract infections:* Pneumonia and lung abscess caused by *Streptococcus pneumoniae*, other streptococci (excluding enterococci, eg, *S. faecalis*), *Staphylococcus aureus* (penicillinase/non-penicillinase-producing), *Escherichia coli*, *Klebsiella* species, *Haemophilus influenzae* and *Bacteroides* species.

CEFOXITIN SODIUM

➤*Urinary tract infections:* Caused by *E. coli, Klebsiella* sp., *Proteus mirabilis,* indole-positive *Proteus* (ie, *Morganella morganii* and *P. vulgaris*) and *Providencia* sp. (including *P. rettgeri*). Uncomplicated gonorrhea caused by *Neisseria gonorrhoeae* (penicillinase/non-penicillinase-producing).

➤*Intra-abdominal infections:* Peritonitis and intra-abdominal abscess caused by *E. coli, Klebsiella* sp., *Bacteroides* sp. including *B. fragilis* and *Clostridium* sp.

➤*Gynecological infections:* Endometritis, pelvic cellulitis and pelvic inflammatory disease caused by *E. coli, N. gonorrhoeae* (penicillinase/non-penicillinase-producing), *Bacteroides* sp. including the *B. fragilis* group, *Clostridium* sp., *Peptococcus* sp., *Peptostreptococcus* sp. and group B streptococci.

➤*Septicemia:* Caused by *S. pneumoniae, S. aureus* (penicillinase/non-penicillinase-producing), *E. coli, Klebsiella* sp. and *Bacteroides* sp. including *B. fragilis.*

➤*Bone/joint infections:* Caused by *S. aureus* (penicillinase/non-penicillinase-producing).

➤*Skin and skin structure infections:* Caused by *S. aureus* (penicillinase/non-penicillinase-producing), *S. epidermidis,* streptococci (excluding enterococci, eg, *S. faecalis), E. coli, P. mirabilis, Klebsiella* sp., *Bacteroides* sp. including the *B. fragilis* group, *Clostridium* sp., *Peptococcus* sp. and *Peptostreptococcus* sp.

➤*Perioperative prophylaxis:* This may reduce the incidence of certain postoperative infections following surgical procedures (eg, vaginal hysterectomy, GI surgery, transurethral prostatectomy) classified as contaminated or potentially contaminated and in those in whom operative site infection would present serious risk (eg, prosthetic arthroplasty). In cesarean section, intraoperative (after clamping umbilical cord) and postoperative use may reduce incidence of postoperative infections.

Give cefoxitin 30 to 60 minutes before the operation, to achieve effective levels in the wound during the procedure. Prophylactic administration should usually be stopped within 24 hours.

Administration and Dosage

➤*Adult:* The dosage range is 1 to 2 g every 6 to 8 hours. Determine dosage and route of administration by susceptibility of the causative organisms, severity of infection and the patient's condition (see table for dosage guidelines). Maintain antibiotic therapy for group A β-hemolytic streptococcal infections for ≥ 10 days to guard against the risk of rheumatic fever or glomerulonephritis.

Cefoxitin Dosage Guidelines		
Type of infection	Daily dosage	Frequency and route
Uncomplicated (pneumonia, urinary tract, cutaneous)[1]	3 to 4 g	1 g every 6 to 8 hours IV
Moderately severe or severe	6 to 8 g	1 g every 4 hours or 2 g every 6 to 8 hours IV
Infections commonly requiring higher dosage (eg, gas gangrene)	12 g	2 g every 4 hours or 3 g every 6 hours IV

[1] Including patients in whom bacteremia is absent or unlikely.

➤*Uncomplicated gonorrhea:* 2 g IM with 1 g oral probenecid given concurrently or ≤ 30 minutes before cefoxitin.

➤*Prophylactic use, surgery:* Administer 2 g IV 30 to 60 minutes prior to surgery followed by 2 g every 6 hours after the first dose for ≤ 24 hours.

➤*Prophylactic use, cesarean section:* Administer 2 g IV as soon as the umbilical cord is clamped. If a three-dose regimen is used, give the second and third 2 g dose IV, 4 and 8 hours after the first dose.

➤*Prophylactic use, transurethral prostatectomy:* Administer 1 g prior to surgery; 1 g every 8 hours for ≤ 5 days.

➤*Renal function impairment:*
Adults – Initial loading dose is 1 to 2 g. Maintenance doses:

Maintenance Cefoxitin Dosage in Renal Impairment			
Renal function	Ccr (ml/min)	Dose (g)	Frequency (hrs)
Mild impairment	50-30	1-2	8-12
Moderate impairment	29-10	1-2	12-24
Severe impairment	9-5	0.5-1	12-24

Maintenance Cefoxitin Dosage in Renal Impairment			
Renal function	Ccr (ml/min)	Dose (g)	Frequency (hrs)
Essentially no function	< 5	0.5-1	24-48

When only serum creatinine level is available, use the following to obtain creatinine clearance. Serum creatinine should represent steady-state renal function.

Males: $\dfrac{\text{Weight (kg)} \times (140 - \text{age})}{72 \times \text{serum creatinine (mg/dL)}} = \text{Ccr}$

Females: $0.85 \times \text{above value}$

Hemodialysis: Administer a loading dose of 1 to 2 g after each hemodialysis. Give the maintenance dose as indicated in the table above.

Infants and children ≥ 3 months – 80 to 160 mg/kg/day divided every 4 to 6 hours. Use higher dosages for more severe or serious infections. Do not exceed 12 g/day.
Prophylactic use (≥ 3 months): 30 to 40 mg/kg/dose every 6 hours.
Renal function impairment: Modify consistent with recommendations for adults.

➤*CDC recommended treatment schedules for acute pelvic inflammatory disease (PID)†:*
Acute PID – 2 g IV every 6 hours plus 100 mg doxycycline IV or orally every 12 hours.

➤*Preparation of solution:*

Preparation of Cefoxitin Solution			
Package size	Diluent to add (ml)	≈ Withdrawable volume (ml)	≈ Concentration (mg/ml)
1 g vial (IM)	2	2.5	400
2 g vial (IM)	4	5	400
1 g vial (IV)	10	10.5	95
2 g vial (IV)	10 or 20	11.1 or 21	180 or 95
1 g infusion bottle (IV)	50 or 100	50 or 100	20 or 10
2 g infusion bottle (IV)	50 or 100	50 or 100	40 or 20
10 g bulk (IV)	43 or 93	49 or 98.5	200 or 100

IV use – Reconstitute 1 g with ≥ 10 ml of Sterile Water for Injection, and 2 g with 10 to 20 ml. May reconstitute 10 g vial with 43 or 93 ml Sterile Water for Injection or any solutions listed under IV Compatibility and Stability. Benzyl alcohol as a preservative has caused toxicity in neonates. This has not occurred in infants > 3 months of age, but they may also be at risk. Do not use benzyl alcohol in infants.

IM use – Reconstitute each g with 2 ml Sterile Water for Injection or 2 ml 0.5% lidocaine HCl (without epinephrine) to minimize IM injection discomfort.

➤*Administration of solution:*

IV administration – This is preferable for patients with bacteremia, bacterial septicemia or other severe or life-threatening infections, or for patients who are poor risks because of lowered resistance from debilitating conditions (malnutrition, trauma, surgery, diabetes, heart failure, malignancy), particularly if shock is present or impending.

Intermittent IV administration – 1 or 2 g in 10 ml of Sterile Water for Injection over 3 to 5 minutes; may also give over longer periods through an existing system. Temporarily discontinue administration of any other solutions at the same site.

Continuous IV infusion – For higher doses, add solution to an IV container of 5% Dextrose Injection, 0.9% Sodium Chloride Injection, 5% Dextrose and 0.9% Sodium Chloride Injection or 5% Dextrose Injection w/0.02% Sodium Bicarbonate Solution.

➤*Storage/Stability:* Store dry powder at < 30°C (86°F). Avoid exposure to temperatures > 50°C (122°F). The dry material, as well as solutions, darkens depending on storage conditions; product potency, however, is not adversely affected.

Premixed frozen – For IV use only. Store at ≤ –20°C (–4°F). Maintains satisfactory potency after thawing for 24 hours at room temperature and 21 days if stored under refrigeration (2° to 8°C; 36° to 46°F). Discard any unused thawed solutions. Do not refreeze.

Admixture incompatibility – Do not add solutions of cefoxitin to aminoglycoside solutions because of potential interaction; administer separately to the same patient. After time periods listed in the table, discard unused solution.

Stability/Storage for Diluents of Cefoxitin					
Diluent	24 hrs at room temp.	Refrigeration		Freezer	
		48 hours	1 week	26 weeks	30 weeks
Sterile Water for Injection	✓[1,2,3,4]	✓[2,4]	✓[1,3]		✓[1,3]
Bacteriostatic Water for Injection	✓[1,3]		✓[1,3]		✓[1,3]
0.9% Sodium Chloride Injection	✓[1,4,5,6]	✓[4,5,6]	✓[1]	✓[5,6]	✓[1]

† *Morbidity and Mortality Weekly Report* 1997 Jan 23;47 (Suppl RR-1);82.

CEFOXITIN SODIUM

Stability/Storage for Diluents of Cefoxitin					
Diluent	24 hrs at room temp.	Refrigeration		Freezer	
		48 hours	1 week	26 weeks	30 weeks
5% Dextrose Injection	✔[1,4,6]	✔[4,6]	✔[1]	✔[6]	✔[1]
10% Dextrose Injection	✔[4]	✔[4]			
Lactated Ringer's	✔[4,6]	✔[4,6]		✔[6]	
5% Dextrose in Lactated Ringer's	✔[4]	✔[4]			
Neut (Sodium Bicarbonate)	✔[4]	✔[4]			
Normosol-M in D5W	✔[4]	✔[4]			
Ionosol B with 5% Dextrose	✔[4]	✔[4]			
10% Mannitol	✔[4]	✔[4]			
5% Dextrose and 0.9% NaCl	✔[4]	✔[4]			
5% Dextrose with 0.02% Sodium Bicarbonate Solution	✔[4]	✔[4]			
5% Dextrose w/ 0.2% or 0.45% NaCl	✔[4]	✔[4]			
Ringer's Injection	✔[4]	✔[4]			
5% or 10% Invert Sugar in Water	✔[4]	✔[4]			
10% Invert Sugar in Saline	✔[4]	✔[4]			
5% Sodium Bicarbonate Injection	✔[4]	✔[4]			
M/6 Sodium Lactate Solution	✔[4]	✔[4]			
Polyonic M56 in 5% Dextrose	✔[4]	✔[4]			
2.5% and 5% Mannitol	✔[4]	✔[4]			
Isolyte E	✔[4]	✔[4]			
Isolyte E with 5% Dextrose	✔[4]	✔[4]			
0.5% or 1% Lidocaine without Epinephrine	✔[3]		✔[3]		✔[3]

[1] When reconstituted to 1 g/10 ml.
[2] After reconstitution and subsequent storage in plastic syringes.
[3] After reconstitution for IM use.
[4] After reconstitution and further dilution in 50 to 1000 ml.
[5] After storage in IV bags, plastic tubing, drip chambers, volume control devices.
[6] After storage in IV bags.

CEFUROXIME

Rx	**Cefuroxime Axetil** (Ranbaxy)	**Tablets:** (as axetil) 125 mg	(RX 750). Blue, capsule shape. In 60s and 100s.
Rx	**Ceftin** (GlaxoWellcome)		(Glaxo 395). White. Capsule shape. Film coated. In 20s and UD 100s.
Rx	**Cefuroxime Axetil** (Ranbaxy)	**Tablets:** (as axetil) 250 mg	(RX 751). Blue, capsule shape. In 20s, 60s, and 100s.
Rx	**Ceftin** (GlaxoWellcome)		(Glaxo 387). Light blue. Capsule shape. Film coated. In 10s, 20s, 60s and UD 100s.
Rx	**Cefuroxime Axetil** (Ranbaxy)	**Tablets:** (as axetil) 500 mg	(RX 752). Blue, capsule shape. In 20s, 60s, and 100s.
Rx	**Ceftin** (GlaxoWellcome)		(Glaxo 394). Dark blue. Capsule shape. Film coated. In 20s, 60s and UD 50s.
Rx	**Ceftin** (GlaxoWellcome)	**Suspension:** 125 mg/5 ml (as axetil) when reconstituted	Sucrose. Tutti-frutti flavor. In 50 and 100 ml bottles.
		250 mg/5 ml (as axetil) when reconstituted	Sucrose. Tutti-frutti flavor. In 50 and 100 ml bottles.
Rx	**Cefuroxime Sodium** (Various)	**Powder for Injection:**[1] 750 mg (as sodium).	In 10 ml vials and 100 ml piggyback vials.
Rx	**Zinacef** (GlaxoWellcome)		In vials, infusion pack and *ADD-Vantage* vials.
Rx	**Cefuroxime Sodium** (Various)	**Powder for Injection:**[1] 1.5 g (as sodium)	In 20 ml vials and 100 ml piggyback vials.
Rx	**Zinacef** (GlaxoWellcome)		In vials, infusion packs and *ADD-Vantage* vials.
Rx	**Cefuroxime Sodium** (Various)	**Powder for Injection:**[1] 7.5 g (as sodium)	In pharmacy bulk package.
Rx	**Zinacef** (GlaxoWellcome)		In pharmacy bulk package.
Rx	**Zinacef** (GlaxoWellcome)	**Injection:**[1] 750 mg (as sodium)	Premixed, frozen. In 50 ml.
		1.5 g (as sodium)	Premixed, frozen. In 50 ml.

[1] Contains 2.4 mEq sodium/g.

For complete prescribing information, refer to the Cephalosporins group monograph.

Indications

➤*Oral:*

Tablets –

Pharyngitis and tonsillitis: Caused by *S. pyogenes* (group A β-hemolytic streptococci).

Otitis media (acute bacterial): Caused by *S. pneumoniae, H. influenzae* (β-lactamase-producing strains), *M. catarrhalis* (β-lactamase-producing strains) and *S. pyogenes.*

Acute bacterial maxillary sinusitis: Caused by *S. pneumoniae* or *H. influenzae* (non-β-lactamase-producing strains only).

Acute bacterial exacerbations of chronic bronchitis and secondary bacterial infections of acute bronchitis: Caused by *S. pneumoniae, H. influenzae* (β-lactamase-negative strains) or *H. parainfluenzae* (β-lactamase-negative strains).

Urinary tract infections (uncomplicated): Caused by *E. coli* or *K. pneumoniae.*

Skin and skin structure infections (uncomplicated): Caused by *S. aureus* (β-lactamase-producing strains) and *S. pyogenes.*

Uncomplicated gonorrhea (urethral and endocervical): Caused by penicillinase- and non-penicillinase-producing strains of *N. gonorrhoeae* and uncomplicated rectal gonorrhea in females caused by non-penicillinase-producing strains of *Neisseria gonorrheae.*

Early Lyme disease (Erythema migrans): Caused by *Borrelia burgdorferi.*

Suspension – Treatment of children 3 months to 12 years of age.

Pharyngitis/Tonsillitis: Caused by *S. pyogenes.*

Otitis media (acute bacterial): Caused by *S. pneumoniae, H. influenzae* (including β-lactamase-producing strains), *M. catarrhalis* (including β-lactamase-producing strains) or *S. pyogenes.*

Impetigo: Caused by *S. aureus* (including β-lactamase-producing strains) or *S. pyogenes.*

CEFUROXIME

Note – Penicillin IM is the usual drug of choice in treatment and prevention of streptococcal infections, including prophylaxis of rheumatic fever. Cefuroxime axetil generally eradicates streptococci from the nasopharynx; however, substantial data establishing efficacy in subsequent prevention of rheumatic fever are not available.

➤ *Parenteral:*

Lower respiratory infections – These include pneumonia caused by *S. pneumoniae, H. influenzae* (including ampicillin-resistant), *Klebsiella* sp., *S. aureus* (penicillinase/ non-penicillinase-producing), *S. pyogenes, E. coli.*

Urinary tract infections – Caused by *E. coli* and *Klebsiella* sp.

Skin and skin structure infections – Caused by *S. aureus* (penicillinase/non-penicillinase-producing), *S. pyogenes, E. coli, Klebsiella* sp. and *Enterobacter* sp.

Septicemia – Caused by *S. aureus* (penicillinase/non-penicillinase-producing), *S. pneumoniae, E. coli, H. influenzae* (including ampicillin-resistant strains) and *Klebsiella* sp.

Meningitis – Caused by *S. pneumoniae, H. influenzae* (including ampicillin-resistant strains), *N. meningitidis* and *S. aureus* (penicillinase/non-penicillinase-producing).

Gonorrhea – Uncomplicated and disseminated gonococcal infections caused by *N. gonorrhoeae* (penicillinase/non-penicillinase-producing) in both males and females.

Bone/joint infections – Caused by *S. aureus* (penicillinase/non-penicillinase-producing).

Mixed infections – Clinical microbiological studies in skin and skin structure infections frequently reveal the growth of susceptible strains of both aerobic and anaerobic organisms. Cefuroxime has been used successfully in these mixed infections in which several organisms have been isolated. In certain cases of confirmed or suspected gram-positive or gram-negative sepsis, or in patients with other serious infections in which the causative organism has not been identified, the drug may be used concomitantly with an aminoglycoside. The recommended doses of both antibiotics may be given, depending on the severity of the infection and on the patient's condition.

Preoperative prophylaxis – May reduce incidence of certain postoperative infections in patients undergoing surgical procedures (eg, vaginal hysterectomy) classified as clean-contaminated or potentially contaminated. Stop prophylaxis within 24 hours. Preoperative use is effective during open heart surgery when operative site infections present a serious risk. For these patients, continue therapy at least 48 hours after procedure ends. If infection is present, obtain culture specimens; institute appropriate therapy.

Administration and Dosage

➤ *Oral:* Tablets and suspension are NOT bioequivalent and are NOT substitutable on a mg/mg basis.

Tablets – The tablets may be given without regard to meals.

Dosage for Cefuroxime Axetil Tablets

Population/Infection	Dosage	Duration (days)
Adults (≥ 13 years)		
Pharyngitis/tonsillitis	250 mg bid	10
Acute bacterial exacerbations of chronic bronchitis[1]	250 or 500 mg bid	10
Secondary bacterial infections of acute bronchitis		5-10
Uncomplicated skin and skin structure infections	250 or 500 mg bid	10
Uncomplicated urinary tract infections	125 or 250 mg bid	7 to 10
Uncomplicated gonorrhea	1000 mg once	single dose
Early Lyme disease	500 mg bid	20
Children who can swallow tablets whole[2]		
Pharyngitis/tonsillitis	125 mg bid	10
Acute otitis media	250 mg bid	10

[1] Safety and efficacy of drug administered < 10 days in patients with acute exacerbations of chronic bronchitis have not been established.
[2] Do not exceed adult recommended doses.

Suspension – Must be administered with food. Shake well each time before using. The suspension may be administered to children ranging in age from 3 months to 12 years, according to dosages in the following table:

Dosage for Cefuroxime Axetil Suspension

Infection (*infants and children, 3 months to 12 years*)	Dosage	Daily maximum dose	Duration (days)
Pharyngitis/tonsillitis	20 mg/kg/day divided bid	500 mg	10
Acute otitis media	30 mg/kg/day divided bid	1000 mg	10
Impetigo	30 mg/kg/day divided bid	1000 mg	10

Renal function impairment: Because cefuroxime is renally eliminated, its half-life will be prolonged in patients with renal failure.

Reconstitution of suspension: Shake the bottle to loosen the powder. Add the total amount of water for reconstitution (see table below). Invert the bottle and vigorously rock the bottle from side to side so that water rises through the powder. Once the sound of the powder against the bottle disappears, turn the bottle upright and vigorously shake it in a diagonal direction.

Amount of Water for Reconstitution of Cefuroxime Suspension

Bottle size	Water required for reconstitution
50 ml	20 ml
100 ml	37 ml
200 ml	74 ml

Each teaspoonful (5 ml) contains the equivalent of 125 mg cefuroxime axetil.

➤ *Parenteral:*

Dosage –

Adults: 750 mg to 1.5 g IM or IV every 8 hours, usually for 5 to 10 days.

Cefuroxime Dosage Guidelines

Type of Infection	Daily Dosage (g)	Frequency
Uncomplicated urinary tract, skin and skin structure, disseminated gonococcal, uncomplicated pneumonia	2.25	750 mg every 8 hours
Severe or complicated	4.5	1.5 g every 8 hours
Bone and joint	4.5	1.5 g every 8 hours
Life-threatening or caused by less susceptible organisms	6	1.5 g every 6 hours
Bacterial meningitis	9	≤ 3 g every 8 hours
Uncomplicated gonococcal	1.5 g IM[1]	Single dose

[1] Administered at 2 different sites together with 1 g oral probenecid.

• *Preoperative prophylaxis* – For clean-contaminated or potentially contaminated surgical procedures, administer 1.5 g IV prior to surgery (≈ ½ to 1 hour before). Thereafter, give 750 mg IV or IM every 8 hours when the procedure is prolonged.

For preventive use during open heart surgery, give 1.5 g IV at the induction of anesthesia and every 12 hours thereafter for a total of 6 g.

• *Renal function impairment* – Reduce dosage.

Parenteral Cefuroxime Dosage in Renal Impairment (Adults)

Creatinine clearance (ml/min)	Dose and frequency
> 20	750 mg to 1.5 g every 8 hours
10 to 20	750 mg every 12 hours
< 10	750 mg every 24 hours[1]

[1] Because cefuroxime is dialyzable, give patients on hemodialysis a further dose at the end of the dialysis.

When only serum creatinine is available, refer to the following formula:

$$\text{Males:} \quad \frac{\text{Weight (kg)} \times (140 - \text{age})}{72 \times \text{serum creatinine (mg/dL)}} = \text{Ccr}$$

Females: $0.85 \times$ above value

Creatinine clearance is ml/min/1.73 m^2.

Infants and children (> 3 months): 50 to 100 mg/kg/day in equally divided doses every 6 to 8 hours. Use 100 mg/kg/day (not to exceed the maximum adult dose) for more severe or serious infections.

• *Bone and joint infections* – 150 mg/kg/day (not to exceed maximum adult dose) in equally divided doses every 8 hours.

• *Bacterial meningitis* – Initially, 200 to 240 mg/kg/day IV in divided doses every 6 to 8 hours.

Renal function impairment: Modify dosage frequency consistent with adult guidelines.

➤ *Administration:*

IV – May be preferable for patients with bacterial septicemia or other severe or life-threatening infections, or for patients who may be poor risks because of lowered resistance, particularly if shock is present or impending.

Direct intermittent IV: Slowly inject solution into a vein over 3 to 5 minutes or give it through the tubing by which the patient receives other IV solutions.

Intermittent IV infusion with a Y–type administration set: Dose through the tubing by which the patient is receiving other IV solutions. However, during infusion, temporarily discontinue administration of other solutions at the same site.

Continuous IV infusion: A solution may be added to an IV bottle containing one of the following fluids: 0.9% Sodium Chloride Injection; 5% or 10% Dextrose Injection; 5% Dextrose and 0.45% or 0.9% Sodium Chloride Injection; 1/6M Sodium Lactate Injection.

IM – Give by deep IM injection into a large muscle mass. Prior to IM injection, aspiration is necessary to avoid injection into a blood vessel.

CEFUROXIME

	Kefurox			Zinacef		
Strength	Diluent to add (ml)	Volume to be withdrawn (ml)	Approximate concentration (mg/ml)	Diluent to add (ml)	Volume to be withdrawn	Approximate concentration (mg/ml)
			Preparation of Cefuroxime Solution			
750 mg vial	3.6 (IM)	3.6[1]	220	3 (IM)	Total[1]	220
750 mg vial	9 (IV)	8	100	8 (IV)	Total	90
1.5 g vial	14 (IV)	Total	100	16 (IV)	Total	90
750 mg infusion pack	50 (IV)	—	15	100 (IV)	—	7.5
750 mg infusion pack	100 (IV)	—	7.5			
1.5 g infusion pack	50 (IV)	—	30	100 (IV)	—	15
1.5 g infusion pack	100 (IV)	—	15			
750 mg bottle	50 (IV)	—	15			
750 mg bottle	100 (IV)	—	7.5			
1.5 g bottle	50 (IV)	—	30			
1.5 g bottle	100 (IV)	—	15			
750 mg ADD-Vantage	50 (IV)	—	15			
750 mg ADD-Vantage	100 (IV)	—	7.5			
1.5 g ADD-Vantage	50 (IV)	—	30			
1.5 g ADD-Vantage	100 (IV)	—	15			
7.5 g pharmacy bulk package				77 (IV)	Amount needed[2]	95

[1] Cefuroxime sodium is a suspension at IM concentrations.

[2] 8 ml of solution contains 750 mg cefuroxime; 16 ml of solution contains 1.5 g cefuroxime.

Use Sterile Water for Injection, 5% Dextrose in Water, 0.9% Sodium Chloride or any solution listed in the Compatibility/Stability IV section. If Sterile Water for Injection is used, reconstitute with ≈ 20 ml/g to avoid a hypotonic solution.

►*Admixture compatibility/stability:* Discard unused solutions after specified time periods.

IV – When the 750 mg, 1.5 g and 7.5 g pharmacy bulk vials are reconstituted as directed with Sterile Water for Injection, the solutions for IV administration maintain potency for 24 hours at room temperature and for 48 hours (750 mg and 1.5 g vials) and for 7 days (pharmacy bulk vial) when refrigerated at 5°C (41°F). More dilute solutions such as 750 mg or 1.5 g plus 100 ml Sterile Water for Injection, 5% Dextrose Injection or 0.9% Sodium Chloride Injection maintain potency for 24 hours at room temperature and for 7 days refrigerated.

These solutions may be further diluted to concentrations between 1 and 30 mg/ml in the following solutions and will lose ≤ 10% activity for 24 hours at room temperature or for ≥ 7 days under refrigeration: 0.9% Sodium Chloride Injection; 1/6M Sodium Lactate Injection; Ringer's Injection; Lactated Ringer's Injection; 5% Dextrose and 0.225%, 0.45% or 0.9% Sodium Chloride Injection; 5% or 10% Dextrose Injection; 10% Invert Sugar in Water for Injection.

The following are compatible for 24 hours at room temperature when admixed in IV infusion: Heparin (10 and 50 units/ml) in 0.9% Sodium Chloride Injection and Potassium Chloride (10 and 40 mEq/L) in 0.9% Sodium Chloride Injection.

Sodium bicarbonate injection is not recommended for dilution.

Premixed, frozen solution: Thaw at room temperature. Do not force thaw by immersion in water bath or by microwave irradiation. Components of the solution may precipitate in the frozen state and will dissolve upon reaching room temperature with little or no agitation. Potency is not affected. Mix after solution has reached room temperature. Do not add supplementary medication. The thawed solution is stable for 28 days under refrigeration (5°C; 41°F) or for 24 hours at room temperature (25°C; 77°F). Do not refreeze.

IM – When reconstituted with Sterile Water for Injection, suspensions for IM injection maintain satisfactory potency for 24 hours at room temperature and for 48 hours when refrigerated at 5°C (41°F).

Frozen, reconstituted –
Zinacef: Reconstitute 750 mg or 1.5 or 7.5 g vial as directed for IV administration. Immediately withdraw total contents of 750 mg or 1.5 g vial or 8 or 16 ml from the 7.5 g bulk vial and add to a *Viaflex Mini-bag* containing 50 or 100 ml of 0.9% Sodium Chloride Injection or 5% Dextrose Injection and freeze. Frozen solutions are stable for 6 months when stored at −20°C (−4°F). Thaw frozen solutions at room temperature. Do not refreeze. Do not force thaw by immersion in water bath, or by microwave irradiation. Thawed solutions may be stored for 24 hours at room temperature or 7 days in refrigerator.

►*Incompatibility:* Do not add cefuroxime to aminoglycoside solutions. However, each may be administered separately to the same patient.

►*Storage/Stability:*

Parenteral – Store cefuroxime in the dry state between 15° and 30°C (59° and 86°F) and protect from light. Powder, solutions and suspensions tend to darken, depending on storage conditions, without adversely affecting the product's potency.

Premixed, frozen – Do not store at > −20°C (−4°F).

Suspension – Shake the oral suspension well before each use. Store reconstituted suspension between 2° and 25°C (36° and 77°F), either in the refrigerator or at room temperature. Discard after 10 days.

Tablets – Store between 15° and 30°C (59° and 86°F). Protect from excessive moisture.

Patient Information

The tablet should be swallowed whole, not crushed, because the crushed tablet has a strong, persistent, bitter taste. Children who cannot swallow the tablet while should receive the oral suspension. Discontinuation of therapy due to taste or problems of administering this drug occurred in 1.4% of children given the oral suspension. Complaints about taste (which may impair compliance) occurred in 5% of children.

CEFTRIAXONE SODIUM

Rx	**Rocephin** (Roche)	**Powder for Injection:**[1] 250 mg	In vials.
		500 mg	In vials.
		1 g	In vials, piggyback vials and *ADD-Vantage* vials.
		2 g	In vials, piggyback vials and *ADD-Vantage* vials.
		10 g	In bulk containers.
		Injection:[1] 1 g	Dextrose. Premixed, frozen. In 50 ml plastic containers.
		2 g	Dextrose. Premixed, frozen. In 50 ml plastic containers.

[1] Contains 3.6 mEq sodium/g.

For complete prescribing information, refer to the Cephalosporins group monograph.

Indications

►*Lower respiratory tract infections:* Caused by *Streptococcus pneumoniae, Staphylococcus aureus, Haemophilus influenzae, H. parainfluenzae, Klebsiella pneumoniae, Serratia marcescens, Escherichia coli, E. aerogenes, Proteus mirabilis.*

►*Skin and skin structure infections:* Caused by *S. aureus, S. epidermidis, S. pyogenes,* viridans group streptococci, *E. coli, Enterobacter cloacae, K. oxytoca, K. pneumoniae, P. mirabilis, Pseudomonas aeruginosa, Morganella morganii, S. marcescens, Acinetobacter calcoaceticus, Bacteroides fragilis, Peptostreptococcus sp.*

►*Urinary tract infections (complicated and uncomplicated):* Caused by *E. coli, P. mirabilis, P. vulgaris, M. morganii* and *K. pneumoniae.*

CEFTRIAXONE SODIUM

➤*Uncomplicated gonorrhea (cervical/urethral and rectal):* Caused by *Neisseria gonorrhoeae*, including both penicillinase/non-penicillinase-producing strains (considered treatment of choice) and pharyngeal gonorrhea caused by non-penicillinase-producing strains of *N. gonorrhoeae*.

➤*Pelvic inflammatory disease:* Caused by *N. gonorrhoeae*.

➤*Bacterial septicemia:* Caused by *S. aureus, S. pneumoniae, E. coli, H. influenzae* and *K. pneumoniae*.

➤*Bone and joint infections:* Caused by *S. aureus, S. pneumoniae, E. coli, P. mirabilis, K. pneumoniae* and *Enterobacter* sp.

➤*Intra-abdominal infections:* Caused by *E. coli, K. pneumoniae, B. fragilis, Clostridium* sp. (most strains of *C. difficile* are resistant), *Peptostreptococcus* sp.

➤*Meningitis:* Caused by *H. influenzae, N. meningitidis* and *S. pneumoniae*. Has been used successfully in a limited number of cases of meningitis and shunt infections caused by *S. epidermidis* and *E. coli*.

➤*Prophylaxis:* The use of a single preoperative dose may reduce the incidence of postoperative infections in patients undergoing surgical procedures classified as contaminated or potentially contaminated (eg, vaginal or abdominal hysterectomy) and in surgical patients for whom infection at the operative site would present serious risk (eg, coronary artery bypass surgery). Ceftriaxone is as effective as cefazolin in preventing infection following coronary artery bypass surgery.

➤*Unlabeled uses:* Ceftriaxone 2 g/day IV for 14 to 28 days is effective in treating neurologic complications, arthritis and carditis associated with Lyme disease in patients refractory to penicillin G.

Administration and Dosage

Administer IV or IM. Continue for ≥ 2 days after signs and symptoms of infection have disappeared. Usual duration is 4 to 14 days; in complicated infections, longer therapy may be required. For *S. pyogenes*, continue for ≥ 10 days.

➤*Adults:* Usual daily dose is 1 to 2 g once a day (or in equally divided doses twice a day) depending on the type and severity of the infection. Do not exceed total daily dose of 4 g.

Uncomplicated gonococcal infections – Give a single IM dose of 250 mg.

Surgical prophylaxis – Give a single 1 g dose IV 0.5 to 2 hours before surgery.

➤*Children:* To treat serious infections other than meningitis, administer 50 to 75 mg/kg/day (not to exceed 2 g) in divided doses every 12 hours.

Meningitis – 100 mg/kg/day (not to exceed 4 g). Thereafter, a total daily dose of 100 mg/kg/day (not to exceed 4 g/day) is recommended. May give daily dose once per day or in equally divided doses every 12 hours. Usual duration is 7 to 14 days.

Skin and skin structure infections – Give 50 to 75 mg/kg once daily (or in equally divided doses twice daily), not to exceed 2 g.

Renal/hepatic function impairment – No dosage adjustment is necessary; however, monitor blood levels. In patients with both hepatic dysfunction and significant renal disease, the dose should not exceed 2 g/day without closely monitoring serum concentrations.

➤*CDC recommended treatment schedules for chancroid, gonorrhea and acute pelvic inflammatory disease (PID)†:*

Chancroid (Haemophilus ducreyi infection) – 250 mg IM as a single dose.

Gonococcal infections –
  Uncomplicated: 125 mg IM in a single dose plus 1 g azithromycin in single oral dose or 100 mg doxycycline twice a day for 7 days.
  Conjunctivitis: 1 g IM single dose.
  Disseminated: 1 g IM or IV every 24 hours.
  Meningitis/Endocarditis: 1 to 2 g IV every 12 hours for 10 to 14 days (meningitis) or for ≥ 4 weeks (endocarditis).

Reconstitution of Ceftriaxone

	Vial/Bottle dosage size	Amount of diluent to add (ml)	Resultant concentration (mg/ml)
IM[1]	250 mg	0.9	250
	500 mg	1.8	250
	1 g	3.6	250
	2 g	7.2	250

Reconstitution of Ceftriaxone

	Vial/Bottle dosage size	Amount of diluent to add (ml)	Resultant concentration (mg/ml)
IV[2]	250 mg	2.4	100
	500 mg	4.8	100
	1 g	9.6	100
	2 g	19.2	100
Piggyback[3]	1 g	10	
	2 g	20	

[1] If required, use more dilute solutions. Inject well within the body of a large muscle.
[2] Administer by intermittent infusion. Concentrations between 10 and 40 mg/ml are recommended; however, lower concentrations may be used.
[3] After reconstitution, further dilute to 50 or 100 ml with appropriate IV diluent.

➤*10 g bulk container:* This dosage size is not for direct administration. Reconstitute with 95 ml of an appropriate IV diluent. Before parenteral administration, withdraw the required amount, then further dilute to the desired concentration.

➤*Admixture compatibility:* Do not physically mix with other antimicrobial drugs because of possible incompatibility.

➤*Storage/Stability:* Protect from light. After reconstitution, protection from normal light is not necessary.

IM – Solutions remain stable (loss of potency < 10%) for these time periods:

Storage/Stability of Ceftriaxone (IM)

Diluent	Concentration (mg/ml)	Storage	
		Room temp (25°C)	Refrigerated (4°C)
Sterile Water for Injection	100	3 days	10 days
	250	24 hours	3 days
0.9% Sodium Chloride Solution	100	3 days	10 days
	250	24 hours	3 days
5% Dextrose Solution	100	3 days	10 days
	250	24 hours	3 days
Bacteriostatic Water and 0.9% Benzyl Alcohol	100	24 hours	10 days
	250	24 hours	3 days
1% Lidocaine Solution (without epinephrine)	100	24 hours	10 days
	250	24 hours	3 days

IV – At concentrations of 10, 20 and 40 mg/ml, solutions stored in glass or PVC containers and IV solutions at concentrations of 100 mg/ml in the IV piggyback glass containers remain stable (loss of potency < 10%) for the following time periods:

Storage/Stability of Ceftriaxone (IV)

Diluent	Storage	
	Room temp (25°C)	Refrigerated (4°C)
Sterile Water	3 days	10 days
0.9% Sodium Chloride Solution	3 days	10 days
5% or 10% Dextrose Solution	3 days	10 days
5% Dextrose and 0.9% Sodium Chloride Solution[1]	3 days	Incompatible
5% Dextrose and 0.45% Sodium Chloride Solution	3 days	Incompatible

[1] Data available for 10 to 40 mg/ml concentrations in this diluent in PVC containers only.

The following IV solutions are stable at room temperature (25°C; 77°F) for 24 hours at concentrations between 10 and 40 mg/ml: Sodium Lactate (PVC container), 10% Invert Sugar (glass container), 5% Sodium Bicarbonate (glass container), *Freamine* III (glass container), *Normosol-M* in 5% Dextrose (glass and PVC containers), *Ionosol-B* in 5% Dextrose (glass container), 5% or 10% Mannitol (glass container).

Solutions reconstituted with 5% Dextrose or 0.9% Sodium Chloride solution at concentrations between 10 mg/ml and 40 mg/ml, and then frozen (−20°C; −4°F) in PVC or polyolefin containers, remain stable for 26 weeks. Thaw frozen solutions at room temperature before use. After thawing, discard unused portions. Do not refreeze.

† *Morbidity and Mortality Weekly Report* 1997 Jan 23; 47 (No. RR-1):19,61,64-5.

CEFOPERAZONE SODIUM

Rx	Cefobid (Roerig)	Powder for Injection:[1] 1 g	In vials and piggyback units.
		2 g	In vials and piggyback units.
		Injection:[1] 1 g	Premixed, frozen. In 50 ml plastic containers.[2]
		2 g	Premixed, frozen. In 50 ml plastic containers.[3]
		10 g	Pharmacy bulk package.

[1] Contains 1.5 mEq sodium/g.
[2] With 2.3 g dextrose hydrous.

[3] With 1.8 g dextrose hydrous.

For complete prescribing information, refer to the Cephalosporins group monograph.

Indications

➤*Respiratory tract infections:* Caused by *Streptococcus pneumoniae, Haemophilus influenzae, Staphylococcus aureus* (penicillinase/non-penicillinase-producing), *S. pyogenes* (group A β-hemolytic streptococci), *Pseudomonas aeruginosa, Klebsiella pneumoniae, Escherichia coli, Proteus mirabilis* and *Enterobacter* sp.

➤*Peritonitis and other intra-abdominal infections:* Caused by *E. coli, P. aeruginosa,* enterococci, anaerobic gram-negative bacilli (including *Bacteroides fragilis*).

➤*Bacterial septicemia:* Caused by *S. pneumoniae, S. agalactiae, S. aureus,* enterococci, *P. aeruginosa, E. coli, Klebsiella* sp., *Proteus* sp. (indole-positive and indole-negative), *Clostridium* sp. and anaerobic gram-positive cocci.

➤*Skin and skin structure infections:* Caused by *S. aureus* (penicillinase/non-penicillinase-producing), *S. pyogenes, P. aeruginosa* and enterococci.

➤*Pelvic inflammatory disease, endometritis:* Including other female genital tract infections caused by *N. gonorrhoeae, S. epidermidis, S. agalactiae, E. coli, Clostridium* sp., enterococci, *Bacteroides* sp. (including *B. fragilis*), anaerobic gram-positive cocci.

➤*Urinary tract infections:* Caused by enterococci, *E. coli* and *P. aeruginosa.*

Administration and Dosage

Administer IM or IV.

Usual adult dose is 2 to 4 g/day administered in equally divided doses every 12 hours.

In severe infections, or infections caused by less sensitive organisms, the total daily dose or frequency may be increased. Patients have been successfully treated with a total daily dosage of 6 to 12 g divided into 2, 3 or 4 administrations ranging from 1.5 to 4 g/dose. A total daily dose of 16 g by constant infusion has been given without complications. Steady-state serum concentrations were ≈ 150 mcg/ml.

➤*Hepatic disease or biliary obstruction:* Cefoperazone is extensively excreted in bile. The serum half-life is increased 2- to 4-fold in patients with hepatic disease or biliary obstruction. In general, total daily dosage > 4 g should not be necessary. If higher dosages are used, monitor serum concentrations.

➤*Renal function impairment:* Because renal excretion is not the main route of elimination, patients with renal failure require no adjustment in dosage when usual doses are administered. When high doses are used, monitor serum drug concentrations.

Hemodialysis – The half-life is reduced slightly during hemodialysis. Thus, schedule dosing to follow a dialysis period. In patients with both hepatic dysfunction and significant renal disease, do not exceed 1 to 2 g/day without monitoring serum concentration.

➤*IV administration:*

Vials – In general, concentrations of between 2 and 50 mg/ml are recommended. Vials of sterile powder may be initially reconstituted with a minimum of 2.8 ml diluent per g of cefoperazone. Use any compatible diluent listed appropriate for IV administration. Reconstitute, using 5 ml of compatible diluent per g of cefoperazone. Withdraw the entire quantity for further dilution and administer via an IV administration system using one of the following methods:

  Piggyback units:
  • *Intermittent infusion* – Further dilute reconstituted cefoperazone in 20 to 40 ml of diluent per g and administer over 15 to 30 minutes.
  • *Continuous infusion* – After dilution to a final concentration of between 2 and 25 mg/ml, use cefoperazone for continuous infusion.

➤*IM administration:* Any suitable diluent listed may be used to prepare solutions for IM injection. Where concentrations ≥ 250 mg/ml are to be administered, prepare solutions using 0.5% Lidocaine HCl Injection.

After reconstitution, the following volumes and concentrations will be obtained:

Volume and Concentration Following Reconstitution of Cefoperazone			
Package size	Concentration (mg/ml)	Diluent to add (ml)	Withdrawable volume (ml)
1 g vial	333	2.6	3
	250	3.8	4

Volume and Concentration Following Reconstitution of Cefoperazone			
Package size	Concentration (mg/ml)	Diluent to add (ml)	Withdrawable volume (ml)
2 g vial	333	5	6
	250	7.2	8

➤*Preparation of solution:* Reconstitute powder for IV or IM use with any compatible solution for infusion mentioned below. After reconstitution, allow any foaming to dissipate to permit visual inspection for complete solubilization. Vigorous prolonged agitation may be needed to solubilize cefoperazone in higher concentrations (> 333 mg/ml). Maximum solubility of cefoperazone is ≈ 475 mg/ml compatible diluent.

IV use – Reconstitute with 5% Dextrose Injection; 5% Dextrose and Lactated Ringer's Injection; 5% Dextrose and 0.2% or 0.9% Sodium Chloride Injection; 10% Dextrose Injection; Lactated Ringer's Injection; 0.9% Sodium Chloride Injection; *Normosol M* and 5% Dextrose Injection; *Normosol R.*

IM use – Reconstitute with Bacteriostatic Water for Injection (benzyl alcohol or parabens); 0.5% Lidocaine HCl Injection; Sterile Water for Injection.

Do not use preparations containing benzyl alcohol in neonates.

➤*Storage / Stability:* The following parenteral diluents and approximate concentrations of cefoperazone provide stable solutions under the following conditions for the indicated time periods. After indicated time periods, discard unused portions.

Compatibility, Stability and Storage of Cefoperazone					
			Freezer		
Diluent	24 hrs room temperature (15° to 25°C)	5 days refrigeration (2° to 8°C)	3 weeks (-20° to -10°C)	5 weeks (-20° to -10°C)	≈ concentration (mg/ml)
Bacteriostatic Water for Injection (benzyl alcohol or parabens)	✔	✔			300
5% Dextrose Injection	✔	✔	✔[1]		2-50
5% Dextrose & Lactated Ringer's Inj.	✔				2-50
5% Dextrose & 0.2% or 0.9% Sodium Chloride Injection	✔	✔	✔[2]		2-50
10% Dextrose Injection	✔				2-50
Lactated Ringer's Injection	✔	✔			2
0.5% Lidocaine HCl Injection	✔	✔			300
0.9% Sodium Chloride Injection	✔	✔		✔[3]	2-300
Normosol M & 5% Dextrose Injection	✔	✔			2-50
Normosol R	✔	✔			2-50
Sterile Water for Injection	✔	✔		✔	300

[1] The 50 mg/ml injection only.
[2] The 2 mg/ml injection only.
[3] The 300 mg/ml injection only.

Thaw frozen samples at room temperature before use. After thawing, discard unused portions. Do not refreeze.

Sterile powder – Prior to reconstitution, protect sterile powder from light and store at ≤ 25°C (77°F). After reconstitution, protection from light is not necessary.

Frozen solution – Do not store at > 20°C (–4°F). After thawing, solution is stable for 10 days at 5°C (4°F) and for 48 hours at room temperature. Do not refreeze.

Admixture incompatibility – Do not mix cefoperazone directly with an aminoglycoside. If concomitant therapy is necessary, use sequential intermittent IV infusion provided that separate secondary IV tubing is used and the primary IV tubing is irrigated between doses. Administer cefoperazone prior to the aminoglycoside.

CEFOTAXIME SODIUM

Rx	Claforan (Hoechst Marion Roussel)	**Powder for Injection:**[1] 500 mg	In vials, packages of 10.
		1 g	In vials, packages of 10s, 25s, 50s. Infusion bottles in 10s. *ADD-Vantage* system vials in 25s.
		2 g	In vials, packages of 10s, 25s, 50s. Infusion bottles in 10s. *ADD-Vantage* system vials in 25s.
		10 g	In bottles.
		Injection:[1] 1 g	Premixed, frozen. In 50 ml, package of 12s.
		2 g	Premixed, frozen. In 50 ml, package of 12s.

[1] Contains 2.2 mEq sodium/g.

Complete prescribing information for these products begins in the Cephalosporins group monograph.

Indications

➤*Lower respiratory tract infections:* Including pneumonia caused by *Streptococcus pneumoniae*, *S. pyogenes* (group A streptococci) and other streptococci (excluding enterococci [eg, *S. faecalis*]), *Staphylococcus aureus* (penicillinase/non-penicillinase-producing), *Escherichia coli*, *Klebsiella* sp., *Haemophilus influenzae* (including ampicillin-resistant strains), *H. parainfluenzae*, *Proteus mirabilis*, *Serratia marcescens* and *Enterobacter* sp., indole-positive *Proteus* and *Pseudomonas* sp.

➤*Urinary tract infections:* Caused by *Enterococcus* sp., *S. epidermidis*, *S. aureus* (penicillinase/non-penicillinase-producing), *Citrobacter* sp., *Enterobacter* species, *E. coli*, *Klebsiella* sp., *P. mirabilis*, *P. vulgaris*, *P. inconstans* group B, *Morganella morganii*, *Providencia rettgeri*, *S. marcescens* and *Pseudomonas* sp. Also, uncomplicated gonorrhea caused by *Neisseria gonorrhoeae*, including penicillinase-producing strains.

➤*Gynecological infections:* Including pelvic inflammatory disease, endometritis and pelvic cellulitis caused by *S. epidermidis*, streptococci, Enterococcus, *Enterobacter* sp., *Klebsiella* sp., *E. coli*, *P. mirabilis*, *Bacteroides* species (including *B. fragilis*), *Clostridium* sp., anaerobic cocci (including *Peptostreptococcus*, *Peptococcus*) and *Fusobacterium* sp. (including *F. nucleatum*).

➤*Bacteremia/Septicemia:* Caused by *E. coli*, *Klebsiella* sp., *S. marcescens*, *S. aureus* and streptococci.

➤*Skin and skin structure infections:* Caused by *S. aureus* (penicillinase/non-penicillinase-producing), *S. epidermidis*, *S. pyogenes* (group A streptococci) and other streptococci, *Enterococcus*, *Acinetobacter* sp., *Citrobacter* sp., *E. coli*, *Enterobacter*, *Klebsiella* sp., *P. mirabilis*, *M. morganii*, *P. rettgeri*, *P. vulgaris*, *Pseudomonas* sp., *S. marcescens*, *Bacteroides* sp. and anaerobic cocci (including *Peptostreptococcus*, *Peptococcus*).

➤*Intra-abdominal infections:* Including peritonitis caused by streptococci, *E. coli*, *Klebsiella* sp., *Bacteroides* sp. and anaerobic cocci, including *Peptostreptococcus* and *Peptococcus* sp., *P. mirabilis* and *Clostridium* sp.

➤*Bone or joint infections:* Caused by *S. aureus* (penicillinase/non-penicillinase-producing strains), streptococci, *Pseudomonas* sp. and *P. mirabilis*.

➤*CNS infections (eg, meningitis and ventriculitis):* Caused by *N. meningitidis*, *H. influenzae*, *S. pneumoniae*, *K. pneumoniae* and *E. coli*.

Although many strains of enterococci (eg, *S. faecalis*) and *Pseudomonas* species are resistant to cefotaxime in vitro, it has been used successfully in treating patients with infections caused by susceptible organisms.

➤*Perioperative prophylaxis:* This may reduce the incidence of certain postoperative infections in patients undergoing surgical procedures (eg, abdominal or vaginal hysterectomy, GI and GU surgery) that are classified as contaminated or potentially contaminated. Effective perioperative use depends on the time of administration. For patients undergoing GI surgery, preoperative bowel preparation by mechanical cleansing, as well as with a nonabsorbable antibiotic (eg, neomycin), is recommended.

Cesarean section – Intraoperative (after clamping the umbilical cord) and postoperative use may reduce the incidence of certain postoperative infections.

If there are signs of infection, obtain specimens for identification of the causative organism so that appropriate therapy may be instituted.

Concomitant aminoglycoside therapy – In certain cases of confirmed or suspected gram-positive or gram-negative sepsis, or other serious infections in which the causative organism has not been identified, cefotaxime may be used concomitantly with an aminoglycoside. The dosage recommended for both antibiotics depends on the severity of the infection and the patient's condition. Monitor renal function, especially if higher dosages of the aminoglycosides are used or if therapy is prolonged, because of the potential nephrotoxicity and ototoxicity of aminoglycoside antibiotics. Some β-lactam antibiotics also have a certain degree of nephrotoxicity. Although not noted when cefotaxime was given alone, nephrotoxicity may be potentiated if it is used concomitantly with an aminoglycoside.

Administration and Dosage

➤*Adults:* Administer IV or IM. The maximum daily dosage should not exceed 12 g. Determine dosage and route of administration by susceptibility of the causative organisms, severity of the infection and the patient's condition (see table for dosage guidelines).

Cefotaxime Dosage Guidelines for Adults		
Type of infection	Daily dosage (g)	Frequency and route
Gonococcal urethritis/cervicitis in males and females	0.5	0.5 g IM (single dose)
Rectal gonorrhea in females	0.5	0.5 g IM (single dose)
Rectal gonorrhea in males	1	1 g IM (single dose)
Uncomplicated infections	2	1 g every 12 hours IM or IV
Moderate-to-severe	3 to 6	1 to 2 g every 8 hours IM or IV
Infections commonly needing higher dosage (eg, septicemia)	6 to 8	2 g every 6 to 8 hours IV
Life-threatening infections	≤ 12	2 g every 4 hours IV

Perioperative prophylaxis – 1 g IV or IM, 30 to 90 minutes prior to surgery.

Cesarean section – Administer the first 1 g dose IV as soon as the umbilical cord is clamped. Administer the second and third doses as 1 g IV or IM at 6 and 12 hour intervals after the first dose.

Pediatric – It is not necessary to differentiate between premature and normal gestational age infants. The following dosage recommendations may serve as a guide:

Cefotaxime Dosage Guidelines in Pediatric Patients			
Age	Weight (kg)	Dosage schedule	Route
0 to 1 week	—	50 mg/kg every 12 hours	IV
1 to 4 weeks	—	50 mg/kg every 8 hours	IV
1 month to 12 years	< 50[1]	50 to 180 mg/kg/day in 4 to 6 divided doses[2]	IV or IM

[1] For children ≥ 50 kg, use adult dosage. Do not exceed adult recommended doses.
[2] Use higher doses for more severe or serious infections including meningitis.

➤*Renal function impairment:* Determine dosage by degree of renal impairment, severity of infection and susceptibility of the causative organism. In patients with estimated creatinine clearances of < 20 ml/min/1.73 m^2, reduce dosage by 50%.

When only serum creatinine is available, the following formula may be used to convert this value into creatinine clearance. The serum creatinine should represent steady-state renal function.

$$\text{Males:} \quad \frac{\text{Weight (kg)} \times (140 - \text{age})}{72 \times \text{serum creatinine (mg/dL)}} = \text{Ccr}$$

Females: $0.85 \times$ above value

➤*CDC recommended treatment schedules for gonorrhea†:*
Disseminated gonococcal infection – Give 1 g IV every 8 hours.

Gonococcal ophthalmia in adults – For penicillinase-producing *Neisseria gonorrhoeae* (PPNG), give 500 mg, IV, four times per day.

➤*IV administration:* The IV route is preferable for patients with bacteremia, bacterial septicemia, peritonitis, meningitis, or other severe or life-threatening infections, or for patients who may be poor risks because of lowered resistance resulting from debilitating conditions such as malnutrition, trauma, surgery, diabetes, heart failure or malignancy, particularly if shock is present or impending.

Intermittent IV – 1 or 2 g in 10 ml of Sterile Water for Injection over 3 to 5 minutes; may also be given over a longer period of time through the tubing system by which the patient may be receiving other IV solutions. However, temporarily discontinue administration of other solutions at the same site.

Continuous IV infusion – May add to IV bottles containing solutions discussed below.

† *Morbidity and Mortality Weekly Report* 1997 (Jan 23); 47 (Supp RR-1):64.

CEFOTAXIME SODIUM

▶*IM administration:* Inject well within the body of a relatively large muscle (ie, gluteus maximus). Aspiration is necessary. Divide doses of 2 g and administer in different IM sites.

▶*Preparation of solution:* Use the following table as a guide for reconstitution:

| Volume and Concentration Following Reconstitution of Cefotaxime ||||
Package size	Diluent to add (ml)	≈ Withdrawable volume (ml)	≈ Concentration (mg/ml)
500 mg vial	2 (IM)	2.2	230
1 g vial	3 (IM)	3.4	300
2 g vial	5 (IM)	6	330
500 mg vial	10 (IV)	10.2	50
1 g vial	10 (IV)	10.4	95
2 g vial	10 (IV)	11	180
1 g infusion	50-100	50-100	20-10
2 g infusion	50-100	50-100	40-20
10 g bottle	47	52	200
10 g bottle	97	102	100

Shake to dissolve. Solutions range in color from light yellow to amber, depending on concentration, diluent used and length and condition of storage. A solution of 1 g cefotaxime in 14 ml of Sterile Water for Injection is isotonic.

IV – Reconstitute with at least 10 ml of Sterile Water for Injection. Infusion bottles may be reconstituted with 50 or 100 ml of 0.9% Sodium Chloride Injection or 5% Dextrose Injection.

IM – Reconstitute with Sterile Water or Bacteriostatic Water for Injection.

▶*Compatibility:* Reconstituted solutions may be further diluted up to 1000 ml with the following solutions and will maintain potency for 24 hours at room temperature and ≥ 5 days under refrigeration: 0.9% Sodium Chloride; 5% or 10% Dextrose; 5% Dextrose and 0.2%, 0.45% or 0.9% Sodium Chloride; Lactated Ringer's Solution; Sodium Lactate Injection (M/6); 10% Invert Sugar; 8.5% *Travasol* Injection without Electrolytes.

▶*Admixture incompatibility:* Do not admix with aminoglycoside solutions. If cefotaxime and aminoglycosides are to be administered to the same patient, administer separately.

▶*Storage / Stability:*

Powder – Store cefotaxime in the dry state < 30°C (86°F). The dry material, as well as the solutions, tends to darken depending on storage conditions; protect from elevated temperatures and excessive light.

Frozen solutions – Thawed solutions are stable for 24 hours at room temperature (≤ 22°C; 72°F) or for 10 days under refrigeration (≤ 5°C; 4°F).

IV bags – Solutions of cefotaxime in 0.9% Sodium Chloride Injection and 5% Dextrose Injection in IV bags are stable for 24 hours at room temperature, 5 days under refrigeration and 13 weeks frozen.

Thaw frozen samples at room temperature or under refrigeration before use; do not heat. After the periods mentioned above, discard any unused solutions or frozen material. Do not refreeze.

Cefotaxime solutions exhibit maximum stability in the pH 5 to 7 range. Do not use with diluents having a pH > 7.5 (eg, Sodium Bicarbonate Injection).

Solutions reconstituted as described above maintain potency for 24 hours at room temperature (≤ 22°C; 72°F), for 10 days under refrigeration (≤ 5°C; 4°F) and for ≥ 13 weeks frozen. After reconstitution and subsequent storage in original containers and disposable plastic syringes, cefotaxime is stable for 24 hours at room temperature, 5 days under refrigeration and 13 weeks frozen.

CEFTIZOXIME SODIUM

Rx	**Cefizox** (Fujisawa)	**Powder for Injection:**[1,2] 500 mg	In 10 ml single-dose fliptop vials.
		1 g	In 20 ml single-dose fliptop vials and 100 ml piggyback vials.
		2 g	In 20 ml single-dose fliptop vials and 100 ml piggyback vials.
		10 g	In pharmacy bulk package.
		Injection:[2] 1 g	Frozen, premixed. In 50 ml single-dose plastic containers.
		2 g	Frozen, premixed. In 50 ml single-dose plastic containers.

[1] Contains 2.6 mEq sodium/g.   [2] As sodium.

For complete prescribing information, refer to the Cephalosporins group monograph.

Indications

▶*Lower respiratory tract infections:* Caused by *Streptococcus* sp. (including *S. pneumoniae,* but excluding enterococci), *Klebsiella* sp., *Proteus mirabilis, Escherichia coli, Haemophilus influenzae* (including ampicillin-resistant strains), *Staphylococcus aureus* (penicillinase/non-penicillinase-producing), *Serratia* sp., *Enterobacter* sp. and *Bacteroides* sp.

▶*Urinary tract infections:* Caused by *S. aureus* (penicillinase/non-penicillinase-producing), *E. coli, Pseudomonas* sp. (including *P. aeruginosa*), *P. mirabilis, P. vulgaris, Providencia rettgeri, Morganella morganii, Klebsiella* sp., *Serratia* sp. including *S. marcescens* and *Enterobacter* sp.

▶*Gonorrhea:* Uncomplicated cervical and urethral gonorrhea caused by *N. gonorrhoeae.*

▶*Pelvic inflammatory disease (PID):* Caused by *N. gonorrhoeae, E. coli* or *S. agalactiae.*

▶*Intra-abdominal infections:* Caused by *E. coli, S. epidermidis, Streptococcus* sp. (excluding enterococci), *Enterobacter* sp., *Klebsiella* sp., *Bacteroides* sp., including *B. fragilis,* and anaerobic cocci, including *Peptococcus* sp. and *Peptostreptococcus* sp.

▶*Septicemia:* Caused by *Streptococcus* sp. (including *S. pneumoniae,* but excluding enterococci), *S. aureus* (penicillinase/non-penicillinase-producing), *E. coli, Bacteroides* sp. (including *B. fragilis*), *Klebsiella* sp. and *Serratia* sp.

▶*Skin and skin structure infections:* Caused by *S. aureus* (penicillinase/non-penicillinase-producing), *S. epidermidis, E. coli, Klebsiella* sp., *Streptococcus* sp. (including *S. pyogenes,* but excluding enterococci), *P. mirabilis, Serratia* sp., *Enterobacter* sp., *Bacteroides* sp. (including *B. fragilis* and anaerobic cocci, including *Peptococcus* sp. and *Peptostreptococcus* sp.).

▶*Bone and joint infections:* Caused by *S. aureus* (penicillinase/non-penicillinase-producing), *Streptococcus* sp. (excluding enterococci), *P. mirabilis, Bacteroides* sp. and anaerobic cocci, including *Peptococcus* sp. and *Peptostreptococcus* sp.

▶*Meningitis:* Caused by *H. influenzae.* Used to treat limited cases of meningitis caused by *S. pneumoniae.*

Administration and Dosage

▶*Adults:* Usual dosage is 1 or 2 g every 8 to 12 hours. Individualize dosage.

Ceftizoxime Dosage Guidelines in Adults		
Type of infection	Daily dose (g)	Frequency and route
Uncomplicated urinary tract	1	500 mg every 12 hours IM or IV
PID[1]	6	2 g every 8 hours IV
Other sites	2-3	1 g every 8 to 12 hours IM or IV
Severe or refractory	3-6	1 g every 8 hours IM or IV 2 g every 8 to 12 hours IM[1] or IV
Life-threatening [2]	9-12	3 to 4 g every 8 hours IV

[1] Dosages ≤ 2 g every 4 hours have been given.
[2] Divide 2 g IM doses and give in different large muscle masses.

▶*Urinary tract infections:* Because of the serious nature of urinary tract infections caused by *P. aeruginosa* and because many strains of *Pseudomonas* species are only moderately susceptible to ceftizoxime, higher dosage is recommended. Institute other therapy if the response is not prompt.

▶*Gonorrhea, uncomplicated:* A single 1 g IM injection is the usual dose.

▶*Life-threatening infections:* The IV route may be preferable for patients with bacterial septicemia, localized parenchymal abscesses (such as intra-abdominal abscess), peritonitis or other severe or life-threatening infections.

In those patients with normal renal function, the IV dosage is 2 to 12 g/day. In conditions such as bacterial septicemia, 6 to 12 g/day IV may be given initially for several days, and the dosage gradually reduced according to clinical response and laboratory findings.

▶*Pediatric:*

Children (≥ 6 months) – 50 mg/kg every 6 to 8 hours. Dosage may be increased to 200 mg/kg/day. Do not exceed the maximum adult dose for serious infection.

▶*Renal function impairment:* Requires modification of dosage. Following an initial loading dose of 500 mg to 1 g IM or IV, use the maintenance dosing schedule in the following table. Determine further dosing by therapeutic monitoring, severity of the infection and susceptibility of the causative organisms.

CEFTIZOXIME SODIUM

When only serum creatinine is available, calculate creatinine clearance from the formula below. The serum creatinine should represent steady-state renal function.

Males: $\dfrac{\text{Weight (kg)} \times (140 - \text{age})}{72 \times \text{serum creatinine (mg/dL)}} = \text{Ccr}$

Females: $0.85 \times$ above value

Hemodialysis – No additional supplemental dosing is required following hemodialysis; give the dose (according to the table below) at the end of dialysis.

Ceftizoxime Dosage in Adults with Renal Impairment			
Renal function	Creatinine clearance (ml/min)	Less severe infections	Life-threatening infections
Mild impairment	79-50	500 mg q 8 h	750 mg to 1.5 g q 8 h
Moderate-to-severe impairment	49-5	250 to 500 mg q 12 h	500 mg to 1 g q 12 h
Dialysis patients	4-0	500 mg q 48 h or 250 mg q 24 h	500 mg to 1 g q 48 h or 500 mg q 24 h

➤*IM injection:* Inject well within the body of a large muscle.

➤*IV administration:* Direct (bolus) injection, slowly over 3 to 5 minutes, directly or through tubing for patients receiving parenteral fluids (see list below). For intermittent or continuous infusion, dilute reconstituted ceftizoxime in 50 to 100 ml of one of the following: NaCl Injection; 5% or 10% Dextrose Injection; 5% Dextrose and 0.9%, 0.45% or 0.2% NaCl Injection; Ringer's Injection; Lactated Ringer's Injection; 5% Sodium Bicarbonate in Sterile Water for Injection; 5% Dextrose in Lactated Ringer's Injection (only when reconstituted with 4% Sodium Bicarbonate Injection); Invert Sugar 10% in Sterile Water for Injection.

➤*Preparation of solution:* Reconstitute with Sterile Water for Injection. Shake well.

Volume and Concentration Following Reconstitution of Ceftizoxime			
Package size	Diluent to add (ml)	≈ Available volume (ml)	≈ Concentration (mg/ml)
500 mg	1.5 (IM)	1.8	280
1 g vial	3 (IM)	3.7	270
2 g vial[1]	6 (IM)	7.4	270
500 mg	5 (IV)	5.3	95
1 g vial	10 (IV)	10.7	95
2 g vial	20 (IV)	21.4	95
10 g vial	30 (bulk vial)	37	1 g/3.5 ml
	45 (bulk vial)	51	1 g/5 ml

[1] Divide 2 g IM doses and give in different large muscle masses.

Piggyback vials – Reconstitute with 50 to 100 ml of any IV solution listed above. Shake well. Administer as a single dose with primary IV fluids.

A solution of 1 g ceftizoxime in 13 ml Sterile Water for Injection is isotonic.

Frozen injection – Thaw container at room temperature. Do not introduce additives into the solution.

➤*Storage/Stability:* After reconstitution or dilution in the IV fluids above, these solutions are stable for 24 hours at room temperature and for 96 hours if refrigerated (5°C; 41°F).

After thawing the frozen injection, the solution is stable for 24 hours at room temperature or for 10 days if refrigerated. Do not refreeze.

CEFOTETAN DISODIUM

Rx	Cefotan (Zeneca)	Powder for Injection:[1] 1 g	In *ADD-Vantage* and piggyback vials.[2]
		2 g	In *ADD-Vantage* and piggyback vials.[2]
		10 g	In 100 ml vials
		Injection: 1 g/50 ml	Dextrose. Frozen, iso-osmotic, premixed. In 50 ml single-dose *Galaxy* containers.
		2 g/50 ml	Dextrose. Frozen, iso-osmotic, premixed. In 50 ml single-dose *Galaxy* containers.

[1] Contains 3.5 mEq sodium/g.

[2] Reconstitute only with sodium chloride 0.9% or dextrose injection 5% in the 50, 100 or 250 ml flexible diluent containers.

For complete prescribing information, refer to the Cephalosporins group monograph.

Indications

➤*Urinary tract infections:* Caused by *Escherichia coli*, *Klebsiella* sp. (including *K. pneumoniae*) and *Proteus* sp. (including *P. vulgaris*, *Providencia rettgeri* and *Morganella morganii*).

➤*Lower respiratory tract infections:* Caused by *Streptococcus pneumoniae*, *Staphylococcus aureus* (penicillinase/non-penicillinase-producing), *H. influenzae* (including ampicillin-resistant strains), *Klebsiella* sp. (including *K. pneumoniae*), *Proteus mirabilis*, *Serratia marcescens* and *E. coli*.

➤*Skin/Skin structure infections:* Caused by *S. aureus* (penicillinase/non-penicillinase-producing), *S. epidermidis*, *S. pyogenes*, *Streptococcus* sp. (excluding enterococci), *Klebsiella* pneumonia, *Peptococcus niger*, *Peptostreptococcus* sp. and *E. coli*.

➤*Gynecologic infections:* Caused by *S. aureus* (including penicillinase/non-penicillinase-producing), *S. epidermidis*, *Streptococcus* sp. (excluding enterococci), *S. agalactiae*, *E. coli*, *P. mirabilis*, *N. gonorrhoeae*, *Bacteroides* sp. (excluding *B. distasonis*, *B. ovatus*, *B. thetaiotaomicron*), *Fusobacterium* sp. and gram-positive anaerobic cocci (including *Peptococcus* and *Peptostreptococcus* sp.).

➤*Intra-abdominal infections:* Caused by *E. coli*, *Klebsiella* sp. (including *K. pneumoniae*), *Streptococcus* sp. (excluding enterococci), *Bacteroides* sp. (excluding *B. distasonis*, *B. ovatus*, *B. thetaiotaomicron*) and *Clostridium* sp.

➤*Bone and joint infections:* Caused by *S. aureus*.

➤*Concomitant antibiotic therapy:* If cefotetan and an aminoglycoside are used concomitantly, carefully monitor renal function, especially if higher dosages of the aminoglycoside are to be administered or if therapy is prolonged, because of the potential nephrotoxicity and ototoxicity of aminoglycosides. Although to date, nephrotoxicity has not been noted when cefotetan was given alone, it is possible that nephrotoxicity may be potentiated if used concomitantly with an aminoglycoside.

➤*Perioperative prophylaxis:* Preoperative administration may reduce the incidence of certain postoperative infections in patients undergoing surgical procedures classified as clean-contaminated or potentially contaminated (eg, cesarean section, abdominal or vaginal hysterectomy, transurethral surgery, GI and biliary tract surgery).

If there are signs and symptoms of infection, obtain specimens for identification of causative organism so that appropriate therapeutic measures may be initiated.

Administration and Dosage

➤*Adults:* The usual dosage is 1 or 2 g IV or IM every 12 hours for 5 to 10 days. Determine proper dosage and route of administration by the condition of the patient, severity of the infection and susceptibility of the causative organism.

General Cefotetan Dosage Guidelines		
Type of Infection	Daily Dose	Frequency and Route
Urinary tract	1 to 4 g	500 mg every 12 hrs IV or IM
		1 or 2 g every 24 hrs IV or IM
		1 or 2 g every 12 hrs IV or IM
Skin/Skin structure		
Mild-to-moderate[2]	2 g	2 g q 24 hrs IV
		1 g q 12 hrs IV or IM
Severe	4 g	2 g q 12 hrs IV
Other Sites	2 to 4 g	1 or 2 g every 12 hrs IV or IM
Severe	4 g	2 g every 12 hrs IV
Life-threatening	6 g[1]	3 g every 12 hrs IV

[1] Maximum daily dosage should not exceed 6 g.
[2] *Klebsiella pneumoniae* skin and skin structure infections should be treated with 1 or 2 g every 12 hours IV or IM.

➤*Prophylaxis:* To prevent postoperative infection in clean contaminated or potentially contaminated surgery in adults, give a single 1 or 2 g IV dose 0.5 to 1 hour prior to surgery. In patients undergoing cesarean section, give the dose as soon as the umbilical cord is clamped.

➤*Renal function impairment:* Reduce the dosage schedule using these guidelines:

Cefotetan Dosage in Renal Impairment		
Ccr (ml/min)	Dose	Frequency
> 30	usual recommended dose[1]	every 12 hours
10-30	usual recommended dose[1]	every 24 hours
< 10	usual recommended dose[1]	every 48 hours

[1] Determined by type/severity of infection, susceptibility of causative organism.

Alternatively, the dosing interval may remain constant at 12 hour intervals, but reduce dose by ½ for patients with a creatinine clearance of 10 to 30 ml/min, and by ¼ for patients with a creatinine clearance of < 10 ml/min.

CEFOTETAN DISODIUM

When only serum creatinine is available, use the following formula to estimate creatinine clearance. Serum creatinine level should represent steady-state renal function.

$$\text{Males:} \quad \frac{\text{Weight (kg)} \times (140 - \text{age})}{72 \times \text{serum creatinine (mg/dL)}} = \text{Ccr}$$

Females: $0.85 \times$ above value

Dialysis – Cefotetan is dialyzable; for patients undergoing intermittent hemodialysis, give ¼ of the usual recommended dose every 24 hours on days between dialysis and ½ the usual recommended dose on the day of dialysis.

➤*IV:* The IV route is preferable for patients with bacteremia, bacterial septicemia or other severe or life-threatening infections, or for patients who may be poor risks because of lowered resistance resulting from such debilitating conditions as malnutrition, trauma, surgery, diabetes, heart failure or malignancy, particularly if shock is present or impending.

Intermittent IV administration – Inject a solution containing 1 or 2 g in Sterile Water for Injection over 3 to 5 minutes. Using an infusion system, the solution may be given over a longer period through the tubing system by which the patient may be receiving other IV solutions. Butterfly or scalp vein-type needles are preferred. However, during infusion of cefotetan, temporarily discontinue the administration of other solutions at the same site.

➤*IM:* As with all IM preparations, inject well within the body of a relatively large muscle such as the upper outer quadrant of the buttock (ie, gluteus maximus).

➤*Preparation of solution:*
For IV use – Reconstitute with Sterile Water for Injection.

For IM use – Reconstitute with Sterile Water for Injection, Bacteriostatic Water for Injection, 0.5% or 1% Lidocaine HCl, or Sodium Chloride Injection 0.9%.

Volume and Concentration Following Reconstitution of Cefotetan			
Vial size (g)	Amount of diluent to add (ml)	≈ Withdrawable volume (ml)	≈ Average concentration (mg/ml)
IV			
1	10	10.5	95
2	10-20	11-21	182-95
IM			
1	2	2.5	400
2	3	4	500

Infusion bottles (100 ml) – May be reconstituted with 50 to 100 ml of 5% Dextrose Solution or 0.9% Sodium Chloride Solution.

➤*Admixture incompatibility:* Do not admix with solutions containing aminoglycosides. If cefotetan and aminoglycosides are to be administered to the same patient, they must be administered separately and not as a mixed injection.

➤*Storage/Stability:* Do not store vials at > 22°C (72°F); protect from light.

Reconstituted as described above, cefotetan maintains potency for 24 hours at room temperature (25°C; 77°F), for 96 hours refrigerated (5°C; 40°F) and for ≥ 1 week frozen. After reconstitution and subsequent storage in disposable glass or plastic syringes, cefotetan is stable for 24 hours at room temperature and 96 hours refrigerated.

Thaw frozen samples at room temperature before use. After the periods mentioned above, discard any unused solutions or frozen materials. Do not refreeze.

CEFTAZIDIME

Rx	**Fortaz** (GlaxoWellcome)	**Powder for Injection:** 500 mg	In vials.[1]
Rx	**Ceptaz** (GlaxoWellcome)	**Powder for Injection:** 1 g	In vials and infusion packs.[2]
Rx	**Fortaz** (GlaxoWellcome)		In vials, *ADD-Vantage* vials and infusion packs.[1]
Rx	**Tazicef** (SmithKline Beecham/Bristol-Myers Squibb)		In vials, *ADD-Vantage* vials and piggyback vials.[1]
Rx	**Tazidime** (Eli Lilly)		In 20 ml, 100 ml and *ADD-Vantage* vials.[2]
Rx	**Ceptaz** (GlaxoWellcome)	**Powder for Injection:** 2 g	In vials and infusion packs.[2]
Rx	**Fortaz** (GlaxoWellcome)		In vials, *ADD-Vantage* vials and infusion packs.[1]
Rx	**Tazicef** (SmithKline Beecham/Bristol-Myers Squibb)		In vials, *ADD-Vantage* vials and piggyback vials.[1]
Rx	**Tazidime** (Eli Lilly)		In 50 ml, 100 ml and *ADD-Vantage* vials.[2]
Rx	**Fortaz** (GlaxoWellcome)	**Powder for Injection:** 6 g	In bulk package.[1]
Rx	**Tazicef** (SmithKline Beecham/Bristol-Myers Squibb)		In bulk package.[1]
Rx	**Tazidime** (Eli Lilly)		In 100 ml vial.[2]
Rx	**Fortaz** (GlaxoWellcome)	**Injection:** 1 g	Premixed, frozen. In 50 ml.[3]
		2 g	Premixed, frozen. In 50 ml.[4]
Rx	**Tazicef** (SmithKline Beecham/Bristol-Myers Squibb)	**Injection:** 1 g	In *Galaxy* containers.
		2 g	In *Galaxy* containers.

[1] Contains 2.3 mEq sodium/g.
[2] As pentahydrate with L-arginine.
[3] With 2.2 g dextrose hydrous.
[4] With 1.6 g dextrose hydrous.

For complete prescribing information, refer to the Cephalosporins group monograph.

Indications

➤*Lower respiratory tract infections (including pneumonia):* Caused by *Pseudomonas aeruginosa* and other *Pseudomonas* sp.; *Haemophilus influenzae* (including ampicillin-resistant strains); *Klebsiella* sp.; *Enterobacter* sp.; *Proteus mirabilis*; *Escherichia coli*; *Serratia* sp.; *Citrobacter* sp.; *Streptococcus pneumoniae*; *Staphylococcus aureus* (methicillin-susceptible strains).

➤*Skin and skin structure infections:* Caused by *P. aeruginosa*; *Klebsiella* sp.; *E. coli*; *Proteus* sp. (including *P. mirabilis* and indole-positive *Proteus*); *Enterobacter* sp.; *Serratia* sp.; *S. aureus* (methicillin-susceptible strains); *S. pyogenes* (group A β–hemolytic streptococci).

➤*Urinary tract infections:* Both complicated and uncomplicated infections caused by *P. aeruginosa*; *Enterobacter* sp.; *Proteus* sp. (including *P. mirabilis* and indole-positive *Proteus*); *Klebsiella* sp.; *E. coli*.

➤*Bacterial septicemia:* Caused by *P. aeruginosa*; *Klebsiella* sp.; *H. influenzae*; *E. coli*; *Serratia* sp.; *S. pneumoniae*; *S. aureus* (methicillin-susceptible strains).

➤*Bone and joint infections:* Caused by *P. aeruginosa*; *Klebsiella* sp.; *Enterobacter* sp.; *S. aureus* (methicillin-susceptible strains).

➤*Gynecological infections:* Including endometritis, pelvic cellulitis and other infections of the female genital tract caused by *E. coli*.

➤*Intra-abdominal infections:* Including peritonitis caused by *E. coli*; *Klebsiella* sp.; *S. aureus* (methicillin-susceptible strains); polymicrobial infections caused by aerobic and anaerobic organisms and *Bacteroides* species (many strains of *B. fragilis* are resistant).

➤*CNS infections:* Including meningitis caused by *H. influenzae* and *Neisseria meningitidis*. Ceftazidime has also been used successfully in a limited number of cases of meningitis caused by *P. aeruginosa* and *S. pneumoniae*.

➤*Concomitant antibiotic therapy:* Ceftazidime may be used concomitantly with other antibiotics (eg, aminoglycosides, vancomycin and clindamycin) in severe and life-threatening infections and in the immunocompromised patient. Dose depends on the severity of the infection and the patient's condition.

Administration and Dosage

Determine dosage and route by the susceptibility of the causative organisms, severity of infection and patient's condition and renal function.

Ceftazidime Dosage Guidelines		
Patient/Infection site	Dose	Frequency
Adults Usual recommended dose	1 g IV or IM	q 8-12 hrs
Uncomplicated urinary tract infections	250 mg IV or IM	q 12 hrs
Complicated urinary tract infections	500 mg IV or IM	q 8-12 hrs
Uncomplicated pneumonia; mild skin and skin structure infections	500 mg to 1 g IV or IM	q 8 hrs
Bone and joint infections	2 g IV	q 12 hrs

CEFTAZIDIME

Ceftazidime Dosage Guidelines		
Patient/Infection site	Dose	Frequency
Serious gynecological and intra-abdominal infections	2 g IV	q 8 hrs
Meningitis		
Very severe life-threatening infections, especially in immunocompromised patients		
Pseudomonal lung infections in cystic fibrosis patients w/normal renal function[1]	30 to 50 mg/kg IV to a max 6 g/day	q 8 hrs
Neonates (0 to 4 weeks)[2]	30 mg/kg IV	q 12 hrs
Infants and children (1 month to 12 years)[2]	30 to 50 mg/kg IV to 6 g/day[3]	q 8 hrs

[1] Although clinical improvement has been shown, bacteriological cures cannot be expected in patients with chronic respiratory disease and cystic fibrosis.
[2] Do not exceed adult recommended doses.
[3] Reserve the higher dose for immunocompromised children or children with cystic fibrosis or meningitis.

►*Hepatic function impairment:* No dosage adjustment is required.

►*Renal function impairment:* Ceftazidime is excreted by the kidneys, almost exclusively by glomerular filtration. In patients with impaired renal function (GFR < 50 ml/min), reduce dosage to compensate for slower excretion. In patients with suspected renal insufficiency, give an initial loading dose of 1 g. Estimate GFR to determine the appropriate maintenance dose.

Ceftazidime Dosage in Renal Impairment		
Creatinine clearance (ml/min)	Recommended unit dose of ceftazidime	Frequency of dosing
31-50	1 g	q 12 hrs
16-30	1 g	q 24 hrs
6-15	500 mg	q 24 hrs
≤ 5	500 mg	q 48 hrs

When only serum creatinine is available, use the following formula to estimate creatinine clearance. Serum creatinine should represent steady-state renal function.

$$\text{Males:} \quad \frac{\text{Weight (kg)} \times (140 - \text{age})}{72 \times \text{serum creatinine (mg/dL)}} = \text{Ccr}$$

Females: $0.85 \times$ above value

In patients with severe infections who would normally receive ceftazidime 6 g/day were it not for renal insufficiency, the unit dose given in the table above may be increased by 50% or the dosing frequency increased appropriately. Determine further dosing by therapeutic monitoring, severity of the infection and susceptibility of the causative organism.

In children, as for adults, adjust creatinine clearance for body surface area or lean body mass, and reduce the dosing frequency in cases of renal insufficiency.

Dialysis – Give a 1 g loading dose, followed by 1 g after each hemodialysis period.

Ceftazidime can also be used in patients undergoing intraperitoneal dialysis (IPD) and continuous ambulatory peritoneal dialysis (CAPD). Give a loading dose of 1 g, followed by 500 mg every 24 hours. In addition to IV use, ceftazidime (except the L-arginine formulation) can be incorporated in the dialysis fluid at a concentration of 250 mg per 2 L of dialysis fluid.

Preparation of Ceftazidime Solutions			
Package size	Diluent to add (ml)	≈ Available volume (ml)	≈ Ceftazidime concentration (mg/ml)
IM			
500 mg vial	1.5	1.8	280
1 g vial	3	3.6	280
IV			
500 mg vial	5	5.3	100
1 g vial	10	10.6	90-100
2 g vial	10	11.2	170-180
Infusion pack			
1 g vial	100[1]	100	10
2 g vial	100[1]	100	20

Preparation of Ceftazidime Solutions			
Package size	Diluent to add (ml)	≈ Available volume (ml)	≈ Ceftazidime concentration (mg/ml)
Bulk package			
6 g vial	26	30	200
10 g vial	40	Amount needed	200

[1] Note: Addition should be in two stages (see *IV infusion*).

Inject IV or deeply IM into a large muscle mass such as the upper outer quadrant of the gluteus maximus or lateral part of the thigh.

►*IM:* Reconstitute with one of the following diluents: Sterile or Bacteriostatic Water for Injection or 0.5% or 1% Lidocaine HCl Injection. Refer to the Preparation of Ceftazidime Solutions table.

►*IV:* This route is preferable for patients with bacterial septicemia, bacterial meningitis, peritonitis or other severe or life-threatening infections, or for patients who may be poor risks because of lowered resistance resulting from malnutrition, trauma, surgery, diabetes, heart failure or malignancy, particularly if shock is present or impending.

Direct intermittent IV administration – Reconstitute ceftazidime as directed in the table with Sterile Water for Injection. Slowly inject directly into the vein over a period of 3 to 5 minutes or give through the tubing of an administration set while the patient is also receiving one of the compatible IV fluids.

IV infusion – Reconstitute the 1 or 2 g infusion pack with 100 ml Sterile Water for Injection or one of the compatible IV fluids. Alternatively, reconstitute the 500 mg, 1 or 2 g vial and add an appropriate quantity of the resulting solution to an IV container with one of the compatible IV fluids.

Intermittent IV infusion (Y-type) – Can be accomplished with compatible solutions. However, during infusion of ceftazidime solution, discontinue other solution.

►*Admixture incompatibility:* Do not add aminoglycoside antibiotics to ceftazidime. Give separately.

►*Storage/Stability:*

IM – When reconstituted as directed with Sterile or Bacteriostatic Water for Injection or 0.5% or 1% Lidocaine HCl Injection, the solution maintains potency for 24 hours (18 hours for arginine formulation) at room temperature or for 7 days if refrigerated. Solutions in Sterile Water for Injection, frozen immediately after reconstitution in the original container, are stable for 3 months (6 months for arginine formulation) at –20°C (–4°F). Once thawed, do not refreeze. Thawed solutions may be stored for 8 hours (< 12 hours for arginine formulation) at room temperature or 4 days (7 days for arginine formulation) in a refrigerator.

IV – When reconstituted as directed with Sterile Water for Injection, the solution maintains potency for 24 hours (18 hours for arginine formulation) at room temperature or for 7 days under refrigeration. Solutions in Sterile Water for Injection in the original container or in 0.9% Sodium Chloride or 5% Dextrose Injection in PVC small volume containers, frozen immediately after reconstitution, are stable for 3 months (6 months for arginine formulation) at –20°C (–4°F). For larger volumes, when it is necessary to warm the frozen product (to a maximum of 40°C; 104°F), avoid heating after thawing is complete. Once thawed, do not refreeze. Store thawed solutions for 8 to 24 hours (≤ 12 hours for arginine formulation) at room temperature or for 4 days (7 days for arginine formulation) in a refrigerator.

Ceftazidime is compatible with the more common IV infusion fluids. Solutions at concentrations between 1 mg/ml and 40 mg/ml in the following infusion fluids may be stored for up to 18 to 24 hours at room temperature or 7 to 10 days if refrigerated: 0.9% Sodium Chloride; 1/6M Sodium Lactate; Ringer's; Lactated Ringer's; 5% or 10% Dextrose; 5% Dextrose and 0.225%, 0.45% or 0.9% Sodium Chloride; 10% Invert Sugar in Water; *Normosol M* in 5% Dextrose.

Ceftazidime is less stable in Sodium Bicarbonate Injection than in other IV fluids. It is not recommended as a diluent. Solutions in 5% Dextrose and 0.9% Sodium Chloride Injection are stable for ≥ 6 hours at room temperature in plastic tubing, drip chambers and volume control devices of common IV infusion sets.

Ceftazidime at a concentration of 4 mg/ml is compatible for 24 hours at room temperature or 7 days under refrigeration in 0.9% Sodium Chloride Injection or 5% Dextrose Injection when admixed with: Cefuroxime 3 mg/ml; heparin ≤ 50 units/ml; or potassium chloride ≤ 40 mEq/L.

CEFEPIME HCl

Rx	Maxipime (Dura)	Powder for Injection:[1] 500 mg	In 15 ml vial.
		1 g	In 15 ml vials, *ADD-Vantage* vials, and 100 ml piggyback bottles.
		2 g	In 20 ml vials, *ADD-Vantage* vials, and 100 ml piggyback bottles.

[1] Contains arginine.

For complete prescribing information, refer to the Cephalosporins group monograph.

Indications

►*Uncomplicated and complicated urinary tract infections:* Those (including pyelonephritis) caused by *Escherichia coli* or *Klebsiella pneumoniae*, when the infection is severe or caused by *E. coli, K. pneumoniae,* or *Proteus mirabilis,* when the infection is mild-to-moderate, including cases associated with concurrent bacteremia with these microorganisms.

►*Uncomplicated skin and skin structure infections:* Caused by *Staphylococcus aureus* (methicillin-susceptible strains only) or *Streptococcus pyogenes.*

►*Pneumonia (moderate-to-severe):* Caused by *S. pneumoniae,* including cases associated with concurrent bacteremia, *Pseudomonas aeruginosa, K. pneumoniae,* or *Enterobacter* sp.

►*Empiric therapy for febrile neutropenic patients:* As monotherapy for empiric treatment of febrile neutropenic patients. In patients at high risk for severe infection (including patients with a history of recent bone marrow transplantation, with hypotension at presentation, with an underlying hematologic malignancy, or with severe or prolonged neutropenia), antimicrobial monotherapy may not be appropriate. Insufficient data exist to support the efficacy of cefepime monotherapy in such patients.

►*Complicated intra-abdominal infections:* In combination with metronidazole for complicated intra-abdominal infections caused by *E. coli,* viridans group streptococci, *P. aeruginosa, K. pneumoniae, Enterobacter* species, or *Bacteroides fragilis.*

►*Pediatric patients (2 months to 16 years of age):* Treatment of uncomplicated and complicated urinary tract infections (including pyelonephritis), uncomplicated skin and skin structure infections, pneumonia, and as empiric therapy for febrile neutropenic patients.

Administration and Dosage

►*Approved by the FDA:* January 18, 1996.

Recommended Dosage Schedule for Cefepime

Site and type of infection	Dose	Frequency	Duration (days)
Mild-to-moderate uncomplicated or complicated urinary tract infections, including pyelonephritis, caused by *E. coli, K. pneumoniae,* or *P. mirabilis.*[1]	0.5 to 1 g IV/IM[2]	q 12 hrs	7 to 10
Severe uncomplicated or complicated urinary tract infections, including pyelonephritis, caused by *E. coli* or *K. pneumoniae.*[1]	2 g IV	q 12 hrs	10
Moderate-to-severe pneumonia caused by *S. pneumoniae,*[1] *Pseudomonas aeruginosa, Klebsiella pneumoniae,* or *Enterobacter* sp.	1 to 2 g IV	q 12 hrs	10
Moderate-to-severe uncomplicated skin and skin structure infections caused by *S. aureus* or *S. pyogenes.*	2 g IV	q 12 hrs	10
Empiric therapy for febrile neutropenic patients.	2 g IV	q 8 hrs	7[3]

Recommended Dosage Schedule for Cefepime

Site and type of infection	Dose	Frequency	Duration (days)
Complicated intra-abdominal infections (used in combination with metronidazole) caused by *E. coli,* viridans group streptococci, *P. aeruginosa, K. pneumoniae, Enterobacter* species, or *B. fragilis.*	2 g IV	q 12 hrs	7 to 10

[1] Including cases associated with concurrent bacteremia.
[2] IM route of administration is indicated only for mild-to-moderate, uncomplicated, or complicated UTIs caused by *E. coli* when the IM route is a more appropriate route of drug administration.
[3] Or until resolution of neutropenia. In patients whose fever resolves but who remain neutropenic for > 7 days, the need for continued antimicrobial therapy should be reevaluated frequently.

►*Renal function impairment:* In patients with impaired renal function (creatinine clearance ≤ 60 ml/min), adjust the dose of cefepime to compensate for the slower rate of renal elimination. The recommended initial dose should be the same as in patients with normal renal function.

In patients undergoing hemodialysis, ≈ 68% of the total amount of cefepime present in the body at the start of dialysis will be removed during a 3-hour dialysis period. A repeat dose, equivalent to the initial dose, should be given at the completion of each dialysis session.

In elderly patients, adjust dosage and administration in the presence of renal insufficiency.

In patients undergoing continuous ambulatory peritoneal dialysis, administer cefepime at normal recommended doses at a dosage interval of every 48 hours.

Recommended Cefepime Maintenance Schedule in Patients with Renal Impairment

Creatinine clearance (ml/min)	Recommended maintenance schedule			
> 60	500 mg q 12 hrs[1]	1 g q 12 hrs	2 g q 12 hrs	2 g q 8 hrs
30 to 60	500 mg q 24 hrs	1 g q 24 hrs	2 g q 24 hrs	2 g q 12 hrs
11 to 29	500 mg q 24 hrs	500 mg q 24 hrs	1 g q 24 hrs	2 g q 24 hrs
< 11	250 mg q 24 hrs	250 mg q 24 hrs	500 mg q 24 hrs	1 g q 24 hrs

[1] Normal recommended dosing schedule.

When only serum creatinine is available, the following formula may be used to estimate creatinine clearance. The serum creatinine should represent steady state of renal function:

$$\text{Males:} \quad \frac{\text{Weight (kg)} \times (140 - \text{age})}{72 \times \text{serum creatinine (mg/dL)}} = \text{Ccr}$$

Females: 0.85 × above value

►*IV administration:* Administer over ≈ 30 minutes. Reconstitute with 50 or 100 ml of a compatible IV fluid. Cefepime is compatible at concentrations of 1 to 40 mg/ml with 0.9% Sodium Chloride Injection, 5% and 10% Dextrose Injection, M/6 Sodium Lactate Injection, 5% Dextrose and 0.9% Sodium Chloride Injection, Lactated Ringers and 5% Dextrose Injection, *Normosol-R* or *Normosol-M* in 5% Dextrose injection.

Cefepime Admixture Stability

Cefepime concentration (mg/ml)	Admixture and concentration	IV Infusion solutions	Stability time for RT/L[1] (20° to 25°C) (hours)	Stability time for refrigeration (2° to 8°C)
40	Amikacin 6 mg/ml	NS[2] or D5W[3]	24	7 days
40	Ampicillin 1 mg/ml	D5W[3]	8	8 hours
40	Ampicillin 10 mg/ml	D5W[3]	2	8 hours
40	Ampicillin 1 mg/ml	NS[2]	24	48 hours
40	Ampicillin 10 mg/ml	NS[2]	8	48 hours
4	Ampicillin 40 mg/ml	NS[2]	8	8 hours
4 to 40	Clindamycin phosphate 0.25 to 6 mg/ml	NS[2] or D5W[3]	24	7 days
4	Heparin 10 to 50 units/ml	NS[2] or D5W[3]	24	7 days
4	Potassium chloride 10 to 40 mEq/L	NS[2] or D5W[3]	24	7 days
4	Theophylline 0.8 mg/ml	D5W[3]	24	7 days

CEFEPIME HCl

Cefepime Admixture Stability				
Cefepime concentration (mg/ml)	Admixture and concentration	IV Infusion solutions	Stability time for RT/L[1] (20° to 25°C) (hours)	Stability time for refrigeration (2° to 8°C)
1 to 4	na	*Aminosyn II* 4.25% with electrolytes and calcium	8	3 days
0.125 to 0.25	na	*Inpersol* with 4.25% dextrose	24	7 days

[1] Ambient room temperature and light.
[2] 0.9% sodium chloride injection.
[3] 5% dextrose injection.

Admixture compatibility/incompatibility – Intermittent IV infusion with a Y-type administration set can be accomplished with compatible solutions; however, during infusion of a solution containing cefepime, it is desirable to discontinue the other solution.

Solutions of cefepime, like those of most β-lactam antibiotics, should not be added to solutions of ampicillin at a concentration > 40 mg/ml, and should not be added to metronidazole, vancomycin, gentamicin, tobramycin, netilmicin sulfate, or aminophylline because of potential interaction. However, if concurrent therapy with cefepime is indicated, each of these antibiotics can be administered separately.

➤*IM administration:* Reconstitute cefepime with the following diluents: Sterile Water for Injection, 0.9% Sodium Chloride, 5% Dextrose Injection, 0.5% or 1% lidocaine HCl, or Sterile Bacteriostatic Water for Injection with parabens or benzyl alcohol.

➤*Pediatric dosing:* The usual recommended daily dosage in pediatric patients up to 40 kg in weight is 50 mg/kg/dose administered every 12 hours (every 8 hours for febrile neutropenic patients), for 7 to 10 days, depending on the indication and severity of infection. The maximum dose for pediatric patients (2 months to 16 years of age) should not exceed the recommended adult dose.

Renal impairment – Data in pediatric patients with impaired renal function are not available; however, because cefepime pharmacokinetics are similar in adult and pediatric patients, changes in dosing regimen similar to those in adults are recommended for pediatric patients.

➤*Storage/Stability:* Store reconstituted solutions at controlled room temperature 20° to 25°C (68° to 77°F) for 24 hours or store in the refrigerator at 2° to 8°C (36° to 46°F) for 7 days. Store cefepime in the dry state between 2° and 25°C (36° and 77°F). Protect from light.

CEFDITOREN PIVOXIL

Rx **Spectracef** (Purdue) **Tablets:** 200 mg cefditoren (as cefditoren pivoxil) Mannitol. (TAP 200 mg). White, elliptical. Film-coated. In 20s and 60s.

For complete prescribing information, refer to the Cephalosporins group monograph.

Indications

For the treatment of mild-to-moderate infections in adults and adolescents (≥ 12 years of age) that are caused by susceptible strains of the designated microorganisms in the conditions listed below.

➤*Acute bacterial exacerbation of chronic bronchitis:* Acute bacterial exacerbation of chronic bronchitis caused by *Haemophilus influenzae* (including β-lactamase-producing strains), *Haemophilus parainfluenzae* (including β-lactamase-producing strains), *Streptococcus pneumoniae* (penicillin-susceptible strains only), or *Moraxella catarrhalis* (including β-lactamase-producing strains).

➤*Pharyngitis/Tonsillitis:* Pharyngitis/tonsillitis caused by *S. pyogenes.* Cefditoren is effective in the eradication of *S. pyogenes* from the oropharynx. Cefditoren has not been studied for the prevention of rheumatic fever following *S. pyogenes* pharyngitis/tonsillitis. Only IM penicillin has been demonstrated to be effective for the prevention of rheumatic fever.

➤*Uncomplicated skin and skin structure infections:* Uncomplicated skin and skin structure infections caused by *Staphylococcus aureus* (including β-lactamase-producing strains) or *S. pyogenes.*

Administration and Dosage

➤*Approved by the FDA:* August 29, 2001.

Cefditoren Dosage and Administration in Adults and Adolescents ≥ 12 Years of Age[1]		
Type of infection	Dosage	Duration (days)
Acute bacterial exacerbation of chronic bronchitis	400 mg BID	
Pharyngitis/Tonsillitis	200 mg BID	10
Uncomplicated skin and skin structure infections		

[1] Take with meals.

➤*Renal impairment:* No dose adjustment is necessary for patients with mild renal impairment (Ccr 50 to 80 mL/min/1.73 m^2). It is recommended that ≤ 200 mg twice daily be administered to patients with moderate renal impairment (Ccr 30 to 49 mL/min/1.73 m^2) and 200 mg every day be administered to patients with severe renal impairment (Ccr < 30 mL/min/1.73 m^2). The appropriate dose in patients with end-stage renal disease has not been determined.

➤*Storage/Stability:* Store at 25°C (77°F); excursions permitted to 15° to 30°C (59° to 86°F). Protect from light and moisture. Dispense in a tight, light-resistant container.

Contraindications

Known allergy to the cephalosporin class of antibiotics or any of its components.

Cefditoren is contraindicated in patients with carnitine deficiency or inborn errors of metabolism that may result in clinically significant carnitine deficiency because use of cefditoren causes renal excretion of carnitine.

Cefditoren contains sodium caseinate, a milk protein. Do not administer cefditoren to patients with milk protein hypersensitivity (not lactose intolerance).

Drug Interactions

➤*Antacids:* It is not recommended that cefditoren be taken concomitantly with antacids.

➤*H$_2$-receptor antagonists:* It is not recommended that cefditoren be taken concomitantly with H$_2$-receptor antagonists.

MEROPENEM

Rx	Merrem IV (Zeneca)	Powder for Injection: 500 mg	In 20 and 100 ml vials and 15 ml *ADD-Vantage* vials.
		1 g	In 30 and 100 ml vials and 15 ml *ADD-Vantage* vials.

Indications

For the treatment of the following infections when caused by susceptible strains of the designated microorganisms:

➤*Intra-abdominal infections:* Complicated appendicitis and peritonitis caused by viridans group streptococci, *E. coli, K. pneumoniae, P. aeruginosa, B. fragilis, B. thetaiotaomicron* and *Peptostreptococcus* sp.

➤*Bacterial meningitis (pediatric patients ≥ 3 months only):* Bacterial meningitis caused by *S. pneumoniae, H. influenzae* (β- lactamase and non-β-lactamase-producing strains) and *N. meningitidis.*

Administration and Dosage

➤*Approved by the FDA:* June 2, 1996.

➤*Adults:* 1 g by IV administration every 8 hours. Give over ≈ 15 to 30 minutes or as an IV bolus injection (5 to 20 ml) over ≈ 3 to 5 minutes.

➤*Renal function impairment:* Reduce dosage in patients with creatinine clearance < 50 ml/min.

Recommended Meropenem IV Dosage Schedule for Adults with Impaired Renal Function

Creatinine clearance (ml/min)	Dose (dependent on type of infection)	Dosing interval
26 to 50	recommended dose (1000 mg)	every 12 hours
10 to 25	one-half recommended dose	every 12 hours
< 10	one-half recommended dose	every 24 hours

When only serum creatinine is available, the following formula (Cockcroft and Gault equation) may be used to estimate creatinine clearance.

$$\text{Males:} \quad \frac{\text{Weight (kg)} \times (140 - \text{age})}{72 \times \text{serum creatinine (mg/dL)}} = \text{Ccr}$$

Females: 0.85 × above value

➤*Use in pediatric patients:* For pediatric patients from ≥ 3 months of age, the meropenem dose is 20 or 40 mg/kg every 8 hours (maximum dose is 2 g every 8 hours), depending on the type of infection (intra-abdominal or meningitis). Administer pediatric patients weighing > 50 kg 1 g every 8 hours for intra-abdominal infections and 2 g every 8 hours for meningitis. Give over ≈ 15 to 30 minutes or as an IV bolus injection (5 to 20 ml) over ≈ 3 to 5 minutes.

Recommended Meropenem IV Dosage Schedule for Pediatrics with Normal Renal Function

Type of infection	Dose (mg/kg)	Dosing interval
Intra-abdominal	20	every 8 hours
Meningitis	40	every 8 hours

➤*Storage / Stability:*

Admixture compatibility / stability – Do not mix with solutions containing other drugs.

Stability of Solutions of Meropenem for Infusion

Solution	Number of hours stable at controlled room temperature 15° to 25°C (59° to 77°F)	Number of hours stable at 4°C (39°F)
0.9% Sodium Chloride Injection	4	24
5% Dextrose Injection	1	4
10% Dextrose Injection	1	2
5% Dextrose and 0.9% Sodium Chloride Injection	1	2
5% Dextrose and 0.2% Sodium Chloride Injection	1	4
0.15% Potassium Chloride in 5% Dextrose Injection	1	6
0.02% Sodium Bicarbonate in 5% Dextrose Injection	1	6
5% Dextrose Injection in *Normosol-M*	1	8
5% Dextrose Injection in Ringers Lactate Injection	1	4
2.5% Dextrose and 0.45% Sodium Chloride Injection	3	12
2.5% Mannitol Injection	2	16
Ringers Injection	4	24
Ringers Lactate Injection	4	12
Sodium Lactate Injection 1/6 N	2	24
5% Sodium Bicarbonate Injection	1	4
Sterile Water for Injection	2	12

Store at controlled room temperature (20° to 25°C [68° to 77°F]).

Actions

➤*Pharmacology:* Meropenem is a broad-spectrum carbapenem antibiotic. The bactericidal activity of meropenem results from the inhibition of cell-wall synthesis. Meropenem readily penetrates the cell wall of most gram-positive and gram-negative bacteria to reach penicillin-binding-protein (PBP) targets.

➤*Pharmacokinetics:* Meropenem has dose-dependent kinetics. At the end of a 30-minute IV infusion of a single dose of meropenem in normal volunteers, mean peak plasma concentrations are ≈ 23 mcg/ml (range: 14 to 26 mcg/ml) for the 500 mg dose and 49 mcg/ml (range: 39 to 68 mcg/ml) for the 1 g dose. A 5-minute IV bolus injection of meropenem in normal volunteers results in mean peak plasma concentrations of ≈ 45 mcg/ml (range: 18 to 65 mcg/ml) for the 500 mg dose and 112 mcg/ml (range: 83 to 140 mcg/ml) for the 1 g dose.

Following IV doses of 500 mg, mean plasma concentrations of meropenem usually decline to ≈ 1 mcg/ml at 6 hours after administration.

In subjects with normal renal function, the elimination half-life of meropenem is ≈ 1 hour. Meropenem is excreted by the kidney with a half-life of 0.8 to 1.24 hours; 65% to 83% of the dose is recovered in the urine as meropenem and 20% to 28% as the inactive open β-lactam metabolite. Urinary concentrations of meropenem > 10 mcg/ml are maintained for ≤ 5 hours after a 500 mg dose. No meropenem accumulation in plasma or urine was observed with regimens using 500 mg administered every 8 hours or 1 g administered every 6 hours in volunteers with normal renal function.

Plasma protein binding of meropenem is ≈ 2%. There is one metabolite that is microbiologically inactive. The volume of meropenem distribution is 15.7 to 26.68 L. Meropenem penetrates well into most body fluids and tissues, including cerebrospinal fluid, achieving concentrations matching or exceeding those required to inhibit most susceptible bacteria. After a single IV dose of meropenem, the highest mean meropenem concentrations were found in tissues and fluids at 1 hour (0.5 to 1.5 hours) after the start of infusion, except where indicated in the tissues and fluids listed in the table below.

Meropenem Concentrations in Selected Tissues (Highest Concentrations Reported)

Tissue	IV dose (g)	Mean [mcg/ml or mcg/g][1]	Range [mcg/ml or mcg/g]
Endometrium	0.5	4.2	1.7-10.2
Myometrium	0.5	3.8	0.4-8.1
Ovary	0.5	2.8	0.8-4.8
Cervix	0.5	7	5.4-8.5
Fallopian tube	0.5	1.7	0.3-3.4
Skin	0.5, 1	3.3, 5.3	0.5-12.6, 1.3-16.7
Colon	1	2.6	2.5-2.7
Bile	1	14.6 (3 h)	4-25.7
Gall bladder	1	-	3.9
Interstitial fluid	1	26.3	20.9-37.4
Peritoneal fluid	1	30.2	7.4-54.6
Lung	1	4.8 (2 h)	1.4-8.2
Bronchial mucosa	1	4.5	1.3-11.1
Muscle	1	6.1 (2 h)	5.3-6.9
Fascia	1	8.8	1.5-20
Heart valves	1	9.7	6.4-12.1
Myocardium	1	15.5	5.2-25.5
CSF (inflamed)	20 mg/kg[2] 40 mg/kg[3]	1.1 (2 h) 3.3 (3 h)	0.2-2.8 0.9-6.5
CSF (uninflamed)		0.2 (2 h)	0.1-0.3

[1] At 1 hour unless otherwise noted.
[2] In pediatric patients 5 months to 8 years of age.
[3] In pediatric patients 1 month to 15 years of age.

The pharmacokinetics of meropenem in pediatric patients ≥ 2 years of age are essentially similar to those in adults. In children 6 months to 12 years of age, meropenem 10 mg/kg IV produced a mean peak concentration of 28.7 mg/L, and 20 mg/kg IV produced a mean peak concentration of 60.2 mg/L. The half-life was 1 to 1.11 hours and volume of distribution was 0.4 to 0.5 L/kg. Urinary recovery of meropenem averaged 65% of the administered dose. Compared with adults, volume of distribution and clearance were increased, while half-life and amount eliminated unchanged in the urine were similar. In infants and children ages 2 months to 12 years administered meropenem 10 to 40 mg/kg in a pharmacokinetic study, no age- or dose-dependent effects on pharmacokinetic parameters were observed. Mean half-life was 1.13 hours, mean volume of distribution at steady-state was 0.43 L/kg, mean residence time was 1.57 hours, clearance was 5.63 ml/min/kg and renal clearance was 2.53 ml/min/kg. Approximately 55% of the administered dose was recovered in the urine unchanged 12 hours after administration. The elimination half-life is slightly prolonged (1.5 hours) in pediatric patients 3 months to 2 years of age.

MEROPENEM

Pharmacokinetic studies with meropenem in patients with renal insufficiency have shown that the plasma clearance of meropenem correlates with creatinine clearance. In patients with moderate renal dysfunction (Ccr 30 to 80 ml/min), mean half-life has been prolonged to 1.93 to 3.36 hours. In patients with greater dysfunction (Ccr 2 to 30 mg/min), mean half-life has been further prolonged to 3.82 to 5.73 hours. Patients undergoing hemodialysis (patients with end-stage renal disease) had mean predialysis half-lives of 7 to 10 hours. Hemodialysis shortened elimination half-life to 1.4 to 2.9 hours during the dialysis period. Dosage adjustments are necessary in subjects with renal impairment (see Adminstration and Dosage). A pharmacokinetic study with meropenem in elderly patients with renal insufficiency has shown a reduction in plasma clearance of meropenem that correlates with age-associated reduction in creatinine clearance. The mean terminal half-life is prolonged slightly to 1.27 hours. A pharmacokinetic study with meropenem in patients with hepatic impairment has shown that there are no effects of liver disease on the pharmacokinetics of meropenem.

➤*Microbiology:* Its strongest affinities are toward PBP 2, 3 and 4 of *Escherichia coli* and *Pseudomonas aeruginosa*; and PBPs 1, 2 and 4 of *Staphylococcus aureus*. Bactericidal concentrations (defined as a 3 $\log_{10}$ reduction in cell counts within 12 to 24 hours) are typically 1 to 2 times the bacteriostatic concentrations of meropenem, with the exception of *Listeria monocytogenes*, against which lethal activity is not observed.

Meropenem has significant stability to hydrolysis by β-lactamases of most categories, both penicillinases and cephalosporinases produced by gram-positive and gram-negative bacteria, with the exception of matallo-β-lactamases. Do not use to treat methicillin-resistant staphylococci. Cross resistance is sometimes observed with strains resistant to other carbapenems. In vitro tests show meropenem to act synergistically with aminoglycoside antibiotics against some isolates of *P. aeruginosa*.

Meropenem has been shown to be active against most strains of the following microorganisms, both in vitro and in clinical infections as described in the Indications section.

Gram-positive aerobes – *Streptococcus pneumoniae* (excluding penicillin-resistant strains); Viridans group streptococci. Note: Penicillin-resistant strains had meropenem MIC_{90} values of 1 or 2 mcg/ml; this value is above the 0.12 mcg/ml susceptible breakpoint for this species.

Gram-negative aerobes – *E. coli*; *Haemophilus influenzae* (β-lactamase and non-β-lactamase-producing); *Klebsiella pneumoniae*; *Neisseria meningitidis*; *P. aeruginosa*.

Anaerobes – *Bacteroides fragilis*; *B. thetaiotaomicron*; *Peptostreptococcus* sp.

The following in vitro data are available, but their clinical significance is unknown.

Meropenem exhibits in vitro minimum inhibitory concentrations (MICs) of 0.12 mcg/ml against most (≥ 90%) strains of *S. pneumoniae*, ≤ 0.5 mcg/ml against most (≥ 90%) strains of *H. influenzae* and ≤ 4 mcg/ml against most (≥ 90%) strains of the other microorganisms in the following list; however, the safety and effectiveness of meropenem in treating clinical infections due to these microorganisms have not been established in adequate and well controlled clinical trials.

Gram-positive aerobes – *S. aureus* (β-lactamase and non-β-lactamase producing); *S. epidermidis* (β-lactamase and non-β-lactamase producing). Note: Staphylococci that are resistant to methicillin/oxacillin must be considered resistant to meropenem.

Gram-negative aerobes – *Acinetobacter* sp.; *Aeromonas hydrophila*; *Campylobacter jejuni*; *Citrobacter diversus*; *Citrobacter freundii*; *Enterobacter cloacae*; *H. influenzae* (ampicillin-restant, non-β-lactamase producing strains [BLNAR strains]); *Hafnia alvei*; *K. oxytoca*; *Moraxella catarrhalis* (β-lactamase and non-β-lactamase producing strains); *Morganella morganii*; *Pasteurelia multocida*; *Proteus mirabilis*; *P. vulgaris*; *Salmonella* sp.; *Serratia marcescens*; *Shigella* sp.; *Yersinia enterocolitica*.

Anaerobes – *Bacteroides distasonis*; *B. ovatus*; *B. uniformis*; *B. ureolyticus*; *B. vulgatus*; *Clostridium difficile*; *C. perfringens*; *Eubacterium lentum*; *Fusobacterium* sp.; *Prevotella bivia*; *Prevotella intermedia*; *Prevotella melaninogenica*; *Prophyromonas asaccharolytica*; *Propionibacterium acnes*.

➤*Clinical trials:*

Intra-abdominal infection – Meropenem was compared with imipenem/cilastatin in the treatment of intra-abdominal infection requiring surgery. Patients with diffuse or local peritonitis of moderate severity, complicated in most cases by gangrenous appendicitis, stomach perforation or gallbladder disease, were treated with either meropenem or imipenem/cilastatin. Both agents were administered IV at a dosage of 1 g every 8 hours. Therapy was continued for a mean of 7.7 days in the meropenem group and 8.6 days in the imipenem/cilastatin group. Surgical excision and drainage was performed on the first day of therapy or before the start of this antibiotic regimen. Therapy was judged successful in all patients evaluated in both groups. No cases of post-operative wound infection or superinfection at other sites were observed.

Meningitis – Meropenem 40 mg/kg every 8 hours was compared with cefotaxime 75 to 100 mg/kg every 8 hours in 190 children aged 3 months to 14 years with bacterial meningitis. Concurrent dexamethasone was administered to 185 patients. Among patients with no preexisting neurological abnormalities prior to antimicrobial therapy, cure without audiological or neurological sequelae occurred in 79% of meropenem-treated patients and 83% of cefotaxime-treated patients. Among patients with preexisting neurological abnormalities, cure without audiological or neurological sequelae occurred in 47% of the meropenem-treated patients and 60% of the cefotaxime-treated patients. At the end of therapy, among patients without middle ear effusion, hearing impairment was evident in 33% of meropenem-treated patients and 28% of cefotaxime-treated patients. The severity of impairment was similar in the two groups. Bacterial eradication among patients with culture-proven meningitis was 100% in both groups.

Contraindications

Hypersensitivity to any component of this product or to other drugs in the same class or in patients who have demonstrated anaphylactic reactions to β-lactams.

Warnings

➤*Pseudomembranous colitis:* This has been reported with nearly all antibacterial agents, including meropenem and may range in severity from mild to life-threatening. Therefore, it is important to consider this diagnosis in patients who develop diarrhea subsequent to the administration of antibacterial agents.

After the diagnosis of pseudomembranous colitis has been established, initiate appropriate therapeutic measures. Mild cases of pseudomembranous colitis usually respond to drug discontinuation alone. In moderate-to-severe cases, give consideration to management with fluids and electrolytes, protein supplementation and treatment with an antibacterial drug clinically effective against *C. difficile* colitis.

➤*Hypersensitivity reactions:* Serious and occasionally fatal hypersensitivity (anaphylactic) reactions have been reported in patients receiving therapy with β-lactams. These reactions are more likely to occur in individuals with a history of sensitivity to multiple allergens.

There have been reports of individuals with a history of penicillin hypersensitivity who have experienced severe hypersensitivity reactions when treated with other β-lactams. If an allergic reaction to meropenem occurs, discontinue the drug immediately. Serious anaphylactic reactions require immediate emergency treatment with epinephrine, oxygen, intravenous steroids and airway management, including intubation. Other therapy may also be administered as indicated. Refer to Management of Acute Hypersensitivity Reactions.

➤*Renal function impairment:* In patients with renal dysfunction, thrombocytopenia has been observed but no clinical bleeding was reported. (See Administration and Dosage.)

➤*Pregnancy:* Category B. Reproductive studies have been performed with meropenem in rats at doses of ≤ 1000 mg/kg/day, and cynomolgus monkeys at doses of ≤ 360 mg/kg/day. These studies revealed no evidence of impaired fertility or harm to the fetus because of meropenem, although there were slight changes in body weight. However, there are no adequate and well controlled studies in pregnant women. Because animal reproduction studies are not always predictive of human response, use this drug during pregnancy only if clearly needed.

➤*Lactation:* It is not known whether this drug is excreted in breast milk. Because many drugs are excreted in breast milk, use caution when administering to a nursing woman.

➤*Children:* The safety and efficacy of meropenem have not been established for children < 3 months of age (see Administration and Dosage).

Precautions

➤*Monitoring:* While meropenem possesses the characteristic low toxicity of the β-lactam group of antibiotics, periodic assessment of organ system functions, including renal, hepatic and hematopoietic is advisable during prolonged therapy.

➤*Seizures:* This and other CNS adverse experiences have been reported during treatment with meropenem. These adverse experiences have occurred most commonly in patients with CNS disorders (eg, brain lesions or history of seizures) or with bacterial meningitis or compromised renal function.

➤*Superinfection:* As with other broad-spectrum antibiotics, prolonged use of meropenem may result in overgrowth of nonsusceptible organisms. Repeated evaluation of the patient is essential. If superinfection does occur during therapy, take appropriate measures.

Drug Interactions

➤*Probenicid:* This competes with meropenem for active tubular secretion and thus inhibits the renal excretion of meropenem. This led to statistically significant increases in the elimination half-life (38%) and in the extent of systemic exposure (56%). Therefore, the coadministration of probenecid with meropenem is not recommended.

MEROPENEM

Adverse Reactions

➤*Cardiovascular:* Heart failure, heart arrest, tachycardia, hypertension, myocardial infarction, pulmonary embolus, bradycardia, hypotension, syncope (< 1%).

➤*CNS:* Insomnia, agitation/delirium, confusion, dizziness, nervousness, paresthesia, hallucinations, somnolence, anxiety, depression (< 1%); seizures (0.5%).

➤*Dermatologic:* Urticaria, sweating (< 1%).

➤*GI:* Oral moniliasis, anorexia, cholestatic jaundice/jaundice, flatulence, ileus (< 1%).

➤*GU:* Dysuria, kidney failure, presence of urine red blood cells (< 1%).

➤*Hematologic:* Increased platelets, increased eosinophils, prolonged prothrombin time, prolonged partial thromboplastin time, decreased platelets, positive direct or indirect Coombs test, decreased hemoglobin, decreased hematocrit, decreased WBC, shortened prothrombin time, shortened partial thromboplastin time, anemia (< 1%).

➤*Hepatic:* Increased ALT, AST, alkaline phosphatase, LDH and bilirubin (< 1%).

➤*Local:* Inflammation at the injection site (3%); phlebitis/thrombophlebitis (1.2%); injection site reaction (1.1%); pain at the injection site (0.4%); edema at the injection site (0.2%).

➤*Metabolic / Nutritional:* Peripheral edema, hypoxia (< 1%).

➤*Renal:* Increased creatinine and BUN (< 1%).

➤*Respiratory:* Respiratory disorder, dyspnea (< 1%).

➤*Systemic:* Diarrhea (5%); nausea, vomiting (3.9%); headache (2.8%); rash (1.7%); pruritus (1.6%); apnea (1.2%); constipation (1.2%); bleeding events (GI hemorrhage, melena, epistaxis, hemoperitoneum) (0.7%).

➤*Miscellaneous:* Pain, abdominal pain, chest pain, sepsis, shock, fever, abdominal enlargement, back pain, hepatic failure (< 1%).

Children –

  Bacterial infection: Diarrhea (4.3%); rash (1.4%); vomiting (1%).

  Meningitis: Rash (mostly diaper area moniliasis), diarrhea (3.5%); oral moniliasis (2%); glossitis (1%).

  Laboratory abnormalities: Those seen in pediatric-aged patients are similar to those reported in adult patients.

Overdosage

Overdosing might occur if large doses are given to patients with reduced renal function. The largest dose of meropenem administered in clinical trials has been 2 g given IV every 8 hours. At this dosage, no adverse pharmacological effects or increased safety risks have been observed. In the event of an overdose, discontinue meropenem and give general supportive treatment until renal elimination takes place. Meropenem and its metabolite are readily dialyzable and effectively removed by hemodialysis.

IMIPENEM-CILASTATIN

Rx	Primaxin I.V. (Merck)	**Powder for Injection**: 250 mg imipenem equivalent and 250 mg cilastatin equivalent. Contains 0.8 mEq sodium.	In vials, infusion bottles, and *ADD-Vantage* vials.
		500 mg imipenem equivalent and 500 mg cilastatin equivalent. Contains 1.6 mEq sodium.	In vials, infusion bottles, and *ADD-Vantage* vials.
Rx	Primaxin I.M. (Merck)	**Powder for Injection**: 500 mg imipenem equivalent and 500 mg cilastatin equivalent. Contains 1.4 mEq sodium.	In vials.
		750 mg imipenem equivalent and 750 mg cilastatin equivalent. Contains 2.1 mEq sodium.	In vials.

Indications

➤*IV:* Treatment of serious infections caused by susceptible strains of the designated microorganisms in the conditions listed below:

Lower respiratory tract infections – Staphylococcus aureus (penicillinase-producing), *Escherichia coli, Klebsiella* sp., *Enterobacter* sp., *Haemophilus influenzae, Haemophilus parainfluenzae, Acinetobacter* sp., *Serratia marcescens.*

Urinary tract infections (complicated and uncomplicated) – Enterococcus faecalis, S. aureus (penicillinase-producing), E. coli, Klebsiella sp., Enterobacter sp., Proteus vulgaris, Providencia rettgeri, M. morganii, P. aeruginosa.

Intra-abdominal infections – E. faecalis, S. aureus (penicillinase-producing), Staphylococcus epidermidis, E. coli, Klebsiella sp., Enterobacter sp., Proteus sp., Morganella morganii, P. aeruginosa, Citrobacter sp., Clostridium sp., Bacteroides sp. including B. fragilis, Fusobacterium sp., Peptococcus sp., Peptostreptococcus sp., Eubacterium sp., Propionibacterium sp., Bifidobacterium sp.

Gynecologic infections – E. faecalis; S. aureus (penicillinase-producing), S. epidermidis, Streptococcus agalactiae (group B streptococcus), E. coli , Klebsiella sp., Proteus sp., Enterobacter sp., Bifidobacterium sp., Bacteroides sp. including B. fragilis, Gardnerella vaginalis; Peptococcus sp., Peptostreptococcus sp., Propionibacterium sp.

Bacterial septicemia – E. faecalis, S. aureus (penicillinase-producing), E. coli, Klebsiella sp., P. aeruginosa, Serratia sp., Enterobacter sp., Bacteroides sp.

Bone and joint infections – E. faecalis; S. aureus (penicillinase-producing), S. epidermidis, Enterobacter sp., P. aeruginosa.

Skin and skin structure infections – E. faecalis, S. aureus (penicillinase-producing), S. epidermidis, E. coli, Klebsiella sp., Enterobacter sp., P. vulgaris, P. rettgeri, M. morganii, P. aeruginosa, Serratia sp., Citrobacter sp., Acinetobacter sp., Bacteroides sp., Fusobacterium sp., Peptococcus sp., Peptostreptococcus sp.

Endocarditis – S. aureus (penicillinase-producing).

Polymicrobic infections – Including those in which S. pneumoniae (pneumonia, septicemia), S. pyogenes (skin and skin structure) or non-penicillinase-producing S. aureus is one of the causative organisms. However, these monobacterial infections are usually treated with narrower spectrum antibiotics (eg, penicillin G). Although clinical improvement has been observed in patients with cystic fibrosis, chronic pulmonary disease, and lower respiratory tract infections caused by P. aeruginosa, bacterial eradication may not be achieved.

➤*IM:* Treatment of serious infections of mild-to-moderate severity where IM therapy is appropriate. Not intended for severe or life-threatening infections, including bacterial sepsis or endocarditis, or in major physiological impairments (eg, shock).

Lower respiratory tract infections – Including pneumonia and bronchitis as an exacerbation of COPD that are caused by S. pneumoniae and H. influenzae.

Intra-abdominal infections – Including acute gangrenous or perforated appendicitis and appendicitis with peritonitis that are caused by group D streptococcus including E. faecalis; Streptococcus (viridans group); E. coli; Klebsiella pneumoniae; P. aeruginosa; Bacteroides sp. including B. fragilis, B. distasonis, B. intermedius, and B. thetaiotaomicron; Fusobacterium sp; Peptostreptococcus sp.

Skin and skin structure infections – Including abscesses, cellulitis, infected skin ulcers, and wound infections caused by S. aureus (including penicillinase-producing strains); Streptococcus pyogenes; group D streptococcus including E. faecalis; Acinetobacter sp. including A. calcoaceticus; Citrobacter sp; E. coli; Enterobacter cloacae; K. pneumoniae; P. aeruginosa; Bacteroides sp. including B. fragilis.

Gynecologic infections – Including postpartum endomyometritis that are caused by group D streptococcus such as E. faecalis; E. coli; K. pneumoniae; B. intermedius; Peptostreptococcus sp.

Infections resistant to other antibiotics (eg, cephalosporins, penicillins, aminoglycosides) have responded to treatment with imipenem.

Administration and Dosage

Dosage recommendations represent the quantity of imipenem to be administered. An equivalent amount of cilastatin is also present in the solution.

Base the initial dosage on the type or severity of infection and administer in equally divided doses. Base subsequent dosing on severity of illness, degree of susceptibility of the pathogen(s), renal function, weight, and creatinine clearance.

➤*IV:* Give a 125, 250, or 500 mg dose by IV infusion over 20 to 30 min. Infuse a 750 mg or 1 g dose over 40 to 60 min. If nausea develops, slow the infusion rate.

Because of high antimicrobial activity, do not exceed 50 mg/kg/day or 4 g/day, whichever is lower. There is no evidence that higher doses provide greater efficacy.

Imipenem-Cilastatin IV Dosing Schedule for Adults with Normal Renal Function				
Type or severity of infection	Fully susceptible organisms[1]	Total daily dose	Moderately susceptible organisms, primarily some strains of P. aeruginosa	Total daily dose
Mild	250 mg q 6 hr	1 g	500 mg q 6 hr	2 g
Moderate	500 mg q 8 hr or 500 mg q 6 hr	1.5 or 2 g	500 mg q 6 hr or 1 g q 8 hr	2 or 3 g
Severe, life-threatening	500 mg q 6 hr	2 g	1 g q 8 hr or 1 g q 6 hr	3 or 4 g
Uncomplicated UTI	250 mg q 6 hr	1 g	250 mg q 6 hr	1 g
Complicated UTI	500 mg q 6 hr	2 g	500 mg q 6 hr	2 g

[1] Including gram-positive and -negative aerobes and anaerobes

IMIPENEM-CILASTATIN

Renal function impairment or body weight < 70 kg – Patients with creatinine clearance (Ccr) ≤ 70 ml/min/1.73 m² for IV require dosage adjustment (see table). Safety and efficacy of patients with Ccr < 20 ml/min/1.73 m² (for IM administration) have not been studied.

Serum creatinine alone may not be a sufficiently accurate measure of renal function. Ccr may be estimated from the following equation:

$$\text{Males:} \quad \frac{\text{Weight (kg)} \times (140 - \text{age})}{72 \times \text{serum creatinine (mg/dL)}} = \text{Ccr}$$

Females: 0.85 × above value

From the IV Dosing Schedule for Adults with Normal Renal Function table, determine a total daily dose based on type of infection and organism. Then, using the table below, find the appropriate reduced dosing schedule according to the patient's weight and Ccr.

Reduced IV Dosage in Adult Patients with Impaired Renal Function or Body Weight < 70 kg

Body weight / Ccr (ml/min/1.73 m²)	≥ 70 kg	60 kg	50 kg	40 kg	30 kg
If total daily dose for normal renal function is 1 g/day, use:					
≥ 71	250 q 6 hr	250 q 8 hr	125 q 6 hr	125 q 6 hr	125 q 8 hr
41-70	250 q 8 hr	125 q 6 hr	125 q 6 hr	125 q 8 hr	125 q 8 hr
21-40	250 q 12 hr	250 q 12 hr	125 q 8 hr	125 q 8 hr	125 q 12 hr
6-20	250 q 12 hr	125 q 12 hr	125 q 12 hr	125 q 12 hr	125 q 12 hr
If total daily dose for normal renal function is 1.5 g/day, use:					
≥ 71	500 q 8 hr	250 q 6 hr	250 q 6 hr	250 q 8 hr	125 q 6 hr
41-70	250 q 6 hr	250 q 8 hr	250 q 8 hr	125 q 6 hr	125 q 8 hr
21-40	250 q 8 hr	250 q 8 hr	250 q 12 hr	125 q 8 hr	125 q 8 hr
6-20	250 q 12 hr	250 q 12 hr	250 q 12 hr	125 q 12 hr	125 q 12 hr
If total daily dose for normal renal function is 2 g/day, use:					
≥ 71	500 q 6 hr	500 q 8 hr	250 q 6 hr	250 q 6 hr	250 q 8 hr
41-70	500 q 8 hr	250 q 6 hr	250 q 6 hr	250 q 8 hr	125 q 6 hr
21-40	250 q 6 hr	250 q 8 hr	250 q 8 hr	250 q 12 hr	125 q 8 hr
6-20	250 q 12 hr	250 q 12 hr	250 q 12 hr	250 q 12 hr	125 q 12 hr
If total daily dose for normal renal function is 3 g/day, use:					
≥ 71	1000 q 8 hr	750 q 8 hr	500 q 6 hr	500 q 8 hr	250 q 6 hr
41-70	500 q 6 hr	500 q 8 hr	500 q 8 hr	250 q 6 hr	250 q 8 hr
21-40	500 q 8 hr	500 q 8 hr	250 q 6 hr	250 q 8 hr	250 q 8 hr
6-20	500 q 12 hr	500 q 12 hr	250 q 12 hr	250 q 12 hr	250 q 12 hr
If total daily dose for normal renal function is 4 g/day, use:					
≥ 71	1000 q 6 hr	1000 q 8 hr	750 q 8 hr	500 q 6 hr	500 q 8 hr
41-70	750 q 8 hr	750 q 8 hr	500 q 6 hr	500 q 8 hr	250 q 6 hr
21-40	500 q 6 hr	500 q 8 hr	500 q 8 hr	250 q 6 hr	250 q 8 hr
6-20	500 q 12 hr	500 q 12 hr	500 q 12 hr	250 q 12 hr	250 q 12 hr

Pediatric Dosing Guidelines (≥ 3 months old)

≥ 3 months old (non-CNS infections)
15 to 25 mg/kg/dose every 6 hours
Maximum daily dose for fully susceptible organisms is 2 g/day, and for infections with moderately susceptible organisms (primarily some strains of *P. aeruginosa*) is 4 g/day (based on adults studies).
Higher doses (≤ 90 mg/kg/day in older children) have been used in cystic fibrosis patients.

Pediatric Dosing Guidelines (≤ 3 months old)

≤ 3 months old (weighing ≥ 1500 g; non-CNS infections)
< 1 week old: 25 mg/kg every 12 hours
1 to 4 weeks old: 25 mg/kg every 8 hours
4 weeks to 3 months old: 25 mg/kg every 6 hours

Give doses ≤ 500 mg by IV infusion over 15 to 30 minutes. Give doses > 500 mg by IV infusion over 40 to 60 minutes.

Imipenem-cilastatin IV is not recommended in pediatric patients with CNS infections because of the risk of seizures and in pediatric patients < 30 kg with impaired renal function, as no data are available.

➤*IM:* Total daily IM dosages > 1500 mg/day are not recommended.

Duration of therapy depends on the type and severity of the infection. Generally, continue for ≥ 2 days after signs and symptoms of infection have resolved. Safety and efficacy of treatment > 14 days have not been established.

Administer by deep IM injection into a large muscle mass (such as the gluteal muscles or lateral part of the thigh) with a 21-gauge 2-inch needle. Aspiration is necessary to avoid inadvertent injection into a blood vessel.

Imipenem-Cilastatin IM Dosage Guidelines in Adults

Type/Location of infection	Severity	Dosage regimen
Lower respiratory tract Skin and skin structure Gynecologic	Mild/Moderate	500 or 750 mg q 12 hr depending on the severity of infection
Intra-abdominal	Mild/Moderate	750 mg q 12 hr

Children – In mild-to-moderate infections the recommended dose is 10 to 15 mg/kg every 6 hours.

Hemodialysis – Imipenem-cilastatin is cleared by hemodialysis. Administer after hemodialysis and at 12-hour intervals timed from the end of that dialysis session. For patients on hemodialysis, imipenem-cilastatin is recommended only when the benefits outweigh the potential risk of seizures. There is inadequate information to recommend usage for patients undergoing peritoneal dialysis. Carefully monitor dialysis patients, especially those with CNS diseases.

➤*Preparation of solution:*

IV – Reconstitute contents of infusion bottles with 100 ml diluent (see Compatibility).

IM – Prepare with 1% lidocaine HCl solution (without epinephrine). Prepare the 500 mg vial with 2 ml and the 750 mg vial with 3 ml lidocaine HCl.

➤*Compatibility:* Do not mix with or physically add to antibiotics. However, it may be administered concomitantly with other antibiotics (eg, aminoglycosides).

Diluents – Imipenem-cilastatin in infusion bottles and vials, reconstituted as directed with the following diluents, maintains satisfactory potency for 4 hours at room temperature and for 24 hours when refrigerated (5°C; 41°F): 0.9% Sodium Chloride Injection; 5% or 10% Dextrose Injection; 5% Dextrose and 0.9% Sodium Chloride Injection; 5% Dextrose Injection with 0.225% or 0.45% saline solution; 5% Dextrose Injection with 0.15% potassium chloride solution; Mannitol 5% and 10%. Do not freeze solutions.

IMIPENEM-CILASTATIN

➤*Storage / Stability:* Store dry powder at < 25°C (77°F).

Actions

➤*Pharmacology:* This product is a formulation of imipenem, a thienamycin antibiotic, and cilastatin sodium, the inhibitor of dehydropeptidase 1, which inactivates imipenem when it is administered alone. Cilastatin thereby increases urinary recovery of imipenem and decreases possible renal toxicity associated with excessive intracellular antibiotic accumulation. The bactericidal activity of imipenem results from the inhibition of cell wall synthesis with a high affinity for penicillin binding proteins (PBPs) 1A, 1B, 2, 4, 5, and 6 of *Escherichia coli* and 1A, 1B, 2, 4, and 5 of *Pseudomonas aeruginosa*. The lethal effect is related to binding to PBP 2 and PBP 1B.

➤*Pharmacokinetics:*

Absorption / Distribution –

IV: IV infusion over 20 minutes results in peak plasma levels of imipenem antimicrobial activity of 14 to 24 mcg/ml for the 250 mg dose, 21 to 58 mcg/ml for the 500 mg dose, and 41 to 83 mcg/ml for the 1 g dose. Plasma levels declined to ≤ 1 mcg/ml in 4 to 6 hours. Peak plasma levels of cilastatin following a 20-minute IV infusion range from 15 to 25 mcg/ml for the 250 mg dose, 31 to 49 mcg/ml for the 500 mg dose, and 56 to 88 mcg/ml for the 1 g dose.

The plasma half-life of each component is ≈ 1 hour. Protein binding is 20% for imipenem and 40% for cilastatin. Urine imipenem concentrations > 10 mcg/ml can be maintained for up to 8 hours at the 500 mg dose.

After a 1 g dose, the following average levels (mcg/ml or mcg/g) of imipenem were measured (usually 1 hour post-dose except where indicated) in the following tissues and fluids: Peritoneal 23.9 (2 hours); pleural 22; interstitial 16.4; fallopian tubes 13.6; endometrium 11.1; lung 5.6; bile 5.3 (2.25 hours); myometrium 5; skin, fascia 4.4; vitreous humor 3.4 (3.5 hours); aqueous humor 2.99 (2 hours); CSF (inflamed) 2.6 (2 hours); bone 2.6; sputum 2.1; CSF (uninflamed) 1 (4 hours).

IM: Following IM administration of 500 or 750 mg doses, peak plasma levels of imipenem antimicrobial activity occur within 2 hours and average 10 and 12 mcg/ml, respectively. For cilastatin, peak plasma levels average 24 and 33 mcg/ml, respectively, and occur within 1 hour. When compared with IV administration, imipenem is ≈ 75% bioavailable following IM administration while cilastatin is ≈ 95% bioavailable. The absorption of imipenem from the IM injection site continues for 6 to 8 hours while that for cilastatin is essentially complete within 4 hours. This prolonged absorption of imipenem following IM use results in an effective plasma half-life of ≈ 2 to 3 hours and plasma levels which remain above 2 mcg/ml for at least 6 or 8 hours following a 500 or 750 mg dose, respectively. This plasma profile for imipenem permits IM administration every 12 hours with no accumulation of cilastatin and only slight accumulation of imipenem.

Imipenem urine levels remain above 10 mcg/ml for the 12-hour dosing interval following IM administration of 500 or 750 mg doses. Total urinary excretion of imipenem and cilastatin averages 50% and 75%, respectively, following either dose.

Metabolism / Excretion – Imipenem, when administered alone, is metabolized in the kidneys by dehydropeptidase 1 resulting in relatively low levels in urine. Cilastatin, an inhibitor of this enzyme, prevents renal metabolism of imipenem. Within 10 hours of administration, ≈ 70% of imipenem and cilastatin is recovered in urine.

➤*Microbiology:* Imipenem has in vitro activity against a wide range of gram-positive and gram-negative organisms. It has a high degree of stability in the presence of β-lactamases, including penicillinases and cephalosporinases produced by gram-negative and gram-positive bacteria. It is a potent inhibitor of β-lactamases from certain gram-negative bacteria resistant to many β-lactam antibiotics (eg, *Pseudomonas aeruginosa*, *Serratia* sp., *Enterobacter* sp.).

In vitro, imipenem is active against most strains of clinical isolates in the following microorganisms: Gram-positive aerobes; streptococcus; gram-negative aerobes; gram-positive anaerobes; gram-negative anaerobes.

In vitro tests show imipenem to act synergistically with aminoglycoside antibiotics against some isolates of *Pseudomonas aeruginosa*.

Contraindications

Hypersensitivity to any component of this product.

➤*IM:* Hypersensitivity to local anesthetics of the amide type and in patients with severe shock or heart block due to the use of lidocaine HCl diluent.

➤*IV:* Patients with meningitis (safety and efficacy have not been established).

Warnings

➤*Benzyl alcohol:* As a preservative, it has been associated with toxicity in neonates. While toxicity has not been demonstrated in children > 3 months old, small pediatric patients in this age range may also be at risk for benzyl alcohol toxicity. Therefore, do not use diluents containing benzyl alcohol when imipenem-cilastatin IV is constituted for administration to pediatric patients in this age range.

➤*Resistance:* As with other β-lactam antibiotics, some strains of *Pseudomonas aeruginosa* may develop resistance fairly rapidly during treatment with imipenem-cilastatin. During therapy of *P. aeruginosa* infections, perform periodic susceptibility testing when clinically appropriate.

➤*Pseudomembranous colitis:* Consider this diagnosis in patients who present with diarrhea because it has occurred with nearly all antibacterial agents. Treatment with antibacterial agents alters the normal flora of the colon and may permit overgrowth of clostridia. Studies show that a toxin produced by *Clostridium difficile* is a primary cause of "antibiotic-associated colitis." Initiate therapeutic measures after the diagnosis of pseudomembranous colitis has been established. Mild cases respond to the discontinuation of the drug alone. In moderate-to-severe cases, consider management with fluids and electrolytes, protein supplementation, and treatment with an antibacterial drug effective against *C. difficile* colitis.

➤*Hypersensitivity reactions:* Serious and occasionally fatal hypersensitivity (anaphylactic) reactions have occurred with β-lactam therapy and are more apt to occur in people with a sensitivity history to multiple allergens. Patients with a history of penicillin hypersensitivity have experienced severe reactions when treated with another β-lactam. If a reaction occurs, discontinue the drug. Serious reactions require immediate emergency measures (see Management of Acute Hypersensitivity Reactions).

➤*Renal function impairment:* Do not give imipenem-cilastatin IV to patients with creatinine clearance (Ccr) of ≤ 5 ml/min/1.73 m² unless hemodialysis is instituted within 48 hours. For patients on hemodialysis, imipenem-cilastatin IV is recommended only when the benefit outweighs the potential risk of seizures.

➤*Pregnancy:* Category C. There are no adequate and well controlled studies in pregnant women. Use only when potential benefits outweigh potential hazards.

➤*Lactation:* It is not known whether this drug is excreted in breast milk. Exercise caution when administering to a nursing woman.

➤*Children:*

IM – Safety and efficacy in children < 12 years old have not been established.

IV – Use in neonates to 16 years of age (with non-CNS infections) is supported by evidence from adequate and well controlled studies. IV use is not recommended in pediatric patients with CNS infections because of the risk of seizures, or in pediatric patients < 30 kg with impaired renal function as no data are available.

Precautions

➤*Monitoring:* While imipenem-cilastatin has the characteristic low toxicity of the β-lactam group of antibiotics, periodically assess organ system functions, including renal, hepatic, and hematopoietic, during prolonged therapy.

➤*CNS:* Adverse experiences (eg, myoclonic activity, confusional states, seizures) have occurred with the IV formulation, especially when recommended dosages were exceeded. They are most common in patients with CNS disorders (eg, brain lesions, history of seizures) who may also have compromised renal function. However, CNS adverse experiences have been reported in patients who had no recognized or documented underlying CNS disorder or compromised renal function. Closely adhere to recommended dosage and dosage schedules, especially in patients with known factors that predispose to convulsive activity. Continue anticonvulsants in patients with a known seizure disorder. If focal tremors, myoclonus, or seizures occur, neurologically evaluate patient, institute anticonvulsants, re-examine the dose, and determine whether to decrease dosage or discontinue the drug. If these effects occur with the IM formulation, discontinue the drug.

➤*Cross-allergenicity:* Use caution when administering to patients with a history of penicillin allergy due to a possible cross-sensitivity to imipenem-cilastatin.

➤*Superinfection:* Use of antibiotics (especially prolonged or repeated therapy) may result in bacterial or fungal overgrowth of nonsusceptible organisms. Such overgrowth may lead to secondary infection. Take appropriate measures if superinfection occurs.

Drug Interactions

Imipenem-Cilastatin Drug Interactions			
Precipitant Drug	Object Drug*		Description
Cyclosporine	Imipenem-Cilastatin	↑	The CNS side effects of both agents may be increased possibly because of additive or synergistic toxicity.
Imipenem-Cilastatin	Cyclosporine	↑	
Imipenem-Cilastatin	Ganciclovir	↑	Generalized seizures have occurred with coadministration. Do not use concomitantly.
Probenecid	Imipenem	↑	Coadministration results in only minimal increases in imipenem levels and half-life; do not give probenecid concurrently.

* ↑ = Object drug increased.

IMIPENEM-CILASTATIN

Adverse Reactions

➤ *IV*:

Lab test abnormalities –

Hepatic: Increased AST, ALT, alkaline phosphatase, bilirubin, and LDH.

Hemic: Increased eosinophils, monocytes, lymphocytes, basophils; decreased neutrophils, agranulocytosis, hemoglobin, hematocrit; increased/decreased WBCs and platelets; positive Coombs' test; abnormal prothrombin time.

Electrolytes: Decreased serum sodium; increased potassium and chloride.

Renal: Increased BUN and creatinine.

Urinalysis: Presence of protein, RBCs, WBCs, casts, bilirubin, or urobilinogen.

Cardiovascular – Hypotension (0.4%); palpitations, tachycardia (< 0.2%).

CNS – Fever (0.5%); seizures (0.4%); dizziness (0.3%); somnolence (0.2%); encephalopathy, tremor, confusion, myoclonus, paresthesia, vertigo, headache, psychic disturbances including hallucinations (< 0.2%).

Dermatologic – Rash (0.9%); pruritus (0.3%); urticaria (0.2%); erythema multiforme, Stevens-Johnson syndrome, angioneurotic edema, toxic epidermal necrolysis, flushing, cyanosis, skin texture changes, candidiasis, hyperhidrosis, pruritus vulvae (< 0.2%).

GI – Nausea (2%); diarrhea (1.8%); vomiting (1.5%); pseudomembranous colitis, hemorrhagic colitis, hepatitis, jaundice, staining of the teeth or tongue, gastroenteritis, abdominal pain, glossitis, tongue papillar hypertrophy, heartburn, pharyngeal pain, increased salivation (< 0.2%).

Hematologic – Pancytopenia, bone marrow depression, thrombocytopenia, neutropenia, leukopenia, hemolytic anemia (< 0.2%).

Local – Phlebitis/thrombophlebitis (3.1%); pain (0.7%) and erythema at injection site (0.4%); vein induration (0.2%); infused vein infection (0.1%).

Respiratory – Chest discomfort, dyspnea, hyperventilation, thoracic spine pain (< 0.2%).

Miscellaneous – Hearing loss, tinnitus, polyarthralgia, taste perversion, asthenia/weakness, drug fever, oliguria/anuria, polyuria, acute renal failure, urine discoloration (< 0.2%).

Pediatric patients ≥ 3 months old: Diarrhea (3.9%); rash, phlebitis (2.2%); gastroenteritis, vomiting, IV site irritation, urine discoloration (1.1%).

Newborn to 3 months old: Convulsions (5.9%); diarrhea (3%); oliguria/anuria (2.2%); oral candidiasis, rash, tachycardia (1.5%).

➤ *IM*:

Lab test abnormalities –

Hemic: Decreased hemoglobin and hematocrit; eosinophilia; increased/decreased WBCs and platelets; decreased erythrocytes; increased prothrombin time.

Hepatic: Increased AST, ALT, alkaline phosphatase and bilirubin.

Renal: Increased BUN and creatinine.

Urinalysis: Presence of RBCs, WBCs, casts and bacteria in the urine.

Miscellaneous – Pain at the injection site (1.2%); nausea, diarrhea (0.6%); rash (0.4%); vomiting (0.3%).

Overdosage

In the case of overdosage, discontinue the drug. Treat symptomatically and institute supportive measures as required. Refer to General Management of Acute Overdosage. Imipenem-cilastatin is hemodializable; however, usefulness of this procedure in the overdosage setting is questionable.

ERTAPENEM

Rx	Invanz (Merck)	**Powder, lyophilized:** 1.046 g ertapenem sodium (equivalent to 1 g ertapenem)	175 mg sodium bicarbonate, sodium hydroxide. In vials.

Indications

For the treatment of adult patients with the following moderate to severe infections caused by susceptible strains of the designated microorganisms.

➤ *Complicated intra-abdominal infections:* Due to *Escherichia coli, Clostridium clostridioforme, Eubacterium lentum, Peptostreptococcus* sp., *Bacteroides fragilis, B. distasonis, B. ovatus, B. thetaiotaomicron,* or *B. uniformis.*

➤ *Complicated skin and skin structure infections:* Due to *Staphylococcus aureus* (methicillin-susceptible strains only), *Streptococcus pyogenes, E. coli,* or *Peptostreptococcus* sp.

➤ *Community-acquired pneumonia:* Due to *Streptococcus pneumoniae* (penicillin-susceptible strains only), including cases with concurrent bacteremia, *Haemophilus influenzae* (beta-lactamase-negative strains only), or *Moraxella catarrhalis.*

➤ *Complicated urinary tract infections, including pyelonephritis:* Due to *E. coli,* including cases with concurrent bacteremia, or *Klebsiella pneumoniae.*

➤ *Acute pelvic infections, including postpartum endomyometritis, septic abortion, and postsurgical gynecologic infections:* Due to *Streptococcus agalactiae, E. coli, B. fragilis, Porphyromonas asaccharolytica, Peptostreptococcus* sp., or *Prevotella bivia.*

Obtain appropriate specimens for bacteriological examination in order to isolate and identify the causative organisms and to determine their susceptibility to ertapenem. Therapy with ertapenem may be initiated empirically before results of these tests are known; once results become available, adjust antimicrobial therapy accordingly.

Administration and Dosage

➤ *Approved by the FDA:* November 29, 2001.

1 g given once a day.

Ertapenem may be administered by IV infusion for up to 14 days or IM injection for up to 7 days. When administered IV, infuse ertapenem over a period of 30 minutes.

IM administration of ertapenem may be used as an alternative to IV administration in the treatment of those infections for which IM therapy is appropriate.

Do not mix or co-infuse ertapenem with other medications. Do not use diluents containing dextrose (α-D-glucose).

Ertapenem Dosage Guidelines for Adults with Normal Renal Function[1] and Body Weight		
Infection[2]	Daily dose (IV or IM)	Recommended duration of total antimicrobial treatment
Complicated intra-abdominal infections	1 g	5 to 14 days
Complicated skin and skin structure infections	1 g	7 to 14 days

Ertapenem Dosage Guidelines for Adults with Normal Renal Function[1] and Body Weight		
Infection[2]	Daily dose (IV or IM)	Recommended duration of total antimicrobial treatment
Community-acquired pneumonia	1 g	10 to 14 days[3]
Complicated urinary tract infections, including pyelonephritis	1 g	10 to 14 days[3]
Acute pelvic infections, including postpartum endomyometritis, septic abortion, and postsurgical gynecologic infections	1 g	3 to 10 days

[1] Defined as creatinine clearance (Ccr) > 90 mL/min/1.73 m^2.
[2] Due to the designated pathogens (see Indications).
[3] Duration includes a possible switch to an appropriate oral therapy after ≥ 3 days of parenteral therapy once clinical improvement has been demonstrated.

➤ *Renal insufficiency:* Ertapenem may be used for the treatment of infections in patients with renal insufficiency. In patients whose Ccr is > 30 mL/min/1.73 m^2, no dosage adjustment is necessary. Patients with advanced renal insufficiency (Ccr ≤ 30 mL/min/1.73 m^2) and end-stage renal insufficiency (Ccr ≤ 10 mL/min/1.73 m^2) should receive 500 mg daily.

➤ *Hemodialysis:* When patients on hemodialysis are given the recommended daily dose of 500 mg of ertapenem within 6 hours prior to hemodialysis, a supplementary dose of 150 mg is recommended following the hemodialysis session. If ertapenem is given ≥ 6 hours prior to hemodialysis, no supplementary dose is needed. There are no data in patients undergoing peritoneal dialysis or hemofiltration.

When only the serum creatinine is available, the following formula may be used to estimate creatinine clearance. The serum creatinine should represent a steady state of renal function.

$$\text{Males:} \quad \frac{\text{Weight (kg)} \times (140 - \text{age})}{72 \times \text{serum creatinine (mg/dL)}} = \text{Ccr}$$

Females: 0.85 × above value

➤ *Preparation of solution:*

Preparation for IV administration – Do not mix or co-infuse ertapenem with other medications. Do not use diluents containing dextrose (α-D-glucose).

Ertapenem must be reconstituted and then diluted prior to administration.

1.) Reconstitute the contents of a 1 g vial of ertapenem with 10 mL of one of the following: Water for Injection, 0.9% Sodium Chloride Injection, or Bacteriostatic Water for Injection.

2.) Shake well to dissolve, and immediately transfer contents of the reconstituted vial to 50 mL of 0.9% Sodium Chloride Injection.

3.) Complete the infusion within 6 hours of reconstitution.

ERTAPENEM

Preparation for IM administration – Ertapenem for injection must be reconstituted prior to administration.

1.) Reconstitute the contents of a 1 g vial of ertapenem with 3.2 mL of 1% lidocaine HCl injection (without epinephrine). Shake vial thoroughly to form solution.
2.) Immediately withdraw the contents of the vial, and administer by deep IM injection into a large muscle mass (such as the gluteal muscles or lateral part of the thigh).
3.) Use the reconstituted IM solution within 1 hour after preparation. Note: Do not administer the reconstituted solution IV.

Visually inspect parenteral drug products for particulate matter and discoloration prior to use whenever solution and container permit. Solutions of ertapenem range from colorless to pale yellow. Variations of color within this range do not affect the potency of the product.

➤ *Storage / Stability:*

Before reconstitution – Do not store lyophilized powder above 25°C (77°F).

Reconstituted and infusion solutions – The reconstituted solution, immediately diluted in 0.9% Sodium Chloride Injection, may be stored at room temperature (25°C; 77°F) and used within 6 hours or stored for 24 hours under refrigeration (5°C; 41°F) and used within 4 hours after removal from refrigeration. Do not freeze ertapenem solutions.

Actions

➤ *Pharmacokinetics:*

Absorption – Ertapenem, reconstituted with 1% lidocaine HCl injection (in saline without epinephrine), is almost completely absorbed following IM administration at the recommended dose of 1 g. The mean bioavailability is ≈ 90%. Following 1 g daily IM administration, mean peak plasma concentrations (C_{max}) are achieved in ≈ 2.3 hours (T_{max}).

Distribution – Ertapenem is highly bound to human plasma proteins, primarily albumin. In healthy young adults, the protein binding of ertapenem decreases as plasma concentrations increase, from ≈ 95% bound at an approximate plasma concentration of < 100 mcg/mL to ≈ 85% bound at an approximate plasma concentration of 300 mcg/mL.

The apparent volume of distribution at steady state of ertapenem is ≈ 8.2 L.

The concentration of ertapenem in breast milk from 5 lactating women with pelvic infections (5 to 14 days postpartum) was measured at random time points daily for 5 consecutive days following the last 1 g dose of IV therapy (3 to 10 days of therapy). The concentration of ertapenem in breast milk within 24 hours of the last dose of therapy in all 5 women ranged from < 0.13 (lower limit of quantitation) to 0.38 mcg/mL; peak concentrations were not assessed. By day 5 after discontinuation of therapy, the level of ertapenem was undetectable in the breast milk of 4 women and below the lower limit of quantitation (< 0.13 mcg/mL) in 1 woman.

Metabolism – In healthy young adults, after infusion of 1 g IV radiolabeled ertapenem, the plasma radioactivity consists predominantly (94%) of ertapenem. The major metabolite of ertapenem is the inactive ring-opened derivative formed by hydrolysis of the beta-lactam ring.

In vitro studies in human liver microsomes indicate that ertapenem does not inhibit metabolism mediated by any of the following cytochrome P450 (CYP) isoforms: 1A2, 2C9, 2C19, 2D6, 2E1, and 3A4.

In vitro studies indicate that ertapenem does not inhibit P-glycoprotein-mediated transport of digoxin or vinblastine and that ertapenem is not a substrate for P-glycoprotein-mediated transport.

Excretion – Ertapenem is eliminated primarily by the kidneys. The mean plasma half-life in healthy young adults is ≈ 4 hours, and the plasma clearance is ≈ 1.8 L/hour.

Following the administration of 1 g IV radiolabeled ertapenem to healthy young adults, ≈ 80% is recovered in urine and 10% in feces. Of the 80% recovered in urine, ≈ 38% is excreted as unchanged drug and ≈ 37% as the ring-opened metabolite.

In healthy young adults given a 1 g IV dose, the mean percentage of the administered dose excreted in urine was 17.4% during 0 to 2 hours postdose, 5.4% during 4 to 6 hours postdose, and 2.4% during 12 to 24 hours postdose.

Plasma concentrations – Average plasma concentrations (mcg/mL) of ertapenem following a single 30-minute infusion of a 1 g IV dose and administration of a single 1 g IM dose in healthy young adults are presented in the following table.

Plasma Concentrations of Ertapenem After Single-Dose Administration									
	Average plasma concentrations (mcg/mL)								
Dose/Route	0.5 hr	1 hr	2 hr	4 hr	6 hr	8 hr	12 hr	18 hr	24 hr
1 g IV[1]	155	115	83	48	31	20	9	3	1
1 g IM	33	53	67	57	40	27	13	4	2

[1] Infused at a constant rate over 30 minutes.

The area under the plasma concentration-time curve (AUC) of ertapenem increased less-than-dose proportionally based on total ertapenem concentrations over the 0.5 to 2 g dose range, whereas the AUC increased greater-than-dose proportionally based on unbound ertapenem concentrations. Ertapenem exhibits nonlinear pharmacokinetics because of concentration-dependent plasma protein binding at the proposed therapeutic dose.

There is no accumulation of ertapenem following multiple IV or IM 1 g daily doses in healthy adults.

Special populations –

Renal insufficiency: Total and unbound fractions of ertapenem pharmacokinetics were investigated in 26 adult subjects (31 to 80 years of age) with varying degrees of renal impairment. No dosage adjustment is necessary in patients with Ccr ≥ 31 mL/min/1.73 m². The recommended dose of ertapenem in patients with Ccr ≤ 30 mL/min/1.73 m² is 0.5 g every 24 hours. Following a single 1 g IV dose given immediately prior to a 4-hour hemodialysis session in 5 patients with end-stage renal insufficiency, ≈ 30% of the dose was recovered in the dialysate. A supplementary dose of 150 mg is recommended if ertapenem is administered within 6 hours prior to hemodialysis.

➤ *Microbiology:* Ertapenem has in vitro activity against gram-positive and gram-negative aerobic and anaerobic bacteria. The bactericidal activity of ertapenem results from the inhibition of cell wall synthesis and is mediated through ertapenem binding to penicillin-binding proteins (PBPs). In *E. coli*, it has strong affinity toward PBPs 1a, 1b, 2, 3, 4, and 5 with preference for PBPs 2 and 3. Ertapenem is stable against hydrolysis by a variety of beta-lactamases, including penicillinases, cephalosporinases, and extended spectrum beta-lactamases (ESBL). Ertapenem is hydrolyzed by metallo-beta-lactamases.

Ertapenem has been shown to be active against most strains of the following microorganisms in vitro and in clinical infections.

Aerobic gram-positive microorganisms
    S. aureus (methicillin-susceptible strains only)
    S. agalactiae
    S. pneumoniae (penicillin-susceptible strains only)
    S. pyogenes
    Note: Methicillin-resistant staphylococci and *Enterococcus* sp. are resistant to ertapenem.

Aerobic gram-negative microorganisms
    E. coli
    H. influenzae (beta-lactamase-negative strains only)
    K. pneumoniae
    M. catarrhalis

Anaerobic microorganisms
    B. fragilis
    B. distasonis
    B. ovatus
    B. thetaiotaomicron
    B. uniformis
    C. clostridioforme
    E. lentum
    Peptostreptococcus species
    P. asaccharolytica
    P. bivia

The following in vitro data are available, but their clinical significance is unknown.

At least 90% of the following microorganisms exhibit an in vitro minimum inhibitory concentration (MIC) less than or equal to the susceptible breakpoint for ertapenem; however, the safety and effectiveness of ertapenem in treating clinical infections due to these microorganisms have not been established in adequate and well-controlled clinical studies:

Aerobic gram-positive microorganisms
    S. pneumoniae (penicillin-intermediate strains only)

Aerobic gram-negative microorganisms
    Citrobacter freundii
    Citrobacter koseri
    Enterobacter aerogenes
    Enterobacter cloacae
    H. influenzae (beta-lactamase-positive strains)
    H. parainfluenzae
    Klebsiella oxytoca (excluding ESBL-producing strains)
    Morganella morganii
    Proteus mirabilis
    Proteus vulgaris
    Serratia marcescens

Anaerobic microorganisms
    Clostridium perfringens
    Fusobacterium sp.

➤ *Clinical trials:*

Complicated intra-abdominal infections – Ertapenem was evaluated in adults for the treatment of complicated intra-abdominal infections in a clinical trial. The combined clinical and microbiologic success rates in the microbiologically evaluable population at 4 to 6 weeks post-therapy (test of cure) were 83.6% (163/195) for ertapenem and 80.4% (152/189) for piperacillin/tazobactam.

Complicated skin and skin structure infections – Ertapenem was evaluated in adults for the treatment of complicated skin and skin structure infections in a clinical trial. The clinical success rates at 10 to

ERTAPENEM

21 days posttherapy (test of cure) were 83.9% (141/168) for ertapenem and 85.3% (145/170) for piperacillin/tazobactam.

Community-acquired pneumonia – Ertapenem was evaluated in adults for the treatment of community-acquired pneumonia in 2 clinical trials. In the first study, the primary efficacy parameter was the clinical success rate in the clinically evaluable population, and success rates were 92.3% (168/182) for ertapenem and 91% (183/201) for ceftriaxone at 7 to 14 days posttherapy (test of cure). In the second study, the primary efficacy parameter was the clinical success rate in the microbiologically evaluable population, and success rates were 91% (91/100) for ertapenem and 91.8% (45/49) for ceftriaxone at 7 to 14 days posttherapy (test of cure).

Complicated urinary tract infections, including pyelonephritis – Ertapenem was evaluated in adults for the treatment of complicated urinary tract infections, including pyelonephritis, in 2 clinical trials. The microbiological success rates (combined studies) at 5 to 9 days post-therapy (test of cure) were 89.5% (229/256) for ertapenem and 91.1% (204/224) for ceftriaxone.

Acute pelvic infections, including endomyometritis, septic abortion, and postsurgical gynecological infections – Ertapenem was evaluated in adults for the treatment of acute pelvic infections in a clinical trial. The success rates in the evaluable population at 2 to 4 weeks posttherapy (test of cure) were 93.9% (153/163) for ertapenem and 91.5% (140/153) for piperacillin/tazobactam.

Contraindications

Ertapenem is contraindicated in patients with known hypersensitivity to any component of this product or to other drugs in the same class or in patients who have demonstrated anaphylactic reactions to beta-lactams.

Because of the use of lidocaine HCl as a diluent, ertapenem administered IM is contraindicated in patients with a known hypersensitivity to local anesthetics of the amide type.

Warnings

➤*Seizures:* Seizures and other CNS adverse experiences have been reported during treatment with ertapenem.

➤*Pseudomembranous colitis:* Pseudomembranous colitis has been reported with nearly all antibacterial agents, including ertapenem, and may range in severity from mild to life-threatening. Therefore, it is important to consider this diagnosis in patients who present with diarrhea subsequent to the administration of antibacterial agents.

Treatment with antibacterial agents alters the normal flora of the colon and may permit overgrowth of clostridia. Studies indicate that a toxin produced by *Clostridium difficile* is a primary cause of antibiotic-associated colitis.

After the diagnosis of pseudomembranous colitis has been established, initiate therapeutic measures. Mild cases of pseudomembranous colitis usually respond to drug discontinuation alone. In moderate to severe cases, consider management with fluids and electrolytes, protein supplementation, and treatment with an antibacterial drug clinically effective against *C. difficile* colitis.

➤*Hypersensitivity reactions:* Serious and occasionally fatal hypersensitivity (anaphylactic) reactions have been reported in patients receiving therapy with beta-lactams. These reactions are more likely to occur in individuals with a history of sensitivity to multiple allergens. There have been reports of individuals with a history of penicillin hypersensitivity who have experienced severe hypersensitivity reactions when treated with another beta-lactam. Before initiating therapy with ertapenem, careful inquiry should be made concerning previous hypersensitivity reactions to penicillins, cephalosporins, other beta-lactams, and other allergens. If an allergic reaction to ertapenem occurs, discontinue the drug immediately. Serious anaphylactic reactions require immediate emergency treatment with epinephrine, oxygen, IV steroids, and airway management, including intubation. Other therapy also may be administered as indicated.

➤*Elderly:* This drug is known to be substantially excreted by the kidney, and the risk of toxic reactions to this drug may be greater in patients with impaired renal function. Because elderly patients are more likely to have decreased renal function, take care in dose selection; it may be useful to monitor renal function.

➤*Pregnancy: Category B.* In mice given 700 mg/kg/day, slight decreases in average fetal weights and an associated decrease in the average number of ossified sacrocaudal vertebrae were observed. Ertapenem crosses the placental barrier in rats.

There are no adequate and well-controlled studies in pregnant women. Because animal reproduction studies are not always predictive of human response, use this drug during pregnancy only if clearly needed.

➤*Lactation:* Ertapenem is excreted in breast milk. Exercise caution when ertapenem is administered to a nursing woman. Administer ertapenem to nursing mothers only when the expected benefit outweighs the risk.

➤*Children:* Safety and effectiveness in pediatric patients have not been established. Therefore, use in patients < 18 years of age is not recommended.

Precautions

➤*Monitoring:* As with other antibiotics, prolonged use of ertapenem may result in overgrowth of nonsusceptible organisms. Repeated evaluation of the patient's condition is essential. If superinfection occurs during therapy, take appropriate measures.

While ertapenem possesses toxicity similar to the beta-lactam group of antibiotics, periodic assessment of organ system function, including renal, hepatic, and hematopoietic, is advisable during prolonged therapy.

➤*Special risk:* During clinical investigations in adult patients treated with ertapenem (1 g once a day), seizures, irrespective of drug relationship, occurred in 0.5% of patients during study therapy plus 14-day follow-up period. These experiences have occurred most commonly in patients with CNS disorders (eg, brain lesions or history of seizures) or compromised renal function. Close adherence to the recommended dosage regimen is urged, especially in patients with known factors that predispose to convulsive activity. Continue anticonvulsant therapy in patients with known seizure disorders. If focal tremors, myoclonus, or seizures occur, evaluate patients neurologically, place them on anticonvulsant therapy if not already instituted, and reexamine the dosage of ertapenem to determine whether it should be decreased or the antibiotic discontinued. Dosage adjustment of ertapenem is recommended in patients with reduced renal function.

Drug Interactions

When ertapenem is coadministered with probenecid (500 mg by mouth every 6 hours), probenecid competes for active tubular secretion and reduces the renal clearance of ertapenem. Based on total ertapenem concentrations, probenecid increased the AUC by 25% and reduced the plasma and renal clearances by 20% and 35%, respectively. The half-life increased from 4 to 4.8 hours. Because of the small effect on half-life, the coadministration with probenecid to extend the half-life of ertapenem is not recommended.

Other than with probenecid, no specific clinical drug interaction studies have been conducted.

Adverse Reactions

Clinical studies enrolled 1954 patients treated with ertapenem; in some of the clinical studies, parenteral therapy was followed by a switch to an appropriate oral antimicrobial. Most adverse experiences reported in these clinical studies were described as mild to moderate in severity. Ertapenem was discontinued because of adverse experiences in 4.7% of patients. The following table shows the incidence of adverse experiences reported in ≥ 1% of patients in these studies. The most common drug-related adverse experiences in patients treated with ertapenem, including those who were switched to therapy with an oral antimicrobial, were diarrhea (5.5%), infused vein complication (3.7%), nausea (3.1%), headache (2.2%), vaginitis (2.1%), phlebitis/thrombophlebitis (1.3%), and vomiting (1.1%).

Incidence of Adverse Experiences Reported During Study Therapy Plus 14-Day Follow-Up in ≥ 1% of Patients Treated with Ertapenem in Clinical Studies (%)				
Adverse events	Ertapenem[1] 1 g daily (n = 802)	Piperacillin/ Tazobactam[1] 3.375 g q6h (n = 774)	Ertapenem[2] 1 g daily (n = 1152)	Ceftriaxone[2] 1 or 2 g daily (n = 942)
Cardiovascular				
Chest pain	1.5	1.4	1	2.5
Hypertension	1.6	1.4	0.7	1
Hypotension	2	1.4	1	1.2
Tachycardia	1.6	1.3	1.3	0.7
CNS				
Altered mental status[3]	5.1	3.4	3.3	2.5
Anxiety	1.4	1.3	0.8	1.2
Dizziness	2.1	3	1.5	2.1
Headache	5.6	5.4	6.8	6.9
Insomnia	3.2	5.2	3	4.1
Dermatologic				
Erythema	1.6	1.7	1.2	1.2
Extravasation	1.9	1.7	0.7	1.1
Infused vein complication	7.1	7.9	5.4	6.7
Phlebitis/ Thrombo- phlebitis	1.9	2.7	1.6	2
Pruritus	2	2.6	1	1.9
Rash	2.5	3.1	2.3	1.5
GI				
Abdominal pain	3.6	4.8	4.3	3.9
Acid regurgitation	1.6	0.9	1.1	0.6
Constipation	4	5.4	3.3	3.1
Diarrhea	10.3	12.1	9.2	9.8
Dyspepsia	1.1	0.6	1	1.6

ERTAPENEM

Incidence of Adverse Experiences Reported During Study Therapy Plus 14-Day Follow-Up in ≥ 1% of Patients Treated with Ertapenem in Clinical Studies (%)

Adverse events	Ertapenem[1] 1 g daily (n = 802)	Piperacillin/ Tazobactam[1] 3.375 g q6h (n = 774)	Ertapenem[2] 1 g daily (n = 1152)	Ceftriaxone[2] 1 or 2 g daily (n = 942)
Nausea	8.5	8.7	6.4	7.4
Oral candidiasis	0.1	1.3	1.4	1.9
Vomiting	3.7	5.3	4	4
Respiratory				
Cough	1.6	1.7	1.3	0.5
Dyspnea	2.6	1.8	1	2.4
Pharyngitis	0.7	1.4	1.1	0.6
Rales/Rhonchi	1.1	1	0.5	1
Respiratory distress	1	0.4	0.2	0.2
Miscellaneous				
Asthenia/ Fatigue	1.2	0.9	1.2	1.1
Death	2.5	1.6	1.3	1.6
Edema/Swelling	3.4	2.5	2.9	3.3
Fever	5	6.6	2.3	3.4
Leg pain	1.1	0.5	0.4	0.3
Vaginitis	1.4	1	3.3	3.7

[1] Includes Phase IIb/III complicated intra-abdominal infections, complicated skin and skin structure infections, and acute pelvic infections studies.
[2] Includes Phase IIb/III community-acquired pneumonia and complicated urinary tract infections and Phase IIa studies.
[3] Includes agitation, confusion, disorientation, decreased mental acuity, changed mental status, somnolence, stupor.

In patients treated for complicated intra-abdominal infections, death occurred in 4.7% (15/316) of patients receiving ertapenem and 2.6% (8/307) of patients receiving comparator drug. These deaths occurred in patients with significant comorbidity or severe baseline infections. Deaths were considered unrelated to study drugs by investigators.

In clinical studies, seizure was reported during study therapy plus 14-day follow-up period in 0.5% of patients treated with ertapenem, 0.3% of patients treated with piperacillin/tazobactam, and 0% of patients treated with ceftriaxone.

Additional adverse experiences that were reported with ertapenem with an incidence of > 0.1% within each body system are listed below.

►*Cardiovascular:* Heart failure; hematoma; cardiac arrest; bradycardia; arrhythmia; atrial fibrillation; heart murmur; ventricular tachycardia; asystole; subdural hemorrhage.

►*CNS:* Nervousness; seizure; tremor; depression; hypesthesia; spasm; paresthesia; aggressive behavior; vertigo.

►*Dermatologic:* Sweating; dermatitis; desquamation; flushing; urticaria; injection site induration; injection site pain.

►*GI:* Abdominal distention; GI hemorrhage; anorexia; flatulence; *C. difficile*-associated diarrhea; stomatitis; dysphagia; hemorrhoids; ileus; cholelithiasis; duodenitis; esophagitis; gastritis; jaundice; mouth ulcer; pancreatitis; pyloric stenosis.

►*GU:* Oliguria/Anuria; vaginal pruritus; hematuria; urinary retention; bladder dysfunction; vaginal candidiasis; vulvovaginitis.

►*Respiratory:* Pleural effusion; hypoxemia; bronchoconstriction; pharyngeal discomfort; epistaxis; pleuritic pain; asthma; hemoptysis; hiccoughs; voice disturbance.

►*Miscellaneous:* Pain; chills; septicemia; septic shock; dehydration; gout; malaise; necrosis; candidiasis; weight loss; facial edema; flank pain; syncope; taste perversion; renal insufficiency.

►*Lab test abnormalities:* In repeat-dose studies in rats, treatment-related neutropenia occurred at every dose level tested, including the lowest dose (2 mg/kg; 12 mg/m²).

Laboratory adverse experiences that were reported during therapy in ≥ 1% of patients treated with ertapenem in clinical studies are presented in the following table. Drug-related laboratory adverse experi-

ences that were reported during therapy in ≥ 1% of patients treated with ertapenem, including those who were switched to therapy with an oral antimicrobial, in clinical studies were ALT increased (6%), AST increased (5.2%), serum alkaline phosphatase increased (3.4%), platelet count increased (2.8%), and eosinophils increased (1.1%). Ertapenem was discontinued because of laboratory adverse experiences in 0.3% of patients.

Incidence[1] of Specific Laboratory Adverse Experiences Reported During Study Therapy Plus 14-Day Follow-Up in ≥ 1% of Patients Treated with Ertapenem in Clinical Studies (%)

Adverse laboratory experiences	Ertapenem[2] 1 g daily (n[3]= 766)	Piperacillin/ Tazobactam[2] 3.375 g q6h (n[3]= 755)	Ertapenem[4] 1 g daily (n[3]= 1122)	Ceftriaxone[4] 1 or 2 g daily (n[3]= 920)
ALT increased	8.8	7.3	8.3	6.9
AST increased	8.4	8.3	7.1	6.5
Serum albumin decreased	1.7	1.5	0.9	1.6
Serum alkaline phosphatase increased	6.6	7.2	4.3	2.8
Serum creatinine increased	1.1	2.7	0.9	1.2
Serum glucose increased	1.2	2.3	1.7	2
Serum potassium decreased	1.7	2.8	1.8	2.4
Serum potassium increased	1.3	0.5	0.5	0.7
Total serum bilirubin increased	1.7	1.4	0.6	1.1
Eosinophils increased	1.1	1.1	2.1	1.8
Hematocrit decreased	3	2.9	3.4	2.4
Hemoglobin decreased	4.9	4.7	4.5	3.5
Platelet count decreased	1.1	1.2	1.1	1
Platelet count increased	6.5	6.3	4.3	3.5
Segmented neutrophils decreased	1	0.3	1.5	0.8
Prothrombin time increased	1.2	2	0.3	0.9
WBC decreased	0.8	0.7	1.5	1.4
Urine RBCs increased	2.5	2.9	1.1	1
Urine WBCs increased	2.5	3.2	1.6	1.1

[1] Number of patients with laboratory adverse experiences/Number of patients with the laboratory test.
[2] Includes Phase IIb/III complicated intra-abdominal infections, complicated skin and skin structure infections, and acute pelvic infections studies.
[3] Number of patients with ≥ 1 laboratory tests.
[4] Includes Phase IIb/III community-acquired pneumonia and complicated urinary tract infections and Phase IIa studies.

Additional laboratory adverse experiences that were reported during therapy in > 0.1% but < 1% of patients treated with ertapenem in clinical studies include the following: Increases in BUN, direct and indirect serum bilirubin, serum sodium, monocytes, PTT, or urine epithelial cells; decreases in serum bicarbonate.

Overdosage

►*Symptoms:* No specific information is available on the treatment of overdosage with ertapenem. Intentional overdosage with ertapenem is unlikely. IV administration of ertapenem at a dose of 2 g over 30 minutes or 3 g over 1 to 2 hours in healthy volunteers resulted in an increased incidence of nausea. In clinical studies, inadvertent administration of three 1 g doses of ertapenem in a 24-hour period resulted in diarrhea and transient dizziness in 1 patient.

►*Treatment:* In the event of an overdose, discontinue ertapenem and give general supportive treatment until renal elimination takes place.

Ertapenem can be removed by hemodialysis; the plasma clearance of the total fraction of ertapenem was increased 30% in subjects with end-stage renal insufficiency when hemodialysis (4-hour session) was performed immediately following administration. However, no information is available on the use of hemodialysis to treat overdosage.

AZTREONAM

Rx	Azactam (Squibb)	Powder for Injection (lyophilized cake): 500 mg[1]	In single-dose 15 ml vials.
		1 g[1]	In single-dose 15 ml vials and single-dose 100 ml infusion bottles.
		2 g[1]	In 30 ml single-dose vials and single-dose 100 ml infusion bottles.

[1] With ≈ 780 mg L–arginine per gram aztreonam.

Indications

Treatment of the following infections caused by susceptible gram-negative microorganisms:

➤*Urinary tract infections (complicated and uncomplicated):* Including pyelonephritis and cystitis (initial and recurrent) caused by *E. coli, K. pneumoniae, P. mirabilis, P. aeruginosa, E. cloacae, K. oxytoca, Citrobacter* sp., and *S. marcescens.*

➤*Lower respiratory tract infections:* Including pneumonia and bronchitis, caused by *E. coli, K. pneumoniae, P. aeruginosa, H. influenzae, P. mirabilis, Enterobacter* sp., and *S. marcescens.*

➤*Septicemia:* Caused by *E. coli, K. pneumoniae, P. aeruginosa, P. mirabilis, S. marcescens,* and *Enterobacter* sp.

➤*Skin and skin structure infections:* Including those associated with postoperative wounds, ulcers, and burns caused by *E. coli, P. mirabilis, S. marcescens, Enterobacter* sp., *P. aeruginosa, K. pneumoniae,* and *Citrobacter* sp.

➤*Intra-abdominal infections:* Including peritonitis caused by *E. coli, Klebsiella* sp.. including *K. pneumoniae, Enterobacter* sp. including *E. cloacae, P. aeruginosa, Citrobacter* sp. including *C. freundii,* and *Serratia* sp. including *S. marcescens.*

➤*Gynecologic infections:* Including endometritis and pelvic cellulitis, caused by *E. coli, K. pneumoniae, Enterobacter* sp. including *E. cloacae,* and *P. mirabilis.*

➤*Surgery:* For adjunctive therapy to surgery to manage infections caused by susceptible organisms.

➤*Concurrent initial therapy:* This with other antimicrobials and aztreonam is recommended before the causative organism(s) is known in seriously ill patients who are also at risk of having an infection due to gram-positive aerobic pathogens. If anaerobic organisms are also suspected, initiate therapy concurrently with aztreonam.

➤*Unlabeled uses:* 1 g IM may be beneficial for acute uncomplicated gonorrhea in patients with penicillin-resistant gonococci, as an alternative to spectinomycin.

Administration and Dosage

Give IM or IV. Individualize dosage.

Aztreonam Dosage Guide (Adults)

Type of infection	Dose[1]	Frequency (hours)
Urinary tract infection	500 mg or 1 g	8 or 12
Moderately severe systemic infections	1 or 2 g	8 or 12
Severe systemic or life-threatening infections	2 g	6 or 8

[1] Maximum recommended dose is 8 g/day.

Aztreonam Dosage Guide (Children)

Type of infection	Dose[1]	Frequency (hours)
Mild-to-moderate infections	30 mg/kg	8
Moderate-to-severe infections	30 mg/kg	6 or 8

[1] Maximum recommended dose is 120 mg/kg/day.

➤*IV route:* This is recommended for patients requiring single doses > 1 g or those with bacterial septicemia, localized parenchymal abscess (eg, intra-abdominal abscess), peritonitis, or other severe systemic or life-threatening infections. For infections due to *P. aeruginosa,* a dosage of 2 g every 6 or 8 hours is recommended, at least upon therapy initiation.

➤*Duration:* Therapy duration depends on the severity of infection. Generally, continue aztreonam for ≥ 48 hours after the patient becomes asymptomatic or evidence of bacterial eradication has been obtained. Persistent infections may require treatment for several weeks. Do not use doses smaller than those indicated.

➤*Children:* Administer aztreonam intravenously to pediatric patients with normal renal function. There are insufficient data regarding IM administration to pediatric patients or dosing in pediatric patients with renal impairment.

➤*Renal function impairment:* Prolonged aztreonam serum levels may occur in patients with transient or persistent renal insufficiency. Therefore, reduce dosage by 50% in patients with estimated creatinine clearances (Ccr) between 10 and 30 ml/min/1.73 m² after an initial loading dose of 1 g or 2 g.

When only the serum creatinine concentration is available, the following formula may be used to approximate creatinine clearance. The serum creatinine should represent steady-state renal function.

Males:
$$\frac{\text{Weight (kg)} \times (140 - \text{age})}{72 \times \text{serum creatinine (mg/dL)}} = \text{Ccr}$$

Females: $0.85 \times$ above value

In patients with severe renal failure (creatinine clearance < 10 ml/min/1.73 m²), such as those supported by hemodialysis, give 500 mg, 1 g, or 2 g initially. The maintenance dose should be 25% of the usual initial dose given at the usual fixed interval of 6, 8, or 12 hours. For serious or life-threatening infections, in addition to the maintenance doses, give 12.5% of the initial dose after each hemodialysis session.

➤*Elderly:* Renal status is a major determinant of dosage in the elderly. Serum creatinine may not be an accurate determinant of renal status. Therefore, obtain estimates of Ccr and make appropriate dosage modifications.

➤*IV:* Bolus injection may be used to initiate therapy. Slowly inject directly into a vein or into the tubing of a suitable administration set over 3 to 5 minutes.

Infusion – With any intermittent infusion of aztreonam and another drug not pharmaceutically compatible, flush the common delivery tube before and after delivery of aztreonam with an infusion solution compatible with both drug solutions. Do not deliver the drugs simultaneously. Complete the infusion within 20 to 60 minutes. With a Y-type administration set, give careful attention to the calculated volume of aztreonam solution required so that the entire dose will be infused. If a volume-control administration set is used to deliver an initial dilution of aztreonam during use, the final aztreonam dilution should provide a concentration ≤ 2% w/v.

➤*IM:* Inject deeply into a large muscle mass (eg, upper outer quadrant of gluteus maximus or lateral thigh). Aztreonam is well tolerated; do not admix with local anesthetics.

➤*Preparation of solutions:* Upon the addition of the diluent to the container, shake the contents immediately and vigorously. Constituted solutions are not for multiple-dose use. Discard unused solution. Constituted aztreonam yields a colorless to light straw-yellow solution that may develop a slight pink tint on standing (potency is not affected).

IV solutions –

For bolus injection: Constitute the contents of the 15 or 30 ml vial with 6 to 10 ml Sterile Water for Injection.

For infusion – Constitute the contents of the 100 ml bottle to a final concentration ≤ 2% w/v (≥ 50 ml of any infusion solution listed below per gram of aztreonam). Most solutions may be frozen in the original container immediately after constitution.

If the contents of a 15 to 30 ml capacity vial are to be transferred to an appropriate infusion solution, each gram of aztreonam should be initially constituted with at least 3 ml Sterile Water for Injection.

Diluents: Further dilute with 1 of the following IV infusion solutions: Sodium Chloride Injection, 0.9%; Ringer's or Lactated Ringer's Injection; Dextrose Injection, 5% or 10%; Dextrose and Sodium Chloride Injection, 5%:0.9%, 5%:0.45%, or 5%:0.2%; Sodium Lactate Injection (M/6 Sodium Lactate); *Ionosol B* and 5% Dextrose; *Isolyte E* or *Isolyte E* with 5% Dextrose; *Isolyte M* with 5% Dextrose; *Normosol R; Normosol R* and 5% Dextrose; *Normosol M* and 5% Dextrose; Mannitol Injection, 5% or 10%; Lactated Ringer's and 5% Dextrose Injection; *Plasma-Lyte M* and 5% Dextrose; *10% Travert* Injection; *10% Travert and Electrolyte No. 1, 2,* or *3* Injection.

IM solutions – Constitute the contents of aztreonam for injection 15 or 30 ml capacity vial with ≥ 3 ml of an appropriate diluent per gram aztreonam. The following diluents may be used: Sterile Water for Injection; Bacteriostatic Water for Injection (with benzyl alcohol or methyl- and propylparabens); Sodium Chloride Injection, 0.9%; Bacteriostatic Sodium Chloride Injection (with benzyl alcohol).

➤*Admixture compatibilities:* IV infusion solutions of aztreonam prepared with NaCl Injection 0.9% or Dextrose Injection 5%, to which clindamycin, gentamicin, tobramycin, or cefazolin have been added, are stable for ≤ 48 hours at room temperature or 7 days refrigerated. Ampicillin admixtures with aztreonam in NaCl Injection 0.9% are stable for 24 hours at room temperature and 48 hours under refrigeration; stability in Dextrose Injection 5% is 2 hours at room temperature and 8 hours refrigerated. Aztreonam-cloxacillin and aztreonam-vancomycin admixtures are stable in *Dianeal 137* (peritoneal dialysis solution) with 4.25% Dextrose for ≤ 24 hours at room temperature.

➤*Admixture incompatibilities:* Aztreonam is incompatible with nafcillin sodium, cephradine, and metronidazole. Other admixtures are not recommended because compatibility data are not available.

➤*Storage/Stability:* Use solutions for IV infusion at concentrations ≤ 2% w/v within 48 hours following constitution if kept at controlled room temperature (15° to 30°C; 59° to 86°F) or within 7 days if refrigerated (2° to 8°C; 36° to 46°F). Frozen infusion solutions may be stored for ≤ 3 months at -20°C (-4°F). Use frozen solutions that have been

AZTREONAM

thawed and maintained at controlled room temperature or by overnight refrigeration within 24 or 72 hours, respectively, after removal from the freezer. Do not refreeze solutions. After preparation, promptly use solutions at concentrations exceeding 2% w/v, except those prepared with Sterile Water for Injection or NaCl Injection; use the 2 excepted solutions ≤ 48 hours if stored at controlled room temperature or within 7 days if refrigerated.

Actions

➤*Pharmacology:* Aztreonam, a synthetic bactericidal antibiotic, belongs to a class of antibiotics identified as monobactams. The monobactams have a monocyclic β-lactam nucleus and are structurally different from other β-lactams (eg, penicillins, cephalosporins, cephamycins). Aztreonam has a wide spectrum of activity against gram-negative aerobic pathogens. The bactericidal action results from the inhibition of bacterial cell-wall synthesis because of the high affinity of aztreonam for penicillin-binding protein 3 (PBP 3).

➤*Pharmacokinetics:*

Absorption/Distribution – Single 30-minute IV infusions of 500 mg, 1 g, and 2 g doses in healthy subjects produced peak serum levels of 54, 90, and 204 mcg/ml, respectively, immediately after administration; at 8 hours, serum levels were 1, 3, and 6 mcg/ml, respectively.

Following single IM injections of 500 mg and 1 g, maximum serum concentrations occur at ≈ 1 hour.

The serum half-life averaged 1.7 hours (range, 1.5 to 2) in subjects with normal renal function, independent of the dose and route. In healthy subjects, based on a 70 kg person, the serum clearance is 91 ml/min and renal clearance is 56 ml/min. The apparent mean volume of distribution at steady state averaged 12.6 L.

Elderly: The average elimination half-life appears slightly longer in healthy elderly males.

Renal/hepatic impairment: In patients with impaired renal function, the serum half-life is prolonged. Serum half-life is slightly prolonged in patients with hepatic impairment because the liver is a minor pathway of excretion.

Body fluids: The concentration in breast milk at 2 hours after a single 1 g IV dose (6 patients) was 0.2 mcg/ml; in amniotic fluid at 6 to 8 hours after a single 1 g IV dose (5 patients) it was 2 mcg/ml. The concentration in peritoneal fluid obtained 1 to 6 hours after multiple 2 g IV doses ranged between 12 and 90 mcg/ml in 7 of 8 patients studied.

Metabolism/Excretion – After IM injection of single 500 mg and 1 g doses, urinary levels were ≈ 500 and 1200 mcg/ml, respectively, in the first 2 hours, declining to 180 and 470 mcg/ml in the 6- to 8-hour specimens. Aztreonam is excreted in the urine equally by active tubular secretion and glomerular filtration. In an IV or IM dose, ≈ 60% to 70% was recovered in the urine by 8 hours; recovery was complete by 12 hours. About 12% of a single IV dose was recovered in the feces.

IV or IM administration of a single 500 mg or 1 g dose every 8 hours for 7 days to healthy subjects produced no apparent accumulation; serum protein binding averaged 56% and was independent of dose.

➤*Microbiology:* Aztreonam exhibits potent and specific activity in vitro against a wide spectrum of gram-negative aerobic pathogens including *Pseudomonas aeruginosa.* Aztreonam does not induce β-lactamase activity, and its molecular structure confers a high degree of resistance to hydrolysis by β-lactamases; therefore, it is usually active against gram-negative aerobic organisms. Aztreonam is effective in clinical infections against most strains of the following organisms: *Escherichia coli; Enterobacter* sp.; *Klebsiella pneumoniae* and *K. oxytoca; Proteus mirabilis; P. aeruginosa; Serratia marcescens; Haemophilus influenzae,* including ampicillin-resistant and other penicillinase-producing strains; *Citrobacter* sp.

While in vitro studies have demonstrated susceptibility to aztreonam in most of these strains, clinical efficacy for infections other than those included in the indications section has not been documented such as the following: *Neisseria gonorrhoeae* (including penicillinase-producing strains); *P. vulgaris; Morganella morganii* (formerly *Proteus morganii*); *Providencia* species including *P. stuartii* and *P. rettgeri; Pseudomonas* sp.; *Shigella* sp.; *Pasteurella multocida; Yersinia enterocolitica; Aeromonas hydrophila; N. meningitidis.*

Aztreonam and aminoglycosides are synergistic in vitro against most strains of *P. aeruginosa,* many strains of Enterobacteriaceae, and other gram-negative aerobic bacilli.

Aztreonam has little effect on the anaerobic intestinal microflora in in vitro studies. *Clostridium difficile* and its cytotoxin were not found in animal models following administration of aztreonam.

Contraindications

Hypersensitivity to aztreonam or any other component in the formulation.

Warnings

➤*Pseudomembranous colitis:* This has been reported with nearly all antibacterial agents, including aztreonam, and may range in severity from mild to life-threatening. Therefore, it is important to consider this diagnosis in patients who develop diarrhea subsequent to the administration of antibacterial agents.

Initiate therapeutic measures after the diagnosis of pseudomembranous colitis has been established. Mild cases usually respond to drug discontinuation alone. In moderate-to-severe cases, consider management with fluids and electrolytes, protein supplementation, and treatment with an antibacterial drug clinically effective against *C. difficile* colitis.

➤*Epidermal necrolysis:* Rare cases of toxic epidermal necrolysis have been reported in association with aztreonam in patients undergoing bone marrow transplant with multiple risk factors including graft-vs-host disease, sepsis, radiation therapy, and other concomitantly administered drugs associated with toxic epidermal necrolysis.

➤*Hypersensitivity reactions:* Make careful inquiry for a history of hypersensitivity reactions. Administer with caution to patients who have had hypersensitivity reactions to penicillins, cephalosporins, or carbapenems. If an allergic reaction to aztreonam occurs, discontinue the drug and institute supportive treatment. Refer to Management of Acute Hypersensitivity Reactions. Cross-sensitivity of aztreonam with other penicillins or β-lactam antibiotics is rare.

➤*Renal/Hepatic function impairment:* Appropriate monitoring is recommended.

➤*Pregnancy: Category B.* Aztreonam crosses the placenta and enters fetal circulation. There are no adequate and well-controlled studies in pregnant women. Use during pregnancy only if clearly needed.

➤*Lactation:* Aztreonam is excreted in breast milk in concentrations that are < 1% of maternal serum (see Pharmacokinetics). Consider temporary discontinuation of nursing.

➤*Children:* Safety and efficacy of IV aztreonam have been established children 9 months to 16 years of age. Sufficient data are not available for pediatric patients < 9 months of age or for treatment of the following indications/pathogens: Septicemia and skin and skin-structure infections (where the skin infection is due to *H. influenzae* type b). In pediatric patients with cystic fibrosis, higher doses of aztreonam may be warranted.

Precautions

➤*Superinfection:* Use of antibiotics (especially prolonged or repeated therapy) may result in bacterial (including gram-positive *S. aureus* and *S. faecalis*) or fungal overgrowth of nonsusceptible organisms. Such overgrowth may lead to a secondary infection. Take appropriate measures if superinfection occurs.

Drug Interactions

Aztreonam Drug Interactions			
Precipitant drug	Object drug[*]		Description
Probenecid Furosemide	Aztreonam	↑	Concomitant administration causes clinically insignificant increases in aztreonam serum levels.
Antibiotics (eg, cefoxitin, imipenem)	Aztreonam	↓	Antibiotics may induce high levels of β-lactamase in vitro in some gram-negative aerobes such as *Enterobacter* and *Pseudomonas* sp, resulting in antagonism to many β-lactam antibiotics including aztreonam. Do not use β-lactamase-inducing antibiotics concurrently with aztreonam.
Aztreonam	Aminoglycosides	↑	If an aminoglycoside is used concurrently with aztreonam, especially if high dosages of the former are used or if therapy is prolonged, monitor renal function because of potential nephrotoxicity and ototoxicity of aminoglycoside antibiotics.

[*] ↑ = Object drug increased.   ↓ = Object drug decreased.

AZTREONAM

Adverse Reactions

➤*Children:* Adverse reactions in children including rash, diarrhea, and fever were comparable to those in the adult population. Pain occurred in 1.5% of patients while erythema, induration, and phlebitis had an incidence of 0.5%.

➤*Cardiovascular:* Hypotension, transient ECG changes (ventricular bigeminy and PVC), flushing (< 1%).

➤*CNS:* Seizure, confusion, headache, vertigo, paresthesia, insomnia, dizziness (< 1%).

➤*Dermatologic:* Rash (1% to 1.3%); toxic epidermal necrolysis, purpura, erythema multiforme, exfoliative dermatitis, urticaria, petechiae, pruritus, diaphoresis (< 1%).

➤*GI:* Diarrhea, nausea, vomiting (1% to 1.3%); abdominal cramps, *C. difficile*-associated diarrhea (including pseudomembranous colitis, GI bleeding; symptoms may occur during or after antibiotic treament) (< 1%).

➤*Hematologic:* Pancytopenia, neutropenia, thrombocytopenia, anemia, eosinophilia, leukocytosis, thrombocytosis (< 1%).

➤*Hypersensitivity:* Anaphylaxis, angioedema, bronchospasm (< 1%).

➤*Local:* Phlebitis/thrombophlebitis following IV administration (1.9%); discomfort/swelling at the injection site following IM administration (2.4%).

➤*Special senses:* Tinnitus, diplopia, mouth ulcer, altered taste, numb tongue, sneezing, nasal congestion, halitosis (< 1%).

➤*Miscellaneous:* Vaginal candidiasis, vaginitis, breast tenderness, weakness, muscular aches, fever, malaise, chest pain, dyspnea, wheezing, hepatitis, jaundice (< 1%).

➤*Lab test abnormalities:* Elevations of AST, ALT, and alkaline phosphatase, hepatobiliary dysfunction, increases in prothrombin and partial thromboplastin times, positive Coombs test, and increases in serum creatinine (< 1%).

Children – Of patients < 2 years of age receiving 30 mg/kg every 6 hours, 11.6% experienced neutropenia; of patients > 2 years of age receiving 50 mg/kg every 6 hours, 15% to 20% had elevations of AST and ALT > 3 times the upper limit of normal. The increased frequency of these reported laboratory adverse events may be due either to increased severity of illness treated or higher doses of aztreonam administered.

Overdosage

If necessary, clear aztreonam from the serum by hemodialysis or peritoneal dialysis.

CHLORAMPHENICOL

Rx	**Chloramphenicol Sodium Succinate** (Various)	**Powder for Injection:** 100 mg/ml (as sodium succinate) when reconstituted	1 g in 15 ml vials.
Rx	**Chloromycetin Sodium Succinate** (Parke-Davis)		2.25 mEq sodium per g. In 1 g vials.

WARNING

Serious and fatal blood dyscrasias (aplastic anemia, hypoplastic anemia, thrombocytopenia and granulocytopenia) occur after chloramphenicol administration. Aplastic anemia, which later terminated in leukemia, has been reported. Blood dyscrasias have occurred after both short-term and prolonged therapy. Chloramphenicol must not be used when less potentially dangerous agents are effective. *It must not be used to treat trivial infections (ie, influenza, colds, throat infections), infections other than indicated, or as prophylaxis for bacterial infections.*

It is essential that adequate blood studies be performed during treatment. While blood studies may detect early peripheral blood changes, such as leukopenia, reticulocytopenia or granulocytopenia before they become irreversible, such studies cannot be relied upon to detect bone marrow depression prior to development of aplastic anemia. To facilitate appropriate studies and observation, patients should be hospitalized.

Indications

➤*Serious infections:* Those for which less potentially dangerous drugs are ineffective or contraindicated caused by susceptible strains of *Salmonella* species; *H. influenzae*, specifically, meningeal infections; rickettsiae; lymphogranuloma-psittacosis group; various gram-negative bacteria causing bacteremia, meningitis or other serious gram-negative infections; infections involving anaerobic organisms, when *Bacteroides fragilis* is suspected; other susceptible organisms which have been demonstrated to be resistant to all other appropriate antimicrobial agents.

If presumptive therapy is initiated, perform in vitro sensitivity tests concurrently, so that the drug may be discontinued if less potentially dangerous agents are indicated.

➤*Acute infections:* Those caused by *S. typhi.* Chloramphenicol is a drug of choice. In treatment of typhoid fever, some authorities recommend that chloramphenicol be used at therapeutic levels for 8 to 10 days after the patient becomes afebrile, to lessen the possibility of relapse. It is not recommended for the routine treatment of the typhoid "carrier state."

➤*Cystic fibrosis regimens:*

Administration and Dosage

➤*Therapeutic concentrations:* These generally should be maintained as follows: Peak 10 to 20 mcg/ml; trough 5 to 10 mcg/ml.

➤*Monitoring:* It is important to monitor serum levels because of the variability of chloramphenicol's pharmacokinetics. Monitor serum concentrations weekly; monitor more often in patients with hepatic dysfunction, in therapy > 2 weeks or with potentially interacting drugs (see Drug Interactions).

➤*Adults:* 50 mg/kg/day in divided doses every 6 hours for typhoid fever and rickettsial infections. Exceptional infections (ie, meningitis, brain abscess) due to moderately resistant organisms may require dosage up to 100 mg/kg/day to achieve blood levels inhibiting the pathogen; decrease high doses as soon as possible.

Renal/hepatic function impairment – This reduces the ability to metabolize and excrete the drug. Impaired metabolic processes require that doses be adjusted based on drug concentration in the blood. An initial loading dose of 1 g followed by 500 mg every 6 hours has been recommended in impaired hepatic function.

➤*Children:* 50 to 75 mg/kg/day in divided doses every 6 hours has been recommended for most indications. For meningitis, 50 to 100 mg/kg/day in divided doses every 6 hours has been recommended.

➤*Newborns:* (See Gray syndrome under Adverse Reactions.) 25 mg/kg/day in 4 doses every 6 hours usually produces and maintains adequate concentrations in blood and tissues. Give increased dosage demanded by severe infections only to maintain the blood concentration within an effective range. After the first 2 weeks of life, full-term infants ordinarily may receive up to 50 mg/kg/day in 4 doses every 6 hours.

Neonates (< 2 kg) – 25 mg/kg once daily.

Neonates from birth to 7 days (> 2 kg) – 25 mg/kg once daily.

Neonates over 7 days (> 2 kg) – 50 mg/kg/day in divided doses every 12 hours.

These dosage recommendations are extremely important because blood concentration in all premature and full-term infants < 2 weeks of age differs from that of other infants due to variations in the maturity of the metabolic functions of the liver and kidneys. When these functions are immature (or seriously impaired in adults), the drug is found in high concentrations which tend to increase with succeeding doses.

➤*Infants and children with immature metabolic processes:* 25 mg/kg/day usually produces therapeutic concentrations. In this group particularly, carefully monitor the concentration of drug in the blood.

➤*IV administration:* Chloramphenicol sodium succinate is intended for IV use only; it is ineffective when given IM. It must be hydrolyzed to its active form, and there is a lag in achieving adequate blood levels following infusion. Administer IV as a 10% solution injected over at least 1 minute. Prepare by adding 10 ml of an aqueous diluent (eg, Water for Injection or 5% Dextrose Injection). Substitute oral dosage as soon as feasible.

Actions

➤*Pharmacology:* Chloramphenicol binds to 50 S ribosomal subunits of bacteria and interferes with or inhibits protein synthesis. In vitro, chloramphenicol exerts mainly a bacteriostatic effect on a wide range of gram-negative and gram-positive bacteria.

➤*Pharmacokinetics:*

Absorption – Chloramphenicol base is absorbed rapidly from the intestinal tract and is 75% to 90% bioavailable. In adults, at doses of 1 g every 6 hours for 8 doses, the average peak serum level was 11.2 mcg/ml 1 hour after the first dose, and 18.4 mcg/ml after the fifth 1 g dose. Mean serum levels ranged from 8 to 14 mcg/ml over the 48 hour period.

The inactive prodrug, chloramphenicol palmitate, is rapidly hydrolyzed to active chloramphenicol base. Bioavailability is approximately 80% for the palmitate ester. The bioavailability of the IV succinate is approximately 70%. Hydrolysis of the succinate is probably by esterases of the liver, kidney and lungs. Approximately 30% is eliminated in the urine as unhydrolyzed ester.

Distribution – The therapeutic range for total serum chloramphenicol concentration is: Peak, 10 to 20 mcg/ml; trough, 5 to 10 mcg/ml. The drug is approximately 60% bound to plasma proteins. Because of the significantly greater concentration of free drug in the serum of premature infants, the therapeutic range for total serum concentration of chloramphenicol may be lower.

Chloramphenicol diffuses rapidly, but its distribution is not uniform. Highest concentrations are found in liver and kidney, and lowest concentrations are found in brain and cerebrospinal fluid (CSF). However, chloramphenicol enters the CSF, even in the absence of meningeal inflammation, appearing in concentrations 45% to 99% of those found in the blood. Measurable levels are also detected in pleural and ascitic fluids, saliva, milk and in the aqueous and vitreous humors. Transport across the placental barrier occurs with somewhat lower concentrations in the cord blood of newborns than in maternal blood.

Metabolism/Excretion – Total urinary excretion of chloramphenicol ranges from 68% to 99% over 3 days. From 5% to 15% is excreted as free chloramphenicol; the remainder consists of inactive metabolites via the liver, principally the glucuronide. Since the glucuronide is excreted rapidly, most chloramphenicol detected in the blood is in the active free form. Small amounts of active drug are found in bile and feces.

The elimination half-life of chloramphenicol is approximately 4 hours, and correlates well with serum bilirubin concentration. Protein binding and clearance are decreased in patients with severe liver dysfunction, leading to potentially toxic serum concentrations of free drug.

➤*Microbiology:* Chloramphenicol is effective against a wide range of gram-positive and -negative bacteria, and is active in vitro against rickettsiae, the lymphogranuloma-psittacosis group and *Vibrio cholerae.* It is particularly active against *Salmonella typhi* and *Haemophilus influenzae.*

Contraindications

History of hypersensitivity to, or toxicity from, chloramphenicol.

Chloramphenicol must not be used to treat trivial infections (ie, colds, influenza, throat infections), infections other than indicated, or as prophylaxis for bacterial infections.

Warnings

➤*Blood dyscrasias:* See Warning Box. Serious and fatal blood dyscrasias (aplastic anemia, hypoplastic anemia, thrombocytopenia and granulocytopenia) occur. An irreversible type of marrow depression leading to aplastic anemia with a high rate of mortality is characterized by appearance of bone marrow aplasia or hypoplasia weeks or months after therapy. Peripherally, pancytopenia is most often observed, but only one or two of the three major cell types (erythrocytes, leukocytes and platelets) may be depressed. This complication appears unrelated to administration route. One estimate based on 149 cases stated that the route was oral in 83%, parenteral in 14% and rectal in 3%. Several cases of aplastic anemia have been associated with chloramphenicol ophthalmic ointment.

CHLORAMPHENICOL

A dose-related reversible type of bone marrow depression may occur and is associated with sustained serum levels at peak ≥ 25 mcg/ml, trough ≥ 10 mcg/ml. This type of marrow depression is characterized by vacuolization of the erythroid cells, a decrease in red cell iron uptake, an increase in circulating serum iron with saturation of iron-binding globulin (usually within 6 to 10 days) and reduction of reticulocytes (usually within 5 to 7 days) and leukopenia; it responds promptly to withdrawal of the drug.

➤*Renal/Hepatic function impairment:* Excessive blood levels may result from the use of the recommended dose in patients with impaired liver or kidney function, including that due to immature metabolic processes in the infant. Adjust dosage accordingly or, preferably, determine the blood concentration at appropriate intervals.

➤*Pregnancy:* There are no studies to establish the safety of this drug in pregnancy. Since it readily crosses the placental barrier, cautious use is particularly important during pregnancy at term or during labor because of potential toxic effects on the fetus (gray syndrome).

➤*Lactation:* Chloramphenicol appears in breast milk with a milk: plasma ratio of 0.5. Use with caution, if at all, during lactation, because of the possibility of toxic effects on the nursing infant.

➤*Children:* Use with caution and in reduced dosages in premature and full-term infants to avoid gray syndrome toxicity. (See Adverse Reactions.) Monitor drug serum levels carefully during therapy of the newborn.

Precautions

➤*Hematology:* Evaluate baseline and periodic blood studies approximately every 2 days during therapy. Discontinue the drug upon appearance of reticulocytopenia, leukopenia, thrombocytopenia, anemia or any other findings attributable to chloramphenicol. Such studies do not exclude the possible later appearance of the irreversible type of bone marrow depression. Avoid concurrent therapy with other drugs that may cause bone marrow depression.

Avoid repeated courses if at all possible. Do not continue treatment longer than required to produce a cure.

➤*Acute intermittent porphyria or glucose-6-phosphate dehydrogenase deficiency:* Use with caution in patients with these conditions.

➤*Superinfection:* Use of antibiotics (especially prolonged or repeated therapy) may result in bacterial or fungal overgrowth of nonsusceptible organisms. Such overgrowth may lead to a secondary infection. Take appropriate measures if superinfection occurs.

Drug Interactions

Chloramphenicol Drug Interactions

Precipitant drug	Object drug*		Description
Barbiturates	Chloramphenicol	↓	Decreased chloramphenicol serum levels may occur, and barbiturate clearance may be decreased, resulting in increased levels or toxicity.
Chloramphenicol	Barbiturates	↑	
Rifampin	Chloramphenicol	↓	Concomitant administration may reduce serum chloramphenicol levels, presumably through hepatic enzyme induction.
Chloramphenicol	Anticoagulants	↑	Anticoagulant action may be enhanced.
Chloramphenicol	Cyclophospha-mide	↓	Decreased or delayed activation of cyclophosphamide may occur, although it is unclear if a significant decrease in its effect would occur.
Chloramphenicol	Hydantoins	↑	Serum hydantoin levels may be increased, possibly resulting in toxicity. In addition, chloramphenicol levels may be increased or decreased.
Hydantoins	Chloramphenicol	↔	

Chloramphenicol Drug Interactions

Precipitant drug	Object drug*		Description
Chloramphenicol	Iron salts	↑	Serum iron levels may be increased.
Chloramphenicol	Penicillins	↔	Synergistic effects may develop in the treatment of certain microorganisms, but antagonism may also occur.
Chloramphenicol	Sulfonylureas	↑	Clinical manifestations of hypoglycemia may occur with concurrent use.
Chloramphenicol	Vitamin B$_{12}$	↓	Hematologic effects of vitamin B$_{12}$ may be decreased in patients with pernicious anemia by concurrent chloramphenicol.

*↑ = Object drug increased. ↓ = Object drug decreased. ↔ = Undetermined effect.

Adverse Reactions

➤*CNS:* Headache; mild depression; mental confusion; delirium. Optic and peripheral neuritis have been reported, usually following long-term therapy; if this occurs, promptly withdraw the drug.

➤*GI:* Nausea; vomiting; glossitis; stomatitis; diarrhea; enterocolitis (low incidence).

➤*Hematologic:* (see Warnings).

Blood dyscrasias – The most serious adverse effect is bone marrow depression.

Aplastic anemia – It is estimated to occur in 1:40,000 cases (range 1:19,000 to 1:200,000). There have been reports of aplastic anemia attributed to the drug which later terminated in leukemia.

Hemoglobinuria – Paroxysmal nocturnal hemoglobinuria has been reported.

➤*Hypersensitivity:* Fever; macular and vesicular rashes; angioedema; urticaria; anaphylaxis. Herxheimer reactions have occurred during therapy for typhoid fever.

➤*Miscellaneous:*

Gray syndrome – Toxic reactions including fatalities (approximately 40%) have occurred in the premature infant and newborn; the signs and symptoms associated with these reactions have been referred to as the "gray syndrome". The following summarizes the clinical and laboratory studies:

• In most cases, therapy was instituted within the first 48 hours of life.
• Symptoms first appeared after 3 to 4 days of treatment with high doses.
• Symptoms appeared in the following order: Abdominal distension with or without emesis; progressive pallid cyanosis; vasomotor collapse, frequently accompanied by irregular respiration; death within a few hours of onset. Other initial symptoms may include refusal to suck, loose green stools, flaccidity, ashen color, decrease in temperature and refractory lactic acidosis. Death occurs in approximately 40% of the patients within 2 days of initial symptoms.
• Progression of symptoms was accelerated with higher doses.
• Serum level studies revealed unusually high drug concentrations (≥ 40 mcg/ml after repeated doses) with doses in excess of 25 mg/kg/day in newborns.
• Termination of therapy upon early evidence of associated symptoms frequently reversed the process with complete recovery.
• Preexisting liver dysfunction may be a significant risk factor.

Patient Information

Preferably taken on an empty stomach at least 1 hour before or 2 hours after meals. Take with food if GI upset occurs.

Take at evenly spaced intervals (every 6 hours) around the clock.

Notify physician if fever, sore throat, tiredness or unusual bleeding or bruising occurs.

NALIDIXIC ACID

Rx	**NegGram** (Sanofi Winthrop)	**Caplets**: 250 mg	Scored. In 56s.
		500 mg	Scored. In 56s and 500s.
		1 g	Scored. In 100s.
		Suspension: 250 mg per 5 ml	Saccharin, sorbitol. Raspberry flavor. In 480 ml.

Indications

➤*Urinary tract infections:* Caused by susceptible gram-negative microorganisms, including the majority of Proteus strains, *Klebsiella* and *Enterobacter* species and *E. coli.*

Administration and Dosage

Underdosage (< 4 g/day) during initial treatment may predispose to emergence of bacterial resistance.

➤*Adults:*

Initial therapy – 1 g 4 times/day (total dose 4 g/day) for 1 or 2 weeks.

Prolonged therapy – May be reduced to 2 g/day after the initial treatment period.

➤*Children (3 months to ≤ 12 years of age):*

Initial therapy – 55 mg/kg/day (25 mg/lb/day) in 4 equally divided doses.

Prolonged therapy – May be reduced to 33 mg/kg/day (15 mg/lb/day).

Do not administer to infants < 3 months of age.

Actions

➤*Pharmacology:* Nalidixic acid, a bactericidal agent, appears to interfere with DNA polymerization.

➤*Pharmacokinetics:*

Absorption/Distribution – Nalidixic acid is well absorbed; peak serum levels of 20 to 40 mcg/ml are attained 1 to 2 hours after an oral 1 g dose. The drug concentrates in renal tissue and seminal fluid; it does not penetrate prostatic tissue.

Metabolism/Excretion – Hepatic metabolism to hydroxynalidixic acid (activity similar to nalidixic acid) and inactive conjugates is followed by rapid renal excretion. Protein binding is ≈ 93% to 97% for nalidixic acid and 63% for hydroxynalidixic acid. Approximately 2% to 3% of nalidixic acid and 13% of hydroxynalidixic acid appear in the urine. Plasma half-life in normal renal function is 1.5 hours; half-life in urine is about 6 hours. Renal failure significantly affects renal clearance of nalidixic acid, increasing serum concentrations and decreasing urine levels of parent and metabolites. Approximately 4% of nalidixic acid is excreted in the feces.

➤*Microbiology:* Nalidixic acid is bactericidal and has marked antibacterial activity over the urinary pH against gram-negative bacteria (eg, *Proteus mirabilis, P. morganii, P. vulgaris, Providencia rettgeri, Escherichia coli, Enterobacter* and *Klebsiella* species). *Pseudomonas* strains are generally resistant. Conventional chromosomal resistance to full dosage emerges in ≈ 2% to 14% of patients during treatment.

Contraindications

Hypersensitivity to nalidixic acid; history of convulsive disorders.

Warnings

➤*CNS:* Brief convulsions, increased intracranial pressure and toxic psychosis (rare) usually occur from overdosage or with predisposing factors, such as epilepsy, cerebral vascular insufficiency, parkinsonism, mental instability or cerebral arteriosclerosis. They usually rapidly disappear upon drug discontinuation. If these reactions occur, discontinue use and institute therapeutic measures. If CNS symptoms do not disappear within 48 hours, perform diagnostic procedures even if risky to the patient. In infants and children receiving therapeutic doses, intracranial hypertension, increased intracranial pressure with bulging anterior fontanelle, papilledema and headache have occasionally occurred. A few cases of sixth cranial nerve palsy were reported. Signs and symptoms usually disappear rapidly upon discontinuation.

➤*Hematologic:* Nalidixic acid has caused hemolytic anemia in patients with or without glucose–6–phosphate dehydrogenase deficiency (G-6-PD).

➤*Renal function impairment:* Therapeutic concentrations in the urine, without increased toxicity due to drug accumulation in the blood, have occurred in patients on full dosage with creatinine clearances as low as 2 to 8 ml/min. However, exercise caution.

➤*Pregnancy: Category B.* Safe use during the first trimester has not been established. The drug has been used during the last two trimesters without apparent ill effects on mother or child. No drug-linked congenital defects have been reported.

Labor and delivery – Use caution when giving nalidixic acid in the days prior to delivery because of the theoretical risk that exposure in utero may lead to significant blood levels in the neonate immediately after birth. Advise patients using nalidixic acid during pregnancy to discontinue use at the first sign of labor.

➤*Lactation:* Data are scant; reported milk:plasma ratios are 0.08 to 0.13. Milk levels of 4 mcg/ml have been noted. Although the amounts are small, hemolytic anemia has been reported in one infant whose mother received 1 g nalidixic acid, 4 times/day.

➤*Children:* Nalidixic acid and related drugs can produce erosions of the cartilage in weight-bearing joints and other signs of arthropathy in animals. No joint lesions have been reported in humans; however, use care in prepubertal children.

Precautions

➤*Monitoring:* Perform periodic blood counts and renal and liver function tests if treatment is continued for > 2 weeks.

➤*Resistance:* If bacterial resistance emerges, it is usually within 48 hours, permitting rapid change to another drug. If clinical response is unsatisfactory or if relapse occurs, repeat cultures and sensitivity tests. Underdosage (< 4 g/day for adults) may predispose to resistance. Cross-resistance with cinoxacin has occurred.

➤*Special risk:* Use with caution in liver disease, epilepsy or severe cerebral arteriosclerosis patients.

➤*Photosensitivity:* Photosensitization (photoallergy or phototoxicity) may occur; therefore, caution patients to take protective measures (ie, sunscreens, protective clothing) against exposure to sunlight or ultraviolet light (eg, tanning beds) until tolerance is determined.

Drug Interactions

➤*Anticoagulants:* Nalidixic acid may enhance the anticoagulant effects by displacing significant amounts of these drugs from serum albumin binding sites.

➤*Drug/Lab test interactions:* Urinary metabolites of nalidixic acid liberate glucuronic acid and produce false-positive **urinary glucose** results when Benedict's or Fehling's solutions or *Clinitest* reagent tablets are used. Avoid this problem by using *Clinistix* or *Tes-Tape.* **Urinary 17–keto and ketogenic steroids** may be falsely elevated due to an interaction between nalidixic acid and the m–dinitrobenzene used in the assay. In such cases, use the Porter-Silber method.

Adverse Reactions

➤*CNS:* Drowsiness; weakness; headache; dizziness; vertigo; toxic psychosis, brief convulsions (rare); intracranial hypertension; increased intracranial pressure with bulging anterior fontanel, papilledema and headache; sixth cranial nerve palsy in children and infants (see Warnings).

➤*GI:* Abdominal pain; nausea; vomiting; diarrhea.

➤*Hypersensitivity:* Rash; pruritus; urticaria; angioedema; eosinophilia; arthralgia with joint stiffness and swelling; anaphylactoid reaction (rare).

➤*Hematologic:* Thrombocytopenia, leukopenia or hemolytic anemia, sometimes associated with G-6-PD deficiency (rare).

➤*Ophthalmic:* Reversible subjective visual disturbances occur infrequently (generally with each dose during the first few days) and include overbrightness of lights, change in color perception, focusing difficulty, decrease in visual acuity and double vision. They usually disappear promptly with reduced dosage or discontinuation.

➤*Miscellaneous:* Cholestatic jaundice, cholestasis, paresthesia, metabolic acidosis (rare).

Photosensitivity – Reactions (eg, erythema and painful bullae on exposed skin surfaces) usually resolve completely in 2 weeks to 2 months after discontinuing the drug. However, bullae may continue to appear with successive exposures to sunlight or with mild skin trauma for up to 3 months after discontinuation.

Overdosage

➤*Symptoms:* Toxic psychosis, convulsions, increased intracranial pressure, metabolic acidosis, vomiting, nausea and lethargy may occur in patients taking more than the recommended dosage.

➤*Treatment:* Reactions are short lived (2 to 3 hours) because the drug is rapidly excreted. If overdosage is noted early, gastric lavage is indicated. If absorption has occurred, increase fluid administration and have supportive measures available. Anticonvulsants may be indicated in severe cases.

Patient Information

May cause GI upset; take with food.

May produce drowsiness, dizziness or blurred vision; observe caution while driving or performing other tasks requiring alertness, coordination or physical dexterity.

Avoid prolonged exposure to sunlight; photosensitivity may occur.

If seizures, psychotic behavior (eg, hallucinations, incoherent speech, confusion) or severe headaches occur while on nalidixic acid, contact the physician immediately.

CINOXACIN

| Rx | **Cinoxacin** (Biocraft) | **Capsules**: 250 mg | (Biocraft 163). Blue/yellow. In 40s and 100s. |
| Rx | **Cinoxacin** (Various, eg, Moore, Rugby) | **Capsules**: 500 mg | In 50s and 100s. |

Indications

➤*Urinary tract infections:* Treatment of initial and recurrent urinary tract infections in adults caused by the following susceptible microorganisms: *E. coli, P. mirabilis, P. vulgaris, Klebsiella* sp. (including *K. pneumoniae*) and *Enterobacter* sp.

Effective in preventing urinary tract infections for up to 5 months in women with a history of recurrent urinary tract infections.

Administration and Dosage

The usual adult dosage is 1 g/day, in 2 or 4 divided doses for 7 to 14 days. Although susceptible organisms may be eradicated within a few days after therapy has begun, the full treatment course is recommended.

➤*Renal function impairment:* A reduced dosage must be employed. After an initial dose of 500 mg, use the following maintenance dosage schedule:

Cinoxacin Maintenance Dosage Guide for Renal Impairment		
Creatinine clearance (ml/min/1.73 m^2)	Renal Function	Dosage
> 80	Normal	500 mg bid
80-50	Mild impairment	250 mg tid
50-20	Moderate impairment	250 mg bid
< 20	Marked impairment	250 mg daily

Administration of cinoxacin to anuric patients is not recommended.

When only serum creatinine is available, use the following formula to convert this value into creatinine clearance. The serum creatinine should represent a steady-state of renal function.

$$\text{Males:} \quad \frac{\text{Weight (kg)} \times (140 - \text{age})}{72 \times \text{serum creatinine (mg/dL)}} = \text{Ccr}$$

Females: $0.85 \times$ above value

➤*Preventive therapy:* A single dose of 250 mg at bedtime for up to 5 months has been shown to be effective in women with a history of recurrent urinary tract infections.

Actions

➤*Pharmacology:* Cinoxacin, a synthetic organic acid chemically related to nalidixic acid, inhibits DNA replication. The drug is active within the range of urinary pH.

➤*Pharmacokinetics:*

Absorption/Distribution – Cinoxacin is rapidly absorbed after oral administration. Mean peak plasma concentrations of 15 mcg/ml occur ≈ 2 hours after a single 500 mg dose and detectable levels persist 10 to 12 hours. Food decreases peak serum concentrations by about 30%, although the total extent of absorption is not altered. It is > 60% protein bound.

Metabolism/Excretion – Average urine concentrations of 300 mcg/ml occur within 4 hours; urine concentrations usually exceed the MIC (ie, 10 to 30 mcg/ml). The mean serum half-life is 1 to 1.5 hours with normal renal function; renal failure increases half-life. Oral cinoxacin is 97% excreted in the urine within 24 hours. Approximately 60% of cinoxacin is excreted unchanged, 40% as inactive metabolites.

➤*Microbiology:* Cinoxacin has in vitro activity against a wide variety of aerobic gram-negative bacilli, particularly strains of *Enterobacteriaceae*. It is active against most strains of the following organisms: *Escherichia coli, Klebsiella* sp., *Enterobacter* sp. *Proteus mirabilis* and *P. vulgaris*.

Cinoxacin is NOT active against *Pseudomonas*, enterococci or staphylococci. Cross-resistance with nalidixic acid has been demonstrated. Conventional chromosomal resistance to cinoxacin has been reported in ≈ 4% of patients treated with recommended doses; bacterial resistance to cinoxacin has not been shown to be transferable via R-factor (plasmids).

Contraindications

Hypersensitivity to cinoxacin or other quinolones.

Warnings

➤*Convulsions and abnormal EEGs:* These have been reported in a few patients receiving quinolone class antimicrobials. Convulsions, increased intracranial pressure and toxic psychoses have also occurred in patients receiving other drugs in this class.

Quinolones may also cause CNS stimulation with tremors, restlessness, lightheadedness, confusion or hallucinations. If these reactions occur in patients receiving cinoxacin, discontinue the drug and institute appropriate measures. As with all quinolones, use with caution in patients with known or suspected CNS disorders (eg, severe cerebral arteriosclerosis, epilepsy) that predispose to seizures.

➤*Hypersensitivity reactions:* Serious and occasionally fatal hypersensitivity (anaphylactic) reactions, some following the first dose, have occurred in patients receiving quinolone class antimicrobials. Some reactions were accompanied by cardiovascular collapse, loss of consciousness, tingling, pharyngeal or facial edema, dyspnea, urticaria and itching. Only a few patients had a history of previous hypersensitivity reactions. If an allergic reaction to cinoxacin occurs, discontinue the drug. Refer to Management of Acute Hypersensitivity Reactions.

➤*Renal function impairment:* Since cinoxacin is primarily eliminated by the kidney, decrease dosage in patients with reduced renal function. Administration is not recommended for anuric patients.

➤*Pregnancy: Category B.* There are no adequate and well controlled studies in pregnant women. Since cinoxacin causes arthropathy in immature animals (see Children), its use during pregnancy is not recommended.

➤*Lactation:* It is not known whether cinoxacin is excreted in breast milk. Because other drugs in this class are excreted in breast milk and because of the potential for serious adverse reactions in nursing infants, discontinue nursing or discontinue the drug, taking into account the importance of the drug to the mother.

➤*Children:* Safety and efficacy of use in adolescents and children < 18 years of age have not been established. Cinoxacin and other quinolones have produced erosions of the cartilage in weight-bearing joints and other signs of arthropathy in immature animals of various species.

Precautions

➤*Monitoring:* As with any potent drug, periodic assessment of organ system function, including renal, hepatic and hematopoietic function is advisable during prolonged therapy.

➤*Crystalluria:* Although not expected to occur with usual cinoxacin doses, patients should be well hydrated; avoid alkalinization of urine.

➤*Hazardous tasks:* Patients should use caution while driving or performing other tasks requiring alertness, coordination or physical dexterity.

➤*Photosensitivity:* Photosensitization (photoallergy or phototoxicity) may occur; therefore, caution patients to take protective measures (ie, sunscreens, protective clothing) against exposure to sunlight or ultraviolet light (eg, tanning beds) until tolerance is determined.

Drug Interactions

Probenecid pretreatment will block tubule secretion of cinoxacin, and thus, will reduce the elimination rate, increase half-life, decrease urine concentrations by 20% and double serum concentrations.

Also consider drug interactions listed with the Fluoroquinolones (see monograph in Anti-Infectives chapter).

➤*Drug/Food interactions:* Food decreases peak serum cinoxacin by ≈ 30%, although total extent of absorption is not altered.

Adverse Reactions

The overall incidence of adverse reactions is approximately 4%.

➤*CNS:* Headache, dizziness (1%); insomnia, drowsiness, tingling sensation, photophobia, tinnitus (< 1%).

➤*GI:* Nausea (< 3%); anorexia, vomiting, abdominal cramps/pain, diarrhea, perineal burning, distorted taste sensation (1%).

➤*Hematologic:* Thrombocytopenia (rare).

➤*Hypersensitivity:* Rash, urticaria, pruritus, edema, angioedema, eosinophilia (< 3%); anaphylactoid reactions (rare); toxic epidermal necrolysis (very rare); erythema multiforme; Stevens-Johnson syndrome.

CINOXACIN

▶*Lab test abnormalities:* Laboratory values reported to be abnormally elevated were, in order of frequency – BUN, AST, ALT, serum creatinine, alkaline phosphatase and reduction in hematocrit/hemoglobin (each ≤ 1%).

Overdosage

▶*Symptoms:* Anorexia, nausea, vomiting, epigastric distress and diarrhea may follow an overdose of cinoxacin. The severity of epigastric distress and the diarrhea are dose-related. Headache, dizziness, insomnia, photophobia, tinnitus and a tingling sensation have occurred in some patients. If other symptoms are present, they are probably secondary to an underlying disease state, an allergic reaction or the ingestion of a second medication with toxicity.

▶*Treatment:* Patients who have ingested an overdose of cinoxacin shoud be kept well hydrated to prevent crystalluria. Protect the patient's airway and support ventilation and perfusion. Meticulously monitor and maintain, within acceptable limits, the patient's vital signs, blood gases, serum electrolytes, etc. Absorption of drugs from the GI tract may be decreased by giving activated charcoal, which, in many cases, is more effective than emesis or lavage. Forced diuresis, peritoneal dialysis, hemodialysis or charcoal hemoperfusion have not been established as beneficial for a cinoxacin overdose. Refer to General Management of Acute Overdosage.

Patient Information

May be taken without regard to meals, but drink fluids liberally.

May cause dizziness; observe caution while driving or performing other tasks requiring alertness, coordination or physical dexterity.

Avoid excessive sunlight during therapy. If phototoxicity occurs, discontinue therapy.

Indications

For specific approved indications, refer to individual drug monographs.

►*Unlabeled uses:*

Ciprofloxacin – Ciprofloxacin has been used in children with cystic fibrosis for periods of 10 days to 6 months without documented adverse effects or intolerance.

Trovafloxacin – Trovafloxacin is being evaluated as therapy for bacterial meningitis in children. Also, multidrug-resistant gram negative meningitis in neonates and immunocompromised children.

Trovafloxacin, gatifloxacin, and moxifloxacin – Trovafloxacin, gatifloxacin, and moxifloxacin are effective against multidrug-resistant strains of *S. pneumoniae* and, therefore, may be used in pediatric patients who fail initial treatment for acute otitis media and sinusitis.

Ciprofloxacin and norfloxacin – Ciprofloxacin and norfloxacin have been used for the treatment of gastroenteritis in children.

Mycobacterial infections – In children, atypical mycobacterial infections have been satisfactorily treated with ciprofloxacin as part of combination therapy; in vitro, gatifloxacin has been shown to be active against *M. leprae*.

Fluoroquinolones – Fluoroquinolones are used as empiric therapy for low-risk febrile neutropenic pediatric patients. Regimens including fluoroquinolones for tuberculosis have been shown to be equivalent to standard antituberculosis regimens, and these agents are currently suggested for the management of multidrug-resistant infections or in patients with adverse reactions to other agents. The outcome of regimens including quinolones has been poorer in HIV-seropositive patients. Ciprofloxacin and ofloxacin are the quinolones most often evaluated and recommended in mycobacterial diseases.

Actions

►*Pharmacology:* The fluoroquinolones are synthetic, broad-spectrum antibacterial agents that inhibit DNA gyrase and topoisomerase IV. DNA gyrase is an essential enzyme that is involved in the replication, transcription, and repair of bacterial DNA. Topoisomerase IV is an enzyme known to play a key role in the partitioning of the chromosomal DNA during bacterial cell division. The basic molecule has been modified at the N-1 position, with different groups added to the C-6, C-7, and C-8 positions. The addition of a fluorine atom at position C-6 enhances DNA gyrase inhibitory activity and provides activity against *staphylococci*; addition of a second fluorine group at position C-8 increases absorption and longer half-life; the addition of a piperazine group at position C-7 provides the best gram-negative activity; ring alkylation improves gram-positive activity and half-life; substitution of a methyl group for the piperazine group increases absorption and a longer half-life; and addition of acyclopropyl group at position N-1 and amino group at position C-5 and a fluorine group at C-8 increases activity against mycoplasma and chlamydia.

►*Pharmacokinetics:*

Pharmacokinetics of Fluoroquinolones							
Fluoroquinolone	Bio-availability (%)	Max urine concentration (mcg/mL) (dose)	Mean peak plasma concentration (mcg/mL) (dose)	Area under curve (AUC) (mcg·hr/mL) (dose)	Protein binding (%)	t½ (hr)	Urine recovery unchanged (%)
Ciprofloxacin Oral	≈ 70-80	> 200 (250 mg)	1.2 (250 mg) 2.4 (500 mg) 4.3 (750 mg) 5.4 (1000 mg)	4.8 (250 mg) 11.6 (500 mg) 20.2 (750 mg) 30.8 (1000 mg)	20-40	≈ 4	≈ 40-50
IV		> 200 (200 mg) > 400 (400 mg)	4.4 (400 mg)	4.8 (200 mg) 11.6 (400 mg)		≈ 5-6	≈ 50-70
Enoxacin	≈ 90	nd[1]	0.93 (200 mg) 2 (400 mg)		≈ 40	3-6	> 40
Gatifloxacin[2] Oral	≈ 96		≈ 2 (200 mg single dose) ≈ 3.8 (400 mg single dose) ≈ 4.2 (400 mg multiple dose)	≈ 14.2 (200 mg single dose) ≈ 33 (400 mg single dose) ≈ 34.4 (400 mg multiple dose)	≈ 20	≈ 7.8 (400 mg single dose) ≈7.1 (400 mg multiple dose)	≈ 73.8 (200 mg single dose) ≈72.4 (400 mg single dose) ≈ 80.2 (400 mg multiple dose)
IV			≈ 2.2 (200 mg single dose) ≈ 2.4 (200 mg multiple dose) ≈ 5.5 (400 mg single dose) ≈ 4.6 (400 mg multiple dose)	≈ 15.9 (200 mg single dose) ≈ 16.8 (200 mg multiple dose) ≈ 35.1 (400 mg single dose) ≈ 35.4 (400 mg multiple dose)		≈ 11.1 (200 mg single dose) ≈ 12.3 (200 mg multiple dose) ≈ 7.4 (400 mg single dose) ≈ 13.9 (400 mg multiple dose)	≈ 71.7 (200 mg single dose) ≈ 72.4 (200 mg multiple dose) ≈ 62.3 (400 mg single dose) ≈ 83.5 (400 mg multiple dose)
Levofloxacin	≈ 99		≈ 2.8-11.5 (single dose oral or IV) ≈ 5.7-12.1 (multiple dose oral or IV)	≈ 27.2-110 (single dose oral or IV) ≈ 47.5-108 (multiple dose oral or IV)	≈ 24-38	≈ 6.3-7.5 (single dose oral or IV) ≈ 7-8.8 (multiple dose oral or IV)	≈ 87 (oral)
Lomefloxacin	≈ 95-98	> 300 (400 mg)	0.8 (100 mg) 1.4 (200 mg) 3.2 (400 mg)	5.6 (100 mg) 10.9 (200 mg) 26.1 (400 mg)	≈ 10	≈ 8	≈ 65
Moxifloxacin	≈ 90		4.5 (400 mg)	≈ 48 (400 mg)	≈ 50	≈ 12	≈ 20
Norfloxacin	30-40	≥ 200 (400 mg)	0.8 (200 mg) 1.5 (400 mg) 2.4 (800 mg)		10-15	3-4	26-32
Ofloxacin Oral	≈ 98	≈ 220 (200 mg)	1.5 (200 mg) 2.4 (300 mg) 2.9 (400 mg) 4.6 (400 mg steady-state)	14.1 (200 mg) 21.2 (300 mg) 31.4 (400 mg) 61 (400 mg steady-state)	≈ 32	≈ 9	65-80
IV		nd[1]	2.7 (200 mg) 4 (400 mg)	43.5 (400 mg)	≈ 32	5-10	≈ 65
Sparfloxacin	92	> 12 (400 mg)[3]	≈ 1.3 (400 mg)	≈ 34 (400 mg)	≈ 45	≈ 20	≈ 10
Trovafloxacin/Alatrofloxacin[2] Trovafloxacin Single-dose	≈ 88 (oral)		≈ 1 (100 mg) ≈ 2.1 (200 mg)	≈ 11.2 (100 mg) ≈ 26.7 (200 mg)	≈ 76	9.1 (100 mg) 9.6 (200 mg)	≈ 6 (oral)
Multiple dose		≈ 12.1 (200 mg)	≈ 1.1 (100 mg) ≈ 3.1 (200 mg)	≈ 11.8 (100 mg) ≈ 34.4 (200 mg)		10.5 (100 mg) 12.2 (200 mg)	
Alatrofloxacin[4] Single-dose			≈ 2.7 (200 mg) ≈ 3.6 (300 mg)	≈ 28.1 (200 mg) ≈ 46.1 (300 mg)		9.4 (200 mg) 11.2 (300 mg)	
Multiple dose			≈ 3.1 (200 mg) ≈ 4.4 (300 mg)	≈ 32.2 (200 mg) ≈ 46.3 (300 mg)		11.7 (200 mg) 12.7 (300 mg)	

[1] nd = no data.
[2] Single dose: AUC (0-∞); Multiple dose: AUC (0-24).
[3] Following a 400 mg loading dose of sparfloxacin, the mean urine concentration 4 hours postdose was in excess of 12 mcg/mL.
[4] Trovafloxacin equivalents.

Norfloxacin –

Absorption/Distribution: Absorption is rapid. Food or dairy products may decrease absorption. Steady-state norfloxacin levels will be attained within 2 days of dosing. Urinary concentrations of ≥ 200 mcg/mL are attained 2 to 3 hours after a single 400 mg dose.

Mean urinary concentrations of norfloxacin remain above 30 mcg/mL for at least 12 hours following a 400 mg dose. Norfloxacin is least soluble at urinary pH of 7.5; greater solubility occurs at pHs above and below this value.

Metabolism/Excretion: Norfloxacin is eliminated through metabolism, biliary excretion, and renal excretion. Renal excretion occurs by glomerular filtration and tubular secretion, as evidenced by the high rate of renal clearance ($\approx$ 275 mL/min). Within 24 hours of administration, 5% to 8% of the dose is recovered in the urine as 6 less-active metabolites. Fecal recovery accounts for another 30%. In healthy elderly volunteers (65 to 75 years of age), norfloxacin is eliminated more slowly because of decreased renal function. Drug absorption appears unaffected. Disposition of norfloxacin in patients with creatinine clearance (Ccr) rates > 30 mL/min/1.73 m^2 is similar to that in healthy volunteers. In patients with Ccr rates $\leq$ 30 mL/min/1.73 m^2, the renal elimination decreases so that the effective serum half-life is 6.5 hours; dosage alteration is necessary. See Administration and Dosage.

Enoxacin –
Absorption: Peak plasma levels are achieved in 1 to 3 hours. Effect of food on absorption has not been studied. In elderly, mean peak plasma concentrations are 50% higher than in young adults.

Distribution: Enoxacin diffuses into the cervix, fallopian tube, and myometrium at levels $\approx$ 1 to 2 times those in plasma, and into the kidney and prostate at levels $\approx$ 2 to 4 times plasma levels.

Metabolism: Five metabolites have been identified in the urine and account for 15% to 20% of a dose. Some isozymes of the cytochrome P450 hepatic microsomal enzyme system are inhibited by enoxacin, resulting in significant drug interactions with some agents (see Drug Interactions).

Excretion: Clearance is reduced in renal impairment; dosage adjustment is necessary (see Administration and Dosage).

Ciprofloxacin –
Absorption/Distribution: Ciprofloxacin is rapidly and well absorbed from the GI tract after oral administration with no substantial loss by first-pass metabolism. When given concomitantly with food, there is a delay in the absorption of the drug, resulting in peak concentrations that are closer to 2 hours after dosing rather than 1 hour. However, the overall absorption is not substantially affected. Maximum serum concentrations are attained 1 to 2 hours after oral dosing. Mean concentrations 12 hours after dosing with 250, 500, or 750 mg are 0.1, 0.2, and 0.4 mcg/mL, respectively. Following 60-minute IV infusions of 200 and 400 mg, mean maximum serum concentrations achieved were 2.1 and 4.6 mcg/mL, respectively; concentrations at 12 hours were 0.1 and 0.2 mcg/mL, respectively. Ciprofloxacin is widely distributed throughout the body. Tissue concentrations often exceed serum concentrations in men and women, particularly in genital tissue. The drug diffuses into the cerebrospinal fluid (CSF); however, CSF concentrations are generally < 10% of peak serum concentrations.

Metabolism/Excretion: Four metabolites have been identified in urine which, together, account for $\approx$ 15% of an oral dose. The metabolites have antimicrobial activity, but are less active than unchanged ciprofloxacin. After IV administration, 3 metabolites have been identified in urine, which account for $\approx$ 10% of the IV dose. After a 250 mg oral dose, urine concentrations usually exceed 200 mcg/mL during the first 2 hours and are $\approx$ 30 mcg/mL at 8 to 12 hours after dosing. Following a 200 or 400 mg IV dose, urine concentrations usually exceed 200 and 400 mcg/mL, respectively, during the first 2 hours and are generally > 15 and > 30 mcg/mL, respectively, at 8 to 12 hours after dosing. Urinary ciprofloxacin excretion is virtually complete within 24 hours after dosing. Renal clearance is $\approx$ 300 mL/min; active tubular secretion plays a significant role. Although bile concentrations are several-fold higher than serum after oral dosing, only a small amount is recovered from the bile. Approximately 20% to 35% of an oral dose is recovered from feces within 5 days after dosing. In patients with reduced renal function, the half-life is slightly prolonged; dosage adjustments may be required. See Administration and Dosage.

Ofloxacin –
Absorption/Distribution: Maximum serum concentrations are achieved 1 to 2 hours after an oral dose. The amount absorbed increases proportionally with the dose. Elimination is biphasic; half-lives are $\approx$ 4 to 5 hours and 20 to 25 hours, although accumulation at steady state can be estimated using a half-life of 9 hours. Steady-state concentrations are achieved after 4 doses and are $\approx$ 40% higher than concentrations after single doses. Ofloxacin is widely distributed to body tissues and fluids.

Metabolism/Excretion: Ofloxacin has a pyridobenzoxazine ring that appears to decrease the extent of parent compound metabolism; < 5% of a dose is recovered in the urine as the desmethyl or N-oxide metabolites. Elimination is mainly by renal excretion; 4% to 8% is excreted in the feces. A longer plasma half-life of $\approx$ 6.4 to 7.4 hours was observed in elderly subjects, compared with 4 to 5 hours for young subjects. Slower elimination is observed in elderly subjects as compared with younger subjects, which may be attributable to the reduced renal function and renal clearance observed in the elderly subjects. Because ofloxacin is known to be substantially excreted by the kidney, and elderly patients are more likely to have decreased renal function, dosage adjustment is necessary for elderly patients with impaired renal function as recommended for all patients. Clearance is reduced in patients with renal function impairment (Ccr $\leq$ 50 mL/min); dosage adjustment is necessary. See Administration and Dosage.

Lomefloxacin –
Absorption/Distribution: Absorption is rapid. Following coadministration with food, rate of absorption is delayed (time to reach maximum plasma concentration delayed by 41%, maximum concentration

decreased by 18%), and the extent of absorption (AUC) is decreased by 12%. At 24 hours postdose, single doses of 200 or 400 mg result in mean plasma levels of 0.1 and 0.24 mcg/mL, respectively. Steady-state concentrations are achieved within 48 hours of initiating once-daily dosing. The mean urine concentration exceeds 35 mcg/mL for $\geq$ 24 hours after dosing. Urine pH appears to affect the solubility of lomefloxacin, with solubilities ranging from 7.8 mg/mL at pH 5.2, to 2.4 mg/mL at pH 6.5, and 3.03 mg/mL at pH 8.12.

Metabolism/Excretion: Mean renal clearance is 145 mL/min in subjects with normal renal function, which may indicate tubular secretion. Approximately 9% of a dose is recovered in the urine as the glucuronide metabolite; 4 other metabolites have been identified and account for < 0.5% of the dose. Approximately 10% of a dose is recovered unchanged in the feces. In healthy elderly volunteers, plasma clearance was reduced by $\approx$ 25% and the AUC was increased by $\approx$ 33%, which may be caused by decreased renal function in this population. In patients with Ccr between 10 and 40 mL/min/1.73 m^2, the mean AUC after a single dose increased 335% over the AUC in patients with Ccr > 80 mL/min/1.73 m^2, and mean half-life increased to 21 hours. In patients with Ccr < 10 mL/min/1.73 m^2, AUC increased 700% and half-life increased to 45 hours. Adjustment of dosage is necessary. See Administration and Dosage.

Trovafloxacin/Alatrofloxacin –
Absorption: Trovafloxacin is well absorbed from the GI tract after oral administration. Serum concentrations of trovafloxacin are dose-proportional after oral administration of trovafloxacin in the dose range of 30 to 1000 mg or after IV administration of alatrofloxacin in the dose range of 30 to 400 mg (trovafloxacin equivalents). Steady state concentrations are achieved by the third daily oral or IV dose of trovafloxacin with an accumulation factor of $\approx$ 1.3 times the single dose concentrations. Oral absorption of trovafloxacin is not altered by concomitant food intake; therefore, it can be administered without regard to meals. The systemic exposure to trovafloxacin (AUC) administered, as crushed tablets via nasogastric tube into the stomach were identical to that of orally administered intact tablets. Administration of concurrent enteral feeding solutions had no effect on the absorption of trovafloxacin given via nasogastric tube into the stomach. When trovafloxacin was administered as crushed tablets into the duodenum via nasogastric tube, the AUC and peak serum concentrations (C$_{max}$) were reduced by 30% relative to the orally administered intact tablets. Time-to-peak serum level (T$_{max}$) was also decreased from 1.7 to 1.1 hours.

Distribution: The mean plasma protein bound fraction is $\approx$ 76% and is concentration-independent. Trovafloxacin is widely distributed throughout the body. Rapid distribution of trovafloxacin into tissue results in significantly higher trovafloxacin concentrations in most target tissues than in plasma or serum.

Metabolism: Trovafloxacin is metabolized by conjugation (the role of cytochrome P450 oxidative metabolism of trovafloxacin is minimal). Thirteen percent of administered dose appears in the urine in the form of ester glucuronide and 9% appears in the feces as the N-acetyl metabolite (2.5% of the dose is found in the serum as the active N-acetyl metabolite). Other minor metabolites (eg, diacid, sulfamate, hydroxycarboxylic acid) have been identified in urine and feces in small amounts (< 4% of the administered dose).

Excretion: Approximately 50% of the oral dose is excreted unchanged (43% in the feces and 6% in the urine). After multiple 200 mg doses, cumulative urinary trovafloxacin concentrations were $\approx$ 12.1 mcg/mL.

Levofloxacin –
Absorption: Levofloxacin is rapidly and completely absorbed after oral administration. Peak plasma concentrations are usually attained 1 to 2 hours after oral dosing. Levofloxacin pharmacokinetics are linear and predictable after single and multiple oral/IV dosing regimens. Steady-state is reached within 48 hours following a 500 or 750 mg once-daily dosage regimen. The mean peak and trough concentrations attained following multiple once-daily oral dosage regimens were $\approx$ 5.7 and 0.5 mcg/mL after the 500 mg doses, and 8.6 and 1.1 mcg/mL after the 750 mg doses, respectively. The mean peak and trough plasma concentrations attained following multiple once-daily IV regimens were $\approx$ 6.4 and 0.6 mcg/mL after the 500 mg doses and 12.1 and 1.3 mcg/mL after the 750 mg doses, respectively. Oral administration of 500 mg levofloxacin tablet with food slightly prolongs the time to peak concentration by $\approx$ 1 hour and slightly decreases the peak concentration by $\approx$ 14%. Therefore, levofloxacin tablets can be administered without regard to food. The plasma concentration profile of levofloxacin after IV administration is similar and comparable in extent of exposure (AUC) to that observed for levofloxacin tablets when equal doses (mg/mg) are administered. Therefore, the oral and IV routes of administration can be considered interchangeable.

Distribution: The mean volume of distribution of levofloxacin generally ranges from 74 to 112 L after single and multiple 500 or 750 mg doses, indicating widespread distribution into body tissues. It reaches peak levels in skin tissues and in blister fluid at $\approx$ 3 hours after dosing. Levofloxacin also penetrates well into the lung tissues. Lung tissue concentrations were generally 2- to 5-fold higher than plasma concentrations. Levofloxacin is mainly bound to serum albumin and is independent of the drug concentration.

Metabolism: Levofloxacin undergoes limited metabolism and is primarily excreted as unchanged drug in the urine. Less than 4% of the dose was recovered in the feces in 72 hours. Less than 5% of an administered dose was recovered in the urine as the desmethyl and N-oxide metabolites. These metabolites have little relevant pharmacological activity.

Excretion: Levofloxacin is excreted largely as unchanged drug in the urine. The mean apparent total body clearance and renal clearance range from ≈ 144 to 226 mL/min and 96 to 142 mL/min, respectively. Renal clearance in excess of the glomerular filtration rate suggest the tubular secretion of levofloxacin occurs in addition to glomerular filtration.

Sparfloxacin –

Absorption: Sparfloxacin is well absorbed following oral administration. Steady-state concentration was achieved on the first day by giving a loading dose that was double the daily dose. Maximum plasma concentrations for the initial oral 400 mg loading dose were typically achieved between 3 to 6 hours following administration with a mean value of ≈ 4 hours. Maximum plasma concentrations for a 200 mg dose were also achieved between 3 to 6 hours after administration with a mean of ≈ 4 hours. Oral absorption of sparfloxacin is unaffected by administration with milk or food, including high-fat meals.

Distribution: Upon reaching general circulation, it distributes well into the body. The volume of distribution is 3.9 L/kg. It has low plasma protein binding. It penetrates well into body fluids and tissues. The concentrations in the lower respiratory tract tissues and fluids generally exceed the corresponding plasma concentrations.

Metabolism: Sparfloxacin is metabolized by the liver, primarily by phase II glucuronidation, to form a glucuronide conjugate. It does not utilize or interfere with cytochrome P450.

Excretion: The total body clearance and renal clearance of sparfloxacin were 11.4 and 1.5 L/hr respectively. It is excreted in the feces (50%) and urine (50%). The half-life is independent of the administered dose, suggesting the sparfloxacin elimination kinetics is linear.

Moxifloxacin –

Absorption: Moxifloxacin is well absorbed from the GI tract. Coadministration with a high-fat meal (eg, 500 calories from fat) does not affect the absorption of moxifloxacin. Consumption of 1 cup of yogurt with moxifloxacin does not significantly affect the extent or rate of systemic absorption (AUC). The C_{max} is attained 1 to 3 hours after oral dosing. The mean trough concentration is ≈ 0.95 mcg/mL. Plasma concentrations increase proportionally. Steady state is achieved after ≥ 3 days with a 400 mg once-daily regimen.

Distribution: The volume of distribution ranges from 1.7 to 2.7 L/kg. Moxifloxacin is widely distributed throughout the body, with tissue concentrations often exceeding plasma concentrations. The rates of elimination of moxifloxacin from tissue generally parallel the elimination from plasma.

Metabolism/Excretion: Moxifloxacin is metabolized via glucuronide and sulfate conjugation. The cytochrome P450 system is not involved and is not affected by moxifloxacin. The sulfate conjugate (M1) accounts for ≈ 38% of the dose and is eliminated primarily in the feces. Approximately 14% of an oral or IV dose are converted to a glucuronide conjugate (M2), which is excreted exclusively in the urine. A total of 95% of an oral dose is excreted as either unchanged drug or known metabolites. The mean apparent total body clearance and renal clearance are ≈ 12 L/hr and 2.6 L/hr, respectively.

Gatifloxacin –

Absorption: Gatifloxacin is well absorbed from the GI tract after oral administration and can be given without regard to food. Peak plasma concentrations usually occur 1 to 2 hours after oral dosing. The oral and IV routes of administration can be considered interchangeable since the pharmacokinetics of gatifloxacin after 1 hour IV administration are similar to those observed for orally administered gatifloxacin when equal doses are administered. Gatifloxacin pharmacokinetics are linear and time-independent at doses ranging from 200 to 800 mg administered over a period of up to 14 days. Steady-state concentrations are achieved by the third daily oral or IV dose. The mean steady-state peak and trough plasma concentrations attained are ≈ 4.2 mcg/mL and 0.4 mcg/mL, respectively for oral administration 4.6 mcg/mL and 0.4 mcg/mL, respectively for IV administration.

Distribution: Serum protein binding is ≈ 20% and is concentration-independent. Concentrations of gatifloxacin in saliva were approximately equal to those in plasma. The mean volume of distribution of gatifloxacin at steady-state ranged from 1.5 to 2 L/kg. Gatifloxacin was widely distributed throughout the body into many body tissues and fluids. Rapid distribution of gatifloxacin into tissues results in higher gatifloxacin concentrations in most target tissues than in serum.

Metabolism: Gatifloxacin undergoes limited biotransformation in humans with < 1% of the dose excreted in the urine as ethylenediamine and methylethylenediamine metabolites. It does not inhibit cytochrome P450.

Excretion: Gatifloxacin is excreted as unchanged drug primarily by the kidney. Less than 1% of the dose is recovered in the urine as 2 metabolites. The mean elimination half-life ranges from 7 to 14 hours and is independent of dose and route of administration. Renal clearance is independent of dose with mean value ranging from 124 to 161 mL/min. Gatifloxacin undergoes glomerular filtration and tubular secretion. It may also undergo minimal biliary or intestinal elimination, since 5% of the dose was recovered in the feces as unchanged drug.

➤*Microbiology:*

Organisms Generally Susceptible to Fluoroquinolones In Vitro

Organism	Ciprofloxacin	Enoxacin	Gatifloxacin	Levofloxacin	Lomefloxacin	Moxifloxacin	Norfloxacin	Ofloxacin	Sparfloxacin	Trovafloxacin/ Alatrofloxacin
Acinetobacter anitritus									✓[1]	
Acinetobacter iwoffi	✓[1]		✓[1]	✓[1]					✓[1]	
Acinetobacter calcoaceticus								✓[1]		
Aeromonas hydrophilia	✓[1]	✓[1]			✓[1]					
Bacteroides distasonis										✓[1]
Bacteroides ovatus										✓[1]
Bordetella pertussis				✓[1]				✓[1]		
Campylobacter jejuni	✓[2]									
Chlamydia trachamotis								✓		
Citrobacter diversus	✓	✓[1]	✓[1]	✓[1]	✓		✓[1]	✓	✓[1]	
Citrobacter freundii	✓		✓[1]		✓[1]	✓[1]	✓	✓[1]		✓[1]
Citrobacter koseri		✓[1]	✓[1]							
Enterobacter cloacae	✓	✓	✓[1]	✓	✓	✓[1]	✓	✓[1]	✓	
Enterobacter aerogenes	✓[1]	✓[1]	✓[1]	✓[1]	✓[1]		✓	✓	✓[1]	✓[1]
Enterobacter agglomerans				✓[1]	✓[1]		✓[1]			
Enterobacter sakazakii				✓[1]						
Escherichia coli	✓	✓	✓	✓	✓	✓[1]	✓	✓	✓	✓
Edwardsiella tarda	✓[1]						✓[1]			
Fusobacterium sp.						✓[1]				
Gardenella vaginalis								✓		✓
Haemophilus ducreyi		✓[1]					✓[1]	✓[1]		
Haemophilus influenzae	✓		✓	✓	✓	✓		✓	✓	✓
Haemophilus parainfluenzae	✓		✓	✓	✓[1]	✓		✓		
Hafnia alvei				✓[1]						
Klebsiella pneumoniae	✓	✓	✓	✓	✓	✓	✓	✓	✓	✓
Klebsiella oxytoca	✓[1]	✓[1]	✓[1]	✓[1]	✓[1]	✓[1]	✓[1]	✓[1]	✓[1]	
Klebsiella ozaenae		✓[1]			✓[1]					
Moraxella-catarrhalis	✓[2]		✓	✓	✓	✓		✓[1]	✓	✓
Morganella morganii	✓	✓[1]	✓[1]	✓[1]	✓[1]	✓	✓[1]	✓[1]	✓[1]	✓[1]
Mycoplasma hominis								✓[1]		✓[1]
Neisseria gonorrhoeae	✓[2]	✓	✓				✓	✓		
Pasteurella multocida	✓[1]									
Prevotella sp.						✓[1]				✓
Proteus mirabilis	✓	✓	✓	✓	✓	✓[1]	✓	✓	✓[1]	✓
Proteus vulgaris	✓	✓[1]	✓[1]	✓[1]	✓[1]		✓	✓[1]	✓[1]	✓[1]
Providencia alcalifaciens		✓[1]			✓[1]		✓[1]			
Providencia rettgeri	✓			✓[1]	✓[1]		✓[1]	✓[1]		
Providencia stuartii	✓	✓[1]		✓[1]			✓[1]	✓[1]		
Pseudomonas aeruginosa	✓	✓		✓[3]	✓[4]		✓	✓[3]		✓
Pseudomonas fluorescens				✓[1]			✓[1]			
Pseudomonas stutzeri							✓[1]			
Salmonella sp.	✓[5]		✓	✓		✓		✓	✓	✓
Salmonella typhi	✓									
Salmonella enteritidis	✓[1]									
Serratia marcescens	✓	✓[1]		✓[1]	✓[1]		✓	✓[1]		
Serratia proteomaculans		✓[1]			✓[1]					
Shigella sp.	✓[5]		✓	✓		✓		✓	✓	✓
Shigella boydii	✓[2]									
Shigella dysenteriae	✓[2]									
Shigella flexneri	✓[2]									
Shigella sonnei	✓[2]									
Ureoplasma urealtycium							✓[1]	✓[1]		✓[1]
Vibrio parahemolyticus	✓[1]									
Vibrio vulnificus	✓[1]									
Vibrio cholerae	✓[1]									
Yersinia enterocolitica	✓[1]									

Gram-negative

	Organism	Ciprofloxacin	Enoxacin	Gatifloxacin	Levofloxacin	Lomefloxacin	Moxifloxacin	Norfloxacin	Ofloxacin	Sparfloxacin	Trovafloxacin/ Alatrofloxacin
	Organisms Generally Susceptible to Fluoroquinolones In Vitro										
Gram-positive	Staphylococcus aureus methicillin susceptible	✓		✓	✓	✓[1]	✓	✓[6]	✓	✓[6]	✓
	Staphylococcus aureus methicillin resistant					✓[1]					
	Staphylococcus epidermidis methicillin susceptible	✓[6]	✓[6]	✓	✓[1]	✓[1]		✓[6]	✓[1]	✓	✓
	Staphylococcus epidermidis methicillin resistant			✓		✓[1]					
	Staphylococcus hemolyticus	✓									
	Staphylococcus hominis	✓									
	S. saprophyticus	✓	✓	✓[1]	✓	✓					
	Streptococci pyogenes	✓		✓[1]	✓		✓[1]	✓	✓[1]		
	Streptococcus viridans				✓[1]					✓[1]	✓
	Streptococcus group c/f, g				✓[1]					✓[1]	✓
	Streptococcus milleri				✓[1]						
	S. agalactiae				✓[1]						
	Enteroccus faecalis	✓[7]			✓[7]		✓	✓		✓[1]	✓
	Penicillin susceptible			✓	✓		✓	✓	✓		✓[7]
	Penicillin resistant			✓[1]	✓		✓[1]	✓[1]	✓[1]	✓[1]	✓[1]
Atypical bacteria	Legionella pneumophilia	✓[1]		✓	✓	✓[1]	✓[1]		✓[1]	✓[1]	✓[1]
	Mycoplasma pneumoniae			✓	✓		✓		✓[1]	✓	
	Chlamydia pneumoniae			✓	✓	✓	✓		✓[1]	✓	
Anaerobe bacteria	Bacteroides fragilis										
	Peptostreptococcus sp.			✓[1]			✓[1]				✓
	Clostridium perfringes				✓[1]			✓	✓[1]		✓[1]

[1] Exhibits in vitro MIC of ≤ 1 mcg/mL (ciprofloxacin, sparfloxacin); ≤ 2 mcg/mL (enoxacin, gatifloxacin, levofloxacin, lomefloxacin, moxifloxacin, ofloxacin, and trovafloxacin); ≤ 4 mcg/mL norfloxacin against most (≥ 90%) strains of microorganisms; however, the safety and effectiveness in treating clinical infections due to these microorganisms have not been established in adequate and well-controlled clinical trials.
[2] Oral ciprofloxacin.
[3] As with other drugs in this class, some strains of P. aeruginosa may develop resistance fairly rapidly during treatment.
[4] Urinary tract only.
[5] See following text for individual microorganisms.
[6] Does not specify susceptible or resistant.
[7] Many strains are moderately susceptible.

Ciprofloxacin – Most strains of streptococci are only moderately susceptible, as are *Mycobacterium tuberculosis*, *M. fortuitum*, and *Chlamydia trachomatis* (moderate activity). Some strains of *Pseudomonas aeruginosa* may develop resistance fairly rapidly.

Ciprofloxacin does not cross-react with other antimicrobial agents such as beta-lactams or aminoglycosides; however, additive activity may result when it is combined with beta-lactams, aminoglycosides, clindamycin, or metronidazole.

Most strains of *Burkholderia cepacia* and some strains of *Stenotrophomonas maltophilia* are resistant to ciprofloxacin as are most anaerobic bacteria, including *Bacteroides fragilis* and *Clostridium difficile*.

Enoxacin – Many strains of *Streptococcus* species and anaerobes are usually resistant to enoxacin.

The activity of enoxacin against *Treponema pallidum* has not been evaluated; however, other quinolones are not active against *T. pallidum*.

Gatifloxacin – The activity of gatifloxacin against *T. pallidum* has not been evaluated; however, other quinolones are not active against *T. pallidum*.

Levofloxacin – As with other drugs in this class, some strains of *P. aeruginosa* may develop resistance fairly rapidly during treatment with levofloxacin.

Norfloxacin – *Ureoplasma urealyticum* is susceptible in vitro. Resistance to norfloxacin due to spontaneous mutation in vitro is rare (< 1%). Development of resistance is greatest in the following: *P. aeruginosa*; *Klebsiella pneumoniae*; *Acinetobacter* sp.; enterococcus sp. Norfloxacin is not generally active against obligate anaerobes.

Norfloxacin has not been shown to be active against *T. pallidum*.

Ofloxacin – The following organisms are susceptible in vitro:
Anaerobes: *Clostridium perfringens*; *Gardnerella vaginalis*.
Other: *Chlamydia pneumoniae*; *C. trachomatis*; *Mycoplasma pneumoniae*; *M. hominis*; *U. urealyticum*.

Many strains of other streptococcal sp, enterococcus sp, and anaerobes are resistant. It is not active against *T. pallidum*. Although cross-resistance has been observed between ofloxacin and other fluoroquinolones, some organisms resistant to other quinolones may be susceptible to ofloxacin.

Lomefloxacin – Most group A, B, D, and G streptococci, *S. pneumoniae*, *Pseudomonas cepacia*, *U. urealyticum*, *M. hominis* and anaerobic bacteria are resistant.

Cross-resistance has occurred between lomefloxacin and other quinolone-class antimicrobial agents, but not between lomefloxacin and other antimicrobials, such as aminoglycosides, penicillins, tetracyclines, cephalosporins, or sulfonamides. Lomefloxacin is active in vitro against some strains of cephalosporin- and aminoglycoside-resistant gram-negative bacteria.

Trovafloxacin/Alatrofloxacin – *M. tuberculosis* and *M. avium-intracellulare* complex organisms are commonly resistant to trovafloxacin. The activity of trovafloxacin against *T. pallidum* have not been evaluated; however, other quinolones are not active against *T. pallidum*.

Contraindications

Hypersensitivity to fluoroquinolones or the quinolone group; tendinitis or tendon rupture associated with quinolone use; patients receiving disopyramide and amiodarone as well as other QT_c-prolonging antiarrhythmic drugs reported to cause torsade de pointes, such as class IA antiarrhythmic agents (eg, quinidine, procainamide), class III antiarrhythmic agents (eg, sotalol), and bepridil (**sparfloxacin**); patients with known QT_c prolongation or in patients being treated concomitantly with medications known to produce an increase in the QT_c interval or torsades de pointes (**sparfloxacin**); patients whose lifestyle or employment will not permit compliance with required safety precautions concerning phototoxicity (**sparfloxacin**).

Warnings

➤*Phototoxicity:* Moderate-to-severe phototoxic reactions have occurred in patients exposed to direct or indirect sunlight or to artificial ultraviolet light (eg, sunlamps) during or following treatment with **lomefloxacin**, **sparfloxacin**, **ofloxacin**, or **trovafloxacin/alatrofloxacin**. These reactions also have occurred in patients exposed to shaded or diffused light, including exposure through glass. Advise patients to discontinue therapy of any fluoroquinolone antibiotic at the first signs or symptoms of a phototoxicity reaction such as a sensation of skin burning, redness, swelling, blisters, rash, itching, or dermatitis.

These reactions have occurred with and without the use of sunscreens or sunblocks and with single doses of lomefloxacin. In a few cases, recovery was prolonged for several weeks. As with some other types of phototoxicity, there is the potential for exacerbation of the reaction on re-exposure to sunlight or artificial ultraviolet light prior to complete recovery from the reaction. In rare cases, reactions have recurred up to several weeks after stopping therapy.

Avoid direct exposure to direct or indirect sunlight (even when using sunscreens or sunblocks) while taking lomefloxacin and other fluoroquinolones for several days following therapy. Discontinue therapy at first signs or symptoms of phototoxicity.

➤*Hepatic failure:* **Trovafloxacin/alatrofloxacin**-associated liver enzyme abnormalities, symptomatic hepatitis, jaundice, and liver failure (including rare reports of acute hepatic necrosis with eosinophilic infiltration, liver transplantation, or death) have been reported with short- and long-term drug exposure in men and women. Use exceeding 2 weeks in duration is associated with a significantly increased risk of serious liver injury. Liver injury also has been reported following trovafloxacin/alatrofloxacin re-exposure. Clinicians should monitor liver function tests (eg, AST, ALT, bilirubin) in recipients who develop signs or symptoms consistent with hepatitis. Clinicians should consider discontinuing the drug in those patients who develop liver function test abnormalities (see Warning Box in Trovafloxacin/Alatrofloxacin monograph).

➤*Hypotension:* Life-threatening hypotension has been reported with **alatrofloxacin** administration. This has occurred in patients receiving alatrofloxacin either at the recommended rate of infusion or if given more rapidly. Hypotension may be potentiated with the concomitant administration of anesthetic agents. Alatrofloxacin should be only administered by slow IV infusion over a period of 60 minutes. Monitor blood pressure closely during infusion.

➤*Cardiac toxicity:* **Moxifloxacin** and **gatifloxacin** have been shown to prolong the QT interval of the electrocardiogram in some patients. Avoid in patients with known prolongation of the QT interval, patients with uncorrected hypokalemia, and patients receiving class IA (eg, quinidine, procainamide) or class III (eg, amiodarone, sotalol) antiarrhythmic agents, due to the lack of clinical experience with these drugs in these patient populations.

Increases in the QT$_c$ interval have been observed in healthy volunteers treated with **sparfloxacin**. After a single loading dose of 400 mg, a mean increase in the QT$_c$ interval of 11 msec (2.9%) is seen; at steady-state the mean increase is 7 msec (1.9%). The magnitude of the QT$_c$ effect does not increase with repeated administration, and the QT$_c$ returns to baseline within 48 hours of the last dose.

Avoid the concomitant prescription of medications known to prolong the QT$_c$ interval (eg, erythromycin, terfenadine, astemizole, cisapride, pentamidine, tricyclic antidepressants, some antipsychotics including phenothiazines). **Sparfloxacin** is not recommended for use in patients with proarrhythmic conditions (eg, hypokalemia, significant bradycardia, CHF, myocardial ischemia, atrial fibrillation).

➤*Convulsions:* Increased intracranial pressure, convulsions, and toxic psychosis have occurred. CNS stimulation may also occur, which may lead to tremor, restlessness, lightheadedness, confusion, dizziness, depression, hallucinations, and rarely, suicidal thoughts or acts. Use with caution in patients with known or suspected CNS disorders (eg, severe cerebral arteriosclerosis, epilepsy) or other factors that predispose to seizures or lower the seizure threshold, or in the presence of other risk factors that may predispose to seizures or lower the seizure threshold (eg, certain drug therapy, renal dysfunction). If these reactions occur, stop the drug, and institute appropriate measures.

➤*Tendon rupture/Tendinitis:* Ruptures of the shoulder, hand, and Achilles tendons that required surgical repair or resulted in prolonged disability have been reported with fluoroquinolone antimicrobials. Discontinue therapy if the patient experiences pain, inflammation, or rupture of a tendon. Patients should rest and refrain from exercise until the diagnosis of tendinitis or tendon rupture has been confidently excluded. Tendon rupture can occur at any time during or after therapy.

➤*Syphilis:* **Ofloxacin**, **ciprofloxacin**, **norfloxacin**, **gatifloxacin**, **trovafloxacin**, and **enoxacin** are not effective for syphilis. High doses of antimicrobial agents for short periods of time to treat gonorrhea may mask or delay symptoms of incubating syphilis. All patients should have a serologic test for syphilis at the time of gonorrhea diagnosis. Patients treated with ofloxacin, ciprofloxacin, norfloxacin, gatifloxacin, trovafloxacin, and enoxacin should have a follow-up serologic test after 3 months.

➤*Chronic bronchitis due to S. pneumoniae:* **Lomefloxacin** is not indicated for the empiric treatment of acute bacterial exacerbation of chronic bronchitis when it is probable that *S. pneumoniae* is a causative pathogen because it exhibits in vitro resistance to lomefloxacin. Use only if sputum gram stain demonstrates an adequate quality of specimen and there is a predominance of gram-negative and not gram-positive organisms.

➤*Pseudomonas aeruginosa:* In clinical trials of complicated UTIs due to *P. aeruginosa*, 12 of 16 patients had the microorganism eradicated from the urine after therapy with **lomefloxacin**. No patients had concomitant bacteremia. Serum levels of lomefloxacin do not reliably exceed the MIC of *Pseudomonas* isolates. The safety and efficacy of lomefloxacin in treating patients with *Pseudomonas* bacteremia have not been established.

➤*Pseudomembranous colitis:* This has been reported with nearly all antibacterial agents, including fluoroquinolones, and may range from mild to life-threatening in severity. Therefore, it is important to consider this diagnosis in patients who present with diarrhea subsequent to the administration of antibacterial agents. After the diagnosis of pseudomembranous colitis has been established, initiate therapeutic measures. Mild cases of pseudomembranous colitis usually respond to

discontinuation of drug alone. In moderate-to-severe cases, consider management with fluid and electrolytes, protein supplementation, and treatment with an antibacterial drug clinically effective against *C. difficile* colitis.

➤*Hypersensitivity reactions:* Serious and occasionally fatal reactions have occurred in patients receiving quinolone therapy, some following the first dose. Some reactions were accompanied by cardiovascular collapse, loss of consciousness, tingling, pharyngeal or facial edema, dyspnea, urticaria, and itching. If an allergic reaction occurs, discontinue the drug. Refer to Management of Acute Hypersensitivity Reactions.

➤*Renal function impairment:* Alteration in dosage regimen is necessary. See Administration and Dosage.

The pharmacokinetic parameters of **moxifloxacin** are not significantly altered by mild, moderate, or severe renal impairment. No dosage adjustment is necessary in patients with renal impairment.

Total **gatifloxacin** clearance was reduced 57% in moderate renal insufficiency and 77% with severe renal insufficiency following administration of a single oral 400 mg dose. Systemic exposure was ≈ 2 times higher in moderate renal insufficiency and 4 times higher in severe renal insufficiency. Reduce the dose of gatifloxacin in patients with a Ccr < 40 mL/min, including patients requiring hemodialysis or continuous ambulatory peritoneal dialysis (CAPD).

In patients with renal impairment, the terminal elimination half-life is lengthened. Single or multiple doses of **sparfloxacin** in patients with varying degrees of renal impairment typically produce plasma concentrations that are twice those observed in patients with normal renal function. Adjust the dosage accordingly.

The pharmacokinetics of **trovafloxacin** are not affected by renal impairment. Trovafloxacin serum concentrations are not significantly altered in subjects with severe renal insufficiency (Ccr < 20 mL/min), including patients on hemodialysis.

Clearance of **levofloxacin** is substantially reduced and plasma elimination half-life is prolonged in patients with impaired renal function, requiring dosage adjustments in such patients to avoid accumulation. Neither hemodialysis nor CAPD is effective in removal of levofloxacin from the body, indicating that supplemental doses of levofloxacin are not required following hemodialysis or CAPD.

➤*Hepatic function impairment:* The oral clearance of **trovafloxacin** in mild and moderate cirrhosis is reduced ≈ 30%, which corresponds to prolongation of half-life by 2 to 2.5 hours (25% to 30%) increase. There are no data in patients with severe cirrhosis. Dosage adjustment is recommended in patients with mild-to-moderate cirrhosis.

➤*Carcinogenesis:* Mice exposed to UVA light while receiving **lomefloxacin** developed a phototoxic response. Time to development of skin tumors was 16 weeks; with other quinolones and UVA light, times to skin tumor development ranged from 28 to 52 weeks. Well-differentiated squamous cell carcinomas developed in 92% of mice, which were nonmetastatic and endophytic. Lomefloxacin alone did not result in skin or systemic tumors.

In a study of repeated exposure (5 days/week for 40 weeks) of hairless albino mice to a low dose of solar simulated UV radiation, skin tumors were induced with a median onset time of 43 weeks. As expected for this model, gross appearance of the tumors in this study was consistent with squamous cell carcinoma or its precursors. When **sparfloxacin** (6 or 12.5 mg/kg/day) was administered by the oral route, the median tumor onset time was reduced to 38 and 32 weeks, respectively. This reduction in median onset time was similar to that observed when mice were exposed to a higher dose of solar-simulated UV radiation alone. At a dose level of 12.5 mg/kg/day, mice had skin sparfloxacin concentrations of ≈ 1.8 mcg/g. Following a 400 mg dose of sparfloxacin, skin levels measured in human subjects averaged 5.5 mcg/g. A similar effect on the time to the development of skin tumors has been observed in this mouse strain with some other fluoroquinolone antibiotics. The clinical significance of these findings to humans is unknown.

➤*Fertility impairment:* Decreased spermatogenesis and subsequent impaired fertility was noted in male rats given oral **enoxacin** doses of 1000 mg/kg. This dose is ≈ 13-fold greater than the highest human clinical daily oral dose of 16 mg/kg, assuming a 50 kg person and based on a mg/m^2 basis.

➤*Elderly:* **Norfloxacin** is eliminated more slowly because of decreased renal function; absorption appears unaffected. The apparent half-life of **ofloxacin** is 6.4 to 7.4 hours, compared with 4 to 5 hours in younger adults; absorption is unaffected. **Lomefloxacin** plasma clearance was reduced by ≈ 25% and the AUC was increased by ≈ 33% in the elderly, which may be due to decreased renal function in this population. **Enoxacin** plasma concentrations are 50% higher in the elderly than in young adults.

➤*Pregnancy:* Category C. There are no adequate and well-controlled studies in pregnant women. Use during pregnancy only if the potential benefit justifies the potential risk to the fetus.

Norfloxacin – Produces embryonic loss in monkeys when given in doses 10 times the maximum human dose.

Ciprofloxacin, moxifloxacin, sparfloxacin, gatifloxacin, levofloxacin, trovafloxacin/alatrofloxacin, and norfloxacin – Caused lameness in immature dogs due to permanent cartilage lesions, and caused arthropathy in immature animals.

Ofloxacin – Doses equivalent to 10 to 50 times the recommended maximum dose were fetotoxic (ie, decreased fetal body weight, increased fetal mortality) in rats and rabbits, and minor skeletal variations occurred in rats; it also caused arthropathy in immature animals.

Lomefloxacin – Increased incidence of fetal loss in monkeys at ≈ 3 to 6 times the recommended human dose. In rabbits, maternal toxicity and associated fetotoxicity, decreased placental weight and variations of the coccygeal vertebrae occurred at doses 2 times the recommended human dose.

Enoxacin – The IV infusion of enoxacin into pregnant rabbits at doses of 10 to 50 mg/kg caused dose-related maternal toxicity (eg, venous irritation, weight loss) and fetal toxicity (increased postimplantation loss and stunted fetuses). At 50 mg/kg, the incidence of fetal malformations was significantly increased in the presence of overt maternal and fetal toxicity.

➤*Lactation:* **Norfloxacin** was not detected in breast milk following the administration of 200 mg to nursing mothers; however, this was a low dose. **Ciprofloxacin** is excreted in breast milk. **Ofloxacin**, as a single 200 mg dose, resulted in breast milk concentrations in nursing females that were similar to those found in plasma. **Levofloxacin** has not been measured in breast milk. Based upon data from ofloxacin, it can be presumed that levofloxacin will be excreted in breast milk. **Sparfloxacin** is excreted in breast milk. **Gatifloxacin** and **moxifloxacin** are excreted in the breast milk of rats. **Trovafloxacin** is excreted in breast milk and was found in measurable concentrations in the breast milk of lactating subjects. It is not known whether **lomefloxacin**, **gatifloxacin**, or **enoxacin** are excreted in breast milk. Because of the potential for serious adverse reactions in nursing infants, decide whether to discontinue nursing or to discontinue the drug, taking into account the importance of the drug to the mother.

➤*Children:* Safety and efficacy of **gatifloxacin**, **levofloxacin**, **moxifloxacin**, **norfloxacin**, **trovafloxacin**, **lomefloxacin**, **enoxacin**, **sparfloxacin**, and **ofloxacin** in children < 18 years of age have not been established. **Ciprofloxacin**, **sparfloxacin**, **enoxacin**, **trovafloxacin**, **gatifloxacin**, **levofloxacin**, **moxifloxacin**, **lomefloxacin**, and **ofloxacin** cause arthropathy and osteochondrosis in immature animals. Administration of **norfloxacin**, **moxifloxacin**, and **ciprofloxacin** caused lameness in immature dogs due to permanent cartilage lesions.

Precautions

➤*Monitoring:* Periodic assessment of organ system functions, including renal, hepatic, and hematopoietic, is advisable during prolonged therapy.

Symptomatic pancreatitis has been reported with **trovafloxacin/alatrofloxacin** therapy. Monitor pancreatic tests in patients who develop symptoms consistent with pancreatitis.

➤*Crystalluria:* Needle-shaped crystals were found in the urine of some volunteers who received either placebo or 800 or 1600 mg **norfloxacin**. While crystalluria is not expected to occur under usual conditions with 400 mg twice daily, do not exceed the daily recommended dosage. Crystalluria related to **ciprofloxacin** has occurred only rarely in humans because human urine is usually acidic. Advise the patient to drink sufficient fluids to ensure proper hydration and adequate urinary output. Avoid alkalinity of the urine and do not exceed the recommended daily dose.

➤*Hemolytic reactions:* Rarely, hemolytic reactions have been reported in patients with latent or actual defects in glucose-6-phosphate dehydrogenase activity who take quinolone antibacterial agents, including **norfloxacin**.

➤*Myasthenia gravis:* Quinolones may exacerbate the signs of myasthenia gravis and lead to life-threatening weakness of the respiratory muscles. Exercise caution when using quinolones in patients with myasthenia gravis.

➤*Blood glucose abnormalities:* As with other quinolones, disturbances of blood glucose, including symptomatic hyper- and hypoglycemia, have been reported, usually in diabetic patients receiving concomitant treatment with an oral hypoglycemic agent (eg, glyburide/glibenclamide) or with insulin. In these patients, careful monitoring of blood glucose is recommended. If a hypoglycemic reaction occurs, initiate appropriate therapy immediately.

➤*Phototoxicity:* Reactions, moderate to severe, have occurred in patients who are exposed to direct sunlight while receiving some drugs in this class. See Warnings.

➤*Superinfection:* Use of antibiotics (especially prolonged or repeated therapy) may result in bacterial or fungal overgrowth of nonsusceptible organisms. Such overgrowth may lead to a secondary infection. Take appropriate measures if superinfection occurs.

Drug Interactions

Fluoroquinolone Drug Interactions			
Precipitant drug	Object drug[*]		Description
Sparfloxacin Gatifloxacin Moxifloxacin	Antiarrhythmic agents (amiodarone, bretylium, disopyramide, procainamide, quinidine, sotalol)	↓	The risk of life-threatening cardiac arrhythmias including torsades de pointes may be increased. The mechanism is unknown. Sparfloxacin is contraindicated in patients receiving class IA and III antiarrhythmic agents.
Sparfloxacin	Astemizole Terfenadine[1]	↑	Sparfloxacin is contraindicated in patients receiving astemizole.
Sparfloxacin	Bepridil Erythromycin Phenothiazine Tricyclic antidepressants	↑	The risk of life-threatening cardiac arrhythmias, including torsades de pointes may be increased. Sparfloxacin is contraindicated in drugs that prolong the QT$_c$ interval.
Cisapride	Sparfloxacin	↑	The rate of sparfloxacin absorption may be accelerated. The risk of cardiovascular side effects may be increased. Sparfloxacin is contraindicated in patients receiving other QT$_c$-prolonging drugs or drugs reported to cause torsades de pointes.
Fluoroquinolones (eg, ciprofloxacin, enoxacin, norfloxacin, ofloxacin)	Theophyllines	↑	Administration of theophylline with ciprofloxacin has decreased theophylline clearance and increased plasma levels and symptoms of toxicity, including seizures.
Sucralfate	Fluoroquinolones	↓	Decreased GI absorption of quinolones. Avoid simultaneous use; administer sucralfate ≥ 6 hours after the quinolone.
Iron salts	Fluoroquinolones	↓	GI absorption of certain quinolones may be decreased by formation of an iron-quinolone complex. Avoid coadministration of these drugs.
Didanosine	Quinolones	↓	The magnesium and aluminum cations in the buffers present in didanosine tablets decrease the GI absorption of quinolones via chelation. Avoid simultaneous use.
Antacids	Quinolones	↓	Decreased GI absorption of quinolones resulting in decreased serum levels. Avoid simultaneous use.
Ofloxacin	Procainamide	↑	Plasma procainamide concentrations may be increased. Monitor plasma procainamide concentrations and adjust dose accordingly.
Ciprofloxacin Enoxacin Norfloxacin	Caffeine	↑	The hepatic metabolism of caffeine is decreased by certain quinolones; therefore, the pharmacologic effects of caffeine may be increased.
Ciprofloxacin Norfloxacin	Cyclosporine	↑	Increased cyclosporine toxicity. The mechanism is unknown.
Bismuth subsalicylate	Enoxacin	↓	Enoxacin bioavailability is decreased when bismuth subsalicylate is given within 60 minutes after enoxacin. Avoid concurrent use.
Cimetidine	Fluoroquinolones	↑	Cimetidine may interfere with the elimination of the fluoroquinolones.
Nitrofurantoin	Norfloxacin	↓	Antibacterial effect of norfloxacin in the urinary tract may be antagonized.
Probenecid	Norfloxacin Gatifloxacin Lomefloxacin	↑	Diminished urinary excretion of the quinolones have been reported during the concomitant administration with probenecid.
Enoxacin	Digoxin	↑	Digoxin serum levels may be increased. Monitor digoxin levels.

Fluoroquinolone Drug Interactions

Precipitant drug	Object drug*		Description
Fluoroquino-lones (eg, enoxa-cin, levofloxa-cin, norfloxacin)	Anticoagulants	↑	Quinolones (enoxacin) decrease the clearance of the R-warfarin, the less active isomer of racemic warfarin. Enoxacin does not affect the clearance of the active S-iso-mer, and changes in clotting time have not been observed when coadministered. Nevertheless, monitor the prothrombin time when given concomitantly.
NSAIDs	Fluoroquino-lones (eg, ofloxacin, levo-floxacin, enoxa-cin)	↑	The concurrent administration of NSAIDs with a quinolone may increase the risk of CNS stimula-tion and convulsive seizures. Sei-zures have been reported in patients taking enoxacin and NSAIDs.
Morphine	Trovafloxacin	↓	Concomitant administration of IV morphine and oral trovafloxacin resulted in a 36% decrease in trovafloxacin AUC and a 46% decrease in C_{max}.

Fluoroquinolone Drug Interactions

Precipitant drug	Object drug*		Description
Azlocillin	Ciprofloxacin	↑	The clearance of ciprofloxacin is decreased by azlocillin resulting in a higher and prolonged cipro-floxacin serum concentration.

* ↑ = Object drug increased.   ↓ = Object drug decreased.
[1] Withdrawn from market.

▶*Drug/Lab test interactions:* **Sparfloxacin** therapy may produce false-negative culture results for *Mycobacterium tuberculosis* by sup-pression of mycobacterial growth.

▶*Drug/Food interactions:* Food may decrease the absorption of **norfloxacin**. Food delays the absorption of **ciprofloxacin**, resulting in peak concentrations that are closer to 2 hours after dosing rather than 1 hour; however, overall absorption is not substantially affected. Dairy products such as milk and yogurt reduce the absorption of ciprofloxa-cin; avoid concurrent use. The bioavailability of ciprofloxacin may also be decreased by enteral feedings. Food delays the rate of absorption of **lomefloxacin** (time-to-reach maximum plasma concentration delayed by 41%, maximum concentration decreased by 18%) and decreases the extent of absorption (AUC) by 12%.

Adverse Reactions

Fluoroquinolone Adverse Reactions (%)

	Adverse reaction	Ciprofloxacin[1]	Enoxacin[2]	Gatifloxacin	Levofloxacin	Lomefloxacin	Moxifloxacin	Norfloxacin[2]	Ofloxacin[1]	Sparfloxacin	Trovafloxacin/ Alatrofloxacin[1]
CNS	Headache	1.2	≤ 2	3	0.1-6.4	3.6	2	2-2.8	1-9	4.2-8.1	1-5
	Dizziness	< 1	≤ 3	3	0.3-2.7	2.1	3	1.7-2.6	1-5	2-3.8	2-11
	Fatigue/Lethargy/Malaise	< 1	< 1		< 1-1.2	< 1	> 0.05-< 1	0.3-1	1-3	< 1	< 1
	Somnolence/Drowsiness	< 1	< 1	< 0.1	< 1	< 1	> 0.05-< 1	0.3-1	1-3	< 1-1.5	< 1
	Depression	< 1	< 1	< 0.1	< 1	< 1		0.1-0.2	< 1	< 1	< 1
	Insomnia	< 1	1	≥ 0.1-< 3	0.5-4.6	< 1	> 0.05-< 1	0.3-1	3-7	1.9	< 1
	Seizures/Convulsions[3]	< 1	< 1	< 0.1	< 1	< 1		✔[4]	< 1		< 1
	Confusion	≤ 1	< 1	< 0.1	< 1	< 1	> 0.05-< 1	✔[4]			
	Psychotic reactions	< 1	< 0.1					✔[4]			
	Paresthesia	< 1	< 1	≥ 0.1-< 3	< 1	< 1			< 1	< 1	< 1
	Hallucinations	< 1	< 0.1	< 0.1	< 1		> 0.05-< 1		✔[4]		
Dermatologic	Photosensitivity[3]	< 1	< 1			2.3				1.1	< 1-2
	Rash	1.1	≤ 1	≥ 0.1-< 3	0.3-1.2	< 1	> 0.05-< 1	0.3-1	1-3	1.8-3.3	< 1-2
	Pruritus	< 1	1	< 0.1	0.4-1.3	< 1	> 0.05-< 1	0.3-1	1-3	1.8-3.3	
	Toxic epidermal necrolysis	< 1	< 1					✔[4]			
	Stevens-Johnson syndrome	< 1	< 1					✔[4]			
	Exfoliative dermatitis	< 1						✔[4]	✔[3]		
	Hypersensitivity[3]	< 1				< 1		✔[4]			
GI	Nausea	5.2	2-8	8	1.3-7.2	3.5	8	2.6-4.2	3-10	4.3-7.6	4-8
	Abdominal pain/discomfort/cramping	≤ 1-1.7	≤ 2	≥ 0.1-< 3	0.4-2.5	1.2	> 0.05-≤ 2	0.3-1.6	1-3	1.8-2.4	1
	Diarrhea	2.3	1-2	4	1-5.6	1.4	6	0.3-1	1-4	3.2-4.6	2
	Vomiting	≤ 1-2	2-9	≥ 0.1-< 3	0.2-2.3	< 1	2	0.3-1	1-4	< 1-1.3	1-3
	Dry/painful mouth	< 1	< 1		< 1	< 1	> 0.05-< 1	0.3-1	1-3	< 1-1.4	
	Dyspepsia/Heartburn	< 1	1	≥ 0.1-< 3	0.3-2.4	< 1	1	0.3-1	< 1	1.6-2.3	
	Constipation	< 1	< 1	≥ 0.1-< 3	0.1-3.2	< 1	> 0.05-< 1	0.3-1	1-3	< 1	
	Flatulence	< 1	< 1	< 0.1	0.4-1.5	< 1		0.3-1	1-3	< 1-1.1	< 1
	Pseudomembranous colitis[3]	< 1	< 0.1	< 0.1	< 1	✔[4]		✔[4]	✔[3]		< 1
Miscellaneous	Visual disturbances	< 1	< 1						0.1-0.2	1-3	
	Hearing loss	< 1						✔[4]	< 1		
	Vaginitis	< 1	< 1	6	0.7-1.8	< 1	> 0.05-< 1		1-5	< 1	< 1-2
	Hypertension	< 1		< 0.1	< 1	< 1	> 0.05-< 1		< 1	< 1	< 1
	Palpitations	< 1	< 1	≥ 0.1-< 3	< 1		> 0.05-< 1		< 1	< 1	
	Syncope	< 1	< 1		< 1	< 1			< 1		< 1
	Chills	< 1	< 1	≥ 0.1-< 3	< 1	< 1	> 0.05-< 1	0.1-0.2	< 1	< 1	
	Edema	< 1	< 1	< 0.1	< 1	< 1		0.1-0.2	< 1		< 1
	Fever	< 1	< 1	≥ 0.1-< 3	< 1			0.3-1	1-3	< 1	< 1

Fluoroquinolone Adverse Reactions (%)

Abnormal laboratory values:

Adverse reaction	Ciprofloxacin[1]	Enoxacin[2]	Gatifloxacin	Levofloxacin	Lomefloxacin	Moxifloxacin	Norfloxacin[2]	Ofloxacin[1]	Sparfloxacin	Trovafloxacin/ Alatrofloxacin[1]
↑ ALT/↑ AST	1.9/1.7	≥ 1	< 1		≤ 0.4		1.4/1.4-1.6			≥ 1
↑ Alkaline phosphatase	0.8	< 1	< 1		0.1			≥ 1	2-2.3	≥ 1
↑ LDH	0.4			< 1			1.1	≥ 1	< 1	≥ 1
↑ or ↓ Bilirubin	0.3	< 1	< 1		0.1	≥ 2	↙[4]		< 1	
Eosinophilia	0.6	< 1			0.1					
Leukopenia	0.4	< 1		< 1	0.1	> 0.05-< 1	0.6-1.5	≥ 1		≥ 1
↑ or ↓ Platelets	0.1	< 1			0.1	> 0.05-< 1	1.4	≥ 1		
Pancytopenia	0.1				< 1		1		< 1	≥ 1
↑ ESR/Lymphocytopenia					< 0.1					
Neutropenia		< 1						≥ 1		
↑ Serum creatinine	1.1		< 1				1.4	≥ 1		
↑ BUN	0.9				0.1		↙[4]	≥ 1		
Crystalluria/Cylinduria/Candiduria	↙[4]						↙[4]	≥ 1		≥ 1
Hematuria	↙[4]						↙[4]	≥ 1		
Glucosuria/Pyuria								≥ 1		
Proteinuria/Albuminuria		< 1					↙[4]	≥ 1		
↑ γ-glutamyltransferase	< 0.1				< 0.1		1	≥ 1		
↑ Serum amylase	< 0.1		< 1		< 0.1					
↑ Uric acid	< 0.1								< 1	
↑ or ↓ Blood glucose	< 0.1			2.2	< 0.1					
↓ Hemoglobin/Hematocrit	< 0.1	< 1			< 0.1	≥ 2	0.6	≥ 1	< 1	
↑ or ↓ Potassium	↙[4]	< 1			0.1					≥ 1
Anemia	< 0.1				< 0.1				< 1	
Bleeding/↑ PT	< 0.1				< 0.1			≥ 1		
↑ Monocytes	< 0.1				0.2					
Leukocytosis	< 0.1	< 1		< 1	0.1				< 1	
↑ Triglycerides/Cholesterol	↙[4]							≥ 1		

[1] Includes data for oral and IV formulations.
[2] From single- and multiple-dose studies.
[3] See Warnings or Precautions.
[4] ↙ = Adverse reaction observed; incidence not reported.

Other adverse reactions listed only for the individual agents:

►*Ciprofloxacin:*

Cardiovascular – Cardiovascular collapse, arrhythmia, tachycardia, cardiac murmur, hypotension (≤ 1%); angina pectoris, atrial flutter, cardiopulmonary arrest, cerebral thrombosis, MI, ventricular ectopy (< 1%); postural hypotension.

CNS – Restlessness (1.1%); paranoia, toxic psychosis, dysphasia, phobia, depersonalization, unresponsiveness, lightheadedness, anxiety, weakness, manic reaction (≤ 1%); nightmares, irritability, tremor, ataxia, anorexia (< 1%).

Dermatologic – Anaphylactic reactions, erythema multiforme, vasculitis, angioedema, edema of the lips, face, neck, conjunctivae, hands or lower extremities, purpura, cutaneous candidiasis, vesicles, increased perspiration; urticaria, flushing, hyperpigmentation, erythema nodosum (< 1%).

GI – Ileus, jaundice, *C. difficile*-associated diarrhea, pancreatitis, hepatic necrosis, oral ulceration, anorexia (≤ 1%); painful oral mucosa (< 1%).

GU – Renal calculi, hemorrhagic cystitis, frequent urination, gynecomastia, candiduria, crystalluria, cylindruria, hematuria, albuminuria (≤ 1%); acidosis, interstitial nephritis, renal failure, polyuria, urinary retention, urethral bleeding (< 1%); vaginal candidiasis.

Hypersensitivity – Hyperpigmentation (< 1%)

Musculoskeletal – Arthralgia, jaw, arm, or back pain, joint stiffness, neck and chest pain, achiness, flare-up of gout (≤ 1%).

Respiratory – Respiratory arrest, respiratory distress, pleural effusion (≤ 1%); bronchospasm, dyspnea, epistaxis, hemoptysis, hiccoughs, laryngeal/pulmonary edema, pulmonary embolism (< 1%).

Special senses – Nystagmus, decreased visual acuity, blurred vision, anosmia (≤ 1%); bad taste in mouth, eye pain, tinnitus, diplopia (< 1%).

Miscellaneous – Thrombophlebitis, injection site burning, pain, pruritus, paresthesia, erythema, swelling (≤ 1%); oral candidiasis, intestinal perforation, GI bleeding, (< 1%); exacerbation of myasthenia gravis; dysphasia; agranulocytosis; cholestatic jaundice.

►*Enoxacin:*

CNS – Nervousness, anxiety, tremor, agitation, myoclonus, depersonalization, hypertonia (≤ 1%).

Dermatologic – Urticaria, hyperhidrosis, mycotic infection, erythema multiforme (< 1%).

GI – Anorexia, bloody stools, gastritis, stomatitis (< 1%).

GU – Vaginal moniliasis, urinary incontinence, renal failure (< 1%).

Lab test abnormalities – Thrombocytosis, hyperkalemia (< 1%).

Respiratory – Dyspnea, cough, epistaxis (< 1%).

Special senses – Vertigo (3%); unusual taste (1%); tinnitus, conjunctivitis (< 1%).

Miscellaneous – Asthenia, back/chest pain, myalgia, arthralgia, tachycardia, vasodilation, purpura (< 1%); hyperkinesia, amnesia, ataxia, hypotonia, psychosis, emotional lability (< 0.1%).

►*Gatifloxacin:*

CNS – Abnormal dream, tremor, vasodilatation, vertigo (≥ 0.1% to < 3%); abnormal thinking, agitation, alcohol intolerance, anorexia, anxiety, ataxia, depersonalization, euphoria, hostility, migraine, nervousness, panic attack, paranoia, psychosis, stress (< 0.1%).

Cardiovascular – Bradycardia, breast pain, substernal chest pain, tachycardia (< 0.1%).

Dermatologic – Cheilitis, dry skin, ecchymosis, epistaxis, face edema, hyperesthesia, lymphadenopathy, maculopapular rash, vesiculobullous rash (< 0.1%).

Endocrine – Diabetes mellitus, hyperglycemia, hypoglycemia (< 0.1%).

GI – Glossitis, oral moniliasis, stomatitis, mouth ulcer (≥ 0.1% to < 3%); colitis, dysphagia, gastritis, GI hemorrhage, gingivitis, halitosis, hematemesis, mouth edema, rectal hemorrhage, thirst, tongue edema (< 0.1%).

GU – Dysuria, hematuria (≥ 0.1% to < 3%); metrorrhagia (< 0.1%).

Musculoskeletal – Arthralgia, arthritis, asthenia, bone pain, hypertonia, leg cramp, myalgia, myasthenia, neck pain (< 0.1%).

Respiratory – Dyspnea, pharyngitis (≥ 0.1% to < 3%); asthma (bronchospasm), cyanosis, hyperventilation (< 0.1%).

Special senses – Abnormal vision, taste perversion, tinnitus (≥ 0.1% to < 3%); ear pain, eye pain, parosmia, ptosis, taste loss (< 0.1%).

Miscellaneous – Local injection site reaction (redness at injection site) (5%); allergic reaction, back pain, chest pain, peripheral edema, sweating (≥ 0.1% to < 3%); electrolyte abnormalities (< 1%).

►*Levofloxacin:*

Cardiovascular – Cardiac failure, circulatory failure, hypotension, arrhythmia, atrial fibrillation, bradycardia, cardiac arrest, heart block, supraventricular tachycardia, tachycardia, ventricular fibrillation, angina pectoris, coronary thrombosis, MI, postural hypotension (< 1%).

CNS – Abnormal coordination, coma, hyperkinesia, hypertonia, hypoaesthesia, involuntary muscle contractions, paralysis, speech disorder, stupor, tremor, vertigo (< 1%).

Dermatologic – Erythema nodosum, genital pruritus, increased sweating, skin disorder, skin exfoliation, skin ulceration (< 1%); rash erythematous (0.1%); urticaria (< 1% to 0.1%).

GI – Dysphagia, gastroenteritis, GI hemorrhage, pancreatitis, tongue edema (< 1%).

GU – Abnormal renal function, acute renal failure, face edema, hematuria (< 1%).

Hematologic – Abnormal platelets, embolism (blood clot), epistaxis, purpura, thrombocytopenia, anemia (< 1%).

Hepatic – Abnormal hepatic function, cholelithiasis, hepatic coma, jaundice (< 1%).

Lab test abnormalities – Granulocytopenia, lymphadenopathy, WBC abnormal (not otherwise specified) (< 1%).

Metabolic/Nutritional – Aggravated diabetes mellitus, dehydration, hyperglycemia, hyperkalemia, hypoglycemia, hypokalemia, weight decrease (< 1%).

Musculoskeletal – Arthralgia, arthritis, arthrosis, muscle weakness, myalgia, osteomyelitis, rhabdomyolysis, synovitis, tendinitis (< 1%).

Psychiatric – Abnormal dreaming, aggressive reaction, agitation, anorexia, anxiety, delirium, emotional lability, impaired concentration, impotence, manic reaction, mental deficiency, paranoia, sleep disorder, withdrawal syndrome (< 1%); nervousness (0.1% to < 1%).

Respiratory – ARDS, asthma, coughing, dyspnea, hemoptysis, hypoxia, pleural effusion, respiratory insufficiency (< 1%).

Special senses – Taste perversion (0.2% to 1%); ear disorder (not otherwise specified), tinnitus, abnormal vision, conjunctivitis, diplopia (< 1%).

Miscellaneous – Injection site reaction (3.5%); decreased lymphocytes (2.2%); injection site pain (1.7%); pain (1.4%); sinusitis (1.3%); chest pain (1.2%); back pain, injection site inflammation (1.1%); rhinitis (0.2% to 1%); asthenia, rigors, substernal chest pain, carcinoma, parosmia, ejaculation failure, cerebrovascular disorder, phlebitis (< 1%); fungal infection (0.1% to < 1%); genital moniliasis (0.2% to < 1%); moniliasis (0.1%).

➤*Lomefloxacin:*
Cardiovascular – Hypotension, tachycardia, bradycardia, arrhythmia, extrasystoles, cyanosis, cardiac failure, angina pectoris, MI, pulmonary embolism, cerebrovascular disorder, cardiomyopathy, phlebitis (< 1%).

CNS – Coma, hyperkinesia, tremor, vertigo, nervousness, anorexia, anxiety, agitation, increased appetite, depersonalization, paranoid reaction, paroniria, twitching, hypertonia, confusion, abnormal thinking, concentration impairment (< 1%).

Dermatologic – Urticaria, eczema, skin exfoliation, skin disorder, bullous eruption, acne, skin discoloration, skin ulceration, angioedema (< 1%).

GI – GI inflammation/bleeding, dysphagia, tongue discoloration, stomatitis (< 1%).

GU – Dysuria, hematuria, strangury, micturition disorder, anuria, leukorrhea, intermenstrual bleeding, perineal pain, vaginal moniliasis, orchitis, epididymitis, menstrual disorder (< 1%).

Hematologic – Thrombocythemia, thrombocytopenia, anemia (< 1%).

Respiratory – Dyspnea, respiratory tract infection, epistaxis, respiratory disorder, bronchospasm, cough, increased sputum, stridor, rhinitis, pharyngitis, respiratory depression (< 1%).

Special senses – Earache, tinnitus, conjunctivitis, eye pain, abnormal lacrimation, taste perversion (< 1%).

Miscellaneous – Flushing, increased sweating, back/chest pain, asthenia, facial edema, influenza-like symptoms, decreased heat tolerance, purpura, lymphadenopathy, increased fibrinolysis, thirst, gout, hypoglycemia, leg cramps, arthralgia, myalgia, hot flashes, abnormal liver function, hyperglycemia, viral infection, moniliasis, fungal infection, allergic reaction, anaphylactoid reaction (< 1%); abnormalities of urine specific gravity or serum electrolytes (≤ 0.1%); increased albumin, macrocytosis (< 0.1%).

➤*Moxifloxacin:*
Cardiovascular – Vasodilatation, tachycardia, peripheral edema, hypotension, chest pain (> 0.05% to < 1%).

CNS – Nervousness, anxiety, depersonalization, hypertonia, incoordination, tremor, vertigo, paresthesia (> 0.05% to < 1%).

Dermatologic – Sweating, urticaria, dry skin (> 0.05% to < 1%).

GI – Oral moniliasis, anorexia, stomatitis, gastritis, glossitis, GI disorder, cholestatic jaundice, GGTP increased (> 0.05% to < 1%).

GU – Vaginal moniliasis, cystitis, kidney function abnormal (> 0.05% to < 1%).

Hematologic/Lymphatic – Prothrombin time decrease/increase, thrombocythemia, thrombocytopenia (> 0.05% to < 1%).

Lab test abnormalities – Abnormal liver function test (1%); increased MCH, neutrophils, WBCs, PT ratio, ionized calcium, chloride, albumin, globulin (≥ 2%); decreases in RBCs, neutrophils, eosinophils, basophils, PT ratio, glucose, pO₂, amylase (≥ 2%).

Metabolic/Nutritional – Hyperglycemia, hyperlipidemia, lactic dehydrogenase increased (> 0.05% to < 1%).

Musculoskeletal – Arthralgia, myalgia (> 0.05% to < 1%).

Respiratory – Asthma, dyspnea, cough increased, pneumonia, pharyngitis, rhinitis, sinusitis (> 0.05% to < 1%).

Special senses – Taste perversion (1%); tinnitus, amblyopia (> 0.05% to < 1%).

Miscellaneous – Asthenia, moniliasis, pain, lab test abnormal (not specified), allergic reaction, leg pain, pelvic pain, back pain, infection, hand pain (> 0.05% to < 1%).

➤*Norfloxacin (single- and multiple-dose studies):*
Cardiovascular – Chest pain, MI, palpitation (0.1% to 0.2%).

CNS – Myoclonus; tingling of the fingers (0.3% to 1%); anxiety, sleep disturbances (0.1% to 0.2%).

Dermatologic – Erythema multiforme; erythema, urticaria (0.1% to 0.2%).

GI – Hepatitis; pancreatitis; stomatitis; anorexia, anal/rectal pain, loose stools (0.3% to 1%); abdominal swelling, bitter taste, anorexia, mouth ulcer, renal colic (0.1% to 0.2%).

Musculoskeletal – Arthralgia; back pain (0.3% to 1%); bursitis (0.1% to 0.2%).

Miscellaneous – Hyperhidrosis (0.3% to 1%); asthenia (0.3% to 1.3%); allergies, dysmenorrhea, pruritus ani (0.1% to 0.2%).

➤*Ofloxacin:*
Cardiovascular – Chest pain (1% to 3%); vasodilation, cardiac arrest, hypotension (< 1%).

CNS – Sleep disorders, nervousness (1% to 3%); anxiety, cognitive change, dream abnormality, euphoria, vertigo, tremor (< 1%).

Dermatologic – Angioedema, urticaria, vasculitis (< 1%).

GU – Vaginal discharge (1% to 3%); external genital pruritus in women (1% to 6%); burning/irritation/pain/rash of female genitalia, dysmenorrhea, menorrhagia, metrorrhagia, urinary frequency/pain/retention, dysuria (< 1%).

Respiratory – Cough, rhinorrhea, respiratory arrest (< 1%).

Special senses – Dysgeusia (1% to 3%); photophobia, tinnitus, decreased hearing acuity (< 1%).

Miscellaneous – Decreased appetite, GI distress, pharyngitis, trunk pain (1% to 3%); hyperglycemia, hypoglycemia (≥ 1%); arthralgia, asthenia, diaphoresis, myalgia, thirst, vasculitis, weight loss, extremity pain, epistaxis, pain (< 1%).

➤*Sparfloxacin:*
Cardiovascular – QT$_c$ interval prologation (1.3%); chest pain, electrocardiogram abnormal, tachycardia, sinus bradycardia, PR interval shortened, angina pectoris, arrhythmia, atrial fibrillation, atrial flutter, complete AV block, first degree AV block, second degree AV block, cardiovascular disorder, hemorrhage, migraine, peripheral vascular disorder, supraventricular extrasystoles, ventricular extrasystoles, postural hypotension (< 1%).

CNS – Hypesthesia, nervousness, abnormal dreams, tremor, anxiety, hyperesthesia, hyperkinesia, sleep disorder, hypokinesia, vertigo, abnormal gait, agitation, lightheadedness, emotional lability, euphoria, abnormal thinking, amnesia, twitching (< 1%).

Dermatologic – Photosensitivity reaction (3.6% to 7.9%); rash, cellulitis, face edema, maculopapular rash, dry skin, herpes simplex, sweating, urticaria, vesiculobullous rash, exfoliative dermatitis, acne, alopecia, angioedema, contact dermatitis, fungal dermatitis, furunculosis, pustular rash, skin discoloration, herpes zoster, petechial rash (< 1%).

GI – Anorexia, gingivitis, oral moniliasis, stomatitis, tongue disorder, tooth disorder, gastroenteritis, increased appetite, mouth ulceration (< 1%).

GU – Dysuria, breast pain, dysmenorrhea, hematuria, menorrhagia, nocturia, polyuria, urinary tract infection, kidney pain, leukorrhea, metrorrhagia, vulvovaginal disorder (< 1%).

Hematologic – Cyanosis, ecchymosis, lymphadenopathy (< 1%).

Lab test abnormalities – Elevated white blood cells (1.1%); increased/decreased white blood cells, increased aPTT, increased blood urea nitrogen, increased calcium, increased creatinine, increased eosinophils, increased serum lipase, increased neutrophils, increased urine glucose, increased urine protein, increased urine red blood cells, increased urine white blood cells, decreased albumin, decreased creatinine clearance, decreased hematocrit, decreased hemoglobin, decreased lymphocytes, decreased phosphorus, decreased red blood cells, decreased sodium (< 1%).

Metabolic/Nutritional – Gout, peripheral edema, thirst (< 1%).

Musculoskeletal – Arthralgia, arthritis, joint disorder, myalgia, neck pain, rheumatoid arthritis (< 1%).

Respiratory – Asthma, epistaxis, pneumonia, rhinitis, pharyngitis, bronchitis, hemoptysis, sinusitis, cough increased, dyspnea, laryngismus, lung disorder, pleural disorder (< 1%).

Special senses – Taste perversion (1.4%); ear pain, amblyopia, photophobia, tinnitus, conjunctivitis, diplopia, abnormality of accommodation, blepharitis, ear disorder, eye pain, lacrimation disorder, otitis media (< 1%).

Miscellaneous – Vaginal moniliasis (2.8%); asthenia (1.7%); vasodilatation (1%); generalized pain, allergic reaction, back pain, accidental injury, anaphylactoid reaction, infection, mucous membrane disorder (< 1%).

▶*Trovafloxacin / Alatrofloxacin:*

CNS – Lightheadedness (< 1% to 4%); paresthesia, vertigo, hypesthesia, ataxia, dysphonia, hypertonia, migraine, involuntary muscle contractions, speech disorder, encephalopathy, abnormal gait, hyperkinesia, hypokinesia, tongue paralysis, abnormal coordination, tremor, dyskinesia (< 1%).

Cardiovascular – Peripheral edema, chest pain, thrombophlebitis, hypotension, palpitation, periorbital edema, tachycardia, angina pectoris, bradycardia, peripheral ischemia, dizziness postural (< 1%).

Dermatologic – Pruritus ani, skin disorder, skin ulceration, angioedema, dermatitis, fungal dermatitis, photosensitivity, seborrhea, skin exfoliation, urticaria (< 1%).

GI – Altered bowel habits, constipation, *Clostridium difficile*-associated diarrhea, dyspepsia, loose stools, gastritis, dysphagia, increased appetite, gastroenteritis, rectal disorder, colitis, enteritis, eructation, GI disorder, melena, hiccough, gingivitis, stomatitis, altered saliva, tongue disorder, tongue edema, tooth disorder, cheilitis, halitosis (< 1%).

GU – Leukorrhea (female), menstrual disorder, balanoposthitis (male), dysuria, micturition frequency, interstitial nephritis, acute renal failure, abnormal renal function, urinary incontinence (< 1%).

Hematologic – Anemia, granulocytopenia, unspecified hemorrhage, leukopenia, decreased prothrombin, thrombocythemia, thrombocytopenia (< 1%).

Hepatic – Increased hepatic enzymes, abnormal hepatic function, bilirubinemia, discolored feces, jaundice (< 1%).

Lab test abnormalities – Decreased/increased WBC, decreased protein and albumin, increased creatinine, decreased sodium, bicarbonate (≥ 1%).

Metabolic / Nutritional – Hyperglycemia, thirst (< 1%).

Musculoskeletal – Arthralgia, muscle cramps, myalgia, muscle weakness, skeletal pain, tendinitis, arthropathy, back pain (< 1%).

Psychiatric – Anxiety, anorexia, agitation, nervousness, amnesia, impaired concentration, depersonalization, dreaming abnormal, emotional lability, euphoria, impotence, decreased libido (male), paroniria, abnormal thinking (< 1%).

Respiratory – Dyspnea, rhinitis, sinusitis, bronchospasm, coughing, epistaxis, respiratory insufficiency, upper respiratory tract infection, respiratory disorder, asthma, hemoptysis, hypoxia, stridor (< 1%).

Special senses – Taste perversion, eye pain, abnormal vision, conjunctivitis, photophobia, conjunctival hemorrhage, hyperacusis, scotoma, tinnitus, visual field defect, diplopia, xerophthalmia (< 1%).

Miscellaneous – Application/injection/insertion site reaction (2% to 5%); application/injection/insertion site device complications, inflammation, pain, asthenia, moniliasis, hot flushes, chills, infection (bacterial, fungal), malaise, sepsis, alcohol intolerance, allergic reaction, anaphylactoid reaction, drug (other) toxicity/reaction, weight increase/decrease, flushing, increased sweating, dry mouth, cold clammy skin, increased saliva (< 1%).

Overdosage

▶*Symptoms:* One patient developed oliguric acute renal failure following ingestion of 21 g of **ciprofloxacin** (serum concentration, 12 mcg/mL). The patient responded to prednisone therapy.

Information on overdosage with **ofloxacin** is limited. One incident of accidental overdosage has been reported. In this case, an adult female received 3 g of ofloxacin IV over 45 minutes. A blood sample obtained 15 minutes after the completion of the infusion revealed an ofloxacin level of 39.3 mcg/mL. In 7 hours, the level had fallen to 16.2 mcg/mL and by 24 hours to 2.7 mcg/mL. During the infusion, the patient developed drowsiness, nausea, dizziness, hot and cold flushes, subjective facial swelling and numbness, slurring of speech, and mild to moderate disorientation. All complaints, except the dizziness, subsided within 1 hour after discontinuation of the infusion. The dizziness, most bothersome while standing, resolved in ≈ 9 hours. Laboratory testing reportedly revealed no clinically significant changes in routine parameters in this patient.

Levofloxacin exhibits a low potential for acute toxicity. Mice, rats, dogs, and monkeys exhibited the following clinical signs after receiving a single high dose of levofloxacin: Ataxia, ptosis, decreased locomotor activity, dyspnea, prostration, tremors, and convulsions. Doses in excess of 1500 mg/kg orally and 250 mg/kg IV produced significant mortality in rodents. In the event of an acute overdosage, the stomach should be emptied. Observe the patient and maintain appropriate hydration. Levofloxacin is not efficiently removed by hemodialysis or peritoneal dialysis.

In case of overdosage, monitor the patient in a suitably equipped medical facility and advise to avoid sun exposure for 5 days. ECG monitoring is recommended because of the possible prolongation of the QT_c interval. There is no known antidote for **sparfloxacin** overdosage. It is not known whether sparfloxacin is dialyzable.

▶*Treatment:* Empty the stomach by inducing vomiting or by gastric lavage. Observe patient carefully and give symptomatic and supportive treatment. Maintain adequate hydration. Refer to General Management of Acute Overdosage.

Only a small amount of **ciprofloxacin** (< 10%) is removed from the body after hemodialysis or peritoneal dialysis. In the event of acute **moxifloxacin** overdosage, the stomach should be emptied and ECG monitoring is recommended because of the possible prolongation of the QT interval. Carefully observe the patient and give supportive treatment. Adequate hydration must be maintained. It is not known whether moxifloxacin is dialyzable. **Ofloxacin, enoxacin, norfloxacin, gatifloxacin, levofloxacin, trovafloxacin,** and **lomefloxacin** are not efficiently removed by dialysis.

Patient Information

Drink fluids liberally.

Do not take antacids containing magnesium, calcium, or aluminum or products containing citric acid buffered with sodium citrate, iron, magnesium, zinc, or didanosine chewable/buffered tablets or buffered solution, or the pediatric powder for oral solution simultaneously or within 6 hours before or 2 hours (8 hours with **moxifloxacin**) after dosing.

Take **norfloxacin** and **enoxacin** 1 hour before or 2 hours after meals. **Ciprofloxacin, ofloxacin, trovafloxacin/alatrofloxacin, levofloxacin, moxifloxacin, gatifloxacin,** and **lomefloxacin** can be taken without regard to meals.

Sparfloxacin can be taken with food, milk, or caffeine-containing products.

Ciprofloxacin may increase the effects of theophylline and caffeine. There is a possibility of caffeine accumulation when products containing caffeine are consumed while taking quinolones.

May cause dizziness or lightheadedness; observe caution while driving or performing other tasks requiring alertness, coordination, or physical dexterity. CNS stimulation may occur (eg, tremor, restlessness, confusion); use with caution in patients predisposed to seizures or with other CNS disorders.

Hypersensitivity reactions may occur, even following the first dose; discontinue the drug at the first sign of skin rash or other allergic reaction.

Avoid excessive sunlight/artificial ultraviolet light; discontinue drug if phototoxicity occurs. Avoid re-exposure to sunlight and ultraviolet light. Reactions may recur up to several weeks after stopping therapy. See Warnings.

Discontinue treatment and inform physician if experiencing pain, inflammation, or rupture of a tendon, and to rest and refrain from exercise until the diagnosis of tendinitis or tendon rupture has been confidently excluded.

Discontinue **levofloxacin, ofloxacin,** or **gatifloxacin** and consult a physician if patient is diabetic and being treated with insulin or an oral hypoglycemic agent and a hypoglycemic reaction occurs.

Patients should notify their physician if they are taking warfarin; concurrent administration of warfarin and **levofloxacin** has been associated with increases of the International Normalized Ratio (INR) or prothrombin time and clinical episodes of bleeding.

Convulsions have been reported in patients taking quinolones. Notify physician before taking quinolones if there is a history of this condition.

Discontinue **trovafloxacin/alatrofloxacin** therapy and inform physician immediately if symptoms suggestive of hepatic dysfunction including fatigue, anorexia, vomiting, abdominal pain, jaundice, dark urine, or pale stool develop.

Inform physician if development of symptoms suggestive of pancreatitis including abdominal pain or nausea and vomiting occurs.

Gatifloxacin and **moxifloxacin** may produce changes in the electrocardiogram (QT_c interval prolongation).

Avoid **gatifloxacin** and **moxifloxacin** in patients receiving Class IA (eg, quinidine, procainimide) or Class III (eg, amiodarone, sotalol) antiarrhythmic agents.

Use **gatifloxacin** and **moxifloxacin** with caution in patients receiving drugs that may affect the QT_c interval such as cisapride, erythromycin, antipsychotics, and tricyclic antidepressants.

Inform physician of any personal or family history of QT_c prolongation or proarrhythmic condition such as recent hypokalemia, significant bradycardia, or recent myocardial ischemia.

Inform physician of any other medications when taken concurrently with fluoroquinolones, including OTC medications.

Contact the physician if palpitations or fainting spells occur while taking **gatifloxacin** or **moxifloxacin**.

CIPROFLOXACIN

Rx	**Ciprofloxacin** (Dr. Reddy's)	**Tablets:** 100 mg	(R125). White, oval-shape. Film-coated. In 6s.
Rx	**Cipro** (Bayer)		(CIPRO 100). Yellowish. Film-coated. In *Cipro Cystitis Pack* 6s.
Rx	**Ciprofloxacin** (Various, eg, Barr, Dr. Reddy's)	**Tablets:** 250 mg	In 50s, 100s, 500s, and UD 10s.
Rx	**Cipro** (Bayer)		(CIPRO 250). Yellowish. Film-coated. In 50s, 100s, and UD 100s.
Rx	**Ciprofloxacin** (Various, eg, Barr, Dr. Reddy's)	**Tablets:** 500 mg	In 50s, 100s, 500s, and UD 10s.
Rx	**Cipro** (Bayer)		(CIPRO 500). Yellowish, capsule shape. Film-coated. In 50s, 100s, and UD 100s.
Rx	**Ciprofloxacin** (Various, eg, Barr, Dr. Reddy's)	**Tablets:** 750 mg	In 50s, 100s, 500s, and UD 10s.
Rx	**Cipro** (Bayer)		(CIPRO 750). Yellowish, capsule shape. Film-coated. In 50s, 100s, and UD 100s.
Rx	**Cipro XR** (Bayer)	**Tablets, extended-release:** 500 mg	(BAYER C500 QD). Yellowish, oblong. Film-coated. In 50s and 100s.
		1000 mg	(BAYER C1000 QD). Yellowish, oblong. Film-coated. In 50s, 100s, and UD 30s.
Rx	**Ciprofloxacin** (Barr)	**Powder for oral suspension, oral:** 250 mg/5 mL (5%) (when reconstituted)	Sucrose. Strawberry flavor. Contains a bottle of microcapsules, diluent, and a teaspoon.
Rx	**Cipro** (Bayer)		Sucrose. Strawberry flavor. Contains a bottle of microcapsules, diluent, and a teaspoon.
Rx	**Ciprofloxacin** (Barr)	500 mg/5 mL (10%) (when reconstituted)	Sucrose. Strawberry flavor. Contains a bottle of microcapsules, diluent, and a teaspoon.
Rx	**Cipro** (Bayer)		Sucrose. Strawberry flavor. Contains a bottle of microcapsules, diluent, and a teaspoon.
Rx	**Cipro I.V.** (Bayer)	**Injection:** 200 mg	Lactic acid. In 20 mL vials (1%), 100 mL in 5% dextrose flexible containers (0.2%), and 120 mL bulk packages.
		400 mg	Lactic acid. In 40 mL vials (1%), 200 mL in 5% dextrose flexible containers (0.2%), and 120 mL bulk packages.

For complete prescribing information, refer to the Fluoroquinolones group monograph.

Indications

For the treatment of infections caused by susceptible strains of the designated microorganisms in the conditions listed below:

➤*Immediate-release (IR) tablets, oral suspension, IV:*

Acute sinusitis – Caused by *Haemophilus influenzae, Streptococcus pneumoniae,* or *Moraxella catarrhalis.*

Lower respiratory tract infections – Caused by *Escherichia coli, Klebsiella pneumoniae* (including subspecies *pneumoniae* [IV only]), *Enterobacter cloacae, Proteus mirabilis, Pseudomonas aeruginosa, H. influenzae, Haemophilus parainfluenzae,* or *S. pneumoniae.* Treatment of acute exacerbations of chronic bronchitis from *M. catarrhalis.* Note: Ciprofloxacin is not a drug of first choice in the treatment of presumed or confirmed pneumonia secondary to *S. pneumoniae.*

Nosocomial pneumonia (IV only) – Caused by *H. influenzae* or *K. pneumoniae.*

Skin and skin structure infections – Caused by *E. coli, K. pneumoniae* (subspecies *pneumoniae* [IV only]), *E. cloacae, P. mirabilis, Proteus vulgaris, Providencia stuartii, Morganella morganii, Citrobacter freundii, P. aeruginosa, Staphylococcus aureus* (methicillin-susceptible), *Staphylococcus epidermidis,* or *Streptococcus pyogenes.*

Bone / Joint infections – Caused by *E. cloacae, Serratia marcescens,* and *P. aeruginosa.*

Urinary tract infections – Caused by *E. coli* (including cases with secondary bacteremia [IV only]), *K. pneumoniae, E. cloacae, S. marcescens, P. mirabilis, Providencia rettgeri, M. morganii, Citrobacter diversus, C. freundii, P. aeruginosa, S. epidermidis, Enterococcus faecalis,* or *Staphylococcus saprophyticus.*

Acute uncomplicated cystitis in females (IR tablets, oral suspension only) – Caused by *E. coli* or *S. saprophyticus.*

Chronic bacterial prostatitis – Caused by *E. coli* or *P. mirabilis.*

Empirical therapy for febrile neutropenic patients (IV only) – In combination with piperacillin sodium.

Complicated intra-abdominal infections (used in combination with metronidazole) – Caused by *E. coli, P. aeruginosa, P. mirabilis, K. pneumoniae,* or *B. fragilis.*

Infectious diarrhea (IR tablets, oral suspension only) – Caused by *E. coli* (enterotoxigenic strains), *Campylobacter jejuni, Shigella boydii, S. dysenteriae, S. flexneri,* or *S. sonnei* when antibacterial therapy is indicated.

Typhoid fever (enteric fever) (IR tablets, oral suspension only) – Caused by *Salmonella typhi.* Note: Efficacy in the eradication of the chronic typhoid carrier state has not been demonstrated.

Sexually transmitted diseases (IR tablets, oral suspension only) – Uncomplicated cervical and urethral gonorrhea caused by *Neisseria gonorrhoeae.*

Inhalational anthrax (postexposure) – To reduce the incidence or progression of disease following exposure to aerosolized *Bacillus anthracis.*

➤*Extended-release (XR) tablets (only):*

Uncomplicated urinary tract infections (acute cystitis) – Caused by *E. coli, P. mirabilis, E. faecalis,* or *S. saprophyticus.*

Complicated urinary tract infections – Caused by *E. coli, P. mirabilis, P. aeruginosa,* or *K. pneumoniae.*

Acute uncomplicated pyelonephritis – Caused by *E. coli.*

➤*Unlabeled uses: Multi-drug resistant tuberculosis, alternative regimen for tularemia, alternative regimen for cutaneous and GI anthrax, alternative therapy for the plague*

Asymptomatic N. meningitidis – Has been effective in single doses of 500 or 750 mg orally.

Chancroid (Haemophilus ducreyi infection) – 500 mg orally 2 times/day for 3 days.

Disseminated gonorrhea (alternative regimen) – 400 mg IV every 12 hours for 24 to 48 hours after improvement begins, then 500 mg orally twice daily for 7 days.

Granuloma inguinale (alternative regimen) – 750 mg orally 2 times/day for at least 3 weeks.

Uncomplicated gonococcal infections of the pharynx – 500 mg PO in a single dose (plus 1 g azithromycin PO or 100 mg doxycycline orally 2 times/day for 7 days, if chlamydial infection is not ruled out).

Administration and Dosage

➤*Approved by the FDA:* 1987.

XR tablets may be taken with meals that include milk; however, avoid coadministration with dairy products alone or with calcium-fortified products because decreased absorption is possible. A 2-hour window between substantial calcium intake (more than 800 mg) and dosing with XR tablets is recommended. Swallow the XR tablet whole; do not split, crush, or chew.

XR and IR tablets are not interchangeable.

Administer ciprofloxacin at least 2 hours before or 6 hours after magnesium/aluminum antacids, sucralfate, didanosine chewable/buffered tablets or pediatric powder for oral solution, or other products containing calcium, iron, or zinc.

CIPROFLOXACIN

Ciprofloxacin Dosage Guidelines					
Location of infection	Type or severity	Unit dose	Frequency	Daily dose	Usual durations[1]
Urinary tract	acute uncomplicated	100 or 250 mg (500 mg XR)	q 12 h (q 24 h XR)	200 or 500 mg (500 mg XR)	3 days
	mild/moderate	250 mg (200 mg IV)	q 12 h	500 mg (400 mg IV)	7 to 14 days
	severe/complicated[2]	500 mg (400 mg IV) (1000 mg XR)	q 12 h	1000 mg (800 mg IV) (1000 mg XR)	7 to 14 days
Pyelonephritis	acute uncomplicated	1000 mg XR	q 24 h	1000 mg XR	7 to 14 days
Lower respiratory tract Bone and joint Skin and skin structure	mild/moderate	500 mg (400 mg IV)	q 12 h	1000 mg (800 mg IV)	7 to 14 days ≥ 4 to 6 weeks (bone and joint only)
	severe/complicated	750 mg (400 mg IV)	q 12 h (q 8 h)	1500 mg (1200 mg)	7 to 14 days ≥ 4 to 6 weeks (bone and joint only)
Nosocomial pneumonia	mild/moderate/severe	400 mg IV	q 8 h	1200 mg IV	10 to 14 days
Intra-abdominal[3]	complicated	500 mg (400 mg IV)	q 12 h	1000 mg (800 mg IV)	7 to 14 days
Acute sinusitis	mild/moderate	500 mg (400 mg IV)	q 12 h	1000 mg (800 mg IV)	10 days
Chronic bacterial prostatitis	mild/moderate	500 mg (400 mg IV)	q 12 h	1000 mg (800 mg IV)	28 days
Empirical therapy in febrile neutropenic patients	severe: ciprofloxacin + piperacillin	400 mg IV 50 mg/kg IV	q 8 h q 4 h	1200 mg IV not to exceed 24 g/day	7 to 14 days
Infectious diarrhea	mild/moderate/severe	500 mg	q 12 h	1000 mg	5 to 7 days
Typhoid fever	mild/moderate	500 mg	q 12 h	1000 mg	10 days
Urethral/Cervical gonococcal infections	uncomplicated	250 mg	single dose	250 mg	single dose
Inhalational anthrax (postexposure)[4]	adult	500 mg (400 mg IV)	q 12 h	1000 mg (800 mg IV)	60 days
	pediatric	15 mg/kg/dose, not to exceed 500 mg/dose (10 mg/kg/IV dose, not to exceed 400 mg/IV dose)	q 12 h	not to exceed 1000 mg (not to exceed 800 mg IV)	60 days

[1] Generally continue ciprofloxacin for at least 2 days after the signs and symptoms of infection have disappeared, except for inhalational anthrax (postexposure).
[2] Including secondary bacteremia from *E. coli* (IV only).
[3] Used in conjunction with metronidazole.
[4] Begin drug administration as soon as possible after suspected or confirmed exposure.

This indication is based on a surrogate endpoint, ciprofloxacin serum concentrations achieved in humans, reasonably likely to predict clinical benefit. Total duration of ciprofloxacin administration (IV, IR, and suspension) for inhalational anthrax (postexposure) is 60 days.

The duration of treatment depends upon the severity of infection. Generally, continue ciprofloxacin for at least 2 days after the signs and symptoms of infection have disappeared. The usual duration is 7 to 14 days; however, for severe and complicated infections, more prolonged therapy may be required. Bone and joint infections may require treatment for at least 4 to 6 weeks. Infectious diarrhea may be treated for 5 to 7 days. Treat typhoid fever for 10 days. Treat chronic bacterial prostatitis for 28 days.

➤*Renal function impairment :*

IR tablets/suspension – The following table provides dosage guidelines; however, monitoring of serum drug levels provides the most reliable basis for dosage adjustment:

Ciprofloxacin Dosage in Renal Function Impairment	
Ccr (mL/min)	Dose
> 50 (IR, suspension); > 30 (IV)	See usual dosage
30 to 50 (IR, suspension)	250 to 500 mg q 12 h
5 to 29	250 to 500 mg q 18 h (IR, suspension); 200 to 400 mg q 18 to 24 h (IV)
Hemodialysis or peritoneal dialysis (IR, suspension)	250 to 500 mg q 24 h (after dialysis)

In patients with severe infections and severe renal impairment, a unit dose of 750 mg may be administered orally at the intervals noted in the table; however, carefully monitor patients and measure serum ciprofloxacin concentration periodically. Peak concentrations (1 to 2 hours after dosing) generally should range from 2 to 4 mcg/mL. For patients with changing renal function or with renal impairment and hepatic insufficiency, measurement of serum concentrations will provide additional guidance for adjusting dosage.

XR tablets – No dosage adjustment is required for patients with uncomplicated urinary tract infections receiving 500 mg ciprofloxacin XR. In patients with complicated urinary tract infections and acute uncomplicated pyelonephritis who have a Ccr of less than 30 mL/min, reduce the dose of XR tablets from 1000 to 500 mg/day. For patients on hemodialysis or peritoneal dialysis, administer XR tablets after the dialysis procedure is completed.

➤*CDC recommended treatment schedules for uncomplicated gonorrhea:* 500 mg orally in a single dose plus 1 g azithromycin orally in a single dose or 100 mg doxycycline orally twice a day for 7 days, if chlamydial infection is not ruled out.

➤*IV:* Administer by IV infusion over 60 minutes. Slow infusion of a dilute solution into a large vein will minimize patient discomfort and reduce the risk of venous irritation.

Vials – Prepare the IV dose by aseptically withdrawing the appropriate volume of concentrate from the vials. Dilute before use with a suitable IV solution to a final concentration of 1 to 2 mg/mL (see IV admixture compatibility/stability).

IV admixture compatibility/stability – Stable for up to 14 days under refrigeration or at room temperature when diluted with 0.9% sodium chloride injection, 5% dextrose injection, sterile water for injection, 10% dextrose for injection, 5% dextrose and 0.225% sodium chloride for injection, 5% dextrose and 0.45% sodium chloride for injection, or lactated Ringer's for injection. If a Y-type IV infusion set or a piggyback method is used, temporarily discontinue the administration of any other solutions during the ciprofloxacin infusion.

➤*IV to oral switch:* Patients whose therapy is started with ciprofloxacin IV may be switched to ciprofloxacin tablets or oral suspension when clinically indicated. Equivalent dosing regimens are indicated in the table below:

Equivalent AUC Dosing Regimens	
Ciprofloxacin oral dosage[1]	Equivalent ciprofloxacin IV dosage
250 mg tablet q 12 h	200 mg IV q 12 h
500 mg tablet q 12 h	400 mg IV q 12 h
750 mg tablet q 12 h	400 mg IV q 8 h

[1] IR tablets and oral suspension only.

➤*Storage/Stability:*

IR tablets – Store below 30°C (86°F).

XR tablets – Store at 25°C (77°F); excursions permitted to 15° to 30°C (59° to 86°F).

Oral suspension – Prior to reconstitution, store below 25°C (77°F); protect from freezing. Following reconstitution, store below 30°C (86°F) for 14 days; protect from freezing.

IV – Store vials between 5° to 30°C (41° to 86°F) and flexible containers between 5° to 25°C (41° to 77°F). Protect from light, excessive heat, and freezing.

GATIFLOXACIN

Rx	Tequin (Bristol-Myers Squibb)	Tablets: 200 mg	(BMS TEQUIN 200). White, almond shape. Film-coated. In 30s and blister pack 100s.
		400 mg	(BMS TEQUIN 400). White, almond shape. Film-coated. In 50s, blister pack 100s, and carton of 3 *Teq-Paqs* (5 tablets each).
		Injection (concentrate): 400 mg (10 mg/mL)	Preservative-free. In single-use 40 mL vials in 5% dextrose.
		Injection (premix): 200 mg (2 mg/mL)	Preservative-free. In premixed 100 mL flexible containers in 5% dextrose.
		400 mg (2 mg/mL)	Preservative-free. In premixed 200 mL flexible containers in 5% dextrose.

For complete prescribing information, refer to the Fluoroquinolones group monograph.

Indications

For the treatment of infections caused by the susceptible strains of the designated microorganisms in the conditions listed below:

➤*Acute bacterial exacerbation of chronic bronchitis:* Caused by *Streptococcus pneumoniae, Haemophilus influenzae, Haemophilus parainfluenzae, Moraxella catarrhalis,* or *Staphylococcus aureus.*

➤*Acute sinusitis:* Caused by *S. pneumoniae* or *H. influenzae.*

➤*Community-acquired pneumonia:* Caused by *S. pneumoniae, H. influenzae, H. parainfluenzae, M. catarrhalis, S. aureus, Mycoplasma pneumoniae, Chlamydia pneumoniae,* or *Legionella pneumophila.*

➤*Uncomplicated skin and skin structure infections (simple abscesses, furuncles, folliculitis, wound infections, cellulitis):* Caused by *S. aureus* (methicillin-susceptible strains only) or *Streptococcus pyogenes.*

➤*Uncomplicated urinary tract infections (UTIs; cystitis):* Caused by *Escherichia coli, Klebsiella pneumoniae,* or *Proteus mirabilis.*

➤*Complicated UTIs:* Caused by *E. coli, K. pneumoniae,* or *P. mirabilis.*

➤*Pyelonephritis:* Caused by *E. coli.*

➤*Uncomplicated urethral and cervical gonorrhea:* Caused by *Neisseria gonorrhoeae.*

➤*Acute, uncomplicated rectal infections in women:* Caused by *N. gonorrhoeae.*

Administration and Dosage

➤*Approved by the FDA:* December 17, 1999.

Administer gatifloxacin without regard to food, including milk and dietary supplements containing calcium. Administer once every 24 hours.

➤*Oral:* Administer oral gatifloxacin at least 4 hours before the administration of ferrous sulfate; dietary supplements containing zinc, magnesium, or iron (such as multivitamins); aluminum/magnesium-containing antacids; or didanosine buffered tablets, buffered solution, or buffered powder for oral suspension.

When switching from IV to oral dosage administration, no dosage adjustment is necessary. Patients whose therapy is started with the injection may be switched to tablets when clinically indicated.

Gatifloxacin Dosage Guidelines		
Infection[1]	Daily dose (mg)[2]	Duration
Acute bacterial exacerbation of chronic bronchitis	400	5 days
Acute sinusitis	400	10 days
Community-acquired pneumonia	400	7 to 14 days
Uncomplicated skin and skin structure infections	400	7 to 10 days
Uncomplicated UTIs (cystitis)	400	Single dose
	or 200	3 days
Complicated UTIs	400	7 to 10 days
Acute pyelonephritis	400	7 to 10 days
Uncomplicated urethral gonorrhea in men; endocervical and rectal gonorrhea in women	400	Single dose

[1] Caused by the designated pathogens (see Indications).
[2] For oral or IV routes of administration.

➤*Renal function impairment:* Because gatifloxacin is eliminated primarily by renal excretion, a dosage modification of gatifloxacin is recommended for patients with Ccr less than 40 mL/min, including patients on hemodialysis and on continuous ambulatory peritoneal dialysis (CAPD). The recommended dosage of gatifloxacin follows:

Recommended Dosage of Gatifloxacin in Adult Patients with Renal Impairment		
Ccr	Initial dose (mg)	Subsequent dose[1]
≥ 40 mL/min	400	400 mg/day
< 40 mL/min	400	200 mg/day
Hemodialysis	400	200 mg/day
Continuous peritoneal dialysis	400	200 mg/day

[1] Start subsequent dose on day 2 of dosing.

Administer gatifloxacin after a dialysis session for patients on hemodialysis.

Uncomplicated UTIs and gonorrhea – Single 400 mg dose regimen (for the treatment of uncomplicated UTIs and gonorrhea) and 200 mg once daily for 3 days regimen (for the treatment of uncomplicated UTIs) require no dosage adjustment in patients with impaired renal function.

➤*IV administration:* Administer injection by IV infusion only. It is not intended for IM, intrathecal, intraperitoneal, or SC administration.

Administer by IV infusion over a period of 60 minutes. Caution: Avoid rapid or bolus IV infusion.

Preparation for IV administration – Single-use vials must be further diluted with an appropriate solution prior to IV administration. The concentration of the resulting diluted solution should be 2 mg/mL prior to administration.

Compatible IV solutions – Because a hypotonic solution results, do not use water for injection as a diluent when preparing a 2 mg/mL solution from the concentrated solution of gatifloxacin (10 mg/mL). Any of the following IV solutions may be used to prepare a 2 mg/mL gatifloxacin solution: 5% dextrose injection, 0.9% sodium chloride injection, 5% dextrose and 0.9% sodium chloride injection, lactated Ringer's and 5% dextrose injection, 5% sodium bicarbonate injection, *Plasma-Lyte 56* and 5% dextrose injection, and M/6 sodium lactate injection.

Gatifloxacin solution at 2 mg/mL also is compatible with 20 mEq/L KCl in 5% dextrose and 0.45% sodium chloride injection.

Visually inspect this IV drug product for particulate matter prior to dilution and administration. Discard samples containing visible particles. Because no preservative or bacteriostatic agent is present in this product, aseptic technique must be used in preparation of the final IV solution. Because the vials are for single-use only, discard any unused portion remaining in the vial.

Because only limited data are available on the compatibility of gatifloxacin IV injection with other IV substances, do not add additives or other medications to gatifloxacin injection in single-use vials or infuse simultaneously through the same IV line.

If the same IV line is used for sequential infusion of different drugs, flush the line before and after infusion of gatifloxacin injection with an infusion solution compatible with gatifloxacin injection and with any other drug(s) administered via this common line.

If gatifloxacin is to be given concomitantly with another drug, give each drug separately in accordance with the recommended dosage and route of administration for each drug.

Premix – Gatifloxacin injection also is available in ready-to-use 100 and 200 mL flexible bags containing a dilute solution of 200 or 400 mg gatifloxacin in 5% dextrose. No further dilution is necessary.

Because the premix flexible bags are for single use only, discard any unused portion.

Instructions for the use of gatifloxacin injection premix in flexible containers –
To open:
1.) Tear outer wrap at the notch and remove solution container.
2.) Check the container for minute leaks by squeezing the inner bag firmly. If leaks are found or if the seal is not intact, discard the solution, as the sterility may be compromised.
3.) Use only if solution is clear and light yellow to greenish-yellow.
4.) Use sterile equipment.
5.) Warning: Do not use flexible containers in series connections. Such use could result in air embolism caused by residual air being drawn from the primary container before administration of the fluid from the secondary container is complete.

GATIFLOXACIN

Preparation for administration:

1.) Close flow control clamp of administration set.
2.) Remove cover from port at bottom of container.
3.) Insert piercing pin of administration set into port with a twisting motion until the pin is firmly seated. Note: See full directions on administration set carton.
4.) Suspend container from hanger.
5.) Squeeze and release drip chamber to establish proper fluid level in chamber during infusion of gatifloxacin injection premix in flexible containers.
6.) Open flow control clamp to expel air from set. Close clamp.
7.) Regulate rate of administration with flow control clamp.

➤*Storage / Stability:*

Tablets and injection – Store at 25°C (77°F); excursions permitted to 15° to 30°C (59° to 86°F). Do not freeze premix bags.

Injection – When diluted in a compatible IV fluid to a concentration of 2 mg/mL gatifloxacin, it is stable for 14 days when stored at 20° to 25°C (68° to 77°F) or when stored under refrigeration at 2° to 8°C (36° to 46°F).

Gatifloxacin injection, when diluted to a concentration of 2 mg/mL in a compatible IV fluid except for 5% sodium bicarbonate injection, may be stored up to 6 months at -25° to -10°C (-13° to 14°F). Frozen solution may be thawed at controlled room temperature. Solutions that have been thawed are stable for 14 days after removal from the freezer when stored between 20° to 25°C (68° to 77°F) or when stored under refrigeration between 2° to 8°C (36° to 46°F). Do not refreeze solutions.

Stability of gatifloxacin injection as supplied: When stored under recommended conditions, gatifloxacin injection, as supplied in 40 mL vials and in 100 and 200 mL flexible containers, is stable through the expiration date printed on the label.

LEVOFLOXACIN

Rx	Levaquin (Ortho-McNeil)	**Tablets:** 250 mg	(LEVAQUIN 250). Terra cotta pink, rectangular. Film-coated. In 50s and UD 100s.
		500 mg	(LEVAQUIN 500). Peach, rectangular. Film-coated. In 50s and UD 100s.
		750 mg	(LEVAQUIN 750). White, rectangular. Film-coated. In 20s and UD 5s and 100s.
		Injection (concentrate): 500 mg (25 mg/mL)	Preservative-free. In single-use 20 mL vials in water for injection.
		750 mg (25 mg/mL)	Preservative-free. In single-use 30 mL vials in water for injection.
		Injection (premix): 250 mg (5 mg/mL)	Preservative-free. In 50 mL premix flexible containers in 5% dextrose solution.
		500 mg (5 mg/mL)	Preservative-free. In 100 mL premix flexible containers in 5% dextrose solution.
		750 mg (5 mg/mL)	Preservative-free. In 150 mL premix flexible containers in 5% dextrose solution.

For complete prescribing information, refer to the Fluoroquinolones group monograph.

Indications

For the treatment of adults 18 years of age and older with mild, moderate, and severe infections caused by susceptible strains of the designated microorganisms in the following conditions:

➤*Acute bacterial exacerbation of chronic bronchitis:* Caused by *Staphylococcus aureus, Streptococcus pneumoniae, Haemophilus influenzae, H. parainfluenzae,* or *Moraxella catarrhalis.*

➤*Acute maxillary sinusitis:* Caused by *S. pneumoniae, H. influenzae,* or *M. catarrhalis.*

➤*Acute pyelonephritis (mild to moderate):* Caused by *Escherichia coli.*

➤*Chronic bacterial prostatitis:* Caused by *E. coli, Enterococcus faecalis,* or *S. epidermidis.*

➤*Pneumonia, community-acquired:* Caused by *S. aureus, S. pneumoniae* (including penicillin-resistant strains, MIC value for penicillin greater than or equal to 2 mcg/mL), *H. influenzae, H. parainfluenzae, Klebsiella pneumoniae, M. catarrhalis, Chlamydia pneumoniae, Legionella pneumophila,* or *Mycoplasma pneumoniae.*

➤*Pneumonia, nosocomial:* Caused by methicillin-susceptible *S. aureus, Pseudomonas aeruginosa, Serratia marcescens, E. coli, K. pneumoniae, H. influenzae,* or *S. pneumoniae.* Use adjunctive therapy as clinically indicated. Combination therapy with an antipseudomonal β-lactam is recommended when *P. aeruginosa* is a documented or presumptive pathogen.

➤*Skin and skin structure infections (SSSIs), complicated:* Caused by methicillin-susceptible *S. aureus, E. faecalis, S. pyogenes,* or *Proteus mirabilis.*

➤*SSSIs, uncomplicated (mild to moderate):* Including abscesses, cellulitis, furuncles, impetigo, pyoderma, or wound infections caused by *S. aureus* or *S. pyogenes.*

➤*Urinary tract infections (UTIs), complicated (mild to moderate):* Caused by *E. faecalis, Enterobacter cloacae, E. coli, K. pneumoniae, P. mirabilis,* or *P. aeruginosa.*

➤*UTIs, uncomplicated (mild to moderate):* Caused by *E. coli, K. pneumoniae,* or *S. saprophyticus.*

➤*Unlabeled uses:* Anthrax, traveler's diarrhea, multidrug resistant tuberculosis, surgical prophylaxis for transrectal prostate biopsy.

Epididymitis (alternative regimen) – 500 mg/day orally for 10 days.

Gonococcal infections, disseminated (alternative regimen) – 250 mg once daily IV for 24 to 48 hours (after improvement begins, then 500 mg/day orally for 7 days).

Gonococcal infections, uncomplicated, of the cervix, urethra, and rectum – 250 mg orally in a single dose plus 1 g azithromycin as a single oral dose or 100 mg doxycycline orally 2 times/day for 7 days if chlamydial infection is not ruled out.

Nongonococcal urethritis (alternative regimen) – 500 mg/day for 7 days.

Pelvic inflammatory disease (PID) (alternative regimen) – 500 mg IV once daily or 500 mg/day orally for 14 days.

Administration and Dosage

Administer levofloxacin injection only by IV infusion. It is not for IM, intrathecal, intraperitoneal, or SC administration.

Caution: Avoid rapid or bolus IV infusion. Infuse levofloxacin injection IV slowly over a period of not less than 60 or 90 minutes, depending on the dosage.

Single-use vials require dilution prior to administration.

The usual dose of levofloxacin tablets/injection is 250 or 500 mg administered orally or by slow infusion over 60 minutes every 24 hours, or 750 mg administered orally or by slow infusion over 90 minutes every 24 hours, as indicated by infection and described in the following dosing table. Administer oral doses at least 2 hours before or 2 hours after antacids containing magnesium or aluminum, as well as sucralfate, metal cations such as iron and multivitamin preparations with zinc, or didanosine (chewable/buffered tablets or pediatric powder for oral solution).

Levofloxacin Dosing with Normal Renal Function (Ccr > 80 mL/min)				
Infection[1]	Unit dose	Frequency	Duration[2]	Daily dose
Acute bacterial exacerbation of chronic bronchitis	500 mg	q 24 h	7 days	500 mg
Acute maxillary sinusitis	500 mg	q 24 h	10 to 14 days	500 mg
Acute pyelonephritis	250 mg	q 24 h	10 days	250 mg
Chronic bacterial prostatitis	500 mg	q 24 h	28 days	500 mg
Pneumonia, community-acquired	500 mg	q 24 h	7 to 14 days	500 mg
	750 mg[3]	q 24 h	5 days	750 mg
Pneumonia, nosocomial	750 mg	q 24 h	7 to 14 days	750 mg
SSSI, complicated	750 mg	q 24 h	7 to 14 days	750 mg
SSSI, uncomplicated	500 mg	q 24 h	7 to 10 days	500 mg
UTI, complicated	250 mg	q 24 h	10 days	250 mg
UTI, uncomplicated	250 mg	q 24 h	3 days	250 mg

[1] Caused by the designated pathogens (see Indications).
[2] Sequential therapy (IV to oral) may be instituted at the discretion of the physician.
[3] Efficacy of this alternative regimen has only been documented for infections caused by penicillin-susceptible *S. pneumoniae, H. influenzae, H. parainfluenzae, M. pneumoniae,* and *C. pneumoniae.*

➤*Renal function impairment:*

Levofloxacin Dosing with Renal Function Impairment		
Renal status	Initial dose	Subsequent dose
Acute bacterial exacerbation of chronic bronchitis/ community-acquired pneumonia/acute maxillary sinusitis/ uncomplicated SSSI/chronic bacterial prostatitis		
Ccr 50 to 80 mL/min	No dosage adjustment required	
Ccr 20 to 49 mL/min	500 mg	250 mg q 24 h
Ccr 10 to 19 mL/min	500 mg	250 mg q 48 h
Hemodialysis	500 mg	250 mg q 48 h

LEVOFLOXACIN

Levofloxacin Dosing with Renal Function Impairment		
Renal status	Initial dose	Subsequent dose
CAPD[1]	500 mg	250 mg q 48 h
Complicated SSSI/nosocomial pneumonia/community-acquired pneumonia		
Ccr 50 to 80 mL/min	No dosage adjustment required	
Ccr 20 to 49 mL/min	750 mg	750 mg q 48 h
Ccr 10 to 19 mL/min	750 mg	500 mg q 48 h
Hemodialysis	750 mg	500 mg q 48 h
CAPD[1]	750 mg	500 mg q 48 h
Complicated UTI/acute pyelonephritis		
Ccr ≥ 20 mL/min	No dosage adjustment required	
Ccr 10 to 19 mL/min	250 mg	250 mg q 48 h
Uncomplicated UTI	No dosage adjustment required	

[1] CAPD = chronic ambulatory peritoneal dialysis.

➤*Preparation for IV administration:*

Levofloxacin injection in single-use vials – Levofloxacin injection is supplied in single-use vials containing a concentrated levofloxacin solution with the equivalent of 500 mg (20 mL vial) and 750 mg (30 mL vial) levofloxacin in water for injection. The 20 and 30 mL vials each contain 25 mg levofloxacin/mL. These single-use vials must be further diluted with an appropriate solution prior to IV administration (see Compatible IV solutions). The concentration of the resulting diluted solution should be 5 mg/mL prior to administration.

Because no preservative or bacteriostatic agent is present in this product, aseptic technique must be used in preparation of the final IV solution. Because the vials are for single use only, discard any unused portion remaining in the vial. When used to prepare two 250 mg doses from the 20 mL vial containing 500 mg levofloxacin, withdraw the full content of the vial at once using a single-entry procedure, and prepare and store a second dose for subsequent use (see Stability of levofloxacin injection following dilution).

Levofloxacin Dosing Preparation			
Desired dosage strength	Withdraw volume from appropriate vial	Volume of diluent	Infusion time (minutes)
250 mg	10 mL (20 mL vial)	40 mL	60
500 mg	20 mL (20 mL vial)	80 mL	60
750 mg	30 mL (30 mL vial)	120 mL	90

For example, to prepare a 500 mg dose using the 20 mL vial (25 mg/mL), withdraw 20 mL and dilute with a compatible IV solution to a total volume of 100 mL.

Compatible IV solutions: Any of the following IV solutions may be used to prepare a 5 mg/mL levofloxacin solution: 0.9% sodium chloride injection; D_5W; 5% dextrose/0.9% NaCl injection; 5% dextrose in Lactated Ringer's; *Plasma-Lyte 56/5%* dextrose, injection; 5% dextrose, 0.45% sodium chloride, and 0.15% potassium chloride injection; sodium lactate injection (M/6).

Because only limited data are available on the compatibility of levofloxacin IV injection with other IV substances, do not add additives or other medications to levofloxacin injection in single-use vials or infuse simultaneously through the same IV line. If the same IV line is used for sequential infusion of several different drugs, flush the line before and after infusion of levofloxacin injection with an infusion solution compatible with levofloxacin injection and with any other drug(s) administered via this common line.

Premix in single-use flexible containers – Levofloxacin injection also is supplied in flexible containers containing a premixed, ready-to-use levofloxacin solution in D_5W for single-use. The fill volume is either 50 or 100 mL for the 100 mL flexible container or 150 mL for the 150 mL container. No further dilution of these preparations is necessary. Consequently, each 50, 100, and 150 mL premix flexible container already contains a dilute solution with the equivalent of 250, 500, and 750 mg levofloxacin in D_5W.

Because the premix flexible containers are for single use only, discard any unused portion.

Instructions for the use of levofloxacin injection premix in flexible containers:

• *To open –*
1.) Tear outer wrap at the notch and remove solution container.
2.) Check the container for minute leaks by squeezing the inner bag firmly. If leaks are found or if the seal is not intact, discard the solution because the sterility may be compromised.
3.) Do not use if the solution is cloudy or a precipitate is present.
4.) Use sterile equipment.
5.) Warning: Do not use flexible containers in series connections. Such use could result in air embolism caused by residual air being drawn from the primary container before administration of the fluid from the secondary container is complete.

• *Preparation for administration –*
1.) Close flow control clamp of administration set.
2.) Remove cover from port at bottom of container.
3.) Insert piercing pin of administration set into port with a twisting motion until the pin is firmly seated. Note: See full directions on administration set carton.
4.) Suspend container from hanger.
5.) Squeeze and release drip chamber to establish proper fluid level in chamber during infusion of levofloxacin injection in premix flexible containers.
6.) Open flow control clamp to expel air from set. Close clamp.
7.) Regulate rate of administration with flow control clamp.

➤*Storage/Stability:*

Tablets – Store at 15° to 30°C (59° to 86°F) in a well-closed container.

Injection –

Single-use vials: Store at controlled room temperature (15° to 30°C; 59° to 86°F) and protect from light.

Premix: Store at or below 25°C (77°F); however, brief exposures up to 40°C (104°F) do not adversely affect the product. Avoid excessive heat, and protect from freezing and light.

Stability of levofloxacin injection as supplied: When stored under recommended conditions, levofloxacin injection, as supplied in 20 and 30 mL vials, or 100 mL and 150 mL flexible containers, is stable through the expiration date printed on the label.

Stability of levofloxacin injection following dilution: When diluted in a compatible IV fluid to a concentration of 5 mg/mL, it is stable for 72 hours when stored at or below 25°C (77°F) and for 14 days when stored under refrigeration at 5°C (41°F) in plastic IV containers. Solutions that are diluted in a compatible IV solution and frozen in glass bottles or plastic IV containers are stable for 6 months when stored at -20°C (-4°F). Thaw frozen solutions at room temperature 25°C (77°F) or in a refrigerator at 8°C (46°F). Do not force thaw by microwave irradiation or water bath immersion. Do not refreeze after initial thawing.

LOMEFLOXACIN HCl

Rx	**Maxaquin** (Biovail)	**Tablets:** 400 mg	Lactose. (Maxaquin 400). White, oval, scored. Film-coated. In 20s.

For complete prescribing information, refer to the Fluoroquinolones group monograph.

Indications

For the treatment of adults with mild to moderate infections caused by susceptible strains of the designated microorganisms in the following conditions:

➤*Lower respiratory tract infections:*

Acute bacterial exacerbation of chronic bronchitis – Caused by *Haemophilus influenzae* or *Moraxella catarrhalis.* Lomefloxacin is not indicated for the empiric treatment of acute bacterial exacerbation of chronic bronchitis when it is probable that *Streptococcus pneumoniae* is a causative pathogen.

➤*Urinary tract infections (UTIs):*

Uncomplicated (cystitis) – Caused by *Escherichia coli, Klebsiella pneumoniae, Proteus mirabilis,* or *Staphylococcus saprophyticus.*

Complicated – Caused by *E. coli, K. pneumoniae, P. mirabilis, Pseudomonas aeruginosa, Citrobacter diversus,* or *Enterobacter cloacae.* Safety and efficacy of lomefloxacin in treating patients with pseudomonas bacteremia have not been established.

➤*Preoperative prevention of infection:* Preoperative prevention of infection in the following conditions:

Transrectal prostate biopsy – To reduce the incidence of UTIs in the early and late postoperative periods (3 to 5 days and 3 to 4 weeks post-surgery).

Transurethral surgical procedures – To reduce the incidence of UTIs in the early postoperative period (3 to 5 days postsurgery).

Do not use in minor urologic procedures for which prophylaxis is not indicated (eg, simple cystoscopy, retrograde pyelography).

Administration and Dosage

➤*Approved by the FDA:* February 21, 1992.

Risk of reaction to solar UVA light may be reduced by taking lomefloxacin at least 12 hours before exposure to the sun (eg, in the evening). Lomefloxacin may be taken without regard to meals. Sucralfate and antacids containing magnesium or aluminum, or didanosine chewable/buffered tablets or the pediatric powder for oral solution should not be taken within 4 hours before or 2 hours after taking lomefloxacin.

LOMEFLOXACIN HCl

Recommended Daily Dose of Lomefloxacin				
Body system	Infection	Dose	Frequency	Duration
Lower respiratory tract	Acute bacterial exacerbation of chronic bronchitis	400 mg	once daily	10 days
Urinary tract	Uncomplicated cystitis caused by *K. pneumoniae*, *P. mirabilis*, or *S. saprophyticus*	400 mg	once daily	10 days
	Uncomplicated cystitis in females caused by *E. coli*	400 mg	once daily	3 days
	Complicated UTI	400 mg	once daily	14 days

➤*Renal function impairment:* Lomefloxacin is primarily eliminated by renal excretion. Modification of dosage is recommended in patients with renal dysfunction. In patients with a Ccr greater than 10 but less than 40 mL/min/1.73 m^2, the recommended dosage is an initial loading dose of 400 mg followed by daily maintenance doses of 200 mg (½ tablet) once daily for the duration of treatment. It is suggested that serial determinations of lomefloxacin levels be performed to determine any necessary alteration in the appropriate next dosing interval.

➤*Dialysis patients:* Hemodialysis removes only a negligible amount of lomefloxacin (3% in 4 hours). Hemodialysis patients should receive an initial loading dose of 400 mg followed by maintenance doses of 200 mg (½ tablet) once daily for the duration of treatment.

➤*Preoperative prevention:*

Transrectal prostate biopsy – The recommended dose for transrectal prostate biopsy is a single 400 mg dose 1 to 6 hours prior to the procedure.

Transurethral surgical procedures – A single 400 mg dose 2 to 6 hours prior to surgery when oral preoperative prophylaxis for transurethral surgical procedures is considered appropriate.

➤*Storage/Stability:* Store at 15° to 25°C (59° to 77°F).

MOXIFLOXACIN HCl

Rx	**Avelox** (Bayer)	**Tablets:** 400 mg	Lactose. (BAYER M400). Red, oblong. Film-coated. In 30s, UD 50s, and *ABC* packs of 5.
Rx	**Avelox I.V.** (Bayer)	**Injection (premix):** 400 mg	With 0.8% sodium chloride. Preservative-free. In 250 mL flexible bags.[1]

[1] No further dilution of this preparation is necessary.

For complete prescribing information, refer to the Fluoroquinolones group monograph.

Indications

For the treatment of adults at least 18 years of age with infections caused by susceptible strains of the designated microorganisms in the conditions listed below.

➤*Acute bacterial sinusitis:* Caused by *Streptococcus pneumoniae*, *Haemophilus influenzae*, or *Moraxella catarrhalis*.

➤*Acute bacterial exacerbation of chronic bronchitis:* Caused by *S. pneumoniae*, *H. influenzae*, *H. parainfluenzae*, *Klebsiella pneumoniae*, *Staphylococcus aureus*, or *M. catarrhalis*.

➤*Community-acquired pneumonia:* Caused by *S. pneumoniae* (including penicillin-resistant strains, MIC value for penicillin 2 mcg/mL or more), *H. influenzae*, *Mycoplasma pneumoniae*, *Chlamydia pneumoniae*, *M. catarrhalis*, *K. pneumoniae*, *S. aureus*.

➤*Uncomplicated skin and skin structure infections:* Caused by *S. aureus* or *Streptococcus pyogenes*.

Administration and Dosage

➤*Approved by the FDA:* December 10, 1999.

The dose of moxifloxacin is 400 mg (orally or as an IV infusion) once every 24 hours.

Moxifloxacin Dosage Guidelines			
Infection[1]	Daily dose (mg)	Frequency	Duration (days)
Acute bacterial sinusitis	400	q 24 h	10
Acute bacterial exacerbation of chronic bronchitis	400	q 24 h	5
Community-acquired pneumonia	400	q 24 h	7 to 14
Uncomplicated skin and skin structure infections	400	q 24 h	7

[1] Caused by the designated pathogens (see Indications).

Administer oral doses of moxifloxacin at least 4 hours before or 8 hours after antacids containing magnesium or aluminum, sucralfate, metal cations such as iron, multivitamin preparations with zinc, or didanosine (chewable/buffered tablets or pediatric powder for oral solution).

Moxifloxacin may be administered without regard to food.

➤*Switching from IV to oral dosing:* When switching from IV to oral dosage administration, no dosage adjustment is necessary. Patients whose therapy is started with IV moxifloxacin may be switched to the oral dosage form when clinically indicated at the discretion of the physician.

➤*IV:* Administer IV moxifloxacin by IV infusion only. It is not intended for IM, intrathecal, intraperitoneal, or SC administration.

Administer by IV infusion over a period of 60 minutes by direct infusion or through a Y-type IV infusion set that may already be in place. Avoid rapid or bolus IV infusion.

Because only limited data are available on the compatibility of moxifloxacin IV injection with other IV substances, do not add additives or other medications to IV moxifloxacin or infuse simultaneously through the same IV line. If the same IV line is used for sequential infusion of other drugs, or if the "piggyback" method of administration is used, flush the line before and after infusion of moxifloxacin IV with an infusion solution compatible with moxifloxacin IV as well as with other drug(s) administered via this common line.

Moxifloxacin IV is compatible with the following IV solutions at ratios from 1:10 to 10:1:
• 0.9% sodium chloride injection
• 1M sodium chloride injection
• 5% dextrose injection
• Sterile water for injection
• 10% dextrose for injection
• Lactated Ringer's for injection

➤*Storage/Stability:*

Tablets – Store at 25°C (77°F); excursions permitted to 15° to 30°C (59° to 86°F). Avoid high humidity.

IV – Store at 25°C (77°F); excursions permitted to 15° to 30°C (59° to 86°F). Do not refrigerate. Since the premix flexible containers are for single use only, discard any unused portion.

GEMIFLOXACIN MESYLATE

Rx	**Factive** (Genesoft)	**Tablets:** 320 mg (as base)	(GE 320). White to off-white, oval, scored. Film-coated. In unit of use 5s and 7s and hospital pack 30s.

For complete prescribing information, refer to the Fluoroquinolones group monograph.

Indications

For the treatment of infections caused by susceptible strains of the designated microorganisms in the conditions listed below.

➤*Acute bacterial exacerbation of chronic bronchitis:* Caused by *Streptococcus pneumoniae*, *Haemophilus influenzae*, *Haemophilus parainfluenzae*, or *Moraxella catarrhalis*.

➤*Community-acquired pneumonia (of mild to moderate severity):* Caused by *S. pneumoniae* (including multi-drug resistant strains [MDRSP†]), *H. influenzae*, *M. catarrhalis*, *Mycoplasma pneumoniae*, *Chlamydia pneumoniae*, or *Klebsiella pneumoniae*.†

Administration and Dosage

➤*Approved by the FDA:* April 4, 2003.

Gemifloxacin can be taken with or without food and should be swallowed whole with a liberal amount of liquid. The recommended dose of gemifloxacin is 320 mg daily, according to the following table.

Gemifloxacin Dosage Guidelines		
Indication	Dose (mg/d)	Duration (days)
Acute bacterial exacerbation of chronic bronchitis	320	5

† MDRSP includes isolates previously known as PRSP (penicillin-resistant *Streptococcus pneumoniae*) and are strains resistant to two or more of the following antibiotics: penicillin, second generation cephalosporins (eg, cefuroxime), macrolides, tetracyclines, and trimethoprim/sulfamethoxazole.

GEMIFLOXACIN MESYLATE

Gemifloxacin Dosage Guidelines		
Indication	Dose (mg/d)	Duration (days)
Community-acquired pneumonia (of mild to moderate severity)	320	7

Recommended Doses for Patients with Impaired Renal Function	
Creatinine clearance (mL/min)	Dose
> 40	See usual dosage
≤ 40	160 mg q 24 h

Patients requiring routine hemodialysis or continuous ambulatory peritoneal dialysis (CAPD) should receive 160 mg every 24 hours.

➤*Renal function impairment:* Dose adjustment in patients with Ccr greater than 40 mL/min is not required. Modification of the dosage is recommended for patients with Ccr 40 mL/min or less.

➤*Storage/Stability:* Store at 25°C (77°F); excursions permitted to 15° to 30°C (59° to 86°F). Protect from light.

NORFLOXACIN

Rx	Noroxin (Merck)	**Tablets:** 400 mg	(MSD 705 Noroxin). Dark pink, oval. Film coated. In 100s and UD 20s and 100s.

For complete prescribing information, refer to the Fluoroquinolones group monograph.

Indications

For the treatment of adults with the following infections caused by susceptible strains of the designated microorganisms in the conditions listed below:

➤*Urinary tract infections:* Uncomplicated infections (including cystitis) caused by *Enterococcus faecalis, Escherichia coli, Klebsiella pneumoniae, Proteus mirabilis, Pseudomonas aeruginosa, Staphylococcus epidermidis, Staphylococcus saprophyticus, Citrobacter freundii, Enterobacter aerogenes, Enterobacter cloacae, Proteus vulgaris, Staphylococcus aureus,* or *Staphylococcus agalactiae*; complicated infections caused by *E. faecalis, E. coli, K. pneumoniae, P. mirabilis, P. aeruginosa,* or *Serratia marcescens.*

➤*Sexually transmitted diseases:* Uncomplicated urethral and cervical gonorrhea caused by *Neisseria gonorrhoeae.*

➤*Prostatitis:* Due to *E. coli.*

Administration and Dosage

➤*Approved by the FDA:* 1986.

Take ≥ 1 hour before or ≥ 2 hours after meals or ingestion of milk or other dairy products. Take with a glass of water. Hydrate patients well.

Recommended Norfloxacin Dosage					
Infection	Description	Dose	Frequency	Duration	Daily dose
Urinary tract infections (UTI)	Uncomplicated (cystitis) due to *E. coli, K. pneumoniae,* or *P. mirabilis*	400 mg	q 12 h	3 days	800 mg
	Uncomplicated due to other indicated organisms	400 mg	q 12 h	7-10 days	800 mg
	Complicated	400 mg	q 12 h	10-21 days	800 mg
Sexually transmitted diseases	Uncomplicated gonorrhea	800 mg	single dose	1 day	800 mg
Prostatitis	Acute or chronic	400 mg	q 12 h	28 days	800 mg

➤*Renal function impairment:* In patients with a Ccr rate ≤ 30 mL/min/1.73 m², administer 400 mg once daily for the duration given above.

When only the serum creatinine is known, the following formula may be used to estimate Ccr. The serum creatinine should represent a steady state of renal function.

Males: $\dfrac{\text{Weight (kg)} \times (140 - \text{age})}{72 \times \text{serum creatinine (mg/dL)}} = \text{Ccr}$

Females: 0.85 × above value

➤*Elderly:* Dose based on normal or impaired renal function.

➤*CDC recommended treatment schedules for gonorrhea†:* Gonococcal infections, uncomplicated – 800 mg as a single dose (alternative regimen to ciprofloxacin or ofloxacin).

OFLOXACIN

Rx	Ofloxacin (Various, eg, Par, Ranbaxy)	**Tablets:** 200 mg	In 50s and 100s.
Rx	Floxin (Ortho-McNeil)		Lactose. (Floxin 200). Lt. yellow. Film coated. In 50s and UD 6s and 100s.
Rx	Ofloxacin (Various, eg, Par, Ranbaxy)	**Tablets:** 300 mg	In 50s and 100s.
Rx	Floxin (Ortho-McNeil)		Lactose. (Floxin 300). White. Film coated. In 50s and UD 100s.
Rx	Ofloxacin (Various, eg, Par, Ranbaxy)	**Tablets:** 400 mg	In 100s.
Rx	Floxin (Ortho-McNeil)		Lactose. (Floxin 400). Pale gold. Film coated. In 100s and UD 100s.

¹ Preservative free.

For complete prescribing information, refer to the Fluoroquinolones group monograph.

Indications

For the treatment of adults with the following infections caused by susceptible strains of the designated microorganisms.

➤*Lower respiratory tract infections:* Acute bacterial exacerbations of chronic bronchitis or community-acquired pneumonia due to *Haemophilus influenzae* or *Streptococcus pneumoniae.*

➤*Sexually transmitted diseases:* See Warnings. Acute, uncomplicated urethral and cervical gonorrhea due to *Neisseria gonorrhoeae*; nongonococcal urethritis and cervicitis due to *Chlamydia trachomatis*; mixed infections of urethra and cervix due to both organisms. Acute pelvic inflammatory disease (including severe infection) caused by *C. trachomatis* or *N. gonorrhoeae.*

➤*Skin and skin structure infections (uncomplicated):* Due to *Staphylococcus aureus, Streptococcus pyogenes,* or *Proteus mirabilis.*

➤*Urinary tract infections:* Uncomplicated cystitis due to *Citrobacter diversus, Enterobacter aerogenes, Escherichia coli, Klebsiella pneumoniae, P. mirabilis,* or *Pseudomonas aeruginosa*; complicated UTIs due to *E. coli, K. pneumoniae, P. mirabilis, C. diversus,* or *P. aeruginosa.*

➤*Prostatitis:* Due to *E. coli.*

Administration and Dosage

➤*Approved by the FDA:* December 28, 1990.

Usual daily dose is 200 to 400 mg every 12 hours as described in the following table:

OFLOXACIN

Ofloxacin Dosage Guidelines[1]					
Infection	Description	Dose	Frequency	Duration	Daily dose
Lower respiratory tract	Exacerbation of chronic bronchitis	400 mg	q 12 h	10 days	800 mg
	Community acquired pneumonia	400 mg	q 12 h	10 days	800 mg
Sexually transmitted diseases	Acute, uncomplicated urethral and cervical gonorrhea	400 mg	single dose	1 day	400 mg
	Cervicitis/urethritis due to *C. trachomatis*	300 mg	q 12 h	7 days	600 mg
	Cervicitis/urethritis due to *C. trachomatis* and *N. gonorrhoeae*	300 mg	q 12 h	7 days	600 mg
	Acute pelvic inflammatory disease	400 mg	q 12 h	10 to 14 days	800 mg
Skin and skin structure	Uncomplicated	400 mg	q 12 h	10 days	800 mg
Urinary tract	Uncomplicated cystitis due to *E. coli* or *K. pneumoniae*	200 mg	q 12 h	3 days	400 mg
	Uncomplicated cystitis due to other organisms	200 mg	q 12 h	7 days	400 mg
	Complicated UTIs	200 mg	q 12 h	10 days	400 mg
Prostatitis	Due to *E. coli*	300 mg	q 12 h	6 weeks	600 mg

[1] Due to the designated pathogens (see Indications).

Do not take antacids containing calcium, magnesium, or aluminum; sucralfate; divalent or trivalent cations such as iron; multivitamins containing zinc; or didanosine chewable/buffered tablets or the pediatric powder for oral solution 2 hours before or 2 hours after taking ofloxacin.

➤*Renal function impairment:* Adjust dosage in patients with a Ccr value of ≤ 50 mL/min. After a normal initial dose, adjust the dosing interval as follows:

Ofloxacin Dosage in Impaired Renal Function		
Creatinine clearance (mL/min)	Maintenance dose	Frequency
20 to 50	usual recommended unit dose	q 24 hr
< 20	½ usual recommended unit dose	q 24 hr

When only the serum creatinine is known, the following formula may be used to estimate Ccr. Serum creatinine should represent a steady state of renal function.

Males: $\dfrac{\text{Weight (kg)} \times (140 - \text{age})}{72 \times \text{serum creatinine (mg/dL)}} = \text{Ccr}$

Females: $0.85 \times$ above value

➤*Chronic hepatic impairment (cirrhosis):* The excretion of ofloxacin may be reduced in patients with severe liver function disorders (eg, cirrhosis with or without ascites). Do not exceed a maximum dose of 400 mg/day.

➤*CDC recommended treatment schedules for chlamydia, epididymitis, pelvic inflammatory disease (PID), and gonorrhea†:*
Chlamydia – 300 mg orally 2 times a day for 7 days (alternative regimen).

Epididymitis – 300 mg orally 2 times a day for 10 days.

PID, outpatient – 400 mg orally 2 times a day for 14 days plus metronidazole.

Gonococcal infections, uncomplicated – 400 mg orally in a single dose plus doxycycline or azithromycin.

➤*Storage/Stability:* Store below 30°C (86°F) in airtight containers.

SPARFLOXACIN

Rx	**Zagam** (Bertek)	**Tablets:** 200 mg	(B 11). White. Film coated. In 55s and blister pack 11s.

For complete prescribing information, refer to the Fluoroquinolones group monograph.

Indications

For the treatment of adults 18 years of age and older with the following infections caused by susceptible strains of the designated microorganisms in the conditions listed below:

➤*Community-acquired pneumonia:* Caused by *Chlamydia pneumoniae, Haemophilus influenzae, Haemophilus parainfluenzae, Moraxella catarrhalis, Mycoplasma pneumoniae,* or *Streptococcus pneumoniae.*

➤*Acute bacterial exacerbations of chronic bronchitis:* Caused by *C. pneumoniae, Enterobacter cloacae, H. influenzae, H. parainfluenzae, Klebsiella pneumoniae, M. catarrhalis, Staphylococcus aureus,* or *S. pneumoniae.*

Administration and Dosage

➤*Approved by the FDA:* December 20, 1996.

Sparfloxacin can be taken with or without food. Antacids containing magnesium or aluminum or sucralfate or didanosine chewable/buffered tablets or the pediatric powder for oral solution may be taken 4 hours after sparfloxacin administration.

The recommended daily dose of sparfloxacin in patients with normal renal function is two 200 mg tablets taken on the first day as a loading dose. Thereafter, take one 200 mg tablet every 24 hours for a total of 10 days of therapy (11 tablets).

➤*Renal function impairment:* The recommended daily dose of sparfloxacin in patients with renal impairment (creatinine clearance less than 50 mL/min) is two 200 mg tablets taken on the first day as a loading dose. Thereafter, take one 200 mg tablet every 48 hours for a total of 9 days of therapy (6 tablets).

† CDC 1998 Sexually Transmitted Diseases Treatment Guidelines. *Morbidity and Mortality Weekly Report* 1998 Jan 23;47 (RR-1):1–118.

TROVAFLOXACIN MESYLATE/ALATROFLOXACIN MESYLATE

Rx	Trovan	Tablets: 100 mg trovafloxacin mesylate	(Pfizer 378). Blue. Film coated. In 30s and UD 40s.
	(Pfizer)	200 mg trovafloxacin mesylate	(Pfizer 379). Blue, oval. Film coated. In 30s and UD 40s.
		Solution for Injection: 5 mg/mL alatrofloxacin mesylate	Preservative free. In 40 and 60 mL single-use vials.

WARNING

Trovafloxacin has been associated with serious liver injury leading to liver transplantation or death. Trovafloxacin-associated liver injury has been reported with short-term and long-term drug exposure. Trovafloxacin use exceeding 2 weeks in duration is associated with a significantly increased risk of serious liver injury. Liver injury has also been reported following trovafloxacin re-exposure. Reserve trovafloxacin for use in patients with serious, life- or limb-threatening infections who receive their initial therapy in an inpatient health care facility (eg, hospital, long-term nursing care facility). Do not use trovafloxacin when safer, alternative antimicrobial therapy will be effective.

Indications

For the treatment of patients initiating therapy in inpatient health care facilities (eg, hospitals, long term nursing care facilities) with serious, life- or limb-threatening infections caused by susceptible strains of the designated microorganisms in the conditions listed below:

➤*Nosocomial pneumonia:* Caused by *Escherichia coli, Pseudomonas aeruginosa, Haemophilus influenzae,* or *Staphylococcus aureus.* As with other antimicrobials, where *P. aeruginosa* is a documented or presumptive pathogen, combination therapy with either an aminoglycoside or aztreonam may be clinically indicated.

➤*Community-acquired pneumonia:* Caused by *Streptococcus pneumoniae, H. influenzae, S. aureus, Klebsiella pneumoniae, Mycoplasma pneumoniae, Moraxella catarrhalis, Legionella pneumophila,* or *Chlamydia pneumoniae.*

➤*Complicated intra-abdominal infections (including postsurgical infections):* Caused by *E. coli, Bacteroides fragilis,* Viridans group streptococci, *P. aeruginosa, K. pneumoniae, Peptostreptococcus* sp., or *Prevotella* sp.

➤*Gynecologic and pelvic infections (including endomyometritis, parametritis, septic abortion, and postpartum infections):* Caused by *E. coli, B. fragilis,* Viridans group streptococci, *Enterococcus faecalis, Streptococcus agalactiae, Peptostreptococcus* sp., *Prevotella* sp., or *Gardnerella vaginalis.*

➤*Complicated skin and skin structure infections (including diabetic foot infections):* Caused by *S. aureus, S. agalactiae, P. aeruginosa, Enterococcus faecalis, E. coli,* or *Proteus mirabilis.* Note: This drug has not been studied in the treatment of osteomyelitis.

Administration and Dosage

➤*Approved by the FDA:* December 18, 1997.

Administer oral doses ≥ 2 hours before or 2 hours after antacids containing magnesium or aluminum, as well as sucralfate, citric acid buffered with sodium citrate, metal cations (eg, ferrous sulfate), and didanosine (chewable/buffered tablets or pediatric powder for oral solution).

Administer alatrofloxacin only by IV infusion. Do not administer by IM, intrathecal, intraperitoneal, or SC routes.

Single-use vials require dilution prior to administration.

➤*Patients already receiving IV morphine:* If trovafloxacin is taken on an empty stomach, administer IV morphine ≥ 2 hours later. If trovafloxacin is taken with food, administer IV morphine ≥ 4 hours later.

Trovafloxacin/Alatrofloxacin Dosage Guidelines

Infection[1]/ Location and type	Daily unit dose and route of administration	Frequency	Total duration
Nosocomial pneumonia[2]	300 mg IV[3] followed by 200 mg oral	q 24 hr	10 to 14 days
Community-acquired pneumonia	200 mg oral or 200 mg IV followed by 200 mg oral	q 24 hr	7 to 14 days
Complicated intra-abdominal infections, including post-surgical infections	300 mg IV[3] followed by 200 mg oral	q 24 hr	7 to 14 days
Gynecologic and pelvic infections	300 mg IV[3] followed by 200 mg oral	q 24 hr	7 to 14 days
Skin and skin structure infections, complicated, including diabetic foot infections	200 mg oral or 200 mg IV followed by 200 mg oral	q 24 hr	10 to 14 days

[1] Due to the designated pathogens (see Indications).
[2] As with other antimicrobials, where *P. aeruginosa* is a documented or presumptive pathogen, combination therapy with either an aminoglycoside or aztreonam may be clinically indicated.
[3] Where the 300 mg IV dose is indicated, decrease therapy to 200 mg as soon as clinically indicated.

Do not administer trovafloxacin for > 2 weeks. Only administer for > 2 weeks if the treating physician believes the benefits to the individual patient clearly outweigh the risks of longer-term treatment.

➤*Renal function impairment:* No dosage adjustment is necessary in patients with impaired renal function. Trovafloxacin is eliminated primarily by biliary excretion. Trovafloxacin is not efficiently removed by hemodialysis.

➤*Chronic hepatic disease (cirrhosis):* The following table provides dosing guidelines for patients with mild or moderate cirrhosis (Child-Pugh class A/B). There are no data in patients with severe cirrhosis (Child-Pugh class C).

Trovafloxacin/Alatrofloxacin Dosage in Chronic Hepatic Disease

Indicated dose (normal hepatic function)	Chronic hepatic disease dose
300 mg IV	200 mg IV
200 mg IV or oral	100 mg IV or oral

➤*IV administration:* After dilution with an appropriate diluent, administer by IV infusion over a period of 60 minutes. Avoid rapid or bolus IV infusion.

Alatrofloxacin is supplied in single-use vials containing a concentrated solution of alatrofloxacin mesylate in water for injection (equivalent to 200 or 300 mg as trovafloxacin). Each milliliter contains alatrofloxacin mesylate equivalent to 5 mg trovafloxacin. These single-use IV vials must be further diluted with an appropriate solution prior to IV administration.

➤*Preparation of injection:* Prepare the IV dose by aseptically withdrawing the appropriate volume of concentrate from the vials of alatrofloxacin IV. Dilute with a suitable IV solution to a final concentration of 1 to 2 mg/mL (see Compatible IV solutions). Infuse the resulting solution over 60 minutes by direct infusion or through a Y-type IV infusion set that may already be in place.

Because the vials are for single-use only, discard any unused solution.

Alatrofloxacin IV dosage may be prepared according to the following chart:

Preparation of Desired Alatrofloxacin Dosage

Dosage strength (mg) (trovafloxacin equivalent)	Volume to withdraw (mL)	Diluent volume (mL)	Total volume (mL)	Infusion conc. (mg/mL)
100	20	30	50	2
100	20	80	100	1
200	40	60	100	2
200	40	160	200	1
300	60	90	150	2
300	60	240	300	1

For example, to prepare a 200 mg dose at an infusion concentration of 2 mg/mL (as trovafloxacin), 40 mL alatrofloxacin is withdrawn from a vial and diluted with 60 mL of a compatible IV fluid to produce a total infusion solution volume of 100 mL.

➤*Admixture incompatibility:* Only limited data are available; do not add additives or other medications to alatrofloxacin IV through the same IV line. If the same IV line is used for sequential infusion of different drugs, flush the line before and after infusion of alatrofloxacin with an infusion solution compatible with alatrofloxacin and with any other drugs administered via this common line. If alatrofloxacin is given concomitantly with another drug, give each drug separately.

Do not dilute alatrofloxacin with 0.9% sodium chloride injection (normal saline), alone or in combination with other diluents. A precipitate may form under these conditions. In addition, do not dilute alatrofloxacin with lactated Ringer's.

➤*Compatible IV solutions:* 5% dextrose injection; 0.45% sodium chloride injection; 5% dextrose and 0.45% sodium chloride injection; 5% dextrose and 0.2% sodium chloride injection; lactated Ringer's and 5% dextrose injection.

Normal saline, 0.9% sodium chloride injection, can be used for flushing IV lines prior to or after administration of alatrofloxacin.

➤*Storage/Stability:*

Injection – When diluted with the preceding IV solutions to concentrations of 0.5 to 2 mg/mL (as trovafloxacin), the solution is physically and chemically stable for ≤ 7 days when refrigerated and ≤ 3 days at room temperature stored in glass bottles or plastic (PVC type) IV containers.

Store IV solution at 15° to 30°C (59° to 86°F). Protect from light. Do not freeze.

Refer to the Gastrointestinal Agents chapter for additional information regarding tetracycline use in periodontitis.

Indications

Refer to individual agents for more specific information.

➤*Gram-negative organisms:* Haemophilus ducreyi (chancroid); Francisella tularensis (tularemia); Yersinia pestis (plague); Bartonella bacilliformis (bartonellosis); Campylobacter fetus; Vibrio cholerae (cholera); Brucella sp. (brucellosis, may be in conjunction with streptomycin); Calymmatobacterium granulomatis (granuloma inguinale).

➤*Infections caused by the following miscellaneous microorganisms:* Rickettsiae (Rocky Mountain spotted fever, typhus fever and the typhus group, Q fever, rickettsialpox, and tick fevers); Mycoplasma pneumoniae (PPLO, Eaton agent, respiratory tract infections); Chlamydia trachomatis (lymphogranuloma venereum, trachoma [infectious agent not always eliminated], inclusion conjunctivitis, uncomplicated urethral, endocervical, or rectal infections); Chlamydia psittaci (psittacosis [ornithosis]); Borrelia sp. (relapsing fever); Ureaplasma urealyticum (nongonococcal urethritis).

➤*Following susceptibility testing (resistance has been documented):* Escherichia coli; Enterobacter aerogenes; Acinetobacter sp.; Haemophilus influenzae (respiratory tract infections); Klebsiella sp. (respiratory and urinary infections); Streptococcus pneumoniae (upper respiratory tract infections); S. pyogenes, S. pneumoniae, Mycoplasma pneumoniae (Eaton agent), and Klebsiella sp. (lower respiratory tract infections); Staphylococcus aureus, S. pyogenes (skin and skin structure infections); Bacteroides and Shigella sp.

➤*Alternative therapy for the following infections when penicillin is contraindicated:* Uncomplicated gonorrhea due to Neisseria gonorrhoeae; syphilis due to Treponema pallidum; yaws due to T. pertenue; Listeria monocytogenes; anthrax due to Bacillus anthracis; Vincent's infection due to Fusobacterium fusiforme; actinomycosis due to Actinomyces sp.; Clostridium sp.

➤*Acute intestinal amebiasis:* Due to Entamoeba histolytica as adjunct to amebicides.

➤*Severe acne (tetracycline, doxycycline, minocycline only):* As adjunctive therapy.

➤*Anthrax, including inhalational anthrax (doxycline only):* To reduce the incidence or progression of disease following exposure to aerosolized Bacillus anthracis.

➤*Malaria (doxycycline only):* Prophylaxis of malaria due to Plasmodium falciparum in short-term travelers (less than 4 months) to areas with chloroquine and/or pyrimethamine-sulfadoxine resistant strains.

➤*Neisseria meningitidis (minocycline only):* Treatment of asymptomatic meningococcal carriers of N. meningitidis.

➤*Note:* Do not use tetracyclines for streptococcal disease unless organism has been shown to be susceptible. Tetracyclines are not the drugs of choice in treatment of any type of staphylococcal infection.

➤*Unlabeled uses:*

Tetracycline – In conjunction with metronidazole for the treatment of extraintestinal amebiasis caused by E. histolytica; gonococcal arthritis; early Lyme disease; malaria; ocular rosacea; adjunctive therapy for peptic ulcers due to Helicobacter pylori (500 mg 4 times/day).

Doxycycline – Treament of malaria (100 mg twice daily for 7 days in combination with other antimalarial agents), pleural malignant effusions, alternative agent for nocardiosis in patients who cannot take sulfa medications, ocular rosacea, treatment of traveler's diarrhea, prophylaxis of pneumothorax.

  Lyme disease:
  • *Tick bite from endemic area* – 200 mg once.
  • *Early Lyme disease* – 100 mg twice daily for 14 to 21 days.
  • *Carditis (first degree AV block)* – 100 mg twice daily for 14 to 21 days.
  • *Facial nerve paralysis* – 100 mg twice daily for 14 to 21 days.
  • *Arthritis* – 100 mg twice daily for 30 to 60 days.
  CDC recommended treatment schedules for sexually transmitted diseases:
  • *Granuloma inguinale (donovanosis)* – 100 mg twice daily for at least 3 weeks.

• *Early syphilis* – 100 mg twice daily for 14 days.
• *Latent syphilis* – 100 mg twice daily fo 28 days.
• *Chlamydial infections* –
  Adults and children (8 years of age and older): 100 mg twice daily for 7 days.
• *Pelvic inflammatory disease* – 100 mg orally or IV every 12 hours plus cefotetan 2 g IV every 12 hours or cefoxitin 2 g IV every 6 hours. May discontinue parenteral therapy after 24 hours; continue oral therapy with doxycycline for a total of 14 days.
• *Epididymitis most likely caused by gonococcal or chlamydial infection* – 100 mg twice daily for 10 days plus a single dose of ceftriaxone 250 mg IM.
• *Sexual assault prophylaxis* – 100 mg twice daily for 7 days plus ceftriaxone and metronidazole.

Minocycline – Treatment of early rheumatoid arthritis, gallbladder infections caused by E. coli, alternative agent for nocardiosis in patients who cannot take sulfa medications, chronic malignant pleural effusion.

Demeclocycline – Treatment of the syndrome of inappropriate antidiuretic hormone (SIADH).

Oxytetracycline – Peptic ulcers (eradication of H. pylori).

Administration and Dosage

Avoid rapid IV administration. Thrombophlebitis may result from prolonged IV therapy.

Continue therapy at least 24 to 48 hours after symptoms and fever subside. Treat all infections caused by group A β-hemolytic streptococci for 10 days or more.

Take on an empty stomach, at least 2 hours before or after meals. Absorption and peak plasma levels may be reduced when administered with meals or with dairy products, including milk.

Administer oral tetracyclines with plenty of fluids.

Actions

➤*Pharmacology:* The tetracyclines are bacteriostatic. They exert their antimicrobial effect by reversibly binding to the 30S subunit of the bacterial ribosome, preventing the binding of aminoacyl transfer RNA and thus inhibiting protein synthesis and thus cell growth. Tetracyclines are active against a wide range of gram-positive and gram-negative organisms and have similar antimicrobial spectra, and cross-resistance is common.

➤*Pharmacokinetics:*

Absorption/Distribution – Tetracyclines are adequately but incompletely absorbed from the GI tract. The percentage absorbed when taken on an empty stomach is lowest for **oxytetracycline**, **demeclocycline**, and **tetracycline**, and highest for **doxycycline** and **minocycline**. The extent of absorption is usually decreased by the presence of divalent and trivalent cations and to a variable degree by milk or food (see Drug Interactions). Tetracyclines are bound to plasma proteins in varying degrees.

Penetration of the tetracyclines into most body fluids and tissues is excellent. Tetracyclines are distributed in varying amounts into bile, liver, lung, kidney, prostate, urine, CSF, synovial fluid, mucosa of the maxillary sinus, brain, sputum, and bone. Inflammation of the meninges is not required for passage into the CSF, but concentrations may increase in the presence of inflamed meninges. Tetracyclines cross the placenta and enter the fetal circulation and amniotic fluid.

Metabolism/Excretion – The tetracyclines are concentrated in the bile by the liver. They are excreted in the urine and feces at high concentrations in a biologically active form. Because renal clearance of tetracyclines is by glomerular filtration, excretion is significantly affected by the state of renal function. The renal clearance of **demeclocycline** has been shown to be about half of that of tetracycline. The urinary and fecal recovery of **minocycline** is one half to one third that of other tetracyclines, and minocycline also appears to undergo some metabolism, largely to 9-hydroxyminocycline. **Doxycycline** appears to be excreted extensively by the digestive tract.

Tetracycline Pharmacokinetics						
Tetracyclines	Absorption (%)	C_{max} (mcg/mL)	T_{max} (h)	Protein binding (%)	Serum half-life (h)	Excreted in urine (%)
Demeclocycline	60 to 80	1.5 to 1.7[1]	3 to 4[1]	35 to 90	16	nd[*]
Doxycycline	90 to 100	2.6 (hyclate)[2] 3.61 (monohydrate)[2] 3.6 (IV)[3]	2 (hyclate)[2] 2.6 (monohydrate)[2]	80 to 95	18 to 22	40
Minocycline	90 to 100	2.1 to 5.1[4]	1 to 4	75	11 to 22 (oral) 15 to 23 (IV)	5 to 10
Oxytetracycline	60 to 80	nd	2 to 4	20 to 40	6 to 12	10 to 35
Tetracycline	60 to 80	nd	2 to 4	20 to 65	6 to 12	20 to 55

[*] nd = no data
[1] 300 mg single oral dose.
[2] 200 mg single oral dose.
[3] 200 mg administered IV over 2 hours.
[4] Single oral dose of two 100 mg pellet-filled capsules.

➤*Microbiology:*

Organisms Generally Susceptible to Tetracyclines[1]					
Organism	Demeclocycline	Doxycycline	Minocycline	Oxytetracycline	Tetracycline
Gram-positive					
Actinomyces sp.	✓	✓	✓	✓	✓
Alpha-hemolytic streptococci (Viridans group)		✓	✓		✓
Bacillus anthracis	✓	✓	✓	✓	✓
Clostridium sp.	✓	✓	✓	✓	✓
Enterococcus faecalis[2,3]		✓	✓	✓	✓
E. faecium		✓	✓		✓
Listeria monocytogenes	✓	✓	✓	✓	✓
Propionibacterium acnes		✓	✓		✓
Staphylococcus aureus[4]	✓	✓	✓	✓	
Streptococcus pneumoniae[2]	✓	✓	✓	✓	✓
S. pyogenes[2,5]	✓	✓	✓	✓	✓
Treponema pallidum	✓	✓	✓	✓	✓
T. pertenue	✓	✓	✓	✓	✓
Gram-negative					
Acinetobacter sp.[2]	✓	✓	✓	✓	✓
Bacteroides sp.[2]	✓	✓	✓	✓	✓
Bartonella bacilliformis	✓	✓	✓	✓	✓
Borrelia recurrentis	✓	✓	✓	✓	✓
Brucella sp.	✓	✓	✓	✓	✓
Calymmatobacterium granulomatis	✓	✓	✓	✓	✓
Campylobacter fetus	✓	✓	✓	✓	✓
Enterobacter aerogenes[2]	✓	✓	✓	✓	✓
Escherichia coli[2]	✓	✓	✓	✓	✓
Francisella tularensis	✓	✓	✓	✓	✓
Fusobacterium fusiforme	✓	✓	✓	✓	✓
Haemophilus ducreyi	✓	✓	✓	✓	✓
H. influenzae[2]	✓	✓	✓	✓	✓
Klebsiella sp.[2]	✓	✓	✓	✓	✓
Neisseria gonorrhoeae	✓	✓	✓	✓	✓
N. meningitides	✓	✓	✓	✓	✓
Shigella sp.[2]	✓	✓	✓	✓	✓
Vibrio cholerae	✓	✓	✓	✓	✓
Yersinia pestis	✓	✓	✓	✓	✓
Miscellaneous					
Balantidium coli		✓	✓		✓
Chlamydia psittaci	✓	✓	✓	✓	✓
C. trachomatis	✓	✓	✓	✓	✓
Entamoeba sp.	✓	✓	✓	✓	✓
Mycobacterium marinum			✓		
Mycoplasma pneumoniae	✓	✓	✓	✓	✓
Plasmodium falciparum[6]		✓			
Rickettsiae sp.	✓	✓	✓	✓	✓
Ureaplasma urealyticum		✓	✓		✓

[1] Cross-resistance of these organisms to tetracyclines is common.
[2] Because many strains of gram-negative micro-organisms have been shown to be resistant to tetracyclines, culture and susceptibility testing are recommended.
[3] Up to 74% of *Enterococcus faecalis* have been found to be resistant to tetracyclines.
[4] Tetracyclines are not the drugs of choice in the treatment of any type of staphylococcal infections.
[5] Up to 44% of *Streptococcus pyogenes* have been found to be resistant to tetracycline drugs.
[6] Doxycycline has been found to be active against the asexual erythrocytic form of *Plasmodium falciparum* but not against the gametocytes of *P. falciparum*.

Contraindications

Hypersensitivity to any of the tetracyclines or components of product formulations.

Warnings

➤*Malaria prophylaxis (doxycycline only):* **Doxycycline** offers substantial but not complete suppression of the asexual stages of *Plasmodium* strains. It does not suppress *P. falciparum*'s sexual blood stage gametocytes and therefore patients completing this prophylactic regimen may still transmit the infection to mosquitos outside endemic areas. Advise patients taking doxycycline for malaria prophylaxis of when prophylaxis should begin and end; that no present-day antimalarial, including doxycycline, guarantees protection against malaria; and to avoid being bitten by mosquitos by wearing protective clothing, using effective insect-repellent, mosquito nets, etc.

➤*Pseudomembranous colitis:* Treatment with antibacterial agents alters the normal flora of the colon and may permit overgrowth of clostridia. Pseudomembranous colitis has been reported with nearly all antibacterial agents and may range in severity from mild to life-threatening. It is important to consider this diagnosis in patients who present with diarrhea following subsequent administration of antibacterial agents. Once the diagnosis is established, initiate therapeutic measures. Mild cases usually respond to discontinuation of the drug. Moderate to severe cases may require management with fluids, electrolytes, protein supplementation, and treatment with an antibacterial agent effective against *Clostridium difficile* colitis.

➤*Parenteral therapy:* Reserve for situations in which oral therapy is not indicated. Institute oral therapy as soon as possible. If given IV over prolonged periods, thrombophlebitis may result. IM use produces lower blood levels than recommended oral dosages. If high blood levels are needed rapidly, administer IV.

➤*Nephrogenic diabetes insipidus:* Administration of **demeclocycline** has resulted in appearance of the diabetes insipidus syndrome (eg, polyuria, polydipsia, weakness) in some patients on long-term therapy. The syndrome has been shown to be nephrogenic, dose-dependent, and reversible on discontinuation of therapy.

➤*Hypersensitivity reactions:* Sensitivity reactions are more likely to occur on patients with a history of allergy, asthma, hay fever, or urticaria. Use tetracyclines with caution in these patients. Cross-sensitivity among the tetracyclines is extremely common.

➤*Renal function impairment:* Use tetracyclines with caution in patients with impaired renal function.

If renal impairment exists, even usual doses may lead to excessive systemic accumulation of the tetracyclines (with the exception of **doxycycline**) and possible liver toxicity. Use lower than usual doses; if therapy is prolonged, drug serum level determinations may be advisable. Concurrent use of tetracycline and methoxyflurane has resulted in fatal renal toxicity.

The antianabolic action of tetracyclines may cause an increase in blood urea nitrogen. In significantly impaired renal function, higher serum tetracycline levels may lead to azotemia, hyperphosphatemia, and acidosis. This does not seem to occur with doxycycline.

➤*Hepatic function impairment:* Use tetracyclines with caution in patients with impaired liver function.

In the presence of renal dysfunction, and particularly in pregnancy, IV tetracycline more than 2 g/day has been associated with death secondary to liver failure. When need for intensive treatment outweighs its potential dangers (especially during pregnancy or in known or suspected renal and liver impairment), monitor renal and liver function tests. Serum tetracycline concentrations should not exceed 15 mcg/mL. Do not prescribe other potentially hepatotoxic drugs concomitantly.

Hepatotoxicity has been reported with **minocycline**; therefore, minocycline should be used with caution in patients with hepatic dysfunction and in conjunction with other hepatotoxic drugs.

The hazard of liver toxicity is of particular importance in parenteral administration to pregnant or postpartum patients with pyelonephritis.

➤*Carcinogenesis:* There has been evidence of oncogenic activity in studies with **oxytetracycline** (adrenal and pituitary tumors) in rats and **minocycline** (thyroid tumors) in rats and dogs.

➤*Mutagenesis:* **Tetracycline** and **oxytetracycline** have produced positive mutagenic results in mammalian cell assays in vitro.

➤*Fertility impairment:* **Minocycline** has been shown to impair fertility in male rats.

➤*Pregnancy:* Category D. Tetracyclines readily cross the placenta and are found in fetal tissues and can have toxic effects on the developing fetus (retardation of skeletal development). Evidence of embryotoxicity has also been noted in animals treated early in pregnancy.

A case-control study (18,515 mothers of infants with congenital anomalies and 32,804 mothers of infants with no congenital anomalies) shows a weak but marginally statistically significant association with total malformations and use of **doxycycline** any time during pregnancy. Sixty-three (0.19%) of the controls and 56 (0.3%) of the cases were treated with doxycycline. This association was not seen when the analysis was confined to maternal treatment during the period of organogenesis with the exception of a marginal relationship with neural tube defect based on only 2 exposed cases.

➤*Lactation:* Tetracyclines are excreted in breast milk. Milk:plasma ratios vary between 0.25 and 1.5. Because of the potential for serious adverse reactions, decide whether to discontinue nursing or discontinue the drug.

➤*Children:* Generally, do not use tetracyclines in children under 8 years of age (except for anthrax, including inhalational), unless other drugs are not likely to be effective or are contraindicated.

Teeth – The use of tetracyclines during the period of tooth development (from the last half of pregnancy through 8 years of age) may cause permanent discoloration (yellow, gray, brown) of teeth. This adverse reaction is more common during long-term use of the drugs, but has been observed following repeated short-term courses. Enamel hypoplasia has also been reported.

Bone – Tetracyclines form a stable calcium complex in any bone-forming tissue. Decreased fibula growth rate occurred in premature infants given 25 mg/kg oral tetracycline every 6 hours. This was reversible when the drug was discontinued.

Precautions

➤*Monitoring:* In sexually transmitted diseases when coexistent syphilis is suspected, perform darkfield examination before starting treatment and repeat the blood serology monthly for at least 4 months.

In long-term therapy, perform periodic laboratory evaluation of organ systems, including hematopoietic, renal, and hepatic studies.

➤*CNS effects:* In adults, pseudotumor cerebri (benign intracranial hypertension) has been associated with tetracycline use. Usual clinical manifestations are headache and blurred vision. Bulging fontanels have been associated with tetracycline use in infants. While both con-

ditions and related symptoms usually resolve soon after tetracycline discontinuation, the possibility for permanent sequelae exists.

➤*Outdated products:* Under no circumstances should outdated tetracyclines be administered; the degradation products of tetracyclines are highly nephrotoxic and have, on occasion, produced a Fanconi-like syndrome.

➤*Hazardous tasks:* Lightheadedness, dizziness, or vertigo may occur with tetracyclines. Advise patients to observe caution while driving or performing other tasks requiring alertness. These symptoms may disappear during therapy and always disappear rapidly when the drug is discontinued.

➤*Superinfection:* Use of antibiotics (especially prolonged or repeated therapy) may result in bacterial or fungal overgrowth of nonsusceptible organisms. Such overgrowth may lead to a secondary infection. Take appropriate measures if superinfection occurs. Superinfection of the bowel by staphylococci may be life-threatening.

➤*Photosensitivity:* Photosensitivity manifested by an exaggerated sunburn reaction has been observed in some individuals taking tetracyclines. Advise patients who are apt to be exposed to direct sunlight or ultraviolet light that this reaction can occur with tetracycline drugs, and discontinue treatment at the first evidence of skin erythema.

Exaggerated sunburn reactions are characterized by severe burns of exposed surfaces, resulting from direct exposure to sunlight during therapy with moderate or large doses. Phototoxic reactions are most frequent with demeclocycline, and occur less frequently with the other tetracyclines.

➤*Sulfite sensitivity:* Some of these products contain sulfites that may cause allergic-type reactions (eg, anaphylactic symptoms, life-threatening or less severe asthmatic episodes) in certain susceptible people. The **oxytetracycline** injection solution contains sodium formaldehyde sulfoxylate, which serves as an antioxidant. Upon oxidation, this compound can form a potential sulfiting agent. The overall prevalence of sulfite sensitivity in the general population is unknown and probably low. It is seen more frequently in asthmatic or atopic nonasthmatic people. Specific products containing sulfites are identified in the product listings.

Drug Interactions

Tetracycline Drug Interactions			
Precipitant drug	Object drug*		Description
Antacids (containing aluminum, calcium or magnesium salts) Iron salts Zinc salts	Tetracyclines	↓	Tetracyclines administered with aluminum, calcium, magnesium, iron, or zinc salts form an insoluble chelate, thereby decreasing the absorption and serum levels of the tetracycline. Administer tetracyclines at least 2 hours before or after these agents.
Barbiturates	Doxycycline	↓	Barbiturates increase the hepatic metabolism of doxycycline, therefore decreasing doxycycline's half-life and serum levels. Adjust doxycycline dose as needed. Consider using an alternative tetracycline.
Bismuth salts	Tetracyclines	↓	Coadministration of bismuth salts in liquid formulations may decrease the serum levels of tetracyclines. Give the bismuth salt 2 hours after the tetracycline.
Carbamazepine	Doxycycline	↓	Carbamazepine may decrease the half-life and serum levels of doxycycline due to increased hepatic metabolism. Adjust doxycycline dose as needed. Consider using an alternative tetracycline.
Cholestyramine Colestipol	Tetracyclines	↓	Coadministration may decrease or delay the absorption of tetracyclines, therefore decreasing the serum concentrations. Adjust the tetracycline dose if needed.
Phenytoin Rifamycins	Doxycycline	↓	Phenytoin and rifamycins appear to induce the metabolism of doxycycline causing the half-life to be significantly decreased. Increased doxycycline dosage may be needed.
Urinary alkalinizers (eg, sodium lactate, potassium citrate)	Tetracyclines	↓	Coadministration may result in increased excretion of the tetracyclines and decreased serum levels. Separate administration by 3 to 4 hours; however, this may not be effective and an increase in tetracycline dose may be necessary if the pH of the urine remains increased.

Tetracycline Drug Interactions			
Precipitant drug	Object drug*		Description
Tetracyclines	Anticoagulants, oral	↑	The action of oral anticoagulants may be increased because of the elimination of vitamin K-producing gut bacteria by tetracyclines. Monitor coagulation parameters and adjust anticoagulant dose as needed.
Tetracyclines	Contraceptives, oral	↓	Tetracyclines may interfere with the enterohepatic recirculation of certain contraceptive steroids, leading to reduced efficacy. Although infrequently reported, contraceptive failure is possible.
Tetracyclines	Digoxin	↑	Coadministration may result in increased serum levels of digoxin in a small subset of patients (≈ 10%). Monitor digoxin levels and signs of toxicity.
Tetracyclines	Insulin	↑	The ability of insulin to produce hypoglycemia may be potentiated. In diabetic patients, monitor blood glucose concentrations closely and tailor the insulin regimen as needed.
Tetracyclines	Isotretinoin	↑	Isotretinoin use has been associated with a number of cases of pseudotumor cerebri, some of which involved coadministration of tetracyclines. Therefore, avoid concomitant use.
Tetracyclines	Methoxyflurane	↑	Coadministration may enhance the risk for renal toxicity; deaths have been reported. Do not coadminister. If possible seek alternative agents.
Tetracyclines	Penicillins	↓	The bacteriostatic action of tetracyclines may interfere with the bactericidal activity of penicillins. Consider avoiding this combination if at all possible.
Tetracyclines	Theophyllines	↑	The incidence of adverse reactions to theophyllines may be increased. Monitor theophylline levels and adjust dose as needed.

* ↑ = Object drug increased.   ↓ = Object drug decreased.

➤*Drug/Lab test interactions:* During **doxycycline** or **minocycline** therapy, false elevations of urinary catecholamine levels may occur because of interference with the fluorescence test.

➤*Drug/Food interactions:* The administration of **demeclocycline**, **oxytetracycline**, and **tetracycline** with milk and dairy products forms poorly absorbed chelates. A number of studies have reported the serum levels of these tetracyclines, when administered with milk products, to be 50% to 80% lower. Administer the interacting tetracyclines at least 2 hours before or after meals. The inhibitory effect of food and milk on the absorption of **doxycycline** and **minocycline** is considerably less than that observed with the other tetracycline derivatives. These 2 drugs are often administered without regard to meals; but the potential risk of decreased drug efficacy must be weighed against the benefit of treating the infection. The administration of doxycycline with a high-fat meal has been shown to delay the time to peak plasma concentrations by an average 1 hour 20 minutes. Peak plasma concentrations of doxycycline were also decreased by up to 20% with simultaneous ingestion of dairy products or a high-fat, high-protein meal. The peak plasma concentration of minocycline was slightly decreased and delayed by 1 hour when administered with food, compared to dosing under fasting conditions.

Adverse Reactions

The following adverse reactions have been reported with the tetracyclines.

➤*Oral:*

CNS – Dizziness, headache, bulging fontanel, pseudotumor cerebri, convulsions, hypesthesia, paresthesia, sedation, vertigo; myasthenic syndrome (**demeclocycline**; rare).

Dermatologic – Maculopapular and erythematous rashes, photosensitivity, fixed drug eruptions, balanitis, erythema multiforme, Stevens-Johnson syndrome, skin and mucus membrane pigmentation, alopecia, erythema nodosum, hyperpigmentation of the nails, pruritus, toxic epidermal necrolysis, vasculitis; exfoliative dermatitis (rare).

GI – Anorexia, nausea, vomiting, diarrhea, glossitis, dysphagia, enterocolitis, inflammatory lesions (with monilial overgrowth) in the anogenital region, esophageal ulcerations, pancreatitis, dyspepsia, stomatitis, enamel hypoplasia, pseudomembranous colitis, esophagitis; bulky loose stools, sore throat, black hairy tongue, hoarseness (**tetracycline**).

Due to oral **minocycline** and **doxycycline**'s virtually complete absorption, side effects of the lower bowel, particularly diarrhea, have been infrequent.

Hematologic – Anemia, hemolytic anemia, thrombocytopenia, neutropenia, eosinophilia.

Hepatic – Increased liver enzymes, hepatic toxicity, hyperbilirubinemia, hepatic cholestasis; hepatic failure, hepatitis (rare).

Hypersensitivity – Urticaria, angioneurotic edema, pericarditis, anaphylaxis, anaphylactoid purpura, systemic lupus erythematous exacerbation, polyarthralgia, pulmonary infiltrates with eosinophilia.

Musculoskeletal – Arthralgia, arthritis, bone discoloration, myalgia, joint stiffness and swelling.

Renal – Dose-related increase in BUN, acute renal failure, interstitial nephritis; nephrogenic diabetes insipidus (**demeclocycline**).

Respiratory – Cough, dyspnea, bronchospasm, asthma exacerbation.

Miscellaneous – Brown-black microscopic discoloration of thyroid glands (prolonged therapy), tooth discoloration, lupus-like syndrome, fever, secretion discoloration, vulvovaginitis, tinnitus, decreased hearing, serum sickness-like syndrome.

➤*Parenteral:*

CNS – Headache, convulsions, dizziness, hypesthesia, paresthesia, sedation, vertigo, bulging fontanels, pseudotumor cerebri.

Dermatologic – Maculopapular and erythematous rashes, photosensitivity, alopecia, erythema nodosum, hyperpigmentation of the nails, pruritus, toxic epidermal necrolysis, vasculitis, fixed drug eruptions, balanitis, erythema multiforme, Stevens-Johnson syndrome, skin and mucus membrane pigmentation, injection site erythema and injection site pain; exfoliative dermatitis (rare).

GI – Anorexia, nausea, vomiting, diarrhea, glossitis, dysphagia, enterocolitis, inflammatory lesions (with monilial overgrowth) in the anogenital region, dyspepsia, stomatitis, enamel hypoplasia, pseudomembranous colitis, pancreatitis.

Hematologic – Hemolytic anemia, thrombocytopenia, neutropenia, eosinophilia, agranulocytosis, leukopenia, pancytopenia.

Hepatic – Hyperbilirubinemia, hepatic cholestasis, increased liver enzymes, jaundice, hepatitis, liver failure.

Hypersensitivity – Urticaria, angioneurotic edema, anaphylaxis, anaphylactoid purpura, pericarditis, exacerbation of systemic lupus erythematous, myocarditis, pulmonary infiltrates.

Musculoskeletal – Arthralgia, arthritis, bone discoloration, myalgia, joint stiffness and swelling, polyarthralgia.

Renal – Dose-related increase in BUN; interstitial nephritis, acute renal failure (**minocycline**).

Respiratory – Cough, dyspnea, bronchospasm, asthma exacerbation.

Miscellaneous – Brown-black microscopic discoloration of thyroid glands (prolonged therapy); tooth discoloration, vulvovaginitis, tinnitus, hypersensitivity syndrome (cutaneous reaction, eosinophilia, and one or more of the following: Hepatitis, pneumonitis, nephritis, myocarditis, pericarditis, fever, lymphadenopathy), lupus-like syndrome, serum sickness-like syndrome, fever, secretion discoloration.

Overdosage

➤*Symptoms:* Dizziness, nausea, and vomiting are the most commonly seen adverse events in overdosage situations.

➤*Treatment:* Discontinue medication and institute appropriate symptomatic treatment and supportive measures. Tetracyclines are not significantly removed by hemodialysis or peritoneal dialysis.

Patient Information

Take on an empty stomach, at least 2 hours before or after meals. Take with full glass of water (240 mL).

Avoid simultaneous dairy products (milk, cheese), antacids, laxatives, or iron-containing products. If these items must be taken, take at least 2 hours before or 2 hours after tetracyclines.

Concurrent use of tetracyclines with oral contraceptives may render oral contraceptives less effective (see Drug Interactions).

Avoid prolonged exposure to sunlight or sunlamps; may cause photosensitivity.

Caution patients who experience CNS symptoms about driving vehicles or using hazardous machinery while receiving therapy.

Unused supplies of tetracycline antibiotics should be discarded by the expiration date.

TETRACYCLINE HCl

Rx	Tetracycline (Various, eg, Ivax)	Capsules: 250 mg	In 100s, 1000s, and UD 100s.
Rx	Sumycin '250' (Par)		Mineral oil, lactose. (SQUIBB 655). Pink. In 100s and 1000s.
Rx	Tetracycline HCl (Various, eg, Ivax)	Capsules: 500 mg	In 100s, 1000s, and UD 100s.
Rx	Sumycin '500' (Par)		Mineral oil, lactose. (SQUIBB 763). Pink/White. In 100s and 500s.
Rx	Sumycin Syrup (Par)	Oral Suspension: 125 mg/5 mL	Saccharin, sodium metabisulfite, sorbitol, sucrose. Fruit flavor. In 473 mL.

Complete prescribing information for these products begins in the Tetracyclines group monograph.

Indications

➤*Gram-negative organisms: Haemophilus ducreyi* (chancroid); *Francisella tularensis* (tularemia); *Yersinia pestis* (plague); *Bartonella bacilliformis* (bartonellosis); *Campylobacter fetus*; *Vibrio cholerae* (cholera); *Brucella* sp. (in conjunction with streptomycin); *Calymmatobacterium granulomatis* (granuloma inguinale).

➤*Infections caused by the following miscellaneous organisms: Rickettsiae* (Rocky Mountain spotted fever, typhus fever and the typhus group, Q fever, rickettsialpox, tick fevers); *Mycoplasma pneumoniae* (respiratory tract infections); *Chlamydia trachomatis* (lymphogranuloma venereum, trachoma [infectious agent not always eliminated], inclusion conjunctivitis, uncomplicated urethral, endocervical, or rectal infections); *Chlamydia psittaci* (psittacosis [ornithosis]); *Borellia* sp. (relapsing fever); *Ureaplasma urealyticum* (nongonococcal urethritis).

➤*Following susceptibility testing (resistance has been documented): Escherichia coli*; *Enterobacter aerogenes*; *Acinetobacter* sp.; *Haemophilus influenzae* (upper respiratory tract infections); *Klebsiella* sp. (respiratory and urinary tract infections); *Streptococcus pneumoniae* (upper respiratory infections); *Streptococcus pyogenes*, *S. pneumoniae*, *Mycoplasma pneumoniae* (Eaton agent), and *Klebsiella* sp. (lower respiratory tract infections); *Staphylococcus aureus*, *S. pyogenes* (skin and skin structure infections); *Bacteroides* and *Shigella* sp.

➤*Alternative therapy for the following infections when penicillin is contraindicated:* Uncomplicated gonorrhea due to *Neisseria gonorrhoeae*; syphilis due to *Treponema pallidum*; yaws due to *Treponema pertenue*; *Listeria monocytogenes*; anthrax due to *Bacillus anthracis*; Vincent's infection due to *Fusobacterium fusiforme*; actinomycosis due to *Actinomyces* sp.; *Clostridium* sp.

➤*Acute intestinal amebiasis:* As adjunct to amebicides.

➤*Severe acne:* As adjunctive therapy.

➤*Note:* Do not use tetracyclines for streptococcal disease unless the organism has been shown to be susceptible. Tetracyclines are not the drugs of choice in treatment of any type of staphylococcal infection.

Administration and Dosage

Take with plenty of fluids. Food and some dairy products interfere with the absorption of tetracycline.

➤*Adults:* Usual dose: 1 to 2 g/day in 2 or 4 equal doses.

Mild to moderate infections – 500 mg 2 times/day or 250 mg 4 times/day.

Severe infections – 500 mg 4 times/day.

➤*Children (over 8 years of age):* Daily dose is 10 to 20 mg/lb (25 to 50 mg/kg) in 4 equally divided doses.

➤*Brucellosis:* 500 mg 4 times/day for 3 weeks, accompanied by 1 g streptomycin IM twice/day the first week, and once daily the second week.

➤*Syphilis:*

Sumycin only – A total of 30 to 40 g in equally divided doses over 10 to 15 days. Perform close follow-up and laboratory tests.

All except Sumycin –
  Early (less than 1 year): 500 mg 4 times/day for 15 days.
  More than 1 year duration: 500 mg 4 times/day for 30 days.

CDC recommended treatment schedules for syphilis (penicillin-allergic patients)† –
  Early: 500 mg 4 times/day for 14 days.
  More than 1 year's duration: 500 mg 4 times/day for 28 days.

➤*Uncomplicated gonorrhea:* 500 mg every 6 hours for 7 days.

➤*Uncomplicated urethral, endocervical, or rectal infections in adults caused by C. trachomatis:* 500 mg 4 times/day for at least 7 days.

➤*Severe acne (long-term therapy):* Initially, 1 g/day in divided doses. For maintenance, give 125 to 500 mg/day. (Alternate-day or intermittent therapy may be adequate in some patients.)

➤*Streptococcal infections:* Treat streptococcal infections for at least 10 days.

➤*Concomitant therapy:* Absorption is impaired by antacids containing aluminum, calcium, or magnesium, and preparations containing iron, zinc, or sodium bicarbonate.

➤*Renal function impairment:* Decrease recommended dosages and/or extend dosing intervals in patients with renal impairment.

➤*Storage/Stability:* Keep tightly closed. Protect from light; avoid excessive heat. Store below 30°C (86°F).

Under no circumstances should outdated tetracyclines be administered, as the degradation of tetracyclines are highly nephrotoxic and have, on occasion, produced a Fanconi-like syndrome.

DEMECLOCYCLINE HCl

Rx	Demeclocycline HCl (Impax)	Tablets: 150 mg	Lactose. (G 2111). In 100s and 500s.
Rx	Declomycin (ESP Pharma)		(LL D11). Red. Film-coated. In 100s.
Rx	Demeclocycline HCl (Impax)	Tablets: 300 mg	Lactose. (G 2122). In 48s, 100s, and 500s.
Rx	Declomycin (ESP Pharma)		(LL D12). Red. Film-coated. In 48s.

Complete prescribing information for these products begins in the Tetracyclines group monograph.

Indications

➤*Gram-negative organisms: Haemophilus ducreyi* (chancroid); *Francisella tularensis*; *Yersinia pestis*; *Bartonella bacilliformis*; *Campylobacter fetus*; *Vibrio cholerae*; *Brucella* sp. (in conjunction with streptomycin); *Calymmatobacterium granulomatis* (granuloma inguinale).

➤*Infections caused by the following miscellaneous organisms: Rickettsiae* (Rocky Mountain spotted fever, typhus fever and the typhus group, Q fever, rickettsialpox, tick fevers); *Mycoplasma pneumoniae* (PPLO, Eaton agent); *Chlamydia trachomatis* (lymphogranuloma venereum, trachoma [infectious agent not always eliminated], inclusion conjunctivitis); *Chlamydia psittaci* (psittacosis [ornithosis]); *Calymmatobacterium granulomatis* (granuloma inguinale); *Borellia recurrentis* (relapsing fever); *Bacteroides* sp.

➤*Following susceptibility testing (resistance has been documented): Escherichia coli*; *Enterobacter aerogenes*; *Acinetobacter* sp.; *Haemophilus influenzae* (respiratory tract infections); *Klebsiella* sp. (respiratory and urinary tract infections); *Streptococcus pneumoniae* (upper respiratory infections); *Streptococcus pyogenes*, *S. pneumoniae*, *Mycoplasma pneumoniae* (Eaton agent) and *Klebsiella* sp. (lower respiratory tract infections); *Staphylococcus aureus* (skin and skin structure

infections); *Streptococcus pyogenes*; *Shigella* sp.

➤*Alternative therapy for the following infections when penicillin is contraindicated: Neisseria gonorrhoeae*; syphilus due to *Treponema pallidum*; yaws due to *Treponema pertenue*; *Listerial monocytogenes*; anthrax due to *Bacillus anthracis*; Vincent's infection due to *Fusobacterium fusiforme*; *Actinomyces* sp.; *Clostridium* sp.

➤*Acute intestinal amebiasis:* As an adjunct to amebicides.

Administration and Dosage

Take with plenty of fluids. Foods and some dairy products interfere with absoprtion; take demeclocycline at least 1 hour before or 2 hours after meals or dairy products.

➤*Adults:*

Daily dose – 4 divided doses of 150 mg each or 2 divided doses of 300 mg each.

➤*Children (over 8 years of age):*

Usual daily dose – 3 to 6 mg/lb (6.6 to 13.2 mg/kg), depending upon the severity of the disease, divided into 2 or 4 doses.

➤*Gonorrhea patients sensitive to penicillin:* Initially, 600 mg; follow with 300 mg every 12 hours for 4 days to a total of 3 g.

† *MMWR.* 2002 May 10;51 (No. RR-6):1-84.

DEMECLOCYCLINE HCl

➤*Streptococcal infections:* Treat streptococcal infections for at least 10 days.

➤*Concomitant therapy:* Absorption is impaired by antacids containing aluminum, calcium, or magnesium, and by preparations containing iron. Take demeclocycline at least 1 hour before or 2 hours after these products.

➤*Renal/Hepatic function impairment:* Administer tetracyclines cautiously with renal or hepatic impairment; reduce the recommended dosage and/or extend the dosing interval.

➤*Storage/Stability:* Store at controlled room temperature 20° to 25°C (68° to 77°F).

DOXYCYCLINE

Rx	Doxycycline (Various, eg, Ivax, Watson)	**Tablets:** 100 mg (as hyclate)	In 50s, 100s, 200s, 500s and UD 100s.
Rx	Vibra-Tabs (Pfizer)		(VIBRA-TABS PFIZER 099). Salmon. Film-coated. In 50s.
Rx	Doxycycline (Various, eg, Ivax, Watson)	**Capsules:** 50 mg (as hyclate)	In 50s and 500s.
Rx	Vibramycin (Pfizer)		(VIBRA PFIZER 094). White/Lt. blue. In 50s.
Rx	Doxycycline (Various, eg, Ivax, Watson)	**Capsules:** 100 mg (as hyclate)	In 50s, 500s, and UD 100s.
Rx	Vibramycin (Pfizer)		(VIBRA PFIZER 095). Lt. blue. In 50s.
Rx	Doryx (Warner Chilcott)	**Capsules, coated pellets:** 75 mg (as hyclate)	(DORYX 75). Orange/Green. In 60s.
		100 mg (as hyclate)	(DORYX WC). Dk. yellow/lt. blue. In 50s.
Rx	Adoxa (Bioglan)	**Tablets:** 50 mg (as monohydrate)	(B 728). Yellow. Film-coated. In 100s.
		Tablets: 75 mg (as monohydrate)	(B 730). Lt. orange. Film-coated. In 100s and 500s.
		100 mg (as monohydrate)	(B 729). Yellow. Film-coated. In 50s and 250s.
Rx	Monodox (Oclassen)	**Capsules:** 50 mg (as monohydrate)	(MONODOX 50 M 260). White/ yellow. In 100s.
		100 mg (as monohydrate)	(MONODOX 100 M 259). Yellow/brown. In 50s and 250s.
Rx	Vibramycin (Pfizer)	**Powder for Oral Suspension:** 25 mg (as monohydrate) per 5 mL when reconstituted	Parabens, sucrose. Raspberry flavor. In 60 mL.
Rx	Vibramycin (Pfizer)	**Syrup:** 50 mg (as calcium) per 5 mL	Parabens, sodium metabisulfite, sorbitol. Apple-raspberry flavor. In 473 mL.
Rx	Doxycycline (Various, eg, Bedford)	**Powder for Injection, lyophilized:** 100 mg (as hyclate)	In vials.
Rx	Doxy 100 (APP)		300 mg mannitol. In vials.
Rx	Doxy 200 (APP)	**Powder for Injection, lyophilized:** 200 mg (as hyclate)	600 mg mannitol. In vials.

Complete prescribing information for these products begins in the Tetracyclines group monograph.

Indications

➤*Gram-negative organisms:* Haemophilus ducreyi (chancroid); Francisella tularensis (tularemia); Yersinia pestis (plague); Bartonella bacilliformis (bartonellosis); Campylobacter fetus; Vibrio cholerae (cholera); Brucella sp. (in conjunction with streptomycin); Calymmatobacterium granulomatis (granuloma inguinale).

➤*Infections caused by the following miscellaneous organisms:* Rickettsiae (Rocky Mountain spotted fever, typhus fever and the typhus group, Q fever, rickettsialpox, tick fevers); Mycoplasma pneumoniae (respiratory tract infections); Chlamydia trachomatis (lymphogranuloma venereum, trachoma [infectious agent not always eliminated], inclusion conjunctivitis, uncomplicated urethral, endocervical, or rectal infections); Chlamydia psittaci (psittacosis [ornithosis]); Borellia recurrentis (relapsing fever); Ureaplasma urealyticum (nongonococcal urethritis).

➤*Following susceptibility testing (resistance has been documented):* Escherichia coli; Enterobacter aerogenes; Acinetobacter sp.; Haemophilus influenzae (respiratory tract infections); Klebsiella sp. (respiratory and urinary tract infections); Streptococcus pneumoniae (upper respiratory infections); Shigella sp.

➤*Alternative therapy for the following infections when penicillin is contraindicated:* Uncomplicated gonorrhea due to Neisseria gonorrhoeae; syphilis due to Treponema pallidum; yaws due to Treponema pertenue; listeriosis due to Listeria monocytogenes; Vincent's infection due to Fusobacterium fusiforme; actinomycosis due to Actinomyces israelii; infections due to Clostridium sp.

➤*Acute intestinal amebiasis:* As adjunct to amebicides.

➤*Severe acne:* As adjunctive therapy.

➤*Anthrax, including inhalational anthrax:* To reduce the incidence or progression of disease following exposure to aerosolized Bacillus anthracis.

➤*Malaria:* Prophylaxis of malaria due to Plasmodium falciparum in short-term travelers (less than 4 months) to areas with chloroquine and/or pyrimethamine-sulfadoxine resistant strains.

➤*Note:* Tetracyclines should not be used for streptococcal disease unless organism had been shown to be susceptible. Tetracyclines are not the drugs of choice in treatment of any type of staphylococcal infection.

Administration and Dosage

➤*Oral:* When used in streptococcal infections, continue therapy for 10 days. Take with plenty of water. Absorption and peak plasma levels may be reduced when administered with meals or with dairy products, including milk.

Adults –
  Usual dose: 200 mg on the first day of treatment (100 mg every 12 hours); follow with a maintenance dose of 100 mg/day. The maintenance dose may be administered as a single dose or as 50 mg every 12 hours.
  More severe infections (particularly chronic urinary tract infections): 100 mg every 12 hours.

Children (over 8 years of age) –
  100 lb or less (less than 45 kg): 2 mg/lb (4.4 mg/kg) divided into 2 doses on the first day of treatment; follow with 1 mg/lb (2.2 mg/kg) given as a single daily dose or divided into 2 doses on subsequent days.
  More severe infections: Up to 2 mg/lb (4.4 mg/kg) may be used.
  For children over 100 lb (45 kg): Use the usual adult dose.

Uncomplicated gonococcal infection in adults (except anorectal infections in men) – 100 mg twice daily for at least 7 days.
  Single visit dose: Immediately give 300 mg; follow with 300 mg in 1 hour, which should be administered with plenty of water.

Nongonococcal urethritis – 100 mg twice daily for 7 days.

Syphilis –
  Early (except Adoxa, Doryx, Monodox): 100 mg twice daily for 2 weeks.
  More than 1 year duration (except Adoxa, Doryx, Monodox): 100 mg twice daily for 4 weeks.
  Primary and secondary (Adoxa, Doryx, Monodox only): 300 mg/day in divided doses for at least 10 days.

Uncomplicated urethral, endocervical or rectal infections in adults caused by C. trachomatis – 100 mg twice daily for at least 7 days.

Acute epididymo-orchitis caused by N. gonorrhoeae or C. trachomatis – 100 mg twice daily for at least 10 days.

Malaria prophylaxis (except Adoxa, Doryx, Monodox) – Begin prophylaxis 1 to 2 days prior to travel to an endemic area, continue during travel and for 4 weeks after returning from travel.
  Adults: 100 mg/day.
  Children (over 8 years of age): 2 mg/kg once daily up to 100 mg/day.

Inhalation anthrax (post-exposure) –
  Adults and children (100 lb [45 kg] or more): 100 mg twice daily for 60 days.
  Children (less than 100 lb [45 kg]): 1 mg/lb (2.2 mg/kg) twice daily for 60 days.

➤*Parenteral:* Do not inject IM or SC. Avoid rapid administration. Switch to oral therapy as soon as possible. The duration of IV infusion may vary with the dose (100 to 200 mg/day), but is usually 1 to 4 hours. A recommended minimum infusion time for 100 mg of a 0.5 mg/mL solution is 1 hour. Continue therapy for at least 24 to 48 hours after symptoms and fever have subsided. Therapeutic antibacterial serum activity usually persists for 24 hours following recommended dosage.

Adults – The usual dosage is 200 mg IV on the first day of treatment,

DOXYCYCLINE

administered in 1 or 2 infusions. Subsequent daily dosage is 100 to 200 mg, depending upon the severity of infection, with 200 mg administered in 1 or 2 infusions.

Primary and secondary syphilis: 300 mg/day for at least 10 days.

Children (over 8 years of age) –

Up to 100 lb (45 kg): Give 2 mg/lb (4.4 mg/kg) on the first day of treatment, in 1 or 2 infusions. Subsequent daily dosage is 1 to 2 mg/lb (2.2 to 4.4 mg/kg) given as 1 or 2 infusions, depending on the severity of the infection.

Over 100 lb (45 kg): Use the usual adult dose.

➤*Preparation of solution:* To prepare a solution containing 10 mg/mL, reconstitute the contents of the vial with 10 mL (for the 100 mg/vial) or 20 mL (for the 200 mg/vial) of sterile water for injection or any of the IV infusion solutions listed below. Dilute the 100 mg vial further with 100 to 1000 mL (or 200 to 2000 mL for the 200 mg vial) of the following IV solutions: sodium chloride injection; 5% dextrose injection; Ringer's injection; 10% invert sugar in water; Lactated Ringer's injection; 5% dextrose in Lactated Ringer's; *Normosol-M* in D5-W; *Normosol-R* in D5-W; *Plasma-Lyte 56* in 5% dextrose; *Plasma-Lyte 148* in 5% dextrose. This will result in the recommended concentrations of 0.1 to 1 mg/mL. Concentrations lower than 0.1 mg/mL or higher than 1 mg/mL are not recommended.

When diluted with sodium chloride injection; 5% dextrose injection; Ringer's injection; invert sugar, 10% in water; *Normosol-M* in D5-W (Abbott); *Normosol-R* in D5-W (Abbott); *Plasma-Lyte 56* in 5% dextrose (Travenol); or *Plasma-Lyte 148* in 5% dextrose (Travenol), infusion of the solution (about 1 mg/mL) or lower concentrations (not less than 0.1 mg/mL) must be completed within 12 hours after reconstitution to ensure adequate stability.

Reconstituted solutions (1 to 0.1 mg/mL) may also be stored up to 72 hours prior to start of infusion, if refrigerated and protected from sunlight and artificial light.

When diluted with Lactated Ringer's injection, or dextrose 5% in Lactated Ringer's, infusion of the solution (about 1 mg/mL) or lower concentrations (not less than 0.1 mg/mL) must be completed within 6 hours after reconstitution to ensure adequate stability.

➤*CDC recommended treatment schedules for sexually transmitted diseases†:*

Granuloma inguinale (donovanosis) – 100 mg twice daily for at least 3 weeks.

Syphilis in patients allergic to penicillins –
Early syphilis: 100 mg twice daily for 14 days.
Latent syphilis: 100 mg twice daily for 28 days.

Chlamydial infections –
Adults and children (8 years of age or older): 100 mg twice daily for 7 days.

Pelvic inflammatory disease – 100 mg orally or IV every 12 hours plus 2 g cefotetan IV every 12 hours or 2 g cefoxitin IV every 6 hours. May discontinue parenteral therapy after 24 hours; continue oral therapy with doxycycline for a total of 14 days.

Epididymitis most likely caused by gonococcal or chlamydial infection – 100 mg twice daily for 10 days plus a single dose of 250 mg ceftriaxone IM.

Sexual assault prophylaxis – 100 mg twice daily for 7 days plus ceftriaxone and metronidazole.

Lymphogranuloma venereum – 100 mg twice daily for at least 21 days.

Nongonococcal urethritis – 100 mg twice daily for 7 days.

➤*Storage/Stability:*

Injection – Store lyophilized powder at controlled room temperature at or below 25°C (77°F). May store reconstituted solutions (1 to 0.1 mg/mL) for 72 hours under refrigeration. Solutions at a concentration of 10 mg/mL in sterile water for injection can be stored for up to 8 weeks at −20°C, if frozen immediately after reconstitution. Discard any unused portion after that period. Protect from light.

Capsules/Tablets – Store at room temperature 15° to 30°C (59° to 86°F). Dispense in tight, light-resistant and child-resistant containers.

MINOCYCLINE

Rx	**Dynacin** (Medicis)	**Tablets:** 50 mg (as HCl)	Lactose. (DYN-50 747). White, capsule shape. Film coated. In 100s and 1000s.
		75 mg (as HCl)	Lactose. (DYN-75 748). Gray, capsule shape. Film coated. In 100s and 1000s.
		100 mg (as HCl)	Lactose. (DYN-100 749). Dark gray, capsule shape. Film coated. In 50s and 1000s.
Rx	**Minocycline HCl** (Various, eg, Danbury, Global, Ranbaxy, Teva)	**Capsules:** 50 mg (as HCl)	In 100s.
Rx	**Dynacin** (Medicis)		(0497 DYNACIN 50 mg). White. In 100s, 500s, and 1000s.
	Minocycline HCl (Various, eg, Global, Ranbaxy)	**Capsules:** 75 mg (as HCl)	In 100s.
Rx	**Dynacin** (Medicis)		(0499 DYNACIN 75 mg). Lt. gray. In 100s and 1000s.
Rx	**Minocycline HCl** (Various, eg, Danbury, Global, Ranbaxy, Teva)	**Capsules:** 100 mg (as HCl)	In 50s.
Rx	**Dynacin** (Medicis)		(0498 DYNACIN 100 mg). Dk. gray/white. In 50s, 500s, and 1000s.
Rx	**Minocin** (Lederle)	**Capsules, pellet filled:** 50 mg (as HCl)	(M45 Lederle 50 mg). Yellow/Green. In 100s.
		100 mg (as HCl)	(M46 Lederle 100 mg). Lt. green/Green. In 50s.
		Oral suspension: 50 mg (as HCl)/5 mL	5% alcohol, parabens, EDTA, saccharin. Custard flavor. In 60 ml.
Rx	**Minocin** (Lederle)	**Powder for injection, cryodesiccated:** 100 mg	In vials.

Complete prescribing information for these products begins in the Tetracyclines group monograph.

Indications

➤*Gram-negative organisms:* Haemophilus ducreyi (chancroid); Francisella tularensis (tularemia); Yersinia pestis (plague); Bartonella bacilliformis (bartonellosis); Campylobacter fetus; Vibrio cholerae (cholera); Brucella sp. (in conjunction with streptomycin); Neisseria gonorrhoeae (uncomplicated urethritis in men).

➤*Infections caused by the following miscellaneous organisms:* Rickettsiae (Rocky Mountain spotted fever, typhus fever and the typhus group, Q fever, rickettsialpox, tick fevers); Mycoplasma pneumoniae (respiratory tract infections); Chlamydia trachomatis (lymphogranuloma venereum, trachoma [infectious agent not always eliminated], inclusion conjunctivitis); Chlamydia psittaci (psittacosis [ornithosis]); Borellia recurrentis (relapsing fever); Ureaplasma urealyticum (nongonococcal urethritis).

➤*Following susceptibility testing (resistance has been documented):* Escherichia coli; Enterobacter aerogenes; Acinetobacter and Shigella sp.; Haemophilus influenzae (respiratory tract infections); Klebsiella sp. (respiratory and urinary tract infections); Streptococcus pneumoniae (upper respiratory infections); Staphylococcus aureus (skin and skin structure infections).

➤*Alternative therapy for the following infections when penicillin is contraindicated:* Neisseria gonorrhoeae infections; syphilis due to Treponema pallidum; yaws due to Treponema pertenue; listeriosis due to Listeria monocytogenes; anthrax due to Bacillus anthracis; Vincent's infection due to Fusobacterium fusiforme; actinomycosis due to Actinomyces israelii; infections due to Clostridium sp.

➤*Acute intestinal amebiasis:* As adjunct to amebicides.

➤*Severe acne:* As adjunctive therapy.

➤*Neisseria meningitidis:* Treatment of asymptomatic meningococcal carriers of N. meningitidis.

➤*Note:* Do not use tetracyclines for streptococcal disease unless the organism has been shown to be susceptible. Tetracyclines are not the drugs of choice in treatment of any type of staphylococcal infection.

Administration and Dosage

➤*Oral:* May be taken with or without food. Take with plenty of fluids.

Usual dosage –

Adults: 200 mg initially, followed by 100 mg every 12 hours. If more frequent doses are preferred, give 100 or 200 mg initially; follow with 50 mg, 4 times/day.

Children (over 8 years of age): Initially, 4 mg/kg; follow with 2 mg/kg every 12 hours.

† *MMWR.* 2002 May 10;51 (No. RR-6):1-84.

MINOCYCLINE

Syphilis – Administer usual dose over a period of 10 to 15 days. Close follow-up, including laboratory tests, is recommended.

Uncomplicated urethral infections in adults caused by C. trachomatis or Ureaplasma urealyticum – 100 mg every 12 hours for at least 7 days.

Uncomplicated gonococcal urethritis in men – 100 mg every 12 hours for 5 days.

Uncomplicated gonococcal infections except urethritis and anorectal infections in men – 200 mg initially, followed by 100 mg every 12 hours for at least 4 days, with posttherapy cultures within 2 to 3 days.

Meningococcal carrier state – 100 mg every 12 hours for 5 days.

Unlabeled use –

Mycobacterium marinum infections: Although optimal doses are not established, 100 mg every 12 hours for 6 to 8 weeks has been successful in a limited number of cases.

➤*Parenteral:* Administer diluted injections immediately. Avoid rapid administration. Switch to oral therapy as soon as possible.

Adults – 200 mg followed by 100 mg every 12 hours; do not exceed 400 mg in 24 hours.

Children (over 8 years of age) – Initially, usual pediatric dose is 4 mg/kg, followed by 2 mg/kg every 12 hours, not to exceed the usual adult dose.

➤*Preparation of solution:* Initially reconstitute the powder with 5 mL of sterile water for injection and then further dilute to 500 to 1000 mL with either sodium chloride injection, dextrose injection, dextrose and sodium chloride injection, Ringer's injection or Lactated Ringer's injection, but not in other solutions containing calcium (a precipitate may form) especially in neutral and alkaline solutions.

Incompatibilities – Do not mix IV minocycline before or during administration with any solutions containing the following: Adrenocorticotropic hormone (ACTH), aminophylline, amobarbital sodium, amphotericin B, bicarbonate infusion mixtures, calcium gluconate or chloride, carbenicillin, cephalothin sodium, cefazolin sodium, chloramphenicol succinate, colistin sulfate, heparin sodium, hydrocortisone sodium succinate, iodine sodium, methicillin sodium, novobiocin, penicillin, pentobarbital, phenytoin sodium, polymyxin, prochlorperazine, sodium ascorbate, sulfadiazine, sulfisoxazole, thiopental sodium, vitamin K (sodium bisulfate or sodium salt), whole blood.

➤*Renal function impairment:* Decrease the recommended dosage and/or increase the dosing intervals in patients with renal impairment. Do not exceed 200 mg *Minocin* in 24 hours in patients with renal impairment.

➤*Storage / Stability:*

Capsules / Suspension – Store at controlled room temperature 15° to 30°C (59° to 86°F). Do not freeze. Protect from light, moisture, and excessive heat.

Injection – Store powder at controlled room temperature 20° to 25°C (68° to 77°F). Protect from light, moisture, and excessive heat. Store diluted injection (500 to 1000 mL) at room temperature up to 24 hours; discard any unused portions after that period.

OXYTETRACYCLINE

Rx	Terramycin (Roerig/Pfizer)	Injection: 50 mg/mL with 2% lidocaine	In 2 mL single-dose amps and 10 mL multidose vials.
		125 mg/mL with 2% lidocaine	In 2 mL single-dose amps.

Complete prescribing information for these products begins in the Tetracyclines group monograph.

Indications

➤*Gram-negative organisms: Haemophilus ducreyi* (chancroid); *Francisella tularensis* (tularemia); *Yersinia pestis* (plague); *Bartonella bacilliformis* (bartonellosis); *Campylobacter fetus; Vibrio cholerae* (cholera); *Brucella* sp. (in conjunction with streptomycin); *Calymmatobacterium granulomatis* (granuloma inguinale).

➤*Infections caused by the following miscellaneous organisms: Rickettsiae* (Rocky Mountain spotted fever, typhus fever and the typhus group, Q fever, rickettsialpox, tick fevers); *Mycoplasma pneumoniae* (PPLO, Eaton agent); *Chlamydia trachomatis* (lymphogranuloma venereum, trachoma [infectious agent not always eliminated], inclusion conjunctivitis); *Chlamydia psittaci* (psittacosis [ornithosis]); *Borellia recurrentis* (relapsing fever); *Bacteroides* sp.

➤*Following susceptibility testing (resistance has been documented): Escherichia coli; Enterobacter aerogenes; Haemophilus influenzae* (respiratory tract infections); *Klebsiella* sp. (respiratory and urinary tract infections); *Streptococcus* sp.; *Staphylococcus aureus* (skin and skin structure infections); *Acinetobacter* and *Shigella* sp.

➤*Alternative therapy for the following infections when penicillin is contraindicated: Neisseria gonorrhoeae;* syphilis due to *Treponema pallidum;* yaws due to *Treponema pertenue; Listeria monocytogenes; Bacillus anthracis;* Vincent's infection due to *Fusobacterium fusiforme; Actinomyces* sp.; *Clostridium* sp.

➤*Acute intestinal amebiasis:* As adjunct to amebicides.

➤*Note:* Do not use tetracyclines for streptococcal disease unless the organism has been shown to be susceptible. Tetracyclines are not the drugs of choice in treatment of any type of staphylococcal infection.

Administration and Dosage

Reserve IM therapy for situations where oral therapy is not feasible. IM administration produces lower blood levels than oral administration. Switch to oral therapy as soon as possible. If rapid, high blood levels are needed, administer oxytetracycline IV.

The preferred sites of IM injection are the upper outer quadrant of the buttock or mid-lateral thigh in adults and mid-lateral thigh in children.

Treat Group A beta-hemolytic streptococci infections for at least 10 days.

➤*Adults:* The usual daily dose is 250 mg administered IM once every 24 hours or 300 mg given in divided doses at 8 to 12 hour intervals.

➤*Children (over 8 years of age):* 15 to 25 mg/kg, up to a maximum of 250 mg per single daily IM injection. Dosage may be divided and given at 8 to 12 hour intervals.

➤*Renal function impairment:* Decrease recommended dosage and/or extend dosing intervals in patients with renal impairment.

➤*Storage / Stability:* Store below 40°C (104°F), preferably between 15° and 30°C (59° and 86°F). Avoid freezing.

Adverse Reactions

General Indications for Macrolides[1]					
Indication	Azithromycin	Clarithromycin	Dirithromycin	Erythromycin	Troleandomycin
Adults					
Pharyngitis/Tonsillitis	✔	✔	✔		
Respiratory tract infections				✔	✔
Acute maxillary sinusitis		✔			
Acute bacterial exacerbation of chronic bronchitis		✔	✔		
Skin and skin structure infections[2]	✔	✔	✔	✔	
Pertussis (whooping cough)				✔	
Diphtheria				✔	
Erythrasma				✔	
Intestinal amebiasis				✔	
Uncomplicated urethral, endo-cervical, or rectal infections				✔	
Urogenital infections during pregnancy				✔	
Nongonococcal urethritis				✔	
Primary syphilis				✔	
Legionnaire's disease				✔	
Rheumatic fever				✔	
Bacterial endocarditis				✔	
Listeria monocytogenes				✔	
Pneumonia		✔			✔
Community-acquired pneumonia	✔		✔		
Disseminated bacterial infections (TWAR strain)		✔			
Prevention of disseminated Mycobacterium avium complex in patients with advanced HIV infection		✔			
Chronic obstructive pulmonary disease	✔				
Genital ulcer disease	✔				
Pelvic inflammatory disease	✔			✔	
Urethritis/Cervicitis	✔				
Secondary bacterial infection of acute bronchitis			✔		
Children					
Pharyngitis/Tonsillitis	✔	✔			
Pneumonia		✔			
Community-acquired pneumonia	✔				
Acute maxillary sinusitis		✔			
Acute otitis media	✔	✔			
Skin and skin structure infections[2]		✔			
Disseminated mycobacterial infections		✔			
Prevention of disseminated Mycobacterium avium complex disease in patients with advanced HIV infection		✔			
Conjunctivitis of the newborn				✔	
Pneumonia of infancy				✔	

[1] Causative organisms may vary for each indication for specific macrolides. Refer to individual monographs for this information.

[2] Abscesses usually require surgical drainage.

►*Note:* The usual drug of choice in the treatment and prevention of streptococcal infections and the prophylaxis of rheumatic fever is penicillin oral/IM. Azithromycin, clarithromycin, and dirithromycin are generally effective in the eradication of *Streptococcus pyogenes* from the nasopharynx; however, data establishing the efficacy of clarithromycin and dirithromycin in the subsequent prevention of rheumatic fever are not available at present. Because some strains are resistant to azithromycin, perform susceptibility tests when patients are treated with azithromycin.

Injectable benzathine penicillin G or oral penicillin V is considered by the American Heart Association to be the drug of choice in the treatment and prevention of streptococcal pharyngitis. For patients allergic to penicillin, erythromycin and azithromycin are effective alternatives. Erythromycin is also an alternative agent for long-term prophylaxis of rheumatic fever in patients allergic to penicillin or sulfadiazine.

►*Helicobacter pylori double therapy:* Clarithromycin in combination with omeprazole or ranitidine bismuth citrate is indicated for the treatment of patients with an active duodenal ulcer associated with *H. pylori* infection.

►*Helicobacter pylori triple therapy:* Clarithromycin, lansoprazole, and amoxicillin as combination triple therapy for the treatment of *H. pylori* infection and duodenal ulcer disease (active or 1-year history of duodenal ulcer) to eradicate *H. pylori*.

►Unlabeled uses:

Azithromycin –
  Uncomplicated gonococcal infections of the cervix, urethra, and rectum: Caused by *N. gonorrhoeae.*†
    Gonococcal pharyngitis: Caused by *N. gonorrhoeae.*
    Chlamydial infections: Caused by *C. trachomatis.*

Erythromycin –
  Treponema pallidum: Early syphilis (primary or secondary) for nonpregnant patients for whom compliance with therapy and follow-up can be ensured. In treatment of primary syphilis, examine spinal fluid before treatment and as part of the follow-up after therapy. The use of erythromycin for the treatment of in utero syphilis is not recommended.
    Campylobacter jejuni: Erythromycin has been used successfully in prolonged diarrhea associated with campylobacter enteritis.
    Lymphogranuloma venereum: Genital, inguinal, or anorectal.
    Granuloma inguinale: Caused by *Calymmatobacterium granulomatis.*
    Haemophilus ducreyi (chancroid): Treat until ulcers or lymph nodes are healed.

Prior to elective colorectal surgery, to reduce wound complications, erythromycin base with oral neomycin is a popular preoperative combination.

Other uses, as alternative to penicillins, include: Anthrax; Vincent's gingivitis; erysipeloid; tetanus; actinomycosis; *Nocardia* infections (with a sulfonamide); *Eikenella corrodens* infections; *Borrelia* infections (including early Lyme disease).

Actions

►*Pharmacology:* Macrolide antibiotics, which include azithromycin, clarithromycin, dirithromycin, erythromycin, and troleandomycin, reversibly bind to the P site of the 50S ribosomal subunit of susceptible organisms and may inhibit RNA-dependent protein synthesis by stimulating the dissociation of peptidyl t-RNA from ribosomes. They may be bacteriostatic or bactericidal, depending on such factors as drug concentration.

Rearrangement of erythromycin's 9-oxime derivative, followed by reduction and N-methylation, yields the ring-expanded derivative azithromycin, an azalide. Alkylation of the hydroxyl group at C-6 yields clarithromycin. The classical erythromycins A, B, C, and D and oleandomycin are 14-membered macrolides; azithromycin is a 15-membered-ring macrolide. Troleandomycin is a synthetically derived acetylated ester of the macrolide oleandomycin.

Macrolides are weak bases; their activity increases in alkaline pH. Macrolides enter pleural fluid, ascitic fluid, middle-ear exudates, and sputum. When meninges are inflamed, macrolides may enter the CSF. They are used for respiratory, genital, GI tract, and skin and soft tissue infections, especially when beta-lactam antibiotics or tetracyclines are contraindicated.

Erythromycin base, the active form, is marketed in acid-resistant enteric coated form to retard gastric inactivation. Converting the base to its acid-stable salt (stearate), ester (ethyl succinate and propionate), or salt of an ester (estolate) also improves oral bioavailability. For IV injection, a relatively water-soluble salt, lactobionate, is available.

Dirithromycin is a pro-drug. Available as an enteric coated tablet, it is converted non-enzymatically during intestinal absorption into the microbiologically active moiety erythromycylamine.

►*Pharmacokinetics:* Despite differing structures, macrolides have similar antibacterial spectrum, mechanisms of action and resistance, but relatively different pharmacokinetics (see table). Macrolides distribute readily into body tissues and fluids. Because of high intracellular concentrations, tissue levels are higher than serum levels.

Various Pharmacokinetic Parameters of Macrolides

Macrolide	Route of administration	Protein binding (%)	Bioavailability (%)	Effect of food	C_{max}* (mcg/ml)	T_{max}* (hr)	Half-life (hr)	Metabolism	Elimination
Azithromycin	Oral IV	51 (0.02 mcg/L) 7 (2 mcg/L)	≈ 40	Food increases absorption, C_{max} by 23% and suspension by 56%; take on empty stomach.	0.5 1.14[3] 3.63[4]	2.2	68[1]	Some hepatic but mainly excreted unchanged	6% excreted unchanged in urine; primarily excreted unchanged in bile
Clarithromycin	Oral	40-70	≈ 50	Food delays onset of absorption and formation of metabolite; does not affect extent of bioavailability. Take without regard to meals.	1-3	2-3	3-7	Metabolized to active metabolite (14-OH clarithromycin)	Primarily renal; rate approximates normal GFR
Dirithromycin	Oral	15-30[2]	≈ 10	Take with food or within an hour of having eaten.	0.3-0.4[2]	3.9-4.1[2]	2-36	Nonenzymatic conversion to erythromycylamine	81%-97% fecal/hepatic[2]
Erythromycin	Oral IV	70-80 (96 estolate)	> 35	Base or stearate: Take on an empty stomach. Estolate, ethylsuccinate, delayed release base: Take without regard to meals.	0.3-2	1.6	1.6	Hepatic; demethylation	< 5% (oral) and 12% to 15% (IV) excreted unchanged in urine; significant quantity excreted in bile
Troleandomycin	Oral				2	2			20% excreted in urine; significant quantity excreted in bile

* C_{max} = Maximum concentration; T_{max} = Time to reach maximum concentration.
[1] Average terminal half-life.
[2] Value listed for erythromycylamine, the active moiety.
[3] At a concentration of 1 mg/ml.
[4] At a concentration of 2 mg/ml.

Children – In 2 clinical studies, **azithromycin** for oral suspension was dosed at 10 mg/kg on day 1, followed by 5 mg/kg on days 2 through 5 to 2 groups of children (ages 1 to 5 years and 5 to 15 years, respectively). The mean pharmacokinetic parameters at day 5 were C_{max} = 0.216 mcg/ml, T_{max} = 1.9 hours and AUC_{0-24} = 1.822 mcg•hr/ml for the 1- to 5-year-old group. Mean pharmacokinetic parameters at day 5 for the 5- to 15-year olds were C_{max} = 0.383 mcg/ml, T_{max} = 2.4 hours and AUC_{0-24} = 3.109 mcg•hr/ml.

† CDC 1998 Guidelines for Treatment of Sexually Transmitted Diseases. *MMWR* 1998 Jan 23;47(No. 441):1-117.

►*Microbiology:*

Organisms (✓ = generally susceptible)	Azithromycin	Clarithromycin	Dirithromycin	Erythromycin	Troleandomycin[1]
Gram-positive aerobes					
Staphylococcus aureus	✓	✓	✓	✓	
Streptococcus pyogenes	✓	✓	✓		✓
Streptococcus pneumoniae	✓	✓	✓	✓	✓
Streptococcus agalactiae	✓	✓	✓	✓	
Streptococcus sp.	✓	✓	✓	✓	
Streptococcus viridans	✓	✓	✓	✓	
Listeria monocytogenes				✓	
Corynebacterium diphtheriae				✓	
Corynebacterium minutissimum				✓	
Gram-negative aerobes					
Haemophilus influenzae	✓	✓	✓	†[2]	
Haemophilus ducreyi	✓				
Moraxella catarrhalis	✓	✓	✓	✓	
Bordetella pertussis	✓	✓		✓	
Legionella pneumophila	✓	✓	✓	✓	
Neisseria gonorrhoeae	✓	✓		✓	
Pasteurella multocida		✓			
Anaerobes					
Prevotella (formerly Bacteroides) bivius	✓				
Prevotella (formerly Bacteroides) melaninogenicus		✓			
Clostridium perfringens		✓			
Propionibacterium acnes		✓	✓		
Peptococcus niger		✓			
Peptostreptococcus sp.	✓				
Other					
Borrelia burgdorferi	✓				
Chlamydia trachomatis	✓	✓		✓	
Mycobacterium kansasii		✓			
Mycoplasma pneumoniae	✓	✓	✓	✓	
Treponema pallidum	✓			✓	
Ureaplasma urealyticum	✓			✓	
Entamoeba histolytica				✓	
Chlamydia pneumoniae (TWAR strain)	✓	✓			
Mycoplasma hominis	✓				
Mycobacterium avium		✓			
Mycobacterium intracellulare		✓			
Helicobacter pylori		✓			
Clostridium tetani				✓	

[1] Data is limited for troleandomycin.
[2] Many strains resistant to erythromycin alone; may be susceptible to erythromycin plus a sulfonamide.

Contraindications

Hypersensitivity to any of the macrolide antibiotics; patients receiving astemizole, cisapride, or pimozide; known, suspected, or potential bacteremias (dirithromycin); preexisting liver disease (erythromycin estolate).

Warnings

►*Pseudomembranous colitis:* This has occurred with nearly all antibacterial agents and may range in severity from mild to life-threatening. Therefore, it is important to consider this diagnosis in patients who present with diarrhea subsequent to the administration of antibacterial agents.

Treatment with antibacterial agents alters the normal flora of the colon and may permit overgrowth of clostridia. Studies indicate that a toxin produced by *Clostridium difficile* is a primary cause of "antibiotic-associated colitis."

After the diagnosis of pseudomembranous colitis has been established, initiate therapeutic measures. Mild cases of pseudomembranous colitis usually respond to discontinuation of the drug alone. In moderate-to-severe cases, give consideration to management with fluids and electrolytes, protein supplementation and treatment with an antibacterial drug effective against *C. difficile* colitis. When colitis does not improve after discontinuation, or when it is severe, oral vancomycin or metronidazole is the drug of choice; rule out other causes.

►*Acute porphyria:* Do not use **clarithromycin** in combination with ranitidine bismuth citrate in patients with a history of acute porphyria.

►*Pneumonia:* Do not use oral **azithromycin** in patients with pneumonia who are judged to be inappropriate for oral therapy because of moderate-to-severe illness or risk factors such as any of the following: Nosocomially acquired infections; known or suspected bacteremia; conditions requiring hospitalization; cystic fibrosis; significant underlying health problems that may compromise patients' ability to respond to their illness (including immunodeficiency or functional asplenia); elderly or debilitated patients.

►*Cardiac effects:* Ventricular arrhythmias, including ventricular tachycardia and torsades de pointes, in individuals with prolonged QT intervals have been reported with macrolide antibiotics; however, it has not occurred with **azithromycin**.

►*Bacteremias:* Do not use **dirithromycin** in patients with known, suspected, or potential bacteremias because serum levels are inadequate to provide antibacterial coverage of the blood stream.

►*Hepatotoxicity:* **Erythromycin** administration has been associated with the infrequent occurrence of cholestatic hepatitis. This effect is most common with erythromycin estolate; however, it has also occurred with other erythromycin salts. Laboratory findings include abnormal hepatic function, peripheral eosinophilia, and leukocytosis. Symptoms may include malaise, nausea, vomiting, abdominal cramps, and fever. Jaundice may or may not be present. In some instances, severe abdominal pain may simulate the pain of biliary colic, pancreatitis, perforated ulcer, or an acute abdominal surgical problem. In other instances, clinical symptoms and results of liver function tests have resembled findings in extrahepatic obstructive jaundice. Although initial symptoms have developed after a few days of treatment, they generally have followed 1 or 2 weeks of continuous therapy. Symptoms reappear promptly, usually within 48 hours after the drug is readministered to sensitive patients. The syndrome seems to result from a form of sensitization, occurs chiefly in adults, and is reversible when medication is discontinued.

Troleandomycin has been associated with allergic cholestatic hepatitis. Some patients receiving troleandomycin for > 2 weeks or in repeated courses have developed jaundice accompanied by right upper quadrant pain, fever, nausea, vomiting, eosinophilia, and leukocytosis. These have reversed on drug discontinuance. Readministration reproduces hepatotoxicity, often within 24 to 48 hours. Monitor liver function tests and discontinue drug if abnormalities develop.

►*Myasthenia gravis:* **Erythromycin** may aggravate the weakness of patients with myasthenia gravis.

►*Hypersensitivity reactions:* Rare serious allergic reactions, including angioedema, anaphylaxis, and dermatologic reactions including Stevens-Johnson syndrome and toxic epidermal necrolysis have occurred in patients on **azithromycin** therapy. Although rare, fatalities have occurred. Despite initially successful symptomatic treatment of the allergic symptoms, when symptomatic therapy was discontinued, the allergic symptoms recurred soon thereafter in some patients without further azithromycin exposure. These patients required prolonged periods of observation and symptomatic treatment. The relationship of these episodes to the long tissue half-life of azithromycin and subsequent prolonged exposure to antigen is unknown at present.

If an allergic reaction occurs with azithromycin, discontinue and institute appropriate therapy. Physicians should be aware that reappearance of the allergic symptoms may occur when symptomatic therapy is discontinued.

Serious allergic reactions, including anaphylaxis, have occurred with **erythromycin**. Refer to Management of Acute Hypersensitivity Reactions.

►*Renal/Hepatic function impairment:* **Clarithromycin** is principally excreted via the liver and kidney and may be administered without dosage adjustment to patients with hepatic impairment and normal renal function. However, in the presence of severe renal impairment (creatinine clearance [Ccr] < 30 ml/min) with or without coexisting hepatic impairment, the dosage should be halved or the dosing intervals doubled. Clarithromycin in combination with ranitidine bismuth citrate therapy is not recommended in patients with Ccr < 25 ml/min.

Because **azithromycin** and **troleandomycin** are principally eliminated via the liver, exercise caution when administering to patients with impaired hepatic function. There are no data regarding azithromycin usage in patients with renal impairment; thus, exercise caution when prescribing azithromycin in these patients.

The mean peak plasma concentration (C_{max}) and AUC of **dirithromycin** with renal impairment tended to increase as creatinine clearance decreased; however, based on data available to date, no dosage adjustment should be necessary in patients with impaired renal function, including dialysis patients. In patients with mild (Child's Grade A) hepatic impairment, mean peak serum concentration, AUC, and volume of distribution of dirithromycin increased somewhat with multiple-dose administration; however, based on the magnitude of these changes, no dosage adjustment should be necessary in patients with mildly impaired hepatic function. The pharmacokinetics of dirithromycin in patients with moderate or severe hepatic function impairment (Child's Grade B or greater) have not been studied. Because dirithromycin/erythromycylamine is principally eliminated via the liver, administer dirithromycin to such patients only when absolutely necessary.

Erythromycin is principally excreted by the liver. Exercise caution in administering to patients with impaired hepatic function. There have been reports of hepatic dysfunction with or without jaundice.

▶*Elderly:* Maximum concentrations and AUC of **clarithromycin** and 14-OH clarithromycin are increased. These changes in pharmacokinetics parallel known age-related decreases in renal function. In clinical trials, elderly patients did not have an increased incidence of adverse events when compared to younger patients. Consider dosage adjustment in elderly patients with severe renal impairment.

Pharmacokinetic parameters in older volunteers (65 to 85 years old) were similar to those in younger volunteers (18 to 40 years old) for the 5-day therapeutic regimen of **azithromycin**. Dosage adjustment does not appear to be necessary for older patients with normal renal and hepatic function receiving treatment with this dosage regimen.

While C_{max} and AUC of **dirithromycin** tended to increase with age, neither was statistically or clinically significantly altered with age. Therefore, based on these pharmacokinetic results, no dosage adjustment should be necessary in elderly patients.

▶*Pregnancy:* (*Category B:* **Azithromycin**, **erythromycin**; *Category C:* **Clarithromycin**, **dirithromycin**, **troleandomycin**). Clarithromycin has adverse effects on pregnancy outcome or embryo-fetal development in monkeys, rats, mice, and rabbits. Animal studies with dirithromycin demonstrated that fetal weight was significantly depressed at 8 times the maximum recommended human dose with an increased occurrence of incomplete ossification. Erythromycin crosses the placental barrier but fetal levels are low. There are no adequate and well controlled studies in pregnant women. Do not use clarithromycin in pregnant women except in clinical circumstances when no alternative therapy is appropriate. If pregnancy occurs while taking this drug, apprise the patient of the hazard to the fetus. Use clarithromycin and dirithromycin during pregnancy only if the potential benefit justifies the potential risk to the fetus. Use azithromycin and erythromycin only when clearly needed.

▶*Lactation:* **Erythromycin** is excreted in breast milk and may concentrate (observed milk:plasma ratio of 0.5). Although no infant adverse effects are reported, potential problems for the nursing infant include modification of bowel flora, pharmacological effects, and interference with fever work-ups. Erythromycin is considered compatible with breastfeeding by the American Academy of Pediatrics. It is not known whether **clarithromycin**, **dirithromycin**, or **azithromycin** is excreted in breast milk. Exercise caution when administering to a nursing woman.

▶*Children:* Safety and efficacy of **clarithromycin** in children < 6 months of age have not been established. The safety of clarithromycin has not been studied in MAC patients < 20 months of age.

Safety and efficacy of **azithromycin** for IV injection in children or adolescents < 16 years have not been established. In controlled clinical studies, azithromycin has been administered to children (6 months to 16 years of age) by the oral route.

Safety and efficacy of **azithromycin** in children < 6 months of age have not been established for acute otitis media or community-acquired pneumonia.

Safety and efficacy of **azithromycin** in children < 2 years of age have not been established for pharyngitis/tonsillitis.

Safety and efficacy of **dirithromycin** in children < 12 years of age have not been established.

Precautions

▶*Local IV site reactions:* This has been reported with the IV administration of **azithromycin**. The incidence and severity of these reactions were the same when 500 mg was given over 1 hour (2 mg/ml as 250 ml infusion) or over 3 hours (1 mg/ml as 500 ml infusion). All volunteers who received infusate concentrations > 2 mg/ml experienced local IV site reactions; therefore, avoid higher concentrations.

▶*Superinfection:* Use of antibiotics (especially prolonged or repeated therapy) may result in bacterial or fungal overgrowth of nonsusceptible organisms. Such overgrowth may lead to a secondary infection. Appropriate measures should be taken if superinfection occurs.

Drug Interactions

Macrolide Antibiotic Drug Interactions			
Precipitant Drug	Object Drug*		Description
Antacids	Macrolides Azithromycin Dirithromycin Erythromycin	↔	Aluminum- and magnesium-containing antacids reduce peak serum levels but not the extent of azithromycin absorption. When given immediately following antacids, dirithromycin absorption is slightly enhanced. When given immediately prior to antacids, the elimination rate constant of erythromycin may be slightly decreased.
Fluconazole	Macrolides Clarithromycin	↑	Coadministration led to increases in mean steady-state trough levels (33%) and AUC (18%) of clarithromycin.
H₂ antagonists	Macrolides Dirithromycin	↑	When given immediately after H₂ antagonists, dirithromycin absorption is slightly enhanced.
Macrolides Clarithromycin	Ranitidine bismuth citrate	↔	Coadministration resulted in increased plasma ranitidine levels (57%), increased plasma bismuth trough concentrations (48%), and increased 14-OH clarithromycin plasma levels (31%). These effects do not appear to be clinically important.
Ranitidine bismuth citrate	Macrolides Clarithromycin		
Pimozide	Macrolides Azithromycin Clarithromycin Dirithromycin Erythromycin	↑	Coadministration is contraindicated. Two sudden deaths have occurred when clarithromycin was added to ongoing pimozide therapy.
Rifamycins Rifabutin Rifampin	Macrolides Clarithromycin Erythromycin Troleandomycin	↓	The antimicrobial effects of the macrolide antibiotic may be decreased while the frequency of GI adverse effects may be increased.
Macrolides Erythromycin	Alfentanil	↑	Alfentanil clearance may be decreased and the elimination half-life increased.
Macrolides Clarithromycin Erythromycin	Anticoagulants, oral	↑	Anticoagulant effects may be potentiated. Until more data are available, it is prudent to monitor anticoagulant function in patients receiving anticoagulants and any macrolide antibiotic.
Macrolides Clarithromycin Erythromycin Troleandomycin	Benzodiazepines Alprazolam Diazepam Midazolam Triazolam	↑	The plasma levels of certain benzodiazepines may be elevated, increasing and prolonging the CNS depressant effects. Azithromycin and dirithromycin would not be expected to interact.
Macrolides Erythromycin	Bromocriptine	↑	Bromocriptine serum levels may be elevated, resulting in an increase in the pharmacologic and adverse effects.
Macrolides Clarithromycin Erythromycin Troleandomycin	Buspirone	↑	Plasma buspirone concentrations may be elevated, increasing the pharmacologic and adverse effects. Azithromycin and dirithromycin would not be expected to interact.
Macrolides Clarithromycin Erythromycin Troleandomycin	Carbamazepine	↑	Increased concentrations of carbamazepine may occur. Azithromycin and dirithromycin would not be expected to interact.
Macrolides Clarithromycin Erythromycin Troleandomycin	Cisapride	↑	Coadministration of these drugs is contraindicated. Serious cardiac arrhythmias including ventricular tachycardia, ventricular fibrillation, torsades de pointes, and QT interval prolongation may occur. Azithromycin and dirithromycin would not be expected to interact with cisapride.
Macrolides Azithromycin Clarithromycin Erythromycin Troleandomycin	Cyclosporine	↑	Elevated cyclosporine concentrations with increased risk of toxicity (nephrotoxicity, neurotoxicity) may occur. Azithromycin and dirithromycin would not be expected to interact. However, a single case report implied that azithromycin may interact with cyclosporine.

Macrolide Antibiotic Drug Interactions

Precipitant Drug	Object Drug[*]		Description
Macrolides Clarithromycin Erythromycin	Digoxin	↑	Serum digoxin concentrations may be elevated because of the effect of the antibiotic on gut flora that metabolize digoxin in ≈ 10% of patients. Carefully monitor patients receiving digoxin and any macrolide antibiotic.
Macrolides Clarithromycin Erythromycin	Disopyramide	↑	Disopyramide plasma levels may be increased. Arrhythmias and increased QT$_c$ intervals have occurred.
Macrolides Clarithromycin Erythromycin Troleandomycin	Ergot alkaloids	↑	Acute ergot toxicity characterized by severe peripheral vasospasm and dysesthesia has occurred. Carefully monitor patients receiving ergot alkaloids and any macrolide antibiotic.
Macrolides Erythromycin	Felodipine	↑	Felodipine plasma levels may be elevated, increasing pharmacologic and adverse effects.
Macrolides Erythromycin	Fluoroquino-lones Grepafloxacin Sparfloxacin	↑	Sparfloxacin is contraindicated with erythromycin while grepafloxacin is contraindicated unless appropriate cardiac monitoring can be ensured (eg, hospitalized patients). Risk of life-threatening cardiac arrhythmias, including torsades de pointes, may be increased with coadministration.
Macrolides Azithromycin Clarithromycin Erythromycin	HMG-CoA reductase inhibitors	↑	The risk of severe myopathy or rhabdomyolysis may be increased.
Macrolides Erythromycin	Lincosamides	↓	Under some conditions, coadministration may be antagonistic.
Macrolides Erythromycin Troleandomycin	Methylprednisolone	↑	The clearance of methylprednisolone is greatly reduced. This has been used as a therapeutic advantage to reduce the dose.
Macrolides Clarithromycin	Omeprazole	↑	Coadministration may result in increased plasma levels of omeprazole, clarithromycin, and 14-OH clarithromycin.
Omeprazole	Macrolides Clarithromycin		
Macrolides Troleandomycin	Oral contraceptives	↑	Concurrent use may result in increased risk of intrahepatic cholestasis caused by decreased metabolism and accumulation of the contraceptive.
Macrolides Erythromycin	Penicillins	↔	Both antagonism and synergism have occurred with coadministration.
Macrolides Clarithromycin Erythromycin Troleandomycin	Tacrolimus	↑	Concurrent use may be associated with elevated serum tacrolimus levels, increasing the risk of side effects (eg, nephrotoxicity). Azithromycin and dirithromycin would not be expected to interact.
Macrolides Clarithromycin Erythromycin Troleandomycin	Theophylline	↑	Concurrent use may be associated with increased serum theophylline levels. Azithromycin and dirithromycin would not be expected to interact. Monitor serum theophylline levels in patients receiving theophylline and any macrolide antibiotic. In addition, plasma erythromycin levels may be decreased.
Theophylline	Macrolides Erythromycin	↓	
Macrolides Erythromycin	Vinblastine	↑	Risk of vinblastine toxicity (eg, constipation, myalgia, neutropenia) may be increased.
Macrolides Clarithromycin	Zidovudine	↔	Peak serum zidovudine concentrations may be increased or decreased.

[*] ↑ = Object drug increased. ↓ = Object drug decreased. ↔ = Undetermined clinical effect.

➤ *Drug/Lab test interactions:* **Erythromycin** interferes with the fluorometric determination of urinary catecholamines.

Erythromycin may interfere with AST determinations if azone-fast violet B or diphenylhydrazine colorimetric determinations are used.

➤ *Drug/Food interactions:* Food delays both the onset of **clarithromycin** absorption and the formation of 14-OH clarithromycin (the active metabolite) but does not affect the extent of bioavailability of the tablets. Following administration of the suspension, both the mean peak serum levels and extent of absorption were either decreased or increased when administered to adults or children, respectively. How-ever, clarithromycin tablets and oral suspension may be given without regard to meals.

When **azithromycin** suspension was administered with food, the rate of absorption was increased by 56% while the extent of absorption (AUC) was unchanged. Administration of azithromycin tablets with food increased C$_{max}$ by 23% with no change in AUC.

Administer **dirithromycin** with food or within an hour of eating. The effect of food on bioavailability was evaluated after administration of two 250 mg tablets 1 or 4 hours before food and immediately after a standard breakfast. Results indicated an increase in absorption of erythromycylamine when dirithromycin was administered after food, while a significant decrease in C$_{max}$ (33%) and AUC (31%) occurred when administered 1 hour before food. Dietary fat had little or no effect on the bioavailability of dirithromycin.

Antimicrobial effectiveness of **erythromycin** stearate and certain formulations of erythromycin base may be reduced. Take ≥ 2 hours before or after a meal. Erythromycin estolate and ethylsuccinate and the base in a delayed release form may be administered without regard to meals.

Adverse Reactions

The majority of side effects with **clarithromycin** observed in clinical trials were of a mild and transient nature. Less than 3% of adult patients without mycobacterial infections and < 2% of children without mycobacterial infections discontinued therapy because of drug-related side effects.

Most side effects with **azithromycin** are mild-to-moderate in severity and are reversible upon discontinuation of the drug. Approximately 0.7% of the patients (adults and children) from the multiple-dose clinical trials discontinued therapy because of treatment-related side effects. Approximately 1.2% of patients discontinued IV therapy and a total of 2.4% discontinued IV or oral therapy because of clinical or laboratory side effects. Most of the side effects leading to discontinuation were related to the GI tract (eg, nausea, vomiting, diarrhea, abdominal pain). Rare, but potentially serious side effects, were angioedema and cholestatic jaundice. In clinical trials conducted in patients with pelvic inflammatory disease, in which 1 to 2 IV doses were given, 2% of women who received monotherapy with azithromycin and 4% who received azithromycin plus metronidazole discontinued therapy because of clinical side effects.

Eighty-seven of 3299 (2.6%) patients discontinued **dirithromycin** because of adverse reactions. Thirty-five (40%) of the 87 patients who discontinued therapy did so because of nausea or abdominal pain.

Macrolide Adverse Reactions (> 1%)

Adverse reaction	Azithro-mycin	Clarithro-mycin	Dirithro-mycin	Erythro-mycin	Troleando-mycin
GI					
Abdominal pain/discomfort	1.9-7	2	9.7	7.5	✔[1]
Abnormal taste	—	3	> 0.1-< 1	—	—
Anorexia	1.9	—	> 0.1-< 1	✔	—
Diarrhea/loose stools	4.3-14	3	7.7	7.3	✔
Dyspepsia	≤ 1	2	2.6	2.1	—
Flatulence	≤ 1	—	1.5	1.5	—
GI disorder	—	—	1.6	1.4	—
Nausea	3-18	3	8.3	7.5	✔
Vomiting	≤ 7	—	3	2.8	✔
Injection site reactions					
Local inflammation	3.1	—	—	—	—
Pain	6.5	—	—	—	—
Lab test abnormalities					
ALT elevated	1-6	< 1	> 0.1-< 1	—	—
AST elevated	1-6	< 1	> 0.1-< 1	—	—
Bicarbonate decreased	—	—	1.4	2	—
BUN elevated	< 1	4	—	—	—
Eosinophils increased	—	—	1.2	0.6	—
GGT elevated	1-2	< 1	> 0.1-< 1	—	—
LDH elevated	≤ 3	< 1	—	—	—
Platelet count increased	—	—	3.8	4.8	—
Potassium elevated	1-2	—	2.6	—	—
Segmented neutrophils increased	—	—	1.2	1.3	—
Serum CPK elevated	1-2	—	1.2	0.9	—
Serum creatinine elevated	≤ 6	< 1	> 0.1-< 1	—	—
Total bilirubin elevated	≤ 3	< 1	> 0.1-< 1	—	—
Miscellaneous					
Asthenia	—	—	2	1.9	—
Dizziness	≤ 1	—	2.3	2.3	—
Dyspnea	—	—	1.2	1.2	—
Headache	≤ 1	2	8.6	8.2	—
Increased cough	—	—	1.5	2.6	—
Pain (non-specific)	—	—	2.2	1.6	—
Pruritus	1.9	—	1.2	1	—

Macrolide Adverse Reactions (> 1%)					
Adverse reaction	Azithro-mycin	Clarithro-mycin	Dirithro-mycin	Erythro-mycin	Troleando-mycin
Rash	1.9	—	1.4	2.6	✔
Vaginitis	≤ 2.8	—	0.4	0.6	—
Children					
Abdominal pain	1.9-3	3	—	—	—
Diarrhea/loose stools	2-6	6	—	—	—
Headache	≤ 1	2	—	—	—
Nausea	1-2	—	—	—	—
Rash	≤ 1.6	3	—	—	—
Vomiting	1-5	6	—	—	—

[1] ✔ = Event occurred, but incidence is unknown.

The following adverse reactions occurred at an incidence unknown or ≤ 1%:

Azithromycin – Mucositis; oral moniliasis; melena; cholestatic jaundice; gastritis; chest pain; palpitations; fatigue; somnolence; vertigo; monilia; nephritis; angioedema; photosensitivity; bronchospasm; taste perversion; elevated serum alkaline phosphatase; leukopenia; neutropenia; elevated blood glucose; elevated phosphate; decreased platelet count. Laboratory test abnormalities appeared to be reversible.

Children: Hyperkinesia; dizziness; agitation; nervousness; insomnia; fatigue; fever; malaise; dyspepsia; constipation; anorexia; flatulence; gastritis; conjunctivitis; chest pain; pruritus; urticaria.

Significant abnormalities occurring in children during clinical trials were reported at a frequency of < 1% but were similar in type to the adult pattern.

Clarithromycin – Elevated alkaline phosphatase; elevated prothrombin time; decreased WBC.

Dirithromycin – Abnormal stools; constipation; gastritis; anorexia; dry mouth; dysphagia; gastroenteritis; mouth ulceration; palpitations; anxiety; depression; nervousness; paresthesias; somnolence; peripheral edema; sweating; syncope; thirst; tinnitus; tremor; vasodilation; dysmenorrhea; urinary frequency; vaginal moniliasis; allergic reaction; amblyopia; dehydration; edema; epistaxis; eye disorder; fever; flu syndrome; hemoptysis; hyperventilation; malaise; myalgia; myasthenia; neck pain; insomnia; increased leukocytes; elevated alkaline phosphatase; decreased platelet count; decreased albumin; decreased chloride; decreased hematocrit; decreased hemoglobin; decreased lymphocytes; decreased segmented neutrophils; decreased phosphorus; decreased serum alkaline phosphatase; decreased serum uric acid; decreased total protein; increased basophils; increased calcium; increased lymphocytes; increased hematocrit; increased hemoglobin; increased monocytes; increased phosphorus; increased uric acid.

Erythromycin – Pseudomembranous colitis; anorexia; ventricular arrhythmias; hepatotoxicity; urticaria; bullous eruptions; eczema; erythema multiforme; Stevens-Johnson syndrome; toxic epidermal necrolysis; allergic reaction; anaphylaxis; insomnia; increased leukocytes.

Local: Venous irritation and phlebitis have occurred with parenteral administration of erythromycin, but the risk of such reactions may be reduced if the infusion is given slowly, in dilute solution, by continuous IV infusion or intermittent infusion over 20 to 60 minutes.

Special senses: There have been isolated reports of reversible hearing loss with erythromycin occurring chiefly in patients with renal or hepatic insufficiency, in the elderly and in those receiving high doses (> 4 g/day). In rare instances involving IV use, the ototoxic effect has been irreversible.

Troleandomycin – Urticaria; anaphylaxis.

Overdosage

➤*Symptoms:* The toxic symptoms following an overdose of a macrolide antibiotic may include nausea, vomiting, epigastric distress, and diarrhea.

Hearing loss may occur with **erythromycin**, especially in patients with renal insufficiency.

➤*Treatment:* Forced diuresis, peritoneal dialysis, hemodialysis, or hemoperfusion have not been established as beneficial for an overdose of **dirithromycin**. Hemodialysis has been shown to be ineffective in hastening the elimination of erythromycylamine from plasma in patients with chronic renal failure.

Treatment includes usual supportive measures. Refer to General Management of Acute Overdosage. Induce prompt elimination of unabsorbed drug. Control allergic reactions with conventional therapy as indicated. Hemodialysis and peritoneal dialysis are not particularly effective.

Patient Information

Clarithromycin may be given without regard to meals and may be taken with milk.

Caution patients to take **azithromycin** *suspension* ≥ 1 hour prior to a meal or ≥ 2 hours after a meal. Azithromycin *tablets* can be taken with or without food.

Take **dirithromycin** with food or within 1 hour of eating.

Take **erythromycin** on an empty stomach (≥ 1 hour before or 2 hours after meals); if GI upset occurs, take with food. Erythromycin estolate, ethylsuccinate and certain brands of erythromycin base enteric coated tablets may be taken without regard to meals; consult the current package literature. Take each erythromycin dose with an adequate amount of water (180 to 240 ml).

Take **erythromycin** and **troleandomycin** at evenly spaced intervals during the day, preferably around the clock. Complete full course of therapy; take until gone.

Caution patients not to take aluminum- and magnesium-containing antacids and oral **azithromycin** simultaneously.

Patients should discontinue the drug immediately and contact a physician if any signs of an allergic reaction occur.

Do not cut, chew, or crush the tablets.

Notify physician if nausea, vomiting, diarrhea or stomach cramps, severe abdominal pain, yellow discoloration of the skin or eyes, darkened urine, pale stools, or unusual tiredness occurs with **erythromycin**.

Shake the suspension well before each use. Do not refrigerate.

CLARITHROMYCIN

Rx	Biaxin (Abbott)	**Tablets:** 250 mg	(KT). Yellow, oval. Film-coated. In 60s and *ABBO-PAC* UD 100s.
		500 mg	(KL). Yellow, oval. Film-coated. In 60s and *ABBO-PAC* UD 100s.
		Granules for oral suspension when reconstituted: 125 mg/5 mL	Sucrose. Fruit punch flavor. In 50 and 100 mL.
		250 mg/5 mL	Sucrose. Fruit punch flavor. In 50 and 100 mL.
Rx	Biaxin XL (Abbott)	**Tablets, extended-release:** 500 mg	Lactose. (KJ). Yellow, oval. Film-coated. In 60s and *BIAXIN XL PAC* blister pack 4 × 14s.

For complete prescribing information, refer to the Macrolides group monograph.

Indications

➤*Tablets and granules:* For the treatment of mild-to-moderate infections caused by susceptible strains of the designated microorganisms in the following conditions.

Adults –

Pharyngitis/Tonsillitis: Caused by *Streptococcus pyogenes.*

• *Note* – The usual drug of choice in the treatment and prevention of streptococcal infections and the prophylaxis of rheumatic fever is penicillin oral/IM. Clarithromycin is generally effective in the eradication of *S. pyogenes* from the nasopharynx; however, data establishing the efficacy of clarithromycin in the subsequent prevention of rheumatic fever are not available at present.

Acute maxillary sinusitis: Caused by *Haemophilus influenzae, Moraxella catarrhalis,* or *S. pneumoniae.*

Acute bacterial exacerbation of chronic bronchitis: Caused by *H. influenzae, H. parainfluenzae, M. catarrhalis,* or *S. pneumoniae.*

Community-acquired pneumonia: Caused by *H. influenzae, Mycoplasma pneumoniae, S. pneumoniae,* or *Chlamydia pneumoniae* (TWAR strain).

Uncomplicated skin and skin structure infections: Caused by *Staphylococcus aureus* or *S. pyogenes.* Abscesses usually require surgical drainage.

Disseminated mycobacterial infections: Caused by *Mycobacterium avium* or *M. intracellulare.*

Prevention of disseminated Mycobacterium Avium Complex (MAC) disease: In patients with advanced HIV infection.

Helicobacter pylori dual therapy: Clarithromycin in combination with omeprazole or ranitidine bismuth citrate is indicated for the treatment of patients with an active duodenal ulcer associated with *H. pylori* infection. Regimens that contain clarithromycin as the single antimicrobial agent are more likely to be associated with the development of clarithromycin resistance among patients who fail therapy. In patients who fail therapy, susceptibility testing should be done if possible. The eradication of *H. pylori* has been demonstrated to reduce the risk of duodenal ulcer recurrence.

Helicobacter pylori triple therapy: Clarithromycin, lansoprazole or omeprazole, and amoxicillin as combination triple therapy for the treatment of *H. pylori* infection and duodenal ulcer disease (active or 5-year history of duodenal ulcer) to eradicate *H. pylori.*

CLARITHROMYCIN

Children –

Pharyngitis / Tonsillitis: Caused by *S. pyogenes.*

Community-acquired pneumonia: Caused by *M. pneumoniae, S. pneumoniae,* or *C. pneumoniae* (TWAR) strain.

Acute maxillary sinusitis: Caused by *H. influenzae, M. catarrhalis,* or *S. pneumoniae.*

Acute otitis media: Caused by *H. influenzae, M. catarrhalis,* or *S. pneumoniae.*

Uncomplicated skin and skin structure infections: Caused by *S. aureus* or *S. pyogenes.* Abscesses usually require surgical drainage.

Disseminated mycobacterial infections: Caused by *M. avium* or *M. intracellulare.*

Prevention of disseminated MAC disease: In patients with advanced HIV infection.

➤*Extended-release tablets:* Treatment of adults with mild to moderate infection caused by susceptible strains of the designated microorganisms in the conditions listed below.

Acute maxillary sinusitis – Caused by *H. influenzae, M. catarrhalis, S. pneumoniae.*

Acute bacterial exacerbation of chronic bronchitis – Caused by *H. influenzae, H. parainfluenzae, M. catarrhalis,* or *S. pneumoniae.*

Community-acquired pneumonia – Caused by *H. influenzae, H. parainfluenzae, M. catarrhalis, S. pneumoniae, C. pneumoniae* (TWAR), or *M. pneumoniae.*

Administration and Dosage

➤*Approved by the FDA:* October 31, 1991.

Tablets and granules may be given with or without food. Take the extended-release tablets with food.

➤*Adults:*

Clarithromycin Dosage Guidelines

Infection	Tablets		Extended-release tablets	
	Dosage (q 12 hr)	Duration (days)	Dosage (q 24 hr)	Duration (days)
Pharyngitis/Tonsillitis	250 mg	10	-	-
Acute maxillary sinusitis	500 mg	14	2 × 500 mg	14
Acute exacerbation of chronic bronchitis caused by:				
H. parainfluenzae	500 mg	7	2 × 500 mg	7
S. pneumoniae	250 mg	7 to 14	2 × 500 mg	7
M. catarrhalis	250 mg	7 to 14	2 × 500 mg	7
H. influenzae	500 mg	7 to 14	2 × 500 mg	7
Community-acquired pneumonia caused by:				
S. pneumoniae	250 mg	7 to 14	2 × 500 mg	7
M. pneumoniae	250 mg	7 to 14	2 × 500 mg	7
H. influenzae	250 mg	7	2 × 500 mg	7
H. parainfluenzae	-	-	2 × 500 mg	7
M. catarrhalis	-	-	2 × 500 mg	7
C. pneumoniae	250 mg	7 to 14	2 × 500 mg	7
Uncomplicated skin and skin structure infection	250 mg	7 to 14	-	-

➤*H. pylori eradication to reduce the risk of duodenal ulcer recurrence:*

Triple therapy –

Clarithromycin / Lansoprazole / Amoxicillin: 500 mg clarithromycin, 30 mg lansoprazole, and 1 g amoxicillin every 12 hours for 10 or 14 days.

Clarithromycin / Omeprazole / Amoxicillin: 500 mg clarithromycin, 20 mg omeprazole, and 1 g amoxicillin every 12 hours for 10 days. In patients with an ulcer present at the time of initiation of therapy, an additional 18 days of omeprazole 20 mg once daily is recommended for ulcer healing and symptom relief.

Dual therapy –

Clarithromycin / Omeprazole: 500 mg clarithromycin 3 times/day (every 8 hours), and 40 mg omeprazole once daily (every morning) for 14 days. An additional 14 days of 20 mg omeprazole once daily is recommended for ulcer healing and symptom relief.

Clarithromycin / Ranitidine bismuth citrate: 500 mg clarithromycin 2 times/day (every 12 hours) or 3 times/day (every 8 hours), and 400 mg ranitidine bismuth citrate given 2 times/day (every 12 hours) for 14 days. An additional 14 days of ranitidine bismuth citrate 2 times/day is recommended for ulcer healing and symptom relief. This combination is not recommended in patients with a creatinine clearance < 25 mL/min.

➤*Mycobacterial infections:* Recommended as the primary agent for the treatment of disseminated MAC. Use in combination with other antimycobacterial drugs that have shown in vitro activity against MAC or clinical benefit in MAC treatment. Continue clarithromycin therapy for life if clinical and mycobacterial improvements are observed.

Dosage (treatment and prevention) –

Adults: 500 mg twice daily.

Children: 7.5 mg/kg twice daily up to 500 mg twice daily. Doses recommended for pediatric prophylaxis are derived from MAC treatment studies in children. Refer to the Pediatric Dosage table for dosing recommendations.

➤*Children:* Usual recommended daily dosage is 15 mg/kg/day divided every 12 hours for 10 days.

Pediatric Clarithromycin Dosage Guidelines (Based on Body Weight)

Weight		Dose (q 12 hr)	125 mg/5 mL (q 12 hr)	250 mg/5 mL (q 12 hr)
kg	lbs			
9	20	62.5 mg	2.5 mL	1.25 mL
17	37	125 mg	5 mL	2.5 mL
25	55	187.5 mg	7.5 mL	3.75 mL
33	73	250 mg	10 mL	5 mL

Dosing calculated on 7.5 mg/kg q 12 hr

➤*Renal / Hepatic function impairment:* May be administered without dosage adjustment in the presence of hepatic impairment if there is normal renal function. In the presence of severe renal impairment (Ccr < 30 mL/min) with or without coexisting hepatic impairment, halve the dose or double the dosing interval.

➤*Reconstitution of granules:* The following table indicates the volume of water to be added when constituting.

Clarithromycin Granule Reconstitution

Total volume after constitution (mL)	Clarithromycin concentration after constitution	Amount of water to be added (mL)
50	125 mg/5 mL	27
100	125 mg/5 mL	55
50	250 mg/5 mL	27
100	250 mg/5 mL	55

Add half the volume of water to the bottle and shake vigorously. Add the remainder of water to the bottle and shake.

➤*Storage / Stability:*

Tablets and granules – Store at controlled room temperature in a well-closed container. Protect the 250 mg tablets from light.

Extended-release tablets – Store the extended-release tablets at 20° to 25°C (68° to 77°F); excursions permitted to 15° to 30°C (59° to 86°F).

Reconstituted suspension – Shake well before each use. Keep tightly closed. Do not refrigerate. After mixing, store at 15° to 30°C (59° to 86°F), and use within 14 days.

AZITHROMYCIN

Rx	Zithromax (Pfizer)	**Tablets:** 250 mg (as dihydrate)	Lactose. (PFIZER 306). Pink, capsule shape. Film coated. In 30s, UD 50s, and *Z-Pak* 6s.
		500 mg (as dihydrate)	Lactose. (Pfizer ZTM500). Pink, capsule shape. Film coated. In 30s, UD 50s, and *TRI-PAK* 3s.
		600 mg (as dihydrate)	Lactose. (PFIZER 308). White, oval. Film coated. In 30s.
		Powder for Injection, lyophilized: 500 mg	In 10 mL vials and 10 mL vials with 1 *Vial-Mate* adaptor.
		Powder for Oral Suspension: 100 mg/5 mL	Sucrose. In 300 mg bottles.
		200 mg/5 mL	Sucrose. In 600, 900, and 1200 mg bottles.
		1 g/packet (as dihydrate)	Sucrose. In single-dose packets of 3s and 10s.

For complete prescribing information, refer to the Macrolides group monograph.

Indications

For the treatment of patients with infections caused by susceptible strains of the designated microorganisms in the specific conditions listed below:

➤*Adults:*

Oral –

Chronic obstructive pulmonary disease (COPD): In patients with acute bacterial exacerbations of COPD caused by *Haemophilus influenzae, Moraxella catarrhalis,* or *Streptococcus pneumoniae.*

Community-acquired pneumonia: In patients appropriate for oral therapy with community-acquired pneumonia of mild severity caused

AZITHROMYCIN

by *H. influenzae*, *Chlamydia pneumoniae*, *Mycoplasma pneumoniae*, or *S. pneumoniae*.

• *Note* – Azithromycin should not be used in patients with pneumonia who are judged to be inappropriate for oral therapy because of moderate to severe illness or risk factors such as any of the following: Patients with cystic fibrosis, nosocomially acquired infections, known or suspected bacteremia, patients requiring hospitalization, elderly or debilitated patients, or those with significant underlying health problems that may compromise their ability to respond to their illness (including immunodeficiency or functional asplenia).

Genital ulcer disease: In men with genital ulcer disease caused by *Haemophilus ducreyi* (chancroid).

Azithromycin, at the recommended dose, should not be relied upon to treat gonorrhea and syphilis. Antimicrobial agents used in high doses for short periods of time to treat nongonococcal urethritis may mask or delay the symptoms of incubating gonorrhea and syphilis. All patients with sexually transmitted urethritis or cervicitis should have a serologic test for syphilis and appropriate cultures for gonorrhea performed at the time of diagnosis. Initiate appropriate antimicrobial therapy and follow-up tests for these diseases if infection is confirmed.

Pharyngitis/Tonsillitis: As an alternative to first-line therapy in patients with pharyngitis/tonsillitis caused by *Streptococcus pyogenes* in individuals who cannot use first-line therapy.

Skin/Skin structure infections: In patients with uncomplicated skin and skin structure infections caused by *Staphylococcus aureus*, *S. pyogenes*, or *Streptococcus agalactiae*. Abscesses usually require surgical drainage.

Urethritis/Cervicitis: In patients with urethritis and cervicitis caused by *Chlamydia trachomatis* or *Neisseria gonorrhoeae*.

Prophylaxis of disseminated Mycobacterium avium complex (MAC) disease: Azithromycin taken alone or in combination with rifabutin at its approved dose is indicated for the prevention of disseminated MAC disease in people with advanced HIV infection.

Treatment of disseminated MAC disease: Azithromycin taken in combination with ethambutol is indicated for the treatment of disseminated MAC infections in people with advanced HIV infection.

IV –

Community-acquired pneumonia: In patients requiring initial IV therapy with community-acquired pneumonia caused by *C. pneumoniae*, *H. influenzae*, *S. pneumoniae*, *M. pneumoniae*, *Legionella pneumophila*, *M. catarrhalis*, *S. aureus*.

Pelvic inflammatory disease: In patients requiring initial IV therapy with pelvic inflammatory disease caused by *C. trachomatis*, *N. gonorrhoeae*, or *Mycoplasma hominis*. If anaerobic microorganisms are suspected of contributing to the infection, administer an antimicrobial agent with anaerobic activity in combination with azithromycin.

➤*Children:*
Oral –

Acute otitis media: In children 6 months of age and over with acute otitis media caused by *H. influenzae*, *M. catarrhalis*, or *S. pneumoniae*.

Community-acquired pneumonia: In children 6 months of age and over with community-acquired pneumonia caused by *C. pneumoniae*, *H. influenzae*, *M. pneumoniae*, or *S. pneumoniae* in patients appropriate for oral therapy.

• *Note:* – Azithromycin should not be used in pediatric patients with pneumonia who are judged to be inappropriate for oral therapy because of moderate to severe illness or risk factors such as any of the following: Patients with cystic fibrosis, nosocomially acquired infections, known or suspected bacteremia, patients requiring hospitalization, or those with significant underlying health problems that may compromise their ability to respond to their illness (including immunodeficiency or functional asplenia).

Pharyngitis/Tonsillitis: In children ≥ 2 years of age with pharyngitis/ tonsillitis caused by *S. pyogenes* in individuals who cannot use first-line therapy.

IV – IV azithromycin is not for use in children < 16 years of age.

➤*Note:* Penicillin IM is the usual drug of choice in the treatment of *S. pyogenes* infections and the prophylaxis of rheumatic fever. Azithromycin often is effective in the eradication of susceptible strains of *S. pyogenes* from the nasopharynx. Because some strains are resistant to azithromycin, perform susceptibility tests when patients are treated with azithromycin.

➤*Unlabeled uses:* Helicobacter pylori infections, *Bartonella* infection, Lyme disease, toxoplasmosis, babesiosis, granuloma inguinale (donovanosis), cryptosporidiosis.

Chlamydial infections – Caused by *C. trachomatis*. CDC treatment recommendations are 1 g azithromycin orally in a single dose. Alternatives include doxycycline, erythromycin base, erythromycin ethylsuccinate, or ofloxacin.

For children with chlamydial infection who weigh ≥ 45 kg but < 8 years of age, CDC treatment recommendations are 1 g azithromycin orally in a single dose.

For children ≥ 8 years of age with chlamydial infection, CDC treatment recommendations are 1 g azithromycin orally in a single dose. Doxycycline is an alternative to azithromycin.

Uncomplicated gonococcal infections of the cervix, urethra, and rectum – Caused by *N. gonorrhoeae*. CDC treatment recommendations are 1 g azithromycin orally in a single dose in combination with 1 of the following: Cefixime, ceftriaxone, ciprofloxacin, or ofloxacin. Doxycycline is an alternative to azithromycin.

Uncomplicated gonococcal infection of the pharynx – CDC treatment recommendations are 1 g azithromycin orally in a single dose in combination with 1 of the following: Ceftriaxone, ciprofloxacin, or ofloxacin. Doxycycline is an alternative to azithromycin.

Prophylaxis after a sexual assault – CDC treatment recommendations are 1 g azithromycin orally in a single dose plus ceftriaxone and metronidazole. Doxycycline is an alternative to azithromycin.

Administration and Dosage

➤*Approved by the FDA:* November 1991.

Tablets and oral suspension can be taken with or without food; however, increased tolerability has been observed when tablets are taken with food. Single-dose 1 g packets are not for pediatric use.

➤*Renal function impairment:* No dosage adjustment is recommended for subjects with renal impairment (GFR at least 80 mL/min). The mean AUC_{0-120} was similar in subjects with GFR 10 to 80 mL/min compared with subjects with normal renal function, whereas it increased 35% in subjects with GFR less than 10 mL/min compared with subjects with normal renal function. Exercise caution when azithromycin is administered to subjects with severe renal impairment.

➤*Oral:*
Adults –

Mild to moderate acute bacterial exacerbations of COPD in patients 16 years of age and older: 500 mg/day for 3 days or 500 mg as a single dose on the first day followed by 250 mg once daily on days 2 through 5.

Community-acquired pneumonia of mild severity, pharyngitis/tonsillitis (as second-line therapy), and uncomplicated skin and skin structure infections in patients 16 years of age and older: 500 mg as a single dose on the first day followed by 250 mg once daily on days 2 through 5.

Genital ulcer disease caused by H. ducreyi (chancroid): Single 1 g dose.

Nongonococcal urethritis/cervicitis caused by C. trachomatis: Single 1 g dose.

Gonococcal urethritis/cervicitis caused by N. gonorrhoeae: Single 2 g dose.

Prevention of disseminated MAC infections: 1200 mg taken once weekly. This dose of azithromycin may be combined with the approved dosage regimen of rifabutin.

Treatment of disseminated MAC infections: Take 600 mg/day in combination with ethambutol at the recommended daily dose of 15 mg/kg. Other antimycobacterial drugs that have shown in vitro activity against MAC may be added to the regimen of azithromycin plus ethambutol at the discretion of the physician or health care provider.

Children –

Acute otitis media: 30 mg/kg oral suspension given as a single dose or 10 mg/kg once daily for 3 days or 10 mg/kg as a single dose on the first day, followed by 5 mg/kg on days 2 through 5.

Community-acquired pneumonia: 10 mg/kg oral suspension as a single dose on the first day followed by 5 mg/kg on days 2 through 5.

Azithromycin Pediatric Dosage Guidelines for Otitis Media and Community-Acquired Pneumonia (≥ 6 months of age) 5-Day Regimen[1],[2]							
Weight		Amount of 100 mg/5 mL suspension		Amount of 200 mg/5 mL suspension		Total mL per treatment course	Total mg per treatment course
kg	lbs	Day 1	Days 2 to 5	Day 1	Days 2 to 5		
5	11	2.5 mL	1.25 mL			7.5 mL	150 mg
10	22	5 mL	2.5 mL			15 mL	300 mg
20	44			5 mL	2.5 mL	15 mL	600 mg
30	66			7.5 mL	3.75 mL	22.5 mL	900 mg
40	88			10 mL	5 mL	30 mL	1200 mg
≥ 50	≥ 110			12.5 mL	6.25 mL	37.5 mL	1500 mg

[1] Dosing calculated on 10 mg/kg on day 1, followed by 5 mg/kg on days 2 to 5.
[2] Effectiveness of the 1- or 3-day regimen in children with community-acquired pneumonia has not been established.

Azithromycin Pediatric Dosage Guidelines for Otitis Media: 3-Day Regimen[1]					
Weight		Amount of 100 mg/5 mL suspension	Amount of 200 mg/5 mL suspension	Total mL per treatment course	Total mg per treatment course
kg	lbs	Day 1 to 3	Day 1 to 3		
5	11	2.5 mL		7.5 mL	150 mg
10	22	5 mL		15 mL	300 mg
20	44		5 mL	15 mL	600 mg
30	66		7.5 mL	22.5 mL	900 mg
40	88		10 mL	30 mL	1200 mg

AZITHROMYCIN

Azithromycin Pediatric Dosage Guidelines for Otitis Media: 3-Day Regimen[1]				
Weight		Amount of 100 mg/5 mL suspension	Amount of 200 mg/5 mL suspension	Total mL per treatment course	Total mg per treatment course
kg	lbs	Day 1 to 3	Day 1 to 3		
≥ 50	≥ 110		12.5 mL	37.5 mL	1500 mg

[1] Dosing calculated on 10 mg/kg/day.

Azithromycin Pediatric Dosage Guidelines for Otitis Media: 1-Day Regimen[1]				
Weight		Amount of 200 mg/5 mL suspension	Total mL per treatment course	Total mg per treatment course
kg	lbs	Day 1		
5	11	3.75 mL	3.75 mL	150 mg
10	22	7.5 mL	7.5 mL	300 mg
20	44	15 mL	15 mL	600 mg
30	66	22.5 mL	22.5 mL	900 mg
40	88	30 mL	30 mL	1200 mg
≥ 50	≥ 110	37.5 mL	37.5 mL	1500 mg

[1] Dosing calculated on 30 mg/kg as a single dose.

Pharyngitis/Tonsillitis: 12 mg/kg once daily for 5 days. See the following table.

Azithromycin Pediatric Dosage Guidelines for Pharyngitis/Tonsillitis: 5-Day Regimen (≥ 2 years of age)[1]				
Weight		Amount of 200 mg/5 mL suspension	Total mL per treatment course	Total mg per treatment course
kg	lbs	Day 1 to 5		
8	18	2.5 mL	12.5 mL	500 mg
17	37	5 mL	25 mL	1000 mg
25	55	7.5 mL	37.5 mL	1500 mg
33	73	10 mL	50 mL	2000 mg
40	88	12.5 mL	62.5 mL	2500 mg

[1] Dosing calculated on 12 mg/kg/day for 5 days.

➤*IV:*

Adults – Infuse injections over a period of ≥ 60 minutes. The infusate concentration and rate of infusion for azithromycin for injection should be 1 mg/mL over 3 hours or 2 mg/mL over 1 hour. Do not administer azithromycin for injection as a bolus or IM injection.

Community-acquired pneumonia: 500 mg as a single daily dose IV for ≥ 2 days. Follow IV therapy by the oral route at a single daily dose of 500 mg to complete a 7- to 10-day course of therapy.

Pelvic inflammatory disease: 500 mg as a single daily dose IV for 1 or 2 days. Follow IV therapy by the oral route at a single daily dose of 250 mg to complete a 7-day course of therapy. If anaerobic microorganisms are suspected of contributing to the infection, administer an antimicrobial agent with anaerobic activity with azithromycin.

➤*Preparation for IV administration:* Prepare the initial solution of azithromycin for injection by adding 4.8 mL of Sterile Water for Injection to the 500 mg vial and shaking the vial until all of the drug is dissolved. Because azithromycin for injection is supplied under vacuum, it is recommended that a standard 5 mL (nonautomated) syringe be used to ensure that the exact amount of 4.8 mL of sterile water is dispensed. Each mL of reconstituted solution contains 100 mg azithromycin. To provide azithromycin over a concentration range of 1 to 2 mg/mL, transfer 5 mL of the 100 mg/mL azithromycin solution into the appropriate amount of any of the diluents listed below:

Normal Saline (0.9% sodium chloride); ½ Normal Saline (0.45% sodium chloride); 5% Dextrose in Water; Lactated Ringer's Solution; 5% Dextrose in ½ Normal Saline (0.45% sodium chloride) with 20 mEq KCl; 5% Dextrose in Lactated Ringer's Solution; 5% Dextrose in ⅓ Normal Saline (0.3% sodium chloride); 5% Dextrose in ½ Normal Saline (0.45% sodium chloride); *Normosol-M* in 5% Dextrose; *Normosol-R* in 5% Dextrose.

➤*Preparation for administration of single 1 g packet:* Thoroughly mix the entire contents of the packet with approximately 60 mL (2 oz) of water. Drink the entire contents immediately; add an additional 60 mL of water, mix, and drink to ensure complete consumption of dosage. Do not use the single-dose packet to administer doses other than 1000 mg of azithromycin. This packet is not for pediatric use.

➤*Storage/Stability:*

Tablets – Store tablets between 15° to 30°C (59° to 86°F).

Oral suspension – Store dry powder below 30°C (86°F). Store single-dose packets between 5° and 30°C (41° and 86°F). Store reconstituted oral suspension between 5° and 30°C (41° and 86°F) and use within 10 days. Discard after full dosing is completed.

IV – Diluted solution for injection is stable for 24 hours when stored ≤ 30°C or 86°F or for 7 days refrigerated at 5°C (41°F).

DIRITHROMYCIN

Rx	**Dynabac** (Muro)	**Tablets, delayed release:** 250 mg	Enteric coated. (DYNABAC UC5364). White, elliptical. In 60s and *D5-Pak* of 10.

For complete prescribing information, refer to the Macrolides group monograph.

Indications

For the treatment of individuals ≥ 12 years of age with mild to moderate infections caused by susceptible strains of the designated micro-organisms in the specific conditions listed below:

➤*Acute bacterial exacerbations of chronic bronchitis:* Caused by *Haemophilus influenzae*, *Moraxella catarrhalis*, or *Streptococcus pneumoniae* (see Warnings).

➤*Secondary bacterial infection of acute bronchitis:* Caused by *M. catarrhalis* or *S. pneumoniae.*

➤*Community-acquired pneumonia:* Caused by *Legionella pneumophila*, *Mycoplasma pneumoniae*, or *S. pneumoniae.*

➤*Pharyngitis/Tonsillitis:* Caused by *Streptococcus pyogenes.*

The usual drug of choice in the treatment and prevention of streptococcal infections and the prophylaxis of rheumatic fever is penicillin. Dirithromycin generally is effective in the eradication of *S. pyogenes* from the nasopharynx; however, data establishing the efficacy of dirithromycin in the subsequent prevention of rheumatic fever are not available at present.

➤*Uncomplicated skin and skin structure infections:* Caused by *Staphylococcus aureus* (methicillin-susceptible strains) or *S. pyogenes.* Abscesses usually require surgical drainage (see Warnings).

Administration and Dosage

➤*Approved by the FDA:* June 1995.

Administer with food or within 1 hour of having eaten. Do not cut, crush, or chew the tablets.

Recommended Dosage Schedule for Dirithromycin (≥ 12 years of age)			
Infection (mild to moderate severity)	Dose	Frequency	Duration (days)
Acute bacterial exacerbations of chronic bronchitis caused by *H. influenzae*, *M. catarrhalis*, or *S. pneumoniae.*	500 mg	once a day	5 to 7
Secondary bacterial infection of acute bronchitis caused by *M. catarrhalis* or *S. pneumoniae.*	500 mg	once a day	7
Community-acquired pneumonia caused by *L. pneumophila*, *M. pneumoniae*, or *S. pneumoniae.*	500 mg	once a day	14
Pharyngitis/tonsillitis caused by *S. pyogenes.*	500 mg	once a day	10
Uncomplicated skin and skin structure infections caused by *S. aureus* (methicillin-susceptible) or *S. pyogenes.*	500 mg	once a day	5 to 7

➤*Storage/Stability:* Store at controlled room temperature 15° to 30°C (59° to 86°F).

Erythromycin

Indications

Indicated for treatment of infections caused by susceptible strains of the designated microorganisms in the diseases listed below:

➤*Upper respiratory tract infections:* Mild to moderate severity caused by: *Streptococcus pyogenes* (group A beta-hemolytic streptococci), *Streptococcus pneumoniae*, or *Haemophilus influenzae* (with concomitant sulfonamides because not all strains of *H. influenzae* are susceptible at the erythromycin concentrations ordinarily achieved).

➤*Lower respiratory tract infections:* Mild to moderate severity caused by *S. pyogenes* (group A beta-hemolytic streptococci) or *S. (diplococcus) pneumoniae.*

➤*Note:* Injectable benzathine penicillin G is considered by the American Heart Asssociation to be the drug of choice in the treatment and prevention of streptococcal pharyngitis and in long-term prophylaxis of rheumatic fever. When oral medication is preferred for treatment of the above conditions, penicillin G, V, or erythromycin are alternate drugs of choice.

➤*Respiratory tract infections:* Caused by *Mycoplasma pneumoniae* (Eaton's agent).

➤*Skin/Skin structure infections:* Mild to moderate severity caused by *S. pyogenes*; *Staphylococcus aureus* (resistant staphylococci may emerge during treatment).

➤*Pertussis (whooping cough):* Caused by *Bordetella pertussis.* Effective in eliminating the organism from the nasopharynx of infected patients. May be helpful in the prophylaxis of pertussis in exposed susceptible individuals.

➤*Diphtheria:* Adjunct to antitoxin in infections caused by *Corynebacterium diphtheriae*, to prevent establishment of carriers and to eradicate the organism in carriers.

➤*Erythrasma:* Treatment of infections caused by *Corynebacterium minutissimum.*

➤*Intestinal amebiasis:* Caused by *Entamoeba histolytica* (oral erythromycin only). Extra-enteric amebiasis requires treatment with other agents.

➤*Pelvic inflammatory disease (PID), acute:* Caused by *Neisseria gonorrhoeae*: Erythromycin lactobionate IV followed by oral erythromycin as an alternative to penicillin in patients with a history of penicillin sensitivity.

➤*Conjunctivitis of the newborn, pneumonia of infancy, urogenital infections during pregnancy:* Caused by *Chlamydia trachomatis.*

➤*Uncomplicated urethral, endocervical, or rectal infections in adults:* Caused by *C. trachomatis* when tetracyclines are contraindicated or not tolerated.

➤*Nongonococcal urethritis:* Caused by *Ureaplasma urealyticum* when tetracyclines are contraindicated or not tolerated.

➤*Primary syphilis:* Caused by *Treponema pallidum*: Erythromycin (oral only) as an alternative to penicillin in penicillin-allergic patients.

➤*Legionnaire's disease:* Caused by *Legionella pneumophila.* Although no controlled clinical efficacy studies have been conducted, in vitro and limited preliminary clinical data suggest effectiveness.

➤*Rheumatic fever:* Prevention of initial or recurrent attacks as an alternative in patients who are allergic to penicillins or sulfonamides.

➤*Bacterial endocarditis:* Caused by alpha-hemolytic streptococci, viridans group: Prevention as an alternative in patients allergic to penicillins.

➤*Listeria monocytogenes infections:* Listeria monocytogenes infections.

➤*Unlabeled uses:*

T. pallidum – Early syphilis (primary or secondary) for nonpregnant patients for whom compliance with therapy and follow-up can be ensured. In treatment of primary syphilis, examine spinal fluid before treatment and as part of the follow-up after therapy. The use of erythromycin for the treatment of in utero syphilis is not recommended.

Campylobacter jejuni – Erythromycin has been used successfully in prolonged diarrhea associated with campylobacter enteritis.

Lymphogranuloma venereum – Genital, inguinal, or anorectal.

Granuloma inguinale – Caused by *Calymmatobacterium granulomatis.*

Haemophilus ducreyi (chancroid) – Treat until ulcers or lymph nodes are healed.

Prior to elective colorectal surgery, to reduce wound complications, erythromycin base with oral neomycin is a popular preoperative combination.

Other uses, as alternative to penicillins, include the following: Anthrax; Vincent's gingivitis; erysipeloid; tetanus; actinomycosis; *Nocardia* infections (with a sulfonamide); *Eikenella corrodens* infections; *Borrelia* infections (including early Lyme disease).

Administration and Dosage

➤*Oral:* Dosages and product strengths are expressed as erythromycin base equivalents. Because of differences in absorption and biotransformation, varying quantities of each salt form are required to produce the same free erythromycin serum levels. For example, expressed in base equivalents, 400 mg erythromycin ethylsuccinate produces the same free erythromycin serum levels as 250 mg of erythromycin base, stearate, or estolate.

Optimal serum levels of erythromycin are reached when erythromycin base or stearate is taken in the fasting state or immediately before meals. Erythromycin ethylsuccinate, estolate, and enteric-coated erythromycin may be administered without regard to meals.

Urine alkalinization (pH 8.5) increases erythromycin's gram-negative antibacterial activity; several investigators suggest coadministration of urinary alkalinizers (eg, sodium bicarbonate) and erythromycin for urinary tract infections.

Usual dosage –

Adults: 250 mg (or 400 mg ethylsuccinate) every 6 hours taken 1 hour before meals, or 500 mg every 12 hours, or 333 mg every 8 hours. May increase up to 4 g/day, according to severity of infection. If twice daily dosage is desired, the recommended dose is 500 mg every 12 hours. Twice daily dosing is not recommended when doses > 1 g/day are administered.

Children: 30 to 50 mg/kg/day (15 to 25 mg/lb/day) in divided doses. Proper dosage is determined by age, weight, and severity of infection. When twice daily dosing is desired, half of the total daily dose may be taken every 12 hours. For more severe infections, dosage may be doubled.

Erythromycin Uses and Dosages	
Indication (Organism)	Dosage (Stated as erythromycin base)
Labeled uses:	
Upper respiratory tract infections of mild to moderate severity	
S. pyogenes (group A beta-hemolytic streptococcus)	250 to 500 mg 4 times/day or 20 to 50 mg/kg/day for children (not to exceed the adult dose) in divided doses for 10 days.
S. pneumoniae	250 to 500 mg every 6 hours.
H. influenzae (used concomitantly with a sulfonamide)	Erythromycin ethylsuccinate: 50 mg/kg/day for children (not to exceed 6 g/day). Sulfisoxazole: 150 mg/kg/day. Combination given for 10 days.
Lower respiratory tract infections of mild to moderate severity	
S. pyogenes (group A beta-hemolytic streptococcus)	250 to 500 mg 4 times/day or 20 to 50 mg/kg/day for children (not to exceed the adult dose) in divided doses for 10 days.
S. pneumoniae	250 to 500 mg every 6 hours.
Respiratory tract infections	
M. pneumoniae (Eaton agent, PPLO)	500 mg every 6 hours for 5 to 10 days. Treat severe infections for up to 3 weeks.
Skin and skin structure infections of mild to moderate severity	
S. pyogenes	250 to 500 mg 4 times/day or 20 to 50 mg/kg/day for children (not to exceed the adult dose) in divided doses for 10 days.
S. aureus (resistant organisms may emerge)	250 mg every 6 hours or 500 mg every 12 hours, maximum 4 g/day.
Pertussis (whooping cough)	
B. pertussis: Effective in eliminating the organism from the nasopharynx of infected patients. May be helpful in prophylaxis of pertussis in exposed individuals.	40 to 50 mg/kg/day for children (not to exceed the adult dose) in divided doses for 5 to 14 days, or 500 mg 4 times/day for 10 days.
Diphtheria	
C. diphtheriae: Adjunct to antitoxin to prevent establishment of carriers and to eradicate organism in carriers.	500 mg every 6 hours for 10 days.

Erythromycin

Erythromycin Uses and Dosages	
Indication (Organism)	Dosage (Stated as erythromycin base)
Erythrasma *C. minutissimum*	250 mg 3 times/day for 21 days.
Intestinal amebiasis *E. histolytica*: Oral erythromycin only.	Adults: 250 mg 4 times/day for 10 to 14 days. Children: 30 to 50 mg/kg/day in divided doses for 10 to 14 days.
Pelvic inflammatory disease (PID), acute *N. gonorrhoeae*: Erythromycin lactobionate IV followed by oral erythromycin.[1]	500 mg IV every 6 hours for 3 days, then 250 mg orally every 6 hours for 7 days.
Conjunctivitis of the newborn, pneumonia of infancy, urogenital infections during pregnancy *C. trachomatis*	50 mg/kg/day for children (not to exceed the adult dose) in 4 divided doses for 10 to ≥ 14 days (conjunctivitis) or ≥ 21 days (pneumonia); 500 mg 4 times daily for 7 days or 250 mg 4 times daily on an empty stomach for ≥ 14 days (urogenital infections).
Urethral, endocervical, or rectal infections, uncomplicated *C. trachomatis*[1]	500 mg ≥ 4 times/day for 7 days or 250 mg 4 times/day for 14 days if patient cannot tolerate high-dose erythromycin.[2]
Nongonococcal urethritis *U. urealyticum*[1]	500 mg 4 times/day for at least 7 days or 250 mg orally 4 times/day for 14 days if patient cannot tolerate high-dose erythromycin.[2]
Primary syphilis *T. pallidum*: Oral only[1]	20 to 40 g in divided doses over 10 to 15 days.
Legionnaire's disease *L. pneumophila*: No controlled clinical efficacy studies have been conducted, but data suggest effectiveness	1 to 4 g/day in divided doses for 10 to 14 days.
Rheumatic fever *S. pyogenes* (group A beta-hemolytic streptococci): Prevention of initial or recurrent attacks.[1]	250 mg 2 times daily.
Bacterial endocarditis (in penicillin-allergic patients with valvular heart disease who are to undergo dental procedures or surgical procedures of the upper respiratory tract. *Alpha-hemolytic streptococcus* (viridans)[1]	Adults: 1 g 1 to 2 hours prior to procedure, then 500 mg 6 hours after initial dose.[3] Children: 20 mg/kg 2 hours prior to procedure, then 10 mg/kg 6 hours after initial dose.[3]
Listeria monocytogenes	Adults: 250 mg every 6 hours or 500 mg every 12 hours, maximum 4 g/day.
Unlabeled uses: *Campylobacter jejuni*: Has been successful in severe or prolonged diarrhea associated with *Campylobacter enteritis* or enterocolitis.[2]	500 mg 4 times a day for 7 days.
Lymphogranuloma venereum: Genital, inguinal, or anorectal.[2]	500 mg 4 times a day for 21 days.
Haemophilus ducreyi (chancroid): Treat until ulcers or lymph nodes are healed.[2]	500 mg 4 times a day for 7 days.
Treponema pallidum: Early syphilis (primary or secondary)	500 mg 4 times a day for 14 days.
Prior to elective colorectal surgery, to reduce wound complications	Combination of erythromycin base and neomycin is a popular preoperative preparation.
Clostridium tetani: Tetanus[1]	500 mg every 6 hours for 10 days.
Granuloma inguinale *Calymmatobacterium granulomatis*[2,4]	500 mg orally 4 times daily for ≥ 21 days.

[1] Use as alternative drug in penicillin or tetracycline hypersensitivity or when penicillin or tetracycline are contraindicated or not tolerated.

[2] CDC 1998 Guidelines for Sexually Transmitted Diseases Treatment. *Morbidity and Mortality Weekly Report* 1998 Jan 23;47(No. 441):1-117.

[3] American Heart Association statement. *JAMA* 1990;264:2919-2922.

[4] Use as alternate therapy to trimethoprim-sulfamethoxazole or doxycycline.

➤*Parenteral:*

Erythromycin IV – This is indicated when oral use is impossible, or when severity of the infection requires immediate high serum levels. Replace IV therapy with oral as soon as possible.

Continuous infusion: This is preferable, but intermittent infusion in 20- to 60-minute periods at intervals of ≤ 6 hours is also effective. Because of irritative properties of erythromycin, IV push is unacceptable.

Severe infections – 15 to 20 mg/kg/day. Higher doses, up to 4 g/day, may also be given for severe infections.

Preparation of solution –

Vials: Prepare the initial solution by adding 10 ml Sterile Water for Injection, USP, to the 500 mg vial or 20 ml Sterile Water for Injection, USP, to the 1 g vial. Use only Sterile Water for Injection, USP, as other diluents may cause precipitation during reconstitution. Do not use diluents containing preservatives or inorganic salts. Note: When the product is reconstituted as directed above, the resulting solution contains an effective microbial preservative. After reconstitution, each ml contains 50 mg erythromycin activity.

Add the initial dilution to one of the following diluents before administration to give a concentration of 1 g/L (1 mg/ml) erythromycin activity for continuous infusion or 1 to 5 mg/ml for intermittent infusion: 0.9% Sodium Chloride Injection, USP; Lactated Ringer's Injection, USP; *Normosol-R*.

The following solutions may also be used providing they are first buffered with 4% sodium bicarbonate or *Neut* by adding 1 ml of the 4% Sodium Bicarbonate Injection or *Neut* per 100 ml of solution: 5% Dextrose Injection, USP; 5% Dextrose and Lactated Ringer's Injection; 5% Dextrose and 0.9% Sodium Chloride Injection, USP.

Piggyback vial: Add 100 ml 0.9% Sodium Chloride Injection, USP; or Lactated Ringer's Injection, USP; or *Normosol-R* to the dispensing vial. Immediately after adding diluent, shake the product to aid dissolution. Lack of immediate agitation will greatly increase time required for complete dissolution. May also be reconstituted with 100 ml of the following solutions to which 1 ml of 4% Sodium Bicarbonate Injection or *Neut* has first been added: 5% Dextrose Injection, USP; 5% Dextrose and Lactated Ringer's Injection; 5% Dextrose and 0.9% Sodium Chloride Injection, USP; *Normosol-M* and 5% Dextrose Injection; *Normosol-R* and 5% Dextrose Injection.

The 4% sodium bicarbonate injection or *Neut* must be added to these solutions so that their pH is in the optimum range for erythromycin lactobionate stability. Acidic solutions of erythromycin lactobionate are unstable and lose their potency rapidly. A pH of ≥ 5.5 is desirable for the final diluted solution of erythromycin lactobionate.

➤*Storage/Stability:* The *initial* solution is stable for 2 weeks if refrigerated or for 24 hours at room temperature. Completely administer the final diluted solution within 8 hours in order to ensure proper potency because it is not suitable for storage.

Use the solution in the piggyback vial within 8 hours if stored at room temperature and 24 hours if stored in the refrigerator. If the solution is to be frozen, freeze at -10° to -20°C (14° to -4°F) within 4 hours of preparation. Frozen solution may be stored for 30 days. Thaw the frozen solution in the refrigerator and use within 8 hours after thawing is completed. Thawed solution must not be refrozen.

Erythromycin

ERYTHROMYCIN BASE

Rx	E-Mycin (Knoll)	Tablets, enteric coated: 250 mg	Lactose, sucrose. (E-MYCIN 250 mg). Orange. Convex. In 40s, 100s, 500s, and UD 100s.
Rx	Ery-Tab (Abbott)		Delayed release. (EC). Pink. In 100s, 500s, and UD 100s.
Rx	E-Base Caplets and Tablets (Barr)	Tablets, enteric coated: 333 mg	Delayed release. (E-Base/333 barr). White. In 100s, 500s, and 1000s.
Rx	Ery-Tab (Abbott)		Delayed release. (EH). White. In 100s, 500s, and UD 100s.
Rx	PCE Dispertab (Abbott)	Tablets with polymer coated particles: 333 mg	Lactose. (PCE). White with pink speckles. Oval. In 60s.
Rx	E-Base (Barr)	Tablets, enteric coated: 500 mg	(E-Base/500 mg barr). White. Capsule shape. In 100s and 500s.
Rx	Ery-Tab (Abbott)		Delayed release. Pink. In 100s and UD 100s.
Rx	PCE Dispertab (Abbott)	Tablets with polymer coated particles: 500 mg	(EK). White. Oval. In 100s.
Rx	Erythromycin Filmtabs (Abbott)	Tablets, film coated: 250 mg	(ES). Pink. Capsule shape. In 100s, 500s, and UD 100s.
Rx	Erythromycin Filmtabs (Abbott)	Tablets, film coated: 500 mg	Pink. Capsule shape. In 100s.
Rx	Eryc (Warner Chilcott)	Capsules, delayed release: 250 mg	(Eryc/WC 696). Clear and orange. In 100s.
Rx	Erythromycin Base (Various, eg, Abbott, UDL)		In 60s, 100s, and 500s.

Complete prescribing information begins in the Erythromycin group monograph.

ERYTHROMYCIN ESTOLATE

Rx	Erythromycin Estolate (Various, eg, Alpharma)	Suspension: 125 mg (as base)/5 ml	In 480 ml.
Rx	Erythromycin Estolate (Various, eg, Alpharma)	Suspension: 250 mg (as base)/5 ml	In 480 ml.

Complete prescribing information begins in the Erythromycin group monograph.

ERYTHROMYCIN STEARATE

Rx	Erythromycin Stearate (Various, eg, Barr, Mylan)	Tablets, film coated: 250 mg (as base)	In 100s, 500s, and 1000s.
Rx	Erythrocin Stearate (Abbott)		(ES). In 100s and 500s.
Rx	Erythromycin Stearate (Various, eg, Barr, Mylan)	Tablets, film coated: 500 mg (as base)	In 100s, 500s, and UD 100s.
Rx	Erythrocin Stearate (Abbott)		(ET). In 100s, 500s, 1000s, and Abbo-Pac 100s.

Complete prescribing information begins in the Erythromycin group monograph.

ERYTHROMYCIN ETHYLSUCCINATE

Rx	Erythromycin Ethylsuccinate (Various, eg, Abbott, Mylan)	Tablets: 400 mg (as base)	In 100s and 500s.
Rx	E.E.S. 400 (Abbott)		Sugar. (EE). Pink. Film coated. In 100s, 500s, and 1000s.
Rx	Erythromycin Ethylsuccinate (Various, eg, Abbott, Barre-National, Rugby)	Suspension: 200 mg (as base)/5 ml	In 480 ml.
Rx	E.E.S. 200 (Abbott)		Sucrose. Parabens. Fruit flavor. In 100 and 480 ml.
Rx	Erythromycin Ethylsuccinate (Various, eg, Abbott, Barre-National, Rugby, Schein)	Suspension: 400 mg (as base)/5 ml	In 480 ml.
Rx	E.E.S. 400 (Abbott)		Sucrose. Parabens. Orange flavor. In 100 and 480 ml.
Rx	EryPed Drops (Abbott)	Suspension: 100 mg (as base)/2.5 ml	Sucrose. Fruit flavor. In 50 ml.
Rx	EryPed 200 (Abbott)	Powder for Oral Suspension: 200 mg (as base)/5 ml when reconstituted	Sucrose. Fruit flavor. In 100, 200 ml, UD 5 ml (100s).
Rx	E.E.S. Granules (Abbott)		Sucrose. Cherry flavor. In 100 and 200 ml.
Rx	EryPed 400 (Abbott)	Powder for Oral Suspension: 400 mg (as base)/5 ml when reconstituted	Sucrose. Banana flavor. In 60, 100, 200, and UD 5 ml (100s).

Complete prescribing information begins in the Erythromycin group monograph.

Ingredients

Expressed in base equivalents, 400 mg erythromycin ethylsuccinate produces the same free erythromycin serum levels as 250 mg of erythromycin base, stearate, or estolate.

ERYTHROMYCIN LACTOBIONATE

Rx	Erythromycin Lactobionate (Various)	Powder for Injection: 500 mg (as base)	In vials and piggyback vials.
		1 g (as base)	In vials.
Rx	Erythrocin (Abbott)	Powder for injection: 500 mg (as base)	In ADD-Vantage vials.
		1 g (as base)	In ADD-Vantage vials.

Complete prescribing information begins in the Erythromycin group monograph.

ERYTHROMYCIN GLUCEPTATE

Rx	Ilotycin Gluceptate (Lilly)	Injection: 1 g erythromycin (as base)/vial	In 30 ml vials.

Complete prescribing information begins in the Erythromycin group monograph.

TELITHROMYCIN

Rx   **Ketek** (Aventis)   **Tablets:** 400 mg

Lactose. (H3647 400). Lt. orange, oval. Film-coated. In 60s, blister pack 10s, and UD 100s.

Indications

For the treatment of infections caused by susceptible strains of the designated microorganisms in the conditions listed below for patients 18 years of age and older.

➤*Acute bacterial exacerbation of chronic bronchitis:* Caused by *Streptococcus pneumoniae, Haemophilus influenzae,* or *Moraxella catarrhalis.*

➤*Acute bacterial sinusitis:* Caused by *S. pneumoniae, H. influenzae, M. catarrhalis,* or *Staphylococcus aureus.*

➤*Community-acquired pneumonia:* Of mild to moderate severity caused by *S. pneumoniae* (including multidrug resistant isolates (MDRSP), *H. influenzae, M. catarrhalis, Chlamydophila pneumoniae,* or *Mycoplasma pneumoniae.*

Administration and Dosage

➤*Approved by the FDA:* April 1, 2004.

The dose of telithromycin tablets is 800 mg taken orally once every 24 hours. Telithromycin can be administered with or without food.

Telithromycin Dosage			
Infection	Daily dose	Frequency of administration	Duration of treatment
Acute bacterial exacerbation of chronic bronchitis	800 mg oral (2 tablets of 400 mg)	Once daily	5 days
Acute bacterial sinusitis	800 mg oral (2 tablets of 400 mg)	Once daily	5 days
Community-acquired pneumonia	800 mg oral (2 tablets of 400 mg)	Once daily	7 to 10 days

➤*Renal Function Impairment:* In the presence of severe renal impairment (Ccr less than 30 mL/min), including patients who need dialysis, the dose of telithromycin has not been established.

➤*Storage/Stability:* Store at 25°C (77°F); excursions permitted to 15° to 30°C (59° to 86°F).

Actions

➤*Pharmacology:* Telithromycin belongs to the ketolide class of antibacterials and is structurally related to the macrolide family of antibiotics.

Telithromycin blocks protein synthesis by binding to domains II and V of 23S rRNA of the 50S ribosomal subunit. By binding at domain II, telithromycin retains activity against gram-positive cocci in the presence of resistance mediated by methylases (erm genes) that alter the domain V binding site of telithromycin. Telithromycin also may inhibit the assembly of nascent ribosomal units.

➤*Pharmacokinetics:*

Absorption/Distribution – Following oral administration, telithromycin reached maximal concentration at about 1 hour (0.5 to 4 hours).

It has an absolute bioavailability of 57% in young and elderly subjects. The rate and extent of absorption are unaffected by food intake, thus, telithromycin tablets can be given without regard to food.

In healthy adult subjects, peak plasma telithromycin concentrations of approximately 2 mcg/mL are attained at a median of 1 hour after an 800 mg oral dose. Steady-state plasma concentrations are reached within 2 to 3 days of once daily dosing with 800 mg telithromycin. The pharmacokinetics of telithromycin after administration of single and multiple (7 days) once-daily 800 mg doses to healthy adult subjects are shown in the following table:

Mean Telithromycin Pharmacokinetic Parameters		
Parameter	Single dose (n = 18)	Multiple dose (n = 18)
C_{max} (mcg/mL)	1.9	2.27
T_{max} (hr; median value)	1	1
$AUC_{(0\ to\ 24)}$ (mcg·hr/mL)	8.25	12.5
Terminal $t_{1/2}$ (hr)	7.16	9.81
C_{24hr}[1] (mcg/mL)	0.03	0.07

[1] C_{24hr} = Plasma concentration at 24 hours postdose

In a patient population, mean peak and trough plasma concentrations were 2.9 mcg/mL (n = 219) and 0.2 mcg/mL (n = 204), respectively, after 3 to 5 days of 800 mg telithromycin once daily.

Total in vitro protein binding is approximately 60% to 70% and is primarily caused by human serum albumin. The volume of distribution of telithromycin after IV infusion is 2.9 L/kg. Telithromycin concentrations in bronchial mucosa, epithelial lining fluid, and alveolar macrophages after 800 mg once daily dosing for 5 days in patients are displayed in the following table.

Telithromycin Concentrations After 800 mg Once Daily for 5 Days				
	Hours postdose	Mean concentration (mcg/mL)		
		Tissue or fluid	Plasma	Tissue/Plasma ratio
Bronchial mucosa	2	3.88[a]	1.86	2.11
	12	1.41[a]	0.23	6.33
	24	0.78[a]	0.08	12.11
Epithelial lining fluid	2	14.89	1.86	8.57
	12	3.27	0.23	13.8
	24	0.84	0.08	14.41
Alveolar macrophages	2	65	1.07	55
	8	100	0.605	180
	24	41	0.073	540

[a] Units in mg/kg.

Telithromycin concentration in white blood cells (WBCs) exceeds the concentration in plasma and is eliminated more slowly from WBCs than from plasma. Mean WBC concentrations of telithromycin peaked at 72.1 mcg/mL at 6 hours and remained at 14.1 mcg/mL 24 hours after 5 days of repeated dosing of 600 mg once daily. After 10 days, repeated dosing of 600 mg once daily, WBC concentrations remained at 8.9 mcg/mL 48 hours after the last dose.

Metabolism/Excretion – In total, metabolism accounts for approximately 70% of the dose. In plasma, the main circulating compound after administration of an 800 mg radiolabeled dose was parent compound, representing 56.7% of the total radioactivity. The main metabolite represented 12.6% of the AUC of telithromycin. Three other plasma metabolites were quantified, each representing 3% or less of the AUC of telithromycin. It is estimated that approximately 50% of its metabolism is mediated by CYP450 3A4 and the remaining 50% is CYP450-independent.

The systemically available telithromycin is eliminated by multiple pathways as follows: 7% of the dose is excreted unchanged in feces by biliary and/or intestinal secretion; 13% of the dose is excreted unchanged in urine by renal excretion; and 37% of the dose is metabolized by the liver. Following oral dosing, the mean terminal elimination half-life is 10 hours.

Special populations –

Hepatic function impairment: An increase in renal elimination was observed in hepatically impaired patients indicating that this pathway may compensate for some of the decrease in metabolic clearance. No dosage adjustment is recommended because of hepatic impairment.

Renal function impairment: In a multiple-dose study, 36 subjects with varying degrees of renal impairment received 400, 600, or 800 mg telithromycin once daily for 5 days. There was a 1.4-fold increase in $C_{max,SS}$, and a 1.9-fold increase in $AUC_{(0-24hr)SS}$ at 800 mg multiple doses in the severely renally impaired group (Ccr less than 30 mL/min) compared with healthy volunteers. Renal excretion may serve as a compensatory elimination pathway for telithromycin in situations where metabolic clearance is impaired. Patients with severe renal impairment are prone to conditions that may impair their metabolic clearance.

In a single-dose study in patients with end-stage renal failure on hemodialysis (n = 10), the mean C_{max} and AUC values were similar to normal healthy subjects when telithromycin was given 2 hours postdialysis. However, the effect of dialysis on removing telithromycin from the body has not been studied.

No dose has been established in severely renal impaired patients including those who need dialysis.

Multiple insufficiencies: The effects of coadministration of ketoconazole in 12 subjects (60 years of age and older) with impaired renal function were studied (Ccr 24 to 80 mL/min). In this study, when severe renal insufficiency (Ccr less than 30 mL/min, n = 2) and concomitant impairment of CYP3A4 metabolism pathway were present, telithromycin exposure (AUC_{0-24}) was increased by approximately 4- to 5-fold compared with the exposure in healthy subjects with normal renal function receiving telithromycin alone. In the presence of severe renal impairment (Ccr less than 30 mL/min), no dose has been established.

Elderly: Pharmacokinetic data show that there is an increase of 1.4-fold in AUC in 20 patients 65 years of age and older with community-acquired pneumonia in a phase 3 study, and a 2-fold increase in AUC in 14 subjects 65 years of age and older compared with subjects younger than 65 years of age in a phase 1 study. No dosage adjustment is required based on age alone.

➤*Microbiology:* Telithromycin concentrates in phagocytes where it exhibits activity against intracellular respiratory pathogens. In vitro, telithromycin has been shown to demonstrate concentration-dependent bactericidal activity against isolates of *S. pneumoniae* (including MDRSP). MDRSP is multidrug resistant *S. pneumoniae* that includes isolates known as penicillin-resistant *S. pneumonia* (PRSP), and are isolates resistant to 2 or more of the following antimicrobials: Peni-

TELITHROMYCIN

cillin, second generation cephalosporins (eg, cefuroxime), macrolides, tetracyclines, and trimethoprim/sulfamethoxazole.

Resistance – *S. aureus* and *S. pyogenes* with the constitutive macrolide-lincosamide-streptogramin B ($cMLS_B$) phenotype are resistant to telithromycin.

Mutants of *S. pneumoniae* derived in the laboratory by serial passage in subinhibitory concentrations of telithromycin have demonstrated resistance based on L22 riboprotein mutations (telithromycin MICs are elevated but still within the susceptible range), 1 of 2 reported mutations affecting the L4 riboprotein, and production of K-peptide. The clinical significance of these laboratory mutants is not known. Telithromycin does not induce resistance through methylase gene expression in erythromycin-inducibly resistant bacteria, a function of its 3-keto moiety. Telithromycin has not been shown to induce resistance to itself.

Contraindications

A history of hypersensitivity to telithromycin and/or any components of the product or any macrolide antibiotic. Coadministration of telithromycin with cisapride or pimozide is contraindicated.

Warnings

➤*Pseudomembranous colitis:* Pseudomembranous colitis has been reported with nearly all antibacterial agents, including telithromycin, and may range in severity from mild to life threatening. Therefore, it is important to consider this diagnosis in patients who present with diarrhea subsequent to the administration of any antibacterial agents.

Treatment with antibacterial agents alters the flora of the colon and may permit overgrowth of clostridia. Studies indicate that toxin-producing strains *Clostridium difficile* are the primary cause of antibiotic-associated colitis.

After the diagnosis of pseudomembranous colitis has been established, initiate therapeutic measures. Mild cases of pseudomembranous colitis usually respond to drug discontinuation alone. In moderate to severe cases, consider management with fluids and electrolytes, protein supplementation, and treatment with an antibacterial drug clinically effective against *C. difficile* colitis.

➤*Cardiac effects:* Telithromycin has the potential to prolong the QTc interval of the electrocardiogram in some patients. QTc prolongation may lead to an increased risk for ventricular arrhythmias, including torsades de pointes. Thus, avoid telithromycin in patients with congenital prolongation of the QTc interval, and in patients with ongoing proarrhythmic conditions such as uncorrected hypokalemia or hypomagnesemia, clinically significant bradycardia, and in patients receiving Class IA (eg, quinidine and procainamide) or Class III (eg, dofetilide) antiarrhythmic agents. No cardiovascular morbidity or mortality attributable to QTc prolongation occurred with telithromycin treatment in 4,780 patients in clinical efficacy trials, including 204 patients having a prolonged QTc at baseline.

➤*Myasthenia gravis:* Exacerbations of myasthenia gravis have been reported in patients with myasthenia gravis treated with telithromycin. This has sometimes occurred within a few hours after intake of the first dose of telithromycin. Reports have included life-threatening acute respiratory failure with a rapid onset in patients with myasthenia gravis treated for respiratory tract infections with telithromycin. Telithromycin is not recommended in patients with myasthenia gravis unless no other therapeutic alternatives are available. If other therapeutic alternatives are not available, patients with myasthenia gravis taking telithromycin must be closely monitored. Patients must be advised that if they experience exacerbation of their symptoms, they should discontinue treatment of telithromycin and immediately seek medical attention. Institute supportive measures as medically necessary.

➤*Renal/Hepatic function impairment:* Hepatic dysfunction, including increased liver enzymes and hepatitis, with or without jaundice, has been reported with the use of telithromycin. These events were generally reversible. Exercise caution in patients with a history of hepatitis/jaundice associated with the use of telithromycin (see Adverse Reactions).

Telithromycin is principally excreted via the liver and kidney. Telithromycin may be administered without dosage adjustment in the presence of hepatic impairment. In the presence of severe renal impairment (Ccr less than 30 mL/min), the dose of telithromycin has not been established.

➤*Elderly:* Efficacy and safety in elderly patients 65 years of age and older were generally similar to that observed in younger patients, however, greater sensitivity of some older individuals cannot be ruled out. No dosage adjustment is required based on age alone.

➤*Pregnancy: Category C.* At doses higher than 900 mg/m^2 and 240 mg/m^2 in rats and rabbits, respectively, maternal toxicity may have resulted in delayed fetal maturation. There are no adequate and well-controlled studies in pregnant women. Use telithromycin during pregnancy only if the potential benefit justifies the potential risk to the fetus.

➤*Lactation:* Telithromycin is excreted in the breast milk of rats. Telithromycin also may be excreted in human milk. Because many drugs are excreted in human milk, exercise caution when telithromycin is given to a nursing mother.

➤*Children:* The safety and effectiveness of telithromycin in pediatric patients has not been established.

Precautions

Prescribing telithromycin in the absence of a proven or strongly suspected bacterial infection or a prophylactic indication is unlikely to provide benefit to the patient and increases the risk of the development of drug-resistant bacteria.

➤*Visual disturbances:* Telithromycin may cause visual disturbances particularly in slowing the ability to accommodate and the ability to release accommodation. Visual disturbances included blurred vision, difficulty focusing, and diplopia. Most events were mild to moderate; however, severe cases have been reported. Caution patients about the potential effects of these visual disturbances on driving a vehicle, operating machinery, or engaging in other potentially hazardous activities (see Adverse Reactions).

Drug Interactions

➤*Cytochrome P450:* Telithromycin is a strong inhibitor of the cytochrome P450 3A4 system. Coadministration of telithromycin tablets and a drug primarily metabolized by the cytochrome P450 3A4 enzyme system may result in increased plasma concentration of the drug coadministered with telithromycin that could increase or prolong both the therapeutic and adverse effects. Therefore, appropriate dosage adjustments may be necessary for the drug coadministered with telithromycin.

Telithromycin Drug Interactions			
Precipitant drug	Object drug		Description
Itraconazole Ketoconazole	Telithromycin	↑	Coadministration with itraconazole resulted in an increase in telithromycin C_{max} and AUC 22% and 54%, respectively. Coadministration with ketoconazole resulted in an increase in telithromycin C_{max} and AUC by 51% and 95%, respecitvely.
Rifampin Phenytoin Carbamazepine Phenobarbital	Telithromycin	↓	Coadministration of rifampin and telithromycin resulted in a decrease in telithromycin C_{max} and AUC of 79% and 86%, respectively. Avoid coadministration. Coadministration with other CYP 3A4 inducers (eg, phenytoin, carbamazepine, phenobarbital) also is likely to result in subtherapeutic levels of telithromycin and loss of effect.
Telithromycin	Cisapride	↑	Coadministration resulted in a 95% increase in cisapride peak plasma concentrations, resulting in significant increases in QTc interval. Coadministration is contraindicated.
Telithromycin	Digoxin	↑	Coadministration resulted in a 73% and 21% increase in digoxin plasma peak and trough levels, respectively. Monitor digoxin levels and side effects during use with telithromycin therapy.
Telithromycin	Ergot alkaloids	↑	Acute ergot toxicity characterized by severe peripheral vasospasm and dysesthesia has occurred when an ergot alkaloid was given with a macrolide. Without further data, the coadministration of telithromycin and ergot alkaloids is not recommended.
Telithromycin	Metoprolol	↑	Coadministration resulted in an approximate 38% increase in metoprolol C_{max} and AUC, however, there was no effect on metoprolol elimination half-life. Coadminister with caution in heart failure patients.
Telithromycin	Midazolam	↑	Coadministration resulted in an increase in midazolam AUC. Monitor closely and adjust midazolam dose as needed. Use with caution with other benzodiazepines that are metabolized by CYP3A4 and undergo a high first-pass effect (eg, triazolam).
Telithromycin	Pimozide	↑	Coadministration may lead to increased pimozide plasma levels. Coadministration is contraindicated.

TELITHROMYCIN

Telithromycin Drug Interactions			
Precipitant drug	Object drug		Description
Telithromycin	HMG-CoA Reductase Inhibitors Simvastatin Atorvastatin Lovastatin	↑	Coadministration resulted in a 5.3- and 8.9-fold increase in simvastatin C_{max} and AUC, respectively. Avoid concurrent use of simvastatin, atorvastatin, or lovastatin with telithromycin.
Telithromycin	Sotalol	↓	Coadministration resulted in a decrease in sotalol C_{max} and AUC of 34% and 20%, respectively.
Telithromycin	Theophylline	↑	Coadministration resulted in an approximate 16% and 17% increase in theophylline C_{max} and AUC, respectively. Coadministration may worsen GI effects such as nausea and vomiting. Take telithromycin and theophylline 1 hour apart to decrease the risk of GI side effects.

Adverse Reactions

In phase 3 clinical trials, 4,780 patients (n = 2,702 in controlled trials) received daily oral doses of 800 mg once daily for 5 days or 7 to 10 days. Most adverse events were mild to moderate in severity. In the combined phase 3 studies, discontinuation because of treatment-emergent adverse events occurred in 4.4% of telithromycin-treated patients and 4.3% of combined comparator-treated patients. Most discontinuations in the telithromycin group were because of treatment-emergent adverse events in the GI body system, primarily diarrhea (0.9% for telithromycin vs 0.7% for comparators) and nausea (0.7% for telithromycin vs 0.5% for comparators). All and possibly related treatment-emergent adverse events (TEAEs) occurring in controlled clinical studies in 2% or more of all patients are included below:

Telithromycin Adverse Events (%)				
Adverse reaction[a]	All TEAEs		Possibly related TEAEs	
	Telithromycin (n = 2,702)	Comparator[b] (n = 2,139)	Telithromycin (n = 2,702)	Comparator[b] (n = 2,139)
Diarrhea	10.8	8.6	10	8
Dizziness (excluding vertigo)	3.7	2.7	2.8	1.5
Dysgeusia	1.6	3.6	1.5	3.6
Headache	5.5	5.8	2	2.5
Loose stools	2.3	1.5	2.1	1.4
Nausea	7.9	4.6	7	4.1
Vomiting	2.9	2.2	2.4	1.4

[a] Based on a frequency of all and possibly related treatment-emergent adverse events of 2% or more in telithromycin or comparator groups.
[b] Includes comparators from all controlled phase 3 studies.

The following events judged by investigators to be at least possibly drug related were observed infrequently (0.2% or more and less than 2%).

➤*CNS:* Dry mouth, increased sweating, insomnia, somnolence, vertigo.

➤*GI:* Abdominal distention, abdominal pain, anorexia, constipation, dyspepsia, flatulence, gastritis, gastroenteritis, GI upset, glossitis, oral candidiasis, stomatitis, upper abdominal pain, watery stools.

➤*GU:* Vaginal candidiasis, vaginitis, vaginosis fungal.

➤*Hepatic:* Hepatitis, with or without jaundice occurred in 0.07% of patients treated with telithromycin and was reversible (see Precautions).

➤*Lab test abnormalities:* Increased platelet count. Increased transaminases, increased liver enzymes (eg, ALT, AST) were usually asymptomatic and reversible. ALT elevations more than 3 times the ULN were observed in 1.6% and 1.7% of patients treated with telithromycin and comparators, respectively.

➤*Special senses:* Visual adverse events most often included blurred vision, diplopia, or difficulty focusing. Most events were mild to moderate; however, severe cases have been reported. Some patients discontinued therapy because of these adverse events. Visual adverse events were reported as having occurred after any dose during treatment, but most visual adverse events (65%) occurred following the first or second dose. Visual events lasted several hours and recurred upon subsequent dosing in some patients. For patients who continued treatment, some resolved on therapy while others continued to have symptoms until they completed the full course of treatment.

Females and patients younger than 40 years of age experienced a higher incidence of telithromycin-associated visual adverse events.

➤*Miscellaneous:* Fatigue, rash.

➤*Other possible adverse reactions (less than 0.2%):*
Miscellaneous – Anxiety, bradycardia, eczema, elevated blood bilirubin, erythema multiforme, flushing, hypotension, increased blood alkaline phosphatase, increased eosinophil count, paresthesia, pruritus, urticaria.

➤*Postmarketing:* In addition to adverse events reported from clinical trials, the following events have been reported from worldwide postmarketing experience with telithromycin.

Hepatic – Hepatic dysfunction, including increased liver enzymes, and hepatocellular and/or cholestatic hepatitis, with or without jaundice has been infrequently reported. This hepatic dysfunction may be severe and is usually reversible.

Hypersensitivity – Face edema, rare reports of severe allergic reactions, including angioedema and anaphylaxis.

Musculoskeletal – Muscle cramps, rare reports of exacerbation of myasthenia gravis.

Miscellaneous – Atrial arrhythmias.

Overdosage

In the event of acute overdosage, empty the stomach by gastric lavage. Carefully monitor the patient (eg, ECG, electrolytes) and give symptomatic and supportive treatment. Maintain adequate hydration. The effectiveness of hemodialysis in an overdose situation with telithromycin is unknown.

Patient Information

Telithromycin may cause problems with vision particularly when looking quickly between objects close by and objects far away. These events include blurred vision, difficulty focusing, and objects looking doubled. Visual problems were reported as having occurred after any dose during treatment, but most occurred following the first or second dose. These problems lasted several hours and in some patients came back with the next dose.

If visual difficulties occur, advise patients to:
• Avoid driving a motor vehicle, operating heavy machinery, or engaging in otherwise hazardous activities.
• Avoid quick changes in viewing between objects in the distance and objects nearby to decrease the effects of these visual difficulties.
• Contact their physician if these visual difficulties interfere with their daily activities.

Also advise patients:
• To use antibacterial drugs including telithromycin only to treat bacterial infections. These drugs do not treat viral infections (eg, the common cold). When telithromycin is prescribed to treat a bacterial infection, patients should be told that although it is common to feel better early in the course of therapy, the medication should be taken exactly as directed.
• Skipping doses or not completing the full course of therapy may 1) decrease the effectiveness of the immediate treatment and 2) increase the likelihood that bacteria will develop resistance and will not be treatable by telithromycin or other antibacterial drugs in the future.
• Telithromycin has the potential to produce changes in the ECG (QTc interval prolongation) and to report any fainting occurring during drug treatment.
• To avoid telithromycin if receiving Class 1A (eg, quinidine, procainamide) or Class III (eg, dofetilide) antiarrhythmic agents.
• To inform their physician of any personal or family history of QTc prolongation or proarrhythmic conditions such as uncorrected hypokalemia, or clinically significant bradycardia.
• Telithromycin is not recommended in patients with myasthenia gravis. Patients should inform their physician if they have myasthenia gravis.
• To avoid simvastatin, lovastatin, or atorvastatin if receiving telithromycin. If telithromycin is prescribed, stop therapy with simvastatin, lovastatin, or atorvastatin during the course of treatment.
• Telithromycin can be taken with or without food.

SPECTINOMYCIN

Rx   **Trobicin** (Upjohn)   **Powder for Injection:** 400 mg (as HCl) per ml when   In 2 g vial w/ 3.2 ml diluent (w/ 0.9% benzyl alcohol).
                                                        reconstituted

Indications

➤*Gonorrhea:* Acute gonorrheal urethritis and proctitis in the male and acute gonorrheal cervicitis and proctitis in the female due to susceptible strains of *N. gonorrhoeae.* Treat men and women with recent exposure to gonorrhea as those with gonorrhea.

Administration and Dosage

For IM use only. Shake vials vigorously immediately after adding diluent and before withdrawing dose. Inject 5 ml (2 g) IM deep into upper outer quadrant of gluteal muscle. Also recommended for treatment after failure of previous antibiotic therapy. In geographic areas where antibiotic resistance is prevalent, initial treatment with 4 g (10 ml) IM is preferred, and may be divided between 2 gluteal injection sites.

➤*CDC recommended treatment schedules for gonorrhea†:*
Uncomplicated urethral, endocervical or rectal gonococcal infections, alternative regimen – For patients who cannot take cephalosporins or fluoroquinolones, the preferred alternative is spectinomycin 2 g IM as a single dose.

Children ≥ 45 kg (100 lbs) should receive adult regimens. Children < 45 kg with uncomplicated vulvovaginitis, cervicitis, urethritis, pharyngitis or proctitis and who cannot tolerate ceftriaxone may receive a single 40 mg/kg IM dose (max: 2 g).

Gonococcal infections in pregnancy – Treat pregnant women allergic to cephalosporins with a single 2 g IM dose of spectinomycin.

Disseminated gonococcal infection – Spectinomycin 2 g IM every 12 hours may be used as an alternative to fluoroquinolones in patients allergic to β-lactams.

➤*Storage / Stability:* Store reconstituted suspension at controlled room temperature 20° to 25°C (68° to 77°F) and use within 24 hours.

Actions

➤*Pharmacology:* Spectinomycin, structurally different from related aminoglycosides, inhibits protein synthesis in bacterial cells. Site of action is 30S ribosomal subunit.

➤*Pharmacokinetics:* Rapidly absorbed after IM injection. A 2 g injection produces average peak serum concentrations of 100 mcg/ml at 1 hour; a 4 g injection, 160 mcg/ml at 2 hours. Eight hours after a 2 or 4 g injection, plasma concentrations are 15 and 31 mcg/ml, respectively. The majority is excreted in urine in biologically active form.

Contraindications

Hypersensitivity to spectinomycin.

Warnings

➤*Syphilis:* Not effective for syphilis. Antibiotics used to treat gonorrhea may mask or delay symptoms of incubating syphilis. All patients with gonorrhea should have a serologic test for syphilis at time of diagnosis and a follow-up test after 3 months.

➤*Pharyngeal infections:* Use spectinomycin only in patients intolerant to cephalosporins or quinolones. Because spectinomycin is unreliable (52% effective) against pharyngeal infections, evaluate cultures 3 to 5 days after treatment to verify eradication.

➤*Pregnancy: Category B.* Safety for use during pregnancy has not been established.

➤*Lactation:* It is not known whether spectinomycin is excreted in breast milk. Use caution when administering to a nursing woman.

➤*Children:* Safety and efficacy have not been established.

Precautions

➤*Monitoring:* Monitor clinical effectiveness to detect resistance by *N. gonorrhoeae.*

➤*Benzyl alcohol:* The diluent provided with this product contains benzyl alcohol which has been associated with a fatal gasping syndrome in infants.

➤*Hypersensitivity:* A few cases of anaphylaxis or anaphylactoid reactions have been reported. Have epinephrine immediately available. Refer to Management of Acute Hypersensitivity Reactions.

Adverse Reactions

In single- and multiple-dose studies in healthy volunteers, a reduction in urine output was noted; however, renal toxicity has not been demonstrated.

Single-dose – Sore injection site; urticaria; dizziness; nausea; chills; fever; insomnia.

Multiple-dose – Decrease in hemoglobin, hematocrit and creatinine clearance; elevation of alkaline phosphatase, BUN and ALT.

† CDC 1998 Sexually Transmitted Diseases Treatment Guidelines. *Morbidity and Mortality Weekly Report* 1998 Jan 23;47 (No. RR-1):1–116.

QUINUPRISTIN/DALFOPRISTIN

| *Rx* | **Synercid**
(Monarch) | **Injection, lyophilized:** 500 mg (150 mg quinupristin; 350 mg dalfopristin)/10 ml | In 10 ml vials. |

WARNING

One of quinupristin/dalfopristin's approved indications is for the treatment of patients with serious or life-threatening infections associated with vancomycin-resistant *Enterococcus faecium* (VREF) bacteremia. Quinupristin/dalfopristin has been approved for marketing in the US for this indication under the FDA's accelerated approval regulations that allow marketing of products for use in life-threatening conditions when other therapies are not available. Approval of drugs for marketing under these regulations is based upon a demonstrated effect on a surrogate endpoint that is likely to predict clinical benefit.

Approval of this indication is based upon quinupristin/dalfopristin's ability to clear VREF from the bloodstream with clearance of bacteremia considered to be a surrogate endpoint. No results from well-controlled clinical studies confirm the validity of this surrogate marker. However, a study to verify the clinical benefit of therapy with quinupristin/dalfopristin on traditional clinical endpoints (such as cure of the underlying infection) is presently underway.

Indications

➤*Life-threatening infections:* Treatment of patients with serious or life-threatening infections associated with vancomycin-resistant *Enterococcus faecium* (VREF) bacteremia.

➤*Complicated skin and skin structure infections:* Caused by *Staphylococcus aureus* (methicillin-susceptible) or *Streptococcus pyogenes.*

Administration and Dosage

➤*Approved by the FDA:* September 21, 1999.

Administer by IV infusion in 5% Dextrose in Water solution over a 60-minute period (see Warnings). The recommended dosage for the treatment of infections is described in the table below. An infusion pump or device may be used to control the rate of infusion. If necessary, central venous access (eg, PICC) can be used to administer quinupristin/dalfopristin to decrease the incidence of venous irritation.

Indication	Dose
Vancomycin-resistant *Enterococcus faecium*	7.5 mg/kg q8hr
Complicated skin and structure infection	7.5 mg/kg q12hr

The minimum recommended treatment duration for complicated skin and skin structure infections is 7 days. For vancomycin-resistant *E. faecium* infection, base treatment duration on the site and severity of the infection.

➤*Special populations:*

Elderly – No dosage adjustment is required.

Renal insufficiency – No dosage adjustment is required for use in patients with renal impairment or patients undergoing peritoneal dialysis.

Hepatic insufficiency – Data from clinical trials suggest that the incidence of adverse effects in patients with chronic liver insufficiency or cirrhosis was comparable to that in patients with normal hepatic function. Pharmacokinetic data in patients with hepatic cirrhosis (Child Pugh A or B) suggest that dosage reduction may be necessary, but exact recommendations cannot be made at this time.

Pediatric patients (< 16 years of age) – Based on a limited number of pediatric patients treated under emergency-use conditions, no dosage adjustment of quinupristin/dalfopristin is required.

➤*Preparation and administration of solution:*

1.) Reconstitute the single dose vial by slowly adding 5 ml of 5% Dextrose in Water or Sterile Water for Injection.

2.) Gently swirl the vial by manual rotation without shaking to ensure dissolution of contents while limiting foam formation.

3.) Allow the solution to sit for a few minutes until all the foam has disappeared. The resulting solution should be clear. Vials reconstituted in this manner will give a solution of 100 mg/ml. Caution: further dilution required before infusion.

4.) According to the patient's weight, add the reconstituted solution to 250 ml of 5% Dextrose solution (≈ 2 mg/ml). An infusion volume of 100 ml may be used for central line infusions.

5.) If moderate-to-severe venous irritation occurs following peripheral administration of quinupristin/dalfopristin diluted in 250 ml of Dextrose 5% in Water, consider increasing the infusion volume to 500 or 750 ml, changing the infusion site, or infusing by a peripherally inserted central catheter (PICC) or a central venous catheter.

6.) Administer the desired dose by IV infusion over 60 minutes.

➤*Admixture incompatibility:* Do not dilute with saline solutions because quinupristin/dalfopristin is not compatible with these agents.

Do not mix quinupristin/dalfopristin with or physically add to other drugs except for the following drugs, for which compatibility by Y-site injection has been established.

Y-Site Injection Compatibility of Quinupristin/Dalfopristin at 2 mg/ml Concentration	
Admixture and concentration	IV infusion solutions for admixture
Aztreonam 20 mg/ml	D5W[1]
Ciprofloxacin 1 mg/ml	D5W
Fluconazole 2 mg/ml	Used as the undiluted solution
Haloperidol 0.2 mg/ml	D5W
Metoclopramide 5 mg/ml	D5W
Potassium Chloride 40 mEq/L	D5W

[1] D5W = 5% Dextrose Injection.

If quinupristin/dalfopristin is to be given concomitantly with another drug, give each drug separately in accordance with the recommended dosage and route of administration for each drug.

With intermittent infusion of quinupristin/dalfopristin and other drugs through a common IV line, flush the line before and after administration with 5% Dextrose in Water solution.

➤*Storage/Stability:*

Before reconstitution – Refrigerate the unopened vials at 2° to 8°C (36° to 46°F).

Reconstituted and infusion solutions – Because quinupristin/dalfopristin contains no antibacterial preservative, reconstitute under strict aseptic conditions (eg, Laminar Air Flow Hood). Dilute the reconstituted solution within 30 minutes. Vials are for single use. The storage time of the diluted solution should be as short as possible to minimize the risk of microbial contamination. Stability of the diluted solution prior to the infusion is established as 5 hours at room temperature or 54 hours if refrigerated 2° to 8°C (36° to 46°F). Do not freeze the solution.

Actions

➤*Pharmacology:* Quinupristin/dalfopristin, a streptogramin antibacterial agent for IV administration, is a sterile, lyophilized formulation of 2 semisynthetic pristinamycin derivatives, quinupristin (derived from pristinamycin I) and dalfopristin (derived from pristinamycin IIA).

The streptogramin components of quinupristin/dalfopristin are present in a ratio of 30 parts quinupristin to 70 parts dalfopristin. These 2 components act synergistically so that quinupristin/dalfopristin's microbiologic in vitro activity is greater than that of the components individually. Quinupristin's and dalfopristin's metabolites also contribute to the antimicrobial activity of quinupristin/dalfopristin. In vitro synergism of the major metabolites with the complementary parent compound has been demonstrated.

Quinupristin/dalfopristin is bacteriostatic against *E. faecium* and bactericidal against strains of methicillin-susceptible and methicillin-resistant staphylococci.

The site of action of quinupristin and dalfopristin is the bacterial ribosome. Dalfopristin inhibits the early phase of protein synthesis while quinupristin inhibits the late phase of protein synthesis.

The mode of action differs from that of other classes of antibacterial agents such as β-lactams, aminoglycosides, glycopeptides, quinolones, macrolides, lincosamides, and tetracyclines. There is no cross resistance between quinupristin/dalfopristin and these agents when tested by the minimum inhibitory concentration (MIC) method.

In non-comparative studies, emerging resistance to quinupristin/dalfopristin during treatment of VREF infections occurred. Resistance to quinupristin/dalfopristin is associated with resistance to both components.

➤*Pharmacokinetics:* Quinupristin and dalfopristin are the main active components circulating in the plasma. They are converted to several active major metabolites: 2 conjugated metabolites for quinupristin (1 with glutathione and 1 with cysteine) and 1 non-conjugated metabolite for dalfopristin (formed by drug hydrolysis).

Pharmacokinetic profiles of quinupristin and dalfopristin in combination with their metabolites were determined using a bioassay following multiple 60-minute infusions in 2 groups of healthy young adult male volunteers. Each group received 7.5 mg/kg of quinupristin/dalfopristin IV every 12 hours or every 8 hours for a total of 9 or 10 doses, respectively. The pharmacokinetic parameters were proportional with every-12-hour and every-8-hour dosing: Those of the every-8-hour regimen are shown in the following table:

QUINUPRISTIN/DALFOPRISTIN

Mean Steady-State Pharmacokinetic Parameters of Quinupristin and Dalfopristin in Combination with Their Metabolites (Dose = 7.5 mg/kg q8h; n = 10)			
	C$_{max}$ (mcg/ml)	AUC (mcg•hr/ml)	t$_{\frac{1}{2}}$ (hr)
Quinupristin and metabolites	3.2	7.2	3.07
Dalfopristin and metabolite	7.96	10.57	1.04

The clearances of unchanged quinupristin and dalfopristin are similar (0.72 L/hr/kg), and the steady-state volume of distribution is 0.45 and 0.24 L/kg, respectively. The elimination half-life of quinupristin and dalfopristin is ≈ 0.85 and 0.7 hours, respectively. The protein binding is moderate.

Penetration of unchanged quinupristin and dalfopristin in noninflammatory blister fluid corresponds to ≈ 19% and 11%, respectively, of that estimated in plasma. The penetration into blister fluid of quinupristin and dalfopristin in combination with their major metabolites was in total ≈ 40% compared with that in plasma.

In vitro, the transformation of the parent drugs into their major active metabolites occurs by non-enzymatic reactions and is not dependent on cytochrome-P450 or glutathione-transferase enzyme activities. Quinupristin/dalfopristin is a major inhibitor of the activity of cytochrome P450 3A4 isoenzyme (see Warnings). Quinupristin/dalfopristin can interfere with the metabolism of other drug products that are associated with QTc prolongation. However, electrophysiologic studies confirm that quinupristin/dalfopristin does not itself induce QTc prolongation (see Warnings).

Fecal excretion constitutes the main elimination route for both parent drugs and their metabolites (75% to 77% of dose). Urinary excretion accounts for ≈ 15% of the quinupristin dose and 19% of the dalfopristin dose. Preclinical data in rats demonstrated that ≈ 80% of the dose is excreted in the bile and suggest that in humans, biliary excretion is probably the principal route for fecal elimination.

Special populations –

Renal function impairment: In patients with creatinine clearance 6 to 28 ml/min, the AUC of quinupristin and dalfopristin in combination with their major metabolites increased ≈ 40% and 30%, respectively.

In patients undergoing continuous ambulatory peritoneal dialysis, dialysis clearance for quinupristin, dalfopristin, and their metabolites is negligible. The plasma AUC of unchanged quinupristin and dalfopristin increased ≈ 20% and 30%, respectively. Because of the high molecular weight of both components, it is unlikely to be removed by hemodialysis.

Hepatic function impairment: In patients with hepatic dysfunction (Child-Pugh scores A and B), the terminal half-life of quinupristin and dalfopristin was not modified. However, the AUC of quinupristin and dalfopristin in combination with their major metabolites increased ≈ 180% and 50%, respectively (see Administration and Dosage).

Obesity (body mass index ≥ 30): In obese patients, the C$_{max}$ and AUC of quinupristin increased ≈ 30% and those of dalfopristin ≈ 40%.

➤*Microbiology:* Quinupristin/dalfopristin is active against most strains of the following microorganisms both in vitro and in clinical infections.

Aerobic gram-positive microorganisms – Enterococcus faecium (vancomycin-resistant and multi-drug resistant strains only); *Staphylococcus aureus* (methicillin-susceptible strains); *Streptococcus pyogenes*.

Note: Quinupristin/dalfopristin is not active against *Enterococcus faecalis*. Differentiation of enterococcal species is important to avoid misidentification of *E. faecalis* as *E. faecium*.

The combination of quinupristin and dalfopristin exhibits in vitro minimum inhibitory concentrations (MICs) of ≤ 1 mcg/ml against most (≥ 90%) isolates of the following microorganisms; however, the safety and effectiveness of quinupristin/dalfopristin in treating clinical infections due to these microorganisms have not been established in adequate and well-controlled clinical trials.

Aerobic gram-positive microorganisms – Corynebacterium jeikeium; *Staphylococcus aureus* (methicillin-resistant strains); *S. epidermidis* (including methicillin-resistant strains); *Streptococcus agalactiae*.

In vitro combination testing of quinupristin/dalfopristin with aztreonam, cefotaxime, ciprofloxacin, and gentamicin against *Enterobacteriaceae* and *Pseudomonas aeruginosa* did not show antagonism.

In vitro combination testing of quinupristin/dalfopristin with prototype drugs of the following classes did not show antagonism: Aminoglycosides (gentamicin), β-lactams (cefepime, ampicillin, and amoxicillin), glycopeptides (vancomycin), quinolones (ciprofloxacin), tetracyclines (doxycycline), and chloramphenicol against enterococci and staphylococci.

➤*Clinical trials:*

Complicated skin and skin structure infections – Two randomized, open-label, controlled clinical trials of quinupristin/dalfopristin (7.5 mg/kg every 12 hours IV) in the treatment of complicated skin and skin structure infections were performed. The comparator drug was oxacillin (2 g every 6 hr IV) in the first study and cefazolin (1 g every 8 hr IV) in the second study; however, in both studies vancomycin (1 g every 12 hr IV) could be substituted for the specified comparator if the

causative pathogen was suspected or confirmed to be methicillin-resistant staphylococcus or if the patient was allergic to penicillins, cephalosporins, or carbapenems.

The following table shows the clinical success rate (combined results from 2 clinical trials) in the clinically evaluable population. Because of the small numbers of patients in the subsets, statistical conclusions could not be reached.

Quinupristin/Dalfopristin vs Comparator for Skin/Skin Structure Infections		
Infection type	Cured or improved (%)	
	Quinupristin/Dalfopristin	Comparator
Erysipelas (cellulitis)	63.4	55.8
Post-operative infections	36.8	57.1
Traumatic wound infection	60	60

Contraindications

Hypersensitivity to quinupristin/dalfopristin or prior hypersensitivity to other streptogramins (eg, pristinamycin, virginiamycin).

Warnings

➤*Pseudomembranous colitis:* Pseudomembranous colitis has been reported with nearly all antibacterial agents, including quinupristin/dalfopristin, and may range in severity from mild to life-threatening. Therefore, consider this diagnosis in patients who present with diarrhea subsequent to the administration of antibacterial agents. After the diagnosis of pseudomembranous colitis has been established, initiate therapeutic measures. Mild cases usually respond to drug discontinuation alone. In moderate-to-severe cases, consider managing with fluids and electrolytes, protein supplementation, and treatment with an antibacterial drug clinically effective against *C. difficile* colitis.

➤*Hepatic function impairment:* Following a single 1-hour infusion of quinupristin/dalfopristin (7.5 mg/kg) to patients with hepatic insufficiency, plasma concentrations were significantly increased. However, the effect of dose reduction or increase in dosing interval on the pharmacokinetics of quinupristin/dalfopristin in these patients has not been studied. Therefore, no recommendations can be made at this time regarding the appropriate dose modification.

➤*Mutagenesis:* Dalfopristin was associated with the production of structural chromosome aberrations when tested in the Chinese hamster ovary cell chromosome aberration assay. Quinupristin/dalfopristin were negative in this assay.

➤*Elderly:* In phase 3 comparative trials, 37% of patients were ≥ 65 years of age, and in the phase 3 non-comparative trials, 29% of patients were ≥ 65 years of age. There were no apparent differences in the frequency, type, or severity of related adverse reactions, including cardiovascular events, between elderly and younger individuals.

➤*Pregnancy: Category B.* There are no adequate and well-controlled studies in pregnant women. Use during pregnancy only if clearly needed.

➤*Lactation:* In lactating rats, quinupristin/dalfopristin was excreted in milk. It is not known whether quinupristin/dalfopristin is excreted in human breast milk. Exercise caution when administering to a breastfeeding woman.

➤*Children:* Quinupristin/dalfopristin has been used in a limited number of pediatric patients under emergency-use conditions at a dose of 7.5 mg/kg every 8 or 12 hours. However, the safety and efficacy in patients < 16 years of age have not been established.

Precautions

➤*Venous irritation:* Following completion of a peripheral infusion, flush the vein with 5% Dextrose in Water solution to minimize venous irritation. Do not flush with saline or heparin after quinupristin/dalfopristin administration because of incompatibility concerns. If moderate-to-severe venous irritation occurs following peripheral administration of quinupristin/dalfopristin diluted in 250 ml of Dextrose 5% in Water, consider increasing the infusion volume to 500 or 750 ml, changing the infusion site, or infusing by a peripherally inserted central catheter (PICC) or a central venous catheter. In clinical trials, concomitant administration of hydrocortisone or diphenhydramine did not appear to alleviate venous pain or inflammation.

➤*Rate of infusion:* In animal studies, toxicity was higher when quinupristin/dalfopristin was administered as a bolus compared with slow infusion. However, the safety of an IV bolus has not been studied in humans. Clinical trial experience has been exclusively with an IV duration of 60 minutes and, thus, other infusion rates cannot be recommended.

➤*Arthralgias/Myalgias:* Episodes of arthralgia and myalgia, some severe, have been reported in patients treated with quinupristin/dalfopristin. In some patients, improvement has been noted with a reduction in dose frequency to every 12 hours. In those patients available for follow-up, symptoms resolved following discontinuation of treatment. The etiology of these myalgias and arthralgias is under investigation.

➤*Hyperbilirubinemia:* Elevations of total bilirubin > 5 times the upper limit of normal were noted in ≈ 25% of patients in the noncom-

QUINUPRISTIN/DALFOPRISTIN

parative studies. In some patients, isolated hyperbilirubinemia (primarily conjugated) can occur during treatment, possibly resulting from competition between quinupristin/dalfopristin and bilirubin for excretion. In the comparative trials, elevations in ALT and AST occurred at a similar frequency in both the quinupristin/dalfopristin and comparator groups.

➤*Superinfection:* Use of antibiotics (especially prolonged or repeated therapy) may result in bacterial or fungal overgrowth of nonsusceptible organisms. Such overgrowth may lead to a secondary infection. Appropriate measures should be taken if superinfection occurs.

Drug Interactions

➤*Cytochrome P450 3A4 inhibition:* It is reasonable to expect that the concomitant administration of quinupristin/dalfopristin and other drugs primarily metabolized by the cytochrome P450 3A4 enzyme system may result in increased plasma concentrations of these drugs that could increase or prolong their therapeutic effect or increase adverse reactions (see the following table). Therefore, coadministration with drugs that are cytochrome P450 3A4 substrates and possess a narrow therapeutic window requires caution and monitoring of these drugs whenever possible. Avoid concomitant medications metabolized by the cytochrome P450 3A4 enzyme system that may prolong the QTc interval.

Twenty-four subjects given quinupristin/dalfopristin 7.5 mg/kg every 8 hours for 2 days and 300 mg of cyclosporine on day 3 showed an increase of 63% in the AUC of cyclosporine, a 30% increase in C_{max}, a 77% increase in the half-life, and a 34% decrease in clearance. Perform therapeutic level monitoring of cyclosporine when cyclosporine must be used concomitantly with quinupristin/dalfopristin.

Concomitant administration of quinupristin/dalfopristin and nifedipine (repeated oral doses) and midazolam (IV bolus dose) in healthy volunteers led to elevated plasma concentrations of these drugs. The C_{max} increased by 18% and 14% (median values) and the AUC increased by 44% and 33% for nifedipine and midazolam, respectively.

Selected Drugs That are Predicted to Have Plasma Concentrations Increased by Quinupristin/Dalfopristin[1]
Anti-HIV (NNRTIs and protease inhibitors): Delavirdine, nevirapine, indinavir, ritonavir
Antineoplastic agents: Vinca alkaloids (eg, vinblastine), docetaxel, paclitaxel
Benzodiazepines: Midazolam, diazepam
Calcium channel blockers: Dihydropyridines (eg, nifedipine), verapamil, diltiazem
Cholesterol-lowering agents: HMG-CoA reductase inhibitors
GI motility agents: Cisapride
Immunosuppressive agents: Cyclosporine, tacrolimus
Steroids: Methylprednisolone
Other: Carbamazepine, quinidine, lidocaine, disopyramide

[1] This list of drugs is not all inclusive.

Adverse Reactions

➤*Comparative trials:* Safety data are available from 5 comparative clinical studies (n = 1099 quinupristin/dalfopristin; n = 1095 comparator). One of the deaths in the comparative studies was assessed as possibly related to quinupristin/dalfopristin. The most frequent reasons for discontinuation because of drug-related adverse reactions were as follows:

Patients Discontinuing Quinupristin/Dalfopristin Therapy (%): All Comparative Studies		
Type	Quinupristin/Dalfopristin (n = 1099)	Comparator (n = 1095)
Venous	9.2	2
Non-venous	9.6	4.3
Rash	1	0.5
Nausea	0.9	0.6
Vomiting	0.5	0.5
Pain	0.5	0
Pruritus	0.5	0.3

Quinupristin/Dalfopristin Adverse Reactions (≥ 1%): All Comparative Studies		
Adverse reaction	Quinupristin/Dalfopristin (n = 1099)	Comparator (n = 1095)
Inflammation at infusion site	42	25
Pain at infusion site	40	23.7
Edema at infusion site	17.3	9.5
Infusion site reaction	13.4	10.1
Nausea	4.6	7.2
Diarrhea	2.7	3.2

Quinupristin/Dalfopristin Adverse Reactions (≥ 1%): All Comparative Studies		
Adverse reaction	Quinupristin/Dalfopristin (n = 1099)	Comparator (n = 1095)
Vomiting	2.7	3.8
Rash	2.5	1.4
Thrombophlebitis	2.4	0.3
Headache	1.6	0.9
Pruritus	1.5	1.1
Pain	1.5	0.1

Additonal adverse reactions that were possibly or probably related to quinupristin/dalfopristin with an incidence < 1% are listed below.

Cardiovascular – Palpitation; phlebitis.

CNS – Anxiety; confusion; dizziness; hypertonia; insomnia; leg cramps; paresthesia; vasodilation.

Dermatologic – Maculopapular rash; sweating; urticaria.

GI – Constipation; dyspepsia; oral moniliasis; pancreatitis; pseudomembranous enterocolitis; stomatitis.

GU – Hematuria; vaginitis.

Metabolic – Gout; peripheral edema.

Musculoskeletal – Arthralgia; myalgia; myasthenia.

Respiratory – Dyspnea; pleural effusion.

Miscellaneous – Abdominal pain; worsening of underlying illness; allergic reaction; chest pain; fever; infection.

Patients Discontinuing Quinupristin/Dalfopristin Therapy (%): Skin/Skin Structure Studies		
Type	Quinupristin/Dalfopristin (n = 1099)	Comparator[1] (n = 1095)
Venous	12	2
Non-venous	11.8	4
Rash	2	0.9
Nausea	1.1	0
Vomiting	0.9	0
Pain	0.9	0
Pruritus	0.9	0.5

[1] Comparator regimens were oxacillin/vancomycin or cefazolin/vancomycin.

Quinupristin/Dalfopristin Adverse Reactions (%): Skin/Skin Structure Studies		
	Quinupristin/Dalfopristin (n = 1099)	Comparator (n = 1095)
Venous	68	32.7
Pain at infusion site	44.7	17.8
Inflammation at infusion site	38.2	14.7
Edema at infusion site	18	7.2
Infusion site reaction	11.6	3.6
Non-venous	24.7	13.1
Nausea	4	2
Vomiting	3.7	1
Rash	3.1	1.3
Pain	3.1	0.2

There were 8 (1.7%) episodes of thrombus or thrombophlebitis in the quinupristin/dalfopristin arms and none in the comparator arms.

Lab test abnormalities – The following table shows the percentage of patients exhibiting laboratory values above or below the clinically relevant "critical" values during treatment phase.

Lab Test Abnormalities: Quinupristin/Dalfopristin vs Comparator (≥ 0.1%): All Comparative Studies			
Parameter	Critically high or low value	Quinupristin/Dalfopristin critically high or low	Comparator critically high or low
AST	> 10 × ULN	0.9	0.2
ALT	> 10 × ULN	0.4	0.4
Total bilirubin	> 5 × ULN	0.9	0.2
Conjugated bilirubin	> 5 × ULN	3.1	1.3
LDH	> 5 × ULN	2.6	2.1
Alkaline phosphatase	> 5 × ULN	0.3	0.7
Gamma-GT	> 10 × ULN	1.9	1
CPK	> 10 × ULN	1.6	1.4
Creatinine	≥ 440 mcmol/L	0.1	0.1
BUN	≥ 35.5 mmol/L	0.3	1.2
Blood glucose	> 22.2 mmol/L	1.3	1.3

QUINUPRISTIN/DALFOPRISTIN

Lab Test Abnormalities: Quinupristin/Dalfopristin vs Comparator (≥ 0.1%): All Comparative Studies			
Parameter	Critically high or low value	Quinupristin/ Dalfopristin critically high or low	Comparator critically high or low
	< 2.2 mmol/L	0.1	0.1
Bicarbonates	> 40 mmol/L	0.3	0.5
	< 10 mmol/L	0.5	0.5
CO_2	> 50 mmol/L	0	0
	< 15 mmol/L	0.2	0
Sodium	> 160 mmol/L	0	0
	< 120 mmol/L	0.5	0.3
Potassium	> 6 mmol/L	0.3	0.6
	< 2 mmol/L	0	0.1
Hemoglobin	< 8 g/dl	2.6	1.6
Hematocrit	> 60%	0.2	0
Platelets	> 1,000,000/mm³	0.2	0.2
	< 50,000/mm³	0.6	0.7

➤*Noncomparative trials:* Approximately 33% of patients discontinued therapy in these trials because of adverse events. However, the discontinuation rate because of adverse reactions assessed by the investigator as possibly or probably related to quinupristin/dalfopristin therapy was ≈ 5%.

There were 3 prospectively designed non-comparative clinical trials in patients (n = 972) treated with quinupristin/dalfopristin. One of these studies (301) had more complete documentation than the other two (398 and 398B). The most common events probably or possibly related to therapy were the following.

Quinupristin/Dalfopristin Adverse Reactions (%): Noncomparative Studies	
Adverse reaction	
Arthralgia	4.3-7.8
Arthralgia and myalgia	3.3-7.4
Nausea	2.8-4.9
Myalgia	0.95-5.1

The percentage of patients who experienced severe related arthralgia and myalgia was 3.3% and 3.1%, respectively. The percentage of patients who discontinued treatment because of related arthralgia and myalgia was 2.3% and 1.8%, respectively.

Lab test abnormalities – The most frequently observed abnormalities in laboratory studies were in total and conjugated bilirubin, with increases > 5 times the ULN, regardless of relationship to quinupristin/dalfopristin, reported in 25% and 34.6% of patients, respectively. The percentage of patients who discontinued treatment because of increased total and conjugated bilirubin was 2.7% and 2.3%, respectively. Notably, 46.5% and 59% of patients had high baseline total and conjugated bilirubin levels before study entry.

Miscellaneous – Serious adverse reactions in clinical trials, including non-comparative studies, considered possibly or probably related to quinupristin/dalfopristin administration with an incidence of < 0.1% include the following: Acidosis; anaphylactoid reaction; apnea; arrhythmia; bone pain; cerebral hemorrhage; cerebrovascular accident; coagulation disorder; convulsion; dysautonomia; encephalopathy; grand mal convulsion; hemolysis; hemolytic anemia; heart arrest; hepatitis; hypoglycemia; hyponatremia; hypoplastic anemia; hypoventilation; hypovolemia; hypoxia; jaundice; mesenteric arterial occlusion; neck rigidity; neuropathy; pancytopenia; paraplegia; pericardial effusion; pericarditis; respiratory distress syndrome; shock; skin ulcer; supraventricular tachycardia; syncope; tremor; ventricular extrasystoles; ventricular fibrillation. Cases of hypotension and GI hemorrhage were reported in < 0.2% of patients.

Overdosage

There are 4 reports of patients receiving quinupristin/dalfopristin at doses up to 3 times that recommended (7.5 mg/kg). No adverse events were considered possibly or probably related to quinupristin/dalfopristin overdose. Signs of acute overdosage may include dyspnea, emesis, tremors, and ataxia as seen in animals given extremely high doses (50 mg/kg) of quinupristing/dalfopristin. Carefully observe patients who receive an overdose, and give them supportive treatment. Refer to the General Management of Acute Overdosage. Quinupristin/dalfopristin is not removed by peritoneal dialysis or by hemodialysis.

DAPTOMYCIN

Rx	**Cubicin** (Cubist)	**Powder for injection, lyophilized:** 250 mg	Preservative-free. In single-use vials.
		500 mg	Preservative-free. In single-use vials.

Indications

➤ *Complicated skin and skin structure infections:* For the treatment of complicated skin and skin structure infections caused by susceptible strains of the following gram-positive microorganisms: *Staphylococcus aureus* (including methicillin-resistant strains), *Streptococcus pyogenes*, *Streptococcus agalactiae*, *Streptococcus dysgalactiae* subsp. *equisimilis*, and *Enterococcus faecalis* (vancomycin-susceptible strains only). Combination therapy may be clinically indicated if the documented or presumed pathogens include gram-negative or anaerobic organisms.

Administration and Dosage

➤ *Approved by the FDA:* September 12, 2003.

➤ *Complicated skin and skin structure infections:* Administer daptomycin 4 mg/kg over a 30-minute period by IV infusion in 0.9% sodium chloride injection once every 24 hours for 7 to 14 days. In phase 1 and 2 clinical studies, creatine phosphokinase (CPK) elevations appeared to be more frequent when daptomycin was dosed more frequently than once daily. Therefore, do not dose daptomycin more frequently than once a day.

➤ *Renal function impairment:* Because daptomycin is eliminated primarily by the kidney, a dosage modification is recommended for patients with creatinine clearance (Ccr) less than 30 mL/min, including patients receiving hemodialysis or continuous ambulatory peritoneal dialysis (CAPD). When possible, administer daptomycin following hemodialysis on hemodialysis days.

Daptomycin Dosage in Adult Patients with Renal Impairment	
Creatinine clearance	Dosage regimen
≥ 30 mL/min	4 mg/kg once every 24 hours
< 30 mL/min, including hemodialysis or CAPD	4 mg/kg once every 48 hours

➤ *Preparation for administration:* Reconstitute the contents of a daptomycin 250 mg vial with 5 mL of 0.9% sodium chloride injection. Reconstitute the contents of a daptomycin 500 mg vial with 10 mL of 0.9% sodium chloride injection. Dilute reconstituted daptomycin further with 0.9% sodium chloride injection to be administered by IV infusion over a period of 30 minutes.

➤ *Compatibilities:* Daptomycin is compatible with 0.9% sodium chloride injection and lactated Ringer's injection.

➤ *Incompatibilities:* Daptomycin is not compatible with dextrose-containing diluents. Do not add additives or other medications to daptomycin single-use vials or infuse simultaneously through the same IV line. If the same IV line is used for sequential infusion of several different drugs, flush the line with a compatible infusion solution before and after infusion with daptomycin.

➤ *Storage/Stability:* Store original packages at refrigerated temperatures (2° to 8°C; 36° to 46°F); avoid excessive heat. Reconstituted solution is stable in the vial for 12 hours at room temperature or up to 48 hours if stored under refrigeration (2° to 8°C; 36° to 46°F). The diluted solution is stable in the infusion bag for 12 hours at room temperature or 48 hours if stored under refrigeration. The combined time (vial and infusion bag) at room temperature should not exceed 12 hours; the combined time (vial and infusion bag) under refrigeration should not exceed 48 hours.

Actions

➤ *Pharmacology:* Daptomycin is an antibacterial agent of a new class of antibiotics, the cyclic lipopeptides. The mechanism of action of daptomycin is distinct from any other antibiotic. Daptomycin binds to bacterial membranes and causes a rapid depolarization of membrane potential. The loss of membrane potential leads to inhibition of protein, DNA, and RNA synthesis, which results in bacterial cell death. Daptomycin is a natural product that has clinical utility in the treatment of infections caused by aerobic gram-positive bacteria. The in vitro spectrum of daptomycin activity encompasses most clinically relevant gram-positive pathogenic bacteria. Daptomycin retains potency against antibiotic-resistant gram-positive bacteria, including isolates resistant to methicillin, vancomycin, and linezolid.

Daptomycin exhibits rapid, concentration-dependent bactericidal activity against gram-positive organisms in vitro. This has been demonstrated both by time-kill curves and by MBC/MIC ratios using broth dilution methodology.

In vitro studies have demonstrated additive or indifferent interactions of daptomycin with other antibiotics. Antagonism, as determined by kill-curve studies, has not been observed. In vitro synergistic interactions occurred with aminoglycosides and β-lactam antibiotics against some isolates of staphylococci and enterococci, including some MRSA isolates.

➤ *Pharmacokinetics:*

Absorption – The mean pharmacokinetic parameters of daptomycin on day 7 following the IV administration of 4, 6, and 8 mg/kg once daily to healthy young adults (mean age, 35.8 years) are summarized in the following table.

Mean Daptomycin Pharmacokinetic Parameters in Healthy Volunteers on Day 7								
Dose mg/kg	C_{max} (mcg/mL)	T_{max}[1] (h)	AUC_{0-24} (mcg•h/ mL)	$t_{1/2}$ (h)	V_d (L/kg)	CL_T (mL/h/ kg)	CL_R (mL/h/ kg)	Ae_{24} %
4 (n = 6)	57.8	0.8	494	8.1	0.096	8.3	4.8	53
6 (n = 6)	98.6	0.5	747	8.9	0.104	8.1	4.4	47.4
8 (n = 6)	133	0.5	1130	9	0.092	7.2	3.7	52.1

[1] Median (minimum, maximum).
CL_T = Systemic clearance.
CL_R = Renal clearance.
Ae_{24} = Percent of dose recovered in urine over 24 hours as unchanged daptomycin following the first dose.

Daptomycin pharmacokinetics are nearly linear and time-independent at doses up to 6 mg/kg administered once daily for 7 days. Steady-state concentrations are achieved by the third daily dose. The mean steady-state trough concentrations (days 4 to 8) attained following administration of 4, 6, and 8 mg/kg once daily are 5.9, 9.4, and 14.9 mcg/mL, respectively.

Distribution – Daptomycin is reversibly bound to human plasma proteins, primarily to serum albumin, in a concentration-independent manner. The mean serum protein binding of daptomycin was approximately 92% in healthy adults after the administration of 4 or 6 mg/kg. Serum protein binding was not altered as a function of daptomycin concentration, dose, or number of doses received.

In clinical studies, mean serum protein binding in subjects with Ccr greater than or equal to 30 mL/min was comparable to that observed in healthy subjects with normal renal function. However, there was a trend toward decreasing serum protein binding among subjects with Ccr less than 30 mL/min (87.6%), including hemodialysis patients (85.9%) and CAPD patients (83.5%). The protein binding of daptomycin in subjects with hepatic impairment (Child-Pugh B) was similar to healthy adult subjects. The apparent volume of distribution of daptomycin at steady state in healthy adult subjects was approximately 0.09 L/kg.

Metabolism – It is unlikely that daptomycin will inhibit or induce the metabolism of drugs metabolized by the CYP 450 system. It is unknown whether daptomycin is a substrate of the CYP 450 system.

In 5 healthy young adults, after infusion of radiolabeled ^{14}C-daptomycin, the plasma total radioactivity was similar to the concentration determined by microbiological assay. Inactive metabolites of daptomycin have been detected in the urine, as determined by the difference in total radiolabeled concentrations and microbiologically active concentrations. The site of metabolism has not been identified.

Excretion – Daptomycin is excreted primarily by the kidney. In a mass balance study of 5 healthy subjects using radiolabeled daptomycin, approximately 78% of the administered dose was recovered from urine based on total radioactivity (approximately 52% of the dose based on microbiologically active concentrations) and 5.7% of the dose was recovered from feces (collected for up to 9 days), based on total radioactivity.

Because renal excretion is the primary route of elimination, dosage adjustment is necessary in patients with severe renal insufficiency (Ccr less than 30 mL/min) (see Administration and Dosage).

Special populations –

Renal function impairment: Following the administration of a single 4 mg/kg IV dose of daptomycin, the plasma clearance (CL_T) was reduced and the systemic exposure ($AUC_{0-\infty}$) was increased with decreasing renal function (see the following table). The mean $AUC_{0-\infty}$ was not markedly different for subjects and patients with Ccr 30 to 80 mL/min as compared to those with normal renal function (Ccr greater than 80 mL/min). The mean $AUC_{0-\infty}$ values for subjects and patients with Ccr less than 30 mL/min and hemodialysis (dosed post-dialysis)/CAPD subjects were approximately 2- and 3-times higher, respectively, than the values in individuals with normal renal function. The mean C_{max} ranged from 59.6 mcg/mL to 69.6 mcg/mL in subjects with Ccr greater than or equal to 30 mL/min while those with Ccr less than 30 mL/min ranged from 41.1 mcg/mL to 57.7 mcg/mL. In 11 non-infected adult subjects undergoing dialysis, approximately 15% and 11% of the administered dose was removed by 4 hours of hemodialysis and 48 hours of CAPD, respectively. Administer daptomycin following the completion of hemodialysis on hemodialysis days (see Administration and Dosage).

DAPTOMYCIN

Mean Daptomycin Pharmacokinetic Parameters in Patients with Renal Function Impairment[1]				
Renal function (Ccr)[2]	$AUC_{0-\infty}$ (mcg·h/mL)	$t_{1/2}$ (h)	V_{SS} (L/kg)	CL_T (mL/h/kg)
Normal (Ccr > 80 mL/min) (n = 165)	417	9.39	0.13	10.9
Mild renal impairment (Ccr 50 - 80 mL/min) (n = 64)	466	10.75	0.12	9.9
Moderate renal impairment (Ccr 30 - < 50 mL/min) (n = 24)	560	14.7	0.15	8.5
Severe renal impairment (Ccr < 30 mL/min) (n = 8)	925	27.83	0.2	5.9
Hemodialysis and CAPD (n = 21)	1244	29.81	0.15	3.7

[1] Following a single 30-minute IV infusion of 4 mg/kg to infected patients and noninfected subjects with varying degrees of renal function.
[2] Ccr estimated using the Cockroft-Gault equation with actual body weight.

Elderly: Following administration of a single IV 4 mg/kg dose, the mean total clearance of daptomycin was reduced approximately 35% and the mean $AUC_{0-\infty}$ increased approximately 58% in elderly subjects compared with young healthy subjects. There were no differences in C_{max}. No dosage adjustment is warranted for elderly patients with normal (for age) renal function.

Obesity: The pharmacokinetics of daptomycin were evaluated in 6 moderately obese (body mass index [BMI] 25 to 39.9 kg/m²) and 6 extremely obese (BMI at least 40 kg/m²) subjects and controls matched for age, sex, and renal function. Following administration of a single IV 4 mg/kg dose based on total body weight, the plasma clearance of daptomycin increased approximately 18% in moderately obese subjects and 46% in extremely obese subjects compared with nonobese controls. The $AUC_{0-\infty}$ of daptomycin increased approximately 30% in moderately obese and 31% in extremely obese subjects compared with nonobese controls. The differences were most likely caused by differences in the renal clearance of daptomycin. No dosage adjustment of daptomycin is warranted in obese subjects.

➤*Clinical trials:* Adult patients with clinically documented complicated skin and skin structure infections were enrolled in 2 randomized, multinational, multi-center, investigator-blind studies comparing daptomycin (4 mg/kg/day IV) with either vancomycin (1 g/day IV) or a semi-synthetic penicillin (ie, nafcillin, oxacillin, cloxacillin, or flucloxacillin; 4 to 12 g/day IV). Patients known to have bacteremia at baseline were excluded. Patients could switch to oral therapy after a minimum of 4 days of IV treatment if clinical improvement was demonstrated.

The efficacy endpoints in both studies were the clinical success rates in the intent-to-treat (ITT) population and in the clinically evaluable (CE) population. In study 9801, clinical success rates in the ITT population were 62.5% (165/264) in patients treated with daptomycin and 60.9% (162/266) in patients treated with comparator drugs. Clinical success rates in the CE population were 76% (158/208) in patients treated with daptomycin and 76.7% (158/206) in patients treated with comparator drugs. In study 9901, clinical success rates in the ITT population were 80.4% (217/270) in patients treated with daptomycin and 80.5% (235/292) in patients treated with comparator drugs. Clinical success rates in the CE population were 89.9% (214/238) in patients treated with daptomycin and 90.4% (226/250) in patients treated with comparator drugs.

Contraindications

Known hypersensitivity to daptomycin.

Warnings

➤*Pseudomembranous colitis:* Pseudomembranous colitis has been reported with nearly all antibacterial agents, including daptomycin, and may range in severity from mild to life-threatening. Therefore, it is important to consider this diagnosis in patients who present with diarrhea subsequent to the administration of any antibacterial agent.

Treatment with antibacterial agents alters the normal flora of the colon and may permit overgrowth of clostridia. Studies indicated that a toxin produced by *Clostridium difficile* is a primary cause of "antibiotic-associated colitis."

If a diagnosis of pseudomembranous colitis has been established, initiate appropriate therapeutic measures. Mild cases of pseudomembranous colitis usually respond to drug discontinuation alone. In moderate to severe cases, consider management with fluids and electrolytes, protein supplementation, and treatment with an antibacterial agent clinically effective against *C. difficile*.

➤*Elderly:* In the two phase 3 clinical studies in patients with complicated skin and skin structure infections (cSSSI), lower clinical success rates were seen in patients 65 years of age and older compared with those younger than 65 years of age. In addition, treatment-emergent adverse events were more common in patients 65 years of age and older than in patients younger than 65 years of age in both cSSSI studies.

➤*Pregnancy: Category B.* There are no adequate and well-controlled studies in pregnant women. Daptomycin should be used in pregnancy only if clearly needed.

➤*Lactation:* It is not known if daptomycin is excreted in human milk. Exercise caution when administering daptomycin to nursing women.

➤*Children:* Safety and efficacy of daptomycin in patients younger than 18 years of age have not been established.

Precautions

➤*Monitoring:* Monitor CPK levels weekly in patients who receive daptomycin. Monitor patients who develop unexplained elevations in CPK while receiving daptomycin more frequently.

➤*Skeletal muscle effects:* In phase 3 cSSSI trials, elevations in serum CPK were reported as clinical adverse events in 15/534 (2.8%) daptomycin-treated patients, compared with 10/558 (1.8%) comparator-treated patients. Skeletal muscle effects associated with daptomycin were observed in animals.

Monitor patients receiving daptomycin for the development of muscle pain or weakness, particularly of the distal extremities. Monitor CPK levels weekly in patients who receive daptomycin. Monitor patients who develop unexplained elevations in CPK while receiving daptomycin more frequently. Among patients with abnormal CPK (greater than 500 U/L) at baseline, 2/19 (10.5%) treated with daptomycin and 4/24 (16.7%) treated with comparator developed further increases in CPK while on therapy. In this same population, no patients developed myopathy. Daptomycin-treated patients with baseline CPK greater than 500 U/L (n = 19) did not experience an increased incidence of CPK elevations or myopathy relative to those treated with comparator (n = 24).

Discontinue daptomycin in patients with unexplained signs and symptoms of myopathy in conjunction with CPK elevation greater than 1000 U/L (approximately 5 × ULN), or in patients without reported symptoms who have marked elevations in CPK (10 × ULN or greater). In addition, consider temporarily suspending agents associated with rhabdomyolysis, such as HMG-CoA reductase inhibitors, in patients receiving daptomycin.

➤*Neuropathy:* In a small number of patients in phase 1 and 2 studies, administration of daptomycin was associated with decreases in nerve conduction velocity and with adverse events (eg, paresthesias, Bell palsy), possibly reflective of peripheral or cranial neuropathy. Nerve conduction deficits were also detected in a similar number of comparator subjects in these studies.

In phase 3 cSSSI and community-acquired pneumonia (CAP) studies, 7/989 (0.7%) daptomycin-treated patients and 7/1018 (0.7%) comparator-treated patients experienced paresthesias. New or worsening peripheral neuropathy was not diagnosed in any of these patients. In animals, effects of daptomycin on peripheral nerves were observed. Therefore, physicians should be alert to the possibility of signs and symptoms of neuropathy in patients receiving daptomycin.

➤*Superinfection:* The use of antibiotics may promote the overgrowth of nonsusceptible organisms. Should superinfection occur during therapy, take appropriate measures.

Drug Interactions

➤*Warfarin:* Coadministration of daptomycin (6 mg/kg/day for 5 days) and warfarin (25 mg single oral dose) had no significant effect on the pharmacokinetics of either drug, and the international normalized ratio (INR) was not significantly altered. As experience with the coadministration of daptomycin and warfarin is limited to volunteer studies, monitor anticoagulant activity in patients receiving daptomycin and warfarin for the first several days after initiating daptomycin therapy.

➤*HMG-CoA reductase inhibitors:* Inhibitors of HMG-CoA reductase may cause myopathy, which is manifested as muscle pain or weakness associated with elevated levels of CPK. There were no reports of skeletal myopathy in a placebo-controlled phase 1 trial in which 10 healthy subjects on stable simvastatin therapy were treated concurrently with daptomycin (4 mg/kg once every 24 hours) for 14 days. Experience with coadministration of HMG-CoA reductase inhibitors and daptomycin in patients is limited, therefore, consider temporarily suspending use of HMG-CoA reductase inhibitors in patients receiving daptomycin.

Adverse Reactions

Daptomycin Adverse Events (≥ 2%)		
Adverse event	Daptomycin (n = 534)	Comparator[1] (n = 558)
Cardiovascular		
Hypotension	2.4	1.4
Hypertension	1.1	2
CNS		
Headache	5.4	5.4
Insomnia	4.5	5.4
Dizziness	2.2	2

DAPTOMYCIN

Daptomycin Adverse Events (≥ 2%)		
Adverse event	Daptomycin (n = 534)	Comparator[1] (n = 558)
Dermatologic		
Rash	4.3	3.8
Pruritus	2.8	3.8
GI		
Constipation	6.2	6.8
Nausea	5.8	9.5
Diarrhea	5.2	4.3
Vomiting	3.2	3.8
Dyspepsia	0.9	2.5
Lab test abnormalities		
Abnormal liver function tests	3	1.6
Elevated CPK	2.8	1.8
Musculoskeletal		
Limb pain	1.5	2
Arthralgia	0.9	2.2
Miscellaneous		
Injection-site reactions	5.8	7.7
Fungal infections	2.6	3.2
Urinary tract infections	2.4	0.5
Renal failure	2.2	2.7
Anemia	2.1	2.3
Dyspnea	2.1	1.6
Fever	1.9	2.5

[1] Comparators included vancomycin (1 g IV twice daily) and semi-synthetic penicillins (ie, nafcillin, oxacillin, cloxacillin, flucloxacillin; 4 to 12 g/day in divided doses).

In phase 3 studies of CAP, the death rate and rates of serious cardiorespiratory adverse events were higher in daptomycin-treated patients than in comparator-treated patients. These differences were caused by a lack of therapeutic effectiveness of daptomycin in the treatment of CAP in patients experiencing these adverse events. Additional adverse events that occurred in 1% to 2% of patients in either daptomycin- or comparator-treatment groups in the cSSSI studies are as follows: Edema, cellulitis, hypoglycemia, elevated alkaline phosphatase, cough, back pain, abdominal pain, hypokalemia, hyperglycemia, decreased appetite, anxiety, chest pain, sore throat, cardiac failure, confusion, and Candida infections. These events occurred at rates ranging from 0.2% to 1.7% in daptomycin-treated patients and at rates of 0.4% to 1.8% in comparator-treated patients.

Additional drug-related adverse events (possibly or probably related) that occurred in less than 1% of patients receiving daptomycin in cSSSI trials are as follows:

➤*CNS:* Vertigo; mental status change; paresthesias.

➤*GI:* Abdominal distension; flatulence; stomatitis; jaundice; increased serum lactate dehydrogenase.

➤*Hematologic / Lymphatic:* Leukocytosis; thrombocytopenia; thrombocytosis; eosinophilia; increased international normalized ratio.

➤*Metabolic / Nutritional:* Hypomagnesemia; increased serum bicarbonate; electrolyte disturbance.

➤*Musculoskeletal:* Myalgia; muscle cramps; muscle weakness; osteomyelitis.

➤*Special senses:* Taste disturbance; eye irritation.

➤*Miscellaneous:* Fatigue; weakness; rigors; discomfort; jitteriness; flushing; hypersensitivity; supraventricular arrhythmias; eczema.

➤*Laboratory test abnormalities:*

Creatine Phosphokinase (CPK) Elevations in Phase 3 cSSSI Studies (%)[1]				
	All patients		Patients with normal CPK at baseline	
	Daptomycin (n = 430)	Comparator (n = 459)	Daptomycin (n = 374)	Comparator (n = 392)
No increase	90.7	91.1	91.2	91.1
Maximum value > 1 × ULN[2]	9.3	8.9	8.8	8.9
> 2 × ULN	4.9	4.8	3.7	3.1
> 4 × ULN	1.4	1.5	1.1	1
> 5 × ULN	1.4	0.4	1.1	0
> 10 × ULN	0.5	0.2	0.2	0

[1] Elevations in CPK observed in patients treated with daptomycin or comparator were not clinically or statistically significantly different (*P* < 0.05).
[2] ULN (upper limit of normal) is defined as 200 U/L.

In clinical trials, 0.2% of patients treated with daptomycin had symptoms of muscle pain or weakness associated with CPK elevations greater than 4 times the ULN. The symptoms resolved within 3 days and CPK returned to normal within 7 to 10 days after discontinuing treatment (see Precautions). In phase 3 comparator-controlled trials, there was no clinically or statistically significant difference (*P* < 0.05) in the frequency of CPK elevations between patients treated with daptomycin and those treated with comparator. CPK elevations in both groups were generally related to medical conditions, for example, skin and skin structure infection, surgical procedures, or IM injections, and were not associated with muscle symptoms.

Overdosage

In the event of overdosage, supportive care is advised with maintenance of glomerular filtration. Daptomycin is slowly cleared from the body by hemodialysis (approximately 15% recovered over 4 hours) or by peritoneal dialysis (approximately 11% recovered over 48 hours).

VANCOMYCIN

Rx	Vancocin (Eli Lilly)	**Pulvules:** 125 mg	(3125 Vancocin HCl 125 mg). Blue and brown. In *Identi-Dose* 20s.
		250 mg	(3126 Vancocin HCl 250 mg). Blue and lavender. In *Identi-Dose* 20s.
Rx	**Vancomycin HCl** (ESI Lederle)	**Powder for Oral Solution:** 1 g	In bottles.
Rx	**Vancomycin HCl** (Various, eg, Abbott, American Pharmaceutical Partners[1], ESI Lederle)	**Powder for Injection:** 500 mg	In vials.
Rx	**Vancocin** (Eli Lilly)		In 10 ml vials and 15 ml *ADD-Vantage* vials.
Rx	**Vancoled** (Lederle)		In vials.
Rx	**Vancomycin HCl** (Various, eg, Abbott, American Pharmaceutical Partners[1], ESI Lederle)	**Powder for Injection:** 1 g	In vials.
Rx	**Vancoled** (Lederle)		In vials.
Rx	**Vancomycin HCl** (American Pharm. Partners[1])	**Powder for Injection:** 5 g	In 100 ml vials.
Rx	**Vancoled** (Lederle)		In pharmacy bulk package.
Rx	**Vancomycin HCl** (American Pharm. Partners[1])	**Powder for Injection:** 10 g	In vials.
Rx	**Vancocin** (Eli Lilly)		In 100 ml vials.

[1] American Pharmaceutical Partners, Inc., 2045 North Cornell Ave., Melrose Park, IL 60160 (888) 386-1300.

Indications

➤*Parenteral:* Serious or severe infections not treatable with other antimicrobials, including the penicillins and cephalosporins.

Severe staphylococcal infections (including methicillin-resistant staphylococci) – In patients who cannot receive or who have failed to respond to penicillins and cephalosporins, or who have infections with resistant staphylococci. Infections may include endocarditis, bone infections, lower respiratory tract infections, septicemia, and skin and skin structure infections.

Endocarditis –
Staphylococcal: Vancomycin is effective alone.
Streptococcal: Vancomycin is effective alone or in combination with an aminoglycoside for endocarditis caused by *S. viridans* or *S. bovis.* It is only effective in combination with an aminoglycoside for endocarditis caused by enterococci (eg, *S. faecalis*).
Diphtheroid: Vancomycin is effective for diphtheroid endocarditis, and has been used successfully with rifampin, an aminoglycoside or both in early onset prosthetic valve endocarditis caused by *S. epidermidis* or diphtheroids.
Prophylactic: Although no controlled clinical efficacy studies have been conducted, IV vancomycin has been suggested for prophylaxis against bacterial endocarditis in penicillin-allergic patients who have congenital heart disease or rheumatic or other acquired or valvular heart disease when these patients undergo dental procedures or surgical procedures of the upper respiratory tract.

Pseudomembranous colitis/staphylococcal enterocolitis caused by C. difficile – The parenteral form may be administered orally; parenteral use alone is unproven. The oral use of parenteral vancomycin is not effective for other infections.

➤*Oral:* Staphylococcal enterocolitis and antibiotic-associated pseudomembranous colitis produced by *C. difficile.* The parenteral product may also be given orally for these infections. Oral vancomycin is *not* effective for other types of infection.

Administration and Dosage

➤*Oral:*

Adults – 500 mg to 2 g/day given in 3 or 4 divided doses for 7 to 10 days.

Alternatively, dosages of 125 mg 3 or 4 times daily for *C. difficile* colitis may be as effective as the 500 mg dose regimen.

Children – 40 mg/kg/day in 3 or 4 divided doses for 7 to 10 days. Do not exceed 2 g/day.

Preparation of solution – Add 115 ml distilled or deionized water to the 10 g container. Each 6 ml of solution provides ≈ 500 mg vancomycin.

The contents of the 1 g vial may be mixed with distilled or deionized water (20 ml). When reconstituted, each 5 ml contains ≈ 250 mg vancomycin. Mix thoroughly to dissolve.

The appropriate oral solution dose may be diluted in 1 oz of water and given to the patient to drink. Common flavoring syrups may be added to the solution to improve the taste for oral administration. The diluted material may be administered via nasogastric tube.

➤*Parenteral:* Administer each dose over at least 60 minutes. Intermittent infusion is the preferred administration method.

Adults – 500 mg IV every 6 hours or 1 g every 12 hours.

Children – 10 mg/kg per dose given every 6 hours.

Infants and neonates – Initial dose of 15 mg/kg, followed by 10 mg/kg every 12 hours for neonates in the first week of life and every 8 hours thereafter up to the age of 1 month.

Preparation of solution – Reconstitute by adding 10 ml Sterile Water for Injection to the 500 mg vial or 20 ml to the 1 g vial. Further dilution is required.

Dilute reconstituted solutions containing 500 mg or 1 g vancomycin with at least 100 or 200 ml, respectively, of diluent.

Compatible diluents – 5% Dextrose Injection, 5% Dextrose Injection and 0.9% NaCl, Lactated Ringer's Injection, Lactated Ringer's and 5% Dextrose Injection, *Normosol-M* and 5% Dextrose, 0.9% NaCl Injection, *Isolyte E,* and Acetated Ringer's Injection.

➤*Prevention of bacterial endocarditis†:*
GU/GI procedures (high-risk, penicillin-allergic patients) – 1 g IV over 1 to 2 hours (children, 20 mg/kg) plus gentamicin 1.5 mg/kg IV or IM for both adult (not to exceed 120 mg) and children. Complete injection or infusion within 30 minutes of starting procedure.

(Moderate-risk, penicillin-allergic patients) – 1 g IV over 1 to 2 hours (children 20 mg/kg). Complete infusion within 30 minutes of starting procedure.

➤*Renal function impairment:* Adjust dosage; check serum levels regularly. In premature infants and the elderly, dosage reduction may be necessary caused by decreasing renal function.

For most patients, if creatinine clearance (Ccr) can be measured or estimated accurately, the dosage may be calculated by using the following table.

Vancomycin Dosage in Impaired Renal Function	
Ccr (ml/min)	Dose (mg/24 hr)
100	1545
90	1390
80	1235
70	1080
60	925
50	770
40	620
30	465
20	310
10	155

The table is not valid for functionally anephric patients on dialysis. For such patients, give a loading dose of 15 mg/kg to achieve therapeutic serum levels promptly and a maintenance dose of 1.9 mg/kg/24 hr. In patients with marked renal impairment, it may be more convenient to give maintenance doses of 250 to 1000 mg once every several days rather than administering the drug on a daily basis. In anuria a dose of 1000 mg every 7 to 10 days has been recommended.

When only serum creatinine is available, use the formula below to calculate estimated Ccr. Serum creatinine should represent a steady state of renal function.

Males: $\dfrac{\text{Weight (kg)} \times (140 - \text{age})}{72 \times \text{serum creatinine (mg/dL)}} = \text{Ccr}$

Females: $0.85 \times$ above value

➤*Storage/Stability:* Oral and parenteral solutions are stable for 14 days if refrigerated after initial reconstitution. After further dilution, the parenteral solution is stable for 24 hours at room temperature and for 2 months under refrigeration (< 6% loss of potency) after dilution with Dextrose 5% or Sodium Chloride 0.9%.

Actions

➤*Pharmacology:* Vancomycin is a tricyclic glycopeptide antibiotic which inhibits cell-wall biosynthesis. It also alters bacterial-cell-membrane permeability and RNA synthesis.

† American Heart Association Statement. *JAMA* 1997;277:1794-1801.

VANCOMYCIN

➤*Pharmacokinetics:*

Absorption / Distribution – Systemic absorption of oral vancomycin is generally poor, although clinically significant serum concentrations have occurred in patients with active *C. difficile*-induced colitis. With doses of 2 g daily, very high concentrations of drug can be found in the feces (> 3100 mg/kg) and very low concentrations (< 1 mcg/ml) can be found in the serum of patients with normal renal function who have pseudomembranous colitis.

Parenteral: In subjects with normal kidney function, multiple IV dosing of 1 g (15 mg/kg) infused over 60 minutes produces mean plasma concentrations of ≈ 63 mcg/ml immediately after the completion of infusion, ≈ 23 mcg/ml 2 hours after infusion, and ≈ 8 mcg/ml 11 hours after the end of the infusion. Multiple dosing of 500 mg infused over 30 minutes produces mean plasma concentrations of ≈ 49 mcg/ml at the completion of infusion, ≈ 19 mcg/ml 2 hours after infusion, and ≈ 10 mcg/ml 6 hours after infusion. The plasma concentrations during multiple dosing are similar to those after a single dose. Vancomycin IV penetrates inflamed meninges at levels about 15% of those found in serum (mean, 2.5 mcg/ml in adults, 3.1 mcg/ml in infants). In the presence of inflammation, it also penetrates into pleural, pericardial, ascitic, and synovial fluids, urine, peritoneal dialysis fluid, atrial appendage tissue, and bile (≈ 15%). It is ≈ 55% protein bound.

Metabolism / Excretion – In the first 24 hours, ≈ 75% of a dose is excreted in urine by glomerular filtration. Urine concentrations of 90 to 300 mcg/ml are achieved 1 hour after a 500 mg IV dose. Creatinine clearance is linearly associated with vancomycin clearance. Elimination half-life is 4 to 6 hours in adults and 2 to 3 hours in children. Accumulation occurs in renal failure. Serum half-life in anephric patients is ≈ 7.5 days. About 60% of an intraperitoneal dose administered during peritoneal dialysis is absorbed systemically in 6 hours. Serum concentrations of ≈ 10 mcg/ml are achieved by intraperitoneal injection of 30 mg/kg. In anephric patients, the drug is slowly eliminated by unknown routes and mechanisms. Vancomycin is not significantly removed by hemodialysis or continuous ambulatory peritoneal dialysis, although there have been reports of increased clearance with hemoperfusion and hemofiltration.

➤*Microbiology:* At clinically achievable concentrations, vancomycin is active only against gram-positive bacteria. In vitro, at concentrations of 0.5 to 5 mcg/ml, it is active against many strains of streptococci, staphylococci, *Clostridium difficile*, *Corynebacterium*, *Listeria monocytogenes*, *Lactobacillus* sp., *Actinomyces* sp., *Clostridium* sp., and *Bacillus* sp. It is bacteriostatic against enterococci. Vancomycin is not active in vitro against gram-negative bacilli, mycobacteria, or fungi.

No cross-resistance between vancomycin and any other antibiotic has been reported.

The combination of vancomycin and an aminoglycoside acts synergistically in vitro against many strains of *S. aureus*, nonenterococcal group D streptococci, enterococci, and *Streptococcus* sp. (viridans group).

Contraindications

Hypersensitivity to vancomycin.

Warnings

➤*Ototoxicity:* This has occurred in patients receiving vancomycin. It may be transient or permanent. It has occurred mostly in patients who have been given excessive doses, who have an underlying hearing loss, or who are receiving concomitant therapy with another ototoxic agent, such as an aminoglycoside. Serial tests of auditory function may be helpful in order to minimize the risk of ototoxicity.

➤*Hypotension:* Rapid bolus administration (eg, over several minutes) may be associated with exaggerated hypotension, including shock, and, rarely, cardiac arrest. To avoid hypotension, administer in a dilute solution over not less than 60 minutes. Stopping the infusion usually results in prompt cessation of these reactions. Frequently monitor blood pressure and heart rate.

➤*Pseudomembranous colitis:* In rare instances, pseudomembranous colitis has occurred due to *C. difficile* developing in patients who received IV vancomycin.

➤*Reversible neutropenia:* This has occurred in patients receiving vancomycin. Periodically monitor the leukocyte count of patients on prolonged therapy or those receiving concomitant drugs that may cause neutropenia.

➤*Tissue irritation:* Vancomycin is irritating to tissue and must be given by a secure IV route of administration. Pain, tenderness, and necrosis occur with IM injection or inadvertent extravasation. Thrombophlebitis may occur, the frequency and severity of which can be minimized by administering the drug slowly as a dilute solution (2.5 to 5 g/L) and by rotating the sites of infusion. The safety and efficacy of vancomycin administration by the intrathecal (intralumbar or intraventricular) routes have not been assessed.

Reports have revealed that administration of sterile vancomycin by the intraperitoneal route during continuous ambulatory peritoneal dialysis (CAPD) has resulted in a syndrome of chemical peritonitis. This syndrome has ranged from a cloudy dialysate alone to a cloudy dialysate accompanied by variable degrees of abdominal pain and fever. This syndrome appears to be short-lived after discontinuation of intraperitoneal vancomycin.

➤*Nephrotoxicity:* The risk of toxicity may be appreciably increased by high serum concentrations or prolonged therapy. Factors that may increase the risk of nephrotoxicity include use in elderly and neonatal patients and concomitant use with other nephrotoxic drugs.

➤*Renal function impairment:* Because of its nephrotoxicity, use carefully in renal insufficiency.

➤*Elderly:* Total systemic and renal clearance of vancomycin may be reduced in the elderly. The natural decrement of glomerular filtration with increasing age may lead to elevated vancomycin serum concentrations if dosage is not adjusted. Adjust dosage schedules in elderly patients.

➤*Pregnancy: Category C; Category B* (pulvules only). In a controlled clinical study, the potential ototoxic and nephrotoxic effects of vancomycin on infants were evaluated when the drug was administered to pregnant women for serious staphylococcal infections complicating IV drug abuse. Vancomycin was found in cord blood. No sensorineural hearing loss or nephrotoxicity attributable to the drug was noted. One infant whose mother received vancomycin in the third trimester experienced conductive hearing loss that was not attributable to administration of the drug. Because the number of patients treated in this study was limited, and the drug was administered only in the second and third trimesters, it is not known whether vancomycin can cause fetal harm. Give to a pregnant woman only if clearly needed.

➤*Lactation:* Vancomycin is excreted in breast milk. Exercise caution when administering the drug to a nursing woman. Because of the potential for adverse events, decide whether to discontinue nursing or to discontinue the drug, taking into account the importance of the drug to the mother.

➤*Children:* In premature and full-term neonates it may be appropriate to confirm desired vancomycin serum concentrations. Concomitant administration of vancomycin and anesthetic agents has been associated with erythema and histamine-like flushing (see Drug Interactions).

Precautions

➤*Monitoring:* Perform auditory function serial tests and monitor serum levels. When monitoring vancomycin serum levels, draw a peak concentration 1.5 to 2.5 hours after the completion of a 1–hour infusion and a trough concentration within 1 hour of the next scheduled dose. Peak levels are generally expected to be in the 30 to 40 mcg/ml range and trough levels in the 10 to 15 mcg/ml range. The relationship between vancomycin levels and ototoxicity and nephrotoxicity is not well established.

➤*Systemic absorption:* Clinically significant serum concentrations may occur in some patients who have taken multiple oral doses for active *C. difficile*-induced pseudomembranous colitis or who have inflammatory disorders of the intestinal mucosa; the risk is greater with the presence of renal impairment.

➤*Red Man (or Redneck) syndrome:* This is characterized by a sudden and profound fall in blood pressure with or without a maculopapular rash over the face, neck, upper chest, and extremities. The reaction appears to be at least partially mediated through a histaminergic response.

The reaction is usually stimulated by a too rapid IV infusion (dose given over a few minutes), but it has been reported rarely when given as recommended (up to a 2–hour administration) and following oral or intraperitoneal administration. This is not an allergic-type reaction. The onset may occur anytime within a few minutes of starting an IV infusion, to a short time after infusion completion. The rash generally resolves several hours after termination of administration.

Monitor blood pressure throughout the infusion; if treatment is necessary, fluids, antihistamines, or corticosteroids may be beneficial. Pretreatment with either H_1 blockers, H_2 blockers, or both may protect against the hypotension that may occur. Also, desensitization may be useful in managing certain refractory hypersensitivity cases by using sequential increments of vancomycin over several days, allowing for adminstration of therapeutic doses.

➤*Superinfection:* Use of antibiotics (especially prolonged therapy) may result in overgrowth of non-susceptible organisms. Such overgrowth may lead to a secondary infection. Take appropriate measures if superinfection occurs.

Drug Interactions

Vancomycin Drug Interactions			
Precipitant drug	Object drug[*]		Description
Vancomycin	Aminoglycosides	↑	The risk of nephrotoxicity may be increased above that associated with aminoglycoside use alone.
Vancomycin	Anesthetics	↑	Concomitant use has been associated with erythema and histamine-like flushing in children.
Vancomycin	Neurotoxic/ Nephrotoxic agents	↑	Concurrent or sequential systemic or topical use requires careful monitoring.
Vancomycin	Nondepolarizing muscle relaxants	↑	Neuromuscular blockade may be enhanced.

[*] ↑ = Object drug increased.

VANCOMYCIN

Adverse Reactions

➤*Hematologic:* Neutropenia (appears to be promptly reversible when the drug is discontinued), usually starting ≥ 1 week after onset of therapy or after a total dosage of > 25 g; thrombocytopenia (rare).

➤*Renal:* Renal failure (rare), principally manifested by increased serum creatinine or BUN concentrations especially in patients given large doses. Interstitial nephritis (rare), mostly in patients who were given aminoglycosides concomitantly or who had preexisting kidney dysfunction; when vancomycin was discontinued, azotemia resolved in most patients.

➤*Special senses:* Hearing loss (most patients had kidney dysfunction or a preexisting hearing loss or were receiving concomitant treatment with an ototoxic drug); vertigo, dizziness, tinnitus (rare).

➤*Miscellaneous:* Anaphylaxis, drug fever, nausea, chills, eosinophilia, rashes (including exfoliative dermatitis), Stevens-Johnson syndrome (infrequent); toxic epidermal necrolysis; vasculitis (rare).

Chemical peritonitis has been reported following intraperitoneal administration of vancomycin (see Warnings).

Parenteral – Hypotension; wheezing; dyspnea; urticaria; pruritus; inflammation at the site of injection; Redneck or Red Man syndrome (see Precautions). These reactions usually resolve within 20 minutes but may persist for several hours.

Overdosage

Supportive care is advised with maintenance of glomerular filtration. Vancomycin is poorly removed by dialysis. Hemofiltration and hemoperfusion with polysulfone resin have increased vancomycin clearance.

Patient Information

Complete full course of therapy; do not discontinue therapy without notifying physician.

LINEZOLID

Rx	Zyvox (Pharmacia)	Tablets: 400 mg[1]	(ZYVOX 400mg). White, oblong. Film-coated. In 20s, 100s, and UD 30s.
		600 mg[2]	(ZYVOX 600mg). White, capsule-shape. Film-coated. In 20s, 100s, and UD 30s.
		Powder for oral suspension: 100 mg/5 mL[3]	Sucrose, aspartame, mannitol, 20 mg phenylalanine. Orange flavor. In 240 mL.
		Injection: 2 mg/mL[4]	Sodium citrate. In 100, 200, and 300 mL single-use, ready to use bags.

[1] Sodium content is 1.95 mg/400 mg tablet (0.1 mEq/tablet).
[2] Sodium content is 2.92 mg/600 mg tablet (0.1 mEq/tablet).
[3] Sodium content is 8.52 mg/5 mL (0.4 mEq/5 mL).

[4] Sodium content is 0.38 mg/mL (5 mEq/300 mL bag, 3.3 mEq/200 mL bag, 1.7 mEq/100 mL bag).

Indications

➤*Vancomycin-resistant Enterococcus faecium infections:* For the treatment of vancomycin-resistant *E. faecium* infections including cases with concurrent bacteremia.

➤*Nosocomial pneumonia:* For the treatment of nosocomial pneumonia caused by *Staphylococcus aureus* (methicillin-susceptible and -resistant strains) or *Streptococcus pneumoniae* (penicillin-susceptible strains). Combination therapy may be indicated if the documented or presumptive pathogens include gram-negative organisms.

➤*Complicated skin and skin-structure infections:* For the treatment of complicated skin and skin-structure infections, including diabetic foot infections without concomitant osteomyelitis, caused by *S. aureus* (methicillin-susceptible and -resistant strains), *S. pyogenes*, or *S. agalactiae.* It has not been studied in the treatment of decubitus ulcers. Combination therapy may be clinically indicated if the documented or presumptive pathogens include gram-negative organisms.

➤*Uncomplicated skin and skin-structure infections:* For the treatment of uncomplicated skin and skin-structure infections caused by *S. aureus* (methicillin-susceptible strains only) or *S. pyogenes.*

➤*Community-acquired pneumonia:* For the treatment of community-acquired pneumonia caused by *S. pneumoniae* (penicillin-susceptible strains only), including cases with concurrent bacteremia, or *S. aureus* (methicillin-susceptible strains only).

Because of concerns about inappropriate use of antibiotics leading to an increase in resistant organisms, carefully consider alternatives before initiating treatment with linezolid in the outpatient setting.

Administration and Dosage

➤*Approved by the FDA:* April 18, 2000.

Administer without regard to meals.

Linezolid Dosage Guidelines

Infection[1]	Dosage and route of administration — Pediatric patients[2] (birth through 11 years of age)	Dosage and route of administration — Adults and adolescents (12 years and older)	Recommended duration of treatment (consecutive days)
Complicated skin and skin-structure infections	10 mg/kg IV or oral[3] q 8 h	600 mg IV or oral[3] q 12 h	10 to 14
Community-acquired pneumonia, including concurrent bacteremia			
Nosocomial pneumonia			
Vancomycin-resistant Enterococcus faecium infections, including concurrent bacteremia	10 mg/kg IV or oral[3] q 8 h	600 mg IV or oral[3] q 12 h	14 to 28
Uncomplicated skin and skin-structure infections	< 5 yrs: 10 mg/kg oral[3] q 8 h; 5 to 11 yrs: 10 mg/kg oral[3] q 12 h	*Adults:* 400 mg oral[3] q 12 h; *Adolescents:* 600 mg oral[3] q 12 h	10 to 14

[1] Due to the designated pathogens.
[2] Neonates younger than 7 days: Most preterm neonates younger than 7 days of age (gestational age less than 34 weeks) have lower systemic linezolid clearance values and larger AUC values than many full-term neonates and older infants. Initiate these neonates with a dosing regimen of 10 mg/kg twice daily. Consider the use of 10 mg/kg 3 times daily regimen in neonates with a suboptimal clinical response. Give all neonatal patients 10 mg/kg 3 times daily by 7 days of life.
[3] Oral dosing using either linezolid tablets or linezolid for oral suspension.

Treat adult patients with methicillin-resistant *S. aureus* (MRSA) infection with linezolid 600 mg/12 hours.

No dose adjustment is necessary when switching from IV to oral administration. Patients who are started on IV therapy may be switched to either tablets or oral suspension when clinically indicated.

➤*IV administration:* Administer over a period of 30 to 120 minutes. Do not use an IV infusion bag in series connections. Do not introduce additives into this solution. Do not administer concomitantly with another drug; administer each drug separately.

➤*Compatible IV solutions:* 5% dextrose injection, 0.9% NaCl injection; lactated Ringer's injection.

➤*Admixture incompatibilities:* Physical incompatibilities resulted when linezolid IV injection was combined with the following drugs during simulated Y-site administration: Amphotericin B, chlorpromazine HCl, diazepam, pentamidine isethionate, erythromycin lactobionate, phenytoin sodium, and trimethoprim-sulfamethoxazole. Additionally, chemical incompatibility resulted when linezolid IV injection was combined with ceftriaxone sodium.

If the same IV line is used for sequential infusion of several drugs, flush the line before and after infusion of IV injection with an infusion solution compatible with linezolid IV injection and with any other drugs administered via this common line.

➤*Storage/Stability:*

Tablets – Store at 25°C (77°F); excursions permitted to 15° to 30°C (59° to 86°F). Protect from light. Keep bottles tightly closed to protect from moisture.

IV – Keep the infusion bags in the overwrap until ready to use. Store at room temperature. Protect from freezing. Linezolid IV injection may exhibit a yellow color that can intensify over time without adversely affecting potency.

Oral suspension – Store reconstituted suspension at room temperature. Store at room temperature. Use within 21 days after reconstitution.

Actions

➤*Pharmacology:* Linezolid binds to a site on the bacterial 23S ribosomal RNA of the 50S subunit and thus inhibits protein synthesis. The results of time-kill studies have shown linezolid to be bacteriostatic against *Enterococci* and *Staphylococci.* For *Streptococci*, linezolid was found to be bactericidal for the majority of strains.

Linezolid is a synthetic antibacterial agent of oxazolidinones, which has clinical utility in the treatment of infections caused by aerobic gram-positive bacteria. The in vitro spectrum of activity of linezolid also includes certain gram-negative bacteria and anaerobic bacteria. Linezolid inhibits bacterial protein synthesis through a mechanism of action different from that of other antibacterial agents; therefore, cross-resistance between linezolid and other classes of antibiotics is unlikely.

Mean Pharmacokinetic Parameters of Linezolid in Adults

Dose of linezolid	C_{max} (mcg/mL)	C_{min} (mcg/mL)	T_{max} (h)	AUC (mcg•h/mL)	$t_{1/2}$ (h)	CL (mL/min)
400 mg tablet						
single dose[1]	8.10	—	1.52	55.10	5.20	146
every 12 hours	11.00	3.08	1.12	73.40	4.69	110
600 mg tablet						
single dose	12.70	—	1.28	91.40	4.26	127
every 12 hours	21.20	6.15	1.03	138.00	5.40	80
600 mg IV injection[2]						
single dose	12.90	—	0.50	80.20	4.40	138
every 12 hours	15.10	3.68	0.51	89.70	4.80	123
600 mg oral suspension						
single dose	11.00	—	0.97	80.80	4.60	141

[1] Data dose-normalized from 375 mg.
[2] Date dose-normalized from 625 mg; IV dose was given as 0.5-hour infusion.

➤*Pharmacokinetics:*

Absorption – Linezolid is rapidly and extensively absorbed after oral dosing with an absolute bioavailability of approximately 100%. The half-life is 4.4 to 5.5 hours. Steady state is achieved after 3 days of twice-daily dosing. Peak concentrations are reached within 1 to 2 hours. The time to reach the maximum concentration is delayed from 1.5 hours to 2.2 hours and C_{max} is decreased by about 17% when high-fat food is given with linezolid.

Distribution – The plasma protein binding of linezolid is approximately 31% and is concentration-independent. The volume of distribution of linezolid at steady state averaged 40 to 50 L in healthy adult volunteers.

Metabolism – Linezolid is primarily metabolized by oxidation of the morpholine ring, which results in 2 inactive ring-opened carboxylic acid

LINEZOLID

metabolites: The aminoethoxyacetic acid metabolite (A) and the hydroxyethyl glycine metabolite (B). Formation of metabolite B is mediated by a nonenzymatic chemical oxidation mechanism in vitro. Linezolid is not an inducer of cytochrome P450 (CYP) in rats, and it has been demonstrated from in vitro studies that linezolid is not detectably metabolized by human cytochrome P450 and it does not inhibit the activities of clinically significant human CYP isoforms (eg, 1A2, 2C9, 2C19, 2D6, 2E1, 3A4).

Excretion – Nonrenal clearance accounts for approximately 65% of the total clearance of linezolid. Under steady-state conditions, approximately 30% of the dose appears in the urine as linezolid, 40% as metabolite B, and 10% as metabolite A. The renal clearance of linezolid is low (average, 40 mL/min) and suggests net tubular reabsorption. Virtually no linezolid appears in the feces, while approximately 6% of the dose appears in the feces as metabolite B and 3% as metabolite A.

A small degree of nonlinearity in clearance was observed with increasing doses of linezolid, which appears to be caused by lower renal and nonrenal clearance of linezolid at higher concentrations. However, the difference in clearance was small and was not reflected in the apparent elimination half-life.

Special populations –

Children: The C_{max} and the volume of distribution (V_{ss}) of linezolid are similar regardless of age in pediatric patients. However, clearance of linezolid varies as a function of age. With the exclusion of preterm neonates less than 1 week of age, clearance is most rapid in the youngest age groups ranging from older than 1 week old to 11 years of age, resulting in lower single-dose AUC and shorter half-life as compared with adults. As age of pediatric patients increases, the clearance of linezolid gradually decreases, and by adolescence mean clearance values approach those observed for the adult population. There is wider intersubject variability in linezolid clearance and AUC across all pediatric age groups as compared with adults. Similar mean daily AUC values were observed in pediatric patients from birth to 11 years of age dosed every 8 hours relative to adolescents or adults dosed every 12 hours.

Recommendations for the dosage regimen for preterm neonates younger than 7 days of age (gestational age less than 34 weeks) are based on pharmacokinetic data from 9 preterm neonates. Most of these preterm neonates have lower systemic linezolid clearance values and larger AUC values than many full-term neonates and older infants. Therefore, initiate these preterm neonates with a dosing regimen of 10 mg/kg twice daily. Consideration may be given to the use of a 10 mg/kg 3 times daily regimen in neonates with a suboptimal clinical response. Give all neonatal patients 10 mg/kg 3 times daily by 7 days of life.

Gender: Females have a slightly lower volume of distribution of linezolid than males. Plasma concentrations are higher in females than in males, which is partly due to body weight differences. After a 600 mg dose, mean oral clearance is approximately 38% lower in females than in males. However, there are no significant gender differences in mean apparent elimination-rate constant or half-life. Thus, drug exposure in females is not expected to substantially increase beyond levels known to be well tolerated. Therefore, dose adjustment by gender does not appear to be necessary.

Renal function impairment: The pharmacokinetics of the parent drug, linezolid, are not altered in patients with any degree of renal insufficiency; however, the two primary metabolites of linezolid may accumulate in patients with renal insufficiency, with the amount of accumulation increasing with the severity of renal dysfunction. The clinical significance of accumulation of these two metabolites has not been determined in patients with severe renal insufficiency. Given the absence of information on the clinical significance of accumulation of the primary metabolites, weigh the use of linezolid in patients with renal insufficiency against the potential risks of accumulation of these metabolites. Linezolid and the two metabolites are eliminated by dialysis. No information is available on the effect of peritoneal dialysis on the pharmacokinetics of linezolid. Approximately 30% of a dose was eliminated in a 3-hour dialysis session beginning 3 hours after the dose of linezolid was administered; therefore, give linezolid after hemodialysis.

►*Microbiology:* In clinical trials, resistance to linezolid developed in 6 patients infected with *E. faecium* (4 patients received 200 mg twice daily, lower than the recommended dose, and 2 patients received 600 mg twice daily). In a compassionate-use program, resistance to linezolid developed in 8 patients with *E. faecium* and in 1 patient with *E. faecalis*. All patients had either unremoved prosthetic devices or undrained abscesses. In vitro studies have shown that point mutations in the 23S rRNA are associated with linezolid resistance. Reports of vancomycin-resistant *E. faecium* becoming resistant to linezolid during its clinical use have been published. In one report, nosocomial spread of vancomycin- and linezolid-resistant *E. faecium* occurred. There has been a report of *S. aureus* (methicillin-resistant) developing resistance to linezolid during its clinical use.

In vitro studies have demonstrated additivity or indifference between linezolid and vancomycin, gentamicin, rifampin, imipenem-cilastatin, aztreonam, ampicillin, or streptomycin.

Linezolid has been shown to be active against most isolates of the following microorganisms, both in vitro and in clinical infections (see Indications).

Aerobic and facultative gram-positive microorganisms – *E. faecium* (vancomycin-resistant strains only); *S. aureus* (including methicillin-resistant strains); *S. agalactiae*; *S. pneumoniae* (penicillin-susceptible strains only); *S. pyogenes*.

►*Clinical trials:*

Nosocomial pneumonia – Adult patients with clinically and radiologically documented nosocomial pneumonia were enrolled in a randomized, double-blind trial. Patients were treated for 7 to 21 days. One group received linezolid IV injection 600 mg twice daily, and the other group received vancomycin 1 g twice daily IV. Both groups received concomitant aztreonam (1 to 2 g three times daily IV), which could be continued if clinically indicated. The cure rates in clinically evaluable patients were 57% for linezolid-treated patients and 60% for vancomycin-treated patients. The cure rates in clinically evaluable patients with ventilator-associated pneumonia were 47% for linezolid-treatd patients and 40% for vancomycin-treated patients. The cure rates in the modified intent to treat (MITT) analysis were 57% in linezolid-treated patients and 46% in vancomycin-treated patients.

Complicated skin and skin-structure infections – Adult patients with clinically documented complicated skin and skin-structure infections were enrolled in a randomized trial comparing study medications administered IV followed by medications given orally for a total of 10 to 21 days of treatment. One group of patients received linezolid IV injection 600 mg twice daily followed by linezolid tablets 600 mg twice daily; the other group received oxacillin 2 g 4 times daily IV followed by dicloxacillin 500 mg 4 times daily orally. The cure rates in clinically evaluable patients were 90% in linezolid-treated patients and 85% in oxacillin-treated patients. The cure rates in the MITT analysis were 86% in linezolid-treated patients and 82% in oxacillin-treated patients.

A separate study provided additional experience with the use of linezolid in the treatment of methicillin-resistant *S. aureus* (MRSA) infections. This was a randomized, open-label trial in hospitalized adult patients with documented or suspected MRSA infection.

One group of patients received linezolid IV injection 600 mg twice daily followed by linezolid tablets 600 mg twice daily. The other group of patients received vancomycin 1 g twice daily IV. Both groups were treated for 7 to 28 days, and could receive concomitant aztreonam or gentamycin if clinically indicated. The cure rates in microbiologically evaluable patients with MRSA skin and skin-structure infection were 79% for linezolid-treated patients and 73% for vancomycin-treated patients.

Diabetic foot infections – Adult diabetic patients with clinically documented complicated skin and skin-structure infections (diabetic foot infections) were enrolled in a randomized, open-label trial comparing study medications administered IV or orally for a total of 14 to 28 days of treatment. One group of patients received linezolid 600 mg twice daily IV or orally; the other group received ampicillin/sulbactum 1.5 to 3 g IV or amoxicillin/clavulanate 500 to 875 mg two or three times daily orally. Patients in the comparator group could also be treated with vancomycin 1 g twice daily IV if MRSA was isolated from the foot infection. Patients in either treatment group who had gram-negative bacilli isolated from the infection site could also receive aztreonam 1 to 2 g 2 to 3 times daily IV. In the intent-to-treat (ITT) population, the cure rates were 68.5% in linezolid-treated patients and 64% in comparator-treated patients. The cure rates in the clinically evaluable patients (excluding those with indeterminate and missing outcomes) were 83% and 73% in the linezolid- and comparator-treated patients, respectively.

Pediatric patients infections due to gram-positive organisms – A safety and efficacy study provided experience on the use of linezolid in pediatric patients for the treatment of nosocomial pneumonia, complicated skin and skin-structure infections, catheter-related bacteremia, bacteremia of unidentified source, and other infections caused by gram-positive bacterial pathogens, including methicillin-resistant and -susceptible *S. aureus* and vancomycin-resistant *E. faecium*. Pediatric patients ranging in age from birth to 11 years of age with infections caused by the documented or suspected gram-positive organisms were enrolled in a randomized, controlled trial. One group of patients received linezolid IV injection 10 mg/kg three times daily followed by linezolid for oral suspension 10 mg/kg three times daily. A second group received vancomycin 10 to 15 mg/kg IV every 6 to 24 hours, depending on age and renal clearnace. Patients who had confirmed vancomycin-resistant *Enterococcus* infections were placed in a third arm of the study and received linezolid 10 mg/kg three times daily IV and/or orally. All patients were treated for a total of 10 to 28 days. In the ITT population, there were 206 patients randomized to linezolid and 102 patients randomized to vancomycin. The cure rates in ITT patients were 81% in patients randomized to linezolid and 83% in patients randomized to vancomycin. The cure rates in clinically evaluable patients were 91% in linezolid-treated patients and 91% in vancomycin-treated patients. The cure rates in MITT patients were 80% in patients randomized to linezolid and 90% in patients randomized to vancomycin.

LINEZOLID

Contraindications

Hypersensitivity to linezolid or any of the other product components.

Warnings

➤*Myelosuppression:* Myelosuppression (including anemia, leukopenia, pancytopenia, and thrombocytopenia) has been reported in patients receiving linezolid. In cases where the outcome is known when linezolid was discontinued, the affected hematologic parameters rose toward pretreatment levels. Monitor complete blood counts weekly in patients who receive linezolid, particularly in those who receive linezolid for more than 2 weeks, those with preexisting myelosuppression, those receiving concomitant drugs that produce bone marrow suppression, or those with a chronic infection who have received previous or concomitant antibiotic therapy. Consider discontinuation of therapy with linezolid in patients who develop or have worsening myelosuppression.

➤*Pseudomembranous colitis:* Pseudomembranous colitis has been reported with nearly all antibacterial agents, including linezolid, and may range in severity from mild to life-threatening. Mild cases usually respond to drug discontinuation alone. In moderate to severe cases, consider management with fluids and electrolytes, protein supplementation, and treatment with an antibacterial agent clinically effective against *Clostridium difficile*.

➤*Fertility impairment:* Linezolid did not affect the fertility or reproductive performance of adult female rats. It reversibly decreased fertility and reproductive performance in adult male rats when given at doses of 50 mg/kg/day or more, with exposures approximately equal to or greater than the expected human exposure level (exposure comparisons are based on AUCs). The reversible fertility effects were mediated through altered spermatogenesis. Affected spermatids contained abnormally formed and oriented mitochondria and were nonviable. Epithelial cell hypertrophy and hyperplasia in the epididymis was observed in conjunction with decreased fertility. Similar epididymal changes were not seen in dogs.

In sexually mature male rats exposed to linezolid as juveniles, mildly decreased fertility was observed following treatment with linezolid through most of their period of sexual development (50 mg/kg/day from days 7 to 36 of age, and 100 mg/kg/day from days 37 to 55 of age), with exposures up to 1.7-fold greater than mean AUCs observed in pediatric patients from 3 months to 11 years of age.

➤*Pregnancy: Category C.* There are no adequate and well-controlled studies in pregnant women. Use during pregnancy only if the potential benefit justifies the potential risk to the fetus.

In mice, embryo and fetal toxicities were seen only at doses that caused maternal toxicity (clinical signs and reduced body weight gain). A dose of 450 mg/kg/day correlated with increased postimplantational embryo death, including total litter loss, decreased fetal body weights, and an increased incidence of costal cartilage fusion.

In rats, mild fetal toxicity was observed at 15 and 50 mg/kg/day. The effects consisted of decreased fetal body weights and reduced ossification of sternebrae, a finding often seen in association with decreased fetal body weights. Slight maternal toxicity, in the form of reduced body weight gain, was seen at 50 mg/kg/day.

When female rats were treated with 50 mg/kg/day (approximately equivalent to the estimated human exposure based on AUCs) of linezolid during pregnancy and lactation, survival of pups was decreased on postnatal days 1 to 4. Male and female pups permitted to mature to reproductive age, when mated, showed an increase in preimplantation loss.

➤*Lactation:* Linezolid and its metabolites are excreted in the milk of lactating rats. Concentrations in milk were similar to those in maternal plasma. It is not known whether linezolid is excreted in human breast milk. Exercise caution when administering to a nursing woman.

➤*Children:* Safety and efficacy in children have been established in pediatric patients from birth to 11 years of age.

In limited clinical experience, 83% of pediatric patients with infections due to gram-positive pathogens with MIC of 4 mcg/mL treated with linezolid had clinical cures. However, pediatric patients exhibit wider variability in linezolid clearance and AUC compared with adults. In pediatric patients with a suboptimal clinical response, particularly those with pathogens with MIC of 4 mcg/mL, consider lower systemic exposure, site and severity of infection, and the underlying medical condition when assessing clinical response.

Precautions

➤*Duration of therapy:* The safety and efficacy of linezolid formulations given for more than 28 days have not been evaluated in controlled clinical trials.

➤*Phenylketonurics:* Each 5 mL of the 100 mg/5 mL oral suspension contains 20 mg phenylalanine. The other linezolid formulations do not contain phenylalanine. Advise phenylketonuric patients to contact their physician or pharmacist.

➤*Lactic acidosis:* Lactic acidosis has been reported with the use of linezolid. In reported cases, patients experienced repeated episodes of nausea and vomiting. Patients who develop recurrent nausea or vomiting, unexplained acidosis, or a low bicarbonate level while receiving linezolid should receive immediate medical evaluation.

Drug Interactions

➤*CYP450:* Linezolid is not detectably metabolized by human cytochrome P450 and it does not inhibit the activities of clinically significant human CYP isoforms. Therefore, no CYP450-induced drug interactions are expected with linezolid.

Linezolid Drug Interactions			
Precipitant drug	Object drug[*]		Description
Linezolid	Adrenergic agents (eg, dopamine and epinephrine)	↑	Linezolid is a reversible, nonselective inhibitor of monoamine oxidase. Therefore, linezolid has the potential for interaction with adrenergic agents. Reduce and titrate initial doses of adrenergic agents, such as dopamine and epinephrine, to achieve the desired response.
Linezolid	Serotonergic agents (eg, fluoxetine, paroxetine, sertraline)	↑	Linezolid has the potential for interaction with serotonergic agents. Because there is limited experience with administration of linezolid and serotonergic agents, physicians should be alert to the possibility of signs and symptoms of serotonin syndrome (eg, hyperpyrexia, cognitive dysfunction) in patients receiving concomitant therapy.

[*] ↑ = Object drug increased.

➤*Drug/Food interactions:* Advise patients to avoid large quantities of foods or beverages with high tyramine content while taking linezolid. Quantities of tyramine consumed should be less than 100 mg/meal. Foods high in tyramine content include those that may have undergone protein changes by aging, fermentation, pickling, or smoking to improve flavor, such as aged cheeses (0 to 15 mg tyramine/oz); fermented or air-dried meats (0.1 to 8 mg tyramine/oz); soy sauce (5 mg tyramine/1 tsp); tap beers (4 mg tyramine/12 oz); red wines (0 to 6 mg tyramine/8 oz). The tyramine content of any protein-rich food may be increased if stored for long periods or improperly refrigerated.

Adverse Reactions

➤*Thrombocytopenia:* Linezolid has been associated with thrombocytopenia when used in doses up to and including 600 mg twice daily for up to 28 days. In phase 3 comparator-controlled trials, the percentage of patients who developed a substantially low platelet count (defined as less than 75% of lower limit of normal and/or baseline) was 2.4% (range, 0.3% to 10%) with linezolid and 1.5% (range, 0.4% to 7%) with a comparator. In a study of hospitalized pediatric patients ranging from birth through 11 years of age, the percentage of patients who developed a substantially low platelet count (defined as less than 75% of lower limit of normal and/or baseline) was 12.9% with linezolid and 13.4% with vancomycin. In an outpatient study of pediatric patients from 5 through 17 years of age, the percentage of patients who developed a substantially low platelet count was 0% with linezolid and 0.4% with cefadroxil. Thrombocytopenia associated with the use of linezolid appears to be dependent on duration of therapy (generally more than 2 weeks of treatment). The platelet counts for most patients returned to the normal range/baseline during the follow-up period. No related clinical adverse events were identified in phase 3 clinical trials in patients developing thrombocytopenia. Bleeding events were identified in thrombocytopenic patients in a compassionate use program for linezolid; the role of linezolid in these events cannot be determined.

➤*Adults:* The most common adverse events in patients treated with linezolid were diarrhea (2.8% to 11%), headache (0.5% to 11.3%), and nausea (3.4% to 9.6%).

Adverse Events Reported in ≥ 2% of Adult Patients in Comparator-Controlled Clinical Trials with Linezolid (%)		
Adverse event	Linezolid (n = 2046)	All comparators[1] (n = 2001)
CNS		
Headache	6.5	5.5
Insomnia	2.5	1.7
Dizziness	2	1.9
GI		
Diarrhea	8.3	6.3
Nausea	6.2	4.6
Vomiting	3.7	2
Constipation	2.2	2.1
Miscellaneous		
Fever	1.6	2.1
Rash	2	2.2

[1] Comparators included cefpodoxime proxetil 200 mg PO twice daily; ceftriaxone 1 g IV twice daily; clarithromycin 250 mg PO twice daily; dicloxacillin 500 mg PO 4 times daily; oxacillin 2 g IV 4 times daily; vancomycin 1 g IV twice daily.

LINEZOLID

Other adverse events reported included oral moniliasis, vaginal moniliasis, hypertension, dyspepsia, localized abdominal pain, pruritus, and tongue discoloration.

Drug-Related Adverse Events Occurring in > 1% of Adult Patients Treated with Linezolid in Comparator-Controlled Clinical Trials (%)		
	Uncomplicated skin and skin-structure infections	All other indications
Adverse event	Linezolid 400 mg PO q 12 h (n = 548)	Linezolid 600 mg q 12 h (n = 1498)
1 drug-related adverse event	25.4	20.4
Discontinuation due to drug-related adverse events[1]	3.5	2.1
CNS		
Headache	2.7	1.9
Dizziness	1.1	0.4
GI		
Diarrhea	5.3	4
Nausea	3.5	3.3
Vomiting	0.9	1.2
Abnormal liver function	0.4	1.3
Special senses		
Taste alteration	1.8	0.9
Tongue discoloration	1.1	0.2
Miscellaneous		
Vaginal moniliasis	1.6	1
Fungal infection	1.5	0.1
Oral moniliasis	0.4	1.1

[1] The most commonly reported drug-related adverse events leading to discontinuation in patients treated with linezolid were nausea, headache, diarrhea, and vomiting.

▶*Pediatric:* In a study of hospitalized pediatric patients (birth through 11 years of age) with gram-positive infections who were randomized 2:1 (linezolid:vancomycin), mortality was 6% in the linezolid arm and 3% in the vancomycin arm. However, given the severe underlying illness in the patient population, no causality could be established.

Adverse Events Reported in Pediatric Patients Treated with Linezolid in Comparator-Controlled Clinical Trials (%)[1]		
	Uncomplicated skin and skin-structure infections[2]	All other indications[3]
Adverse event	Linezolid (n = 248)	Linezolid (n = 215)
CNS		
Headache	2.4 to 6.5	0.9
Vertigo	1.2	0
Convulsion	0	2.8
GI		
Diarrhea	5.7 to 7.8	3.8 to 10.8
Vomiting	1.2 to 2.9	1.9 to 9.4
Nausea	3.3 to 3.7	1.4 to 1.9
Dyspnea	0	3.3
Oral moniliasis	0	0.9
Generalized abdominal pain	1.6 to 2.4	0.9
Localized abdominal pain	1.6 to 2.4	0.5
Gastrointestinal bleeding	0	2.3
Loose stools	1.2 to 1.6	1.9 to 2.3
Respiratory		
Upper respiratory infection	3.7	4.2
Pharyngitis	2.9	0.5
Pneumonia	0	2.8
Cough	2.4	0.9
Dermatologic		
Rash	0.4 to 1.6	1.4 to 7
Reaction at site of injection or of vascular catheter	0	3.3
Skin disorder	2.0	0.9
Pruritus at nonapplication site	0.4	0
Hematologic		
Anemia	0	1.4 to 5.6
Thrombocytopenia	0	4.7
Eosinophilia	0.4	1.4
Thrombocythemia	0	2.8
Miscellaneous		
Fever	2.9	0.5 to 14.1
Sepsis	0	8

Adverse Events Reported in Pediatric Patients Treated with Linezolid in Comparator-Controlled Clinical Trials (%)[1]		
	Uncomplicated skin and skin-structure infections[2]	All other indications[3]
Adverse event	Linezolid (n = 248)	Linezolid (n = 215)
Trauma	3.3	2.8
Anaphylaxis	0	0
Hypokalemia	0	2.8
Apnea	0	2.3
Generalized edema	0	2.3
Localized pain	2	0.9

[1] Data from pooled trials; not necessarily comparable.
[2] Patients 5 through 11 years of age received linezolid 10 mg/kg PO twice daily. Patients 12 years or older received linezolid 600 mg PO twice daily.
[3] Patients from birth through 11 years of age received linezolid 10 mg/kg IV/PO 3 times daily.

▶*Lab test abnormalities:*
Adults –

Adult Patients Who Experienced At Least One Substantially Abnormal Laboratory Value in Comparator-Controlled Clinical Trials with Linezolid (%)		
	Uncomplicated skin and skin-structure infections	All other indications
Laboratory assay		
Hematology[1]		
Hemoglobin (g/dL)	0.9	7.1
Platelet count ($\times 10^3/mm^3$)	0.7	3
WBC ($\times 10^3/mm^3$)	0.2	2.2
Neutrophils ($\times 10^3/mm^3$)	0	1.1
Serum chemistry[2]		
AST (U/L)	1.7	5
ALT (U/L)	1.7	9.6
LDH (U/L)	0.2	1.8
Alkaline phosphatase (U/L)	0.2	3.5
Lipase (U/L)	2.8	4.3
Amylase (U/L)	0.2	2.4
Total bilirubin (mg/dL)	0.2	0.9
BUN (mg/dL)	0.2	2.1
Creatinine (mg/dL)	0.2	0.2

[1] < 75% (< 50% for neutrophils) of Lower Limit of Normal (LLN) for values normal at baseline; < 75% (< 50% for neutrophils) of LLN of baseline for values abnormal at baseline.
[2] > 2 × Upper Limit of Normal (ULN) for values normal at baseline;> 2 × ULN and > 2 × baseline for values abnormal at baseline.

Pediatric –

Pediatric Patients Who Experience At Least One Substantially Abnormal Laboratory Value in Comparator-Controlled Clinical Trials with Linezolid (%)		
	Uncomplicated skin and skin-structure infections[1]	All other indications[2]
Laboratory assay	Linezolid	Linezolid
Hematology[3]		
Hemoglobulin (g/dL)	0	15.7
Platelet count ($\times 10^3/mm^3$)	0	12.9
WBC ($\times 10^3/mm^3$)	0.8	12.4
Neutrophils $\times 10^3/mm^3$)	1.2	5.9
Serum chemistry[4]		
ALT (U/L)	0	10.1
Lipase (U/L)	0.4	—
Anylase (U/L)	—	0.6
Total bilirubin (mg/dL)	—	6.3
Creatinine (mg/dL)	0.4	2.4

[1] Patients 5 through 11 years of age received linezolid 10 mg/kg PO twice daily. Patients 12 years or older received linezolid 600 mg PO twice daily.
[2] Patients from birth through 11 years of age received linezolid 10 mg/kg IV/PO three times daily.
[3] < 75% (< 50% for neutrophils) of LLN for values normal at baseline; < 75% (< 50% for neutrophils) of LLN and < 75% (< 50% for neutrophils, < 90% for hemogloblin if baseline < LLN) of baseline for values abnormal at baseline.
[4] > 2 × ULN for values normal at baseline; > 2 × ULN and > 2 (> 1.5 for total bilirubin) × baseline for values abnormal at baseline.

▶*Postmarketing:* Myelosuppression (including anemia, leukopenia, pancytopenia, and thrombocytopenia), neuropathy (eg, peripheral, optic), and lactic acidosis have been reported with the use of linezolid. Although these reports have primarily been in patients treated for longer than the maximum recommended duration of 28 days, these events have also been reported in patients receiving shorter courses of therapy.

LINEZOLID

Overdosage

➤*Treatment:* In the event of overdosage, supportive care is advised, with maintenance of glomerular filtration. Hemodialysis may facilitate more rapid elimination of linezolid. In a phase 1 clinical trial, approximately 30% of a dose of linezolid was removed during a 3-hour hemodialysis session beginning 3 hours after the dose of linezolid was administered. Data are not available for removal of linezolid with peritoneal dialysis or hemoperfusion. Clinical signs of acute toxicity in animals included decreased activity and ataxia in rats and vomiting and tremors in dogs treated with 3000 mg/kg/day and 2000 mg/kg/day, respectively.

Patient Information

Advise patients that linezolid may be taken with or without food.

Advise patients to inform their physician if they have a history of hypertension.

Avoid large quantities of food or beverages with high tyramine content while taking linezolid. Quantities of tyramine consumed should be less than 100 mg/meal. Foods high in tyramine content include those that may have undergone protein changes by aging, fermentation, pickling, or smoking to improve flavor, such as aged cheeses (0 to 15 mg tyramine/oz); fermented or air-dried meats (0.1 to 8 mg tyramine/oz); sauerkraut (8 mg tyramine/8 oz); soy sauce (5 mg tyramine/1 tsp); tap beers (4 mg tyramine/12 oz); red wines (0 to 6 mg tyramine/8 oz). The tyramine content of any protein-rich food may be increased if stored for long periods or improperly refrigerated.

Inform physician if taking medications containing pseudoephedrine, such as cold remedies and decongestants.

Inform physician if taking serotonin reuptake inhibitors or other antidepressants.

Each 5 mL of the 100 mg/5 mL oral suspension contains 20 mg phenylalanine. The other formulations do not contain phenylalanine.

WARNING

These agents can cause severe and possibly fatal colitis, characterized by severe persistent diarrhea, severe abdominal cramps, and possibly the passage of blood and mucus. Endoscopic examination may reveal pseudomembranous colitis. Toxin(s) produced by *Clostridia* is a primary cause of antibiotic-associated colitis.

When significant diarrhea occurs, discontinue the drug or, if necessary, continue only with close observation of the patient. Large bowel endoscopy is recommended.

Mild colitis may respond to stopping drug. Promptly manage moderate-to-severe cases with fluid, electrolyte, and protein supplements as indicated. Systemic corticosteroids and corticosteroid retention enemas may help relieve the colitis. Also consider other causes such as previous sensitivities to drugs or other allergens.

Antiperistaltic agents such as opiates and diphenoxylate with atropine may prolong or aggravate the condition. Diarrhea, colitis, and pseudomembranous colitis can begin up to several weeks following cessation of therapy.

Vancomycin is effective in antibiotic-associated pseudomembranous colitis produced by *C. difficile.* (See individual monograph for complete information.)

Reserve for serious infections where less toxic antimicrobial agents are inappropriate (see Indications). Do not use in patients with nonbacterial infections (ie, most upper respiratory tract infections).

Indications

➤*Serious infections:* Treatment of serious infections due to susceptible strains of streptococci, pneumococci, and staphylococci. Reserve use for penicillin-allergic patients or when penicillin is inappropriate. Because of the risk of colitis (see Warning Box), consider the nature of the infection and the suitability of less toxic alternatives (eg, erythromycin).

For specific indications, refer to individual monographs.

Actions

➤*Pharmacology:* **Lincomycin** and **clindamycin** (7-deoxy, 7-chloro derivative of lincomycin), known collectively as lincosamides, bind exclusively to the 50S subunit of bacterial ribosomes and suppress protein synthesis. Cross-resistance has been demonstrated between these two agents. Clindamycin is preferred because it is better absorbed and more potent.

➤*Pharmacokinetics:* Administration with food markedly impairs **lincomycin** (but not **clindamycin**) oral absorption. Both agents achieve significant tissue penetration; lincomycin may reach cerebrospinal fluid (CSF) concentration 40% of serum levels with inflamed meninges, but neither crosses well if meninges are normal.

Lincomycin – Levels above the MIC for most gram-positive organisms are maintained with oral doses of 500 mg for 6 to 8 hours and for 14 hours after a 600 mg IV infusion. Following a 600 mg IM dose, detectable levels persist for 24 hours.

Clindamycin – Serum levels exceed MIC for most indicated organisms ≥ 6 hours after recommended doses. Maintain levels above in vitro MIC for most indicated organisms by giving clindamycin phosphate every 8 to 12 hours to adults, every 6 to 8 hours to children, or by continuous IV infusion. Equilibrium is reached by dose 3.

Select Pharmacokinetic Parameters of Lincosamides

Lincosamides	Bioavailability (%)	Mean peak serum level (mcg/mL)	Time to peak serum level (hours)	Protein binding (%)	Half-life (hours)	Elimination (%) Hepatic	Elimination (%) Unchanged in urine (range)	Elimination (%) Feces
Clindamycin[1]								
Oral	90	2.5	0.75	≈ 90	2.4 to 3[3]	> 90	10	3.6
IM		6 to 9	1 to 3					
IV		7 to 14	0[2]					
Lincomycin								
Oral	20 to 30	1.8 to 5.3	2 to 4	57-72	4.4 to 6.4	> 90	4 (1 to 31)	40
IM		9.3 to 18.5	0.5				17.3 (2 to 25)	
IV		15.9 to 20.9	0				13.8 (5 to 30)	

[1] Clindamycin palmitate and phosphate are rapidly hydrolyzed to the base.
[2] By end of infusion, peak levels are reached.
[3] Increased slightly in patients with markedly reduced renal or hepatic function.

➤*Microbiology:*

Organisms Generally Susceptible to Lincosamides

	Microorganism	Lincosamides Lincomycin	Lincosamides Clindamycin
✔ = generally susceptible			
Gram-positive	*Staphylococcus aureus*	✔	✔
	S. epidermidis[1]	✔	✔
	S. albus	✔	
	Streptococcus pneumoniae	✔	✔
	S. pyogenes	✔	✔
	β-hemolytic streptococci	✔	
	S. viridans	✔	✔
	Pneumococci		✔
	Corynebacterium diphtheriae	✔	✔
	Diplococcus pneumoniae	✔	
	Corynebacterium acnes	✔	
	Nocardia asteroides	✔	✔
Anaerobes	*Bacteroides* sp.	✔	✔[2]
	Fusobacterium sp.		✔
	Propionibacterium (same as *C. acnes*)	✔	✔
	Eubacterium sp.	✔	✔
	Actinomyces sp.	✔	✔
	Peptococcus sp.	✔	✔
	Peptostreptococcus sp.	✔	✔
	Microaerophilic streptococci		✔
	Clostridium perfringens	✔	✔
	C. tetani	✔	✔
	Veillonella sp.		✔

[1] Penicillinase and nonpenicillinase.
[2] Including *B. fragilis* and *B. melaninogenicus.*

Contraindications

Hypersensitivity to lincosamides; treatment of minor bacterial or viral infections.

Warnings

➤*Meningitis:* **Clindamycin** does not diffuse adequately into CSF; not for meningitis.

➤*Hypersensitivity reactions:* Use with caution in patients with a history of asthma or significant allergies. If hypersensitivity occurs, discontinue the drug and institute emergency treatment. Refer to Management of Acute Hypersensitivity Reactions.

➤*Renal/Hepatic function impairment:* Cautiously give **clindamycin** to patients with severe renal or hepatic disease accompanied by severe metabolic aberrations; monitor serum clindamycin levels during high-dose therapy. Use of **lincomycin** in preexisting liver disease is not recommended unless special circumstances so indicate.

➤*Elderly:* Older patients with associated severe illness may not tolerate diarrhea well; carefully monitor these patients for changes in bowel frequency.

➤*Pregnancy: Category B* (**clindamycin**). Safety has not been established. **Clindamycin** and **lincomycin** cross the placenta in amounts ≈ 50% and 25% of maternal serum levels, respectively.

➤*Lactation:* **Clindamycin** appears in breast milk in ranges of 0.7 to 3.8 mcg/mL following doses of 150 mg orally to 600 mg IV. **Lincomycin** appears in breast milk in ranges of 0.5 to 2.4 mcg/mL. Breastfeeding is probably best discontinued when taking these agents to avoid potential problems in the infant. However, the American Academy of Pediatrics considers clindamycin to be compatible with breastfeeding.

➤*Children:* **Lincomycin** is not indicated for use in the newborn. When **clindamycin** is administered to newborns and infants, monitor organ system functions. Each mL of clindamycin and lincomycin contains 9.45 mg benzyl alcohol (see Precautions).

Precautions

➤*Monitoring:* For prolonged therapy, perform liver/kidney function tests, blood counts.

➤*IV infusion:* Do NOT inject IV undiluted as a bolus; infuse over ≥ 10 to 60 minutes as directed in Administration and Dosage.

➤*GI disease:* Use cautiously in patients with GI disease, particularly colitis.

➤*Benzyl alcohol:* Some of these products contain benzyl alcohol which has been associated with fatal "gasping syndrome" in premature infants.

➤*Superinfection:* Use of antibiotics may result in bacterial or fungal overgrowth of nonsusceptible organisms, particularly yeasts. Such overgrowth may lead to a secondary infection. Take appropriate measures if superinfection occurs.

➤*Tartrazine sensitivity:* Some products contain tartrazine, which may cause allergic-type reactions (including bronchial asthma) in susceptible individuals. Although incidence of tartrazine sensitivity in the general population is low, it is frequently seen in patients who also have aspirin hypersensitivity. Refer to product listings.

Drug Interactions

Lincosamide Drug Interactions			
Precipitant drug	Object drug*		Description
Erythromycin	Lincosamides	↓	Antagonism has occurred in vitro between clindamycin and erythromycin.
Kaolin-Pectin	Lincosamides	↓	GI absorption is decreased for lincomycin and delayed for clindamycin when they are administered with kaolin-pectin antidiarrheals.
Lincosamides	Neuromuscular blockers	↑	The actions of the nondepolarizing neuromuscular blockers may be enhanced, possibly contributing to profound and severe respiratory depression.

* ↑ = Object drug increased. ↓ = Object drug decreased.

➤*Drug/Food interactions:* Food impairs the absorption of **lincomycin**; do not take anything by mouth (except water) for 1 to 2 hours before and after lincomycin. **Clindamycin** absorption is not affected by food.

Adverse Reactions

➤*Cardiovascular:* Hypotension, cardiopulmonary arrest after too rapid IV use (rare).

➤*GI:* Diarrhea (clindamycin 2% to 20%); pseudomembranous colitis (clindamycin 0.01% to 10%; more frequent with oral administration); nausea; vomiting; abdominal pain, esophagitis (clindamycin); unpleasant or metallic taste (following higher doses of IV clindamycin); glossitis, stomatitis, pruritus ani (lincomycin).

➤*Hematologic:* Neutropenia; leukopenia; agranulocytosis; thrombocytopenic purpura; aplastic anemia, pancytopenia (rare) (lincomycin).

➤*Hepatic:* Jaundice; liver function test abnormalities (serum transaminase elevations).

➤*Hypersensitivity:* Skin rashes, urticaria, erythema multiforme, some cases resembling Stevens-Johnson syndrome (rare); anaphylaxis; maculopapular rash, generalized morbilliform-like rash (clindamycin); angioneurotic edema, serum sickness (lincomycin).

➤*Local:* Pain following injection. Induration and sterile abscess have occurred after IM injection and thrombophlebitis after IV infusion with clindamycin; give deep IM injections and avoid prolonged use of IV catheters.

➤*Renal:* Dysfunction has been characterized by azotemia, oliguria, and proteinuria (rare).

➤*Special senses:* Tinnitus, vertigo (lincomycin).

➤*Miscellaneous:* Transient eosinophilia, polyarthritis (rare) (clindamycin); vaginitis, exfoliative, vesiculobullous dermatitis (rare) (lincomycin).

Patient Information

May cause diarrhea; notify physician if this occurs. Do not treat diarrhea without notifying the physician.

Take each dose with a full glass of water. Complete full course of therapy.

Do not take anything by mouth (except water) for 1 to 2 hours before and after lincomycin. Clindamycin may be taken without regard to meals.

LINCOMYCIN

Rx	Lincocin (Upjohn)	**Capsules:** 500 mg (as HCl)	Lactose. Powder blue and dark blue. In 100s.
Rx	Lincocin (Upjohn)	**Injection:** 300 mg (as HCl)/ml	In 2 and 10 ml vials.[1]

[1] With 9.45 mg benzyl alcohol per ml.

For complete prescribing information, refer to the Lincosamides group monograph.

Indications

➤*Serious infections:* Treatment of serious infections due to susceptible strains of streptococci, pneumococci, and staphylococci resistant to other antibiotics. Administer concomitantly with other antimicrobial agents when indicated.

Administration and Dosage

If significant diarrhea occurs during therapy, this antibiotic should be discontinued.

➤*Oral:* Take at least 1 to 2 hours before or after eating to ensure optimum absorption.

Adults –
Serious infections: 500 mg every 8 hours.
More severe infections: ≥ 500 mg every 6 hours. With β-hemolytic streptococcal infections, continue treatment for at least 10 days to diminish the likelihood of subsequent rheumatic fever or glomerulonephritis.

Children > 1 month of age –
Serious infections: 30 mg/kg/day (15 mg/lb/day) divided into 3 or 4 equal doses.
More severe infections: 60 mg/kg/day (30 mg/lb/day) divided into 3 or 4 equal doses.

➤*IM:* IM administration is well tolerated.

Adults –
Serious infections: 600 mg every 24 hours.
More severe infections: 600 mg every 12 hours or more often.

Children > 1 month of age –
Serious infections: 10 mg/kg (5 mg/lb) every 24 hours.
More severe infections: 10 mg/kg (5 mg/lb) every 12 hours or more often.

➤*IV:* Dilute to 1 g/100 mL (minimum) and infuse over a period of at least 1 hour. Severe cardiopulmonary reactions have occurred when given at greater than the recommended concentration and rate. IV administration in 250 to 500 mL of 5% Dextrose in Water or Normal Saline produces no local irritation or phlebitis.

Lincomycin Infusion Rates		
Dose	Volume diluent (mL)	Time (hr)
600 mg	100	1
1 g	100	1
2 g	200	2
3 g	300	3
4 g	400	4

Adults – Determine dose by the severity of the infection.
Serious infections: 600 mg to 1 g every 8 to 12 hours.
Severe to life-threatening situations: Doses of 8 g/day have been given.
Maximum recommended dose: 8 g/day.

Children > 1 month of age – Infuse 10 to 20 mg/kg/day (5 to 10 mg/lb/day), depending on severity of infection, in divided doses as described above for adults.

➤*Subconjunctival injection:* 75 mg/0.25 mL injected subconjunctivally results in ocular fluid levels of antibiotic (lasting for at least 5 hours) with MICs sufficient for most susceptible pathogens.

➤*Renal function impairment:* When required, an appropriate dose is 25% to 30% of that recommended for patients with normal renal function.

➤*Admixture compatibilities/incompatibilities:* Compatible and incompatible determinations are physical observations only, not chemical determinations. Lincomycin is incompatible with novobiocin, kanamycin, and phenytoin sodium.

IV compatible solutions – Lincomycin is compatible with the following solutions for 24 hours at room temperature (unless otherwise indicated): Infusion solutions - 5% and 10% Dextrose in Water, 5% and 10% Dextrose in Saline, Ringer's Solution, Sodium Lactate; ⅙ Molar, *Travert 10% – Electrolyte No. 1*, Dextran in 6% Saline; vitamins in infusion solutions – B-Complex, B-Complex with ascorbic acid; antibiotics in infusion solutions - Penicillin G sodium (satisfactory for 4 hours), cephalothin, tetracycline HCl, cephaloridine, colistimethate (satisfactory for 4 hours), ampicillin, methicillin, chloramphenicol, polymyxin B sulfate.

CLINDAMYCIN

Rx	**Clindamycin HCl** (Various, eg, Danbury)	**Capsules:** 75 mg (as HCl)	In 100s.
Rx	**Cleocin** (Upjohn)		(CLEOCIN 75 mg). Tartrazine, lactose. Green. In 100s.
Rx	**Clindamycin HCl** (Various, eg, Compumed, Zenith-Goldline)	**Capsules:** 150 mg (as HCl)	In 100s.
Rx	**Cleocin** (Upjohn)		(CLEOCIN 150 mg). Tartrazine, lactose. Light blue and green. In 16s, 100s, and UD 100s.
Rx	**Clindamycin HCl** (Ranbaxy)	**Capsules:** 300 mg (as HCl)	Lactose. In 16s and 100s.
Rx	**Cleocin** (Upjohn)		(CLEOCIN 300 mg). Lactose. Light blue. In 16s, 100s, and UD 100s.
Rx	**Cleocin Pediatric** (Upjohn)	**Granules for Oral Solution:** 75 mg/5 mL (as palmitate)	Sucrose, parabens. In 100 mL.
Rx	**Clindamycin Phosphate** (Various, eg, Abbott)	**Injection:** 150 mg (as phosphate) per mL	In 2, 4, 6, 60, and 100 mL vials.
Rx	**Cleocin Phosphate** (Upjohn)		In 2, 4, and 6 mL vials[1] and 4 and 6 mL *ADD-Vantage* vials[1], 50 mL Galaxy plastic containers, and 60 mL pharmacy bulk package.

[1] With benzyl alcohol and EDTA.

For complete prescribing information, refer to the Lincosamides group monograph.

Indications

➤*Anaerobes:* Serious respiratory tract infections such as empyema, anaerobic pneumonitis, and lung abscess; serious skin and soft tissue infections; septicemia, intra-abdominal infections such as peritonitis and intra-abdominal abscess (typically resulting from anaerobic organisms resident in the normal GI tract); infections of the female pelvis and genital tract such as endometritis, nongonococcal tubo-ovarian abscess, pelvic cellulitis, and postsurgical vaginal cuff infection.

➤*Streptococci and staphylococci:* Serious respiratory tract infections; serious skin and soft tissue infections; septicemia (parenteral only); acute staphylococcal hematogenous osteomyelitis (parenteral only).

➤*Pneumococci:* Serious respiratory tract infections.

➤*Adjunctive therapy:* In the surgical treatment of chronic bone and joint infections due to susceptible organisms.

➤*Unlabeled uses:* Clindamycin (1200 to 2400 mg/day) may be beneficial as an alternative to sulfonamides in combination with pyrimethamine in the acute treatment of CNS toxoplasmosis in AIDS patients.

Clindamycin (600 mg 4 times/day IV or 900 mg 3 times/day IV) with primaquine may be beneficial in *Pneumocystis carinii* pneumonia.

Clindamycin is effective in the treatment of *Chlamydia trachomatis* infections in women. See CDC recommendations for acute PID in the Dosage section.

Clindamycin 300 mg twice daily for 7 days is effective in bacterial vaginosis due to *Gardnerella vaginalis* and may be an alternative to metronidazole.

Administration and Dosage

If significant diarrhea occurs during therapy, this antibiotic should be discontinued.

➤*Anaerobic infections:* Use parenteral form initially. May be followed by oral therapy.

➤*β-hemolytic streptococcal infections:* Continue treatment for at least 10 days.

➤*Oral:* Take with a full glass of water or with food to avoid esophageal irritation. Clindamycin absorption is not affected by food.

Adults –
 Serious infections: 150 to 300 mg every 6 hours.
 More severe infections: 300 to 450 mg every 6 hours.

Children –
 Clindamycin HCl:
 • *Serious infections –* 8 to 16 mg/kg/day divided into 3 or 4 equal doses.
 • *More severe infections –* 16 to 20 mg/kg/day divided into 3 or 4 equal doses.
 Clindamycin palmitate HCl:
 • *Serious infections –* 8 to 12 mg/kg/day divided into 3 or 4 equal doses.
 • *Severe infections –* 13 to 25 mg/kg/day divided into 3 or 4 equal doses. In children weighing ≤ 10 kg, administer 37.5 mg 3 times daily as the minimum dose.

➤*Parenteral:* May be administered IM or IV. Single IM injections ≥ 600 mg are not recommended.

Adults –
 Serious infections: Due to aerobic gram-positive cocci and the more sensitive anaerobes: 600 to 1200 mg/day in 2 to 4 equal doses.
 More severe infections: Particularly those due to *B. fragilis, Peptococcus* sp. or *Clostridium* sp. other than *C. perfringens*: 1.2 to 2.7 g/day in 2 to 4 equal doses. For more serious infections, these doses may have to be increased.
 In life-threatening situations: Due to aerobes or anaerobes, doses of 4.8 g/day have been given IV to adults.

Children (> 1 month of age to 16 years) – 20 to 40 mg/kg/day in 3 or 4 equal doses, depending on the severity of infection.

Alternatively, children may be dosed based on body surface area:
 Serious infections: 350 mg/m²/day;
 more serious infections: 450 mg/m²/day.

Neonates (< 1 month of age) – 15 to 20 mg/kg/day in 3 to 4 equal doses.

➤*CDC recommendation for acute pelvic inflammatory disease†* : 900 mg IV every 8 hours plus gentamicin loading dose 2 mg/kg IV or IM, followed by 1.5 mg/kg every 8 hours. Parenteral therapy may be discontinued 24 hours after a patient improves.

After discharge from hospital, continue with oral doxycycline 100 mg 2 times a day for 10 to 14 days total. Alternatively, continue with oral clindamycin 450 mg 4 times daily for 14 days.

➤*Dilution and infusion rates:* Dilute clindamycin phosphate prior to IV administration to a concentration of not more than 18 mg/mL.

Clindamycin Infusion Rates		
Dose (mg)	Diluent (mL)	Time (min)
300	50	10
600	50	20
900	50-100	30
1200	100	40

Do not administer > 1200 mg in a single 1 hour infusion.

Alternate Clindamycin Dosing Regimen		
To maintain serum clindamycin levels	Rapid infusion rate	Maintenance infusion rate
> 4 mcg/mL	10 mg/min for 30 min	0.75 mg/min
> 5 mcg/mL	15 mg/min for 30 min	1 mg/min
> 6 mcg/mL	20 mg/min for 30 min	1.25 mg/min

➤*Admixture compatibility/incompatibility:* Compatible at room temperature for 24 hours in IV solutions containing sodium chloride, glucose, calcium, potassium, vitamin B complex, cephalothin, kanamycin, gentamicin, penicillin, and carbenicillin. Incompatible with ampicillin, phenytoin sodium, barbiturates, aminophylline, magnesium, sulfate, and calcium gluconate.

➤*Storage/Stability:* Store unreconstituted palmitate product at room temperature 15° to 30°C (59° to 86°F). Do NOT refrigerate reconstituted solution; it may thicken and be difficult to pour when chilled. Solution is stable for 2 weeks at room temp.

Clindamycin phosphate is stable in 0.9% Sodium Chloride Injection, 5% Dextrose in Water Injection and Lactated Ringer's Solution, in both glass and polyvinyl chloride containers, at concentrations of 6, 9, and 12 mg/mL for 8 weeks frozen (−10°C), 32 days refrigerated (4°C) and 16 days at room temperature (25°C). A concentration of 18 mg/mL in 5% Dextrose in Water Injection, in polyvinyl chloride containers, is stable for 16 days at room temperature.

† CDC 1998 Sexually Transmitted Diseases Treatment Guidelines. *Morbidity and Mortality Weekly Report* 1998 Jan 23;47(No. RR-1):1-116.

WARNING

Toxicity: Aminoglycosides are associated with significant nephrotoxicity or ototoxicity. These agents are excreted primarily by glomerular filtration; thus, the serum half-life will be prolonged and significant accumulation will occur in patients with impaired renal function. Toxicity may develop even with conventional doses, particularly in patients with prerenal azotemia or impaired renal function.

Ototoxicity: Neurotoxicity, manifested as both auditory (cochlear) and vestibular ototoxicity, can occur with any of these agents. Auditory changes are irreversible, usually bilateral and may be partial or total. Risk of hearing loss increases with the degree of exposure to either high peak or high trough serum concentrations and continues to progress after drug withdrawal. The risk is greater in patients with renal impairment and with preexisting hearing loss. High frequency deafness usually occurs first and can be detected by audiometric testing. When feasible, obtain serial audiograms. There may be no clinical symptoms to warn of developing cochlear damage. Tinnitus or vertigo may occur, and are evidence of vestibular injury. Other manifestations of neurotoxicity may include numbness, skin tingling, muscle twitching and convulsions. Total or partial irreversible bilateral deafness may occur after drug discontinuation. Aminoglycoside-induced ototoxicity is usually irreversible. Vestibular toxicity is more predominant with gentamicin and streptomycin; auditory toxicity is more common with kanamycin, and amikacin. Tobramycin affects both functions equally. Relative ototoxicity is: Streptomycin = Kanamycin > Amikacin = Gentamicin = Tobramycin. Kanamycin, amikacin and streptomycin appear in this relative comparison based on high dose (kanamycin, amikacin) and antituberculosis (streptomycin) therapy.

Renal toxicity: This may be characterized by decreased creatinine clearance, cells or casts in the urine, decreased urine specific gravity, oliguria, proteinuria or evidence of nitrogen retention (increasing BUN, nonprotein nitrogen [NPN] or serum creatinine). Renal damage is usually reversible. The relative nephrotoxicity of these agents is estimated to be: Kanamycin = Amikacin = Gentamicin > Tobramycin> Streptomycin.

Monitoring: Closely observe all patients treated with aminoglycosides. Monitoring renal and eighth cranial nerve function at onset of therapy is essential for patients with known or suspected renal impairment and also in those whose renal function is initially normal, but who develop signs of renal dysfunction. Evidence of renal impairment or ototoxicity requires drug discontinuation or appropriate dosage adjustments. When feasible, monitor drug serum concentrations. Avoid concomitant use with other ototoxic, neurotoxic or nephrotoxic drugs. Other factors which may increase risk of toxicity are dehydration and advanced age.

Indications

The indications for specific agents are listed in individual drug monographs on the following pages. Reserve these drugs for treatment of infections caused by organisms not sensitive to less toxic agents. Safety for treatment periods > 14 days has not been established.

➤*Unlabeled uses:* In cystic fibrosis patients, the use of inhaled aminoglycosides may be beneficial in certain populations (eg, younger patients). Clinical outcome is not improved but deterioration of pulmonary function tests may be slowed or prevented.

Administration and Dosage

➤*Synergism:* In vitro studies indicate that aminoglycosides combined with penicillins or cephalosporins act synergistically against some strains of gram-negative organisms and enterococci (*Streptococcus faecalis*). Aminoglycosides may exhibit a synergistic effect when combined with carbenicillin or ticarcillin for *Pseudomonas* infections. Tests for antibiotic synergy are necessary. See also Admixture Incompatibility and Drug Interactions.

➤*Admixture incompatibility:* Beta-lactam antibiotics (eg, penicillins, cephalosporins) may inactivate aminoglycosides when admixed. Ticarcillin and carbenicillin are the worst β-lactam offenders; tobramycin and gentamicin are more susceptible than amikacin. This is most likely to occur: When the agents are mixed in the same container; during the aminoglycoside assay procedure; and in poor renal function. Concomitant cephalosporins may also falsely elevate creatinine determinations.

Ticarcillin and carbenicillin may also decrease aminoglycoside serum levels (see Overdosage).

Inactivation of tobramycin has not occurred in patients with normal renal function if they are given the drugs by separate routes. Kanamycin and methicillin inactivate each other in vitro, but this has not been seen in patients who receive them by different routes.

Guard against in vitro inactivation of aminoglycosides by β-lactam antibiotics in patients on combination therapy: 1) Place sample on ice immediately after drawing the specimen; test immediately. If testing is delayed, freeze serum as soon as possible; 2) draw the aminoglycoside level when the β-lactam antibiotic is at its trough level; 3) inactivation can still occur when the specimen is frozen (eg, kanamycin and ampicillin). If samples are to be frozen for a long period of time, inactivate the penicillin with penicillinase prior to freezing.

➤*Dosing interval:* Although further studies are needed, preliminary evidence indicates that aminoglycosides may be administered on a once daily basis without compromising efficacy and without increasing the potential for nephrotoxicity and ototoxicity. It is possible that the incidence of nephrotoxicity may even be decreased.

Actions

➤*Pharmacology:* Aminoglycosides are bactericidal antibiotics used primarily in the treatment of gram-negative infections. They irreversibly bind to the 30S subunit of bacterial ribosomes, blocking the recognition step in protein synthesis and causing misreading of the genetic code. The ribosomes separate from messenger RNA; cell death ensues.

➤*Pharmacokinetics:*

Absorption – Absorption from the GI tract is poor. Aminoglycosides are occasionally used orally for enteric infections (see Aminoglycosides, Oral monograph). Absorption from IM injection is rapid, with peak blood levels achieved within 1 hour.

Distribution – Aminoglycosides are widely distributed in extracellular fluids; peak serum concentrations may be lower than usual in patients whose extracellular fluid volume is expanded (eg, patients with edema or ascites). These drugs cross the placental barrier. Concentrations are found in bile, tissues, sputum, bronchial secretions and synovial, interstitial, peritoneal, abscess and pleural fluids. Concentrations in renal cortex are several times higher than usual serum levels. Aminoglycosides exhibit low protein binding, except for streptomycin. They do not achieve significant cerebrospinal fluid (CSF) levels in healthy patients. Although penetration is enhanced in the presence of inflamed meninges, only low levels are achieved. When intrathecal gentamicin is given with systemic gentamicin, CSF levels are substantially increased, depending on location of injection. Peak CSF concentrations following intralumbar administration generally occur 1 to 6 hours after injection.

Newborn infants, postpartum females and patients with ascites, spinal cord injury and cystic fibrosis may have an enlarged apparent volume of distribution. Obesity will artificially contract the apparent volume of distribution because adipose tissue contains less water than lean body mass of equal weight.

Excretion – Done by glomerular filtration, largely as unchanged drug; thus, high urine levels are attained. Probenecid does not affect renal tubular transport. The serum half-lives of all the agents are between 2 to 3 hours in patients with normal renal function. Approximately 53% to 98% of a single IV dose is excreted in the urine in 24 hours. However, when renal function is impaired, significant accumulation and subsequent toxicity may occur rapidly if dosage is not adjusted. The serum half-life is longer in young infants, as the immature renal system is unable to excrete these drugs rapidly; during the first days of life, the half-life may exceed 5 to 6 hours. Prolonged half-life may also be noted in the elderly. In severely burned patients, the half-life may be significantly decreased and result in serum concentrations lower than anticipated. Febrile and anemic states may be associated with a shorter serum half-life; dosage adjustment is usually not necessary. Aminoglycosides are removed by hemodialysis (4 to 6 hours removes approximately 50%) and peritoneal dialysis (range, removal of 23% in 8 hours to only 4% in 22 hours).

Serum levels – Because of the narrow range between therapeutic and toxic serum levels, careful attention to dosage calculations is essential, especially in patients with renal impairment, geriatric and female patients, those requiring high peak serum levels, patients on prolonged (> 10 days) therapy, patients with unstable renal function or those undergoing dialysis, those with abnormal extracellular fluid volume, or with prior exposure to ototoxic or nephrotoxic drugs. Age markedly affects peak concentration in children; it is generally lower in young children and infants. Monitor drug serum levels. Peak levels indicate therapeutic levels. Trough serum level determinations (just before next dose) best indicate drug accumulation. Obtain serum levels within 48 hours of start of therapy and every 3 to 4 days assuming stable renal function; also, levels are indicated when dose is changed or in changing renal function. Generally, to measure peak levels, draw a serum sample about 30 minutes after IV infusion or 1 hour after an IM dose. For trough levels, obtain serum samples at 8 hours or just prior to the next dose.

	Various Pharmacokinetic Parameters of the Aminoglycosides					
	Half-life (hrs)		Therapeutic serum levels (peak) (mcg/ml)	Toxic serum levels (mcg/ml)		Dose (mg/kg/day) (normal Ccr)
Aminoglycoside	Normal	ESRD		Peak[1]	Trough[2]	
Amikacin	2-3	24-60	16-32	> 35	> 10	15
Gentamicin	2	24-60	4-8	> 12	> 2	3-5
Kanamycin	2-3	24-60	15-40	> 35	> 10	15
Netilmicin	2-2.7	40	6-10	> 16	> 4	3-6.5
Streptomycin	2.5	100	20-30	> 50	—	15
Tobramycin	2-2.5	24-60	4-8	> 12	> 2	3-5

[1] Measured 1 hour after IM administration.
[2] Measured immediately prior to next dose.

➤*Microbiology:* The bactericidal activity of aminoglycosides is through inhibition of bacterial protein synthesis. One-way cross resistance is frequently noted. Three mechanisms for the development of bacterial resistance to aminoglycosides have been identified: Alteration of the drug target site (the bacterial ribosome); reduction or elimination of transport of the drug into the bacterial cell; inactivation of the drug by enzymatic modification (aminoglycoside inactivating enzymes; most significant).

Perform culture and sensitivity testing. Treat susceptible organisms with less toxic agents, especially if renal function is compromised. Resistance develops slowly, except with streptomycin. Development of streptomycin resistance may be a single step process and may occur rapidly. Most streptococci species (particularly group D), including *S. pneumoniae*, anaerobic organisms (including *Bacteroides* sp. and *Clostridia* sp.) and anaerobic cocci are resistant to aminoglycosides.

Organisms Generally Susceptible to Aminoglycosides							
	Organisms	Amikacin	Gentamicin	Kanamycin	Netimicin	Streptomycin	Tobramycin
Gram-positive	*Mycobacterium tuberculosis*	✓¹				✓²	
	Staphylococci	✓³	✓³		✓³		✓
	S. aureus	✓	✓	✓³	✓³		✓
	S. epidermidis			✓	✓		
	Streptococci					✓²	
	S. faecalis		✓²		✓²	✓²	✓²
Gram-negative	*Acinetobacter* sp.		✓	✓	✓		
	Brucella sp.					✓	
	Citrobacter sp.	✓	✓	✓	✓	✓	✓
	Enterobacter sp.	✓	✓	✓	✓	✓	✓
	Escherichia coli	✓	✓	✓	✓	✓	✓
	Hemophilus influenzae	✓		✓		✓²	
	Hemophilus ducreyi					✓	
	Klebsiella sp.	✓	✓	✓	✓	✓²	✓
	Morganella morganii						✓
	Neisseria sp.	✓		✓	✓	✓	
	Proteus sp.	✓⁴	✓⁴	✓⁴	✓	✓	✓⁴
	Providencia sp.	✓	✓	✓	✓	✓	✓
	Pseudomonas sp.	✓					
	P. aeruginosa	✓	✓²		✓	✓	✓
	Salmonella sp.	✓	✓	✓	✓	✓	✓
	Serratia sp.	✓	✓	✓	✓	✓	✓
	Shigella sp.	✓	✓	✓	✓	✓	✓
	Yersinia (Pasteurella) pestis	✓	✓	✓	✓	✓	✓

[1] ✓ = generally susceptible
[2] Usually used concomitantly with other anti-infectives.
[3] Penicillinase-producing and nonpenicillinase-producing.
[4] Indole-positive and indole-negative.

Contraindications

Previous reactions to these agents. With the exception of the use of streptomycin in tuberculosis, these agents are generally not indicated in long-term therapy because of the ototoxic and nephrotoxic hazards of extended administration.

Warnings

➤*Burn patients:* In patients with extensive burns, altered pharmacokinetics may result in reduced serum concentrations of aminoglycosides. In such patients, measurement of serum concentration is especially important for dosage determination.

➤*Hypomagnesemia:* This may occur in more than ⅓ of patients whose oral diet is restricted or who are eating poorly.

➤*Neuromuscular blockade:* Neurotoxicity can occur after intrapleural and interperitoneal installation of large doses of an aminoglycoside; however, the reaction has followed IV, IM and oral administration. Aminoglycosides may aggravate muscle weakness because of a potential curare-like effect on the neuromuscular junction. Use with caution in patients with neuromuscular disorders (eg, myasthenia gravis, parkinsonism, infant botulism).

Neuromuscular blockade resulting in respiratory paralysis has occurred with aminoglycosides, especially if given with or soon after anesthesia or muscle relaxants (see Drug Interactions).

During or following gentamicin therapy, paresthesias, tetany, positive Chvostek and Trousseau signs, and mental confusion have been described in patients with hypomagnesemia, hypocalcemia and hypo-

kalemia. When this occurred in infants, tetany and muscle weakness occurred. Both adults and infants required appropriate corrective electrolyte therapy.

Use caution in newborns of mothers on magnesium sulfate; these hypermagnesemic infants may experience respiratory arrest after receiving aminoglycosides.

➤*Nephrotoxicity:* This may occur. Risk factors include the elderly, patients with a history of renal impairment who are treated for longer periods or with higher doses than those recommended, a recent course of aminoglycosides (within 6 weeks), concurrent use of other nephrotoxic agents, frequent dosing, potassium depletion and decreased intravascular volume. Adverse renal effects can occur in patients with initially normal renal function. Of patients receiving an aminoglycoside for several days or more, approximately 8% to 26% will develop mild renal impairment which is generally reversible.

Since renal function may alter appreciably during therapy, test renal function daily or more frequently. Examine urine for increased excretion of protein and for presence of cells and casts, keeping in mind the effects of the primary illness on these tests. Obtain one or more of the following laboratory measurements at the onset of therapy, frequently during therapy and at, or shortly after, the end of therapy: Creatinine clearance (Ccr) rate (either carefully measured or estimated from published nomograms or equations based on patient's age, sex, body weight and serial creatinine concentrations; preferred over BUN); serum creatinine concentration (preferred over BUN); BUN. More frequent testing is desirable if renal function is changing. If signs of renal irritation appear such as casts, white or red cells and albumin, increase hydration; a dosage reduction may be desirable (see Administration and Dosage for individual agents). These signs usually disappear when treatment is completed. However, if azotemia or a progressive decrease of urine output occurs, stop treatment. Reduce dosage if other evidence of renal dysfunction occurs (decreased Ccr or urine specific gravity, or increased BUN, creatinine or oliguria).

The risk of toxic reactions is low in well hydrated patients with normal renal function who do not receive **gentamicin** or **kanamycin** injections at higher doses or for longer periods of time than recommended.

Hydration – These drugs reach high concentrations in the renal system; keep patients well hydrated to minimize chemical irritation of tubules. Well hydrated patients with normal renal function have low risk of nephrotoxic reactions if recommended dosage is not exceeded.

Streptomycin, given to patients with preexisting renal insufficiency, calls for extreme caution. In severely uremic patients, a single dose may produce high blood levels for several days and the cumulative effect may produce ototoxic sequelae. Alkalinize the urine to minimize or prevent renal irritation.

➤*Elderly:* These patients may have reduced renal function that is not evident in the results of routine screening tests, such as BUN or serum creatinine. A Ccr determination may be more useful. Monitoring of renal function and drug levels during treatment is particularly important in such patients.

➤*Pregnancy: Category D* (amikacin, gentamicin, kanamycin, tobramycin). Aminoglycosides can cause fetal harm when given to pregnant women. These agents cross the placenta. Fetal serum levels may reach 16% to 50% of maternal levels. There are reports of total irreversible bilateral congenital deafness in children whose mothers received **streptomycin** during pregnancy. Prolonged use of **gentamicin** during pregnancy may result in otological damage to the fetus. Serious side effects to the mother, fetus or newborn have not been reported with other aminoglycosides, but the potential for harm exists. Although there is no clearly defined risk, such experience cannot exclude the possibility of infrequent or subtle damage to the fetus. If these drugs are used during pregnancy, or if the patient becomes pregnant while taking these drugs, apprise her of the potential hazards to the fetus.

➤*Lactation:* Small amounts of **streptomycin** and **kanamycin** are excreted in breast milk. Decide whether to discontinue nursing or discontinue the drug, taking into account the importance of the drug to the mother.

➤*Children:* Use with caution in premature infants and neonates because of their renal immaturity and the resulting prolongation of serum half-life of these drugs.

A syndrome of apparent CNS depression, characterized by stupor and flaccidity to coma and deep respiratory depression, has been reported in very young infants given **streptomycin** in doses greater than those recommended. Do not exceed recommended doses in infants.

Precautions

➤*Monitoring:* Collect urine specimens for examination during therapy (see Nephrotoxicity). Monitor peak and trough serum concentrations periodically to assure adequate levels and to avoid potentially toxic levels. Also monitor serum calcium, magnesium and sodium (see Adverse Reactions).

Eighth cranial nerve function testing – Serial audiometric tests are suggested, particularly when renal function is impaired or prolonged aminoglycoside therapy is required; also repeat such tests periodically after treatment if there is evidence of a hearing deficit or vestibular abnormality before or during therapy, or when consecutive or concomitant use of other potentially ototoxic drugs is unavoidable. Discontinue therapy if tinnitus or subjective hearing loss develops, or if follow-up audiograms show loss of high frequency perception. Aminoglycoside-induced ototoxicity is usually irreversible.

Factors that may increase risk of aminoglycoside-induced ototoxicity include renal impairment (especially if dialysis is required), excessive dosage, dehydration, concomitant administration of ethacrynic acid or furosemide, or previous use of other ototoxic drugs.

Cochlear damage is usually manifested initially by small changes in audiometric test results at the high frequencies and may not be associated with subjective hearing loss; vestibular dysfunction is usually manifested by nystagmus, vertigo, nausea, vomiting or acute Meniere's syndrome.

➤ *Intrathecal gentamicin:* A patient with multiple sclerosis for 7 years was given intra-lumbar gentamicin; disseminated microscopic brainstem lesions were found at autopsy. Tissue rarefaction and marked swelling of axis cylinders with occasional calcification, loss of oligodendroglia and astroglia and poor inflammatory response were seen. Use of excessive (40 to 160 mg) doses of intrathecal gentamicin has produced neuromuscular disturbances (eg, ataxia, paresis, incontinence).

➤ *Cross-allergenicity:* Occurrence among the aminoglycosides has been demonstrated and depends largely on inactivation by bacterial enzymes.

➤ *Syphilis:* In the treatment of sexually transmitted disease, if concomitant syphilis is suspected, perform a darkfield examination before treatment is started. Perform monthly serologic tests for at least 4 months.

➤ *Topical use:* Aminoglycosides are quickly and almost totally absorbed when applied topically in association with surgical procedures, except to the urinary bladder. Irreversible deafness, renal failure, and death due to neuromuscular blockade have occurred following irrigation of both small and large surgical fields with an aminoglycoside preparation. Consider potential toxicity.

➤ *Benzyl alcohol:* This is contained in some of these products as a preservative and has been associated with a fatal "gasping syndrome" in premature infants.

➤ *Superinfection:* Use of antibiotics (especially prolonged or repeated therapy) may result in bacterial or fungal overgrowth of nonsusceptible organisms. Such overgrowth may lead to a secondary infection. Take appropriate measures if this occurs.

➤ *Sulfite sensitivity:* Some products contain sulfites that may cause allergic-type reactions including anaphylactic symptoms and life-threatening/less severe asthmatic episodes in susceptible persons. Overall prevalence in general population is unknown and probably low. It is more frequent in asthmatics or atopic nonasthmatics.

Drug Interactions

Aminoglycoside Drug Interactions

Precipitant drug	Object drug*		Description
Cephalosporins Enflurane Methoxyflurane Vancomycin	Aminoglyco-sides	↑	Risk of nephrotoxicity may increase above that with aminoglycoside alone. Monitor patients. With cephalosporins, bactericidal activity against certain pathogens may be enhanced (see Administration).
Indomethacin IV	Aminoglyco-sides	↑	In preterm infants, the use of indomethacin for closure of patent ductus arteriosus resulted in aminoglycoside accumulation in one study.
Loop diuretics	Aminoglyco-sides	↑	Auditory toxicity appears to increase during concomitant use. Hearing loss of varying degrees may occur; it may be irreversible. Monitor patients.
Penicillins	Aminoglyco-sides	↑	Synergism of these agents is well documented; however, certain penicillins may inactivate certain aminoglycosides. The problem may be greatest in vitro (see Administration).
Aminoglyco-sides	Neuromuscular blockers, depo-larizing and non-depolarizing	↑	The neuromuscular blocking effects are enhanced by aminoglycosides. Prolonged respiratory depression may occur.
Aminoglyco-sides	Polypeptide anti-biotics	↑	Concurrent use of thes agents may increase the risk of respiratory paralysis and renal dysfunction.

* ↑ = Object drug increased

Adverse Reactions

Aminoglycoside Adverse Reactions (%)

	Adverse Reaction	Amikacin	Gentamicin	Kanamycin	Netimicin	Streptomycin	Tobramycin
Central/Peripheral nervous system	Headache	rare	✔[1]	rare	< 0.1		✔
	Encephalopathy		✔		✔		
	Confusion		✔				
	Fever		✔		0.1	✔	✔
	Lethargy		✔				✔
	Disorientation				< 0.1		✔
	Neuromuscular block-ade[2]	✔		✔	✔		✔
	Paresthesia	rare		rare	< 0.1		
	Convulsions		✔		✔		
	Muscle twitching		✔		✔		
	Myasthenia gravis-like syndrome		✔		✔		
	Numbness		✔		✔		
	Peripheral neuropathy		✔		✔		
	Skin tingling		✔		✔		
GI	Vomiting	rare	✔	rare	< 0.1	✔	✔
	Nausea	rare	✔	rare		✔	✔
	Diarrhea			rare	< 0.1		✔
Hematologic	Anemia	rare	✔		< 0.1		✔
	Eosinophilia	rare	✔		0.4	✔	✔
	Leukopenia		✔		< 0.1		✔
	Thrombocytopenia		✔		< 0.1	✔	
	Granulocytopenia		✔				
Hyper-sensitivity	Rash	rare	✔	rare	≤ 0.5	✔	✔
	Urticaria		✔			✔	✔
	Itching		✔		≤ 0.5		✔
	Anaphylaxis/Anaphy-lactoid reaction		✔		✔		
Lab test abnormalities	Increased AST/ALT		✔		1.5		✔
	Increased bilirubin		✔		1.5		✔
	Increased serum LDH		✔				
Renal[1]	Oliguria	✔	✔	✔	✔		✔
	Proteinuria	✔	✔	✔	✔		✔
	Rising serum creati-nine[2]	✔	✔	✔	✔		✔
	Casts	✔	✔		✔		✔
	Rising BUN[2]	✔	✔	✔	✔		✔
	Red and white cells in urine		✔	✔	✔		✔
	Azotemia	✔		✔		✔	
	Rising NPN[2]		✔				✔
	Decreasing Ccr		✔		✔		
Special senses	Dizziness		✔		✔		✔
	Tinnitus		✔		✔		✔
	Vertigo		✔		✔	✔	✔
	Roaring in ears		✔				✔
	Hearing loss/deafness	✔	✔	✔[3]		✔	✔
	Loss of balance	✔		✔[3]			
	Visual disturbances/blurred vision		✔		< 0.1		
Miscellaneous	Apnea	✔	✔	✔	✔	✔	✔
	Drug fever	rare		rare			
	Pain/Irritation at injec-tion site		✔	✔	≈ 0.4		✔
	Hypotension	rare	✔		< 0.1		
	Acute muscular paralysis	✔		✔			
	Decreased serum Ca, Na, K, Mg[2]		✔				✔

[1] ✔ = Reported; no incidence given
[2] See Warnings.
[3] Partially reversible to irreversible bilateral hearing loss.

➤ *Renal:*

Renal function changes – These are usually reversible upon discontinuation. See Warnings.

➤ *Other adverse reactions listed only for the individual agents:*

➤ *Amikacin:* Arthralgia, tremor (rare).

➤ *Gentamicin:*

CNS – Acute organic brain syndrome; depression; pseudotumor cerebri; respiratory depression.

GI – Decreased appetite; hypersalivation; stomatitis; weight loss.

Hematologic – Increased and decreased reticulocyte count; transient agranulocytosis.

Hypersensitivity – Generalized burning; laryngeal edema; purpura.

Miscellaneous – Alopecia; hypertension; joint pain; pulmonary fibrosis; splenomegaly; subcutaneous atrophy or fat necrosis (rare); transient hepatomegaly; leg cramps; increased CSF protein; arachnoiditis or burning at injection site after intrathecal administration (see Warnings); a Fanconi-like syndrome, with aminoaciduria and metabolic acidosis.

➤*Kanamycin:* Granular casts; "malabsorption syndrome" characterized by an increase in fecal fat, decrease in serum carotene and fall in xylose absorption (prolonged therapy).

➤*Streptomycin:*
Neurotoxic: Facial, circumoral or peripheral paresthesia; muscular weakness.

Hypersensitivity – Angioneurotic edema; exfoliative dermatitis.

Miscellaneous – Amblyopia; hemolytic anemia; hepatic necrosis; myocarditis; pancytopenia; serum sickness; toxic epidermal necrolysis.

➤*Tobramycin:* Cylindruria; delirium; leukocytosis.

Overdosage

➤*Symptoms:* The severity of the signs and symptoms following overdose are dependent on the dose administered, patient's renal function, state of hydration and age, and whether or not other medications with similar toxicities are being administered concurrently. Toxicity may occur in patients treated > 10 days or in patients with reduced renal function where dose has not been appropriately adjusted.

Nephrotoxicity following the parenteral administration of an aminoglycoside is most closely related to the area under the curve. Nephrotoxicity is more likely if trough concentrations fail to fall below the intended concentration. Patients who are elderly, have abnormal renal function, are receiving other nephrotoxic drugs or are volume depleted are at greater risk for developing acute tubular necrosis. Auditory and vestibular toxicities have been associated with aminoglycoside overdose. These toxicities occur in patients treated > 10 days, in patients

with abnormal renal function, in dehydrated patients, or in patients receiving medications with additive auditory toxicities. These patients may not have signs or symptoms or may experience dizziness, tinnitus, vertigo and a loss of high-tone acuity as ototoxicity progresses. Ototoxic signs and symptoms may not begin to occur until long after the drug has been discontinued.

Neuromuscular blockade or respiratory paralysis may occur following aminoglycoside administration. Neuromuscular blockade, respiratory failure and prolonged respiratory paralysis may occur more commonly in patients with myasthenia gravis or Parkinson's disease. Prolonged respiratory paralysis may also occur in patients receiving neuromuscular blockers. If neuromuscular blockade occurs, it may be reversed by the administration of calcium salts but mechanical assistance may be necessary.

If an aminoglycoside were ingested, toxicity would be less likely because they are poorly absorbed from an intact GI tract.

➤*Treatment:* The initial intervention is to establish an airway and ensure oxygenation and ventilation. Initiate resuscitative measures promptly if respiratory paralysis occurs. Adequately hydrate patients, and carefully monitor fluid balance, Ccr and plasma levels.

Peritoneal dialysis or hemodialysis will aid in removal from the blood. This is especially important if renal function is, or becomes, compromised. Hemodialysis is preferable because it is more efficient in reducing serum levels. Complexation with ticarcillin or carbenicillin (12 to 30 g/day) appears as effective as hemodialysis in lowering excessive aminoglycoside serum concentrations. In newborns, consider exchange transfusions.

Range of Aminoglycoside Half-Lives (Hours) During Dialysis[1]			
Aminoglycosides	Interdialysis	Hemodialysis	Peritoneal dialysis
Kanamycin	40-96	5	12
Gentamicin	21-59	6-11	5-29
Tobramycin	27-70	3-10	10-37
Amikacin	28-87	4-7	18-29
Netilmicin	24-52	5	—

[1] Patient renal function creatinine clearance ≤ 5 ml/min.

STREPTOMYCIN SULFATE

Rx	Streptomycin Sulfate (Pfizer)	**Injection:** 400 mg/ml	In 2.5 ml amps.
Rx	Streptomycin Sulfate (Pharma-Tek)	**Lyophilized Cake/Powder for Injection:** 200 mg/ml	In 1g vials.

For complete prescribing information, refer to the Aminoglycosides group monograph. SPECIAL NOTE: See Warning Box in the group monograph concerning toxicity.

Indications

➤*Mycobacterium tuberculosis:* The Advisory Council for the Elimination of TB, the American Thoracic Society and the CDC recommend that either streptomycin or ethambutol be added as a fourth drug in a regimen containing isoniazid, rifampin and pyrazinamide for initial treatment of TB unless the likelihood of INH or rifampin resistance is very low. Reassess the need for a fourth drug when susceptibility testing results are known.

Streptomycin is also indicated for therapy of TB when one or more of the above drugs is contraindicated because of toxicity or intolerance. The management of TB has become more complex as a consequence of increasing rates of drug resistance and concomitant HIV infection. Additional consultation from TB experts may be desirable. Refer also to the introduction in the Antituberculous Drugs section.

➤*Nontuberculous infections:* Use only in infections caused by organisms shown to be susceptible, and when less potentially hazardous therapeutic agents are ineffective or contraindicated. Organisms usually sensitive include: *Pasteurella pestis* (plague); *Francisella tularensis* (tularemia); *Brucella, Calymmatobacterium granulomatis* (donovanosis, granuloma inguinale); *Haemophilus ducreyi* (chancroid); *H. influenzae* (in respiratory, endocardial and meningeal infections with another agent); *Klebsiella pneumoniae* pneumonia (with another agent); *E. coli, Proteus* sp., *A. aerogenes, K. pneumoniae* and *Enterococcus faecalis* in urinary tract infections; *Streptococcus* viridans and *E. faecalis* (in endocardial infections with penicillin); gram-negative bacilli (in bacteremia, with another agent).

➤*Unlabeled uses:* Streptomycin 11 to 13 mg/kg/24 hrs IV or 15 mg/kg/day IM may be used as part of a multiple-drug regimen (generally three to five agents) for *Mycobacterium avium* complex, a common infection in AIDS patients.

Administration and Dosage

Administer by the IM route.

➤*Tuberculosis:* The standard regimen for the treatment of drug-susceptible TB has been 2 months of INH, rifampin and pyrazinamide followed by 4 months of INH and rifampin (patients with concomitant TB and HIV infection may require treatment for a longer period). When streptomycin is added to this regimen because of suspected or proven drug resistance, the recommended dosing for streptomycin is as follows:

Streptomycin Dosing for TB			
	Daily	Twice weekly	Thrice weekly
Children	20-40 mg/kg max 1 g	25-30 mg/kg max 1.5 g	25-30 mg/kg max 1.5 g
Adults	15 mg/kg max 1 g	25-30 mg/kg max 1.5 g	25-30 mg/kg max 1.5 g

Streptomycin is usually administered daily as a single IM injection. Give a total dose of ≤ 120 g over the course of therapy unless there are no other therapeutic options. In patients > 60 years of age, use a reduced dosage. Therapy with streptomycin may be terminated when toxic symptoms have appeared, when impending toxicity is feared, when organisms become resistant, or when full treatment effect has been obtained. The total period of drug treatment of TB is a minimum of 1 year.

➤*Tularemia:* 1 to 2 g daily in divided doses for 7 to 14 days until the patient is afebrile for 5 to 7 days.

➤*Plague:* 2 g daily in two divided doses for minimum of 10 days.

➤*Bacterial endocarditis:*
Streptococcal – Streptomycin may be used for 2 week treatment concomitantly with penicillin in penicillin-sensitive alpha and non-hemolytic streptococcal endocarditis (penicillin MIC ≤ 0.1 mcg/ml): 1 g twice daily for 1 week, 0.5 g twice daily for the second week. If patient is > 60 years of age, give 0.5 g twice daily for the entire 2 week period.

Enterococcal – 1 g twice daily for 2 weeks and 0.5 g twice daily for 4 weeks in combination with penicillin. Ototoxicity may require termination of streptomycin prior to completion of the 6–week course of treatment.

➤*Concomitant agents:* For use with other agents to which infecting organism is also sensitive, streptomycin is a secondary choice for treatment of gram-negative bacillary bacteremia, meningitis and pneumonia; brucellosis; granuloma inguinale; chancroid; UTI.

➤*Adults:* 1 to 2 g in divided doses every 6 to 12 hours for moderate to severe infections. Doses should generally not exceed 2 g per day.

➤*Children:* 20 to 40 mg/kg/day (8 to 20 mg/lb/day) in divided doses every 6 to 12 hours. (Take particular care to avoid excessive dosage in children.)

➤*Preparation of solution (lyophilized cake/powder for injection):* Add Water for Injection in an amount to yield the desired concentration as indicated in the following table:

STREPTOMYCIN SULFATE

Preparation of Streptomycin Solution from Lyophilized Cake/Powder	
Desired concentration (mg/ml)	Amount of solvent (ml)
≈200	4.2
≈250	3.2
≈400	1.8

➤*Storage/Stability:*
Injection – Store under refrigeration at 2° to 8°C (36° to 46°F).
Cake/Powder for injection – Store under controlled room temperature 15° to 30°C (59° to 86°F). Protect from light. Sterile reconstituted solution may be stored at room temperature for 1 week without significant loss of potency.

KANAMYCIN SULFATE

Rx	**Kanamycin Sulfate** (Various, eg, Smith & Nephew)	**Injection:** 500 mg	In 2 ml vials.[1]
Rx	**Kantrex** (Apothecon)		In 2 ml vials.[2]
Rx	**Kanamycin Sulfate** (Various, eg, Smith & Nephew)	**Injection:** 1 g	In 2 ml vials.[1]
Rx	**Kantrex** (Apothecon)		In 3 ml vials.[2]
Rx	**Kanamycin Sulfate** (Various, eg, Smith & Nephew)	**Pediatric Injection:** 75 mg	In 2 ml vials.[1]
Rx	**Kantrex** (Apothecon)		In 2 ml vials.[2]

[1] May contain sulfites.

[2] With sodium bisulfite.

For complete prescribing information, refer to the Aminoglycosides group monograph. SPECIAL NOTE: See Warning Box in the group monograph concerning toxicity.

WARNING

Carefully observe elderly patients, patients with preexisting tinnitus or vertigo or known subclinical deafness, those having received prior ototoxic drugs, and patients receiving a total dose of > 15 g kanamycin sulfate for signs of eighth nerve damage. Loss of hearing may occur, even with normal renal function.

Indications

Consider initial therapy for one or more of the following: *Escherichia coli, Proteus* sp. (both indole-positive and indole-negative), *Enterobacter aerogenes, Klebsiella pneumoniae, Serratia marcescens* and *Acinetobacter* sp. May be used as initial therapy with a penicillin or cephalosporin before obtaining results of susceptibility testing. Not the drug of choice for staphylococcal infections; may be indicated for initial therapy of severe infections where the strain is thought to be susceptible in patients allergic to other antibiotics, or in mixed staphylococcal/gram-negative infections.

Not indicated in long-term therapy (eg, tuberculosis) because of the toxic hazard associated with extended administration.

➤*Unlabeled uses:* Kanamycin 11 to 13 mg/kg/24 hours IV or 15 mg/kg/day IM may be used as part of a multiple-drug regimen (generally three to five agents) for Mycobacterium avium complex, a common infection in AIDS patients.

Administration and Dosage

Do not exceed a total of 1.5 g/day by any route.

➤*IM:* Inject deeply into the upper outer quadrant of the gluteal muscle. For adults or children, 7.5 mg/kg every 12 hours (15 mg/kg/day). If continuously high blood levels are desired, give the daily dose of 15 mg/kg in equally divided doses every 6 or 8 hours. Usual treatment duration is 7 to 10 days. Doses of 7.5 mg/kg give mean peak levels of 22 mcg/ml. At 8 hours after a 7.5 mg/kg dose, mean serum levels are 3.2 mcg/ml.

Uncomplicated infections should respond in 24 to 48 hours. If a clinical response does not occur within 3 to 5 days, stop therapy and reevaluate. Failure may be due to resistance of the organism or the presence of septic foci requiring surgical drainage.

➤*IV:* Do not admix with other antibacterial agents; administer separately.

Adults – Do not exceed 15 mg/kg/day. Give slowly. Prepare by adding contents of 500 mg vial to 100 to 200 ml sterile diluent (Normal Saline or 5% Dextrose in Water) or the contents of a 1 g vial to 200 to 400 ml of sterile diluent. Give over 30 to 60 minutes. Divide daily dose into 2 to 3 equal doses.

Children – Use sufficient diluent to infuse the drug over 30 to 60 minutes.

➤*Renal failure:* Follow therapy by appropriate serum assays. If not feasible, reduce frequency of administration. Calculate the dosage interval with the following formula: Serum creatinine (mg/dl) × 9 = dosage interval (in hours).

➤*Intraperitoneal (following exploration for peritonitis or after peritoneal contamination due to fecal spill during surgery):* 500 mg diluted in 20 ml sterile distilled water instilled through a polyethylene catheter into the wound. If possible, postpone instillation until patient has recovered from anesthesia and muscle relaxants. Absorption after intraperitoneal instillation is similar to IM use. After a single instillation of 250 or 500 mg, peak serum levels of 13.5 and 24 mcg/ml, respectively, occurred in one study.

➤*Aerosol treatment:* 250 mg 2 to 4 times a day. Withdraw 250 mg (1 ml) from 500 mg vial, dilute with 3 ml Normal Saline and nebulize.

➤*Other routes:* Concentrations of 0.25% have been used as irrigating solutions in abscess cavities, pleural space, peritoneal and ventricular cavities.

➤*Storage/Stability:* Darkening of vials during shelf life does not indicate loss of potency.

GENTAMICIN

Rx	**Gentamicin Sulfate** (Various, eg, Fujisawa, Major, Moore, Taylor)	**Injection:** 40 mg per ml (as sulfate)	In 2 and 20 ml vials and 1.5 and 2 ml cartridge-needle units.
Rx	**Garamycin** (Schering)		In 2 and 20 ml vials.[1]
Rx	**Pediatric Gentamicin Sulfate** (Fujisawa)	**Injection:** 10 mg per ml (as sulfate)	In 2 ml vials.

[1] With parabens, EDTA and sodium bisulfite.

For complete prescribing information, refer to the Aminoglycosides, Parenteral group monograph. SPECIAL NOTE: See Warning Box in the group monograph concerning toxicity.

Indications

Treatment of serious infections caused by susceptible strains of *Pseudomonas aeruginosa, Proteus* sp. (indole-positive and indole-negative), *Escherichia coli, Klebsiella* sp., *Enterobacter* sp., *Serratia* sp., *Citrobacter* sp. and *Staphylococcus* sp. (coagulase-positive and coagulase-negative).

Effective in bacterial neonatal sepsis; bacterial septicemia; serious bacterial infections of the CNS (meningitis), urinary tract, respiratory tract, GI tract (including peritonitis), skin, bone and soft tissue (including burns).

Not indicated in uncomplicated initial episodes of urinary tract infections, unless causative organisms are susceptible to these antibiotics and are not susceptible to antibiotics with less potential for toxicity. Perform bacterial cultures.

➤*Gram-negative infections:* Consider as initial therapy in suspected or confirmed gram-negative infections; therapy may be started before obtaining results of susceptibility testing, but continue therapy based on susceptibility test results, infection severity and the concepts in the Warning Box.

➤*Unknown causative organisms:* In serious infections, administer gentamicin as initial therapy in conjunction with a penicillin or cephalosporin before obtaining results of susceptibility tests. Following identification of the organism and its susceptibility, continue appropriate antibiotic therapy.

➤*Combination therapy:* Effective in combination with carbenicillin for the treatment of life-threatening infections caused by *P. aeruginosa*. Also effective when combined with a penicillin for treatment of endocarditis caused by group *D. streptococci*. In the neonate with suspected bacterial sepsis or staphylococcal pneumonia, penicillin is usually indicated concomitantly with gentamicin.

➤*Staphylococcal infections:* While not the antibiotic of first choice, consider gentamicin when penicillins or other less toxic drugs are contraindicated, when bacterial susceptibility tests and clinical judgment indicate its use and in mixed infections caused by susceptible strains of staphylococci and gram-negative organisms.

➤*Intrathecal administration:* This is indicated as adjunctive therapy to systemic gentamicin sulfate in the treatment of serious CNS infections (meningitis, ventriculitis) caused by susceptible *Pseudomonas* sp. Perform bacteriologic tests to determine that the causative

GENTAMICIN

organisms are susceptible to gentamicin.

➤*Unlabeled uses:* An alternative regimen for pelvic inflammatory disease is gentamicin 2 mg/kg IV followed by 1.5 mg/kg 3 times daily (normal renal function) plus clindamycin 600 mg IV 4 times daily. Continue for at least 4 days and at least 48 hours after patient improves; then continue clindamycin 450 mg orally 4 times daily for 10 to 14 days total therapy.

Administration and Dosage

➤*Monitoring:* Because of the potential for toxicity, serum level monitoring is recommended when the drug is used in patients with impaired renal function, when doses in excess of 3 mg/kg/day are used, or when the drug is used in any patient in whom altered pharmacokinetics are suspected (ie, patients with extensive burns).

Generally, the peak concentration (at 30 to 60 minutes after IM injection or immediately after a slow IV infusion) is expected to be in the range of 4 to 6 mcg/ml. When monitoring peak concentrations, avoid prolonged levels > 12 mcg/ml. When monitoring trough concentrations (just prior to the next dose), avoid levels > 2 mcg/ml. When determining the adequacy of a serum level for a particular patient, consider susceptibility of the causative organism, infection severity and the status of the patient's host-defense mechanisms.

➤*Dosage:* May be given IM or IV. For patients with serious infections and normal renal function, give 3 mg/kg/day in 3 equal doses every 8 hours. For patients with life-threatening infections, administer up to 5 mg/kg/day in 3 or 4 equal doses. Reduce dosage to 3 mg/kg/day as soon as clinically indicated.

Obese patients – Base dosage on an estimate of lean body mass.

Children – 6 to 7.5 mg/kg/day (2 to 2.5 mg/kg every 8 hours).

Infants and neonates – 7.5 mg/kg/day (2.5 mg/kg every 8 hours).

Premature or full term neonates (≤ 1 week of age) – 5 mg/kg/day (2.5 mg/kg every 12 hours). A regimen of either 2.5 mg/kg every 18 hours or 3 mg/kg every 24 hours may also provide satisfactory peak and trough levels in preterm infants < 32 weeks gestational age.

➤*Duration of therapy:* This is usually 7 to 10 days. In difficult and complicated infections, a longer course of therapy may be necessary. In such cases, monitor renal, auditory and vestibular function, since toxicity is more apt to occur with treatment extended beyond 10 days. Reduce dosage if clinically indicated.

➤*Prevention of bacterial endocarditis:*

In dental, oral or upper respiratory tract procedures (alternate regimen)† – 1 to 2 g (50 mg/kg for children) ampicillin plus 1.5 mg/kg (2 mg/kg for children) gentamicin not to exceed 80 mg, both IM or IV one-half hour prior to procedure, followed by 1.5 g (25 mg/kg for children) amoxicillin 6 hours after initial dose or repeat parenteral dose 8 hours after initial dose.

GU or GI procedures (standard regimen) – 2 g (50 mg/kg for children) ampicillin plus 1.5 mg/kg (2 mg/kg for children) gentamicin not to exceed 80 mg, both IM or IV one-half hour prior to procedure followed by 1.5 mg (25 mg/kg for children) amoxicillin.

➤*Renal function impairment:* Adjust dosage; whenever possible, monitor serum concentrations of gentamicin. One method of dosage adjustment is to increase the interval between the doses administered.

Rule of eights – The serum creatinine concentration roughly correlates with the serum half-life of gentamicin. Creatinine clearance is better, but still roughly correlates with serum aminoglycoside levels. Approximate the interval between doses (in hours) by multiplying the serum creatinine level (mg/dl) by 8. For example, a patient weighing 60 kg with a serum creatinine level of 2 mg/dl could be given 60 mg (1 mg/kg) every 16 hours (2 x 8).

In patients with serious systemic infections and renal impairment, administer the antibiotic more frequently, but in reduced dosage. Mea-

sure serum concentrations of gentamicin so that appropriate levels result. Peak and trough concentrations, measured intermittently during therapy, will provide optimal guidance for adjusting dosage.

After the usual initial dose, a rough guide for determining reduced dosage at 8 hour intervals is to divide the normally recommended dose by the serum creatinine level. For example, after an initial dose of 60 mg (1 mg/kg), a patient weighing 60 kg with a serum creatinine level of 2 mg/dl could be given 30 mg every 8 hours (60 ÷ 2).

The status of renal function may change over the course of the infectious process. Deteriorating renal function may require a greater reduction in dosage than that specified in the above guidelines for patients with stable renal impairment. The above dosage schedules are not rigid recommendations, but are provided as rough guides to dosage when the measurement of gentamicin serum levels is not feasible.

Several predictive methods and published nomograms have been compared, none of which performed as well as individualized pharmacokinetic dosing with serum levels.

Hemodialysis – The amount of gentamicin removed from the blood may vary depending on several factors, including the dialysis method used. An 8 hour hemodialysis may reduce serum concentrations of gentamicin by approximately 50%. The recommended dosage at the end of each dialysis period is 1 to 1.7 mg/kg, depending on the severity of infection. In children, administer a dose of 2 to 2.5 mg/kg.

➤*IV:* The dose for IV and IM administration is identical; IV administration is useful for treating patients with bacterial septicemia or those in shock. It may also be the preferred route for some patients with CHF, hematologic disorders, severe burns or reduced muscle mass. A 1 to 2 mg/kg loading dose may be used, followed by a maintenance dose.

For intermittent IV administration in adults, dilute a single dose in 50 to 200 ml sterile isotonic saline or in a sterile solution of 5% Dextrose in Water. In infants and children, the volume of diluent should be less. Infuse over a period of ½ to 2 hours.

Admixture incompatibility – Do not physically premix gentamicin with other drugs; administer separately in accordance with route and dosage schedule.

➤*Intrathecal:* Administer only the 2 mg/ml intrathecal preparation without preservatives.

Dosage will vary depending upon factors such as age and weight of the patient, site of injection, degree of obstruction to CSF flow and the amount of CSF estimated to be present. In general, the recommended dose for infants and children ≥ 3 months of age is 1 to 2 mg once a day. For adults, administer 4 to 8 mg once a day.

Continue administration as long as sensitive organisms are demonstrated in the CSF. Since the intralumbar or intraventricular dose is administered immediately after specimens are taken for laboratory study, continue treatment for at least 1 day after negative results have been obtained from CSF cultures or stained smears.

The suggested method for administering the intrathecal injection into the lumbar area is as follows: Perform the lumbar puncture and remove a specimen of the spinal fluid for laboratory tests, then insert the syringe containing gentamicin into the hub of the spinal needle. Allow a quantity of CSF (≈ 10% of the estimated total CSF volume) to flow into the syringe and mix with the gentamicin. Inject the resultant solution over a period of 3 to 5 minutes with the bevel of the needle directed upward.

If the CSF is grossly purulent, or if it is unobtainable, dilute gentamicin with sterile normal saline before injection.

May also be administered directly into the subdural space or directly into the ventricles, including administration by use of an implanted reservoir.

TOBRAMYCIN

Rx	**Tobramycin Sulfate Pediatric** (Various, eg, Abbott, Apothecon)	**Injection:** 10 mg/ml	In 2 ml vials.
Rx	**Nebcin Pediatric** (Eli Lilly)		In 2 ml vials.[1]
Rx	**Nebcin** (Eli Lilly)		In 6 and 8 ml *ADD-Vantage* vials.[1]
Rx	**Tobramycin Sulfate** (Various, eg, Abbott, Apothecon)	**Injection:** 40 mg/ml	In 1.5 and 2 ml syringes and 2 and 30 ml vials.
Rx	**Nebcin** (Eli Lilly)	**Powder for injection:** 1.2 g	In 1.2 g vials.
Rx	**TOBI** (PathoGenesis)	**Nebulizer solution:** 300 mg/5 ml	In 5 ml ampules.[2]

[1] With phenol, disodium EDTA, sodium bisulfite. May also contain sulfuric acids or sodium hydroxide.

[2] With sodium chloride, sulfuric acid and sodium hyd oxide.

Information beginning in the Aminoglycoside group monograph must be considered when using these products. SPECIAL NOTE: See Warning Box concerning aminoglycoside toxicity.

Indications

➤*Bacterial infections (parenteral):* Treatment of serious bacterial infections caused by susceptible strains of *Pseudomonas aeruginosa,*

---

† American Heart Association statement. *JAMA* 1990;264:2919-2922.

TOBRAMYCIN

Escherichia coli, Proteus sp. (indole-positive and indole-negative) including *P. mirabilis, Morganella morganii* and *P. vulgaris, Providencia* sp. including *Klebsiella-Enterobacter-Serratia* group, *Citrobacter* sp. and staphylococci including *S. aureus* (coagulase-positive and coagulase-negative).

Septicemia (neonates, children, adults) – Caused by *P. aeruginosa, E. coli, Klebsiella* sp.

Lower respiratory tract infections – Caused by *P. aeruginosa, Klebsiella* sp., *Enterobacter* sp., *Serratia* sp., *E. coli, S. aureus* (penicillinase- and nonpenicillinase-producing).

Serious CNS infections (meningitis) – Caused by susceptible organisms.

Intra-abdominal infections, including peritonitis – Caused by *E. coli, Klebsiella* sp. and *Enterobacter* sp.

Skin, bone and skin structure infections – Caused by *P. aeruginosa, Proteus* sp., *E. coli, Klebsiella* sp., *Enterobacter* sp. and *S. aureus*.

Complicated and recurrent urinary tract infections (UTIs) – Caused by *P. aeruginosa, Proteus* sp. (indole-positive and indole-negative), *E. coli, Klebsiella* sp., *Enterobacter* sp., *Serratia* sp., *S. aureus, Providencia* sp., *Citrobacter* sp. Not for uncomplicated initial episodes of UTIs unless the organisms are not susceptible to less toxic antibiotics.

Tobramycin may be considered in serious staphylococcal infections when penicillin or other potentially less toxic drugs are contraindicated and when bacterial susceptibility testing and clinical judgment indicate its use.

In patients in whom serious life-threatening gram-negative infection is suspected, including those in whom concurrent therapy with a penicillin or cephalosporin and an aminoglycoside may be indicated, initiate tobramycin before susceptibility study results are obtained. Base decision to continue therapy on these results, infection severity and concepts discussed in Warning Box.

➤*Cystic fibrosis (nebulizer solution):* Management of cystic fibrosis patients with *Pseudomonas aeruginosa.*

Administration and Dosage

➤*Bacterial infections (parenteral):*

Dosage – Use the patient's ideal body weight for dosage calculation; for obese patients, use patient's estimated lean body weight plus 40% of the excess as the basic weight on which to calculate mg/kg dosing. Following 1 mg/kg IM, peak serum concentrations reach ≈ 4 mcg/ml and measurable levels persist for ≤ 8 hours. Therapeutic peak levels range from 4 to 6 mcg/ml. Peak and trough serum concentrations should be measured. Serum concentrations of the drug given by IV infusion over 1 hour are similar to those obtained by IM use.

Duration – Usual duration of treatment is 7 to 10 days. A longer course may be necessary in difficult and complicated infections. In such cases, monitor renal, auditory and vestibular functions; toxicity can occur when treatment extends > 10 days.

Monitoring – Serum concentrations, both peak and trough, should be monitored to ensure adequate levels and avoid toxicity; avoid prolonged peak concentrations > 12 mcg/ml or troughs > 2 mcg/ml). Examine urine for decreased specific gravity and for increased excretion of protein, cells and casts.

Cystic fibrosis: Serum levels of parenterally administered tobramycin in patients with cystic fibrosis may be reduced because of altered pharmacokinetics. An initial dosing regimen of 10 mg/kg/day in four equally divided doses is recommended as a guide. Tobramycin serum levels should be measured directly during treatment because of wide interpatient variability.

Adults – Administer 3 mg/kg/day IV or IM in three equal doses every 8 hours for serious infections or ≤ 5 mg/kg/day IV or IM in three or four equal doses for life-threatening infections reduced to 3 mg/kg/day as soon as clinically indicated. To prevent increased toxicity caused by excessive blood levels, do not exceed 5 mg/kg/day, unless serum levels are monitored.

Children – Administer 6 to 7.5 mg/kg/day in 3 or 4 equally divided doses (2 to 2.5 mg/kg every 8 hours or 1.5 to 1.9 mg/kg every 6 hours).

Premature or full-term neonates (≤ 1 week of age) – Administer ≤ 4 mg/kg/day in 2 equal doses every 12 hours. Preliminary data suggest that 2.5 mg/kg every 18 hours or 3 mg/kg every 24 hours may achieve safe and effective peak and trough serum concentrations in newborn infants weighing < 1 kg at birth.

Renal function impairment – Whenever possible, determine serum concentrations. Following a loading dose of 1 mg/kg, adjust subsequent dosage, either with reduced doses administered at 8-hour intervals or with normal doses given at prolonged intervals. Both of these methods are suggested as guides when serum levels of tobramycin cannot be measured directly. They are based on either creatinine clearance (Ccr; preferred) or serum creatinine, because these values correlate with the half-life of tobramycin. Use the dosage schedules derived from either method with careful clinical and laboratory observations of the patient; modify as necessary. These calculation methods may be misleading in patients who have undergone severe wasting and in the elderly. Do not use either method when dialysis is performed.

Reduced dosage at 8-hour intervals: When the Ccr is ≤ 70 ml/min or when serum creatinine is known, determine the amount of the reduced dose by multiplying the normal dose by the percent of normal dose from the accompanying nomogram.

REDUCED DOSAGE NOMOGRAM†

Creatinine Clearance (ml/min/1.73 m²)

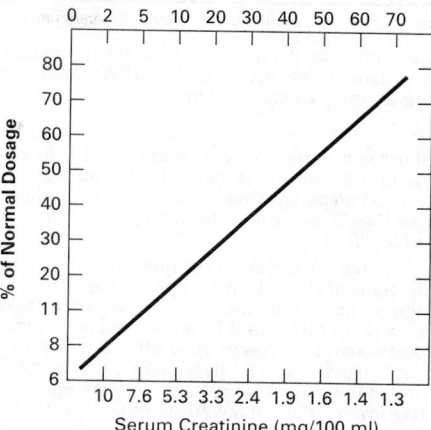

†Scales have been adjusted to facilitate dosage calculations.

An alternate rough guide for determining reduced dosage at 8-hour intervals (for patients whose steady-state serum creatinine values are known) is to divide the normally recommended dose by the patient's serum creatinine.

Normal dosage at prolonged intervals: If the Ccr is not available and the patient's condition is stable, determine a dosage frequency (in hours) for the normal dosage by multiplying the patient's serum creatinine by 6.

Hemodialysis: This removes ≈ 50% of a dose in 6 hours. In anephric patients maintained by regular dialysis, the usual dose of 1.5 to 2 mg/kg given after every dialysis usually maintains therapeutic, nontoxic serum levels. In patients receiving intermittent peritoneal dialysis, patients dialyzed twice weekly should receive a 1.5 to 2 mg/kg loading dose followed by 1 mg/kg every 3 days. Where dialysis occurs every 2 days, give a 1.5 mg/kg loading dose after the first dialysis and 0.75 mg/kg after each subsequent dialysis.

IV administration – The IV dose is the same as the IM dose. The usual volume of diluent (0.9% Sodium Chloride Injection or 5% Dextrose Injection) for adult doses is 50 to 100 ml. For children, the volume of diluent should be proportionately less than for adults. Infuse the diluted solution over a period of 20 to 60 minutes. Infusion periods of < 20 minutes are not recommended because peak serum levels may exceed 12 mcg/ml.

Admixture incompatibility: Do not physically premix with other drugs. Administer separately according to the recommended dose and route.

➤*Cystic fibrosis (nebulizer solution):* Recommended dosage for adults and children ≥ 6 years of age is 300 mg twice a day in repeating cycles of 28 days on drug/28 days off drug. Do not adjust dosage by age or weight. Take as close to 12 hours apart as possible; do not take < 6 hours apart. Administer by inhalation over a 10- to 15-minute period, using a hand-held *PARI LC PLUS* reusable nebulizer with a *DeVilbiss Pulmo-Aide* compressor. Do not dilute or mix with dornase alfa in the nebulizer. Instruct patients on multiple therapies to take them first, followed by tobramycin. Bronchospasm, which can occur with inhalation of tobramycin, may be reduced if inhalation of tobramycin nebulization solution follows bronchodilator therapy.

Inhale while sitting or standing upright and breathing normally through the mouthpiece of the nebulizer. Nose clips may help the patient breathe through the mouth.

Safety and efficacy have not been demonstrated in patients < 6 years of age, patients with FEV_1 < 25% or > 75% predicted or patients colonized with *Burkholderia cepacia.*

Monitoring – In patients with normal renal function, serum tobramycin concentrations are ≈ 1 mcg/ml 1 hour after dose administration and do not require routine monitoring. Monitoring of serum concentrations in patients with renal dysfunction or patients treated with concomitant parenteral tobramycin may reduce the risk of toxicity.

➤*Storage/Stability:* Refrigerate at 2° to 8°C (36° to 46°F). Upon removal from the refrigerator, or if refrigeration is unavailable, tobramycin pouches (opened or unopened) may be stored at room temperature (≤ 25°C [77°F]) for ≤ 28 days.

Do not expose ampules to intense light. The solution in the ampule may darken with age if not stored in the refrigerator; however, this does not indicate any change in the quality of the product as long as it is stored with the recommended storage conditions.

AMIKACIN SULFATE

Rx	Amikacin (Various, eg, Bedford Labs, Elkins-Sinn)	Injection: 250 mg/ml	In 2 and 4 ml vials[1].
Rx	Amikin (Apothecon)		In 2 and 4 ml vials[2] and 2 ml disp syringes.[2]
	Amikacin (Various, eg, Gensia)	Pediatric Injection: 50 mg/ml	0.13% sodium metabisulfite, 0.5% sodium citrate dihydrate. In 2 and 4 ml vials.
Rx	Amikin (Apothecon)		In 2 ml vials.[2]

[1] May contain sodium metabisulfite, sodium citrate dihydrate or sulfuric acid.

[2] With sodium bisulfite and sulfuric acid.

Information beginning in the Aminoglycosides group monograph must be considered when using these products. SPECIAL NOTE: See Warning Box concerning aminoglycoside toxicity.

Indications

➤*Organisms:* Short-term treatment of serious infections caused by susceptible strains of gram-negative bacteria, including *Pseudomonas* sp., *Escherichia coli, Proteus* sp. (indole-positive and indole-negative), *Providencia* sp., *Klebsiella* sp., *Enterobacter* sp., *Serratia* sp. and *Acinetobacter* (*Mima-Herellea*) sp.

➤*Infections:* Effective in bacterial septicemia (including neonatal sepsis); in serious infections of the respiratory tract, bones and joints, CNS (including meningitis) and skin and soft tissue; in intra-abdominal infections (including peritonitis); and in burns and postoperative infections (including postvascular surgery). Also effective in serious complicated and recurrent urinary tract infections (UTIs) caused by these organisms. Not indicated in uncomplicated initial episodes of UTIs unless the causative organisms are not susceptible to antibiotics having less toxicity.

➤*Suspected gram-negative infections:* Consider amikacin as initial therapy in suspected gram-negative infections; therapy may be instituted before obtaining the results of susceptibility testing. It is effective in infections caused by gentamicin- or tobramycin-resistant strains of gram-negative organisms, particularly *P. rettgeri, P. stuartii, S. marcescens* and *P. aeruginosa.* Continue therapy based on susceptibility test results, infection severity, patient response and the concepts discussed in the Warning Box.

➤*Staphylococcal infections:* Consider as initial therapy under certain conditions in the treatment of known or suspected staphylococcal disease, such as: Severe infections where the causative organism may be either a gram-negative bacterium or a staphylococcus; infections caused by susceptible strains of staphylococci in patients allergic to other antibiotics; and in mixed staphylococcal/gram-negative infections.

➤*Neonatal sepsis:* In severe infections, concomitant therapy with a penicillin-type drug may be indicated because of the possibility of infections caused by gram-positive organisms, such as streptococci or pneumococci.

➤*Unlabeled uses:* Intrathecal/intraventricular administration has been suggested at 8 mg/24 hours.

Amikacin 15 mg/kg/day IV in divided doses every 8 to 12 hours may be used as part of a multiple-drug regimen (generally three to five agents) for *Mycobacterium avium* complex, a common infection in AIDS patients.

Administration and Dosage

➤*Monitoring:* The patient's renal status should be monitored. Evidence of impairment in renal, vestibular or auditory function requires drug discontinuation or dosage adjustment. Examine urine for increased protein excretion, the presence of cells and casts and decreased specific gravity. Monitor serum concentrations and avoid prolonged peak concentrations > 35 mcg/ml. In healthy adult volunteers, average peak serum concentrations of about 12, 16 and 21 mcg/ml are obtained 1 hour after IM administration of 250 mg (3.7 mg/kg), 375 mg (5 mg/kg) and 500 mg (7.5 mg/kg) single doses, respectively. At 10 hours, serum levels are about 0.3, 1.2 and 2.1 mcg/ml, respectively.

➤*Adults, children and older infants:* Use the patient's ideal body weight for dosage calculation. Administer IM or IV. Administer 15 mg/kg/day divided into 2 or 3 equal doses at equally divided intervals. Treatment of heavier patients should not exceed 1.5 g/day. In uncomplicated UTIs, use 250 mg twice daily.

Neonates – A loading dose of 10 mg/kg is recommended, followed by 7.5 mg/kg every 12 hours. Preliminary IM studies in newborns of different weights (< 1.5 kg, 1.5 to 2 kg, > 2 kg) at a dose of 7.5 mg/kg revealed that, like other aminoglycosides, serum half-life values were correlated inversely with postnatal age and renal clearances of amikacin. Lower dosages may be safer during the first 2 weeks of life.

➤*Duration:* The usual duration of treatment is 7 to 10 days. Do not exceed 15 mg/kg/day. If treatment beyond 10 days is considered, monitor amikacin serum levels and renal, auditory and vestibular functions daily. Uncomplicated infections caused by sensitive organisms should respond in 24 to 48 hours. If definite clinical response does not occur within 3 to 5 days, stop therapy and reevaluate. Failure of the infection to respond may be because of resistance of the organism or to the presence of septic foci requiring surgical drainage.

➤*Renal function impairment:* Whenever possible, monitor serum concentrations. Adjust doses in patients with impaired renal function by administering normal doses at prolonged intervals or by administering reduced doses at a fixed interval. Both methods are based on the patient's creatinine clearance (Ccr; preferred) or serum creatinine values, since these have been found to correlate with aminoglycoside half-lives. Use these dosage schedules in conjunction with clinical and laboratory observations of the patient, and modify as necessary. These methods of dosage calculation may be misleading in patients who have undergone severe wasting and in the elderly. Neither method should be used when dialysis is being performed.

Normal dosage at prolonged intervals – If the Ccr is not available and the patient's condition is stable, calculate a dosage interval (in hours) for the normal dose by multiplying the patient's serum creatinine by 9.

Reduced dosage at fixed time intervals – Measure serum concentrations to assure accurate administration and to avoid concentrations > 35 mcg/ml. Initiate therapy by administering a normal dose, 7.5 mg/kg, as a loading dose.

To determine maintenance doses administered every 12 hours, reduce the loading dose in proportion to the reduction in the patient's Ccr:

$$\text{Maintenance dose every 12 hours} = \frac{\text{observed Ccr (mL/min)}}{\text{normal Ccr (mL/min)}} \times \text{calculated loading dose (mg)}$$

An alternate rough guide for determining reduced dosage at 12 hour intervals (for patients whose steady-state serum creatinine values are known) is to divide the normally recommended dose by the patient's serum creatinine.

Several predictive methods and published nomograms have been compared for gentamicin, none of which performed as well as individualized pharmacokinetic dosing with serum levels. This would probably also be true for amikacin.

Dialysis – Approximately half the normal mg/kg dose can be given after hemodialysis; in peritoneal dialysis, a parenteral dose of 7.5 mg/kg is given, and then amikacin is instilled in peritoneal dialysate at a concentration desired in serum.

➤*IV administration:* Dose is identical to IM dose.

Adults – Single doses of 500 mg (7.5 mg/kg), administered as an infusion over a period of 30 minutes, produced a mean peak serum concentration of 38 mcg/ml at the end of the infusion, and levels of 24, 18 and 0.75 mcg/ml at 30 minutes, 1 hour and 10 hours postinfusion, respectively. Repeated infusions of 7.5 mg/kg every 12 hours were well tolerated and caused no drug accumulation.

Preparation of solution – Prepare the solution for IV use by adding the contents of a 500 mg vial to 100 or 200 ml of sterile diluent. Administer the solution to adults over 30 to 60 minutes. Do not exceed 15 mg/kg/day, and divide into either 2 or 3 equal doses at equal intervals.

Infants – In pediatric patients, the amount of fluid used will depend on the amount ordered for the patient. It should be a sufficient amount to infuse the amikacin over 30 to 60 minutes. Infants should receive a 1 to 2 hour infusion.

➤*Admixture compatibility:* Amikacin is stable for 24 hours at room temperature at concentrations of 0.25 and 5 mg/ml in the following solutions: 5% Dextrose Injection; 5% Dextrose and 0.2% Sodium Chloride Injection; 5% Dextrose and 0.45% Sodium Chloride Injection; 0.9% Sodium Chloride Injection; Lactated Ringer's Injection; *Normosol M* in 5% Dextrose Injection (or *Plasma-Lyte 56* Injection in 5% Dextrose in Water); *Normosol R* in 5% Dextrose Injection (or *Plasma-Lyte 148* Injection in 5% Dextrose in Water).

➤*Admixture incompatibility:* Do not physically premix amikacin with other drugs; administer separately.

For more complete information on aminoglycosides, refer to the Aminoglycosides, Parenteral group monograph. SPECIAL NOTE: See Warning Box in Aminoglycosides, Parenteral group monograph concerning toxicity.

Indications

Suppression of intestinal bacteria.

Hepatic coma.

See individual monographs for specific information.

Actions

➤*Pharmacokinetics:* Oral aminoglycosides are poorly absorbed; therefore use only for suppression of GI bacterial flora. The small absorbed fraction is rapidly excreted with normal kidney function. The unabsorbed drug is eliminated unchanged in the feces. Most intestinal bacteria are rapidly eliminated with bacterial suppression persisting for 48 to 72 hours. Nonpathogenic yeasts and occasionally resistant strains of *Enterobacter aerogenes* replace the intestinal bacteria.

Contraindications

Presence of intestinal obstruction; hypersensitivity to aminoglycosides.

Warnings

➤*Increased absorption:* Although negligible amounts are absorbed through intact mucosa, consider the possibility of increased absorption from ulcerated or denuded areas.

➤*Nephrotoxicity/Ototoxicity:* Because of reported cases of deafness and potential nephrotoxic effects, closely observe patients. Perform urine and blood examinations and audiometric tests prior to and during extended therapy, especially in those with hepatic or renal disease. If renal insufficiency develops, reduce dosage or discontinue the drug. Refer to the Warning Box in the Aminoglycosides, Parenteral monograph concerning aminoglycoside toxicity.

➤*Pregnancy:* Safety for use during pregnancy has not been established. Use only when clearly needed and when the potential benefits outweigh the potential hazards.

Neomycin – Category D. Aminoglycosides can cause fetal harm when administered to a pregnant woman. Aminoglycosides cross the placenta. Although serious side effects to fetus or newborn have not been reported in the treatment of pregnant women, the potential for harm exists. If neomycin is used during pregnancy, or if the patient becomes pregnant while taking this drug, apprise the patient of the potential hazard to the fetus.

➤*Lactation:* Neomycin is excreted in cow milk following a single IM injection. It is not known whether neomycin is excreted in human breast milk. Other aminoglycosides are excreted in human breast milk. Because of the potential for serious adverse reactions from the aminoglycosides in nursing infants, decide whether to discontinue nursing or to discontinue the drug, taking into account the importance of the drug to the mother.

➤*Children:* The safety and efficacy of oral neomycin in patients < 18 years of age have not been established. If treatment is necessary, use with caution; do not exceed a treatment period of 3 weeks because of absorption from the GI tract.

Precautions

➤*Muscular disorders:* Use with caution in patients with muscular disorders such as myasthenia gravis or parkinsonism; these drugs may aggravate muscle weakness because of their potential curare-like effect on neuromuscular junction.

➤*GI effects:*

Neomycin – Orally administered neomycin increases fecal bile acid excretion and reduces intestinal lactase activity.

Paromomycin – Use with caution in individuals with ulcerative lesions of the bowel to avoid renal toxicity through inadvertent absorption.

➤*Superinfection:* Use of antibiotics (especially prolonged or repeated therapy) may result in bacterial or fungal overgrowth of nonsusceptible organisms. Such overgrowth may lead to a secondary infection. Take appropriate measures if superinfection occurs.

Drug Interactions

Oral Aminoglycoside Drug Interactions			
Precipitant drug	Object drug*		Description
Aminoglycosides	Anticoagulants	↑	A small rise in warfarin-induced hypoprothrombinemia may occur, possibly due to interference in absorption of dietary vitamin K by aminoglycosides.
Aminoglycosides	Digoxin	↓	Rate and extent of digoxin absorption may be reduced; however, in a small number of patients (< 10%), this may be off-set by a reduction in digoxin's metabolism.
Aminoglycosides	Methotrexate	↓	Methotrexate's absorption and bioavailability may be decreased.
Aminoglycosides	Neuromuscular blockers - Depolarizing and non-depolarizing	↑	The actions of the neuromuscular blockers may be enhanced; prolonged respiratory depression may occur.
Aminoglycosides	Polypeptide antibiotics	↑	Concurrent use may increase the risk of respiratory paralysis and renal dysfunction.
Aminoglycosides	Vitamin A	↓	Serum retinol and plasma carotene levels may be decreased.

* ↑ = Object drug increased.   ↓ = Object drug decreased.

Adverse Reactions

Nausea, vomiting and diarrhea are most common. The "malabsorption syndrome" characterized by increased fecal fat, decreased serum carotene and fall in xylose absorption has occurred with prolonged therapy. *Clostridium difficile*-associated colitis has occurred following neomycin therapy. Nephrotoxicity and ototoxicity have occurred following prolonged and high dosage therapy in hepatic coma.

Overdosage

Because of low absorption, it is unlikely that acute overdosage would occur with oral neomycin sulfate. However, prolonged administration could result in sufficient systemic drug levels to produce neurotoxicity, ototoxicity or nephrotoxicity. Hemodialysis will remove neomycin sulfate from the blood.

Patient Information

Complete full course of therapy; take until gone. May cause nausea, vomiting or diarrhea.

Notify physician if ringing in the ears, hearing impairment or rash, problems urinating or dizziness occurs.

Drink plenty of fluids.

➤*Neomycin:* Before administering the drug, inform patients or members of their families of possible toxic effects on the eighth cranial nerve. The possibility of acute toxicity increases in premature infants and neonates.

KANAMYCIN SULFATE

Rx	**Kantrex** (Apothecon)	**Capsules:** 500 mg (as sulfate)	Lactose. In 20s & 100s.

For complete prescribing information, refer to the Aminoglycosides, Oral group monograph.

Indications

➤*Suppression of intestinal bacteria:* For short-term adjunctive therapy.

➤*Hepatic coma:* Prolonged administration is effective adjunctive therapy by reduction of the ammonia-forming bacteria in the intestinal tract. The subsequent reduction in blood ammonia has resulted in neurologic improvement.

Administration and Dosage

➤*Suppression of intestinal bacteria:* As an adjunct to mechanical cleansing of the large bowel in short-term therapy – 1 g every hour for 4 hours, followed by 1 g every 6 hours for 36 to 72 hours.

➤*Hepatic coma:* 8 to 12 g/day in divided doses.

NEOMYCIN SULFATE

Rx	Neomycin Sulfate (Various, eg, Goldline)	**Tablets**: 500 mg	In 100s.
Rx	Neo-fradin (Pharma-Tek)	**Oral solution**: 125 mg per 5 ml	Parabens. In 480 ml.

Refer to the general discussion of these products in the Aminoglycosides, Oral group monograph.

Indications

➤*Suppression of bowel intestinal bacteria (eg, preoperative preparation of the bowel):* It is given concurrently with enteric coated erythromycin.

➤*Hepatic coma:* Administration has been effective adjunctive therapy in hepatic coma by reduction of the ammonia-forming bacteria in the intestinal tract. The subsequent reduction in blood ammonia has resulted in neurologic improvement.

➤*Unlabeled uses:* Many studies have documented lipid-lowering efficacy of neomycin. Alone, it reduced LDL cholesterol levels by 24%. Combined with niacin, it reduced LDL cholesterol level to below the 90th percentile in 92% of patients.

Administration and Dosage

➤*Preoperative prophylaxis for elective colorectal surgery:*

Recommended Bowel Preparation Regimen (Proposed Surgery Time 8 am)[1]			
Therapy	Day 3 before surgery	Day 2 before surgery	Day 1 before surgery
Diet	Minimum residue or clear liquid	Minimum residue or clear liquid	Clear liquid
Bisacodyl, 1 oral cap	6 pm (–62 hrs)		
Magnesium sulfate, 30 ml of a 50% solution orally		10 am (–46 hrs). Repeat at 2 pm (–42 hrs) and 6 pm (–38 hrs).	10 am (–22 hrs). Repeat at 2 pm (–18 hrs).
Enema		7 pm (–37 hrs) & 8 pm (–36 hrs). Repeat hourly until no solid feces return with last enema.	None
Supplemental IV fluids			As needed
Neomycin and erythromycin tablets, 1 g each, orally			1 pm (–19 hrs). Repeat at 2 pm (–18 hrs) and 11 pm (–9 hrs).

[1] On day of surgery, patient should evacuate rectum at 6:30 am (–1½ hrs) for 8 am procedure.

➤*Hepatic coma (as adjunct):* The following regimen has been used: Withdraw protein from diet; avoid diuretics; supportive therapy, including transfusions, as needed.

Adults – 4 to 12 g/day in divided doses.

Children – 50 to 100 mg/kg/day in divided doses. Continue treatment over a period of 5 to 6 days; during this time, return protein to the diet incrementally. Chronic hepatic insufficiency may require up to 4 g/day over an indefinite period.

PAROMOMYCIN SULFATE

Rx	Humatin (Parke-Davis)	**Capsules**: 250 mg paromomycin (as sulfate)	In 16s.

Refer to the general discussion of these products in the Aminoglycosides, Oral group monograph.

Indications

➤*Intestinal amebiasis (acute and chronic):* Note: Paromomycin is not effective in extraintestinal amebiasis. (See monograph in Amebicides section of this chapter.)

➤*Hepatic coma:* As adjunctive therapy.

➤*Unlabeled uses:* Has been recommended for other parasitic infections — *Dientamoeba fragilis* (25 to 30 mg/kg/day in 3 doses for 7 days); *Diphyllobothrium latum, Taenia saginata, T. solium, Dipylidium caninum* (adults: 1 g every 15 min for 4 doses; pediatric: 11 mg/kg every 15 min for 4 doses); *Hymenolepis nana* (45 mg/kg/day for 5 to 7 days).

Administration and Dosage

➤*Intestinal amebiasis:*

Adults and children – Usual dose is 25 to 35 mg/kg/day, in 3 doses with meals for 5 to 10 days.

➤*Management of hepatic coma:*

Adults – Usual dose is 4 g/day in divided doses at regular intervals for 5 to 6 days.

COLISTIMETHATE SODIUM

Rx **Coly-Mycin M**   **Injection (lyophilized cake):** 150 mg colistin (as colistimethate sodium) for reconstitution   In vials.
(Parke-Davis)

Indications

Treatment of acute or chronic infections due to sensitive strains of certain gram-negative bacilli. Particularly indicated when the infection is caused by sensitive strains of *P. aeruginosa*. Clinically effective in treatment of infections due to the following gram-negative organisms: *E. aerogenes, E. coli, K. pneumoniae* and *P. aeruginosa*. Pending results of bacteriologic cultures and sensitivity tests, colistimethate may be used to initiate therapy in serious infections that are suspected to be due to gram-negative organisms.

Administration and Dosage

For IM or IV use.

➤*Adults and children:* 2.5 to 5 mg/kg/day in 2 to 4 divided doses for patients with normal renal function, depending upon the severity of the infection. Reduce the daily dose in the presence of any renal impairment.

Suggested Modification of Colistimethate Dosage Schedules for Adults with Impaired Renal Function						
Renal function			Dosage			
Degree of impairment	Plasma creatinine (mg/dl)	Urea clearance % (of normal)	Dose[1] (mg)	Frequency (times per day)	Total daily dose (mg)	Approx. daily dose (mg/kg)
Normal	0.7 - 1.2	80 - 100	100 - 150	4 to 2	300	5
Mild	1.3 - 1.5	40 - 70	75 - 115	2	150 - 230	2.5 - 3.8
Moderate	1.6 - 2.5	25 - 40	66 - 150	2 or 1	133 - 150	2.5
Severe	2.6 - 4	10 - 25	100 - 150	q 36 h	100	1.5

[1] Suggested unit dose is 2.5 to 5 mg/kg; increase time interval between injections in presence of impaired renal function.

➤*IV administration:*

Direct intermittent administration – Inject one-half the total daily dose over a period of 3 to 5 minutes every 12 hours.

Continuous infusion – Slowly inject one-half the daily dose over 3 to 5 minutes. Add the remaining half of the total daily dose of colistimethate to one of the following: 0.9% Sodium Chloride; 5% Dextrose in Water; 5% Dextrose with 0.9% Sodium Chloride; 5% Dextrose with 0.45% Sodium Chloride; 5% Dextrose with 0.225% Sodium Chloride; Lactated Ringer's solution. Swirl gently to avoid frothing.

Administer by slow IV infusion starting 1 to 2 hours after the initial dose over the next 22 to 23 hours in the presence of normal renal function. In the presence of impaired renal function, reduce infusion rate. Choice of IV solution and volume to be employed are dictated by requirements of fluid and electrolyte management.

➤*Storage/Stability:* Freshly prepare any infusion solution containing colistimethate and use for no longer than 24 hours.

Actions

➤*Pharmacokinetics:* Higher initial blood levels are obtained following IV administration. Blood levels peak at between 5 and 10 mcg/ml between 2 and 3 hours after IM administration. Serum half-life is 2 to 3 hours.

Average urinary levels range from about 270 mcg/ml at 2 hours to about 15 mcg/ml at 8 hours after IV administration and from about 200 to 25 mcg/ml during a similar period following IM administration.

➤*Microbiology:* Colistimethate has bactericidal activity against the following gram-negative bacilli: *Enterobacter aerogenes, Escherichia coli, Klebsiella pneumoniae* and *Pseudomonas aeruginosa.*

Contraindications

Hypersensitivity to colistimethate sodium; infections due to *Proteus* or *Neisseria* species.

Warnings

➤*Maximum dosage:* Do not exceed 5 mg/kg/day in patients with normal renal function.

➤*Neurologic effects:* May occur transiently. These include circumoral paresthesias or numbness, tingling or formication of the extremities, generalized pruritus, vertigo, dizziness and slurring of speech. Warn patients not to drive vehicles or use hazardous machinery while on therapy. Dosage reduction may alleviate symptoms. Therapy need not be discontinued, but observe such patients carefully. Overdosage can result in renal insufficiency, muscle weakness and apnea.

➤*Renal function impairment:* Since colistimethate is eliminated mainly by renal excretion, use with caution when the possibility of impaired renal function exists. Consider the decline in renal function with advanced age.

When actual renal impairment is present, use colistimethate with extreme caution; reduce the dosage in proportion to the extent of the impairment. Administration of amounts in excess of renal excretory capacity will lead to high serum levels. This can result in further impairment of renal function, initiating a cycle which, if not recognized, can lead to acute renal insufficiency, renal shutdown and further concentration of the antibiotic to toxic levels in the body. Interference with nerve transmission at neuromuscular junctions may occur and result in muscle weakness and apnea.

Signs indicating the development of impaired renal function are diminishing urine output and rising BUN or serum creatinine. If present, discontinue therapy immediately. If a life-threatening situation exists, reinstate therapy at a lower dosage after blood levels have fallen.

➤*Pregnancy:* Colistimethate sodium is transferred across the placental barrier, and blood levels of about 1 mcg/ml are obtained in the fetus following IV administration to the mother. Safety for use during pregnancy has not been established. Use only when clearly needed and when the potential benefits outweigh the potential hazards.

Precautions

➤*Respiratory effects:* Respiratory arrest has occurred following IM administration. Impaired renal function increases the possibility of apnea and neuromuscular blockade, generally because of failure to follow recommended guidelines, overdosage, failure to reduce dose commensurate with degree of renal impairment or concomitant use of other antibiotics or drugs with neuromuscular blocking potential. If apnea occurs, treat with assisted respiration, oxygen and calcium chloride injections.

➤*Nephrotoxicity:* A decrease in urine output or increase in BUN or serum creatinine can be signs of nephrotoxicity, which is probably a dose-dependent effect. These manifestations are reversible following discontinuation. Increases of BUN have occurred at dose levels of 1.6 to 5 mg/kg/day. Values returned to normal following cessation.

Drug Interactions

Colistimethate Drug Interactions			
Precipitant drug	Object drug[*]		Description
Aminoglyco-sides	Colistimethate	↑	Concurrent use may increase the risk of respiratory paralysis and renal dysfunction.
Cephalothin	Colistimethate	↑	Concurrent use may increase the risk of renal dysfunction.
Colistimethate	Nondepolar-izing muscle relaxants	↑	Neuromuscular blockade may be enhanced.

[*] ↑ = Object drug increased.

Adverse Reactions

Respiratory arrest (see Precautions); decreased urine output or increased BUN or serum creatinine (see Precautions); paresthesia; tingling of the extremities or the tongue; generalized itching or urticaria; drug fever; GI upset; vertigo; slurring of speech. The subjective symptoms reported by the adult may not be manifest in infants or young children, thus requiring close attention to renal function.

POLYMYXIN B SULFATE

Rx	Polymyxin B Sulfate (Bedford)	Injection: 500,000 units	In vials.

WARNING

When this drug is given intramuscularly or intrathecally, administer only to hospitalized patients to provide constant physician supervision.

Carefully determine renal function; reduce dosage in patients with renal damage and nitrogen retention. Patients with nephrotoxicity due to polymyxin B sulfate usually show albuminuria, cellular casts and azotemia. Diminishing urine output and a rising BUN are indications to discontinue therapy.

Neurotoxic reactions may be manifested by irritability, weakness, drowsiness, ataxia, perioral paresthesia, numbness of the extremities and blurring of vision. These are usually associated with high serum levels found in patients with impaired renal function or nephrotoxicity. Avoid concurrent use of other nephrotoxic and neurotoxic drugs, particularly kanamycin, streptomycin, paromomycin, colistin, tobramycin, neomycin and gentamicin.

The drug's neurotoxicity can result in respiratory paralysis from neuromuscular blockade, especially when the drug is given soon after anesthesia or muscle relaxants.

Indications

Acute infections caused by susceptible strains of *Pseudomonas aeruginosa*. It may be used topically and subconjunctively in the treatment of infections of the eye caused by susceptible strains of *P. aeruginosa*.

It may be indicated (when less toxic drugs are ineffective or contraindicated) in serious infections caused by susceptible strains of the following organisms: *Haemophilus influenzae* (meningeal infections); *Escherichia coli* (urinary tract infections); *Enterobacter aerogenes* (bacteremia); *Klebsiella pneumoniae* (bacteremia).

➤*Note:* In meningeal infections, administer polymyxin B sulfate only intrathecally.

Administration and Dosage

➤*IV:* Dissolve 500,000 units polymyxin B sulfate in 300 to 500 ml of 5% Dextrose in Water for continuous IV drip.

Adults and children – 15,000 to 25,000 units/kg/day in individuals with normal renal function. Reduce this amount from 15,000 units/kg downward for individuals with renal impairment. Infusions may be given every 12 hours; however, the total daily dose must not exceed 25,000 units/kg/day.

Infants – Those with normal renal function may receive up to 40,000 units/kg/day.

➤*IM:* Not recommended routinely because of severe pain at injection sites, particularly in infants and children. Dissolve 500,000 units in 2 ml sterile distilled water (Water for Injection, USP) or sterile physiologic saline (Sodium Chloride Injection) or 1% procaine HCl solution.

Adults and children – 25,000 to 30,000 units/kg/day. Reduce dosage in the presence of renal impairment. Dosage may be divided and given at either 4 or 6 hour intervals.

Infants – Those with normal renal function may receive up to 40,000 units/kg/day.

Note: Doses as high as 45,000 units/kg/day have been used in limited clinical studies in treating premature and newborn infants for sepsis caused by *Pseudomonas aeruginosa*.

➤*Intrathecal:* A treatment of choice for *P. aeruginosa* meningitis. Dissolve 500,000 units in 10 ml sterile physiologic saline for a concentration of 50,000 units/ml.

Adults and children (> 2 years of age) – 50,000 units once daily intrathecally for 3 to 4 days, then 50,000 units once every other day for at least 2 weeks after cultures of the CSF are negative and glucose content has returned to normal.

Children (< 2 years of age) – 20,000 units once daily, intrathecally for 3 to 4 days or 25,000 units once every other day. Continue with a dose of 25,000 units once every other day for at least 2 weeks after cultures of the CSF are negative and glucose content has returned to normal.

➤*Storage/Stability:* Refrigerate and discard any unused portion after 72 hours.

Actions

➤*Pharmacology:* Polymyxin is bactericidal against almost all gram-negative bacilli except the *Proteus* group; it increases the permeability of bacterial cell membranes.

➤*Pharmacokinetics:* Polymyxin B sulfate is not absorbed from the normal GI tract. Since the drug loses 50% of its activity in the presence of serum, active blood levels are low. Repeated injections may give a cumulative effect. Levels tend to be higher in infants and children. Tissue diffusion is poor; the drug does not pass blood-brain barrier into cerebrospinal fluid (CSF). Drug is excreted slowly by kidneys. In therapeutic dosage, it causes some nephrotoxicity with slight tubule damage.

➤*Microbiology:* All gram-positive bacteria, fungi and gram-negative cocci, *Neisseria gonorrhoeae* and *N. meningitidis*, are resistant.

Contraindications

Hypersensitivity to the polymyxins.

Warnings

➤*Pregnancy:* Safety for use during pregnancy has not been established.

Precautions

➤*Monitoring:* Determine baseline renal function prior to therapy. Frequently monitor renal function and drug levels during therapy. The use of doses higher than those recommended is dangerous and potentially fatal. In doses of 3 mg/kg/day (30,000 units), polymyxin B may cause nephrotoxicity in patients with normal renal function, but lower doses may cause renal damage in patients with preexisting renal impairment.

➤*Superinfection:* Use of antibiotics (especially prolonged or repeated therapy) may result in bacterial or fungal overgrowth of nonsusceptible organisms. Such overgrowth may lead to a secondary infection. Take appropriate measures if this occurs.

Drug Interactions

Polymyxin B Drug Interactions			
Precipitant drug	Object drug*		Description
Aminoglyco-sides	Polymyxin B	↑	Concurrent use may increase the risk of respiratory paralysis and renal dysfunction.
Polymyxin B	Nondepolarizing muscle relaxants	↑	Neuromuscular blockade may be enhanced.

* ↑ = Object drug increased.

Adverse Reactions

➤*Nephrotoxic:* Albuminuria; cylindruria; azotemia; rising blood levels without increase in dosage.

➤*Neurotoxic:* Facial flushing; dizziness progressing to ataxia; drowsiness; peripheral paresthesias (circumoral and stocking-glove); apnea due to concurrent use of curariform muscle relaxants, other neurotoxic drugs or inadvertent overdosage.

Meningeal irritation with intrathecal administration (eg, fever, headache, stiff neck and increased cell count and protein in CSF).

➤*Miscellaneous:* Drug fever; urticarial rash; severe pain or thrombophlebitis at injection sites.

BACITRACIN

Rx	**Bacitracin USP** (Various, eg, Upjohn)	**Powder for Injection:** 50,000 units	In vials.
Rx	**Baci-IM** (Pharma-Tek)		In vials.

WARNING

Nephrotoxicity: Parenteral (IM) bacitracin may cause renal failure due to tubular and glomerular necrosis. Restrict use to infants with staphylococcal pneumonia and empyema when due to organisms shown to be susceptible. Use only where laboratory facilities are adequate and constant supervision is possible.

Carefully determine renal function prior to therapy, and daily during therapy. Do not exceed the recommended daily dose, and maintain fluid intake and urinary output at proper levels to avoid renal toxicity. If renal toxicity occurs, discontinue the drug. Avoid the concurrent use of other nephrotoxic drugs, particularly streptomycin, kanamycin, polymyxin B, colistin and neomycin.

Indications

Limit use of IM bacitracin to the treatment of infants with pneumonia and empyema caused by staphylococci shown to be sensitive to the drug (see Warning Box).

➤*Unlabeled uses:* Oral use in antibiotic-associated colitis has been successful.

Administration and Dosage

IM use only. Give in upper outer quadrant of buttocks, alternating sides and avoiding multiple injections in the same region because of transient pain following injection.

➤*Infants < 2.5 kg:* 900 units/kg/24 hours, in 2 or 3 divided doses.

➤*Infants > 2.5 kg:* 1000 units/kg/24 hours, in 2 or 3 divided doses.

➤*Preparation of solutions:* Dissolve in Sodium Chloride Injection containing 2% procaine HCl. Antibiotic concentration in solution should not be < 5000 units/ml nor > 10,000 units/ml. Do not use diluents containing parabens; cloudy solutions and precipitate formation have occurred. Reconstitution of the 50,000 unit vial with 9.8 ml of diluent will result in a concentration of 5000 units/ml.

➤*Storage/Stability:* Refrigerate the unreconstituted product at 2° to 8°C (36° to 46°F). Solutions are stable for 1 week when refrigerated at 2° to 8°C (36° to 46°F).

Actions

➤*Pharmacology:* Bacitracin exerts pronounced antibacterial action in vitro against a variety of gram-positive and a few gram-negative organisms. However, among systemic diseases, only staphylococcal infections qualify for consideration of bacitracin therapy. Bacitracin is assayed against a standard, and its activity is expressed in units, with 1 mg having a potency of not less than 50 units.

➤*Pharmacokinetics:* Absorption after IM injection is rapid and complete. A dose of 200 or 300 units/kg every 6 hrs gives serum levels of 0.2 to 2 mcg/ml in individuals with normal renal function. It is widely distributed in all body organs and is demonstrable in ascitic and pleural fluids. It is excreted slowly by glomerular filtration.

Contraindications

Hypersensitivity or toxic reaction to bacitracin.

Precautions

➤*Fluid intake:* Maintain adequate fluid intake orally, or if necessary, parenterally.

➤*Superinfection:* Use of antibiotics (especially prolonged or repeated therapy) may result in bacterial or fungal overgrowth of nonsusceptible organisms. Such overgrowth may lead to a secondary infection. Take appropriate measures if this occurs.

Drug Interactions

Bacitracin Drug Interactions			
Precipitant drug	Object drug*		Description
Aminoglyco-sides	Bacitracin	↑	Concurrent use may increase risk of respiratory paralysis and renal dysfunction.
Bacitracin	Nondepolarizing muscle relaxants	↑	Neuromuscular blockade may be enhanced.

* ↑ = Object drug increased

Adverse Reactions

Albuminuria; cylindruria; azotemia; rising blood levels without increase in dosage; nausea and vomiting; pain at injection site; skin rashes.

RIFAXIMIN

Rx Xifaxan (Salix)	**Tablets:** 200 mg	EDTA. (Sx). Pink, biconvex. Film-coated. In 30s.

Indications

➤*Traveler's diarrhea:* For the treatment of patients 12 years of age and older with traveler's diarrhea caused by noninvasive strains of *Escherichia coli.*

Do not use in patients with diarrhea complicated by fever, blood in the stool, or diarrhea caused by pathogens other than *E. coli.*

Administration and Dosage

➤*Approved by the FDA:* May 25, 2004.

Administer orally with or without food. The recommended dose is one 200 mg tablet taken 3 times/day for 3 days.

➤*Storage/Stability:* Store at 20° to 25°C (68° to 77°F); excursions permitted to 15° to 30°C (59° to 86°F).

Actions

➤*Pharmacology:* Rifaximin acts by binding to the beta-subunit of bacterial DNA-dependent RNA polymerase resulting in inhibition of bacterial RNA synthesis. Rifaximin is a structural analog of rifampin. Organisms with high rifaximin minimum inhibitory concentration (MIC) values also have elevated MIC values against rifampin. Cross-resistance between rifaximin and other classes of antimicrobials has not been studied.

Rifaximin has been shown to be active against *E. coli* (enterotoxigenic and enteroaggregative strains) in clinical studies of infectious diarrhea.

➤*Pharmacokinetics:*

Absorption – Rifaximin is not suitable for treating systemic bacterial infections because less than 0.4% of the drug is absorbed after oral administration. The mean pharmacokinetic parameters of rifaximin in 14 healthy subjects after a single oral 400 mg dose given as 2 × 200 mg doses under fed and fasting conditions are summarized in the following table.

Rifaximin (Single 400 mg Dose) Mean Pharmacokinetic Parameters (N = 14)		
Parameter	Fasting	Fed
C_{max} (ng/mL)	3.8	9.63
T_{max} (h)	1.21	1.9
Half-life (h)	5.85	5.95
AUC (ng•h/mL)	18.35	34.7
Excreted in urine (%)	0.023	0.051

Rifaximin can be administered with or without food. Systemic absorption of rifaximin was low in the fasting state and when administered within 30 minutes of a high-fat breakfast.

Distribution – Animal pharmacokinetic studies have demonstrated that 80% to 90% of orally administered rifaximin is concentrated in the gut with less than 0.2% in the liver and kidney, and less than 0.01% in other tissues. In adults with infectious diarrhea treated with 800 mg/day rifaximin for 3 days, concentrations of rifaximin in stools averaged approximately 8,000 mcg/g the day after treatment ended.

Metabolism – In an in vitro hepatocyte induction model, rifaximin was shown to induce cytochrome P450 3A4 (CYP3A4), an isoenzyme that rifampin is known to induce.

Excretion – Rifaximin is excreted primarily in the feces. After oral administration of 400 mg rifaximin to healthy volunteers, approximately 97% of the dose was recovered in feces, almost entirely as unchanged drug, and 0.32% was recovered in the urine.

Contraindications

Hypersensitivity to rifaximin, any of the rifamycin antimicrobial agents, or any of the components in rifaximin.

Warnings

➤*Diarrhea:* Tablets were not found to be effective in patients with diarrhea complicated by fever and/or blood in the stool or diarrhea caused by pathogens other than *E. coli.* Rifaximin is not effective in cases of traveler's diarrhea caused by *Campylobacter jejuni.* The effectiveness of rifaximin in traveler's diarrhea caused by *Shigella* spp. and *Salmonella* spp. has not been proven. Do not use in patients where *C. jejuni, Shigella* spp., or *Salmonella* spp. may be suspected as causative pathogens.

Discontinue rifaximin if diarrhea symptoms get worse or persist more than 24 to 48 hours and consider an alternative antibiotic therapy.

➤*Pseudomembranous colitis:* Pseudomembranous colitis has been reported with nearly all antibacterial agents and may range in severity from mild to life-threatening. Therefore, it is important to consider this diagnosis in patients who present with diarrhea subsequent to the administration of antibacterial agents.

Treatment with antibacterial agents alters the normal flora of the colon and may permit overgrowth of clostridia. Studies indicate that a toxin produced by *Clostridium difficile* is the primary cause of antibiotic-associated colitis.

After the diagnosis of pseudomembranous colitis has been established, initiate therapeutic measures. Mild cases of pseudomembranous colitis usually respond to drug discontinuation alone. In moderate to severe cases, consider management with fluids and electrolytes, protein supplementation, and treatment with an antibacterial drug clinically effective against *C. difficile.*

➤*Pregnancy: Category C.* Rifaximin was teratogenic in rats at doses of 150 to 300 mg/kg (approximately 2.5 to 5 times the clinical dose adjusted for body surface area) and in rabbits at doses of 62.5 to 1,000 mg/kg (approximately 2 to 33 times the clinical dose adjusted for body surface area). These effects include the following: Agnathia, brachygnathia, cleft palate, eye partially open, hemorrhage, incomplete ossification, increased thoracolumbar vertebrae, jaw shortening, and small eyes. There are no adequate and well-controlled studies in pregnant women. Use rifaximin during pregnancy only if the potential benefit outweighs the potential risk to the fetus.

➤*Lactation:* It is not known whether rifaximin is excreted in human milk. Decide whether to discontinue nursing or to discontinue the drug, taking into account the importance of the drug to the mother.

➤*Children:* The safety and efficacy of rifaximin in pediatric patients younger than 12 years of age of age have not been established.

Precautions

➤*Superinfection:* The use of antibiotics may promote the overgrowth of nonsusceptible organisms. Take appropriate measures if superinfection occurs during therapy.

Adverse Reactions

Rifaximin Adverse Reactions (≥ 2%)		
Adverse reaction	Rifaximin 600 mg/day (N = 320)	Placebo (N = 228)
GI		
Abdominal pain NOS[a]	7.2	10.1
Constipation	3.8	3.5
Defecation urgency	5.9	9.2
Flatulence	11.3	19.7
Nausea	5.3	8.3
Rectal tenesmus	7.2	8.8
Vomiting NOS[a]	2.2	1.8
Miscellaneous		
Headache	9.7	9.2
Pyrexia	3.1	4.4

[a] NOS = not otherwise specified.

The following adverse events also have been reported in less than 2% of patients taking rifaximin. The following includes adverse events regardless of causal relationship to drug exposure.

➤*CNS:* Abnormal dreams, dizziness, insomnia, loss of taste, migraine (NOS), syncope.

➤*Dermatologic:* Clamminess, rash (NOS), sunburn, sweating increased.

➤*Hematologic:* Lymphocytosis, monocytosis, neutropenia.

➤*GI:* Abdominal distension, anorexia, blood in stool, diarrhea (NOS), dry lips, dry throat, fecal abnormality (NOS), gingival disorder (NOS), inguinal hernia (NOS), stomach discomfort.

➤*GU:* Blood in urine, choluria, dysuria, hematuria, polyuria, proteinuria, urinary frequency.

➤*Metabolic:* Dehydration, weight decreased.

➤*Musculoskeletal:* Arthralgia, muscle spasms, myalgia, neck pain.

RIFAXIMIN

➤*Respiratory:* Dyspnea (NOS), nasal passage irritation, nasopharyngitis, pharyngitis, pharyngolaryngeal pain, respiratory tract infection (NOS), rhinitis (NOS), rhinorrhea, upper respiratory tract infection (NOS).

➤*Special senses:* Ear pain, motion sickness, tinnitus.

➤*Miscellaneous:* Aspartate aminotransferase increased, chest pain, dysentery (NOS), fatigue, hot flashes (NOS), malaise, pain (NOS), weakness.

➤*Postmarketing:* Hypersensitivity reactions, including allergic dermatitis, angioneurotic edema, pruritus, rash, and urticaria have been identified during foreign postapproval use of rifaximin. Because these events are reported voluntarily from a population of uncertain size, it is not always possible to estimate their frequency or establish a causal relationship to drug exposure.

Overdosage

➤*Symptoms:* In clinical studies at doses higher than the recommended dose (greater than 600 mg/day), adverse events were similar to the recommended dose (200 mg 3 times/day) and to placebo.

➤*Treatment:* In the case of overdosage, discontinue rifaximin, treat symptomatically, and institute supportive measures as required.

Patient Information

Advise patients that rifaximin may be taken with or without food.

Advise patients to discontinue rifaximin and seek medical care if their diarrhea persists for more than 24 to 48 hours or worsens, or if they have fever and/or blood in the stool.

METRONIDAZOLE

Rx	**Metronidazole** (Various, eg, Mutual, Teva, UDL)	**Tablets:** 250 mg	In 25s, 100s, 250s, and 500s.
Rx	**Flagyl** (Pharmacia)		(SEARLE 1831 FLAGYL 250). Blue. Film-coated. In 50s, 100s, and 2500s.
Rx	**Metronidazole** (Various, eg, Mutual, Teva, UDL)	**Tablets:** 500 mg	In 25s, 50s, 100s, and 500s.
Rx	**Flagyl** (Pharmacia)		(FLAGYL 500). Blue, oblong. Film-coated. In 50s, 100s, and 500s.
Rx	**Metronidazole** (Able)	**Tablets, extended-release:** 750 mg	Lactose, polydextrose. (A352). Yellow, oval. Film coated. In 30s, 100s, 500s, and 1000s.
Rx	**Flagyl ER** (Pharmacia)		Lactose. (SEARLE 1961 FLAGYL ER). Blue, oval. Film-coated. In 30s.
Rx	**Metronidazole** (Able)	**Capsules:** 375 mg	(A 353). Yellow and grey. In 30s, 50s, 100s, 500s, and 1000s.
Rx	**Flagyl 375** (Pharmacia)		(375 mg Flagyl). Iron gray/lt. green. In 50s and UD 100s.
Rx	**Flagyl IV** (Pharmacia)	**Powder for Injection, lyophilized:** 500 mg	In single-dose vials.[1]
Rx	**Metronidazole** (B. Braun)	**Injection:** 5 mg/mL	In 100 mL vials.
Rx	**Flagyl IV RTU** (Pharmacia)		In 100 mL single-dose plastic containers.[2]

[1] 415 mg mannitol per vial. [2] 14 mEq sodium per vial.

Metronidazole is also available for topical and intravaginal use. For further information refer to the individual monographs in the Dermatologicals chapter. It also is used orally as an amebicide; refer to the individual monograph in the Amebicides section of this chapter.

WARNING
Metronidazole is carcinogenic in rodents. Avoid unnecessary use.

Indications

➤*Anaerobic infections:* Treatment of serious infections caused by susceptible anaerobic bacteria. Effective in *Bacteroides fragilis* infections resistant to clindamycin, chloramphenicol, and penicillin.

Intra-abdominal infections – Peritonitis, intra-abdominal abscess and liver abscess caused by *Bacteroides* sp. including the *B. fragilis* group (*B. fragilis, B. distasonis, B. ovatus, B. thetaiotaomicron, B. vulgatus*), *Clostridium* sp., *Eubacterium* sp., *Peptostreptococcus* sp., and *Peptococcus niger*.

Skin and skin structure infections – Caused by *Bacteroides* sp. including the *B. fragilis* group, *Clostridium* sp., *Peptococcus niger*, *Peptostreptococcus* sp., and *Fusobacterium* sp.

Gynecologic infections – Endometritis, endomyometritis, tubo-ovarian abscess, and postsurgical vaginal cuff infection caused by *Bacteroides* sp. including the *B. fragilis* group, *Clostridium* sp., *Peptococcus niger*, and *Peptostreptococcus* sp.; bacterial vaginosis (*Flagyl ER* only).

Bacterial septicemia – Caused by *Bacteroides* sp. including the *B. fragilis* group and *Clostridium* sp.

Bone and joint infections – Caused by *Bacteroides* sp. including the *B. fragilis* group, as adjunctive therapy.

CNS infections – Meningitis and brain abscess caused by *Bacteroides* sp. including the *B. fragilis* group.

Lower respiratory tract infections – Pneumonia, empyema, and lung abscess caused by *Bacteroides* sp. including the *B. fragilis* group.

Endocarditis – Caused by *Bacteroides* sp. including the *B. fragilis* group.

Metronidazole also is indicated for amebiasis and trichomoniasis, intravaginally for bacterial vaginosis, and topically for acne rosacea (see individual monographs).

➤*Prophylaxis:* Preoperative, intraoperative, and postoperative IV metronidazole may reduce the incidence of postoperative infection in patients undergoing elective colorectal surgery, which is classified as contaminated or potentially contaminated.

Discontinue within 12 hours after surgery. If there are signs of infection, obtain specimens for cultures to identify the causative organisms.

➤*Unlabeled uses:*

Hepatic encephalopathy – Metronidazole (800 mg/day) for 1 week has comparable efficacy to neomycin.

Crohn's disease – Metronidazole (250 mg 4 times/day) plus ciprofloxacin (500 mg twice/day) has been useful for patients with active acute-phase Crohn's disease.

Diarrhea associated with Clostridium difficile – Metronidazole (500 mg 3 times/day or 250 mg 4 times/day) has similar rates of efficacy compared with vancomycin.

Helicobacter pylori – Metronidazole is useful in eradicating *H. pylori* but should be used in combination therapy.

Recurrent and persistent urethritis – The CDC recommends metronidazole 2 g orally in a single dose plus erythromycin for 7 days.

Bacterial vaginosis – Per CDC recommendations, metronidazole 500 mg twice/day for 7 days or 2 g orally in a single dose. *Flagyl ER* is approved for this use.

Pelvic inflammatory disease – As an alternative parenteral regimen, the CDC recommends metronidazole 500 mg IV every 8 hours combined with ofloxacin alone or ciprofloxacin plus doxycycline. For oral therapy, metronidazole 500 mg twice/day is given with ofloxacin for 14 days.

Prophylaxis after sexual assault – CDC guidelines recommend metronidazole 2 g orally in a single dose plus ceftriaxone and either azithromycin or doxycycline.

Administration and Dosage

➤*Anaerobic bacterial infections:* In the treatment of most serious anaerobic infections, metronidazole is usually administered IV initially.

IV –

Loading dose: 15 mg/kg infused over 1 hour (≈ 1 g for a 70 kg adult).

Maintenance dose: 7.5 mg/kg infused over 1 hour every 6 hours (≈ 500 mg for a 70 kg adult). Administer the first maintenance dose 6 hours following the initiation of loading dose. Do not exceed a maximum of 4 g in 24 hours.

Administer by slow IV drip infusion only, either as continuous or intermittent infusion. Do not use equipment containing aluminum (eg, needles, cannulae). If used with a primary IV fluid system, discontinue the primary solution during infusion. Do not give by direct IV bolus injection because of the low pH (0.5 to 2) of the reconstituted product. The drug must be further diluted and neutralized for infusion. Do not introduce additives into the solution.

➤*Oral:* Following IV therapy, use oral metronidazole when conditions warrant. The usual adult oral dosage is 7.5 mg/kg every 6 hours (≈ 500 mg for a 70 kg adult). Do not exceed a maximum of 4 g in 24 hours.

➤*Duration:* The usual duration of therapy is 7 to 10 days; however, infections of the bone and joints, lower respiratory tract, and endocardium may require longer treatment.

➤*Bacterial vaginosis:*

7-day course of treatment – 750 mg ER once daily by mouth for 7 consecutive days.

Take *Flagyl ER* tablets under fasting conditions, ≥ 1 hour before or 2 hours after meals. The optimum extended-release characteristics are obtained when taken under fasting conditions.

➤*Prophylaxis:* To prevent postoperative infection in contaminated or potentially contaminated colorectal surgery, the recommended adult dosage is 15 mg/kg infused over 30 to 60 minutes and completed ≈ 1 hour before surgery; followed by 7.5 mg/kg infused over 30 to 60 minutes at 6 and 12 hours after the initial dose.

Complete administration of the initial preoperative dose ≈ 1 hour before surgery so that adequate drug levels are present in the serum and tissues at the time of initial incision, and administer, if necessary, at 6-hour intervals to maintain effective drug levels. Limit prophylactic use to the day of surgery only, following the above guidelines.

➤*Hepatic disease:* These patients metabolize metronidazole slowly; accumulation of metronidazole and its metabolites occurs. Therefore, reduce doses below those usually recommended. Monitor plasma metronidazole levels and observe for toxicity.

➤*Renal disease:* Do not specifically reduce the dose in anuric patients, because accumulated metabolites may be rapidly removed by dialysis.

➤*Elderly:* Dosage adjustment may be necessary; monitor serum levels.

➤*Preparation of parenteral solution:* NOTE: Order of mixing is important. (1) Reconstitution; (2) dilution in IV solution; (3) pH neutralization with sodium bicarbonate injection.

Aluminum-containing equipment – Do not use with metronidazole IV.

METRONIDAZOLE

Reconstitution – Add 4.4 mL of one of the following diluents to the vial and mix thoroughly: Sterile Water for Injection; Bacteriostatic Water for Injection; 0.9% Sodium Chloride Injection; Bacteriostatic 0.9% Sodium Chloride Injection. The resultant volume is 5 mL with an approximate concentration of 100 mg/mL.

The pH of the reconstituted product will be between 0.5 to 2; the solution is clear, and pale yellow to yellow-green in color. Do not use if cloudy or precipitated.

Dilution in IV solutions – Add the properly reconstituted product to a glass or plastic IV container. Do not exceed a concentration of 8 mg/mL. Use any of the following: 0.9% Sodium Chloride Injection; 5% Dextrose Injection; Lactated Ringer's Injection.

Neutralization for IV infusion – Prior to administration, neutralize the IV solution containing metronidazole with ≈ 5 mEq sodium bicarbonate injection for each 500 mg used. Mix thoroughly. The pH of the neutralized IV solution will be ≈ 6 to 7. Carbon dioxide gas will be generated with neutralization. It may be necessary to relieve gas pressure within the container.

When the contents of one vial (500 mg) are diluted and neutralized to 100 mL, the resultant concentration is 5 mg/mL. Do not exceed an 8 mg/mL concentration in the neutralized IV solution; neutralization will decrease aqueous solubility and precipitation may occur. Do not refrigerate neutralized solutions; precipitation may occur.

➤*Ready-to-use:* Do not use plastic containers in series connections; it could result in air embolism because of residual air (≈ 15 mL) being drawn from the primary container before administration of the fluid from the secondary container is complete.

➤*Storage/Stability:* Reconstituted *Flagyl IV* is stable for 96 hours when stored < 30°C (86°F) in room light. Use diluted and neutralized IV solutions within 24 hours. Store ready-to-use solution at 15° to 30°C (59° to 86°F); protect from light.

Store *Flagyl ER* in a dry place at 25°C (77°F); excursions permitted to 15° to 30°C (59° to 86°F). Dispense in a well-closed container with a child-resistant closure.

Actions

➤*Pharmacology:* Metronidazole, a nitroimidazole, is active against various anaerobic bacteria and protozoa. It is believed to act in 4 phases: a) Enter into the bacterium cell; b) reduce the nitro group; c) invoke cytotoxicity on the reduced product; and d) liberate inactive end products. The redox intermediate intracellular metabolites are believed to target the RNA, DNA, or cellular proteins of the organisms.

➤*Pharmacokinetics:*

Absorption – Disposition of metronidazole in the body is similar for oral and IV dosage forms. Metronidazole is well absorbed after oral administration. Peak serum levels occur at ≈ 1 to 2 hours.

Distribution – Plasma concentrations of metronidazole are proportional to the administered dose. Metronidazole is the major component appearing in the plasma, with lesser quantities of the 2-hydroxymethyl metabolite also being present. Metronidazole also appears in CSF, saliva, and breast milk in concentrations similar to those found in plasma. Bactericidal concentrations of metronidazole also have been detected in pus from hepatic abscesses. Less than 20% of the circulating metronidazole is bound to plasma proteins.

Metabolism – The parent compound and the metabolite possess in vitro bactericidal activity against most strains of anaerobic bacteria. The metabolites that appear in the urine result primarily from side-chain oxidation and the glucuronide conjugation, with unchanged metronidazole accounting for ≈ 20% of the total.

Excretion – The major route of elimination of metronidazole and its metabolites is via the urine (60% to 80% of the dose), with fecal excretion accounting for 6% to 15% of the dose. Renal clearance is ≈ 10 mL/min/1.73 m². The average elimination half-life in healthy humans is 8 hours.

Special populations –

Hepatic insufficiency: Plasma clearance of metronidazole is decreased in patients with decreased liver function.

Children: In one study, newborn infants appeared to demonstrate diminished capacity to eliminate metronidazole. The elimination half-life, measured during the first 3 days of life, was inversely related to gestational age.

➤*Microbiology:* Metronidazole is active in vitro against most obligate anaerobes but does not appear to possess activity against facultative anaerobes or obligate aerobes. It is generally bactericidal against susceptible organisms, at concentrations equal to or slightly higher than the minimal inhibitory concentrations (MICs). Metronidazole is active against anaerobic gram-negative bacilli, including *Bacteroides* sp. (eg, *B. fragilis, B. distasonis, B. ovatus, B. thetaiotaomicron, B. vulgatus*); *Fusobacterium* sp.; anaerobic gram-positive bacilli, including *Clostridium* sp. and susceptible strains of *Eubacterium*; anaerobic gram-positive cocci, including *Peptococcus niger*, and *Peptostreptococcus* sp.; protozoal parasites, including *Trichomonas vaginalis, Entamoeba histolytica, Giardia lamblia*, and *Balantidium coli*.

Perform bacteriologic studies to determine the causative organisms and their susceptibility; however, therapy may be started while awaiting these results.

Contraindications

Hypersensitivity to metronidazole or other nitroimidazole derivatives; pregnancy (first trimester in patients with trichomoniasis; see Warnings).

Warnings

➤*Neurologic effects:* Seizures and peripheral neuropathy (characterized by numbness or paresthesia of an extremity) have occurred. Appearance of abnormal neurologic signs demands prompt discontinuation of therapy. Administer metronidazole with caution to patients with CNS diseases.

➤*Hepatic function impairment:* Patients with severe hepatic disease metabolize metronidazole slowly. Accumulation of the drug and its metabolites may occur. Cautiously administer doses below those usually recommended.

➤*Carcinogenesis:* Metronidazole has shown evidence of carcinogenic activity with chronic oral administration in rodents. Prominent among the effects in the mouse was the promotion of pulmonary tumorigenesis. Malignant lymphomas and pulmonary neoplasms are also increased with lifetime feeding of the drug to mice. In several long-term studies in rats, there was an increase in the incidence of neoplasms, particularly mammary and hepatic tumors, among female rats. Also, metronidazole has shown mutagenic activity in a number of in vitro assay systems.

➤*Elderly:* Because the pharmacokinetics of metronidazole may be altered in the elderly, monitoring of serum levels may be necessary to adjust the dosage accordingly.

➤*Pregnancy:* Category B. Metronidazole crosses the placenta and enters fetal circulation rapidly. Do not administer to pregnant patients during the first trimester. There are no adequate and well-controlled studies in pregnant women. Use during pregnancy only if clearly needed.

Restrict metronidazole for trichomoniasis in the second and third trimesters to those in whom local alternative treatment has been inadequate to control symptoms.

➤*Lactation:* Because of the potential for tumorigenicity, shown for metronidazole in mouse and rat studies, decide whether to discontinue nursing or to discontinue the drug, taking into account the importance of the drug to the mother. Metronidazole is secreted in breast milk in concentrations similar to those found in plasma.

➤*Children:* Safety and efficacy in children have not been established, except for the treatment of amebiasis. Newborns demonstrate a diminished capacity to eliminate metronidazole. The elimination half-life is inversely related to gestational age. In infants whose gestational ages were between 28 and 40 weeks, the corresponding elimination half-lives ranged from 109 to 22.5 hours.

Precautions

➤*Crohn's disease:* These patients are known to have an increased incidence of GI and certain extraintestinal cancers. There have been some reports in the medical literature of breast and colon cancer in Crohn's disease patients who have been treated with metronidazole at high doses for extended periods of time. A cause and effect relationship has not been established (see Unlabeled Uses).

➤*Candidiasis:* Known or previously unrecognized candidiasis may present more prominent symptoms during therapy and requires treatment with a candicidal agent.

➤*Hematologic effects:* Metronidazole is a nitroimidazole; use with care in patients with evidence or history of blood dyscrasia. Mild leukopenia has been seen during administration; however, no persistent hematologic abnormalities attributable to the drug have been observed. Perform total and differential leukocyte counts before and after therapy.

Drug Interactions

Metronidazole Drug Interactions			
Precipitant drug	Object drug*		Description
Barbiturates Phenytoin	Metronidazole	↓	Coadministration may accelerate the elimination of metronidazole, resulting in reduced plasma levels.
Cimetidine	Metronidazole	↑	Decreased metronidazole clearance and increased serum levels may occur; however, data conflict.
Metronidazole	Anticoagulants	↑	The anticoagulant effect of warfarin may be enhanced.
Metronidazole	Disulfiram	↑	Concurrent use may result in an acute psychosis or confusional state. Do not give metronidazole to patients who have taken disulfiram within the last 2 weeks.

METRONIDAZOLE

Metronidazole Drug Interactions			
Precipitant drug	Object drug*		Description
Metronidazole	Ethanol	↑	A disulfiram-like reaction including symptoms of flushing, palpitations, tachycardia, nausea, vomiting, etc, may occur with concurrent use. Although the risk for most patients may be slight, caution is advised. Do not consume alcohol during therapy and for ≥ 1 to 3 days afterward.
Metronidazole	Hydantoins	↑	The total clearance of phenytoin may be decreased and its elimination half-life prolonged.
Metronidazole	Lithium	↑	In patients stabilized on relatively high lithium doses, short-term metronidazole has been associated with increased lithium levels and toxicity in some cases.

*↑ = Object drug increased. ↓ = Object drug decreased.

►*Drug/Lab test interactions:* The drug may interfere with chemical analyses for AST, ALT, LDH, triglycerides, and hexokinase glucose. Zero values may occur.

►*Drug/Food interactions:* Relative to the fasting state, the rate of metronidazole absorption from the extended-release tablet is increased in the fed state resulting in alteration of the extended-release characteristics.

Adverse Reactions

Adverse Reactions Irrespective of Treatment Causality (≥ 2%)		
Adverse reaction	Flagyl ER 7 days (n = 267) (%)	Vaginal preparation (n = 285) (%)
CNS		
Headache	18	15
Dizziness	4	1
GI		
Nausea	10	3
Tast perversion (metallic taste)	9	0
Abdominal pain	4	5
Diarrhea	4	1
Dry mouth	2	1
GU		
Vaginitis	15	12
Genital pruritus	5	9
Abnormal urine	3	1
Dysmenorrhea	3	2
Urinary tract infection	2	6
Respiratory		
Upper respiratory tract infection	4	4
Rhinitis	4	4
Sinusitis	3	2
Pharyngitis	3	1

Adverse Reactions Irrespective of Treatment Causality (≥ 2%)		
Adverse reaction	Flagyl ER 7 days (n = 267) (%)	Vaginal preparation (n = 285) (%)
Miscellaneous		
Bacterial infection	7	6
Influenza-like symptoms	6	7
Moniliasis	3	3

►*Cardiovascular:* Flattening of the T-wave may be seen in ECG tracings.

►*CNS:* Seizures and peripheral neuropathy, the latter characterized mainly by numbness or paresthesia of an extremity; dizziness; vertigo; incoordination; ataxia; confusion; irritability; depression; weakness; insomnia; headache; syncope.

►*GI:* Nausea, sometimes accompanied by headache, anorexia, and occasional vomiting; diarrhea; epigastric distress; abdominal cramping; constipation; proctitis; sharp, unpleasant metallic taste; a modification of the taste of alcoholic beverages; furry tongue, glossitis, stomatitis (these may be associated with a sudden overgrowth of *Candida*).

►*GU:* Dysuria; cystitis; polyuria; incontinence; sense of pelvic pressure; proliferation of *Candida* in the vagina; dyspareunia; decreased libido. Darkened urine (dark brown color) has been reported. The pigment appears to be a metabolite of metronidazole and it seems to have no clinical significance.

►*Hematologic:* Reversible neutropenia (leukopenia); reversible thrombocytopenia (rare).

►*Hypersensitivity:* Urticaria; erythematous rash; flushing; nasal congestion; dryness of the mouth (or vagina or vulva); fever.

►*Local:* Thrombophlebitis after IV infusion can be minimized or eliminated by avoiding prolonged use of indwelling IV catheters.

►*Miscellaneous:* Fever; fleeting joint pains, sometimes resembling "serum sickness." Rare cases of pancreatitis, which generally abated on withdrawal of the drug, have been reported.

Overdosage

►*Symptoms:* Nausea, vomiting, and ataxia. Neurotoxic effects (seizures and peripheral neuropathy) have been reported after 5 to 7 days of 6 to 10.4 g every other day. Single oral doses up to 15 g have been reported in suicide attempts and accidental overdoses. Use of doses higher than those recommended (27 mg/kg 3 times a day for 20 days and a 75 mg/kg loading dose followed by 7.5 mg/kg maintenance doses) have been used with no adverse effects.

►*Treatment:* No specific antidote for metronidazole overdose exists. Treatment consists of usual supportive measures. Refer to General Management of Acute Overdosage.

Patient Information

Avoid alcoholic beverages.

Take *Flagyl ER* under fasting conditions ≥ 1 hour before or 2 hours after meals.

Specifically warn patients about seizures and peripheral neuropathy and tell them to stop the drug and immediately report any neurological symptoms to their physician.

Complete full course of therapy; take until gone. May cause darkening of urine.

An unpleasant metallic taste may be noticeable.

In addition to the sulfonamides listed on the following pages, other preparations that contain sulfonamides include: Ophthalmic; vaginal; burn preparations (eg, mafenide, silver sulfadiazine). Sulfasalazine is indicated for ulcerative colitis and rheumatoid arthritis and is described in other sections. See individual monographs or sections.

Indications

Sulfonamide Indications		
Indications	Sulfadiazine	Sulfisoxazole
Chancroid	✓	✓
Inclusion conjunctivitis	✓	✓
Malaria[1]	✓	✓
Meningitis, *Haemophilus influenzae*	✓	✓
Meningitis, meningococcal[2]	✓	✓
Nocardiosis	✓	✓
Otitis media, acute[3]	✓	✓
Rheumatic fever	✓	
Toxoplasmosis[4]	✓	
Trachoma	✓	✓
Urinary tract infections[5] (pyelonephritis, cystitis)	✓	✓

[1] As adjunctive therapy because of chloroquine-resistant strains of *Plasmodium falciparum*.

[2] When the organism is susceptible and for prophylaxis when sulfonamide-sensitive group A strains prevail.

[3] Caused by *H. influenzae* when used with penicillin.

[4] As adjunctive therapy with pyrimethamine.

[5] In the absence of obstructive uropathy or foreign bodies when caused by *Escherichia coli, Klebsiella-Enterobacter, Staphylococcus aureus, Proteus mirabilis,* and *P. vulgaris*.

Administration and Dosage

See individual products for specific guidelines based on indication.

➤*CDC recommended treatment schedules for sexually transmitted diseases†:*

Lymphogranuloma venereum – As an alternative regimen to doxycycline, sulfisoxazole 500 mg 4 times/day for 21 days or equivalent sulfonamide course.

Chlamydia trachomatic infections – As an alternative regimen to doxycycline or azithromycin (or if erythromycin is not tolerated), sulfisoxazole 500 mg 4 times/day for 10 days or equivalent sulfonamide course.

Actions

➤*Pharmacology:* Sulfonamides exert their bacteriostatic action by competitive antagonism of para-aminobenzoic acid (PABA), an essential component in folic acid synthesis. Microorganisms that require exogenous folic acid and do not synthesize folic acid are not susceptible to the action of sulfonamides.

➤*Pharmacokinetics:*

Absorption/Distribution – The oral sulfonamides are readily absorbed from the GI tract. Approximately 70% to 100% of an oral dose is absorbed. These agents are distributed throughout all body tissues and readily enter the cerebrospinal fluid, pleura, synovial fluids, the eye, the placenta, and the fetus. Sulfonamides are bound to plasma proteins in varying degrees. "Free" sulfonamide serum levels of 5 to 15 mg/dL may be therapeutically effective for most infections. Avoid levels > 20 mg/dL.

Metabolism – Metabolism occurs in the liver by conjugation and acetylation to inactive metabolites. Individuals who are are slow acetylators have an increased risk of toxicity from sulfonamide accumulation.

Excretion – Renal excretion is mainly by glomerular filtration. Some of the acetylated metabolites are less soluble and may contribute to crystalluria and renal complications. To prevent the possibility of crystalluria, alkalinization of the urine and adequate fluid intake are recommended when using the less soluble sulfonamides (eg, sulfadiazine). Small amounts are eliminated in the feces, and in bile, breast milk, and other secretions.

➤*Microbiology:* Sulfonamides have a broad antibacterial spectrum that includes both gram-positive and gram-negative organisms.

Resistance – Organisms that produce excessive amounts of PABA develop resistance. The increasing frequency of resistant organisms is a limitation to the usefulness of the sulfonamides alone, especially in the treatment of chronic and recurrent urinary tract infections. Cross-resistance between sulfonamides is common once resistance develops. Minimize resistance by initiating treatment promptly with adequate doses and continuing for a sufficient period. In vitro sensitivity tests are not always reliable; carefully coordinate the test with bacteriologic and clinical response.

Contraindications

Hypersensitivity to sulfonamides or chemically related drugs (eg, sulfonylureas, thiazide and loop diuretics, carbonic anhydrase inhibitors, sunscreens with PABA, local anesthetics); pregnancy at term, lactation (see Warnings); infants < 2 months of age (except in congenital toxoplasmosis as adjunct with pyrimethamine).

Warnings

➤*Deaths:* Those associated with the administration of sulfonamides have been reported from hypersensitivity reactions, hepatocellular necrosis, agranulocytosis, aplastic anemia, and other blood dyscrasias. Sore throat, fever, pallor, purpura, or jaundice may be early indications of serious blood disorders. Perform complete blood counts.

➤*Group A beta-hemolytic streptococcal infections:* Do not use for treatment of these infections. In an established infection, they will not eradicate the streptococcus and will not prevent sequelae, such as rheumatic fever and glomerulonephritis.

➤*Hypersensitivity reactions:* May cause cholestatic jaundice.

➤*Renal function impairment:* Use with caution. The frequency of renal complications is considerably lower in patients receiving the more soluble sulfonamides (sulfisoxazole). Maintain adequate fluid intake (2 to 3 L/day) to prevent crystalluria and stone formation.

➤*Hepatic function impairment:* Cholestatic jaundice occurs in 0.5% to 1% of patients because of hypersensitivity or idiosyncrasy.

➤*Pregnancy: Category C.* Safety for use during pregnancy is not established. Sulfonamides cross the placenta; fetal levels average 70% to 90% of maternal serum levels. Significant levels may persist in the neonate if these drugs are given near term; jaundice, hemolytic anemia and kernicterus may occur. Teratogenicity (eg, tracheoesophageal fistula, cataracts) has occurred in some animal species. Do not use at term.

➤*Lactation:* Sulfonamides are excreted in breast milk in low concentrations. Milk:plasma ratios for sulfonamides are as low as 0.5 to 0.6. According to the American Academy of Pediatrics, breastfeeding and sulfonamide use are compatible because sulfonamide excretion into breast milk does not pose a significant risk to the healthy full-term neonate. However, do not nurse premature infants or those with hyperbilirubinemia or G-6-PD deficiency.

➤*Children:* Do not use in infants < 2 months of age (except for congenital toxoplasmosis as adjunctive therapy with pyrimethamine).

Precautions

➤*Monitoring:* Monitor blood counts frequently, especially during prolonged administration. Perform microscopic urinalyses once a week when a patient is treated for > 2 weeks. Use urine cultures to confirm eradication of bacteriuria.

➤*Allergy or asthma:* Give with caution to patients with severe allergy or bronchial asthma.

➤*Hemolytic anemia:* Frequently dose-related, this may occur in G-6-PD deficient individuals.

➤*Photosensitivity:* Photosensitization (photoallergy or phototoxicity) may occur; therefore, caution patients to take protective measures (eg, sunscreens, protective clothing) against exposure to ultraviolet light or sunlight until tolerance is determined.

† *Morbidity and Mortality Weekly Report* 1993 Sep 24;42 (No. RR-14):i-102.

Drug Interactions

Sulfonamide Drug Interactions

Precipitant Drug	Object Drug*		Description
Sulfonamides	Anticoagulants, oral	↑	Warfarin's anticoagulation action may be enhanced. Hemorrhage could occur.
Sulfisoxazole	Barbiturate anesthetics	↑	The anesthetic effects of thiopental may be enhanced.
Sulfonamides	Cyclosporine	↓	Cyclosporine concentrations are decreased, and the risk of nephrotoxicity may be increased.
Sulfonamides	Hydantoins	↑	Serum hydantoin levels may be increased.
Sulfonamides	Methotrexate	↑	The risk of methotrexate-induced bone marrow suppression may be enhanced.
Sulfonamides	Sulfonylureas	↑	Increased sulfonylurea half-lives and hypoglycemia may occur.
Sulfonamides	Tolbutamide	↑	The half-life of tolbutamide may be prolonged when administered with sulfamethizole.
Sulfonamides	Uricosuric agents	↑	Potentiation of uricosuric action may be noted.
Diuretics (eg, thiazide)	Sulfonamides	↑	Coadministration may cause an increased incidence of thrombocytopenia with purpura.
Indomethacin	Sulfonamides	↑	Sulfonamides may be displaced from plasma albumin resulting in increased free-drug concentrations.
Methenamine	Sulfonamides	↑	An insoluble precipitate may form in acidic urine when sulfamethizole is used concomitantly with methenamine mandelate.
Probenecid	Sulfonamides	↑	Sulfonamides may be displaced from plasma albumin resulting in increased free-drug concentrations.
Salicylates	Sulfonamides	↑	Sulfonamides may be displaced from plasma albumin resulting in increased free-drug concentrations.

* ↑ = Object drug increased. ↓ = Object drug decreased.

Adverse Reactions

➤*CNS:* Headache; peripheral neuropathy; mental depression; convulsions; ataxia; hallucinations; tinnitus; vertigo; insomnia; apathy; drowsiness; polyneuritis; neuritis; optic neuritis; transient myopia.

➤*GI:* Nausea; emesis; abdominal pains; diarrhea; anorexia; pancreatitis; stomatitis; hepatitis; hepatocellular necrosis; pseudomembranous enterocolitis; glossitis.

➤*Hematologic:* Agranulocytosis; aplastic anemia; thrombocytopenia; leukopenia; hemolytic anemia; purpura; hypoprothrombinemia; neutropenia; eosinophilia; methemoglobinemia.

➤*Hypersensitivity:* Stevens-Johnson type erythema multiforme; generalized skin eruptions; allergic myocarditis; epidermal necrolysis; urticaria; periarteritis nodosum; serum sickness; pruritus; exfoliative dermatitis; anaphylactoid reactions; periorbital edema; conjunctival, scleral injection; photosensitization; arthralgia; allergic myocarditis; transient pulmonary changes with eosinophilia and decreased pulmonary function.

➤*Renal:* Crystalluria; elevated creatinine; toxic nephrosis with oliguria and anuria.

➤*Miscellaneous:* Drug fever; chills; pyrexia; L.E. phenomenon. Reports of adverse effects in breastfeeding infants are rare.

The sulfonamides bear chemical similarities to some goitrogens, diuretics (acetazolamide and thiazides) and oral hypoglycemic agents. Goiter production, diuresis and hypoglycemia have occurred rarely in patients receiving sulfonamides. Cross-sensitivity may exist with these agents (see Contraindications).

Overdosage

➤*Symptoms:*
GI – Anorexia; colic; nausea; vomiting.
CNS – Dizziness; headache; drowsiness; unconsciousness; vertigo.
Pyrexia, hematuria and crystalluria have been reported. Blood dyscrasias and jaundice are late manifestations of overdosage.

➤*Treatment:* Discontinue the drug immediately. Within 1 or 2 days after discontinuation, the less serious symptoms disappear; grave symptoms require 1 to 3 weeks for remission. Empty the stomach if large doses have been ingested. Alkalinize the urine to enhance solubility and excretion. Force fluids if kidney function is normal, up to 4 L/day, to increase excretion. Monitor renal function with appropriate blood chemistries including electrolytes closely and in the acute period. Follow hematologic parameters over the next 10 days to 2 weeks after the overdose ingestion. Methemoglobinuria can be acutely reversed with IV 1% methylene blue.

Patient Information

Complete full course of therapy.

Take with a full glass of water (2 to 3 L/day).

Avoid prolonged exposure to sunlight; photosensitivity may occur. If outside, wear protective clothing and apply sunscreen to exposed areas.

Notify physician if any of the following occurs: Blood in urine, rash, ringing in ears, difficulty in breathing, fever, sore throat or chills.

SULFADIAZINE

Rx	**Sulfadiazine** (Various, eg, Eon, Major, Rugby, UDL, Zenith-Goldline)	**Tablets**: 500 mg	In 100s, 1000s and UD 100s.

For complete prescribing information, refer to the Sulfonamides group monograph.

Administration and Dosage

➤*Adults:*
Loading dose – 2 to 4 g.
Maintenance dose – 2 to 4 g/day in 3 to 6 divided doses.
➤*Children (> 2 months):*
Loading dose – 75 mg/kg (or 2 g/m²).
Maintenance dose – 150 mg/kg/day (4 g/m²/day) in 4 to 6 divided doses.

Maximum dose – 6 g/day.

Contraindicated in infants < 2 months old (except in congenital toxoplasmosis as an adjunct with pyrimethamine).

➤*Other recommended doses for toxoplasmosis (for 3 to 4 weeks) include:*
Infants (< 2 months) – 25 mg/kg/dose 4 times daily.
Children (> 2 months) – 25 to 50 mg/kg/dose 4 times daily.

➤*Prevention of recurrent attacks of rheumatic fever:* Patients > 30 kg (> 66 lbs) – 1 g/day; < 30 kg (< 66 lbs) – 0.5 g/day.

SULFISOXAZOLE

Rx	**Sulfisoxazole** (Various, eg, Geneva, Moore, Rugby)	**Tablets**: 500 mg	In 100s and 1000s.
Rx	**Gantrisin Pediatric** (Roche)	**Suspension**: 500 mg/5 ml	0.3% alcohol, parabens, sugar, sucrose. Raspberry flavor. In 480 ml.

For complete prescribing information, refer to the Sulfonamides group monograph.

Administration and Dosage

➤*Loading dose:* 2 to 4 g.
➤*Maintenance dose:* 4 to 8 g/day in 4 to 6 divided doses.
➤*Children and infants (> 2 months):*

Initial dose – 75 mg/kg.

Maintenance dose – 150 mg/kg/day (4 g/m²/day) in 4 to 6 divided doses (max, 6 g/day).

Contraindicated in infants < 2 months old (except in congenital toxoplasmosis as an adjunct with pyrimethamine).

NITROFURANTOIN

Rx   **Furadantin** (Dura) | **Oral Suspension:** 25 mg per 5 ml | Saccharin, sorbitol. In 60 and 470 ml.

Indications

➤*Urinary tract infections:* Treatment of urinary tract infections due to susceptible strains of *E. coli*, enterococci, *S. aureus* (not for treatment of pyelonephritis or perinephric abscesses) and certain strains of *Klebsiella* and *Enterobacter* species.

Administration and Dosage

Give with food or milk to improve drug absorption and, in some patients, tolerance. Continue for at least 1 week, or for at least 3 days after sterile urine is obtained. Continued infection indicates need for reevaluation.

➤*Adults:* 50 to 100 mg 4 times/day with meals and at bedtime. For long-term suppressive therapy, reduce dosage (50 to 100 mg at bedtime).

➤*Children:* 5 to 7 mg/kg/24 hrs given in 4 divided doses. For long-term suppressive therapy, doses as low as 1 mg/kg/24 hrs, given in single or in 2 divided doses, may be adequate. Contraindicated in children less than 1 month of age.

The following table is based on an average weight in each range receiving 5 to 6 mg/kg of body weight per 24 hours, given in four divided doses. It can be used to calculate an average dose of oral suspension (5 mg/ml).

Nitrofurantoin Dosage in Children Based on Body Weight		
Body weight		No. of teaspoonsful 4 times a day
lbs	kg	
15 to 26	7 to 11	½ (2.5 ml)
27 to 46	12 to 21	1 (5 ml)
47 to 68	22 to 30	1½ (7.5 ml)
69 to 91	31 to 41	2 (10 ml)

Actions

➤*Pharmacology:* Nitrofurantoin is a synthetic nitrofuran that is bacteriostatic in low concentrations (5 to 10 mcg/ml) and bactericidal in higher concentrations. Nitrofurantoin may inhibit acetylcoenzyme A, interfering with bacterial carbohydrate metabolism. It may also disrupt bacterial cell wall formation.

➤*Pharmacokinetics:*

Absorption/Distribution – Well absorbed from the GI tract after oral administration. The macrocrystalline form is absorbed more slowly due to slower dissolution and causes less GI distress. Bioavailability of micro- and macrocrystalline forms is enhanced by concomitant ingestion of food. Therapeutic serum and tissue concentrations are not achieved after usual oral doses, except in the urinary tract. Protein binding is about 60%.

Metabolism/Excretion – Approximately 50% to 70% of the drug is rapidly metabolized by body tissues. The plasma half-life is about 20 minutes in healthy individuals and increases to 60 minutes in the anephric patient. In patients with impaired renal function, nitrofurantoin accumulates in the serum. Renal excretion is via glomerular filtration and tubular secretion. About 30% to 50% of a dose is excreted unchanged in the urine. Usual doses produce urinary levels of 50 to 250 mcg/ml in patients with normal renal function. If creatinine clearance is < 40 ml/min, antibacterial concentrations attained in the urine are inadequate, and the subsequent elevated blood levels increase the danger of toxicity. Antibacterial activity is greater in an acidic urine. Acid urine enhances tubular reabsorption of nitrofurantoin, enhancing antibacterial activity in the renal tissues and lowering urinary concentrations. However, do not alkalinize urine to increase urinary concentration of nitrofurantoin, because the antimicrobial activity is decreased at a higher pH.

➤*Microbiology:* The MIC in urine for most susceptible organisms is ≤ 32 mcg/ml. Resistant species generally have an MIC of ≥ 100 mcg/ml. Most gram-negative bacilli and gram-positive cocci associated with urinary tract infections are susceptible, including: *Escherichia coli*, *Klebsiella* and *Enterobacter* sp., enterococci (eg, *Enterococcus faecalis*), *Staphylococcus aureus* and *S. saprophyticus*. Some strains of *Enterobacter* and *Klebsiella* sp. are resistant. Most strains of *Proteus* and *Serratia* species are resistant. It has no activity against *Pseudomonas* sp. Susceptible bacteria do not readily develop resistance to nitrofurantoin during therapy. However, plasmid-mediated, transferable resistance has been demonstrated. Although in vitro susceptibility of *Salmonella*, *Shegella*, *Neisseria*, *Streptococcus pyogenes*, *S. pneumoniae*, *Corynebacterium* and many anaerobes has been demonstrated, nitrofurantoin is of little clinical importance for infections caused by these organisms.

Contraindications

Renal function impairment (creatinine clearance < 60 ml/min), anuria or oliguria (treatment is much less effective and carries an increased risk of toxicity because of impaired excretion of the drug); hypersensitivity to nitrofurantoin.

Pregnant patients at term, during labor and delivery, or when the onset of labor is imminent, and in infants under 1 month of age (possibility of hemolytic anemia due to immature enzyme systems [glutathione instability]).

Warnings

➤*Pulmonary reactions:*

Acute – Manifested by sudden onset of dyspnea, chest pain, cough, fever and chills, pulmonary infiltration with consolidation or pleural effusion on x-ray; elevated sedimentation rate and eosinophilia are also present. Resolution of clinical and radiological abnormalities occurs within 24 to 48 hours after discontinuation. Rechallenge is dangerous and will produce similar symptoms.

Subacute/chronic – Associated with prolonged therapy. These reactions are characterized by insidious development of dyspnea, nonproductive cough and malaise after 1 to 6 months or more of therapy. Pulmonary function tests demonstrate a restrictive pattern. Radiographs show an interstitial pneumonitis. Usually, symptoms regress with discontinuation of the drug over weeks to months. Pulmonary function may be permanently impaired, even after cessation of nitrofurantoin. Death has been reported.

➤*Hemolysis:* Hemolytic anemia of the primaquine sensitivity type has been induced by nitrofurantoin. The hemolysis appears to be linked to a glucose-6-phosphate dehydrogenase (G-6-PD) deficiency in the red blood cells of affected patients. At any sign of hemolysis, discontinue the drug. Hemolysis ceases when the drug is withdrawn.

➤*Hepatic reactions:* Those including hepatitis, cholestatic jaundice, chronic active hepatitis, and hepatic necrosis, occur rarely. Fatalities have been reported. The onset of chronic active hepatitis may be insidious. Periodically monitor patients receiving long-term therapy for changes in liver function. If hepatitis occurs, withdraw the drug and take appropriate measures.

➤*Pregnancy:* Category B. In mice, at doses of 19 and 68 times the human dose, induction of papillary adenomas, growth retardation and a low incidence of minor and common malformations occurred. Safety for use during pregnancy has not been established. Use in women of childbearing potential only when clearly needed and when the potential benefits outweigh the potential hazards to the fetus. Do not give to pregnant patients with G-6-PD deficiency because of the risk of hemolysis in the mother and fetus, although fetal hemolysis has not been documented. Contraindicated in pregnant women at term.

Labor and delivery – Nitrofurantoin use is contraindicated during labor and delivery. See Contraindications.

➤*Lactation:* Nitrofurantoin is excreted into breast milk in very low concentrations. Concentrations of 0.3 to 0.5 mcg/ml were reported in two women who received 100 mg nitrofurantoin every 6 hours for 1 day followed by either 100 or 200 mg the next morning. However, infants with G-6-PD deficiency may be adversely affected. Safety for use in the nursing mother has not been established.

➤*Children:* Contraindicated in infants < 1 month of age. (See Contraindications.)

Precautions

➤*Monitoring:* Obtain specimens for culture and susceptibility testing prior to and during drug administration.

➤*Peripheral neuropathy:* This may occur and may become severe or irreversible. Fatalities have been reported. Predisposing conditions such as renal impairment, anemia, diabetes, electrolyte imbalance, vitamin B deficiency and debilitating disease may enhance such occurrences.

➤*Superinfection:* Use of antibiotics (especially prolonged or repeated therapy) may result in bacterial or fungal overgrowth of nonsusceptible organisms. Such overgrowth may lead to a secondary infection. Appropriate measures should be taken if superinfection occurs.

Drug Interactions

Nitrofurantoin Drug Interactions			
Precipitant drug	Object drug*		Description
Anticholinergics	Nitrofurantoin	↑	Anticholinergic drugs increase nitrofurantoin bioavailability by delaying gastric emptying and increasing absorption.
Magnesium salts	Nitrofurantoin	↓	Magnesium salts may delay or decrease the absorption of nitrofurantoin.
Uricosurics	Nitrofurantoin	↑	Administration of high doses of probenecid with nitrofurantoin decreases renal clearance and increases serum levels of nitrofurantoin. The result could be increased toxic effects.

* ↑ = Object drug increased. ↓ = Object drug decreased.

NITROFURANTOIN

➤*Drug/Lab test interactions:* A false-positive reaction for glucose in the urine may occur. This has been observed with Benedict's and Fehling's solutions but not with the glucose enzymatic test.

➤*Drug/Food interactions:* Bioavailability of nitrofurantoin is increased by food.

Adverse Reactions

➤*CNS:* Peripheral neuropathy (see Precautions); headache; dizziness; nystagmus; drowsiness; asthenia; vertigo; confusion; depression; euphoria, psychotic reactions (rare).

➤*Dermatologic:* Exfoliative dermatitis and erythema multiforme (including Stevens-Johnson syndrome) have been reported rarely; maculopapular, erythematous or eczematous eruption; pruritus; urticaria; angioedema.

➤*GI:* Anorexia, nausea, emesis (most frequent); abdominal pain, diarrhea parotitis, pancreatitis (less frequent).

➤*Hematologic:* Glucose-6–phosphate dehydrogenase deficiency anemia (see Warnings); granulocytopenia; agranulocytosis; leukopenia; thrombocytopenia; eosinophilia; megaloblastic anemia; hemolytic anemia. In most cases, these hematologic abnormalities resolved following cessation of therapy. Aplastic anemia (rare).

➤*Hepatic:* Hepatic reactions, including hepatitis, cholestatic jaundice, chronic active hepatitis and hepatic necrosis (rare).

➤*Hypersensitivity:* Anaphylaxis; asthmatic attack in patients with history of asthma; drug fever; arthralgia; myalgia; chills; sialadenitis.

➤*Lab test abnormalities:* Increased AST, increased ALT, decreased hemoglobin, increased serum phosphorus.

➤*Pulmonary:* Sensitivity reactions (acute, subacute or chronic) are documented with outcomes ranging from complete resolution to death. See Warnings.

➤*Miscellaneous:* Transient alopecia; superinfections in GU tract by resistant organisms; benign sintracranial hypertension; changes in ECG; collapse; cyanosis; a lupus-like syndrome associated with pulmonary reactions; muscular aches.

Overdosage

➤*Symptoms:* Occasional incidents of acute overdosage of nitrofurantoin have not resulted in any specific symptoms other than vomiting.

➤*Treatment:* Induction of emesis is recommended. There is no specific antidote, but a high fluid intake should be maintained to promote urinary excretion of the drug. It is dialyzable.

Patient Information

Complete full course of therapy; do not discontinue without notifying physician.

May cause GI upset; take with food or milk.

May cause brown discoloration of the urine.

Notify physician if fever, chills, cough, chest pain, difficult breathing, skin rash, numbness or tingling of the fingers or toes, or intolerable GI upset occurs.

NITROFURANTOIN MACROCRYSTALS

Rx	Macrodantin (Procter & Gamble Pharm)	Capsules: 25 mg	(Macrodantin 25 mg 0149–0007). White. In 100s.
Rx	Nitrofurantoin (Various, eg, Goldline, Major, Moore, Rugby, URL, Warner Chilcott, Zenith)	Capsules: 50 mg	In 100s, 500s and 1000s.
Rx	Macrodantin (Procter & Gamble Pharm.)		(Macrodantin 50 mg 0149–0008). Yellow/white. In 100s, 1000s, and UD 100s.
Rx	Nitrofurantoin (Various, eg, Goldline, Major, Moore, Rugby, URL, Warner Chilcott, Zenith)	Capsules: 100 mg	In 100s, 500s and 1000s.
Rx	Macrodantin (Procter & Gamble Pharm)		(Macrodantin 100 mg 0149–0009). Yellow. In 100s, 500s, 1000s and UD 100s.
Rx	Macrobid (Procter & Gamble Pharm)	Capsules: 100 mg (as 25 mg macrocrystals, 75 mg monohydrate)	(Macrobid). Sugar, lactose. Black and yellow. In 100s.

Actions

➤*Pharmacology:* The large crystal size improves GI tolerance.

FURAZOLIDONE

Rx	Furoxone (Procter & Gamble Pharm.)	Tablets: 100 mg	Sucrose. (Eaton 072). Green, scored. In 20s and 100s.

Indications

Specific and symptomatic treatment of bacterial or protozoal diarrhea and enteritis caused by susceptible organisms.

➤*Unlabeled uses:* Furazolidone 7.5 mg/kg plus oral rehydration therapy for 5 days was more effective than oral rehydration therapy alone in the treatment of acute infantile diarrhea (when fecal leukocytes were present) in children 3 to 73 months of age.

Furazolidone appears effective in the treatment of typhoid fever in adults (800 mg/day for 14 days) and for the treatment of giardiasis in children (67 to 266 mg/day for 10 days).

Furazolidone may also be useful in treating traveler's diarrhea, cholera and bacteremic salmonellosis.

Administration and Dosage

Dosage is based on an average dose of 5 mg/kg/day given in 4 equally divided doses. Do not exceed 8.8 mg/kg/day due to the possibility of nausea and emesis. If these are severe, reduce dosage.

➤*Adults:* 100 mg 4 times daily.

➤*Children:*

(≥ *5 years of age*) – 25 to 50 mg 4 times daily (tablet or liquid).

(*1 to 4 years*) – 17 to 25 mg 4 times daily (liquid).

(*1 month to 1 year*) – 8 to 17 mg 4 times daily (liquid).

If satisfactory clinical response is not obtained within 7 days, the pathogen is refractory to furazolidone; discontinue the drug. Adjunctive therapy with other antibacterial agents or bismuth salts is not contraindicated.

Actions

➤*Pharmacology:* Furazolidone exerts bactericidal activity via interference with several bacterial enzyme systems, minimizing the development of resistant organisms. It neither significantly alters the normal bowel flora nor results in fungal overgrowth.

➤*Pharmacokinetics:* There are limited data in humans. Previously it was thought that very little drug was absorbed following oral administration. However, recent data indicate significant absorption. It is rapidly and extensively metabolized, possibly in the intestine. Colored metabolites are excreted in the urine.

➤*Microbiology:* Its broad antibacterial spectrum covers the majority of GI tract pathogens, including *Escherichia coli*, staphylococci, *Salmonella*, *Shigella* and *Proteus* species, *Aerobacter aerogenes*, *Vibrio cholerae* and *Giardia lamblia*.

Contraindications

Do not administer to infants < 1 month of age.

Prior sensitivity to furazolidone.

Warnings

➤*Pregnancy: Category C.* Safety for use during pregnancy has not been established. Use only when clearly needed and when the potential benefits outweigh the potential hazards to the fetus. Theoretically, furazolidone could produce hemolytic anemia in a glucose-6-phosphate dehydrogenase (G-6-PD) deficient neonate if given at term.

➤*Lactation:* Safety for use in the nursing mother has not been established. Drug concentration in breast milk has not been determined.

Precautions

➤*Orthostatic hypotension and hypoglycemia:* These may occur.

➤*Hemolysis:* This may occur in G-6-PD deficient individuals.

➤*Hypertensive crisis:* When considering the administration of larger than recommended doses, or for > 5 days, consider the possibility of hypertensive crises.

➤*Monoamine oxidase (MAO) inhibition:* Furazolidone inhibits the enzyme MAO. Doses of 400 mg/day for 5 days increased tyramine and amphetamine sensitivity two- to threefold. (See Drug Interactions.) Use caution if administering with other MAOIs.

FURAZOLIDONE

Drug Interactions

Furazolidone Drug Interactions			
Precipitant drug	Object drug*		Description
Furazolidone	Alcohol	↑	A disulfiram-like reaction (eg, facial flushing, light-headedness, weakness, lacrimation) has occurred. (See Adverse Reactions.)
Furazolidone	Anorexiants	↑	Increased sensitivity to the pressor response of the anorexiants due to MAO inhibition.
Furazolidone	Levodopa	↑	Both the efficacy and adverse effects of levodopa may be increased, specifically hypertensive crisis. This may occur for several weeks after stopping furazolidone.
Furazolidone	Meperidine	↑	Effects are difficult to characterize, but may include agitation, seizures, diaphoresis, fever and progress to coma and apnea.
Furazolidone	Sympatho-mimetics (indirect and mixed)	↑	Increased pressor sensitivity to the indirect- and mixed-acting sympathomimetics due to MAO inhibition. Direct-acting agents are not affected.
Furazolidone	Tricyclic antidepessants	↑	Variable effects, including hypertension, hyperpyrexia, seizures, tachycardia; acute psychosis has occurred.

* ↑ = Object drug increased.

➤*Drug/Food interactions:* Patients taking furazolidone may experience marked elevation of blood pressure, hypertensive crisis or hemorrhagic strokes if foods high in amine content are consumed concurrently or after therapy. For a list of foods, see the MAOI group monograph.

Adverse Reactions

➤*CNS:* Headache; malaise.

➤*GI:* Colitis; proctitis; anal pruritus; staphylococcic enteritis. Nausea or emesis occurs occasionally and may be minimized or eliminated by reducing or withdrawing the drug.

➤*Hematologic:* May cause mild reversible intravascular hemolysis in G-6-PD deficient patients. Observe patients closely; discontinue the drug if there is any indication of hemolysis.

Do not administer to infants < 1 month of age because of possible hemolytic anemia due to immature enzyme systems (glutathione instability).

➤*Hypersensitivity:* Hypotension; urticaria; fever; arthralgia; vesicular morbilliform rash. These reactions subsided following withdrawal of the drug.

➤*Miscellaneous:*

Disulfiram-like reaction – Rarely, individuals have exhibited a disulfiram-like reaction to alcohol characterized by flushing, fever, dyspnea, and in some instances, chest tightness. All symptoms disappeared within 24 hours with no lasting ill effects. During 9 years of clinical use, 43 cases have been reported (14 under experimental conditions with doses in excess of those recommended). Three experienced hypotension necessitating active therapy. Norepinephrine may be used for hypotensive episodes, since it is not potentiated by furazolidone. Avoid indirectly acting pressor agents. Avoid ingestion of alcohol in any form during therapy and for 4 days thereafter.

Other – Renal or hepatic toxicity have not been significant with furazolidone.

Patient Information

Avoid ingestion of alcohol during and within 4 days after furazolidone therapy (a disulfiram-like reaction may occur; see Adverse Reactions).

Avoid foods containing tyramine, especially if therapy extends beyond 5 days (see Drug Interactions).

Avoid over-the-counter or prescription medications containing sympathomimetic drugs (eg, cold and hay fever remedies, anorexiants).

Medication may color the urine brown.

May cause nausea, vomiting or headache. Notify physician if these symptoms become severe.

Indications

➤*Urinary tract infections:* Prophylaxis or suppression/elimination of frequently recurring urinary tract infections when long-term therapy is considered necessary. Use only after eradication of the infection by other appropriate antimicrobial agents.

Actions

➤*Pharmacology:* In acid urine, methenamine is hydrolyzed to ammonia and formaldehyde, which is bactericidal. Methenamine does not liberate formaldehyde in the serum. The acid salts (mandelate and hippurate) help maintain a low urine pH.

➤*Pharmacokinetics:*

Absorption – Methenamine is readily absorbed following oral administration; 10% to 30% of the drug will be hydrolyzed by the gastric juices unless it is protected by an enteric coating.

Metabolism/Excretion – Approximately 10% to 25% of methenamine is metabolized in the liver and has a half-life of 3 to 6 hours. Generation of formaldehyde depends upon urinary pH, the concentration of methenamine and the duration that the urine is retained in the bladder. Peak concentrations of formaldehyde occur at a urine pH of ≤ 5.5 and are seen approximately 2 hours after a dose of methenamine hippurate and 3 to 8 hours after a dose of methenamine mandelate. A urinary formaldehyde concentration of > 25 mcg/ml is necessary for antimicrobial activity. Steady-state urinary formaldehyde concentrations are achieved in 2 to 3 days. Formaldehyde levels range from 1 to 85 mcg/ml, and decrease with increasing pH, urinary volume or flow rate.

In some instances, supplementary urine acidification may be desirable, especially in infections caused by urea-splitting organisms (which raise the urine pH). Ingestion of acidifying agents (eg, mandelic acid, hippuric acid, ammonium chloride, monobasic sodium phosphate) or acid-producing foods (eg, cranberries, plums, prunes) aid in maintaining an acid urine; however, effects may be negligible. Ammonium chloride 8 to 12 g/day, methionine 8 to 15 g/day and cranberry juice 1200 to 4000 ml/day, have all been recommended, but with marginal results. There is no reliable oral urinary acidifier at present. Monitor urine pH.

Excretion occurs via glomerular filtration and tubular secretion. Approximately 90% of the methenamine moiety is excreted in the urine within 24 hours. The influence of renal dysfunction on the pharmacology of methenamine is unknown.

➤*Microbiology:* The nonspecific antibacterial action of formaldehyde is effective against gram-positive and gram-negative organisms and fungi. *Escherichia coli*, enterococci and staphylococci are usually susceptible. *Enterobacter aerogenes* and *Proteus vulgaris* are generally resistant. Urea-splitting organisms (eg, *Proteus, Pseudomonas*) may be resistant since they raise the pH of the urine inhibiting the release of formaldehyde. An effective urine concentration of formaldehyde must persist for a minimum of 2 hours.

Methenamine is effective clinically against most common urinary tract pathogens since most bacteria are sensitive to free formaldehyde concentrations of 20 mcg/ml.

Methenamine is particularly suited for therapy of chronic infections, since bacteria and fungi do not develop resistance to formaldehyde.

Contraindications

Renal insufficiency; severe dehydration; severe hepatic insufficiency (because it facilitates ammonia production in the intestine); use alone for acute infections with parenchymal involvement causing systemic symptoms; hypersensitivity to the drug; concurrent sulfonamides since an insoluble precipitate may form with formaldehyde in the urine.

Warnings

➤*Pregnancy: Category C.* Safe use of methenamine in early pregnancy has not been established. Safety in the last trimester is suggested, but not proven. Methenamine passes into the fetus, but there is no evidence that methenamine salts cause fetal abnormalities. It is not known whether the drug can cause fetal harm when administered to a pregnant woman or can affect reproduction capacity. Give to pregnant women only if clearly needed.

➤*Lactation:* Methenamine passes into breast milk; levels are about equivalent to maternal serum and peak in 1 hour. One estimate revealed that an infant would receive about 0.15 to 0.4 mg methenamine/feeding. No adverse effects on the nursing infant have been reported.

Precautions

➤*Large doses:* (8 g daily for 3 to 4 weeks). These have caused bladder irritation, painful and frequent micturition, proteinuria and gross hematuria.

➤*Acid urine pH:* This should be maintained, especially when treating infections due to urea-splitting organisms such as *Proteus* and strains of *Pseudomonas*. When acidification is contraindicated or unattainable (as with some urea-splitting bacteria) the drug is not recommended.

➤*Serum transaminases:* These have elevated mildly during treatment in a few instances and returned to normal while patients were still receiving methenamine hippurate. Perform liver function studies periodically on patients receiving methenamine hippurate, especially those with liver dysfunction.

➤*Gout:* Methenamine salts may cause precipitation of urate crystals in the urine.

➤*Tartrazine sensitivity:* Some of these products contain tartrazine, which may cause allergic-type reactions (including bronchial asthma) in certain susceptible individuals. Although the overall incidence of tartrazine sensitivity in the general population is low, it is frequently seen in patients who also have aspirin hypersensitivity. Specific products containing tartrazine are identified in the product listings.

Drug Interactions

Methenamine Drug Interactions			
Precipitant drug	Object drug*		Description
Sulfonamides	Methenamine	↓	An insoluble precipitate between the sulfonamide and formaldehyde may form in the urine.
Urinary alkalinizers	Methenamine	↓	Alkalinizing agents may decrease the efficacy of methenamine by inhibiting its conversion to formaldehyde.

* ↓ = Object drug decreased.

➤*Drug/Lab test interactions:* Methenamine may interfere with laboratory urine determinations of **17-hydroxycorticosteroids, catecholamines** and **vanillylmandelic acid** (false increases); and **5-hydroxyindoleacetic acid** (false decrease).

Methenamine taken during pregnancy can interfere with laboratory tests of **urine estriol** (resulting in unmeasurably low values) when an acid hydrolysis procedure is used. This is due to the presence in the urine of methenamine or formaldehyde. Use enzymatic hydrolysis in place of acid hydrolysis.

Adverse Reactions

➤*Overall incidence:* Approximately 1% to 7%.

➤*Dermatologic:* Pruritus (rare); urticaria; erythematous eruptions; rash.

➤*GI:* Nausea; vomiting; cramps; stomatitis; anorexia.

➤*GU:* Bladder irritation, dysuria, proteinuria, hematuria, urinary frequency/urgency, crystalluria (large doses).

➤*Miscellaneous:* Headache, dyspnea, lipoid pneumonitis, generalized edema (rare).

Overdosage

➤*Treatment:* Immediately after ingestion of an overdose, further absorption of the drug may be minimized by inducing vomiting or by gastric lavage, followed by administration of activated charcoal. Force fluids, either oral or parenteral, to tolerance.

Patient Information

It may be necessary to attempt to acidify the urine (eg, ascorbic acid, cranberry juice).

Take with food to minimize GI upset.

Drink sufficient fluids to ensure adequate urine flow.

Avoid excessive intake of alkalinizing foods (milk products) or medication (bicarbonate, acetazolamide).

Complete full course of therapy; take until gone.

Notify physician if skin rash, painful urination or intolerable GI upset occurs.

METHENAMINE HIPPURATE

Rx	Hiprex (Hoechst Marion Roussel)	Tablets: 1 g	Tartrazine, saccharin. (Merrell 277). Yellow, scored. In 100s.
Rx	Urex (3M Pharm)		Saccharin. (3M Urex). White, scored. In 100s.

Complete prescribing information for these products begins in the Methenamine monograph.

Administration and Dosage

➤*Adults and children > 12 years of age:* 1 g twice daily.

➤*Children (6 to 12 years of age):* 0.5 to 1 g twice daily.

METHENAMINE MANDELATE

Rx	**Mandelamine** (Warner Chilcott)	**Tablets**: 0.5 g	(166). Brown. Film coated. In 100s.
Rx	**Mandelamine** (Warner Chilcott)	**Tablets**: 1 g	(167). Purple. Film coated. In 100s.
Rx	**Methenamine Mandelate** (Various, eg, Major)	**Tablets, enteric coated**: 0.5 g	In 100s and 1000s.
Rx	**Methenamine Mandelate** (Various, eg, Rugby)	**Tablets, enteric coated**: 1 g	In 100s and 1000s.
Rx	**Methenamine Mandelate** (Various, eg, Barre-National)	**Suspension**: 0.5 g/5 ml	In 480 ml.

Complete prescribing information for these products begins in the Methenamine monograph.

►*Children (6 to 12 years of age):* 0.5 g, 4 times daily.

►*Children (< 6 years of age):* 0.25 g/30 lb (14 kg), 4 times daily.

Administration and Dosage

►*Adults:* 1 g 4 times daily, after meals and at bedtime.

METHENAMINE COMBINATIONS

Rx	**Trac Tabs 2X** (Hyrex)	**Tablets**: 120 mg methenamine, 30 mg phenyl salicylate, 0.06 mg atropine sulfate, 0.03 mg hyoscyamine sulfate, 7.5 mg benzoic acid, 6 mg methylene blue *Dose*: 1 or 2 tablets 4 times daily	In 100s and 1000s.
Rx	Uretron D/S (A. G. Marin[1])	**Tablets**: 120 mg methenamine, 36.2 mg phenyl salicylate, 0.12 mg hyoscyamine sulfate, 10.8 mg methylene blue, 40.8 mg sodium biphosphate *Dose*: Adults - 1 qid followed by liberal fluid intake; *older children* - individualize dosing	Parabens, sucrose. (URETRON D/S). Purple. Sugar-coated. In 100s.
Rx	**Urelle** (Pharmelle[2])	**Tablets**: 81 mg methenamine, 32.4 mg phenyl salicylate, 10.8 mg methylene blue, 40.8 mg sodium phosphate monobasic, 0.12 mg hyoscyamine sulfate *Dose*: Adults - 1 qid followed by liberal fluid intake; *older children* - individualize dosing	Sugar, mineral oil. (P-002). Blue. Sugar-coated. In 90s.
Rx	**Prosed/DS** (Star)	**Tablets**: 81.6 mg methenamine, 36.2 mg phenyl salicylate, 10.8 mg methylene blue, 9 mg benzoic acid, 0.06 mg atropine sulfate, 0.06 mg hyoscyamine sulfate *Dose*: 1 tablet 4 times daily	Parabens, sugar. (Prosed/DS). Dark blue. Sugar coated. In 100s and 1000s.
Rx	**Uritact DS** (Cypress)	**Tablets**: 81.6 mg methenamine, 36.2 mg phenyl salicylate, 10.8 mg methylene blue, 9 mg benzoic acid, 0.06 mg atropine sulfate, 0.06 mg hyoscyamine sulfate *Dose*: 1 tablet 4 times daily with liquid	Alcohol-free. (CYP 516). Light blue, capsule shape. In 100s.
Rx	**Uro Blue** (R. A. McNeil[3])	**Tablets**: 81.6 mg methenamine, 40.8 mg sodium biphosphate, 36.2 mg phenyl salicylate, 10.8 mg methylene blue, 0.12 mg hyoscyamine sulfate *Dose*: 1 tablet 4 times daily followed by liberal fluid intake	Sucrose, parabens. (MD-20). Purple, oval. Sugar-coated. In 100s.
Rx	**Urogesic Blue** (Edwards)		Sucrose, parabens. (MD-20). Purple. Oval. Sugar coated. In 100s.
Rx	**Urimax** (Integrity)	**Tablets, delayed release**: 81.6 mg methenamine, 40.8 mg sodium biphosphate, 36.2 mg phenyl salicylate, 10.8 mg methylene blue, 0.12 mg hyoscyamine sulfate *Dose*: 1 tablet 4 times daily	(Urimax). Magenta. Film coated. In 100s.
Rx	**Urimar-T** (Marnel)	**Tablets**: 81.6 mg methenamine, 40.8 mg sodium biphosphate, 36.2 mg phenyl salicylate, 10.8 mg methylene blue, 0.12 mg hyoscyamine sulfate *Dose*: 1 tablet 4 times daily	In 100s.
Rx	**Uroquid-Acid No. 2** (Beach)	**Tablets**: 500 mg methenamine mandelate, 500 mg sodium acid phosphate monohydrate *Dose*: Initial - 2 tablets 4 times daily Maintenance - 2 to 4 tablets daily in divided doses	(Beach 1114). Yellow. Film coated. Capsule shape. In 100s.
Rx	**Urisedamine** (PolyMedica)	**Tablets**: 500 mg methenamine mandelate, 0.15 mg hyoscyamine *Dose*: 2 tablets 4 times daily Children (≥ 6 years) – Reduce dosage in proportion to age and weight	Sucrose. (W2210). Light blue. Capsule shape. In 100s.
Rx	**Atrosept** (Geneva)	**Tablets**: 40.8 mg methenamine, 18.1 mg phenyl salicylate, 0.03 mg atropine sulfate, 0.03 mg hyoscyamine (as sulfate), 4.5 mg benzoic acid, 5.4 mg methylene blue *Dose*: Adults – 2 tablets 4 times daily	(220). Deep blue. Sugar coated. In 100s and 1000s.
Rx	**Dolsed** (American Urologicals)	Children (≥ 6 years) – Reduce dosage in proportion to age and weight	(Dolsed). Deep blue. Sugar coated. In 100s and 1000s.
Rx	**UAA** (Econo Med)		(UAA). Blue. Sugar coated. In 100s and 1000s.
Rx	**Uridon Modified** (Rugby)		Blue. Sugar coated. In 100s and 1000s.
Rx	**Urinary Antiseptic No. 2** (Various)		In 100s and 1000s.
Rx	**Urised** (PolyMedica)		(W 2183). Purple. Sugar coated. In 100s and 500s.
Rx	**Uritin** (Various, eg, Goldline)		In 1000s.
Rx	**MHP-A** (Cypress)	**Tablets**: 40.8 mg methenamine, 18.1 mg phenyl salicylate, 0.03 mg atropine sulfate, 0.03 mg hyoscyamine sulfate, 4.5 mg benzoic acid, 5.4 mg methylene blue *Dose*: Adults – 2 qid Children (≥ 6 years) – Dosage must be individualized by physician.	(CYP515). Green. In 100s.
Rx	**Uriseptic** (SDA Labs[4])	**Tablets**: 40.8 mg methenamine, 18.1 mg phenyl salicylate, 0.03 mg atropine sulfate, 0.03 mg hyoscyamine sulfate, 4.5 mg benzoic acid, 5.4 mg methylene blue *Dose*: Adults – 2 qid followed by liberal fluid intake Children (≥ 6 years) – Individualize dosage	Dk. blue. Film-coated. In 100s.
otc	**Cystex** (Numark)	**Tablets**: 162 mg methenamine, 162.5 mg sodium salicylate, 32 mg benzoic acid *Dose*: Adults and children > 16 years old – 2 tablets 4 times daily with meals and at bedtime	In 40s and 100s.

[1] A. G. Marin Pharmaceuticals, 1730 N.W. 79th Avenue, Miami, FL 33126; 305-593-5333, fax 305-593-8333.

[2] Pharmelle L.L.C., 890 N. Lafayette, Florissant, MO 63031; 314-830-4950, 877-577-2577.

[3] R. A. McNeil Company, 1210 E. Dallas Road, Chattanooga, TN 37405; 423-265-8240, 800-755-3038; fax 423-265-7373.

[4] SDA Laboratories, 280 Railroad Avenue, Greenwich, CT 06830; 203-861-0005, fax 203-861-0006.

TRIMETHOPRIM (TMP)

Rx	**Trimethoprim** (Various, eg, Biocraft, Moore, Parmed, Rugby, Schein)	**Tablets**: 100 mg	In 14s, 30s, 100s and UD 100s.
Rx	**Proloprim** (GlaxoWellcome)		(Proloprim 09A). White, scored. In 100s.
Rx	**Trimethoprim** (Various, eg, Biocraft, Moore, Rugby)	**Tablets**: 200 mg	In 100s.
Rx	**Proloprim** (GlaxoWellcome)		(Proloprim 200). Yellow, scored. In 100s.
Rx	**Primsol** (Ascent Pediatrics)	**Solution, oral**: 50 mg/5 ml	Parabens, sorbitol. Alcohol free. Bubble gum flavor. In 473 ml.

Indications

For the treatment of initial uncomplicated UTIs due to susceptible strains including: *E. coli*, *P. mirabilis*, *K. pneumoniae*, *Enterobacter* species, and coagulase-negative *Staphylococcus* species, including *S. saprophyticus*.

Perform culture and susceptibility tests. May initiate therapy prior to obtaining test results.

Administration and Dosage

➤*Adults:* 100 mg every 12 hours or 200 mg every 24 hours for 10 days.

➤*Renal impairment:* If creatinine clearance is 15 to 30 ml/min, give 50 mg every 12 hours. If it is < 15 ml/min, use is not recommended.

➤*Children:* Effectiveness has not been established.

➤*Storage / Stability:* Protect the 200 mg tablet from light.

Actions

➤*Pharmacology:* Trimethoprim blocks production of tetrahydrofolic acid from dihydrofolic acid by binding to and reversibly inhibiting the enzyme dihydrofolate reductase. This binding is much stronger for the bacterial enzyme than for the corresponding mammalian enzyme. Bacterial biosynthesis of nucleic acids and proteins is blocked by trimethoprim's interference with the normal bacterial metabolism of folinic acid.

➤*Pharmacokinetics:*

Absorption / Distribution – Oral trimethoprim is rapidly absorbed. Mean peak serum levels of approximately 1 mcg/ml occur 1 to 4 hours after a single 100 mg dose. Approximately 44% is serum protein bound. Urine concentrations are considerably higher than blood concentrations. After a single oral dose of 100 mg, urine levels ranged from 30 to 160 mcg/ml during the 0 to 4 hour period and declined to approximately 18 to 91 mcg/ml during the 8 to 24 hour period.

Metabolism / Excretion – Trimethoprim is metabolized less than 20%. The half-life is 8 to 10 hours. Elimination is delayed in patients with renal function impairment and half-life is prolonged. Excretion is chiefly by the kidneys through glomerular filtration and tubular secretion. After oral administration, 50% to 60% is excreted in the urine within 24 hours; ≈ 80% is unmetabolized, and ≈ 4% is detectable in feces.

➤*Microbiology:* In vitro, the spectrum of antibacterial activity includes common urinary tract pathogens except *Pseudomonas aeruginosa*.

Using the dilution method for determining the minimum inhibitory concentrations (MIC), the MIC for susceptible organisms is ≤ 8 mcg/ml. Resistant species have an MIC of ≥ 16 mcg/ml.

Representative Trimethoprim MICs For Susceptible Organisms	
Bacteria	Trimethoprim MIC (mcg/ml)
Escherichia coli	0.05-1.5
Proteus mirabilis	0.5-1.5
Klebsiella pneumoniae	0.5-5
Enterobacter species	0.5-5
Staphylococcus species (coagulase-negative)	0.15-5

Normal vaginal and fecal flora are the source of most pathogens causing urinary tract infections (UTIs). Concentrations in vaginal secretions are consistently greater (1.6 fold) than those in serum. Sufficient trimethoprim is excreted in the feces to markedly reduce or eliminate susceptible organisms. Dominant fecal organisms (non-*Enterobacteriaceae*, *Bacteroides* and *Lactobacillus* species), are generally not susceptible.

Trimethoprim acts synergistically with sulfonamides, blocking sequential steps in the biosynthesis of folic acid. See trimethoprim-sulfamethoxazole monograph.

Contraindications

Hypersensitivity to trimethoprim; megaloblastic anemia due to folate deficiency.

Warnings

➤*Hematologic effects:* Trimethoprim rarely interferes with hematopoiesis, especially in large doses or for prolonged periods. Sore throat, fever, pallor, or purpura may be early indications of serious blood disorders; obtain complete blood counts. Discontinue drug if the count of any formed blood element is significantly reduced.

➤*Renal / Hepatic function impairment:* Use with caution.

➤*Pregnancy: Category C.* Teratogenic in small animals at 40 times the human dose; increased fetal loss occurred with 6 times the human therapeutic dose.

Trimethoprim crosses the placenta, producing similar levels in fetal and maternal serum and in amniotic fluid. In a report of 186 pregnancies in which the mother received either placebo or trimethoprim/sulfamethoxazole, the incidence of congenital abnormalities was 4.5% (3 of 66) for placebo and 3.3% (4 of 120) for the drug combination. There were no abnormalities in 10 children exposed during the first trimester or in 35 children exposed to trimethoprim/sulfamethoxazole at conception or shortly after.

Trimethoprim may interfere with folic acid metabolism; use only when potential benefits outweigh potential hazards to the fetus.

➤*Lactation:* Following 160 mg twice daily for 5 days, milk concentrations ranged from 1.2 to 2.4 mcg/ml; observed milk:plasma ratios were 1.25. Because it may interfere with folic acid metabolism, use caution when administering to nursing women.

➤*Children:* Safety for use in infants < 2 months has not been established. The efficacy for use in children < 12 has not been established.

Precautions

➤*Folate deficiency:* Use with caution. Folates may be administered concomitantly without interfering with antibacterial action.

Drug Interactions

Phenytoin's pharmacologic effects may be increased by coadministration of trimethoprim, apparently due to inhibition of hepatic metabolism.

Adverse Reactions

➤*Dermatologic:* Rash (3% to 7%); pruritus; exfoliative dermatitis. In high-dose studies, an increased incidence of mild to moderate maculopapular, morbilliform and pruritic rashes occurred 7 to 14 days after therapy began.

➤*GI:* Epigastric distress; nausea; vomiting; glossitis.

➤*Hematologic:* Thrombocytopenia; leukopenia; neutropenia; megaloblastic anemia; methemoglobinemia.

➤*Miscellaneous:* Fever; elevation of serum transaminase and bilirubin; increased BUN and serum creatinine levels.

Overdosage

➤*Acute:*

Symptoms – After ingestion of ≥ 1 g, nausea, vomiting, dizziness, headaches, mental depression, confusion, and bone marrow depression may occur (see Chronic Overdosage).

Treatment – Gastric lavage and general supportive measures. Urine acidification increases renal elimination. Peritoneal dialysis is not effective and hemodialysis is only moderately effective.

➤*Chronic:*

Symptoms – Use at high doses or for extended periods may cause bone marrow depression manifested as thrombocytopenia, leukopenia or megaloblastic anemia.

Treatment – Discontinue use and give leucovorin, 3 to 6 mg IM daily for 3 days, or as required to restore normal hematopoiesis. Alternatively, 5 to 15 mg daily of oral leucovorin has been recommended.

Patient Information

Take for full course of therapy until medication is gone.

TRIMETREXATE GLUCURONATE

Rx **Neutrexin** (US Bioscience) **Powder for Injection, lyophilized:** 25 mg trimetrexate In 5 ml vials with or without 50 mg leucovorin.

WARNING

Trimetrexate must be used with concurrent leucovorin (leucovorin protection) to avoid potentially serious or life-threatening toxicities (see Precautions and Administration and Dosage).

Indications

As an alternative therapy with concurrent leucovorin administration (leucovorin protection) for the treatment of moderate-to-severe *Pneumocystis carinii* pneumonia (PCP) in immunocompromised patients, including patients with acquired immunodeficiency syndrome (AIDS), who are intolerant of, or are refractory to trimethoprim-sulfamethoxazole therapy or for whom TMP-SMZ is contraindicated.

➤*Unlabeled uses:* Trimetrexate is being investigated for treatment of non-small cell lung, prostate and colorectal cancer.

Administration and Dosage

➤*Approved by the FDA:* December 17, 1993.

Trimetrexate must be given with concurrent leucovorin (leucovorin protection) to avoid potentially serious or life-threatening toxicities. Leucovorin must be given daily during trimetrexate treatment and for 72 hours past the last trimetrexate dose.

Trimetrexate is administered at a dose of 45 mg/m^2 once daily by IV infusion over 60 to 90 minutes. Leucovorin may be administered IV at a dose of 20 mg/m^2 over 5 to 10 minutes every 6 hours for a total daily dose of 80 mg/m^2, or orally as 4 doses of 20 mg/m^2 spaced equally throughout the day. Round up the oral dose to the next higher 25 mg increment. The recommended course of therapy is 21 days of trimetrexate and 24 days of leucovorin.

➤*Dosage modifications:*

Hematologic toxicity – Modify trimetrexate and leucovorin doses based on the worst hematologic toxicity according to the following table. If leucovorin is given orally, round up doses to the next higher 25 mg increment.

	Dose Modifications for Hematologic Toxicity			
Toxicity Grade	Neutrophils per mm^3	Platelets per mm^3	Trimetrexate	Leucovorin
1	> 1,000	> 75,000	45 mg/m^2 once daily	20 mg/m^2 every 6 hours
2	750-1000	50,000-75,000	45 mg/m^2 once daily	40 mg/m^2 every 6 hours
3	500-749	25,000-49,999	22 mg/m^2 once daily	40 mg/m^2 every 6 hours
4	< 500	< 25,000	Day 1-9 discontinue Day 10-21 interrupt up to 96 hours[1]	40 mg/m^2 every 6 hours

[1] If Grade 4 hematologic toxicity occurs prior to day 10, discontinue trimetrexate. Administer leucovorin (40 mg/m^2 every 6 hours) for an additional 72 hours. If Grade 4 hematologic toxicity occurs at day 10 or later, trimetrexate may be held up to 96 hours to allow counts to recover. If counts recover to Grade 3 within 96 hours, administer trimetrexate at a dose of 22 mg/m^2 and maintain leucovorin at 40 mg/m^2 every 6 hours. When counts recover to Grade 2 toxicity, trimetrexate dose may be increased to 45 mg/m^2, but the leucovorin dose should be maintained at 40 mg/m^2 for the duration of treatment. If counts do not improve to ≤ Grade 3 toxicity within 96 hours, discontinue trimetrexate. Administer leucovorin at a dose of 40 mg/m^2 every 6 hours for 72 hours following the last dose of trimetrexate.

Hepatic toxicity – Transient elevations of transaminases and alkaline phosphatase have occurred in trimetrexate patients. Treatment interruption is advisable if transaminase levels or alkaline phosphatase levels increase to > 5 times the upper limit of normal range.

Renal toxicity – Interruption of trimetrexate is advisable if serum creatinine levels increase to > 2.5 mg/dl and the elevation is considered secondary to trimetrexate.

Other toxicities – Interruption of treatment is advisable in patients with severe mucosal toxicity that interferes with oral intake. Discontinue treatment for fever (oral temperature ≥ 40.5°C [105°F]) that cannot be controlled with antipyretics. Leucovorin therapy must extend for 72 hours past the last dose of trimetrexate.

➤*Reconstitution and dilution:* Reconstitute with 2 ml of 5% Dextrose Injection or Sterile Water for Injection to yield a concentration of 12.5 mg/ml (complete dissolution should occur within 30 seconds). The reconstituted product will appear as a pale greenish-yellow solution and must be inspected visually for particulate matter prior to dilution. Do not use if cloudiness or precipitate is observed. Filter this solution (0.22 mcM) prior to dilution. Do not reconstitute with solutions containing either chloride ion or leucovorin, since precipitation occurs instantly.

Further dilute reconstituted solution with 5% Dextrose Injection to yield a final concentration of 0.25 to 2 mg/ml. Administer the diluted solution by IV infusion over 60 minutes. The IV line must be flushed thoroughly with at least 10 ml of 5% Dextrose Injection before and after administering trimetrexate.

Trimetrexate and leucovorin solutions must be administered separately. Leucovorin protection may be administered prior to or following trimetrexate. In either case the IV line must be flushed thoroughly with at least 10 ml of 5% Dextrose Injection between infusions. Dilute leucovorin according to the manufacturer's instructions and administer over 5 to 10 minutes every 6 hours.

➤*Handling and disposal:* If trimetrexate contacts the skin or mucosa, immediately and thoroughly wash with soap and water. Procedures for proper disposal of cytotoxic drugs should be considered.

➤*Storage/Stability:* Store vials at controlled room temperature and protect from exposure to light. After reconstitution, the solution is stable under refrigeration or at room temperature for up to 24 hours. Do not freeze reconstituted solution. Discard the unused portions after 24 hours.

Actions

➤*Pharmacology:* Trimetrexate, a 2.4-diaminoquinazoline, non-classical folate antagonist, is a synthetic inhibitor of the enzyme dihydrofolate reductase (DHFR). In vitro, trimetrexate is a competitive inhibitor of DHFR from bacterial, protozoan and mammalian sources. DHFR catalyzes the reduction of intracellular dihydrofolate to the active coenzyme, leading directly to interference with thymidylate biosynthesis, as well as inhibition of folate-dependent formyltransferases, and indirectly to inhibition of purine biosynthesis. The end result is disruption of DNA, RNA and protein synthesis, with consequent cell death. Leu-

covorin (folinic acid) is readily transported into mammalian cells by an active, carrier-mediated process and can be assimilated into cellular folate pools following its metabolism. In vitro, leucovorin provides a source of reduced folates necessary for normal cellular biosynthetic processes. Because the *Pneumocystis carinii* organism lacks the reduced folate carrier-mediated transport system, leucovorin is prevented from entering the organism. Therefore, at concentrations achieved with therapeutic doses of trimetrexate plus leucovorin, the selective transport of trimetrexate, but not leucovorin, into the *P. carinii* organism allows the concurrent administration of leucovorin to protect normal host cells from the cytotoxicity of trimetrexate without inhibiting the antifolate's inhibition of *P. carinii*. It is not known if considerably higher doses of leucovorin would affect trimetrexate's effect on *P. carinii*.

➤*Pharmacokinetics:* Trimetrexate pharmacokinetics were assessed in six patients with acquired immunodeficiency syndrome (AIDS) who had *P. carinii* pneumonia (PCP; n = 4) or toxoplasmosis (n = 2). Trimetrexate was administered IV as a bolus injection at a dose of 30 mg/m^2/day every 6 hours for 21 days. Clearance was 38 ± 15 ml/min/m^2 and volume of distribution at steady state (Vd$_{ss}$) was 20 ± 8 L/m^2. The plasma concentration time profile declined in a biphasic manner over 24 hours with a terminal half-life of 11 ± 4 hours.

The pharmacokinetics of trimetrexate without the concomitant administration of leucovorin have been evaluated in cancer patients with advanced solid tumors using various dosage regimens. Following the single-dose administration of 10 to 130 mg/m^2 to 37 patients, plasma concentrations were obtained for 72 hours. The alpha phase half-life was 57 ± 28 minutes, followed by a terminal phase with a half-life of 16 ± 3 hours. The plasma concentrations in the remaining patients exhibited a triphasic decline with half-lives of 8.6 ± 6.5 minutes, 2.4 ± 1.3 hours and 17.8 ± 8.2 hours.

Trimetrexate clearance in cancer patients has been reported as 53 ± 41 ml/min (n = 14) and 32 ± 18 ml/min/m^2 (n = 23) following single-dose administration. After a 5 day infusion to 16 patients, plasma clearance was 30 ± 8 ml/min/m^2.

Renal clearance in cancer patients has varied from about 4 ± 2 to 10 ± 6 ml/min/m^2 and 10% to 30% is excreted unchanged in the urine. Considering the free fraction of trimetrexate, active tubular secretion may possibly contribute to the renal clearance. Renal clearance has been associated with urine flow, suggesting the possibility of tubular reabsorption as well.

The Vd$_{ss}$ of trimetrexate in cancer patients after single-dose administration and for whom plasma concentrations were obtained for 72 hours was 36.9 ± 17.6 L/m^2 (n = 23) and 0.62 ± 0.24 L/kg (n = 14). Following a constant infusion for 5 days, Vd$_{ss}$ was 32.8 ± 16.6 L/m^2.

There have been inconsistencies in the reporting of trimetrexate protein binding. The in vitro plasma protein binding of trimetrexate using ultrafiltration is approximately 95% over the concentration range of 18.75 to 1000 ng/ml. There is a suggestion of capacity-limited binding (saturable binding) at concentrations> 1000 ng/ml, with free fraction progressively increasing to about 9.3% as concentration is increased to

TRIMETREXATE GLUCURONATE

15 mcg/ml. Other reports have declared trimetrexate to be > 98% bound at concentrations of 0.1 to 10 mcg/ml; however, specific free fractions were not stated. The free fraction of trimetrexate also has been reported to be about 15% to 16% at a concentration of 60 ng/ml, increasing to about 20% at a concentration of 6 mcg/ml.

Trimetrexate metabolism in man has not been characterized. Preclinical data strongly suggest that the major metabolic pathway is oxidative O-demethylation, followed by conjugation to either glucuronide or the sulfate. N-demethylation and oxidation is a related minor pathway. Preliminary findings in humans indicate the presence of a glucuronide conjugate with DHFR inhibition and a demethylated metabolite in urine. Data suggest the presence of one or more metabolites with DHFR inhibition activity.

Fecal recovery of trimetrexate over 48 hours after IV administration ranged from 0.09% to 7.6% of the dose as determined by DHFR inhibition and 0.02% to 5.2% of the dose as determined by HPLC.

The pharmacokinetics of trimetrexate have not been determined in patients with renal insufficiency or hepatic dysfunction.

➤*Microbiology:* Trimetrexate inhibits, in a dose-related manner, in vitro growth of the trophozoite stage of rat *P. carinii* cultured on human embryonic lung fibrolast cells. Leucovorin alone did not alter either the growth of the trophozoites or the anti-pneumocystis activity of trimetrexate. Resistance to trimetrexate's antimicrobial activity against *P. carinii* has not been studied.

➤*Clinical trials:*

Trimetrexate vs trimethoprim-sulfamethoxazole (TMP-SMZ) – This double-blind, randomized trial was designed to compare the safety and efficacy of trimetrexate/leucovorin (TMTX/LV) to that of TMP-SMZ for the treatment of histologically confirmed, moderate-to-severe PCP in patients with AIDS. Of the 220 patients with histologically confirmed PCP, 109 were randomized to receive TMTX/LV (45 mg/m² of TMTX daily for 21 days plus 20 mg/m² of LV every 6 hours for 24 days), and 111 to TMP-SMZ (5 mg/kg TMP plus 25 mg/kg SMZ 4 times daily for 21 days). Response to therapy, defined as alive and off ventilatory support at completion of therapy, without a requirement for a change in anti-pneumocystis therapy, or addition of supraphysiologic doses of steroids, occurred in 50% of patients in each treatment group. The observed mortality in the TMTX/LV treatment group was approximately twice that in the TMP-SMZ treatment group. Thirty of 109 (27%) patients treated with TMTX/LV and 18 of 111 (16%) patients receiving TMP-SMZ died during the 21 day treatment course or 4 week follow-up period. Twenty-seven of 30 deaths in the TMTX/LV arm were attributed to PCP; all 18 deaths in the TMP-SMZ arm were attributed to PCP. A significantly smaller proportion of patients who received TMTX/LV compared to TMP-SMZ failed therapy due to toxicity (10% vs 25%), and a significantly greater proportion of patients failed due to lack of efficacy (40% vs 24%). Six patients (12%) who responded to TMTX/LV relapsed during the 1 month follow-up period; no patient responding to TMP-SMZ relapsed during this period.

Treatment IND – The FDA granted a Treatment IND for trimetrexate with leucovorin protection in February 1988 to make trimetrexate therapy available to HIV-infected patients with histologically confirmed PCP who had disease refractory to, or who were intolerant of TMP-SMZ or IV pentamidine. Of the 577 evaluable patients, 227 patients were intolerant of both TMP-SMZ and pentamidine (IST; patients intolerant of both standard therapies), 146 were intolerant of one therapy and refractory to the other (RIST; patients refractory to one therapy and intolerant of the other) and 204 were refractory to both therapies (RST; refractory to both standard therapies). This was a very ill patient population; 38% required ventilatory support at entry. These studies did not have concurrent control groups. The overall survival rate 1 month after completion of TMTX/LV as salvage therapy was 48%. Patients who had not responded to treatment with both TMP-SMZ and pentamidine, of whom 63% required mechanical ventilation at entry, achieved a survival rate of 25% following treatment with TMTX/LV. Survival was 67% in patients who were intolerant to both TMP-SMZ and pentamidine. In the Treatment IND, 12% of patients discontinued TMTX/LV for toxicity.

Contraindications

Clinically significant sensitivity to trimetrexate, leucovorin or methotrexate.

Warnings

➤*Concurrent leucovorin:* Trimetrexate must be used with concurrent leucovorin to avoid potentially serious or life-threatening complications including bone marrow suppression, oral and GI mucosal ulceration, and renal and hepatic dysfunction. Leucovorin therapy must extend for 72 hours past the last dose of trimetrexate. Inform patients that failure to take the recommended dose and duration of leucovorin can lead to fatal toxicity. Closely monitor patients for the development of serious hematologic adverse reactions (see Precautions and Administration and Dosage).

➤*Hypersensitivity reactions:* An anaphylactoid reaction has occurred in a cancer patient receiving trimetrexate as a bolus injection.

➤*Fertility impairment:* No studies have been conducted to evaluate the potential of trimetrexate to impair fertility. However, during standard toxicity studies conducted in mice and rats, degeneration of the testes and spermatocytes, including the arrest of spermatogenesis, was observed.

➤*Pregnancy: Category D.* Trimetrexate can cause fetal harm when administered to a pregnant woman. Trimetrexate is fetotoxic and teratogenic in rats and rabbits. Rats administered 1.5 and 2.5 mg/kg/day IV on gestational days 6 to 15 showed substantial postimplantation loss and severe inhibition of maternal weight gain; 0.5 and 1 mg/kg/day on gestational days 6 to 15 retarded normal fetal development and was teratogenic. Rabbits given daily doses of 2.5 and 5 mg/kg/day on gestational days 6 to 18 resulted in significant maternal and fetotoxicity; 0.1 mg/kg/day was teratogenic in the absence of significant maternal toxicity. These effects were observed using doses 1/20 to 1/2 the equivalent human therapeutic dose based on a mg/m² basis. Teratogenic effects included skeletal, visceral, ocular and cardiovascular abnormalities. If trimetrexate is used during pregnancy, or if the patient becomes pregnant while taking this drug, apprise the patient of the potential hazard to the fetus. Advise women of childbearing potential to avoid becoming pregnant.

➤*Lactation:* It is not known if trimetrexate is excreted in breast milk. Because of the potential for serious adverse reactions in nursing infants, it is recommended that breastfeeding be discontinued if the mother is treated with trimetrexate.

➤*Children:* Safety and efficacy of trimetrexate for the treatment of histologically confirmed PCP has not been established for patients < 18 years of age. Under the Compassionate Use Protocol, two children (9 and 15 months of age) were treated with trimetrexate and leucovorin using a dose of 45 mg/m²/day of trimetrexate for 21 days and 20 mg/m²/day of leucovorin for 24 days. There were no serious or unexpected adverse effects.

Precautions

➤*Monitoring:* Mild elevations in transaminase and alkaline phosphatase have been observed and are usually not cause for modifications of therapy (see Administration and Dosage). Patients receiving trimetrexate with leucovorin protection should be seen frequently by a physician. Perform blood tests at least twice a week during therapy to assess the following parameters: Hematology (absolute neutrophil counts [ANC], platelets); renal function (serum creatinine, BUN); hepatic function (AST, ALT, alkaline phosphatase).

➤*Seizures:* These have been reported rarely (<1%) in AIDS patients receiving trimetrexate; however, a causal relationship has not been established.

➤*Pulmonary conditions:* Trimetrexate has not been evaluated clinically for the treatment of concurrent pulmonary conditions such as bacterial, viral or fungal pneumonia or mycobacterial diseases. In vitro activity has been observed against *Toxoplasma gondii, Mycobacterium avium* complex, gram-positive cocci and gram-negative rods. If clinical deterioration is observed in patients, carefully evaluate them for other possible causes of pulmonary disease and treat with additional agents as appropriate.

➤*Special risk:* Patients receiving trimetrexate may experience hematologic, hepatic, renal and GI toxicities. Use caution in treating patients with impaired hematologic, renal or hepatic function. Treat and carefully monitor patients who require concomitant therapy with nephrotoxic, myelosuppressive or hepatotoxic drugs with trimetrexate at the discretion of the physician. To allow for full therapeutic doses of trimetrexate, discontinue treatment with zidovudine during trimetrexate therapy. Trimetrexate-associated myelosuppression, stomatitis and GI toxicities can generally be ameliorated by adjusting the dose of leucovorin.

Drug Interactions

Since trimetrexate is metabolized by a P450 enzyme system, drugs that induce or inhibit this drug metabolizing enzyme system may elicit important drug interactions that may alter trimetrexate plasma concentrations. Agents that might be coadministered with trimetrexate in AIDS patients for other indications that could elicit this activity include erythromycin, rifampin, rifabutin, ketoconazole and fluconazole. In vitro, cimetidine caused a significant reduction in trimetrexate metabolism and acetaminophen altered the relative concentration of trimetrexate metabolites, possibly by competing for sulfate metabolites. In vitro, nitrogen substituted imidazole drugs (eg, clotrimazole, ketoconazole, miconazole) were potent, non-competitive inhibitors of trimetrexate metabolism. Carefully monitor patients being treated with these drugs and receiving concurrent trimetrexate.

Adverse Reactions

Because many patients who participated in clinical trials had complications of advanced HIV disease, it is difficult to distinguish adverse events caused by trimetrexate from those resulting from underlying medical conditions. Laboratory toxicities were generally manageable with dose modification of trimetrexate/leucovorin (see Administration and Dosage). Of the patients receiving TMP-SMZ, 29% discontinued therapy due to adverse events vs 10% of patients treated with TMTX/LV. Hematologic toxicity was the principal dose-limiting side effect. An anaphylactoid reaction occurred in a cancer patient receiving trimetrexate as a bolus injection.

TRIMETREXATE GLUCURONATE

Adverse reaction	Trimetrexate Adverse Reactions (%)	
	TMTX/LV (n = 109)	TMP-SMZ (n = 111)
Non-laboratory:		
Fever	8.3	12.6
Rash/Pruritus	5.5	12.6
Nausea/Vomiting	4.6	13.5
Confusion	2.8	2.7
Fatigue	1.8	0
Hematologic toxicity:		
Neutropenia ($\leq$ 1000/mm^3)	30.3	33.3
Thrombocytopenia ($\leq$ 75,000/mm^3)	10.1	15.3
Anemia (Hgb < 8 g/dl)	7.3	9
Hepatotoxicity:		
Increased AST (> 5 x ULN)	13.8	9
Increased ALT (> 5 x ULN)	11	
Increased alkaline phosphatase (> 5 x ULN)	4.6	11.7
Increased bilirubin (2.5 x ULN)	1.8	2.7
Renal:		0.9
Increased serum creatinine (> 3 x ULN)	0.9	1.8
Electrolyte imbalance:		
Hyponatremia	4.6	9
Hypocalcemia	1.8	0
Number of patients with $\geq$ 1 adverse event	53.2	54.1

Overdosage

▶*Symptoms:* Trimetrexate administered without concurrent leucovorin can cause lethal complications. There has been no extensive experience in humans receiving single IV doses of trimetrexate > 90 mg/m^2/day with concurrent leucovorin. The toxicities seen at this dose were primarily hematologic.

▶*Treatment:* In the event of overdose, stop trimetrexate and administer leucovorin at a dose of 40 mg/m^2 every 6 hours for 3 days.

METHYLENE BLUE

| Rx | Methblue 65 (Manne Co) | Tablets: 65 mg | In 100s and 1000s. |
| Rx | Urolene Blue (Star) | | In 100s and 1000s. |

Indications

➤*GU antiseptic:* A mild genitourinary antiseptic for cystitis and urethritis. However, other agents have replaced methylene blue for this purpose.

➤*Diagnostic:* Used as a diagnostic agent and indicator dye.

➤*Methemoglobinemia:* For treatment of idiopathic and drug-induced methemoglobinemia

➤*Antidote:* Antidote for cyanide poisoning (see individual monograph in the Endocrine/Metabolic chapter).

➤*Unlabeled uses:* May be useful in the management of patients with oxalate and phosphate urinary tract calculi.

Administration and Dosage

Take 65 to 130 mg 3 times daily after meals with a full glass of water.

Actions

➤*Pharmacology:* Methylene blue is a dye that is a weak germicide and is used as a mild genitourinary antiseptic. However, its use in these conditions is now obsolete; it has largely been replaced by other agents. It is primarily bacteriostatic; bactericidal properties are very mild.

This compound has an oxidation-reduction action and a tissue staining property. In high concentrations, methylene blue converts the ferrous iron of reduced hemoglobin to the ferric form; as a result, methemoglobin is produced. This action is the basis for the antidotal action of methylene blue in cyanide poisoning (see monograph in the Endocrine/Metabolic chapter). In contrast, low concentrations of methylene blue are capable of hastening the conversion of methemoglobin to hemoglobin. Oral absorption is reported to be 53% to 97% (74% average).

Contraindications

Renal insufficiency; patients allergic to methylene blue; glucose–6–phosphate dehydrogenase (G-6-PD) deficient patients (methylene blue may induce hemolysis).

Adverse Reactions

Turns the urine and sometimes the stool and skin blue-green. May cause bladder irritation, and in some cases, nausea, vomiting and diarrhea. Large doses may cause fever.

Patient Information

Take after meals with a glass of water.

May discolor the urine, skin or stool blue-green.

FOSFOMYCIN TROMETHAMINE

| Rx | Monurol (Forest) | Granules: 3 g | In single-dose packets. |

Indications

➤*Uncomplicated urinary tract infections:* Treatment of uncomplicated urinary tract infections (acute cystitis) in women caused by susceptible strains of *E. coli* and *E. faecalis.* Fosfomycin is not indicated for the treatment of pyelonephritis or perinephric abscess.

Administration and Dosage

➤*Approved by the FDA:* December 19, 1996.

The recommended dosage for women ≥ 18 years of age for uncomplicated urinary tract infection (acute cystitis) is one packet of fosfomycin. Fosfomycin may be taken with or without food.

Do not take in its dry form. Always mix fosfomycin with water before ingesting.

Pour the entire contents of a single-dose packet of fosfomycin into 90 to 120 ml (3 to 4 ounces) of water and stir to dissolve. Do not use hot water. Take immediately after dissolving in water.

Actions

➤*Pharmacology:* Fosfomycin is a synthetic, broad-spectrum bactericidal antibiotic for oral administration.

Fosfomycin has in vitro activity against a broad range of gram-positive and gram-negative aerobic microorganisms which are associated with uncomplicated urinary tract infections. Fosfomycin is bactericidal in urine at therapeutic doses. The bactericidal action of fosfomycin is because of its inactivation of the enzyme enolpyruvyl transferase, thereby irreversibly blocking the condensation of uridine diphosphate-N-acetylglucosamine with p-enolpyruvate, one of the first steps in bacterial cell wall synthesis. It also reduces adherence of bacteria to uroepithelial cells.

➤*Pharmacokinetics:*

Absorption – Fosfomycin is rapidly absorbed following oral administration and converted to the free acid fosfomycin. Absolute oral bioavailability under fasting conditions is 37%. After a single 3 g dose, the mean maximum serum concentration (C_{max}) achieved was 26.1 mcg/ml within 2 hours. The oral bioavailability is reduced to 30% under fed conditions. Following a single 3 g oral dose with a high-fat meal, the mean C_{max} achieved was 17.6 mcg/ml within 4 hours.

Distribution – The mean apparent steady-state volume of distribution is 136.1 L following oral administration. It is not bound to plasma proteins.

Fosfomycin is distributed to the kidneys, bladder wall, prostate and seminal vesicles. Following a 50 mg/kg dose to patients undergoing urological surgery for bladder carcinoma, the mean concentration in the bladder, taken at a distance from the neoplastic site, was 18 mcg/g of tissue at 3 hours after dosing. Fosfomycin crosses the placental barrier.

Excretion – Fosfomycin is excreted unchanged in both urine and feces. Following oral administration, the mean total body clearance and mean renal clearance were 16.8 and 6.3 L/hr, respectively. Approximately 38% of a 3 g dose is recovered from urine and 18% is recovered from feces. Following IV administration, the mean total body clearance and mean renal clearance of fosfomycin were 6.1 L/hr and 5.5 L/hr, respectively.

A mean urine fosfomycin concentration of 706 mcg/ml was attained within 2 to 4 hours after a single oral 3 g dose under fasting conditions.

The mean urinary concentration was 10 mcg/ml in samples collected 72 to 84 hours following a single oral dose.

Following a 3 g dose administered with a high fat meal, a mean urine concentration of 537 mcg/ml was attained within 6 to 8 hours. Although the rate of urinary excretion was reduced under fed conditions, the cumulative amount of fosfomycin excreted in the urine was the same, 1118 mg (fed) vs 1140 mg (fasting). Further, urinary concentrations ≥ 100 mcg/ml were maintained for the same duration, 26 hours, indicating that fosfomycin can be taken without regard to food. Following oral administration, the mean half-life for elimination ($t_{1/2}$) is 5.7 hours.

Renal function impairment – In five patients undergoing hemodialysis, the $t_{1/2}$ of fosfomycin during hemodialysis was 40 hours. In patients with varying degrees of renal impairment (creatinine clearances varying from 54 or 7 ml/min), the $t_{1/2}$ increased from 11 hours to 50 hours. The percent of fosfomycin recovered in urine decreased from 32% to 11% indicating that renal impairment significantly decreases the excretion of fosfomycin.

➤*Microbiology:* There is generally no cross-resistance between fosfomycin and other classes of antibacterial agents such as beta-lactams and aminoglycosides.

Fosfomycin has been shown to be active against most strains of the following microorganisms, both in vitro and in clinical infections:

Aerobic gram-positive microorganisms – *Enterococcus faecalis.*

Aerobic gram-negative microorganisms – *Escherichia coli.*

Fosfomycin exhibits in vitro minimum inhibitory concentrations of ≤ 64 mcg/ml against most (≥ 90%) strains of the following microorganisms; however, the safety and effectiveness of fosfomycin in treating clinical infections caused by these microorganisms has not been established in adequate and well controlled clinical trials:

Aerobic gram-positive microorganisms – *Enterococcus faecium.*

Aerobic gram-negative microorganisms – *Citrobacter diversus; Citrobacter freundii; Enterobacter aerogenes; Klebsiella oxytoca; Klebsiella pneumoniae; Proteus mirabilis; Proteus vulgaris; Serratia marcescens.*

➤*Clinical trials:* In controlled studies of acute cystitis, a single dose of fosfomycin was compared with three other oral antibiotics. Based on differences in microbiologic eradication rates at 5 to 11 days post-therapy, fosfomycin was inferior to ciprofloxacin and trimethoprim/sulfamethoxazole and equivalent to nitrofurantoin.

Contraindications

Known hypersensitivity to the drug.

Warnings

➤*Elderly:* Based on limited data regarding 24–hour urinary drug concentrations, no differences in urinary excretion of fosfomycin have been observed in elderly subjects. No dosage adjustment is necessary in the elderly. There were no clinically significant differences in the bacteriological effectiveness or safety profiles of fosfomycin for women > 65 years of age.

➤*Pregnancy: Category B.* When administered IM as the sodium salt at a dose of 1 g to pregnant women, fosfomycin crosses the placental barrier. However, there are no adequate and well controlled studies in pregnant women. Use this drug during pregnancy only if clearly needed.

FOSFOMYCIN TROMETHAMINE

➤*Lactation:* It is not known whether fosfomycin is excreted in breast milk. Decide whether to discontinue nursing or to discontinue the drug, taking into account the importance of the drug to the mother.

➤*Children:* Safety and efficacy in children ≤ 12 years of age have not been established.

Precautions

➤*Acute cystitis:* Do not use more than one single dose of fosfomycin to treat a single episode of acute cystitis. Repeated daily doses of fosfomycin did not improve the clinical success or microbiological eradication rates compared with single dose therapy, but did increase the incidence of adverse events.

Drug Interactions

➤*Metoclopramide:* When coadministered with fosfomycin, metoclopramide lowers the serum concentration and urinary excretion of fosfomycin. Other drugs that increase GI motility may produce similar effects.

Adverse Reactions

Adverse Reactions in Fosfomycin and Comparator Populations (%)				
Adverse reaction	Fosfomycin (n = 1233)	Nitrofurantoin (n = 374)	Trimethoprim/ Sulfamethox- azole (n = 428)	Ciprofloxacin (n = 445)
Diarrhea	9	6.4	2.3	3.1
Vaginitis	5.5	5.3	4.7	6.3
Rhinitis	4.5	-	-	-
Nausea	4.1	7.2	8.6	3.4
Headache	3.9	5	5.4	3.4
Back pain	3	-	-	-
Dysmenorrhea	2.6	-	-	-
Pharyngitis	2.5	-	-	-
Abdominal pain	2.2	+	+	1.7
Rash	1.4	+	+	1.1
Dizziness	1.3	1.8	2.3	2.2
Dyspepsia	1.1	2.1	0.7	1.1

Adverse Reactions in Fosfomycin and Comparator Populations (%)				
Adverse reaction	Fosfomycin (n = 1233)	Nitrofurantoin (n = 374)	Trimethoprim/ Sulfamethox- azole (n = 428)	Ciprofloxacin (n = 445)
Asthenia	1.1	0.3	0.5	0

+ Occurs, but significance is unknown.

The following adverse events occurred in clinical trials at a rate of < 1%: Abnormal stools, anorexia, constipation, dry mouth, dysuria, ear disorder, fever, flatulence, flu syndrome, hematuria, infection, insomnia, lymphadenopathy, menstrual disorder, migraine, myalgia, nervousness, paresthesia, pruritus, ALT increased, skin disorder, somnolence, vomiting, unilateral optic neuritis (one patient).

Postmarketing experience – Angioedema, aplastic anemia, asthma (exacerbation), cholestatic jaundice, hepatic necrosis, toxic megacolon (all rare).

➤*Lab test abnormalities:* Increased eosinophil count, increased or decreased WBC count, increased bilirubin, increased ALT, increased AST, increased alkaline phosphatase, decreased hematocrit, decreased hemoglobin, increased and decreased platelet count. The changes were generally transient and were not clinically significant.

Overdosage

In acute toxicology studies, oral administration of high doses of fosfomycin up to 5 g/kg were well-tolerated in mice and rats, produced transient and minor incidences of watery stool in rabbits, and produced diarrhea with anorexia in dogs 2 to 3 days after single-dose administration. These doses represent 50 to 125 times the human therapeutic dose.

There have been no reported cases of overdosage. In the event of overdosage, treatment should be symptomatic and supportive. Refer to General Management of Acute Overdosage.

Patient Information

Fosfomycin can be taken with or without food.

Symptoms should improve in 2 to 3 days after taking fosfomycin; if not improved, the patient should contact their health care provider.

Do not take in its dry form. Always mix fosfomycin with water before ingesting.

TRIMETHOPRIM AND SULFAMETHOXAZOLE (Co-Trimoxazole; TMP-SMZ)

Rx	**Trimethoprim and Sulfamethoxazole** (Various, eg, Geneva, Goldline, Lemmon, Moore, Rugby, Schein, URL)	**Tablets:** 80 mg trimethoprim and 400 mg sulfamethoxazole	In 100s and 500s.
Rx	**Bactrim** (Roche)		(Bactrim-Roche). Lt. green, scored. Capsule shape. In 100s.
Rx	**Septra** (Monarch)		(Septra Y2B). Pink, scored. In 100s.
Rx	**Trimethoprim and Sulfamethoxazole DS** (Various, eg, Goldline, Geneva, Lemmon, Moore, Rugby, Schein, URL)	**Tablets, Double Strength:** 160 mg trimethoprim and 800 mg sulfamethoxazole	In 100s and 500s.
Rx	**Bactrim DS** (Roche)		(Bactrim-DS Roche). White. Capsule shape. In 100s, 250s and 500s.
Rx	**Septra DS** (Monarch)		(Septra DS O2C). Pink, scored. Oval. In 100s, 250s and UD 100s.
Rx	**Trimethoprim and Sulfamethoxazole** (Various, eg, Goldline, Lemmon, Moore, Rugby)	**Oral Suspension:** 40 mg trimethoprim and 200 mg sulfamethoxazole per 5 ml	In 150, 200 and 480 ml.[1]
Rx	**Cotrim Pediatric** (Lemmon)		Cherry flavor. In 473 ml.[2]
Rx	**Septra** (Monarch)		Cherry flavor in 20, 100, 150, 200 and 473 ml.[3] Grape flavor in 473 ml.[3]
Rx	**Sulfatrim** (Various, eg, URL)		In 473 ml.
Rx	**Trimethoprim and Sulfamethoxazole** (Various, eg, Sanofi)	**Injection:** 80 mg/ml sulfamethoxazole, 16 mg/ml trimethoprim per 5 ml	In 5 ml *Carpuject*.
Rx	**Bactrim IV** (Roche)	**Injection:** 80 mg trimethoprim and 400 mg sulfamethoxazole per 5 ml	In 10 and 30 ml multiple-dose vials.[4]
Rx	**Septra IV** (Monarch)		In 5 ml vials and 10 and 20 ml multiple-dose vials.[4]

[1] With 0.3% alcohol, saccharin, sorbitol, sucrose, parabens, EDTA.
[2] With ≤ 0.5% alcohol, saccharin, sorbitol.
[3] With 0.26% alcohol, 0.1% methylparaben, 0.1% sodium benzoate, saccharin, sorbitol.
[4] With 40% propylene glycol, 10% ethyl alcohol, 0.3% diethanolamine, 0.1% sodium metabisulfite and 1% benzyl alcohol.

See also individual monographs for trimethoprim and sulfonamides.

Indications

➤*Oral and parenteral:*
Urinary tract infections (UTIs) due to susceptible strains of E. coli, Klebsiella and Enterobacter species, M. morganii, P. mirabilis and P. vulgaris – Treat initial uncomplicated UTIs with a single antibacterial agent.

Parenteral therapy is indicated in severe or complicated infections when oral therapy is not feasible.

Shigellosis enteritis – Caused by susceptible strains of *S. flexneri* and *S. sonnei* in children and adults.

Pneumocystis carinii pneumonia (PCP) – Treatment of PCP in children and adults.

➤*Oral:*
Pneumocystis carinii pneumonia – Prophylaxis against PCP in individuals who are immunosuppressed and considered to be at increased risk.

Acute otitis media in children – Due to susceptible strains of *H. influenzae* or *S. pneumoniae*. There are limited data on the safety of repeated use in children < 2 years of age. Not indicated for prophylactic use or prolonged administration.

Acute exacerbations of chronic bronchitis in adults – Due to susceptible strains of *H. influenzae* and *S. pneumoniae*.

Travelers' diarrhea in adults – Due to susceptible strains of enterotoxigenic *E. coli*.

➤*Unlabeled uses:* Treatment of cholera and salmonella-type infections and nocardiosis.

TMP 40 mg and SMZ 200 mg daily at bedtime, a minimum of 3 times weekly or postcoitally has been used to prevent recurrent UTIs in females.

Low-dose TMP–SMZ has been studied in the prophylaxis of neutropenic patients with *P. carinii* infections or leukemia patients to reduce the incidence of gram-negative rod bacteremia.

Prophylaxis with TMP-SMZ (320/1600 mg/day) appears beneficial in reducing the incidence of bacterial infection (especially of the urinary tract and blood) following renal transplantation, and may provide protection against *P. carinii* pneumonia.

Treatment of acute and chronic prostatitis – 160 mg TMP/800 mg SMZ twice daily has been used for chronic bacterial prostatitis for up to 12 weeks.

Administration and Dosage

Administration and Dosage of TMP-SMZ	
Organisms/Infections	Dosage
Urinary tract infections, shigellosis and acute otitis media:	
Adults:	160 mg TMP/800 mg SMZ every 12 hours for 10 to 14 days (5 days for shigellosis).

Administration and Dosage of TMP-SMZ	
Organisms/Infections	Dosage
Children (≥ 2 months of age):	8 mg/kg TMP/40 mg/kg SMZ per day given in 2 divided doses every 12 hours for 10 days (5 days for shigellosis).

Guideline for proper dosage:

Weight (kg)	Dose every 12 hours:	
	Teaspoonfuls	Tablets
10	1 (5 ml)	-
20	2 (10 ml)	1
30	3 (15 ml)	1½
40	4 (20 ml)	2 (or 1 double strength tablet)

Patients with impaired renal function Ccr (ml/min):	Recommended dosage regimen:
> 30	Usual regimen
15-30	½ usual regimen
< 15	Not recommended
IV: Adults and children > 2 months with normal renal function for severe UTIs and shigellosis.	8 to 10 mg/kg/day (based on TMP) in 2 to 4 divided doses every 6, 8 or 12 hours for up to 14 days for severe UTIs and 5 days for shigellosis.
Travelers' diarrhea in adults:	160 mg TMP/800 mg SMZ every 12 hrs for 5 days.
Acute exacerbations of chronic bronchitis in adults:	160 mg TMP/800 mg SMZ every 12 hrs for 14 days.
Pneumocystis carinii pneumonia: Treatment:	15 to 20 mg/kg TMP/100 mg/kg SMZ per day in divided doses every 6 hours for 14 to 21 days.

Guideline for proper dosage in children

Weight (kg)	Dose every 6 hours:	
	Teaspoonfuls	Tablets
8	1 (5 ml)	-
16	2 (10 ml)	1
24	3 (15 ml)	1½
32	4 (20 ml)	2 (or 1 double strength tablet)

IV for adults and children > 2 months:	15 to 20 mg/kg/day (based on TMP) in 3 or 4 divided doses every 6 to 8 hours for up to 14 days.
Prophylaxis: Adults:	160 mg TMP/800 mg SMZ given orally every 24 hours.

TRIMETHOPRIM AND SULFAMETHOXAZOLE (Co-Trimoxazole; TMP-SMZ)

Administration and Dosage of TMP-SMZ		
Organisms/Infections	Dosage	
Children:	150 mg/m^2 TMP/ 750 mg/m^2 SMZ per day given orally in equally divided doses twice a day, on 3 consecutive days per week. The total daily dose should not exceed 320 mg TMP/1600 mg SMZ.	
Guideline for proper dosage in children	Dose every 12 hours	
Body surface area (m^2)	Teaspoonfuls	Tablets
0.26	½ (2.5 ml)	-
0.53	1 (5 ml)	½
1.06	2 (10 ml)	1

[1] Also recommended by the Public Service Task Force on Antipneumocystis Prophylaxis. CDC 1993 Sexually Transmitted Diseases Treatment Guidelines. *Morbidity and Mortality Weekly Report* 1993 Sep 24;42 (No. RR-14):1–102.

➤*Parenteral:*

IV – Administer over 60 to 90 minutes. Avoid rapid infusion or bolus injection. Do not give IM. When administered by an infusion device, thoroughly flush all lines used to remove any residual TMP-SMZ. The following infusion systems have been tested and found satisfactory: Unit-dose glass containers; unit-dose polyvinyl chloride; polyolefin containers.

Preparation of solution – Infusion must be diluted; add the contents of each 5 ml amp to 125 ml of 5% Dextrose in Water. Do not mix with other drugs or solutions. Do not refrigerate and use within 6 hours. If a dilution of 5 ml per 100 ml D5W is desired, use within 4 hours. When fluid restriction is desirable, add each 5 ml amp to 75 ml of D5W. Mix solution just prior to use and administer within 2 hours. If solution is cloudy or precipitates after mixing, discard and prepare fresh solution.

➤*Storage/Stability:* Store infusion at room temperature (15° to 30°C; 59° to 86°F). Do not refrigerate. Protect from light. After initial entry into the multi-dose vials, use the remaining contents within 48 hours.

Actions

➤*Pharmacology:* Sulfamethoxazole (SMZ) inhibits bacterial synthesis of dihydrofolic acid by competing with para-aminobenzoic acid. Trimethoprim (TMP) blocks the production of tetrahydrofolic acid by inhibiting the enzyme dihydrofolate reductase. Thus, this combination blocks two consecutive steps in the bacterial biosynthesis of essential nucleic acids and proteins. In vitro, bacterial resistance develops more slowly with this combination than with either drug alone.

➤*Pharmacokinetics:*

Absorption/Distribution – TMP-SMZ is rapidly and completely absorbed following oral administration. Peak plasma levels occur in 1 to 4 hours following oral administration and 1 to 1.5 hours after IV infusion. The 1:5 ratio of TMP to SMZ achieves an approximate 1:20 ratio of peak serum concentrations. Detectable amounts of TMP-SMZ are present in the blood 24 hours after administration. During 3 days of administration of 160 mg TMP/800 mg SMZ twice daily, the mean steady-state plasma TMP concentration was 1.72 mcg/ml. The steady-state mean plasma levels of free and total SMZ were 57.4 mcg/ml and 68 mcg/ml, respectively. Approximately 44% of TMP and 70% of SMZ are protein bound. Both distribute to sputum, vaginal fluid and middle ear fluid, pass the placental barrier, and are excreted in breast milk; TMP also distributes to bronchial secretion. Two to three times the serum concentration of TMP is achieved in prostatic fluid. Therapeutic concentrations are achieved in vaginal secretions, cerebrospinal fluid, pulmonary tissue, pleural effusion, bile, sputa and aqueous humor. It is also detectable in breast milk, amniotic fluid and fetal serum. Following oral administration, the half-lives of TMP (8 to 11 hours) and SMZ (10 to 12 hours) are similar. Following IV administration, the mean plasma half-life was 11.3 ± 0.7 hours for TMP and 12.8 ± 1.8 hours for SMZ. Patients with severely impaired renal function exhibit an increase in the half-lives of both components, requiring dosage regimen adjustment.

Metabolism/Excretion – TMP is metabolized to a relatively small extent; SMZ undergoes biotransformation to inactive compounds. The metabolism of SMZ occurs predominantly by N_4-acetylation, although the glucuronide conjugate has been identified. The principal metabolites of TMP are the 1- and 3-oxides and the 3'- and 4'-hydroxy derivatives. The free forms are the therapeutically active forms.

Excretion is chiefly by the kidneys through both glomerular filtration and tubular secretion. Urine concentrations are considerably higher than serum concentrations. Concurrent administration does not affect the excretion pattern of either drug. The average percentage of the dose recovered in urine from 0 to 72 hours after a single oral dose is 84.5% for total sulfonamide and 66.8% for free TMP. Of the total sulfonamide, 30% is excreted as free SMZ, with the remaining as N_4-acetylated metabolite.

➤*Microbiology:* The antibacterial activity of TMP-SMZ includes the common urinary tract pathogens except *Pseudomonas aeruginosa*. The following are usually susceptible: *Escherichia coli*, *Klebsiella* and *Enterobacter* sp., *Morganella morganii*, *Proteus mirabilis* and indole-positive *Proteus* sp. including *P. vulgaris*. The following pathogens isolated from middle ear exudate and bronchial secretions are usually susceptible: *Haemophilus influenzae* (including ampicillin-resistant strains), *Streptococcus pneumoniae*, *Shigella flexneri* and *S. sonnei*.

Contraindications

Hypersensitivity to trimethoprim or sulfonamides; megaloblastic anemia due to folate deficiency; pregnancy at term and lactation (see Warnings); infants < 2 months old.

The sulfonamides are chemically similar to some goitrogens, diuretics (acetazolamide and the thiazides) and oral hypoglycemic agents. Goiter production, diuresis and hypoglycemia occur rarely in patients receiving sulfonamides. Cross-sensitivity may exist with these agents.

Warnings

➤*Streptococcal pharyngitis:* Do not use to treat streptococcal pharyngitis. Patients with group A β-hemolytic streptococcal tonsillopharyngitis have a greater incidence of bacteriologic failure with this combination than with penicillin.

➤*Hematologic effects:* Sulfonamide-associated deaths, although rare, have occurred from hypersensitivity of the respiratory tract, Stevens-Johnson syndrome, toxic epidermal necrolysis, fulminant hepatic necrosis, agranulocytosis, aplastic anemia and other blood dyscrasias. Both TMP and SMZ can interfere with hematopoiesis. In elderly patients receiving diuretics (primarily thiazides), an increased incidence of thrombocytopenia with purpura occurred. Discontinue the drug at the first appearance of skin rash or any sign of adverse reaction. Rash, sore throat, fever, arthralgia, cough, shortness of breath, pallor, purpura or jaundice may be early indications of serious reactions. Obtain complete blood counts frequently. If significant reduction in the count of any formed blood element is noted, discontinue therapy.

IV use at high doses or for extended periods of time may cause bone marrow depression manifested as thrombocytopenia, leukopenia or megaloblastic anemia. If signs of bone marrow depression occur, give leucovorin as needed to restore normal hematopoiesis. Oral leucovorin, 5 to 15 mg/day has been recommended.

➤*Pneumocystis carinii pneumonitis in patients with AIDS:* Because of their unique immune dysfunction, AIDS patients may not tolerate or respond to TMP-SMZ. The incidence of side effects, particularly rash, fever, leukopenia, elevated aminotransferase values, hyperkalemia and hyponatremia in these patients is greatly increased compared with non-AIDS patients.

Adverse effects are generally less severe in patients receiving TMP-SMZ for prophylaxis. A history of mild intolerance to TMP-SMZ in AIDS patients does not appear to predict intolerance of subsequent secondary prophylaxis. However, if a patient develops skin rash or any sign of adverse reaction, re-evaluate therapy.

➤*Renal/Hepatic function impairment:* Use with caution. Maintain adequate fluid intake to prevent crystalluria and stone formation. Perform urinalyses and renal function tests during therapy, particularly in impaired renal function.

➤*Elderly:* There may be an increased risk of severe adverse reactions, particularly when complicating conditions exist (eg, impaired kidney or liver function, concomitant use of other drugs). Severe skin reactions, generalized bone marrow suppression or a decrease in platelets (with or without purpura) are the most frequently reported severe adverse reactions. In those concurrently receiving certain diuretics, primarily thiazides, an increased incidence of thrombocytopenia with purpura has occurred. Make appropriate dosage adjustments for impaired kidney function.

➤*Pregnancy: Category C.* Do not use at term. Sulfonamides readily cross the placenta. Fetal levels average 70% to 90% of maternal levels. Toxicities observed in the neonate include jaundice, hemolytic anemia and kernicterus. Trimethoprim crosses the placenta, producing similar levels in fetal and maternal serum. There are no large, well controlled studies; however, in one study of 186 pregnancies where the mother received either placebo or oral TMP-SMZ, the incidence of congenital abnormalities was 4.5% (3 of 66) in those who received placebo and 3.3% (4 of 120) in those receiving TMP-SMZ. There were no abnormalities in 10 children whose mothers received the drug during the first trimester or in 35 children whose mothers had taken the drug at conception or shortly thereafter.

Because TMP-SMZ may interfere with folic acid metabolism, use during pregnancy only if the potential benefits outweigh the potential hazards to the fetus.

➤*Lactation:* TMP-SMZ is not recommended in the nursing period because sulfonamides are excreted in breast milk and may cause kernicterus. Premature infants and infants with hyperbilirubinemia or G-6-PD deficiency are also at risk for adverse effects.

➤*Children:* Not recommended for infants < 2 months old. See Indications.

TRIMETHOPRIM AND SULFAMETHOXAZOLE (Co-Trimoxazole; TMP-SMZ)

Precautions

➤*Extravascular infiltration:* If local irritation and inflammation due to extravascular infiltration of the infusion occurs, discontinue the infusion and restart at another site.

➤*Benzyl alcohol:* This is contained in some of these products as a preservative and has been associated with a fatal "gasping syndrome" in premature infants.

➤*Special risk:* Use with caution in patients with possible folate deficiency (eg, elderly patients, chronic alcoholics, anticonvulsant therapy, malabsorption syndrome, patients in malnutrition states), severe allergy or bronchial asthma. In G-6-PD deficient individuals, hemolysis may occur; it is frequently dose-related.

➤*Superinfection:* Use of antibiotics (especially prolonged or repeated therapy) may result in bacterial or fungal overgrowth of nonsusceptible organisms. Such overgrowth may lead to a secondary infection. Take appropriate measures if this occurs.

➤*Sulfite sensitivity:* Sulfites may cause allergic-type reactions (eg, hives, itching, wheezing, anaphylaxis) in susceptible persons. Although the prevalence of sulfite sensitivity in the general population is probably low, it is more frequent in asthmatics or atopic nonasthmatic persons. Products containing sulfites are identified in the product listings.

Drug Interactions

TMP-SMZ Drug Interactions			
Precipitant drug	Object drug*		Description
TMP-SMZ	Anticoagulants	↑	The prothrombin time of warfarin may be prolonged. Monitor coagulation tests and adjust dosage as required.
TMP-SMZ	Cyclosporine	↓	A decrease in the therapeutic effect of cyclosporine and an increased risk of nephrotoxicity have occurred.
TMP-SMZ	Dapsone	↑	Increased serum levels of both dapsone and TMP may occur.
Dapsone	TMP-SMZ	↑	
TMP-SMZ	Diuretics	↑	In elderly patients, concomitant use has increased incidence of thrombocytopenia with purpura.
TMP-SMZ	Hydantoins	↑	Phenytoin's hepatic clearance may be decreased and the half-life prolonged.
TMP-SMZ	Methotrexate	↑	Sulfonamides can displace methotrexate (MTX) from plasma protein binding sites, thus increasing free MTX concentrations; bone marrow depressant effects may be potentiated.
TMP-SMZ	Sulfonylureas	↑	The hypoglycemic response may be increased.
TMP-SMZ	Zidovudine	↑	The serum levels of zidovudine may be increased due to a decreased renal clearance.

* ↑ = Object drug increased. ↓ = Object drug decreased.

➤*Drug/Lab test interactions:* Trimethoprim can interfere with a serum methotrexate assay as determined by the competitive binding protein technique (CBPA) when a bacterial dihydrofolate reductase is used as the binding protein. No interference occurs if methotrexate is measured by a radioimmunoassay.

TMP-SMZ may interfere with the Jaffe alkaline picrate reaction assay for creatinine, resulting in overestimations of about 10% in the range of normal values.

Adverse Reactions

➤*Parenteral therapy:* Local reaction, pain and slight irritation on IV administration (infrequent); thrombophlebitis (rare).

➤*Most common:* GI disturbances (nausea, vomiting, anorexia); allergic skin reactions (eg, rash, urticaria).

➤*CNS:* Headache; mental depression; convulsions; ataxia; hallucinations; tinnitus; vertigo; insomnia; apathy; fatigue; weakness; nervousness; aseptic meningitis; peripheral neuritis.

➤*GI:* Glossitis; anorexia; stomatitis; nausea; emesis; abdominal pain; diarrhea; pseudomembranous enterocolitis; hepatitis (including cholestatic jaundice and hepatic necrosis); pancreatitis; elevation of serum transaminase and bilirubin.

➤*GU:* Renal failure; interstitial nephritis; BUN and serum creatinine elevation; toxic nephrosis with oliguria and anuria; crystalluria.

➤*Hematologic:* Agranulocytosis; aplastic, hemolytic or megaloblastic anemia; thrombocytopenia; leukopenia; neutropenia; hypoprothrombinemia; eosinophilia; methemoglobinemia; hyperkalemia; hyponatremia.

➤*Hypersensitivity:* Erythema multiforme; Stevens-Johnson syndrome; generalized skin eruptions; rash; toxic epidermal necrolysis; urticaria; serum sickness-like syndrome; pruritus; exfoliative dermatitis; anaphylactoid reactions; conjunctival and scleral injection; photosensitization; allergic myocarditis; angioedema; drug fever; chills; Henoch-Schoenlein purpura; systemic lupus erythematosus; generalized allergic reactions; periarteritis nodosa.

➤*Musculoskeletal:* Arthralgia; myalgia.

➤*Respiratory:* Pulmonary infiltrates.

Overdosage

➤*Symptoms:*

Acute – Signs and symptoms observed with either TMP or SMZ alone include: Anorexia; colic; nausea; vomiting; dizziness; headache; drowsiness; unconsciousness; pyrexia; hematuria; crystalluria; depression; confusion; blood dyscrasias and jaundice (late manifestations).

Chronic – High doses or use for extended periods may cause bone marrow depression manifested as thrombocytopenia, leukopenia or megaloblastic anemia. Give leucovorin; 5 to 15 mg/day has been recommended.

➤*Treatment:* Treatment includes usual supportive measures. Refer to General Management of Acute Overdosage. Perform gastric lavage or emesis, force oral fluids and administer IV fluids if urine output is low and renal function is normal. Acidifying urine will increase renal elimination of TMP. Monitor patient with blood counts and appropriate blood chemistries, including electrolytes. If significant blood dyscrasia or jaundice occurs, institute specific therapy for these complications. Peritoneal dialysis is not effective and hemodialysis is only moderately effective in eliminating TMP and SMZ.

Patient Information

Complete full course of therapy. Take each oral dose with a full glass of water.

Maintain adequate fluid intake.

Notify physician immediately if sore throat, fever, chills, pale skin, yellowing of skin or eyes, rash or unusual bleeding or bruising occurs.

ERYTHROMYCIN ETHYLSUCCINATE AND SULFISOXAZOLE

Rx	**Erythromycin and Sulfisoxazole** (Various, eg, Barr, Goldline, Harber, Lederle, Moore, Rugby, URL)	**Granules for Oral Suspension:** Erythromycin ethylsuccinate (equivalent to 200 mg erythromycin activity) and sulfisoxazole acetyl (equivalent to 600 mg sulfisoxazole) per 5 ml when reconstituted	In 100, 150 and 200 ml.
Rx	**Eryzole** (Alra)		Sucrose. Strawberry flavor. In 100, 150 and 200 ml.
Rx	**Pediazole** (Ross)		Sucrose. Strawberry-banana flavor. In 100, 150, 200 and 250 ml.

For complete information on each of the components, refer to Erythromycin and Sulfisoxazole individual monographs.

Indications

➤*Children:* Acute otitis media caused by susceptible strains of *Haemophilus influenzae*.

Administration and Dosage

Do not administer to infants < 2 months old; systemic sulfonamides are contraindicated in this age group.

➤*Acute otitis media:* 50 mg/kg/day erythromycin and 150 mg/kg/day (to a maximum of 6 g/day), sulfisoxazole. Give in equally divided doses 4 times daily for 10 days. Administer without regard to meals. The following dosage schedule is recommended:

Erythromycin/Sulfisoxazole Dosage Based on Weight		
Weight		Dose (every 6 hours)
kg	lb	
< 8	< 18	Adjust dosage by body weight
8	18	2.5 ml
16	35	5 ml
24	53	7.5 ml
> 45	> 100	10 ml

FLUCYTOSINE (5-FC; 5-Fluorocytosine)

Rx	Ancobon (ICN)	**Capsules:** 250 mg	Talc, lactose, and parabens. (Ancobon 250 ICN). Green and gray. In 100s.
		500 mg	Talc, lactose, and parabens. (Ancobon 500 ICN). White and gray. In 100s.

WARNING

Use with extreme caution in patients with renal impairment. Close monitoring of hematologic, renal, and hepatic status of all patients is essential.

Indications

For treatment of serious infections caused by susceptible strains of *Candida* or *Cryptococcus*.

With the exception of urinary tract infection (UTI), use flucytosine in combination with amphotericin B for the treatment of systemic candidiasis and cryptococcosis because of rapid emergence of resistance to flucytosine in *Candida* and *Cryptococcus* isolates in patients receiving flucytosine alone.

➤*Candida:* Septicemia, endocarditis, and UTIs have been effectively treated. Limited trials in pulmonary infections justify the use of flucytosine.

➤*Cryptococcus:* For the treatment of meningitis and pulmonary infections. Good responses in septicemias and UTIs have occurred although studies are limited.

Administration and Dosage

The usual dosage is 50 to 150 mg/kg/day in divided doses at 6-hour intervals. To reduce or avoid nausea or vomiting, take capsules a few at a time over a 15-minute period. Use a lower initial dose if BUN or serum creatinine is elevated, or if there are other signs of renal impairment (see Warnings).

➤*Storage/Stability:* Store at 25°C (77°F); excursions permitted to 15° to 30°C (59° to 86°F).

Actions

➤*Pharmacology:* Flucytosine has in vitro and in vivo activity against *Candida* and *Cryptococcus*. Although the exact mechanism is unknown, it has been reported that flucytosine acts directly on fungal organisms by competitive inhibition of purine and pyrimidine uptake and indirectly by intracellular metabolism to 5-fluorouracil. The 5-fluorouracil is extensively incorporated into fungal RNA and inhibits synthesis of DNA and RNA. The result is unbalanced growth and death of the fungal organism. It is rarely used alone; generally, it is used in combination with amphotericin B for synergistic antifungal activity (see Drug Interactions).

➤*Pharmacokinetics:*

Absorption/Distribution – Flucytosine is well absorbed after oral use with peak blood levels of 30 to 40 mcg/mL reached within 2 hours. After 5 days of continuous therapy, median peak levels in infants were 19.6, 27.7, and 83.9 mcg/mL at doses of 25, 50, and 100 mg/kg, respectively. Mean time to peak serum levels were approximately 2.5 hours, similar to that observed in adult patients. It is well distributed into aqueous humor and other body fluids and tissues; CSF concentrations are approximately 65% to 90% of serum levels. Bioavailability is 78% to 89%. Plasma protein binding is minimal. Toxicity occurs at blood levels higher than 100 mcg/mL.

Metabolism/Excretion – More than 90% of the dose is excreted unchanged in the urine by glomerular filtration; a small portion is found unchanged in the feces. Serum half-life is 2.4 and 4.8 hours in patients with normal renal function; half-life increases significantly, up to an average of 85 hours, in patients with renal failure. The median half-life observed in infants was 7.4 hours, approximately double that seen in adults. The drug is removed rapidly by hemodialysis.

Fungal resistance –

Cryptococcus: Any isolate with an MIC greater than 12.5 mcg/mL is considered resistant. In vitro resistance has developed in originally susceptible strains during therapy. It is recommended that clinical cultures for susceptibility testing be taken initially and at weekly intervals during therapy. Reserve the initial culture as a reference in susceptibility testing of subsequent isolates.

Candida: As high as 40% to 50% of the pretreatment clinical isolates of *Candida* have been reported to be resistant to flucytosine. It is recommended that susceptibility studies be performed as early as possible and be repeated during therapy. An MIC value greater than 100 mcg/mL is considered resistant.

Contraindications

Hypersensitivity to flucytosine.

Warnings

➤*Bone marrow depression:* Give with extreme caution to patients with bone marrow depression. Patients may be more prone to bone marrow depression if they have a hematologic disease, are being treated with radiation or marrow-suppressant drugs, or have a history of treatment with such drugs or radiation. Bone marrow toxicity can be irreversible and may lead to death in immunosuppressed patients. Frequently monitor hepatic function and the hematopoietic system during therapy.

➤*Renal function impairment:* Give with extreme caution; drug accumulation may occur. Monitor blood levels to determine the adequacy of renal excretion in such patients. Adjust dosage to prevent progressive accumulation of the drug and to maintain the blood levels at less than 100 mcg/mL.

➤*Pregnancy:* Category C. Flucytosine is teratogenic in rats at 40 mg/kg/day. At higher doses (700 mg/kg/day) cleft lip and palate and micrognathia were reported. There are no adequate and well-controlled studies in pregnant women. Use only if the potential benefit justifies the potential risk to the fetus.

➤*Lactation:* It is not known whether this drug is excreted in breast milk. Because of potential serious adverse reactions in nursing infants, decide whether to discontinue nursing or the drug, taking into account the importance of the drug to mother.

➤*Children:* Safety and efficacy in children have not been established. Hypokalemia and acidemia were reported in one patient who received flucytosine in combination with amphotericin B, and anemia was observed in a second patient who received flucytosine alone. Transient thrombocytopenia was noted in 2 additional patients, one of whom also received amphotericin B.

Precautions

➤*Monitoring:* Before therapy is initiated, determine electrolytes and hematological and renal status of the patient (see Warnings). Because renal impairment can cause accumulation of the drug, monitor blood concentrations and renal function during therapy. Monitor hematologic status (WBC and platelet count) and liver function (alkaline phosphatase, ALT, and AST) at frequent intervals during treatment.

➤*Photosensitivity:* Photosensitization (photoallergy or phototoxicity) may occur; therefore, caution patients to take protective measures (ie, sunscreens, protective clothing) against exposure to sunlight or ultraviolet light (eg, tanning beds) until tolerance is determined.

Drug Interactions

Drugs that impair glomerular filtration may prolong the half-life of flucytosine.

➤*Amphotericin B:* Amphotericin B may increase the therapeutic action and toxicity of flucytosine.

➤*Cytosine:* Cytosine may inactivate the antifungal activity of flucytosine.

➤*Drug/Lab test interactions:* Determine measurement of serum creatinine levels by the Jaffe reaction, because flucytosine does not interfere with the determination of creatinine values by this method.

Adverse Reactions

➤*Cardiovascular:* Cardiac arrest; myocardial toxicity; ventricular dysfunction.

➤*CNS:* Ataxia; confusion; convulsions; fatigue; hallucinations; headache; hearing loss; paresthesia; parkinsonism; peripheral neuropathy; psychosis; pyrexia; sedation; vertigo; weakness.

➤*Dermatologic:* Photosensitivity; pruritus; rash; urticaria.

➤*GI:* Abdominal pain; anorexia; bilirubin elevation; diarrhea; dry mouth; duodenal ulcer; emesis; GI hemorrhage; hepatic dysfunction; elevation of hepatic enzymes; acute hepatic injury with possible fatal outcome in debilitated patients; jaundice; nausea; ulcerative colitis.

➤*GU:* Azotemia; creatinine and BUN elevation; crystalluria; renal failure.

FLUCYTOSINE (5-FC; 5-Fluorocytosine)

➤*Hematologic:* Agranulocytosis; aplastic anemia; anemia; eosinophilia; leukopenia; pancytopenia; thrombocytopenia.

➤*Respiratory:* Chest pain; dyspnea; respiratory arrest.

➤*Miscellaneous:* Allergic reactions; hypoglycemia; hypokalemia; Lyell syndrome.

Overdosage

➤*Symptoms:* There is no experience with intentional overdosage. It is reasonable to expect pronounced manifestations of known clinical adverse reactions. Prolonged serum concentration in excess of 100 mcg/mL may be associated with an increased incidence of toxicity, especially GI (diarrhea, nausea, vomiting), hematologic (leukopenia, thrombocytopenia), and hepatic (hepatitis).

➤*Treatment:* Prompt gastric lavage or emetic use is recommended. Maintain adequate fluid intake by IV route if necessary, because flucytosine is excreted unchanged in the renal tract. Hemodialysis rapidly reduced serum concentrations in anuric patients. Monitor hematologic parameters frequently, and monitor liver and kidney function. If any abnormalities appear in any of these parameters, institute appropriate therapeutic measures. Refer to General Management of Acute Overdosage.

Patient Information

May cause GI upset (eg, nausea, vomiting, diarrhea). Inform patient that this can be reduced or avoided by taking capsules a few at a time over a 15-minute period. Instruct patient to notify physician if effects become intolerable.

Inform patients that lab tests will be required while taking this medication and to be sure to keep appointments.

Advise patients that this drug may cause photosensitivity (sensitivity to sunlight). Advise them to avoid prolonged exposure to the sun and other ultraviolet light (eg, tanning beds) and to use sunscreens and wear protective clothing until tolerance is determined.

Indications

➤*Ringworm infections:* Treatment of ringworm infections of the skin, hair, and nails, namely the folowing: Tinea corporis, tinea pedis, tinea cruris, tinea barbae, tinea capitis, tinea unguium (onychomycosis) when caused by ≥ 1 of the following fungi: *Trichophyton rubrum, T. tonsurans, T. mentagrophytes, T. interdigitalis, T. verrucosum, T. megninii, T. gallinae, T. crateriform, T. sulphureum, T. schoenleinii, Microsporum audouinii, M. canis, M. gypseum,* and *Epidermophyton floccosum.*

➤*Note:* Prior to therapy, identify the types of fungi responsible for the infection. Use of this drug is not justified in minor or trivial infections that will respond to topical agents alone.

Griseofulvin is NOT effective in bacterial infections; candidiasis (moniliasis); histoplasmosis; actinomycosis; sporotrichosis; chromoblastomycosis; coccidioidomycosis; North American blastomycosis; cryptococcosis (torulosis); tinea versicolor; nocardiosis.

Administration and Dosage

Accurate diagnosis of the infecting organism is essential.

➤*Duration of therapy:* Continue medication until the infecting organism is completely eradicated, as indicated by appropriate clinical or laboratory examination. Representative treatment periods are as follows: Tinea capitis, 4 to 6 weeks; tinea corporis, 2 to 4 weeks; tinea pedis, 4 to 8 weeks; tinea unguium (depending on rate of growth) – fingernails, ≥ 4 months; toenails, ≥ 6 months.

➤*Hygiene:* Observe good hygiene to control sources of infection or reinfection. Concomitant use of appropriate topical agents is usually required, particularly in treatment of tinea pedis. In some forms of athlete's foot, yeasts and bacteria may be involved, as well as fungi. Griseofulvin will not eradicate the bacterial or monilial infection.

➤*Adults:*

Tinea corporis, tinea cruris, tinea capitis – A single or divided daily dose of 330 to 375 mg ultramicrosize will give a satisfactory response in most patients.

Tinea pedis, tinea unguium – 660 to 750 mg ultramicrosize per day in divided doses.

➤*Children:* Approximately 7.3 mg ultramicrosize/kg/day (3.3 mg/lb/day) is an effective dose for most children. The following dosage schedule is suggested:

Griseofulvin Dosage for Children Based on Weight		
Weight		Daily dose (mg)
lb	kg	ultramicrosize
30 to 50	13.6 to 22.6	82.5 to 165
> 50	> 22.6	165 to 330

Clinical experience indicates that a single daily dose is effective in children with tinea capitis.

Children (≤ 2 years of age) – Dosage not established.

➤*Storage/Stability:*

Tablets – Store between 2° and 30°C (36° and 86°F).

Capsules – Store at room temperature, ≈ 25°C (77°F). Dispense in a well-closed container.

Oral suspension – Store at room temperature in a tight, light-resistant container.

Actions

➤*Pharmacology:* Griseofulvin, an antibiotic derived from a species of *Penicillium,* is deposited in the keratin precursor cells, which are gradually exfoliated and replaced by noninfected tissue; it has a greater affinity for diseased tissue. The drug is tightly bound to the new keratin, which becomes highly resistant to fungal invasions.

➤*Pharmacokinetics:* The peak serum level found in fasting adults given 0.5 g griseofulvin microsize occurred at ≈ 4 hours and ranged between 0.5 to 1.5 mcg/ml. Some individuals are consistently "poor absorbers" and tend to attain lower blood levels at all times. The serum level may be increased by giving the drug with a high-fat meal. GI absorption varies considerably among individuals because of insolubility of the drug in aqueous media of the upper GI tract. The efficiency of GI absorption of the ultramicrocrystalline formulation is ≈ 1.5 times that of conventional microsized griseofulvin. This factor permits the oral intake of ⅔ as much ultramicrocrystalline griseofulvin as the microsized form; however, there is no evidence this confers any significant clinical differences in regard to safety and efficacy.

➤*Microbiology:* Griseofulvin is fungistatic with in vitro activity against species of *Microsporum, Epidermophyton,* and *Trichophyton.* It has no effect on bacteria or other fungi.

Contraindications

Hypersensitivity to griseofulvin; porphyria; hepatocellular failure.

Warnings

➤*Prophylaxis:* Safety and efficacy for prophylaxis of fungal infections have not been established.

➤*Hypersensitivity reactions:* Hypersensitivity reactions (eg, skin rashes, urticaria, angioneurotic edema, erythema multiforme-like reactions) may occur and necessitate withdrawal of therapy. Institute appropriate countermeasures; refer to Management of Acute Hypersensitivity Reactions.

➤*Carcinogenesis:* Chronic feeding of griseofulvin to mice at levels ranging from 0.5% to 2.5% of the diet resulted in the development of liver tumors. Smaller particle sizes resulted in an enhanced effect. Thyroid tumors developed in male rats receiving griseofulvin at levels of 2%, 1%, and 0.2% of the diet.

In subacute toxicity studies, griseofulvin produced hepatocellular necrosis in mice, but not in other species. Griseofulvin produced disturbances in porphyrin metabolism, a colchicine-like effect on mitosis and cocarcinogenicity with methylcholanthrene in cutaneous tumor induction in laboratory animals.

➤*Fertility impairment:* Because griseofulvin has demonstrated harmful effects in vitro on the genotype bacteria, plants, and fungi, males should wait ≥ 6 months after completing therapy before fathering a child. Females should avoid risk of pregnancy while receiving griseofulvin.

➤*Pregnancy:* Category C. Griseofulvin was embryotoxic and teratogenic in rats. Rare cases of conjoined twins have been reported in patients taking griseofulvin during the first trimester of pregnancy. Do not give to pregnant women or women contemplating pregnancy.

Precautions

➤*Prolonged therapy:* Closely observe patients on prolonged therapy. Periodically monitor renal, hepatic, and hematopoietic function.

➤*Penicillin cross-sensitivity:* This is possible because griseofulvin is derived from species of *Penicillium;* however, known penicillin-sensitive patients have been treated without difficulty.

➤*Lupus erythematosus:* Lupus-like syndromes or exacerbation of lupus erythematosus have occurred in patients receiving griseofulvin.

➤*Photosensitivity:* Caution patients to take protective measures (eg, sunscreens, protective clothing) against exposure to ultraviolet light or sunlight.

Photosensitivity reactions may aggravate lupus erythematosus.

Drug Interactions

Griseofulvin Drug Interactions			
Precipitant drug	Object drug*		Description
Griseofulvin	Anticoagulants	↓	Griseofulvin may decrease the hypoprothrombinemic activity of warfarin; patients may require anticoagulant dosage adjustment.
Griseofulvin	Contraceptives, oral	↓	Loss of contraceptive effectiveness may occur, possibly leading to breakthrough bleeding, amenorrhea, or unintended pregnancy.
Griseofulvin	Cyclosporine	↓	Cyclosporine levels may be reduced, resulting in a decrease in pharmacologic effects.
Griseofulvin	Salicylates	↓	Serum salicylate concentrations may be decreased.
Barbiturates	Griseofulvin	↓	Serum griseofulvin levels may be decreased.

* ↓ = Object drug decreased.

Adverse Reactions

➤*Most common:* Hypersensitivity reactions such as skin rashes and urticaria (see Warnings).

➤*Occasional:* Oral thrush; nausea; vomiting; epigastric distress; diarrhea; headache; fatigue; dizziness; insomnia; mental confusion; impairment of performance of routine activities.

➤*Rare:* Angioneurotic edema and erythema multiforme-like drug reactions may occur.

Griseofulvin interferes with porphyrin metabolism. Proteinuria; nephrosis; leukopenia; hepatic toxicity; GI bleeding; menstrual irregularities; paresthesias of the hands and feet after extended therapy have occurred. Discontinue administration if granulocytopenia occurs.

Rarely, serious reactions occur with griseofulvin. They are usually associated with high dosages, long periods of therapy, or both.

Patient Information

Beneficial effects may not be noticeable for some time; continue taking medication for entire course of therapy.

Photosensitivity reactions may occur; avoid prolonged exposure to sunlight or sunlamps.

Notify physician if fever, sore throat, or skin rash occurs.

Griseofulvin

GRISEOFULVIN MICROSIZE

Rx	**Fulvicin U/F** (Schering-Plough)	**Tablets:** 250 mg	(948). White, scored. In 60s and 250s.
Rx	**Fulvicin U/F** (Schering-Plough)	**Tablets:** 500 mg	(496). White, scored. In 60s and 250s.

For complete prescribing information refer to the griseofulvin group monograph.

GRISEOFULVIN ULTRAMICROSIZE

Rx	**Gris-PEG** (Pedinol)	**Tablets:** 125 mg	Lactose, parabens. (Gris-PEG 125). White, elliptical, scored. Film-coated. In 100s.
		250 mg	Parabens. (Gris-PEG 250). White, capsule shape, scored. Film-coated. In 100s and 500s.

For complete prescribing information refer to the griseofulvin group monograph.

Administration and Dosage

The efficiency of GI absorption of griseofulvin ultramicrosize is ≈ 1.5 times that of conventional microsized griseofulvin. This factor permits the oral intake of ⅔ as much ultramicrosize as the microsize form, but there is no evidence that this confers any significant clinical difference in regard to safety and efficacy.

AMPHOTERICIN B DESOXYCHOLATE

Rx	Amphotericin B (Pharma-Tek)	**Powder for Injection:** 50 mg (as desoxycholate)	In vials.
Rx	Amphocin (Gensia Sicor)		In vials.
Rx	Fungizone Intravenous (Apothecon)		In vials.

Indications

➤*Fungal infections, systemic:* Intended to treat the following potentially life-threatening invasive fungal infections: Aspergillosis; cryptococcosis (torulosis); North American blastomycosis; systemic candidiasis; coccidioidomycosis; histoplasmosis; zygomycosis including mucormycosis caused by susceptible species of *Mucor, Rhizopus,* and *Absidia* sp.; infections caused by related susceptible species of *Conidiobolus* and *Basidiobolus;* sporotrichosis.

➤*Leishmaniasis:* For treatment of American mucocutaneous leishmaniasis but not as primary therapy.

➤*Unlabeled uses:* Prophylaxis of fungal infection in patients with bone marrow transplantation (0.1 mg/kg/day); for the treatment of primary amoebic meningoencephalitis caused by *Naegleria fowleri;* subconjunctival or intravitreal injection in ocular aspergillosis; as a bladder irrigation for candidal cystitis; as chemoprophylaxis by low-dose IV, intranasal, or nebulized administration in immunocompromised patients at risk of aspergillosis; intrathecally for patients with severe meningitis unresponsive to IV therapy; intra-articularly or IM for coccidioidal arthritis.

Administration and Dosage

Individualize and adjust dosage based on patient's clinical status (eg, cardiorenal function, reaction to test dose, site, and severity of infection). If administered through an existing IV line, flush with 5% Dextrose for Injection prior to and following infusion; otherwise administer via a separate line.

➤*Fungal infection, systemic:*

Suggested Indication-Specific Dosage Regimens for Amphotericin B Desoxycholate		
Fungal infection, systemic	Treatment regimen	Dose[1] (mg/kg/day)
Aspergillosis	up to 3.6 g total dose	1 to 1.5
Blastomycosis	4 to 12 weeks	0.5 to 0.6
Candidiasis	4 to 12 weeks	0.5 to 1
Coccidioidomycosis	4 to 12 weeks	0.5 to 1
Cryptococcosis	4 to 12 weeks	0.5 to 0.7
Histoplasmosis	4 to 12 weeks	0.5 to 0.6
Mucormycosis	4 to 12 weeks	1 to 1.5
Rhinocerebral phycomycosis	3 to 4 g total dose	0.25 to 0.3 up to 1 to 1.5
Sporotrichosis	up to 2.5 g total dose	0.5

[1] Some of these dosages are not FDA-approved.

Because patient tolerance varies greatly, a test dose may be preferred: 1 mg in 20 ml of 5% Dextrose delivered IV over 20 to 30 minutes. Record patient's temperature, pulse, respiration, and blood pressure every 30 minutes for 2 to 4 hours.

The recommended initial dose is 0.25 to 0.3 mg/kg/day prepared as 0.1 mg/ml infusion and delivered slowly over 2 to 6 hours. Depending on the patient's cardiorenal status, dosage may be gradually increased by 5 to 10 mg/day up to a total dose of 0.5 to 0.7 mg/kg/day. Some mycoses may require total doses up to 1 to 1.5 mg/kg/day. Do not exceed a total daily dose of 1.5 mg/kg; overdoses can result in cardiorespiratory arrest. Alternate daily dosing is recommended for total daily doses of 1.5 mg/kg. In patients with impaired cardiorenal function or a severe reaction to the test dose, initiate therapy with smaller daily doses (eg, 5 to 10 mg). An in-line membrane filter of ≥ 1 micron mean pore diameter may be used.

➤*Leishmaniasis:* 0.5 mg/kg/day administered on alternate days for 14 doses has been effective but is not recommended as primary therapy.

➤*Rhinocerebral phycomycosis:* A cumulative dose of ≥ 3 g amphotericin B is recommended. Although a total dose of 3 to 4 g will infrequently cause lasting renal impairment, it is a reasonable minimum where there is clinical evidence of deep tissue invasion. Rhinocerebral phycomycosis usually follows a rapidly fatal course; therapy must be more aggressive than that for more indolent mycoses.

➤*Unlabeled:*

Cystitis, candidal – Irrigate bladder with a 50 mcg/ml solution, instilled periodically or continuously for 5 to 10 days.

Meningitis, coccidioidal or cryptococcal – Administer intrathecally at initial doses of 0.025 mg, gradually increased to the maximum tolerable dose. The usual dose is 0.25 to 1 mg every 2 to 5 days.

Paracoccidioidomycosis – Administer 0.4 to 0.5 mg/kg/day slow IV infusion; treat for 4 to 12 weeks.

➤*Preparation of infusion solutions:* Do not dilute or reconstitute with saline solutions or mix with other drugs or electrolytes. The use of any solution other than those recommended or the presence of a bacteriostatic agent (eg, benzyl alcohol) may cause precipitation of amphotericin B.

For initial concentration of 5 mg/ml, rapidly inject 10 ml Sterile Water for Injection without a bacteriostatic agent directly into the lyophilized cake, using a sterile needle (minimum diameter: 20-gauge). Shake the vial immediately until the colloidal solution is clear. The infusion solution, providing 0.1 mg/ml, is then obtained by further dilution (1:50) with 5% Dextrose for Injection of pH above 4.2.

Ascertain the pH of each container of Dextrose for Injection before use. Commercial Dextrose Injection usually has a pH > 4.2; however, if it is < 4.2, add 1 or 2 ml of buffer to the Dextrose Injection before it is infused to dilute the concentrated solution of amphotericin B. The recommended buffer has the following composition: Dibasic sodium phosphate (anhydrous) 1.59 g; monobasic sodium phosphate (anhydrous) 0.96 g with Water for Injection, dilute to 100 ml.

Sterilize the buffer before adding to the Dextrose Injection, either by filtration through a bacterial retentive stone, mat, or membrane or by autoclaving for 30 minutes at 15 lb pressure and 121°C (249.8°F).

➤*Storage / Stability:* Refrigerate vials; protect against light. Store the concentrate (after reconstitution) in the dark at room temperature for 24 hours or refrigerate for 1 week with minimal loss of potency and clarity. Discard any unused material. Use solutions prepared for IV infusions promptly; protect solution from light during administration.

Actions

➤*Pharmacology:* Amphotericin B is a polyene antibiotic produced by a strain of *Streptomyces nodosus* that is fungistatic or fungicidal, depending on the concentration obtained in body fluids and on the susceptibility of the fungus. It acts by binding to sterols (primarily ergosterol) in the fungal cell membrane with a resultant change in membrane permeability, allowing leakage of a variety of intracellular components. It can also bind to the cholesterol component of the mammalian cell leading to cytotoxicity.

➤*Pharmacokinetics:* An initial IV infusion of 1 to 5 mg/day, gradually increased to 0.4 to 0.6 mg/kg/day, produces peak plasma concentrations of ≈ 0.5 to 2 mcg/ml. Amphotericin B is highly protein bound (> 90%) and is poorly dialyzable. Approximately 66% of concurrent plasma concentrations have been detected in fluids from inflamed pleura, peritoneum, synovium, and aqueous humor; concentrations in the CSF seldom exceed 2.5% of those in the plasma; little amphotericin B penetrates into vitreous humor or normal amniotic fluid. Complete details of tissue distribution are not known.

Metabolic pathways of amphotericin B are not known. It has a relatively short initial serum half-life of 24 hours, followed by a second elimination phase with a half-life of ≈ 15 days. The drug is slowly excreted by the kidneys with 2% to 5% as the biologically active form. After treatment is discontinued, amphotericin B can be detected in the urine for ≥ 7 weeks. The cumulative urinary output over 7 days amounts to ≈ 40% of the infused drug.

Children – In a small study of 12 children 4 months to 14 years of age infused with 0.25 to 1.5 mg/kg/day of amphotericin B, plasma levels ranged from 0.78 to 10.02 mcg/ml and were independent of dose. The mean elimination half-life was 18.1 hours. An inverse relationship between age and total clearance was observed indicating that children > 9 years of age may require lower doses.

➤*Microbiology:*

Amphotericin B desoxycholate – Amphotericin B desoxycholate is active in vitro against many species of fungi. *Histoplasma capsulatum, Coccidioides immitis, Candida* sp., *Blastomyces dermatitidis, Rhodotorula* sp., *Cryptococcus neoformans, Sporothrix schenckii, Mucor mucedo,* and *Aspergillus fumigatus* are inhibited by concentrations ranging from 0.03 to 1 mcg/ml in vitro. It has no effect on bacteria, rickettsiae, and viruses.

Contraindications

Hypersensitivity to amphotericin B or any other component of the formulation unless the condition requiring treatment is life-threatening and amenable only to amphotericin B therapy.

Warnings

➤*Fatal fungal diseases:* Amphotericin B is frequently the only effective treatment for potentially fatal fungal diseases. Balance its possible

AMPHOTERICIN B DESOXYCHOLATE

lifesaving effect against its dangerous side effects.

►*Nephrotoxicity:* Renal damage is a limiting factor for the use of amphotericin B. Renal dysfunction usually improves upon interruption of therapy, dose reduction, or increased dosing interval; however, some permanent impairment often occurs, especially in patients receiving large doses (> 5 g) or receiving other nephrotoxic agents (eg, aminoglycosides, cyclosporine, pentamidine). Decreased glomerular filtration rate and renal blood flow, increased serum creatinine, and renal tubular dysfunction are prominent.

Sodium loading may be effective in reducing nephrotoxicity, but this may be a problem in patients with cardiac or hepatic disease. In some patients, hydration and sodium repletion prior to amphotericin B administration may reduce the risk of developing nephrotoxicity. Supplemental alkali medication may decrease renal tubular acidosis complications.

Lipid formulations of amphotericin B have been shown to reduce the severe kidney toxicity of amphotericin B and are indicated in patients with renal impairment or when unacceptable toxicity precludes the use of amphotericin B desoxycholate in effective doses.

In a randomized, double-blind study of 4 mg/kg/day amphotericin B cholesteryl and 0.8 mg/kg/day amphotericin B desoxycholate as empiric treatment in febrile neutropenic patients, it was demonstrated that in patients with normal baseline renal function the incidence of nephrotoxicity was significantly lower with amphotericin B cholesteryl than with amphotericin B desoxycholate.

►*Infusion reactions:* Acute reactions including fever, shaking chills, hypotension, anorexia, vomiting, nausea, headache, and tachypnea are common 1 to 3 hours after starting an IV infusion. These reactions are usually more severe with the first few doses of amphotericin B and usually diminish with subsequent doses. Acute infusion-related reactions can be managed by pretreatment with antihistamines and corticosteroids or by reducing the rate of infusion and by prompt administration of antihistamines and corticosteroids. Avoid rapid IV infusion because it has been associated with hypotension, hypokalemia, arrhythmias, bronchospasm, and shock.

►*Leukoencephalopathy:* This has been reported following use of amphotericin B. The literature has suggested that total body irradiation may be a predisposition.

►*Rhinocerebral phycomycosis:* A fulminating disease, this generally occurs in association with diabetic ketoacidosis. Diabetic control must be instituted before successful treatment with amphotericin B can be accomplished. Pulmonary phycomycosis, which is more common in association with hematologic malignancies, is often an incidental finding at autopsy.

►*Hypersensitivity reactions:* Anaphylaxis has been reported with amphotericin B. If severe respiratory distress occurs, discontinue the infusion immediately. Do not give further infusions. Have cardiopulmonary resuscitation facilities available during administration.

►*Renal function impairment:* Use amphotericin B desoxycholate with care in patients with reduced renal function; frequent monitoring is recommended (see Precautions). Lipid formulations have been reported to overcome most problems of chronic nephrotoxicity, even in patients with impaired renal function following previous treatment with amphotericin B desoxycholate.

►*Pregnancy: Category B.* Systemic fungal infections have been successfully treated in pregnant women with amphotericin B without obvious effects to the fetus, but the number of cases reported has been small. Adequate and well-controlled studies have not been conducted; therefore, use during pregnancy only if clearly needed.

►*Lactation:* It is not known whether amphotericin B is excreted in breast milk. Because of the potential for serious adverse reactions in nursing infants, decide whether to discontinue breastfeeding or discontinue treatment, taking into account the importance of the drug to the mother.

►*Children:* Safety and efficacy of amphotericin B desoxycholate in children have not been established. Systemic fungal infections have been successfully treated in children without reports of unusual side effects. Limit administration to the least amount compatible with an effective therapeutic regimen.

Pediatric patients < 16 years of age (n = 97) with systemic fungal infections have been treated with amphotericin B cholesteryl at daily mg/kg doses similar to those given in adults and had significantly less renal toxicity than the desoxycholate formulation (12% vs 52%).

Precautions

►*Monitoring:* Monitor renal function frequently during amphotericin B therapy. It is also advisable to monitor liver function, serum electrolytes (particularly magnesium and potassium), blood counts and hemoglobin concentrations on a regular basis. Use laboratory test results as a guide to subsequent dose adjustments. Monitor complete blood count and prothrombin time as medically indicated.

Testing dose – Record the patient's temperature, pulse, respiration, and blood pressure every 30 minutes for 2 to 4 hours after administration.

►*Resistance:* Variants with reduced susceptibility to amphotericin B have been isolated from several fungal species after serial passage in cell culture media containing the drug and from some patients receiving prolonged therapy with amphotericin B desoxycholate. The relevance of drug resistance to clinical outcome has not been established.

►*Therapy interruption:* Whenever amphotericin B desoxycholate therapy is interrupted for > 7 days, resume therapy with the lowest dosage level (eg, 0.25 mg/kg) and increase gradually (see Administration and Dosage).

►*Pulmonary reactions:* Pulmonary reactions characterized by acute dyspnea, hypoxemia, and interstitial infiltrates have been observed in neutropenic patients receiving amphotericin B and leukocyte transfusions. Although pulmonary toxicity has occurred in association with either agent used alone, it was more frequent when amphotericin B was given after or during initiation of leukocyte transfusions. Administer amphotericin B cautiously in patients receiving leukocyte transfusions, and separate the infusion as far as possible from the time of a leukocyte transfusion.

►*Lab test abnormalities:* Serum electrolyte, liver function, renal function, and other test abnormalities have been reported, including the following: Hypomagnesemia, hyperkalemia, hypokalemia, hypercalcemia, hypocalcemia, hypophosphatemia; increased AST, ALT, GGT, bilirubin, alkaline phosphatase, LDH, BUN, and serum creatinine; acidosis, hyperamylasemia, hypoglycemia, hyperglycemia, and hyperuricemia.

Drug Interactions

Amphotericin B Drug Interactions			
Precipitant drug	Object drug*		Description
Antineoplastic agents	Amphotericin B	↑	Concurrent administration may enhance the potential for renal toxicity, bronchospasm, and hypotension.
Azole antifungals	Amphotericin B	↓	In vitro animal studies suggest that imidazoles may induce fungal resistance to amphotericin B. Administer with caution, especially in immunocompromised patients.
Corticosteroids and corticotropin	Amphotericin B	↑	Concurrent administration may potentiate hypokalemia and predispose patients to cardiac dysfunction. Do not give unless necessary to control adverse reactions.
Zidovudine	Amphotericin B	↑	Increases in myelotoxicity and nephrotoxicity were observed in dogs administered zidovudine concomitantly with amphotericin B desoxycholate.
Amphotericin B	Cyclosporine	↑	The risk of renal toxicity is increased with concomitant administration. Severe muscle tremors were reported in 1 patient.
Cyclosporine	Amphotericin B		
Amphotericin B	Digitalis glycosides	↑	Concurrent administration may induce hypokalemia and may potentiate digitalis toxicity.
Amphotericin B	Flucytosine	↑	A synergistic relationship with amphotericin B has been reported. Flucytosine toxicity may be increased by increasing its cellular uptake or impairing renal excretion.
Amphotericin B	Nephrotoxic agents	↑	Concomitant administration may enhance risk of drug-induced renal toxicity. Use caution when administering concomitantly. Monitor renal function intensively.
Nephrotoxic agents	Amphotericin B		
Amphotericin B	Skeletal muscle relaxants	↑	Amphotericin B-induced hypokalemia may enhance the curariform effect of skeletal muscle relaxants. Monitor serum potassium levels closely.
Amphotericin B	Thiazides	↑	Electrolyte depletion may be intensified, particularly hypokalemia. Monitor potassium levels.

* ↑ = Object drug increased. ↓ = Object drug decreased.

Adverse Reactions

►*Prevention of adverse reactions:* Most patients will exhibit some intolerance, often at less than full therapeutic dosage. Severe reactions may be lessened by giving aspirin, antipyretics (eg, acetaminophen),

AMPHOTERICIN B DESOXYCHOLATE

antihistamines, and antiemetics before the infusion and by maintaining sodium balance. Administration on alternate days may decrease anorexia and phlebitis. Small doses of IV adrenal corticosteroids given prior to or during the infusion may decrease febrile reactions. Keep the dosage and duration of such corticosteroid therapy to a minimum (see Drug Interactions). In 3 patients, dantrolene was a successful adjunctive agent for the prophylaxis (50 mg oral) and treatment (50 mg IV) of amphotericin B-induced rigors. Adding a small amount of heparin to the infusion (500 to 2000 units), removal of needle after infusion, rotation of infusion sites, administration through a large central vein, and using a pediatric scalp-vein needle may lessen the incidence of thrombophlebitis. Extravasation may cause chemical irritation. Meperidine 25 to 50 mg IV has been shown in some patients to decrease the duration of shaking chills, and fever that may accompany infusion of amphotericin B.

➤*Cardiovascular:* Hypotension (most common); cardiac arrest, cardiac failure, arrhythmias including ventricular fibrillation, hypertension.

➤*CNS:* Headache (most common); convulsions, tinnitus, transient vertigo, peripheral neuropathy, encephalopathy, other neurologic symptoms.

➤*Dermatologic:* Rash, particularly maculopapular; pruritus.

➤*GI:* Anorexia, nausea, vomiting, dyspepsia, diarrhea, cramping, epigastric pain (most common); acute liver failure, hepatitis, melena, jaundice, hemorrhagic gastroenteritis.

➤*Hematologic:* Normochromic anemia, normocytic anemia (most common); agranulocytosis, coagulation defects, thrombocytopenia, leukopenia, eosinophilia, leukocytosis.

➤*Lab test abnormalities:* Hypomagnesemia, hypokalemia, hyperkalemia, hypocalcemia; elevated AST, ALT, CGT, bilirubin, alkaline phosphatase, BUN, and serum creatinine.

➤*Special senses:* Hearing loss, visual impairment, diplopia.

➤*Renal:* Decreased renal function and renal function abnormalities including the following: Azotemia, hypokalemia, hyposthenuria, renal tubular acidosis, and nephrocalcinosis. These usually improve with interruption of therapy. However, permanent damage is often related to a large total dose (> 5 g) or receiving other nephrotoxic agents (most common); acute renal failure, anuria, oliguria.

➤*Respiratory:* Tachypnea (most common); shock, pulmonary edema, hypersensitivity pneumonitis, dyspnea, bronchospasm, wheezing.

➤*Miscellaneous:* Fever (sometimes with shaking or chills usually occurring within 15 to 20 minutes after initiation of treatment), malaise, weight loss, pain at injection site with or without phlebitis or thrombophlebitis, generalized pain including muscle and joint pain (most common); flushing, anaphylactoid and other allergic reactions.

Overdosage

Amphotericin B overdose has been reported to cause cardiorespiratory arrest. If overdose is suspected, discontinue therapy, monitor clinical status, and administer supportive therapy. Refer to General Management of Acute Overdosage. Amphotericin B desoxycholate is not hemodialyzable.

AMPHOTERICIN B, LIPID-BASED

Rx	**Abelcet** (Enzon)	**Suspension for Injection:** 100 mg/20 ml (as lipid complex)	In 10 and 20 ml single-use vials with 5-micron filter needles.
Rx	**Amphotec** (Sequus Pharmaceuticals)	**Powder for Injection:** 50 mg (as cholesteryl)	In 20 ml single-use vials.
		100 mg (as cholesteryl)	In 50 ml single-use vials.
Rx	**AmBisome** (Fujisawa)	**Powder for Injection:** 50 mg (as liposomal)	Sucrose. In single-dose vials with 5-micron filter.

WARNING

Use primarily for treatment of patients with progressive and potentially fatal fungal infections. Do not use to treat noninvasive forms of fungal disease such as oral thrush, vaginal candidiasis, and esophageal candidiasis in patients with normal neutrophil counts.

Indications

➤*Fungal infections, systemic:* For use in patients refractory to conventional amphotericin B desoxycholate therapy or when renal impairment or unacceptable toxicity precludes the use of the desoxycholate formulation for the treatment of invasive fungal infections (lipid complex); for the treatment of invasive aspergillosis (cholesteryl); for the treatment of infections caused by *Aspergillus, Candida,* or *Cryptococcus* sp. (liposomal).

➤*Fungal infections, empirical:* For empirical treatment in febrile, neutropenic patients with presumed fungal infection (*AmBisome* only).

➤*Cryptococcal meningitis in HIV:* Treatment of cryptococcal meningitis in HIV-infected patients (*AmBisome* only).

➤*Leishmaniasis:* For treatment of visceral leishmaniasis (*AmBisome* only).

➤*Unlabeled uses:* Prophylaxis of fungal infection in patients with bone marrow transplantation (0.1 mg/kg/day); for the treatment of primary amoebic meningoencephalitis caused by *Naegleria fowleri;* subconjunctival or intravitreal injection in ocular aspergillosis; as a bladder irrigation for candidal cystitis; as chemoprophylaxis by low-dose IV, intranasal, or nebulized administration in immunocompromised patients at risk of aspergillosis; intra-articularly or IM for coccidioidal arthritis.

Administration and Dosage

Individualize and adjust dosage based on patient's clinical status (eg, cardiorenal function, reaction to test dose, site, and severity of infection). If administered through an existing IV line, flush with 5% Dextrose for Injection prior to and following infusion; otherwise administer via a separate line.

➤*Fungal infection, empirical:* Administer 3 mg/kg/day of liposomal amphotericin B for empirical fungal infections using a controlled infusion device over ≈ 120 minutes; infusion time may be reduced to 60 minutes if well tolerated or increased if patient experiences discomfort.

➤*Fungal infection, systemic:*

Abelcet – The recommended dose is 5 mg/kg/day prepared as a 1 mg/ml infusion and delivered at a rate of 2.5 mg/kg/hour. For pediatric patients and patients with cardiovascular disease, the drug may be diluted to a final concentration of 2 mg/ml. If the infusion exceeds 2 hours, mix the contents by shaking the infusion bag every 2 hours. Do not use an in-line filter.

Amphotec – A test dose is advisable (eg, 10 ml of final preparation containing 1.6 to 8.3 mg infused over 15 to 30 min). The recommended dose is 3 to 4 mg/kg/day prepared as a 0.6 mg/ml (range, 0.16 to 0.83 mg/ml) infusion delivered at a rate of 1 mg/kg/hr. Do not filter or use an in-line filter.

AmBisome – The recommended dose is 3 to 5 mg/kg/day prepared as a 1 to 2 mg/ml infusion delivered initially over 120 minutes; infusion time may be reduced to 60 minutes if well tolerated or increased if patient experiences discomfort. Lower infusion concentrations of 0.2 to 0.5 mg/ml may be appropriate for infants and small children to provide sufficient volume for infusion. An in-line membrane filter of ≥ 1 micron mean pore diameter may be used.

➤*Cryptococcal meningitis in HIV:*

AmBisome – Administer 6 mg/kg/day using a controlled infusion device over ≈ 120 minutes; infusion time may be reduced to 60 minutes if well tolerated or increased if patient experiences discomfort.

➤*Leishmaniasis:*

AmBisome – Administer 3 mg/kg/day on days 1 through 5, 14, and 21 to immunocompetent patients; a repeat course of therapy may be useful if parasitic clearance is not achieved. Administer 4 mg/kg/day on days 1 through 5, 10, 17, 24, 31, and 38 to immunosuppressed patients; seek expert advice regarding further therapy if parasitic clearance is not achieved.

➤*Unlabeled uses:*

Cystitis, candidal – Irrigate bladder with a 50 mcg/ml solution, instilled periodically or continuously for 5 to 10 days.

Paracoccidioidomycosis – Administer 0.4 to 0.5 mg/kg/day slow IV infusion; treat for 4 to 12 weeks.

➤*Preparation of infusion solutions:* Do not dilute or reconstitute with saline solutions or mix with other drugs or electrolytes. The use of any solution other than those recommended or the presence of a bacteriostatic agent (eg, benzyl alcohol) may cause precipitation of amphotericin B.

Abelcet – Shake the vial gently until there is no yellow sediment at the bottom. Withdraw the appropriate dose from the required number of vials into ≥ 1 sterile 20 ml syringes using an 18-gauge needle. Remove the needle from each syringe and replace with a 5-micron filter needle. Each filter needle may be used to filter the content of up to 4 vials. Insert the filter needle of the syringe into an IV bag containing 5% Dextrose for Injection, and empty the contents of the syringe into the bag for a final concentration of 1 mg/ml (2 mg/ml for pediatric and cardiovascular patients).

Amphotec – Reconstitute with Sterile Water for Injection. Do not use saline or dextrose for reconstitution. Using a sterile syringe and a 20-gauge needle, rapidly add the following volumes to the vial to provide a liquid containing 5 mg/ml. Shake gently by hand, rotating the vial until all solids have dissolved. Note that the fluid may be opalescent or clear. For 50 mg/vial add 10 ml Sterile Water for Injection; for the 100 mg/vial add 20 ml Sterile Water for Injection.

AMPHOTERICIN B, LIPID-BASED

For infusion, further dilute the reconstituted liquid to a final concentration of $\approx$ 0.6 mg/ml (range, 0.16 to 0.83 mg/ml).

AmBisome – Add 12 ml of Sterile Water for Injection to each vial to yield 4 mg/ml. Immediately shake the vial vigorously for 30 seconds to completely disperse the drug until a yellow, translucent suspension is formed. Calculate total dose needed, withdraw appropriate amount of reconstituted solution into sterile syringe, attach the 5-micron filter provided, and inject contents of syringe through filter needle into an appropriate volume of 5% Dextrose (use only 1 filter needle per vial) to yield a final concentration of 1 to 2 mg/ml. Concentrations of 0.2 to 0.5 mg/ml may be more appropriate for infants and small children.

➤*Admixture incompatibility:* Do not dilute or reconstitute with saline solutions or mix with other drugs or electrolytes. The use of any solution other than those recommended or the presence of a bacteriostatic agent (eg, benzyl alcohol) may cause precipitation of amphotericin B. If administered through an existing IV line, flush with 5% Dextrose for Injection prior to and following infusion; otherwise administer via a separate line.

➤*Storage/Stability:*

Abelcet – Prior to admixture, store at 2° to 8°C (36° to 46°F). Protect from exposure to light. Do not freeze. Retain in the carton until time of use. The admixture may be stored for ≤ 48 hours at 2° to 8°C (36° to 46°F) and an additional 6 hours at room temperature.

Amphotec – Store unopened vials at 15° to 30°C (59° to 86°F). After reconstitution, refrigerate at 2° to 8°C (36° to 46°F), and use within 24 hours. Do not freeze. After further dilution with 5% Dextrose for Injection, refrigerate (2° to 8°C; 36° to 46°F), and use within 24 hours.

AmBisome – Refrigerate unopened vials at 2° to 8°C (36° to 46°F). Store reconstituted product concentrate at 2° to 8°C for ≤ 24 hours. Do not freeze. Use within 6 hours of dilution with 5% Dextrose.

Actions

➤*Pharmacology:* Amphotericin B is a polyene antibiotic produced by a strain of *Streptomyces nodosus* that is fungistatic or fungicidal, depending on the concentration obtained in body fluids and on the susceptibility of the fungus. It acts by binding to sterols (primarily ergosterol) in the fungal cell membrane with a resultant change in membrane permeability, allowing leakage of a variety of intracellular components. It can also bind to the cholesterol component of the mammalian cell, leading to cytotoxicity.

Liposomal encapsulation or incorporation in a lipid complex can substantially affect a drug's functional properties relative to those of the unencapsulated or nonlipid-associated drug. Lipid-based formulations increase the circulation time and alter the biodistribution of the associated amphotericin. Because drugs complexed with lipid vehicles have a longer residence time in the vasculature, they are able to localize and reach greater concentrations in regions with increased capillary permeability (eg, solid tumors, infection, inflammation) compared with regions of normal tissue, which are essentially impermeable to lipid-complexed drugs. This opportunistic method of increasing the localization of drugs to diseased sites is referred to as passive targeting and allows drug levels to be increased several times higher than those allowable with the free drug. Increasing drug levels at the site of action and reducing levels in normal tissues offers 2 distinct clinical advantages: An increased therapeutic index and an altered toxicity profile relative to the free drug.

In addition, different lipid-based formulations with a common active ingredient may vary from one another in the chemical composition (eg, phospholipid and cholesterol content) and physical form of the lipid component (eg, sphere, disc, ribbon). Such differences may affect functional properties of these drug products.

➤*Pharmacokinetics:*

Lipid-based formulations – The pharmacokinetics of lipid-based amphotericin B products are nonlinear. Steady-state volume of distribution (Vss) and total plasma clearance (CL) increase with escalating doses, resulting in less than proportional increases in plasma concentration over a given dose range.

The increased volume of distribution probably reflects uptake by tissues. The long terminal elimination half-life for the cholesteryl (*Amphotec*), lipid complex (*Abelcet*), and liposomal (*AmBisome*) formulations probably reflects a slow redistribution from tissues. Mean trough levels for each of these formulations remain relatively constant with repeated dosing, indicating little accumulation in plasma. The following table presents pharmacokinetic parameters at steady state for lipid-based formulations of amphotericin B; the assay used to measure serum levels did not distinguish between free and complexed amphotericin B.

	AmBisome 1 mg/kg/day (n = 7)	AmBisome 2.5 mg/kg/day (n = 7)	AmBisome 5 mg/kg/day (n = 9)	Amphotec 3 mg/kg/day (predicted)[2]	Amphotec 4 mg/kg/day (predicted)[2]	Abelcet 5 mg/kg/day (n = varied)[3]
Pharmacokinetic Parameters of Lipid-Based Amphotericin B Formulations[1]						
Parameter						
C_{max} (mcg/ml)	≈ 12.2	≈ 31.4	≈ 83	2.6	2.9	≈ 1.7
AUC (mcg/ml•hr)	≈ 60	≈ 197	≈ 555	29	36	≈ 14
t½ (hours)	≈ 7	≈ 6.3	≈ 6.8	27.5 (100 to 153)[4]	28.2 (100 to 153)[4]	≈ 173.4
Vss (L/kg)	≈ 0.14	≈ 0.16	≈ 0.1	3.8	4.1	≈ 131
CL (ml/hr/kg)	≈ 17	≈ 22	≈ 11	105	112	≈ 436

[1] Data are pooled from separate studies and are not necessarily comparable.
[2] Values based on the population model developed from 51 bone marrow transplant patients with systemic fungal infections given *Amphotec* 0.5 to 8 mg/kg/day.
[3] Data obtained from various studies in patients with mucocutaneous leishmaniasis or cancer with presumed or proven fungal infections.
[4] Based on total amphotericin B levels measured within a 24-hour dosing interval (for up to 49 days after dosing).

Following a 1 mg/kg/hour infusion, ≈ 25% of the total amphotericin B concentration measured in plasma was in the amphotericin B cholesteryl complex, dropping to ≈ 9.3% at 1 hour and ≈ 7.5% at 24 hours after the end of the infusion.

Children – In a small study of 12 children 4 months to 14 years of age infused with 0.25 to 1.5 mg/kg/day of amphotericin B, plasma levels ranged from 0.78 to 10.02 mcg/ml and were independent of dose. The mean elimination half-life was 18.1 hours. An inverse relationship between age and total clearance was observed indicating that children > 9 years of age may require lower doses.

➤*Microbiology: Abelcet* is active in animal models against *Aspergillus fumigatus, Candida albicans, C. guillermondi, C. stellatoideae, C. tropicalis, Cryptococcus* sp., *Coccidioidomyces* sp., *Histoplasma* sp., and *Blastomyces* sp.

Amphotec is active in vitro against *Aspergillus, Candida* sp., and other fungi. In animal models, it has shown additional activity against *Coccidioides immitis, Cryptococcus neoformans,* and *Leishmania* sp.

AmBisome has shown in vitro activity against *Aspergillus* sp. (*A. fumigatus, A. flavus*), *Candida* sp. (*C. albicans, C. krusei, C. lusitaniae, C. parapsilosis, C. tropicalis*), *Cryptococcus neoformans,* and *Blastomyces dermatitidis*. In animal models, it has shown additional activity against *Coccidioides immitis, Histoplasma capsulatum, Paracoccidioides brasiliensis, Leishmania donovani,* and *Leishmania infantum*.

Contraindications

Hypersensitivity to amphotericin B or any other component of the formulation unless the condition requiring treatment is life-threatening and amenable only to amphotericin B therapy.

Warnings

➤*Fatal fungal diseases:* Amphotericin B is frequently the only effective treatment for potentially fatal fungal diseases. Balance its possible life-saving effect against its dangerous side effects.

➤*Nephrotoxicity:* Lipid formulations of amphotericin B reduced the severe kidney toxicity of amphotericin B and are indicated in patients with renal impairment or when unacceptable toxicity precludes use of amphotericin B desoxycholate in effective doses.

In a randomized, double-blind study of amphotericin B cholesteryl (*Amphotec* 4 mg/kg/day) and amphotericin B desoxycholate (0.8 mg/kg/day) as empiric treatment in febrile neutropenic patients, it was demonstrated that in patients with normal baseline renal function the incidence of nephrotoxicity was significantly lower with amphotericin B cholesteryl than with amphotericin B desoxycholate.

In a randomized, double-blind study of amphotericin B liposomal (*AmBisome*) in neutropenic patients, the incidence of nephrotoxicity is summarized in the following table.

Nephrotoxicity in Neutropenic Patients Taking *AmBisome* (%)			
	AmBisome		Amphotericin B lipid complex 5 mg/kg/day
	3 mg/kg/day	5 mg/kg/day	Both	
Total patients	85	81	166	78
Patients with nephrotoxicity				
1.5 × baseline serum creatinine value	29.4	25.9	27.7	62.8
2 × baseline serum creatinine value	14.1	14.8	14.5	42.3

AMPHOTERICIN B, LIPID-BASED

►*Infusion reactions:* Acute reactions including fever, shaking chills, hypotension, anorexia, vomiting, nausea, headache, and tachypnea are common 1 to 3 hours after starting an IV infusion. These reactions are usually more severe with the first few doses of amphotericin B and usually diminish with subsequent doses. Acute infusion-related reactions can be managed by pretreatment with antihistamines and corticosteroids or by reducing the rate of infusion and by prompt administration of antihistamines and corticosteroids. Avoid rapid IV infusion because it has been associated with hypotension, hypokalemia, arrhythmias, bronchospasm, and shock.

►*Leukoencephalopathy:* Leukoencephalopathy has been reported following use of amphotericin B; total body irradiation may be a predisposition.

►*Hypersensitivity reactions:* Anaphylaxis has been reported with amphotericin B. If severe respiratory distress occurs, discontinue the infusion immediately. Do not give further infusions. Have cardiopulmonary resuscitation facilities available during administration.

►*Renal function impairment:* Use amphotericin B with care in patients with reduced renal function; frequent monitoring is recommended (see Precautions). Lipid formulations have been reported to overcome most problems of chronic nephrotoxicity, even in patients with impaired renal function following previous treatment with amphotericin B desoxycholate.

►*Elderly:* A total of 188 patients > 65 years of age have been treated with lipid-based formulations of amphotericin B with no reports of unexpected adverse events.

►*Pregnancy: Category B.* Systemic fungal infections have been successfully treated in pregnant women with amphotericin B without obvious effects to the fetus, but the number of cases reported has been small. Adequate and well-controlled studies have not been conducted; therefore, use during pregnancy only if clearly needed.

►*Lactation:* It is not known whether amphotericin B is excreted in breast milk. Because of the potential for serious adverse reactions in nursing infants, decide whether to discontinue breastfeeding or discontinue treatment, taking into account the importance of the drug to the mother.

►*Children:* Pediatric patients < 16 years of age (n = 97) with systemic fungal infections have been treated with amphotericin B cholesteryl (*Amphotec*) at daily mg/kg doses similar to those given adults and had significantly less renal toxicity than the desoxycholate formulation (12% vs 52%); 273 pediatric patients age 1 month to 16 years of age with presumed fungal infections, confirmed systemic fungal infections, or with visceral leishmaniasis have been successfully treated with liposomal amphotericin B (*AmBisome*); 111 children < 16 years of age, including 11 patients < 1 year of age, have been treated with amphotericin B lipid complex (*Abelcet*) at 5 mg/kg/day and 5 children with hepatosplenic candidiasis were effectively treated with 2.5 mg/kg/day. Safety and efficacy in patients < 1 month of age have not been established.

Precautions

►*Monitoring:* Monitor renal function frequently during amphotericin B therapy. Monitor liver function, serum electrolytes (particularly magnesium and potassium), blood counts, and hemoglobin concentrations on a regular basis. Use laboratory test results as a guide to subsequent dose adjustments. Monitor complete blood count and prothrombin time as medically indicated.

Testing dose – Record the patient's temperature, pulse, respiration, and blood pressure every 30 minutes for 2 to 4 hours after administration.

►*Resistance:* Variants with reduced susceptibility to amphotericin B have been isolated from several fungal species after serial passage in cell culture media containing the drug and from some patients receiving prolonged therapy with amphotericin B desoxycholate. The relevance of drug resistance to clinical outcome has not been established.

►*Pulmonary reactions:* Pulmonary reactions characterized by acute dyspnea, hypoxemia, and interstitial infiltrates have been observed in neutropenic patients receiving amphotericin B and leukocyte transfusions. Although pulmonary toxicity has occurred in association with either agent used alone, it was more frequent when amphotericin B was given after or during initiation of leukocyte transfusions. Administer amphotericin B cautiously in patients receiving leukocyte transfusions and separate the infusion as far as possible from the time of leukocyte transfusion.

►*Lab test abnormalities:* Serum electrolyte, liver function, renal function, and other test abnormalities have been reported, including the following: Hypomagnesemia, hyperkalemia, hypokalemia, hypercalcemia, hypocalcemia, hypophosphatemia; increased AST, ALT, GGT, bilirubin, alkaline phosphatase, LDH, BUN, and serum creatinine; acidosis, hyperamylasemia, hypoglycemia, hyperglycemia, and hyperuricemia.

Drug Interactions

Amphotericin B Drug Interactions			
Precipitant drug	Object drug*		Description
Antineoplastic agents	Amphotericin B	↑	Concurrent administration may enhance the potential for renal toxicity, bronchospasm, and hypotension.
Corticosteroids and corticotropin	Amphotericin B	↑	Concurrent administration may potentiate hypokalemia and predispose patient to cardiac dysfunction. Do not give unless necessary to control adverse reactions.
Zidovudine	Amphotericin B	↑	Increases in myelotoxicity and nephrotoxicity were observed in dogs administered zidovudine concomitantly with amphotericin B desoxycholate or lipid complex.
Amphotericin B	Cyclosporine	↑	The risk of renal toxicity is increased with concomitant administration. Severe muscle tremors were reported in 1 patient.
Cyclosporine	Amphotericin B		
Amphotericin B	Digitalis glycosides	↑	Concurrent administration may induce hypokalemia and may potentiate digitalis toxicity.
Amphotericin B	Flucytosine	↑	A synergistic relationship with amphotericin B has been reported. Flucytosine toxicity may be increased by increasing its cellular uptake or impairing renal excretion.
Azole antifungals	Amphotericin B	↓	In vitro animal studies suggest that imidazoles may induce fungal resistance to amphotericin B. Administer with caution, especially in immunocompromised patients.
Nephrotoxic agents	Amphotericin B	↑	Concomitant administration may enhance risk of drug-induced renal toxicity. Use caution when administering concomitantly. Monitor renal function intensively.
Amphotericin B	Nephrotoxic agents		
Amphotericin B	Skeletal muscle relaxants	↑	Amphotericin B-induced hypokalemia may enhance the curariform effect of skeletal muscle relaxants. Monitor serum potassium levels closely.
Amphotericin B	Thiazides	↑	Electrolyte depletion may be intensified, particularly hypokalemia. Monitor potassium levels.

* ↑ = Object drug increased. ↓ = Object drug decreased.

Adverse Reactions

►*Prevention of adverse reactions:* Most patients will exhibit some intolerance, often at less than full therapeutic dosage. Severe reactions may be lessened by giving aspirin, antipyretics (eg, acetaminophen), antihistamines, and antiemetics before the infusion and by maintaining sodium balance. Administration on alternate days may decrease anorexia and phlebitis. Small doses of IV adrenal corticosteroids given prior to or during the infusion may decrease febrile reactions. Keep the dosage and duration of such corticosteroid therapy to a minimum (see Drug Interactions). In 3 patients, dantrolene was a successful adjunctive agent for the prophylaxis (50 mg oral) and treatment (50 mg IV) of amphotericin B-induced rigors. Adding a small amount of heparin to the infusion (500 to 2000 units), removal of needle after infusion, rotation of infusion sites, administration through a large central vein, and using a pediatric scalp-vein needle may lessen the incidence of thrombophlebitis. Extravasation may cause chemical irritation. In some patients meperidine (25 to 50 mg IV) has been shown to decrease the duration of shaking chills and fever that may accompany infusion of amphotericin B.

Polyene Antifungals

AMPHOTERICIN B, LIPID-BASED

Amphotericin B, Lipid-Based Adverse Reactions (%)[1]			
Adverse reaction	Abelcet (5 mg/kg/day)	Amphotec (3 to 6 mg/kg/day)	AmBisome[2]
Cardiovascular			
Hypotension	8	10-12	14.3
Cardiac arrest	6	1-5	2-10
Hypertension	5	7	7.9
Chest pain	3	≥ 5	12
Tachycardia	—	9-10	13.4
CNS			
Headache	6	4-5	19.8
Anxiety	—	1-5	13.7
Confusion	—	1-5	11.4
Insomnia	—	≥ 5	17.2
Dermatologic			
Rash	4	≥ 5	24.8
Pruritus	✔	≥ 5	10.8
Sweating	—	≥ 5	7
GI			
Nausea	9	7-8	39.7
Vomiting	8	6-11	31.8
Diarrhea	6	≥ 5	30.3
Abdominal pain	4	≥ 5	19.8
GI hemorrhage	4	1-5	9.9
Nausea/Vomiting	3	4-7	—
Hematologic			
Thrombocytopenia	5	1-6	2-10
Anemia	4	≥ 5	2-10
Leukopenia	4	1-5	—
Bilirubinemia	4	—	—
Metabolic/Nutritional			
Creatine, increased	11	12-21[3]	22.4
BUN, increased	5	1-5	21
Hyperbilirubinemia	—	3-19	18.1
Alkaline phosphatase, increased	✔	3-7	22.2
ALT, increased	✔	1-5	14.6
AST, increased	✔	1-5	12.8
Liver function test abnormality		4-11	2-10
Hypokalemia	5	8-26	42.9
Hypomagnesemia	✔	4-6	20.4
Hyperglycemia	✔	1-6	23
Hypernatremia	—	1-5	4.1
Hypocalcemia	✔	≥ 5	18.4
Hypervolemia	—	1-5	12.2
Peripheral edema	—	≥ 5	14.6
Edema	—	≥ 5	14.3
Respiratory			
Respiratory failure	8	—	2-10
Dyspnea	7	5-9	23
Respiratory disorder	4	1-5	2-10
Hypoxia	—	5-9	7.6
Cough increased	—	≥ 5	17.8
Epistaxis	—	≥ 5	14.9
Lung disorder	—	≥ 5	17.8
Pleural effusion	—	1-5	12.5
Rhinitis	—	≥ 5	11.1
Miscellaneous			
Chills	18	50-77	47.5
Fever	14	33-55	—
Multiple organ failure	11	—	—
Sepsis	7	≥ 5	14
Infection	5	1-5	11.1
Pain	5	≥ 5	14
Kidney failure	5	1-5	2-10
Chills and fever	—	3-7	—
Asthenia	—	1-5	13.1
Back pain	—	≥ 5	12
Blood product transfusion reaction	—	—	18.4
Hematuria		≥ 5	14

[1] Data are pooled from separate studies and are not necessarily comparable.
[2] Incidence of ≥ 10%.
[3] Includes patients with "abnormal kidney function," which was associated with an increase in creatinine.
* ✔ = occurred, no incidence figure reported.

➤*Abelcet:* The following adverse reactions have also been reported in patients using *Abelcet,* but the causal association between these adverse reactions and *Abelcet* is uncertain.

Cardiovascular – Cardiac failure, MI, cardiomyopathy, arrhythmias including ventricular fibrillation.

CNS – Convulsions, peripheral neuropathy, transient vertigo, encephalopathy, cerebrovascular accident, extrapyramidal syndrome and other neurologic symptoms.

Dermatologic – Maculopapular rash, exfoliative dermatitis, erythema multiforme.

GI – Melena, dyspepsia, cramping, epigastric pain.

GU – Oliguria, decreased renal function, anuria, renal tubular acidosis, impotence, dysuria.

Hematologic – Coagulation defects, leukocytosis, blood dyscrasias including eosinophilia.

Hepatic – Acute liver failure, hepatitis, jaundice, venoocclusive liver disease, hepatomegaly, cholangitis, cholecystitis.

Lab test abnormalities – Hyperkalemia, hypercalcemia, increased LDH, increased BUN, hyperamylasemia, hypoglycemia, hyperuricemia, hypophosphatemia.

Musculoskeletal – Myasthenia, bone pain, muscle pain, joint pain.

Respiratory – Bronchospasm, wheezing, asthma, pulmonary edema, hemoptysis, pulmonary embolus, tachypnea, pleural effusion.

Special senses – Deafness, tinnitus, visual impairment, hearing loss, diplopia.

Miscellaneous – Malaise, weight loss, injection site reactions including inflammation, anaphylactoid and other allergic reactions, shock, thrombophlebitis, anorexia, acidosis.

➤*Amphotec:* The following adverse events also occured in *Amphotec* patients, but the causal relationship is uncertain.

Cardiovascular – Hemorrhage, postural hypotension (≥ 5%); arrhythmia, atrial fibrillation, bradycardia, CHF, phlebitis, shock, supraventricular tachycardia, syncope, vasodilation, venoocclusive liver disease, ventricular extrasystoles (1% to < 5%).

CNS – Dizziness, somnolence, abnormal thinking, tremor (≥ 5%); agitation, convulsion, depression, hallucinations, hypertonia, nervousness, neuropathy, paresthesia, psychosis, speech disorder, stupor (1% to < 5%).

Dermatologic – Maculopapular rash (≥ 5%); acne, alopecia, petechial rash, skin discoloration, skin disorder, skin nodule, skin ulcer, urticaria, vesiculobullous rash (1% to < 5%).

GI – Dry mouth, hematemesis, jaundice, stomatitis (≥ 5%); anorexia, bloody diarrhea, constipation, dyspepsia, fecal incontinence, gamma glutamyl transpeptidase increase, GI disorder, gingivitis, glossitis, hepatic failure, melena, mouth ulceration, oral moniliasis, rectal disorder (1% to < 5%).

GU – Albuminuria, dysuria, glycosuria, oliguria, urinary incontinence, urinary retention, urinary tract disorder (1% to < 5%).

Hematologic/Lymphatic – Coagulation disorder, prothrombin decreased (≥ 5%); ecchymosis, increased fibrinogen, hypochromic anemia, leukocytosis, petechia, decreased thromboplastin (1% to < 5%).

Metabolic/Nutritional – Hypophosphatemia, peripheral edema, weight gain (≥ 5%); acidosis, dehydration, hyponatremia, hyperkalemia, hyperlipemia, hypoglycemia, hypoproteinemia, lactic dehydrogenase increased, weight loss (1% to < 5%).

Musculoskeletal – Arthralgia, myalgia (1% to < 5%).

Respiratory – Apnea, asthma, hyperventilation (≥ 5%); hemoptysis, lung edema, pharyngitis, sinusitis (1% to < 5%).

Special senses – Eye hemorrhage (≥ 5%); amblyopia, deafness, ear disorder, tinnitus (1% to < 5%).

Miscellaneous – Abdomen enlarged, face edema, injection site inflammation, mucous membrane disorder (≥ 5%); accidental injury, allergic reaction, death, hypothermia, immune system disorder, injection site pain, injection site reaction, neck pain (1% to < 5%).

➤*AmBisome:* The following adverse reactions occurred in 2% to 10% of *AmBisome* patients receiving chemotherapy or bone marrow transplantation.

Cardiovascular – Arrhythmia, atrial fibrillation, bradycardia, cardiomegaly, hemorrhage, postural hypertension, valvular heart disease, vascular disorder, flushing.

CNS – Agitation, coma, convulsions, cough, depression, dysesthesia, dizziness, hallucinations, nervousness, paresthesia, somnolence, thinking abnormality, tremor.

Dermatologic – Alopecia, dry skin, herpes simplex, injection site inflammation, purpura, skin discoloration, skin disorder, skin ulcer, urticaria, vesiculobullous rash.

GI – Anorexia, constipation, dry mouth, dry nose, dyspepsia, dysphagia, eructation, fecal incontinence, flatulence, GI hemorrhage, hemor-

AMPHOTERICIN B, LIPID-BASED

rhoids, gum or oral hemorrhage, hematemesis, hepatocellular damage, hepatomegaly, mucositis, rectal disorder, stomatitis, ulcerative stomatitis, venoocclusive disease.

GU – Abnormal renal function, acute renal failure, dysuria, toxic nephropathy, urinary incontinence, vaginal hemorrhage.

Hematologic/Lymphatic – Coagulation disorder, ecchymosis, fluid overload, petechia, decreased prothrombin, increased prothrombin.

Metabolic/Nutritional – Acidosis, increased amylase, hyperchloremia, hyperkalemia, hypermagnesemia, hyperphosphatemia, hyponatremia, hypophosphatemia, hypoproteinemia, increased lactate dehydrogenase, increased nonprotein nitrogen, respiratory alkalosis.

Musculoskeletal – Arthralgia, bone pain, dystonia, myalgia, rigors.

Respiratory – Asthma, atelectasis, hemoptysis, hiccough, hyperventilation, influenza-like symptoms, lung edema, pharyngitis, pneumonia, sinusitis.

Special senses – Conjunctivitis, dry eyes, eye hemorrhage.

Miscellaneous – Abdomen enlarged, allergic reaction, cellulitis, cell-mediated immunological reaction, face edema, graft-vs-host disease, malaise, neck pain.

Postmarketing – The following have been reported during postmarketing surveillance: Angioedema, erythema, urticaria, cyanosis/hypoventilation, pulmonary edema, agranulocytosis, hemorrhagic cystitis.

Overdosage

➤*Symptoms:* Amphotericin B overdose has been reported to cause cardio-respiratory arrest. Amphotericin B lipid complex at doses of 7 to 13 mg/kg and repeated daily doses of liposomal amphotericin B up to 7.5 mg/kg have been administered without serious adverse reactions.

➤*Treatment:* If overdose is suspected, discontinue therapy, monitor clinical status, and administer supportive therapy. Refer to General Management of Acute Overdosage. Amphotericin B lipid complex and cholesteryl are not hemodialyzable.

NYSTATIN, ORAL

Rx	**Nystatin** (Various, eg, Major, Teva)	**Tablets:** 500,000 units	In 100s.
Rx	**Mycostatin** (Apothecon)		Lactose. (Squibb 580). Light brown, biconvex. Film-coated. In 100s.

For information on nystatin oral suspension and troches for the treatment of oral candidiasis, refer to the monograph in the Mouth and Throat Products section in the Gastrointestinal Agents chapter.

Indications

➤*Nonesophageal membrane GI candidiasis:* Treatment of nonesophageal membrane GI candidiasis.

Administration and Dosage

One to 2 tablets (500,000 to 1,000,000 units) 3 times daily. Continue treatment for ≥ 48 hours after clinical cure to prevent relapse.

Actions

➤*Pharmacology:* A polyene antibiotic with fungistatic and fungicidial activity, nystatin acts by binding to sterols in the cell membrane of susceptible *Candida* species with a resultant change in membrane permeability, allowing leakage of intracellular components. Nystatin exhibits no appreciable activity against bacteria, protozoa, or viruses.

➤*Pharmacokinetics:* GI absorption is insignificant. Most orally administered nystatin is passed unchanged in the stool. In patients with renal insufficiency receiving oral therapy with conventional dosage forms, significant plasma concentrations of nystatin may occasionally occur.

Contraindications

Hypersensitivity to nystatin or any of its components.

Warnings

➤*Pregnancy:* Category C. It is not known whether nystatin can cause fetal harm when administered to a pregnant woman or can affect reproduction capacity. Use only if potential benefits outweigh potential risks to the fetus.

➤*Lactation:* It is not known whether nystatin is excreted in breast milk. Exercise caution when administering nystatin to a nursing woman.

Adverse Reactions

Nystatin is well tolerated, even during prolonged administration.

➤*Dermatologic:* Rash, including urticaria, Stevens-Johnson syndrome (rare).

➤*GI:* Diarrhea (including 1 case of bloody diarrhea), nausea, vomiting, GI upset/disturbances.

➤*Miscellaneous:* Tachycardia, bronchospasm, facial swelling, and nonspecific myalgia (rare).

Overdosage

Oral doses > 5 million units have produced GI distress and nausea.

Patient Information

Continue therapy for ≥ 2 days after symptoms have resolved.

KETOCONAZOLE

Rx	**Ketoconazole** (Various, eg, Mutual, Mylan, Novopharm, Taro, Teva)	**Tablets**: 200 mg	In 30s, 50s, 100s, 250s, 500s, 1000s, blister packs of 10, and UD 30s, 50s, and 100s.
Rx	**Nizoral** (Janssen)		(Janssen/Nizoral). White, scored. In 100s.

For information on topical ketoconazole, refer to the individual monograph in the Dermatological Anti-infectives section.

> ### WARNING
>
> Ketoconazole has been associated with hepatic toxicity, including some fatalities. Closely monitor patients and inform them of the risk (see Warnings).

Indications

Treatment of the following systemic fungal infections: Candidiasis, chronic mucocutaneous candidiasis, oral thrush, candiduria, blastomycosis, coccidioidomycosis, histoplasmosis, chromomycosis, and paracoccidioidomycosis.

➤*Severe recalcitrant cutaneous dermatophyte infections:* Treatment of severe recalcitrant cutaneous dermatophyte infections not responding to topical therapy or oral griseofulvin or in patients unable to take griseofulvin.

Do not use ketoconazole tablets for fungal meningitis because it penetrates poorly into the CSF.

➤*Unlabeled uses:* Ketoconazole has been used successfully in the treatment of onychomycosis (caused by *Trichophyton* and *Candida* sp.); pityriasis versicolor (tinea versicolor); tinea pedis, corporis, and cruris (200 to 400 mg/day); tinea capitis (3.3 to 6.6 mg/kg/day); and vaginal candidiasis.

High-dose (800 to 1200 mg/day) ketoconazole has shown some success in treating CNS fungal infections.

Ketoconazole in doses of 400 mg every 8 hours has been used in the treatment of advanced prostate cancer (see Warnings).

Ketoconazole 800 to 1200 mg/day has been used to effectively treat Cushing's syndrome because of its ability to inhibit adrenal steroidogenesis.

Administration and Dosage

➤*Approved by the FDA:* December 31, 1985.

Prior to starting therapy, determine laboratory and clinical documentation of infection. Continue therapy until tests indicate that active fungal infection has subsided.

➤*Adults:* Initially, 200 mg once daily. In very serious infections, or if clinical response is insufficient, increase dose to 400 mg once daily.

➤*Children:*

(*> 2 years of age*) – 3.3 to 6.6 mg/kg/day as a single daily dose.

(*< 2 years of age*) – Daily dosage has not been established.

Inadequate treatment periods may yield poor response and lead to early recurrence of clinical symptoms. Minimum treatment for candidiasis is 1 or 2 weeks and 6 months for the other indicated systemic mycoses. Chronic mucocutaneous candidiasis usually requires maintenance therapy.

Minimum treatment of recalcitrant dermatophyte infections is 4 weeks in cases involving glabrous skin. Palmar and plantar infections may respond more slowly. Apparent cures may subsequently recur after discontinuation of therapy in some cases.

➤*Storage/Stability:* Store at 15° to 30°C (59° to 86°F). Protect from moisture.

Actions

➤*Pharmacology:* Ketoconazole, an imidazole broad-spectrum antifungal agent, impairs the synthesis of ergosterol, the main sterol of fungal cell membranes, allowing increased permeability and leakage of cellular components.

➤*Pharmacokinetics:*

Absorption/Distribution – Bioavailability depends on an acidic pH for dissolution and absorption (see Precautions). Mean peak plasma levels of 3.5 mcg/ml occur 1 to 2 hours after a 200 mg oral dose taken with a meal. Administration with food may decrease absorption. In vitro, plasma protein binding is ≈ 99%, mainly to albumin. At recommended doses, CSF penetration is negligible. Detectable concentrations are achieved in urine, saliva, sebum, and cerumen.

Metabolism/Excretion – The drug undergoes extensive hepatic metabolism to inactive metabolites. Plasma elimination is biphasic; half-life is 2 hours during the first 10 hours; 8 hours thereafter. The major excretory route is enterohepatic. Approximately 13% of the dose is excreted in the urine, of which 2% to 4% is unchanged drug. The major route of excretion is through the bile into the intestinal tract.

Renal failure does not alter ketoconazole dosing requirements; the drug does not appear to be dialyzable.

➤*Microbiology:* Active against clinical infections caused by *Blastomyces dermatitidis*, *Candida* sp., *Coccidioides immitis*, *Histoplasma capsulatum*, *Paracoccidioides brasiliensis*, *Phialophora* sp., *Trichophyton* sp., *Epidermophyton* sp., and *Microsporum* sp. In animals, activity has been demonstrated against *Malassezia furfur* and *Cryptococcus neoformans*.

Contraindications

Hypersensitivity to ketoconazole. Do not use for the treatment of fungal meningitis because of poor penetration into the CSF (see Unlabeled Uses).

Concomitant administration of ketoconazole with oral triazolam is contraindicated.

Warnings

➤*Hepatotoxicity:* Hepatotoxicity primarily of the hepatocellular type has been associated with ketoconazole including rare fatalities. The incidence has been ≈ 1:10,000 exposed patients, but this probably represents under-reporting. The median duration of therapy in patients who developed symptomatic hepatotoxicity was ≈ 28 days, although the range extended to as low as 3 days. The hepatic injury is usually reversible upon discontinuation of treatment. Several cases of hepatitis have occurred in children.

Prompt recognition of liver injury is essential. Measure liver function (eg, AST, ALT, alkaline phosphatase, bilirubin) before starting treatment and frequently during treatment. Carefully monitor patients receiving ketoconazole concurrently with other potentially hepatotoxic drugs, particularly those patients requiring prolonged therapy or those with a history of liver disease.

Most of the reported cases of hepatic toxicity have to date been in patients treated for onychomycosis. Of 180 patients worldwide developing idiosyncratic liver dysfunction during ketoconazole therapy, 61.3% had onychomycosis and 16.8% had chronic recalcitrant dermatophytoses.

Transient minor elevations in liver enzymes have occurred. Discontinue drug if these persist or worsen, or are accompanied by symptoms of possible liver injury.

➤*Prostatic cancer:* In clinical trials involving 350 patients with metastatic prostatic cancer, 11 deaths were reported within 2 weeks of starting high-dose ketoconazole (1200 mg/day). It is not known whether death was related to therapy. High ketoconazole doses are known to suppress adrenal corticosteroid secretion.

➤*Hypersensitivity reactions:* Anaphylaxis occurs rarely after the first dose. Hypersensitivity reactions, including urticaria, have been reported. Refer to Management of Acute Hypersensitivity Reactions.

➤*Pregnancy: Category C.* Teratogenic effects (syndactylia and oligodactylia), embryotoxic effects and dystocia have been seen in animals at 80 mg/kg/day (10 times the maximum recommended human dose). There are no adequate and well-controlled studies in pregnant women. Use only if the potential benefit justifies the potential risk to the fetus.

➤*Lactation:* Ketoconazole is excreted in breast milk. Administer to nursing mothers only if the potential benefits outweigh the potential risks to the infant.

➤*Children:* Safety for use in children < 2 years of age has not been established. Do not use in pediatric patients unless the potential benefits outweigh the risks.

Precautions

➤*Hormone levels:* Ketoconazole lowers serum testosterone. Testosterone levels are impaired with doses of 800 mg/day and abolished by 1600 mg/day. Once therapy has been discontinued, levels return to baseline values. It also decreases ACTH-induced corticosteroid serum levels at similar high doses. Closely follow the recommended dose of 200 to 400 mg/day.

➤*Gastric acidity:* Ketoconazole requires acidity for dissolution and absorption. If antacids, anticholinergics, or H₂ blockers are needed, give ≥ 2 hours after administration. With achlorhydria, dissolve each tablet in a 4 ml aqueous solution of 0.2 N HCl. Use a glass or plastic straw to avoid contact with teeth. Follow with a glass of water.

Drug Interactions

Ketoconazole is a potent inhibitor of the cytochrome P450 3A4 enzyme system. Coadministration of ketoconazole with other drugs metabolized by the same enzyme system may result in increased plasma concentrations of the drugs that could increase or prolong both therapeutic and adverse effects. Unless otherwise specified, dosage adjustment may be necessary.

KETOCONAZOLE

Ketoconazole Drug Interactions			
Precipitant drug	Object drug[*]		Description
Antacids	Ketoconazole	↓	Increased gastric pH may inhibit keto-conazole absorption. Consider giving antacids ≥ 2 hours after ketoconazole.
Didanosine	Ketoconazole	↓	The therapeutic effects of ketoconazole may be decreased. The buffers in didanosine chewable tablets decrease the absorption of ketoconazole.
Ketoconazole	Protease inhibitors Indinavir Ritonavir Saquinavir	↑	Plasma protease inhibitors concentrations may be elevated, increasing the risk of toxicity. Ketoconazole may inhibit the hepatic metabolism of protease inhibitors.
Ketoconazole	Tricyclic antidepressants	↑	Serum tricyclic antidepressant concentrations may be elevated, resulting in an increase in therapeutic and adverse effects.
Ketoconazole	Carbamazepine	↑	Plasma concentrations of carbamazepine may be elevated, increasing clinical and adverse effects. Ketoconazole may inhibit the metabolism of carbamazepine.
Sucralfate	Ketoconazole	↓	The therapeutic effects of ketoconazole may be reduced. The mechanism of action is unkown but likely because of a decrease in ketoconazole bioavailability. When clinical situation permits, administer ketoconazole ≥ 2 hours before sucralfate.
Proton pump inhibitors	Ketoconazole	↓	The effects of ketoconazole may be decreased. The bioavailability of ketoconazole may be decreased because of a possible reduction in tablet dissolution in the presence of a high gastric pH.
Ketoconazole	Quinidine	↑	Serum quinidine levels may be elevated, increasing therapeutic and toxic effects. Ketoconazole may inhibit quinidine metabolism.
Ketoconazole	Sulfonylureas	↑	Serum sulfonylurea concentrations may be elevated increasing the hypoglycemic effect.
Ketoconazole	Benzodiazepines	↑	Increased and prolonged serum levels, CNS depression, and psychomotor impairment with certain benzodiazepines are possible for several days after stopping ketoconazole. Concomitant administration of ketoconazole with oral triazolam is contraindicated.
Ketoconazole	Buspirone	↑	Plasma buspirone concentrations may be elevated, increasing pharmacologic and adverse effects.
Ketoconazole	Contraceptives, oral	↔	The therapeutic efficacy of oral contraceptives may be reduced. In addition, elevated ethinyl estradiol blood levels may occur. The mechanism of action is unknown. Inform women of the possible increased risk of oral contraceptive failure. Consider an alternative method of contraception.
Ketoconazole	Donepezil	↑	Donepezil plasma concentration and side effects may be increased.
Ketoconazole	HMG-CoA Reductase Inhibitors	↑	Increased plasma levels and side effects of HMG-CoA reductase inhibitors may occur. Rhabdomyolysis has been reported. If concurrent administration cannot be avoided, consider reducing the HMG-CoA reductase inhibitor dose.
Ketoconazole	Nisoldipine	↑	Nisoldipine concentrations may be elevated, increasing pharmacologic and adverse effects.

Ketoconazole Drug Interactions			
Precipitant drug	Object drug[*]		Description
Ketoconazole	Tacrolimus	↑	Plasma concentrations may be elevated, increasing the risk of toxicity because of inhibition of tacrolimus gut metabolism.
Ketoconazole	Vinca alkaloids	↑	Increased risk of vinca alkaloid toxicity has occurred because of inhibition of vinca alkaloid metabolism (CYP3A4) by ketoconazole.
Ketoconazole	Zolpidem	↑	Plasma concentrations and the therapeutic effects of zolpidem may be increased.
Histamine H$_2$ antagonists	Ketoconazole	↓	Increased gastric pH may inhibit ketoconazole absorption.
Isoniazid	Ketoconazole	↓	Bioavailability of ketoconazole may be decreased.
Rifampin	Ketoconazole	↓	Decreased serum levels of either drug may occur. Avoid concurrent use if possible.
Ketoconazole	Warfarin	↑	The anticoagulant response may be enhanced secondary to inhibition of warfarin metabolism.
Ketoconazole	Corticosteroids	↑	Corticosteroid bioavailability may be increased and clearance may be decreased, possibly resulting in toxicity.
Ketoconazole	Cyclosporine	↑	Increased cyclosporine concentrations may occur because of inhibition of metabolism, resulting in toxicity. Because the effect on cyclosporine levels is consistent and predictable, this interaction has been used beneficially to decrease cyclosporine dosage in some patients.
Ketoconazole	Theophyllines	↓	Decreased absorption of theophylline may occur, resulting in decreased theophylline serum levels.

[*] ↑ = Object drug increased   ↓ = Object drug decreased   ↔ = Undertermined clinical effect

Adverse Reactions

Most reactions are mild, transient, and rarely require discontinuation. In contrast, the rare occurrences of hepatic dysfunction require special attention.

➤*CNS:* Headache, dizziness, somnolence, photophobia (< 1%).

➤*GI:* Nausea/vomiting (3% to 10%); abdominal pain (1.2%); diarrhea (< 1%); hepatotoxicity.

➤*Psychiatric:* Suicidal tendencies, severe depression (rare).

➤*Miscellaneous:* Pruritus (1.5%); fever, chills, impotence, gynecomastia, thrombocytopenia, leukopenia, hemolytic anemia, bulging fontanelles, impotence (< 1%). Hypersensitivity including urticaria (see Warnings). Oligospermia has occurred at dosages above those approved but not at dosages ≤ 400 mg/day; sperm counts were obtained infrequently at these dosages.

Overdosage

Institute supportive measures, including gastric lavage with sodium bicarbonate. Refer to General Management of Acute Overdosage.

Patient Information

Do not take with antacids; if antacids are required, delay administration by 2 hours.

May produce headache and dizziness.

Notify physician of any signs or symptoms suggesting liver dysfunction (eg, unusual fatigue, anorexia, nausea, vomiting, jaundice, dark urine, pale stools), or if abdominal pain, fever, or diarrhea become pronounced.

VORICONAZOLE

Rx	Vfend (Roerig)	**Tablets:** 50 mg	Lactose. (Pfizer VOR50). White. Film-coated. In 30s.
		200 mg	Lactose. (Pfizer VOR200). White, capsule shape. Film-coated. In 30s.
		Powder for injection, lyophilized:[a] 200 mg	Preservative-free. In single-use vials.
		Powder for oral suspension: 45 g (40 mg/mL after reconstitution)	Sucrose. Orange flavor. In 100 mL high density polyethylene bottles w/ a 5 mL oral dispenser and a press-in bottle adaptor.

[a] Contains IV vehicle of 3200 mg sulfobutyl ether beta-cyclodextrin sodium (SBECD).

Indications

➤*Esophageal candidiasis:* For the treatment of esophageal candidiasis.

➤*Invasive aspergillosis:* For the treatment of invasive aspergillosis. In clinical trials, the majority of isolates recovered were *Aspergillus fumigatus*. There were a small number of cases of culture-proven disease caused by species of *Aspergillus* other than *A. fumigatus*.

➤*Serious fungal infections:* For the treatment of serious fungal infections caused by *Scedosporium apiospermum* (asexual form of *Pseudallescheria boydii*) and *Fusarium* sp. including *Fusarium solani*, in patients intolerant of, or refractory to, other therapy.

Administration and Dosage

➤*Approved by the FDA:* May 28, 2002.

Correct electrolyte disturbances (eg, hypokalemia, hypomagnesemia, hypocalcemia) prior to initiation of voriconazole therapy.

➤*Invasive aspergillosis and serious fungal infections:* Initiate therapy with the specified loading dose regimen of IV voriconazole to achieve plasma concentrations on day 1 that are close to steady state. On the basis of high oral bioavailability, switching between IV and oral administration is appropriate when clinically indicated. Base duration of therapy on the severity of the patient's underlying disease, recovery from immunosuppression, and clinical response.

For the treatment of adults with invasive aspergillosis and infections caused by *Fusarium* sp. and *S. apiospermum*, the recommended dosing regimen of voriconazole is as follows: Loading dose of 6 mg/kg IV every 12 hours for 2 doses, followed by a maintenance dose of 4 mg/kg IV every 12 hours.

Once the patient can tolerate medication given by mouth, the tablet form or oral suspension of voriconazole may be used. Give patients who weigh more than 40 kg an oral maintenance dose of 200 mg voriconazole every 12 hours. Give adult patients who weigh less than 40 kg an oral maintenance dose of 100 mg every 12 hours.

Dosage adjustment – If patient response is inadequate, the oral maintenance dose may be increased from 200 mg every 12 hours to 300 mg every 12 hours. For adult patients weighing less than 40 kg, the oral maintenance dose may be increased from 100 mg every 12 hours to 150 mg every 12 hours.

If patients are unable to tolerate treatment, reduce the IV maintenance dose to 3 mg/kg every 12 hours and the oral maintenance dose by 50 mg steps to a minimum of 200 mg every 12 hours (or to 100 mg every 12 hours for adult patients weighing less than 40 kg).

➤*Esophageal candidiasis (oral only):* Recommended dosing regimen is an oral dose of 200 mg every 12 hours for patients who weigh 40 kg or more. Adult patients who weigh less than 40 kg should receive an oral dose of 100 mg every 12 hours. Treat patients for a minimum of 14 days and for at least 7 days following resolution of symptoms.

➤*Coadministration with phenytoin:* Phenytoin may be coadministered with voriconazole if the maintenance dose of voriconazole is increased to 5 mg/kg IV every 12 hours, or from 200 to 400 mg every 12 hours orally (100 to 200 mg every 12 hours orally in adult patients weighing less than 40 kg).

➤*Hepatic function impairment:* In the clinical program, patients were included who had baseline liver function tests (ALT, AST) up to 5 times the upper limit of normal. No dose adjustment is necessary in patients with this degree of abnormal liver function, but continued monitoring of liver function tests for further elevations is recommended (see Warnings).

It is recommended that the standard loading dose regimens be used but that the maintenance dose be halved in patients with mild to moderate hepatic cirrhosis (Child-Pugh class A and B).

➤*Renal function impairment:*

Oral – No adjustment is necessary for oral dosing in patients with mild to severe renal impairment.

IV – In patients with moderate or severe renal insufficiency (Ccr below 50 mL/min), accumulation of the IV vehicle, SBECD, occurs. Administer oral voriconazole to these patients, unless an assessment of the benefit/risk to the patient justifies the use of IV voriconazole. Closely monitor serum creatinine levels in these patients, and, if increases occur, consider changing to oral voriconazole therapy.

➤*IV administration:* Voriconazole IV for injection requires reconstitution to 10 mg/mL and subsequent dilution to 5 mg/mL or less prior to administration as an infusion. Infuse at a maximum rate of 3 mg/kg/h over 1 to 2 hours. Not for IV bolus injection.

Reconstitution – The powder is reconstituted with 19 mL of water for injection to obtain an extractable volume of 20 mL of clear concentrate containing 10 mg/mL of voriconazole. Use of a standard 20 mL (nonautomated) syringe is recommended to ensure that the exact amount (19 mL) of water for injection is dispensed. Discard the vial if a vacuum does not pull the diluent into the vial. Shake the vial until all of the powder is dissolved.

Dilution – Voriconazole must be infused over 1 to 2 hours at a concentration of 5 mg/mL or less. Therefore, further dilute the required volume of the 10 mg/mL voriconazole concentrate as follows (appropriate diluents listed below):

1.) Calculate the volume of 10 mg/mL voriconazole concentrate required based on the patient's weight (see following table).
2.) In order to allow the required volume of voriconazole to be added, withdraw and discard at least an equal volume of diluent from the infusion bag or bottle. The volume of diluent remaining in the bag or bottle should be such that when the 10 mg/mL voriconazole concentrate is added, the final concentration is not less than 0.5 mg/mL nor greater than 5 mg/mL.
3.) Using a suitable size syringe and aseptic technique, withdraw the required volume of voriconazole concentrate from the appropriate number of vials and add to the infusion bag or bottle. Discard partially used vials.

The final voriconazole solution must be infused over 1 to 2 hours at a maximum rate of 3 mg/kg/h.

Required Volumes of 10 mg/mL Voriconazole Concentrate			
Body weight (kg)	Volume of voriconazole concentrate (10 mg/mL) required:		
	3 mg/kg dose (number of vials)	4 mg/kg dose (number of vials)	6 mg/kg dose (number of vials)
30	9 mL (1)	12 mL (1)	18 mL (1)
35	10.5 mL (1)	14 mL (1)	21 mL (2)
40	12 mL (1)	16 mL (1)	24 mL (2)
45	13.5 mL (1)	18 mL (1)	27 mL (2)
50	15 mL (1)	20 mL (1)	30 mL (2)
55	16.5 mL (1)	22 mL (2)	33 mL (2)
60	18 mL (1)	24 mL (2)	36 mL (2)
65	19.5 mL (1)	26 mL (2)	39 mL (2)
70	21 mL (2)	28 mL (2)	42 mL (3)
75	22.5 mL (2)	30 mL (2)	45 mL (3)
80	24 mL (2)	32 mL (2)	48 mL (3)
85	25.5 mL (2)	34 mL (2)	51 mL (3)
90	27 mL (2)	36 mL (2)	54 mL (3)
95	28.5 mL (2)	38 mL (2)	57 mL (3)
100	30 mL (2)	40 mL (2)	60 mL (3)

The reconstituted solution can be diluted with the following: 0.9% sodium chloride, lactated Ringer's, 5% dextrose and lactated Ringer's, 5% dextrose and 0.45% sodium chloride, 5% dextrose, 5% dextrose and 20 mEq potassium chloride, 0.45% sodium chloride, 5% dextrose and 0.9% sodium chloride.

➤*Admixture incompatibilities:* Voriconazole IV must not be infused into the same line or cannula concomitantly with other drug infusions, including parenteral nutrition (eg, *Aminofusin 10% Plus*). *Aminofusin 10% Plus* is physically incompatible, with an increase in subvisible particulate matter after 24 hours storage at 4°C (39°F).

Infusions of blood products must not occur simultaneously with voriconazole IV.

Infusions of total parenteral nutrition may occur simultaneously with voriconazole IV.

Voriconazole IV must not be diluted with 4.2% sodium bicarbonate infusion. The mildly alkaline nature of this diluent caused slight degradation of voriconazole after 24 hours storage at room temperature. Although refrigerated storage is recommended following reconstitution, use of this diluent is not recommended as a precautionary measure. Compatibility with other concentrations is unknown.

➤*Oral administration:* Take voriconazole tablets or oral suspension at least 1 hour before or 1 hour following a meal.

VORICONAZOLE

Reconstitution of oral suspension – Tap the bottle to release the powder. Add 46 mL of water to the bottle. Shake the closed bottle vigorously for about 1 minute. Remove the child-resistant cap, and push the bottle adaptor into the neck of the bottle. Replace the cap. Write the date of expiration of the reconstituted suspension on the bottle label (the shelf-life of the reconstituted suspension is 14 days at controlled room temperature 15° to 30°C [59° to 86°F]).

Instructions for use – Shake the closed bottle of reconstituted suspension for approximately 10 seconds before each use. Administer the reconstituted oral suspension only using the oral dispenser supplied with each pack.

Incompatibilities – Do not mix voriconazole for oral suspension and the 40 mg/mL reconstituted oral suspension with any other medication or additional flavoring agent. It is not intended that the suspension be further diluted with water or other vehicles.

➤*Storage/Stability:* Store tablets and powder for injection at 15° to 30°C (59° to 86°F).

Voriconazole for injection is a single-dose, unpreserved, sterile lyophile. Use product immediately following reconstitution. If not used immediately, in-use storage times should not be longer than 24 hours at 2° to 8°C (37° to 46°F). Discard any unused solution. Use only clear solutions without particles.

Store voriconazole powder for oral suspension at 2° to 8°C (37° to 46°F) (in a refrigerator) before reconstitution. The shelf-life of the powder for oral suspension is 18 months. Store the reconstituted suspension at 15° to 30°C (59° to 86°F). Do not refrigerate or freeze. Keep the container tightly closed. The shelf-life of the reconstituted suspension is 14 days. Discard any remaining suspension 14 days after reconstitution.

Actions

➤*Pharmacology:* Voriconazole is a triazole antifungal agent. The primary mode of action of voriconazole is the inhibition of fungal cytochrome P450-mediated 14 alpha-lanosterol demethylation, an essential step in fungal ergosterol biosynthesis. The accumulation of 14 alpha-methyl sterols correlates with the subsequent loss of ergosterol in the fungal cell wall and may be responsible for the antifungal activity of voriconazole. Voriconazole has been shown to be more selective for fungal cytochrome P450 enzymes than for various mammalian cytochrome P450 enzyme systems.

➤*Pharmacokinetics:*

Absorption – The pharmacokinetic properties of voriconazole are similar following administration by the IV and oral routes. Based on a population pharmacokinetic analysis of pooled data in healthy subjects (N = 207), the oral bioavailability of voriconazole is estimated to be 96% (CV 13%). Bioequivalence was established between the 200 mg tablet and the 40 mg/mL oral suspension when administered as a 400 mg loading dose every 12 hours followed by a 200 mg maintenance dose every 12 hours. Maximum plasma concentration (C_{max}) is achieved 1 to 2 hours after dosing.

The pharmacokinetics of voriconazole are nonlinear because of the saturation of its metabolism. The interindividual variability of voriconazole pharmacokinetics is high. Greater than proportional increase in exposure is observed with increasing dose. On average, it is estimated that increasing the oral dose in healthy subjects from 200 mg every 12 hours to 300 mg every 12 hours leads to a 2.5-fold increase in exposure (AUC), while increasing the IV dose from 3 mg/kg every 12 hours to 4 mg/kg every 12 hours produces a 2.3-fold increase in exposure (see the following table).

Population Pharmacokinetic Parameters of Voriconazole in Volunteers				
	200 mg oral q 12 h	300 mg oral q 12 h	3 mg/kg IV q 12 h	4 mg/kg IV q 12 h
AUC[a] (mcg•h/mL) (CV%)	19.86 (94%)	50.32 (74%)	21.81 (100%)	50.4 (83%)

[a] Mean AUC values are predicted from population pharmacokinetic analysis of data from 236 volunteers.

When the recommended IV or oral loading dose regimens are administered to healthy subjects, peak plasma concentrations close to steady state are achieved within the first 24 hours of dosing. Without the loading dose, accumulation occurs during twice-daily multiple dosing with steady-state peak plasma voriconazole concentrations being achieved by day 6 in the majority of subjects (see the following table).

Pharmacokinetic Parameters of Voriconazole from Loading Dose and Maintenance Dose Regimens (Individual Studies in Volunteers)				
	400 mg q 12 h on day 1, 200 mg q 12 h on days 2 through 10 (n = 17)		6 mg/kg IV[a] q 12 h on day 1, 3 mg/kg IV q 12 h on days 2 through 10 (n = 9)	
	Day 1, first dose	Day 10	Day 1, first dose	Day 10
AUC[b] (mcg•h/mL) (CV%)	9.31 (38%)	11.13 (103%)	13.22 (22%)	13.25 (58%)
C_{max} (mcg/mL) (CV%)	2.3 (19%)	2.08 (62%)	4.7 (22%)	3.06 (31%)

[a] IV infusion over 60 minutes.
[b] AUC values are calculated over dosing interval of 12 hours. Pharmacokinetic parameters for loading and maintenance doses summarized for same cohort of volunteers.

Steady-state trough plasma concentrations with voriconazole are achieved after approximately 5 days of oral or IV dosing without a loading dose regimen. However, when an IV loading dose regimen is used, steady-state trough plasma concentrations are achieved within 1 day.

Distribution – The volume of distribution at steady state for voriconazole is estimated to be 4.6 L/kg, suggesting extensive distribution into tissues. Plasma protein binding is estimated to be 58% and was shown to be independent of plasma concentrations achieved following single and multiple oral doses of 200 or 300 mg (approximate range, 0.9 to 15 mcg/mL). Varying degrees of hepatic and renal insufficiency do not affect the protein binding of voriconazole.

Metabolism – In vitro studies showed that voriconazole is metabolized by the human hepatic cytochrome P450 enzymes CYP2C19, CYP2C9, and CYP3A4. In vivo studies indicated that CYP2C19 is significantly involved in the metabolism of voriconazole. The major metabolite of voriconazole is the N-oxide, which accounts for 72% of the circulating radiolabeled metabolites in plasma. Because the metabolite has minimal antifungal activity, it does not contribute to the overall efficacy of voriconazole.

Excretion – Voriconazole is eliminated via hepatic metabolism with less than 2% of the dose excreted unchanged in the urine. After administration of a single radiolabeled dose of oral or IV voriconazole, preceded by multiple oral or IV dosing, approximately 80% to 83% of the radioactivity is recovered in the urine. The majority (more than 94%) of the total radioactivity is excreted in the first 96 hours after oral and IV dosing. As a result of nonlinear pharmacokinetics, the terminal half-life of voriconazole is dose dependent and therefore not useful in predicting the accumulation or elimination of voriconazole.

Special populations:

Race: CYP2C19 exhibits genetic polymorphism. For example, 15% to 20% of Asian populations may be expected to be poor metabolizers. For Caucasians and Blacks, the prevalence of poor metabolizers is 3% to 5%. Studies conducted in healthy Caucasian and Japanese subjects have shown that poor metabolizers have, on average, a 4-fold higher voriconazole exposure (AUC) than their homozygous extensive metabolizer counterparts. Subjects who are heterozygous extensive metabolizers have, on average, a 2-fold higher voriconazole exposure than their homozygous extensive metabolizer counterparts.

Gender: In a multiple oral dose study, the mean C_{max} and AUC for healthy young females were 83% and 113% higher, respectively, than in healthy young males (18 to 45 years of age) after tablet dosing. In a similar study, after dosing with the oral suspension, the mean AUC for healthy young females was 45% higher than in healthy young males, whereas the mean C_{max} was comparable between genders. The steady state trough voriconazole concentrations (C_{min}) seen in females were 100% and 91% higher than in males receiving the tablet and the oral suspension, respectively. No dosage adjustment based on gender is necessary.

Elderly: In an oral, multiple-dose study, the mean C_{max} and AUC in healthy elderly males (65 years of age and older) were 61% and 86% higher, respectively, than in young males (18 to 45 years of age). No significant differences in the mean C_{max} and AUC were observed between healthy elderly females (65 years of age and older) and healthy young females (18 to 45 years of age). No dosage adjustment is necessary for the elderly.

Hepatic function impairment: After a single oral dose (200 mg) of voriconazole in 8 patients with mild (Child-Pugh class A) and 4 patients with moderate (Child-Pugh class B) hepatic insufficiency, the mean systemic exposure (AUC) was 3.2-fold higher than in age and weight matched controls with normal hepatic function. There was no difference in mean C_{max} between the groups. When only the patients with mild (Child-Pugh class A) hepatic insufficiency were compared with controls, there was still a 2.3-fold increase in the mean AUC in the group with hepatic insufficiency compared with controls.

VORICONAZOLE

It is recommended that the standard loading dose regimens be used but that the maintenance dose be halved in patients with mild to moderate hepatic cirrhosis (Child-Pugh class A and B) receiving voriconazole. No pharmacokinetic data are available for patients with severe hepatic cirrhosis (Child-Pugh class C) (see Administration and Dosage).

Renal function impairment: In patients with moderate renal dysfunction (Ccr 30 to 50 mL/min), accumulation of the IV vehicle, SBECD, occurs. The mean AUC and C_{max} of SBECD were increased by 4-fold and almost 50%, respectively, in the moderately impaired group compared with the normal control group.

Avoid IV voriconazole in patients with moderate or severe renal impairment (Ccr below 50 mL/min), unless an assessment of the benefit/risk to the patient justifies the use of IV voriconazole (see Administration and Dosage).

A pharmacokinetic study in subjects with renal failure undergoing hemodialysis showed that voriconazole is dialyzed with clearance of 121 mL/min. The IV vehicle, SBECD, is hemodialyzed with clearance of 55 mL/min. A 4-hour hemodialysis session does not remove a sufficient amount of voriconazole to warrant dose adjustment.

➤*Microbiology:* Voriconazole has demonstrated in vitro activity against *Aspergillus* sp. (*A. fumigatus, A. flavus, A. niger, A. terreus*), *Candida* sp. (*C. albicans, C. glabrata, C. krusei*), *Scedosporium apiospermum*, and *Fusarium* sp., including *F. solani*.

Cross-resistance: Fungal isolates exhibiting reduced susceptibility to fluconazole or itraconazole also may show reduced susceptibility to voriconazole, suggesting that cross-resistance can occur among these azoles. The relevance of cross-resistance and clinical outcome has not been fully characterized. Clinical cases where azole cross-resistance is demonstrated may require alternative antifungal therapy.

➤*Clinical trials:*

Invasive aspergillosis – The efficacy of voriconazole compared with amphotericin B in the primary treatment of acute invasive aspergillosis was demonstrated in 277 patients treated for 12 weeks. The majority of study patients had underlying hematologic malignancies, including bone marrow transplantation. The study also included patients with solid organ transplantation, solid tumors, and AIDS. The patients were mainly treated for definite or probable invasive aspergillosis of the lungs. Other aspergillosis infections included disseminated disease, CNS infections, and sinus infections.

Voriconazole was administered IV with a loading dose of 6 mg/kg every 12 hours for the first 24 hours, followed by a maintenance dose of 4 mg/kg every 12 hours for a minimum of 7 days. Therapy could then be switched to the oral formulation at a dose of 200 mg every 12 hours. Median duration of IV voriconazole therapy was 10 days (range, 2 to 90 days). After IV voriconazole therapy, the median duration of oral voriconazole therapy was 76 days (range, 2 to 232 days).

Patients in the comparator group received conventional amphotericin B as a slow infusion at a daily dose of 1 to 1.5 mg/kg/day. Median duration of IV amphotericin therapy was 12 days (range, 1 to 85 days). Treatment was then continued with other licensed antifungal therapy (OLAT), including itraconazole and lipid amphotericin B formulations. Although initial therapy with conventional amphotericin B was to be continued for at least 2 weeks, actual duration of therapy was at the discretion of the investigator.

A satisfactory global response at 12 weeks (complete or partial resolution of all attributable symptoms, signs, radiographic/bronchoscopic abnormalities present at baseline) was seen in 53% of voriconazole-treated patients compared with 32% of amphotericin B-treated patients. A benefit of voriconazole compared with amphotericin B on patient survival at day 84 was seen with a 71% survival rate on voriconazole compared with 58% on amphotericin B.

Esophageal candidiasis – The efficacy of 200 mg oral voriconazole twice daily compared with 200 mg/day oral fluconazole in the primary treatment of esophageal candidiasis was demonstrated in a study in immunocompromised patients with endoscopically proven esophageal candidiasis. Patients were treated for a median of 15 days (range, 1 to 49 days). Outcome was assessed by repeat endoscopy at end of treatment (EOT). A successful response was defined as a normal endoscopy at EOT or at least a 1 grade improvement over baseline endoscopic score. For patients in the intent-to-treat (ITT) population with only a baseline endoscopy, a successful response was defined as symptomatic cure or improvement at EOT compared with baseline. Voriconazole and fluconazole (200 mg/day) showed comparable efficacy rates against esophageal candidiasis, as presented in the following table.

Success Rates In Patients Treated for Esophageal Candidiasis			
Population	Voriconazole	Fluconazole	Difference % (95% CI)[a]
PP[b]	98.2%	95%	3.2 (−1.1, 7.5)
ITT[c]	87.5%	89.5%	−2 (−8.3, 4.3)

[a] Confidence Interval for the difference (Voriconazole − Fluconazole) in success rates.
[b] PP (Per Protocol) patients had confirmation of *Candida* esophagitis by endoscopy, received at least 12 days of treatment, and had a repeat endoscopy at EOT.
[c] ITT patients without endoscopy or clinical assessment at EOT were treated as failures.

Known hypersensitivity to voriconazole or its excipients. Use caution when prescribing voriconazole to patients with hypersensitivity to other azoles.

Coadministration of the CYP3A4 substrates, cisapride, pimozide, or quinidine with voriconazole is contraindicated because increased plasma concentrations of these drugs can lead to QT prolongation and rare occurrences of torsades de pointes.

Coadministration of voriconazole with sirolimus, rifampin, carbamazepine, long-acting barbiturates, rifabutin, ergot alkaloids (ergotamine and dihydroergotamine), ritonavir (400 mg every 12 hours), or efavirenz.

Warnings

➤*Visual disturbances:* If treatment continues beyond 28 days, the effect of voriconazole on visual function is not known. If treatment continues beyond 28 days, monitor visual function including visual acuity, visual field, and color perception.

The mechanism of action of the visual disturbance is unknown, although the site of action is most likely to be within the retina. In a study of healthy volunteers investigating the effect of 28-day treatment with voriconazole on retinal function, voriconazole caused a decrease in the electroretinogram (ERG) waveform amplitude, a decrease in the visual field, and an alteration in color perception. The ERG measures electrical currents in the retina. The effects were noted early in administration of voriconazole and continued through the course of study drug dosing. Fourteen days after end of dosing, ERG, visual fields, and color perception returned to normal.

➤*Hepatic toxicity:* In clinical trials, there have been uncommon cases of serious hepatic reactions during treatment with voriconazole (eg, clinical hepatitis, cholestasis, and fulminant hepatic failure, including fatalities). Instances of hepatic reactions were noted to occur primarily in patients with serious underlying medical conditions (predominantly hematological malignancy). Hepatic reactions, including hepatitis and jaundice, have occurred among patients with no other identifiable risk factors. Liver dysfunction usually has been reversible on discontinuation of therapy.

Evaluate liver function tests at the start of and during the course of voriconazole therapy. Monitor patients who develop abnormal liver function tests during voriconazole therapy for the development of more severe hepatic injury. Patient management should include laboratory evaluation of hepatic function (particularly liver function tests and bilirubin). Discontinuation of voriconazole must be considered if clinical signs and symptoms consistent with liver disease develop that may be attributable to voriconazole.

➤*Hepatic function impairment:* It is recommended that the standard loading dose regimens be used but that the maintenance dose be halved in patients with mild to moderate hepatic cirrhosis (Child-Pugh class A and B) receiving voriconazole.

Voriconazole has not been studied in patients with severe cirrhosis (Child-Pugh class C). Voriconazole has been associated with elevations in liver function tests and clinical signs of liver damage, such as jaundice, and only should be used in patients with severe hepatic insufficiency if the benefit outweighs the potential risk. Patients with hepatic insufficiency must be monitored carefully for drug toxicity.

➤*Renal function impairment:* In patients with moderate to severe renal dysfunction (Ccr below 50 mL/min), accumulation of the IV vehicle, SBECD, occurs. Administer oral voriconazole to these patients unless an assessment of the benefit/risk to the patient justifies the use of IV voriconazole. Closely monitor serum creatinine levels in these patients, and if increases occur, consider changing to oral voriconazole therapy.

➤*Galactose intolerance:* Voriconazole tablets contain lactose and should not be given to patients with rare hereditary problems of galactose intolerance, Lapp lactase deficiency, or glucose-galactose malabsorption.

➤*Carcinogenesis:* Two-year carcinogenicity studies were conducted in rats and mice. Rats were given oral doses of 6, 18, or 50 mg/kg voriconazole, or 0.2, 0.6, or 1.6 times the recommended maintenance dose (RMD) on a mg/m² basis. Hepatocellular adenomas were detected in females at 50 mg/kg and hepatocellular carcinomas were found in males at 6 and 50 mg/kg. Mice were given oral doses of 10, 30, or 100 mg/kg voriconazole, or 0.1, 0.4, or 1.4 times the RMD on a mg/m² basis. In mice, hepatocellular adenomas were detected in males and females and hepatocellular carcinomas were detected in males at 1.4 times the RMD of voriconazole.

➤*Mutagenesis:* Voriconazole demonstrated clastogenic activity (mostly chromosome breaks) in human lymphocyte cultures in vitro.

➤*Fertility impairment:* Voriconazole produced a reduction in the pregnancy rates of rats dosed at 50 mg/kg, or 1.6 times the RMD. This was statistically significant only in the preliminary study and not in a larger fertility study.

➤*Elderly:* The AUC and C_{max} were increased in elderly males compared with young males. Voriconazole plasma concentrations in the eld-

VORICONAZOLE

erly patients were approximately 80% to 90% higher than those in younger patients after either IV or oral administration. However, the overall safety profile of the elderly patients was similar to that of the young, so no dosage adjustment is recommended.

➤*Pregnancy: Category D.* Voriconazole can cause fetal harm when administered to pregnant women.

Voriconazole was teratogenic in rats (ie, cleft palates, hydronephrosis/hydroureter) from 10 mg/kg (0.3 times the RMD on a mg/m² basis) and embryotoxic in rabbits at 100 mg/kg (6 times the RMD). Other effects in rats included reduced ossification of sacral and caudal vertebrae, skull, pubic and hyoid bone, super numerary ribs, anomalies of the sternebrae, and dilation of the ureter/renal pelvis. Plasma estradiol in pregnant rats was reduced at all dose levels. Voriconazole treatment in rats produced increased gestation length and dystocia, which were associated with increased perinatal pup mortality at the 10 mg/kg dose. The effects seen in rabbits were increased embryomortality, reduced fetal weight, and increased incidence of skeletal variations, cervical ribs, and extra sternebral ossification sites.

If this drug is used during pregnancy, or if the patient becomes pregnant while taking this drug, apprise the patient of the potential hazard to the fetus. Women of childbearing potential should use effective contraception during treatment.

➤*Lactation:* The excretion of voriconazole in breast milk has not been investigated. Voriconazole should not be used by nursing mothers unless the benefit clearly outweighs the risk.

➤*Children:* Safety and effectiveness in pediatric patients under 12 years of age have not been established.

Precautions

➤*Monitoring:* Patient management should include laboratory evaluation of renal (particularly serum creatinine) and hepatic function (particularly liver function tests and bilirubin).

Evaluate liver function tests at the start of and during the course of voriconazole therapy. Monitor patients who develop abnormal liver function tests during voriconazole therapy for the development of more severe hepatic injury.

Correct electrolyte disturbances (eg, hypokalemia, hypomagnesemia, hypocalcemia) prior to initiation of voriconazole therapy.

➤*Cardiovascular:* Some azoles, including voriconazole, have been associated with prolongation of the QT interval on the electrocardiogram. During clinical development and postmarketing surveillance, there have been rare cases of torsades de pointes in patients taking voriconazole. These reports involved seriously ill patients with multiple confounding risk factors such as history of cardiotoxic chemotherapy, cardiomyopathy, hypokalemia, and concomitant medications that may have been contributory.

Administer voriconazole with caution to patients with these potentially proarrhythmic conditions.

Before starting voriconazole, make rigorous attempts to correct potassium, magnesium, and calcium.

➤*Infusion-related reactions:* During infusion of the IV formulation of voriconazole in healthy subjects, anaphylactoid-type reactions, including flushing, fever, sweating, tachycardia, chest tightness, dyspnea, faintness, nausea, pruritus, and rash, have occurred uncommonly. Symptoms appeared immediately upon initiating the infusion. Consider stopping the infusion if these reactions occur.

➤*Renal toxicity:* Acute renal failure has been observed in severely ill patients undergoing treatment with voriconazole. Patients being treated with voriconazole are likely to be treated concomitantly with nephrotoxic medications and have concurrent conditions that may result in decreased renal function.

Monitor patients for the development of abnormal renal function. This should include laboratory evaluation, particularly serum creatinine.

➤*Dermatological reactions:* Patients have rarely developed serious cutaneous reactions, such as Stevens-Johnson syndrome, during treatment with voriconazole. If patients develop a rash, monitor them closely and consider discontinuing voriconazole. Voriconazole has been infrequently associated with photosensitivity skin reaction, especially during long-term therapy. It is recommended that patients avoid strong, direct sunlight during voriconazole therapy.

Drug Interactions

➤*CYP450:* Voriconazole is metabolized by CYP2C19, CYP2C9, and CYP3A4. The affinity of voriconazole is highest for CYP2C19, followed by CYP2C9, and is appreciably lower for CYP3A4. Inhibitors or inducers of these 3 enzymes may increase or decrease voriconazole systemic exposure (plasma concentrations), respectively.

Voriconazole inhibits the metabolic activity of CYP2C19, CYP2C9, and CYP3A4. The inhibition potency of voriconazole for CYP3A4 was significantly less than that of 2 other azoles, ketoconazole and itracona-

zole. The major metabolite of voriconazole, the voriconazole N-oxide, inhibits the metabolic activity of CYP2C9 and CYP3A4 to a greater extent than that of CYP2C19. There is potential for voriconazole and its major metabolite to increase the systemic exposure (plasma concentration) of other drugs metabolized by these CYP450 enzymes.

Voriconazole Drug Interactions			
Precipitant drug	Object drug*		Description
Barbiturates, long acting Carbamazepine	Voriconazole	↓	Coadministration may decrease voriconazole plasma concentrations caused by CYP450 induction. Coadministration is contraindicated.
Cimetidine	Voriconazole	↑	Cimetidine increased voriconazole C$_{max}$ and AUC by an average of 18% and 23%, respectively. No dosage adjustment is required.
Nonnucleoside reverse transcriptase inhibitors (NNRTIs) (ie, delavirdine, nevirapine)	Voriconazole	↑↓	Coadministration may induce or inhibit the metabolism of voriconazole. Monitor for toxicity and effectiveness of voriconazole. Voriconazole also may inhibit the metabolism of an NNRTI. Monitor for drug toxicity. Coadministration with efavirenz is contraindicated.
Voriconazole	NNRTIs (ie, delavirdine, efavirenz)	↑	
Phenytoin	Voriconazole	↓	Phenytoin may decrease the C$_{max}$ and AUC of voriconazole by 50% and 70%, respectively (see Administration and Dosage for dosing recommendations). Voriconazole may increase the C$_{max}$ and AUC of phenytoin up to 2 times. Monitor for adverse reactions and phenytoin plasma concentrations.
Voriconazole	Phenytoin	↑	
Protease inhibitors (ie, ritonavir, saquinavir, amprenavir, nelfinavir)	Voriconazole	↓	Voriconazole may inhibit the metabolism of protease inhibitors, and the metabolism of voriconazole may be inhibited or induced by protease inhibitors. Monitor closely for toxicity. Coadministration with indinavir showed no significant effects on voriconazole or indinavir exposure. Ritonavir decreased voriconazole AUC and C$_{max}$ by approximately 82% and 66%, respectively. Coadministration with ritonavir (400 mg every 12 hours) is contraindicated.
Voriconazole	Protease inhibitors (ie, ritonavir, saquinavir, amprenavir, nelfinavir)	↑	
Proton pump inhibitors (ie, omeprazole)	Voriconazole	↑	Omeprazole may increase the C$_{max}$ and AUC of voriconazole by an average of 15% and 40%, respectively. No dosage adjustment of voriconazole is recommended. Voriconazole may increase the C$_{max}$ and AUC of omeprazole by an average of 2 and 4 times, respectively. When initiating voriconazole in patients already receiving omeprazole doses of 40 mg or greater, reduce the dose of omeprazole by 50%. Voriconazole also may inhibit the metabolism of other proton pump inhibitors that are CYP2C19 substrates.
Voriconazole	Proton pump inhibitors (ie, omeprazole)		
Rifampin Rifabutin	Voriconazole	↓	Voriconazole plasma concentrations are significantly reduced during coadministration. Voriconazole may increase the C$_{max}$ and AUC of rifabutin by an average of 3 and 4 times, respectively. Coadministration is contraindicated.
Voriconazole	Rifabutin	↑	
Voriconazole	Benzodiazepines (ie, midazolam, triazolam, alprazolam)	↑	Voriconazole may increase the plasma concentrations of benzodiazepines that are metabolized by CYP3A4 (ie, alprazolam, midazolam, triazolam,). Adjust benzodiazepine dose if needed.
Voriconazole	Calcium channel blockers	↑	Voriconazole may increase plasma concentrations of calcium channel blockers that are metabolized by CYP3A4 (ie, felodipine). Adjust calcium channel blocker dose if needed.

VORICONAZOLE

Voriconazole Drug Interactions

Precipitant drug	Object drug*		Description
Voriconazole	Cisapride Pimozide Quinidine	↑	Voriconazole may inhibit the metabolism of these drugs. Increased plasma concentration may lead to QT prolongation and rare occurrences of torsades de pointes. Coadministration is contraindicated.
Voriconazole	Coumarin anti-coagulants (ie, warfarin)	↑	Coadministration significantly increased maximum prothrombin time approximately 2 times. Closely monitor coagulation tests and adjust warfarin dose accordingly. Voriconazole also may increase the PT in patients receiving other coumarin anticoagulants.
Voriconazole	Cyclosporine	↑	Coadministration of oral voriconazole increased cyclosporine C_{max} and AUC an average of 1.1 and 1.7 times, respectively. When initiating voriconazole therapy in patients already receiving cyclosporine, reduce the dose of cyclosporine to 50% of the original dose. Frequently monitor cyclosporine levels during coadministration and when voriconazole is discontinued.
Voriconazole	Ergot alkaloids	↑	Voriconazole may increase the plasma concentrations of ergot alkaloids (ie, ergotamine, dihydroergotamine) and lead to ergotism. Coadministration is contraindicated.
Voriconazole	HMG-CoA reductase inhibitors (ie, lovastatin)	↑	Voriconazole has been shown to inhibit lovastatin metabolism. Voriconazole may increase the plasma concentrations of statins that are metabolized by CYP3A4. Consider dosage adjustment of the statin during coadministration.
Voriconazole	Prednisolone	↑	Voriconazole may increase the C_{max} and AUC of prednisolone by an average 11% and 34%, respectively. No dosage adjustment recommended.
Voriconazole	Sirolimus	↑	Voriconazole can significantly increase the C_{max} and AUC of sirolimus an average of 7-fold and 11-fold, respectively. Coadministration is contraindicated.
Voriconazole	Sulfonylureas	↑	Voriconazole may increase plasma concentrations of sulfonylureas. Monitor for hypoglycemia. Dose adjustment of the sulfonylurea is recommended.
Voriconazole	Tacrolimus	↑	Voriconazole can significantly increase the C_{max} and AUC of tacrolimus by an average of 2-fold and 3-fold, respectively. When initiating voriconazole therapy in patients already receiving tacrolimus, reduce the dose of tacrolimus to 33% of the original dose. Frequently monitor tacrolimus levels during coadministration and when voriconazole is discontinued.
Voriconazole	Vinca alkaloids (ie, vincristine, vinblastine)	↑	Coadministration may increase the plasma concentrations of the vinca alkaloids and lead to neurotoxicity. Consider adjusting the dose of the vinca alkaloid and monitor for toxicity.

* ↓ = Object drug decreased. ↑ = Object drug increased.

▶*Drug/Food interactions:* When multiple doses of voriconazole are administered with high-fat meals, the mean C_{max} and AUC are reduced 34% and 24%, respectively when administered as a tablet and by 58% and 37% respectively when administered as the oral suspension (see Administration and Dosage).

Adverse Reactions

The most frequently reported adverse events (all causalities) in the therapeutic trials were visual disturbances, fever, rash, vomiting, nausea, diarrhea, headache, sepsis, peripheral edema, abdominal pain, and respiratory disorder. The treatment-related adverse events that most often led to discontinuation of voriconazole therapy were elevated liver function tests, rash, and visual disturbances.

Voriconazole Adverse Reactions (%)

Adverse reaction	All studies Voriconazole (N = 1493)	Oral Voriconazole (N = 200)	Oral Fluconazole (N = 191)	IV/Oral Voriconazole (N = 196)	IV/Oral Ampho B[a] (N = 185)
Cardiovascular					
Hypertension	1.9	0	0	0.5	1.1
Hypotension	1.7	0.5	0	0.5	1.6
Tachycardia	2.5	0	0	2.6	2.7
Vasodilation	1.5	0	0	1	1.1
CNS					
Dizziness	1.3	0	1	2.6	0
Hallucinations	2.5	0	0	5.1	0.5
Headache	3.2	0	0.5	3.6	4.3
Dermatologic					
Maculopapular rash	1.1	1.5	0	0.5	0
Pruritus	1.1	0	0	1	1.1
Rash	5.8	1.5	0.5	6.6	3.8
Hemic/Lymphatic					
Anemia	0.1	0	0	0	2.7
Leukopenia	0.3	0	0	0.5	0
Pancytopenia	0.1	0	0	0	0
Thrombocytopenia	0.5	0	0.5	1	1.1
GI					
Abdominal pain	1.7	0	0	2.6	3.2
Cholestatic jaundice	1.1	1.5	0	2	0
Diarrhea	1.1	0	0	1.5	3.2
Dry mouth	1	0	0.5	1.5	0
Jaundice	0.2	0.5	0	0	0
Liver function test abnormal	2.7	3	1	4.6	2.2
Nausea	5.9	1	1.6	7.1	15.7
Vomiting	4.8	1	0.5	5.6	9.7
GU					
Acute kidney failure	0.5	0	0	0	5.9
Kidney function abnormal	0.5	0.5	0.5	2	21.6
Metabolic/Nutritional					
Alkaline phosphatase increased	3.6	5	1.6	3.1	2.2
ALT increased	1.8	3	1	1.5	0.5
AST increased	1.9	4	1	0.5	0
Bilirubinemia	0.8	0.5	0	0.5	1.6
Creatinine increased	0.3	0.5	0	0	31.9
Hepatic enzymes increased	1.9	1.5	0	3.6	2.7
Hypomagnesemia	1.1	0	0	1	5.4
Hypokalemia	1.6	0	0	0.5	19.5
Peripheral edema	1.1	0.5	0	3.6	4.9
Special senses					
Abnormal vision	20.6	15.5	4.2	28.1	0.5
Chromatopsia	1.3	1	0	1	0
Eye hemorrhage	0.2	0	0	0	0
Photophobia	2.4	2.5	1	3.6	0
Miscellaneous					
Chills	4.1	0.5	0	0	19.5
Chest pain	0.9	0	0	2	1.1
Fever	6.2	0	0	3.6	13.5

[a] Amphotericin B followed by OLAT.

▶*Cardiovascular:* Atrial arrhythmia, atrial fibrillation, AV block complete, bigeminy, bradycardia, bundle branch block, cardiomegaly, cardiomyopathy, cerebral hemorrhage, cerebral ischemia, cerebrovascular accident, CHF, deep thrombophlebitis, endocarditis, extrasystoles, heart arrest, MI, nodal arrhythmia, palpitation, phlebitis, postural hypotension, pulmonary embolus, QT interval prolonged, supraventricular tachycardia, syncope, thrombophlebitis, vasodilation, ventricular arrhythmia, ventricular fibrillation, ventricular tachycardia (including torsades de pointes) (less than 1%).

VORICONAZOLE

➤*CNS:* Abnormal dreams, acute brain syndrome, agitation, akathisia, amnesia, anxiety, ataxia, brain edema, coma, confusion, convulsion, delirium, dementia, depersonalization, depression, encephalitis, encephalopathy, euphoria, extrapyramidal syndrome, grand mal convulsion, Guillain-Barré syndrome, hypertonia, hypesthesia, insomnia, intracranial hypertension, neuralgia, neuropathy, paresthesia, psychosis, somnolence, suicidal ideation, tremor, vertigo (less than 1%).

➤*Dermatologic:* In clinical trials, rashes considered related to therapy were reported by 6% of voriconazole-treated patients. The majority of rashes were of mild to moderate severity. Cases of photosensitivity reactions appear to be more likely to occur with long-term treatment. Patients have rarely developed serious cutaneous reactions, including Stevens-Johnson syndrome, toxic epidermal necrolysis, and erythema multiforme during treatment with voriconazole. If patients develop a rash, monitor closely and consider discontinuing voriconazole. It is recommended that patients avoid strong, direct sunlight during voriconazole therapy.

Alopecia, angioedema, contact dermatitis, discoid lupus erythematosus, dry skin, eczema, erythema multiforme, exfoliative dermatitis, fixed drug eruption, furunculosis, herpes simplex, melanosis, photosensitivity skin reaction, psoriasis, skin discoloration, skin disorder, Stevens-Johnson syndrome, sweating, toxic epidermal necrolysis, urticaria (less than 1%).

➤*Endocrine:* Adrenal cortex insufficiency, diabetes insipidus, hyperthyroidism, hypothyroidism (less than 1%).

➤*GI:* Abdomen enlarged, anorexia, cheilitis, cholecystitis, cholelithiasis, constipation, duodenal ulcer perforation, duodenitis, dyspepsia, dysphagia, enlarged liver, esophageal ulcer, esophagitis, flatulence, gastroenteritis, GI hemorrhage, GGT/LDH elevated, gingivitis, glossitis, gum hemorrhage, gum hyperplasia, hematemesis, hepatic coma, hepatic failure, hepatitis, intestinal perforation, intestinal ulcer, melena, mouth ulceration, pancreatitis, parotid gland enlargement, periodontitis, proctitis, pseudomembranous colitis, rectal disorder, rectal hemorrhage, stomach ulcer, stomatitis, tongue edema (less than 1%).

➤*GU:* Anuria, blighted ovum, creatinine clearance decreased, dysmenorrhea, dysuria, epididymitis, glycosuria, hemorrhagic cystitis, hematuria, hydronephrosis, impotence, kidney pain, kidney tubular necrosis, libido decreased, metrorrhagia, nephritis, nephrosis, oliguria, scrotal edema, urinary incontinence, urinary retention, urinary tract infection, uterine hemorrhage, vaginal hemorrhage (less than 1%).

➤*Hematologic/Lymphatic:* Agranulocytosis, anemia (ie, macrocytic, megaloblastic, microcytic, normocytic), aplastic anemia, bleeding time increased, cyanosis, disseminated intravascular coagulation, ecchymosis, enlarged spleen, eosinophilia, hemolytic anemia, hypervolemia, lymphadenopathy, lymphangitis, marrow depression, petechia, purpura, thrombotic thrombocytopenic purpura (less than 1%).

➤*Lab test abnormalities:* The overall incidence of clinically significant transaminase abnormalities in the voriconazole clinical program was 13.4% of patients treated with voriconazole. Increased incidence of liver function test abnormalities may be associated with higher plasma concentrations or doses. The majority of abnormal liver function tests either resolve during treatment without dose adjustment or following dose adjustment, including discontinuation of therapy.

Voriconazole vs Amphotericin B Laboratory Test Abnormalities

	Criteria[a]	Voriconazole n[b]/N[c] (%)	Amphotericin B[d] n/N (%)
Total bilirubin	> 1.5 x ULN[e]	35/180 (19.4)	46/173 (26.6)
AST	> 3 x ULN	21/180 (11.7)	18/174 (10.3)
ALT	> 3 x ULN	34/180 (18.9)	40/173 (23.1)
Alkaline phosphatase	> 3 x ULN	29/181 (16)	38/173 (22)
Creatinine	> 1.3 x ULN	39/182 (21.4)	102/177 (57.6)
Potassium	< 0.9 x LLN[f]	30/181 (16.6)	70/178 (39.3)

[a] Without regard to baseline value.
[b] n = Number of patients with a clinically significant abnormality while on study therapy.
[c] N = Total number of patients with at least 1 observation of the given lab test while on study therapy.
[d] Amphotericin B followed by other licensed antifungal therapy.
[e] ULN = upper limit of normal.
[f] LLN = lower limit of normal.

Voriconazole vs Fluconazole Laboratory Test Abnormalities

	Criteria[a]	Voriconazole n[b]/N[c] (%)	Fluconazole n/N (%)
Total bilirubin	> 1.5 x ULN[d]	8/185 (4.3)	7/186 (3.8)
AST	> 3 x ULN	38/187 (20.3)	15/186 (8.1)
ALT	> 3 x ULN	20/187 (10.7)	12/186 (6.5)
Alkaline phosphatase	> 3 x ULN	19/187 (10.2)	14/186 (7.5)

[a] Without regard to baseline value.
[b] n = Number of patients with a clinically significant abnormality while on study therapy.
[c] N = Total number of patients with at least 1 observation of the given lab test while on study therapy.
[d] ULN = upper limit of normal.

➤*Metabolic/Nutritional:* Albuminuria, BUN increased, creatine phosphokinase increased, edema, glucose tolerance decreased, hypercalcemia, hypercholesteremia, hyperglycemia, hyperkalemia, hypermagnesemia, hypernatremia, hyperuricemia, hypocalcemia, hypoglycemia, hyponatremia, hypophosphatemia, uremia (less than 1%).

➤*Musculoskeletal:* Arthralgia, arthritis, bone necrosis, bone pain, leg cramps, myalgia, myasthenia, myopathy, osteomalacia, osteoporosis (less than 1%).

➤*Ophthalmic:* Voriconazole treatment-related visual disturbances are common. In clinical trials, approximately 30% of patients experienced altered/enhanced visual perception, blurred vision, color vision change, or photophobia. The visual disturbances were generally mild and rarely resulted in discontinuation. Visual disturbances may be associated with higher plasma concentrations or doses.

Abnormality of accommodation, blepharitis, color blindness, conjunctivitis, corneal opacity, diplopia, eye pain, dry eyes, keratitis, keratoconjunctivitis, mydriasis, night blindness, nystagmus, oculogyric crisis, optic atrophy, optic neuritis, papilledema, retinal hemorrhage, retinitis, scleritis, uveitis, visual field defect (less than 1%).

➤*Respiratory:* Cough increased, dyspnea, epistaxis, hemoptysis, hypoxia, lung edema, pharyngitis, pleural effusion, pneumonia, respiratory disorder, respiratory distress syndrome, respiratory tract infection, rhinitis, sinusitis, voice alteration (less than 1%).

➤*Special senses:* Deafness, ear pain, otitis externa, taste loss, taste perversion, tinnitus (less than 1%).

➤*Miscellaneous:* Allergic reaction, anaphylactoid reaction, ascites, asthenia, back pain, cellulitis, face edema, flank pain, flu syndrome, graft vs host reaction, granuloma, infection, bacterial infection, fungal infection, injection site pain, injection site infection/inflammation, mucous membrane disorder, multi-organ failure, pain, pelvic pain, peritonitis, sepsis, substernal chest pain (less than 1%).

Overdosage

➤*Symptoms:* In clinical trials, there were 3 cases of accidental overdose. All occurred in pediatric patients who received up to 5 times the recommended IV dose of voriconazole. A single adverse event of photophobia of 10 minutes duration was reported.

The minimum lethal oral dose in mice and rats was 300 mg/kg (equivalent to 4 and 7 times the RMD, based on body surface area). At this dose, clinical signs observed in mice and rats included salivation, mydriasis, titubation (loss of balance while moving), depressed behavior, prostration, partially closed eyes, and dyspnea. Other signs in mice were convulsions, corneal opacification, and swollen abdomen.

➤*Treatment:* There is no known antidote for voriconazole. Voriconazole is hemodialyzed with clearance of 121 mL/min. The IV vehicle, SBECD, is hemodialyzed with clearance of 55 mL/min. In an overdose, hemodialysis may assist in the removal of voriconazole and SBECD from the body.

Patient Information

Advise patients to take oral voriconazole at least 1 hour before or 1 hour following a meal.

Advise patients not to drive at night while taking voriconazole. Voriconazole may cause changes to vision, including blurring or photophobia.

Advise patients to avoid potentially hazardous tasks, such as driving or operating machinery if they perceive any changes in vision.

Advise patients to avoid strong, direct sunlight during voriconazole therapy.

Women of childbearing potential should use effective contraception during treatment.

FLUCONAZOLE

Rx	Fluconazole (Mayne)	Injection: 2 mg/mL	In 100 and 200 mL.
Rx	Diflucan (Pfizer)	Tablets: 50 mg	(Diflucan 50 Roerig). Pink, trapezoid shape. In 30s.
		100 mg	(Diflucan 100 Roerig). Pink, trapezoid shape. In 30s and UD 100s.
		150 mg	(Diflucan 150 Roerig). Pink, oval. In UD 1s.
		200 mg	(Diflucan 200 Roerig). Pink, trapezoid shape. In 30s and UD 100s.
		Powder for oral suspension: 10 mg/mL when reconstituted	Sucrose. Orange flavor. In 350 mg.
		40 mg/mL when reconstituted	Sucrose. Orange flavor. In 1400 mg.
		Injection: 2 mg/mL	In 100 or 200 mL bottles or *Viaflex Plus* (available with NaCl[1] or dextrose diluents).[2]

[1] Contains 9 mg/mL NaCl.

[2] Contains 56 mg/mL dextrose, hydrous.

Indications

▶*Candidiasis:* For the treatment of oropharyngeal and esophageal candidiasis. In open, noncomparative trials of small numbers of patients, fluconazole was effective in the treatment of candidal urinary tract infections, peritonitis, and systemic candidal infections including candidemia, disseminated candidiasis, and pneumonia.

▶*Vaginal candidiasis:* Vaginal candidiasis (vaginal yeast infections due to *Candida*).

▶*Prophylaxis:* To decrease the incidence of candidiasis in patients undergoing bone marrow transplantation who receive cytotoxic chemotherapy and/or radiation therapy.

▶*Cryptococcal meningitis:* Treatment of cryptococcal meningitis.

Administration and Dosage

▶*Approved by the FDA:* January 29, 1990.

▶*Single dose:*

Vaginal candidiasis – 150 mg as a single oral dose.

▶*Multiple dose:* Because oral absorption is rapid and almost complete, the daily dose of fluconazole is the same for oral and IV administration. In general, a loading dose of twice the daily dose is recommended on the first day of therapy to achieve plasma levels close to steady state by the second day of therapy.

For infections other than vaginal candidiasis, base the daily dose on the infecting organism and patient response to therapy. Continue treatment until clinical parameters or lab tests indicate that active fungal infection has subsided. An inadequate treatment period may lead to recurrence of active infection. Patients with AIDS and cryptococcal meningitis or recurrent oropharyngeal candidiasis usually require maintenance therapy to prevent relapse.

Oropharyngeal candidiasis – 200 mg on the first day, followed by 100 mg once daily. Clinical evidence of oropharyngeal candidiasis generally resolves within several days, but continue treatment for at least 2 weeks to decrease likelihood of relapse.

Esophageal candidiasis – 200 mg on the first day, followed by 100 mg once daily. Doses up to 400 mg/day may be used based on the patient's response. Treat patients with esophageal candidiasis for a minimum of 3 weeks and for 2 weeks or more following resolution of symptoms.

Candidiasis, other – For candidal urinary tract infections (UTIs) and peritonitis, 50 to 200 mg/day has been used. For systemic candidal infections (including candidemia, disseminated candidiasis, and pneumonia), optimal dosage and duration have not been determined, although doses 400 mg/day or less have been used.

Prevention of candidiasis in bone marrow transplant – 400 mg once daily. In patients anticipated to have severe granulocytopenia (less than 500 neutrophils/mm^3), start fluconazole prophylaxis several days before anticipated onset of neutropenia, and continue 7 days after neutrophil count rises above 1000 cells/mm^3.

Cryptococcal meningitis – 400 mg on the first day followed by 200 mg once daily. A dosage of 400 mg once daily may be used based on the patient's response to therapy. The duration of treatment for initial therapy of cryptococcal meningitis is 10 to 12 weeks after the cerebrospinal fluid (CSF) becomes culture negative. The dosage of fluconazole for suppression of relapse of cryptococcal meningitis in patients with AIDS is 200 mg once daily.

▶*Children:* The following dose equivalency table provides equivalent exposure in pediatric and adult patients.

Equivalent Fluconazole Dosage in Children vs Adults	
Children	Adults
3 mg/kg	100 mg
6 mg/kg	200 mg
12 mg/kg[1]	400 mg

[1] Some older children may have clearances similar to that of adults. Absolute doses more than 600 mg/day are not recommended.

Neonates – Experience in neonates is limited to pharmacokinetic studies in premature newborns. Based on the prolonged half-life seen in premature newborns (gestational age, 26 to 29 weeks), administer the same dosage (mg/kg) to neonates in the first 2 weeks of life as in older children, but administer every 72 hours. After the first 2 weeks, dose neonates once daily.

Oropharyngeal candidiasis – The recommended dosage is 6 mg/kg on the first day, followed by 3 mg/kg once daily. Administer treatment for at least 2 weeks to decrease the likelihood of relapse.

Esophageal candidiasis – The recommended dosage is 6 mg/kg on the first day followed by 3 mg/kg once daily. Doses up to 12 mg/kg/day may be used based on the patient's response to therapy. Treat patients with esophageal candidiasis for a minimum of 3 weeks and for at least 2 weeks following the resolution of symptoms.

Systemic Candida infections – For the treatment of candidemia and disseminated *Candida* infections, daily doses of 6 to 12 mg/kg/day have been used in an open, noncomparative study of a small number of children.

Cryptococcal meningitis – The recommended dosage is 12 mg/kg on the first day, followed by 6 mg/kg once daily. A dosage of 12 mg/kg once daily may be used based on medical judgment of the patient's response to therapy. The recommended duration of treatment for initial therapy of cryptococcal meningitis is 10 to 12 weeks after the CSF becomes culture negative. For suppression of cryptococcal meningitis relapse in children with AIDS, the recommended dose is 6 mg/kg once daily.

▶*Renal function impairment:* Fluconazole is cleared primarily by renal excretion as unchanged drug. A 3-hour hemodialysis session decreases plasma levels by approximately 50%. There is no need to adjust single-dose therapy for vaginal candidiasis in patients with impaired renal function. In patients with impaired renal function who will receive multiple doses, give an initial loading dose of 50 to 400 mg. After the loading dose, base the daily dose on the following table:

Fluconazole Dose in Impaired Renal Function	
Creatinine clearance (mL/min)	Percentage of recommended dose
> 50	100
≤ 50 (no dialysis)	50
Patients receiving regular hemodialysis	100 after each dialysis

These are suggested dose adjustments based on pharmacokinetics following administration of multiple doses. Further adjustment may be needed depending upon clinical condition.

When serum creatinine is the only measure of renal function available, use the following formula to estimate the creatinine clearance.

Males: $\dfrac{\text{Weight (kg)} \times (140 - \text{age})}{72 \times \text{serum creatinine (mg/dL)}} = \text{Ccr}$

Females: $0.85 \times$ above value

Children – Although the pharmacokinetics of fluconazole have not been studied in children with renal insufficiency, dosage reduction in children with renal insufficiency parallels the adult recommendation. The following formula may be used to estimate Ccr in children:

$$\text{K†} \times \frac{\text{linear length or height (cm)}}{\text{serum creatinine (mg/100 mL)}}$$

▶*Directions for mixing oral suspension:* To reconstitute, add 24 mL distilled water or purified water to fluconazole bottle and shake vigorously to suspend powder. Each bottle will deliver 35 mL of suspension. The concentrations of the reconstituted suspensions are 10 mg/mL (350 mg bottle) and 40 mg/mL (1400 mg bottle). Shake well before using.

▶*Injection:* Fluconazole injection has been used safely for up to 14 days of IV therapy. Administer the IV infusion of fluconazole at a maximum rate of approximately 200 mg/hr given as a continuous infusion. Fluconazole injections are intended only for IV administration. Do not use if the solution is cloudy, contains a precipitate, or if the seal is not intact.

† (Where K = 0.55 for children older than 1 year of age and 0.45 for infants).

FLUCONAZOLE

Directions for IV use of Viaflex Plus plastic containers – Do not remove unit from overwrap until ready for use. The overwrap is a moisture barrier. The inner bag maintains the sterility of the product. Do not use plastic containers in series connections; such use could result in air embolism because of residual air being drawn from the primary container before administration of the fluid from the secondary container is completed.

To open, tear overwrap down side at slit and remove solution container. Some opacity of the plastic may be observed because of moisture absorption during the sterilization process. This is normal and does not affect the solution quality or safety. The opacity will diminish gradually. After removing overwrap, check for minute leaks by squeezing inner bag firmly. If leaks are found, discard solution as sterility may be impaired.

Admixture incompatibility – Do not add supplementary medication.

▶*Storage / Stability:*

Oral suspension – Store reconstituted suspension between 5° and 30°C (41° and 86°F). Discard unused portion after 2 weeks. Protect from freezing.

Tablets – Store below 30°C (86°F).

Injection –
    Viaflex Plus plastic containers: Store between 5° and 25°C (41° and 77°F). Brief exposure to temperatures up to 40°C (104°F) does not adversely affect the product. Protect from freezing.
    Glass bottles: Store between 5° and 30°C (41° and 86°F). Protect from freezing.

Actions

▶*Pharmacology:* Fluconazole is a synthetic triazole antifungal agent. Fluconazole is a highly selective inhibitor of fungal cytochrome P450 and sterol C-14 alpha-demethylation. Mammalian cell demethylation is much less sensitive to fluconazole inhibition. The subsequent loss of normal sterols correlates with the accumulation of 14 alpha-methyl sterols in fungi and may be responsible for the fungistatic activity of fluconazole.

Doses of 200 to 400 mg once daily for up to 2 weeks in healthy volunteers were associated with small, inconsistent effects on testosterone and endogenous corticosteroid concentrations and the ACTH-stimulated cortisol response.

▶*Pharmacokinetics:*

Absorption / Distribution – The pharmacokinetic properties of fluconazole are similar following administration by the IV or oral routes. In healthy volunteers, the bioavailability of oral fluconazole is more than 90% compared with IV administration. Bioequivalence was established between the 100 mg tablet and both suspension strengths when administered as a single 200 mg dose.

Peak plasma concentrations (C_{max}) in fasting healthy volunteers occur between 1 and 2 hours. A single oral 400 mg dose leads to a mean C_{max} of 6.72 mcg/mL (range, 4.12 to 8.08 mcg/mL); after single oral doses of 50 to 400 mg, plasma concentrations and AUC are dose-proportional. A single 150 mg oral dose to 10 lactating women resulted in a mean C_{max} of 2.61 mcg/mL (range, 1.57 to 3.65 mcg/mL).

Steady-state concentrations are reached within 5 to 10 days following oral doses of 50 to 400 mg given once daily. Administration of a loading dose (day 1) of twice the usual daily dose results in plasma concentrations close to steady state by day 2. The apparent volume of distribution approximates that of total body water. Plasma protein binding is low (11% to 12%). Following either single or multiple oral doses for up to 14 days, fluconazole penetrates into all body fluids studied (see table).

Tissue/Fluid Concentration of Fluconazole	
Tissue or fluid	Concentration[1] (tissue/plasma ratio)
CSF[2]	0.5 to 0.9
Saliva	1
Sputum	1
Blister fluid	1
Urine	10
Normal skin	10
Nails	1
Blistered skin	2
Vaginal tissue	1
Vaginal fluid	0.4 to 0.7

[1] Relative to plasma concentrations in subjects with normal renal function.
[2] Variable degree of meningeal inflammation.

Metabolism / Excretion – In healthy volunteers fluconazole is cleared primarily by renal excretion with approximately 80% of the dose appearing in the urine unchanged and with approximately 11% as metabolites. The terminal plasma elimination half-life is approximately 30 hours (range, 20 to 50) after oral administration.

Special populations –

Renal function impairment: The pharmacokinetics of fluconazole are markedly affected by reduction in renal function. There is an inverse relationship between the elimination half-life and creatinine clearance. The dose may need to be reduced in patients with impaired renal function (see Administration and Dosage). A 3-hour hemodialysis session decreases plasma concentrations by approximately 50%.

▶*Microbiology:* Fluconazole exhibits in vitro activity against *Cryptococcus neoformans* and *Candida* sp. Fungistatic activity also has been demonstrated in normal and immunocompromised animal models for systemic and intracranial fungal infections because of *C. neoformans* and for systemic infections because of *Candida albicans*. There have been reports of cases of superinfection with *Candida* species other than *C. albicans*, which are often inherently nonsusceptible to fluconazole (eg, *Candida krusei*). Such cases may require alternative antifungal therapy.

As with other azole antifungal agents, most fungi show a higher apparent sensitivity to fluconazole in vivo than in vitro. Activity has been demonstrated against fungal infections caused by *Aspergillus flavus* and *Aspergillus fumigatus* in mice. Fluconazole is active in animal models of endemic mycoses, including 1 model of *Blastomyces dermatitidis* pulmonary infections, 1 model of *Coccidioides immitis* intracranial infections, and several models of *Histoplasma capsulatum* pulmonary infection.

▶*Clinical trials:*

Cryptococcal meningitis – Fluconazole (200 mg/day) was compared with amphotericin B (0.3 mg/kg/day) for cryptococcal meningitis in AIDS patients. Mortality among high-risk patients was 33% and 40% for amphotericin B and fluconazole, respectively, with overall deaths 14% and 18%, respectively.

Vaginal candidiasis – In two studies of patients with vaginal candidiasis, the results of the 150 mg single-dose fluconazole regimen were comparable to the control regimen (clotrimazole or miconazole intravaginally for 7 days) at the 1-month post-treatment evaluation. The therapeutic cure rate (complete resolution of signs and symptoms [clinical cure] along with a negative KOH examination and negative culture for *Candida* [microbiologic eradication]) was 55% for both groups. Approximately 75% of patients had acute vaginitis and achieved 80% clinical cure, 67% mycologic eradication, and 59% therapeutic cure with fluconazole, which was comparable with controls. The remaining 25% of patients had recurrent vaginitis (4 or more episodes within 12 months) and achieved 57% clinical cure, 47% mycologic eradication, and 40% therapeutic cure; the numbers are too small to make a meaningful comparison.

Contraindications

Hypersensitivity to fluconazole or any excipients in the product. There is no information regarding cross hypersensitivity between fluconazole and other azole antifungal agents; use with caution in patients hypersensitive to other azoles. Coadministration with cisapride.

Warnings

▶*Hepatic injury:* Fluconazole has been associated with rare cases of serious hepatic toxicity. In cases of fluconazole-associated hepatotoxicity, no obvious relationship to total daily dose, duration of therapy, sex, or age of the patient has been observed. Fluconazole hepatotoxicity has usually, but not always, been reversible upon discontinuation of therapy. Monitor patients who develop abnormal liver function tests during fluconazole therapy for the development of more severe hepatic injury. Discontinue fluconazole if clinical signs and symptoms consistent with liver disease develop that may be attributable to fluconazole.

▶*Anaphylaxis:* Anaphylaxis has occurred, rarely.

▶*Dermatologic changes:* Patients rarely have developed exfoliative skin disorders during treatment with fluconazole. In patients with serious underlying diseases (predominantly AIDS and malignancy), exfoliative skin disorders rarely have resulted in fatal outcomes. Closely monitor patients who develop rashes during treatment with fluconazole, and discontinue the drug if lesions progress.

▶*Carcinogenesis:* Male rats treated with 5 and 10 mg/kg/day had an increased incidence of hepatocellular adenomas.

▶*Fertility impairment:* Onset of parturition was slightly delayed in rats at 20 mg/kg orally. With doses of 5, 20, and 40 mg/kg, dystocia and prolongation of parturition were observed in a few dams at 20 mg/kg (approximately 5 to 15 times the recommended human dose) and 40 mg/kg but not at 5 mg/kg. The effects on parturition in rats are consistent with the species-specific, estrogen-lowering property produced by high doses of fluconazole. Such a hormone change has not been observed in women treated with fluconazole.

▶*Pregnancy: Category C.* Fluconazole was administered orally to pregnant rabbits during organogenesis in 2 studies at 5, 10, and 20 mg/kg and at 5, 25, and 75 mg/kg, respectively. Maternal weight gain was impaired at all dose levels and abortions occurred at 75 mg/kg (approximately 20 to 60 times the recommended human dose); no adverse fetal effects were detected. In several studies in which pregnant rats were treated orally with fluconazole during organogenesis, maternal weight gain was impaired and placental weights were increased at 25 mg/kg. There were no fetal effects at 5 or 10 mg/kg;

FLUCONAZOLE

increases in fetal anatomical variants (eg, supernumerary ribs, renal pelvis dilation) and delays in ossification were observed at 25 and 50 mg/kg and higher doses. At doses ranging from 80 mg/kg (approximately 20 to 60 times the recommended human dose) to 320 mg/kg, embryolethality in rats was increased and fetal abnormalities included wavy ribs, cleft palate, and abnormal craniofacial ossification. These effects are consistent with the inhibition of estrogen synthesis in rats and may be a result of known effects of lowered estrogen on pregnancy, organogenesis, and parturition.

There are no adequate and well-controlled studies in pregnant women. Use in pregnancy only if the potential benefit justifies the possible risk to the fetus.

►*Lactation:* Fluconazole is excreted in breast milk at concentrations similar to plasma. Therefore, the use of fluconazole in nursing mothers is not recommended.

►*Children:* In a noncomparative study of children with serious systemic fungal infections, most of which were candidemia, the efficacy of fluconazole was similar to that reported for the treatment of candidemia in adults. The efficacy of fluconazole for the suppression of cryptococcal meningitis was successful in 4 of 5 children treated in a compassionate-use study of fluconazole for the treatment of life-threatening or serious mycoses. The safety profile of fluconazole in children has been studied in 577 children 1 day to 17 years of age who received doses ranging from 1 to 15 mg/kg/day for 1 to 1616 days. Efficacy of fluconazole has not been established in infants younger than 6 months of age. A small number of patients (29) ranging in age from 1 day to 6 months have been treated safely with fluconazole.

Precautions

►*Vaginal candidiasis:* Weigh the convenience and efficacy of the single-dose regimen for treatment of vaginal yeast infections against the acceptability of a higher incidence of adverse reactions with fluconazole (26%) vs intravaginal agents (16%).

Drug Interactions

►*CYP450 system:* Fluconazole is an inhibitor of CYP3A4 and CYP2C9. Use with caution with drugs metabolized by these enzymes.

Fluconazole Drug Interactions

Precipitant drug	Object drug*		Description
Cimetidine	Fluconazole	↓	Cimetidine resulted in a reduction in fluconazole AUC and C_{max}.
Hydrochloro-thiazide	Fluconazole	↑	Concomitant use resulted in a significant increase in fluconazole C_{max} and AUC, which can be attributed to reduced renal clearance.
Rifampin	Fluconazole	↓	Rifampin enhances the metabolism of concurrently administered fluconazole. Depending on the clinical circumstances, give consideration when increasing the dose of fluconazole when administered with rifampin.
Fluconazole	Alfentanil	↑	The pharmacologic and adverse effects of alfentanil may be increased. Possible inhibition of alfentanil metabolism (CYP3A4) by fluconazole may occur. Monitor for prolonged or recurrent respiratory depression. It may be necessary to administer a lower dose of alfentanil.
Fluconazole	Benzodiazepines	↑	Increased and prolonged serum levels, CNS depression, and psychomotor impairment with certain benzodiazepines may occur, possibly lasting for several days after stopping fluconazole.
Fluconazole	Buspirone	↑	Plasma buspirone concentrations may be elevated because of inhibition of buspirone metabolism. The pharmacologic and adverse effects of buspirone may be increased. Adjust the dose of buspirone as needed.
Fluconazole	Carbamazepine	↑	Plasma concentrations of carbamazepine may be elevated, increasing clinical and adverse effects because of possible inhibition of carbamazepine metabolism (CYP3A4) by fluconazole. Monitor carbamazepine concentrations.
Fluconazole	Cisapride	↑	Concurrent use may increase cisapride concentrations and cardiotoxicity may occur. Coadministration is contraindicated.

Fluconazole Drug Interactions

Precipitant drug	Object drug*		Description
Fluconazole	Contraceptives, oral	↔	Concurrent use with an OC containing ethinyl estradiol/levonorgestrel produced an overall mean increase in the levels of the OC components; however, in some cases there were decreases ≤ 47% and 33% of ethinyl estradiol and levonorgestrel levels, respectively.
Fluconazole	Corticosteroids	↑	The effects of corticosteroids may be enhanced, resulting in increased toxicity because of inhibition of corticosteroid metabolism. Adjust corticosteroid dose as needed.
Fluconazole	Cyclosporine	↑	Significant increases in cyclosporine C_{max}, C_{min}, and AUC values and a significant decrease in oral clearance occurred following fluconazole use.
Fluconazole	Haloperidol	↑	Concurrent use may increase haloperidol plasma concentrations, increasing the risk of side effects. Adjust haloperidol dose as needed.
Fluconazole	HMG-CoA reductase inhibitors	↑	Coadministration causes increased plasma levels of the HMG-CoA reductase inhibitors. Rhabdomyolysis has been reported. If concurrent use can not be avoided, consider reducing the dose of the HMG-CoA reductase inhibitor. Pravastatin levels appear to be the least affected by concurrent use.
Fluconazole	Losartan	↑	The antihypertensive and adverse effects of losartan may be increased because of possible inhibition of metabolism (CYP2D9) of losartan by fluconazole. Monitor blood pressure.
Fluconazole	Nisoldipine	↑	Serum nisoldipine concentrations may be elevated, increasing pharmacologic and adverse effects. Fluconazole, especially > 200 mg/day, may inhibit CYP3A4.
Fluconazole	Phenytoin	↑	Coadministration resulted in an increase of phenytoin AUC values. Monitor phenytoin levels and adjust dose as needed.
Fluconazole	Protease inhibitors	↑	Concurrent use may elevate protease inhibitor levels, increasing the risk of toxicity. Adjust protease inhibitor dose as needed.
Fluconazole	Rifabutin	↑	Coadministration may increase rifabutin levels. Cases of uveitis have been reported in patients receiving both drugs. Monitor closely.
Fluconazole	Sirolimus	↑	Plasma sirolimus concentrations may be elevated because of an inhibition of sirolimus gut metabolism.
Fluconazole	Sulfonylureas	↑	Fluconazole reduces the metabolism of sulfonylureas and increases the plasma concentrations of these agents. Carefully monitor blood glucose concentrations and adjust the sulfonylurea dose as necessary when these agents are coadministered.
Fluconazole	Tacromilus	↑	There have been reports of nephrotoxicity in patients when these agents were coadministered. Carefully monitor.
Fluconazole	Theophylline	↑	Theophylline AUC, C_{max}, and half-life were significantly increased, and clearance was decreased.
Fluconazole	Tolterodine	↑	Concurrent use may increase tolterodine plasma levels. Adjust tolterodine dose as needed. Do not give more than 1 mg of tolterodine twice daily when coadministered with azole antifungals.

FLUCONAZOLE

Fluconazole Drug Interactions			
Precipitant drug	Object drug*		Description
Fluconazole	Tricyclic antide-pressants (ie, amitriptyline, nortriptyline)	↑	Serum tricyclic antidepressant (TCA) concentrations may be elevated, resulting in an increase in therapeutic and adverse effects including cardiac arrhythmia. Inhibition of TCA metabolism is suspected (CYP2C9 by fluconazole). Adjust the TCA dose as needed.
Fluconazole	Vinca alkaloids (eg, vincristine)	↑	The risk of vinca alkaloid toxicity (eg, constipation, myalgia, neutropenia) may be increased. Avoid coadministration of these agents whenever possible.
Fluconazole	Warfarin	↑	The anticoagulant effect of warfarin may be increased. A single warfarin dose after 14 days of fluconazole resulted in an increase in the PT response. Monitor PT and INR frequently.
Fluconazole	Zidovudine	↑	There was a significant increase in zidovudine AUC following fluconazole administration.
Fluconazole	Zolpidem	↑	Plasma concentrations and therapeutic effects of zolpidem may be increased. The dose of zolpidem may need to be decreased during coadministration of azole antifungal agents.

↑ = Object drug increased. ↓ = Object drug decreased. ⟷ = Undetermined clinical effect.

Adverse Reactions

▶*Patients receiving single doses:* In 448 patients with vaginal candidiasis receiving single 150 mg doses, the overall incidence of adverse reactions was 26%. In 422 patients receiving active comparative agents, the incidence was 16%. Effects reported with fluconazole were the following: Headache (13%); nausea (7%); abdominal pain (6%); diarrhea (3%); dyspepsia, dizziness, taste perversion (1%); angioedema, anaphylactic reaction (rare). Most reactions were mild to moderate in severity.

▶*Patients receiving multiple doses:* Of the more than 4000 patients treated with fluconazole in clinical trials for up to 7 days, 16% experienced adverse events. Treatment was discontinued in 1.5% of patients because of adverse clinical events and in 1.3% of patients because of

laboratory test abnormalities. Clinical adverse events were reported more frequently in HIV-infected patients (21%) than in non-HIV infected patients (13%); however, the patterns in both patient groups were similar. The proportions of patients discontinuing therapy because of clinical adverse events were similar in the 2 groups (1.5%).

The following adverse events have occurred: Nausea (3.7%); headache (1.9%); skin rash (1.8%); vomiting, abdominal pain (1.7%); diarrhea (1.5%); seizures; exfoliative skin disorders (including Stevens-Johnson syndrome and toxic epidermal necrolysis) (see Warnings); alopecia; leukopenia; thrombocytopenia; hypercholesterolemia; hypertriglyceridemia; hypokalemia; serious hepatic reactions (see Warnings).

▶*Lab test abnormalities:* In 2 comparative trials a statistically significant increase was observed in median AST levels from a baseline value of 30 to 41 IU/L in 1 trial and 34 to 66 IU/L in the other. The overall rate of serum transaminase elevations of more than 8 times the upper limit of normal was approximately 1% in fluconazole-treated patients in clinical trials. These elevations occurred in patients with severe underlying disease (predominantly AIDS or malignancies) most of whom were receiving multiple concomitant medications, including many known to be hepatotoxic. The incidence of abnormally elevated serum transaminases was greater in patients taking fluconazole concomitantly with 1 or more of the following medications: Rifampin, phenytoin, isoniazid, valproic acid, or oral sulfonylurea hypoglycemic agents.

Overdosage

▶*Symptoms:* There has been 1 reported case of overdosage; a patient 42 years of age infected with HIV developed hallucinations and exhibited paranoid behavior after reportedly ingesting 8.2 g of fluconazole. The patient's condition resolved within 48 hours. In mice and rats receiving very high doses of fluconazole, clinical effects included decreased motility and respiration, ptosis, lacrimation, salivation, urinary incontinence, loss of righting reflex, and cyanosis; death was sometimes preceded by clonic convulsions.

▶*Treatment:* In the event of overdose, institute symptomatic treatment with supportive measures and gastric lavage if clinically indicated. Refer to General Management of Acute Overdosage.

Fluconazole is largely excreted in urine. A 3-hour hemodialysis session decreases plasma levels by approximately 50%.

Patient Information

Use of this medicine has been associated with rare cases of serious liver damage.

Do not take this medicine if you are breastfeeding.

Shake the suspension well before using.

Discard unused portion of the reconstituted suspension after 2 weeks.

ITRACONAZOLE

Rx	**Sporanox** (Janssen)	**Capsules:** 100 mg	Sucrose, sugar, FD&C No. 1 and No. 2. (Janssen Sporanox 100). Blue/pink. In 30s, UD 30s, and *PulsePak* 28s.
Rx	**Sporanox** (Ortho Biotech)	**Injection:** 10 mg/mL	Kit: 25 mL amp, 50 mL bag of 0.9% NaCl injection, and 1 filtered infusion set.
		Oral solution: 10 mg/mL	Saccharin, sorbitol. Cherry/caramel flavor. In 150 mL.

WARNING

CHF: Do not administer itraconazole for the treatment of onychomycosis in patients with evidence of ventricular dysfunction, such as CHF or a history of CHF. Discontinue if signs and symptoms of CHF occur during treatment. If signs and symptoms of CHF occur during treatment, reassess the continued use of itraconazole. When itraconazole was administered IV to dogs and healthy human volunteers, negative inotropic effects were seen.

Drug interactions: Coadministration of cisapride, pimozide, dofetilide, or quinidine with itraconazole is contraindicated. Itraconazole is a potent inhibitor of the cytochrome P450 3A4 isoenzyme system and may raise plasma concentrations of drugs metabolized by this pathway. Serious cardiovascular events, including QT prolongation, torsades de pointes, ventricular tachycardia, cardiac arrest, and/or sudden death have occurred in patients taking itraconazole concomitantly with cisapride, pimozide, or quinidine, which are inhibitors of the cytochrome P450 3A4 system (see Contraindications, Warnings, and Drug Interactions).

Indications

▶*Aspergillosis (capsules and injection):* Treatment of pulmonary and extrapulmonary aspergillosis in nonimmunocompromised or immunocompromised patients who are intolerant of or who are refractory to amphotericin B therapy.

▶*Blastomycosis (capsules and injection):* Treatment of pulmonary and extrapulmonary blastomycosis in nonimmunocompromised or immunocompromised patients.

▶*Febrile neutropenia, empiric (oral solution and injection):* For empiric therapy of febrile neutropenic (ETFN) patients with suspected fungal infections.

▶*Histoplasmosis (capsules and injection):* Treatment of histoplasmosis, including chronic cavitary pulmonary disease and disseminated, nonmeningeal histoplasmosis in nonimmunocompromised or immunocompromised patients.

▶*Onychomycosis (capsules only):* Treatment of onychomycosis of the toenail with or without fingernail involvement and onychomycosis of the fingernail because of dermatophytes (*Tinea unguium*) in nonimmunocompromised patients.

▶*Oropharyngeal/esophageal candidiasis (oral solution only):* Treatment of oropharyngeal or esophageal candidiasis.

▶*Unlabeled uses:* Itraconazole solution (200 mg/day) is recommended as an alternative to fluconazole as secondary prevention of oropharyngeal, vaginal, or esophageal candidiasis in HIV-infected patients who have severe or frequent recurrences; itraconazole capsules (200 mg/day) have been used as an alternative to fluconazole for primary prevention of cryptococcosis in adults with advanced HIV disease (CD4 counts less than 50 cells/mcL) and are recommended as an alternate to fluconazole for lifelong secondary prevention of cryptococcal disease in HIV-infected adults; itraconazole capsules (200 mg/day) are recommended as first-line agent in the primary prevention of histoplasmosis in adults with advanced HIV disease (CD4 counts less than 100 cells/mcL) and live in endemic areas (rate greater than or equal to 10 cases per 100 patient-years) and also as first-line agent for lifelong secondary prophylaxis (200 mg twice daily); itraconazole capsules (200 mg twice daily) are recommended as an alternate agent to fluconazole for lifelong secondary prevention of coccidioidomycosis in HIV-infected adults; oral itraconazole also is recommended for secondary prevention of histoplasmosis (first line; 2 to 5 mg/kg every 12 to

ITRACONAZOLE

48 hours), cryptococcal disease (alternate therapy; 2 to 5 mg/kg every 12 to 24 hours), and coccidioidomycosis (alternate therapy; 2 to 5 mg/kg every 12 to 48 hours) in children with HIV; oral itraconazole (2 to 5 mg/kg every 12 to 24 hours) is recommended for primary prevention of histoplasmosis (first-line agent) and cryptococcal disease (alternate therapy) in children with HIV, severe immunosuppression, and live in endemic areas (histoplasmosis).

Administration and Dosage

➤*Approved by the FDA:* September 11, 1992.

When itraconazole therapy may be indicated, isolate and identify the type of organism responsible for the infection; however, therapy may be initiated prior to obtaining these results when clinically warranted.

Do not use capsules and oral solution interchangeably.

➤*Capsules:* Take with a full meal to ensure maximal absorption.

Aspergillosis – A daily dose of 200 to 400 mg is recommended.

Blastomycosis / histoplasmosis – 200 mg once daily. If there is no obvious improvement or there is evidence of progressive fungal disease, increase the dose in 100 mg increments to a maximum of 400 mg/day. Give doses above 200 mg/day in 2 divided doses.

Life-threatening situations – Although clinical studies did not provide for a loading dose, it is recommended, based on pharmacokinetic data, that a loading dose of 200 mg 3 times/day be given for the first 3 days of treatment.

Continue treatment for a minimum of 3 months and until clinical parameters and laboratory tests indicate that the active fungal infection has subsided. An inadequate period of treatment may lead to recurrence of active infection.

Treatment of onychomycosis (fingernails only) – Two treatment pulses, each consisting of 200 mg twice daily for 1 week. The pulses are separated by a 3-week period without itraconazole.

Treatment of onychomycosis (toenails with or without fingernail involvement) – 200 mg/day for 12 weeks.

➤*Oral solution:* Take without food, if possible.

Esophageal candidiasis – 100 mg/day for a minimum treatment of 3 weeks. Continue treatment for 2 weeks following resolution of symptoms. Doses up to 200 mg/day may be used based on medical judgment of the patient's response to therapy. Vigorously swish the solution in the mouth (10 mL at a time) for several seconds and swallow.

ETFN patients with suspected fungal infections – After approximately 14 days of IV therapy, continue treatment with oral solution 200 mg twice daily until resolution of clinically significant neutropenia. The safety and efficacy of itraconazole use exceeding 28 days in ETFN is not known.

Oropharyngeal candidiasis – 200 mg/day for 1 to 2 weeks. Vigorously swish the solution in the mouth (10 mL at a time) for several seconds and swallow. For patients with oropharyngeal candidiasis unresponsive/refractory to treatment with fluconazole tablets, the recommended dose of itraconazole is 100 mg twice daily. Expect clinical response in 2 to 4 weeks. Patients may be expected to relapse shortly after discontinuing therapy. Limited data on the safety of long-term use (more than 6 months) of the oral solution are available at this time.

➤*Injection:* Use only the components provided in the kit. Do not substitute.

Admixture incompatibility – The compatibility of itraconazole injection with diluents other than 0.9% sodium chloride injection (normal saline) is not known. Do not dilute with 5% dextrose injection or with lactated Ringer's injection alone or in combination with any other diluent. Not for IV bolus injection.

Preparation / Administration – Use only a dedicated infusion line for administration of itraconazole injection. Do not introduce concomitant medication in the same bag or through the same line used for itraconazole injection. Other medications may be administered after flushing the line/catheter with 0.9% sodium chloride injection as described below and removing and replacing the entire infusion line. Alternatively use another lumen in the case of a multilumen catheter.

Add the full contents (25 mL) of the injection ampule into the infusion bag provided, which contains 50 mL of 0.9% sodium chloride injection. Mix gently after the solution is completely transferred. Using a flow control device, infuse 60 mL of the dilute solution (3.33 mg/mL = 200 mg itraconazole, pH approximately 4.8) IV over 60 minutes, using an extension line and the infusion set provided. After administration, flush the infusion set with 15 to 20 mL of 0.9% sodium chloride injection over 30 seconds to 15 minutes, via the 2-way stopcock. Do not use bacteriostatic sodium chloride injection. Discard the entire infusion line.

Blastomycosis, histoplasmosis, and aspergillosis – 200 mg IV twice daily for 4 doses, followed by 200 mg/day. Infuse each IV dose over 1 hour.

For the treatment of blastomycosis, histoplasmosis, and aspergillosis, itraconazole can be given as oral capsules or IV. The safety and efficacy of the injection administered for more than 14 days are not known.

Continue total itraconazole therapy (injection followed by capsules) for a minimum of 3 months and until clinical parameters and laboratory tests indicate that the active fungal infection has subsided. An inadequate period of treatment may lead to recurrence of active infection.

Renal function impairment: Do not use in patients with Ccr below 30 mL/min.

ETFN patients with suspected fungal infections – 200 mg twice daily for 4 doses, followed by 200 mg once daily for up to 14 days. Infuse each IV dose over 1 hour. Continue treatment with 200 mg itraconazole oral solution (20 mL) twice daily until resolution of clinically significant neutropenia. The safety and efficacy of itraconazole use exceeding 28 days in ETFN is not known.

➤*Storage / Stability:*

Capsules – Store at controlled room temperature, 15° to 25°C (59° to 77°F). Protect from light and moisture.

Oral solution – Store at or below 25°C (77°F). Do not freeze.

Injection – Store at or below 25°C (77°F). Protect from light and freezing. After reconstitution, refrigerate the diluted itraconazole injection at 2° to 8°C (36° to 46°F) or store at room temperature 15° to 25°C (59° to 77°F) for up to 48 hours when protected from direct light. During administration, exposure to normal room light is acceptable.

Actions

➤*Pharmacology:* Itraconazole is a synthetic triazole antifungal agent. In vitro, itraconazole inhibits the cytochrome P450-dependent synthesis of ergosterol, which is a vital component of fungal membranes.

➤*Pharmacokinetics:*

Absorption / Distribution –

Capsules: The oral bioavailability of itraconazole is maximal when itraconazole capsules are taken with a full meal. Absorption of itraconazole under fasted conditions in individuals with AIDS or volunteers taking gastric acid section suppressors (eg, H_2 receptor antagonists) was increased when itraconazole capsules were administered with a cola beverage. The plasma protein binding of itraconazole is 99.8%.

The pharmacokinetics of itraconazole were studied in 6 healthy male volunteers who received, in a crossover design, single 100 mg doses of the itraconazole capsule, with or without a full meal. The same 6 volunteers also received 50 or 200 mg with a full meal in a crossover design.

Mean Pharmacokinetics of Various Dosages of Itraconazole Capsules				
	50 mg (fed)	100 mg (fed)	100 mg (fasted)	200 mg (fed)
C_{max} (ng/mL)	45	132	38	289
T_{max} (hours)	3.2	4	3.3	4.7
$AUC_{0-\infty}$ (ng•h/mL)	567	1899	722	5211

Doubling the itraconazole dose results in a 3-fold increase in plasma concentrations.

The following table represents data from a crossover pharmacokinetics study in which 27 healthy male volunteers each took a single 200 mg dose of the itraconazole capsules with or without a full meal.

Mean Pharmacokinetic Parameters of a Single 200 mg Itraconazole Capsule				
	Itraconazole capsules (fed)	Itraconazole capsules (fasted)	Hydroxy-itraconazole (fed)	Hydroxy-itraconazole (fasted)
C_{max} (ng/mL)	239	140	397	286
T_{max} (hours)	4.5	3.9	5.1	4.5
$AUC_{0-\infty}$ (ng•h/mL)	3423	2094	7978	5191
$t_{1/2}$ (hours)	21	21	12	12

Steady-state concentrations were reached within 15 days following doses of 50 to 400 mg/day. Values given in the following table are data at steady state from a pharmacokinetics study in which 27 healthy male volunteers took 200 mg itraconazole capsules twice daily (with a full meal) for 15 days.

ITRACONAZOLE

Mean Steady-State Pharmacokinetic Parameters for 200 mg Itraconazole Capsules		
	Itraconazole (fed)	Hydroxyitraconazole
C_{max} (ng/mL)	2282	3488
C_{min} (ng/mL)	1855	3349
T_{max} (hours)	4.6	3.4
AUC_{0-12} (ng•h/mL)	22,569	38,572
$t_{1/2}$ (hours)	64	56

Oral solution: The absolute bioavailability of itraconazole administered as a nonmarketed solution formulation under fed condition was 55% in 6 healthy male volunteers. However, the bioavailability of the oral solution is increased under fasted conditions reaching higher maximum plasma concentrations in a shorter period of time. Unlike itraconazole capsules, administer itraconazole solution without food. The bioavailability of the solution relative to the capsules is expected to be increased further when these 2 formulations are administered under conditions that optimize their systemic absorption. Therefore, it is recommended not to use the oral solution and capsules interchangeably.

Presented in the following table are the steady-state (day 15) pharmacokinetic parameters for itraconazole oral solution under fasted and fed conditions.

Mean Pharmacokinetic Parameters for Itraconazole Oral Solution				
	Itraconazole (fasted)	Itraconazole (fed)	Hydroxy-itraconazole (fasted)	Hydroxy-itraconazole (fed)
C_{max} (ng/mL)	1963	1435	2055	1781
T_{max} (hours)	2.5	4.4	5.3	4.3
AUC_{0-24} (ng•h/mL)	29,271	22,815	45,184	38,823
$t_{1/2}$ (hours)	39.7	37.4	27.3	26.1

Injection:

The pharmacokinetics of itraconazole injection (200 mg twice daily for 2 days then 200 mg/day for 5 days) followed by oral dosing of itraconazole capsules were studied in patients with advanced HIV infection. Steady-state plasma concentrations were reached after the fourth dose for itraconazole and by the seventh dose for hydroxyitraconazole. Steady-state plasma concentrations were maintained by administration of 200 mg twice daily itraconazole capsules. Pharmacokinetic parameters for itraconazole and hydroxyitraconazole are presented in the following table.

Mean Itraconazole Pharmacokinetic Parameters				
	Injection day 7 (n = 29)		Capsules, 200 mg bid day 36 (n = 12)	
Parameter	Itraconazole	Hydroxy-itraconazole	Itraconazole	Hydroxy-itraconazole
C_{max} (ng/mL)	2856	1906	2010	2614
t_{max} (hour)	1.08	8.53	3.92	5.92
AUC_{0-12h} (ng•h/mL)	-	-	18,768	28,516
AUC_{0-24h} (ng•h/mL)	30,605	42,445	-	-

Following IV administration, the volume of distribution of itraconazole averaged 796 ± 185 L.

Metabolism/Excretion – Itraconazole is metabolized predominantly by the cytochrome P450 3A4 isoenzyme system (CYP3A4), resulting in the formation of several metabolites including hydroxyitraconazole, the major metabolite. Itraconazole may undergo saturable metabolism with multiple dosing.

Fecal excretion of the parent drug varies between 3% to 18% of the dose. Renal excretion of the parent drug is less than 0.03% of the dose. About 40% is excreted as inactive metabolites in the urine. No single excreted metabolite represents more than 5% of the dose.

Injection: Itraconazole total plasma clearance was approximately 381 mL/min following IV administration. Approximately 80% to 90% of hydroxypropyl-β-cyclodextrin is eliminated through the kidneys.

Special populations –

Renal function impairment: Plasma concentrations of itraconazole in subjects with mild to moderate renal insufficiency were comparable with those obtained in healthy subjects. Following a single IV dose of 200 mg to subjects with severe renal impairment (Ccr 19 mL/min or less), clearance of hydroxypropyl-β-cyclodextrin was reduced 6-fold compared with subjects with normal renal function. Do not use itraconazole injection in patients with a Ccr less than 30 mL/min. Itraconazole is not removed by dialysis.

Hepatic function impairment: Carefully monitor patients with impaired hepatic function. Consider the prolonged elimination half-life of itraconazole observed in a clinical trial with itraconazole capsules in cirrhotic patients when deciding to initiate therapy with other medications metabolized by CYP3A4 (see Warning Box, Contraindications, and Drug Interactions).

Decreased cardiac contractility: When itraconazole was administered IV to anesthetized dogs, a dose-related, negative inotropic effect was documented. In a healthy volunteer study of itraconazole injection, transient, asymptomatic decreases in left ventricular ejection fraction (LVEF) were observed; these resolved before the next infusion 12 hours later. Discontinue if signs or symptoms of CHF appear during administration.

Cystic fibrosis: Seventeen cystic fibrosis patients, 7 to 28 years of age, were administered 2.5 mg/kg itraconazole oral solution twice daily for 14 days in a pharmacokinetic study. Steady-state trough concentrations greater than 250 ng/mL were achieved in 6 of 11 patients at least 16 years of age but in none of the 5 patients younger than 16 years of age. Large variability was observed in the pharmacokinetic data (%CV for trough concentrations = 98% and 70% for patients 16 years of age or older and patients younger than 16 years of age, respectively; %CV for AUC = 75% and 58% for patients 16 years of age or older and patients younger than 16 years of age, respectively). If a patient with cystic fibrosis does not respond to itraconazole oral solution, consider switching to alternative therapy.

►*Microbiology:* Itraconazole exhibits in vitro activity against *Blastomyces dermatitidis*, *Histoplasma capsulatum* and *duboisii*, *Aspergillus flavus* and *fumigatus*, *Candida albicans*, and *Cryptococcus neoformans*. Itraconazole also exhibits varying in vitro activity against *Sporothrix schenckii*, *Trichophyton* sp., *Candida krusei*, and other *Candida* sp. The bioactive metabolite hydroxyitraconazole has not been evaluated against *H. capsulatum* and *B. dermatitidis*.

Resistance – Several in vitro studies have reported that some fungal clinical isolates, including *Candida* species, with reduced susceptibility to 1 azole antifungal agent also may be less susceptible to other azole derivatives. The finding of cross-resistance is dependent upon a number of factors, including the species evaluated, its clinical history, the particular azole compounds compared, and the type of susceptibility test that is performed. The relevance of these in vitro susceptibility data to clinical outcome remains to be elucidated.

►*Clinical trials:*

ETFN patients – An open, randomized trial compared the efficacy and safety of itraconazole (IV followed by oral solution) with amphotericin B for empiric therapy in 384 febrile, neutropenic patients with hematologic malignancies who had suspected fungal infections. Patients received either itraconazole (injection 200 mg twice daily for 2 days followed by 200 mg once daily for up to 14 days, followed by oral solution 200 mg twice daily) or amphotericin B (total daily dose of 0.7 to 1 mg/kg body weight). The longest treatment duration was 28 days. An outcome assignment of success required (a) patient survival with resolution of fever and neutropenia within 28 days of treatment, (b) absence of emergent fungal infections, (c) no discontinuation of therapy because of toxicity or lack of efficacy, and (d) treatment for 3 or more days. The success rate using an intent-to-treat analysis was 47% for the itraconazole group and 38% for the amphotericin B arm.

Overview of Efficacy (Intent-to-Treat Population)		
Efficacy parameters	Itraconazole (N = 179) (%)	Amphotericin B (N = 181) (%)
Success	84 (47)	68 (38)
Unevaluable[1]	24 (13)	44 (24)
Failure	71 (40)	69 (38)
Reason for failure		
Intolerance after > 3 days of antifungal medication	12	37
Persistent fever	20	7
Change in antifungal medication due to fever	13	1
Emergent fungal infection	10	9
Documented bacterial or viral infection	7	8
Insufficient response	6	5

ITRACONAZOLE

Overview of Efficacy (Intent-to-Treat Population)		
Efficacy parameters	Itraconazole (N = 179) (%)	Amphotericin B (N = 181) (%)
Deterioration of signs and symptoms	2	0
Death after > 3 days of antifungal medication	1	2
Resolution of fever	131 (73)	127 (70)
Survival	161 (90)	156 (86)

[1] Treatment duration 3 days or less (including patients who died within 3 days, withdrew because of adverse events or were deemed ineligible because of a confirmed pretreatment infection).

Oropharyngeal candidiasis – Two randomized, controlled studies for the treatment of oropharyngeal candidiasis have been conducted (N = 344). In one trial, clinical response to either 7 or 14 days of 200 mg/day itraconazole oral solution was similar to fluconazole tablets and averaged 84% across all arms. Response to 14 days therapy of itraconazole oral solution was associated with a lower relapse rate than 7 days of itraconazole therapy. In another trial, the clinical response rate for itraconazole oral solution was similar to clotrimazole troches and averaged approximately 71% across both arms. Ninety-two percent of the patients in these studies were HIV seropositive.

Esophageal candidiasis – A double-blind, randomized study (n = 119, 111 of whom were HIV seropositive) compared 100 mg/day itraconazole oral solution to 100 mg/day fluconazole tablets. The dose of each was increased to 200 mg/day for patients not responding initially. Treatment continued for 2 weeks following resolution of symptoms, for a total duration of treatment of 3 to 8 weeks. Clinical response was not significantly different between the 2 study arms. Eleven percent of itraconazole-treated patients and 21% fluconazole-treated patients were escalated to the 200 mg dose in this trial. Of the subgroup of patients who responded and entered a follow-up phase (n = 88), approximately 23% relapsed across both arms within 4 weeks.

Contraindications

➤*CHF:* Do not administer itraconazole for the treatment of onychomycosis in patients with evidence of ventricular dysfunction such as CHF or a history of CHF.

Coadministration of pimozide, quinidine, dofetilide, cisapride, triazolam, or oral midazolam; HMG-CoA reductase inhibitors metabolized by the CYP3A4 enzyme system (eg, lovastatin, simvastatin) (see Warning Box and Drug Interactions); hypersensitivity to the drug or its excipients (there is no information regarding cross-hypersensitivity between itraconazole and other azole antifungal agents; use caution in prescribing to patients with hypersensitivity to other azoles); treatment of onychomycosis in pregnant women or in women contemplating pregnancy.

Warnings

➤*Cystic fibrosis:* If a patient with cystic fibrosis does not respond to itraconazole oral solution, consider switching to alternative therapy (see Actions).

➤*HIV infection:* Because hypochlorhydria has been reported in HIV-infected patients, the absorption of itraconazole may be decreased in these patients. Administration with a cola beverage has been shown to increase itraconazole absorption in these patients.

➤*Cardiac dysrhythmias:* Life-threatening cardiac dysrhythmias or sudden death have occurred in patients using cisapride, pimozide, or quinidine concomitantly with itraconazole and/or other CYP3A4 inhibitors. Concomitant administration of these drugs with itraconazole is contraindicated.

➤*CHF:* Do not administer itraconazole for the treatment of onychomycosis in patients with evidence of ventricular dysfunction such as CHF or a history of CHF. Do not use itraconazole capsules for other indications in patients with evidence of ventricular dysfunction unless the benefit clearly outweighs the risk.

In preliminary data from a healthy volunteer study (n = 12) with itraconazole injection, a transient, asymptomatic decrease of the LVEF was observed; this resolved before the next infusion 12 hours later.

Itraconazole has been shown to have a negative inotropic effect, and has been associated with reports of CHF. Do not use itraconazole in patients with CHF or with a history of CHF unless the benefit clearly outweighs the risk. This individual benefit/risk assessment should consider factors such as the severity of the indication, the dosing regimen, and the individual risk factors for CHF. These risk factors include cardiac disease, such as ischemic and valvular disease; significant pulmonary disease, such as chronic obstructive pulmonary disease (COPD); and renal failure and other edematous disorders. Inform such patients of the signs and symptoms of CHF, treat with caution, and monitor for signs and symptoms of CHF during treatment; if such signs and symptoms do occur during treatment, discontinue itraconazole.

Cases of CHF, peripheral edema, and pulmonary edema have been reported in the postmarketing period among patients being treated for onychomycosis and/or systemic fungal infections.

➤*Hepatotoxicity:* Itraconazole has been associated with rare cases of serious hepatoxicity, including liver failure and death. Some of these cases had neither pre-existing liver disease nor a serious underlying medical condition, and some of these cases developed within the first week of treatment. If clinical signs or symptoms develop that are consistent with liver disease, discontinue treatment and perform liver function testing. Continued itraconazole use or reinstitution of treatment with itraconazole is strongly discouraged unless there is a serious or life-threatening situation where the expected benefit exceeds the risk.

In patients with elevated or abnormal liver enzymes or active liver disease, or who have experienced liver toxicity with other drugs, treatment with itraconazole is strongly discouraged unless there is a serious or life-threatening situation where the expected benefit exceeds the risk. Perform liver function monitoring in patients with pre-existing hepatic function abnormalities or those who have experienced liver toxicity with other medications, and consider in all patients receiving itraconazole. Immediately stop treatment and conduct liver function testing in patients who develop signs and symptoms suggestive of liver dysfunction.

➤*Bioequivalency:* Do not use itraconazole capsules and oral solution interchangeably. Drug exposure is greater with the oral solution than with the capsules when the same dose of drug is given. In addition, the topical effects of mucosal exposure may be different between the 2 formulations. Only the oral solution has been demonstrated effective for oral and/or esophageal candidiasis.

➤*Renal function impairment:* Do not use itraconazole injection in patients with severe renal dysfunction (Ccr less than 30 mL/min) because of prolonged elimination of hydroxypropyl-β-cyclodextrin.

➤*Carcinogenesis:* Male rats treated with 25 mg/kg/day (3.1 times the maximum recommended human dose [MRHD]) had a slightly increased incidence of soft tissue sarcoma. These sarcomas may have been a consequence of hypercholesterolemia, which is a response of rats to chronic itraconazole administration. Female rats treated with 50 mg/kg/day (6.25 times the MRHD) had an increased incidence of lung squamous cell carcinoma.

The oral solution and injection contain the excipient hydroxypropyl-β-cyclodextrin, which produced pancreatic adenocarcinomas in rats. These findings were not observed in mice. The clinical relevance of these findings is unknown.

➤*Elderly:* In general, use caution in dose selection for an elderly patient, reflecting the greater frequency of decreased hepatic, renal, or cardiac function, and of concomitant disease or other drug therapy.

➤*Pregnancy: Category C.* There are no studies in pregnant women. Use itraconazole for systemic fungal infections in pregnancy only if the benefit outweighs the potential risk. Do not administer itraconazole for the treatment of onychomycosis to pregnant patients or to women contemplating pregnancy.

Itraconazole was found to cause a dose-related increase in maternal toxicity, embryotoxicity, and teratogenicity in rats at dosage levels of approximately 40 to 160 mg/kg/day (5 to 20 × MRHD), and in mice at dosage levels of approximately 80 mg/kg/day (10 × MRHD). In rats, the teratogenicity consisted of major skeletal defects; in mice, it consisted of encephaloceles and/or macroglossia.

Women of childbearing age – Do not administer itraconazole to women of childbearing potential for the treatment of onychomycosis unless they are using effective measures to prevent pregnancy and they begin therapy on the second or third day following the onset of menses. Continue effective contraception throughout itraconazole therapy and for 2 months following the end of treatment.

➤*Lactation:* Itraconazole is excreted in breast milk; therefore, weigh the benefits for the mother against the potential risk to the infant. The US Public Health Service Centers for Disease Control and Prevention advises HIV-infected women not to breastfeed to avoid potential transmission of HIV to uninfected infants.

➤*Children:* Safety and efficacy have not been established. Patients 3 to 16 years of age have been treated with 100 mg/day itraconazole capsules for systemic fungal infections. No serious adverse effects were reported. Itraconazole oral solution was given to 26 pediatric patients, 6 months to 12 years of age. Itraconazole was dosed at 5 mg/kg once daily for 2 weeks, and no serious unexpected adverse events were reported.

Itraconazole, when administered to rats, produced bone toxicity. While no such toxicity has been reported in adult patients, the long-term effect of itraconazole in children is unknown.

Precautions

➤*Monitoring:* Monitor liver function in patients with pre-existing hepatic function abnormalities or those who have experienced liver toxicity with other medications; consider monitoring in all patients. Stop treatment immediately and conduct liver function testing in patients who develop signs and symptoms suggestive of liver dysfunction.

ITRACONAZOLE

➤*Neuropathy:* Discontinue if neuropathy occurs that may be attributable to itraconazole capsules or oral solution.

➤*Decreased gastric acidity:* Under fasted condition, itraconazole absorption was decreased in the presence of decreased gastric acidity. The absorption of itraconazole may be decreased with coadministration of antacids or gastric acid secretion suppressors. Studies conducted under fasted conditions demonstrated that administration with 8 oz of a cola beverage resulted in increased absorption of itraconazole in AIDS patients with relative or absolute achlorhydria. This increase relative to the effects of a full meal is unknown (see Actions).

Drug Interactions

➤*Cytochrome P450 system:* Itraconazole and its major metabolite, hydroxyitraconazole, are inhibitors of the cytochrome CYP3A4 enzyme system. Coadministration of itraconazole and drugs primarily metabolized by the cytochrome P450 3A4 enzyme system may result in increased plasma concentrations of the object drug, potentially increasing or prolonging therapeutic and adverse effects, including potentially serious or life-threatening adverse effects. Therefore, monitor plasma concentrations and adjust dosage accordingly or discontinue concomitant medications metabolized by the CYP3A4 enzyme system as medically indicated.

Inducers of CYP3A4 may decrease the plasma concentrations of itraconazole. Itraconazole may not be effective in patients concomitantly taking itraconazole with one of these drugs. Therefore, administration of these drugs with itraconazole is not recommended.

Other inhibitors of CYP3A4 may increase the plasma concentrations of itraconazole. Closely monitor patients who must take itraconazole concomitantly with one of these drugs for signs or symptoms of increased or prolonged pharmacologic effects of itraconazole.

Itraconazole Drug Interactions

Precipitant drug	Object drug*		Description
Antacids Proton pump inhibitors H₂-antagonists	Itraconazole	↓	Absorption of itraconazole capsules is impaired when gastric acidity is decreased. Administer at least 1 hour before or 2 hours after itraconazole capsules. Administer itraconazole with a cola beverage when coadministering with H₂-antagonists or other gastric acid suppressors.
Didanosine	Itraconazole	↓	The therapeutic effects of itraconazole may be decreased. Administer itraconazole ≥ 2 hours before didanosine chewable tablets.
Macrolide antibiotics Erythromycin Clarithromycin	Itraconazole	↑	Macrolide antibiotics may increase plasma itraconazole concentrations through inhibition of CYP3A4.
Nevirapine	Itraconazole	↓	Coadministration may lead to decreased itraconazole plasma levels and, therefore, is not recommended.
Phenobarbital	Itraconazole	↓	Decreased itraconazole plasma concentrations may occur with coadministration.
Itraconazole	Alfentanil	↑	Pharmacologic and adverse effects may be increased. Use caution when administering concurrently.
Itraconazole	Amphotericin B	↓	Studies suggest that amphotericin B activity may be suppressed by prior azole antifungal therapy. Clinical significance is unknown.
Itraconazole	Benzodiazepines Triazolam Oral midazolam Alprazolam Diazepam	↑	Increased and prolonged serum levels, CNS depression, and psychomotor impairment with certain benzodiazepines may occur, possibly several days after stopping itraconazole. Concurrent use of triazolam and oral midazolam is contraindicated.
Itraconazole	Buspirone	↑	Plasma buspirone concentrations may be elevated, increasing the pharmacologic and adverse effects. In patients receiving an azole antifungal agent when buspirone is started, it may be prudent to start with a conservative dose of buspirone.
Itraconazole	Busulfan	↑	Itraconazole may inhibit busulfan metabolism.

Itraconazole Drug Interactions

Precipitant drug	Object drug*		Description
Itraconazole	Calcium channel blockers	↑	Concomitant administration may increase negative inotropic effects. Itraconazole may inhibit the metabolism of calcium channel blockers such as dihydropyridines (eg, felodipine, nisoldipine, nifedipine) and verapamil. Edema also has been reported with concomitant therapy. Coadminister with caution.
Itraconazole	Carbamazepine	↑	Plasma concentrations of carbamazepine may be elevated, increasing clinical and adverse effects. Monitor serum levels. Decreased itraconazole plasma concentrations may occur with coadministration.
Carbamazepine	Itraconazole	↓	
Itraconazole	Cisapride	↑	Increased cisapride concentrations with cardiotoxicity may occur. Azole antifungal agents are contraindicated in patients receiving cisapride.
Itraconazole	Corticosteroids	↑	The effects of corticosteroids may be enhanced, possibly resulting in increased toxicity. Patients may require a reduction of the corticosteroid dose.
Itraconazole	Cyclosporine	↑	Increased cyclosporine levels may occur. Monitor cyclosporine levels and serum creatinine when azole antifungal therapy is added or discontinued.
Itraconazole	Digoxin	↑	Serum digoxin concentrations may be increased, enhancing its pharmacologic and adverse effects. Monitor plasma digoxin concentrations and observe the patient for signs of digoxin toxicity. Adjust digoxin dose accordingly.
Itraconazole	Docetaxel	↑	Itraconazole may inhibit docetaxel metabolism.
Itraconazole	Dofetilide	↑	Elevated dofetilide plasma concentrations may occur with increased risk of ventricular arrhythmias, including torsades de pointes. Administration with itraconazole is contraindicated.
Itraconazole	Haloperidol	↑	Haloperidol concentrations may be elevated, increasing the risk of side effects.
Itraconazole	HMG-CoA reductase inhibitors Simvastatin Lovastatin	↑	Increased plasma levels and side effects of HMG-CoA reductase inhibitors may occur. Rhabdomyolysis has been reported. If concurrent administration of these agents cannot be avoided, consider reducing the HMG-CoA reductase inhibitor dose. Coadministration with lovastatin and simvastatin is contraindicated.
Itraconazole	Hydantoins (eg, phenytoin)	↑	The pharmacologic effects of itraconazole may be decreased while those of hydantoins may be increased. Avoid concomitant use if possible.
Hydantoins (eg, phenytoin)	Itraconazole	↓	
Itraconazole	Methylprednisolone	↑	Itraconazole may inhibit methylprednisolone metabolism.
Itraconazole	Oral hypoglycemic agents	↑	Severe hypoglycemia has been reported in those receiving concomitant therapy. Monitor blood glucose levels carefully.
Itraconazole	Pimozide	↑	Concomitant use may increase pimozide plasma concentrations, resulting in serious cardiac effects. Administration with itraconazole is contraindicated.
Itraconazole	Protease inhibitors	↑	Protease inhibitor concentrations may be elevated, increasing the risk of toxicity. Consider reducing the dose of the protease inhibitor during concurrent administration with the azole antifungals. Plasma concentrations of itraconazole may be increased.
Protease inhibitors Indinavir Ritonavir	Itraconazole		

ITRACONAZOLE

Itraconazole Drug Interactions			
Precipitant drug	Object drug*		Description
Itraconazole	Quinidine	↑	Quinidine concentrations may be elevated, increasing the risk of serious cardiovascular events. Coadministration is contraindicated.
Itraconazole	Rifamycins Rifabutin Rifampin Rifapentine Isoniazid	↑	Itraconazole levels may be decreased. Itraconazole may increase rifabutin plasma levels and toxicity. Monitor antimicrobial activity, and adjust the dosage as needed if coadministration cannot be avoided.
Rifamycins Rifabutin Rifampin Rifapentine Isoniazid	Itraconazole	↓	
Itraconazole	Sirolimus	↑	Coadministration may lead to increased sirolimus plasma levels.
Itraconazole	Tacrolimus	↑	Tacrolimus concentrations may be elevated, increasing the toxicity risk.
Itraconazole	Tolterodine	↑	Tolterodine plasma concentrations may be elevated. The manufacturer of tolterodine states that patients receiving azole antifungals should not receive more than 1 mg tolterodine twice daily.
Itraconazole	Trimetrexate	↑	Itraconazole may inhibit trimetrexate metabolism.
Itraconazole	Vinca alkaloids	↑	Vinca alkaloid toxicity (constipation, myalgia, neutropenia) may be increased. Avoid concurrent administration of these agents if possible.
Itraconazole	Warfarin	↑	The anticoagulant effect of warfarin may be increased. Monitor prothrombin time (PT) and international normalized ratio (INR) values every 2 days when adding or discontinuing an azole antifungal agent. Adjust warfarin dose accordingly.
Itraconazole	Zolpidem	↑	Plasma concentrations and therapeutic effects of zolpidem may be increased. Monitor the clinical response of the patient. The dose of zolpidem may need to be decreased.

* ↑ = Object drug increased. ↓ = Object drug decreased.

►*Drug/Food interactions:* When itraconazole capsules are administered, cola/food may increase itraconazole levels. To ensure optimal itraconazole absorption, take capsules immediately after meals. Oral bioavailability is maximal when itraconazole oral solution is taken without food. Grapefruit juice may reduce plasma levels and the therapeutic effects of itraconazole. Avoid coadministration with grapefruit products.

Adverse Reactions

Itraconazole has been associated with rare cases of serious hepatotoxicity, including liver failure and death. Some of these cases had neither pre-existing liver disease nor a serious underlying medical condition. If clinical signs or symptoms develop that are consistent with liver disease, discontinue treatment and perform liver function tests. Reassess the risks and benefits of itraconazole use.

►*Capsules:*

Adverse events in the treatment of systemic fungal infections – Adverse event data were derived from 602 patients treated for systemic fungal disease in US clinical trials who were immunocomprised or receiving multiple concomitant medications. Treatment was discontinued in 10.5% of patients due to adverse events. The median duration before discontinuation of therapy was 81 days (range, 2 to 776 days). The table lists adverse events reported by at least 1% of patients.

Itraconazole Adverse Events During Clinical Trials of Systemic Fungal Infections ≥ 1%	
Adverse reaction	Incidence (N = 602)
CNS	
Dizziness	2
Headache	4
Libido decreased	1
Somnolence	1

Itraconazole Adverse Events During Clinical Trials of Systemic Fungal Infections ≥ 1%	
Adverse reaction	Incidence (N = 602)
Dermatologic	
Pruritus	3
Rash[1]	9
GI	
Abdominal pain	2
Anorexia	1
Diarrhea	3
Nausea	11
Vomiting	5
Miscellaneous	
Albuminuria	1
Edema	4
Fatigue	3
Fever	3
Hepatic function abnormal	3
Hypertension	3
Hypokalemia	2
Impotence	1
Malaise	1

[1] Rash tends to occur more frequently in immunocompromised patients receiving immunosuppressive medications.

Adverse events infrequently reported in all studies included adrenal insufficiency, constipation, depression, gastritis, gynecomastia, insomnia, male breast pain, menstrual disorder, and tinnitus.

Adverse events reported in toenail onychomycosis clinical trials – Patients in these trials were on a continuous dosing regimen of 200 mg once daily for 12 consecutive weeks.

Itraconazole Adverse Events in Clinical Trials of Onychomycosis of the Toenail (≥ 1%)	
Adverse reaction	Incidence (n = 112)
Cardiovascular	
Hypertension	2
Orthostatic hypotension	1
CNS	
Abnormal dreaming	2
Asthenia	4
Dizziness	2
Headache	10
Malaise	1
Tremor	2
Vertigo	1
GI	
Abdominal pain	4
Appetite increased	2
Constipation	2
Diarrhea	4
Dyspepsia	4
Flatulence	4
Gastritis	2
Gastroenteritis	2
Nausea	3
GU	
Cystitis	3
Urinary tract infection	3
Respiratory	
Pharyngitis	2
Rhinitis	9
Sinusitis	7
Upper respiratory tract infection	8
Miscellaneous	
Fever	2
Herpes zoster	2
Injury	7
Liver function abnormality	3
Myalgia	3
Pain	2
Rash	4
Vasculitis	1

ITRACONAZOLE

Patients Temporarily or Permanently Discontinuing Itraconazole Treatment of Onychomycosis of the Toenail Because of an Adverse Event	
Adverse reaction	Incidence (%)
Elevated liver enzymes > 2 times the ULN	4
GI disorder	4
Headache	1
Hypertension	2
Malaise	1
Myalgia	1
Orthostatic hypotension	1
Rash	3
Vasculitis	1
Vertigo	1

Adverse events reported in fingernail onychomycosis clinical trials – Patients in these trials were on a pulse regimen consisting of two 1-week treatment periods of 200 mg twice daily, separated by a 3-week period without drug.

Itraconazole Adverse Events in Clinical Trials of Onychomycosis of the Fingernail (≥ 1%)	
Adverse reaction	Incidence (n = 37)
CNS	
Anxiety	3
Depression	3
Headache	8
Malaise	3
Dermatologic	
Pruritus	5
Rash	3
GI	
Abdominal pain	3
Constipation	3
Dyspepsia	3
Gingivitis	3
Nausea	5
Ulcerative stomatitis	3
Respiratory	
Rhinitis	5
Sinusitis	3
Miscellaneous	
Bursitis	3
Fatigue	3
Hypertriglyceridemia	3
Injury	3
Pain	3

Patients Temporarily or Permanently Discontinuing Itraconazole Treatment of Onychomycosis of the Fingernail Because of Adverse Events (%)	
Adverse reaction	Incidence Itraconazole (N = 37)
Hypertriglyceridemia	3
Rash/Pruritus	3

The following adverse events occurred with an incidence of at least 1% (N = 37): Headache (8%); nausea, pruritus, rhinitis (5%); abdominal pain, anxiety, bursitis, constipation, depression, dyspepsia, fatigue, gingivitis, hypertriglyceridemia, injury, malaise, pain, rash, sinusitis, ulcerative stomatitis (3%).

➤*Oral solution:*

Adverse events reported in ETFN patients – Adverse events considered at least possibly drug related in a clinical trial of empiric therapy in 384 febrile, neutropenic patients (192 treated with itraconazole and 192 with amphotericin B) with suspected fungal infections are listed in the following table. Patients received a regimen of itraconazole injection followed by itraconazole oral solution. The dose of itraconazole injection was 200 mg twice daily for the first 2 days followed by a single daily dose of 200 mg for the remainder of the IV treatment period. The majority of patients received between 7 and 14 days of itraconazole injection. The dose of itraconazole oral solution was 200 mg (20 mL) twice daily for the remainder of therapy.

Itraconazole Oral Solution Adverse Events (≥ 2%)		
Adverse reaction	Itraconazole (N = 192)	Amphotericin B (N = 192)
Cardiovascular		
Hypertension	0	2
Hypotension	1	3
Tachycardia	1	3
Dermatological		
Rash	5	3
Sweating increased	2	1
GI		
Abdominal pain	3	3
Diarrhea	10	9
Nausea	11	15
Vomiting	7	10
Hepatic		
ALT increased	3	1
AST increased	2	1
Bilirubinemia	6	3
Hepatic function abnormal	3	2
Jaundice	2	1
Metabolic		
Alkaline phosphatase increased	2	2
BUN increased	1	6
Fluid overload	1	3
Hypocalcemia	1	2
Hypokalemia	9	28
Hypomagnesemia	2	4
LDH increased	2	0
Serum creatinine increased	3	25
Miscellaneous		
Dyspnea	1	3
Edema	2	2
Fever	0	7
Headache	2	2
Renal function abnormal	1	12
Rigors	1	34

The following additional adverse events considered at least possibly related occurred in between 1% and 2% of patients who received itraconazole injection and oral solution: Constipation, dizziness, erythematous rash, gamma-GT increased, hypophosphatemia, pruritus, pulmonary infiltration, and tremor.

Adverse events reported in oropharyngeal or esophageal candidiasis trials – US adverse experience data are derived from 350 immunocompromised patients (332 HIV seropositive/AIDS) treated for oropharyngeal or esophageal candidiasis. The table below lists adverse events reported by at least 2% of patients treated with itraconazole oral solution in US clinical trials. Data on patients receiving comparator agents in these trials are included for comparison.

Summary of Adverse Events of Itraconazole Treated Patients in US Clinical Trials (Total) (≥ 2%)				
	Itraconazole			
Adverse reaction	Total (n = 350[1])	All controlled studies (n = 272)	Fluconazole (n = 125)	Clotrimazole (n = 81)
CNS				
Depression	2	1	0	1
Dizziness	2	2	4	1
Headache	4	4	6	6
Dermatologic				
Increased sweating	3	4	6	1
Rash	4	5	4	6
Skin disorder, unspecified	2	2	2	1
GI				
Abdominal pain	6	4	7	7
Constipation	2	2	1	0
Diarrhea	11	10	10	4
Nausea	11	10	11	5
Vomiting	7	6	8	1
Respiratory				
Coughing	4	4	10	0
Dyspnea	2	3	5	1
Pneumonia	2	2	0	0
Sinusitis	2	2	4	0
Sputum increased	2	3	3	1
Miscellaneous				
Chest pain	3	3	2	0

ITRACONAZOLE

Summary of Adverse Events of Itraconazole Treated Patients in US Clinical Trials (Total) (≥ 2%)				
	Itraconazole			
Adverse reaction	Total (n = 350[1])	All controlled studies (n = 272)	Fluconazole (n = 125)	Clotrimazole (n = 81)
Fatigue	2	1	2	0
Fever	7	6	8	5
Pain	2	2	4	0
Pneumocystis carinii infection	2	2	2	0

[1] Of the 350 patients, 209 were treated for oropharyngeal candidiasis in controlled studies, 63 were treated for esophageal candidiasis in controlled studies and 78 were treated for oropharyngeal candidiasis in an open study.

Other adverse events (less than 2%): Abnormal vision, adrenal insufficiency, asthenia, back pain, dehydration, dyspepsia, dysphagia, flatulence, gynecomastia, hematuria, hemorrhoids, hot flushes, implantation complication, infection unspecified, injury, insomnia, male breast pain, myalgia, pharyngitis, pruritus, rhinitis, rigors, ulcerative stomatitis, taste perversion, tinnitus, upper respiratory tract infection, and weight decrease.

►*Injection:* Adverse events considered at least possibly drug-related are listed in the following table and are based on the experience of 360 patients treated with itraconazole injection. Nearly all patients were neutropenic or were otherwise immunocompromised and were treated empirically for febrile episodes, for documented systemic fungal infections, or in trials to determine pharmacokinetics.

Itraconazole Injection Adverse Reactions (≥ 1%)				
		Comparative studies		
Adverse reaction	Itraconazole injection (n = 360)	Itraconazole injection (n = 234)	IV Fluconazole (N = 32)	IV Amphotericin B (N = 202)
CNS				
Dizziness	1	2	0	1
Headache	2	2	0	3
Dermatologic				
Rash	3	3	3	3
Sweating increased	1	2	0	0
GI				
Abdominal pain	2	2	0	3
Constipation	0	1	3	0
Diarrhea	6	6	3	9
Jaundice	1	2	0	0
Nausea	8	9	0	15
Vomiting	4	6	0	10
Lab test abnor malities				
ALT increased	2	3	3	1
AST increased	1	2	0	0
Alkaline phosphatase, increased	1	2	3	2
BUN increased	0	1	0	7
Bilirubinemia	4	6	9	3
Hepatic function abnormal	1	2	0	2
Hypokalemia	5	8	0	29

Itraconazole Injection Adverse Reactions (≥ 1%)				
		Comparative studies		
Adverse reaction	Itraconazole injection (n = 360)	Itraconazole injection (n = 234)	IV Fluconazole (N = 32)	IV Amphotericin B (N = 202)
Hypomagnesemia	1	1	0	5
Serum creatinine increased	2	2	3	26
Miscellaneous				
Abnormal renal function	1	1	0	11
Application site reaction	4	0	0	0
Pain	1	2	0	0
Tachycardia	0	1	0	3
Vein disorder	3	0	0	0

►*Postmarketing experience:* Worldwide postmarketing experiences with the use of itraconazole include adverse events of GI origin, such as abdominal pain, constipation, diarrhea, dyspepsia, nausea, and vomiting. Other reported adverse events include allergic reactions (eg, anaphylaxis, angioedema, pruritus, rash, urticaria); alopecia, CHF and pulmonary edema, dizziness, headache, hepatitis, hypertriglyceridemia, hypokalemia, liver failure, menstrual disorders, neutropenia, peripheral edema, peripheral neuropathy, reversible increases in hepatic enzymes, and Stevens-Johnson syndrome.

Overdosage

►*Symptoms:* There is limited experience of overdosage with itraconazole. In patients taking either 1000 mg itraconazole oral solution or up to 3000 mg itraconazole capsules, or twice-daily dosing for 4 days with itraconazole injection, the adverse event profile was similar to that observed at recommended doses.

►*Treatment:* Itraconazole is not removed by dialysis. In the event of accidental overdosage, employ supportive measures, including gastric lavage with sodium bicarbonate. Refer to General Management of Acute Overdosage.

Patient Information

Instruct patients to contact a physician at once if swelling of the legs or difficulty breathing occurs.

Instruct patients to report any signs and symptoms that may suggest liver problems so that the appropriate laboratory testing can be done. Such signs may include fatigue, appetite loss, nausea, and/or vomiting, yellowing of the skin or eyes, dark urine, or pale stool.

Instruct patients to contact a physician before taking any concomitant medications with this medicine to ensure there are no potential drug interactions.

Instruct patients with previous conditions to talk with their health care provider before taking this medication.

Instruct patients not to use oral solution and capsules interchangeably.

►*Capsules:* Advise patients that before taking this medicine for a nail infection, they must have nail specimens and certain lab tests performed to confirm that they have a nail infection.

Instruct patients to take this medicine with a full meal.

►*Oral solution:* Instruct patients to take without food, if possible.

Instruct patients to swish solution vigorously in the mouth for several seconds and swallow.

TERBINAFINE HCl

Rx   Lamisil (Novartis)   **Tablet:** 250 mg   (Lamisil 250). White to yellow-tinged white, biconvex. In 30s and 100s.

WARNING

Rare cases of hepatic failure, some leading to death or liver transplant, have occurred with the use of terbinafine for the treatment of onychomycosis in individuals with and without preexisting liver disease. In the majority of liver cases reported in association with terbinafine use, the patients had serious underlying systemic conditions and an uncertain causal relationship with terbinafine. Terbinafine is not recommended for patients with chronic or active liver disease. Before prescribing terbinafine, assess preexisting liver disease. Hepatotoxicity may occur in patients with and without preexisting liver disease. Pretreatment serum transaminase (ALT and AST) tests are advised for all patients before taking terbinafine.

Indications

➤*Onychomycosis:* Treatment of onychomycosis of the toenail or fingernail because of dermatophytes (tinea unguium).

Prior to initiating treatment, obtain appropriate nail specimens for laboratory testing (KOH preparation, fungal culture, or nail biopsy) to confirm the diagnosis of onychomycosis.

Administration and Dosage

➤*Approved by the FDA:* May 10, 1996.

➤*Onychomycosis:*

Fingernail – 250 mg/day for 6 weeks.

Toenail – 250 mg/day for 12 weeks.

The optimal clinical effect is seen months after mycological cure and cessation of treatment. This is related to the period required for outgrowth of healthy nail.

➤*Storage/Stability:* Store tablets below 25°C (77°F) in a tight container. Protect from light.

Actions

➤*Pharmacology:* Terbinafine HCl is a synthetic allylamine derivative and is hypothesized to act by inhibiting squalene epoxidase, thus blocking the biosynthesis of ergosterol, an essential component of fungal cell membranes.

➤*Pharmacokinetics:*

Absorption/Distribution – Terbinafine is well absorbed (greater than 70%). As a result of first-pass metabolism, the bioavailability is approximately 40%. Peak plasma concentrations of 1 mcg/mL appear within 2 hours after a single 250 mg dose; the area under the plasma concentration-time curve (AUC) is approximately 4.56 mcg•hr/mL. An increase in the AUC of terbinafine of less than 20% is observed when terbinafine is taken with food.

Metabolism/Excretion – Prior to excretion, terbinafine is extensively metabolized. No metabolites have been identified that have antifungal activity similar to terbinafine. Approximately 70% of the administered dose is eliminated in the urine.

Special populations – In patients with renal impairment (creatinine clearance less than or equal to 50 mL/min) or hepatic cirrhosis, the clearance of terbinafine is decreased by approximately 50%. In plasma, terbinafine is more than 99% bound to plasma proteins with no specific binding sites. At steady-state, in comparison to a single dose, the peak concentration of terbinafine is 25% higher and plasma AUC increases by a factor of 2.5; the increase in plasma AUC is consistent with an effective half-life of approximately 36 hours. A terminal half-life of 200 to 400 hours may represent the slow elimination of terbinafine from tissues such as skin and adipose.

➤*Microbiology:* Terbinafine is active against most strains of the following organisms both in vitro and in clinical infections: *Trichophyton mentagrophytes* and *T. rubrum*. In vitro, terbinafine exhibits satisfactory MICs against most strains of the following organisms which can infect the nail; however, safety and efficacy of terbinafine in treating clinical infections caused by the following organisms have not been established: *Epidermophyton floccosum*, *Candida albicans*, and *Scopulariopsis brevicaulis*.

Contraindications

Hypersensitivity to terbinafine or any component of the product.

Warnings

➤*Hepatic failure:* Rare cases of liver failure, some leading to death or liver transplant, have occurred with the use of terbinafine for the treatment of onychomycosis in individuals with and without preexisting liver disease.

The severity of hepatic events and/or their outcome may be worse in patients with active or chronic liver disease. Discontinue treatment with terbinafine if biochemical or clinical evidence of liver injury develops.

➤*Ophthalmic:* Changes in the ocular lens and retina have been reported. The clinical significance of these changes is unknown.

➤*Neutropenia:* Isolated cases of severe neutropenia have been reported but were reversible with discontinuation of treatment with or without supportive therapy. If clinical signs and symptoms suggest a secondary infection, obtain a complete blood count (CBC). If the neutrophil count is 1000 cells/mm^3 or less, discontinue treatment and start supportive management.

➤*Dermatologic:* There have been isolated reports of serious skin reactions (eg, Stevens-Johnson syndrome, toxic epidermal necrolysis). If progressive skin rash occurs, discontinue treatment.

➤*Renal function impairment:* In patients with renal impairment (creatinine clearance 50 mL/min or less), the use of terbinafine has not been adequately studied, and therefore, is not recommended.

➤*Hepatic function impairment:* Terbinafine is not recommended for patients with chronic or active liver disease. Before prescribing terbinafine tablets, assess preexisting liver disease. Hepatotoxicity may occur in patients with and without preexisting liver disease.

➤*Pregnancy:* Category B. There are no adequate and well-controlled studies in pregnant women. Because treatment of onychomycosis can be postponed until after pregnancy is completed, it is recommended that terbinafine tablets not be initiated during pregnancy.

➤*Lactation:* After oral administration, terbinafine is present in the breast milk of nursing mothers. The ratio of terbinafine in milk to plasma is 7:1. Treatment with terbinafine is not recommended in nursing mothers.

➤*Children:* Safety and efficacy in children have not been established.

Precautions

➤*Monitoring:*

Immunodeficiency – Consider monitoring CBC in patients receiving treatment for more than 6 weeks in patients with known or suspected immunodeficiency.

Hepatic – Pretreatment serum transaminase (ALT and AST) tests are advised for all patients before taking terbinafine. Warn patients to immediately report to their physician any symptoms of persistent nausea, anorexia, fatigue, vomiting, right upper abdominal pain or jaundice, dark urine, or pale stools. Patients with these symptoms should discontinue taking oral terbinafine, and the patient's liver function should be immediately evaluated.

Drug Interactions

Terbinafine inhibits CYP2D6-mediated metabolism. This may be of clinical relevance for compounds predominantly metabolized by this enzyme, such as tricyclic antidepressants, beta blockers, selective serotonin reuptake inhibitors (SSRIs), and monoamine oxidase inhibitors (MAOIs) type B, if they have a narrow therapeutic window.

Terbinafine Drug Interactions			
Precipitant drug	Object drug*		Description
Cimetidine	Terbinafine	↑	Terbinafine clearance is decreased 33% by cimetidine.
Rifampin	Terbinafine	↓	Terbinafine clearance is increased 100% by rifampin.
Terbinafine	Caffeine	↑	Terbinafine decreases the clearance of caffeine by 19%.
Terbinafine	Cyclosporine	↓	Terbinafine increases the clearance of cyclosporine by 15%.
Terbinafine	Dextromethorphan	↑	Plasma dextromethorphan concentrations may be elevated, increasing the pharmacologic and adverse effects. Terbinafine inhibits dextromethorphan metabolism via the cytochrome P450 2D6 enzyme.

* ↑ = Object drug increased. ↓ = Object drug decreased.

Adverse Reactions

Terbinafine Adverse Reactions (%)		
Adverse reaction	Terbinafine (n = 465)	Placebo (n = 137)
Dermatologic		
Rash	5.6	2.2
Pruritus	2.8	1.5
Urticaria	1.1	0
GI		
Diarrhea	5.6	2.9
Dyspepsia	4.3	2.9
Abdominal pain	2.4	1.5
Nausea	2.6	2.9
Flatulence	2.2	2.2

TERBINAFINE HCl

Terbinafine Adverse Reactions (%)		
Adverse reaction	Terbinafine (n = 465)	Placebo (n = 137)
Miscellaneous		
Liver enzyme abnormalities[1]	3.3	1.4
Headache	12.9	9.5
Taste disturbance	2.8	0.7
Visual disturbance	1.1	1.5

[1] Liver enzyme abnormalities 2 times or more the upper limit of the normal range.

➤*Other (rare):* Idiosyncratic and symptomatic hepatic injury and more rarely, cases of liver failure, some leading to death or liver transplant, serious skin reactions, severe neutropenia, thrombocytopenia, and allergic reactions (including anaphylaxis) have occurred. Uncommonly, terbinafine may cause taste disturbance (including taste loss), which usually recovers within several weeks after discontinuation of the drug. There have been isolated reports of prolonged (more than 1 year) taste disturbance. Rarely, taste disturbances associated with oral terbinafine have been reported to be severe enough to result in decreased food intake leading to significant and unwanted weight loss.

Other adverse reactions that have been reported include malaise, fatigue, vomiting, arthralgia, myalgia, and hair loss.

Clinical adverse effects reported spontaneously since the drug was marketed include altered prothrombin time (prolongation and reduction) in patients concomitantly treated with warfarin and terbinafine tablets and agranulocytosis (rare).

Overdosage

➤*Symptoms:* Clinical experience regarding overdosage with terbinafine is limited. Doses up to 5 g (20 times the therapeutic daily dose) have been taken without inducing serious adverse reactions. Symptoms of overdose included the following: Nausea, vomiting, abdominal pain, dizziness, rash, frequent urination, and headache.

Patient Information

Continue taking this medication for the recommended length of treatment.

Immediately report to physician any symptoms of persistent nausea, anorexia, jaundice, dark urine, or pale stools.

CASPOFUNGIN ACETATE

Rx **Cancidas** (Merck)

Powder for injection, lyophilized: 50 mg	In single-use vials.
70 mg	In single-use vials.

Indications

➤*Invasive aspergillosis:* For the treatment of invasive aspergillosis in patients who are refractory to or intolerant of other therapies (eg, amphotericin B, lipid formulations of amphotericin B, or itraconazole). Caspofungin has not been studied as initial therapy for invasive aspergillosis.

Administration and Dosage

➤*Approved by the FDA:* January 29, 2001.

➤*Invasive aspergillosis:* A single 70 mg loading dose should be administered on day 1, followed by 50 mg daily thereafter. Administer by slow IV infusion of ≈ 1 hour. Duration of treatment should be based upon the severity of the patient's underlying disease, recovery from immunosuppression, and clinical response. The efficacy of a 70 mg dose regimen in patients who are not clinically responding to the 50 mg daily dose is not known. Limited safety data suggests that an increase in dose to 70 mg daily is well tolerated. The safety and efficacy of doses > 70 mg have not been adequately studied.

➤*Hepatic insufficiency:* Patients with mild hepatic insufficiency (Child-Pugh score 5 to 6) do not need a dosage adjustment. However, for patients with moderate hepatic insufficiency (Child-Pugh score 7 to 9), after the initial 70 mg loading dose, caspofungin 35 mg daily is recommended. There is no clinical experience in patients with severe hepatic insufficiency (Child-Pugh score > 9; see Pharmacokinetics).

➤*IV admixture incompatibility:* Do not mix or co-infuse caspofungin with other medications. Do not use diluents containing dextrose (α-D-glucose).

➤*Preparation of solution:*

Preparation of the 70 mg day 1 loading dose infusion –
1.) Equilibrate the refrigerated vial of caspofungin to room temperature.
2.) Aseptically add 10.5 mL of 0.9% Sodium Chloride Injection to the vial.
3.) Aseptically transfer 10 mL of reconstituted caspofungin to an IV containing 250 mL 0.9% Sodium Chloride Injection. (If a 70 mg vial is unavailable, see alternative infusion preparation methods).

Preparation of the daily 50 mg infusion –
1.) Equilibrate the refrigerated vial of caspofungin to room temperature.
2.) Aseptically add 10.5 mL of 0.9% Sodium Chloride Injection to the vial.
3.) Aseptically transfer 10 mL of reconstituted caspofungin to an IV containing 250 mL 0.9% Sodium Chloride Injection. (If a reduced infusion volume is medically necessary, see alternative infusion preparation methods.)

Alternative infusion preparation methods –

Preparation of 70 mg day 1 loading dose from two 50 mg vials: Reconstitute two 50 mg vials with 10.5 mL of diluent each (see Preparation of the daily 50 mg infusion). Aseptically transfer a total of 14 mL of the reconstituted caspofungin from the 2 vials to 250 mL of 0.9% Sodium Chloride Injection.

Preparation of 50 mg daily doses at reduced volume: When medically necessary, the 50 mg daily doses can be prepared by adding 10 mL of reconstituted caspofungin to 100 mL of 0.9% Sodium Chloride Injection (see Preparation of the daily 50 mg infusion).

Preparation of a 35 mg daily dose for patients with moderate hepatic insufficiency – Reconstitute one 50 mg vial (see Preparation of the daily 50 mg infusion). Aseptically transfer 7 mL of the reconstituted caspofungin from the vial to 250 mL of 0.9% Sodium Chloride Injection or, if medically necessary, to 100 mL of 0.9% Sodium Chloride Injection.

Preparation notes –
1.) The white to off-white cake will dissolve completely. Mix gently until a clear solution is obtained.
2.) Visually inspect the reconstituted solution for particulate matter or discoloration during reconstitution and prior to infusion. Do not use if the solution is cloudy or has precipitated.
3.) Caspofungin is formulated to provide the full labeled vial dose (70 or 50 mg) when 10 mL is withdrawn from the vial.

Caspofungin Concentrations			
Dose	Reconstituted solution concentration	Infusion volume	Infusion solution concentration
70 mg initial dose	7.2 mg/mL	260 mL	0.28 mg/mL
50 mg daily dose	5.2 mg/mL	260 mL	0.2 mg/mL
70 mg initial dose[1] (from 2 50 mg vials)	5.2 mg/mL	264 mL	0.28 mg/mL

Caspofungin Concentrations			
Dose	Reconstituted solution concentration	Infusion volume	Infusion solution concentration
50 mg daily dose[1] (reduced volume)	5.2 mg/mL	110 mL	0.47 mg/mL
35 mg daily dose[1] (from 1 50 mg vial) for moderate hepatic insufficiency	5.2 mg/mL or 5.2 mg/mL	257 mL or 107 mL	0.14 mg/mL or 0.34 mg/mL

[1] See preceding text for these special situations.

➤*Storage/Stability:*

Vials – Store the lyophilized vials at 2° to 8°C (36° to 46°F).

Reconstituted concentrate – Reconstituted caspofungin may be stored at ≤ 25°C (≤ 77°F) for 1 hour prior to the preparation of the patient infusion solution.

Diluted product – The final patient infusion solution in the IV bag or bottle can be stored at ≤ 25°C (≤ 77°F) for 24 hours.

Actions

➤*Pharmacology:* Caspofungin acetate is the first of a new class of antifungal drugs (glucan synthesis inhibitors) that inhibit the synthesis of β (1,3)-D-glucan, an integral component of the fungal cell wall.

➤*Pharmacokinetics:*

Distribution – Plasma concentrations of caspofungin decline in a polyphasic manner following single 1-hour IV infusions. A short α-phase occurs immediately postinfusion, followed by an β-phase (half-life of 9 to 11 hours) that characterizes much of the profile and exhibits clear log-linear behavior from 6 to 48 hours postdose, during which the plasma concentration decreases 10-fold. An additional, longer half-life phase, γ-phase (half-life of 40 to 50 hours) also occurs. Distribution, rather than excretion or biotransformation, is the dominant mechanism influencing plasma clearance. Caspofungin is extensively bound to albumin (≈ 97%), and distribution into red blood cells is minimal. Mass balance results showed that ≈ 92% of the administered radioactivity was distributed to tissues by 36 to 48 hours after a single 70 mg dose of [3H] caspofungin acetate. There is little excretion or biotransformation of caspofungin during the first 30 hours after administration.

Metabolism – Caspofungin is slowly metabolized by hydrolysis and N-acetylation. Caspofungin also undergoes spontaneous chemical degradation to an open-ring peptide compound, L-747969. At later time points (5 to 20 days postdose), there is a low level (3 to 7 picomoles/mg protein, or 0.6% to 1.3% of administered dose) of covalent binding of radiolabel in plasma following single-dose administration of [3H] caspofungin acetate, which may be due to 2 reactive intermediates formed during the chemical degradation of caspofungin to L-747969. Additional metabolism involves hydrolysis into constitutive amino acids and their degradates, including dihydroxyhomotyrosine and N-acetyl-dihydroxyhomotyrosine. These 2 tyrosine derivatives are found only in urine, suggesting rapid clearance of these derivatives by the kidneys.

Excretion – In a single-dose radiolabeled pharmacokinetic study, plasma, urine, and feces were collected over 27 days. Plasma concentrations of radioactivity and of caspofungin were similar during the first 24 to 48 hours postdose; thereafter, drug levels fell more rapidly. Radiolabel remained quantifiable through day 27; whereas caspofungin concentrations fell below the limit of quantitation after 6 to 8 days postdose. After single IV administration of [3H] caspofungin acetate, excretion of caspofungin and its metabolites in humans were 35% of dose in feces and 41% of dose in urine. A small amount of caspofungin is excreted unchanged in urine (≈ 1.4% of dose). Renal clearance of parent drug is low (≈ 0.15 mL/min) and total clearance of caspofungin is 12 mL/min.

Special populations –

Renal insufficiency: In a clinical study of single 70 mg doses, caspofungin pharmacokinetics were similar in volunteers with mild renal insufficiency (creatinine clearance [Ccr] 50 to 80 mL/min) and control subjects. Moderate (Ccr 31 to 49 mL/min), advanced (Ccr 5 to 30 mL/min), and end-stage (Ccr < 10 mL/min and dialysis dependent) renal insufficiency moderately increased caspofungin plasma concentrations after single-dose administration (range, 30% to 49% for AUC). However, in patients with invasive aspergillosis who received multiple daily doses of 50 mg caspofungin, there was no significant effect of mild to advanced renal impairment on caspofungin trough concentrations. No dosage adjustment is necessary for patients with renal insufficiency. Caspofungin is not dialyzable, thus supplementary dosing is not required following hemodialysis.

Hepatic insufficiency: Plasma concentrations of caspofungin after a single 70 mg dose in patients with mild hepatic insufficiency (Child-Pugh score 5 to 6) were increased by ≈ 55% in AUC compared to healthy control subjects. In a 14-day multiple-dose study (70 mg on day

CASPOFUNGIN ACETATE

1 followed by 50 mg daily thereafter), plasma concentrations in patients with mild hepatic insufficiency were increased modestly (19% to 25% in AUC) on days 7 and 14 relative to healthy control subjects. No dosage adjustment is recommended for patients with mild hepatic insufficiency. Patients with moderate hepatic insufficiency (Child-Pugh score 7 to 9) who received a single 70 mg dose of caspofungin had an average plasma caspofungin increase of 76% in AUC compared to control subjects. A dosage reduction is recommended for patients with moderate hepatic insufficiency (see Administration and Dosage). There is no clinical experience in patients with severe hepatic insufficiency (Child-Pugh score > 9).

Microbiology – Caspofungin inhibits the synthesis of β (1,3)-D-glucan, an essential component of the cell wall of susceptible filamentous fungi. β (1,3)-D-glucan is not present in mammalian cells. Caspofungin has shown activity in regions of active cell growth of the hyphae of *Aspergillus fumigatus*.

Caspofungin exhibits in vitro activity against *A. fumigatus, A. flavus,* and *A. terreus.*

Contraindications

Hypersensitivity to any component of this product.

Warnings

➤*Concomitant use with cyclosporine:* Concomitant use of caspofungin with cyclosporine is not recommended unless the potential benefit outweighs the potential risk to the patient. In 1 clinical study, 3 of 4 healthy subjects who received caspofungin 70 mg on days 1 through 10, and also received two 3 mg/kg doses of cyclosporine 12 hours apart on day 10, developed transient elevations of ALT on day 11 that were 2 to 3 times the upper limit of normal (ULN). In a separate panel of subjects in the same study, 2 of 8 who received caspofungin 35 mg daily for 3 days and cyclosporine (two 3 mg/kg doses administered 12 hours apart) on day 1 had small increases in ALT (slightly above the ULN) on day 2. In both groups, elevations in AST paralleled ALT elevations, but were of lesser magnitude (see Adverse Reactions). Hence, concomitant use of caspofungin with cyclosporine is not recommended until multiple-dose use in patients is studied.

➤*Hepatic function impairment:* Patients with mild hepatic insufficiency (Child-Pugh score 5 to 6) do not need a dosage adjustment. For patients with moderate hepatic insufficiency (Child-Pugh score 7 to 9), after the initial 70 mg loading dose, caspofungin 35 mg daily is recommended. There is no clinical experience in patients with severe hepatic insufficiency (Child-Pugh score > 9).

➤*Pregnancy: Category C.* Caspofungin was shown to be embryotoxic in rats and rabbits. Findings included incomplete ossification of the skull and torso and an increased incidence of cervical rib in rats. An increased incidence of incomplete ossifications of the talus/calcaneus was seen in rabbits. Caspofungin also produced increases in resorptions in rats and rabbits and peri-implantation losses in rats. These findings were observed at doses that produced exposures similar to those seen in patients treated with a 70 mg dose. Caspofungin crossed the placental barrier in rats and rabbits and was detected in the plasma of fetuses of pregnant animals dosed with caspofungin. There are no adequate and well-controlled studies in pregnant women. Caspofungin should be used during pregnancy only if the potential benefit justifies the potential risk to the fetus.

➤*Lactation:* Caspofungin was found in the milk of lactating, drug-treated rats. It is not known whether caspofungin is excreted in human milk. Because many drugs are excreted in human milk, caution should be exercised when caspofungin is administered to a nursing woman.

➤*Children:* Safety and efficacy in pediatric patients have not been established.

Drug Interactions

Caspofungin Drug Interactions

Precipitant drug	Object drug*		Description
Caspofungin	Tacrolimus	↓	Concomitant administration produced a decrease in the AUC of tacrolimus by ≈ 20%, C_{max} by 16%, and 12-hour blood concentration by 26%. Monitor tacrolimus blood concentrations and adjust dose accordingly.
Cyclosporine	Caspofungin	↑	Cyclosporine increased the AUC of caspofungin by ≈ 35%. Concurrent use also produced transient elevations in ALT and AST.
Inducers of drug clearance or mixed inducer/inhibitors (efavirenz, nelfinavir, nevirapine, phenytoin, rifampin, dexamethasone, or carbamazepine)	Caspofungin	↓	Coadministration may result in clinically meaningful reductions in caspofungin concentrations. When coadministering caspofungin with those listed, an increase in the daily dose of caspofungin to 70 mg, following the usual 70 mg loading dose, should be considered in patients who are not clinically responding.

*↓ = Object drug decreased. ↑ = Object drug increased.

Adverse Reactions

Caspofungin Adverse Reactions (%)

Adverse reaction	50 mg[1]	50 to 70 mg[2]
Cardiovascular		
Infused vein complications	2.9	1.5 to 12
Phlebitis/thrombophlebitis	-	11.3 to 15.7
Tachycardia	-	< 2
Vasculitis	-	< 2
CNS		
Headache	-	6 to 11.3
Insomnia	-	< 2
Paresthesia	-	≤ 3.1
Tremor	-	< 2
Dermatologic		
Flushing	2.9	-
Erythema	-	< 2
Induration	-	≤ 3.1
Pruritus	-	≤ 2.5
Rash	-	≤ 4.6
Sweating	-	< 2
GI		
Nausea	2.9	2.5 to 6
Vomiting	2.9	1.2 to 3.1
Abdominal pain	-	≤ 3.6
Anorexia	-	< 2
Diarrhea	-	1.3 to 3.6
Hematologic/Lymphatic		
Eosinophils increased	3.2	3.1
Anemia	-	≤ 3.8
Hematocrit decreased	-	1.5 to 11.1
Hemoglobin decreased	-	3.1 to 12.3
Neutrophils decreased	-	1.9 to 3.1
Platelet count decreased	-	1.5 to 3.1
Prothrombin time increased	-	1.3 to 1.5
WBC count decreased	-	4.6 to 6.2

CASPOFUNGIN ACETATE

Caspofungin Adverse Reactions (%)		
Adverse reaction	50 mg[1]	50 to 70 mg[2]
Lab test abnormalities		
ALT increased	-	10.6 to 10.8
AST increased	-	10.8 to 13
Direct serum bilirubin increased	-	≤ 0.6
Serum albumin decreased	-	4.6 to 8.6
Serum alkaline phosphatase increased	2.9	7.7 to 10.5
Serum bicarbonate decreased	-	≤ 0.9
Serum creatinine increased	-	≤ 1.5
Serum potassium decreased	2.9	3.7 to 10.8
Serum uric acid increased	-	≤ 0.6
Total serum protein decreased	-	≤ 3.1
Urine pH increased	-	≤ 0.8
Urine protein increased	4.9	≤ 1.2
Urine RBCs increased	2.2	1.1 to 3.8
Urine WBCs increased	-	≤ 7.7
Metabolic		
Edema/swelling	-	< 2
Edema, facial	-	≤ 3.1
Musculoskeletal		
Myalgia	-	≤ 3.1
Back pain	-	< 2
Musculoskeletal pain	-	< 2

Caspofungin Adverse Reactions (%)		
Adverse reaction	50 mg[1]	50 to 70 mg[2]
Miscellaneous		
Asthenia/fatigue	-	< 2
Fever	2.9	3.6 to 26.2
Chills	-	≤ 2.5
Flu-like illness	-	≤ 3.1
Malaise	-	< 2
Pain	-	≤ 4.6
Warm sensation	-	< 2
Anaphylaxis	-	< 2
Tachypnea	-	< 2

[1] Adverse reactions in patients with invasive aspergillosis. Patients received 70 mg on day 1, then 50 mg daily for the remainder of their treatment.
[2] Adverse reactions derived from Phase II and Phase III studies among patients treated for off-label indications.

► *Hypersensitivity:* Possible histamine-mediated symptoms have been reported in clinical studies including isolated reports of rash, facial swelling, pruritus, or sensation of warmth. One case of anaphylaxis characterized by dyspnea, stridor, and worsening of rash during initial administration of caspofungin was reported.

Overdosage

In clinical studies, the highest dose was 100 mg administered as a single dose to 5 patients. This dose was generally well tolerated. No overdosages have been reported. Caspofungin is not dialyzable. The minimum lethal dose of caspofungin in rats was 50 mg/kg, a dose that is equivalent to 10 times the recommended daily dose based on relative body surface area comparison.

Cinchona Alkaloid

QUININE SULFATE

Rx	**Quinine Sulfate** (Various, eg, Moore)	**Capsules:** 200 mg	In 100s, 500s, and 1000s.
		260 mg	In 100s, 500s, and 1000s.
		325 mg	In 100s, 500s, and 1000s.
Rx	**Quinine Sulfate** (Various, eg, Moore, Zenith Goldline)	**Tablets:** 260 mg	In 100s, 500s, and 1000s.

Indications

➤*Chloroquine-resistant falciparum malaria:* Either alone, with pyrimethamine and a sulfonamide, or with a tetracycline. It is also considered alternative therapy for chloroquine-sensitive strains of *P. falciparum*, *P. malariae*, *P. ovale*, and *P. vivax*. Mefloquine and clindamycin may also be used with quinine depending on where the malaria was acquired (eg, Southeast Asia, Bangladesh, East Africa).

➤*Unlabeled uses:* Nocturnal recumbency leg cramps, prevention and treatment. Dose: 260 to 300 mg at bedtime.

Administration and Dosage

➤*Adults:* 260 to 650 mg 3 times a day for 6 to 12 days.

➤*Children:* 10 mg/kg every 8 hours for 5 to 7 days.

➤*Storage/Stability:* Dispense in a tight, light-resistant container as defined in the USP. Use child-resistant closure. Store at controlled room temperature 15° to 30°C (59° to 86°F). Protect from light.

Actions

➤*Pharmacology:* Quinine, a cinchona alkaloid, acts primarily as a blood schizonticide. Its antimalarial action is unclear. It was once believed to be due to the intercalation of the quinoline moiety into the DNA of the parasite, thereby reducing the effectiveness of DNA to act as a template, as well as depression of the oxygen uptake and carbohydrate metabolism of plasmodia. More recently it is thought that pH elevation in intracellular organelles of the parasites by quinine plays a role in the mechanism.

Quinine has a skeletal muscle relaxant effect, increasing the refractory period by direct action on the muscle fiber, decreasing the excitability of the motor end-plate by a curariform action, and affecting the distribution of calcium within the muscle fiber. It also has oxytocic effects. It is an optical isomer of quinidine, and has cardiovascular effects similar to quinidine.

➤*Pharmacokinetics:*

Absorption – Quinine is readily absorbed orally, mainly from the upper small intestine. Absorption is almost complete, even in patients with marked diarrhea. Peak plasma concentrations occur within 1 to 3 hours after a single oral dose. Chronic administration of 1 g/day produces an average plasma concentration of 7 mcg/mL.

Tinnitus and hearing impairment rarely occur at plasma concentrations of < 10 mcg/mL. However, an occasional patient may have some evidence of cinchonism such as tinnitus (see Warnings).

Distribution – Quinine is ≈ 70% to 85% protein bound. The concentration of the alkaloid in cerebrospinal fluid is only 2% to 7% of that in the plasma. However, it can cross the placenta and readily reach fetal tissues.

Metabolism/Excretion – The cinchona alkaloids are primarily metabolized in the liver; < 5% is excreted unaltered in the urine. There is no accumulation in the body upon continued administration. Half-life is 4 to 5 hours. After termination of therapy, the plasma level falls rapidly and only a negligible concentration is detectable after 24 hours.

The metabolites are excreted in the urine, many as hydroxy derivatives; small amounts also appear in the feces, gastric juice, bile, and saliva. Renal excretion of quinine is twice as rapid when the urine is acidic as when it is alkaline; greater tubular reabsorption of the alkaloidal base occurs in an alkaline medium.

The pharmacokinetics of quinine are affected by malarial infection, with volume of distribution, and systemic clearance decreasing. Also, protein binding increases to > 90% in patients with cerebral malaria, in pregnant patients and in children.

Contraindications

Hypersensitivity to quinine; glucose-6-phosphate dehydrogenase (G-6-PD) deficiency; optic neuritis; tinnitus; history of blackwater fever and thrombocytopenic purpura (associated with previous quinine ingestion); pregnancy (see Warnings).

Warnings

➤*Cinchonism:* Repeated doses or overdosage of quinine may precipitate cinchonism. The mildest symptoms include tinnitus, headache, nausea, and slightly disturbed vision, which usually subside rapidly upon discontinuation of the drug. When quinine is continued or after large single doses, symptoms also involve the GI tract, the nervous and cardiovascular systems, and the skin.

➤*Tinnitus and impaired hearing:* These may occur at plasma quinine concentrations > 10 mcg/mL, a level not normally attained with quinine 260 to 520 mg/day. In a hypersensitive patient, as little as 300 mg may produce tinnitus.

➤*Glucose-6-phosphate dehydrogenase (G-6-PD) deficiency:* In patients with G-6-PD deficiency, primaquine should only be administered if essential and under close supervision. A weekly, as opposed to daily, regimen is recommended to reduce the risk of hemolysis.

➤*Hemolysis (with the potential for hemolytic anemia):* This has been associated with a G-6-PD deficiency in patients taking quinine. Stop therapy immediately if hemolysis appears.

➤*Cardiac disease:* Use with caution in patients with cardiac arrhythmias; quinine has quinidine-like activity. In patients with atrial fibrillation, quinine use requires the same precautions as those for quinidine. May cause cardiotoxicity.

➤*Hypersensitivity reactions:* Discontinue quinine if there is any evidence of hypersensitivity. Cutaneous flushing, pruritus, skin rashes, fever, gastric distress, dyspnea, ringing in the ears, and visual impairment may occur, particularly with only small doses of quinine. Extreme flushing of the skin accompanied by intense, generalized pruritus is most common. Hemoglobinuria and asthma are idiosyncratic. Refer to Management of Acute Hypersensitivity Reactions.

➤*Pregnancy: Category X.* Quinine has an oxytocic action that appears to occur only with doses that are higher than those recommended. It also crosses the placenta. Congenital malformations have occurred primarily with large doses (30 g) for attempted abortion. In about 50%, the malformation was deafness related to auditory nerve hypoplasia. Other abnormalities were limb anomalies, visceral defects, and visual changes.

➤*Lactation:* Quinine is excreted in breast milk in small amounts. Although no adverse effects have been reported in the nursing infant, rule out patients at risk for G-6-PD deficiency before breastfeeding.

Drug Interactions

Quinine Drug Interactions			
Precipitant drug	Object drug *		Description
Antacids, aluminum-containing	Quinine	↓	Aluminum-containing antacids may delay or decrease absorption of concurrent quinine.
Cimetidine	Quinine	↑	Cimetidine may reduce quinine's oral clearance and increase its elimination half-life.
Mefloquine	Quinine	↑	Do not use concurrently with quinine. If these agents are to be used in the initial treatment of severe malaria, delay mefloquine administration ≥ 12 hours after the last dose of quinine. ECG abnormalities or cardiac arrest may occur. The risk of convulsions may also be increased with coadministration.
Rifamycins (rifabutin, rifampin)	Quinine	↓	Rifamycins, potent inducers of hepatic microsomal enzymes, increased the hepatic clearance of quinine. Enzyme induction can persist for several days following discontinuation of the rifamycin.
Urinary alkalinizers (eg, acetazolamide, sodium bicarbonate)	Quinine	↑	Urinary alkalinizers administered concurrently with quinine may increase quinine blood levels with potential for toxicity.
Quinine	Anticoagulants, oral	↑	Quinine may depress the hepatic enzyme system that synthesizes the vitamin K-dependent clotting factors and thus may enhance the action of warfarin and other oral anticoagulants.
Quinine	Digoxin	↑	Digoxin serum concentrations may be increased by concurrent quinine. Monitor digoxin levels periodically.
Quinine	Neuromuscular blocking agents (depolarizing and nondepolarizing)	↑	The neuromuscular blockade of these agents may be potentiated by quinine, and may result in respiratory difficulties.
Quinine	Succinylcholine	↑	Quinidine may produce a decrease in plasma cholinesterase activity, resulting in a slowed metabolic rate for succinylcholine.

* ↑ = Object drug increased.   ↓ = Object drug decreased.

QUININE SULFATE

➤*Drug/Lab test interactions:* Elevated values for urinary 17-ketogenic steroids may occur with the Zimmerman method.

Adverse Reactions

➤*Cardiovascular:* Anginal symptoms.

➤*CNS:* Tinnitus (see Warnings); deafness; vertigo; headache; fever; apprehension; restlessness; confusion; syncope; excitement; delirium; hypothermia; convulsions; dizziness.

➤*GI:* Nausea; vomiting; epigastric pain; hepatitis; GI disturbance.

➤*Hematologic:* Acute hemolysis; hemolytic anemia; thrombocytopenic purpura; agranulocytosis; hypoprothrombinemia.

➤*Hypersensitivity:* Cutaneous rashes (urticarial, papular, scarlatinal); pruritus; flushing; sweating; facial edema; asthmatic symptoms. See Warnings.

➤*Ophthalmic:* Visual disturbances, including disturbed color vision and perception; photophobia; blurred vision with scotomata; night blindness; amblyopia; diplopia; diminished visual fields; mydriasis; optic atrophy.

➤*Miscellaneous:* Cinchonism (see Warnings). Vasculitis; hypoglycemia; lichenoid photosensitivity.

Overdosage

➤*Symptoms:* The more common signs and symptoms are tinnitus, dizziness, skin rash, and GI disturbance (intestinal cramping). With higher doses, cardiovascular and CNS effects may occur, including headache, fever, vomiting, apprehension, confusion, and convulsions. Other effects are listed in Adverse Reactions.

Fatalities with quinine have occurred from single oral doses of 2 to 8 g; a single fatality reported with a dose of 1.5 g may reflect an idiosyncratic effect. Several cases of blindness following large overdoses of quinine, with partial recovery of vision in each instance, have been reported.

➤*Treatment:* Employ gastric lavage or induce emesis. Support blood pressure and maintain renal function; provide mechanical ventilation if needed. Use sedatives, oxygen and other supportive measures as necessary. Maintain fluid and electrolyte balance with IV fluids. Refer to General Management of Acute Overdosage.

Urinary acidification will promote renal excretion of quinine; however, in the presence of hemoglobinuria, acidification of the urine may augment renal blockade. Quinine is readily dialyzable by hemodialysis or hemoperfusion.

Angioedema or asthma may require epinephrine, corticosteroids, or antihistamines.

In the acute phase of toxic amaurosis caused by quinine, IV vasodilators may have a salutory effect. Stellate block also has been used effectively for quinine-associated blindness. Residual visual impairment occasionally yields to vasodilators.

Patient Information

Take with food or after meals to minimize GI irritation.

Medication may cause diarrhea, nausea, stomach cramps or pain, vomiting, or ringing in the ears; notify physician if these become pronounced.

May produce blurred vision, vertigo, restlessness, confusion, or dizziness; patients should observe caution while driving or performing other tasks requiring alertness.

Stop the drug if there is any evidence of allergy such as flushing, itching, rash, fever, stomach pain, difficult breathing, ringing in the ears, or vision problems.

MEFLOQUINE HCl

Rx	Mefloquine HCl (Geneva)	Tablets: 250 mg	(GP 118). White, scored. In 25s.
Rx	Lariam (Roche)		Lactose. (LARIAM 250 ROCHE). White, scored. In UD 25s.

Indications

➤*Treatment of acute malaria infections:* Mild to moderate acute malaria caused by mefloquine-susceptible strains of *Plasmodium falciparum* (both chloroquine-susceptible and resistant strains) or *P. vivax.* There are insufficient clinical data to document mefloquine's effect in malaria caused by *P. ovale* or *P. malariae.*

➤*Prevention of malaria:* Prophylaxis of *P. falciparum* and *P. vivax* malarial infections, including prophylaxis of chloroquine-resistant strains of *P. falciparum.*

Administration and Dosage

➤*Treatment of mild to moderate malaria in adults caused by P. vivax or mefloquine-susceptible strains of P. falciparum:* 5 tablets (1250 mg) as a single dose. Do not take on an empty stomach. Give with at least 240 mL (8 oz) water.

If a full treatment course has been administered without clinical cure, give alternative treatment. Similarly, if previous prophylaxis with mefloquine has failed, do not use mefloquine for curative treatment.

Patients given mefloquine for acute *P. vivax* malaria are at high risk of relapse; mefloquine does not eliminate exoerythrocytic (hepatic phase) parasites. To avoid such relapse, subsequently treat with 8-aminoquinolone (eg, primaquine).

➤*Treatment of mild to moderate malaria in pediatric patients caused by mefloquine-susceptible strains of P. falciparum:* 20 to 25 mg/kg for nonimmune patients. Splitting the total curative dose into 2 doses taken 6 to 8 hours apart may reduce the occurrence or severity of adverse effects. Experience with mefloquine in infants less than 3 months of age or weighing less than 5 kg is limited. Do not take the drug on an empty stomach and administer with ample water. For very young patients, the dose may be crushed, mixed with water or sugar water and may be administered via an oral syringe.

If a full treatment course has been administered without clinical cure, give alternative treatment. Similarly, if previous prophylaxis with mefloquine has failed, do not use mefloquine for curative treatment.

In pediatric patients, the administration of mefloquine for the treatment of malaria has been associated with early vomiting. In some cases, early vomiting has been cited as a possible cause of treatment failure. If a significant loss of drug product is observed or suspected because of vomiting, administer a second full dose of mefloquine to patients who vomit less than 30 minutes after receiving the drug. If vomiting occurs 30 to 60 minutes after a dose, give an additional half dose. If vomiting recurs, closely monitor the patient and consider alternative malaria treatment if improvement is not observed within a reasonable period of time.

The safety and effectiveness of mefloquine to treat malaria in pediatric patients below 6 months of age have not been established.

➤*Malaria prophylaxis:* Initiate prophylactic drug use 1 week prior to departure to an endemic area. The same day of the week must be used for each subsequent dose. To reduce risk of development of malaria after return from an endemic area, continue prophylaxis for 4 additional weeks. Do not take on an empty stomach. Administer with at least 240 mL (8 oz) water.

Concomitant medications – In certain cases (eg, when a traveler is taking other medication), it may be desirable to start prophylaxis 2 to 3 weeks prior to departure in order to ensure that the combination of drugs is well tolerated.

Adults – 250 mg once weekly.

Children – The following doses have been extrapolated from the recommended adult dose. Neither the pharmacokinetics nor the clinical efficacy of these doses have been determined in children owing to the difficulty of acquiring this information in pediatric subjects. The recommended prophylactic dose is 3 to 5 mg/kg once weekly. One 250 mg mefloquine tablet should be taken once weekly in pediatric patients weighing over 45 kg. In pediatric patients weighing less than 45 kg, the weekly dose decreases in proportion to body weight: More than 30 kg to 45 kg, ¾ tablet; more than 20 kg to 30 kg, ½ tablet; up to 20 kg, ¼ tablet.

Experience with mefloquine in infants less than 3 months of age or weighing less than 5 kg is limited.

➤*Storage/Stability:* Store at 15° to 30°C (59° to 86°F).

Actions

➤*Pharmacology:* Mefloquine is an antimalarial agent that acts as a blood schizonticide. Its exact mechanism of action is unknown. It is a structural analog of quinine.

➤*Pharmacokinetics:* Studies of healthy males showed a significant lag time after administration; terminal elimination half-life varied widely (13 to 24 days) with a mean of about 3 weeks. Mefloquine is a mixture of enantiomeric molecules whose rates of release, absorption, transport, action, degradation, and elimination may differ.

Additional studies showed slightly greater drug concentrations for longer periods. Absorption half-life was 0.36 to 2 hours; terminal elimination half-life was 15 to 33 days. Concentrations of the primary metabolite surpassed the concentrations of mefloquine. In multiple-dose studies, mean metabolite-to-mefloquine ratio at steady state ranged between 2.3 and 8.6.

Total drug clearance, which is essentially all hepatic, is about 30 mL/min. Volume of distribution, about 20 L/kg, indicates extensive distribution. The drug is highly bound (98%) to plasma proteins and concentrated in blood erythrocytes, the target cells in malaria, at a relatively constant erythrocyte-to-plasma concentration ratio of approximately 2.

The pharmacokinetics of mefloquine in patients with compromised renal and hepatic function have not been studied.

Microbiology – Strains of *P. falciparum* resistant to mefloquine have been reported.

Contraindications

Hypersensitivity to mefloquine or related compounds (eg, quinine, quinidine). Mefloquine should not be prescribed for prophylaxis in patients with active depression, recent history of depression, generalized anxiety disorder, psychosis, schizophrenia or other major psychiatric disorders, or a history of convulsions.

Warnings

➤*Acute P. vivax malaria:* Patients with acute *P. vivax* malaria treated with mefloquine are at high risk of relapse because mefloquine does not eliminate exoerythrocytic (hepatic phase) parasites. To avoid relapse, after initial treatment of the acute infection with mefloquine, patients should subsequently be treated with an 8-aminoquinoline (eg, primaquine).

➤*Infection caused by P. falciparum:* In case of life-threatening, serious, or overwhelming malarial infections caused by *P. falciparum,* treat patients with an IV antimalarial drug. Following completion of IV treatment, mefloquine may be given orally to complete the course of therapy.

➤*Psychiatric disturbances:* Mefloquine should not be prescribed for prophylaxis in patients with active depression, recent history of depression, generalized anxiety disorder, psychosis, schizophrenia, or other major psychiatric disorders, or with a history of convulsions. During prophylactic use, if signs of acute anxiety, depression, restlessness, or confusion are noticed, these may be considered prodromal to a more serious event. In these cases, discontinue the drug and substitute an alternative medication.

Mefloquine may cause psychiatric symptoms in a number of patients, ranging from anxiety, paranoia, and depression to hallucinations and psychotic behavior. On occasions, these symptoms have been reported to continue long after mefloquine has been stopped. Rare cases of suicidal ideation and suicide have been reported, although no relationship to drug administration has been confirmed. To minimize the chances of these adverse events, mefloquine should not be taken for prophylaxis in patients with active depression or with a recent history of depression, generalized anxiety disorder, psychosis, or schizophrenia or other major psychiatric disorders. Use mefloquine with caution in patients with a previous history of depression.

➤*Hepatic function impairment:* In patients with impaired liver function, the elimination of mefloquine may be prolonged, leading to higher plasma levels.

➤*Fertility impairment:* Fertility studies in rats at doses of 5, 20, and 50 mg/kg/day of mefloquine have demonstrated adverse effects on fertility in males at the high dose of 50 mg/kg/day and in females at doses of 20 and 50 mg/kg/day. Histopathological lesions were noted in the epididymides from male rats at doses of 20 and 50 mg/kg/day.

➤*Pregnancy: Category C.* Mefloquine is teratogenic in rats and mice at a dose of 100 mg/kg/day. In rabbits, 160 mg/kg/day was embryotoxic and teratogenic and 80 mg/kg/day was teratogenic but not embryotoxic. There are no adequate and well-controlled studies in pregnant women. However, clinical experience with mefloquine has not revealed any embryotoxic or teratogenic effect. Use during pregnancy only if potential benefit justifies potential risk to the fetus. Warn women of childbearing potential traveling to areas where malaria is endemic against becoming pregnant and to practice reliable contraceptive measures during prophylaxis.

➤*Lactation:* Mefloquine is excreted in breast milk. Based on a study in a few subjects, low concentrations (3% to 4%) of mefloquine were excreted in breast milk following a dose equivalent to 250 mg of the free base. Because of the potential for serious adverse reactions in nursing infants from mefloquine, decide whether to discontinue the drug, taking into account the importance of the drug to the mother.

➤*Children:* Use of mefloquine to treat acute uncomplicated *P. falciparum* malaria in pediatric patients is supported by evidence from adequate and well-controlled studies of mefloquine in adults with addi-

MEFLOQUINE HCl

tional data from published open-label and comparative trials using mefloquine to treat malaria caused by *P. falciparum* in patients younger than 16 years of age. The safety and effectiveness of mefloquine for the treatment of malaria in pediatric patients below 6 months of age have not been established.

In several studies, the administration of mefloquine for the treatment of malaria was associated with early vomiting in pediatric patients. Early vomiting was cited in some reports as a possible cause of treatment failure. If a second dose is not tolerated, monitor the patient closely and consider alternative malaria treatment if improvement is not observed within a reasonable period of time.

Precautions

➤*Monitoring:* This drug has been administered for periods longer than 1 year. If it is to be given for a prolonged period, perform periodic evaluations including liver function tests.

➤*Epilepsy:* In patients with epilepsy, mefloquine may increase the risk of convulsions. Therefore, prescribe the drug only for curative treatment in such patients and only if there are compelling medical reasons for its use.

➤*Cardiac disease:* Parenteral animal studies show that mefloquine, a myocardial depressant, possesses 20% of the antifibrillatory action of quinidine and produces 50% of the increase in the PR interval reported with quinine. Mefloquine's effect on the compromised cardiovascular system has not been evaluated. However, transitory and clinically silent ECG alterations have been reported during mefloquine use. Alterations include sinus bradycardia, sinus arrhythmia, first-degree AV block, prolongation of the QT_c interval, and abnormal T waves. Weigh the benefits of therapy against possible adverse effects in cardiac disease patients.

➤*Ocular lesions:* These were observed in rats fed mefloquine daily for 2 years. All surviving rats given 30 mg/kg/day had ocular lesions in both eyes characterized by retinal degeneration, opacity of the lens, and retinal edema. Similar but less severe lesions were observed in 80% of female and 22% of male rats fed 12.5 mg/kg/day for 2 years. At doses of 5 mg/kg/day, only corneal lesions were observed (9% of rats studied). Periodic ophthalmic examinations are recommended.

➤*Hazardous tasks:* Exercise caution with regard to activities requiring alertness and fine motor coordination, such as when driving, piloting aircraft, or operating hazardous machinery; dizziness, a loss of balance, or other disorders of the central or peripheral nervous system have occurred during and following the use of mefloquine. These effects may occur after therapy is discontinued because of the drug's long half-life.

Drug Interactions

Mefloquine Drug Interactions			
Precipitant drug	Object drug*		Description
Beta-adrenergic blockers (propranolol)	Mefloquine	↑	There is one report of cardiopulmonary arrest with full recovery in a patient taking propranolol.
Chloroquine	Mefloquine	↑	The risk of convulsions may be increased with concomitant mefloquine.
Halofantrine	Mefloquine	↑	Do not give halofantrine with or subsequently to mefloquine because of the danger of a potentially fatal prolongation of the QT_c interval.
Mefloquine	Bacterial vaccines, live attenuated (ie, oral live typhoid vaccines)	↓	When mefloquine is taken concurrently with oral live typhoid vaccines, attenuation of immunization cannot be excluded. Vaccinations with attenuated live bacteria should therefore be completed at least 3 days before the first dose of mefloquine.
Mefloquine	Quinine or Quinidine	↑	Coadministration may produce ECG abnormalities. If these agents are to be used in the initial treatment of severe malaria, delay mefloquine administration at least 12 hours after the last dose of quinine or quinidine. The risk of convulsions also may be increased with concurrent mefloquine and quinine.
Mefloquine	Anticonvulsants (eg, valproic acid, carbamazepine, phenobarbital, phenytoin)	↓	Monitor anticonvulsant blood levels and adjust the dosage as necessary. Coadministration may reduce seizure control by lowering the plasma levels of the anticonvulsant.

* ↑ = Object drug increased.   ↓ = Object drug decreased.

Adverse Reactions

At doses used for acute malaria, symptoms possibly attributable to the drug cannot be distinguished from symptoms usually attributable to the disease itself. Because of its long half-life, adverse reactions may occur or persist up to several weeks after the last dose.

➤*Prophylaxis of malaria:* Vomiting (3%); dizziness, syncope, extrasystoles (less than 1%).

➤*Treatment of malaria:* The most frequently observed adverse reactions included: Dizziness; myalgia; nausea; fever; headache; vomiting; chills; diarrhea; skin rash; abdominal pain; fatigue; loss of appetite; tinnitus. Side effects occurring in less than 1% included: Bradycardia; hair loss; emotional problems; pruritus; asthenia; transient emotional disturbances; telogen effluvium (loss of resting hair); seizures.

➤*Postmarketing:* The most frequently reported adverse events are nausea, vomiting, loose stools or diarrhea, abdominal pain, dizziness or vertigo, loss of balance, and neuropsychiatric events such as headache, somnolence, and sleep disorders (insomnia, abnormal dreams). These are usually mild and may decrease despite continued use.

Occasionally, more severe neuropsychiatric disorders have been reported such as: Sensory and motor neuropathies (eg, paresthesia, tremor, ataxia), convulsions, agitation or restlessness, anxiety, depression, mood changes, panic attacks, forgetfulness, confusion, hallucinations, aggression, psychotic or paranoid reactions, encephalopathy. Rare cases of suicidal ideation and suicide have been reported, although no relationship to drug administration has been confirmed.

Postmarketing surveillance indicates that the same adverse experiences are reported during prophylaxis, as well as acute treatment.

Cardiovascular – Circulatory disturbances (hypotension, hypertension, flushing, syncope), chest pain, tachycardia or palpitation, bradycardia, irregular pulse, extrasystoles, AV block, other transient cardiac conduction alterations (infrequent).

Dermatologic – Rash, exanthema, erythema, urticaria, pruritus, edema, hair loss, erythema multiforme, Stevens-Johnson syndrome (infrequent).

Musculoskeletal – Muscle weakness, muscle cramps, myalgia, arthralgia (infrequent).

➤*Lab test abnormalities:* Decreased hematocrit; transient elevation of transaminases; leukopenia; thrombocytopenia. These alterations were observed in patients with acute malaria who received treatment doses of the drug and were attributed to the disease itself. During prophylactic mefloquine to indigenous populations in malaria-endemic areas, the following occasional alterations in lab values were observed: Transient elevation of transaminases; leukocytosis; thrombocytopenia.

➤*Miscellaneous:* Visual disturbances, vestibular disorders (including tinnitus and hearing impairment), dyspnea, asthenia, malaise, fatigue, fever, sweating, chills, dyspepsia, loss of appetite (infrequent).

Overdosage

Induce vomiting or perform gastric lavage, as appropriate. Monitor cardiac function (if possible by ECG) and neurologic and psychiatric status for at least 24 hours. Provide symptomatic and intensive supportive treatment as required, particularly for cardiovascular disturbances. See a physician immediately because of the potential cardiotoxic effect. Treat vomiting or diarrhea with standard fluid therapy. Refer to General Management of Acute Overdosage.

Patient Information

➤*Hazardous tasks:* May produce dizziness; patients should observe caution while driving or performing other tasks requiring alertness and physical dexterity.

Advise patients that when used as prophylaxis, the first dose of mefloquine should be taken 1 week prior to departure.

Advise patients if they experience psychiatric symptoms such as acute anxiety, depression, restlessness or confusion, these may be considered prodromal to a more serious event. In these cases, the drug must be discontinued and an alternative medication should be substituted.

Advise patients that no chemoprophylactic regimen is 100% effective, and protective clothing, insect repellants, and bednets are important components of malaria prophylaxis.

DOXYCYCLINE

Refer to the Tetracyclines group monograph and the individual doxycycline monograph for more information.

Indications

➤*Malaria prophylaxis:* Prophylaxis of malaria caused by *Plasmodium falciparum* in short-term travelers (fewer than 4 months) to areas with chloroquine and/or pyrimethamine-sulfadoxine-resistant strains.

Administration and Dosage

Begin doxycycline prophylaxis 1 to 2 days before travel to malarious areas and continue daily during travel in the malarious area and for 4 weeks after the traveler leaves the area.

➤*Adults:* 100 mg once daily.

➤*Children over 8 years of age:* 2 mg/kg/day up to adult dose of 100 mg/day.

4-Aminoquinoline Compounds

Indications

➤*Malaria:* Prophylaxis and treatment of acute attacks of malaria caused by *Plasmodium vivax, P. malariae, P. ovale,* and susceptible strains of *P. falciparum.* Chloroquine phosphate is the drug of choice in this situation. Chloroquine HCl is used when oral therapy is not feasible. For radical cure of *P. vivax* and *P. malariae* malaria, concomitant primaquine therapy is required.

➤*Unlabeled uses:* Chloroquine has been used to suppress rheumatoid arthritis and in the treatment of systemic and discoid lupus erythematosus, scleroderma, pemphigus, lichen planus, polymyositis, sarcoidosis, and porphyria cutanea tarda.

For other uses, refer to individual product monographs.

Actions

➤*Pharmacology:* Chloroquine's exact mechanism of action is not known, but several mechanisms have been suggested. It concentrates in parasite acid vesicles and raises internal pH. The "non-weak base effect" inhibits parasite growth at extracellular drug concentrations; this may occur due to active chloroquine-concentrating mechanism in parasite acid vesicles. Another mechanism may involve ferriprotoporphyrin IX aggregates, which are released by parasitized erythrocytes during hemoglobin degradation and serve as chloroquine receptors, causing membrane damage with lysis of parasites or erythrocytes. Chloroquine also may influence hemoglobin digestion or interfere with parasite/nucleoprotein synthesis.

➤*Pharmacokinetics:* Absorbed readily from GI tract, peak plasma levels are reached in 1 to 6 hours. Plasma protein binding is 55%. Drug concentrates in liver, spleen, kidney and brain and is strongly bound in melanin-containing cells such as in eyes and skin. Chloroquine is eliminated very slowly and may persist in tissues for a prolonged period. Up to 70% of a dose may be excreted unchanged in urine and up to 25% as a metabolite. Renal excretion is enhanced by urinary acidification.

➤*Microbiology:* Active against the erythrocytic forms of *P. vivax* and *malariae* and most strains of *P. falciparum* (but not the gametocytes of *P. falciparum*).

These drugs do not prevent relapses or infection of *P. vivax* or *malariae* malaria; not effective against exoerythrocytic parasite forms. Highly effective in suppressing *P. vivax* or *malariae* malaria, terminating acute attacks and significantly lengthening interval between treatment and relapse. In *P. falciparum* malaria, they abolish acute attack and completely cure infection unless due to resistant strain. Hydroxychloroquine is not effective against chloroquine-resistant *P. falciparum* strains.

Contraindications

Retinal or visual field changes; hypersensitivity; long-term therapy in children (hydroxychloroquine). Consider an exception in acute malarial attacks caused by *Plasmodia* strains susceptible only to 4-aminoquinolines.

Warnings

➤*Resistance:* Certain strains of *P. falciparum* are resistant to 4-aminoquinoline compounds; normally adequate doses fail to prevent or cure malaria or parasitemia.

➤*Retinopathy:* Irreversible retinal damage has occurred with long-term or high dosages. Retinopathy may be dose-related. During prolonged therapy, perform baseline and periodic ophthalmologic exams. If there is any indication of abnormality in visual acuity/field or retinal macular areas or any visual symptoms not explainable by difficulties of accommodation or corneal opacities, stop drug immediately; observe for possible progression. Retinal changes/visual disturbances may progress after therapy cessation.

➤*Glucose-6-phosphate dehydrogenase (G-6-PD) deficiency:* Use with caution in patients with G-6-PD deficiencies.

➤*Muscular weakness:* Periodically question and examine patients who are on long-term therapy; test knee and ankle reflexes to detect muscular weakness. If weakness occurs, discontinue therapy.

➤*Psoriasis or porphyria:* Use of these drugs may exacerbate these conditions. Do not use in these conditions unless the benefit outweighs the possible hazard.

➤*Hepatic function impairment:* These drugs concentrate in liver; use with caution in hepatic disease or alcoholism, or in conjunction with hepatotoxic drugs.

➤*Pregnancy:* Use only when clearly needed and when potential benefits outweigh potential hazards to the fetus.

➤*Lactation:* Safety for use has not been established; these agents are excreted in breast milk. A nursing infant may consume ≈ 0.55% of a 300 mg maternal dose over 24 hours. One study determined the milk:blood ratio of the nursing mother to be 0.358.

➤*Children:* Children are especially sensitive to the 4-aminoquinoline compounds. Fatalities following accidental ingestion of relatively small doses and sudden deaths from parenteral chloroquine have been recorded. Do not exceed a single dose of 5 mg base/kg of chloroquine HCl in infants or children.

Precautions

➤*Monitoring:* Perform periodic CBCs during prolonged therapy. If any severe blood disorder not attributable to the disease appears, consider discontinuing therapy. Measure G-6-PD in susceptible individuals prior to initiating therapy. Although probably safe when given in normal therapeutic doses, these compounds may induce hemolysis in G-6-PD deficient individuals in the presence of infection or stressful conditions. An acute drop in hematocrit, hemoglobin, and red blood cell count may occur.

Drug Interactions

4-Aminoquinoline Drug Interactions			
Precipitant drug	Object drug *		Description
Cimetidine	Chloroquine	↑	Cimetidine may reduce the oral clearance rate and metabolism of chloroquine
Chloroquine	Kaolin or magnesium trisilicate	↓	GI absorption of chloroquine may be decreased by coadministration of these agents.

* ↑ = Object drug increased. ↓ = Object drug decreased.

Adverse Reactions

➤*Cardiovascular:* Hypotension; ECG changes (particularly inversion or depression of the T wave, widening of QRS complex); cardiomyopathy (rare).

➤*CNS:* Mild, transient headache; psychic stimulation; psychotic episodes, convulsions (rare).

➤*GI:* Anorexia; nausea; vomiting; diarrhea; abdominal cramps.

➤*Ophthalmic:* Irreversible retinal damage (see Warnings); visual disturbances (blurred vision, difficulty of focusing or accommodation); nyctalopia; scotomatous vision with field defects of paracentral, pericentral ring types and typically temporal scotomas (eg, difficulty reading with words tending to disappear, seeing half an object, misty vision, fog before eyes).

➤*Miscellaneous:* Agranulocytosis; hair loss; pruritus; neuromyopathy, blood dyscrasias, lichen planus-like eruptions, skin/mucosal pigment changes, pleomorphic skin eruptions. A few cases of a nerve-type deafness have occurred after prolonged high doses.

Overdosage

➤*Symptoms:* Symptoms may occur within 30 minutes in overdosage (or rarely with lower doses in hypersensitive patients) and consist of headache, drowsiness, visual disturbances, nausea, vomiting, cardiovascular collapse, and convulsions followed by sudden and early respiratory and cardiac arrest. Respiratory depression, cardiovascular collapse, shock, convulsions, and death have occurred with overdose of parenteral chloroquine HCl, especially in infants and children. The ECG may reveal atrial standstill, nodal rhythm, prolonged intraventricular conduction and bradycardia progressing to ventricular fibrillation or arrest. In a retrospective study, it was determined that ingestion of > 5 g of chloroquine was an accurate predictor of fatal outcome in adults.

➤*Treatment:* Treatment is symptomatic; the stomach must be immediately evacuated by emesis or gastric lavage until the stomach is completely emptied. After lavage, activated charcoal (a dose not less than 5 times estimated dose ingested) may inhibit further absorption if given within 30 minutes of ingestion.

Control convulsions before attempting gastric lavage. If due to cerebral stimulation, cautious administration of a short-acting barbiturate may be tried. Treat anoxia-induced convulsions by oxygen, mechanical ventilation or, in shock with hypotension, by vasopressor therapy. Tracheal intubation or tracheostomy may be necessary. Peritoneal dialysis and exchange transfusions have been suggested.

For at least 6 hours, closely observe an asymptomatic patient who survives the acute phase. Force fluids and acidify the urine with 8 g ammonium chloride in divided doses (for adults) to help promote excretion.

In 1 study, 10 of 11 patients who ingested > 5 g of chloroquine survived after treatment with diazepam and epinephrine for several days along with mechanical ventilation. The use of diazepam has also been successful in other reports.

Patient Information

May cause GI upset; take with food. Complete full course of therapy.

Report visual disturbances or difficulty in hearing or ringing in ears to physician.

Keep out of reach of children; overdosage is especially dangerous in children.

Medication may cause diarrhea, loss of appetite, nausea, stomach pain or vomiting, muscle weakness, or rash. Notify physician if pronounced or bothersome.

CHLOROQUINE PHOSPHATE

Rx	Chloroquine Phosphate (Various, eg, CMC, Gallipot)	Tablets: 250 mg (equiv. to 150 mg base)	In 100s and 1000s.
Rx	Aralen Phosphate (Sanofi Synthelabo)	Tablets: 500 mg (equiv. to 300 mg base)	(W/A77). Pink. Film coated. In 25s.

Indications

▶*Malaria:* Prophylaxis and treatment of acute attacks of malaria due to *P. vivax, P. malariae, P. ovale* and susceptible strains of *P. falciparum.*

▶*Amebiasis:* Also used for treatment of extraintestinal amebiasis (see Amebicides section).

Administration and Dosage

Chloroquine phosphate 500 mg is equivalent to 300 mg chloroquine base and 400 mg hydroxychloroquine sulfate.

Children's doses, expressed in mg/kg, should not exceed the recommended adult dose.

▶*Suppression:*

Adults – 300 mg (base) weekly, on the same day each week. Begin 1 to 2 weeks prior to exposure; continue for 4 weeks after leaving endemic area.

If suppressive therapy is not begun prior to exposure, double the initial loading dose (adults - 600 mg base; children - 10 mg base/kg) and give in 2 divided doses, 6 hours apart.

Children – Administer 5 mg base/kg weekly, up to a maximum adult dose of 300 mg base.†

Children's Chloroquine Dose Based on Age	
Age (years)	Chloroquine base equivalent
< 1	37.5 mg
1 to 3	75 mg
4 to 6	100 mg
7 to 10	150 mg
11 to 16	225 mg

▶*CDC recommended schedule for chloroquine as an alternative to mefloquine†:* Travelers to areas of risk where chloroquine-resistant *P. falciparum* is endemic and for whom mefloquine is contraindicated may elect to use an alternative regimen. Chloroquine alone taken weekly is recommended for travelers who cannot use mefloquine or doxycycline, especially pregnant women and children < 15 kg. In addition, give these travelers a single treatment dose of sulfadoxine/pyrimethamine to keep during travel and to take promptly in the event of a febrile illness during their travel when professional medical care is not readily available. Continue weekly chloroquine prophylaxis after presumptive treatment with sulfadoxine/pyrimethamine.

▶*Acute attack:*

Chloroquine Phosphate Dose in Acute Malarial Attack			
		Dosage (in mg of base)	
Dose	Time	Adults	Children
Initial dose	Day 1	600 mg	10 mg/kg
2nd dose	6 hours later	300 mg	5 mg/kg
3rd dose	Day 2	300 mg	5 mg/kg
4th dose	Day 3	300 mg	5 mg/kg

CHLOROQUINE HCl

Rx	Aralen HCl (Sanofi Winthrop)	Injection: 50 mg (equiv. to 40 mg base)/ml	In 5 ml amps.

Indications

▶*Malaria:* Treatment of malaria when oral therapy is not feasible.

▶*Amebiasis:* Also used for treatment of extraintestinal amebiasis (see Amebicides section).

Administration and Dosage

Chloroquine HCl 50 mg is equivalent to 40 mg chloroquine base.

▶*Adults:* 160 to 200 mg base (4 to 5 ml) IM initially; repeat in 6 hours if necessary. Do not exceed 800 mg (base) total dose in the first 24 hours. Begin oral dosage as soon as possible and continue for 3 days until ≈ 1.5 g base has been administered.

Other suggested dosages include 2.5 mg base/kg every 4 hours or 3.5 mg/kg every 6 hours; repeat if necessary, maximum 25 mg/kg/day.

▶*Children:* Infants and children are extremely susceptible to overdosage. Severe reactions and deaths have occurred. The recommended single dose is 5 mg base/kg; repeat in 6 hours. Do not exceed 10 mg/kg/24 hours.

HYDROXYCHLOROQUINE SULFATE

Rx	Hydroxychloroquine Sulfate (Various, eg, Copley, Geneva, Moore, Royce, Zenith)	Tablets: 200 mg (equiv. to 155 mg base)	White. In 100s, 500s.
Rx	Plaquenil Sulfate (Winthrop)		(PLAQUENIL). In 100s.

Indications

▶*Malaria:* Prophylaxis and treatment of acute attacks of malaria due to *P. vivax, P. malariae, P. ovale* and susceptible strains of *P. falciparum.*

▶*Lupus erythematosus and rheumatoid arthritis:* Also used for the treatment of discoid and systemic lupus erythematosus and rheumatoid arthritis (see monograph in Antirheumatic Agents section in the Biologicals chapter).

Administration and Dosage

Hydroxychloroquine sulfate 200 mg is equivalent to 155 mg hydroxychloroquine base and 250 mg chloroquine phosphate.

▶*Children's doses:* Expressed in mg/kg, these should not exceed the recommended adult dose.

▶*Suppression:*

Adults – 310 mg base weekly on the same day each week. Begin 1 to 2 weeks prior to exposure; continue for 4 weeks after leaving endemic area.

If suppressive therapy is not begun prior to exposure, double the initial loading dose (adults – 620 mg base; children – 10 mg base/kg) and give in 2 doses, 6 hours apart.

Children – Administer 5 mg base/kg weekly, up to a maximum adult dose.

Children's Hydroxychloroquine Dose Based on Age	
Age (years)	Hydroxychloroquine base equivalent
< 1	37.5 mg
1 to 3	75 mg
4 to 6	100 mg
7 to 10	150 mg
11 to 16	225 mg

▶*Acute attack:*

Hydroxychloroquine Dose in Acute Malarial Attack			
		Dosage (mg of base)	
Dose	Time	Adults	Children
Initial dose	Day 1	620 mg	10 mg/kg
2nd dose	6 hours later	310 mg	5 mg/kg
3rd dose	Day 2	310 mg	5 mg/kg
4th dose	Day 3	310 mg	5 mg/kg

An alternative method, using a single dose of 620 mg base, has also been proven effective.

† *Morbidity and Mortality Weekly Report* 1990 (Mar 9);39 (RR-3):1–10.

8–Aminoquinoline Compound

PRIMAQUINE PHOSPHATE

Rx	Primaquine Phosphate (Various, eg, Quality Care, Sanofi Winthrop)	**Tablets:** 26.3 mg (equivalent to 15 mg base)	Lactose. In 20s and 100s.
Rx	**Primaquine Phosphate** (Various, eg, Medisca, Palisades)	**Powder**	In 5, 25, 100, and 500 g

Indications

➤*P. Vivax malaria:* Recommended only for the radical cure of *P. vivax* malaria, the prevention of relapse in *P. vivax* malaria or following the termination of chloroquine phosphate suppressive therapy in an area where *P. vivax* malaria is endemic.

Administration and Dosage

Primaquine phosphate 26.3 mg is equivalent to 15 mg primaquine base.

Patients suffering from an attack of *P. vivax* malaria or having parasitized red blood cells should receive a course of chloroquine phosphate which quickly destroys the erythrocytic parasites and terminates the paroxysm. Administer primaquine concurrently to eradicate the exoerythrocytic parasites in a dosage of 15 mg (base) daily for 14 days.

➤*CDC recommended treatment schedule†:* Begin therapy during the last 2 weeks of, or following a course of, suppression with chloroquine or a comparable drug.

Adults – 26.3 mg (15 mg base) daily for 14 days.

Children – 0.5 mg/kg/day (0.3 mg base/kg/day); for 14 days.

Actions

➤*Pharmacology:* An 8-aminoquinoline, primaquine is structurally similar to the 4-aminoquinolines but possesses markedly different antimalarial activities.

Primaquine may disrupt the parasite's mitochondria and bind to native DNA. The resulting structural changes create a major disruption in the metabolic process. The gametocyte and exoerythrocyte forms are inhibited. Some gametocytes are destroyed while others are rendered incapable of undergoing maturation division in the mosquito gut. By eliminating tissue (exoerythrocyte) infection, primaquine prevents development of blood (erythrocytic) forms responsible for relapses in *P. vivax* malaria.

➤*Pharmacokinetics:* After oral administration, peak plasma concentrations of primaquine are reached in 1 to 3 hours. Primaquine, as compared to other antimalarials, is found in relatively low concentrations in the tissues. Highest concentrations are in the liver, lungs, brain, heart and skeletal muscle.

Primaquine is rapidly metabolized to a carboxylic acid derivative and then to further metabolites which have varying degrees of activity. Approximately 1% is excreted unchanged in the urine.

➤*Microbiology:* Active against *Plasmodium vivax*, *P. ovale* and the gametocytial forms of *P. falciparum*.

Contraindications

Concomitant administration of quinacrine and primaquine (see Drug Interactions); the acutely ill suffering from systemic disease manifested by tendency to granulocytopenia (eg, rheumatoid arthritis and lupus erythematosus); concurrent administration of other potentially hemolytic drugs or bone marrow depressants.

Warnings

➤*Hemolytic reactions (moderate to severe):* May occur in the following groups of people while receiving primaquine: Glucose-6-phosphate dehydrogenase (G-6-PD) deficient patients; individuals with idiosyncratic reactions (manifested by hemolytic anemia, methemoglobinemia or leukopenia); individuals with nicotinamide adenine dinucleotide (NADH) methemoglobin reductase deficiency; or individuals with a family or personal history of favism. Discontinue if marked darkening of the urine or sudden decrease in hemoglobin concentration or leukocyte count occurs.

➤*Pregnancy:* Safety for use during pregnancy has not been established. Use only when clearly needed and when potential benefits outweigh potential hazards to the fetus.

Precautions

➤*Monitoring:* Anemia, methemoglobinemia and leukopenia have occurred following large doses; do not exceed recommended dose. Perform routine blood examinations (particularly blood cell counts and hemoglobin determinations) during therapy.

Drug Interactions

➤*Quinacrine:* May potentiate the toxicity of antimalarial compounds which are structurally related to primaquine. Do not administer primaquine to patients who have recently received quinacrine.

Adverse Reactions

➤*GI:* Nausea; vomiting; epigastric distress; abdominal cramps.

➤*Hematologic:* Leukopenia; hemolytic anemia in G-6-PD deficient individuals; methemoglobinemia in NADH methemoglobin reductase deficient individuals.

Overdosage

➤*Symptoms:* Abdominal cramps; vomiting; burning, epigastric distress; CNS and cardiovascular disturbances; cyanosis; methemoglobinemia; moderate leukocytosis or leukopenia; anemia. The most striking symptoms are granulocytopenia and acute hemolytic anemia in sensitive persons. Acute hemolysis occurs, but patients recover completely if the dosage is discontinued.

➤*Treatment:* Symptomatic.

Patient Information

Complete full course of therapy.

If GI upset occurs, may be taken with food. If stomach upset (nausea, vomiting or stomach pain) continues, notify physician.

Notify physician if a darkening of the urine occurs.

---

† *Morbidity and Mortality Weekly Report* 1990 Mar 9;39(No. RR-3):1-10.

Folic Acid Antagonist

PYRIMETHAMINE

| Rx | **Daraprim** (GlaxoSmithKline) | **Tablets:** 25 mg | Lactose. (Daraprim A3A). White, scored. In 100s. |

Indications

➤*Chemoprophylaxis of malaria:* In susceptible strains of plasmodia only. It is not suitable as a prophylactic agent for travelers to most areas because of prevalent resistance worldwide.

➤*Toxoplasmosis:* Use with a sulfonamide; synergism exists with this combination.

➤*Acute malaria:* In conjunction with a sulfonamide (eg, sulfadoxine) to initiate transmission control and suppression for susceptible strains of plasmodia. Fast-acting schizonticides (chloroquine, quinine) are preferable for the treatment of acute malaria.

Administration and Dosage

Administer with food to minimize vomiting.

➤*Chemoprophylaxis of malaria:* Do not exceed recommended dosage.

Adults and children (older than 10 years of age) – 25 mg once weekly.

Children (4 to 10 years of age) – 12.5 mg once weekly.

Infants and children (younger than 4 years of age) – 6.25 mg once weekly.

➤*Treatment of acute malaria:* Recommended in areas where only susceptible plasmodia exist. Not recommended for use alone to treat acute malaria. Fast-acting schizonticides (chloroquine, quinine) are indicated for treatment of acute malaria. However, concomitant pyrimethamine, 25 mg daily for 2 days, with a sulfonamide will initiate transmission control and suppression of nonfalciparum malaria.

If pyrimethamine must be used alone in semi-immune people, dose as follows:

Adults and children (older than 10 years of age) – 50 mg daily for 2 days.

Children (4 to 10 years of age) – 25 mg daily for 2 days.

Follow with once weekly regimen described in the chemoprophylaxis regimen above. Extend regimens to include suppression through any characteristic periods of early recrudescence and late relapse for at least 10 weeks in each case.

➤*Toxoplasmosis:* At the dosage required, there is marked variation in tolerance. Young patients may tolerate higher doses than older patients. Coadministration of folinic acid (leucovorin) is strongly recommended in all patients. The dosage of pyrimethamine required for the treatment of toxoplasmosis is 10 to 20 times the recommended antimalaria dosage and approaches the toxic level (see Warnings).

Adults – Initial dose is 50 to 75 mg daily with 1 to 4 g of a sulfonamide of the sulfapyrimidine type (eg, sulfadoxine). Continue for 1 to 3 weeks, depending on response and tolerance. Dosage for each drug may then be reduced by one half and continued for an additional 4 or 5 weeks.

Children – Dosage is 1 mg/kg/day divided into 2 equal daily doses; after 2 to 4 days, reduce to one half and continue for approximately 1 month. The usual pediatric sulfonamide dosage is used in conjunction with pyrimethamine.

Convulsive disorders – Use lower initial dose to avoid potential CNS toxicity.

➤*Storage/Stability:* Store at 15° to 25°C (59° to 77°F) in a dry place and protect from light.

Actions

➤*Pharmacology:* Pyrimethamine is a folic acid antagonist; its therapeutic action is based on differential requirement between host and parasite for nucleic acid precursors involved in growth as it selectively inhibits plasmodial dihydrofolate reductase. Pyrimethamine inhibits the enzyme dihydrofolate reductase, which catalyzes the reduction of dihydrofolate to tetrahydrofolate. This activity is highly selective against plasmodia and *Toxoplasma gondii*. It does not destroy gametocytes but arrests sporogony in the mosquito. Pyrimethamine possesses blood schizonticidal and some tissue schizonticidal activity against human malaria parasites. The action of pyrimethamine against *T. gondii* is greatly enhanced when used in conjunction with sulfonamides.

➤*Pharmacokinetics:* Pyrimethamine is well absorbed after oral use. Peak plasma concentrations occur in 2 to 6 hours. Plasma half-life is approximately 4 days; suppressive concentrations are maintained for approximately 2 weeks (but lower in malaria patients). It is approximately 87% plasma protein-bound. Several metabolites appear in the urine.

Contraindications

Hypersensitivity to the drug or any components of the formulation; megaloblastic anemia caused by folate deficiency.

Warnings

➤*Folic acid deficiency:* The dosage of pyrimethamine required for the treatment of toxoplasmosis is 10 to 20 times the recommended antimalaria dosage and approaches the toxic level. If signs of folate defi-

ciency develop, reduce dosage or discontinue drug according to patient response. Folinic acid (leucovorin) may be given in a dosage of 5 to 15 mg/day (oral, IM, or IV) until normal hematopoiesis is restored. Use with caution in possible folate deficiency (eg, malabsorption syndrome, alcoholism, pregnancy, phenytoin usage).

➤*Accidental ingestion:* Keep pyrimethamine out of the reach of infants and children as they are extremely susceptible to adverse effects from an overdose. Deaths in pediatric patients have been reported after accidental ingestion.

➤*Hypersensitivity reactions:* Occasionally severe hypersensitivity reactions (eg, Stevens-Johnson syndrome, toxic epidermal necrolysis, erythema multiforme, and anaphylaxis) have occurred, particularly if given with a sulfonamide (see Adverse Reactions). Refer to Management of Acute Hypersensitivity Reactions.

➤*Renal/Hepatic function impairment:* Use with caution.

➤*Carcinogenesis:* Data in 2 humans indicate that pyrimethamine may be carcinogenic: A 51-year-old female who developed chronic granulocytic leukemia after taking pyrimethamine for 2 years for toxoplasmosis, and a 56-year-old patient who developed reticulum cell sarcoma after 14 months of pyrimethamine for toxoplasmosis. Pyrimethamine has been reported to produce a significant increase in the number of lung tumors in mice when given intraperitoneally at doses of 25 mg/kg.

➤*Mutagenesis:* Pyrimethamine has been shown to be mutagenic in the L5178Y/TK +/- mouse lymphoma assay in the absence of exogenous metabolic activation. Human blood lymphocytes cultured in vitro had structural chromosome aberrations induced by pyrimethamine.

➤*Elderly:* Dose selection for an elderly patient should be cautious, usually starting at the low end of the dosing range, reflecting the greater frequency of decreased hepatic, renal, or cardiac function, and of concomitant disease or other drug therapy.

➤*Pregnancy: Category C.* Pyrimethamine has been shown to be teratogenic in rats when given in oral doses 7 times the human dose for chemoprophylaxis of malaria or 2.5 times the human dose for treatment of toxoplasmosis. At these doses in rats, there was a significant increase in abnormalities such as cleft palate, brachygnathia, oligodactyly, and microphthalmia. Pyrimethamine also has been shown to produce terata such as meningocele in hamsters and cleft palate in miniature pigs when given in oral doses 170 and 5 times the human dose, respectively, for chemoprophylaxis of malaria or for treatment of toxoplasmosis. There are no adequate and well-controlled studies in pregnant women. Use pyrimethamine during pregnancy only if the potential benefit justifies the potential risk to the fetus. Coadministration of folinic acid is strongly recommended when treating toxoplasmosis during pregnancy.

➤*Lactation:* Pyrimethamine is excreted in breast milk. Because of the potential for serious adverse reactions in nursing infants from pyrimethamine and from concurrent use of a sulfonamide with pyrimethamine for treatment of some patients with toxoplasmosis, decide whether to discontinue nursing or discontinue the drug, taking into account the importance of the drug to the mother.

➤*Children:* See Administration and Dosage.

Precautions

➤*Monitoring:* For toxoplasmosis, perform semiweekly blood counts, including platelet counts. Because of the long half-life of pyrimethamine, daily monitoring of peripheral blood counts is recommended for up to several weeks after an overdose until normal hematological values are restored.

➤*G-6-PD:* Large doses of pyrimethamine may precipitate hemolytic anemia in patients with glucose-6-phosphate dehydrogenase deficiency.

Drug Interactions

➤*Antifolate drugs or agents associated with myelosuppression (eg, proguanil, zidovudine, cytostatic agents [eg, methotrexate], sulfonamides, trimethoprim-sulfamethoxazole):* Concurrent use of antifolic acids and pyrimethamine may increase the risk of bone marrow suppression. Discontinue pyrimethamine if signs of folate deficiency develop. Administer folinic acid (leucovorin) until normal hematopoiesis is restored (see Warnings).

➤*Lorazepam:* Mild hepatotoxicity has been reported when lorazepam and pyrimethamine were coadministered.

Adverse Reactions

➤*GI:* Anorexia, vomiting (large doses); atrophic glossitis. Vomiting may be minimized by giving with meals; it usually disappears promptly upon dosage reduction.

➤*Hematologic:* Megaloblastic anemia, leukopenia, thrombocytopenia, pancytopenia, hematuria.

➤*Hypersensitivity:* Hypersensitivity reactions, occasionally severe (eg, Stevens-Johnson syndrome, toxic epidermal necrolysis, erythema

PYRIMETHAMINE

multiforme, anaphylaxis), and hyperphenylalaninemia have occurred particularly when coadministered with a sulfonamide.

➤*Miscellaneous:* Rhythm disorders; pulmonary eosinophilia (rare).

Overdosage

➤*Symptoms:* Following the ingestion of 300 mg or more of pyrimethamine, GI and/or CNS signs may be present, including convulsions. Initial GI symptoms include abdominal pain, nausea, and severe and repeated vomiting possibly including hematemesis. CNS toxicity is manifested by initial excitability; generalized and prolonged convulsions, which may be followed by respiratory depression; circulatory collapse; and death within a few hours. Neurological symptoms appear rapidly (30 minutes to 2 hours after drug ingestion), suggesting that in gross overdosage, pyrimethamine has a direct toxic effect on the CNS.

Fatal dose is variable; the smallest reported fatal single dose is 375 mg. There are reports of children who have recovered after taking 375 to 625 mg.

➤*Treatment:* There is no specific antidote for pyrimethamine. Gastric lavage is effective. Use parenteral diazepam to control convulsions. Administer folinic acid (leucovorin) within 2 hours of ingestion to counteract effects on the hematopoietic system. Because of the long half-life of pyrimethamine, daily monitoring of peripheral blood counts is recommended for up to several weeks after the overdose until normal hematological values are restored. Treatment includes usual supportive measures. Refer to General Management of Acute Overdosage.

Patient Information

May cause anorexia or vomiting; inform patients to take with food or meals.

At first appearance of a skin rash, inform patients to discontinue the drug and immediately seek medical attention.

Warn patients that the appearance of sore throat, pallor, purpura, or glossitis may be early indications of serious disorders that require seeking medical treatment.

Warn women of childbearing potential against becoming pregnant.

Advise patients to keep medication out of the reach of children.

Advise patients not to exceed recommended doses.

Coadministration of folinic acid (leucovorin) is strongly recommended in all patients when used for the treatment of toxoplasmosis.

SULFADOXINE AND PYRIMETHAMINE

| Rx | **Fansidar** (Roche) | **Tablets:** 500 mg sulfadoxine and 25 mg pyrimethamine | Lactose, talc. (FANSIDAR ROCHE). Scored. In UD 25s. |

WARNING

Fatalities associated with the administration of sulfadoxine and pyrimethamine have occurred because of severe reactions, including Stevens-Johnson syndrome and toxic epidermal necrolysis. Discontinue sulfadoxine and pyrimethamine prophylaxis at the first appearance of skin rash, if a significant reduction in the count of any formed blood elements is noted, or upon the occurrence of active bacterial or fungal infections.

Indications

➤*Malaria:* For the treatment of *Plasmodium falciparum* malaria for those patients in whom chloroquine resistance is suspected.

➤*Malaria prophylaxis:* For travelers to areas where chloroquine-resistant *P. falciparum* malaria is endemic (strains of *P. falciparum* may be encountered that have developed resistance to sulfadoxine and pyrimethamine therapy).

➤*Unlabeled uses:* Sulfadoxine and pyrimethamine combination has been used in the prophylaxis of *Pneumocystis carinii* infection.

Administration and Dosage

➤*Acute attack of malaria:* A single dose of the following number of sulfadoxine and pyrimethamine tablets is used in sequence with quinine or alone:

Sulfadoxine and Pyrimethamine Dosing for an Acute Malaria Attack	
Age	Dosing
Adults	2 to 3 tablets
9 to 14 years of age	2 tablets
4 to 8 years of age	1 tablet
< 4 years of age	½ tablet

➤*Malaria prophylaxis:* Take the first dose of sulfadoxine and pyrimethamine 1 or 2 days before departure to an endemic area; continue administration during the stay and for 4 to 6 weeks after return.

Sulfadoxine and Pyrimethamine Dosing for Malaria Prophylaxis		
Age	Once weekly	Once every 2 weeks
Adults	1 tablet	2 tablets
9 to 14 years of age	¾ tablet	1½ tablets
4 to 8 years of age	½ tablet	1 tablet
< 4 years of age	¼ tablet	½ tablet

Actions

➤*Pharmacology:* Sulfadoxine and pyrimethamine combination is an antimalarial agent that acts by reciprocal potentiation of its 2 components, achieved by a sequential blockade of 2 enzymes involved in the biosynthesis of folinic acid within the parasites. It is effective against certain strains of *P. falciparum* that are resistant to chloroquine.

➤*Pharmacokinetics:*

Absorption / Distribution – Both sulfadoxine and pyrimethamine are absorbed orally. Following a single tablet administration, sulfadoxine peak plasma concentrations of 51 to 76 mcg/mL were achieved in 2.5 to 6 hours, and the pyrimethamine peak plasma concentrations of 0.13 to 0.4 mcg/mL were achieved in 1.5 to 8 hours. Both drugs appear in the breast milk of nursing mothers.

Metabolism / Excretion – Both sulfadoxine and pyrimethamine are excreted mainly by the kidney. The apparent elimination half-life of sulfadoxine ranged from 100 to 231 hours (mean, 169 hours), whereas pyrimethamine half-lives ranged from 54 to 148 hours (mean, 111 hours).

Contraindications

Prophylactic use in patients with severe renal insufficiency, marked liver parenchymal damage, or blood dyscrasias; hypersensitivity to pyrimethamine or sulfonamides; patients with documented megaloblastic anemia caused by folate deficiency; infants younger than 2 months of age; pregnancy at term and during the nursing period.

Warnings

➤*Death:* Fatalities associated with the administration of sulfonamides, although rare, have occurred caused by severe reactions, including fulminant hepatic necrosis, agranulocytosis, aplastic anemia, and other blood dyscrasias (see Warning Box).

➤*Leukopenia:* Sulfadoxine and pyrimethamine prophylactic regimen has been reported to cause leukopenia during a treatment of 2 months or longer. This leukopenia is generally mild and reversible.

➤*Renal / Hepatic function impairment:* Administer with caution to patients with impaired renal or hepatic function. Perform a urinalysis with microscopic examination and renal function tests during therapy for patients who have impaired renal function.

➤*Mutagenesis:* Pyrimethamine was found to be mutagenic in laboratory animals and also in human bone marrow following 3 or 4 consecu-

tive daily doses totaling 200 to 300 mg. Testicular changes have been observed in rats treated with 105 mg/kg/day of sulfadoxine and pyrimethamine and with 15 mg/kg/day of pyrimethamine alone.

➤*Fertility impairment:* The pregnancy rate of female rats was not affected following their treatment with 10.5 mg/kg/day, but was significantly reduced at dosages of 31.5 mg/kg/day or higher, a dosage approximately 30 times or more the weekly human prophylactic dose.

➤*Elderly:* Dose selection for an elderly patient should be cautious, usually starting at the low end of the dosing range, reflecting the greater frequency of decreased hepatic, renal, or cardiac function, and of concomitant disease or other drug therapy. This drug is known to be substantially excreted by the kidney, and the risk of toxic reactions to this drug may be greater in patients with impaired renal function. Because elderly patients are more likely to have decreased renal function, use caution in dose selection and monitor renal function.

➤*Pregnancy:* Category C. Sulfadoxine and pyrimethamine therapy is contraindicated during pregnancy at term. It has been shown to be teratogenic in rats when given in weekly doses approximately 12 times the weekly human prophylactic dose. Teratogenicity studies with pyrimethamine plus sulfadoxine (1:20) in rats showed the minimum oral teratogenic dose to be approximately 0.9 mg/kg pyrimethamine plus 18 mg/kg sulfadoxine. In rabbits, no teratogenic effects were noted at oral doses as high as 20 mg/kg pyrimethamine plus 400 mg/kg sulfadoxine.

There are no adequate and well-controlled studies in pregnant women. However, because of the teratogenic effect shown in animals and because pyrimethamine plus sulfadoxine may interfere with folic acid metabolism, use during pregnancy only if the potential benefit justifies the potential risk to the fetus. Warn women of childbearing potential who are traveling to areas where malaria is endemic against becoming pregnant.

➤*Lactation:* Sulfadoxine and pyrimethamine therapy is contraindicated in the nursing period because sulfonamides cross the placenta and are excreted in breast milk, which may result in kernicterus.

➤*Children:* Do not give to infants younger than 2 months of age because of inadequate development of the glucuronide-forming enzyme system.

Precautions

➤*Monitoring:* Periodic blood counts and analysis of urine for crystalluria are desirable during prolonged prophylaxis.

➤*Folic acid deficiency:* Discontinue therapy if signs of folic acid deficiency develop. Folinic acid (leucovorin) may be administered in doses of 5 to 15 mg/day IM, for 3 days or longer for depressed platelet or white blood cell counts in patients with drug-induced folic acid deficiency when recovery is too slow.

➤*Special risk:* Administer with caution to patients with possible folate deficiency and to those with severe allergy or bronchial asthma. As with some sulfonamide drugs, in glucose-6-phosphate dehydrogenase-deficient individuals, hemolysis may occur.

Drug Interactions

➤*Chloroquine:* There have been reports that may indicate an increase in incidence and severity of adverse reactions when chloroquine is used with sulfadoxine and pyrimethamine tablets as compared with the use of the sulfadoxine and pyrimethamine tablets alone.

➤*Antifolic drugs:* Do not use antifolic drugs (eg, sulfonamides or trimethoprim-sulfamethoxazole combinations) while the patient is receiving sulfadoxine and pyrimethamine tablets for antimalarial prophylaxis.

➤*Goitrogens, diuretics, hypoglycemic agents:* The sulfonamides bear certain chemical similarities to some goitrogens, diuretics (acetazolamide and the thiazides), and oral hypoglycemic agents. Diuresis and hypoglycemia have occurred rarely in patients receiving sulfonamides. Cross-sensitivity may exist with these agents.

Adverse Reactions

➤*CNS:* Headache; peripheral neuritis; mental depression; convulsions; ataxia; hallucinations; tinnitus; vertigo; insomnia; apathy; fatigue; muscle weakness; nervousness.

➤*GI:* Glossitis; stomatitis; nausea; emesis; abdominal pains; hepatitis; hepatocellular necrosis; diarrhea; pancreatitis.

➤*Hematologic:* Agranulocytosis; aplastic anemia; megaloblastic anemia; thrombopenia; leukopenia; hemolytic anemia; purpura; hypoprothrombinemia; methemoglobinemia; eosinophilia.

➤*Hypersensitivity:* Erythema multiforme; Stevens-Johnson syndrome; generalized skin eruptions; toxic epidermal necrolysis; urticaria; serum sickness; pruritus; exfoliative dermatitis; anaphylactoid reactions; periorbital edema; conjunctival and scleral injection; photosensitization; arthralgia; allergic myocarditis.

➤*Miscellaneous:* Pulmonary infiltrates; drug fever; chills; toxic nephrosis with oliguria and anuria; periarteritis nodosa; LE phenomenon.

SULFADOXINE AND PYRIMETHAMINE

Overdosage

➤*Symptoms:* Acute intoxication may be manifested by anorexia, vomiting, and CNS stimulation (including convulsions), followed by megaloblastic anemia, leukopenia, thrombocytopenia, glossitis, and crystalluria.

➤*Treatment:* In acute intoxication, emesis and gastric lavage followed by purges may be of benefit. Adequately hydrate the patient to prevent renal damage. Monitor the renal and hematopoietic systems for at least 1 month after overdosage. If the patient is having convulsions, the use of a parenteral barbiturate is indicated. Administer folinic acid (leucovorin) 5 to 15 mg/day IM for 3 days or longer for depressed platelet or white blood cell counts.

Patient Information

Advise the patient to immediately seek medical attention and discontinue therapy at first appearance of rash. Adequate fluid intake must be maintained in order to prevent crystalluria and stone formation.

Instruct the patient to seek medical attention and discontinue prophylactic therapy if sore throat, fever, arthralgia, cough, shortness of breath, pallor, purpura, jaundice, or glossitis develop.

Caution women against becoming pregnant and not to breastfeed their infants during therapy or prophylactic treatment.

ATOVAQUONE AND PROGUANIL HCl

Rx	**Malarone** (Glaxo Wellcome)	**Tablets:** 250 mg atovaquone/ 100 mg proguanil HCl	(GX CM3). Pink, biconvex. Film-coated. In 100s.
Rx	**Malarone Pediatric** (Glaxo Wellcome)	**Tablets:** 62.5 mg atovaquone/ 25 mg proguanil HCl	(GX CG7). Pink, biconvex. Film-coated. In 100s.

Indications

➤*Malaria prevention:* Prophylaxis of *Plasmodium falciparum* malaria, including areas where chloroquine resistance has been reported.

➤*Malaria treatment:* Treatment of acute, uncomplicated *P. falciparum* malaria. Atovaquone and proguanil have been shown to be effective in regions where the drugs chloroquine, halofantrine, mefloquine, and amodiaquine may have unacceptable failure rates, presumably because of drug resistance.

Administration and Dosage

➤*Approved by the FDA:* July 21, 2000.

Take the daily dose at the same time each day with food or milk. In the event of vomiting within 1 hour after dosing, take a repeat dose.

➤*Malaria prophylaxis:* Start prophylactic treatment with atovaquone/proguanil 1 or 2 days before entering a malaria-endemic area and continue daily during the stay and for 7 days after return.

Adults – Take 1 tablet (adult strength = 250 mg atovaquone/100 mg proguanil) per day.

Children – The dosage for prevention of malaria in pediatric patients is based upon body weight (see table below).

Dosage of Atovaquone/Proguanil for Prevention of Malaria in Pediatric Patients		
Weight (kg)	Atovaquone/ Proguanil total daily dose	Dosage regimen
11-20	62.5 mg/25 mg	1 pediatric tablet daily
21-30	125 mg/50 mg	2 pediatric tablets as a single daily dose
31-40	187.5 mg/75 mg	3 pediatric tablets as a single daily dose
> 40	250 mg/100 mg	1 tablet (adult strength) as a single daily dose

➤*Treatment of acute malaria:*

Adults – 4 tablets (adult strength; total daily dose 1 g atovaquone/ 400 mg proguanil) as a single daily dose for 3 consecutive days.

Children – The dosage for treatment of acute malaria in pediatric patients is based upon body weight (see table below).

Dosage of Atovaquone/Proguanil for Treatment of Acute Malaria in Pediatric Patients		
Weight (kg)	Atovaquone/ Proguanil total daily dose	Dosage regimen
11-20	250 mg/100 mg	1 tablet (adult strength) daily for 3 consecutive days
21-30	500 mg/200 mg	2 tablets (adult strength) as a single daily dose for 3 consecutive days
31-40	750 mg/300 mg	3 tablets (adult strength) as a single daily dose for 3 consecutive days
> 40	1 g/400 mg	4 tablets (adult strength) as a single daily dose for 3 consecutive days

Actions

➤*Pharmacology:* Atovaquone and proguanil is a fixed-dose combination of the antimalarial agents atovaquone and proguanil. The constituents of the combination interfere with 2 different pathways involved in the biosynthesis of pyrimidines required for nucleic acid replication. Atovaquone is a selective inhibitor of parasite mitochondrial electron transport. Proguanil primarily exerts its effect by means of the metabolite cycloguanil, a dihydrofolate reductase inhibitor. Inhibition of dihydrofolate reductase in the malaria parasite disrupts deoxythymidylate synthesis.

Atovaquone and cycloguanil (an active metabolite of proguanil) are active against the erythrocytic and exoerythrocytic stages of *Plasmo-*dium spp. Enhanced efficacy of the combination compared with either atovaquone or proguanil alone was demonstrated in clinical studies in immune and nonimmune patients.

Drug resistance – Strains of *P. falciparum* with decreased susceptibility to atovaquone or proguanil/cycloguanil alone can be selected in vitro or in vivo. The combination of atovaquone and proguanil may not be effective for treatment of recrudescent malaria that develops after prior therapy with the combination.

➤*Pharmacokinetics:*

Absorption – Atovaquone is a highly lipophilic compound with low aqueous solubility. The bioavailability of atovaquone shows considerable interindividual variability.

Dietary fat taken with atovaquone increases the rate and extent of absorption, increasing AUC 2 to 3 times and C_{max} 5 times over fasting. The absolute bioavailability of the tablet formulation of atovaquone when taken with food is 23%. Take atovaquone and proguanil tablets with food or milk. Proguanil is extensively absorbed regardless of food intake.

Distribution – Atovaquone is highly protein bound (> 99%) over the concentration range of 1 to 90 mcg/ml. The apparent volume of distribution of atovaquone after oral administration is ≈ 3.5 L/kg.

Proguanil is 75% protein bound. The apparent volume of distribution is ≈ 42 L/kg. In human plasma, the binding of atovaquone and proguanil was unaffected by the presence of the other.

Metabolism – In a study where atovaquone was administered to healthy volunteers,> 94% of the dose was recovered unchanged in the feces over 21 days. There was little or no excretion of atovaquone in the urine (< 0.6%). There is indirect evidence that atovaquone may undergo limited metabolism; however, a specific metabolite has not been identified. Between 40% to 60% of proguanil is excreted by the kidneys. Proguanil is metabolized to cycloguanil (primarily via CYP2C19) and 4-chlorophenylbiguanide. The main routes of elimination are hepatic biotransformation and renal excretion.

Excretion – The elimination half-life of atovaquone is ≈ 2 to 3 days in adult patients. The mean oral clearance of atovaquone is ≈ 0.04 L/hr/kg. The mean oral clearance of proguanil is 3.22 L/hr/kg. The elimination half-life of proguanil is 12 to 21 hours in adult and pediatric patients, but may be longer in individuals who are slow metabolizers.

Special populations –
Children: The pharmacokinetics of proguanil and cycloguanil are similar in adult and pediatric patients. However, the elimination half-life of atovaquone is shorter in pediatric patients (1 to 2 days) than in adult patients (2 to 3 days).

Renal function impairment: The pharmacokinetics of atovaquone and proguanil combination have not been studied in patients with renal impairment. Because proguanil and cycloguanil are eliminated primarily via the renal route, the clinical implication of treating patients with severe renal dysfunction with the combination is unknown.

Contraindications

Hypersensitivity to atovaquone, proguanil, or any component of the formulation.

For prophylaxis of *P. falciparum* malaria in patients with severe renal impairment (creatinine clearance less than 30 mL/min).

Warnings

➤*Renal function impairment:* Administer with caution to patients with severe pre-existing renal failure because proguanil is eliminated by renal excretion.

➤*Pregnancy: Category C.* Falciparum malaria carries a higher risk of morbidity and mortality in pregnant women than in the general population. Maternal death and fetal loss are known complications of falciparum malaria in pregnancy. In pregnant women who must travel to malaria-endemic areas, personal protection against mosquito bites should always be employed (see Patient Information) in addition to antimalarials.

ATOVAQUONE AND PROGUANIL HCl

In rabbits, atovaquone caused maternal toxicity at plasma concentrations that were ≈ 0.6 to 1.3 times the estimated human exposure during treatment of malaria. Adverse fetal effects in rabbits, including decreased fetal body lengths and increased early resorption and post-implantation losses, were observed only in the presence of maternal toxicity. Concentrations of atovaquone in rabbit fetuses averaged 30% of the concurrent maternal plasma concentrations.

While there are no adequate and well-controlled studies of atovaquone or proguanil in pregnant women, the combination may be used if the potential benefit justifies the potential risk to the fetus. The proguanil component acts by inhibiting the parasitic dihydrofolate reductase (see Pharmacology). However, there are no clinical data indicating that folate supplementation diminishes drug efficacy, and for women of childbearing age receiving folate supplements to prevent neural tube birth defects, such supplements may be continued while taking the atovaquone/proguanil combination.

➤*Lactation:* It is not known whether atovaquone is excreted in breast milk. In a rat study, atovaquone concentrations in the milk were 30% of the concurrent atovaquone concentrations in the maternal plasma. Proguanil is excreted in breast milk in small quantities. Exercise caution when the atovaquone/proguanil combination is administered to a nursing woman.

➤*Children:* Safety and efficacy for the treatment and prophylaxis of malaria in pediatric patients who weigh < 11 kg have not been established.

Precautions

➤*Cerebral malaria:* Atovaquone/Proguanil combination has not been evaluated for the treatment of cerebral malaria or other severe manifestations of complicated malaria, including hyperparasitemia, pulmonary edema, or renal failure. Patients with severe malaria are not candidates for oral therapy.

➤*Diarrhea/Vomiting:* Absorption of atovaquone may be reduced in patients with diarrhea or vomiting. If atovaquone and proguanil combination is used in patients who are vomiting (see Administration and Dosage), closely monitor parasitemia and consider the use of an antiemetic. Vomiting occurred in ≤ 19% of pediatric patients given treatment doses. In the controlled clinical trials, 15.3% of adults who were treated with atovaquone/proguanil received an antiemetic. Of these patients, 98.3% were successfully treated. In patients with severe or persistent diarrhea or vomiting, alternative antimalarial therapy may be required.

➤*Relapse:* Parasite relapse occurred commonly when *Plasmodium vivax* malaria was treated with atovaquone/proguanil alone. In the event of recrudescent *P. falciparum* infections after treatment with or failure of chemoprophylaxis with atovaquone/proguanil, treat patients with a different blood schizonticide.

Drug Interactions

Atovaquone is highly protein bound (> 99%) but does not displace other highly protein-bound drugs in vitro. Proguanil is metabolized primarily by CYP2C19. Potential pharmacokinetic interactions with other substrates or inhibitors of this pathway are unknown.

Atovaquone/Proguanil Drug Interactions			
Precipitant drug	Object drug*		Description
Tetracycline	Atovaquone	↓	Concomitant treatment with tetracycline has been associated with ≈ 40% reduction in plasma concentrations of atovaquone. Closely monitor parasitemia in patients receiving tetracycline.
Metoclopramide	Atovaquone	↓	Concomitant treatment with metoclopramide has been associated with decreased bioavailability of atovaquone. Use only if other antiemetics are not available.
Rifampin	Atovaquone	↓	Concomitant administration of rifampin is known to reduce atovaquone levels by ≈ 50%. The concomitant administration of these agents is not recommended. The mechanism of this interaction is unknown.

* ↓ = Object drug decreased.

➤*Drug/Food interactions:* Dietary fat taken with atovaquone increases the rate and extent of absorption, increasing AUC 2 to 3 times and C_{max} 5 times over fasting. The absolute bioavailability of the tablet formulation of atovaquone when taken with food is 23%. Take atovaquone and proguanil tablets with food or milk. Proguanil is extensively absorbed regardless of food intake.

Adverse Reactions

The type and severity of adverse reactions associated with the individual components of atovaquone and proguanil may be expected. The higher treatment doses of the combination were less tolerated than the lower prophylactic doses.

Malaria prophylaxis – Among subjects who received atovaquone/proguanil for prophylaxis of malaria, adverse reactions occurred in similar proportions of subjects receiving the combination or placebo. The most commonly reported adverse experiences possibly attributable to atovaquone/proguanil or placebo were headache and abdominal pain. Prophylaxis was discontinued prematurely because of a treatment-related adverse experience in 3 of 381 adults and 0 of 125 pediatric patients.

Malaria treatment – Among adults who received atovaquone/proguanil for malaria treatment, attributable adverse experiences that occurred in ≥ 5% of patients were abdominal pain (17%); nausea, vomiting (12%); headache (10%); diarrhea, asthenia (8%); anorexia, dizziness (5%). Treatment was discontinued prematurely because of an adverse experience in 4 of 436 adults.

Among pediatric patients who received atovaquone/proguanil for malaria treatment, attributable adverse experiences that occurred in ≥ 5% of patients were vomiting (10%) and pruritus (6%). Vomiting occurred in 43 of 319 (13%) pediatric patients who did not have symptomatic malaria but were given treatment doses of atovaquone/proguanil for 3 days in a clinical trial. The design of this clinical trial required that any patient who vomited be withdrawn from the trial. Among pediatric patients with symptomatic malaria treated with the combination, treatment was discontinued prematurely because of adverse experience in 1 of 116 (0.9%).

➤*Lab test abnormalities:* Abnormalities in laboratory tests reported in clinical trials were limited to elevations of transaminases in malaria patients being treated with atovaquone/proguanil. The frequency of these abnormalities varied substantially across studies of treatment and were not observed in the randomized portions of the prophylaxis trials.

In one phase III trial of malaria treatment in Thai adults, early elevations of AST and ALT were observed to occur more frequently in patients treated with atovaquone/proguanil compared with patients treated with an active control drug. Rates for patients who had normal baseline levels of these clinical laboratory parameters were: Day 7 – ALT 26.7% vs 15.6%; AST 16.9% vs 8.6%. By day 14 of this 28-day study, the frequency of transaminase elevations equalized across the 2 groups.

In this and other studies in which transaminase elevations occurred, they were noted to persist for ≤ 4 weeks following treatment with atovaquone/proguanil for malaria. None were associated with untoward clinical events.

Adverse Reactions of Atovaquone/Proguanil Combination for Prophylaxis of Malaria					
	Patients with adverse experiences (%) (Patients with adverse experiences attributable to therapy [%])				
	Adults			Children and adolescents	
Adverse reaction	Placebo (n = 206)	Atovaquone/ Proguanil[1] (n = 206)	Atovaquone/ Proguanil[2] (n = 381)	Placebo (n = 140)	Atovaquone/ Proguanil (n = 125)
Headache	27 (7)	22 (3)	17 (5)	21 (14)	19 (14)
Fever	13 (1)	5 (0)	3 (0)	11 (< 1)	6 (0)
Myalgia	11 (0)	12 (0)	7 (0)	0 (0)	0 (0)
Abdominal pain	10 (5)	9 (4)	6 (3)	29 (29)	33 (31)
Cough	8 (< 1)	6 (< 1)	4 (1)	9 (0)	9 (0)
Diarrhea	8 (3)	6 (2)	4 (1)	3 (1)	2 (0)
Upper respiratory tract infection	7 (0)	8 (0)	5 (0)	0 (0)	< 1 (0)
Dyspepsia	5 (4)	3 (2)	2 (1)	0 (0)	0 (0)
Back pain	4 (0)	8 (0)	4 (0)	0 (0)	0 (0)
Gastritis	3 (2)	3 (3)	2 (2)	0 (0)	0 (0)
Vomiting	2 (< 1)	1 (< 1)	< 1 (< 1)	6 (6)	7 (7)
Flu syndrome	1 (0)	2 (0)	4 (0)	6 (0)	9 (0)
Any adverse event	65 (32)	54 (17)	49 (17)	62 (41)	60 (42)

[1] Subjects receiving the recommended dose of atovaquone and proguanil in placebo-controlled trials.
[2] Subjects receiving the recommended dose of atovaquone and proguanil in any trial.

Overdosage

There have been no reports of overdosage from the administration of atovaquone/proguanil combination tablets.

➤*Atovaquone:* There is no known antidote for atovaquone, and it is currently unknown if atovaquone is dialyzable. The median lethal dose is higher than the maximum oral dose tested in mice and rats (1825 mg/kg/day). Overdoses ≤ 31,500 mg of atovaquone have been reported. In one such patient who also took an unspecified dose of dap-

ATOVAQUONE AND PROGUANIL HCl

sone, methemoglobinemia occurred. Rash also has been reported after overdose.

➤*Proguanil:* Overdoses of proguanil as large as 1500 mg have been followed by complete recovery, and doses as high as 700 mg twice daily have been taken for over 2 weeks without serious toxicity. Adverse events occasionally associated with proguanil doses of 100 to 200 mg/day, such as epigastric discomfort and vomiting, would be likely to occur with overdose. There also are reports of reversible hair loss and scaling of the skin on the palms or soles, reversible aphthous ulceration, and hematologic side effects.

Patient Information

Instruct patients to do the following:

- Take atovaquone/proguanil combination tablets at the same time each day with food or milk.
- Take a repeat dose of the combination if vomiting occurs within 1 hour after dosing.
- Consult a health care professional regarding alternative forms of prophylaxis if prophylaxis with atovaquone/proguanil is prematurely discontinued for any reason.
- Include protective clothing, insect repellants, and bednets as important components of malaria prophylaxis.
- No chemoprophylactic regimen is 100% effective; therefore, patients should seek medical attention for any febrile illness that occurs during or after return from a malaria-endemic area and inform their health care professional that they may have been exposed to malaria.
- *Falciparum* malaria carries a higher risk of death and serious complications in pregnant women than in the general population. Pregnant women anticipating travel to malarious areas should discuss the risks and benefits of such travel with their physicians (see Pregnancy section).

Antituberculosis drugs have been described in terms of the following 3 areas of activity: Bactericidal activity, sterilizing activity, and drug resistance prevention. Isoniazid is the most potent bactericidal antituberculosis agent, although rifampin and streptomycin have some bactericidal activity. Rifampin and pyrazinamide are the most potent sterilizing drugs for tuberculosis. Drugs that eliminate all bacterial populations and do not allow the emergence of resistant organisms prevent drug resistance.

Standard treatment regimens are divided into the following 2 phases: An initial phase, during which agents are used to kill rapidly multiplying populations of *Mycobacterium tuberculosis* and to prevent the emergence of drug resistance, followed by a continuation phase, during which sterilizing drugs kill the intermittently dividing populations.

The initial phase of the regimen must contain ≥ 3 of the following drugs: Isoniazid, rifampin, and pyrazinamide, along with either ethambutol or streptomycin if the local resistance pattern to isoniazid is not documented or is > 4%.

➤*Directly observed therapy (DOT):* Adherence to the treatment regimen can be achieved by DOT, the "gold standard." The health care provider watches the patient swallow each dose of medication. This allows for monitoring the number of doses that an individual has taken.

DOT may be given intermittently (2 to 3 times/week) or daily. Intermittent therapy was introduced when it was shown in controlled clinical trials that therapeutic serum levels of the various antituberculosis drugs were maintained even when medications were given only 2 or 3 times/week. Intermittent regimens do not have more toxic effects than daily regimens; allow drug administration to be adapted to local conditions. All intermittent regimens must involve DOT.

Recommended Drugs for the Treatment of Tuberculosis in Children and Adults[1]							
	Daily dose[2]		Maximum daily dose in children and adults	Twice weekly dose		3 times/week dose	
Drug	Children	Adults		Children	Adults	Children	Adults
Initial treatment							
Isoniazid	10 to 20 mg/kg PO or IM	5 mg/kg PO or IM	300 mg	20 to 40 mg/kg max 900 mg	15 mg/kg max 900 mg	20 to 40 mg/kg max 900 mg	15 mg/kg max 900 mg
Rifampin	10 to 20 mg/kg PO	10 mg/kg PO	600 mg	10 to 20 mg/kg max 600 mg	10 mg/kg max 600 mg	10 to 20 mg/kg max 600 mg	10 mg/kg max 600 mg
Pyrazinamide	15 to 30 mg/kg PO	15 to 30 mg/kg PO	2 g	50 to 70 mg/kg max 4 g	50 to 70 mg/kg max 4 g	50 to 70 mg/kg max 3 g	50 to 70 mg/kg max 3 g
Streptomycin	20 to 40 mg/kg IM	15 mg/kg IM	1 g[3]	25 to 30 mg/kg IM max 1.5 g	25 to 30 mg/kg IM max 1.5 g	25 to 30 mg/kg max 1.5 g	25 to 30 mg/kg max 1.5 g
Ethambutol	15 to 25 mg/kg PO	15 to 25 mg/kg PO	—	50 mg/kg	50 mg/kg	25 to 30 mg/kg	25 to 30 mg/kg
Rifapentine	—	—	—	—	600 mg PO	—	—
Second-line treatment							
Cycloserine	15 to 20 mg/kg PO	15 to 20 mg/kg PO	1 g	—	—	—	—
Ethionamide	15 to 20 mg/kg PO	15 to 20 mg/kg PO	1 g	—	—	—	—
Capreomycin	15 to 30 mg/kg IM	15 to 30 mg/kg IM	1 g	—	—	—	—
Kanamycin	15 to 30 mg/kg IM or IV	15 to 30 mg/kg IM or IV	1 g	—	—	—	—
Ciprofloxacin	—	1000 to 1500 mg PO	1500 mg	—	—	—	—
Ofloxacin	—	800 mg PO	800 mg	—	—	—	—
Levofloxacin	—	500 to 750 mg PO	750 mg	—	—	—	—
Sparfloxacin	—	200 mg PO	200 mg	—	—	—	—
P-aminosalicyclic acid	150 mg/kg PO	150 mg/kg PO	12 g	—	—	—	—
Rifabutin	—	300 to 450 mg PO	—	—	—	—	—

[1] For detailed dosing information and frequency, see individual monographs.
[2] Doses based on weight. Adjust as weight changes.
[3] In people ≥ 60 years of age, limit the daily dose of streptomycin to 0.5 g IM.

➤*Treatment regimens:* Treatment for tuberculosis is a long-term process. Begin treatment as soon as possible after diagnosis. Combination therapy is required. The CDC recommends at least a 3-drug regimen with rifampin, isoniazid, and pyrazinamide for a minimum of 2 months, followed by rifampin and isoniazid for 4 months in areas with a low incidence of tuberculosis. Administer streptomycin or ethambutol for the first 2 months in areas with a high incidence of tuberculosis.

➤*Retreatment:* Retreatment is necessary when treatment fails because of noncompliance or inadequate drug treatment. Retreatment regimens include ≥ 4 drugs; however, depending on disease progression and the bacteriostatic or bactericidal activity of the drug, ≤ 7 drugs can be used. Retreatment drug regimens most commonly include the second-line agents of ethionamide, aminosalicylic acid, cycloserine, and capreomycin, as well as ofloxacin and ciprofloxacin.

Therapy includes 2 or 3 agents not given previously when current susceptibility data are unavailable. Add to the initial 4-drug regimen of isoniazid, rifampin, pyrazinamide, and ethambutol or streptomycin, ≥ 2 drugs to which the organism is susceptible on the basis of local resistance patterns. The ineffective agents may be discontinued once susceptibility test results are available.

Individualize treatment on the basis of the susceptibility pattern of the infecting organism when re-treating patients known to be infected with drug-resistant isolates. Include in this regimen ≥ 3 new drugs to which the organism is susceptible. Continue therapy until sputum cultures convert to negative and then continue therapy for an additional 12 months with 2 drugs. Treatment may be continued for 24 months after sputum culture conversion.

➤*HIV:* The initial phase of a 6-month tuberculosis regimen consists of isoniazid, rifabutin, pyrazinamide, and ethambutol for patients receiving therapy with protease inhibitors or nonnucleoside reverse transcriptase inhibitors. These drugs are administered a) daily for at least the first 2 weeks, followed by twice weekly dosing for 6 weeks or b) daily for 8 weeks to complete the 2-month induction phase. The second phase of treatment consists of rifabutin and isoniazid administered twice weekly or daily for 4 months.

Patients for whom the use of rifamycins is limited or contraindicated for any reason (eg, patient/clinician decision not to combine antiretroviral therapy with rifabutin, intolerance to rifamycins), the initial phase of a 9-month tuberculosis regimen consists of isoniazid, streptomycin, pyrazinamide, and ethambutol administered a) daily for at least the first 2 weeks, followed by twice weekly dosing for 6 weeks or b) daily for 8 weeks to complete the 2-month induction phase. The second phase of treatment consists of isoniazid, streptomycin, and pyrazinamide administered 2 to 3 times/week for 7 months.

The preferred option for patients who are not candidates for antiretroviral therapy or for whom a decision is made not to combine the initiation of tuberculosis therapy with antiretroviral therapy is to administer a 6-month regimen of isoniazid, rifampin, pyrazinamide, and ethambutol or streptomycin. These drugs are administered a) daily for at least the first 2 weeks, followed by 2 or 3 times/week dosing for 6 weeks or b) daily for 8 weeks to complete the 2-month induction phase. The second phase of treatment consists of isoniazid and rifampin administered daily or 2 to 3 times/week for 4 months. Isoniazid, rifampin, pyrazinamide, and ethambutol or streptomycin can be administered 3 times/week for 6 months.

Do not use tuberculosis regimens consisting of isoniazid, ethambutol, and pyrazinamide (ie, 3-drug regimens that do not contain a rifamycin, an aminoglycoside [eg, streptomycin, amikacin, kanamycin], or capreomycin) for the treatment of patients with HIV-related tuberculosis. The minimum duration of therapy is 18 months (or 12 months after documented culture conversion) if these regimens are used for the treatment of tuberculosis.

Administer pyridoxine (vitamin B_6) 25 to 50 mg daily or 50 to 100 mg twice weekly to all HIV-infected patients who are undergoing tuberculosis treatment with isoniazid to reduce the occurrence of isoniazid-induced side effects in the central and peripheral nervous system.

Because the MMWR's most recent recommendations for the use of antiretroviral therapy strongly advise against interruptions of therapy, and because alternative tuberculosis treatments that do not contain rifampin are available, previous antituberculosis therapy options that involved stopping protease inhibitor therapy to allow the use of rifampin are no longer recommended.

►*Pregnancy:* Do not delay treatment for suspected or confirmed tuberculosis during pregnancy. The best therapeutic choices with the least danger to the fetus appear to be combinations of isoniazid, ethambutol, and rifampin. Pyrazinamide and streptomycin are not recommended during pregnancy because of possible teratogenic effects.

Administer pyridoxine to all pregnant women receiving tuberculosis treatment to prevent peripheral neuropathy as a result of taking isoniazid. In pregnant women, delay prophylaxis until after delivery.

►*Multidrug resistance:* The most recent cultures should undergo susceptibility testing to all antituberculosis drugs if cultures remain positive after 3 to 4 months of treatment. The patient may continue to receive the most recent treatment regimen, if his or her condition is clinically stable, while awaiting results of drug susceptibility testing. Alternatively, add ≥ 2 new drugs to the original medications if the patient is acutely ill. Administer an aminoglycoside or capreomycin as one of the medications, because these drugs lead to earlier sputum conversion.

►*Chemoprophylaxis:* Administer isoniazid to adults in a daily dose of 300 mg for 1 year. Administer 10 mg/kg to a maximum daily dose of 300 mg for 1 year to children. Consider prophylactic therapy for the following: Those exposed to tuberculosis but who have no evidence of infection; those with infection (positive tuberculin test: > 5 mm [HIV infected] or 10 mm [not immunocompromised] of induration to 5 units purified protein derivative [PPD]) and no apparent disease; those with a history of tuberculosis but in whom the disease is presently "inactive;" and anergic people from populations at risk for tuberculosis. Prophylaxis with isoniazid is contraindicated for patients who have had reactions to the drug or have active hepatic disease. There are insufficient data on the advisability of prophylaxis with alternative drugs such as rifampin.

ISONIAZID (Isonicotinic acid hydrazide; INH)

Rx	Isoniazid (Various, eg, Barr, Eon, Paddock, UDL)	**Tablets:** 100 mg	In 30s, 100s, and 1000s.
Rx	Isoniazid (Various, eg, Barr, Eon, Major, UDL)	**Tablets:** 300 mg	In 30s, 60s, 100s, 200s, and 1000s.
Rx	Isoniazid (Carolina Medical)	**Syrup:** 50 mg/5 ml	Sorbitol. Orange flavor. In pt.
Rx	Nydrazid (Apothecon)	**Injection:** 100 mg/ml	In 10 ml vials.[1]

[1] With 0.25% chlorobutanol.

Refer to the general discussion in the Antituberculosal Agents Introduction.

WARNING

Severe and sometimes fatal hepatitis associated with isoniazid therapy may occur or develop even after many months of treatment. The risk of developing hepatitis is age-related. Approximate case rates by age are < 1 per 1000 for people < 20 years of age, 3 per 1000 for people 20 to 34, 12 per 1000 for people 35 to 49, 23 per 1000 for people 50 to 64, and 8 per 1000 for people > 65 years of age. Risk of hepatitis increases with daily alcohol consumption. Precise fatality rates for isoniazid-related hepatitis is not available; however, in 13,838 people taking isoniazid, there were 8 deaths among 174 cases of hepatitis.

Carefully monitor and interview patients at monthly intervals. For people > 35 years of age, in addition to a monthly symptom review, measure hepatic enzymes (specifically AST and ALT) prior to starting isoniazid therapy and periodically throughout treatment. Isoniazid-associated hepatitis usually occurs during the first 3 months of treatment. Enzyme levels generally return to normal despite continuance of the drug, but in some cases, progressive liver dysfunction occurs. Other factors associated with an increased risk of hepatitis include daily use of alcohol, chronic liver disease, and injection drug use. A report suggests an increased risk of fatal hepatitis associated with isoniazid among women, particularly black and Hispanic women. The risk may also be increased during the postpartum period. Consider more careful monitoring in these groups, possibly including more frequent laboratory monitoring. If abnormalities of liver function exceed 3 to 5 times the upper limit of normal, consider discontinuation of isoniazid. Liver function tests are not a substitute for a clinical evaluation at monthly intervals or for the prompt assessment of signs or symptoms of adverse reactions occurring between regularly scheduled evaluations. Instruct patients to report immediately signs or symptoms consistent with liver damage or other adverse effects. These include any or the following: Unexplained anorexia, nausea, vomiting, dark urine, icterus, rash, persistent paresthesias of the hands and feet, persistent fatigue, weakness or fever of > 3 days duration or abdominal tenderness, especially right upper quadrant discomfort. If these symptoms appear, or if signs suggestive of hepatic damage are detected, discontinue isoniazid promptly because continued use of the drug in such cases may cause a more severe form of liver damage.

Treat patients with tuberculosis who have hepatitis attributed to isoniazid with appropriate alternative drugs. Reinstitute isoniazid after symptoms and laboratory abnormalities have become normal. Restart the drug in very small doses; gradually increase doses and withdraw immediately if there is any indication of recurrent liver involvement.

Defer preventive treatment in people with acute hepatic diseases.

Indications

►*Treatment of tuberculosis:* Isoniazid is recommended for all forms of tuberculosis in which organisms are susceptible. However, active tuberculosis must be treated with multiple concomitant antituberculosis medications to prevent the emergence of drug resistance.

►*Prophylaxis:* Isoniazid is recommended as preventive therapy for the following groups, regardless of age. (Note: the criterion for a positive reaction to a skin test [in millimeters of induration] for each group is given in parentheses).

HIV – People with human immunodeficiency virus (HIV) infection (≥ 5 mm) and people with risk factors for HIV infection whose HIV infection status is unknown but who are suspected of having HIV infection.

Preventive therapy may be considered for HIV-infected people who are tuberculin-negative but belong to groups in which the prevalence of tuberculosis infection is high. Candidates for preventive therapy who have HIV infection should have a minimum of 12 months of therapy.

Close contacts of people with newly diagnosed infectious tuberculosis – Close contacts of people with newly diagnosed infectious tuberculosis (≥ 5 mm). In addition, tuberculin-negative (< 5 mm) children and adolescents who have been close contacts of infectious people within the past 3 months are candidates for preventive therapy until a repeat tuberculin skin test is done 12 weeks after contact with the infectious source. If the repeat skin test is positive (> 5 mm), continue therapy.

Recent converters – Recent converters, as indicated by a tuberculin skin test (≥ 10 mm increase within a 2-year period for those < 35 years of age; ≥ 15 mm increase for those ≥ 35 years of age). All infants and children < 4 years of age with a > 10 mm skin test are included in this category.

Abnormal chest radiographs – People with abnormal chest radiographs that show fibrotic lesions likely to represent old healed tuberculoses (≥ 5 mm). Candidates for preventive therapy who have fibrotic pulmonary lesions consistent with healed tuberculosis or who have pulmonary silicosis should have 12 months of isoniazid or 4 months of isoniazid and rifampin, concomitantly.

Intravenous drug users – IV drug users known to be HIV-seronegative (> 10 mm).

Increased risk of tuberculosis – People with the following medical conditions that have been reported to increase the risk of tuberculosis (≥ 10 mm): Silicosis; diabetes mellitus; prolonged therapy with adrenocorticosteroids; immunosuppressive therapy; some hematologic and reticuloendothelial disease, such as leukemia or Hodgkin's disease; end-stage renal disease; clinical situations associated with substantial rapid weight loss or chronic undernutrition (including intestinal bypass surgery for obesity, the postgastrectomy state [with or without weight loss], chronic peptic ulcer disease, chronic malabsorption syndromes, and carcinomas of the oropharynx and upper GI tract that prevent adequate nutritional intake). Candidates for preventive therapy who have fibrotic pulmonary lesions consistent with healed tuberculosis or who have pulmonary silicosis should have 12 months of isoniazid or 4 months of isoniazid and rifampin, concomitantly.

ISONIAZID (Isonicotinic acid hydrazide; INH)

Adults < 35 years of age with tuberculin skin test reaction of ≥ 10 mm – Additionally in the absence of any of the above risk factors, people < 35 years of age with a tuberculin skin test reaction of ≥ 10 mm are also appropriate candidates for preventive therapy if they are a member of any of the following high-incidence groups:

1.) Foreign-born people from high-prevalence countries who never received BCG vaccine.
2.) Medically underserved low-income populations, including high-risk racial or ethnic minority populations, especially blacks, Hispanics, and Native Americans.
3.) Residents of long-term care facilities (eg, correctional institutions, nursing homes, mental institutions).

Children < 4 years of age – Children who are < 4 years of age are candidates for isoniazid preventive therapy if they have > 10 mm induration from a purified protein derivative (PPD) Mantoux tuberculin skin test.

Adults < 35 years of age with a tuberculin skin test reaction of ≥ 15 mm – People < 35 years of age who a) have none of the above risk factors; b) belong to none of the high-incidence groups; and c) have a tuberculin skin test reaction of ≥ 15 mm are appropriate candidates for preventive therapy.

The risk of hepatitis must be weighed against the risk of tuberculosis in positive tuberculin reactors > 35 years of age. However, the use of isoniazid is recommended for those with the additional risk factors listed above and on an individual basis in situations where there is likelihood of serious consequences to contacts who may become infected.

Administration and Dosage

Do not administer with food.

IM administration is intended for use whenever oral administration is not possible.

➤*Treatment of tuberculosis:* Use in conjunction with other effective antituberculosis agents. If the bacilli become resistant, therapy must be changed to agents to which the bacilli are susceptible.

Usual parenteral dosage (depending on the regimen) –
   Adults: 5 mg/kg (≤ 300 mg daily) in a single dose, or 15 mg/kg (≤ 900 mg daily) 2 to 3 times weekly.
   Children: 10 to 15 mg/kg (≤ 300 mg daily) in a single dose, or 20 to 40 mg/kg (≤ 900 mg/day) 2 to 3 times weekly.

Patients with pulmonary tuberculosis without HIV infection – There are 3 regimen options for the initial treatment of tuberculosis in children and adults:

1.) Option 1: Daily isoniazid, rifampin, and pyrazinamide for 8 weeks followed by 16 weeks of isoniazid and rifampin daily or 2 to 3 times weekly. Add ethambutol or streptomycin to the initial regimen until sensitivity to isoniazid and rifampin is demonstrated. The addition of a fourth drug is optional if the relative prevalence of isoniazid-resistant *Mycobacterium tuberculosis* isolates in the community is ≤ 4%.
2.) Option 2: Daily isoniazid, rifampin, pyrazinamide, and streptomycin or ethambutol for 2 weeks followed by twice weekly administration of the same drugs for 6 weeks, subsequently twice weekly isoniazid and rifampin for 16 weeks.
3.) Option 3: 3 times weekly with isoniazid, rifampin, pyrazinamide, and ethambutol or streptomycin for 6 months.

A health care worker should directly observe all regimens given 2 or 3 times weekly at time of administration (directly observed therapy [DOT]).

The above treatment guidelines apply only when the disease is caused by organisms that are susceptible to the standard antituberculous agents. Because of the impact of resistance to isoniazid and rifampin on the response to therapy, it is essential that physicians initiating therapy for tuberculosis be familiar with the prevalence of drug resistance in their communities. It is suggested that ethambutol not be used in children whose visual acuity cannot be monitored.

Pulmonary tuberculosis and HIV infection – The response of the immunologically impaired host to treatment may not be as satisfactory as that of a person with normal host responsiveness. For this reason, therapeutic decisions for the impaired host must be individualized. Because patients co-infected with HIV may have problems with malabsorption, screening of antimycobacterial drug levels (especially in patients with advanced HIV disease) may be necessary to prevent the emergence of multi-drug resistant tuberculosis (MDRTB).

Extrapulmonary tuberculosis – The basic principles that underlie the treatment of pulmonary tuberculosis also apply to extrapulmonary forms of the disease. Although there have not been the same kinds of carefully conducted controlled trials of treatment of extrapulmonary tuberculosis as for pulmonary disease, increasing clinical experience indicates that 6- to 9-month short-course regimens are effective. Because of the insufficient data, miliary tuberculosis, bone/joint tuberculosis, and tuberculosis meningitis in infants and children should receive 12-month therapy.

Bacteriologic evaluation of extrapulmonary tuberculosis may be limited by the relative inaccessibility of the sites of disease. Thus, response to treatment often must be judged on the basis of clinical and radiographic findings.

The use of adjunctive therapies such as surgery and corticosteroids is more commonly required in extrapulmonary tuberculosis than in pulmonary disease. Surgery may be necessary to obtain specimens for diagnosis and to treat such processes as constrictive pericarditis and spinal cord compression from Pott's disease. Corticosteroids have been shown to be of benefit in preventing cardiac constriction from tuberculous pericarditis and in decreasing the neurologic sequelae of all stages of tuberculosis meningitis, especially when administered early in the course of the disease.

Pregnant women with tuberculosis – The options listed above must be adjusted for the pregnant patient. Streptomycin interferes with in utero development of the ear and may cause congenital deafness. Routine use of pyrazinamide is also not recommended in pregnancy because of inadequate teratogenicity data. The initial treatment regimen should consist of isoniazid and rifampin. Include ethambutol unless primary isoniazid resistance is unlikely (isoniazid resistance rate is documented to be < 4%).

MDRTB – MDRTB (ie, resistance to at least isoniazid and rifampin) presents difficult treatment problems. Treatment must be individualized and based on susceptibility studies. In such cases, consultation with an expert in tuberculosis is recommended.

➤*Preventive treatment:* Before isoniazid preventive therapy is initiated, bacteriologically positive or radiographically progressive tuberculosis must be excluded. Perform appropriate evaluations if extrapulmonary tuberculosis is suspected.

Adults (> 30 kg) – 300 mg/day in a single dose.

Infants and children – 10 mg/kg/day (≤ 300 mg total) in a single dose.

In situations where adherence with daily preventative therapy cannot be assured, administer 20 to 30 mg/kg (not to exceed 900 mg) twice weekly under the direct observation of a health care worker.

Continuous administration of isoniazid for a sufficient period is an essential part of the regimen, because relapse rates are higher if chemotherapy is stopped prematurely. In the treatment of tuberculosis, resistant organisms may multiply and the emergence of resistant organisms may necessitate a change in the regimen.

➤*Directly observed therapy (DOT):* A major cause of drug-resistant tuberculosis is patient non-compliance with treatment. The use of DOT can help assure patient compliance with drug therapy. DOT is the observation of the patient by a health care provider or other responsible person as the patient ingests antituberculosis medications. DOT can be achieved with daily, twice weekly, or 3 times weekly regimens, and is recommended for all patients.

For following patient compliance: the Potts-Cozart test, a simple colorimetric method of checking for isoniazid in the urine, is a useful tool for assuring patient compliance, which is essential for effective tuberculosis control. Additionally, isoniazid test strips are also available to check patient compliance.

➤*Pyridoxine (B₆):* Concomitant administration of 10 to 25 mg/day pyridoxine is recommended in the malnourished and in those predisposed to neuropathy (eg, alcoholics, diabetics). See Adverse Reactions.

Administer pyridoxine (vitamin B_6) 25 to 50 mg daily or 50 to 100 mg twice weekly to all HIV-infected patients who are undergoing tuberculosis treatment with isoniazid to reduce the occurrence of isoniazid-induced side effects in the central and peripheral nervous system.

Actions

➤*Pharmacology:* Isoniazid inhibits the synthesis of mycoloic acids, an essential component of the bacterial cell wall. At therapeutic levels, isoniazid is bactericidal against actively growing intracellular and extracellular *M. tuberculosis* organisms.

Pyridoxine (vitamin B_6) deficiency is sometimes observed in adults taking high doses of INH, and probably is due to the drug's competition with pyridoxal phosphate for the enzyme apotryptophanase.

➤*Pharmacokinetics:*

Absorption – Within 1 to 2 hours after oral administration, isoniazid produces peak blood levels that decline to ≤ 50% within 6 hours. However, the rate and extent of absorption is decreased by food.

Distribution – INH readily diffuses into all body fluids (including cerebrospinal, pleural, and ascitic), tissues, organs, and excreta (saliva, sputum, feces). It also passes through the placental barrier and into breast milk in concentrations comparable to those in plasma.

Metabolism – Isoniazid is metabolized primarily by acetylation and dehydrazination. The rate of acetylation is genetically determined. Approximately 50% of blacks and whites are "slow acetylators" and the rest are "rapid acetylators;" the majority of Alaskan natives and Asians are "rapid acetylators." The rate of acetylation does not significantly alter the effectiveness of INH. However, slow acetylation may lead to higher blood levels of the drug, and thus to an increase in toxic reactions.

ISONIAZID (Isonicotinic acid hydrazide; INH)

Excretion – Approximately 50% to 70% of a dose of isoniazid is excreted in the urine in 24 hours.

➤*Microbiology:* Two standardized in vitro susceptibility methods are available for testing isoniazid against *M. tuberculosis* organisms. The agar proportion method (CDC or NCCLS M24-P) uses middlebrook 7H10 medium impregnated with isoniazid at 2 final concentrations, 0.2 and 1 mcg/ml. MIC_{99} values are calculated by comparing the quantity of organisms growing in the medium containing drug to the control cultures. Mycobacterial growth in the presence of drug ≥ 1% of the control indicates resistance.

The radiometric broth method employs the BACTEC 460 machine to compare the growth index from untreated control cultures to cultures grown in the presence of 0.2 and 1 mcg/ml of isoniazid. Strict adherence to the manufacturer's instructions for sample processing and data interpretation is required for this assay.

M. tuberculosis isolates with an MIC_{99} ≤ 0.2 mcg/ml are considered to be susceptible to isoniazid. Susceptibility test results obtained by the 2 different methods discussed above cannot be compared unless equivalent drug concentrations are evaluated.

The clinical relevance of in vitro susceptibility for mycobacterium species other than *M. tuberculosis* using either the BACTEC or the proportion method has not been determined.

Contraindications

Severe hypersensitivity reactions, including drug-induced hepatitis; previous isoniazid-associated hepatic injury or other severe adverse reactions (eg, drug fever, chills, arthritis, acute liver disease of any etiology).

Warnings

➤*Hypersensitivity reactions:* Stop all drugs and evaluate at the first sign of a hypersensitivity reaction. If isoniazid must be reinstituted, give only after symptoms have cleared. Restart the drug in very small and gradually increasing doses and withdraw immediately if there is any indication of recurrent hypersensitivity reaction. Refer to Management of Acute Hypersensitivity Reactions.

➤*Renal/Hepatic function impairment:* Monitor patients with active chronic liver disease or severe renal dysfunction.

➤*Carcinogenesis:* Isoniazid induces pulmonary tumors in a number of strains of mice.

➤*Pregnancy: Category C.* Isoniazid exerts an embryocidal effect in both rats and rabbits when given orally during pregnancy. Isoniazid was not teratogenic in reproduction studies in mammalian species (mice, rats, and rabbits). There are no adequate and well-controlled studies in pregnant women. Use isoniazid as a treatment for active tuberculosis during pregnancy because the benefit justifies the potential risk to the fetus. Weigh the benefit of preventive therapy against a possible risk to the fetus. Start preventive treatment generally after delivery because of the increased risk of tuberculosis for new mothers.

Because isoniazid is known to cross the placental barrier, carefully observe neonates of isoniazid-treated mothers for any evidence of adverse effects.

Refer to the Antituberculosal Drugs Introduction for treatment regimens suggested during pregnancy.

➤*Lactation:* The small concentrations of isoniazid in breast milk do not produce toxicity in the nursing newborn; therefore, do not discourage breast feeding. However, because levels of isoniazid are so low in breast milk, they cannot be relied upon for prophylaxis or therapy in nursing infants.

Precautions

➤*Monitoring:* Carefully monitor isoniazid in the following:
1.) Daily users of alcohol. Daily ingestion of alcohol may be associated with a higher incidence of positive isoniazid hepatitis.
2.) Patients with active chronic liver disease or severe renal dysfunction.
3.) Patients > 35 years of age.
4.) Concurrent use of any chronically administered medication.
5.) History of previous discontinuation of isoniazid.
6.) Existence of peripheral neuropathy or conditions predisposing to neuropathy.
7.) Pregnancy.
8.) Injection drug use.
9.) Women belonging to minority groups, particularly in the postpartum period.
10.) HIV seropositive patients.

Laboratory tests – Because there is a higher frequency of isoniazid-associated hepatitis among certain patient groups (including age > 35, daily users of alcohol, chronic liver disease, injection drug use, and women belonging to minority groups, particularly in the postpartum period), obtain transaminase measurements prior to starting and monthly during preventative therapy, or more frequently as needed. If any of the values exceed 3 to 5 times the upper limit of normal, temporarily discontinue isoniazid and consider restarting therapy.

➤*Periodic ophthalmologic examinations:* During isoniazid therapy, periodic examinations are recommended when visual symptoms occur.

➤*Pyridoxine administration:* This is recommended in individuals likely to develop peripheral neuropathies secondary to INH therapy (see Adverse Reactions). Prophylactic doses of 10 to 25 mg of pyridoxine daily have been recommended.

Drug Interactions

Isoniazid Drug Interactions			
Precipitant drug	Object drug*		Description
Rifampin	Isoniazid	↑	Hepatotoxicity may occur at a rate higher than either agent alone. If alterations in liver function tests occur, consider discontinuation of one or both of these agents.
Isoniazid	Acetaminophen	↑	Hepatotoxicity has been reported due to inhibition of acetaminophen metabolism. Monitor patient for acetaminophen toxicity.
Isoniazid	Carbamazepine	↑	Isoniazid hepatotoxicity may result due to carbamazepine increasing isoniazid degradation to hepatotoxic metabolites. Carbamazepine toxicity may result due to inhibition of carbamazepine metabolism by isoniazid. Monitor serum carbamazepine concentrations, monitor liver function, and adjust doses as necessary.
Carbamazepine	Isoniazid	↑	
Isoniazid	Chlorzoxazone	↑	Plasma concentrations of chlorzoxazone may be elevated, increasing therapeutic and adverse effects. Adjust the dose of chlorzoxazone as appropriate.
Isoniazid	Disulfiram	↑	The coadministration of disulfiram and isoniazid may result in acute behavioral and coordination changes. The mechanism is unknown; possible excess dopaminergic activity may occur. If acute behavioral or coordination changes develop during concurrent administration of disulfiram and isoniazid, the disulfiram dose may need to be decreased or the drug discontinued.
Isoniazid	Enflurane	↑	In rapid isoniazid acetylators, high output renal failure may occur due to nephrotoxic concentrations of inorganic fluoride. Monitor renal function in patients receiving this combination, particularly those who are rapid acetylators.
Isoniazid	Hydantoins (eg, phenytoin)	↑	Serum hydantoin levels may be increased, producing an increase in the pharmacologic and toxic effects of hydantoins. In usual therapeutic doses, phenytoin toxicity appears to be most significant in patients who are slow acetylators of isoniazid. Monitor serum hydantoin levels and observe for toxicity.
Isoniazid	Ketoconazole	↓	The therapeutic benefit of ketoconazole may be attenuated. Avoid concomitant use if possible. Monitoring of ketoconazole serum levels or antifungal activity may be necessary.
Isoniazid	Theophylline	↑	Isoniazid may increase theophylline plasma levels. Also a slight decrease in isoniazid elimination has been noted. Monitor and adjust the dose as necessary.
Theophylline	Isoniazid	↑	

* ↑ = Object drug increased.   ↓ = Object drug decreased.

➤*Drug/Food interactions:* Because isoniazid has some monoamine oxidase inhibitor activity, an interaction may occur with tyramine-containing foods (see Monoamine Oxidase Inhibitors group monograph).

Adverse Reactions

The most frequent adverse reactions are those affecting the nervous system and the liver.

➤*CNS:* Peripheral neuropathy, the most common toxic effect, is dose-related, occurs most often in the malnourished and in those predisposed to neuritis (eg, alcoholics, diabetics), and is usually preceded by paresthesias of the feet and hands. The incidence is higher in "slow acetylators."

ISONIAZID (Isonicotinic acid hydrazide; INH)

Other neurotoxic effects uncommon with conventional doses: Convulsions; toxic encephalopathy; optic neuritis and atrophy; memory impairment; toxic psychosis.

➤*GI:* Nausea; vomiting; epigastric distress.

➤*Hepatic:* Elevated serum transaminase levels (AST, ALT); bilirubinemia; bilirubinuria; jaundice; occasionally, severe and sometimes fatal hepatitis. The common prodromal symptoms are anorexia, nausea, vomiting, fatigue, malaise, and weakness. Mild and transient elevation of serum transaminase levels occurs in 10% to 20% of patients taking isoniazid. This abnormality usually appears in the first 1 to 3 months of treatment, but can develop at any time during therapy. Enzyme levels return to normal in most instances, and there is no need to discontinue medication. Occasionally, progressive liver damage with accompanying symptoms may occur. In such cases, discontinue the drug immediately. If the AST value exceeds 3 to 5 times the upper limit of normal, strongly consider discontinuation of isoniazid. The frequency of progressive liver damage increases with age. It is rare in individuals < 20 years of age, but is seen in as many as 2.3% of those patients > 50 years of age.

➤*Hematologic:* Agranulocytosis; hemolytic, sideroblastic or aplastic anemia; thrombocytopenia; eosinophilia.

➤*Hypersensitivity:* Fever; skin eruptions (morbilliform, maculopapular, purpuric or exfoliative); lymphadenopathy; vasculitis. (See Warnings.)

➤*Metabolic/Nutritional:* Pyridoxine deficiency; pellagra; hyperglycemia; metabolic acidosis; gynecomastia.

➤*Miscellaneous:* Rheumatic syndrome and systemic lupus erythematosus-like syndrome. Local irritation has been observed at the site of IM injection.

Overdosage

➤*Symptoms:* Symptoms occur within 30 minutes to 3 hours. Nausea, vomiting, dizziness, slurred speech, blurred vision, and visual hallucinations (including bright colors and strange designs) are among the early manifestations. With marked overdosage, respiratory distress and CNS depression, progressing rapidly from stupor to profound coma, are to be expected along with severe, intractable seizures. Severe metabolic acidosis, acetonuria, and hyperglycemia are typical laboratory findings.

➤*Treatment:* Untreated or inadequately treated cases of gross isoniazid overdosage, 80 to 150 mg/kg, can cause neurotoxicity and be fatal, but good response has been reported in most patients brought under adequate treatment within the first few hours after drug ingestion.

Asymptomatic patient – Absorption of drug from the GI tract may be decreased by giving activated charcoal. Also employ gastric emptying in the asymptomatic patient. Safeguard the patient's airway when employing these procedures. Treat patients who acutely ingest > 80 mg/kg of isoniazid with IV pyridoxine on a gram per gram basis equal to the isoniazid dose. If an unknown amount of isoniazid is ingested, consider an initial dose of 5 g of pyridoxine given over 30 to 60 minutes in adults, or 80 mg/kg of pyridoxine in children.

Symptomatic patient – Ensure adequate ventilation, support cardiac output, and protect the airway while treating seizures and attempting to limit absorption. If the dose of isoniazid is known, treat the patient initially with a slow IV bolus of pyridoxine, over 3 to 5 minutes, on a gram per gram basis, equal to the isoniazid dose. If the quantity of isoniazid ingestion is unknown, then consider an initial IV bolus of pyridoxine of 5 g in the adult or 80 mg/kg in the child. If seizures continue, the dosage of pyridoxine may be repeated. It would be rare that > 10 g of pyridoxine would need to be given. The maximum safe dose of pyridoxine in isoniazid intoxication is not known. If the patient does not respond to pyridoxine, diazepam may be administered. Use phenytoin cautiously, because isoniazid interferes with the metabolism of phenytoin.

General – Obtain blood samples for immediate determination of gases, electrolytes, BUN, glucose, and other tests; type and crossmatch blood in preparation for possible hemodialysis.

Rapid control of metabolic acidosis – Patients with this degree of isoniazid intoxication are likely to have hypoventilation. The administration of sodium bicarbonate under these circumstances can cause exacerbation of hypercarbia. Ventilation must be monitored carefully by measuring blood carbon dioxide levels and supported mechanically if there is respiratory insufficiency.

Dialysis – Both peritoneal dialysis and hemodialysis have been used in the management of isoniazid overdosage. These procedures are probably not required if control of seizures and acidosis is achieved with pyridoxine, diazepam, and bicarbonate.

Patient Information

Take as directed. Do not discontinue except on the advice of a physician.

Avoid certain foods (eg, fish [skipjack, tuna], and perhaps tyramine-containing products) (see Monoamine Oxidase Inhibitor group monograph).

Notify physician of weakness, fatigue, loss of appetite, nausea and vomiting, yellowing of skin or eyes, darkening of urine, or numbness or tingling in hands and feet.

ISONIAZID COMBINATIONS

Rx	Rifater (Aventis)	Tablets: 120 mg rifampin, 50 mg isoniazid, 300 mg pyrazinamide	(Rifater). Sugar-coated. Light beige. In 60s.
Rx	Rifamate (Aventis)	Capsules: 300 mg rifampin and 150 mg isoniazid	(RIFAMATE). Red. In 60s.

Refer to the general discussion in the Antituberculosal Agents Introduction.

Indications

➤*ISONIAZID:* Bacteriocidal against *Mycobacterium tuberculosis.* See individual monograph.

➤*PYRAZINAMIDE:* Acts against *M. tuberculosis.* See individual monograph.

➤*RIFAMPIN:* Bactericidal against *M. tuberculosis.* See individual monograph.

RIFAMPIN

Rx	Rifampin (Various, eg, Eon)	Capsules: 150 mg	In 30s and 100s.
Rx	Rifadin (Aventis)		(Rifadin 150). Maroon and scarlet. In 30s.
Rx	Rifampin (Various, eg, Eon, UDL)	Capsules: 300 mg	In 30s, 60s, 100s, and 500s.
Rx	Rifadin (Aventis)		(Rifadin 300). Maroon and scarlet. In 30s, 60s, and 100s.
Rx	Rimactane (Novartis)		(Ciba 154). Scarlet and caramel. In 30s, 60s, and 100s.
Rx	Rifadin (Aventis)	Powder for Injection: 600 mg	In vials.

Refer to the general discussion in the Antituberculosal Agents Introduction.

Indications

Obtain bacteriologic cultures before starting therapy to confirm the susceptibility of the organism to rifampin; repeat cultures throughout therapy to monitor treatment response. Because rapid emergence of resistance can occur, perform culture and susceptibility tests in the event of persistent positive cultures during the course of treatment. If test results show resistance to rifampin and the patient is not responding to therapy, modify the drug regimen.

➤*Tuberculosis:*

Oral – Oral treatment is for all forms of tuberculosis. A 3-drug regimen consisting of rifampin, isoniazid, and pyrazinamide is recommended in the initial phase of short-course therapy that is usually continued for 2 months. The Advisory Council for the Elimination or Tuberculosis, the American Thoracic Society, and Centers for Disease Control and Prevention recommend that either streptomycin or ethambutol be added as a fourth drug in a regimen containing isoniazid (INH), rifampin, and pyrazinamide for initial treatment of tuberculosis unless the likelihood of INH resistance is very low. Reassess the need for a fourth drug when the results of susceptibility testing are known. If community rates of INH resistance are currently < 4%, an initial treatment regimen with < 4 drugs may be considered.

Following the initial phase, continue treatment with rifampin and isoniazid for ≥ 4 months. Continue treatment for longer if the patient is still sputum- or culture-positive, if resistant organisms are present, or if the patient is HIV positive.

IV – The IV form is for initial treatment and retreatment of tuberculosis when the drug cannot be taken by mouth.

➤*Neisseria meningitidis carriers:* For treatment of asymptomatic carriers of *N. meningitidis* to eliminate meningococci from the nasopharynx. Not indicated for the treatment of meningococcal infection.

To avoid indiscriminate use, perform diagnostic laboratory procedures, including serotyping and susceptibility testing. Reserve the drug for situations in which the risk of meningococcal meningitis is high.

➤*Unlabeled uses:* Rifampin has a broad antibacterial spectrum. Use in monotherapy is limited to *Haemophilus influenzae* type B. Rifampin, in combination with other effective agents, has been used in combina-

RIFAMPIN

tion for the following: To clear pharyngeal carriage of group A beta-hemolytic streptococcus; eradicate pharyngeal carriage of group b streptococci (GBS) in infants who have had recurrent GBS sepsis; treat manifestations of cat scratch disease caused by *Bartonella henselae*; treat resistant *Streptococcus pneumoniae meningitis*; treat severe staphylococcal bone and joint infections; treat prosthetic valve endocarditis due to coagulase-negative staphylococci; treat Aspergillus; treat Leprosy. Rifampin, in combination with other agents, has also shown activity against *S. pneumoniae, Staphylococcus aureus, Staphylococcus epidermidis, C. jeikeium, L. monocytogenes, N. gonorrhoeae, M. catarrhalis, F. tularensis, Brucella* sp, *N. meningitides,* and *Chlamydia trachomatis*. Rifampin has been used for prophylaxis in high-risk, close contacts of patients infected with *Neisseria meningitidis*. Dosage in adults is 600 mg every 12 hours for 2 days; dosage in children > 1 month is 10 mg/kg (maximum dose 600 mg) every 12 hours for 2 days; dosage in infants ≤ 1 month is 5 mg/kg every 12 hours for 2 days.

Administration and Dosage

Rifampin can be administered by the oral route or by IV infusion. IV doses are the same as oral.

➤*Oral:* Administer once daily, either 1 hour before or 2 hours after meals with a full glass of water.

Data is not available to determine dosage for children < 5 years of age (*Rimactane*).

For pediatric and adult patients in whom capsule swallowing is difficult or when lower doses are needed, a rifampin suspension can be prepared (see Preparation of extemporaneous oral suspension).

➤*Rifampin IV:* For IV infusion only. Must not be administered by IM or SC route. Avoid extravasation during injection; local irritation and inflammation because of extravascular infiltration of the infusion have been observed. If these occur, discontinue the infusion and restart at another site.

➤*Oral and IV:*

Tuberculosis –

Adults: 10 mg/kg in a single daily administration not to exceed 600 mg once daily.

Children: 10 to 20 mg/kg, not to exceed 600 mg/day.

Use with at least one other antituberculous agent. In general, continue therapy until bacterial conversion and maximal improvement have occurred. This information is best explained by the regimens that follow.

➤*The 2-month regimen:* According to the MMWR, the 2-month daily regimen of rifampin and pyrazinamide is recommended on the basis of a prospective randomized trial of treatment of latent tuberculosis infection (LTBI) in HIV-infected people that demonstrated the 2-month regimen to be similar in safety and efficacy to a 12-month regimen of isoniazid. Although this regimen has not been evaluated in HIV-uninfected people with LTBI, the efficacy is not expected to differ significantly. However, the drug toxicities may be increased. Two randomized prospective trials of intermittent dosing of rifampin and pyrazinamide for 2 and 3 months respectively, have been reported in HIV-infected people; in neither case was the sample size adequate to conclude with certainty that efficacy was equivalent to daily dosing.

➤*The 4-month regimen:* According to the MMWR, rifampin given daily for 3 months has resulted in better protection than placebo in treatment of LTBI in non-HIV patients with silicosis in a randomized prospective trial. However, because the patients receiving rifampin had a high rate of active tuberculosis (4%), experts have concluded that a 4-month regimen would be more prudent when using rifampin alone. This option may be useful for patients who cannot tolerate isoniazid or pyrazinamide.

➤*The 6-month regimen:* Ordinarily this consists of an initial 2-month phase of rifampin, isoniazid, and pyrazinamide and, if clinically indicated, streptomycin or ethambutol, followed by 4 months of rifampin and isoniazid. Reassess the need for a fourth drug when the results of susceptibility testing are known. If community rates of INH resistance are currently < 4%, an initial treatment regimen with < 4 drugs may be considered. Continue treatment for > 6 months if the patient is still sputum- or culture-positive, if resistant organisms are present, or if the patient is HIV positive.

➤*Meningococcal carriers:* Once daily for 4 consecutive days in the following doses:

Adults – 600 mg (two 300 mg capsules) in a single daily administration.

Children – 10 to 20 mg/kg, not to exceed 600 mg/day.

The following dosage has also been recommended:

Adults – 600 mg every 12 hours for 2 days.

Children (≥ 1 month of age) – 10 mg/kg (not to exceed 600 mg/dose) every 12 hours for 2 days.

Children (< 1 month of age) – 5 mg/kg every 12 hours for 2 days.

➤*Preparation/Stability of solution for IV infusion:* Reconstitute the lyophilized powder by transferring 10 ml of Sterile Water for Injection to a vial containing 600 mg of rifampin for injection. Swirl vial gently to completely dissolve the antibiotic. The resultant solution contains rifampin 60 mg/ml and is stable at room temperature for 24 hours. Withdraw a volume equivalent to the amount of rifampin calculated to be administered and add to 500 ml of infusion medium. Mix well and infuse at a rate allowing for complete infusion in 3 hours. In some cases, the amount of rifampin calculated to be administered may be added to 100 ml of infusion medium and infused in 30 minutes. Dilutions in Dextrose 5% for Injection are stable at room temperature for up to 4 hours and should be prepared and used within this time. Precipitation of rifampin from the infusion solution may occur beyond this time. Dilutions in normal saline are stable at room temperature for up to 24 hours and should be prepared and used within this time. Other infusion solutions are not recommended.

➤*Incompatibilities:* Physical incompatibility (precipitate) was observed with undiluted (5 mg/ml) and diluted (1 mg/ml in normal saline) diltiazem HCl and rifampin (6 mg/ml in normal saline) during simulated Y-site administration.

➤*Preparation of extemporaneous oral suspension:* Preparation of suspension (to contain rifampin 10 mg/ml) – 1) Empty the contents of 4 rifampin 300 mg (or 8 rifampin 150 mg) capsules into a 4 oz amber glass bottle. 2) Add 20 ml of simple syrup (*Syrup NF*, Humco Laboratories), *Syrpalta syrup* (Emerson Laboratories), or *Raspberry syrup* (Humco Laboratories). Shake vigorously. 3) Add 100 ml of simple syrup. Shake again.

➤*Storage/Stability:* The extemporaneously prepared oral suspension is stable for 4 weeks when stored at room temperature or in a refrigerator (2° to 8°C; 36° to 46°F).

Actions

➤*Pharmacology:* Rifampin inhibits DNA-dependent RNA polymerase activity in susceptible cells. Specifically, it interacts with bacterial RNA polymerase but does not inhibit the mammalian enzyme. Cross-resistance has only been shown with other rifamycins. Rifampin at therapeutic levels has demonstrated bactericidal activity against intracellular and extracellular *Mycobacterium tuberculosis* organisms.

➤*Pharmacokinetics:*

Absorption/Distribution – Rifampin, 600 mg administered orally, is almost completely absorbed and achieves mean peak plasma levels within 1 to 4 hours. The peak level averages at 7 mcg/ml but may vary from 4 to 32 mcg/ml. In children, mean peak serum levels range from 3.5 to 15 mcg/ml. Absorption of rifampin is reduced by ≈ 30% when the drug is ingested with food.

Metabolism – Rifampin is metabolized in the liver by deacetylation; the metabolite is still active against *M. tuberculosis*. It undergoes enterohepatic circulation; however, the deacetylated metabolite is poorly absorbed. The half-life is ≈ 3 hours after a 600 mg oral dose, up to 5.1 hours after a 900 mg oral dose. With repeated administration, the half-life decreases and averages ≈ 2 to 3 hours.

Excretion – Elimination occurs mainly through the bile and, to a much lesser extent, the urine. Dosage adjustment is not necessary in renal failure, but is with hepatic dysfunction. Rifampin is not significantly removed by hemodialysis.

IV – Following administration of a 300 or 600 mg IV dose in 12 volunteers, mean peak plasma concentrations were 9 and 17 mcg/ml, respectively. The average plasma concentrations remained detectable for 8 and 12 hours, respectively. The elimination of the larger dose was not as rapid. Volumes of distribution at steady state were ≈ 0.66 and ≈ 0.64 L/kg for the 300 and 600 mg IV doses, respectively. After repeated once daily infusions of 600 mg in 5 patients for 7 days, concentrations decreased from 5.8 mcg/ml 8 hours after the infusion on day 1 to 2.6 mcg/ml 8 hours after the infusion on day 7.

Special populations –

Children:

• *Oral –* In 1 study, pediatric patients 6 to 58 months of age were given rifampin suspended in simple syrup or as dry powder mixed with applesauce at a dose of 10 mg/kg body weight. Peak serum concentrations of ≈ 10.7 and ≈ 11.5 mcg/ml were obtained 1 hour after preprandial ingestion of the drug suspension and the applesauce mixture, respectively. After the administration of either preparation, the half-life of rifampin averaged 2.9 hours. It should be noted that in other studies in pediatric populations, at doses of 10 mg/kg body weight, mean peak serum concentrations of 3.5 to 15 mcg/ml have been reported.

• *IV –* In children 0.25 to 12.8 years of age (n = 12), the mean peak serum concentration was 26 mcg/ml following a 300 mg/m² infusion, 11.7 to 41.5 mcg/ml 1 to 4 days after initiation of therapy, and 13.6 to 37.4 mcg/ml 5 to 14 days after initiation of therapy. The half-life was 1.17 to 3.19 hours.

➤*Microbiology:* Rifampin has bactericidal activity against slow and intermittently growing *M. tuberculosis* organisms. It also has significant activity against *N. meningitidis* isolates (see Indications). In the treatment of tuberculosis and the meningococcal carrier state, the small number of resistant cells present within large populations of susceptible cells can rapidly become predominant. In addition, resistance to rifampin has been determined to occur as single-step mutations of the DNA-dependent RNA polymerase. Since resistance can emerge rapidly, perform appropriate susceptibility tests in the event of persistent positive cultures. Rifampin has been shown to be active against most

RIFAMPIN

strains of the following microorganisms, both in vitro and in clinical infections as described in Indications: *N. meningitidis* and *M. tuberculosis*.

Rifampin has initial in vitro activity against the following microorganisms; however, clinical efficacy has not been established: *M. leprae*; *Haemophilus influenzae*; *S. aureus* (including methacillin resistant *S. aureus*); *S. epidermidis*.

Contraindications

Hypersensitivity to any rifamycin.

Warnings

➤*Hepatotoxicity:* There have been fatalities associated with jaundice in patients with liver disease or patients receiving rifampin concomitantly with other hepatotoxic agents. Since an increased risk may exist for individuals with liver disease, weigh benefits against risk of further liver damage. Carefully monitor liver function, especially AST and ALT, prior to therapy and then every 2 to 4 weeks during therapy. Withdraw rifampin if signs of hepatocellular damage occur.

➤*Hyperbilirubinemia:* This results from competition between rifampin and bilirubin for excretory pathways of the liver at the cell level can occur in the early days of treatment. An isolated report showing a moderate rise in bilirubin or transaminase level is not in itself an indication to interrupt treatment. Make the decision based on repeat tests and the patient's clinical condition.

➤*Porphyria:* Isolated reports have associated porphyria exacerbation with rifampin administration.

➤*Meningococci resistance:* The possibility of rapid emergence of resistant meningococci restricts use to short-term treatment of asymptomatic carrier state. Rifampin is not to be used for treatment of meningococcal disease.

➤*Hypersensitivity reactions:* These reactions have occurred during intermittent therapy or when treatment was resumed following accidental or intentional interruption and were reversible with rifampin discontinuation and appropriate therapy. Refer to Management of Acute Hypersensitivity Reactions (see Adverse Reactions).

➤*Carcinogenesis:* A few cases of accelerated growth of lung carcinoma have occurred in humans, but a causal relationship has not been established. An increase in the incidence of hepatomas in female mice (of a strain known to be particularly susceptible to the spontaneous development of hepatomas) was observed when rifampin was administered in doses of 2 to 10 times the average daily human dose for 60 weeks. Rifampin possesses immunosuppressive potential in animals and humans. Antitumor activity in vitro has also occurred.

➤*Pregnancy:* Category C. The effect of rifampin (alone or in combination with other antituberculous drugs) on the human fetus is not known. Rifampin crosses the placental barrier and appears in cord blood. It is teratogenic in rodents given oral doses of 15 to 25 times the human dose. An increase in congenital malformations, primarily spina bifida and cleft palate, has occurred in the offspring of rodents given oral doses of 150 to 250 mg/kg/day. Imperfect osteogenesis and embryotoxicity occurred in rabbits given doses up to 20 times the usual human daily dose. When administered during the last few weeks of pregnancy, rifampin can cause postnatal hemorrhages in the mother and infant for which treatment with vitamin K may be indicated. Carefully weigh possible teratogenic potential in women capable of bearing children against benefits of therapy (also see Antituberculosal Drugs introduction).

Carefully observe neonates of rifampin-treated mothers for any adverse effects.

➤*Lactation:* Rifampin is excreted in breast milk. Decide whether to discontinue nursing or discontinue the drug, taking into account the importance of the drug to the mother.

➤*Children:* Safety and efficacy in pediatric patients have not been established.

Precautions

➤*Monitoring:* Perform baseline measurements of hepatic enzymes, bilirubin, serum creatinine, a complete blood count, and a platelet count (or estimate) in adults treated for tuberculosis with rifampin. Baseline tests are unnecessary in pediatric patients unless a complicating condition is known or clinically suspected.

➤*Intermittent therapy:* May be used if the patient cannot or will not self-administer drugs on a daily basis. Closely monitor patients on intermittent therapy for compliance, and caution against intentional or accidental interruption of prescribed therapy because of increased risk of serious adverse reactions.

➤*Red discoloration of body fluids:* Urine, sputum, sweat, and tears may be red-orange colored. Soft contact lenses may be permanently stained. Advise patients of these possibilities.

➤*Thrombocytopenia:* This reaction has occurred, primarily with high dose intermittent therapy, but has also been noted after resumption of interrupted treatment. It rarely occurs during well-supervised daily therapy. This effect is reversible if the drug is discontinued as soon as purpura occurs. Cerebral hemorrhage and fatalities have occurred when rifampin administration has continued or resumed after appearance of purpura.

Drug Interactions

➤*Cytochrome P450:* Rifampin is known to induce certain cytochrome P450 enzymes. Administration of rifampin with drugs that undergo biotransformation through these metabolic pathways may accelerate elimination of coadministered drugs. To maintain optimum therapeutic blood levels, dosages of drugs metabolized by these enzymes may require adjustment when starting or stopping concomitantly administered rifampin.

Rifampin Drug Interactions			
Precipitant drug	Object drug*		Description
Aminosalicylic acid, oral	Rifampin	↓	Aminosalicylic acid decreases the effect of rifampin. Give the combination of these 2 agents at an interval of 8 to 12 hours apart.
Halothane	Rifampin	↑	Hepatotoxicity and hepatic encephalopathy have been reported.
Rifampin	Antiarrhythmics (eg, amiodarone, disopyramide, mexiletine, propafenone, quinidine, tocainide)	↓	Serum concentrations of antiarrhythmics may be decreased because of CYP3A4 induction by rifampin. Closely monitor serum concentrations when starting or stopping rifampin.
Rifampin	ACE inhibitors (eg, enalapril)	↓	The pharmacologic effects of enalapril may be decreased, resulting in a decrease in antihypertensive control. The mechanism by which this occurs is unknown. Monitor the patient's blood pressure; consider an alternative antihypertensive if blood pressure remains uncontrolled.
Rifampin	Anticoagulants	↓	Rifampin decreases the anticoagulation activity of warfarin because of increased hepatic microsomal enzyme metabolism. Increased dosage of anticoagulants may be needed. Monitor coagulation parameters closely when rifampin is discontinued.
Rifampin	Azole antifungals (eg, fluconazole, itraconazole, ketoconazole)	↓	Rifampin may induce the metabolism of azole antifungal agents. Ketoconazole may interfere with rifampin absorption decreasing serum rifampin levels. If concurrent use cannot be avoided, monitor and adjust the dosages as needed.
Azole antifungals (eg, fluconazole, itraconazole, ketoconazole)	Rifampin	↓	
Rifampin	Barbiturates	↓	Rifampin may stimulate liver microsomal enzymes resulting in more rapid degradation of barbiturates. When rifampin is added to the regimen of a patient receiving a barbiturate, monitor the patient for changes in clinical status and plasma barbiturate levels. The barbiturate dosage may need to be raised.
Rifampin	Benzodiazepines (eg, diazepam, midazolam, triazolam)	↓	The pharmacologic effects of diazepam, midazolam, and triazolam may be decreased because of increased metabolism of benzodiazepines. Monitor the clinical response to the benzodiazepine when starting or stopping rifampin.
Rifampin	Beta blockers (eg, bisoprolol, metoprolol, propranolol)	↓	The pharmacologic effects of certain beta blockers (eg, bisoprolol, metoprolol, propranolol) may be reduced possibly because of increased hepatic metabolism from enzyme induction by rifampin. A 3- to 4-week washout period may be necessary for the enzyme induction effect to diminish. Close monitoring of therapeutic response is essential.
Rifampin	Buspirone	↓	Buspirone plasma concentrations and pharmacologic effects may be decreased because of induction of first-pass metabolism (CYP3A4) by rifampin. Escalation of buspirone dose may be necessary.

RIFAMPIN

Rifampin Drug Interactions			
Precipitant drug	Object drug*		Description
Rifampin	Chloramphenicol	↓	Chloramphenicol metabolism may be increased because of induction of hepatic microsomal enzymes by rifampin.
Rifampin	Contraceptives, oral	↓	Reduced oral contraceptive efficacy and an increased incidence of menstrual abnormalities may occur. Advise patients to use an additional form of birth control while receiving rifampin therapy.
Rifampin	Corticosteroids	↓	The pharmacologic effects of corticosteroids may be decreased. Lack of effect may occur within a few days of adding rifampin and reverse 2 to 3 weeks following discontinuation. Avoid coadministration.
Rifampin	Cyclosporine	↓	The immunosuppressive effects of cyclosporine may be reduced 2 days following the initiation of rifampin and persist for 1 to 3 weeks after discontinuation. Cyclosporine bioavailability is decreased because of induction of intestinal cytochrome P450 enzymes. Increased doses may be necessary; avoid this combination if possible.
Rifampin	Delavirdine	↓	Rifampin may increase the metabolism of delavirdine by enzyme induction thereby decreasing the plasma concentrations. Avoid concurrent use.
Rifampin	Digoxin	↓	Rifampin coadministration may decrease the serum concentration of digoxin. An increased digoxin dosage may be necessary.
Rifampin	Doxycycline	↓	Rifampin may decrease the serum concentration and half-life of doxycycline, possibly reducing the therapeutic effect. Monitor the clinical response.
Rifampin	Estrogens	↓	Rifampin may impair the effectiveness of estrogens by inducing drug metabolism, decreasing AUC, and half-life. Consider alternate methods of contraception.
Rifampin	Fluoroquinolones	↓	Rifampin may accelerate the metabolism of fluoroquinolones. It may be necessary to adjust the dosage of a fluoroquinolone.
Rifampin	Haloperidol	↓	Rifampin may decrease the plasma concentration and clinical effectiveness of halperidol. When adding or discontinuing rifamycin therapy, carefully monitor the clinical response of the patient. Adjust the haloperidol dose as indicated.
Rifampin	Hydantoins	↓	Serum hydantoin levels may be decreased because of rifampin increasing hepatic enzyme metabolism. Monitor serum hydantoin levels and observe the patient.
Rifampin	Isoniazid	↑	Hepatotoxicity may occur at a rate higher than with either agent alone. If alterations in liver function tests occur, consider discontinuation of one or both agents.
Isoniazid	Rifampin	↑	
Rifampin	Losartan	↓	Rifampin may increase the metabolism of losartan. Observe the clinical response of the patient when starting or stopping rifampin.
Rifamycins	Macrolide antibiotics (eg, clarithromycin)	↓	The metabolism of rifampin may be inhibited, while the metabolism of the macrolide antibiotic may be increased. Monitor for increased side effects and a decrease in the response to the macrolide antibiotic.
Macrolide antibiotics (eg, clarithromycin)	Rifamycins	↑	
Rifampin	Narcotic analgesics (eg, methadone, morphine)	↓	Patients may experience withdrawal symptoms. Rifampin primarily appears to stimulate the hepatic metabolism of methadone. A higher dose of narcotic analgesics may be required during concurrent administration of rifampin.
Rifampin	Nifedipine	↓	The therapeutic effects of nifedipine may be reduced. Monitor blood pressure and angina symptoms. Adjust the nifedipine dose accordingly or consider a different antihypertensive medication.
Rifampin	Ondansetron	↓	Plasma concentrations of ondansetron may be reduced. Consider use of an alternative antiemetic.
Rifampin	Progestins	↓	Rifampin may increase the elimination rate of progestin-containing oral contraceptives. Avoid coadministration.
Rifampin	Protease inhibitors (eg, indinavir, nelfinavir, ritonavir)	↓	Rifampin may increase the metabolism of protease inhibitors while protease inhibitors may decrease rifampin metabolism. Avoid concomitant use.
Protease inhibitors (eg, indinavir, nelfinavir, ritonavir)	Rifampin	↑	
Rifampin	Quinine derivatives	↓	Rifampin increases the hepatic clearance of quinine derivatives. Enzyme induction can persist for several days following discontinuation of rifampin. Addition of rifampin to stable quinine derivative regimens may require increased doses of quinine derivatives to maintain the desired therapeutic effect. Withdrawal of rifampin may result in quinine derivative dose-related toxicity. Monitor quinine derivative serum levels and the ECG.
Rifampin	Sulfapyridine	↓	Plasma concentrations of sulfapyridine may be reduced following the concomitant administration of sulfasalazine and rifampin. This finding may be the result of alteration in the colonic bacteria responsible for the reduction of sulfasalazine to sulfapyridine and mesalamine.
Rifampin	Sulfones	↓	The pharmacologic effect of dapsone may be decreased because of increased metabolism of dapsone. Higher doses of dapsone may be necessary.
Rifampin	Sulfonylureas	↓	Rifampin may decrease the half-life and serum levels while increasing the clearance of tolbutamide and chlorpropamide, possibly resulting in hyperglycemia. Closely monitor blood glucose and possibly increase the sulfonylurea dose.
Rifampin	Tacrolimus	↓	The immunosuppressive effects of tacrolimus may be reduced as early as 2 days following the initiation of rifampin. Closely monitor tacrolimus whole blood concentrations when starting or stopping rifampin.
Rifampin	Theophylline	↓	The addition of rifampin may result in decreased theophylline levels and exacerbation of pulmonary symptoms. Monitor thophylline levels.
Rifampin	Thyroid hormones	↓	Thyroid stimulating hormone (TSH) levels may be increased, resulting in hypothyroidism. Monitor thyroid status in patients receiving both drugs.
Rifampin	Tricyclic antidepressants (TCAs)	↓	TCA levels may decrease because of increased hepatic metabolism of TCAs. Consider monitoring TCA concentrations when starting, stopping, or altering the rifampin dose.
Rifampin	Verapamil	↓	There is an increase in first-pass hepatic metabolism resulting in a lowered bioavailability of oral verapamil. Use IV verapamil or substitute another agent for either verapamil or rifampin.
Rifampin	Zidovudine	↓	The pharmacologic effects of zidovudine may be decreased possibly because of increased hepatic metabolism.
Rifampin	Zolpidem	↓	Plasma concentrations and therapeutic effects of zolpidem may be reduced. Monitor the clinical response of the patient.

* ↓ = Object drug decreased.   ↑ = Object drug increased.

RIFAMPIN

➤*Enzyme induction properties:* Rifampin has enzyme induction properties that can enhance the metabolism of endogenous substrates including adrenal hormones, thyroid hormones, and vitamin D. Rifampin and isoniazid have been reported to alter vitamin D metabolism. In some cases, reduced levels of circulating 25-hydroxy vitamin D and 1,25-dihydroxy vitamin D have been accompanied by reduced serum calcium and phosphate, and elevated parathyroid hormone.

➤*Drug/Lab test interactions:* Therapeutic levels of rifampin inhibit standard assays for serum folate and vitamin B_{12}. Consider alternative methods when determining folate and vitamin B_{12} concentrations in the presence of rifampin.

Hepatitis or shock-like syndrome with hepatic involvement and abnormal liver function tests have been reported.

Transient abnormalities in liver function tests (eg, elevation in serum bilirubin, alkaline phosphatase, and serum transaminases), and reduced biliary excretion of contrast media used for visualization of the gallbladder have also been observed. Therefore, perform these tests before the morning dose of rifampin.

➤*Drug/Food interactions:* Food interferes with the absorption of rifampin, possibly resulting in increased peak plasma concentrations. Take on an empty stomach, either 1 hour before or 2 hours after a meal, with a full glass of water.

Adverse Reactions

High doses of rifampin (> 600 mg) given once or twice weekly have resulted in a high incidence of adverse reactions including: The "flu-like" syndrome (eg, fever, chills, malaise); hematopoietic reactions (eg, leukopenia, thrombocytopenia, acute hemolytic anemia); cutaneous, GI and hepatic reactions; shortness of breath; shock; renal failure. Recent studies indicate that regimens using twice-weekly doses of rifampin 600 mg plus isoniazid 15 mg/kg are much better tolerated.

➤*CNS:* Headache; ataxia; drowsiness; fatigue; dizziness; inability to concentrate; mental confusion; psychoses; generalized numbness; behavioral changes (rare).

➤*Dermatologic:* Rash; flushing; itching (with or without rash).

➤*GI:* Heartburn; epigastric distress; anorexia; nausea; vomiting; gas; cramps; diarrhea; jaundice; pseudomembranous colitis.

➤*Hematologic:* Transient leukopenia; hemolytic anemia; decreased hemoglobin; hemolysis; disseminated intravascular coagulation; thrombocytopenia (see Precautions).

➤*Hepatic:* Hepatitis or shock-like syndrome with hepatic involvement (rare); abnormal liver function tests; transient abnormalities in liver function tests (elevations in serum bilirubin, BSP, alkaline phosphatase, serum transaminases). Perform BSP test prior to the morning dose of rifampin to avoid false-positive results.

➤*Hypersensitivity:* Pruritus; urticaria; pemphigoid reaction; erythema multiforme including Stevens-Johnson syndrome; toxic epidermal necrolysis; vasculitis; eosinophilia; sore mouth; sore tongue; conjunctivitis. Rarely hemolysis, hemoglobinuria, hematuria, renal insufficiency, or acute renal failure have occurred.

➤*Musculoskeletal:* Ataxia; muscular weakness; pain in extremities; myopathy.

➤*Renal:* Interstitial nephritis; acute tubular necrosis.

➤*Miscellaneous:* Visual disturbances; menstrual disturbances; fever; elevations in BUN and serum uric acid; adrenal insufficiency in patients with compromised adrenal function; edema of face and extremities; shortness of breath; wheezing; decrease in blood pressure; shock; flu syndrome (eg, fever, chills, headache, dizziness, bone pain).

Overdosage

➤*Symptoms:* The minimum acute lethal or toxic dose is not well established. However, nonfatal acute overdoses in adults have been reported with doses ranging from 9 to 12 g rifampin. Fatal acute overdoses in adults have been reported with doses ranging from 14 to 60 g. Alcohol or a history of alcohol abuse was involved in some of the fatal and nonfatal reports. Nonfatal overdoses in pediatric patients ages 1 to 4 years of age or 100 mg/kg for 1 to 2 doses has been reported.

Nausea, vomiting, abdominal pain, pruritus, headache, and increasing lethargy will probably occur shortly after ingestion; unconsciousness may occur with severe hepatic disease. Transient increases in liver enzymes or bilirubin may occur. Brownish-red or orange discoloration of skin, urine, sweat, saliva, tears, and feces is proportional to amount ingested. Facial or periorbital edema has also been reported in pediatric patients. Hypotension, sinus tachycardia, ventricular arrhythmias, seizures, and cardiac arrest were reported in some fatal cases. Liver enlargement, possibly with tenderness, can develop within a few hours after severe overdosage, and jaundice may develop rapidly. Hepatic involvement may be more marked in patients with prior impairment of hepatic function. Other physical findings remain essentially normal.

Direct and total bilirubin levels may increase rapidly with severe overdosage; hepatic enzyme levels may be affected, especially with prior impairment of hepatic function. A direct effect on the hematopoietic system, electrolyte levels, or acid-base balance is unlikely.

➤*Treatment:* Nausea and vomiting are likely to be present. Gastric lavage is probably preferable to inducing emesis. Instill activated charcoal slurry into stomach after evacuation of gastric contents to help absorb any remaining drug in GI tract. Antiemetic medication may be required to control severe nausea or vomiting.

Forced diuresis (with measured intake and output) will promote excretion of the drug. Hemodialysis may be of value in some patients. Bile drainage may be indicated in the presence of serious impairment of hepatic function lasting > 24 to 48 hours; extracorporeal hemodialysis may be required. In patients with previously adequate hepatic function, reversal of liver enlargement, and impaired hepatic excretory function probably will be noted within 72 hours, with rapid return toward normal thereafter.

Patient Information

Take on an empty stomach, ≥ 1 hour before or 2 hours after meals, with a full glass of water.

Take medication on a regular basis; avoid missing doses. Do not discontinue therapy except on advice of physician.

Advise patient that the reliability of oral or other systemic hormonal contraceptive may be affected; give consideration to using alternative contraceptive measures.

Medication may cause a reddish-orange discoloration of urine, stools, saliva, tears, sweat, and sputum. This is to be expected and is not harmful. It may also permanently discolor soft contact lenses.

Notify physician if fever, loss of appetite, malaise, nausea, vomiting, darkened urine, or yellowish discoloration of skin or eyes occurs.

RIFABUTIN

| Rx | Mycobutin (Pharmacia & Upjohn) | Capsules: 150 mg | (MYCOBUTIN/PHARMACIA & UPJOHN). Opaque red/brown. In 100s. |

Refer to the general discussion in the Antituberculosal Agents Introduction.

Indications

➤*Mycobacterium avium complex (MAC):* Prevention of disseminated MAC disease in patients with advanced HIV infection.

Administration and Dosage

➤*Approved by the FDA:* December 23, 1992.

➤*Usual dose:* 300 mg once daily. For those patients with a propensity to nausea, vomiting, or other GI upset, administration of rifabutin at doses of 150 mg twice daily taken with food may be useful.

Actions

➤*Pharmacology:* Rifabutin, an antimycobacterial agent, is a semisynthetic ansamycin antibiotic derived from rifamycin S. Rifabutin inhibits DNA-dependent RNA polymerase in susceptible strains of *Escherichia coli* and *Bacillus subtilis* but not in mammalian cells. In resistant strains of *E. coli*, rifabutin, like rifampin, does not inhibit this enzyme. It is not known whether rifabutin inhibits DNA-dependent RNA polymerase in *Mycobacterium avium* or in *M. intracellulare*, which comprise MAC.

➤*Pharmacokinetics:* Following a single oral dose of 300 mg to healthy adult volunteers, rifabutin was readily absorbed from the GI tract with mean peak plasma levels (C_{max}) of 375 ng/ml (range, 141 to 1033 ng/ml) attained in 3.3 hours (T_{max} range, 2 to 4 hours). Plasma concentrations post-C_{max} declined in an apparent biphasic manner.

Kinetic dose-proportionality has been established over the 300 to 600 mg dose range in healthy adult volunteers and in early symptomatic human immunodeficiency virus (HIV)-positive patients over a 300 to 900 mg dose range. Rifabutin was slowly eliminated from plasma in healthy adult volunteers, presumably because of distribution-limited elimination, with a mean terminal half-life of 45 hours (range, 16 to 69 hours). Although the systemic levels of rifabutin following multiple dosing decreased by 38%, its terminal half-life remained unchanged. Rifabutin, because of its high lipophilicity, demonstrates a high propensity for distribution and intracellular tissue uptake. Estimates of apparent steady-state distribution volume (9.3 L/kg) in HIV-positive patients, following IV dosing, exceed total body water by ≈ 15-fold. Substantially higher intracellular tissue levels than those seen in plasma have been observed. The lung to plasma concentration ratio, obtained at 12 hours, was ≈ 6.5 in 4 surgical patients. Mean rifabutin steady-state trough levels (24 hours post-dose) ranged from 50 to 65 ng/ml in HIV-positive patients and in healthy adult volunteers. About 85% of the drug is bound in a concentration-independent manner to plasma proteins over a concentration range of 0.05 to 1 mcg/ml.

Mean systemic clearance in healthy adult volunteers following a single oral dose was 0.69 L/hr/kg (range, 0.46 to 1.34 L/hr/kg); renal and biliary clearance of unchanged drug each contribute ≈ 5%. About 30% of the dose is excreted in the feces; 53% of the oral dose is excreted in the urine, primarily as metabolites. Of the 5 metabolites that have been identified, 25-O-desacetyl and 31-hydroxy are the most predominant, and show a plasma metabolite:parent area under the curve ratio of

RIFABUTIN

0.1:0.07, respectively. The 25-O-desacetyl metabolite has an activity equal to the parent drug and contributes ≤ 10% to the total antimicrobial activity.

Absolute bioavailability assessed in HIV-positive patients averaged 20%. At least 53% of the orally administered dose is absorbed from the GI tract. The bioavailability from the capsule dosage form, relative to a solution, was 85% in healthy adult volunteers. High-fat meals slow the rate without influencing the extent of absorption. The overall pharmacokinetics are modified only slightly by alterations in hepatic function or age. Compared with healthy volunteers, steady-state kinetics are more variable in elderly patients (> 70 years of age) and in symptomatic HIV-positive patients. Somewhat reduced drug distribution and faster drug elimination in compromised renal function may result in decreased drug concentrations.

➤*Microbiology:* Rifabutin has demonstrated in vitro activity against MAC organisms isolated from both HIV-positive and HIV-negative people. The vast majority of isolates from MAC-infected, HIV-positive people are *M. avium*, whereas from HIV-negative people, ≈ 40% of the MAC isolates are *M. intracellulare*. Rifabutin has in vitro activity against many strains of *M. tuberculosis*.

Cross-resistance between rifampin and rifabutin is commonly observed with *M. tuberculosis* and *M. avium* complex isolates. Isolates of *M. tuberculosis* resistant to rifampin are likely to be resistant to rifabutin.

Susceptibility of MAC Strains to Rifampin and Rifabutin					
Susceptibility to rifampin (mcg/ml)	Number of strains	% of strains susceptible/resistant to different concentrations of rifabutin (mcg/ml)			
		Susceptible to 0.5	Resistant to 0.5 only	Resistant to 1	Resistant to 2
Susceptible to 1	30	100	0	0	0
Resistant to 1 only	163	88.3	11.7	0	0
Resistant to 5	105	38	57.1	2.9	2
Resistant to 10	225	20	50.2	19.6	10.2
Total	523	49.5	36.7	9	4.8

Contraindications

Hypersensitivity to this drug or to any other rifamycins.

Warnings

➤*Active tuberculosis:* Do not administer rifabutin prophylaxis to patients with active tuberculosis. Tuberculosis in HIV-positive patients is common and may present with atypical or extrapulmonary findings. Patients are likely to have a nonreactive purified protein derivative (PPD) despite active disease. In addition to chest X-ray and sputum culture, the following studies may be useful in the diagnosis of tuberculosis in the HIV-positive patient: Blood culture, urine culture, or biopsy of a suspicious lymph node.

Immediately evaluate patients who develop complaints consistent with active tuberculosis while on rifabutin prophylaxis, so that those with active disease may be given an effective combination regimen of anti-tuberculosis medications. Administration of single-agent rifabutin to patients with active tuberculosis is likely to lead to the development of tuberculosis that is resistant to rifabutin and rifampin.

There is no evidence that rifabutin is effective prophylaxis against *M. tuberculosis*. Patients requiring prophylaxis against both *M. tuberculosis* and *M. avium* complex may be given isoniazid and rifabutin concurrently.

➤*Fertility impairment:* Fertility was impaired in male rats given 160 mg/kg (32 times the recommended human daily dose).

➤*Pregnancy: Category B.* In rats given 200 mg/kg/day (40 times the recommended human daily dose) there was a decrease in fetal viability. In rats, 40 mg/kg/day caused an increase in fetal skeletal variants. In rabbits, 80 mg/kg/day caused maternotoxicity and an increase in fetal skeletal anomalies. There are no adequate and well-controlled studies in pregnant women. Use in pregnant women only if the potential benefit justifies the potential risk to the fetus.

➤*Lactation:* It is not known whether rifabutin is excreted in breast milk. Because of the potential for serious adverse reactions in nursing infants, decide whether to discontinue nursing or discontinue the drug, taking into account the importance of the drug to the mother.

➤*Children:* Safety and efficacy in children have not been established. Limited safety data are available from treatment use in 22 HIV-positive children with MAC who received rifabutin in combination with ≥ 2 other antimycobacterials for periods from 1 to 183 weeks. Mean doses (mg/kg) for these children were the following: 18.5 (range, 15 to 25) for infants 1 year of age; 8.6 (range, 4.4 to 18.8) for children 2 to 10 years of age; and 4 (range, 2.8 to 5.4) for adolescents 14 to 16 years of age. There is no evidence that doses > 5 mg/kg/day are useful. Adverse experiences were similar to those observed in the adult population, and included leukopenia, neutropenia, and rash. Doses of rifabutin may be administered mixed with foods such as applesauce.

Precautions

➤*Monitoring:* Because rifabutin may be associated with neutropenia, and more rarely thrombocytopenia, consider obtaining hematologic studies periodically in patients receiving prophylaxis.

➤*Red discoloration of body fluids:* Urine, feces, saliva, sputum, perspiration, tears, and skin may be brown-orange colored with rifabutin and some of its metabolites. Soft contact lenses may be permanently stained. Alert patients treated with rifabutin about these possibilities.

Drug Interactions

➤*CYP450:* Rifabutin has liver enzyme-inducing properties. The related drug, rifampin, is known to reduce the activity of a number of other drugs. Because of the structural similarity of rifabutin and rifampin, rifabutin may be expected to have similar interactions. However, unlike rifampin, rifabutin appears not to affect the acetylation of isoniazid. Rifabutin appears to be a less potent enzyme inducer than rifampin. The significance of this finding for clinical drug interactions is not known. Dosage adjustment of other drugs may be necessary if they are given concurrently with rifabutin. For further information, refer to the Rifampin monograph.

Rifabutin Drug Interactions			
Precipitant drug	Object drug*		Description
Rifamycins	Anticoagulants	↓	Rifampin decreases the anticoagulation action of warfarin. Increased doses of anticoagulants may be needed when rifamycins are administered concomitantly.
Rifamycins	Azole antifungal agents (eg, ketoconazole, itraconazole)	↓	Plasma levels of azole antifungal agents may be decreased, reducing antifungal activity. Ketoconazole may decrease serum rifamycin levels. Itraconazole may increase rifabutin plasma levels and toxicity. If concurrent use cannot be avoided, monitor antimicrobial activity, and adjust doses as needed.
Azole antifungal agents (eg, ketoconazole, itraconazole)	Rifamycins	↔	
Rifamycins	Benzodiazepines	↓	The pharmacologic effects of certain benzodiazepines may be decreased. Monitor the clinical response to the benzodiazepines when starting or stopping the rifamycin.
Rifamycins	Beta blockers	↓	The pharmacologic effects of certain beta blockers may be reduced by rifampin. May need a 3- to 4-week wash-out period for the enzyme induction effect to disappear. Closely monitor therapeutic response (eg, blood pressure).
Rifamycins	Buspirone	↓	Buspirone plasma concentrations and pharmacologic effects may be decreased. Escalation of buspirone dose may be necessary. Buspirone concentrations may increase following discontinuation of concomitantly administered rifamycins.
Rifamycins	Corticosteroids	↓	The pharmacologic effects of corticosteroids may be markedly decreased with initiation of rifampin therapy. This appears to occur within a few days of adding rifampin and to reverse 2 to 3 weeks following its administration. Double corticosteroid dosage after the addition of rifampin 300 mg/day.
Rifamycins	Cyclosporine	↓	Immunosuppressive effects of cyclosporine may be reduced as early as 2 days following rifamycin initiation. Avoid this combination if possible; otherwise, frequently monitor.
Rifamycins	Delavirdine	↓	Rifamycins decrease delavirdine plasma concentrations. Avoid concurrent use if possible.
Rifamycins	Doxycycline	↓	Rifamycins may decrease the serum concentration of doxycycline. Monitor the clinical response. Streptomycin does not appear to decrease doxycycline concentrations.
Rifamycins	Hydantoins	↓	Serum hydantoin levels may be decreased, resulting in a decreased pharmacologic hydantoin effect. Monitor hydantoin levels.

RIFABUTIN

Rifabutin Drug Interactions			
Precipitant drug	Object drug*		Description
Rifamycins	Indinavir	↓	Rifamycins may decrease indinavir serum concentrations. In addition, indinavir may elevate serum rifabutin concentrations, increasing the risk of rifabutin toxicity. It is recommended to reduce the rifabutin dose by 50% when administered with indinavir.
Indinavir	Rifamycins	↑	
Rifamycins	Losartan	↓	Losartan plasma concentrations may be reduced, decreasing antihypertensive effects. Observe the clinical response when rifamycin is started or stopped and adjust therapy as needed.
Rifamycins	Macrolide antibiotics (eg, clarithromycin, erythromycin)	↓	The antimicrobial effects of macrolide antibiotics may be decreased. The frequency of GI adverse reactions may be increased.
Rifamycins	Methadone	↓	The actions of methadone may be reduced, requiring higher doses of methadone during rifampin administration. Patients receiving methadone treatment may experience withdrawal symptoms.
Rifamycins	Morphine	↓	The analgesic effects of morphine may be decreased.
Rifamycins	Nelfinavir	↓	Rifamycins may decrease nelfinavir serum concentrations, decreasing the pharmacologic effects. Avoid concomitant rifampin and nelfinavir administration.
Rifamycins	Quinine, Quinidine	↓	Addition of rifamycins to stable quinine derivative regimens may require increased doses of quinine derivative to maintain the desired therapeutic effect. Monitor quinine derivative serum levels and the ECG.
Rifamycins	Theophylline, Aminophylline	↓	The addition of rifamycin may cause decreased theophylline levels and exacerbation of pulmonary symptoms. Monitor theophylline levels and the patient's response.
Rifamycins	Tricyclic antidepressants	↓	Tricyclic antidepressant (TCA) levels may be decreased, resulting in a decrease in pharmacologic effects. Consider monitoring the TCA concentrations when starting, discontinuing, or altering the rifamycin dose.
Rifamycins	Zolpidem	↓	Plasma concentrations and therapeutic effects of zolpidem may be reduced. Monitor the clinical response, possibly increasing the dose of zolpidem during concomitant administration of rifamycins.

* ↓ = Object drug decreased.   ↑ = Object drug increased.   ↔ = Undetermined clinical effect.

➤ *Drug/Food interactions:* High-fat meals slow the rate of absorption without influencing the extent.

Adverse Reactions

Rifabutin is generally well tolerated. Discontinuation of therapy because of an adverse event was required in 16% of patients receiving rifabutin vs 8% with placebo. Primary reasons for discontinuation were rash (4%), GI intolerance (3%), and neutropenia (2%).

Rifabutin Adverse Reactions (%)		
Adverse reaction	Rifabutin (n = 566)	Placebo (n = 580)
GI		
Nausea	6	5
Diarrhea	3	3
Nausea/vomiting	3	2
Dyspepsia	3	1
Eructation	3	1
Anorexia	2	2
Flatulence	2	1
Vomiting	1	1
Miscellaneous		
Discolored urine	30	6
Rash	11	8
Abdominal pain	4	3
Headache	3	5
Taste perversion	3	1
Fever	2	1
Myalgia	2	1
Pain	1	2
Asthenia	1	1
Chest pain	1	1
Insomnia	1	1

Other adverse reactions include the following: Flu-like syndrome, hepatitis, hemolysis, arthralgia, myositis, chest pressure or pain with dyspnea, skin discoloration (< 1%); seizure, paresthesia, aphasia, confusion, non-specific T-wave changes on ECG (> 1%; etiologic role not established).

Rifabutin Lab Test Abnormalities		
Lab test abnormalities	Rifabutin (n = 566)	Placebo (n = 580)
Increased alkaline phosphatase (> 450 U/L)	< 1	3
Increased AST (> 150 U/L)	7	12
Increased ALT (> 150 U/L)	9	11
Anemia (Hgb < 8 g/dl)	6	7
Eosinophilia	1	1
Leukopenia (WBC < 1500/mm³)	17	16
Neutropenia (ANC < 750/mm³)	25	20
Thrombocytopenia (platelets < 50,000/mm³)	5	4

Neutropenia – The incidence of neutropenia in patients treated with rifabutin was significantly greater than in patients treated with placebo. Although thrombocytopenia was not significantly more common among rifabutin-treated patients, it has been clearly linked to thrombocytopenia in rare cases. One patient developed thrombotic thrombocytopenic purpura, which was attributed to rifabutin.

Uveitis – When rifabutin was administered at doses from 1050 to 2400 mg/day, generalized arthralgia and uveitis occurred. These adverse experiences abated when rifabutin was discontinued.

Uveitus is rare when rifabutin is used as a single agent at 300 mg/day for prophylaxis of MAC in HIV-infected people, even with the concomitant use of fluconazole and/or macrolide antibiotics. However, if higher doses of rifabutin are administered in combination with these agents, the incidence of uveitis is higher.

Patients who developed uveitis had mild to severe symptoms that resolved after treatment with corticosteroids and/or mydriatic eye drops; however, in some severe cases, resolution of symptoms occurred after several weeks.

When uveitis occurs, temporary discontinuance of rifabutin and ophthalmologic evaluation are recommended. In most mild cases, rifabutin may be restarted; however, if signs or symptoms recur, discontinue use of rifabutin.

Overdosage

➤ *Treatment:* While there is no experience in the treatment of overdose with rifabutin, clinical experience with rifamycins suggest that gastric lavage to evacuate gastric contents (within a few hours of overdose), followed by instillation of an activated charcoal slurry into the stomach, may help absorb any remaining drug from the GI tract.

Rifabutin is 85% protein bound and distributed extensively into tissues. It is not primarily excreted via the urinary route (< 10% as unchanged drug); therefore, neither hemodialysis nor forced diuresis is expected to enhance the systemic elimination of unchanged rifabutin from the body in a patient with rifabutin overdose.

Patient Information

Advise patients of the signs and symptoms of both MAC and tuberculosis, and instruct them to consult their physician if they develop new complaints consistent with either of these diseases. In addition, because rifabutin may rarely be associated with myositis and uveitis, advise patients to notify their physician if they develop signs or symptoms suggesting either of these disorders.

Urine, feces, saliva, sputum, perspiration, tears, and skin may be brown-orange colored with rifabutin and some of its metabolites. Soft contact lenses may be permanently stained. Warn patients of these possibilities.

Advise patients using oral contraceptives to consider changing to nonhormonal methods of birth control because rifabutin, like rifampin, may decrease their efficacy.

ETHAMBUTOL HCl

Rx	Myambutol (Dura)	Tablets: 100 mg	(LL M6). White, film coated. Convex. In 100s.
		400 mg	(LL M7). White, scored, film coated. Convex. In 100s, 1000s, and UD 10s.

Refer to the general discussion in the Antituberculosal Agents Introduction.

Indications

Pulmonary tuberculosis: Use in conjunction with ≥ 1 other antituberculous drug. In patients who have not received previous antituberculous therapy (ie, initial treatment), the most frequently used regimens have been the following: Ethambutol plus isoniazid; ethambutol plus isoniazid plus streptomycin.

In patients who have received previous therapy, mycobacterial resistance to other drugs used in initial therapy is frequent. In retreatment patients, combine ethambutol with ≥ 1 of the second-line drugs not previously administered to the patient, and to which bacterial susceptibility has been indicated. Antituberculous drugs used with ethambutol have included cycloserine, ethionamide, pyrazinamide, viomycin, and other drugs. Isoniazid, aminosalicylic acid, and streptomycin also have been used in multiple drug regimens. Alternating drug regimens also have been used.

Administration and Dosage

Do not use ethambutol alone. Administer once every 24 hours only. Absorption is not significantly altered by administration with food. Continue therapy until bacteriological conversion has become permanent and maximal clinical improvement has occurred.

Initial treatment: In patients who have not received previous antituberculous therapy, administer 15 mg/kg (7 mg/lb) of body weight as a single oral dose once every 24 hours. Isoniazid has been administered concurrently in a single, daily oral dose.

Retreatment: In patients who have received previous antituberculous therapy, administer 25 mg/kg (11 mg/lb) of body weight as a single oral dose once every 24 hours. Concurrently administer ≥ 1 other antituberculous drug to which the organisms have been demonstrated to be susceptible by in vitro tests. Suitable drugs usually include those not previously used in the treatment of the patient. After 60 days of administration, decrease the dose to 15 mg/kg and administer as a single oral dose once every 24 hours.

During the period when a patient is receiving a daily dose of 25 mg/kg, monthly eye examinations are advised (see Precautions).

Ethambutol Weight-Dose Table

Weight range		Daily dose (mg)
kg	lbs	
15 mg/kg (7 mg/lb) schedule		
< 37	< 85	500
37-43	85-94.5	600
43-50	95-109.5	700
50-57	110-124.5	800
57-64	125-139.5	900
64-71	140-154.5	1000
71-79	155-169.5	1100
79-84	170-184.5	1200
84-90	185-199.5	1300
90-97	200-214.5	1400
> 97	≥ 215	1500
25 mg/kg (11 mg/lb) schedule		
< 38	< 85	900
38-42	85-92.5	1000
42-45.5	93-101.5	1100
45.5-50	102-109.5	1200
50-54	110-118.5	1300
54-58	119-128.5	1400
58-62	129-136.5	1500
62-67	137-146.5	1600
67-71	147-155.5	1700
71-75	156-164.5	1800
75-79	165-173.5	1900
79-83	174-182.5	2000
83-87	183-191.5	2100
87-91	192-199.5	2200
91-95	200-209.5	2300
95-99	210-218.5	2400
> 99	≥ 219	2500

Children: Not recommended for use in children < 13 years of age.

Actions

Pharmacology: Ethambutol diffuses into actively growing mycobacterium cells such as tubercle bacilli. It inhibits the synthesis of ≥ 1 metabolites, thus causing impairment of cell metabolism, arrest of multiplication, and cell death. No cross-resistance with other agents has been demonstrated.

Pharmacokinetics:

Absorption/Distribution – Following a single oral dose of 25 mg/kg, ethambutol attains a peak of 2 to 5 mcg/ml in serum 2 to 4 hours after administration. Serum levels are similar after prolonged dosing. The serum level is undetectable 24 hours after the last dose except in some patients with abnormal renal function.

Excretion – Approximately 50% of unchanged drug is excreted in the urine, 8% to 15% as metabolites and 20% to 22% unchanged in the feces. Marked accumulation may occur with renal insufficiency. Ethambutol is not significantly removed by hemodialysis.

Microbiology: Ethambutol is effective against strains of *Mycobacterium tuberculosis*, but does not seem to be active against fungi, viruses, or other bacteria. *M. tuberculosis* strains previously unexposed to ethambutol have been uniformly sensitive to concentrations of ≤ 8 mcg/ml, depending on the nature of the culture media. When used alone for treatment of tuberculosis, tubercle bacilli from these patients have developed resistance by in vitro susceptibility tests; the development of resistance has been unpredictable and appears to occur in a stepwise manner. Ethambutol has reduced incidence of mycobacterial resistance to isoniazid when used concurrently.

Contraindications

Hypersensitivity to ethambutol; known optic neuritis, unless clinical judgment determines that it may be used.

Warnings

Renal function impairment: Patients with decreased renal function require reduced dosage (as determined by serum levels) because this drug is excreted by the kidneys.

Pregnancy: Category B. The effects of combinations of ethambutol with other antituberculous drugs on the fetus are not known. Administration to pregnant patients has produced no detectable effect upon the fetus; use only when clearly needed and when the potential benefits outweigh the potential hazards to the fetus.

In fetuses born of mice treated with high doses of ethambutol during pregnancy, a low incidence of cleft palate, exencephaly, and abnormality of the vertebral column were observed. Minor abnormalities of the cervical vertebra were seen in newborn rats treated with high doses of ethambutol during pregnancy. Rabbits receiving high doses during pregnancy gave birth to 2 fetuses with monophthalmia, 1 with a shortened right forearm accompanied by bilateral wrist-joint contracture and 1 with hare lip and cleft palate.

Children: Not recommended for use in children < 13 years of age.

Precautions

Monitoring: Perform periodic assessment of renal, hepatic, and hematopoietic systems during long-term therapy.

Visual effects: This drug may have adverse effects on vision. The effects are generally reversible when the drug is discontinued promptly. In rare cases, recovery may be delayed for up to ≥ 1 year, and the effect may possibly be irreversible. Patients have received the drug again without recurrence of loss of visual acuity. Acuity changes may be unilateral or bilateral; therefore, each eye must be tested separately and both eyes tested together. Perform testing before beginning therapy and periodically during drug administration (monthly when a patient is receiving > 15 mg/kg/day). Use Snellen eye charts for testing of visual acuity. Physical examination should include ophthalmoscopy, finger perimetry, and testing of color discrimination.

In patients with visual defects such as cataracts, recurrent inflammatory conditions of the eye, optic neuritis, and diabetic retinopathy, the evaluation of changes in visual acuity is more difficult; the variations in vision may be because of underlying disease conditions. In such patients, consider the relationship between benefits expected and possible visual deterioration, because evaluation of visual changes is difficult.

Advise patients to report promptly any change in visual acuity. If evaluation confirms visual change and fails to reveal other causes, discontinue the drug and reevaluate the patient at frequent intervals. Consider progressive decreases in visual acuity during therapy to be because of the drug.

Patients developing visual abnormality during treatment may show subjective visual symptoms before, or simultaneously with, the demonstration of decreases in visual acuity; periodically question all patients receiving ethambutol about blurred vision and other subjective eye symptoms.

ETHAMBUTOL HCl

Drug Interactions

➤*Aluminum salts:* May delay and reduce the absorption of ethambutol. Separate their administration by several hours.

Adverse Reactions

➤*CNS:* Malaise; headache; dizziness; mental confusion; disorientation; possible hallucinations. Numbness and tingling of the extremities because of peripheral neuritis have occurred infrequently.

➤*GI:* Anorexia; nausea; vomiting; GI upset; abdominal pain.

➤*Hypersensitivity:* Anaphylactoid reactions; dermatitis; pruritus.

➤*Metabolic:* Elevated serum uric acid levels; precipitation of acute gout.

➤*Ophthalmic:* May produce decreases in visual acuity, which appear to be because of optic neuritis and to be related to dose and duration of treatment (see Precautions).

➤*Miscellaneous:* Fever; joint pain; pulmonary infiltrates; eosinophilia; transient impairment of liver function as indicated by abnormal liver function tests.

Patient Information

May cause stomach upset; take with food.

Notify physician if changes in vision (eg, blurring, red-green color blindness) or skin rash occurs.

PYRAZINAMIDE

| *Rx* | **Pyrazinamide** (UDL & ESI) | **Tablets:** 500 mg | (P36 LL). White, scored. In UD 100s. |

Refer to the general discussion in the Antituberculosal Agents Introduction.

Indications

➤*Tuberculosis:* Initial treatment of active tuberculosis in adults and children when combined with other antituberculous agents.

The current CDC recommendation for drug-susceptible initial treatment of active tuberculosis disease is a 6-month regimen consisting of isoniazid, rifampin, and pyrazinamide given for 2 months, followed by isoniazid and rifampin for 4 months.

➤*Treatment failure:* After treatment failure with other primary drugs in any form of active tuberculosis.

Administration and Dosage

Administer pyrazinamide with other effective antituberculous drugs for the initial 2 months of a ≥ 6-month treatment regimen for drug-susceptible patients. Treat patients who are known or suspected to have drug-resistant disease with regimens individualized to their situation.

➤*HIV infection:* Patients with concomitant HIV infection may require longer courses of therapy. Be alert to any revised recommendations from the CDC for this group of patients.

➤*Usual dose:* 15 to 30 mg/kg orally once daily. Do not exceed 2 g/day when given as a daily regimen.

➤*Alternative dosing:* Alternatively, a twice weekly dosing regimen (50 to 70 mg/kg twice weekly based on lean body weight) has been developed to promote patient compliance on an outpatient basis. In studies evaluating the twice weekly regimen, doses of pyrazinamide in excess of 3 g twice weekly have been administered without an increased incidence of adverse reactions.

➤*Storage/Stability:*

Suspension – Pyrazinamide 100 mg/ml was stable in a suspension containing simple syrup or 0.5% methylcellulose with simple syrup during a 2-month storage period in glass or plastic bottles at 4° to 25°C (40° to 77°F).

Actions

➤*Pharmacology:* Pyrazinamide, the pyrazine analog of nicotinamide, is an antituberculous agent. Pyrazinamide may be bacteriostatic or bactericidal against *Mycobacterium tuberculosis* depending on the concentration of the drug attained at the site of infection. The mechanism of action is unknown.

➤*Pharmacokinetics:*

Absorption/Distribution – Pyrazinamide is well absorbed from the GI tract and attains peak plasma concentrations within 2 hours. Plasma concentrations generally range from 30 to 50 mcg/ml with doses of 20 to 25 mg/kg. It is widely distributed in body tissues and fluids including the liver, lungs, and cerebrospinal fluid. Pyrizinamide is ≈ 10% bound to plasma proteins.

Metabolism/Excretion – The half-life is 9 to 10 hours; it may be prolonged in patients with impaired renal or hepatic function. Pyrazinamide is hydrolyzed in the liver to its major active metabolite, pyrazinoic acid. Pyrazinoic acid is hydroxylated to the main excretory product, 5-hydroxypyrazinoic acid.

Approximately 70% of an oral dose is excreted in urine, mainly by glomerular filtration, within 24 hours. Pyrazinamide is significantly dialyzed and should be dosed after hemodialysis.

Contraindications

Severe hepatic damage; hypersensitivity; acute gout.

Warnings

➤*Combination therapy:* Use only in conjunction with other effective antituberculous agents. Individualize regimens to treat patients with drug-resistant disease.

➤*Hyperuricemia:* Pyrazinamide inhibits renal excretion of urates, frequently resulting in hyperuricemia, which is usually asymptomatic. Patients started on pyrazinamide should have baseline serum uric acid determinations. Discontinue the drug and do not resume if signs of hyperuricemia accompanied by acute gouty arthritis appear.

➤*Renal function impairment:* It does not appear that patients with impaired renal function require a reduction in dose. However, it may be prudent to select doses at the low end of the dosing range.

➤*Hepatic function impairment:* Patients started on pyrazinamide should have baseline liver function determinations. Closely follow patients with preexisting liver disease or those at an increased risk for drug-related hepatitis (eg, alcohol abusers). Discontinue pyrazinamide and do not resume if signs of hepatocellular damage appear.

➤*Elderly:* In general, use caution when selecting a dose for an elderly patient. Start at the low end of the dosing range to reflect the greater frequency of decreased hepatic or renal function and of concomitant disease or other drug therapy.

➤*Pregnancy: Category C.* It is not known whether pyrazinamide can cause fetal harm when administered to a pregnant woman or can affect reproduction capacity. Give to a pregnant woman only if clearly needed.

➤*Lactation:* Pyrazinamide has been found in small amounts in breast milk. Therefore, it is advised that pyrazinamide be used with caution in nursing mothers, taking into account the risk-benefit of this therapy.

➤*Children:* Pyrazinamide regimens employed in adults are probably equally effective in children. Pyrazinamide appears to be well tolerated in children.

Precautions

➤*Monitoring:* Determine baseline liver function studies (especially ALT and AST) and uric acid levels prior to therapy. Perform appropriate laboratory testing at periodic intervals and if any clinical signs or symptoms occur during therapy.

➤*HIV infection:* In patients with concomitant HIV infection, be aware of current CDC recommendations. It is possible these patients may require a longer course of treatment.

➤*Diabetes mellitus:* Use with caution in patients with a history of diabetes mellitus, as management may be more difficult.

➤*Primary resistance of M. tuberculosis:* Primary resistance to pyrazinamide is uncommon. In cases with known or suspected drug resistance, perform in vitro susceptibility tests with recent cultures of *M. tuberculosis* against pyrazinamide and the usual primary drugs. There are few reliable in vitro tests for pyrazinamide resistance. A reference laboratory capable of performing these studies must be employed.

Drug Interactions

➤*Drug/Lab test interactions:* Pyrazinamide has been reported to interfere with *Acetest* and *Ketostix* urine tests to produce a pink-brown color.

Adverse Reactions

➤*GI:* Nausea; vomiting; anorexia.

➤*Hematologic/Lymphatic:* Thrombocytopenia and sideroblastic anemia with erythroid hyperplasia, vacuolation of erythrocytes, increased serum iron concentration and adverse effects on blood clotting mechanisms (rare).

➤*Hepatic:* The principal adverse effect is a hepatic reaction (see Warnings). Hepatotoxicity appears to be dose-related, and may appear at any time during therapy.

➤*Miscellaneous:* Mild arthralgia and myalgia (frequent); hypersensitivity reactions including rashes, urticaria, pruritus; fever, acne, photosensitivity, porphyria, dysuria, interstitial nephritis (rare); gout (see Warnings).

Overdosage

Overdosage experience is limited. In 1 case report of overdose, abnormal liver function tests developed. These spontaneously reverted to normal when the drug was stopped. Employ clinical monitoring and supportive therapy. Pyrazinamide is dialyzable. Refer to General Management of Acute Overdosage.

PYRAZINAMIDE

Patient Information

Instruct patients to notify their physician promptly if they experience any of the following: Fever, loss of appetite, malaise, nausea and vomiting, darkened urine, yellowish discoloration of the skin and eyes, pain or swelling of the joints.

Compliance with the full course of therapy must be emphasized; stress the importance of not missing any doses.

ETHIONAMIDE

Rx	Trecator-SC (Wyeth-Ayerst)	Tablets: 250 mg	(Wyeth 4130). Reddish-orange. Sugar coated. In 100s.

Refer to the general discussion in the Antituberculosal Agents Introduction.

Indications

►*Tuberculosis:* For the treatment of active tuberculosis in patients with *Mycobacterium tuberculosis* resistant to isoniazid or rifampin, or when there is intolerance on the part of the patient to other drugs. Its use alone in the treatment of tuberculosis results in the rapid development of resistance. Therefore, it is essential to give a suitable companion drug or drugs, the choice being based on the results of susceptibility tests. If the susceptibility tests indicate that the patient's organism is resistant to one of the first-line antituberculosis drugs (eg, isoniazid, rifampin) yet susceptible to ethionamide, accompany ethionamide by ≥ 1 drug to which the *M. tuberculosis* isolate is known to be susceptible. If the tuberculosis is resistant to both isoniazid and rifampin yet susceptible to ethionamide, accompany ethionamide by ≥ 2 other drugs to which the *M. tuberculosis* isolate is known to be susceptible. Directly observed therapy is recommended for all patients receiving treatment for tuberculosis.

Administration and Dosage

Administer with ≥ 1 other effective antituberculous drug.

►*Average adult dose:* 15 to 20 mg/kg/day taken once daily up to a maximum of 1 g/day. If GI intolerance develops, administer in divided doses after meals. Also to reduce GI intolerance, initiate therapy at 250 mg/day and titrate to optimal dose as tolerated by the patient. A regimen of 250 mg daily for 1 or 2 days, followed by 250 mg twice daily for 1 or 2 days with a subsequent increase to 1 g in 3 or 4 divided doses.

►*Children:* A dose of 10 to 20 mg/kg/day in 2 to 3 divided doses given after meals or 15 mg/kg/24 hours as a single daily dose has been recommended. As with adults, ethionamide may be administered to pediatric patients once daily.

►*HIV infection:* In patients with concomitant tuberculosis and HIV infection, malabsorption syndrome may be present. Suspect drug malabsorption in patients who adhere to therapy, but who fail to respond appropriately. In such cases, consider therapeutic drug monitoring.

Concomitant administration of pyridoxine is recommended.

►*Length of therapy:* Base duration of treatment on individual clinical response. In general, continue therapy until bacteriological conversion has become permanent and maximal clinical improvement has occurred.

Actions

►*Pharmacology:* Ethionamide may be bacteriostatic or bactericidal in action, depending on the concentration of the drug attained at the site of infection and the susceptibility of the infecting organism. The exact mechanism of action of ethionamide has not been fully elucidated, but the drug appears to inhibit peptide synthesis in susceptible organisms.

►*Pharmacokinetics:*

Absorption / Distribution – Ethionamide is essentially completely absorbed following oral administration and is not subjected to any appreciable first pass metabolism.

The drug is ≈ 30% bound to plasma proteins. Ethionamide is rapidly and widely distributed into body tissues and fluids, with concentrations in plasma and various organs being approximately equal. Significant concentrations also are present in cerebrospinal fluid.

Metabolism / Excretion – Ethionamide is extensively metabolized to active and inactive metabolites with < 1% excreted as the free form in urine. Metabolism is presumed to occur in the liver, and thus far the following 6 metabolites have been isolated: 2-ethylisonicotinamide, carbamoyl-dihydropyridine, thiocarbamoyl-dihydropyridine, S-oxocarbamoyl dihydropyridine, 2-ethylthioiso-nicotinamide, ethionamide sulfoxide. The sulfoxide metabolite has been demonstrated to have antimicrobial activity against *M. tuberculosis*. Ethionamide has a plasma elimination half-life of ≈ 2 hours after oral dosing.

Monitoring – Normal serum concentrations of 1 to 5 mcg/ml are usually seen 2 hours following doses of 250 to 500 mg. These concentrations approximate the therapeutic range for this drug when the therapeutic range is defined by those serum concentrations associated with a high probability of success and a low probability of dose-related toxicity.

►*Microbiology:* Ethionamide exhibits bacteriostatic activity against extracellular and intracellular *M. tuberculosis* organisms. The development of ethionamide-resistant *M. tuberculosis* isolates can be obtained by repeated subculturing in liquid or on solid media containing increasing concentrations of ethionamide. Multi-drug-resistant strains of *M. tuberculosis* may have acquired resistance to both isoniazid and ethionamide. However, the majority of *M. tuberculosis* isolates that are resistant to one are usually susceptible to the other. There is no evidence of cross-resistance between ethionamide and para-aminosalicylic acid (PAS), streptomycin, or cycloserine. However, limited data suggest that cross-resistance may exist between ethionamide and thiosemicarbazones (ie, thiacetazone) as well as isoniazid.

Ethionamide administered orally initially decreased the number of culturable *M. tuberculosis* organisms from the lungs of H37Rv-infected mice. Drug resistance developed with continued ethionamide monotherapy but did not occur when mice received ethionamide in combination with streptomycin or isoniazid.

Contraindications

Hypersensitivity to ethionamide; severe hepatic impairment.

Warnings

►*Resistance:* The use of ethionamide alone in the treatment of tuberculosis results in rapid development of resistance. Therefore, it is essential to give a suitable companion drug or drugs, the choice being based on the results of susceptibility testing. However, therapy may be initiated prior to receiving the results of susceptibility tests as deemed appropriate by the physician. Administer ethionamide with ≥ 1, sometimes 2, other drugs to which the organism is known to be susceptible. The drugs that have been used as companion agents are rifampin, ethambutol, pyrazinamide, cycloserine, kanamycin, streptomycin, and isoniazid.

►*Compliance:* Patient compliance is essential to the success of the antituberculosis therapy and to prevent the emergence of drug-resistant organisms. Therefore, patients should adhere to the drug regimen for the full duration of treatment. It is recommended that directly observed therapy be practiced when patients are receiving antituberculous medication. Additional consultation from experts in the treatment of drug-resistant tuberculosis is recommended when patients develop drug-resistant organisms.

►*Pregnancy: Category C.* Teratogenic effects have been demonstrated in small animals receiving doses in excess of those recommended in humans. There are no adequate and well-controlled studies in pregnant women. However, because of these animal studies, it must be recommended that ethionamide be withheld from women who are pregnant, or who are likely to become pregnant while under therapy, unless the prescribing physician considers it to be an essential part of the treatment.

►*Lactation:* Because no information is available on the excretion of ethionamide in breast milk, administer to nursing mothers only if the benefits outweigh the risks. Monitor for adverse effects those newborns who are being breastfed by mothers who are taking ethionamide.

►*Children:* Because of the fact that pulmonary tuberculosis resistant to primary therapy is rarely found in neonates, infants, and children, investigations have been limited in these age groups. Do not use in pediatric patients < 12 years of age except when the organisms are definitely resistant to primary therapy and systemic dissemination of the disease, or other life-threatening complications of tuberculosis, is judged to be imminent.

Precautions

►*Monitoring:* Make determinations of serum transaminase (AST, ALT) prior to therapy and monitor monthly. If serum transaminases become elevated during therapy, ethionamide and the companion antituberculosis drug or drugs may be discontinued temporarily until the laboratory abnormalities have resolved. Then reintroduce ethionamide and the companion antituberculosis medications sequentially to determine which drug (or drugs) is (are) responsible for the hepatotoxicity.

Determine blood glucose prior to and periodically throughout therapy with ethionamide. Diabetic patients should be particularly alert for episodes of hypoglycemia. Periodic monitoring of thyroid function tests is recommended as hypothyroidism, with or without goiter, has been reported with ethionamide therapy.

Ethionamide may potentiate the adverse effects of the other antituberculous drugs administered concomitantly (see Drug Interactions). Perform ophthalmologic examinations (including ophthalmoscopy) before and periodically during therapy.

Drug Interactions

►*Antituberculosis agents:* Ethionamide has been found to temporarily raise serum concentrations of isoniazid. Ethionamide may potentiate the adverse effects of other antituberculous drugs administered

ETHIONAMIDE

concomitantly. In particular, convulsions have been reported when ethionamide is administered with cycloserine; take special care when the treatment regimen includes both of these drugs. Avoid excessive ethanol ingestion because a psychotic reaction has been reported.

Adverse Reactions

➤*CNS:* Psychotic disturbances (including depression); drowsiness; dizziness; headache; restlessness; peripheral neuritis. Concurrent administration of pyridoxine has been recommended to prevent or relieve neurotoxic effects.

➤*GI:* Nausea, vomiting, diarrhea, abdominal pain, excessive salivation, metallic taste, stomatitis, anorexia, and weight loss are most common (50% of patients are unable to tolerate doses of 1 g). GI effects may be minimized by decreasing dosage, changing the time of drug administration, or by the concurrent administration of an antiemetic agent.

➤*Hepatic:* Transient increases in serum bilirubin, AST, and ALT; hepatitis (with or without jaundice).

➤*Ophthalmic:* Blurred vision; diplopia; optic neuritis.

➤*Miscellaneous:* Postural hypotension; skin rash; photosensitivity; acne; thrombocytopenia; purpura; hypoglycemia; pellagra-like syndrome; gynecomastia; impotence; increased difficulty managing diabetes mellitus.

Patient Information

May cause stomach upset, loss of appetite, metallic taste, or salivation. Notify physician if these effects persist or are severe. Taking with food may help reduce GI upset.

➤*Diabetic patients:* Monitor blood glucose throughout therapy and be alert for episodes of hypoglycemia.

AMINOSALICYLIC ACID (p-aminosalicylic acid; 4-aminosalicylic acid)

Rx	Paser (Jacobus Pharm)	Granules, delayed-release: 4 g	In packets.

Refer to the general discussion in the Antituberculosal Agents Introduction.

Indications

➤*Tuberculosis:* Treatment of tuberculosis in combination with other active agents. It is most commonly used in patients with multi-drug resistant tuberculosis (MDR-TB) or in situations when therapy with isoniazid and rifampin is not possible due to a combination of resistance and intolerance. When aminosalicylic acid is added to the treatment regimen in patients with proven or suspected drug resistance, it should be accompanied by ≥ 1 and preferably 2 other new agents of which the patient's organism is known or expected to be susceptible.

Administration and Dosage

➤*Tuberculosis:* The adult dosage of 4 g (1 packet) 3 times/day, or correspondingly smaller doses in children, is to be taken without chewing by sprinkling on applesauce or yogurt or by swirling in the glass to suspend the granules in an acidic drink such as tomato or orange juice or food such as applesauce or yogurt. The coating will last ≥ 2 hours.

Do not use if packet is swollen or the granules have lost their tan color, turning dark brown or purple.

➤*Storage / Stability:* Store at < 15°C (< 59°F) in a refrigerator or freezer. The packets may be stored at room temperature for short periods of time. Avoid excessive heat.

Actions

➤*Pharmacology:* Aminosalicylic acid is bacteriostatic against *Mycobacterium tuberculosis.* It inhibits the onset of bacterial resistance to streptomycin and isoniazid. The mechanism of action has been postulated to be inhibition of folic acid synthesis (but without potentiation with antifolic compounds) or inhibition of synthesis of the cell wall component, mycobactin, thus reducing iron uptake by *M. tuberculosis.*

Enteric-coated – After 2 hours in simulated gastric fluid, 10% of unprotected aminosalicylic acid is decarboxylated to form meta-aminophenol, a known hepatotoxin. The acid-resistant coating of the granules protects against degradation in the stomach.

The small granules are designed to escape the usual restriction on gastric emptying of large particles. Under neutral conditions, such as those found in the small intestine or in neutral foods, the acid-resistant coating is dissolved within 1 minute. Care must be taken in the administration of these granules to protect the acid-resistant coating by maintaining the granules in an acidic food during dosage administration. Patients who have neutralized gastric acid with antacids will not need to protect the acid-resistant coating with an acidic food because acid is not present to spoil the drug. Antacids are not necessary for aminosalicylic acid consumed with an acidic food.

Because aminosalicylic acid granules are protected by an enteric coating, absorption does not commence until they leave the stomach; the soft skeletons of the granules remain and may be seen in the stool.

➤*Pharmacokinetics:*

Absorption / Distribution – In a single 4 g pharmacokinetic study with food in normal volunteers, the initial time to a 2 mcg/ml serum level of aminosalicylic acid was 2 hours (range, 45 minutes to 24 hours); the median time to peak was 6 hours (range, 1.5 to 24 hours); the mean peak level was 20 mcg/ml (range, 9 to 35 mcg/ml); a level of 2 mcg/ml was maintained for an average of 7.9 hours (range, 5 to 9 hours); a level of 1 mcg/ml was maintained for an average of 6.8 hours (range, 6 to 11.5 hours). Approximately 50 to 60% of aminosalicylic acid is protein bound; binding is reported to be reduced 50% in kwashiorkor.

Excretion – 80% of aminosalicylic acid is excreted in the urine by glomerular filtration, with ≥ 50% of the dosage excreted in acetylated form.

➤*Microbiology:* The aminosalicylic acid MIC for *M. tuberculosis* in 7H11 agar was < 1 mcg/ml for 9 strains including 3 multidrug resistant strains, but 4 and 8 mcg/ml for 2 other multidrug resistant strains. The 90% inhibition in 7H12 broth (Bactec) showed little dose response but was interpreted as being ≤ 0.12 to 0.25 mcg/ml for 8 strains, of which 3

were multi-resistant, 0.5 mcg/ml for 1 resistant strain, questionable for 4 non-resistant strains, and > 1 mcg/ml for 1 non-resistant and 3 resistant strains. Aminosalicylic acid is not active in vitro against *M. avium.*

Contraindications

Hypersensitivity to any component of this medication; severe renal disease.

Warnings

➤*Hepatitis:* In one retrospective study of 7492 patients on rapidly absorbed aminosalicylic acid preparations, drug-induced hepatitis occurred in 38 patients (0.5%); in these 38, the first symptom usually appeared within 3 months of the start of therapy with a rash as the most common event followed by fever and much less frequently by GI disturbances of anorexia, nausea, or diarrhea. Only 1 patient was diagnosed on routine biochemistry.

Premonitory symptoms in 90% of these 38 patients preceded jaundice by a few days to several weeks with the mean time of onset 33 days (range, 7 to 90 days). Half of the adverse reactions occurred during the third, fourth, or fifth weeks. When aminosalicylic acid-induced hepatitis was diagnosed, hepatomegaly was invariably present with lymphadenopathy in 46%, leukocytosis in 79%, and eosinophilia in 55%. Prompt recognition with discontinuation led to the recovery of all 38 patients. If recognized in the premonitory stage, the reaction is reported to "settle" in 24 hours and no jaundice ensues. From other reported studies, failure to recognize the reaction can result in a mortality of ≤ 21%. The patient must be monitored carefully during the first 3 months of therapy and treatment must be discontinued immediately at the first sign of a rash, fever, or other premonitory signs of intolerance.

➤*Hypersensitivity reactions:* Stop all drugs at the first sign suggesting a hypersensitivity reaction. They may be restarted one at a time in very small but gradually increasing doses to determine whether the manifestations are drug-induced and, if so, which drug is responsible.

Desensitization has been accomplished successfully in 15 of 17 patients starting with 10 mg aminosalicylic acid given as a single dose. The dosage is doubled every 2 days until reaching a total of 1 g, after which the dosage is divided to follow the regular schedule of administration. If a mild temperature rise or skin reaction develops, the increment is to be dropped back 1 level or the progression held for 1 cycle. Reactions are rare after a total dosage of 1.5 g.

➤*Renal function impairment:* Patients with severe renal disease will accumulate aminosalicylic acid and its acetyl metabolite but will continue to acetylate, thus leading exclusively to the inactive acetylated form; deacetylation, if any, is not significant.

The half-life of free aminosalicylic acid in renal disease is 30.8 minutes in comparison to 26.4 minutes in normal volunteers, but the half-life of the inactive metabolite is 309 minutes in uremic patients in comparison to 51 minutes in normal volunteers. Although aminosalicylic acid passes dialysis membranes, the frequency of dialysis usually is not comparable to the half-life of 50 minutes for the free acid. Patients with end-stage renal disease should not receive aminosalicylic acid.

➤*Hepatic function impairment:* Patients with hepatic disease may not tolerate aminosalicylic acid as well as normal patients, even though the metabolism in patients with hepatic disease has been reported to be comparable to that in normal volunteers.

➤*Pregnancy: Category C.* Aminosalicylic acid has been reported to produce occipital malformations in rats when given at doses within the human dose range. Although there probably is a dose reponse, the frequency of abnormalities was comparable to controls at the highest level tested (2 times the human dose). When administered to rabbits at 5 mg/kg throughout all 3 trimesters, no teratologic or embryocidal effects were seen. Literature reports on aminosalicylic acid in pregnant women always report coadministration of other medications. Because there are no adequate and well-controlled studies of aminosalicylic acid in humans, give aminosalicylic acid granules to a pregnant woman only if clearly needed.

AMINOSALICYLIC ACID (p-aminosalicylic acid; 4-aminosalicylic acid)

▶*Lactation:* After administration of a different preparation of amino-salicylic acid to 1 patient, the maximum concentration in the breast milk was 1 mcg/ml at 3 hours with a half-life of 2.5 hours; the maximum maternal plasma concentration was 70 mcg/ml at 2 hours.

Precautions

▶*Malabsorption syndrome:* A malabsorption syndrome can develop in patients on aminosalicylic acid but is usually not complete. The complete syndrome includes steatorrhea, an abnormal small bowel pattern on x-ray, villus atrophy, depressed cholesterol, reduced D-xylose, and iron aborption. Triglyceride absorption is always normal.

▶*Lab test abnormalities:* Aminosalicylic acid has been reported to interfere technically with the serum determinations of albumin by dye-binding AST by the azoene dye method and with qualitative urine tests for ketones, bilirubin, urobilinogen, or porphobilinogen.

Crystalluria may develop and can be prevented by the maintenance of urine at a neutral or alkaline pH.

Drug Interactions

Aminosalicylic Acid Drug Interactions			
Precipitant	Object drug*		Description
Aminosalicylic acid	Isoniazid	↑	Aminosalicylic acid at a dose of 12 g in a rapidly available form has been reported to produce a 20% decrease in the acetylation of INH, especially in fast acetylators. The effect is dose related and, while it has not been studied with the current delayed-release formulation, the lower serum levels with this preparation will result in a reduced effect on the acetylation of INH. Special precautions are not deemed necessary.
Aminosalicylic acid	Digoxin	↓	Oral absorption of digoxin may be reduced when given concomitantly with aminosalicylic acid. Monitor serum digoxin levels.
Aminosalicylic acid	Vitamin B$_{12}$	↓	Aminosalicylic acid impairs the absorption of vitamin B$_{12}$. Consider vitamin B$_{12}$ therapy for patients on aminosalicylic acid therapy > 1 month.

* ↑ = Object drug increased. ↓ = Object drug decreased.

Adverse Reactions

▶*GI:* The most common side effect is GI intolerance manifested by nausea, vomiting, diarrhea, and abdominal pain.

▶*Hypersensitivity:* Fever, skin eruptions of various types, including exfoliative dermatitis, infectious mononuclosis-like, or lymphoma-like syndrome, leukopenia, agranulocytosis, thrombocytopenia, Coombs' positive hemolytic anemia, jaundice, hepatitis, pericarditis, hypoglycemia, optic neuritis, encephalopathy, Leoffler's syndrome, vasculitis, and a reduction in prothrombin.

Overdosage

Overdosage has not been reported.

Patient Information

Advise patients that the first signs of hypersensitivity include a rash, often followed by fever, and much less frequently, GI disturbances of anorexia, nausea, or diarrhea. If such symptoms develop, immediately cease taking the medication and arrange for prompt clinical visit.

Poor compliance in taking anti-tuberculosis medication often leads to treatment failure, and not infrequently, to the development of resistance of the organisms in the individual patient.

Advise patients that the skeleton of the granules may be seen in the stool.

Instruct patients to sprinkle the granules on acidic foods, such as applesauce or yogurt, or to suspend them in a fruit drink, which will protect the coating; the granules sink and will have to be swirled. The coating will last ≥ 2 hours in either system. Satisfactory juices tested to date include the following: Tomato, orange, grapefruit, grape, cranberry, apple, fruit punch.

Store aminosalicylic acid in the refrigerator or freezer. It may be stored at room temperature for short periods of time.

Do not use if the packets are swollen or the granules have lost their tan color and are dark brown or purple. The patient should inform the pharmacist or physician immediately and return the medication.

CYCLOSERINE

Rx	Seromycin Pulvules (Dura)	Capsules: 250 mg	(51479 019). Red/gray. In 40s.

Refer to the general discussion in the Antituberculosal Agents Introduction.

Indications

▶*Active pulmonary and extrapulmonary tuberculosis:* Treatment of active pulmonary and extrapulmonary tuberculosis (including renal disease) when organisms are susceptible, after failure of adequate treatment with the primary medications. Use in conjunction with other effective chemotherapy.

▶*Acute urinary tract infections:* May be effective in the treatment of acute urinary tract infections caused by susceptible strains of gram-positive and gram-negative bacteria, especially *Enterobacter* sp. and *Escherichia coli*. It is usually less effective than other antimicrobial agents in the treatment of urinary tract infections caused by bacteria other than mycobacteria. Consider using only when the more conventional therapy has failed and when the organism has demonstrated sensitivity.

Administration and Dosage

Administer 500 mg to 1 g daily in divided doses monitored by blood levels. The usual initial dosage is 250 mg twice daily at 12-hour intervals for the first 2 weeks. Do not exceed 1 g/day.

Pyridoxine 200 to 300 mg/day may prevent the neurotoxic effects.

Actions

▶*Pharmacology:* Inhibits cell-wall synthesis in susceptible strains of gram-positive and gram-negative bacteria and in *Mycobacterium tuberculosis*.

▶*Pharmacokinetics:*

Absorption/Distribution – When given orally, cycloserine is rapidly absorbed, reaching peak plasma concentrations in 4 to 8 hours. Concentrations in the cerebrospinal fluid, pleural fluid, fetal blood, and breast milk levels are similar to plasma. Detectable amounts also are found in ascitic fluid, bile, sputum, amniotic fluid, and lung and lymph tissues.

Metabolism/Excretion – Approximately 35% of the drug is metabolized into unknown substances; 50% of the drug is excreted in 12 hours with maximum excretion occurring 2 to 6 hours after administration. About 65% of the drug is recoverable in the urine in 72 hours.

Contraindications

Hypersensitivity to cycloserine; epilepsy; depression, severe anxiety, or psychosis; severe renal insufficiency; excessive concurrent use of alcohol.

Warnings

▶*CNS toxicity:* Discontinue the drug or reduce dosage if patient develops symptoms of CNS toxicity, such as convulsions, psychosis, somnolence, depression, confusion, hyperreflexia, headache, tremor, vertigo, paresis, or dysarthria. The risk of convulsions is increased in chronic alcoholics.

▶*Allergic dermatitis:* Discontinue the drug or reduce dosage if patient develops allergic dermatitis.

▶*Toxicity:* This is closely related to excessive blood levels (> 30 mcg/ml), which are because of high dosage or inadequate renal clearance. The ratio of toxic dose to effective dose in tuberculosis is small.

▶*Renal function impairment:* Patients will accumulate cycloserine and may develop toxicity if the dosage regimen is not modified in renal function impairment. Do not give cycloserine to patients with severe impairment.

▶*Pregnancy: Category C.* It is not known whether this drug can cause fetal harm when administered to a pregnant woman or can affect reproduction capacity. Use only if clearly needed.

▶*Lactation:* Because of the potential for serious adverse reactions in nursing infants, decide whether to discontinue nursing or to discontinue the drug, taking into account the importance of the drug to the mother.

▶*Children:* Safety and dosage have not been established for pediatric use.

Precautions

▶*Monitoring:* Monitor patients by hematologic, renal excretion, blood level, and liver function studies.

Determine blood levels weekly for patients having reduced renal function, for individuals receiving > 500 mg/day, and for those with symptoms of toxicity. Adjust dosage to maintain blood level < 30 mcg/ml.

CYCLOSERINE

▶*Obtain cultures:* Determine susceptibility before treatment.

▶*Anticonvulsant drugs or sedatives:* May be effective in controlling symptoms of CNS toxicity, such as convulsions, anxiety, and tremor. Closely observe patients receiving > 500 mg/day for such symptoms. The value of pyridoxine in preventing CNS toxicity from cycloserine has not been proven.

▶*Anemia:* Administration has been associated in a few cases with vitamin B_{12} or folic acid deficiency, megaloblastic anemia, and sideroblastic anemia. If evidence of anemia develops, institute appropriate studies and therapy.

Drug Interactions

▶*Alcohol:* Incompatible with cycloserine; alcohol increases the possibility and risk of epileptic episodes.

▶*Ethionamide:* Concurrent administration of ethionamide has been reported to potentiate neurotoxic side effects.

▶*Isoniazid:* Isoniazid in combination with cycloserine may result in increased cycloserine CNS side effects, most notably dizziness or drowsiness.

Adverse Reactions

▶*Cardiovascular:* Sudden development of CHF has been reported (in patients receiving 1 to 1.5 g of cycloserine daily).

▶*CNS:* These symptoms appear to be related to dosages > 500 mg/day: Convulsions; drowsiness and somnolence; headache; tremor; dysarthria; vertigo; confusion and disorientation with loss of memory; psychoses, possibly with suicidal tendencies, character changes, hyperirritability, aggression; paresis; hyperreflexia; paresthesias; major and minor (localized) clonic seizures; coma.

▶*Miscellaneous:* Elevated transaminase, especially in patients with pre-existing liver disease; skin rash; allergy (not related to dosage).

Overdosage

▶*Symptoms:* Acute toxicity can occur if > 1 g is ingested; chronic toxicity is dose-related and can occur if > 500 mg/day is administered. Toxic effects may include drowsiness, mental confusion, headache, vertigo, hyperirritability, paresthesias, dysarthrias, and psychosis. Paresis, convulsions, and coma may occur after larger doses.

▶*Treatment:* Management includes supportive therapy. Charcoal may be more effective than emesis or lavage; consider charcoal instead of or in addition to gastric emptying. Repeated doses of charcoal over time may hasten elimination of some drugs that have been absorbed. Safeguard the patient's airway when employing gastric emptying or charcoal. Hemodialysis removes the drug from the bloodstream; reserve for patients with life-threatening toxicity. Pyridoxine 200 to 300 mg/day may treat the neurotoxic effects. Refer to General Management of Acute Overdosage.

Patient Information

May cause drowsiness. Observe caution when driving or performing other tasks requiring alertness. Avoid excessive alcohol consumption.

Notify physician if mental confusion, dizziness, headache, or tremors occur.

STREPTOMYCIN SULFATE

Rx	Streptomycin Sulfate (Pharma-Tek)	Cake, lyophilized: 1 g	In vials.

Also refer to the streptomycin sulfate monograph in the Aminoglycosides, Parenteral section.

WARNING

The risk of severe neurotoxic reactions is sharply increased in patients with impaired renal function or prerenal azotemia. These include disturbances of vestibular and cochlear function, optic nerve dysfunction, peripheral neuritis, arachnoiditis, and encephalopathy. The incidence of clinically detectable, irreversible vestibular damage is particularly high in patients treated with streptomycin.

Monitor renal function carefully; patients with renal impairment and/or nitrogen retention should receive reduced doses. Do not exceed peak serum concentrations of 20 to 25 mcg/mL in individuals with kidney damage.

Avoid concurrent or sequential use of other neurotoxic and/or nephrotoxic drugs with streptomycin sulfate, including the following: Neomycin, kanamycin, gentamicin, cephaloridine, paromomycin, viomycin, polymyxin B, colistin, tobramycin, cyclosporine.

The neurotoxicity of streptomycin can result in respiratory paralysis from neuromuscular blockage, especially when the drug is given soon after the use of anesthesia or muscle relaxants. Reserve the administration of streptomycin in parenteral form for patients where adequate laboratory and audiometric testing facilities are available during therapy.

Indications

▶*Mycobacterium tuberculosis:* Add streptomycin or ethambutol as a fourth drug in a regimen containing isoniazid (INH), rifampin, and pyrazinamide for initial treatment of tuberculosis unless the likelihood of INH or rifampin resistance is very low. Reassess the need for a fourth drug when the results of susceptibility testing are known. In the past, when the national rate of primary drug resistance to INH was known to be less than 4% and was stable or declining, therapy with 2 to 3 drug regimens was considered adequate. If community rates of INH resistance are currently less than 4%, an initial treatment regimen with fewer than 4 drugs may be considered.

Streptomycin also is indicated for therapy of tuberculosis when one or more of the above drugs is contraindicated because of toxicity or intolerance.

For more indications, please see the streptomycin sulfate monograph in the Aminoglycosides, Parenteral section.

Administration and Dosage

▶*Approved by the FDA:* June 30, 1998.

▶*Skin sensitivity:* Take care handling streptomycin for injection to avoid skin sensitivity reactions. As with all IM preparations, inject streptomycin sulfate injection well within the body of a relatively large muscle and take care to minimize the possibility of damage to peripheral nerves.

▶*IM route only:* Only use the deltoid area if well developed, such as in certain adults and older children, and then only with caution to avoid radial nerve injury. Do not give IM injections into the lower or mid-third of the upper arm. As with all IM injections, aspiration is necessary to help avoid inadvertent injection into a blood vessel.

Alternate injection sites. As higher doses or more prolonged therapy with streptomycin may be indicated for more severe or fulminating infections (eg, endocarditis, meningitis), always take adequate measures to be immediately aware of any toxic signs or symptoms occurring in the patient as a result of streptomycin therapy.

Adults – The preferred IM injection site is the upper outer quadrant of the buttock (ie, gluteus maximus) or the mid-lateral thigh.

Children – It is recommended that IM injections be given preferably in the mid-lateral muscles of the thigh. In infants and small children, use the periphery of the upper outer quadrant of the gluteal region only when necessary, such as in burn patients, in order to minimize the possibility of damage to the sciatic nerve.

▶*Tuberculosis:* The standard regimen for the treatment of drug-susceptible tuberculosis has been 2 months of INH, rifampin, and pyrazinamide followed by 4 months of INH and rifampin (patients with concomitant infection with tuberculosis and HIV may require an extended treatment period). When streptomycin is added to this regimen because of suspected or proven drug resistance, the recommended dosing for streptomycin is as follows:

Streptomycin Recommended Dosing			
Patient	Daily	Twice weekly	3 times/week
Children	20 to 40 mg/kg; max, 1 g	25 to 30 mg/kg; max, 1.5 g	25 to 30 mg/kg; max, 1.5 g
Adults	15 mg/kg; max, 1 g	25 to 30 mg/kg; max, 1.5 g	25 to 30 mg/kg; max, 1.5 g

Streptomycin usually is administered daily as a single IM injection. Give a total dose of not more than 120 g over the course of therapy unless there are no other therapeutic options. In patients older than 60 years of age, reduce dosage because of the risk of increased toxicity (see Warning Box).

Therapy with streptomycin may be terminated when toxic symptoms have appeared, when impending toxicity is feared, when organisms become resistant, or when full treatment effect has been obtained. The total period of drug treatment of tuberculosis is a minimum of 1 year; however, indications for terminating therapy with streptomycin may occur at any time as noted above.

▶*Preparation:* The dry lyophilized cake is dissolved by adding water for injection in an amount to yield the desired concentration as indicated in the following table:

Concentration of Streptomycin Sulfate	
Approximate concentration (mg/mL)	Volume of solvent (mL)
200	4.2
250	3.2
400	1.8

▶*Storage/Stability:* Sterile reconstituted solutions can be stored at room temperature for 1 week. Protect from light. Store dry powder at room temperature (15° to 30°C; 59° to 86°F).

Actions

▶*Pharmacology:* Streptomycin sulfate is a bactericidal antibiotic. It acts by interfering with normal protein synthesis.

STREPTOMYCIN SULFATE

➤*Pharmacokinetics:* Following IM injection of 1 g of streptomycin as the sulfate, a peak serum level of 25 to 50 mcg/mL is reached within 1 hour, diminishing slowly to about 50% after 5 to 6 hours.

Appreciable concentrations are found in all organ tissues except the brain. Significant amounts have been found in pleural fluid and tuberculous cavities. Streptomycin passes through the placenta with serum levels in the cord blood similar to maternal levels. Small amounts are excreted in milk, saliva, and sweat.

Streptomycin is excreted by glomerular filtration. In patients with normal kidney function, between 29% and 89% of a single 600 mg dose is excreted in the urine within 24 hours. Any reduction of glomerular function results in decreased excretion of the drug and a concurrent rise in serum and tissue levels.

Contraindications

Hypersensitivity to streptomycin sulfate or any other aminoglycoside.

Warnings

➤*Ototoxicity:* Both vestibular and auditory dysfunction can follow the administration of streptomycin. The degree of impairment is directly proportional to the dose and duration of streptomycin administration, the age of the patient, the level of renal function, and the amount of underlying existing auditory dysfunction. The ototoxic effects of the aminoglycosides, including streptomycin, are potentiated by the coadministration of ethacrynic acid, mannitol, furosemide, and possibly other diuretics.

The vestibulotoxic potential of streptomycin exceeds that of its capacity for cochlear toxicity. Vestibular damage is heralded by headache, nausea, vomiting, and disequilibrium. Early cochlear injury is demonstrated by the loss of high frequency hearing. Appropriate monitoring and early discontinuation of the drug may permit recovery prior to irreversible damage to the sensorineural cells.

➤*Renal function impairment:* Exercise extreme caution in selecting a dosage regimen in the presence of pre-existing renal insufficiency. In severely uremic patients, a single dose may produce high blood levels for several days and the cumulative effect may produce ototoxic sequelae. When streptomycin must be given for prolonged periods of time, alkalinization of the urine may minimize or prevent renal irritation.

➤*Pregnancy: Category D.* Streptomycin can cause fetal harm when administered to a pregnant woman. Because streptomycin readily crosses the placental barrier, caution in use of the drug is important to prevent ototoxicity in the fetus. If this drug is used during pregnancy, or if the patient becomes pregnant while taking this drug, apprise the patient of the potential hazard to the fetus.

➤*Lactation:* Because of the potential for serious adverse reactions in nursing infants from streptomycin, decide whether to discontinue nursing or to discontinue the drug, taking into account the importance of the drug to the mother.

➤*Children:*

Infants – A syndrome of apparent CNS depression, characterized by stupor and flaccidity, occasionally coma, and deep respiratory depression, has been reported in young infants in whom streptomycin dosage had exceeded the recommended limits. Thus, do not give infants streptomycin in excess of the recommended dosage.

Precautions

➤*Monitoring:* Baseline and periodic caloric stimulation tests and audiometric tests are advisable with extended streptomycin therapy. Tinnitus, roaring noises, or a sense of fullness in the ears indicates need for audiometric examination, termination of streptomycin therapy, or both.

➤*Superinfection:* As with other antibiotics, use of this drug may result in overgrowth of nonsusceptible organisms, including fungi. If superinfection occurs, institute appropriate therapy.

Drug Interactions

The ototoxic effects of the aminoglycosides, including streptomycin, are potentiated by the coadministration of ethacrynic acid, furosemide, mannitol, and possibly other diuretics.

Adverse Reactions

The following reactions are common: Vestibular ototoxicity (eg, nausea, vomiting, vertigo); paresthesia of face; rash; fever; urticaria; angioneurotic edema; eosinophilia.

The following reactions are less frequent: Cochlear ototoxicity (deafness); exfoliative dermatitis; anaphylaxis; azotemia; leukopenia; thrombocytopenia; pancytopenia; hemolytic anemia; muscular weakness; amblyopia.

Vestibular dysfunction – Vestibular dysfunction resulting from the parenteral administration of streptomycin is cumulatively related to the total daily dose. When 1.8 to 2 g/day are given, symptoms are likely to develop in a large percentage of patients (especially in the elderly or patients with impaired renal function) within 4 weeks. Therefore, it is recommended that caloric and audiometric tests be done prior to, during, and following intensive therapy with streptomycin in order to facilitate detection of any vestibular dysfunction and/or impairment of hearing that may occur.

Vestibular symptoms generally appear early and usually are reversible with early detection and cessation of streptomycin administration. Two to 3 months after stopping the drug, gross vestibular symptoms usually disappear, except from the relative inability to walk in total darkness or on very rough terrain.

Nephrotoxicity – Although streptomycin is the least nephrotoxic of the aminoglycosides, nephrotoxicity does occur rarely. Exercise clinical judgment as to termination of therapy when side effects occur.

CAPREOMYCIN

Rx	**Capastat Sulfate** (Dura)	**Powder for Injection:** 1 g (as sulfate)/vial.	In 10 mL vials.

Refer to the general discussion in the Antituberculosal Agents Introduction.

> ### WARNING
>
> Undertake the use of capreomycin in patients with renal insufficiency or pre-existing auditory impairment with great caution. Weigh the risk of additional eighth nerve impairment or renal injury against benefits to be derived from therapy.
>
> Because other parenteral antituberculous agents (eg, streptomycin, viomycin) also have similar and sometimes irreversible toxic effects, particularly on eighth cranial nerve and renal function, simultaneous administration of these agents with capreomycin is not recommended. Use concurrent nonantituberculous drugs (eg, polymyxin A sulfate, colistin sulfate, amikacin, gentamicin, tobramycin, vancomycin, kanamycin, neomycin) that have ototoxic or nephrotoxic potential only with great caution.
>
> *Pregnancy:* The safety of capreomycin in pregnancy has not been determined
>
> *Children:* Safety and effectiveness in pediatric patients have not been established.

Indications

➤*Tuberculosis:* Intended for use concomitantly with other antituberculous agents in pulmonary infections caused by capreomycin-susceptible strains of *Mycobacterium tuberculosis* when the primary agents (eg, isoniazid, rifampin) have been ineffective or cannot be used because of toxicity or the presence of resistant tubercle bacilli.

Perform susceptibility studies to determine the presence of a capreomycin-susceptible strain of *M. tuberculosis*.

Administration and Dosage

May be administered IM or IV following reconstitution. Always administer in combination with ≥ 1 other antituberculous agent to which the patient's strain of tubercle bacilli is susceptible.

➤*Preparation of solution:* Dissolve vial contents (1 g) in 2 mL of 0.9% sodium chloride injection or sterile water for injection. Allow 2 to 3 minutes for complete dissolution. For administration of a 1 g dose, give the entire contents of the vial. For dosages < 1 g, the following dilution table may be used.

Preparation of Capreomycin Solution		
Diluent added to 1 g, 10 mL vial	Volume of solution	Concentration[1] (approx.)
2.15 mL	2.85 mL	350 mg/mL
2.63 mL	3.33 mL	300 mg/mL
3.3 mL	4 mL	250 mg/mL
4.3 mL	5 mL	200 mg/mL

[1] Stated in terms of milligram of capreomycin activity.

➤*IV:* For IV infusion, further dilute reconstituted capreomycin solution in 100 mL of 0.9% sodium chloride injection and administer over 60 minutes.

➤*IM:* Give reconstituted capreomycin by deep IM injection into a large muscle mass; superficial injections may be associated with increased pain and sterile abscesses.

➤*Usual dose:* 1 g/day (not to exceed 20 mg/kg/day) given IM or IV for 60 to 120 days, followed by 1 g by either route 2 or 3 times weekly.

Maintain therapy for tuberculosis for 12 to 24 months. If facilities for administering injectable medication are not available, a change to oral therapy is indicated upon the patient's release from the hospital.

➤*Renal function impairment:* Reduce the dosage based on Ccr using the guidelines in the table. These dosages are designed to achieve a mean steady-state capreomycin level of 10 mcg/L.

CAPREOMYCIN

Capreomycin Dosage in Renal Function Impairment

Ccr (mL/min)	Capreomycin clearance (L/kg/h × 10⁻²)	Half-life (h)	Dose[1] (mg/kg) for the following dosing intervals		
			24 h	48 h	72 h
0	0.54	55.5	1.29	2.58	3.87
10	1.01	29.4	2.43	4.87	7.30
20	1.49	20.0	3.58	7.16	10.7
30	1.97	15.1	4.72	9.45	14.2
40	2.45	12.2	5.87	11.7	—
50	2.92	10.2	7.01	14	—
60	3.40	8.8	8.16	—	—
80	4.35	6.8	10.4[2]	—	—
100	5.31	5.6	12.7[2]	—	—
110	5.78	5.2	13.9[2]	—	—

[1] Initial maintenance dose estimates are given for optional dosing intervals; longer dosing intervals are expected to provide greater peak and lower trough serum capreomycin levels than shorter dosing intervals.

[2] The usual dosage for patients with normal renal function is 1 g/day, not to exceed 20 mg/kg/day, for 60 to 120 days, then 1 g 2 to 3 times/week.

➤ *Storage / Stability:* The solution may acquire a pale straw color and darken with time, but this is not associated with loss of potency or the development of toxicity. After reconstitution, solutions may be refrigerated for up to 24 hours.

Actions

➤ *Pharmacology:* A polypeptide antibiotic isolated from *Streptomyces capreolus*.

➤ *Pharmacokinetics:*

Absorption – Capreomycin sulfate is not absorbed in significant quantities from the GI tract and must be administered parenterally. The AUC is similar for single-dose capreomycin (1 g) administered IM and by IV (over 1 hour) routes of administration. Capreomycin peak concentrations after IV infusion were ≈ 30% higher than after IM administration.

Distribution – Peak serum concentrations following IM administration of 1 g are achieved in 1 to 2 hours. Low serum concentrations are present at 24 hours. Doses of 1 g/day for ≥ 30 days produce no significant accumulation in subjects with normal renal function.

Excretion – Capreomycin is excreted essentially unaltered; 52% is excreted in the urine within 12 hours. Urine concentrations average 1.68 mcg/mL during the 6 hours following a 1 g dose.

➤ *Microbiology:* Active against human strains of *M. tuberculosis*.

Cross-resistance – Frequent cross-resistance occurs between capreomycin and viomycin. Varying degrees of cross-resistance between capreomycin and kanamycin and neomycin have occurred. No cross-resistance has been observed between capreomycin and isoniazid, aminosalicylate sodium, cycloserine, streptomycin, ethionamide, or ethambutol.

Contraindications

Hypersensitivity to capreomycin.

Warnings

➤ *Hypersensitivity reactions:* These have occurred when capreomycin and other antituberculous drugs were given concomitantly. Refer to General Management of Acute Hypersensitivity Reactions.

➤ *Renal function impairment:* Dosage reduction is necessary. See Administration and Dosage.

➤ *Pregnancy:* Category C. Well-controlled studies have not been performed in pregnant women. Use only if clearly needed and when potential benefits justify potential risks to the fetus. Safety for use during pregnancy has not been established.

➤ *Lactation:* It is not known whether this drug is excreted in breast milk. Therefore, exercise caution when administering capreomycin to nursing mothers.

➤ *Children:* Safety and efficacy for use in infants and children have not been established.

Precautions

➤ *Neuromuscular blockade:* A partial neuromuscular blockade was demonstrated after large IV doses of capreomycin. This action was enhanced by ether anesthesia (as has been reported for neomycin) and was antagonized by neostigmine.

➤ *Ototoxicity:* Perform audiometric measurements and assessment of vestibular function prior to initiation of therapy and at regular intervals during treatment.

➤ *Nephrotoxicity:* Perform regular tests of renal function throughout treatment, and reduce dose in patients with renal impairment. Renal injury with tubular necrosis, elevation of BUN or serum creatinine, and abnormal urinary sediment has been noted. Monitor renal function both before therapy is started and on a weekly basis during treatment. Slight elevation of the BUN or serum creatinine has been observed in a significant number of patients receiving prolonged therapy. The appearance of casts, red cells, and white cells in the urine has been noted in a high percentage of these cases.

Elevation of the BUN > 30 mg/dl or any other evidence of decreasing renal function with or without a rise in BUN level should indicate careful evaluation of the patient; reduce the dosage or withdraw the drug. The clinical significance of abnormal urine sediment and slight elevation in the BUN (or serum creatinine) during long-term therapy has not been established.

➤ *Hypokalemia:* May occur during therapy; therefore, determine serum potassium levels frequently.

Drug Interactions

➤ *Aminoglycosides:* Administration with capreomycin may increase the risk of respiratory paralysis and renal dysfunction.

➤ *Nondepolarizing neuromuscular blocking agents:* Neuromuscular blockade may be enhanced by concurrent capreomycin because of a synergistic effect on myoneural function.

Adverse Reactions

➤ *Hematologic:* Leukocytosis and leukopenia have been observed. The majority of patients treated have had eosinophilia exceeding 5% while receiving daily injections of capreomycin. This subsided with reduction of the capreomycin dosage to 2 or 3 g weekly.

Rare cases of thrombocytopenia have occurred.

➤ *Hepatic:* Serial tests of liver function have demonstrated a decrease in bromosulfophthalein excretion without change in AST or ALT in the presence of preexisting liver disease. Abnormal results in liver function tests have occurred in many people receiving capreomycin in combination with other antituberculous agents that are also known to cause changes in hepatic function. The role of capreomycin is not clear; however, periodic determinations of liver function are recommended.

➤ *Hypersensitivity:* Urticaria and maculopapular skin rashes were associated in some cases with febrile reactions (see Warnings).

➤ *Miscellaneous:* Pain and induration and excessive bleeding at the injection sites; sterile abscesses.

Nephrotoxicity – In 36% of 722 patients treated with capreomycin, elevation of the BUN > 20 mg/dl has been observed. In many instances, there was also depression of PSP excretion and abnormal urine sediment. In 10% of this series, the BUN elevation exceeded 30 mg/dl.

Toxic nephritis was reported in 1 patient with tuberculosis and portal cirrhosis who was treated with capreomycin (1 g) and aminosalicylic acid daily for 1 month. This patient developed renal insufficiency and oliguria and died. Autopsy showed subsiding acute tubular necrosis.

Electrolyte disturbances resembling Bartter's syndrome occurred in 1 patient.

Ototoxicity – Subclinical auditory loss was noted in ≈ 11% of patients. This has been a 5- to 10-decibel loss in the 4000 to 8000 cycles/second range. Clinically apparent hearing loss occurred in 3% of 722 subjects. Some audiometric changes were reversible. Other cases with permanent loss were not progressive following withdrawal of capreomycin.

Tinnitus and vertigo have also occurred.

Overdosage

➤ *Symptoms:* Nephrotoxicity following the parenteral administration of capreomycin is most closely related to the area under the curve of the serum concentration vs time graph. The elderly patient, patients with abnormal renal function or dehydration, and patients receiving other nephrotoxic drugs are at much greater risk for developing acute tubular necrosis.

Damage to the auditory and vestibular divisions of cranial nerve VIII has been associated with capreomycin given to patients with abnormal renal function or dehydration and in those receiving medications with additive auditory toxicities. These patients often experience dizziness, tinnitus, vertigo, and a loss of high-tone acuity.

Neuromuscular blockade or respiratory paralysis may occur following rapid IV infusion. If capreomycin is ingested, toxicity would be unlikely because it is poorly absorbed (< 1%) from an intact GI system.

Hypokalemia, hypocalcemia, hypomagnesemia, and an electrolyte disturbance resembling Bartter's syndrome have been reported to occur in patients with capreomycin toxicity. The SC median lethal dose in mice was 514 mg/kg.

➤ *Treatment:* Protect the patient's airway and support ventilation and perfusion. Meticulously monitor and maintain, within acceptable limits, the patient's vital signs, blood gases, serum electrolytes, etc. Absorption of drugs from the GI tract may be decreased by giving activated charcoal, which, in many cases, is more effective than emesis or lavage; consider charcoal instead of or in addition to gastric emptying. Repeated doses of charcoal over time may hasten elimination of some drugs that have been absorbed. Safeguard the patient's airway when employing gastric emptying or charcoal. Carefully hydrate patients who have received an overdose of capreomycin and have normal renal function to maintain a urine output of 3 to 5 mL/kg/hr. Carefully monitor fluid balance, electrolytes, and creatinine clearance.

Hemodialysis may be effectively used to remove capreomycin in patients with significant renal disease.

RIFAPENTINE

Rx	**Priftin** (Aventis)	**Tablets:** 150 mg	Pink. Film coated. In 32s.

Refer to the general discussion in the Antituberculosal Agents Introduction.

Indications

➤*Tuberculosis:* For the treatment of pulmonary tuberculosis (TB). Rifapentine must always be used in conjunction with ≥ 1 other antituberculosis drug to which the isolate is susceptible.

Administration and Dosage

➤*Approved by the FDA:* June 26, 1998.

Do not use rifapentine alone. Concomitant administration of pyridoxine (vitamin B_6) is recommended in the malnourished, in those predisposed to neuropathy (eg, alcoholics, diabetics), and in adolescents.

➤*Tuberculosis:*

Intensive phase – 600 mg (four 150 mg tablets twice weekly) with an interval of ≥ 3 days (72 hours) between doses continued for 2 months. May be given with food if stomach upset, nausea, or vomiting occurs.

Administer rifapentine in combination as part of an appropriate regimen that includes daily companion drugs. Compliance with all drugs in the intensive phase (ie, rifapentine, isoniazid, pyrazinamide, ethambutol, streptomycin), especially on days when rifapentine is not administered, is imperative to ensure early sputum conversion and protection against relapse. The Advisory Council for the Elimination of Tuberculosis, the American Thoracic Society (ATS), and the Centers for Disease Control and Prevention (CDC) also recommend that either streptomycin or ethambutol be added to the regimen unless the likelihood of isoniazid resistance is very low.

Continuation phase – Continue treatment with rifapentine once weekly for 4 months in combination with isoniazid or an appropriate agent for susceptible organisms. If the patient is still sputum-smear- or culture-positive, if resistant organisms are present, or if the patient is HIV-positive, follow ATS/CDC treatment guidelines.

Actions

➤*Pharmacology:* Rifapentine is a rifamycin-derivative antibiotic and has a similar profile of microbiological activity to rifampin. It is a cyclopentyl rifamycin that inhibits DNA-dependent RNA polymerase in susceptible strains of *Mycobacterium tuberculosis* but not in mammalian cells. At therapeutic levels, rifapentine exhibits bactericidal activity against intracellular and extracellular *M. tuberculosis* organisms. Rifapentine and the 25-desacetyl metabolite accumulate in human monocyte-derived macrophages with intracellular/extracellular ratios of ≈ 24:1 and 7:1, respectively.

➤*Pharmacokinetics:*

Absorption/Distribution – The absolute bioavailability of rifapentine has not been determined; relative bioavailability to an oral solution after a single 600 mg dose is 70%. Maximum levels were achieved in 5 to 6 hours. Food increased the area under the plasma concentration-time curve (AUC) and C_{max} in healthy volunteers and in asymptomatic HIV-infected volunteers (see Drug Interactions). Steady-state conditions were achieved by day 10 following daily administration of 600 mg. The estimated apparent volume of distribution is ≈ 70 L. In healthy volunteers, rifapentine and 25-desacetyl rifapentine (active metabolite) were 97.7% and 93.2% bound to plasma proteins, respectively, mainly to albumin. Similar extent of protein binding was observed in healthy volunteers, asymptomatic HIV-infected subjects, and hepatically impaired subjects.

Select Pharmacokinetic Parameters of Rifapentine

Pharmacokinetic parameter	Rifapentine[1] (n = 12)	25-desacetyl rifapentine[1] (n = 12)
C_{max} (mcg/ml)	≈ 15.05	≈ 6.26
AUC (0-72 hr) (mcg•hr/ml)	≈ 319.54	≈ 215.88
t½ (hr)	≈ 13.19	≈ 13.35
T_{max} (hr)	≈ 4.83	≈ 11.25
Cl_{po} (L/hr)	≈ 2.03	–

[1] Mean values, day 10.

Metabolism/Excretion – Rifapentine is hydrolyzed by an esterase enzyme to form a microbiologically active 25-desacetyl rifapentine. Rifapentine and 25-desacetyl rifapentine account for 99% of total drug in plasma. Plasma AUC and C_{max} values of the 25-desacetyl rifapentine metabolite are 50% and 33% those of rifapentine, respectively. Based upon relative in vitro activities and AUC values, rifapentine and 25-desacetyl rifapentine potentially contribute 62% and 38% to the clinical activities against *M. tuberculosis*, respectively. Eighty-seven percent of the total dose was recovered in the urine (17%) and feces (70%); > 80% was excreted within 7 days.

Special populations –

Gender: The estimated apparent oral clearance of rifapentine for males and females was ≈ 2.51 and ≈ 1.69 L/hr, respectively. The clinical significance of the difference in the estimated apparent oral clearance is not known.

Contraindications

Hypersensitivity to any of the rifamycins (eg, rifampin, rifabutin).

Warnings

➤*Compliance:* Poor compliance with the dosage regimen, particularly daily administered nonrifamycin drugs in the intensive phase, was associated with late sputum conversion and a high relapse rate. Therefore, emphasize compliance with the full course of therapy, and stress the importance of not missing any doses.

➤*Hyperbilirubinemia:* Resulting from competition for excretory pathways between rifapentine and bilirubin, this cannot be excluded, because competition between the related drug rifampin and bilirubin can occur. An isolated report showing a moderate rise in bilirubin or transaminase level is not an indication to interrupt treatment; rather, repeat tests, noting trends in the levels, and consider them in conjunction with the patient's clinical condition.

➤*Pseudomembranous colitis:* This has occurred with various antibiotics, including other rifamycins. Diarrhea, particularly if severe or persistent, occurring during treatment or in the initial weeks following treatment may be symptomatic of *Clostridium difficile*-associated disease, of which the most severe form is pseudomembranous colitis. If pseudomembranous colitis is suspected, stop rifapentine immediately and treat the patient with supportive and specific treatment without delay (eg, oral vancomycin). Products inhibiting peristalsis are contraindicated in this clinical situation.

➤*HIV-infected patients:* Experience is limited. In an ongoing CDC tuberculosis trial, 5 of 30 HIV-infected patients randomized to once-weekly rifapentine (plus isoniazid) in the continuation phase and who completed treatment, relapsed. Four of these patients developed rifampin mono-resistant (RMR) tuberculosis. Each RMR patient had late-stage HIV infection, low CD4 counts, and extrapulmonary disease and documented coadministration of azole antifungals. These findings are consistent with the literature in which an emergence of RMR tuberculosis in HIV-infected tuberculosis patients has been reported in recent years. Further study in this sub-population is warranted. As with other antituberculous treatments, when rifapentine is used in HIV-infected patients, employ a more aggressive regimen (eg, more frequent dosing). Based on the CDC trial results to date, once-weekly dosing during the continuation phase of treatment is not recommended.

➤*Hepatic function impairment:* Because antituberculous multidrug treatments, including the rifamycin class, are associated with serious hepatic events, only give patients with abnormal liver tests or liver disease rifapentine in cases of necessity and then with caution and under strict medical supervision. In these patients, carefully monitor liver tests (especially serum transaminases) prior to therapy and then every 2 to 4 weeks during therapy. If signs of liver disease occur or worsen, discontinue rifapentine.

➤*Pregnancy: Category C.* Rifapentine is teratogenic in rats and rabbits. When given in doses 0.6 times the human dose during the period of organogenesis, rat pups showed cleft palates, right aortic arch, increased incidence of delayed ossification, and increased number of ribs. Rabbits treated with doses between 0.3 and 1.3 times the human dose displayed major malformations including ovarian agenesis, pes varus, arhinia, microphthalmia, and irregularities of the ossified facial tissues. Rifapentine was also associated with increased resorption rate and postimplantation loss, decreased mean fetus weight, and increased number of stillborn pups.

There are no adequate and well-controlled studies in pregnant women. Use during pregnancy only if the potential benefit justifies the potential risk to the fetus.

When administered during the last few weeks of pregnancy, rifampin can cause postnatal hemorrhages in the mother and infant that may be treated with vitamin K. Evaluate appropriate clotting parameters in patients and infants who receive rifapentine during the last few weeks of pregnancy.

➤*Lactation:* Rifapentine was associated with slightly increased rat pup mortality during lactation. It is not known whether rifapentine is excreted in human breast milk. Because of the potential for serious adverse reactions in nursing infants, decide whether to discontinue nursing or discontinue the drug, taking into account the importance of the drug to the mother.

➤*Children:* Safety and efficacy in children < 12 years of age have not been established.

Precautions

➤*Monitoring:* Obtain baseline measurements of hepatic enzymes, bilirubin, a complete blood count, and a platelet count (or estimate). Assess patients at least monthly during therapy, and specifically question patients concerning symptoms associated with adverse reactions. Follow up on patients with abnormalities, including laboratory testing, if necessary. Routine laboratory monitoring for toxicity in people with normal baseline measurements is generally not necessary.

RIFAPENTINE

▶*Resistance:* M. tuberculosis organisms resistant to other rifamycins are likely to be resistant to rifapentine. A high level of cross resistance between rifampin and rifapentine has been demonstrated with M. tuberculosis strains. Cross resistance does not appear between rifapentine and nonrifamycin antimycobacterial agents such as isoniazid and streptomycin.

▶*Red discoloration of body fluids:* Rifapentine may produce a predominately red-orange discoloration of body tissues or fluids (eg, skin, teeth, tongue, urine, feces, saliva, sputum, tears, sweat, cerebrospinal fluid). Contact lenses may become permanently stained.

Drug Interactions

▶*Indinavir:* Indinavir C_{max} decreased by 55%, while AUC was reduced by 70% with concomitant rifapentine. Clearance of indinavir increased by 3-fold in the presence of rifapentine, while half-life did not change. Use rifapentine with extreme caution, if at all, in patients who are also taking protease inhibitors.

▶*Cytochrome P450:* Rifapentine is an inducer of cytochromes P450 3A4 and P450 2C8/9 and may increase the metabolism of other coadministered drugs that are metabolized by these enzymes. Induction studies have suggested rifapentine induction potential may be less than rifampin but more potent than rifabutin.

Rifampin may accelerate the metabolism and reduce the activity of the following drugs; therefore, rifapentine may interact similarly. Dosage adjustments of these drugs may be necessary. *Note:* Advise patients using oral or other systemic hormonal contraceptives to change to nonhormonal methods of birth control.

Amitriptyline	Doxycycline	Phenytoin
Barbiturates	Fluconazole	Progestins
Beta blockers	Fluoroquinolones	Quinidine
Buspirone	Haloperidol	Quinine
Cardiac glycosides	Indinavir	Ritonavir
Chloramphenicol	Itraconazole	Saquinavir
Clarithromycin	Ketoconazole	Sildenafil
Clofibrate	Levothyroxine	Sulfonylureas
Corticosteroids	Methadone	Tacrolimus
Cyclosporine	Mexiletine	Theophylline
Dapsone	Morphine	Tocainide

Delavirdine	Nelfinavir	Verapamil
Diazepam	Nifedipine	Warfarin
Diltiazem	Nortriptyline	Zidovudine
Disopyramide	Oral contraceptives	Zolpidem

▶*Drug/Lab test interactions:* Therapeutic concentrations of rifampin have been shown to inhibit standard microbiological assays for serum **folate** and **vitamin B$_{12}$**. Consider similar drug-laboratory interactions for rifapentine; consider alternative assay methods.

▶*Drug/Food interactions:* Food (850 total calories: 33 g protein, 55 g fat and 58 g carbohydrate) increased AUC and C_{max} in healthy volunteers by 43% and 44%, respectively, and in asymptomatic HIV-infected volunteers by 51% and 53%, respectively.

Adverse Reactions

Three patients (2 rifampin combination therapy patients and 1 rifapentine combination therapy patient) were discontinued in the intensive phase as a result of hepatitis with increased liver function tests (eg, ALT, AST, LDH, bilirubin). Concomitant medications for all 3 patients included isoniazid, pyrazinamide, ethambutol, and pyridoxine. The 2 rifampin patients and 1 rifapentine patient recovered without sequelae.

The overall occurrence rate of treatment-related adverse events was higher in males with the rifapentine combination regimen (50%) vs the rifampin combination regimen (43%), while in females the overall rate was greater in the rifampin combination group (68%) compared with the rifapentine combination group (59%). However, there were higher frequencies of treatment-related hematuria and ALT increases for female patients in both treatment groups compared with those for male patients.

Adverse events associated with rifampin may also occur with rifapentine. The effects of enzyme induction to increase metabolism may result in decreased concentration of endogenous substrates, including adrenal hormones, thyroid hormones, and vitamin D.

The following table presents treatment-related adverse events that occurred in ≥ 1% of patients deemed by the investigators to be at least possibly related to any of the 4 drugs in the regimens (rifapentine/rifampin, isoniazid, pyrazinamide, or ethambutol). Hyperuricemia was the most frequently reported event that was assessed as treatment related and was most likely related to the pyrazinamide.

Rifapentine Combination vs Rifampin Combination Adverse Reactions (≥ 1%)						
	Intensive phase[1]		Continuation phase[2]		Total	
Adverse reaction	Rifapentine combination (n = 361)	Rifampin combination (n = 361)	Rifapentine combination (n = 321)	Rifampin combination (n = 306)	Rifapentine combination (n = 361)	Rifampin combination (n = 361)
CNS						
Headache	0.8	1.1	0.3	1	1.1	1.9
Dizziness	1.1	0	0	0.3	1.1	0.3
Dermatologic						
Rash	2.5	5.5	1.2	1	3.6	6.1
Acne	1.4	0.8	0.6	0.3	1.9	1.1
Rash, maculopapular	1.1	0.8	0	0	1.1	0.8
GI						
Anorexia	1.7	2.2	0.9	1.3	2.2	2.8
Nausea	1.9	0.6	0	0.3	1.9	0.8
Vomiting	1.1	1.7	0.3	0.3	1.4	1.9
Dyspepsia	0.8	1.4	0.6	1	1.1	2.2
Diarrhea	1.1	0	0	0	1.1	0
Hemoptysis	0.6	0	0.6	0	1.1	0
GU						
Pyuria	3.3	2.8	1.9	0.7	4.2	3.3
Proteinuria	4.2	2.8	0.6	0.3	4.7	3
Hematuria	2.8	3	1.2	1	3.6	3.9
Urinary casts	3	0.8	1.2	0	3.9	0.8
Hematologic						
Neutropenia	1.9	2.5	3.7	2.9	5	5
Lymphopenia	3.9	3.6	0.9	0.3	4.4	3.9
Anemia	1.9	2.5	0.6	0.3	2.5	2.8
Leukopenia	1.1	1.1	0.9	1.6	1.9	2.2
Thrombocytosis	1.1	0.6	0	0	1.1	0.6
Miscellaneous						
Hyperuricemia[3]	21.3	15.2	0	0	21.3	15.2
Hypertension	0.8	0	0.3	0.3	1.1	0.3
Pruritus	2.2	4.2	0.3	0.3	2.5	4.4
Arthralgia	2.5	1.9	0	0	2.5	1.9
Pain	1.9	1.4	0	0.3	1.9	1.7

RIFAPENTINE

Rifapentine Combination vs Rifampin Combination Adverse Reactions (≥ 1%)					
	Intensive phase[1]		Continuation phase[2]		Total	
Adverse reaction	Rifapentine combination (n = 361)	Rifampin combination (n = 361)	Rifapentine combination (n = 321)	Rifampin combination (n = 306)	Rifapentine combination (n = 361)	Rifampin combination (n = 361)
Lab test abnormalities						
ALT increased	3.9	4.7	1.6	2.3	5.3	6.6
AST increased	3.3	4.4	1.6	2.3	4.4	6.4

[1] Intensive phase consisted of therapy with either rifapentine or rifampin combined with isoniazid, pyrazinamide, and ethambutol administered daily (rifapentine twice weekly for 60 days).

[2] Continuation phase consisted of therapy with either rifapentine or rifampin combined with isoniazid for 120 days. Rifapentine patients were dosed once weekly; rifampin patients were dosed twice weekly. Events recorded in this phase include those reported ≤ 3 months after continuation phase therapy was completed.

[3] Most likely related to pyrizinamide.

Treatment-related adverse events of moderate or severe intensity in < 1% of rifapentine combination therapy patient areas follows:

➤*Dermatologic:* Urticaria; skin discoloration.

➤*GI:* Constipation; esophagitis; gastritis; pancreatitis.

➤*Hematologic:* Thrombocytopenia; neutrophilia, leukocytosis; purpura; hematoma.

➤*Hepatic:* Bilirubinemia; hepatitis.

➤*Metabolic/Nutritional:* Hyperkalemia; hypovolemia; alkaline phosphatase increased; LDH increased.

➤*Musculoskeletal:* Gout; arthrosis.

➤*Miscellaneous:* Peripheral edema; fatigue; aggressive reaction.

Overdosage

There is no experience with the treatment of acute overdosage with rifapentine at doses > 1200 mg/dose. Single oral doses ≤ 1200 mg have been administered without serious adverse events. The only adverse events reported with the 1200 mg dose were heartburn, headache, and increased urinary frequency. In clinical trials, tuberculosis patients ranging from 20 to 74 years of age accidentally received continuous daily doses of rifapentine 600 mg. Some patients received continuous daily dosing for ≤ 20 days without evidence of serious adverse effects. One patient experienced a transient elevation in ALT and glucose (the latter attributed to preexisting diabetes); a second patient experienced slight pruritus.

➤*Treatment:* While there is no experience with the treatment of acute overdosage with rifapentine, clinical experience with rifamycins suggests that gastric lavage to evacuate gastric contents (within a few hours of overdose), followed by instillation of an activated charcoal slurry into the stomach, may help adsorb any remaining drug from the GI tract. Neither hemodialysis nor forced diuresis is expected to enhance the systemic elimination of unchanged rifapentine from a patient with rifapentine overdose.

Patient Information

Inform patients that rifapentine may produce a reddish discoloration of the urine, sweat, sputum, and tears and that contact lenses may be permanently stained.

Advise the patient that the reliability of oral or other systemic hormonal contraceptives may be affected and to use alternative contraceptive measures.

Advise patients with a propensity to nausea, vomiting, or GI upset to take rifapentine with food.

Instruct patients to notify their physician promptly if they experience any of the following: Fever, appetite loss, malaise, nausea and vomiting, darkened urine, yellowish discoloration of the skin and eyes, pain or swelling of the joints.

Emphasize compliance with the full course of therapy, and stress the importance of not missing any doses of the daily administered companion medications in the intensive phase (see Administration and Dosage and Warnings).

The agents listed in this group are recommended for the following disorders (see individual monographs):

		Iodoquinol	Emetine HCl
Intestinal amebiasis:	*Extraintestinal amebiasis:*	Metronidazole	Chloroquine
Paromomycin	Metronidazole	Emetine HCl	

PAROMOMYCIN

Rx	Humatin (Parke-Davis)	Capsules: 250 mg paromomycin (as sulfate)	In 16s.

Indications

Acute and chronic intestinal amebiasis.

Adjunctive therapy in the management of hepatic coma.

Not indicated in extraintestinal amebiasis because it is not absorbed.

➤*Unlabeled uses:* Has been recommended for other parasitic infections — *Dientamoeba fragilis* (25 to 30 mg/kg/day in 3 doses for 7 days); *Diphyllobothrium latum, Taenia saginata, T. solium, Dipylidium caninum* (adults: 1 g every 15 minutes for 4 doses; pediatric: 11 mg/kg every 15 minutes for 4 doses); *Hymenolepsis nana* (45 mg/kg/day for 5 to 7 days).

Administration and Dosage

➤*Intestinal amebiasis:*

Adults and children – 25 to 35 mg/kg/day in 3 divided doses with meals for 5 to 10 days.

➤*Management of hepatic coma:*

Adults – 4 g daily in divided doses administered at regular intervals for 5 to 6 days.

Actions

➤*Pharmacology:* Paromomycin is an amebicidal and antibacterial aminoglycoside obtained from a strain of *Streptomyces rimosus*, and is active in intestinal amebiasis. Its in vitro and in vivo antibacterial activity closely parallels that of neomycin; complete cross-resistance exists between paromomycin, kanamycin and neomycin. Effective against enteric bacteria *Salmonella* and *Shigella*.

➤*Pharmacokinetics:*

Absorption – GI absorption of paromomycin is poor; almost 100% of the drug is recovered in the stool.

Contraindications

Hypersensitivity reactions to paromomycin; intestinal obstruction.

Precautions

➤*Ototoxicity and renal damage:* Inadvertent absorption through ulcerative bowel lesions may result in eighth cranial nerve damage and renal damage.

➤*Superinfection:* Use of antibiotics (especially prolonged or repeated therapy) may result in bacterial or fungal overgrowth of nonsusceptible organisms. Such overgrowth may lead to secondary infections. Take appropriate measures if superinfection occurs.

Drug Interactions

Because paromomycin is an aminoglycoside, consider the interactions that may occur with the other oral aminoglycosides as potentially occurring with paromomycin as well (see Aminoglycosides, Oral section).

Adverse Reactions

➤*GI:* Doses > 3 g daily have reportedly produced nausea, abdominal cramps, and diarrhea.

Patient Information

Complete full course of therapy.

May cause nausea, vomiting, or diarrhea.

Notify physician if ringing in the ears, hearing impairment, or dizziness occurs.

IODOQUINOL (Diiodohydroxyquin)

Rx	Yodoxin (Glenwood)	Tablets: 210 mg	In 100s and 1000s.
		650 mg	In 100s and 1000s.
		Powder	In 25 g.

Indications

Treatment of intestinal amebiasis.

Not indicated for treatment of chronic diarrhea, particularly in children, because of potential association with optic atrophy and permanent loss of vision.

Administration and Dosage

➤*Adults:* 650 mg 3 times daily after meals for 20 days.

➤*Children:* 40 mg/kg daily (maximum 650 mg/dose) in 3 divided doses for 20 days. Do not exceed 1.95 g in 24 hours for 20 days.

Actions

➤*Pharmacology:* Iodoquinol is effective against the trophozoites and cysts of *Entamoeba histolytica* located in the large intestine. Because it is poorly absorbed in the GI tract, the drug can reach high concentrations in the intestinal lumen, and produce its potent amebicidal effect precisely at the site of infection, without significant systemic absorption (≈ 8%). This is useful for the prevention of extraintestinal (liver, lung) complications of amebic dysentery. The drug is not effective in amebic hepatitis and amebic abscess of the liver.

Contraindications

Hypersensitivity to any 8-hydroxyquinoline (eg, iodoquinol, iodochlorhydroxyquin) or iodine-containing preparations; hepatic damage.

Warnings

➤*Optic neuritis, optic atrophy, and peripheral neuropathy:* These have occurred following prolonged high dosage therapy; avoid long-term therapy.

➤*Pregnancy:* Safety for use during pregnancy and in the nursing mother has not been established.

Precautions

Use with caution in patients with thyroid disease.

Drug Interactions

➤*Drug/Lab test interactions:* Protein bound iodine levels may be increased during treatment and interfere with the results of certain **thyroid** function tests. These effects may persist for as long as 6 months after discontinuance of therapy.

Adverse Reactions

➤*Dermatologic:* Various forms of skin eruptions (acneiform, papular, pustular, bullae, vegetating, or tuberous iododerma); urticaria; pruritus.

➤*GI:* Nausea; vomiting; abdominal cramps; diarrhea; pruritus ani.

➤*Miscellaneous:* Fever; chills; headache; vertigo; enlargement of thyroid. Optic neuritis, optic atrophy, and peripheral neuropathy have occurred in association with prolonged high dosage 8-hydroxyquinoline therapy.

Patient Information

Complete full course of therapy.

May cause nausea, vomiting, diarrhea, or GI upset.

METRONIDAZOLE

Rx	Metronidazole (Various, eg, Baxter, Geneva, Goldline, Lederle, Lemmon, Moore, Rugby, Schein)	Tablets: 250 mg	In 100s, 250s, 500s, 1000s and UD 32s and 100s.
Rx	Flagyl (Searle)		(Searle 1831 Flagyl 250). Blue. Film coated. In 50s, 100s, 250s, 1000s, 2500s and UD 100s.
Rx	Metric 21 (Fielding)		In 100s.
Rx	Protostat (Ortho)		(Ortho 1570). White, scored. Capsule shape. In 100s.
Rx	Metronidazole (Various, eg, Baxter, Geneva, Lederle, Lemmon, Rugby, Schein)	Tablets: 500 mg	In 100s, 200s, 250s, 500s and UD 32s and 100s.
Rx	Flagyl (Searle)		(Flagyl 500). Blue. Film coated. Oblong. In 50s, 100s, 500s and UD 100s.
Rx	Protostat (Ortho)		(Ortho 1571). White, scored. Capsule shape. In 50s.
Rx	Metronidazole (Able)	Capsules: 375 mg	(A 353). Yellow and grey. In 30s, 50s, 100s, 500s, and 1000s.
Rx	Flagyl 375 (Searle)		(375 Flagyl). Gray/light green. In 50s, 100s and UD 100s.

The following is an abbreviated monograph for metronidazole. Complete prescribing information begins in the full monograph in the Antibiotics section.

WARNING

Metronidazole has been shown to be carcinogenic in rodents. Avoid unnecessary use.

Indications

▶*Amebiasis:* Treatment of acute intestinal amebiasis (amebic dysentery) and amebic liver abscess. In amebic liver abscess, therapy does not obviate the need for aspiration or drainage of pus.

▶*Trichomoniasis, symptomatic:* Treatment in females and males when the presence of the trichomonad has been confirmed by appropriate laboratory procedures (wet smears or cultures).

▶*Trichomoniasis, asymptomatic:* Treatment of asymptomatic females with endocervicitis, cervicitis or cervical erosion. Since there is evidence that presence of the trichomonad can interfere with accurate assessment of abnormal cytological smears, perform additional smears after eradication of the parasite.

▶*Treatment of asymptomatic partners: T. vaginalis* infection is a sexually transmitted disease. Therefore, in order to prevent reinfection, simultaneously treat asymptomatic sexual partners of treated patients if the organism has been found to be present. Since there can be difficulty in isolating the organism from the asymptomatic male carrier, negative smears and cultures cannot be relied upon. Women may become reinfected if the male partner is not treated. Therefore, it may be advisable to treat an asymptomatic male partner with a negative culture or when no culture has been attempted.

▶*Anaerobic bacterial infections:* Refer to the use of metronidazole as an antibiotic in the Anti-Infectives chapter.

▶*Unlabeled uses:* The CDC has recommended the use of oral metronidazole for *Gardnerella vaginalis* (500 mg twice daily for 7 days) and for giardiasis (alternative to quinacrine; 250 mg 3 times daily for 7 days).

Administration and Dosage

▶*Amebiasis:*

Acute intestinal amebiasis (acute amebic dysentery) – 750 mg 3 times daily for 5 to 10 days.

Amebic liver abscess – 500 or 750 mg 3 times daily for 5 to 10 days.

Children – 35 to 50 mg/kg/24 hours (maximum 750 mg/dose) in 3 divided doses for 10 days.

▶*Trichomoniasis:*

1 day treatment – 2 g given either as a single dose or in 2 divided doses of 1 g each given in the same day.

7 day course of treatment –
Adults: 250 mg 3 times daily for 7 consecutive days;
Children: 5 mg/kg/dose 3 times daily for 7 days.

Cure rates, as determined by vaginal smears, signs and symptoms, may be higher after a 7 day course of treatment than after the 1 day treatment regimen. Individualize dosage. Single dose treatment can assure compliance, especially if administered under supervision, in those patients who cannot be relied upon to continue the 7 day regimen. A 7 day course of treatment may minimize reinfection of the female long enough to treat sexual contacts. Further, some patients may tolerate one course of therapy better than the other.

Do not treat pregnant patients during the first trimester – If treated during the second or third trimester in those whom local palliative treatment has been inadequate to control symptoms, do not use the 1 day course of therapy as it results in higher serum levels which reach the fetal circulation.

When repeat courses of drug are required, 4 to 6 weeks should elapse between courses and reconfirm presence of trichomonad by appropriate laboratory measures. Perform total and differential leukocyte counts before and after retreatment.

Patients with severe hepatic disease metabolize metronidazole slowly, with resultant accumulation of metronidazole and its metabolites in the plasma. Accordingly, cautiously administer doses below those usually recommended. Monitor plasma metronidazole levels and toxicity.

Do not specifically reduce the dose of metronidazole in anuric patients since accumulated metabolites may be rapidly removed by dialysis.

Actions

▶*Microbiology:* Metronidazole is a nitroimidazole that possesses direct trichomonacidal and amebicidal activity against *Trichomonas vaginalis* and *Entamoeba histolytica.* The in vitro minimal inhibitory concentration (MIC) for most strains of these organisms is ≤ 1 mcg/ml. Metronidazole's mechanism of antiprotozoal action is unknown.

Patient Information

May cause GI upset; take with food.

Complete full course of therapy; take until gone.

Avoid alcoholic beverages.

May cause darkening of urine.

An unpleasant metallic taste may be noticeable.

During treatment for trichomoniasis, it is recommended that the patient refrain from sexual intercourse or the male partner wear a condom to avoid reinfection.

CHLOROQUINE PHOSPHATE

Rx	Chloroquine Phosphate (Various, eg, Danbury)	Tablets: 250 mg (equiv. to 150 mg base)	In 20s, 22s, 30s, 100s, 1000s, UD 100s.
Rx	Aralen Phosphate (Sanofi Winthrop)	Tablets: 500 mg (equiv. to 300 mg base)	(W/A77). In 25s.

For complete prescribing information, see 4–Aminoquinoline Compounds in the Antimalarial Preparations section.

Indications

Treatment of extraintestinal amebiasis.

Administration and Dosage

▶*Adults:* 1 g (600 mg base) daily for 2 days, followed by 500 mg (300 mg base) daily for at least 2 to 3 weeks. Treatment is usually combined with an effective intestinal amebicide.

CHLOROQUINE HCl

Rx	Aralen HCl (Sanofi Winthrop)	Injection: 50 mg (equiv. to 40 mg base) per ml	In 5 ml amps.

For complete prescribing information, refer to the 4–Aminoquinoline Compounds in the Antimalarial Preparations section.

Indications

Treatment of extraintestinal amebiasis when oral therapy is not feasible.

Administration and Dosage

▶*Adults:* 4 to 5 ml (200 to 250 mg; 160 to 200 mg base) IM daily for 10 to 12 days. Substitute or resume oral administration as soon as possible.

FOSCARNET SODIUM (Phosphonoformic acid; PFA)

| Rx | Foscavir (Astra) | Injection: 24 mg/ml | In 250 and 500 ml bottles. |

WARNING

Renal impairment is the major toxicity of foscarnet. Continual assessment of a patient's risk, frequent monitoring of serum creatinine with dose adjustment for changes in renal function and adequate hydration with administration are imperative (see Administration and Dosage).

Seizures, related to alterations in plasma minerals and electrolytes, have been associated with foscarnet treatment. Therefore, patients must be carefully monitored for such changes and their potential sequelae. Mineral and electrolyte supplementation may be required.

Foscarnet is indicated for use only in immunocompromised patients with CMV retinitis and mucocutaneous acyclovir-resistant HSV infections (see Indications).

Indications

➤*CMV retinitis:* Treatment of CMV retinitis in patients with AIDS.

➤*Combination:* Combination therapy with ganciclovir for patients who have relapsed after monotherapy with either drug.

➤*HSV infections:* Treatment of acyclovir-resistant mucocutaneous HSV infections in immunocompromised patients.

Administration and Dosage

➤*Caution:* Do not administer by rapid or bolus IV injection. Toxicity may be increased as a result of excessive plasma levels. Take care to avoid unintentional overdose; carefully control the rate of infusion by using an infusion pump. In spite of the use of an infusion pump, overdoses have occurred.

Hydration may reduce the risk of nephrotoxicity. It is recommended that 750 to 1000 ml of normal saline or 5% dextrose solution should be given prior to the first infusion of foscarnet to establish diuresis. With subsequent infusions, 750 to 1000 ml of hydration fluid should be given with 90 to 120 mg/kg of foscarnet and 500 ml with 40 to 60 mg/kg of foscarnet. Hydration fluid may need to be decreased if clinically warranted. After the first dose, the hydration fluid should be administered concurrently with each infusion of foscarnet.

Administer by controlled IV infusion, either by using a central venous line or a peripheral vein. The standard 24 mg/ml solution may be used without dilution when using a central venous catheter for infusion. When a peripheral vein catheter is used, dilute the 24 mg/ml solution to 12 mg/ml with 5% Dextrose in Water or with a Normal Saline Solution prior to administration to avoid local irritation of peripheral veins. Because the dose is calculated on the basis of body weight, it may be desirable to remove and discard any unneeded quantity from the bottle before starting with the infusion to avoid overdosage.

➤*Induction treatment:*

CMV retinitis – The recommended initial dose for patients with normal renal function is either 90 mg/kg (1.5- to 2-hour infusion) every 12 hours or 60 mg/kg over a minimum of 1 hour every 8 hours for 2 to 3 weeks depending on clinical response.

HSV infections – The recommended initial dose for acyclovir-resistant HSV patients with normal renal function is 40 mg/kg (minimum 1 hour infusion) either every 8 or 12 hours for 2 to 3 weeks or until healed.

An infusion pump must be used to control the rate of infusion. Adequate hydration is recommended to establish diuresis, both prior to and during treatment to minimize renal toxicity (see Warnings), provided there are no clinical contraindications.

➤*Maintenance treatment:* 90 to 120 mg/kg/day (individualized for renal function) given as an IV infusion over 2 hours. Because the superiority of the 120 mg/kg/day has not been established in controlled trials and given the likely relationship of higher plasma foscarnet levels to toxicity, it is recommended that most patients be started on maintenance treatment with a dose of 90 mg/kg/day. Escalation to 120 mg/kg/day may be considered should early reinduction be required because of retinitis progression. Some patients who show excellent tolerance to foscarnet may benefit from initiation of maintenance treatment at 120 mg/kg/day earlier in their treatment. An infusion pump must be used to control the rate of infusion with all doses. Again, hydration to establish diuresis both prior to and during treatment is recommended to minimize renal toxicity.

Patients who experience progression of retinitis while receiving maintenance therapy may be retreated with the induction and maintenance regimens given above.

➤*Renal function impairment:* Use with caution in patients with abnormal renal function because reduced plasma clearance of foscarnet will result in elevated plasma levels. In addition, foscarnet has the potential to further impair renal function (see Warnings). Safety and efficacy data for patients with baseline serum creatinine levels> 2.8 mg/dL or measured 24-hour creatinine clearances < 50 ml/min are limited. Carefully monitor renal function at baseline and during induction and maintenance therapy with appropriate dose adjustments. If Ccr falls below the limits of the dosing nomograms (0.4 ml/min/kg) during therapy, discontinue foscarnet and monitor the patient daily until resolution of renal impairment is ensured.

Dose adjustment – Individualize foscarnet dosing according to the patient's renal function status. Refer to the table below for recommended doses and adjust the dose as indicated.

To use this dosing guide, actual 24 hour Ccr (ml/min) must be divided by body weight (kg) or the estimated Ccr in ml/min/kg can be calculated from serum creatinine (mg/dl) using the following formula (modified Cockcroft and Gault equation):

Males: $\dfrac{\text{Weight (kg)} \times (140 - \text{age})}{72 \times \text{serum creatinine (mg/dL)}} = \text{Ccr}$

Females: $0.85 \times \text{above value}$

Foscarnet Dosing Guide Based on Ccr for Induction

Ccr (ml/min/kg)	HSV: Equivalent to		CMV: Equivalent to	
	40 mg/kg q 12 hr	40 mg/kg q 8 hr	60 mg/kg q 8 hr	90 mg/kg q 12 hr
> 1.4	40 q 12 hr	40 q 8 hr	60 q 8 hr	90 q 12 hr
> 1 to 1.4	30 q 12 hr	30 q 8 hr	45 q 8 hr	70 q 12 hr
> 0.8 to 1	20 q 12 hr	35 q 12 hr	50 q 12 hr	50 q 12 hr
> 0.6 to 0.8	35 q 24 hr	25 q 12 hr	40 q 12 hr	80 q 24 hr
> 0.5 to 0.6	25 q 24 hr	40 q 24 hr	60 q 24 hr	60 q 24 hr
≥ 0.4 to 0.5	20 q 24 hr	35 q 24 hr	50 q 24 hr	50 q 24 hr
< 0.4	Not recommended	Not recommended	Not recommended	Not recommended

Foscarnet Dosing Guide Based on Ccr for Maintenance

Ccr (ml/min/kg)	CMV: Equivalent to	
	90 mg/kg/day	120 mg/kg/day
> 1.4	90 q 24 hr	120 q 24 hr
> 1 to 1.4	70 q 24 hr	90 q 24 hr
> 0.8 to 1	50 q 24 hr	65 q 24 hr
> 0.6 to 0.8	80 q 48 hr	105 q 48 hr
> 0.5 to 0.6	60 q 48 hr	80 q 48 hr
≥ 0.4 to 0.5	50 q 48 hr	65 q 48 hr
< 0.4	Not recommended	Not recommended

➤*Admixture incompatibility:* Other drugs and supplements can be administered to a patient receiving foscarnet. However, take care to ensure that foscarnet is only administered with Normal Saline or 5% Dextrose Solution and that no other drug or supplement is administered concurrently via the same catheter. Foscarnet is chemically incompatible with 30% Dextrose Solution, amphotericin B and solutions containing calcium such as Ringer's Lactate and TPN. Physical incompatibility with other IV drugs includes: Acyclovir sodium, diphenhydramine, dobutamine, droperidol, ganciclovir, gentamicin, haloperidol, isethionate, morphine sulfate, trimetrexate, pentamidine, vancomycin, trimethoprim/sulfamethoxazole, diazepam, midazolam, digoxin, phenytoin, leucovorin and prochlorperazine. Because of foscarnet's chelating properties, a precipitate can potentially occur when divalent cations are administered concurrently in the same catheter.

➤*Storage/Stability:* Store at room temperature 15° to 30°C (59° to 86°F) and do not freeze. At a concentration of 12 mg/ml in Normal Saline Solution, foscarnet is stable for 30 days at 5°C (41°F).

Actions

➤*Pharmacology:* Foscarnet is an organic analog of inorganic pyrophosphate that inhibits replication of known herpes viruses in vitro including cytomegalovirus (CMV) and herpes simplex virus types 1 and 2 (HSV-1, HSV-2).

Foscarnet exerts its antiviral activity by a selective inhibition at the pyrophosphate binding site on virus-specific DNA polymerases at concentrations that do not affect cellular DNA polymerases. Foscarnet does not require activation (phosphorylation) by thymidine kinase or other kinases, and therefore is active in vitro against HSV mutants deficient in thymidine kinase and CMV UL97 mutants. HSV strains resistant to acyclovir or CMV strains resistant to ganciclovir may be sensitive to foscarnet. However, acyclovir or ganciclovir resistant mutants with alterations in the viral DNA polymerase may be resistant

FOSCARNET SODIUM (Phosphonoformic acid; PFA)

to foscarnet and may not respond to therapy with foscarnet. The combination of foscarnet and ganciclovir has enhanced activity in vitro.

The quantitative relationship between the in vitro susceptibility of human CMV or herpes simplex virus 1 and 2 to foscarnet and clinical response to therapy has not been established and virus sensitivity testing has not been standardized.

Resistance – All foscarnet resistant mutants are known to be generated through mutation in the viral DNA polymerase gene. CMV strains with double mutations conferring resistance to both foscarnet and ganciclovir have been isolated from patients with AIDS. Consider the possibility of viral resistance in patients who show poor clinical response or experience persistent viral excretion during therapy.

▶*Pharmacokinetics:* Foscarnet is 14% to 17% bound to plasma protein at plasma drug concentrations of 1 to 1000 mcM.

The foscarnet terminal half-life determined by urinary excretion was 87.5 ± 41.8 hours, possibly because of release of foscarnet from bone. Postmortem data on several patients in European clinical trials provide evidence that foscarnet does accumulate in bone in humans; however, the extent to which this occurs has not been determined. In animal studies (mice), 40% of an IV dose of foscarnet was deposited in bone in young animals and 7% was deposited in adult animals.

Foscarnet Pharmacokinetic Characteristics		
Parameter	60 mg/kg q 8 h	90 mg/kg q 12 h
C_{max} at steady-state (mcM)	589	623
C_{trough} at steady-state (mcM)	114	63
Volume of distribution (L/kg)	0.41	0.52
Plasma half-life (hr)	4	3.3
Systemic clearance (L/hr)	6.2	7.1
Renal clearance (L/hr)	5.6	6.4
CSF: plasma ratio	0.69[1]	0.68[2]

[1] 50 mg/kg q 8 h for 28 days, samples taken 3 hrs after end of 1 hr infusion.
[2] 90 mg/kg q 12 h for 28 days, samples taken 1 hr after end of 2 hr infusion.

Approximately 80% to 90% of IV foscarnet is excreted unchanged in the urine of patients with normal renal function. Both tubular secretion and glomerular filtration account for urinary elimination of foscarnet.

Renal function impairment –

Pharmacokinetic Parameters After a Single 60 mg/kg Dose of Foscarnet in Four Groups of Adults with Varying Degrees of Renal Function				
Parameter	Group 1 (n=6)	Group 2 (n=6)	Group 3 (n=6)	Group 4 (n=4)
Creatinine clearance (ml/min)	108	68	34	70
Foscarnet CL (ml/min/kg)	2.13	1.33	0.45	0.43
Foscarnet half-life (hr)	1.93	3.35	13	25.3

Group 1 patients had normal renal function, defined as a creatinine clearance (Ccr) of > 80 ml/min, Group 2 Ccr was 50 to 80 ml/min, Group 3 Ccr was 25 to 49 ml/min and Group 4 Ccr was 10 to 24 ml/min.

Total systemic clearance (CL) of foscarnet decreased and half-life increased with diminishing renal function (as expressed by creatinine clearance). Based on these observations, it is necessary to modify the dosage of foscarnet in patients with renal impairment.

▶*Clinical trials:*

CMV retinitis – A prospective, randomized, controlled clinical trial was conducted in 24 patients with AIDS and CMV retinitis. Patients received induction treatment of 60 mg/kg every 8 hours for 3 weeks, followed by maintenance treatment with 90 mg/kg/day until retinitis progression (appearance of a new lesion or advancement of the border of a posterior lesion > 750 microns in diameter). The 13 patients randomized to treatment with foscarnet had a significant delay in progression of CMV retinitis compared with untreated controls. Median times to retinitis progression from study entry were 93 days (range, 21 to > 364) and 22 days (range, 7 to 42), respectively.

In another prospective clinical trial of CMV retinitis in AIDS patients, 33 were treated with 2 to 3 weeks of foscarnet induction (60 mg/kg 3 times daily) and then randomized to two maintenance dose groups, 90 and 120 mg/kg/day. Median times from study entry to retinitis progression were 96 days (range, 14 to > 176) and 140 days (range, 16 to > 233), respectively. This was not statistically significant.

In another study, 107 patients with newly diagnosed CMV retinitis were randomized to treatment with foscarnet (induction 60 mg/kg twice a day for 2 weeks, maintenance 90 mg/kg once daily) and 127 were randomized to treatment with ganciclovir (induction 5 mg/kg twice a day, maintenance 5 mg/kg once daily). The median time to progression on the two drugs was similar (foscarnet 59 days and ganciclovir 56 days).

Relapsed CMV retinitis – A randomized, open-label comparison of foscarnet or ganciclovir monotherapy to the combination of both drugs for the treatment of persistently active or relapsed CMV retinitis in patients with AIDS was conducted. Subjects were randomized to one of three treatments: Foscarnet 90 mg/kg twice a day induction followed by 120 mg/kg once daily maintenance (Fos), ganciclovir 5 mg/kg twice a

day induction followed by 10 mg/kg once daily maintenance (Gcv) or the combination of the two drugs, consisting of continuation of the subject's current therapy and induction dosing of the other drug followed by maintenance with foscarnet 90 mg/kg once daily plus ganciclovir 5 mg/kg once daily. Assessment of retinitis progression was performed by masked evaluation of retinal photographs. The median times to retinitis progression or death were 39 days for the foscarnet group, 61 days for the ganciclovir group and 105 days for the combination group. For the alternative endpoint of retinitis progression (censoring on death) the median times were 39 days for the foscarnet group, 61 days for the ganciclovir group and 132 days for the combination group. Because of censoring on death, the latter analysis may overestimate the treatment effect. Treatment modifications caused by toxicity were more common in the combination group than in the foscarnet or ganciclovir monotherapy groups.

HSV infections – A prospective, comparative trial was conducted in 25 AIDS patients with mucocutaneous, acyclovir-resistant HSV infections. Fourteen patients were randomized to either foscarnet (n = 8) at a dose of 40 mg/kg 3 times daily or vidarabine (n = 6) at a dose of 15 mg/kg/day; eleven patients received foscarnet without being randomized. Lesions in the eight patients randomized to foscarnet healed after 11 to 25 days; seven of the eleven nonrandomized patients treated with foscarnet had healed lesions in 10 to 30 days. Vidarabine was discontinued because of intolerance or poor therapeutic response. Five of these patients were subsequently treated with foscarnet and two had healed lesions in 15 and 24 days. In a second prospective, randomized trial, 40 AIDS patients and three bone marrow transplant recipients with mucocutaneous, acyclovir-resistant HSV infections were randomized to receive foscarnet at a dose of either 40 mg/kg twice daily or three times daily. Fifteen of the 43 patients had healing of their lesions in 11 to 72 days with no difference in response between the two treatment groups.

Contraindications

Hypersensitivity to foscarnet.

Warnings

▶*Mineral and electrolyte imbalances:* Foscarnet has been associated with changes in serum electrolytes including hypocalcemia (15%), hypophosphatemia (8%), hyperphosphatemia (6%), hypomagnesemia (15%) and hypokalemia (16%). Foscarnet is associated with a dose-related decrease in ionized calcium, which may not be reflected in total serum calcium. This effect is most likely related to foscarnet's chelation of divalent metal ions such as calcium. Therefore, advise patients to report symptoms of low ionized calcium such as perioral tingling, numbness in the extremities and paresthesias. Be prepared to treat these as well as severe manifestations of electrolyte abnormalities, such as tetany, cardiac disturbances and seizures. The rate of infusion may affect the decrease in ionized calcium; slowing the rate may decrease or prevent symptoms.

Particular caution and careful management of serum electrolytes is advised in patients with altered calcium or other electrolyte levels before treatment and especially in those with neurologic or cardiac abnormalities and those receiving other drugs known to influence minerals and electrolytes.

▶*Accidental exposure:* Accidental skin and eye contact with foscarnet sodium solution may cause local irritation and burning sensation. If accidental contact occurs, flush the exposed area with water.

▶*Seizures:* Foscarnet was associated with seizures in 18/189 (10%) of AIDS patients in five controlled studies. Several cases were associated with death. Three cases were associated with overdoses of foscarnet (see Overdosage). Risk factors associated with seizures include impaired baseline renal function, low total serum calcium and underlying CNS conditions.

▶*Other CMV infections:* Safety and efficacy have not been established for the treatment of other CMV infections (eg, pneumonitis, gastroenteritis); congenital or neonatal CMV disease; non-immunocompromised individuals.

▶*Other HSV infections:* Safety and efficacy have not been established for treatment of other HSV infections (eg, retinitis, encephalitis); congenital or neonatal HSV disease; or HSV in non-immunocompromised individuals.

▶*Nephrotoxicity:* The major toxicity of foscarnet is renal impairment, which occurs to some degree in most patients. Approximately 33% of patients with AIDS and CMV retinitis who received IV foscarnet without adequate hydration in clinical studies developed significant impairment of renal function, manifested by a rise in serum creatinine concentration to ≥ 2 mg/dl. Therefore, use foscarnet with caution in all patients, especially those with a history of renal function impairment. Patients vary in their sensitivity to foscarnet-induced nephrotoxicity, and initial renal function may not be predictive of the potential for drug-induced renal impairment.

Renal impairment is most likely to become clinically evident during the second week of induction therapy but may occur at any time during treatment; therefore, monitor renal function carefully (see Monitoring).

Elevations in serum creatinine are usually reversible following discontinuation or dose adjustment. Because of foscarnet's potential to cause renal impairment, dose adjustment based on serum creatinine is nec-

FOSCARNET SODIUM (Phosphonoformic acid; PFA)

essary. Hydration may reduce the risk of nephrotoxicity. It is recommended that 750 to 1000 ml of normal saline or 5% dextrose solution be given prior to the first infusion of foscarnet to establish diuresis. With subsequent infusions, 750 to 1000 ml of hydration fluid should be given with 90 to 120 mg/kg of foscarnet, and 500 ml with 40 to 60 mg/kg of foscarnet. Hydration fluid may need to be decreased if clinically warranted. After the first dose, administer the hydration fluid concurrently with each infusion of foscarnet.

➤*Mutagenesis:* Foscarnet showed genotoxic effects in the BALB/3T3 in vitro transformation assay at concentrations > 0.5 mcg/ml and an increased frequency of chromosome aberrations in the sister chromatid exchange assay at 1000 mcg/ml. A high dose of foscarnet (350 mg/kg) caused an increase in micronucleated polychromatic erythrocytes in vivo in mice at doses that produced exposures (AUC) comparable to that anticipated clinically.

➤*Elderly:* No studies of the efficacy or safety of foscarnet in people > 65 years of age have been conducted. Because these individuals frequently have reduced glomerular filtration, pay particular attention to assessing renal function before and during administration.

➤*Pregnancy: Category C.* Daily SC doses up to 75 mg/kg administered to rabbits and 150 mg/kg administered to rats during gestation caused an increase in the frequency of skeletal anomalies/variations. On the basis of estimated drug exposure (as measured by AUC), the 150 mg/kg dose in rats and 75 mg/kg dose in rabbits were ≈ 1/8 (rat) and 1/3 (rabbit) the estimated maximal daily human exposure. These studies are inadequate to define the potential teratogenicity at levels to which women will be exposed. There are no adequate and well controlled studies in pregnant women. Use during pregnancy only if clearly needed.

➤*Lactation:* In lactating rats administered 75 mg/kg, foscarnet was excreted in maternal milk at concentrations three times higher than peak maternal blood concentrations. It is not known whether foscarnet is excreted in breast milk. Exercise caution if foscarnet is administered to a nursing woman.

➤*Children:* The safety and efficacy of foscarnet in children have not been studied. Foscarnet is deposited in teeth and bone, and deposition is greater in young and growing animals. Foscarnet adversely affects development of tooth enamel in mice and rats. The effects of this deposition on skeletal development have not been studied. Because deposition in human bone also occurs, it is likely that it does so to a greater degree in developing bone in children. Administer to children only after careful evaluation and only if the potential benefits for treatment outweigh the risks.

Precautions

➤*Monitoring:*

Renal – The majority of patients will experience some decrease in renal function due to foscarnet administration. Therefore, it is recommended that Ccr, either measured or estimated using the modified Cockcroft and Gault equation based on serum creatinine, be determined at baseline, 2 to 3 times/week during induction therapy and at least once every 1 to 2 weeks during maintenance therapy, with foscarnet dose adjusted accordingly (see Administration and Dosage). More frequent monitoring may be required for some patients. It is also recommended that a 24 hour Ccr be determined at baseline and periodically thereafter to ensure correct dosing. Discontinue foscarnet if Ccr drops to < 0.4 ml/min/kg.

Electrolytes – Because of foscarnet's propensity to chelate divalent metal ions and alter levels of serum electrolytes, closely monitor patients for such changes. It is recommended that a schedule similar to that recommended for serum creatinine (see above) be used to monitor serum calcium, magnesium, potassium and phosphorus. Particular caution is advised in patients with decreased total serum calcium or other electrolyte levels before treatment, as well as in patients with neurologic or cardiac abnormalities, and in patients receiving other drugs known to influence serum calcium levels. Correct any clinically significant metabolic changes. Patients who experience mild (eg, perioral numbness or paresthesias) or severe symptoms (eg, seizures) of electrolyte abnormalities should have serum electrolyte and mineral levels assessed as close in time to the event as possible. Carefully monitor electrolytes, including calcium and magnesium (see Monitoring).

Careful monitoring and appropriate management of electrolytes, calcium, magnesium and creatinine are of particular importance in patients with conditions that may predispose them to seizures (see Warnings).

➤*Toxicity/local irritation:* Infuse solutions containing foscarnet only into veins with adequate blood flow to permit rapid dilution and distribution and avoid local irritation (see Administration and Dosage). Local irritation and ulcerations of penile epithelium have occurred in male patients receiving foscarnet, possibly related to the presence of the drug in urine. One case of vulvovaginal ulceration has occurred. Adequate hydration with close attention to personal hygiene may minimize the occurrence of such events.

➤*Granulocytopenia:* This has been reported in 17% of patients receiving foscarnet in controlled studies; however, only 1% (2/189) were terminated from these studies because of neutropenia.

➤*Anemia:* Occurred in 33% of patients.

Drug Interactions

Foscarnet Drug Interactions

Precipitant drug	Object drug*		Description
Nephrotoxic drugs (eg, aminoglycosides, amphotericin B, IV pentamidine)	Foscarnet	↑	Because of foscarnet's tendency to cause renal impairment, avoid the use of foscarnet in combination with potentially nephrotoxic drugs unless the potential benefits outweigh the risks to the patient.
Foscarnet	Ganciclovir	↔	The pharmacokinetics of foscarnet and ganciclovir were not altered in 13 patients receiving either concomitant therapy or daily alternating therapy for maintenance of CMV disease.
Foscarnet	Pentamidine	↑	Concomitant treatment of four patients with foscarnet and IV pentamidine may have caused hypocalcemia; one patient died with severe hypocalcemia. Toxicity associated with concomitant use of aerosolized pentamidine has not been reported.
Foscarnet	Calcium	↓	Foscarnet decreases serum levels of ionized calcium. Exercise particular caution when other drugs known to influence serum calcium levels are used concurrently.

* ↑ = Object drug increased. ↓ = Object drug decreased. ↔ = Undetermined effect.

Adverse Reactions

The most frequently reported events were: Fever (65%); nausea (47%); anemia (33%); diarrhea (30%); abnormal renal function, decreased Ccr (27%); vomiting, headache (26%); seizure (10%) (see Warnings and Precautions).

Adverse events categorized as "severe" were: Death (14%); abnormal renal function (14%); marrow suppression (10%); anemia (9%); seizures (7%). Although death was specifically attributed to foscarnet in only one case, other complications of foscarnet (eg, renal impairment, electrolyte abnormalities, seizures) may have contributed to patient deaths (see Warnings and Precautions).

➤*Cardiovascular:* Hypertension, palpitations, ECG abnormalities including sinus tachycardia, first degree sinus AV block and non-specific ST-T segment changes, hypotension, flushing, cerebrovascular disorder (1% to 5%); cardiac arrest, arrhythmias (< 1%).

➤*CNS:* Headache, paresthesia, dizziness, involuntary muscle contractions, hypoesthesia, neuropathy, seizures (including grand mal; see Warnings) (≥ 5%); tremor, ataxia, dementia, stupor, generalized spasms, sensory disturbances, meningitis, aphasia, abnormal coordination, leg cramps, EEG abnormalities (1% to 5%); coma (< 1%).

➤*Dermatologic:* Rash, increased sweating (≥ 5%); pruritus, skin ulceration, seborrhea, erythematous rash, maculopapular rash, skin discoloration (1% to 5%).

➤*Endocrine:* Antidiuretic hormone disorders (< 1%).

➤*GI:* Anorexia, nausea, diarrhea, vomiting, abdominal pain (≥ 5%); constipation, dysphagia, dyspepsia, rectal hemorrhage, dry mouth, melena, flatulence, ulcerative stomatitis, pancreatitis (1% to 5%); increased amylase (< 1%).

➤*GU:* Alterations in renal function, including increased serum creatinine, decreased Ccr and abnormal renal function (see Warnings) (≥ 5%); albuminuria, dysuria, polyuria, urethral disorder, urinary retention, urinary tract infections, acute renal failure, nocturia (1% to 5%); hematuria (< 1%).

➤*Hematologic:* Anemia, granulocytopenia, leukopenia (≥ 5%); thrombocytopenia, platelet abnormalities, thrombosis, WBC abnormalities, lymphadenopathy (1% to 5%); pancytopenia (< 1%).

➤*Hepatic:* Abnormal A-G ratio, abnormal hepatic function, increased AST and ALT (1% to 5%).

Injection site – 7

Injection site pain or inflammation (1% to 5%).

➤*Metabolic/Nutritional:* Mineral/electrolyte imbalances (see Warnings), including hypokalemia, hypocalcemia, hypomagnesemia, hypo- or hyperphosphatemia (≥ 5%); hyponatremia, decreased weight, increased alkaline phosphatase, increased LDH, increased BUN, acidosis, cachexia, thirst (1% to 5%); dehydration, increased creatine phosphokinase, hypoproteinemia (< 1%).

➤*Musculoskeletal:* Arthralgia, myalgia (1% to 5%).

Neoplasms – Lymphoma-like disorder, sarcoma (1% to 5%).

➤*Psychiatric:* Depression, confusion, anxiety (≥ 5%); insomnia, somnolence, nervousness, amnesia, agitation, aggressive reaction, hallucination (1% to 5%).

FOSCARNET SODIUM (Phosphonoformic acid; PFA)

►*Respiratory:* Coughing, dyspnea (≥ 5%); pneumonia, sinusitis, pharyngitis, rhinitis, respiratory disorders or insufficiency, pulmonary infiltration, stridor, pneumothorax, hemoptysis, bronchospasm (1% to 5%).

►*Special senses:* Vision abnormalities (≥ 5%); taste perversions, eye abnormalities, eye pain, conjunctivitis (1% to 5%).

►*Miscellaneous:* Fever, fatigue, rigors, asthenia, malaise, pain, infection, sepsis, death (≥ 5%); back/chest pain, edema, influenza-like symptoms, bacterial/fungal infections, facial edema, moniliasis, abscess (1% to 5%).

Overdosage

►*Symptoms:* In controlled clinical trials, overdosage was reported in 10 patients. All 10 patients experienced adverse events, and all except 1 made a complete recovery. One patient died after receiving a total daily dose of 12.5 g for 3 days instead of the intended 10.9 g. The patient suffered a grand mal seizure, became comatose, and died 3 days later. The cause of death was listed as respiratory/cardiac arrest. The other 9 patients received doses ranging from 1.14 to 8 times their recommended doses with an average of 4 times their recommended doses. Overall, 3 patients had seizures, 3 had renal function impairment, 4 had paresthesias either in limbs or periorally, and 5 had documented electrolyte disturbances primarily involving calcium and phosphate.

►*Treatment:* There is no specific antidote. Hemodialysis and hydration may be of benefit in reducing drug plasma levels in patients who receive an overdosage, but these have not been evaluated in a clinical trial setting. Observe the patient for signs and symptoms of renal impairment and electrolyte imbalance. Institute medical treatment if clinically warranted. Refer to General Management of Acute Overdosage.

Patient Information

►*CMV retinitis:* Foscarnet is not a cure for CMV retinitis; patients may continue to experience progression of retinitis during or following treatment. Regular ophthalmologic examinations are necessary.

►*HSV infections:* Foscarnet is not a cure for HSV infections. While complete healing may occur, relapse occurs in most patients. Because relapse may be due to acyclovir-sensitive HSV, sensitivity testing of the viral isolate is advised. Repeated treatment with foscarnet has led to development of resistance associated with poorer response. In this case, sensitivity testing of the viral isolate is also advised.

The major toxicities of foscarnet are renal impairment, electrolyte disturbances, and seizures; dose modifications and possibly discontinuation may be required.

Close monitoring while on therapy is essential. Advise patients of the importance of perioral tingling, numbness in the extremities, or paresthesias during or after infusion as possible symptoms of electrolyte abnormalities. Should such symptoms occur, stop the infusion, obtain appropriate laboratory samples for assessment of electrolyte concentrations, and consult a physician before resuming treatment. The rate of infusion must be ≤ 1 mg/kg/min.

The potential for renal impairment may be minimized by accompanying administration with hydration adequate to establish and maintain diuresis during dosing.

GANCICLOVIR (DHPG)

Rx	**Ganciclovir** (Ranbaxy)	**Capsules:** 250 mg	(RX 636). Green. In 180s.
Rx	**Cytovene** (Roche)		(Roche Cytovene 250 mg). Green. In 180s.
Rx	**Ganciclovir** (Ranbaxy)	**Capsules:** 500 mg	(RX 637). Yellow/Green. In 180s.
Rx	**Cytovene** (Roche)		(Roche Cytovene 500 mg). Yellow/green. In 180s.
Rx	**Cytovene** (Roche)	**Powder for injection, lyophilized:** 500 mg/vial ganciclovir (as sodium)	46 mg sodium. In 10 mL vials.

WARNING

The clinical toxicity of ganciclovir includes granulocytopenia, anemia, and thrombocytopenia. In animal studies, ganciclovir was carcinogenic, teratogenic, and caused aspermatogenesis.

Ganciclovir IV is indicated for use only in the treatment of cytomegalovirus (CMV) retinitis in immunocompromised patients and for the prevention of CMV disease in transplant patients at risk for CMV disease.

Ganciclovir capsules are indicated only for prevention of CMV disease in patients with advanced HIV infection at risk for CMV disease, for maintenance treatment of CMV retinitis in immunocompromised patients, and for prevention of CMV disease in solid organ transplant recipients.

Because oral ganciclovir is associated with a risk of more rapid rate of CMV retinitis progression, use as maintenance treatment only in those patients for whom this risk is balanced by the benefit associated with avoiding daily IV infusions.

Indications

►*IV:*

CMV retinitis – Treatment of CMV retinitis in immunocompromised patients, including patients with AIDS.

CMV disease – Prevention of CMV disease in transplant recipients at risk for CMV disease.

►*Oral:*

CMV retinitis – Alternative to the IV formulation for maintenance treatment of CMV retinitis in immunocompromised patients, including patients with AIDS, in whom retinitis is stable following appropriate induction therapy, and for whom the risk of more rapid progression is balanced by the benefit associated with avoiding daily IV infusions.

CMV disease – Prevention of CMV disease in solid organ transplant recipients and in individuals with advanced HIV infection at risk for developing CMV disease.

►*Unlabeled uses:* Ganciclovir may be beneficial in CMV pneumonia in organ transplant patients, CMV gastroenteritis in patients with irritable bowel disease, and CMV pneumonitis in patients.

Administration and Dosage

►*Approved by the FDA:* 1989.

Do not exceed the recommended dose.

►*IV:* Do not administer by rapid or bolus IV injection. The toxicity may be increased as a result of excessive plasma levels. Do not exceed the recommended infusion rate. IM or SC injection of reconstituted ganciclovir may result in severe tissue irritation because of high pH.

►*CMV retinitis (normal renal function):*

Induction – The recommended initial dose is 5 mg/kg (given IV at a constant rate over 1 hour) every 12 hours for 14 to 21 days. Do not use oral ganciclovir for induction treatment.

Maintenance –

   IV: Following induction treatment, the recommended maintenance dose is 5 mg/kg given as a constant rate IV infusion over 1 hour once daily 7 days per week, or 6 mg/kg once daily 5 days/week.

   Oral: Following induction treatment, the recommended maintenance dose of oral ganciclovir is 1000 mg 3 times daily with food. Alternatively, the dosing regimen of 500 mg 6 times daily every 3 hours with food, during waking hours, may be used.

For patients who experience progression of CMV retinitis while receiving maintenance treatment with either formulation of ganciclovir, reinduction treatment is recommended.

►*Prevention of CMV disease in transplant recipients with normal renal function:*

IV – The recommended initial dose of IV ganciclovir for patients with normal renal function is 5 mg/kg (given IV at a constant rate over 1 hour) every 12 hours for 7 to 14 days, followed by 5 mg/kg once daily 7 days/week or 6 mg/kg once daily 5 days/week.

Oral – The recommended prophylactic dosage is 1000 mg 3 times daily with food.

The duration of treatment with ganciclovir in transplant recipients is dependent on the duration and degree of immunosuppression. In controlled clinical trials in bone marrow allograft recipients, IV ganciclovir treatment was continued until day 100 to 120 post-transplantation. CMV disease occurred in several patients who discontinued treatment with IV ganciclovir prematurely. In heart allograft recipients, the onset of newly diagnosed CMV disease occurred after treatment with IV ganciclovir was stopped at day 28 post-transplant, suggesting that continued dosing may be necessary to prevent late occurrence of CMV disease in this patient population.

►*Prevention of CMV disease in patients with advanced HIV infection and normal renal function:* The recommended dose of ganciclovir capsules is 1000 mg 3 times daily with food.

►*Renal impairment:*

IV – Refer to the following table for recommended doses and adjust the dosing interval as indicated.

IV Ganciclovir Dose in Renal Impairment				
Ccr (mL/min)	Ganciclovir induction dose (mg/kg)	Dosing interval (hours)	Ganciclovir maintenance dose (mg/kg)	Dosing interval (hours)
≥ 70	5	12	5	24
50 to 69	2.5	12	2.5	24
25 to 49	2.5	24	1.25	24

GANCICLOVIR (DHPG)

IV Ganciclovir Dose in Renal Impairment					
Ccr (mL/min)	Ganciclovir induction dose (mg/kg)	Dosing interval (hours)	Ganciclovir maintenance dose (mg/kg)	Dosing interval (hours)
10 to 24	1.25	24	0.625	24
< 10	1.25	3 times/week following hemodialysis	0.625	3 times/week following hemodialysis

Hemodialysis: Dosing for patients undergoing hemodialysis should not exceed 1.25 mg/kg 3 times/week, following each hemodialysis session. Give shortly after completion of the hemodialysis session, because hemodialysis reduces plasma levels by ≈ 50%.

Oral – In patients with renal impairment, modify the dose of oral ganciclovir as follows:

Oral Ganciclovir Dose in Renal Impairment	
Ccr (mL/min)	Ganciclovir doses
≥ 70	1000 mg TID or 500 mg q 3 hr, 6×/day
50 to 69	1500 mg QD or 500 mg TID
25 to 49	1000 mg QD or 500 mg BID
10 to 24	500 mg QD
< 10	500 mg 3 times/week, following hemodialysis

➤*Patient monitoring:* Because of the frequency of granulocytopenia, anemia, and thrombocytopenia, it is recommended that complete blood counts (CBCs) and platelet counts be performed frequently, especially in patients in whom ganciclovir or other nucleoside analogs have previously resulted in cytopenia, or in whom neutrophil counts are < 1000/mcL at the beginning of treatment. Patients should have serum creatinine or creatinine clearance (Ccr) values followed carefully to allow for dosage adjustment in renally impaired patients.

➤*Reduction of dose:* Dose reductions are required with IV therapy and should be considered with oral therapy for patients with renal impairment and for those with neutropenia, anemia, or thrombocytopenia. Do not administer in severe neutropenia (ANC < 500/mcL) or severe thrombocytopenia (platelets < 25,000/mcL).

➤*Preparation of IV solution:* Each 10 mL clear glass vial contains ganciclovir sodium equivalent to 500 mg ganciclovir and 46 mg of sodium. Prepare the contents of the vial for administration in the following manner:

Reconstituted solution –
1.) Reconstitute lyophilized ganciclovir by injecting 10 mL of Sterile Water for Injection into the vial. Do not use bacteriostatic water for injection containing parabens; it is incompatible with ganciclovir and may cause precipitation.
2.) Shake the vial to dissolve the drug.
3.) Visually inspect the reconstituted solution for particulate matter and discoloration prior to proceeding with infusion solution. Discard the vial if particulate matter or discoloration is observed.
4.) Reconstituted solution in the vial is stable at room temperature for 12 hours. Do not refrigerate.

Infusion solution – Based on patient weight, remove the appropriate volume of the reconstituted solution (ganciclovir concentration 50 mg/mL) from the vial and add to an acceptable (see below) infusion fluid (typically 100 mL) for delivery over the course of 1 hour. Infusion concentrations > 10 mg/mL are not recommended. The following infusion fluids have been determined to be chemically and physically compatible with ganciclovir IV solution: 0.9% Sodium Chloride, 5% Dextrose, Ringer's Injection, and Lactated Ringer's Injection.

IV ganciclovir, when reconstituted with sterile water for injection, further diluted with 0.9% Sodium Chloride Injection, stored refrigerated at 5°C (41°F) in polyvinyl chloride (PVC) bags, remains physically and chemically stable for 14 days.

➤*Handling and disposal:* Exercise caution in the handling and preparation of ganciclovir. Solutions of IV ganciclovir are alkaline (pH 11). Avoid direct contact with the skin or mucous membranes of the powder contained in ganciclovir capsules or of ganciclovir IV solutions. If such contact occurs, wash thoroughly with soap and water; rinse eyes thoroughly with plain water. Do not open or crush ganciclovir capsules.

Because ganciclovir shares some of the properties of antitumor agents (eg, carcinogenicity, mutagenicity), give consideration to handling and disposal according to guidelines issued for antineoplastic drugs.

➤*Storage/Stability:* Store vials at temperatures < 40°C (104°F). Store capsules between 5° and 25°C (41° and 77°F). Reconstituted solution in the vial is stable at room temperature for 12 hours. Do not refrigerate.

The infusion solution must be used within 24 hours of dilution to reduce the risk of bacterial contamination. Refrigerate the infusion solution. Freezing is not recommended.

Actions

➤*Pharmacology:* Ganciclovir, a synthetic guanine derivative active against CMV, is an acyclic nucleoside analog of 2′-deoxyguanosine that inhibits replication of herpes viruses in vivo. Ganciclovir has been shown to be active against CMV and herpes simplex virus in human clinical studies.

The median concentration of ganciclovir that inhibits the replication of either laboratory strains or clinical isolates of CMV (IC_{50}) has ranged from 0.02 to 3.48 mcg/mL. The relationship of in vitro sensitivity of CMV to ganciclovir and clinical response has not been established. Ganciclovir inhibits mammalian cell proliferation in vitro at higher concentrations; CIC_{50} values range from 30 to 725 mcg/mL. Bone marrow-derived colony-forming cells are more sensitive with CIC_{50} values ranging from 0.028 to 0.7 mcg/mL.

➤*Pharmacokinetics:*

Absorption – The absolute bioavailability of oral ganciclovir under fasting conditions was ≈ 5% and following food it was 6% to 9%. When given with a meal containing 602 calories and 46.5% fat, the steady-state area under serum concentration vs time curve (AUC) increased and there was a significant prolongation of time to peak serum concentrations (see Drug Interactions).

At the end of a 1-hour IV infusion of 5 mg/kg, total AUC ranged between 22.1 and 26.8 mcg•hr/mL and C_{max} ranged between 8.27 and 9 mcg/mL.

Distribution – The steady-state volume of distribution after IV administration was 0.74 L/kg. Cerebrospinal fluid concentrations obtained 0.25 to 5.67 hours postdose in 3 patients who received 2.5 mg/kg ganciclovir IV every 8 or 12 hours ranged from 0.31 to 0.68 mcg/mL, representing 24% to 70% of the respective plasma concentrations. Binding to plasma proteins was 1% to 2% over ganciclovir concentrations of 0.5 and 51 mcg/mL.

For ganciclovir capsules, no correlation was observed between AUC and reciprocal weight (range, 55 to 128 kg); oral dosing according to weight is not required.

Metabolism – Following oral administration of a single 1000 mg dose, 86% of the administered dose was recovered in the feces, and 5% was recovered in the urine. No metabolite accounted for > 1% to 2% recovered in urine or feces.

Excretion – When administered IV, ganciclovir exhibits linear pharmacokinetics over the range of 1.6 to 5 mg/kg. When administered orally, it exhibits linear kinetics up to a total daily dose of 4 g/day. Renal excretion of unchanged drug by glomerular filtration and active tubular secretion is the major route of elimination. In patients with normal renal function, 91.3% of IV ganciclovir was recovered unmetabolized in the urine. Systemic clearance of IV ganciclovir was 3.52 mL/min/kg while renal clearance was 3.2 mL/min/kg, accounting for 91% of the systemic clearance. After oral administration, steady state is achieved within 24 hours. Renal clearance following oral administration was 3.1 mL/min/kg. Half-life was 3.5 hours following IV administration and 4.8 hours following oral use.

Special populations –
Renal function impairment: Because the major elimination pathway for ganciclovir is renal, dosage reductions according to Ccr are required for the IV formulation and should be considered for oral ganciclovir (see Administration and Dosage). The pharmacokinetics following IV administration were evaluated in 10 immunocompromised patients with renal impairment who received doses ranging from 1.25 to 5 mg/kg.

IV Ganciclovir Pharmacokinetics in Patients with Renal Impairment			
Estimated Ccr (mL/min)	Dose (mg/kg)	Clearance (mL/min)	Half-life (hours)
50 to 79 (n = 4)	3.2 to 5	128	4.6
25 to 49 (n = 3)	3 to 5	57	4.4
< 25 (n = 3)	1.25 to 5	30	10.7

The pharmacokinetics of ganciclovir following oral administration were evaluated in 44 patients who were either solid organ transplant recipients or HIV positive. Apparent oral clearance of ganciclovir decreased and $AUC_{0-24\ hr}$ increased with diminishing renal function (as expressed by Ccr). Based on these observations, it is necessary to modify the dosage of ganciclovir in patients with renal impairment (see Administration and Dosage).

Hemodialysis reduces plasma concentrations of ganciclovir by ≈ 50% after IV and oral administration.

Race: The effects of race were studied in subjects receiving a dose regimen of 1000 mg every 8 hours. Although the numbers of blacks (16%) and Hispanics (20%) were small, there appeared to be a trend towards a lower steady-state C_{max} and $AUC_{0-8\ hr}$ in these subpopulations as compared with whites.

Children: At an IV dose of 4 or 6 mg/kg in 27 neonates (ages 2 to 49 days), the pharmacokinetic parameters were, respectively, C_{max} of 5.5 and 7 mcg/mL, systemic clearance of 3.14 and 3.56 mL/min/kg, and half-life of 2.4 hours for both.

Ganciclovir pharmacokinetics also were studied in 10 pediatric patients from 9 months to 12 years of age. The pharmacokinetic characteristics of ganciclovir were the same after single and multiple (every 12 hour) IV doses (5 mg/kg). The steady-state volume of distribution was 0.64 ±

GANCICLOVIR (DHPG)

0.22 L/kg, C_{max} was 7.9 ± 3.9 mcg/mL, systemic clearance was 4.7 ± 2.2 mL/min/kg, and $t_{1/2}$ was 2.4 ± 0.7 hours. The pharmacokinetics of IV ganciclovir in pediatric patients are similar to those observed in adults.

➤*Clinical trials:* In a controlled, randomized study, immediate treatment with ganciclovir IV was compared with delayed treatment in 42 patients with AIDS and peripheral CMV retinitis; 35 of 42 patients (13 in the immediate-treatment group and 22 in the delayed-treatment group) were included in the analysis of time to retinitis progression. Based on masked assessment of fundus photographs, the mean (95% CI) and median (95% CI) times to progression of retinitis were 66 days (39, 94) and 50 days (40, 84), respectively, in the immediate-treatment group compared to 19 days (11, 27) and 13.5 days (8, 18), respectively, in the delayed-treatment group.

Contraindications

Hypersensitivity to ganciclovir or acyclovir.

Warnings

➤*CMV disease:* Safety and efficacy have not been established for congenital or neonatal CMV disease, treatment of established CMV disease other than retinitis, or use in nonimmunocompromised individuals. The safety and efficacy of oral ganciclovir have not been established for treating any manifestation of CMV disease other than maintenance treatment of CMV retinitis.

➤*Diagnosis of CMV retinitis:* The diagnosis should be made by indirect ophthalmoscopy. Other conditions in the differential diagnosis of CMV retinitis include candidiasis, toxoplasmosis, histoplasmosis, retinal scars, and cotton wool spots, any of which may produce a retinal appearance similar to CMV. The diagnosis may be supported by a culture of CMV from urine, blood, throat, but a negative CMV culture does not rule out CMV retinitis.

➤*Retinal detachment:* This has been observed in subjects with CMV retinitis both before and after initiation of therapy with ganciclovir. Its relationship to therapy is unknown. Retinal detachment occurred in 11% of patients treated with IV ganciclovir and in 8% of patients treated with oral ganciclovir. Patients with CMV retinitis should have frequent ophthalmologic evaluations to monitor the status of their retinitis and to detect any other retinal pathology.

➤*Hematologic:* Do not administer if the absolute neutrophil count is < 500 cells/mcL or the platelet count is < 25,000 cells/mcL. Granulocytopenia (neutropenia), anemia, and thrombocytopenia have been observed in patients treated with ganciclovir. The frequency and severity of these events vary widely in different patient populations (see Adverse Reactions). Therefore, use with caution in patients with preexisting cytopenias or with a history of cytopenic reactions to other drugs, chemicals, or irradiation. Granulocytopenia usually occurs during the first or second week of treatment, but may occur at any time during treatment. Cell counts usually begin to recover within 3 to 7 days after discontinuing drug. Colony-stimulating factors have increased neutrophil and WBC counts in patients receiving IV ganciclovir for CMV retinitis.

➤*Renal function impairment:* Use ganciclovir with caution. Half-life and plasma/serum concentrations of ganciclovir will be increased because of reduced renal clearance (see Administration and Dosage).

If renal function is impaired, dosage adjustments are required for ganciclovir IV and should be considered for oral ganciclovir. Base such adjustments on measured or estimated Ccr values.

Hemodialysis reduces plasma levels of ganciclovir by ≈ 50%.

➤*Carcinogenesis:* In mice given daily oral doses of 1000 mg/kg, there was a significant increase in the incidence of tumors in the preputial gland of males, nonglandular mucosa of the stomach of males and females, and reproductive tissues (ovaries, uterus, mammary glands, clitoral gland, vagina) and liver in females. A slight increased incidence of tumors occurred in the preputial and harderian glands (males), nonglandular mucosa (males and females) of the stomach, and liver (females) in mice given 20 mg/kg/day. No carcinogenic effect was observed in mice administered ganciclovir at 1 mg/kg/day (estimated as 0.01 times the human dose based on AUC comparison). Except for histiocytic sarcoma of the liver, ganciclovir-induced tumors were generally of epithelial or vascular origin. Although the forestomach, preputial, clitoral, and harderian glands of mice do not have human counterparts, ganciclovir should be considered a potential carcinogen in humans.

➤*Mutagenesis:* Because of the mutagenic and teratogenic potential of ganciclovir, advise women of childbearing potential to use effective contraception during treatment. Similarly, advise men to practice barrier contraception during and for ≥ 90 days following treatment with ganciclovir.

Ganciclovir increased mutations in mouse lymphoma cells and DNA damage in human lymphocytes in vitro at concentrations between 50 to 500 and 250 to 2000 mcg/mL, respectively. In the mouse micronucleus assay, ganciclovir was clastogenic at doses of 150 and 500 mg/kg (IV) (2.8 to 10 times human exposure based on AUC), but not 50 mg/kg (exposure approximately comparable to the human based on AUC). Ganciclovir was not mutagenic in the Ames Salmonella assay at concentrations of 500 to 5000 mcg/mL.

➤*Fertility impairment:* Animal data indicate that ganciclovir causes inhibition of spermatogenesis and subsequent infertility. These effects were reversible at lower doses and irreversible at higher doses. Although data in humans have not been obtained regarding this effect, it is considered probable that ganciclovir, at the recommended doses, causes temporary or permanent inhibition of spermatogenesis. Animal data also indicate that suppression of fertility in females may occur.

Ganciclovir caused decreased mating behavior, decreased fertility, and an increased incidence of embryolethality in female mice following IV doses of 90 mg/kg/day (≈ 1.7 times the mean drug exposure in humans following the dose of 5 mg/kg, based on AUC comparisons). Ganciclovir caused decreased fertility in male mice and hypospermatogenesis in mice and dogs following daily oral or IV administration of doses ranging from 0.2 to 10 mg/kg. Systemic drug exposure (AUC) at the lowest dose showing toxicity in each species ranged from 0.03 to 0.1 times the AUC of the recommended human IV dose.

➤*Elderly:* The pharmacokinetic profile in elderly patients has not been established. Because elderly individuals frequently have a reduced glomerular filtration rate, pay particular attention to assessing renal function before and during administration of ganciclovir (see Administration and Dosage).

➤*Pregnancy: Category C.* Ganciclovir is embryotoxic in rabbits and mice following IV administration and teratogenic in rabbits. Fetal resorptions were present in ≥ 85% of rabbits and mice administered 2 times the human exposure. Effects observed in rabbits included the following: Fetal growth retardation, embryolethality, teratogenicity, and maternal toxicity. Teratogenic changes included cleft palate, anophthalmia/microphthalmia, aplastic organs (kidney and pancreas), hydrocephaly and brachygnathia. In mice, effects observed were maternal/fetal toxicity and embryolethality.

Daily IV doses administered to female mice prior to mating, during gestation, and during lactation caused hypoplasia of the testes and seminal vesicles in the month-old male offspring, as well as pathologic changes in the nonglandular region of the stomach.

Ganciclovir may be teratogenic or embryotoxic at dose levels recommended for human use. There are no adequate and well-controlled studies in pregnant women. Use during pregnancy only if the potential benefits justify the potential risk to the fetus.

➤*Lactation:* It is not known whether ganciclovir is excreted in breast milk. However, because carcinogenic and teratogenic effects occurred in animals treated with ganciclovir, the possibility of serious adverse reactions from ganciclovir in nursing infants is considered likely. Instruct mothers to discontinue nursing if they are receiving ganciclovir. The minimal interval before nursing can safely be resumed after the last dose of ganciclovir is unknown.

➤*Children:* Safety and efficacy in children have not been established. The use of ganciclovir in children warrants extreme caution regarding the probability of long-term carcinogenicity and reproductive toxicity. Administer to children only after careful evaluation and only if the potential benefits of treatment outweigh the risks. Oral ganciclovir has not been studied in children < 13 years of age.

There has been very limited clinical experience using IV ganciclovir for the treatment of CMV retinitis in patients < 12 years of age. Two children (9 and 5 years of age) showed improvement or stabilization of retinitis for 23 and 9 months, respectively. These children received induction treatment with 2.5 mg/kg 3 times daily followed by maintenance therapy with 6 to 6.5 mg/kg once a day, 5 to 7 days per week. When retinitis progressed during once-daily maintenance therapy, both children were treated with the 5 mg/kg twice-daily regimen. Two other children (2.5 and 4 years of age) who received similar induction regimens showed only partial or no response to treatment. Another child, a 6-year-old with T-cell dysfunction, showed stabilization of retinitis for 3 months while receiving continuous infusions of IV ganciclovir at doses of 2 to 5 mg/kg/day. Continuous infusion treatment was discontinued due to granulocytopenia.

Eleven of the 72 patients in the placebo-controlled trial in bone marrow transplant recipients were children, ranging from 3 to 10 years of age (5 treated with IV ganciclovir and 6 with placebo). Five of the pediatric patients treated with ganciclovir received 5 mg/kg IV twice daily for up to 7 days; 4 patients went on to receive 5 mg/kg once daily up to day 100 post-transplant. Results were similar to those observed in adult transplant recipients treated with IV ganciclovir. Two of the 6 placebo-treated pediatric patients developed CMV pneumonia vs none of the 5 treated with ganciclovir. The spectrum of adverse events in the pediatric group was similar to that observed in the adult patients.

Precautions

➤*Monitoring:* Because of the frequency of neutropenia, anemia, and thrombocytopenia in patients receiving ganciclovir, it is recommended that CBCs and platelet counts be performed frequently, especially in patients in whom ganciclovir or other nucleoside analogs have previously resulted in cytopenia, or in whom neutrophil counts are < 1000 cells/mcL at the beginning of treatment. Patients should have serum creatinine or Ccr values followed carefully to allow for dosage adjustments in renally impaired patients (see Administration and Dosage).

➤*Large doses/Rapid infusion:* In clinical studies, the maximum single dose administered was 6 mg/kg by IV infusion over 1 hour.

GANCICLOVIR (DHPG)

Larger doses have resulted in increased toxicity. It is likely that more rapid infusions would also result in increased toxicity (see Overdosage).

➤*Phlebitis/Pain at injection site:* Reconstituted solutions of IV ganciclovir have a high pH (pH 11). Despite further dilution in IV fluids, phlebitis or pain may occur at the site of IV infusion. Take care to infuse solutions containing ganciclovir only into veins with adequate blood flow to permit rapid dilution and distribution.

➤*Hydration:* Since ganciclovir is excreted by the kidneys and normal clearance depends on adequate renal function, administration of ganciclovir should be accompanied by adequate hydration.

Drug Interactions

Ganciclovir Drug Interactions			
Precipitant drug	Object drug*		Description
Ganciclovir	Cytotoxic drugs	↑	Cytotoxic drugs that inhibit replication of rapidly dividing cell populations such as bone marrow, spermatogonia, and germinal layers of skin and GI mucosa may have additive toxicity when administered concomitantly with ganciclovir. Therefore, consider the concomitant use of drugs such as dapsone, pentamidine, flucytosine, vincristine, vinblastine, adriamycin, amphotericin B, trimethoprim/sulfamethoxazole combinations, or other nucleoside analogs only if potential benefits outweigh the risks.
Imipenem-cilastatin	Ganciclovir	↑	Generalized seizures occurred in patients who received ganciclovir and imipenem-cilastatin. Do not use these drugs concomitantly unless the potential benefits outweigh the risks.
Nephrotoxic drugs	Ganciclovir	↑	Increases in serum creatinine were observed following concurrent use of ganciclovir and either cyclosporine or amphotericin B.
Probenecid	Ganciclovir	↑	Ganciclovir AUC increased 53% (range, -14% to 299%) in the presence of probenecid. Renal clearance of ganciclovir decreased 22% (range, -54% to -4%), which is consistent with an interaction involving competition for renal tubular secretion.
Ganciclovir	Didanosine	↑	Steady-state didanosine AUC increased 111% (range, 10% to 493%) when didanosine was administered either 2 hours prior to or simultaneously with ganciclovir. A decrease in steady-state ganciclovir AUC of 21% (range, -44% to 5%) was observed when didanosine was administered 2 hours prior to administration of ganciclovir, but ganciclovir AUC was not affected by the presence of didanosine when the 2 drugs were administered simultaneously.
Didanosine	Ganciclovir	↓	
Ganciclovir	Zidovudine	↑	Mean steady-state ganciclovir AUC decreased 17% (range, -52% to 23%) in the presence of zidovudine (100 mg every 4 hours [n = 12]). Steady-state zidovudine AUC increased 19% (range, -11% to 74%) in the presence of ganciclovir. Because both drugs can cause neutropenia and anemia, some patients will not tolerate combination therapy at full dosage.
Zidovudine	Ganciclovir	↓	

* ↑ = Object drug increased. ↓ = Object drug decreased.

➤*Drug/Food interactions:* When ganciclovir was administered orally with food at a total daily dose of 3 g/day (either 500 mg every 3 hours 6 times daily or 1000 mg 3 times daily), the steady-state absorption as measured by AUC and C_{max} were similar following both regimens. When ganciclovir capsules were given with a meal containing 602 calories and 46.5% fat at a dose of 1000 mg every 8 hours to 20 HIV-positive subjects, the steady-state AUC increased by 22% (range, -6% to 68%) and there was a significant prolongation of time to peak serum concentrations (T_{max}) from 1.8 to 3 hours and a higher C_{max} (0.85 vs 0.96 mcg/mL).

Adverse Reactions

➤*AIDS patients:* Three controlled, randomized, phase 3 trials comparing ganciclovir IV with ganciclovir capsules for maintenance treatment of CMV retinitis have been completed. During these trials, ganciclovir (both doseforms) was prematurely discontinued in 9% of subjects because of adverse events. In a placebo-controlled, randomized, phase 3 trial of ganciclovir capsules for prevention of CMV disease in patients with AIDS, treatment was prematurely discontinued because of adverse events, new or worsening intercurrent illnesses, or laboratory abnormalities in 19.5% of subjects treated with ganciclovir capsules and 16% of the subjects receiving placebo.

Selected Laboratory Abnormalities in Trials for Treatment of CMV Retinitis in Oral vs IV Ganciclovir Treatment (%)[1]		
Adverse reaction	Oral (3000 mg/day)[2] (n = 320)	IV (5 mg/kg/day)[3] (n = 175)
Neutropenia (ANC/mcL)		
< 500	18	25
500 to < 750	17	14
750 to < 1000	19	26
Anemia hemoglobin (g/dL)		
< 6.5	2	5
6.5 to < 8	10	16
8 to < 9.5	25	26
Maximum serum creatinine		
≥ 2.5 mg/dL	1	2
≥ 1.5 to < 2.5	12	14

[1] Pooled data from treatment studies, ICM 1653, Study ICM 1774, and Study AVI 034.
[2] Mean time on therapy = 91 days, including allowed reinduction treatment periods.
[3] Mean time on therapy = 103 days, including allowed reinduction treatment periods.

Selected Adverse Reactions Oral vs IV Ganciclovir for Maintenance Treatment of CMV Retinitis (%)		
Adverse reaction	Oral (3000 mg/day) (n = 326)	IV (5 mg/kg/day) (n = 179)
GI		
Diarrhea	41	44
Anorexia	15	14
Vomiting	13	13
Hemic/Lymphatic		
Leukopenia	29	41
Anemia	19	25
Thrombocytopenia	6	6
Miscellaneous		
Fever	38	48
Infection	9	13
Neuropathy	8	9
Chills	7	10
Sepsis	4	15
Sweating	11	12
Pruritus	6	5
Catheter-related[1]		
Total catheter events	6	22
Catheter infection	4	9
Catheter sepsis	1	8

[1] Some of these events also appear under other body systems.

➤*Transplant recipients:*

Granulocytopenia/Thrombocytopenia with IV Ganciclovir in Transplant Recipients (%)				
	Heart allograft[1]		Bone marrow allograft[2]	
Hematologic effect	Ganciclovir (n = 76)	Placebo (n = 73)	Ganciclovir IV (n = 57)	Control (n = 55)
Neutropenia				
Minimum ANC < 500/mcL	4	3	12	6
Minimum ANC 500 to 1000/mcL	3	8	29	17
Total ANC ≤ 1000/mcL	7	11	41	23
Thrombocytopenia				
Platelet count < 25,000/mcL	3	1	32	28
Platelet count 25,000 to 50,000/mcL	5	3	25	37
Total platelet ≤ 50,000/mcL	8	4	57	65

[1] Mean duration of treatment = 28 days.
[2] Mean duration of treatment = 45 days.

GANCICLOVIR (DHPG)

Elevated Serum Creatinine with IV Ganciclovir in Transplant Recipients (%)						
	Heart allograft		Bone marrow allograft[1]			
Maximum serum creatinine levels	Ganciclovir IV (n = 76)	Placebo (n = 73)	Ganciclovir IV (n = 20)	Control (n = 20)	Ganciclovir IV (n = 37)	Placebo (n = 35)
Serum creatinine ≥ 2.5 mg/dL	18	4	20	0	0	0
Serum creatinine ≥ 1.5 to < 2.5 mg/dL	58	69	50	35	43	44

[1] Results of 2 clinical trials.

In 3 out of 4 trials, patients receiving ganciclovir had elevated serum creatinine levels when compared to those receiving placebo. Most patients in these studies also received cyclosporine. Careful monitoring of renal function during therapy with ganciclovir is essential, especially for those patients receiving concomitant agents that may cause nephrotoxicity.

➤*Other adverse reactions:*
Cardiovascular – Phlebitis, hypertension, vasodilation.

CNS – Abnormal dreams, abnormal thinking, anxiety, confusion, depression, dizziness, insomnia, seizures, somnolence, tremor.

Dermatologic – Alopecia, dry skin.

GI – Aphthous stomatitis, abnormal liver function test, dyspepsia, constipation, eructation, dry mouth.

GU – Ccr decreased, kidney failure, kidney function abnormal, urinary frequency.

Metabolic/Nutritional – Increased creatinine, AST, ALT; weight loss.

Musculoskeletal – Arthralgia, leg cramps, myalgia, myasthenia.

Respiratory – Cough increased, dyspnea.

Special senses – Abnormal vision, taste perversion, tinnitus, vitreous disorder.

Miscellaneous – Asthenia, headache, injection site inflammation, pain, abdomen enlarged, chest pain, edema, malaise, pancytopenia.

The following adverse reactions may be fatal: Pancreatitis, sepsis, GI perforation, and multiple organ failure.

Postmarketing – Acidosis, allergic reaction, anaphylactic reaction, arthritis, bronchospasm, cardiac arrest, cardiac conduction abnormality, cataracts, cholelithiasis, cholestasis, congenital anomaly, dry eyes, dysphasia, elevated triglyceride levels, encephalopathy, exfoliative dermatitis, extrapyramidal reaction, facial palsy, hallucinations, hemolytic anemia, hemolytic uremic syndrome, hepatic failure, hepatitis, hypercalcemia, hyponatremia, inappropriate serum ADH, infertility, intestinal ulceration, intracranial hypertension, irritability, loss of memory, loss of sense of smell, myelopathy, oculomotor nerve paralysis, peripheral ischemia, pulmonary fibrosis, renal tubular disorder, rhabdomyolysis, Stevens-Johnson syndrome, stroke, testicular hypotrophy, torsades de pointes, vasculitis, ventricular tachycardia.

➤*Children:* The spectrum of adverse reactions reported in 120 immunocompromised pediatric clinical trial participants with serious CMV infections receiving IV ganciclovir were similar to those reported in adults. Granulocytopenia (17%) and thrombocytopenia (10%) were the most common adverse events reported.

Sixteen pediatric patients (8 months to 15 years of age) with life- or sight-threatening CMV infections were evaluated in an open-label, IV ganciclovir solution, pharmacokinetics study. Adverse events reported for > 1 pediatric patient were as follows: Hypokalemia (25%); abnormal kidney function, sepsis, thrombocytopenia (19%); leukopenia, coagulation disorder, hypertension, pneumonia, immune system disorder (13%).

Overdosage

➤*IV:* The following have been reported after IV ganciclovir overdosage: Irreversible pancytopenia, GI symptoms, acute renal failure. Other adverse effects reported following IV ganciclovir overdosage include persistent bone marrow suppression, reversible neutropenia or granulocytopenia, hepatitis, renal toxicity, seizures.

➤*Oral:* There have been no reports of overdosage with oral ganciclovir. Doses as high as 6000 mg/day did not result in overt toxicity other than transient neutropenia.

➤*Treatment:* Dialysis may be useful in reducing serum concentrations. Maintain adequate hydration. Consider the use of hematopoietic growth factors.

Patient Information

➤*HIV-positive patients with CMV retinitis:* Ganciclovir is not a cure for CMV retinitis, and immunocompromised patients may continue to experience progression of retinitis during or following treatment. Advise patients to have regular ophthalmologic examinations at a minimum of every 4 to 6 weeks while being treated. Some patients will require more frequent follow-up.

The major toxicities of ganciclovir are granulocytopenia (neutropenia), anemia, and thrombocytopenia. Dose modifications may be required, including discontinuation. Emphasize the importance of close monitoring of blood counts while on therapy. Inform patients that ganciclovir has been associated with increases in serum creatinine.

Advise patients to take oral ganciclovir with food to maximize bioavailability.

➤*All HIV-positive patients:* HIV-positive patients may be receiving zidovudine. Treatment with zidovudine and ganciclovir may not be tolerated by some patients and may result in severe granulocytopenia (neutropenia). Patients with AIDS may be receiving didanosine. Counsel patients that concurrent treatment with ganciclovir and didanosine can significantly increase didanosine serum concentrations.

Advise patients that ganciclovir has caused decreased sperm production in animals and may cause infertility. Advise women of childbearing potential that ganciclovir causes birth defects in animals and should not be used during pregnancy; use effective contraception during ganciclovir treatment. Similarly, advise men to practice barrier contraception during and for ≥ 90 days following ganciclovir treatment.

Although there is no information, consider ganciclovir a potential carcinogen.

➤*Transplant recipients:* Counsel transplant recipients regarding the high frequency of impaired renal function, particularly in patients receiving concomitant administration of nephrotoxic agents such as cyclosporine and amphotericin B.

VALGANCICLOVIR HCl

Rx	Valcyte (Roche)	Tablets: 450 mg (as base)	(VGC 450). Pink. In 60s.

WARNING

The clinical toxicity of valganciclovir, which is metabolized to ganciclovir, includes granulocytopenia, anemia, and thrombocytopenia. In animal studies, ganciclovir was carcinogenic, teratogenic, and caused aspermatogenesis.

Indications

➤*Cytomegalovirus (CMV) retinitis:* For the treatment of CMV retinitis in patients with acquired immunodeficiency syndrome (AIDS).

➤*CMV disease:* For the prevention of CMV disease in kidney, heart, and kidney-pancreas transplant patients at high risk (Donor CMV seropositive/Recipient CMV seronegative [(D+/R−)]).

Administration and Dosage

➤*Approved by the FDA:* March 30, 2001.

Strict adherence to dosage recommendations is essential to avoid overdose. Valganciclovir tablets cannot be substituted for ganciclovir capsules on a one-to-one basis.

➤*CMV retinitis:*

Induction – 900 mg (two 450 mg tablets) twice daily for 21 days with food.

Maintenance – Following induction treatment, or in patients with inactive CMV retinitis, the recommended dosage is 900 mg (two 450 mg tablets) once daily with food.

➤*Prevention of CMV disease:* 900 mg (two 450 mg tablets) once daily with food starting within 10 days of transplantation until 100 days posttransplantation.

➤*Renal impairment:* Monitor serum creatinine or creatinine clearance levels carefully. Dosage adjustment is required according to creatinine clearance, as shown in the table below. Increased monitoring for cytopenias may be warranted in patients with renal impairment.

Valganciclovir in Renal Impairment		
Ccr[1] (mL/min)	Induction dose	Maintenance/prevention dose
≥ 60	900 mg twice daily	900 mg once daily
40 to 59	450 mg twice daily	450 mg once daily
25 to 39	450 mg once daily	450 mg every 2 days
10 to 24	450 mg every 2 days	450 mg twice weekly

[1] Estimated creatinine clearance.

➤*Hemodialysis patients:* Do not prescribe valganciclovir to patients receiving hemodialysis.

➤*Handling and disposal:* Exercise caution in the handling of valganciclovir tablets. Do not break or crush tablets. Because valganciclovir is considered a potential teratogen and carcinogen in humans, observe caution in handling broken tablets. Avoid direct contact of broken or crushed tablets with skin or mucous membranes. If such contact occurs, wash thoroughly with soap and water, and rinse eyes thoroughly with plain water.

VALGANCICLOVIR HCl

Because ganciclovir shares some of the properties of antitumor agents (ie, carcinogenicity and mutagenicity), consider handling and disposing according to guidelines issued for antineoplastic drugs.

▶*Storage/Stability:* Store at 25°C (77°F); excursions permitted to 15° to 30°C (59° to 86°F).

Actions

▶*Pharmacology:* Valganciclovir is an L-valyl ester (prodrug) of ganciclovir that exists as a mixture of 2 diastereomers. After oral administration, both diastereomers are rapidly converted to ganciclovir by intestinal and hepatic esterases. Ganciclovir is a synthetic analog of 2′-deoxyguanosine, which inhibits replication of human cytomegalovirus in vitro and in vivo.

In CMV-infected cells, ganciclovir is initially phosphorylated to ganciclovir monophosphate by the viral protein kinase pUL97. Further phosphorylation occurs by cellular kinases to produce ganciclovir triphosphate, which is then slowly metabolized intracellularly (half-life, 18 hours). As the phosphorylation is largely dependent on the viral kinase, phosphorylation of ganciclovir occurs preferentially in virus-infected cells. The virustatic activity of ganciclovir is caused by inhibition of viral DNA synthesis by ganciclovir triphosphate.

Antiviral activity – Sensitivity test results, expressed as the concentration of drug required to inhibit the growth of virus in cell culture by 50% (IC_{50}), vary greatly depending upon a number of factors. Thus, the IC_{50} of ganciclovir that inhibits human CMV replication in vitro (laboratory and clinical isolates) has ranged from 0.02 to 5.75 mcg/mL. Ganciclovir inhibits mammalian cell proliferation (IC_{50}) in vitro at higher concentrations ranging from 10.21 to more than 250 mcg/mL. Bone marrow-derived colony-forming cells are more sensitive (IC_{50} = 0.69 to 3.06 mcg/mL).

Viral resistance – Viruses resistant to ganciclovir can arise after prolonged treatment with valganciclovir by selection of mutations in either the viral protein kinase gene (UL97) responsible for ganciclovir monophosphorylation or in the viral polymerase gene (UL54). A virus with mutations in the UL97 gene is resistant to ganciclovir alone, whereas a virus with mutations in the UL54 gene may show cross-resistance to other antivirals with a similar mechanism of action.

The current working definition of CMV resistance to ganciclovir in in vitro assays is IC_{50} at least 1.5 mcg/mL. CMV resistance to ganciclovir has been observed in individuals with AIDS and CMV retinitis who have never received ganciclovir therapy. Viral resistance has also been observed in patients receiving prolonged treatment for CMV retinitis with ganciclovir. Consider the possibility of viral resistance in patients who show poor clinical response or experience persistent viral excretion during therapy.

▶*Pharmacokinetics:*

Absorption – Valganciclovir is well absorbed from the GI tract and rapidly metabolized in the intestinal wall and liver to ganciclovir. The absolute bioavailability of ganciclovir from valganciclovir tablets following administration with food was approximately 60%. Ganciclovir median T_{max} following administration of 450 to 2625 mg valganciclovir tablets ranged from 1 to 3 hours. Dose proportionality with respect to ganciclovir AUC following administration of valganciclovir tablets was demonstrated only under fed conditions. Systemic exposure to the prodrug, valganciclovir, is transient and low, and the AUC_{24} and C_{max} values are approximately 1% and 3% of those of ganciclovir, respectively.

The AUC for ganciclovir administered as valganciclovir tablets is comparable to the ganciclovir AUC for IV ganciclovir. Ganciclovir C_{max} following valganciclovir administration is 40% lower than following IV ganciclovir administration.

Distribution – Plasma protein binding of ganciclovir is 1% to 2% over concentrations of 0.5 and 51 mcg/mL. When ganciclovir was administered IV, the steady-state volume of distribution of ganciclovir was approximately 0.703 L/kg (n = 69).

Metabolism – Valganciclovir is rapidly hydrolyzed to ganciclovir; no other metabolites have been detected. No metabolite of orally administered radiolabeled ganciclovir (1000 mg single dose) accounted for more than 1% to 2% of the radioactivity recovered in the feces or urine.

Excretion – The major route of elimination of valganciclovir is by renal excretion as ganciclovir through glomerular filtration and active tubular secretion. Systemic clearance of IV administered ganciclovir was approximately 3.07 mL/min (n = 68) while renal clearance was approximately 2.99 mL/min/kg (n = 16).

The terminal half-life of ganciclovir following oral administration of valganciclovir tablets to healthy or HIV-positive/CMV-positive subjects was approximately 4.08 hours (n = 73), and that following administration of IV ganciclovir was approximately 3.81 hours (n = 69). In heart, kidney, kidney-pancreas, and liver transplant patients, the terminal elimination half-life of ganciclovir following oral administration of valganciclovir was approximately 6.48 hours and following oral administration of ganciclovir was approximately 8.56 hours.

Mean Ganciclovir Pharmacokinetic[1] Measures in Healthy Volunteers and HIV-Positive/CMV-Positive Adults at Maintenance Dosage			
Formulation	Valganciclovir	Ganciclovir IV	Ganciclovir
Dosage	900 mg once daily with food	5 mg/kg once daily	100 mg three times daily with food
$AUC_{0-24\ hr}$ (mcg·hr/mL)	≈ 29.1 (n = 57)	≈ 26.5 (n = 68)	Range of means 12.3 to 19.2 (n = 94)
C_{max} (mcg/mL)	≈ 5.61 (n = 58)	≈ 9.46 (n = 68)	Range of means 0.955 to 1.4 (n = 94)
Absolute oral bioavailability (%)	≈ 59.4 (n = 32)	Not applicable	Range of means ≈ 6.22 to ≈ 8.53 (n = 32)
Elimination $t_{1/2}$ (h)	≈ 4.08 (n = 73)	≈ 3.81 (n = 69)	Range of means 3.86 to 5.03 (n = 61)
Renal clearance (mL/min/kg)	≈ 3.21 (n = 20)	≈ 2.99 (n = 16)	Range of means 2.67 to 3.98 (n = 30)

[1] Data were obtained from single- and multiple-dose studies in healthy volunteers, HIV-positive patients, and HIV-positive/CMV-positive patients with and without retinitis. Patients with CMV retinitis tended to have higher ganciclovir plasma concentrations than patients without CMV retinitis.

Mean Ganciclovir Pharmacokinetic Measures in Solid Organ Transplant Recipients						
Parameter	Heart transplant recipients		Kidney transplant recipients[1]		Liver transplant patients	
Formulation and dosage	VAL[2] 900 mg/ day (n = 17)	GAN[3] 3000 mg/ day (n = 13)	VAL 900 mg/ day (n = 68)	GAN 3000 mg/ day (n = 36)	VAL 900 mg/ day (n = 75)	GAN 3000 mg/ day (n = 33)
AUC (0-24 h) (mcg·h/mL)	≈ 40.2	≈ 26.6	≈ 48.2	≈ 31.3	≈ 46	≈ 24.9
C_{max} (mcg/mL)	≈ 4.9	≈ 1.4	≈ 5.3	≈ 1.5	≈ 5.4	≈ 1.3
Elimination $t_{1/2}$ (h)	≈ 6.58	≈ 8.47	≈ 6.77	≈ 9.44	≈ 6.18	≈ 7.68

[1] Includes kidney-pancreas.
[2] VAL = valganciclovir.
[3] GAN = ganciclovir.

Special populations –

Renal function impairment: Because the major elimination pathway for ganciclovir is renal, dosage reductions according to creatinine clearance are required for valganciclovir tablets. For dosing instructions in patients with renal impairment, refer to Administration and Dosage.

The pharmacokinetics of ganciclovir from a single oral dose of 900 mg valganciclovir tablets were evaluated in 24 otherwise healthy individuals with renal impairment.

Pharmacokinetics of Ganciclovir from a Single Oral Dose of 900 mg Valganciclovir Tablets (n = 6)			
Estimated creatinine clearance (mL/min)	Mean apparent clearance (mL/min)	Mean AUC (mcg·h/mL)	Mean $t_{1/2}$ (hours)
51 to 70	249	49.5	4.85
21 to 50	136	91.9	10.2
11 to 20	45	223	21.8
≤ 10	12.8	366	67.5

Decreased renal function results in decreased clearance of ganciclovir from valganciclovir and a corresponding increase in terminal half-life. Therefore, dosage adjustment is required for patients with impaired renal function.

Hemodialysis – Hemodialysis reduces plasma concentrations of ganciclovir by approximately 50% following valganciclovir administration. Patients receiving hemodialysis (Ccr less than 10 mL/min) cannot use valganciclovir tablets because the daily dose of valganciclovir tablets required for these patients is less than 450 mg (see Administration and Dosage).

▶*Clinical trials:*

Induction therapy of CMV retinitis – In a randomized, open-label controlled study, 160 AIDS patients and newly diagnosed CMV retinitis patients were randomized to receive treatment with either valganciclovir tablets (900 mg twice daily for 21 days, then 900 mg once daily for 7 days) or with IV ganciclovir solution (5 mg/kg twice daily for 21 days, then 5 mg/kg once daily for 7 days). The median baseline HIV-1 RNA was 4.9 $\log_{10}$, and the median CD4 cell count was 23 cells/mm[3]. A determination of CMV retinitis progression by the masked review of retinal photographs taken at baseline and week 4 was the primary outcome measurement of the 3-week induction therapy. The table below provides the outcomes at 4 weeks.

Week 4 Masked Review of Retinal Photographs		
Determination of CMV retinitis progression at Week 4	Ganciclovir (n = 80)	Valganciclovir (n = 80)
Progressor	7	7
Nonprogressor	63	64
Death	2	1

VALGANCICLOVIR HCl

Week 4 Masked Review of Retinal Photographs		
Determination of CMV retinitis progression at Week 4	Ganciclovir (n = 80)	Valganciclovir (n = 80)
Discontinuations because of adverse events	1	2
Failed to return	1	1
CMV not confirmed at baseline or no interpretable baseline photos	6	5

Prevention of CMV disease in heart, kidney, kidney-pancreas, and liver transplantation – A double-blind, double-dummy active comparator study was conducted in 372 heart, liver, kidney, and kidney-pancreas transplant patients at high-risk for CMV disease (D+/R−). Patients were randomized (2 valganciclovir:1 oral ganciclovir) to receive either valganciclovir (900 mg once daily) or oral ganciclovir (1000 mg 3 times/day) starting within 10 days of transplantation until day 100 posttransplant. The proportion of patients who developed CMV disease, including CMV syndrome and/or tissue-invasive disease during the first 6 months posttransplant was similar between the valganciclovir arm (12.1%, n = 239) and the oral ganciclovir arm (15.2%, n = 125). However, in liver transplant patients, the incidence of tissue-invasive CMV disease was significantly higher in the valganciclovir group compared with the ganciclovir group. Mortality at 6 months was 3.7% (9/244) in the valganciclovir group and 1.6% (2/126) in the oral ganciclovir group.

Contraindications

Hypersensitivity to valganciclovir or ganciclovir.

Warnings

➤*Liver transplant patients:* In liver transplant patients, there was a significantly higher incidence of tissue-invasive CMV disease in the valganciclovir-treated group compared with the oral ganciclovir group. Valganciclovir is not indicated for use in liver transplant patients.

➤*Toxicity:* The clinical toxicity of valganciclovir, which is metabolized to ganciclovir, includes granulocytopenia, anemia, and thrombocytopenia. In animal studies, ganciclovir was carcinogenic, teratogenic, and caused aspermatogenesis.

➤*Hematologic:* Do not administer valganciclovir tablets if the absolute neutrophil count is less than 500 cells/mm^3, the platelet count is less than 25,000/mm^3, or the hemoglobin is less than 8 g/dL.

Severe leukopenia, neutropenia, anemia, thrombocytopenia, pancytopenia, bone marrow depression, and aplastic anemia have been observed in patients treated with valganciclovir tablets (and ganciclovir) (see Precautions and Adverse Reactions).

Therefore, use valganciclovir tablets with caution in patients with pre-existing cytopenias, or in those who have received or are receiving myelosuppressive drugs or irradiation. Cytopenia may occur at any time during treatment and may increase with continued dosing. Cell counts usually begin to recover within 3 to 7 days of discontinuing the drug.

➤*Renal function impairment:* Because ganciclovir is excreted by the kidneys, normal clearance depends on adequate renal function. If renal function is impaired, dosage adjustments are required for valganciclovir. Base such adjustments on measured or estimated creatinine clearance values (see Administration and Dosage). For patients on hemodialysis (Ccr less than 10 mL/min), it is recommended that ganciclovir be used (in accordance with the dose-reduction algorithm cited in Administration and Dosage in the ganciclovir package insert) rather than valganciclovir (see Administration and Dosage).

➤*Carcinogenesis:* No long-term carcinogenicity studies have been conducted with valganciclovir. However, after oral administration, valganciclovir is rapidly and extensively converted to ganciclovir. Therefore, like ganciclovir, valganciclovir is a potential carcinogen.

Ganciclovir was carcinogenic in mice at oral doses approximately 0.1 and 1.4 times the mean drug exposure in humans based on AUC following the recommended IV dose of 5 mg/kg. At the higher dose, there was a significant increase in the incidence of tumors of the preputial gland in males, forestomach (nonglandular mucosa) in males and females, and reproductive tissues (ovaries, uterus, mammary gland, clitoral gland, and vagina) and liver in females. At the lower dose, a slightly increased incidence of tumors was noted in the preputial and harderian glands in males, forestomach in males and females, and liver in females. Consider ganciclovir a potential carcinogen in humans.

➤*Mutagenesis:* Valganciclovir increases mutations in mouse lymphoma cells. In the mouse micronucleaus assay, valganciclovir was clastogenic. Valganciclovir was not mutagenic in the Ames Salmonella assay. Ganciclovir increased mutations in mouse lymphoma cells and DNA damage in human lymphocytes in vitro. In the mouse micronucleus assay, ganciclovir was clastogenic. Ganciclovir was not mutagenic in the Ames Salmonella assay.

➤*Fertility impairment:* Animal data indicate that administration of ganciclovir causes inhibition of spermatogenesis and subsequent infertility. These effects were reversible at lower doses and irreversible at higher doses. It is considered probable that in humans, valganciclovir at the recommended doses may cause temporary or permanent inhibition of spermatogenesis. Animal data also indicate that suppression of fertility in females may occur.

Valganciclovir is converted to ganciclovir and therefore is expected to have similar reproductive toxicity effects as ganciclovir. Ganciclovir caused decreased mating behavior, decreased fertility, and an increased incidence of embryolethality in female mice following IV doses approximately 1.7 times the mean drug exposure in humans following the dose of 5 mg/kg, based on AUC comparisons. Ganciclovir caused decreased fertility in male mice and hypospermatogenesis in mice and dogs following daily oral or IV administration. Systemic drug exposure (AUC) at the lowest dose showing toxicity in each species ranged from 0.03 to 0.1 times the AUC of the recommended human IV dose. Valganciclovir caused similar effects on spermatogenesis in mice, rats, and dogs. It is considered likely that ganciclovir (and valganciclovir) could cause inhibition of human spermatogenesis.

Because of the mutagenic and teratogenic potential of ganciclovir, advise women of childbearing potential to use effective contraception during treatment. Similarly, advise men to practice barrier contraception during and for at least 90 days following treatment with valganciclovir.

➤*Elderly:* The pharmacokinetic characteristics of valganciclovir in elderly patients have not been established. Since elderly individuals frequently have a reduced glomerular filtration rate, pay particular attention to assessing renal function before and during administration of valganciclovir.

➤*Pregnancy:* Category C. Valganciclovir is converted to ganciclovir and therefore is expected to have reproductive toxicity effects similar to ganciclovir. Ganciclovir has been shown to be embryotoxic in rabbits and mice following IV administration, and teratogenic in rabbits. Fetal resorptions were present in at least 85% of rabbits and mice when they were administered doses that were twice the human exposure based on AUC comparisons. Effects observed in rabbits included: Fetal growth retardation, embryolethality, teratogenicity, or maternal toxicity. Teratogenic changes included cleft palate, anophthalmia/microphthalmia, aplastic organs (kidney and pancreas), hydrocephaly, and brachygnathia. In mice, effects observed were maternal/fetal toxicity and embryolethality.

Daily IV doses administered to female mice prior to mating, during gestation, and during lactation caused hypoplasia of the testes and seminal vesicles in the month-old male offspring, as well as pathologic changes in the nonglandular region of the stomach. The drug exposure in mice as estimated by the AUC was approximately 1.7 times the human AUC.

Valganciclovir may be teratogenic or embryotoxic at dose levels recommended for human use. There are no adequate and well-controlled studies in pregnant women. Use valganciclovir tablets during pregnancy only if the potential benefit justifies the potential risk to the fetus.

Data obtained using an ex vivo human placental model show that ganciclovir crosses the placenta and that simple diffusion is the most likely mechanism of transfer. The transfer was not saturable over a concentration range of 1 to 10 mg/mL and occurred by passive diffusion.

➤*Lactation:* It is not known whether ganciclovir or valganciclovir is excreted in human milk. Because valganciclovir caused granulocytopenia, anemia, and thrombocytopenia in clinical trials and ganciclovir was mutagenic and carcinogenic in animal studies, the possibility of serious adverse events from ganciclovir in nursing infants is possible. Because of the potential for serious adverse events in nursing infants, instruct mothers not to breastfeed if they are receiving valganciclovir tablets. In addition, the Centers for Disease Control and Prevention recommend that HIV-infected mothers not breastfeed their infants to avoid risking postnatal transmission of HIV.

➤*Children:* Safety and efficacy of valganciclovir in pediatric patients have not been established.

Precautions

➤*Monitoring:* Because of the frequency of neutropenia, anemia, and thrombocytopenia in patients receiving valganciclovir tablets, it is recommended that complete blood counts and platelet counts be performed frequently, especially in patients in whom ganciclovir or other nucleoside analogs have previously resulted in leukopenia, or in whom neutrophil counts are less than 1000 cells/mm^3 at the beginning of treatment. Increased monitoring for cytopenias may be warranted if therapy with oral ganciclovir is changed to oral valganciclovir because of increased plasma concentrations of ganciclovir after valganciclovir administration.

Increased serum creatinine levels have been observed in trials evaluating valganciclovir tablets. Carefully monitor serum creatinine or creatinine clearance values to allow for dosage adjustments in renally impaired patients. The mechanism of impairment of renal function is not known.

VALGANCICLOVIR HCl

Drug Interactions

There were no in vivo drug interaction studies conducted with valganciclovir. However, because valganciclovir is rapidly and extensively converted to ganciclovir, interactions associated with ganciclovir will be expected for valganciclovir tablets.

Ganciclovir Drug Interactions			
Precipitant drug	Object drug*		Description
Didanosine	Ganciclovir	↓	Steady-state didanosine AUC increased 111% (range, 10% to 493%) when didanosine was administered either 2 hours prior to or simultaneously with ganciclovir. Closely monitor for didanosine toxicity. A decrease in steady-state ganciclovir AUC of 21% (range, -44% to 5%) was observed when didanosine was administered 2 hours prior to administration of ganciclovir, but ganciclovir AUC was not affected by the presence of didanosine when the 2 drugs were administered simultaneously.
Ganciclovir	Didanosine	↑	
Imipenem-cilastatin	Ganciclovir	↑	Generalized seizures occurred in patients who received ganciclovir and imipenem-cilastatin. Do not administer these drugs concomitantly unless the potential benefits outweigh the risks.
Nephrotoxic drugs	Ganciclovir	↑	Increases in serum creatinine were observed following concurrent use of ganciclovir and either cyclosporine or amphotericin B.
Probenecid	Ganciclovir	↑	Ganciclovir AUC increased 53% (range, -14% to 299%) in the presence of probenecid. Renal clearance of ganciclovir decreased 22% (range, -54% to -4%), which is consistent with an interaction involving competition for renal tubular secretion. Monitor for ganciclovir toxicity.
Trimethoprim	Ganciclovir	↑	Coadministration resulted in decreased ganciclovir renal clearance and increased t$_{1/2}$.
Zalcitabine	Ganciclovir	↑	Zalcitabine 0.75 mg administered 2 hours before ganciclovir resulted in an increase in ganciclovir AUC by 13%.
Zidovudine	Ganciclovir	↓	Mean steady-state ganciclovir AUC decreased 17% (range, -52% to 23%) in the presence of zidovudine. Zidovudine AUC increased 19% (range, -11% to 74%) in the presence of ganciclovir. Because both drugs can cause neutropenia and anemia, many patients will not tolerate combination therapy at full dosage.
Ganciclovir	Zidovudine	↑	
Ganciclovir	Cytotoxic drugs	↑	Cytotoxic drugs that inhibit replication of rapidly dividing cell populations such as bone marrow, spermatogonia, and germinal layers of skin and GI mucosa may have additive toxicity when administered concomitantly with ganciclovir. Therefore, consider the concomitant use of drugs such as dapsone, pentamidine, flucytosine, vincristine, vinblastine, adriamycin, amphotericin B, trimethoprim/sulfamethoxazole combinations, or other nucleoside analogs only if potential benefits outweigh the risks.

* ↑ = Object drug increased. ↓ = Object drug decreased.

►*Drug/Food interactions:* When valganciclovir tablets were administered with a high-fat meal containing approximately 600 total calories (31.1 g fat, 51.6 g carbohydrates, and 22.2 g protein) at a dose of 875 mg once daily to 16 HIV-positive subjects, the steady-state ganciclovir AUC increased by 30% (95% CI 12% to 51%), and the C$_{max}$ increased by 14% (95% CI −5% to 36%), without any prolongation in time to peak plasma concentrations (T$_{max}$). Administer valganciclovir tablets with food.

Adverse Reactions

Valganciclovir vs Ganciclovir Selected Adverse Events (%)		
Adverse reaction	Valganciclovir (n = 79)	Ganciclovir IV (n = 79)
Anemia	8	8
Catheter-related infection	3	11
Diarrhea	16	10
Headache	9	5
Nausea	8	14
Neutropenia	11	13

Valganciclovir Adverse Reactions Occurring in CMV Retinitis Patients (≥ 5%)	
Adverse reaction	Patients (n = 370)
CNS	
Headache	22
Insomnia	16
Paresthesia	8
Peripheral neuropathy	9
GI	
Abdominal pain	15
Diarrhea	41
Nausea	30
Vomiting	21
Hematologic/Lymphatic	
Anemia	26
Neutropenia	27
Thrombocytopenia	6
Lab test abnormalities	
Anemia: Hemoglobin g/dL	
< 6.5	7
6.5 to < 8	13
8 to < 9.5	16
Neutropenia: ANC/mm^3	
< 500	19
500 to < 750	17
750 to < 1000	17
Serum creatinine: mg/dL	
> 2.5	3
> 1.5 to 2.5	12
Thrombocytopenia: Platelets/mm^3	
< 25,000	4
25,000 to < 50,000	6
50,000 to < 100,000	22
Miscellaneous	
Pyrexia	31
Retinal detachment	15

Adverse Events Reported in ≥ 5% of Selected Organ Transplant Patients		
Adverse reaction	Valganciclovir (n=244)	Oral ganciclovir (n=126)
CNS		
Headache	22	27
Insomnia	20	16
Tremors	28	25
GI		
Diarrhea	30	29
Nausea	23	23
Vomiting	16	14
Lab test abnormalities		
Anemia (Hemoglobulin g/dL)		
< 6.5	1	2
6.5 to < 8	5	7
8 to < 9.5	31	25
Neutropenia (ANC/mm^3)		
< 500	5	3
500 to < 750	3	2
750 to < 1000	5	2
Serum creatinine (mg/dL)		
> 2.5	14	21
> 1.5 to 2.5	45	47
Thrombocytopenia (Platelets/mm^3)		
< 25,000	0	2
25,000 to < 50,000	1	3

VALGANCICLOVIR HCl

Adverse Events Reported in ≥ 5% of Selected Organ Transplant Patients		
Adverse reaction	Valganciclovir (n=244)	Oral ganciclovir (n=126)
50,000 to < 100,000	18	21
Miscellaneous		
Graft rejection	24	30
Hypertension	18	15
Leukopenia	14	7
Pyrexia	13	14

➤*Other adverse events:*

CNS – Agitation; confusion; convulsion; depression; dizziness (excluding vertigo); hallucinations; paresthesia; psychosis.

Dermatologic – Acne; dermatitis; pruritus.

GI – Abdominal distention; abdominal pain; ascites; constipation; dyspepsia.

GU – Decreased creatinine clearance; dysuria; renal impairment; urinary tract infection.

Hematologic/Lymphatic – Anemia; aplastic anemia; bone marrow depression; neutropenia; pancytopenia; potential life-threatening bleeding associated with thrombocytopenia.

Hypersensitivity – Valganciclovir hypersensitivity.

Metabolic – Appetite decreased; dehydration; hyperglycemia; hyperkalemia; hypocalcemia; hypokalemia; hypomagnesemia; hypophosphatemia.

Musculoskeletal – Arthralgia; back pain; limb pain; muscle cramps.

Respiratory – Cough; dyspnea; pharyngitis/nasopharyngitis; pleural effusion; rhinorrhea; upper respiratory tract infection.

Miscellaneous – Abnormal hepatic function; edema; fatigue; hypotension; increased wound drainage; local and systemic infections and sepsis; pain; peripheral edema; postoperative complications; postoperative pain; postoperative wound infection; weakness; wound dehiscence.

Refer to the ganciclovir package insert for postmarketing adverse reactions associated with ganciclovir.

Overdosage

➤*Symptoms:*

Valganciclovir – One adult developed fatal bone marrow depression (medullary aplasia) after several days of dosing that was at least 10-fold greater than recommended for the patient's estimated degree of renal impairment.

It is expected that valganciclovir overdose could possibly result in increased renal toxicity.

Reports of overdoses with IV ganciclovir have been received from clinical trials and during postmarketing experience. The majority of patients experienced at least 1 of the following adverse events: Pancytopenia, bone marrow depression, medullary aplasia, leukopenia, neutropenia, granulocytopenia, hepatitis, liver function disorder, worsening of hematuria in a patient with pre-existing renal impairment, acute renal failure, elevated creatinine, abdominal pain, diarrhea, vomiting, generalized tremor, convulsion.

➤*Treatment:* Because ganciclovir is dialyzable, dialysis may be useful in reducing serum concentrations in patients who have received an overdose of valganciclovir tablets. Maintain adequate hydration. Consider the use of hematopoietic growth factors.

Patient Information

Valganciclovir tablets cannot be substituted for ganciclovir capsules on a one-to-one basis. Advise patients switching from ganciclovir capsules to valganciclovir tablets that taking more than the prescribed valganciclovir can result in overdosage.

Valganciclovir is changed to ganciclovir once it is absorbed into the body. Inform patients that major toxicities associated with ganciclovir include granulocytopenia (neutropenia), anemia, and thrombocytopenia and that dose modifications may be required, including discontinuation. Emphasize the importance of close monitoring of blood counts while on therapy. Inform patients that ganciclovir has been associated with elevations in serum creatinine.

Instruct patients to take valganciclovir tablets with food to maximize bioavailability.

Advise patients ganciclovir has caused decreased sperm production in animals and may cause decreased fertility in humans. Advise women of childbearing potential that ganciclovir causes birth defects in animals and should not be used during pregnancy. Because of the potential for serious adverse events in nursing infants, instruct mothers not to breastfeed if they are receiving valganciclovir tablets. Advise women of childbearing potential to use effective contraception during valganciclovir treatment. Similarly, advise men to practice barrier contraception during and for at least 90 days following treatment with valganciclovir tablets.

Although there is no information from human studies, advise patients that ganciclovir should be considered a potential carcinogen.

Convulsions, sedation, dizziness, ataxia, or confusion have been reported with the use of valganciclovir tablets or ganciclovir. If they occur, such effects may affect tasks requiring alertness, including the patient's ability to drive and operate machinery.

Tell patients that ganciclovir is not a cure for CMV retinitis, and that they may continue to experience progression of retinitis during or following treatment. Advise patients to have ophthalmologic follow-up examinations at a minimum of every 4 to 6 weeks while being treated with valganciclovir tablets. Some patients will require more frequent follow-up.

Antiherpes Virus Agents

ACYCLOVIR (Acycloguanosine)

Rx	**Acyclovir** (Various, eg, Dixon-Shane, Mylan, PAR, Purepac, Teva, Zenith-Goldline)	**Tablets:** 400 mg	In 100s, 500s, and 1000s.
Rx	**Zovirax** (GlaxoWellcome)		(Zovirax). White, shield shape. In 100s.
Rx	**Acyclovir** (Various, eg, Dixon-Shane, Mylan, PAR, Purepac, Teva, Zenith-Goldline)	**Tablets:** 800 mg	In 100s and 500s.
Rx	**Zovirax** (GlaxoWellcome)		(Zovirax 800 mg). Blue, oval. In 100s and UD 100s.
Rx	**Acyclovir** (Various, eg, Dixon-Shane, Mylan, PAR, Purepac, Teva, Zenith-Goldline)	**Capsules:** 200 mg	In 100s.
Rx	**Zovirax** (GlaxoWellcome)		Lactose. (Wellcome Zovirax 200). Blue. In 100s and UD 100s.[1]
Rx	**Acyclovir** (Various, eg, Alpharma, Xactdose)	**Suspension:** 200 mg/5 mL	In 473 mL.
Rx	**Zovirax** (GlaxoWellcome)		Banana flavor. In 473 mL.[2]
Rx	**Acyclovir** (Various, eg, Bertek, APP)	**Injection:** 50 mg/mL (as sodium)	In cartons of 10.
Rx	**Acyclovir** (Various, eg, Abbott, Bedford, Gensia Sicor, Novaplus)	**Powder for injection:** 500 mg/vial (as sodium)	In 10 mL vials.
		1000 mg/vial (as sodium)	In 20 mL vials.
Rx	**Zovirax** (GlaxoWellcome)	**Powder for injection, lyophilized:** 500 mg/vial (as sodium)[3]	In 10 mL vials.
		1000 mg/vial (as sodium)[4]	In 20 mL vials.

[1] May contain parabens.
[2] With 0.1% methylparaben, 0.02% propylparaben, and sorbitol.
[3] Contains 49 mg of sodium.
[4] Contains 98 mg of sodium.

Indications

➤*Neonatal herpes simplex virus infection:* Treatment of neonatal herpes infections.

➤*Parenteral:* Treatment of initial and recurrent mucosal and cutaneous herpes simplex virus types 1 and 2 (HSV-1 and HSV-2) and varicella-zoster virus (VZV/shingles) infections in immunocompromised patients.

Herpes simplex encephalitis.

Severe initial clinical episodes of genital herpes in patients who are not immunocompromised.

➤*Oral:* Treatment of initial episodes and management of recurrent episodes of genital herpes.

Acute treatment of herpes zoster (shingles) and chickenpox (varicella).

➤*Unlabeled uses:* Prophylaxis of mucocutaneous HSV infection in immunosuppressed HSV-seropositive patients (oral and IV); prophylaxis of VZV in transplant and chemotherapy patients (oral); high-dose IV acyclovir may reduce the risk of CMV infection in CMV-seropositive patients undergoing bone-marrow transplantation; high dose oral acyclovir may reduce the risk of CMV infection in certain patients undergoing solid-organ transplantation.

Administration and Dosage

➤*Approved by the FDA:* 1984.

➤*Parenteral:* Avoid rapid or bolus IV injection. Avoid IM or SC injection. Initiate therapy as soon as possible following onset of signs and symptoms. For IV infusion only. Administer over at least 1 hour to prevent renal tubular damage.

Do not exceed a maximum dose equivalent of 20 mg/kg every 8 hours for any patient.

IV Acyclovir Dosage/Management Guidelines		
	Dosage	
Indication	**Adults**	**Children (< 12 years)**
Mucosal and cutaneous HSV infections in immunocompromised patients	5 mg/kg infused at a constant rate over 1 hour every 8 hours (15 mg/kg/day) for 7 days[1]	10 mg/kg[2] infused at a constant rate over 1 hour every 8 hours for 7 days
VZV (shingles) infections in immunocompromised patients[2]	10 mg/kg infused at a constant rate over 1 hour every 8 hours for 7 days	20 mg/kg infused at a constant rate over at least 1 hour every 8 hours for 7 days
Herpes simplex encephalitis	10 mg/kg infused at a constant rate over at least 1 hour every 8 hours for 10 days	20 mg/kg infused at a constant rate over at least 1 hour every 8 hours for 10 days[3]
Neonatal HSV infections	NA	10 mg/kg infused at a constant rate over 1 hour every 8 hours for 10 days[4]

[1] For severe initial clinical episodes of herpes genitalis, use the same dose for 5 days.
[2] Base dosage for obese patients on ideal body weight (10 mg/kg).
[3] Children 3 months to 12 years of age.
[4] Children birth to 3 months. Doses of 15 or 20 mg/kg infused at a constant rate over 1 hour every 8 hours have been used; however, safety and efficacy of these doses are unknown.

CDC recommendations for neonatal herpes infections –
Disseminated and CNS disease: 20 mg/kg IV every 8 hours for 21 days.
Mucocutaneous disease: 20 mg/kg IV every 8 hours for 14 days.

Renal function impairment, acute or chronic – Adjust the dosing interval as indicated below:

Parenteral Acyclovir Dosage in Renal Function Impairment		
Creatinine clearance (mL/min/1.73 m²)	Percent of recommended dose	Dosing interval (hours)
> 50	100%	8
25 to 50	100%	12
10 to 25	100%	24
0 to 10	50%	24

Hemodialysis – The mean plasma half-life of acyclovir during hemodialysis is approximately 5 hours; a 60% decrease in plasma concentrations follows a 6-hour dialysis period. Therefore, administer a dose after each dialysis.

Preparation of IV solution – Dissolve the contents of the 500 or 1000 mg vial in 10 or 20 mL sterile water for injection, respectively, to yield a final concentration of 50 mg/mL acyclovir (pH approximately 11). Shake the vial well to assure complete dissolution before measuring and transferring each individual dose. Do not use bacteriostatic water for injection containing benzyl alcohol or parabens.

Add the calculated dose to an appropriate IV solution at a volume selected for administration during each 1 hour infusion. Infusion concentrations of approximately 7 mg/mL or lower are recommended. In clinical studies, the average 70 kg adult received between 60 and 150 mL of fluid per dose. Higher concentrations (eg, 10 mg/mL) may produce phlebitis or inflammation at the injection site upon inadvertent extravasation. The addition of acyclovir to biologic or colloidal fluids (eg, blood products, protein solutions) is not recommended.

➤*Oral:*

Herpes simplex – For severe disease that requires hospitalization (eg, disseminated infection, pneumonitis, hepatitis, meningitis, encephalitis) IV acyclovir therapy is recommended.
Initial genital herpes: 200 mg every 4 hours, 5 times daily for 10 days.
Chronic suppressive therapy for recurrent disease: 400 mg 2 times daily for up to 12 months, followed by re-evaluation. Re-evaluate the frequency and severity of the patient's HSV after 1 year of therapy to assess the need for continuation of therapy; frequency and severity of episodes of untreated genital herpes may change over time.
Intermittent therapy: 200 mg every 4 hours, 5 times daily for 5 days. Initiate therapy at the earliest sign or symptom (prodrome) of recurrence.

CDC guidelines recommend the following oral regimens –
First initial clinical episode of genital herpes: 400 mg 3 times daily for 7 to 10 days or 200 mg 5 times daily for 7 to 10 days.
Episodic therapy for recurrent genital herpes: 400 mg 3 times a day or 200 mg 5 times a day for 5 days.

Herpes zoster, acute treatment – 800 mg every 4 hours, 5 times daily for 7 to 10 days.

Chickenpox – Initiate treatment at earliest sign or symptom. There are no data about the efficacy of therapy initiated more than 24 hours after onset of signs and symptoms.
Adults and children (greater than 40 kg): 800 mg 4 times daily for 5 days.
Children (2 years and older; 40 kg or less): 20 mg/kg 4 times daily for 5 days.

ACYCLOVIR (Acycloguanosine)
Renal impairment, acute or chronic –

Oral Acyclovir Dosage in Renal Function Impairment			
Normal dosage regimen (5x daily)	Creatinine clearance (mL/min/1.73 m²)	Adjusted dosage regimen	
		Dose (mg)	Dosing interval
200 mg every 4 hours	> 10	200	Every 4 hours, 5x daily
	0 to 10	200	Every 12 hours
400 mg every 12 hours	> 10	400	Every 12 hours
	0 to 10	200	Every 12 hours
800 mg every 4 hours	> 25	800	Every 4 hours, 5x daily
	10 to 25	800	Every 8 hours
	0 to 10	800	Every 12 hours

Hemodialysis – For patients that require hemodialysis, adjust dosing schedule so that a dose is administered after each dialysis. No supplemental dose is necessary after peritoneal dialysis.

➤*Bioequivalence:* Acyclovir suspension was shown to be bioequivalent to acyclovir capsules, and one 800 mg acyclovir tablet was shown to be bioequivalent to four 200 mg acyclovir capsules.

➤*Storage / Stability:*

Injection – Use reconstituted solution within 12 hours. Once diluted for administration, use each dose within 24 hours. Refrigeration of reconstituted solutions may result in formation of a precipitate which redissolves at room temperature.

Store unopened vials at 15° to 25°C (59° to 77°F).

Capsules, tablets, suspension – Store at 15° to 25°C (59° to 77°F). Protect tablets and capsules from moisture.

Actions

➤*Pharmacology:* A synthetic purine nucleoside analog, acyclovir has in vitro and in vivo inhibitory activity against HSV-1, HSV-2, and VZV (shingles).

The inhibitory activity of acyclovir is highly selective because of its affinity for the enzyme thymidine kinase (TK) encoded by HSV and VZV. This viral enzyme converts acyclovir into acyclovir monophosphate, a nucleotide analog. The monophosphate is further converted into diphosphate by cellular guanylate kinase and into triphosphate by a number of cellular enzymes. In vitro, acyclovir triphosphate stops replication of herpes viral DNA. This is accomplished in the following 3 ways: 1) competitive inhibition of viral DNA polymerase; 2) incorporation into, and termination of, the growing viral DNA chain; and 3) inactivation of the viral DNA polymerase. The greater antiviral activity of acyclovir against HSV compared with VZV is because of its more efficient phosphorylation by the viral TK.

Drug resistance – Resistance of HSV and VZV to acyclovir can result from qualitative and quantitative changes in the viral TK and/or DNA polymerase. Clinical isolates of HSV and VZV with reduced susceptibility to acyclovir have been recovered from immunocompromised patients, especially with advanced HIV infection. While most of the acyclovir-resistant mutants isolated thus far from immunocompromised patients have been found to be TK-deficient mutants, other mutants involving the viral TK gene (TK partial and TK altered) and DNA polymerase have been isolated. TK-negative mutants may cause severe disease in infants and immunocompromised adults. Consider the possibility of viral resistance to acyclovir in patients who show poor clinical response during therapy.

➤*Pharmacokinetics:*

Absorption / Distribution – Proportionality between dose and plasma levels is seen after single doses or at steady-state after multiple dosing. When acyclovir was administered to adults at 5 mg/kg by 1 hour infusions every 8 hours, mean steady-state peak and trough concentrations were 9.8 mcg/mL (5.5 to 13.8 mcg/mL) and 0.7 mcg/mL (0.2 to 1 mcg/mL), respectively. When acyclovir was administered to adults at 10 mg/kg by 1 hour infusions every 8 hours, mean steady-state peak and trough concentrations were 22.9 mcg/mL (14.1 to 44.1 mcg/mL) and 1.9 mcg/mL (0.5 to 2.9 mcg/mL), respectively. Absorption is unaffected by food. Bioavailability is between 10% and 20% and decreases with increasing doses. Concentrations achieved in CSF are approximately 50% of plasma values. Plasma protein binding is 9% to 33%. Acyclovir distributes widely in body fluids including vesicular fluid, aqueous humor, and cerebrospinal fluid. Acyclovir is concentrated in breast milk, amniotic fluid, and placenta.

Metabolism / Excretion – Renal excretion of unchanged drug following IV use accounts for 62% to 91% of the dose. The only major urinary metabolite is 9-carboxymethoxymethylguanine; this may account for up to 14% of the dose in patients with normal renal function.

Half-life and total body clearance depend on renal function:

Acyclovir Half-Life and Total Body Clearance Based on Renal Function		
Creatinine clearance (mL/min/1.73 m²)	Half-life (h)	Total body clearance (mL/min/1.73 m²)
> 80	2.5	327
50 to 80	3	248
15 to 50	3.5	190
0 (Anuric)	19.5	29

Special populations –

Elderly: Acyclovir plasma concentrations are higher in elderly patients compared with younger adults. This may be in part because of age-related renal function changes.

Microbiology – Using plaque-reduction assays, the IC$_{50}$ against HSV isolates ranges from 0.02 to 13.5 mcg/mL for HSV-1 and from 0.01 to 9.9 mcg/mL for HSV-2. The IC$_{50}$ for acyclovir against most laboratory strains and clinical isolates of VZV ranges from 0.12 to 10.8 mcg/mL. Acyclovir also demonstrates activity against the Oka vaccine strain of VZV with a mean IC$_{50}$ of 1.35 mcg/mL.

➤*Clinical trials:*

Herpes simplex encephalitis – Sixty-two patients 6 months to 79 years of age with brain biopsy-proven herpes simplex encephalitis were randomized to receive either acyclovir IV (10 mg/kg every 8 hours) or vidarabine (15 mg/kg/day) for 10 days. Overall mortality at 12 months for patients treated with acyclovir IV was 25% compared with 59% for patients treated with vidarabine. The proportion of patients treated with acyclovir functioning normally or with only mild sequelae was 32% compared with 12% of patients treated with vidarabine.

Patients less than 30 years of age and those who had the least severe neurologic involvement at time of entry into the study had the best outcome with treatment with acyclovir IV.

Neonatal herpes simplex virus infection – Two hundred two infants with neonatal herpes simplex infections were randomized to receive either 10 mg/kg acyclovir IV every 8 hours or 30 mg/kg/day vidarabine for 10 days.

Mortality at 1 Year		
HSV disease classification	Treatment group	
	Acyclovir IV (n = 107)	Vidarabine (n = 95)
SEM[1]	0/54	0/31
CNS[2]	5/35	5/36
DISS[3]	11/18	14/28

[1] SEM refers to localized infection with disease limited to skin, eye, and/or mouth.
[2] CNS refers to infection of the CNS with compatible neurologic and CSF findings.
[3] DISS refers to visceral organ involvement such as hepatitis or pneumonitis with or without CNS involvement.

Rates of neurologic sequelae at 1 year were comparable between the treatment groups.

Contraindications

Hypersensitivity to acyclovir or any component of the formulation or to valacyclovir.

Warnings

➤*Pregnancy: Category B.* There are no adequate and well-controlled studies in pregnant women. Use during pregnancy only if the potential benefit outweighs the potential risk to the fetus. Potential uses in pregnancy would be for life-threatening disseminated HSV infections to reduce the maternal, fetal, and infant mortality of these infections. Oral acyclovir treatment of primary genital HSV infections also appears to prevent adverse fetal outcomes, such as prematurity, intrauterine growth retardation, and neonatal HSV infection.

➤*Lactation:* Acyclovir concentrations in breast milk in women following oral administration have ranged from 0.6 to 4.1 times corresponding plasma levels. These concentrations would potentially expose the breastfeeding infant to a dose of acyclovir up to 0.3 mg/kg/day. Exercise caution when administering to a breastfeeding woman.

➤*Children:* Safety and efficacy of oral acyclovir in children under 2 years of age have not been established.

Precautions

➤*Genital herpes:* Inform patients acyclovir is not a cure for genital herpes. There are no data evaluating whether acyclovir will prevent transmission of infection to others. Avoid contact with lesions, or avoid intercourse when lesions and/or symptoms are present to prevent infecting partners. Genital herpes can also be transmitted in the absence of symptoms through asymptomatic viral shedding. If medical management of a genital herpes recurrence is indicated, advise patients to initiate therapy at the first sign or symptom of an episode.

ACYCLOVIR (Acycloguanosine)

➤*Herpes zoster infections:* There are no data on treatment initiated more than 72 hours after the onset of the rash. Initiate treatment as soon as possible after diagnosis. In clinical trials, treatment was most effective when started within the first 48 hours of rash onset.

➤*Chickenpox:* Although chickenpox in otherwise healthy children is usually a self-limited disease of mild to moderate severity, adolescents and adults tend to have more severe disease. Treatment was initiated within 24 hours of the typical chickenpox rash in the controlled studies; there is no information regarding the effects of treatment begun later in the disease course. IV acyclovir is indicated for the treatment of varicella-zoster infections in immunocompromised patients.

➤*Do not exceed:* Do not exceed the recommended dosage, frequency, or length of treatment. Base dosage adjustments on estimated creatinine clearance.

➤*Renal function impairment:* Renal failure, sometimes fatal, has been observed with acyclovir therapy. Dosage adjustment is recommended in patients with renal impairment (see Administration and Dosage). Use caution when coadministering acyclovir with other potentially nephrotoxic agents since this may increase the risk of renal impairment and/or the risk of reversible CNS symptoms.

Precipitation of acyclovir crystals in renal tubules can occur if the maximum solubility of free acyclovir (2.5 mg/mL at 37°C in water) is exceeded or if the drug is administered by bolus injection. Ensuing renal tubular damage can produce acute renal failure.

Occurrence of renal failure depends also on the patient's state of hydration, other treatments, and the rate of drug administration. Concomitant use of other nephrotoxic agents, pre-existing renal disease, and dehydration make further renal impairment with acyclovir more likely.

➤*Thrombotic thrombocytopenic purpura/hemolytic uremic syndrome (TTP/HUS):* TTP/HUS which has resulted in death, has occurred in immunocompromised patients receiving acyclovir therapy.

➤*Mutagenesis:* Acyclovir was tested in 16 in vitro and in vivo genetic toxicity assays. Acyclovir was positive in 5 of the assays.

➤*Fertility impairment:* At doses of 50 mg/kg/day SC in rats and rabbits (11 to 22 times and 16 to 31 times human levels, respectively) implantation efficacy was decreased. Also, in a rat peri- and postnatal study of 50 mg/kg/day SC there was a statistically significant decrease in group mean numbers of corpora lutea, total implantation sites, and live fetuses. Testicular atrophy and aspermatogenesis were observed in rats and dogs at doses higher than 50 mg/kg/day IV or 60 mg/kg/day orally.

➤*Elderly:* A clinical trial of patients 50 years of age or older reported an increased incidence of adverse effects, particularly nausea, vomiting, dizziness, and CNS effects including somnolence, hallucinations, confusion, and coma. In general, use caution in dose selection for the elderly to reflect the greater frequency of renal impairment, concomitant diseases, and drugs.

➤*Hydration:* Accompany IV infusion by adequate hydration.

➤*Encephalopathic changes:* Approximately 1% of patients receiving acyclovir IV have manifested encephalopathic changes characterized by either lethargy, obtundation, tremors, confusion, hallucinations, agitation, seizures, or coma. Use with caution in those patients who have underlying neurologic abnormalities; those with serious renal, hepatic, or electrolyte abnormalities or significant hypoxia.

➤*Photosensitivity:* Photosensitive rash may occur; therefore, caution patients to take protective measures (ie, sunscreens, protective clothing) against exposure to ultraviolet light or sunlight until tolerance is determined.

Drug Interactions

Acyclovir Drug Interactions			
Precipitant drug	Object drug*		Description
Probenecid	Acyclovir	↑	Acyclovir bioavailability and terminal plasma half-life may be increased, and renal clearance may be decreased.
Acyclovir	Theophyllines	↑	Coadministration may result in increased theophylline plasma concentrations; monitor plasma levels and side effects. Adjust theophylline dose as necessary.
Acyclovir	Hydantoins Valproic acid	↓	Plasma levels of hydantoins and valproic acid may be decreased with coadministration of acyclovir.

* ↑ = Object drug increased.   ↓ = Object drug decreased.

Adverse Reactions

➤*Parenteral:*

Frequency at least 1% – Inflammation or phlebitis at injection site (approximately 9%); transient elevations of serum creatinine or BUN (5% to 10%, the higher incidence usually occurring following rapid [less than 10 minutes] IV infusion); nausea or vomiting (approximately 7%); itching, rash, hives (approximately 2%); elevation of transaminases (1% to 2%).

Frequency less than 1% – Anemia; hematuria; anorexia; neutropenia; thrombocytopenia; thrombocytosis; leukocytosis; neutrophilia.

➤*Oral:*

Oral Acyclovir Adverse Reactions (Treatment of Herpes Simplex)			
Body system	Short-term administration	Long-term administration	Intermittent administration
CNS	-	-	Headache (2.2%)
GI	Nausea/vomiting (2.7%)	Nausea (4.8%); diarrhea (2.4%)	Diarrhea (2.7%); nausea (2.4%)

Oral Acyclovir Adverse Reactions (Treatment of Herpes Zoster and Chickenpox)				
	Herpes zoster		Chickenpox	
Adverse reaction	Acyclovir	Placebo	Acyclovir	Placebo
Malaise	11.5%	11.1%	—	—
Diarrhea	—	—	3.2%	2.2%

➤*Postmarketing:* Because they are reported voluntarily from a population of unknown size, estimates of frequency cannot be made. These events have been chosen for inclusion because of either their seriousness, frequency of reporting, potential causal connection to acyclovir/acyclovir IV, or a combination of these factors.

Cardiovascular – Hypotension (IV).

CNS – Aggressive behavior; agitation; ataxia; coma; confusion; decreased consciousness (oral); delirium; dizziness; encephalopathy; hallucinations; obtundation (IV); paresthesia; psychosis; seizure; somnolence; tremors. These symptoms may be marked, particularly in older adults or in patients with renal impairment.

Dermatologic – Alopecia; erythema multiforme; photosensitive rash; pruritus; rash; Stevens-Johnson syndrome; toxic epidermal necrolysis; urticaria. Severe local inflammatory reactions, including tissue necrosis, have occurred following infusion of acyclovir IV into extravascular tissues.

GI – Diarrhea; GI distress; nausea.

Hematologic/Lymphatic – Anemia (oral); disseminated intravascular coagulation (IV); hemolysis (IV); leukocytoclastic vasculitis; leukopenia; lymphadenopathy; thrombocytopenia (oral).

Hepatic – Elevated LFTs; hepatitis; hyperbilirubinemia; jaundice.

Musculoskeletal – Myalgia.

Renal – Renal failure; elevated blood urea nitrogen; elevated creatinine; hematuria (oral).

Special senses – Visual abnormalities.

Miscellaneous – Anaphylaxis; angioedema; fever; headache; pain; peripheral edema.

Overdosage

➤*Symptoms:* Precipitation of acyclovir in renal tubules may occur when the solubility (2.5 mg/mL) in the intratubular fluid is exceeded.

Parenteral – Overdosage has occurred with bolus injections, or inappropriately high doses, and in patients whose fluid and electrolyte balance was not properly monitored. Elevations in BUN, serum creatinine, and subsequent renal failure resulted.

Oral – Overdoses involving ingestion of up to 100 capsules (20 g) have been reported. Adverse events that have been reported in association with overdosage include agitation, coma, seizures, and lethargy.

➤*Treatment:* Acyclovir is dialyzable. A 6-hour hemodialysis results in a 60% decrease in plasma acyclovir concentration. Peritoneal dialysis appears less efficient in removing acyclovir from the blood. In the event of acute renal failure and anuria, the patient may benefit from hemodialysis until renal function is restored.

Patient Information

Avoid sexual intercourse when visible herpes lesions are present.

Oral acyclovir does not eliminate latent HSV virus and is not a cure.

Do not exceed recommended dosage.

Notify a physician if frequency and severity of recurrences do not improve.

May cause photosensitivity (sensitivity to sunlight). Avoid prolonged exposure to the sun and other ultraviolet light. Use sunscreens and wear protective clothing until tolerance is determined.

FAMCICLOVIR

Rx	**Famvir** (Novartis)	**Tablets:** 125 mg	Lactose. (Famvir 125). White. Film coated. In 30s.
		250 mg	Lactose. (Famvir 250). White. Film coated. In 30s.
		500 mg	Lactose. (Famvir 500). White, oval. Film coated. In 30s and UD 50s.

Indications

➤*Acute herpes zoster:* Treatment of acute herpes zoster (shingles).

➤*Genital herpes:* Treatment or suppression of recurrent episodes of genital herpes.

➤*Herpes simplex:* Treatment of recurrent mucocutaneous herpes simplex infections in HIV-infected patients.

➤*Unlabeled uses:* Management of initial episodes of herpes genitalis, dose: 250 mg 3 times/day for 7 to 10 days.

Administration and Dosage

➤*Approved by the FDA:* June 29, 1994.

➤*Herpes zoster:* 500 mg every 8 hours for 7 days. Promptly initiate therapy as soon as herpes zoster is diagnosed.

➤*Genital herpes (recurrent episodes):* 125 mg twice /day for 5 days. Initiate therapy at the first sign or symptom if medical management of a genital herpes recurrence is indicated.

The efficacy of famciclovir has not been established when treatment is initiated more than 6 hours after onset of symptoms or lesions.

➤*Suppression of recurrent genital herpes:* 250 mg twice /day for up to 1 year. The safety and efficacy of famciclovir therapy beyond 1 year of treatment have not been established.

➤*HIV-infected patients:* For recurrent orolabial or genital herpes simplex infection, the recommended dosage is 500 mg twice daily for 7 days.

In patients with reduced renal function, dosage reduction is recommended.

➤*Renal function impairment:*

Famciclovir Dosage in Renal Function Impairment	
Creatinine clearance (mL/min)	Dose regimen
Herpes zoster	
≥ 60	500 mg every 8 hours
40 to 59	500 mg every 12 hours
20 to 39	500 mg every 24 hours
< 20	250 mg every 24 hours
Recurrent genital herpes	
≥ 40	125 mg every 12 hours
20 to 39	125 mg every 24 hours
< 20	125 mg every 24 hours
Suppression of recurrent genital herpes	
≥ 40	250 mg every 12 hours
20 to 39	125 mg every 12 hours
< 20	125 mg every 24 hours
Recurrent orolabial and genital herpes simplex infection in HIV-infected patients	
≥ 40	500 mg every 12 hours
20 to 39	500 mg every 24 hours
< 20	250 mg every 24 hours

➤*Hemodialysis patients:* The recommended dosage to be administered following each dialysis treatment is presented in the table below for each indication.

Recommended Dosage Following Dialysis Treatment	
Herpes zoster	250 mg
Recurrent genital herpes	125 mg
Suppression of recurrent genital herpes	125 mg
Recurrent orolabial and genital herpes simplex infection in HIV-infected patients	250 mg

➤*Storage / Stability:* Store between 15° and 30°C (59° and 86°F).

Actions

➤*Pharmacology:* Famciclovir undergoes rapid biotransformation to the active antiviral compound penciclovir, which has inhibitory activity against herpes simplex virus types 1 (HSV-1) and 2 (HSV-2) and varicella zoster virus (VZV). In cells infected with HSV-1, HSV-2, or VZV, viral thymidine kinase phosphorylates penciclovir to a monophosphate form that, in turn, is converted to penciclovir triphosphate by cellular kinases. In vitro studies demonstrate that penciclovir triphosphate inhibits HSV-2 polymerase competitively with deoxyguanosine triphosphate. Consequently, herpes viral DNA synthesis and, therefore, replication are selectively inhibited.

➤*Pharmacokinetics:*

Absorption / Distribution – The absolute bioavailability of famciclovir is approximately 77%. The AUC is 8.6 mcg•hr/mL. C_{max} is 3.3 mcg/mL and T_{max} is 0.9 hours after a single 500 mg dose of famciclovir.

The volume of distribution (Vd) was approximately 1.08 L/kg following a single IV dose of penciclovir at 400 mg administered as a 1-hour IV infusion. Penciclovir is less than 20% bound to plasma proteins over the concentration range of 0.1 to 20 mcg/mL. The blood/plasma ratio of penciclovir is approximately 1.

Penciclovir C_{max} decreased approximately 50% and T_{max} was delayed by 1.5 hours when a capsule formulation of famciclovir was administered with food (nutritional content was approximately 910 Kcal and 26% fat). There was no effect on the extent of availability (AUC) of penciclovir. There was an 18% decrease in C_{max} and a delay in T_{max} of about 1 hour when famciclovir was given 2 hours after a meal as compared with its administration 2 hours before a meal because there was no effect on the extent of systemic availability of penciclovir, it appears that famciclovir can be taken without regard to meals.

Metabolism – Following oral administration, famciclovir is deacetylated and oxidized to form penciclovir. Metabolites that are inactive include 6-deoxy penciclovir, monoacetylated penciclovir, and 6-deoxy monoacetylated penciclovir. Little or no famciclovir is detected in plasma or urine. The conversion of 6-deoxy penciclovir to penciclovir is catalyzed by aldehyde oxidase.

Excretion – Following the oral administration of a single 500 mg dose of radiolabeled famciclovir, 73% and 27% of administered radioactivity were recovered in urine and feces over 72 hours, respectively. Penciclovir accounted for 82% and 6-deoxy penciclovir accounted for 7% of the radioactivity excreted in the urine. Approximately 60% of administered dose was collected in urine in the first 6 hours.

After IV administration of penciclovir, the mean total plasma clearance of penciclovir was approximately 36.6 L/hr. Penciclovir renal clearance accounted for 74.5% of total plasma clearance.

Renal clearance of penciclovir following the oral administration of a single 500 mg dose of famciclovir was approximately 27.7 L/hr.

The plasma elimination half-life of penciclovir was approximately 2 hours after IV administration of penciclovir and approximately 2.3 hours after oral administration of 500 mg famciclovir. The half-life in 7 patients with herpes zoster was approximately 3 hours.

Renal function impairment – Apparent plasma clearance, renal clearance, and the plasma-elimination rate constant of penciclovir decreased linearly with reductions in renal function. After the administration of a single 500 mg famciclovir oral dose to healthy volunteers and to volunteers with varying degrees of renal insufficiency.

Pharmacokinetics of Famciclovir in Patients with Renal Function Impairment				
Parameter (mean)	C_{CR}[1] ≥ 60 (mL/min; n = 15)	C_{CR} 40-59 (mL/min; n = 5)	C_{CR} 20-39 (mL/min; n = 4)	C_{CR} < 20 (mL/min; n = 3)
C_{CR} (mL/min)	88.1	49.3	26.5	12.7
CL_R (L/hr)	30.1	13[2]	4.2	1.6
CL/F[3] (L/hr)	66.9	27.3	12.8	5.8
Half-life (hr)	2.3	3.4	6.2	13.4

[1] C_{CR} is measured CCr.
[2] n = 4.
[3] CL/F consists of bioavailability factor and famciclovir to penciclovir conversion factor.

A dosage adjustment is recommended for patients with renal insufficiency (see Administration and Dosage).

Hepatic function impairment – Well compensated chronic liver disease (eg, chronic hepatitis, chronic ethanol abuse, primary biliary cirrhosis) had no effect on the extent of availability (AUC) of penciclovir following a single dose of 500 mg famciclovir. However, there was a 44% decrease in penciclovir mean maximum plasma concentration and the time to maximum plasma concentration was increased by 0.75 hours in patients with hepatic insufficiency compared with healthy volunteers. No dosage adjustment is recommended for patients with well compensated hepatic impairment. The pharmacokinetics of penciclovir have not been evaluated in patients with severe uncompensated hepatic impairment.

Elderly – Based on cross-study comparisons, mean penciclovir AUC was 40% larger and penciclovir renal clearance was 22% lower after the oral administration of famciclovir in elderly volunteers (65 to 79 years of age) compared with younger volunteers. Some of this difference may be because of differences in renal function between the 2 groups.

Gender – AUC of penciclovir was approximately 9.3 mcg•hr/mL and approximately 11.1 mcg•hr/mL in males and females, respectively. Penciclovir renal clearance was approximately 28.5 L/hr and approximately 21.8 L/hr, respectively. These differences were attributed to differences in renal function between the 2 groups.

FAMCICLOVIR

➤*Microbiology:* In cell culture studies, penciclovir has antiviral activity against the herpes viruses HSV-1, HSV-2, and VZV.

Resistance – Penciclovir-resistant mutants of HSV and VZV can result from qualitative changes in viral thymidine kinase or DNA polymerase. The most commonly encountered acyclovir-resistant mutants that are deficient in viral thymidine kinase also are resistant to penciclovir. Consider the possibility of viral resistance to penciclovir in patients who show poor clinical response during therapy.

➤*Clinical trials:*

Herpes zoster – A double-blind controlled trial in 545 otherwise healthy patients with uncomplicated herpes zoster treated within 72 hours of initial lesion appearance compared 250 mg famciclovir 3 times/day, 500 mg famciclovir 3 times/day, 750 mg famciclovir 3 times/day, and 800 mg acyclovir 5 times/day for 7 days. Patients treated with famciclovir and acyclovir had comparable times to full lesion crusting and times to loss of acute pain. There were no statistically significant differences in the time to loss of post-therapeutic neuralgia between famciclovir and acyclovir treated groups.

Recurrent mucocutaneous herpes simplex infection in HIV-infected patients – A randomized, double-blind, multicenter study compared famciclovir 500 mg twice daily for 7 days with oral acyclovir 400 mg 5 times/day for 7 days in HIV-infected patients with recurrent mucocutaneous HSV infection treated within 48 hours of lesion onset. Approximately 40% of patients had a CD_4 count below 200 cells/mm^3, 54% of patients had anogenital lesions, and 35% had orolabial lesions. Famciclovir therapy was comparable with oral acyclovir in reducing new lesion formation and in time to complete healing.

Contraindications

Hypersensitivity to famciclovir, its components, and penciclovir cream.

Warnings

➤*Renal function impairment:* Dosage adjustment is recommended when administering famciclovir to patients with CCr values less than 60 mL/min. (see Administration and Dosage).

➤*Carcinogenesis:* A significant increase in the incidence of mammary adenocarcinoma was seen in female rats receiving 600 mg/kg/day. No increases in tumor incidence were reported for male rats treated at doses up to 240 mg/kg/day or in female mice at doses up to 600 mg/kg/day.

➤*Mutagenesis:* Famciclovir induced increases in polyploidy in human lymphocytes in vitro in the absence of chromosomal damage (1200 mcg/mL). Penciclovir was positive in the L5178Y mouse lymphoma assay for gene mutation/chromosomal aberrations. In human lymphocytes, penciclovir caused chromosomal aberrations in the absence of metabolic activation (250 mcg/mL). Penciclovir caused an increased incidence of micronuclei in mouse bone marrow in vivo when administered IV at doses highly toxic to bone marrow (500 mg/kg), but not when administered orally.

➤*Fertility impairment:* Testicular toxicity was observed in rats, mice, and dogs following repeated administration of famciclovir or penciclovir. Testicular changes included atrophy of the seminiferous tubules, reduction in sperm count, and/or increased incidence of sperm with abnormal morphology or reduced motility. The degree of toxicity to male reproduction was related to dose and duration of exposure.

➤*Pregnancy: Category B.* There are no adequate and well-controlled studies in pregnant women. Use during pregnancy only if the benefit to the mother clearly exceeds the potential risk to the fetus.

➤*Lactation:* It is not known whether famciclovir is excreted in breast milk. Following oral administration of famciclovir to lactating rats, penciclovir was excreted in breast milk at concentrations higher than those seen in the plasma. Decide whether to discontinue breastfeeding or to discontinue the drug, taking into account the importance of the drug to the mother.

➤*Children:* Safety and efficacy in children less than 18 years of age have not been established.

Drug Interactions

The conversion of 6-deoxy penciclovir to penciclovir is catalyzed by aldehyde oxidase. Interactions with other drugs metabolized by this enzyme could potentially occur.

Concurrent use with probenecid or other drugs significantly eliminated by active renal tubular secretion may result in increased plasma concentrations of penciclovir.

➤*Drug/Food interactions:* When famciclovir was administered with food, penciclovir C_{max} decreased approximately 50%. Because the systemic availability of penciclovir (AUC) was not altered, it appears that famciclovir may be taken without regard to meals.

Adverse Reactions

The most frequent adverse events associated with famciclovir were headache and nausea.

Famciclovir Adverse Reactions (%)

Adverse reaction	Herpes zoster		Genital herpes		Genital herpes-suppression	
	Famciclovir (n = 273)	Placebo (n = 146)	Famciclovir (n = 640)	Placebo (n = 225)	Famciclovir (n = 458)	Placebo (n = 63)
CNS						
Headache	22.7	17.8	23.6	16.4	39.3	42.9
Migraine	0.7	0.7	1.3	0.4	3.1	0
Paresthesia	2.6	0	1.3	0	0.9	0
Dermatologic						
Pruritus	3.7	2.7	0.9	0	2.2	0
Rash	0.4	0.7	0.6	0.4	3.3	1.6
GI						
Nausea	12.5	11.6	10	8	7.2	9.5
Diarrhea	7.7	4.8	4.5	7.6	9	9.5
Abdominal pain	1.1	3.4	3.9	5.8	7.9	7.9
Flatulence	1.5	0.7	1.9	2.2	4.8	1.6
Vomiting	4.8	3.4	1.3	0.9	3.1	1.6
Miscellaneous						
Fatigue	4.4	3.4	6.3	4.4	4.8	3.2
Dysmenorrhea	0	0.7	2.2	1.3	7.6	6.3

Selected Laboratory Abnormalities (%) Studies[1]

Parameter	Famcyclovir (n = 660)	Placebo (n = 210)
Anemia (< 0.8 × NRL[2])	0.1	0
Leukopenia (< 0.75 × NRL[2])	1.3	0.9
Neutropenia (< 0.8 × NRL[2])	3.2	1.5
AST (> 2 × NRH[3])	2.3	1.2
ALT (> 2 × NRH[3])	3.2	1.5
Total bilirubin (>1.5 × NRH[3])	1.9	1.2
Serum creatine (> 1.5 × NRH[3])	0.2	0.3
Amylase (> 1.5 × NRH[3])	1.5	1.9
Lipase (>1.5 × NRH[3])	4.9	4.7

[1] Percentage of patients with laboratory abnormalities that were increased or decreased from baseline and were outside of specified ranges.
[2] NRH = Normal Range High.
[3] NRL = Normal Range Low.

➤*HIV-infected patients:* In HIV-infected patients, the most frequently reported adverse events for famciclovir (500 mg twice daily) and acyclovir (400 mg, 5 times/day), respectively, were headache (16.7% vs 15.4%), nausea (10.7% vs 12.6%), diarrhea (6.7% vs 10.5%), vomiting (4.7% vs 3.5%), fatigue (4% vs 2.1%), and abdominal pain (3.3% vs 5.6%).

➤*Postmarketing:* Confusion (eg, delirium, disorientation, confusional state) has been reported. Most of these spontaneous reports have occurred in the elderly.

Overdosage

Give appropriate symptomatic and supportive therapy. Penciclovir is removed by hemodialysis.

Patient Information

May be taken without regard to meals.

➤*Herpes zoster:* Begin medication as soon as herpes zoster is diagnosed.

➤*Genital herpes:* Inform patients that famciclovir is not a cure for genital herpes. There are no data evaluating whether famciclovir will prevent transmission of infection to others. As genital herpes is a sexually transmitted disease, advise patients to avoid contact with lesions or avoid intercourse when lesions or symptoms are present to prevent infection of partners. Genital herpes also can be transmitted in the absence of symptoms through asymptomatic viral shedding.

Begin medication at the first sign or symptom (eg, pain, tenderness, burning, itching, tingling, vesicles, ulcers, crusts) if medical management of genital herpes recurrence is indicated. The effectiveness of famciclovir has not been established when treatment is started more than 6 hours after onset of symptoms or lesions.

VALACYCLOVIR HCl

Rx	Valtrex (GlaxoSmithKline)	**Tablets:** 500 mg	FD&C Blue No. 2 Lake. (VALTREX 500 mg). Blue, capsule shape. Film-coated. In 30s and UD 100s.
		1 g	FD&C Blue No. 2 Lake. (VALTREX 1 gram). Blue, capsule shape. Film-coated. In 21s.

Indications

➤*Herpes zoster:* For the treatment of herpes zoster (shingles).

➤*Genital herpes:* For the treatment or suppression of genital herpes in immunocompetent individuals and for the suppression of recurrent genital herpes in HIV-infected individuals.

When valacyclovir is used as suppressive therapy in immunocompetent individuals with genital herpes, the risk of heterosexual transmission to susceptible partners is reduced. Instruct patients to use safer sex practices with suppressive therapy (see current Centers for Disease Control and Prevention *Sexually Transmitted Disease Treatment Guidelines*).

➤*Herpes labialis:* For the treatment of herpes labialis (cold sores).

➤*Unlabeled uses:* For the prophylaxis of cytomegalovirus (CMV) disease in patients who have undergone stem-cell or renal transplantation received from a seropositive donor; however, its use in patients with AIDS for CMV prophylaxis is not recommended because of a trend of increasing deaths associated with its use in this population.

Administration and Dosage

➤*Approved by the FDA:* June 23, 1995.

Valacyclovir may be given without regard to meals.

➤*Herpes zoster:* One gram 3 times/day for 7 days. Initiate therapy at the earliest sign or symptom of herpes zoster; it is most effective when started within 48 hours of the onset of zoster rash. No data are available on efficacy of treatment started more than 72 hours after rash onset.

➤*Genital herpes:*

Initial episodes – One gram twice daily for 10 days. There are no data on the effectiveness of treatment when initiated more than 72 hours after the onset of signs and symptoms. Therapy was most effective when administered within 48 hours of the onset of signs and symptoms.

Recurrent episodes – 500 mg twice daily for 3 days. If medical management of a genital herpes recurrence is indicated, advise patients to initiate therapy at the first sign or symptom of an episode. There are no data on the efficacy of treatment when initiated more than 24 hours after the onset of signs or symptoms.

Suppressive therapy – The recommended dosage for chronic suppressive therapy of recurrent genital herpes is 1 g once daily in immunocompetent patients. In patients with a history of 9 or fewer recurrences per year, an alternative dose is 500 mg once daily. The safety and efficacy of therapy with valacyclovir beyond 1 year have not been established.

Transmission – The recommended dosage of valacyclovir for reduction of transmission of genital herpes in patients with a history of 9 or fewer recurrences per year is 500 mg once daily for the source partner. Counsel patients to use safer sex practices in combination with suppressive therapy with valacyclovir. The efficacy of reducing transmission beyond 8 months in discordant couples has not been established.

➤*HIV-infected patients:* In HIV-infected patients with CD4 cell count at least 100 cells/mm[3], the recommended dosage of valacyclovir for chronic suppressive therapy of recurrent genital herpes is 500 mg twice daily. The safety and efficacy of therapy with valacyclovir beyond 6 months in patients with HIV infection have not been established.

➤*Herpes labialis:* The recommended dosage of valacyclovir for the treatment of cold sores is 2 g twice daily for 1 day taken approximately 12 hours apart. Initiate therapy at the earliest symptom of a cold sore (eg, tingling, itching, burning). There are no data on the effectiveness of treatment initiated after the development of clinical signs of a cold sore (eg, papule, vesicle, ulcer). Therapy beyond 1 day does not appear to provide additional clinical benefit.

➤*Renal function impairment:*

Valacyclovir Dosage Adjustments for Renal Impairment				
	Normal dosage (Ccr ≥ 50)	Ccr (mL/min)		
Indication		30 to 49	10 to 29	< 10
Herpes zoster	1 g q 8 h	1 g q 12 h	1 g q 24 h	500 mg q 24 h
Genital herpes				
Initial treatment	1 g q 12 h	No reduction	1 g q 24 h	500 mg q 24 h
Recurrent episodes	500 mg q 12 h	No reduction	500 mg q 24 h	500 mg q 24 h
Suppressive therapy	1 g q 24 h	No reduction	500 mg q 24 h	500 mg q 24 h
Suppressive therapy (≤ 9 recurrences/yr)	500 mg q 24 h	No reduction	500 mg q 48 h	500 mg q 48 h

Valacyclovir Dosage Adjustments for Renal Impairment				
	Normal dosage (Ccr ≥ 50)	Ccr (mL/min)		
Indication		30 to 49	10 to 29	< 10
Suppressive therapy in HIV-infected patients	500 mg q 12 h	No reduction	500 mg q 24 h	500 mg q 24 h
Herpes labialis (cold sores) (do not exceed 1 day of treatment)	Two 2 g doses taken ≈ 12 h apart	Two 1 g doses taken ≈ 12 h apart	Two 500 mg doses taken ≈ 12 h apart	500 mg single dose

➤*Hemodialysis:* During hemodialysis, the half-life of acyclovir after administration of valacyclovir is approximately 4 hours. About 33% of acyclovir in the body is removed by dialysis during a 4-hour hemodialysis session. Give patients requiring hemodialysis the recommended dose of valacyclovir after hemodialysis.

➤*Peritoneal dialysis:* Supplemental doses of valacyclovir should not be required following chronic ambulatory peritoneal dialysis (CAPD) or continuous arteriovenous hemofiltration/hemodialysis (CAVHD).

➤*Storage/Stability:* Store at 15° to 25°C (59° to 77°F).

Actions

➤*Pharmacology:* Valacyclovir is the hydrochloride salt of L-valyl ester of the antiviral drug acyclovir. Valacyclovir is rapidly converted to acyclovir, which has demonstrated in vitro and in vivo antiviral activity against herpes simplex virus types 1 (HSV-1) and 2 (HSV-2) and varicella-zoster virus (VZV).

The inhibitory activity of acyclovir is highly selective because of its affinity for the enzyme thymidine kinase (TK). This viral enzyme converts acyclovir into acyclovir monophosphate, a nucleotide analog. The monophosphate is further converted into diphosphate by cellular guanylate kinase and into triphosphate by a number of cellular enzymes. In vitro, acyclovir triphosphate stops replication of herpes viral DNA in the following 3 ways: 1) Competitive inhibition of viral DNA polymerase; 2) incorporation and termination of the growing viral DNA chain; and 3) inactivation of the viral DNA polymerase. The greater antiviral activity of acyclovir against HSV compared with VZV is because of its more efficient phosphorylation by the viral TK.

➤*Pharmacokinetics:*

Absorption/Distribution – After oral administration, valacyclovir is rapidly absorbed from the GI tract and nearly completely converted to acyclovir and L-valine by first-pass intestinal and/or hepatic metabolism. The absolute bioavailability of acyclovir after administration of valacyclovir is approximately 54.5% following a 1 g oral dose of valacyclovir.

There was a lack of dose proportionality in acyclovir C_{max} and AUC after single-dose administration of 100, 250, 500, and 750 mg and 1 g valacyclovir to 8 healthy volunteers. The approximate mean C_{max} was 0.83, 2.15, 3.28, 4.17, and 5.65 mcg/mL, respectively, and the approximate mean AUC was 2.28, 5.76, 11.59, 14.11, and 19.52 h•mcg/mL, respectively. There also was a lack of dose proportionality in acyclovir C_{max} and AUC after the multiple-dose administration of 250 mg, 500 mg, and 1 gram of valacyclovir 4 times/day for 11 days in parallel groups of 8 healthy volunteers. The approximate mean C_{max} was 2.11, 3.69, and 4.96 mcg/mL, respectively, and the approximate mean AUC was 5.66, 9.88, and 15.7 h•mcg/mL, respectively.

The binding of valacyclovir to human plasma proteins ranged from 13.5% to 17.9%.

Metabolism – Valacyclovir is converted to acyclovir and L-valine by first-pass intestinal and/or hepatic metabolism. Acyclovir is converted to a small extent to inactive metabolites by aldehyde oxidase and by alcohol and aldehyde dehydrogenase. Neither valacyclovir nor acyclovir is metabolized by cytochrome P450 enzymes. Plasma concentrations of unconverted valacyclovir are low and transient, generally becoming nonquantifiable by 3 hours after administration. Peak plasma valacyclovir concentrations are generally less than 0.5 mcg/mL at all doses. After single-dose administration of 1 g, average plasma valacyclovir concentrations were 0.5, 0.4, and 0.8 mcg/mL in patients with hepatic dysfunction, renal insufficiency, and in healthy volunteers who received concomitant cimetidine and probenecid, respectively.

Excretion – The pharmacokinetic disposition of acyclovir delivered by valacyclovir is consistent with previous experience from IV and oral acyclovir. Following oral administration of a single 1 g valacyclovir dose to 4 healthy subjects, 45.6% and 47.12% were recovered in urine and feces, respectively, over 96 hours. Acyclovir accounted for 88.6% excreted in the urine. Renal clearance of acyclovir after a single 1 g valacyclovir dose to 12 healthy volunteers was approximately 255 mL/

VALACYCLOVIR HCl

min, which represents 41.9% of total acyclovir apparent plasma clearance.

The plasma elimination half-life of acyclovir typically averaged 2.5 to 3.3 hours in volunteers with normal renal function.

Special populations –

End-stage renal disease (ESRD): Following valacyclovir administration to volunteers with ESRD, the average acyclovir half-life was approximately 14 hours. During hemodialysis, the acyclovir half-life was approximately 4 hours. Approximately 33% of acyclovir was removed by dialysis during a 4-hour hemodialysis session. Apparent plasma clearance of acyclovir in dialysis patients and healthy volunteers was approximately 86.3 and approximately 679.16 mL/min/ 1.73 m^2, respectively. A dosage reduction is recommended in patients with renal impairment (see Administration and Dosage).

Elderly: After single-dose administration of 1 g valacyclovir in healthy elderly volunteers, the half-life of acyclovir was approximately 3.11 hours compared with approximately 2.91 hours in healthy volunteers. Dosage reduction may be required in elderly patients, depending on the underlying renal status of the patient (see Administration and Dosage).

Hepatic function impairment: Administration of valacyclovir to patients with moderate (biopsy-proven cirrhosis) or severe (with and without ascites and biopsy-proven cirrhosis) liver disease indicated that the rate but not the extent of conversion of valacyclovir to acyclovir was reduced, and the acyclovir half-life was not affected. Dosage modification is not recommended for patients with cirrhosis.

➤*Microbiology:*

Drug resistance – Consider the possibility of viral resistance to valacyclovir (and, therefore, to acyclovir) in patients who show poor clinical response during therapy.

➤*Clinical trials:*

Herpes zoster – In 2 randomized, double-blind clinical trials in immunocompetent patients with localized herpes zoster, valacyclovir was compared with placebo in patients younger than 50 years of age and with acyclovir in patients older than 50 years of age. All patients were treated within 72 hours of appearance of zoster rash. In patients younger than 50 years of age, the median time to cessation of new lesion formation was 2 days for those treated with valacyclovir, compared with 3 days for those treated with placebo. In patients older than 50 years of age, the median time to cessation of new lesions was 3 days in patients treated with valacyclovir or acyclovir. In patients younger than 50 years of age, no difference was found in the duration of pain after healing (postherpetic neuralgia) between the recipients of valacyclovir and placebo. In patients older than 50 years of age who reported pain after healing (postherpetic neuralgia), the median duration of pain after healing in days was 40, 43, and 59 for 7-day valacyclovir, 14-day valacyclovir, and 7-day acyclovir, respectively.

Genital herpes infections –

Initial episode: In a double-blind trial, 643 immunocompetent adults with first-episode genital herpes who presented within 72 hours of symptom onset were randomized to receive 10 days of 1 g valacyclovir twice daily (n = 323) or 200 mg acyclovir 5 times/day (n = 320). For both treatment groups, the median time to lesion healing was 9 days, to cessation of pain was 5 days, and to cessation of viral shedding was 3 days.

Suppressive therapy: Immunocompetent adults with a history of 6 or more recurrences per year were enrolled into a double-blind, placebo- and active-controlled study. Outcomes for the overall study population are shown in the table below.

	Recurrence Rates in Immunocompetent Adults at 6 and 12 Months (%)					
	6 months			12 months		
Treatment	Valacyclovir 1 g qd (n = 269)	Acyclovir 400 mg bid (n = 267)	Placebo (n = 134)	Valacyclovir 1 g qd (n = 269)	Acyclovir 400 mg bid (n = 267)	Placebo (n = 134)
Recurrence-free	55	54	7	34	34	4
Recurrences	35	36	83	46	46	85
Unknowns[1]	10	10	10	19	19	10

[1] Includes lost to follow-up, discontinuations because of adverse events, and consent withdrawn.

Subjects with 9 or fewer recurrences per year showed comparable results with valacyclovir 500 mg once/day.

Hypersensitivity or intolerance to valacyclovir, acyclovir, or any component of the formulation.

Warnings

➤*Thrombotic thrombocytopenic purpura/hemolytic uremic syndrome (TTP/HUS):* TTP/HUS has been reported, in some cases resulting in death, in patients with advanced HIV disease and also in allogeneic bone marrow and renal transplant recipients participating in clinical trials of valacyclovir at doses of 8 grams/day.

➤*Renal function impairment:* Dosage reduction is recommended when administering valacyclovir to patients with renal impairment (see Administration and Dosage). Acute renal failure and CNS symptoms have been reported in patients with underlying renal disease who have received inappropriately high doses for their level of renal function. Exercise similar caution when administering valacyclovir to elderly patients and patients receiving potentially nephrotoxic agents.

Give special attention when prescribing valacyclovir for cold sores in patients with impaired renal function. Treatment should not exceed 1 day. Therapy beyond 1 day does not provide additional clinical benefit.

Precipitation of acyclovir in renal tubules may occur when the solubility (2.5 mg/mL) is exceeded in the intratubular fluid. In the event of acute renal failure and anuria, the patient may benefit from hemodialysis until renal function is restored (see Administration and Dosage).

➤*Mutagenesis:* In the mouse lymphoma assay, valacyclovir was not mutagenic in the absence of metabolic activation. In the presence of metabolic activation (76% to 88% conversion to acyclovir), valacyclovir was mutagenic. Valacyclovir was mutagenic in a mouse micronucleus assay.

➤*Elderly:* The pharmacokinetics of acyclovir following single- and multiple-dose oral administration of valacyclovir in elderly volunteers varied with renal function. Dosage reduction may be required in elderly patients, depending on the underlying renal status of the patient (see Administration and Dosage).

Elderly patients also are more likely to have renal or CNS adverse events. With respect to CNS adverse events observed during clinical practice, agitation, hallucinations, confusion, delirium, and encephalopathy were reported more frequently in elderly patients.

➤*Pregnancy: Category B.* There are no adequate and well-controlled studies of valacyclovir or acyclovir in pregnant women. A prospective epidemiologic registry of acyclovir use during pregnancy was established in 1984 and completed in April 1999. There were 749 pregnancies followed in women exposed to systemic acyclovir during the first trimester of pregnancy, resulting in 756 outcomes. The occurrence rate of birth defects approximates that found in the general population. However, the small size of the registry is insufficient to evaluate the risk for less common defects or to permit reliable or definitive conclusions regarding the safety of acyclovir in pregnant women and their developing fetuses. Use valacyclovir during pregnancy only if the potential benefit justifies the potential risk to the fetus.

➤*Lactation:* There is no experience with valacyclovir. However, acyclovir concentrations have been documented in breast milk in 2 women following oral administration of acyclovir and ranged from 0.6 to 4.1 times corresponding plasma levels. These concentrations would expose the breastfeeding infant to a dose of acyclovir as high as 0.3 mg/kg/day. Administer valacyclovir to a breastfeeding mother with caution and only when indicated.

➤*Children:* Safety and efficacy in prepubertal pediatric patients have not been established.

Drug Interactions

➤*Cimetidine/Probenecid:* After a combination of cimetidine and probenecid, acyclovir C$_{max}$ and AUC increased following a single 1 g dose of valacyclovir 8% and 32%, respectively, following a single 800 mg dose of cimetidine, 22% and 49%, respectively, following a 1 g dose of probenecid, or by 30% and 78%, respectively, following a combination of cimetidine and probenecid. These effects are primarily caused by a reduction in renal clearance of acyclovir. These effects are not considered to be of clinical significance in subjects with normal renal function and no dosage adjustment is recommended.

VALACYCLOVIR HCl

Adverse Reactions

Adverse reaction	Valacyclovir Adverse Reactions (%)				
	Herpes zoster	Genital herpes treatment		Genital herpes suppression	
	1 g tid	1 g bid	500 mg bid	1 g/day	500 mg/day
CNS					
Headache	14	16	15	35	38
Dizziness	3	3	2	4	2
Depression	—	1	0	7	5
GI					
Nausea	15	6	5	11	11
Vomiting	6	1	< 1	3	3
Abdominal pain	3	2	1	11	9
Lab test abnormalities					
Leukopenia (WBCs < 0.75 × LLN[1])	1.3	0.7	0.6	0.7	0.8
AST (> 2 × ULN[2])	1	1	—[3]	4.1	3.8
Thrombocytopenia (platelet count < 100,000/mm^3)	1	0.3	0.1	0.4	1.1
Hemoglobin (< 0.8 × LLN)	0.8	0.3	0.2	0	0.8
Serum creatinine (> 1.5 × ULN)	0.2	0.7	0	0	0
Miscellaneous					
Dysmenorrhea	—	< 1	< 1	8	5
Arthralgia	—	< 1	< 1	6	5

[1] LLN = Lower limit of normal.
[2] ULN = Upper limit of normal.
[3] Data were not collected prospectively.

➤*Herpes labialis:* In clinical studies for the treatment of cold sores, the adverse events reported by patients receiving valacyclovir (n = 609) or placebo (n = 609) included headache (14% valacyclovir vs 10% placebo) and dizziness (2% vs 1%). Also in clinical studies for treatment of cold sores, the frequencies of abnormal ALT (greater than 2 × ULN) were 1.8% for patients receiving valacyclovir compared with 0.8% for placebo. Other laboratory abnormalities (hemoglobin, WBCs, alkaline phosphatase, and serum creatinine) occurred with similar frequencies in the 2 groups.

➤*General herpes suppression in HIV-infected patients:* In HIV-infected patients, frequently reported adverse events for valacyclovir (500 mg twice daily) included, headache (13%), fatigue (8%), and rash (8%). Postrandomization laboratory abnormalities that were reported more frequently in valacyclovir subjects vs placebo included elevated alkaline phosphatase (4%), elevated ALT (14%), elevated AST (16%), decreased neutrophil counts (18%), and decreased platelet counts (3%).

➤*Reduction of transmission:* In a clinical study for the reduction of transmission of genital herpes, the adverse events reported by patients receiving valacyclovir 500 mg once daily (n = 73) included headache (29%), nasopharyngitis (16%), and upper respiratory tract infection (9%).

➤*Postmarketing:*
Cardiovascular – Hypertension; tachycardia.

CNS – Aggressive behavior; agitation; ataxia; coma; confusion; decreased consciousness; dysarthria; encephalopathy; mania; psychosis, including auditory and visual hallucinations; seizures; tremors.

Dermatologic – Erythema multiforme; rashes including photosensitivity; alopecia.

GI – Diarrhea; hepatitis.

Hypersensitivity – Acute hypersensitivity reactions including anaphylaxis, angioedema, dyspnea, pruritus, rash, and urticaria.

Lab test abnormalities – Liver enzyme abnormalities; elevated creatinine; thrombocytopenia; aplastic anemia.

Miscellaneous – Facial edema; visual abnormalities; renal failure; leukocytoclastic vasculitis; TTP/HUS.

Overdosage

Precipitation of acyclovir in renal tubules may occur when the solubility (2.5 mg/mL) is exceeded in the intratubular fluid. In the event of acute renal failure and anuria, the patient may benefit from hemodialysis until renal function is restored.

Patient Information

➤*Herpes zoster:* There are no data on treatment initiated more than 72 hours after onset of the zoster rash. Advise patients to initiate treatment as soon as possible after a diagnosis of herpes zoster.

➤*Genital herpes:* Inform patients that valacyclovir is not a cure for genital herpes. Because genital herpes is a sexually transmitted disease, advise patients to avoid contact with lesions and to avoid intercourse when lesions or symptoms are present to avoid infecting others. Genital herpes is frequently transmitted in the absence of symptoms through asymptomatic viral shedding. If medical management of herpes recurrence is indicated, advise patients to initiate therapy at the first sign or symptom of an episode.

Counsel patients to use safer sex practices in combination with suppressive therapy with valacyclovir. Advise infected patients to notify sex partners that they might be infected even if they have no symptoms. Type-specific serologic testing of asymptomatic partners of persons with genital herpes can determine whether risk for HSV-2 acquisition exists.

Valacyclovir has not been shown to reduce transmission of sexually transmitted infections other than HSV-2.

There are no data on the effectiveness of treatment initiated more than 72 hours after the onset of signs and symptoms of a first episode of genital herpes or more than 24 hours after the onset of signs and symptoms of a recurrent episode.

➤*Cold sores:* Advise patients to initiate treatment at the earliest symptom of a cold sore (eg, tingling, itching, burning). There are no data on the effectiveness of treatment initiated after the development of clinical signs of a cold sore (eg, papule, vesicle, ulcer). Instruct patients not to exceed 1 day (2 doses) for cold sore treatment and to take their doses approximately 12 hours apart. Inform patients that valacyclovir is not a cure for cold sores.

May cause photosensitive rash. Instruct patients to avoid prolonged exposure to the sun and other ultraviolet light and to use sunscreens and wear protective clothing until tolerance is determined.

AMANTADINE HCl

Rx	Symmetrel (Endo)	Tablets: 100 mg	(SYMMETREL). Orange, triangular. In 100s and 500s.
Rx	Amantadine HCl (Various, eg, Banner, Geneva, Major, Martec, UDL, URL)	Capsules: 100 mg	In 100s, 500s, and UD 100s.
Rx	Amantadine HCl (Various, eg, Alpharma, Endo, Morton Grove)	Syrup: 50 mg/5 mL	May contain sorbitol and parabens. In 480 mL.
Rx	Symmetrel (Endo)		Sorbitol and parabens. In 480 mL.

Amantadine is also used as an antiparkinson agent. For information regarding this use, refer to amantadine in the Antiparkinson Agents section.

Indications

➤*Influenza A viral infection:* Amantadine is indicated for the prophylaxis and treatment of signs and symptoms of infection caused by various strains of influenza A virus.

Prophylaxis – Chemoprophylaxis against signs and symptoms of influenza A virus infection when early vaccination is not feasible or when the vaccine is contraindicated or not available. Following vaccination during an influenza A outbreak, consider amantadine prophylaxis for the 2- to 4-week time period required to develop an antibody response.

Treatment – Treatment of uncomplicated respiratory tract illness caused by influenza A virus strains, especially when administered early in the course of illness.

➤*Prophylaxis recommendations:*
1.) High-risk patients vaccinated after influenza outbreak has begun: Consider prophylaxis until immunity from the influenza vaccine has developed (this may take up to 2 weeks).
2.) Caretakers of those at high risk: Consider prophylaxis for unvaccinated caretakers of high-risk patients during peak influenza activity.
3.) Patients with immune deficiency: Consider prophylaxis for high-risk patients who are expected to have inadequate antibody response to influenza vaccine (eg, HIV).
4.) Other: Consider prophylaxis in high-risk patients who should not be vaccinated. Prophylaxis may also be offered to those patients who desire to avoid influenza illness.

➤*Parkinsonism and drug-induced extrapyramidal reactions:* See amantadine in the Antiparkinson Agents section.

Administration and Dosage

➤*Prophylaxis:* Start dosing in anticipation of an influenza A outbreak and before or after contact with individuals with influenza A virus respiratory tract illness. Continue for ≥ 10 days following known exposure. If used in conjunction with influenza vaccine, then administer for 2 to 4 weeks after the vaccine has been given. When the vaccine is unavailable or contraindicated, give amantadine for the duration of known influenza A in the community because of repeated and unknown exposure.

➤*Treatment:* Start treatment as soon as possible, preferably within 24 to 48 hours after onset of signs and symptoms, and continue for 24 to 48 hours after disappearance of signs and symptoms.

➤*Dosage:*

Amantadine Dosage by Patient Age and Renal Function	
Renal function	Dosage
No recognized renal disease	
1 to 9 yrs[1]	4.4 to 8.8 mg/kg/day given once daily or divided twice daily, not to exceed 150 mg/day
9 to 12 yrs	100 mg twice daily
13 to 64 yrs	200 mg once daily or divided twice daily
≥ 65 yrs	100 mg once daily
Renal function impairment – Creatinine clearance (mL/min/1.73 m²)	
30 to 50	200 mg 1st day; 100 mg daily thereafter
15 to 29	200 mg 1st day; then 100 mg on alternate days
< 15	200 mg every 7 days
Hemodialysis patients	200 mg every 7 days

[1] Use in children < 1 year of age has not been evaluated adequately.

➤*Dosage adjustments:* For adults < 65 years of age, if CNS effects develop in a once-daily dosage, a split dosage schedule may reduce such complaints.

➤*Special risk patients:* Dose may need reduction in patients with CHF, peripheral edema, orthostatic hypotension, or impaired renal function.

➤*Storage/Stability:* Store at 25°C (77°F), excursions permitted to 15° to 30°C (59° to 86°F). Dispense in a tight container with a child-resistant closure (as required).

Actions

➤*Pharmacology:* Inhibits the replication of influenza A virus isolates from each of the subtypes (ie, H1N1, H2N2, H3N3). It has very little or no activity against influenza B virus isolates. Amantadine's antiviral activity is not completely understood. Its mode of action appears to be the prevention of the release of infectious viral nucleic acid into the host cell. Amantadine does not appear to interfere with the immunogenicity of inactivated influenza A virus vaccine.

Amantadine is 70% to 90% effective in preventing illnesses caused by type A influenza viruses.

➤*Pharmacokinetics:*

Absorption/Distribution – Amantadine is well absorbed orally. Maximum plasma concentrations are directly related to dose for doses up to 200 mg/day. Doses > 200 mg/day may result in a greater than proportional increase in maximum plasma concentrations. Administration of 100 mg orally resulted in a mean maximum plasma concentration of ≈ 0.22 mcg/mL. The time to peak concentration was ≈ 3.3 hours. After IV administration, the volume of distribution was 3 to 8 L/kg, suggesting tissue binding.

Metabolism/Excretion – Amantadine is primarily excreted unchanged in the urine by glomerular filtration and tubular secretion. After administration of 100 mg orally, the apparent oral clearance was ≈ 0.28 L/hr/kg, and the half-life was ≈ 17 hours.

Special populations –
Elderly: The apparent oral plasma clearance of amantadine is reduced and the plasma half-life and plasma concentrations are increased in healthy elderly individuals ≥ 60 years of age. Whether these changes are caused by decline in renal function or other age-related factors is not known.
Renal function impairment: The clearance is significantly reduced in adult patients with renal insufficiency. The elimination half-life increases ≥ 2- to 3-fold when creatinine clearance is < 40 mL/min/1.73 m² and averages 8 days in patients on chronic maintenance hemodialysis. Amantadine is removed in negligible amounts by hemodialysis.

Contraindications

Hypersensitivity to amantadine or to any of the other ingredients.

Warnings

➤*Deaths:* Deaths have been reported from overdose with amantadine (see Overdosage).

➤*Suicide attempts:* Suicide attempts, some of which have been fatal, have been reported in patients treated with amantadine, many of whom received short courses for influenza treatment or prophylaxis. Suicide attempts and suicidal ideation have been reported in patients with and without prior history of psychiatric illness. Amantadine can exacerbate mental problems in patients with a history of psychiatric disorders or substance abuse. Patients who attempt suicide may exhibit abnormal mental states, which include disorientation, confusion, depression, personality changes, agitation, aggressive behavior, hallucinations, paranoia, other psychotic reactions, and somnolence or insomnia. Because of the possibility of serious adverse effects, observe caution when prescribing amantadine to patients being treated with drugs having CNS effects, or for whom the potential risks outweigh the benefit of treatment.

➤*Seizures and other CNS effects:* Closely observe patients with a history of epilepsy or other seizures for increased seizure activity. Caution patients who note CNS effects or blurring of vision against driving or working in situations where alertness and adequate motor coordination are important.

➤*CHF or peripheral edema:* Closely follow patients with a history of CHF or peripheral edema as there are patients who developed CHF while receiving amantadine.

➤*Glaucoma:* Because amantadine has anticholinergic effects and may cause mydriasis, do not give to patients with untreated angle closure glaucoma.

➤*Other:* Exercise care when administering to patients with a history of recurrent eczematoid rash, or to patients with psychosis or severe psychoneurosis not controlled by chemotherapeutic agents.

➤*Renal function impairment:* Amantadine is mainly excreted in the urine and accumulated in the plasma and body when renal function declines. Reduce the dose in those with renal impairment. Hemodialysis does not remove significant amounts of amantadine.

➤*Hepatic function impairment:* Exercise care when administering amantadine to patients with liver disease.

➤*Elderly:* Reduce dose in patients ≥ 65 years of age.

➤*Pregnancy: Category C.* Amantadine has been reported to be teratogenic in rats at 50 mg/kg/day and embryotoxic at 100 mg/kg/day (estimated human equivalent dose of 7.1 mg/kg/day and 14.2 mg/kg/day, respectively, based on body surface area conversion). Tetralogy of Fallot and tibial hemimelia (normal karyotype) occurred in an infant exposed to amantadine during the first trimester of pregnancy (100 mg PO for

AMANTADINE HCl

7 days during the 6th and 7th week of gestation). Cardiovascular maldevelopment (single ventricle with pulmonary atresia) was associated with maternal exposure to amantadine (100 mg/day) administered during the first 2 weeks of pregnancy. Use amantadine during pregnancy only if the potential benefit justifies the potential risk to the embryo or fetus.

➤*Lactation:* Amantadine is excreted in breast milk. Use is not recommended in nursing mothers.

➤*Children:* Safety and efficacy for use in neonates and infants < 1 year of age have not been established.

Precautions

➤*Abrupt withdrawal:* Do not discontinue amantadine abruptly in patients with Parkinson's disease because a few patients have experienced a parkinsonian crisis (a sudden marked clinical deterioration) when this medication was suddenly stopped. Abrupt discontinuation may also precipitate delirium, agitation, delusions, hallucinations, paranoid reaction, stupor, anxiety, depression, and slurred speech.

➤*Neuroleptic malignant syndrome (NMS):* Sporadic cases of possible NMS have been reported in association with dose reduction or withdrawal of amantadine therapy. Therefore, observe patients carefully when the dosage of amantadine is reduced abruptly or discontinued, especially if the patient is receiving neuroleptics.

Drug Interactions

Coadministration of amantadine and thioridazine has been reported to worsen the tremor in elderly Parkinson's disease patients.

Amantadine Drug Interactions			
Precipitant drug	Object drug*		Description
Anticholinergic agents	Amantadine	↑	Concurrent administration may potentiate the anticholinergic-like side effects of amantadine. Consider reducing the dose of the anticholinergic agent if atropine-like effects appear.
Quinidine Quinine	Amantadine	↑	Coadministration was shown to reduce renal clearance of amantadine.
Triamterene Thiazide diuretics	Amantadine	↑	Coadministration resulted in a higher plasma amantadine concentration.
Trimethoprim/ sulfamethoxazole	Amantadine	↑	Coadministration may impair renal clearance of amantadine, resulting in higher plasma concentrations.
Amantadine	CNS stimulants	↑	Careful observation is required during concomitant administration.

* ↑ = Object drug increased.

Adverse Reactions

➤*CNS:* Dizziness, lightheadedness, insomnia (5% to 10%); depression, anxiety, irritability, hallucinations, confusion, ataxia, headache, somnolence, nervousness, dream abnormality, agitation, fatigue (1% to 5%); psychosis, slurred speech, euphoria, thinking abnormality, amnesia, hyperkinesia, decreased libido (0.1% to 1%); convulsions, suicide attempt, suicide, suicidal ideation (< 0.1%).

➤*GI:* Nausea (5% to 10%); anorexia, dry mouth, constipation, diarrhea (1% to 5%); vomiting (0.1% to 1%).

➤*Cardiovascular:* Orthostatic hypotension (1% to 5%); CHF, hypertension (0.1% to 1%).

➤*Special senses:* Visual disturbance, including punctate subepithelial or other corneal opacity, corneal edema, decreased visual acuity, sensitivity to light, optic nerve palsy (0.1% to 1%); oculogyric episodes (< 0.1%).

➤*Dermatologic:* Livedo reticularis (1% to 5%); skin rash (0.1% to 1%); eczematoid dermatitis (< 0.1%).

➤*Miscellaneous:* Peripheral edema, dry nose (1% to 5%); weakness, urinary retention, dyspnea (0.1% to 1%); leukopenia, neutropenia (< 0.1%).

➤*Postmarketing:* The following adverse reactions were reported during postmarketing experience:

Cardiovascular – Cardiac arrest; arrhythmias, including malignant arrhythmias; hypotension; tachycardia.

CNS – Coma; stupor; delirium; hypokinesia; hypertonia; delusions; aggressive behavior; paranoid reaction; manic reaction; involuntary muscle contractions; gait abnormalities; paresthesia; EEG changes; tremor. Abrupt discontinuation may also precipitate delirium, agitation, delusions, hallucinations, paranoid reaction, anxiety, depression, slurred speech.

Lab test abnormalities – Elevated CPK, BUN, serum creatinine, alkaline phosphatase, LDH, bilirubin, GGT, AST, and ALT.

Respiratory – Acute respiratory failure; pulmonary edema; tachypnea.

Miscellaneous – Dysphagia; leukocytosis; keratitis; mydriasis; pruritus; diaphoresis; NMS; allergic reactions, including anaphylactic reactions; edema; fever.

Overdosage

➤*Symptoms:* Deaths have been reported from overdose with amantadine. The lowest reported acute lethal dose was 1 g. Acute toxicity may be attributable to the anticholinergic effects of amantadine. Drug overdose has resulted in cardiac, respiratory, renal, or CNS toxicity. Cardiac dysfunction includes arrhythmia, tachycardia, and hypertension. Pulmonary edema and respiratory distress (including adult respiratory distress syndrome) have been reported; renal dysfunction, including increased BUN, decreased creatinine clearance, and renal insufficiency can occur. CNS effects that have been reported include insomnia, anxiety, agitation, aggressive behavior, hypertonia, hyperkinesia, ataxia, gait abnormality, tremor, confusion, disorientation, depersonalization, fear, delirium, hallucinations, psychotic reactions, lethargy, somnolence, and coma. Seizures may be exacerbated in patients with prior history of seizure disorders. Hyperthermia has also been observed.

➤*Treatment:* There is no specific antidote. Employ general supportive measures along with immediate gastric lavage. Refer to General Management of Acute Overdosage. Monitor blood pressure, pulse, respiration, temperature, electrolytes, urine pH, and urinary output. Observe the patient for hyperactivity and convulsions; administer sedatives and anticonvulsants if required. Give appropriate antiarrhythmic and vasopressor therapy when warranted.

Hemodialysis does not remove significant amounts of amantadine.

Patient Information

Blurry vision or impaired mental acuity may occur.

Gradually increase physical activity as the symptoms of Parkinson's disease improve.

Avoid excessive alcohol usage because it may increase the potential for CNS effects such as dizziness, confusion, lightheadedness, and orthostatic hypotension.

Avoid getting up suddenly from a sitting or lying position. If dizziness or lightheadedness occurs, notify a physician.

Notify physician if mood/mental changes, swelling of extremities, difficulty urinating, or shortness of breath occur.

Do not take more medication than prescribed because of the risk of overdose. If there is no improvement in a few days, or if medication appears less effective after a few weeks, discuss with a physician.

Consult physician before discontinuing medication.

Seek medical attention immediately if it is suspected that an overdose of medication has been taken.

CIDOFOVIR

Rx　Vistide (Gilead Sciences)	Injection: 75 mg/mL	Preservative free. In 5 mL single-use vials.

WARNING

Renal impairment is the major toxicity of cidofovir. Cases of acute renal failure resulting in dialysis or contributing to death have occurred with as few as 1 or 2 doses of cidofovir. To minimize possible nephrotoxicity, IV prehydration with normal saline and administration of probenecid must be used with each cidofovir infusion. Monitor renal function (serum creatinine and urine protein) within 48 hours prior to each dose of cidofovir and modify the dose for changes in renal function as appropriate. Cidofovir is contraindicated in patients who are receiving other nephrotoxic agents.

Neutropenia has been observed in association with cidofovir treatment. Monitor neutrophil counts during cidofovir therapy.

Cidofovir is indicated only for the treatment of cytomegalovirus (CMV) retinitis in patients with acquired immunodeficiency syndrome (AIDS).

In animal studies, cidofovir was carcinogenic, teratogenic, and caused hypospermia.

Indications

➤*CMV retinitis:* For the treatment of CMV retinitis in patients with AIDS.

Administration and Dosage

➤*Approved by the FDA:* June 26, 1996.

Do not administer by intraocular injection.

The recommended dosage, frequency, or infusion rate must not be exceeded. Cidofovir must be diluted in 100 mL 0.9% normal saline solution prior to administration. To minimize potential nephrotoxicity, probenecid and IV saline prehydration must be administered with each cidofovir infusion.

➤*Induction treatment:* The recommended dose of cidofovir for patients with a serum creatinine of ≤ 1.5 mg/dL, a calculated creatinine clearance (Ccr) > 55 mL/min, and a urine protein < 100 mg/dL (equivalent to < 2+ proteinuria) is 5 mg/kg body weight (given as an IV infusion at a constant rate over 1 hour) administered once weekly for 2 consecutive weeks. Because serum creatinine in patients with advanced AIDS and CMV retinitis may not provide a complete picture of the patient's underlying renal status, it is important to utilize the Cockcroft-Gault formula to more precisely estimate Ccr. As Ccr is dependent on serum creatinine and patient weight, it is necessary to calculate clearance prior to initiation of cidofovir. Calculate Ccr (mL/min) according to the following formula:

$$\text{Males:} \quad \frac{\text{Weight (kg)} \times (140 - \text{age})}{72 \times \text{serum creatinine (mg/dL)}} = \text{Ccr}$$

Females: 0.85 × above value

➤*Maintenance treatment:* The recommended maintenance dose of cidofovir is 5 mg/kg body weight (given as an IV infusion at a constant rate over 1 hour) administered once every 2 weeks.

➤*Probenecid:* Probenecid must be administered orally with each cidofovir dose. Administer 2 g 3 hours prior to the cidofovir dose and administer 1 g at 2 hours and again at 8 hours after completion of the 1-hour cidofovir infusion (for a total of 4 g).

Ingestion of food prior to each dose of probenecid may reduce drug-related nausea and vomiting. Administration of an antiemetic may reduce the potential for nausea associated with probenecid ingestion. In patients who develop allergic or hypersensitivity reactions to probenecid, consider the use of an appropriate prophylactic or therapeutic antihistamine or acetaminophen.

Zidovudine should either be temporarily discontinued or decreased by 50% when coadministered with probenecid on the day of cidofovir infusion.

➤*Hydration:* Patients must receive a total of 1 L of 0.9% normal saline solution IV with each infusion of cidofovir. Infuse the saline solution over a 1- to 2-hour period immediately before the cidofovir infusion. Patients who can tolerate the additional fluid load should receive a second liter. If administered, initiate the second liter of saline at the start of the cidofovir infusion or immediately afterwards, and infuse over a 1- to 3-hour period.

➤*Changes in renal function during therapy:* For increases in serum creatinine (0.3 to 0.4 mg/dL), reduce the cidofovir dose from 5 mg/kg to 3 mg/kg. Discontinue cidofovir therapy for an increase in serum creatinine of ≥ 0.5 mg/dL above baseline or development of ≥ 3+ proteinuria.

➤*Preexisting renal impairment:* Cidofovir is contraindicated in patients with a serum Ccr > 1.5 mg/dL, a calculated Ccr of ≤ 55 mL/min, or a urine protein ≥ 100 mg/dL (equivalent to ≥ 2+ proteinuria).

➤*Handling and disposal:* Because of the mutagenic properties of cidofovir, adequate precautions, including the use of appropriate safety equipment are recommended for the preparation, administration, and disposal of cidofovir. If cidofovir contacts the skin, wash membranes and flush thoroughly with water.

➤*Storage / Stability:* Store at controlled room temperature 20° to 25°C (68° to 77°F).

Admixtures may be stored under refrigeration (2° to 8°C; 36° to 46°F) for ≤ 24 hours. Allow refrigerated admixtures to equilibrate to room temperature prior to use. Discard partially used vials.

Actions

➤*Pharmacology:* Cidofovir is a nucleotide analog. Cidofovir suppresses CMV replication by selective inhibition of viral DNA synthesis. Biochemical data support selective inhibition of CMV DNA polymerase by cidofovir diphosphate, the active intracellular metabolite of cidofovir. Cidofovir diphosphate inhibits herpes virus polymerases at concentrations that are 8- to 600-fold lower than those needed to inhibit human cellular DNA polymerases alpha, beta, and gamma. Incorporation of cidofovir into the growing viral DNA chain results in reductions in the rate of viral DNA synthesis.

Resistance – CMV isolates with reduced susceptibility to cidofovir have been selected in vitro in the presence of high concentrations of cidofovir. IC_{50} values for selected resistant isolates ranged from 7 to 15 mcM.

Consider the possibility of viral resistance for patients who show a poor clinical response or experience recurrent retinitis progression during therapy.

Cross resistance – Cidofovir-resistant isolates selected in vitro following exposure to increasing concentrations of cidofovir were assessed for susceptibility to ganciclovir and foscarnet. All were cross-resistant to ganciclovir, but remained susceptible to foscarnet. Ganciclovir or ganciclovir/foscarnet-resistant isolates that are cross-resistant to cidofovir have been obtained from drug-naive patients and from patients following ganciclovir or ganciclovir/foscarnet therapy. To date, the majority of ganciclovir-resistant isolates are UL97 gene product (phosphokinase) mutants and remain susceptible to cidofovir. However, reduced susceptibility to cidofovir has been reported for DNA polymerase mutants of CMV that are resistant to ganciclovir. To date, all clinical isolates that exhibit high level resistance to ganciclovir, because of mutations in the DNA polymerase and UL97 genes, have been shown to be cross-resistant to cidofovir. Cidofovir is active against some, but not all, CMV isolates that are resistant to foscarnet. The incidence of foscarnet-resistant isolates that are resistant to cidofovir is not known.

➤*Pharmacokinetics:* Cidofovir must be administered with probenecid. Renal tubular secretion contributes to the elimination of cidofovir.

Cidofovir Pharmacokinetic Parameters Following 3 and 5 mg/kg Infusions With and Without Probenecid				
	Cidofovir administered without probenecid		Cidofovir administered with probenecid	
Parameters	3 mg/kg	5 mg/kg	3 mg/kg	5 mg/kg
AUC (mcg·hr/mL)	≈ 20	28.3	≈ 25.7	≈ 40.8
C_{max} (end of infusion) (mcg/mL)	≈ 7.3	11.5	≈ 9.8	≈ 19.6
Vd_{ss} (mL/kg)	≈ 537		≈ 410	
Clearance (mL/min/1.73 m²)	≈ 179		≈ 148	
Renal clearance (mL/min/1.73 m²)	≈ 150		≈ 98.6	

In vitro, cidofovir was < 6% bound to plasma or serum proteins over the cidofovir concentration range 0.25 to 25 mcg/mL. CSF concentrations of cidofovir following IV infusion of cidofovir 5 mg/kg with concomitant probenecid and IV hydration were undetectable (< 0.1 mcg/mL, assay detection threshold) at 15 minutes after the end of a 1-hour infusion in 1 patient whose corresponding serum concentration was 8.7 mcg/mL.

Contraindications

Initiation of therapy in patients with a serum creatinine of > 1.5 mg/dL, a calculated Ccr of ≤ 55 mL/min, or a urine protein ≥ 100 mg/dL (equivalent to ≥ 2+ proteinuria); patients receiving agents with a nephrotoxic potential (such agents must be discontinued ≥ 7 days prior to starting cidofovir therapy); hypersensitivity to cidofovir; a history of clinically severe hypersensitivity to probenecid or other sulfa-containing medications; direct intraocular injection.

Warnings

➤*Other CMV infections:* The safety and efficacy of cidofovir have not been established for treatment of other CMV infections (eg, pneumonitis, gastroenteritis), congenital or neonatal CMV disease, or CMV disease in non-HIV-infected individuals.

➤*Direct intraocular injection:* May be associated with iritis, ocular hypotony, and permanent impairment of vision.

➤*Nephrotoxicity:* Dose-dependent nephrotoxicity is the major dose-limiting toxicity related to cidofovir administration. Monitor renal func-

CIDOFOVIR

tion (serum creatinine and urine protein) within 48 hours prior to each dose of cidofovir. Dose adjustment or discontinuation is required for changes in renal function while on therapy. Proteinuria may be an early indicator of cidofovir-related nephrotoxicity. Continued administration of cidofovir may lead to additional proximal tubular cell injury that may result in glycosuria; decreases in serum phosphate, uric acid, and bicarbonate; elevations in serum creatinine; or acute renal failure, in some cases, resulting in the need for dialysis. Patients with these adverse events occurring concurrently and meeting a criteria of Fanconi's syndrome have been reported. Renal function that did not return to baseline after drug discontinuation has been observed in clinical studies of cidofovir.

Because of the potential for increased nephrotoxicity, doses greater than the recommended dose must not be administered and the frequency or rate of administration must not be exceeded.

➤*Hematological toxicity:* Neutropenia may occur during cidofovir therapy. Monitor neutrophil count while receiving cidofovir therapy.

➤*Metabolic acidosis:* Decreased serum bicarbonate associated with proximal tubule injury and renal wasting syndrome (including Fanconi's syndrome) have been reported in patients receiving cidofovir. Cases of metabolic acidosis in association with liver dysfunction and pancreatitis resulting in death have been reported in patients receiving cidofovir.

➤*Decreased intraocular pressure (OPV)/ocular hypotony:* Decreased OPV may occur during cidofovir therapy, and in some instances has been associated with decreased visual acuity. Monitor OPV during cidofovir therapy.

➤*Renal function impairment:* Initiation of therapy with cidofovir is contraindicated in patients with baseline serum creatinine > 1.5 mg/dL or Ccr ≤ 55 mL/min or a urine protein ≥ 100 mg/dL (equivalent to ≥ 2+ proteinuria).

➤*Carcinogenesis:* Mammary adenocarcinomas have occurred in rats, and Zymbal's gland carcinomas have occurred in rats at high doses.

➤*Fertility impairment:* Studies showed inhibition of spermatogenesis in rats and monkeys. However, no adverse effects on fertility or reproduction were seen following once weekly IV injections of cidofovir in male rats for 13 consecutive weeks.

➤*Elderly:* No studies of the safety and efficacy of cidofovir in patients > 60 years of age have been conducted. Because elderly individuals frequently have reduced glomerular filtration, pay particular attention to assessing renal function before and during cidofovir administration.

➤*Pregnancy:* Category C. Cidofovir was embryotoxic (reduced fetal body weights) in rats and in rabbits. An increased incidence of fetal external, soft tissue, and skeletal anomalies (meningocele, short snout, and short maxillary bones) occurred in rabbits. There are no adequate and well-controlled studies in pregnant women. Use cidofovir during pregnancy only if the potential benefit justifies the potential risk to the fetus.

➤*Lactation:* It is not known whether cidofovir is excreted in breast milk. Since many drugs are excreted in breast milk and because of the potential for adverse reactions as well as the potential for tumorigenicity shown for cidofovir in animal studies, do not administer cidofovir to nursing women. The US Public Health Service Centers for Disease Control and Prevention advises HIV-infected women not to breastfeed to avoid postnatal transmission of HIV to a child who may not be infected.

➤*Children:* Safety and efficacy in children have not been studied. The use of cidofovir in children with AIDS warrants extreme caution because of the risk of long-term carcinogenicity and reproductive toxicity. Administer cidofovir to children only after careful evaluation and only if the potential benefits of treatment outweigh the risks.

Precautions

➤*Monitoring:* Monitor serum creatinine and urine protein within 48 hours prior to each dose, and white blood cell counts with differential prior to each dose. In patients with proteinuria, administer IV hydration and repeat the test. Periodically monitor intraocular pressure, visual acuity, and ocular symptoms.

➤*Uveitis/Iritis:* Uveitis or iritis was reported in clinical trials and during postmarketing in patients receiving cidofovir therapy. Consider treatment with topical corticosteroids with or without topical cycloplegic agents. Monitor patients for signs and symptoms of uveitis/iritis during cidofovir therapy.

Drug Interactions

➤*Nephrotoxic agents:* Concomitant administration of cidofovir and agents with nephrotoxic potential (eg, IV aminoglycosides [eg, tobramycin, gentamicin, amikacin], amphotericin B, foscarnet, IV pentamidine, vancomycin, and nonsteroidal anti-inflammatory agents) is contraindicated. Such agents must be discontinued ≥ 7 days prior to starting therapy with cidofovir.

Adverse Reactions

In clinical trials, cidofovir was withdrawn because of adverse events in 39% of patients treated with 5 mg/kg every other week as maintenance therapy.

Cidofovir Serious Clinical Adverse Events or Laboratory Abnormalities Occurring in > 5% of Patients	
Adverse reaction	Cidofovir 5 mg/kg (n = 135)
Proteinuria (≥ 100 mg/dL)	50
Neutropenia (≤ 500 cells/mm³)	24
Decreased intraocular pressure[1]	24
Decreased serum bicarbonate (≤ 16 mEq/L)	16
Fever	14
Infection	12
Creatinine elevation (≥ 2 mg/dL)	12
Pneumonia	9
Dyspnea	8
Nausea with vomiting	7

[1] Defined as decreased intraocular pressure (IOP) to ≤ 50% that at baseline. Based on 70 patients receiving 5 mg/kg maintenance dosing to whom baseline and follow-up IOP determinations were recorded.

Cidofovir Adverse Reactions (> 15%)	
Adverse reaction	Cidofovir 5 mg/kg (n = 115)
Any adverse reaction	100
Proteinuria (≥ 30 mg/dL)	88
Nausea/Vomiting	69
Fever	58
Neutropenia (< 750 cells/mm³)	43
Asthenia	43
Headache	30
Rash	30
Infection	28
Alopecia	27
Diarrhea	26
Pain	25
Creatinine elevation (> 1.5 mg/dL)	24
Anemia	24
Anorexia	23
Dyspnea	23
Chills	22
Increased cough	19
Oral moniliasis	18

The following additional list of adverse reactions/intercurrent illnesses have been observed in clinical studies of cidofovir and are listed below regardless of causal relationship to cidofovir. Evaluation of these reports was difficult because of the diverse manifestations of the underlying disease and because most patients received numerous concomitant medicines.

➤*Cardiovascular:* Cardiomyopathy; cardiovascular disorder; CHF; hypertension; hypotension; migraine; pallor; peripheral vascular disorder; phlebitis; postural hypotension; shock; syncope; tachycardia; vascular disorder; edema.

➤*CNS:* Abnormal dreams; abnormal gait; acute brain syndrome; agitation; amnesia; anxiety; ataxia; cerebrovascular disorder; confusion; convulsion; delirium; dementia; depression; dizziness; drug dependence; dry mouth; encephalopathy; facial paralysis; hallucinations; hemiplegia; hyperesthesia; hypertonia; hypotony; incoordination; increased libido; insomnia; myoclonus; nervousness; neuropathy; paresthesia; personality disorder; somnolence; speech disorder; tremor; twitching; vasodilation; vertigo.

➤*Dermatologic:* Acne; angioedema; dry skin; eczema; exfoliative dermatitis; furunculosis; herpes simplex; nail disorder; pruritus; rash; seborrhea; skin discoloration; skin disorder; skin hypertrophy; skin ulcer; sweating; urticaria.

➤*GI:* Cholangitis; colitis; constipation; esophagitis; dyspepsia; dysphagia; fecal incontinence; flatulence; gastritis; GI hemorrhage; gingivitis; hepatitis; hepatomegaly; hepatosplenomegaly; jaundice; abnormal liver function; liver damage; liver necrosis; melena; pancreatitis; proctitis; rectal disorder; stomatitis; aphthous stomatitis; tongue discoloration; mouth ulceration; tooth caries.

➤*GU:* Decreased Ccr; dysuria; glycosuria; hematuria; kidney stone; mastitis; metrorrhagia; nocturia; polyuria; prostatic disorder; toxic nephropathy; urethritis; urinary casts; urinary incontinence; urinary retention; urinary tract infection.

➤*Hematologic:* Hypochromic anemia; leukocytosis; leukopenia; lymphadenopathy; lymphoma-like reaction; pancytopenia; splenic disorder; splenomegaly; thrombocytopenia; thrombocytopenic purpura.

In clinical trials, at the 5 mg/kg maintenance dose, a decrease in absolute neutrophil count to ≤ 500 cells/mm³ occurred in 24% of patients. Granulocyte colony stimulating factor (GCSF) was used in 39% of patients.

➤*Metabolic:* Cachexia; dehydration; hypercalcemia; hyperglycemia; hyperkalemia; hyperlipidemia; hypocalcemia; hypoglycemia; hypoglycemic reaction; hypokalemia; hypomagnesemia; hyponatremia; hypophosphatemia; hypoproteinemia; increased alkaline phosphatase;

CIDOFOVIR

increased BUN; increased lactic dehydrogenase; increased AST; increased ALT; peripheral edema; respiratory alkalosis; thirst; weight loss; weight gain.

A diagnosis of Fanconi's syndrome, as manifested by multiple abnormalities of proximal renal tubular function, was reported in 1% of patients. Decreases in serum bicarbonate to ≤ 16 mEq/L occurred in 16% of cidofovir-treated patients. Cases of metabolic acidosis in association with liver dysfunction and pancreatitis resulting in death have been reported in patients receiving cidofovir.

➤*Musculoskeletal:* Arthralgia; arthrosis; bone necrosis; bone pain; joint disorder; leg cramps; myalgia; myasthenia; pathological fracture.

➤*Ophthalmic:* Among the subset of patients monitored for IOP changes, a ≥ 50% decrease from baseline IOP was reported in 17 of 70 (24%) patients at the 5 mg/kg maintenance dose. Severe hypertony (IOP of 0 to 1 mm Hg) has been reported in 3 patients. Uveitis or iritis has been reported in clinical trials and during postmarketing in patients receiving cidofovir therapy. Uveitis or iritis was reported in 15 of 135 (11%) patients receiving 5 mg/kg maintenance dosing.

➤*Renal:* Renal toxicity, as manifested by ≥ 2+ proteinuria, serum creatinine elevations of ≥ 0.4 mg/dL, or decreased Ccr ≤ 55 mL/min, occurred in 79 of 135 (59%) patients receiving cidofovir at a maintenance dose of 5 mg/kg every other week. Maintenance dose reductions from 5 to 3 mg/kg because of proteinuria or serum creatinine elevations were made in 12 of 41 (29%) of patients who had not received prior therapy for CMV retinitis and in 19 of 74 (26%) patients who had received prior therapy for CMV retinitis.

➤*Respiratory:* Asthma; bronchitis; epistaxis; hemoptysis; hiccough; hyperventilation; hypoxia; increased sputum; larynx edema; lung disorder; pharyngitis; pneumothorax; rhinitis; sinusitis.

➤*Special senses:* Abnormal vision; amblyopia; blindness; cataract; conjunctivitis; corneal lesion; corneal opacity; diplopia; dry eyes; ear disorder; ear pain; eye disorder; eye pain; hearing loss; hyperacusis; iritis; keratitis; miosis; otitis externa; otitis media; refraction disorder; retinal detachment; retinal disorder; taste perversion; tinnitus; uveitis; visual field defect.

➤*Miscellaneous:* Abdominal pain; accidental injury; adrenal cortex insufficiency; AIDS; allergic reaction; back pain; catheter blocked; cellulitis; chest pain; chills and fever; cryptococcosis; cyst; death; face edema; flu-like syndrome; hypothermia; injection site reaction; malaise; mucous membrane disorder; neck pain; overdose; photosensitivity reaction; sarcoma; sepsis.

Overdosage

Two cases of cidofovir overdose have been reported. These patients received single doses of cidofovir at 16.3 and 17.4 mg/kg, respectively, with concomitant oral probenecid and IV hydration. In both cases, the patients were hospitalized and received oral probenecid (1 g 3 times daily) and vigorous IV hydration with normal saline for 3 to 5 days. Significant changes in renal function were not observed in either patient.

Patient Information

Advise patients that cidofovir is not a cure for CMV retinitis, and that they may continue to experience progression of retinitis during and following treatment. Advise patients receiving cidofovir to have regular follow-up ophthalmologic examinations. Patients also may experience other manifestations of CMV disease despite cidofovir therapy.

HIV-infected patients may continue taking antiretroviral therapy. However, because probenecid reduces metabolic clearance of zidovudine, advise those taking zidovudine to temporarily discontinue zidovudine administration or decrease their zidovudine dose by 50% on days of cidofovir administration only.

Inform patients of the major toxicity of cidofovir, namely renal impairment, and that dose modification, including reduction, interruption, and possibly discontinuation, may be required. Emphasize close monitoring of renal function (routine urinalysis and serum creatinine) while on therapy.

Emphasize the importance of completing a full course of probenecid with each cidofovir dose. Warn patients of potential adverse events caused by probenecid (eg, headache, nausea, vomiting, hypersensitivity reactions). Hypersensitivity/allergic reactions may include rash, fever, chills, and anaphylaxis. Administration of probenecid after a meal or use of antiemetics may decrease the nausea. Prophylactic or therapeutic antihistamines or acetaminophen may be used to ameliorate hypersensitivity reactions.

Advise patients that cidofovir causes tumors, primarily mammary adenocarcinomas, in rats. Cidofovir should be considered a potential carcinogen in humans. Advise women of the limited enrollment of women in clinical trials with cidofovir.

Cidofovir caused reduced testes weight and hypospermia in animals. Such changes may occur in humans and cause infertility. Advise women of childbearing potential that cidofovir is embryotoxic in animals and not to use the drug during pregnancy. Women of childbearing potential should use effective contraception during and for 1 month following treatment. Men should practice barrier contraceptive methods during and for 3 months following treatment.

RIBAVIRIN

Rx	**Copegus** (Roche)	**Tablets**: 200 mg	(RIB 200 ROCHE). Lt. pink to pink, oval. Film-coated. In 168s.
Rx	**Rebetol** (Schering)	**Capsules**: 200 mg	Lactose. (REBETOL 200 mg). White. In 42s, 56s, 70s, and 84s.
Rx	**Virazole** (ICN)	**Lyophilized powder for aerosol reconstitution**: 6 g ribavirin/100 mL vial. Contains 20 mg/mL when reconstituted with 300 mL sterile water.	In vials.

WARNING

Capsules/Tablets: Ribavirin monotherapy is not effective for the treatment of chronic hepatitis C virus infection and should not be used alone for this indication.

The primary toxicity of ribavirin is hemolytic anemia, which may result in worsening of cardiac disease that has led to fatal and non-fatal MIs. Do not treat patients with a history of significant or unstable cardiac disease with ribavirin.

Significant teratogenic and/or embryocidal effects have been demonstrated in all animal species exposed to ribavirin. In addition, ribavirin has a multiple-dose half-life of 12 days, and it may persist in nonplasma compartments for as long as 6 months. Therefore, ribavirin therapy is contraindicated in women who are pregnant and in the male partners of women who are pregnant. Extreme care must be taken to avoid pregnancy during therapy and for 6 months after completion of treatment in female patients and in female partners of male patients who are taking ribavirin. At least 2 reliable forms of effective contraception must be used during treatment and during the 6-month posttreatment follow-up period.

Aerosol: Use of aerosolized ribavirin in patients requiring mechanical ventilator assistance should be undertaken only by physicians and support staff familiar with the specific ventilator being used and this mode of administration of the drug. Strict attention must be paid to procedures that have been shown to minimize the accumulation of drug precipitate, which can result in mechanical ventilator dysfunction and associated increased pulmonary pressures.

Sudden deterioration of respiratory function has been associated with initiation of aerosolized ribavirin use in infants. Carefully monitor respiratory function during treatment. If initiation of aerosolized ribavirin treatment appears to produce sudden deterioration of respiratory function, stop treatment and reinstitute only with extreme caution, continuous monitoring, and consideration of concomitant administration of bronchodilators (see Warnings).

Ribavirin aerosol is not indicated for use in adults. Physicians and patients should be aware that ribavirin has been shown to produce testicular lesions in rodents and to be teratogenic in all animal species in which adequate studies have been conducted (rodents and rabbits).

Indications

▶*Tablets:*

Chronic hepatitis C – In combination with peginterferon alfa-2a for the treatment of adults with chronic hepatitis C virus infection who have compensated liver disease and have not been previously treated with interferon alpha. Patients in whom efficacy was demonstrated included patients with compensated liver disease and histological evidence of cirrhosis (Child-Pugh class A).

▶*Capsules:*

Chronic hepatitis C – In combination with interferon alfa-2b injection for the treatment of chronic hepatitis C in patients with compensated liver disease previously untreated with alpha interferon or who have relapsed following alpha interferon therapy.

In combination with peginterferon alfa-2b injection for the treatment of chronic hepatitis C in patients with compensated liver disease who have not been previously treated with interferon alpha and are at least 18 years of age.

The safety and efficacy of ribavirin capsules with interferons other than interferon alfa-2b or peginterferon alfa-2b products have not been established.

▶*Aerosol:*

Severe lower respiratory tract infections – Treatment of hospitalized infants and young children with severe lower respiratory tract infections caused by respiratory syncytial virus (RSV). Many children with mild lower respiratory tract involvement will require shorter hospitalization than would be required for a full course of therapy (3 to 7 days) and should not be treated with the drug.

▶*Unlabeled uses:*

Aerosol – Influenza A or B viral infection, pneumonia caused by adenovirus, severe lower respiratory tract infection in adults.

Administration and Dosage

▶*Tablets:* The daily dose of ribavirin tablets is 800 to 1200 mg administered orally in 2 divided doses with food. Individualize the dose depending on baseline disease characteristics (eg, genotype), reponse to therapy, and tolerability of the regimen.

The recommended duration of treatment for patients previously untreated with ribavirin and interferon is 24 to 48 weeks.

Peginterferon alfa-2a and Ribavirin Tablet Dosing Recomendations			
Genotype[1]	Peginterferon alfa-2a dose	Ribavirin tablet dose	Duration
Genotype 1, 4	180 mcg	< 75 kg = 1000 mg	48 wk
		≥ 75 kg = 1200 mg	48 wk
Genotype 2, 3	180 mcg	800 mg	24 wk

[1] Genotypes non-1 showed no increased response to treatment beyond 24 weeks. Data on genotypes 5 and 6 are insufficient for dosing recommendations.

Dose modifications – If severe adverse reactions or laboratory abnormalities develop during combination ribavirin tablets/peginterferon alfa-2a therapy, modify or discontinue the dose, if appropriate, until the adverse reactions abate. If intolerance persists after dose adjustment, discontinue ribavirin tablet/peginterferon alfa-2a therapy.

Administer ribavirin tablets with caution to patients with pre-existing cardiac disease. Assess patients before commencement of therapy and appropriately monitor them during therapy. If there is any deterioration of cardiovascular status, stop therapy.

Ribavirin Tablet Dosage Modification Guidelines		
Laboratory values	Reduce only ribavirin tablet dose to 600 mg/day[1] if:	Discontinue ribavirin tablets if:
Hemoglobin in patients with no cardiac disease	< 10 g/dL	< 8.5 g/dL
Hemoglobin in patients with history of stable cardiac disease	≥ 2 g/dL decrease in hemoglobin during any 4-wk treatment period	< 12 g/dL despite 4 wk at reduced dose

[1] One 200 mg tablet in the morning and two 200 mg tablets in the evening.

Once ribavirin tablets have been withheld because of a laboratory abnormality or clinical manifestation, an attempt may be made to restart ribavirin tablets at 600 mg/day and further increase the dose to 800 mg/day depending upon the physician's judgement. However, it is not recommended that ribavirin tablets be increased to the original assigned dose (1000 to 1200 mg).

Renal impairment – Do not use ribavirin tablets in patients with creatinine clearance (Ccr) less than 50 mL/min.

▶*Capsules:* The recommended dose of ribavirin capsules depends on the patient's body weight and are provided in the table below:

Recommended Dosing for Ribavirin Capsules	
Body weight	Ribavirin capsules
≤ 75 kg	2 × 200 mg capsules AM, 3 × 200 mg capsules PM daily PO
> 75 kg	3 × 200 mg capsules AM, 3 × 200 mg capsules PM daily PO

Ribavirin capsules may be administered without regard to food, but should be administered in a consistent manner with respect to food intake.

Treatment duration – The recommended duration of treatment for patients previously untreated with interferon is 24 to 48 weeks. Individualize the duration of the patient's treatment depending on baseline disease characteristics, response to therapy, and tolerability of the regimen. Assess virologic response after 24 weeks of treatment. Consider treatment discontinuation in any patient who has not achieved a hepatitic C virus (HCV)-RNA below the limit of detection of the assay by 24 weeks. There are no safety and efficacy data on treatment for longer than 48 weeks in the previously untreated patient population.

Therapy relapse – In patients who relapse following interferon therapy, the recommended duration of treatment is 24 weeks. There are no safety and efficacy data on treatment for longer than 24 weeks in the relapsed patient population.

Ribavirin capsules/Peginterferon alfa-2b combination therapy – The recommended dose of ribavirin capsules is 800 mg/day in 2 divided doses: 2 capsules (400 mg) in the morning with food and 2 capsules (400 mg) in the evening with food.

Dose modifications – If severe adverse reactions or laboratory abnormalities develop during combination therapy, modify or discontinue the dose, if appropriate, until the adverse reactions abate. If intolerance persists after dose adjustment, discontinue combination therapy.

A permanent dose reduction is required for patients with a history of stable cardiovascular disease if the hemoglobin decreases by 2 g/dL or more during any 4-week period. In addition, discontinue combination therapy in patients with a cardiac history if the hemoglobin remains less than 12 g/dL after 4 weeks on a reduced dose.

It is recommended that patients whose hemoglobin level falls below 10 g/dL have their ribavirin dose reduced to 600 mg/day (1 × 200 mg

RIBAVIRIN

capsule AM, 2 × 200 mg capsules PM). Permanently discontinue ribavirin therapy in patients whose hemoglobin level falls below 8.5 g/dL.

Ribavirin Guidelines for Dose Modifications and Discontinuation for Anemia Based on Hemoglobin Levels		
Laboratory values	Dose reduction ribavirin capsules 600 mg/day	Permanent discontinuation of ribavirin treatment
Hemoglobin in patients with no cardiac history	< 10 g/dL	< 8.5 g/dL
Hemoglobin in patients with a cardiac history	≥ 2 g/dL decrease during any 4-wk period during treatment	< 12 g/dL after 4 wk of dose reduction

Special populations: Do not use ribavirin in patients with Ccr less than 50 mL/min. Administer ribavirin with caution to patients with pre-existing cardiac disease. Assess patients before commencement of therapy and appropriately monitor them during therapy. Stop therapy if there is any deterioration of cardiovascular status.

►*Aerosol:* For aerosol administration only. Ribavirin aerosol is not to be administered with any other aerosol-generating device or together with other aerosolized medications.

The recommended treatment regimen is 20 mg/mL as the starting solution in the drug reservoir of the Small Particle Aerosol Generator (SPAG-2) unit. Treatment is carried out for 12 to 18 hours/day for 3 to 7 days.

Mechanically ventilated infants – The recommended dose and administration schedule for infants who require mechanical ventilation is the same as for those who do not. Either a pressure or volume cycle ventilator may be used in conjunction with the SPAG-2. In either case, suction endotracheal tubes every 1 to 2 hours and monitor pulmonary pressures frequently (every 2 to 4 hours). For both pressure and volume ventilators, heated wire connective tubing and bacteria filters in series in the expiratory limb of the system (which must be changed frequently, eg, every 4 hours) must be used to minimize the risk of ribavirin precipitation in the system and the subsequent risk of ventilator dysfunction. Use water column pressure release valves in the ventilator circuit for pressure-cycled ventilators. They also may be used with volume-cycled ventilators.

Nonmechanically ventilated infants – The aerosol is delivered to an infant oxygen hood from the SPAG-2 aerosol generator. Administration by face mask or oxygen tent may be necessary if a hood cannot be used. However, the volume and condensation area are larger in a tent, and this may alter the drug's delivery dynamics.

Reconstitution – Reconstitute drug with a minimum of 75 mL sterile water for injection or inhalation in the original 100 mL vial. Shake well. Transfer to the clean, sterilized 500 mL SPAG-2 reservoir and further dilute to a final volume of 300 mL with sterile water for injection or inhalation. The final concentration should be 20 mg/mL.

Important: This water should not have any antimicrobial agent or other substance added. Discard solutions placed in the SPAG-2 unit at least every 24 hours and when the liquid level is low before adding newly reconstituted solution. Using the recommended drug concentration of 20 mg/mL ribavirin as the starting solution in the SPAG-2 unit's drug reservoir, the average aerosol concentration for a 12-hour period is 190 mcg/L of air.

►*Storage/Stability:*
Capsules/Tablets – Store at 25°C (77°F); excursions are permitted between 15° and 30°C (59° and 86°F). Keep bottle tightly closed.

Aerosol – Store lyophilized drug powder at 15° to 25°C (59° to 78°F) in a dry place. Reconstituted solutions may be stored under sterile conditions at room temperature (20° to 30°C, 68° to 86°F) for 24 hours.

Actions

►*Pharmacology:*
Capsules/Tablets – Ribavirin is a synthetic nucleoside analog. The mechanism by which the combination of ribavirin and an interferon product exerts its effect against the hepatitis C virus has not been fully established.

Aerosol –
Antiviral effects: Ribavirin has antiviral activity in vitro against RSV, influenza A and B viruses, and herpes simplex virus. The mechanism of action is unknown. Reversal of the in vitro antiviral activity by guanosine or xanthosine suggests that ribavirin may act as an analog of these cellular metabolites.

Immunologic effects: Neutralizing antibody responses to RSV were decreased in aerosolized ribavirin-treated infants compared with placebo-treated infants. In rats, ribavirin resulted in lymphoid atrophy of the thymus, spleen, and lymph nodes. Humoral immunity was reduced in guinea pigs and ferrets. Cellular immunity was mildly depressed in animal studies. Clinical significance of these observations is unknown.

►*Pharmacokinetics:*
Absorption:
Tablets: After administration of 1200 mg/day with food for 12 weeks, the $AUC_{0-12 h}$ was 25,361 ng•h/mL and C_{max} was 2748 ng/mL. The average time to reach C_{max} was 2 hours. There is extensive accumulation after multiple dosing (twice daily) such that the C_{max} at steady state was 4-fold higher than that of a single dose.

Capsules: Ribavirin was rapidly and extensively absorbed following oral administration. However, because of first-pass metabolism, the absolute bioavailability averaged 64%.

Aerosol: Ribavirin administered by aerosol is absorbed systemically. Four pediatric patients inhaling ribavirin aerosol by face mask for 2.5 hours/day for 3 days had plasma concentrations ranging from 0.44 to 1.55 mcM (mean, 0.76 mcM). The plasma half-life was 9.5 hours. Three pediatric patients inhaling ribavirin aerosol by face mask or mist tent for 20 hours/day for 5 days had plasma concentrations ranging from 1.5 to 14.3 mcM (mean, 6.8 mcM).

Distribution –
Capsules: Upon multiple oral dosing, based on $AUC_{12 h}$, a 6-fold accumulation of ribavirin was observed in plasma. Following oral dosing with 600 mg twice daily, steady-state was reached by about 4 weeks, with mean steady-state plasma concentrations of 2200 ng/mL.

Aerosol: After aerosol use, peak plasma concentrations are less than the concentration that reduced RSV plaque formation in tissue culture by 85% to 98%. Respiratory tract secretions are likely to contain ribavirin in concentrations many-fold higher than those required to reduce plaque formation. However, RSV is an intracellular virus, and it is unknown whether plasma concentrations or respiratory secretion concentrations of the drug better reflect intracellular concentrations in the respiratory tract. Accumulation of drug and/or metabolites in red blood cells may occur, plateauing in red cells in about 4 days. Accumulation gradually declines with an apparent half-life of 40 days. Accumulation following inhalation is not well defined.

Metabolism –
Capsules: Ribavirin has 2 pathways of metabolism: (1) a reversible phosphorylation pathway in nucleated cells; and (2) a degradative pathway involving deribosylation and amide hydrolysis to yield a triazole carboxylic acid metabolite.

Excretion –
Tablets: The terminal half-life following a single dose administration is approximately 120 to 170 hours. The total apparent clearance is about 26 L/h.

Capsules: Ribavirin and its triazole carboxamide and triazole carboxylic acid metabolites are excreted renally. After oral administration of 600 mg ribavirin, about 61% and 12% was eliminated in the urine and feces, respectively, in 336 hours. Unchanged ribavirin accounted for 17% of the administered dose. Upon discontinuaton of dosing, the mean half-life was 298 hours, which probably reflects slow elimination from nonplasma compartments.

Special populations –
Capsules:
• *Renal dysfunction –* The pharmacokinetics of ribavirin were assessed after administration of a single oral dose (400 mg) of ribavirin to non-HCV-infected subjects with varying degrees of renal dysfunction. The mean AUC value was 3-fold greater in subjects with Ccr values between 10 to 30 mL/min when compared with control subjects (Ccr more than 90 mL/min). In subjects with Ccr values between 30 to 60 mL/min, AUC was 2-fold greater when compared with control subjects. The increased AUC appears to be because of reduction of renal and nonrenal clearance in these patients. Phase III efficacy trials included subjects with Ccr values more than 50 mL/min. The multiple-dose pharmacokinetics of ribavirin cannot be accurately predicted in patients with renal dysfunction. Ribavirin is not effectively removed by hemodialysis. Do not treat patients with Ccr less than 50 mL/min with ribavirin.

• *Hepatic dysfunction –* The mean C_{max} values increased with severity of hepatic dysfunction and was 2-fold greater in subjects with severe hepatic dysfunction when compared with control subjects.

►*Clinical trials:*
Peginterferon alfa-2a/Ribavirin tablets combination – The safety and effectiveness of peginterferon alfa-2a in combination with ribavirin tablets for the treatment of hepatitis C virus infection were assessed in a randomized controlled clinical trial.

In study 1, patients were randomized to receive peginterferon alfa-2a 180 mcg SC once weekly (QW) with oral placebo, peginterferon alfa-2a 180 mcg QW with ribavirin tablets 1000 mg PO (body weight less than 75 kg) or 1200 mg PO (body weight 75 kg or more) or interferon alfa-2b 3 MIU SC 3 times/week (TIW) plus ribavirin 1000 mg or 1200 mg PO). All patients received 48 weeks of therapy followed by 24 weeks of treatment-free follow-up. Peginterferon alfa-2a in combination with ribavirin tablets resulted in a higher sustained virologic response (SVR) (defined as undetectable HCV RNA at the end of the 24-week treatment-free follow-up period) compared with peginterferon alfa-2a alone or interferon alfa-2b and ribavirin. In all treatment arms, patients with viral genotype 1, regardless of viral load, had a lower response rate to peginterferon alfa-2a in combination with ribavirin tablets compared with patients with other viral genotypes.

RIBAVIRIN

Sustained Virologic Response to Combination Therapy (%)			
	Interferon alfa-2b + ribavirin 1000 or 1200 mg	Peginterferon alfa-2a + placebo	Peginterferon alfa-2a + ribavirin tablets 1000 or 1200 mg
All patients	44	29	53
Genotype 1	36	20	44
Genotypes 2-6	59	46	70

Difference in overall treatment response (peginterferon alfa-2a/ribavirin tablet combination vs interferon alfa-2b/ribavirin) was 9%.

Ribavirin capsules/Peginterferon alfa 2b – A randomized study compared treatment with 2 peginterferon alfa-2b/ribavirin capsule regimens (peginterferon alfa-2b 1.5 mcg/kg SC QW/ribavirin capsules 800 mg/day PO [in divided doses]; peginterferon alfa-2b 1.5 mcg/kg SC QW for 4 weeks, then 0.5 mcg/kg SC QW for 44 weeks/ribavirin capsules 1000/1200 mg/day PO [in divided doses]) with interferon alfa-2b (3 MIU SC TIW/ribavirin capsules 1000/1200 mg/day PO [in divided doses]) in 1530 adults with chronic hepatitis C, interferon naive-patients were treated for 48 weeks and followed for 24 weeks posttreatment.

Response to treatment was defined as undetectable HCV RNA at 24 weeks posttreatment.

Rates of Response to Combination Treatment (%)		
	Peginterferon alfa-2b 1.5 mg/kg QW Ribavirin capsules 800 mg QD	Interferon alfa-2b 3 MIU TIW Ribavirin capsules 1000/1200 mg QD
Overall response[1]	52	46
Genotype 1	41	33
Genotype 2-6	75	73

[1] Difference in overall treatment response is 6% with 95% confidence interval of (0.18, 11.63) adjusted for viral genotype and presence of cirrhosis at baseline.

The response rate to peginterferon alfa-2b 1.5→0.5 mcg/kg/ribavirin capsules was essentially the same as the response to interferon alfa-2b/ribavirin capsules.

Patients with viral genotype 1, regardless of viral load, had a lower reponse rate to peginterferon alfa-2b (1.5 mcg/kg)/ribavirin capsules combination therapy compared with patients with other viral genotypes.

Contraindications

▶*Tablets/Capsules:* Hypersensitivity to the drug or any component of the tablet; women who are pregnant; men whose female partners are pregnant; patients with hemoglobinopathies (eg, thalassemia major or sickle-cell anemia).

Ribavirin may cause birth defects and/or death of the exposed fetus. Ribavirin capsules are contraindicated in women who are pregnant or in men whose female partners are pregnant (see Warnings). It also is contraindicated in patients with a history of hypersensitivity to ribavirin or any component of the capsule.

Do not treat patients with hemoglobinopathies (eg, thalassemia major, sickle-cell anemia) with ribavirin capsules.

Ribavirin tablets/Peginterferon alfa-2a – Ribavirin tablets/peginterferon alfa-2a combination therapy is contraindicated in patients with autoimmune hepatitis and hepatic decompensation (Child-Pugh class B and C) before or during treatment.

Ribavirin capsules/Interferon alfa-2b – Patients with autoimmune hepatitis must not be treated with combination ribavirin capsules/interferon alfa-2b therapy because using these medicines can make the hepatitis worse.

▶*Aerosol:* Hypersensitivity to the drug or its components; pregnancy or the potential for pregnancy during exposure to the drug (see Warnings).

Warnings

▶*Monotherapy (capsules/tablets):* Based on results of clinical trials, ribavirin monotherapy is not effective for the treatment of chronic hepatitis C virus infection. Therefore, ribavirin must not be used alone. The safety and efficacy of ribavirin capsules have been established only when used with interferon alfa-2b as interferon alfa-2b/ribavirin capsule combination therapy or with peginterferon alfa-2b injection. The safety and efficacy of ribavirin tablets have been established only when used with pegylated interferon alfa-2a.

▶*Combination therapy adverse events (capsules/tablets):* There are significant adverse events caused by ribavirin capsules/interferon alfa-2b or peginterferon alfa-2b therapy, and ribavirin tablets/peginterferon alfa-2a therapy, including severe depression and suicidal ideation, hemolytic anemia, suppression of bone marrow function, autoimmune and infectious disorders, pulmonary dysfunction, pancreatitis, and diabetes. Review the interferon alfa-2b/ribavirin capsule

combination therapy, peginterferon alfa-2b, and peginterferon alfa-2a package inserts in their entirety prior to initiation of combination treatment for additional safety information.

▶*Pancreatitis (capsules/tablets/aerosol):* Suspend ribavirin, interferon alfa-2b, peginterferon alfa-2b, or peginterferon alfa-2a therapy in patients with signs and symptoms of pancreatitis and discontinue in patients with confirmed pancreatitis.

▶*Renal function impairment (capsules/tablets):* Do not use in patients with Ccr less than 50 mL/min.

▶*Assisted ventilation (aerosol):* Some subjects requiring assisted ventilation have experienced serious difficulties because of inadequate ventilation and gas exchange. Drug precipitation within the ventilatory apparatus, including the endotracheal tube, has resulted in increased positive and expiratory pressure and increased positive inspiratory pressure. Accumulation of fluid in tubing (rain out) also has been noted.

▶*Pulmonary effects:*

Aerosol – Pulmonary function significantly deteriorated during ribavirin aerosol treatment in all 6 adults with chronic obstructive lung disease and in 4 of 6 asthmatic adults. Dyspnea and chest soreness also occurred in the latter group. In the original study population of approximately 200 infants who received aerosolized ribavirin, several serious adverse events occurred in severely ill infants with life-threatening underlying diseases, many of whom required assisted ventilation. The role of ribavirin in these events is undetermined. Additional reports of worsening of respiratory status, bronchospasm, pulmonary edema, hypoventilation, cyanosis, dyspnea, bacterial pneumonia, pneumothorax, apnea, atelectasis, and ventilator dependence have occurred. Sudden deterioration of respiratory function has been associated with initiation of aerosolized ribavirin aerosol use in infants. If ribavirin aerosol treatment produces sudden deterioration of respiratory function, stop treatment and reinstitute only with extreme caution, continuous monitoring, and consideration of concomitant administration of bronchodilators.

Capsules/Tablets – Pulmonary symptoms, including dyspnea, pulmonary infiltrates, pneumonitis, and pneumonia have been reported during therapy with ribavirin and interferon. Occasional cases of fatal pneumonia have occurred. In addition, sarcoidosis or the exacerbation of sarcoidosis has been reported. If there is evidence of pulmonary infiltrates or pulmonary function impairment, closely monitor the patient and if appropriate, discontinue treatment.

▶*Hemolytic anemia:*

Capsules/Tablets – The primary toxicity of ribavirin is hemolytic anemia (hemoglobin less than 10 g/dL), which was observed in about 10% of ribavirin capsules/interferon alfa-2b-treated patients and about 13% in ribavirin tablets/peginterferon alfa-2a-treated patients in clinical trials (see Adverse Reactions). The anemia associated with ribavirin occurs within 1 to 2 weeks of initiation of therapy. Because the initial drop in hemoglobin may be significant, it is advised that hemoglobin or hematocrit be obtained pretreatment and at week 2 and 4 of therapy, or more frequently if clinically indicated. Then follow patients as clinically appropriate.

Aerosol – Although anemia has not been reported with aerosol use, it occurs frequently with experimental oral and IV ribavirin, and most infants treated with the aerosol have not been evaluated 1 to 2 weeks posttreatment when anemia is likely. Cases of anemia, reticulocytosis, and hemolytic anemia associated with aerosolized ribavirin use have been reported in postmarketing reporting systems. All have been reversible with discontinuation of the drug.

▶*Cardiovascular effects:*

Capsules/Tablets – Fatal and nonfatal MIs have been reported in patients with anemia caused by ribavirin. Assess patients for underlying cardiac disease before initiation of ribavirin therapy and appropriately monitor them during therapy. If there is any deterioration of cardiovascular status, suspend or discontinue therapy (see Administration and Dosage). Because cardiac disease may be worsened by drug-induced anemia, patients with a history of significant or unstable cardiac disease should not use ribavirin.

Aerosol – Events associated with aerosolized ribavirin have included cardiac arrest, hypotension, bradycardia, and digitalis toxicity. Bigeminy, bradycardia, and tachycardia have been described in patients with underlying congenital heart disease.

▶*Coadministration with nucleoside analogs (didanosine):*

Tablets – Coadministration of ribavirin and didanosine is not recommended. Reports of fatal hepatic failure, as well as peripheral neuropathy, pancreatitis, and symptomatic hyperlactatemia/lactic acidosis have been reported in clinical trials.

▶*Carcinogenesis:*

Capsules – Ribavirin has produced positive findings in multiple in vitro and animal in vivo genotoxicity assays, and should be considered a potential carcinogen.

Aerosol – Chronic feeding of ribavirin to rats at doses of 16 to 100 mg/kg/day (estimated human equivalent of 2.3 to 14.3 mg/kg/day, based on body surface area adjustment for adults) suggest that ribavirin may induce benign mammary, pancreatic, pituitary, and adrenal tumors.

RIBAVIRIN

▶*Mutagenesis:*

Tablets – The in vitro mouse lymphoma assay demonstrated mutagenic activity. Results from studies showed clastogenic activity in the in vivo mouse micronucleus assay at oral doses up to 2000 mg/kg.

Capsules – Ribavirin demonstrated increased incidences of mutation and cell transformation in multiple genotoxicity assays. Mutagenic activity was observed in the mouse lymphoma assay and at doses of 20 to 200 mg/kg (estimated human equivalent of 1.67 to 16.7 mg/kg, based on body surface area adjustment for a 60 kg adult; 0.1 to 1 times the maximum recommended human 24-hour dose of ribavirin) in a mouse micronucleus assay.

Aerosol – An increased incidence of cell transformations and mutations was shown in mouse fibroblasts and lymphoma cells at concentrations of 0.015 and 0.03 to 5 mg/mL, respectively. Increased incidence of mutation rates (3 to 4 times) were observed at concentrations between 3.75 and 10 mg/mL in vitro and mouse micronucleus assay was clastogenic at IV doses of 20 to 200 mg/kg.

▶*Fertility impairment:*

Capsules / Tablets – Use ribavirin with caution in fertile men. In studies in mice to evaluate the time course and reversibility of ribavirin-induced testicular degeneration at doses of 15 to 150 mg/kg/day (estimated human equivalent of 1.25 to 12.5 mg/kg/day, based on body surface area adjustment for a 60 kg adult; 0.1 to 0.8 times the maximum human 24-hour dose of ribavirin) administered for 3 or 6 months, abnormalities in sperm occurred. Upon cessation of treatment, essentially total recovery from ribavirin-induced testicular toxicity was apparent within 1 or 2 spermatogenesis cycles.

Aerosol – Doses administered to mice between 35 and 150 mg/kg/day resulted in significant seminiferous tubule atrophy, decreased sperm concentrations, and increased numbers of sperm with abnormal morphology. Partial recovery of sperm production was apparent 3 to 6 months following dose cessation. Testicular lesions (tubular atrophy) in adult rats at oral dose levels as low as 16 mg/kg/day was shown.

▶*Elderly:*

Capsules – In clinical trials, elderly subjects had a higher frequency of anemia (67%) than did younger patients (28%) (see Warnings).

In general, cautiously administer ribavirin capsules to elderly patients, starting at the lower end of the dosing range, reflecting the greater frequency of decreased hepatic or cardiac function and of concomitant disease or other drug therapy.

Take care in dose selection because elderly patients often have decreased renal function. Monitor renal function and make dosage adjustments accordingly. Do not use ribavirin in elderly patients with Ccr less than 50 mL/min.

▶*Pregnancy: Category X.* Ribavirin has demonstrated significant teratogenic effects (ie, malformation of skull, palate, eye, jaw, limbs, skeleton, GI tract) and/or embryocidal potential in all animal species in which adequate studies have been conducted. The incidence and severity of teratogenic effects increased with escalation of the drug dose. Although clinical studies have not been performed, ribavirin may cause fetal harm in humans.

Capsules / Tablets – Ribavirin may cause birth defects or death of the exposed fetus. Extreme care must be taken to avoid pregnancy in female patients and in female partners of male patients. Ribavirin has demonstrated significant teratogenic and/or embryocidal effects in all animal species in which adequate studies have been conducted. These effects occurred at doses as low as one-twentieth of the recommended human dose of ribavirin. Do not start ribavirin therapy until a report of a negative pregnancy test has been obtained immediately prior to planned initiation of therapy. Instruct male and female patients to use at least 2 forms of effective contraception during treatment and during the 6-month period after treatment has been stopped based on a multiple-dose half-life of ribavirin of 12 days. Pregnancy testing should occur monthly during ribavirin therapy and for 6 months after therapy has stopped.

Patients or partners of patients should immediately report any pregnancy that occurs during treatment or within 6 months after treatment cessation to their physician. Physicians should report such cases for ribavirin capsules by calling (800) 727-7064 and for ribavirin tablets by calling (800) 526-6367.

▶*Lactation:*

Capsules / Tablets – It is not known whether ribavirin is excreted in human milk. Because of the potential for serious adverse reactions from the drug in nursing infants, decide whether to discontinue nursing or to delay or discontinue ribavirin.

Aerosol – Ribavirin is toxic to lactating animals and their offspring. It is not known whether the drug is excreted in human breast milk.

▶*Children:*

Capsules / Tablets – Safety and efficacy have not been established in children under 18 years of age (ribavirin tablets).

Precautions

▶*Monitoring:*

Capsules / Tablets – The following laboratory tests are recommended for all patients treated with ribavirin prior to beginning treatment and then periodically thereafter:
- Standard hematologic tests: Including hemoglobin (pretreatment, week 2, and week 4 of therapy, and as clinically appropriate) (see Warnings), complete and differential white blood cell counts, and platelet count.
- Blood chemistries: Liver function tests and TSH.
- Pregnancy: Including monthly monitoring for women of childbearing potential and for 6 months after discontinuing therapy.
- ECG

Consider acceptable baseline values for initiation of ribavirin tablets and peginterferon alfa-2a therapy: Platelet count 90,000 cell/mm^3 or more; absolute neutrophil count (ANC) 1500 cells/mm^3 or more; TSH and T_4 within normal limits or adequately controlled thyroid function; ECG.

Aerosol – Monitor respiratory and fluid status; sudden deterioration of respiratory function has been associated with initiation of aerosolized ribavirin. Carefully monitor respiratory function during treatment.

▶*HIV or HBV coinfection:*

Capsules / Tablets – The safety and efficacy of ribavirin and interferon alfa-2b or peginterferon alfa-2a combination therapy for the treatment of hepatitis C have not been established in patients coinfected with HIV or HBV.

▶*Hepatitis C:*

Capsules / Tablets – The safety and efficacy of ribavirin and interferon alfa-2b or peginterferon alfa-2a combination therapy for the treatment of hepatitis C in patients who have received liver or other organ transplants have not been established.

▶*Other infections:*

Capsules / Tablets – The safety and efficacy of ribavirin and peginterferon alfa-2a, interferon alfa-2b, and peginterferon alfa-2b combination therapy for the treatment of HIV infection, adenovirus RSV, parainfluenza, or influenza infections have not been established. Do not use ribavirin for these indications.

▶*Health care personnel information:*

Aerosol – Health care workers directly providing care to patients receiving aerosolized ribavirin should be aware that ribavirin is teratogenic in all animal species in which adequate studies have been conducted (rodents and rabbits). No reports of teratogenesis in offspring of mothers who were exposed to aerosolized ribavirin during pregnancy have been confirmed, but no controlled studies have been conducted in pregnant women. Studies of environmental exposure in treatment settings have shown that the drug can disperse into the immediate bedside area during routine patient care activities with highest ambient levels closest to the patient and extremely low levels outside of the immediate bedside area. Adverse reactions resulting from actual occupational exposure in adults are described below. Some studies have documented ambient drug concentrations at the bedside that could potentially lead to systemic exposures above those considered safe for exposure during pregnancy.

It is good practice to avoid unnecessary occupational exposure to chemicals wherever possible. Health care workers who are pregnant should consider avoiding direct care of patients receiving aerosolized ribavirin. If close patient contact cannot be avoided, take precautions to limit exposure. These include the following: Administration of ribavirin in negative pressure rooms; adequate room ventilation (at least 6 air exchanges/hour); the use of ribavirin aerosol scavenging devices; turning off the SPAG-2 device for 5 to 10 minutes prior to prolonged patient contact; wearing appropriately fitted respirator masks (surgical masks do not provide adequate filtration of ribavirin particles). Further information is available from the National Institute for Occupational Safety and Health's Hazard Evaluation and Technical Assistance Branch and additional recommendations have been published in an Aerosol Consensus Statement by the American Respiratory Care Foundation and the American Association for Respiratory Care.

Drug Interactions

▶*Antacids:*

Capsules – Coadministration with an antacid containing magnesium, aluminum, and simethicone (*Mylanta*) resulted in a 14% decrease in mean ribavirin AUC. The clinical relevance of results from this single-dose study is unknown.

▶*Nucleoside analogs:*

Tablets – Ribavirin has shown in vitro to inhibit phosphorylation of zidovudine and stavudine, which could lead to decreased antiretroviral activity. Avoid concomitant use.

▶*Drug / Food interactions:*

Capsules / Tablets – Both AUC and C_{max} increased by 70% when ribavirin capsules were administered with a high-fat meal. For ribavirin tablets, the absorption was slowed (T_{max} was doubled) and the AUC and C_{max} increased by 42% and 66%, respectively, when taken with a

RIBAVIRIN

high-fat meal. There are insufficient data to address the clinical relevance of these results.

Adverse Reactions

➤**Aerosol:**

Cardiovascular – Cardiac arrest, hypotension, bradycardia, digitalis toxicity, bigeminy, bradycardia, and tachycardia have been described in patients with underlying disease.

Hematologic – There are postmarketing reports of anemia (type unspecified), reticulocytosis, and hemolytic anemia.

Respiratory – Worsening of respiratory status, bronchospasm, pulmonary edema, hypoventilation, cyanosis, dyspnea, bacterial pneumonia, pneumothorax, apnea, atelectasis, and ventilator dependence have occurred.

Miscellaneous – Rash; conjunctivitis; seizures and asthenia have been reported with experimental IV ribavirin.

Deaths – During or shortly after treatment with aerosolized ribavirin, deaths occurred in 20 patients treated with ribavirin (12 of these patients were being treated for RSV infections). Several cases have been characterized as "possibly related" to ribavirin by the treating physician; these were in infants who experienced worsening respiratory status related to bronchospasm while being treated with the drug. Several other cases have been attributed to mechanical ventilator malfunction in which ribavirin precipitation within the ventilator apparatus led to excessively high pulmonary pressures and diminished oxygenation.

Health care workers – Headache (51%); conjunctivitis (32%); rhinitis, nausea, rash, dizziness, pharyngitis, lacrimation (10% to 20%). Several cases of bronchospasm and/or chest pain also were reported, usually in individuals with known underlying reactive airway disease. There are several case reports of damage to contact lenses after prolonged close exposure to aerosolized ribavirin. Most signs and symptoms reported as having occurred in exposed health care workers resolved within minutes to hours of discontinuing close exposure to aerosolized ribavirin.

➤**Capsules:** The primary toxicity of ribavirin is hemolytic anemia. Reductions in hemoglobin levels occurred within the first 1 to 2 weeks of oral therapy. Cardiac and pulmonary events associated with anemia occurred in about 10% of patients (see Warnings).

Combination therapy – In clinical trials, 19% and 6% of previously untreated and relapse patients, respectively, discontinued therapy because of adverse events in the combination arms compared with 13% and 3% in the interferon arms. Selected treatment-emergent adverse events that occurred in the US studies with 5% or more incidence are provided in the table below by treatment group. In general, the selected treatment-emergent adverse events reported with lower incidence in the international studies as compared with the US studies with the exception of asthenia, influenza-like symptoms, nervousness, and pruritus.

Selected Adverse Events: Previously Untreated and Relapse Patients (%)

	US previously untreated study				US relapse study	
	24 wk of treatment		48 wk of treatment		24 wk of treatment	
Adverse reaction[1]	Interferon alfa-2b plus ribavirin capsules (N = 228)	Interferon alfa-2b plus placebo (N = 231)	Interferon alfa-2b plus ribavirin capsules (N = 228)	Interferon alfa-2b plus placebo (N = 225)	Interferon alfa-2b plus ribavirin capsules (N = 77)	interferon alfa-2b plus placebo (N = 76)
CNS						
Dizziness	17	15	23	19	26	21
Headache	63	63	66	67	66	68
GI						
Anorexia	27	16	25	19	21	14
Dyspepsia	14	6	16	9	16	9
Nausea	38	35	46	33	47	33
Vomiting	11	10	9	13	12	8
Musculo-skeletal						
Arthralgia	30	27	33	36	29	29
Musculo-skeletal pain	20	26	28	32	22	28
Myalgia	61	57	64	63	61	58
Psychiatric						
Impaired concentration	11	14	14	14	10	12
Depression	32	25	36	37	23	14
Emotional lability	7	6	11	8	12	8
Insomnia	39	27	39	30	26	25
Irritability	23	19	32	27	25	20
Nervousness	4	2	4	4	5	4

Selected Adverse Events: Previously Untreated and Relapse Patients (%)

	US previously untreated study				US relapse study	
	24 wk of treatment		48 wk of treatment		24 wk of treatment	
Adverse reaction[1]	Interferon alfa-2b plus ribavirin capsules (N = 228)	Interferon alfa-2b plus placebo (N = 231)	Interferon alfa-2b plus ribavirin capsules (N = 228)	Interferon alfa-2b plus placebo (N = 225)	Interferon alfa-2b plus ribavirin capsules (N = 77)	interferon alfa-2b plus placebo (N = 76)
Respiratory						
Dyspnea	19	9	18	10	17	12
Sinusitis	9	7	10	14	12	7
Dermato-logic						
Alopecia	28	27	32	28	27	26
Injection site inflammation	13	10	12	14	6	8
Injection site reaction	7	9	8	9	5	3
Pruritus	21	9	19	8	13	4
Rash	20	9	28	8	21	5
Miscellaneous						
Asthenia	9	4	9	9	10	4
Chest pain	5	4	9	8	6	7
Fatigue	68	62	70	72	60	53
Fever	37	35	41	40	32	36
Influenza-like symptoms	14	18	18	20	13	13
Rigors	40	32	42	39	43	37
Taste perversion	7	4	8	4	6	5

[1] Patients reporting 1 or more adverse event. A patient may have reported more than 1 adverse event within a body system/organ class category.

In addition, the following spontaneous adverse events have been reported during the marketing surveillance of ribavirin capsules/interferon alfa-2b therapy: Hearing disorder and vertigo.

Ribavirin capsules/Peginterferon alfa-2b combination therapy: Overall in clinical trials, 14% of patients receiving ribavirin capsules/peginterferon alfa-2b combination therapy discontinued therapy compared with 13% treated with the ribavirin capsules in combination with interferon alfa-2b. The most common reasons for discontinuation of therapy were related to psychiatric, systemic (eg, fatigue, headache), or GI adverse events. Adverse events that occurred in clinical trials at more then 5% incidence are provided below.

Adverse Events with Ribavirin Capsules and Peginterferon Alfa-2b Combination Therapy Compared with Ribavirin Capsules and Interferon Alfa-2b Combination Therapy (> 5%)

Adverse reaction[1]	Peginterferon alfa-2b/ Ribavirin capsules (N = 511)	Interferon alfa-2b/ Ribavirin capsules (N = 505)
CNS		
Agitation	8	5
Anxiety/Emotional lability/Irritabiltiy	47	47
Concentration impaired	17	21
Depression	31	34
Dizziness	21	17
Insomnia	40	41
Nervousness	6	6
Dermatologic		
Alopecia	36	32
Flushing	4	3
Pruritus	29	28
Rash	24	23
Skin dry	24	23
Sweating increased	11	7
GI		
Abdominal pain	13	13
Anorexia	32	27
Constipation	5	5
Diarrhea	22	17
Dyspepsia	9	8
Nausea	43	33
Vomiting	14	12
Hematologic		
Anemia	12	17
Leukopenia	6	5
Neutropenia	26	14
Thrombocytopenia	5	2

RIBAVIRIN

Adverse Events with Ribavirin Capsules and Peginterferon Alfa-2b Combination Therapy Compared with Ribavirin Capsules and Interferon Alfa-2b Combination Therapy (> 5%)

Adverse reaction[1]	Peginterferon alfa-2b/ Ribavirin capsules (N = 511)	Interferon alfa-2b/ Ribavirin capsules (N = 505)
Musculoskeletal		
Arthralgia	34	28
Musculoskeletal pain	21	19
Myalgia	56	50
Resistance mechanism		
Infection, fungal	6	1
Infection, viral	12	12
Respiratory		
Coughing	23	16
Dyspnea	26	24
Pharyngitis	12	13
Rhinitis	8	6
Sinusitis	6	5
Special senses		
Conjunctivitis	4	5
Taste perversion	9	4
Vision blurred	5	6
Miscellaneous		
Chest pain	8	7
Fatigue/Asthenia	66	63
Fever	46	33
Headache	62	58
Hepatomegaly	4	4
Hypothyroidism	5	4
Injection site inflammation	25	18
Injection site reaction	58	36
Malaise	4	6
Menstrual disorder	7	6
Mouth dry	12	8
Right upper quadrant pain	12	6
Rigors	48	41
Weight decrease	29	20

[1] Patients reporting 1 or more adverse events. A patient may have reported more than 1 adverse event within a body system/organ class category.

►*Tablets:*

Ribavirin tablets/Peginterferon alfa-2a combination therapy: The most common life-threatening or fatal events induced or aggravated by ribavirin tablets/peginterferon alfa-2a combination therapy were depression, suicide, relapse of drug abuse/overdose, and bacterial infections; each occurred at a frequency of less than 1%.

The most commonly reported adverse reactions were psychiatric reactions, including depression, irritability, anxiety, and flu-like symptoms such as fatigue, pyrexia, myalgia, headache, and rigors.

The most common reasons for discontinuation of therapy were psychiatric, flu-like syndrome (eg, lethargy, fatigue, headache), dermatologic, and GI disorders.

The most common reason for dose modification in patients receiving combination therapy was for laboratory abnormalities; neutropenia (20%) and thrombocytopenia (4%) for peginterferon alfa-2a and anemia (22%) for ribavirin tablets.

Peginterferon alfa-2a dose was reduced in 12% of patients receiving 1000 to 1200 mg ribavirin tablets for 48 weeks and in 7% of patients receiving 800 mg ribavirin tablets for 24 weeks. Ribavirin tablet dose was reduced in 21% of patients receiving 1000 to 1200 mg for 48 weeks and 12% in patients receiving 800 mg for 24 weeks.

Adverse Reactions Occurring in Patients in Hepatitis C Clinical Trials (≥ 5%)

Adverse reaction	Peginterferon alfa-2a 180 mcg + 1000 or 1200 mg ribavirin tablet 48 wk (N = 451)	Interferon alfa-2b + 1000 or 1200 mg ribavirin capsules 48 wk (N = 443)
CNS		
Concentration impairment	10	13
Depression	20	28
Dizziness (excluding vertigo)	14	14
Headache	43	49
Insomnia	30	37

Adverse Reactions Occurring in Patients in Hepatitis C Clinical Trials (≥ 5%)

Adverse reaction	Peginterferon alfa-2a 180 mcg + 1000 or 1200 mg ribavirin tablet 48 wk (N = 451)	Interferon alfa-2b + 1000 or 1200 mg ribavirin capsules 48 wk (N = 443)
Irritability/ Anxiety/ Nervousness	33	38
Memory impairment	6	5
Mood alteration	5	6
Dermatologic		
Alopecia	28	33
Dermatitis	16	13
Dry skin	10	13
Eczema	5	4
Injection site reaction	23	16
Pruritus	19	18
Rash	8	5
Sweating increased	6	5
GI		
Abdominal pain	8	9
Anorexia	24	26
Diarrhea	11	10
Dry mouth	4	7
Dyspepsia	6	5
Nausea/Vomiting	25	29
Weight decrease	10	10
Hematologic		
Anemia	11	11
Lymphopenia	14	12
Neutropenia	27	8
Thrombocytopenia	5	< 1
Musculoskeletal		
Arthralgia	22	23
Back pain	5	5
Myalgia	40	49
Respiratory		
Cough	10	7
Dyspnea	13	14
Dyspnea exertional	4	7
Miscellaneous		
Fatigue/Asthenia	65	68
Hypothyroidism	4	5
Overall resistance mechanism disorders	12	10
Pain	10	9
Pyrexia	41	55
Rigors	25	37
Vision blurred	5	2

The most common serious adverse event (3%) was bacterial infection (eg, sepsis, osteomyelitis, endocarditis, pyelonephritis, pneumonia). Others that occurred at a frequency of less than 1% included the following: Suicide, suicidal ideation, psychosis, aggression, anxiety, drug abuse and drug overdose, angina, hepatic dysfunction, fatty liver, cholangitis, arrhythmia, diabetes mellitus, autoimmune phenomena (eg, hyperthyroidism, hypothyroidism, sarcoidosis, systemic lupus erythematosus, rheumatoid arthritis), peripheral neuropathy, aplastic anemia, peptic ulcer, GI bleeding, pancreatitis, colitis, corneal ulcer, pulmonary embolism, coma, myositis, cerebral hemorrhage.

►*Laboratory values:*

Hemoglobin – Hemoglobin decreases among patients receiving ribavirin therapy began at week 1, with stabilization by week 4. Hemoglobin values returned to pretreatment levels within 4 to 8 weeks of cessation of therapy in most patients.

Ribavirin capsules induced a decrease in hemoglobin levels in approximately two-thirds of patients. Hemoglobin levels decreased to less than 11 g/dL in about 30% of patients. Severe anemia (less than 8 g/dL) occurred in less than 1% of patients. Dose modification was required in 9% and 13% of patients in the peginterferon alfa-2b/ribavirin capsules and interferon alfa-2b/ribavirin capsules groups.

Hemoglobin less than 10 g/dL was observed in 13% of ribavirin tablets and peginterferon alfa-2a combination-treated patients in clinical trials. The maximum drop in hemoglobin occurred during the first 8 weeks of initiation of ribavirin therapy (see Warnings).

Bilirubin and uric acid – Increases in bilirubin and uric acid, associated with hemolysis, were noted in clinical trials. Most were moderate biochemical changes and were reversed within 4 weeks after treatment discontinuation.

RIBAVIRIN

In the peginterferon alfa-2b/ribavirin capsule combination trial, 10% to 14% of patients developed hyperbilirubinemia and 33% to 38% developed hyperuricemia in association with hemolysis. Six patients developed mild to moderate gout.

Selected Hematologic Values During Treatment with Ribavirin Capsules Plus Interferon Alfa-2b: Previously Untreated and Relapse Patients (%)

	US previously untreated study				US relapse study	
	24 wk of treatment		48 wk of treatment		24 wk of treatment	
	Interferon alfa-2b plus ribavirin capsules (n = 228)	Interferon alfa-2b plus placebo (n = 231)	Interferon alfa-2b plus ribavirin capsules (n = 228)	Interferon alfa-2b plus placebo (n = 225)	Interferon alfa-2b plus ribavirin capsules (n = 77)	Interferon alfa-2b plus placebo (n = 76)
Hemoglobin (g/dL)						
9.5 to 10.9	24	1	32	1	21	3
8 to 9.4	5	0	4	0	4	0
6.5 to 7.9	0	0	0	0.4	0	0
< 6.5	0	0	0	0	0	0
Leukocytes (x 10^9/L)						
2 to 2.9	40	20	38	23	45	26
1.5 to 1.9	4	1	9	2	5	3
1 to 1.4	0.9	0	2	0	0	0
< 1	0	0	0	0	0	0
Neutrophils (x 10^9/L)						
1 to 1.49	30	32	31	44	42	34
0.75 to 0.99	14	15	14	11	16	18
0.5 to 0.74	9	9	14	7	8	4
< 0.5	11	8	11	5	5	8
Platelets (x 10^9/L)						
70 to 99	9	11	11	14	6	12
50 to 69	2	3	2	3	0	5
30 to 49	0	0.4	0	0.4	0	0
< 30	0.9	0	1	0.9	0	0
Total bilirubin (mg/dL)						
1.5 to 3	27	13	32	13	21	7
3.1 to 6	0.9	0.4	2	0	3	0
6.1 to 12	0	0	0.4	0	0	0
> 12	0	0	0	0	0	0

Selected Hematologic Values During Treatment with Ribavirin Capsules Plus Peginterferon alfa-2b (%)

	Ribavirin capsules + peginterferon alfa-2b (N = 511)
Hemoglobin (g/dL)	
9.5 to 10.9	26
8 to 9.4	3
6.5 to 7.9	0.2
< 6.5	0
Leukocytes (× 10^9/L)	
2 to 2.9	46
1.5 to 1.9	24
1 to 1.4	5
< 1	0
Neutrophils (× 10^9/L)	
1 to 1.49	33
0.75 to 0.99	25
0.5 to 0.74	18
< 0.5	4
Platelets (× 10^9/L)	
70 to 99	15

Selected Hematologic Values During Treatment with Ribavirin Capsules Plus Peginterferon alfa-2b (%)

	Ribavirin capsules + peginterferon alfa-2b (N = 511)
50 to 69	3
30 to 49	0.2
< 30	0
Total bilirubin (mg/dL)	
1.5 to 3	10
3.1 to 6	0.6
6.1 to 12	0
> 12	0
ALT	
2 × baseline	0.6
2.1 to 5 × baseline	3
5.1 to 10 × baseline	0
> 10 × baseline	0

Overdosage

►*Capsules:* Acute ingestion of up to 20 g ribavirin, and ingestion of interferon alfa-2b up to 120 million units, and SC doses of up to 10 times the recommended dose have been reported. Primary effects observed were increased severity of adverse effects. However, hepatic enzyme abnormalities, renal failure, hemorrhage, and MI were observed with doses exceeding recommended single SC doses of interferon alfa-2b. There is no specific antidote known for interferon alfa-2b and ribavirin overdose, nor is hemodialysis and peritoneal dialysis effective.

►*Aerosol:* No overdosage with ribavirin by aerosol administration has been reported in humans. The LD$_{50}$ in mice is 2 g orally and is associated with hypoactivity and GI symptoms (estimated human equivalent dose of 0.17 g/kg, based on body surface area conversion). Refer to General Management of Acute Overdosage.

Patient Information

►*Capsules/Tablets:* Inform patients that ribavirin may cause birth defects or death of the exposed fetus. Ribavirin must not be used by women who are pregnant or by men whose female partners are pregnant. Extreme care must be taken to avoid pregnancy in female patients and female partners of male patients taking ribavirin. Do not initiate ribavirin until a report of a negative pregnancy test has been obtained immediately prior to initiation of therapy. Patients must perform a pregnancy test monthly during therapy and for 6 months posttherapy. Women of childbearing potential must be counseled about use of effective contraception (2 reliable forms) prior to initiating therapy. Patients (male and female) must be advised of the teratogenic/embryocidal risks and must be instructed to practice effective contraception during ribavirin therapy and for 6 months posttherapy. Advise patients (male and female) to notify the physician immediately in the event of a pregnancy (see Contraindications and Warnings). Physicians should report such cases by calling (800) 727-7064 for ribavirin capsules and (800) 526-6367 for ribavirin tablets.

Inform patients receiving ribavirin of the benefits and risks associated with treatment, directed in its appropriate use, and referred to the patient medication guide. Inform patients that the effect of treatment of hepatitis C infection on transmission is not known, and that they should take appropriate precautions to prevent transmission of the hepatitis C virus.

Advise the patient that laboratory evaluations are required prior to starting therapy and periodically thereafter (see Precautions). Advise patients to be well hydrated, especially during the initial stages of treatment.

Caution patients who develop dizziness, confusion, somnolence, and fatigue to avoid driving or operating machinery. Advise patients to take ribavirin tablets with food.

RIMANTADINE HCl

Rx	**Flumadine** (Forest)	**Tablets:** 100 mg	(FLUMADINE 100 FOREST). Orange, oval. Film-coated. In 100s.
		Syrup: 50 mg/5 mL	Saccharin, sorbitol, parabens. Raspberry flavor. In 240 mL.

Indications

►*Adults:* Prophylaxis and treatment of illness caused by various strains of influenza A virus.

►*Children:* Prophylaxis against influenza A virus.

►*Prophylaxis recommendations:*

1.) High-risk patients vaccinated after influenza outbreak has begun: Consider prophylaxis until immunity from the influenza vaccine has developed (this may take up to 2 weeks).

2.) Caretakers of those at high risk: Consider prophylaxis for unvaccinated caretakers of high-risk patients during peak influenza activity.

3.) Patients with immune deficiency: Consider prophylaxis for high-risk patients who are expected to have inadequate antibody response to influenza vaccine (eg, HIV).

4.) Other: Consider prophylaxis in high-risk patients who should not be vaccinated. Prophylaxis may also be offered to those patients who desire to avoid influenza illness.

Administration and Dosage

►*Approved by the FDA:* September 17, 1993.

►*Prophylaxis:*

Adults – The recommended dose of rimantadine is 100 mg twice daily. In patients with severe hepatic dysfunction, renal failure (Ccr ≤ 10 mL/min), and elderly nursing home patients, a dose reduction to 100 mg daily is recommended.

RIMANTADINE HCl

Children (< 10 years of age) – Administer once daily at a dose of 5 mg/kg, not exceeding 150 mg. For children ≥ 10 years of age, use the adult dose.

➤*Treatment:*

Adults – The recommended dose is 100 mg twice daily. In patients with severe hepatic dysfunction, renal failure (Ccr ≤ 10 mL/min), and elderly nursing home patients, a dose reduction to 100 mg daily is recommended. Initiate therapy as soon as possible, preferably within 48 hours after onset of signs and symptoms of influenza A infection. Continue therapy for ≈ 7 days from the initial onset of symptoms.

➤*Renal function impairment:* Because of the potential for accumulation of rimantadine metabolites during multiple dosing, monitor patients with any degree of renal insufficiency for adverse effects, making dosage adjustments as necessary.

➤*Storage/Stability:* Store tablets and syrup at 15° to 30°C (59° to 86°F).

Actions

➤*Pharmacology:* Rimantadine is a synthetic antiviral agent. The mechanism of action is not fully understood. It appears to exert its inhibitory effect early in the viral replicative cycle, possibly inhibiting the uncoating of the virus. Genetic studies suggest that a virus protein specified by the virion M_2 gene plays an important role in the susceptibility of influenza A virus to inhibition by rimantadine.

Rimantadine is safe and effective in preventing signs and symptoms of infection caused by various strains of influenza A virus. Early vaccination on an annual basis as recommended by the CDC's Immunization Practices Advisory Committee is the method of choice in the prophylaxis of influenza unless vaccination is contraindicated, not available, or not feasible. Because rimantadine does not completely prevent the host immune response to influenza A infection, individuals who take this drug may still develop immune responses to natural disease or vaccination and may be protected when later exposed to antigenically related viruses. Following vaccination during an influenza outbreak, consider rimantadine prophylaxis for the 2- to 4-week time period required to develop an antibody response. However, the safety and effectiveness of prophylaxis have not been demonstrated for > 6 weeks.

Consider rimantadine therapy for adults who develop an influenza-like illness during known or suspected influenza A infection in the community. When administered within 48 hours after onset of signs and symptoms of infection caused by influenza A virus strains, rimantadine reduces the duration of fever and systemic symptoms.

➤*Pharmacokinetics:* There are no data establishing a correlation between plasma concentration and antiviral effect. The tablet and syrup formulations of rimantadine are equally absorbed after oral administration. The mean peak plasma concentration after a single 100 mg dose was ≈ 74 ng/mL (range, 45 to 138 ng/mL). The time to peak concentration was ≈ 6 hours in healthy adults (age, 20 to 44 years). The single-dose elimination half-life in this population was ≈ 25.4 hours (range, 13 to 65 hours). The single-dose elimination half-life in a group of healthy 71- to 79-year-old subjects was ≈ 32 hours (range, 20 to 65 hours). The in vitro human plasma protein binding is ≈ 40% over typical plasma concentrations. Albumin is the major binding protein.

After the administration of 100 mg twice daily to healthy volunteers (18 to 70 years of age) for 10 days, area under the curve (AUC) values were ≈ 30% greater than predicted from a single dose. Plasma trough levels at steady state ranged between 118 and 468 ng/mL. In a comparison of 3 groups of healthy older subjects (50 to 60, 61 to 70, and 71 to 79 years of age), the 71- to 79-year-old group had average AUC values, peak concentrations, and elimination half-life values at steady state that were 20% to 30% higher than the other 2 groups. Steady-state concentrations in elderly nursing home patients (68 to 102 years of age) were 2- to 4-fold higher than those seen in healthy young and elderly adults.

Special populations –

Children: In a group (n = 10) of children (4 to 8 years of age) who were given a single dose (6.6 mg/kg) of syrup, plasma concentrations ranged from 446 to 988 ng/mL at 5 to 6 hours and from 170 to 424 ng/mL at 24 hours. In some children, the drug was detected in plasma 72 hours after the last dose.

Following oral administration, rimantadine is extensively metabolized in the liver with < 25% of the dose excreted in the urine as unchanged drug. Three hydroxylated metabolites have been found in plasma. These metabolites, an additional conjugated metabolite, and parent drug account for ≈ 74% of a single 200 mg dose excreted in urine over 72 hours.

Hepatic function impairment – In a group of patients with chronic liver disease, the majority of whom were stabilized cirrhotics, the pharmacokinetics of rimantadine were not appreciably altered following a single 200 mg oral dose compared with 6 healthy subjects. After administration of a single 200 mg dose to patients with severe hepatic dysfunction, AUC was ≈ 3-fold larger, elimination half-life was ≈ 2-fold longer, and apparent clearance was ≈ 50% lower when compared with historic data from healthy subjects.

Renal function impairment – Studies of the effects of renal insufficiency on the pharmacokinetics of rimantadine have given inconsistent results. Following administration of a single 200 mg oral dose to 8 patients with a Ccr of 31 to 50 mL/min and 6 patients with Ccr of 11 to 30 mL/min, the apparent clearance was 37% and 16% lower, respectively, and plasma metabolite concentrations were higher when compared with healthy subjects (n = 9, Ccr > 50 mL/min). After a single 200 mg oral dose was given to 8 hemodialysis patients (Ccr 0 to 10 mL/min), there was a 1.6-fold increase in the elimination half-life and a 40% decrease in apparent clearance compared with healthy subjects. Hemodialysis did not contribute to the clearance of rimantadine.

➤*Microbiology:* Rimantadine is inhibitory to the in vitro replication of influenza A virus isolates from each of the 3 antigenic subtypes (H1N1, H2N2, and H3N2) that have been isolated from humans. Rimantadine has little or no activity against influenza B virus. Rimantadine does not interfere with the immunogenicity of inactivated influenza A vaccine. A quantitative relationship between the in vitro susceptibility of influenza A virus to rimantadine and clinical response to therapy has not been established. Rimantadine-resistant strains of influenza A virus have emerged among freshly isolated epidemic strains in closed settings where rimantadine has been used. Resistant viruses have been shown to be transmissible and to cause typical influenza illness.

Contraindications

Hypersensitivity to drugs of the adamantane class, including rimantadine and amantadine.

Warnings

➤*Renal/Hepatic function impairment:* The safety and pharmacokinetics of rimantadine in renal and hepatic insufficiency have only been evaluated after single-dose administration. In a single-dose study of patients with anuric renal failure, the apparent clearance was ≈ 40% lower and the elimination half-life was 1.6-fold greater than that in healthy controls. In a study of 14 people with chronic liver disease (mostly stabilized cirrhotics), no alterations in the pharmacokinetics were observed after a single dose of rimantadine. However, the apparent clearance of rimantadine following a single dose to 10 patients with severe liver dysfunction was 50% lower than that reported for healthy subjects. Because of the potential for accumulation of rimantadine and its metabolites in plasma, exercise caution when patients with renal or hepatic insufficiency are treated with rimantadine.

➤*Pregnancy:* Category C. There are no adequate and well-controlled studies in pregnant women. Rimantadine crosses the placenta in mice. Rimantadine is embryotoxic in rats when given at a dose of 200 mg/kg/day (11 times the recommended human dose), which consisted of increased fetal resorption; this dose also produced a variety of maternal effects including ataxia, tremors, convulsions, and significantly reduced weight gain. In rabbits, there was evidence of a developmental abnormality in the form of a change in the ratio of fetuses with 12 or 13 ribs. This ratio is normally about 50:50 in a litter but was 80:20 after rimantadine treatment. In pregnant rats using doses of 30, 60, and 120 mg/kg/day (1.7, 3.4, and 6.8 times the recommended human dose), maternal toxicity during gestation was noted at the 2 higher doses of rimantadine, and at the highest dose there was an increase in pup mortality during the first 2 to 4 days postpartum. Decreased fertility of the F1 generation was also noted for the 2 higher doses. For these reasons, use during pregnancy only if the potential benefit justifies the risk to the fetus.

➤*Lactation:* Do not administer rimantadine to nursing mothers because of the adverse affects noted in offspring of rats treated with rimantadine during the nursing period. Rimantadine is concentrated in rat milk in a dose-related manner: 2 to 3 hours following administration of rimantadine, rat breast milk levels were ≈ 2 times those observed in serum.

➤*Children:* In children, rimantadine is recommended for the prophylaxis of influenza A. Safety and efficacy of rimantadine in the treatment of symptomatic influenza infection in children have not been established. Prophylaxis studies with rimantadine have not been performed in children < 1 year of age.

Precautions

➤*Seizures:* An increased incidence of seizures has been reported in patients with a history of epilepsy who received the related drug amantadine. In clinical trials, the occurrence of seizure-like activity was observed in a small number of patients with a history of seizures who were not receiving anticonvulsant medication while taking rimantadine. If seizures develop, discontinue the drug.

➤*Resistance:* Consider transmission of rimantadine-resistant virus when treating patients whose contacts are at high risk for influenza A illness. Influenza A virus strains resistant to rimantadine can emerge during treatment and may be transmissible and cause typical influenza illness. Of patients with initially sensitive virus upon treatment with rimantadine, 10% to 30% shed rimantadine-resistant virus. Clinical response, although slower in those patients, was not significantly different from those who did not shed resistant virus.

RIMANTADINE HCl

Drug Interactions

Rimantadine Drug Interactions			
Precipitant drug	Object drug[*]		Description
Acetaminophen	Rimantadine	↓	Coadministration with acetaminophen reduced the peak concentration and AUC values for rimantadine by ≈ 11%.
Aspirin	Rimantadine	↓	Peak plasma and AUC of rimantadine were reduced ≈ 10% when coadministered with aspirin.
Cimetidine	Rimantadine	↑	When a single 100 mg dose of rimantadine was administered 1 hour after cimetidine (300 mg 4 times/day) in healthy adults, the apparent total rimantadine clearance was reduced by 18%.

[*] ↑ = Object drug increased. ↓ = Object drug decreased.

Adverse Reactions

The most frequently reported adverse events involved GI and CNS. Rates increased significantly using higher-than-recommended doses. In most cases, symptoms resolved rapidly with discontinuation of treatment.

Adverse Reactions: Rimantadine vs Placebo (%)		
Adverse reaction	Rimantadine (n = 1027)	Placebo (n = 986)
CNS		
Insomnia	2.1	0.9
Dizziness	1.9	1.1
Headache	1.4	1.3
Asthenia	1.4	0.5
Nervousness	1.3	0.6
Fatigue	1	0.9
GI		
Nausea	2.8	1.6
Vomiting	1.7	0.6
Anorexia	1.6	0.8
Dry mouth	1.5	0.6
Abdominal pain	1.4	0.8

Adverse Reactions: Rimantadine vs Amantadine (%)			
Adverse reaction	Rimantadine 200 mg/day (n = 145)	Placebo (n = 143)	Amantadine 200 mg/day (n = 148)
Insomnia	3.4	0.7	7
Nervousness	2.1	0.7	2.8

Adverse Reactions: Rimantadine vs Amantadine (%)			
Adverse reaction	Rimantadine 200 mg/day (n = 145)	Placebo (n = 143)	Amantadine 200 mg/day (n = 148)
Impaired concentration	2.1	1.4	2.1
Dizziness	0.7	0	2.1
Depression	0.7	0.7	3.5
Total % with adverse reactions	6.9	4.1	14.7
Total % withdrawn because of adverse reactions	6.9	3.4	14

➤*Cardiovascular:* Pallor, palpitation, hypertension, cerebrovascular disorder, cardiac failure, pedal edema, heart block, tachycardia, syncope (< 0.3%).

➤*CNS:* Impairment of concentration, ataxia, somnolence, agitation, depression (0.3% to 1%); gait abnormality, euphoria, hyperkinesia, tremor, hallucination, confusion, convulsions (< 0.3%); agitation, diaphoresis, hypesthesia.

➤*GI:* Diarrhea, dyspepsia (0.3% to 1%); constipation, dysphagia, stomatitis.

➤*Respiratory:* Dyspnea (0.3% to 1%); bronchospasm, cough (< 0.3%).

➤*Special senses:* Tinnitus (0.3% to 1%); taste loss/change, parosmia (< 0.3%); eye pain, increased lacrimation.

➤*Miscellaneous:* Rash (0.3% to 1%); nonpuerperal lactation (< 0.3%); increased micturition frequency, fever, rigors.

Elderly – Geriatric subjects who received 200 or 400 mg of rimantadine daily for 1 to 50 days experienced considerably more CNS and GI adverse events than comparable geriatric subjects receiving placebo. CNS events, including dizziness, headache, anxiety, asthenia, and fatigue occurred up to 2 times more often in subjects treated with rimantadine than in those treated with placebo. GI symptoms, particularly nausea, vomiting, and abdominal pain occurred at least twice as frequently in subjects receiving rimantadine than in those receiving placebo. The GI symptoms appeared to be dose-related.

Overdosage

As with any overdose, administer supportive therapy as indicated. Overdoses of a related drug, amantadine, have been reported with adverse reactions consisting of agitation, hallucinations, cardiac arrhythmia, and death. The administration of IV physostigmine (a cholinergic agent) at doses of 1 to 2 mg in adults and 0.5 mg in children repeated as needed as long as the dose did not exceed 2 mg/hr has been reported anecdotally to be beneficial in patients with CNS effects from overdoses of amantadine. Refer to General Management of Acute Overdosage.

ZANAMIVIR

Rx	**Relenza** (GlaxoSmithKline)	**Blisters of powder for inhalation:** 5 mg	20 mg lactose. In 4 blisters with 5 *Rotadisks* and 1 *Diskhaler*.

Indications

➤*Influenza treatment:* For the treatment of uncomplicated acute illness caused by influenza A and B virus in adults and pediatric patients 7 years of age and older who have been symptomatic for no more than 2 days.

Zanamivir is not recommended for treatment of patients with underlying airways disease such as asthma or chronic obstructive pulmonary disease (COPD) (see Warnings).

Administration and Dosage

➤*Approved by the FDA:* July 27, 1999.

Zanamivir is for administration to the respiratory tract by oral inhalation only, using the *Diskhaler* device provided. Instruct patients in the use of the delivery system. Include a demonstration whenever possible. If zanamivir is prescribed for children, it should be used only under adult supervision and instruction, and the supervising adult should first be instructed by a health care professional.

The recommended dose of zanamivir for the treatment of influenza in patients 7 years of age and older is 2 inhalations (one 5 mg blister per inhalation for a total dose of 10 mg) twice daily (approximately 12 hours apart) for 5 days. Take 2 doses on the first day of treatment whenever possible, provided there is at least 2 hours between doses. On subsequent days, take doses approximately 12 hours apart (eg, morning and evening) at approximately the same time each day. There are no data on the effectiveness of treatment with zanamivir when initiated more than 2 days after the onset of signs or symptoms.

Instruct patients scheduled to use an inhaled bronchodilator at the same time as zanamivir to use their bronchodilator before taking zanamivir (see Warnings).

➤*Storage/Stability:* Store at 25°C (77°F); excursions permitted to 15° to 30°C (59° to 86°F). Do not puncture any *Rotadisk* blister until taking a dose using the *Diskhaler*.

Actions

➤*Pharmacology:* The proposed mechanism of action of zanamivir is via inhibition of influenza virus neuraminidase with the possibility of alteration of virus particle aggregation and release.

Drug resistance – Influenza viruses with reduced susceptibility to zanamivir have been recovered in vitro by passage of the virus in the presence of increasing concentrations of the drug. Genetic analysis of these viruses showed that the reduced susceptibility in vitro to zanamivir is associated with mutations that result in amino acid changes in the viral neuraminidase or viral hemagglutinin or both.

In an immunocompromised patient infected with influenza B virus, a variant virus emerged after treatment with an investigational nebulized solution of zanamivir for 2 weeks. Analysis of this variant showed a hemagglutinin mutation that resulted in a reduced affinity for human cell receptors and a mutation in the neuraminidase active site that reduced the enzyme's activity to zanamivir by 1000-fold.

Cross-resistance – Cross-resistance has been observed between zanamivir-resistant and oseltamivir-resistant influenza virus mutants generated in vitro.

➤*Pharmacokinetics:*

Absorption – Approximately 4% to 17% of the inhaled dose is systemically absorbed. Peak serum concentrations ranged from 17 to 142 ng/mL within 1 to 2 hours following a 10 mg dose. The AUC ranged from 111 to 1364 ng•h/mL.

The amount of drug delivered to the respiratory tract per inhalation will depend on patient factors such as inspiratory flow. Under standardized in vitro testing, *Rotadisk* delivers 4 mg zanamivir from the

ZANAMIVIR

Diskhaler device when tested at a pressure drop of 3 kPa (corresponding to a flow rate of approximately 62 to 65 L/min) for 3 seconds.

Distribution – Zanamivir has limited plasma protein binding (less than 10%).

Metabolism – Zanamivir is renally excreted as unchanged drug. No metabolites have been detected.

Excretion – The serum half-life of zanamivir following oral inhalation ranges from 2.5 to 5.1 hours. It is excreted unchanged in the urine with excretion of a single dose completed within 24 hours. Total clearance ranges from 2.5 to 10.9 L/h. Unabsorbed drug is excreted in the feces.

Special populations –

Renal function impairment: Systemic exposure is limited after inhalation (see Absorption). After a single IV dose of 2 or 4 mg of zanamivir in volunteers with mild/moderate or severe renal impairment, respectively, significant decreases in renal clearance (total clearance: healthy 5.3 L/h, mild/moderate 2.7 L/h, and severe 0.8 L/h; median values) and significant increases in half-life (healthy 3.1 h, mild/moderate 4.7 h, and severe 18.5 h; median values) and systemic exposure were observed. Safety and efficacy have not been documented in the presence of severe renal insufficiency.

Contraindications

Hypersensitivity to any component of the formulation.

Warnings

➤*Underlying respiratory disease:* Safety and efficacy have not been demonstrated in patients with underlying chronic pulmonary disease. In particular, zanamivir has not been shown to be effective and may carry risk in patients with severe or decompensated COPD or asthma, and serious adverse events have been reported in such patients. Therefore, zanamivir is not generally recommended for treatment of patients with underlying airways disease such as asthma or COPD.

Bronchospasm was documented following administration of zanamivir in 1 of 13 patients with mild or moderate asthma (but without acute influenza-like illness) in a phase 1 study. In interim results from an ongoing treatment study in patients with acute influenza-like illness superimposed on underlying asthma or COPD, more patients on zanamivir than on placebo experienced greater than 20% decline in FEV_1 or peak expiratory flow rate. If treatment with zanamivir is considered for a patient with underlying airways disease, carefully weigh the potential risks and benefits. If a decision is made to prescribe zanamivir for such a patient, this should be done only under conditions of careful monitoring of respiratory function, close observation, and appropriate supportive care including availability of fast-acting bronchodilators.

Some patients have experienced bronchospasm or decline in lung function when treated with zanamivir. Many, but not all, of these patients had underlying airways disease such as asthma or COPD. Because of the risk of serious adverse events and because efficacy has not been demonstrated in this population, zanamivir generally is not recommended for treatment of patients with underlying airways disease. Some patients with serious adverse events during zanamivir treatment have had fatal outcomes, although causality was difficult to assess.

Discontinue zanamivir in any patient who develops bronchospasm or decline in respiratory function; immediate treatment and hospitalization may be required. Some patients without prior pulmonary disease also may have respiratory abnormalities from acute respiratory infection that could resemble adverse drug reactions or increase patient vulnerability to adverse drug reactions.

➤*Pregnancy:* Category C. An embryo/fetal study in a different strain of rat was conducted using SC administration of zanamivir 3 times/day at doses of 1, 9, or 80 mg/kg during days 7 to 17 of pregnancy. There was an increase in the incidence rates of a variety of minor skeleton alterations and variants in the exposed offspring in this study. Based on AUC measurements, the high dose in the study produced an exposure greater than 1000 times the human exposure at the proposed clinical dose. However, the individual incidence rate of each skeletal alteration or variant, in most instances, remained within the background rates of the historical occurrence in the strain studied.

Zanamivir crosses the placenta in rats and rabbits. In these animals, fetal blood concentrations of zanamivir were significantly lower than zanamivir concentrations in the maternal blood.

There are no adequate and well-controlled studies in pregnant women. Use during pregnancy only if the potential benefit justifies the potential risk to the fetus.

➤*Lactation:* Studies in rats have demonstrated that zanamivir is excreted in milk. However, it is not known whether zanamivir is excreted in human milk. Exercise caution when zanamivir is administered to a nursing mother.

➤*Children:* Safety and efficacy of zanamivir have not been established in pediatric patients younger than 7 years of age. Carefully evaluate the ability of young children to use the delivery system if prescription of zanamivir is considered. When zanamivir is prescribed for children, use only under adult supervision and with attention to proper use of the delivery system.

Precautions

➤*Start of treatment:* No data are available to support safety or efficacy in patients who begin treatment after 48 hours of symptoms.

➤*Repeated courses:* Safety and efficacy of repeated treatment courses have not been studied.

➤*Allergic reactions:* Allergic-like reactions, including oropharyngeal edema and serious skin rashes, have been reported in postmarketing experience with zanamivir. Stop zanamivir and institute appropriate treatment if an allergic reaction occurs or is suspected.

➤*Bacterial infections:* Serious bacterial infections may begin with influenza-like symptoms or may coexist with or occur as complications during the course of influenza. Zanamivir has not been shown to prevent such complications.

➤*Other illness:* There is no evidence for efficacy of zanamivir in any illness caused by agents other than influenza virus A and B.

➤*Prevention of influenza:* Safety and efficacy of zanamivir have not been established for prophylactic use to prevent influenza. Use of zanamivir should not affect the evaluation of individuals for annual influenza vaccination in accordance with guidelines of the Centers for Disease Control and Prevention Advisory Committee on Immunization Practices.

➤*High-risk patients:* Safety and efficacy have not been demonstrated in patients with high-risk underlying medical conditions. No information is available regarding treatment of influenza in patients with any medical condition sufficiently severe or unstable to be considered at imminent risk of requiring inpatient management.

Drug Interactions

Zanamivir is not a substrate nor does it affect cytochrome P450 (CYP) isoenzymes (CYP1A1/2, 2A6, 2C9, 2C18, 2D6, 2E1, and 3A4) in human liver microsomes.

Adverse Reactions

Zanamivir Adverse Reactions in Adults and Adolescents (%)			
	Zanamivir		Placebo (lactose vehicle[2]) (n = 1520)
Adverse reaction	10 mg bid inhaled (n = 1132)	All dosing regimens[1] (n = 2289)	
GI			
Diarrhea	3	3	4
Nausea	3	3	3
Vomiting	1	1	2
Respiratory			
Nasal signs and symptoms	2	3	3
Bronchitis	2	2	3
Cough	2	2	3
Sinusitis	3	2	2
Ear, nose, and throat infections	2	1	2
Miscellaneous			
Dizziness	2	1	< 1
Headaches	2	2	3

[1] Includes studies where zanamivir was administered intranasally (6.4 mg 2 to 4 times/day in addition to inhaled preparation) or inhaled more frequently (qid) than the currently recommended dose.

[2] Because the placebo consisted of inhaled lactose powder, which is also the vehicle for the active drug, some adverse events occurring at similar frequencies in different treatment groups could be related to lactose-vehicle inhalation.

Additional adverse reactions occurring in less than 1.5% of patients receiving zanamivir included malaise, fatigue, fever, abdominal pain, myalgia, arthralgia, and urticaria.

➤*Lab test abnormalities:* The most frequent laboratory abnormalities in phase 3 treatment studies included elevations of liver enzymes and CPK, lymphopenia, and neutropenia. These were reported in similar proportions of zanamivir and lactose-vehicle placebo recipients with acute influenza-like illness.

➤*Clinical trials in pediatric patients:*

Adverse Events During Treatment in Pediatric Patients (%)[1]		
Adverse reaction	Zanamivir 10 mg bid inhaled (n = 291)	Placebo (lactose vehicle[2]) (n = 318)
Respiratory		
Ear, nose, and throat infections	5	5
Ear, nose, and throat hemorrhage	< 1	2
Asthma	< 1	2
Cough	< 1	2

ZANAMIVIR

Adverse Events During Treatment in Pediatric Patients (%)[1]		
Adverse reaction	Zanamivir 10 mg bid inhaled (n = 291)	Placebo (lactose vehicle[2]) (n = 318)
GI		
Vomiting	2	3
Diarrhea	2	2
Nausea	< 1	2

[1] Includes a subset of patients receiving zanamivir for treatment of influenza in a prophylaxis study.
[2] Because the placebo consisted of inhaled lactose powder, which is also the vehicle for the active drug, some adverse events occurring at similar frequencies in different treatment groups could be related to lactose-vehicle inhalation.

In 1 of the 2 studies described in the table above, some additional information is available from children 5 to 12 years of age without acute influenza-like illness who received an investigational prophylaxis regimen of zanamivir; 132 children received zanamivir and 145 children received placebo. Among these children, nasal signs and symptoms (zanamivir 20%, placebo 9%), cough (zanamivir 16%, placebo 8%), and throat/tonsil discomfort and pain (zanamivir 11%, placebo 6%) were reported more frequently with zanamivir than placebo. In a subset with chronic respiratory disease, lower respiratory adverse events (described as asthma, cough, or viral respiratory infections that could include influenza-like symptoms) were reported in 7 of 7 zanamivir recipients and 5 of 12 placebo recipients.

➤*Postmarketing:* In addition to adverse events reported from clinical trials, the following adverse events have been identified during post-marketing use of zanamivir. Because they are reported voluntarily from a population of unknown size, estimates of frequency cannot be made. These events have been chosen for inclusion because of a combination of their seriousness, frequency of reporting, or potential causal connection to zanamivir: Allergic or allergic-like reaction, including oropharyngeal edema (see Precautions); arrhythmias; bronchospasm, dyspnea (see Warnings); facial edema; rash, including serious cutaneous reactions; seizures; syncope.

Overdosage

There have been no reports of overdosage from administration. Doses of zanamivir up to 64 mg/day have been administered by nebulizer. Additionally, doses of up to 1200 mg/day for 5 days have been administered IV. Adverse effects were similar to those seen in clinical studies at the recommended dose.

Patient Information

Instruct patients in use of the delivery system. Include a demonstration whenever possible. For the proper use of zanamivir, have the patient read and carefully follow the accompanying Patient's Instructions for Use. Effective and safe use of zanamivir requires proper use of the *Diskaler* to inhale the drug.

Advise patients to finish the entire 5-day course of treatment even if they start to feel better sooner.

Advise patients that the use of zanamivir for treatment of influenza has not been shown to reduce the risk of transmission of influenza to others.

Advise patients of the risk of bronchospasm, especially in the setting of underlying airways disease, and to stop zanamivir and contact their physician if they experience increased respiratory symptoms during treatment such as worsening wheezing, shortness of breath, or other signs or symptoms of bronchospasm. If a decision is made to prescribe zanamivir for a patient with asthma or COPD, make the patient aware of the risks and advise them to have a fast-acting bronchodilator available. Advise patients scheduled to take inhaled bronchodilators at the same time as zanamivir to use their bronchodilators before taking zanamivir.

OSELTAMIVIR PHOSPHATE

Rx	**Tamiflu** (Roche)	**Capsules:** 75 mg (as base)	Talc. (ROCHE 75 mg). Grey/yellow. In blister pack 10s.
		Powder for oral suspension: 12 mg/mL after reconstitution (as base)	Sorbitol, saccharin. Tutti-frutti flavor. In 25 mL with bottle adapter and oral dispenser.

Indications

➤*Influenza infection:*

Treatment – For the treatment of uncomplicated acute illness caused by influenza infection in patients 1 year of age and older who have been symptomatic for no more than 2 days.

Prophylaxis – For prophylaxis of influenza in adults and adolescents 13 years of age and older.

Oseltamivir is not a substitute for early vaccination on an annual basis as recommended by the Centers for Disease Control and Prevention Advisory Committee on Immunization Practices.

Administration and Dosage

➤*Approved by the FDA:* October 27, 1999.

Oseltamivir may be taken with or without food. However, when taken with food, tolerability may be enhanced in some patients.

➤*Treatment of influenza:*

Adults and adolescents (13 years of age and older) – The recommended oral dose of oseltamivir is 75 mg twice daily for 5 days. Begin treatment within 2 days of onset of symptoms of influenza.

Children (1 year of age and older) – The recommended oral dose of oseltamivir oral suspension for children or adults who cannot swallow a capsule is as follows:

Oseltamivir Oral Suspension Dosing			
Body weight (kg)	Body weight (lbs)	Recommended dose for 5 days	Volume per recommended dose
≤ 15	≤ 33	30 mg twice daily	2.5 mL (½ tsp)
> 15 to 23	> 33 to 51	45 mg twice daily	3.8 mL (¾ tsp)
> 23 to 40	> 51 to 88	60 mg twice daily	5 mL (1 tsp)
> 40	> 88	75 mg twice daily	6.2 mL (1¼ tsp)

An oral dosing dispenser with 30, 45, and 60 mg graduations is provided with the oral suspension; the 75 mg dose can be measured using a combination of 30 and 45 mg. It is recommended that patients use this dispenser.

➤*Influenza prophylaxis:* The recommended oral dose of oseltamivir for influenza prophylaxis in adults and adolescents 13 years of age and older following close contact with an infected individual is 75 mg once daily for at least 7 days. Begin therapy within 2 days of exposure. The recommended dose for prophylaxis during a community outbreak of influenza is 75 mg once daily. Safety and efficacy have been demonstrated for up to 6 weeks. The duration of protection lasts for as long as dosing is continued.

➤*Renal function impairment:* For plasma concentrations of oseltamivir carboxylate predicted to occur following various dosing schedules in patients with renal impairment, see Pharmacokinetics.

Influenza treatment – Dose adjustment is recommended for patients with creatinine clearance (Ccr) between 10 and 30 mL/min receiving oseltamivir for treatment of influenza. In these patients, it is recommended that the dose be reduced to 75 mg oseltamivir once daily for 5 days. No recommended dosing regimens are available for patients undergoing routine hemodialysis and continuous peritoneal dialysis treatment with end-stage renal disease.

Influenza prophylaxis – For prophylaxis of influenza, dose adjustment is recommended for patients with Ccr between 10 and 30 mL/min receiving oseltamivir. In these patients, it is recommended that the dose be reduced to 75 mg every other day or 30 mg oseltamivir oral suspension every day. No recommended dosing regimens are available for patients undergoing routine hemodialysis and continuous peritoneal dialysis treatment with end-stage renal disease.

➤*Preparation of oral suspension:* It is recommended that oseltamivir oral suspension be reconstituted by the pharmacist prior to dispensing to the patient:
1.) Tap the closed bottle several times to loosen the powder.
2.) Measure 23 mL of water into a graduated cylinder.
3.) Add the total amount of water for reconstitution to the bottle and shake the closed bottle well for 15 seconds.
4.) Remove the child-resistant cap and push bottle adapter into the neck of the bottle.
5.) Close bottle with child-resistant cap tightly. This will assure the proper seating of the bottle adapter in the bottle and child-resistant status of the cap.

The reconstituted oral suspension should be used within 10 days of preparation; the pharmacist should write the date of expiration of the reconstituted suspension on a pharmacy label. The patient package insert and oral dispenser should be dispensed to the patient.

➤*Storage/Stability:*

Capsules/Dry powder for suspension – Store at 25°C (77°F); excursions permitted to 15° to 30°C (59° to 86°F).

Reconstituted suspension – Store at 25°C (77°F); excursions permitted to 15° to 30°C (59° to 86°F); or under refrigeration at 2° to 8°C (36° to 46°F). Do not freeze.

Actions

➤*Pharmacology:* Oseltamivir is an ethyl ester prodrug requiring ester hydrolysis for conversion to the active form, oseltamivir carboxylate. The proposed mechanism of action of oseltamivir is via inhibition of influenza virus neuraminidase with the possibility of alteration of virus particle aggregation and release.

OSELTAMIVIR PHOSPHATE

Drug resistance – Influenza A virus isolates with reduced susceptibility to oseltamivir carboxylate has been recovered in vitro by passage of virus in the presence of increasing concentrations of oseltamivir carboxylate. Genetic analysis of these isolates show that reduced susceptibility to oseltamivir carboxylate is associated with mutations that result in amino acid changes in the viral neuraminidase or viral hemagglutinin or both.

In clinical studies of naturally acquired infection with influenza virus, 1.3% of posttreatment isolates in adults and adolescents and 8.6% in children from 1 to 12 years of age showed emergence of influenza variants with decreased neuraminidase susceptibility to oseltamivir carboxylate.

Genotypic analysis of these variants showed a specific mutation in the active site of neuraminidase compared with pretreatment isolates. The contribution of resistance because of alterations in the viral hemagglutinin has not been fully evaluated.

Cross-resistance – Cross-resistance between zanamivir-resistant influenza mutants and oseltamivir-resistant influenza mutants has been observed in vitro. Because of limitations in the assays available to detect drug-induced shifts in virus susceptibility, an estimate of the incidence of oseltamivir resistance and possible cross-resistance to zanamivir in clinical isolates cannot be made. However, 1 of the 3 oseltamivir-induced mutations in the viral neuraminidase from clinical isolates is the same as 1 of the 3 mutations observed in zanamivir-resistant virus.

➤*Pharmacokinetics:*

Absorption – Oseltamivir is readily absorbed from the GI tract after oral administration and is extensively converted predominantly by hepatic esterases to oseltamivir carboxylate. At least 75% of an oral dose reaches the systemic circulation as oseltamivir carboxylate. Exposure to oseltamivir is less than 5% of the total exposure after oral dosing.

The mean C_{max} of oseltamivir and oseltamivir carboxylate were 65.2 ng/mL and 348 ng/mL, respectively, after multiple doses of 75 mg twice daily. The mean $AUC_{(0-12\ h)}$ for oseltamivir was 112 ng•h/mL and 2719 ng•h/mL for oseltamivir carboxylate.

Plasma concentrations of oseltamivir carboxylate are proportional to doses up to 500 mg given twice daily.

Coadministration with food has no significant effect on the peak plasma concentration and the area under the plasma concentration time curve of oseltamivir carboxylate.

Distribution – The volume of distribution of oseltamivir carboxylate following IV administration in 24 subjects ranged between 23 and 26 L.

The binding of oseltamivir carboxylate to human plasma protein is low (3%). The binding of oseltamivir to human plasma protein is 42%.

Metabolism – Oseltamivir is extensively converted to oseltamivir carboxylate by esterases located predominantly in the liver. Neither oseltamivir nor oseltamivir carboxylate is a substrate for, or inhibitor of, cytochrome P450 isoforms.

Excretion – Absorbed oseltamivir is primarily (more than 90%) eliminated by conversion to oseltamivir carboxylate. Plasma concentrations of oseltamivir declined with a half-life of 1 to 3 hours in most subjects after oral administration. Oseltamivir carboxylate is not further metabolized and is eliminated in the urine. Plasma concentrations of oseltamivir carboxylate declined with a half-life of 6 to 10 hours in most subjects after oral administration. Oseltamivir carboxylate is eliminated entirely (more than 99%) by renal excretion. Renal clearance (18.8 L/h) exceeds glomerular filtration rate (7.5 L/h) indicating that tubular secretion occurs in addition to glomerular filtration. Less than 20% of an oral dose is eliminated in feces.

Special populations –

Renal function impairment: Administration of 100 mg oseltamivir twice daily for 5 days to patients with various degrees of renal impairment showed that exposure to oseltamivir carboxylate is inversely proportional to declining renal function. Dose adjustment is recommended for patients with serum Ccr less than 30 mL/min. Oseltamivir carboxylate exposures in patients with normal and abnormal renal function administered various dose regimens of oseltamivir are described in the following table.

Oseltamivir Carboxylate Exposures in Patients with Normal and Reduced Serum Ccr							
	Normal renal function			Impaired renal function			
				Ccr < 10 mL/min		Ccr > 10 and < 30 mL/min	
Parameter	75 mg qd	75 mg bid	150 mg bid	CAPD 30 mg/ week	Hemodialysis 30 mg alternate HD cycle	75 mg/ day	75 mg alternate days	30 mg/ day
C_{max}	259[1]	348[1]	705[1]	766	850	1638	1175	655
C_{min}	39[1]	138[1]	288[1]	62	48	864	209	346
AUC_{48}	7476[1]	10,876[1]	21,864[1]	17,381	12,429	62,636	21,999	25,054

[1] Observed values. All other values are predicted.

Children: Pediatric patients 12 years of age or younger cleared both the prodrug and the active metabolite faster than adult patients, resulting in a lower exposure for a given mg/kg dose. The pharmacokinetics of oseltamivir in pediatric patients older than 12 years of age are similar to those in adult patients.

Elderly: Exposure to oseltamivir carboxylate at steady state was 25% to 35% higher in geriatric patients (range, 65 to 78 years of age) compared with young adults given comparable doses of oseltamivir. Dose adjustments are not required for geriatric patients for either treatment or prophylaxis.

Contraindications

Hypersensitivity to any of the components of the product.

Warnings

➤*Renal function impairment:* Dose adjustment is recommended for patients with a serum Ccr less than 30 mL/min (see Administration and Dosage).

➤*Mutagenesis:* Although found to be nonmutagenic in other tests, oseltamivir was found to be positive in a Syrian hamster embryo (SHE) cell transformation test.

➤*Pregnancy: Category C.* There are insufficient human data upon which to base an evaluation of risk of oseltamivir to pregnant women or the developing fetus. Studies for effects on embryo-fetal development were conducted in rats (50, 250, and 1500 mg/kg/day) and rabbits (50, 150, and 500 mg/kg/day) by the oral route. Relative exposures at these doses were respectively, 2, 13, and 100 times the human exposure in the rat and 4, 8, and 50 times the human exposure in the rabbit. Pharmacokinetic studies indicated that fetal exposure was seen in both species. In the rat study, minimal maternal toxicity was reported in the 1500 mg/kg/day group. In the rabbit study, slight and marked maternal toxicities were observed respectively, in the 150 and 500 mg/kg/day groups. There was a dose-dependent increase in the incidence rates of a variety of minor skeletal abnormalities and variants in the exposed offspring in these studies. However, the individual incidence rate of each skeletal abnormality or variant remained within the background rates of occurrence in the species studied.

Because there are no adequate and well-controlled studies of oseltamivir in pregnant women, use during pregnancy only if the potential benefit justifies the potential risk to the fetus.

➤*Lactation:* In lactating rats, oseltamivir and oseltamivir carboxylate are excreted in the milk. It is not known whether oseltamivir or oseltamivir carboxylate is excreted in human milk. Therefore, use oseltamivir only if the potential benefit for the lactating mother justifies the potential risk to the breastfed infant.

➤*Children:* Safety and efficacy for treatment in children younger than 1 year of age have not been established. The safety and efficacy of oseltamivir for prophylaxis in children younger than 13 years of age have not been established.

Precautions

➤*Bacterial infections:* Serious bacterial infections may begin with influenza-like symptoms or may coexist with or occur as complications during the course of influenza. Oseltamivir has not been shown to prevent such complications.

➤*Other illnesses:* There is no evidence for efficacy of oseltamivir in any illness caused by agents other than influenza viruses types A and B.

➤*Start of treatment:* Efficacy of oseltamivir in patients who begin treatment after 40 hours of symptoms has not been established.

➤*High-risk patients:* Efficacy of oseltamivir in subjects with chronic cardiac disease or respiratory disease has not been established. No difference in the incidence of complications was observed between the treatment and placebo groups in this population. No information is available regarding treatment of influenza in patients with any medical condition sufficiently severe or unstable to be considered an imminent risk of requiring hospitalization.

➤*Prevention of influenza:* Use of oseltamivir should not affect the evaluation of individuals for annual influenza vaccination in accordance with guidelines of the Centers for Disease Control and Prevention Advisory Committee on Immunization Practices.

➤*Repeated courses:* Safety and efficacy of repeated treatment courses have not been established.

Drug Interactions

➤*Probenecid:* Coadministration of probenecid results in an approximate 2-fold increase in exposure to oseltamivir carboxylate because of a decrease in active anionic tubular secretion in the kidney.

Adverse Reactions

➤*Adults:*

Treatment studies: A total of 1171 patients who participated in adult phase 3 controlled clinical trials for the treatment of influenza were treated with oseltamivir. The most frequently reported adverse events in these studies were nausea and vomiting. These events were generally of mild to moderate degree and usually occurred on the first 2 days of administration. Less than 1% of subjects discontinued prematurely from clinical trials because of nausea and vomiting.

Adverse events that occurred with an incidence of at least 1% in 1440 patients taking placebo or oseltamivir 75 mg twice daily in adult phase 3 treatment studies appear in the following table. This summary

OSELTAMIVIR PHOSPHATE

includes 945 healthy young adults and 495 at-risk patients (elderly patients and patients with chronic cardiac or respiratory disease). Those events reported numerically more frequently in patients taking oseltamivir compared with placebo were nausea, vomiting, bronchitis, insomnia, and vertigo.

Oseltamivir Adverse Reactions (%)

Adverse reaction	Treatment		Prophylaxis	
	Oseltamivir 75 mg bid (n = 724)	Placebo (n = 716)	Oseltamivir 75 mg qd (n = 1480)	Placebo (n = 1434)
Nausea (without vomiting)	9.9	5.6	7	3.9
Vomiting	9.4	2.9	2.1	1
Diarrhea	6.6	9.8	3.2	2.6
Bronchitis	2.3	2.1	0.7	1.2
Abdominal pain	2.2	2.2	2	1.6
Dizziness	2.1	3.5	1.6	1.5
Headache	1.8	2	20.1	17.5
Cough	1.2	1.7	5.6	6
Insomnia	1.1	0.8	1.2	1
Vertigo	1	0.6	0.3	0.2
Fatigue	1	1	7.9	7.5

Additional adverse events occurring in less than 1% of patients receiving oseltamivir included unstable angina, anemia, pseudomembranous colitis, humerus fracture, pneumonia, pyrexia, and peritonsillar abscess.

Prophylaxis studies: A total of 3434 subjects (adolescents, healthy adults, and elderly) participated in phase 3 prophylaxis studies, of whom 1480 received the recommended dose of 75 mg once daily for up to 6 weeks. Adverse events were qualitatively very similar to those seen in the treatment studies, despite a longer duration of dosing (see table above). Events reported more frequently in subjects receiving oseltamivir compared with subjects receiving placebo in prophylaxis studies, and more commonly than in treatment studies, were aches and pains, rhinorrhea, dyspepsia, and upper respiratory tract infections. However, the difference in incidence between oseltamivir and placebo for these events was less than 1%. There were no clinically relevant differences in the safety profile of the 942 elderly subjects who received oseltamivir or placebo, compared with the younger population.

►*Children:*

Treatment studies: A total of 1032 pediatric patients 1 to 12 years of age (including 698 otherwise healthy pediatric patients 1 to 12 years of age and 334 asthmatic pediatric patients 6 to 12 years of age) participated in phase 3 studies of oseltamivir given for the treatment of influenza. A total of 515 pediatric patients received treatment with oseltamivir oral suspension.

Adverse events occurring in more than 1% of pediatric patients receiving oseltamivir treatment are listed in the following table. The most frequently reported adverse event was vomiting. Other events reported more frequently by pediatric patients treated with oseltamivir included abdominal pain, epistaxis, ear disorder, and conjunctivitis. These events generally occurred once and resolved despite continued dosing. They did not cause discontinuation of drug in the vast majority of cases.

The adverse event profile in adolescents is similar to that described for adult patients and pediatric patients 1 to 12 years of age.

Adverse Events During Treatment in > 1% of Pediatric Patients Enrolled in Phase 3 Trials of Oseltamivir Treatment of Naturally Acquired Influenza (%)

Adverse reaction	Oseltamivir 2 mg/kg twice daily (n = 515)	Placebo (n = 517)
Vomiting	15	9.3
Diarrhea	9.5	10.6
Otitis media	8.7	11.2
Abdominal pain	4.7	3.9
Asthma (including aggravated)	3.5	3.7
Nausea	3.3	4.3
Epistaxis	3.1	2.5
Pneumonia	1.9	3.3
Ear disorder	1.7	1.2
Sinusitis	1.7	2.5
Bronchitis	1.6	2.1
Conjunctivitis	1	0.4
Dermatitis	1	1.9
Lymphadenopathy	1	1.5
Tympanic membrane disorder	1	1.2

Postmarketing: The following adverse reactions have been identified during postmarketing use of oseltamivir. Because these reactions are reported voluntarily from a population of uncertain size, it is not possible to reliably estimate their frequency or establish a causal relationship to oseltamivir exposure: Rash; swelling of the face or tongue; toxic epidermal necrolysis; hepatitis; abnormal liver function tests; arrhythmia; seizure; confusion; aggravation of diabetes.

Overdosage

At present, there has been no experience with overdose. Single doses of up to 1000 mg of oseltamivir have been associated with nausea and/or vomiting.

Patient Information

Instruct patients to begin treatment with oseltamivir as soon as possible after the first appearance of flu symptoms.

Instruct the patient to shake oseltamivir oral suspension well before each use and to use the constituted oral suspension within 10 days of preparation.

Instruct patients to take any missed doses as soon as they remember, except if it is near the next scheduled dose (within 2 hours), and then to continue to take oseltamivir at the usual times.

Oseltamivir is not a substitute for a flu shot. Advise patients to continue receiving an annual flu shot according to guidelines on immunization practices.

ADEFOVIR DIPIVOXIL

Rx	Hepsera (Gilead Sciences)	Tablets: 10 mg	Lactose. (10 GILEAD). White. In 30s.

WARNING

Severe acute exacerbations of hepatitis have been reported in patients who have discontinued anti-hepatitis B therapy, including therapy with adefovir dipivoxil. Closely monitor hepatic function in patients who discontinue anti-hepatitis B therapy. If appropriate, resumption of anti-hepatitis B therapy may be warranted (see Warnings).

In patients at risk of or having underlying renal dysfunction, chronic administration of adefovir dipivoxil may result in nephrotoxicity. Closely monitor these patients for renal function and adjust dose as required (see Warnings and Administration and Dosage).

Human immunodeficiency virus (HIV) resistance may emerge in chronic hepatitis B patients with unrecognized or untreated HIV infection treated with anti-hepatitis B therapies, such as therapy with adefovir dipivoxil, that may have activity against HIV (see Warnings).

Lactic acidosis and severe hepatomegaly with steatosis, including fatal cases, have been reported with the use of nucleoside analogs alone or in combination with other antiretrovirals (see Warnings).

Indications

►*Chronic hepatitis B:* Treatment of chronic hepatitis B in adults with evidence of active viral replication and evidence of persistent elevations in serum aminotransferases (ALT or AST) or histologically active disease.

This indication is based on histological, virological, biochemical, and serological responses in adult patients with HBeAg-positive and HBeAg-negative chronic hepatitis B with compensated liver function, and in adult patients with clinical evidence of lamivudine-resistant hepatitis B virus with compensated or decompensated liver function.

Administration and Dosage

►*Approved by the FDA:* September 20, 2002.

The recommended dose of adefovir dipivoxil in chronic hepatitis B patients with adequate renal function is 10 mg once daily taken orally without regard to food. The optimal duration of treatment is unknown.

►*Dose adjustment in renal impairment:* Significantly increased drug exposures were seen when adefovir dipivoxil was administered to patients with renal impairment. Adjust the dosing interval of adefovir dipivoxil in patients with baseline creatinine clearance (Ccr) less than 50 mL/min using the following suggested guidelines.

Dosing Interval Adjustment of Adefovir Dipivoxil in Patients with Renal Impairment

	Ccr (mL/min)[1]			
	≥ 50	20 to 49	10 to 19	Hemodialysis patients
Recommended dose and dosing interval	10 mg q 24 h	10 mg q 48 h	10 mg q 72 h	10 mg q 7 days following dialysis

[1] Ccr calculated by Cockcroft-Gault method using lean or ideal body weight.

ADEFOVIR DIPIVOXIL

The pharmacokinetics of adefovir have not been evaluated in nonhemodialysis patients with Ccr below 10 mL/min; therefore, no dosing recommendation is available for these patients.

➤*Storage/Stability:* Store in original container at 25°C (77°F), excursions permitted to 15° to 30°C (59° to 86°F).

Actions

➤*Pharmacology:* Adefovir is an acyclic nucleotide analog of adenosine monophosphate. Adefovir is phosphorylated to the active metabolite, adefovir diphosphate, by cellular kinases. Adefovir diphosphate inhibits HBV DNA polymerase (reverse transcriptase) by competing with the natural substrate deoxyadenosine triphosphate and by causing DNA chain termination after its incorporation into viral DNA. The inhibition constant (K_i) for adefovir diphosphate for HBV DNA polymerase was 0.1 mcM. Adefovir diphosphate is a weak inhibitor of human DNA polymerases α and γ with K_i values of 1.18 mcM and 0.97 mcM, respectively.

➤*Pharmacokinetics:*

Absorption – Adefovir dipivoxil is a diester prodrug of the active moiety adefovir. Based on a cross-study comparison, the approximate oral bioavailability of adefovir from a 10 mg single dose of adefovir dipivoxil is 59%.

Following oral administration of a 10 mg single dose of adefovir dipivoxil to chronic hepatitis B patients (n = 14), the peak adefovir plasma concentration (C_{max}) was approximately 18.4 ng/mL and occurred between 0.58 and 4 hours (median = 1.75 hours) postdose. The adefovir area under the plasma concentration-time curve ($AUC_{0-\infty}$) was approximately 220 ng•h/mL. Plasma adefovir concentrations declined in a biexponential manner.

Adefovir may be taken without regard to food.

Distribution – In vitro binding of adefovir to human plasma or human serum proteins is less than or equal to 4% over the adefovir concentration range of 0.1 to 25 mcg/mL. The volume of distribution at steady-state following IV administration of 1 or 3 mg/kg/day is approximately 392 and 352 mL/kg, respectively.

Metabolism/Elimination – Terminal elimination half-life is approximately 7.48 hours. Following oral administration, adefovir dipivoxil is rapidly converted to adefovir. Forty-five percent of the dose is recovered as adefovir in the urine over 24 hours at steady state following 10 mg oral doses of adefovir dipivoxil. Adefovir is renally excreted by a combination of glomerular filtration and active tubular secretion.

Special populations –

Renal impairment: In subjects with moderately or severely impaired renal function or with end-stage renal disease (ESRD) requiring hemodialysis, C_{max}, AUC, and half-life ($T_{\frac{1}{2}}$) were increased compared with subjects with normal renal function. It is recommended that the dosing interval of adefovir dipivoxil be modified in these patients.

The pharmacokinetics of adefovir in nonchronic hepatitis B patients with varying degrees of renal impairment are described in the following table. In this study, subjects received a 10 mg single dose of adefovir dipivoxil.

Pharmacokinetic Parameters of Adefovir in Patients with Varying Degrees of Renal Function				
Renal function group	Unimpaired	Mild	Moderate	Severe
Baseline Ccr (mL/min)	> 80 (n = 7)	50 to 80 (n = 8)	30 to 49 (n = 7)	10 to 29 (n = 10)
C_{max} (ng/mL)	≈ 17.8	≈ 22.4	≈ 28.5	≈ 51.6
$AUC_{0-\infty}$ (ng•h/mL)	≈ 201	≈ 266	≈ 455	≈ 1240
CL/F (mL/min)	≈ 469	≈ 356	≈ 237	≈ 91.7
CL_{renal} (mL/min)	≈ 231	≈ 148	≈ 83.9	≈ 37

Contraindications

Previously demonstrated hypersensitivity to any of the components of the product.

Warnings

➤*Exacerbations of hepatitis after discontinuation of treatment:* Severe acute exacerbation of hepatitis has been reported in patients who have discontinued anti-hepatitis B therapy, including therapy with adefovir dipivoxil. Monitor patients who discontinue adefovir dipivoxil at repeated intervals over a period of time for hepatic function. If appropriate, resumption of anti-hepatitis B therapy may be warranted.

➤*Nephrotoxicity:* Nephrotoxicity characterized by a delayed onset of gradual increases in serum creatinine and decreases in serum phosphorus historically was shown to be the treatment-limiting toxicity of adefovir dipivoxil therapy at substantially higher doses in HIV-infected patients (60 and 120 mg/day) and in chronic hepatitis B patients (30 mg/day). Chronic administration of adefovir dipivoxil (10 mg once daily) may result in nephrotoxicity. The overall risk of nephrotoxicity in patients with adequate renal function is low. However, this is of special importance in patients at risk of or having underlying renal dysfunction and patients taking concomitant nephrotoxic agents (eg, cyclo-

sporine, tacrolimus, aminoglycosides, vancomycin, nonsteroidal anti-inflammatory drugs).

➤*Lactic acidosis/severe hepatomegaly with steatosis:* Lactic acidosis and severe hepatomegaly with steatosis, including fatal cases, have been reported with the use of nucleoside analogs alone or in combination with antiretrovirals. A majority of these cases have been in women. Obesity and prolonged nucleoside exposure may be risk factors. Exercise particular caution when administering nucleoside analogs to any patient with known risk factors for liver disease; however, cases also have been reported in patients with no known risk factors. Suspend treatment with adefovir dipivoxil in any patient who develops clinical or laboratory findings suggestive of lactic acidosis or pronounced hepatotoxicity (which may include hepatomegaly and steatosis even in the absence of marked transaminase elevations).

➤*Elderly:* Exercise caution when prescribing to elderly patients because they have greater frequency of decreased renal or cardiac function caused by concomitant disease or other drug therapy.

➤*Pregnancy: Category C.* There are no adequate and well-controlled studies in pregnant women. Because animal reproduction studies are not always predictive of human response, use adefovir dipivoxil during pregnancy only if clearly needed and after careful consideration of the risks and benefits.

To monitor fetal outcomes of pregnant women exposed to adefovir dipivoxil, a pregnancy registry has been established. Health care providers are encouraged to register patients by calling 1-800-258-4263.

There are no studies in pregnant women and no data on the effect of adefovir dipivoxil on transmission of hepatitis B virus from mother to infant. Therefore, use appropriate infant immunizations to prevent neonatal acquisition of hepatitis B virus.

➤*Lactation:* It is not known whether adefovir is excreted in human milk. Instruct mothers not to breastfeed if they are taking adefovir dipivoxil.

Precautions

➤*Monitoring:*

Renal function – It is important to monitor renal function for all patients during treatment with adefovir dipivoxil, particularly for those with pre-existing or other risks for renal impairment. Patients with renal insufficiency at baseline or during treatment may require dose adjustment. Carefully evaluate the risks and benefits of adefovir dipivoxil treatment prior to discontinuing adefovir dipivoxil in a patient with treatment-emergent nephrotoxicity.

HIV resistance – Prior to initiating adefovir dipivoxil, offer HIV antibody testing to all patients. Treatment with anti-hepatitis B therapies, such as adefovir dipivoxil, that have activity against HIV in a chronic hepatitis B patient with unrecognized or untreated HIV infection may result in emergence of HIV resistance.

Drug coadministration – Closely monitor patients for adverse events when adefovir dipivoxil is coadministered with drugs that are excreted renally or with other drugs known to affect renal function.

Drug Interactions

When adefovir dipivoxil was coadministered with ibuprofen 800 mg 3 times/day, increases in adefovir C_{max} (33%), AUC (23%), and urinary recovery were observed. This increase appears to be caused by higher oral bioavailability, not a reduction in renal clearance of adefovir.

Because adefovir is eliminated by the kidney, coadministration of adefovir dipivoxil with drugs that reduce renal function or compete for active tubular secretion may increase serum concentrations of adefovir or these coadministered drugs.

Adverse Reactions

Assessment of adverse reactions is based on 2 studies in which 522 patients with chronic hepatitis B received double-blind treatment with adefovir dipivoxil (n = 294) or placebo (n = 228) for 48 weeks. With extended therapy in the second 48-week treatment period, 492 patients were treated for up to 109 weeks, with a median time on treatment of 49 weeks.

Treatment-Related Adverse Reactions (Grades 1 to 4) Reported in ≥ 3% of All Treated Patients (%)		
Adverse reaction	Adefovir dipivoxil 10 mg (n = 294)	Placebo (n = 228)
Asthenia	13	14
Headache	9	10
Abdominal pain	9	11
Nausea	5	8
Flatulence	4	4
Diarrhea	3	4
Dyspepsia	3	2

ADEFOVIR DIPIVOXIL

Grade 3 to 4 Laboratory Abnormalities Reported in ≥ 1% of All Treated Patients (%)		
Adverse reaction	Adefovir dipivoxil 10 mg (n = 294)	Placebo (n = 228)
ALT (> 5 × ULN)	20	41
Hematuria (≥ 3+)	11	10
AST (> 5 × ULN)	8	23
Creatine kinase (> 4 × ULN)	7	7
Amylase (> 2 × ULN)	4	4
Glycosuria (≥ 3+)	1	3

In patients with adequate renal function, increases in serum creatinine of greater than or equal to 0.3 mg/dL from baseline were observed in 4% of patients treated with adefovir dipivoxil 10 mg/day compared with 2% of patients in the placebo group by week 48. No patients developed a serum creatinine increase greater than or equal to 0.5 mg/dL from baseline by week 48. By week 96, 10% and 2% of adefovir dipivoxil-treated patients, by Kaplan-Meier estimate, had increases in serum creatinine greater than or equal to 0.3 mg/dL and greater than or equal to 0.5 mg/dL from baseline, respectively (no placebo-controlled results were available for comparison beyond week 48). Of the 29 of 492 patients with elevations in serum creatinine greater than or equal

to 0.3 mg/dL from baseline, 20 out of 29 resolved on continued treatment (less than or equal to 0.2 mg/dL from baseline), 8 of 29 remained unchanged, and 1 of 29 resolved on discontinuing treatment.

➤*Special-risk patients:* The most common treatment-related adverse events reported in pre- and post-liver transplantation patients treated with adefovir dipivoxil with a 2% frequency or higher include the following:

GI: Nausea; vomiting; diarrhea; flatulence; hepatic failure.
GU: Increases in creatinine; renal failure; renal insufficiency.
Respiratory: Increased cough; pharyngitis; sinusitis.
Miscellaneous: Asthenia; abdominal pain; headache; fever; pruritus; rash; increases in ALT and AST; abnormal liver function.

Overdosage

➤*Symptoms:* Doses of adefovir dipivoxil 500 mg/day for 2 weeks and 250 mg/day for 12 weeks have been associated with GI side effects.

➤*Treatment:* If overdose occurs, the patient must be monitored for evidence of toxicity, and standard supportive treatment applied as necessary. Following a single 10 mg dose of adefovir dipivoxil, a 4-hour hemodialysis session removed approximately 35% of the adefovir dose.

Patient Information

Advise patients to review the patient pamphlet carefully before starting adefovir and to read and check for new information each time adefovir is dispensed. The patient pamphlet does not take the place of talking with the prescribing physician.

SAQUINAVIR

Rx	**Invirase** (Roche)	**Capsules:** 200 mg (as mesylate)	Lactose. (ROCHE 0245). Lt. brown/green. In 270s.
Rx	**Fortovase** (Roche)	**Capsules, soft gelatin:** 200 mg	(ROCHE 0246). Beige. In 180s.

> ### WARNING
>
> Saquinivir mesylate capsules (*Invirase*) and saquinavir soft gelatin capsules (*Fortovase*) are not bioequivalent and cannot be used interchangeably. When using saquinavir as part of an antiviral regimen, *Fortovase* is the recommended formulation. In rare circumstances, *Invirase* may be considered if it is to be combined with antiretrovirals that significantly inhibit saquinavir's metabolism (see Pharmacology).

Indications

➤*Human immunodeficiency virus (HIV) infection:* In combination with antiretroviral agents for the treatment of HIV infection.

This indication is based on a study that showed a reduction in mortality and AIDS-defining clinical events for patients who received *Invirase* in combination with zalcitabine compared with patients who received either drug alone and also on studies that showed increased saquinavir concentrations and improved antiviral activity for *Fortovase* 1200 mg 3 times daily vs *Invirase* 600 mg 3 times daily.

Administration and Dosage

➤*Approved by the FDA:* December 6, 1995.

Saquinavir soft gelatin capsules (*Fortovase*) and saquinavir mesylate capsules (*Invirase*) are not bioequivalent and cannot be used interchangeably. When using saquinavir as part of an antiviral regimen, *Fortovase* is the recommended formulation. In rare circumstances, *Invirase* may be considered if it is to be combined with antiretrovirals that significantly inhibit saquinavir's metabolism.

➤*Invirase:* Three 200 mg capsules 3 times daily taken within 2 hours after a full meal in combination with a nucleoside analog.

Use saquinavir mesylate only in combination with an active antiretroviral nucleoside analog regimen. Base concomitant therapy on a patient's prior drug exposure.

➤*Fortovase:* Six 200 mg capsules, 3 times daily with a meal or up to 2 hours after a meal. When used in combination with nucleoside analogs, the dosage of saquinavir should not be reduced, as this will lead to greater than dose-proportional decreases in saquinavir plasma levels.

➤*Dose adjustment for combination therapy with saquinavir:* For toxicities that may be associated with saquinavir, interrupt therapy. Saquinavir mesylate at doses < 600 mg 3 times daily are not recommended because lower doses have not shown antiviral activity. For recipients of combination therapy with saquinavir and other retrovirals, base dose adjustment of the other retrovirals on the known toxicity profile of the individual drug.

➤*Storage/Stability:*

Invirase – Store at 15° to 30°C (59° to 86°F) in tightly closed bottles.

Fortovase – Refrigerate at 2° to 8°C (36° to 46°F) in tightly closed bottles.

Refrigerated capsules remain stable until the expiration date printed on the label. Once brought to room temperature (≤ 25°C [77°F]), use capsules within 3 months.

Actions

➤*Pharmacology:* Saquinavir is an inhibitor of HIV protease. HIV protease cleaves viral polyprotein precursors to generate functional proteins in HIV-infected cells. The cleavage is essential for maturation of infectious virus. Saquinavir is a peptide-like substrate analog that inhibits the activity of HIV protease and prevents the cleavage of viral polyproteins.

➤*Pharmacokinetics:*

Absorption/Distribution – Saquinavir exhibits a low absolute bioavailability of 4% following a single dose of *Invirase* after a high-fat breakfast (48 g protein, 60 g carbohydrate, 57 g fat, 1006 kcal). This is considered to be the result of incomplete absorption and extensive first-pass metabolism. However, the relative bioavailability is ≈ 331% when saquinavir is administered as *Fortovase* compared with *Invirase*.

In HIV-infected patients, multiple dosing yields steady-state AUC values ≈ 2.5 times higher than a single *Invirase* dose and 80% higher than a single *Fortovase* dose. AUCs and peak levels in these patients are about twice those observed in healthy volunteers. Greater than dose-proportional increases in plasma levels occur following single and multiple doses when saquinavir is administered as *Fortovase*.

The mean steady-state Vd following 12 mg IV is 700 L, suggesting saquinavir partitions into tissues. Saquinavir is ≈ 98% bound to plasma proteins over a concentration range of 15 to 700 ng/mL. CSF levels are negligible.

Metabolism/Excretion – In vitro, the metabolism of saquinavir is cytochrome P450-mediated with specific isoenzyme, CYP3A4, responsible for > 90% of the hepatic metabolism. In vitro, saquinavir is rapidly metabolized to a range of mono- and dihydroxylated inactive compounds; within 5 days of oral dosing, 88% and 1% were recovered in feces and urine, respectively. In studies, 13% of circulating radioactivity in plasma was attributed to unchanged drug after oral administration and the remainder attributed to saquinavir metabolites. Following IV administration, 66% of circulating radioactivity was attributed to unchanged drug, suggesting that saquinavir undergoes extensive first-pass metabolism.

Systemic clearance of saquinavir was rapid, 1.14 L/h/kg after IV doses of 6, 36, and 72 mg. The mean residence time of saquinavir was 7 hours.

Special populations –

Fortovase:

• *Renal or hepatic function impairment* – Saquinavir pharmacokinetics in patients with hepatic or renal insufficiency has not been investigated. Only 1% of saquinavir is excreted in urine, so the impact of renal impairment on saquinavir elimination should be minimal.

➤*Microbiology:*

Antiviral activity in vitro – In cell culture, saquinavir demonstrated additive to synergistic effects against HIV in double and triple combination regimens with reverse transcriptase inhibitors zidovudine (AZT), zalcitabine (ddC), and didanosine (ddI) (*Invirase* and *Fortovase*), and lamivudine, stavudine, and nevirapine (*Fortovase* only) without enhanced cytotoxicity.

Cross-resistance to other antiretrovirals – The potential for HIV cross-resistance between protease inhibitors has not been fully explored; therefore, it is unknown what effect saquinavir therapy will have on the activity of subsequent protease inhibitors. Varying degrees of cross-resistance among protease inhibitors have been observed. Continued administration of saquinavir therapy following loss of viral suppression may increase the likelihood of cross-resistance to other protease inhibitors.

➤*Clinical trials:*

Advanced patients without prior AZT therapy – A study compared saquinavir mesylate doses of 75, 200, and 600 mg 3 times daily in combination with AZT 200 mg 3 times daily to saquinavir 600 mg 2 times daily alone and AZT alone. In analyses of average CD4 changes over 16 weeks, treatment with the combination of saquinavir 600 mg 3 times daily plus AZT produced greater CD4 cell increases than AZT monotherapy. The CD4 changes of AZT in combination with doses of saquinavir < 600 mg 3 times daily were no greater than that of AZT alone.

Advanced patients with prior AZT therapy – Patients (mean baseline CD4 = 165) with prolonged AZT treatment (median, 713 days) were randomized to receive either saquinavir mesylate 600 mg 3 times daily plus ddC and AZT, saquinavir 600 mg 3 times daily plus AZT or ddC plus AZT. In analyses of average CD4 changes over 24 weeks, the triple combination produced greater increases in CD4 cell counts compared with that of ddC plus AZT. There were no significant differences in CD4 changes among patients receiving saquinavir plus AZT and ddC plus AZT.

Fortovase vs Invirase: At week 16 of one study (n = 171), 60 patients on the *Fortovase* arm compared with 30 patients on the *Invirase* arm had plasma HIV RNA levels below the limit of assay quantification. Mean changes from baseline in CD4 cell counts and plasma HIV-RNA levels between the 2 treatment arms were statistically indistinguishable.

Contraindications

Clinically significant hypersensitivity to saquinavir or any components in the capsules; coadministration with cisapride, triazolam, midazolam, or ergot derivatives.

Warnings

➤*Diabetes mellitus, new onset:* Exacerbation of pre-existing diabetes mellitus and hyperglycemia have been reported during postmarketing surveillance in HIV-infected patients receiving protease inhibitor therapy. Some patients required initiation or dose adjustments of insulin or oral hypoglycemic agents. In some cases, diabetic ketoacidosis has occurred. Hyperglycemia persisted in some patients who discontinued protease inhibitor therapy. Because these events have been reported voluntarily during clinical practice, estimates of frequency cannot be made and a causal relationship between protease inhibitor therapy and these events has not been established.

➤*Hepatic function impairment:* Exercise caution when administering to patients with hepatic insufficiency because saquinavir is principally metabolized by the liver, and patients with baseline liver function tests > 5 times the normal upper limit were not included in clinical studies. Exacerbation of chronic liver dysfunction, including portal hypertension, in patients with underlying hepatitis B or C, cirrhosis, or other underlying liver abnormalities have been reported.

SAQUINAVIR

➤*Elderly:* In general, take caution when dosing *Fortovase* in elderly patients because of the greater frequency of decreased hepatic, renal, or cardiac function, and of concomitant disease or other drug therapy.

➤*Pregnancy: Category B.* Use during pregnancy after taking into account the importance of the drug to the mother.

Antiretroviral pregnancy registry – To monitor maternal-fetal outcomes of pregnant women exposed to antiretroviral medications, including saquinavir, an Antiretroviral Pregnancy Registry has been established. Physicians are encouraged to register patients by calling (800) 258-4263.

➤*Lactation:* It is not known whether saquinavir is excreted in breast milk. Because of the potential for HIV transmission and the potential for serious adverse reactions in nursing infants, instruct mothers not to breastfeed if they are receiving antiretroviral medications, including saquinavir.

The Centers for Disease Control and Prevention recommends that HIV-infected women not breastfeed to avoid postnatal transmission of HIV.

➤*Children:* Safety and efficacy in HIV-infected children or adolescents < 16 years of age have not been established.

Precautions

➤*Monitoring:* Perform clinical chemistry tests prior to initiating saquinavir therapy and at appropriate intervals thereafter. Elevated nonfasting triglyceride levels have been observed in patients in saquinavir trials. Periodically monitor triglyceride levels during therapy.

➤*General:* Saquinavir soft gelatin capsules (*Fortovase*) and saquinavir mesylate capsules (*Invirase*) are not bioequivalent and cannot be used interchangeably. Only *Fortovase* should be used for the initiation of saquinavir therapy (see Administration and Dosage) because *Fortovase* capsules provide greater bioavailability and efficacy than *Invirase*. For patients taking *Invirase* capsules with a viral load below the limit of quantification, a switch to *Fortovase* is recommended to maintain a virologic response. For patients taking *Invirase* capsules who have not had an adequate response or are failing therapy, if saquinavir resistance is clinically suspected, then do not use *Fortovase*. If resistance to saquinavir is not clinically suspected, consider a switch to *Fortovase*.

➤*Hemophilia:* There have been reports of spontaneous bleeding in patients with hemophilia A and B treated with protease inhibitors. In some patients additional factor VIII was required. In the majority of reported cases, treatment with protease inhibitors was continued or restarted. A causal relationship between protease inhibitor therapy and these episodes has not been established.

➤*Fat redistribution:* Redistribution/Accumulation of body fat, including central obesity, dorsocervical fat enlargement (buffalo hump), peripheral wasting, breast enlargement, and "cushingoid appearance" have been observed in patients receiving protease inhibitors. A causal relationship between protease inhibitor therapy and these events has not been established and the long-term consequences are unknown.

➤*Use with HMG-CoA reductase inhibitors:* Concomitant use of saquinavir with lovastatin or simvastatin is not recommended. Exercise caution if HIV protease inhibitors, including saquinavir, are used concurrently with other HMG-CoA reductase inhibitors that are also metabolized by the CYP3A4 pathway (eg, atorvastatin, cerivastatin). Because increased concentrations of statins can, in rare cases, cause severe adverse events such as myopathy, including rhabdomyolysis, this risk may be increased when HIV protease inhibitors, including saquinavir, are used in combination with these drugs.

➤*Toxicity:* If serious or severe toxicity occurs during treatment with saquinavir, interrupt therapy until the etiology of the event is identified or the toxicity resolves. At that time, consider resumption of treatment with full-dose saquinavir.

Drug Interactions

Saquinavir Drug Interactions			
Precipitant drug	Object drug*		Description
CYP3A4 inducers (eg, phenobarbital, phenytoin, dexamethasone, carbamazepine)	Saquinavir	↓	Coadministration may reduce saquinavir plasma concentrations.

Saquinavir Drug Interactions			
Precipitant drug	Object drug*		Description
Delavirdine	Saquinavir	↑	Coadministration of delavirdine with *Invirase* resulted in a 5-fold increase in saquinavir plasma AUC. There are limited safety and no efficacy data available on the use of this combination. In a small, preliminary study, hepatocellular enzyme elevations occurred in 13% of subjects during the first several weeks of the delavirdine and saquinavir combination (6% Grade 3 or 4). Frequently monitor hepatocellular changes if this combination is prescribed.
Ketoconazole	Saquinavir	↑	Coadministration results in a 130% increase in saquinavir mesylate AUC.
Nevirapine	Saquinavir	↓	Coadministration of nevirapine with saquinavir mesylate resulted in a 24% decrease in saquinavir plasma AUC. There are no safety and efficacy data available from the use of this combination.
Rifamycins	Saquinavir	↓	Coadministration of rifampin decreases the steady-state AUC and C_{max} of saquinavir by ≈ 80%. Steady-state AUC of saquinavir is decreased by ≈ 40% when saquinavir is coadministered with rifabutin.
Ritonavir	Saquinavir	↑	Following ≈ 4 weeks of a combination regimen of saquinavir 400 mg or 600 mg bid and ritonavir 400 mg or 600 mg bid in HIV-infected patients, saquinavir AUC values were ≥ 17-fold greater than historical AUC values from patients who received saquinavir 600 mg tid without ritonavir. When used in combination therapy for ≤ 24 weeks, doses > 400 mg bid of either ritonavir or saquinavir were associated with an increase in adverse events. Plasma exposures achieved with *Invirase* 400 mg bid and ritonavir 400 mg bid are similar to those achieved with *Fortovase* 400 mg bid and ritonavir 400 mg bid.
Clarithromycin	Saquinavir	↑	Coadministration resulted in a 177% increase in saquinavir plasma AUC, a 45% increase in clarithromycin AUC, and a 24% decrease in clarithromycin 14-OH metabolite AUC.
Saquinavir	Clarithromycin	↑	
Indinavir	Saquinavir	↑	Coadministration of indinavir with *Fortovase* (1200 mg single dose) resulted in a 364% increase in saquinavir plasma AUC. There are no safety and efficacy data available from the use of this combination.
Nelfinavir	Saquinavir	↑	Coadministration of nelfinavir with *Fortovase* resulted in an 18% increase in nelfinavir plasma AUC and a 392% increase in saquinavir plasma AUC. There are no safety and efficacy data available on the use of this combination. If nelfinavir is used in combination with *Invirase* at the recommended dose of 600 mg tid, no dose adjustments are needed.
Saquinavir	Nelfinavir	↑	
Saquinavir	CYP3A metabolized drugs (cisapride, ergot derivatives, midazolam, triazolam)	↑	Competition for CYP3A4 by saquinavir could result in inhibition of the metabolism of these drugs and create the potential for serious or life-threatening reactions such as cardiac arrhythmias or prolonged sedation. Other compounds that are substrates of CYP3A4 (eg, calcium channel blockers, clindamycin, dapsone, quinidine, triazolam) may have elevated plasma concentrations when administered with *Invirase*; therefore, monitor patients for toxicities associated with such drugs.

SAQUINAVIR

Saquinavir Drug Interactions			
Precipitant drug	Object drug*		Description
Saquinavir	Sildenafil	↑	In healthy volunteers, coadministration of saquinavir, a CYP3A4 inhibitor, at steady state (1200 mg tid) with sildenafil (100 mg single dose) resulted in a 140% increase in sildenafil C_{max} and a 210% increase in sildenafil AUC. Sildenafil had no effect on saquinavir pharmacokinetics. When sildenafil is administered concomitantly with saquinavir, consider a starting dose of 25 mg sildenafil.

* ↑ = Object drug increased. ↓ = Object drug decreased.

➤*Drug/Food interactions:* The mean 24-hour AUC after a single 600 mg oral dose in healthy volunteers was increased from 24 to 161 ng•h/mL under fasting conditions when saquinavir was given following a high-fat breakfast. Saquinavir 24-hour AUC and C_{max} following the administration of a higher calorie meal (943 kcal, 54 g fat) were on average 2 times higher than after a lower calorie, lower fat meal (355 kcal, 8 g fat). The effect of food persists for ≤ 2 hours.

Adverse Reactions

The majority of adverse events were of mild intensity. The most frequently reported treatment-emergent adverse events among patients receiving saquinavir in combination with other antiretroviral agents were dyspepsia (*Fortovase*), diarrhea, abdominal discomfort, and nausea (*Fortovase* and *Invirase*).

Rare occurrences of the following serious adverse experiences have been reported during clinical trials with *Fortovase*: Confusion; ataxia and weakness; acute myeloblastic leukemia; hemolytic anemia; attempted suicide; Stevens-Johnson syndrome; seizures; severe cutaneous reaction associated with increased liver function tests; isolated elevation of transaminases; thrombophlebitis; headache; thrombocytopenia; exacerbation of chronic liver disease with Grade 4 elevated liver function tests; jaundice, ascites, and right and left upper quadrant abdominal pain; pancreatitis leading to death; intestinal obstruction; portal hypertension; peripheral vasoconstriction; drug fever; nephrolithiasis; acute renal insufficiency; thrombocytopenia and intracranial hemorrhage leading to death; and bullous skin eruption and polyarthritis.

Saquinavir Adverse Reactions of At Least Moderate Intensity (≥ 2%)			
	Study 1 (48 weeks)	Study 2 (16 weeks) (Naive patients)	
Adverse event	Fortovase + TOC[1] (n = 442)	Invirase + 2 RTIs[2] (n = 81)	Fortovase + 2 RTIs[2] (n = 90)
CNS			
Headaches	5	4.9	8.9
Depression	2.7	-	-
Insomnia	-	1.2	5.6
Anxiety	-	2.5	2.2
Libido disorder	-	-	2.2
Dermatologic			
Eczema	-	2.5	-
Rash	-	2.5	-
Verruca	-	-	2.2
GI			
Diarrhea	19.9	12.3	15.6
Nausea	10.6	13.6	17.8
Abdominal discomfort	8.6	4.9	13.3
Dyspepsia	8.4	-	8.9
Flatulence	5.7	7.4	12.2
Vomiting	2.9	1.2	4.4
Abdominal pain	2.3	1.2	7.8
Constipation	-	-	3.3
Miscellaneous			
Fatigue	4.8	6.2	6.7
Pain	-	3.7	3.3
Taste alteration	-	1.2	4.4

[1] Antiretroviral treatment of choice.
[2] Reverse transcriptase inhibitor.

Marked Laboratory Abnormalities with Saquinavir[1]				
		Study 1 (48 weeks)	Study 2 (16 weeks) (Naive patients)	
Lab test abnormality	Limit	Fortovase + TOC[2] (n = 442)	Invirase + 2 RTIs[3] (n = 81)	Fortovase + 2 RTIs[3] (n = 90)
Biochemistry				
Alkaline phosphatase	> 5 x ULN[4]	0.5	0	0
Calcium (high)	> 12.5 mg/dL	0.2	0	0
Creatine kinase	> 4 x ULN	7.8	0	4.8
Gamma GT	> 5 x ULN	5.7	2.6	7.1
Glucose (low)	< 40 mg/dL	6.4	2.5	3.5
Glucose (high)	> 250 mg/dL	1.4	1.3	1.2
Phosphate	< 1.5 mg/dL	0.5	0	0
Potassium (high)	> 6.5 mEq/L	2.7	0	1.2
Serum amylase	> 2 x ULN	1.9	ND[5]	ND[5]
AST	> 5 x ULN	4.1	0	1.2
ALT	> 5 x ULN	5.7	1.3	2.3
Sodium (high)	> 157 mEq/L	0.7	0	0
Total bilirubin	> 2.5 x ULN	1.6	0	0
Hematology				
Hemoglobin	< 7 g/dL	0.7	0	1.2
Absolute neutrophil count	< 750 mm^3	2.9	2.9	1.2
Platelets	< 50,000 mm^3	0.9	2.5	0

[1] ACTG Grade 3 or above.
[2] Antiretroviral treatment of choice.
[3] Reverse transcriptase inhibitor.
[4] ULN = Upper limit of normal range.
[5] ND = Not done.

The following table lists clinical adverse events that occurred in ≥ 2% of patients receiving saquinavir mesylate (SAQ) 600 mg tid alone or in combination with AZT or ddC in 2 trials. Median duration of treatment in NV14255/ACTG229 (triple combination study) was 48 weeks; median duration of treatment in NV14256 (double combination study) was ≈ 1 year.

Adverse Reactions Considered at Least Possibly Related to Study Drug or of Unknown Relationship and of Moderate, Severe, or Life-Threatening Intensity, Occurring in ≥ 2% of Patients						
	Triple combination (NV14255/ACTG229)			Double combination (NV14256)		
Adverse event	SAQ + AZT (n = 99)	SAQ + ddc + AZT (n = 98)	ddC + AZT (n = 100)	ddC (n = 325)	SAQ (n = 327)	SAQ + ddC (n = 318)
CNS						
Headache	2	2	2	3.4	2.4	0.9
Paresthesia	2	3.1	4	1.2	0.3	0.3
Extremity numbness	2	1	4	1.5	0.6	0.9
Dizziness	-	2	1	-	0.3	-
Peripheral neuropathy	-	1	2	11.4	3.1	11.3
GI						
Diarrhea	3	1	-	0.9	4.9	4.4
Abdominal discomfort	2	3.1	4	0.9	0.9	0.9
Nausea	-	3.1	3	1.5	2.4	0.9
Dyspepsia	1	1	2	0.6	0.9	0.9
Abdominal pain	2	1	2	0.6	1.2	0.3
Mucosa damage	-	-	4	-	-	0.3
Buccal mucosa ulceration	-	2	2	6.2	2.1	3.8
Miscellaneous						
Asthenia	6.1	9.2	10	-	0.3	-
Appetite disturbances	-	1	2	-	-	-
Rash	-	-	3	1.5	2.1	1.3
Pruritus	-	-	2	-	0.6	-
Musculoskeletal pain	2	2	4	0.6	0.6	0.6
Myalgia	1	-	3	0.6	0.3	0.3

The following table shows the percentages of patients with marked laboratory abnormalities in studies NV14255/ACTG229 and NV14256. Marked laboratory abnormalities are defined as Grade 3 or 4 abnormality in a patient with a normal baseline value or a Grade 4 abnormality in a patient with a Grade 1 abnormality at baseline (ACTG Grading System).

SAQUINAVIR

	Percentage of Patients by Treatment Group with Marked[1] Laboratory Abnormalities					
	Triple combination (NV14255/ACTG229)			Double combination (NV14256)		
Laboratory abnormality	SAQ + AZT (n = 99)	SAQ + ddC + AZT (n = 98)	ddc + AZT (n = 100)	ddC (n = 325)	SAQ (n = 327)	SAQ + ddC (n = 318)
Calcium (high)	1	0	0	< 1	0	0
Calcium (low)	-	-	-	< 1	< 1	0
Creatine phosphokinase (high)	10	12	7	6	3	7
Glucose (high)	0	0	0	< 1	1	1
Glucose (low)	0	0	0	5	5	5
Phosphate (low)	2	1	0	0	< 1	< 1
Potassium (high)	0	0	0	2	2	3
Potassium (low)	0	0	0	0	1	0
Serum amylase (high)	2	1	1	2	1	1
AST (high)	2	2	0	2	2	3
ALT (high)	0	3	1	2	2	2
Sodium (high)	-	-	-	0	0	< 1
Sodium (low)	-	-	-	0	< 1	0
Total bilirubin (high)	1	0	0	0	< 1	1
Uric acid	0	0	1	Not assessed	Not assessed	Not assessed
Hematology						
Neutrophils (low)	2	2	8	1	1	1
Hemoglobin (low)	0	0	1	< 1	< 1	0
Platelets (low)	0	0	2	1	1	< 1

[1] Marked laboratory abnormality is defined as a shift from Grade 0 to ≥ Grade 3, or from Grade 1 to Grade 4 (ACTG Grading System).

Other adverse reactions (< 2%) are listed below.

➤*Cardiovascular:* Cyanosis; heart murmur; stroke; heart rate disorder; heart valve disorder; hypertension; hypotension; syncope; vein distended.

➤*CNS:* Ataxia; confusion; lightheaded feeling; myelopolyradiculoneuritis; prickly sensation; unconsciousness; convulsions; dysarthria; dysesthesia; hyperesthesia; hyperreflexia; hyporeflexia; face numbness; malaise; cerebral hemorrhage; dizziness; neuropathy; extremities numbness; paresthesias; peripheral neuropathy; paresis; poliomyelitis; progressive multifocal leukoencephalopathy; spasms; tremor.

➤*Dermatologic:* Acne; dermatitis; seborrheic dermatitis; alopecia; chalazion; nail disorder; papillomatosis; papular rash; pruritus; psoriasis; pruritic rash; red face; eczema; erythema; folliculitis; furunculosis; hair changes; hot flushes; photosensitivity reaction; skin pigment changes; maculopapular rash; skin disorder/nodule/syndrome/ulceration; sweating increased; urticaria; verruca; xeroderma.

➤*GI:* Abdominal distention; buccal mucosa ulceration; canker sores (oral); esophageal ulceration; fecal incontinence; gastroesophageal reflux; pruritus ani; pyrosis; toothache; GI ulcer; sclerosing cholangitis; cholelithiasis; abdominal colic; esophagitis; infectious diarrhea; stomach upset; cheilitis; frequent bowel movements; constipation; dyspepsia; flatulence; diarrhea; dysphagia; eructation; bloodstained/discolored feces; dry mouth; gastralgia; gastritis; GI inflammation; gingivitis; glossitis; rectal hemorrhage; hemorrhoids; melena; pelvic pain; painful defecation; pancreatitis; parotid disorder; salivary glands disorder; stomatitis; tooth disorder; vomiting.

➤*GU:* Prostate enlarged; impotence; vaginal discharge; micturition disorder; renal calculus; urinary tract bleeding/infection; epididymitis; erectile impotence; menstrual disorder; menstrual irregularity; nocturia; penis disorder; renal colic.

➤*Hematologic:* Anemia; microhemorrhages; neutropenia; dermal bleeding; pancytopenia; splenomegaly; thrombocytopenia; hemorrhage.

➤*Hepatic:* Hepatitis; hepatomegaly; hepatosplenomegaly; jaundice; liver enzyme disorder.

➤*Metabolic:* Dehydration; diabetes mellitus; hyperglycemia; weight increase; weight decrease; hypoglycemia; hypothyroidism; thirst; triglyceride increase.

➤*Musculoskeletal:* Arthralgia; arthritis; back pain; muscle cramps; musculoskeletal disorders; stiffness; tissue changes; trauma; leg cramps; weakness generalized; facial pain; lumbago; myalgia; myopathy; jaw pain; leg pain; musculoskeletal pain; creatine phosphokinase increased.

➤*Psychiatric:* Agitation; amnesia; anxiety attack; psychosis; anxiety; depression; behavior disturbances; excessive dreaming; euphoria; hallucination; insomnia; reduced intellectual ability; irritability; lethargy; libido disorder; overdose effect; suicide attempt; psychic disorder; somnolence; speech disorder.

➤*Respiratory:* Bronchitis; cough; dyspnea; epistaxis; hemoptysis; laryngitis; pharyngitis; pneumonia; respiratory disorder; rhinitis; sinusitis; upper respiratory tract infection; bronchial asthma; allergic atopic rhinitis; pulmonary disease.

➤*Special senses:* Blepharitis; earache; dry eye syndrome; ear pressure; eye irritation; decreased hearing; otitis; taste alteration; conjunctivitis; cytomegalovirus retinitis; unpleasant taste; tinnitus; visual disturbance; xerophthalmia.

➤*Miscellaneous:* Allergic reaction; anorexia; decreased appetite; appetite disturbances; body pain; Kaposi's sarcoma; molluscum contagiosum; parasitic infestation; chest pain; edema; fever; fatigue; intoxication; asthenia; olfactory disorder; moniliasis; night sweats; cellulitis; external parasites; retrosternal pain; shivering; wasting syndrome; abscess; angina tonsillaris; candidiasis; herpes simplex; herpes zoster; infection (bacterial/mycotic/staphylococcal); influenza; lymphadenopathy; tumor; redistribution/accumulation of body fat (see Precautions); trauma.

Overdosage

Overdosage with *Fortovase* has not been reported. There were 2 patients who had overdoses with saquinavir mesylate. No acute toxicities or sequelae were noted in 1 patient who ingested 8 g saquinavir mesylate as a single dose. The patient was treated with induction of emesis within 2 to 4 hours after ingestion. The second patient ingested 2.4 g of saquinavir mesylate in combination with 600 mg of ritonavir and experienced pain in the throat that lasted for 6 hours and then resolved. In an exploratory Phase II study with saquinavir mesylate at 7200 mg/day, no serious toxicities were reported through the first 25 weeks of treatment.

Patient Information

Inform patients that saquinavir is not a cure for HIV infection and that they may continue to acquire illnesses associated with advanced HIV infection, including opportunistic infections.

Tell patients that the long-term effects of saquinavir are unknown at this time. Inform them that saquinavir therapy has not been shown to reduce the risk of transmitting HIV to others through sexual contact or blood contamination.

Advise patients that saquinavir should be taken within 2 hours after a full meal. When saquinavir mesylate is taken without food, concentrations of saquinavir in the blood are substantially reduced and may result in no antiviral activity.

Saquinavir may interact with some drugs; therefore, advise patients to report to their physician the use of any other prescription or nonprescription medication.

Advise patients of the importance of taking their medication every day as prescribed to achieve maximum benefit. Patients should not alter the dose or discontinue therapy without consulting their physician. If a dose is missed, patients should take the next dose as soon as possible. However, the patient should not double the next dose.

Advise patients that saquinavir, like other protease inhibitors, is recommended for use in combination with active antiretroviral therapy. Greater activity has been observed when new antiretroviral therapies are begun at the same time as saquinavir. As with all protease inhibitors, adherence to the prescribed regimen is strongly recommended. Base concomitant therapy on a patient's prior drug exposure.

Advise patients of proper storage of *Fortovase* capsules. Refrigerated (2° to 8°C; 36° to 46°F) capsules of *Fortovase* remain stable until the expiration date printed on the label. Once brought to room temperature (≤ 25°C; 77°F), use capsules within 3 months.

Inform patients that redistribution or accumulation of body fat may occur in patients receiving protease inhibitors and that the cause and long-term health effects of these conditions are not known at this time.

RITONAVIR

| *Rx* | **Norvir** (Abbott) | **Capsules, soft gelatin:** 100 mg | Ethanol. (100 DS). White. In 120s. |
| | | **Oral solution:** 80 mg/mL | Saccharin, ethanol. Peppermint or caramel flavors. In 240 mL. |

WARNING

Coadministration of ritonavir with certain sedative hypnotics, antiarrhythmics, or ergot alkaloid preparations may result in potentially serious or life-threatening adverse events because of possible effects of ritonavir on the hepatic metabolism of certain drugs (see Contraindications and Drug Interactions).

Indications

▶*HIV infection:* In combination with other antiretroviral agents for the treatment of HIV infection.

Administration and Dosage

▶*Approved by the FDA:* March 6, 1996.

▶*Adults:* The recommended dosage is 600 mg twice daily. Use of a dose titration schedule may help to reduce treatment-emergent adverse events while maintaining appropriate ritonavir plasma levels. Start ritonavir at no less than 300 mg twice daily and increase at 2 to 3 days intervals by 100 mg twice daily. If saquinavir and ritonavir are used in combination, reduce the dosage of saquinavir by 400 mg twice daily. The optimum dosage of ritonavir (400 or 600 mg twice daily) in combination with saquinavir has not been determined; however, the combination regimen was better tolerated in patients who received ritonavir 400 mg twice daily.

▶*Children:* Use ritonavir in combination with other antiretroviral agents. The recommended dosage of ritonavir is 400 mg/m² twice daily by mouth and should not exceed 600 mg twice daily. Start ritonavir at 250 mg/m² and increase at 2- to 3-day intervals by 50 mg/m² twice daily. If patients do not tolerate 400 mg/m² twice daily because of adverse events, the highest tolerated dose may be used for maintenance therapy in combination with other antiretroviral agents; however, consider alternative therapy. When possible, administer dose using a calibrated dosing syringe.

Pediatric Dosage Guidelines

Body surface area[1] (m²)	Twice-daily dose 250 mg/m²	Twice-daily dose 300 mg/m²	Twice-daily dose 350 mg/m²	Twice-daily dose 400 mg/m²
0.25	0.8 mL (62.5 mg)	0.9 mL (75 mg)	1.1 mL (87.5 mg)	1.25 mL (100 mg)
0.5	1.6 mL (125 mg)	1.9 mL (150 mg)	2.2 mL (175 mg)	2.5 mL (200 mg)
1	3.1 mL (250 mg)	3.75 mL (300 mg)	4.4 mL (350 mg)	5 mL (400 mg)
1.25	3.9 mL (312.5 mg)	4.7 mL (375 mg)	5.5 mL (437.5 mg)	6.25 mL (500 mg)
1.5	4.7 mL (375 mg)	5.6 mL (450 mg)	6.6 mL (525 mg)	7.5 mL (600 mg)

[1] Body surface area can be calculated with the following equation:

$$\text{BSA (m}^2) = \sqrt{\frac{\text{ht (cm)} \times \text{wt (kg)}}{3600}}$$

▶*Dosing guidelines:* Alert patients that frequently observed adverse events, such as mild to moderate GI disturbances and paresthesias, may diminish as therapy is continued. In addition, patients initiating combination regimens with ritonavir and nucleosides may improve GI tolerance by initiating ritonavir alone and subsequently adding nucleosides before completing 2 weeks of ritonavir monotherapy.

If possible, take with food. Patients may improve the taste of ritonavir oral solution by mixing with chocolate milk, *Ensure,* or *Advera* within 1 hour of dosing. The effects of antacids on the absorption of ritonavir have not been studied.

▶*Storage/Stability:* Store capsules in a refrigerator between 2° and 8°C (36° and 46°F). Refrigeration of ritonavir capsules by the patient is recommended, but not required if used within 30 days and stored < 25°C (77°F). Protect from light and excessive heat.

Store ritonavir solution at room temperature 20° to 25°C (68° to 77°F). Do not refrigerate. Shake well before each use. Use by expiration date. Store and dispense in the original container. Avoid exposure to excessive heat. Keep cap tightly closed.

Actions

▶*Pharmacology:* Ritonavir is a peptidomimetic inhibitor of both the HIV-1 and HIV-2 proteases. Inhibition of HIV protease renders the enzyme incapable of processing the *gag-pol* polyprotein precursor, which leads to production of noninfectious immature HIV particles.

Among protease inhibitors, variable cross-resistance has been recognized. One ZDV-resistant HIV isolate tested in vitro retained full susceptibility to ritonavir. Serial HIV isolates obtained from 6 patients during ritonavir therapy showed a decrease in ritonavir susceptibility in vitro but did not demonstrate a concordant decrease in susceptibility to saquinavir in vitro when compared with matched baseline isolates. However, isolates from 2 of these patients demonstrated decreased susceptibility to indinavir in vitro (8-fold). Cross-resistance between ritonavir and reverse transcriptase inhibitors is unlikely because of the different enzyme targets involved.

▶*Pharmacokinetics:* After a 600 mg dose of oral solution, peak concentrations of ritonavir were achieved ≈ 2 and 4 hours after dosing under fasting and nonfasting (514 KCal: 9% fat, 12% protein and 79% carbohydrate) conditions, respectively. When the oral solution was given under nonfasting conditions, peak ritonavir concentrations decreased 23% and the extent of absorption decreased 7% relative to fasting conditions. Dilution of the oral solution within 1 hour of administration with 240 mL of chocolate milk, *Advera,* or *Ensure* did not significantly affect the extent and rate of ritonavir absorption. After a single 600 mg dose under nonfasting conditions in 2 separate studies, the capsule and oral solution formulations yielded mean areas under the plasma concentration-time curve (AUCs) of ≈ 121.7 and ≈ 129 mcg•hr/mL, respectively. Relative to fasting conditions, the extent of absorption of ritonavir from the capsule formulation was 13% higher when administered with a meal (615 KCal: 14.5% fat, 9% protein, and 76% carbohydrate).

Nearly all of the plasma radioactivity after a single oral 600 mg dose of ¹⁴C-ritonavir oral solution was attributed to unchanged ritonavir. Five ritonavir metabolites have been identified in urine and feces. The isopropylthiazole oxidation metabolite (M-2) is the major metabolite and has antiviral activity similar to that of the parent drug; however, the concentrations of this metabolite in plasma are low. Studies utilizing human liver microsomes have demonstrated that cytochrome P450 3A (CYP3A) is a major isoform involved in ritonavir metabolism, although CYP2D6 also contributes to the formation of M-2.

In a study of 5 subjects receiving a 600 mg dose of oral solution, ≈ 11.3% of the dose was excreted into the urine; ≈ 3.5% of the dose excreted was unchanged parent drug. In that study, ≈ 86.4% of the dose was excreted in the feces with ≈ 33.8% of the dose excreted as unchanged parent drug.

Ritonavir Pharmacokinetic Characteristics

Parameter	Values (mean)	Parameter	Values (mean)
C_{max} SS[1]	≈ 11.2 mcg/mL	CL/F[2]	≈ 4.6 L/hr
C_{trough} SS[1]	≈ 3.7 mcg/mL	CL_R	< 0.1 L/hr
V_β/F[2]	≈ 0.41 L/kg	RBC/Plasma ratio	0.14
CL/F SS[1]	≈ 8.8 L/h	Percent bound[3]	98% to 99%

[1] SS = Steady state; ritonavir doses of 600 mg q 12 hr.
[2] Single ritonavir 600 mg dose.
[3] Primarily bound to human serum albumin and alpha-1 acid glycoprotein over the ritonavir concentration range of 0.01 to 30 mcg/mL.

Special populations –

Children: The pharmacokinetic profile of ritonavir in pediatric patients < 2 years of age has not been established. Steady-state pharmacokinetics were evaluated in 37 HIV-infected patients ages 2 to 14 years receiving doses ranging from 250 mg/m² twice daily to 400 mg/m² twice daily. Across dose groups, ritonavir steady-state oral clearance (CL/F/m²) was ≈ 1.5 times faster in pediatric patients than in adult subjects. Ritonavir concentrations obtained after 350 to 400 mg/m² twice daily in pediatric patients were comparable to those obtained in adults receiving 600 mg (≈ 330 mg/m²) twice daily.

Contraindications

Hypersensitivity to the drug or any of its ingredients.

Do not administer ritonavir concurrently with any of the following listed drugs because competition for primarily CYP3A by ritonavir could result in inhibition of the metabolism of these drugs and create the potential for serious or life-threatening reactions such as cardiac arrhythmias, prolonged or increased sedation, and respiratory depression:

Postmarketing reports indicate that coadministration of ritonavir with ergotamine or dihydroergotamine has been associated with acute ergot toxicity characterized by peripheral vasospasm and ischemia of the extremities.

Drugs Contraindicated with Ritonavir[1]

Drug class	Drugs within class
Antiarrhythmics	Amiodarone, bepridil, flecainide, propafenone, quinidine
Antimigraines	Dihydroergotamine, ergotamine
Sedative/Hypnotics	Midazolam, triazolam
GI motility agents	Cisapride
Neuroleptics	Pimozide

[1] This list may not be all inclusive; see Drug Interactions for more information.

RITONAVIR

Warnings

Allergic reactions: Allergic reactions including urticaria, mild skin eruptions, bronchospasm, and angioedema have been reported. Rare cases of anaphylaxis and Stevens-Johnson syndrome also have been reported.

Pancreatitis: Pancreatitis has been observed in patients receiving ritonavir therapy, including those who developed hypertriglyceridemia. In some cases, fatalities have been observed. Patients with advanced HIV disease may be at increased risk of elevated triglycerides and pancreatitis.

Consider pancreatitis if clinical symptoms (eg, nausea, vomiting, abdominal pain) or abnormalities in laboratory values (such as increased serum lipase or amylase values) suggestive of pancreatitis occur. Evaluate patients who exhibit these signs or symptoms and discontinue ritonavir if a diagnosis of pancreatitis is made.

Diabetes mellitus/Hyperglycemia: New-onset diabetes mellitus, exacerbation of pre-existing diabetes mellitus, and hyperglycemia have been reported during postmarketing surveillance in HIV-infected patients receiving protease inhibitors. Some patients required either initiation or dose adjustments of insulin or oral hypoglycemic agents for treatment of these events. In some cases, diabetic ketoacidosis has occurred. In those patients who discontinued protease inhibitor therapy, hyperglycemia persisted in some cases. Because these events have been reported voluntarily during clinical practice, estimates of frequency cannot be made and a causal relationship between protease inhibitor therapy and these events has not been established.

Hepatic function impairment: Hepatic transaminase elevations exceeding 5 times the upper limit of normal, clinical hepatitis, and jaundice have occurred in patients receiving ritonavir alone or in combination with other antiretroviral drugs. There may be an increased risk for transaminase elevations in patients with underlying hepatitis B or C. Therefore, exercise caution when administering ritonavir to patients with pre-existing liver diseases, liver enzyme abnormalities, or hepatitis. Consider increased AST/ALT monitoring in these patients, especially during the first 3 months of ritonavir treatment.

There have been postmarketing reports of hepatic dysfunction, including some fatalities. These have generally occurred in patients taking multiple concomitant medications or with advanced AIDs.

Ritonavir is principally metabolized by the liver. Exercise caution when administering this drug to patients with impaired hepatic function.

Pregnancy: Category B. Developmental toxicity observed in rats (eg, early resorptions, decreased fetal body weight, ossification delays, developmental variations) occurred at a maternally toxic dosage at an exposure equivalent to ≈ 30% of that achieved with the proposed therapeutic dose. A slight increase in the rate of cryptorchidism was also noted in rats at an exposure ≈ 22% of that achieved with the proposed therapeutic dose. Developmental toxicity observed in rabbits (eg, resorptions, decreased litter size, decreased fetal weights) also occurred at a maternally toxic dosage equivalent to 1.8 times the proposed therapeutic dose.

There are no adequate and well-controlled studies in pregnant women. Use during pregnancy only if clearly needed.

Lactation: It is not known whether this drug is excreted in breast milk. Exercise caution when administering to a nursing woman. The US Public Health Service Centers for Disease Control and Prevention advises HIV-infected women not to breastfeed to avoid postnatal transmission of HIV to a child who may not be infected.

Children: The safety and pharmacokinetic profile of ritonavir in pediatric patients < 2 years of age has not been established. In HIV-infected patients 2 to 16 years of age, the adverse event profile seen during a clinical trial and postmarketing experience was similar to that for adult patients. The evaluation of the antiviral activity of ritonavir in pediatric patients in clinical trials is ongoing.

Precautions

Resistance/Cross-resistance: Varying degrees of cross-resistance among protease inhibitors have been observed. Continued administration of ritonavir therapy following loss of viral suppression may increase the likelihood of cross-resistance to other protease inhibitors.

Hemophilia: There have been reports of increased bleeding, including spontaneous skin hematomas and hemarthrosis, in patients with hemophilia type A and B treated with protease inhibitors. In some patients, additional factor VIII was given. In > 50% of the reported cases, treatment with protease inhibitors was continued and reintroduced. A causal relationship has not been established.

Fat redistribution: Redistribution/accumulation of body fat including central obesity, dorsocervical fat enlargement (buffalo hump), peripheral wasting, breast enlargement, and "cushingoid appearance" have been observed in patients receiving protease inhibitors. The mechanism and long-term consequences of these events are currently unknown. A causal relationship has not been established.

Lipid disorders: Treatment with ritonavir alone or in combination with saquinavir has resulted in substantial increases in the concentration of total triglycerides and cholesterol. Perform triglyceride and cholesterol testing prior to initiating ritonavir and at periodic intervals during therapy. Manage lipid disorders as clinically appropriate.

Lab test abnormalities: Ritonavir has been associated with alterations in triglycerides, AST, ALT, GGT, CPK, and uric acid. Perform appropriate laboratory testing prior to initiating ritonavir therapy and at periodic intervals or if any clinical signs and symptoms occur during therapy.

Drug Interactions

CYP450: Ritonavir has been found to be an inhibitor of cytochrome P450 3A (CYP3A) in vitro and in vivo. Agents that are extensively metabolized by CYP3A and have high first-pass metabolism appear to be the most susceptible to large increases in AUC (> 3-fold) when coadministered with ritonavir. Ritonavir also inhibits CYP2D6 to a lesser extent. Coadministration of substrates of CYP2D6 with ritonavir could result in increases (up to 2-fold) in the AUC of the other agent, possibly requiring a proportional dosage reduction. Ritonavir also appears to induce CYP3A as well as other enzymes, including glycuronosyl transferase, CYP1A2, possibly CYP2C9.

Ritonavir Drug Interactions			
Precipitant drug	Object drug*		Description
Azole antifungals	Ritonavir	↑	Plasma ritonavir concentrations may be elevated, increasing the risk of toxicity.
Clarithromycin	Ritonavir	↑	Coadministration for 4 days increased the ritonavir AUC by 12% and C_{max} by 15%, and the clarithromycin AUC increased by 77% and C_{max} by 31%.
Ritonavir	Clarithromycin	↑	
Didanosine	Ritonavir	↔	Coadministration for 4 days decreased the didanosine AUC by 13% and the C_{max} by 16%. Dosing of didanosine and ritonavir should be separated by 2.5 hours to avoid formulation incompatibility.
Ritonavir	Didanosine	↓	
Interleukins	Ritonavir	↑	Ritonavir concentrations may be elevated, increasing the risk of toxicity.
Rifamycins (eg, rifabutin, rifampin)	Ritonavir	↓	Rifamycins may decrease ritonavir serum concentrations.
St. John's Wort	Ritonavir	↓	Coadministration decreased the ritonavir AUC by 57% and the C_{max} by 28%.
Ritonavir	Antiarrhythmic agents (eg, amiodarone, bepridil, flecainide, encainide, propafenone)	↑	Increases in serum antiarrhythmic agent concentrations may occur, increasing risk of toxicity. Concurrent use of ritonavir with amiodarone, bepridil, flecainide, propafenone, or encainide is contraindicated.
Ritonavir	Benzodiazepines (eg, alprazolam, flurazepam, triazolam)	↑	Possibly severe sedation and respiratory depression may occur. Certain benzodiazepines are contraindicated in patients taking ritonavir.
Ritonavir	Bupropion	↑	Increased serum bupropion concentrations may occur, increasing bupropion toxicity. Ritonavir is contraindicated in patients taking bupropion.
Ritonavir	Clozapine	↑	Increases of serum concentrations may occur, possibly increasing clozapine toxicity.
Ritonavir	Desipramine	↑	Concurrent use increased the desipramine AUC by 145% and the C_{max} by 22%. Dosage reduction and concentration monitoring of desipramine is recommended.
Ritonavir	Disulfiram Metronidazole	↑	Ritonavir formulations contain alcohol, which can produce reactions when coadministered with disulfiram or other drugs that produce disulfiram-like reactions.
Ritonavir	Ergot alkaloids	↑	The risk of ergot toxicity may be increased. Coadministration is contraindicated.
Ritonavir	Ethinyl estradiol	↓	Coadministration decreased the ethinyl estradiol AUC by 40% and the C_{max} by 32%.

RITONAVIR

Ritonavir Drug Interactions			
Precipitant drug	Object drug*		Description
Ritonavir	Indinavir	↑	Indinavir plasma concentrations may be elevated, increasing the pharmacologic effect and adverse effects.
Ritonavir	Narcotic analgesics (eg, propoxyphene, methadone, fentanyl, meperidine)	↑↓	Plasma concentrations of propoxyphene and fentanyl may be increased, possibly causing toxicity. The pharmacologic effects of methadone may be decreased. Meperidine levels may decrease, possibly decreasing efficacy but increasing neurologic toxicity. Concurrent use of propoxyphene or meperidine is contraindicated.
Ritonavir	Piroxicam	↑	Large increases in serum piroxicam concentrations may occur, increasing piroxicam toxicity. Concomitant use is contraindicated.
Ritonavir	Quinidine	↑	Large increases in serum quinidine concentrations may occur, increasing the risk of quinidine toxicity. Concurrent use is contraindicated.
Ritonavir	Rifamycins (eg, rifabutin, rifampin)	↑	Ritonavir may elevate serum rifabutin concentrations, increasing the risk of hematologic toxicity of rifabutin. Decrease rifabutin dose by ≥ 75%.
Ritonavir	Saquinavir	↑	Ritonavir extensively inhibits the metabolism of saquinavir, resulting in increased saquinavir plasma concentrations.
Ritonavir	Sildenafil	↑	Elevated sildenafil plasma concentrations may occur, resulting in severe and potentially fatal hypotension.
Ritonavir	Theophylline	↓	Coadministration decreased the theophylline AUC by 43% and the C_{max} by 27%.
Ritonavir	Zolpidem	↑	Possibly severe sedation and respiratory depression may occur. Coadministration is contraindicated.

* ↑ = Object drug increased. ↓ = Object drug decreased. ↔ = Undetermined effect.

Drugs Contraindicated with Ritonavir[1]	
Drug class	Drugs within class
Antiarrhythmics	Amiodarone, bepridil, flecainide, propafenone, quinidine
Antimigraines	Dihydroergotamine, ergotamine
Sedative/Hypnotics	Midazolam, triazolam
GI motility agents	Cisapride
Neuroleptics	Pimozide

[1] This list may not be all inclusive; see Drug Interaction table for more information.

➤ *Predicted drug interactions:* Use with caution. Dose decrease of the following coadministered drugs may be needed.

Drugs in which Plasma Concentrations may be Increased by Coadministration with Ritonavir	
Drug class	Examples within drug class
Analgesics, narcotic	Tramadol, propoxyphene
Antiarrhythmics	Disopyramide, lidocaine, mexilitine
Anticonvulsants	Carbamazepine, clonazepam, ethosuximide
Antidepressants	Bupropion, nefazodone, SSRIs, tricyclics
Antiemetics	Dronabinol
Antiparasitics	Quinine
β-blockers	Metoprolol, timolol
Calcium channel blockers	Diltiazem, nifedipine, verapamil
Hypolipidemics, HMG-CoA reductase inhibitors[1]	Atorvastatin, cerivastatin, lovastatin, simvastatin
Immunosuppressants	Cyclosporine, tacrolimus
Neuroleptics	Perphenazine, risperidone, thioridazine
Sedative/Hypnotics	Clorazepate, diazepam, estazolam, flurazepam, zolpidem
Steroids	Dexamethasone, prednisone
Stimulants	Methamphetamine

[1] Coadministration with lovastatin and simvastatin is not recommended.

➤ *Predicted drug interactions:* Use with caution. Dose increase of following coadministered drugs may be necessary.

Drugs in which Plasma Concentrations may be Decreased by Coadministration with Ritonavir	
Drug class	Examples within drug class
Anticoagulants	Warfarin
Anticonvulsants	Phenytoin, divalproex, lamotrigine
Antiparasitics	Atovaquone

➤ *Postmarketing experience with drug interactions:* Cardiac and neurologic events have been reported when ritonavir has been coadministered with disopyramide, mexiletine, nefazodone, fluoxetine, and beta blockers. The possibility of drug interaction cannot be excluded.

➤ *Drug/Food interactions:* When the oral solution was given under nonfasting conditions, peak ritonavir concentrations decreased 23% and extent of absorption decreased 7% relative to fasting conditions. Extent of absorption of ritonavir from the capsule was 15% higher when given with a meal relative to fasting conditions. The manufacturer recommends taking ritonavir with meals, if possible.

Adverse Reactions

The most frequent clinical adverse events, other than asthenia, among patients receiving ritonavir were GI and neurological disturbances including nausea, diarrhea, vomiting, anorexia, abdominal pain, taste perversion, and circumoral and peripheral paresthesias.

Ritonavir Adverse Events (≥ 2%)[1]						
	Naive patients[2]			Advanced patients[3]		Protease inhibitor-naive patients[4]
Adverse reaction	Ritonavir + zidovudine (n = 116)	Ritonavir (n = 117)	Zidovudine (n = 119)	Ritonavir (n = 541)	Placebo (n = 545)	Ritonavir + saquinavir (n = 141)
Cardiovascular						
Syncope	0.9	1.7	0.8	0.6	0	2.1
Vasodilation	3.4	1.7	0.8	1.7	0	3.5
CNS						
Anxiety	0.9	0	0.8	1.7	0.9	2.1
Circumoral paresthesia	5.2	3.4	0	6.7	0.4	6.4
Confusion	0	0.9	0	0.6	0.6	2.1
Depression	1.7	1.7	2.5	1.7	0.7	7.1
Dizziness	5.2	2.6	3.4	3.9	1.1	8.5
Headache	7.8	6	6.7	6.5	5.7	4.3
Insomnia	3.4	2.6	0.8	2	1.8	2.8
Paresthesia	5.2	2.6	0	3	0.4	2.1
Peripheral paresthesia	0	6	0.8	5	1.1	5.7
Somnolence	2.6	2.6	0	2.4	0.2	0
Thinking abnormal	2.6	0	0.8	0.9	0.4	0.7
Dermatologic						
Rash	0.9	0	0.8	3.5	1.5	0.7
Sweating	3.4	2.6	1.7	1.7	1.1	2.8

RITONAVIR

Ritonavir Adverse Events (≥ 2%)[1]						
	Naive patients[2]			Advanced patients[3]		Protease inhibitor-naive patients[4]
Adverse reaction	Ritonavir + zidovudine (n = 116)	Ritonavir (n = 117)	Zidovudine (n = 119)	Ritonavir (n = 541)	Placebo (n = 545)	Ritonavir + saquinavir (n = 141)
GI						
Anorexia	8.6	1.7	4.2	7.8	4.2	4.3
Constipation	3.4	0	0.8	0.2	0.4	1.4
Diarrhea	25	15.4	2.5	23.3	7.9	22.7
Dyspepsia	2.6	0	1.7	5.9	1.5	0.7
Fecal incontinence	0	0	0	0	0	2.8
Flatulence	2.6	0.9	1.7	1.7	0.7	3.5
Local throat irritation	0.9	1.7	0.8	2.8	0.4	1.4
Nausea	46.6	25.6	26.1	29.8	8.4	18.4
Vomiting	23.3	13.7	12.6	17.4	4.4	7.1
Musculoskeletal						
Arthralgia	0	0	0	1.7	0.7	2.1
Myalgia	1.7	1.7	0.8	2.4	1.1	2.1
Miscellaneous						
Abdominal pain	5.2	6	5.9	8.3	5.1	2.1
Asthenia	28.4	10.3	11.8	15.3	6.4	16.3
Fever	1.7	0.9	1.7	5	2.4	0.7
Malaise	5.2	1.7	3.4	0.7	0.2	2.8
Nocturia	0	0	0	0.2	0	2.8
Pain (unspecified)	0.9	1.7	0.8	2.2	1.8	4.3
Pharyngitis	0.9	2.6	0	0.4	0.4	1.4
Taste perversion	17.2	11.1	8.4	7	2.2	5
Weight loss	0	0	0	2.4	1.7	0

[1] Includes those adverse events at least possibly related to study drug or of unknown relationship and excludes concurrent HIV conditions.
[2] The median duration of treatment for patients randomized to regimens containing ritonavir was 9.1 months.
[3] The median duration of treatment for patients randomized to regimens containing ritonavir was 9.4 months.
[4] The median duration of treatment for patients in the ongoing study was 48 weeks.

Laboratory Abnormalities with Ritonavir Therapy (> 3%)							
		Naive patients			Advanced patients		Protease inhibitor-naive patients
Variable	Limit	Ritonavir + zidovudine	Ritonavir	Zidovudine	Ritonavir	Placebo	Ritonavir + saquinavir
Chemistry values	High						
Cholesterol	(> 240 mg/dL)	30.7	44.8	9.3	36.5	8	65.2
CPK	(> 1000 IU/L)	9.6	12.1	11	9.1	6.3	9.9
GGT	(> 300 IU/L)	1.8	5.2	1.7	19.6	11.3	9.2
AST	(> 180 IU/L)	5.3	9.5	2.5	6.4	7	7.8
ALT	(> 215 IU/L)	5.3	7.8	3.4	8.5	4.4	9.2
Triglycerides	(> 800 mg/dL)	9.6	17.2	3.4	33.6	9.4	23.4
Triglycerides	(> 1500 mg/dL)	1.8	2.6	-	12.6	0.4	11.3
Triglycerides fasting	(>1500 mg/dL)	1.5	1.3	-	9.9	0.3	-
Uric acid	(> 12 mg/dL)	-	-	-	3.8	0.2	1.4
Hematology values	Low						
Hematocrit	(< 30%)	2.6	-	0.8	17.3	22	0.7
Hemoglobin	(< 8 g/dL)	0.9	-	-	3.8	3.9	-
Neutrophils	(≤ 0.5 × 10⁹/L)	-	-	-	6	8.3	-
RBC	(< 3 × 10¹²/L)	1.8	-	5.9	18.6	24.4	-
WBC	(< 2.5 × 10⁹/L)	-	0.9	6.8	36.9	59.4	3.5

[1] ULN = upper limit of the normal range.

⋅ Indicates no events reported.

➤*Cardiovascular:* Cardiovascular disorder, cerebral ischemia, cerebral venous thrombosis, hypertension, hypotension, migraine, MI, palpitation, peripheral vascular disorder, phlebitis, postural hypotension, tachycardia, vasospasm (< 2%).

➤*CNS:* Abnormal dreams, abnormal gait, agitation, amnesia, aphasia, ataxia, coma, convulsions, dementia, depersonalization, emotional lability, euphoria, grand mal convulsions, hallucinations, hyperesthesia, hyperkinesia, hypesthesia, incoordination, libido decreased, manic reaction, nervousness, neuralgia, neuropathy, paralysis, peripheral neuropathy, peripheral sensory neuropathy, peripheral neuropathic pain, personality disorder, sleep disorder, speech disorder, stupor, subdural hematoma, tremor, vertigo, vestibular disorder (< 2%).

➤*Dermatologic:* Acne, contact dermatitis, dry skin, eczema, erythema multiforme, exfoliative dermatitis, folliculitis, fungal dermatitis, furunculosis, maculopapular rash, molluscum contagiosum, onychomycosis, pruritus, psoriasis, pustular rash, seborrhea, skin discoloration, skin disorder, skin hypertrophy, skin melanoma, urticaria, vesiculobullous rash (< 2%).

➤*GI:* Abnormal stools, bloody diarrhea, cheilitis, cholestatic jaundice, colitis, dry mouth, dysphagia, eructation, esophageal ulcer, esophagitis, gastritis, gastroenteritis, GI disorder, GI hemorrhage, gingivitis, hepatic coma, hepatitis, hepatomegaly, hepatosplenomegaly, ileitis, liver damage, melena, mouth ulcer, pancreatitis, pseudomembranous colitis, rectal disorder, rectal hemorrhage, sialadenitis, stomatitis, tenesmus, thirst, tongue edema, ulcerative colitis (< 2%).

➤*GU:* Acute kidney failure, breast pain, cystitis, dysuria, hematuria, impotence, kidney calculus, kidney failure, kidney function abnormal, kidney pain, menorrhagia, penis disorder, polyuria, urethritis, urinary frequency, urinary retention, urinary tract infection, vaginitis (< 2%).

➤*Hematologic/Lymphatic:* Acute myeloblastic leukemia, anemia, ecchymosis, leukopenia, lymphadenopathy, lymphocytosis, myeloproliferative disorder, thrombocytopenia (< 2%).

➤*Metabolic/Nutritional:* Albuminuria, alcohol intolerance, avitaminosis, BUN increased, dehydration, diabetes mellitus, edema, enzymatic abnormality, facial edema, glycosuria, gout, hypercholesterolemia, peripheral edema, xanthomatosis (< 2%).

➤*Musculoskeletal:* Arthritis, arthrosis, bone disorder, bone pain, extraocular palsy, joint disorder, leg cramps, muscle cramps, muscle weakness, myositis, twitching (< 2%).

➤*Respiratory:* Asthma, bronchitis, dyspnea, epistaxis, hiccough, hypoventilation, increased cough, interstitial pneumonia, larynx edema, lung disorder, rhinitis, sinusitis (< 2%).

➤*Special senses:* Abnormal electro-oculogram, abnormal electroretinogram, abnormal vision, amblyopia/blurred vision, blepharitis, conjunctivitis, diplopia, ear pain, eye disorder, eye pain, hearing

RITONAVIR

impairment, increased cerumen, iritis, parosmia, photophobia, taste loss, tinnitus, uveitis, visual field defect, vitreous disorder (< 2%).

➤*Miscellaneous:* Abdomen enlarged, accidental injury, adrenal cortex insufficiency, allergic reaction, back pain, cachexia, chest pain, chills, facial pain, flu syndrome, hormone level altered, hypothermia, neck pain, neck rigidity, pelvic pain, photosensitivity reaction, substernal chest pain (< 2%).

Postmarketing – There have been postmarketing reports of seizure. Cause and effect relationship has not been established.

Dehydration, usually associated with GI symptoms and sometimes resulting in hypotension, syncope, or renal insufficiency has been reported. Syncope, orthostatic hypotension, and renal insufficiency have also been reported without known dehydration.

Redistribution/Accumulation of body fat has been reported. There have been reports of increased bleeding in patients with hemophilia A or B. (See Precautions.)

Overdosage

➤*Symptoms:* One patient in clinical trials took ritonavir 1500 mg/day for 2 days. The patient reported paresthesias that resolved after the dose was decreased.

The approximate lethal dose was found to be > 20 times the related human dose in rats and 10 times the related human dose in mice.

➤*Treatment:* Consists of general supportive measures including monitoring of vital signs and observation of the clinical status of the patient. If indicated, eliminate unabsorbed drug by emesis or gastric lavage; observe usual precautions to maintain the airway. Administration of activated charcoal also may be used to aid in the removal of unabsorbed drug. Ritonavir is extensively metabolized by the liver and is highly protein bound. Dialysis is unlikely to aid in removal of the drug.

Patient Information

A statement to patients and health care providers is included on the product's bottle label: Alert: Find out about medicines that should not be taken with ritonavir. A patient package insert for ritonavir is available.

Advise patients to take ritonavir with food.

Ritonavir is not a cure for HIV infection. Patients may continue to acquire illnesses associated with advanced HIV infection, including opportunistic infections.

Inform patients that redistribution or accumulation of body fat may occur in patients receiving protease inhibitors and that the cause and long-term health effects of these conditions are not known at this time.

Long-term effects are unknown at this time. Ritonavir has not been shown to reduce the risk of transmitting HIV through sexual contact or blood contamination.

Take ritonavir every day as prescribed. Do not alter the dose or discontinue ritonavir without consulting a doctor. If a dose is missed, take the next dose as soon as possible. However, if a dose is skipped, do not double the next dose.

Ritonavir interacts with some drugs when taken together. Report the use of any other medications, including prescription and nonprescription drugs or herbal products (particularly St. John's Wort), to a physician (see Drug Interactions).

The taste of ritonavir oral solution may be improved by mixing it with chocolate milk, *Ensure,* or *Advera* within 1 hour of dosing. If possible, take ritonavir with food.

INDINAVIR SULFATE

Rx	Crixivan (Merck)	Capsules: 100 mg[1]	Lactose. (CRIXIVAN 100 mg). White. In unit-of-use 180s.
		200 mg[1]	Lactose. (CRIXIVAN 200 mg). White. In unit-of-use 360s.
		333 mg[1]	Lactose. (CRIXIVAN 333 mg). White. In unit-of-use 135s.
		400 mg[1]	Lactose. (CRIXIVAN 400 mg). White. In unit dose 42s, and unit-of-use 18s, 90s, 120s, and 180s.

[1] Corresponding to 125, 250, 416.3, and 500 mg indinavir sulfate, respectively.

Indications

➤*HIV infection:* Treatment of HIV infection in combination with other antiretroviral agents.

Administration and Dosage

➤*Approved by the FDA:* March 13, 1995.

➤*Adults:* The recommended dosage is 800 mg (two 400 mg capsules) orally every 8 hours.

Administer at intervals of 8 hours. For optimal absorption, administer without food, but with water, 1 hour before or 2 hours after a meal or administer with other liquids such as skim milk, juice, coffee or tea, or with a light meal (eg, dry toast with jelly, juice, and coffee with skim milk and sugar; or corn flakes, skim milk, and sugar).

To ensure adequate hydration, it is recommended that adults drink ≥ 1.5 L (≈ 48 oz) of liquids during the course of 24 hours.

➤*Delavirdine:* Consider dose reduction of indinavir to 600 mg every 8 hours when administering delavirdine 400 mg 3 times/day.

➤*Didanosine:* If indinavir and didanosine are administered concomitantly, administer them ≥ 1 hour apart on an empty stomach.

➤*Efavirenz:* Dose increase of indinavir to 1000 mg every 8 hours is recommended when concurrently administering efavirenz.

➤*Itraconazole:* Dose reduction of indinavir to 600 mg every 8 hours is recommended when concurrently administering itraconazole 200 mg twice daily.

➤*Ketoconazole:* Dose reduction of indinavir to 600 mg every 8 hours is recommended when concurrently administering ketoconazole.

➤*Rifabutin:* Dose reduction of rifabutin to half the standard dose and a dose increase of indinavir to 1000 mg (three 333 mg capsules) every 8 hours are recommended when rifabutin and indinavir are coadministered.

➤*Cirrhosis:* Reduce the dosage of indinavir to 600 mg every 8 hours in patients with mild to moderate hepatic insufficiency caused by cirrhosis.

➤*Nephrolithiasis/Urolithiasis:* In addition to adequate hydration, medical management in patients who experience nephrolithiasis may include temporary interruption of therapy (eg, 1 to 3 days) or discontinuation of therapy.

➤*Storage/Stability:* Store in a tightly closed container at room temperature, 15° to 30°C (59° to 86°F). Protect from moisture. Indinavir capsules are sensitive to moisture. Dispense and store in the original container. Keep the desiccant in the original bottle.

Actions

➤*Pharmacology:* Indinavir is an inhibitor of the human immunodeficiency virus (HIV) protease. HIV protease is an enzyme required for the proteolytic cleavage of the viral polyprotein precursors into the individual functional proteins found in infectious HIV. Indinavir binds to the protease active site and inhibits the activity of the enzyme. This inhibition prevents cleavage of the viral polyproteins resulting in the formation of immature noninfectious viral particles. The relationship between in vitro susceptibility of HIV to indinavir and inhibition of HIV replication in humans has not been established.

Drug resistance – Isolates of HIV with reduced susceptibility to the drug have been recovered from some patients treated with indinavir. Viral resistance was correlated with the accumulation of mutations that resulted in the expression of amino acid substitutions in the viral protease. Eleven amino acid residue positions, at which substitutions are associated with resistance, have been identified. Resistance was mediated by the coexpression of multiple and variable substitutions at these positions. In general, higher levels of resistance were associated with the coexpression of greater numbers of substitutions.

Cross-resistance – Cross-resistance was noted between indinavir and the protease inhibitor ritonavir. Varying degrees of cross-resistance have been observed between indinavir and other HIV-protease inhibitors.

➤*Pharmacokinetics:*

Absorption – Indinavir was rapidly absorbed in the fasted state with a time to peak plasma concentration (T_{max}) of ≈ 0.8 hours. A greater than dose-proportional increase in indinavir plasma concentrations was observed over the 200 to 1000 mg dose range. At a dosing regimen of 800 mg every 8 hours, steady-state area under the plasma concentration-time curve (AUC) was ≈ 30,691 nM•hour, peak plasma concentration (C_{max}) was ≈ 12,617 nM and plasma concentration 8 hours postdose (trough) was ≈ 251 nM. High-calorie, fat, and protein meals decrease the AUC and C_{max} (see Drug Interactions).

Distribution – Indinavir was ≈ 60% bound to human plasma proteins over a concentration range of 81 to 16,300 nM.

Metabolism – Following a 400 mg dose of ^{14}C-indinavir, ≈ 83% and ≈ 19% of the total radioactivity was recovered in feces and urine, respectively; radioactivity due to parent drug in feces and urine was 19.1% and 9.4%, respectively. Seven metabolites have been identified, 1 glucuronide conjugate and 6 oxidative metabolites. In vitro studies indicate that cytochrome P450 3A4 (CYP3A4) is the major enzyme responsible for formation of the oxidative metabolites.

Excretion – Less than 20% of indinavir is excreted unchanged in the urine. Mean urinary excretion of unchanged drug was ≈ 10.4% and ≈ 12% following a single 700 and 1000 mg dose, respectively. Indinavir

INDINAVIR SULFATE

was rapidly eliminated with a half-life of ≈ 1.8 hours. Significant accumulation was not observed after multiple dosing at 800 mg every 8 hours.

Special populations –

Hepatic function impairment: Patients with mild to moderate hepatic insufficiency and clinical evidence of cirrhosis had evidence of decreased metabolism of indinavir resulting in ≈ 60% higher mean AUC following a single 400 mg dose. The half-life of indinavir increased to ≈ 2.8 hours. Indinavir pharmacokinetics have not been studied in patients with severe hepatic insufficiency.

➤*Clinical trials:* Study ACTG 320 was a multicenter, randomized, double-blind clinical endpoint trial to compare the effect of indinavir in combination with zidovudine and lamivudine with that of zidovudine plus lamivudine on the progression to an AIDS-defining illness (ADI) or death. Results are shown in the table below.

Results from Study ACTG 320		
	Number of patients with AIDS-defining illness or death (%)	
Endpoint	IDV + ZDV + L (n = 577)	ZDV + L (n = 579)
HIV progression or death	6.1	10.9
Death[1]	1.7	3.3

[1] The number of deaths is inadequate to assess the impact of indinavir on survival. IDV = indinavir, ZDV = zidovudine, L = lamivudine.

Study 028, a double-blind, multicenter, randomized, clinical endpoint trial compared the effects of indinavir plus zidovudine with those of indinavir alone or zidovudine alone on the progression to an ADI or death, and on surrogate marker responses. Results are shown in the table below.

Results from Study 028			
	Number of patients with AIDS-defining illness or death (%)		
Endpoint	IDV + ZDV (n = 332)	IDV (n = 332)	ZDV (n = 332)
HIV progression or death	6.3	8.1	18.7
Death[1]	2.4	1.5	3.3

[1] The number of deaths is inadequate to assess the impact of indinavir on survival. IDV = indinavir, ZDV = zidovudine.

Contraindications

Hypersensitivity to any component of the product.

➤*Concomitant agents:* Do not administer indinavir concurrently with cisapride, triazolam, midazolam, pimozide, or ergot derivatives. Inhibition of CYP3A4 by indinavir could result in elevated plasma concentrations of these drugs, potentially causing serious or life-threatening events.

Warnings

➤*Nephrolithiasis / Urolithiasis:* Nephrolithiasis/Urolithiasis has occurred with indinavir. The frequency of nephrolithiasis/urolithiasis is substantially higher in pediatric patients (29%) than in adult patients (9.3%). In some cases, nephrolithiasis/urolithiasis has been associated with renal insufficiency or acute renal failure. If signs or symptoms of nephrolithiasis/urolithiasis occur, (including flank pain, with or without hematuria or microscopic hematuria), temporary interruption (eg, 1 to 3 days) or discontinuation of therapy may be considered. Adequate hydration is recommended in all patients treated with indinavir (see Administration and Dosage). Of the patients treated with indinavir who developed nephrolithiasis/urolithiasis, 3.1% were reported to develop hydronephrosis and 3.1% underwent stent placement. Following the acute episode, 3.6% of patients discontinued therapy.

➤*Hemolytic anemia:* Acute hemolytic anemia, including cases resulting in death, has been reported in patients treated with indinavir. Once a diagnosis is apparent, institute appropriate measures for the treatment of hemolytic anemia, including discontinuation of indinavir.

➤*Hyperglycemia:* New-onset diabetes mellitus, exacerbation of preexisting diabetes mellitus, and hyperglycemia have been reported during postmarketing surveillance in HIV-infected patients receiving protease inhibitor therapy. Some patients required either initiation or dose adjustments of insulin or oral hypoglycemic agents for treatment of these events. In some cases, diabetic ketoacidosis has occurred. In those patients who discontinued protease inhibitor therapy, hyperglycemia persisted in some cases. Because these events have been reported voluntarily during clinical practice, estimates of frequency cannot be made and a causal relationship between protease inhibitor therapy and these events has not been established.

➤*Hepatic function impairment:* Hepatitis including cases resulting in hepatic failure and death has been reported in patients treated with indinavir. Because the majority of these patients had confounding medical conditions or were receiving concomitant therapy(ies), a causal relationship between indinavir and these events has not been established.

Patients with hepatic insufficiency because of cirrhosis should have the dosage of indinavir lowered because of decreased metabolism (see Administration and Dosage).

➤*Pregnancy: Category C.* Treatment-related increases over controls in the incidence of supernumerary ribs (at doses at or below those in humans) and of cervical ribs (at doses comparable to or slightly greater than those in humans) were seen in rats.

There are no adequate and well-controlled studies in pregnant women. Use during pregnancy only if the potential benefit justifies the potential risk to the fetus.

To monitor maternal fetal outcomes of pregnant women exposed to indinavir, an antiretroviral pregnancy registry has been established. Physicians are encouraged to register patients by calling (800) 258-4263.

➤*Lactation:* Studies in lactating rats have demonstrated that indinavir is excreted in milk. Although it is not known whether indinavir is excreted in human breast milk, there exists the potential for adverse effects from indinavir in nursing infants. Instruct mothers to discontinue nursing if they are receiving indinavir. This is consistent with the recommendation by the US Public Health Service Centers for Disease Control and Prevention that HIV-infected mothers not breastfeed their infants to avoid risking postnatal transmission of HIV.

➤*Children:* The optimal dosing regimen for use of indinavir in pediatric patients has not been established. A dose of 500 mg/m² every 8 hours has been studied in uncontrolled studies of 70 children, 3 to 18 years of age. The pharmacokinetic profiles of indinavir at this dose were not comparable to profiles previously observed in adults receiving the recommended dose. Although viral suppression was observed in some of the 32 children who were followed on this regimen through 24 weeks, a substantially higher rate of nephrolithiasis was reported when compared with adult historical data. Physicians considering the use of indinavir in pediatric patients without other protease inhibitor options should be aware of the limited data available in this population and the increased risk of nephrolithiasis.

Precautions

➤*Hyperbilirubinemia:* Indirect hyperbilirubinemia has occurred frequently during treatment with indinavir and has infrequently been associated with increases in serum transaminases. It is not known whether indinavir will exacerbate the physiologic hyperbilirubinemia seen in neonates.

Asymptomatic hyperbilirubinemia (total bilirubin ≥ 2.5 mg/dL), reported predominantly as elevated indirect bilirubin, has occurred in ≈ 14% of patients. In < 1%, this was associated with elevations in ALT or AST.

➤*Hemophilia:* There have been reports of spontaneous bleeding in patients with hemophilia A and B treated with protease inhibitors. In some patients, additional factor VIII was required. In many of the reported cases, treatment with protease inhibitors was continued or restarted. A causal relationship between protease inhibitor therapy and these episodes has not been established.

➤*Fat redistribution:* Redistribution/Accumulation of body fat including central obesity, dorsocervical fat enlargement (buffalo hump), peripheral wasting, breast enlargement, and "cushingoid appearance" have been observed in patients receiving protease inhibitors. The mechanism and long-term consequences of these events are currently unknown. A causal relationship has not been established.

Drug Interactions

Indinavir Drug Interactions			
Precipitant drug	Object drug*		Description
Azole antifungals	Indinavir	↑	Plasma indinavir concentrations may be elevated, increasing the risk of toxicity.
Didanosine	Indinavir	↓	The therapeutic effects of indinavir may be decreased.
Delavirdine	Indinavir	↑	Indinavir plasma concentrations may be elevated, increasing the pharmacologic and adverse effects.
Efavirenz	Indinavir	↓	Because of a decrease in the plasma concentrations of indinavir, a dosage increase of indinavir is recommended when indinavir and efavirenz are coadministered.
Interleukins	Indinavir	↑	Indinavir concentrations may be elevated, increasing the risk of toxicity.
Rifamycins (eg, rifabutin, rifampin)	Indinavir	↓	Rifamycins may decrease indinavir serum concentrations.
St. John's Wort	Indinavir	↓	Coadministration decreased the indinavir AUC by 57% and the C_{max} by 28%.

INDINAVIR SULFATE

Indinavir Drug Interactions			
Precipitant drug	Object drug*		Description
Indinavir	Amiodarone	↑	Increases in serum amiodarone concentrations may occur, increasing risk of toxicity. Concurrent use of indinavir with amiodarone is contraindicated.
Indinavir	Benzodiazepines (eg, alprazolam; flurazepam; triazolam)	↑	Possibly severe sedation and respiratory depression may occur. Certain benzodiazepines are contraindicated in patients taking indinavir.
Indinavir	Cisapride	↑	Increased cisapride plasma concentrations with cardiotoxicity may occur.
Indinavir	Ergot alkaloids	↑	The risk of ergot toxicity may be increased. Coadministratioin is contraindicated.
Indinavir	Fentanyl	↑	Plasma concentrations of fentanyl may be increased and the half-life prolonged, possibly causing toxicity.
Indinavir	Rifamycins (eg, rifabutin, rifampin)	↑	Indinavir may elevate serum rifabutin concentrations, increasing the risk of hematologic toxicity of rifabutin.
Indinavir	Ritonavir	↑	Ritonavir plasma concentrations may be elevated, increasing the pharmacologic effect and adverse effects.
Indinavir	Sildenafil	↑	Elevated sildenafil plasma concentrations may occur, resulting in severe and potentially fatal hypotension.

* ↑ = Object drug increased. ↓ = Object drug decreased.

➤ *Drug / Food interactions:* Administration of indinavir with a meal high in calories, fat, and protein (784 kcal, 48.6 g fat, 31.3 g protein) resulted in a ≈ 77% reduction in AUC and an ≈ 84% reduction in C_{max}. Administration with lighter meals (eg, a meal of dry toast with jelly, apple juice, and coffee with skim milk and sugar or a meal of corn flakes, skim milk, and sugar) resulted in little or no change in AUC, C_{max}, or trough concentration.

Adverse Reactions

Adverse Reactions: Indinavir vs Zidovudine (≥ 2%)			
Adverse reaction	Indinavir (n = 332)	Indinavir + zidovudine (n = 332)	Zidovudine (n = 332)
CNS			
Headache	5.4	9.6	6
Dizziness	3	3.9	0.9
Somnolence	2.4	3.3	3.3
Dermatologic			
Pruritus	4.2	2.4	1.8
Rash	1.2	0.6	2.4
GI			
Nausea	11.7	31.9	19.6
Abdominal pain	16.6	16	12
Diarrhea	3.3	3	2.4
Vomiting	8.4	17.8	9
Acid regurgitation	2.7	5.4	1.8
Anorexia	2.7	5.4	3
Dyspepsia	1.5	2.7	0.9
Jaundice	1.5	2.1	0.3
GU			
Nephrolithiasis/Urolithiasis[1]	8.7	7.8	2.1
Dysuria	1.5	2.4	0.3
Respiratory			
Cough	1.5	0.3	0.6
Difficulty breathing/Dyspnea/ Shortness of breath	0	0.6	0.3
Miscellaneous			
Appetite increase	2.1	1.5	1.2
Asthenia/Fatigue	2.1	4.2	3.6
Fever	1.5	1.5	2.1
Malaise	2.1	2.7	1.8
Taste perversion	2.7	8.4	1.2
Back pain	8.4	4.5	1.5
Anemia	0.6	1.2	2.1

[1] Including renal colic, and flank pain with and without hematuria.

Adverse Reactions: Indinavir, Zidovudine, and Lamivudine vs Zidovudine and Lamivudine (≥ 2%)		
Adverse reactions	Indinavir + zidovudine + lamivudine (n = 571)	Zidovudine + lamivudine (n = 575)
CNS		
Headache	2.4	2.8
Dizziness	0.5	0.7
Dermatologic		
Pruritus	0.5	0
Rash	1.1	0.5
GI		
Nausea	2.8	1.4
Diarrhea	0.9	1.2
Vomiting	1.4	1.4
Acid regurgitation	0.4	0
Anorexia	0.5	0.2
GU		
Nephrolithiasis/ Urolithiasis[1]	2.6	0.3
Dysuria	0.4	0.2
Respiratory		
Cough	1.6	1
Difficulty breathing/ Dyspnea/Shortness of breath	1.8	1
Miscellaneous		
Abdominal pain	1.9	0.7
Asthenia/Fatigue	2.4	4.5
Fever	3.8	3
Anemia	2.4	3.5
Back pain	0.9	0.7
Taste perversion	0.2	0

[1] Including renal colic, and flank pain with and without hematuria.

Indinavir vs Zidovudine: Selected Lab Test Abnormalities (%)			
Lab test abnormalities	Indinavir (n = 329)	Indinavir + zidovudine (n = 320)	Zidovudine (n = 330)
Hematology			
Decreased hemoglobin < 7 g/dL	0.6	0.9	3.3
Decreased platelet count < 50,000/mm³	0.9	0.9	1.8
Decreased neutrophil < 750/mm³	2.4	2.2	6.7
Blood chemistry			
Increased ALT >500% ULN[1]	4.9	4.1	3
Increased AST > 500% ULN	3.7	2.8	2.7
Total serum bilirubin > 250% ULN	11.9	9.7	0.6
Increased serum amylase> 200% ULN	2.1	1.9	1.8
Increased glucose > 250 mg/dL	0.9	0.9	0.6
Increased creatinine > 300% ULN	0	0	0.6

[1] Upper limit of the normal range.

Indinavir + Zidovudine + Lamivudine vs Zidovudine + Lamivudine: Selected Lab Test Abnormalities (%)		
Lab test abnormalities	Indinavir + zidovudine + lamivudine (n = 571)	Zidovudine + lamivudine (n = 575)
Hematology		
Decreased hemoglobin < 7 g/dL	2.4	3.5
Decreased platelet count < 50,000/mm³	0.2	0.9
Decreased neutrophils < 750/mm³	5.1	14.6
Blood chemistry		
Increased ALT > 500% ULN[1]	2.6	2.6
Increased AST > 500% ULN	3.3	2.8
Total serum bilirubin > 250% ULN	6.1	1.4
Increased serum amylase > 200% ULN	0.9	0.3

INDINAVIR SULFATE

Indinavir + Zidovudine + Lamivudine vs Zidovudine + Lamivudine: Selected Lab Test Abnormalities (%)		
Lab test abnormalities	Indinavir + zidovudine + lamivudine (n = 571)	Zidovudine + lamivudine (n = 575)
Increased glucose > 250 mg/dL	1.6	1.9
Increased creatinine > 300% ULN	0.2	0

[1] Upper limit of normal range.

➤*Postmarketing experience:*

Cardiovascular – MI; angina pectoris; cerebrovascular disorder.

CNS – Oral paresthesia; depression.

Dermatologic – Rash, including erythema multiforme and Stevens-Johnson syndrome; hyperpigmentation; alopecia; ingrown toenails or paronychia; pruritus.

GI – Liver function abnormalities; hepatitis, including reports of hepatic failure (see Warnings); pancreatitis; jaundice; abdominal distention; dyspepsia.

GU – Nephrolithiasis/Urolithiasis, in some cases resulting in renal insufficiency or acute renal failure (see Warnings); interstitial nephritis sometimes with indinavir crystal deposits; in some patients, the interstitial nephritis did not resolve following discontinuation of indinavir; crystalluria; dysuria.

Hematologic – Increased spontaneous bleeding in patients with hemophilia (see Precautions); acute hemolytic anemia (see Warnings).

Hypersensitivity – Anaphylactoid reactions; urticaria.

Lab test abnormalities – Increased serum triglycerides; increased serum cholesterol.

Metabolic/Nutritional – New onset diabetes mellitus, exacerbation of pre-existing diabetes mellitus, hyperglycemia (see Warnings).

Miscellaneous – Arthralgia; redistribution/accumulation of body fat (see Precautions).

Overdosage

There have been > 60 reports of acute or chronic human overdosage (up to 23 times the recommended total daily dose of 2400 mg) with indinavir. The most commonly reported symptoms were renal (eg, nephrolithiasis/urolithiasis, flank pain, hematuria) and GI (eg, nausea, vomiting, diarrhea).

It is not known whether indinavir is dialyzable by peritoneal or hemodialysis.

Patient Information

A statement to patients and health care providers is included on the product's bottle label. Alert: Find out about medicines that should not be taken with indinavir. A patient package insert for indinavir is available.

Indinavir is not a cure for HIV and patients may continue to develop opportunistic infections and other complications associated with HIV disease. Indinavir has not been shown to reduce the incidence or frequency of such illnesses. The long-term effects of indinavir are unknown. Indinavir has not been shown to reduce the risk of transmission of HIV to others through sexual contact or blood contamination.

Advise patients to remain under the care of a physician when using indinavir and not to modify or discontinue treatment without first consulting the physician. Therefore, if a dose is missed, patients should take the next dose at the regularly scheduled time and should not double this dose.

Indinavir may interact with some drugs; therefore, advise patients to report to their doctor the use of any other prescription, nonprescription medication, or herbal products, particularly St. John's wort.

For optimal absorption, administer indinavir without food, but with water, 1 hour before or 2 hours after a meal. Alternatively, administer with other liquids such as skim milk, juice, coffee or tea, or with a light meal (eg, dry toast with jelly, juice, and coffee with skim milk and sugar; or corn flakes, skim milk, and sugar). Ingestion of indinavir with a meal high in calories, fat, and protein reduces the absorption of indinavir.

Advise patients receiving sildenafil that they may be at an increased risk of sildenafil-associated adverse events including hypotension, visual changes, and priapism, and should promptly report any symptoms to their doctors.

Inform patients that redistribution or accumulation of body fat may occur in patients receiving protease inhibitors and that the cause and long-term health effects of these conditions are not known at this time.

Indinavir capsules are sensitive to moisture. Instruct patients to store indinavir in the original container and to keep the desiccant in the bottle.

NELFINAVIR MESYLATE

Rx	**Viracept** (Agouron)	**Tablets:** 250 mg (as base)	(Viracept 250 mg). Lt. blue, capsule shape. In 270s and 300s.
		625 mg (as base)	(V 625). White, oval. In 120s.
		Powder: 50 mg/g (as base)	Aspartame,[1] sucrose. In multiple-dose bottles containing 144 g powder with 1 g scoop.

[1] 11.2 mg/g phenylalanine

Indications

➤*HIV:* For the treatment of HIV infection in combination with other antiretroviral agents.

➤*Unlabeled uses:* Used as part of a 3-drug regimen for occupational HIV postexposure prophylaxis in cases where there is an increased risk for transmission; for HIV infection in neonates; twice daily dosing for HIV infection in children older than 6 years of age.

Administration and Dosage

➤*Approved by the FDA:* March 14, 1997.

Take with a meal. Patients unable to swallow the 250 or 625 mg tablets may dissolve the tablets in a small amount of water. Once dissolved, patients should mix the cloudy liquid well and consume it immediately. The glass should be rinsed with water and the rinse swallowed to ensure the entire dose is consumed.

➤*Adults:* The recommended dose is 1250 mg (five 250 mg tablets or two 625 mg tablets) twice daily or 750 mg (three 250 mg tablets) 3 times/day.

➤*Pediatric patients 2 to 13 years of age:* 20 to 30 mg/kg/dose, 3 times/day. Doses as high as 45 mg/kg every 8 hours have been used.

The recommended pediatric dose of nelfinavir to be administered 3 times/day is described in the following table:

Pediatric Dose of Nelfinavir to be Administered 3 Times/Day				
Body weight		Number of level 1 g scoops	Number of level teaspoons	Number of 250 mg tablets
kg	lbs			
7 to < 8.5	15.5 to < 18.5	4	1	-
8.5 to < 10.5	18.5 to < 23	5	1 ¼	-
10.5 to < 12	23 to < 26.5	6	1 ½	-

Pediatric Dose of Nelfinavir to be Administered 3 Times/Day				
Body weight		Number of level 1 g scoops	Number of level teaspoons	Number of 250 mg tablets
kg	lbs			
12 to < 14	26.5 to < 31	7	1 ¾	-
14 to < 16	31 to < 35	8	2	-
16 to < 18	35 to < 39.5	9	2 ¼	-
18 to < 23	39.5 to < 50.5	10	2 ½	2
≥ 23	≥ 50.5	15	3 ¾	3

Oral powder – The oral powder may be mixed with a small amount of water, milk, formula, soy formula, soy milk, or dietary supplement; once mixed, the entire contents must be consumed in order to obtain the full dose. Acidic food or juice (eg, orange juice, apple juice, apple sauce) are not recommended because of a bitter taste. Do not reconstitute with water in its original container.

➤*Storage/Stability:* Store tablets and powder at 15° to 30°C (59° to 86°F). Once mixed, the oral powder may be refrigerated for up to 6 hours. Keep container tightly closed. Dispense in original container.

Actions

➤*Pharmacology:* Nelfinavir is an inhibitor of the HIV-1 protease. Inhibition of the viral protease prevents cleavage of the gagpol polyprotein resulting in the production of immature, non-infectious virus.

The antiviral activity of nelfinavir in vitro has been demonstrated in acute and/or chronic HIV infections in lymphoblastoid cell lines, peripheral blood lymphocytes, and monocytes/macrophages. Nelfinavir was found to be active against several laboratory strains and clinical isolates of HIV-1 and the HIV-2 strain ROD. The EC_{95} (95% effective concentration) of nelfinavir ranged from 7 to 196 nM. Drug combination studies with protease inhibitors showed nelfinavir had antagonistic interactions with indinavir, additive interactions with ritonavir or saquinavir, and synergistic interactions with amprenavir and lopinavir.

NELFINAVIR MESYLATE

Minimal to no cellular cytotoxicity was observed with any of these protease inhibitors alone or in combination with nelfinavir. In combination with reverse transcriptase inhibitors, nelfinavir demonstrated additive (didanosine or stavudine) to synergistic (zidovudine, lamivudine, zalcitabine, abacavir, tenofovir, delavirdine, efavirenz, or nevirapine) antiviral activity in vitro without enhanced cytotoxicity.

Drug resistance – One or more virus protease mutations at amino acid positions 30, 35, 36, 46, 71, 77, and 88 were detected in greater than 10% of patients with evaluable isolates. The overall incidence of the D30N mutation in the viral protease of evaluable isolates (n = 157) from patients receiving nelfinavir monotherapy or nelfinavir in combination with zidovudine and lamivudine or stavudine was 54.8%. The overall incidence of other mutations associated with primary protease inhibitor resistance was 9.6% for the L90M substitution, whereas substitutions at 48, 82, or 84 were not observed. Nine isolates showed reduced susceptibility (5- to 93-fold) to nelfinavir in vitro and all 9 isolates possessed 1 or more mutations in the viral protease gene. Amino acid position 30 appeared to be the most frequent mutation site.

Cross-resistance – Patient-derived recombinant HIV isolates containing the D30N mutation (n = 4) and demonstrating high-level (more than 10-fold) nelfinavir-resistance remained susceptible (less than 2.5-fold resistance) to saquinavir, indinavir, lopinavir, and amprenavir in vitro. Patient-derived recombinant HIV isolates containing the L90M mutation (n = 8) demonstrated moderate to high-level resistance to nelfinavir and had varying levels of susceptibility to saquinavir, indinavir, lopinavir, and amprenavir in vitro. Most patient-derived recombinant isolates with phenotypic and genotypic evidence of reduced susceptibility (more than 2.5-fold) to lopinavir, amprenavir, saquinavir, and/or indinavir demonstrated high-level cross-resistance to nelfinavir in vitro. Mutations associated with resistance to other protease inhibitors (eg, G48V, V82A/F/T, I84V, L90M) appeared to confer high-level cross-resistance to nelfinavir. Following ritonavir therapy, 6 of 7 clinical isolates with decreased ritonavir susceptibility (8- to 113-fold) in vitro compared with baseline also exhibited decreased susceptibility to nelfinavir in vitro (5- to 40-fold).

➤*Pharmacokinetics:*

Absorption / Distribution – The pharmacokinetic parameters of nelfinavir are summarized in the table below.

Summary of Pharmacokinetic Data in HIV-Positive Patients with Multiple Dosing of 1250 mg BID for 28 days and 750 mg TID for 28 days[1]				
Regimen	AUC_{24} (mg•h/L)	C_{max} (mg/L)	C_{trough} morning (mg/L)	C_{trough} afternoon or evening (mg/L)
1250 mg BID	52.8	4	2.2	0.7
750 mg TID	43.6	3	1.4	1

[1] Data are expressed as the mean.

The apparent volume of distribution following oral administration of nelfinavir was 2 to 7 L/kg. Nelfinavir in serum is extensively protein-bound (more than 98%). In healthy volunteers receiving a single 1250 mg dose, the 625 mg tablet was not bioequivalent to the 250 mg tablet formulation. Under fasted conditions (n = 27), the AUC and C_{max} were 34% and 24% higher, respectively, for the 625 mg tablets. In a relative bioavailability assessment under fed conditions (n = 28), the AUC was 24% higher for the 625 mg tablet; the C_{max} was comparable for both formulations. In healthy volunteers receiving a single 750 mg dose under fed conditions, nelfinavir concentrations were similar following administration of the 250 mg tablet and oral powder.

Effect of food: Maximum plasma concentrations and area under the plasma concentration-time curve (AUC) were 2- to 3-fold higher under fed conditions compared with fasting.

Metabolism / Excretion – Unchanged nelfinavir comprised 82% to 86% of the total plasma radioactivity after a single oral 750 mg dose of ^{14}C-nelfinavir. In vitro, multiple cytochrome P450 enzymes including CYP3A and CYP2C19 are responsible for metabolism of nelfinavir. One major and several minor oxidative metabolites were found in plasma. The major oxidative metabolite has in vitro antiviral activity comparable with the parent drug. The terminal half-life in plasma was typically 3.5 to 5 hours. The majority (87%) of an oral 750 mg dose was recovered in the feces and consisted of numerous oxidative metabolites (78%) and unchanged nelfinavir (22%). Only 1% to 2% of the dose was recovered in the urine, of which unchanged nelfinavir was the major component.

➤*Clinical trials:* A randomized, double-blind study that evaluated the combination of nelfinavir 750 mg TID and/or efavirenz 600 mg qd with 2 NRTIs (either didanosine [ddI] + d4T, ddI + 3TC, or d4T + 3TC) in patients with prolonged prior nucleoside exposure. Mean baseline CD4 cell count was 389 cells/mm[3] and mean baseline plasma HIV RNA was 3.9 log_{10} copies/mL (7954 copies/mL).

The percent of patients with plasma HIV RNA of fewer than 500 copies/mL at 48 weeks was 42%, 62%, and 72% for the nelfinavir (n = 66), efavirenz (n = 65), and nelfinavir + efavirenz (n = 64) treatment groups, respectively. The 4-drug combination of nelfinavir + efavirenz +

2 NRTIs was more effective in suppressing plasma HIV RNA in these patients than either 3-drug regimen.

Contraindications

Hypersensitivity to any component of the product. Coadministration of nelfinavir is contraindicated with drugs that are highly dependent on CYP3A for clearance and for which elevated plasma concentrations are associated with serious and/or life-threatening events (eg, amiodarone, quinidine, ergot derivatives, pimozide, midazolam, triazolam, lovastatin, simvastatin; see Drug Interactions).

Warnings

➤*Diabetes mellitus / hyperglycemia:* New-onset diabetes mellitus, exacerbation of pre-existing diabetes mellitus and hyperglycemia have been reported during postmarketing surveillance in HIV-infected patients receiving protease inhibitor therapy. Some patients required either initiation or dose adjustments of insulin or oral hypoglycemic agents for treatment of these events. In some cases, diabetic ketoacidosis has occurred. In those patients who discontinued protease inhibitor therapy, hyperglycemia persisted in some cases. Because these events have been reported voluntarily during clinical practice, estimates of frequency cannot be made and a causal relationship between protease inhibitor therapy and these events has not been established.

➤*Phenylketonurics:* Nelfinavir oral powder contains 11.2 mg phenylalanine per g of powder.

➤*Renal function impairment:* Because less than 2% of nelfinavir is excreted in the urine, the impact of renal impairment on nelfinavir elimination should be minimal.

➤*Hepatic function impairment:* Nelfinavir is principally metabolized by the liver. Exercise caution when administering this drug to patients with hepatic impairment.

➤*Carcinogenesis:* Thyroid follicular cell adenomas and carcinomas were increased in male rats at 300 mg/kg/day and higher and in female rats at 1000 mg/kg/day. The systemic exposures (C_{max}) at 300 and 1000 mg/kg/day were 1- to 3-fold, respectively, of those measured in humans at the recommended therapeutic dose (750 mg TID or 1250 mg BID).

➤*Pregnancy: Category B.* There are no adequate and well-controlled studies in pregnant women. Use during pregnancy only if clearly needed.

To monitor maternal-fetal outcomes of pregnant women exposed to nelfinavir and other antiretroviral agents, an Antiretroviral Pregnancy Registry has been established. Physicians are encouraged to register patients by calling (800) 258-4263.

➤*Lactation:* The Centers for Disease Control and Prevention advises HIV-infected women not to breastfeed to avoid postnatal transmission of HIV to a child who may not yet be infected. Nelfinavir is excreted in the breast milk of rats. It is not known whether nelfinavir is excreted in human breast milk. Do not breastfeed if receiving nelfinavir.

➤*Children:* A similar adverse event profile was seen during the pediatric clinical trial as in adult patients. The evaluation of the antiviral activity of nelfinavir in pediatric patients is ongoing.

The safety, efficacy, and pharmacokinetics of nelfinavir have not been evaluated in children under 2 years of age (see Administration and Dosage).

Precautions

➤*Fat redistribution:* Redistribution/accumulation of body fat including central obesity, dorsocervical fat enlargement (buffalo hump), peripheral wasting, facial wasting, breast enlargement, and "cushingoid appearance" have been observed in patients receiving antiretroviral therapy. The mechanism and long-term consequences of these events are currently unknown. A causal relationship has not been established.

➤*Hemophilia:* There have been reports of increased bleeding, including spontaneous skin hematomas and hemarthrosis, in patients with hemophilia type A and B treated with protease inhibitors. In some patients, additional factor VIII was given. In more than half of the reported cases, treatment with protease inhibitors was continued or reintroduced. A causal relationship has not been established.

Drug Interactions

➤*CYP450:* Nelfinavir is an inhibitor of CYP3A (cytochrome P450 3A). Coadministration of nelfinavir and drugs primarily metabolized by CYP3A may result in increased plasma concentrations of the other drug, which could increase or prolong its therapeutic and adverse effects. Exercise caution when inhibitors of CYP3A, including nelfinavir, are coadministered with drugs that are metabolized by CYP3A and that prolong the QT interval. Nelfinavir is metabolized by CYP3A and CYP2C19. Coadministration of nelfinavir and drugs that induce CYP3A and CYP2C19 may decrease nelfinavir plasma concentrations and reduce its therapeutic effect. Coadministration of nelfinavir and drugs that inhibit CYP3A or CYP2C19 may increase nelfinavir plasma concentrations.

NELFINAVIR MESYLATE

Nelfinavir Drug Interactions			
Precipitant drug	Object drug[*]		Description
Anticonvulsants (ie, carbamazepine, phenobarbital)	Nelfinavir	↓	Concurrent use may decrease nelfinavir plasma concentrations.
Azithromycin	Nelfinavir	↓	Coadministration resulted in a decrease in the AUC and C_{max} of nelfinavir by 15% and 10%, respectively.
Nelfinavir	Azithromycin	↑	Coadministration resulted in an increase in the AUC of 112% and C_{max} of 136% of azithromycin. Dose adjustment is not recommended; closely monitor for liver enzyme abnormalities and hearing impairment.
Azole antifungals	Nelfinavir	↑	May inhibit the metabolism of protease inhibitors. Ketoconazole increased nelfinavir AUC and C_{max} by 35% and 25%, respectively. Monitor for protease inhibitor toxicity and adjust dose as needed.
Efavirenz Delavirdine	Nelfinavir	↑	Coadministration resulted in an increase in the AUC and C_{max} of nelfinavir, 107% and 88% with delavirdine, and 20% and 21% with efavirenz, respectively.
Nelfinavir	Efavirenz Delavirdine	↓	Coadministration caused a decrease in the AUC and C_{max} of efavirenz of 12% and 12%, respectively, and delavirdine of 31% and 27%, respectively.
Indinavir	Nelfinavir	↑	Coadministration resulted in an 83% increase in nelfinavir AUC and a 51% increase in indinavir AUC.
Nelfinavir	Indinavir		
Interleukins	Nelfinavir	↑	May inhibit protease inhibitor metabolism. May be necessary to adjust protease inhibitor dose.
Nevirapine	Nelfinavir	↓	Increased hepatic metabolism of the protease inhibitor is suspected. Monitor protease inhibitor blood levels and adjust dose as necessary.
Rifabutin	Nelfinavir	↓	Coadministration resulted in a 32% decrease in nelfinavir AUC and a 207% increase in rifabutin AUC. It is recommended that the dose of rifabutin be reduced to one half the usual dose when administered with nelfinavir.
Nelfinavir	Rifabutin	↑	
Rifampin	Nelfinavir	↓	Coadministration resulted in an 83% decrease in nelfinavir AUC. Do not coadminister nelfinavir with rifampin.
Ritonavir	Nelfinavir	↑	Coadministration resulted in a 152% increase in nelfinavir AUC and very little change in ritonavir AUC.
Saquinavir	Nelfinavir	↑	Coadministration resulted in an 18% increase in nelfinavir AUC and a 392% increase in saquinavir AUC. If used in combination, no dose adjustments are needed.
Nelfinavir	Saquinavir		
St. John's wort	Nelfinavir	↓	Increased metabolism of the protease inhibitor is suspected and may lead to loss of virologic response and possible resistance to nelfinavir. Avoid coadministration.
Nelfinavir	Didanosine	↔	It is recommended that didanosine be administered on an empty stomach; administer nelfinavir (with food) 1 hour after or > 2 hours before didanosine.
Nelfinavir	HMG-CoA reductase inhibitors (atorvastatin, lovastatin, simvastatin)	↑	Coadministration resulted in an increase in the C_{max} and AUC of simvastatin (517% and 505%) and atorvastatin (122% and 74%). Concomitant administration with nelfinavir is contraindicated due to potential for serious reactions such as risk of myopathy including rhabdomyolysis.

Nelfinavir Drug Interactions			
Precipitant drug	Object drug[*]		Description
Nelfinavir	Lamivudine	↑	Coadministration resulted in an increase in lamivudine's AUC and C_{max} by 10% and 31%, respectively.
Nelfinavir	Oral contraceptives	↓	Coadministration resulted in a 47% decrease in ethinyl estradiol and an 18% decrease in norethindrone plasma levels. Use alternate or additional contraceptive measures during nelfinavir therapy.
Nelfinavir	Phenytoin	↓	Coadministration resulted in a decrease in the AUC and C_{max} of phenytoin, 29% and 21%, respectively. Monitor phenytoin plasma levels and adjust dose as necessary.
Nelfinavir	Pimozide	↑	Coadministration is contraindicated due to potential for serious or life-threatening reactions such as cardiac arrhythmias.
Nelfinavir	Zidovudine	↓	Coadministration of zidovudine with nelfinavir resulted in a 35% decrease in zidovudine AUC.
Nelfinavir	Antiarrhythmics (amiodarone, quinidine)	↑	Protease inhibitors may inhibit the metabolism via cytochrome P450 3A4 isoenzyme. Coadministration with nelfinavir is contraindicated.
Nelfinavir	Benzodiazepines	↑	Possibly severe sedation and respiratory depression caused by the inhibition of the metabolism of benzodiazepines that undergo oxidation. Midazolam and triazolam are contraindicated in patients receiving nelfinavir.
Nelfinavir	Cisapride	↑	Protease inhibitors may inhibit the metabolism of cisapride via cytochrome P450 3A4 isoenzyme.
Nelfinavir	Ergot alkaloids	↑	Protease inhibitors may inhibit the metabolism of ergot alkaloids via cytochrome P450 3A4 isoenzyme. Coadministration with nelfinavir is contraindicated due to potential for serious or life-threatening reactions, such as acute ergot toxicity characterized by peripheral vasospasm and ischemia of the extremities and other tissues.
Nelfinavir	Fentanyl	↑	Possible inhibition of metabolism of fentanyl. Closely monitor respiratory function if coadministered. A reduction in the fentanyl dose may be necessary.
Nelfinavir	Methadone	↓	Increased metabolism of methadone is suspected. Coadministration resulted in a decrease of the AUC and C_{max} of methadone, 47% and 46%, respectively. Monitor for withdrawal symptoms and adjust dose as necessary.
Nelfinavir	Sildenafil	↑	Inhibition of sildenafil metabolism. Coadminister with extreme caution; sildenafil should not exceed a maximum single dose of 25 mg/48 hours when used concomitantly.
Nelfinavir	Tacrolimus Sirolimus	↑	Plasma concentrations of the immunosuppressants may be increased with concomitant administration. Carefully monitor renal function and immunosuppressant concentrations when starting, stopping, or changing the dose of a protease inhibitor and adjust the dose of the immunosuppressant as necessary.

[*] ↑ = Object drug increased. ↓ = Object drug decreased. ↔ = Undetermined clinical effect.

►*Drug/Food interactions:* Following coadministration with food, nelfinavir C_{max} and AUC were 2- to 3-fold higher compared with the fasting state.

Adverse Reactions

The most frequently reported adverse event among patients receiving nelfinavir was diarrhea, which was generally of mild to moderate intensity. The frequency of nelfinavir-associated diarrhea may be increased

NELFINAVIR MESYLATE

in patients receiving the 625 mg tablet because of the increased bioavailability of this formulation.

	Nelfinavir Adverse Reactions, Moderate or Severe Intensity[1]				
	Treatment up to 24 weeks			Treatment up to 48 weeks	
Adverse reaction	Placebo + ZDV[2]/3TC[3] (n = 101)	500 mg TID nelfinavir + ZDV[2]/3TC[3] (n = 97)	750 mg TID nelfinavir + ZDV[2]/3TC[3] (n = 100)	1250 mg BID nelfinavir + d4T[4]/3TC[3] (n = 344)	750 mg TID nelfinavir + d4T[4]/3TC[3] (n = 210)
GI					
Diarrhea	3%	14%	20%	20%	15%
Nausea	4%	3%	7%	3%	3%
Flatulence	0%	5%	2%	1%	1%
Hematologic abnormalities[5]					
Hemoglobin	6%	3%	2%	0%	0%
Neutrophils	4%	3%	5%	2%	1%
Lymphocytes	1%	6%	1%	1%	0%
Laboratory abnormalities[5]					
ALT	6%	1%	1%	2%	1%
AST	4%	1%	0%	2%	1%
Creatine kinase	7%	2%	2%	NA	NA
Miscellaneous					
Rash	1%	1%	3%	2%	1%

[1] Includes those adverse events at least possibly related to study drug or of unknown relationship and excludes concurrent HIV conditions.
[2] ZDV = Zidovudine.
[3] 3TC = Lamivudine.
[4] d4T = Stavudine.
[5] Marked laboratory abnormalities are defined as a shift from grade 0 at baseline to at least grade 3 or from grade 1 to grade 4.

Other adverse reactions occurring in less than 2% of patients include the following:

➤*CNS:* Anxiety; depression; dizziness; emotional lability; headache; hyperkinesia; insomnia; migraine; paresthesia; seizures; sleep disorder; somnolence; suicidal ideation.

➤*Dermatologic:* Dermatitis; folliculitis; fungal dermatitis; maculopapular rash; pruritus; sweating; urticaria.

➤*GI:* Abdominal pain; anorexia; dyspepsia; epigastric pain; GI bleeding; hepatitis; mouth ulceration; pancreatitis; vomiting.

➤*GU:* Kidney calculus; sexual dysfunction; urine abnormality.

➤*Hematologic/Lymphatic:* Anemia; leukopenia; thrombocytopenia.

➤*Metabolic/Nutritional:* Increases in alkaline phosphatase, amylase, creatine phosphokinase, lactic dehydrogenase, AST, ALT, gamma glutamyl transpeptidase; hyperlipidemia; hyperuricemia; hypoglycemia; dehydration; abnormal liver function tests ; hyperglycemia.

➤*Musculoskeletal:* Arthralgia; arthritis; cramps; myalgia; myasthenia; myopathy.

➤*Respiratory:* Dyspnea; pharyngitis; rhinitis; sinusitis.

➤*Special senses:* Acute iritis; eye disorder.

➤*Miscellaneous:* Accidental injury; allergic reaction; asthenia; back pain; fever; malaise; pain; redistribution/accumulation of body fat.

➤*Postmarketing:*

Cardiovascular – QT$_c$ prolongation; torsade de pointes.

Metabolic/Nutritional – Bilirubinemia; metabolic acidosis.

Miscellaneous – Hypersensitivity reactions (including bronchospasm, moderate to severe rash, fever, and edema); jaundice.

Overdosage

There is no specific antidote for overdose with nelfinavir. If indicated, eliminate unabsorbed drug by emesis or gastric lavage, or administer activated charcoal. Because nelfinavir is highly protein bound, dialysis is unlikely to be of benefit.

Patient Information

For optimal absorption, advise patients to take nelfinavir with food.

The most frequent adverse event associated with nelfinavir is diarrhea, which can usually be controlled with nonprescription drugs such as loperamide.

Instruct patients taking oral contraceptives to use alternate or additional contraceptive measures.

Inform patients that nelfinavir is not a cure for HIV infection and that they may continue to acquire illnesses associated with advanced HIV infection, including opportunistic infections.

Advise patients to take nelfinavir and other antiretroviral therapy every day as prescribed. Patients should not alter the dose or discontinue therapy without consulting their doctor. If a dose is missed, patients should take the dose as soon as possible and then return to their normal schedule. However, if a dose is skipped, the patient should not double the next dose.

Inform patients that there are currently no data demonstrating that nelfinavir therapy can reduce the risk of transmitting HIV to others through sexual contact or blood contamination.

Inform patients that redistribution or accumulation of body fat may occur in patients receiving antiretroviral therapy and that the cause and long-term health effects of these conditions are not known at this time.

Nelfinavir may interact with some drugs; therefore, advise patients to report to their doctor the use of any other prescription or nonprescription medication, or herbal products, particularly St. John's wort.

Advise patients receiving sildenafil and nelfinavir that they may be at an increased risk of sildenafil-associated adverse events, including hypotension, visual changes, and prolonged penile erection, and that they should report promptly any symptoms to their doctor.

Instruct patients not to breastfeed if they are receiving nelfinavir.

FOSAMPRENAVIR CALCIUM

Rx	**Lexiva** (GlaxoSmithKline)	**Tablets:** 700 mg (equivalent to 600 mg amprenavir)	(GX LL7). Pink, capsule shape. Film-coated. In 60s.

Indications

➤*HIV infection:* In combination with other antiretroviral agents for the treatment of human immunodeficiency virus (HIV) infection in adults.

Administration and Dosage

➤*Approved by the FDA:* October 21, 2003.

Fosamprenavir may be taken with or without food. Consult the full monograph for ritonavir when using this agent in combination with fosamprenavir.

➤*Therapy-naive patients:* The recommended oral dose of fosamprenavir alone or in combination with ritonavir is as follows: Fosamprenavir 1400 mg twice daily (without ritonavir); fosamprenavir 1400 mg once daily plus ritonavir 200 mg once daily; fosamprenavir 700 mg twice daily plus ritonavir 100 mg twice daily.

➤*Protease inhibitor (PI)-experienced patients:* The recommended oral dose is fosamprenavir 700 mg twice daily plus ritonavir 100 mg twice daily. Once-daily administration of fosamprenavir plus ritonavir is not recommended in PI-experienced patients.

➤*Adjustment of ritonavir dose when fosamprenavir plus ritonavir are administered with efavirenz:* An additional 100 mg/day (300 mg total) of ritonavir is recommended when efavirenz is administered with fosamprenavir plus ritonavir once daily.

➤*Hepatic function impairment:* Use fosamprenavir with caution, at a reduced dosage of 700 mg twice daily, in patients with mild or moderate hepatic impairment (Child-Pugh score ranging from 5 to 8) receiving fosamprenavir without concurrent ritonavir. Do not use fos-

FOSAMPRENAVIR CALCIUM

amprenavir in patients with severe hepatic impairment (Child-Pugh score ranging from 9 to 12) because the dose cannot be reduced below 700 mg. There are no data on the use of fosamprenavir in combination with ritonavir in patients with any degree of hepatic impairment.

►*Storage / Stability:* Store at controlled room temperature of 25°C (77°F); excursions permitted to 15° to 30°C (59° to 86°F). Keep container tightly closed.

Actions

►*Pharmacology:* Fosamprenavir is a prodrug of amprenavir, an inhibitor of HIV protease. Fosamprenavir is rapidly converted to amprenavir by cellular phosphatases in vivo. Amprenavir is an inhibitor of HIV-1 protease. Amprenavir binds to the active site of HIV-1 protease and thereby prevents the processing of viral Gag and Gag-Pol polyprotein precursors, resulting in the formation of immature noninfectious viral particles.

►*Pharmacokinetics:*

Absorption – Fosamprenavir is a prodrug that is rapidly hydrolyzed to amprenavir by enzymes in the gut epithelium as it is absorbed. After administration of a single dose of fosamprenavir to HIV-1-infected patients, the time to peak amprenavir concentration (T_{max}) occurred between 1.5 and 4 hours (median 2.5 hours). The absolute oral bioavailability of amprenavir after administration of fosamprenavir in humans has not been established.

Administration of a single 1400 mg dose of fosamprenavir in the fed state compared with the fasted state was associated with no significant changes in amprenavir C_{max}, T_{max}, or $AUC_{0-\infty}$.

The pharmacokinetic parameters of amprenavir after administration of fosamprenavir (with and without concomitant ritonavir) are shown in the table below.

Mean Steady-State Plasma Amprenavir Pharmacokinetic Parameters				
Regimen	C_{max} (mcg/mL)	T_{max} (hours)[1]	AUC_{24} (mcg•h/mL)	C_{min} (mcg/mL)
Fosamprenavir 1400 mg bid	4.82	1.3	33	0.35
Fosamprenavir 1400 mg qd plus ritonavir 200 mg qd	7.24	2.1	69.4	1.45
Fosamprenavir 700 mg bid plus ritonavir 100 mg bid	6.08	1.5	79.2	2.12

[1] Data shown are median (range).

Distribution – In vitro, amprenavir is approximately 90% bound to plasma proteins, primarily to alpha$_1$-acid glycoprotein. In vitro, concentration-dependent binding was observed over the concentration range of 1 to 10 mcg/mL, with decreased binding at higher concentrations. The partitioning of amprenavir into erythrocytes is low but increases as amprenavir concentrations increase, reflecting the higher amount of unbound drug at higher concentrations.

Metabolism – After oral administration, fosamprenavir is rapidly and almost completely hydrolyzed to amprenavir and inorganic phosphate prior to reaching the systemic circulation. This occurs in the gut epithelium during absorption. Amprenavir is metabolized in the liver by the cytochrome P450 3A4 (CYP3A4) enzyme system. The 2 major metabolites result from oxidation of the tetrahydrofuran and aniline moieties. Glucuronide conjugates of oxidized metabolites have been identified as minor metabolites in urine and feces.

Excretion – Excretion of unchanged amprenavir in urine and feces is minimal. Approximately 14% and 75% of an administered single dose of ^{14}C-amprenavir can be accounted for as metabolites in urine and feces, respectively. Two metabolites accounted for more than 90% of the radiocarbon in fecal samples. The plasma elimination half-life of amprenavir is approximately 7.7 hours.

Special populations –

Hepatic function impairment: The pharmacokinetics of amprenavir after administration of fosamprenavir have not been studied in patients with hepatic insufficiency. Based on amprenavir capsule data (see amprenavir monograph for further information), patients with impaired hepatic function receiving fosamprenavir without concurrent ritonavir may require dosage reduction. There are no data on the use of fosamprenavir in combination with ritonavir in patients with any degree of hepatic impairment (see Warnings and Administration and Dosage).

►*Microbiology:*

Antiviral activity in vitro – Fosamprenavir has little or no antiviral activity in vitro. The in vitro antiviral activity observed with fosamprenavir is not measurable because of trace amounts of amprenavir (see amprenavir monograph for further information).

Resistance – HIV-1 isolates with a decreased susceptibility to amprenavir have been selected in vitro and obtained from patients treated with fosamprenavir. Genotypic analysis of isolates from amprenavir-treated patients showed mutations in the HIV-1 protease gene, resulting in amino acid substitutions primarily at positions V32I, M46I/L, I47V, I50V, I54L/M, and I84V, as well as mutations in the p7/p1 and p1/p6 Gag and Gag-Pol polyprotein precursor cleavage sites. Some of

these amprenavir resistance-associated mutations also have been detected in HIV-1 isolates from antiretroviral-naive patients treated with fosamprenavir. Of the 488 antiretroviral-naive patients treated with fosamprenavir or fosamprenavir/ritonavir, 61 patients (29 receiving fosamprenavir and 32 receiving fosamprenavir/ritonavir) with virologic failure (plasma HIV-1 RNA greater than 1000 copies/mL on 2 occasions on or after week 12) were genotyped. Five of the 29 antiretroviral-naive patients (17%) receiving fosamprenavir without ritonavir had evidence of genotypic resistance to amprenavir: I54L/M (n = 2), I54L + L33F (n = 1), V32I + I47V (n = 1), and M46I + I47V (n = 1). No amprenavir-associated mutations were detected in antiretroviral-naive patients treated with fosamprenavir/ritonavir.

Cross-resistance – Varying degrees of cross-resistance among HIV-1 PI have been observed. An association between virologic response at 48 weeks (HIV-1 RNA level less than 400 copies/mL) and PI-resistance mutations detected in baseline HIV-1 isolates from PI-experienced patients receiving fosamprenavir/ritonavir twice daily (n = 88) or lopinavir/ritonavir twice daily (n = 85) in study APV30003 is shown in the table below. The majority of subjects had previously received either 1 (47%) or 2 (36%) PIs, most commonly nelfinavir (57%) and indinavir (53%). Of the 102 subjects with baseline phenotypes receiving twice-daily fosamprenavir/ritonavir, 54% (55) had resistance to at least 1 PI with 98% (54) of those having resistance to nelfinavir. Of 97 subjects with baseline phenotypes in the lopinavir/ritonavir arm, 60% (58) had resistance to at least 1 PI with 97% (56) of those having resistance to nelfinavir.

Responders at Week 48 by Presence of Baseline PI Resistance-Associated Mutations (%)[1]		
PI-mutations[2]	Fosamprenavir/ ritonavir bid (n = 88)	Lopinavir/ ritonavir bid (n = 85)
D30N	95	89
N88D/S	91	100
L90M	52	59
M46I/L	50	50
V82A/F/T/S	22	35
I54V	18	55
I84V	17	40

[1] Interpret results with caution because the subgroups were small.
[2] Most patients had more than 1 PI resistance-associated mutation at baseline.

The virologic response based upon baseline phenotype was assessed. Baseline isolates from PI-experienced patients responding to fosamprenavir/ritonavir twice daily had a median shift in susceptibility to amprenavir relative to a standard wild-type reference strain of 0.7 (range, 0.1 to 5.4, n = 62), and baseline isolates from individuals failing therapy had a median shift in susceptibility of 1.9 (range, 0.2 to 14, n = 29). Because this was a select patient population, these data do not constitute definitive clinical susceptibility break points. Additional data are needed to determine clinically relevant break points for fosamprenavir.

Isolates from 15 of the 20 patients receiving twice-daily fosamprenavir/ritonavir and experiencing virologic failure/ongoing replication were subjected to genotypic analysis. The following amprenavir resistance-associated mutations were found either alone or in combination: V32I, M46I/L, I47V, I50V, I54L/M, and I84V.

►*Clinical trials:*

Therapy-naive patients – APV30001 was a randomized, open-label study comparing treatment with fosamprenavir (1400 mg twice daily) vs nelfinavir (1250 mg twice daily) in 249 antiretroviral treatment-naive patients. Both groups of patients also received abacavir (300 mg twice daily) and lamivudine (150 mg twice daily). Through 48 weeks of therapy, 65% of patients in the fosamprenavir group and 52% in the nelfinavir group were responders (ie, patients achieved and maintained confirmed HIV-1 RNA less than 400 copies/mL). The median increases from baseline in CD4+ cell counts were 201 cells/mm^3 in the group receiving fosamprenavir and 216 cells/mm^3 in the nelfinavir group.

APV30002 was a randomized, open-label study comparing treatment with fosamprenavir (1400 mg once daily) plus ritonavir (200 mg once daily) vs nelfinavir (1250 mg twice daily) in 649 treatment-naive patients. Both treatment groups also received abacavir (300 mg twice daily) and lamivudine (150 mg twice daily). Through 48 weeks of therapy, 69% in the fosamprenavir/ritonavir group and 68% in the nelfinavir group responded to therapy (ie, patients achieved and maintained confirmed HIV-1 RNA less than 400 copies/mL). The median increases from baseline in CD4+ cell counts were 203 cells/mm^3 in the group receiving fosamprenavir and 207 cells/mm^3 in the nelfinavir group.

PI-experienced patients: APV30003 was a randomized, open-label, multicenter study comparing 2 different regimens of fosamprenavir plus ritonavir (fosamprenavir 700 mg twice daily plus ritonavir 100 mg twice daily or fosamprenavir 1400 mg once daily plus ritonavir 200 mg once daily) vs lopinavir/ritonavir (400 mg/100 mg twice daily) in 315 patients who had experienced virologic failure to 1 or 2 prior PI-containing regimens). The proportions of patients who achieved and

FOSAMPRENAVIR CALCIUM

maintained confirmed HIV-1 RNA less than 400 copies/mL (secondary efficacy endpoint) were 58% with twice-daily fosamprenavir/ritonavir and 61% with lopinavir/ritonavir. Through 48 weeks of therapy, the median increases from baseline in CD4+ cell counts were 81 cells/mm³ with twice-daily fosamprenavir/ritonavir and 91 cells/mm³ with lopinavir/ritonavir. This study was not large enough to reach a definitive conclusion that fosamprenavir/ritonavir and lopinavir/ritonavir are clinically equivalent. Once-daily administration of fosamprenavir plus ritonavir is not recommended for PI-experienced patients (see Administration and Dosage).

Contraindications

Previously demonstrated clinically significant hypersensitivity to any of the components of this product or to amprenavir; coadministration with dihydroergotamine, ergonovine, ergotamine, methylergonovine, cisapride, pimozide, midazolam, or triazolam.

If fosamprenavir is coadministered with ritonavir, the antiarrhythmic agents flecainide and propafenone also are contraindicated.

Warnings

➤*Drug interactions:* Serious and/or life-threatening drug interactions could occur between fosamprenavir and amiodarone, lidocaine (systemic), tricyclic antidepressants, and quinidine. Concentration monitoring of these agents is recommended if these agents are used concomitantly with fosamprenavir (see Contraindications and Drug Interactions).

➤*Skin reactions:* Severe or life-threatening skin reactions, including 1 case of Stevens-Johnson syndrome among 700 patients treated with fosamprenavir, were reported in less than 1% of patients treated with fosamprenavir in the clinical studies. Discontinue treatment with fosamprenavir for severe or life-threatening rashes and moderate rashes accompanied by systemic symptoms.

Skin rash (without regard to causality) occurred in approximately 19% of patients treated with fosamprenavir in the pivotal efficacy studies. Rashes usually were maculopapular and of mild or moderate intensity, some with pruritus. Rash had a median onset of 11 days after initiation of fosamprenavir and had a median duration of 13 days. Skin rash led to discontinuation of fosamprenavir in less than 1% of patients. In some patients with mild or moderate rash, dosing with fosamprenavir was often continued without interruption; if interrupted, reintroduction of fosamprenavir generally did not result in rash recurrence.

➤*Hemolytic anemia:* Acute hemolytic anemia has been reported in a patient treated with amprenavir.

➤*Diabetes mellitus/hyperglycemia:* New-onset diabetes mellitus, exacerbation of preexisting diabetes mellitus, and hyperglycemia have been reported during postmarketing surveillance in HIV-infected patients receiving PI therapy. Some patients required either initiation or dose adjustments of insulin or oral hypoglycemic agents for treatment of these events. In some cases, diabetic ketoacidosis has occurred. In those patients who discontinued PI therapy, hyperglycemia persisted in some cases. Because these events have been voluntarily reported during clinical practice, estimates of frequency cannot be made and causal relationships between PI therapy and these events have not been established.

➤*Hepatic function impairment:* Fosamprenavir is principally metabolized by the liver; therefore, exercise caution when administering fosamprenavir to patients with hepatic impairment because amprenavir concentrations may be increased (see Actions). Patients with impaired hepatic function receiving fosamprenavir without concurrent ritonavir may require dose reduction (see Administration and Dosage). There are no data on the use of fosamprenavir in combination with ritonavir in patients with any degree of hepatic impairment.

Patients with underlying hepatitis B or C or marked elevations in transaminases prior to treatment may be at increased risk for developing transaminase elevations. Conduct appropriate laboratory testing prior to initiating therapy with fosamprenavir and closely monitor patients during treatment.

➤*Carcinogenesis:* Carcinogenicity studies of fosamprenavir in rats and mice are in progress; however, results are available from carcinogenicity studies with amprenavir. Amprenavir was evaluated for carcinogenic potential by oral gavage administration to mice and rats for up to 104 weeks. Results showed an increase in the incidence of benign hepatocellular adenomas and an increase in the combined incidence of hepatocellular adenomas plus carcinoma in males of both species at the highest doses tested. Female mice and rats were not affected. These observations were made at systemic exposures equivalent to approximately 2 (mice) and 4 (rats) times the human exposure (based on $AUC_{0-24\,h}$ measurement) at the recommended dose of 1200 mg twice daily.

➤*Elderly:* In general, dose selection for an elderly patient should be cautious, reflecting the greater frequency of decreased hepatic, renal, or cardiac function, and of concomitant disease or other drug therapy.

➤*Pregnancy:* Category C. Administration of fosamprenavir to pregnant rats and rabbits produced no major effects on embryo-fetal development; however, the incidence of abortion was increased in rabbits. Systemic exposures ($AUC_{0-24\,h}$) to amprenavir at these dosages were

0.8 (rabbits) to 2 (rats) times the exposures in humans following administration of the maximum recommended human dose (MRHD) of fosamprenavir alone or 0.3 (rabbits) to 0.7 (rats) times the exposures in humans following administration of the MRHD of fosamprenavir in combination with ritonavir. In contrast, administration of amprenavir was associated with abortions and an increased incidence of minor skeletal variations resulting from deficient ossification of the femur, humerus, and trochlea in pregnant rabbits at the tested dose; approximately one-twentieth the exposure seen at the recommended human dose.

The mating and fertility of the F_1 generation born to female rats given fosamprenavir was not different from control animals; however, fosamprenavir did cause a reduction in both pup survival and body weights. Surviving F_1 female rats showed an increased time to successful mating, an increased length of gestation, a reduced number of uterine implantation sites per litter, and reduced gestational body weights compared with control animals. Systemic exposure ($AUC_{0-24\,h}$) to amprenavir in the F_0 pregnant rats was approximately 2 times higher than exposures in humans following the administration of the MRHD of fosamprenavir alone or approximately the same as those seen in humans following administration of the MRHD of fosamprenavir in combination with ritonavir.

There are no adequate and well-controlled studies in pregnant women. Use fosamprenavir during pregnancy only if the potential benefit justifies the potential risk to the fetus.

Antiretroviral pregnancy registry – To monitor maternal-fetal outcomes of pregnant women exposed to fosamprenavir, an Antiretroviral Pregnancy Registry has been established. Physicians are encouraged to register patients by calling 1-800-258-4263.

➤*Lactation:* The Centers for Disease Control and Prevention recommend that HIV-infected mothers not breastfeed their infants to avoid risking postnatal transmission of HIV. Although it is not known if amprenavir is excreted in human milk, amprenavir is secreted into the milk of lactating rats. Because of both the potential for HIV transmission and the potential for serious adverse reactions in nursing infants, instruct mothers not to breastfeed if they are receiving fosamprenavir.

➤*Children:* The safety and efficacy of fosamprenavir have not been established in pediatric patients.

Precautions

➤*Sulfa sensitivity:* Use fosamprenavir with caution in patients with a known sulfonamide allergy. Fosamprenavir contains a sulfonamide moiety. The potential for cross-sensitivity between drugs in the sulfonamide class and fosamprenavir is unknown. In a clinical study of fosamprenavir used as the sole PI, rash occurred in 2 of 10 patients (20%) with a history of sulfonamide allergy compared with 42 of 126 patients (33%) with no history of sulfonamide allergy. In 2 clinical studies of fosamprenavir plus low-dose ritonavir, rash occurred in 8 of 50 patients (16%) with a history of sulfonamide allergy compared with 50 of 412 patients (12%) with no history of sulfonamide allergy.

➤*Hemophilia:* There have been reports of spontaneous bleeding in patients with hemophilia A and B treated with PI. In some patients, additional factor VIII was required. In many of the reported cases, treatment with PI was continued or restarted. A causal relationship between PI therapy and these episodes has not been established.

➤*Opportunistic infections:* During the initial phase of treatment, patients responding to antiretroviral therapy may develop an inflammatory response to indolent or residual opportunistic infections such as *Mycobacterium avium* complex, cytomegalovirus, *Pneumocystis carinii*, and tuberculosis that may necessitate further evaluation and treatment.

➤*Fat redistribution:* Redistribution/accumulation of body fat including central obesity, dorsocervical fat enlargement (buffalo hump), peripheral wasting, facial wasting, breast enlargement, and "cushingoid appearance" have been observed in patients receiving antiretroviral therapy, including fosamprenavir. The mechanism and long-term consequences of these events are currently unknown. A causal relationship has not been established.

➤*Lipid elevations:* Treatment with fosamprenavir plus ritonavir has resulted in increases in the concentration of triglycerides. Perform triglyceride and cholesterol testing prior to initiating therapy with fosamprenavir and at periodic intervals during therapy. Manage lipid disorders as clinically appropriate.

➤*Resistance/Cross-resistance:* Because the potential for HIV cross-resistance among PI has not been fully explored, it is unknown what effect therapy with fosamprenavir will have on the activity of subsequently administered PI. Fosamprenavir has been studied in patients who have experienced treatment failure with PI.

Drug Interactions

Because amprenavir is the active metabolite of fosamprenavir, please refer to the amprenavir monograph for other possible drug interactions. Amprenavir is metabolized by CYP3A4 and is an inhibitor (and possibly an inducer) of CYP3A4. Coadministration of fosamprenavir and drugs that induce CYP3A4, such as rifampin, may decrease amprenavir concentrations and reduce its therapeutic effect. Coadministration

FOSAMPRENAVIR CALCIUM

of fosamprenavir and drugs that inhibit CYP3A4 may increase amprenavir concentrations and increase the incidence of adverse effects.

➤*CYP450 system:* The potential for drug interactions with fosamprenavir changes when fosamprenavir is coadministered with the potent CYP3A4 inhibitor ritonavir. Because ritonavir is a CYP2D6 inhibitor, clinically significant interactions with drugs metabolized by CYP2D6 are possible when coadministered with fosamprenavir plus ritonavir.

Fosamprenavir Drug Interactions

Precipitant drug	Object drug[*]		Description
Fosamprenavir	Amiodarone Lidocaine (systemic) Quinidine	↑	Coadminister with caution because of potential serious and/or life-threatening reactions. Monitor concentrations if available.
Fosamprenavir	Amitriptyline Imipramine	↑	Therapeutic concentration monitoring is recommended for the tricyclic antidepressants when coadministered.
Fosamprenavir	Benzodiazepines	↑	Coadministration with midazolam or triazolam is contraindicated because of serious and/or life-threatening reactions such as prolonged or increased sedation or respiratory depression. Alprazolam, clorazepate, diazepam, and flurazepam may have increased serum concentrations, which could increase their activity.
Fosamprenavir	Calcium channel blockers	↑	Concurrent use may increase bepridil concentrations, possibly causing life-threatening reactions such as cardiac arrhythmias. Use with caution. The concentrations of other calcium channel blockers may be increased when given with fosamprenavir.
Fosamprenavir	Cisapride Pimozide	↑	Coadministration is contraindicated because of potential for serious and/or life-threatening reactions such as cardiac arrhythmias.
Fosamprenavir	Contraceptives, oral	↓	Coadministration of fosamprenavir with ethinyl estradiol/norethindrone may alter the hormonal levels. Alternative nonhormonal methods of contraception are recommended.
Fosamprenavir	Cyclosporine Tacrolimus	↑	Therapeutic concentration monitoring of immunosuppressants is recommended with coadministration.
Fosamprenavir	Ergot derivatives	↑	Coadministration is contraindicated because of potential for serious and/or life-threatening reactions such as acute ergot toxicity (peripheral vasospasm and ischemia of the extremities and other tissues).
Fosamprenavir	HMG-CoA reductase inhibitors	↑	Fosamprenavir may increase serum concentrations of atorvastatin, lovastatin, and simvastatin, which could increase their toxicity such as myopathy including rhabdomyolysis. Avoid administration with lovastatin or simvastatin, use ≤ 20 mg/day of atorvastatin with careful monitoring, or use fluvastatin, pravastatin, or rosuvastatin.
HMG-CoA reductase inhibitors Atorvastatin	Fosamprenavir	↓	Administration of atorvastatin with fosamprenavir produced a decrease in amprenavir C_{max} and AUC.
Fosamprenavir	Ketoconazole Itraconazole	↑	Coadministration may lead to increase in ketoconazole or itraconazole adverse events. Dose reduction of ketoconazole or itraconazole may be necessary in patients who are receiving more than 400 mg/day of ketoconazole or itraconazole.
Fosamprenavir	Methadone	↓	Dosage of methadone may need to be increased with coadministration.

Fosamprenavir Drug Interactions

Precipitant drug	Object drug[*]		Description
Fosamprenavir	Rifabutin	↑	Monitor for neutropenia weekly when coadministered. When coadministered, a dosage reduction of rifabutin by at least half the usual dose is recommended. When coadministered with fosamprenavir plus ritonavir, a dosage reduction of rifabutin by at least 75% of the usual dose is recommended (max dose of 150 mg every other day or 3 times/week).
Fosamprenavir	Sildenafil Vardenafil	↑	Use with caution. When coadministered, decreased doses of sildenafil (25 mg every 48 hours) and vardenafil (2.5 mg every 24 hours) are recommended with increased monitoring for adverse events. When vardenafil is coadministered with fosamprenavir plus ritonavir, decrease vardenafil dose to no more than 2.5 mg every 72 hours.
Fosamprenavir	Warfarin	↔	Concentrations of warfarin may be affected. Monitor INR.
Fosamprenavir plus ritonavir	Flecainide Propafenone	↑	Coadministration may increase the plasma concentrations of the antiarrhythmics and cause serious and/or life-threatening reactions such as cardiac arrhythmias. Coadministration is contraindicated.
Antacids	Fosamprenavir	↓	Coadministration resulted in a decrease in the amprenavir C_{max} and AUC by 35% and 18%, respectively.
Efavirenz	Fosamprenavir with or without ritonavir	↓	Coadministration led to decreases in fosamprenavir concentrations. An additional 100 mg/day of ritonavir is recommended when efavirenz is administered with fosamprenavir plus ritonavir once daily. No change in dose is necessary when efavirenz is administered with fosamprenavir plus ritonavir twice daily.
Efavirenz plus ritonavir	Fosamprenavir plus ritonavir	↑	Coadministration led to increases in amprenavir C_{max} and AUC by 18% and 11%, respectively.
Indinavir Nelfinavir	Fosamprenavir	↑	Coadministration has led to increases in amprenavir concentrations.
Lopinavir plus ritonavir	Fosamprenavir plus ritonavir	↓	Coadministration decreased amprenavir C_{max} and AUC but increased lopinavir C_{max} and AUC.
Fosamprenavir plus ritonavir	Lopinavir plus ritonavir	↑	
Nevirapine Saquinavir	Fosamprenavir	↓	Coadministration has led to decreases in amprenavir concentrations.
Ranitidine	Fosamprenavir	↓	Coadministration led to decreases in amprenavir C_{max} and AUC by 51% and 30%, respectively.
Rifampin St. John's wort Delavirdine Carbamazepine Phenobarbital Phenytoin Dexamethasone Histamine H_2- receptor antagonists Proton pump inhibitors	Fosamprenavir	↓	Coadministration may result in loss of virologic response and possible resistance to fosamprenavir and/or other PI. Rifampin decreases plasma levels of amprenavir by approximately 90% after coadministration. Avoid administration with rifampin, St. John's wort, and delavirdine.

[*] ↑ = Object drug increased. ↓ = Object drug decreased. ↔ = Undetermined clinical effect.

Adverse Reactions

Fosamprenavir was studied in 700 patients in phase 3 controlled clinical studies. The most common treatment-emergent adverse events in clinical studies of fosamprenavir were diarrhea, nausea, vomiting, headache, and rash (see Warnings) and were generally mild to moderate in severity. Treatment discontinuation because of adverse events occurred in 6.4% of patients receiving fosamprenavir and in 5.9% of patients receiving comparator treatments.

Protease Inhibitors

FOSAMPRENAVIR CALCIUM

► *Antiretroviral-naive patients:*

Adverse Reactions in Antiretroviral-Naive Patients (%)							
	Fosamprenavir 1400 mg bid[1] (n = 166)		Nelfinavir 1250 mg bid[1] (n = 83)		Fosamprenavir 1400 mg qd/ ritonavir 200 mg qd[1] (n = 322)		Nelfinavir 1250 mg bid[1] (n = 327)
Adverse reaction	Moderate/severe drug-related	All grades[2]	Moderate/severe drug-related	All grades[2]	Moderate/severe drug-related	All grades[2]	Moderate/severe drug-related	All grades[2]
CNS								
Headache	2	19	4	20	3	21	3	27
Fatigue	2	10	1	7	4	18	2	13
Depressive/ mood disorders	1	8	0	8	< 1	8	0	6
Paresthesia, oral	0	2	0	0	< 1	10	0	< 1
Dermatologic								
Rash	8	35	2	19	3	17	2	21
Pruritus	0	7	0	11	< 1	7	1	9
GI								
Nausea	7	39	4	24	7	37	5	27
Diarrhea	5	34	18	63	10	52	18	72
Vomiting	2	16	4	17	6	20	4	13
Abdominal pain	1	5	0	8	2	11	2	11

[1] All patients also received abacavir and lamivudine twice daily.
[2] Includes adverse events of all grades regardless of causality reported in more than 5% of patients.

Laboratory abnormalities –

Grade 3/4 Laboratory Abnormalities Reported in ≥ 2% of Antiretroviral-Naive Adult Patients[1]				
Laboratory abnormality	Fosamprenavir 1400 mg bid[2] (n = 166)	Nelfinavir 1250 mg bid[2] (n = 83)	Fosamprenavir 1400 mg qd/ ritonavir 200 mg qd[2] (n = 322)	Nelfinavir 1250 mg bid[2] (n = 327)
Serum lipase (> 2 × ULN)	8	4	6	4
AST (> 5 × ULN)	6	6	6	7
ALT (> 5 × ULN)	6	5	8	8
Hypertriglyceridemia[3] (> 750 mg/dL)	0	1	6	2
Neutropenia (< 750 cells/mm³)	3	6	3	4

[1] The incidence of grade 3 or 4 hyperglycemia in antiretroviral-naive patients who received fosamprenavir in the pivotal studies was less than 1%.
[2] All patients also received abacavir and lamivudine twice daily.
[3] Fasting specimens.
ULN = Upper limit of normal.

► *Protease inhibitor-experienced patients:*

Fosamprenavir Adverse Reactions Reported in Protease Inhibitor-Experienced Patients (%)				
	Fosamprenavir 700 mg bid/ ritonavir 100 mg bid[1] (n = 106)		Lopinavir 400 mg bid/ ritonavir 100 mg bid[1] (n = 103)	
Adverse reaction	Moderate/severe drug-related	All grades[2]	Moderate/severe drug-related	All grades[2]
CNS				
Headache	4	27	2	20
Depressive/ mood disorders	< 1	11	< 1	10
Fatigue	< 1	9	< 1	14
Paresthesia, oral	0	< 1	0	0
Dermatologic				
Rash	3	9	0	22
Pruritus	< 1	8	0	3
GI				
Diarrhea	13	38	11	47
Nausea	3	20	9	31
Vomiting	3	10	5	17

Fosamprenavir Adverse Reactions Reported in Protease Inhibitor-Experienced Patients (%)				
	Fosamprenavir 700 mg bid/ ritonavir 100 mg bid[1] (n = 106)		Lopinavir 400 mg bid/ ritonavir 100 mg bid[1] (n = 103)	
Adverse reaction	Moderate/severe drug-related	All grades[2]	Moderate/severe drug-related	All grades[2]
Abdominal pain	< 1	11	2	9

[1] All patients also received 2 reverse transcriptase inhibitors.
[2] Includes adverse events of all grades regardless of causality reported in more than 5% of patients.

Laboratory abnormalities –

Grade 3/4 Laboratory Abnormalities Reported in ≥ 2% of Protease Inhibitor-Experienced Adult Patients		
Laboratory abnormality	Fosamprenavir 700 mg bid/ ritonavir 100 mg bid[1] (n = 104)	Lopinavir 400 mg bid/ ritonavir 100 mg bid[1] (n = 103)
Hypertriglyceridemia[2] (> 750 mg/dL)	11[3]	6[3]
Serum lipase (> 2 × ULN)	5	12
ALT (> 5 × ULN)	4	4
AST (> 5 × ULN)	4	2
Hyperglycemia (> 251 mg/dL)	2[3]	2[3]

[1] All patients also received 2 reverse transcriptase inhibitors.
[2] Fasting specimens.
[3] n = 100 for fosamprenavir/ritonavir, n = 98 for lopinavir/ritonavir.
ULN = Upper limit of normal.

Overdosage

There is no known antidote for fosamprenavir. It is not known whether amprenavir can be removed by peritoneal dialysis or hemodialysis. If overdosage occurs, monitor the patient for evidence of toxicity and apply standard supportive treatment as necessary.

Patient Information

A patient information sheet for fosamprenavir is available for patient information.

Inform patients that fosamprenavir is not a cure for HIV infection and that they may continue to develop opportunistic infections and other complications associated with HIV disease. The long-term effects of fosamprenavir are unknown at this time. Inform patients that there are currently no data demonstrating that therapy with fosamprenavir can reduce the risk of transmitting HIV to others.

Inform patients that sustained decreases in plasma HIV-1 RNA have been associated with a reduced risk of progression to AIDS and death. Advise patients to remain under the care of a physician while using fosamprenavir and to take fosamprenavir every day as prescribed. Fosamprenavir must always be used in combination with other antiretroviral drugs.

Instruct patients not to alter the dose or discontinue therapy without consulting their physician. If a dose is missed, advise patients to take the dose as soon as possible and then return to their normal schedule. However, if a dose is skipped, instruct patients not to double the next dose.

Advise patients to inform their health care provider if they have a sulfa allergy. The potential for cross-sensitivity between drugs in the sulfonamide class and fosamprenavir is unknown.

Fosamprenavir may interact with many drugs; therefore, advise patients to report to their health care provider the use of any other prescription or nonprescription medication or herbal products, particularly St. John's wort.

Advise patients receiving phosphodiesterase type 5 (PDE5) inhibitors that they may be at an increased risk of PDE5 inhibitor-associated adverse events, including hypotension, visual changes, and priapism, and to promptly report any symptoms to their health care provider.

Instruct patients receiving hormonal contraceptives to use alternative contraceptive measures during therapy with fosamprenavir because hormonal levels may be altered.

Inform patients that redistribution or accumulation of body fat may occur in patients receiving antiretroviral therapy, including fosamprenavir, and that the cause and long-term health effects of these conditions are not known at this time.

AMPRENAVIR

Rx	Agenerase (GlaxoSmithKline)	Capsules:	50 mg[1]	(GX CC1). Off-white to cream. Oblong. In 480s.
			150 mg[2],[3]	(GX CC2). Off-white to cream. Oblong. In 240s.
		Oral solution:	15 mg/mL[4],[5]	Grape/bubblegum/peppermint flavor. In 240 mL.

[1] With D-sorbitol, d-alpha tocopheryl polyethylene glycol 1000 succinate (TPGS), 19 mg propylene glycol.
[2] With D-sorbitol, TPGS, 57 mg propylene glycol.

[3] Contains 109 IU vitamin E (in the form of TPGS). The total amount of vitamin E in the recommended daily adult dose of amprenavir is 1744 IU.
[4] With acesulfame potassium, saccharin, 550 mg propylene glycol.
[5] Each mL of amprenavir oral solution contains 46 IU vitamin E in the form of TPGS.

WARNING

Because of the potential risk of toxicity from the large amount of the excipient propylene glycol, amprenavir oral solution is contraindicated in infants and children below 4 years of age, pregnant women, patients with hepatic or renal failure, and patients treated with disulfiram or metronidazole (see Contraindications and Warnings).

Use amprenavir oral solution only when amprenavir capsules or other protease inhibitor formulations are not therapeutic options.

Indications

►*HIV infection:* In combination with other antiretroviral agents for the treatment of HIV-1 infection.

Administration and Dosage

►*Approved by the FDA:* April 16, 1999.

Amprenavir may be taken with or without food; however, a high-fat meal decreases the absorption of amprenavir and should be avoided (see Drug Interactions). Advise adult and pediatric patients not to take supplemental vitamin E because the vitamin E content of amprenavir capsules and oral solution exceeds the Reference Daily Intake (adults, 30 IU; pediatrics, approximately 10 IU).

Amprenavir capsules and oral solution are not interchangeable on a milligram per milligram basis (see Pharmacokinetics).

►*Adults:* The recommended oral dose of amprenavir capsules for adults is 1200 mg (eight 150 mg capsules) twice daily in combination with other antiretroviral agents.

Concomitant therapy – If amprenavir and ritonavir are used in combination, the recommended dosage regimens are the following: Amprenavir 1200 mg with ritonavir 200 mg once daily or amprenavir 600 mg with ritonavir 100 mg twice daily.

►*Children:*

Capsules – For adolescents (13 to 16 years of age), the recommended dose is 1200 mg (eight 150 mg capsules) twice daily in combination with other antiretroviral agents. For patients between 4 and 12 years of age or for patients 13 to 16 years of age with weight of less than 50 kg, the recommended dose is 20 mg/kg twice daily or 15 mg/kg 3 times daily (to a maximum daily dose of 2400 mg) in combination with other antiretroviral agents.

Oral solution – Consider switching patients from amprenavir oral solution to capsules as soon as they are able to take the capsule formulation.

The recommended dose for patients between 4 and 12 years of age or for patients 13 to 16 years of age weighing less than 50 kg is 22.5 mg/kg (1.5 mL/kg) twice daily or 17 mg/kg (1.1 mL/kg) 3 times daily (to a maximum daily dose of 2800 mg) in combination with other antiretroviral agents. The recommended dose for patients between 13 and 16 years of age and weighing 50 kg or more or for patients older than 16 years of age is 1400 mg twice daily.

Concomitant therapy – Concomitant use of amprenavir oral solution and ritonavir oral solution is not recommended because the large amount of propylene glycol in amprenavir oral solution and ethanol in ritonavir oral solution may compete for the same metabolic pathway for elimination.

►*Hepatic function impairment:*

Capsules – Use with caution in patients with moderate or severe hepatic impairment. Patients with a Child-Pugh score ranging from 5 to 8 should receive a reduced dose of amprenavir capsules of 450 mg twice daily, and patients with a Child-Pugh score ranging from 9 to 12 should receive a reduced dose of amprenavir capsules of 300 mg twice daily.

Oral solution – Amprenavir oral solution is contraindicated in patients with hepatic failure (see Contraindications). Patients with hepatic impairment are at increased risk of propylene glycol-associated adverse events (see Warnings). Use amprenavir oral solution with caution in patients with hepatic impairment. Based on a study with amprenavir capsules, adult patients with a Child-Pugh score ranging from 5 to 8 should receive a reduced dose of amprenavir oral solution of 513 mg (34 mL) twice daily, and adult patients with a Child-Pugh score ranging from 9 to 12 should receive a reduced dose of amprenavir oral solution of 342 mg (23 mL) twice daily.

►*Renal function impairment:* Amprenavir oral solution is contraindicated in patients with renal failure (see Contraindications).

►*Storage/Stability:* Store at controlled room temperature of 25°C (77°F).

Actions

►*Pharmacology:* Amprenavir is an inhibitor of human immunodeficiency virus (HIV)-1 protease. Amprenavir binds to the active site of HIV-1 protease and thereby prevents the processing of viral gag and gag-pol polyprotein precursors, resulting in the formation of immature noninfectious viral particles.

►*Pharmacokinetics:*

Absorption – Amprenavir was rapidly absorbed after oral administration in HIV-1-infected patients with a time to peak concentration (T_{max}) typically between 1 and 2 hours after a single oral dose.

Increases in the area under the plasma concentration vs time curve (AUC) after single oral doses between 150 and 1200 mg were slightly greater than dose-proportional. Increases in AUC were dose-proportional after 3 weeks of amprenavir therapy with doses from 300 to 1200 mg twice daily. The pharmacokinetic parameters after administration of amprenavir 1200 mg twice daily for 3 weeks to HIV-infected subjects are shown in the following table.

Average Pharmacokinetic Parameters after Amprenavir Capsules 1200 mg Twice Daily (n = 54)					
C_{max} (mcg/mL)	T_{max} (h)	AUC_{0-12} (mcg•h/mL)	C_{avg} (mcg/mL)	C_{min} (mcg/mL)	CL/F (mL/min/kg)
7.66	1	17.7	1.48	0.32	19.5

Amprenavir oral solution was 14% less bioavailable compared with the capsules. Administration of a single 1200 mg dose in the fed state (standardized high-fat meal) compared with the fasted state was associated with changes in C_{max}, T_{max}, and AUC (see Drug Interactions).

Distribution – The apparent volume of distribution is approximately 430 L in healthy adult subjects. In vitro binding is approximately 90% to plasma proteins. The high affinity binding protein for amprenavir is alpha$_1$-acid glycoprotein (AAG). The partitioning of amprenavir into erythrocytes is low but increases as amprenavir concentrations increase, reflecting the higher amount of unbound drug at higher concentrations.

Metabolism – Amprenavir is metabolized in the liver by the cytochrome CYP3A4 enzyme system. The 2 major metabolites result from oxidation of the tetrahydrofuran and aniline moieties. Glucuronide conjugates of oxidized metabolites have been identified as minor metabolites in urine and feces.

Amprenavir oral solution contains a large amount of propylene glycol, which is hepatically metabolized by the alcohol and aldehyde dehydrogenase enzyme pathway. Alcohol dehydrogenase (ADH) is present in the human fetal liver at 2 months of gestational age, but its activity is only 3% that of adults. Although the data are limited, it appears that by 12 to 30 months of postnatal age, ADH activity is equal to or greater than that observed in adults. Additionally, certain patient groups (females, Asians, Eskimos, Native Americans) may be at increased risk of propylene glycol-associated adverse events because of diminished ability to metabolize propylene glycol.

Excretion – Excretion of unchanged amprenavir in urine and feces is minimal. Approximately 14% and 75% of an administered single dose of ^{14}C-amprenavir can be accounted for as radiocarbon in urine and feces, respectively. Two metabolites accounted for more than 90% of the radiocarbon in fecal samples. The plasma elimination half-life of amprenavir ranged from 7.1 to 10.6 hours.

Special populations –

Children: The pharmacokinetics of amprenavir have been studied after single or repeat doses of amprenavir in 84 pediatric patients. Twenty HIV-1-infected children ranging from 4 to 12 years of age received single doses of 5 to 20 mg/kg using 25 or 150 mg capsules. The C_{max} of amprenavir increased less than proportionally with dose. The $AUC_{0-\infty}$ increased proportionally at doses between 5 and 20 mg/kg. Amprenavir is 14% less bioavailable from the liquid formulation than from the capsules; therefore, amprenavir capsules and oral solution are not interchangeable on a mg per mg basis.

AMPRENAVIR

Average Pharmacokinetic Parameters in Children 4 to 12 Years of Age Receiving 20 mg/kg Twice Daily or 15 mg/kg 3 Times Daily of Amprenavir Oral Solution

Dose	n	C_{max} (mcg/mL)	T_{max} (h)	AUC_{ss}[1] (mcg•h/mL)	C_{avg} (mcg/mL)	C_{min} (mcg/mL)	CL/F (mL/min/kg)
20 mg/kg bid	20	6.77	1.1	15.46	1.29	0.24	29
15 mg/kg tid	17	3.99	1.4	8.73	1.09	0.27	32

[1] AUC is 0 to 12 hours for twice daily and 0 to 8 hours for 3 times daily; therefore, the C_{avg} is a better comparison of the exposures.

Hepatic function impairment: Amprenavir capsules have been studied in adult patients with impaired hepatic function using a single 600 mg oral dose. The $AUC_{0-\infty}$ was significantly greater in patients with moderate cirrhosis (25.76 ± 14.68 mcg•h/mL) compared with healthy volunteers (12 ± 4.38 mcg•h/mL). The $AUC_{0-\infty}$ and C_{max} were significantly greater in patients with severe cirrhosis ($AUC_{0-\infty}$, 38.66 ± 16.08 mcg•h/mL; C_{max}, 9.43 ± 2.61 mcg/mL) compared with healthy volunteers ($AUC_{0-\infty}$, 12 ± 4.38 mcg•h/mL; C_{max}, 4.9 ± 1.39 mcg/mL).

➤*Microbiology:*

Antiviral activity in vitro – The in vitro antiviral activity of amprenavir was evaluated against HIV-1 IIIB in both acutely and chronically infected lymphoblastic cell lines and in peripheral blood lymphocytes. The 50% inhibitory concentration of amprenavir ranged from 0.012 to 0.08 mcM in acutely infected cells and was 0.41 mcM in chronically infected cells (1 mcM = 0.5 mcg/mL). Amprenavir exhibited synergistic anti-HIV-1 activity in combination with abacavir, zidovudine, didanosine, or saquinavir, and additive anti-HIV-1 activity in combination with indinavir, nelfinavir, and ritonavir in vitro. These drug combinations have not been adequately studied in humans. The relationship between in vitro anti-HIV-1 activity of amprenavir and the inhibition of HIV-1 replication in humans has not been defined.

Resistance – HIV-1 isolates with a decreased susceptibility to amprenavir have been selected in vitro and obtained from patients treated with amprenavir. Phenotypic analysis of HIV-1 isolates from 21 nucleoside reverse transcriptase inhibitor- (NRTI-) experienced, protease inhibitor-naive patients treated with amprenavir in combination with NRTIs for 16 to 48 weeks identified isolates from 15 patients that exhibited a 4- to 17-fold decrease in susceptibility to amprenavir in vitro compared with wild-type virus. Clinical isolates that exhibited a decrease in amprenavir susceptibility harbored 1 or more amprenavir-associated mutations. The clinical relevance of the genotypic and phenotypic changes associated with amprenavir therapy is under evaluation.

Cross-resistance – Varying degrees of HIV-1 cross-resistance among protease inhibitors have been observed. Five of 15 amprenavir-resistant isolates exhibited 4- to 8-fold decrease in susceptibility to ritonavir. However, amprenavir-resistant isolates were susceptible to either indinavir or saquinavir.

➤*Clinical trials:* A randomized, open-label multicenter study compared treatment with amprenavir capsule (1200 mg twice daily) plus NRTIs vs indinavir (800 mg every 8 hours) plus NRTIs in 504 NRTI-experienced, protease inhibitor-naive patients, median age 37 years of age (range, 20 to 71 years of age), 72% Caucasian, 80% male, with a median CD4 cell count of 404 cells/mm³ (range, 9 to 1706 cells/mm³) and a median plasma HIV-1 RNA level of 3.93 $\log_{10}$ copies/mL (range, 2.6 to 7.01 $\log_{10}$ copies/mL) at baseline. Through 48 weeks of therapy, the median CD4 cell count increase from baseline in the amprenavir group was significantly lower than in the indinavir group, 97 cells/mm³ vs 144 cells/mm³, respectively. There also was a significant difference in the proportions of patients with plasma HIV-1 RNA levels less than 400 copies/mL through 48 weeks.

Amprenavir Capsules vs Indinavir: Outcomes of Randomized Treatment Through Week 48 (%)

Outcome	Amprenavir capsules (n = 254)	Indinavir (n = 250)
HIV-1 RNA < 400 copies/mL[2]	30	49
HIV-1 RNA ≥ 400 copies/mL[1],[2]	38	26
Discontinued because of adverse events[2]	16	12
Discontinued because of other reasons[2],[3]	16	13

[1] Virological failures at or before week 48.
[2] Considered to be treatment failure in the analysis.
[3] Includes discontinuations because of consent withdrawal, loss to follow-up, protocol violations, noncompliance, pregnancy, never treated, and other reasons.

Contraindications

Concurrent use with cisapride, dihydroergotamine, ergotamine, ergonovine, methylergonovine, pimozide, midazolam, and triazolam. Coadministration of amprenavir is contraindicated with drugs that are highly dependent on CYP3A4 for clearance and for which elevated plasma concentrations are associated with serious and/or life-threatening events.

If amprenavir is coadministered with ritonavir, the antiarrhythmic agents flecainide and propafenone also are contraindicated.

Hypersensitivity to any of the components of this product.

➤*Oral solution:* Because of the potential risk of toxicity from the large amount of the excipient propylene glycol, amprenavir oral solution is contraindicated in infants and children below 4 years of age, pregnant women, patients with renal or hepatic failure, and patients treated with disulfiram or metronidazole.

Warnings

➤*Drug interactions:* See also Contraindications and Drug Interactions.

Serious and/or life-threatening drug interactions could occur between amprenavir and amiodarone, lidocaine (systemic), tricyclic antidepressants, and quinidine. Concentration monitoring of these agents is recommended if these agents are used concomitantly with amprenavir.

➤*Oral solution:* Because of the potential risk of toxicity from the large amount of the excipient propylene glycol, amprenavir oral solution is contraindicated in infants and children below 4 years of age, pregnant women, patients with hepatic or renal failure, and patients treated with disulfiram or metronidazole.

Because of the possible toxicity associated with the large amount of propylene glycol and the lack of information on chronic exposure to large amounts of propylene glycol, use amprenavir oral solution only when amprenavir capsules or other protease inhibitor formulations are not therapeutic options. Certain ethnic populations (Asians, Eskimos, Native Americans) and women may be at increased risk of propylene glycol-associated adverse events because of diminished ability to metabolize propylene glycol; no data are available on propylene glycol metabolism in these groups.

Closely monitor patients who require treatment with amprenavir oral solution for propylene glycol-associated adverse events, including seizures, stupor, tachycardia, hyperosmolality, lactic acidosis, renal toxicity, and hemolysis. Switch patients from amprenavir oral solution to amprenavir capsules as soon as they are able to take the capsule formulation.

Concurrent use of amprenavir oral solution and ritonavir oral solution is not recommended because the large amount of propylene glycol in amprenavir oral solution and ethanol in ritonavir oral solution may compete for the same metabolic pathway for elimination.

Use of alcoholic beverages is not recommended in patients treated with amprenavir oral solution.

➤*Skin reactions:* Severe and life-threatening skin reactions, including Stevens-Johnson syndrome, have occurred in patients treated with amprenavir (see Adverse Reactions).

➤*Hemolytic anemia:* Acute hemolytic anemia occurred in a patient treated with amprenavir.

➤*Diabetes mellitus/hyperglycemia:* New-onset diabetes mellitus, exacerbation of pre-existing diabetes mellitus, and hyperglycemia have been reported during postmarketing surveillance in HIV-infected patients receiving protease inhibitor therapy. Some patients required initiation or dose adjustments of insulin or oral hypoglycemic agents for treatment of these events. In some cases, diabetic ketoacidosis has occurred. In those patients who discontinued protease inhibitor therapy, hyperglycemia persisted in some cases.

➤*Renal function impairment:* Amprenavir oral solution is contraindicated in patients with renal failure. Patients with renal impairment are at increased risk of propylene glycol-associated adverse events. Additionally, because metabolites of the excipient propylene glycol in amprenavir oral solution may alter acid-base balance, monitor patients with renal impairment for potential adverse events. Use amprenavir oral solution with caution in patients with renal impairment. The impact of renal impairment on amprenavir elimination has not been studied. The renal elimination of unchanged amprenavir represents less than 3% of the administered dose.

➤*Hepatic function impairment:* Amprenavir is principally metabolized by the liver. Amprenavir, when used alone and in combination with low-dose ritonavir, has been associated with elevations of AST and ALT in some patients. Exercise caution when administering this drug to patients with hepatic impairment (see Administration and Dosage). Conduct appropriate laboratory testing prior to initiating therapy with amprenavir and at periodic intervals during treatment.

Amprenavir oral solution is contraindicated in patients with hepatic failure. Patients with hepatic impairment are at increased risk of propylene glycol-associated adverse events. Use amprenavir oral solution with caution in patients with hepatic impairment.

➤*Carcinogenesis:* Amprenavir was evaluated for carcinogenic potential by oral gavage administration to mice and rats for up to 104 weeks. Daily doses of 50, 275 to 300, and 500 to 600 mg/kg/day were administered to mice and doses of 50, 190, and 750 mg/kg/day were adminis-

AMPRENAVIR

tered to rats. Results showed an increase in the incidence of benign hepatocellular adenomas and an increase in the combined incidence of hepatocellular adenomas plus carcinoma in males of both species at the highest doses tested. Female mice and rats were not affected. These observations were made at systemic exposures equivalent to approximately 2 times (mice) and 4 times (rats) the human exposure (based on AUC_{0-24h} measurement) at the recommended dose of 1200 mg twice daily.

➤*Elderly:* In general, dose selection for an elderly patient should be cautious, reflecting the greater frequency of decreased hepatic, renal, or cardiac function, and of concomitant disease or other drug therapy.

➤*Pregnancy: Category C.* In pregnant rabbits, amprenavir administration was associated with abortions and an increased incidence of 3 minor skeletal variations resulting from deficient ossification of the femur, humerus trochlea, and humerus. Systemic exposure at the highest tested dose was approximately 5% of the exposure seen at the recommended human dose. In rat fetuses, thymic elongation and incomplete ossification of bones were attributed to amprenavir. Both findings were seen at systemic exposures that were 50% of that associated with the recommended human dose.

Pre- and postnatal development studies were performed in rats dosed from day 7 of gestation to day 22 of lactation. Reduced body weights (10% to 20%) were observed in the offspring. The systemic exposure associated with this finding was approximately twice the exposure in humans following administration of the recommended human dose. The subsequent development of these offspring, including fertility and reproductive performance, was not affected by the maternal administration of amprenavir.

Amprenavir oral solution is contraindicated during pregnancy because of the potential risk of toxicity to the fetus from the high propylene glycol content. Therefore, if amprenavir is used in pregnant women, use the capsule formulation.

There are no adequate and well-controlled studies in pregnant women. Use during pregnancy only if the potential benefit justifies the potential risk to the fetus.

Antiretroviral pregnancy registry – To monitor maternal-fetal outcomes of pregnant women exposed to amprenavir, an Antiretroviral Pregnancy Registry has been established. Physicians are encouraged to register patients by calling (800) 258-4263.

➤*Lactation:* The Centers for Disease Control and Prevention recommend that HIV-infected mothers not breastfeed their infants to avoid risking postnatal transmission of HIV. Although it is not known if amprenavir is excreted in breast milk, amprenavir is secreted into the milk of lactating rats. Because of both the potential for HIV transmission and any possible adverse effects of amprenavir, instruct mothers not to breastfeed if they are receiving amprenavir.

➤*Children:* Two hundred fifty-one patients 4 years of age and above have received amprenavir as single or multiple doses in studies. An adverse event profile similar to that seen in adults was seen in pediatric patients. The safety, efficacy, and pharmacokinetics of amprenavir capsules have not been evaluated in pediatric patients below 4 years of age.

Amprenavir oral solution is contraindicated in infants and children below 4 years of age because of the potential risk of toxicity from the excipient propylene glycol (see Contraindications and Warnings). ADH, which metabolizes propylene glycol, is present in the human fetal liver at 2 months of gestational age, but its activity is only 3% of that of adults. Although the data are limited, it appears that by 12 to 30 months of postnatal age, ADH activity is equal to or greater than that observed in adults.

Precautions

➤*Doseform interchangeability:* Amprenavir capsules and oral solution are not interchangeable on a mg per mg basis (see Pharmacokinetics).

➤*Sulfonamide cross-sensitivity:* Amprenavir is a sulfonamide. The potential for cross-sensitivity between drugs in the sulfonamide class and amprenavir is unknown. Treat patients with a known sulfonamide allergy with caution.

➤*Vitamin E:* Formulations of amprenavir provide high daily doses of vitamin E. The effects of long-term, high-dose vitamin E administrations in humans is not well characterized and has not been specifically studied in HIV-infected individuals. High vitamin E doses may exacerbate the blood coagulation defect of vitamin K deficiency caused by anticoagulant therapy or malabsorption.

➤*Hemophilia:* There have been reports of spontaneous bleeding in patients with hemophilia A and B treated with protease inhibitors. In some patients, additional factor VIII was required. In many of the reported cases, treatment with protease inhibitors was continued or restarted.

➤*Fat redistribution:* Redistribution/accumulation of body fat including central obesity, dorsocervical fat enlargement (buffalo hump), peripheral wasting, facial wasting, breast enlargement, and "cushin-

goid appearance" have been observed in patients receiving antiretroviral therapy. The mechanism and long-term consequences of these events are currently unknown.

➤*Lipid elevations:* Treatment with amprenavir alone or in combination with ritonavir has resulted in increases in the concentration of total cholesterol and triglycerides. Perform triglyceride and cholesterol testing prior to initiation of therapy with amprenavir and at periodic intervals during treatment. Manage lipid disorders as clinically appropriate.

➤*Resistance/Cross-resistance:* Because the potential for HIV cross-resistance among protease inhibitors has not been fully explored, it is unknown what effect amprenavir therapy will have on the activity of subsequently administered protease inhibitors.

Drug Interactions

➤*CYP450 system:* Amprenavir is metabolized by the cytochrome P450 enzyme system. Amprenavir inhibits CYP3A4. Use caution when coadministering medications that are substrates, inhibitors, or inducers of CYP3A4, or potentially toxic medications that are metabolized by CYP3A4.

Amprenavir Drug Interactions			
Precipitant drug	Object drug*		Description
Abacavir	Amprenavir	↑	Concurrent use may increase amprenavir's C_{max}, AUC, and C_{min}.
Aldesleukin	Amprenavir	↑	Amprenavir concentration may be elevated.
Antacids	Amprenavir	↓	It is advisable that antacids not be taken at the same time as amprenavir because of potential interference with absorption. It is recommended to separate administration by at least 1 hour.
Anticonvulsants Carbamazepine Phenobarbital Phenytoin	Amprenavir	↓	Carbamazepine, phenobarbital, and phenytoin induce CYP3A4 and may decrease amprenavir concentrations. Amprenavir may increase carbamazepine plasma concentrations.
Amprenavir	Anticonvulsants Carbamazepine	↑	
Amprenavir	Pimozide	↑	Contraindicated because of potential for serious and/or life-threatening reactions such as cardiac arrhythmias.
Azole antifungals Fluconazole Itraconazole Ketoconazole	Amprenavir	↑↓	Itraconazole may increase amprenavir serum concentrations, and ketoconazole may increase amprenavir's AUC and decrease its C_{max}. Amprenavir may increase ketoconazole's C_{max} and AUC. Dose reduction of ketoconazole or itraconazole may be needed for patients receiving more than 400 mg ketoconazole or itraconazole per day.
Amprenavir	Azole antifungals Itraconazole Ketoconazole	↑	
Clarithromycin	Amprenavir	↑	Clarithromycin may increase amprenavir's C_{max}, AUC, and C_{min}. Concurrent use may slightly decrease clarithromycin's C_{max}.
Amprenavir	Clarithromycin	↓	
Dexamethasone	Amprenavir	↓	Use with caution. Amprenavir concentrations may be decreased.
Didanosine (buffered formulation only)	Amprenavir	↓	Coadministration may decrease amprenavir concentrations. Take amprenavir at least 1 hour before or after the buffered formulation of didanosine.
Disulfiram Metronidazole	Amprenavir (oral solution)	↑	Coadministration is contraindicated because of the potential risk for toxicity from the large amount of the excipient, propylene glycol, in the amprenavir oral solution.
Ethanol	Amprenavir	↑	Concurrent use is not recommended because the large amount of propylene glycol and ethanol may compete for the same metabolic pathway for elimination.
Indinavir	Amprenavir	↑	Concurrent use may increase amprenavir's C_{max}, AUC, and C_{min}, and decrease indinavir's C_{max}, AUC, and C_{min}.
Amprenavir	Indinavir	↓	
Methadone	Amprenavir	↓	Amprenavir plasma concentrations may be decreased; consider alternate antiretroviral therapy. Methadone plasma concentrations may be decreased; therefore, the dosage of methadone may need to be increased.
Amprenavir	Methadone	↓	

Protease Inhibitors

AMPRENAVIR

Amprenavir Drug Interactions			
Precipitant drug	Object drug*		Description
Nelfinavir	Amprenavir	⟷	Concurrent use may decrease amprenavir's C_{max} and increase its C_{min}, and nelfinavir's C_{max}, AUC, and C_{min} may be increased.
Amprenavir	Nelfinavir	↑	
NNRTIs Delavirdine Efavirenz Nevirapine	Amprenavir	↑↓	NNRTIs have the potential to increase (delavirdine) or decrease (efavirenz, nevirapine) amprenavir serum concentrations. Delavirdine serum concentrations may be decreased when given with amprenavir.
Rifamycins	Amprenavir	↓	Coadministration with rifabutin results in a 15% decrease in amprenavir AUC and a 193% increase in rifabutin AUC. A dosage reduction of rifabutin to at least half the recommended dose is required during concurrent use. Perform a CBC weekly and as clinically indicated to monitor for neutropenia. Rifampin should not be coadministered because it reduces amprenavir plasma concentrations and AUC by ≈ 90%.
Amprenavir	Rifabutin	↑	
Ritonavir	Amprenavir	↑	Concurrent use may increase amprenavir's AUC and C_{min} and decrease ritonavir's C_{max}, AUC, and C_{min}. Reduce the amprenavir dose when given with ritonavir capsules (see Administration and Dosage). Concurrent use of amprenavir oral solution and ritonavir oral solution is not recommended (see Warnings).
Amprenavir	Ritonavir	↓	
Saquinavir	Amprenavir	↓	Concurrent use may decrease amprenavir's C_{max}, AUC, and C_{min}, and increase saquinavir's C_{max} and decrease its AUC and C_{min}.
Amprenavir	Saquinavir	↑↓	
St. John's wort	Amprenavir	↓	St. John's wort may increase the metabolism (CYP3A4) of amprenavir, thus decreasing the concentration and clinical efficacy of amprenavir.
Zidovudine	Amprenavir	↑	Concurrent use may increase amprenavir's AUC and zidovudine's C_{max} and AUC.
Amprenavir	Zidovudine		
Amprenavir	Antiarrhythmics Amiodarone Lidocaine (systemic) Quinidine	↑	Serious or life-threatening interactions could occur between amprenavir and amiodarone, lidocaine, or quinidine. Concentration monitoring is recommended.
Amprenavir	Benzodiazepines	↑	Do not use amprenavir and midazolam or triazolam concurrently. Coadministration may result in competitive inhibition of these benzodiazepines and cause serious or life-threatening adverse events. Alprazolam, clorazepate, diazepam, and flurazepam may have increased serum concentrations, which could increase their activity.
Amprenavir	Calcium channel blockers	↑	Concurrent use of amprenavir and bepridil may increase bepridil concentrations. Increased bepridil exposure may be associated with life-threatening reactions such as cardiac arrhythmias. Use with caution. The concentrations of amlodipine, diltiazem, felodipine, isradipine, nifedipine, nicardipine, nimodipine, nisoldipine, or verapamil may be increased when given with amprenavir.
Amprenavir	Cisapride	↑	Do not use concurrently. Coadministration may result in increased cisapride concentrations and cause serious or life-threatening adverse events, such as cardiac arrhythmias.

Amprenavir Drug Interactions			
Precipitant drug	Object drug*		Description
Amprenavir	Contraceptives, oral	↑	Concurrent use of amprenavir with ethinyl estradiol/norethindrone may decrease amprenavir AUC and C_{min} and also increase the AUC and C_{min} of the oral contraceptive. Alternative methods of nonhormonal contraception are recommended.
Contraceptives, oral	Amprenavir	↓	
Amprenavir	Cyclosporine Tacrolimus	↑	The concentration of the immunosuppressant may be increased. Monitor therapeutic concentration. Protease inhibitor concentrations also may be increased. This may occur within 3 days of concurrent therapy. Monitor the clinical response to the protease inhibitor.
Cyclosporine	Amprenavir		
Amprenavir	Ergot alkaloids	↑	Contraindicated because of potential for serious and/or life-threatening reactions such as acute ergot toxicity characterized by peripheral vasospasm and ischemia of the extremities and other tissues.
Amprenavir	Fentanyl	↑	Fentanyl plasma concentrations may be increased and the half-life prolonged. Monitor closely; dosage reduction may be needed.
Amprenavir	HMG-CoA reductase inhibitors	↑	Amprenavir may increase serum concentrations of atorvastatin, lovastatin, and simvastatin, which could increase their toxicity, such as myopathy including rhabdomyolysis. Use the lowest possible dose with careful monitoring.
Amprenavir	Sildenafil	↑	Amprenavir may inhibit sildenafil's metabolism (CYP3A4), increasing the concentration of sildenafil and possibly resulting in severe and potentially fatal hypotension. Use sildenafil with caution at reduced doses of 25 mg every 48 hours with increased monitoring.
Amprenavir	Tricyclic antidepressants Amitriptyline Imipramine	↑	Concentrations of the tricyclic antidepressant may be increased. Therapeutic concentration monitoring is recommended.
Amprenavir	Warfarin	⟷	Plasma warfarin concentrations may be affected. Coadministration requires monitoring of international normalized ratio (INR).

* ↑ = Object drug increased. ↓ = Object drug decreased. ⟷ = Undetermined clinical effect.

▶*Drug/Food interactions:* The relative bioavailability of amprenavir capsules was assessed in the fasting and fed states in healthy volunteers (standardized high-fat meal: 967 kcal, 67 g fat, 33 g protein, 58 g carbohydrate). Administration of a single 1200 mg dose of amprenavir in the fed state compared with the fasted state was associated with changes in C_{max} (fed: 6.18 ± 2.92 mcg/mL, fasted: 9.72 ± 2.75 mcg/mL), T_{max} (fed: 1.51 ± 0.68, fasted: 1.05 ± 0.63), and $AUC_{0-\infty}$ (fed: 22.06 ± 11.6 mcg•h/mL, fasted: 28.05 ± 10.1 mcg•h/mL). Amprenavir may be taken with or without food but should not be taken with a high-fat meal.

Adverse Reactions

In clinical studies, adverse events leading to amprenavir discontinuation occurred primarily during the first 12 weeks of therapy and were mostly because of GI events (nausea, vomiting, diarrhea, abdominal pain/discomfort) that were mild to moderate in severity.

Selected Clinical Amprenavir Adverse Reactions of All Grades in Adults (> 5%)				
	Therapy-naive patients		NRTI-experienced patients	
Adverse reaction	Amprenavir/ Lamivudine/ Zidovudine (n = 113)	Lamivudine/ Zidovudine (n = 109)	Amprenavir/ NRTI (n = 245)	Indinavir/ NRTI (n = 241)
CNS				
Paresthesia, oral/ perioral	26	6	31	2
Paresthesia, peripheral	10	4	14	10

AMPRENAVIR

Selected Clinical Amprenavir Adverse Reactions of All Grades in Adults (> 5%)				
	Therapy-naive patients		NRTI-experienced patients	
Adverse reaction	Amprenavir/ Lamivudine/ Zidovudine (n = 113)	Lamivudine/ Zidovudine (n = 109)	Amprenavir/ NRTI (n = 245)	Indinavir/ NRTI (n = 241)
GI				
Nausea	74	50	43	35
Diarrhea or loose stools	39	35	60	41
Vomiting	34	17	24	20
Taste disorders	10	6	2	8
Miscellaneous				
Rash	27	6	20	15
Depressive or mood disorders	16	4	9	13

Amprenavir Selected Laboratory Abnormalities of All Grades in Adults (≥ 5%)				
	Therapy-naive patients		NRTI-experienced patients	
Laboratory abnormality (nonfasting specimens)	Amprenavir/ Lamivudine/ Zidovudine (n = 111)	Lamivudine/ Zidovudine (n = 108)	Amprenavir/ NRTI (n = 237)	Indinavir/ NRTI (n = 239)
Hyperglycemia (> 116 mg/dL)	45	31	53	58
Hypertriglyceridemia (> 213 mg/dL)	41	27	56	52
Hypercholesterolemia (> 283 mg/dL)	7	3	13	15

➤*Dermatologic:* In all multidose studies in HIV-infected patients, skin rash occurred in 22% of patients treated with amprenavir. Rashes were usually maculopapular of mild or moderate intensity, some with pruritus. Rashes had a median onset of 11 days after amprenavir initiation and a median duration of 10 days. Rashes led to amprenavir discontinuation in approximately 3% of patients. With mild or moderate rash, amprenavir dosing was often continued without interruption; if interrupted, reintroduction of amprenavir generally did not result in rash recurrence. Severe or life-threatening rash (Grade 3 or 4), including Stevens-Johnson syndrome, occurred in approximately 1% of recipients of amprenavir). Discontinue therapy for severe or life-threatening rashes and for moderate rashes accompanied by systemic symptoms.

➤*Miscellaneous:* In Phase 3 studies, 2 patients developed de novo diabetes mellitus, 1 patient developed a dorsocervical fat enlargement (buffalo hump), and 9 patients developed fat redistribution.

Treatment with amprenavir in combination with ritonavir has resulted in increases in the concentration of total cholesterol and triglycerides (see Precautions).

Pediatric patients – An adverse event profile similar to that seen in adults was seen in pediatric patients.

Overdosage

There is no known antidote for amprenavir. It is not known whether amprenavir can be removed by peritoneal dialysis or hemodialysis. If overdosage occurs, monitor the patient for evidence of toxicity and standard supportive treatment applied as necessary. Refer to the General Management of Acute Overdosage.

Patient Information

A Patient Package Insert (PPI) for amprenavir is available for patient information.

Amprenavir oral solution is contraindicated in infants and children below 4 years of age, pregnant women, patients with hepatic or renal failure, and patients treated with disulfiram or metronidazole. Amprenavir oral solution should be used only when amprenavir capsules or other protease inhibitor formulations are not therapeutic options.

Caution patients treated with amprenavir capsules against switching to amprenavir oral solution because of the increased risk of adverse events from the large amount of propylene glycol in the oral solution.

Women, Asians, Eskimos, or Native Americans, as well as patients who have hepatic or renal insufficiency, should be informed that they may be at increased risk of adverse events from the large amount of propylene glycol in amprenavir oral solution.

Inform patients that amprenavir is not a cure for HIV infection and that they may continue to develop opportunistic infections and other complications associated with HIV disease. The long-term effects of amprenavir are unknown at this time. Tell patients that there are currently no data demonstrating that therapy with amprenavir can reduce the risk of transmitting HIV to others through sexual contact.

Instruct patients to remain under the care of a physician while using amprenavir. Advise patients to take amprenavir every day as prescribed. Amprenavir must always be used in combination with other antiretroviral drugs. Instruct patients not to alter the dose or discontinue therapy without consulting their physician. If a dose is missed, advise patients to take the dose as soon as possible and then return to their normal schedule. However, if a dose is skipped, tell the patient not to double the next dose.

Advise patients to inform their doctors if they have a sulfa allergy. The potential for cross-sensitivity between drugs in the sulfonamide class and amprenavir is unknown.

Amprenavir may interact with many drugs; therefore, advise patients that they must report to their doctor the use of any other prescription or nonprescription medication or herbal products, particularly St. John's wort.

Instruct patients taking antacids (or the buffered formulation of didanosine) to take amprenavir at least 1 hour before or after antacid (or the buffered formulation of didanosine) use.

Advise patients that drinking alcoholic beverages is not recommended while taking amprenavir oral solution.

Advise patients receiving sildenafil that they may be at an increased risk of sildenafil-associated adverse events including hypotension, visual changes, and priapism, and to promptly report any symptoms to their doctor.

Instruct patients not to use hormonal contraceptives because some birth control pills (those containing ethinyl estradiol/norethindrone) have been found to decrease the concentration of amprenavir. Instruct patients receiving hormonal contraceptives to use alternate contraceptive measures during therapy with amprenavir.

Avoid high-fat meals because they may decrease the absorption of amprenavir. Amprenavir may be taken with meals of normal fat content.

Inform patients that redistribution or accumulation of body fat may occur in patients receiving antiretroviral therapy and that the cause and long-term health effects of these conditions are not known at this time.

Advise adult and pediatric patients not to take supplemental vitamin E because the vitamin E content of amprenavir capsules and oral solution exceeds the Reference Daily Intake (adults, 30 IU; pediatrics, approximately 10 IU).

ATAZANAVIR SULFATE

Rx	**Reyataz** (Bristol-Myers Squibb Virology)	**Capsules:** 100 mg (as base)	Lactose, n-butyl alcohol, dehydrated alcohol. (BMS 100 mg 3623). Blue/White. In 60s.
		150 mg (as base)	Lactose, n-butyl alcohol, dehydrated alcohol. (BMS 150 mg 3624). Blue/Powder blue. In 60s.
		200 mg (as base)	Lactose, n-butyl alcohol, dehydrated alcohol. (BMS 200 mg 3631). Blue. In 60s.

Indications

➤*HIV infection:* In combination with other antiretroviral agents for the treatment of HIV-1 infection.

Administration and Dosage

➤*Approved by the FDA:* June 20, 2003.

➤*Dosage:* The recommended dose is 400 mg (two 200 mg capsules) once daily taken with food.

➤*Concomitant therapy:* When coadministered with efavirenz, it is recommended that 300 mg atazanavir and 100 mg ritonavir be given with 600 mg efavirenz (all as a single daily dose with food). Do not coadminister atazanavir without ritonavir with efavirenz.

When coadministered with didanosine buffered formulations, give atazanavir (with food) 2 hours before or 1 hour after didanosine.

For these drugs and other antiretroviral agents (eg, ritonavir, saquinavir) for which dosing modifications may be appropriate, see the Drug Interactions table.

➤ *Hepatic function impairment:* Give with extreme caution in patients with mild to moderate hepatic insufficiency. Consider a dose reduction to 300 mg once daily for patients with moderate hepatic insufficiency (Child-Pugh Class B). Do not use atazanavir in patients with severe hepatic insufficiency (Child-Pugh Class C).

➤*Storage/Stability:* Store at 25°C (77°F); excursions permitted to 15° to 30°C (59° to 86°F).

ATAZANAVIR SULFATE

Actions

▶*Pharmacology:* Atazanavir is an azapeptide HIV-1 protease inhibitor. The compound selectively inhibits the virus-specific processing of viral Gag and Gag-Pol polyproteins in HIV-1 infected cells, thus preventing formation of mature virions.

▶*Pharmacokinetics:*

Absorption –

Atazanavir Steady-State Pharmacokinetics in the Fed State After 400 mg Once Daily		
Parameter	Healthy subjects (n = 14)	HIV-infected patients (n = 13)
C_{max} (ng/mL) Mean	5358	3152
T_{max} (h) Median	2.5	2
AUC (ng•h/mL) Mean	29,303	22,262
$t\text{-}\frac{1}{2}$ (h) Mean	7.9	6.5
C_{min} (ng/mL) Mean	218	273

Atazanavir is rapidly absorbed with a T_{max} of approximately 2.5 hours. Atazanavir demonstrates nonlinear pharmacokinetics with greater than dose-proportional increases in AUC and C_{max} values over the dose range of 200 to 800 mg once daily. Steady-state is achieved between days 4 and 8, with an accumulation of approximately 2.3-fold.

Distribution – Atazanavir is 86% bound to human serum proteins, and protein binding is independent of concentration. Atazanavir binds to both alpha-1-acid glycoprotein (AAG) and albumin to a similar extent (89% and 86%, respectively). In a multiple-dose study in HIV-infected patients dosed with atazanavir 400 mg once daily with a light meal for 12 weeks, atazanavir was detected in the cerebrospinal fluid and semen. The cerebrospinal fluid/plasma ratio for atazanavir (n = 4) ranged between 0.0021 and 0.0226 and seminal fluid/plasma ratio (n = 5) ranged between 0.11 and 4.42.

Metabolism – Atazanavir is extensively metabolized in humans. The major biotransformation pathways of atazanavir in humans consisted of mono-oxygenation and dioxygenation. Other minor biotransformation pathways for atazanavir or its metabolites consisted of glucuronidation, N-dealkylation, hydrolysis, and oxygenation with dehydrogenation. Two minor metabolites of atazanavir in plasma have been characterized. Neither metabolite demonstrated in vitro antiviral activity. In vitro studies using human liver microsomes suggested that atazanavir is metabolized by CYP3A.

Excretion – Following a single 400 mg dose of atazanavir, 79% and 13% was recovered in the feces and urine, respectively. Unchanged drug accounted for approximately 20% and 7% of the administered dose in the feces and urine, respectively. The mean elimination half-life of atazanavir in healthy volunteers (n = 214) and HIV-infected adult patients (n = 13) was approximately 7 hours at steady-state following a dose of 400 mg/day with a light meal.

Effect of food – Administration of atazanavir with food enhances bioavailability and reduces pharmacokinetic variability. Administration of a single 400 mg dose of atazanavir with a light meal (357 kcal, 8.2 g fat, 10.6 g protein) resulted in a 70% increase in AUC and a 57% increase in C_{max} relative to the fasting state. Administration of a single 400 mg dose of atazanavir with a high-fat meal (721 kcal, 37.3 g fat, 29.4 g protein) resulted in a mean increase in AUC of 35% with no change in C_{max} relative to the fasting state. Administration of atazanavir with either a light meal or high-fat meal decreased the coefficient of variation of AUC and C_{max} by approximately 50% compared with the fasting state.

Special populations –

Hepatic function impairment: Atazanavir is metabolized and eliminated primarily by the liver. Atazanavir has been studied in adult subjects with moderate to severe hepatic impairment (14 Child-Pugh B and 2 Child-Pugh C subjects) after a single 400 mg dose. The mean $AUC_{0-\infty}$ was 42% greater in subjects with impaired hepatic function than in healthy volunteers. The mean half-life of atazanavir in hepatically impaired subjects was 12.1 hours compared with 6.4 hours in healthy volunteers. Increased concentrations of atazanavir are expected in patients with moderately or severely impaired hepatic function.

▶*Microbiology:*

Antiviral activity in vitro – Atazanavir exhibits anti-HIV-1 activity with a mean 50% effective concentration (EC_{50}) in the absence of human serum of 2 to 5 nM against a variety of laboratory and clinical HIV-1 isolates grown in peripheral blood mononuclear cells, macrophages, CEM-SS cells, and MT-2 cells. Two-drug combination studies with atazanavir showed additive to antagonistic antiviral activity in vitro with abacavir and the NNRTIs (delavirdine, efavirenz, and nevirapine) and additive antiviral activity in vitro with the protease inhibitors (aprenavir, indinavir, lopinavir, nelfinavir, ritonavir, and saquinavir) and NRTIs (didanosine, lamivudine, stavudine, tenofovir, zalcitabine, and zidovudine) without enhanced cytotoxicity.

Cross-resistance – Atazanavir susceptibility was evaluated in vitro using a diverse panel of 551 clinical isolates from patients without prior atazanavir exposure. These isolates exhibited resistance to at least 1 approved protease inhibitor, with resistance defined as 2.5-fold or greater change in EC_{50} relative to a reference strain. Greater than 80% of the isolates resistant to 1 or 2 protease inhibitors (with the majority resistant to nelfinavir) retained susceptibility to atazanavir despite the presence of key mutations (eg, D30N) associated with protease inhibitor resistance. Of 104 isolates displaying nelfinavir-specific resistance, 84 retained susceptibility to atazanavir. There was a clear trend toward decreased atazanavir susceptibility as isolates exhibited resistance to multiple protease inhibitors. Baseline phenotypic and genotypic analyses of clinical isolates from atazanavir clinical trials of protease inhibitor-experienced subjects showed that isolates cross resistant to multiple protease inhibitors were also highly cross resistant (61% to 95%) to atazanavir. Greater than 90% of the isolates containing mutations I84V or G48V were resistant to atazanavir. Greater than 60% of isolates containing L90M, A71V/T, M46I, or a change at V82 were resistant to atazanavir, and 38% of isolates containing a D30N mutation in addition to other changes were resistant to atazanavir. Atazanavir-resistant isolates were highly cross resistant (51% to 100%) to other protease inhibitors (amprenavir, indinavir, lopinavir, nelfinavir, ritonavir, and saquinavir). The I50L and I50V substitutions yielded selective resistance to atazanavir and amprenavir, respectively, and did not appear to confer cross-resistance.

Resistance – Atazanavir-resistant isolates have been obtained from patients experiencing virologic failure on atazanavir therapy. There were 14 atazanavir-resistant isolates from studies of treatment-naïve patients (n = 96 evaluable isolates) that showed decreases in susceptibility levels from baseline, and all had an I50L substitution emerge on atazanavir therapy (after an average of 50 weeks of therapy) often in combination with an A71V mutation. Phenotypic analysis of the isolates containing the signature mutation I50L showed atazanavir-specific resistance, which coincided with increased susceptibility to other protease inhibitors (amprenavir, indinavir, lopinavir, nelfinavir, ritonavir, and saquinavir). In contrast, 89% (32 of 36) of atazanavir-resistant isolates from studies of treatment-experienced patients (n = 67 evaluable isolates) treated with atazanavir (n = 26) or atazanavir plus saquinavir (n = 10) showed no evidence of the emergence of the I50L substitution. Instead, these isolates displayed decreased susceptibility to multiple protease inhibitors. These mutations included I84V, L90M, A71V/T, N88S/D, and M46I, which conferred atazanavir resistance and reduced the clinical response to atazanavir. Generally, if protease inhibitor mutations were present in the HIV-1 of the patient at baseline, atazanavir resistance developed through mutations associated with resistance to other protease inhibitors instead of the I50L mutation. These mutations conferred high cross-resistance to other protease inhibitors with 100% of the isolates resistant to nelfinavir, more than 80% of the isolates resistant to indinavir, ritonavir, and saquinavir, and more than 35% of the isolates resistant to amprenavir and lopinavir. Genotypic and/or phenotypic analysis of baseline virus may aid in determining atazanavir susceptibility before initiation of atazanavir therapy.

▶*Clinical trials:* Study AI424-034 was a randomized, double-blind, multicenter trial comparing 400 mg atazanavir once daily to 600 mg efavirenz once daily, each in combination with a fixed-dose combination of 150 mg lamivudine and 300 mg zidovudine given twice daily in 810 antiretroviral treatment-naïve patients.

Through 48 weeks of therapy, the proportion of responders among patients with high viral loads (ie, baseline HIV RNA 100,000 or more copies/mL) was comparable for the atazanavir and efavirenz arms. The mean increase from baseline in CD4 cell count was 176 cells/mm^3 for the atazanavir arm and 160 cells/mm^3 for the efavirenz arm.

Study AI424-008 was a 48-week, randomized multicenter trial blinded to dose of atazanavir, comparing atazanavir at 2 dose levels (400 and 600 mg once daily) with nelfinavir (1250 mg twice daily), each in combination with stavudine (40 mg) and lamivudine (150 mg) given twice daily in 467 antiretroviral treatment-naïve patients.

Through 48 weeks of therapy, the mean increase from baseline in CD4 cell count was 234 cells/mm^3 for the atazanavir 400 mg arm and 211 cells/mm^3 for the nelfinavir arm.

Contraindications

Known hypersensitivity to atazanavir or any of its ingredients.

Coadministration of atazanavir is contraindicated with drugs (eg, midazolam, triazolam, ergot derivatives, cisapride, pimozide) that are highly dependent on CYP3A for clearance and for which elevated plasma concentrations are associated with serious and/or life-threatening events.

Warnings

▶*PR interval prolongation:* Concentration- and dose-dependent prolongation of the PR interval in the electrocardiogram has been observed in healthy volunteers receiving atazanavir. In a placebo-controlled study, the mean (±SD) maximum change in PR interval from

ATAZANAVIR SULFATE

the predose value was 24 (±15) msec following oral dosing with 400 mg atazanavir (n = 65) compared with 13 (±11) msec following dosing with placebo (n = 67). The PR interval prolongations in this study were asymptomatic.

In healthy volunteers and in patients, abnormalities in atrioventricular (AV) conduction were asymptomatic and limited to first-degree AV block with rare exceptions (see Overdosage). In clinical trials, asymptomatic first-degree AV block was observed in 5.9% of atazanavir-treated patients (n = 920), 5.2% of lopinavir/ritonavir-treated patients (n = 252), 10.4% of nelfinavir-treated patients (n = 48), and in 3% of efavirenz-treated patients (n = 329). There has been no second- or third-degree AV block. Because of limited clinical experience, use atazanavir with caution in patients with pre-existing conduction system disease (eg, marked first-degree AV block or second- or third-degree AV block).

In a pharmacokinetic study between 400 mg atazanavir once daily and 180 mg diltiazem once daily, a CYP3A substrate, there was a 2-fold increase in the diltiazem plasma concentration and an additive effect on the PR interval. When used in combination with atazanavir, consider a 50% dose reduction of diltiazem and recommend ECG monitoring (See Drug Interactions).

➤*Diabetes mellitus/hyperglycemia:* New-onset diabetes mellitus, exacerbation of pre-existing diabetes mellitus, and hyperglycemia have been reported during postmarketing surveillance in HIV-infected patients receiving protease inhibitor therapy. Some patients required either initiation or dose adjustments of insulin or oral hypoglycemia agents for treatment of these events. In some cases, diabetic ketoacidosis has occurred. In those patients who discontinued protease inhibitor therapy, hyperglycemia persisted in some cases. Because these events have been reported voluntarily during clinical practice, estimates of frequency cannot be made and a causal relationship between protease inhibitor therapy and these events has not been established.

➤*Hepatic function impairment:* Atazanavir is principally metabolized by the liver; exercise caution when administering this drug to patients with hepatic impairment because atazanavir concentrations may be increased (see Administration and Dosage). Patients with underlying hepatitis B or C viral infections or marked elevations in transaminases prior to treatment may be at increased risk for developing further transaminase elevations or hepatic decompensation.

➤*Elderly:* In general, exercise appropriate caution in the administration and monitoring of atazanavir in elderly patients reflecting the greater frequency of decreased hepatic, renal, or cardiac function, and of concomitant disease or other drug therapy.

➤*Pregnancy: Category B.* In the pre- and postnatal development assessment in rats, atazanavir, at maternally toxic drug exposure levels 2 times those at the human clinical dose, caused body weight loss or weight gain suppression in the offspring.

Hyperbilirubinemia occurred frequently during treatment with atazanavir. It is not known whether atazanavir administered to the mother during pregnancy will exacerbate physiological hyperbilirubinemia and lead to kernicterus in neonates and young infants. In the prepartum period, consider additional monitoring and alternative therapy to atazanavir.

There are no adequate and well-controlled studies in pregnant women. Cases of lactic acidosis syndrome, sometimes fatal, and symptomatic hyperlactatemia have been reported in patients (including pregnant women) receiving atazanavir in combination with nucleoside analogs, which are known to be associated with increased risk of lactic acidosis syndrome. Use atazanavir during pregnancy only if the potential benefit justifies the potential risk to the fetus.

Antiretroviral pregnancy registry – To monitor maternal-fetal outcomes of pregnant women exposed to atazanavir, an antiretroviral pregnancy registry has been established. Physicians are encouraged to register patients by calling (800) 258-4263.

➤*Lactation:* The Centers for Disease Control and Prevention recommend that HIV-infected mothers not breastfeed their infants to avoid risking postnatal transmission of HIV.

It is not known whether atazanavir is secreted in human breast milk. A study in lactating rats has demonstrated that atazanavir is secreted in breast milk. Because of both the potential for HIV transmission and the potential for serious adverse reactions in breastfeeding infants, instruct mothers not to breastfeed if they are receiving atazanavir.

➤*Children:* Do not administer atazanavir to pediatric patients below 3 months of age because of the risk of kernicterus.

Precautions

➤ *Hyperbilirubinemia:* Most patients taking atazanavir experience asymptomatic elevations in indirect (unconjugated) bilirubin related to inhibition of UDP-glucuronosyl transferase (UGT). This hyperbilirubinemia is reversible upon discontinuation of atazanavir. Evaluate hepatic transaminase elevations that occur with hyperbilirubinemia for alternative etiologies. No long-term safety data are available for patients experiencing persistent elevations in total bilirubin more than $5 \times$ ULN. Alternative antiretroviral therapy to atazanavir may be considered if jaundice or scleral icterus associated with bilirubin elevations

presents cosmetic concerns for patients. Dose reduction of atazanavir is not recommended since long-term efficacy of reduced doses has not been established.

➤*Resistance/Cross-resistance:* Various degrees of cross-resistance among protease inhibitors have been observed. Resistance to atazanavir may not preclude the subsequent use of other protease inhibitors.

➤*Hemophilia:* There have been reports of increased bleeding, including spontaneous skin hematomas and hemarthrosis in patients with hemophilia type A and B treated with protease inhibitors. In some patients additional factor VIII was given. In more than half of the reported cases, treatment with protease inhibitors was continued or reintroduced. A causal relationship between protease inhibitor therapy and these events has not been established.

➤*Lactic acidosis syndrome:* Cases of lactic acidosis syndrome (LAS), sometimes fatal, and symptomatic hyperlactatemia have been reported in patients receiving atazanavir in combination with nucleoside analogs, which are known to be associated with increased risk of LAS. Female gender and obesity are also known risk factors for LAS. The contribution of atazanavir to the risk of development of LAS has not been established.

➤ *Fat redistribution:* Redistribution/accumulation of body fat including central obesity, dorsocervical fat enlargement (buffalo hump), peripheral wasting, facial wasting, breast enlargement, and cushingoid appearance have been observed in patients receiving antiretroviral therapy. The mechanism and long-term consequences of these events are currently unknown. A causal relationship has not been established.

➤*Photosensitivity:* Photosensitization may occur; therefore, caution patients to take protective measures (ie, sunscreens, protective clothing) against exposure to ultraviolet light or sunlight until tolerance is determined.

Drug Interactions

➤*CYP450:* Atazanavir is an inhibitor of CYP3A, CYP1A2, CYP2C9, and UGT1A1. Coadministration of atazanavir and drugs primarily metabolized by CYP3A (eg, calcium channel blockers, HMG-CoA reductase inhibitors, immunosuppressants, and sildenafil) or UGT1A1 (eg, irinotecan) may result in increased plasma concentrations of the other drug that could increase or prolong its therapeutic and adverse effects.

Atazanavir Drug Interactions			
Precipitant drug	Object drug*		Description
Rifampin	Atazanavir	↓	Rifampin decreases plasma concentrations and AUC of most protease inhibitors by ≈ 90%, possibly resulting in loss of therapeutic effect and development of resistance. Coadministration is not recommended.
Atazanavir	Irinotecan	↑	Atazanavir inhibits UGT and may interfere with the metabolism of irinotecan, resulting in increased irinotecan toxicities. Coadministration is not recommended.
Atazanavir	Benzodiazepines (midazolam, triazolam)	↑	Contraindicated because of potential for serious and/or life-threatening events such as prolonged or increased sedation or respiratory depression.
Atazanavir	Ergot derivatives (dihydroergotamine, ergotamine)	↑	Contraindicated because of potential for serious and/or life-threatening events such as acute ergot toxicity.
Atazanavir	Cisapride	↑	Contraindicated because of potential for serious and/or life-threatening events such as cardiac arrhythmias.
Atazanavir	HMG-CoA Reductase inhibitors (lovastatin, simvastatin, atorvastatin)	↑	Atazanavir may increase serum concentrations of HMG-CoA reductase inhibitors, which could increase their toxicity, including rhabdomyolysis. Do not coadminister with simvastatin or lovastatin.
Atazanavir	Indinavir	↑	Both atazanavir and indinavir are associated with indirect (unconjugated) hyperbilirubinemia. Coadministration is not recommended.
Indinavir	Atazanavir		
Atazanavir	Pimozide	↑	Contraindicated because of increased serum pimozide concentrations and increased toxicity such as cardiac arrhythmias.
Proton pump inhibitors	Atazanavir	↓	Coadministration is not recommended because of expected substantial decreases in atazanavir concentrations and decreased therapeutic effect.

Protease Inhibitors

ATAZANAVIR SULFATE

Atazanavir Drug Interactions			
Precipitant drug	Object drug*		Description
St. John's wort	Atazanavir	↓	Concurrent use may be expected to reduce plasma concentrations of atazanavir. This may result in loss of therapeutic effect and development of resistance. Concurrent use is not recommended.
Didanosine (buffered formulation only)	Atazanavir	↓	Coadministration may decrease atazanavir concentrations. Take atazanavir (with food) 2 h before or 1 h after the buffered formulation of didanosine. Because didanosine EC capsules are to be given on an empty stomach and atazanavir is to be given with food, administer at different times.
Efavirenz	Atazanavir	↓	If atazanavir is to be coadministered with efavirenz, which decreases atazanavir exposure, it is recommended that 300 mg atazanavir with 100 mg ritonavir be coadministered with 600 mg efavirenz (all as a single daily dose with food). Atazanavir without ritonavir should not be coadministered with efavirenz.
Atazanavir	Saquinavir	↑	Appropriate dosing recommendations for this combination, with respect to efficacy and safety, have not been established.
Ritonavir	Atazanavir	↔	Coadministration of atazanavir and ritonavir is currently under clinical investigation. If atazanavir is coadministered with ritonavir, it is recommended that 300 mg atazanavir once daily be given with 100 mg ritonavir once daily with food.
Antacids and buffered medications	Atazanavir	↓	Reduced plasma concentrations of atazanavir are expected if antacids, including buffered medications, are administered with atazanavir. Administer atazanavir 2 h before or 1 h after these medications.
Atazanavir	Antiarrhythmics (eg, amiodarone, systemic lidocaine, quinidine)	↑	Concurrent use of atazanavir with antiarrhythmics have the potential to produce serious and/or life-threatening adverse events. Concentration monitoring of the antiarrhythmic agent is recommended if they are used concomitantly.
Atazanavir	Warfarin	↑	Coadministration has the potential to produce serious and/or life-threatening bleeding and has not been studied. It is recommended that INR be monitored.
Atazanavir	Tricyclic antidepressants	↑	Concentrations of the tricyclic antidepressant may be increased. Concentration monitoring of the tricyclic antidepressant is recommended.
Atazanavir	Rifabutin	↑	Concentrations of rifabutin may be increased. A rifabutin dose reduction of up to 75% (eg, 150 mg every other day or 3 times/wk) is recommended.
Atazanavir	Calcium channel blockers (eg, bepridil, diltiazem, felodipine, nicardipine, verapamil)	↑	Atanazavir has the potential to prolong the PR interval in some patients. Caution is warranted. Administration with bepridil is not recommended. Consider a dose reduction of diltiazem by 50% and consider dose titration of other calcium channel blockers. ECG monitoring is recommended.
Atazanavir	Sildenafil	↑	Coadministration may result in an increase in sildenafil-associated adverse events, including hypotension, visual changes, and priapism. Use sildenafil with caution at a reduced dose of 25 mg every 48 h and monitor for adverse events.

Atazanavir Drug Interactions			
Precipitant drug	Object drug*		Description
H₂-receptor antagonists	Atazanavir	↓	Reduced plasma concentrations of atazanavir are expected if coadministered with H₂-receptor antagonists. This may result in loss of therapeutic effect and development of resistance. Administer atazanavir 12 h apart from H₂-receptor antagonists.
Atazanavir	Immunosuppressants (cyclosporine, sirolimus, tacrolimus)	↑	Coadministration may result in increased plasma concentrations of the immunosuppressant. Therapeutic concentration monitoring is recommended for the immunosuppressant agents when coadministered with atazanavir.
Clarithromycin	Atazanavir	↑↓	Increased concentrations of clarithromycin may cause QTc prolongations; therefore, consider a dose reduction of clarithromycin of 50% when it is administered with atazanavir. In addition, concentrations of the active metabolite 14-OH clarithromycin are significantly reduced; consider alternative therapy for indications other than infections because of *Mycobacterium avium* complex.
Atazanavir	Clarithromycin		
Atazanavir	Contraceptives, oral (ethinyl estradiol and norethindrone)	↑	Mean concentrations of ethinyl estradiol and norethindrone are increased when administered with atazanavir. Exercise caution and use the lowest effective dose of each oral contraceptive component.

* ↑ = Object drug increased. ↓ = Object drug decreased. ↔ = Undetermined clinical effect.

➤ *Drug/Food interactions:* Administration of atazanavir with food enhances bioavailability and reduces pharmacokinetic variability. Administration of atazanavir with either a light meal or high-fat meal decreased the coefficient of variation of AUC and C_{max} by approximately one-half compared with the fasting state.

Adverse Reactions

Atazanavir Adverse Events of Moderate or Severe Intensity Reported in Adult Treatment-Naive Patients (%)[1]				
	Phase III study AI424-034		Phase II studies AI424-007, -008	
Adverse reaction	64 weeks[2] atazanavir 400 mg once daily + lamivudine + zidovudine[4] (n = 404)	64 weeks[2] efavirenz 600 mg once daily + lamivudine + zidovudine[4] (n = 401)	120 weeks[2,3] atazanavir 400 mg once daily + stavudine + lamivudine or stavudine + didanosine (n = 279)	73 weeks[2,3] nelfinavir 750 mg tid or 1250 mg bid + stavudine + lamivudine or stavudine + didanosine (n = 191)
CNS				
Depression	4	5	8	3
Dizziness	3	8	1	-
Headache	14	13	10	8
Insomnia	3	5	1	< 1
Peripheral neurologic symptoms	1	2	8	7
GI				
Abdominal pain	6	5	10	8
Diarrhea	6	7	8	25
Jaundice/scleral icterus	7	< 1	8	-
Nausea	16	13	10	6
Vomiting	6	8	8	7
Miscellaneous				
Arthralgia	< 1	2	4	4
Back pain	2	5	6	3
Fatigue	2	2	3	2
Fever	4	6	5	5
Increased cough	3	4	5	1
Lipodystrophy	1	1	8	3
Pain	3	2	1	3
Rash	9	13	10	3
Lab abnormalities				
AST (≥ 5.1 × ULN[5]s)	2	2	7	5
ALT (≥ 5.1 × ULN[5])	4	3	9	7

ATAZANAVIR SULFATE

Atazanavir Adverse Events of Moderate or Severe Intensity Reported in Adult Treatment-Naive Patients (%)[1]			
	Phase III study AI424-034		Phase II studies AI424-007, -008
Adverse reaction	64 weeks[2] atazanavir 400 mg once daily + lamivudine + zidovudine[4] (n = 404)	64 weeks[2] efavirenz 600 mg once daily + lamivudine + zidovudine[4] (n = 401)	120 weeks[2,3] atazanavir 400 mg once daily + stavudine + lamivudine or stavudine + didanosine (n = 279)	73 weeks[2,3] nelfinavir 750 mg tid or 1250 mg bid + stavudine + lamivudine or stavudine + didanosine (n = 191)
Total bilirubin (≥ 2.6 × ULN[5])	35	< 1	47	3
Amylase (≥ 2.1 × ULN[5])	-	-	14	10
Lipase (≥ 2.1 × ULN[5])	< 1	1	4	5
Hemoglobin (< 8.0 g/dL)	5	3	< 1	4
Neutrophils (< 750 cells/mm[3])	7	9	3	7

[1] Based on regimen(s) containing atazanavir.
[2] Median time on therapy.
[3] Includes long-term follow-up.
[4] As a fixed-dose combination: 150 mg lamivudine, 30 mg zidovudine twice daily.
[5] ULN = upper limit of normal.

➤*Cardiovascular:* Heart arrest; heart block; hypertension; myocarditis; palpitation; syncope; vasodilation.

➤*CNS:* Abnormal dream; abnormal gait; agitation; amnesia; anxiety; confusion; convulsion; decreased libido; emotional lability; hallucination; hostility; hyperkinesia; hypesthesia; increased reflexes; nervousness; psychosis; sleep disorder; somnolence; suicide attempt; twitch.

➤*Dermatologic:* Alopecia; cellulitis; dermatophytosis; dry skin; eczema; nail disorder; pruritus; seborrhea; urticaria; vesiculobullous rash.

➤*GI:* Acholia; anorexia; aphthous stomatitis; colitis; constipation; dental pain; dyspepsia; enlarged abdomen; esophageal ulcer; esophagitis; flatulence; gastritis; gastroenteritis; GI disorder; hepatitis; hepatomegaly; hepatosplenomegaly; increased appetite; liver damage; liver fatty deposit; mouth ulcer; pancreatitis; peptic ulcer.

➤*GU:* Abnormal urine; amenorrhea; crystalluria; decreased male fertility; gynecomastia; hematuria; impotence; kidney calculus; kidney failure; kidney pain; menstrual disorder; oliguria; pelvic pain; polyuria; proteinuria; urinary frequency; urinary tract infection.

➤*Lab test abnormalities:*

Grade 3-4 Lab Abnormalities Reported in ≥ 2% Adult Treatment-Experienced Patients[1]				
	Phase III study AI424-043		Phase III study AI424-045	
Lab value	24 weeks[2] atazanavir 400 mg once daily + 2 NRTIs (n = 144)	24 weeks[2] lopinavir + ritonavir (400/100 mg) bid[3] + 2 NRTIs (n = 146)	15 weeks[2] atazanavir 300 mg once daily + ritonavir 100 mg once daily + tenofovir + NRTI (n = 119)	12 weeks[2] atazanavir 400 mg once daily + saquinavir[4] 1200 mg once daily + tenofovir + NRTI (n = 110)	13 weeks[2] lopinavir + ritonavir (400/100 mg) bid[3] + tenofovir + NRTI (n = 118)
AST (≥ 5.1 × ULN)	3	1	< 1	2	< 1
ALT (≥ 5.1 × ULN)	6	1	3	3	3
Total bilirubin (≥ 2.6 × ULN)	22	-	40	13	-
Lipase (≥ 2.1 × ULN)	4	3	4	<1	6
Platelets (< 50,000/mm[3])	-	-	< 1	4	< 1
Neutrophils (< 750 cells/mm[3])	5	3	4	5	4

[1] Based on regimen(s) containing atazanavir.
[2] Median time on therapy.
[3] As a fixed-dose combination.
[4] Soft gelatin capsules.

➤*Hepatic:* Monitor LFTs in patients with a history of hepatitis B or C. In studies AI424-008 and AI424-034, 74 patients treated with 400 mg atazanavir once daily, 58 who received efavirenz, and 12 who received nelfinavir were seropositive for hepatitis B and/or C at study entry. AST

levels more than 5 times the ULN developed in 9% of atazanavir-treated patients, 5% of the efavirenz-treated patients, and 17% of the nelfinavir-treated patients. ALT levels more than 5 × ULN developed in 15% of the atazanavir-treated patients, 14% of the efavirenz-treated patients, and 17% of the nelfinavir-treated patients. Within atazanavir and control regimens, no difference in frequency of bilirubin elevations was noted between seropositive and seronegative patients.

➤*Lipids:*

Lipid Values, Mean Change from Baseline, Study AI424-034						
	Atazanavir[1]			Efavirenz[2]		
	Baseline	Week 48		Baseline	Week 48	
	mg/dL (n = 383)[4]	mg/dL (n = 283)[4]	Change[3] (n = 272)[4]	mg/dL (n = 378)[4]	mg/dL (n = 264)[4]	Change[3] (n = 253)[4]
LDL-cholesterol[5]	98	98	+ 1%	98	114	+ 18%
HDL-cholesterol	39	43	+ 13%	38	46	+ 24%
Total-cholesterol	164	168	+ 2%	162	195	+ 21%
Triglycerides[5]	138	124	− 9%	129	168	+ 23%

[1] Atazanavir 400 mg once daily with the fixed-dose combination: 150 mg lamivudine, 300 mg zidovudine twice daily.
[2] Efavirenz 600 mg once daily with the fixed-dose combination: 150 mg lamivudine, 300 mg zidovudine twice daily.
[3] The change from baseline is the mean of within-patient changes from baseline for patients with both baseline and week 48 values and is not a simple difference of the baseline and week 48 mean values.
[4] Number of patients with LDL-cholesterol measured.
[5] Fasting.

Lipid Values, Mean Change from Baseline, Study AI424-043						
	Atazanavir[1]			Lopinavir + Ritonavir[2]		
	Baseline	Week 24		Baseline	Week 24	
	mg/dL (n = 143)[4]	mg/dL (n = 123)[4]	Change[3] (n = 123)[4]	mg/dL (n = 144)[4]	mg/dL (n = 107)[4]	Change[3] (n = 106)[4]
LDL-cholesterol[5,6]	106	95	− 6%	103	107	+ 5%
HDL-cholesterol	39	41	+ 12%	37	45	+ 18%
Total-cholesterol	181	170	− 2%	175	201	+ 17%
Triglycerides[6]	192	193	− 2%	192	262	+ 55%

[1] Atazanavir 400 mg once daily + 2 NRTIs.
[2] Lopinavir + ritonavir (400/100 mg) bid + 2 NRTIs.
[3] The change from baseline is the mean of within-patient changes from baseline for patients with both baseline and week 24 values and is not a simple difference of the baseline and week 24 mean values.
[4] Number of patients with LDL-cholesterol measured.
[5] Protocol-defined coprimary safety outcome measure.
[6] Fasting.

➤*Metabolic/Nutritional:* Buffalo hump; dehydration; diabetes mellitus; dyslipidemia; gout; lactic acidosis; lipohypertrophy; obesity; weight decrease; weight gain.

➤*Musculoskeletal:* Bone pain; extremity pain; muscle atrophy; myalgia; myasthenia; myopathy.

➤*Respiratory:* Dyspnea; hiccough; hypoxia.

➤*Special senses:* Otitis; taste perversion; tinnitus.

➤*Miscellaneous:* Allergic reaction; angioedema; asthenia; burning sensation; chest pain; dysplasia; ecchymosis; edema; facial atrophy; generalized edema; heat sensitivity; infection; malaise; overdose; pallor; peripheral edema; photosensitivity; purpura; substernal chest pain; sweating.

Overdosage

➤*Symptoms:* Human experience of acute overdose with atazanavir is limited. Single doses up to 1200 mg have been taken by healthy volunteers without symptomatic untoward effects. A single self-administered overdose of 29.2 g atazanavir in an HIV-infected patient (73 times the 400 mg recommended dose) was associated with asymptomatic bifascicular block and PR interval prolongation. These events resolved spontaneously. At high doses that lead to high drug exposures, jaundice caused by indirect (unconjugated) hyperbilirubinemia (without associated liver function test changes) or PR interval prolongation may be observed.

➤*Treatment:* Treatment of overdosage consists of general supportive measures, including monitoring of vital signs and ECG, and observations of the patient's clinical status. If indicated, achieve elimination of unabsorbed atazanavir by emesis or gastric lavage. Administration of activated charcoal may also be used to aid removal of unabsorbed drug. There is no specific antidote for overdose with atazanavir. Since atazanavir is extensively metabolized by the liver and is highly protein bound, dialysis is unlikely to be beneficial in significant removal of this medicine

ATAZANAVIR SULFATE

Patient Information

Tell patients that sustained decreases in plasma HIV RNA have been associated with a reduced risk of progression to AIDS and death.

Advise patients to take atazanavir with food every day and take other concomitant antiretroviral therapy as prescribed. Take atazanavir with food to enhance absorption.

Atazanavir must always be used in combination with other antiretroviral drugs.

Do not alter the dose or discontinue therapy without consulting a physician. If a dose of atazanavir is missed, take the dose as soon as possible and then return to the normal schedule. However, if a dose is skipped, do not double the next dose.

Inform patients that atazanavir is not a cure for HIV infection, and they may continue to develop opportunistic infections and other complications associated with HIV disease. Tell patients that there are currently no data demonstrating that therapy with atazanavir can reduce the risk of transmitting HIV to others through sexual contact.

Atazanavir may interact with some drugs; therefore, advise patients to report to their doctor the use of any other prescription, nonprescription medication, or herbal products, particularly St. John's wort.

Advise patients receiving sildenafil and atazanavir that they may be at an increased risk of sildenafil-associated adverse effects including hypotension, visual changes, and prolonged penile erection. Advise patients to promptly report any symptoms to a physician.

Inform patients that atazanavir may produce changes in the electrocardiogram (PR prolongation). Advise patients to consult a physician if symptoms such as dizziness or light-headedness are experienced.

Inform patients that asymptomatic elevations in indirect bilirubin have occurred in patients receiving atazanavir. This may be accompanied by yellowing of the skin or whites of the eyes. Alternative antiretroviral therapy may be considered if the patient has cosmetic concerns.

Inform patients that redistribution or accumulation of body fat may occur in patients receiving antiretroviral therapy including protease inhibitors, and the cause and long-term effects of these conditions are not known at this time. It is unknown whether long-term use of atazanavir will result in a lower incidence of lipodystrophy than with other protease inhibitors.

May cause photosensitivity (sensitivity to sunlight). Avoid prolonged exposure to the sun and other ultraviolet light. Use suncreens and wear protective clothing until tolerance is determined.

LOPINAVIR/RITONAVIR

Rx	Kaletra (Abbott)	Capsules, soft gelatin: 133.3 mg lopinavir/ 33.3 mg ritonavir	Sorbitol. (PK). Orange. In 180s.
		Solution, oral: 80 mg lopinavir/20 mg ritonavir per mL	42.4% alcohol, menthol, corn syrup, saccharin, peppermint oil. Cotton candy or vanilla flavors. In 160 mL bottles with dosing cup.

Indications

➤*HIV infection:* In combination with other antiretroviral agents for the treatment of HIV infection. This indication is based on analyses of plasma HIV RNA levels and CD4 cell counts in a controlled study of lopinavir/ritonavir combination of 48 weeks duration and in smaller uncontrolled dose-ranging studies of 72 weeks duration. At present, there are no results from controlled trials evaluating the effect on clinical progression of HIV.

Administration and Dosage

➤*Approved by the FDA:* September 15, 2000.

➤*Adults:* The recommended dosage is 400/100 mg of lopinavir/ ritonavir (3 capsules or 5 mL) twice daily with food.

Concomitant therapy with efavirenz or nevirapine – Consider a dose increase to 533/133 mg lopinavir/ritonavir (4 capsules or 6.5 mL) twice daily with food when used in combination with efavirenz or nevirapine in treatment-experienced patients where reduced susceptibility to lopinavir is clinically suspected (by treatment history or laboratory evidence).

➤*Children (6 months to 12 years of age):* The recommended dosage of lopinavir/ritonavir oral solution is 12/3 mg/kg for those weighing 7 to less than 15 kg and 10/2.5 mg/kg for those 15 to 40 kg (approximately equivalent to 230/57.5 mg/m^2) twice daily with food, up to a maximum dose of 400/100 mg in children greater than 40 kg (5 mL or 3 capsules) twice daily. It is preferred that the prescriber calculate the appropriate milligram dose for each individual child 12 years of age and younger and determine the corresponding volume of solution or number of capsules.

Lopinavir/Ritonavir Pediatric Dosage Without Efavirenz or Nevirapine		
Weight (kg)[1]	Dose (mg/kg)[2]	Volume of oral solution BID (80 mg lopinavir/20 mg ritonavir per mL)
7 to < 15	12 mg/kg BID	
7 to 10		1.25 mL
> 10 to < 15		1.75 mL
15 to 40	10 mg/kg BID	
15 to 20		2.25 mL
> 20 to 25		2.75 mL
> 25 to 30		3.5 mL
> 30 to 35		4 mL
> 35 to 40		4.75 mL
> 40	Adult dose	5 mL (or 3 capsules)

[1] Note: Use adult dosage recommendation for children above 12 years of age.
[2] Dosing based on the lopinavir component of lopinavir/ritonavir solution (80 mg/20 mg per mL).

Concomitant therapy with efavirenz or nevirapine – Consider a dose increase of lopinavir/ritonavir oral solution to 13/3.25 mg/kg for those weighing 7 to less than 15 kg and 11/2.75 mg/kg for those 15 to 45 kg (approximately equivalent to 300/75 mg/m^2) twice daily with food, up to a maximum dose of 533/133 mg in children over 45 kg twice daily when used in combination with efavirenz or nevirapine in treatment-experienced children 6 months to 12 years of age in which reduced susceptibility to lopinavir is clinically suspected (by treatment history or laboratory evidence).

Lopinavir/Ritonavir Pediatric Dosage with Efavirenz or Nevirapine		
Weight (kg)[1]	Dose (mg/kg)[2]	Volume of oral solution BID (80 mg lopinavir/20 mg ritonavir per mL)
7 to < 15	13 mg/kg BID	
7 to 10		1.5 mL
> 10 to < 15		2 mL
15 to 45	11 mg/kg BID	
15 to 20		2.5 mL
> 20 to 25		3.25 mL
> 25 to 30		4 mL
> 30 to 35		4.5 mL
> 35 to 40		5 mL (or 3 capsules)
> 40 to 45		5.75 mL
> 45	Adult dose	6.5 mL (or 4 capsules)

[1] Note: Use adult dosage recommendation for children over 12 years of age.
[2] Dosing based on the lopinavir component of lopinavir/ritonavir solution (80 mg/20 mg per mL).

➤*Storage/Stability:* Store capsules and oral solution at 2° to 8°C (36° to 46°F) until dispensed. Avoid exposure to excessive heat. Under refrigeration, the capsules and solution remain stable until the expiration date printed on the label. If stored at room temperature up to 25°C (77°F), use within 2 months.

Actions

➤*Pharmacology:* Lopinavir, an HIV protease inhibitor, prevents cleavage of the Gag-Pol polyprotein, resulting in the production of immature, noninfectious viral particles. As coformulated in the lopinavir/ritonavir combination, ritonavir inhibits the CYP3A-mediated metabolism of lopinavir, providing increased lopinavir plasma levels.

➤*Pharmacokinetics:*

Absorption – Administration of a single 400/100 mg dose of lopinavir/ ritonavir with a moderate-fat meal was associated with a mean increase of 48% and 23% in lopinavir AUC and C$_{max}$, respectively, relative to fasting. For lopinavir/ritonavir oral solution, the corresponding increases in lopinavir AUC and C$_{max}$ were 80% and 54%, respectively. Relative to fasting, administration of lopinavir/ritonavir with a high-fat meal increased lopinavir AUC and C$_{max}$ by 97% and 43%, respectively, for capsules, and 130% and 56%, respectively, for oral solution. To enhance bioavailability and minimize pharmacokinetic variability, take lopinavir/ritonavir with food.

Distribution – At steady state, lopinavir is approximately 98% to 99% bound to plasma proteins. Lopinavir binds to alpha-1-acid glycoprotein (AAG) and albumin, but has a higher affinity for AAG. At steady state, lopinavir protein binding remains constant over the range of observed concentrations after 400/100 mg lopinavir/ritonavir twice daily, and is similar between healthy volunteers and HIV-positive patients.

Metabolism – In vitro experiments with human hepatic microsomes indicate that lopinavir primarily undergoes oxidative metabolism. Lopinavir is extensively metabolized by the hepatic cytochrome P450 system, almost exclusively by the CYP3A isozyme. Ritonavir is a potent CYP3A inhibitor that inhibits the metabolism of lopinavir, and therefore increases plasma levels of lopinavir. At least 13 lopinavir oxidative metabolites have been identified in man. Ritonavir has been shown to induce metabolic enzymes, resulting in the induction of its own metabolism. Pre-dose lopinavir concentrations decline with time during multiple dosing, stabilizing after approximately 10 to 16 days.

Across studies, administration of lopinavir/ritonavir 400/100 mg twice daily yields mean steady-state lopinavir plasma concentrations 15- to 20-fold higher than those of ritonavir in HIV-infected patients. The plasma levels of ritonavir are less than 7% of those obtained after the ritonavir dose of 600 mg twice daily. The in vitro antiviral 50% effective concentration (EC$_{50}$) of lopinavir is approximately 10-fold lower than that of ritonavir. Therefore, the antiviral activity of lopinavir/ritonavir combination is due to lopinavir.

Excretion – Following a 400/100 mg ^{14}C-lopinavir/ritonavir dose, approximately 10.4% and approximately 82.6% of an administered dose of ^{14}C-lopinavir can be accounted for in urine and feces, respectively, after 8 days. Unchanged lopinavir accounted for approximately 2.2% and 19.8% of the administered dose in urine and feces, respectively. After multiple dosing, less than 3% of the lopinavir dose is excreted unchanged in the urine. The half-life of lopinavir over a 12-hour dosing interval averaged 5 to 6 hours, and the apparent oral clearance (CL/F) of lopinavir is 6 to 7 L/h.

➤*Microbiology:*

Antiviral activity in vitro – The in vitro antiviral activity of lopinavir against laboratory HIV strains and clinical HIV isolates was evaluated in acutely infected lymphoblastic cell lines and peripheral blood lymphocytes, respectively. In the absence of human serum, the mean EC$_{50}$ of lopinavir against 5 different HIV-1 laboratory strains ranged from 10 to 27 nM (0.006 to 0.017 mcg/mL, 1 mcg/mL = 1.6 mcM) and ranged from 4 to 11 nM (0.003 to 0.007 mcg/mL) against several HIV-1 clinical isolates (n = 6). In the presence of 50% human serum, the mean EC$_{50}$ of lopinavir against these 5 laboratory strains ranged from 65 to 289 nM (0.04 to 0.18 mcg/mL), representing a 7- to 11-fold attenuation. Combination drug activity studies with lopinavir and other protease inhibitors or reverse transcriptase inhibitors have not been completed.

Resistance – HIV-1 isolates with reduced susceptibility to lopinavir have been selected in vitro. The presence of ritonavir does not appear to influence the selection of lopinavir-resistant viruses in vitro.

The selection of resistance to lopinavir/ritonavir in antiretroviral treatment-naive patients has not yet been characterized. In a Phase III study of 653 antiretroviral treatment-naive patients, plasma viral isolates from each patient on treatment with plasma HIV greater than 400 copies/mL at week 24, 32, 40, and/or 48 were analyzed. No evidence of resistance to lopinavir/ritonavir was observed in 37 evaluable lopinavir/ritonavir-treated patients. Evidence of genotypic resistance to nelfinavir, defined as the presence of the D30N and/or L90M mutation in HIV protease, was observed in 25/76 (33%) of evaluable nelfinavir-treated patients. The selection of resistance to lopinavir/ritonavir in antiretroviral treatment-naive pediatric patients appears to be consistent with that seen in adult patients.

LOPINAVIR/RITONAVIR

Resistance to lopinavir/ritonavir has been noted to emerge in patients treated with other protease inhibitors prior to lopinavir/ritonavir therapy. In Phase II studies of 227 antiretroviral treatment-naive and protease inhibitor-experienced patients, isolates from 4 of 23 patients with quantifiable (greater than 400 copies/mL) viral RNA following treatment for 12 to 100 weeks displayed significantly reduced susceptibility to lopinavir compared with the corresponding baseline viral isolates. Three of these patients previously had received treatment with a single protease inhibitor (nelfinavir, indinavir, or saquinavir) and 1 patient had received treatment with multiple protease inhibitors (indinavir, saquinavir, and ritonavir). All 4 of these patients had at least 4 mutations associated with protease inhibitor resistance immediately prior to lopinavir/ritonavir therapy. Following viral rebound, isolates from these patients all contained additional mutations, some of which are recognized to be associated with protease inhibitor resistance. However, there are insufficient data at this time to identify lopinavir-associated mutational patterns in isolates from patients on lopinavir/ritonavir therapy. The assessment of these mutational patterns is under study.

Cross-resistance (preclinical studies) – Varying degrees of cross-resistance have been observed among protease inhibitors. Little information is available on the cross-resistance of viruses that developed decreased susceptibility to lopinavir during therapy.

The in vitro activity of lopinavir against clinical isolates from patients previously treated with a single protease inhibitor was determined. Isolates that displayed greater than 4-fold reduced susceptibiltiy to nelfinavir (n = 13) and saquinavir (n = 4) displayed less than 4-fold reduced susceptibility to lopinavir. Isolates with greater than 4-fold reduced susceptibility to indinavir (n = 16) and ritonavir (n = 3) displayed a mean of 5.7- and 8.3-fold reduced susceptibility to lopinavir, respectively. Isolates from patients previously treated with 2 or more protease inhibitors showed greater reductions in susceptibility to lopinavir.

Contraindications

Hypersensitivity to any of its ingredients, including ritonavir.

Coadministration of lopinavir/ritonavir is contraindicated with drugs that are highly dependent on CYP3A or CYP2D6 for clearance and for which elevated plasma concentrations are associated with serious and/or life-threatening events (see Drug Interactions). These drugs include the following: Flecainide, propafenone, dihydroergotamine, ergonovine, ergotamine, methylergonovine, pimozide, midazolam, cisapride, triazolam.

Warnings

➤*Hepatic function impairment:* Lopinavir/ritonavir is principally metabolized by the liver; therefore, exercise caution when administering this drug to patients with hepatic impairment because lopinavir concentrations may be increased. Patients with underlying hepatitis B or C or marked elevations in transaminases prior to treatment may be at increased risk for developing further transaminase elevations or hepatic decompensation. There have been postmarketing reports of hepatic dysfunction, including some fatalities. These have generally occurred in patients with advanced HIV disease taking multiple concomitant medications in the setting of underlying chronic hepatitis or cirrhosis. A causal relationship with lopinavir/ritonavir therapy has not been established. Consider increased AST/ALT monitoring in these patients, especially during the first several months of lopinavir/ritonavir treatment.

➤*Carcinogenesis:* In male mice, at levels of 50, 100, or 200 mg/kg/day of ritonavir, there was a dose-dependent increase in the incidence of both adenomas and combined adenomas and carcinomas in the liver. Based on AUC measurements, the exposure for males at the high dose was approximately 4-fold that of the exposure in humans with the recommended therapeutic dose (400/100 mg lopinavir/ritonavir twice daily). There were no carcinogenic effects seen in females at the dosages tested. The exposure for females at the high dose was approximately 9-fold that of the exposure in humans. In rats dosed at levels of 7, 15, or 30 mg/kg/day, there were no carcinogenic effects. In this study, the exposure at the high dose was approximately 0.7-fold that of the exposure in humans with 400/100 mg lopinavir/ritonavir twice-daily regimen. Based on the exposures achieved in the animal studies, the significance of the observed effects is not known.

➤*Elderly:* Exercise appropriate caution in the administration and monitoring of lopinavir/ritonavir in elderly patients, reflecting the greater frequency of decreased hepatic, renal, or cardiac function and of concomitant disease or other drug therapy.

➤*Pregnancy: Category C.* There are no adequate and well-controlled studies in pregnant women. Use lopinavir/ritonavir during pregnancy only if the potential benefit justifies the potential risk to the fetus. To monitor maternal-fetal outcomes of pregnant women exposed to lopinavir/ritonavir, an antiretroviral pregnancy registry has been established. Physicians are encouraged to register patients by calling (800) 258-4263.

➤*Lactation:* The Centers for Disease Control and Prevention recommend that HIV-infected mothers not breastfeed their infants to avoid risking postnatal transmission of HIV. Studies in rats have demonstrated that lopinavir is secreted in breast milk. It is not known whether lopinavir is secreted in human milk. Because of both the potential for HIV transmission and the potential for serious adverse reactions in nursing infants, instruct mothers not to breastfeed if they are receiving lopinavir/ritonavir.

➤*Children:* The safety and pharmacokinetic profiles of lopinavir/ritonavir in children under 6 months of age have not been established. In HIV-infected patients 6 months to 12 years of age, the adverse event profile seen during a clinical trial was similar to that for adult patients. The evaluation of the antiviral activity of lopinavir/ritonavir in pediatric patients in clinical trials is ongoing.

Precautions

➤*Pancreatitis:* Pancreatitis has been observed in patients receiving lopinavir/ritonavir therapy, including those who developed marked triglyceride elevations. Fatalities have been observed. Although a causal relationship to lopinavir/ritonavir has not been established, marked triglyceride elevation is a risk factor for development of pancreatitis. Patients with advanced HIV disease may be at increased risk of elevated triglycerides and pancreatitis, and patients with a history of pancreatitis may be at increased risk for recurrence during therapy.

Consider pancreatitis if clinical symptoms (nausea, vomiting, abdominal pain) or abnormalities in laboratory values (eg, increased serum lipase, amylase values) suggestive of pancreatitis should occur. Evaluate patients who exhibit these signs or symptoms and suspend lopinavir/ritonavir or other antiretroviral therapy as clinically appropriate.

➤*Diabetes mellitus/hyperglycemia:* New-onset diabetes mellitus, exacerbation of pre-existing diabetes mellitus, and hyperglycemia have been reported during postmarketing surveillance in HIV-infected patients receiving protease inhibitor therapy. Some patients required initiation or dose adjustments of insulin or oral hypoglycemic agents for treatment of these events. In some cases, diabetic ketoacidosis has occurred. In those patients who discontinued protease inhibitor therapy, hyperglycemia persisted in some cases. Because these events have been reported voluntarily during clinical practice, estimates of frequency cannot be made. A causal relationship between protease inhibitor therapy and these events has not been established.

➤*Resistance/Cross-resistance:* Various degrees of cross-resistance among protease inhibitors have been observed. The effect of lopinavir/ritonavir therapy on the efficacy of subsequently administered protease inhibitors is under investigation.

➤*Hemophilia:* There have been reports of increased bleeding, including spontaneous skin hematomas and hemarthrosis, in patients with hemophilia type A and B treated with protease inhibitors. In some patients, additional factor VIII was given. In more than 50% of the reported cases, treatment with protease inhibitors was continued or reintroduced. A causal relationship between protease inhibitor therapy and these events has not been established.

➤*Fat redistribution:* Redistribution/accumulation of body fat including central obesity, dorsocervical fat enlargement (buffalo hump), peripheral wasting, facial wasting, breast enlargement, and "cushingoid appearance" have been observed in patients receiving antiretroviral therapy. The mechanism and long-term consequences of these events are currently unknown. A causal relationship has not been established.

➤*Lipid elevations:* Treatment with lopinavir/ritonavir has resulted in large increases in the concentration of total cholesterol and triglycerides. Perform triglyceride and cholesterol testing prior to initiating therapy and at periodic intervals during therapy. Manage lipid disorders as clinically appropriate.

Drug Interactions

➤*CYP 450:* Lopinavir/ritonavir is an inhibitor of the P450 isoform CYP3A in vitro. Coadministration of the combination and drugs primarily metabolized by CYP3A may result in increased plasma concentrations of the other drug, which could increase or prolong its therapeutic and adverse effects.

Lopinavir/ritonavir inhibits CYP2D6 in vitro, but to a lesser extent than CYP3A. Clinically significant drug interactions with drugs metabolized by CYP2D6 are possible with the combination at the recommended dose, but the magnitude is not known. Lopinavir/ritonavir does not inhibit CYP2C9, CYP2C19, CYP2E1, CYP2B6, or CYP1A2 at clinically relevant concentrations.

Lopinavir/ritonavir has been shown in vivo to induce its own metabolism and to increase the biotransformation of some drugs metabolized by cytochrome P450 enzymes and by glucuronidation.

Lopinavir/ritonavir is metabolized by CYP3A. Drugs that induce CYP3A activity would be expected to increase the clearance of lopinavir, resulting in lowered plasma concentrations of lopinavir. Although not noted with concurrent ketoconazole, coadministration of lopinavir/ritonavir and other drugs that inhibit CYP3A may increase lopinavir plasma concentrations.

LOPINAVIR/RITONAVIR

Lopinavir and Ritonavir Drug Interactions			
Precipitant drug	Object drug*		Description
Anticonvulsants (eg, carbamazepine, pheno-barbital, phenytoin)	Lopinavir	↓	Use with caution. Lopinavir/Ritonavir may be less effective because of decreased lopinavir plasma concentrations in patients taking these agents concomitantly.
Azole antifungals	Ritonavir	↑	Plasma ritonavir concentrations may be elevated, increasing the risk of toxicity.
Corticosteroids (eg, dexa-methasone)	Lopinavir	↓	Use with caution. Lopinavir/Ritonavir may be less effective because of decreased lopinavir plasma concentrations in patients taking these agents concomitantly.
Delavirdine	Lopinavir	↔	Appropriate doses of the combination with respect to safety and efficacy have not been established.
Efavirenz Nevirapine	Lopinavir Ritonavir	↓	Plasma levels and clinical efficacy may be reduced. Consider a dose increase of lopinavir/ritonavir to 533/133 mg (4 capsules or 6.5 mL) twice daily taken with food when used in combination with efavirenz or nevirapine in patients where reduced susceptibility to lopinavir is clinically suspected (by treatment history or laboratory evidence) (see Administration and Dosage). Note: Efavirenz and nevirapine induce the activity of CYP3A and thus have the potential to decrease plasma concentrations of other protease inhibitors when used in combination with lopinavir/ritonavir.
Rifabutin	Ritonavir	↓	Rifamycins may decrease ritonavir serum concentrations.
Rifampin	Lopinavir Ritonavir	↓	May lead to loss of virologic response and possible resistance to lopinavir/ritonavir or to the protease inhibitors class or other coadministered antiretroviral agents when administered with rifampin. Avoid coadministration.
St. John's wort (Hypericum perforatum)	Lopinavir Ritonavir	↓	Concomitant use of lopinavir/ritonavir and St. John's wort or products containing St. John's wort, is not recommended. Coadministration of protease inhibitors, including lopinavir/ritonavir with St. John's wort, is expected to substantially decrease protease inhibitor concentrations and may result in suboptimal levels of lopinavir and lead to loss of virologic response and possible resistance to lopinavir or to the protease inhibitors class.
Lopinavir	Atovaquone	↔	Clinical significance is unknown; however, increase in atovaquone doses may be needed.
Lopinavir	Calcium channel blockers, dihydropyridine (eg, felo-dipine, nifedipine, nicardi-pine)	↑	Caution is warranted and clinical monitoring of patients is recommended.
Lopinavir	HMG-CoA reductase inhibitors (eg, atorvastatin, lovastatin, simvastatin)	↑	Use lowest possible dose of atorvastatin with careful monitoring, or consider other HMG-CoA reductase inhibitors such as pravastatin or fluvastatin in combination with lopinavir/ritonavir. Avoid coadministration because of potential for serious reactions, such as risk of myopathy including rhabdomyolysis.
Lopinavir	Ketoconazole Itraconazole	↑	High doses of ketoconazole or itraconazole (> 200 mg/day) are not recommended.
Lopinavir	Pimozide	↑	Contraindicated because of potential serious and/or life-threatening reactions (eg, cardiac arrhythmias).
Lopinavir Ritonavir	Antiarrhythmics (eg, fle-cainide, propafenone, amiodarone, bepridil, lido-caine [systemic], quini-dine)	↑	Amiodarone, flecainide, and propafenone are contraindicated because of the potential for serious and/or life-threatening reactions such as cardiac arrhythmia. Caution is warranted and therapeutic concentration monitoring is recommended for antiarrhythmics when coadministered with lopinavir/ritonavir, if available.
Lopinavir Ritonavir	Cisapride	↑	Contraindicated because of potential for serious and/or life-threatening reactions such as cardiac arrhythmias.
Lopinavir Ritonavir	Clarithromycin	↑	Clarithromycin AUC increased by 77% and C_{max} by 31% with coadministration of ritonavir. For patients with renal impairment, consider the following dosage adjustments: For patients with Ccr 30 to 60 mL/min, reduce the dose of clarithromycin by 50%. For patients with Ccr < 30 mL/min, reduce the dose of clarithromycin by 75%. No dose adjustment for patients with normal renal function is necessary.
Lopinavir Ritonavir	Disulfiram Metronidazole	↑	Lopinavir/Ritonavir oral solution contains alcohol, which can produce disulfiram-like reactions when coadministered with disulfiram or other drugs that produce this reaction (eg, metronidazole).
Lopinavir Ritonavir	Ergot derivatives (eg, dihydroergotamine, ergonovine, ergotamine, methylergonovine)	↑	Contraindicated because of potential for serious and/or life-threatening reactions, such as acute ergot toxicity characterized by peripheral vasospasm and ischemia of the extremities and other tissues.
Lopinavir Ritonavir	HIV protease inhibitors (amprenavir, indinavir, saquinavir)	↔	Amprenavir 750 mg BID and indinavir 600 mg BID, when coadministered with lopinavir/ritonavir 400/100 mg BID, may produce a similar AUC, lower C_{max}, and higher C_{min} compared with their respective established clinical dosing regimens. Saquinavir 800 mg BID, when coadministered with lopinavir/ritonavir 400/100 mg BID, may produce a similar AUC and higher C_{min} to its respective established clinical dosing regimen (no comparative information regarding C_{max}). The clinical significance of the lower C_{max} and higher C_{min} is unknown. Appropriate doses of amprenavir, indinavir, and saquinavir in combination with lopinavir/ritonavir with respect to safety and efficacy have not been established.
Lopinavir Ritonavir	Immunosuppressants (eg, cyclosporine, tacrolimus, rapamycin)	↑	Therapeutic concentration monitoring is recommended for immunosuppressant agents when coadministered with lopinavir/ritonavir.
Lopinavir Ritonavir	Midazolam Triazolam	↑	Contraindicated because of potential serious and/or life-threatening reactions such as prolonged or increased sedation or respiratory depression.
Lopinavir Ritonavir	Narcotic analgesics (eg, propoxyphene, metha-done, fentanyl, meperi-dine)	↓	Dosage of methadone may need to be increased when coadministered with lopinavir/ritonavir. Plasma concentrations of propoxyphene and fentanyl may be increased possibly, causing toxicity. Meperidine levels may decrease, possibly decreasing efficacy but increasing neurologic toxicity. Concurrent use of propoxyphene or meperidine is contraindicated with ritonavir.
Lopinavir Ritonavir	Oral contraceptives (eg, ethinyl estradiol)	↓	Use alternative or additional contraceptive measures when estrogen-based oral contraceptives and lopinavir/ritonavir are coadministered.
Lopinavir Ritonavir	Rifabutin and rifabutin metabolite	↑	Dosage reduction of rifabutin by at least 75% of the usual dose of 300 mg/day is recommended (ie, a maximum dose of 150 mg every other day or 3 times/week). Increased monitoring for adverse events is warranted in patients receiving the combination. Further dosage reduction of rifabutin may be necessary.
Lopinavir Ritonavir	Sildenafil	↑	Use with caution at reduced doses of 25 mg sildenafil every 48 hours with increased monitoring for adverse events.

LOPINAVIR/RITONAVIR

Lopinavir and Ritonavir Drug Interactions			
Precipitant drug	Object drug*		Description
Lopinavir Ritonavir	Warfarin	↓	The anticoagulant effect of warfarin may be decreased. Carefully monitor the international normalized ratio when starting or stopping a protease inhibitor.
Ritonavir	Bupropion	↑	Increased serum bupropion concentrations may occur, increasing bupropion toxicity. Ritonavir is contraindicated in patients taking bupropion.
Ritonavir	Clozapine	↑	Increases of serum concentrations may occur, possibly increasing clozapine toxicity.
Ritonavir	Desipramine	↑	Concurrent use increased the desipramine AUC by 145% and the C_{max} by 22%. Dosage reduction and concentration monitoring of desipramine is recommended.
Ritonavir	Piroxicam	↑	Large increases in serum piroxicam concentrations may occur, increasing piroxicam toxicity. Concomitant use is contraindicated.
Ritonavir	Quinidine	↑	Large increases in serum quinidine concentrations may occur, increasing the risk of quinidine toxicity. Concurrent use is contraindicated.
Ritonavir	Theophylline	↓	Coadministration decreased the theophylline AUC by 43% and the C_{max} by 27%.
Ritonavir	Zolpidem	↓	Possibly severe sedation and respiratory depression may occur. Coadministration is contraindicated.

* ↑ = Object drug increased.   ↓ = Object drug decreased.   ↔ = Undetermined clinical effect.

➤*Drug / Food interactions:*

Didanosine – It is recommended that didanosine be administered on an empty stomach; therefore, give didanosine 1 hour before or 2 hours after lopinavir/ritonavir (give with food).

Adverse Reactions

The most common adverse event associated with lopinavir/ritonavir therapy was diarrhea (generally of mild to moderate severity).

Lopinavir/Ritonavir Adverse Reactions of Moderate or Severe Intensity in Adult Patients (≥ 2%)			
	Antiretroviral-naive patients			Protease inhibitor-experienced patients
Adverse reaction	Lopinavir/Ritonavir 400/100 mg BID + d4T* + 3TC* (N = 326)[1]	Nelfinavir 750 mg TID + d4T* + 3TC* (N = 327)[1]	Lopinavir/Ritonavir BID[2] + d4T* + 3TC* (N = 84)[3]	Lopinavir/Ritonavir BID[4] + NNRTI + NRTIs* (N = 186)
CNS				
Headache	2.5	1.8	7.1	1.6
Insomnia	1.5	1.2	2.4	1.1
GI				
Abdominal pain	4	3.1	4.8	1.6
Abnormal stools	0	0.3	6	1.6
Diarrhea	15.6	17.1	23.8	15.6
Dyspepsia	2.1	0.3	1.2	0.5
Nausea	6.7	4.6	15.5	2.7
Vomiting	2.5	2.4	4.8	1.6
Miscellaneous				
Asthenia	4	3.4	7.1	5.4
Pain	0.6	0	2.4	1.6
Rash	0.6	1.5	3.6	2

* d4T = stavudine; 3TC = lamivudine; NRTIs = nucleoside reverse transcriptase inhibitors; NNRTI = nonnucleoside reverse transcriptase inhibitor
[1] Study performed over the course of 48 weeks.
[2] Includes adverse event data from dose group I (400/100 mg BID only [N = 16]) and dose group II (400/100 mg BID [N = 35] and 400/200 mg BID [N = 33]). Within dosing groups, moderate to severe nausea of probable/possible relationship to lopinavir/ritonavir occurred at a higher rate in the 400/200 mg dose arm compared with the 400/100 mg dose arm in group II.

[3] Study performed over the course of 72 weeks.
[4] Includes adverse event data from patients receiving 400/100 mg BID, 400/200 mg BID, and 533/133 mg BID for 16 to 72 weeks. All 186 patients received lopinavir/ritonavir in combination with NRTIs and either nevirapine or efavirenz.

Adverse events occurring in less than 2% of adult patients receiving lopinavir/ritonavir are as follows:

➤*Cardiovascular:* Deep vein thrombosis; hypertension; palpitation; thrombophlebitis; vasculitis.

➤*CNS:* Abnormal dreams; agitation; amnesia; anxiety; ataxia; confusion; depression; dizziness; dyskinesia; emotional lability; encephalopathy; hypertonia; libido decreased; nervousness; neuropathy; paresthesia; peripheral neuritis; somnolence; abnormal thinking; tremor; migraine; facial paralysis.

➤*Dermatologic:* Acne; alopecia; dry skin; exfoliative dermatitis; furunculosis; maculopapular rash; nail disorder; pruritus; skin benign neoplasm; skin discoloration; sweating; eczema; seborrhea; skin ulcer.

➤*Endocrine:* Cushing syndrome; hypothyroidism; diabetes mellitus.

➤*GI:* Anorexia; cholecystitis; constipation; dry mouth; dyspepsia; dysphagia; enterocolitis; eructation; esophagitis; fecal incontinence; flatulence; gastritis; gastroenteritis; GI disorder; hemorrhagic colitis; increased appetite; pancreatitis; sialadenitis; stomatitis; ulcerative stomatitis; enlarged abdomen; mouth ulceration.

➤*GU:* Abnormal ejaculation; gynecomastia; hypogonadism (male); kidney calculus; urine abnormality.

➤*Hematologic / Lymphatic:* Anemia; leukopenia; lymphadenopathy.

LOPINAVIR/RITONAVIR

➤*Lab test abnormalities:*

		Grade 3 to 4 Lopinavir/Ritonavir Lab Test Abnormalities in Adult Patients (≥ 2%)			
		Antiretroviral-naive patients			Antiretroviral-experienced patients
Variable	Limit[1]	Lopinavir/Ritonavir 400/100 mg BID + d4T* + 3TC* (N = 326)[2]	Nelfinavir 750 mg TID + d4T* + 3TC* (N = 327)[2]	Lopinavir/Ritonavir BID[3] + d4T* + 3TC* (N = 84)[4]	Lopinavir/Ritonavir BID[5] + NNRTI* + NRTIs* (N = 186)
Glucose	> 250 mg/dL	2.2	1.6	2.4	4.4
Uric acid	> 12 mg/dL	2.2	1.6	3.6	0.5
AST	> 180 U/L	2.2	4.1	9.5	5.5
ALT	> 215 U/L	3.8	3.8	8.3	7.1
GGT	> 300 U/L	N/A	N/A	3.6	24.6[6]
Total cholesterol	> 300 mg/dL	9	5	14.3	28.4
Triglycerides	> 750 mg/dL	9.3	1.3	10.7	28.4
Amylase	> 2 × ULN	3.2	2.2	4.8	4.9
Inorganic phosphorus	< 1.5 mg/dL	0	0	0	2.2
Neutrophils	0.75 × 10⁹/L	0.6	2.5	2.4	2.7

* d4T = stavudine; 3TC = lamivudine; NRTIs = nucleoside reverse transcriptase inhibitors; NNRTI = nonnucleoside reverse transcriptase inhibitor; N/A = not applicable
[1] ULN = upper limit of normal range.
[2] Study performed over the course of 48 weeks.
[3] Includes clinical laboratory data from dose group I (400/100 mg BID only [N = 16]) and dose group II (400/100 mg BID [N = 35] and 400/200 mg BID [N = 33]).
[4] Study performed over the course of 72 weeks.
[5] Includes clinical laboratory data from patients receiving 400/100 mg BID, 400/200 mg BID, and 533/133 mg BID for 16 to 72 weeks. All 186 patients received lopinavir/ritonavir in combination with NRTIs and either nevirapine or efavirenz.
[6] GGT was only measured in 69 patients receiving 400/100 mg BID or 400/200 mg BID in combination with nevirapine.

➤*Metabolic / Nutritional:* Avitaminosis; dehydration; edema; glucose tolerance, decreased; lactic acidosis; obesity; peripheral edema; weight loss; weight gain.

➤*Musculoskeletal:* Arthralgia; arthrosis; myalgia.

➤*Respiratory:* Bronchitis; dyspnea; lung edema; sinusitis; rhinitis.

➤*Special senses:* Abnormal vision; eye disorder; otitis media; taste perversion; tinnitus.

➤*Miscellaneous:* Back pain; chest pain; substernal chest pain; chills; drug interaction; drug level increased; face edema; fever; flu syndrome; malaise; viral infection; cyst; hypertrophy; bacterial infection; varicose vein.

➤*Postmarketing:* Redistribution/Accumulation of body fat has been reported (see Precautions).

➤*Children:* The adverse event profile seen during a clinical trial was similar to that for adults. Rash (3%) was the only drug-related clinical adverse event of moderate or severe intensity in 2% or more of pediatric patients enrolled.

		Grade 3 to 4 Lopinavir/Ritonavir Lab Test Abnormalities in Children (≥ 2%)
Variable	Limit[1]	Lopinavir/Ritonavir BID + RTIs* (N = 100)
Sodium, high	> 149 mEq/L	3
Total bilirubin	≥ 3 × ULN	3
AST	> 180 U/L	8
ALT	> 215 U/L	7
Total cholesterol	> 300 mg/dL	3
Amylase	> 2.5 × ULN	7[2]
Sodium, low	< 130 mEq/L	3
Platelet count	< 50 × 10⁹/L	4
Neutrophils	< 0.4 × 10⁹/L	2

* RTIs = reverse transcriptase inhibitors
[1] ULN = upper limit of normal range.
[2] Subjects with Grade 3 to 4 amylase confirmed by elevations in pancreatic amylase.

Overdosage

Lopinavir/ritonavir oral solution contains 42.4% alcohol (v/v). Accidental ingestion of the product by a young child could result in significant alcohol-related toxicity and could approach the potential lethal dose of alcohol.

➤*Treatment:* Treatment of overdose with lopinavir/ritonavir should consist of general supportive measures, including monitoring of vital signs and observation of the clinical status of the patient. There is no specific antidote for overdose with lopinavir/ritonavir. If indicated, elimination of unabsorbed drug should be achieved by emesis or gastric lavage. Administration of activated charcoal also may be used to aid in removal of unabsorbed drug. Because lopinavir/ritonavir is highly protein bound, dialysis is unlikely to be beneficial in significant removal of the drug. Refer to Management of Acute Overdosage.

Patient Information

A patient package insert for lopinavir/ritonavir is available for patient information.

Inform patients that sustained decreases in plasma HIV RNA have been associated with a reduced risk of progression to AIDS and death. Patients should remain under the care of a physician while using lopinavir/ritonavir. Advise patients to take lopinavir/ritonavir and other concomitant antiretroviral therapy every day as prescribed. It must always be used in combination with other antiretroviral drugs. Patients should not alter the dose or discontinue therapy without consulting their doctor. If a dose is missed, patients should take the dose as soon as possible and then return to their normal schedule. However, if a dose is skipped, the patient should not double the next dose.

Inform patients that lopinavir/ritonavir is not a cure for HIV infection and that they may continue to develop opportunistic infections and other complications associated with HIV disease. The long-term effects of lopinavir/ritonavir are unknown at this time. There are currently no data demonstrating that therapy with lopinavir/ritonavir can reduce the risk of transmitting HIV to others through sexual contact.

Lopinavir/ritonavir may interact with some drugs; therefore, advise patients to report to their doctor the use of any other prescription or nonprescription medication or herbal product, particularly St. John's wort.

Patients taking didanosine should take didanosine 1 hour before or 2 hours after lopinavir/ritonavir.

Advise patients receiving sildenafil that they may be at an increased risk of sildenafil-associated adverse events, including hypotension, visual changes, and sustained erection, and to promptly report any symptoms to their doctor.

Instruct patients receiving estrogen-based hormonal contraceptives to use additional or alternate contraceptive measures during therapy.

Take with food to enhance absorption.

Inform patients that redistribution or accumulation of body fat may occur in patients receiving antiretroviral therapy, including protease inhibitors, and that the cause and long-term health effects of these conditions are not known at this time.

Nucleotide Analog Reverse Transcriptase Inhibitor

TENOFOVIR DISOPROXIL FUMARATE (PMPA)

Rx	**Viread** (Gilead Sciences)	**Tablets**: 300 mg (equivalent to 245 mg tenofovir disoproxil)	Lactose. (GILEAD 4331 300). Light blue, almond shape. Film-coated. In 30s.

WARNING

Lactic acidosis and severe hepatomegaly with steatosis, including fatal cases, have been reported with the use of nucleoside analogs alone or in combination with other antiretrovirals (see Warnings).

Indications

➤*HIV infection:* In combination with other antiretroviral agents for the treatment of HIV-1 infection.

Administration and Dosage

➤*Approved by the FDA:* October 26, 2001.

➤*Dosage:* 300 mg once daily taken orally without regard to food.

➤*Renal function impairment:* Significantly increased drug exposures occurred when tenofovir was administered to patients with moderate to severe renal impairment. Adjust the dosing interval of tenofovir in patients with baseline creatinine clearance (Ccr) less than 50 mL/min using the recommendations in the following table. The safety and effectiveness of these dosing interval adjustment recommendations have not been clinically evaluated, therefore, closely monitor clinical response to treatment and renal function in these patients.

Tenofovir Dosage Adjustment for Patients with Altered Ccr				
	Ccr (mL/min)[a]			Hemodialysis patients
	≥ 50	30 to 49	10 to 29	
Recommended 300 mg dosing interval	Every 24 hours	Every 48 hours	Twice a week	Every 7 days or after a total of ≈ 12 hours of dialysis[b]

[a] Calculated using ideal (lean) body weight.
[b] Generally once weekly assuming 3 hemodialysis sessions/week of approximately 4-hours duration. Administer tenofovir following completion of dialysis.

The pharmacokinetics of tenofovir have not been evaluated in nonhemodialysis patients with Ccr less than 10 mL/min; therefore, no dosing recommendation is available for these patients.

➤*Storage/Stability:* Store at 25°C (77°F); excursions permitted to 15° to 30°C (59° to 86°F).

Actions

➤*Pharmacology:* Tenofovir disoproxil fumarate is an acyclic nucleoside phosphonate diester analog of adenosine monophosphate. Tenofovir disoproxil fumarate requires initial diester hydrolysis for conversion to tenofovir and subsequent phosphorylations by cellular enzymes to form tenofovir diphosphate. Tenofovir diphosphate inhibits the activity of HIV-1 reverse transcriptase by competing with the natural substrate deoxyadenosine 5'-triphosphate and, after incorporation into DNA, by DNA chain termination.

➤*Pharmacokinetics:*

Absorption – The oral bioavailability of tenofovir in fasted patients is approximately 25%. Following oral administration of a single 300 mg dose of tenofovir disoproxil to HIV-1 infected patients in the fasted state, maximum serum concentrations (C_{max}) are achieved in approximately 1 hour. C_{max} and AUC values are approximately 296 ng/mL and approximately 2287 ng•h/mL, respectively.

Administration of tenofovir disoproxil following a high-fat meal increases the oral bioavailability with an increase in tenofovir $AUC_{0-\infty}$ of approximately 40% and an increase in C_{max} of approximately 14%. Food delays the time to C_{max} by approximately 1 hour. C_{max} and AUC of tenofovir are approximately 326 ng/mL and approximately 3324 ng•h/mL following multiple doses of tenofovir 300 mg/day in the fed state.

Distribution – In vitro binding of tenofovir to human plasma or serum proteins is less than 0.7% and 7.2%, respectively. The volume of distribution at steady state is approximately 1.3 L/kg and 1.2 L/kg following IV administration of tenofovir 1 and 3 mg/kg, respectively.

Metabolism/Excretion – In vitro studies indicate that neither tenofovir disoproxil nor tenofovir are substrates of CYP450 enzymes. Following IV administration of tenofovir, approximately 70% to 80% of the dose is recovered in the urine as unchanged tenofovir within 72 hours of dosing. Following a single oral dose of tenofovir, the terminal elimination half-life is approximately 17 hours. After multiple oral doses of tenofovir 300 mg/day (under fed conditions), approximately 32% of the administered dose is recovered in urine over 24 hours. Tenofovir is eliminated by a combination of glomerular filtration and active tubular secretion. There may be competition for elimination with other compounds that are also renally eliminated.

Special populations –
Renal function impairment: In patients with Ccr less than 50 mL/min or with end-stage renal disease requiring dialysis, C_{max} and AUC of tenofovir were increased to approximately 372 to 601 ng/mL and

6008 to 15,984 ng•h/mL, respectively. It is recommended that the dosing interval be modified in these patients.

Tenofovir is efficiently removed by hemodialysis with an extraction coefficient of approximately 54%. Following a single 300 mg dose, a 4-hour hemodialysis session removed approximately 10% of the administered tenofovir dose (see Administration and Dosage).

➤*Microbiology:*

Antiviral activity in vitro – In drug combination studies of tenofovir with nucleoside and non-nucleoside reverse transcriptase inhibitors, and protease inhibitors, additive to synergistic effects were observed.

Drug resistance – HIV-1 isolates with reduced susceptibility to tenofovir have been selected in vitro. These viruses expressed a K65R mutation in reverse transcriptase and showed a 3- to 4-fold reduction in susceptibility to tenofovir.

Tenofovir-resistant isolates of HIV-1 have also been recovered from some patients treated with tenofovir in combination with certain antiretroviral agents. In treatment-naive patients treated with tenofovir + lamivudine + efavirenz, viral isolates from 24% of patients with virologic failure showed reduced susceptibility to tenofovir. In treatment-experienced patients, 4.6% of the tenofovir-treated patients with virologic failure showed reduced susceptibility to tenofovir. Genotypic analysis of the resistant isolates showed a mutation in the HIV-1 reverse transcriptase gene resulting in the K65R amino acid substitution.

Cross-resistance – Cross-resistance among certain reverse transcriptase inhibitors has been recognized. The K65R mutation selected by tenofovir also is selected in some HIV-1 infected subjects treated with abacavir, didanosine, or zalcitabine. HIV isolates with this mutation also show reduced susceptibility to emtricitabine and lamivudine. Therefore, cross-resistance among these drugs may occur in patients whose virus harbors the K65R mutation. HIV-1 isolates from patients (n = 20) whose HIV-1 expressed a mean of 3 zidovudine-associated reverse transcriptase mutations (M41L, D67N, K70R, L210W, T215Y/F, or K219Q/E/N), showed a 3.1-fold decrease in the susceptibility to tenofovir. Multinucleoside resistant HIV-1 with a T69S double insertion mutation in the reverse transcriptase showed reduced susceptibility to tenofovir.

➤*Clinical trials:* Data through 48 weeks are reported for a double-blind, active-controlled multicenter study comparing tenofovir (300 mg QD) administered in combination with lamivudine and efavirenz vs stavudine, lamivudine, and efavirenz in 600 antiretroviral-naive patients. The mean baseline CD4 cell count was 279 cells/mm³ and median baseline plasma HIV-1 RNA was 77,600 copies/mL. Forty-three percent of patients had baseline viral loads greater than 100,000 copies/mL and 39% had CD4 cell counts lower than 200 cells/mL. Achievement of plasma HIV-1 RNA concentrations of less than 400 copies/mL at week 48 was similar between the 2 treatment groups. Through 48 weeks of therapy, 76% and 79% of patients in the tenofovir and stavudine arms, respectively, achieved HIV-1 RNA less than 50 copies/mL. The mean increase from baseline in CD4 cell count was 169 cells/mm³ for the tenofovir arm and 167 cells/mm³ for the stavudine arm.

Contraindications

Previously demonstrated hypersensitivity to any of the components of the product.

Warnings

➤*Coinfection:* It is recommended that all patients with HIV be tested for the presence of hepatitis B virus (HBV) before initiating antiretroviral therapy. Tenofovir is not indicated for the treatment of chronic HBV infection and the safety and efficacy of tenofovir have not been established in patients coinfected with HBV and HIV. Exacerbations of HBV have been reported in patients after the discontinuation of tenofovir. Closely monitor patients coinfected with HBV and HIV with both clinical and laboratory follow-up for at least several months after stopping tenofovir treatment.

➤*Lactic acidosis/severe hepatomegaly with steatosis:* Lactic acidosis and severe hepatomegaly with steatosis, including fatal cases, have been reported with the use of nucleoside analogs alone or in combination with other antiretrovirals. A majority of these cases have been in women. Obesity and prolonged nucleoside exposure may be risk factors. Exercise particular caution when administering nucleoside analogs to any patient with known risk factors for liver disease. Cases also have been reported in patients with no known risk factors. Suspend treatment with tenofovir in any patient who develops clinical or laboratory findings suggestive of lactic acidosis or pronounced hepatotoxicity, which may include hepatomegaly and steatosis even in the absence of marked transaminase elevations (see Warning Box).

➤*Virologic failure:* A high rate of early virologic failure and emergence of nucleoside reverse transcriptase inhibitor (NRTI) resistance mutations have been observed in studies of HIV-infected treatment-naive patients receiving once-daily 3-drug combination therapies with either lamivu-

TENOFOVIR DISOPROXIL FUMARATE (PMPA)

dine, abacavir, and tenofovir or didanosine, lamivudine and tenofovir. Overall, these studies demonstrate a lower response rate in patients on a triple NRTI regimen and indicate that patients who achieve viral suppression on a triple NRTI regimen have a higher rate of virologic failure. Based on the results of these studies, it is recommended not to use abacavir and lamivudine or didanosine and lamivudine in combination with tenofovir as a triple antiretroviral therapy when considering a new treatment regimen for therapy-naive or pretreated patients with HIV infection. Closely monitor any patient currently controlled with either of these combinations and consider modification of therapy. Also closely monitor for signs of treatment failure any time one of these triple NRTI combinations is used with other antiretroviral agents.

➤*Renal function impairment:* Tenofovir is principally eliminated by the kidney. Dosing interval adjustment is recommended in all patients with Ccr less than 50 mL/min (see Administration and Dosage). No safety data are available in patients with renal dysfunction who received tenofovir using these dosing guidelines.

Renal impairment, including cases of acute renal failure and Fanconi syndrome (renal tubular injury with severe hypophosphatemia), has been reported in association with the use of tenofovir (see Adverse Reactions, Postmarketing). The majority of these cases occurred in patients with underlying systemic or renal disease or in patients taking nephrotoxic agents; however, some cases occurred in patients without identified risk factors.

Avoid tenofovir with concurrent or recent use of a nephrotoxic agent. Carefully monitor patients at risk for, or with a history of, renal dysfunction and patients receiving concomitant nephrotoxic agents for changes in serum creatinine and phosphorus.

➤*Mutagenesis:* Tenofovir was mutagenic in the in vitro mouse lymphoma assay and negative in an in vitro bacterial mutagenicity test (Ames test). In an in vivo mouse micronucleus assay, tenofovir was negative when administered to male mice.

➤*Fertility impairment:* There was an alteration of the estrous cycle in female rats at a dose equivalent to 19 times the human dose based on body surface area.

➤*Elderly:* In general, be cautious with dose selection for the elderly patient, keeping in mind the greater frequency of decreased hepatic, renal, or cardiac function, and of concomitant disease or other drug therapy.

➤*Pregnancy:* Category B. There are no adequate and well-controlled studies in pregnant women. Use during pregnancy only if clearly needed.

Antiretroviral Pregnancy Registry – To monitor fetal outcomes of pregnant women exposed to tenofovir, an Antiretroviral Pregnancy Registry has been established. Health care providers are encouraged to register patients by calling (800) 258-4263.

➤*Lactation:* The Centers for Disease Control and Prevention recommend that HIV-infected mothers not breastfeed their infants to avoid risking postnatal transmission of HIV. Studies in rats have demonstrated that tenofovir is secreted in milk. It is not known whether tenofovir is excreted in human milk. Because of the potential for HIV transmission and the potential for serious adverse reactions, instruct mothers not to breastfeed if they are receiving tenofovir.

➤*Children:* Safety and efficacy in pediatric patients have not been established.

Precautions

➤*Bone toxicity:* In a 48-week, active-controlled study, percent decreases in bone mineral density (BMD) from mean baseline were greater in patients receiving tenofovir plus lamivudine plus efavirenz (spine, −3.3%; hip, −3.2%) compared with patients receiving stavudine plus lamivudine plus efavirenz (spine, −2%; hip, −1.8%). The proportion of patients who met a protocol defined value of BMD loss (5% decrease in spine or 7% decrease in hip) was higher in the tenofovir group than the stavudine group. In addition, there were significant increases in levels of 4 biochemical markers of bone metabolism in the tenofovir group relative to the stavudine group, suggesting increased bone turnover. Serum parathyroid hormone levels also were higher in the tenofovir group. Except for bone specific alkaline phosphatase, these changes resulted in values that remained within the normal range. There was 1 bone fracture reported in the tenofovir group, compared with 4 in the stavudine group. The clinical significance of the changes in BMD and biochemical markers is unknown and follow-up is continuing to assess long-term impact.

Bone monitoring should be considered for HIV infected patients who have a history of pathologic bone fracture or are at substantial risk for osteopenia. Supplementation with calcium and vitamin D may be considered for HIV-associated osteopenia or osteoporosis. If bone abnormalities are suspected, obtain appropriate consultation.

➤*Fat redistribution:* Redistribution and accumulation of body fat including central obesity, dorsocervical fat enlargement (buffalo hump), peripheral wasting, facial wasting, breast enlargement, and "cushingoid appearance" have been observed in patients receiving antiretroviral therapy. The mechanism and long-term consequences of these events are currently unknown. A causal relationship has not been established.

Drug Interactions

➤*Drugs eliminated by the kidneys:* Tenofovir is primarily excreted by the kidneys by a combination of glomerular filtration and active tubular secretion. Coadministration of tenofovir with drugs that are eliminated by active tubular secretion may increase serum concentrations of tenofovir and/or the coadministered drug because of competition for this elimination pathway. Some examples include, but are not limited to, adefovir dipivoxil, cidofovir, acyclovir, valacyclovir, ganciclovir, and valganciclovir. Drugs that decrease renal function also may increase serum concentrations of tenofovir.

Tenofovir Drug Interactions			
Precipitant drug	Object drug[*]		Description
Indinavir	Tenofovir	↑	Coadministration increased tenofovir $C_{max} \approx 14\%$ but AUC remained unchanged.
Lopinavir/Ritonavir	Tenofovir	↑	Concurrent use increased tenofovir AUC by 32%.
Tenofovir	Abacavir	↑	Concurrent use increased abacavir C_{max} by 12% but AUC remained unchanged.
Tenofovir	Atazanavir	↓	Coadministration of tenofovir and unboosted atazanavir resulted in decreased concentrations of atazanavir, which may lead to loss or lack of response and possible resistance.
Tenofovir	Didanosine (buffered formulation or enteric coated)	↑	The C_{max} and AUC of didanosine (buffered formulation or enteric coated) increased when given with tenofovir. Increases in didanosine concentrations could potentiate adverse events, including pancreatitis and neuropathy.
Tenofovir	Indinavir	↓	The C_{max} of indinavir decreased $\approx 11\%$ but AUC remained unchanged.
Tenofovir	Lamivudine	↓	Concurrent use decreased lamivudine C_{max} by 24% but AUC remained unchanged.

[*] ↑ = Object drug increased. ↓ = Object drug decreased.

Adverse Reactions

➤*Treatment-experienced patients:* The most common adverse events that occurred in patients receiving tenofovir with other antiretroviral agents in clinical trials were mild to moderate GI events such as nausea, diarrhea, vomiting, and flatulence. Less than 1% discontinued participation in the clinical studies because of GI adverse events.

Tenofovir Adverse Events (Grades 2-4) (≥ 3%)			
	Tenofovir (n = 368) (week 0-24)	Placebo (n = 182) (week 0-24)	Tenofovir (n = 368) (week 0-48)	Placebo crossover to tenofovir (n = 170) (week 24-48)
CNS				
Asthenia	7	6	11	1
Headache	5	5	8	2
Depression	4	3	8	4
Peripheral neuropathy[a]	3	3	5	2
Insomnia	3	2	4	4
Dizziness	1	3	3	1
GI				
Diarrhea	11	10	16	11
Nausea	8	5	11	7
Abdominal pain	4	3	7	6
Vomiting	4	1	7	5
Anorexia	3	2	4	1
Dyspepsia	3	2	4	2
Flatulence	3	1	4	1
Skin and appendages				
Rash event[b]	5	4	7	1
Sweating	3	2	3	1
Miscellaneous				
Pain	7	7	12	4
Back pain	3	3	4	2
Myalgia	3	3	4	1
Chest pain	3	1	3	2
Fever	2	2	4	2
Weight loss	2	1	4	2
Pneumonia	2	0	3	2

[a] Peripheral neuropathy includes peripheral neuritis and neuropathy.
[b] Rash event includes rash, pruritus, maculopapular rash, urticaria, vesiculobullous rash, and pustular rash.

Nucleotide Analog Reverse Transcriptase Inhibitor

TENOFOVIR DISOPROXIL FUMARATE (PMPA)

Lab test abnormalities –

	Tenofovir (n = 368) (week 0-24)	Placebo (n = 182) (week 0-24)	Tenofovir (n = 368) (week 0-48)	Placebo crossover to tenofovir (n = 170) (week 24-48)
Any ≥ grade 3 laboratory abnormality	25	38	35	34
Triglycerides (> 750 mg/dL)	8	13	11	9
Creatine kinase (M: > 990 U/L) (F:> 845 U/L)	7	14	12	12
Serum amylase (> 175 U/L)	6	7	7	6
Urine glucose (≥ 3+)	3	3	3	2
AST (M: > 180 U/L) (F: > 170 U/L)	3	3	4	5
ALT (M: > 215 U/L) (F: > 170 U/L)	2	2	4	5
Serum glucose (> 250 U/L)	2	4	3	3
Neutrophils (< 750 mg/dL)	1	1	2	1

Table title: Tenofovir Grade 3/4 Laboratory Abnormalities (≥ 1%)

►*Treatment-naive patients:* Adverse reactions seen in treatment-naive patients were generally consistent, with the addition of dizziness, with those seen in treatment-experienced patients. Mild adverse events (grade 1) were common and included dizziness, diarrhea, and nausea.

Tenofovir Adverse Events (Grades 2-4) (≥ 3%)	Tenofovir plus 3TC plus EFV (N = 299)	d4T plus 3TC plus EFV (N = 301)
CNS		
Headache	10	11
Depression	7	5
Insomnia	4	6
Abnormal dreams	3	3
Dizziness	3	5
Paresthesia	2	3
Peripheral neuropathy[a]	1	4
GI		
Diarrhea	6	6
Nausea	5	6
Abdominal pain	4	8
Dyspepsia	3	2
Vomiting	3	6
Miscellaneous		
Rash event[b]	15	11
Pain	7	6
Fever	5	6
Back pain	4	3
Asthenia	3	5
Pneumonia	3	3
Arthralgia	2	4

[a] Peripheral neuropathy includes peripheral neuritis and neuropathy.
[b] Rash event includes rash, pruritus, maculopapular rash, urticaria, vesiculobullous rash, and pustular rash.

Lab test abnormalities –

	Tenofovir plus 3TC plus EFV (N = 299)	d4T plus 3TC plus EFV (N = 301)
Any ≥ grade 3 laboratory abnormality	28	31
Creatine kinase (M: > 990 U/L) (F: > 845 U/L)	8	9
Serum amylase (> 175 U/L)	7	6
AST (M: > 180 U/L) (F: > 170 U/L)	4	5
ALT (M: > 215 U/L) (F: > 170 U/L)	4	4
Hematuria (> 100 RBC/HPF)	4	4
Neutrophil (< 750/mm³)	3	1
Triglyceride (> 750 mg/dL)	2	8

Table title: Tenofovir Grade 3/4 Laboratory Abnormalities (≥ 1%)

►*Postmarketing:* Pancreatitis; hypophosphatemia; lactic acidosis; dyspnea; increased creatinine; renal insufficiency; kidney failure; Fanconi syndrome; allergic reaction; abdominal pain; acute renal failure; proximal tubulopathy; proteinuria; acute tubular necrosis.

Overdosage

Limited clinical experience at doses higher than the therapeutic dose of tenofovir 300 mg is available. In a study, tenofovir disoproxil fumarate 600 mg was administered to 8 patients orally for 28 days. No severe adverse reactions were reported. The effects of higher doses are not known.

If overdose occurs, monitor the patient for evidence of toxicity and apply standard supportive treatment as necessary. Tenofovir is efficiently removed by hemodialysis with an extraction coefficient of approximately 54%. Following a single 300 mg dose of tenofovir, a 4-hour hemodialysis session removed approximately 10% of the administered tenofovir dose.

Patient Information

Tenofovir does not cure HIV infection or AIDS. The long-term effects of tenofovir are not known at this time. People taking tenofovir may still get opportunistic infections or other conditions that happen with HIV infection.

Tenofovir does not reduce the risk of passing HIV to others through sexual contact or blood contamination. Instruct the patient to continue to practice safe sex and to not use or share dirty needles.

Instruct patients not to breastfeed if they are taking tenofovir.

Instruct the patient to take tenofovir with or without a meal.

The most common side effects of tenofovir are diarrhea, nausea, vomiting, and flatulence.

Changes in body fat have been seen in some patients taking anti-HIV medicine.

DIDANOSINE (ddl; dideoxyinosine)

Rx	Videx (Bristol-Myers Squibb)	Tablets, buffered, chewable/dispersible[1]: 25 mg	(VIDEX 25). Off-white to light orange/yellow, mottled. Orange flavor. In 60s.
		50 mg	(VIDEX 50). Off-white to light orange/yellow, mottled. Orange flavor. In 60s.
		100 mg	(VIDEX 100). Off-white to light orange/yellow, mottled. Orange flavor. In 60s.
		200 mg	(VIDEX 200). Off-white to light orange/yellow, mottled. Orange flavor. In 60s.
Rx	Videx EC (Bristol-Myers Squibb)	Capsules, delayed-release (with enteric-coated beadlets): 125 mg	(BMS 125 mg 6671). White. In 30s and 60s.
		200 mg	(BMS 200 mg 6672). White. In 30s and 60s.
		250 mg	(BMS 250 mg 6673). White. In 30s and 60s.
		400 mg	(BMS 400 mg 6674). White. In 30s and 60s.
Rx	Videx (Bristol-Myers Squibb)	Powder for oral solution, buffered[2]: 100 mg	In single-dose packets.
		250 mg	In single-dose packets.
		Powder for oral solution, pediatric: 2 g	In 4 oz bottles.
		4 g	In 8 oz bottles.

[1] Buffered with calcium carbonate and magnesium hydroxide. With aspartame, sorbitol, magnesium stearate, and phenylalanine (see Precautions).

[2] Buffered with dibasic sodium phosphate, sodium citrate, and citric acid. Total sodium content 1380 mg/packet. With sucrose.

WARNING

Fatal and nonfatal pancreatitis has occurred during therapy with didanosine alone or in combination regimens in treatment-naive and treatment-experienced patients, regardless of degree of immunosuppression. Suspend didanosine in patients with suspected pancreatitis, and discontinue therapy in patients with confirmed pancreatitis (see Warnings).

Lactic acidosis and severe hepatomegaly with steatosis, including fatal cases, have been reported with the use of nucleoside analogs alone or in combination, including didanosine and other antiretrovirals. Fatal lactic acidosis has been reported in pregnant women who received the combination of didanosine and stavudine with other antiretroviral agents. The combination of didanosine and stavudine should be used with caution during pregnancy and is recommended only if the potential benefit clearly outweighs the potential risk (see Warnings).

Indications

➤HIV infection:

Didanosine (Videx) – In combination with other antiretroviral agents for treatment of HIV-1 infection.

Didanosine EC (Videx EC) – In combination with other antiretroviral agents for treatment of HIV-1 infection in adults whose management requires once-daily administration of didanosine or an alternative didanosine formulation. There are limited data to date to support the long-term durability of response with a once-daily regimen of didanosine.

Administration and Dosage

➤*Approved by the FDA:* October 1991.

➤*Dosage:*

Didanosine (Videx) – Administer all didanosine formulations on an empty stomach, at least 30 minutes before or 2 hours after eating. For either a once-daily or twice-daily regimen, patients must take at least 2 of the appropriate strength tablets at each dose to provide adequate buffering and prevent gastric acid degradation of didanosine. Because of the need for adequate buffering, use the 200 mg strength buffered tablet only as a component of the once-daily regimen. To reduce the risk of GI side effects, patients should take no more than 4 tablets at each dose.

➤*Adults:*

Didanosine (Videx) – The preferred dosing frequency of didanosine buffered is twice daily because there is more evidence to support the effectiveness of this dosing regimen. Once-daily dosing should be considered only for adult patients whose management requires once-daily dosing of didanosine.

Didanosine EC (Videx EC) – Didanosine EC should be administered on an empty stomach and should be swallowed intact.

Adult Didanosine Dosing

Patient weight (kg)	Tablets[1]	Buffered powder[2]	Enteric-coated capsules
≥ 60	400 mg qd or 200 mg bid	250 mg bid	400 mg qd
< 60	250 mg qd or 125 mg bid	167 mg bid	250 mg qd

[1] Use the 200 mg strength tablet only as a component of the once-daily regimen.
[2] Not suitable for once-daily dosing except for patients with renal impairment.

➤Children:

Didanosine (Videx) – The recommended dose of didanosine in pediatric patients is 120 mg/m[2] twice daily. There are no data on once-daily dosing of didanosine in pediatric patients.

Didanosine EC (Videx EC) – Didanosine EC has not been studied in pediatric patients. Please consult the complete prescribing information for didanosine buffered formulation and pediatric powder for oral solution for dosage and administration of didanosine to pediatric patients.

➤*Dose adjustment:* If clinical and laboratory signs suggest pancreatitis, promptly suspend dose and carefully evaluate the possibility of pancreatitis. Discontinue in patients with confirmed pancreatitis.

Based on data with buffered didanosine formulations, patients with symptoms of peripheral neuropathy may tolerate a reduced dose after resolution of these symptoms following drug discontinuation. If neuropathy recurs after resumption of didanosine, consider permanent discontinuation.

Renal function impairment – In adult patients with impaired renal function, adjust the dose of didanosine to compensate for the slower rate of elimination.

Recommended Dose (mg) of Didanosine by Body Weight in Renal Function Impairment

Creatinine clearance (mL/min)	≥ 60 kg			< 60 kg		
	Tablet (mg)[1]	Buffered powder (mg)[2]	Enteric-coated capsules	Tablet (mg)[1]	Buffered powder (mg)[2]	Enteric-coated capsules
≥ 60	400 qd or 200 bid	250 bid	400 mg qd	250 qd or 125 bid	167 bid	250 mg qd
30 to 59	200 qd or 100 bid	100 bid	200 mg qd	150 qd or 75 bid	100 bid	125 mg qd
10 to 29	150 qd	167 qd	125 mg qd	100 qd	100 qd	125 mg qd
< 10	100 qd	100 qd	125 mg qd	75 qd	100 qd	—[3]

[1] Didanosine chewable/dispersible buffered tablets. Two didanosine tablets must be taken with each dose; different strengths of tablets may be combined to yield the recommended dose.
[2] Didanosine buffered powder for oral solution.
[3] Didanosine EC capsules are not suitable for patients < 60 kg with Ccr < 10 mL/min. An alternate didanosine formulation should be used.

Didanosine (Videx): Urinary excretion is also a major route of didanosine elimination in pediatric patients; therefore, the clearance of didanosine may be altered in children with renal impairment. Although there are insufficient data to recommend a specific dose adjustment in this patient population, consider a reduction in the dose or an increase in the interval between doses.

Patients requiring continuous ambulatory peritoneal dialysis (CAPD) or hemodialysis –

Didanosine (Videx): It is recommended that ¼ of the total daily dose of didanosine be administered once daily. For patients with Ccr < 10 mL/min, it is not necessary to administer a supplemental dose of didanosine following hemodialysis.

Didanosine EC (Videx EC): For patients ≥ 60 kg, administer 125 mg once daily. Didanosine EC is not suitable for use in patients < 60 kg with Ccr < 10 mL/min. It is not necessary to administer a supplemental dose of didanosine EC following hemodialysis.

➤*Method of preparation:*

Adults –

Chewable/Dispersible buffered tablets: To provide adequate buffering, thoroughly chew at least 2 of the appropriate strength tablets, but no more than 4 tablets, or disperse in ≥ 1 oz of water prior to consumption. To disperse tablets, add 2 tablets to ≥ 1 oz of water. Stir until a uniform

DIDANOSINE (ddI; dideoxyinosine)

dispersion forms, and drink entire dispersion immediately. If additional flavoring is desired, the dispersion may be diluted with 1 oz of clear apple juice. Stir the further diluted dispersion just prior to consumption. The dispersion with clear apple juice is stable at room temperature (17° to 23°C; 62° to 73°F) for up to 1 hour.

Buffered powder for oral solution:

1.) Open packet carefully and pour contents into ≈ 4 oz of water. Do not mix with fruit juice or other acid-containing liquid.
2.) Stir until the powder completely dissolves (≈ 2 to 3 minutes).
3.) Drink the entire solution immediately.

Children –

Chewable/Dispersible buffered tablets: Chew tablets or manually crush or disperse 1 or 2 tablets in water prior to consumption, as described for adults.

Pediatric powder for oral solution: Prior to dispensing, the pharmacist must constitute dry powder with Purified Water to an initial concentration of 20 mg/mL and immediately mix the resulting solution with antacid to a final concentration of 10 mg/mL as follows:

• *20 mg/mL initial solution –* Reconstitute the product to 20 mg/mL by adding 100 or 200 mL Purified Water to the 2 or 4 g of powder, respectively, in the product bottle. Prepare final admixture as described below.

• *10 mg/mL final admixture –*

1.) Immediately mix 1 part of the 20 mg/mL initial solution with 1 part of either *Mylanta Double Strength Liquid, Extra Strength Maalox Plus Suspension,* or *Maalox TC Suspension* for a final dispensing concentration of 10 mg/mL didanosine. For patient home use, dispense the admixture in flint-glass or plastic bottles with child-resistant closures. This admixture is stable for 30 days under refrigeration at 2° to 8°C (36° to 46°F).
2.) Instruct the patient or caregiver to shake the admixture thoroughly prior to use and to store the tightly closed container in the refrigerator at 2° to 8°C (36° to 46°F) for up to 30 days.

➤*Spill, leak, and disposal procedure:* Avoid generating dust during clean-up of powdered products; use wet mop or damp sponge. Clean surface with soap and water as necessary. Contain larger spills.

➤*Storage/Stability:*

Tablets – Store at 15° to 30°C (59° to 86°F) in tightly closed bottles. If dispersed in water, dose may be held for ≤ 1 hour at ambient temperature.

Enteric-coated capsules – Store at 25°C (77°F) in tightly closed bottles. Excursions permitted between 15° and 30°C (59° and 86°F).

Powder for oral solution – Store at 15° to 30°C (59° to 86°F).
Buffered: After dissolving in water, solution may be stored at ambient room temperature for ≤ 4 hours.
Pediatric: Admixtures may be stored ≤ 30 days in a refrigerator (2° to 8°C; 36° to 46°F). Discard unused portion after 30 days.

Actions

➤*Pharmacology:* Didanosine is a synthetic purine nucleoside analog of deoxyadenosine, in which the 3'-hydroxyl group is replaced by hydrogen. Intracellularly, it is converted by cellular enzymes to the active metabolite, dideoxyadenosine 5'-triphosphate. It inhibits the activity of HIV-1 reverse transcriptase by competing with the natural substrate, deoxyadenosine 5'-triphosphate, and by incorporation into viral DNA causing termination of viral DNA chain elongation.

➤*Pharmacokinetics:*

Effect of food on oral absorption –

Tablets: Didanosine C_{max} and AUC were decreased by ≈ 55% when didanosine tablets were administered up to 2 hours after a meal. Administration of didanosine tablets up to 30 minutes before a meal did not result in any significant changes in bioavailability.

Enteric-coated capsules: In the presence of food, C_{max} and AUC for didanosine capsules were reduced by ≈ 46% and 19%, respectively, compared to the fasting state. Take didanosine capsules on an empty stomach.

The pharmacokinetic parameters of didanosine are summarized in the table below. Didanosine is rapidly absorbed, with peak plasma concentrations generally observed from 0.25 to 1.5 hours following oral dosing. Increases in plasma didanosine concentrations were dose proportional over the range 50 to 400 mg. Steady-state pharmacokinetic parameters did not differ significantly from values observed after a single dose. Plasma protein binding of didanosine in vitro was low (< 5%). Based on data from in vitro and animal studies, it is presumed that the metabolism of didanosine in humans occurs by the same pathways responsible for the elimination of endogenous purines.

Pharmacokinetic Parameters of Didanosine in Adult and Pediatric Patients		
Parameter	Adult patients[1]	Pediatric patients
Oral bioavailability	≈ 42%	≈ 25%
Apparent volume of distribution[2]	≈ 1.08 L/kg	≈ 28 L/m²
CSF[3]-plasma ratio[4]	≈ 21%	46% (range, 12% to 85%)

Pharmacokinetic Parameters of Didanosine in Adult and Pediatric Patients		
Parameter	Adult patients[1]	Pediatric patients
Systemic clearance[2]	≈ 13 mL/min/kg	≈ 516 mL/min/m²
Renal clearance[5]	≈ 5.5 mL/min/kg	≈ 240 mL/min/m²
Elimination half-life[5]	≈ 1.5 hr	≈ 0.8 hr
Urine recovery of didanosine[5]	≈ 18%	≈ 18%

[1] Administered as buffered formulation.
[2] Following IV administration.
[3] CSF = cerebrospinal fluid.
[4] Following IV administration in adults and IV or oral administration in pediatric patients.
[5] Following oral administration.

Children – The pharmacokinetics of didanosine administered as *Videx EC* has not been studied in pediatric patients.

Comparison of didanosine formulations – In didanosine EC (*Videx EC*), the active ingredient, didanosine, is protected against degradation by stomach acid by the use of an enteric coating on the beadlets in the capsule. The enteric coating dissolves when the beadlets empty into the small intestine, the site of drug absorption. With buffered formulations of didanosine, administration with antacid provides protection from degradation by stomach acid.

In healthy volunteers, as well as subjects infected with HIV, the area under the plasma concentration-time curve (AUC) is equivalent for didanosine administered as the *Videx EC* formulation relative to a buffered tablet formulation. The peak plasma concentration (C_{max}) of didanosine administered as *Videx EC*, is reduced ≈ 40% relative to didanosine buffered tablets. The time to the peak concentration (T_{max}) increases from ≈ 0.67 hours for didanosine buffered tablets to 2 hours of *Videx EC*.

Renal insufficiency – Modify didanosine dose in patients with reduced creatinine clearance and in patients receiving maintenance hemodialysis. The absolute bioavailability of didanosine is not affected in patients requiring dialysis.

Mean Pharmacokinetic Parameters of Didanosine Following a Single Oral Dose of a Buffered Formulation					
	Creatinine clearance (mL/min)				
Parameter	≥ 90 (n = 12)	60 to 90 (n = 6)	30 to 59 (n = 6)	10 to 29 (n = 3)	Dialysis patients (n = 11)
Ccr[1] (mL/min)	≈ 112	≈ 68	≈ 46	≈ 13	ND[2]
CL/F[3] (mL/min)	≈ 2164	≈ 1566	≈ 1023	≈ 628	≈ 543
CL$_R$[4] (mL/min)	≈ 458	≈ 247	≈ 100	≈ 20	< 10
t½ (hr)	≈ 1.42	≈ 1.59	≈ 1.75	≈ 2	≈ 4.1

[1] Ccr = creatinine clearance.
[2] ND = not determined due to anuria.
[3] CL/F = apparent oral clearance.
[4] CL$_R$ = renal clearance.

➤*Microbiology:*

In vitro HIV susceptibility – Didanosine has in vitro anti-HIV-1 activity in a variety of HIV-infected lymphoblastic cell lines and monocyte/macrophage cell cultures. The concentration of drug necessary to inhibit viral replication 50% ranges from 2.5 to 10 mcM (1 mcM = 0.24 mcg/mL) in lymphoblastic cell lines and from 0.01 to 0.1 mcM in monocyte/macrophage cell cultures.

Drug resistance – HIV-1 isolates with reduced sensitivity to didanosine have been selected in vitro and were also obtained from patients treated with didanosine. Genetic analysis of isolates from didanosine-treated patients showed mutations in the reverse transcriptase gene that resulted in the amino acid substitutions. Phenotypic analysis of HIV-1 isolates from 60 patients (some with prior zidovudine treatment) receiving 6 to 24 months of didanosine monotherapy showed that isolates from 10 of 60 patients exhibited an average of a 10-fold decrease in susceptibility to didanosine in vitro compared to baseline isolates. Clinical isolates that exhibited a decrease in didanosine susceptibility harbored ≥ 1 didanosine-associated mutations. The clinical relevance of genotypic and phenotypic changes associated with didanosine therapy has not been established.

Cross-resistance – HIV-1 isolates from 2 of 39 patients receiving combination therapy for up to 2 years with zidovudine and didanosine exhibited decreased susceptibility to zidovudine, didanosine, zalcitabine, stavudine, and lamivudine in vitro.

➤*Clinical trials:*

Didanosine (Videx) –

Combination therapy: START 2 was a multicenter, randomized, open-label study comparing didanosine/stavudine/indinavir to zidovudine/lamivudine/indinavir in 205 treatment-naive patients. Both regimens resulted in a similar magnitude of suppression of HIV RNA levels and

DIDANOSINE (ddI; dideoxyinosine)

increases in CD4 cell counts through 48 weeks.

Monotherapy: The efficacy of didanosine was demonstrated in 2 randomized, double-blind studies comparing didanosine to zidovudine. In treatment-naive patients, the rate of HIV disease progression or death was similar between the treatment groups; mortality rates were 26% for didanosine patients and 21% for zidovudine patients. Of the patients who had received previous zidovudine treatment, those treated with didanosine had a lower rate of HIV disease progression or death (32%) compared to those treated with zidovudine (41%); however, survival rates were similar between the treatment groups.

The efficacy of didanosine in pediatric patients was demonstrated in a randomized, double-blind, controlled study. Patients treated with didanosine or didanosine plus zidovudine had lower rates of HIV disease progression or death compared to those treated with zidovudine alone.

Studies have demonstrated that the clinical benefit of monotherapy with antiretrovirals, including didanosine, was time-limited.

Contraindications

Clinically significant hypersensitivity to any of the components of the formulations.

Warnings

➤*Pancreatitis:* Fatal and nonfatal pancreatitis has occurred during didanosine therapy used alone or in combination regimens in treatment-naive and treatment-experienced patients regardless of degree of immunosuppression (see Warning Box). Suspend didanosine in patients with signs or symptoms of pancreatitis and discontinue in patients with confirmed pancreatitis. Patients treated with didanosine in combination with stavudine, with or without hydroxyurea, may be at increased risk for pancreatitis. When treatment with life-sustaining drugs known to cause pancreatic toxicity is required, suspension of didanosine is recommended. In patients with risk factors for pancreatitis, use didanosine with extreme caution and only if clearly indicated. Closely follow patients with advanced HIV infection who are at increased risk of pancreatitis, especially the elderly. Patients with renal impairment may be at greater risk for pancreatitis if treated without dose adjustment.

The frequency of pancreatitis is dose-related. In phase 3 studies with buffered formulations, incidence ranged from 1% to 10% with high dose and 1% to 7% with recommended dose.

In pediatric studies with pediatric powder for oral solution, pancreatitis occurred in 3% of patients treated at entry doses < 300 mg/m²/day and in 13% treated at higher doses. In pediatric patients with symptoms similar to pancreatitis, suspend didanosine until the diagnosis is excluded and discontinue in pediatric patients with confirmed pancreatitis.

➤*Lactic acidosis / Severe hepatomegaly with steatosis:* Lactic acidosis and severe hepatomegaly with steatosis, including fatal cases, have been reported with the use of nucleoside analogs alone or in combination, including didanosine and other antiretrovirals. A majority of these cases have been in women. Obesity and prolonged nucleoside exposure may be risk factors. Fatal lactic acidosis has been reported in pregnant women who received the combination of didanosine and stavudine with other antiretroviral agents. The combination of didanosine and stavudine should be used with caution during pregnancy and is recommended only if the potential benefit clearly outweighs the potential risk (see Pregnancy). Exercise particular caution when administering didanosine to any patient with known risk factors for liver disease; however, cases have also been reported in patients with no known risk factors. Suspend treatment with didanosine in any patient who develops clinical or laboratory findings suggestive of lactic acidosis or pronounced hepatotoxicity (which may include hepatomegaly and steatosis even in the absence of marked transaminase elevations).

➤*Retinal changes and optic neuritis:* Retinal changes and optic neuritis have been reported in adult and pediatric patients. Consider periodic retinal examinations for patients receiving didanosine.

➤*Peripheral neuropathy:* Peripheral neuropathy, manifested by numbness, tingling, or pain in the hands or feet, has been reported in patients receiving didanosine therapy. Peripheral neuropathy has occurred more frequently in patients with advanced HIV disease, in patients with a history of neuropathy, or in patients being treated with neurotoxic drug therapy, including stavudine.

➤*Myopathy:* Evidence of a dose-limiting skeletal muscle toxicity has been observed in mice and rats (but not in dogs) following long-term (> 90 days) dosing with didanosine at doses that were ≈ 1.2 to 12 times the estimated human exposure. Human myopathy has been associated with administration of other nucleoside analogs.

➤*Renal function impairment:* Patients with renal impairment (creatinine clearance < 60 mL/min) may be at greater risk of toxicity from didanosine because of decreased drug clearance; a dose reduction is recommended. The magnesium content of each buffered tablet (8.6 mEq) may present an excessive magnesium load to patients with significant renal impairment, particularly after prolonged dosing.

➤*Hepatic function impairment:* It is unknown if hepatic impairment significantly affects didanosine pharmacokinetics. Therefore, monitor these patients closely for evidence of didanosine toxicity.

➤*Mutagenesis:* Didanosine was positive in the following genetic toxicology assays: 1) The *Escherichia coli* tester strain WP2 uvrA bacterial mutagenicity assay; 2) the L5178Y/TK+/-mouse lymphoma mammalian cell gene mutation assay; 3) the in vitro chromosomal aberrations assay in cultured human peripheral lymphocytes; 4) the in vitro chromosomal aberrations assay in Chinese Hamster Lung cells; and 5) the BALB/c 3T3 in vitro transformation assay. No evidence of mutagenicity was observed in an Ames *Salmonella* bacterial mutagenicity assay or in rat and mouse in vivo micronucleus assays.

➤*Elderly:* In an expanded access program using a buffered formulation of didanosine for the treatment of advanced HIV infection, patients ≥ 65 years of age had a higher frequency of pancreatitis (10%) than younger patients (5%). Clinical studies of didanosine did not include sufficient numbers of subjects ≥ 65 years old to determine whether they respond differently than younger subjects. Didanosine is known to be substantially excreted by the kidney, and the risk of toxic reactions to this drug may be greater in patients with impaired renal function. Because elderly patients are more likely to have decreased renal function, care should be taken in dose selection. In addition, renal function should be monitored and dosage adjustments should be made accordingly (see Administration and Dosage).

➤*Pregnancy: Category B.* At ≈ 12 times the estimated human exposure, didanosine was slightly toxic to female rats and their pups during mid- and late lactation. These rats showed reduced food intake and body weight gains but the physical and functional development of the offspring was not impaired and there were no major changes in the F2 generation. There are no adequate and well-controlled studies in pregnant women. Use during pregnancy only if the potential benefit justifies the potential risk.

Fatal lactic acidosis has been reported in pregnant women who received the combination of didanosine and stavudine with other antiretroviral agents. It is unclear if pregnancy augments the risk of lactic acidosis/hepatic steatosis syndrome reported in nonpregnant individuals receiving nucleoside analogs (see Lactic acidosis/Severe hepatomegaly with steatosis). The combination of didanosine and stavudine should be used with caution during pregnancy and is recommended only if the potential benefit clearly outweighs the potential risk. Health care providers caring for HIV-infected pregnant women receiving didanosine should be alert for early diagnosis of lactic acidosis/hepatic steatosis syndrome.

To monitor maternal-fetal outcomes of pregnant women exposed to didanosine and other antiretroviral agents, an Antiretroviral Pregnancy Registry has been established. Physicians are encouraged to register patients by calling (800) 258-4263.

➤*Lactation:* The CDC recommends that HIV-infected mothers not breastfeed their infants to avoid risking postnatal transmission of HIV. It is not known if didanosine is excreted in human milk. Because of the potential for HIV transmission and for serious adverse reactions in nursing infants, mothers should be instructed not to breastfeed if they are receiving didanosine.

➤*Children:* Safety and efficacy of didanosine EC have not been established in pediatric patients (see Administration and Dosage).

Precautions

➤*Frequency of dosing:* The preferred dosing frequency of didanosine is twice daily because there is more evidence to support the effectiveness of this dosing frequency. Once daily dosing should be considered only for adult patients whose management requires once daily dosing of didanosine.

➤*Phenylketonuria:* Didanosine chewable/dispersible buffered tablets contain 73 mg phenylalanine per 2-tablet dose (36.5 mg phenylalanine per tablet).

➤*Sodium-restricted diets:* Each single-dose packet of buffered powder for oral solution contains 1380 mg sodium.

➤*Hyperuricemia:* Didanosine has been associated with asymptomatic hyperuricemia; consider suspending treatment if clinical measures aimed at reducing uric acid levels fail.

Drug Interactions

Didanosine Drug Interactions			
Precipitant drug	Object drug*		Description
Allopurinol	Didanosine	↑	The AUC of didanosine was increased ≈ 4-fold when 300 mg/day allopurinol was coadministered with a single 200 mg dose of didanosine to 2 patients with renal impairment. Coadministration of these 2 drugs is not recommended.

DIDANOSINE (ddI; dideoxyinosine)

Didanosine Drug Interactions			
Precipitant drug	Object drug*		Description
Ganciclovir	Didanosine	↑	Administration of didanosine 2 hours prior to or concurrent with oral ganciclovir was associated with an increase in the steady-state AUC of didanosine. A decrease in the steady-state AUC of ganciclovir was observed when didanosine was administered 2 hours prior to ganciclovir, but not when the 2 drugs were administered simultaneously.
Didanosine	Ganciclovir	↓	
Methadone	Didanosine	↓	Administration of a single 200 mg dose of didanosine with chronic methadone dosing decreased the AUC and C_{max} of didanosine by 41% and 59%, respectively.
Didanosine	Antacids	↑	Concomitant administration of antacids containing magnesium or aluminum with didanosine chewable/dispersible tablets and pediatric powder may potentiate adverse events associated with the antacid components.
Didanosine	Antifungal agents	↓	The therapeutic effects of azole antifungal agents may be decreased. The buffers in didanosine chewable tablets appear to decrease the absorption of azole antifungal agents. Administer the azole antifungal drugs ≥ 2 hours before chewable tablets.
Didanosine	Antiretroviral drugs	↓	Significant decreases in the AUC of delavirdine and indinavir occurred following simultaneous administration of these agents with didanosine. To avoid this interaction, give delavirdine or indinavir 1 hour prior to dosing with didanosine. The pharmacokinetics of nelfinavir are not altered to a clinically significant degree when it is administered with a light meal 1 hour after didanosine.
Didanosine	Fluoroquinolones	↓	Plasma concentrations of some quinolone antibiotics are decreased when administered with antacids containing magnesium, calcium, or aluminum. Therefore, if concurrent use cannot be avoided, give the quinolone ≥ 2 hours before or 6 hours after didanosine.
Didanosine	Stavudine	↑	Combination therapy of didanosine, stavudine, and other antiretrovirals has caused fatal lactic acidosis in women. Peripheral neuropathy has occurred more frequently in patients treated with neurotoxic drugs, including stavudine.

* ↑ = Object drug increased.   ↓ = Object drug decreased.

Coadministration of didanosine buffered tablets, buffered powder for oral solution, and pediatric powder for oral solution with drugs that are known to cause peripheral neuropathy or pancreatitis or patients who have a history of neuropathy or neurotoxic drug therapy may have increased risk of toxicities. Closely observe patients who receive these drugs or have a history of neuropathy or neurotoxic drug therapy.

▶Drug/Food interactions:

Tablets – Didanosine C_{max} and AUC were decreased by ≈ 55% when didanosine buffered tablets were administered up to 2 hours after a meal. Administration of didanosine buffered tablets up to 30 minutes before a meal did not result in any significant changes in bioavailability. Take didanosine on an empty stomach, ≥ 30 minutes before or 2 hours after eating.

Adverse Reactions

A serious toxicity of didanosine is pancreatitis, which may be fatal (see Warnings). Other important toxicities include lactic acidosis/severe hepatomegaly with steatosis; retinal changes and optic neuritis; and peripheral neuropathy (see Warnings and Precautions).

When didanosine is used in combination with other agents with similar toxicities, the incidence of these toxicities may be higher than when didanosine is used alone. Thus, patients treated with didanosine in combination with stavudine, with or without hydroxyurea, may be at increased risk for pancreatitis and liver function abnormalities (see

Warnings). Patients treated with didanosine in combination with stavudine may also be at increased risk for peripheral neuropathy (see Precautions).

Didanosine Adverse Reactions from Monotherapy Studies (%)				
	Study 1		Study 2	
Adverse reactions	Buffered didanosine (n = 197)	Zidovudine (n = 212)	Buffered didanosine (n = 298)	Zidovudine (n = 304)
Diarrhea	19	15	28	21
Peripheral neurologic symptoms/Neuropathy	17	14	20	12
Rash/Pruritus	7	8	9	5
Abdominal pain	13	8	7	8
Pancreatitis	7	3	6	2

Lab Test Abnormalities from Didanosine Monotherapy Studies (%)				
	Study 1		Study 2	
Parameter	Buffered didanosine (n = 197)	Zidovudine (n = 212)	Buffered didanosine (n = 298)	Zidovudine (n = 304)
AST (> 5 × ULN[1])	9	4	7	6
ALT (> 5 × ULN)	9	6	6	6
Alkaline phosphatase (> 5 × ULN)	4	1	1	1
Amylase (≥ 1.4 × ULN)	17	12	15	5
Uric acid (> 12 mg/dL)	3	1	2	1

[1] ULN = upper limit of normal.

Didanosine Adverse Reactions from Combination Therapy Studies (%)[1]				
	Study A1454-148		Study A1454-152	
Adverse reaction	Buffered didanosine + stavudine + nelfinavir (n = 482)	Zidovudine + lamivudine + nelfinavir (n = 248)	Didanosine EC + stavudine + nelfinavir (n = 255)	Zidovudine/ lamivudine[2] + nelfinavir (n = 250)
Nausea	28	40	21	35
Headache	21	30	20	16
Diarrhea	70	60	54	56
Rash	13	16	10	10
Vomiting	12	14	13	18
Peripheral neurologic symptoms/Neuropathy	26	6	20	8
Pancreatitis	1	—[3]	< 1	—[3]

[1] Median duration of treatment 48 weeks.
[2] Zidovudine/lamivudine combination tablet.
[3] This event not observed in this study arm.

Pancreatitis resulting in death was observed in 1 patient who received a buffered didanosine formulation + stavudine + nelfinavir in 1 study, and in 1 patient who received didanosine + stavudine + indinavir in another study. In addition, pancreatitis resulting in death was observed in 2 of 68 patients who received didanosine + stavudine + indinavir + hydroxyurea in another clinical trial. In an early access program, pancreatitis resulting in death occurred in 1 patient receiving didanosine EC capsules + stavudine + hydroxyurea + ritonavir + indinavir + efavirenz (see Warnings).

Selected Laboratory Abnormalities from Combination Studies of Didanosine Dosed Once Daily (%)								
	Study A1454-152[1]				Study A1454-148[2]			
	Didanosine EC + stavudine + nelfinavir (n = 255)		Zidovudine/ lamivudine[3] + nelfinavir (n = 250)		Didanosine buffered tablets + stavudine + nelfinavir (n = 482)		Zidovudine + lamivudine + nelfinavir (n = 248)	
Parameter	Grades 3-4[4]	All grades	Grades 3-4[4]	All grades	Grades 3-4[4]	All grades	Grades 3-4[4]	All grades
AST	4	40	4	17	3	42	2	23
ALT	4	39	4	20	3	37	3	24
Lipase	3	18	< 1	8	7	17	2	11
Bilirubin	< 1	7	< 1	3	< 1	7	< 1	3

[1] Median duration of treatment 43 weeks in the didanosine EC + stavudine + nelfinavir group and 39 weeks in the zidovudine/lamivudine + nelfinavir group.
[2] Median duration of treatment 48 weeks.
[3] Zidovudine/lamivudine combination tablet.
[4] > 5 × ULN for AST and ALT, ≥ 2.1 × ULN for lipase, and ≥ 2.6 × ULN for bilirubin (ULN = upper limit or normal).

▶*Didanosine buffered formulations:* The following events have been identified during postapproval use of didanosine buffered formulations. Because they are reported voluntarily from a population of unknown size, esimates of frequency cannot be made. These events

Nucleoside Reverse Transcriptase Inhibitors

DIDANOSINE (ddI; dideoxyinosine)

have been chosen for inclusion because of seriousness, frequency of reporting, causal connection to didanosine, or a combination of these factors.

GI – Anorexia; dyspepsia; flatulence; dry mouth; abdominal pain.

Hematologic – Anemia; leukopenia; thrombocytopenia.

Hepatic – Lactic acidosis and hepatic steatosis (see Warnings); hepatitis; liver failure.

Metabolic/Nutritional – Diabetes mellitus; hypoglycemia; hyperglycemia; elevated serum alkaline phosphatase, serum amylase, serum GGT, and serum uric acid levels.

Musculoskeletal – Myalgia (with or without increases in creatine phosphokinase); rhabdomyolysis, including acute renal failure and hemodialysis; arthralgia; myopathy.

Special senses – Retinal depigmentation and optic neuritis (see Warnings).

Miscellaneous – Alopecia; anaphylactoid reaction; asthenia; chills/fever; pain; pancreatitis (including fatal cases); sialoadenitis; parotid gland enlargement; dry eyes.

➤*Children:*

Miscellaneous – Adverse events and laboratory abnormalities reported to occur in the pediatric patients with pediatric powder for oral solution were generally similar to adverse events and laboratory abnormalities reported in adult patients.

In pediatric studies with pediatric powder for oral solution, pancreatitis occurred in 3% of patients treated at entry doses < 300 mg/m^2/day and in 13% of patients treated at higher doses.

Retinal changes and optic neuritis have been reported in pediatric patients with pediatric powder for oral solution.

Overdosage

There is no known antidote for overdosage. Experience in Phase I studies in which buffered formulations of didanosine were initially administered at doses 10 times the currently recommended dose, tox-

icities included pancreatitis, peripheral neuropathy, diarrhea, hyperuricemia, and hepatic dysfunction. Didanosine is not dialyzable by peritoneal dialysis, although there is some clearance by hemodialysis.

Patient Information

Inform patients that pancreatitis, a serious toxicity of didanosine when used alone and in combination regimens, has been fatal.

Advise patients that peripheral neuropathy, manifested by numbness, tingling, or pain in the hands or feet, may develop during therapy with didanosine. Counsel patients that peripheral neuropathy occurs with greatest frequency in patients with advanced HIV disease or a history of peripheral neuropathy, and that dose modification or discontinuation of didanosine may be required if toxicity develops.

Inform patients that when didanosine is used in combination with other agents with similar toxicities, the incidence of adverse events may be higher than when didanosine is used alone. Follow these patients closely.

Caution patients about the use of medications or other substances, including alcohol, that may exacerbate didanosine toxicities.

Didanosine is not a cure for HIV infection, and patients may continue to develop HIV-associated illnesses, including opportunistic infections. Therefore, counsel patients to remain under the care of a physician when using didanosine. Advise patients that didanosine therapy has not been shown to reduce the risk of HIV transmission to others through sexual contact or blood contamination. Inform patients that the long-term effects of didanosine are unknown at this time.

Inform patients that the preferred dosing frequency of didanosine is twice daily because there is more evidence to support the effectiveness of this dosing frequency. Consider once-daily dosing only for adult patients whose management requires once-daily dosing of didanosine.

Advise patients that to ensure proper acid neutralization in the stomach they must take ≥ 2 of the appropriate strength didanosine buffered tablets at each dose. To reduce the risk of GI side effects from excess antacid, patients should take no more than 4 didanosine buffered tablets at each dose.

LAMIVUDINE (3TC)

Rx	Epivir-HBV (GlaxoSmithKline)	**Tablets:** 100 mg		(GX CG5). Butterscotch color, capsule shape. Film-coated. In 60s.
Rx	Epivir (GlaxoSmithKline)	**Tablets:** 150 mg		(GX CJ7 150). White, diamond shape. Film-coated. In 60s.
		300 mg		(GX EJ7). Gray, diamond shape. Film-coated. In 30s.
Rx	Epivir-HBV (GlaxoSmithKline)	**Oral solution:** 5 mg/mL		Parabens, sucrose. Strawberry-banana flavor. In 240 mL.
Rx	Epivir (GlaxoSmithKline)	**Oral solution:** 10 mg/mL		Parabens, sucrose. Strawberry-banana flavor. In 240 mL.

WARNING

Lactic acidosis and severe hepatomegaly with steatosis, including fatal cases, have been reported with the use of nucleoside analogs alone or in combination, including lamivudine and other antiretroviral agents (see Warnings).

Offer human immunodeficiency virus (HIV) counseling and testing to patients before beginning *Epivir-HBV* and periodically during treatment (see Warnings) because *Epivir-HBV* tablets and oral solution contain a lower dose of the same active ingredient (lamivudine) as the *Epivir* tablets and oral solution used to treat HIV infection. If treatment with *Epivir-HBV* is prescribed for chronic hepatitis B for a patient with unrecognized or untreated HIV infection, rapid emergence of HIV resistance is likely because of subtherapeutic dose and inappropriate monotherapy.

Epivir tablets and oral solution (used to treat HIV infection) contain a higher dose of the active ingredient (lamivudine) than *Epivir-HBV* tablets and oral solution (used to treat chronic hepatitis B). Patients with HIV infection should receive only dosing forms appropriate for the treatment of HIV (see Warnings).

Indications

➤*HIV infection (Epivir):* In combination with other antiretroviral agents for the treatment of HIV infection.

➤*Chronic hepatitis B (Epivir-HBV):* Treatment of chronic hepatitis B associated with evidence of hepatitis B viral replication and active liver inflammation.

Administration and Dosage

➤*Approved by the FDA:* November 17, 1995.

Administer with or without food.

➤*HIV infection:*

Adults – 300 mg/day, administered as either 150 mg twice daily or 300 mg once daily, in combination with other antiretroviral agents.

Children (3 months up to 16 years of age) – 4 mg/kg twice daily (up to a maximum of 150 mg twice a day) administered with other antiretroviral agents.

Renal function impairment – Adjust lamivudine dose in accordance with renal function. Insufficient data are available to recommend a dosage of lamivudine in dialysis. Although there are insufficient data to recommend a specific dose adjustment of lamivudine in pediatric patients with renal impairment, consider a reduction in the dose and/or an increase in the dosing interval.

Adjustment of Lamivudine Dosage in HIV-Infected Adult and Adolescent Patients with Renal Function Impairment	
Ccr (mL/min)	Recommended lamivudine dosage
≥ 50	150 mg twice daily or 300 mg once daily
30 to 49	150 mg once daily
15 to 29	150 mg first dose, then 100 mg once daily
5 to 14	150 mg first dose, then 50 mg once daily
< 5	50 mg first dose, then 25 mg once daily

➤*Chronic hepatitis B:*

Adults – 100 mg once daily. Safety and efficacy of treatment beyond 1 year have not been established and the optimum duration of treatment is not known.

Children (2 to 17 years of age) – 3 mg/kg once daily up to a maximum daily dose of 100 mg. Safety and effectiveness of treatment beyond 1 year have not been established, and the optimum duration of treatment is not known.

HIV coinfection – The formulation and dosage of lamivudine in *Epivir-HBV* are not appropriate for patients dually infected with hepatitis B virus (HBV) and HIV. If lamivudine is administered to such patients, use the higher dosage indicated for HIV therapy as part of an appropriate combination regimen.

Renal function impairment – Adjust the dose of lamivudine in accordance with renal function. No additional dosing of *Epivir-HBV* is required after routine (4-hour) hemodialysis. Insufficient data are available to recommend a dosage of *Epivir-HBV* in patients undergoing peritoneal dialysis. Although there are insufficient data to recommend a specific dose adjustment of lamivudine in pediatric patients with renal impairment, consider a reduction in the dose.

LAMIVUDINE (3TC)

Adjustment of Lamivudine Dosage in Chronic Hepatitis B Adult Patients with Renal Function Impairment	
Ccr (mL/min)	Recommended lamivudine dosage
≥ 50	100 mg once daily
30 to 49	100 mg first dose, then 50 mg once daily
15 to 29	100 mg first dose, then 25 mg once daily
5 to 14	35 mg first dose, then 15 mg once daily
< 5	35 mg first dose, then 10 mg once daily

➤*Storage/Stability:*

Epivir – Store oral solution at 25°C (77°F) tightly closed. Store tablets at 25°C (77°F); excursions permitted to 15° to 30° C (59° to 86°F).

Epivir-HBV – Store between 20° and 25°C (68° and 77°F) tightly closed.

Actions

➤*Pharmacology:* Lamivudine is a synthetic nucleoside analog with activity against HIV-1 and HBV. Lamivudine is phosphorylated intracellularly to lamivudine triphosphate (L-TP). The principal mode of action of L-TP is the inhibition of HIV-1 reverse transcriptase (RT) via DNA chain termination after incorporation of the nucleoside analog into viral DNA. Incorporation of the monophosphate form into viral DNA by HBV polymerase results in DNA chain termination. L-TP also inhibits the RNA- and DNA-dependent DNA polymerase activities of HIV-1 reverse transcriptase.

➤*Pharmacokinetics:*

Absorption/Distribution – Lamivudine is rapidly absorbed after oral administration in HIV- and HBV-infected patients and intracellularly phosphorylated to its active metabolite, L-TP. Absolute bioavailability as demonstrated in HIV-infected patients is approximately 86% for the 150 mg tablet and approximately 87% for the 10 mg/mL oral solution. Absorption is slower and C_{max} is approximately 40% lower in the fed vs the fasted state; however, no significant difference in AUC is evident. Although the solution demonstrates a slightly higher C_{max} than the tablet, no significant difference exists in AUC; therefore, the solution and tablet may be used interchangeably.

The apparent volume of distribution (V_d) is approximately 1.3 L/kg after IV administration, suggesting distribution into extravascular spaces; V_d is independent of dose and body weight. Binding of lamivudine to human plasma proteins is low (less than 36%). In vitro studies showed that, over the concentration range of 0.1 to 100 mcg/mL, the amount of lamivudine associated with erythrocytes ranged from 53% to 57% and was independent of concentration. AUC and C_{max} increase in proportion to dose. Following 2 mg/kg twice-daily doses in HIV-infected patients and 100 mg single daily doses to HBV-infected patients, steady-state peak concentrations are 1.5 and 1.28 mcg/mL, respectively. T_{max} reported in HBV-infected patients was 0.5 to 2 hours.

Metabolism/Excretion – Metabolism is a minor route of elimination; the only known metabolite is the trans-sulfoxide metabolite. The mean elimination half-life of lamivudine ranges from 5 to 7 hours. In HIV-infected patients, total clearance is approximately 398.5 mL/min in serum sampling 24 hours after dosing. The majority of the dose is eliminated in the urine as unchanged drug.

Special populations:

• *Children* – In HIV-infected pediatric patients approximately 4 months to 16 years of age and chronic hepatitis B pediatric patients 2 to 12 years of age, lamivudine was rapidly absorbed with a T_{max} of 0.5 to 1 hour and an absolute bioavailability of 66%. After 8 mg/kg/day, C_{max} was approximately 1.1 mcg/mL and half-life was approximately 2 hours (vs 3.7 hours in adults). Weight-corrected oral clearances were highest at 2 years of age and declined from 2 to 12 years of age, where values were then similar to those seen in adults. Total exposure to lamivudine, as reflected by mean AUC values, was comparable between pediatric patients receiving 8 mg/kg/day and adults receiving 4 mg/kg/day. In 8 patients, CSF lamivudine concentrations (0.04 to 0.3 mcg/mL) ranged from 5.6% to 30.9% of the concentration in a simultaneous serum sample.

• *Renal function impairment* – Exposure (AUC), C_{max}, and half-life increased with diminishing renal function. Apparent total oral clearance (Cl/F) of lamivudine decreased as Ccr decreased. T_{max} was not significantly affected by renal function. Based on these observations, modify the lamivudine dosage in patients with renal impairment (see Administration and Dosage). The effects of renal impairment on lamivudine pharmacokinetics in pediatric patients are not known.

➤*Microbiology:*

Drug resistance – In patients receiving lamivudine monotherapy or combination therapy with zidovudine, HIV-1 isolates from most patients became phenotypically and genotypically resistant to lamivudine within 12 weeks. In some patients harboring zidovudine-resistant virus at baseline, phenotypic sensitivity to zidovudine was restored by 12 weeks of treatment. Combination therapy with lamivudine plus zidovudine delayed the emergence of mutations conferring resistance to zidovudine. In HIV-1-infected MT-4 cells, lamivudine in combination with zidovudine had synergistic antiretroviral activity.

Cross-resistance – Lamivudine resistant HIV-1 mutants were cross-resistant to didanosine and zalcitabine. In some patients treated with zidovudine plus didanosine or zalcitabine, isolates resistant to multiple reverse transcriptase inhibitors, including lamivudine, have emerged.

Contraindications

Clinically significant hypersensitivity to any of the components of the products.

Warnings

➤*Lactic acidosis/severe hepatomegaly with steatosis:* Lactic acidosis and severe hepatomegaly with steatosis, including fatal cases, have occurred with the use of antiretroviral nucleoside analogs alone or in combination, including lamivudine and other antiretrovirals, and in some patients receiving lamivudine therapy for hepatitis B. A majority of these cases have been in women. Obesity and prolonged nucleoside exposure may be risk factors. Exercise caution when administering lamivudine to any patient, particularly to those with known risk factors for liver disease; however, cases also have been reported in patients with no known risk factors. Suspend treatment with lamivudine in any patient who develops clinical or laboratory findings suggestive of lactic acidosis or pronounced hepatotoxicity, which may include hepatomegaly and steatosis even in the absence of marked transaminase elevations.

➤*Differences between lamivudine-containing products/risk of emergence of resistant HIV:* Epivir-HBV tablets and oral solution contain a lower dose of the same active ingredient (lamivudine) as Epivir tablets and oral solution, lamivudine/zidovudine tablets (Combivir), and abacavir/lamivudine/zidovudine tablets (Trizivir) used to treat HIV infection. The formulation and dosage of lamivudine in Epivir-HBV are not appropriate for patients infected with both HBV and HIV. Lamivudine has not been adequately studied for the treatment of chronic hepatitis B in patients dually infected with HIV and HBV. If treatment with Epivir-HBV is prescribed for chronic hepatitis B for a patient with unrecognized or untreated HIV infection, rapid emergence of HIV resistance is likely to result because of the subtherapeutic dose and the inappropriateness of monotherapy HIV treatment. If a decision is made to administer lamivudine to patients dually infected with HIV and HBV, use Epivir tablets or oral solution or Combivir (lamivudine/zidovudine) tablets as a part of an appropriate combination regimen. Do not administer Combivir concomitantly with Epivir, Epivir-HBV, Retrovir, or Trizivir.

➤*Posttreatment exacerbations of hepatitis:* Clinical and laboratory evidence of exacerbations of hepatitis have occurred after discontinuation of lamivudine (these have been primarily detected by serum ALT elevations in addition to the re-emergence of HBV DNA commonly observed after stopping treatment). Although most events appear to have been self-limited, fatalities have been reported in some cases. Similar events have been reported from postmarketing experience after changes from lamivudine-containing HIV treatment regimens to non-lamivudine-containing regimens in patients infected with both HIV and HBV. The causal relationship to the discontinuation of lamivudine treatment is unknown. Closely monitor patients with clinical and laboratory follow-up for at least several months after stopping treatment. There is insufficient evidence to determine whether reinitiation of therapy alters the course of posttreatment exacerbations of hepatitis.

➤*Renal function impairment:* Reduction of the dosage of lamivudine is recommended for patients with impaired renal function (see Administration and Dosage).

➤*Elderly:* Because elderly patients are more likely to have decreased renal function, monitor renal function carefully and make dosage adjustments accordingly (see Administration and Dosage).

➤*Pregnancy: Category C.* Some evidence of early embryolethality was seen in the rabbit at exposure levels similar to those observed in humans, but there was no indication of this effect in the rat at HBV doses up to 60 times that in humans. Studies in pregnant rats and rabbits showed that lamivudine is transferred to the fetus through the placenta. Lamivudine concentrations generally were similar in maternal, neonatal, and cord serum samples. In a subset of subjects from whom amniotic fluid specimens were obtained following natural rupture of membranes, amniotic fluid concentrations of lamivudine were typically greater than 2 times the maternal serum levels. Use during pregnancy only if the potential benefits outweigh the risks. There are no data regarding effect on vertical transmission. Lamivudine has not affected the transmission of HBV from mother to infant; immunize infants appropriately to prevent neonatal acquisition of HBV.

Antiretroviral pregnancy registry – To monitor maternal-fetal outcomes of pregnant women exposed to lamivudine, an Antiretroviral Pregnancy Registry has been established. Physicians are encouraged to register patients by calling (800) 258-4263.

➤*Lactation:* A study in lactating rats showed that lamivudine concentrations in milk were slightly greater than those in plasma. Lamivudine also is excreted in human milk. The CDC recommends that HIV-infected mothers not breastfeed their infants to avoid risking postnatal transmission of HIV infection. Instruct mothers not to breastfeed if they are receiving lamivudine.

LAMIVUDINE (3TC)

➤*Children:*

Hepatitis B – Safety and efficacy in pediatric patients under 2 years of age have not been established.

HIV infection – The safety and effectiveness of twice-daily lamivudine in combination with other antiretroviral agents have been established in pediatric patients 3 months of age and older. Lamivudine clearance was substantially reduced in 1-week-old neonates relative to pediatric patients (over 3 months of age) studied previously. There is insufficient information to establish the time course of changes in clearance between the immediate neonatal period and the age ranges over 3 months of age.

Total exposure to lamivudine, as reflected by mean AUC values, was comparable between pediatric patients receiving an 8 mg/kg/day dose and adults receiving a 4 mg/kg/day dose.

Pancreatitis – Pancreatitis has been observed in antiretroviral nucleoside-experienced pediatric patients receiving lamivudine. Use lamivudine with caution in pediatric patients with a history of prior antiretroviral nucleoside exposure, a history of pancreatitis, or other significant risk factors for the development of pancreatitis. Stop lamivudine treatment immediately if clinical signs, symptoms, or lab abnormalities suggestive of pancreatitis occur (see Adverse Reactions).

Precautions

➤*Monitoring:*

Epivir-HBV – Monitor patients regularly during treatment. The safety and efficacy of treatment with *Epivir-HBV* beyond 1 year have not been established. During treatment, combinations of events such as return of persistently elevated ALT, increasing levels of HBV DNA over time after an initial decline below assay limit, progression of clinical signs or symptoms of hepatic disease, and/or worsening of hepatic necroinflammatory findings may be considered as potentially reflecting loss of therapeutic response. Consider such observations when determining the advisability of continuing therapy.

➤*Emergence of resistance-associated HBV mutations:* In controlled clinical trials, YMDD-mutant HBV was detected in patients with on-lamivudine reappearance of HBV DNA after an initial decline below the assay limit. These mutations can be detected by assay and have been associated with reduced susceptibility to lamivudine in vitro. Lamivudine-treated patients with YMDD-mutant HBV at 52 weeks showed diminished treatment responses in comparison to lamivudine-treated patients without evidence of YMDD mutations, including lower rates of HBeAg seroconversion and HBeAg loss (no greater than placebo recipients), more frequent return of positive HBV DNA by assay, and more frequent ALT elevations. In controlled trials, when patients developed YMDD-mutant HBV, they had a rise in HBV DNA and ALT from their own previous on-treatment levels. Progression of hepatitis B, including death, has been reported in some patients with YMDD-mutant HBV, including patients from the liver transplant setting and from other clinical trials. The long-term clinical significance of YMDD-mutant HBV is not known. Increased clinical and laboratory monitoring may aid in treatment decisions if emergence of viral mutants is suspected.

➤*Fat redistribution:* Redistribution/Accumulation of body fat including central obesity, dorsocervical fat enlargement (buffalo hump), peripheral wasting, facial wasting, breast enlargement, and "cushingoid appearance" have been observed in patients receiving antiretroviral therapy. The mechanism and long-term consequences of these events are currently unknown. A causal relationship has not been established.

➤*Special risk:* Safety and efficacy of *Epivir-HBV* have not been established in patients with decompensated liver disease or organ transplants; pediatric patients under 2 years of age (use appropriate infant immunizations to prevent neonatal acquisition of HBV); patients dually infected with HBV and HCV, hepatitis delta, or HIV; or other populations not included in the principal Phase III controlled studies.

Drug Interactions

➤*Trimethoprim/Sulfamethoxazole:* Coadministration resulted in an increase of approximately 44% in lamivudine AUC, a decrease of approximately 29% in oral clearance, and a decrease of approximately 30% in renal clearance. No change in the dose of either drug is recommended.

➤*Zalcitabine:* Lamivudine and zalcitabine may inhibit the intracellular phosphorylation of one another. Therefore, use of lamivudine in combination with zalcitabine is not recommended.

Adverse Reactions

➤*HIV infection:* In clinical trials using lamivudine as part of a combination regimen for treatment of HIV infection, several clinical adverse events occurred more often in lamivudine-containing treatment arms than in comparator arms. These included nasal signs and symptoms (20% vs 11%), dizziness (10% vs 4%), and depressive disorders (9% vs 4%). Pancreatitis was observed in 3 of 656 adult patients (fewer than 0.5%) who received lamivudine in controlled clinical trials. Laboratory abnormalities reported more often in lamivudine-containing arms included neutropenia and elevations of liver function tests (also more frequent in lamivudine-containing arms for a retrospective analysis of HIV/HBV dually infected patients in 1 study), and amylase elevations.

Selected Adverse Reactions of Lamivudine in HIV-Infected Adults (%)		
Adverse reaction	Lamivudine 150 mg bid plus zidovudine (n = 251)	Zidovudine[1] (n = 230)
CNS		
Headache	35	27
Neuropathy	12	10
Insomnia and other sleep disorders	11	7
Dizziness	10	4
Depressive disorders	9	4
GI		
Nausea	33	29
Diarrhea	18	22
Nausea and vomiting	13	12
Anorexia or decreased appetite	10	7
Abdominal pain	9	11
Abdominal cramps	6	3
Dyspepsia	5	5
Musculoskeletal		
Musculoskeletal pain	12	10
Myalgia	8	6
Arthralgia	5	5
Respiratory		
Nasal signs and symptoms	20	11
Cough	18	13
Miscellaneous		
Malaise and fatigue	27	23
Fever or chills	10	12
Rash	9	6

[1] Either zidovudine monotherapy or zidovudine in combination with zalcitabine.

Lab test abnormalities –

Lamivudine Lab Test Abnormalities in HIV-Infected Adults (%)				
	24-week surrogate endpoint study[1]		Clinical endpoint study[1]	
Test (threshold level)	Lamivudine + zidovudine	Zidovudine[2]	Lamivudine + current therapy	Placebo + current therapy[3]
Absolute neutrophil count (< 750/mm³)	7.2	5.4	15	13
Hemoglobin (< 8 g/dL)	2.9	1.8	2.2	3.4
Platelets (< 50,000/mm³)	0.4	1.3	2.8	3.8
ALT (> 5 × ULN[4])	3.7	3.6	3.8	1.9
AST (> 5 × ULN[4])	1.7	1.8	4	2.1
Bilirubin (> 2.5 × ULN[4])	0.8	0.4	ND[5]	ND[5]
Amylase (> 2 × ULN[4])	4.2	1.5	2.2	1.1

[1] Median duration of study was 12 months.
[2] Either zidovudine monotherapy or zidovudine in combination with zalcitabine.
[3] Current therapy was zidovudine, zidovudine plus didanosine, or zidovudine plus zalcitabine.
[4] ULN = Upper limit of normal.
[5] ND = Not done.

Miscellaneous – In small, uncontrolled studies in which pregnant women were given lamivudine alone or in combination with zidovudine beginning in the last few weeks of pregnancy (see Warnings), reported adverse events included anemia, urinary tract infections, and complications of labor and delivery. In postmarketing experience, liver function abnormalities and pancreatitis have been reported in women who received lamivudine in combination with other antiretroviral drugs during pregnancy. It is not known whether risks of adverse events associated with lamivudine are altered in pregnant women compared with other HIV-infected patients.

➤*Chronic hepatitis B:*

Selected Adverse Reactions of Lamivudine in Adults with Chronic Hepatitis B (%)		
Adverse reaction	Lamivudine (n = 332)	Placebo (n = 200)
GI		
Abdominal discomfort and pain	16	17
Nausea and vomiting	15	17
Diarrhea	14	12
Musculoskeletal		
Myalgia	14	17
Arthralgia	7	5
Special senses		
Ear, nose, and throat infections	25	21
Sore throat	13	8

Nucleoside Reverse Transcriptase Inhibitors

LAMIVUDINE (3TC)

Selected Adverse Reactions of Lamivudine in Adults with Chronic Hepatitis B (%)		
Adverse reaction	Lamivudine (n = 332)	Placebo (n = 200)
Miscellaneous		
Malaise and fatigue	24	28
Headache	21	21
Fever or chills	7	9
Rash	5	5
Lab test abnormalities		
ALT (> 3 × baseline)	11	13
Albumin (< 2.5 g/dL)	0	1
Amylase (> 3 × baseline)	< 1	2
Serum lipase (≥ 2.5 × ULN)[1,2]	10	7
CPK (≥ 7 × baseline)	9	5
Neutrophils (< 750/mm³)	0	< 1
Platelets < 50,000/mm³	4	3

[1] Includes observations during and after treatment in 2 placebo-controlled trials.
[2] ULN = Upper limit of normal.

Posttreatment ALT Elevations with Lamivudine in Patients with Hepatitis B		
	Patients with ALT elevations/ Patients with observations (%)[1]	
Abnormal value	Lamivudine	Placebo
ALT ≥ 2 × baseline value	27	19
ALT ≥ 3 × baseline value[2]	21	8
ALT ≥ 2 × baseline value and absolute ALT > 500 IU/L	15	7
ALT ≥ 2 × baseline value and bilirubin > 2 × ULN[3] and ≥ 2 × baseline value	0.7	0.9

[1] Each patient may be represented in ≥ 1 category.
[2] Comparable to a Grade 3 toxicity in accordance with modified WHO criteria.
[3] ULN = Upper limit of normal.

➤*Children:*

Miscellaneous – Pancreatitis, fatal in some cases, has been observed in antiretroviral nucleoside-experienced pediatric HIV patients receiving lamivudine alone or in combination with other antiretroviral agents. In 1 study, 14% of patients developed pancreatitis while receiving monotherapy with lamivudine. Three of these patients died of complications of pancreatitis. In a second study, 18% of patients developed pancreatitis. Pancreatitis was not observed in 236 patients randomized to lamivudine plus zidovudine. Pancreatitis was observed in 1 patient in this study who received open-label lamivudine in combination with zidovudine and ritonavir following discontinuation of didanosine monotherapy.

In several studies, paresthesias and peripheral neuropathies were reported in fewer than 1% to 15%.

In early open-label studies of lamivudine in children with HIV, peripheral neuropathy, and neutropenia were reported, and pancreatitis was observed in 14% to 15% of patients.

Limited short-term safety information is available from 2 small, uncontrolled studies in South Africa in neonates receiving lamivudine with or without zidovudine for the first week of life following maternal treatment starting at week 38 or 36 of gestation. Adverse events reported in these neonates included increased liver function tests, anemia, diarrhea, electrolyte disturbances, hypoglycemia, jaundice and hepatomegaly, rash, respiratory infections, sepsis, and syphilis; 3 neonates died (1 from gastroenteritis with acidosis and convulsions, 1 from traumatic injury, and 1 from unknown causes). Two other nonfatal gastroenteritis or diarrhea cases were reported, including 1 with convulsions; 1 infant had transient renal insufficiency associated with dehydration. The absence of control groups further limits assessments of causality, but it should be assumed that perinatally exposed infants may be at risk for adverse events comparable to those reported in pediatric and adult HIV-infected patients treated with lamivudine-containing combination regimens. Long-term effects of in utero and infant lamivudine exposure are not known.

Adverse Reactions in HIV-Infected Pediatric Patients (≥ 5%)		
Adverse reaction	Lamivudine + zidovudine (n = 236)	Didanosine (n = 235)
GI		
Hepatomegaly	11	11
Nausea and vomiting	8	7
Diarrhea	8	6
Stomatitis	6	12
Splenomegaly	5	8

Adverse Reactions in HIV-Infected Pediatric Patients (≥ 5%)		
Adverse reaction	Lamivudine + zidovudine (n = 236)	Didanosine (n = 235)
Respiratory		
Cough	15	18
Abnormal breath sounds/wheezing	7	9
Special senses		
Nasal discharge or congestion	8	11
Ear signs or symptoms[1]	7	6
Miscellaneous		
Fever	25	32
Skin rashes	12	14
Lymphadenopathy	9	11

[1] Includes pain, discharge, erythema, or swelling of an ear.

Selected Lab Test Abnormalities in HIV-Infected Pediatric Patients (%)		
Test (threshold level)	Lamivudine + zidovudine	Didanosine
Absolute neutrophil count (< 400/mm³)	8	3
Hemoglobin (< 7 g/dL)	4	2
Platelets (< 50,000/mm³)	1	3
ALT (> 10 × ULN[1])	1	3
AST (> 10 × ULN[1])	2	4
Lipase (> 2.5 × ULN[1])	3	3
Total amylase (> 2.5 × ULN[1])	3	3

[1] ULN = Upper limit of normal.

➤*Postmarketing surveillance:*

Miscellaneous – The following events have been identified during postapproval use of lamivudine. Because they are reported voluntarily from a population of unknown size, estimates of frequency cannot be made. The following events have been chosen for inclusion because of their seriousness, frequency of reporting, or potential causal connection to lamivudine: Hyperglycemia, weakness, lactic acidosis, anaphylaxis, urticaria, rhabdomyolysis, peripheral neuropathy, alopecia, pruritus, rash, anemia, pure red cell aplasia, lymphadenopathy, splenomegaly, pancreatitis, paresthesia, abnormal breath sounds/wheezing, posttreatment exacerbation of hepatitis B (see Warnings and Precautions), stomatitis; hepatic steatosis, muscle weakness, CPK elevation, redistribution/accumulation of body fat, severe anemias progressing on therapy (*Epivir*).

Overdosage

One case of an adult ingesting 6 g of lamivudine was reported; there were no clinical signs or symptoms noted and hematologic tests remained normal. Two cases of pediatric overdose were reported. One case was a single dose of 7 mg/kg of lamivudine; the second case involved use of 5 mg/kg of lamivudine twice daily for 30 days. There were no clinical signs or symptoms noted in either case. It is not known whether lamivudine can be removed by peritoneal dialysis or hemodialysis. There is no known antidote for lamivudine.

Patient Information

Lamivudine is not a cure for HIV infection or hepatitis B; patients may continue to experience illnesses associated with HIV infection, including opportunistic infections. Have patients remain under the care of a physician when using lamivudine.

Advise patients that the use of lamivudine does not reduce the risk of transmission of HIV or HBV to others through sexual contact or blood contamination.

Advise patients to discuss any new symptoms or concurrent medications with their physician.

Advise patients that long-term effects of lamivudine are unknown at this time.

Advise chronic hepatitis B patients that the long-term benefits of lamivudine are unknown at this time; the relationship of initial treatment response to outcomes such as hepatocellular carcinoma and decompensated cirrhosis is unknown. Inform chronic hepatitis B patients that deterioration of liver disease has occurred in some cases if treatment was discontinued and that they should discuss any change in regimen with their physician. Inform patients that emergence of resistant hepatitis B virus and worsening of disease can occur during treatment and that they should promptly report any new symptoms to their physician.

Advise patients of the importance of taking lamivudine exactly as it is prescribed and on a regular dosing schedule and to avoid missing doses.

Lamivudine tablets and oral solution are for oral ingestion only.

Advise parents to monitor pediatric patients for symptoms of pancreatitis (eg, abdominal pain, nausea, fever).

LAMIVUDINE (3TC)

Inform patients that redistribution or accumulation of body fat may occur in patients receiving antiretroviral therapy and that the cause and long-term health effects of these conditions are not known at this time.

Counsel patients on the importance of testing for HIV to avoid inappropriate therapy and development of resistant HIV; offer HIV counseling and testing before starting *Epivir-HBV* and periodically during therapy.

Advise patients that *Epivir-HBV* tablets and oral solution contain a lower dose of the same active ingredient (lamivudine) as *Epivir* oral solution and tablets, *Combivir* (lamivudine/zidovudine) tablets, and *Trizivir* (abacavir/lamivudine/zidovudine) tablets. If a decision is made to include lamivudine in the HIV treatment regimen of a patient dually infected with HIV and HBV, the formulation and dosage of lamivudine in *Epivir* (not *Epivir-HBV*) should be used. Advise patients to not take *Epivir-HBV* concurrently with *Epivir*, *Combivir*, or *Trizivir*. Patients infected with both HBV and HIV who are planning to change their HIV treatment regimen to a regimen that does not include *Epivir*, *Combivir*, or *Trizivir* should discuss continued therapy for hepatitis B with their physician.

STAVUDINE (d4T)

Rx	Zerit (BMS Virology)	Capsules: 15 mg	Lactose. (BMS 1964 15). Lt. yellow/dark red. In 60s.
		20 mg	Lactose. (BMS 1965 20). Lt. brown. In 60s.
		30 mg	Lactose. (BMS 1966 30). Lt. orange/dk. orange. In 60s.
		40 mg	Lactose. (BMS 1967 40). Dk. orange. In 60s.
		Powder for oral solution: 1 mg/mL when reconstituted	Sucrose, parabens. Dye-free. Fruit flavor. In 200 mL.
Rx	Zerit XR (BMS Virology)	Capsules, extended-release: 37.5 mg	Lactose. (BMS 37.5 mg 1555). Red/Yellow. In 30s.
		50 mg	Lactose. (BMS 50 mg 1556). Orange. In 30s.
		75 mg	Lactose. (BMS 75 mg 1557). Red. In 30s.
		100 mg	Lactose. (BMS 100 mg 1558). Yellow. In 30s.

WARNING

Lactic acidosis and severe hepatomegaly with steatosis, including fatal cases, have been reported with the use of nucleoside analogs alone or in combination, including stavudine and other antiretrovirals (see Warnings). Fatal lactic acidosis has been reported in pregnant women who received the combination of stavudine and didanosine with other antiretroviral agents. Use the combination of stavudine and didanosine with caution during pregnancy; use is recommended only if the potential benefit clearly outweighs the potential risk (see Warnings).

Fatal and nonfatal pancreatitis have occurred during therapy when stavudine was part of a combination regimen that included didanosine, with or without hydroxyurea, in both treatment-naive and treatment-experienced patients, regardless of degree of immunosuppression (see Warnings).

Indications

►*HIV infection:* For the treament of HIV-1 infection in combination with other antiretroviral agents.

Administration and Dosage

►*Approved by the FDA:* June 24, 1994.

May be taken without regard to meals.

►*Stavudine immediate-release:*

Adults – The recommended dose based on body weight is as follows:
Patients weighing 60 kg or greater: 40 mg every 12 hours.
Patients weighing less than 60 kg: 30 mg every 12 hours.

Children – The recommended dose for newborns from birth to 13 days of age is 0.5 mg/kg/dose given every 12 hours. The recommended dose for pediatric patients at least 14 days of age and weighing less than 30 kg is 1 mg/kg/dose, given every 12 hours. Pediatric patients weighing 30 kg or greater should receive the recommended adult dosage.

Dosage adjustment in renal function impairment – Stavudine may be administered to adult patients with impaired renal function. The following schedule is recommended:

Stavudine Dosage in Adults with Renal Function Impairment		
Creatinine clearance (mL/min)	Recommended stavudine dose by patient weight	
	≥ 60 kg	< 60 kg
> 50	40 mg every 12 hours	30 mg every 12 hours
26 to 50	20 mg every 12 hours	15 mg every 12 hours
10 to 25	20 mg every 24 hours	15 mg every 24 hours

Because urinary excretion is a major route of elimination of stavudine in pediatric patients, the clearance may be altered in children with renal impairment. Although there are insufficient data to recommend a specific dose adjustment in this patient population, consider a reduction in the dose or an increase in the interval between doses.

Hemodialysis patients – The recommended dose is 20 mg every 24 hours (60 kg or more) or 15 mg every 24 hours (less than 60 kg) administered after the completion of hemodialysis and at the same time of day on nondialysis days.

►*Extended-release capsules:*

Adults – The recommended daily dose is based on body weight and is administered in a once-daily schedule as follows:
Patients weighing 60 kg or more: 100 mg once daily.
Patients weighing less than 60 kg: 75 mg once daily

For patients who have difficulty swallowing intact capsules, the capsule can be carefully opened and the contents mixed with 30 mL of yogurt or applesauce. Patients should be cautioned not to chew or crush the beads while swallowing.

Children – Extended-release stavudine has not been studied in pediatric patients.

Renal impairment – Extended-release stavudine has not been studied in patients with renal impairment.

►*Dosage adjustment in peripheral neuropathy:* Monitor patients for the development of peripheral neuropathy, which is usually characterized by numbness, tingling, or pain in the feet or hands. These symptoms may be difficult to detect in young children. If these symptoms develop, interrupt stavudine therapy. Symptoms may resolve if therapy is withdrawn promptly. In some cases, symptoms may worsen temporarily following discontinuation of therapy. Switching the patient to an alternate treatment regimen should be considered. If switching to an alternate regimen is not suitable and if symptoms resolve satisfactorily, resumption of treatment may be considered at 50% of the recommended dose using the following dosage schedule:

Patients weighing 60 kg or greater –
Immediate-release: 20 mg every 12 hours.
Extended-release: 50 mg once daily.

Patients weighing less than 60 kg –
Immediate-release: 15 mg every 12 hours.
Extended-release: 37.5 mg once daily.

If peripheral neuropathy recurs after resumption of stavudine, consider permanent discontinuation.

►*Preparation of stavudine oral solution:* Prior to dispensing, reconstitute the dry powder with purified water to a concentration of 1 mg/mL of solution as follows:
1.) Add 202 mL of purified water to the container.
2.) Shake container vigorously until the powder dissolves completely. Constitution in this way produces 200 mL (deliverable volume) of 1 mg/mL stavudine solution. The solution may appear slightly hazy.
3.) Dispense solution in original container with measuring cup provided. Instruct patient to shake the container vigorously prior to measuring each dose and to store the tightly closed container in a refrigerator at 36° to 46°F (2° to 8°C). Discard any unused portion after 30 days.

►*Storage/Stability:*

Capsules (immediate-release) – Store in tightly closed containers at 15° to 30°C (59° to 86°F).

Capsules (extended-release) – Store in tightly closed containers at 25°C (77°F); excursions between 15° and 30°C (59° and 86°F) are permitted.

Oral solution – Protect from excessive moisture and store in a tightly closed container at 15° to 30°C (59° to 86°F). After reconstitution, store stavudine for oral solution under refrigeration (2° to 8°C; 36° to 46°F) in tightly closed containers. Discard any unused portion after 30 days.

Actions

►*Pharmacology:* Stavudine is a synthetic thymidine nucleoside analog active against HIV. It inhibits the replication of HIV in human cells in vitro. Stavudine is phosphorylated by cellular kinases to stavudine

STAVUDINE (d4T)

triphosphate, which exerts antiviral activity and inhibits HIV replication by 2 known mechanisms:

1.) It inhibits HIV reverse transcriptase by competing with the natural substrate deoxythymidine triphosphate; and

2.) It inhibits viral DNA synthesis by its incorporation into viral DNA. This causes DNA chain elongation termination because stavudine lacks the 3'-hydroxyl group necessary for DNA elongation. Stavudine triphosphate also inhibits cellular DNA polymerase beta and gamma, and markedly reduces mitochondrial DNA synthesis.

➤*Pharmacokinetics:*

Absorption – The pharmacokinetics of stavudine have been evaluated in HIV-infected adult and pediatric patients (see table below). Peak plasma concentrations (C_{max}) and area under the plasma concentration-time curve (AUC) increased in proportion to dose after single and multiple doses ranging from 0.03 to 4 mg/kg. There was no significant accumulation of stavudine with repeated administration every 6, 8, or 12 hours.

Following oral administration, stavudine is rapidly absorbed, with peak plasma concentrations occurring within 1 hour after dosing. The systemic exposure to stavudine is the same following administration as capsules or solution.

In a crossover study in healthy volunteers, equivalent values for stavudine AUC (total daily exposure) were observed for the extended-release and immediate-release formulations. AUC increased proportionally with dose in the oral dose range of 37.5 to 100 mg.

In parallel groups of HIV-infected patients, stavudine exposure was on average 23% lower following administration of 100 mg once daily of the extended-release formulation compared with 40 mg twice daily of the immediate-release formulation. The maximum plasma concentration (C_{max}) for the extended-release capsule is 43% of the value for the immediate-release capsule, and the time to reach C_{max} (T_{max}) is approximately 3 hours for the extended-release capsule compared with 1 hour for the immediate-release capsule. No significant accumulation of stavudine was observed after repeated administration of the extended-release capsule every 24 hours.

Pharmacokinetic Parameters of Stavudine in HIV-Infected Adults, Extended Release vs Immediate-Release: Absorption		
Parameter	Extended-release 100 mg qd, mean ± SD (n = 19[1])	Immediate-release 40 mg bid, mean ± SD (n = 8[1])
AUC (ng•h/mL)	1966 ± 629	2568 ± 454
C_{max} (ng/mL)	228 ± 62	536 ± 148
C_{min} (ng/mL)	24 ± 17	8 ± 9

[1] Parallel groups for extended release and immediate release formulation in HIV-infected adults.

Distribution – Binding to serum proteins was negligible over the concentration range of 0.01 to 11.4 mcg/mL. Stavudine distributes equally between red blood cells and plasma.

Excretion – Renal elimination accounted for approximately 40% of the overall clearance regardless of the route of administration; there is active tubular secretion in addition to glomerular filtration. The remaining 60% of the drug is presumably eliminated by endogenous pathways. The elimination half-life of stavudine is 1.6 hours.

Pharmacokinetic Parameters of Stavudine in Adult and Pediatric HIV-Infected Patients		
Parameter	Adult patients	Pediatric patients
Oral bioavailability	≈ 86.4%	≈ 76.9%
Volume of distribution[1]	≈ 58 L	≈ 0.73 L/kg
Apparent oral volume of distribution[2]	≈ 66 L	not determined
Ratio of CSF:plasma concentrations (as %)[3]	not determined	≈ 59
Total body clearance[1]	≈ 8.3 mL/min/kg	≈ 9.75 mL/min/kg
Apparent oral clearance[2]	≈ 8 mL/min/kg	≈ 13.75 mL/min/kg
Elimination half-life, IV dose[1]	≈ 1.15 h	≈ 1.11 h
Elimination half-life, oral dose[2]	≈ 1.44 h	≈ 0.96 h
Urinary recovery of stavudine (% of dose)[2]	≈ 39	≈ 34

[1] Following 1 hour IV infusion.
[2] Following single oral dose.
[3] Following multiple oral doses.

Special populations –

Renal insufficiency: The apparent oral clearance of stavudine decreased and the terminal elimination half-life increased as Ccr decreased. C_{max} and T_{max} were not significantly affected by reduced renal function. The mean ± SD hemodialysis clearance value of stavudine was 120 ± 18 mL/min (n = 12); the mean ± SD percentage of the stavudine dose recovered in the dialysate, timed to occur between 2 and 6 hours postdose, was 31% ± 5%. Based on these observations, adjust dosage in patients with reduced Ccr and in patients receiving maintenance hemodialysis. The extended release formulation should not be used in patients with creatinine clearance of 50 mL/min or less. (See Administration and Dosage.)

Pharmacokinetic Parameter Values for Single 40 mg Oral Dose of Immediate-Release Stavudine				
	Creatinine clearance			
	> 50 mL/min (n = 10)	26 to 50 mL/min (n = 5)	9 to 25 mL/min (n = 5)	Hemodialysis patients[1] (n = 11)
Ccr (mL/min)	≈ 104	≈ 41	≈ 17	NA[2]
CL/F[3] (mL/min)	≈ 335	≈ 191	≈ 116	≈ 105
CL_R[4] (mL/min)	≈ 167	≈ 73	≈ 17	NA
$T_{1/2}$[5] (h)	≈ 1.7	≈ 3.5	≈ 4.6	≈ 5.4

[1] Determined while patients were off dialysis.
[2] Not applicable.
[3] Apparent oral clearance.
[4] Renal clearance.
[5] Terminal elimination half-life.

➤*Microbiology:*

In vitro HIV susceptibility – The in vitro antiviral activity of stavudine was measured in peripheral blood mononuclear cells, monocytic cells, and lymphoblastoid cell lines. The concentration of drug necessary to inhibit viral replication by 50% (IC_{50}) ranged from 0.009 to 4 mcM against laboratory and clinical isolates of HIV-1. The relationship between in vitro susceptibility of HIV to stavudine and the inhibition of HIV replication in humans has not been established.

Drug resistance – HIV isolates with reduced susceptibility to stavudine have been selected in vitro and also were obtained from patients treated with stavudine. Phenotypic analysis of HIV isolates from stavudine-treated patients revealed in 3 of 20 paired isolates, a 4- to 12-fold decrease in susceptibility to stavudine in vitro. The genetic basis for these susceptibility changes has not been identified. The clinical relevance of changes in stavudine susceptibility has not been established.

Cross-resistance – Five of 11 stavudine post-treatment isolates developed moderate resistance to zidovudine (9- to 196-fold), and 3 of those 11 isolates developed moderate resistance to didanosine (7- to 29-fold). The clinical relevance of these findings is unknown.

➤*Clinical trials:*

Combination therapy – The combination use of stavudine is based on the results of clinical studies in HIV-infected patients in double- and triple-combination regimens with other antiretroviral agents.

One of these studies was a multicenter, randomized, open-label study comparing immediate-release stavudine (40 mg twice daily) plus lamivudine plus indinavir to zidovudine plus lamivudine plus indinavir in 202 treatment-naive patients. Both regimens resulted in a similar magnitude of inhibition of HIV RNA levels and increases in CD4 cell counts through 48 weeks.

Monotherapy – The efficacy of immediate-release stavudine was demonstrated in a randomized, double-blind study comparing stavudine with zidovudine in 822 patients with a spectrum of HIV-related symptoms. The outcome in terms of progression of HIV disease and death was similar for both drugs.

Contraindications

Clinically significant hypersensitivity to stavudine or to any components of the formulation.

Warnings

➤*Lactic acidosis/severe hepatomegaly with steatosis/hepatic failure:* Lactic acidosis and severe hepatomegaly with steatosis, including fatal cases, have been reported with the use of nucleoside analogs alone or in combination, including stavudine and other antiretrovirals. Longitudinal cohort and retrospective studies suggest that this infrequent event may be more often associated with antiretroviral combinations containing stavudine. Female gender, obesity, and prolonged nucleoside exposure may be risk factors. Fatal lactic acidosis has been reported in pregnant women who received the combination of stavudine and didanosine with other antiretroviral agents. Use the combination of stavudine and didanosine with caution during pregnancy; it is recommended only if the potential benefit clearly outweighs the potential risk (see Pregnancy). In addition, deaths attributed to hepatotoxicity have occurred in patients receiving the combination of stavudine, didanosine, and hydroxyurea. Exercise caution when administering stavudine to any patient with known risk factors for liver disease; however, cases also have been reported in patients with no known risk factors. Generalized fatigue, digestive symptoms (eg, nausea, vomiting, abdominal pain, sudden unexplained weight loss), respiratory symptoms (eg, tachypnea, dyspnea), or neurologic symptoms (eg, motor weakness) might be indicative of the development of symptomatic hyperlactatemia or lactic acidosis syndrome. Suspend treatment with stavudine in any patient who develops clinical or laboratory findings suggestive of symptomatic hyperlactatemia, lactic acidosis, or pronounced hepatotoxicity (which may include hepatomegaly and steatosis

STAVUDINE (d4T)

even in the absence of marked transaminase elevations). An increased risk of hepatotoxicity, which may be fatal, may occur in patients treated with stavudine in combination with didanosine and hydroxyurea compared with when stavudine is used alone. Closely monitor patients treated with this combination for signs of liver toxicity.

➤*Neurologic symptoms:* Motor weakness has been reported rarely. Most of these cases occurred in the setting of lactic acidosis. The evolution of motor weakness may mimic the clinical presentation of Guillain-Barré syndrome (including respiratory failure). Symptoms may continue or worsen following discontinuation of therapy.

Stavudine therapy has been associated with peripheral neuropathy, which can be severe and is dose-related. Peripheral neuropathy is manifested by numbness, tingling, or pain in the hands or feet. Peripheral neuropathy has occurred more frequently in patients with advanced HIV disease, a history of neuropathy, or concurrent neurotoxic drug therapy, including didanosine (see Adverse Reactions).

Monitor patients for development of neuropathy. Stavudine-related peripheral neuropathy may resolve if therapy is withdrawn promptly. Symptoms may worsen temporarily following therapy discontinuation. Switching the patient with peripheral neuropathy to an alternate treatment regimen should be considered. If switching to an alternative regimen is not suitable and if symptoms resolve satisfactorily, resumption of treatment may be considered at 50% of the dose (see Administration and Dosage). If neuropathy recurs after resumption of stavudine, consider permanent discontinuation.

➤*Pancreatitis:* Fatal and nonfatal pancreatitis have occurred during therapy when stavudine was part of a combination regimen that included didanosine, with or without hydroxyurea, in treatment-naive and treatment-experienced patients, regardless of degree of immunosuppression. Suspend the combination of stavudine and didanosine (with or without hydroxyurea) and any other agents that are toxic to the pancreas in patients with suspected pancreatitis. Undertake reinstitution of stavudine after a confirmed diagnosis of pancreatitis with particular caution and close patient monitoring. The new regimen should not contain either didanosine or hydroxyurea.

➤*Fat redistribution:* Redistribution/accumulation of body fat including central obesity, dorsocervical fat enlargement (buffalo hump), peripheral wasting, facial wasting, breast enlargement, and "cushingoid appearance" have been observed in patients receiving antiretroviral therapy. The mechanism and long-term consequences of these events are currently unknown. A causal relationship has not been established.

➤*Carcinogenesis:* Benign and malignant liver tumors in mice and rats and malignant urinary bladder tumors in male rats occurred at levels of exposure 250 (mice) and 732 (rats) times the human exposure at the recommended clinical dose.

➤*Mutagenesis:* Stavudine produced positive results in the in vitro human lymphocyte clastogenesis and mouse fibroblast assays and in the in vivo mouse micronucleus test. In the in vitro assays, stavudine elevated the frequency of chromosome aberrations in human lymphocytes and increased the frequency of transformed foci in mouse fibroblast cells. In the in vivo micronucleus assay, stavudine was clastogenic in bone marrow cells following oral stavudine administration to mice at dosages of 600 to 2000 mg/kg/day for 3 days.

➤*Elderly:* Clinical studies of stavudine did not include sufficient numbers of patients 65 years of age and older to determine whether they respond differently than younger patients. Greater sensitivity of some older individuals to the effects of stavudine cannot be ruled out.

In a monotherapy expanded access program for patients with advanced HIV infection, peripheral neuropathy or peripheral neuropathic symptoms were observed in 15 of 40 (38%) elderly patients receiving stavudine immediate-release 40 mg twice daily and 8 of 51 (16%) elderly patients receiving 20 mg twice daily. Of the approximately 12,000 patients enrolled in the expanded access program, peripheral neuropathy or peripheral neuropathic symptoms developed in 30% of patients receiving 40 mg twice daily and 25% of patients receiving 20 mg twice daily. Closely monitor elderly patients for signs and symptoms of peripheral neuropathy.

Stavudine is known to be substantially excreted by the kidneys, and the risk of toxic reactions to this drug may be greater in patients with impaired renal function. Because elderly patients are more likely to have decreased renal function, it may be useful to monitor renal function. Stavudine immediate-release with dose adjustment is recommended for patients with Ccr of 50 mL/min or less (see Administration and Dosage).

➤*Pregnancy: Category C.* In rat fetuses, the incidence of a common skeletal variation, unossified or incomplete ossification of sternebra, was increased at 399 times human exposure. A slight postimplantation loss was noted at 216 times the human exposure. An increase in early rat neonatal mortality (birth to 4 days of age) occurred at 399 times the human exposure. A study in rats showed that stavudine is transferred to the fetus through the placenta. The concentration in fetal tissue was about 50% that in maternal plasma. There are no adequate and well-controlled studies in pregnant women. Use stavudine during pregnancy only if the potential benefit justifies the potential risk.

Fatal lactic acidosis has been reported in pregnant women who received the combination of stavudine and didanosine with other antiretroviral agents. It is unclear if pregnancy augments the risk of lactic acidosis/hepatic steatosis syndrome reported in nonpregnant individuals receiving nucleoside analogs (see Lactic acidosis/severe hepatomegaly with steatosis/hepatic failure). Use the combination of stavudine and didanosine with caution during pregnancy; it is recommended only if the potential benefit clearly outweighs the potential risk. Health care providers caring for HIV-infected pregnant women receiving stavudine should be alert for early diagnosis of lactic acidosis/hepatic steatosis syndrome.

To monitor maternal-fetal outcomes of pregnant women exposed to stavudine and other antiretroviral agents, an Antiretroviral Pregnancy Registry has been established. Physicians are encouraged to register patients by calling (800) 258-4263.

➤*Lactation:* The CDC recommends that HIV-infected mothers not breastfeed their infants to avoid risking postnatal transmission of HIV. Studies in lactating rats demonstrated that stavudine is excreted in milk. Although it is not known whether stavudine is excreted in human milk, there exists the potential for adverse effects from stavudine in nursing infants. Because of the potential for HIV transmission and the potential for serious adverse reactions in nursing infants, instruct mothers not to breastfeed if they are receiving stavudine.

➤*Children:* Use of immediate-release stavudine in pediatric patients is supported by evidence from adequate and well-controlled studies of stavudine in adults with additional pharmacokinetic and safety data in pediatric patients. The safety and efficacy of the extended-release form in pediatric patients have not been established.

Drug Interactions

Stavudine Drug Interactions			
Precipitant drug	Object drug[*]		Description
Didanosine Hydroxyurea	Stavudine	↑	Coadministration may increase the risk for lactic acidosis, hepatotoxicity, pancreatitis, or peripheral neuropathy (see Warnings).
Doxorubicin Ribavirin	Stavudine	↓	Phosphorylation of stavudine is inhibited at relevant concentrations by doxorubicin and ribavirin. Coadministration should be undertaken with caution.
Methadone	Stavudine	↓	Coadministration produced a 25% decrease in AUC and a 44% decrease in peak drug concentration of stavudine.
Zidovudine	Stavudine	↓	Zidovudine may competitively inhibit the intracellular phosphorylation of stavudine. Coadministration is not recommended.

[*] ↑ = Object drug increased. ↓ = Object drug decreased.

Adverse Reactions

Fatal lactic acidosis has occurred in patients treated with stavudine in combination with other antiretroviral agents. Patients with suspected lactic acidosis should immediately suspend therapy with stavudine. Consider permanent discontinuation of stavudine for patients with confirmed lactic acidosis.

Stavudine therapy rarely has been associated with motor weakness, occurring predominantly in the setting of lactic acidosis. If motor weakness develops, discontinue stavudine.

Stavudine therapy also has been associated with peripheral sensory neuropathy, which can be severe, is dose related, and occurs more frequently in patients being treated with neurotoxic drug therapy, including didanosine, in patients with advanced HIV infection, or in patients who have previously experienced peripheral neuropathy (see Administration and Dosage and Warnings).

When stavudine is used in combination with other agents with similar toxicities, the incidence of adverse events may be higher than when stavudine is used alone. Pancreatitis, peripheral neuropathy, and liver function abnormalities occur more frequently in patients treated with the combination of stavudine and didanosine, with or without hydroxyurea. Fatal pancreatitis and hepatotoxicity may occur more frequently in patients treated with stavudine in combination with didanosine and hydroxyurea (see table below, Warnings).

➤*Immediate-release:*

Stavudine Adverse Reactions in Monotherapy Study[1] (%)		
Adverse reaction	Stavudine (40 mg bid) (n = 412)	Zidovudine (200 mg tid) (n = 402)
Headache	54	49
Diarrhea	50	44
Peripheral neurologic symptoms/neuropathy	52	39

STAVUDINE (d4T)

Stavudine Adverse Reactions in Monotherapy Study[1] (%)		
Adverse reaction	Stavudine (40 mg bid) (n = 412)	Zidovudine (200 mg tid) (n = 402)
Rash	40	35
Nausea and vomiting	39	44
Laboratory test abnormalities[2]		
AST (> 5 × ULN[3])	11	10
ALT (> 5 × ULN[3])	13	11
Amylase (≥ 1.4 × ULN[3])	14	13

[1] Median duration of stavudine therapy = 79 weeks; median duration of zidovudine therapy = 53 weeks.
[2] Data presented for patients for whom laboratory evaluations were performed.
[3] ULN = Upper limit of normal.

Pancreatitis was observed in 3 of the 412 adult patients who received stavudine in a controlled monotherapy study.

Selected clinical adverse events that occurred in antiretroviral-naive adult patients receiving stavudine from 2 controlled combination studies are provided below.

Stavudine Adverse Reactions in Combination Therapy Studies[1] (%)				
	Study 1		Study 2	
Adverse reaction	Stavudine + lamivudine + indinavir (n = 100)[2]	Zidovudine + lamivudine + indinavir (n = 102)	Stavudine + didanosine + indinavir (n = 102)[2]	Zidovudine + lamivudine + indinavir (n = 103)
Nausea	43	63	53	67
Diarrhea	34	16	45	39
Headache	25	26	46	37
Rash	18	13	30	18
Vomiting	18	33	30	35
Peripheral neurologic symptoms/ neuropathy	8	7	21	10

[1] Study 2 compared 2 triple-combination regimens in 205 treatment-naive patients. Patients received either stavudine (40 mg twice daily) plus didanosine plus indinavir or zidovudine plus lamivudine plus indinavir.
[2] Duration of stavudine therapy = 48 weeks.

Selected Stavudine Lab Test Abnormalities in Combination Studies (Grades 3 to 4) (%)				
	Study 1		Study 2	
Parameter	Stavudine + lamivudine + indinavir (n = 100)	Zidovudine + lamivudine + indinavir (n = 102)	Stavudine + didanosine + indinavir (n = 102)	Zidovudine + lamivudine + indinavir (n = 103)
Bilirubin (> 2.6 x ULN)	7	6	16	8
AST (> 5 × ULN)	5	2	7	7
ALT (> 5 × ULN)	6	2	8	5
GGT (> 5 × ULN)	2	2	5	2
Lipase (> 2 x ULN)	6	3	5	5
Amylase (> 2 x ULN)	4	< 1	8	2

Stavudine Lab Test Abnormalities in Combination Studies (All Grades) (%)				
	Study 1		Study 2	
Parameter	Stavudine + lamivudine + indinavir (n = 100)	Zidovudine + lamivudine + indinavir (n = 102)	Stavudine + didanosine + indinavir (n = 102)	Zidovudine + lamivudine + indinavir (n = 103)
Total bilirubin	65	60	68	55
AST	42	20	53	20
ALT	40	20	50	18
GGT	15	8	28	12
Lipase	27	12	26	19
Amylase	21	19	31	17

Postmarketing – The following events have been identified during postapproval use of stavudine. Because they are reported voluntarily from a population of unknown size, estimates of frequency cannot be made. These events have been chosen for inclusion because of their seriousness, frequency of reporting, causal connection to stavudine, or a combination of these factors.

CNS: Insomnia; severe motor weakness (most often reported in the setting of lactic acidosis).
Hematologic: Anemia; leukopenia; thrombocytopenia.
Hepatic: Symptomatic hyperlactatemia/lactic acidosis and hepatic steatosis; hepatitis; liver failure.

Miscellaneous: Abdominal pain; allergic reaction; anorexia; chills/fever; redistribution/accumulation of body fat; myalgia; pancreatitis (including fatal cases).

Children: Adverse reactions and serious laboratory abnormalities in pediatric patients from birth through adolescence were similar in type and frequency to those seen in adult patients.

►*Extended-release:* In the pooled database from 2 studies and an ongoing long-term follow-up study for patients completing these 2 trials (median duration of therapy 56 weeks, ranging up to 120 weeks), the rates of discontinuation of therapy because of adverse events were 5% for the extended-release stavudine capsules regimen and 7% for stavudine immediate-release. In clinical trials, less than 1% of 486 patients treated with stavudine extended-release for a median duration of 56 weeks (ranging up to 120 weeks) discontinued therapy because of peripheral neuropathy.

Selected Clinical Adverse Events[1] of Any Severity from Combination Studies of Stavudine Extended-Release (Pooled Data) (%)[2]		
Adverse event	Stavudine extended-release + lamivudine + efavirenz (n = 466)	Stavudine immediate-release + lamivudine + efavirenz (n = 467)
CNS		
Dizziness	30	30
PNS[3]/Neuropathy	16	19
Abnormal dreams	13	14
Somnolence	8	8
Insomnia	8	5
Abnormal thinking	3	2
Depression	2	1
GI		
Diarrhea	10	10
Nausea	10	9
Dyspepsia	4	3
Vomiting	3	4
Miscellaneous		
Headache	12	8
Fatigue	6	4
Lipodystrophy	3	4
Rash	16	12
Pruritus	4	4
Lab abnormalities		
AST (> 5 × ULN[4])	2	3
ALT (> 5 × ULN)	8	3
Lipase (> 2.1 × ULN)	4	3
Total bilirubin (> 2.6 × ULN)	< 1	0
Neutropenia (ANC[5] < 750/mm³)	5	5
Anemia (hemoglobin < 6 g/dL)	< 1	< 1
Thrombocytopenia (platelets < 50,000/mm³)	1	2

[1] Considered by the investigator to be of possible, probable, or unknown relationship to any component of the drug regimen.
[2] Patients received stavudine extended-release 100 mg once daily or stavudine immediate-release 40 mg twice daily each in combination with lamivudine 150 mg twice daily and efavirenz 600 mg once daily. Median duration of treatment was 56 weeks (ranging up to 120 weeks).
[3] PNS = Peripheral neurologic symptoms (includes neuropathy, paresthesia, and peripheral neuritis).
[4] ULN = Upper limit of normal
[5] ANC = absolute neutrophil count

In clinical trials, lactic acidosis syndrome/symptomatic hyperlactatemia (LAS/SHL), sometimes fatal, was reported. LAS/SHL occurred in 3 of 466 patients treated with stavudine extended-release and in 6 of 467 patients treated with stavudine immediate-release. The overall incidence of LAS/SHL for these trials was 8.8/1000 patient years.

Elevations in liver function tests or progression of liver disease, sometimes fatal, that resulted in discontinuation of study drug were observed in 3 of 466 patients in the extended-release stavudine arm and 3 of 467 patients in the immediate-release arm of clinical trials. All 6 patients were coinfected with hepatitis B or C.

Pancreatitis was observed in 1 of 466 patients treated with stavudine extended-release and 4 of 467 treated with immediate-release in clinical trials. Pancreatitis resulting in death was observed in patients treated with stavudine plus didanosine with or without hydroxyurea in controlled clinical studies and in postmarketing reports.

Overdosage

Experience with adults treated with the immediate-release formulation at 12 to 24 times the recommended daily dosage revealed no acute toxicity. Complications of chronic overdosage include peripheral neuropathy and hepatic toxicity. Stavudine can be removed by hemodialysis; the hemodialysis clearance of stavudine is approximately 120 mL/min. It is not known whether stavudine is eliminated by peritoneal dialysis.

STAVUDINE (d4T)

Patient Information

Inform patients that stavudine is not a cure for HIV infection and that they may continue to acquire illnesses associated with HIV infection, including opportunistic infections. Advise patients to remain under a physician's care when using stavudine.

Advise patients of the importance of adherence to any antiretroviral regimen, including those that contain stavudine.

Inform patients of the importance of early recognition of symptoms of symptomatic hyperlactatemia or lactic acidosis, which include unexplained weight loss, abdominal discomfort, nausea, vomiting, fatigue, dyspnea, and motor weakness. Patients in whom these symptoms develop should seek medical attention immediately.

Inform patients that an important toxicity of stavudine is peripheral neuropathy. They should be aware that the symptoms include tingling, pain, or numbness in the hands or feet. Counsel patients that this toxicity occurs with greatest frequency in patients with advanced HIV disease or a history of peripheral neuropathy. Advise them to report these symptoms to their physician and that dose changes or discontinuation may be necessary if toxicity develops. Also caution them about the use of other medications that may exacerbate peripheral neuropathy.

Instruct caregivers of young children receiving therapy regarding detection and reporting of peripheral neuropathy.

Inform patients that when stavudine is used in combination with other agents with similar toxicities, the incidence of adverse events may be higher than when stavudine is used alone. An increased risk of pancreatitis, which may be fatal, may occur in patients treated with the combination of stavudine and didanosine, with or without hydroxyurea. Closely monitor patients treated with this combination for symptoms of pancreatitis. An increased risk of hepatotoxicity, which may be fatal, may occur in patients treated with stavudine in combination with didanosine and hydroxyurea. Closely monitor patients treated with this combination for signs of liver toxicity.

Inform patients that the CDC recommends that HIV-infected mothers not nurse newborn infants to reduce the risk of postnatal transmission of HIV infection.

Tell patients that the long-term effects of stavudine are unknown at this time. Advise them that therapy has not been shown to reduce the risk of transmission of HIV to others through sexual contact or blood contamination.

Inform patients that redistribution or accumulation of body fat may occur in patients receiving antiretroviral therapy and that the cause and long-term health effects of these conditions are not known at this time.

ZALCITABINE (Dideoxycytidine; ddC)

Rx	**Hivid** (Roche)	**Tablets:** 0.375 mg	Lactose. (Hivid 0.375 Roche). Beige, oval. Film-coated. In 100s.
		0.75 mg	Lactose. (Hivid 0.750 Roche). Gray, oval. Film-coated. In 100s.

WARNING

The use of zalcitabine has been associated with significant clinical adverse reactions, some of which are potentially fatal. Zalcitabine can cause severe peripheral neuropathy; therefore use with extreme caution in patients with pre-existing neuropathy. Zalcitabine may also rarely cause pancreatitis; immediately suspend therapy in patients who develop any symptoms suggestive of pancreatitis while using zalcitabine until this diagnosis is excluded.

Lactic acidosis and severe hepatomegaly with steatosis, including fatal cases, have been reported with the use of antiretroviral nucleoside analogs alone or in combination, including zalcitabine. In addition, rare cases of hepatic failure and death considered possibly related to underlying hepatitis B and zalcitabine have been reported (see Warnings).

Indications

➤*Combination therapy with antiretrovirals:* For the treatment of human immunodeficiency virus (HIV) infection.

Administration and Dosage

➤*Approved by the FDA:* June 19, 1992.

➤*Combination therapy with antiretrovirals:* The recommended regimen is one 0.75 mg tablet of zalcitabine orally every 8 hours (2.25 mg zalcitabine total daily dose) in combination with other antiretroviral agents.

Advise patients that zalcitabine is recommended for use in combination with active antiretroviral therapy. Greater activity has been observed when new antiretroviral therapies are started at the same time as zalcitabine. Base concomitant therapy on a patient's prior drug exposure. Refer to the complete product information for each of the other antiretroviral agents for the recommended doses of these agents.

➤*Renal function impairment:* Dosage reduction is recommended: Ccr 10 to 40 mL/min, 0.75 mg every 12 hours; Ccr < 10 mL/min, 0.75 mg every 24 hours.

➤*Dose adjustment:*

Combination therapy – For toxicities likely to be associated with zalcitabine (eg, peripheral neuropathy, severe oral ulcers, pancreatitis, elevated liver function tests, especially in patients with chronic hepatitis B; see Warnings and Precautions), interrupt or reduce dose. For severe toxicities or those persisting after dose reduction, interrupt zalcitabine therapy. For recipients of combination therapy with zalcitabine and other antiretrovirals, base dose adjustments or interruption for either drug on the known toxicity profile of the individual drugs.

Peripheral neuropathy – Patients developing moderate discomfort with signs or symptoms of peripheral neuropathy should stop zalcitabine. Zalcitabine-associated peripheral neuropathy may continue to worsen despite interruption of therapy. Reintroduce the drug at 50% dose (0.375 mg every 8 hours) only if all findings related to peripheral neuropathy have improved to mild symptoms. Permanently discontinue the drug when patients experience severe discomfort related to peripheral neuropathy or moderate discomfort progresses. If other moderate to severe clinical adverse reactions or lab abnormalities (eg, increased liver function tests) occur, interrupt zalcitabine (or both zalcitabine and the other potential causative agent(s) in combination therapy) until the adverse reaction abates. Carefully reintroduce zalcitabine or the other agent at lower doses if appropriate. If adverse reactions recur, discontinue therapy. The minimum effective dose of zalcitabine in combination with zidovudine for the treatment of adults with advanced HIV infection has not been established.

Hematologic toxicities – Significant toxicities, such as anemia (hemoglobin < 7.5 g/dL or reduction of > 25% of baseline) or granulocytopenia (granulocyte count of < 750/mm^3 or reduction of > 50% from baseline), may require a treatment interruption of zalcitabine and zidovudine until evidence of marrow recovery is observed (see Warnings). For less severe anemia or granulocytopenia, a reduction in the daily dose of zidovudine in those patients receiving combination therapy may be adequate. In patients who develop significant anemia, dose modification does not necessarily eliminate the need for transfusion. If marrow recovery occurs following dose modification, gradual increases in dose may be appropriate depending on hematologic indices and patient intolerance.

➤*Storage/Stability:* Store at 15° to 30°C (59° to 86°F) in tightly closed bottle.

Actions

➤*Pharmacology:* Zalcitabine, active against HIV, is a synthetic pyrimidine nucleoside analog of the naturally occurring nucleoside deoxycytidine in which the 3′-hydroxyl group is replaced by hydrogen. Within cells, zalcitabine is converted to the active metabolite, dideoxycytidine 5′-triphosphate (ddCTP), by cellular enzymes. ddCTP inhibits the activity of the HIV-reverse transcriptase by competing for utilization of the natural substrate, deoxycytidine 5′-triphosphate (dCTP), and by its incorporation into viral DNA. The lack of a 3′-OH group in the incorporated nucleoside analog prevents the formation of the 5′ to 3′ phosphodiester linkage essential for DNA chain elongation and, therefore, the viral DNA growth is terminated. The active metabolite, ddCTP, is also an inhibitor of cellular DNA polymerase-beta and mitochondrial DNA polymerase-gamma and has been reported to be incorporated into the DNA of cells in culture.

➤*Pharmacokinetics:*

Adults –

Absorption/Distribution: Following oral administration to HIV-infected patients, the mean absolute bioavailability of zalcitabine was > 80%. The absorption rate of a 1.5 mg oral dose was reduced when administered with food. This resulted in a 39% decrease in mean maximum plasma concentrations (C_{max}) from 25.2 to 15.5 ng/mL, and a 2-fold increase in time to achieve C_{max} from a mean of 0.8 hours under fasting conditions to 1.6 hours when the drug was given with food. The extent of absorption was decreased by 14% (from 72 to 62 ng•h/mL).

The steady-state volume of distribution following IV administration of a 1.5 mg dose averaged 0.534 L/kg. Cerebrospinal fluid obtained from 9 patients at 2 to 3.5 hours following 0.06 or 0.09 mg/kg IV infusion showed measurable concentrations of zalcitabine. The CSF:Plasma concentration ratio ranged from 9% to 37% (mean, 20%), demonstrating drug penetration through the blood-brain barrier.

Metabolism/Excretion: Zalcitabine is phosphorylated intracellularly to zalcitabine triphosphate, the active substrate for HIV-reverse transcriptase. Concentrations of zalcitabine triphosphate are too low for quantitation. Zalcitabine does not undergo a significant degree of metabolism by the liver. Renal excretion appears to be the primary route of elimination, and it accounted for ≈ 60% of an orally administered dose within 24 hours after dosing. The mean elimination half-life is 2 hours and generally ranges from 1 to 3 hours. Total body clearance

ZALCITABINE (Dideoxycytidine; ddC)

following an IV dose averages 285 mL/min. Approximately 10% of a dose appears in the feces.

Special populations:

• *Renal function impairment* – In patients with impaired kidney function, prolonged elimination of zalcitabine may be expected. Results from 7 patients with renal impairment (estimated Ccr < 55 mL/min) indicate that the half-life was prolonged (up to 8.5 hours) in these patients compared with those with normal renal function. C_{max} was higher in some patients after a single dose. In patients with normal renal function, the pharmacokinetics of zalcitabine were not altered during 3 times/day multiple dosing. Accumulation of drug in plasma during this regimen was negligible. The drug was < 4% bound to plasma proteins, indicating that drug interactions involving binding-site displacement are unlikely (see Drug Interactions).

Children – Limited pharmacokinetic data have been reported for 5 HIV-positive children using doses of 0.03 and 0.04 mg/kg administered orally every 6 hours. The mean bioavailability of zalcitabine in this study was 54% and mean apparent systemic clearance was 150 mL/min/m^2.

➤*Microbiology:*

Drug resistance – The emergence of HIV isolates with reduced susceptibility (resistance) to zalcitabine has been demonstrated in a small number of patients who received monotherapy by 1 year of therapy. Combination therapy of zalcitabine plus zidovudine does not appear to prevent the emergence of zidovudine-resistant isolates.

➤*Clinical trials:*

Monotherapy – Zalcitabine was compared with didanosine for treatment of advanced HIV infection (mean CD4 cell count, 37 cells/mm^3) in patients who were intolerant to zidovudine or had disease progression while receiving zidovudine. Zalcitabine was at least as effective as didanosine in terms of time to an AIDS-defining event or death, while for survival alone the results favored zalcitabine.

Combination therapy – The use of zalcitabine in combination with AZT is based on the clinical results from study ACTG 175, a randomized, double-blind controlled trial. A total of 2467 HIV-infected adults (mean baseline CD4 count = 352 cells/mm^3) with no prior AIDS-defining event enrolled with the following demographics: Male (82%), Caucasian (70%), mean age 35 years, asymptomatic HIV infection (81%) and prior antiretroviral use (57%, mean duration = 89.5 weeks). The overall mean duration of study treatment was 99 weeks. The incidence of AIDS-defining events or death is shown in the table below:

First AIDS-Defining Event or Death and Death Only by Study Arm and Antiretroviral Experience in ACTG 175					
		Treatment			
Antiretroviral experience	Event	AZT 200 mg tid	AZT 200 mg tid + ddI 200 mg bid	AZT 200 mg tid + ddC 0.75 mg tid	ddI 200 mg bid
Overall	n	619	613	615	620
	AIDS/Death	16%	11%	12%	11%
	Death only	9%	5%	7%	5%
Naive	n	269	263	267	268
	AIDS/Death	12%	8%	6%	9%
	Death only	7%	4%	3%	4%
Experienced	n	350	350	348	352
	AIDS/Death	18%	13%	17%	14%
	Death only	10%	6%	9%	5%

Contraindications

Hypersensitivity to zalcitabine or any excipients of the product.

Warnings

Significant clinical adverse reactions, some of which are potentially fatal, have been reported with zalcitabine. Patients with decreased CD$_4$ cell counts appear to have an increased incidence of adverse events.

➤*Peripheral neuropathy:* The major clinical toxicity is peripheral neuropathy, which may occur in ≤ 33% of patients with advanced disease treated with zalcitabine. The incidence in patients with less advanced disease is lower.

Zalcitabine-related peripheral neuropathy is a sensorimotor neuropathy characterized initially by numbness and burning dysesthesia involving the distal extremities. These symptoms may be followed by sharp shooting pains or severe continuous burning pain if the drug is not withdrawn. The neuropathy may progress to severe pain requiring narcotic analgesics and is potentially irreversible. In some patients, symptoms of neuropathy may initially progress despite discontinuation of zalcitabine. With prompt discontinuation, the neuropathy is usually slowly reversible.

There are no data regarding the use of zalcitabine in patients with preexisting peripheral neuropathy because these patients were excluded from clinical trials; therefore, use with extreme caution in these patients. Avoid zalcitabine in individuals with moderate or severe peripheral neuropathy, as evidenced by symptoms accompanied by objective findings.

Zalcitabine should be used with caution in patients with a risk of developing peripheral neuropathy: Patients with low CD4 cell counts (CD4 < 50 cells/mm^3), diabetes, weight loss, or patients receiving zalcitabine concomitantly with drugs that have the potential to cause peripheral neuropathy (see Drug Interactions). Careful monitoring is strongly recommended for these individuals.

Stop zalcitabine promptly if signs or symptoms of peripheral neuropathy occurs, such as when moderate discomfort from numbness, tingling, burning, or pain of the extremities progresses, or any related symptoms occur that are accompanied by an objective finding (see Administration and Dosage).

➤*Pancreatitis:* Pancreatitis, fatal in some cases, has been observed with zalcitabine administration. Pancreatitis is an uncommon complication of zalcitabine therapy, occurring in up to 1.1% of patients.

Closely follow patients with a history of pancreatitis or known risk factors for the development of pancreatitis while on zalcitabine. In 528 patients with a history of pancreatitis or increased amylase, 5.3% developed pancreatitis and an additional 4.4% developed asymptomatic elevated serum amylase.

Stop treatment immediately if clinical signs or symptoms (eg, nausea, vomiting, abdominal pain) or if abnormalities in lab values (eg, hyperamylasemia associated with dysglycemia, rising triglyceride level, decreasing serum calcium) suggestive of pancreatitis occur. If clinical pancreatitis develops, it is recommended that zalcitabine be permanently discontinued. Interrupt treatment if therapy with another drug known to cause pancreatitis is required (see Drug Interactions).

➤*Lactic acidosis/Severe hepatomegaly with steatosis/Hepatic toxicity:* Lactic acidosis and severe hepatomegaly with steatosis, including fatal cases, have been reported with the use of nucleoside analogs alone or in combination, including zalcitabine and other antiretrovirals. A majority of these cases have been in women. Obesity and prolonged nucleoside exposure may be risk factors. Exercise particular caution when administering zalcitabine to any patient with known risk factors for liver disease; however, cases have also been reported in patients with no known risk factors. Treatment with zalcitabine should be suspended in any patient who develops clinical or laboratory findings suggestive of lactic acidosis or pronounced hepatotoxicity (which may include hepatomegaly and steatosis even in the absence of marked transaminase elevations).

In addition, rare cases of hepatic failure and death considered possibly related to underlying hepatitis B and zalcitabine have been reported. Treatment with zalcitabine in patients with preexisting liver disease, liver enzyme abnormalities, a history of ethanol abuse, or hepatitis should be approached with caution. Suspend treatment with zalcitabine in any patient who develops clinical or laboratory findings suggestive of pronounced hepatotoxicity. In clinical trials, drug interruption was recommended if liver function tests exceeded > 5 times the upper limit of normal.

➤*Hematologic toxicities:* In patients with poor bone marrow reserve, particularly those patients with advanced symptomatic HIV disease, frequent monitoring of hematologic indices is recommended to detect serious anemia or granulocytopenia. In patients who experience hematologic toxicity, reduction in hemoglobin may occur as early as 2 to 4 weeks after initiation of therapy and granulocytopenia usually occurs after 6 to 8 weeks of therapy.

➤*Oral ulcers:* Severe oral ulcers occurred in ≤ 3% of patients in 2 trials. Less severe oral ulcerations occurred at higher frequencies in other clinical trials.

➤*Esophageal ulcers:* Infrequent cases of esophageal ulcers have been attributed to zalcitabine therapy. Consider interruption of therapy in patients who develop esophageal ulcers that do not respond to specific treatment for opportunistic pathogens in order to assess a possible relationship to zalcitabine.

➤*Cardiomyopathy/CHF:* These have occurred with the use of nucleoside analogs in AIDS patients; infrequent cases have occurred in patients receiving zalcitabine. Approach treatment with caution in patients with baseline cardiomyopathy or history of CHF.

➤*Anaphylactoid reaction:* There has been 1 report of an anaphylactoid reaction occurring in a patient receiving both zalcitabine and zidovudine. In addition, there have been several reports of hypersensitivity reactions (anaphylactic reactions or urticaria without other signs of anaphylaxis).

➤*Renal function impairment:* Patients with renal impairment (estimated Ccr < 55 mL/min) may be at a greater risk of toxicity because of decreased drug clearance. Dosage reduction is recommended (see Administration and Dosage).

➤*Carcinogenesis:* Zalcitabine was administered orally by dietary admixture to mice at dosages of 3, 83, or 250 mg/kg/day for 2 years. Plasma exposures (as measured by AUC) at these doses were 6- to 704-fold greater than the systemic exposure in humans with the therapeutic dose. Zalcitabine was administered orally by dietary admixture to

ZALCITABINE (Dideoxycytidine; ddC)

rats at dosages of 3, 28, 83, or 250 mg/kg/day. At the highest dose tested, the systemic exposure to zalcitabine was 833 times the systemic exposure in humans with the therapeutic dose.

A significant increase in thymic lymphoma in all zalcitabine dose groups and Harderian gland (a gland of the eye of rodents) adenoma in the 2 highest dose groups was observed in female mice after 2 years of dosing. No increase in tumor incidence was observed in rats or male mice treated with zalcitabine. In an independent study, administration of zalcitabine to mice at a dose of 1000 mg/kg/day for 3 months induced an increased incidence of thymic lymphoma. A high rate of spontaneous lymphoreticular neoplasms have previously been noted in this strain of mice.

➤*Mutagenesis:* Zalcitabine was positive in a cell transformation assay and induced chromosomal aberrations in vitro in human peripheral blood lymphocytes. Oral doses of zalcitabine at 2500 and 4500 mg/kg were clastogenic in the mouse micronucleus assay.

➤*Fertility impairment:* Fertility and reproductive performance were assessed in rats at plasma concentrations up to 2142 times those achieved with the maximum recommended human dose (MRHD) based on AUC measurements. The highest dose was associated with embryolethality and evidence of teratogenicity. The next lower dose studied (plasma concentrations equivalent to 485 times the MRHD) was associated with a lower frequency of embryotoxicity, but no teratogenicity. The fertility of F_1 males was significantly reduced at a calculated dose of 2142 (but not 485) times the MRHD (based on AUC measurements) in a teratology study in which rat mothers were dosed on gestation days 7 to 15.

➤*Elderly:* Clinical studies of zalcitabine did not include sufficient numbers of subjects ≥ 65 years of age to determine whether they respond differently from younger subjects. In general, dose selection for an elderly patient should be cautious, reflecting the greater frequency of decreased hepatic, renal, or cardiac function, and of concomitant disease or other drug therapy. Zalcitabine is known to be substantially excreted by the kidney, and the risk of toxic reactions to this drug may be greater in patients with impaired renal function. Because elderly patients are more likely to have decreased renal function, take care in dose selection. In addition, monitor renal function and make dosage adjustments accordingly (see Renal Function Impairment and Administration and Dosage).

➤*Pregnancy: Category C.* Zalcitabine has been shown to be teratogenic in mice at calculated exposure levels of 1365 and 2730 times that of the MRHD (based on AUC measurements). In rats, zalcitabine was teratogenic at a calculated exposure level of 2142 times the MRHD, but not at an exposure level of 485 times the MRHD. In a perinatal and postnatal study in the rat, a high incidence of hydrocephalus was observed in the F_1 offspring derived from litters of dams treated with 1071 (but not 485) times the MRHD (based on AUC measurements). There are no adequate and well-controlled studies in pregnant women. Use during pregnancy only if the potential benefit justifies the potential risk to the fetus. Fertile women should not receive zalcitabine unless they are using an effective contraceptive during therapy. If pregnancy occurs, physicians are encouraged to report such cases by calling 800-526-6367.

➤*Lactation:* It is not known whether zalcitabine is excreted in breast milk. Decide whether to discontinue nursing or the drug, taking into account the importance of the drug to the mother. It is currently recommended in the US that HIV-infected women do not breastfeed infants regardless of the use of antiretroviral agents.

The US Public Health Service Centers for Disease Control and Prevention advises HIV-infected women not to breastfeed to avoid postnatal transmission of HIV to a child who may not yet be infected.

➤*Children:* Safety and efficacy of zalcitabine in HIV-infected children < 13 years of age have not been established.

Precautions

➤*Monitoring:* Perform complete blood counts and clinical chemistry tests prior to initiating therapy and at appropriate intervals thereafter. Perform baseline testing of serum amylase and triglyceride levels in individuals with a history of elevated amylase, pancreatitis, ethanol abuse, who are on parenteral nutrition, or who are otherwise at high risk of pancreatitis. Carefully monitor for signs or symptoms suggestive of peripheral neuropathy, particularly in individuals with a low CD4 cell count or who are at a greater risk of developing peripheral neuropathy while on therapy (see Warnings).

The duration of clinical benefit from antiretroviral therapy may be limited. Consider alterations in antiretroviral therapy in cases of disease progression, either clinical or as demonstrated by viral rebound (increase in HIV RNA after initial decline).

➤*Lymphoma:* High doses of zalcitabine for 3 months in mice (resulting in plasma concentrations > 1000 times those seen in patients taking the recommended doses) induced an increased incidence of thymic lymphoma. Although the pathogenesis of the effect is unclear, predisposition to chemically induced thymic lymphoma and high rates of spontaneous lymphoreticular neoplasms have previously been noted in this strain of mice.

The incidence of lymphomas was reviewed in 13 comparative studies conducted by Roche, the NIAID and the NCI, as well as 7 Roche expanded-access studies that included zalcitabine. In 1 study, ACTG 155, a statistically significant increased rate of lymphomas was seen in patients receiving zalcitabine or combination zalcitabine and zidovudine compared to zidovudine alone (rates of 0, 1.3, and 2.3 per 100 person years for zidovudine, zalcitabine, and combination zalcitabine and zidovudine, respectively; log rank p-value = 0.01, pooling zalcitabine, and combination zalcitabine and zidovudine vs zidovudine, p-value = 0.003.) Based on review of the literature, the incidence of lymphomas in HIV-infected patients with advanced disease on zidovudine monotherapy would be expected to be ≈ 1 to 2 per 100 person years of follow-up.

None of the other comparative studies evaluated showed a statistically significant difference in rates of lymphomas in patients receiving zalcitabine. In a large, controlled clinical trial (ACTG 175) zalcitabine in combination with zidovudine was not associated with an increase in the incidence of lymphoma over that seen with zidovudine monotherapy (6 of 615 and 9 of 619, respectively).

Lymphoma has been identified as a consequence of HIV infection. This most likely represents a consequence of prolonged immunosuppression; however, an association between the occurrence of lymphoma and antiviral therapy cannot be excluded.

➤*HIV infection complications:* Patients receiving zalcitabine or any other antiretroviral therapy may continue to develop opportunistic infections and other complications of HIV infection, and should remain under close clinical observation by physicians experienced in the treatment of patients with associated HIV diseases.

Drug Interactions

Zalcitabine Drug Interactions			
Precipitant drug	Object drug*		Description
Amphotericin, foscarnet, aminoglycosides	Zalcitabine	↑	These drugs may increase the risk of developing peripheral neuropathy or other zalcitabine-associated adverse events by interfering with the renal clearance of zalcitabine (and thereby raising systemic exposure). Patients who require the use of 1 of these drugs with zalcitabine should have frequent clinical and laboratory monitoring with dosage adjustment for any significant change in renal function.
Antacids (aluminum and magnesium-containing)	Zalcitabine	↓	Zalcitabine absorption is moderately reduced (≈ 25%) when coadministered with magnesium/aluminum-containing antacids. Do not ingest simultaneously.
Antiretroviral nucleoside analogs Chloramphenicol Cisplatin Dapsone Didanosine Disulfiram Ethionamide Glutethimide Gold Hydralazine Iodoquinol Isoniazid Metronidazole Nitrofurantoin Phenytoin Ribavirin Vincristine	Zalcitabine	↑	These drugs have been associated with peripheral neuropathy. Avoid concomitant use when possible. Concomitant use of zalcitabine with didanosine is not recommended.
Cimetidine	Zalcitabine	↑	Concomitant use decreases zalcitabine elimination, most likely by inhibition of renal tubular secretion. Monitor for signs of toxicity and reduce zalcitabine dose if warranted.
Doxorubicin	Zalcitabine	↓	Doxorubicin caused a decrease in zalcitabine phosphorylation (> 50% inhibition of total phosphate formation) in U937/Molt 4 cells. Although there may be decreased zalcitabine activity because of lessened active metabolite formation, the clinical relevance of these in vitro results are not known.
Metoclopramide	Zalcitabine	↓	Zalcitabine bioavailability is mildly reduced (≈ 10%).

ZALCITABINE (Dideoxycytidine; ddC)

Zalcitabine Drug Interactions			
Precipitant drug	Object drug*		Description
Pentamidine (and other agents that have potential to cause pancreatitis)	Zalcitabine	↑	Interrupt treatment when the use of a drug that has the potential to cause pancreatitis is required. Death because of fulminant pancreatitis possibly related to zalcitabine and IV pentamidine was reported. If IV pentamidine is required to treat *Pneumocystis carinii* pneumonia, interrupt treatment with zalcitabine.
Probenecid	Zalcitabine	↑	Concomitant use decreases zalcitabine elimination, most likely by inhibition of renal tubular secretion. Monitor for signs of toxicity and reduce the zalcitabine dose if warranted.

* ↑ = Object drug increased. ↓ = Object drug decreased.

➤*Drug/Food interactions:* The absorption rate of a 1.5 mg dose is reduced when administered with food resulting in a 39% decrease in mean C_{max} and a 2-fold increase in time to achieve C_{max}. The extent of absorption is decreased by 14%.

Adverse Reactions

Zidovudine Adverse Reactions: Zalcitabine vs Didanosine[1] (%)		
Adverse reaction	Zalcitabine 0.75 mg q 8 h (n = 237)	Didanosine 250 mg q 12 h (n = 230)
CNS		
Convulsions	1.3	2.2
Peripheral neuropathy[2]	28.3	13
Depression	0.4	0
Headache	2.1	1.3
GI		
Abdominal pain	3	7
Oral lesions/Stomatitis	3	0
Vomiting/Nausea	3.4	7
Diarrhea/Constipation	2.5	17.4
Miscellaneous		
Abnormal hepatic function	8.9	7
Fatigue	3.8	2.6
Rash/Pruritus/Urticaria	3.4	3.9
Fever	1.7	0.4
Pancreatitis	0	1.7
Painful/Swollen joints	0.4	0

[1] Grade 2 adverse events possibly or probably related to treatment or unassessable were included if study drug dosage was changed or interrupted. Patients were AZT intolerant or had experienced AZT treatment failure.
[2] Study included patients who were dose-adjusted for Grade 2 events.

Additional clinical adverse experiences associated with zalcitabine that occurred in < 1% of patients in study CPCRA 002 (at least possibly related; Grade 3 or higher), study ACTG 175 (any relationship; Grade 3/4) or in other clinical studies are listed below by body system. Several of these events occurred in slightly higher rates in other studies. The incidence of adverse experiences varied in different studies, generally being lower in patients with less advanced disease.

➤*Cardiovascular:* Abnormal cardiac movement, arrhythmia, atrial fibrillation, cardiac failure, cardiac dysrhythmias, cardiomyopathy, heart racing, hypertension, palpitation, subarachnoid hemorrhage, syncope, tachycardia, ventricular ectopy (< 1%).

➤*CNS:* Abnormal coordination, aphasia, ataxia, Bell's palsy, confusion, decreased concentration, decreased neurological function, disequilibrium, dizziness, dysphonia, facial nerve palsy, focal motor seizures, grand mal seizure, hyperkinesia, hypertonia, hypokinesia, memory loss, migraine, neuralgia, neuritis, paralysis, seizures, speech disorder, status epilepticus, stupor, tremor, twitch, vertigo (< 1%).

➤*Dermatologic:* Acne, alopecia, bullous eruptions, carbuncle/furuncle, cellulitis, cold sore, dermatitis, dry skin, dry rash, desquamation, erythematous rash, exfoliative dermatitis, finger inflammation, flushing, follicular rash, impetigo, increased sweating, infection, itchy rash, lip blisters/lesions, macular/papular rash, maculopapular rash, moniliasis, mucocutaneous/skin disorder, nail disorder, photosensitivity reaction, pruritic disorder, pruritus, skin disorder/lesions/fissure/ulcer, urticaria (< 1%).

➤*Endocrine:* Abnormal triglycerides, abnormal lipase, altered serum glucose, decreased bicarbonate, diabetes mellitus, glycosuria, gout, hot flushes, hypercalcemia, hyperkalemia, hyperlipidemia, hypernatremia, hyperuricemia, hypocalcemia, hypoglycemia, hypokalemia, hypomagnesemia, hyponatremia, hypophosphatemia, increased nonprotein nitrogen, lactic acidosis (< 1%).

➤*GI:* Abdominal bloating or cramps, acute pancreatitis, anal/rectal pain, anorexia, bloody or black stools, bleeding gums, colitis, dental abscess, dry mouth, dyspepsia, dysphagia, enlarged abdomen, epigastric pain, eructation, esophageal pain, esophageal ulcers, esophagitis, flatulence, gagging with pills, gastritis, GI hemorrhage, gingivitis, glossitis, gum disorder, heartburn, hemorrhagic pancreatitis, hemorrhoids, increased saliva, left quadrant pain, melena, mouth lesion, odynophagia, painful sore gums, painful swallowing, pancreatitis, rectal hemorrhage, rectal mass, rectal ulcers, salivary gland enlargement, sore tongue, sore throat, tongue disorder, tongue ulcer, toothache, unformed/loose stools (< 1%).

➤*GU:* Abnormal renal function, acute renal failure, albuminuria, bladder pain, dysuria, frequent urination, genital lesion/ulcer, increased blood urea nitrogen, increased creatinine, micturition frequency, nocturia, pain on urination, painful penis sore, penile edema, polyuria, renal cyst, renal calculus, testicular swelling, toxic nephropathy, urinary retention, vaginal itch, vaginal ulcer, vaginal pain/discharge, vaginal/cervix disorder (< 1%).

➤*Hematologic:* Absolute neutrophil count alteration, anemia, epistaxis, decreased hematocrit, granulocytosis, hemoglobinemia, leukopenia, neutrophilia, platelet alteration, purpura, thrombus, unspecified hematologic toxicity, white blood cell alteration (< 1%).

➤*Hepatic:* Abnormal lactate dehydrogenase, bilirubinemia, cholecystitis, decreased alkaline phosphatase, hepatitis, hepatocellular damage, hepatomegaly, increased alkaline phosphatase, jaundice (< 1%).

➤*Musculoskeletal:* Arthralgia, arthritis, arthropathy, arthrosis, back pain, backache, bone pains/aches, bursitis, cold extremities, extremity pain, joint pain, joint inflammation, leg cramps, muscle aches, muscle weakness, muscle disorder, muscle stiffness, muscle cramps, myalgia, myopathy, myositis, neck pain, rib pain, stiff neck (< 1%).

➤*Psychiatric:* Acute psychotic disorder, acute stress reaction, agitation, amnesia, anxiety, confusion, decreased motivation, decreased sexual desire, decreased concentration, dementia, depersonalization, emotional lability, euphoria, hallucination, impaired concentration, insomnia, manic reaction, mood swings, nervousness, paranoid state, somnolence, suicide attempt (< 1%).

➤*Respiratory:* Acute nasopharyngitis, chest congestion, coughing, cyanosis, difficulty breathing, dry nasal mucosa, dyspnea, flu-like symptoms, hemoptysis, nasal discharge, pharyngitis, rales/rhonchi, respiratory distress, sinus congestion, sinus pain, sinusitis, wheezing (< 1%).

➤*Special senses:* Abnormal/blurred/decreased vision, dry/burning eyes, decreased taste, ear pain/problem/blockage, eye abnormality/inflammation/itching/pain/irritation/redness/hemorrhage, fluid in ears, hearing loss, increased tears, loss of taste, mucopurulent conjunctivitis, parosmia, photophobia, smell dysfunction, taste perversion, tinnitus, unequal-sized pupils, xerophthalmia, yellow sclera (< 1%).

➤*Miscellaneous:* Asthenia, cachexia, chest tightness or pain, chills, cutaneous/allergic reaction, debilitation, difficulty moving, dry mouth, edema, facial pain or swelling, flank pain, hypersensitivity reactions (see Warnings), lymphadenopathy, malaise, night sweats, pain, pelvic/groin pain, rigors, abnormal weight decrease (< 1%).

➤*Lab test abnormalities:*

Zalcitabine Laboratory Test Abnormalities (%)		
Lab test abnormality	Zalcitabine 0.75 mg q 8 h (n = 237)	Didanosine 250 mg q 12 h (n = 230)
Anemia (< 7.5 g/dL)	8.4	7.4
Leukopenia (< 1500/mm³)	13.1	9.6
Neutropenia (< 750/mm³)	16.9	11.7
Eosinophilia (> 1000 or 25%)	2.5	1.7
Thrombocytopenia (< 50,000/mm³)	1.3	4.8
AST (> 5 × ULN)	7.6	5.7
CPK elevation (> 4 × ULN)[1]	0.8	0
Bilirubin (> 2.5 × ULN)	0.8	0.9
Amylase (> 2 × ULN)	5.1	3.9
Hyperglycemia[1] (> 250 mg/dL)	0	1.7

[1] Grade 3 or higher.

Overdosage

➤*Acute:* Inadvertent pediatric overdoses have occurred with doses up to 1.5 mg/kg. The children had prompt gastric lavage and treatment with activated charcoal and had no sequelae. Mixed overdoses including zalcitabine and other drugs have led to drowsiness and vomiting or increased GGT or creatine phosphokinase. There is no experience with

ZALCITABINE (Dideoxycytidine; ddC)

acute overdosage at higher doses and sequelae are unknown. There is no known antidote. It is not known whether zalcitabine is dialyzable by peritoneal dialysis or hemodialysis.

➤*Chronic:* In a study in which zalcitabine was administered at doses 25 times (0.25 mg/kg every 8 hours) the currently recommended dose, 1 patient discontinued zalcitabine after 1.5 weeks of treatment subsequent to the development of a rash and fever.

In early phase I studies, all patients receiving zalcitabine at ≈ 6 times the current total daily recommended dose experienced peripheral neuropathy by week 10; 80% who received ≈ 2 times the current total daily recommended dose experienced peripheral neuropathy by week 12.

Patient Information

Zalcitabine is not a cure for HIV infection; patients may continue to develop illnesses associated with advanced HIV infection including opportunistic infections. Because it is frequently difficult to determine whether symptoms are caused by drug effect or underlying disease, encourage patients to report all changes in their condition to their physician. Use of zalcitabine or other antiretroviral drugs does not preclude the ongoing need to maintain practices designed to prevent transmission of HIV.

Tell patients that there are currently no data demonstrating that zalcitabine therapy can reduce the risk of transmitting HIV to others through sexual contact or blood contamination.

Advise patients to take zalcitabine every day as prescribed. Patients should not alter the dose or discontinue therapy without consulting with their physician. If a dose is missed, patients should take the dose as soon as possible and then return to their normal schedule. However, if a dose is skipped, the patient should not double the next dose.

Instruct patients that the major toxicity of zalcitabine is peripheral neuropathy. Pancreatitis and hepatic toxicity are other serious and potentially life-threatening toxicities. Advise patients of the early symptoms of these conditions and instruct them to promptly report these symptoms to their physician. Because development of peripheral neuropathy appears dose-related, advise patients to follow prescribed dose.

Women of childbearing age should use effective contraception while on zalcitabine.

ZIDOVUDINE (Azidothymidine; AZT; Compound S)

Rx	Retrovir (GlaxoSmithKline)	Tablets: 300 mg	(GX CW3 300). White. Film-coated. In 60s.
		Capsules: 100 mg	(Wellcome Y9C 100). White with blue band. In 100s and UD 100s.
		Syrup: 50 mg/5 mL	0.2% sodium benzoate, sucrose. Strawberry flavor. In 240 mL.
		Injection: 10 mg/mL	In 20 mL single-use vial.

WARNING

Zidovudine has been associated with hematologic toxicity, including neutropenia and severe anemia, particularly in patients with advanced human immunodeficiency (HIV) disease (see Warnings). Prolonged use of zidovudine has been associated with symptomatic myopathy.

Lactic acidosis and severe hepatomegaly with steatosis, including fatal cases, have been reported with the use of nucleoside analogs alone or in combination, including zidovudine and other antiretrovirals (see Warnings).

Indications

➤*HIV infection:* In combination with other antiretroviral agents for the treatment of HIV infection.

Maternal-fetal HIV transmission – Prevention of maternal-fetal HIV transmission as part of a regimen that includes oral zidovudine beginning between 14 and 34 weeks of gestation, IV zidovudine during labor, and administration of zidovudine syrup to the neonate after birth. The efficacy of this regimen for preventing HIV transmission in women who have received zidovudine for a prolonged period before pregnancy has not been evaluated. The safety of zidovudine for the mother or fetus during the first trimester of pregnancy has not been assessed.

Administration and Dosage

➤*Approved by the FDA:* March 19, 1987.

➤*HIV infection:*

Adults (oral) – Recommended dose is 600 mg/day in divided doses in combination with other antiretroviral agents.

Adults (IV) – Recommended IV dose is 1 mg/kg infused over 1 hour. Administer this dose 5 to 6 times daily (5 to 6 mg/kg/day). Patients should receive zidovudine IV infusion only until oral therapy can be administered. The IV dosing regimen equivalent to the oral administration of 100 mg every 4 hours is approximately 1 mg/kg IV every 4 hours. Avoid rapid infusion or bolus injection. Do not give IM.

Children (oral) – Recommended dose in children 6 weeks to 12 years of age is 160 mg/m^2 every 8 hours (480 mg/m^2/day up to a maximum of 200 mg every 8 hours) in combination with other antiretroviral agents.

➤*Maternal-Fetal HIV transmission:* Recommended dosing regimen to pregnant women (greater than 14 weeks of pregnancy) and their neonates is as follows:

Maternal dosing (oral) – 100 mg orally 5 times per day until the start of labor.

Maternal dosing (IV) – During labor and delivery, administer IV zidovudine at 2 mg/kg (total body weight) over 1 hour followed by a continuous IV infusion of 1 mg/kg/h (total body weight) until clamping of the umbilical cord.

Neonatal dosing (oral) – 2 mg/kg orally every 6 hours starting within 12 hours after birth and continuing through 6 weeks of age.

Neonatal dosing (IV) – Neonates unable to receive oral dosing may

be given zidovudine IV at 1.5 mg/kg, infused over 30 minutes, every 6 hours.

➤*Dose adjustment:* Significant anemia (hemoglobin of less than 7.5 g/dL or reduction of greater than 25% from baseline) and/or significant neutropenia (granulocyte count of less than 750 cells/mm^3 or reduction of greater than 50% from baseline) may require a dose interruption until evidence of marrow recovery is observed. In patients who develop significant anemia, dose interruption does not necessarily eliminate the need for transfusion. If marrow recovery occurs following dose interruption, resumption in dose may be appropriate using adjunctive measures such as epoetin alfa at recommended doses, depending on hematologic indices such as serum erythropoietin level and patient tolerance.

For patients experiencing pronounced anemia while receiving chronic coadministration of zidovudine and some of the drugs (eg, fluconazole, valproic acid), zidovudine dose adjustment may be considered.

Renal function impairment – In end-stage renal disease patients maintained on hemodialysis or peritoneal dialysis, recommended dosing is 100 mg every 6 to 8 hours.

Hepatic function impairment – Because zidovudine is primarily eliminated by hepatic metabolism, a reduction in the daily dose may be necessary in these patients. Frequent monitoring for hematologic toxicities is advised.

➤*IV:*

Preparation – Dilute prior to administration. Remove the calculated dose from the vial; add to 5% dextrose injection to achieve a concentration of no greater than 4 mg/mL.

IV admixture incompatibility – Admixture in biologic or colloidal fluids (eg, blood products, protein solutions) is not recommended.

➤*Storage/Stability:*

Oral – Store at 15° to 25°C (59° to 77°F). Protect capsules from moisture.

IV – After dilution, the solution is physically and chemically stable for 24 hours at room temperature and 48 hours if refrigerated at 2° to 8°C (36° to 46°F). As an additional precaution, administer the diluted solution within 8 hours if stored at 25°C (77°F) or 24 hours if refrigerated at 2° to 8°C (36° to 46°F) to minimize the potential administration of a microbially contaminated solution. Store undiluted vials at 15° to 25°C (59° to 77°F) and protect from light.

Actions

➤*Pharmacology:* Zidovudine is a synthetic nucleoside analog of the naturally occurring nucleoside thymidine, in which the 3′-hydroxy(-OH) group is replaced by an azido(-N$_3$) group. Within cells, zidovudine is converted to the active metabolite zidovudine 5′-triphosphate (AztTP) by the sequential action of the cellular enzymes. Zidovudine 5′-triphosphate inhibits the activity of the HIV reverse transcriptase by competing for utilization with the natural substrate deoxythymidine 5′-triphosphate (dTTP) and by its incorporation into viral DNA. The lack of a 3′-OH group in the incorporated nucleoside analog prevents the formation of the 5′ to 3′ phosphodiester linkage essential for DNA chain elongation and, therefore, the viral DNA growth is terminated. The active metabolite AztTP is also a weak inhibitor of the cellular DNA polymerase-alpha and mitochondrial polymerase-gamma and has

ZIDOVUDINE (Azidothymidine; AZT; Compound S)

been reported to be incorporated into the DNA of cells in culture.

▶*Pharmacokinetics:*

Adults – Following oral administration, zidovudine is rapidly absorbed and extensively distributed, with peak serum concentrations occurring within 0.5 to 1.5 hours. Zidovudine is primarily eliminated by hepatic metabolism. The major metabolite of zidovudine is 3'-azido-3'-deoxy-5'-O-β-D-glycopyranuronosylthymidine (GZDV). GZDV AUC is about 3-fold greater than the zidovudine AUC. Urinary recovery of zidovudine and GZDV accounts for 14% and 74%, respectively, of the dose following oral administration. A second metabolite, 3'-amino-3'-deoxythymidine (AMT), has been identified in the plasma following single-dose IV administration of zidovudine.

Zidovudine Pharmacokinetic Parameters in Fasting Adult Patients	
Parameter	Mean value
Oral bioavailability (%)	≈ 64
Apparent volume of distribution (L/kg)	≈ 1.6
Plasma protein binding (%)	< 38
CSF:plasma ratio[1]	0.6 (0.04 to 2.62)
Systemic clearance (L/h/kg)	≈ 1.6
Renal clearance (L/h/kg)	≈ 0.34
Elimination half-life (h)[2]	0.5 to 3 (oral); 1.1 (IV)

[1] Median (range).
[2] Approximate range.

Adults with impaired renal function – Zidovudine clearance was decreased resulting in increased zidovudine and GZDV half-life and AUC in patients with impaired renal function. A dose adjustment should not be necessary for patients with creatinine clearance (Ccr) greater than or equal to 15 mL/min.

Zidovudine Pharmacokinetics Parameters in Patients with Severe Renal Impairment		
Parameter	Control subjects (normal renal function) (n = 6)	Patients with renal impairment (n = 14)
Ccr (mL/min)	≈ 120	≈ 18
Zidovudine AUC (ng•h/mL)	≈ 1400	≈ 3100
Zidovudine half-life (h)	≈ 1	≈ 1.4

Hemodialysis and peritoneal dialysis appeared to have a negligible effect on the removal of zidovudine, whereas GZDV elimination was enhanced. A dosage adjustment is recommended for patients undergoing hemodialysis or peritoneal dialysis.

Patients younger than 3 months of age – The half-life was about 13 hours. In neonates 14 days of age or less, bioavailability was greater, total body clearance was slower, and half-life was longer than in pediatric patients more than 14 days old.

Zidovudine Pharmacokinetic Parameters in Pediatric Patients			
Parameter	Birth to 14 days of age	14 days to 3 months of age	3 months to 12 years of age
Oral bioavailability (%)	≈ 89	≈ 61	≈ 65
CSF:Plasma ratio	no data	no data	≈ 0.68 (0.03 to 3.25)[1] (oral); ≈ 0.26[1] (IV)
CL (L/h/kg)	≈ 0.65	≈ 1.14	≈ 1.85
Elimination half-life (h)	≈ 3.1	≈ 1.9	≈ 1.5

[1] Median (range).

▶*Microbiology:*

In vitro HIV susceptibility – The in vitro anti-HIV activity of zidovudine was assessed by infecting cell lines of lymphoblastic and monocytic origin and peripheral blood lymphocytes with laboratory and clinical isolates of HIV. Zidovudine showed antiviral activity in all acutely infected cell lines; however, activity was substantially less in chronically infected cell lines. In drug combination studies with zalcitabine, didanosine, lamivudine, saquinavir, indinavir, ritonavir, nevirapine, delavirdine, or interferon-alpha, zidovudine showed additive to synergistic activity in cell culture. The relationship between the in vitro susceptibility of HIV to reverse transcriptase inhibitors and the inhibition of HIV replication in humans has not been established.

Drug resistance – Reduced sensitivity has been recovered from patients treated with zidovudine. Genetic analysis of the isolates showed mutations that result in 5 amino acid substitutions in the viral reverse transcriptase. Higher levels of resistance were associated with greater numbers of mutations with 215 mutation being the most significant.

Cross-resistance – The potential for cross-resistance between HIV reverse transcriptase inhibitors and protease inhibitors is low because of the different enzyme targets involved. Combination therapy with zidovudine plus zalcitabine or didanosine does not appear to prevent the emergence of zidovudine-resistant isolates. Combination therapy with zidovudine plus lamivudine delayed the emergence of mutations conferring resistance to zidovudine. In some patients harboring zidovu-

dine-resistant virus, combination therapy with zidovudine plus lamivudine restored phenotypic sensitivity to zidovudine by 12 weeks of treatment. HIV isolates with multidrug resistance to zidovudine, didanosine, zalcitabine, stavudine, and lamivudine were recovered from a small number of patients treated for at least 1 year with the combination of zidovudine and didanosine or zalcitabine.

▶*Clinical trials:*

Combination therapy in adults – Zidovudine in combination with other antiretroviral agents has been shown to be superior to monotherapy for 1 or more of the following endpoints: Delaying death, delaying development of AIDS, increasing CD4 cell counts, decreasing plasma HIV RNA. In a multicenter, randomized, double-blind, placebo-controlled trial comparing zidovudine 600 mg/day plus lamivudine 300 mg/day to zidovudine plus lamivudine plus indinavir 800 mg 3 times daily, the incidence of AIDS-defining events or death was lower in the triple-drug-containing arm compared with the 2-drug-containing arm (6.1% vs 10.9%, respectively).

Pediatric patients – In a multicenter, randomized, double-blind study comparing lamivudine plus zidovudine to didanosine monotherapy, the mean baseline CD4 cell count was 868 cells/mm^3 and the mean baseline plasma HIV RNA was 5 $\log_{10}$ copies/mL. The median duration that patients remained on study was approximately 10 months. Results are summarized in the following table.

Zidovudine Patients Reaching a Primary Clinical Endpoint (Disease Progression or Death) (%)		
Endpoint	Lamivudine plus zidovudine (n = 236)	Didanosine (n = 235)
HIV disease progression or death (total)	6.4	15.7
Physical growth failure	3	2.6
CNS deterioration	1.7	5.1
CDC Clinical Category C	0.8	3.4
Death	0.8	4.7

Contraindications

Potentially life-threatening allergic reactions to any of the components of the product.

Warnings

▶*Hematologic effects:* Use with extreme caution in patients who have bone marrow compromise evidenced by granulocyte count less than 1000 cells/mm^3 or hemoglobin less than 9.5 g/dL. Anemia and neutropenia are the most significant adverse events observed. There have been reports of pancytopenia that was reversible in most instances after discontinuance of the drug.

Frequent blood counts are strongly recommended for advanced HIV disease patients. Periodic blood counts are recommended for asymptomatic and early HIV disease. However, significant anemia, in many cases requiring dose adjustment, discontinuation of zidovudine, and/or blood transfusions has occurred during treatment with zidovudine alone or in combination with other antiretrovirals.

▶*Myopathy and myositis:* With pathological changes similar to that produced by HIV disease, these have been associated with prolonged use of zidovudine.

▶*Lactic acidosis / severe hepatomegaly with steatosis:* Lactic acidosis and severe hepatomegaly with steatosis, including fatal cases, have been reported with the use of nucleoside analogs alone or incombination, including zidovudine and other antiretrovirals. A majority of these cases have been in women. Obesity and prolonged exposure to antiretroviral nucleoside analogs may be risk factors. Exercise particular caution when administering zidovudine to any patient with known risk factors for liver disease; however, cases also have been reported in patients with no known risk factors. Suspend treatment with zidovudine in any patient who develops clinical or laboratory findings suggestive of lactic acidosis or pronounced hepatotoxicity (which may include hepatomegaly and steatosis even in the absence of marked transaminase elevations).

▶*Combination therapy:* Lamivudine/zidovudine and abacavir/lamivudine/zidovudine are combination product tablets that contain zidovudine as one of their components. Do not administer zidovudine concomitantly with lamivudine/zidovudine or abacavir/lamivudine/zidovudine.

▶*Renal / Hepatic function impairment:* Zidovudine is eliminated from the body primarily by renal excretion following metabolism in the liver (glucuronidation). In patients with severely impaired renal function (Ccr less than 15 mL/min), dosage reduction is recommended. Although data are limited, zidovudine concentrations appear to be increased in patients with severely impaired hepatic function, which may increase the risk of hematologic toxicity (see Administration and Dosage).

▶*Carcinogenesis:* In mice, 7 late-appearing (after 19 months) vaginal neoplasms (5 nonmetastasizing squamous cell carcinomas, 1 squamous cell papilloma, 1 squamous polyp) occurred in animals given the highest dose of zidovudine; 1 squamous cell papilloma occurred with the middle dose. In rats, 2 late-appearing (after 20 months) nonmetastasiz-

ZIDOVUDINE (Azidothymidine; AZT; Compound S)

ing vaginal squamous cell carcinomas occurred in animals given the highest dose.

A second study administered zidovudine at maximum tolerated doses of 12.5 or 25 mg/day to pregnant mice from days 12 through 18 of gestation. There was an increase in the number of tumors in the lung, liver, and female reproductive tracts in the offspring of mice receiving the higher dose level of zidovudine.

➤*Mutagenesis:* Zidovudine was mutagenic in a mouse lymphoma assay, positive in an in vitro cell transformation assay, clastogenic in a cytogenic assay using cultured human lymphocytes, and positive in mouse and rat micronucleus tests after repeated doses.

➤*Elderly:* Make dose selection for an elderly patient with caution, reflecting the greater frequency of decreased hepatic, renal, or cardiac function and of concomitant disease or other drug therapy.

➤*Pregnancy: Category C.* Oral teratology studies in rats and rabbits at doses up to 500 mg/kg/day revealed no evidence of teratogenicity with zidovudine. Zidovudine treatment resulted in embryo/fetal toxicity as evidenced by an increase in the incidence of fetal resorptions in rats given 150 or 450 mg/kg/day and rabbits given 500 mg/kg/day. The doses used in the teratology studies resulted in peak zidovudine plasma concentrations (after one half of the daily dose) in rats 66 to 226 times and in rabbits 12 to 87 times mean steady-state peak human plasma concentrations (after one sixth of the daily dose) achieved with the recommended daily dose (100 mg every 4 hours). In an additional teratology study in rats, a dose of 3000 mg/kg/day (very near the oral median lethal dose in rats of 3683 mg/kg) caused marked maternal toxicity and an increase in the incidence of fetal malformations. This dose resulted in peak zidovudine plasma concentrations 350 times peak human plasma concentrations. (Estimated AUC in rats at this dose level was 300 times the daily AUC in humans given 600 mg/day.) No evidence of teratogenicity was seen in this experiment at doses of 600 mg/kg/day or less.

A randomized, double-blind, placebo-controlled trial was conducted in HIV-infected pregnant women to determine the utility of zidovudine for the prevention of maternal-fetal HIV-transmission. Congenital abnormalities occurred with similar frequency between neonates born to mothers who received zidovudine and neonates born to mothers who received placebo. Abnormalities were problems in embryogenesis (prior to 14 weeks) or were recognized on ultrasound before or immediately after initiation of study drug.

Antiretroviral pregnancy registry – To monitor maternal-fetal outcomes of pregnant women exposed to zidovudine, an Antiretroviral Pregnancy Registry has been established. Physicians are encouraged to register patients by calling (800) 258-4263.

➤*Lactation:* The Centers for Disease Control and Prevention recommend that HIV-infected women not breastfeed to avoid postnatal transmission of HIV.

Zidovudine is excreted in breast milk. Because of the potential for HIV transmission and for serious adverse reactions in nursing infants, instruct mothers not to breastfeed if they are receiving zidovudine.

➤*Children:* Zidovudine has been studied in HIV-infected pediatric patients over 3 months of age who had HIV-related symptoms or who were asymptomatic with abnormal laboratory values indicating significant HIV-related immunosuppression. Zidovudine also has been studied in neonates perinatally exposed to HIV.

Precautions

➤*Monitoring:* Hematologic toxicities appear to be related to pretreatment bone marrow reserve and to dose and duration of therapy. In patients with poor bone marrow reserve, particularly in patients with advanced symptomatic HIV disease, frequent monitoring of hematologic indices is recommended to detect serious anemia or neutropenia. In patients who experience hematologic toxicity, reduction in hemoglobin may occur as early as 2 to 4 weeks, and neutropenia usually occurs after 6 to 8 weeks.

Drug Interactions

Zidovudine Drug Interactions			
Precipitant drug	Object drug*		Description
Acetaminophen	Zidovudine	↓	Acetaminophen may decrease the AUC of zidovudine.
Atovaquone	Zidovudine	↑	Atovaquone appears to inhibit glucuronidation of zidovudine, thus increasing zidovudine concentrations and decreasing clearance.
Bone marrow suppressive/ cytotoxic agents (eg, interferon-alpha, interferon-beta-1b)	Zidovudine	↑	Coadministration may increase the hematologic toxicity of zidovudine.

Zidovudine Drug Interactions			
Precipitant drug	Object drug*		Description
Clarithromycin	Zidovudine	↔	Peak serum zidovudine concentrations may be increased or decreased.
Doxorubicin	Zidovudine	↓	Avoid coadministration. An antagonistic relationship has been demonstrated.
Fluconazole	Zidovudine	↑	Concurrent use may increase the zidovudine AUC.
Ganciclovir	Zidovudine	↑	Concomitant use may increase zidovudine plasma levels and AUC, thus increasing risk of life-threatening hematologic toxicities.
Methadone	Zidovudine	↑	Zidovudine serum concentrations and AUC may be elevated, increasing the risk of side effects.
Nelfinavir/ Ritonavir	Zidovudine	↓	Zidovudine AUC is decreased.
Probenecid	Zidovudine	↑	Probenecid may increase zidovudine AUC by inhibiting glucuronidation or reducing renal excretion. Some patients have developed symptoms consisting of myalgia, malaise or fever, and maculopapular rash.
Rifamycins	Zidovudine	↓	The AUC of zidovudine may be decreased.
Stavudine, ribavirin	Zidovudine	↓	Avoid concomitant use because some nucleoside analogs affect viral replication and may antagonize antiviral activity of zidovudine against HIV.
Trimethoprim	Zidovudine	↑	Serum levels of zidovudine and its metabolite may be increased, especially in patients with impaired hepatic glucuronidation from liver disease or drug inhibition.
Valproic acid	Zidovudine	↑	Concurrent use may inhibit glucuronide metabolism, thus increasing zidovudine AUC.
Zidovudine	Phenytoin	↔	Phenytoin levels have been reported to increase, decrease or not change with concurrent use. In addition, zidovudine clearance was decreased by phenytoin.
Phenytoin	Zidovudine	↑	

* ↑ = Object drug increased. ↓ = Object drug decreased. ↔ = Undetermined clinical effect.

Adverse Reactions

➤*Adults:* The frequency and severity of adverse events associated with the use of zidovudine are greater in patients with more advanced infection at the time of initiation of therapy.

Zidovudine Adverse Reactions (≥ 5%) in Patients with Asymptomatic HIV Infection		
Adverse reaction	Zidovudine 500 mg/day (n = 453)	Placebo (n = 428)
GI		
Nausea	51.4	29.9
Anorexia	20.1	10.5
Vomiting	17.2	9.8
Constipation	6.4[1]	3.5
Miscellaneous		
Headache	62.5	52.6
Malaise	53.2	44.9
Asthenia	8.6[1]	5.8

[1] Not statistically significant vs placebo.

Other adverse events observed in clinical studies were abdominal cramps, abdominal pain, arthralgia, chills, dyspepsia, fatigue, hyperbilirubinemia, insomnia, musculoskeletal pain, myalgia, and neuropathy.

Lab test abnormalities –

Zidovudine Frequencies of Selected (Grade 3/4) Laboratory Abnormalities in Adult Patients with Asymptomatic HIV Infection (%)		
Adverse reaction	Zidovudine 500 mg/day (n = 453)	Placebo (n = 428)
Anemia (Hgb < 8 g/dL)	1.1	0.2
Granulocytopenia (< 750 cells/mm³)	1.8	1.6
Thrombocytopenia (platelets < 50,000/mm³)	0	0.5
ALT (> 5 × ULN[1])	3.1	2.6

ZIDOVUDINE (Azidothymidine; AZT; Compound S)

Zidovudine Frequencies of Selected (Grade 3/4) Laboratory Abnormalities in Adult Patients with Asymptomatic HIV Infection (%)		
Adverse reaction	Zidovudine 500 mg/day (n = 453)	Placebo (n = 428)
AST (> 5 × ULN[1])	0.9	1.6

[1] ULN = Upper limit of normal.

➤*Children:* Adverse reactions during therapy with lamivudine 4 mg/kg twice daily plus zidovudine 160 mg/m^2 3 times daily compared with didanosine in therapy-naive (56 days or less of antiretroviral therapy) pediatric patients are listed in the table below.

Zidovudine Adverse Reactions in Pediatric Patients (≥ 5%)		
Adverse reaction	Zidovudine plus lamivudine (n = 236)	Didanosine (n = 235)
GI		
Hepatomegaly	11	11
Nausea and vomiting	8	7
Diarrhea	8	6
Stomatitis	6	12
Splenomegaly	5	8
Respiratory		
Cough	15	18
Abnormal breath sounds/wheezing	7	9
Special senses		
Signs or symptoms of ears[1]	7	6
Nasal discharge or congestion	8	11
Miscellaneous		
Fever	25	32
Skin rashes	12	14
Lymphadenopathy	9	11

[1] Includes pain, discharge, erythema, or swelling of an ear.

Additional adverse reactions reported in pediatric patients were CHF, decreased reflexes, ECG abnormality, edema, hematuria, left ventricular dilation, macrocytosis, nervousness/irritability, and weight loss.

The clinical adverse reactions reported among adult recipients of zidovudine may also occur in pediatric patients.

Lab test abnormalities – Laboratory abnormalities experienced by therapy-naive (56 days or less of antiretroviral therapy) pediatric patients are listed in the following table.

Zidovudine Frequencies of Selected (Grade 3/4) Laboratory Abnormalities in Pediatric Patients (%)		
Test (abnormal level)	Lamivudine plus zidovudine	Didanosine
Neutropenia (ANC[1] < 400 cells/mm^3)	8	3
Anemia (Hgb < 7 g/dL)	4	2
Thrombocytopenia (platelets < 50,000/mm^3)	1	3
ALT (> 10 × ULN[2])	1	3
AST (> 10 × ULN[2])	2	4
Lipase (> 2.5 × ULN[2])	3	3
Total amylase (> 2.5 × ULN[2])	3	3

[1] ANC = Absolute neutrophil count.
[2] ULN = Upper limit of normal.

➤*Prevention of maternal-fetal transmission of HIV:*

Hematologic – The most commonly reported adverse reactions were anemia (hemoglobin less than 9 g/dL) and neutropenia (less than 1000 cells/mm^3). Anemia occurred in 22% of the neonates who received zidovudine. No neonates with anemia required transfusion and all hemoglobin values spontaneously returned to normal within 6 weeks after completion of therapy. Neutropenia was reported in 21% of the neonates in the group that received zidovudine.

➤*Postmarketing:* The following events have been identified during the use of zidovudine in clinical practice. Because they are reported voluntarily from a population of unknown size, estimates of frequency cannot be made. These events have been chosen for inclusion because of

their seriousness, frequency of reporting, potential causal connection to zidovudine, or a combination of these factors.

Cardiovascular – Vasodilation; syncope; cardiomyopathy.

CNS – Anxiety; confusion; depression; emotional lability; nervousness; syncope; loss of mental acuity; vertigo; dizziness; paresthesia; somnolence; mania; seizures.

Dermatologic – Acne; pruritus; urticaria; skin/nail pigmentation changes; rash; sweating; Stevens-Johnson syndrome; toxic epidermal necrolysis.

GI – Constipation; dysphagia; edema of the tongue; eructation; flatulence; bleeding gums; rectal hemorrhage; mouth ulcer; diarrhea; oral mucosa pigmentation.

GU – Dysuria; polyuria; urinary frequency; urinary hesitancy; gynecomastia.

Hematologic – Aplastic anemia; hemolytic anemia; leukopenia; lymphadenopathy; pancytopenia with marrow hypoplasia; pure red cell aplasia.

Hepatic – Hepatitis; hepatomegaly with steatosis; jaundice; lactic acidosis; pancreatitis.

Musculoskeletal – Arthralgia; muscle spasm; tremor; twitch; increased CPK; increased LDH; myopathy; myositis with pathological changes (similar to that produced by HIV disease); rhabdomyolysis.

Respiratory – Cough; epistaxis; pharyngitis; rhinitis; sinusitis; hoarseness; dyspnea.

Special senses – Amblyopia; hearing loss; photophobia; taste perversion; macular edema.

Miscellaneous – Body odor; chills; edema of the lip; flu-like syndrome; hyperalgesia; generalized/back/chest pain; lymphadenopathy; sensitization reactions including anaphylaxis, angioedema, vasculitis.

Overdosage

Cases of acute overdoses in children and adults have occurred with doses up to 50 g. No specific symptoms or signs have been identified following acute overdosage with zidovudine apart from those listed as adverse reactions such as fatigue, headache, vomiting, and occasional reports of hematological disturbances. All patients recovered without permanent sequelae. Hemodialysis and peritoneal dialysis appear to have a negligible effect on zidovudine while elimination of its primary metabolite, GZDV, is enhanced.

Patient Information

Zidovudine is not a cure for HIV infections; patients may continue to acquire illnesses associated with HIV infection, including opportunistic infections. Patients should seek medical care for any significant change in their health status.

The major toxicities of zidovudine are neutropenia and/or anemia that may require transfusions or discontinuation. Frequency and severity of these toxicities are greater in patients with more advanced disease and in those who initiate therapy later in the course of their infection. It is extremely important to follow blood counts closely while on therapy, especially patients with advanced symptomatic HIV disease.

Warn patients about the use of other medications (eg, ganciclovir, interferon-alpha) that may exacerbate the toxicity of zidovudine (see Drug Interactions).

Advise patients to contact their physician if they experience shortness of breath, muscle weakness, symptoms of hepatitis or pancreatitis, or any other unexpected adverse reaction. Inform patients that nausea and vomiting may also occur.

Long-term effects of zidovudine are unknown at this time.

Zidovudine therapy has not been shown to reduce the risk of transmission of HIV to others through sexual contact or blood contamination.

Advise pregnant women considering use of the drug to prevent maternal-fetal transmission of HIV that transmission may still occur in some cases despite therapy. Long-term consequences of in utero and infant exposure are unknown, including the possible risk of cancer. Advise HIV-infected pregnant women not to breastfeed to avoid postnatal transmission of HIV to a child who may not yet be infected.

➤*Oral:* Take exactly as prescribed. Do not share medication; do not exceed the recommended dose.

ABACAVIR SULFATE

Rx	Ziagen (GlaxoSmithKline)	Tablets: 300 mg	(GX 623). Yellow, capsule shape. Film-coated. In 60s and UD blister packs of 60s.
		Oral solution: 20 mg/mL	Parabens, saccharin, sorbitol. Strawberry-banana flavor. In 240 mL.

WARNING

Fatal hypersensitivity reactions have been associated with abacavir therapy. Discontinue abacavir in patients developing signs or symptoms of hypersensitivity (eg, fever, rash, fatigue; GI symptoms such as nausea, vomiting, diarrhea, abdominal pain; respiratory symptoms such as pharyngitis, dyspnea, cough) as soon as a hypersensitivity reaction is suspected. To avoid a delay in diagnosis and minimize the risk of a life-threatening hypersensitivity reaction, permanently discontinue abacavir therapy if hypersensitivity cannot be ruled out, even when other diagnoses are possible (eg, acute onset respiratory diseases, gastroenteritis, reactions to other medications). Do not restart abacavir following a hypersensitivity reaction because more severe symptoms will recur within hours and may include life-threatening hypotension and death. Severe or fatal hypersensitivity reactions can occur within hours after reintroduction of abacavir in patients who have no identified history or unrecognized symptoms of hypersensitivity to abacavir therapy (see Warnings).

Lactic acidosis and severe hepatomegaly with steatosis, including fatal cases, have been reported with the use of nucleoside analogs alone or in combination, including abacavir and other antiretrovirals (see Warnings).

Indications

➤HIV infection: In combination with other antiretroviral agents for the treatment of HIV-1 infection.

Administration and Dosage

➤Approved by the FDA: December 17, 1998.

Dispense the Medication Guide and Warning Card that provide information about recognition of hypersensitivity reactions with each new prescription and refill.

Always use abacavir in combination with other antiretroviral agents. Do not add abacavir as a single agent when antiretroviral regimens are changed because of loss of virologic response.

Abacavir may be taken with or without food.

➤Adults: 300 mg twice daily in combination with other antiretroviral agents.

➤Children (3 months to 16 years of age): 8 mg/kg twice daily (up to a maximum of 300 mg twice daily) in combination with other antiretroviral agents.

➤Dose adjustment in hepatic impairment: The recommended dose of abacavir in patients with mild hepatic impairment (Child-Pugh score 5 to 6) is 200 mg twice daily. To enable dose reduction, abacavir oral solution (10 mL twice daily) should be used for the treatment of these patients. The safety, efficacy, and pharmacokinetic properties of abacavir have not been established in patients with moderate to severe hepatic impairment; therefore, abacavir is contraindicated in these patients.

➤Storage/Stability:

Tablets – Store at controlled room temperature 20° to 25°C (68° to 77°F).

Oral solution – Store at controlled room temperature 20° to 25°C (68° to 77°F). Do not freeze. May be refrigerated.

Actions

➤Pharmacology: Abacavir is a carbocyclic synthetic nucleoside analog. Intracellularly, abacavir is converted by cellular enzymes to the active metabolite carbovir triphosphate. Carbovir triphosphate is an analog of deoxyguanosine-5′-triphosphate (dGTP). Carbovir triphosphate inhibits the activity of HIV-1 reverse transcriptase (RT) by competing with the natural substrate dGTP and by its incorporation into viral DNA. The lack of a 3′-OH group in the incorporated nucleoside analog prevents the formation of the 5′ to 3′ phosphodiester linkage essential for DNA chain elongation; therefore, the viral DNA growth is terminated.

➤Pharmacokinetics:

Absorption – Abacavir was rapidly and extensively absorbed after oral administration. The mean absolute bioavailability of the tablet was 83%. The steady-state peak serum concentration (C_{max}) was approximately 3 mcg/mL and $AUC_{(0-12h)}$ was approximately 6.02 mcg•h/mL. There was no significant difference in systemic exposure (AUC_{∞}) in the fed and fasting states; therefore, abacavir tablets may be administered with or without food. Systemic exposure to abacavir was comparable after administration of oral solution and tablets. Therefore, these products may be used interchangeably.

Distribution – The apparent volume of distribution after IV administration of abacavir was approximately 0.86 L/kg, suggesting that abacavir distributes into extravascular space. In 3 subjects, the CSF to $AUC_{(0-6h)}$ ratio ranged from 27% to 33%. Total blood and plasma drug-related radioactivity concentrations were identical, demonstrating that abacavir readily distributes into erythrocytes. Binding to human plasma proteins was approximately 50% and was independent of concentration.

Metabolism – Abacavir is not significantly metabolized by cytochrome P450 enzymes. In vitro experiments reveal that abacavir does not inhibit human CYP3A4, CYP2D6, or CYP2C9 activity at clinically relevant concentrations. The primary routes of elimination are metabolism by alcohol dehydrogenase (to form the 5′-carboxylic acid) and glucuronyl transferase (to form the 5′-glucuronide). The metabolites do not have antiviral activity.

Excretion – Of the 99% of the total abacavir dose recovered, 1.2% was excreted in the urine as abacavir, 30% as the 5′-carboxylic acid metabolite, 36% as the 5′-glucuronide metabolite, and 15% as unidentified minor metabolites in the urine. Fecal elimination accounted for 16% of the dose. In single-dose studies, the observed elimination half-life was approximately 1.54 h. After IV administration, total clearance was approximately 0.8 L/h/kg.

Special populations –

Adults with hepatic function impairment: The pharmacokinetics of abacavir have been studied in patients with mild hepatic impairment (Child-Pugh score 5 to 6). Results showed that there was a mean increase of 89% in the abacavir AUC, and an increase of 58% in the half-life of abacavir after a single dose of 600 mg. The AUCs of the metabolites were not modified by mild liver disease; however, the rates of formation and elimination of the metabolites were decreased. A dose of 200 mg (provided by 10 mL abacavir oral solution) administered twice daily is recommended for patients with mild liver disease. The safety, efficacy, and pharmacokinetics of abacavir have not been studied in patients with moderate or severe hepatic impairment; therefore abacavir is contraindicated in these patients.

Children: The pharmacokinetics of abacavir have been studied after single or repeat doses of abacavir in 68 pediatric patients. Following multiple-dose administration of abacavir 8 mg/kg twice daily, steady-state $AUC_{(0-12h)}$ and C_{max} were approximately 9.8 mcg•h/mL and approximately 3.71 mcg/mL, respectively.

➤Microbiology:

Antiviral activity in vitro – Abacavir has synergistic activity in combination with amprenavir, nevirapine, and zidovudine, and additive activity in combination with didanosine, lamivudine, stavudine, and zalcitabine in vitro. These drug combinations have not been adequately studied in humans. The relationship between in vitro susceptibility of HIV to abacavir and the inhibition of HIV replication in humans has not been established.

Drug resistance – HIV-1 isolates with reduced sensitivity to abacavir have been selected in vitro and also were obtained from patients treated with abacavir. Genetic analysis of isolates from abacavir-treated patients showed point mutations in the reverse transcriptase gene that resulted in amino acid substitutions. Phenotypic analysis of HIV-1 isolates that harbored abacavir-associated mutations from 17 patients after 12 weeks of monotherapy exhibited a 3-fold decrease in susceptibility to abacavir in vitro.

Cross-resistance – In vitro, recombinant laboratory strains of HIV-1 (HXB2) containing multiple reverse transcriptase mutations conferring abacavir resistance exhibited cross-resistance to lamivudine, didanosine, and zalcitabine.

➤Clinical trials:

Therapy-naive adults – In a multicenter, double-blind, controlled study, 562 HIV-infected, therapy-naïve adults with a preentry plasma HIV-1 RNA greater than 10,000 copies/mL were randomized to receive abacavir (300 mg twice daily) plus lamivudine/zidovudine (150/300 mg twice daily) or indinavir (800 mg 3 times daily) plus lamivudine/zidovudine twice daily. The median pretreatment CD4 cell count was 360 cells/mm³ and the median plasma HIV-1 RNA was 4.8 $\log_{10}$ copies/mL. Proportions of patients with plasma HIV-1 RNA less than 400 copies/mL through 48 weeks of treatment are summarized below.

Abacavir Outcomes of Randomized Treatment Through Week 48 (%)		
Outcome	Abacavir/ Lamivudine/ Zidovudine (n = 282)	Indinavir/ Lamivudine/ Zidovudine (n = 280)
HIV RNA < 400 copies/mL	46	47
HIV RNA ≥ 400 copies/mL[1]	29	28
CDC Class C event	2	< 1
Discontinued because of adverse reactions	9	11
Discontinued because of other reasons[2]	6	6
Randomized but never initiated treatment	7	5

[1] Includes viral rebound and failure to achieve confirmed fewer than 400 copies/mL by week 48.

[2] Includes consent withdrawn, lost to follow-up, protocol violations, those with missing data, and other.

ABACAVIR SULFATE

Therapy-experienced children – A randomized, double-blind study compared abacavir 8 mg/kg twice daily, lamivudine 4 mg/kg twice daily, and zidovudine 180 mg/m^2 twice daily vs lamivudine 4 mg/kg twice daily and zidovudine 180 mg/m^2 twice daily. Patients had a baseline CD4 cell percent greater than 15% (median, 27%) and a median baseline plasma HIV-1 RNA of 4.6 log$_{10}$ copies/mL. Eighty percent and 55% of patients had prior therapy with zidovudine and lamivudine, respectively, most often in combination. Proportions of patients with plasma HIV-1 RNA levels of 10,000 or less and fewer than 400 copies/mL, respectively, were followed through 24 weeks of treatment. After 16 weeks of therapy, the median CD4 increases from baseline were 69 cells/mm^3 in the group receiving abacavir and 9 cells/mm^3 in the control group.

Contraindications

Previously demonstrated hypersensitivity to any of the components of the product associated with fatal hypersensitivity reactions (see Warnings and Warning Box).

Moderate or severe hepatic impairment (Child-Pugh score greater than 6).

Warnings

➤*Lactic acidosis/severe hepatomegaly with steatosis:* Lactic acidosis and severe hepatomegaly with steatosis, including fatal cases, have been reported with the use of nucleoside analogs alone or in combination, including abacavir and other antiretrovirals. A majority of these cases have been in women. Obesity and prolonged nucleoside exposure may be risk factors. Exercise particular caution when administering abacavir to any patient with known risk factors for liver disease; however, cases have been reported in patients with no known risk factors. Suspend treatment in any patient who develops clinical or laboratory findings suggestive of lactic acidosis or pronounced hepatotoxicity (which may include hepatomegaly and steatosis even in the absence of marked transaminase elevations).

➤*Hypersensitivity reactions:* Fatal hypersensitivity reactions have been associated with abacavir therapy. Discontinue abacavir in patients developing signs or symptoms of hypersensitivity (eg, fever, rash, fatigue; GI symptoms such as nausea, vomiting, diarrhea, abdominal pain; respiratory symptoms such as pharyngitis, dyspnea, cough) as soon as a hypersensitivity reaction is first suspected; seek medical evaluation immediately. To avoid a delay in diagnosis and minimize the risk of a life-threatening hypersensitivity reaction, permanently discontinue abacavir if hypersensitivity cannot be ruled out, even when other diagnoses are possible (eg, acute onset respiratory diseases, gastroenteritis, or reactions to other medications). Carefully consider the diagnosis of hypersensitivity reaction for patients presenting with symptoms of acute onset respiratory diseases, even if alternative respiratory diagnoses (pneumonia, bronchitis, pharyngitis, or flu-like illness) are possible. Do not restart abacavir following a hypersensitivity reaction because more severe symptoms will recur within hours and may include life-threatening hypotension and death. Severe or fatal hypersensitivity reactions can occur within hours of reintroduction of abacavir in patients with no identified history or unrecognized symptoms of hypersensitivity to abacavir therapy (see Adverse Reactions).

When abacavir therapy has been discontinued for reasons other than symptoms of a hypersensitivity reaction, and if reinitiation of therapy is under consideration, evaluate the reason for discontinuation to ensure that the patient did not have symptoms of a hypersensitivity reaction. Do not reintroduce abacavir therapy if hypersensitivity cannot be ruled out. If symptoms of hypersensitivity are not identified, undertake reintroduction with continued monitoring for symptoms of a hypersensitivity reaction. Advise patients that a hypersensitivity reaction can occur with reintroduction of abacavir, and that abacavir reintroduction should be undertaken only if medical care can be readily accessed by the patient or others.

Hypersensitivity reaction registry – To facilitate reporting of hypersensitivity reactions and collection of information on each case, an Abacavir Hypersensitivity Registry has been established. Physicians are encouraged to register patients by calling (800) 270-0425.

➤*Carcinogenesis:* Single doses of abacavir 55, 110, and 330 mg/kg/day in mice and 30, 120, and 600 mg/kg/day in rats were administered. Results showed an increase in the incidence of malignant and nonmalignant tumors. Malignant tumors occurred in the preputial gland of males and the clitoral gland of females of both species and in the liver of female rats. In addition, nonmalignant tumors also occurred in the liver and thyroid gland of female rats. These observations were made at systemic exposures in the range of 6 to 32 times the human exposure.

➤*Mutagenesis:* Abacavir induced chromosomal aberrations in the presence and absence of metabolic activation in an in vitro cytogenetic study in human lymphocytes. Abacavir was mutagenic in the absence of metabolic activation, although it was not mutagenic in the presence of metabolic activation in an L5178Y mouse lymphoma assay. At systemic exposures approximately 9 times higher than in humans at the therapeutic dose, abacavir was clastogenic in males and not clastogenic in females in an in vivo mouse bone marrow micronucleus assay.

➤*Elderly:* Clinical studies of abacavir did not include sufficient numbers of patients 65 years of age and older to determine whether they respond differently than younger patients. In general, exercise caution in dose selection for an elderly patient, reflecting the greater frequency of decreased hepatic, renal, or cardiac function, and of concomitant disease or other drug therapy.

➤*Pregnancy: Category C.* There are no adequate and well-controlled studies in pregnant women. Use during pregnancy only if the potential benefits outweigh the risk. Studies in pregnant rats showed that abacavir is transferred to the fetus through the placenta. Developmental toxicity (depressed fetal body weight and reduced crown-rump length) and increased incidences of fetal anasarca and skeletal malformations were observed when rats were treated with abacavir at doses of 1000 mg/kg (35 times the human exposure based on AUC) during organogenesis. In a fertility study, evidence of toxicity to the developing embryo and fetuses (increased resorptions, decreased fetal body weights) occurred only at 500 mg/kg/day. The offspring of female rats treated with 500 mg/kg/day (beginning at embryo implantation and ending at weaning) showed increased incidence of stillbirth and lower body weights throughout life.

Antiretroviral pregnancy registry – To monitor maternal-fetal outcomes of pregnant women exposed to abacavir, an Antiretroviral Pregnancy Registry has been established. Physicians are encouraged to register patients by calling (800) 258-4263.

➤*Lactation:* The Centers for Disease Control and Prevention recommend that HIV-infected mothers not breastfeed their infants to avoid risking postnatal transmission of HIV infection.

Although it is not known if abacavir is excreted in breast milk, abacavir is present in the milk of lactating rats. Because of the potential for HIV transmission and any possible adverse effects, instruct mothers not to breastfeed if they are receiving abacavir.

➤*Children:* Use of abacavir is safe and effective in pediatric patients 3 months to 13 years of age and is supported by pharmacokinetic studies and evidence from adequate and well-controlled studies of abacavir in adults and pediatric patients.

Precautions

➤*Cross-resistance:* In clinical trials, patients with prolonged prior nucleoside reverse transcriptase inhibitor (NRTI) exposure or who had HIV-1 isolates that contained multiple mutations conferring resistance to NRTIs had limited response to abacavir. Consider the potential for cross-resistance between abacavir and other NRTIs when choosing new therapeutic regimens in therapy-experienced patients.

➤*Fat redistribution:* Redistribution/accumulation of body fat including central obesity, dorsocervical fat enlargement (buffalo hump), peripheral wasting, facial wasting, breast enlargement, and "cushingoid appearance" have been observed in patients receiving antiretroviral therapy. The mechanism and long-term consequences of these events are currently unknown. A causal relationship has not been established.

Drug Interactions

➤*Ethanol:* Ethanol decreases the elimination of abacavir, causing an increase in overall exposure because of their common metabolic pathway. Coadministration of ethanol 0.7 g/kg and abacavir 600 mg resulted in a 41% increase in abacavir AUC$_\infty$ and a 26% increase in abacavir half-life.

➤*Methadone:* Coadministration increased oral methadone clearance by 22% (90% CI 6% to 42%). This alteration will not result in a methadone dose modification in the majority of patients; however, an increased methadone dose may be required in a small number of patients.

Adverse Reactions

➤*Adults:*

Selected Adverse Reactions of Abacavir in Therapy-Naïve Adults (Study 1) (≥ 5%)		
Adverse reaction	Abacavir/Lamivudine/Zidovudine[1] (n = 83)	Lamivudine/Zidovudine[2] (n = 81)
GI		
Nausea	47	41
Nausea and vomiting	16	11
Diarrhea	12	11
Loss of appetite/anorexia	11	10
Miscellaneous		
Insomnia and other sleep disorders	7	5

[1] Regimen was abacavir 300 mg twice daily, lamivudine 150 mg twice daily, and zidovudine 300 mg twice daily for 16 weeks.
[2] Regimen was lamivudine 150 mg twice daily and zidovudine 300 mg twice daily for 16 weeks.

ABACAVIR SULFATE

Selected Adverse Reactions of Abacavir in Therapy-Naïve Adults (Study 2) ($\geq$ 5%)		
Adverse reaction	Abacavir/Lamivudine/Zidovudine[1] (n = 262)	Indinavir/Lamivudine/Zidovudine[2] (n = 264)
GI		
Nausea	60	61
Nausea and vomiting	30	27
Diarrhea	26	27
Loss of appetite/anorexia	15	11
Miscellaneous		
Malaise and/or fatigue	44	41
Headache	28	25
Fever and/or chills	20	13
Insomnia and other sleep disorders	13	12

[1] Regimen was abacavir 300 mg twice daily, lamivudine 150 mg twice daily, and zidovudine 300 mg twice daily for 48 weeks.
[2] Regimen was indinavir 800 mg 3 times daily, lamivudine 150 mg twice daily, and zidovudine 300 mg twice daily for 48 weeks.

Five subjects in the abacavir arm of the study experienced worsening of preexisting depression compared with none in the indinavir arm.

►*Children:*

Selected Adverse Reactions of Abacavir in Therapy-Experienced Children ($\geq$ 5%)		
Adverse reaction	Abacavir/Lamivudine/Zidovudine[1] (n = 102)	Lamivudine/Zidovudine[2] (n = 103)
GI		
Nausea and vomiting	38	18
Diarrhea	16	15
Loss of appetite/anorexia	9	2
Miscellaneous		
Fever	19	12
Headache	16	12
Rash	11	8

[1] Regimen was abacavir 8 mg/kg twice daily, lamivudine 4 mg/kg twice daily, and zidovudine 180 mg/m[2] twice daily for 16 weeks.
[2] Regimen was lamivudine 4 mg/kg twice daily and zidovudine 180 mg/m[2] twice daily for 16 weeks.

►*Hypersensitivity:* Fatal hypersensitivity reactions have been associated with abacavir therapy (see Warnings and Warning Box).

In clinical studies, approximately 5% of adult and pediatric patients receiving abacavir developed a hypersensitivity reaction. This reaction is characterized by the appearance of symptoms indicating multi-organ/body system involvement. Symptoms usually appear within the first 6 weeks of treatment, although these reactions may occur at any time during therapy. Frequently observed signs and symptoms include fever, rash, fatigue, and GI symptoms (eg, nausea, vomiting, diarrhea, abdominal pain). Other signs and symptoms include malaise, lethargy, myalgia, arthralgia, edema, myolysis, pharyngitis, cough, abnormal chest x-ray findings (predominantly infiltrates, which can be localized), dyspnea, headache, and paresthesia. Some patients who experienced a hypersensitivity reaction were initially thought to have acute onset or worsening respiratory disease. The diagnosis of hypersensitivity reaction should be carefully considered for patients presenting with symptoms of acute onset respiratory diseases, even if alternative respiratory diagnoses (eg, pneumonia, bronchitis, pharyngitis, flu-like illness) are possible. Physical findings include lymphadenopathy, mucous membrane lesions (conjunctivitis and mouth ulcerations), and rash. The rash usually appears maculopapular or urticarial but may be variable in appearance. Hypersensitivity reactions have occurred without rash. Anaphylaxis, liver failure, renal failure, hypotension, adult respiratory distress syndrome, respiratory failure, and death have occurred in association with hypersensitivity reactions. Symptoms worsen with continued therapy but often resolve upon discontinuation of therapy.

Risk factors that may predict the occurrence or severity of hypersensitivity to abacavir have not been identified.

►*Miscellaneous:* Other adverse events observed in the expanded-access program were pancreatitis and increased gamma-glutamyltransferase (GGT).

►*Lab test abnormalities:* Anemia; neutropenia; liver function test abnormalities; CPK or creatinine elevations; mild elevations of blood glucose; triglyceride elevations (all grades were more common on the abacavir arm [25%] than on the placebo arm [11%]); hyperglycemia and disorders of lipid metabolism (occurred with similar frequency in the abacavir and indinavir treatment arms).

►*Postmarketing:* Because they are reported voluntarily from a population of unknown size, estimates of frequency cannot be made. These events have been chosen for inclusion because of their seriousness, frequency of reporting, potential causal connection to abacavir, or a combination of these factors.

Dermatologic – Suspected Stevens-Johnson syndrome (SJS) and toxic epidermal necrolysis (TEN) have been reported in patients receiving abacavir primarily in combination with medications known to be associated with SJS and TEN, respectively. Because of the overlap of clinical signs and symptoms between hypersensitivity to abacavir and SJS and TEN and the possibility of multiple drug sensitivities in some patients, discontinue abacavir and do not restart in such cases. There also have been reports of erythema multiforme with abacavir use.

Miscellaneous – Redistribution/accumulation of body fat (see Precautions).

Overdosage

There is no known antidote for abacavir. It is not known whether abacavir can be removed by peritoneal dialysis or hemodialysis.

Patient Information

Advise patients of the possibility of a hypersensitivity reaction to abacavir that may result in death. Instruct patients to discontinue abacavir and seek medical evaluation immediately if they develop signs or symptoms of hypersensitivity (eg, fever, rash, fatigue; GI symptoms such as nausea, vomiting, diarrhea, abdominal pain; respiratory symptoms such as sore throat, shortness of breath, cough). Instruct patients not to reintroduce abacavir without medical consultation and to undertake reintroduction of abacavir only if medical care can be readily accessed by the patient or others.

Give the Medication Guide to patients and instruct them to read it thoroughly because it provides written information including hypersensitivity reactions. Dispense with each new prescription and refill. Provide a Warning Card for the patient with each prescription summarizing the symptoms of the abacavir hypersensitivity reaction. Instruct patients to carry this card with them.

Inform patients that abacavir is not a cure for HIV infection and they may continue to experience illnesses associated with HIV infection, including opportunistic infections. Advise patients to remain under the care of a physician when using abacavir. Advise patients that the use of abacavir has not been shown to reduce the risk of transmission of HIV to others through sexual contact or blood contamination.

Inform patients that redistribution or accumulation of body fat may occur in patients receiving antiretroviral therapy and that the cause and long-term health effects of these conditions are not known at this time.

Advise patients that the long-term effects of abacavir are unknown at this time. Instruct patients that abacavir tablets and oral solution are for oral ingestion only.

Advise patients of the importance of taking abacavir exactly as it is prescribed.

Advise patients to talk to their doctor if they have liver problems. Some patients with liver disease should not take abacavir.

Nucleoside Reverse Transcriptase Inhibitors

EMTRICITABINE

Rx	Emtriva (Gilead Sciences)	Capsules: 200 mg	(200 mg GILEAD). Blue/White. In 30s.

WARNING

Lactic acidosis and severe hepatomegaly with steatosis, including fatal cases, have been reported with the use of nucleoside analogs alone or in combination with other antiretrovirals (see Warnings).

Indications

➤*HIV infection:* In combination with other antiretroviral agents for the treatment of HIV-1 infection in adults.

Administration and Dosage

➤*Approved by the FDA:* July 2, 2003.

➤*Adults:* 200 mg once daily taken orally with or without food.

➤*Renal function impairment:* The dosing interval of emtricitabine should be adjusted in patients with baseline creatinine clearance less than 50 mL/min using the following guidelines (see table). The safety and effectiveness of these dosing interval adjustment guidelines have not been clinically evaluated. Therefore, clinical response to treatment and renal function should be closely monitored in these patients.

Emtricitabine Dosing Interval Adjustment in Patients with Renal Impairment

	Creatinine clearance (mL/min)			
	≥ 50	30 to 49	15 to 29	< 15 (including patients requiring hemodialysis)[1]
Recommended dose and dosing interval	200 mg q 24 h	200 mg q 48 h	200 mg q 72 h	200 mg q 96 h

[1] Hemodialysis patients: If dosing on day of dialysis, give dose after dialysis.

➤*Storage/Stability:* Store at 25°C (77°F); excursions permitted to 15° to 30°C (59° to 86°F).

Actions

➤*Pharmacology:* Emtricitabine, a synthetic nucleoside analog of cytosine, is phosphorylated by cellular enzymes to form emtricitabine 5'-triphosphate. Emtricitabine 5'-triphosphate inhibits the activity of the HIV-1 reverse transcriptase by competing with the natural substrate deoxycytidine 5'-triphosphate and by being incorporated into nascent viral DNA, which results in chain termination. Emtricitabine 5'-triphosphate is a weak inhibitor of mammalian DNA polymerase α, β, ε, and mitochondrial DNA polymerase γ.

➤*Pharmacokinetics:*

Absorption – Emtricitabine is rapidly and extensively absorbed following oral administration with peak plasma concentrations occurring at 1 to 2 hours postdose. Following multiple dose oral administration of emtricitabine to 20 HIV-infected subjects, the mean ($\pm$ SD) steady-state plasma emtricitabine peak concentration (C_{max}) was 1.8 ± 0.7 mcg/mL and the area under the plasma concentration-time curve (AUC) over a 24-hour dosing interval was 10 ± 3.1 h•mcg/mL. The mean steady-state plasma trough concentration at 24 hours postdose was 0.09 mcg/mL. The mean absolute bioavailability of emtricitabine was 93%.

The multiple dose pharmacokinetics of emtricitabine are dose-proportional over a dose range of 25 to 200 mg.

Effects of food: Emtricitabine may be taken with or without food. Emtricitabine systemic exposure (AUC) was unaffected while C_{max} decreased by 29% when emtricitabine was administered with food (an approximately 1000 kcal high-fat meal).

Distribution – In vitro binding of emtricitabine to human plasma proteins was less than 4% and independent of concentration over the range of 0.02 to 200 mcg/mL. At peak plasma concentration, the mean plasma to blood drug concentration ratio was approximately 1 and the mean semen to plasma drug concentration ratio was approximately 4.

Metabolism/Excretion – In vitro studies indicate that emtricitabine is not an inhibitor of human CYP450 enzymes. Following administration of emtricitabine, complete recovery of the dose was achieved in urine (approximately 86%) and feces (approximately 14%). Of the dose, 13% was recovered in urine as 3 putative metabolites. The biotransformation of emtricitabine includes oxidation of the thiol moiety to form the 3'-sulfoxide diastereomers (approximately 9% of dose) and conjugation with glucuronic acid to form 2'-O-glucuronide (approximately 4% of dose). The plasma emtricitabine half-life is approximately 10 hours. The renal clearance of emtricitabine is greater than the estimated creatinine clearance, suggesting elimination by both glomerular filtration and active tubular secretion. There may be competition for elimination with other compounds that are also renally eliminated.

Special populations –

Renal function impairment: The pharmacokinetics of emtricitabine are altered in patients with renal impairment. In patients with creatinine clearance less than 50 mL/min or with end-stage renal disease (ESRD) requiring dialysis, C_{max} and AUC of emtricitabine were increased due to a reduction in renal clearance (see table below). It is recommended that the dosing interval for emtricitabine be modified in patients with creatinine clearance less than 50 mL/min or in patients with ESRD who require dialysis (See Administration and Dosage).

Emtricitabine Mean Pharmacokinetic Parameters in Patients with Renal Function Impairment

Creatinine clearance (mL/min)	> 80 (n = 6)	50 to 80 (n = 6)	30 to 49 (n = 6)	< 30 (n = 5)	ESRD < 30 (n = 5)[1]
Baseline creatinine clearance (mL/min)	107	59.8	40.9	22.9	8.8
C_{max} (mcg/mL)	2.2	3.8	3.2	2.8	2.8
AUC (h•mcg/mL)	11.8	19.9	25	34	53.2
CL/F (mL/min)	302	168	138	99	64
CLr (mL/min)	213.3	121.4	68.6	29.5	NA

[1] ESRD patients requiring dialysis.

Hemodialysis treatment removes approximately 30% of the emtricitabine dose over a 3-hour dialysis period starting within 1.5 hours of emtricitabine dosing (blood flow rate of 400 mL/min and a dialysate flow rate of 600 mL/min). It is not known whether emtricitabine can be removed by peritoneal dialysis.

➤*Microbiology:*

Antiviral activity in vitro – In drug combination studies of emtricitabine with nucleoside reverse transcriptase inhibitors (abacavir, lamivudine, stavudine, tenofovir, zalcitabine, zidovudine), nonnucleoside reverse transcriptase inhibitors (NNRTIs; delavirdine, efavirenz, nevirapine), and protease inhibitors (amprenavir, nelfinavir, ritonavir, saquinavir), additive to synergistic effects were observed. Most of these drug combinations have not been studied in humans.

Drug resistance – Emtricitabine-resistant isolates of HIV have been selected in vitro. Genotypic analysis of these isolates showed that the reduced susceptibility to emtricitabine was associated with a mutation in the HIV reverse transcriptase gene at codon 184, which resulted in an amino acid substitution of methionine by valine or isoleucine (M184V/I).

Emtricitabine-resistant isolates of HIV have been recovered from some patients treated with emtricitabine alone or in combination with other antiretroviral agents. In a clinical study, viral isolates from 37.5% of treatment-naïve patients with virologic failure showed reduced susceptibility to emtricitabine. Genotypic analysis of these isolates showed that the resistance was due to M184V/I mutations in the HIV reverse transcriptase gene.

Cross-resistance – Cross-resistance among certain nucleoside analog reverse transcriptase inhibitors has been recognized. Emtricitabine-resistant isolates (M184V/I) were cross-resistant to lamivudine and zalcitabine but retained sensitivity to abacavir, didanosine, stavudine, tenofovir, zidovudine, and NNRTIs (delavirdine, efavirenz, and nevirapine). HIV-1 isolates containing the K65R mutation, selected in vivo by abacavir, didanosine, tenofovir, and zalcitabine, demonstrated reduced susceptibility to inhibition by emtricitabine. Viruses harboring mutations conferring reduced susceptibility to stavudine and zidovudine or didanosine remained sensitive to emtricitabine. HIV-1 containing the K103N mutation associated with resistance to NNRTIs was susceptible to emtricitabine.

➤*Clinical trials:* A 48-week double-blind, active-controlled multicenter study compared emtricitabine (200 mg QD) administered in combination with didanosine and efavirenz versus stavudine, didanosine, and efavirenz in 571 antiretroviral naïve patients. The mean increase from baseline in CD4 cell count was 168 cells/mm^3 for the emtricitabine arm and 134 cells/mm^3 for the stavudine arm.

A 48-week open-label, active-controlled multicenter study compared emtricitabine 200 mg every day to lamivudine in combination with stavudine or zidovudine and a protease inhibitor or NNRTI in 440 patients who were on a lamivudine-containing triple-antiretroviral drug regimen for at least 12 weeks prior to study entry and had HIV-1 RNA 400 copies/mL or fewer. Patients were randomized 1:2 to continue therapy with lamivudine 150 mg twice daily or to switch to emtricitabine 200 mg every day. All patients were maintained on their stable background regimen. The mean increase from baseline in CD4 cell count was 29 cells/mm^3 for the emtricitabine arm and 61 cells/mm^3 for the lamivudine arm.

Contraindications

Previously demonstrated hypersensitivity to any of the components of the products.

Warnings

➤*Lactic acidosis/Severe hepatomegaly with steatosis:* Lactic acidosis and severe hepatomegaly with steatosis, including fatal cases, have been reported with the use of nucleoside analogs alone or in combination, including emtricitabine and other antiretrovirals. A majority

EMTRICITABINE

of these cases have been in women. Obesity and prolonged nucleoside exposure may be risk factors. However, cases have been reported in patients with no known risk factors. Treatment with emtricitabine should be suspended in any patient who develops clinical or laboratory findings suggestive of lactic acidosis or pronounced hepatotoxicity (which may include hepatomegaly and steatosis even in the absence of marked transaminase elevations).

➤*Posttreatment exacerbation of hepatitis:* It is recommended that all patients with HIV be tested for the presence of chronic hepatitis B virus (HBV) before initiating antiretroviral therapy. Exacerbations of hepatitis B have been reported in patients after the discontinuation of emtricitabine. Patients coinfected with HIV and HBV should be closely monitored with both clinical and laboratory follow-up for at least several months after stopping treatment.

➤*Renal function impairment:* Emtricitabine is principally eliminated by the kidney. Reduction of the dosage of emtricitabine is recommended for patients with impaired renal function (see Pharmacokinetics and Administration and Dosage).

➤*Elderly:* Dose selection for elderly patients should be cautious, keeping in mind the greater frequency of decreased hepatic, renal, or cardiac function, and of concomitant disease or other drug therapy.

➤*Pregnancy: Category B.* The incidence of fetal variations and malformations was not increased in embryofetal toxicity studies performed with emtricitabine in mice at exposures (AUC) approximately 60-fold higher and in rabbits at approximately 120-fold higher than human exposures at the recommended daily dose. However, there are no adequate and well-controlled studies in pregnant women. Emtricitabine should be used during pregnancy only if clearly needed.

Antiretroviral pregnancy registry – To monitor fetal outcomes of pregnant women exposed to emtricitabine, an antiretroviral pregnancy registry has been established. Health care providers are encouraged to register patients by calling (800) 258-4263.

➤*Lactation:* The Centers for Disease Control and Prevention recommend that HIV-infected mothers not breastfeed their infants to avoid risking postnatal transmission of HIV. It is not known whether emtricitabine is secreted into human milk. Because of both the potential for HIV transmission and the potential for serious adverse reactions in nursing infants, mothers should be instructed not to breastfeed if they are receiving emtricitabine.

➤*Children:* Safety and effectiveness in pediatric patients have not been established.

Precautions

➤*Fat redistribution:* Redistribution/accumulation of body fat including central obesity, dorsocervical fat enlargement (buffalo hump), peripheral wasting, facial wasting, breast enlargement, and "cushingoid appearance" have been observed in patients receiving antiretroviral therapy. The mechanism and long-term consequences of these events are unknown. A causal relationship has not been established.

Adverse Reactions

The most common adverse events that occurred in patients receiving emtricitabine with other antiretroviral agents in clinical trials were headache, diarrhea, nausea, and rash, which were generally of mild to moderate severity. Approximately 1% of patients discontinued participation in the clinical studies due to these events. All adverse events were reported with similar frequency in emtricitabine and control treatment groups with the exception of skin discoloration, which was reported with higher frequency in the emtricitabine treated group.

Skin discoloration, manifested by hyperpigmentation on the palms and/or soles was generally mild and asymptomatic. The mechanism and clinical significance are unknown.

Emtricitabine Adverse Events (≥ 3%)			
	Study 1		Study 2
Adverse event	Emtricitabine + Zidovudine or Stavudine + NNRTI or PI (n = 294)	Lamivudine + Zidovudine or Stavudine + NNRTI or PI (n = 146)	Emtricitabine + Didanosine + Efavirenz (n = 286)	Stavudine + Didanosine + Efavirenz (n = 285)
CNS				
Abnormal dreams	2	< 1	11	19
Depressive disorders	6	10	9	13
Dizziness	4	5	25	26
Headache	13	6	22	25
Insomnia	7	3	16	21
Neuropathy/ Peripheral neuritis	4	3	4	13
Paresthesia	5	7	6	12

Emtricitabine Adverse Events (≥ 3%)			
	Study 1		Study 2
Adverse event	Emtricitabine + Zidovudine or Stavudine + NNRTI or PI (n = 294)	Lamivudine + Zidovudine or Stavudine + NNRTI or PI (n = 146)	Emtricitabine + Didanosine + Efavirenz (n = 286)	Stavudine + Didanosine + Efavirenz (n = 285)
GI				
Abdominal pain	8	11	14	17
Diarrhea	23	18	23	32
Dyspepsia	4	5	8	12
Nausea	18	12	13	23
Vomiting	9	7	9	12
Laboratory test abnormalities				
Percentage with grade 3 or 4 laboratory abnormality	31	28	34	38
ALT (> 5 x ULN[1])	2	1	5	6
AST (> 5 x ULN)	3	< 1	6	9
Bilirubin (> 2.5 x ULN)	1	2	< 1	< 1
Creatine kinase (> 4 x ULN)	11	14	12	11
Neutrophils (< 750 mm³)	5	3	5	7
Pancreatic amylase (> 2 x ULN)	2	2	< 1	1
Serum amylase (> 2 x ULN)	2	2	5	10
Serum glucose (< 40 or > 250 mg/dL)	3	3	2	3
Serum lipase (> 2 x ULN)	< 1	< 1	1	2
Triglycerides (> 750 mg/dL)	10	8	9	6
Musculoskeletal				
Arthralgia	3	4	5	6
Myalgia	4	4	6	3
Respiratory				
Increased cough	14	11	14	8
Rhinitis	18	12	12	10
Miscellaneous				
Asthenia	16	10	12	17
Rash event[2]	17	14	30	33

[1] ULN = upper limit of normal.
[2] Rash event includes rash, pruritus, maculopapular rash, urticaria, vesiculobullous rash, pustular rash, and allergic reaction.

Overdosage

There is no known antidote for emtricitabine. Limited clinical experience is available at doses higher than the therapeutic dose of emtricitabine. In one clinical pharmacology study, single doses of emtricitabine 1200 mg were administered to 11 patients. No severe adverse reactions were reported.

The effects of higher doses are not known. If overdose occurs, the patient should be monitored for signs of toxicity, and standard supportive treatment applied as necessary.

Hemodialysis treatment removes approximately 30% of the emtricitabine dose over a 3-hour dialysis period starting within 1.5 hours of emtricitabine dosing (blood flow rate of 400 mL/min and a dialysate flow rate of 600 mL/min). It is not known whether emtricitabine can be removed by peritoneal dialysis.

Patient Information

Emtricitabine is not a cure for HIV infection and patients may continue to experience illnesses associated with HIV infection, including opportunistic infections.

Advise patients that the use of emtricitabine has not been shown to reduce the risk of transmission of HIV to others through sexual contact or blood contamination.

Advise patients that the long-term effects of emtricitabine are unknown.

Advise patients that it is important to take emtricitabine with combination therapy on a regular dosing schedule to avoid missing doses.

Advise patients that redistribution or accumulation of body fat may occur in patients receiving antiretroviral therapy and that the cause and long-term health effects of these conditions are not known.

Nucleoside Analog Reverse Transcriptase Inhibitor Combination

LAMIVUDINE/ZIDOVUDINE (3TC/ZDV, 3TC/AZT)

Rx **Combivir** (GlaxoSmithKline) | **Tablets:** 150 mg lamivudine/300 mg zidovudine | (GXFC3). White, capsule shape. Film-coated. In 60s and UD 120s.

Consult the complete prescribing information for each agent, lamivudine and zidovudine, prior to administration of lamivudine/zidovudine combination tablets.

> ## WARNING
>
> Zidovudine, one of the two active ingredients in this product, has been associated with hematologic toxicity (eg, neutropenia, severe anemia) especially in patients with advanced human immunodeficiency virus (HIV). Prolonged use has been associated with symptomatic myopathy (see zidovudine Warnings section).
>
> Lactic acidosis and severe hepatomegaly with steatosis, including fatal cases, have been reported with use of nucleoside analogs alone or in combination, including lamivudine, zidovudine, and other antiretrovirals (see zidovudine Warnings section).

Indications

➤*HIV infection:* In combination with other antiretrovirals for the treatment of HIV infection.

Administration and Dosage

➤*Approved by the FDA:* September 26, 1997.

➤*Adults and children at least 12 years of age:* One tablet (150 mg lamivudine/300 mg zidovudine) orally twice daily without regard to food.

➤*Renal function impairment:* Because it is a fixed-dose combination, do not prescribe lamivudine/zidovudine for patients requiring dosage adjustment, such as those with reduced renal function (Ccr less than 50 mL/min) or those experiencing dose-limiting adverse events.

➤*Hepatic function impairment:* A reduction in the daily dose of zidovudine may be necessary in patients with mild to moderate hepatic function impairment or liver cirrhosis. Because lamivudine/zidovudine is a fixed-dose combination that cannot be adjusted for this patient population, it is not recommended for patients with impaired hepatic function.

➤*Storage/Stability:* Store between 2° and 30° C (36° and 86°F).

Actions

➤*Pharmacology:* Lamivudine/Zidovudine combination tablets contain 2 synthetic nucleoside analog reverse transcriptase inhibitors with activity against HIV. Lamivudine, in combination with zidovudine, has exhibited synergistic antiretroviral activity. Refer to lamivudine and zidovudine individual monographs for a complete explanation of mechanisms of action.

➤*Pharmacokinetics:* One combination lamivudine/zidovudine (150 mg/300 mg) tablet is bioequivalent to a 150 mg lamivudine tablet plus a 300 mg zidovudine tablet. Following oral administration, lamivudine and zidovudine each are rapidly absorbed, extensively distributed, and exhibit low binding to plasma protein (less than 38%). Select pharmacokinetic parameters for lamivudine and zidovudine individually are listed in the following table. Refer to specific monographs for a more thorough discussion of the pharmacokinetics for each agent.

Select Pharmacokinetic Parameters for Lamivudine and Zidovudine[1]						
	Bioavailability (%)	V_d (L/kg)	CSF:Plasma ratio	Clearance (L/h/kg)	Renal clearance (L/h/kg)	t½ (h)
Lamivudine	≈ 86	≈ 1.3	≈ 0.12	≈ 0.33	≈ 0.22	5 to 7
Zidovudine	≈ 64	≈ 1.6	≈ 0.6	≈ 1.6	≈ 0.34	0.5 to 3

[1] In adults.

Contraindications

Previously demonstrated clinically significant hypersensitivity to any of the components of this product.

Because this product is a fixed-dose combination doseform, avoid use in patients requiring dosage reduction (see Warnings).

Warnings

➤*Fixed-dose combination:* Lamivudine/zidovudine tablets are a fixed-dose combination doseform. Avoid use in patients requiring lamivudine or zidovudine dosage reduction including children under 12 years of age, renally impaired patients with Ccr less than 50 mL/min, or those experiencing dose-limiting adverse effects.

➤*Hematologic:* Use lamivudine/zidovudine with caution in patients who have bone marrow compromise evidenced by granulocyte count less than 1000 cells/mm^3 or hemoglobin less than 9.5 g/dL.

➤*Lactic acidosis/severe hepatomegaly with steatosis:* Lactic acidosis and severe hepatomegaly with steatosis, including fatal cases, have been reported with the use of nucleoside analogs alone or in combination, including lamivudine, zidovudine, and other antiretrovirals. A majority of these cases have been in women. Obesity and prolonged nucleoside exposure may be risk factors. Exercise caution when administering lamivudine/zidovudine to any patient with known risk factors for liver disease; however, cases have been reported in patients with no known risk factors. Suspend treatment with lamivudine/zidovudine in any patient who develops clinical or laboratory findings suggestive of lactic acidosis or pronounced hepatotoxicity (which may include hepatomegaly and steatosis even in the absence of marked transaminase elevations).

➤*Pregnancy:* Category C. There are no adequate and well-controlled studies in pregnant women. Use lamivudine/zidovudine combination tablets during pregnancy only if the potential benefits outweigh the risks. Refer to lamivudine and zidovudine individual monographs for more information.

Antiretroviral pregnancy registry – To monitor maternal-fetal outcomes of pregnant women exposed to lamivudine/zidovudine combination tablets or other antiretroviral agents, an Antiretroviral Pregnancy Registry has been established. Physicians are encouraged to register patients by calling (800) 258-4263.

Precautions

➤*Monitoring:* Blood counts are recommended frequently for patients with advanced HIV disease and periodically for patients with asymptomatic or early HIV disease.

Nucleoside Analog Reverse Transcriptase Inhibitor Combination

ABACAVIR SULFATE/LAMIVUDINE/ZIDOVUDINE

Rx	Trizivir (GlaxoSmithKline)	**Tablets:** 300 mg abacavir sulfate/150 mg lamivudine/ 300 mg zidovudine	(GX LL1). Blue-green, capsule shape. Film-coated. In 60s.

Consult the complete prescribing information for each agent, abacavir, lamivudine, and zidovudine, prior to administration of abacavir/lamivudine/zidovudine combination tablets.

WARNING

This product contains 3 nucleoside analogs (abacavir sulfate, lamivudine, and zidovudine) and is intended only for patients whose regimen would otherwise include these 3 components.

Abacavir sulfate has been associated with fatal hypersensitivity reactions (see abacavir Warnings section). Patients developing signs or symptoms of hypersensitivity (eg, fever; skin rash; fatigue; GI symptoms such as nausea, vomiting, diarrhea, or abdominal pain; respiratory symptoms such as pharyngitis, dyspnea, or cough) should discontinue abacavir/lamivudine/zidovudine as soon as a hypersensitivity reaction is suspected. To avoid a delay in diagnosis and minimize the risk of a life-threatening hypersensitivity reaction, permanently discontinue abacavir/lamivudine/zidovudine if hypersensitivity cannot be ruled out, even when other diagnoses are possible (eg, acute onset respiratory diseases, gastroenteritis, or reactions to other medications).

Do not restart abacavir following a hypersensitivity reaction to abacavir because more severe symptoms will recur within hours and may include life-threatening hypotension and death.

Severe or fatal hypersensitivity reactions can occur within hours after reintroduction of abacavir in patients who have no identified history or unrecognized symptoms of hypersensitivity to abacavir therapy (see abacavir Warnings and Adverse Reactions sections).

Zidovudine has been associated with hematologic toxicity including neutropenia and severe anemia, particularly in patients with advanced HIV disease (see zidovudine Warnings section). Prolonged use of zidovudine has been associated with symptomatic myopathy.

Lactic acidosis and severe hepatomegaly with steatosis, including fatal cases, have been reported with the use of nucleoside analogs alone or in combination, including abacavir, lamivudine, zidovudine, and other antiretrovirals (see Warnings sections in individual monographs).

There are limited data on the use of this triple-combination regimen in patients with higher viral load levels (more than 100,000 copies/mL) at baseline.

Indications

▶*HIV infection:* For use alone or in combination with other antiretroviral agents for the treatment of HIV-1 infection.

Administration and Dosage

▶*Approved by the FDA:* November 14, 2000.

Dispense a Medication Guide and Warning Card that provide information about recognition of hypersensitivity reactions with each new prescription or refill. To facilitate reporting hypersensitivity reactions and collection of information on each case, an Abacavir Hypersensitivity Registry has been established. Physicians should register patients by calling (800) 270-0425.

▶*Adults and adolescents (40 kg or greater):* 1 tablet twice daily. Not recommended in adults or adolescents who weigh less than 40 kg because it is a fixed-dose tablet. May be taken without regard to food.

▶*Dose adjustment:* Because it is a fixed-dose tablet, do not prescribe for patients requiring dosage adjustments such as those with creatinine clearance less than 50 mL/min or those experiencing dose-limiting adverse events.

▶*Storage/Stability:* Store at 25°C (77°F); excursions permitted to 15° to 30°C (59° to 86°F).

Actions

▶*Pharmacology:* The combination tablets contain the following 3 synthetic nucleoside analog reverse transcriptase inhibitors with activity against HIV: Abacavir sulfate, lamivudine, and zidovudine. Refer to abacavir, lamivudine, and zidovudine individual monographs for a complete explanation of mechanisms of action.

▶*Pharmacokinetics:* Following oral administration, abacavir, lamivudine, and zidovudine are rapidly absorbed and extensively distributed. Binding of abacavir to human plasma proteins is about 50%; binding of lamivudine and zidovudine to plasma proteins are low.

The pharmacokinetic properties of abacavir, lamivudine, and zidovudine in fasting patients are summarized below.

Pharmacokinetic Parameters for Abacavir, Lamivudine, and Zidovudine in Adults			
Parameter	Abacavir	Lamivudine	Zidovudine
Oral bioavailability (%)	≈ 86	≈ 86	≈ 64
Apparent volume of distribution (L/kg)	≈ 0.86	≈ 1.3	≈ 1.6
Systemic clearance (L/h/kg)	≈ 0.8	≈ 0.33	≈ 1.6
Renal clearance (L/h/kg)	≈ 0.007	≈ 0.22	≈ 0.34
Elimination half-life (h)[1]	≈ 1.45	5 to 7	0.5 to 3

[1] Approximate range.

Contraindications

Abacavir sulfate has been associated with fatal hypersensitivity reactions. Do not restart abacavir following a hypersensitivity reaction to abacavir (see Warning Box).

Abacavir/lamivudine/zidovudine tablets are contraindicated in patients with previously demonstrated hypersensitivity to any of the components of the product.

Warnings

▶*Lactic acidosis/severe hepatomegaly with steatosis:* Lactic acidosis and severe hepatomegaly with steatosis, including fatal cases, have been reported with the use of nucleoside analogs alone or in combination, including abacavir, lamivudine, zidovudine, and other antiretrovirals. A majority of these cases have been in women. Obesity and prolonged nucleoside exposure may be risk factors. Exercise particular caution when administering abacavir/lamivudine/zidovudine to any patient with known risk factors for liver disease; however, cases have also been reported in patients with no known risk factors. Suspend treatment in any patient who develops clinical or laboratory findings suggestive of lactic acidosis or pronounced hepatotoxicity (which may include hepatomegaly and steatosis even in the absence of marked transaminase elevations).

▶*Hypersensitivity reactions:* This combination contains abacavir sulfate, which has been associated with fatal hypersensitivity reactions. Patients developing signs or symptoms of hypersensitivity (eg, fever; skin rash; fatigue; GI symptoms such as nausea, vomiting, diarrhea, or abdominal pain; respiratory symptoms such as pharyngitis, dyspnea, or cough) should discontinue abacavir/lamivudine/zidovudine tablets as soon as a hypersensitivity reaction is first suspected, and should seek medical evaluation immediately. To avoid a delay in diagnosis and minimize the risk of a life-threatening hypersensitivity reaction, permanently discontinue abacavir/lamivudine/zidovudine tablets if hypersensitivity cannot be ruled out, even when other diagnoses are possible (eg, acute onset respiratory diseases, gastroenteritis, reactions to other medications). Do not restart abacavir/lamivudine/zidovudine tablets following a hypersensitivity reaction to abacavir because more severe symptoms will recur within hours and may include life-threatening hypotension and death.

Severe or fatal hypersensitivity reactions can occur within hours after reintroduction of abacavir/lamivudine/zidovudine tablets in patients who have no identified history or unrecognized symptoms of hypersensitivity to abacavir therapy (see abacavir Warnings section).

▶*Hematologic effects:* Because the combination contains zidovudine, use with caution in patients who have bone marrow compromise evidenced by granulocyte count less than 1000 cells/mm³ or hemoglobin less than 9.5 g/dL. Frequent blood counts are strongly recommended in patients with advanced HIV disease who are treated with this product. For HIV-infected individuals and patients with asymptomatic or early HIV disease, periodic blood counts are recommended.

▶*Fixed-dose combination:* This combination contains fixed doses of 3 nucleoside analogs, abacavir, lamivudine, and zidovudine; do not administer concomitantly with abacavir, lamivudine, or zidovudine.

▶*Pregnancy: Category C.* There are no adequate and well-controlled studies in pregnant women. Use abacavir/lamivudine/zidovudine combination tablets during pregnancy only if the potential benefits outweigh the risks. Refer to abacavir, lamivudine, and zidovudine individual monographs for more information.

Antiretroviral pregnancy registry – To monitor maternal-fetal outcomes of pregnant women exposed to abacavir/lamivudine/zidovudine combination tablets or other antiretroviral agents, an Antiretroviral Pregnancy Registry has been established. Physicians are encouraged to register patients by calling (800) 258-4263.

NEVIRAPINE

Rx	**Viramune** (Boehringer Ingelheim)	**Tablets**: 200 mg	Lactose. (54 193). White. Oval. In 60s, 100s, and UD 100s.
		Oral suspension: 50 mg/5 mL (as hemihydrate)	Parabens, sorbitol, sucrose. In 240 mL.

WARNING

Severe, life-threatening, and, in some cases, fatal hepatotoxicity, including fulminant and cholestatic hepatitis, hepatic necrosis, and hepatic failure, has been reported in patients treated with nevirapine. In some cases, patients presented with nonspecific prodromal signs or symptoms of hepatitis and progressed to hepatic failure. These events are often associated with rash. Women and patients with higher CD4 counts are at increased risk of these hepatic events. Women with CD4 counts greater than 250 cells/mm³, including pregnant women receiving chronic treatment for HIV infection, are at considerably higher risk of these events. Advise patients with signs or symptoms of hepatitis to discontinue nevirapine and seek medical evaluation immediately (see Warnings).

Severe, life-threatening skin reactions, including fatal cases, have occurred in patients treated with nevirapine. These have included cases of Stevens-Johnson syndrome, toxic epidermal necrolysis, and hypersensitivity reactions characterized by rash, constitutional findings, and organ dysfunction. Patients developing signs or symptoms of severe skin reactions or hypersensitivity reactions must discontinue nevirapine and seek medical evaluation immediately (see Warnings).

It is essential that patients be monitored intensively during the first 18 weeks of nevirapine therapy to detect potentially life-threatening hepatotoxicity or skin reactions. The greatest risk of severe rash or hepatic events (often associated with rash) occurs in the first 6 weeks of therapy. However, the risk of any hepatic event, with or without rash, continues past this period and monitoring should continue at frequent intervals. In some cases, hepatic injury has progressed despite discontinuation of treatment. Do not restart nevirapine following severe hepatic, skin, or hypersensitivity reactions. In addition, strictly follow the 14-day lead-in period with 200 mg/day nevirapine dosing (see Warnings).

Indications

➤*Human Immunodeficiency Virus type 1 (HIV-1) infection:* In combination with other antiretroviral agents for the treatment of HIV-1 infection.

Administration and Dosage

➤*Approved by the FDA:* June 21, 1996.

➤*Adults:*

Initial therapy – One 200 mg tablet daily for 14 days. Use this lead-in period because it has been found to lessen the frequency of rash.

Maintenance – One 200 mg tablet twice daily in combination with other antiretroviral agents.

➤*Children:*

2 months up to 8 years of age – 4 mg/kg once daily for 14 days followed by 7 mg/kg twice daily.

8 years of age and older – 4 mg/kg once daily for 14 days followed by 4 mg/kg twice daily.

Do not exceed a total daily dose of 400 mg for any patient.

➤*Dosage adjustment:* Discontinue nevirapine if patients experience severe rash or a rash accompanied by constitutional findings (see Warnings). Patients experiencing rash during the 14-day lead-in period of 200 mg/day (4 mg/kg/day in pediatric patients) should not have their nevirapine dose increased until the rash has resolved.

If clinical hepatitis occurs, permanently discontinue nevirapine and do not restart after recovery.

➤*Hepatic function impairment:* Exercise caution when nevirapine is administered to patients with moderate hepatic impairment. Do not administer nevirapine to patients with severe hepatic impairment.

➤*Renal function impairment:* An additional 200 mg dose of nevirapine following each dialysis treatment is indicated in patients requiring dialysis. Patients with Ccr 20 mL/min or greater do not require an adjustment in nevirapine dosing.

➤*Suspension:* Gently shake nevirapine suspension prior to administration. It is important to administer the entire measured dose of suspension by using an oral dosing syringe or dosing cup. If a dosing cup is used, thoroughly rinse with water and administer the rinse to the patient.

➤*Missed doses:* Patients who interrupt nevirapine dosing for more than 7 days should restart the recommended dosing, using one 200 mg tablet daily (4 mg/kg/day in pediatric patients) for the first 14 days (lead-in), followed by one 200 mg tablet twice daily (4 or 7 mg/kg twice daily, according to age, for pediatric patients).

➤*Storage/Stability:* Store tablets and oral suspension at 15° to 30°C (59° to 86°F).

Actions

➤*Pharmacology:* Nevirapine is a nonnucleoside reverse transcriptase inhibitor (NNRTI) with activity against HIV-1. Nevirapine is structurally a member of the dipyridodiazepinone chemical class of compounds.

Nevirapine binds directly to reverse transcriptase (RT) and blocks the RNA-dependent and DNA-dependent DNA polymerase activities by causing a disruption of the enzyme's catalytic site. The activity of nevirapine does not compete with template or nucleoside triphosphates. HIV-2 RT and eukaryotic DNA polymerases (such as human DNA polymerases α, β, γ, or δ) are not inhibited by nevirapine.

In vitro HIV susceptibility – In cell culture, nevirapine demonstrated additive to synergistic activity against HIV-1 in drug combination regimens with zidovudine (ZDV), didanosine (ddI), stavudine (d4T), lamivudine (3TC), saquinavir, and indinavir.

Resistance – HIV-1 isolates with reduced susceptibility (100- to 250-fold) to nevirapine emerge in vitro. Genotypic analysis showed mutations in the HIV-1 RT gene depending upon the virus strain and cell line employed. Time to emergence of nevirapine resistance in vitro was not altered when selection included nevirapine in combination with several other NNRTIs.

Phenotypic and genotypic changes in HIV-1 isolates from patients treated with either nevirapine (n = 24) or nevirapine and zidovudine (n = 14) were monitored in phase I/II trials over 1 to approximately 12 weeks. After 1 week of nevirapine monotherapy, isolates from 3/3 patients had decreased susceptibility to nevirapine in vitro; 1 or more of the RT mutations were detected in HIV-1 isolates from some patients as early as 2 weeks after therapy initiation. By week 8 of nevirapine monotherapy, 100% of the patients tested (n = 24) had HIV-1 isolates with a greater than 100-fold decrease in susceptibility to nevirapine in vitro compared with baseline, and had 1 or more of the nevirapine-associated RT resistance mutations; 19 of 24 patients (80%) had isolates with Y181C mutations regardless of dose. Nevirapine plus zidovudine combination therapy did not alter the emergence rate of nevirapine-resistant virus or the magnitude of nevirapine resistance in vitro.

Cross-resistance – Rapid emergence of HIV-1 strains that are cross-resistant to NNRTIs has been observed in vitro. Nevirapine-resistant HIV-1 isolates were cross-resistant to the NNRTIs efavirenz and delavirdine. However, nevirapine-resistant isolates were susceptible to the nucleoside analogs zidovudine and didanosine. Similarly, zidovudine-resistant isolates were susceptible to nevirapine in vitro.

➤*Pharmacokinetics:*

Absorption – Nevirapine is readily absorbed (more than 90%) after oral administration in healthy volunteers and in adults with HIV-1 infection. Absolute bioavailability was approximately 93% for a 50 mg tablet and approximately 91% for oral solution. Peak plasma nevirapine concentrations of approximately 2 mcg/mL (7.5 mcM) were attained within 4 hours following a single 200 mg dose. Following multiple doses, nevirapine peak concentrations appear to increase linearly in the dose range of 200 to 400 mg/day. Steady-state trough nevirapine concentrations of approximately 4.5 mcg/mL were attained at 400 mg/day. Nevirapine tablets and suspension have been shown to be comparably bioavailable and interchangeable at doses up to 200 mg.

Distribution – Nevirapine is highly lipophilic and essentially nonionized at physiologic pH. Following IV administration to healthy adults, the volume of distribution of nevirapine was approximately 1.21 L/kg, suggesting that nevirapine is widely distributed. Nevirapine readily crosses the placenta and is found in breast milk. Nevirapine is approximately 60% bound to plasma proteins in the plasma concentration range of 1 to 10 mcg/mL. Nevirapine concentrations in human cerebrospinal fluid (CSF) were approximately 45% of concentrations in plasma; this ratio is approximately equal to the fraction not bound to plasma protein.

Metabolism/Excretion – In vivo studies in humans and in vitro studies with human liver microsomes have shown that nevirapine is extensively biotransformed via cytochrome P450 (oxidative) metabolism to several hydroxylated metabolites. In vitro studies with human liver microsomes suggest that oxidative metabolism of nevirapine is mediated primarily by cytochrome P450 isozymes from the CYP3A4 and CYP2B6 families, although other isozymes may have a secondary role. In a mass balance/excretion study in 8 healthy male volunteers dosed to steady state with 200 mg nevirapine given twice daily followed by a single 50 mg dose of ¹⁴C-nevirapine, approximately 91.4% of the dose was recovered, with urine (approximately 81.3%) representing the primary route of excretion compared with feces (approximately 10.1%). Greater than 80% of the radioactivity in urine was made up of glucuronide conjugates of hydroxylated metabolites. Thus, cytochrome P450 metabolism, glucuronide conjugation, and urinary excretion of glucuronidated metabolites represent the primary route of nevirapine biotransformation and elimination. Only a small fraction (less than 5%) of the radioactivity in urine (representing less than 3% of the total dose)

NEVIRAPINE

was made up of parent compound; therefore, renal excretion plays a minor role in elimination of the parent compound.

Nevirapine is an inducer of hepatic cytochrome P450 metabolic enzymes 3A4 and 2B6. Nevirapine induces CYP3A4 and CYP2B6 by approximately 20% to 25%, as indicated by erythromycin breath-test results and urine metabolites. Autoinduction of CYP3A4- and CYP2B6-mediated metabolism leads to an approximately 1.5- to 2-fold increase in the apparent oral clearance of nevirapine as treatment continues from a single dose to 2 to 4 weeks of dosing with 200 to 400 mg/day. Autoinduction also results in a corresponding decrease in the terminal phase half life of nevirapine in plasma from approximately 45 hours (single dose) to approximately 25 to 30 hours following multiple dosing with 200 to 400 mg/day.

Special populations –

Renal function impairment: Subjects requiring dialysis exhibited a 44% reduction in nevirapine AUC over a 1-week exposure period. There also was evidence of accumulation of nevirapine hydroxy-metabolites in plasma in subjects requiring dialysis. An additional 200 mg dose following each dialysis treatment is indicated.

Hepatic function impairment: A significant increase in the AUC of nevirapine observed in 1 patient with Child-Pugh class B and ascites suggests that patients with worsening hepatic function and ascites may be at risk of accumulating nevirapine in the systemic circulation. Because nevirapine induces its own metabolism with multiple dosing, a single-dose study may not reflect the impact of hepatic impairment on multiple-dose pharmacokinetics. Do not administer nevirapine to patients with severe hepatic impairment (see Warnings).

Children: Nevirapine apparent clearance adjusted for body weight was at least 2-fold greater in children younger than 8 years of age compared with adults.

Contraindications

Hypersensitivity to any of the components contained in the tablet or the oral suspension.

Warnings

▶*Skin reactions/Hypersensitivity:* Severe, life-threatening skin reactions, including fatal cases, have been reported with nevirapine treatment, occurring most frequently during the first 6 weeks of therapy. These have included cases of Stevens-Johnson syndrome, toxic epidermal necrolysis, and hypersensitivity reactions characterized by rash, constitutional findings, and organ dysfunction. Instruct patients developing signs or symptoms of severe skin reactions or hypersensitivity reactions (including, but not limited to, severe rash or rash accompanied by fever, general malaise, fatigue, muscle or joint aches, blisters, oral lesions, conjunctivitis, facial edema, and/or hepatitis, eosinophilia, granulocytopenia, lymphadenopathy, and renal dysfunction) to permanently discontinue nevirapine and seek medical evaluation immediately. Do not restart nevirapine following severe skin rash or hypersensitivity reaction. Some of the risk factors for developing serious cutaneous reactions include failure to follow the initial dosing of 200 mg/day during the 14-day lead-in period and delay in stopping the nevirapine treatment after the onset of the initial symptoms. If rash is observed during this lead-in period, dose escalation should not occur until the rash has resolved. Closely monitor patients if isolated rash of any severity occurs.

If patients present with a suspected nevirapine-associated rash, perform liver function tests. Permanently discontinue patients with rash-associated AST or ALT elevations.

Women appear to be at higher risk than men of developing rash with nevirapine.

In a clinical trial, concomitant prednisone use (40 mg/day for the first 14 days of nevirapine administration) was associated with an increase in incidence and severity of rash during the first 6 weeks of nevirapine therapy. Therefore, use of prednisone to prevent nevirapine-associated rash is not recommended.

▶*Hepatotoxicity:* Severe, life-threatening, and in some cases fatal hepatotoxicity, including fulminant and cholestatic hepatitis, hepatic necrosis, and hepatic failure, have been reported in patients treated with nevirapine. In clinical trials, the risk of hepatic events regardless of severity was greatest in the first 6 weeks of therapy. The risk continued to be greater in the nevirapine groups compared with controls through 18 weeks of treatment. However, hepatic events may occur at any time during treatment. In some cases, patients presented with non-specific, prodromal signs or symptoms of fatigue, malaise, anorexia, nausea, jaundice, liver tenderness, or hepatomegaly with or without initially abnormal serum transaminase levels. Some of these events have progressed to hepatic failure with transaminase elevation, with or without hyperbilirubinemia, prolonged partial thromboplastin time, or eosinophilia. Rash and fever accompanied some of these hepatic events. Patients with signs or symptoms of hepatitis must be advised to discontinue nevirapine and immediately seek medical evaluation, which should include liver function tests.

In addition, serious hepatotoxicity (including liver failure requiring transplantation in 1 instance) has been reported in HIV-uninfected individuals receiving multiple doses of nevirapine in the setting of post-exposure prophylaxis, an unapproved use.

Increased AST or ALT levels and/or coinfection with hepatitis B or C at the start of antiretroviral therapy are associated with a greater risk of hepatic adverse events.

The patients at greatest risk of hepatic events, including potentially fatal events, are women with high CD4 counts.

In general, women have a 3-fold higher risk than men for symptomatic, often rash-associated, hepatic events (5.8% vs 2.2%), and patients with higher CD4 counts at initiation of nevirapine therapy are at higher risk for symptomatic hepatic events with nevirapine. In a retrospective review, women with CD4 counts greater than 250 cells/mm³ had a 12-fold higher risk of symptomatic hepatic adverse events compared with women with CD4 counts less than 250 cells/mm³ (11.0% vs 0.9%). An increased risk was observed in men with CD4 counts greater than 400 cells/mm³ (6.3% vs 2.3% for men with CD4 counts less than 400 cells/mm³).

Because increased nevirapine levels and nevirapine accumulation may be observed in patients with serious liver disease, do not administer to patients with severe hepatic impairment.

If clinical hepatitis occurs, permanently discontinue nevirapine and do not restart after recovery. In some cases, hepatic injury progresses despite discontinuation of treatment.

Physicians and patients should be vigilant for the appearance of signs or symptoms of hepatitis, such as fatigue, malaise, anorexia, nausea, jaundice, bilirubinuria, acholic stools, liver tenderness, or hepatomegaly. Consider the diagnosis of hepatotoxicity in this setting, even if liver function tests are initially normal or alternative diagnoses are possible.

▶*Resistant virus:* Resistant virus emerges rapidly and uniformly when nevirapine is administered as monotherapy. Therefore, always administer nevirapine in combination with other antiretroviral agents.

▶*Renal function impairment:* In patients undergoing chronic hemodialysis, an additional 200 mg dose following each dialysis treatment is indicated. Nevirapine metabolites may accumulate in patients receiving dialysis; however, the clinical significance of this accumulation is not known.

▶*Hepatic function impairment:* Patients with moderate hepatic impairment and ascites may be at risk of accumulating nevirapine in the systemic circulation. Exercise caution when nevirapine is administered to patients with moderate hepatic impairment. Do not administer nevirapine to patients with severe hepatic impairment.

▶*Carcinogenesis:* Mice were dosed with 0, 50, 375, or 750 mg/kg/day for 2 years. Hepatocellular adenomas and carcinomas were increased at all doses in males and at the 2 high doses in females. In studies in which rats were administered nevirapine at doses of 0, 3.5, 17.5, or 35 mg/kg/day for 2 years, an increase in hepatocellular adenomas was seen in males at all doses and in females at the high dose.

▶*Fertility impairment:* Evidence of impaired fertility was seen in female rats at doses providing systemic exposure, based on AUC, approximately equivalent to that provided with the recommended clinical dose of nevirapine.

▶*Elderly:* Dose selection for an elderly patient should be cautious, reflecting the greater frequency of decreased hepatic, renal, or cardiac function, and of concomitant disease or other drug therapy.

▶*Pregnancy:* Category C. In rats, a significant decrease in fetal body weight occurred at doses providing systemic exposure approximately 50% higher, based on AUC, than that seen at the recommended human clinical dose. There are no adequate and well-controlled studies in pregnant women. Administer during pregnancy only if the potential benefit justifies the risk to the fetus.

Antiretroviral pregnancy registry – To monitor maternal-fetal outcomes of pregnant women exposed to nevirapine, an Antiretroviral Pregnancy Registry has been established. Physicians are encouraged to register patients by calling (800) 258-4263.

▶*Lactation:* The Centers for Disease Control and Prevention recommend that HIV-infected mothers not breastfeed their infants to avoid risking postnatal transmission of HIV. Nevirapine is excreted in breast milk. Instruct mothers not to breastfeed if they are receiving nevirapine.

▶*Children:* Nevirapine apparent clearance adjusted for body weight was at least 2-fold greater in children younger than 8 years of age compared with adults.

Precautions

▶*Monitoring:* The first 18 weeks of therapy with nevirapine are a critical period during which intensive patient monitoring is required to detect potentially life-threatening hepatic events and skin reactions. The optimal frequency of monitoring during this time period has not been established. Some experts recommend clinical and laboratory monitoring more often than once a month, and in particular, monitoring of liver function tests at baseline, prior to dose escalation and at 2 weeks post-dose escalation. After the initial 18-week period, continue

NEVIRAPINE

frequent clinical and laboratory monitoring throughout nevirapine treatment. Immediately perform liver function tests if a patient experiences signs or symptoms suggestive of hepatitis, hypersensitivity reaction, and/or rash.

➤*Fat redistribution:* Redistribution/accumulation of body fat, including central obesity, dorsocervical fat enlargement (buffalo hump), peripheral wasting, facial wasting, breast enlargement, and "cushingoid appearance," has been observed in patients receiving antiretroviral therapy. The mechanism and long-term consequences of these events are currently unknown. A causal relationship has not been established.

Drug Interactions

➤*CYP450 system:* Nevirapine induces hepatic CYP3A4 and 2B6. Coadministration of nevirapine and drugs primarily metabolized by CYP3A4 or CYP2B6 may result in decreased plasma concentrations of these drugs and attenuate their therapeutic effects. Nevirapine may also inhibit this system. Nevirapine may interact with some drugs; therefore, advise patients to report to their health care provider the use of any other prescription, nonprescription medication, or herbal products, particularly St. John's wort.

Nevirapine Drug Interactions

Precipitant drug	Object drug*		Description
Fluconazole	Nevirapine	↑	Nevirapine concentrations may be increased. Use with caution.
Rifamycins (eg, rifampin, rifabutin)	Nevirapine	↓	Nevirapine plasma concentrations may be reduced and, therefore, should not be used with rifampin. When treating tuberculosis, use rifabutin instead. Rifabutin and its metabolite concentrations are moderately increased when coadministered with nevirapine. Use this combination with caution. Rifampin AUC also may increase slightly.
Nevirapine	Rifamycins (eg, rifampin, rifabutin)	↑	
St. John's wort	Nevirapine	↓	Nevirapine concentrations may be reduced because of increased hepatic metabolism. Coadministration is not recommended.
Nevirapine	Clarithromycin	↑↓	Clarithromycin exposure may be decreased; however, the active metabolite concentration may be increased. Consider an alternative to clarithromycin such as azithromycin.
Nevirapine	Contraceptives, oral	↓	Reduced oral contraceptive efficacy may occur. An alternative nonhormonal or additional method of contraception is recommended.
Nevirapine	Efavirenz	↓	Efavirenz plasma concentration may be decreased. Appropriate dose for this combination has not been established.
Nevirapine	Ketoconazole	↓	Ketoconazole plasma concentrations may be decreased. Do not coadminister.
Nevirapine	Methadone	↓	Methadone levels may be decreased. Adjust methadone dose as needed. Narcotic withdrawal syndrome has been reported.
Nevirapine	Protease inhibitors	↓	Nevirapine may decrease plasma levels and clinical efficacy of protease inhibitors. An increase in indinavir and saquinavir dose may be required. A dose increase of lopinavir/ritonavir to 533/133 mg twice daily with food is recommended.
Nevirapine	Warfarin	↓	The anticoagulant effect of warfarin may be decreased. Monitor coagulation parameters and adjust warfarin dose as needed.
Nevirapine	Zidovudine	↓	Coadministration decreased zidovudine AUC and C_{max} 28% and 30%, respectively.

* ↑ = Object drug increased. ↓ = Object drug decreased.

There may be potential pharmacokinetic interactions between nevirapine and other drug classes that are metabolized by the CYP450 system (see the following table). Use with caution. Dose adjustment of coadministered drug may be needed because of possible decreases in clinical effect.

Potential Nevirapine Drug Interactions

Drug class	Examples of drugs
Antiarrhythmics	Amiodarone, disopyramide, lidocaine
Anticonvulsants	Carbamazepine, clonazepam, ethosuximide
Antifungals	Itraconazole
Calcium channel blockers	Diltiazem, nifedipine, verapamil
Cancer chemotherapy	Cyclophosphamide
Ergot alkaloids	Ergotamine
Immunosuppressants	Cyclosporine, tacrolimus, sirolimus
Motility agents	Cisapride
Opiate agonists	Fentanyl

Adverse Reactions

The most serious adverse reactions associated with nevirapine are clinical hepatitis/hepatic failure, Stevens-Johnson syndrome, toxic epidermal necrolysis, and hypersensitivity reactions. Clinical hepatitis/hepatic failure may be isolated or associated with signs of hypersensitivity that may include severe rash or rash accompanied by fever, general malaise, fatigue, muscle or joint aches, blisters, oral lesions, conjunctivitis, facial edema, and/or hepatitis, eosinophilia, granulocytopenia, lymphadenopathy, and renal dysfunction.

Moderate or Severe Adverse Reactions in Nevirapine-Treated Adults (> 2%)

	Trial 1090[a]		Trial 1037, 1038, 1046[b]	
Adverse reaction	Nevirapine (n = 1121)	Placebo (n = 1128)	Nevirapine (n = 253)	Placebo (n = 203)
Any adverse reaction	14.5	11.1	31.6	13.3
GI				
Abdominal pain	0.1	0.4	2	0
Diarrhea	0.2	0.8	2	0.5
Nausea	0.5	1.1	8.7	3.9
Lab test abnormalities				
ALT > 250 U/L	5.3	4.4	14	4
AST > 250 U/L	3.7	2.5	7.6	1.5
Bilirubin > 2.5 mg/dL	1.7	2.2	1.7	1.5
Hemoglobin < 8 g/dL	3.2	4.1	0	0
Neutrophils < 750/mm³	13.3	13.5	3.6	1
Platelets < 50,000/mm³	1.3	1	0.4	1.5
Miscellaneous				
Abnormal LFTs	1.2	0.9	6.7	1.5
Fatigue	0.2	0.3	4.7	3.9
Granulocytopenia	1.8	2.8	0.4	0
Headache	0.7	0.4	3.6	0.5
Myalgia	0.2	0	1.2	2
Rash	5.1	1.8	6.7	1.5

[a] Background therapy included lamivudine for all patients and combinations of nucleoside reverse transcriptase inhibitors and protease inhibitors. Patients had CD4 cell counts less than 200 cells/mm³. Median exposure was 58 weeks for the nevirapine group and 52 weeks for the placebo group.
[b] Background therapy included zidovudine and zidovudine plus didanosine; nevirapine monotherapy was administered in some patients. Patients had CD4 cell counts at least 200 cells/mm³. Median exposure was 28 weeks for both groups.

Dermatologic – The most common clinical toxicity of nevirapine is rash. Severe or life-threatening rash occurred in approximately 2% of nevirapine-treated patients, most frequently within the first 6 weeks of therapy. Rashes are usually mild to moderate; maculopapular, erythematous, cutaneous eruptions, with or without pruritus, located on the trunk, face, and extremities. Women tend to be at higher risk for development of nevirapine-associated rash.

A Risk of Rash in Nevirapine-Treated Adults[a] (%)

	Nevirapine (n = 1374)	Placebo (n = 1331)
Through 6 weeks of treatment[b]		
Rash events of all grades[c]	14.8	5.9
Grade 1[c]	8.5	4.2
Grade 2[c]	4.8	1.6
Grade 3 or 4[c]	1.5	0.1
Through 52 weeks of treatment[b]		
Rash events of all grades[c]	24	14.9
Grade 1[c]	15.5	10.8
Grade 2[c]	7.1	3.9
Grade 3 or 4[c]	1.7	0.2
Proportion of patients who discontinued treatment because of rash	4.3	1.2

[a] Trials 1037, 1038, 1046, 1090.
[b] Percent based on Kaplan-Meier probability estimates.
[c] NCI grading system: Grade 1: Erythema, pruritus. Grade 2: Diffuse maculopapular rash, dry desquamation. Grade 3: Vesiculation, moist desquamation, ulceration. Grade 4: Erythema multiforme, Stevens-Johnson syndrome, toxic epidermal necrolysis, necrosis requiring surgery, exfoliative dermatitis.

NEVIRAPINE

Hepatic – Severe and life-threatening hepatotoxicity and fatal fulminant hepatitis have been reported in patients treated with nevirapine. Hepatic adverse events have been reported to occur more frequently during the first 18 weeks of treatment, but such events may occur at any time during treatment.

In controlled clinical trials, clinical hepatic events regardless of severity occurred in 4% (range, 2.5% to 11%) of patients who received nevirapine and 1.2% of patients in control groups. Transaminase elevations (ALT or AST greater than 5 times ULN) were observed in 8.8% of patients receiving nevirapine and 6.2% of patients in control groups in clinical trials.

Lab abnormalities – Asymptomatic elevations in gamma-glutamyl-transferase (GGT) occur frequently but are not a contraindication to continue nevirapine therapy in the absence of elevations in other liver function tests. Other laboratory abnormalities (bilirubin, anemia, neutropenia, thrombocytopenia) were observed with similar frequencies in clinical trials comparing nevirapine and control regimens.

Postmarketing –
CNS: Paresthesia, somnolence.
Dermatological: Allergic reactions including anaphylaxis, angioedema, bullous eruptions, ulcerative stomatitis, and urticaria have all been reported. In addition, hypersensitivity syndrome and hypersensitivity reactions with rash associated with constitutional findings such as blistering, conjunctivitis, facial edema, fatigue, fever, general malaise, muscle or joint aches, oral lesions, or significant hepatic abnormalities plus 1 or more of the following: Eosinophilia, granulocytopenia, hepatitis, lymphadenopathy, and/or renal dysfunction have been reported with the use of nevirapine.
Hematologic: Anemia, eosinophilia, neutropenia.
Hepatic: Fulminant and cholestatic hepatitis, hepatic failure, hepatic necrosis, jaundice.
Miscellaneous: Arthralgia, drug withdrawal, fever, redistribution/accumulation of body fat, vomiting.

Children – The most frequently reported adverse events related to nevirapine in pediatric patients were similar to those observed in adults, with the exception of granulocytopenia, which was more commonly observed in children. In a double-blind, placebo-controlled trial, 2 patients were reported to experience Stevens-Johnson syndrome or Stevens-Johnson/toxic epidermal necrolysis transition syndrome. Cases of allergic reaction, including 1 case of anaphylaxis, also were reported.

Lab Test Abnormalities in Nevirapine-Treated Children (n = 37) (%)	
Decreased hemoglobin (< 8 g/dL)	
Decreased neutrophils (< 750/mm³)	38
Decreased platelets (< 50,000/mm³)	11
Increased alkaline phosphatase (> 2 times ULNª)	51
Increased ALT (> 250 U/L)	11
Increased amylase (> 2 times ULN)	16
Increased AST (> 250 U/L)	14
Increased GGT (> 450 U/L)	11
Increased mean cell volume (> 100 fL)	35
Increased total bilirubin (> 2.5 mg/dL)	19

ª ULN = Upper limit of normal.

Overdosage

There is no known antidote for nevirapine overdosage. Cases of overdose at doses ranging from 800 to 1800 mg/day for up to 15 days have been reported. Patients have experienced events including edema, erythema nodosum, fatigue, fever, headache, insomnia, nausea, pulmonary infiltrates, rash, vertigo, vomiting, and weight decrease. All events subsided following discontinuation of nevirapine.

Patient Information

There is a possibility of severe liver disease or skin reactions associated with nevirapine that may result in death. Instruct patients who develop signs or symptoms of liver disease or skin reactions to seek medical attention immediately, including performance of laboratory monitoring. Symptoms of liver disease include acholic stools, anorexia, fatigue, hepatomegaly, jaundice, liver tenderness, malaise, or nausea. Symptoms of severe skin or hypersensitivity reactions include rash accompanied by fever, general malaise, fatigue, muscle or joint aches, blisters, oral lesions, conjunctivitis, facial edema, and/or hepatitis.

Intensive clinical and laboratory monitoring, including liver function tests, is essential during the first 18 weeks of therapy with nevirapine to detect potentially life-threatening hepatotoxicity. However, liver disease can occur after this period; therefore, continue monitoring at frequent intervals throughout nevirapine treatment.

The majority of rashes associated with nevirapine occur within the first 6 weeks of initiation of therapy. If any rash occurs during the 2-week lead-in period, do not escalate the nevirapine dose until the rash resolves. Advise patients who experience severe rash or hypersensitivity reactions to discontinue nevirapine and consult a physician. Do not restart nevirapine following severe skin rash or hypersensitivity reaction. Women tend to be at higher risk for development of nevirapine-associated rash.

Instruct patients not to use oral contraceptives or other hormonal methods of birth control as the sole method of contraception, because nevirapine may lower the plasma levels of these medications. Additionally, when oral contraceptives are used for hormonal regulation during nevirapine therapy, monitor the therapeutic effect of the hormonal therapy.

Nevirapine therapy has not been shown to reduce the risk of transmission of HIV-1 to others through sexual contact or blood contamination. Nevirapine is not a cure for HIV-1 infection; patients may continue to experience illnesses associated with advanced HIV-1 infection, including opportunistic infections.

Nevirapine may interact with some drugs; therefore, instruct patients to report the use of any other prescription, nonprescription medication, or herbal products, particularly St. John's wort, to their doctor.

Redistribution or accumulation of body fat may occur in patients receiving antiretroviral therapy. The cause and long-term health effects of these conditions are not known at this time.

Instruct patients to gently shake the oral suspension before use and to use an oral dosing syringe or dosing cup to measure the right dose. After they drink the medicine, instruct patients to rinse the dosing cup with water and drink the rinse to make sure they get all the medicine. If the dose is less than 5 mL (1 teaspoon), instruct the patient to use the syringe.

If patients stop taking nevirapine for more than 7 days, instruct them to ask how much to take before starting again. Patients may need to start with a once-a-day dose.

DELAVIRDINE MESYLATE

Rx	**Rescriptor** (Agouron)	**Tablets:** 100 mg	Lactose. (U 3761). White, capsule shape. In 360s.
		200 mg	Lactose. (RESCRIPTOR 200 mg). White, capsule shape. In 180s.

WARNING

Delavirdine tablets are indicated for the treatment of HIV-1 infection in combination with appropriate antiretroviral agents when therapy is warranted. This indication is based on surrogate marker changes in clinical studies. Clinical benefit was not demonstrated for delavirdine based on survival or incidence of AIDS-defining clinical events in a completed trial comparing delavirdine plus didanosine with didanosine monotherapy.

Resistant virus emerges rapidly when delavirdine is administered as monotherapy. Therefore, always administer delavirdine in combination with appropriate antiretroviral therapy.

Indications

➤*Human immunodeficiency virus-1 (HIV-1):* For the treatment of HIV-1 infection in combination with appropriate antiretroviral agents when therapy is warranted.

Administration and Dosage

➤*Approved by the FDA:* April 4, 1997.

The recommended dosage for delavirdine is 400 mg (four 100 mg or two 200 mg tablets) 3 times daily. Use delavirdine in combination with appropriate other antiretroviral therapy. Consult the complete prescribing information for other antiretroviral agents for information on dosage and administration.

The 100 mg delavirdine tablets may be dispersed in water prior to consumption. To prepare a dispersion, add four 100 mg tablets to ≥ 3 ounces of water, allow to stand for a few minutes, and then stir until a uniform dispersion occurs. Consume the dispersion promptly. Rinse the glass and swallow the rinse to ensure the entire dose is consumed. Take the 200 mg tablets intact because they are not readily dispersed in water.

Administer delavirdine with or without food. Patients with achlorhydria should take delavirdine with an acidic beverage (eg, orange or cranberry juice). However, the effect of an acidic beverage on the absorption of delavirdine in patients with achlorhydria has not been investigated.

➤*Storage/Stability:* Store at controlled room temperature 20° to 25°C (68° to 77°F). Keep container tightly closed. Protect from high humidity.

DELAVIRDINE MESYLATE

Actions

►*Pharmacology:* Delavirdine is a non-nucleoside reverse transcriptase inhibitor (NNRTI) of HIV-1. Delavirdine binds directly to reverse transcriptase (RT) and blocks RNA-dependent and DNA-dependent DNA polymerase activities. Delavirdine does not compete with template: primer or deoxyribonucleoside triphosphates. HIV-2 RT and human cellular DNA polymerases α, γ, or δ are not inhibited by delavirdine. In addition, HIV-1 group O, a group of highly divergent strains that are uncommon in North America, may not be inhibited by delavirdine.

In vitro HIV-1 susceptibility – In drug combination studies of delavirdine with zidovudine, didanosine, zalcitabine, lamivudine, interferon-α, and protease inhibitors, additive to synergistic anti-HIV-1 activity was observed in cell culture. The relationship between the in vitro susceptibility of HIV-1 RT inhibitors and the inhibition of HIV replication in humans has not been established.

Drug resistance – Phenotypic analyses of isolates from patients treated with delavirdine as monotherapy showed a 50- to 500-fold reduction in sensitivity in 14 of 15 patients by week 8 of therapy. Genotypic analyses of HIV-1 isolates from patients receiving delavirdine plus zidovudine combination therapy (n = 19) showed mutations in 16 of 19 isolates by week 24 of therapy. In a separate study, an average 86-fold increase in the zidovudine sensitivity of patient isolates (n = 24) was observed after 24 weeks on delavirdine and zidovudine combination therapy. The clinical relevance of the phenotypic and the genotypic changes associated with delavirdine therapy has not been determined.

Cross-resistance – Rapid emergence of HIV strains that are cross-resistant to certain NNRTIs has been observed in vitro. Delavirdine may confer cross-resistance to other non-nucleoside reverse transcriptase inhibitors when used alone or in combination.

The potential for cross-resistance between delavirdine and protease inhibitors is low because of the different enzyme targets involved. The potential for cross-resistance between NNRTIs and nucleoside analog RT inhibitors is low because of different binding sites on the viral RT and distinct mechanisms of action.

►*Pharmacokinetics:*

Absorption – Delavirdine is rapidly absorbed following oral administration, with peak plasma concentrations occurring at $\approx$ 1 hour. Following administration of delavirdine 400 mg 3 times daily (n = 67, HIV-1-infected patients), the mean steady-state peak plasma concentration (C_{max}) was 35 mcmol (range, 2 to 100 mcmol), systemic exposure (AUC) was 180 mcmol•hr (range, 5 to 515 mcmol•hr), and trough concentration (C_{min}) was 15 mcmol (range, 0.1 to 45 mcmol). The single-dose bioavailability of delavirdine tablets relative to an oral solution was 85% (n = 16, non-HIV-infected subjects). The single-dose bioavailability of delavirdine tablets (100 mg strength) was increased by $\approx$ 20% when a slurry of drug was prepared by allowing delavirdine tablets to disintegrate in water before administration. The bioavailability of the 200 mg strength delavirdine tablets has not been evaluated when administered as a slurry because they are not readily dispersed in water.

Distribution – Delavirdine is extensively bound ($\approx$ 98%) to plasma proteins, primarily albumin. CSF concentrations of delavirdine averaged 0.4% of the corresponding plasma delavirdine concentrations; this represents $\approx$ 20% of the fraction not bound to plasma proteins. Steady-state delavirdine concentrations in saliva and semen were $\approx$ 6% and 2%, respectively, of the corresponding plasma delavirdine concentrations collected at the end of a dosing interval.

Metabolism / Excretion – Delavirdine is extensively converted to several inactive metabolites. Delavirdine is primarily metabolized by cytochrome P450 3A (CYP3A), but in vitro data suggest that delavirdine may also be metabolized by CYP2D6. The major metabolic pathways for delavirdine are N-desalkylation and pyridine hydroxylation. Delavirdine exhibits nonlinear steady-state elimination pharmacokinetics, with apparent oral clearance decreasing by $\approx$ 22-fold as the total daily dose of delavirdine increases from 60 to 1200 mg/day. In a study of ^{14}C-delavirdine in 6 healthy volunteers who received multiple doses of delavirdine tablets 300 mg 3 times daily, $\approx$ 44% of the radiolabeled dose was recovered in feces and $\approx$ 51% was excreted in urine; < 5% of the dose was recovered unchanged in urine. The apparent plasma half-life of delavirdine increases with dose; mean half-life following 400 mg 3 times daily is 5.8 hours (range, 2 to 11 hours).

In vitro and in vivo studies have shown that delavirdine reduces CYP3A activity and inhibits its own metabolism. In vitro studies have also shown that delavirdine reduces CYP2C9 and CYP2C19 activity. Inhibition of CYP3A by delavirdine is reversible within 1 week after discontinuation of drug.

Gender – Following administration of delavirdine (400 mg every 8 hours), median delavirdine AUC was 31% higher in female patients (n = 12) than in male patients (n = 55).

Contraindications

Hypersensitivity to any of the components of the formulation.

Warnings

►*Cytochrome P450 inhibition:* Coadministration of delavirdine tablets with sedative hypnotics, antiarrhythmics, calcium channel blockers, ergot alkaloid preparations, amphetamines, cisapride, and sildenafil may result in potentially serious or life-threatening adverse events caused by possible effects of delavirdine on the hepatic metabolism of certain drugs metabolized by CYP3A and CYP2C9 (see Drug Interactions).

►*Hepatic function impairment:* Delavirdine is metabolized primarily by the liver. Therefore, exercise caution when administering to patients with impaired hepatic function.

►*Pregnancy:* Category C. Delavirdine has been shown to be teratogenic in rats. Doses of 200 and 400 mg/kg/day administered during the period of organogenesis caused maternal toxicity, embryotoxicity, and abortions in rabbits. No adequate and well-controlled studies in pregnant women have been conducted. Use during pregnancy only if the potential benefit justifies the potential risk to the fetus. Of 7 unplanned pregnancies reported in premarketing clinical studies, 3 were ectopic pregnancies and 3 pregnancies resulted in healthy live births. One infant was born prematurely with a small muscular ventricular septal defect to a patient who received $\approx$ 6 weeks of treatment with delavirdine and zidovudine early in the course of the pregnancy.

►*Lactation:* Delavirdine was excreted in the milk of lactating rats at a concentration 3 to 5 times that of rat plasma. The U.S. Public Health Services Centers for Disease Control and Prevention advises HIV-infected women not to breastfeed in order to avoid postnatal transmission of HIV to a child who may not yet be infected.

►*Children:* Safety and efficacy of delavirdine in combination with other antiretroviral agents have not been established in HIV-1-infected individuals < 16 years of age.

Precautions

►*Monitoring:* Hepatocellular enzymes (ALT/AST) should be monitored frequently if delavirdine is prescribed with saquinavir (see Drug Interactions).

►*Resistance / Cross-resistance:* Non-nucleoside reverse transcriptase inhibitors, when used alone or in combination, may confer cross-resistance to other non-nucleoside reverse transcriptase inhibitors.

►*Skin rash:* Skin rash attributable to delavirdine has occurred in 18% of patients in combination regimens in clinical trials who received delavirdine 400 mg 3 times daily. In 2 separate studies, 42% to 50% of patients treated with delavirdine 400 mg 3 times daily experienced rash compared with 24% to 32% of patients receiving monotherapy with zidovudine or didanosine, respectively. Of the patients treated with delavirdine 400 mg 3 times daily, 4.3% discontinued treatment because of rash.

Dose titration did not significantly reduce the incidence of rash. Rash was typically diffuse, maculopapular, erythematous, and often pruritic. Skin rash was more common in patients with lower CD4 cell counts and usually occurred within 1 to 3 weeks (median, 11 days) of treatment. Rash classified as severe was observed in 3.6% of patients. In most cases, the duration of the rash was < 2 weeks and did not require dose reduction or discontinuation of delavirdine. Most patients were able to resume therapy after rechallenge with delavirdine following a treatment interruption caused by rash. The distribution of the rash was mainly on the upper body and proximal arms, with decreasing intensity of the lesions on the neck and face and progressively less on the rest of the trunk and limbs. Erythema multiforme and Stevens-Johnson syndrome were rarely seen and resolved after withdrawal of delavirdine.

Any patient experiencing severe rash or rash accompanied by symptoms such as fever, blistering, oral lesions, conjunctivitis, swelling, or muscle or joint aches should discontinue delavirdine and consult a physician. Occurrence of a delavirdine-related rash after 1 month of therapy is uncommon unless prolonged interruption of treatment with delavirdine occurs. Symptomatic relief has been obtained using diphenhydramine, hydroxyzine, or topical corticosteroids.

►*Animal toxicology:* Toxicities among various organs and organ systems in rats, mice, rabbits, dogs, and monkeys were observed following the administration of delavirdine. Necrotizing vasculitis was the most significant toxicity that occurred in dogs. Vasculitis in dogs was not reversible during a 2.5 month recovery period; however, partial resolution of the vascular lesion characterized by reduced inflammation, diminished necrosis and intimal thickening occurred during this period. Other major target organs included the GI tract, endocrine organs, liver, kidneys, bone marrow, lymphoid tissue, lung, and reproductive organs.

DELAVIRDINE MESYLATE

Drug Interactions

Delavirdine Drug Interactions

Precipitant drug	Object drug*		Description
Antacids	Delavirdine	↓	Separate administration by ≥ 1 hour because antacids may reduce absorption of delavirdine.
Anticonvulsants (eg, phenytoin, phenobarbital, carbamazepine)	Delavirdine	↓	Coadministration not recommended because anticonvulsants may decrease plasma delavirdine concentrations.
Clarithromycin	Delavirdine	↑	Clarithromycin may increase plasma delavirdine concentrations.
Didanosine	Delavirdine	↓	Coadministration reduces AUC of both drugs by 20%. Separate administration times by ≥ 1 hour.
Delavirdine	Didanosine		
Fluoxetine, ketoconazole	Delavirdine	↑	These drugs may increase trough plasma delavirdine concentrations by ≈ 50%.
H₂ receptor antagonists	Delavirdine	↓	H₂ antagonists increase gastric pH and may decrease absorption of delavirdine. Although the effect on delavirdine absorption is unknown, chronic use is not recommended.
Rifabutin, rifampin	Delavirdine	↓	Coadministration not recommended because plasma delavirdine concentrations may be decreased.
Saquinavir	Delavirdine	↓	Coadministration with saquinavir may decrease delavirdine AUC. Monitor ALT/AST closely when coadministering.
Delavirdine	Amprenavir	↑	Plasma concentrations of amprenavir may be increased.
Delavirdine	Benzodiazepines (eg, alprazolam, midazolam, triazolam)	↑	Alprazolam, midazolam, and triazolam plasma concentrations may be increased.
Delavirdine	Cisapride	↑	Plasma concentrations of cisapride may be increased.
Delavirdine	Clarithromycin, dapsone, rifabutin	↑	Rifabutin, clarithromycin, or dapsone plasma concentrations of may be increased.
Delavirdine	Dihydropyridine calcium channel blockers	↑	Delavirdine may increase plasma concentrations of nifedipine and other dihydropyridine calcium channel blockers.
Delavirdine	Ergot derivatives	↑	Coadministration is not recommended because of increased risk for ergot toxicity.
Delavirdine	Indinavir	↑	Delavirdine inhibits metabolism of indinavir. When coadministered, reduce indinavir dose to 600 mg 3 times daily.
Delavirdine	Quinidine	↑	Plasma concentrations of quinidine may be increased.
Delavirdine	Saquinavir	↑	Saquinavir AUC increased 5-fold when coadministered with delavirdine. Monitor ALT/AST closely when coadministered.
Delavirdine	Sildenafil	↑	Delavirdine may increase sildenafil plasma concentration. Do not exceed a single 25 mg dose of sildenafil in a 48-hour period.
Delavirdine	Warfarin	↑	Plasma concentrations of warfarin may be increased.

* ↑ = Object drug increased. ↓ = Object drug decreased.

Adverse Reactions

Adverse Events of Moderate or Severe Intensity in ≥ 2% of Patients Receiving Delavirdine (%)[1]

	Study 0017		Study 0021	
Adverse reaction	Didanosine[2] 200 mg bid (n = 591)	Delavirdine 400 mg tid + didanosine[2] 200 mg bid (n = 594)	Zidovudine 200 mg tid (n = 271)	Delavirdine 400 mg tid + zidovudine 200 mg tid (n = 287)
Dermatologic				
Rash	3	9.8	1.5	12.5
Maculopapular rash	2	6.6	1.1	4.5

Adverse Events of Moderate or Severe Intensity in ≥ 2% of Patients Receiving Delavirdine (%)[1]

	Study 0017		Study 0021	
Adverse reaction	Didanosine[2] 200 mg bid (n = 591)	Delavirdine 400 mg tid + didanosine[2] 200 mg bid (n = 594)	Zidovudine 200 mg tid (n = 271)	Delavirdine 400 mg tid + zidovudine 200 mg tid (n = 287)
Pruritus	1.7	2.2	1.5	3.1
GI				
Nausea	3.4	4.9	6.6	10.8
Diarrhea	4.4	4.5	2.2	3.5
Vomiting	1.2	2.4	1.1	2.8
Metabolic/Nutritional				
Increased ALT	3.6	5.2	0.7	2.4
Increased AST	3	4.5	0.7	1.7
Miscellaneous				
Headache	4.7	5.6	4.8	5.6
Fatigue	2.7	2.9	4.8	5.2

[1] Includes those adverse events at least possibly related to study drug or of unknown relationship and excludes concurrent HIV conditions.
[2] Dose adjusted body weight < 60 kg = 125 mg twice a day; ≥ 60 kg = 200 mg twice a day.

Adverse reactions occurring in < 2% of patients include:

►*Cardiovascular:* Bradycardia; pallor; palpitation; postural hypotension; syncope; tachycardia; vasodilation.

►*CNS:* Abnormal coordination; agitation; amnesia; anxiety; change in dreams; cognitive impairment; confusion; decreased libido; depressive symptoms; disorientation; dizziness; emotional lability; hallucination; hyperesthesia; hyperreflexia; hypesthesia; impaired concentration; insomnia; manic symptoms; migraine; muscle cramps; nervousness; neuropathy; nightmares; nystagmus; paralysis; paranoid symptoms; paresthesia; restlessness; somnolence; tingling; tremor; vertigo; weakness.

►*Dermatologic:* Dermal leukocytoblastic vasculitis; dermatitis; desquamation; diaphoresis; dry skin; erythema; erythema multiforme; folliculitis; fungal dermatitis; alopecia; nail disorder; petechial rash; seborrhea; skin disorders; skin nodules; Stevens-Johnson syndrome; urticaria; vesiculobullous rash.

►*GI:* Anorexia; aphthous stomatitis; bloody stools; colitis; constipation; decreased appetite; diarrhea (*Clostridium difficile*); diverticulitis; duodenitis; dry mouth; dyspepsia; dysphagia; enteritis; esophagitis; fecal incontinence; flatulence; gagging; gastritis; gastroesophageal reflux; GI bleeding; GI disorders; gingivitis; gum hemorrhage; increased appetite; increased saliva; increased thirst; mouth ulcers; nonspecific hepatitis; pancreatitis; rectal disorder; sialoadenitis; stomatitis; tongue edema or ulceration.

►*GU:* Breast enlargement; calculi of the kidney; epididymitis; hematuria; hemospermia; impotence; kidney pain; metrorrhagia; nocturia; polyuria; proteinuria; vaginal moniliasis.

►*Hematologic/Lymphatic:* Anemia; bruise; ecchymosis; eosinophilia; granulocytosis; neutropenia; pancytopenia; petechia; prolonged partial thromboplastin time; purpura; spleen disorder; thrombocytopenia.

►*Metabolic/Nutritional:* Alcohol intolerance; bilirubinemia; hyperkalemia; hyperuricemia; hypocalcemia; hyponatremia; hypophosphatemia; increased gamma glutamyl transpeptidase; increased lipase; increased serum alkaline phosphatase; increased serum amylase; increased serum creatine phosphokinase; increased serum creatinine; peripheral edema; weight increase or decrease.

►*Musculoskeletal:* Arthralgia or arthritis of single and multiple joints; bone disorders; bone pain; leg cramps; muscular weakness; myalgia; tendon disorders; tenosynovitis; tetany.

►*Respiratory:* Bronchitis; chest congestion; cough; dyspnea; epistaxis; laryngismus; pharyngitis; rhinitis; sinusitis.

►*Special senses:* Blepharitis; conjunctivitis; diplopia; dry eyes; ear pain; photophobia; taste perversion; tinnitus.

►*Miscellaneous:* Abdominal cramps; abdominal distention; abdominal pain (generalized or localized); allergic reaction; angioedema; asthenia; back pain; chest pain; chills; edema (generalized or localized); epidermal cyst; fever; flank pain; flu syndrome; lethargy; lip edema; malaise; neck rigidity; pain (generalized or localized); sebaceous cyst; trauma; upper respiratory tract infection.

DELAVIRDINE MESYLATE

➤*Lab test abnormalities:*

Frequency of Clinically Important Laboratory Abnormalities with Delavirdine (%)[1]				
	Study 0017		Study 0021	
Laboratory test	Didanosine[2] (n = 591)	Delavirdine 400 mg tid + didanosine[2] (n = 594)	Zidovudine 200 mg tid (n = 271)	Delavirdine 400 mg tid + zidovudine 200 mg tid (n = 287)
Neutropenia (Absolute neutrophil count < 750/mm³)	6.7	5.7	7.7[3]	3.5
Anemia (Hgb < 7 g/dL)	0.2	0.7	1.1	1
Thrombocytopenia (platelets < 50,000/mm³)	1.4	1.5	0	0
ALT (> 5 × ULN[4])	4.6	6.7	3.7	3.8
AST (> 5 × ULN[4])	4.9	5.6	3	2.1
Bilirubin (> 2.5 × ULN[4])	0.7	0.5	0.4	1
Amylase (> 2 × ULN[4])	6.5	5.2	1.1	0

[1] Percentage based on number of patients for which data on that laboratory test was available.
[2] Dose adjusted by body weight < 60 kg = 125 mg bid; ≥ 60 kg = 200 mg bid.
[3] Significant (p < 0.05) delavirdine + zidovudine vs zidovudine.
[4] ULN = Upper limit of normal.

Overdosage

No reports of overdose with delavirdine are available. Several patients have received up to 850 mg 3 times daily for up to 6 months with no serious drug-related medical events.

➤*Treatment:* Treatment of overdosage with delavirdine should consist of general supportive measures, including monitoring of vital signs and observation of the patient's clinical status. There is no specific antidote for overdosage with delavirdine. If indicated, achieve elimination of unabsorbed drug by emesis or gastric lavage. Because delavirdine is extensively metabolized by the liver and is highly protein bound, dialysis is unlikely to be beneficial in significant removal of the drug (refer to General Management of Acute Overdosage).

Patient Information

Inform patients that delavirdine is not a cure for HIV-1 infection and that they may continue to acquire illnesses associated with HIV-1 infection, including opportunistic infections. Treatment with delavirdine has not been shown to reduce the incidence or frequency of such illnesses. Advise patients to remain under the care of a physician when using delavirdine.

Advise patients that the long-term effects of treatment with delavirdine are unknown at this time. Advise them that the use of delavirdine has not been shown to reduce the risk of transmitting HIV-1.

Instruct patients that the major adverse event of delavirdine is rash, and advise them to promptly notify their physician should rash occur. The majority of rashes associated with delavirdine occur within 1 to 3 weeks after initiating treatment with delavirdine. The rash normally resolves in 3 to 14 days and may be treated symptomatically while therapy with delavirdine is continued. Any patient experiencing severe rash or rash accompanied by symptoms such as fever, blistering, oral lesions, conjunctivitis, swelling, or muscle or joint aches should discontinue medication and consult a physician.

Inform patients to take delavirdine every day as prescribed. Patients should not alter the dose of delavirdine without consulting their physician. If a dose is missed, patients should take the next dose as soon as possible. However, if a dose is skipped, the patient should not double the next dose.

Patients with achlorhydria should take delavirdine with an acidic beverage (eg, orange or cranberry juice). However, the effect of an acidic beverage on the absorption of delavirdine in patients with achlorhydria has not been investigated.

Advise patients that delavirdine may be taken with or without food.

Advise patients taking delavirdine and antacids to take them ≥ 1 hour apart.

Because delavirdine may interact with certain drugs, advise patients to report to their physician or pharmacist the use of any prescription or *otc* medications or dietary supplements.

EFAVIRENZ

Rx	Sustiva (Bristol-Myers Squibb Oncology/Immunology)	Capsules: 50 mg	Lactose. (SUSTIVA 50 mg). Gold/white. In 30s.
		100 mg	Lactose. (SUSTIVA 100 mg). White. In 30s.
		200 mg	Lactose. (SUSTIVA 200 mg). Gold. In 90s.
		Tablets: 600 mg	Lactose. (SUSTIVA). Yellow, capsule shape. Film-coated. In 30s and UD blister 100s.

Indications

➤*HIV infection:* In combination with other antiretroviral agents for the treatment of human immunodeficiency virus type 1 (HIV-1) infection.

Administration and Dosage

➤*Approved by the FDA:* September 17, 1998.

➤*Adults:* The recommended dosage is 600 mg once daily in combination with a protease inhibitor or nucleoside analog reverse transcriptase inhibitors (NRTIs). It is recommended that efavirenz be taken on an empty stomach, preferably at bedtime. The increased efavirenz concentration observed following administration of efavirenz with food may lead to an an increase in frequency of adverse events.

In order to improve the tolerability of nervous system side effects, bedtime dosing is recommended.

➤*Concomitant antiretroviral therapy:* Efavirenz must be given in combination with other antiretroviral medications (see Warnings).

➤*Children:* It is recommended that efavirenz be taken on an empty stomach, preferably at bedtime. The following table describes the recommended dose for pediatric patients ≥ 3 years of age and weighing between 10 and 40 kg (22 and 88 lbs). The recommended dosage for pediatric patients weighing > 40 kg (88 lbs) is 600 mg once daily.

Pediatric Dose of Efavirenz to be Administered Once Daily		
Body weight		Efavirenz dose (mg)
kg	lbs	
10 to < 15	22 to < 33	200
15 to < 20	33 to < 44	250
20 to < 25	44 to < 55	300
25 to < 32.5	55 to < 71.5	350
32.5 to < 40	71.5 to < 88	400
≥ 40	≥ 88	600

➤*Storage/Stability:* Store efavirenz capsules and tablets at 25°C (77°F); excursions permitted to 15° to 30°C (59° to 86°F).

Actions

➤*Pharmacology:* Efavirenz is a non-nucleoside reverse transcriptase inhibitor (NNRTI) of HIV-1. Its activity is mediated predominantly by noncompetitive inhibition of HIV-1 reverse transcriptase (RT). It does not inhibit HIV-2 RT and human cellular DNA polymerases alpha, beta, gamma, and delta. Efavirenz demonstrated synergistic activity against HIV-1 in cell culture when combined with zidovudine (ZDV), didanosine, or indinavir (IDV).

Resistance – HIV-1 isolates with reduced susceptibility to efavirenz compared with baseline can emerge in vitro.

Cross-resistance – Rapid emergence of HIV-1 strains that are cross-resistant to NNRTIs has been observed in vitro. Thirteen clinical isolates previously characterized as efavirenz-resistant were also phenotypically resistant to nevirapine and delavirdine in vitro compared with baseline. Clinically derived ZDV-resistant HIV-1 isolates tested in vitro retained susceptibility to efavirenz. Cross-resistance between efavirenz and HIV protease inhibitors is unlikely because of the different enzyme targets involved.

➤*Pharmacokinetics:*

Absorption – In HIV-infected patients at steady state, mean C_{max}, mean C_{min}, and mean AUC were dose-proportional following 200, 400, and 600 mg daily doses. Time-to-peak plasma concentrations were ≈ 3 to 5 hours and steady-state plasma concentrations were reached in 6 to 10 days. In 35 patients receiving efavirenz 600 mg once daily, steady-state C_{max} was ≈ 12.9 mcmol, steady-state C_{min} was ≈ 5.6 mcmol, and AUC was ≈ 184 mcmol•hr.

Distribution – Efavirenz is highly protein-bound (≈ 99.5% to 99.75%), predominantly to albumin. In HIV-1-infected patients (n = 9) who received efavirenz 200 to 600 mg once daily for ≥ 1 month, CSF concentrations ranged from 0.26% to 1.19% (mean 0.69%) of the corresponding plasma concentration. This proportion is ≈ 3-fold higher than the non-protein-bound (free) fraction in plasma.

Metabolism – Efavirenz is principally metabolized by the cytochrome P450 system to hydroxylated metabolites with subsequent glucuronidation of these hydroxylated metabolites. These metabolites are essentially inactive against HIV-1. In vitro studies suggest that CYP3A4 and CYP2B6 are the major isozymes responsible for efavirenz metabolism.

EFAVIRENZ

Efavirenz induces P450 enzymes, resulting in the induction of its own metabolism. Multiple doses of 200 to 400 mg/day for 10 days resulted in a lower than predicted extent of accumulation (22% to 42% lower) and a shorter terminal half-life of 40 to 55 hours (single-dose half-life, 52 to 76 hours).

Excretion – Efavirenz has a terminal half-life of 52 to 76 hours after single doses and 40 to 55 hours after multiple doses. A 1-month mass balance/excretion study was conducted using 400 mg/day with a ^{14}C-labeled dose administered on day 8. Approximately 14% to 34% of the radiolabel was recovered in the urine and 16% to 61% was recovered in the feces. Nearly all of the urinary excretion of the radiolabeled drug was in the form of metabolites. Less than 1% is excreted unchanged in the urine. Efavirenz accounted for the majority of the total radioactivity measured in feces.

Food – Administration of a single 600 mg dose of efavirenz capsules with a high fat/high caloric meal or a reduced fat/normal caloric meal was associated with a mean increase of 22% and 17% in efavirenz AUC_∞ and a mean increase of 39% and 51% in efavirenz C_{max}, respectively, relative to the exposures achieved when given under fasted conditions. Administration of a single 600 mg efavirenz tablet with a high fat/high caloric meal was associated with a 28% increase in mean AUC_∞ of efavirenz and a 79% increase in mean C_{max} of efavirenz relative to the exposures achieved under fasted conditions.

Contraindications

Do not administer concurrently with cisapride, midazolam, triazolam, or ergot derivatives. Competition for CYP3A4 by efavirenz could result in inhibition of metabolism of these drugs and create the potential for serious or life-threatening adverse events (eg, cardiac arrhythmias, prolonged sedation, respiratory depression) (see Drug Interactions).

Clinically significant hypersensitivity to any components of the product.

Warnings

➤*Monotherapy:* Resistant virus emerges rapidly when NNRTIs are administered as monotherapy. Therefore, efavirenz must not be used as a single agent to treat HIV or added on as a sole agent to a failing regimen. The choice of new antiretroviral agents to be used in combination with efavirenz should take into consideration the potential for viral cross-resistance.

➤*Psychiatric symptoms:* Serious psychiatric adverse experiences have been reported in patients treated with efavirenz. Patients with a prior history of psychiatric disorders appear to be at greater risk for serious psychiatric adverse experiences. There also have been occasional postmarketing reports of death by suicide, delusions, and psychosis-like behavior, although a causal relationship to the use of efavirenz cannot be determined from these reports. Patients with serious psychiatric adverse experiences should seek immediate medical evaluation to assess the possibility that the symptoms may be related to the use of efavirenz, and if so, to determine whether the risks of continued therapy outweigh the benefits (see Adverse Reactions).

➤*CNS symptoms:* Inform patients that common symptoms were likely to improve with continued therapy and were not predictive of subsequent onset of the less frequent psychiatric symptoms. Dosing at bedtime improves the tolerability of these nervous system symptoms.

Alert patients to the potential for additive CNS effects when efavirenz is used concomitantly with alcohol or psychoactive drugs.

➤*Pregnancy: Category C.* Malformations have been observed in 3 of 20 fetuses/infants from efavirenz-treated cynomolgus monkeys (vs 0 of 20 concomitant controls) in a developmental toxicity study. The pregnant monkeys were dosed throughout pregnancy (postcoital days 20 to 150) with efavirenz 60 mg/kg daily, a dose that resulted in plasma drug concentration similar to those in humans given 600 mg/day of efavirenz. Anencephaly and unilateral anophthalmia were observed in 1 fetus, micro-ophthalmia was observed in another fetus, and cleft palate was observed in a third fetus. Efavirenz crosses the placenta in cynomolgus monkeys and produces fetal blood concentrations similar to maternal blood concentrations. Because teratogenic effects have been seen in primates at efavirenz exposures similar to those seen in the clinic at the recommended dose, advise women to avoid pregnancy. Always use barrier contraception in combination with other methods of contraception (eg, oral or other hormonal contraceptives). Women of childbearing potential should undergo pregnancy testing prior to initiation of efavirenz.

There are no adequate and well-controlled studies in pregnant women. Use during pregnancy only if the potential benefit justifies the potential risk to the fetus, such as in pregnant women without other therapeutic options.

Antiretroviral Pregnancy Registry – To monitor fetal outcomes of pregnant women exposed to efavirenz, an Antiretroviral Pregnancy Registry has been established. Physicians are encouraged to register patients by calling (800) 258-4263.

➤*Lactation:* The Centers for Disease Control and Prevention recommend that HIV-infected mothers not breastfeed their infants to avoid risking postnatal transmission of HIV infection. Studies in rats have demonstrated that efavirenz is excreted in breast milk. Instruct mothers not to breastfeed during efavirenz treatment.

➤*Children:* Study ACTG 382 is an ongoing open-label 48-week study in 57 NRTI-experienced pediatric patients to characterize the safety, pharmacokinetics, and antiviral activity of efavirenz in combination with nelfinavir (20 to 30 mg/kg 3 times/day) and NRTIs. Mean age was 8 years (range, 3 to 16). Efavirenz has not been studied in pediatric patients < 3 years of age or who weigh < 13 kg (29 lbs). The type and frequency of adverse experiences generally were similar to those of adult patients with the exception of a higher incidence of rash, which was reported in 46% of pediatric patients compared with 26% of adults. A higher frequency of Grade 3 or 4 rash was reported in 5% of pediatric patients compared with 0.9% of adults. The pharmacokinetics of efavirenz in pediatric patients were similar to the pharmacokinetics in adults who received 600 mg daily doses of efavirenz.

Precautions

➤*Skin rash:* In controlled clinical trials, 26% of patients treated with 600 mg efavirenz experienced new onset skin rash compared with 17% of patients treated in control groups. Rash associated with blistering, moist desquamation, or ulceration occurred in 0.9% of patients treated with efavirenz. The incidence of Grade 4 rash (eg, erythema multiforme, Stevens-Johnson syndrome) in patients treated with efavirenz in all studies and expanded access was 0.1%. The median time to onset of rash in adults was 11 days and the median duration, 16 days. The discontinuation rate for rash in clinical trials was 1.7%. Discontinue use in patients developing severe rash associated with blistering, desquamation, mucosal involvement, or fever. Appropriate antihistamines or corticosteroids may improve the tolerability and hasten the resolution of rash.

Rash was reported in 46% of children treated with efavirenz capsules. One child experienced Grade 3 rash (confluent rash with fever), and 2 children had Grade 4 rash (erythema multiforme). The median time to onset of rash in children was 8 days. Consider prophylaxis with appropriate antihistamines prior to initiating therapy in children.

➤*Hepatic enzymes:* Monitor liver enzymes in patients with known or suspected history of hepatitis B or C infection and in patients treated with other medications associated with liver toxicity. In patients with persistent elevations of serum transaminases to > 5 times the upper limit of the normal range, the benefit of continued therapy needs to be weighed against the unknown risks of significant liver toxicity. Because of the extensive cytochrome P450-mediated metabolism of efavirenz and limited clinical experience in patients with hepatic impairment, exercise caution in administering efavirenz to these patients.

➤*Cholesterol:* Consider monitoring of cholesterol and triglycerides in patients treated with efavirenz.

➤*Fat redistribution:* Redistribution/accumulation of body fat including central obesity, dorsocervical fat enlargement (buffalo hump), peripheral wasting, facial wasting, breast enlargement, and "cushingoid appearance" have been observed in patients receiving antiretroviral therapy. The mechanism and long-term consequences of these events are currently unknown. A causal relationship has not been established.

Drug Interactions

➤*P450 system:* Efavirenz induces CYP3A4 in vivo. Other compounds that are substrates of CYP3A4 may have decreased plasma concentrations when coadministered with efavirenz. Drugs that induce CYP3A4 activity (eg, phenobarbital, rifampin, rifabutin) would be expected to increase the clearance of efavirenz resulting in lowered plasma concentrations.

In vitro, efavirenz inhibits 2C9, 2C19, and 3A4 isozymes in the range of observed efavirenz plasma concentrations. Coadministration with drugs primarily metabolized by these isozymes may result in altered plasma concentrations of the coadministered drug. Therefore, appropriate dose adjustments may be necessary for these drugs.

Efavirenz Drug Interactions			
Precipitant drug	Object drug*		Description
Phenytoin Phenobarbital Carbamazepine	Efavirenz	↓	Potential for reduction in anticonvulsant or efavirenz plasma levels; periodically monitor anticonvulsant plasma levels.
Efavirenz	Phenytoin Phenobarbital Carbamazepine		
Rifampin	Efavirenz	↓	Decreased efavirenz plasma concentrations may occur; the clinical significance is unknown.
Rifabutin	Efavirenz	↓	Rifabutin would be expected to increase the clearance of efavirenz caused by CYP3A4 induction. Coadministration also may decrease rifabutin concentration. Increase daily dose of rifabutin by 50%. Consider doubling the rifabutin dose when rifabutin is given 2 to 3 times/week.
Efavirenz	Rifabutin		

EFAVIRENZ

Efavirenz Drug Interactions

Precipitant drug	Object drug*		Description
Ritonavir	Efavirenz	↑	With concurrent use, the concentration for each drug was increased. The combination was associated with a higher frequency of adverse clinical experiences (eg, dizziness, nausea, paresthesia) and laboratory abnormalities (elevated liver enzymes). Monitoring of liver enzymes is recommended.
Efavirenz	Ritonavir		
St. John's wort (*Hypericum perforatum*)	Efavirenz	↓	Expected to substantially decrease plasma levels of efavirenz; although, the drug combination has not been studied.
Efavirenz	Amprenavir	↓	Efavirenz has the potential to decrease serum concentrations of amprenavir.
Efavirenz	Benzodiazepines (midazolam, triazolam), cisapride, ergot derivatives	↑	Do not coadminister. Competition for CYP3A4 by efavirenz could result in serious or life-threatening adverse events (eg, cardiac arrhythmias, prolonged sedation, respiratory depression).
Efavirenz	Clarithromycin	↔	Clarithromycin plasma levels decreased while clarithromycin hydroxymetabolite levels increased. The clinical significance of these changes is unknown. No dose adjustment of efavirenz is recommended. Consider alternatives to clarithromycin, such as azithromycin. Other macrolide antibiotics have not been studied.
Efavirenz	Ethinyl estradiol	↔	The AUC of a single dose of ethinyl estradiol was increased; no significant changes were observed in C_{max}. The clinical significance is unknown. Because the interaction with oral contraceptives has not been fully characterized, use a reliable method of barrier contraception in addition to oral contraception.
Efavirenz	Indinavir	↓	Coadministration decreased indinavir AUC and C_{max}. Therefore, increase the indinavir dose from 800 to 1000 mg every 8 hours when efavirenz and indinavir are coadministered.
Efavirenz	Itraconazole Ketoconazole	↓	Although no drug interaction studies have been conducted, efavirenz has the potential to decrease plasma concentrations of itraconazole and ketoconazole.
Efavirenz	Methadone	↓	Coadministration decreased methadone AUC and C_{max}. Monitor for withdrawal symptoms and increase methadone dose as needed.
Efavirenz	Nelfinavir	↑	The AUC and C_{max} of nelfinavir are increased with coadministration. No dose adjustment is necessary.
Efavirenz	Saquinavir	↓	Coadministration decreased saquinavir AUC and C_{max} by 62% and 50%, respectively. Do not use saquinavir with efavirenz as the sole protease inhibitor.
Efavirenz	Warfarin	↔	Plasma concentrations and effects potentially increased or decreased by efavirenz.

* ↑ = Object drug increased. ↓ = Object drug decreased. ↔ = Undetermined clinical effect.

►*Drug/Lab test interactions:*
Cannabinoid test interaction – False-positive urine cannabinoid test results have been reported in uninfected volunteers who received efavirenz. False-positive test results have been observed only with the CEDIA DAU Multi-Level THC assay used for screening and have not been observed with tests used for confirmation of positive results. Efavirenz does not bind to cannabinoid receptors.

►*Drug/Food interactions:* Food increases efavirenz concentrations and may increase the frequency of adverse events (see Administration and Dosage).

Adverse Reactions

The most significant adverse events with efavirenz are nervous system symptoms, psychiatric symptoms, and rash.

►*CNS:* Fifty-three percent of patients receiving efavirenz reported central nervous system symptoms compared with 25% of patients receiving control regimens. These symptoms included, but were not limited to, dizziness (28.1%), insomnia (16.3%), impaired concentration (8.3%), somnolence (7%), abnormal dreams (6.2%), and hallucinations (1.2%). These symptoms were severe in 2% of patients and 2.1% of patients discontinued therapy as a result. These symptoms usually begin during the first or second day of therapy and generally resolve after the first 2 to 4 weeks of therapy. After 4 weeks of therapy, the prevalence of nervous system symptoms of at least moderate severity ranged from 5% to 9% in patients treated with regimens containing efavirenz and from 3% to 5% in patients treated with a control regimen.

The following table lists the frequency of symptoms of different degrees of severity, and gives the discontinuation rates, in clinical trials for ≥ 1 of the following nervous system symptoms: Dizziness, insomnia, impaired concentration, somnolence, abnormal dreaming, euphoria, confusion, agitation, amnesia, hallucinations, stupor, abnormal thinking, depersonalization.

Patients with ≥ 1 Selected Nervous System Symptoms (%)[1]

Symptom severity	Efavirenz 600 mg once daily (n = 1008)	Control groups (n = 635)
Symptoms of any severity	52.7	24.6
Mild symptoms[2]	33.3	15.6
Moderate symptoms[3]	17.4	7.7
Severe symptoms[4]	2	1.3
Treatment discontinuation as a result of symptoms	2.1	1.1

[1] Includes events reported regardless of causality.
[2] "Mild" – Symptoms that do not interfere with patient's daily activities.
[3] "Moderate" – Symptoms that may interfere with patient's daily activities.
[4] "Severe" – Events that interrupt patient's usual daily activities.

►*Psychiatric:* Serious psychiatric adverse experiences have been reported in patients treated with efavirenz. In controlled trials of 1008 patients treated with regimens containing efavirenz for an average of 1.6 years and 635 patients treated with control regimens for an average of 1.3 years, the frequency of specific serious psychiatric events among patients who received efavirenz or control regimens, respectively, were: severe depression (1.6%, 0.6%), suicidal ideation (0.6%, 0.3%), nonfatal suicide attempts (0.4%, 0%), aggressive behavior (0.4%, 0.3%), paranoid reactions (0.4%, 0.3%), and manic reactions (0.1%, 0%). Patients with a history of psychiatric disorders appear to be at greater risk of these serious psychiatric adverse experiences, with the frequency of each of the above events ranging from 0.3% for manic reactions to 2% for severe depression and suicidal ideation. There also have been occasional postmarketing reports of death by suicide, delusions, and psychosis-like behavior, although a causal relationship to the use of efavirenz cannot be determined from these reports.

►*Dermatologic:* Rashes are usually mild to moderate maculopapular skin eruptions that occur within the first 2 weeks of initiating therapy. Rash is more common in children and more often of higher grade (ie, more severe). In most patients, rash resolves with continuing therapy within 1 month. Efavirenz can be reinitiated in patients interrupting therapy because of rash. Consider use of appropriate antihistamines or corticosteroids when it is restarted. Discontinue in patients developing severe rash associated with blistering, desquamation, mucosal involvement, or fever (see Precautions).

Patients with Treatment-Emergent Rash with Efavirenz Administration (%)

Symptom severity	Description of rash grade[1]	Efavirenz 600 mg once daily (Adults; n = 1008)	Efavirenz (Children; n = 57)	Control groups (Adults; n = 635)
Rash of any grade	—	26.3	45.6	17.5
Grade 1 rash	Erythema, pruritus	10.7	8.8	9.8
Grade 2 rash	Diffuse maculopapular rash, dry desquamation	14.7	31.6	7.4
Grade 3 rash	Vesiculation, moist desquamation, ulceration	0.8	1.8	0.3

EFAVIRENZ

	Patients with Treatment-Emergent Rash with Efavirenz Administration (%)			
Symptom severity	Description of rash grade[1]	Efavirenz 600 mg once daily (Adults; n = 1008)	Efavirenz (Children; n = 57)	Control groups (Adults; n = 635)
Grade 4 rash	Erythema multiforme, Stevens-Johnson syndrome, toxic epidermal necrolysis, necrosis requiring surgery, exfoliative dermatitis	0.1	3.5	0
Treatment discontinuation as a result of rash	—	1.7	8.8	0.3

[1] NCI Grading System.

➤ *GI:* A few cases of pancreatitis have been described, although a causal relationship with efavirenz has not been established.

Adverse Reactions of Moderate or Severe Intensity in ≥ 2% Patients Receiving Efavirenz (%)[1]						
	Study 006 lamivudine (LAM), NNRTI, and protease inhibitor-naive patients			Study ACTG 364 NRTI-experienced, NNRTI and protease inhibitor-naive patients		
Adverse reaction	Efavirenz[2] + ZDV/LAM (n = 412)	Efavirenz[2] + Indinavir (n = 415)	Indinavir + ZDV/LAM (n = 401)	Efavirenz[2] + nelfinavir + NRTIs (n = 64)	Efavirenz[2] + NRTIs (n = 65)	Nelfinavir + NRTIs (n = 66)
CNS						
Dizziness	8	8	3	2	6	6
Headache	7	4	4	5	2	3
Insomnia	6	7	3	0	0	2
Concentration impaired	5	2	0	0	0	0
Abnormal dreams	3	1	0	—	—	—
Somnolence	3	2	2	0	0	0
Depression	2	1	0	3	0	5
Nervousness	2	2	0	2	0	2
Anxiety	1	3	0	—	—	—
Dermatologic						
Rash	13	20	7	9	5	9
Pruritus	0	1	1	9	5	9
GI						
Nausea	12	7	25	3	2	2
Vomiting	7	6	14	—	—	—
Diarrhea	6	8	6	14	3	9
Dyspepsia	3	3	5	0	0	2
Abdominal pain	1	2	4	3	3	3
Anorexia	1	0	1	0	2	2
Miscellaneous						
Fatigue	7	5	8	0	2	3
Increased sweating	2	1	0	0	0	0
Pain	1	1	5	13	6	17

[1] Includes adverse events at least possibly related to study drug or of unknown relationship for Study 006. Includes all adverse events regardless of relationship to study drug for Study ACTG 364.

[2] Efavirenz provided as 600 mg once daily.
[3] IDV = indinavir.

In Study 006, lipodystrophy was reported in 2.3% of patients treated with efavirenz + IDV, 0.7% of patients treated with efavirenz + ZDV + LAM and 1% of patients treated with IDV + ZDV + LAM.

➤ *Lab test abnormalities:*

Hepatic enzymes – Three percent of patients treated with 600 mg of efavirenz in controlled clinical trials developed AST and ALT levels > 5 times the upper limit of normal range. Similar elevations in AST and ALT were seen in patients treated with control regimen.

In 156 patients treated with 600 mg efavirenz who were seropositive for hepatitis B or C, 7% (vs 5% of control group) developed AST levels and 8% (vs 4% of control group) developed ALT levels > 5 times the upper limit of normal. Elevations of GGT to > 5 times the upper limit of the normal range were observed in 4% of all patients treated with 600 mg efavirenz and in 10% (vs 1.5% to 2% of control group) of patients seropositive for hepatitis B or C. Isolated elevations of GGT in patients receiving efavirenz may reflect enzyme induction not associated with liver toxicity. Monitor liver function tests in patients with a history of hepatitis B or C (see Precautions).

Lipids – Increases in total cholesterol of 10% to 20% have been observed in some uninfected volunteers receiving efavirenz. In patients treated with efavirenz + ZDV + LAM, increases in nonfasting total cholesterol and HDL of ≈ 20% and 25%, respectively, were observed. In patients treated with efavirenz + IDV, increases in nonfasting cholesterol and HDL of ≈ 40% and 35%, respectively, were observed. However, the significance of these findings is unknown. The effect of efavirenz on triglycerides and LDL cholesterol in patients receiving therapy has not been well characterized.

Serum amylase – Asymptomatic elevations in serum amylase > 1.5 times the upper limit of normal were seen in 10% of patients treated with efavirenz and in 6% of patients treated with control regimens. The clinical significance of asymptomatic increases in serum amylase is unknown.

➤ *Postmarketing experience:*

Cardiovascular – Flushing; palpitations.

CNS – Abnormal coordination; ataxia; convulsions; hypesthesia; paresthesia; neuropathy; tremor.

Dermatologic – Erythema multiforme; nail disorders; skin discoloration; Stevens-Johnson syndrome.

GI – Hepatitis; constipation; malabsorption; hepatic enzyme increase; hepatic failure.

Musculoskeletal – Arthralgia; myalgia; myopathy.

Psychiatric – Aggressive reactions; agitation; delusions; emotional lability; mania; neurosis; paranoia; psychosis; suicide.

Special senses – Abnormal vision; tinnitus.

Miscellaneous – Allergic reaction; asthenia; redistribution/accumulation of body fat; gynecomastia; hypercholesterolemia; hypertriglyceridemia; dyspnea.

➤ *Children:* Clinical adverse experiences observed in ≥ 10% of 57 pediatric patients 3 to 16 years of age who received efavirenz capsules, nelfinavir, and ≥ 1 NRTIs were the following: Rash (46%), diarrhea/loose stools (39%), fever (21%), cough (16%), dizziness/lightheadedness/fainting (16%); ache/pain/discomfort (14%), nausea/vomiting (12%), head-

EFAVIRENZ

ache (11%). The incidence of nervous system symptoms was 18%. One patient experienced Grade 3 rash, 2 patients had Grade 4 rash, and 5 patients (9%) discontinued because of rash.

Overdosage

►*Symptoms:* Some patients accidentally taking 600 mg twice daily have reported increased nervous system symptoms. One patient experienced involuntary muscle contractions.

►*Treatment:* Overdose treatment consists of general supportive measures, including monitoring of vital signs and observation of the patient's clinical status. Administration of activated charcoal may be used to aid removal of unabsorbed drug. There is no specific antidote for overdose with efavirenz. Because it is highly protein-bound, dialysis is unlikely to significantly remove the drug from blood. Refer to General Management of Acute Overdosage.

Patient Information

Inform patients that efavirenz is not a cure for HIV infection and that they may continue to develop opportunistic infections and other complications associated with HIV disease. Inform patients that there are currently no data demonstrating that efavirenz therapy can reduce the risk of transmitting HIV to others through sexual contact or blood contamination.

Advise patients to take efavirenz every day as prescribed on an empty stomach, preferably at bedtime. Taking efavirenz with food increases efavirenz concentrations and may increase the frequency of adverse events. Dosing at bedtime may improve the tolerability of nervous system symptoms. It must always be used in combination with other antiretroviral drugs. Patients should remain under the care of a physician while taking efavirenz.

Inform patients that CNS symptoms are commonly reported in the first weeks of therapy in patients taking efavirenz and that it may cause dizziness, impaired concentration, insomnia, abnormal dreams, or drowsiness. These symptoms are likely to improve with continued therapy. Dosing at bedtime improves the tolerability of these symptoms. Alert patients to the potential for additive CNS effects when used concomitantly with alcohol or psychoactive drugs. Instruct patients to avoid potentially hazardous tasks such as driving or operating machinery or other tasks requiring coordination or physical dexterity if they experience these symptoms.

Inform patients that serious psychiatric symptoms including severe depression, suicide attempts, aggressive behavior, delusions, paranoia, and psychosis-like symptoms also have been infrequently reported in patients receiving efavirenz. Inform patients that if they experience severe psychiatric adverse experiences, they should seek immediate medical evaluation to assess the possibility that the symptoms may be related to the use of efavirenz, and if so, to determine whether discontinuation of efavirenz may be required. Also advise patients to inform their physician of any history of mental illness or substance abuse.

Inform patients that one of the most common side effects is rash, which usually goes away without any change in treatment. In a small number of patients, rash may be serious. Advise patients to contact their physician promptly if they develop a rash.

Because malformations have been observed in fetuses from efavirenz-treated animals, advise patients to avoid becoming pregnant while receiving therapy. Instruct women to notify their physician if they become pregnant while taking efavirenz. Always use a reliable form of barrier contraception in combination with other methods of contraception, including oral or other hormonal contraception because the effects of efavirenz on hormonal contraceptives are not fully characterized.

Efavirenz may interact with some drugs; therefore, advise patients to report the use of any prescription or nonprescription medication, as well as any natural product, particularly St. John's wort, to their physician.

Inform patients that redistribution or accumulation of body fat may occur in patients receiving antiretroviral therapy and that the cause and long-term health effects of these conditions are not known at this time.

ENFUVIRTIDE

Rx	Fuzeon (Hoffman-La Roche)	**Powder for injection, lyophilized:** 108 mg ($\approx$ 90 mg/mL when reconstituted)	Preservative-free. Convenience Kit contains: Single-use vials, syringes, diluent, and alcohol wipes.

Indications

▶*HIV-1 infection:* In combination with other antiretroviral agents for the treatment of HIV-1 infection in treatment-experienced patients with evidence of HIV-1 replication despite ongoing antiretroviral therapy.

Administration and Dosage

▶*Approved by the FDA:* March 13, 2003.

▶*Adults:* 90 mg (1 mL) twice daily injected SC into the upper arm, anterior thigh, or abdomen.

▶*Children:* No data are available to establish a dose recommendation of enfuvirtide in pediatric patients below 6 years of age. In pediatric patients 6 through 16 years of age, the recommended dosage is 2 mg/kg twice daily up to a maximum dose of 90 mg twice daily injected SC into the upper arm, anterior thigh, or abdomen. Monitor weight periodically and adjust the enfuvirtide dose accordingly.

Enfuvirtide Pediatric Dosing Guidelines			
Weight		Dose per bid injection (mg/dose)	Injection volume (90 mg enfuvirtide per mL)
Kilograms (kg)	Pounds (lb)		
11 to 15.5	24 to 34	27	0.3 mL
15.6 to 20	> 34 to 44	36	0.4 mL
20.1 to 24.5	> 44 to 54	45	0.5 mL
24.6 to 29	> 54 to 64	54	0.6 mL
29.1 to 33.5	> 64 to 74	63	0.7 mL
33.6 to 38	> 74 to 84	72	0.8 mL
38.1 to 42.5	> 84 to 94	81	0.9 mL
≥ 42.6	> 94	90	1 mL

▶*Administration:* Give each injection at a site different from the preceding injection site, and only where there is no current injection site reaction from an earlier dose. Do not inject enfuvirtide into moles, scar tissue, bruises, or the navel.

Patients should contact their health care provider for any questions regarding the administration of enfuvirtide. Information about the self-administration of enfuvirtide also may be obtained by calling the toll-free number 1-877-4-FUZEON (1-877-438-9366) or at the enfuvirtide website, http://www.fuzeon.com.

▶*Preparation for administration:* Enfuvirtide must only be reconstituted with 1.1 mL of sterile water for injection.

Enfuvirtide contains no preservatives. Once reconstituted, inject enfuvirtide immediately or keep refrigerated in the original vial; use within 24 hours. The subsequent dose can be reconstituted in advance, stored in the refrigerator in the original vial, and used within 24 hours. Bring refrigerated reconstituted solution to room temperature before injection and visually inspect the vial again to ensure that the contents are fully dissolved in the solution and that the solution is clear, colorless, and without bubbles or particulate matter. Suitable for single use only; unused portions must be discarded.

▶*Storage/Stability:* Store at 25°C (77°F); excursions permitted to 15° to 30°C (59° to 86°F). Store reconstituted solution under refrigeration at 2° to 8°C (36° to 46°F); use within 24 hours.

Actions

▶*Pharmacology:* Enfuvirtide is an inhibitor of the fusion of HIV-1 with CD4+ cells. Enfuvirtide interferes with the entry of HIV-1 into cells by inhibiting fusion of viral and cellular membranes. Enfuvirtide binds to the first heptad-repeat (HR1) in the gp41 subunit of the viral envelope glycoprotein and prevents the conformational changes required for the fusion of viral and cellular membranes.

▶*Pharmacokinetics:*

Absorption – Following a 90 mg single SC injection of enfuvirtide into the abdomen in 12 HIV-1 infected subjects, the mean (±SD) C_{max} was 4.59 ± 1.5 mcg/mL, AUC was 55.8 ± 12.1 mcg•h/mL, and the median T_{max} was 8 hours (range, 3 to 12 hours). The absolute bioavailability (using a 90 mg IV dose as a reference) was 84.3% ± 15.5%. Following 90 mg twice daily dosing of enfuvirtide SC in combination with other antiretroviral agents in 11 HIV-1 infected subjects, the mean (±SD) steady-state C_{max} was 5 ± 1.7 mcg/mL, C_{trough} was 3.3 ± 1.6 mcg/mL, AUC_{0-12h} was 48.7 ± 19.1 mcg•h/mL, and the median T_{max} was 4 hours (range, 4 to 8 hours).

Absorption of the 90 mg dose was comparable when injected into the subcutaneous tissue of the abdomen, thigh, or arm.

Distribution – The mean (±SD) steady-state volume of distribution after IV administration of a 90 mg dose of enfuvirtide (N = 12) was 5.5 ± 1.1 L.

Enfuvirtide is approximately 92% bound to plasma proteins in HIV-infected plasma over a concentration range of 2 to 10 mcg/mL. It is bound predominantly to albumin and, to a lower extent, to α-1 acid glycoprotein.

Metabolism/Excretion – As a peptide, enfuvirtide is expected to undergo catabolism to its constituent amino acids, with subsequent recycling of the amino acids in the body pool.

Mass balance studies to determine elimination pathway(s) of enfuvirtide have not been performed in humans.

An M3 metabolite is detected in human plasma following administration of enfuvirtide, with an AUC ranging from 2.4% to 15% of the enfuvirtide AUC.

Following a 90 mg single SC dose of enfuvirtide (N = 12) the mean ± SD elimination half-life of enfuvirtide is 3.8 ± 0.6 hours and the mean ± SD apparent clearance was 24.8 ± 4.1 mL/h/kg. Following 90 mg twice daily dosing of enfuvirtide SC in combination with other antiretroviral agents in 11 HIV-1 infected subjects, the mean ± SD apparent clearance was 30.6 ± 10.6 mL/h/kg.

Special populations –

Renal insufficiency: Analysis of plasma concentration data from subjects in clinical trials indicated that the clearance of enfuvirtide is not affected in patients with creatinine clearance greater than 35 mL/min. The effect of creatinine clearance less than 35 mL/min on enfuvirtide clearance is unkown.

Gender: Analysis of plasma concentration data from subjects in clinical trials indicated that the clearance of enfuvirtide is 20% lower in females than males after adjusting for body weight. No dose adjustment is recommended for gender.

Weight: Enfuvirtide clearance decreases with decreased body weight irrespective of gender. Relative to the clearance of a 70 kg male, a 40 kg male will have 20% lower clearance and a 110 kg male will have a 26% higher clearance. Relative to a 70 kg male, a 40 kg female will have a 36% lower clearance and a 110 kg female will have the same clearance. No dose adjustment is recommended for weight.

Pediatric patients: The pharmacokinetics of enfuvirtide have been studied in 18 pediatric subjects 6 through 16 years of age at a dose of 2 mg/kg. Enfuvirtide pharmacokinetics were determined in the presence of concomitant medications including antiretroviral agents. A dose of 2 mg/kg twice daily (maximum 90 mg twice daily) provided enfuvirtide plasma concentrations similar to those obtained in adult patients receiving 90 mg twice daily.

In the 18 pediatric subjects receiving the 2 mg/kg twice daily dose, the mean ± SD steady-state AUC was 53.6 ± 21.4 mcg•h/mL, C_{max} was 5.9 ± 2.2 mcg/mL, C_{trough} was 3 ± 1.5 mcg/mL, and apparent clearance was 40 ± 14 mL/h/kg.

▶*Microbiology:*

Antiviral activity in vitro – Enfuvirtide exhibited additive to synergistic effects in cell culture assays when combined with individual members of various antiretroviral classes, including zidovudine, lamivudine, nelfinavir, indinavir, and efavirenz.

Drug resistance – In clinical trials, HIV-1 isolates with reduced susceptibility to enfuvirtide have been recovered from subjects treated with enfuvirtide in combination with other antiretroviral agents.

Cross-resistance – HIV-1 clinical isolates resistant to nucleoside analog reverse transcriptase inhibitors (NRTIs), nonnucleoside analog reverse transcriptase inhibitors (NNRTIs), and protease inhibitors (PIs) were susceptible to enfuvirtide in cell culture.

▶*Clinical trials:* Studies T20-301 and T20-302 are ongoing, randomized, controlled, open-label, multicenter trials in HIV-1 infected subjects. Subjects were required to have either (1) viremia despite 3 to 6 months prior therapy with an NRTI, NNRTI, and PI or (2) viremia and documented resistance or intolerance to at least one member in each of the NRTI, NNRTI, and PI classes.

All subjects received an individualized background regimen consisting of 3 to 5 antiretroviral agents selected on the basis of the subject's prior treatment history and baseline genotypic and phenotypic viral resistance measurements. Subjects were then randomized at a 2:1 ratio to enfuvirtide 90 mg twice daily with background regimen or background regimen alone.

Outcomes of Randomized Treatment at Week 24		
Outcomes	Enfuvirtide 90 mg bid + background regimen N = 661	Background regimen N = 334
HIV-1 RNA log change from baseline (log$_{10}$ copies/mL)[1]	-1.52	-0.73
CD4 + cell count change from baseline (cells/mm^3)[2]	+71	+35

ENFUVIRTIDE

Outcomes of Randomized Treatment at Week 24		
Outcomes	Enfuvirtide 90 mg bid + background regimen N = 661	Background regimen N = 334
HIV RNA ≥ 1 log below baseline	342 (52%)	86 (26%)
HIV RNA < 400 copies/mL	247 (37%)	54 (16%)
HIV RNA < 50 copies/mL	151 (23%)	30 (9%)
Discontinued because of adverse reactions/labs[3]	40 (6%)	12 (4%)
Discontinued because of injection site reactions[3]	20 (3%)	N/A
Discontinued because of other reasons[3,4,5]	36 (5%)	14 (4%)

[1] Based on results from pooled data of T20–301 and T20–302 on ITT population (week 24 viral load for subjects who were lost to follow-up, discontinued therapy, or switched from their original randomization, is replaced by their baseline value).
[2] Last value carried forward.
[3] Percentages based on safety population enfuvirtide + background (N = 663) and background (N = 337).
[4] As per the judgment of the investigator.
[5] Includes discontinuations from loss to follow-up, treatment refusal, and other reasons.

Contraindications

Enfuvirtide is contraindicated in patients with known hypersensitivity to enfuvirtide or any of its components (see Warnings).

Warnings

➤*Local injection site reactions:* The most common adverse events associated with enfuvirtide use are local injection site reactions. Manifestations may include pain and discomfort, induration, erythema, nodules and cysts, pruritus, and ecchymosis. Nine percent of patients had local reactions that required analgesics or limited usual activities (see Adverse Reactions). Reactions are often present at more than one injection site. Patients must be familiar with the enfuvirtide injection instructions in order to know how to inject enfuvirtide appropriately and how to monitor carefully for signs or symptoms of cellulitis or local infection.

➤*Pneumonia:* An increased rate of bacterial pneumonia was observed in subjects treated with enfuvirtide in the phase 3 clinical trials compared with the control arm. Because of this finding, carefully monitor patients with HIV infection for signs and symptoms of pneumonia, especially if they have underlying conditions that may predispose them to pneumonia. Risk factors for pneumonia included low initial CD4 cell count, high initial viral load, IV drug use, smoking, and a prior history of lung disease (see Adverse Reactions).

➤*Hypersensitivity reactions:* Hypersensitivity reactions have been associated with enfuvirtide therapy and may recur on rechallenge. Hypersensitivity reactions have included individually and in combination: Rash, fever, nausea and vomiting, chills, rigors, hypotension, and elevated serum liver transaminases. Other adverse events that may be immune mediated and have been reported in subjects receiving enfuvirtide include primary immune complex reaction, respiratory distress, glomerulonephritis, and Guillain-Barre syndrome. Patients developing signs and symptoms suggestive of a systemic hypersensitivity reaction should discontinue enfuvirtide and should seek medical evalution immediately. Do not restart therapy with enfuvirtide following systemic signs and symptoms consistent with a hypersensitivity reaction. Risk factors that may predict the occurrence or severity of hypersensitivity to enfuvirtide have not been identified.

➤*Pregnancy:* Category B. Because animal reproduction studies are not always predictive of human response, use this drug during pregnancy only if clearly needed.

Antiretroviral pregnancy registry – To monitor maternal-fetal outcomes of pregnant women exposed to enfurviride and other antiretroviral drugs, an antiretroviral pregnancy registry has been established. Physicians are encouraged to register patients by calling 1-800-258-4263.

➤*Lactation:* The Centers for Disease Control and Prevention recommends that HIV-infected mothers not breastfeed their infants to avoid the risk of postnatal transmission of HIV. It is not known whether enfuvirtide is excreted in human milk. Because of the potential for HIV transmission and the potential for serious adverse reactions in nursing infants, mothers should be instructed not to breastfeed if they are receiving enfuvirtide.

➤*Children:* The safety and pharmacokinetics of enfuvirtide have not been established in pediatric subjects below 6 years of age. Limited efficacy data are available in pediatric subjects 6 years of age and older.

Thirty-five HIV-1 infected pediatric subjects 6 through 16 years of age have received enfuvirtide in 2 open-labeled, single-arm clinical trials. Adverse experiences were similar to those observed in adult patients.

Precautions

➤*Non-HIV infected individuals:* There is a theoretical risk that enfuvirtide use may lead to the production of antienfuvirtide antibodies that cross react with HIV gp41. This could result in a false positive HIV test with an ELISA assay; a confirmatory western blot test would be expected to be negative. Enfuvirtide has not been studied in non-HIV infected individuals.

Adverse Reactions

➤*Local injection site reactions:* Local injection site reactions were the most frequent adverse events associated with the use of enfuvirtide. In Phase 3 clinical studies (T20-301 and T20-302), 98% of subjects had at least 1 local injection site reaction (ISR). Three percent of subjects discontinued treatment with enfuvirtide because of ISRs. Eighty-six percent of subjects experienced their first ISR during the initial week of treatment. The majority of ISRs were associated with mild to moderate pain at the injection site, erythema, induration, and the presence of nodules or cysts. For most subjects the severity of signs and symptoms associated with ISRs did not change during the 24 weeks of treatment. In 17% of subjects, an individual ISR lasted for longer than 7 days. Because of the frequency and duration of individual ISRs, 23% of subjects had 6 or more ongoing ISRs at any given time. Individual signs and symptoms characterizing local ISRs are summarized in the following table. Infection at the injection site (including abscess and cellulitis) was reported in 1% of subjects.

Local Injection Site Reactions (N = 663)			
Event category	Any severity grade (%)	Grade 3 reactions (%)	Grade 4 reactions (%)
Pain/Discomfort[1]	95	9	0
Induration[2]	89	41	16
Erythema[3]	89	22	10
Nodules and cysts[4]	76	26	0
Pruritus[5]	62	4	N/A
Ecchymosis[6]	48	8	5

[1] Grade 3 = severe pain requiring analgesics (or narcotic analgesics for ≤ 72 hours) and/or limiting usual activities. Grade 4 = severe pain requiring hospitalization or prolongation of hospitalization, resulting in death, or persistent or significant disability/incapacity, or life-threatening, or medically significant.
[2] Grade 3 = ≥ 25 mm but < 50 mm; Grade 4 = ≥ 50 mm average diameter.
[3] Grade 3 = ≥ 50 mm but < 85 mm average diameter; Grade 4 = ≥ 85 mm average diameter.
[4] Grade 3 = ≥ 3 cm; Grade 4 = if draining.
[5] Grade 3 = refractory to topical treatment or requiring oral or parenteral treatment; Grade 4 = not applicable.
[6] Grade 3 = > 3 cm but ≤ 5 cm; Grade 4 = > 5 cm.

➤*Other adverse events:* Hypersensitivity reactions have been attributed to enfuvirtide (less than or equal to 1%) and in some cases have recurred upon rechallenge (see Warnings).

The events most frequently reported in subjects receiving enfuvirtide plus background regimen, excluding injection site reactions, were diarrhea (26.8%), nausea (20.1%), and fatigue (16.1%). These events were also commonly observed in subjects who received background regimen alone: Diarrhea (33.5%), nausea (23.7%), and fatigue (17.4%).

Treatment-emergent adverse events (% of subjects), excluding ISRs, from phase 3 studies are summarized for adult subjects, regardless of severity and causality, in the following table. Only events occurring in 2% or more of subjects and at a higher rate in subjects treated with enfuvirtide are summarized in the following table. Events that occurred at a higher rate in the control arms are not displayed.

Selected Enfuvirtide Adverse Reactions[1] in ≥ 2% of Adults (%)		
Adverse event	Enfuvirtide + background regimen (N = 663)	Background regimen (N = 334)
CNS		
Anxiety	5.7	3
Depression	8.6	7.2
Insomnia	11.3	8.7
Peripheral neuropathy	8.9	6.3
Taste disturbance	2.4	1.5
GI		
Anorexia	2.6	1.8
Appetite decrease	6.3	2.4
Constipation	3.9	2.7
Pancreatitis	2.4	0.9
Upper abdominal pain	3	2.7
Infections		
Sinusitis	6.2	2.1
Herpes simplex	5	3.9
Skin papilloma	4.2	1.5
Influenza	3.9	1.8

ENFUVIRTIDE

Selected Enfuvirtide Adverse Reactions[1] in ≥ 2% of Adults (%)

Adverse event	Enfuvirtide + background regimen (N = 663)	Background regimen (N = 334)
Miscellaneous		
Asthenia	5.7	4.2
Conjunctivitis	2.4	0.9
Cough	7.4	5.4
Influenza-like illness	2.3	0.9
Lymphadenopathy	2.3	0.3
Myalgia	5	2.4
Pruritus NOS[2]	5.1	4.2
Weight decreased	6.5	5.1

[1] Excludes injection site reactions.
[2] NOS = Not otherwise specified.

An increased rate of bacterial pneumonia was observed in subjects treated with enfuvirtide in the phase 3 clinical trials compared with the control arm (4.68 pneumonia events per 100 patient-years versus 0.61 events per 100 patient-years, respectively). Approximately half of the study subjects with pneumonia required hospitalization. One subject death in the enfuvirtide arm was attributed to pneumonia.

▶*Less common events:* The following adverse events have been reported in 1 or more subjects; however, a causal relationship to enfuvirtide has not been established.

CNS – Guillain-Barre syndrome (fatal); sixth nerve palsy.

GU – Renal insufficiency (glomerulonephritis); renal failure.

Hematologic – Thrombocytopenia; neutropenia; fever.

Miscellaneous – Hyperglycemia; hypersensitivity reaction; pneumonia; worsening abacavir.

Lab test abnormalities –

Enfuviritide Lab Test Abnormalities in ≥ 2% of Adults (%)

Laboratory parameters	Grading	Enfuvirtide + background regimen (N = 663)	Background regimen (N = 334)
Eosinophilia			
1 to 2 × ULN (0.7 × 10^9/L)	0.7 to 1.4 × 10^9/L	8.3	1.5
> 2 × ULN (0.7 × 10^9/L)	> 1.4 × 10^9/L	1.8	0.9
Amylase (U/L)			
Grade 3	> 2 to 5 × ULN	6.2	3.6
Grade 4	> 5 × ULN or clinical pancreatitis	0.9	0.6
Lipase (U/L)			
Grade 3	> 2 to 5 × ULN	5.9	3.6
Grade 4	> 5 × ULN	2.3	1.8
Triglycerides (mmol/L)			
Grade 3	> 1000 mg/dL	8.9	7.2
ALT			
Grade 3	> 5 to 10 × ULN	3.5	2.1
Grade 4	> 10 × ULN	0.9	0.6
AST			
Grade 3	> 5 to 10 × ULN	3.6	3
Grade 4	> 10 × ULN	1.2	0.6

Enfuviritide Lab Test Abnormalities in ≥ 2% of Adults (%)

Laboratory parameters	Grading	Enfuvirtide + background regimen (N = 663)	Background regimen (N = 334)
Creatine phosphokinase (U/L)			
Grade 3	> 5 to 10 × ULN	5.9	3.6
Grade 4	> 10 × ULN	2.3	3.6
GGT (U/L)			
Grade 3	> 5 to 10 × ULN	3.5	3.3
Grade 4	> 10 × ULN	2.4	1.8
Hemoglobin (g/dL)			
Grade 3	6.5 to 7.9 g/dL	1.5	0.9
Grade 4	< 6.5 g/dL	0.6	0.6

* ULN = Upper limit of normal.

Overdosage

There are no reports of human experience of acute overdose with enfuvirtide. The highest dose administered to 12 subjects in a clinical trial was 180 mg as a single SC dose. There is no specific antidote for overdose with enfuvirtide. Treatment of overdose should consist of general supportive measures.

Patient Information

Inform patients that injection site reactions commonly occur. Familiarize patients with the enfuvirtide injection instructions on how to appropriately inject enfuvirtide and how to carefully monitor for signs or symptoms of cellulitis or local infection. Instruct patients when to contact their health care provider about these reactions.

Inform patients that an increased rate of bacterial pneumonia was observed in subjects treated with enfuvirtide in phase 3 clinical trials compared with the control arm. Advise patients to seek medical evaluation immediately if they develop signs or symptoms suggestive of pneumonia (cough with fever, rapid breathing, shortness of breath) (see Warnings).

Advise patients of the possibility of a hypersensitivity reaction to enfuvirtide. Advise patients to discontinue therapy and immediately seek medical evaluation if they develop signs/symptoms of hypersensitivity.

Enfuvirtide is not a cure for HIV-1 infection; patients may continue to contract illnesses associated with HIV-1 infection. The long-term effects of enfuvirtide are unknown at this time. Enfuvirtide therapy has not been shown to reduce the risk of transmitting HIV-1 to others through sexual contact or blood contamination.

Enfuvirtide must be taken as part of a combination antiretroviral regimen.

Inform patients to contact their health care provider if they are pregnant, plan to become pregnant, or become pregnant while taking this medication.

Advise patients to inform their health care provider if they are breastfeeding.

Advise patients to contact their health care provider immediately if they stop or change the dose of enfuvirtide or any other drug in their antiretroviral regimen.

Tell patients that they can obtain more information on the self-administration of enfuvirtide at http://www.fuzeon.com or by calling 1-877-4-FUZEON (1-877-438-9366).

Advise patients to talk to their health care provider before driving or operating machinery if the patients experience dizziness while taking enfuvirtide.

DAPSONE (DDS)

Rx	Dapsone (Jacobus)	**Tablets:** 25 mg	(Jacobus 25 102). White, scored. In 100s.
		100 mg	(Jacobus 100 101). White, scored. In 100s.

Indications

➤*Dermatitis herpetiformis:* Treatment of dermatitis herpetiformis.

➤*Leprosy:* All forms of leprosy (Hansens disease) except for cases of proven dapsone resistance.

➤*Unlabeled uses:* Treatment of relapsing polychondritis; prophylaxis of malaria; inflammatory bowel disorders; Leishmaniasis; *Pneumocystis carinii* pneumonia; rheumatic/connective tissue disorders (eg, rheumatoid arthritis, lupus erythematosus); brown recluse spider bites. Doses used generally range from 50 to 200 mg/day.

Administration and Dosage

➤*Dermatitis herpetiformis:* Individualize dosage. Start with 50 mg daily in adults and correspondingly smaller doses in children. If full control is not achieved within the range of 50 to 300 mg daily, higher doses may be tried. Reduce dosage to a minimum maintenance level as soon as possible. In responsive patients, there is a prompt reduction in pruritus followed by clearance of skin lesions. There is no effect on the GI component of the disease.

Dapsone levels are influenced by acetylation rates. Patients with high acetylation rates or who are receiving treatment affecting acetylation may require a dosage adjustment.

Maintenance dosage may be reduced or eliminated by following a strict gluten-free diet. The average time for dosage reduction is 8 months with a range of 4 months to 2½ years and for dosage elimination 29 months with a range of 6 months to 9 years.

➤*Leprosy:* To reduce a secondary dapsone resistance, the World Health Organization (WHO) Expert Committee on Leprosy and the United States Public Health Service (USPHS)† recommend therapy be commenced and maintained at full dosage (100 mg/day) without interruption in combination with ≥ 1 antileprosy drugs (with correspondingly smaller doses for children).

Bacteriologically negative tuberculoid and indeterminate disease – An adult dosage of 100 mg daily with 6 months of rifampin 600 mg/day is recommended. Under WHO, daily rifampin may be replaced by 600 mg rifampin monthly, if supervised. After all signs of clinical activity are controlled (usually after an additional 6 months), continue dapsone therapy a minimum of 3 years for tuberculoid and indeterminate patients.

Lepromatous and borderline patients – Administer dapsone (100 mg/day) for 2 years with rifampin 600 mg daily. Under WHO, daily rifampin may be replaced by 600 mg rifampin monthly, if supervised. One may elect the concurrent administration of a third antileprosy drug, usually clofazimine 50 to 100 mg daily or ethionamide 250 to 500 mg daily. Dapsone 100 mg daily is continued 3 to 10 years until all signs of clinical activity are controlled with skin scrapings and biopsies negative for 1 year. Continue Dapsone for an additional 10 years for borderline patients and for life for lepromatous patients.

Suspect secondary dapsone resistance whenever a lepromatous or borderline lepromatous patient receiving dapsone treatment relapses clinically and bacteriologically. If such cases show no response to regular and supervised dapsone therapy within 3 to 6 months, consider dapsone resistance confirmed clinically. Determination of drug sensitivity after prior arrangement is available without charge from USPHS.† Treat patients with proven dapsone resistance with other drugs.

➤*Children:* The recommended dosage is 1 to 2 mg/kg/day for a minimum of 3 years; maximum is usual adult dosage of 100 mg/day.

Actions

➤*Pharmacology:* Dapsone (4,4-diaminodiphenylsulphone; DDS), a sulfone, is bactericidal as well as bacteriostatic against *Mycobacterium leprae*. The mechanism of action in dermatitis herpetiformis has not been established.

➤*Pharmacokinetics:*

Absorption/Distribution – Dapsone is rapidly and nearly completely absorbed from the GI tract; peak plasma concentrations are reached in 4 to 8 hours. Daily administration of 200 mg for at least 8 days is necessary to achieve a plateau level of 0.1 to 7 mcg/mL (average, 2.3). Approximately 70% to 90% of dapsone is plasma protein bound. Its main metabolite is monoacetyl dapsone (MADDS), which is nearly 100% protein bound. Enterohepatic circulation accounts for appreciable tissue levels of dapsone 3 weeks after therapy is discontinued.

Metabolism/Excretion – Dapsone is acetylated in the liver, and the degree of acetylation is genetically determined. The plasma half-life ranges from 10 to 50 hours (average, 28 hours). Repeat tests in the same individual show the clearance rate to be constant. Daily administration (50 to 100 mg) in leprosy patients will provide blood levels in excess of the usual minimum inhibitory concentration even for patients with a short dapsone half-life.

About 70% to 85% is excreted in urine as conjugates and unidentified water-soluble metabolites. Excretion of the drug is slow and a constant blood level can be maintained with the usual dosage.

Contraindications

Hypersensitivity to dapsone or its derivatives.

Warnings

➤*Hematologic effects:* Deaths associated with dapsone administration have been reported from agranulocytosis, aplastic anemia, and other blood dyscrasias. Sore throat, fever, pallor, purpura, or jaundice may occur.

Severe anemia – Treat prior to initiation of therapy and monitor hemoglobin. Hemolysis and methemoglobin may be poorly tolerated by patients with severe cardiopulmonary disease.

➤*Hypersensitivity reactions:* Cutaneous reactions (especially bullous) include exfoliative dermatitis, toxic erythema, erythema multiforme, toxic epidermal necrolysis, morbilliform and scarlatiniform reactions, urticaria, and erythema nodosum. These are some of the most serious and rare complications of dapsone therapy. They are directly because of drug sensitization. If new or toxic dermatologic reactions occur, promptly discontinue sulfone therapy and institute appropriate therapy.

Sulfone syndrome – This is an unusual and potentially fatal hypersensitivity reaction. It consists of fever, malaise, jaundice with hepatic necrosis, exfoliative dermatitis, lymphadenopathy, methemoglobinemia, and hemolytic anemia.

Leprosy reactional states including cutaneous – These are not hypersensitivity reactions to dapsone and do not require discontinuation (see Precautions).

➤*Carcinogenesis:* Dapsone is carcinogenic (sarcomagenic) in small animals.

➤*Pregnancy: Category C.* Extensive but uncontrolled experience and 2 published surveys in pregnant women have not shown that dapsone increases the risk of fetal abnormalities if administered during all trimesters. Because of the lack of controlled studies, use during pregnancy only if necessary.

In general, for leprosy, the USPHS† recommends maintenance of dapsone. Dapsone has been important for the management of some pregnant dermatitis herpetiformis patients. It is generally not considered to have an effect on the later growth, development, and functional maturation of the child.

➤*Lactation:* Dapsone is excreted in breast milk in substantial amounts. Hemolytic reactions can occur in neonates. Because of the potential for tumorigenicity shown in animal studies, discontinue nursing or discontinue the drug.

Precautions

➤*Monitoring:* Perform blood counts weekly for the first month, monthly for 6 months, and semi-annually thereafter. If a significant reduction in leukocytes, platelets, or hematopoiesis occurs, discontinue dapsone; follow the patient intensively.

➤*Hemolysis:* Hemolysis and Heinz body formation may be exaggerated in individuals with glucose-6-phosphate dehydrogenase (G-6-PD) deficiency, methemoglobin reductase deficiency, or hemoglobin M. This reaction is frequently dose-related. Give dapsone with caution to these patients or patients exposed to other agents or conditions such as infection or diabetic ketosis capable of producing hemolysis.

➤*Hepatic effects:* Toxic hepatitis and cholestatic jaundice have been reported early in therapy. Hyperbilirubinemia may occur more often in G-6-PD deficient patients. When feasible, baseline and subsequent monitoring of liver function is recommended. If abnormal, discontinue dapsone until the source of the abnormality is established.

➤*Peripheral neuropathy:* This is an unusual complication in non-leprosy patients. Motor loss is predominant. If muscle weakness appears, withdraw dapsone. Recovery on withdrawal is usually substantially complete. The mechanism of recovery is reportedly by axonal regeneration. In leprosy, this complication may be difficult to distinguish from a leprosy reactional state.

➤*Leprosy reactional states:* These are abrupt changes in clinical activity occurring in leprosy with any effective treatment and are classified into 2 groups.

Type 1 (reversal reaction; downgrading) – May occur in borderline or tuberculoid leprosy patients soon after chemotherapy is started, and is presumed to result from a reduction in the antigenic load. The patient has an enhanced delayed hypersensitivity response to residual infection leading to swelling ("reversal") of existing skin and nerve lesions. If severe, or if neuritis is present, use large doses of steroids

DAPSONE (DDS)

and hospitalize the patient. In general, continue antileprosy treatment and therapy to suppress the reaction, using measures such as analgesics, steroids or surgical decompression of swollen nerve trunks. Contact USPHS* for advice in management.

Type 2 (erythema nodosum leprosum; ENL; lepromatous reaction) – Occurs mainly in lepromatous patients and small numbers of borderline patients. Approximately 50% of treated patients show this reaction in the first year. The principal clinical features are fever and tender erythematous skin nodules sometimes associated with malaise, neuritis, orchitis, albuminuria, joint swelling, iritis, epistaxis or depression. Skin lesions can become pustular or ulcerate. Histologically, there is a vasculitis with an intense polymorphonuclear infiltrate. Elevated circulating immune complexes are considered the mechanism of the reaction. If severe, hospitalize patients. In general, antileprosy treatment is continued. Analgesics, steroids and other agents (eg, thalidomide, clofazimine) available from USPHS* are used to suppress the reaction.

➤*Photosensitivity:* Phototoxicity may occur; caution patients to take protective measures (ie, sunscreens, protective clothing) against exposure to ultraviolet light or sunlight until tolerance is determined.

Drug Interactions

Dapsone Drug Interactions			
Precipitant drug	Object drug*		Description
Charcoal, activated	Dapsone	↓	Activated charcoal may decrease dapsone's GI absorption and enterohepatic recycling.
Didanosine	Dapsone	↓	Possible therapeutic failure of dapsone, leading to an increase in infection.
Folic acid antagonists	Dapsone	↑	Folic acid antagonists such as pyrimethamine may increase the likelihood of hematologic reactions. Weekly concomitant use has caused agranulocytosis during the second and third months of therapy.
Para-aminobenzoic acid	Dapsone	↓	Para-aminobenzoic acid may antagonize the effect of dapsone by interfering with the primary mechanism of action.
Probenecid	Dapsone	↑	Probenecid reduces urinary excretion of dapsone metabolites, increasing plasma concentrations.
Rifampin	Dapsone	↓	Rifampin lowers dapsone levels seven to tenfold by accelerating plasma clearance.

Dapsone Drug Interactions			
Precipitant drug	Object drug*		Description
Trimethoprim	Dapsone	↑	Increased serum levels of both drugs may occur, possibly increasing the pharmologic and toxic effects of each drug.
Dapsone	Trimethoprim	↑	

* ↑ = Object drug increased. ↓ = Object drug decreased.

Adverse Reactions

➤*CNS:* Peripheral neuropathy (see Precautions); headache; psychosis; insomnia; vertigo; paresthesia.

➤*Dermatologic:* Drug-induced lupus erythematosus; phototoxicity.

➤*GI:* Nausea; vomiting; abdominal pain; anorexia.

➤*Hematologic:* Dose-related hemolysis is the most common adverse effect, including hemolytic anemia (in patients with or without G-6-PD deficiency). Hemolysis develops in almost every individual treated with 200 to 300 mg dapsone per day. Doses of ≤ 100 mg in healthy individuals and ≤ 50 mg in individuals with G-6-PD deficiency do not cause hemolysis. Almost all patients demonstrate the interrelated changes of a loss of 1 to 2 g hemoglobin, an increase in the reticulocytes (2% to 12%), a shortened red cell life span and a rise in methemoglobin. G-6-PD deficient patients have greater responses.

Hypoalbuminemia without proteinuria has occurred.

➤*Renal:* Albuminuria; the nephrotic syndrome; renal papillary necrosis.

➤*Miscellaneous:* Blurred vision; tinnitus; fever; male infertility; tachycardia; an infectious mononucleosis-like syndrome; pancreatitis; pulmonary eosinophilia.

Overdosage

➤*Symptoms:* Nausea, vomiting and hyperexcitability can appear a few minutes and up to 24 hours after ingestion of an overdose. Methemoglobin-induced depression, convulsions and severe cyanosis require prompt treatment.

➤*Treatment:* Empty the stomach by lavage. In normal and methemoglobin reductase deficient patients, methylene blue, 1 to 2 mg/kg, given slowly IV is the treatment of choice. The effect is complete in 30 minutes, but may have to be repeated if methemoglobin reaccumulates. For nonemergencies, if treatment is needed, methylene blue may be given orally in doses of 3 to 5 mg/kg every 4 to 6 hours. Methylene blue reduction depends on G-6-PD; do not give to fully expressed G-6-PD deficient patients. Hemolysis may be treated by blood transfusions to replace damaged cells. Other supportive measures are oxygen and IV fluids.

Use of activated charcoal in intoxicated patients increased the rate of elimination by 3 to 5 times. The half-life of dapsone and MADDS was reduced by 50%.

Patient Information

May cause photosensitivity; avoid prolonged exposure to sunlight or sunlamps.

CLOFAZIMINE

Rx	Lamprene (Geigy)	Capsules: 50 mg	Brown. In 100s.

Indications

➤*Leprosy:* Treatment of lepromatous leprosy, including dapsone-resistant lepromatous leprosy and lepromatous leprosy complicated by erythema nodosum leprosum.

Combination drug therapy has been recommended for initial treatment of multibacillary leprosy to prevent the development of drug resistance.

Administration and Dosage

Take with meals.

Clofazimine should be used preferably in combination with one or more other antileprosy agents to prevent the emergence of drug resistance.†

➤*Dapsone-resistant leprosy:* Give 100 mg clofazimine/day in combination with one or more other antileprosy drugs for 3 years, followed by monotherapy with 100 mg clofazimine/day. Clinical improvement usually can be detected between the first and third months of treatment and is usually clearly evident by the sixth month.

➤*Dapsone-sensitive multibacillary leprosy:* Combination therapy with two other antileprosy drugs is recommended. Give the triple-drug regimen for at least 2 years and continue, if possible, until negative skin smears are obtained. At this time, monotherapy with an appropriate antileprosy drug can be instituted.

➤*Erythema nodosum leprosum:* Treatment depends on the severity of symptoms. In general, continue basic antileprosy treatment; if nerve injury or skin ulceration is threatened, give corticosteroids. Where prolonged corticosteroid therapy becomes necessary, clofazimine 100 to 200 mg daily for up to 3 months may be useful in eliminating or reducing corticosteroid requirements. Dosages > 200 mg daily are not recommended; taper dosage to 100 mg daily as quickly as possible after the

reactive episode is controlled. Keep patient under medical surveillance.

➤*Storage/Stability:* Store below 86°F; protect from moisture.

Actions

➤*Pharmacology:* Clofazimine exerts a slow bactericidal effect on *Mycobacterium leprae* (Hansen's bacillus). It inhibits mycobacterial growth and binds preferentially to mycobacterial DNA. The drug also exerts anti-inflammatory properties in controlling erythema nodosum leprosum reactions. Precise mechanism of action is unknown.

➤*Pharmacokinetics:*

Absorption/Distribution – Absorption rate ranges from 45% to 62% after oral administration. Average serum concentrations in patients treated with 100 and 300 mg daily were 0.7 and 1 mcg per ml, respectively.

Clofazimine is highly lipophilic and is deposited predominantly in fatty tissue and in the reticuloendothelial system. It is taken up by macrophages.

Metabolism/Excretion – After ingestion of a single 300 mg dose, elimination of unchanged drug and its metabolites in urine in 24 hours was negligible. Clofazimine is retained in the human body for a long time. Half-life after repeated doses is estimated to be at least 70 days. Part of the drug recovered from feces may represent excretion via bile. A small amount is eliminated in sputum, sebum and sweat.

➤*Microbiology:* Measurement of the minimum inhibitory concentration (MIC) of clofazimine against leprosy bacilli in vitro is not yet feasible. Although bacterial killing may begin shortly after starting the drug, it cannot be measured in patient biopsy tissues until approximately 50 days after therapy starts.

† For information about combination drug regimens, contact the Gillis W. Long Hansen's Disease Center, Carville, LA 70721: (800) 642-2477.

CLOFAZIMINE

Clofazimine does not show cross-resistance with dapsone or rifampin. Rarely are microorganisms other than mycobacteria inhibited by the drug.

Warnings

►*GI effects:* Severe abdominal symptoms have necessitated exploratory laparotomies in patients receiving clofazimine. Rare reports have included splenic infarction, bowel obstruction and GI bleeding. Death has been reported following severe abdominal symptoms. Autopsies have revealed crystalline deposits of clofazimine in the intestinal mucosa, liver, gallbladder, bile, spleen, adrenals, subcutaneous fat, mesenteric lymph nodes, muscles, bone and skin.

Use with caution in patients who have GI problems such as abdominal pain and diarrhea. Give dosages of > 100 mg daily for as short a period as possible and only under close medical supervision. If a patient complains of colicky or burning pain in the abdomen, nausea, vomiting or diarrhea, reduce the dose and, if necessary, increase the interval between doses or discontinue the drug.

►*Pregnancy:* Category C. Clofazimine crosses the human placenta. The infant skin was deeply pigmented at birth. No evidence of teratogenicity was found in these infants. There are no adequate and well controlled studies in pregnant women. Use during pregnancy only if clearly needed and when the potential benefits outweigh the potential hazards to the fetus.

There was evidence of fetotoxicity in the mouse at 12 to 25 times the human dose. Skin and fatty tissue of offspring became discolored ≈ 3 days after birth; this was attributed to the presence of the drug in maternal milk.

►*Lactation:* Clofazimine is excreted in breast milk. Do not administer to a nursing woman unless clearly indicated.

►*Children:* Safety and efficacy in children have not been established. Several cases of children treated with clofazimine have been reported in the literature.

Precautions

►*Skin discoloration:* Due to the drug, this may result in depression. Two suicides have been reported in patients receiving clofazimine. For skin dryness and ichthyosis, apply oil to the skin.

Drug Interactions

►*Dapsone:* Preliminary data which suggest that dapsone may inhibit the anti-inflammatory activity of clofazimine have not been confirmed.

If leprosy-associated inflammatory reactions develop in patients being treated with dapsone and clofazimine, it is still advisable to continue treatment with both drugs.

Adverse Reactions

In general, clofazimine is well tolerated when administered in dosages no greater than 100 mg daily. The most consistent adverse reactions are usually dose-related and reversible when the drug is discontinued.

►*CNS:* Dizziness, drowsiness, fatigue, headache, giddiness, neuralgia, taste disorder (< 1%).

►*Dermatologic:* Pigmentation (pink to brownish black) in 75% to 100% of patients within a few weeks of treatment; ichthyosis, dryness (8% to 28%); rash, pruritus (1% to 5%); phototoxicity, erythroderma, acneiform eruptions, monilial cheilosis (< 1%).

►*GI:* Abdominal/epigastric pain, diarrhea, nausea, vomiting, GI intolerance (40% to 50%); bowel obstruction and GI bleeding (see Warnings), anorexia, constipation, weight loss, hepatitis, jaundice, eosinophilic enteritis, enlarged liver (< 1%).

►*Lab test abnormalities:* Elevated albumin, serum bilirubin and AST, eosinophilia, hypokalemia (< 1%).

►*Ophthalmic:* Conjunctival and corneal pigmentation due to clofazimine crystal deposits; dryness; burning; itching; irritation.

►*Psychiatric:* Depression secondary to skin discoloration; two suicides have occurred (< 1%).

►*Miscellaneous:* Splenic infarction (see Warnings), thromboembolism, anemia, cystitis, bone pain, edema, fever, lymphadenopathy, vascular pain, diminished vision (< 1%); discolored urine, feces, sputum or sweat; elevated blood sugar or ESR.

Overdosage

No specific data available. In case of overdose, empty the stomach by inducing vomiting or by gastric lavage. Treatment includes usual supportive measures. Refer to General Management of Acute Overdosage.

Patient Information

Take with meals.

Warn patients that clofazimine may discolor the skin from red to brownish black, as well as discoloring the conjunctivae, lacrimal fluid, sweat, sputum, urine and feces. Skin discoloration, although reversible, may take several months or years to disappear after the conclusion of therapy.

NITAZOXANIDE

Rx **Alinia** (Romark Laboratories)   **Powder for oral suspension:** 100 mg/5 mL   With sugar and 1.48 mg of sucrose per 5 mL. Strawberry flavor. In 60 mL.

Indications

➤*Diarrhea:* For the treatment of diarrhea caused by *Cryptosporidium parvum* or *Giardia lamblia* in pediatric patients 1 through 11 years of age.

Administration and Dosage

➤*Approved by the FDA:* November 22, 2002.

Take nitazoxanide with food.

➤*Children 12 to 47 months of age:* 5 mL every 12 hours for 3 days.

➤*Children 4 to 11 years of age:* 10 mL every 12 hours for 3 days.

➤*Reconstitution:* Prepare a suspension at time of dispensing as follows: The amount of water required for preparation of the suspension is 48 mL. Tap bottle until all powder flows freely. Add approximately one-half of the total amount of water required for reconstitution and shake vigorously to suspend powder. Add remainder of water and again shake vigorously.

➤*Storage/Stability:* Store the unsuspended powder and the reconstituted oral suspension at 25°C (77°F); excursions permitted to 15° to 30°C (59° to 86°F). Keep container tightly closed. The suspension may be stored for 7 days, after which any unused portion must be discarded.

Actions

➤*Pharmacology:* The antiprotozoal activity of nitazoxanide is believed to be due to interference with the pyruvate:ferredoxin oxido-reductase (PFOR) enzyme-dependent electron transfer reaction, which is essential to anaerobic energy metabolism. Studies have shown that the PFOR enzyme from *G. lamblia* directly reduces nitazoxanide by transfer of electrons in the absence of ferredoxin. The DNA-derived PFOR protein sequence of *C. parvum* appears to be similar to that of *G. lamblia.* Interference with the PFOR enzyme-dependent electron transfer reaction may not be the only pathway by which nitazoxanide exhibits its antiprotozoal activity. Nitazoxanide and its metabolite, tizoxanide, are active in vitro in inhibiting the growth of sporozoites and oocysts of *C. parvum* and trophozoites of *G. lamblia.*

➤*Pharmacokinetics:*

Absorption/Distribution – Following oral administration of nitazoxanide, maximum plasma concentrations of the active metabolites tizoxanide and tizoxanide glucuronide are observed within 1 to 4 hours. The parent nitazoxanide is not detected in plasma. In plasma, more than 99% of tizoxanide is bound to proteins.

Mean (± SD) Plasma Pharmacokinetic Parameter Values Following Administration of a Single Dose of Nitazoxanide with Food to Pediatric Subjects

Age	Dose (mg)[1]	Tizoxanide			Tizoxanide glucuronide		
		C_{max} (mcg/mL)	T_{max} (h)[2]	AUC_∞ (mcg·h/mL)	C_{max} (mcg/mL)	T_{max} (h)	AUC_∞ (mcg·h/mL)
12 to 47 mo	100	3.11 (2)	3.5 (2 to 4)	11.7 (4.46)	3.64 (1.16)	4 (3 to 4)	19 (5.03)
4 to 11 y	200	3 (0.99)	2 (1 to 4)	13.5 (3.3)	2.84 (0.97)	4 (2 to 4)	16.9 (5)

[1] Dose: 100 mg/5 mL nitazoxanide, 200 mg/10 mL nitazoxanide.
[2] T_{max} is given as mean (range).

Metabolism/Excretion – Following oral administration in humans, nitazoxanide is rapidly hydrolyzed to an active metabolite, tizoxanide (desacetyl-nitazoxanide). Tizoxanide then undergoes conjugation, primarily by glucuronidation. Tizoxanide is excreted in the urine, bile, and feces, and tizoxanide glucuronide is excreted in urine and bile.

➤*Clinical trials:*

G. lamblia – In a randomized, controlled study in 110 pediatric patients with diarrhea caused by *G. lamblia,* a 3-day course of treatment with nitazoxanide (100 mg twice daily in pediatric patients 24 to 47 months of age; 200 mg twice daily in pediatric patients 4 through 11 years of age) was compared with a 5-day course of treatment with metronidazole (125 mg twice daily in pediatric patients 2 through 5 years of age; 250 mg twice daily in pediatric patients 6 through 11 years of age). Clinical response was evaluated 7 to 10 days following initiation of treatment with a "well" response defined as "no symptoms, no watery stools, and no more than 2 soft stools with no hematochezia within the past 24 hours" or "no symptoms and no unformed stools within the past 48 hours." Seven patients in each treatment group

missed at least 1 dose of medication and 1 in the metronidazole group was lost to follow-up. The following clinical cure rates were obtained.

Pediatric Patients with Diarrhea Caused by *G. lamblia*
Clinical Response Rates 7 to 10 Days Following Initiation of Therapy
Intent to Treat and Protocol Analyses
(%) (number of successes/total)
[95% confidence interval]

Population	Nitazoxanide (3 days)	Metronidazole (5 days)	95% CI diff[1]
Intent-to-treat analysis	85% (47/55)	80% (44/55)	[-9%, 20%]
Per protocol analysis	90% (43/48)	83% (39/47)	[-8%, 21%]

[1] 95% Confidence Interval on the difference in response rates (nitazoxanide-metronidazole).

Contraindications

Prior hypersensitivity to nitazoxanide.

Warnings

➤*Renal/Hepatic function impairment:* The pharmacokinetics of nitazoxanide in patients with compromised renal or hepatic function have not been studied. Therefore, nitazoxanide must be administered with caution to patients with hepatic and biliary disease, to patients with renal disease, and to patients with combined renal and hepatic disease.

➤*Pregnancy: Category B.* Reproduction studies have been performed at doses up to 3200 mg/kg/day in rats (approximately 48 times the clinical dose adjusted for body surface area [BSA]) and 100 mg/kg/day in rabbits (approximately 3 times the clinical dose adjusted for BSA) and have revealed no evidence of impaired fertility or harm to the fetus caused by nitazoxanide. However, there are no adequate and well-controlled studies in pregnant women.

➤*Lactation:* It is not known whether nitazoxanide is excreted in human milk. Because many drugs are excreted in human milk, exercise caution when nitazoxanide is administered to a nursing woman.

➤*Children:* Safety and efficacy in pediatric patients less than 1 year of age or greater than 11 years of age have not been studied.

Drug Interactions

Tizoxanide is highly bound to plasma protein (greater than 99.9%). Therefore, use caution when administering nitazoxanide concurrently with other highly plasma protein-bound drugs with narrow therapeutic indices, as competition for binding sites may occur.

Adverse Reactions

In controlled and uncontrolled studies of 613 HIV-negative pediatric patients who received nitazoxanide, the most frequent adverse events reported regardless of causality assessment were the following: Abdominal pain (7.8%); diarrhea (2.1%); vomiting, headache (1.1%). These typically were mild and transient in nature.

➤*Adverse reactions occurring in less than 1% of patients:*
Dermatologic – Pruritus, sweat.

GI – Nausea, anorexia, flatulence, appetite increase, enlarged salivary glands.

Metabolic/Nutritional – Increased creatinine, increased ALT.

Miscellaneous – Fever, infection, malaise, eye discoloration (pale yellow), rhinitis, dizziness, discolored urine.

Overdosage

Information on nitazoxanide overdosage is not available. In acute studies in rodents and dogs, the oral LD_{50} was higher than 10,000 mg/kg. Single oral doses of up to 4000 mg nitazoxanide in a tablet formulation have been administered to healthy adult volunteers without significant adverse effects. In the event of overdose, gastric lavage may be appropriate soon after oral administration. Carefully observe patients and give symptomatic and supportive treatment.

Patient Information

Shake suspension well before each administration.

Take nitazoxanide with food.

Diabetic patients and caregivers should be aware that the oral suspension contains 1.48 g of sucrose per 5 mL.

TINIDAZOLE

Rx	Tindamax (Presutti)	Tablets: 250 mg	(P L 250). Pink, scored. Film-coated. In 40s and 100s.
		500 mg	(P L 500). Pink, caplet-shaped, scored. Film-coated. In 20s and 60s.

WARNING

Carcinogenicity has been seen in mice and rats treated chronically with another agent in the nitroimidazole class (metronidazole) (see Warnings). Although such data have not been reported for tinidazole, avoid unnecessary use. Reserve tinidazole use for the conditions described in Indications.

Indications

➤*Amebiasis:* For the treatment of intestinal amebiasis and amebic liver abscess caused by *Entamoeba histolytica* in adults and pediatric patients older than 3 years of age. It is not indicated in the treatment of asymptomatic cyst passage.

➤*Giardiasis:* For the treatment of giardiasis caused by *Giardia duodenalis* (also termed *Giardia lamblia*) in adults and pediatric patients older than 3 years of age.

➤*Trichomoniasis:* For the treatment of trichomoniasis caused by *Trichomonas vaginalis* in female and male patients. Identify the organism by appropriate diagnostic procedures. Because trichomoniasis is a sexually transmitted disease with potentially serious sequelae, partners of infected patients should be treated simultaneously in order to prevent reinfection.

Administration and Dosage

➤*Approved by the FDA:* May 17, 2004.

Take tinidazole with food to minimize the incidence of epigastric discomfort and other GI side effects. Food does not affect the oral bioavailability of tinidazole.

Tinidazole Dosing Regimens			
Indication	Adult dose	Pediatric dose ($\geq$ 3 years of age)	Duration of therapy
Amebiasis			
Amebic liver abscess	2 g/day	50 mg/kg/day (up to 2 g)	3 to 5 days
Intestinal	2 g/day	50 mg/kg/day (up to 2 g)	3 days
Giardiasis	2 g	50 mg/kg (up to 2 g)	Single dose
Trichomoniasis	2 g	—	Single dose

➤*Trichomoniasis:* Because trichomoniasis is a sexually transmitted disease, sexual partners should be treated with the same dose and at the same time.

➤*Renal function impairment:* If tinidazole is administered on a day when dialysis is performed, administer an additional dose of tinidazole equivalent to one half the recommended dose after the end of the hemodialysis.

➤*Extemporaneous oral suspension:* Grind four 500 mg oral tablets to a fine powder with a mortar and pestle. Add approximately 10 mL of cherry syrup to the powder and mix until smooth. Transfer the suspension to a graduated amber container. Use several small rinses of cherry syrup to transfer any remaining drug in the mortar to the final suspension for a final volume of 30 mL. The suspension of crushed tablets in artificial cherry syrup (*Humco*) is stable for 7 days at room temperature. When this suspension is used, shake well before each administration.

➤*Storage/Stability:* Store at controlled room temperature 20° to 25°C (68° to 77°F); excursions permitted to 15° to 30°C (59° to 86°F). Protect from light.

Actions

➤*Pharmacology:*

Mechanism of action – Tinidazole is an antiprotozoal agent. The nitro group of tinidazole is reduced by cell extracts of *Trichomonas*. The free nitro radical generated as a result of this reduction may be responsible for the antiprotozoal activity. The mechanism by which tinidazole exhibits activity against *Giardia* and *Entamoeba* species is not known.

Tinidazole demonstrates activity both in vitro and in clinical infections against the following protozoa: *T. vaginalis*, *G. duodenalis* (also termed *G. lamblia*), and *E. histolytica*. Tinidazole does not appear to have activity against most strains of vaginal lactobacilli.

➤*Pharmacokinetics:*

Absorption – After oral administration, tinidazole is rapidly and completely absorbed. A bioavailability study of tinidazole tablets was conducted in adult healthy volunteers. All subjects received a single oral dose of 2 g (four 500 mg tablets) tinidazole following an overnight fast. Oral administration of four 500 mg tablets of tinidazole under fasted conditions produced a mean peak plasma concentration (C_{max}) of 47.7 mcg/mL with a mean time to peak concentration (T_{max}) of 1.6 hours and a mean area under the plasma concentration-time curve ($AUC_{0-\infty}$) of 901.6 mcg•h/mL at 72 hours. Mean plasma levels decreased to 14.3 mcg/mL at 24 hours, 3.8 mcg/mL at 48 hours, and 0.8 mcg/mL at 72 hours following administration. Steady-state conditions are reached in 2½ to 3 days of multi-day dosing. Administration

of tinidazole tablets with food resulted in a delay in T_{max} of approximately 2 hours and a decline in C_{max} of approximately 10% compared with fasted conditions. However, administration of tinidazole with food did not affect AUC or half-life in this study.

In healthy volunteers, administration of crushed tinidazole tablets in artificial cherry syrup, prepared as described above, after an overnight fast had no effect on any pharmacokinetic parameter as compared with tablets swallowed whole under fasted conditions.

Distribution – Tinidazole is distributed into virtually all tissues and body fluids and also crosses the blood-brain barrier. The apparent volume of distribution is approximately 50 L. Plasma protein binding of tinidazole is 12%. Tinidazole crosses the placental barrier and is secreted in breast milk.

Metabolism – Tinidazole, like metronidazole, is significantly metabolized in humans prior to excretion. Tinidazole is partly metabolized by oxidation, hydroxylation, and conjugation. Tinidazole is the major drug-related constituent in plasma after human treatment, along with a small amount of the 2-hydroxymethyl metabolite. Tinidazole is biotransformed mainly by CYP3A4.

Excretion – The plasma half-life of tinidazole is approximately 12 to 14 hours. Tinidazole is excreted by the liver and the kidneys. Tinidazole is excreted in the urine mainly as unchanged drug (approximately 20% to 25% of the administered dose). Approximately 12% of the drug is excreted in the feces.

Special populations –

  Renal function impairment: During hemodialysis, clearance of tinidazole is significantly increased; the half-life is reduced from 12 to 4.9 hours. Approximately 43% of the amount present in the body is eliminated during a 6-hour hemodialysis session.

  Hepatic function impairment: There are no data on tinidazole pharmacokinetics in patients with impaired hepatic function. Reduction of metabolic elimination of metronidazole, a chemically related nitroimidazole, in patients with hepatic dysfunction has been reported in several studies.

Contraindications

Hypersensitivity to tinidazole, any component of the tablet, or other nitroimidazole derivatives; during the first trimester of pregnancy (see Warnings).

Warnings

➤*Neurologic effects:* Convulsive seizures and peripheral neuropathy, the latter characterized mainly by numbness or paresthesia of an extremity, have been reported in patients treated with nitroimidazole drugs including tinidazole and metronidazole. The appearance of abnormal neurologic signs demands the prompt discontinuation of tinidazole therapy. Administer tinidazole with caution to patients with central nervous system diseases.

➤*Hepatic function impairment:* Patients with severe hepatic disease metabolize nitroimidazoles slowly, with resultant accumulation of parent drug in the plasma. Accordingly, for patients with hepatic dysfunction, cautiously administer the usual recommended doses of tinidazole.

➤*Carcinogenesis:* Metronidazole, a chemically related nitroimidazole, has been reported to be carcinogenic in mice and rats but not hamsters. In several studies, metronidazole showed evidence of pulmonary, hepatic, and lymphatic tumorigenesis in mice and mammary and hepatic tumors in female rats.

➤*Mutagenesis:* Tinidazole was mutagenic in the TA 100, *Salmonella typhimurium* tester strain both with and without the metabolic activation system. Mutagenicity results were mixed (positive and negative) in the TA 1535, 1537, and 1538 strains. Tinidazole also was mutagenic in a tester strain of *Klebsiella pneumoniae*. Tinidazole was positive for in vivo genotoxicity in the mouse micronucleus assay.

➤*Fertility impairment:* In a 60-day fertility study, tinidazole reduced fertility and produced testicular histopathology in male rats at a 600 mg/kg/day dose level (approximately 3-fold the highest human therapeutic dose based upon body surface area conversions). Spermatogenic effects resulted from 300 and 600 mg/kg/day dose levels. The no observed adverse effect level for testicular and spermatogenic effects was 100 mg/kg/day (approximately 0.5-fold the highest human therapeutic dose based upon body surface area conversions). This effect is characteristic of agents in the 5-nitroimidazole class.

➤*Elderly:* In general, dose selection for an elderly patient should be cautious, reflecting the greater frequency of decreased hepatic, renal, or cardiac function, and of concomitant disease or other drug therapy.

➤*Pregnancy: Category C.* The use of tinidazole in pregnant patients has not been studied. Because tinidazole crosses the placental barrier and enters fetal circulation, do not administer to pregnant patients in the first trimester. In a study with pregnant rats, a slightly higher incidence of fetal mortality was observed at a maternal dose of 500 mg/kg (2.5-fold the highest human therapeutic dose based upon body surface

TINIDAZOLE

area conversions). The use of tinidazole during pregnancy requires that the potential benefits of the drug be weighed against the possible risks to the mother and the fetus.

➤*Lactation:* Tinidazole is excreted in breast milk in concentrations similar to those seen in serum. Tinidazole can be detected in breast milk for up to 72 hours following administration. Interruption of breastfeeding is recommended during tinidazole therapy and for 3 days following the last dose.

➤*Children:* Other than for use in the treatment of giardiasis and amebiasis in pediatric patients older than 3 years of age, safety and efficacy of tinidazole in pediatric patients have not been established.

Precautions

➤*Candidiasis:* Known or previously unrecognized candidiasis may present more prominent symptoms during therapy with tinidazole and requires treatment with an antifungal agent.

➤*Hematologic effects:* Tinidazole is a nitroimidazole; use with caution in patients with evidence of or history of blood dyscrasia. Tinidazole, like metronidazole, may produce transient leukopenia and neutropenia; however, no persistent hematological abnormalities attributable to tinidazole have been observed in clinical studies. Total and differential leukocyte counts are recommended if retreatment is necessary.

Drug Interactions

Although not studied specifically for tinidazole, the following drug interactions were reported for metronidazole, a chemically related nitroimidazole. Therefore, these drug interactions may occur with tinidazole.

Tinidazole Drug Interactions			
Precipitant drug	Object drug*		Description
Cholestyramine	Tinidazole	↓	Cholestyramine was shown to decrease the oral bioavailability of metronidazole. Thus, consider separating the dosing of cholestyramine and tinidazole.
CYP3A4 inducers (eg, phenobarbital, rifampin, phenytoin)	Tinidazole	↓	CYP3A4 inducers may accelerate the elimination of tinidazole.
CYP3A4 inhibitors (eg, cimetidine, ketoconazole)	Tinidazole	↑	CYP3A4 inhibitors may prolong the half-life and decrease plasma clearance of tinidazole.
Oxytetracycline	Tinidazole	↓	Oxytetracycline was reported to antagonize the therapeutic effect of metronidazole.
Tinidazole	Alcohols	↑	Avoid alcoholic beverages and preparations containing ethanol or propylene glycol during tinidazole therapy and for 3 days after discontinuation. Symptoms such as abdominal cramps, nausea, vomiting, headaches, and flushing may occur.
Tinidazole	Anticoagulants	↑	Tinidazole may enhance the effect of warfarin, resulting in a prolongation of prothrombin time. Adjust the anticoagulant dose as needed during coadministration and up to 8 days after tinidazole discontinuation.
Tinidazole	Cyclosporine Tacrolimus	↑	Several case reports suggest that metronidazole has the potential to increase the levels of cyclosporine and tacrolimus. During tinidazole coadministration, monitor for toxicities.
Tinidazole	Disulfiram	↑	Psychotic reactions have been reported in patients using metronidazole and disulfiram. Although no similar reactions have been reported with tinidazole, do not give tinidazole to patients who have taken disulfiram within the last 2 weeks.
Tinidazole	Fluorouracil	↑	Metronidazole was shown to decrease the clearance of fluorouracil, resulting in toxicities. If concomitant use of tinidazole and fluorouracil cannot be avoided, monitor for toxicities.

Tinidazole Drug Interactions			
Precipitant drug	Object drug*		Description
Tinidazole	Hydantoins (eg, fosphenytoin)	↑	Administration of oral metronidazole with IV fosphenytoin (prodrug of phenytoin) was reported to prolong the half-life and reduce the clearance of phenytoin. Orally administered phenytoin was not affected by metronidazole.
Tinidazole	Lithium	↑	Metronidazole has been reported to increase serum lithium levels. Although it is not known if tinidazole will interact with lithium, consider monitoring lithium and creatinine levels.

* ↑ = Object drug increased. ↓ = Object drug decreased.

➤*Drug/Lab test interactions:* Tinidazole, like metronidazole, may interfere with certain types of determinations of serum chemistry values, such as aspartate aminotransferase (AST), alanine aminotransferase (ALT), lactate dehydrogenase (LDH), triglycerides, and hexokinase glucose. Values of zero may be observed. All of the assays in which interference has been reported involve enzymatic coupling of the assay to oxidation-reduction of nicotinamide adenine dinucleotide. Potential interference is caused by the similarity of absorbance peaks of nicotinamide adenine dinucleotide and tinidazole.

Adverse Reactions

Tinidazole Adverse Reactions (≥ 1%)[a]		
Adverse reaction	2 g dose (n = 3,669)	Multi-day dose (n = 1,765)
Total patients with adverse effects	11	13.8
CNS		
Dizziness	1.1	0.5
Headache	1.3	0.7
Weakness/fatigue/malaise	2.1	1.1
GI		
Anorexia	1.5	2.5
Constipation	0.4	1.4
Dyspepsia/cramps/epigastric discomfort	1.8	1.4
Metallic/bitter taste	3.7	6.3
Nausea	3.2	4.5
Vomiting	1.5	0.9

[a] Data are pooled from separate studies and are not necessarily comparable.

Other adverse effects reported with tinidazole include:

➤*CNS:* Two serious adverse reactions reported include convulsions and transient peripheral neuropathy including numbness and paresthesia. Other CNS reports include ataxia, drowsiness, giddiness, insomnia, vertigo; coma, confusion, depression (rare).

➤*GI:* Diarrhea, stomatitis, tongue discoloration; furry tongue (rare).

➤*GU:* Darkened urine, increased vaginal discharge, oral candidiasis.

➤*Hematologic:* Transient leukopenia, transient neutropenia; reversible thrombocytopenia (rare).

➤*Hypersensitivity:* Angioedema, burning sensation, dryness of mouth, fever, flushing, pruritus, rash, salivation, sweating, thirst, urticaria.

➤*Musculoskeletal:* Arthralgias, arthritis, myalgias.

➤*Respiratory:* Bronchospasm, dyspnea, pharyngitis (rare).

➤*Miscellaneous: Candida* overgrowth, hepatic abnormalities including raised transaminase level, palpitations.

Children – Adverse events reported in pediatric patients taking tinidazole were similar in nature and frequency to adult findings, including abdominal pain, anorexia, diarrhea, nausea, taste change, and vomiting.

Overdosage

➤*Symptoms:* There are no reported overdoses with tinidazole in humans. In acute studies with mice and rats, the LD_{50} for mice generally was more than 3,600 mg/kg for oral administration and more than 2,300 mg/kg for intraperitoneal administration. In rats, the LD_{50} was more than 2,000 mg/kg for both oral and intraperitoneal administration.

➤*Treatment:* There is no specific antidote for the treatment of overdosage with tinidazole; therefore, treatment should be symptomatic and supportive. Gastric lavage may be helpful. Consider hemodialysis because approximately 43% of the amount present in the body is eliminated during a 6-hour hemodialysis session.

Patient Information

Instruct patients to take tinidazole tablets with food.

Advise patients to avoid alcoholic beverages while taking tinidazole and for 3 days afterward.

EFLORNITHINE HCl (DFMO)

Rx　**Ornidyl** (Marion Merrell　　**Injection Concentrate:** 200 mg/ml (as monohydrate)　　　In 100 ml vials.
　　　Dow)

Indications

Treatment of meningoencephalitic stage of *Trypanosoma brucei gambiense* infection (sleeping sickness). Extended follow-up of patients is required to assure adequate further therapy should relapse occur (see Precautions).

Administration and Dosage

➤*Trypanosoma brucei gambiense (sleeping sickness):* Administer 100 mg/kg/dose (46 mg/lb/dose) every 6 hours by IV infusion for 14 days. Administer infusion over a minimum of 45 consecutive minutes. Other drugs should not be administered intravenously during the infusion of eflornithine.

➤*Renal function impairment:* In patients with impaired renal function, dose adjustments are necessary to compensate for the slower excretion of the drug. When only serum creatinine is available, the following formula (Cockcroft's equation) may be used to estimate creatinine clearance. The serum creatinine should represent a steady state of renal function:

Males:　$\dfrac{\text{Weight (kg)} \times (140 - \text{age})}{72 \times \text{serum creatinine (mg/dL)}} = \text{Ccr}$

Females:　$0.85 \times$ above value

➤*Preparation for IV administration:* Eflornithine concentrate is hypertonic and must be diluted with Sterile Water for Injection, USP, before infusion.

Solutions within 10% of plasma tonicity can be produced using 1 part eflornithine concentrate to 4 parts Sterile Water for Injection, USP, by volume as described below.

Using strict aseptic technique, withdraw the entire contents of each 100 ml vial. Inject 25 ml into each of four IV diluent bags, each of which contains 100 ml of Sterile Water, USP. The eflornithine concentration following dilution will be 40 mg/ml (5000 mg of eflornithine in 125 ml total volume).

➤*Storage/Stability:* The diluted drug must be used within 24 hours of preparation. Store bags containing diluted eflornithine at 4°C (39°F) to minimize the risk of microbial proliferation. Store undiluted vial at room temperature, preferably below 30°C (86°F). Protect from freezing and light.

Actions

➤*Pharmacology:* Eflornithine is an antiprotozoal agent for IV injection. Its activity has been attributed to inhibition of the enzyme ornithine decarboxylase. Eflornithine differs from other currently available antiprotozoal drugs in both structure and mode of action. It is a specific, enzyme-activated, irreversible inhibitor of ornithine decarboxylase. In all mammalian and many non-mammalian cells, decarboxylation of ornithine by ornithine decarboxylase is an obligatory step in the biosynthesis of polyamines such as putrescine, spermidine and spermine, which are ubiquitous in living cells and thought to play important roles in cell division and differentiation.

➤*Pharmacokinetics:* Following IV administration to humans, approximately 80% of the administered dose is excreted unchanged in the urine within 24 hours, and the terminal plasma elimination half-life is approximately 3 hours. Eflornithine's excretion through the kidney approximates that of creatinine clearance. Therefore, in patients with impaired renal function, dose adjustments are necessary to compensate for the slower excretion of the drug.

Eflornithine does not bind significantly to human plasma proteins. It crosses the blood-brain barrier and produces cerebrospinal fluid:blood ratios between 0.13 and 0.51 (studies in 5 patients).

➤*Microbiology:* In tissue culture, eflornithine inhibits growth of *Trypanosoma brucei brucei*. This effect is reversed by the addition of polyamine putrescine to the culture medium.

Eflornithine is active in treatment of African trypanosomal infections in various animal models, including *Trypanosoma brucei gambiense* infection in a monkey model.

Warnings

➤*Concentrate:* Must be diluted before use.

➤*Hematologic effects:*

Myelosuppression – The safe and effective use of eflornithine demands thorough knowledge of the natural history of trypanosomiasis due to *T. brucei gambiense* and of the condition of the patient. The most frequent, serious, toxic effect of eflornithine is myelosuppression, which may be unavoidable if successful treatment is to be completed. Base decisions to modify dosage or to interrupt or cease treatment upon the response to treatment, the severity of the observed adverse event(s) and the availability of support facilities.

Anemia – Hemoglobin < 10 g/dl, a decrease of ≥ 2 g/dl hemoglobin during treatment of hematocrit < 35%, or a decrease of > 5% in hematocrit during treatment occurred in about 55% of monitored patients, but was generally found to be reversible upon stopping treatment. Many of these patients were chronically anemic prior to the start of therapy.

Leukopenia ($\leq 4,000\ WBC/mm^3$) – This occurred in about 37% of the patients monitored. The minimum value usually occurred within 8 days of the start of therapy, and the condition usually resolved after discontinuation of therapy.

Thrombocytopenia ($< 100,000\ platelets/mm^3$) – This developed in approximately 14% of the patients in clinical trials. In these patients, thrombocytopenia was reversible with interruption of or after completion of eflornithine therapy.

➤*Seizures:* Eflornithine has been temporally associated with seizures, an adverse event that can also be caused by the underlying disease. Seizures occurred in approximately 8% of patients treated with IV eflornithine in clinical trials. The etiology of the seizures (intrinsic meningoencephalitis or drug or combination) has not been determined. Be aware of the potential for seizure activity.

➤*Occasional hearing impairment:* This has occurred. When feasible, it is recommended that serial audiograms be obtained.

➤*Relapse:* Due to limited data on the risk of relapse after eflornithine therapy for Stage II gambiense trypanosomiasis, physicians are advised to follow their patients for at least 24 months to assure further therapy should relapses occur.

➤*Renal function impairment:* Since approximately 80% of the IV dose is eliminated unchanged in the urine, exercise caution in patients with renal impairment.

➤*Fertility impairment:* Decreased spermatogenetic effects in rats and rabbits were observed at doses equivalent to one-half the recommended human dose and in mice at approximately twice the human dose.

➤*Pregnancy: Category C.* Eflornithine is contragestational in rats, rabbits and mice when given, respectively, in doses 0.5, 0.5 and 2 times the human dose. There are no adequate and well controlled studies in pregnant women. Use during pregnancy only if the potential benefit justifies the potential risk to the fetus. In postnatal studies, retarded development occurred in rat pups on doses slightly higher than the human dose.

➤*Lactation:* It is not known whether this drug is excreted in breast milk. Because of the potential for serious adverse reactions in nursing infants from eflornithine, decide whether to discontinue nursing or to discontinue the drug, taking into account the importance of the drug to the mother.

➤*Children:* Safety and efficacy in children have not been established.

Precautions

➤*Monitoring:* Perform complete blood counts, including platelet counts, before treatment, twice weekly during therapy, and weekly after completion of therapy until hematologic values return to baseline levels.

Adverse Reactions

➤*Most frequent:* Anemia (55%), leukopenia (37%), thrombocytopenia (14%), see Warnings; diarrhea (9%); seizures (8%), see Warnings; hearing impairment (5%), see Warnings; vomiting (5%); alopecia (3%); abdominal pain, anorexia, headache, asthenia, facial edema, eosinophilia (2%); dizziness (1%).

Four percent of patients died during therapy or shortly after completion of treatment. It could not be established whether these deaths were caused by underlying disease or the use of eflornithine.

Overdosage

In mice and rats given intraperitoneal doses of 3 g/kg, moderate CNS depression was observed after 2 to 4 hours. Convulsions were observed in 3 out of 10 rats, and 2 of them died within 3 hours following receipt of the drug.

ATOVAQUONE

Rx   **Mepron** (GlaxoWellcome)   **Suspension:** 750 mg/5 ml   Benzyl alcohol, saccharin. Bright yellow. Citrus flavor. In 210 ml.

Indications

➤*Pneumocystis carinii pneumonia:* Prevention of PCP in patients who are intolerant to trimethoprim-sulfamethoxazole (TMP-SMZ).

Acute oral treatment of mild-to-moderate PCP in patients who are intolerant to trimethoprim-sulfamethoxazole (TMP-SMZ).

Administration and Dosage

➤*Approved by the FDA:* November 25, 1992.

➤*Prevention of PCP:*

Adults and adolescents 13 to 16 years of age – 1500 mg once daily with a meal.

➤*Treatment of mild-to-moderate PCP:*

Adults and adolescents 13 to 16 years of age – 750 mg administered with food twice daily for 21 days (total daily dose 1500 mg).

Failure to administer atovaquone with food may result in lower atovaquone plasma concentrations and may limit response to therapy (see Precautions and Drug Interactions).

➤*Storage/Stability:* Do not freeze.

Actions

➤*Pharmacology:* Atovaquone, an analog of ubiquinone, is an antiprotozoal with antipneumocystis activity. The mechanism of action against *Pneumocystis carinii* has not been fully elucidated. In *Plasmodium* species, the site of action appears to be the cytochrome bc_1 complex (Complex III). Several metabolic enzymes are linked to the mitochondrial electron transport chain via ubiquinone. Inhibition of electron transport by atovaquone will result in indirect inhibition of these enzymes. The ultimate metabolic effects of such blockade may include inhibition of nucleic acid and ATP synthesis.

➤*Pharmacokinetics:*

Absorption – Atovaquone is a highly lipophilic compound with a low aqueous solubility. Bioavailability is highly dependent on formulation and diet. The suspension provides an ≈ 2-fold increase in bioavailability in the fasting or fed state compared with the previously marketed tablet formulation. Absolute bioavailability of a 750 mg dose given under fed conditions in 9 HIV-infected volunteers was 47% (vs 23% with the tablet). Absorption is enhanced ≈ 2-fold when given with food (see Drug Interactions). Plasma concentrations do not increase proportionally with dose; when given with food at doses of 500, 750, and 1000 mg once daily, average steady-state concentrations were 11.7, 12.5, and 13.5 mcg/ml, respectively, and C_{max} concentrations were 15.1, 15.3, and 16.8 mcg/ml.

Distribution – Following IV administration, volume of distribution at steady-state was 0.6 L/kg. Atovaquone is extensively bound to plasma proteins (99.9%). CSF concentrations are < 1% of plasma concentrations.

Metabolism/Excretion – Plasma clearance following IV administration in 9 HIV-infected volunteers was 10.4 ml/min. Half-life was 62.5 hours following IV use and ranged from 67 to 77.6 hours following the suspension. The long half-life is due to presumed enterohepatic cycling and eventual fecal elimination. In healthy volunteers, > 94% of the dose was recovered unchanged in the feces over 21 days; there was little or no excretion in the urine (< 0.6%). There is indirect evidence that atovaquone may undergo limited metabolism; however, a specific metabolite has not been identified.

Children – Preliminary analysis indicates that atovaquone pharmacokinetics are age-dependent. At doses of 10 and 30 mg/kg, children between 2 and 13 years of age had steady-state plasma concentrations of 16.8 and 37.1 mcg/ml, respectively. Children between 3 and 24 months had concentrations of 5.7 and 9.8 mcg/ml, respectively, and at a dose of 45 mg/kg, the concentration was 15.4 mcg/ml. Children between 1 and 3 months of age had concentrations of 5.9 and 27.8 mcg/ml, respectively.

➤*Clinical trials:*

Trimethoprim-sulfamethoxazole (TMP-SMZ) comparative study – In AIDS patients with histologically confirmed mild-to-moderate *Pneumocystis carinii* pneumonia (PCP), 160 received atovaquone (750 mg) and 162 received TMP-SMZ (320/1600 mg), both 3 times daily for 21 days. Therapy success was defined as improved clinical and respiratory measures persisting ≥ 4 weeks after therapy cessation. Failures included lack of response, drug discontinuation because of an adverse experience, and unevaluable patients.

Outcome of Treatment for PCP-Positive Patients: Atovaquone vs TMP-SMZ (%)		
Outcome of therapy	Atovaquone (n = 160)	TMP-SMZ (n = 162)
Therapy success	62	64
Therapy failure		
Lack of response	17	6
Adverse experience	7	20

Outcome of Treatment for PCP-Positive Patients: Atovaquone vs TMP-SMZ (%)		
Outcome of therapy	Atovaquone (n = 160)	TMP-SMZ (n = 162)
Unevaluable	14	10
Required alternate PCP therapy during study	34	34

There was significant difference in mortality rates between the treatment groups: 8% of patients treated with atovaquone and 2.5% receiving TMP-SMZ died during the 21-day treatment course or 8-week follow-up period. Of the 13 patients treated with atovaquone who died, 4 died of PCP and 5 died with a combination of bacterial infections and PCP; bacterial infections did not appear to be a factor in any of the 4 deaths among TMP-SMZ-treated patients.

A correlation between plasma atovaquone concentrations and death was demonstrated; in general, patients with lower plasma concentrations were more likely to die; 63% of the patients with concentrations < 5 mcg/ml died during participation in the study. However, only 2% with day 4 plasma concentrations ≥ 5 mcg/ml died. Failure rate because of lack of response was significantly larger with atovaquone while failure rate because of adverse experiences was significantly larger with TMP-SMZ.

Pentamidine comparative study – One study compared the safety and efficacy of atovaquone with that of pentamidine for the treatment of histologically confirmed mild-to-moderate PCP in AIDS patients. Approximately 80% of the patients had a history of intolerance to trimethoprim or sulfonamides (the primary therapy group) or were experiencing intolerance to TMP-SMZ with treatment of an episode of PCP at the time of enrollment in the study (the salvage treatment group). Patients received either atovaquone 750 mg 3 times daily for 21 days or pentamidine isethionate 3 to 4 mg/kg single IV infusion daily for 21 days.

There was no difference in mortality rates between the treatment groups. Among the 135 patients with confirmed PCP, 14% receiving atovaquone and 14% receiving pentamidine died during the 21-day treatment course or 8-week follow-up period. Of those patients for whom day 4 atovaquone plasma concentrations are available, 60% with concentrations < 5 mcg/ml died during participation in the study. However, only 9% with day 4 plasma concentrations ≥ 5 mcg/ml died.

Outcome of Treatment for PCP-Positive Patients: Atovaquone vs Pentamidine (%)				
	Primary treatment		Salvage treatment	
Outcome of therapy	Atovaquone (n = 56)	Pentamidine (n = 53)	Atovaquone (n = 14)	Pentamidine (n = 11)
Therapy success	57	40	93	64
Therapy failure				
Lack of response	29	17	—	—
Adverse experience	3.6	36	—	27
Unevaluable	11	8	7	9
Required alternate PCP therapy during study	34	55	—	36

PCP prevention – The indication for PCP prevention is based on the results of 2 clinical trials in HIV-infected adult and adolescent patients at risk of PCP (CD4 count < 200 cells/mm^3 or a prior episode of PCP) and intolerant to TMP-SMZ.

Dapsone: In 1057 patients randomized to receive 1500 mg atovaquone suspension once daily (n = 536) or 100 mg dapsone once daily (n = 521), PCP event rates were 15% and 19%, respectively. There was no significant difference in mortality rates between groups.

Aerosolized pentamidine: In 549 patients randomized to receive 1500 mg atovaquone suspension once daily (n = 175), 750 mg atovaquone suspension once daily (n = 188), or 300 mg aerosolized pentamidine once monthly (n = 186), PCP event rates were 23%, 18%, and 17%, respectively. There were no significant differences in mortality rates among the groups.

Contraindications

Development or history of potentially life-threatening allergic reactions to any of the components of the formulation.

Warnings

➤*Severe PCP/Prophylaxis:* Clinical experience has been limited to patients with mild-to-moderate PCP. Treatment of more severe episodes of PCP has not been systematically studied. Atovaquone efficacy in patients who are failing therapy with TMP-SMZ has not been systematically studied.

➤*Hepatic function impairment:* Use caution in patients with severe hepatic impairment, and closely monitor administration.

➤*Elderly:* Atovaquone studies have had insufficient numbers of patients ≥ 65 years of age to determine if they respond differently from younger subjects. Dose selection for an elderly patient should be cautious, reflecting the greater frequency of decreased hepatic, renal, and

ATOVAQUONE

cardiac function and of concomitant disease or other drug therapy in this population.

➤*Pregnancy: Category C.* Atovaquone caused maternal toxicity in rabbits at plasma concentrations that were ≈ ½ the estimated human exposure. Mean fetal body lengths and weights were decreased, and there were higher numbers of early resorption and postimplantation loss per dam. It is not clear whether these effects were caused by atovaquone or were secondary to maternal toxicity. Concentrations of atovaquone in rabbit fetuses averaged 30% of the concurrent maternal plasma concentrations. In a separate study in rats, concentrations in rat fetuses were 18% (middle gestation) and 60% (late gestation) of concurrent maternal plasma concentrations. There are no adequate and well-controlled studies in pregnant women. Use during pregnancy only if the potential benefit justifies the potential risk to the fetus.

➤*Lactation:* It is not known whether atovaquone is excreted in breast milk. Exercise caution when administering atovaquone to a nursing woman. In a rat study, atovaquone concentrations in the milk were 30% of the concurrent atovaquone concentrations in the maternal plasma.

➤*Children:* Safety and efficacy have not been established. In a study of atovaquone suspension in 27 HIV-infected, asymptomatic infants and children between 1 month and 13 years of age, the pharmacokinetics were age-dependent. No treatment-limiting adverse events were observed.

Precautions

➤*Absorption:* The absorption of oral atovaquone is limited but can be significantly increased when the drug is taken with food. Plasma concentrations correlate with the likelihood of successful treatment and survival. Therefore, consider parenteral therapy with other agents for patients who have difficulty taking atovaquone with food (see Drug Interactions). GI disorders may limit absorption of oral drugs. Patients with these disorders also may not achieve plasma concentrations of atovaquone associated with response to therapy in controlled trials.

➤*Concurrent pulmonary conditions:* Based on the spectrum of in vitro antimicrobial activity, atovaquone is not effective therapy for concurrent pulmonary conditions such as bacterial, viral, or fungal pneumonia or mycobacterial diseases. Clinical deterioration in patients may be due to infections with other pathogens, as well as progressive PCP. Carefully evaluate all patients with acute PCP for other possible causes of pulmonary disease and treat with additional agents as appropriate.

Drug Interactions

Atovaquone is highly bound to plasma protein (> 99.9%). Therefore, use caution when administering atovaquone concurrently with other highly plasma protein bound drugs with narrow therapeutic indices, as competition for binding sites may occur. However, the extent of plasma protein binding of atovaquone in human plasma is not affected by the presence of therapeutic concentrations of phenytoin (15 mcg/ml), nor is the binding of phenytoin affected by the presence of atovaquone.

Atovaquone Drug Interactions			
Precipitant drug	Object drug*		Description
Rifamycins	Atovaquone	↓	Concurrent use with rifampin results in a significant decrease in average steady-state plasma concentrations of atovaquone and an increase in average steady-state plasma concentrations of rifampin. The half-life of atovaquone decreased. Rifabutin may interact similarly.
Atovaquone	TMP-SMZ	↔	Coadministration resulted in a 17% and 8% decrease in average steady-state concentrations of TMP and SMZ in plasma, respectively. However, this effect is minor and would not be expected to produce any clinically significant events.
Atovaquone	Zidovudine	↔	In 1 study, concurrent use resulted in a 24% decrease in zidovudine apparent oral clearance, leading to a 35% increase in AUC. The glucuronide metabolite:parent ratio decreased from a mean of 4.5 (zidovudine alone) to 3.1. However, this effect is minor and would not be expected to produce any clinically significant events.

* ↓ = Object drug decreased. ↔ = Clinical significance unknown.

➤*Drug/Food interactions:* Administering atovaquone with food enhances its absorption by ≈ 2-fold. In 1 study, 16 healthy volunteers received a single dose of 750 mg after an overnight fast and following a standard breakfast (23 g fat: 610 kcal). The mean AUC values were 324 and 801 hr•mcg/ml under fasting and fed conditions, respectively. In a multidose study in 19 HIV-infected volunteers receiving atovaquone 500 mg daily, AUC values were 169 and 280 hr•mcg/ml under fasting and fed conditions, respectively; C_{max} was 8.8 and 15.1 mcg/ml, respectively.

Adverse Reactions

Because many patients who participated in clinical trials had complications of advanced HIV disease, it was often difficult to distinguish adverse events caused by atovaquone from those caused by underlying medical conditions. There were no life-threatening or fatal adverse experiences caused by atovaquone.

Adverse Reactions: Atovaquone vs Dapsone for PCP Prevention (%)				
	All patients		Patients not taking either drug at enrollment	
Adverse reactions	Atovaquone (1500 mg/day) (n = 536)	Dapsone (100 mg/day) (n = 521)	Atovaquone (1500 mg/day) (n = 238)	Dapsone (100 mg/day) (n = 249)
Any event	24.4	25.9	20.2	43.4
Rash	6.3	8.8	7.6	16.1
Nausea	4.1	0.6	2.5	0.8
Diarrhea	3.2	0.2	2.1	0.4
Vomiting	2.2	0.6	1.3	0.8
Allergic reaction	1.1	2.9	0.8	4.8
Fever	0.6	2.9	0	5.6
Anemia	0	1.5	0	2

Adverse Reactions: Atovaquone vs Pentamidine for PCP Prevention (%)			
Adverse reactions	Atovaquone (1500 mg/day) (n = 175)	Atovaquone (750 mg/day) (n = 188)	Aerosolized pentamidine (n = 186)
Diarrhea	42	42	35
Rash	39	46	28
Headache	28	31	22
Nausea	26	32	23
Cough increased	25	25	31
Fever	25	31	18
Rhinitis	24	18	17
Asthenia	22	31	31
Infection	22	18	19
Abdominal pain	20	21	20
Dyspnea	15	21	16
Vomiting	15	22	11
Patients discontinuing therapy because of an adverse experience	25	16	7
Patients reporting ≥ 1 adverse experience	98	96	89

Adverse Reactions: Atovaquone vs TMP-SMZ for PCP Treatment (%)		
Adverse reactions	Atovaquone (n = 203)	TMP-SMZ (n = 205)
Rash (including maculopapular)	23	34
Nausea	21	44
Diarrhea	19	7
Headache	16	22
Vomiting	14	35
Fever	14	25
Insomnia	10	9
Asthenia	8	8
Pruritus	5	9
Monilia, oral	5	10
Abdominal pain	4	7
Constipation	3	17
Dizziness	3	8
Patients discontinuing therapy because of an adverse experience	9	24
Patients reporting ≥ 1 adverse experience	63	65

Laboratory Test Abnormalities: Atovaquone vs TMP-SMZ for PCP Treatment (%)		
Lab test abnormality	Atovaquone	TMP-SMZ
Anemia (Hgb < 8 g/dl)	6	7
Neutropenia (ANC < 750 cells/mm³)	3	9
Elevated ALT (> 5 × ULN[1])	6	16
Elevated AST (> 5 × ULN)	4	14
Elevated alkaline phosphatase (> 2.5 × ULN)	8	6
Elevated amylase (> 1.5 × ULN)	7	12
Hyponatremia (< 0.96 × LLN[2])	7	26

[1] ULN = upper limit of normal range
[2] LLN = lower limit of normal range

ATOVAQUONE

Of patients receiving atovaquone, 4% discontinued therapy because of development of rash. The majority of cases of rash among patients were mild and did not require the discontinuation of treatment. The only other clinical adverse experience that led to premature discontinuation by > 1 patient was vomiting (< 1%). The most common adverse experience requiring discontinuation in the TMP-SMZ group was rash (8%). Therapy was prematurely discontinued because of elevations in ALT/AST in 2% of atovaquone patients and 7% with TMP-SMZ.

Adverse Reactions: Atovaquone vs Pentamidine for PCP Treatment (%)

Adverse reactions	Atovaquone (n = 73)	Pentamidine (n = 71)
Fever	40	25
Nausea	22	37
Rash	22	13
Diarrhea	21	31
Insomnia	19	14
Headache	18	28
Vomiting	14	17
Cough	14	1
Abdominal pain	10	11
Pain	10	10
Sweating	10	3
Monilia, oral	10	3
Asthenia	8	14
Dizziness	8	14
Anxiety	7	10
Anorexia	7	10
Sinusitis	7	6
Dyspepsia	5	10
Rhinitis	5	7
Taste perversion	3	13
Hypoglycemia	1	15
Hypotension	1	10
Patients discontinuing therapy because of an adverse experience	7	41
Patients reporting ≥ 1 adverse experience	63	72

Laboratory Test Abnormalities: Atovaquone vs Pentamidine for PCP Treatment (%)

Lab test abnormality	Atovaquone	Pentamidine
Anemia (Hgb < 8 g/dl)	4	9
Neutropenia (ANC < 750 cells/mm³)	5	9
Hyponatremia (< 0.96 × LLN[1])	10	10
Hyperkalemia (> 1.18 × ULN[2])	0	5
Alkaline phosphatase (> 2.5 × ULN)	5	2
Hyperglycemia (> 1.8 × ULN)	9	13
Elevated AST (> 5 × ULN)	0	5
Elevated amylase (> 1.5 × ULN)	8	4
Elevated creatinine (> 1.5 × ULN)	0	7

[1] LLN = lower limit of normal range
[2] ULN = upper limit of normal range

Only 7% of patients discontinued treatment with atovaquone because of adverse events while 41% of patients who received pentamidine discontinued treatment for this reason. Of the 5 patients who discontinued therapy with atovaquone, 3 reported rash (4%). Rash was not severe in any patient. No other reason for discontinuation of atovaquone was cited more than once. The most frequently cited reasons for discontinuation of pentamidine therapy were hypoglycemia (11%) and vomiting (9%).

Laboratory abnormality was the reason for discontinuation of treatment in 2 of 73 patients who received atovaquone. One patient (1%) had elevated creatinine and BUN levels, and 1 patient (1%) had elevated amylase levels. Laboratory abnormalities were the sole or contributing factor in 14 patients who prematurely discontinued pentamidine therapy. In the 71 patients who received pentamidine, laboratory parameters most frequently reported as reasons for discontinuation were hypoglycemia (11%), elevated creatinine levels (6%), and leukopenia (4%).

Patient Information

Stress the importance of taking the prescribed dose. Instruct patients to take their daily doses with meals as the presence of food will significantly improve the absorption of the drug.

PENTAMIDINE ISETHIONATE

Rx	Pentam 300 (American Pharmaceutical Partners)	Injection: 300 mg	In single-dose vials.
Rx	Pentamidine Isethionate (Abbott)	Powder for Injection, lyophilized: 300 mg	In single-dose flip-top vials.
Rx	NebuPent (American Pharmaceutical Partners)	Aerosol: 300 mg	In single dose vials.

Indications

➤*Injection:* Treatment of *Pneumocystis carinii* pneumonia (PCP).

➤*Inhalation:* Prevention of PCP in high-risk, HIV-infected patients defined by one or both of the following criteria:

1) a history of one or more episodes of PCP

2) a peripheral CD4+ (T4 helper/inducer) lymphocyte count ≤ 200 cu mm.

➤*Unlabeled uses:* Pentamidine has been used in the treatment of trypanosomiasis and visceral leishmaniasis.

Administration and Dosage

➤*Injection:*

Adults and children – 4 mg/kg once a day for 14 days administered deep IM or IV only. The benefits and risks of therapy for more than 14 days are not well defined. Dosage in renal failure should be patient-specific. If necessary, reduce dosage, use a longer infusion time or extend the dosing interval.

➤*Preparation of solution:*

IM – Dissolve the contents of 1 vial in 3 ml of Sterile Water for Injection.

IV – Dissolve the contents of 1 vial in 3 to 5 ml of Sterile Water for Injection or 5% Dextrose Injection. Further dilute the calculated dose in 50 to 250 ml of 5% Dextrose solution. Infuse the diluted IV solution over 60 minutes.

➤*Aerosol:*

Prevention of PCP – 300 mg once every 4 weeks administered via the *Respirgard* II nebulizer by Marquest.

Deliver the dose until the nebulizer chamber is empty (approximately 30 to 45 minutes). The flow rate should be 5 to 7 L/min from a 40 to 50 pounds per square inch (PSI) air or oxygen source. Alternatively, a 40 to 50 PSI air compressor can be used with flow limited by setting the flowmeter at 5 to 7 L/min or by setting the pressure at 22 to 25 PSI. Do not use low pressure (less than 20 PSI) compressors.

Reconstitution – The contents of one vial must be dissolved in 6 ml Sterile Water for Injection, USP. It is important to use *only* sterile water; saline solution will cause the drug to precipitate. Place the entire reconstituted contents of the vial into the Respirgard® II nebu-

lizer reservoir for administration. Do not mix the pentamidine solution with any other drugs.

➤*Storage/Stability:*

Injection – IV solutions of 1 and 2.5 mg/ml prepared in 5% Dextrose Injection are stable at room temperature for up to 48 hours. Store dry product between 15° to 30°C (59° to 86°F). Protect from light. Discard unused portion.

Aerosol – Use freshly prepared solutions. After reconstitution with sterile water, the solution is stable for 48 hours in the original vial at room temperature if protected from light. Store dry product at controlled room temperature 15° to 30°C (59° to 86°F).

Actions

➤*Pharmacology:* Pentamidine isethionate, an aromatic diamidine antiprotozoal agent, has activity against *Pneumocystis carinii*. The mode of action is not fully understood. In vitro studies indicate that the drug interferes with nuclear metabolism and inhibits the synthesis of DNA, RNA, phospholipids and protein synthesis.

➤*Pharmacokinetics:*

Absorption/Distribution – Pentamidine is well absorbed after IM administration. It is detectable in the blood briefly, due to extensive tissue binding.

The mean concentrations of pentamidine determined 18 to 24 hours after inhalation therapy were 23.2 ng/ml in bronchoalveolar lavage fluid and 705 ng/ml in sediment after administration of a 300 mg single dose via the *Respirgard* II nebulizer. The mean concentrations of pentamidine determined 18 to 24 hours after a 4 mg/kg IV dose were 2.6 ng/ml in bronchoalveolar lavage fluid and 9.3 ng/ml in sediment. In the patients who received aerosolized pentamidine, the peak plasma levels of pentamidine were at or below the lower limit of detection of the assay (2.3 ng/ml).

Metabolism/Excretion – Approximately ⅓ of the dose is excreted unchanged by the kidneys in the first 6 hours; however, small amounts are found in the urine up to 6 to 8 weeks following administration. Pentamidine may accumulate in renal failure. Following a single 2 hour IV infusion of 4 mg/kg of pentamidine the mean maximum plasma concentration, half-life and clearance were 612 ± 371 ng/ml, 6.4 ± 1.3 hr and 248 ± 91 L/hr respectively.

Plasma concentrations after aerosol administration are substantially lower than those observed after a comparable IV dose. The extent of

PENTAMIDINE ISETHIONATE

pentamidine accumulation and distribution following chronic inhalation therapy are not known.

Contraindications

➤*Injection:* Once the diagnosis of PCP has been established, there are no absolute contraindications to the use of pentamidine.

➤*Inhalation:* Patients with a history of an anaphylactic reaction to inhaled or parenteral pentamidine isethionate.

Warnings

➤*Development of acute PCP:* This still exists in patients receiving pentamidine prophylaxis. Therefore, any patient with symptoms suggestive of the presence of a pulmonary infection, including but not limited to dyspnea, fever or cough, should receive a thorough medical evaluation and appropriate diagnostic tests for possible acute PCP and for other opportunistic and non-opportunistic pathogens. The use of pentamidine may alter the clinical and radiographic features of PCP and could result in an atypical presentation, including but not limited to mild diseases or focal infection.

Prior to initiating pentamidine prophylaxis, evaluate symptomatic patients to exclude the presence of PCP. The recommended dose of pentamidine for the prevention of PCP is insufficient to treat acute PCP.

➤*Fatalities:* Those due to severe hypotension, hypoglycemia and cardiac arrhythmias have been reported, both by the IM and IV routes. Severe hypotension may result after a single dose. Limit administration of the drug to patients in whom *P. carinii* has been demonstrated. Closely monitor patients for serious adverse reactions.

➤*Pregnancy: Category C.* Safety and efficacy for use during pregnancy have not been established. Use only when clearly needed and when the potential benefits outweigh the unknown potential hazards to the fetus.

➤*Lactation:* It is not known whether pentamidine is excreted in breast milk. Because of the potential for serious adverse reactions in nursing infants decide whether to discontinue nursing or to discontinue the drug, taking into account the importance of the drug to the mother.

➤*Children:* Safety and efficacy of inhalation solution have not been established.

Precautions

➤*Use with caution:* In patients with hypertension, hypotension, hypoglycemia, hyperglycemia, hypocalcemia, leukopenia, thrombocytopenia, anemia, hepatic or renal dysfunction, ventricular tachycardia, pancreatitis, Stevens-Johnson syndrome.

➤*Hypotension:* Patients may develop sudden, severe hypotension after a single dose, whether given IV or IM. Therefore, patients receiving the drug should be supine; monitor blood pressure closely during drug administration and several times thereafter until the blood pressure is stable. Have equipment for emergency resuscitation readily available. If pentamidine is administered IV, infuse over 60 minutes.

➤*Hypoglycemia:* Pentamidine-induced hypoglycemia has been associated with pancreatic islet cell necrosis and inappropriately high plasma insulin concentrations. Hyperglycemia and diabetes mellitus, with or without preceding hypoglycemia, have also occurred, sometimes several months after therapy. Therefore, monitor blood glucose levels daily during therapy and several times thereafter.

➤*Pulmonary:* Inhalation of pentamidine isethionate may induce bronchospasm or cough particularly in patients who have a history of smoking or asthma. In clinical trials, cough and bronchospasm were the most frequently reported adverse experiences associated with pentamidine administration (38% and 15%, respectively of patients receiving the 300 mg dose); however less than 1% of the doses were interrupted or terminated due to these effects. For the majority of patients, cough and bronchospasm were controlled by administration of an aerosolized bronchodilator (only 1% of patients withdrew from the study due to treatment-associated cough or bronchospasm). In patients who experience bronchospasm or cough, administration of an inhaled bronchodilator prior to giving each pentamidine dose may minimize recurrence of the symptoms.

Extrapulmonary infection with *P. carinii* has been reported infrequently with inhalation use. Most have been reported in patients who have a history of PCP. Consider the presence of extrapulmonary pneumocystosis when evaluating patients with unexplained signs and symptoms.

➤*Lab test abnormalities:* Perform the following before, during and after therapy:

1.) Daily BUN, serum creatinine and blood glucose.
2.) Complete blood count and platelet counts.
3.) Liver function test, including bilirubin, alkaline phosphatase, AST and ALT.
4.) Serum calcium.
5.) ECG at regular intervals.

Adverse Reactions

➤*Injection:* 244 of 424 (57.5%) patients treated with pentamidine injection developed some adverse reaction. Most of the patients had acquired immunodeficiency syndrome (AIDS). In the following, "severe" refers to life-threatening reactions or reactions that required immediate corrective measures and led to discontinuation of pentamidine.

Severe: Leukopenia (< 1000/cu mm) 2.8%; hypoglycemia (< 25 mg/dl) 2.4%; thrombocytopenia (< 20,000/cu mm) 1.7%; hypotension (< 60 mm Hg systolic) 0.9%; acute renal failure (serum creatinine > 6 mg/dl) 0.5%; hypocalcemia (0.2%); Stevens-Johnson syndrome and ventricular tachycardia (0.2%); fatalities due to severe hypotension, hypoglycemia and cardiac arrhythmias.

Moderate: Elevated serum creatinine (2.4 to 6 mg/dl) 23.1%; sterile abscess, pain or induration at the IM injection site (11.1%); elevated liver function tests (8.7%); leukopenia (7.5%); nausea, anorexia (5.9%); hypotension (4%); fever, hypoglycemia (3.5%); rash (3.3%); bad taste in mouth, confusion/hallucinations (1.7%); anemia (1.2%); neuralgia, thrombocytopenia (0.9%); hyperkalemia, phlebitis (0.7%); dizziness without hypotension (0.5%).

Each of the following was reported in one patient: Abnormal ST segment of ECG, bronchospasm, diarrhea, hypocalcemia and hyperglycemia.

➤*Aerosol:*

Most Frequent: Fatigue, metallic taste, shortness of breath, decreased appetite (53% to 72%); dizziness, rash, cough (31% to 47%); nausea, pharyngitis, chest pain/congestion, night sweats, chills, vomiting, bronchospasm (10% to 23%).

Less frequent: Pneumothorax, diarrhea, headache, anemia (generally associated with zidovudine use), myalgia, abdominal pain, edema (1% to 5%).

Causal relationship unknown: (≤ 1%):

Cardiovascular – Tachycardia; hypotension; hypertension; palpitations; syncope; cerebrovascular accident; vasodilation; vasculitis.

CNS – Tremors; confusion; anxiety; memory loss; seizure; neuropathy; paresthesia; insomnia; hypesthesia; drowsiness; emotional lability; vertigo; paranoia; neuralgia; hallucination; depression; unsteady gait.

Dermatologic – Pruritus; erythema; dry skin; desquamation; urticaria.

GI – Gingivitis; dyspepsia; oral ulcer/abscess; gastritis; gastric ulcer; hypersalivation; dry mouth; splenomegaly; melena; hematochezia; esophagitis; colitis; pancreatitis.

Hematologic – Pancytopenia; neutropenia; eosinophilia; thrombocytopenia.

Hepatic – Hepatitis; hepatomegaly; hepatic dysfunction.

Metabolic – Hypoglycemia; hyperglycemia; hypocalcemia.

Renal – Renal failure; flank pain; nephritis.

Respiratory – Rhinitis; laryngitis; laryngospasm; hyperventilation; hemoptysis; gagging; eosinophilic or interstitial pneumonitis; pleuritis; cyanosis; tachypnea; rales.

Special senses – Eye discomfort; conjunctivitis; blurred vision; blepharitis; loss of taste and smell.

Miscellaneous – Incontinence; miscarriage; arthralgia; allergic reactions; extrapulmonary pneumocystosis.

The following table lists the major parasitic infections, causative organisms and drugs of choice for treatment. For investigational antiparasitic agents available from the Centers for Disease Control, refer to the CDC Anti-Infective Agents monograph.

Major Parasite Infections

	Infection (common name)	Organism	Drug(s) of Choice
Intestinal Nematodes	Ascariasis[1] (Roundworm)	Ascaris lumbricoides	Mebendazole, Pyrantel pamoate or Diethylcarbamazine
	Uncinariasis (Hookworm)	Ancylostoma duodenale Necator americanus	Mebendazole or Pyrantel pamoate[2]
	Strongyloidiasis (Threadworm)	Strongyloides stercoralis	Thiabendazole
	Trichuriasis (Whipworm)	Trichuris trichiura	Mebendazole
	Enterobiasis[3] (Pinworm)	Enterobius vermicularis	Mebendazole, Pyrantel pamoate or Albendazole
	Capillariasis	Capillaria philippinensis	Mebendazole, Thiabendazole or Albendazole
Tissue Nematodes	Trichinosis	Trichinella spiralis	Steroids for severe symptoms plus Thiabendazole, Albendazole, Flubendazole[6] or Mebendazole[2]
	Cutaneous larva migrans (Creeping eruption)	Ancylostoma braziliense and others	Thiabendazole, Albendazole or Ivermectin[4]
	Onchocerciasis (River blindness)	Onchocerca volvulus	Suramin[5], Diethylcarbamazine or Ivermectin[4]
	Dracontiasis (Guinea worm)	Dracunculus medinensis	Thiabendazole or Mebendazole
	Angiostrongyliasis (Rat lungworm)	Angiostrongylus cantonensis	Thiabendazole or Mebendazole
	Loiasis	Loa loa	Diethylcarbamazine
Cestodes	Taeniasis (Beef tapeworm) (Pork tapeworm)	Taenia saginata Taenia solium	Praziquantel[2] or Niclosamide[6] Praziquantel[2], Niclosamide[6] or Albendazole
	Diphyllobothriasis (Fish tapeworm)	Diphyllobothrium latum	Praziquantel[2] or Niclosamide[6]
	Dog tapeworm	Dipylidium caninum	Praziquantel[2]
	Hymenolepiasis (Dwarf tapeworm)	Hymenolepis nana	Praziquantel[2] or Niclosamide[6]
	Hydatid cysts	Echinococcus granulosus	Albendazole or Praziquantel
Trematodes	Schistosomiasis	Schistosoma mansoni	Praziquantel or Oxamniquine
		Schistosoma japonicum	Praziquantel
		Schistosoma haematobium	Praziquantel
		Schistosoma mekongi	Praziquantel
	Hermaphroditic Flukes Fasciolopsiasis (Intestinal fluke)	Fasciolopsis buski	Praziquantel
		Heterophyes heterophyes Metagonimus yokogawai	Praziquantel
	Clonorchiasis (Chinese liver fluke)	Clonorchis sinensis	Praziquantel
	Fascioliasis (Sheep liver fluke)	Fasciola hepatica	Praziquantel or Bithionol[4]
	Opisthorchiasis (Liver fluke)	Opisthorchis viverrini	Praziquantel
	Paragonimiasis (Lung fluke)	Paragonimus westermani	Praziquantel or Bithionol[4] (alternate)

[1] Thiabendazole is also indicated in Ascariasis.
[2] Unlabeled use.
[3] Thiabendazole is also indicated in Enterobiasis.

[4] Available from the CDC.
[5] Available from the CDC, although generally not recommended.
[6] Not available in the US.

Benzimidazoles

MEBENDAZOLE

Rx	**Vermox** (Janssen)	**Tablets, chewable:** 100 mg	(VERMOX JANSSEN). In 12s.
Rx	**Mebendazole** (Copley)		In 12s.

Refer to the general discussion of these products in the Anthelmintics introduction.

Indications

➤*Helminths:* Treatment of *Trichuris trichiura* (whipworm), *Enterobius vermicularis* (pinworm), *Ascaris lumbricoides* (roundworm), *Ancylostoma duodenale* (common hookworm) or *Necator americanus* (American hookworm), in single or mixed infections.

Administration and Dosage

The same dosage schedule applies to children and adults.

Tablets may be chewed, swallowed or crushed and mixed with food. No special procedures, such as fasting or purging, are required.

If the patient is not cured 3 weeks after treatment, a second treatment course is advised.

➤*Trichuriasis, ascariasis and hookworm infection:* One tablet morning and evening on 3 consecutive days. In one study, treatment with a single 500 mg dose was effective against *A. lumbricoides.*

➤*Enterobiasis:* A single tablet given once.

Actions

➤*Pharmacology:* Mebendazole inhibits the formation of the worms' microtubules and irreversibly blocks glucose uptake by the susceptible helminths, thereby depleting endogenous glycogen stored within the parasite that is required for survival and reproduction of the helminth. Mebendazole does not affect blood glucose concentrations in the host.

➤*Pharmacokinetics:* Mebendazole is poorly absorbed (5% to 10%) after oral administration. Peak plasma levels are reached in 2 to 4 hours. Following administration of 100 mg of mebendazole twice daily for 3 consecutive days, plasma levels of mebendazole and its primary metabolite did not exceed 0.03 mcg/ml and 0.09 mcg/ml, respectively. Approximately 2% of the drug is excreted in the urine during the first 24 to 48 hours. Most of the dose is excreted in the feces as unchanged drug or primary metabolites.

➤*Microbiology:* Active against *Trichuris trichiura* (whipworm), *Enterobius vermicularis* (pinworm), *Ascaris lumbricoides* (roundworm), *Ancylostoma duodenale* (common hookworm) and *Necator americanus* (American hookworm). Parasite immobilization and death are slow, and complete clearance from the GI tract may take up to 3 days after treatment. Efficacy varies as a function of such factors as preexisting diarrhea and GI transit time, degree of infection and helminth strains.

Contraindications

Hypersensitivity to mebendazole.

Warnings

➤*Hydatid disease:* There is no evidence that mebendazole is effective for hydatid disease.

➤*Pregnancy: Category C.* Mebendazole was embryotoxic and teratogenic in pregnant rats at single oral doses as low as 10 mg/kg. This drug is not recommended for use in pregnant women. Based on a limited number of women, the incidence of spontaneous abortion, malformation and teratogenesis did not exceed that in the general population. During pregnancy, especially during the first trimester, use mebendazole only if the potential benefit justifies the potential risk to the fetus.

➤*Lactation:* It is not known whether mebendazole is excreted in breast milk. Because many drugs are excreted in breast milk, excercise caution when mebendazole is administered to a nursing woman.

➤*Children:* Safety and efficacy for use in children < 2 years of age have not been established; consider the relative benefit vs risk.

Drug Interactions

➤*Carbamazepine and hydantoins:* May reduce the plasma levels of concomitant mebendazole, possibly decreasing its therapeutic effect.

Adverse Reactions

➤*GI:* Transient abdominal pain and diarrhea have occurred in cases of massive infection and expulsion of worms.

MEBENDAZOLE

➤*Hematologic:* Two patients receiving high doses of mebendazole for echinococcosis developed a severe but reversible neutropenia apparently because of marrow suppression.

➤*Miscellaneous:* Fever, a possible response to drug-induced tissue necrosis, has occurred.

Overdosage

GI complaints lasting up to a few hours may occur. Induce vomiting and purging. Refer to General Management of Acute Overdosage.

Patient Information

Chew or crush tablet and mix with food.

Parasite death may be slow. Removal from digestive tract may take up to 3 days after treatment. Effectiveness depends on factors such as degree of infection or resistance of parasite to treatment, presence of diarrhea and how quickly things pass through the digestive system. Laxative therapy and fasting are not necessary.

If not cured in 3 weeks, a second treatment is recommended.

➤*Pinworm infections:* These are easily spread to others. If one family member has a pinworm infection, treat all family members in close contact with the patient. This decreases the chance of spreading the infection.

Strict hygiene is essential to prevent reinfection. Disinfect toilet facilities daily. Change and launder undergarments, bed linens, towels and nightclothes daily.

THIABENDAZOLE

Rx	Mintezol (Merck)	Tablets, chewable: 500 mg	Lactose, saccharin. (MSD 907). White, scored. Orange flavor. In 36s.
		Oral Suspension: 500 mg/5 ml	Sorbic acid, sorbitol. In 120 ml.

Refer to the general discussion of these products in the Anthelmintics introduction.

Indications

➤*Helminths:* Treatment of strongyloidiasis (threadworm infection), cutaneous larva migrans (creeping eruption) and visceral larva migrans.

Although not indicated as primary therapy, when enterobiasis (pinworm) occurs with any of the conditions listed above, additional therapy is not required for most patients. Use thiabendazole only in the following infestations when more specific therapy is not available or cannot be used or when further therapy with a second agent is desirable: Uncinariasis (hookworm: *Necator americanus* and *Ancylostoma duodenale*); Trichuriasis (whipworm); Ascariasis (large roundworm).

Also indicated for alleviating symptoms of trichinosis during the invasive phase.

Administration and Dosage

➤*< 150 lbs (68 kg):* 10 mg/lb/dose (22 mg/kg/dose).

➤*≥ 150 lbs:* 1.5 g/dose.

The usual dosage schedule for all conditions is 2 doses per day. Maximum daily dose is 3 g after meals if possible.

Dietary restriction, complementary medications and cleansing enemas are not needed.

Thiabendazole Dosage Regimen for Each Indication

Indication	Regimen	Comments
Strongyloidiasis[1] Ascariasis[1] Uncinariasis[1] Trichuriasis[1]	2 doses/day for 2 successive days	May also use single dose of 20 mg/lb (44 mg/kg) but with higher incidence of side effects.
Cutaneous larva migrans (creeping eruption)	2 doses/day for 2 successive days	If active lesions are still present 2 days after end of therapy, a second course is recommended.
Trichinosis[1]	2 doses/day for 2 to 4 successive days. Individualize dosage	Optimal dosage has not been established.
Visceral larva migrans	2 doses/day for 7 successive days	Safety and efficacy data on the 7 day treatment are limited.

[1] Clinical experience with thiabendazole in children weighing < 13.6 kg (30 lbs) is limited.

Actions

➤*Pharmacokinetics:* Thiabendazole is rapidly absorbed and peak plasma concentrations occur within 1 to 2 hours. It is metabolized almost completely and appears in the urine as conjugates. In 48 hours, ≈ 5% of the administered dose is recovered from feces and ≈ 90% from urine. Most is excreted within the first 24 hours.

➤*Microbiology:* Thiabendazole is vermicidal or vermifugal against *Enterobius vermicularis* (pinworm); *Ascaris lumbricoides* (roundworm); *Strongyloides stercoralis* (threadworm); *Necator americanus* and *Ancylostoma duodenale* (hookworm); *Trichuris trichiura* (whipworm); *Ancylostoma braziliense* (dog and cat hookworm); and *Toxocara canis* and *Toxocara cati* (ascarids).

Thiabendazole's effect on larvae of *Trichinella spiralis* that have migrated to muscle is questionable. It suppresses egg or larval production and may inhibit the subsequent development of those eggs or larvae which are passed in the feces. While the exact mechanism is unknown, the drug inhibits the helminth-specific enzyme fumarate reductase. The anthelmintic activity against *Trichuris trichiura* (whipworm) is least predictable.

Contraindications

Hypersensitivity to thiabendazole.

Warnings

➤*CNS effects:* Because CNS side effects may occur, avoid activities requiring mental alertness.

➤*Hypersensitivity reactions:* If hypersensitivity reactions occur, discontinue the drug immediately. Erythema multiforme has been associated with therapy; in severe cases (eg, Stevens-Johnson syndrome), fatalities have occurred. Refer to Management of Acute Hypersensitivity Reactions.

➤*Pregnancy: Category C.* There are no adequate and well controlled studies in pregnant women. Use during pregnancy only if the potential benefit outweighs the risk to the fetus.

➤*Lactation:* It is not known whether this drug is excreted in breast milk. Because of the potential for serious adverse reactions in nursing infants, decide whether to discontinue nursing or drug taking into account importance of drug to mother.

➤*Children:* Safety and efficacy for the treatment of Strongyloidiasis, Ascariasis, Uncinariasis, Trichuriasis and Trichinosis in children weighing < 13.6 kg (30 lbs) has been limited.

Precautions

➤*Monitoring:* Monitor patients with hepatic or renal dysfunction carefully.

➤*Supportive therapy:* This is indicated for anemic, dehydrated or malnourished patients prior to initiation of therapy.

➤*Metabolite:* Some patients may excrete a metabolite that imparts an odor to urine similar to that occurring after ingestion of asparagus.

➤*Thiabendazole:* It is not suitable for the treatment of mixed infections with ascaris because it may cause these worms to migrate. Use only in patients in whom susceptible worm infestation has been diagnosed; do not use prophylactically.

➤*Lab test abnormalities:* Rarely, a transient rise in cephalin flocculation and AST has occurred in patients receiving thiabendazole.

Drug Interactions

➤*Xanthines:* Thiabendazole may compete with these agents for sites of metabolism in the liver, thus elevating the serum levels of the xanthine to potentially toxic levels. Monitor xanthine serum levels and reduce the dose if necessary.

Adverse Reactions

➤*CNS:* Dizziness; weariness; drowsiness; giddiness; headache; numbness; hyperirritability; convulsions; collapse; psychic disturbances.

➤*GI:* Anorexia; nausea; vomiting; diarrhea; epigastric distress; jaundice; cholestasis; parenchymal liver damage.

➤*GU:* Hematuria; enuresis; malodor of the urine; crystalluria.

➤*Hypersensitivity:* Pruritus; fever; facial flush; chills; conjunctival injection ("red eye"); angioedema; anaphylaxis; skin rashes (including perianal); erythema multiforme (including Stevens-Johnson syndrome); lymphadenopathy. (See Warnings.)

THIABENDAZOLE

▶*Special senses:* Tinnitus; abnormal sensation in eyes; xanthopsia (objects appear yellow); blurring of vision; drying of mucous membranes (eg, mouth, eyes).

▶*Miscellaneous:* Appearance of live Ascaris in the mouth and nose; hypotension; transient leukopenia; hyperglycemia.

Overdosage

▶*Symptoms:* Possible transient disturbances of vision and psychic alterations.

▶*Treatment:* There is no specific antidote. Use symptomatic and supportive measures. Induce emesis or carefully perform gastric lavage. Refer to General Management of Acute Overdosage.

Patient Information

May cause stomach upset. Take with food.

▶*Chewable tablets:* Chew thoroughly before swallowing.

Cleansing enemas are not needed after drug therapy.

Duration of therapy varies from 2 or more days depending upon the condition being treated.

Pinworm infections are easily spread to others. If one family member has a pinworm infection, treat all family members in close contact with the patient. This decreases the chance of spreading the infection.

Repeat therapy in 7 days to prevent reinfection.

Strict hygiene is essential to prevent reinfection. Disinfect toilet facilities daily. Change and launder undergarments, bed linens, towels and nightclothes daily.

May produce drowsiness or dizziness. Use caution when driving or performing other tasks requiring alertness.

ALBENDAZOLE

| Rx | **Albenza** (SmithKline Beecham) | **Tablets:** 200 mg | Lactose, saccharin. (SB 5500). Biconvex. In film-coated *Tiltab.* In 112s. |

Refer to the general discussion of these products in the Anthelmintics introduction.

Indications

▶*Neurocysticercosis:* For the treatment of parenchymal neurocysticercosis due to active lesions caused by larval forms of the pork tapeworm, *T. solium.*

▶*Hydatid disease:* For the treatment of cystic hydatid disease of the liver, lung and peritoneum caused by the larval form of the dog tapeworm, *E. granulosus.*

When medically feasible, surgery is considered the treatment of choice for hydatid disease. When administering albendazole in the pre- or post-surgical setting, optimal killing of cyst contents is achieved when three courses of therapy have been given.

Administration and Dosage

Dosing of Albendazole According to the Parasitic Infection			
Indication	Weight	Dose	Duration
Hydatid disease	≥ 60 kg	400 mg twice a day with meals	28-day cycle followed by a 14-day albendazole-free interval, for a total of three cycles[1]
	< 60 kg	15 mg/kg/day given in divided doses twice a day with meals (maximum total daily dose 800 mg)	
Neurocysticercosis	≥ 60 kg	400 mg twice a day with meals	8 to 30 days
	< 60 kg	15 mg/kg/day given in divided doses twice a day with meals (maximum total daily dose 800 mg)	

[1] When administering albendazole in the pre- or post-surgical setting, optimal killing of cyst contents is achieved when three courses of therapy have been given.

Patients being treated for neurocysticercosis should receive appropriate steroid and anticonvulsant therapy as required. Consider oral or IV corticosteroids to prevent cerebral hypertensive episodes during the first week of treatment.

▶*Storage / Stability:* Store between 20° and 25°C (68° and 77°F).

Actions

▶*Pharmacology:* Albendazole's principal mode of action is its inhibitory effect on tubulin polymerization, which results in the loss of cytoplasmic microtubules.

▶*Pharmacokinetics:*

Absorption – Albendazole is poorly absorbed from the GI tract because of its low aqueous solubility. Albendazole concentrations are negligible or undetectable in plasma as it is rapidly converted to the sulfoxide metabolite prior to reaching the systemic circulation. The systemic anthelmintic activity has been attributed to the primary metabolite, albendazole sulfoxide. Oral bioavailability appears to be enhanced when albendazole is coadministered with a fatty meal (estimated fat content 40 g) as evidenced by higher (up to 5–fold on average) plasma concentrations of albendazole sulfoxide as compared with the fasted state.

Maximal plasma concentrations of albendazole sulfoxide are typically achieved 2 to 5 hours after dosing and are on average 1.31 mcg/ml (0.46 to 1.58 mcg/ml) following oral doses of albendazole (400 mg) when administered with a fatty meal. Plasma concentrations of albendazole sulfoxide increase in a dose-proportional manner over the therapeutic dose range following ingestion of a fatty meal (fat content 43.1 g). The mean apparent terminal elimination half-life of albendazole sulfoxide typically ranged from 8 to 12 hours in 25 healthy subjects, as well as in 14 hydatid and 8 neurocysticercosis patients.

Following 4 weeks of treatment with albendazole (200 mg three times daily), 12 patients' plasma concentrations of albendazole sulfoxide were ≈ 20% lower than those observed during the first half of the treatment period, suggesting that albendazole may induce its own metabolism.

Distribution – Albendazole sulfoxide is 70% bound to plasma protein and is widely distributed throughout the body; it has been detected in urine, bile, liver, cyst wall, cyst fluid and cerebral spinal fluid (CSF). Concentrations in plasma were 3– to 10–fold and 2– to 4–fold higher than those simultaneously determined in cyst fluid and CSF, respectively. Limited in vitro and clinical data suggest that albendazole sulfoxide may be eliminated from cysts at a slower rate than observed in plasma.

Metabolism / Excretion – Albendazole is rapidly converted in the liver to the primary metabolite, albendazole sulfoxide, which is further metabolized to albendazole sulfone and other primary oxidative metabolites that have been identified in human urine. Following oral administration, albendazole has not been detected in human urine. Urinary excretion of albendazole sulfoxide is a minor elimination pathway with < 1% of the dose recovered in the urine. Biliary elimination presumably accounts for a portion of the elimination as evidenced by biliary concentrations of albendazole sulfoxide similar to those achieved in plasma.

Special populations –

Renal function impairment: The pharmacokinetics of albendazole in patients with impaired renal function have not been studied. However, because renal elimination of albendazole and its primary metabolite, albendazole sulfoxide, is negligible, it is unlikely that clearance of these compounds would be altered in these patients.

Hepatic function impairment: In patients with evidence of extrahepatic obstruction, the systemic availability of albendazole sulfoxide is increased, as indicated by a 2–fold increase in maximum serum concentration and a 7–fold increase in area under the curve (AUC). The rate of absorption/conversion and elimination of albendazole sulfoxide appeared to be prolonged with mean T_{max} and serum elimination half-life values of 10 hours and 31.7 hours, respectively. Plasma concentrations of parent albendazole were measurable in only one of five patients.

Children: Albendazole sulfoxide pharmacokinetics were similar to those observed in fed adults.

Elderly: Although no studies have investigated the effect of age on albendazole sulfoxide pharmacokinetics, data in 26 hydatid cyst patients (up to 79 years) suggest pharmacokinetics similar to those in young healthy subjects.

▶*Microbiology:* Albendazole is active against the larval forms of *Echinococcus granulosus* and *Taenia solium.*

Contraindications

Hypersensitivity to the benzimidazole class of compound or any components of albendazole.

Warnings

▶*Hepatic function impairment:* Albendazole has been associated with mild to moderate elevations of hepatic enzymes in ≈ 16% of patients. These have returned to normal upon discontinuation of therapy. Perform liver function tests (transaminases) before the start of each treatment. If enzymes are significantly increased, discontinue

ALBENDAZOLE

albendazole therapy. Therapy can be reinstituted when liver enzymes have returned to pretreatment levels, but perform laboratory tests frequently during repeated therapy.

➤*Fertility impairment:* Patients should not become pregnant for at least 1 month following cessation of albendazole therapy.

➤*Elderly:* Experience in patients ≥ 65 years of age is limited. No problems associated with an older population have been observed.

➤*Pregnancy: Category C.* Albendazole has been shown to be teratogenic in animals. There are no adequate and well controlled studies of albendazole administration in pregnant women. Do not use albendazole in pregnant women except in clinical circumstances where no alternative management is appropriate. If a patient becomes pregnant while taking this drug, discontinue albendazole immediately.

➤*Lactation:* It is not known whether albendazole is excreted in breast milk. Because many drugs are excreted in breast milk, use caution when administering to a nursing woman.

➤*Children:* Experience in children < 6 years of age is limited. In hydatid disease, infection in infants and young children is uncommon, but no problems have been encountered in those who have been treated. In neurocysticercosis, infection is more frequently encountered. In studies involving pediatric patients as young as 1 year of age, no significant problems were encountered, and the efficacy appeared similar to the adult population.

Precautions

➤*Monitoring:*

White blood cell count – Albendazole has been shown to cause occasional (< 1% of treated patients) reversible reductions in total white blood cell count. Rarely, more significant reductions may be enountered including granulocytopenia, agranulocytosis or pancytopenia. Perform blood counts at the start of each 28–day treatment cycle and every 2 weeks during each 28–day cycle. Albendazole may be continued if the total white blood cell count decrease appears modest and does not progress.

➤*Coadministration:* Patients being treated for neurocysticercosis should receive appropriate steroid and anticonvulsant therapy as required. Consider oral or IV corticosteroids to prevent cerebral hypertensive episodes during the first week of anticysticeral therapy.

➤*Cysticercosis:* It may, in rare cases, involve the retina. Before initiating therapy for neurocysticercosis, examine the patient for the presence of retinal lesions. If such lesions are visualized, weigh the need for anticysticeral therapy against the possibility of retinal damage caused by albendazole-induced changes to the retinal lesion.

Drug Interactions

Albendazole Drug Interactions			
Precipitant drug	Object drug[*]		Description
Dexamethasone	Albendazole	↑	Steady-state trough concentrations of albendazole sulfoxide were ≈ 56% higher when 8 mg dexamethasone was coadministered with each dose of albendazole (15 mg/kg/day) in eight neurocysticercosis patients.

Albendazole Drug Interactions			
Precipitant drug	Object drug[*]		Description
Praziquantel	Albendazole	↑	Praziquantel (40 mg/kg) increased mean maximum plasma concentration and AUC of albendazole sulfoxide by ≈ 50% in healthy subjects.
Cimetidine	Albendazole	↑	Albendazole sulfoxide concentrations in bile and cystic fluid were increased (≈ 2-fold) in hydatid cyst patients treated with cimetidine.

[*] ↑ = Object drug increased.

Adverse Reactions

Adverse Reaction Incidence in Hydatid Disease and Neurocysticercosis (%)		
Adverse reaction	Hydatid disease	Neurocysticercosis
Abnormal liver function tests	15.6	< 1
Abdominal pain	6	0
Nausea/Vomiting	3.7	6.2
Headache	1.3	11
Dizziness/Vertigo	1.2	< 1
Raised intracranial pressure	0	1.5
Meningeal signs	0	1
Reversible alopecia	1.6	< 1
Fever	1	0

The following adverse reactions were observed at an incidence of < 1%.

➤*Dermatologic:* Rash; urticaria.

➤*Hematologic:* Leukopenia (0.7%); granulocytopenia, pancytopenia, agranulocytosis, thrombocytopenia (rare).

➤*Hypersensitivity:* Allergic reactions.

➤*Renal:* Acute renal failure.

Overdosage

One case of overdosage has been reported with albendazole in a patient who took at least 16 g over 12 hours. No untoward effects were reported. In case of overdosage, symptomatic therapy (eg, gastric lavage and activated charcoal) and general supportive measures are recommended. Refer to General Management of Acute Overdosage.

Patient Information

Albendazole may cause fetal harm; therefore, begin treatment after a negative pregnancy test in women of childbearing age.

Caution women of childbearing age against becoming pregnant while on albendazole or within 1 month of completing treatment.

Take with food.

DIETHYLCARBAMAZINE CITRATE

Rx	**Hetrazan**[1] (Wyeth-Ayerst)	**Tablets:** 50 mg	In 100s.

[1] Hetrazan is available from Wyeth-Ayerst Labs without charge for compassionate use only. For more information, physicians should contact: Wyeth-Ayerst Labs, P.O. Box 8299, Philadelphia, PA 19101; (610) 688–4400.

Refer to the general discussion of these products in the Anthelmintics introduction.

Indications

Treatment of Bancroftian filariasis, onchocerciasis, ascariasis, tropical eosinophilia, loiasis.

Administration and Dosage

➤*Bancroft's filariasis, onchocerciasis and loiasis:* Usual dose is 2 mg/kg 3 times a day immediately following meals. When the disease is in the acute stage, continue treatment for 3 to 4 weeks. Recurrences have been more frequent with smaller doses. When, as a public health measure, it is desirable to treat large numbers of patients known to harbor microfilariae, use the same dosage schedule for 3 to 5 days. Laboratory tests in randomly selected patients are helpful in assessing efficacy of therapy.

➤*Ascariasis:*

Outpatients – 13 mg/kg, given once a day for 7 days, should reduce the number of worms by 85% to 100%. No pretreatment fasting or post-treatment purging is required. Expulsion of ascarids usually begins 1 or 2 days after therapy initiation.

Children – Give 6 to 10 mg/kg 3 times daily for 7 to 10 days. In particularly obstinate cases, an additional course consisting of 10 mg/kg 3 times daily is indicated.

➤*Tropical eosinophilia:* 13 mg/kg/day for 4 to 7 days.

Actions

➤*Pharmacology:* Diethylcarbamazine does not resemble other antiparasitic compounds. It is a synthetic organic compound which is highly specific for several common parasites and does not contain any toxic metallic elements.

The drug is effective against the following organisms: *Wuchereria bancrofti*, *Onchocerca volvulus*, *Loa loa* and *Ascaris lumbricoides*.

Diethylcarbamazine has demonstrated a low order of toxicity in animals.

Precautions

➤*Administration:* Administer carefully to avoid or to control allergic or other untoward reactions.

Adverse Reactions

➤*Wuchereria bancrofti:* Mild reactions are transient but fairly frequent. Headache, lassitude, weakness or general malaise are most common. Nausea, vomiting and skin rash occasionally occur. These effects are not considered serious and do not usually require discontinuation of therapy. However, it may be necessary to stop therapy when severe allergic phenomena appear in conjunction with skin rash. It has not yet been determined what proportion or type of reactions result from the death of the parasites rather than from the influence of the drug.

➤*Onchocerciasis:* Facial edema and pruritus, especially of the eyes, are often encountered. Severe reactions may develop after a single dose when intense infestations are treated. In such cases, only 1 dose should be given on the first day, 2 doses the second day and 3 daily thereafter for 30 days. If very severe reactions occur, discontinue the drug and start antihistamine therapy. After 1 or 2 days, therapy may be resumed, but if severe allergic phenomena again supervene, use the drug only with extreme caution.

➤*Ascariasis:* Giddiness, nausea, vomiting and malaise may occur more frequently following treatment of ascariasis in children who are malnourished or who suffer from various debilitating diseases.

PYRANTEL

otc	**Pin-Rid** (Apothecary)	**Capsules, soft gel:** 180 mg pyrantel pamoate (equiv. to 62.5 mg pyrantel base)	In 24s.
otc	**Reese's Pinworm** (Reese)		(RC P). In 24s.
otc	**Antiminth** (Pfizer Labs)	**Oral Suspension:** 50 mg pyrantel (as pamoate) per ml	Sorbitol. Caramel-currant flavor. In 60 ml.
otc	**Pin-X** (Effcon)	**Liquid:** 50 mg pyrantel (as pamoate) per ml	Sorbitol, parabens. Caramel flavor. In 30 ml.
otc	**Reese's Pinworm** (Reese)		In 30 ml.

Refer to the general discussion of these products in the Anthelmintics introduction.

Indications

➤*Helminths:* Treatment of ascariasis (roundworm infection) and enterobiasis (pinworm infection).

Administration and Dosage

A single dose of 11 mg/kg (5 mg/lb). Maximum total dose is 1 g.

May be administered without regard to ingestion of food or time of day. Purging is not necessary. May be taken with milk or fruit juices.

Actions

➤*Pharmacology:* Pyrantel is a depolarizing neuromuscular blocking agent, resulting in spastic paralysis of the worm. It also inhibits cholinesterases. It is active against *Enterobius vermicularis* (pinworm) and *Ascaris lumbricoides* (roundworm); it is also effective against *Ancylostoma duodenale* (hookworm).

➤*Pharmacokinetics:* Pyrantel is poorly absorbed from the GI tract. Plasma levels of unchanged drug are low. Greater than 50% is excreted in feces as unchanged drug; ≤ 7% of the dose is found in the urine as parent drug and metabolites.

Contraindications

Hepatic disease; pregnancy (see Warnings); hypersensitivity to pyrantel.

Warnings

➤*Pregnancy:* Do not use during pregnancy unless otherwise directed by a physician.

➤*Children:* Safety and efficacy for use in children < 2 years have not been established.

Drug Interactions

➤*Piperazine:* In ascariasis, pyrantel and piperazine are mutually antagonistic; therefore, concomitant use is unwise.

➤*Theophylline:* Serum levels increased in a pediatric patient following pyrantel pamoate administration. Further study is needed.

Adverse Reactions

➤*CNS:* Headache; dizziness; drowsiness; insomnia.

➤*Dermatologic:* Rash.

➤*GI:* Anorexia; nausea; vomiting; abdominal cramps; diarrhea.

Patient Information

A single dose is required. The dose is based on body weight.

May be taken with food, milk, juice or on an empty stomach anytime during the day. Be certain to take the entire dose.

Using a laxative after taking the drug to facilitate removal of the parasites is not necessary.

➤*Pinworm infections:* These are easily spread to others. If one family member has a pinworm infection, treat all family members in close contact with the patient. This decreases the chance of spreading the infection.

Strict hygiene is essential to prevent reinfection. Disinfect toilet facilities daily. Change and launder undergarments, bed linens, towels and nightclothes daily.

A package insert is available for patients containing the following information: Symptoms of pinworm infestations; how to find and identify the pinworm; pinworm life cycle; how it is spread from person to person.

PRAZIQUANTEL

Rx	Biltricide (Bayer)	Tablets: 600 mg	(Bayer LG). White to orange-tinged, oblong, tri-scored. Film-coated. In 6s.

Refer to the general discussion of these products in the Anthelmintics introduction.

Indications

For infections caused by the following: All species of schistosoma (eg, *Schistosoma mekongi, S. japonicum, S. mansoni,* and *S. hematobium*); liver flukes, *Clonorchis sinensis/Opisthorchis viverrini* (approval of this indication was based on studies in which the 2 species were not differentiated).

➤*Unlabeled uses:* Praziquantel has been used in the treatment of neurocysticercosis. It may also be beneficial in the treatment of other tissue flukes (eg, *Opisthorchis felineus, Paragonimus westermani,* and other species, toxemic schisto, Katayama fever), intestinal flukes (eg, *Heterophyes heterophyes, Fasciolopsis buski, Metagonimus yokogawai, Paragonimus westermani*), and intestinal cestodes (eg, *Diphyllobothrium latum, Taenia saginata* and *T. solium, Dipylidium caninum, Hymenolepis nana,* and *H. diminuta*).

Administration and Dosage

➤*Schistosomiasis:* 3 doses of 20 mg/kg as a 1 day treatment.

➤*Clonorchiasis and opisthorchiasis:* 3 doses of 25 mg/kg as a 1 day treatment.

The interval between the doses should not be < 4 and not > 6 hours.

Swallow the tablets unchewed with some liquid during meals. Keeping the tablets or the segments thereof in the mouth may reveal a bitter taste that can produce gagging or vomiting.

Segments are broken off by pressing the score (notch) with thumbnails. If ¼ of a tablet is required, this is best achieved by breaking the segment from the outer end.

Actions

➤*Pharmacology:* Praziquantel increases cell membrane permeability in susceptible worms, resulting in a loss of intracellular calcium, massive contractions, and paralysis of their musculature. The drug further results in vacuolization and disintegration of the schistosome tegument. This effect is followed by attachment of phagocytes to the parasite and death.

➤*Pharmacokinetics:* Praziquantel is rapidly absorbed (80%), reaching maximal serum concentration in 1 to 3 hours. CSF levels are ≈ 14% to 20% the total amount of drug in plasma. It undergoes significant first-pass biotransformation and the elimination half-life is 0.8 to 1.5 hours. Metabolites are excreted primarily in urine.

Contraindications

Previous hypersensitivity to praziquantel; ocular cysticercosis.

Warnings

➤*Ocular cysticercosis:* Because parasite destruction within the eyes may cause irreparable lesions, do not treat ocular cysticercosis with praziquantel.

➤*Pregnancy: Category B.* An increase in the abortion rate was found in rats at 3 times the single human therapeutic dose. There are no adequate and well-controlled studies in pregnant women. Use this drug during pregnancy only if clearly needed.

➤*Lactation:* Praziquantel appeared in breast milk at a concentration of ≈ 25% that of maternal serum. Do not nurse during treatment or the subsequent 72 hours.

➤*Children:* Safety in children < 4 years of age has not been established.

Precautions

➤*Hepatic effects:* Minimal increases in liver enzymes have occurred in some patients.

➤*Cerebral cysticercosis:* When schistosomiasis or fluke infection is found to be associated with cerebral cysticercosis, hospitalize the patient for the duration of treatment.

➤*Hazardous tasks:* May produce dizziness or drowsiness; observe caution while driving or performing other tasks requiring alertness on the day of and the day after treatment.

Drug Interactions

➤*H₂ antagonists:* Plasma concentrations of praziquantel may be elevated, increasing the effectiveness and risk of adverse reactions.

Adverse Reactions

In general, praziquantel is very well tolerated. Side effects are usually mild and transient and do not need treatment but may be more frequent or serious in patients with a heavy worm burden.

In order of severity: Malaise; headache; dizziness; abdominal discomfort (with or without nausea); rising temperature; urticaria (rare). Such symptoms can, however, also result from the infection itself. In patients with liver impairment caused by the infection, no adverse effects occurred that necessitated restriction in use.

Overdosage

In the event of overdose, give a fast-acting laxative.

Patient Information

Take with liquids during meals. Do not chew tablets.

May cause dizziness or drowsiness; observe caution while driving or performing other tasks requiring alertness.

IVERMECTIN

Rx	Stromectol (Merck)	Tablets: 3 mg	(MSD 32) White. In UD 20s.
		6 mg	(MSD 139). White, scored. In UD 10s.

Indications

➤*Strongyloidiasis of the intestinal tract:* Treatment of intestinal (eg, nondisseminated) strongyloidiasis caused by the nematode parasite *Strongyloides stercoralis.*

➤*Onchocerciasis:* Treatment of onchocerciasis caused by the nematode parasite *Onchocerca volvulus.*

Note – Ivermectin has no activity against adult *Onchocerca volvulus* parasites. The adult parasites reside in subcutaneous nodules, which are infrequently palpable. Surgical excision of these nodules (nodulectomy) may be considered in the management of patients with onchocerciasis, since this procedure will eliminate the microfilariae-producing parasites.

➤*Unlabeled uses:* Ivermectin has been found to be effective for the treatment and prophylaxis of infections with Loa loa and *Wucheria bancrofti,* scabies, and human cutaneous larva migrans.

Administration and Dosage

➤*Approved by the FDA:* November 1996.

➤*Strongyloidiasis:* The recommended dosage for the treatment of strongyloidiasis is a single oral dose designed to provide ≈ 200 mcg/kg. Take tablets with water. In general, additional doses are not necessary. Perform follow-up stool examinations to verify eradication of infection.

Dosage Guidelines for Ivermectin for Strongyloidiasis		
	Single oral dose (# of tablets)	
Body weight (kg)	3 mg tablets	6 mg tablets
15 to 24	1	0.5
25 to 35	2	1
36 to 50	3	1.5
51 to 65	4	2

Dosage Guidelines for Ivermectin for Strongyloidiasis		
	Single oral dose (# of tablets)	
Body weight (kg)	3 mg tablets	6 mg tablets
66 to 79	5	2.5
≥ 80	200 mcg/kg	200 mcg/kg

➤*Onchocerciasis:* The recommended dosage for treatment of onchocerciasis is a single oral dose designed to provide ≈ 150 mcg/kg. Take tablets with water. In mass distribution campaigns in international treatment programs, the most commonly used dose interval is 12 months. For the treatment of individual patients, consider retreatment at intervals as short as 3 months.

Dosage Guidelines for Ivermectin for Onchocerciasis		
	Single oral dose (# of tablets)	
Body weight (kg)	3 mg tablets	6 mg tablets
15 to 25	1	0.5
26 to 44	2	1
45 to 64	3	1.5
65 to 84	4	2
≥ 85	150 mcg/kg	150 mcg/kg

➤*Storage/Stability:* Store at < 30°C (86°F).

Actions

➤*Pharmacology:* Ivermectin is a semisynthetic anthelmintic agent. It is derived from the avermectins, a class of highly active broad-spectrum antiparasitic agents isolated from the fermentation products of *Streptomyces avermitilis.*

Compounds of the avermectin class bind selectively and with high affinity to glutamate-gated chloride ion channels that occur in invertebrate nerve and muscle cells. This leads to an increase in the perme-

IVERMECTIN

ability of the cell membrane to chloride ions with hyperpolarization of the nerve or muscle cell, resulting in paralysis and death of the parasite. Compounds of this class may also interact with other ligand-gated chloride channels, such as those gated by the neurotransmitter gamma-aminobutyric acid (GABA).

The selective activity of this class is attributable to the fact that some mammals do not have glutamate-gated chloride channels and that the avermectins have a low affinity for mammalian ligand-gated chloride channels.

➤*Pharmacokinetics:*

Absorption/Distribution – Following oral administration, plasma concentrations are approximately proportional to the dose. In 2 studies, after single 12 mg doses in fasting, healthy volunteers (representing a mean dose of 165 mcg/kg), the mean peak plasma concentrations of the major component (H_2B_{1a}) were 46.6 ng/mL (range, 16.4 to 101.1) and 30.6 ng/mL (range, 13.9 to 68.4), respectively, at ≈ 4 hours after dosing. The apparent plasma half-life of ivermectin is approximately ≥ 16 hours following oral administration. Ivermectin does not readily cross the blood-brain barrier.

Metabolism/Excretion – Ivermectin is metabolized in the liver, and ivermectin or its metabolites are excreted almost exclusively in the feces over an estimated 12 days, with < 1% of the administered dose excreted in the urine.

➤*Microbiology:* Ivermectin is active against various life-cycle stages of many but not all nematodes. It is active against the tissue microfilariae of *Onchocerca volvulus* but not against the adult form. Its activity against *Strongyloides stercoralis* is limited to the intestinal stages.

➤*Clinical trials:*

Strongyloidiasis – Two studies showed the efficacy was significantly greater for ivermectin (a single dose of 170 to 200 mcg/kg) than for albendazole (200 mg twice daily for 3 days). Another study showed ivermectin administered as a single dose of 200 mcg/kg for 1 day was as efficacious as thiabendazole administered at 25 mg/kg twice daily for 3 days.

Contraindications

Hypersensitivity to any component of this product.

Warnings

➤*Mazzotti reaction:* Historical data have shown that microfilaricidal drugs, such as diethylcarbamazine citrate (DEC-C), may cause cutaneous or systemic reactions of varying severity (the Mazzotti reaction) and ophthalmological reactions in patients with onchocerciasis. These reactions are probably caused by allergic and inflammatory responses to the death of microfilariae. Patients treated with ivermectin for onchocerciasis may experience these reactions in addition to clinical adverse reactions possibly, probably, or definitely related to the drug itself.

Oral hydration, recumbency, IV normal saline, or parenteral corticosteroids have been used to treat postural hypotension. Antihistamines or aspirin have been used for most mild-to-moderate Mazzotti reactions.

➤*Pregnancy: Category C.* Ivermectin was teratogenic in mice, rats, and rabbits when given in repeated doses of 0.2, 8.1, and 4.5 times the maximum recommended human dose, respectively (on a mg/m^2/day basis). Teratogenicity was characterized in the 3 species tested by cleft palate; clubbed forepaws were additionally observed in rabbits. There are no adequate and well-controlled studies in pregnant women. Do not use ivermectin during pregnancy because safety in pregnancy has not been established.

➤*Lactation:* Ivermectin is excreted in breast milk in low concentrations. Treat mothers who intend to breastfeed only when the risk of delayed treatment to the mother outweighs the possible risk to the newborn.

➤*Children:* Safety and efficacy in pediatric patients weighing < 15 kg (33 lbs) have not been established.

Precautions

➤*Hyperreactive onchodermatitis:* After treatment with microfilaricidal drugs, patients with hyperreactive onchodermatitis (sowda) may be more likely than others to experience severe adverse reactions, especially edema and aggravation of onchodermatitis.

➤*Loiasis co-infection:* Rarely, patients with onchocerciasis who are also heavily infected with Loa loa may develop a serious or even fatal encephalopathy either spontaneously or following treatment with an effective microfilaricide. This syndrome has been seen very rarely following the use of ivermectin; a cause and effect relationship has not been established. Pretreatment assessment for loiasis and careful posttreatment follow-up should be implemented.

➤*Immunocompromised hosts:* In immunocompromised (including HIV-infected) patients being treated for intestinal strongyloidiasis, repeated courses of therapy may be required. Adequate and well controlled clinical studies have not been conducted in such patients to determine the optimal dosing regimen. Several treatments (eg, at 2-week intervals) may be required, and cure may not be achievable. Control of extra-intestinal strongyloidiasis in these patients is difficult, and suppressive therapy (eg, once per month) may be helpful.

Adverse Reactions

In comparative trials, patients treated with ivermectin experienced more abdominal distention and chest discomfort than patients treated with albendazole. Ivermectin was better tolerated than thiabendazole in comparative studies involving 37 patients treated with thiabendazole.

➤*Strongyloidiasis:*

CNS – Dizziness (2.8%); somnolence, tremor, vertigo (0.9%).

Dermatologic – Pruritus (2.8%); rash, urticaria (0.9%).

GI – Diarrhea, nausea (1.8%); anorexia, constipation, vomiting (0.9%).

Miscellaneous – Asthenia/fatigue, abdominal pain (0.9%).

Lab test abnormalities – Decrease in leukocyte count (3%); elevation in ALT or AST (2%); leukopenia and anemia (1 patient).

➤*Onchocerciasis:*

Mazzotti reaction: Pruritus (27.5%); skin involvement including edema, papular and pustular or frank urticarial rash (22.7%); fever (22.6%); inguinal lymph node enlargement and tenderness (12.6% and 13.9%, respectively); axillary lymph node enlargement and tenderness (11% and 4.4%, respectively); arthralgia/synovitis (9.3%); cervical lymph node enlargement and tenderness (5.3% and 1.2%, respectively); other lymph node enlargement and tenderness (3% and 1.9%, respectively) (see Warnings).

Ophthalmic – Ophthalmological conditions were examined in 963 adult patients before treatment, at day 3, and at months 3 and 6 after treatment with 100 to 200 mcg/kg ivermectin. Changes observed were primarily deterioration from baseline 3 days posttreatment. Most changes either returned to baseline condition or improved over baseline severity at the 3- and 6-month visits. The percentages of patients with worsening of the following conditions at day 3, month 3 and 6, respectively, were Limbitis, 5.5%, 4.8%, and 3.5%, and punctate opacity, 1.8%, 1.8%, and 1.4%.

The following ophthalmological side effects occur because of the disease itself but have also been reported after treatment with ivermectin: Abnormal sensation in the eyes; anterior uveitis; chorioretinitis or choroiditis; conjunctivitis; eyelid edema; keratitis; limbitis. These have rarely been severe or associated with loss of vision and have generally resolved without corticosteroid treatment.

Note – The Mazzotti-type and ophthalmologic reactions associated with the treatment of onchocerciasis or the disease itself would not be expected to occur in strongyloidiasis patients treated with ivermectin.

Miscellaneous – Tachycardia (3.5%); peripheral edema (3.2%); facial edema (1.2%); orthostatic hypotension (1.1%); drug-related headache, myalgia (< 1%); hypotension (mainly orthostatic hypotension); worsening of bronchial asthma. A similar safety profile was observed in an open study in pediatric patients 6 to 13 years of age.

➤*Lab test abnormalities:* Eosinophilia (3%); hemoglobin increase (1%).

Overdosage

➤*Symptoms:* Significant lethality was observed in mice and rats after single oral doses of 25 to 50 mg/kg and 40 to 50 mg/kg, respectively. At these doses, treatment-related signs observed in these animals included ataxia, bradypnea, decreased activity, emesis, mydriasis, ptosis, and tremors.

In accidental intoxication with or significant exposure to unknown quantities of veterinary formulations of ivermectin in humans by ingestion, inhalation, injection, or exposure to body surfaces, the following adverse effects have been reported most frequently: Asthenia, diarrhea, dizziness, edema, headache, nausea, rash, and vomiting. Other adverse effects that have been reported include: Abdominal pain, ataxia, dyspnea, paresthesia, seizure, and urticaria.

➤*Treatment:* In case of accidental poisoning, supportive therapy, if indicated, should include parenteral fluids and electrolytes, respiratory support (oxygen and mechanical ventilation if necessary) and pressor agents if clinically significant hypotension is present. Induce emesis or gastric lavage as soon as possible, followed by purgatives and other routine antipoison measures if needed to prevent absorption of ingested material.

Patient Information

Take ivermectin with water.

➤*Strongyloidiasis:* Remind the patient of the need for repeated stool examinations to document clearance of infection.

➤*Onchocerciasis:* Remind the patient that treatment with ivermectin does not kill the adult *Onchocerca* parasites; therefore, repeated follow-up and retreatment is usually required.

CDC ANTI-INFECTIVE AGENTS

In addition to the commercially available anti-infective agents, the Centers for Disease Control and Prevention (CDC) can supply several investigational agents upon request. These agents may be requested from the Drug Service, Division of Host Factors, Center for Infectious Disease, by calling 404-639-3670, 8:00 am to 4:30 pm EST Monday through Friday; for emergencies (evenings, weekends, or holidays), call 404-639-2888.

Indications

Available CDC Anti-Infective Agents

Generic name	Trade name	Disease/Infestation	Organism
Bithionol	Lorothidol Bitin	Paragonimiasis Fascioliasis	Paragonimus sp. Fasciola hepatica
Dehydroemetine	Mebadin	Extraintestinal amebiasis that fails to respond to metronidazole Amebic dysentery	Entamoeba histolytica
Diethylcarbamazine citrate (DEC)	Hetrazan	Lymphatic filariasis Tropical pulmonary eosinophilia Loiasis	Wuchereria bancrofti Brugia malayi Brugia timori
Melarsoprol	Arsobal Mel B	Trypanosomiasis (African sleeping sickness) with neurologic involvement and for the treatment of early African (Gambian and Rhodesian) sleeping sickness that is resistant to treatment with suramin or pentamidine	Trypanosoma brucei gambiense Trypanosoma brucei rhodesiense
Nifurtimox	Lampit Bayer 2502	Chagas' disease	Trypanosoma cruzi
Sodium antimony gluconate (sodium stibogluconate)	Pentostam	Leishmaniasis (visceral [kala azar], cutaneous [Oriental sore], or mucosal)	Leishmania sp.
Suramin	Fourneau 309 Bayer 205 Germanin Moranyl Belganyl Naphuride Antrypol	Trypanosomiasis (African sleeping sickness) Onchocerciasis (river blindness)	Trypanosoma brucei rhodesiense Trypanosoma brucei gambiense (second-line therapy to pentamidine) Onchocerca volvulus

The following general information applies to all immune sera. For specific information on individual agents, refer to specific monographs:
- Cytomegalovirus Immune Globulin, IV (CMV-IGIV)
- Hepatitis B Immune Globulin (HBIG)
- Immune Globulin, IM (IGIM)
- Immune Globulin, IV (IGIV)
- Lymphocyte Immune Globulin, Antithymocyte Globulin (Equine) (ATG equine)
- Antithymocyte Globulin (Rabbit) (ATG rabbit)
- Rabies Immune Globulin (RIG)
- Rh$_o$(D) Immune Globulin, IM (Rh$_o$[D] IGIM)
- Rh$_o$(D) Immune Globulin, IV (Rh$_o$[D] IGIV)
- Rh$_o$(D) Immune Globulin Micro-dose (Rh$_o$[D] IG Micro-dose)
- Respiratory Syncytial Virus Immune Globulin, IV (RSV-IGIV)
- Tetanus Immune Globulin (TIG)
- Varicella-Zoster Immune Globulin (VZIG)

WARNING

Immune globulin IV (human): IGIV (human) products have been associated with renal dysfunction, acute renal failure, osmotic nephrosis, and death. Patients predisposed to acute renal failure include patients with any degree of pre-existing renal insufficiency, diabetes mellitus, > 65 years of age, volume depletion, sepsis, paraproteinemia, or patients receiving known nephrotoxic drugs. Especially in such patients, administer IGIV products at the minimum concentration available and the minimum rate of infusion practicable. While these reports of renal dysfunction and acute renal failure have been associated with the use of many of the licensed IGIV products, those containing sucrose as a stabilizer accounted for a disproportionate share of the total number. See Precautions and Administration and Dosage sections for important information intended to reduce the risk of acute renal failure. (*Polygam S/D, Gammagard S/D, Gamimune N, Venoglobulin-S,* and *Iveegam* do not contain sucrose).

Antithymocyte globulin (equine): Only physicians experienced in immunosuppressive therapy in the treatment of renal transplant or aplastic anemia patients should use **antithymocyte globulin** (equine).

Treat patients receiving antithymocyte globulin (equine) in facilities equipped and staffed with adequate laboratory and supportive medical resources.

Antithymocyte globulin (rabbit): **Antithymocyte globulin** (rabbit) should only be used by physicians experienced in immunosuppressive therapy for the management of renal transplant patients.

Indications

To provide passive immunization to ≥ 1 infectious diseases. Protection will be of rapid onset, but of short duration (1 to 3 months). See individual monographs for specific indications.

Actions

►*Pharmacology:*

CMV-IGIV – This product contains IgG antibodies representative of the large number of healthy people who contributed to the plasma pools from which the product was derived. The globulin contains a relatively high concentration of antibodies directed against CMV. In people who may be exposed to CMV, this product can raise the relevant antibodies to levels sufficient to attenuate or reduce the incidence of serious CMV disease.

HBIG – HBIG provides passive immunization for individuals exposed to the hepatitis B virus (HBV). The administration of the usual recommended dose of this immune globulin generally results in a detectable level of circulating anti-HBs, which persists for ≈ 2 months or longer.

IGIM – IGIM is a transient source of IgG that specifically and nonspecifically inactivates various bacteria, viruses, and fungi. IgG antibodies activate the complement system, promote opsonization, neutralize microorganisms and their toxins, and participate in antibody-dependent cytolytic reactions.

Hepatitis A: IGIM is 80% to 95% effective in preventing hepatitis A, depending on the temporal relation between administration and exposure and on the severity of exposure.

Measles: IGIM reduces the risk of clinical evidence of measles by an estimated 50%. A lower incidence of measles encephalitis also has been associated with the use of IGIM.

Varicella: IGIM reduces severity of disease, as measured by temperature and the number of pox.

IGIV – IGIV passively supplies a broad spectrum of IgG antibodies against bacterial, viral, parasitic, and mycoplasmic antigens. IGIV antibodies act through a variety of mechanisms, including antimicrobial or antitoxin neutralization. IGIV appears to work by contributing anti-idiotypic antibodies that bind and neutralize pathogenic autoantibodies. There may also be negative feedback and down-regulation of antibody production. Other mechanisms may involve binding to CD5 receptors, interleukin-1a, IL-6, tumor necrosis factor-alpha, and T-cell receptors, suppressing pathogenic cytokines and phagocytes. IGIV also interferes with pathogenic effects of products of complement activation.

ATG equine – ATG equine is a lymphocyte-selective immunosuppressant. It reduces the number of circulating, thymus-dependent lymphocytes that form rosettes with sheep erythrocytes. This antilymphocytic effect is believed to reflect an alteration of the function of the T-lymphocytes, which are responsible, in part, for cell-mediated immunity and are involved in humoral immunity. It also contains low concentrations of antibodies against other formed elements of the blood. In rhesus and cynomolgus monkeys, this drug reduces lymphocytes in the thymus-dependent areas of the spleen and lymph nodes. It also decreases the circulating sheep-erythrocyte-rosetting lymphocytes that can be detected, but ordinarily does not cause severe lymphopenia.

In general, when administered with other immunosuppressive therapy, such as antimetabolites and corticosteroids, the patient's own antibody response to horse gamma globulin is minimal.

Precise methods of determining potency have not been established; thus activity may potentially vary from lot to lot.

In general, ATG equine enables a 1 year graft survival rate of ≥ 80%. Graft and patient survival are dependent on whether the transplanted organ is harvested from a living or deceased host, the degree of antigenic matching, the combination of immunosuppressive drugs delivered, and other factors.

ATG rabbit – The mechanism of action by which polyclonal antilymphocyte preparations suppress immune responses is not fully understood. Possible mechanisms by which ATG rabbit may induce immunosuppression in vivo include: T-cell clearance from the circulation and modulation of T-cell activation, homing, and cytotoxic activities. ATG rabbit includes antibodies against T-cell markers such as CD2, CD3, CD4, CD8, CD11a, CD18, CD25, CD44, CD45, HLA-DR, HLA Class 1 heavy chains, and β2 microglobulin. In vitro, ATG rabbit (concentrations > 0.1 mg/mL) mediates T-cell suppressive effects via inhibition of proliferative responses to several mitogens. In patients, T-cell depletion is usually observed within a day from initiating ATG rabbit therapy. ATG rabbit has not been shown to be effective for treating antibody (humoral) mediated rejections.

RIG – Rabies antibody provides passive protection when given immediately to individuals exposed to rabies virus. RIG of adequate potency was used in conjunction with rabies vaccine of duck embryo origin. When a globulin dose of 20 IU/kg of rabies antibody was given simultaneously with the first dose of vaccine, levels of passive rabies antibody were detected 24 hours after injection in all individuals. There was minimal or no interference with the immune response to the initial and subsequent doses of vaccine, including booster doses. Studies of RIG given with the first of 5 doses of HDCV confirmed that passive immunization with 20 IU/kg of RIG provides maximum circulating antibody with minimum interference of active immunization by HDCV.

Rh$_o$(D) IGIM – Rh$_o$(D) IGIM acts by suppressing the immune response of Rh$_o$(D)-negative individuals to Rh$_o$(D)-positive red blood cells. The mechanism of action of the full dose is not fully understood.

Passive immunization with Rh$_o$(D) prevents the formation of anti-Rh$_o$(D) antibodies in nonsensitized Rh$_o$(D) antigen-negative individuals who receive Rh$_o$(D) antigen-positive red blood cells. Rh$_o$(D) antibody binds circulating antigen, thus preventing stimulation of antigen-sensitive lymphocytes and the resulting production of anti-Rh$_o$(D). Prevention of Rh$_o$(D) sensitization in turn prevents hemolytic disease of the fetus and newborn in subsequent Rh$_o$(D) antigen-positive children.

Rh$_o$(D) IGIV –

Suppression of Rh isoimmunization: Rh$_o$(D) IGIV is used to suppress the immune response of nonsensitized Rh$_o$(D)-negative individuals following Rh$_o$(D)-positive red blood cell exposure by fetomaternal hemorrhage during delivery of an Rh$_o$(D)-positive infant, abortion (spontaneous or induced), amniocentesis, abdominal trauma, or mismatched transfusion. The mechanism of action is not completely understood.

Idiopathic thrombocytopenic purpura (ITP): The mechanism of action is not completely understood, but is thought to be due to the formation of anti-Rh$_o$(D) (anti-D)-coated RBC complexes resulting in Fc receptor blockade, thus sparing antibody-coated platelets.

Rh$_o$(D) IG micro-dose – Rh$_o$(D) IG micro-dose is used to prevent the formation of anti-Rh$_o$(D) antibody in Rh$_o$(D)-negative women who are exposed to the Rh$_o$(D) antigen at the time of spontaneous or induced abortion (up to 12 weeks gestation). Rh$_o$(D) IG micro-dose suppresses the stimulation of active immunity by Rh$_o$(D)-positive fetal erythrocytes that may enter the maternal circulation at the time of termination of the pregnancy.

The amount of anti-Rh$_o$(D) in Rh$_o$(D) IG micro-dose has been shown to effectively prevent material isosensitization to the Rh$_o$(D) antigens following spontaneous or induced abortion occurring up to the 12th week of gestation. After the 12th week of gestation, a standard dose of Rh$_o$(D) IGIM full dose is indicated.

Rh$_o$(D) IG micro-dose acts by suppressing the immune response of Rh-negative individuals to Rh-positive red blood cells. The risk of immunization is related to the number of D-positive red blood cells received. The risk was found to be 3% when 0.1 mL of fetal red blood cells is present in the mother and 65% when 5 mL is present. In the first 12 weeks of gestation, the total volume of red blood cells in the fetus is estimated at < 2.5 mL.

RSV-IGIV – RSV-IGIV is a sterile liquid immunoglobulin G (IgG) containing neutralizing antibody to respiratory syncytial virus (RSV). The immunoglobulin is purified from pooled adult human plasma selected for high titers of neutralizing antibody against RSV. A widely utilized solvent-detergent viral inactivation process is used to decrease the possibility of transmission of bloodborne pathogens. Each milliliter contains 50 ± 10 mg immunoglobulin, primarily IgG, and trace amounts of IgA and IgM.

TIG – TIG is an antibody preparation containing antitoxin that neutralizes the free form of the powerful tetanus exotoxin. TIG does not affect toxin fixed to nerve tissue.

VZIG – VZIG is the globulin fraction of human plasma, primarily immunoglobulin G (IgG) found in routine screening of normal volunteer blood donors. When absorbed into the circulation, the antibodies persist for ≥ 1 month. The precise concentration of varicella-zoster antibodies that must be achieved or maintained in order to attenuate varicella is not known. In the clinical studies demonstrating its efficacy, VZIG was given within 96 hours of chickenpox exposure. It significantly reduces mortality and morbidity from varicella among immunodeficient children.

➤*Pharmacokinetics:* Immunoglobulins are primarily eliminated by catabolism.

CMV-IGIV – The onset of action is rapid. The mean half-life is 21 days, shorter in transplant recipients, where half-lives have been measured as 8 days immediately after transplant, or 13 to 15 days if given ≥ 60 days after transplant. The protective level is unknown.

HBIG – Antibodies appear within 1 to 6 days after IM administration and peak in 3 to 11 days. The mean half-life is 17 to 25 days (range, 6 to 35) and clinical protection typically persists for ≈ 2 months. The protective level of anti-HBs titer is ≥ 10 mIU/mL. The clearance rate was 0.433 ± 0.144 L/day, with a volume of distribution of 15.3 ± 6.2 L.

IGIM – IgG titers peak 2 to 5 days after IM injection. Mean IgG half-life in circulation of people with normal IgG levels is 23 days. Protective levels are 200 mg/100 mL of plasma as a target in immunoglobulin replacement therapy.

IGIV – The onset is rapid. In general, the mean half-life in healthy people is 18 to 25 days, although there is tremendous intersubject variability. Fever or infection may decrease antibody half-life because of increased catabolism or consumption, respectively. In idiopathic thrombocytopenic pupura (ITP), the increase in platelets usually lasts from several days to several weeks, although it may rarely persist for ≥ 1 year. In a group of burn patients, the half-life ranged from 47 to 154 days.

IV administration makes essentially 100% of the dose immediately available in the recipient's circulation. After ≈ 6 days, $\approx 50\%$ of the body pool partitions into the extravascular space, with the balance remaining in the serum.

Expect a rapid fall in serum IgG in the first week after infusion, mainly because of equilibration of IgG between plasma and the extravascular space. The decrease averages 40% of peak level after infusion; within 24 hours, 30% of a single dose is removed from circulation to extravascular fluid, tissue, cells, and catabolism.

ATG equine – Onset is rapid. Peak plasma level of equine IgG occurs after 5 days of infusion at 10 mg/kg/day. Peak values vary depending on recipient's ability to catabolize equine IgG. In a small study, mean peak plasma value was 727 ± 310 mcg/mL. Rosette-forming cells decrease immediately after beginning therapy. Recovery to normal values after therapy cessation is dependent on recipient's catabolic rate and, in some cases, upon length of therapy. Mean half-life is ≈ 5.7 days (range, 2.7 to 8.7 days).

ATG rabbit – After an IV dose of 1.25 to 1.5 mg/kg/day (over 4 hours for 7 to 11 days) 4 to 8 hours post-infusion, ATG rabbit levels were on average 21.5 mcg/mL (10 to 40 mcg/mL) with a half-life of 2 to 3 days after the first dose, and 87 mcg/mL (23 to 170 mcg/mL) after the last dose.

RIG – Adequate levels of antibody appear in serum within 24 hours and peak within 2 to 13 days. Because rabies vaccine takes ≈ 1 week to induce active immunity, the importance of RIG cannot be overemphasized. The mean serum half-life of rabies antibody is 24 days, consistent with the 21-day half-life expected of IgG.

TIG – The efficacy is high, with a rapid onset of action and peak serum titer occurring within 2 to 3 days after IM injection. The mean half-life is 3.5 to 4.5 weeks and adequate antibody titer persists for ≈ 4 weeks. The protective level is 0.01 antitoxin units/mL; 250 units yield at least 0.01 IU/mL of tetanus antitoxin in serum for 4 weeks, an adequate response.

Rh$_o$(D) IGIM (human) – The onset of action is prompt. The mean half-life is 23 to 26 days, with antibody titers $\geq 1:5$ by RFFIT indicative of adequate protection.

Rh$_o$(D) immune globulin, when administered within 72 hours of a full-term delivery of an Rh$_o$(D)-positive infant by an Rh$_o$(D)-negative mother, will reduce the incidence of Rh isoimmunization from between 12% and 13% to between 1% and 2%. The 1% to 2% range is due, for the most part, to isoimmunization during the last trimester of pregnancy.

When treatment is given both antenatally at 28 weeks gestation and postpartum, the Rh immunization rate drops to $\approx 0.1\%$.

When 600 IU (120 mcg) of Rh$_o$(D) IGIV is given to pregnant women, passive anti-Rh$_o$(D) antibodies are not detectable in the circulation for > 6 weeks; therefore, give a dose of 1500 IU (300 mcg) for antenatal administration.

IM vs IV administration: In a clinical study involving Rh$_o$(D)-negative volunteers, 2 subjects were given 600 IU (120 mcg) IM and 2 subjects were given this dose IV. Peak levels (36 to 48 ng/mL) were reached within 2 hours of IV administration; for IM, peak levels (18 to 19 ng/mL) were reached at 5 to 10 days. The calculated areas under the curve were the same for both routes of administration. The half-life was ≈ 24 and 30 days following IV and IM administration, respectively.

Rh$_o$(D) IG micro-dose – Administration of Rh$_o$(D) IG micro-dose within 3 hours following abortion was 100% effective in preventing Rh immunization. Studies showed Rh$_o$(D) IG micro-dose to be effective when given as long as 72 hours after the infusion of Rh-positive red cells. A lesser degree of protection is afforded if the antibody is administered beyond this time period.

RSV-IGIV – The onset of action is rapid with the mean half-life of serum RSV neutralizing antibodies after RSV-IG infusion as 22 to 28 days. The protective level is not established. In one study, monthly doses of 750 mg/kg of RSV-IG attained trough geometric mean serum RSV neutralization antibody titers of $1:297 \pm 38$ (SE) 1 month after the first infusion, $1:477 \pm 85$ 1 month after the second infusion, $1:490 \pm 61$ 1 month after the third infusion, and $1:429 \pm 23$ 1 month after the fourth infusion.

VZIG – Onset of action is prompt, but the duration of protection is unknown. The mean half-life is 21 days. The concentration of varicella-zoster antibodies that must be achieved or maintained in order to attenuate varicella is unknown.

Contraindications

History of systemic allergic reactions following administration of human immunoglobulin preparations.

Allergic response to gamma globulin or anti-immunoglobulin A (IgA) antibodies.

Allergic response to thimerosal.

People with isolated immunoglobulin A (IgA) deficiency. Such people have the potential for developing antibodies to IgA and could have anaphylactic reactions to subsequent administration of blood products that contain IgA.

➤*IGIM:* Patients who have severe thrombocytopenia or any coagulation disorder that would contraindicate IM use.

➤*ATG equine:* Severe prior systemic reaction with the administration of antithymocyte globulin (equine) or other equine immunoglobulin preparations.

➤*ATG rabbit:* In patients with a history of allergy or anaphylaxis to rabbit proteins, or who have an acute viral illness.

➤*RIG (Imogam):* Rabies immune globulin should not be administered in repeated doses once vaccine treatment has been initiated. Repeating the dose may interfere with maximum active immunity expected from the vaccine.

➤*Rh$_o$(D) IGIV:* Anaphylactic or severe systemic reaction to any human immunoglobulin. Rh$_o$(D) immune globulin contains trace amounts of IgA (≈ 5 mcg per 600 IU [120 mcg] vial). Individuals who are deficient in IgA may have the potential for developing IgA antibodies and have anaphylactic reactions. Weigh the potential benefit of treatment with Rh$_o$(D) immune globulin against the potential for hypersensitivity reactions.

➤*Rh$_o$(D) IG micro-dose (MICRhoGAM):* Must not be used for any indication with continuation of pregnancy; not recommended for any indication beyond 12 weeks gestation.

Warnings

➤*Renal risks:* IGIV (Human) products have been reported to be associated with renal dysfunction, acute renal failure, osmotic nephrosis, and death. Patients predisposed to acute renal failure include patients with any degree of pre-existing renal insufficiency, diabetes mellitus, > 65 years of age, volume depletion, sepsis, paraproteinemia, or patients receiving known nephrotoxic drugs. Especially in such patients, IGIV products should be administered at the minimum concentrations available and at the minimum rate of infusion practical. While these reports of renal dysfunction and acute renal failure have been associated with the use of many IGIV products, those containing sucrose as a stabilizer (and given at daily doses of ≥ 400 mg/kg) account for a disproportionate share of the total number. See Precautions and Administration and Dosage sections for important information intended to reduce the risk of acute renal failure.

➤*Bloodborne viral transmission:* Most of these products are made from human plasma and like other plasma products, they carry the possibility for transmission of bloodborne pathogenic agents. The risk of transmission of recognized bloodborne viruses is considered to be low because of the screening of plasma donors, the collection and testing of plasma, through the application of viral elimination/reduction step such as alcohol fractionation, PEG/Bentonite precipitation and solvent-detergent treatment. Despite these measures, such products can still potentially transmit disease; therefore, the risk of infectious agents cannot be totally eliminated. Report all infections thought by the physician to have been possibly transmitted by these products to the manufacturer. Weigh the risks and benefits of the use of this product and discuss these with the patient.

➤*Route of administration:* Administer these agents only as indicated (eg, IM or IV). Inappropriate IV injections may cause a precipitous fall in blood pressure and a picture similar to anaphylaxis (ie, RIG). Administer IM.

➤*Rate of administration:* Except for hypersensitivity reactions, adverse reactions to IGIVs may be related to the rate of administration. Careful adherence to the infusion rate outlined under Administration and Dosage is therefore important. Have loop diuretics available for the management of patients who are at risk for fluid overload. Although systemic allergic reactions are rare (see Adverse Reactions), have epinephrine and diphenhydramine available for treatment of acute allergic symptoms.

➤*Immunoglobulin A deficiency:* People with isolated immunoglobulin A (IgA) deficiency have the potential for developing antibodies to IgA and could have anaphylactic reactions to subsequent administration of blood products that contain IgA.

➤*Aseptic meningitis syndrome (AMS):* Rare occurrences of AMS have been reported in association with IGIV treatment. AMS usually begins within several hours to 2 days following IGIV treatment and is characterized by symptoms including severe headache, drowsiness, fever, photophobia, painful eye movements, muscle rigidity, nausea, and vomiting. Cerebrospinal fluid studies generally demonstrate pleocytosis, predominately granulocytic, and elevated protein levels. Thoroughly evaluate patients exhibiting such signs and symptoms to rule out other causes of meningitis. AMS may occur more frequently in association with high-dose (2 g/kg) IGIV treatment. Discontinuation of IGIV treatment has resulted in remission of AMS within several days without sequelae.

➤*Bleeding complications:* As will all preparations administered by the IM route, bleeding complications may be encountered in patients with thrombocytopenia or other bleeding disorders.

➤*ATG equine:* Only physicians experienced in immunosuppressive therapy in the treatment of renal transplant or aplastic anemia patients should use lymphocyte immune globulin. Treat patients receiving lymphocyte immune globulin in facilities equipped and staffed with adequate laboratory and supportive medical resources.

Discontinuation – Discontinue treatment if any of the following occurs: Anaphylaxis; severe and unremitting thrombocytopenia and severe and unremitting leukopenia in renal transplant patients.

Hemolysis: Clinically significant hemolysis is rare. Treatment may include transfusion of erythrocytes; if necessary, administer IV mannitol, furosemide, sodium bicarbonate, and fluids. Severe and unremitting hemolysis may require discontinuation of therapy.

Thrombocytopenia: Thrombocytopenia is usually transient; platelet counts generally return to adequate levels without discontinuing therapy; platelet transfusions may be necessary in patients with aplastic anemia.

➤*ATG rabbit:* ATG rabbit should only be used by physicians experienced in immunosuppressive therapy for the treatment of renal transplant patients. Medical surveillance is required during ATG rabbit infusion.

Hematologic effects – Thrombocytopenia or neutropenia may result from crossreactive antibodies and is reversible following dose adjustments.

➤*Criteria for Rh$_o$(D) IGIV administration:* The criteria for an Rh-incompatible pregnancy requiring administration of Rh$_o$(D) immune globulin at 28 weeks gestation and within 72 hours after delivery are the following: The mother must be Rh$_o$(D) antigen-negative; the mother is carrying a child whose father is either Rh$_o$(D) antigen-positive or Rh$_o$(D) unknown; the infant is either Rh$_o$(D) antigen-positive or Rh$_o$(D) unknown; and the mother must not be previously sensitized to the Rh$_o$(D) antigen.

Rh$_o$D-negative or splenectomized patients – Do not administer Rh$_o$(D) immune globulin IV to Rh$_o$(D)-negative or splenectomized individuals as its efficacy in these patients has not been demonstrated.

➤*RSV-IGIV:*

Fluid overload – Infants with underlying pulmonary disease may be sensitive to the extra fluid volume. Infusion of RSV-IGIV, particularly in children with bronchopulmonary dysplasia (BPD), may precipitate symptoms of fluid overload. Overall, 8.4% of participants (1% premature and 13% BPD) received new or extra diuretics during the period 24 hours before through 48 hours after at least one of their infusions in the PREVENT trial. RSV-IGIV-related fluid overload was reported in 3 patients (1.2%) and RSV-IGIV-related respiratory distress was reported in 4 patients (1.6%); all had underlying BPD. These children were managed with diuretics or modification of the infusion rate and went on to receive subsequent infusions.

Complications related to fluid volume were recorded as a reason for incomplete or prolonged infusion in 2% of children receiving RSV-IGIV

(2.5% BPD and 1.1% premature) and in 1.5% of children receiving placebo. Children with clinically apparent fluid overload should not be infused with RSV-IGIV.

➤*Anaphylactic reactions:* Anaphylactic reactions (rare) may occur following injection of human immune globulin preparations. Anaphylaxis is more likely if immune globulin is given IV; therefore, except for IGIV, these products must only be given IM. In highly allergic individuals, repeated injections may lead to anaphylactic shock.

➤*Hypersensitivity reactions:* Give with caution to patients with prior systemic allergic reactions following use of human immunoglobulin preparations. Hypersensitivity reactions are rare; the incidence may be increased by use of large IM doses or repeated injections of immune globulin. Have epinephrine available for treatment of acute allergic symptoms. Refer to Management of Acute Hypersensitivity Reactions.

Severe reactions – Severe reactions, such as anaphylaxis or angioneurotic edema, have been reported in association with IV immunoglobulins, even in patients not known to be sensitive to human immunoglobulins or blood products. If hypotension, anaphylaxis, or severe allergic reaction occurs, discontinue infusion and administer epinephrine (1:1000) as required. Administer steroids, assist respiration, and provide other resuscitative measures. If hypotension occurs, stop infusion and stabilize blood pressure with pressors if necessary. Respiratory distress may also indicate anaphylaxis. Pain in the chest, flank, or back may indicate anaphylaxis or hemolysis. Treat appropriately with an antihistamine, epinephrine, corticosteroids, or some combination of the three. Refer to Management of Acute Hypersensitivity Reactions.

Although systemic reactions to immunoglobulin preparations are rare, epinephrine should be available for treatment of acute anaphylactic symptoms.

➤*Pregnancy:* Category C. No studies have been conducted in pregnant patients. Clinical experience suggests no adverse effects on the fetus per se; however, it is not known whether these agents can cause fetal harm.

It should be noted again that *BayRho-D Mini-Dose* is not indicated for use during pregnancy and it should be administered only postabortion or postmiscarriage.

Intact IgG crosses the placenta significantly after 32 weeks gestation.

➤*Lactation:* Safety for use in the nursing mother has not been established. It is not known whether immune globulin is excreted in breast milk.

➤*Children:* Safety and efficacy have not been established in pediatric patients. Do not inject infants with **Rh$_o$(D) IGIV, Rh$_o$(D) IGIM,** or **Rh$_o$(D) IG micro-dose**.

ATG equine has been administered safely to a small number of pediatric renal allograft recipients and pediatric aplastic anemia patients at dosage levels comparable to those used in adults on a mg/kg basis.

RSV-IGIV is indicated for use in children < 24 months of age. However, the safety and efficacy of RSV-IGIV in children with congenital heart disease have not been established. Although equivalent proportions of children in the RSV-IGIV and control groups in one trial had adverse events, a larger number of RSV-IGIV recipients had severe or life-threatening adverse events. These events were most frequently observed in infants with CHD with right to left shunts who underwent cardiac surgery.

IGIV – The safety and efficacy of *Gammar-P I.V.* has not been established in neonates and infants with primary defective antibody syntheses.

High-dose administration of *Panglobulin* in pediatric patients with acute or chronic immune thrombocytopenic purpura did not reveal any pediatric-specific hazard.

Venoglobulin-S:

• *Immunodeficiency* – The safety and effectiveness of *Venoglobulin-S* in the treatment of primary immunodeficiency was established in adults and a limited number of children. No infants or neonates were studied. No differences in dosing were found necessary for pediatric patients, nor were any special precautions required.

• *ITP* – The safety and effectiveness of *Venoglobulin-S* was established in both pediatric and adult populations and included all pediatric age groups except neonates. No differences in dosing were found necessary for pediatric patients, nor were any special precautions required.

• *Kawasaki disease* – The safety and efficacy of *Venoglobulin* was established in pediatric populations containing all age groups except neonates.

Sandoglobulin: High-dose administration of *Sandoglobulin* in pediatric patients with acute or chronic ITP did not reveal any pediatric-specific hazard.

Precautions

➤*Monitoring:* Assure that patients are not volume depleted prior to the initiation of therapy.

Periodic monitoring of renal function tests and urine output is particularly important in patients judged to have a potential increased risk for developing acute renal failure. Renal function, including the measurement of blood urea nitrogen (BUN) or serum creatinine should be assessed prior to the initial infusion, and again at appropriate intervals thereafter. If renal function deteriorates, discontinuation of the product should be considered.

For patients judged to be at risk for developing renal dysfunction, it may be prudent to reduce the amount of product infused per unit time (see specific product inserts for measurements).

Administer **RSV-IGIV** cautiously. During administration, monitor the patient's vital signs frequently for increases in heart rate, respiratory rate, retractions, and rales. A loop diuretic such as furosemide or bumetanide should be available for management of fluid overload.

During **ATG rabbit** therapy, monitoring the lymphocyte count (eg, total lymphocyte or T-cell subset) may help assess the degree of T-cell depletion. For safety, monitor the WBC and platelet counts.

➤*Skin testing:* Skin testing should not be performed. Intradermal injection of concentrated gamma globulin causes a localized area of inflammation that can be misinterpreted as a positive allergic reaction. It is actually localized chemical tissue irritation. Misinterpretation can cause necessary medication to be withheld from a patient not actually allergic to this material. True allergic responses to human gamma globulin given in the prescribed IM manner are extremely rare.

➤*Mercury:* Some of these products contain mercury in the form of ethyl mercury from thimerosal. While there are no definitive data on the toxicity of ethyl mercury, literature suggests that information related to methyl mercury toxicities may be applicable.

➤*Latex sensitivity:* Certain components of some of the packaging of these products contain natural rubber latex, which may cause an allergic reaction in sensitive individuals.

➤*Admixture incompatibilities:* Do not admix with other medications.

➤*Rh$_o$(D) IGIM:*

Hemorrhage – A large fetomaternal hemorrhage late in pregnancy or following delivery may cause a weak mixed field positive D^u test result. If there is any doubt about the mother's Rh type, she should be given Rh$_o$(D) immune globulin. A screening test to detect fetal red blood cells may be helpful in such cases.

If > 15 mL of D-positive fetal red blood cells are present in the mother's circulation, more than a single dose of Rh$_o$(D) immune globulin full dose is required. Failure to recognize this may result in the administration of an inadequate dose.

➤*Rh$_o$D IGIV:* Do not administer Rh$_o$(D) IGIV as immunoglobulin replacement therapy for immune globulin deficiency syndromes.

Treatment of ITP – Following administration of Rh$_o$(D) IGIV, monitor Rh$_o$(D)-positive patients for signs and symptoms of intravascular hemolysis (IVH), clinically compromising anemia, and renal insufficiency. If patients are to be transfused, use Rh$_o$(D)-negative packed RBCs so as not to exacerbate ongoing IVH. Platelet products may contain up to 5 mL of RBCs, thus exercise caution if platelets from Rh$_o$(D)-positive donors are transfused.

Suppression of Rh isoimmunization – Do not administer Rh$_o$(D) IGIV to Rh$_o$(D)-negative individuals who are Rh immunized, as evidenced by an indirect antiglobulin (Coombs') test revealing the presence of anti-Rh$_o$(D) (anti-D) antibody.

Fetomaternal hemorrhage: A large fetomaternal hemorrhage late in pregnancy or following delivery may cause a weak mixed field positive D^u test result. Assess such an individual for a large fetomaternal hemorrhage and adjust the dose of Rh$_o$ (D) immune globulin accordingly. Administer Rh$_o$(D) immune globulin if there is any doubt about the mother's blood type.

Hemoglobin – If a patient has a lower than normal hemoglobin level (< 10 g/dL), give a reduced dose of 125 to 200 IU/kg to minimize the risk of increasing the severity of anemia in the patient. Rh$_o$(D) IGIV must be used with extreme caution in patients with a hemoglobin level that is < 8 g/dL because of the risk of increasing the severity of the anemia (see Administration and Dosage).

➤*ATG equine:*

Infection – Because this agent is ordinarily given with corticosteroids and antimetabolites, monitor patients carefully for leukopenia, thrombocytopenia, or for concurrent infection. If infection occurs, institute adjunctive therapy promptly. On the basis of the clinical circumstances, decide whether therapy will continue.

Concomitant immunosuppressive therapy – Safety and efficacy have been demonstrated in renal transplant patients who received concomitant immunosuppressive therapy and in patients with aplastic anemia.

When the dose of corticosteroids and other immunosuppressants is being reduced, some previously masked reactions to the drug may appear; observe patients carefully during therapy.

Chills and fever – Chills and fever occur frequently. ATG equine may release endogenous leukocyte pyrogens. Prophylactic or therapeutic administration of antihistamines, antipyretics, or corticosteroids generally controls this reaction.

Chemical phlebitis – Chemical phlebitis can be caused by infusion through peripheral veins. Avoid by administering the solution into a high-flow vein. An SC arterialized vein produced by a Brescia fistula is also a useful administration site.

Itching and erythema – Itching and erythema probably result from the drug's effect on blood elements. Antihistamines control the symptoms.

Serum sickness-like symptoms – Serum sickness-like symptoms in aplastic anemia patients have been treated with oral or IV corticosteroids. Resolution of symptoms has generally been prompt and long-term sequelae have not been observed. Prophylactic administration of corticosteroids may decrease the frequency of this reaction.

➤*ATG rabbit:*

Chills and fever – ATG rabbit infusion may produce fever and chills. To minimize these, infuse the first dose over a minimum of 6 hours into a high-flow vein. Also premedication with corticosteroids, acetaminophen, or an antihistamine or slowing the infusion rate may reduce reaction incidence and intensity (see Administration and Dosage).

Prolonged use or overdosage – Prolonged use or overdosage of ATG rabbit in association with other immunosuppressive agents may cause over-immunosuppression resulting in severe infections and may increase the incidence of lymphoma or posttransplant lymphoproliferative disease (PTLD) or other malignancies. Appropriate antiviral, antibacterial, antiprotozoal, or antifungal prophylaxis is recommended.

➤*RSV-IGIV:*

Rate of administration – Except for hypersensitivity reactions, adverse reactions to IGIVs may be related to the rate of administration. Careful adherence to the infusion rate outlined under Administration and Dosage is therefore important. Have loop diuretics available for the management of patients who are at risk for fluid overload. Although systemic allergic reactions are rare (see Adverse Reactions), have epinephrine and diphenhydramine available for treatment of acute allergic symptoms.

Discard after use – RSV-IGIV does not contain a preservative. Enter the single-use vial only once for administration purposes and begin the infusion within 6 hours. Closely adhere to the infusion schedule (see Administration and Dosage). Do not use if the solution is turbid.

➤*Thrombotic events:* There is clinical evidence of a possible association between IGIV administration and the potential for the development of thrombotic events. The exact cause of this is unknown; therefore, exercise caution in the prescribing and infusion of IGIV in patients with a history of and predisposing factors toward cardiovascular disease or thrombotic episodes. Analysis of adverse event reports has indicated that a rapid rate of infusion may be a risk factor for vascular occlusive events.

Drug Interactions

Immune Globulin Drug Interactions			
Precipitant drug	Object drug*		Description
RIG, RSV-IGIV, VZIG, IGIV	Virus vaccines, live (measles/mumps/rubella vaccine)	↓	Antibodies present in immune globulin preparations may interfere with the immune response to live virus vaccines, such as mumps, rubella and particularly, measles. As a general rule, administer live virus vaccines 14 to 30 days before or 6 to 12 weeks after immune globulin administration. Administer live virus vaccines during this interval if corresponding antibody titers are measured 3 months after **RIG** administration. For varicella vaccine, wait 5 months. For a vaccine containing the measles virus, wait 4 months. If live vaccines are given during or within 10 months after **RSV-IGIV** infusion, reimmunization is recommended, if appropriate. Do not administer within 3 months of immune globulin administration [Rh$_o$(D), HBIG, CMV-IGIV, IG, RIG, TIG] because antibodies in the globulin preparation may interfere with the immune response to the live virus vaccinations (eg, measles, mumps, polio, or rubella). It may be necessary to revaccinate people who received immune globulin shortly after live virus vaccination. Live virus vaccines should be deferred until ≈ 5 months after VZIG administration. People who received VZIG within 14 days of live virus vaccination should be revaccinated with the live virus vaccine 5 months later. Use of live vaccines should be deferred for ≈ 6 months after (IGIV) administration.

Immune Globulin Drug Interactions

Precipitant drug	Object drug*		Description
Rho(D), HBIG, CMV-IGIV, IG, TIG	Inactivated vaccines (DPT, Hib, OPV)	↓	Responses to non-live childhood vaccines (eg, DPT) do not appear to be substantially influenced by administration of IGIVs. Limited information available from infants who receive **RSV-IGIV** concurrently with one or more doses of their primary immunization series indicates that antibody responses to diphtheria, tetanus, pertussis and *Haemophilus influenzae* b may be lower in RSV-IGIV recipients than in controls. It is not known whether antibody responses to trivalent oral polio vaccine might be affected. Consider giving a booster dose of these vaccines 3 to 4 months after the last dose of RSV-IGIV in order to ensure immunity to DPT, DtaP, Hib and OPV (oral polio virus).
RIG	Rabies vaccine	↓	Simultaneous administration may slightly delay the antibody response to rabies vaccine; follow CDC recommendations exactly and give no more than the recommended dose of **RIG**.
ATG rabbit	Immunosuppressants	↑	Because **antithymocyte globulin (rabbit)** is administered to patients receiving a standard immunosuppressive regimen, this may predispose patients to over-immunosuppression. Many transplant centers decrease maintenance immunosuppression therapy during the period of antibody therapy. **Antithymocyte globulin (rabbit)** can stimulate the production of antibodies that cross-react with rabbit immune globulins.
ATG equine	Immunosuppressants	↓	When dose of corticosteroids and other immunosuppressants is being reduced, some previously masked reactions to antithymocyte globulin (equine) may appear. Observe patient carefully.

* ↓ = Object drug decreased. ↑ = Object drug increased.

➤*Drug/Lab test interactions:*

Rh₀(D) IGIM – Babies born of women given Rh₀(D) IGIM antepartum may have a weakly positive direct antiglobulin test at birth.

Passively acquired anti-Rh₀(D) may be detected in maternal serum if antibody screening tests are performed subsequent to antepartum or postpartum administration of Rh₀(D) IGIM. This does not preclude further antepartum or postpartum prophylaxis.

Late in pregnancy or following delivery, there may be sufficient fetal red blood cells in the maternal circulation to cause a positive antiglobulin test for weak D(Dᵘ). When there is any doubt as to the patient's Rh type, administer Rh₀(D) IGIM.

Elevated bilirubin levels have been reported in some individuals receiving multiple doses of Rh₀(D) IGIM following mismatched transfusions. This is believed to be due to a relatively rapid rate of foreign red cell destruction. About 25% of a group of 22 individuals who were given multiple doses of Rh₀(D) IGIM to treat mismatched transfusions noted fever, myalgia, and lethargy, and 1 had splenomegaly.

Rh₀(D) IGIV – The presence of passively administered anti-Rh₀(D) antibodies in maternal or fetal blood can lead to a positive direct antiglobulin (Coombs') test. If there is an uncertainty about the mother's Rh group or immune status, administer Rh₀(D) immune globulin to the mother.

In addition to anti-D, Rh₀(D) IGIV contains trace amounts of anti-A, anti-B, anti-C, and anti-E antibodies. Passively acquired anti-A, anti-B, anti-C, and anti-E blood group antibodies may be detectable in direct and indirect antiglobulin (Coombs') tests obtained following Rh₀(D) IGIV administration. Interpretation of direct and indirect antiglobulin tests must be made in the context of the patients' underlying clinical condition and supporting laboratory data.

ATG rabbit – ATG rabbit has not been shown to interfere with any routine clinical laboratory tests that do not use immunoglobulins. ATG rabbit may interfere with antibody-based immunoassays and with cross-match or panel-reactive antibody cytotoxicity assays.

VZIG – Administration of VZIG will result in false-positive tests for immunity to VZV for ≈ 2 months after receiving VZIG. Therefore, do not perform serodiagnostic tests to determine immunity to VZV should within 2 months of VZIG administration.

Adverse Reactions

There is a remote chance of an idiosyncratic or anaphylactic reaction in individuals with hypersensitivity to blood products.

➤*Local:* Tenderness, pain, muscle stiffness at injection site, urticaria, angioedema, ache, erythema, burning; may persist for several hours.

➤*Systemic:* Urticaria; angioedema; malaise, nausea, diarrhea. The most common adverse events were headache, chills, and fever. Less frequently reported reactions include the following: Emesis; chills; fever; fatigue; lightheadedness; abdominal cramping; retching; myalgia; lethargy; chest tightness; nausea. Isolated cases of angioneurotic edema and nephrotic syndrome have occurred.

Systemic reactions associated with administration are extremely rare. Discomfort at the site of injection has been reported and a small number of women have noted a slight elevation in temperature. While sensitization to repeated injections is extremely rare, it has occurred.

Potential reactions for all immune globulin IV products are often related to infusion rate and may include the following: Nausea, vomiting, abdominal cramps, chills, pyrexia, chest tightness, palpitations, tachycardia, blood pressure changes, edema, flushing, diaphoresis, rash, erythema, pruritus, cyanosis, dizziness, headache, backache, or other body aches, anxiety, wheezing (and other respiratory events), myalgia, shaking, fatigue, malaise, and arthralgia, usually beginning within 1 hour of the start of the infusion. Other reactions include feeling of faintness; chest tightness; shortness of breath; dyspnea; chills; headache; mild hemolysis; hypertension; pallor; irritability; pain (chest/hip/back/neck/legs); urticaria (hives); rash (rare).

➤*CMV-IGIV:* Minor reactions such as flushing, chills, muscle cramps, back pain, fever, nausea, vomiting, arthralgia, and wheezing were the most frequent adverse reactions observed during the clinical trials of CMV-IGIV. The incidence of these reactions during the clinical trials was < 6% of all infusions and such reactions were most often related to infusion rates. A decrease in blood pressure was observed in 1 of 1039 infusions in clinical trials. If a patient develops a minor side effect, slow the rate immediately or temporarily interrupt the infusion.

Increases in serum creatinine and BUN have been observed as soon as 1 to 2 days following IGIV infusion. Progression to oliguria or anuria requiring dialysis has been observed. Types of severe renal adverse events that have been seen following IGIV therapy include acute renal failure, acute tubular necrosis, proximal tubular nephropathy, and osmotic nephrosis.

Severe reactions such as angioneurotic edema and anaphylactic shock, although not observed during clinical trials, are a possibility. Clinical anaphylaxis may occur even when the patient is not known to be sensitized to immune globulin products. A reaction may be related to the rate of infusion; therefore, carefully adhere to the infusion rates as outlined under Administration and Dosage. If anaphylaxis or drop in blood pressure occurs, discontinue infusion and use antidote such as diphenhydramine and epinephrine. Refer to the Management of Acute Hypersensitivity Reactions.

➤*IGIV:* Increases in creatinine and BUN have been observed as soon as 1 to 2 days following infusion. Progression to oliguria and anuria requiring dialysis has been observed, although some patients have improved spontaneously following cessation of treatment. Types of severe renal adverse reactions that have been seen following IGIV therapy include the following: acute renal failure, acute tubular necrosis, proximal tubular nephropathy, and osmotic nephrosis.

➤*ATG equine:*

Renal transplantation: Fever (33%); chills, leukopenia (14%); dermatological reactions (eg, rash, pruritus, urticaria, wheal, flare) (13%); thrombocytopenia (11%); arthralgia, chest/back pain, clotted A/V fistula, diarrhea, dyspnea, headache, hypotension, nausea, vomiting, night sweats, pain at the infusion site, peripheral thrombophlebitis, stomatitis (1% to 5%); anaphylaxis, dizziness, weakness, faintness, edema, herpes simplex reactivation, hiccoughs, epigastric pain, hyperglycemia, hypertension, iliac vein obstruction, laryngospasm, localized infection, lymphadenopathy, malaise, myalgia, paresthesia, possible serum sickness, pulmonary edema, renal artery thrombosis, seizures, systemic infection, tachycardia, toxic epidermal necrosis, wound dehiscence (< 1%).

Aplastic anemia: Chills, arthralgia (50%); headache (17%); myalgia (10%); nausea, chest pain (7%); phlebitis (5%); diaphoresis, joint stiffness, periorbital edema, aches, edema, muscle ache, vomiting, agitation/lethargy, listlessness, lightheadedness, seizures, diarrhea, bradycardia, myocarditis, cardiac irregularity, hepatosplenomegaly, encephalitis or postviral encephalopathy, hypotension, CHF, hypertension, burning soles/palms, foot sole pain, lymphadenopathy, postcervical lymphadenopathy, tender lymph nodes, bilateral pleural effusion, respiratory distress, anaphylaxis, proteinuria (< 5%); abnormal tests of liver function (eg, AST, ALT, alkaline phosphatase) and renal function (eg, serum creatinine). In some trials, clinical and laboratory findings of serum sickness were seen in a majority of patients.

Postmarketing experience: Fever (51%); thrombocytopenia (30%); rashes (27%); chills (16%); leukopenia (14%); systemic infection (13%); abnormal renal function tests, serum sickness-like symptoms, dyspnea or apnea, arthralgia, chest/back/flank pain, diarrhea, nausea, vomiting (5% to 10%); hypertension, herpes simplex infection, pain, swelling or redness at the infusion site, eosinophilia, headache, myalgia, leg pains, hypotension, anaphylaxis, tachycardia, edema, localized infection, malaise, seizures, GI bleeding/perforation, deep vein thrombosis, sore mouth/throat, hyperglycemia, acute renal failure, abnormal liver function tests, confusion, disorientation, cough, neutropenia, granulocytopenia, anemia, thrombophlebitis, dizziness, epigastric/stomach pain, lymphadenopathy, pulmonary edema, CHF, abdominal pain, nosebleed, vasculitis, aplasia, pancytopenia, abnormal involuntary movement, tremor, rigidity, sweating, laryngospasm, edema, hemolysis/hemolytic anemia, viral hepatitis, faintness, enlarged/ruptured kidney, paresthesias, renal artery thrombosis (< 5%).

➤*ATG rabbit:* ATG rabbit adverse events are generally manageable or reversible. In the US Phase III controlled clinical trial (n = 163) comparing the efficacy and safety of ATG rabbit and ATG equine, there were no significant differences in clinically significant adverse events between the 2 treatment groups. Malignancies were reported in 3 patients who received ATG rabbit and in 3 patients who received ATG equine during the 1-year follow-up period. These included 2 PTLDs in the ATG rabbit group and 2 PTLDs in the ATG equine group. Infections occurring in both treatment groups during the 3-month follow-up are summarized in the following table. No significant differences were seen between the ATG rabbit and ATG equine groups for all types of infections, and the incidence of CMV infection was equivalent in both groups. (Viral prophylaxis was by the centers discretion during antibody treatment, but all centers used ganciclovir infusion during treatment.)

Antithymocyte Globulin Adverse Reactions (%)		
Adverse reactions	ATG rabbit (n = 82)	ATG equine (n = 81)
Cardiovascular		
Hypertension	36.6	28.4
Tachycardia	26.8	23.5
Respiratory		
Dyspnea	28	19.8
Pneumonia	0	1.2
GI		
Abdominal pain	37.8	27.2
Diarrhea	36.6	32.1
Nausea	36.6	28.4
GI moniliasis	4.9	1.2
Oral moniliasis	3.7	2.5
Gastritis	1.2	0
GU		
Urinary tract infection	18.3	25.9
Vaginitis	0	1.2
Hematologic		
Leukopenia	57.3	29.6
Thrombocytopenia	36.6	44.4
Miscellaneous		
Fever	63.4	63
Chills	57.3	43.2
Pain	46.3	43.2
Headache	40.2	34.6
Peripheral edema	34.1	34.6
Asthenia	26.8	32.1
Hyperkalemia	26.8	18.5
Infection	30.5	23.5
Infection (other)	17.1	13.6
Infection (CMV)	13.4	11.1
Malaise	13.4	3.7
Sepsis	12.2	9.6
Dizziness	8.5	24.7
Herpes simplex	4.9	0
Infection (not specified)	0	2.5
Moniliasis	0	1.2

➤*Rh$_o$(D) IGIV:* Rh$_o$(D) IGIV is administered to Rh$_o$(D) positive patients with ITP. Side effects related to the destruction of Rh$_o$(D)-positive red cells, such as decreased hemoglobin, can be expected. At the recommended initial IV dose of 250 IU/kg, the mean maximum decrease in hemoglobin was 1.7 g/dL (range, +0.4 to -6.1 g/dL). At a reduced dose, ranging from 125 to 200 IU/kg, the mean maximum decrease in hemoglobin was 0.81 g/dL (range, +0.65 to -1.9 g/dL). Only 5 of the 137 (3.7%) patients had a maximum decrease in hemoglobin of > 4 g/dL (range, 4.2 to 6.1 g/dL).

In most cases, the RBC destruction is believed to occur in the spleen. However, signs and symptoms consistent with IVH, including back pain, shaking chills, or hemoglobinuria have been reported, occurring within 4 hours of Rh$_o$(D) IGIV administration.

IVH-related complications that have been reported include death (4 cases reported between May 1996 and April 1999), acute onset or exacerbation of anemia, and acute onset or exacerbation of renal insufficiency. One patient died from complications secondary to IVH-induced exacerbation of anemia after administration of Rh$_o$(D) IGIV for treatment of ITP. Although the primary cause of death in the other 3 ITP patients treated with Rh$_o$(D) IGIV was related to underlying disease, the extent to which IVH-related clinical complications exacerbated their conditions and contributed to their deaths is unknown.

In addition to the adverse reactions described above, the following have been reported infrequently in clinical trials or postmarketing experience, in patients treated for ITP or Rh isoimmunization suppression, and are thought to be temporally associated with Rh$_o$(D) IGIV use: Asthenia, abdominal or back pain, hypotension, pallor, diarrhea, increased LDH, arthralgia, myalgia, dizziness, hyperkinesia, somnolence, vasodilation, pruritus, rash, and sweating.

➤*RSV-IGIV:* RSV-IGIV is generally well tolerated. In the PREVENT trial of RSV-IGIV in children with BPD or prematurity, there was no difference in the proportion of children in the RSV-IGIV and placebo groups who report adverse events.

RSV-IGIV Adverse Reactions (%)		
Adverse Reaction	RSV-IGIV (n = 250)	Placebo (n = 260)
Fever/Pyrexia	6	2
Respiratory distress	2	< 1
Vomiting/Emesis	2	1
Wheezing	2	2
Diarrhea	1	< 1
Rales	1	0
Fluid overload	1	0
Tachycardia/Increased pulse rate	1	0
Rash	1	2
Hypertension	1	0
Hypoxia/Hypoxemia	1	1
Tachypnea	1	< 1
Gastroenteritis	1	< 1
Injection site inflammation	1	1
Overdose effect	1	< 1

Infrequent adverse reactions included: Edema, pallor, hypotension, heart murmur, gagging, cyanosis, sleepiness, cough, rhinorrhea, eczema, cold and clammy skin, conjunctival hemorrhage (< 1%).

Reactions similar to those reported with other IGIVs may occur with RSV-IGIV. These include: Dizziness; flushing; blood pressure changes; anxiety; palpitations; chest tightness; dyspnea; abdominal cramps; pruritus; myalgia; arthralgia. Such reactions are often related to the rate of infusion. Immediate allergic, anaphylactic, or hypersensitivity reactions may be observed (see Warnings). Rarely, aseptic meningitis syndrome (AMS) has been reported in association with IGIV treatment, particularly at high dosage (2 g/kg; see Precautions).

In the PREVENT trial, 3 children developed aseptic meningitis of unknown etiology. In the single-blind, controlled NIAID trial in children with BPD, CHD or prematurity, adverse reactions were reported in 3% of all RSV-IGIV infusions. Five of 160 children were considered to have had mild fluid overload associated with infusion. The remaining adverse reactions consisted of mild decreases in oxygen saturation (n = 8) and fever (n = 5). In the open-label study in children with BPD or prematurity (n = 6), infusion-associated adverse reactions were noted in 14 of 294 (4.8%) infusions. Six adverse events were considered related to infusion, including 4 mild and 2 moderate events. In the CARDIAC study, children with CHD with right to left shunts appeared to have an increased frequency of cardiac surgery and had a greater frequency of severe and life-threatening adverse events associated with cardiac surgery (see Warnings).

Overdosage

Although few data are available, clinical experience with other immune globulin preparations suggests that the major manifestations would be those related to fluid volume overload. Other reactions would include pain and tenderness at the injection site.

➤*ATG equine:* Because of its mode of action and because it is a biologic substance, the maximal tolerated dose of ATG equine solution would be expected to vary from patient to patient. To date, the largest single daily dose administered to a patient, a renal transplant recipient, was 7000 mg administered at a concentration of ≈ 10 mg/mL Sodium Chloride Injection, USP, ≈ 7 times the recommended total dose and infusion concentration. In this patient, administration of ATG equine was not associated with any signs of acute intoxication.

The greatest number of doses (10 to 20 mg/kg/dose) that can be administered to a single patient has not yet been determined. Some renal transplant patients have received up to 50 doses in 4 months, and others have received 28-day courses of 21 doses followed by as many as 3 more courses for the treatment of acute rejection. The incidence of toxicologic manifestations did not increase with any of these regimens.

➤*ATG rabbit:* ATG rabbit overdosage may result in leukopenia or thrombocytopenia, which can be managed with dose reduction (see Administration and Dosage).

➤*Rh$_o$(D) IGIV:* There are no reports of known overdoses in patients being treated for Rh isoimmunization or ITP. In clinical studies with nonpregnant Rh$_o$(D) positive patients with ITP (n = 141) treated with 600 to 32,500 IU (120 to 6500 mcg) of Rh$_o$(D) IGIV, there were no signs or symptoms that warranted medical intervention. However, these same doses were associated with a mild, transient hemolytic anemia.

Patient Information

Instruct patients to report symptoms of decreased urine output, sudden weight gain, fluid retention/edema and/or shortness of breath (which may suggest kidney damage) immediately to their physician.

Instruct patients, parents, or guardians to report any serious adverse reaction to their health care provider.

Patients, parents, or guardians should be fully informed by their health care provider of the benefits and risks of these products.

CYTOMEGALOVIRUS IMMUNE GLOBULIN INTRAVENOUS, HUMAN (CMV-IGIV)

Rx	**CytoGam** (MedImmune)	**Solution for injection:**[1] 50 ± 10 mg/mL	In 20 and 50 mL vials.

[1] Preservative free. 5% sucrose, 1% Albumin (human). Solvent/Detergent treated.

For additional information, refer to the Immune Globulins group monograph.

Indications

▶*Cytomegalovirus (CMV):* For the prophylaxis of cytomegalovirus disease associated with transplantation of kidney, lung, liver, pancreas, and heart. In transplants of these organs other than kidney from CMV seropositive donors into seronegative recipients, consider prophylactic CMV-IGIV in combination with ganciclovir.

▶*Unlabeled uses:* For prevention or attenuation of primary CMV disease in immunosuppressed recipients of organ transplants (eg, bone marrow, liver). Also used in immunocompromised patients with CMV pneumonia or to prevent CMV disease.

Administration and Dosage

The maximum recommended total dosage per infusion is 150 mg/kg, administered according to the following schedule:

Dosage Schedule for CMV-IGIV in Transplantation		
	Dosage (mg/kg)	
Time of infusion	Kidney	Liver, pancreas, lung, heart
Within 72 hours of transplant	150	150
2 weeks posttransplant	100	150
4 weeks posttransplant	100	150
6 weeks posttransplant	100	150
8 weeks posttransplant	100	150
12 weeks posttransplant	50	100
16 weeks posttransplant	50	100

▶*Initial dose:* Administer IV at 15 mg Ig/kg/hr. If no untoward reactions occur after 30 minutes, the rate may be increased to 30 mg Ig/kg/hr; if no untoward reactions occur after a subsequent 30 minutes, the infusion may be increased to 60 mg Ig/kg/hr (volume not to exceed 75 mL/hour). Do not exceed this rate of administration. Monitor the patient closely during and after each rate change.

▶*Subsequent doses:* Administer at 15 mg Ig/kg/hr for 15 minutes. If no untoward reactions occur, increase to 30 mg Ig/kg/hr for 15 minutes and then increase to a maximum rate of 60 mg Ig/kg/hr (volume not to exceed 75 mL/hr). Do not exceed this rate of administration. Monitor the patient closely during each rate change.

Renal insufficiency – Use with caution in patients with pre-existing renal insufficiency and in patients judged to be at increased risk of developing renal insufficiency (including, but not limited to, those with diabetes mellitus, > 65 years of age, volume depletion, paraproteinemia, sepsis, and patients receiving known nephrotoxic drugs). In these cases especially, it is important to ensure that patients are not volume depleted prior to CMV-IGIV infusion. While most cases of renal insufficiency have occurred in patients receiving total doses of ≥ 400 mg Ig/kg, no prospective data are presently available to identify a maximum safe dose, concentration, or rate of infusion in patients determined to be at increased risk of acute renal failure. In the absence of prospective data, do not exceed recommended doses and select the minimum practicable concentration and infusion rate. Infuse the product at a rate of ≤ 180 mg Ig/kg/hr.

Potential adverse reactions are flushing; chills; muscle cramps; back pain; fever; nausea; vomiting; wheezing; drop in blood pressure. Minor adverse reactions have been infusion-rate related. If the patient develops a minor side effect (eg, nausea, back pain, flushing), slow the rate or temporarily interrupt the infusion. If anaphylaxis or drop in blood pressure occurs, discontinue infusion and use an antidote such as diphenhydramine and epinephrine. Refer to Management of Acute Hypersensitivity Reactions.

▶*Infusion:* Begin infusion within 6 hours of entering the vial and complete within 12 hours of entering the vial. Monitor vital signs pre-infusion, midway, and post-infusion, as well as before any rate increase. Administer through an IV line using an administration set that contains an in-line filter (pore size 15 mc) and a constant infusion pump (eg, IVAC pump or equivalent). A smaller in-line filter (0.2 mc) is also acceptable. Predilution of CMV-IGIV before infusion is not recommended. Administer through a separate IV line. If this is not possible, it may be "piggybacked" into a preexisting line if that line contains either Sodium Chloride Injection or one of the following dextrose solutions (with or without NaCl added): 2.5%, 5%, 10%, or 20% Dextrose in Water. If a pre-existing line must be used, do not dilute the CMV-IGIV more than 1:2 with any of the above solutions. Admixtures of CMV-IGIV with any other solutions have not been evaluated.

▶*Storage/Stability:* Store between 2° to 8°C (36° to 46°F). Use within 6 hours after entering the vial.

HEPATITIS B IMMUNE GLOBULIN (HUMAN) (HBIG)

Rx	**BayHep B** (Bayer Pharmaceutical)	**Solution for Injection:**[1] 15% to 18% protein	In 1 and 5 mL single-dose vials and 0.5 mL neonatal single-dose syringe.
Rx	**Nabi-HB** (Nabi)	**Solution for Injection:**[2] 5% ± 1% protein	In 1 and 5 mL single-dose vials.

[1] Preservative free. With 0.21 to 0.32 M glycine. Solvent/Detergent treated.
[2] Preservative free. With 0.15 M glycine. Solvent/Detergent treated.

For additional information, refer to the Immune Globulins group monograph.

Indications

▶*Postexposure prophylaxis in the following situations:*

Acute exposure to blood containing HBsAg – Following either parenteral exposure (eg, accidental "needle-stick"), direct mucous membrane contact (eg, accidental splash), or oral ingestion (eg, pipetting accident) involving HBsAg-positive materials such as blood, plasma, or serum. For inadvertent percutaneous exposure, a regimen of 2 doses of HBIG, given after exposure and a month later, is ≈ 75% effective in preventing hepatitis B in this setting.

Perinatal exposure of infants born to HBsAg-positive mothers – Such infants are at risk of being infected with hepatitis B virus and becoming chronic carriers. The risk is especially great if the mother is HBeAg-positive. For an infant with perinatal exposure to an HBsAg-positive and HBeAg-positive mother, a regimen combining 1 dose of HBIG at birth with the hepatitis B vaccine series started soon after birth is 85% to 95% effective in preventing development of the HBV carrier state. Regimens involving either multiple doses of HBIG alone or the vaccine series alone have 70% to 90% efficacy, while a single dose of HBIG alone has only 50% efficacy.

Sexual exposure to an HBsAg-positive person – Sex partners of HBsAg-positive people are at increased risk of acquiring HBV infection. For sexual exposure to a person with acute hepatitis B, a single dose of HBIG is 75% effective if administered within 2 weeks of last sexual exposure.

Household exposure to people with Acute HBV infection – Because infants have close contact with primary caregivers and they have a higher risk of becoming HBV carriers after acute HBV infection, prophylaxis of an infant < 12 months of age with HBIG and hepatitis B vaccine is indicated if the mother or primary care-give has acute HBV infection.

Administration of HBIG either preceding or concomitant with the commencement of active immunization with hepatitis B vaccine provides for more rapid achievement of protective levels of hepatitis B antibody than when the vaccine alone is administered. Rapid achievement of protective levels of antibody to hepatitis B virus may be desirable in certain clinical situations as in cases of accidental inoculations with contaminated medical instruments. Administration of HBIG either 1 month preceding or at the time of commencement of a program of active vaccination with hepatitis B vaccine has been shown not to interfere with the active immune response to the vaccine.

Administration and Dosage

Give injections IM. IM injections are preferably administered in the anterolateral aspects of the upper thigh and the deltoid muscle of the upper arm. The gluteal region should not be used routinely as an injection site because of the risk of injury to the sciatic nerve. An individual decision as to which muscle is injected must be made for each patient based on the volume of material to be administered. If the gluteal region is used when very large volumes are to be injected or multiple doses are necessary, the central region must be avoided; use only the upper, outer quadrant.

▶*Postexposure prophylaxis:* The recommended dose is 0.06 mL/kg; the usual adult dose is 3 to 5 mL. Administer the appropriate dose as soon after exposure as possible (preferably within 7 days) and repeat 28 to 30 days after exposure.

Recommendations for Hepatitis B Prophylaxis Following Percutaneous or Permucosal Exposure		
	Exposed person	
Source	Unvaccinated	Vaccinated
HBsAg-positive	1. HBIG × 1 immediately[1] 2. Initiate HB vaccine series[2]	1. Test exposed person for anti-HBs. 2. If inadequate antibody,[3] HBIG (× 1) immediately plus HB vaccine booster dose, or 2 doses of HBIG,[1] one as soon as possible after exposure and the second 1 month later.

HEPATITIS B IMMUNE GLOBULIN (HUMAN)

Recommendations for Hepatitis B Prophylaxis Following Percutaneous or Permucosal Exposure		
	Exposed person	
Source	Unvaccinated	Vaccinated
Known source (high risk)	1. Initiate HV vaccine series 2. Test source for HBsAg. If positive, HBIG × 1	1. Test source for HBsAg only if exposed is vaccine nonresponder; if source is HBsAg-positive, give HBIG (× 1) immediately plus HB vaccine booster dose, or 2 doses of HBIG,[1] one as soon as possible after exposure and the second 1 month later.
Low risk HBsAg-positive	Initiate HB vaccine series.	Nothing required.
Unknown source	Initiate HB vaccine series within 7 days of exposure.	Nothing required.

[1] HBIG, dose 0.06 mL/kg IM.
[2] HB vaccine dose 20 mcg IM for adults; 10 mcg IM for infants or children < 10 years of age. First dose within 1 week; second and third doses, 1 and 6 months later.
[3] < 10 sample ratio units (SRU) by radioimmunoassay (RIA), negative by enzyme immunoassay (EIA).

➤*Prophylaxis of infants born to HBsAG- and HBeAg-positive mothers:* The recommended dose for at-risk newborns is 0.5 mL IM into the anterolateral thigh, as soon after birth as possible, preferably within 12 hours. Administer hepatitis B vaccine IM in 3 doses of 0.5 mL of vaccine (10 mcg) each. Give the first dose within 7 days of birth and give concurrently with HBIG but at a separate site. Give the second and third doses of vaccine 1 month and 6 months, respectively, after the first. If administration of the first dose of hepatitis B vaccine is delayed for as long as 3 months, then repeat a 0.5 mL dose of HBIG at 3 months. If hepatitis B vaccine is refused, repeat the 0.5 mL dose of HBIG at 3 and 6 months.

Recommended Schedule of Hepatitis B Immunoprophylaxis to Prevent Perinatal Transmission of Hepatitis B Virus Infection		
	Age of infant	
Administer	Infant born to mother known to be HBsAg positive	Infant born to mother not screened for HBsAg
First vaccination[1] Hepatitis B Immune Globulin (human)[2]	Birth (within 12 hours) Birth (within 12 hours)	Birth (within 12 hours) If mother is found to be HBsAg positive, administer dose to infant as soon as possible, not later than 1 week after birth.

Recommended Schedule of Hepatitis B Immunoprophylaxis to Prevent Perinatal Transmission of Hepatitis B Virus Infection		
	Age of infant	
Administer	Infant born to mother known to be HBsAg positive	Infant born to mother not screened for HBsAg
Second vaccination[1] Third vaccination[1]	1 month 6 months[3]	1 to 2 months 6 months[3]

[1] See manufacturer's recommendations for appropriate dose.
[2] 0.5 mL administered IM at a site different from that used for the vaccine.
[3] See ACIP recommendations.

➤*Sexual exposure to an HBsAg-positive person:* All susceptible people whose sex partners have acute hepatitis B infection should receive a single dose of HBIG (0.06 mL/kg) and should begin the hepatitis B vaccine series if prophylaxis can be started within 14 days of the last sexual contact or if sexual contact with the infected person will continue (see table below). Administering the vaccine with HBIG may improve the efficacy of postexposure treatment. The vaccine has the added advantage of conferring long-lasting protection.

Recommendations for Postexposure Prophylaxis for Sexual Exposure to Hepatitis B			
HBIG		Vaccine	
Dose	Recommended timing	Dose	Recommended timing
0.06 mL/kg IM	Single dose within 14 days of last sexual contact.	1 mL IM	First dose at time of HBIG[1] treatment.

[1] The first dose can be administered the same time as the HBIG dose but at a different site; subsequent doses should be administered as recommended for specific vaccine.

➤*Household exposure to people with acute HBV infection:* Prophylactic treatment with a 0.5 mL dose of HBIG and hepatitis B vaccine is indicated for infants < 12 months of age who have been exposed to a primary care-giver who has acute hepatitis B. Prophylaxis for other household contacts of people with acute HBV infection is not indicated unless they have had identifiable blood exposure to the index patient (eg, sharing toothbrushes or razors). Such exposures should be treated like sexual exposures. If the index patient becomes an HBV carrier, all household contacts should receive hepatitis B vaccine.

HBIG may be administered at the same time (but at a different site), or ≤ 1 month preceding hepatitis B vaccination without impairing the active immune response from hepatitis B vaccination.

➤*Storage/Stability:* Store at 2° to 8°C (36° to 46°F). Do not freeze. Use within 6 hours after the vial has been entered.

IMMUNE GLOBULIN (HUMAN) (IG; IGIM; Gamma Globulin; IgG)

Rx **BayGam** (Bayer) **Solution for Injection:**[1] 15% to 18% protein In 2 and 10 mL single-dose vials.

[1] Preservative-free. With 0.21 to 0.32 M glycine. Solvent/Detergent treated.

For additional information, refer to the Immune Globulins group monograph.

Indications

➤*Hepatitis A:* The prophylactic value of IGIM is greatest when given before or soon after exposure to hepatitis A. Not indicated in individuals with clinical manifestations of hepatitis A or in those exposed > 2 weeks previously.

➤*Measles (Rubeola):* For the prevention or modification of measles in susceptible contacts (one who has not been vaccinated and has not had measles previously) exposed < 6 days previously. May be especially indicated for susceptible household contacts of measles patients, particularly those < 1 year of age, for whom the risk of complications is highest. Do not give with measles vaccine. If a child> 12 months of age has received IGIM, give measles vaccine ≈ 3 months later, when the measles antibody titer will have disappeared.

If a susceptible child exposed to measles is immunocompromised, administer IGIM immediately. Do not give children who are immunocompromised the measles vaccine or any other live viral vaccine.

➤*Immunoglobulin deficiency:* IGIM therapy may prevent serious infection if circulating IgG levels of ≈ 200 mg/dL plasma are maintained. However, it may not prevent chronic infections of external secretory tissues such as the respiratory and GI tracts.

Prophylactic therapy, especially against infections due to encapsulated bacteria, is often effective in Bruton-type, sex-linked congenital agammaglobulinemia, agammaglobulinemia associated with thymoma, and acquired agammaglobulinemia.

➤*Varicella:* Passive immunization against varicella in immunosuppressed patients is best accomplished with varicella-zoster immune globulin. If unavailable, IGIM may be used.

➤*Rubella:* The routine use of IGIM for rubella prophylaxis in early pregnancy is of dubious value and cannot be justified. Some studies suggest that the use of IGIM in susceptible women exposed to rubella can lessen the likelihood of infection and fetal damage. See Administration and Dosage.

Administration and Dosage

For IM injection only, preferably in the anterolateral aspects of the upper thigh and the deltoid muscle of the upper arm. Do not use the gluteal region routinely as an injection site because of the risk of injury to the sciatic nerve. Divide and inject doses> 10 mL into several muscle sites to reduce local pain and discomfort. An individual decision as to which muscle is injected must be made for each patient based on the volume of material to be administered. If the gluteal region is used when very large volumes are to be injected or multiple doses are necessary, avoid the central region; use only the upper outer quadrant.

➤*Hepatitis A:* A dose of 0.02 mL/kg (0.01 mL/lb) is recommended for household and institutional hepatitis A case contacts. The following doses are recommended for people who plan to travel in areas where hepatitis A is common:

IG Dose for Common Hepatitis A Areas	
Length of stay	Dose (mL/kg)
< 3 months	0.02
Prolonged (> 3 months)	0.06 (repeat every 4 to 6 months)

➤*Measles (Rubeola):* To prevent or modify measles in a susceptible person exposed < 6 days previously, give 0.11 mL/lb (0.25 mL/kg). If a susceptible child who is also immunocompromised is exposed to measles, give 0.5 mL/kg (15 mL maximum) immediately.

➤*Immunoglobulin deficiency:* The usual dosage consists of an initial dose of 1.3 mL/kg followed in 3 or 4 weeks by 0.66 mL/kg (≥ 100 mg/kg) to be given every 3 to 4 weeks. Some patients may require more frequent injections.

➤*Varicella:* Give 0.6 to 1.2 mL/kg promptly, if varicella-zoster immune globulin is unavailable.

IMMUNE GLOBULIN (HUMAN) (IG; IGIM; Gamma Globulin; IgG)

➤*Rubella:* Some studies suggest that the use of IG in exposed susceptible women can lessen the likelihood of infection and fetal damage;

therefore, a dose of 0.55 mL/kg may benefit those women who do not consider a therapeutic abortion.

➤*Storage/Stability:* Store between 2° to 8°C (36° to 46°F). Do not freeze.

IMMUNE GLOBULIN INTRAVENOUS (IGIV)

Rx	Flebogamma 5% (Grifols)	Injection: 5% immune globulin (human) (50 mg/mL)[1]	In 10, 50, 100, and 200 mL vials.
Rx	Octagam (Octapharma)	Injection: 5% immune globulin (human) (50 mg/mL)[2]	In 1, 2.5, 5, and 10 g single-use bottles.
Rx	Gamimune N (Bayer)	Injection: 5%[3]	In 10, 50, 100, 200, and 250 mL vials.
		Injection: 10%[4]	In 10, 50, 100, and 200 mL vials.
Rx	Gamunex (Bayer)	Injection: 10% immune globulin (human)[5]	In 10, 25, 50, 100, and 200 mL.
Rx	Polygam S/D (American Red Cross)	Powder for Injection (freeze-dried): 50 mg/mL; 90% gammaglobulin[6]	In 2.5, 5, and 10 g single-use bottles with diluent, transfer device, and administration set.
Rx	Panglobulin NF (American Red Cross)	Powder for injection, lyophilized: 1, 3, 6, 12 g immune globulin IV.[7]	In 1, 3, 6, and 12 g vials.
Rx	Carimune NF (ZLB Bioplasma)	Powder for injection, lyophilized: 1, 3, 6, 12 g immune globulin IV.[7]	In 1, 3, 6, and 12 g vials.
Rx	Panglobulin (American Red Cross)	Powder for Injection, lyophilized: 6 g, 12 g[8]	In vials.
Rx	Venoglobulin-S (Alpha Therapeutic)	Powder for Injection: 5% immune globulin IV (human)[9]	In 50, 100, and 200 mL with sterile IV administration set.
		10% immune globulin IV (human)[10]	In 50, 100, and 200 mL with sterile IV administration set.
Rx	Gammar-P I.V. (Aventis)	Powder for Injection, lyophilized: 5% IgG, 3% human albumin[11]	In 1, 2.5, and 5 g single-dose vials with diluent and 10 g with administration set and diluent. With vented transfer spike. In bulk pack 6s, diluent not supplied.

[1] 50 mg sorbitol, ≤ 6 mg/mL polyethylene glycol, preservative-free.

[2] 100 mg maltose.

[3] Preservative free. In 9% to 11% maltose. Solvent/Detergent treated.

[4] Preservative free. In 0.16 to 0.24 M glycine. Solvent/Detergent treated.

[5] With 0.16 to 0.24 M glycine. Caprylate/Chromatography purified.

[6] Preservative free. With 20 mg glucose, 2 mg polyethylene glycol, 22.5 mg glycine, 1 mcg tri-n-butyl phosphate, 1 mcg octoxynol 9, 100 mcg polysorbate 80, 3 mg albumin (human) per mL. Solvent/Detergent treated.

[7] Preservative free. With 1.67 g sucrose/g protein.

[8] Preservative free. With ≈ 1.67 g sucrose and < 20 mg NaCl per g. Filtrated.

[9] Preservative free. With 50 mg d-sorbitol, ≤ 1.3 mg albumin (human), ≤ 100 mcg polyethylene glycol, ≤ 100 mcg polysorbate 80, and ≤ 10 mcg tri-n-butyl phosphate per mL. Solvent/Detergent treated.

[10] Preservative free. With 50 mg d-sorbitol, ≤ 2.6 mg albumin (human), ≤ 200 mcg polyethylene glycol, ≤ 200 mcg polysorbate 80, and ≤ 20 mcg tri-n-butyl phosphate per mL. Solvent/Detergent treated.

[11] Preservative free. With 5% sucrose, 0.5% NaCl. Heat treated.

For additional information, refer to the Immune Globulins group monograph.

WARNING

Immune globulin IV (human) products have been associated with renal dysfunction, acute renal failure, osmotic nephrosis, and death. Patients predisposed to acute renal failure include patients with any degree of pre-existing renal insufficiency, diabetes mellitus, > 65 years of age, volume depletion, sepsis, paraproteinemia, or patients receiving known nephrotoxic drugs. Especially in such patients, IGIV products should be administered at the minimum concentration available and the minimum rate of infusion practicable. While these reports of renal dysfunction and acute renal failure have been associated with the use of many of the licensed IGIV products, those containing sucrose as a stabilizer accounted for a disproportionate share of the total number.

See Precautions and Administration and dosage sections for important information intended to reduce the risk of acute renal failure.

Indications

➤*Immunodeficiency syndrome:* For the maintenance treatment of patients who are unable to produce sufficient amounts of IgG antibodies. IGIV may be preferred to IM immunoglobulin, especially in patients who require an immediate and substantial increase in IV immunoglobulin levels, in patients with a small muscle mass, and in patients with bleeding tendencies in whom IM injections are contraindicated. It may be used in disease states such as congenital agammaglobulinemia (eg, x-linked agammaglobulinemia), common variable hypogammaglobulinemia, x-linked immunodeficiency with or without hyper IgM, Wiskott-Aldrich syndrome, and severe combined immunodeficiency.

➤*Idiopathic thrombocytopenic purpura (ITP) (Gamimune N, Gammagard S/D, Polygam S/D, Sandoglobulin, Panglobulin, and Venoglobulin-S only):* Some children and adults with ITP have shown a temporary increase in platelet counts upon administration of IGIV. Therefore, consider administration in situations that require a rapid, temporary rise in platelet count (eg, prior to surgery, to control excessive bleeding, as a measure to defer splenectomy). Not all patients will respond. Even in those patients who do respond, do not consider this treatment curative.

Venoglobulin-S is also indicated in cases of chronic (> 6 months duration) ITP to maintain platelet counts > 30,000/mm^3 in children and > 20,000/mm^3 in adults.

➤*B-cell chronic lymphocytic leukemia (CLL) (Gammagard S/D, Polygam S/D):* Prevention of bacterial infections in patients with hypogammaglobulinemia or recurrent bacterial infections associated with B-cell CLL.

➤*Kawasaki disease (Iveegam, Venoglobulin-S, Gammagard S/D, Polygam S/D):* For the prevention of coronary artery aneurysms associated with Kawasaki disease in conjunction with high-dose aspirin (ie, 100 mg/kg/day).

➤*Bone marrow transplantation (BMT) (Gamimune N only):* To decrease the risk of septicemia, interstitial pneumonia of infectious and idiopathic etiologies and acute graft-vs-host disease in patients ≥ 20 years of age in the first 100 days posttransplant.

➤*Pediatric HIV infection (Gamimune N only):* To decrease the frequency of serious and minor bacterial infections and the frequency of hospitalization and to increase the time free of serious bacterial infections. The effect of IGIV in preventing serious bacterial infections was especially apparent in preventing primary bacteremia (including *Streptococcus pneumoniae*) and acute pneumonia.

➤*Primary immune deficiency diseases:*

Octagam – For the treatment of primary immune deficient diseases, such as congenital agammaglobulinemia and hypogammaglobulinemia, common variable immunodeficiency, Wiskott-Aldrich syndrome, and severe combined immunodeficiencies.

Flebogamma – For primary (inherited) humoral immunodeficiency disorders, such as common variable immunodeficiency, X-linked agammaglobulinemia, severe combined immunodeficiency, and Wiskott-Aldrich Syndrome. It is especially useful when rapid replacement of IgG or the attainment of high serum levels of IgG is desired.

Panglobulin NF/Carimune NF – For the maintenance treatment of patients with primary immunodeficiencies, such as common variable immunodeficiency, X-linked agammaglobulinemia, or severe combined immunodeficiency.

➤*Unlabeled uses:* Posttransfusion purpura, Guillain-Barré syndrome, and chronic inflammatory demyelinating polyneuropathy (as an alternative to plasma exchange). IGIV is being investigated in the prevention or treatment of the following diseases: Autoimmune diseases (eg, rhesus hemolytic disease, Factor VIII deficiencies, bullous pemphigoid, rheumatoid arthritis, Sjogren syndrome, type 1 diabetes mellitus), IgG$_4$ subclass deficiencies, intractable epilepsy (possibly caused by IgG$_2$ subclass deficiency), cystic fibrosis, trauma, thermal injury (eg, severe burns), cytomegalovirus infection, neuromuscular disorders, prophylaxis of infections associated with bone marrow transplantation, and GI protection (ie, oral administration).

Administration and Dosage

Administer IV only.

IGIV is well tolerated and less likely to produce side effects if infused at indicated rates.

➤*Gammar-P I.V.:*

Immunodeficiency syndrome – Starting doses of 200 mg/kg body weight every 3 to 4 weeks are recommended in children and adolescents. Slightly higher doses of 200 to 400 mg/kg every 3 to 4 weeks are recommended in adults. Individualize treatment.

IMMUNE GLOBULIN INTRAVENOUS (IGIV)

Rate of administration – 0.01 mL/kg/min, increasing to 0.02 mL/kg/min after 15 to 30 minutes. Most patients tolerate a gradual increase to 0.03 to 0.06 mL/kg/min. For the average 70 kg person, this is equivalent to 2 to 4 mL/min. If adverse reactions develop, slowing the infusion rate will usually eliminate the reaction. Discard any unused solution.

Renal dysfunction – For patients judged to be at increased risk for developing renal dysfunction, it may be prudent to reduce the amount of product (and sucrose stabilizer) infused per unit time by infusing *Gammar-P I.V.* at a rate < 3 mg Ig/kg/min (3 mg sucrose/kg/min) (0.06 mL/kg/min).

No prospective data are presently available to identify a maximum safe dose, concentration, and rate of infusion in patients determined to be at an increased risk of acute renal failure. In the absence of prospective data, recommended doses should not be exceeded and the concentration and infusion rate selected should be the minimum level praticable. Reduction in dose, concentration, or rate of administration in patients at risk of acute renal failure has been proposed in the literature in order to reduce the risk of acute renal failure.

➤*Gamimune N:*

Immunodeficiency syndrome – 100 to 200 mg/kg/month (2 to 4 mL/kg/month). The dosage may be given more frequently or increased as high as 400 mg/kg (8 mL/kg) if the clinical response is inadequate or the level of IgG is insufficient.

ITP – 400 mg/kg for 5 consecutive days or 1000 mg/kg/day for 1 day or 2 consecutive days.
   Maintenance: If platelet count falls to < 30,000/mm^3 or if the patient manifests clinically significant bleeding, 400 mg/kg may be given as a single infusion. If an adequate response does not result, the dose can be increased to 800 to 1000 mg/kg given as a single infusion. Maintenance infusions may be administered intermittently as clinically indicated to maintain a platelet count > 30,000/mm^3.

BMT – 500 mg/kg (10 mL/kg) beginning on days 7 and 2 pretransplant or at the time conditioning therapy for transplantation is begun, then weekly through the 90-day posttransplant period.

Pediatric HIV infection – 400 mg/kg (8 mL/kg) every 28 days.

Rate of administration – 0.01 to 0.02 mL/kg/min for 30 minutes by itself. If the patient does not experience any discomfort, the rate may be increased to a maximum of 0.08 mL/kg/min. If side effects occur, reduce the rate or interrupt the infusion until symptoms subside; resume at a rate tolerable by the patient.

➤*Panglobulin:* Give by a separate infusion line. Do not mix other medications or fluids with the *Panglobulin* preparation. Infuse the product at a rate < 2 mg Ig/kg/min.

Any undissolved particles should respond to careful rotation of the bottle. Avoid foaming. Do not shake.

Filtering of *Panglobulin* is acceptable but not required. Pore sizes of 15 microns or larger will be less likely to slow infusion, especially with higher *Panglobulin* concentrations. Antibacterial filters (0.2 microns) may be used. When reconstitution of *Panglobulin* occurs outside of sterile laminar air flow conditions, administration must begin promptly with partially used vials discarded. When reconstitution is carried out in a sterile laminar flow hood using aseptic technique, administration may begin within 24 hours provided the solution has been refrigerated during that time. Do not freeze *Panglobulin* solution.

Immunodeficiency syndrome –
   Adult and child substitution therapy: The usual dose of *Panglobulin* in immunodeficiency syndromes is 0.2 g/kg of body weight administered once a month IV. If the clinical response is inadequate, the dose may be increased to 0.3 g/kg or the infusion may be repeated more frequently than once a month.

The first infusion in previously untreated agammaglobulinemic or hypogammaglobulinemic patients must be given as a 3% immunoglobulin solution. Start with a flow rate of 10 to 20 drops (0.5 to 1 mL) per minute. After 15 to 30 minutes the rate of infusion may be further increased to 30 to 50 drops (1.5 to 2.5 mL) per minute.

After the first bottle of 3% solution is infused and the patient shows good tolerance, subsequent infusions may be administered at a higher rate or concentration. Such increases should be made gradually allowing 15 to 30 minutes before each increment.

The first infusion of *Panglobulin* in previously untreated agammaglobulinemic and hypogammaglobulinemic patients may lead to systemic side effects. The nature of these effects has not been fully elucidated. Subsequent administration of *Panglobulin* to immunodeficient patients as well as to normal individuals usually does not cause further untoward side effects.

ITP – Initiate 0.4 g/kg of body weight on 2 to 5 consecutive days.
   Acute ITP-childhood: In acute ITP of childhood, if an initial platelet count response to the first 2 doses is adequate (30,000 to 50,000/mcgL), therapy may be discontinued after the second day of the 5-day course.
   Maintenance-chronic ITP: In adults and children, if after induction therapy the platelet count falls to < 30,000/mcgL or the patient manifests clinically significant bleeding, 0.4 g/kg of body weight may be given as a single infusion. If an adequate response does not result, the

dose can be increased to 0.8 to 1 g/kg of body weight given as a single infusion.

➤*Panglobulin NF / Carimune NF:*

Immunodeficiency syndrome – 0.2 g/kg of body weight administered once a month by IV infusion. If the clinical response is inadequate, the dose may be increased to 0.3 g/kg of body weight or the infusion may be repeated more frequently than once a month.

The first infusion in previously untreated agammaglobulinemic or hypogammaglobulinemic patients must be given as a 3% immunoglobulin solution.

Start with a flow rate of 10 to 20 drops (0.5 to 1 mL) per minute. After 15 to 30 minutes the rate of infusion may be further increased to 30 to 50 drops (1.5 to 2.5 mL) per minute. After the first bottle of 3% solution is infused and the patient shows good tolerance, subsequent infusions may be administered at a higher rate or concentration. Such increases should be made gradually allowing 15 to 30 minutes before each increment.

➤*Polygam S/D:*

Immunodeficiency diseases – 100 mg/kg/month. An initial dose of 200 to 400 mg/kg may be administered. Individualize treatment.

B-Cell CLL – 400 mg/kg every 3 to 4 weeks.

Kawasaki disease – For patients with Kawasaki disease, either a single 1 g/kg dose or a dose of 400 mg/kg for four consecutive days beginning within 7 days of the onset of fever, administered concomitantly with appropriate aspirin therapy (80 to 100 mg/kg/day in 4 divided doses is recommended.

ITP – 1 g/kg. A need for additional doses can be determined by clinical response and platelet count. Give ≤ 3 separate doses on alternate days if required.

Rate of administration – Initially 0.5 mL/kg/hr. If rate causes the patient no distress, it may be gradually increased, not to exceed 4 mL/kg/hr. Patients who tolerate the 5% solution at 4 mL/kg/hr can receive the 10% concentration starting at 0.5 mL/kg/hr.

If rate causes the patient no distress, it may be increased, not to exceed 8 mL/kg/hr.

For patients judged to be at risk for developing renal dysfunction, it may be prudent to reduce the amount of product infused per unit time by infusing IGIV at a rate < 13.3 mg Ig/kg/min (< 0.27 mL/kg/min of 5% or < 0.13 mL/kg/min of 10%.

It is recommended that antecubital veins be used especially for 10% solvent, if possible. This may reduce the likelihood of the patient experiencing discomfort at the infusion site.

A rate of administration that is too rapid may cause flushing and changes in pulse rate and blood pressure. Slowing or stopping the infusion usually allows the symptoms to disappear promptly.

Drug interactions – Admixtures of IGIV with other drugs and IV solutions have not been evaluated. It is recommended that *Polygam S/D* be administered separately from other drugs or medications that the patient may be receiving. The product should not be mixed with IGIV from other manufacturers.

Administration – Administer as soon after reconstitution as possible. The reconstituted material should be at room temperature during administration.

Parenteral drugs products should be inspected visually for particulate matter and discoloration prior to administration whenever solution and container permit. Do not use if particulate matter or discoloration is observed.

➤*Octagam / Flebogamma:*

Primary immunodeficiency diseases – 300 to 600 mg/kg body weight administered every 3 to 4 weeks. May be adjusted over time to achieve the desired trough levels and clinical responses.

➤*Venoglobulin-S:*

Immunodeficiency syndrome – 200 mg/kg/month. If clinical response is inadequate or the level of serum IgG achieved is felt to be insufficient, the dose may be increased to 300 to 400 mg/kg/month or the infusion may be repeated more frequently than once per month.

ITP – 2000 mg/kg over ≤ 5 days for induction therapy.
   Maintenance therapy: 1000 mg/kg may be administered as needed to maintain platelet counts of 30,000/mm^3 in children and 20,000/mm^3 in adults or to prevent bleeding episodes in the interval between infusions.

Kawasaki disease – Initiate treatment within 10 days of the onset of symptoms. Give a single dose of 2 g/kg (40 mL/kg) over a 10- to 12-hour period. The treatment regimen should include the administration of aspirin (100 mg/kg/day) until the patient becomes afebrile or through the fourteenth day after the onset of symptoms. Administer 3 to 10 mg/kg/day of aspirin for the following 5 weeks. If symptoms persist or recur due to active Kawasaki Disease, retreatment with the same dose level may be useful.

Rate of administration – Initially 0.01 to 0.02 mL/kg/min or 0.6 to 1.2 mL/kg/hr for the first 30 minutes. If the patient does not experience any discomfort, the rate for the 5% solution may be increased to 0.08 mL/kg/min or 4 mg/kg/min and the rate for the 10% solution may

IMMUNE GLOBULIN INTRAVENOUS (IGIV)

be increased to 0.05 mL/kg/min or 5 mg/kg/min.

➤*Storage/Stability:*

Gamimune N – Store at 2° to 8°C (36° to 46°F). Do not freeze.

Panglobulin – Store at a temperature < 30°C (86°F).

Gammar-P I.V., Polygam S/D, Venoglobulin-S – Store at ≤ 25°C (77°F). Avoid freezing. Administration of *Polygam S/D* should begin ≤ 2 hours after reconstitution. Discard unused solution.

Panglobulin NF/Carimune NF – Store at room temperature not exceeding 30°C (86°F). Do not use after expiration date.

Octagam – May be stored for 24 months at 2° to 8°C (36° to 46°F) or may be stored at temperatures not to exceed 25°C (77°F) for up to 18 months from the date of manufacture. Do not use after expiration date.

Flebogamma – Store at 2° to 25°C (36° to 77°F). Do not freeze. Discard after expiration date.

LYMPHOCYTE IMMUNE GLOBULIN, ANTITHYMOCYTE GLOBULIN (EQUINE) (LIG, ATG, ATG equine)

| *Rx* | **Atgam** (Pharmacia) | **Injection:**[1] 50 mg horse gamma globulin/mL | In 5 mL amps. |

[1] With 0.3 M glycine.

For additional information, refer to the Immune Globulins group monograph.

> ### WARNING
>
> Only physicians experienced in immunosuppressive therapy in the treatment of renal transplant or aplastic anemia patients should use this product.
>
> Treat patients receiving this drug in facilities equipped and staffed with adequate laboratory and supportive medical resources.

Indications

➤*Renal transplantation:* Management of allograft rejection in renal transplant patients. When administered with conventional therapy at the time of rejection, it increases the frequency of resolution of the acute rejection episode.

Also used as an adjunct to other immunosuppressives to delay onset of first rejection episode. Data have not consistently demonstrated improvement in functional graft survival associated with therapy to delay onset of first rejection episode.

➤*Aplastic anemia:* Treatment of moderate-to-severe aplastic anemia in patients unsuited for bone marrow transplantation. When administered with a regimen of supportive care, ATG equine may include partial or complete hematologic remission.

The usefulness of ATG equine has not been demonstrated in patients with aplastic anemia who are suitable candidates for bone marrow transplantation or in patients with aplastic anemia secondary to neoplastic disease, storage disease, myelofibrosis, Fanconi syndrome, or in patients known to have been exposed to myelotoxic agents or radiation.

➤*Unlabeled uses:* As an immunosuppressant in the course of liver, bone-marrow, heart, and other organ transplants; treatment of multiple sclerosis, myasthenia gravis, pure red-cell aplasia, and scleroderma, although efficacy is not definitively established.

Administration and Dosage

➤*Skin testing:* Test patients with an intradermal injection of 0.1 mL of a 1:1000 dilution (5 mcg horse IgG) in normal saline and a saline control. Use only freshly diluted drug for skin testing. The patient, and specifically the skin test, should be observed every 15 to 20 minutes over the first hour after intradermal injection. If this causes a wheal or erythema > 10 mm or both with or without pseudopod formation and itching or a marked local swelling, it should be considered a positive test. A systemic reaction such as a generalized rash, tachycardia, dyspnea, hypotension, or anaphylaxis precludes any additional administration of the drug. The predictive value of this test is not proven; allergic reactions can occur in patients whose skin test is negative. In the presence of a locally positive skin test to lymphocyte immune globulin (equine), serious consideration to alternative forms of therapy should be given. The risk-to-benefit ratio must be carefully weighed. If therapy with lymphocyte immune globulin is deemed appropriate following a locally positive skin test, treatment should be administered in a setting where intensive life support facilities are immediately available and with a physician familiar with the treatment of potentially life-threatening allergic reactions in attendance.

➤*Renal allograft recipients:*
Adults – 10 to 30 mg/kg/day.

Children – 5 to 25 mg/kg/day.

The drug has been used to delay the onset of the first rejection episode and at the time of the first rejection episode. Most patients who received it for the treatment of acute rejection had not received it at the time of transplantation. Usually, it is used concomitantly with azathioprine and corticosteroids. Exercise caution during repeat courses of therapy; carefully observe patients for signs of allergic reactions.

Delaying the onset of renal allograft rejection – Give a fixed dose of 15 mg/kg/day for 14 days, then every other day for 14 days, for a total of 21 doses in 28 days. Administer the first dose within 24 hours before or after the transplant.

Treatment of allograft rejection – The first dose can be delayed until the diagnosis of the first rejection episode. The recommended dose is 10 to 15 mg/kg/day for 14 days. Additional alternate-day therapy up to a total of 21 doses can be given.

➤*Aplastic anemia:* 10 to 20 mg/kg/day for 8 to 14 days. Additional alternate-day therapy up to a total of 21 doses can be given. Because thrombocytopenia can be associated with ATG administration, patients receiving it may need prophylactic platelet transfusions to maintain platelets at clinically acceptable levels.

➤*Infusion instructions:* Inspect parenteral drug products visually for particulate matter and discoloration prior to administration whenever solution and container permit. However, because ATG equine is a gamma globulin product, it can be transparent to slightly opalescent, colorless to faintly pink or brown, and may develop a slight granular or flaky deposit during storage. Do not shake diluted or undiluted solution because excessive foaming or denaturation of the protein may occur.

Dilute in saline solution before IV infusion. Invert the IV saline bottle so undiluted drug does not contact the air inside. Add the total daily dose to a sterile vehicle. Ideally, concentration should not exceed 4 mg/mL. Gently rotate or swirl the diluted solution to effect thorough mixing.

Adding the drug to dextrose solutions is not recommended, as low-salt concentrations can cause precipitation. Highly acidic infusion solutions can also contribute to physical instability over time.

During clinical trials, most investigators infused into a vascular shunt, arterial venous fistula, or a high-flow central vein through an in-line filter with a pore size of 0.2 to 1 micron to prevent inadvertent administration of any insoluble material that may develop in the product during storage. Using high-flow veins will minimize the occurrence of phlebitis and thrombosis.

Allow diluted solution to reach room temperature before infusion. Do not infuse a dose in < 4 hours.

Always keep a tray containing epinephrine, antihistamines, corticosteroids, syringes, and an airway at the patient's bedside while this agent is being administered. Observe the patient continuously for possible allergic reactions throughout the infusion.

➤*Admixture compatibility:* Diluted ATG is physically and chemically stable for up to 24 hours in concentrations of up to 4 mg/mL in 0.9% Sodium Chloride, 5% Dextrose with 0.225% Sodium Chloride, and 5% Dextrose with 0.45% Sodium Chloride.

➤*Storage/Stability:* Refrigerate at 2° to 8°C (36° to 46°F). Do not freeze; discard if frozen. Do not keep in diluted form for > 12 hours (including actual infusion time). Refrigerate diluted solution if prepared prior to time of infusion. Even if refrigerated, total time in dilution should not exceed 24 hours, including infusion time.

ANTITHYMOCYTE GLOBULIN (RABBIT) (ATG Rabbit)

| *Rx* | **Thymoglobulin** (SangStat) | **Powder for Injection, lyophilized:**[1] 25 mg | In 7 mL vials with 5 mL vial of diluent. |

[1] 50 mg glycine, 50 mg mannitol, 10 mg NaCl.

For additional information, refer to the Immune Globulins group monograph.

> ### WARNING
>
> Antithymocyte globulin (rabbit) should only be used by physicians experienced in immunosuppressive therapy for the management of renal transplant patients.

Indications

➤*Acute rejection:* For the treatment of renal transplant acute rejection in conjunction with concomitant immunosuppression.

Administration and Dosage

➤*Approved by the FDA:* December 30, 1998.

➤*Acute renal graft rejection:* Administer 1.5 mg/kg/day for 7 to 14 days using a high-flow vein. Infuse over a minimum of 6 hours for the first infusion and over ≥ 4 hours on subsequent days of therapy. Administer ATG rabbit through an in-line 0.22 mcm filter.

Adjunctive therapy – Administration of antiviral prophylactic therapy is recommended. Premedication with corticosteroids, acetaminophen, or an antihistamine 1 hour prior to the infusion is recommended and may reduce the incidence and intensity of side effects during the infusion.

ANTITHYMOCYTE GLOBULIN (RABBIT) (ATG Rabbit)

Overdosage of ATG rabbit may result in leukopenia or thrombocytopenia. The ATG rabbit dose should be reduced by 50% if the WBC count is between 2000 and 3000 cells/mm^3 or if the platelet count is between 50,000 and 75,000 cells/mm^3. Stopping ATG rabbit treatment should be considered if the WBC count falls below 2000 cells/mm^3 or platelets below 50,000 cells/mm^3.

➤*Preparation for administration:*

Reconstitution – After calculating the number of vials needed, reconstitute ATG rabbit with the supplied diluent, Sterile Water for Injection, USP, immediately before use. Use within 4 hours of reconstitution if kept at room temperature.

Allow ATG rabbit and diluent vials to reach room temperature before reconstituting product. Aseptically remove 5 mL of diluent using a sterile, single-use syringe and inject it slowly into the vial containing ATG rabbit lyophilized powder. Rotate vial gently until powder is completely dissolved. Each reconstituted vial contains 25 mg or 5 mg/mL. Continue to rotate the vial until no particulate matter is visible; discard if particulate matter persists.

Dilution – Transfer the contents of the calculated number of ATG rabbit into the bag of infusion solution (saline or dextrose). Recommended volume: Use 50 mL of infusion solution per vial of ATG rabbit. Mix the solution by inverting the bag gently only once or twice.

Infusion – Follow the manufacturer's instructions for the infusion administration set. Infuse through a 0.22-micron filter into a high-flow vein. Set the flow rate to deliver the dose over a minimum of 6 hours for the first dose and over at least 4 hours for subsequent doses.

➤*Storage / Stability:* Store in refrigerator between (2° to 8°C; 36° to 46°F). Protect from light. Do not freeze. Use reconstituted vials within 4 hours; infusion solutions must be used immediately. Discard any unused drug after infusion.

RABIES IMMUNE GLOBULIN, HUMAN (RIG)

Rx	BayRab[1] (Bayer Pharmaceutical)	Injection: 150 IU/mL	In 2 and 10 mL single-dose vials.
Rx	Imogam Rabies - HT [2] (Aventis Pasteur)		In 2 and 10 mL vials.

[1] Preservative free. With 0.21 to 0.32 M glycine. Solvent/Detergent treated.

[2] Preservative free. With 0.3 M glycine. Heat treated.

Refer to the general discussion for Rabies Prophylaxis in the Treatment Guidelines section of the Appendix.

Indications

➤*Rabies exposure:* RIG is indicated for individuals suspected of exposure to rabies, particularly severe exposure, with one exception: People who have been previously immunized with HDCV rabies vaccine in a pre- or postexposure treatment series should receive only vaccine. People who have received rabies vaccines other than HDCV or RVA vaccines should have confirmed adequate rabies antibody titers if they are to receive only vaccine.

Promptly inject as soon as possible after exposure along with the first dose of vaccine. If initiation of treatment is delayed for any reason, rabies immune globulin and the first dose of vaccine should still be given regardless of the interval between exposure and treatment. Rabies immune globulin may be given up to 8 days after the first dose of vaccine is given.

➤*Rabies prophylaxis:* Rabies antibody provides passive protection when given immediately to individuals exposed to rabies virus. Rabies immune globulin (human) of adequate potency was used in conjunction with rabies vaccine of duck embryo origin. When a globulin dose of 20 IU/kg of rabies antibody was given simultaneously with the first dose of vaccine, levels of passive rabies antibody were detected 24 hours after injection in all individuals. There was minimal or no interference with the immune response to the initial and subsequent doses of vaccine, including booster doses.

Studies of RIG (*Imogam*) given with the first 5 doses of HDCV confirmed that passive immunization with 20 IU/kg of RIG provides maximum circulating antibody with minimum interference of active immunization by HDCV.

Administration and Dosage

For IM administration only, preferably in gluteal muscle (upper, outer quadrant only) or deltoid muscle; do not administer IV. Begin with immediate and thorough washing of all bite wounds and scratches with soap and water. If available, use a virucidal agent such as a povidone-iodine solution to irrigate the wounds. Give RIG 20 IU/kg (0.133 mL/kg) or 9 IU/lb (0.06 mL/lb) as soon as possible after exposure, preferably with the first dose of vaccine. As much as possible of the recommended dose should be infiltrated around the wound if anatomically feasible and the remaining HRIG should be administered IM in the gluteal region. Give 2 injections in the gluteal region if the volume is > 5 mL.

Never administer HRIG in the same syringe or into the same anatomical site as vaccine. Because HRIG may partially suppress active production of antibody, do not give more than recommended dose.

➤*Storage / Stability:* Refrigerate between 2° to 8°C (36° to 46°F). Do not freeze.

Rh$_o$(D) IMMUNE GLOBULIN (Rh$_o$[D] IGIM)

Rx	BayRho-D Full Dose (Bayer Pharmaceutical)	Solution for Injection:[1] 15% to 18% protein	In individual and multiple-pack single-dose syringes with attached needles and vials.
Rx	RhoGAM (Ortho Diagnostics)	Solution for Injection:[2] 5% ± 1% gamma globulin	In packages with prefilled single-dose syringes, package insert, control form, and patient ID card. In 5s, 25s, and 100s.

[1] Preservative free. With 0.21 to 0.32 M glycine. Solvent/Detergent treated.

[2] Preservative free. With 2.9 mg sodium chloride, 0.01% polysorbate 80, 15 mg/mL glycine. Filtrated.

For additional information, refer to the Immune Globulins group monograph.

Indications

➤*Pregnancy and other obstetric conditions:* Rh$_o$(D) IGIM is recommended for the prevention of Rh hemolytic disease of the newborn by its administration to the Rh$_o$(D)-negative mother within 72 hours after birth of a Rh$_o$(D)-positive infant, providing the following criteria are met:

1.) The mother must be Rh$_o$(D) negative and must not already be sensitized to the Rh$_o$(D) factor.
2.) Her child must be Rh$_o$(D) positive, and should have a negative direct antiglobulin test.

If Rh$_o$(D) IGIM is administered antepartum, it is essential that the mother receive another dose of Rh$_o$(D) IGIM after delivery of a Rh$_o$(D) positive infant.

If the father can be determined to be Rh$_o$(D) negative, Rh$_o$(D) IGIM need not be given.

Administer Rh$_o$(D) IGIM within 72 hours to all nonimmunized Rh$_o$(D)-negative women who have undergone spontaneous or induced abortion, following ruptured tubal pregnancy, amniocentesis, or abdominal trauma unless the blood group of the fetus or the father is known to be Rh$_o$(D) negative. If the fetal blood group cannot be determined, one must assume that it is Rh$_o$(D) positive, and Rh$_o$(D) IGIM should be administered to the mother.

➤*Transfusion:* Rh$_o$(D) IGIM may be used to prevent isoimmunization in Rh$_o$(D)-negative individuals who have been transfused with Rh$_o$(D)-positive red blood cells or blood components containing red blood cells.

➤*Unlabeled uses:* A multicenter study showed that escalating doses of a Canadian IV form of Rh$_o$(D) IGIM was effective in treating immune thrombocytopenia purpura in 25 Rh$_o$(D) antigen-positive children.

Administration and Dosage

Never administer Rh$_o$(D) IGIM IV. Inject IM. Never administer to the neonate.

➤*Pregnancy and other obstetric conditions:*

1.) For postpartum prophylaxis, administer 1 vial or syringe of Rh$_o$(D) IGIM (300 mcg) preferably within 72 hours of delivery. Although a lesser degree of protection is afforded if Rh antibody is administered beyond the 72-hour period, Rh$_o$(D) IGIM may still be given. Full term deliveries can vary in their dosage requirements depending on the magnitude of the fetomaternal hemorrhage. One 300 mcg vial or syringe of Rh$_o$(D) IGIM provides sufficient antibody to prevent Rh sensitization if the volume of red blood cells that has entered the circulation is ≤ 15 mL. In instances where a large (> 30 mL of whole blood or 15 mL red blood cells) fetomaternal hemorrhage is suspected, perform a fetal red cell count by an approved laboratory technique (eg, modified Kleihauer-Betke acid elution stain technique) to determine the dosage of immune globulin required. The red blood cell volume of the calculated fetomaternal hemorrhage is divided by 15 mL to obtain the number of vials or syringes of Rh$_o$(D) IGIM for administration. If > 15 mL of red cells is suspected or if the dose calculation results in a fraction, administer the next higher whole number of vials or syringes (eg, if 1.4, give 2 vials or 2 syringes).
2.) For antenatal prophylaxis, one 300 mcg vial or syringe of Rh$_o$(D) IGIM is administered at ≈ 28 weeks' gestation. This must be followed by another 300 mcg dose, preferably within 72 hours following delivery, if the infant is Rh positive.

Rh$_o$(D) IMMUNE GLOBULIN (Rh$_o$[D] IGIM)

3.) Following threatened abortion at any stage of gestation with continuation of pregnancy, it is recommended that 300 mcg of Rh$_o$(D) IGIM be given. If > 15 mL of red cells is suspected due to fetomaternal hemorrhage, the same dose modification in No. 1 applies.

4.) Following miscarriage, abortion, or termination of ectopic pregnancy at or beyond 13 weeks' gestation, it is recommended that 300 mcg of Rh$_o$(D) IGIM be given. If > 15 mL of red cells is suspected due to fetomaternal hemorrhage, the same dose modification in No. 1 applies. If pregnancy is terminated prior to 13 weeks' gestation, where liscensed, a single dose of Rh$_o$(D) IG micro-dose ($\approx$ 50 mcg) may be used instead of Rh$_o$(D) IGIM.

5.) Following amniocentesis at either 15 to 18 weeks' gestation or during the third trimester, or following abdominal trauma in the second or third trimester, it is recommended that 300 mcg of Rh$_o$(D) Immune globulin (human) full dose be administered. If there is a fetomaternal hemorrhage in excess of 15 mL of red cells, the same dose modification in No. 1 applies.

If abdominal trauma, amniocentesis or other adverse event requires the administration of Rh$_o$(D) IGIM at 13 to 18 weeks gestation, another 300 mcg dose should be given at 26 to 28 weeks. To maintain protection throughout pregnancy, the level of passively acquired anti-Rh$_o$(D) should not be allowed to fall below the level required to prevent an immune response to Rh-positive red cells. The half-life of IgG is 23 to 26 days. In any case, a dose of Rh$_o$(D) IGIM should be given within 72 hours after delivery if the baby is Rh positive. If delivery occurs within 3 weeks after the last dose, the postpartum dose may be withheld unless there is a fetomaternal hemorrhage in excess of 15 mL of red blood cells.

➤*Transfusion:* In the case of a transfusion of Rh$_o$(D)-positive red cells to an Rh$_o$(D)-negative recipient, the volume of Rh-positive whole blood administered is multiplied by the hematocrit of the donor unit giving the volume of red blood cells transfused. The volume of red blood cells is divided by 15 mL which provides the number of vials or syringes of Rh$_o$(D) IGIM to be administered

If the dose calculated results in a fraction, the next higher whole number of vials or syringes should be administered (eg, if 1.4, give 2 vials or 2 syringes). Rh$_o$(D) IGIM should be administered within 72 hours after an incompatible transfusion, but preferably as soon as possible.

➤*Injection procedure:* Do not inject IV. Do not inject the neonate. Rh$_o$(D) IGIM is administered IM, preferably in the anterolateral aspects of the upper thigh and the deltoid muscle of the upper arm. The gluteal region should not be used routinely as an injection site because of the risk of injury to the sciatic nerve. If the gluteal region is used, the central region must be avoided; only the upper, outer quadrant should be used.

1.) Single vial or syringe dose — Inject entire contents of the vial or syringe into the individual IM.

2.) Multiple vial or syringe dose
   a.) Calculate the number of vials or syringes of Rh$_o$(D) IGIM to be given.
   b.) The total volume of Rh$_o$(D) IGIM can be given in divided doses at different sites at 1 time or the total dose may be divided and injected at intervals, provided the total dosage is given within 72 hours of the fetomaternal hemorrhage or transfusion.

Parenteral drug products should be inspected visually for particulate matter and discoloration prior to administration, whenever solution and container permit.

Directions for syringe usage:

1.) Remove the prefilled syringe from the package. Lift syringe by barrel, not by plunger.
2.) Twist the plunger rod clockwise until the threads are seated.
3.) With the rubber needle shield secured on the syringe tip, push the plunger rod forward a few millimeters to break any friction seal between the rubber stopper and the glass syringe barrel.
4.) Remove the needle shield and expel air bubbles.
5.) Proceed with hypodermic needle puncture.
6.) Aspirate prior to injection to confirm that the needle is not in a vein or artery.
7.) Inject the medication.
8.) Withdraw the needle and destroy it.

Rh$_o$(D) IMMUNE GLOBULIN IV (HUMAN) (Rh$_o$[D] IGIV)

Rx	**Rhophylac** (ZLB Bioplasma)	**Injection:** 1500 IU (300 mcg)	Preservative-free. In 2 mL pre-filled syringes.
Rx	**WinRho SDF** (Nabi)	**Powder for injection, freeze-dried:**[1] 600 IU (120 mcg)	With 2.5 mL 0.9% Sodium Chloride Injection diluent. In single-dose vials.
		1500 IU (300 mcg)	With 2.5 mL 0.9% Sodium Chloride Injection diluent. In single-dose vials.
		5000 IU (1000 mcg)	With 8.5 mL 0.9% Sodium Chloride Injection diluent. In single-dose vials.

[1] Preservative free. Contains 0.1 M glycine, 0.04 M sodium chloride, 0.01% polysorbate 80. Solvent/Detergent treated.

For additional information, refer to the Immune Globulins group monograph.

Indications

➤*Pregnancy/Other obstetric conditions:* Suppression of Rh isoimmunization in nonsensitized Rh$_o$(D)-negative women within 72 hours after spontaneous or induced abortions, amniocentesis, chorionic villus sampling, ectopic pregnancy or hydatidiform mole, obstetric manipulative procedures, abdominal trauma, transplacental hemorrhage, or in the normal course of pregnancy unless the blood type of the fetus or father is known to be Rh$_o$(D)-negative. In the case of maternal bleeding because of threatened abortion, administer Rh$_o$(D) immune globulin as soon as possible. Suppression of Rh isoimmunization reduces the likelihood of hemolytic disease in an Rh$_o$(D)-positive fetus in present and future pregnancies. The criteria for an Rh-incompatible pregnancy requiring administration of Rh$_o$(D) IGIV at 28 to 30 weeks gestation and within 72 hours after delivery are the following:
• The mother must be Rh$_o$(D) negative,
• The mother is carrying a child whose father is either Rh$_o$(D) positive or Rh$_o$(D) unknown,
• The baby is either Rh$_o$(D) positive or Rh$_o$(D) unknown, and
• The mother must not be previously sensitized to the Rh$_o$(D) factor.

➤*Transfusion:* Suppression of Rh isoimmunization in Rh$_o$(D)-negative female children and female adults in their childbearing years transfused with Rh$_o$(D)-positive RBCs or blood components containing Rh$_o$(D)-positive RBCs. Initiate treatment within 72 hours of exposure. Give treatment (without preceding exchange transfusion) only if the transfused Rh$_o$(D)-positive blood represents less than 20% of the total circulating red cells. A 1500 IU (300 mcg) dose will suppress the immunizing potential of approximately 15 to 17 mL of Rh$_o$(D)-positive RBCs.

➤*Immune thrombocytopenic purpura (ITP) (WinRho SDF only):* Treatment of non-splenectomized Rh$_o$(D)-positive children with chronic or acute ITP, adults with chronic ITP, or children and adults with ITP secondary to HIV infection in clinical situations requiring an increase in platelet count to prevent excessive hemorrhage. The safety and efficacy of Rh$_o$(D) IGIV have not been evaluated in clinical trials for patients with non-ITP causes of thrombocytopenia or in previously splenectomized patients.

Administration and Dosage

➤*Approved by the FDA:* March 24, 1995.

Rh$_o$(D) IGIV may be given IV or IM for the suppression of Rh isoimmunization.

Rh$_o$(D) IGIV must be given IV for the treatment of ITP (WinRho SDF only).

➤*Suppression of Rh isoimmunization:* Administer IM or IV.

Rhophylac – For routine antepartum prevention (at 28 to 30 weeks of gestation), administer 1500 IU (300 mcg). For postpartum prevention (within 72 hours), administer 1500 IU (300 mcg).

WinRho SDF – Administer 1500 IU (300 mcg) at 28 weeks gestation. If Rh$_o$(D) IGIV is administered early in the pregnancy, it is recommended that it be given at 12-week intervals in order to maintain an adequate level of passively acquired anti-Rh.

Administer a 600 IU (120 mcg) dose as soon as possible after delivery of a confirmed Rh$_o$(D) antigen-positive baby and within 72 hours after delivery. In the event that the Rh status of the baby is not known at 72 hours, administer Rh$_o$(D) IGIV to the mother at 72 hours after delivery. If more than 72 hours have elapsed, do not withhold Rh$_o$(D) IGIV, but administer as soon as possible, up to 28 days after delivery.

➤*Other obstetric conditions:* Administer IM or IV.

Rhophylac – Administer as soon as possible within 72 hours of the at-risk event in casess of obstetric complications or invasive procedures.

In case of known or suspected excessive feto-maternal hemorrhage, the number of fetal red blood cells in the maternal circulation should be determined. If excess transpacental bleeding is measured, extra anti-D immunoglobulin (100 IU [20 mcg] for each 1 mL of fetal red blood cells) should be administered, preferably by the IV route. If testing is not feasible and an excessive feto-maternal hemorrhage cannot be excluded, a further 1500 IU (300 mcg) should be administered. A 1500 IU (300 mcg) dose will suppress the immunizing potential of at least 15 mL of Rh$_o$(D)-positive red blood cells.

Obstetric Indications and Recommended Doses of Rh$_o$(D) IGIV (*Rhopylac*)	
Indication	Dose (IM or IV)
Pregnancy	
Routine antepartum prevention (at 28 to 30 weeks of gestation)	1500 IU (300 mcg)
Postpartum prevention (within 72 hrs)	1500 IU (300 mcg)

Rh₀(D) IMMUNE GLOBULIN IV (HUMAN) (Rh₀[D] IGIV)

Obstetric Indications and Recommended Doses of Rh₀ (D) IGIV (*Rhopylac*)	
Indication	Dose (IM or IV)
Obstetric conditions	
Obstetric complications (eg, miscarriage, abortion, threatened abortion, ectopic pregnancy or hydatidiform mole, transplacental hemorrhage) resulting from antepartum hemorrhage	1500 IU (300 mcg)
Invasive procedures during pregnancy (eg, amniocentesis, chorionicbiopsy or obstetric manipulative procedures [eg, external vision, or abdominaltrauma])	1500 IU (300 mcg)

WinRho SDF – Administer 600 IU (120 mcg) immediately after abortion, amniocentesis (after 34 weeks gestation), or any other manipulation late in pregnancy (after 34 weeks gestation) associated with increased risk of Rh isoimmunization. Administer within 72 hours after the event.

Administer a 1500 IU (300 mcg) dose immediately after amniocentesis before 34 weeks gestation or after chorionic villus sampling. Repeat this dose every 12 weeks during the pregnancy. In the case of threatened abortion, administer as soon as possible.

Obstetric Indications and Recommended Doses of Rh₀(D) IGIV (*WinRho SDF*)	
Indication	Dose (IM or IV)
Pregnancy	
28 weeks gestation	1500 IU (300 mcg)
Postpartum (if newborn is Rh positive)	600 IU (120 mcg)
Obstetric conditions	
Threatened abortion at any time	1500 IU (300 mcg)
Amniocentesis and chorionic villus sampling before 34 weeks gestation	1500 IU (300 mcg)
Abortion, amniocentesis, or any other manipulation after 34 weeks gestation	600 IU (120 mcg)

▶*Transfusion:*

Rhoyphylac – The recommended dose is 100 IU (20 mcg) anti-D IgG per 2 mL of transfused Rh₀(D)-positive blood or per 1 mL of Rh₀(D)-positive erythrocyte concentrate.

WinRho SDF – Administer within 72 hours after exposure for treatment of incompatible blood transfusions or massive fetal hemorrhage as outlined in the following table:

Transfusion Indication and Recommended Rh₀(D) IGIV Dosage			
Route	Dose and Frequency	If exposed to Rh₀(D) positive whole blood	If exposed to Rh₀(D) positive red blood cells
IV	3000 IU (600 mcg) every 8 hours until the total dose is administered	45 IU (9 mcg)/mL blood	90 IU (18 mcg)/mL cells
IM	6000 IU (1200 mcg) every 12 hours until the total dose is administered.	60 IU (12 mcg)/mL blood	120 IU (24 mcg)/mL cells

▶*ITP (WinRho SDF only):* Administer IV only.

Initial dose – After confirming the patient is Rh₀(D) positive, an initial dose of 250 IU (50 mcg) per kg as a single injection is recom-

mended. If the patient has a hemoglobin level less than 10 g/dL, give a reduced dose of 125 to 200 IU (25 to 40 mcg) per kg to minimize the risk of increasing the severity of the patient's anemia. The initial dose may be administered as a single dose or in 2 divided doses given on separate days. Monitor all patients to determine clinical response by assessing platelet counts, red cell counts, hemoglobin, and reticulocyte levels (see Precautions).

Subsequent therapy – If subsequent therapy is required to elevate platelet counts, an IV dose of 125 to 300 IU (25 to 60 mcg) per kg is recommended. Determine the frequency and dose used in maintenance therapy by the patient's clinical response by assessing platelet counts, red cell counts, hemoglobin, and reticulocyte levels.

Adequate response to initial dose: If patient responded to the initial dose with a satisfactory increase in platelets, maintenance therapy is 125 to 300 IU/kg (25 to 60 mcg/kg), individualized based on platelet and hemoglobin levels.

Inadequate response to initial dose: If the patient did not respond to the initial dose, administer a subsequent dose based on hemoglobin. If hemoglobin is more than 10 g/dL, redose between 250 and 300 IU/kg (50 to 60 mcg/kg); if hemoglobin is 8 to 10 g/dL, redose between 125 and 200 IU/kg (25 to 40 mcg/kg); if hemoglobin is more than 8 g/dL, use with caution.

▶*Reconstitution/administration: Rhophylac* should be administered by slow IV or IM injection. If large doses (greater than 5 mL) are required and IM injection is chosen, it is advisable to administer them in divided doses at different sites.

IV compatibility –

Treatment of ITP and suppression of Rh isoimmunization: Reconstitute *WinRho SDF* only with the accompanying vial of 0.9% Sodium Chloride Injection. Do not administer concurrently with other products.

IV administration – Aseptically reconstitute *WinRho SDF* with 0.9% Sodium Chloride Injection shortly before use (see following table). Inject the diluent slowly onto the inside wall of the vial, gently swirling until dissolved. Do not shake. Infuse the entire dose into a suitable vein over 3 to 5 minutes. Administer separately from other drugs.

IM administration – Aseptically reconstitute *WinRho SDF* with 0.9% Sodium Chloride Injection shortly before use (see following table). Inject the diluent slowly onto the inside wall of the vial, gently swirling until dissolved. Do not shake. Administer into the deltoid muscle of the upper arm or the anterolateral aspects of the upper thigh. Because of the risk of sciatic nerve injury, do not use the gluteal region as a routine injection site. If the gluteal region is used, use only the upper, outer quadrant.

Reconstitution of *WinRho SDF*	
Vial size	Volume of diluent to be added to vial (mL)
IV injection	
600 IU (120 mcg)	2.5
1500 IU (300 mcg)	2.5
5000 IU (1000 mcg)	8.5
IM injection	
600 IU (120 mcg)	1.25
1500 IU (300 mcg)	1.25
5000 IU (1000 mcg)	8.5[1]

[1] To be administered into several sites.

▶*Storage/Stability:* Store at 2° to 8°C (36° to 46°F). If stored at this temperature, *Rhophylac* has a shelf life of 36 months. Protect from light. Do not freeze. If the reconstituted product is not used immediately, store at room temperature for up to 12 hours. Do not freeze the reconstituted product. Use the product within 12 hours of reconstitution. Discard any unused portion.

RH₀(D) IMMUNE GLOBULIN MICRO-DOSE (Rh₀[D] IG Micro-dose)

Rx	**BayRho-D Mini Dose** (Bayer Pharmaceutical)	**Solution for Injection:**[1] 15% to 18% protein	In single-dose syringes (10s).
Rx	**MICRhoGAM** (Ortho Diagnostics)	**Solution for Injection:**[2] 5% ± 1% gamma globulin	In packages with prefilled single-dose syringes, package insert, injection control form, and patient ID card. In 5s and 25s.

[1] Preservative free. With 0.21 to 0.32 M glycine. Solvent/Detergent treated.

[2] Preservative free. With 2.9 mg/mL NaCl, 0.01% polysorbate 80, 15 mg/mL glycine. Filtrated.

For additional information, refer to the Immune Globulins group monograph.

Indications

Rh₀(D) IG micro-dose is recommended to prevent the isoimmunization of Rh₀(D)-negative women at the time of spontaneous or induced abortion of up to 12 weeks' gestation, provided the following criteria are met:

1.) The mother must be Rh₀(D)-negative and must not already be sensitized to the Rh₀(D) antigen.
2.) The father is not known to be Rh₀(D) negative.
3.) Gestation is ≤ 12 weeks at termination.

▶*Note:* Rh₀(D) immune globulin prophylaxis is not indicated if the fetus or father can be determined to be Rh negative. If the Rh status of the fetus is unknown, the fetus must be assumed to be Rh₀(D) positive, and Rh₀(D) IG micro-dose should be administered to the mother.

For abortions or miscarriages occurring after 12 weeks' gestation, a standard dose of Rh₀(D) immune globulin (human) is indicated.

Administer Rh₀(D) IG micro-dose within 3 hours or as soon as possible after spontaneous passage or surgical removal of the products of conception. However, if Rh₀(D) IG micro-dose is not given within this time period, consideration should still be given to its administration since clinical studies in male volunteers have demonstrated the effectiveness of Rh₀(D) immune globulin in preventing isoimmunization as long as 72 hours after infusion of Rh₀(D)-positive red cells.

RH$_o$(D) IMMUNE GLOBULIN MICRO-DOSE (Rh$_o$[D] IG Micro-dose)

Administration and Dosage

Do not give Rh$_o$(D) IG micro-dose IV. Inject only IM. Administer to women postabortion or postmiscarriage of ≤ 12 weeks gestation. Never administer to the neonate. One vial will suppress the immune response to 2.5 mL of Rh$_o$(D)-positive packed red blood cells or the equivalent (5 mL) of whole blood. One vial contains ≈ 50 mcg immunoglobulin.

Give 1 vial IM as soon as possible after termination of pregnancy. At or beyond 13 weeks gestation, administer a full dose (300 mcg) Rh$_o$(D) immune globulin.

➤ *Storage / Stability:* Store at 2° to 8°C (35° to 46°F). Do not freeze.

RESPIRATORY SYNCYTIAL VIRUS IMMUNE GLOBULIN INTRAVENOUS (HUMAN) (RSV-IGIV)

Rx	RespiGam (MedImmune)	Injection:[1] 50 ± 10 mg immunoglobulin/mL	In single-use 20 and 50 mL vials.

[1] Preservative free. Contains 5% sucrose, 1% albumin (human) and 1 to 1.5 mEq sodium per 50 mL. Solvent/Detergent treated.

For additional information, refer to the Immune Globulins group monograph.

Indications

➤ *Respiratory syncytial virus (RSV):* Prevention of serious lower respiratory tract infection caused by RSV in children < 24 months of age with bronchopulmonary dysplasia (BPD) or a history of premature birth (≤ 35 weeks gestation). RSV-IGIV is safe and effective in reducing the incidence and duration of RSV hospitalization and the severity of RSV illness in these high-risk infants.

➤ *Unlabeled uses:* Consider using RSV-IGIV rather than IGIV during the RSV season in immunocompromised children who receive IGIV monthly.

Administration and Dosage

➤ *Approved by the FDA:* January 18, 1996.

➤ *Renal insufficiency:* Use IGIV products containing sucrose with caution in patients with pre-existing renal insufficiency and in patients judged to be at increased risk for developing renal insufficiency (including, but not limited to those with diabetes mellitus, > 65 years of age, volume depletion, paraproteinemia, sepsis, and patients receiving known nephrotoxic drugs). RSV-IGIV contains sucrose; therefore, it is important to assure that patients are not volume depleted prior to infusion. While most cases of renal insufficiency have occurred in patients receiving total doses of ≥ 400 mg Ig/kg of IGIV products containing sucrose, no prospective data are presently available to identify a maximum safe dose, concentration, or rate of infusion in patients determined to be at increased risk of acute renal failure. In the absence of prospective data, do not exceed recommended doses in patients at increased risk of renal failure and select the minimum practicable concentration and infusion rate.

The maximum recommended total dosage per monthly infusion is 750 mg/kg, administered according to the following schedule:

RSV-IGIV Infusion Schedule	
Time after start of infusion	Rate of infusion (mL/kg of body mass per hour)
0 to 15 minutes	1.5 mL/kg/hr
15 minutes to end of infusion	3.6 mL/kg/hr

Administer RSV-IGIV intravenously at 1.5 mL/kg/hr for 15 minutes. If the clinical condition does not contraindicate a higher rate, increase the rate to 3.6 mL/kg/hr for the remainder of the infusion. *Do not exceed this rate of administration.* Monitor the patient closely during and after each rate change. In especially ill children with BPD, slower rates of infusion may be indicated.

Consider factors such as other clinical illness, how well the child has grown, and the risk of exposure from siblings or daycare when determining whether to use RSV-IGIV. Administer the first dose prior to commencement of the RSV season and subsequent doses monthly throughout the RSV season in order to maintain protection. In the Northern Hemisphere, the RSV season typically commences in November and runs through April. Infuse children from early November through April, unless RSV activity begins earlier or persists later in a community. It is recommended that RSV-IGIV be administered separately from other drugs or medications that the patient may be receiving. It is recommended that children infected with RSV continue to receive monthly doses for the duration of the RSV season.

➤ *Infusion:* Begin infusion within 6 hours and complete within 12 hours after the single-use vial is entered. Assess the patient's vital signs and cardiopulmonary status prior to infusion, before each rate increase, and thereafter, at 30-minute intervals until 30 minutes following completion of the infusion. Administer RSV-IGIV through an IV line using a constant infusion pump (ie, *IVAC* pump or equivalent). Predilution of RSV-IGIV before infusion is not recommended. If possible, administer RSV-IGIV through a separate IV line, although it may be "piggy-backed" into a preexisting line if that line contains one of the following dextrose solutions (with or without sodium chloride): 2.5%, 5%, 10%, or 20% Dextrose in Water. If a preexisting line must be used, the RSV-IGIV should not be diluted more than 1:2 with any of the above-named solutions. An in-line filter with a pore size > 15 micrometers may be used for RSV-IGIV infusions.

➤ *Admixture incompatibility:* It is recommended that RSV-IGIV be administered separately from other drugs or medications that the patient may be receiving.

➤ *Storage / Stability:* Store between 2° and 8°C (36° and 46°F). Do not freeze. Do not shake vial; avoid foaming.

TETANUS IMMUNE GLOBULIN (HUMAN) (TIG)

Rx	BayTet (Bayer Pharmaceutical)	Solution for Injection:[1] 15% to 18% protein	In 250 unit vial and 250 unit syringe.

[1] Preservative free. With 0.21 to 0.32 M glycine. Solvent/Detergent treated.

For additional information, refer to the Immune Globulins group monograph.

Indications

TIG is indicated for prophylaxis against tetanus following injury in patients whose immunization is incomplete or uncertain. It is also indicated, although evidence of effectiveness is limited, in the regimen of treatment of active cases of tetanus.

A thorough attempt must be made to determine whether a patient has completed primary vaccination. Patients with unknown or uncertain previous vaccination histories should be considered to have had no previous tetanus toxoid doses. People who had military service since 1941 can be considered to have received ≥1 dose, and although most of them may have completed a primary series of tetanus toxoid, this cannot be assumed for each individual. Patients who have not completed a primary series may require tetanus toxoid and passive immunization at the time of wound cleaning and debridement.

Administration and Dosage

Good medical care is essential in the prevention of tetanus in fresh wounds. Thorough cleansing and removal of all foreign and necrotic material from the injury is important.

Administer IM. Do not inject IV.

➤ *Prophylaxis:*

Adults and children ≥ 7 years of age – 250 units.

Children < 7 years of age – In small children, the dose may be calculated by the body weight (4 units/kg). However, it may be advisable to administer the entire contents of the vial or syringe (250 units) regardless of the child's size, since theoretically the same amount of toxin will be produced in his body by the infecting tetanus organisms as in an adult.

➤ *Therapy:* Several studies suggest the value of human tetanus antitoxin in the actual treatment of active tetanus using single doses of 3000 to 6000 units in combination with other accepted clinical procedures.

The following table is a summary guide to tetanus prophylaxis in wound management.

Guide to Tetanus Prophylaxis in Wound Management				
History of tetanus immunization (doses)	Clean, minor wounds		All other wounds[1]	
	Td[2]	TIG[3]	Td	TIG
Uncertain or < 3	Yes	No	Yes	Yes
≥ 3[4]	No[5]	No	No[6]	No

[1] Such as, but not limited to, wounds contaminated with dirt, feces, soil, and saliva; puncture wounds; avulsions; and wounds resulting from missiles, crushing, burns, and frostbite.

[2] Adult type tetanus and diphtheria toxoids. If the patient is < 7 years of age, DT or DTP is preferred to tetanus toxoid alone. For people ≥ 7 years of age, Td is preferred to tetanus toxoid alone.

[3] Tetanus immune globulin (human).

[4] If only 3 doses of fluid tetanus toxoid have been received, a fourth dose of toxoid, preferably an adsorbed toxoid, should be given.

[5] Yes, if > 10 years since the last dose.

[6] Yes, if > 5 years since the last dose. (More frequent boosters are not needed and can accentuate side effects.)

➤ *Storage / Stability:* Store between 2° and 8°C (36° and 46°F). Do not freeze.

VARICELLA-ZOSTER IMMUNE GLOBULIN (HUMAN) (VZIG)

| *Rx* | **Varicella-Zoster Immune Globulin (Human)** (American Red Cross)[1] | **Injection:**[2] A sterile 10% to 18% solution of the globulin fraction of human plasma, primarily IgG. | In single dose vials containing 125 units of varicella-zoster virus antibody in ≈ 1.25 mL and 625 units in ≈ 6.25 mL. |

[1] Within MA, VZIG is distributed by the MA Public Health Biologic Laboratories. Outside Mass., distribution is arranged by the American Red Cross Blood Services – Northeast Region through other regional distribution centers. VZIG is distributed free of charge to MA residents.

[2] Preservative free. In 0.3 M glycine. Solvent/Detergent treated.

For additional information, refer to the Immune Globulins group monograph.

Indications

For the passive immunization of exposed, susceptible individuals who are at greater risk of complications from varicella than healthy individuals. High-risk groups include immunocompromised children, newborns of mothers with varicella shortly before or after delivery, premature infants, immunocompromised adults, and normal susceptible adults, and may also include susceptible high-risk infants < 1 year of age.

➤*Immunocompromised children:* For passive immunization of susceptible, immunocompromised children after significant exposure to chickenpox or zoster. These children include those with primary cellular immune deficiency disorders or neoplastic diseases and those currently receiving immunosuppressive treatments.

➤*Newborns of mothers with varicella shortly before or after delivery:* For newborns of mothers who develop chickenpox within 5 days before or within 48 hours after delivery.

➤*Premature infants:* Although the risk of postnatally acquired varicella in the premature infant is unknown, it has been judged prudent to administer VZIG to exposed premature infants of ≥ 28 weeks gestation if their mothers have a negative or uncertain history of varicella. Consider premature infants of < 28 weeks gestation or birth weight of < 1000 g for VZIG regardless of maternal history since they may not yet have acquired transplacental maternal antibody.

➤*Full-term infants < 1 year of age:* Evaluate the decision to administer VZIG to infants < 1 year of age on an individual basis. After careful evaluation of the type of exposure, susceptibility to varicella including maternal history of varicella and zoster, and presence of underlying disease, VZIG may be administered to selected infants.

➤*Immunocompromised adults:* After careful evaluation, which might include the measurement of antibody to varicella-zoster virus by a reliable and sensitive assay such as fluorescent antibody to membrane antigen (FAMA), adults who are believed susceptible should receive VZIG.

➤*Healthy adults:* Evaluate the decision to administer VZIG to an adult on an individual basis. If, after careful evaluation, a healthy adult with significant exposure to varicella is believed susceptible, administer VZIG.

➤*Pregnant women:* To prevent complications of varicella in a susceptible adult patient rather than to prevent intrauterine infection.

Administration and Dosage

Greatest efficacy of treatment is to be expected when begun within 96 hours after exposure. High-risk susceptible patients who are exposed after a prior dose of VZIG should receive another full dose.

➤*Do not inject IV:* Administer by deep IM injection in the gluteal muscle, or in another large muscle mass.

VZIG Dose Based on Weight				
Weight of patient		**Dose**	
Kilograms	Pounds	Units	Number of Vials
0 to 10	0 to 22	125	1 @ 125 units
10.1 to 20	22.1 to 44	250	2 @ 125 units
20.1 to 30	44.1 to 66	375	3 @ 125 units
30.1 to 40	66.1 to 88	500	4 @ 125 units
> 40	> 88	625	1 @ 625 units or 5 @ 125 units

Administer entire contents of each vial. For patients ≤ 10 kg, administer 1.25 mL at a single site. For patients > 10 kg, give no more than 2.5 mL at a single site. Each vial of varicella-zoster virus antibody contains 125 units in a volume of ≈ 1.25 mL and each 625 unit vial contains 625 units of antibody in a volume of ≈ 6.25 mL.

The regimen effectively modifies severity of chickenpox and reduces frequency of death, pneumonia, and encephalitis to < 25% expected without treatment.

➤*Storage/Stability:* Store at 2° to 8°C (36° to 46°F). Do not freeze.

BOTULISM IMMUNE GLOBULIN IV (HUMAN) (BIG-IV)

| *Rx* | **BabyBIG** (California Dept. of Health Services) | **Powder for injection, lyophilized**[1]: 100 ± 20 mg (50 mg/mL when reconstituted) | Preservative-free. In single-dose vial with 2 mL vial of diluent. |

[1] Contains 5% sucrose, 1% albumin (human). Solvent/detergent treated.

For additional information, refer to the Immune Globulins group monograph.

Indications

➤*Infant botulism:* For the treatment of patients younger than 1 year of age with infant botulism caused by toxin type A or B.

Administration and Dosage

➤*Approved by the FDA:* October 23, 2003.

Recommended total dosage is 1 mL/kg (50 mg/kg) given as a single IV infusion as soon as the clinical diagnosis of infant botulism is made.

➤*Special populations:* Use with caution in patients with preexisting renal insufficiency and in patients judged to be at increased risk of developing renal insufficiency (including, but not limited to, those with diabetes mellitus, volume depletion, paraproteinemia, sepsis, or who are receiving known nephrotoxic drugs).

➤*Preparation for administration:* Reconstitute the lyophilized powder with 2 mL of sterile water for injection to obtain a 50 mg/mL solution. A double-ended transfer needle or large syringe is suitable for adding the water for reconstitution. Allow an approximately 30-minute interval for dissolving the powder. Do not shake the vial, as this will cause foaming. Infuse the solution only if it is colorless, free of particulate matter, and not turbid.

➤*Infusion:* Begin infusion within 2 hours after reconstitution is complete and conclude within 4 hours after reconstitution. Continuously monitor vital signs during infusion. Administer BIG-IV intravenously using low-volume tubing and a constant infusion pump (ie, an IVAC pump or equivalent). Predilution of BIG-IV before infusion is not recommended. Administer the product through a separate IV line. If this is not possible, it may be "piggybacked" into a preexisting line if that line contains either sodium chloride injection or one of the following dextrose solutions (with or without NaCl added): 2.5%, 5%, 10%, or 20% dextrose in water. If a preexisting line must be used, do not dilute BIG-IV more than 1:2 with any of the above-named solutions. Admixtures of BIG-IV with any other solutions have not been evaluated. Use of an in-line or syringe-tip sterile, disposable filter (18 mcm) is recommended for the administration of BIG-IV.

➤*Rate of administration:* Begin infusion slowly. Administer BIG-IV intravenously at 0.5 mL per kg body weight per hour (25 mg/kg/h). If no untoward reactions occur after 15 minutes, the rate may be increased to 1 mL/kg/h (50 mg/kg/h). Do not exceed this rate of administration. Closely monitor the patient during and after each rate change. At the recommended rates, infusion of the indicated dose should take 67.5 minutes total elapsed time. Minor adverse reactions experienced by patients treated with IGIV products have been related to the infusion rate. If the patient develops a minor side effect (ie, flushing), slow the rate of infusion or temporarily interrupt the infusion. If anaphylaxis or a significant drop in blood pressure occurs, discontinue the infusion and administer epinephrine.

➤*Storage/Stability:* Store between 2° and 8°C (35.6° to 46.4°F). Use reconstituted BIG-IV within 2 hours. Do not store in the reconstituted state.

PALIVIZUMAB

Rx	Synagis (MedImmune)	Powder for Injection, lyophilized: 50 mg	47 mM histidine, 3 mM glycine, 5.6% mannitol. Preservative-free. In 0.5 mL single-use vials.
		100 mg	47 mM histidine, 3 mM glycine, 5.6% mannitol. Preservative-free. In 1 mL single-use vials.

Indications

➤*Respiratory syncytial virus (RSV):* Prevention of serious lower respiratory tract disease caused by RSV in pediatric patients at high risk of RSV disease. Safety and efficacy were established in infants with bronchopulmonary dysplasia (BPD) and infants with a history of prematurity (35 weeks or less gestational age) and children with hemodynamically significant congenital heart disease (CHD).

Administration and Dosage

➤*Approved by the FDA:* June 19, 1998.

➤*RSV:* The recommended dose of palivizumab is 15 mg/kg. Patients, including those who develop an RSV infection, should receive monthly doses throughout the RSV season. Administer the first dose prior to commencement of the RSV season. In the northern hemisphere, the RSV season typically commences in November and lasts through April, but it may begin earlier or persist later in certain communities.

Palivizumab serum levels are decreased after cardiopulmonary bypass. Administer a dose of palivizumab to patients undergoing cardiopulmonary bypass as soon as possible after the cardiopulmonary bypass procedure (even if sooner than a month from the previous dose). Thereafter, administer doses monthly.

Administer palivizumab in a dose of 15 mg/kg IM, preferably in the anterolateral aspect of the thigh. Do not use the gluteal muscle routinely as an injection site because of the risk of damage to the sciatic nerve.

The dose per month = patient weight (kg) × 15 mg/kg ÷ 100 mg/mL (of palivizumab).

Give injection volumes more than 1 mL as a divided dose.

➤*Preparation for administration:* Slowly add 0.6 mL sterile water for injection to the 50 mg vial or 1 mL of sterile water for injection to the 100 mg vial. Gently swirl the vial for 30 seconds to avoid foaming. Do not shake vial. Let reconstituted palivizumab stand at room temperature for a minimum of 20 minutes until the solution clarifies. Reconstituted palivizumab does not contain a preservative; administer within 6 hours of reconstitution.

➤*Storage/Stability:* Upon receipt and until reconstitution for use, store palivizumab between 2° and 8°C (36° and 46°F) in its original container. Do not freeze. Reconstituted palivizumab does not contain a preservative; administer within 6 hours of reconstitution. Vials are for single-use only; do not re-enter the vial and discard any unused portion. Do not use beyond the expiration date.

Actions

➤*Pharmacology:* Palivizumab is a humanized monoclonal antibody (IgG1κ) produced by recombinant DNA technology, directed to an epitope in the A antigenic site of the F protein of RSV. Palivizumab is a composite of human (95%) and murine (5%) antibody sequences.

Palivizumab exhibits neutralizing and fusion-inhibitory activity against RSV. These activities inhibit RSV replication in laboratory experiments. Although resistant RSV strains may be isolated in laboratory studies, a panel of 57 clinical RSV isolates were all neutralized by palivizumab. Palivizumab serum concentrations of at least 40 mcg/mL reduce pulmonary RSV replication in the cotton rat model of RSV infection by 100-fold. The in vivo neutralizing activity of palivizumab was assessed in a randomized, placebo-controlled study of 35 pediatric patients tracheally intubated because of RSV disease. In these patients, palivizumab significantly reduced the quantity of RSV in the lower respiratory tract compared with control patients.

➤*Pharmacokinetics:* In pediatric patients younger than 24 months of age without CHD, the mean half-life was 20 days and monthly IM doses of 15 mg/kg achieved mean 30-day trough serum drug concentrations of approximately 37 mcg/mL after the first injection, approximately 57 mcg/mL after the second injection, approximately 68 mcg/mL after the third injection, and approximately 72 mcg/mL after the fourth injection. Trough concentrations following the first and fourth palivizumab dose were similar in children with CHD and in noncardiac patients. In pediatric patients given palivizumab for a second season, the mean serum concentrations following the first and fourth injections were approximately 61 and 86 mcg/mL, respectively.

In 139 pediatric patients 24 months of age or younger with hemodynamically significant CHD who received palivizumab and underwent cardiopulmonary bypass for open-heart surgery, the mean serum palivizumab concentration was 98 mcg/mL before bypass and declined to 41 mcg/mL after bypass, a reduction of 58%. The clinical significance of this reduction is unknown.

Contraindications

Pediatric patients with a history of a severe reaction to palivizumab or other components of this product.

Warnings

➤*Hypersensitivity reactions:* Very rare cases of anaphylaxis (less than 1 case per 100,000 patients) have been reported following re-exposure to palivizumab. Rare severe acute hypersensitivity reactions have also been reported on initial exposure or re-exposure to palivizumab. If a severe hypersensitivity reaction occurs, permanently discontinue therapy with palivizumab. If milder hypersensitivity reactions occur, use with caution on readministration of palivizumab. If anaphylaxis or severe allergic reaction occurs, administer appropriate medications (eg, epinephrine 1:1000) and provide supportive care as required. Refer to Management of Acute Hypersensitivity Reactions.

➤*Pregnancy: Category C.* Palivizumab is not indicated for adult usage. It is not known whether palivizumab can cause fetal harm when administered to a pregnant woman or affect reproductive capacity.

➤*Children:* Palivizumab is indicated for use in pediatric patients.

Precautions

➤*Administration:* Palivizumab is for IM use only. As with any IM injection, give with caution to patients with thrombocytopenia or any coagulation disorder.

➤*RSV disease, established:* The safety and efficacy of palivizumab have not been demonstrated for treatment of established RSV disease.

➤*Immunogenicity:* In a clinical trial, the incidence of anti-palivizumab antibody following the fourth injection was 1.1% in the placebo group and 0.7% in the palivizumab group. In pediatric patients receiving palivizumab for a second season, 1 of 56 patients had transient, low titer reactivity. This reactivity was not associated with adverse events or alteration in palivizumab serum concentrations.

Adverse Reactions

The most serious adverse reactions occurring with palivizumab treatment are anaphylaxis and other acute hypersensitivity reactions (see Warnings). The adverse reactions most commonly observed in palivizumab-treated patients were upper respiratory tract infection, otitis media, fever, rhinitis, rash, diarrhea, cough, vomiting, gastroenteritis, and wheezing. Upper respiratory tract infection, otitis media, fever, and rhinitis occurred at a rate of 1% or more in the palivizumab group compared to placebo.

The data described reflect palivizumab exposure for 1641 pediatric patients of 3 days to 24.1 months of age in trials 1 and 2. Among these patients, 496 had bronchopulmonary dysplasia, 506 were premature birth infants less than 6 months of age, and 639 had CHD.

Palivizumab Adverse Reactions (≥ 1%)[1]		
Adverse reaction	Palivizumab (n = 1641)	Placebo (n = 1148)
Upper respiratory tract infection	50.6	47.4
Otitis media	36.4	34.6
Fever	27.1	25.2
Rhinitis	26.8	24.6
Hernia	4.1	2.6
AST increased	3	1.7

[1] Cyanosis (palivizumab [9.1%]/placebo [6.9%]) and arrhythmia (palivizumab [3.1%]/placebo [1.7%]) were reported during trial 2 in CHD patients.

➤*Postmarketing:* Based on experience in over 400,000 patients who have received palivizumab (more than 2 million doses), rare severe acute hypersensitivity reactions have been reported on initial or subsequent exposure. Very rare cases of anaphylaxis (fewer than 1 case per 100,000 patients) have also been reported following re-exposure. None of the reported hypersensitivity reactions were fatal. Hypersensitivity reactions may include dyspnea, cyanosis, respiratory failure, urticaria, pruritus, angioedema, hypotonia, and unresponsiveness. The relationship between these reactions and the development of antibodies to palivizumab is unknown.

Limited information from postmarketing reports suggests that, within a single RSV season, adverse events after a sixth or greater dose of palivizumab are similar in character and frequency to those after the initial 5 doses.

Overdosage

No toxicity was observed in rabbits administered a single IM or SC injection of palivizumab at a dose of 50 mg/kg.

Patient Information

Advise patients to contact their physician immediately if they experience severe allergic reactions (ie, rash, hives, difficulty breathing, tightness in chest, swelling of mouth, face, lips, or tongue).

ANTIVENIN (LATRODECTUS MACTANS) (Black Widow Spider Antivenin) (Equine Origin)

Rx	Antivenin (*Latrodectus mactans*) (Merck)	Powder for Injection: ≥ 6000 antivenin units/vial[1]	In single-use vials with 1 vial diluent (2.5 mL vial of sterile water for injection) and 1 mL vial of normal horse serum[1] (1:10 dilution) for sensitivity testing.

[1] With 1:10,000 thimerosal.

Indications

➤*Envenomations:* For passive, transient protection from toxic effects of bites by the black widow (*Latrodectus mactans*) and similar spiders. Emphasize early use of this antivenin for prompt relief. The best effect occurs with antivenin administration within 4 hours after envenomation.

Administration and Dosage

➤*Sensitivity testing (horse serum):* Prior to treatment with any product prepared from horse serum, carefully review the patient's history emphasizing prior exposure to horse serum or any allergies. Serious sickness and even death could result from the use of horse serum in a sensitive patient. Perform a skin or conjunctival test prior to administration.

Skin test – Inject into (not under) the skin no more than 0.02 mL of the test material (1:10 dilution of normal horse serum in physiologic saline). Evaluate result in 10 minutes. A positive reaction is an urticarial wheal surrounded by a zone of erythema. A control test using sodium chloride injection facilitates interpretation of the results.

Conjunctival test – For adults, instill 1 drop of a 1:10 dilution of horse serum into the conjunctival sac, and for children instill 1 drop of 1:100 dilution. Itching of the eye and reddening of the conjunctiva indicate a positive reaction, usually within 10 minutes.

➤*Adults and children:* Inject 1 vial (2.5 mL) of antivenin IM, preferably in the region of the anterolateral thigh so that a tourniquet may be applied in the event of a systemic reaction. Symptoms usually subside in 1 to 3 hours. Although 1 dose is usually adequate, a second dose may be necessary.

May also be given IV in 10 to 50 mL of saline over 15 minutes. This is the preferred route in severe cases, when the patient is younger than 12 years of age, or in shock. One vial is usually adequate.

➤*Desensitization:* Attempt desensitization only when the administration of antivenin is considered necessary to save a life. Epinephrine must be available in case of untoward reaction.

If the history is positive or the results of the sensitivity tests are mildly or questionably positive, administer antivenin as follows to reduce the risk of an immediate severe allergic reaction:

1.) In separate sterile vials or syringes, prepare 1:10 or 1:100 dilutions of antivenin in sodium chloride for injection.
2.) Allow at least 15 but preferably 30 minutes between injections and only proceed with the next dose if no reactions occurred following the previous dose.
3.) Using a tuberculin syringe, inject SC 0.1, 0.2, and 0.5 mL of the 1:100 dilution at 15- or 30-minute intervals; repeat with the 1:10 dilution, and finally the undiluted antivenin.
4.) If there is a reaction after any of the injections, place a tourniquet proximal to the sites of injection and administer epinephrine 1:1000 (0.3 to 1 mL SC, 0.05 to 0.1 mL IV), proximal to the tourniquet or into another extremity. Wait at least 30 minutes before giving another injection of antivenin, the amount of which should be the same as the last one not evoking a reaction.
5.) If no reaction has occurred after 0.5 mL of undiluted antivenin has been given, it is probably safe to continue the dose at 15-minute intervals until the entire dose has been injected.

➤*Storage/Stability:* Refrigerate at 2° to 8°C (36° to 46°F). Do not freeze. Discard if frozen. Do not expose to excessive heat. When reconstituted, the color of the antivenin ranges from light (straw) to very dark (iced tea), but the color has no effect on potency.

Actions

➤*Pharmacology:* Prepared from blood serum of horses immunized against black widow spider venom. Moderately effective in pain relief and can be life-saving. IV effect is rapid; concentration peaks 2 to 3 days after IM injection. Mean half-life is less than 15 days. Symptoms begin to subside within 1 to 3 hours following administration.

Warnings

➤*Envenomation:*

Symptoms – Local muscular cramps begin from 15 minutes to several hours after bite, usually producing sharp pain similar to that caused by needle puncture. The exact sequence of symptoms depends on location of the bite. Venom acts on the myoneural junctions or nerve endings, causing ascending motor paralysis or destruction of peripheral nerve endings. Muscles most frequently affected first are thigh, shoulder, and back. Later, pain becomes more severe, spreading to the abdomen, and weakness and tremor usually develop. Abdominal muscles assume a board-like rigidity, but tenderness is slight. Respiration is thoracic; patient is restless and anxious. Feeble pulse, cold, clammy skin, labored breathing and speech, light stupor, and delirium may occur. Convulsions may also occur, particularly in small children. Temperature may be normal or slightly elevated. Urinary retention, shock, cyanosis, nausea, vomiting, insomnia, and cold sweats have been reported. The syndrome following the bite of the black widow spider may be confused with any medical or surgical condition with acute abdominal symptoms.

The symptoms of black widow spider bite increase in severity for several hours, perhaps a day, and then very slowly become less severe, gradually passing off in 2 or 3 days, except in fatal cases. Residual symptoms such as general weakness, tingling, nervousness, and transient muscle spasm may persist for weeks or months after recovery from the acute stage.

Supportive therapy – Supportive therapy is indicated by the condition of the patient. If possible, hospitalize the patient. Additional treatment consists of prolonged warm baths and IV injection of 10 mL of calcium gluconate 10%, repeated as necessary to control muscle pain. Morphine may be required to control pain. Barbiturates may be used for extreme restlessness. However, because venom can cause respiratory paralysis, consider this when using morphine or a barbiturate. Adrenocorticosteroids have been used with varying degrees of success. Local treatment of the bite is of no value; nothing is gained by applying a tourniquet or attempting to remove venom by incision and suction.

In otherwise healthy individuals between 16 and 60 years of age, the use of antivenin may be deferred and treatment with muscle relaxants may be considered.

➤*Serum sickness:* Observe patients for serum sickness for an average of 8 to 12 days following administration of antivenin.

➤*Pregnancy: Category C.* It is not known whether the antivenin can cause fetal harm when administered to a pregnant woman or can affect reproduction capacity. Give to a pregnant woman only if clearly needed and when potential benefits outweigh potential hazards to the fetus.

Envenomation has produced spontaneous abortion.

➤*Lactation:* It is not known whether this drug is excreted in breast milk. Use caution when administering to a nursing woman.

➤*Children:* Controlled studies have not been conducted. However, there have been virtually no adverse effects in children receiving this product.

Adverse Reactions

➤*Hypersensitivity:* Anaphylaxis and serum sickness have been reported following use of antivenin.

Patient Information

Advise patients to contact their physician immediately if they experience any signs and symptoms of delayed allergic reactions or serum sickness (eg, rash, pruritus, urticaria, muscle aches, fever) after hospital discharge.

ANTIVENIN (CROTALIDAE) POLYVALENT (Equine Origin)

Rx	Antivenin (Crotalidae) Polyvalent (Wyeth-Ayerst)[1]	Powder for Injection, lyophilized[2]	In single-use vials with 1 vial diluent (10 mL Bacteriostatic Water for Injection, USP).[3]

[1] The manufacturer is in the process of discontinuing this product; however, it will continue to produce the product until an alternative source is identified.

[2] With 0.25% phenol and 0.005% thimerosal.
[3] With 0.001% phenylmercuric nitrate.

Indications

➤*Envenomations:* For treatment of envenomations caused by the bites of crotalids (pit vipers) native to North, Central, and South America, including rattlesnakes (*Crotalus, Sistrurus*); copperhead and cottonmouth (*Agkistrodon*), including *A. halys* of Korea and Japan; the Fer-de-lance and other species of Bothrops; the tropical rattler (*C. durissus* and similar species); the Cantil (*A. bilineatus*); and bushmaster (*Lachesis mutus*) of South and Central America.

Administration and Dosage

➤*Test for sensitivity to horse serum:* Test for sensitivity whenever a product containing horse serum is administered. There is a possibility of a severe immediate reaction. Constant observation for untoward reactions is mandatory. Should any systemic reaction occur, discontinue use and initiate appropriate treatment including a tourniquet, airway, oxygen, epinephrine, an injectable pressor amine, and corticosteroids. See also Management of Acute Hypersensitivity Reactions.

➤*Sensitivity testing (horse serum):* Before administration of any product prepared from horse serum, appropriate measures must be taken in an effort to detect the presence of dangerous sensitivity:

1.) A careful review of the patient's history including any report of the following:
  a.) asthma, hay fever, urticaria, or other allergic manifestations;
  b.) allergic reactions upon exposure to horses;
  c.) prior injections of horse serum.
2.) A suitable test for detection of sensitivity. Perform a skin test in

ANTIVENIN (CROTALIDAE) POLYVALENT (Equine Origin)

every patient prior to administration, regardless of clinical history.

Skin test – Intracutaneously inject 0.02 to 0.03 mL of a 1:10 dilution of Normal Horse Serum or Antivenin. A control test on the opposite extremity, using Sodium Chloride Injection, USP, facilitates interpretation. Use of larger amounts for the skin-test dose increases the likelihood of false-positive reactions, and in the exquisitely sensitive patient, increases the risk of a systemic reaction from the skin-test dose. Use ≥ 1:100 dilution for preliminary skin testing if the history suggests sensitivity. A positive reaction to a skin test occurs within 5 to 30 minutes and is manifested by a wheal with or without pseudopodia and surrounding erythema. In general, the shorter the interval between injection and the beginning of the skin reaction, the greater the sensitivity.

If the history is negative for allergy and the result of a skin test is negative, proceed with administration of antivenin as outlined. If the history is positive, and a skin test is strongly positive, administration may be dangerous, especially if the positive sensitivity test is accompanied by systemic allergic manifestations. In such instances, the risk of administering antivenin must be weighed against the risk of withholding it, keeping in mind that severe envenomation can be fatal.

A negative allergic history and absence of reaction to a properly applied skin test do not rule out the possibility of an immediate reaction. Also, a negative skin test has no bearing on whether or not delayed serum reactions (serum sickness) will occur after administration of the full dose.

Desensitization – If the history is negative, and the skin test is mildly or questionably positive, administer as follows to reduce the risk of a severe immediate systemic reaction:

1.) Prepare, in separate sterile vials or syringes, 1:100 and 1:10 dilutions of antivenin.
2.) Allow ≥ 15 minutes between injections and proceed with the next dose if no reaction follows the previous dose.
3.) Inject SC using a tuberculin-type syringe, 0.1, 0.2, and 0.5 mL of the 1:100 dilution at 15-minute intervals; repeat with the 1:10 dilution, and finally undiluted antivenin.
4.) If a systemic reaction occurs after any injection, place a tourniquet proximal to the site of injections and administer an appropriate dose of epinephrine, 1:1000, proximal to the tourniquet or into another extremity. Wait ≥ 30 minutes before injecting another dose. The amount of the next dose should be the same as the last that did not evoke a reaction.
5.) If no reaction occurs after 0.5 mL of undiluted antivenin has been administered, switch to the IM route and continue doubling the dose at 15-minute intervals until the entire dose has been injected IM or proceed to the IV route as described in Administration and Dosage.

Obviously, if the just-described schedule is used, ≥ 3 to 5 hours would be required to administer the initial dose suggested for a moderate or severe envenomation, and time is an important factor in neutralization of venom in a critically ill patient. Wingert and Wainschel have described a procedure based on the experience of their group, which they have used in some severely envenomated patients who have positive sensitivity tests: 50 to 100 mg of diphenhydramine HCl is given IV followed by slow IV infusion of diluted antivenin for 15 to 20 minutes while carefully observing the patient for symptoms and signs of anaphylaxis; if anaphylaxis does not occur, antivenin is continued, maintaining close observation of the patient. Patients who require antivenin but develop signs of impending anaphylaxis in spite of this or the procedure described earlier, present a difficult problem; seek consultation.

➤*IV route:* IV route is preferred; if shock is present, IV use is mandatory. Administer within 4 hours of bite; it is less effective when given after 8 hours, and may be of questionable value after 12 hours. However, in severe poisonings, administer antivenin even if 24 hours have elapsed since time of bite. Maximum blood levels of antivenin may not be obtained for ≥ 8 hours following IM administration.

➤*Reconstituting dried antivenin:* Withdraw diluent and inject into the vial of antivenin. Gentle agitation will hasten complete dissolution of the lyophilized drug.

For IV drip, prepare a 1:1 to 1:10 dilution of reconstituted drug in Sodium Chloride Injection, USP, or 5% Dextrose Injection, USP. Gently swirl to avoid foaming. Infuse initial 5 to 10 mL over 3 to 5 minutes, while observing patient; if no immediate systemic reactions appear, continue infusion with delivery at the maximum safe rate for IV fluid administration. To determine dilution, type of electrolyte solution, and delivery rate, consider the patient's age, weight, and cardiac status; severity of envenomation; estimated total amount of parenteral fluids needed; and interval between bite and therapy initiation.

➤*Initial dose:* Give entire initial dose as soon as possible based on the best estimate of the severity of envenomation. The following doses are recommended:

No envenomation – No local or systemic manifestations: No dose given.

Minimal envenomation – Local swelling and other local changes; no systemic manifestations; normal laboratory findings: 20 to 40 mL (2 to 4 vials).

Moderate envenomation – Swelling progresses beyond the site of bite; ≥ 1 systemic manifestations; abnormal laboratory findings (eg, decreased hematocrit or platelets): 50 to 90 mL (5 to 9 vials).

Severe envenomation – Marked local response, severe systemic manifestations, significant alteration in laboratory findings: ≥ 100 to 150 mL (≥ 10 to 15 vials).

Base the need for additional antivenin on clinical response to initial dose and continuing assessment of severity of poisoning. If swelling progresses, systemic symptoms increase in severity, or if new manifestations appear, administer an additional 10 to 50 mL (1 to 5 vials) IV.

➤*Children:* Envenomation by large snakes in children or small adults requires larger doses of antivenin. The amount administered to a child is not based on weight (see Warnings).

➤*IM:* Administer into large muscle mass, preferably the gluteal area, taking care to avoid nerve trunks. Never inject into a finger or toe.

➤*Other treatment:* The efficacy of corticosteroids in treatment of envenomation per se or venom shock is not resolved. Do not give corticosteroids simultaneously with antivenin on a routine basis or during the acute state of envenomation; however, their use may be necessary to treat immediate allergic reactions to antivenin, and corticosteroids are the agents of choice for treating serious delayed reactions to antivenin.

Snakes' mouths do not harbor *Clostridium tetani*. However, appropriate tetanus prophylaxis is indicated, since tetanus spores may be carried into the fang puncture wounds by dirt present on skin at time of bite or by nonsterile first-aid procedures.

A broad-spectrum antibiotic in adequate dosage is indicated if local tissue damage is evident.

➤*Storage/Stability:* Store at room temperature, not exceeding 37°C (99°F). The lyophilized form can tolerate 3 freeze/thaw cycles. The product can be stored ≤ 10 days at 45°C (113°F). Use reconstituted solution within 48 hours and dilutions within 12 hours. To avoid foaming and protein degradation, mix by gently swirling rather than shaking.

Actions

➤*Pharmacology:* Concentrated serum globulins from horses immunized with the following venoms: *Crotalus adamanteus* (Eastern diamond rattlesnake), *C. atrox* (Western diamond rattlesnake), *C. durissus terrificus* (tropical rattlesnake, Cascabel), and *Bothrops atrox* (Fer-de-lance). IV effect is rapid; concentration peaks in ≥ 8 hours after IM injection. Mean half-life is < 15 days.

The location of antivenins for rare species and names and telephone numbers of experts on venomous bites can be obtained at any hour from the Arizona Poison Control Center (520-626-6016).

Warnings

➤*Pit viper bites and envenomation:* Symptoms, signs, and severity of snake venom poisoning depend on many factors including species, age, and size of the snake; number and location of bite(s); depth of venom deposit; condition of the snake's fangs and venom glands; length of time the snake "hangs on"; age, general health and size of the victim; timing, type, and efficacy of first-aid treatment rendered to remove venom. In any snake bite, the actual amount of venom introduced is unknown. The type of clothing or leg/footwear through which the snake's fangs pass may affect the amount of venom delivered. Although most North American pit vipers tend to bite and introduce venom superficially, their fangs may get hung up in SC tissues during the biting act and penetrate deeper tissues during the attempt to release the bitten part. In some bites, fangs may penetrate into muscle. In such cases, the usual local superficial manifestations of envenomation may not appear early in the course of poisoning. In bites by some species, systemic evidence of envenomation may be present in the absence of significant local manifestations. It may be difficult to determine the severity of envenomation during the first several hours after a pit viper bite; estimates of severity may need to be revised as poisoning progresses. Not all pit viper bites result in envenomation. In ≈ 20% of rattlesnake bites, the snake may not inject any venom.

➤*Local (fang punctures) signs and symptoms of envenomation:* Swelling – Edema, usually seen around the bite area within 5 minutes, may progress rapidly and involve the entire extremity within an hour. Generally, edema spreads more slowly, usually over a period of ≥ 8 hours. Swelling is usually most severe following envenomation by the Eastern diamondback; less severe after bites by the Western diamondback, prairie, timber, red, Pacific, Mojave, and blacktailed rattlers, the sidewinder, and the cottonmouth; least severe after bites by copperheads, massasauga, and pygmy rattlers.

Ecchymosis and skin discoloration – These effects often appear in the bite area within a few hours. Vesicles may form in a few hours and are usually present at 24 hours. Hemorrhagic blebs and petechiae are common. Necrosis may develop, necessitating amputation.

Pain – Pain frequently begins shortly after a bite by most pit vipers. Pain may be absent after bites by Mojave rattlers.

➤*Systemic signs and symptoms of envenomation:* Weakness; faintness; nausea; sweating; numbness or tingling around the mouth, tongue, scalp, fingers, toes, bite area; muscle fasciculations; hypotension; prolonged bleeding and clotting times; hemoconcentration fol-

ANTIVENIN (CROTALIDAE) POLYVALENT (Equine Origin)

lowed by decrease in erythrocytes; thrombocytopenia; hematuria; proteinuria; vomiting, including hematemesis; melena; hemoptysis; epistaxis.

In fatal poisoning, cause of death is frequently associated with destruction of erythrocytes and changes in capillary permeability, especially of the pulmonary vascular system, leading to pulmonary edema; hemoconcentration usually occurs early, probably as a result of plasma loss secondary to vascular permeability; hemoglobin may fall, and bleeding may occur throughout the body as early as 6 hours after the bite. Renal involvement is common. Mojave rattler venom may cause neuromuscular changes leading to respiratory failure.

Defibrination and disseminated intravascular coagulation syndromes have been associated with envenomation caused by some pit vipers native to the US, and appropriate therapy may be indicated.

➤*Supportive care:* Treat suspected envenomation as a medical emergency. Until careful observation provides clear evidence that envenomation has not occurred or is minimal, follow these procedures: Monitor vital signs frequently. Draw blood as soon as possible for baseline lab studies, including type and cross-match, CBC, hematocrit, platelet count, prothrombin time, clot retraction, bleeding and coagulation times, BUN, electrolytes, and bilirubin. During the first 4 or 5 days after a severe envenomation, perform hemoglobin, hematocrit, and platelet counts several times a day. Obtain urine samples at frequent intervals, with special attention to microscopic examination for presence of erythrocytes. Chart fluid intake and urine output. To monitor progression of edema, measure the circumference of the bitten extremity every 15 to 30 minutes, just proximal to the bite and at ≥ 1 additional points, each several inches closer to the trunk.

Have the following available for immediate use: Oxygen and resuscitation equipment including airway, epinephrine, parenteral antihistamines, and corticosteroids.

Start IV infusions: Use 1 line for supportive therapy, if needed, and the other line for administration of the antivenin and electrolytes.

Treat shock following envenomation like shock from hypovolemia of any cause, including administration of blood products or plasma expanders, as indicated.

Codeine is usually adequate for relieving pain. Sedation with phenobarbital or mild tranquilizers may be used if indicated, but not in the presence of respiratory failure.

Do not pack the bitten extremity in ice, and cryotherapy is contraindicated.

Compartment syndromes may complicate pit viper envenomations, especially those caused by bites on the lower extrimities. Prompt surgical consultion is indicated whenever a closed-compartment syndrome is suspected.

➤*Hypersensitivity reactions:* The immediate reaction (eg, shock, anaphylaxis) usually occurs within 30 minutes. Symptoms and signs include the following: Apprehension; flushing; itching; urticaria; edema of the face, tongue, and throat; cough; dyspnea; cyanosis; vomiting; collapse.

Serum sickness – Serum sickness usually occurs 5 to 24 days after administration. The incubation period may be < 5 days, especially in those who have received horse-serum-containing preparations in the past. The usual symptoms and signs are malaise, fever, urticaria, lymphadenopathy, edema, arthralgia, nausea, and vomiting. Occasionally, neurological manifestations develop, such as meningismus or peripheral neuritis. Peripheral neuritis usually involves the shoulders and arms. Pain and muscle weakness are frequently present, and permanent atrophy may develop.

➤*Pregnancy: Category C.* Use only if clearly needed, with appropriate consideration of the risk-benefit ratio. It is not known if antivenin antibodies cross the placenta. Intact IgG crosses the placenta from the maternal circulation increasingly after 30 weeks gestation.

➤*Lactation:* It is not known if antivenin antibodies are excreted into breast milk. Problems in humans have not been documented.

➤*Children:* Children may require larger doses than adults, because of a child's relatively small volume of body fluid in which to dilute the venom. Do not adjust pediatric doses by the weight of the patient.

Adverse Reactions

➤*Hypersensitivity:* The immediate reaction (eg, shock, anaphylaxis) usually occurs within 30 minutes. Symptoms and signs include the following: Apprehension; flushing; itching; urticaria; edema of the face, tongue, and throat; cough; dyspnea; cyanosis; vomiting; collapse.

Serum sickness – Serum sickness usually occurs 5 to 24 days after administration. The incubation period may be < 5 days, especially in those who have received horse-serum-containing preparations in the past. The usual symptoms and signs are malaise, fever, urticaria, lymphadenopathy, edema, arthralgia, nausea, and vomiting. Occasionally, neurological manifestations develop, such as meningismus or peripheral neuritis. Peripheral neuritis usually involves the shoulders and arms. Pain and muscle weakness are frequently present, and permanent atrophy may develop.

Patient Information

Advise patients to contact their physician immediately if they experience any signs or symptoms of delayed allergic reactions or serum sickness (eg, rash, pruritus, urticaria) after hospital discharge.

CROTALIDAE POLYVALENT IMMUNE FAB (Ovine Origin)

Rx	CroFab (Altana)	Powder for Injection, lyophilized	1 g total protein and thimerosal (0.11 mg mercury)/vial. Diluent not included. In single-use vials.

Indications

➤*Envenomations:* Crotalidae polyvalent immune fab (ovine) is indicated for the management of patients with minimal or moderate North American rattlesnake envenomation. Early use of Crotalidae polyvalent immune fab (ovine) (within 6 hours of snakebite) is advised to prevent clinical deterioration and the occurrence of systemic coagulation abnormalities.

Administration and Dosage

➤*Approved by the FDA:* October 2, 2000.

➤*Preparation for administration:* Reconstitute each vial of Crotalidae polyvalent immune fab (ovine) with 10 mL of Sterile Water for Injection, USP (diluent not included) and mix by continuous gentle swirling. Further dilute the contents of the reconstituted vials in 250 mL of 0.9% Sodium Chloride, USP and mix by gently swirling. Use the reconstituted and diluted product within 4 hours.

➤*Initial dose:* Initiate administration of antivenin as soon as possible after crotalid snakebite in patients who develop signs of progressive envenomation (eg, worsening local injury, coagulation abnormality, systemic signs of envenomation). Crotalidae polyvalent immune fab (ovine) was shown in the clinical studies to be effective when given within 6 hours of snakebite.

The recommended initial dose is 4 to 6 vials. Observe the patient for ≤ 1 hour following the completion of this first dose to determine if initial control of the envenomation has been achieved (as defined by complete arrest of local manifestations, and return of coagulation tests and systemic signs to normal).

Skin testing has not been used in clinical trials of Crotalidae polyvalent immune fab and is not required.

➤*Subsequent doses:* If initial control is not achieved by the first dose, repeat an additional dose of 4 to 6 vials until initial control of the envenomation syndrome has been achieved.

After initial control has been established, additional 2-vial doses every 6 hours for ≤ 18 hours (3 doses) is recommended. Optimal dosing following the 18-hour scheduled dose of Crotalidae polyvalent immune fab (ovine) has not been determined. Additional 2-vial doses may be administered as deemed necessary by the treating physician, based on the patient's clinical course.

➤*IV administration:* Infuse the initial dose of Crotalidae polyvalent immune fab (ovine) diluted in 250 mL of saline IV over 60 minutes. However, the infusion should proceed slowly over the first 10 minutes at a 25 to 50 mL/hour rate with careful observation for any allergic reaction. If no such reaction occurs, the infusion rate may be increased to the full 250 mL/hour rate until completion. Close patient monitoring is necessary.

It has been noted in the literature with the use of other antibody therapies that reactions during the infusion, such as fever, lower back pain, wheezing, and nausea often are related to the rate of infusion and can be controlled by decreasing the rate of administration of the solution.

➤*Treatment for subsequent envenomation:* Patients who receive a course of treatment with a foreign protein such as Crotalidae polyvalent immune fab may become sensitized to it. Therefore, use caution when administering a repeat course of treatment with Crotalidae polyvalent immune fab for a subsequent envenomation episode.

➤*Storage/Stability:* Store at 2° to 8°C (36° to 46°F). Do not freeze. The product must be used within 4 hours after reconstitution.

Actions

➤*Pharmacology:* Crotalidae polyvalent immune fab (ovine) is a venom-specific Fab fragment of immunoglobulin G (IgG) that works by binding and neutralizing venom toxins, facilitating their redistrubution away from target tissues and their elimination from the body.

Crotalidae polyvalent immune fab (ovine) is a preparation of ovine Fab (monovalent) immunoglobulin fragments obtained from the blood of healthy sheep flocks immunized with 1 of the following North American snake venoms: *Crotalus atrox* (Western Diamondback rattlesnake), *Crotalus adamanteus* (Eastern Diamondback rattlesnake), *Crotalus scutulatus* (Mojave rattlesnake), *Agkistrodon piscivorus* (Cottonmouth or Water Moccasin). To obtain the final antivenin product, the 4 different monospecific antivenins are mixed. Each monospecific antivenin is

CROTALIDAE POLYVALENT IMMUNE FAB (Ovine Origin)

prepared by fractionating the immunoglobulin from the ovine serum, digesting it with papain, and isolating the venom-specific Fab fragments on ion exchange and affinitiy chromatography columns.

Contraindications

Known history of hypersensitivity to papaya or papain unless the benefits outweigh the risks and appropriate management for anaphylactic reactions is readily available.

Warnings

➤*Pit viper bites and envenomation:* Symptoms, signs, and severity of snake venom poisoning depend on many factors including species, age, and size of the snake; number and location of bite(s); depth of venom deposit; condition of the snake's fangs and venom glands; length of time the snake "hangs on"; age, general health and size of the victim; timing, type, and efficacy of first-aid treatment rendered to remove venom. In any snake bite, the actual amount of venom introduced is unknown. The type of clothing or leg/footwear through which the snake's fangs pass may affect the amount of venom delivered. Although most North American pit vipers tend to bite and introduce venom superficially, their fangs may get hung up in SC tissues during the biting act and penetrate deeper tissues during the attempt to release the bitten part. In some bites, fangs may penetrate into muscle. In such cases, the usual local superficial manifestations of envenomation may not appear early in the course of poisoning. In bites by some species, systemic evidence of envenomation may be present in the absence of significant local manifestations. It may be difficult to determine the severity of envenomation during the first several hours after a pit viper bite; estimates of severity may need to be revised as poisoning progresses. Not all pit viper bites result in envenomation. In ≈ 20% of rattlesnake bites, the snake may not inject any venom.

➤*Local (fang punctures) signs and symptoms of envenomation:*
Swelling – Edema, usually seen around the bite area within 5 minutes, may progress rapidly and involve the entire extremity within an hour. Generally, edema spreads more slowly, usually over a period of ≥ 8 hours. Swelling is usually most severe following envenomation by the Eastern diamondback; less severe after bites by the Western diamondback, prairie, timber, red, Pacific, Mojave, and blacktailed rattlers, the sidewinder, and the cottonmouth; least severe after bites by copperheads, massasauga, and pygmy rattlers.

Ecchymosis and skin discoloration – Often appear in the bite area within a few hours. Vesicles may form in a few hours and are usually present at 24 hours. Hemorrhagic blebs and petechiae are common. Necrosis may develop, necessitating amputation.

Pain – Frequently begins shortly after a bite by most pit vipers. Pain may be absent after bites by Mojave rattlers.

➤*Systemic signs and symptoms of envenomation:* Weakness; faintness; nausea; sweating; numbness or tingling around the mouth, tongue, scalp, fingers, toes, bite area; muscle fasciculations; hypotension; prolonged bleeding and clotting times; hemoconcentration followed by decrease in erythrocytes; thrombocytopenia; hematuria; proteinuria; vomiting, including hematemesis; melena; hemoptysis; epistaxis.

In fatal poisoning, cause of death is frequently associated with destruction of erythrocytes and changes in capillary permeability, especially of the pulmonary vascular system, leading to pulmonary edema; hemoconcentration usually occurs early, probably as a result of plasma loss secondary to vascular permeability; hemoglobin may fall, and bleeding may occur throughout the body as early as 6 hours after the bite. Renal involvement is common. Mojave rattler venom may cause neuromuscular changes leading to respiratory failure.

Defibrination and disseminated intravascular coagulation syndromes have been associated with envenomation caused by some pit vipers native to the US, and appropriate therapy may be indicated.

➤*Supportive care:* Treat suspected envenomation as a medical emergency. Until careful observation provides clear evidence that envenomation has not occurred or is minimal, follow these procedures: Monitor vital signs frequently. Draw blood as soon as possible for baseline lab studies, including type and cross-match, CBC, hematocrit, platelet count, prothrombin time, clot retraction, bleeding and coagulation times, BUN, electrolytes, and bilirubin. During the first 4 or 5 days after a severe envenomation, perform hemoglobin, hematocrit, and platelet counts several times a day. Obtain urine samples at frequent intervals, with special attention to microscopic examination for presence of erythrocytes. Chart fluid intake and urine output. To monitor progression of edema, measure the circumference of the bitten extremity every 15 to 30 minutes, just proximal to the bite and at ≥ 1 additional points, each several inches closer to the trunk.

Have the following available for immediate use: Oxygen and resuscitation equipment including airway, tourniquet, epinephrine, parenteral antihistamines, and corticosteroids.

Start IV infusions: Use 1 line for supportive therapy, if needed, and the other line for administration of the antivenin and electrolytes.

Treat shock following envenomation like shock from hypovolemia of any cause, including administration of blood products or plasma expanders, as indicated.

Codeine is usually adequate for relieving pain. Sedation with phenobarbital or mild tranquilizers may be used if indicated, but not in the presence of respiratory failure.

Do not pack the bitten extremity in ice, and cryotherapy is contraindicated.

Compartment syndromes may complicate pit viper envenomations, especially those caused by bites on the lower extrimities. Prompt surgical consultion is indicated whenever a closed-compartment syndrome is suspected.

➤*Coagulopathy:* Coagulopathy is a complication noted in many victims of viper envenomation that arises because of the ability of the snake venom to interfere with the blood coagulation cascade. In clinical trials with Crotalidae polyvalent immune fab (ovine), recurrent coagulopathy (the return of a coagulation abnormality after it has been successfully treated with antivenin), characterized by decreased fibrinogen, decreased platelets, and elevated prothrombin time, occurred in ≈ 50% of patients studied. The clinical significance of these recurrent abnormalities is not known. Recurrent coagulation abnormalities were observed only in patients who experienced coagulation abnormalities during their initial hospitalization. Optimal dosing to completely prevent recurrent coagulopathy has not been determined. Because Crotalidae polyvalent immune fab (ovine) has a shorter persistence in the blood than crotalid venoms that can leak from depot sites over a prolonged period of time, repeat dosing to prevent or treat such recurrence may be necessary (see Administration and Dosage).

Recurrent coagulopathy may persist for ≥ 1 to 2 weeks. Monitor patients who experience coagulopathy, because of snakebite during hospitalization for initial treatment, for signs and symptoms of recurrent coagulopathy for up to or ≥ 1 week at the physician's discretion. During this period, the physician should assess carefully the need for retreatment with Crotalidae polyvalent immune fab (ovine) and use of any type of anticoagulant or antiplatelet drug.

➤*Allergy to papain or derivatives:* Papain is used to cleave the whole antibody into Fab and Fc fragments, and trace amounts of papain or inactivated papain residues may be present in Crotalidae polyvalent immune fab (ovine). Patients with allergies to papain, chymopapain, other papaya extracts, or the pineapple enzyme bromelain may also be at risk for an allergic reaction to Crotalidae polyvalent immune fab (ovine). In addition, it has been noted in the literature that some dust mite allergens and some latex allergens share antigenic structures with papain and patients with these allergies may be allergic to papain (see Contraindications).

➤*Hypersensitivity reactions:* The possible risks and side effects that attend the administration of heterologous animal proteins in humans include anaphylactic and anaphylactoid reactions, delayed allergic reactions (late serum reaction or serum sickness), and a possible febrile response to immune complexes formed by animal antibodies and neutralized venom components. Although no patient in the clinical studies of Crotalidae polyvalent immune fab has experienced a severe anaphylactic reaction, consider the possibility of an anaphylactic reaction. Inform the patient of the possibility of an anaphylactic reaction and close patient monitoring and readiness with IV therapy using epinephrine and diphenhydramine HCl is recommended during the infusion of Crotalidae polyvalent immune fab. If an anaphylactic reaction occurs during the infusion, terminate Crotalidae polyvalent immune fab at once and administer appropriate treatment. Patients with known allergies to sheep protein will be particularly at risk for an anaphylactic reaction.

Carefully monitor all patients treated with antivenin for signs and symptoms of an acute allergic reaction (eg, urticaria, pruritus, erythema, angioedema, bronchospasm with wheezing or cough, stridor, laryngeal edema, hypotension, tachycardia) and treat with appropriate emergency medical care (eg, epinephrine, IV antihistamines, albuterol).

Follow-up on all patients for signs and symptoms of delayed allergic reactions or serum sickness (eg, rash, fever, myalgia, arthralgia) and treated appropriately if necessary.

➤*Pregnancy:* Category C. Animal reproduction studies have not been conducted with Crotalidae polyvalent immune fab. It is also not known whether Crotalidae polyvalent immune fab can cause fetal harm when administered to a pregnant woman or can affect reproduction capacity. Give Crotalidae polyvalent immune fab to a pregnant woman only if clearly needed.

Crotalidae polyvalent immune fab contains mercury in the form of ethyl mercury from thimerosal (see Precautions). Although there are limited toxicology data on ethyl mercury, high dose and acute exposures to methyl mercury have been associated with neurological and renal toxicities. Developing fetuses and very young children are most susceptible and, therefore, at greater risk.

➤*Lactation:* It is not known whether Crotalidae polyvalent immune fab is excreted in human breast milk. Because many drugs are excreted in human milk, exercise caution when Crotalidae polyvalent immune fab is administered to a nursing woman.

➤*Children:* Specific studies in pediatric patients have not been conducted. The absolute venom dose following a snakebite is expected to be

CROTALIDAE POLYVALENT IMMUNE FAB (Ovine Origin)

the same in children and adults, therefore, no dosage adjustment for age should be made.

Crotalidae polyvalent immune fab contains mercury in the form of ethyl mercury from thimerosal (see Precautions). Although there are limited toxicology data on ethyl mercury, high dose and acute exposures to methyl mercury have been associated with neurological and renal toxicities. Developing fetuses and very young children are most susceptible and, therefore, at greater risk.

Precautions

➤**Mercury:** Crotalidae polyvalent immune fab (ovine) contains mercury in the form of ethyl mercury from thimerosal. The final product contains up to 104.5 mcg or ≈ 0.11 mg of mercury per vial, which amounts to not more than 1.9 mg of mercury per dose (based on the maximum dose of 18 vials studied in clinical trials of Crotalidae polyvalent immune fab). While there are no definitive data on the toxicity of ethyl mercury, literature suggests that information related to methyl mercury toxicities may be applicable.

Adverse Reactions

The most common adverse events reported in the clinical studies were urticaria and rash. Adverse events involving the skin and appendages (primarily rash, urticaria, and pruritus) were reported in 14 of the 42 patients.

Of the 25 patients who experienced adverse reactions, 3 patients experienced severe or serious adverse reactions. The 1 patient who experienced a serious adverse event had a recurrent coagulopathy because of envenomation, which required rehospitalization and additional antivenin administration. This patient eventually made a complete recovery. The other patients had severe adverse reactions: 1 patient had severe hives following treatment and the other had a severe rash and pruritus several days following treatment. Both patients recovered following treatment with antihistamines and prednisone.

One patient discontinued Crotalidae polyvalent immune fab therapy because of a recurrent coagulation abnormalitiy.

Crotalidae Polyvalent Immune Fab (Ovine) Adverse Reactions	
Adverse reaction	Number of events (n = 42)
CNS	
Circumoral paresthesia	1
General paresthesia	1
Nervousness	1
Dermatologic	
Urticaria	7
Rash	5
Pruritus	3
SC nodule	1
GI	
Nausea	3
Anorexia	1
Hematologic/Lymphatic	
Coagulation disorder	3
Ecchymosis	1
Respiratory	
Asthma	1
Cough	1
Increased sputum	1

Crotalidae Polyvalent Immune Fab (Ovine) Adverse Reactions	
Adverse reaction	Number of events (n = 42)
Miscellaneous	
Back pain	2
Chest pain	1
Cellulitis	1
Wound infection	1
Chills	1
Allergic reaction[1]	1
Serum sickness	1
Hypotension	1
Myalgia	1

[1] Allergic reaction consisted of urticaria, dyspnea, and wheezing in 1 patient.

In the 42 patients treated with Crotalidae polyvalent immune fab (ovine) for minimal or moderate crotalid envenomations, there were 7 events classified as early serum reactions and 5 events classified as late serum reactions; none were serious. In clinical studies, serum reactions consisted mainly of urticaria and rash, and all patients recovered without sequelae.

Early and Late Serum Reactions with Crotalidae Polyvalent Immune Fab (Ovine)	
Serum reactions	Number of events (n = 42)[1]
Early serum reactions	
Urticaria	5
Cough	1
Allergic reaction[2]	1
Late serum reactions	
Rash	2
Pruritus	1
Urticaria	1
Serum sickness[3]	1

[1] 6 of 42 patients experienced an adverse event associated with an early serum reaction and 4 experienced an adverse event associated with a late serum reaction. Two additional patients were considered to have a late serum reaction by the investigator, although no associated adverse event was reported.
[2] Allergic reaction consisted of urticaria, dyspnea, and wheezing in 1 patient.
[3] Serum sickness consisted of severe rash and pruritus in 1 patient.

Overdosage

The maximum amount of Crotalidae polyvalent immune fab (ovine) that can safely be administered in single or multiple doses has not been determined. Doses of up to 18 vials (≈ 13.5 g of protein) have been administered without any observed direct toxic effect.

Patient Information

Advise patients to contact their physician immediately if they experience any signs and symptoms of delayed allergic reactions or serum sickness (eg, rash, pruritus, urticaria) after hospital discharge.

Advise patients to contact their physician immediately if they experience unusual bruising or bleeding (eg, nosebleeds, excessive bleeding after brushing teeth, the appearance of blood in stools or urine, excessive menstrual bleeding, petechiae, excessive bruising or persistent oozing from superficial injuries) after hospital discharge as they may need additional antivenin treatment. Such bruising or bleeding may occur for up to 1 week or longer following initial treatment, and advise patients to follow-up with their physician for monitoring.

ANTIVENIN (MICRURUS FULVIUS) (North American Coral Snake Antivenin) (Equine Origin)

Rx	**Antivenin** (*Micrurus fulvius*)[1] (Wyeth-Ayerst)	**Powder for Injection, lyophilized**[2]	In single-use vials with 1 vial diluent (10 mL Water for Injection).[3]

[1] The manufacturer is in the process of discontinuing this product; however, it will be producing enough antivenin to satisfy demand for several years.

[2] Prior to lyophilization, product contains 0.25% phenol and 0.005% thimerosal.
[3] With 1:100,000 phenylmercuric nitrate.

Indications

➤**Envenomations:** For passive, transient protection from toxic effects of venoms of *Micrurus fulvius fulvius* (Eastern coral snake). Also neutralizes venom of *M. fulvius tenere* (Texas coral snake). If indicated, the best effect results if antivenin administration begins within 4 hours of envenomation.

This antivenin partially neutralizes the venom of *M. dumerilii carinicauda* and minimally neutralizes the venom of *M. spixii*. It may also provide some protection against the venom of *M. nigrocinctus*.

Administration and Dosage

➤**Test for sensitivity to horse serum:** Whenever a product containing horse serum is administered, there is a possibility of a severe immediate reaction. Have appropriate therapeutic agents available (not corticosteroids). See also Management of Acute Hypersensitivity Reactions.

➤**Sensitivity testing (horse serum):** Before administration of any product prepared from horse serum, take appropriate measures in an effort to detect the presence of dangerous sensitivity:

1.) A careful review of the patient's history should be noted, including any report of the following:
  a.) Asthma, hay fever, urticaria, or other allergic manifestations;
  b.) allergic reactions upon exposure to horses;
  c.) prior injections of horse serum.
2.) A suitable test for detection of sensitivity. Perform a skin test in every patient prior to administration, regardless of clinical history.

Skin test – Intracutaneously inject 0.02 to 0.03 mL of a 1:10 dilution of Normal Horse Serum or Antivenin. A control test on the opposite extremity, using Sodium Chloride Injection, USP, facilitates interpretation. Use of larger amounts for the skin-test dose increases the likelihood of false-positive reactions, and in the exquisitely sensitive patient, increases the risk of a systemic reaction from the skin-test dose. A ≥ 1:100 dilution should be used for preliminary skin testing if the history suggests sensitivity. A positive reaction to a skin test occurs within 5 to 30 minutes and is manifested by a wheal with or without pseudopodia and surrounding erythema. In general, the shorter the interval between injection and the beginning of the skin reaction, the greater the sensitivity.

ANTIVENIN (MICRURUS FULVIUS) (North American Coral Snake Antivenin) (Equine Origin)

If the history is negative for allergy and the result of a skin test is negative, proceed with administration of antivenin as outlined. If the history is positive and a skin test is strongly positive, administration may be dangerous, especially if the postitive sensitivity test is accompanied by systemic allergic manifestations. In such instances, the risk of administering antivenin must be weighed against the risk of withholding it, keeping in mind that severe envenomation can be fatal.

A negative allergic history and absence of reaction to a properly applied skin test do not rule out the possibility of an immediate reaction. Also, a negative skin test has no bearing on whether or not delayed serum reactions (serum sickness) will occur after administration of the full dose.

➤*Desensitization:* If the history is negative, and the skin test is mildly or questionably positive, administer as follows to reduce the risk of a severe immediate systemic reaction:

1.) Prepare, in separate sterile vials or syringes, 1:100 and 1:10 dilutions of antivenin.
2.) Allow ≥ 15 minutes between injections and proceed with the next dose if no reaction follows the previous dose.
3.) Inject SC using a tuberculin-type syringe, 0.1, 0.2, and 0.5 mL of the 1:100 dilution at 15-minute intervals; repeat with the 1:10 dilution, and finally undiluted antivenin.
4.) If a systemic reaction occurs after any injection, place a tourniquet proximal to the site of injections and administer an appropriate dose of epinephrine, 1:1000, proximal to the tourniquet or into another extremity. Wait ≥ 30 minutes before injecting another dose. The amount of the next dose should be the same as the last that did not evoke a reaction.
5.) If no reaction occurs after 0.5 mL of undiluted antivenin has been administered, switch to the IM route and continue doubling the dose at 15-minute intervals until the entire dose has been injected IM or proceed to the IV route as described in Administration and Dosage.

➤*Reconstituting dried antivenin:* Withdraw diluent and inject into the vial of antivenin. Gentle agitation will hasten complete dissolution of lyophilized drug. Do not shake.

➤*Antivenin therapy:* If symptoms or signs of envenomation occur or are already present at the time the patient is first seen, give IV antivenin promptly. With vigorous treatment and careful observation, patients with complete respiratory paralysis have recovered.

Start an IV drip of 250 to 500 mL of Sodium Chloride Injection, USP. If the results of appropriate tests have indicated the patient is not dangerously hypersensitive to horse serum and depending on the nature and severity of the signs and symptoms of envenomation, administer the contents of 3 to 5 vials as the initial dose IV by slow injection directly into the IV tubing or by slow IV infusion by adding to the reservoir bottle of the IV drip. In either case, give the first 1 to 2 mL of the antivenin dilution over 3 to 5 minutes and watch the patient carefully for evidence of an allergic reaction. If no signs or symptoms of anaphylaxis appear, continue the injection or infusion. Administer additional antivenin as required. Some envenomed patients may need the contents of > 10 vials.

Adjust the rate of delivery by the severity of signs and symptoms of envenomation and tolerance of antivenin. Nonetheless, until the contents of 3 to 5 vials of antivenin have been given, administer at the maximum safe rate for IV fluids, based on body weight and general condition of the patient. For example, 250 to 500 mL over 30 minutes may be appropriate in a healthy adult, while small children may receive the first 100 mL rapidly, followed by a rate not to exceed 4 mL/min. Response to treatment may be rapid and dramatic.

➤*Storage/Stability:* Store at 2° to 8°C (36° to 46°F). Do not expose to temperatures > 40°C (104°F). Do not freeze diluent. Product can tolerate 10 days in solution at room temperature. Use reconstituted solutions within 48 hours and dilutions within 12 hours. To avoid foaming and protein degradation, mix by gently swirling rather than shaking. Product shelf life expires within 60 months.

Actions

➤*Pharmacology:* Refined, concentrated, lyophilized preparation of serum globulins obtained by fractionating blood from healthy horses immunized with eastern coral snake (*Micrurus fulvius fulvius*) venom.

Two genera of coral snakes inhabit the US: *Micrurus* (including the eastern and Texas varieties), and *Micruroides* (the Arizonan or Sonoran variety). *Micrurus fulvius fulvius* inhabits an area from North Carolina south to Florida and west to the Mississippi River. *Micrurus fulvius tenere* inhabits an area west of the Mississippi River including Louisiana, Arkansas, and Texas. Several other species of coral snake inhabit much of Central and South America, including 3 genera, *Leptomicrurus*, *Micrurus*, and *Micruroides*.

Warnings

➤*Not effective:* Not effective against the venom of *Euryxanthus* (Arizonan or Sonoran coral snake), found only in southeastern Arizona, southwestern New Mexico, and portions of Mexico. Not effective in other snakes not described above.

➤*Envenomation:* Coral snake venom is chiefly paralytic (neurotoxic) and usually causes only minimal to moderate tissue reaction and pain at the bite area. Coral snakebites, like bites by crotalids, are not always followed by envenomation. However, severe and even fatal envenomation from a coral snakebite may be present without significant local tissue reaction.

Symptoms of envenomation – Symptoms usually begin 1 to 7 hours after the bite, but may be delayed for as long as 18 hours. If envenomation occurs, symptoms and signs may progress rapidly and precipitously. Paralysis has been observed 2.5 hours postbite and appears to be of a bulbar type, involving cranial motor nerves. Death from respiratory paralysis has occurred within 4 hours of the bite.

Systemic signs and symptoms – May include euphoria, lethargy, weakness, nausea, vomiting, excessive salivation, ptosis of eyelids, dyspnea, abnormal reflexes, seizures, and motor weakness or paralysis, including complete respiratory paralysis.

Local signs and symptoms – May include scratch marks or fang puncture wounds, no edema to moderate edema, erythema, pain at the bite area, and paresthesia in the bitten extremity.

Supportive therapy – Appropriate tetanus prophylaxis is indicated. Morphine or other narcotics that depress respiration are contraindicated. Use sedatives with extreme caution.

If practical, immobilize victim immediately and completely. If complete immobilization is not practical, splint bitten extremity to limit spread of venom.

Hemoglobinuria has occurred in animals. Therefore, continuous bladder drainage with careful attention to urinary output and blood electrolyte balance is recommended.

➤*Hypersensitivity reactions:* The immediate reaction (eg, shock, anaphylaxis) usually occurs within 30 minutes. Symptoms and signs may include apprehension; flushing; itching; urticaria; edema of the face, tongue, and throat; cough; dyspnea; cyanosis; vomiting; and collapse.

Serum sickness – Serum sickness usually occurs 5 to 24 days after administration. The incubation period may be < 5 days, especially in those who have received horse-serum-containing preparations on the past. The usual symptoms and signs are malaise, fever, urticaria, lymphadenopathy, edema, arthralgia, nausea, and vomiting. Occasionally, neurological manifestations develop, such as meningismus or peripheral neuritis. Peripheral neuritis usually involves the shoulders and arms. Pain and muscle weakness are frequently present, and permanent atrophy may develop.

➤*Pregnancy: Catagory C.* Use only if clearly needed, with appropriate consideration of the risk-benefit ratio. It is not known if antivenom antibodies cross the placenta. Intact IgG crosses the placenta from the maternal circulation increasingly after 30 weeks gestation.

➤*Lactation:* It is not known if antivenom antibodies are excreted into breast milk. Problems in humans have not been documented.

➤*Children:* The pediatric dose is equivalent to the adult dose. Pediatric doses are not adjusted by the weight of the patient.

Adverse Reactions

➤*Hypersensitivity:* The immediate reaction (eg, shock, anaphylaxis) usually occurs within 30 minutes. Symptoms and signs may include apprehension; flushing; itching; urticaria; edema of the face, tongue, and throat; cough; dyspnea; cyanosis; vomiting; and collapse.

Serum sickness – Serum sickness usually occurs 5 to 24 days after administration. The incubation period may be < 5 days, especially in those who have received horse-serum-containing preparations on the past. The usual symptoms and signs are malaise, fever, urticaria, lymphadenopathy, edema, arthralgia, nausea, and vomiting. Occasionally, neurological manifestations develop, such as meningismus or peripheral neuritis. Peripheral neuritis usually involves the shoulders and arms. Pain and muscle weakness are frequently present, and permanent atrophy may develop.

Patient Information

Advise patients to contact their physician immediately if they experience any signs and symptoms of delayed allergic reactions or serum sickness (eg, rash, pruritus, urticaria) after hospital discharge.

In contrast to the immune serums and antitoxins, which contain exogenous antibodies to provide passive immunity, the Agents for Active Immunization include specific antigens that induce the endogenous production of antibodies. Agents that induce active immunity include vaccines and the subset of vaccines called toxoids.

Vaccines contain whole (killed or attenuated live) or partial microorganisms capable of inducing antibody formation, but which are not pathogenic. Toxoids are detoxified by-products derived from organisms that induce disease primarily through the elaboration of exotoxins. Although toxoids are not toxic, they are antigenic, and therefore, stimulate specific antibody production. Active immunization induced through administration of vaccines and toxoids provides prolonged immunity, whereas passive immunization with immune sera or antitoxins is of short duration.

Vaccination with any vaccine may not result in a protective antibody response in all individuals given the vaccine.

The table below indicates the recommended immunization schedule for infants and children. This schedule has been approved by the ACIP, the American Academy of Pediatrics (AAP), and the American Academy of Family Physicians (AAFP). This table is revised annually.

Recommended Childhood Immunization Schedule[a] - United States July to December 2004												
Vaccine	Birth	1 mo	2 mo	4 mo	6 mo	12 mo	15 mo	18 mo	24 mo	4-6 y	11-12 y	13-18 y
Hepatitus B (Hep B)[b]	Hep B-1[c]											
		Hep B-2[c]			Hep B-3[c]					Hep B series[d]		
Diphtheria, tetanus and pertussis (DTaP)[e]			DTaP	DTaP	DTaP		DTaP[c]			DTaP	Td[c]	
Haemophilus influenzae type b (Hib)[f]			Hib	Hib	Hib	Hib[c]						
Polio (IPV)[g]			IPV	IPV		IPV[c,g]				IPV		
Measles, mumps, rubella (MMR)[h]						MMR-1[c]				MMR-2[h]	MMR-2[d]	
Varicella (Var)[i]						Var[c]					Var[d,i]	
Hepatitis A (Hep A)[j]										Hep A series (in selected areas)[c,j]		
Pneumococcal[k]			PCV	PCV	PCV	PCV				PCV[d]	PPV (24 mos to 18 yrs in selected populations)[k]	
Influenza[l]						Influenza (yearly)				Influenza (yearly in selected populations)		

[a] This schedule indicates the recommended age for routine administration of currently licensed childhood vaccines as of April 1, 2004. Additional vaccines may be licensed and recommended during the year. Combination vaccines may be used whenever any components of the combination are indicated and its other components are not contraindicated. Give catch-up immunizations whenever feasible. Consult the manufacturers' package inserts for detailed recommendations. Report clinically significant adverse events that follow vaccination to the Vaccine Adverse Event Reporting System (VAERS). Guidance about how to obtain and complete a VAERS form is available at http://www-.vaers.org or by telephone, (800) 822-7967.

[b] **Infants born to HBsAg-negative mothers** should receive the first dose of Hep B vaccine soon after birth and before hospital discharge or by 2 months of age. Only monovalent Hep B can be used for the birth dose. Monovalent or combination vaccine containing Hep B may be used to complete the series; 4 doses of vaccine may be administered when a birth dose is given. Give the second dose of Hep B vaccine ≥ 4 weeks after the first dose. Administer the third dose ≥ 16 weeks after the first dose and ≥ 8 weeks after the second dose. Do not administer the last dose in the vaccination series (third or fourth dose) before 24 weeks of age. **Infants born to HBsAg-positive mothers** should receive Hep B vaccine and 0.5 mL Hep B immune globulin (HBIG) within 12 hours of birth at separate sites. The second dose is recommended at 1 to 2 months of age and the last dose not before 24 weeks of age. Test these infants for HBsAg and anti-HBs at age 9 to 15 months of age. **Infants born to mothers whose HBsAg status is unknown** should receive Hep B vaccine within 12 hours of birth. Draw aternal blood at the time of delivery to determine the mother's HBsAg status; if the HBsAg test is positive, the infant should receive HBIG as soon as possible (≤ 1 week of age). The second dose is recommended at 1 to 2 months of age. Do not administer the last dose in the vaccination series before 24 weeks of age. **All children and adolescents** (≤ 18 years of age) who have not been immunized against Hep B may begin the series during any visit. Make special efforts to immunize children who were born in or whose parents were born in areas of the world with moderate or high endemicity of Hep B virus infection.

[c] Range of acceptable ages for vaccination.

[d] Vaccines to be assessed and administered if necessary.

[e] The fourth dose of DTaP may be administered as early as 12 months of age, provided 6 months have elapsed since the third dose and the child is unlikely to return at 15 to 18 months of age. Give the final dose in the series at ≥ 4 years of age. Tetanus and diphtheria toxoids (Td) is recommended at 11 to 12 years of age if ≥ 5 years have elapsed since the last dose of DTP, DTaP, or diphtheria and tetanus toxoids (DT). Subsequent routine Td boosters are recommended every 10 years.

[f] Three Hib conjugate vaccines are licensed for infant use. If PRP-OMP (*Pedvax-HIB* or *ComVax*, Merck) is administered at 2 and 4 months of age, a dose at 6 months of age is not required. Do not use DTaP/Hib combination products for primary immunization in infants at 2, 4, or 6 months of age, but use as boosters following any Hib vaccine. Give the final dose in the series at ≥ 12 months of age.

[g] To eliminate the risk of vaccine-associated paralytic polio (VAPP), an all-IPV schedule is now recommended for routine childhood polio vaccination in the US. All children should receive 4 doses of IPV at 2, 4, and 6 to 18 months of age and 4 to 6 years of age.

OPV (if available) may be used only for the following special circumstances: 1) Mass vaccination campaigns to control outbreaks of paralytic polio, 2) unvaccinated children who will be traveling in < 4 weeks to areas where polio is endemic or epidemic, 3) children of parents who do not accept the recommended number of vaccine injections. These children may receive OPV only for the third or fourth dose or both; in this situation, health care providers should administer OPV only after discussing the risks for VAPP with parents or caregivers. During the transition to an all-IPV schedule, recommendations for the use of remaining OPV supplies in physicians' offices and clinics have been issued by the AAP (see *Pediatrics*, December 1999) and the AAFP.

[h] The second dose of MMR vaccine is routinely recommended at 4 to 6 years of age but may be administered during any visit provided ≥ 4 weeks have elapsed since receipt of the first dose and that both doses are administered at or after 12 months of age. Those who have not previously received the second dose should complete the schedule by 11 to 12 years of age.

[i] Var vaccine is recommended at any visit on or after 12 months of age for susceptible children, (ie, those who lack a reliable history of chickenpox as judged by a health care provider) and who have not been immunized. Susceptible people ≥ 13 years of age should receive 2 doses given ≥ 4 weeks apart.

[j] Hep A is included to indicate its recommended use in selected states or regions; consult the local public health authority. (Also see *MMWR*. Oct. 1, 1999;48(RR-12):1-37.) Children and adolescents in these states, regions, and high-risk groups who have not been immunized against Hep A can begin the Hep A vaccination series during any visit. Administer the 2 doses in the series at least 6 months apart.

[k] The heptavalent pneumococcal conjugate vaccine (PCV) is recommended for all children 2 to 23 months of age. It also is recommended for certain children 24 to 59 months of age. Give the final dose in the series at ≥ 12 months of age. Pneumococcal polysaccharide vaccine (PPV) is recommended in addition to PCV for certain high-risk groups. (See *MMWR*. 2000;49[RR-9]:1-38).

[l] Influenza vaccine is recommended annually for children 6 months of age or older with certain risk factors (including, but not limited to asthma, cardiac disease, sickle cell disease, HIV, diabetes), healthcare workers, and household members of people in high-risk groups (see *MMWR*. 2004;53[RR][in press]) and can be administered to all others wishing to obtain immunity. In addition, healthy children 6 to 23 months of age and close contacts of healthy children 0 to 23 months of age are encouraged to receive influenza vaccine if feasible because children in this age group are at substantially increased risk for influenza-related hospitalizations. For healthy people 5 to 49 years of age, the intranasally administered live, attenuated influenza vaccine (LAIV) is an acceptable alternative to the intramuscular trivalent inactivated influenza vaccine (TIV). (See *MMWR*. 2003;52[No. RR-13]:1-8). Children receiving TIV should be administered a dosage appropriate for their age (0.25 mL if 6 to 35 months of age or 0.5 mL if ≥ 3 years of age). Children 8 years of age and younger who are receiving influenza vaccine for the first time should receive 2 doses separated by at least 4 weeks for TIV and at least 6 weeks for LAIV.

Catch-up Schedule for Children 4 Months Through 6 Years of Age Who Start Late or Who Are > 1 Month Behind				
	Minimum interval between doses			
Dose 1 (minimum age)	Dose 1 to dose 2	Dose 2 to dose 3	Dose 3 to dose 4	Dose 4 to dose 5
DTaP (6 wk)	4 wk	4 wk	6 mo	6 mo[a]
IPV (6 wk)	4 wk	4 wk	4 wk[b]	
HepB[c] (birth)	4 wk	8 wk (and 16 wk after dose 1)		
MMR (12 mo)	4 wk[d]			
Varicella (12 mo)				
Hib[e] (6 wk)	**4 wk:** If dose 1 given at < 12 mo of age **8 wk (as final dose):** If dose 1 given at 12 to 14 mo of age **No further doses needed:** If dose 1 given at ≥ 15 mo of age	**4 wk:**[f] If currently < 12 mo of age **8 wk (as final dose):**[f] If currently ≥ 12 mo of age and dose 2 given at < 15 mo of age **No further doses needed:** If previous dose given at ≥ 15 mo of age	**8 wk (as final dose):** This dose only necessary for children 12 mo to 5 y of age who received 3 doses before 12 mo of age	

Catch-up Schedule for Children 4 Months Through 6 Years of Age Who Start Late or Who Are > 1 Month Behind				
Dose 1 (minimum age)	Minimum interval between doses			
	Dose 1 to dose 2	Dose 2 to dose 3	Dose 3 to dose 4	Dose 4 to dose 5
PCV[g] (6 wk)	**4 wk:** If dose 1 given at age < 12 mo and currently < 24 mo of age **8 wk (as final dose):** If dose 1 given at ≥ 12 mo of age or current age is 24 to 59 mo of age **No further doses needed:** For healthy children if dose 1 given at ≥ 24 mo of age	**4 wk:** If currently < 12 mo of age **8 wk (as final dose):** If currently ≥ 12 mo of age **No further doses needed:** For healthy children if previous dose given at ≥ 24 mo of age	**8 wk (as final dose):** This dose only necessary for children 12 mo to 5 y of age who received 3 doses before 12 mo of age	

[a] The fifth dose is not necessary if the fourth dose was given after the fourth birthday.
[b] For children who received an all-IPV or all-OPV series, a fourth dose is not necessary if third dose was given at 4 years of age or older. If both OPV and IPV were given as part of a series, give a total of 4 doses regardless of the child's current age.
[c] All children and adolescents who have not been immunized against Hep B should begin the Hep B vaccination series during any visit. Providers should make special efforts to immunize children who were born in, or whose parents were born in, areas of the world where Hep B virus infection is moderately or highly endemic.
[d] The second dose of MMR is recommended routinely at 4 to 6 years of age, but may be given early if desired.
[e] Vaccine is not generally recommended for children 5 years of age and older.
[f] If current age is less than 12 months of age and first 2 doses were PRP-OMP (*PedvaxHIB* or *ComVax*), give the third (and final) dose at 12 to 15 months of age and at least 8 weeks after the second dose.
[g] Vaccine is not generally recommended for children 5 years of age and older.

Catch-up Schedule for Children 7 Through 18 Years of Age Who Start Late or Who Are > 1 Month Behind		
Minimum interval between doses		
Dose 1 to dose 2	Dose 2 to dose 3	Dose 3 to booster dose
Td: 4 wk	Td: 6 mo	Td:[a] **6 mo:** If dose 1 given at < 12 mo of age and current age < 11 y of age **5 y:** If dose 1 given at ≥ 12 mo of age and dose 3 given at < 7 y of age and current age ≥ 11 y of age **10 y:** If dose 3 given at ≥ 7 y of age
IPV:[b,c] 4 wk	IPV:[b,c] 4 wk	IPV[b,c]
HepB: 4 wk	HepB: 8 wk (and 16 wk after dose 1)	
MMR: 4 wk		
Varicella:[d] 4 wk		

[a] For children 7 to 10 years of age, the interval between the third and booster dose is determined by the age when the first dose was given. For adolescents 11 to 18 years of age, the interval is determined by the age when the third dose was given.
[b] Inactivated polio vaccine (IPV): For children who received an all-IPV or all-oral poliovirus (OPV) series, a fourth dose is not necessary if third dose was given at age ≥ 4 years of age. If both OPV and IPV were given as part of a series, a total of 4 doses should be given, regardless of the child's current age.
[c] Vaccine is not generally recommended for people 18 years of age and older.
[d] Give 2-dose series to all susceptible adolescents 13 years of age and older.

➤**Concomitant vaccination:** Several routine pediatric vaccines may safely and effectively be administered simultaneously at separate injection sites. National authorities recommend simultaneous immunization at separate sites as indicated by age or health risk if return of a vaccine recipient for a subsequent visit is doubtful.

➤**Immunization for other diseases:** Immunization for other diseases is recommended for people with a risk of exposure. Specific immunization requirements and recommendations for international travel can be obtained from the CDC website (http://www.cdc.gov), including their online publication, "Health Information for International Travel." These also can be found in the following publication: Grabenstein JD. *ImmunoFacts: Vaccines & Immunologic Drugs.* St. Louis: Facts and Comparisons, Aug. 2004.

➤**Hypersensitivity to vaccine components:** Vaccine antigens produced in systems containing allergenic substances (ie, embryonated chicken eggs) may cause hypersensitivity reactions, including anaphylaxis. Do not give such vaccines to individuals with known hypersensitivity to these components. Influenza vaccine antigens (whole or split), although prepared in embryonated eggs, are highly purified and are rarely associated with hypersensitivity reactions.

Live virus vaccines prepared by growing viruses in cell cultures are essentially devoid of allergenic substances. On very rare occasions, hypersensitivity reactions to measles vaccine have been reported in individuals with anaphylactic hypersensitivity to gelatin. However, measles vaccine can be given safely to egg-allergic individuals provided the allergies are not manifested by anaphylactic symptoms. The same precautions apply to mumps and varicella vaccines.

Some vaccines contain preservatives (eg, thimerosal) or trace amounts of antibiotics (eg, neomycin) to which patients may be hypersensitive. Such allergies are relevant only if they reflect immediate hypersensitivity (eg, the airway).

Before the injection of any biological, take all precautions known for prevention of allergic or other side effects, including a review of the patient's history regarding possible sensitivity, occurrence of any adverse event-related symptoms or signs to determine any contraindication to immunization, and a knowledge of the recent literature pertaining to the use of the biological concerned. Have epinephrine 1:1000

available for immediate use when this product is injected. Refer to Management of Acute Hypersensitivity Reactions.

➤*Altered immunocompetence:* Microbial replication after administration of live, attenuated vaccines may be enhanced in people with immune deficiency diseases and in those with suppressed capability for immune response (eg, leukemia, lymphoma, generalized malignancy or therapy with corticosteroids, alkylating agents, antimetabolites, radiation). Do not give live, attenuated vaccines to such patients or to a member of a household in which there is a family history of congenital or hereditary immunodeficiency until the immune competence of the recipient is known.

➤*Hep B:* Use a separate, sterilized syringe and needle for each patient to prevent transmission of Hep B virus and other infectious agents from one person to another.

➤*Vaccine reconstitution:* When preparing injections for reconstitution, cleanse the rubber stoppers of both vials with a suitable germicide prior to reconstitution.

➤*Aspirate:* Before delivering the IM or SC dose, aspirate to help avoid inadvertent injection into a blood vessel.

➤*HIV infection:* Special immunization recommendations are appropriate for individuals infected with HIV.

Live bacterial or viral vaccines – Individuals infected with HIV and those who have developed AIDS are theoretically at risk of disseminated infection following immunization with a live, albeit attenuated, bacterial or viral vaccine.

Inactivated vaccines or toxoids – In general, immunization with an inactivated vaccine or toxoid poses no additional risk to people infected with HIV and those who have developed AIDS, but these people may be less likely to develop an adequate immune response to vaccination and may remain susceptible to the disease at issue. While HIV-infected individuals and AIDS patients may develop less than optimal immunity, compared with uninfected people, immunization is often still recommended to confer at least partial protection. Optimally, complete the immunization of HIV-infected individuals before they meet the criteria for AIDS.

Immunization of HIV-infected individuals – In vitro studies demonstrate that proliferating CD4 cells are more susceptible to infection with HIV than nonproliferating cells, raising the possibility that immunization may be a cofactor in exacerbating the progression of HIV infection to AIDS. CDC and WHO continue to recommend immunization of HIV-infected people when the benefits of immunization outweigh the risks of infection.

Summary Recommendations for Routine Immunization of HIV-infected People in the US		
Drug	Known asymptomatic	Symptomatic
DTP/Td	yes	yes
OPV	no	no
e-IPV[a]	yes	yes
MMR	yes	yes[b]
Hib[c]	yes	yes
Pneumococcal	yes	yes
Influenza	yes[b]	yes
BCG	no	no
Cholera	yes	yes
Hepatitis A	yes	yes
Hep B	yes	yes
Meningococcal	yes	yes
Rabies	yes	yes
Typhoid	yes (injection only)	yes (injection only)
Vaccinia	no	no
Varicella[d]	yes	
Yellow fever	yes, if high risk	no

[a] For adults ≥ 18 years of age; use only if indicated.
[b] Consider risk and benefit.
[c] Consider for HIV-infected adults also.
[d] Consult detailed references.

➤*Severe febrile illnesses:* Generally defer immunization of individuals with severe febrile illnesses until they have recovered.

➤*Vaccination during pregnancy:* On the grounds of a theoretical risk to the developing fetus, live, attenuated virus vaccines are not generally given to pregnant women or to those likely to become pregnant within 3 months after receiving vaccine(s). With some of these vaccines, particularly rubella, measles, and mumps, pregnancy is contraindicated. When the vaccine is to be given during pregnancy, waiting until the second or third trimester to minimize any concern over teratogenicity is a reasonable precaution. However, there has been no evidence of congenital rubella syndrome in infants born to susceptible mothers who received rubella vaccine during pregnancy.

Measles, mumps, rubella, or oral polio vaccines may be safely administered to children of pregnant women. Experience to date has not revealed any risks of polio vaccine virus to the fetus.

There is no convincing evidence of risk to the fetus from immunization of pregnant women using inactivated virus vaccines, bacterial vaccines, or toxoids. Give tetanus and Td to inadequately immunized pregnant women because it affords protection against neonatal tetanus. Similarly, Hep B, influenza, and meningococcal vaccines may be indicated during pregnancy.

➤*Adverse events following immunization:* Modern vaccines are extremely safe and effective, but not completely so. Adverse events following immunization have been reported with all vaccines. These range from frequent, minor, local reactions to extremely rare, severe, systemic illness such as paralysis associated with oral polio vaccine.

The health care provider should provide vaccine information required to be given with each vaccine to the patient, parent, or guardian, and inform them of the benefits and risks associated with the vaccine.

Reporting of adverse events – The National Vaccine Injury Compensation Program, established by the National Childhood Vaccine Injury Act of 1986, requires physicians and other health care providers who administer vaccines to maintain permanent vaccination records and to report occurrences of certain adverse events to the US Department of Health and Human Services. Reportable events include those listed in the Act for each vaccine and events specified in the package insert as contraindications to further doses of that vaccine.

Patients, parents, or guardians should report serious adverse reactions to their health care provider, who, in turn, should report the events to the US Department of Health and Human Services (DHHS) through the Vaccine Adverse Event Reporting System (VAERS) at (800) 822-7967.

Encourage reporting by patients, parents, or guardians of all adverse events occurring after vaccine administration. Adverse events following immunization with vaccine should be reported by the health care provider to the DHHS VAERS. Reporting forms and information about reporting requirements or completion of the form can be obtained from VAERS through a toll-free number (800) 822-7967. Health care providers also should report these events to the manufacturer.

Record the date, lot number, and manufacturer of the vaccine as part of the patient's immunization record.

Vaccines, Bacterial

BCG VACCINE

| Rx | BCG Vaccine (Organon) | **Powder for injection, lyophilized:** TICE strain[1] (1 to 8 x 10^8 CFU equivalent to ≈ 50 mg) | In vials.[2] |

[1] Developed at the University of Illinois.   [2] Preservative free.

For additional information, refer to the Agents for Active Immunization introduction. TICE BCG vaccine is also indicated for carcinoma in situ of the bladder. See individual monograph in the Antineoplastics section.

Indications

For the prevention of tuberculosis (TB) in people not previously infected with *Mycobacterium tuberculosis* who are at high risk for exposure. As with any vaccine, immunization with BCG vaccine may not protect 100% of susceptible individuals.

The Advisory Committee on Immunization Practices (ACIP) and the Advisory Committee for the Elimination of Tuberculosis has recommended that BCG vaccination be considered in the following circumstances:

➤*TB exposed tuberculin skin test-negative infants and children:* BCG vaccination is recommended for infants and children with negative tuberculin skin test who are at high risk of intimate and prolonged exposure to persistently untreated or ineffectively treated patients with infectious pulmonary tuberculosis and who cannot be removed from the source of exposure and cannot be placed on long-term preventive therapy, or who are continuously exposed to people with infectious pulmonary tuberculosis who have bacilli resistant to isoniazid and rifampin.

➤*TB exposed health care workers (HCW) in high risk settings:* Consider BCG vaccination of HCWs on an individual basis in settings where a high percentage of TB patients are infected with *M. tuberculosis* strains resistant to both isoniazid and rifampin, transmission of such drug resistant *M. tuberculosis* strains to HCWs and subsequent infection are likely, and comprehensive TB infection control precautions have been implemented and have not been successful. Vaccination should not be required for employment or for assignment of HCWs in specific work areas. Counsel HCWs considered for BCG vaccination regarding the risks and benefits associated with BCG vaccinations and TB preventive therapy.

➤*Exposed HCWs in low risk settings:* BCG vaccination is not recommended for HCWs in settings in which the risk for *M. tuberculosis* transmission is low.

➤*Unlabeled uses:* BCG vaccine induces antibodies that bind to *M. leprae* and may be effective in the prevention of leprosy.

Administration and Dosage

➤*Preparation:* Add 1 mL sterile water for injection at 4° to 25°C (39° to 77°F) to one vial of vaccine. Gently swirl the vial until a homogenous suspension is obtained. Avoid forceful agitation, which may cause clumping of the mycobacteria.

➤*Treatment and schedule:* Vaccination is recommended only for those who are tuberculin negative to a recent skin test with 5 tuberculin units (5TU). The vaccine is administered after fully explaining the risks and benefits to the vaccinee, parent, or guardian. After the vaccine is prepared, the immunizing dose of 0.2 to 0.3 mL is dropped on the cleansed surface of the skin and spread over a 1 × 2 inch area using the edge of the multiple puncture device. The vaccine is administered percutaneously utilizing a sterile multiple-puncture device. While holding the skin taut, press downward on the device, allowing the points to be well buried in the skin for 5 seconds. Do not "rock" the device. After successful puncture, spread vaccine as evenly as possible over the

puncture area with the edge of the device. An additional 1 to 2 drops of BCG vaccine may be added to ensure a very wet vaccination site. No dressing is required; however, it is recommended that the site be kept dry for 24 hours. Advise the patient that the vaccine contains live organisms. Although the vaccine will not survive in a dry state for long, infection of others is possible.

Repeat vaccination for those who remain tuberculin-negative to 5TU of tuberculin after 2 to 3 months.

➤*Children:* In infants under 1 month of age, reduce the dosage of vaccine by 50% by using 2 mL sterile water when reconstituting. If a vaccinated infant remains tuberculin negative to 5TU on skin testing, and if indications for vaccination persist, the infant should receive a full dose after 1 year of age.

➤*Storage/Stability:* Refrigerate the intact vial at 2° to 8°C (36° to 46°F). Protect from light. Do not use after the expiration date printed on the label.

Keep reconstituted vaccine refrigerated; protect from light; use within 2 hours. Freezing of the reconstituted product is not recommended.

Actions

➤*Pharmacology:* BCG vaccine for percutaneous use is an attenuated, live culture preparation of the Bacillus of Calmette and Guerin (BCG) strain of *M. bovis.* The TICE strain was developed at the University of Illinois from a strain originated at the Pasteur Institute.

The greatest known risk factor for developing active TB disease is immunodeficiency, particularly if caused by coinfection with HIV. People infected with HIV are estimated to be over 100 times as likely as uninfected people to develop TB primarily as a result of reactivation of a latent TB infection. Other groups at high risk for devloping TB include foreign-born individuals and people in institutional settings such as correctional facilities, shelters for the homeless, and nursing homes.

Prospective vaccine efficacy trials have shown that the protective benefit of BCG (various strains from different manufacturers) against clinical TB was variable, ranging from 0% to 80%. A recent meta-analysis of data from 14 prospective trials and 12 case-control studies concluded that the overall protective effect of BCG against tuberculosis infection was 50%. Estimates in areas where BCG vaccination is performed at birth indicate that the effectiveness of BCG in preventing childhood TB meningitis or miliary TB exceeds 70%.

Contraindications

Impaired immunologic responses because of HIV infections, congenital immunodeficiency such as chronic granulomatous disease or interferon gamma receptor deficiency, leukemia, lymphoma, or generalized malignancy; immunologic responses that have been suppressed by steroids, alkylating agents, antimetabolites, or radiation; HIV-infected or immunocompromised infants, children, or adults; hypersensitivity or history of hypersensitivity to the product; active tuberculosis. Do not use in infants, children, or adults with severe immune deficiency syndromes.

Warnings

➤*Route of administration:* Do not inject IV, SC, or intradermally. Use percutaneous administration with the multiple puncture device (see Administration and Dosage).

BCG VACCINE

➤*Immune deficiency syndromes:* Administer with caution to people in groups at high risk for HIV infection. Do not vaccinate children with a family history of immune deficiency disease. If they are, consult an infectious disease specialist and administer antituberculous therapy if clinically indicated.

➤*BCG infection:* Symptoms such as fever of 103°F or greater, or acute localized inflammation persisting longer than 2 to 3 days suggest active infections, and evaluation for serious infectious complication should be considered. If a BCG infection is suspected, the physician should consult with an infectious disease expert before therapy is initiated. Treatment should be started without delay. In patients who develop persistent fever or experience an acute febrile illness consistent with BCG infection, 2 or more antimycobacterial agents should be administered while diagnostic evaluation, including cultures, is conducted. Negative cultures do not necessarily rule out infection. The most serious complication of BCG vaccination is disseminated BCG infection. BCG osteitis affecting the epiphyses of the long bones, particularly the epiphyses of the leg can occur from 4 months to 2 years after vaccination. Fatal disseminated BCG disease has occurred at a rate of 0.06 to 1.56 cases per million doses of vaccine administered; these deaths occurred primarily among immunocompromised people.

➤*Hypersensitivity reactions:* Assess the possibility of allergic reactions. Epinephrine injection (1:1000) for the control of immediate allergic reactions must be available should an acute anaphylactic reaction occur.

➤*Pregnancy: Category C.* It is not known whether BCG vaccine can cause fetal harm when administered to a pregnant woman or can affect reproduction capacity. Although no harmful effects to the fetus have been associated with BCG vaccine, its use is not recommended during pregnancy.

➤*Lactation:* It is not known whether BCG vaccine is excreted in breast milk. Because many drugs are excreted in human milk and because of the potential for serious adverse reactions in nursing infants from BCG vaccine, decide whether to discontinue nursing or not to vaccinate, taking into account the importance of tuberculosis vaccination to the mother.

➤*Children:* Take precautions with respect to infants vaccinated with BCG and exposed to individuals with active tuberculosis (see Administration and Dosage).

Precautions

➤*Aseptic technique:* BCG contains live bacteria; use with aseptic technique. Handle and dispose of all equipment, supplies, and receptacles in contact with BCG vaccine as biohazardous.

➤*Normal reaction:* The intensity and duration of the local reaction depends on the depth of penetration of the multiple-puncture device and individual variations in patients' tissue reactions. The initial skin lesions usually appear within 10 to 14 days and consist of small red papules at the site. The papules reach maximum diameter (about 3 mm) after 4 to 6 weeks, after which they may scale and then slowly subside.

After vaccination, it is usually not possible to clearly distinguish between a tuberculin reaction caused by persistent postvaccination sensitivity and one caused by a virulent suprainfection. Caution is advised in attributing a positive skin test to BCG vaccination. Further investigate a sharp rise in the tuberculin reaction since the latest test (except in the immediate postvaccination period).

Drug Interactions

➤*Antimicrobial or immunosuppressive agents:* These may interfere with the development of the immune response; use only under medical supervision.

➤*Vaccine:* Because BCG is a live vaccine, the immune response to the vaccine might be impaired if administered within 30 days of another live vaccine. However, no evidence exists for currently available vaccines to support this concern. Whenever possible, live vaccines administered on different days should be administered at least 30 days apart.

➤*Drug/Lab test interactions:* BCG vaccination results in tuberculin skin test reactivity. Tuberculin skin test reactivity as a result of BCG vaccination cannot be readily differentiated from reactivity following exposure to tuberculosis. BCG vaccination should not be administered to individuals with a positive tuberculin skin test.

Adverse Reactions

All suspected adverse reactions to BCG vaccination should be reported to Organon at (800) 842-3220 and to the Vaccine Adverse Effect Reporting System (VAERS) at (800) 822-7967. These reactions occasionally could occur more than 1 year after vaccination.

Local – Although BCG vaccination often results in local adverse effects, serious or long-term complications are rare. Reactions that can be expected after vaccination include moderate axillary or cervical lymphadenopathy and induration and subsequent pustule formation at the injection site; these reactions can persist for as long as 3 months after vaccination. More severe local reactions include ulceration at the vaccination site, regional suppurative lymphadenitis with draining sinuses, and caseous lesions or purulent drainage at the puncture site; these manifestations might occur within the 5 months after vaccination and could persist for several weeks.

Systemic – Acute, localized irritative toxicities of BCG may be accompanied by systemic manifestations, consistent with a flu-like syndrome. Systemic adverse effects of 1 to 2 days' duration such as fever, anorexia, myalgia, and neuralgia, often reflect hypersensitivity reactions.

Overdosage

Accidental overdosages, if treated immediately with antituberculous drugs, have not led to complications. If vaccination response is allowed to progress, it can still be treated successfully with antituberculous drugs but complications may occur (eg, regional adenitis, lupus vulgaris, SC cold abscesses, ocular lesions).

Patient Information

Keep the vaccination site clean until the local reaction has disappeared.

Following BCG vaccination, no dressing is required; however, it is recommended that the site be loosely covered and kept dry for 24 hours.

The patients should be advised that the vaccine contains live organisms. Although the vaccine will not survive in a dry state for long, infection of others is possible. Following vaccination with BCG, initial skin lesions usually appear within 10 to 14 days and consist of small red papules at the vaccination site. The papules reach a maximum diameter (about 3 mm) after 4 to 6 weeks, after which they may scale and slowly subside.

Patients may experience flu-like symptoms for 24 to 48 hours following BCG vaccination. However, the patients should consult with their physician immediately if they experience fever of 103°F or greater, or acute local reactions persisting longer than 2 to 3 days.

Vaccines, Bacterial

HAEMOPHILUS b CONJUGATE VACCINE

Rx	**HibTITER** (Wyeth-Lederle)	**Injection:** 10 mcg purified *Haemophilus* b saccharide capsular oligosaccharide and ≈ 25 mcg diphtheria CRM$_{197}$ protein/0.5 mL	In 1 and 10 dose vials.[1]
Rx	**ActHIB** (Aventis Pasteur)	**Powder for injection, lyophilized:** 10 mcg purified *Haemophilus* b capsular polysaccharide, 24 mcg tetanus toxoid/0.5 mL	8.5% sucrose. In single-dose vials with 7.5 mL vials of diphtheria and tetanus toxoids and pertussis vaccine as diluents or with 0.6 mL vial containing 0.4% sodium chloride diluent.
Rx	**Liquid PedvaxHIB** (Merck)	**Injection:** 7.5 mcg *Haemophilus* b PRP, 125 mcg *Neisseria meningitidis* OMPC and 225 mcg aluminum (as aluminum hydroxide)/0.5 mL	In single-dose vials.

[1] Multidose vials contain thimerosal 1:10,000.

For additional information, refer to the Agents for Active Immunization introduction.

Indications

For the routine immunization of children 2 months to 71 months of age (*HibTITER, PedvaxHIB*), 2 through 18 months of age (*ActHIB* and *ActHIB* reconstituted with Aventis Pasteur DTP), and 15 to 18 months of age (*ActHIB* reconstituted with *Tripedia* [*TriHIBiT*]) against invasive diseases caused by *Haemophilus influenzae* type b.

Consider children under 24 months of age who have had invasive *H. influenzae* type b (Hib) disease unimmunized. Start vaccination as soon as possible during the convalescent phase of the illness. Complete the schedule according to the child's age.

Conjugate vaccines may be given simultaneously with diphtheria and tetanus toxoids and pertussis vaccine adsorbed (DTP); combined measles, mumps, and rubella vaccine (MMR); oral poliovirus vaccine (OPV); or inactivated poliovirus vaccine (IPV).

Haemophilus b conjugate vaccines will not protect children against *H. influenzae* other than type b or other microorganisms that cause meningitis or septic disease.

Administration and Dosage

Administer IM doses in the outer aspect area of the vastus lateralis (mid-thigh) or deltoid. Do not inject IV.

➤*HibTITER:*

2 to 6 months of age – Three separate IM injections of 0.5 mL given at approximately 2-month intervals.

7 to 11 months of age (previously unvaccinated) – 2 separate IM injections of 0.5 mL given approximately 2 months apart.

12 to 14 months of age (previously unvaccinated) – One IM injection.

All vaccinated children receive a single booster dose at 15 months of age or older, but not less than 2 months after the previous dose. Previously unvaccinated children 15 to 71 months of age receive a single 0.5 mL IM injection.

➤*PedvaxHIB:* Shake well before withdrawal and use.

2 to 14 months of age – Two separate IM injections of 0.5 mL given at 2 months of age and 2 months later (or as soon as possible thereafter). When the primary 2-dose regimen is completed before 12 months of age, a 0.5 mL booster dose is required at 12 to 15 months of age but not earlier than 2 months after the second dose.

At least 15 months of age (previously unvaccinated) – Give a single 0.5 mL IM injection.

➤*ActHIB:* Use only Aventis Pasteur (AP) whole-cell DTP, *Tripedia*, or 0.4% sodium chloride diluent for reconstitution of lyophilized *ActHIB*.

Reconstitution with DTP or Tripedia – Thoroughly agitate the DTP or *Tripedia* vials, withdraw a 0.6 mL dose and inject into the vial of *ActHIB*. After reconstitution and thorough agitation, the combined vaccines will appear whitish in color. Withdraw and administer a 0.5 mL dose IM.

ActHIB/DTP: Use reconstituted vaccine within 24 hours.

ActHIB/Tripedia (TriHIBiT): Use reconstituted vaccine immediately (within 30 minutes).

Reconstitution with 0.4% sodium chloride – Inject the entire volume of diluent in the vial or syringe into the vial of *ActHIB*. Thoroughly agitate to ensure complete reconstitution. Draw back the entire volume of reconstituted vaccine into the syringe before injecting 0.5 mL IM. Vaccine will appear clear and colorless. Use within 24 hours.

ActHIB immunization schedule (previously unvaccinated) –

2 to 6 months of age:

Recommended Immunization Schedule for *ActHIB* **and DTP or** *Tripedia* **for Previously Unvaccinated Children**		
Dose	Age (months)	Immunization
First, second, and third	2, 4, and 6	*ActHIB* reconstituted with DTP or saline diluent (0.4% Sodium Chloride)
Fourth	15 to 18	*ActHIB* reconstituted with DTP or *Tripedia* (*TriHIBiT*) or with saline diluent (0.4% Sodium Chloride)
Fifth	4 to 6	DTP or *Tripedia*

7 to 11 months of age: Two 0.5 mL IM doses of *Haemophilus* b conjugate vaccine at 8-week intervals and a booster dose at 15 to 18 months of age.

12 to 14 months of age: One 0.5 mL IM dose of *Haemophilus* b conjugate vaccine followed by a booster 2 months later.

Vaccination Schedule for Haemophilus b Conjugate Vaccines						
Age at first dose (mo)	*HibTITER*		*PedvaxHIB*		*ActHIB*	
	Primary series	Booster	Primary series	Booster	Primary series	Booster
2-6	3 doses, 2 mo apart	15 mo[1]	2 doses, 2 mo apart	12 to 15 mo[1]	3 doses,[2] 2 mo apart	15-18 mo[3]
7-11	2 doses, 2 mo apart	15 mo[1]	2 doses, 2 mo apart	12 to 15 mo[1]	2 doses, 2 mo apart	15-18 mo[1]
12-14	1 dose	15 mo[1]	2 doses, 2 mo apart	-	1 dose	2 mo after previous dose[1]
15-71	1 dose	-	1 dose	-	-	-

[1] At least 2 months after previous dose.
[2] *ActHIB* reconstituted with DTP or saline diluent.
[3] *ActHIB* reconstituted with DTP, *Tripedia*, or saline diluent.

➤*Storage/Stability:* Store at 2° to 8°C (36° to 46°F). Do not freeze.

Actions

➤*Pharmacology:* The mechanism of action is through induction of specific protective antibodies against type b strains of *Haemophilus influenzae*. Vaccination may decrease nasopharyngeal colonization and produce lower rates of acquisition of colonization by unvaccinated infants.

The immune response depends on the type of cells producing the response and the antigens stimulating the process. Protein antigens induce B lymphocytes to produce antibody, aided by thymus-derived lymphocytes (T-helper cells); thus, they are called thymus-dependent antigens. This immune response is potentially boostable and IgG antibody predominates. In contrast, polysaccharide antigens stimulate B cells directly, without T-cell help, producing a nonboostable response of both IgG and IgM antibodies; these antigens are known as thymus-independent antigens. Linkage of Hib saccharides to a protein can convert the thymus-independent saccharide to a thymus-dependent antigen and can result in an enhanced antibody response to the saccharide and immunologic memory.

IgG$_1$ subclass predominates in the response to *HibTITER* and *Pedvax-HIB*. IgG$_1$ also predominates after administration of *ActHIB* to children under 2 years of age, but IgG$_2$ is induced after vaccination of older children and adults. IgG$_2$ is associated with natural infection. There is some evidence suggesting natural increases in antibody levels over time after vaccination.

ActHIB consists of the *Haemophilus* b capsular polysaccharide (polyribosyl-ribitol-phosphate, PRP), a high molecular weight polymer prepared from the *H. influenzae* type b strain 1482 grown in a semisynthetic medium, covalently bound to tetanus toxoid.

HibTITER (*Haemophilus* b conjugate vaccine [diphtheria CRM$_{197}$ protein conjugate]) is a sterile conjugate of a conjugate of oligosaccharides of the capsular antigen of *H. influenzae* type b (*Haemophilus* b) and diphtheria CRM$_{197}$ protein.

PedvaxHIB (*Haemophilus* b conjugate vaccine [meningococcal protein conjugate]) is a highly purified capsular polysaccharide (polyribosylribitol phosphate or PRP) of *H. influenzae* type b (*Haemophilus* b, Ross strain) that is covalently bound to an outer membrane protein complex (OMPC) of the B11 strain of *Neisseria meningitidis* serogroup B.

Epidemiology – Prior to the introduction of *Haemophilus* b conjugate vaccines, *H. influenzae* type b (Hib) was the most frequent cause of bacterial meningitis and a leading cause of serious, systemic bacterial disease in young children worldwide.

Hib disease occurred primarily in children under 5 years of age in the US prior to the initiation of a vaccine program and was estimated to account for nearly 20,000 cases of invasive infections annually, about 12,000 of which were meningitis. The mortality rate from Hib meningitis is about 5%. In addition, up to 35% of survivors develop neurologic sequelae including seizures, deafness, and mental retardation. Other

HAEMOPHILUS b CONJUGATE VACCINE

invasive diseases caused by this bacterium include cellulitis, epiglottitis, sepsis, pneumonia, septic arthritis, osteomyelitis, and pericarditis.

Prior to the introduction of the vaccine, it was estimated that 17% of all cases of Hib disease occurred in infants under 6 months of age. The peak incidence of Hib meningitis occurs between 6 to 11 months of age. Of all cases, 47% occur by 1 year of age with the remaining 53% occurring over the next 4 years.

Among children under 5 years of age, the risk of invasive Hib disease is increased in certain populations including the following:

Day care attendees
Lower socioeconomic groups
Blacks (especially those who lack the Km(1) immunoglobulin allotype)
Caucasians who lack the G2m(n or 23) immunoglobulin allotype
Native Americans
Household contacts of cases
Individuals with asplenia, sickle cell disease, or antibody deficiency syndromes.

Contraindications

Hypersensitivity to any component of the vaccine, the diluent, or diphtheria toxoid; hypersensitivity to thimerosal in the multidose vials (*HibTITER*). Any contraindication for DTP or *Tripedia* is a contraindication for use of *ActHIB* reconstituted with those respective vaccines.

Warnings

The expected immune response may not be obtained in people with malignancies or those receiving immunosuppressive therapy or who are otherwise immunocompromised.

An acute febrile illness or active infection is reason for delaying vaccination. A minor afebrile illness, such as a mild upper respiratory infection, is not usually reason to defer immunization.

Haemophilus b disease may occur in the week after vaccination, prior to the onset of the protective effects of the vaccine.

➤*Latex allergy:* The stopper of the diluent vial for *ActHIB* contains dry natural latex rubber that may cause allergic reactions; the lyophilized vaccine vial contains no rubber of any kind. Packaging for *HibTITER* contains dry natural rubber; health care professionals should administer *HibTITER* with caution to patients with a possible history of latex sensitivity.

➤*Pregnancy:* Category C. It is not known whether these vaccines can cause fetal harm or affect reproduction capacity; they are not recommended for use in pregnant patients.

➤*Children: PedvaxHIB* is not recommended for use in infants under 6 weeks of age. Safety and efficacy are not established for use in infants under 6 weeks of age (*HibTITER, ActHIB* reconstituted with Aventis Pasteur DTP or 0.4% sodium chloride), under 2 months of age (*Pedvax HIB*), under 15 months of age (*ActHIB* reconstituted with *Tripedia*), or 6 years of age or older (*Pedvax HIB*).

Drug Interactions

➤*Immunosuppressive therapies:* Immunosuppressive therapies, including irradiation, antimetabolites, alkylating agents, cytotoxic drugs, and corticosteroids (used in greater than physiologic doses) may reduce the immune response to vaccines.

➤*Drug/Lab test interactions:* Sensitive tests (eg, *Latex Agglutination Kits*) may detect PRP derived from the vaccine in urine of some vaccinees for up to 30 days following vaccination with *Pedvax HIB*.

Adverse Reactions

➤*Local:* Erythema, swelling, pain/soreness/tenderness.

➤*Systemic:* Fever (above 38°C), irritability, prolonged crying, drowsiness/sleepiness, vomiting, diarrhea. Rash, hives (urticaria), erythema multiforme, convulsions, vomiting/diarrhea, and Guillain-Barré syndrome have been observed following the administration of *Haemophilus b* polysaccharide and *Haemophilus b* conjugate vaccines. However, a cause-and-effect relationship among any of these events and the vaccination has not been established.

➤*Miscellaneous:*

HibTITER – Warmth, appetite loss, rash.

PedvaxHIB – Induration, unusual high-pitched crying, crying, otitis media, rash, upper respiratory infection, lymphadenopathy, angioedema (rare), febrile seizures, sterile injection site abscess.

ActHIB – Lethargy, induration, anorexia.

Patient Information

Provide guidance on measures to be taken if adverse events occur, such as antipyretic measures for elevated temperatures.

HAEMOPHILUS b CONJUGATE VACCINE WITH HEPATITIS B VACCINE

Rx	Comvax (Merck)	Injection: 7.5 mcg *Haemophilus* b PRP, 5 mcg hepatitis B surface antigen/0.5 mL[1]	In 0.5 mL single-dose vials.

[1] With 125 mcg *Neisseria meningitidis* OMPC, approximately 225 mcg aluminum (as aluminum hydroxide), and 35 mcg sodium borate (decahydrate) in 0.9% sodium chloride.

For additional information, refer to the Agents for Active Immunization introduction. For complete prescribing information, refer to the Haemophilus b conjugate vaccine monograph.

Indications

➤*Immunization:* For the routine immunization of children 6 weeks to 15 months of age born of hepatitis B surface antigen (HBsAg) negative mothers against invasive diseases caused by *Haemophilus influenzae* type b and against infection caused by all known subtypes of hepatitis B virus.

Consider children under 24 months of age who have had invasive *H. influenzae* type b (Hib) disease unimmunized. Start vaccination as soon as possible during the convalescent phase of the illness. Complete the schedule according to the child's age.

Conjugate vaccines may be given simultaneously with diphtheria and tetanus toxoids and pertussis vaccine adsorbed (DTP); combined measles, mumps, and rubella vaccine (MMR); oral poliovirus vaccine (OPV); or inactivated poliovirus vaccine (IPV); and with a booster dose of DTaP at approximately 15 months of age, using separate sites and syringes for injectable vaccines.

Haemophilus b conjugate vaccines will not protect children against *H. influenzae* other than type b or other microorganisms that cause meningitis or septic disease.

Administration and Dosage

Administer IM doses in the anterolateral thigh. Do not inject IV, intradermally, or SC. Shake well before withdrawal and use.

➤*Infants born to HBsAg negative mothers:* Three 0.5 mL doses administered IM ideally at 2, 4, and 12 to 15 months of age. If the recommended schedule cannot be followed exactly, the interval between the first 2 doses should be at least 2 months and the interval between the second and third doses should be as close as possible to 8 to 11 months.

➤*Children previously vaccinated with at least 1 dose of either hepatitis B vaccine or Haemophilus b conjugate vaccine:* Children who receive one dose of hepatitis B vaccine at or shortly after birth may receive *Comvax* on the schedule of 2, 4, and 12 to 15 months of age. There are no data to support the use of a 3-dose series of *Comvax* in infants who previously received more than 1 dose of hepatitis B vaccine; however, *Comvax* may be given to children otherwise scheduled to receive concurrent *Recombivax HB* and *PedvaxHIB*.

➤*Children not vaccinated according to recommended schedule:* Consider vaccination schedules on an individual basis. The number of doses of a PRP-OMPC-containing product (ie, *COMVAX, PedvaxHIB*) depends on the age that vaccination is begun. An infant 2 to 10 months of age should receive 3 doses of a product containing PRP-OMPC. An infant 11 to 14 months of age should receive 2 doses of a product containing PRP-OMPC. A child 15 to 71 months of age should receive one dose of a product containing PRP-OMPC. Infants and children, regardless of age, should receive 3 doses of an HBsAg-containing product.

➤*Storage/Stability:* Store at 2° to 8°C (36° to 46°F). Do not freeze.

MENINGOCOCCAL POLYSACCHARIDE VACCINE

| Rx | Menomune-A/C/Y/W-135 (Aventis Pasteur) | **Powder for Injection:** When reconstituted, each 0.5 mL contains 50 mcg "isolated product" from each of groups A, C, Y, and W-135 | Freeze-dried. In single- and 10-dose vials with diluent.[1] |

[1] With lactose (2.5 to 5 mg per dose). Single-dose vial supplied with 0.78 mL preservative-free distilled water diluent. Ten-dose vial supplied with 6 mL diluent with 1:10,000 thimerosal.

For additional information, refer to the Agents for Active Immunization introduction.

Indications

Active immunization against invasive meningococcal disease caused by these serogroups; may be used to prevent and control outbreaks of serogroup C meningococcal disease.

For evaluation and management of suspected outbreaks, it is recommended that the health care workers consult the *MMWR* for guidance.

Routine vaccination is recommended for the following high-risk groups:

1.) Deficiencies in late complement components (C3, C5-C-9).
2.) Functional or actual asplenia.
3.) People with laboratory or industrial exposure to *Neisseria meningitidis* aerosols.
4.) Travelers to, and residents of, hyperendemic areas such as sub-Saharan Africa. For information concerning geographic areas for which vaccination is recommended, contact the CDC at 888-232-3299.

The American College Health Association (ACHA) and the CDC also recommend that college students consider vaccination to reduce the risk for potentially fatal meningococcal disease.

Consider vaccinations for household or institutional contacts of people with meningococcal disease and for medical and laboratory personnel at risk of exposure to meningococcal disease.

Protective antibody levels may be achieved within 7 to 10 days after vaccination.

Meningococcal polysaccharide vaccine is not to be used for treatment of actual infection. Meningococcal polysaccharide vaccine is not indicated for infants and children under 2 years of age except as short-term protection of infants at least 3 months of age against Group A. For people remaining at high risk, especially children who were first vaccinated at less than 4 years of age, revaccination may be indicated (see Administration and Dosage).

aRoutine vaccination is not recommended in the US for the following reasons:

1.) Meningococcal disease is infrequent (about 3000 cases/year).
2.) No vaccine exists for serogroup B, which accounts for about 50% of cases in the US.
3.) Vaccine is not efficacious against group C disease in children under 2 years of age, which account for 28% of the group C cases in the US.

Administration and Dosage

Take special care to avoid injecting the vaccine intradermally, IM, or IV because clinical studies have not been done to establish safety and efficacy of the vaccine using these routes of administration.

The immunizing dose is a single injection of 0.5 mL administered SC.

Simultaneous administration of meningococcal polysaccharide vaccine can be given concurrently with other vaccines at separate sites and separate syringes. However, because of the combined endotoxin content, do not administer the vaccine at the same time as whole-cell pertussis or whole-cell typhoid vaccines (see Drug Interactions). Do not use multiple-dose needle and syringe with jet injector.

➤*Primary immunization:* For adults and children, the vaccine is administered SC as a single 0.5 mL dose. Protective antibody levels may be achieved within 7 to 10 days after vaccination.

➤*Revaccination:* Revaccination of a single 0.5 mL dose administered SC may be indicated for individuals at high risk of infection, particularly children who were first vaccinated when they were under 4 years of age; consider such children for revaccination after 2 or 3 years if they remain at high risk. Although the need for revaccination in older children and adults has not been determined, antibody levels decline rapidly over 2 to 3 years, and if indications still exist for immunization, consider revaccination within 3 to 5 years.

➤*Reconstitution:* Reconstitute the vaccine using only the diluent supplied for this purpose. Draw the volume of diluent shown on the diluent label into a suitable size syringe and inject into the vial containing the vaccine. Shake vial until the vaccine is dissolved. The reconstituted vaccine is a clear colorless liquid.

➤*Storage/Stability:* Store freeze-dried vaccine and reconstituted vaccine, when not in use, between 2° and 8°C (35° to 46°F). Discard remainder of multidose vials of vaccine within 5 days after reconstitution. Use the single-dose vial within 30 minutes after reconstitution.

Actions

➤*Pharmacology:* Meningococcal polysaccharide vaccine is a freeze-dried preparation of the group-specific polysaccharide antigens from *Neisseria meningitidis*, Group A, Group C, Group Y, and Group-W-135.

N. meningitidis is cultivated with Mueller Hinton agar and Watson Scherp media. After reconstitution with diluent as indicated on the label, the 0.5 mL dose is formulated to contain 50 mcg of "isolated product" from each of Groups A, C, Y, and W-135 in an isotonic sodium chloride solution. Each dose of vaccine also is formulated to contain 2.5 to 5 mg lactose added as a stabilizer.

Potency is evaluated by measuring the molecular size of each polysaccharide component using a column chromatography method as standardized by the FDA and WHO for meningococcal polysaccharide vaccine. This vaccine conforms to the WHO requirements.

Vaccine efficacy – The immunogenicity and clinical efficacy of serogroups A and C meningococcal vaccines have been well established. The serogroup A polysaccharide induces antibody in some children as young as 3 months of age, although a response comparable with that among adults is not achieved until 4 or 5 years of age; the serogroup C component is poorly immunogenic in recipients who are under 18 to 24 months of age. The serogroups A and C vaccines have demonstrated estimated clinical efficacies of 85% to 100% in older children and adults and are useful in controlling epidemics. Serogroups Y and W-135 polysaccharides are safe and immunogenic in adults and in children over 2 years of age.

A study performed using 4 lots of meningococcal polysaccharide vaccine in 150 adults showed a 4-fold or greater increase in bactericidal antibodies to all groups in more than 90% of subjects.

A study was conducted in 73 children 2 to 12 years of age. Postimmunization sera were not obtained on 4 children; seroconversion rates were calculated on 69 paired samples. Seroconversion rates as measured by bactericidal antibody were the following: Group A - 72%, Group C - 58%, Group Y - 90%, and Group W-135 - 82%. Seroconversion rates as measured by a 2-fold rise in antibody titers based on Solid Phase Radioimmunoassay were: Group A - 99%, Group C - 99%, Group Y - 97%, and Group W-135 - 89%.

Duration of efficacy – Measurable levels of antibodies against the group A and C polysaccharides decrease markedly during the first 3 years following a single dose of vaccine. This decrease in antibody occurs more rapidly in infants and young children than in adults. Similarly, although vaccine-induced clinical protection probably persists in schoolchildren and adults for at least 3 years, the efficacy of the Group A vaccine in young children may decreased markedly with the passage of time. In a 3-year study, efficacy declined from more than 90% to less than 10% among children who were under 4 years of age at the time of vaccination, whereas among children who were 4 years of age or older when vaccinated, efficacy was 67% 3 years later. In a New Zealand study, children 2 to 13 years of age received a single dose of monovalent group A vaccine, 26% of children 3 to 23 months of age in this study received 2 doses of the vaccine, given approximately 3 months apart. After 2.5 of active surveillance (1987 to 1989) there were no cases of invasive group A disease in children vaccinated at 2 years of age or older.

Contraindications

Acute illness; immediate-type sensitivity to thimerosal or any other component of the vaccine. For individuals sensitive to thimerosal, administer the 1-dose package size and reconstitute with the 0.78 mL vial of diluent that contains no preservatives. Do not use meningococcal polysaccharide vaccine for treatment of actual infection.

Warnings

➤*Latex sensitivity:* Use caution in patients with a possible history of latex sensitivity; the stopper to the vial contains natural latex rubber.

➤*Immunosuppressive therapy:* If the vaccine is used in people receiving immunosuppressive therapy, the expected immune response may not be obtained.

➤*Pregnancy: Category C.* It is not known whether meningococcal polysaccharide vaccine can cause fetal harm when given to a pregnant woman or can affect reproduction capacity. Give meningococcal polysaccharide vaccine to a pregnant woman only if clearly needed.

➤*Lactation:* It is not known whether this drug is excreted in breast milk. Because many drugs are excreted in human milk, exercise caution when meningococcal polysaccharide vaccine is given to a nursing woman.

➤*Children:* Safety and efficacy of meningococcal polysaccharide vaccine in children under 2 years of age have not been established.

Drug Interactions

➤*Immunosuppressants:* If meningococcal polysaccharide vaccine is administered to immunosuppressed people or people receiving immunosuppressive therapy, an adequate immunologic response may not be obtained.

MENINGOCOCCAL POLYSACCHARIDE VACCINE

➤*Other vaccines:* Do not give meningococcal polysaccharide vaccine at the same time as whole-cell pertussis or whole-cell typhoid vaccines due to combined endotoxin content.

Adverse Reactions

Adverse reactions to meningococcal vaccine are mild and consist principally of pain and redness at the injection site for 1 to 2 days. Pain at the injection site is the most commonly reported adverse reaction, and a transient fever might develop in 2% or less of young children.

The following adverse events were reported by 150 adults following vaccination with meningococcal polysaccharide vaccine and occurred within 3 weeks following vaccination. Local reactions resolved within 48 hours and no significant systemic reactions were reported.

➤*Local:* Pain (mild reaction, 2.6%; moderate reaction, 2%), tenderness (mild, 36%; moderate, 9%), diameter (mild, less than 2 in.; moderate, 2 in. or greater), erythema (mild, 3.8%; moderate, 1.2%), induration (mild, 4.4%; moderate, 1.2%).

In a clinical study involving 73 children 2 to 12 years of age who received meningococcal polysaccharide vaccine, local reactions consisting of erythema or tenderness were seen in approximately 40% of the children. In another clinical study involving 53 children 4 to 6 years of age who received meningococcal polysaccharide vaccine, erythema was seen in 89% of the children, swelling in 92%, and tenderness in 64%. None of these reactions were considered serious or necessitated medical intervention.

➤*Systemic:* Headaches (mild, 5.2%; moderate, 1.8%), malaise (mild, 2.5%), chills (mild, 2.5%), oral temperature (mild, 2.6% [100° to 101°F]; moderate, 0.6% [> 101°F]).

On rare occasions, IgA nephropathy has occurred following vaccinations with meningococcal polysaccharide vaccine; however, a cause-and-effect relationship has not been established.

PNEUMOCOCCAL VACCINE, POLYVALENT

| Rx | **Pneumovax 23** (Merck) | **Injection:** 25 mcg each of 23 polysaccharide isolates per 0.5 mL dose | In 1- and 5-dose vials.[1] |
| Rx | **Pnu-Imune 23** (Wyeth-Lederle) | | In 5-dose vials[2] and *Lederject* disp. syringes.[2] |

[1] With 0.25% phenol.

[2] With 0.01% thimerosal.

For additional information, refer to the Agents for Active Immunization introduction.

Indications

For immunization against pneumococcal pneumonia and bacteremia caused by the types of pneumococci included in the vaccine.

➤*Adults†:* Immunocompetent adults at increased risk of pneumococcal disease or its complications because of chronic illnesses (eg, cardiovascular or pulmonary disease, diabetes mellitus, alcoholism, cirrhosis, cerebrospinal fluid [CSF] leaks) or adults ≥ 65 years of age.

Immunocompromised adults at increased risk of pneumococcal disease or its complications (eg, those with splenic dysfunction or anatomic asplenia, Hodgkin's disease, lymphoma, multiple myeloma, chronic renal failure, nephrotic syndrome, conditions such as organ transplantation associated with immunosuppression).

Asymptomatic or symptomatic HIV infection.

➤*Children†:* Children ≥ 2 years of age with chronic illnesses specifically associated with increased risk of pneumococcal disease or its complications (eg, anatomic or functional asplenia [including sickle cell disease], nephrotic syndrome, CSF leaks, and conditions associated with immunosuppression).

Children ≥ 2 years of age with asymptomatic or symptomatic HIV infection.

Note – The CDC states that recurrent upper respiratory diseases, including otitis media and sinusitis, are *not* considered indications for vaccine use in children.

➤*Special groups:* People living in special environments or social settings with an identified increased risk of pneumococcal disease or its complications (eg, certain Native American populations). People > 2 years of age in closed groups (eg, residential schools, nursing homes, other institutions).

Administration and Dosage

Give one 0.5 mL dose. Do not inject IV. Avoid intradermal administration. Administer SC or IM (preferably in the deltoid muscle or lateral mid-thigh).

➤*Storage/Stability:* Refrigerate at 2° to 8°C (36° to 46°F). At room temperature, *Pnu-Imune 23* is stable for several days (≤ 25°C; 77°F) and *Pneumovax 23* is stable for 1 month (≤ 15°C to 30°C; 59°F to 86°F). Do not freeze.

Actions

➤*Pharmacology:* The 23-valent vaccine affords protection against the 23 most prevalent or invasive pneumococcal types, accounting for ≥ 90% of pneumococcal blood isolates and ≥ 85% of all pneumococcal isolates from generally sterile sites.

Because the polysaccharide capsules are immunogenic, they stimulate antipneumococcal antibody production and prevent pneumococcal disease. The vaccine will protect only against the capsular types of pneumococci contained in the vaccine.

Contraindications

Hypersensitivity to any component of the vaccine, including thimerosal.

The occurrence of any type of neurological symptoms or signs following administration of this product is a contraindication to further use.

➤*Immunosuppressive therapy:* Do not attempt immunization of patients < 2 weeks prior to or during treatment with immunosuppressive drugs, irradiation, or initiation of chemotherapy.

➤*Infections:* Defer administration in the presence of any febrile respiratory illness, acute respiratory, or other active infections, except when withholding the agent entails even greater risk.

Warnings

➤*Limited effectiveness: Pneumovax 23* may not be effective in preventing pneumococcal meningitis in patients who have chronic CSF leakage resulting from congenital lesions, skull fractures, or neurosurgical procedures.

When elective splenectomy is considered, give pneumococcal vaccine ≥ 2 weeks before the operation, if possible. Similarly, when cancer chemotherapy or other immunosuppressive therapy is planned, as in candidates for organ or bone marrow transplants, the interval between vaccination and initiation of immunosuppressive therapy should be ≥ 2 weeks.

Although vaccine failures have occurred in some of these groups, especially those who are immunocompromised, vaccination is still recommended for such people because they are at high risk of developing severe disease.

➤*Hypersensitivity reactions:* Epinephrine 1:1000 must be available to control immediate allergic reactions. Refer to Management of Acute Hypersensitivity Reactions.

➤*Pregnancy: Category C.* It is not known whether pneumococcal vaccine can cause fetal harm when administered to a pregnant woman or affect reproduction capacity. Not recommended for use in pregnant women. Give to a pregnant woman only if clearly needed.

➤*Lactation:* It is not known whether this drug is excreted in breast milk. Exercise caution when administering to a nursing woman.

➤*Children:* Safety and efficacy in children < 2 years of age have not been established. Not recommended for children < 2 years of age because they do not respond satisfactorily to the capsular types of the vaccine.

Precautions

➤*History of pneumococcal pneumonia or other pneumococcal infection:* Patients may have high levels of preexisting pneumococcal antibodies, which may result in increased reactions to this vaccine. These reactions are mostly local, but are occasionally systemic. Exercise caution if such patients are considered for vaccination.

➤*Cardiac/pulmonary disease:* Exercise caution in those with severely compromised cardiac or pulmonary function; a systemic reaction could pose a significant risk.

➤*Revaccination:* Early studies have indicated that local reactions (ie, arthus-type reactions) among adults receiving the second dose of 14-valent vaccine within 2 years after the first dose are more severe than those occurring after initial vaccination. However, subsequent studies have suggested that revaccination after intervals of ≥ 4 years is not associated with an increased incidence of adverse side effects.

Routine revaccination of immunocompromised people previously vaccinated with 23-valent polysaccharide vaccine is not recommended. However, 1 revaccination is recommended for people ≥ 2 years of age who are at highest risk of serious pneumococcal infection and those likely to have a rapid decline in pneumococcal antibody levels, provided that ≥ 5 years have passed since receipt of a first dose of pneumococcal vaccine.

† *MMWR.* 1997;46(RR-8):1-24.

PNEUMOCOCCAL VACCINE, POLYVALENT

The highest risk group includes people with functional or anatomic asplenia (eg, sickle cell disease, or splenectomy), HIV infection, leukemia, lymphoma, Hodgkin's disease, multiple myeloma, generalized malignancy, chronic renal failure, nephrotic syndrome, or other conditions associated with immunosuppression (eg, organ or bone marrow transplantation), and those receiving immunosuppressive chemotherapy (including long-term systemic corticosteroids).

For children ≤ 10 years of age at revaccination and at highest risk of severe pneumococcal infection (eg, children with functional or anatomic asplenia, including sickle cell disease or splenectomy, or conditions associated with rapid antibody decline after initial vaccination, including nephrotic syndrome, renal failure, or renal transplantation), the Immunization Practices Advisory Committee (ACIP) recommends that revaccination may be considered 3 years after the previous dose.

If prior vaccination status is unknown for patients in the high risk group, patients should be given pneumococcal vaccine.

All people ≥ 65 years of age who have not received the vaccine within 5 years (and were < 65 years of age at the time of vaccination) should receive another dose of vaccination.

Because data are insufficient concerning the safety of pneumococcal vaccine when administered ≥ 3 times, revaccination following a second dose is not routinely recommended.

The ACIP recommendations regarding immunization are as follows: People who receive the 14-valent vaccine should not be routinely reimmunized with the 23-valent vaccine. However, strongly consider revaccination with 23-valent vaccine for those who received 14-valent vaccine if they are at highest risk of fatal pneumococcal infection (eg, asplenic).

▶*Antibiotic prophylaxis:* In patients who require antibiotic prophylaxis against pneumococcal infection, do not discontinue prophylaxis after vaccination.

Patients with impaired immune responsiveness whether because of the use of immunosuppressive therapy, a genetic defect, human immunodeficiency virus (HIV) infection, or other causes may have a reduced antibody response to active immunization procedures. At least 2 weeks should elapse between immunization and initiation of chemotherapy or immunosuppressive therapy.

Drug Interactions

▶*Concomitant use of influenza virus vaccine:* The ACIP states that pneumococcal vaccine may be administered at the same time as influenza vaccine (by separate injection in the other arm) without an increase in side effects or decreased antibody response to either vaccine. In contrast to pneumococcal vaccine, influenza vaccine is recommended annually for appropriate populations.

▶*Chemotherapy/Radiation:* Avoid vaccination during chemotherapy or radiation therapy. Based on literature reports, pneumococcal vaccine may be given as early as several months following completion of chemotherapy or radiation therapy for neoplastic disease. In Hodgkin disease, immune response to vaccination may be impaired for ≥ 2 years after intensive chemotherapy (with or without radiation). Patients who have received extensive chemotherapy or splenectomy for treatment of Hodgkin disease have been shown to have an impaired serum antibody response to pneumococcal vaccine. In 1 study, administration of the vaccine to patients on immunosuppressive drugs or radiation for Hodgkin disease resulted in reduction of pre-existing antibody levels in several patients. It is unclear whether this effect was caused by the vaccine or to the effects of radiation or chemotherapy. During the 2 years following the completion of chemotherapy or other immunosuppressive therapy, antibody responses improve in some patients as the interval between the end of treatment and pneumococcal vaccination increases.

Adverse Reactions

▶*Local:* Erythema, induration, warmth, swelling, and soreness at the injection site (≈ 72%) occur within 3 days after vaccination.

▶*Systemic:* Low grade fever (< 37.7°C; 100°F) and mild myalgia occur occasionally, usually within 24 hours following vaccination. However, acute febrile reactions (> 38.9°C; 102°F), rash, urticaria, arthritis, adenitis, marked local swelling, and arthralgia have occurred rarely.

Rarely, patients with otherwise stabilized idiopathic thrombocytopenic purpura have experienced a relapse, occurring 2 to 14 days after vaccination, and lasting ≤ 2 weeks.

Systemic reactions of greater severity, duration, or extent are unusual.

Neurological disorders such as paresthesias and acute radiculoneuropathy, including Guillain-Barré syndrome, occur rarely in temporal association with use of pneumococcal vaccine. No cause-and-effect relationship has been established.

Anaphylactoid reactions have been rare.

▶*Miscellaneous:* Asthenia; headache; hemolytic anemia in patients who have had other hematologic disorders; lymphadenitis; malaise; nausea; serum sickness; thrombocytopenia in patients with stabilized idiopathic thrombocytopenic purpura; vomiting.

PNEUMOCOCCAL 7–VALENT CONJUGATE VACCINE (DIPHTHERIA CRM$_{197}$ PROTEIN)

Rx	**Prevnar** (Wyeth Lederle Vaccines)	**Injection:** 2 mcg each of 6 polysaccharide isolates; 4 mcg of 1 polysaccharide isolate per 0.5 mL dose[1]	In 0.5 mL single-dose vials.

[1] Contains 0.125 mg aluminum per dose as aluminum phosphate adjuvant.

For additional information, refer to the Agents for Active Immunization introduction.

Indications

▶*Immunization against Streptococcus pneumoniae:* Active immunization of infants and toddlers against invasive disease caused by *S. pneumoniae* due to the capsular serotypes included in the vaccine (4, 6B, 9V, 14, 18C, 19F, and 23F).

▶*Immunization against otitis media:* Active immunization of infants and toddlers against otitis media caused by serotypes included in the vaccine. However, for vaccine serotypes, protection against otitis media is expected to be substantially lower than protection against invasive disease. Additionally, because otitis media is caused by many organisms other than serotypes of *S. pneumoniae* represented in the vaccine, protection against all causes of otitis media is expected to be low.

This vaccine is not intended to be used for treatment of active infection.

Administration and Dosage

▶*Approved by the FDA:* February 17, 2000.

Administer as one 0.5 mL IM injection. Do not inject IV.

The preferred sites of IM injection are the anterolateral aspect of the thigh in infants or the deltoid muscle of the upper arm in toddlers and young children. Do not inject the vaccine in the gluteal area or areas where there may be a major nerve trunk or blood vessel.

▶*Vaccination schedule:* For infants, the immunization series of pneumococcal 7-valent conjugate vaccine consists of 3 doses of 0.5 mL each, at approximately 2-month intervals, followed by a fourth dose of 0.5 mL at 12 to 15 months of age. The customary age for the first dose is 2 months of age, but it can be given as young as 6 weeks of age. The recommended dosing interval is 4 to 8 weeks. Administer the fourth dose at least 2 months after the third dose.

▶*Previously unvaccinated older infants and children:* For previously unvaccinated older infants and children who are beyond the age of the routine infant schedule, the following schedule applies:

Pneumococcal Vaccine Dosage in Previously Unvaccinated Older Infants and Children	
Age at first dose	Total number of 0.5 mL doses
7 to 11 months of age	3[1]
12 to 23 months of age	2[2]
≥ 24 months through 9 years of age	1

[1] Two doses at least 4 weeks apart; third dose after the 1-year birthday, separated from the second dose by at least 2 months.
[2] Two doses at least 2 months apart.

Safety and immunogenicity data are limited or not available for children in specific high-risk groups for invasive pneumococcal disease (eg, individuals with sickle cell disease, asplenia, HIV infection).

▶*Preparation:* Because this product is a suspension containing an aluminum phosphate adjuvant, shake vigorously immediately prior to use to obtain a uniform suspension prior to withdrawing the dose. Do not use the vaccine if it cannot be resuspended. After shaking, the vaccine appears as a homogeneous, white suspension. Administer immediately after drawing the vaccine up into the syringe.

▶*Storage/Stability:* Refrigerate at 2° to 8°C (36° to 46°F). Do not freeze.

Actions

▶*Pharmacology:* Pneumococcal 7-valent conjugate vaccine is a sterile solution of saccharides of the capsular antigens of *S. pneumoniae* serotypes 4, 6B, 9V, 14, 18C, 19F, and 23F individually conjugated to diphtheria CRM$_{197}$ protein. The polysaccharides are chemically activated to make saccharides, which are directly conjugated to the protein carrier CRM$_{197}$ to form the glycoconjugate. This is effected by reductive amination. CRM$_{197}$ is a nontoxic variant of diphtheria toxin isolated from cultures of *Corynebacterium diphtheriae* strain C7 (β197) grown in a casamino acids and yeast extract-base medium.

Epidemiology – Approximately 90 serotypes of *S. pneumoniae* have been identified based on antigenic differences in their capsular polysaccharides. The distribution of serotypes responsible for disease differ with age and geographic location.

PNEUMOCOCCAL 7–VALENT CONJUGATE VACCINE (DIPHTHERIA CRM$_{197}$ PROTEIN)

Serotypes 4, 6B, 9V, 14, 18C, 19F, and 23F have been responsible for approximately 80% of invasive pneumococcal disease in children under 6 years of age in the United States. These 7 serotypes also accounted for 74% of penicillin-nonsusceptible *S. pneumoniae* (PNSP) and 100% of pneumococci with high-level penicillin resistance isolated from children under 6 years of age with invasive disease during a 1993-1994 surveillance by the Centers for Disease Control and Prevention.

Contraindications

Hypersensitivity to any component of the vaccine, including diphtheria toxoid.

➤*Infections:* Severe or even a moderate febrile illness is sufficient reason to postpone vaccinations. Minor illnesses, such as a mild upper respiratory tract infection, with or without low-grade fever, are not generally contraindications.

Warnings

➤*Efficacy:* This vaccine will not protect against *S. pneumoniae* disease other than that caused by the 7 serotypes included in the vaccine, nor will it protect against other microorganisms that cause invasive infection such as bacteremia and meningitis or noninvasive infections such as otitis media.

Immunization with pneumococcal 7-valent conjugate vaccine does not substitute for routine diphtheria immunization.

➤*Immunosuppressed patients:* Children with impaired immune responsiveness, whether caused by the use of immunosuppressive therapy (including irradiation, corticosteroids, antimetabolites, alkylating agents, and cytotoxic agents), a genetic defect, HIV infection, or other causes, may have reduced antibody response to active immunization (see Drug Interactions).

➤*Immunocompromised patients:* The use of pneumococcal conjugate vaccine does not replace the use of 23-valent pneumococcal polysaccharide vaccination in children at least 24 months of age with sickle cell disease, asplenia, HIV infection, chronic illness, or those who are immunocompromised. Data on sequential vaccination with pneumococcal 7-valent conjugate vaccine followed by 23-valent pneumococcal polysaccharide vaccine are limited. In a randomized study, 23 children at least 2 years of age with sickle cell disease were administered 2 doses of pneumococcal 7-valent conjugate vaccine followed by a dose of polysaccharide vaccine or a single dose of polysaccharide vaccine alone. In this small study, safety and immune responses with the combined schedule were similar to polysaccharide vaccine alone.

➤*Latex sensitivity:* Use caution in patients with a possible history of latex sensitivity; the packaging contains dry natural rubber.

➤*Hypersensitivity reactions:* Epinephrine 1:1000 and other appropriate agents must be available to control immediate allergic reaction. Refer to Management of Acute Hypersensitivity Reactions.

➤*Elderly:* This vaccine is not recommended for use in adult populations. Do not use as a substitute for the pneumococcal polysaccharide vaccine in geriatric populations.

➤*Pregnancy: Category C.* It is not known whether pneumococcal 7-valent conjugate vaccine can cause fetal harm when administered to a pregnant woman or whether it can affect reproductive capacity. Pneumococcal 7-valent conjugate vaccine is not recommended for use in pregnant women.

➤*Lactation:* It is not known whether vaccine antigens or antibodies are excreted in breast milk. This vaccine is not recommended for use in nursing mothers.

➤*Children:* Pneumococcal 7-valent conjugate vaccine has been shown to be usually well-tolerated and immunogenic in infants. The safety and efficacy of pneumococcal 7-valent conjugate vaccine in children under 6 weeks of age or on or after the tenth birthday have not been established. Immune responses elicited by pneumococcal 7-valent conjugate vaccine among infants born prematurely have not been studied. See Administration and Dosage for the recommended pediatric dosage.

Precautions

➤*Route of administration:* Pneumococcal 7-valent conjugate vaccine is for IM use only. Do not administer IV under any circumstances. The safety and immunogenicity for other routes of administration (eg, SC) have not been evaluated. Take special care to prevent injection into or near a blood vessel or nerve.

➤*Postvaccination fever:* Fever and, rarely, febrile seizure have been reported in children receiving pneumococcal 7-valent conjugate vaccine. For children at higher risk of seizures than the general population, acetaminophen or other appropriate antipyretics (dosed according to respective prescribing information) may be administered around the time of vaccination to reduce the possibility of postvaccination fever.

Drug Interactions

➤*Immunosuppressive agents:* Children receiving therapy with immunosuppressive agents (large amounts of corticosteroids, antime-tabolites, alkylating agents, cytotoxic agents) may not respond optimally to active immunization.

Adverse Reactions

Health care professionals should report any suspected adverse events following immunization to the US Department of Health and Human Services (DHHS). The National Vaccine Injury Compensation Program requires that the manufacturer and lot number of the vaccine administered be recorded by the health care professional in the vaccine recipient's permanent medical record (or in a permanent office log or file), along with the date of administration of the vaccine and the name, address, and title of the person administering the vaccine.

The US DHHS established the Vaccine Adverse Event Reporting System (VAERS) to accept all reports of suspected adverse events after the administration of any vaccine including, but not limited to, the reporting of events required by the National Childhood Vaccine Injury Act of 1986. The FDA web site is http://www.fda.gov/cber/vaers/vaers.htm.

The VAERS toll-free number for VAERS forms and information is (800) 822-7967.

Pneumococcal Vaccine Adverse Reactions Within 2 or 3 Days of Administration to Infants as a Primary Series at 2, 4, and 6 Months of Age (%)			
	Pneumococcal 7-valent conjugate vaccine concurrently with DTP-HbOC	Pneumococcal 7-valent conjugate vaccine concurrently with DTaP and HbOC	DTaP and HbOC only
Number of doses	9191[1]	3848[2]	538[3]
GI			
Decreased appetite	24.7	18.1	13.6
Vomiting	16.2	13.4	9.8
Diarrhea	11.4	9.8	4.4
Miscellaneous			
Irritability	69.1	52.5	45.2
Drowsiness	36.9	32.9	27.7
Fever of 38°C (100.4°F) or higher	35.6	21.1	14.2
Restless sleep	25.8	20.6	22.3
Fever of greater than 39°C (102.2°F)	3.1	1.8	0.4
Urticaria-like rash	0.9	0.6	0.3

[1] Total from which reaction data are available varies between reactions from 8874 to 9191 doses.
[2] Total from which reaction data are available varies between reactions from 3121 to 3848 doses.
[3] Total from which reaction data are available varies between reactions from 295 to 538 doses.

Pneumococcal Vaccine Adverse Reactions Within 2 or 3 Days of Administration to Toddlers as a Fourth Dose at 12 to 15 Months of Age (%)			
	Pneumococcal 7-valent conjugate vaccine concurrently with DTP-HbOC	Pneumococcal 7-valent conjugate vaccine concurrently with DTaP and HbOC	Pneumococcal 7-valent conjugate vaccine only
Number of doses	709[1]	270[2]	727[3]
GI			
Decreased appetite	33	21.1	18.3
Diarrhea	12.1	13.7	12.8
Vomiting	9.6	5.6	6.3
Miscellaneous			
Irritability	72.8	45.9	45.8
Fever of ≥ 38°C (100.4°F) or higher	41.9	19.6	13.4
Restless sleep	29.9	21.2	21.2
Drowsiness	21.3	17.5	15.9
Fever of greater than 39°C (102.2°F)	4.5	1.5	1.2
Urticaria-like rash	1.4	0.7	1.2

[1] Total from which reaction data are available varies between reactions from 706 to 709 doses.
[2] Total from which reaction data are available varies between reactions from 269 to 270 doses.
[3] Total from which reaction data are available varies between reactions from 725 to 727 doses.

With vaccines in general, including pneumococcal 7-valent conjugate vaccine, it is not uncommon for patients to note within 48 to 72 hours the following minor reactions at or around the injection site: Edema; pain or tenderness; redness, inflammation, or skin discoloration; mass; local hypersensitivity reaction. Such local reactions are usually self-limited and require no therapy.

As with other aluminum-containing vaccines, a nodule may occasionally be palpable at the injection site for several weeks.

➤*Postmarketing:*

Hypersensitivity – Hypersensitivity reaction including face edema, dyspnea, bronchospasm, anaphylactic/anaphylactoid reaction including shock.

Vaccines, Bacterial

PNEUMOCOCCAL 7-VALENT CONJUGATE VACCINE (DIPHTHERIA CRM$_{197}$ PROTEIN)

Local – Injection site dermatitis; injection site urticaria; injection site pruritus.

Miscellaneous – Lymphadenopathy localized to the region of the injection site; angioneurotic edema; erythema multiforme.

Overdosage

There have been reports of overdose with pneumococcal 7-valent conjugate vaccine, including cases of administration of a higher than recommended dose and cases of subsequent doses administered closer than recommended to the previous dose. Most individuals were asymptomatic. In general, adverse events reported with overdose have also been reported with recommended single doses of pneumococcal 7-valent conjugate vaccine.

Patient Information

Prior to administration of this vaccine, inform the parent, guardian, or other responsible adult of the potential benefits and risks to the patient (see Adverse Reactions and Warnings) and the importance of completing the immunization series unless contraindicated. Instruct parents or guardians to report any suspected adverse reactions to their health care professional. Provide vaccine information prior to each vaccination.

TYPHOID VACCINE

Rx	**Vivotif Berna** (Berna)	**Capsules, enteric-coated:** 2 to 6 x 10^9 colony-forming units of viable *Salmonella typhi* Ty21a and 5 to 50 x 10^9 bacterial cells of nonviable *S. typhi* Ty21a[1]	Salmon/White. In blister pack 4s.
Rx	**Typhim Vi** (Aventis Pasteur)	**Injection:** 25 mcg purified Vi capsular polysaccharide/0.5 mL[2]	In 0.5 mL syringes and 20 and 50 dose vials.

[1] With 26 to 130 mg sucrose, 1 to 5 mg ascorbic acid, 1.4 to 7 mg amino acid mixture, 100 to 180 mg lactose, and 3.6 to 4.4 mg magnesium stearate.

[2] With 4.15 mg NaCl, 0.065 mg disodium phosphate, 0.023 mg monosodium phosphate, 0.5 mL sterile water for injection.

For additional information, refer to the Agents for Active Immunization introduction.

Indications

➤*Oral:* For immunization of adults and children over 6 years of age against disease caused by *Salmonella typhi*. Complete the vaccine regimen at least 1 week before potential exposure to typhoid bacteria.

➤*Parenteral:* For active immunity against typhoid fever for people 2 years of age. Complete the vaccine regimen at least 2 weeks before potential exposure to typhoid bacteria.

Routine immunization against typhoid fever is not recommended in the United States. Selective immunization against typhoid fever is recommended under the following circumstances: 1) Expected intimate exposure to a household contact with typhoid fever or a known carrier; 2) travelers to typhoid-endemic areas (especially Africa, Asia, and South and Central America), especially if prolonged exposure to potentially contaminated food and water is likely, and travelers to areas of the world with a risk of exposure to typhoid fever; and 3) workers in microbiology laboratories with expected frequent contact with *S. typhi*.

➤*Unlabeled uses:* Parenteral typhoid vaccine may offer some cross-protection against *Salmonella paratyphi* A. These bacteria share a common O antigen factor 12 with *S. typhi*.

Administration and Dosage

➤*Oral:*

Primary immunization – One capsule on alternate days (eg, days 1, 3, 5, and 7) swallowed whole about 1 hour before a meal with cold or lukewarm drink, not to exceed body temperature (37°C; 98.6°F). The vaccine capsule should not be chewed; swallow as soon as possible after placing in the mouth. A complete immunization schedule is the ingestion of 4 vaccine capsules as described above. Immunization (ingestion of all 4 doses should be completed at least 1 week prior to potential exposure to *S. typhi*). Unless a complete immunization schedule is followed, an optimum immune response may not be achieved. Not all recipients will be fully protected against typhoid fever. Travelers should take all necessary precautions to avoid contact or ingestion of potentially contaminated food or water.

Booster dose – The optimum booster schedule has not been determined. Efficacy persists for at least 5 years. Further, there is no experience with oral typhoid vaccine as a booster in people previously immunized with parenteral typhoid vaccine. It is recommended that a booster dose consisting of 4 vaccine capsules taken on alternate days be given every 5 years under conditions of repeated or continued exposure to typhoid fever.

➤*Parenteral:*

Primary immunization – For IM use only. Do not inject IV. Indicated only for individuals 2 years of age or older. Give a single 0.5 mL (25 mcg) IM dose. Inject adults in the deltoid muscle. Inject children in the deltoid or vastus lateralis. Do not inject in the gluteal area or where there may be a nerve trunk. There are no published data on safety and efficacy with administration by jet injector.

Booster doses – Give a single 0.5 mL (25 mcg) dose every 2 years under conditions of repeated or continued exposure. Booster doses do not elicit higher antibody levels than primary immunization with the polysaccharide antigen.

➤*Storage/Stability:*

Oral – The oral vaccine is not stable when exposed to ambient temperatures. Ship and store between 2° and 8°C (36° to 46°F). If frozen, thaw capsules before use. Product can tolerate 48 hours at 25°C (77°F). Each package of vaccine has an expiration date. This expiration date is valid only if the product has been maintained at these temperatures.

Parenteral – Store at 2° to 8°C (36° to 46°F). Discard frozen vaccine.

Actions

➤*Pharmacology:*

Oral – Typhoid vaccine live oral Ty21a is a live attenuated vaccine for oral administration. The vaccine contains the attenuated strain *S. typhi* Ty21a. The vaccine strain is grown under controlled conditions and lyophilized. The lyophilized bacteria are filled into gelatin capsules coated with an organic solution to render them resistant to dissolution in stomach acid.

Parenteral – The Vi polysaccharide is extracted from *S. typhi* Ty2 strain. The organism is grown in a semi-synthetic medium without animal proteins. Each single dose of 0.5 mL is formulated to contain 25 mcg of purified Vi polysaccharide in a colorless isotonic phosphate buffered saline (pH 7 ± 0.3).

There are 400 to 600 cases of typhoid fever (also called *typhus abdominalis*) per year diagnosed in the United States. In 62% of these patients (statistics from 1977 to 1979), the disease was acquired outside of the United States, while in 38%, the disease was acquired within the United States. Of the cases acquired in the United States, 23% were associated with typhoid carriers, 24% were due to food outbreaks, 23% were associated with the ingestion of contaminated food or water, 6% were due to household contact with an infected person, and 4% were acquired following exposure to *S. typhi* in a laboratory setting.

Upon ingestion, virulent strains of *S. typhi* are able to pass through the stomach acid barrier, colonize the intestinal tract, penetrate the lumen, and enter the lymphatic system and blood stream, thereby causing disease.

The ability of *S. typhi* to cause disease and to induce a protective immune response is dependent upon the bacteria possessing a complete lipopolysaccharide. The *S. typhi* Ty21a vaccine strain is restricted in its ability to produce a complete lipopolysaccharide. However, a sufficient quantity of complete lipopolysaccharide is synthesized to evoke a protective immune response.

Efficacy –

Oral: Vaccination reduces disease incidence by 60% to 70%.

Parenteral: A 25 mcg dose produced a 4-fold rise in antibody titers in 88% to 96% of healthy American adults. The Vi polysaccharide vaccine reduced disease incidence by 49% to 87% in a trial among adults and children in Nepal. In a pediatric study in South Africa, blood culture-confirmed cases of typhoid fever were reduced 61%, 52%, and 50% in the first, second, and third years, respectively, after a single dose of Vi polysaccharide vaccine.

Efficacy of protective immunity seems to depend on the size of the bacterial inoculum consumed. Counsel travelers to take standard food and water precautions to avoid typhoid fever. Select appropriate antibiotics to treat active infections (eg, chloramphenicol, ampicillin). Consider cholecystectomy or ciprofloxacin therapy for chronic carriers. No evidence indicates that typhoid vaccine is useful in controlling common-source outbreaks. Typhoid vaccine will not prevent infection or disease caused by other species of *Salmonella* or other bacteria that cause enteric disease.

Onset –

Oral: Finish the fourth capsule at least 1 week before travel.

Parenteral: Protective antibody titers develop within 2 weeks after a single dose.

Duration –

Oral: Approximately 5 years.

Parenteral: Approximately 2 years.

Contraindications

Typhoid fever or a chronic typhoid carrier.

➤*Oral:* Hypersensitivity to any component of the vaccine or the capsule. Do not administer the capsules during acute febrile illness or during an acute GI illness (eg, persistent diarrhea or vomiting).

TYPHOID VACCINE

Safety of the vaccine has not been demonstrated in people deficient in their ability to mount a humoral or cell-mediated immune response because of a congenital or acquired immunodeficient state, including treatment with immunosuppressive or antimitotic drugs. Do not administer the vaccine to these people regardless of benefit.

➤*Parenteral:* Hypersensitivity to any component of the vaccine. Defer administration in the presence of acute respiratory or other active infection, or intensive physical activity (particularly when environmental temperatures are high).

Warnings

➤*Immunodeficiency:* If administered to immunosuppressed people or those receiving immunosuppressive therapy, the expected immune response may not be obtained. This includes patients with asymptomatic or symptomatic HIV infection, severe combined immunodeficiency, hypogammaglobulinemia, or agammaglobulinemia, altered immune states because of diseases such as leukemia, lymphoma, or generalized malignancy; or an immune system compromised by treatment with corticosteroids, alkylating drugs, antimetabolites, or radiation.

➤*Hypersensitivity reactions:* Allergic reactions have been reported rarely in postmarketing experience. Epinephrine injection (1:1000) must be immediately available following immunization should anaphylactic or other allergic reactions occur because of any component of the vaccine.

➤*Pregnancy: Category C.* It is not known whether typhoid vaccine can cause fetal harm when administered to pregnant women or can affect reproduction capacity. Give to a pregnant woman only if clearly needed.

➤*Lactation:* There are no data to warrant the use of the product in nursing mothers. It is not known if the vaccine is excreted in breast milk.

➤*Children:*

Oral – Safety and efficacy have not been established for the oral vaccine in children under 6 years of age and is, therefore, not recommended for use in this age group.

Parenteral – Vaccine is not recommended for children under 2 years of age because no safety or efficacy data are available for that age group.

Precautions

➤*Protection:* Not all recipients of typhoid vaccine will be fully protected against typhoid fever. Travelers should take all necessary precautions to avoid contact with or ingestion of potentially contaminated food or water sources.

➤*Latex sensitivity:* The parenteral form of this product contains dry natural latex rubber as follows: The stopper to the vial contains no rubber of any kind. In the case of the syringe, the needle cover contains dry natural latex rubber, but the plunger for the syringe contains no rubber of any kind.

➤*Infection:* Acute infection or febrile illness may be reason for delaying use of typhoid vaccine except when in the opinion of the physician, withholding the vaccine entails a greater risk.

Drug Interactions

Typhoid Vaccine Drug Interactions			
Precipitant drug	Object drug*		Description
Immunosuppressants	Typhoid vaccine	↓	Administration of typhoid vaccine to people receiving immunosuppressant drugs, including high-dose corticosteroids or radiation therapy may result in an insufficient response to immunization. They may remain susceptible despite immunization.
Proguanil	Typhoid vaccine (oral)	↓	Coadministration may decrease the immune response rate. Administer proguanil only if at least 10 days have elapsed since the final dose of the oral typhoid vaccine.

Typhoid Vaccine Drug Interactions		
Precipitant drug	Object drug*	Description
Sulfonamides Antibiotics	Typhoid vaccine (oral) ↓	Do not administer the vaccine to individuals receiving sulfonamides and antibiotics because these agents may be active against the vaccine strain and prevent a sufficient degree of multiplication to occur in order to induce a protective immune response.

* ↓ = Object drug decreased.

Adverse Reactions

Encourage parents and patients to report all adverse events occurring after vaccine administration. The health care provider should report adverse events following immunization with the vaccine to the US Department of Health and Human Services (DHHS) Vaccine Adverse Event Reporting System (VAERS). Reporting forms and information about reporting requirements or completion of the form can be obtained from VAERS through a toll-free number: (800) 822-7967.

➤*Oral:* Reported adverse reactions include the following: Nausea (5.8%), abdominal pain (6.4%), headache (4.8%), fever (3.3%), diarrhea (2.9%), vomiting (1.5%), skin rash (1%), abdominal cramps, or urticaria on the trunk or extremities. One case of nonfatal anaphylactic shock, considered to be an allergic reaction, has been reported. Only the incidence of nausea occurred at a statistically higher frequency in the vaccinated group compared with placebo.

➤*Parenteral:*

Typhoid Vaccine Adverse Reactions Occurring within 48 Hours in Adults (%)			
Adverse reaction	Trial 1 Placebo (N = 54)	Trial 1 Typhoid vaccine (parenteral) (1 lot) (N = 54)	Trial 2 Typhoid vaccine (parenteral) (2 lots combined) (N = 98)
Local			
Tenderness	13	98	96.9
Pain	7.4	40.7	26.5
Induration	0	14.8	5.1
Erythema	0	3.7	5.1
Systemic			
Malaise	14.8	24	4.1
Headache	13	20.4	16.3
Diarrhea	3.7	0	3.1
Nausea	3.7	1.9	8.2
Fever ≥ 100°F	0	1.9	0
Feverish (subjective)	0	11.1	3.1
Myalgia	0	7.4	3.1
Vomiting	0	1.9	0

Patient Information

Advise vaccine recipients to take standard food and water precautions to avoid typhoid fever. Vaccine protection can be overwhelmed by swallowing a large dose of typhoid bacteria.

➤*Oral:* It is essential that all 4 doses of vaccine be taken at the prescribed alternate day interval to obtain a maximal protective immune response.

Vaccine potency is dependent upon storage under refrigeration (2° to 8°C; 36° to 46°F). Store the vaccine under refrigeration at all times. It is essential to replace unused vaccine in the refrigerator between doses.

Swallow the vaccine capsule about 1 hour before a meal with a cold or lukewarm drink, not to exceed body temperature (37°C; 98.6°F). Do not chew the vaccine capsule; swallow as soon as possible.

MEASLES VIRUS VACCINE, LIVE, ATTENUATED

Rx **Attenuvax** (Merck)	**Powder for Injection, lyophilized:** ≥ 1000 $TCID_{50}$ (tissue culture infectious doses) per 0.5 ml dose.	Preservative free. With ≈ 25 mcg neomycin, 14.5 mg sorbitol, 1.9 mg sucrose, 14.5 mg hydrolyzed gelatin, 0.3 mg human albumin, < 1 ppm fetal bovine serum per dose. In single-dose vials with diluent and 50-dose vials with 30 ml diluent.

For information on recommended immunization schedules, refer to the Agents for Active Immunization introduction.

Indications

▶*Note:* Trivalent measles-mumps-rubella (MMR) vaccine is the preferred immunizing agent for most children and many adults.

Selective induction of active immunity against measles. Almost all children and some adults need > 1 dose of MMR.

Vaccination is recommended for susceptible individuals in high-risk groups, such as college students, health care workers, and military personnel.

All children, adolescents, and adults born after 1956 are considered susceptible and should be vaccinated if there are no contraindications.

Prior to international travel, give individuals known to be susceptible to measles, mumps, or rubella either a single-antigen vaccine or a polyvalent vaccine, as appropriate. Trivalent MMR vaccine is preferred for those likely to be susceptible to mumps and rubella. If single-antigen vaccines are not readily available, give travelers trivalent MMR regardless of their immune status to mumps or rubella.

Administration and Dosage

Federal law requires that (1) the manufacturer and lot number of this vaccine, (2) the date of its administration, and (3) the name, address, and title of the person administering the vaccine be documented in the recipient's permanent medical record or in a permanent office log. Certain adverse events must be reported to the VAERS system, 1-800-822-7967.

Trivalent MMR vaccine is the preferred product for most vaccinations.

Inject 0.5 ml of reconstituted vaccine SC into the outer aspect of the upper arm. Do not inject IV. Ensure that the injection does not enter a blood vessel. The recommended age for primary vaccination is 12 to 15 months.

Revaccination with MMR is recommended prior to elementary school entry.

▶*Recommended vaccination schedule:* Children first vaccinated when younger than 12 months of age should receive another dose between 12 to 15 months of age followed by revaccination prior to elementary school entry.

▶*Reconstitution:* Use a sterile syringe free of preservatives, antiseptics, and detergents for each injection or reconstitution, as these substances may inactivate the live virus vaccine. A 25-gauge, ⅝" needle is recommended. Use the 50-dose vial by jet injection only. When reconstituted, the solution is clear yellow.

Single-dose vial – First, withdraw the entire volume of diluent into the syringe to be used for reconstitution. Inject all the diluent in the syringe into the vial of lyophilized vaccine, and agitate to mix thoroughly. If the lyophilized vaccine cannot be dissolved, discard. Withdraw the entire contents into a syringe and inject the total volume of restored vaccine SC.

50-dose vial (available only to government agencies/institutions) – Withdraw the entire contents (30 ml) of diluent vial into the sterile syringe to be used for reconstitution and introduce into the 50-dose vial of lyophilized vaccine. Agitate to ensure thorough mixing. If the lyophilized vaccine cannot be dissolved, discard. Attach the vial to the sterilized multidose jet injector apparatus. Use 0.5 ml of the reconstituted vaccine for SC injection.

Use with other vaccines – Do not administer measles vaccine < 1 month before or after administration of other live viral vaccines unless given simultaneously.

M-M-R II has been administered concurrently with varicella virus vaccine live, and *Haemophilus* b conjugate vaccine (meningococcal protein conjugate) using separate sites and syringes. No impairment of immune response to individual tested vaccine antigens was demonstrated. The type, frequency, and severity of adverse experiences observed with M-M-R II were similar to those seen when each vaccine was given alone.

The ACIP has stated, "Although data are limited concerning the simultaneous administration of the entire recommended vaccine series (ie, DTP, OPV, MMR, Hib, and hepatitis B vaccines), data from numerous studies have indicated no interference between routinely recommended childhood vaccines (either live, attenuated, or killed). These findings support the simultaneous use of all vaccines as recommended."

▶*Storage/Stability:* Before reconstitution, store at ≤ 2° to 8°C (≤ 36° to 46°F). The diluent may be stored in the refrigerator with the lyophilized vaccine or separately at room temperature. Freezing does not harm the vaccine. Protect from light at all times; such exposure may inactivate the virus. Use only the diluent supplied and use as soon as possible after reconstitution. Store reconstituted vaccine in a dark place at 2° to 8°C. Discard if not used within 8 hours. Vaccine powder can tolerate 7 days at room temperature.

Actions

▶*Pharmacology:* Measles virus vaccine is a more attenuated line of measles virus derived from Enders' attenuated Edmonston strain grown in cell cultures of chick embryo. Attenuated measles vaccine induces a modified measles infection in susceptible patients. Fever and rash may appear. Antibodies induced by this infection protect against subsequent infection. The vaccine is highly immunogenic and generally well tolerated. A single injection induces measles hemagglutination-inhibiting antibodies in ≥ 97% of susceptible people. However, a small percentage (1% to 5%) of vaccinees may fail to seroconvert after the primary dose. Vaccine-induced antibody levels persist for ≥ 13 years without substantial decline. Neutralizing and ELISA (enzyme linked immunosorbent assay) antibodies to measles virus are still detectable in most individuals 11 to 13 years after primary vaccination.

Contraindications

Until the immune competence of the intended recipient is demonstrated, do not administer this vaccine to the following: Pregnant women; patients with a history of hypersensitivity reactions to this vaccine or any of its components (see Warnings); patients receiving immunosuppressive therapy; patients with blood dyscrasia, leukemia, lymphoma of any type, or other malignant neoplasms affecting the bone marrow or lymphatic systems; patients with primary or acquired immunodeficiency, any febrile illness or infection, or active untreated TB; patients with a family history of congenital or hereditary immunodeficiency. Do not administer this vaccine during febrile respiratory illness or other active febrile infection. However, the ACIP has recommended that all vaccines can be administered to people with minor illnesses such as diarrhea, mild upper respiratory infection with or without low-grade fever, or other low-grade febrile illness.

Do not vaccinate individuals who are immunosuppressed in association with AIDS or other clinical manifestations of infection with HIV, cellular immune deficiencies, and hypogammaglobulinemic and dysgammaglobulinemic states. Nonetheless, ACIP and AAP recommend that asymptomatic children with HIV infection be vaccinated.

Defer immunization during the course of any acute illness.

Warnings

▶*Hypersensitivity reactions:*

Hypersensitivity to eggs – Traditionally, experts recommended that patients with a history of anaphylactoid or other immediate reactions (eg, hives, swelling of the mouth or throat, difficulty breathing, hypotension, shock) following egg ingestion not be vaccinated. The recommendation had been to give patients suspected of being hypersensitive to egg protein a skin test using a dilution of the vaccine as the antigen and to avoid vaccinating those with adverse reactions to such testing.

More recent information indicates that supposedly egg-allergic patients almost always fail to react to vaccines containing eggs. This includes patients with positive oral egg challenges or egg skin tests. More anaphylaxis has been reported in patients without allergy to eggs than with it. Patients do react severely to M-M-R in extraordinarily rare cases, but egg hypersensitivity does little to predict it. Patients are also not at risk if they have egg allergies that are not anaphylactoid in nature; vaccinate these patients in the usual manner. There is no evidence to indicate that patients with allergies to chickens or feathers are at increased risk of reaction to the vaccine.

Hypersensitivity to neomycin – The AAP states, "Persons who have experienced anaphylactic reactions to topically or systemically administered neomycin should not receive measles vaccine. Most often, however, neomycin allergy manifests as a contact dermatitis, which is a delayed-type (cell-mediated) immune response rather than anaphylaxis. In such persons, an adverse reaction to neomycin in the vaccine would be an erythematous, pruritic nodule or papule, 48 to 96 hours after vaccination. A history of contact dermatitis to neomycin is not a contraindication to receiving measles vaccine."

▶*Elderly:* Most people born in 1956 or earlier are likely to have been infected naturally and generally are considered not susceptible.

▶*Pregnancy: Category C.* It is not known whether the drug can cause fetal harm or can affect reproduction capacity. Therefore, do not give to pregnant women. Avoid pregnancy for 3 months following vaccination.

Contracting natural measles during pregnancy enhances fetal risk. Increased rates of spontaneous abortion, stillbirth, congenital defects, and prematurity have occurred. There are no adequate studies of measles virus vaccine in pregnancy. However, it is assumed that the vaccine strain of virus is also capable of inducing adverse fetal effects for up to 3 months following vaccination.

▶*Lactation:* It is not known whether measles vaccine virus is secreted in breast milk. Exercise caution when administering to a nursing woman.

MEASLES VIRUS VACCINE, LIVE, ATTENUATED

➤*Children:* Attenuated measles vaccine is safe and effective in people ≥ 12 months of age. Younger people may fail to respond due to circulating residual measles antibodies passively transferred from the child's mother. Revaccinate infants vaccinated when < 12 months of age after they reach 15 months of age. There is evidence to suggest that infants immunized when < 1 year old may not develop sustained antibody levels when later reimmunized. Weigh the advantage of early protection against the chance for failure to respond adequately on reimmunization. Trivalent MMR vaccine is the preferred agent for children and many adults.

Children and young adults known to be infected with human immunodeficiency viruses and are not immunosuppressed may be vaccinated. However, monitor closely for vaccine-preventable diseases because immunization may be less effective than for uninfected people.

Precautions

➤*Tuberculosis:* Children under treatment for tuberculosis have not experienced exacerbation of the disease when immunized with measles vaccine.

➤*Cerebral injury/convulsions:* Use caution when administering measles vaccine to people with a history of cerebral injury, individual or family histories of convulsions, or any other conditions in which stress due to fever should be avoided. The physician should be alert to the temperature elevation that may occur following vaccination.

➤*Thrombocytopenia:* Individuals with current thrombocytopenia may develop more severe thrombocytopenia following vaccination. In addition, individuals who experienced thrombocytopenia with the first dose of M-M-R II (or its component vaccines) may develop thrombocytopenia with repeat doses. Serologic status may be evaluated to determine whether or not additional doses of vaccine are needed. Evaluate the risk-to-benefit ratio.

➤*Immunosuppressive therapy:* The immune status of patients about to undergo immunosuppressive therapy should be evaluated. The ACIP has stated that "patients with leukemia in remission who have not received chemotherapy for ≥ 3 months may receive live virus vaccines. Short-term (< 2 weeks), low-to-moderate-dose systemic corticosteroid therapy, topical steroid therapy (eg, nasal, skin), long-term alternate-day treatment with low to moderate doses of short-acting systemic steroid, and intra-articular, bursal, or tendon injection of corticosteroids) are not immunosuppressive in their usual doses and do not contraindicate the administration of measles vaccine."

Drug Interactions

Measles Virus Vaccine Drug Interactions			
Precipitant drug	Object drug*		Description
Immunosuppressants	Measles vaccine	↓	Administration of measles vaccine to patients receiving immunosuppressants, including corticosteroids or radiation therapy, may result in insufficient response to immunization. They may remain susceptible despite immunization.
Immune globulins	Measles vaccine	↓	To avoid inactivation of the attenuated virus, administer the vaccine at least 14 to 30 days before or 6 to 8 weeks after the immune globulin. Alternately, check antibody titers or repeat the vaccine dose 3 months after immune globulin administration. Base the interval on the dose of IgG administered: 3 months for 3 to 10 mg/kg, 4 months for 20 mg/kg, 5 months for 40 mg/kg, 6 months for 60 to 100 mg/kg, 7 months for 160 mg/kg, 8 months for 300 to 400 mg/kg, 10 months for 1 g/kg, 11 months for 2 g/kg.
Interferon	Measles vaccine	↓	Concurrent use may inhibit antibody response to the vaccine.
Vitamin A	Measles vaccine	↓	Simultaneous administration of large doses of vitamin A impaired the response to Schwarz-strain measles vaccine in a group of Indonesian infants at 6 months of age.

Measles Virus Vaccine Drug Interactions			
Precipitant drug	Object drug*		Description
Measles vaccine	Meningococcal vaccine	↓	Reduced seroconversion rate to meningococci may occur with concurrent immunization. If possible, separate these 2 vaccinations by ≥ 1 month.
Measles vaccine	Tuberculin skin test	↓	Measles vaccine may temporarily depress tuberculin skin sensitivity. Administer the test before or simultaneously with the vaccine.
Measles vaccine	Virus vaccines, other	↓	To avoid the hypothetical concern over antigenic competition, give measles vaccine ≥ 1 month before or after other virus vaccines. However, several vaccines may be given simultaneously at separate injection sites (eg, DTP, OPV or e-IPV, MMR, Hib, hepatitis B, varicella, influenza).

* ↓ = Object drug decreased.

➤*Drug/Lab test interactions:* Methacholine inhalation challenge may be falsely positive for a few days after influenza, measles, or other immunization. This effect appears to mimic the bronchospastic effect associated with acute respiratory infections. The effect has been observed in 44% to 90% of asthmatic patients but apparently not among healthy subjects.

Live virus vaccines may cause delayed-hypersensitivity skin tests (eg, tuberculin, histoplasmin) to appear falsely negative. Evaluate such tests carefully. The effect may persist for several weeks after vaccination. ACIP and AAP recommend that tuberculin tests be given prior to live-virus vaccination, simultaneously or ≥ 6 weeks after vaccination.

Adverse Reactions

➤*Cardiovascular:* Syncope, vasculitis.

➤*CNS:* Encephalitis; encephalopathy; measles inclusion body encephalitis (MIBE); subacute sclerosing panencephalitis (SSPE); Buillain-Barre Syndrome (GBS); febrile convulsions; afebrile convulsions or seizures; ataxia; ocular palsies; headache, dizziness; malaise; irritability.

Significant CNS reactions (eg, encephalitis, encephalopathy) occurring within 30 days after vaccination have been temporally associated with measles vaccine very rarely. In no case has it been shown that reactions were actually caused by vaccine. The risk following measles vaccine administration remains far less than that for encephalitis and encephalopathy with natural measles (1 per 2000 reported cases).

Subacute sclerosing panencephalitis (SSPE) has occurred in children who did not have a history of natural measles but received measles vaccine. The association of SSPE cases to measles vaccination is about one case per million doses, far less than that associated with natural measles, 6 to 22 cases per million.

➤*Dermatologic:* Stevens-Johnson syndrome; erythema multiforme; urticaria; rash. Local reactions have occurred, including burning/stinging at injection site; wheal and flare; redness (erythema); swelling; vesiculation at injection site.

➤*Hematologic:* Thrombocytopenia; purpura; lymphadenopathy; leukocytosis.

➤*Hypersensitivity:* Anaphylaxis and anaphylactoid reactions have occurred, as well as related phenomena (eg, angioneurotic edema [including peripheral or facial edema] and bronchial spasm).

➤*Respiratory:* Pneumonitis; cough; rhinitis.

➤*Special senses:* Nerve deafness; otitis media; retinitis; optic neuritis; papillitis; retrobulbar neuritis; conjunctivitis.

➤*Miscellaneous:* Diarrhea; panniculitis; atypical measles; fever. Death from various, and in some cases unknown, causes has been reported rarely following vaccination with measles, mumps, and rubella vaccines; however, a causal relationship has not been established.

RUBELLA VIRUS VACCINE, LIVE

Rx	**Meruvax** II (Merck)	**Powder for Injection**: ≥1000 TCID$_{50}$ (tissue culture infectious doses) of rubella per 0.5 ml dose.	With 25 mcg neomycin. In single dose vials.

For information on recommended immunization schedules, refer to the Agents for Active Immunization introduction.

> ## WARNING
>
> Trivalent measles-mumps-rubella (MMR) vaccine is the preferred immunizing agent for most children and many adults.

Indications

Selective active immunization against rubella. The national rubella immunization program is intended to reduce the occurrence of congenital rubella syndrome (CRS) among offspring of women who contract rubella during pregnancy.

➤*Children:* Vaccination is routinely recommended for individuals from 12 months of age to puberty. Give previously unimmunized children of susceptible pregnant women attenuated rubella (or preferably MMR) vaccine, since an immunized child is less likely to acquire natural rubella and introduce it into the household.

➤*Adolescent or adult males:* Vaccination is a useful procedure in preventing or controlling outbreaks of rubella in circumscribed populations.

➤*Nonpregnant adolescent and adult females:* Immunization of susceptible nonpregnant adolescent and adult females of childbearing potential is indicated, if precautions to avoid pregnancy are observed. When vaccinating postpubertal females, counsel these women to avoid pregnancy for 3 months following vaccination. Vaccinating susceptible postpubertal females confers individual protection against subsequently acquiring rubella infection during pregnancy, which in turn prevents infection of the fetus and CRS. It may be convenient to vaccinate rubella-susceptible women in the immediate postpartum period.

➤*International travel:* Prior to international travel, give individuals known to be susceptible to measles, mumps or rubella either a single-antigen vaccine or a polyvalent vaccine, as appropriate. Trivalent MMR vaccine is preferred for people likely to be susceptible to mumps and rubella. Almost all children and some adults need > 1 dose of MMR vaccine. If single-antigen vaccines are not readily available, give travelers trivalent MMR regardless of their immune status to mumps or rubella.

➤*Unlabeled uses:* Intranasal administration may boost antibody titers, although this route is not confirmed as safe and effective by the FDA and is not commonly employed.

Administration and Dosage

Federal law requires that (1) the manufacturer and lot number of this vaccine, (2) the date of its administration, and (3) the name, address and title of the person administering the vaccine be documented in the recipient's permanent medical record or in a permanent office log. Certain adverse events must be reported to the VAERS system, 1-800-822-7967.

Inject total volume of reconstituted vaccine SC, into the outer aspect of the upper arm. Do not inject IV or administer intranasally.

➤*Storage/Stability:* Prior to and after reconstitution, store at 2° to 8°C (36° to 46°F) and protect from light. To reconstitute, use only the diluent supplied. Use as soon as possible after reconstitution. Discard reconstituted vaccine if not used within 8 hours.

Ship vaccine at ≤ 10°C (50°F); it may be shipped on dry ice.

Actions

➤*Pharmacology:* Attenuated rubella vaccine induces a modified, noncommunicable rubella infection in susceptible people. RA 27/3 strain elicits higher immediate postvaccination hemagglutination-inhibiting (HI), complement-fixing and neutralizing antibody levels than other strains of rubella vaccine and induces a broader profile of circulating antibodies, including anti-theta and anti-iota precipitating antibodies. RA 27/3 strain immunologically simulates natural infection more closely than other rubella virus strains. The increased levels and broader profile of antibodies produced by RA 27/3 strain appear to correlate with greater resistance to subclinical reinfection by the wild virus.

Onset of rubella vaccine is 2 to 6 weeks. It induces HI antibodies in at least 97% of susceptible children. Seroconversion is somewhat less in adults. Disease incidence is typically reduced by 95% in family and classroom cohorts. Antibody levels persist ≥ 10 years in most recipients. Specific rubella HI antibody titer of ≥ 1:8 is considered immune.

Contraindications

Pregnancy (see Warnings); history of a hypersensitivity reaction to this vaccine or any of its components; patients receiving immunosuppressive therapy; blood dyscrasia, leukemia, lymphoma of any type, or other malignant neoplasms affecting the bone marrow or lymphatic systems; primary or acquired immunodeficiency; active untreated tuberculosis; family history of congenital or hereditary immunodeficiency, until the immune competence of the potential vaccine recipient is demonstrated.

Do not vaccinate individuals who are immunosuppressed in association with AIDS or other clinical manifestations of infection with HIV, cellular immune deficiencies, and hypogammaglobulinemic and dysgammaglobulinemic states. Nonetheless, vaccinate asymptomatic children with HIV infection.

Defer immunization during the course of any acute illness.

Warnings

➤*Immunodeficiency:* Do not use in immunodeficient people, including those with congenital or acquired immune deficiencies, whether due to genetics, disease, or drug or radiation therapy. Contains live viruses. Nonetheless, routine immunization of symptomatic and asymptomatic HIV-infected individuals with MMR is recommended.

➤*Hypersensitivity reactions:* Have epinephrine 1:1000 available to control immediate allergic reactions. See also Management of Acute Hypersensitivity Reactions.

➤*Elderly:* Most people born in 1956 or earlier are likely to have been infected naturally and generally are considered not susceptible.

➤*Pregnancy: Category C.* Natural rubella infection of the fetus may result in congenital rubella syndrome. There is evidence suggesting transmission of attenuated rubella virus to the fetus, although the vaccine is not known to cause fetal harm when administered to pregnant women. Nonetheless, do not intentionally give attenuated rubella vaccine to pregnant females. If postpubertal females are vaccinated, counsel these women to avoid pregnancy for 3 months following vaccination. It may be convenient to vaccinate rubella-susceptible women in the immediate postpartum period.

In counseling women who are inadvertently vaccinated when pregnant or who become pregnant within 3 months of vaccination, the following information may be useful. In a 10 year survey of > 700 pregnant women who received rubella vaccine within 3 months before or after conception (of whom 189 received the current RA 27/3 strain), none of the newborns had abnormalities compatible with congenital rubella syndrome.

Generally, most IgG passage across the placenta occurs during third trimester.

➤*Lactation:* Vaccine-strain virus is secreted in breast milk and may be transmitted to infants in this manner. In the infants with serologic evidence of rubella infection, none exhibited severe disease. However, one exhibited mild clinical illness typical of acquired rubella.

➤*Children:* Safe and effective for children ≥ 12 months of age. Vaccination is not recommended for children < 12 months of age, since remaining maternal rubella neutralizing antibody may interfere with the immune response. Trivalent MMR vaccine is the preferred agent for children and many adults.

Drug Interactions

Rubella Virus Vaccine Drug Interactions			
Precipitant drug	Object drug*		Description
Immunosuppressants	Rubella vaccine	↓	Administration of rubella vaccine to patients receiving immunosuppressants, including corticosteroids or radiation therapy, may result in insufficient response to immunization. They may remain susceptible despite immunization.
Immune globulins	Rubella vaccine	↓	To avoid inactivation of the attenuated virus, administer the vaccine at least 14 to 30 days before or 6 to 8 weeks after the immune globulin. Alternately, check antibody titers or repeat the vaccine dose 3 months after IgG.
Interferon	Rubella vaccine	↓	Concurrent use may inhibit antibody response to the vaccine.
Rubella vaccine	Meningococcal vaccine	↓	Reduced seroconversion rate to meningococci may occur with concurrent immunization.
Rubella vaccine	Virus vaccines, other	↓	To avoid the hypothetical concern over antigenic competition, give rubella vaccine after or ≥ 1 month before other virus vaccines. However, several vaccines may be given simultaneously at separate injection sites (eg, DTP, OPV, MMR, Hib, hepatitis B).

* ↓ = Object drug decreased.

Adverse Reactions

Reactions are usually mild and transient. Because the vaccine is slightly acidic, patients may experience burning or stinging of short

RUBELLA VIRUS VACCINE, LIVE

duration at the injection site. Symptoms similar to those seen following natural rubella may occur and include: Regional lymphadenopathy; urticaria; rash; malaise; sore throat; fever; headache; polyneuritis; temporary arthralgia (infrequently associated with inflammation). Local pain, induration and erythema may occur at the injection site. Moderate fever (38° to 39.4°C; 101° to 102.9°F) occurs occasionally, high fever (> 39.4°C or 103°F) less commonly.

Encephalitis and other CNS reactions, erythema multiforme, optic neuritis and polyneuropathy (including Guillain-Barre syndrome) may occur. Because of decreases in platelet counts, thrombocytopenic purpura is a theoretical hazard.

➤*Musculoskeletal:* Chronic arthritis has been associated with natural rubella infection. Only rarely have vaccine recipients developed chronic joint symptoms. Following vaccination in children, reactions in joints are uncommon (≤ 3%) and generally of brief duration. In adult women, incidence rates for arthritis and arthralgia are generally higher (12% to 20%) and the reactions tend to be more marked and of longer duration. Symptoms may persist for months or, on rare occasions, for years. In adolescent girls, the reactions appear to be intermediate in incidence between those seen in children and in adult women. Even in older women (35 to 45 years of age), these reactions are generally well tolerated and rarely interfere with normal activities. Myalgia and paresthesia have been reported rarely. Advise postpubertal females of the frequent occurrence of generally self-limited arthralgia or arthritis beginning 2 to 4 weeks after vaccination.

MUMPS VIRUS VACCINE, LIVE

Rx	**Mumpsvax** (Merck)	**Powder for Injection:** ≥ 20,000 TCID$_{50}$ (tissue culture infectious doses) per 0.5 ml dose.	25 mcg neomycin. In single-dose vials with vials of diluent.

For information on recommended immunization schedules, refer to the Agents for Active Immunization introduction.

> ### WARNING
> Trivalent measles-mumps-rubella (MMR) vaccine is the preferred immunizing agent for most children and many adults.

Indications

Selective active immunization against mumps. Prior to international travel, give individuals known to be susceptible to measles, mumps or rubella either a single-antigen vaccine or a polyvalent vaccine, as appropriate. Trivalent MMR vaccine is preferred for people likely to be susceptible to mumps and rubella.

Almost all children and some adults need > 1 dose of MMR vaccine. If single-antigen vaccines are not readily available, give travelers trivalent MMR regardless of their immune status to mumps or rubella.

Administration and Dosage

Federal law requires that (1) the manufacturer and lot number of this vaccine, (2) the date of its administration, and (3) the name, address and title of the person administering the vaccine be documented in the recipient's permanent medical record or in a permanent office log. Certain adverse events must be reported to the VAERS system, 1-800-822-7967.

➤*Vaccination:* 0.5 ml, for children at 15 months of age and adults. Trivalent MMR vaccine is the preferred product for most vaccinations. Inject total volume of reconstituted vaccine SC, into the outer aspect of the upper arm. Do not inject IV. Use a sterile syringe free of preservatives, antiseptics and detergents. A 25-gauge ⅝-inch needle is recommended.

➤*Booster dose:* If concern exists about mumps immune status, consider revaccination with appropriate monovalent or polyvalent vaccines. Routine MMR is recommended by ACIP as children enter kindergarten or first grade. AAP recommends a routine second vaccination as children enter middle or junior high school.

➤*Storage/Stability:* Prior to and after reconstitution, store at 2° to 8°C (36° to 46°F). Powder can tolerate 5 days room temperature. Protect from light. Reconstitute only with diluent supplied and use as soon as possible. Discard within 8 hours.

Actions

➤*Pharmacology:* Prepared from the Jeryl Lynn (B level) strain grown in cell cultures of chick embryo. Attenuated mumps vaccine produces a modified, noncommunicable mumps infection in susceptible persons. Antibodies induced by this infection protect against subsequent infection. A single dose induced an effective antibody response in ≈ 97% of susceptible children and 93% of susceptible adults.

Mumps vaccine reduced disease incidence 95% in family and classroom cohorts for at least 20 months. Onset occurs in 2 to 3 weeks. Antibody levels persist ≥ 15 years in most recipients, with a rate of decline comparable to natural infection.

The vaccine will not offer protection when given after exposure to natural mumps.

Contraindications

Pregnancy (see Warnings); history of a hypersensitivity reaction to this vaccine or any of its components (eg, eggs); concomitant immunosuppressive therapy; patients with a blood dyscrasia, leukemia, lymphoma of any type, or other malignant neoplasms affecting the bone marrow or lymphatic systems; primary or acquired immunodeficiency; active untreated tuberculosis; family history of congenital or hereditary immunodeficiency, until the immune competence of the potential vaccine recipient is demonstrated.

Do not vaccinate people who are immunosuppressed in association with AIDS or other clinical manifestations of infection with HIV, cellular

immune deficiencies, and hypogammaglobulinemic and dysgammaglobulinemic states. Nonetheless, vaccinate asymptomatic children with HIV infection.

Do not vaccinate people with a history of anaphylactoid or other immediate reactions (eg, hives, swelling of the mouth and throat, difficulty breathing, hypotension, shock) subsequent to egg ingestion since the vaccine is propagated in cell cultures of chick embryo. Skin-test individuals suspected of being hypersensitive to egg protein, using a dilution of the vaccine as the antigen. Do not vaccinate persons with adverse reactions to such testing. People are apparently not at risk if they have egg allergies that are not anaphylactoid in nature; vaccinate such persons in the usual manner. There is no evidence that people with allergies to chickens or feathers are at increased risk of reaction to the vaccine. Defer immunization during the course of any acute illness.

Warnings

➤*Allergy skin testing:* Do not use for delayed hypersensitivity (anergy) skin testing. Use mumps skin test antigen, a killed viral product (see individual monograph).

➤*Hypersensitivity reactions:* Have epinephrine 1:1000 available to control immediate allergic reactions. See also Management of Acute Hypersensitivity Reactions.

Immunodeficiency – Do not use in immunodeficient people, including those with congenital or acquired immune deficiencies, whether due to genetics, disease, or drug or radiation therapy. Contains live viruses. Nonetheless, routine immunization of symptomatic and asymptomatic HIV-infected people with MMR is recommended.

➤*Elderly:* People born prior to 1957 are generally considered immune and need not be vaccinated.

➤*Pregnancy: Category C.* Although mumps virus can infect the placenta and fetus, there is no good evidence that it causes congenital malformations in humans. Attenuated mumps vaccine virus can infect the placenta, but virus has not been isolated from fetal tissues of susceptible women who were vaccinated and underwent elective abortions. Nonetheless, do not intentionally give attenuated mumps vaccine to pregnant females. If postpubertal females are vaccinated, counsel these women to avoid pregnancy for 3 months following vaccination. Generally most IgG passage across the placenta occurs during the third trimester.

➤*Lactation:* It is not known if attenuated mumps virus or corresponding antibodies are excreted in breast milk.

➤*Children:* Mumps vaccine is safe and effective for children ≥ 12 months of age. Vaccination is not recommended for children < 12 months of age since remaining maternal virus neutralizing antibody may interfere with the immune response. Trivalent MMR vaccine is the preferred agent for children and many adults.

Drug Interactions

Mumps Virus Vaccine Drug Interactions		
Precipitant drug	Object drug*	Description
Immunosuppressants	Mumps vaccine ↓	Administration of mumps vaccine to patients receiving immunosuppressants, including corticosteroids or radiation therapy, may result in insufficient response to immunization. They may remain susceptible despite immunization.
Immune globulins	Mumps vaccine ↓	To avoid inactivating attenuated virus, give the vaccine at least 14 to 30 days before or 6 to 8 weeks after immune globulin. Alternately, check antibody titers or repeat the vaccine 3 months after IgG.
Interferon	Mumps vaccine ↓	Concurrent use may inhibit antibody response to the vaccine.

MUMPS VIRUS VACCINE, LIVE

Mumps Virus Vaccine Drug Interactions			
Precipitant drug	Object drug*		Description
Mumps vaccine	Virus vaccines, other	↓	To avoid the hypothetical concern over antigenic competition, give mumps vaccine after or ≥ 1 month before other virus vaccines. However, several vaccines may be given simultaneously at separate injection sites (eg, DTP, OPV, MMR, Hib, hepatitis B).

* ↓ = Object drug decreased.

➤*Drug/Lab test interactions:* Live virus vaccines may cause delayed-hypersensitivity skin tests (eg, tuberculin, histoplasmin) to appear falsely negative. Evaluate such tests knowingly. The effect may persist for several weeks after vaccination. ACIP and AAP recommend that tuberculin tests be given prior to live-virus vaccination, simultaneously, or ≥ 6 weeks after vaccination.

Adverse Reactions

Burning or stinging of short duration at the injection site have occurred. Occasional reactions include mild fever, mild lymphadenopathy or diarrhea. Fever > 39.4°C (> 103°F) is uncommon. Rarely, parotitis and orchitis may occur. In most of these cases, prior exposure to natural mumps was established. Infrequently, optic neuritis may follow vaccination. Allergic reactions at the injection site or erythema multiforme occurred rarely. Very rarely, encephalitis, febrile seizures, nerve deafness and other nervous system reactions have occurred.

RUBELLA AND MUMPS VIRUS VACCINE, LIVE

Rx	**Biavax** II (Merck)	**Powder for Injection:** Mixture of 2 viruses: ≥ 20,000 mumps TCID$_{50}$ (tissue culture infectious doses) and ≥ 1000 rubella TCID$_{50}$ per 0.5 ml dose	25 mcg neomycin. In single-dose vials with diluent.

For information on recommended immunization schedules, refer to the Agents for Active Immunization introduction. Consider the prescribing information for rubella virus vaccine and for mumps virus vaccine when using this product (see individual monographs).

Indications

➤*Children (≥ 12 months of age):* Simultaneous immunization against rubella and mumps.

➤*Infants (< 12 months of age):* Not recommended. Infants may retain maternal rubella and mumps neutralizing antibodies which may interfere with the immune response.

➤*Revaccination:* If concern exists about immune status, consider revaccination with appropriate monovalent or polyvalent vaccines. Routine revaccination with trivalent MMR vaccine is recommended by ACIP as children enter into kindergarten or first grade. AAP recommends a routine second vaccination as children enter into middle school or junior high school. Unnecessary doses of a vaccine are best avoided by ensuring that written documentation of vaccination is preserved and a copy given to each vaccinee or the vaccinee's agent.

Administration and Dosage

➤*Vaccination:* 0.5 ml for children (preferably at 15 months of age) and adults. Trivalent MMR vaccine is the preferred product for most vaccinations. Inject the total volume of reconstituted vaccine SC, preferably into the outer aspect of the upper arm, with a 25-gauge ⅝"-inch needle. Do not inject IV.

➤*Storage/Stability:* Prior to and after reconstitution, store at 2° to 8°C (36° to 46°F) and protect from light. To reconstitute, use only the diluent supplied. Use as soon as possible after reconstitution. Discard within 8 hours.

MEASLES, MUMPS AND RUBELLA VIRUS VACCINE, LIVE

Rx	**M-M-R** II (Merck)	**Powder for injection:** Mixture of 3 viruses: ≥ 1000 measles TCID$_{50}$ (tissue culture infectious doses), ≥ 20,000 mumps TCID$_{50}$ and ≥ 1000 rubella TCID$_{50}$ per 0.5 ml dose.	With 25 mcg neomycin. In single dose vials with diluent.

For information on recommended immunization schedules, refer to the Agents for Active Immunization introduction. Consider the prescribing information for measles (rubeola) virus vaccine, mumps virus vaccine and rubella virus vaccine when using this product (see individual monographs).

Indications

➤*Children (≥ 15 months of age) or adults:* Simultaneous immunization against measles, mumps and rubella.

➤*Infants (< 15 months of age):* May fail to respond to one or all three components of the vaccine due to presence in the circulation of residual measles, mumps or rubella antibody of maternal origin; the younger the infant, the lower the likelihood of seroconversion.

In geographically isolated or other relatively inaccessible populations for whom immunization programs are logistically difficult, and in population groups in which natural measles infection may occur in a significant proportion of infants before 15 months of age, it may be desirable to give the vaccine to infants at an earlier age. Weigh the advantage of early protection against the chance for failure of response; revaccinate these infants after they reach 15 months of age.

➤*Revaccination:* Almost all children and some adults should receive a booster dose of MMR vaccine, in addition to a primary dose given after the age of 12 months. Routine revaccination with trivalent MMR vaccine is recommended by the Advisory Committee on Immunization Practices as children enter into kindergarten or first grade, since this procedure is easier to implement in public health clinics. The American Academy of Pediatrics recommends a routine second vaccination as children enter into middle school or junior high school, a procedure that has epidemiologic advantages.

If concern also exists about immune status to mumps or rubella, consider revaccination with appropriate monovalent or polyvalent vaccines.

Administration and Dosage

➤*Vaccination:* 0.5 ml for children (preferably at 15 months of age) and adults. Inject the total volume of reconstituted vaccine SC into the outer aspect of the upper arm with a 25-gauge ⅝-inch needle. Do not inject IV.

➤*Storage/Stability:* Prior to and after reconstitution, store at 2° to 8°C (36° to 46°F) and protect from light. To reconstitute, use only the diluent supplied. Use as soon as possible after reconstitution. Discard within 8 hours.

POLIOVIRUS VACCINE, INACTIVATED (IPV)

Rx	**IPOL** (Connaught)	**Injection:** Suspension of 3 types of poliovirus (Types 1, 2 and 3) grown in monkey kidney cell cultures	In 0.5 ml single-dose syringe with integrated needle.[1]

[1] Each dose contains 0.5% 2-phenoxyethanol, a maximum of 0.02% formaldehyde and not more than 200 ng streptomycin, 25 ng polymyxin B and 5 ng neomycin.

For additional information, refer to the Agents for Active Immunization introduction.

Indications

For active immunization of infants, children and adults for preventing poliomyelitis. Recommendations on the use of live and inactivated poliovirus vaccines are described in the ACIP (Advisory Committee on Immunization Practices) Recommendations and the 1988 American Academy of Pediatrics Red Book.

➤*Infants, children and adolescents:*

General recommendations – It is recommended that all infants, unimmunized children and adolescents not previously immunized be vaccinated routinely against paralytic poliomyelitis. Inactivated poliovirus vaccine (IPV) should be offered to individuals who have refused poliovirus vaccine live oral trivalent (OPV) or in whom OPV is contraindicated. Adequately inform parents of the risks and benefits of both inactivated and oral polio vaccines so that they can make an informed choice.

OPV should not be used in households with immunodeficient individuals because OPV is excreted in the stool by healthy vaccinees and can infect an immunocompromised household member, which may result in paralytic disease. In a household with an immunocompromised member, use only IPV for all those requiring poliovirus immunization.

Children incompletely immunized – Children of all ages should have their immunization status reviewed and be considered for supplemental immunization as follows for adults. Time intervals between doses longer than those recommended for routine primary immunization do not necessitate additional doses as long as a final total of four doses is reached (see Administration and Dosage).

Previous clinical poliomyelitis (usually due to only a single poliovirus type) or incomplete immunization with OPV are not contraindications to completing the primary series of immunization with IPV.

➤*Adults:*

General recommendations – Routine primary poliovirus vaccination of adults (generally those ≥ 18 years of age) residing in the US is not recommended. Adults who have increased risk of exposure to either vaccine or wild poliovirus and have not been adequately immunized should receive polio vaccination in accordance with the schedule given in the Administration and Dosage section.

POLIOVIRUS VACCINE, INACTIVATED (IPV)

The following categories of adults run an increased risk of exposure to wild polioviruses:

1.) Travelers to regions or countries where poliomyelitis is endemic or epidemic.
2.) Health care workers in close contact with patients who may be excreting polioviruses.
3.) Laboratory workers handling specimens that may contain polioviruses.
4.) Members of communities or specific population groups with disease caused by wild polioviruses.
5.) Incompletely vaccinated or unvaccinated adults in a household with (or other close contacts of) children given OPV provided that immunization of the child can be assured and not unduly delayed. Inform adults of the small OPV related risk to the contact.

➤*Immunodeficiency and altered immune status:* Patients with recognized immunodeficiency are at a greater risk of developing paralysis when exposed to live poliovirus than those with a normal immune system. Under no circumstances should OPV be used in such patients or introduced into a household where such a patient resides.

Use IPV in all patients with immunodeficiency diseases and members of such patients' households when vaccination of such persons is indicated. This includes patients with asymptomatic HIV infection, AIDS or AIDS-related complex, severe combined immunodeficiency, hypogammaglobulinemia or aggammaglobulinemia; altered immune states due to diseases such as leukemia, lymphoma or generalized malignancy; or an immune system compromised by treatment with corticosteroids, alkylating drugs, antimetabolites or radiation. Patients with an altered immune state may develop a protective response against paralytic poliomyelitis after IPV administration.

Administration and Dosage

Administer SC; do not administer IV. In infants and small children, the mid-lateral aspect of the thigh is the preferred site. In adults, administer the vaccine in the deltoid area.

Take care to avoid administering the injection into or near blood vessels and nerves. After aspiration, if blood or any suspicious discoloration appears in the syringe, do not inject; discard contents and repeat procedures using a new dose of vaccine administered at a different site.

➤*Children:*

Primary immunization – A primary series of IPV consists of three 0.5 ml doses administered SC. The interval between the first two doses should be at least 4 weeks, but preferably 8 weeks. The first two doses are usually administered with DTP immunization and are given at 2 and 4 months of age. The third dose should follow at least 6 months but preferably 12 months after the second dose. It may be desirable to administer this dose with MMR and other vaccines, but at a different site, in children 15 to 18 months of age. Give all children who received a primary series of IPV, or a combination of IPV and OPV, a booster dose of OPV or IPV before entering school, unless the first dose of the primary series was administered on or after the fourth birthday. The need to routinely administer additional doses is unknown at this time.

A final total of four doses is necessary to complete a series of primary and booster doses. Children and adolescents with a previously incomplete series of IPV should receive sufficient additional doses to reach this number.

➤*Adults:*

Unvaccinated adults – For unvaccinated adults at increased risk of exposure to poliovirus, a primary series of IPV is recommended. While the responses of adults to primary series have not been studied, the recommended schedule for adults is two doses given at a 1- to 2-month interval and a third dose given 6 to 12 months later. If < 3 months but > 2 months are available before protection is needed, give 3 doses at least 1 month apart. Likewise, if only 1 or 2 months are available, give 2 doses of IPV at least 1 month apart. If < 1 month is available, a single dose of either OPV or IPV is recommended.

Incompletely vaccinated adults – Adults who are at an increased risk of exposure to poliovirus and who have had at least one dose of OPV, < 3 doses of conventional IPV or a combination of conventional IPV or OPV totalling < 3 doses should receive at least 1 dose of OPV or IPV. Give additional doses to complete a primary series if time permits.

Completely vaccinated adults – Adults who are at an increased risk of exposure to poliovirus and who have previously completed a primary series with one or a combination of polio vaccines can be given a dose of either OPV or IPV.

➤*Storage/Stability:* The vaccine is stable if stored in the refrigerator between 2° and 8°C (35° and 46°F). The vaccine must not be frozen.

Actions

➤*Pharmacology:* Poliovirus vaccine, inactivated (IPV) is a sterile suspension of three types of poliovirus: Type 1 (Mahoney), Type 2 (MEF-1), and Type 3 (Saukett). The viruses are grown in cultures of VERO cells, a continuous line of monkey kidney cells (IPOL) or in human diploid cell cultures (*Poliovax*), both by the microcarrier technique. This culture tech-

nique and improvements in purification, concentration and standardization of poliovirus antigen have resulted in a more potent and more consistently immunogenic vaccine than the poliovirus vaccine inactivated which was available in the US prior to 1988. These new methods allow for the production of vaccine that induces antibody responses in most children after administering fewer doses than with vaccine available prior to 1988. Studies in developed and developing countries with similar inactivated poliovirus vaccine produced by the same technology have shown that a direct relationship exists between the antigenic content of the vaccine, the frequency of seroconversion, and resulting antibody titer. Since the *Poliovax* vaccine will be available mainly as a backup to *IPOL*, this monograph will refer to prescribing information for *IPOL*; however, the prescribing information for *Poliovax* closely follows that of *IPOL*.

➤*Clinical trials:* Of 120 infants who received two doses of IPV at 2 and 4 months of age, detectable serum neutralizing antibody was induced after two doses of vaccine in 98.3% (Type 1), 100% (Type 2) and 97.5% (Type 3) of the children. In 83 children receiving three doses at 2, 4 and 12 months of age, detectable serum neutralizing antibodies were detected in 97.6% (Type 1) and 100% (Types 2 and 3) of the children. Paralytic polio has not been reported in association with administration of IPV.

Contraindications

Hypersensitivity to any component of the vaccine, including neomycin, streptomycin and polymyxin B (see Warnings).

Defer vaccination of people with any acute, febrile illness until after recovery; however, minor illnesses such as mild upper respiratory infection, are not in themselves reasons for postponing vaccine administration.

Warnings

➤*Hypersensitivity reactions:* Neomycin, streptomycin, and polymyxin B are used in producing this vaccine. Although purification procedures eliminate measurable amounts of these substances, traces may be present and allergic reactions may occur in people sensitive to these substances. If anaphylaxis or anaphylactic shock occurs within 24 hours of administration of a dose, no further doses should be given. Epinephrine HCl (1:1000) and other appropriate agents should be available to control immediate allergic reactions. Refer to Management of Acute Hypersensitivity Reactions.

➤*Pregnancy: Category C.* It is not known whether IPV can cause fetal harm when administered to a pregnant woman or can affect reproduction capacity. Give to a pregnant woman only if clearly needed.

➤*Children:* Safety and efficacy of IPV have been shown in children > 6 weeks of age (see Administration and Dosage).

Precautions

➤*Patient review:* Before injection of the vaccine, the physician should carefully review the recommendations for product use and the patient's medical history including possible hypersensitivities and side effects that may have occurred following previous doses of the vaccine.

➤*HIV infection:* Concerns have been raised that stimulation of the immune system of a patient with HIV infection by immunization with inactivated vaccines might cause deterioration in immunologic function. However, such effects have not been noted thus far among children with AIDS or among immunosuppressed individuals after immunizations with inactivated vaccines. The potential benefits of immunization of these children outweigh the undocumented risk of such adverse events.

Adverse Reactions

In earlier studies with the vaccine grown in primary monkey kidney cells, transient local reactions at the site of injection have been observed. Erythema, induration and pain occurred in 3.2%, 1% and 13%, respectively, of vaccinees within 48 hours post-vaccination. Temperatures ≥ 39°C (≥ 102°F) were reported in up to 38% of vaccinees. Other symptoms noted included sleepiness, fussiness, crying, decreased appetite and spitting up of feedings. Because IPV was given in a different site but concurrently with Diphtheria and Tetanus Toxoids and Pertussis Vaccine Adsorbed (DTP), systemic reactions could not be attributed to a specific vaccine. However, these systemic reactions were comparable in frequency and severity to that reported for DTP given without IPV.

In another study using IPV in the US, there were no significant local or systemic reactions following injection of the vaccine. There were 7% (6/86), 12% (8/65) and 4% (2/45) of children with temperatures > 100.6°F, following the first, second and third doses, respectively. Most of the children received DTP at the same time as IPV and therefore it was not possible to attribute reactions to a particular vaccine; however, such reactions were not significantly different than when DTP is given alone.

Although no causal relationship between IPV and Guillain-Barré Syndrome (GBS) has been established, GBS has been temporally related to administration of another IPV.

Note: The National Childhood Vaccine Injury Act of 1986 requires the keeping of certain records and the reporting of certain events occurring after the administration of vaccine, including the occurrence of any contraindicating reaction. Poliovirus vaccines are listed vaccines covered by this Act and healthcare providers should ensure that they comply with the terms thereof.

INFLUENZA VIRUS VACCINE

Rx	**Fluzone** (Aventis Pasteur)	**Injection (purified split-virus):** 15 mcg of each of A/Wyoming/03/2003 (H3N2) (A/Fujian/411/2002-like), A/New Caledonia/20/99 (H1N1), and B/Jiangsu/10/2003 (B/Shanghai/361/2002-like) per 0.5 mL	Thimerosal. In 0.25[1] and 0.5 mL prefilled syringes[2] and 5 mL vials.[3]
Rx	**Fluvirin** (Evans Vaccine Ltd.)	**Injection (purified split-virus):** 15 mcg each of A/Wyoming/3/2003/X-147 (A/Fujian/411/2003 (H3N2)-like), A/New Caledonia/20/99 IVR-116, and B/Jiangsu/10/2003 (B/Shanghai/361/2002-like) per 0.5 mL	Thimerosal. In 0.5 mL prefilled syringes.[2]
Rx	**FluMist** (MedImmune Vaccines/Wyeth)	**Intranasal spray:** A/New Caledonia/20/99 (H1N1), A/Wyoming (H3N2), B/Jilin/20/2003	Preservative free. In 0.5 mL prefilled single-use sprayers.

[1] With 0.5 mcg or less mercury per 0.25 mL dose.
[2] With 0.98 mcg or less mercury per 0.5 mL dose.
[3] With 25 mcg mercury per 0.5 mL dose.

For additional information, refer to the Agents for Active Immunization introduction.

Indications

➤*Influenza:* For active immunization against the specific influenza virus strains contained in the formulation. Influenza vaccine is strongly recommended for anyone 6 months of age or older who, because of age or underlying medical conditions, is at increased risk for complications from influenza. Vaccinate health care workers and others (including household members) in close contact with high-risk people. In addition, influenza vaccine may be given to any person 6 months of age or older who wishes to reduce the chance of becoming infected with influenza. (Note: *Fluvirin* is not indicated in children under 4 years of age. *FluMist* is indicated in healthy children and adolescents 5 to 17 years of age and healthy adults 18 to 49 years of age.) The following are guidelines for use of the vaccine in specific groups.

➤*Groups at increased risk of influenza-related complications:*
1.) People 65 years of age or older. Vaccination also is recommended for people 50 to 64 years of age because of increased prevalence of people with high-risk conditions.
2.) Residents of nursing homes and other chronic-care facilities that house people of any age with chronic medical conditions.
3.) Adults and children with chronic disorders of the pulmonary or cardiovascular systems, including asthma.
4.) Adults and children who have required regular medical follow-up or hospitalization during the preceding year because of chronic metabolic diseases (including diabetes mellitus), renal dysfunction, hemoglobinopathies, or immunosuppression (including immunosuppression caused by medications or by human immunodeficiency virus [HIV]).
5.) Children and adolescents (6 months to 18 years of age) who are receiving long-term aspirin therapy and, therefore, may be at risk of developing Reye's syndrome after influenza.
6.) Women who will be pregnant during the influenza season.
7.) Although not recommended by the Advisory Committee on Immunization Practices (ACIP), consider vaccination in people who smoke tobacco products because of increased risk for influenza-related complications.

➤*Groups that can transmit influenza to high-risk people:* People who are clinically or subclinically infected can transmit influenza virus to people at high risk for complications from influenza. Decreasing transmission of influenza from caregivers to people at high risk might reduce influenza-related deaths among people at high risk. Vaccination of health care workers and others in close contact with people at high risk, including household members, is recommended. Therefore, vaccinate the following groups:
1.) Physicians, nurses, and other personnel in hospital and outpatient-care settings, including emergency response workers.
2.) Employees of nursing homes and chronic-care facilities who have contact with patients or residents.
3.) Providers of home care to high-risk people (eg, visiting nurses, volunteer workers).
4.) Household members (including children) of high-risk people.
5.) Employees of assisted living and other residences for people in high-risk groups.

In addition, because children 0 to 23 months of age are at an increased risk for influenza-related hospitalization, vaccination is encouraged for their household contacts and out-of-home caretakers, particularly for contacts of children 0 to 5 months of age because influenza vaccines have not been approved by the FDA for use among children under 6 months of age.

➤*General population:* Any individual wishing to reduce the chance of acquiring an influenza infection. People who provide essential community service and students or other people in institutional settings may be considered for vaccination programs to minimize potential disruption of routine activities during outbreaks.

➤*Children:* Because children 6 to 23 months of age are at substantially increased risk for influenza-related hospitalizations, influenza vaccination of all children in this age group is encouraged when feasible.

➤*People infected with HIV:* Limited information exists regarding the frequency and severity of influenza illness in HIV-infected people, but reports suggest that symptoms may be prolonged and the risk of complications increased for some patients in this group. Because influenza may result in serious illness and complications, vaccination is a prudent precaution and will result in protective antibody titers in many recipients. However, the antibody response to vaccine may be low in people with advanced HIV-related illnesses; a booster dose of vaccine has not improved the immune response for these individuals.

➤*Foreign travelers:* The risk of exposure to influenza during foreign travel varies, depending on season and destination. In the tropics, influenza can occur throughout the year; in the Southern Hemisphere, the season of greatest activity is April through September. People at high risk for complications of influenza who were not vaccinated with influenza vaccine during the preceding fall or winter should consider receiving influenza vaccine before travel if they plan to do any of the following:
• Travel to the tropics,
• travel with large organized tourist groups at any time of the year, or
• travel to the Southern Hemisphere from April through September.

People at high risk who received the previous season's vaccine before travel should be revaccinated with the current vaccine in the following fall or winter. People 50 years of age and older and others at high risk might wish to consult with their physicians before embarking on travel during the summer to discuss the symptoms and risks of influenza and the advisability for carrying antiviral medications for prophylaxis or treatment of influenza.

➤*Pregnancy:* See Warnings.

Administration and Dosage

Do not use remaining 2003 to 2004 vaccine during influenza vaccination for 2004 to 2005.

➤*Fluzone/Fluvirin:* Do not inject IV. Give injections IM, preferably in the deltoid muscle for adults and older children; for infants and young children, the preferred site is the anterolateral aspect of the thigh. Shake well before withdrawing dose (*Fluzone* only).

➤*FluMist:* For nasal use only. Do not administer parenterally.
Administer according to the following schedule:

FluMist Dosing Schedule		
Age group	Vaccination status	Dosage schedule
Children 5 through 8 years of age	Not previously vaccinated with *FluMist*	2 doses (0.5 mL each, 60 days apart ± 14 days) for initial season
Children 5 through 8 years of age	Previously vaccinated with *FluMist*	1 dose (0.5 mL) per season
Children and adults 9 through 49 years of age	Not applicable	1 dose (0.5 mL) per season

For healthy children 5 through 8 years of age who have not previously received *FluMist* vaccine, the recommended dosage schedule for nasal administration is one 0.5 mL dose followed by a second 0.5 mL dose given at least 6 weeks later.

For all other healthy individuals, including children 5 through 8 years of age who have previously received at least 1 dose of *FluMist*, the recommended schedule is 1 dose.

FluMist must be thawed prior to administration. *FluMist* may be thawed by holding the sprayer in the palm of the hand and supporting the plunger rod with the thumb; the vaccine must be administered immediately thereafter. Alternatively, *FluMist* may be thawed in a refrigerator and stored at 2° to 8°C (36° to 46°F) for no more than 24 hours prior to use.

Approximately 0.25 mL (ie, half of the dose from a single *FluMist* sprayer) is administered into each nostril while the recipient is in an upright position. Insert the tip of the sprayer just inside the nose and depress the plunger to spray. The dose divider clip is removed from the sprayer to administer the second half of the dose (approximately 0.25 mL) into the other nostril. Once *FluMist* has been administered, dispose of the used sprayer according to the standard procedures for biohazardous waste products.

➤*Vaccination timing (ACIP guidelines):* Beginning each September, offer influenza vaccines to people at high risk when they are seen by health care providers. Vaccination of children less than 9 years of

INFLUENZA VIRUS VACCINE

age who are receiving the vaccine for the first time should begin in October because they need a booster dose 1 month after the initial dose. The optimal time to vaccinate is usually from October through November because influenza activity in the United States generally peaks between late December and early March. Therefore, although the timing of influenza activity can vary by region, vaccine administered after November is likely to be beneficial in most influenza seasons. Adults develop peak antibody protection against influenza infection 2 weeks after vaccination. Although vaccine generally becomes available in August or September, in some years, vaccine for the upcoming influenza season might not be available until later in the fall. To minimize the possibility that large organized vaccination campaigns will need to be cancelled because vaccine is unavailable, people planning substantial organized vaccination campaigns may consider scheduling these events after mid-October because the availability of vaccine in any location cannot be assured consistently in the early fall. Administering vaccine before October generally should be avoided in facilities such as nursing homes because antibody levels can begin to decline within a few months after vaccination.

Influenza Vaccine Dosage Recommendations by Age Group		
Age	Dosage (mL)	Number of doses
6 to 35 months[1]	0.25	1 or 2[2]
3 to 8 years[1]	0.5	1 or 2[2]
≥ 9 years	0.5	1

[1] *Fluvirin* is indicated only in children 4 years of age and older.
[2] Two doses are recommended for children less than 9 years of age who are receiving influenza virus vaccine for the first time. Allow at least 1 month between doses. If possible, administer the second dose before December.

➤*Storage / Stability:*

Parenteral – Store between 2° to 8°C (36° to 46°F). Freezing destroys potency; do not use vaccine if it has been frozen.

Inhalational – Store at or below -15°C (5°F). Do not refreeze after thawing. Upon receipt, immediately store *FluMist* at -15°C (5°F) or below. *FluMist* may be stored in a non-frost-free freezer to be maintained continuously at -15°C (5°F) or below. Avoid storage of *FluMist* in a frost-free freezer because the temperature could cycle above -15°C (5°F) and can therefore negatively impact the stability of the product. *FluMist* may be thawed in a refrigerator and stored at 2° to 8°C (36° to 46°F) for no more than 24 hours prior to use.

Actions

➤*Pharmacology:* Influenza A viruses are classified into subtypes on the basis of the following 2 surface antigens: Hemagglutinin (H) and neuraminidase (N). A person's immunity to the surface antigens, especially hemagglutinin, reduces the likelihood of infection and severity of disease if infection occurs.

Influenza vaccines are standardized to contain the hemagglutinins of strains (ie, typically 2 type A and 1 type B), representing the influenza viruses likely to circulate in the United States in the upcoming winter. The vaccine is made from highly purified, egg-grown viruses that have been made noninfectious (ie, inactivated). Subvirion and purified surface-antigen preparations are available. Because the vaccine viruses initially are grown in embryonated hens' eggs, the vaccine might contain small amounts of residual egg protein.

The trivalent influenza vaccine prepared for the 2004 to 2005 season will include A/Fujian/411/2002 (H3N2)-like, A/New Caledonia/20/99 (H1N1)-like, and B/Shanghai/361/2002-like antigens (for the A/Fujian/411/2002 (H3N2)-like antigen, manufacturers may use the antigenically equivalent A/Wyoming/3/2003 [H3N2] virus, and for the B/Shanghai/361/2002-like antigen, manufacturers may use the antigenically equivalent B/Jilin/20/2003 virus or B/Jiangsu/10/2003 virus). These viruses will be used because of their growth properties, and because they are representative of influenza viruses likely to circulate in the US during the 2004 to 2005 influenza season.

The influenza vaccine is available as a split-virus (synonymous with subvirion or purified surface antigen) preparation.

FluMist contains live attenuated influenza viruses that replicate in the nasopharynx of the recipient and are shed in respiratory secretions. Assessing the probability that these shed vaccine viruses will be transmitted from a vaccinated individual to a nonvaccinated individual was the primary objective of a prospective, randomized, double-blind, placebo-controlled trial in a daycare setting in Finland. Of *FluMist* recipients, 80% shed at least 1 vaccine strain, with a mean duration of shedding 7.6 days (range, 1 to 21 days). Assuming that a single transmission event occurred (isolation of the Type B vaccine strain), the probability of a young child acquiring vaccine virus following close contact with a single *FluMist* vaccinee in this daycare setting was 0.58%.

Contraindications

Hypersensitivity to any component of the vaccine; hypersensitivity to eggs or egg products or chicken proteins. Before being vaccinated, give a skin test to people suspected of being hypersensitive to egg protein, using the influenza virus vaccine as the antigen. Do not vaccinate people with adverse reactions to such testing. Chemoprophylaxis (with amantadine or rimantadine) may be indicated for prevention of influenza A in such people.

According to the product manufacturers, do not administer the influenza virus vaccine to patients with a history of Guillain-Barré syndrome (GBS). However, the ACIP recommends influenza vaccination in patients with a history of GBS and who are at a high risk for severe complications from influenza (see Precautions).

Defer vaccination in patients with acute febrile illnesses (and/or respiratory illness for at least 72 hours [*FluMist* only]), until their symptoms have abated. Minor illnesses, with or without fever, are not contraindicated in the use of influenza virus vaccine, particularly in children with a mild upper respiratory tract infection or allergic rhinitis.

Delay immunization in patients with an active neurologic disorder characterized by changing neurological findings until stabilized. The occurrence of any neurological symptoms after vaccination is a contraindication for further use.

➤*FluMist:* Under no circumstances should *FluMist* be administered parenterally.

FluMist is contraindicated in children and adolescents 5 to 17 years of age receiving aspirin therapy or aspirin-containing therapy because of the association of Reye syndrome with aspirin and wild-type influenza infection.

As with other live virus vaccines, do not administer *FluMist* to individuals with known or suspected immune deficiency diseases such as combined immunodeficiency, agammaglobulinemia, and thymic abnormalities, and conditions such as HIV infection, malignancy, leukemia, or lymphoma. *FluMist* is also contraindicated in patients who may be immunosuppressed or have altered or compromised immune status as a consequence of treatment with systemic corticosteroids, alkylating drugs, antimetabolites, radiation, or other immunosuppressive therapies.

Warnings

➤*Postvaccination (FluMist):* Due to the possible transmission of vaccine virus, vaccine recipients or their parents/guardians should be advised to avoid close contact (eg, within the same household) with immunocompromised individuals for at least 21 days. Health-care workers should refrain from contact with severely immunosuppressed patients for 7 days after vaccine receipt.

➤*Asthma / Reactive airways disease:* The safety of *FluMist* in individuals with asthma or reactive airways disease has not been established. In a large safety study in children 1 to 17 years of age, children under 5 years of age who received *FluMist* were found to have an increased rate of asthma within 42 days of vaccination when compared to placebo recipients. *FluMist* should not be administered to individuals with a history of asthma or reactive airways disease.

➤*Impaired immune response:* Patients with impaired immune responsiveness, whether caused by the use of immunosuppressive therapy (including irradiation, large amounts of corticosteroids, antimetabolites, alkylating agents, and cytotoxic agents), a genetic defect, HIV infection, AIDS, leukemia, lymphoma, generalized malignancy, or other causes, may have a reduced antibody response to active immunization procedures and may remain susceptible despite immunization. Chemoprophylaxis of influenza A with amantadine or rimantadine may be indicated.

The safety of *FluMist* in individuals with underlying medical conditions that may predispose them to severe disease following wild-type influenza infection has not been established. *FluMist* is not indicated for these individuals. According to the Advisory Committee on Immunization Practices (ACIP), such individuals include, but are not limited to, adults and children with chronic disorders of the cardiovascular and pulmonary systems (including asthma), pregnant women who will be in their second or third trimesters during influenza season; adults and children who required regular medical follow-up or hospitalization during the preceding year because of chronic metabolic diseases (including diabetes), renal dysfunction, or hemoglobinopathies; and adults and children with congenital or acquired immunosuppression caused by underlying disease or immunosuppressive therapy (see Contraindications). IM administered inactivated influenza vaccines are available to immunize high-risk individuals. Severely immunosuppressed persons should not administer *FluMist*.

➤*People infected with HIV:* Limited information exists regarding the frequency and severity of influenza illness or the benefits of influenza vaccination among people with HIV infection. Reports suggest influenza symptoms may be prolonged and the risk for complications increased. Vaccination will benefit many HIV-infected patients. However, in patients with advanced HIV-related illnesses, the antibody response for vaccination may be low; a booster dose has not improved the immune response for these individuals.

➤*Hypersensitivity reactions:* Have epinephrine 1:1000 immediately available. Refer to Management of Acute Hypersensitivity Reactions.

➤*Pregnancy: Category C.* It is not known whether the influenza virus vaccine can cause fetal harm when administered to a pregnant woman. Do not administer *FluMist* to pregnant women. The ACIP recommends parenteral vaccination for women who will be pregnant during influ-

INFLUENZA VIRUS VACCINE

enza season. Vaccinate pregnant women who have medical conditions that increase their risk for complications from influenza before the influenza season, regardless of the pregnancy stage.

A study of influenza vaccination of more than 2000 pregnant women demonstrated no adverse fetal effects associated with parenteral influenza vaccine. However, more data are needed to confirm the safety of vaccination during pregnancy. Some experts prefer to administer influenza vaccine during the second trimester to avoid a coincidental association with spontaneous abortion, which is common in the first trimester, and because exposures to vaccines traditionally have been avoided during the first trimester.

▶*Lactation:*

Parenteral – Influenza vaccine does not affect the safety of breastfeeding for mothers or infants.

Inhalational – It is not known whether *FluMist* is excreted in human milk. Therefore, as some viruses are excreted in human milk and additionally, because of the possibility of shedding of vaccine virus and the close proximity of a nursing infant and mother, exercise caution if *FluMist* is administered to nursing mothers.

▶*Children:* Safety and efficacy of *Fluzone* have not been established in infants under 6 months of age. The safety and efficacy of *Fluvirin* in children under 4 years of age have not been established. The safety of *FluMist* in infants and children under 60 months of age has not been established.

Precautions

▶*Concurrent vaccination:* The target groups for influenza and pneumococcal vaccination overlap considerably. For people at high risk who have not previously been vaccinated with pneumococcal vaccine, health care providers should strongly consider administering pneumococcal and influenza vaccines concurrently. Both vaccines can be administered at the same time, using separate syringes, and at different sites without increasing side effects. However, influenza vaccine is administered each year, whereas pneumococcal vaccine is not. Children at high risk for influenza-related complications, including those 6 to 23 months of age, can receive influenza vaccine at the same time they receive other routine vaccinations.

▶*Seroconversion:* Vaccination may not result in seroconversion in all individuals.

▶*Latex:* Dry, natural latex rubber may be contained in vial stoppers.

▶*GBS:* During 3 of 4 influenza seasons studied from 1977 through 1991, the overall relative risk estimates for GBS after influenza vaccination were elevated slightly, but were not statistically significant in any of these studies. However, in a study of the 1992 to 1993 and 1993 to 1994 seasons, the overall relative risk for GBS was 1.7 (95% confidence intervals = 1 to 2.8; $P = 0.04$) during the 6 weeks following vaccination, representing approximately 1 additional case of GBS per million people vaccinated; the combined number of GBS cases peaked 2 weeks after vaccination. Thus, investigations to date suggest no large increase in GBS associated with influenza vaccines (other than the swine influenza vaccine of 1976) and that if influenza vaccine does pose a risk, it is probably slightly greater than 1 additional case per million people vaccinated. Cases of GBS following influenza infection have been reported, but no epidemiological studies have documented such an association.

The incidence of GBS in the general population is very low, but people with a history of GBS have a substantially greater likelihood of subsequently developing GBS than people without such a history. Thus, the likelihood of coincidentally developing GBS after influenza vaccination is expected to be greater among people with a history of GBS than among people with no history of this syndrome. Whether influenza vaccination specifically might increase the risk for recurrence of GBS is not known.

▶*Gentamicin sensitivity:* Gentamicin was used during *FluMist* preparation; however, the drug is not detectable in the final product by assay procedures.

▶*Neomycin sensitivity:* Neomycin was used during *Fluvirin* preparation; however, the drug is not detectable in the final product by current assay procedures.

▶*Thimerosal sensitivity:* Hypersensitivity reactions to any vaccine component can occur. Although exposure to vaccines containing thimerosal can lead to induction of hypersensitivity, most patients do not develop reactions to thimerosal when it is administered as a component of vaccines, even when patch or intradermal tests for thimerosal indicate hypersensitivity. When reported, hypersensitivity to thimerosal usually has consisted of local, delayed-type hypersensitivity reactions.

Drug Interactions

▶*Aspirin:* Children or adolescents who are receiving aspirin therapy or aspirin-containing therapy should not receive *FluMist* (see Contraindications).

▶*Antivirals:* The concurrent use of *FluMist* with antiviral compounds that are active against influenza A and/or B viruses has not been evaluated. However, based upon the potential for interference between such compounds and *FluMist*, it is advisable not to administer *FluMist* until

48 hours after the cessation of antiviral therapy and that antiviral agents not be administered until 2 weeks after administration of *FluMist* unless medically indicated.

▶*Other vaccines:* The safety and immunogenicity of *FluMist* when administered concurrently with other vaccines have not been determined. Therefore, *FluMist* should not be administered concurrently with other vaccines. Studies of *FluMist* in healthy individuals excluded subjects who received any live virus vaccine within 1 month of enrollment and any inactivated or subunit vaccine within 2 weeks of enrollment; therefore, health care providers should adhere to these intervals when administering *FluMist*.

▶*Drug/Lab test interactions:* Nasopharyngeal secretions or swabs collected from *FluMist* vaccinees may test positive for influenza virus for up to 3 weeks.

Adverse Reactions

Report adverse events following immunization to the US Department of Health and Human Services (DHHS) Vaccine Adverse Event Reporting System (VAERS). Reporting forms and information about reporting requirements or completion of the form can be obtained from VAERS by calling (800) 822-7967.

▶*Parenteral:*

CNS – Neurological disorders temporally associated with influenza vaccination such as unspecified neuritis, encephalitis, peripheral nerve disease, paresthesia, hypesthesia, brachial neuritis, demyelinating disease, labyrinthitis, meningitis, allergic asthma, systemic anaphylaxis, encephalopathy, optic neuritis/neuropathy, partial facial paralysis, and brachial plexus neuropathy have been reported; however, no cause-and-effect has been established. Transverse myelitis has been reported rarely. Clinical reactions began as soon as a few hours and as late as 2 weeks after vaccination; full recovery was almost always reported.

Local – The most frequent side effect (affecting 10% to 64% of patients) was soreness at the injection site that lasted up to 2 days.

Systemic – Fever, malaise, myalgia, and other symptoms occur more often in young children and others who have had no exposure to the influenza virus antigen. These reactions begin 6 to 12 hours after vaccination and persist for 1 to 2 days.

Immediate, presumably allergic responses (eg, hives, angioedema, allergic asthma, systemic anaphylaxis) have occurred rarely and probably resulted from hypersensitivity to some vaccine component, most likely residual egg protein (see Contraindications).

▶*FluMist:*

Children – Runny nose/nasal congestion, sore throat, cough, irritability, headache, chills, vomiting, muscle aches, and decreased activity and a feeling of tiredness/weakness have occurred.

FluMist Adverse Reactions Observed Within 10 Days After Each Dose for Healthy Children 60 to 71 Months of Age (%)[1]				
	Postdose 1		Postdose 2	
Adverse reaction	*FluMist* (n = 214)[2]	Placebo (n = 95)[2]	*FluMist* (n = 161)[2]	Placebo (n = 75)[2]
Any event	65.4	61.4	66.5	53.3
Cough	26.8	32.7	38.5	30.7
Runny rose/nasal congestion	48.1	44.2	46	32
Sore throat	12.6	19.8	9.3	16
Irritability	19.5	16.8	9.9	9.3
Headache	17.8	11.6	6.8	16
Chills	6.1	5.3	2.5	4
Vomiting	4.7	3.2	5.6	12
Muscle aches	6.1	4.2	5	4
Decreased activity	14	12.6	10.6	13.3
Fever[3]				
Temp 1	9.5	9.9	4.3	4
Temp 2	2.2	2	0.6	1.3
Temp 3	0	0	0	0

[1] Note: There were no statistically significant differences in any of these events (p-value > 0.05; Fisher's Exact method.
[2] Number of evaluable subjects (those who returned diary cards) for each event.
[3] Fever: Temp 1 - Oral greater than 100°F, rectal or aural greater than 100.6°F, or axillary greater than 99.6°F; temp 2 - oral greater than 102°F, rectal or aural greater than 102.6°F, or axillary greater than 101.6°F; temp 3 - oral greater than 104°F, rectal or aural greater than 104.6°F, axillary greater than 103.6°F.

Among healthy children 60 to 71 months in the pediatric efficacy study, the events that occurred in at least 1% of *FluMist* recipients and at a higher rate compared with placebo were abdominal pain (3.7% *FluMist* vs 0% placebo), otitis media (1.4% *FluMist* vs 0% placebo), accidental injury (2.3% *FluMist* vs 2.1% placebo), diarrhea (3.7% *FluMist* vs 1.1% placebo), following dose 1 and otitis media (3.1% *FluMist* vs 1.3% placebo) following dose 2. None of these differences were statistically significant.

INFLUENZA VIRUS VACCINE
Adults –

FluMist Adverse Reactions Observed Within 7 Days in Healthy Adults 18 to 49 Years of Age (%)		
Adverse reaction	*FluMist* (N = 2548)[1]	Placebo (N = 1290)[1]
Any event	71.9[2]	62.6
Cough	13.9[2]	10.8
Runny nose	44.5[2]	27.1
Sore throat	27.8[2]	17.1
Headache	40.4	38.4
Chills	8.6[2]	6
Muscle aches	16.7	14.6
Tiredness/weakness	25.7[2]	21.6
Fever		

FluMist Adverse Reactions Observed Within 7 Days in Healthy Adults 18 to 49 Years of Age (%)		
Adverse reaction	*FluMist* (N = 2548)[1]	Placebo (N = 1290)[1]
Oral temp > 100°F	1.5	1.3
Oral temp > 101°F	0.5	0.7
Oral temp > 102°F	0.1	0.2
Oral temp > 103°F	0	0

[1] Denotes statistically significant p-value ≤ 0.05; no adjustments for multiple comparisons; Fisher's Exact Method.
[2] Number of evaluable subjects (those who returned diary cards): 97.9% of *FluMist* recipients and 97.9% of placebo recipients.

For adults 18 to 49 years of age in the adult effectiveness study, nasal congestion (9.2% *FluMist* vs 2.2% placebo), rhinitis (6.3% *FluMist* vs 3.1% placebo), and sinusitis (4.1% *FluMist* vs 2.2% placebo) were reported significantly more often by *FluMist* recipients compared with placebo recipients.

Vaccines, Viral

JAPANESE ENCEPHALITIS VIRUS VACCINE

Rx	JE-VAX (Connaught)	Powder for Injection, lyophilized[1,2]	In single-dose vial with 1.3 ml diluent (sterile water for injection) and 10 dose vial with 11 ml diluent (sterile water for injection).

[1] Potency is determined by immunizing mice with either the test vaccine or the JE Reference Vaccine. Neutralizing antibodies are measured in a plaque-neutralization assay performed on sera from the immunized mice. The potency of the test vaccine must be no less than that of the reference vaccine.

[2] With thimerosal 0.007%. Each 1 ml dose contains ≈ 500 mcg gelatin, < 100 mcg formaldehyde and < 50 ng mouse serum protein.

For additional information, refer to the Agents for Active Immunization introduction.

Indications

For active immunization against Japanese encephalitis (JE) for people > 1 year of age.

Consider JE vaccine in people who plan to reside in or travel to areas where JE is endemic or epidemic during a transmission season. It is not recommended for all people traveling to or residing in Asia. Consider the incidence of JE in the location of intended stay, the conditions of housing, nature of activities, duration of stay and the possibility of unexpected travel to high-risk areas in the decision to administer vaccine. In general, consider vaccinating people spending ≥ 1 month in epidemic or endemic areas during the transmission season, especially if travel will include rural areas. Depending on the epidemic circumstances, consider for persons spending < 30 days whose activities, such as extensive outdoor activities in rural areas, place them at particularly high risk for exposure.

In all instances, travelers are advised to take personal precautions to reduce exposure to mosquito bites. (See Patient Information.)

Consult current CDC advisories with regard to JE epidemicity in specific locales.

Administration and Dosage

➤*Approved by the FDA:* December 10, 1992.

Previously available in the US from 1983 through 1987 on an investigational basis through the CDC.

➤*Primary immunization schedule:*

Adults and children > 3 years of age – The recommended primary immunization series is three SC doses of 1 ml each given on days 0, 7 and 30.

Children 1 to 3 years of age – Give a series of three SC doses of 0.5 ml each on days 0, 7 and 30.

An abbreviated schedule of days 0, 7 and 14 can be used when the longer schedule is impractical because of time constraints. When it is impossible to follow one of the above recommended schedules, two doses given a week apart will induce antibodies in ≈ 80% of vaccinees; however, this two-dose regimen should not be used except under unusual circumstances. Give the last dose at least 10 days before the commencement of international travel to ensure an adequate immune response and access to medical care in the event of delayed adverse reactions.

Infants < 1 year of age – There are no data on the safety and efficacy of JE vaccine. Whenever possible, defer immunization of infants until they are ≥ 1 year of age.

➤*Booster dose:* A booster dose of 1 ml (0.5 ml for children from 1 to 3 years of age) may be given after 2 years. In the absence of firm data on the persistence of antibody after primary immunization, a definite recommendation cannot be made on the spacing of boosters beyond 2 years.

Clean and disinfect the skin at the site of injection first. Shake vial thoroughly before each use. Cleanse top of rubber stopper of the vial with a suitable antiseptic and wipe away all excess before withdrawing vaccine. Inspect visually for extraneous particulate matter or discoloration prior to administration. If either of these conditions exist, do not administer the vaccine.

➤*Concomitant vaccines:* When JE vaccine and any other vaccines are given concurrently, use separate syringes and separate sites.

➤*Reconstitution:* Remove plastic tab of flip-off cap. Do not remove rubber stopper. Cleanse stopper with a suitable disinfectant. Reconstitute only with the supplied 1.3 ml (single-dose vial) or 11 ml (10 dose vial) of diluent (sterile water for injection). Shake vial thoroughly.

➤*Storage/Stability:* Store the vaccine between 2° to 8°C (35° to 46°F). Do not freeze. After reconstitution, store the vaccine between 2° to 8°C and use within 8 hours. Do not freeze reconstituted vaccine.

Actions

➤*Pharmacology:* JE virus vaccine is a sterile, lyophilized vaccine for SC use, prepared by inoculating mice intracerebrally with JE virus ("Nakayama-NIH" strain). JE, a mosquito-borne arboviral Flavivirus infection, is the leading cause of viral encephalitis in Asia. Infection leads to overt encephalitis in 1 of 20 to 1000 cases. Encephalitis usually is severe, resulting in a fatal outcome in 25% of cases and residual neuropsychiatric sequelae in 50% of cases. JE acquired during the first or second trimesters of pregnancy may cause intrauterine infection and miscarriage. Infections that occur during the third trimester of preg-

nancy have not been associated with adverse outcomes in newborns. The virus is transmitted in an enzootic cycle among mosquitoes and vertebrate amplifying hosts, chiefly domestic pigs and, in some areas, wild Ardeid (wading) birds. Viral infection rates in mosquitoes range from < 1% to 3%. JE virus is transmitted seasonally in most areas of Asia. The periods of greatest risk for JE viral transmission may vary regionally and within countries, and from year to year.

In areas where JE is endemic, annual incidence ranges from 1 to 10 per 10,000 people. Cases occur primarily in children < 10 years of age. Seroprevalence studies in these endemic areas indicate nearly universal exposure by adulthood. In addition to children < 10 years, an increase in JE incidence has been observed in the elderly.

➤*Clinical trials:* The efficacy of JE vaccine was demonstrated in a placebo-controlled, randomized clinical trial in Thai children. In this trial, children between 1 and 14 years of age received a monovalent or a bivalent vaccine or tetanus toxoid as a placebo. Immunization consisted of two SC 1 ml doses of vaccine, except in children < 3 years of age who received two 0.5 ml doses. One case (5 cases/100,000) of JE occurred in the monovalent vaccine group, one case (5 cases/100,000) in the bivalent vaccine group and 11 cases (51 cases/100,000) in the placebo group. The observed efficacy of both monovalent and bivalent vaccines was 91% (95% confidence interval, 54% to 98%). Side effects of vaccination, including headache, sore arm, rash, and swelling were reported at rates similar to those in the placebo group, usually < 1%. Symptoms did not increase after the second dose. A schedule of two doses, separated by 7 days, may be appropriate for use in residents of endemic or epidemic areas, where pre-existing exposure to Flaviviruses may contribute to the immune response.

A three-dose vaccination schedule is recommended for US travelers and military personnel, based on the CDC experience and on a controlled immunogenicity trial performed in US military personnel. The CDC experience demonstrated that neutralizing antibody was produced in < 80% of vaccinees following two doses of vaccine in US travelers, and antibody levels declined substantially in most vaccinees within 6 months. In 538 volunteers, two three-dose regimens were evaluated (day 0, 7 and 14 or day 0, 7 and 30). All vaccine recipients demonstrated neutralizing antibodies at 2 and 6 months after initiation of vaccination. The schedule of day 0, 7 and 30 produced higher antibody responses. Of the original study participants, 273 were tested at 12 months post-vaccination and there was no longer a statistical difference in antibody titers between the two vaccination regimens.

The full duration of protection is unknown. Of volunteers completing a three-dose regimen, 252 agreed to receive a booster dose of vaccine 1 year after the primary series. All participants still had antibody 12 months after the booster. Protective levels of neutralizing antibody persisted for 24 months in all 21 people who had not received a booster. Definitive recommendations cannot be given on the timing of booster doses at this time.

Contraindications

Adverse reactions to a prior dose of JE vaccine manifesting as generalized urticaria and angioedema (report patients who develop allergic and unusual adverse events after vaccination through the Vaccine Adverse Event Reporting System [VAERS] at 1-800-822-7967); hypersensitivity to proteins of rodent or neural origin (JE vaccine is produced in mouse brains) or thimerosal.

Warnings

➤*Hypersensitivity reactions:* Adverse reactions to JE vaccine manifesting as generalized urticaria or angioedema may occur within minutes following vaccination. A possibly related reaction has occurred as late as 17 days after vaccination. Most reactions occur within 10 days with the majority occurring within 48 hours. (See Adverse Reactions.) Observe vaccinees for 30 minutes after vaccination and warn about the possibility of delayed generalized urticaria, often in a generalized distribution or angioedema of the extremities, face and oropharynx, especially of the lips. Advise vaccinees to remain in areas where they have ready access to medical care for 10 days after receiving JE vaccine, and instruct them to seek medical attention immediately upon onset of any reaction.

People should not embark on international travel within 10 days of JE vaccine immunization because of the possibility of delayed allergic reactions.

People with a history of urticaria after *Hymenoptera* envenomation, drugs, physical or other provocations or of idiopathic cause appear to have a greater risk of developing reactions to JE vaccine. Consider this history when weighing risks and benefits of the vaccine for an individual patient. When patients with such a history are offered JE vaccine, alert them to their increased risk for reaction and monitor

JAPANESE ENCEPHALITIS VIRUS VACCINE

appropriately. There are no data supporting the efficacy of prophylactic antihistamines or steroids in preventing JE vaccine-related allergic reactions.

Have epinephrine and other medications and equipment to treat anaphylaxis. Refer to Management of Acute Hypersensitivity Reactions.

►*Elderly:* Advanced age may be a risk factor for developing symptomatic illness after infection. Consider this when advising elderly people who plan to visit JE-endemic areas.

►*Pregnancy: Category C.* It is not known whether JE vaccine can cause fetal harm when administered to a pregnant woman. Immunize pregnant women who must travel to an area where risk of JE is high when the theoretical risks of immunization are outweighed by the risk of infection to the mother and developing fetus; JE acquired during the first or second trimesters of pregnancy may cause intrauterine infection and miscarriage. Give to a pregnant woman only if clearly needed.

►*Lactation:* It is not known whether JE vaccine is excreted in breast milk. Exercise caution when administering to a nursing woman.

►*Children:* Safety and efficacy in infants < 1 year of age have not been established. Whenever possible defer immunization of infants until they are ≥ 1 year of age.

Precautions

►*Patient history:* Prior to injection of any vaccine, take all known precautions to prevent adverse reactions. This includes a review of the patient's history with respect to possible sensitivity to this vaccine, a similar vaccine or allergic disorders in general.

►*Transmission of infectious agents:* Use a separate sterile syringe and needle or a disposable unit for each patient to prevent transmission of infectious agents from person to person. Do not recap needles; dispose of properly.

►*Antibody level:* Although substantial neutralizing antibody titers are elicited by JE vaccine, in > 90% of US travelers without history of prior JE immunization or of prior exposure to JE, the precise relationship between antibody level and efficacy has not been established even though these titers persisted for at least 2 years after immunization.

►*Risks:* The decision to administer JE vaccine should balance the risks for exposure to the virus and for developing illness, the availability and acceptability of repellents and other alternative protective measures, and the side effects of vaccination.

►*Research laboratory workers:* Laboratory acquired JE has been reported in 22 cases. JE virus may be transmitted in a laboratory setting through needle sticks and other accidental exposures. Vaccine-derived immunity presumably protects against exposure through these percutaneous routes. Exposure to aerosolized JE virus, and particularly to high concentrations of virus (eg, during viral purification), potentially could lead to infection through mucous membranes and possibly directly into the CNS through the olfactory mucosa. It is unknown whether vaccine-derived immunity protects against such exposures, but immunization is recommended for all laboratory workers with a potential for exposure to infectious JE virus.

As with any vaccine, vaccination with JE vaccine may not result in protection in all individuals. Long-term protection, as demonstrated by persistence of neutralizing antibody for > 2 years, has not yet been shown.

Adverse Reactions

In clinical trials, side effects including headache, sore arm, rash and swelling occurred at rates similar to those in placebo groups, usually < 1%. Overall, 20% of vaccine recipients experience mild to moderate local side effects: Tenderness, redness, swelling (range, < 1% to 31%). Systemic effects include: Fever, headache, malaise, rash, chills, dizziness, muscle pain, nausea, vomiting, abdominal pain (5% to 10%); hives (0.2%); facial swelling (0.1%). Report adverse events to the VAERS system at 1-800-822-7967.

Some adverse reactions to JE vaccine occur within minutes, most within 48 hours, and nearly all within 10 days, although one reaction

occurred 17 days after vaccination. Median time to reaction after a first dose of vaccine was 12 hours; 88% of reactions occurred within 3 days. The interval between a second dose and onset of symptoms was longer (median, 3 days; outer limit, 2 weeks). Symptoms did not increase in frequency or severity with increasing numbers of doses. Reactions occurred after a second or third dose when preceding doses had not evoked a reaction.

Since 1989, an apparently new pattern of adverse reactions has been reported among vaccinees in Europe, North America and Australia. The pattern is characterized by urticaria, often in a generalized distribution, or angioedema of the extremities or face, especially of the lips and oropharynx; three vaccinees developed respiratory distress. Distress or collapse due to hypotension or other causes led to hospitalization in several cases. Most reactions were treated successfully with antihistamines or oral corticosteroids; some patients were hospitalized for IV steroid therapy. Three patients developed erythema multiforme or nodosum and some patients had joint swelling. Some vaccinees complained of generalized itching without objective evidence of rash. Rates of serious allergic reactions (eg, generalized urticaria, angioedema) are ≈ 1 to 104 per 10,000 doses. People with certain allergic histories (eg, urticaria after *Hymenoptera* envenomation, drugs, physical or other provocations, idiopathic cause) appear to be 9.1 times more likely to experience an adverse reaction after vaccination. Due to the possibility of delayed allergic reactions, advise recipients to remain in areas where they have ready access to medical care for 10 days after receiving a dose (see Warnings).

Other serious adverse events reported after vaccination include: (1) A case of Guillain-Barre syndrome although this patient also was diagnosed as having mononucleosis 3 weeks before the onset of weakness; (2) a case of urticaria, hepatitis, eosinophilia and respiratory failure with effusion and infiltrate on chest radiograph 1 week after the second JE dose; (3) a case of respiratory and renal failure, with infiltrate on chest radiograph and AFB in sputum; and (4) a case of newly diagnosed hypertension in a young adult presenting with a headache several hours after receiving a first dose. The etiology of these adverse events is unconfirmed. Sudden death occurred 60 hours after receiving the first dose in a 21-year-old with a history of recurrent hypersensitivity and a prior episode of possible anaphylaxis. This person received a third dose of plague vaccine 12 to 15 hours prior to death. There was no evidence of urticaria or angioedema.

Patient Information

JE vaccine is given to provide immunization against Japanese encephalitis virus. Complete a three-dose immunizing series, except in unusual circumstances. (see Contraindications and Administration and Dosage).

Give to a pregnant woman only if, in the opinion of a physician, withholding the vaccine entails even greater risk.

Report adverse events following JE vaccine through the Vaccine Adverse Event Reporting System (VAERS) at 1-800-822-7967 after immediately contacting the physician.

If the patient has a history of urticaria (hives) following *Hymenoptera* envenomation, drugs, physical or other provocation, or of idiopathic origin, adverse effects are more likely.

Adverse events consisting of arm soreness and local redness can occur shortly after vaccination. Adverse events consisting of headache, rash, edema and generalized urticaria or angioedema may occur shortly after vaccination or up to 17 days (usually within 10 days) following vaccination.

International travel should not be initiated within 10 days of JE vaccination because of the possibility of delayed adverse reactions. Instruct patients to seek medical attention immediately upon onset of any adverse reaction.

Take personal precautions to avoid exposure to mosquito bites by the use of insect repellents and protective clothing. Avoiding outdoor activity, especially during twilight periods and in the evening, will reduce risk even further.

YELLOW FEVER VACCINE

Rx	YF-Vax[1] (Connaught)	**Powder for Injection:** Not less than 5.04 Log$_{10}$ Plaque Forming Units (PFU) per 0.5 ml dose when reconstituted[2]	In single-dose vials with 1 ml diluent, and 5 and 20 dose vials.

[1] Supplied only to designated Yellow Fever Vaccination Centers authorized to issue certificates of Yellow Fever Vaccination.

[2] With gelatin and sorbitol.

For additional information, refer to the Agents for Active Immunization introduction.

Indications

Induction of active immunity against yellow fever virus, primarily among travenlers to yellow fever endemic areas.

The World Health Organization (WHO) requires revaccination every 10 years to maintain travelers' vaccination certificates. US vaccination certificates are valid for 10 years, beginning 10 days after initial vaccination or revaccination.

Administration and Dosage

►*Adults and children:* Administer a single immunizing dose of 0.5 ml SC.

►*Preparation:* Reconstitute the vaccine using only the diluent supplied. The vaccine is slightly opalescent and light orange after reconstitution. Draw the volume of the diluent, shown on the diluent label, into a suitable size syringe and inject into the vial containing the vaccine. Slowly add diluent to vaccine, let set for 1 to 2 minutes and then carefully swirl mixture until suspension is uniform. Avoid vigorous shaking as it tends to cause foaming of the suspension. Use vaccine within 60 minutes of reconstitution.

YELLOW FEVER VACCINE

➤*Storage/Stability:* Yellow fever vaccine is shipped in a container with dry ice; do not use vaccine unless shipping case contains some dry ice on arrival. Maintain vaccine continuously at a temperature between −30° to 5°C (−22° to 41°F). Elevated temperatures reduce half-life. Sterilize and discard all unused rehydrated vaccine and containers after 1 hour. Shelf life is 12 months.

Actions

➤*Pharmacology:* This vaccine is a live, attenuated virus preparation prepared by culturing the 17D strain virus in living chick embryo. Onset of immunity is 7 to 10 days; duration is ≥ 10 years.

Contraindications

Hypersensitivity to the vaccine or to egg or chick embryo protein; pregnant women; children < 6 months (except in high risk areas); any form of immunodeficiency.

Warnings

➤*Immunodeficiency:* Do not use in immunodeficient people, including those with congenital or acquired immune deficiencies, whether due to genetics, disease, or radiation therapy. Contains live viruses. Avoid use in HIV-positive people.

➤*Hypersensitivity reactions:* Yellow fever vaccine is produced in chick embryos; do not administer to individuals hypersensitive to egg or chicken protein. Perform intradermal skin tests with the vaccine and sterile normal saline as a control on all such individuals. Inject 0.02 to 0.03 ml into the volar surface of the forearm. This should raise a noticeable intradermal wheal at each test site.

A positive sensitivity test consists of an urticarial wheal, with or without pseudopods, surrounded by an area of erythema and no response to the control. A positive reaction contraindicates vaccine administration. Have epinephrine 1:1000 and a tourniquet available while performing the sensitivity test.

An intradermal dose of 0.02 ml administered for hypersensitivity testing may induce immunity. However, in such individuals, the presence of specific protective antibodies must be confirmed through evaluation of serum obtained ≈ 4 weeks after skin testing. Contact the state or public health laboratory for assistance.

Immediate hypersensitivity – Immediate hypersensitivity reactions characterized by rash, urticaria or asthma are very rare (< 1 per 1 million) and occur principally in people with histories of egg allergy. Have epinephrine 1:1000 available. Refer to Management of Acute Hypersensitivity Reactions.

➤*Pregnancy: Category C.* Avoid use unless travel to a high-risk area is unavoidable. Generally, most IgG passage across the placenta occurs during the third trimester. Yellow fever vaccine virus crossed the placenta to 1 newborn among 41 mothers unknowingly vaccinated during pregnancy. The child appeared unaffected by infection, but yellow fever virus is known to be neurotropic. Avoid vaccination during pregnancy if at all possible.

➤*Lactation:* It is not known if yellow fever virus or corresponding antibodies are excreted in breast milk. Problems in humans have not been documented.

➤*Children:* The same dose is used for children as for adults. Do not administer to infants < 6 months of age, unless travel to high-risk area is unavoidable, to avoid a risk of encephalitis. Vaccinate pregnant women and infants 6 to 9 months of age only if they must travel and they cannot avoid mosquito bites. Vaccinate infants 4 to 6 months of age only if the risk of infection is high. Use the same dose for children

and adults. Do not vaccinate infants < 4 months of age. They are especially vulnerable to swelling of the brain after vaccination.

Precautions

➤*Blood/Plasma transfusion:* Defer vaccination with yellow fever vaccine for 8 weeks following blood or plasma transfusion.

Drug Interactions

Yellow Fever Vaccine Drug Interactions			
Precipitant drug	Object drug*		Description
Cholera vaccine	Yellow fever vaccine	↓	Concurrent cholera and yellow fever vaccinations impair the immune response to each vaccine. Separate these vaccinations by ≥ 3 weeks, if possible; may be administered on the same day if separation is not feasible.
Yellow fever vaccine	Cholera vaccine		
Hepatitis B vaccine	Yellow fever vaccine	↓	Concurrent vaccination against hepatitis B and yellow fever viruses in 1 study reduced the antibody titer expected from yellow fever vaccine. Separate these vaccinations by 1 month if possible.
Immune globulins	Yellow fever vaccine	↔	Yellow fever vaccine does not interact with US-produced immune globulins, although it may be prudent to maintain an interval of several weeks between these drugs if time permits.
Preservatives	Yellow fever vaccine	↓	Because yellow fever vaccine consists of live viruses, reconstitute it with a diluent that does not contain preservatives. Preservatives may inactivate constituent viruses and render the vaccine ineffective.
Yellow fever vaccine	Immunosuppressants	↓	Like all live viral vaccines, administration to patients receiving immunosuppressant drugs, including steroids, or radiation may predispose patients to disseminated infections or insufficient response to immunization. They may remain susceptible despite immunization.

* ↓ = Object drug decreased. ↔ = Undetermined effect.

Adverse Reactions

Frequent – Fever or malaise, usually appearing 7 to 14 days after administration (10%; treatment is symptomatic); myalgia and headache (2% to 5%). Fewer than 0.2% curtail regular activities.

Rare – Encephalitis has developed in very young infants; only 2 cases have been reported in the US. One death has been reported.

Anaphylaxis – Anaphylaxis may occur, even in individuals with no history of hypersensitivity to any vaccine component (see Warnings).

Patient Information

Advise vaccinated people to take personal precautions to reduce exposure to mosquito bites. Travelers should stay in screened or air conditioned rooms, use insecticidal space sprays as necessary, and use mosquito repellents and protective clothing to avoid mosquito bites.

HEPATITIS B VACCINE, RECOMBINANT

Rx	**Recombivax HB** (Merck)	**Injection (adult formulation):** 10 mcg hepatitis B surface antigen/mL[1]	In 1 mL single-dose vials, 3 mL multi-dose vials, and 1 mL prefilled single-dose syringes.
		Injection (pediatric/adolescent formulation): 5 mcg hepatitis B surface antigen/0.5 mL	Preservative free. In 0.5 mL single-dose vials.
		Injection (dialysis formulation): 40 mcg hepatitis B surface antigen/mL[1]	In 1 mL single-dose vials.
Rx	**Engerix-B** (GlaxoSmithKline)	**Injection (adult formulation):** 20 mcg hepatitis B surface antigen/mL[2]	Preservative free. In single-dose vials.
		Injection (pediatric/adolescent formulation): 10 mcg hepatitis B surface antigen/0.5 mL[3]	Preservative free. In single-dose vials and prefilled syringes.

[1] With thimerosal 50 mcg/mL.
[2] With thimerosal (< 1 mcg mercury).
[3] With thimerosal (< 0.5 mcg mercury).

For additional information, refer to the Agents for Active Immunization introduction.

Indications

▶*Immunization:* For immunization against infection caused by all known subtypes of hepatitis B virus. Because hepatitis D virus (also called the delta agent) can only infect and cause illness in people infected with hepatitis B, immunity to hepatitis B also protects against hepatitis D.

▶*Vaccination:* Vaccination is recommended in people of all ages, especially those at increased risk of exposure with hepatitis B virus.

Health care personnel – Dentists; oral surgeons; physicians; surgeons; podiatrists; nurses; paramedical and ambulance personnel and custodial staff who may be exposed via blood or patient specimens; dental hygienists and nurses; blood bank and plasma fractionation workers; laboratory personnel handling blood, its products, and patient specimens; dental, medical, and nursing students; and hospital cleaning staff who handle potentially infectious waste.

Selected patients and patient contacts – Patients and staff in hemodialysis units and hematology/oncology units; hemodialysis patients and patients with early renal failure before they require hemodialysis; patients requiring frequent or large volume blood transfusions or clotting factor concentrates (eg, people with hemophilia, thalassemia, sickle cell anemia, cirrhosis; residents and staff of institutions for the mentally handicapped; classroom contacts of deinstitutionalized mentally handicapped people who have persistent hepatitis B antigenemia and who show aggressive behavior; household and other intimate contacts of people with persistent hepatitis B antigenemia.

Adolescents – Because a vaccination strategy limited to high-risk individuals has failed to substantially lower the overall incidence of hepatitis B infection, both the Advisory Committee on Immunization Practices (ACIP) and the Committee on Infectious Diseases of the American Academy of Pediatrics (AAP) have endorsed universal infant immunization as part of a comprehensive strategy for the control of hepatitis B infection. These advisory groups further recommend broad-based vaccination of adolescents. All individuals not receiving the hepatitis B vaccine are recommended to be vaccinated at 11 to 12 years of age. In addition, vaccination is recommended in older unvaccinated adolescents at high-risk.

Infants, including those born to hepatitis B surface antigen (HBsAg)-positive mothers whether HBsAg-positive or -negative – CDC, ACIP, and AAP recommend routine vaccination of all infants against hepatitis B.

Populations with high incidence of the disease – Alaskan natives; Pacific Islanders; Indochinese immigrants; Haitian immigrants; refugees from other HBV-endemic areas; all infants of women born in areas where the infection is highly endemic.

Individuals with chronic hepatitis C – Risk factors for hepatitis C are similar to those for hepatitis B. Consequently, immunization with hepatitis B vaccine is recommended for individuals with chronic hepatitis C.

People at increased risk because of their sexual practices – People who have heterosexual activity with multiple partners (eg, > 1 partner in a 6-month period), people who repeatedly contract sexually transmitted diseases, homosexual and bisexual adolescent and adult men, and female prostitutes.

Others at increased risk and people who are exposed to the hepatitis B virus by travel to high-risk areas – Military personnel; international travelers; morticians and embalmers; prisoners; users of illicit injectable drugs; police and fire department personnel who render first aid or medical assistance; adoptees from countries of high HBV endemicity; and any others who through their work or personal lifestyle may be exposed to the hepatitis B virus.

▶*Revaccination (booster doses):*
Adults and children with normal immune status – The antibody response to properly administered vaccine is excellent, and protection lasts for ≥ 10 years. Booster doses are not routinely recommended, nor is routine serologic testing to assess antibody levels in vaccine recipients necessary during this period.

Hemodialysis patients – The vaccine-induced protection is less complete and may persist only as long as antibody levels remain > 10 mIU/mL. Assess the need for booster doses by annual antibody testing; give booster doses when antibody levels are < 10 mIU/mL.

Vaccinated people who experience percutaneous or needle exposure to HBsAg-positive blood – Serologic testing to assess immune status is recommended unless tests previously have indicated adequate antibody levels. If inadequate levels exist, treat with HBIG and a booster dose of vaccine.

Nonresponders – Give additional doses of vaccine to people who do not develop protective levels of anti-HBs antibodies after an initial 3-dose series. Various approaches have been published involving 1 to 3 extra doses, typically at 1- to 5-month intervals. Roughly 30% to 75% of this group will respond to the second vaccination series.

▶*Unlabeled uses:* Hepatitis B vaccination is appropriate for people expected to receive human alpha-1 proteinase inhibitor that is produced from heat-treated, pooled human plasma that may contain the causative agents of hepatitis and other viral diseases.

Administration and Dosage

▶*Route and site:* For IM use. Never inject IV or ID. The deltoid muscle is the preferred site in adults. Injections given in the buttocks frequently are given into fatty tissue instead of muscle and have resulted in a lower seroconversion rate than expected. The anterolateral thigh is the recommended site in infants and young children. May be given SC to people at risk of hemorrhage following IM injection (eg, hemophiliacs). However, the SC route may produce a less than optimal response and an increased incidence of local reactions, including SC nodules, may occur.

Immunization Regimen of Hepatitis B Vaccine				
Age group	Number of doses	Schedule	*Engerix-B* dose	*Recombivax* dose[1]
Infants born of:				
HBsAg-negative mothers	3	0, 1, and 6 months	10 mcg/0.5 mL	5 mcg/0.5 mL
HBsAg-positive mothers[2]	3	0, 1, and 6 months	10 mcg/0.5 mL	5 mcg/0.5 mL
Children and adolescents 1 to 19 years of age	3	0, 1, and 6 months	10 mcg/0.5 mL	5 mcg/0.5 mL
Adolescents 11 to 15 years of age	2	0 and 4 to 6 months	N/A	10 mcg/1 mL[3]
Adults ≥ 20 years of age	3	0, 1, and 6 months	20 mcg/1 mL	10 mcg/1 mL
Adult predialysis and dialysis patients	4	0, 1, 2, and 6 months	40 mcg/2 mL[4]	N/A
	3	0, 1, and 6 months	N/A	40 mcg/1 mL

[1] If the suggested formulation is not available, the appropriate dosage can be achieved from another formulation provided that the total volume of vaccine administered does not exceed 1 mL. However, the dialysis formulation only may be used in adult dialysis patients.
[2] If the mother is determined to be HBsAg-positive within 7 days of delivery, immediately administer HBIG (0.5 mL) in the opposite anterolateral thigh of the infant.
[3] Adolescents (11 to 15 years of age) may receive either of the following regimens: the 3 × 5 mcg (pediatric/adolescent) or the 2 × 10 mcg (adult formulation).
[4] Two × 20 mcg in 1 or 2 injections.

▶*Alternate schedule:*

Engerix-B – Designed for certain populations (eg, neonates born of hepatitis B-infected mothers, others who have or might have been recently exposed to the virus, certain travelers to high-risk areas). On this alternate schedule, an additional dose at 12 months is recommended for prolonged maintenance of protective titers.

Alternate Dosage and Administration Schedules		
Age group	Dose	Schedules
Infants born of:		
HBsAG-positive mothers	10 mcg/0.5 mL	0, 1, 2, 12 months
Children:		

HEPATITIS B VACCINE, RECOMBINANT

Alternate Dosage and Administration Schedules		
Age group	Dose	Schedules
Birth through 10 years of age	10 mcg/0.5 mL	0, 1, 2, 12 months
5 through 10 years of age	10 mcg/0.5 mL	0, 12, 24 months[1]
Adolescents:		
11 through 16 years of age	10 mcg/0.5 mL	0, 12, 24 months[1]
11 through 19 years of age	20 mcg/1 mL	0, 1, 6 months
11 through 19 years of age	20 mcg/1 mL	0, 1, 2, 12 months
Adults (> 19 years of age)	20 mcg/1 mL	0, 1, 2, 12 months

[1] For children and adolescents for whom an extended administration schedule is acceptable based on risk of exposure.

Recombivax HB – An alternate schedule has been recommended outside the product labeling. Give doses at 0, 1, and 2 months to provide rapid induction of immunity. On this alternate schedule, give an additional dose 12 months after the first dose if prolonged protection is needed.

➤*Postexposure prophylaxis:* Also see the HBIG monograph. In response to known or presumed exposure to hepatitis B surface antigen (eg, needlestick; ocular or mucous-membrane exposure; human bites that penetrate the skin; sexual contact; infants born of HBsAg-positive mothers), give previously unvaccinated people postexposure prophylaxis. This consists of 0.06 mL/kg HBIG as soon as possible or within 24 hours after exposure, if possible (within 14 days in the case of sexual contact). Give the appropriate volume of either hepatitis B vaccine based on age within 7 days of exposure, and additional vaccine doses (see above tables).

➤*Revaccination (booster):*

Hemodialysis patients – A booster dose may be considered if the anti-HBs level is < 10 mIU/mL 1 to 2 months after the third dose. Assess need by annual antibody testing. Give 40 mcg when antibody levels decline below 10 mIU/mL.

Other populations (Engerix-B) – Whenever administration of a booster dose is appropriate, the dose of *Engerix-B* is 10 mcg for children ≤ 10 years of age, 20 mcg for adolescents 11 through 19 years of age, and 20 mcg for adults.

➤*Preparation:* Shake well before use to maintain suspension of the vaccine. After thorough agitation, the vaccine is a slightly opaque, white suspension. Use as supplied; no dilution or reconstitution is necessary.

➤*Storage/Stability:* Store at 2° to 8°C (36° to 46°F). Do not freeze; freezing destroys potency. Discard if product has been frozen.

Actions

➤*Pharmacology:* Approximately 140,000 to 320,000 hepatitis B virus infections are reported annually in the US. The infection is acquired through sexual intercourse, perinatal transmission, and parenteral exposure, but horizontal transmission is common among young children. Those individuals at increased risk of infection include the following: IV drug users; sexually active heterosexuals; homosexual men; infants/children of immigrants from disease-endemic areas; low socioeconomic level; sexual/household contacts of infected individuals; infants born to infected mothers; health care workers; hemodialysis patients (see Indications).

In > 95% of healthy adults, infection is self-limited and resolution is indicated by the serologic appearance of anti-HBs. Cellular responses to several viral proteins correlate with disease severity and viral clearance. Clinical features associated with hepatitis B infection include jaundice, fatigue, abdominal pain, anorexia, intermittent nausea, and vomiting. Serious pathologic changes in the liver may result, such as acute massive hepatic necrosis, chronic active hepatitis, cirrhosis of the liver, and an increased risk of developing primary hepatocellular carcinoma.

Currently, there is no specific treatment for acute hepatitis B infection. However, studies have demonstrated that individuals who develop anti-HBs following active infection with the hepatitis B virus are protected against the disease upon re-exposure to the virus. Considering the serious consequences of infection, the recommended strategy is to vaccinate all patients at potential risk of exposure.

The recombinant hepatitis B vaccine is derived from HBsAg produced in yeast cells and are free of association with human blood or blood products. It induces protective anti-HBs antibodies in 95% to 99% of healthy infants, children, and young adults receiving the recommended 3-dose regimen. Lack of responsiveness to the vaccine can be attributed to genetic predisposition (eg, recessive trait associated with the major

histocompatibility complex [MHC]), male gender, obesity, smoking, gluteal vaccination, SC injection, freezing of vaccine, accelerated schedule, age > 40 years, and immunocompromised and immunosuppressed individuals. Antibody titers ≥ 10 mIU/mL against HBsAg are recognized as conferring protection against hepatitis B; seroconversion is defined as antibody titers ≥ 1 mIU/mL. Duration of the protective effect of the vaccine is unknown.

Interchangeability with hepatitis B vaccines – It is possible to interchange the use of vaccines for completion of a series or for booster doses because studies indicate the antibody produced in response to each type of vaccine is comparable. However, the quantity of antigen or the dosage volume will vary.

Contraindications

Anaphylactic hypersensitivity to yeast or any component of the vaccines.

Warnings

➤*Immunosuppressed patients:* As with any vaccine administered to immunosuppressed people or people receiving immunosuppressive therapy, the expected immune response may not be obtained. For individuals receiving immunosuppressive therapy, deferral of vaccination for ≥ 3 months after therapy may be considered.

➤*Unrecognized hepatitis B infection:* Unrecognized hepatitis B infection may be present at the time the vaccine is given, and the vaccine may not prevent hepatitis B in such patients because of the long incubation period. Additionally, it may not prevent infection in individuals who do not achieve protective antibody titers.

➤*Limitations:* No hepatitis B vaccine will protect against hepatitis A, C, and E viruses, or other viruses known to infect the liver.

➤*Hypersensitivity reactions:* Have epinephrine immediately available for use in case of anaphylaxis or anaphylactoid reaction. Refer to Management of Acute Hypersensitivity Reactions.

➤*Pregnancy: Category C.* Problems in vaccination of pregnant women have not been reported and are unlikely. Use if the woman is likely to be exposed to hepatitis B virus during or after pregnancy.

➤*Lactation:* Problems in lactating women have not been reported and are unlikely. Empirical evidence suggests no harm.

➤*Children:* Hepatitis B vaccine is well tolerated and highly immunogenic in infants and children of all ages. Newborns also respond well; maternally transferred antibodies do not interfere with the active immune response to the vaccine.

Precautions

➤*Infection:* Serious active infection, including febrile illness, is reason to delay use of hepatitis B vaccine, except when withholding the vaccine entails a greater risk. Minor illnesses, such as mild upper respiratory infections with or without low-grade fever, are not contraindications.

➤*Special risk patients:* Exercise caution and appropriate care in administering the vaccine to individuals with severely compromised cardiopulmonary status or to others in whom a febrile or systemic reaction could pose a significant risk.

➤*Multiple sclerosis (MS):* Although no causal relationship has been established, rare instances of MS exacerbation have been reported following administration of hepatitis B vaccines and other vaccines. In people with MS, the benefit of immunization for prevention of hepatitis B infection and sequelae must be weighed against the risk of disease exacerbation.

Drug Interactions

➤*Other vaccines:* ACIP states that, in general, simultaneous administration of certain live and inactivated pediatric vaccines has not resulted in impaired antibody responses or increased rates of adverse reactions. Use separate sites and syringes for simultaneous administration of injectable vaccines.

Hepatitis B Vaccine (HBV) Drug Interactions			
Precipitant drug	Object drug*		Description
Immunosuppressants	HBV	↓	Administration of HBV to people receiving immunosuppressant drugs, including high-dose corticosteroids or radiation therapy, may result in an inadequate response to immunization.
HBV	Yellow fever vaccine	↓	In 1 study, concurrent vaccination against hepatitis B and yellow fever viruses reduced the antibody titer otherwise expected from yellow fever vaccine. Separate these vaccines by a month, if possible.

HEPATITIS B VACCINE, RECOMBINANT

Hepatitis B Vaccine (HBV) Drug Interactions			
Precipitant drug	Object drug*		Description
Interleukin-2	HBV	⟷	Natural interleukin 2 may boost systemic immune response to HBsAg in immunodeficient nonresponders to hepatitis B vaccination, but recombinant interleukin 2 did not augment response to hepatitis B vaccine in healthy adults in 1 study.

* ↓ = Object drug decreased. ⟷ = Undetermined clinical effect.

Adverse Reactions

The National Childhood Vaccine Injury Act requires that the manufacturer and lot number of the vaccine administered be recorded by the health care provider in the vaccine recipient's permanent medical record, along with the date of administration of the vaccine and the name, address, and title of the person administering the vaccine. The act further requires the health care provider to report to the US Department of Health and Human Services via the Vaccine Adverse Event Reporting System (VAERS) the occurrence following immunization of any event set forth in the Vaccine Injury Table, including the following: Anaphylaxis or anaphylactic shock within 4 hours, encephalopathy or encephalitis within 72 hours, or any sequelae thereof (including death). In addition, any event considered a contraindication to further doses should be reported. The VAERS toll-free number is 1-800-822-7967.

➤*CNS:* Headache; lightheadedness; vertigo; dizziness; paresthesia; insomnia/disturbed sleep; radiculopathy; encephalitis; somnolence; irritability; agitation; migraine; syncope; paresis; neuropathy including hypesthesia, seizures, Guillain-Barré syndrome, Bell's palsy; transverse myelitis; optic neuritis; MS.

➤*Dermatologic:* Pruritus; rash; urticaria; petechiae; erythema and erythema nodosum; eczema; purpura; herpes zoster; alopecia.

➤*GI:* Nausea; vomiting; abdominal pain/cramps; dyspepsia; constipation; anorexia; diarrhea; abnormal liver function tests.

➤*Hypersensitivity:* Anaphylaxis; Stevens-Johnson syndrome; angioedema; arthritis. An apparent hypersensitivity syndrome (serum-sickness-like) of delayed onset has been reported days to weeks after vaccination, including arthritis (usually transient) and erythema multiforme.

➤*Local:* Injection site soreness; erythema; swelling; warmth; induration; tenderness; pruritus; pain; ecchymosis; nodule formation.

➤*Musculoskeletal:* Arthralgia; myalgia; back, neck, arm, and shoulder pain/stiffness; muscle weakness.

➤*Respiratory:* Upper respiratory tract infection; influenza-like symptoms; bronchospasm including asthma-like symptoms; pharyngitis; rhinitis; cough.

➤*Miscellaneous:* Fatigue; lymphadenopathy; tinnitus; earache; hypotension; dysuria; increased erythrocyte sedimentation rate; systemic lupus erythematosus; lupus-like syndrome; vasculitis; tachycardia/palpitations; hypertension; thrombocytopenia; conjunctivitis; keratitis; visual disturbances; weakness; fever ($\geq$ 37.5°C; 100°F); malaise; sweating; achiness; sensation of warmth; chills; flushing; tingling.

Patient Information

Inform patients, parents, or guardians of the potential benefits and risks of the vaccine and of the importance of completing the immunization series. As with any vaccine, it is important when a subject returns for the next dose in a series that he or she be questioned concerning occurrence of any symptoms or signs of an adverse reaction after a previous dose of the same vaccine. Tell patients, parents, or guardians to report severe or unusual adverse reactions to their health care provider.

HEPATITIS A VACCINE, INACTIVATED

Rx	Havrix (GlaxoSmithKline)	Injection (pediatric formulation): 360 EL.U. of viral antigen/0.5 mL[1]	In single-dose vials.
		Injection (pediatric formulation): 720 EL.U. of viral antigen/0.5 mL[1]	In single-dose vials and prefilled syringes.
		Injection (adult formulation): 1440 EL.U. of viral antigen/1 mL[1]	In single-dose vials.
Rx	Vaqta (Merck)	Injection (pediatric/adolescent): 25 U hepatitis A virus antigen/0.5 mL	In single-dose vials and prefilled syringes.
		Injection (adult): 50 U hepatitis A virus antigen/1 mL	In single-dose vials and prefilled syringes.

[1] EL.U. = ELISA (enzyme linked immunosorbent assay) Units.

For additional information, refer to the Agents for Active Immunization introduction.

Indications

➤*Hepatitis A virus (HAV):* For active immunization of people $\geq$ 2 years of age against disease caused by HAV.

➤*Primary immunization:* Primary immunization should be completed at least 2 weeks prior to expected exposure to HAV. Immunization with hepatitis A vaccine is indicated for those desiring protection against hepatitis A who are, or will be, at increased risk of HAV infection:

Travelers – People traveling to areas of higher endemicity for hepatitis A. These areas include, but are not limited to, Africa, Asia (except Japan), the Mediterranean basin, Eastern Europe, the Middle East, Central and South America, Mexico, and parts of the Caribbean. Consult current CDC advisories with regard to specific locales.

Populations with high incidence of the disease – Native peoples of Alaska and the Americas.

People with chronic liver disease – Alcoholic cirrhosis; chronic hepatitis B; chronic hepatitis C; autoimmune hepatitis; primary biliary cirrhosis.

People exposed to hepatitis A – For those requiring both immediate and long-term protection, hepatitis A vaccine may be administered concomitantly with immune globulin (IG).

People at increased risk because of their employment – Certain institutional workers (eg, caretakers for the developmentally challenged); employees of child day care centers; laboratory workers who handle live hepatitis A virus; handlers of primate animals that may be harboring HAV.

Others at increased risk – People engaging in high-risk sexual activity (such as homosexually active males); users of illicit injectable drugs; residents of a community experiencing an outbreak of hepatitis A; military personnel; people living in or relocating to areas of high endemicity; hemophiliacs and other recipients of therapeutic blood products.

Administration and Dosage

➤*Approved by the FDA:* February 22, 1995 (*Havrix*) and March 29, 1996 (*Vaqta*).

For IM use. Do not inject IV, ID, or SC. In adults, give the injection in the deltoid region. Do not administer in the gluteal region; such injections may result in suboptimal response.

Dosing Regimens for Hepatitis A Vaccine				
Age	Vaccine	Dose	Number of doses	Schedule (in months)
Children (2 to 18 years of age)	Havrix	360 EL.U. (0.5 mL)	3	0, 1, and 6 to 12 mos later
	Havrix	720 EL.U. (0.5 mL)	2	0 and 6 to 12 mos later
	Vaqta	25 U (0.5 mL)	2	0 and 6 to 18 mos later
Adults ($\geq$ 19 years of age)	Havrix	1440 EL.U. (1 mL)	2	0 and 6 to 12 mos later
	Vaqta	50 U (1 mL)	2	0 and 6 to 12 mos later

Do not alternate between the 360 EL.U. and 720 EL.U. doses. Those who receive an initial 360 EL.U. dose should continue on the 360 EL.U. dosing schedule. Likewise, those who receive a single 720 EL.U. primary dose should receive a 720 EL.U. booster dose.

➤*Interchangeability of the booster dose:* A booster dose of *Vaqta* may be given at 6 to 12 months following the initial dose of other inactivated hepatitis A vaccines (eg, *Havrix*).

➤*Preparation:* Shake vial/syringe well before withdrawal and use. With thorough agitation, the vaccine is a turbid white suspension. Discard if it appears otherwise.

Use the vaccine as supplied; no dilution or reconstitution is necessary. Use the full recommended dose of the vaccine.

➤*Storage/Stability:* Store between 2° and 8°C (36° and 46°F). Do not freeze; discard if product has been frozen. Do not dilute to administer.

Actions

➤*Pharmacology:* HAV belongs to the picornavirus family. Only 1 serotype of HAV has been described.

Hepatitis A is highly contagious, and the predominant mode of transmission is person-to-person via the fecal-oral route. Infection has been shown to be spread (1) by contaminated water or food; (2) by infected

HEPATITIS A VACCINE, INACTIVATED

food handlers; (3) after breakdown in usual sanitary conditions or after floods or natural disasters; (4) by ingestion of raw or undercooked shellfish (eg, oysters, clams, mussels) from contaminated waters; (5) during travel to areas of the world with poor hygienic conditions; (6) among institutionalized adults and children; (7) in day care centers where children have not been toilet trained; (8) by parenteral transmission, either through blood transfusions or sharing needles with infected people. Sexual transmission has also been reported.

The level of economic development influences the prevalence of hepatitis A and the age at which it is most likely to occur. In developing countries with poor hygiene and sanitation, ≈ 90% of children are infected by 5 years of age. As conditions improve, the prevalence decreases and the age at which infection occurs increases. Hence, it is more likely to occur in adulthood, when disease is generally more severe and more likely to be fatal. In the US, attack rates for hepatitis A infection are cyclical and vary by population. The rates have increased gradually from 9.2 per 100,000 in 1983 to 14.6 per 100,000 in 1989.

The incubation period for hepatitis A averages 28 days (range, 15 to 50 days). The course of hepatitis A infection is extremely variable, ranging from asymptomatic infection to icteric hepatitis. However, most infected adults (76% to 97%) become symptomatic. Symptoms range from mild and transient to severe and prolonged and may include fever, nausea, vomiting, and diarrhea in the prodromal phase, followed by jaundice in up to 88% of adults, as well as hepatomegaly and biochemical evidence of hepatocellular damage. Recovery is generally complete and followed by protection against HAV infection. However, illness may be prolonged and relapse of clinical illness and viral shedding have been described.

Hepatitis A infection is often asymptomatic in children < 2 years of age, who nonetheless excrete the virus in their stool and thereby serve as a source of infection. In older patients and those with underlying liver disease, it is generally much more severe. This is reflected in mortality rates. While an overall case fatality rate of 0.6% has been reported, death occurs in 2.7% of patients ≥ 49 years of age. While 67% of cases occur in children, > 70% of deaths occur in those > 49 years of age.

There is no chronic carrier state. The virus replicates in the liver and is excreted in bile. The highest concentrations of HAV are found in stools of infected individuals during the 2-week period immediately before the onset of jaundice and decline after jaundice appears. Children and infants may shed HAV for longer periods than adults, possibly lasting as long as several weeks after the onset of clinical illness. Chronic shedding of HAV in feces has not been demonstrated, but relapses of hepatitis A can occur in as many as 20% of patients; fecal shedding of HAV may recur at this time.

Contraindications

Hypersensitivity to any component of the vaccine.

Warnings

➤*Hepatitis:* Hepatitis A vaccine will not prevent hepatitis caused by other agents, such as hepatitis B, C, or E virus or other pathogens known to infect the liver.

➤*Pre-existing infection/antibody development:* Hepatitis A vaccine may not prevent hepatitis A infection in individuals who have an unrecognized hepatitis A infection at the time of vaccination. Additionally, it may not prevent infection in individuals who do not achieve protective antibody titers (although the lowest titer needed to confer protection has not been determined).

➤*Hypersensitivity reactions:* Anaphylaxis/anaphylactoid reactions following commercial use of the vaccine in other countries have been reported rarely. Patients experiencing hypersensitivity reactions after a hepatitis A vaccine injection should not receive further hepatitis A vaccine injections. Have epinephrine available for use in case of anaphylaxis or anaphylactoid reaction.

➤*Pregnancy:* Category C. Safety for use during pregnancy has not been established. Use only when clearly needed.

➤*Lactation:* It is not known whether the vaccine is excreted in breast milk. Exercise caution when administering to a nursing woman.

➤*Children:* Hepatitis A vaccine is well tolerated and highly immunogenic and effective in children ≥ 2 years of age.

Precautions

➤*Acute infection/febrile illness:* Acute infection or febrile illness is reason to delay use of hepatitis A vaccine, except when withholding the vaccine entails a greater risk.

➤*Bleeding disorders:* Administer cautiously to people with thrombocytopenia or a bleeding disorder, as bleeding may occur following IM use.

➤*Immunosuppression:* Immunosuppressed people, those with malignancies, or those receiving immunosuppressive therapy may not obtain the expected immune response. In those with an impaired immune system, adequate anti-HAV response may not be obtained after the primary immunization course. Therefore, such patients may require administration of additional doses of vaccine.

Drug Interactions

➤*Concomitant agents:* Hepatitis A vaccine may be administered concomitantly with IG, although the ultimate antibody titer obtained is likely to be lower than when the vaccine is given alone. *Havrix* has been administered simultaneously with *Engerix-B* without interference with their respective immune responses. When concomitant administration of other vaccines or IG is required, give them with different syringes and at different injection sites.

Adverse Reactions

The US Department of Health and Human Services has established the Vaccine Adverse Events Reporting System (VAERS) to accept reports of suspected adverse events after the administration of any vaccine, including, but not limited to, the reporting of events required by the National Childhood Vaccine Injury Act of 1986. The toll-free number for VAERS forms and information is 1-800-822-7967.

Hepatitis A vaccine is generally well tolerated. The frequency of solicited adverse events tended to decrease with successive doses of hepatitis A vaccine. Most events reported were considered by the subjects as mild and did not last for > 24 hours.

➤*CNS:* Headache; hypertonic episode; insomnia; photophobia; vertigo; convulsions; encephalopathy; dizziness; neuropathy; myelitis; paresthesia; multiple sclerosis; Guillain-Barré syndrome (rare).

➤*Dermatologic:* Pruritus; rash; urticaria; erythema multiforme; hyperhydrosis; generalized erythema; dermatitis; angioedema (rare).

➤*GI:* Anorexia; nausea; abdominal pain; diarrhea; dysgeusia; vomiting.

➤*Local:* Injection site soreness; injection site pain; tenderness; warmth; induration; redness; swelling; hematoma; ecchymosis; injection site pruritus or rash; localized edema (rare).

➤*Musculoskeletal:* Arthralgia; elevation of creatine phosphokinase; myalgia; arm and back pain; stiffness.

➤*Respiratory:* Pharyngitis; cough; other upper respiratory tract infections; nasal congestion; bronchial constriction; asthma; wheezing; dyspnea (rare).

➤*Miscellaneous:* Fatigue; fever (> 37.5°C; 99.5°F); malaise; lymphadenopathy; menstruation disorder; congenital abnormality; jaundice; hepatitis; syncope; anaphylaxis/anaphylactoid reactions; edema; eye irritation/itching; somnolence (rare).

Patient Information

Fully inform patients, parents, or guardians of the benefits and risks of immunization.

Hepatitis A vaccine is indicated in a variety of situations. For people traveling to endemic or epidemic areas, consult current CDC advisories with regard to specific locales.

Travelers should take all necessary precautions to avoid contact with or ingestion of contaminated food or water.

The duration of immunity following a complete schedule of immunization with hepatitis A vaccine has not been established.

HEPATITIS A, INACTIVATED AND HEPATITIS B, RECOMBINANT VACCINE

| Rx | Twinrix (GlaxoSmithKline) | Injection: ≥ 720 EL.U.[1] inactivated hepatitis A, 20 mcg recombinant HBsAg[2] protein/mL[3] | In single-dose vials (1s and 10s). |

[1] EL.U. = ELISA (enzyme linked immunosorbent assay) units.
[2] HBsAg = Hepatitis B surface antigen.
[3] With thimerosal (< 1 mcg mercury).

For additional information, refer to the Agents for Active Immunization introduction and the individual Hepatitis A, Inactivated and Hepatitis B, Recombinant monographs.

Indications

➤*Hepatitis A and B viruses:* For active immunization of people ≥ 18 years of age against disease caused by hepatitis A virus (HAV) and infection by all known subtypes of hepatitis B virus (HBV). As with any vaccine, vaccination with this product may not protect 100% of recipients. As hepatitis D (caused by the delta virus) does not occur in the absence of HBV infection, it can be expected that hepatitis D also will be prevented by vaccination.

Vaccination will not prevent hepatitis caused by other agents, such as hepatitis C virus, hepatitis E virus, or other pathogens known to infect the liver.

Immunization is recommended for all susceptible people ≥ 18 years of age who are or will be at risk of exposure to hepatitis A and B viruses, including, but not limited to, the following: Travelers to areas of high/

HEPATITIS A, INACTIVATED AND HEPATITIS B, RECOMBINANT VACCINE

intermediate endemicity for HAV and HBV (see table) who are at increased risk of HBV infection because of behavioral or occupational factors.

Hepatitis A and B Endemicity by Region		
Geographic region	HAV	HBV
Africa	high	high (most)
Caribbean	high	intermediate
Central America	high	intermediate
South America (temperate)	high	intermediate
South America (tropical)	high	high
South and Southeast Asia[1]	high	high
Middle East[2]	high	high
Eastern Europe	intermediate	intermediate
Southern Europe	intermediate	intermediate
Former Soviet Union	intermediate	intermediate

[1] Japan: Low HAV and intermediate HBV endemicity.
[2] Israel: Intermediate HBV endemicity.

Patients with chronic liver disease – Patients with chronic liver disease, including alcoholic cirrhosis, chronic hepatitis C, autoimmune hepatitis, and primary biliary cirrhosis.

People at risk through their work – Laboratory workers who handle live hepatitis A and hepatitis B viruses, police, and other personnel who render first-aid or medical assistance, workers who come in contact with feces or sewage.

People exposed to HAV and HBV – Health care personnel who render first-aid or emergency medical assistance; personnel employed in day care centers and correctional facilities; residents of drug and alco-

hol treatment centers; staff of hemodialysis units; people living in, or relocating to, areas of high/intermediate endemicity of HAV and who have risk factors for HBV; men who have sex with men; people at increased risk of disease because of their sexual practices; patients frequently receiving blood products, including people who have clotting-factor disorders (hemophiliacs and other recipients of therapeutic blood products); military recruits and other military personnel at increased risk for HBV; users of injectable illicit drugs; individuals who are at increased risk for HBV infection and who are close household contacts of patients with acute or relapsing hepatitis A; individuals who are at increased risk for HAV infection and who are close household contacts of individuals with acute or chronic hepatitis B infection.

Administration and Dosage

➤*Approved by the FDA:* May 11, 2001.

➤*Vaccination schedule:* Primary immunization for adults consists of 3 doses, given on a 0-, 1-, and 6-month schedule.

➤*Administration:* Administer by IM injection. Do not inject IV or ID. In adults, give the injection in the deltoid region. Do not administer in the gluteal region; such injections may result in a suboptimal response.

When concomitant administration of other vaccines or immunoglobulin is required, give with different syringes and at different injection sites.

➤*Preparation:* Shake vial or syringe well before withdrawal and use. Visually inspect parenteral drug products for particulate matter or discoloration prior to administration. With thorough agitation, the vaccine is a slightly turbid white suspension. Discard if it appears otherwise.

Use vaccine as supplied; no dilution or reconstitution is necessary. Use the full recommended dose of the vaccine. After removal of the appropriate volume from a single-dose vial, discard any vaccine remaining in the vial.

➤*Storage/Stability:* Store refrigerated between 2° and 8°C (36° and 46°F). Do not freeze; discard if product has been frozen. Do not dilute to administer.

VARICELLA VIRUS VACCINE

Rx	Varivax (Merck)	**Powder for Injection:** 1350 PFU of Oka/ Merck varicella virus (live)	Sucrose. In single-dose vials of 1s and 10s.

For additional information, refer to the Agents for Active Immunization introduction.

Indications

➤*Varicella:* Vaccination against varicella in individuals ≥ 12 months of age.

Administration and Dosage

For SC administration; the outer aspect of the upper arm (deltoid) is the preferred site of injection. Do not inject IV. During clinical trials, some children received varicella vaccine IM resulting in seroconversion rates similar to those in children who received the vaccine by the SC route. Persistence of antibody and efficacy in those receiving IM injections have not been defined.

➤*Children (1 to 12 years of age):* A single 0.5 mL dose administered SC.

➤*Adults and adolescents (≥ 13 years of age):* A 0.5 mL dose administered SC at elected date and a second 0.5 mL dose 4 to 8 weeks later.

➤*Reconstitution of vaccine:* To reconstitute the vaccine, first withdraw 0.7 mL of diluent into the syringe to be used for reconstitution. Inject all the diluent in the syringe into the vial of lyophilized vaccine and gently agitate to mix thoroughly. Withdraw the entire contents into a syringe, change the needle and inject the total volume (≈ 0.5 mL) of reconstituted vaccine. It is recommended that the vaccine be administered immediately after reconstitution to minimize loss of potency. Discard if reconstituted vaccine is not used within 30 minutes. Caution: Use a sterile syringe free of preservatives, antiseptics, and detergents for each injection or reconstitution of varicella vaccine because these substances may inactivate the vaccine virus. It is important to use a separate sterile syringe and needle for each patient to prevent transmission of infectious agents from one individual to another. To reconstitute the vaccine, use only the diluent supplied, as it is free of preservatives or other antiviral substances that might inactivate the vaccine virus. Do not freeze reconstituted vaccine. Do not give immune globulin (including VZIG) concurrently. When reconstituted, varicella vaccine is a clear, colorless to pale yellow liquid.

➤*Storage/Stability:* Varicella vaccine retains a potency level of ≥ 1500 PFU per dose for at least 18 months in a frostfree freezer with an average temperature of -15°C (5°F) or colder. Varicella vaccine has a minimum potency level of ≈ 1350 PFU 30 minutes after reconstitution at room temperature (20° to 25°C; 68° to 77°F). For information regarding stability at temperatures other than those recommended for storage, call 1-800-9-VARIVAX. During shipment, to ensure that there is no loss of potency, the vaccine must be maintained at a temperature of -20°C (-4°F) or colder. Before reconstitution, store the lyophilized vaccine in a freezer at an average temperature of -15°C (5°F) or colder. Storage in a frostfree freezer with an average temperature of -15°C

(5°F) or colder is acceptable. Before reconstitution, protect from light. Store the diluent separately at room temperature or in the refrigerator.

Actions

➤*Pharmacology:* Varicella virus vaccine is a preparation of the Oka/Merck strain of live, attenuated varicella virus. The virus was initially obtained from a child with natural varicella, then introduced into human embryonic lung cell cultures, adapted to and propagated in embryonic guinea pig cell cultures, and finally propagated in human diploid cell cultures.

Varicella is a highly communicable disease in children, adolescents and adults caused by the varicella-zoster virus. The disease usually consists of 300 to 500 maculopapular or vesicular lesions accompanied by a fever (oral temperature > 37.8°C or > 100°F) in up to 70% of individuals. Approximately 3.5 million cases of varicella occurred annually from 1980 to 1994 in the US with the peak incidence occurring in children 5 to 9 years of age. The incidence rate of chickenpox is 8.3% to 9.1% per year in children 1 to 9 years of age. The attack rate of natural varicella following household exposure among healthy susceptible children was shown to be 87%. Although it is generally a benign, self-limiting disease, varicella may be associated with serious complications (eg, bacterial superinfection, pneumonia, encephalitis, Reye's syndrome) or death.

➤*Clinical trials:*

Children – The majority of subjects who received varicella vaccine and were exposed to wild-type virus were either completely protected from chickenpox or developed a milder form of the disease.

In clinical trials with the current vaccine, it was observed that 0.2% to 1% of vaccinees per year reported breakthrough chickenpox for up to 3 years after single-dose vaccination. This represents an ≈ 93% decrease from the total number of cases expected based on attack rates in children 1 to 9 years of age over this same period (8.3% to 9.1%). In those who developed breakthrough chickenpox postvaccination, the majority experienced mild disease.

Among a subset of vaccinees who were actively followed, 259 were exposed to an individual with chickenpox in a household setting. There were no reports of breakthrough chickenpox in 80% of exposed children; 20% reported a mild form of chickenpox. This represents a 77% reduction in the expected number of cases when compared with the historical attack rate of 87% in unvaccinated individuals following household exposure to chickenpox.

In one trial, a single dose of varicella vaccine protected 96% to 100% of children against chickenpox over a 2-year period. The study enrolled healthy individuals 1 to 14 years of age (vaccine, n = 491; placebo, n = 465). In the first year, 8.5% of placebo recipients contracted chickenpox, while no vaccine recipient did, for a calculated protection rate of 100% during the first varicella season. In the second year, when only a subset

VARICELLA VIRUS VACCINE

of individuals agreed to remain in the blinded study (vaccine, n = 163; placebo, n = 161), 96% protective efficacy was calculated for the vaccine group as compared with placebo.

Adults/Adolescents – In up to 2 years of active follow-up, 17 of 64 (27%) vaccinees reported breakthrough chickenpox following household exposure; of the 17 cases, 12 (71%) reported < 50 lesions, 5 reported 50 to 300 lesions and none reported > 300 lesions with an oral temperature > 100°F. In combined clinical studies of adolescents and adults (n = 1019) who received 2 doses of varicella vaccine and later developed breakthrough chickenpox (42 of 1019), 60% reported < 50 lesions, 38% reported 50 to 300 lesions and 2% reported > 300 lesions and an oral temperature > 100°F.

When compared with the previously reported attack rate of natural varicella of 87% following household exposure among unvaccinated children, this represents an ≈ 70% reduction in the expected number of cases in the household setting.

Immunogenicity – Seroconversion as defined by the acquisition of any detectable varicella antibodies was observed in 97% of vaccinees at ≈ 4 to 6 weeks postvaccination in 6889 susceptible children 12 months to 12 years of age. Rates of breakthrough disease were significantly lower among children having varicella antibody titers > 5 compared with children having titers < 5. Titers > 5 were induced in ≈ 76% of children vaccinated with a single dose of vaccine. In a multicenter study involving susceptible adolescents and adults 13 years of age and older, 2 doses of varicella vaccine administered 4 to 8 weeks apart induced a seroconversion rate of ≈ 75% in 539 individuals 4 weeks after the first dose and of 99% in 479 individuals 4 weeks after the second dose. The average antibody response in vaccinees who received the second dose 8 weeks after the first dose was higher than that in those who received the second dose 4 weeks after the first dose. In another multicenter study involving adolescents and adults, 2 doses of varicella vaccine administered 8 weeks apart induced a seroconversion rate of 94% in 142 individuals 6 weeks after the first dose, 99% in 142 individuals 6 weeks after the first dose and 99% in 122 individuals 6 weeks after the second dose.

Persistence of immune response – Studies in vaccinees examining chickenpox breakthrough rates over 5 years showed the lowest rates (0.2% to 2.9%) in the first 2 years postvaccination, with somewhat higher but stable rates in years 3 through 5. The severity of reported breakthrough chickenpox, as measured by number of lesions and maximum temperature, appeared not to increase with time.

In clinical studies involving healthy children who received 1 dose of vaccine, detectable varicella antibodies were present in 98.8% at 1 year, 98.9% at 2 years, 97.5% at 3 years, and 99.5% at 4 years postvaccination. Antibody levels were present at least 1 year in 97.2% of healthy adolescents and adults who received 2 doses of live varicella vaccine separated by 4 to 8 weeks.

Herpes Zoster – Eight cases of herpes zoster have been reported in children during 44,994 person-years of follow-up in clinical trials, resulting in a calculated incidence of at least 18 cases per 100,000 person-years. One case of herpes zoster has been reported in the adolescent and adult age group during 7826 person-years of follow-up in clinical trials resulting in a calculated incidence of 12.8 cases per 100,000 person-years. All 9 cases were mild and without sequelae.

Contraindications

Hypersensitivity to any component of the vaccine, including gelatin; history of anaphylactoid reaction to neomycin (each dose of reconstituted vaccine contains trace quantities of neomycin); individuals with blood dyscrasia, leukemia, lymphomas of any type, or other malignant neoplasms affecting the bone marrow or lymphatic systems; concomitant immunosuppressive therapy (see Drug Interactions); individuals with primary and acquired immunodeficiency states, including those who are immunosuppressed in association with AIDS or other clinical manifestations of infection with human immunodeficiency virus, cellular immune deficiencies, and hypogammaglobulinemic and dysgammaglobulinemic states; family history of congenital or hereditary immunodeficiency, unless the immune competence of the potential vaccine recipient is demonstrated; active untreated tuberculosis; any febrile respiratory illness or other active febrile infection; pregnancy (see Warnings).

Warnings

➤*Booster doses:* The duration of protection of varicella vaccine is unknown at present and the need for booster doses is not defined. However, a boost in antibody levels has been observed in vaccinees following exposure to natural varicella as well as following a booster dose of varicella vaccine administered 4 to 6 years postvaccination.

In a highly vaccinated population, immunity for some individuals may wane due to lack of exposure to natural varicella as a result of shifting epidemiology. Postmarketing surveillance studies are ongoing to evaluate the need and timing for booster vaccination.

➤*Protection/Prevention:* Vaccination with varicella vaccine may not result in protection of all healthy, susceptible children, adolescents and adults. It is not known whether varicella vaccine given immediately after exposure to natural varicella virus will prevent illness.

➤*Acute lymphoblastic leukemia (ALL):* Children and adolescents with ALL in remission can receive the vaccine under an investigational protocol. More information is available by contacting the varicella vaccine coordinating center: Bio-Pharm Clinical Services, Inc., 4 Valley Square, Blue Bell, PA 19422, (215) 283-0897.

➤*Hypersensitivity reactions:* Have adequate treatment provisions, including epinephrine injection (1:1000), available for immediate use should an anaphylactoid reaction occur. Refer to Management of Acute Hypersensitivity Reactions.

➤*Pregnancy: Category C.* It is not known whether varicella vaccine can cause fetal harm or affect reproduction capacity when administered to a pregnant woman. However, natural varicella is known to sometimes cause fetal harm. Therefore, do not administer varicella vaccine to pregnant females; furthermore, avoid pregnancy for 3 months following vaccination.

➤*Lactation:* It is not known whether varicella vaccine virus is secreted in breast milk. Therefore, because some viruses are secreted in breast milk, exercise caution if varicella vaccine is administered to a nursing woman.

➤*Children:* No clinical data are available on safety or efficacy of varicella vaccine in children < 1 year of age; administration to infants < 1 year of age is not recommended.

Precautions

➤*Reye's syndrome:* Vaccine recipients should avoid use of salicylates for 6 weeks after vaccination with varicella vaccine as Reye's syndrome has been reported following the use of salicylates during natural varicella infections.

➤*Transmission:* Individuals vaccinated with varicella vaccine may potentially be capable of transmitting the vaccine virus to close contacts. Therefore, vaccine recipients should avoid close association with susceptible high-risk individuals (eg, newborns, pregnant women, immunocompromised people). Weigh the potential risk of transmission of vaccine virus against the risk of transmission of natural varicella virus in such circumstances.

Use a separate sterile needle and syringe for administration of each dose of varicella vaccine to prevent transfer of infectious diseases. Properly dispose of needles and do not recap.

➤*Immunodeficiency:* The safety and efficacy of varicella vaccine have not been established in children and young adults who are known to be infected with human immunodeficiency viruses with and without evidence of immunosuppression. Vaccination should be deferred in patients with a family history of congenital or hereditary immunodeficiency until the patient's own immune system has been evaluated.

➤*Injection site:* Do not inject into a blood vessel.

Drug Interactions

Varicella Vaccine Drug Interactions			
Precipitant drug	Object drug*		Description
Immune globulins	Varicella vaccine	⟷	Defer vaccination for at least 5 months following blood or plasma transfusions, or administration of immune globulin or varicella-zoster immune globulin (VZIG). Following administration of varicella vaccine, do not give any immune globulin, including VZIG, for 2 months thereafter unless its use outweighs the benefits of vaccination.
Immunosuppressants	Varicella vaccine	↓	Individuals who are on immunosuppressant drugs are more susceptible to infections than healthy individuals. Vaccination with live attenuated varicella vaccine can result in a more extensive vaccine-associated rash or disseminated disease in individuals on immunosuppressant doses of corticosteroids.
Salicylates	Varicella vaccine	↑	Avoid use of salicylates for 6 weeks after varicella vaccine; Reye's syndrome has been reported following salicylate use during natural varicella infections.

* ↑ = Object drug increased. ↓ = Object drug decreased. ⟷ = Undetermined clinical effect.

➤*Concomitant vaccines:* Results from clinical studies indicate that varicella vaccine can be administered concomitantly with MMR II.

Limited data from an experimental product containing varicella vaccine suggest that varicella vaccine can be administered concomitantly with DTaP and *PedvaxHIB* (haemophilus b conjugate vaccine) using separate sites and syringes. However, there are no data relating to simultaneous administration of varicella vaccine with DTP or OPV.

VARICELLA VIRUS VACCINE

Adverse Reactions

The US Department of Health and Human Services has established a Vaccine Adverse Event Reporting System (VAERS) to accept all reports of suspected adverse events after the administration of any vaccine, including, but not limited to, the reporting of events required by the National Childhood Vaccine Injury Act of 1986. The toll-free number for VAERS forms and information is 1-800-822-7967.

In clinical trials, varicella vaccine was administered to 11,102 healthy children, adolescents and adults; the vaccine was generally well tolerated. In a study of 914 healthy children and adolescents, the only adverse reactions that occurred at a significantly greater rate in vaccine recipients than in placebo recipients were pain and redness at the injection site.

Children (1 to 12 years of age) – In clinical trials involving healthy children monitored for up to 42 days after a single dose of varicella vaccine, the frequency of fever, injection-site complaints, or rashes were reported as follows: Fever (≥ 39°C [102°F], 14.7%); injection site complaints (pain/soreness, swelling, erythema, rash, pruritus, hematoma, induration, stiffness, 19.3%); varicella-like rash (injection site, 3.4%; generalized, 3.8%).

In addition, the most frequently (> 1%) reported adverse experiences, listed in decreasing order of frequency, include the following: Upper respiratory illness; cough; irritability; nervousness; fatigue; disturbed sleep; diarrhea; loss of appetite; vomiting; otitis; diaper rash/contact rash; headache; teething; malaise; abdominal pain; other rash; nausea;

eye complaints; chills; lymphadenopathy; myalgia; lower respiratory illness; allergic reactions (including allergic rash, hives); stiff neck; heat rash/prickly heat; arthralgia; eczema/dry skin/dermatitis; constipation; itching; pneumonitis, febrile seizures (< 1%).

Adults and adolescents (≥ 13 years of age) – In clinical trials involving healthy adolescents, the majority of whom received 2 doses of varicella vaccine and were monitored for up to 42 days after any dose, the frequency of fever, injection-site complaints, or rashes were reported as follows: Fever (≥ 39°C [102°F], 9.5% to 10.2%); injection site complaints (soreness, erythema, swelling, rash, pruritus, pyrexia, hematoma, induration, numbness; 24.4% to 32.5%); varicella-like rash (injection site, 1% to 3%; generalized, 0.9% to 5.5%).

In addition, the most frequently (> 1%) reported adverse experiences, listed in decreasing order of frequency, include the following: Upper respiratory illness; headache; fatigue; cough; myalgia; disturbed sleep; nausea; malaise; diarrhea; stiff neck; irritability; nervousness; lymphadenopathy; chills; eye complaints; abdominal pain; loss of appetite; arthralgia; otitis; itching; vomiting; other rashes; constipation; lower respiratory illness; allergic reactions (including allergic rash, hives); contact rash; cold/canker sore.

Patient Information

Inform the patient, parent or guardian of the benefits and risks of varicella vaccine, and instruct them to report any adverse reactions to their health-care provider.

Avoid pregnancy for 3 months following vaccination.

RABIES VACCINE

Rx	**Imovax Rabies Vaccine (Human Diploid Cell)** (Connaught)	**Powder for Injection:** Freeze-dried suspension of Wistar rabies virus strain PM-1503-3M grown in human diploid cell cultures (inactivated whole virus). Contains ≥ 2.5 IU rabies antigen per ml.	In single dose vial[1] with disposable needle and syringe containing diluent and disposable needle for administration.
Rx	**Imovax Rabies I.D. Vaccine (Human Diploid Cell)[2]** (Connaught)	**Powder for Injection:** Freeze-dried suspension of Wistar rabies virus strain PM-1503-3M grown in human diploid cell cultures. Contains 0.25 IU rabies antigen per 0.1 ml intradermal dose.	In single-dose syringe with 1 vial diluent.[3]
Rx	**RabAvert** (Chiron)	**Powder for Injection:** Freeze-dried fixed-virus strain Flury LEP grown in cultures of chicken fibroblasts. Contains ≥ 2.5 IU rabies antigen per 1 ml intramuscular dose.	Preservative-free. In single-dose vial[4] with 1 vial diluent, 1 disposable syringe, 1 longer needle for reconstitution, 1 smaller needle for injection.
Rx	**Rabies Vaccine (Adsorbed)** (Various, eg, Michigan Department of Public Health, SK-Beecham)	**Injection:** Challenge Virus Standard (CVS) Kissling/MDPH strain	In single-dose 1 ml vial.[5]

[1] With < 100 mg human albumin, < 150 mcg neomycin sulfate and 20 mcg phenol red indicator.
[2] This product is for preexposure use only by the intradermal route.
[3] With < 15 mg human albumin, < 22 mcg neomycin sulfate and 3 mcg phenol red indicator/dose.

[4] With < 3 ng ovalbumin, < 12 mg processed bovine gelatin, 1 mg potassium glutamate, 0.3 mg sodium EDTA, < 1 mcg neomycin, < 20 ng chlortetracycline and < 2 ng amphotericin B/dose.
[5] With ≤ 2 mg/ml aluminum phosphate and 0.01% thimerosal.

Refer to the general discussion in the Rabies Prophylaxis Products introduction.

Indications

►*Preexposure immunization:* Vaccinate persons with greater than usual risk of exposure to rabies virus by reason of occupation or avocation, including veterinarians, certain laboratory workers, animal handlers, forest rangers, spelunkers and persons staying > 1 month in countries (eg, India) where rabies is a constant threat.

►*Postexposure prophylaxis:* If a bite from a carrier animal is unprovoked, the animal is not apprehended and rabies is present in that species in the area, administer RIG and vaccine as indicated. Consider vaccine recipients adequately immunized if they previously completed pre- or postexposure prophylaxis with any current rabies vaccine or have a documented adequate antibody response to duck-embryo rabies vaccine (DEV).

Administration and Dosage

►*Dosage:*

Preexposure prophylaxis – Vaccine doses on days 0, 7 and 21 to 28, and then every 2 to 5 years based on antibody titers. Give 1 ml IM (either *Imovax Rabies Vaccine* or *Rabies Vaccine Adsorbed*) or 0.1 ml ID (*Imovax Rabies ID Vaccine* only).

Postexposure prophylaxis – Do not inject postexposure vaccine intradermally. Give rabies immune globulin (20 IU/kg) as soon after exposure as possible, followed by IM vaccine doses (either manufacturer) on days 0, 3, 7, 14 and 28.

For patients who have previously received preexposure prophylaxis, give 1 ml of either vaccine IM only on days 0 and 3. Do not give RIG.

►*Route and site:* The deltoid area is the only acceptable site for postexposure vaccination of adults and older children. For younger children, use the outer aspect of the thigh. Never administer rabies vaccine in the gluteal area.

Travelers to endemic areas may receive vaccine by the ID route if the 3-dose series can be completed ≥ 30 days before departure; otherwise give the vaccine IM.

HDCV – IM in deltoid muscle or ID. Use only the IM route for postexposure prophylaxis. ID injections given in the lateral aspect of the upper arm are less likely to result in adverse reactions, compared with ID injection in the forearm.

RVA – IM only, in deltoid muscle. Do not inject ID. Vaccinate children in the anterolateral aspect of the thigh muscle.

►*Booster dose:* For occupational or other continuing risk, every 2 to 5 years based on antibody titers, in a single 1 ml IM or 0.1 ml ID injection.

Preexposure booster immunization – Test people who work with live rabies virus in research laboratories or in vaccine production or with diagnostic tests for serum rabies antibody titer every 6 months. Give booster vaccine doses as needed to maintain an adequate titer. Give workers (eg, veterinarians, animal control and wildlife officers in areas where animal rabies is epizootic) booster doses every 2 years or have their serum rabies antibody titer determined every 2 years. If the titer is insufficient, give a booster dose. Veterinarians and similar workers in areas of low rabies endemicity do not require routine booster doses of rabies vaccine after completion of primary preexposure immunization or postexposure prophylaxis.

►*Missed doses:*

Preexposure prophylaxis – Prolonging the interval between doses does not interfere with immunity achieved after the concluding dose of the basic series.

Postexposure prophylaxis – Prolonging the interval between doses may seriously delay achieving protective antibody titers, with potentially fatal consequences.

►*Storage/Stability:* Refrigerate dried vaccine at 2° to 8°C (36° to 46°F). Do not freeze. HDCV can presumably tolerate 30 days at room temperature.

Actions

►*Pharmacology:* Rabies vaccine is available as a human diploid-cell vaccine (HDCV) and an adsorbed vaccine (RVA).

Preexposure immunization – High titer antibody responses of HDCV have been demonstrated. Seroconversion was often obtained with only one dose. With two doses 1 month apart, 100% of recipients developed specific antibody.

RABIES VACCINE

Postexposure immunization – Postexposure immunization efficacy was proven in conjunction with antirabies serum. Individuals severely bitten by rabid dogs and wolves received the vaccine within hours of, and up to 14 days after, the bites. All individuals were fully protected against rabies.

Contraindications

Theoretically, rabies vaccine may be contraindicated in people who have had life-threatening allergic reactions to rabies vaccine or any of its components, but carefully consider a patient's risk of developing rabies before deciding to discontinue vaccination.

Warnings

➤*Serious reactions:* Report any serious reactions immediately to the State Health Department or the manufacturer/distributor of the vaccine.

➤*Guillain-Barré syndrome:* Two cases of acute polyradiculoneuropathy (Guillain-Barré syndrome) that resolved within 12 weeks, and a focal subacute CNS disorder temporally associated with HDCV have been reported.

➤*Immune complex-like reactions:* Recently, a significant increase has been noted in "immune complex-like" reactions (6%) in people receiving booster doses of HDCV. The illness, characterized by onset at 2 to 21 days postbooster, presents with a generalized urticaria and may also include arthralgia, arthritis, angioedema, nausea, vomiting, fever and malaise. In no case were the illnesses life-threatening. This reaction occurred much less frequently in people receiving primary immunization.

➤*Hypersensitivity reactions:* May give antihistamines. Have epinephrine available to counteract anaphylactic reactions. Refer to Management of Acute Hypersensitivity Reactions.

While the concentration of antibiotics in each dose of vaccine is extremely small, people with known hypersensitivity to any of these agents could manifest an allergic reaction.

➤*Pregnancy: Category C.* Give rabies vaccine to a pregnant woman only if clearly needed. Pregnancy is not a contraindication to postexposure therapy. There have been no fetal abnormalities associated with rabies vaccination. If there is substantial risk of rabies exposure, preexposure prophylaxis may also be indicated during pregnancy.

➤*Lactation:* It is not known if rabies vaccine or corresponding antibodies are excreted in breast milk. Problems in humans have not been documented.

➤*Children:* Pediatric and adult doses are the same. Safety and efficacy are established in children. Safe and effective use of the Michigan/SKB vaccine is established for people ≥ 6 years of age.

Precautions

➤*Route of administration:*
Imovax Rabies Vaccine and Rabies Vaccine Adsorbed – Inject IM only in the deltoid area; possible vaccine failure may occur if injected in the gluteal area. Do not inject intradermally (ID).

Imovax Rabies ID Vaccine – Inject intradermally only; do not inject IM.

Drug Interactions

Rabies Vaccine Drug Interactions

Precipitant drug	Object drug[*]		Description
Chloroquine	Rabies vaccine, ID	↓	Long-term therapy with chloroquine may suppress the immune response to low-dose HDCV administered ID. Complete preexposure rabies vaccination 1 to 2 months before chloroquine administration begins. If this is not feasible, perform serologic tests several weeks after vaccination to determine the magnitude of the recipient's antibody response.
Immunosuppressants	Rabies vaccine	↓	Like all inactivated vaccines, administration of rabies vaccine to people receiving immunosuppressants, including high-dose corticosteroids, or radiation therapy, may result in an insufficient response to immunization. They may remain susceptible despite immunization. Do not give immunosuppressives during postexposure therapy unless essential. It may be helpful to test steroid-treated patients for development of antirabies antibodies.
Rabies immune-globulin	Rabies vaccine	↓	Simultaneous administration may slightly delay the antibody response to rabies vaccine. Because of this possibility, follow CDC recommendations exactly and give no more than the recommended dose of RIG.

[*] ↓ = Object drug decreased.

Adverse Reactions

HDCV – Transient pain, erythema, swelling or itching at the injection site (25%). Treat such reactions with simple analgesics.

Mild systemic reactions (20%): Headache, nausea, abdominal pain, muscle aches and dizziness. In general, ID administration results in fewer adverse reactions, except for a slight increase in transient local reactions. Serum-sickness-like reactions occur in 6% of those receiving ID booster doses 2 to 21 days after injection. These reactions may be due to albumin in the vaccine formula rendered allergenic by beta-propiolactone during the manufacturing process.

RVA – Transient pain, redness and swelling at the injection site (65% to 70%). In a few cases, these effects persist 48 hours and may be successfully treated with simple analgesics. Mild, transient constitutional reactions (8% to 10%); headache, nausea, slight fever or fatigue. Serum-sickness-like reaction (< 1%), between 7 and 14 days after booster vaccination, perhaps due to lack of albumin in the vaccine formula.

SMALLPOX VACCINE

Rx	**Dryvax**[1] (Wyeth-Ayerst)	**Powder for Injection:** Dried, calf lymph type live-virus preparation of vaccinia virus.[2] The reconstituted vaccine contains ≈ 100 million infectious vaccinia viruses/mL.	In vials with 1 diluent syringe[3] (0.25 mL), 1 vented needle, 100 bifurcated needles.

[1] Licensed for restricted use and available only from the Centers for Disease Control and Prevention (CDC).
[2] Polymyxin B sulfate, dihydrostreptomycin sulfate, chlortetracycline HCl, and neomycin sulfate are added in trace amounts.
[3] With 50% glycerin and 0.25% phenol.

Indications

➤*Smallpox disease:* Active immunization against smallpox disease.

The Advisory Committee on Immunization Practices (ACIP) recommends vaccination of laboratory workers who directly handle cultures or animals contaminated or infected with non-highly attenuated vaccinia virus, recombinant vaccinia viruses derived from non-highly attenuated vaccinia strains, or other Orthopoxviruses that infect humans (eg, monkeypox, cowpox, vaccinia, variola). The ACIP also recommends that vaccination be considered for health care workers who have contact with clinical specimens, contaminated materials (eg, dressings), or patients receiving vaccinia or recombinant vaccinia viruses. Laboratory and other health care personnel who work with highly attenuated poxvirus strains such as modified vaccinia Ankara (MVA), NYVAC (derived from the Copenhagen vaccinia strain), ALVAC (derived from canarypox virus), and TROVAC (derived from fowlpox virus) do not require routine vaccination.

The Armed Forces continue to recommend the use of smallpox vaccine for certain categories of personnel.

➤*Response to bioterrorism:* Recommendations for use of smallpox vaccine in response to bioterrorism are periodically updated by the CDC; the most recent recommendations can be found at http://www.cdc.gov.

Administration and Dosage

➤*Reconstitution:*
1.) Lift up tab of aluminum seal on vaccine vial. Do not break off or tear down tab.
2.) Place vaccine vial upright on a hard, flat surface. Insert a sterile 21-gauge or smaller needle into the rubber stopper to release the vacuum from the vaccine vial. The needle to release the vacuum is not included in the kit.
3.) To reduce viscosity of cold diluent, warm by holding diluent cartridge in palm of hand for a minute or so.
4.) After attaching the vented needle to the diluent syringe, aseptically insert the vented needle through the rubber stopper into the vaccine vial up to the first hub.
5.) Depress the plunger to ensure the entire volume of diluent is delivered into the vial.
6.) Withdraw diluent syringe/vented needle and discard in biohazard waste container.
7.) Allow vaccine vial to stand undisturbed for 3 to 5 minutes. Then, if necessary, swirl vial gently to effect complete reconstitution.
8.) Record date of reconstitution.

SMALLPOX VACCINE

➤*Route and site:* Do not inject IM, IV, or SC. For conventional smallpox vaccination (scarification) only.

The skin over the insertion of the deltoid muscle or the posterior aspect of the arm over the triceps muscle is the preferred site for smallpox vaccination.

➤*Administration:*

1.) Remove entire aluminum seal from the vaccine vial. Then remove rubber stopper from vaccine vial and aseptically retain stopper (set aside inverted) for subsequent reuse.

2.) Carefully dip bifurcated end of needle into vaccine. Visually confirm that the needle picks up a drop of vaccine in the space between the 2 tips.

3.) Deposit the drop of vaccine onto clean, dry site previously prepared for vaccination. Do not redip needle into vaccine if needle has touched skin.

4.) With the same needle, and using multiple-puncture technique, vaccinate through drop of vaccine. Holding the bifurcated needle perpendicular to the skin, punctures are rapidly made with strokes vigorous enough to allow a trace of blood to appear after 15 to 20 seconds. Two or 3 punctures are recommended for primary vaccination; 15 punctures for revaccination. Any remaining vaccine should be wiped off with dry sterile gauze and the gauze disposed of in a biohazard waste container.

5.) If the vaccine is to be stored for subsequent use, restopper the vial with rubber stopper and store at 2° to 8°C (36° to 46°F). The vaccine may be stored for no more than 15 days after reconstitution.

6.) When next needed, remove vial from refrigerator, gently swirl suspension to ensure resuspension, and then carefully take off stopper cap.

➤*Interpretation of responses:* Inspect the vaccination site 6 to 8 days after vaccination. Two types of responses have been defined by the World Health Organization (WHO) Expert Committee on Smallpox. They are: 1) Major reaction, indicating that virus replication has taken place and vaccination was successful; or 2) equivocal reaction, indicating a possible consequence of immunity capable of suppressing viral multiplication or allergic reactions to an inactive vaccine with production of immunity.

Major reaction – Major reaction is defined as a vesicular or pustular lesion or an area of definite palpable induration or congestion surrounding a central lesion that might be a crust or an ulcer. The inoculation site becomes reddened and pruritic 3 to 4 days after vaccination. A vesicle surrounded by a red areola then forms, which becomes umbilicated and then pustular the 7th to 11th day after vaccination, and the pustule begins to dry, the redness subsides, and the lesion usually becomes crusted between the 14th and 21st days. By the end of approximately the third week, the scab falls off, leaving a permanent scar, which at first is pink in color but eventually becomes flesh-colored. Primary vaccination also may be accompanied by fever, regional lymphadenopathy, and malaise persisting for a few days. Revaccination is considered successful if a vesicular or pustular lesion is present or an area of definite palpable induration or congestion surrounding a central lesion, which may be a scar or ulcer, is present on examination 6 to 8 days after revaccination. Major reactions, especially when there has been an interval of many years since the last successful vaccination, may be accompanied by fever, regional lymphadenopathy, and malaise persisting for a few days.

Equivocal reaction – Equivocal reactions are defined as all responses other than major reactions. If an equivocal reaction is observed, check vaccination procedures and repeat vaccination with vaccine from another vial or vaccine lot, if available. If a repeat vaccination by using vaccine from another vial or vaccine lot fails to produce a major reaction, health care providers should consult the CDC or their state or local health department before giving another vaccination.

➤*Revaccination:* For those in the special-risk categories, as defined by ACIP, revaccination is recommended at appropriate intervals (every 10 years).

➤*Disposal:* The vaccine vial, its stopper, the needle to release the vacuum, the diluent syringe, the vented needle used for reconstitution, the bifurcated needle used for administration, and any gauze or cotton that came in contact with the vaccine should be burned, boiled, or autoclaved before disposal.

➤*Storage/Stability:* Store unreconstituted smallpox vaccine in the refrigerator (2° to 8°C, 36° to 46°F). Do not freeze. Reconstituted smallpox vaccine may be used for 15 days if stored at 2° to 8°C (36° to 46°F) when not in actual use. At time of reconstitution, record date. Do not use the smallpox vaccine after the expiration date regardless of whether it is in the dry or reconstituted form.

Actions

➤*Pharmacology:* Smallpox vaccine, dried, calf lymph type, is a live-virus preparation of vaccinia virus prepared from calf lymph.

Introduction of potent smallpox vaccine containing infectious vaccinia viruses into the superficial layers of the skin results in viral multiplication, immunity, and cellular hypersensitivity. With the primary vaccination, a papule appears at the site of vaccination on about the second to fifth day. This becomes a vesicle on the fifth or sixth day, which becomes pustular, umbilicated, and surrounded by erythema and induration. The maximal area of erythema is attained between the eighth and twelfth day following vaccination (usually the tenth). The erythema and swelling then subside, and a crust forms that comes off about the fourteenth to twenty-first day. At the height of the primary reaction known as the Jennerian response, there is usually regional lymphadenopathy and there may be systemic manifestations of fever and malaise.

Primary vaccination with product at a potency of 100 million pock-forming units (pfu)/mL elicits a 97% response rate by major reaction (see Administration and Dosage) and neutralizing antibody response in children. Immunity wanes after several years, and an allergic sensitization to viral proteins can persist. This allergy is manifested by the appearance of a papule and a small area of redness appearing within the first 24 hours after revaccination; this may be the maximum reaction but not infrequently vesicles appear in 24 to 48 hours with ultimate scabbing. The peak of this type of reaction is passed within 3 days following the application of fully potent vaccine with an antibody rise occurring in roughly half of those who exhibit such a reaction. As immunity wanes, revaccination with potent vaccine elicits this allergic response followed by the changes produced by propagating virus. The lesion may then go through the same course as the primary vaccination or may exhibit an accelerated development of the lesion and its attendant erythema. Viral propagation is assumed to have occurred (and an immune response evoked) when the greatest area of skin involvement (erythema) occurs after the third day following revaccination. Revaccination is considered successful if a vesicular or pustular lesion is present or an area of definite palpable induration or congestion surrounding a central lesion, which may be a scar or ulcer, is present on examination 6 to 8 days after revaccination.

Contraindications

➤*Routine nonemergency vaccine use:* Primary vaccination and revaccination with smallpox vaccine are contraindicated as follows:

1.) For any individuals who are allergic to any component of the vaccine, including polymyxin B sulfate, dihydrostreptomycin sulfate, chlortetracycline HCl, and neomycin sulfate.

2.) Infants less than 12 months of age. The ACIP advises against nonemergency use of smallpox vaccine in children less than 18 years of age.

3.) For individuals of any age with eczema or past history of eczema or for those whose household contacts have eczema, other acute, chronic, or exfoliative skin conditions (eg, atopic dermatitis, wounds, burns, impetigo, varicella zoster), and for siblings or other household contacts of such individuals.

4.) For people of any age receiving therapy with systemic corticosteriods at certain doses (eg, greater than or equal to 2 mg/kg body weight or greater than or equal to 20 mg/day of prednisone for 2 weeks or longer), immunosuppressive drugs (eg, alkylating agents, antimetabolites), or radiation. Do not vaccinate household contacts of such individuals.

5.) For individuals with congenital or acquired deficiencies of the immune system, including individuals infected with the human immunodeficiency virus (HIV). Do not vaccinate household contacts of such individuals.

6.) For individuals with immunosuppression (eg, leukemia, lymphomas of any type, generalized malignancy, solid organ transplantation, hematopoietic stem cell transplantation, cellular or humoral immunity disorders, agammaglobulinemia, other malignant neoplasms affecting the bone marrow or lymphatic systems) or household contacts of such individuals.

7.) During pregnancy, suspected pregnancy, or to household contacts of pregnant women.

➤*Smallpox emergency vaccine use:* There are no absolute contraindications regarding vaccination of a person with a high-risk exposure to smallpox. People at greatest risk for experiencing serious vaccination complications are often those at greatest risk for death from smallpox. If a relative contraindication to vaccination exists, the risk for experiencing serious vaccination complications must be weighed against the risks for experiencing a potentially fatal smallpox infection.

Warnings

➤*Elderly:* There are no published data to support the use of this vaccine in geriatric populations. This vaccine is not recommended for use in geriatric populations in nonemergency conditions. For use in emergency conditions, see Contraindications.

➤*Pregnancy: Category C.* Animal reproduction studies have not been conducted with smallpox vaccine. Do not give smallpox vaccine to pregnant women in routine, nonemergency conditions. For emergency conditions, see Contraindications and Indications. On rare occasions, almost always after primary vaccination, vaccinia virus has been reported to cause fetal infection. Fetal vaccinia usually results in stillbirth or death of the infant shortly after delivery. Vaccinia vaccine is not known to cause congenital malformations.

➤*Lactation:* It is not known whether vaccine antigens or antibodies are excreted in human milk. This vaccine is not recommended for use in a nursing mother in nonemergency conditions. For use in emergency conditions, see Contraindications.

SMALLPOX VACCINE

➤*Children:* The vaccine is considered safe and effective in children. However, smallpox vaccine is not recommended for use in nonemergency situations and is contraindicated for infants less than 12 months of age in nonemergency situations.

Precautions

➤*Complications of vaccine:* The CDC can assist physicians in the diagnosis and management of patients with suspected complications of vaccinia (smallpox) vaccination. Vaccinia Immune Globulin (VIG) is indicated for certain complications of smallpox vaccination. Several antiviral compounds have been shown to have activity against vaccinia virus or other Orthopoxviruses in vitro and in animal models. However, insufficient information exists on which to base recommendations for any antiviral compound to treat postvaccination complications or Orthopoxvirus infections, including smallpox. If VIG is needed or additional information is required, physicians should contact the CDC at (404) 639-3670 or (404) 639-2888.

➤*Latex sensitivity:* The vial stopper contains dry natural rubber that may cause hypersensitivity reactions when handled by, or when the product is administered to, people with known or possible latex sensitivity.

➤*Prevention of contact transmission:* Vaccinia virus may be cultured from the site of primary vaccination beginning at the time of development of a papule (2 to 5 days after vaccination) until the scab separates from the skin lesion (14 to 21 days after vaccination). During this time, care must be taken to prevent spread of the virus to another area of the body or to another person.

Identify individuals susceptible to adverse effects of vaccinia virus (eg, those with eczema or immunodeficiency states, including HIV infection) and take measures to avoid contact with people with active vaccination lesions.

Recently vaccinated health care workers should avoid contact with patients, particularly those with immunodeficiencies, until the scab has separated from the skin at the vaccination site. However, if continued contact with patients is essential and unavoidable, they may continue to have contact with patients, including those with immunodeficiencies, as long as the vaccination site is well covered and good hand-washing technique is maintained by the vaccinee. In this setting, a more occlusive dressing may be required. Semipermeable polyurethane dressings are effective barriers to vaccinia and recombinant vaccinia viruses. However, exudate may accumulate beneath the dressing, and care must be taken to prevent viral contamination when the dressing is removed. In addition, accumulation of fluid beneath the dressing may increase the maceration of the vaccination site. Accumulation of exudate may be decreased by first covering the vaccination with dry gauze, then applying the dressing over the gauze. The dressing should also be changed at least once a day.

The most important measure to prevent inadvertent implantation and contact transmission from vaccinia vaccination is thorough hand washing after changing the bandage or after any other contact with the vaccination site.

Adverse Reactions

The U.S. Department of Health and Human Services has established the Vaccine Adverse Event Reporting System (VAERS) to accept all reports of suspected adverse events of any vaccine. The VAERS toll-free number for VAERS forms and information is (800) 822-7967.

➤*Local:* Generalized rashes (erythematous, urticarial, nonspecific) and secondary pyogenic infections at the site of vaccine applications may occur. Bullous erythema multiforme (Stevens-Johnson syndrome) occurs rarely.

Inadvertent inoculation at other sites is the most frequent complication of vaccinia vaccination, usually resulting from autoinoculation of the vaccine virus transferred from the site of vaccination. The most common sites involved are the face, eyelid, nose, mouth, genitalia, and rectum. Accidental infection (autoinoculation) of the eye may result in blindness.

Generalized vaccinia among people without underlying illnesses is characterized by a vesicular rash of varying extent. The rash is generally self-limited and requires little or no therapy except among patients whose conditions appear to be toxic or who have serious underlying illnesses.

➤*Systemic:* A fever is common after vaccinia vaccination is administered. Up to 70% of children have 1 or more days of temperature of 38°C (100°F) or higher from 4 to 14 days after primary vaccination, and 15% to 20% have temperatures of 39°C (102°F) or higher. After revaccination, 35% of children develop temperatures of 38°C (100°F) or higher, and 5% have temperatures of 39°C (102°F) or higher. Fever is less common in adults than children after vaccination or revaccination.

More severe complications that may follow primary vaccination or revaccination include the following: Postvaccinial encephalitis, encephalomyelitis, encephalopathy, progressive vaccinia (vaccinia necrosum), eczema vaccinatum. Such complications may result in severe disability, permanent neurological sequelae, and/or death. Although a rare event, approximately 1 death per million primary vaccinations and 1 death per 4 million revaccinations have occurred after vaccinia vaccination. Death is most often the result of postvaccinial encephalitis or progressive vaccinia. Death also has been reported in unvaccinated contacts of individuals who have been vaccinated.

➤*Revaccination:* The risk of complications associated with revaccination is low. Complications have occurred, especially in patients with underlying diseases, in patients receiving therapy that impairs immunologic competence, or in subjects who have not been vaccinated for many years. Subjects who have not been vaccinated for many years may respond as primary vaccinees as regards both the local and systemic reaction to vaccine administration and risk of occurrence of the above-mentioned serious complications.

TETANUS TOXOID

For additional information, refer to the Agents for Active Immunization introduction.

WARNING

Trivalent DTP is the preferred immunizing agent for most children up to their seventh birthday. Tetanus and diphtheria toxoids (Td) for adult use is the preferred immunizing agent for most adults and older children. For information about tetanus therapy, refer to the monograph on tetanus immune globulin.

Indications

➤*Tetanus toxoid, adsorbed:* Active immunization of adults and children ≥ 7 years of age against tetanus, wherever combined antigen preparations are not indicated.

Not recommended for immunizing children < 7 years of age. In children > 7 years of age, either diphtheria and tetanus toxoids and acellular pertussis vaccine adsorbed (DTaP) or diphtheria and tetanus toxoids and pertussis vaccine adsorbed (for pediatric use) is recommended. If a contraindication to pertussis immunization exists, the recommended vaccine is diphtheria and tetanus toxoids adsorbed (for pediatric use) (DT).

For the prevention of neonatal tetanus in infants born of unvaccinated pregnant women.

Do not use this vaccination for the treatment of tetanus infection. If passive immunization is required, use tetanus immune globulin (human) (TIG).

➤*Tetanus toxoid, fluid:* For booster injection against tetanus in people ≥ 7 years of age. Not indicated for primary immunization.

Primary immunization schedule for children < 7 years of age should consist of 5 doses of a vaccine containing tetanus toxoid. The initial 3 doses are given as diphtheria and tetanus toxoids and pertussis vaccine adsorbed (DTP). The fourth and fifth doses are DTaP. If the pertussis component is contraindicated, DT (for pediatric use) is recommended. For people ≥ 7 years of age, tetanus and diphtheria toxoids adsorbed (for adult use) (Td) is preferred to tetanus toxoid alone.

For the prevention of neonatal tetanus in infants born of unvaccinated pregnant women.

Do not use this vaccination for the treatment of tetanus infection. If passive immunization is required, use TIG.

Administration and Dosage

The National Childhood Vaccine Injury Act requires that the manufacturer and lot number of the vaccine administered be recorded by the health care provider in the vaccine recipient's permanent medical record (or in a permanent office log or file), along with the date of administration of the vaccine and the name, address, and title of the person administering the vaccine.

➤*Administration:* Shake well. Inject in the area of the lateral midthigh or deltoid. Do not inject into the gluteal area or areas where there may be a major nerve trunk.

➤*Tetanus toxoid, adsorbed:* For primary immunization of people ≥ 7 years of age, a series of three 0.5 mL IM injections is given. The second dose of 0.5 mL IM is given 4 to 8 weeks after the first dose, and the third dose of 0.5 mL IM is given 6 to 12 months after the second dose.

For children ≥ 1 year of age in whom vaccines containing pertussis and diphtheria antigens are contraindicated, 2 doses of 0.5 mL each, 4 to 8 weeks apart, followed by a third dose of 0.5 mL, 6 to 12 months after the second dose are recommended.

For booster injections, a booster dose of 0.5 mL of Td (for adult use) vaccine or tetanus toxoid adsorbed vaccine every 10 years thereafter is recommended.

➤*Tetanus toxoid, fluid:* After the initial immunization series is completed, give a booster dose of 0.5 mL IM every 10 years to maintain adequate immunity.

➤*Tetanus prophylaxis in wound management:* Td is the preferred vaccine for active tetanus immunization in wound management of patients ≥ 7 years of age. This is to enhance diphtheria protection, because a large proportion of adults are susceptible. TIG is the product of choice for passive immunization. Refer to the Diphtheria and Tetanus Toxoids monograph or the Tetanus Immune Globulin monograph.

Tetanus Prophylaxis in Routine Wound Management				
History of adsorbed tetanus toxoid (doses)	Clean, minor wounds		All other wounds[1]	
	Td	TIG[2]	Td	TIG
Unknown or < 3	Yes	No	Yes	Yes
≥ 3	No[3]	No	No[4]	No

[1] Such as, but not limited to, wounds contaminated with dirt, feces, soil, or saliva; puncture wounds; avulsions; and wounds resulting from missiles, crushing burns, and frostbite.
[2] TIG (human).
[3] Yes, if > 10 years since last dose.
[4] Yes, if > 5 years since last dose.

➤*Concomitant vaccines:* Several routine vaccines may safely and effectively be administered simultaneously at separate injection sites (eg, DTP or Td, MMR, Hib, hepatitis B). National authorities recommend simultaneous immunization at separate sites as indicated by age or health risk, if return of a vaccine recipient for a subsequent visit is doubtful.

➤*Storage/Stability:* Store at 2° to 8°C (36° to 46°F). Do not freeze. Discard frozen toxoid.

Actions

➤*Pharmacology:* Adsorbed tetanus toxoid induces specific protective antibodies against the exotoxin excreted by *Clostridium tetani*. The aluminum salt, a mineral adjuvant, prolongs and enhances the antigenic properties of tetanus toxoid by retarding the rate of absorption. Its duration is ≈ 10 years.

While the rate of seroconversion and promptness of antibody response are essentially equivalent for the fluid and adsorbed forms of tetanus toxoid, adsorbed toxoids induce more persistent antitoxin titers. Therefore, adsorbed tetanus toxoid is strongly recommended for primary and booster immunizations. Use fluid tetanus toxoid to immunize the rare patient who is hypersensitive to the aluminum adjuvant. The only other rational use for fluid tetanus toxoid is in compounding dilutions of a reagent for delayed-hypersensitivity skin-testing.

Contraindications

History of systemic allergic or neurologic reactions following a previous dose or hypersensitivity to thimerosal.

Give only passive immunization, using TIG (human), if a contraindication exists in a person who has not completed a primary immunizing course of tetanus toxoid and other than a clean, minor wound is sustained.

Defer elective immunization during the course of any febrile illness or acute infection, or during an outbreak of poliomyelitis. A minor afebrile illness such as a mild upper respiratory tract infection should not preclude immunization.

Warnings

➤*Tetanus infection:* Under no circumstances should tetanus toxoid be used to treat actual tetanus infections. Employ tetanus antitoxin, preferably TIG (human), in all such cases.

➤*Immunodeficiency:* People receiving immunosuppressive therapy, including radiation, corticosteroids, antimetabolites, alkylating agents, and cytotoxic drugs, or with other immunodeficiencies may have a diminished antibody response to active immunization. This is a reason to consider deferring immunization. Nonetheless, routine immunization of symptomatic and asymptomatic HIV-infected people is recommended.

➤*Hypersensitivity reactions:* Take every precaution to prevent and arrest allergic and other untoward reactions. A careful history should review possible sensitivity to the vaccine or similar vaccines, to dry natural latex rubber, or to the type of protein to be injected. Epinephrine 1:1000 and other appropriate agents should be readily available to combat unexpected allergic reactions. Refer to Management of Acute Hypersensitivity Reactions.

People who experience Arthus-type hypersensitivity reactions or temperature > 39.4°C (103°F) after a previous dose of tetanus toxoid usually have very high serum tetanus antitoxin levels and should not be given even emergency doses of tetanus toxoid more frequently than every 10 years, even if they have a wound that is neither clean nor minor.

➤*Elderly:* The elderly develop lower to normal antitoxin levels following tetanus immunization than younger people.

➤*Pregnancy: Category C.* Use only if clearly needed, although Td is preferred. Based on extensive human experience, there is no evidence that tetanus toxoid is teratogenic. Give a previously unimmunized pregnant woman who may deliver her child under nonhygienic conditions 2 doses of Td 4 to 8 weeks apart before delivery, preferably during the last 2 trimesters. Incompletely immunized pregnant women should complete their 3 dose primary series. Give those immunized > 10 years previously a booster dose. It is not known if tetanus toxoid or corresponding antibodies cross the placenta. Generally, most IgG passage across the placenta occurs during the third trimester.

➤*Lactation:* It is not known if tetanus toxoid or corresponding antibodies are excreted in breast milk. It is unlikely that intradermal tetanus toxoid is excreted in breast milk.

➤*Children:* DTaP is the preferred immunizing agent for most children until their seventh birthday. Safety and efficacy of tetanus toxoid in infants < 6 weeks of age have not been established. However, tetanus toxoid is not indicated for children < 7 years of age.

TETANUS TOXOID

Drug Interactions

Tetanus Toxoid Drug Interactions			
Precipitant drug	Object drug*		Description
Immunosuppressants	Tetanus toxoid	↓	Administration of tetanus toxoid to patients receiving immunosuppressants including corticosteroids or radiation therapy, may result in insufficient response to immunization. They may remain susceptible despite immunization.
Chloramphenicol	Tetanus toxoid, adsorbed	↓	Systemic chloramphenicol may impair anamnestic response to tetanus toxoid. Avoid concurrent use.
TIG	Tetanus toxoid, adsorbed	↓	Concurrent use may delay development of active immunity by several days; however, this interaction is not clinically significant and does not preclude concurrent use.

* ↓ = Object drug decreased.

Adverse Reactions

The National Childhood Vaccine Injury Act requires the healthcare provider to report to the US Department of Health and Human Services through the Vaccine Adverse Event Reporting System (VAERS) the occurrence following immunization of any event set forth in the Vaccine Injury Table, including: Anaphylaxis or anaphylactic shock within 4 hours; encephalopathy or encephalitis within 72 hours; shock-collapse or hypotonic-hyporesponsive collapse within 7 days; residual seizure disorder; any acute complication of sequelae (including death) of above events, or any event that would contraindicate further doses of vaccine.

The US Department of Health and Human Services has established VAERS to accept all reports of suspected adverse events after the administration of any vaccine, including but not limited to the reporting of events required by the National Childhood Vaccine Injury Act of 1986. The VAERS toll-free number for forms and information is 800-822-7967.

➤*CNS:* Cochlear lesion; brachial plexus neuropathies; paralysis of the radial nerve; paralysis of the recurrent nerve; accommodation paresis; Guillain-Barré syndrome; EEG disturbances with encephalopathy.

➤*Dermatologic:* Urticaria; rash.

➤*Local:* Redness; warmth; edema; induration with or without tenderness; nodule; sterile abscess formation; SC atrophy.

➤*Miscellaneous:* Malaise; transient fever; chills; pain; hypotension; nausea; myalgia; arthralgia; headaches; Arthus-type hypersensitivity (characterized by severe local reactions, generally starting 2 to 8 hours after injection, particularly in patients who have received multiple prior boosters).

Rarely, anaphylactic reaction and death have been reported after receiving preparations containing tetanus and diphtheria antigens.

TETANUS TOXOID, FLUID

Rx	**Tetanus Toxoid** (Aventis Pasteur)	**Injection:** 4 Lf units tetanus per 0.5 mL dose	In 7.5 mL vials.[1]

[1] With thimerosal.

For complete prescribing information, refer to the Tetanus Toxoid group monograph.

TETANUS TOXOID, ADSORBED

Rx	**Tetanus Toxoid, Adsorbed** (Aventis Pasteur)	**Injection:** 5 Lf units tetanus per 0.5 mL dose	In 5 mL vials.[1]
Rx	**Tetanus Toxoid, Adsorbed, Purogenated** (Lederle)	**Injection:** 5 Lf units tetanus per 0.5 mL dose	In 0.5 mL disposable syringes and 5 mL vials[2]

[1] With aluminum potassium sulfate and thimerosal.
[2] With aluminum phosphate and thimerosal.

For complete prescribing information, refer to the Tetanus Toxoid group monograph.

DIPHTHERIA AND TETANUS TOXOIDS, COMBINED (DT; Td)

For additional information, refer to the Agents for Active Immunization introduction.

> ## WARNING
>
> Trivalent DTP is the preferred immunizing agent for most children. Tetanus and diphtheria toxoids for adult use (Td) is the preferred immunizing agent for most adults and older children.
>
> Specific information about the individual components of this drug appear in the individual monographs on diphtheria toxoid and tetanus toxoid.

Indications

➤*Diphtheria and tetanus toxoids, adsorbed (for pediatric use) (DT):* Active immunization of children ≤ 7 years of age against diphtheria and tetanus. Diphtheria and tetanus toxoids and acellular pertussis, adsorbed (DTaP) is recommended for primary immunization of infants and children ≤ 7 years of age. However, in instances where the pertussis vaccine component is contraindicated, or where the physician decides the pertussis vaccine is not to be administered, use DT.

Start immunization at 6 weeks to 2 months of age and complete before the seventh birthday.

Not to be used for the treatment of diphtheria or tetanus infection. If passive immunization is required, use tetanus immune globulin (TIG) or diphtheria antitoxin.

➤*Diphtheria and tetanus toxoids, adsorbed (for adult use) (Td):* Active immunization of adults and children ≥ 7 years of age against diphtheria and tetanus.

For the prevention of neonatal tetanus and diphtheria in infants born of unvaccinated pregnant women.

Administration and Dosage

The National Childhood Vaccine Injury Act requires that the manufacturer and lot number of the vaccine administered be recorded by the health care provider in the vaccine recipient's permanent medical record (or in a permanent office log or file), along with the date of administration of the vaccine and the name, address, and title of the person administering the vaccine.

Interruption of the recommended schedule with a delay between doses does not interfere with the final immunity achieved, nor does it necessitate starting the series over again, regardless of the length of time elapsed between doses.

➤*Administration:* Shake well. Inject in the area of the anterolateral aspect of the thigh or deltoid. Do not inject into the gluteal area or areas where there may be a major nerve trunk. During the course of primary immunizations, do not make injections more than once at the same site.

➤*Children:*

Infants 6 weeks to 2 months of age – Primary immunization series consists of 4 doses. Administer three 0.5 mL doses IM, 4 to 8 weeks apart; a reinforcing dose is given 6 to 12 months after the third injection.

Children 1 to 6 years of age – Primary immunization series consists of 3 doses. Administer two 0.5 mL doses IM, 4 to 8 weeks apart; a reinforcing dose is given 6 to 12 months after the third injection. In the event the final immunizing dose would be given after the seventh birthday, use Td (for adults).

Vaccinate preterm infants according to their chronological age from birth.

Booster dose: For children 4 to 6 years of age (preferably at time of kindergarten or elementary school entrance), give a booster of 0.5 mL IM. Those who receive all 4 primary immunizing doses before the fourth birthday should receive a single dose of DT just before entering kindergarten or elementary school. This booster dose is not necessary if the fourth dose in the primary series was given after the fourth birthday. Therafter, routine booster immunizations should be Td at intervals of 10 years.

➤*Adults and children ≥ 7 years of age:* Primary immunization series consists of three 0.5 mL IM doses. The second dose is given 4 to 8 weeks after the first dose; and the third dose is given 6 to 12 months after the second dose.

Booster dose – 0.5 mL IM every 10 years to maintain adequate protection.

➤*Wound management:* For tetanus prophylaxis in wound management, refer to the Tetanus Toxoid monograph.

➤*Storage/Stability:* Store between 2° to 8°C (36° to 46°F). Do not freeze.

DIPHTHERIA AND TETANUS TOXOIDS, COMBINED (DT; Td)

Actions

➤*Pharmacology:* These preparations combine diphtheria and tetanus toxins (detoxified by formaldehyde). Adequate immunization is thought to confer protection for at least 10 years. It significantly reduces both the risk of developing diphtheria and tetanus and the severity of clinical illness. However, it does not eliminate carriage of *Corynebacterium diphtheriae* in the pharynx or nose or on the skin. A serum level ≥ 0.01 antitoxin units/mL is generally protective.

Contraindications

Hypersensitivity to any component of the vaccine, including thimerosal.

History of systemic allergic or neurologic reactions following a previous dose.

If a contraindication exists in a person who has not completed a primary immunizing course of tetanus toxoid and other than a clean, minor wound is sustained, give only passive immunization using TIG (human).

Elective immunization should be deferred during the course of any severe, febrile illness or acute infection, or during an outbreak of poliomyelitis. A minor afebrile illness such as a mild upper respiratory tract infection should not preclude immunization.

Patients ≥ 7 years of age (DT only).

Warnings

➤*Infections:* Do not use for treatment of actual tetanus or diphtheria infections.

➤*Immunodeficiency:* People receiving immunosuppressive therapy, including radiation, corticosteroids, antimetabolites, alkylating agents, and cytotoxic drugs, or with other immunodeficiencies may have diminished antibody response to active immunization. This is a reason for deferring primary immunization. Nonetheless, routine immunization of symptomatic and asymptomatic HIV-infected people is recommended.

➤*Hypersensitivity reactions:* Take every precaution to prevent and arrest allergic and other untoward reactions. A careful history should review possible sensitivity to the type of vaccine to be injected and also sensitivity to dry natural latex rubber. Epinephrine 1:1000 and other appropriate agents should be readily available to combat unexpected allergic reactions. Refer to Management of Acute Hypersensitivity Reactions.

➤*Elderly:* The elderly develop lower to normal antitoxin levels following tetanus immunization than younger people.

➤*Pregnancy: Category C.* Use Td only if clearly needed. There is no evidence that tetanus and diphtheria toxoids are teratogenic. Give a previously unimmunized pregnant woman who may deliver her child under nonhygienic conditions 2 doses of Td 4 to 8 weeks apart before delivery, preferably during the last 2 trimesters. Incompletely immunized pregnant women should complete the 3 dose series. Give those immunized > 10 years previously a booster dose. Generally, most IgG passage across the placenta occurs during the third trimester.

➤*Lactation:* It is not known if DT or Td antigens or corresponding antibodies are excreted in breast milk.

➤*Children:* DT is indicated for children > 6 weeks and < 7 years of age in whom pertussis vaccination is contraindicated. DTaP is the preferred immunizing agent for most children up to their seventh birthday. Td is the preferred immunizing agent for most adults and children > 7 years of age.

Drug Interactions

DT/Td Drug Interactions			
Precipitant drug	Object drug*		Description
Immunosuppressants	DT/Td	↓	Like all inactivated vaccines, administration of DT/Td vaccine to people receiving immunosuppressant drugs, including high-dose corticosteroids or radiation, may result in an insufficient response to immunization. They may remain susceptible despite immunization.
DT/Td	Anticoagulants	↑	As with other drugs administered by IM injection, give with caution to people receiving anticoagulants.

* ↑ = Object drug increased.   ↓ = Object drug decreased.

Adverse Reactions

The National Childhood Vaccine Injury Act requires the health care provider to report to the US Department of Health and Human Services through the Vaccine Adverse Event Reporting System (VAERS) the occurrence following immunization of any event set forth in the Vaccine Injury Table, including the following: Anaphylaxis or anaphylactic shock within 4 hours; encephalopathy or encephalitis within 72 hours; shock-collapse or hypotonic-hyporesponsive collapse within 7 days; residual seizure disorder; any acute complication of sequelae (including death) of above events, or any event that would contraindicate further doses of vaccine.

The US Department of Health and Human Services has established VAERS to accept all reports of suspected adverse events after the administration of any vaccine, including but not limited to the reporting of events required by the National Childhood Vaccine Injury Act of 1986. The VAERS toll-free number for forms and information is 800-822-7967.

➤*Cardiovascular:* Hypotension; tachycardia; syncope.

➤*CNS:* Headache; dizziness; cochlear lesion; brachial plexus neuropathies; paralysis of the radial nerve; paralysis of the recurrent nerve; accommodation paresis; polyneuritis; convulsions; transverse myelitis; mononeuritis; polyradiculoneuropathy; acute midbrain syndrome; parasthesia; Guillain-Barré syndrome; EEG disturbances with encephalopathy.

➤*Dermatologic:* Urticaria; rash; pruritus; erythema multiforme; sweating.

➤*GI:* Nausea; anorexia; vomiting.

➤*Hematologic / Lymphatic:* Lymphadenopathy; phlebitis; thrombocytopenic purpura.

➤*Local:* Redness; warmth; edema; induration with or without tenderness; pain; nodule; abscess; SC atrophy; cellulitis.

➤*Musculoskeletal:* Arthralgia; myalgia.

➤*Miscellaneous:* Malaise; transient fever; pain; difficult breathing; irritability; Arthus-type hypersensitivity (characterized by severe local reactions, generally starting 2 to 8 hours after injection, particularly in patients who have received multiple prior boosters).

Rarely, anaphylactic reaction and death have been reported after receiving preparations containing tetanus and diphtheria antigens.

DIPHTHERIA AND TETANUS TOXOIDS, ADSORBED (FOR PEDIATRIC USE)

Rx	Diphtheria & Tetanus Toxoids, Pediatric (Aventis Pasteur)	Injection: 6.7 Lf units diphtheria and 5 Lf units tetanus per 0.5 mL dose	In 5 mL multidose vials.[1]

[1] With aluminum potassium sulfate, thimerosal.

For complete prescribing information, refer to the Diphtheria and Tetanus Toxoids, Combined group monograph.

Administration and Dosage

For use only in patients ≤ 6 years of age.

DIPHTHERIA AND TETANUS TOXOIDS, ADSORBED (FOR ADULT USE)

Contains ≤ 2 Lf units of diphtheria toxoid per 0.5 mL.

Rx	Diphtheria & Tetanus Toxoids, Adult (Aventis Pasteur)	Injection: 2 Lf units diphtheria and 5 Lf units tetanus per 0.5 mL dose	In 5 mL vials and 0.5 mL syringes.[1]
Rx	Diphtheria & Tetanus Toxoids, Adult (Massachusetts Public Health Biologic Labs)	Injection: 2 Lf units diphtheria and 2 Lf units tetanus per 0.5 mL dose	In 5 and 10 mL vials.[2]

[1] With aluminum potassium sulfate, thimerosal.   [2] With aluminum phosphate, thimerosal.

For complete prescribing information, refer to the Diphtheria and Tetanus Toxoids, Combined group monograph.

Toxoids

DIPHTHERIA AND TETANUS TOXOIDS AND ACELLULAR PERTUSSIS VACCINE, ADSORBED (DTaP)

Rx	**Tripedia** (Aventis Pasteur)	**Injection:** 6.7 Lf units diphtheria toxoid, 5 Lf units tetanus toxoid, 46.8 mcg pertussis antigens (≈ 23.4 mcg each of inactivated pertussis toxin and FHA[1]) per 0.5 mL	In preservative-free single-dose[2] and 7.5 mL multidose vials.[3]
Rx	**Daptacel** (Aventis Pasteur)	**Injection:** 15 Lf units diphtheria toxoid, 5 Lf units tetanus toxoid, 10 mcg pertussis toxoid, 5 mcg FHA,[1] 3 mcg pertactin, 5 mcg fimbriae types 2 and 3 per 0.5 mL	In single-dose vials.[4]
Rx	**Infanrix** (SmithKline Beecham)	**Injection:** 25 Lf units diphtheria toxoid, 10 Lf units tetanus toxoid, 25 mcg inactivated pertussis toxin, 25 mcg FHA,[1] 8 mcg pertactin per 0.5 mL	In single-dose vials[5] and disposable *Tip-Lok* syringes.

[1] Filamentous hemagglutinin.
[2] With thimerosal (not more than 0.3 mcg mercury/dose). Also contains gelatin.
[3] With thimerosal (25 mcg mercury/dose), not more than 0.17 mg aluminum and not more than 100 mcg of residual formaldehyde per 0.5 mL dose. Also contains gelatin and polysorbate 80.

[4] With 3.3 mg 2-phenoxyethanol, 0.33 mg of aluminum as the adjuvant, ≤ 0.1 mg residual formaldehyde, and < 50 ng residual glutaraldehyde.
[5] With 2.5 mg 2-phenoxyethanol as a preservative, 4.5 mg sodium chloride, not more than 0.625 mg aluminum by assay, not more than 100 mcg of residual formaldehyde, and not more than 100 mcg of polysorbate 80.

For additional information, refer to the Agents for Active Immunization introduction.

Indications

Active immunization against diphtheria, tetanus, and pertussis simultaneously in infants and children 6 weeks to 7 years of age (prior to the seventh birthday).

Children 7 years of age or older should receive diphtheria and tetanus toxoids (Td) (for adult use).

In instances where the pertussis vaccine component is contraindicated, use diphtheria and tetanus toxoids adsorbed (DT) (for pediatric use) for the remaining doses.

Children who have had well-documented pertussis (ie, positive culture for *Bordetella pertussis* or epidemiologic linkage to a culture-positive case) should complete the vaccination series with at least DT. Some experts recommend including the pertussis component as well (ie, administration of DTaP). Although well-documented pertussis disease is likely to confer immunity against pertussis, the duration of such immunity is unknown.

Not to be used for treatment of pertussis, diphtheria, or tetanus infections. If passive immunization is required, use tetanus immune globulin and/or diphtheria antitoxin.

Administration and Dosage

The National Childhood Vaccine Injury Act requires that the manufacturer and lot number of the vaccine administered be recorded by the health care provider in the vaccine recipient's permanent medical record, along with the date of administration of the vaccine and the name, address, and title of the person administering the vaccine.

Interrupting the recommended schedule or delaying subsequent doses should not interfere with the final immunity achieved with the vaccine and does not require restarting the series. Use Td, rather than DTaP, for any doses needed after a child's seventh birthday.

➤*Administration:* Shake well. Administer IM only. The anterolateral aspect of the thigh (for children under 1 year of age) or the deltoid muscle of the upper arm (for older children) is preferred. Do not inject DTaP in the gluteal area or other areas where there may be a major nerve trunk.

➤*Primary immunization:* The primary series consists of three 0.5 mL IM doses. The customary age for the first dose is 2 months of age, but it may be given as early as 6 weeks of age and up to the seventh birthday. Preterm infants should be vaccinated according to their chronological age from birth.

Vaccination Schedule for DTaP			
Dose	CDC recommendations	*Daptacel*	*Infanrix* or *Tripedia*
Doses 1 to 3	2, 4, and 6 months	2, 4, and 6 months[1]	2, 4, and 6 months[2]
Dose 4	15 to 18 months[3]	17 to 20 months[4]	15 to 20 months[4]
Dose 5	4 to 6 years		4 to 6 years[5]

[1] 6- to 8-week intervals.
[2] 4- to 8-week intervals.
[3] May be administered as early 12 months, provided 6 months have elapsed since the third dose and the child is unlikely to return at age 15 to 18 months.
[4] At least 6 months between the third and fourth doses.
[5] Preferably prior to school entry. If the fourth dose was administered after the fourth birthday, a fifth dose prior to school entry is not necessary.

➤*Booster dose:* When DTaP is given for the primary series, a fourth dose is recommended. The interval between the third and fourth dose should be at least 6 months.

If a child receives whole-cell pertussis DTP for 1 or more doses, DTaP vaccines may be given to complete the series.

Infanrix may be used to complete a DTaP immunization series initiated with *Pediarix*.

➤*Interchangeability of vaccines:* The manufacturers recommend that the same vaccine be given for the vaccination series. The CDC recommends that the same brand of DTaP vaccine be used for all doses of the vaccination series when feasible. However, when this is not possible, use any DTaP vaccine to continue or complete the series. Do not defer vaccination because the previously used brand is not available or is unknown.

➤*Concomitant vaccine administration:* According to the recommendations of the Advisory Committee on Immunization Practices (ACIP) and the American Academy of Family Physicians (AAFP), children aged 12 to 15 months can receive 7 or less injections (DTaP, MMR, varicella, *Haemophilus influenzae* type B [Hib], pneumococcal conjugate, inactivated polio virus [IPV], and hepatitis B vaccines) during a single visit, depending on vaccines given in the first year of life.

When concomitant administration of other vaccines is required, give with different syringes and at different injection sites.

According to the manufacturer, no immunogenicity data are available on the simultaneous administration of *Infanrix* with pneumococcal conjugate vaccine or IPV. No immunogenicity or safety date is available on the simultaneous administration of *Infanrix* with MMR or varicella vaccine.

There are no data available to the manufacturer about the simultaneous administration of *Tripedia* with varicella vaccine, IPV, or pneumococcal conjugate vaccine.

According to the manufacturer, no safety and immunogenicity data are available about the simultaneous administration of *Daptacel* with pneumococcal conjugate vaccine, MMR, and varicella vaccine, and no immunogenicity data are currently available about the simultaneous administration of IPV.

➤*Storage/Stability:* Store at 2° to 8°C (36° to 46°F). Do not freeze. Temperature extremes may adversely affect resuspendability of the vaccine. Discard if vaccine has been frozen. Do not use after expiration date.

Actions

➤*Pharmacology:* These preparations combine diphtheria and tetanus toxoids with acellular pertussis bacterial vaccine. The acellular pertussis antigens are pertussis toxin (PT), FHA, and pertactin. Adequate immunization with diphtheria and tetanus toxoids is thought to confer protection for at least 10 years. However, diphtheria toxoid does not eliminate carriage of *Corynebacterium diphtheriae* in the pharynx or nose or on the skin.

Protection against pertussis persists approximately 4 to 6 years. Serum diphtheria and tetanus antitoxin levels of 0.1 IU/mL and higher are regarded as protective. Efficacy of the pertussis component does not have a well-established correlate of protection.

Contraindications

Not recommended for use in adults or children 7 years of age or older.

Hypersensitivity to any component of the vaccine; history of a serious allergic reaction (eg, anaphylaxis) temporally associated with a previous dose of the vaccine or with any component of the vaccine.

Encephalopathy (eg, coma, decreased level of consciousness, prolonged seizures) within 7 days of administration of a previous dose of DTP or DTaP and is not attributable to another identifiable cause.

Progressive neurologic disorders, including infantile spasms, uncontrolled epilepsy, or progressive encephalopathy. Pertussis vaccine should not be administered to individuals with such conditions until a treatment regimen has been established and the condition has stabilized.

If a contraindication to the pertussis vaccine component occurs, substitute diphtheria and tetanus toxoids for pediatric use (DT) for each of the remaining doses.

Defer elective immunization procedures during an outbreak of poliomyelitis because of the risk of provoking paralysis.

Warnings

➤*Special risk patients:* If any of the following events occurs in temporal relation with the receipt of either whole-cell pertussis DTP or DTaP, carefully consider the decision to administer subsequent doses of vaccine containing the pertussis component. Although these events were once considered contraindications to whole-cell pertussis DTP, there may be circumstances, such as high incidence of pertussis, in which the potential benefits outweigh the possible risks, particularly because the following events have not been proven to cause permanent sequelae:

DIPHTHERIA AND TETANUS TOXOIDS AND ACELLULAR PERTUSSIS VACCINE, ADSORBED (DTaP)

1.) Temperature of at least 40.5°C (105°F) within 48 hours, not caused by another identifiable cause.
2.) Collapse or shock-like state (hypotonic-hyporesponsive episode) within 48 hours.
3.) Persistent, inconsolable crying lasting at least 3 hours, occurring within 48 hours.
4.) Convulsions, with or without fever, occurring within 3 days.

When the decision is made to withhold the pertussis component, continue immunization with DT.

The decision to administer or delay vaccination because of a current or recent febrile illness depends on the severity of symptoms and on the etiology of the disease. All vaccines can be administered to people with mild illness such as diarrhea, mild upper respiratory tract infection with or without low-grade fever, or other low grade febrile illness. However, do not immunize children with moderate or serious illnesses until recovered.

If Guillain-Barré syndrome occurs within 6 weeks of receipt of prior vaccine containing tetanus toxoid, base the decision to give subsequent doses of DTaP or any vaccine containing tetanus toxoid on careful consideration of the potential benefits and possible risks.

►*Immunodeficiency:* People receiving immunosuppressive therapy, including irradiation, antimetabolites, alkylating agents, cytotoxic drugs, and corticosteroids (used in greater than physiologic doses), or with other immunodeficiencies may have diminished antibody response to active immunization. If immunosuppressive therapy will be discontinued shortly, it would be reasonable to defer immunization until the patient has been off therapy for more than 1 month; otherwise, vaccinate the patient while still on therapy. If DTaP vaccine has been administered to people receiving immunosuppressive therapy, a recent injection of immune globulin, or having an immunodeficiency disorder, an adequate immunological response may not be obtained. Nonetheless, routine immunization of symptomatic and asymptomatic HIV-infected people is recommended.

►*Convulsions:* The Advisory Committee on Immunization Practices (ACIP) and the American Academy of Pediatrics (AAP) recognize cases when children with stable CNS disorders, including well-controlled seizures or satisfactorily explained single seizures, may receive acellular pertussis vaccine. The ACIP and AAP do not consider a family history of seizures to be a contraindication to pertussis vaccine. Studies suggest that when given whole-cell pertussis DTP vaccine, infants and children with a history of convulsions in first-degree family members (ie, siblings, parents) have an increased risk for neurologic events, compared with those without such histories.

For children at higher risk for seizures than the general population, an appropriate antipyretic may be administered at the time of vaccination with a vaccine containing an acellular pertussis component (including DTaP) and for the ensuing 24 hours to reduce the possibility of post-vaccination fever.

►*Latex sensitivity:* The stopper of the *Tripedia* and *Daptacel* vials and the tip cap and rubber plunger of the *Infanrix* needleless prefilled syringes contain dry natural latex rubber, which may cause allergic reactions in latex sensitive individuals.

►*Hypersensitivity reactions:* Rarely, an anaphylactic reaction (eg, hives, swelling of the mouth, difficulty breathing, hypotension, shock) has been reported after receiving preparations containing diphtheria, tetanus, and/or pertussis antigens (see Adverse Reactions). Refer to the Management of Acute Hypersensitivity Reactions.

►*Pregnancy: Category C.* DTaP is generally contraindicated after the seventh birthday. It is not known if DTaP antigens or corresponding antibodies cross the placenta. Most IgG passage across the placenta occurs during the third trimester. Not recommended for use in pregnant women.

►*Lactation:* It is not known if DTaP antigens or corresponding antibodies are excreted into breast milk.

►*Children:* Safety and efficacy of DTaP in infants below 6 weeks of age have not been established. DTaP is not recommended for adults and children 7 years of age and older.

Precautions

►*Adverse events:* When an infant or child returns for the next dose in the series, question the parent concerning occurrence of any symptoms or signs of adverse reactions after the previous dose (see Contraindications, Warnings, and Adverse Reactions).

Drug Interactions

►*Immunosuppressants:* Immunosuppressive therapies, including irradiation, antimetabolites, alkylating agents, cytotoxic drugs, and corticosteroids (used in greater than physiologic doses), may reduce the immune response to vaccines. If immunosuppressive therapy will be discontinued shortly, it would be reasonable to defer immunization until the patient has been off therapy for 3 months; otherwise, vaccinate the patient while still on therapy. If DTaP is administered to a person receiving immunosuppressive therapy, or who received a recent injection of immune globulin, or who has an immunodeficiency disorder, an adequate immunologic response may not be obtained.

Adverse Reactions

The National Childhood Vaccine Injury Act requires the health care provider to report to the US Department of Health and Human Services through the Vaccine Adverse Event Reporting System (VAERS) the occurrence following immunization of any event set forth in the Vaccine Injury Table, including the following: Anaphylaxis or anaphylactic shock within 7 days; encephalopathy or encephalitis within 7 days; brachial neuritis within 28 days; any acute complication or sequelae (including death) of above events; any event that would contraindicate further doses of vaccine. The VAERS toll-free number for forms and information is (800) 822-7967.

Adverse Reactions Occurring within 72 Hours after Primary Immunization with *Tripedia*, *Infanrix*, and *Daptacel* (%)[1]

Adverse reaction	Tripedia			Infanrix			Daptacel		
	Dose 1 (2 mo)	Dose 2 (4 mo)	Dose 3 (6 mo)	Dose 1 (2 mo)	Dose 2 (4 mo)	Dose 3 (6 mo)	Dose 1 (2 mo)	Dose 2 (4 mo)	Dose 3 (6 mo)
Local									
Redness (any)	12.6	12.7	19.1	16.6	15.4	26.3	12.5	15.8	19.7
Swelling	8.8	8.2	10.7	12.5	15.4	21	14.3	15.4	17.8
Pain/Tenderness	8.1[2]	3.7[2]	2.3[2]	5[2]	5.1[2]	0.9[2]	30.5	19.6	15.9
GI									
Anorexia	8.1	9.7	9.9	7.5	6	9.6	26.2	14.8	17.8
Vomiting	5.2	1.5	2.3	5.8	6.8	3.5	-	-	-
Miscellaneous									
Fever[3]	0.7	1.4	3.1	0	0.9	3.5	11.9	9.9	9.9
Drowsiness	28.9	17.9	4.6	37.5	19.7	13.2	62	44.8	35.6
Irritability/Fussiness	8.1[4]	7.4[4]	7.6[4]	3.3[4]	7.7[4]	8.8[4]	72	61.2	56.2
Crying ≥ 3 hours	-	-	-	-	-	-	0.3	0	0

[1] Data are pooled from separate studies and are not necessarily comparable.
[2] Moderate or severe; cried or protested to touch or cried when limb was moved.
[3] *Tripedia*: ≥ 38.3°C,> 101°F (rectal); *Infanrix*: ≥ 38.4°C, ≥ 101.1°F (rectal); *Daptacel*: ≥ 38°C, ≥ 100.4°F (rectal).
[4] Moderate or severe; prolonged or persistent crying that could not be comforted and refusal to play.

Adverse Reactions Occurring within 72 Hours after Booster Doses with *Tripedia* and *Infanrix* (%)[1]

Adverse reaction	Tripedia		Infanrix
	Dose 4 (15 to 20 mo)	Dose 5 (4 to 6 yr)	Dose 4 (15 to 20 mo)
Local			
Redness (any)	17.1	33.3	39.5
Swelling	15.9	27.8	32.9
Pain	7.3[2]	11.1[2]	10.5[2]
GI			
Anorexia	8.5	0	11.8
Vomiting	2.4	0	2.6
Miscellaneous			

Adverse Reactions Occurring within 72 Hours after Booster Doses with *Tripedia* and *Infanrix* (%)[1]

Adverse reaction	Tripedia		Infanrix
	Dose 4 (15 to 20 mo)	Dose 5 (4 to 6 yr)	Dose 4 (15 to 20 mo)
Fever[3]	2.4	5.6	6.6
Drowsiness	6.1	5.6	6.6
Irritability/Fussiness[4]	3.7	0	9.2

[1] Data are pooled from separate studies and are not necessarily comparable.
[2] Moderate or severe; cried or protested to touch or cried when limb was moved.
[3] *Tripedia*: ≥ 38.3°C,> 100.1°F (oral); *Infanrix*: ≥ 38.4°C, ≥ 101.1°F (rectal).
[4] Moderate or severe; prolonged or persistent crying that could not be comforted and refusal to play.

DIPHTHERIA AND TETANUS TOXOIDS AND ACELLU-LAR PERTUSSIS VACCINE, ADSORBED (DTaP)

►*CNS:* A review by the Institute of Medicine found a causal relation between tetanus toxoid and brachial neuritis and Guillain Barré syndrome. The following illnesses have been reported as temporally associated with vaccine containing tetanus toxoid: Neurological complications including cochlear lesion, brachial plexus neuropathies, paralysis of the radial nerve, paralysis of the recurrent nerve, accommodation paresis, and EEG disturbances with encephalopathy.

►*Miscellaneous:* Rarely, an anaphylactic reaction (eg, hives, swelling of the mouth, difficulty breathing, hypotension, shock) has been reported after receiving preparations containing diphtheria, tetanus, and/or pertussis antigens.

Arthus-type hypersensitivity reactions, characterized by severe local reactions (generally starting 2 to 8 hours after an injection), may follow receipt of tetanus toxoid. A few cases of peripheral neuropathy have been reported following tetanus toxoid administration, although the evidence is inadequate to accept or reject a causal relation.

►*Postmarketing:* Worldwide voluntary reports of adverse events for *Infanrix* since market introduction are listed below. This list includes adverse events for which 20 or more reports were received with the exception of intussusception, idiopathic thrombocytopenic purpura, thrombocytopenia, anaphylactic reaction, encephalopathy, and hypotonic-hyporesponsive episode for which fewer than 20 reports were received. These latter events are included either because of the seriousness of the event or the strength of causal connection to components of this or other vaccines or drugs.

CNS – Convulsions, crying, encephalopathy, hypotonia, hypotonic-hyporesponsive episode, irritability, somnolence.

Dermatologic – Erythema, pruritus, rash, urticaria.

GI – Diarrhea, intussusception, vomiting.

Hematologic/Lymphatic – Idiopathic thrombocytopenic purpura, lymphadenopathy, thrombocytopenia.

Miscellaneous – Anaphylactic reaction, cellulitis, cyanosis, ear pain, fever, hypersensitivity, injection site reactions, limb swelling, respiratory tract infection, Sudden Infant Death Syndrome.

Patient Information

This medicine is used to immunize children 6 weeks to 7 years of age (before the seventh birthday) against diphtheria, tetanus, and pertus-

sis (whooping cough). It is not to be used to treat diphtheria, tetanus, or patients older than 7 years of age.

Inform the parent or guardian of the importance of completing the pertussis immunization series, unless a contraindication to further immunization exists.

Children with minor illnesses, such as a cold, may be vaccinated. Wait to vaccinate children who are moderately or severely ill until they recover.

Advise the parent or guardian to contact a health care provider at once if the child develops the following signs of encephalopathy within 7 days after receiving a vaccination: Changes in alertness; unresponsiveness; seizure activity.

Advise the parent or guardian to contact a health care provider at once if the child develops a fever of 105°F or more, faints, persistently cries for more than 3 hours within 48 hours of receiving this vaccine, or has a seizure with or without fever within 3 days of receiving this vaccine.

Inform the parent or guardian of the following adverse effects that may occur.

►*Common mild problems that may occur:*
• Fever (up to about 1 child in 4);
• Redness or swelling where the shot was given (up to about 1 child in 4);
• Soreness or tenderness where the shot was given (up to about 1 child in 4).

These problems occur more often after the fourth and fifth doses of the DTaP series than after earlier doses. Sometimes the fourth and fifth dose of DTaP vaccine is followed by swelling of the entire arm or leg in which the shot was given, lasting 1 to 7 days (up to about 1 child in 30).

►*Other mild problems:*
• Fussiness (up to 1 child in 3);
• Tiredness or poor appetite (up to about 1 child in 10);
• Vomiting (up to about 1 child in 50).

These problems generally occur 1 to 3 days after the shot.

Controlling fever is especially important for children who have had seizures, for any reason. It is also important if another family member has had seizures. Reduce fever and pain by giving the child an aspirin-free pain reliever when the shot is given and for the next 24 hours, following the package instructions.

DIPHTHERIA AND TETANUS TOXOIDS, ACELLULAR PERTUSSIS, AND HAEMOPHILUS INFLUENZAE TYPE B CONJUGATE VACCINES (DTaP-HIB)

| *Rx* | **TriHIBit**[1] (Aventis Pasteur) | **Injection:** 10 mcg *Haemophilus influenzae* type b purified capsular polysaccharide conjugated to 24 mcg inactivated tetanus toxoid, 6.7 Lf diphtheria toxoid, 5 Lf tetanus toxoid, 46.8 mcg pertussis antigens per 0.5 mL | Sucrose, trace thimerosal. In vials.[2] |

[1] Supplied as *ActHIB* (*Haemophilus* b conjugate vaccine [tetanus toxoid conjugate]) with *Tripedia* (diphtheria and tetanus toxoids and acellular pertussis vaccine adsorbed [DTaP]).

[2] *ActHIB* single-dose vials of dry lyophilized powder for reconstitution with 0.6 mL single-use vials of *Tripedia.*

For complete prescribing information, refer to the *Haemophilus* b Conjugate Vaccine and the Diphtheria and Tetanus Toxoids and Acellular Pertussis Vaccine monographs. For additional information, also refer to the Agents for Active Immunization introduction.

Indications

For the active immunization of children 15 to 18 months of age who previously have been immunized against diphtheria, tetanus, and pertussis with 3 doses consisting of diphtheria and tetanus toxoids and whole cell pertussis (DTP) or DTaP vaccine and 3 doses or fewer of *ActHIB* within the first year of life for the prevention of invasive diseases caused by *Haemophilus influenzae* type b or by diphtheria, tetanus, and pertussis (refer to *ActHIB* package insert).

Do not administer *TriHIBit* to infants younger than 15 months of age.

Administration and Dosage

Do not administer IV. Administer IM in the outer aspect of the midthigh or deltoid. Do not inject the vaccine into the gluteal area or areas where there may be a nerve trunk.

Recommended Immunization Schedule for *ActHIB* and DTP or *Tripedia* for Previously Unvaccinated Children		
Dose	Age	Immunization
First, second, and third	At 2, 4, and 6 mo	*ActHIB* reconstituted with DTP or saline diluent (0.4% sodium chloride)
Fourth	At 15 to 18 mo	*ActHIB* reconstituted with DTP or *Tripedia* (*TriHIBit*) or with saline diluent (0.4% sodium chloride)
Fifth	At 4 to 6 yr	*Tripedia* or DTP

Vaccinate preterm infants according to their chronological age from birth.

Interruption of the recommended schedule with a delay between doses should not interfere with the final immunity achieved with *ActHIB* reconstituted with DTP or *Tripedia* (*TriHIBit*) or saline diluent (0.4% sodium chloride). There is no need to start the series over again, regardless of the time elapsed between doses.

It is acceptable to administer a booster dose of *TriHIBit* following a primary series of *Haemophilus* b conjugate and whole-cell DTP vaccines or a primary series of a combination vaccine containing whole-cell DTP.

►*Reconstitution:* To prepare *TriHIBit*, clean the *Tripedia* and *ActHIB* vial rubber stoppers with a suitable germicide prior to reconstitution. Thoroughly agitate the vial of *Tripedia*, then withdraw a 0.6 mL dose and inject into the vial of lyophilized *ActHIB*. After reconstitution and thorough agitation, the combined vaccines will appear whitish in color. Withdraw a 0.5 mL dose of the combined vaccines and administer IM. Use vaccine immediately (within 30 minutes) after reconstitution.

►*Storage/Stability:* Store between 2° to 8°C (35° to 46°F). Do not freeze. Temperature extremes may adversely affect vaccine resuspendability. Use vaccine immediately (within 30 minutes) after reconstitution.

DIPHTHERIA AND TETANUS TOXOIDS AND ACELLULAR PERTUSSIS ADSORBED, HEPATITIS B (RECOMBINANT) AND INACTIVATED POLIOVIRUS VACCINE COMBINED

Rx **Pediarix** (SmithKline Beecham)	**Injection:** 25 Lf diphtheria toxoid, 10 Lf tetanus toxoid, 25 mcg inactivated pertussis toxin (PT), 25 mcg filamentous hemagglutinin (FHA), 8 mcg pertactin, 10 mcg hepatitis B surface antigen (HBsAg), 40 D-antigen units (DU) Type 1 poliovirus, 8 DU Type 2 poliovirus, and 32 DU Type 3 poliovirus per 0.5 mL.[1]	Preservatives.[2] In single-dose vials and prefilled syringes.

[1] Each 0.5 mL dose also contains 2.5 mg 2-phenoxyethanol as a preservative, 4.5 mg NaCl, and aluminum adjuvant (not more than 0.85 mg aluminum by assay). Each dose also contains up to 100 mcg of residual formaldehyde and up to 100 mcg of polysorbate 80 (*Tween 80*).

[2] Thimerosal (less than 12.5 ng mercury per dose); neomycin sulfate, polymyxin B (up to 0.05 ng neomycin and up to 0.01 ng polymyxin B per dose); up to 5% yeast protein.

For complete prescribing information, refer to the Diphtheria and Tetanus Toxoids and Acellular Pertussis Vaccine, Hepatitis B Recombinant Vaccine, and Poliovirus Inactivated Vaccine monographs. For additional information, also refer to the Agents for Active Immunization introduction.

Indications

➤*Immunization:* Active immunization against diphtheria, tetanus, pertussis (whooping cough), all known subtypes of hepatitis B virus, and poliomyelitis caused by poliovirus Types 1, 2, and 3 as a 3-dose primary series in infants born of HBsAg-negative mothers, beginning as early as 6 weeks of age.

Do not administer to any infant before the age of 6 weeks or to individuals 7 years of age or older.

➤*Infants born of HBsAg-positive mothers:* Infants should receive hepatitis B immune globulin (human) (HBIG) and monovalent hepatitis B vaccine (recombinant) within 12 hours of birth and should complete the hepatitis B vaccination series according to a particular schedule (see Hepatitis B Vaccine [Recombinant] monograph).

➤*Infants born of mothers of unknown HBsAg status:* Infants should receive monovalent hepatitis B vaccine (recombinant) within 12 hours of birth and should complete the hepatitis B vaccination series according to a particular schedule (see Hepatitis B Vaccine [Recombinant] monograph).

Pediarix will not prevent hepatitis caused by other agents, such as hepatitis A, C, and E viruses, or other pathogens known to infect the liver. As hepatitis D (caused by the delta virus) does not occur in the absence of hepatitis B infection, hepatitis D also will be prevented by vaccination with *Pediarix*.

Vaccination with *Pediarix* may not prevent hepatitis B infection in individuals who had an unrecognized hepatitis B infection at the time of vaccine administration.

When passive protection against tetanus or diphtheria is required, administer tetanus immune globulin or diphtheria antitoxin, respectively.

Pediarix may not protect 100% of individuals receiving the vaccine and is not recommended for treatment of actual infections.

Administration and Dosage

➤*Approved by the FDA:* December 16, 2002.

➤*Administration: Pediarix* contains an adjuvant; therefore, shake vigorously to obtain a homogeneous, turbid, white suspension. Do not use if resuspension does not occur with vigorous shaking. Discard any vaccine remaining in the vial.

Administer by IM injection. The preferred sites are the anterolateral aspects of the thigh or the deltoid muscle of the upper arm. Do not inject the vaccine into the gluteal area or areas where there may be a major nerve trunk. Gluteal injections may result in suboptimal hepatitis B immune response.

Do not administer this product SC or IV.

➤*Primary immunization:* The primary immunization series for *Pediarix* is 3 doses of 0.5 mL, given IM, at 6- to 8-week intervals (preferably 8 weeks). The customary age for the first dose is 2 months of age, but it may be given starting at 6 weeks of age.

Do not administer *Pediarix* to any infant before the age of 6 weeks. Only monovalent hepatitis B vaccine can be used for the birth dose.

➤*Children previously vaccinated with 1 or more doses of hepatitis B vaccine:* Infants born of HBsAg-negative mothers and who received a dose of hepatitis B vaccine at or shortly after birth may be administered 3 doses of *Pediarix* according to the recommended schedule.

➤*Children previously vaccinated with 1 or more doses of Infanrix: Pediarix* may be used to complete the first 3 doses of the DTaP series in infants who have received 1 or 2 doses of *Infanrix* and also are scheduled to receive the other vaccine components of *Pediarix*.

➤*Children previously vaccinated with 1 or more doses of inactivated poliovirus vaccine (IPV): Pediarix* may be used to complete the first 3 doses of the IPV series in infants who have received 1 or 2 doses of IPV and also are scheduled to receive the other vaccine components of *Pediarix*.

➤*Interchangeability of Pediarix and licensed DTaP, IPV, or recombinant hepatitis B vaccines:* It is recommended that *Pediarix* be given for all 3 doses because data are limited regarding the safety and efficacy of using acellular pertussis vaccines from different manufacturers for successive doses of the pertussis vaccination series. *Pediarix* is not recommended for completion of the first 3 doses of the DTaP vaccination series initiated with a DTaP vaccine from a different manufacturer because no data are available regarding the safety or efficacy of using such a regimen.

Pediarix may be used to complete a hepatitis B vaccination series initiated with a licensed hepatitis B vaccine (recombinant) vaccine from a different manufacturer.

Pediarix may be used to complete the first 3 doses of the IPV vaccination series initiated with IPV from a different manufacturer.

➤*Additional dosing information:* If any recommended dose of pertussis vaccine cannot be given, DT (for pediatric use), hepatitis B (recombinant), and IPV should be given as needed to complete the series.

Interruption of the recommended schedule with a delay between doses should not interfere with the final immunity achieved with *Pediarix*. There is no need to start the series over again, regardless of the time elapsed between doses.

The use of reduced volume (fractional doses) is not recommended.

Children who have received a 3-dose primary series of *Pediarix* should receive a fourth dose of IPV at 4 to 6 years of age and a fourth dose of DTaP vaccine at 15 to 18 months of age. Because the pertussis antigen components of *Infanrix* are the same as those components in *Pediarix*, these children should receive *Infanrix* as their fourth dose of DTaP.

➤*Concomitant vaccine administration:* Safety data are available following the first dose of *Pediarix* administered concomitantly, at separate sites, with *Haemophilus* B and pneumococcal conjugate vaccines.

When concomitant administration of other vaccines is required, they should be given with separate syringes and at different injection sites.

➤*Storage / Stability:* Refrigerate between 2° and 8°C (36° and 46°F). Do not freeze. Discard if the vaccine has been frozen.

Indications

Diagnosis of specific allergies, when properly diluted.

Relief of allergic symptoms (eg, hay fever, rhinitis, allergic asthma, insect-sting anaphylaxis) due to specifically identified materials by means of a graduated schedule of doses.

Administration and Dosage

Begin immunotherapy with very small doses; increase progressively until maintenance levels are reached. Dosages vary depending on the type of standardization used. Individualize dosage.

Do not inject IV. SC injection is preferable because it is less painful, allows better delineation of reaction size and slows the absorption rate, thus lowering the likelihood of an anaphylactic reaction. Although IM administration is acceptable, it is more painful and more difficult to assess the local reaction.

➤*Combining allergens:* Do not combine allergens to which the patient is extremely sensitive with allergens for which only a nominal sensitivity is shown. Distinct treatment schedules for each formula are frequently employed. (See Precautions.)

➤*Children:* Dosage is the same as for adults; divide large volume doses among several injection sites.

➤*Diagnostic testing:* Perform puncture (prick) or intradermal testing with appropriate dilutions, employing positive and negative controls. Consult manufacturer's literature for each allergen. Do not conduct test with alum-precipitated allergen extracts.

➤*Therapeutic dosing:* Typical doses are given SC every 3 to 14 days (or 7 to 14 days with alum-precipitated allergen extracts). Progress to the maximum tolerated dose or a weekly maintenance dose. Consult manufacturer's literature for each allergen.

➤*Admixtures:* Limit combinations of allergens so that each allergen will be present at a therapeutic concentration. Do not combine allergens of different standardization types. Stability varies with diluent, storage condition and concentration. Stability will be shortest in the low concentration ranges.

➤*Storage/Stability:* Store between 2° and 8°C (36° to 46°F).

Actions

➤*Pharmacology:* Allergenic extracts are derived individually from various biological sources containing antigens that possess immunologic activity. They are categorized based standardization and doseform. Standardization systems include the following: 1) Standardized by biological activity (in allergenic units, AU), 2) weight-to-volume (w/v) standardized, and 3) protein nitrogen unit (PNU) standardized. Doseforms include: 1) aqueous, 2) glycerinated and 3) alum-precipitated.

The mechanism of action is not completely defined. Specific immunoglobulin G (IgG) appears in the serum following injection of allergenic extracts. IgG competes with specific IgE for a specific antigen. Bound to receptors on mast cell membranes, IgE produces an allergenic reaction by releasing histamine and other agents upon coupling with an antigen. Serum IgE levels decrease over time. Decreased leukocyte sensitivity to allergens and increased numbers of T-suppressor cells for IgE-producing plasma cells are also noted. The histamine release response of circulating basophils to a specific allergen may be reduced in some patients by hyposensitization.

Onset/Duration – Relief of symptoms is dose-related. It is rarely achieved before maintenance dosage levels are reached, which often takes 4 to 6 months, sometimes 12 months. Serum IgG levels remain elevated for weeks to months following injection and vary markedly between individuals.

Contraindications

As initial therapy when an allergen can be environmentally avoided.

Frequent large local reactions or systemic reactions are relative contraindications for continued immunotherapy.

Foodstuff allergen extracts are diagnostic tools; efficacy for hyposensitization immunotherapy has not been demonstrated.

Warnings

➤*Cross-sensitivity:* Cross-immunoreactivity has been documented within botanical genus groups, especially among grasses. Exercise caution in prescribing since the additive effects could precipitate an allergic reaction. Markedly increased exposure to allergens in the environment may have an additive effect when coupled with an allergen extract injection. Dosage reduction may be necessary.

➤*Hypersensitivity reactions:* Anaphylactic reactions may occur with an overdose or in extremely sensitive individuals. Administer allergen extracts only where emergency facilities are immediately available.

Refer to Management of Acute Hypersensitivity Reactions.

➤*Pregnancy: Category C.* Controlled studies of hyposensitization with allergen extracts throughout pregnancy failed to demonstrate any fetal or maternal risk. Because histamine can produce uterine contraction, avoid any reaction that releases significant amounts of histamine, whether from natural allergen exposure or from hyposensitization overdose. IgG crosses the placenta, especially in the third trimester. Administer during pregnancy only if clearly needed and with caution. Although pregnancy is not an indication to stop allergen extract therapy in women receiving maintenance doses without side effects, some allergists empirically decrease the maintenance dose by 50% throughout gestation.

➤*Lactation:* Minimal amounts of IgG are excreted in breast milk. No problems in humans have been documented. Various nutritional, immunologic and other advantages of breastfeeding have been described, especially in children of atopic mothers.

➤*Children:* Dosage for children is generally the same as for adults. The larger dosage volumes may produce relatively greater discomfort. To achieve the total dose required, the volume of the dose may be distributed among several injection sites.

Precautions

➤*Mixed allergens:* Mixed allergens are not to be used for skin testing. In the case of a negative reaction, a mixture fails to indicate whether one of the individual components at the full labeled concentration is capable of evoking a positive reaction. If the patient responds positively, there is no indication which component of the mixture produced the antigenic response. Treatment with nonreactive allergens can lead to sensitization and induction of IgE production.

➤*Combining allergens:* Do not combine allergens to which the patient is extremely sensitive with allergens for which only a nominal sensitivity is shown. Administer separately to individualize and better control dosage.

➤*Seasonal exposure:* Delay the start of immunotherapy until after any period of symptoms from seasonal environmental exposure. Typical allergic symptoms may follow shortly after an injection, particularly when the sum of the antigen load from the environment and from the injection exceeds the patient's antigen tolerance.

➤*Routine immunizations:* While routine immunizations may theoretically exacerbate autoimmune diseases, studies have failed to demonstrate this. Give hyposensitization cautiously to patients with autoimmune diseases and only if the risk from exposure exceeds the risk of exacerbating the underlying condition.

Drug Interactions

➤*Drug/Lab test interactions:* **Histamine H$_1$ antagonists** and **tricyclic antidepressants** may produce a false-negative reaction to cutaneous diagnostic testing with allergen extracts, unless a 72-hour period of antihistamine abstinence is observed. Long-acting antihistamines may interfere for weeks. **H$_2$ antagonists** do not decrease skin-test responsiveness alone, but may enhance suppression synergistically with H$_1$ antihistamines. **Topical corticosteroids** suppress dermal reactivity to allergan extracts locally.

Adverse Reactions

Most serious reactions begin within 30 minutes of an injection. Observe patients for at least 30 minutes after every injection, even once they have achieved maintenance therapy.

➤*Local:* Erythema and swelling at the injection site are common, but not significant unless they persist > 24 hours or exceed the diameter of a nickel (about 2 cm).

➤*Systemic:* Anaphylaxis, including fainting, pallor, bradycardia, hypotension, angioedema, wheezing, cough, conjunctivitis, rhinitis, generalized urticaria (see Warnings).

Patient Information

Comply with full course of therapy. To achieve efficacy, take regularly and in the proper dosage. Medication will not cure allergies, but will help control them.

Notify physician of increased environmental exposure to natural allergens; a dosage reduction may be required.

➤*Missed dose:* Depending on the amount of time elapsed, dosage reduction may be required. Do *not* double the dose to make up for the missed dose. More frequent injections may be necessary to return to maintenance doses.

Notify physician if erythema, swelling or generalized urticaria persists.

Notify physician immediately if fainting, wheezing, hypotension or bradycardia occurs.

AQUEOUS AND GLYCERINATED ALLERGENIC EXTRACTS

Rx	**Allergenic Extracts, Aqueous and Glycerinated** (Various, eg, ALK, Allergy Laboratories, Allermed, ALO, Antigen Laboratories, Center, Greer, Iatric, Meridian, Miles, Nelco)	**Injection:** Over 900 distinct allergens available in these categories: Animal products, foods, grass pollens, insect products, molds, tree pollens, weed pollens and other inhalants	Extracts supplied in various aqueous diluents or with varying concentrations of glycerin. In multidose vials of 2, 5, 10, 20, 30 and 50 ml.

For complete prescribing information, refer to the Allergenic Extracts group monograph.

ALUM-PRECIPITATED ALLERGENIC EXTRACTS

Rx	**Allpyral** (Miles)	**Injection:** Alum-precipitated extracts, prepared by pyridine extraction	In multidose vials of 10 and 30 ml at 5000, 10,000 and 20,000 PNU/ml.
Rx	**Center-Al** (Center)	**Injection:** Alum-precipitated extracts	In multidose vials of 10 and 30 ml at 10,000 and 20,000 PNU/ml.

For complete prescribing information, refer to the Allergenic Extracts group monograph.

HYMENOPTERA VENOM/VENOM PROTEIN

Rx	**Albay, Venomil** (Miles)	**Injection:** Purified venoms of honey bee, wasp, white faced hornet, yellow hornet, yellow jacket and mixed vespids (both hornets and yellow jackets)	In vials of 12, 120 and 550 mcg.
Rx	**Pharmalgen** (ALK)		In vials of 120 and 1100 mcg.

For complete prescribing information, refer to the Allergenic Extracts group monograph.

PEGADEMASE BOVINE

| Rx | Adagen (Enzon) | Injection: 250 units[1]/ml | In 1.5 ml vials.[2] |

[1] One unit of activity is defined as the amount of ADA that converts 1 mcM of adenosine to inosine per minute at 25°C and pH 7.3.

[2] With 1.2 mg monobasic sodium phosphate, 5.58 mg dibasic sodium phosphate, 8.5 mg sodium chloride and water for injection.

Indications

For enzyme replacement therapy for adenosine deaminase (ADA) deficiency in patients with severe combined immunodeficiency disease who are not suitable candidates for or who have failed bone marrow transplantation. Pegademase bovine is recommended for use in infants from birth or in children of any age at the time of diagnosis. It is not intended as a replacement for HLA identical bone marrow transplant therapy, and it is also not intended to replace continued close medical supervision and therapy and the initiation of appropriate diagnostic tests and therapy (eg, antibiotics, nutrition, oxygen, gammaglobulin) as indicated for intercurrent illnesses.

Administration and Dosage

Before prescribing pegademase bovine, the physician should be thoroughly familiar with the details of this prescribing information. For further information concerning the essential monitoring of therapy, contact Enzon, Inc., 20 Kingsbridge Rd., Piscataway, NJ 08854-3998 (732-980-4500).

Pegademase bovine is recommended for use in infants from birth or in children of any age at the time of diagnosis.

➤*Administer:* Administer every 7 days as an IM injection. Individualize the dosage.

First dose – 10 U/kg.

Second dose – 15 U/kg.

Third dose – 20 U/kg.

Usual maintenance dose – 20 U/kg/week. Further increases of 5 U/kg/week may be necessary, but a maximum single dose of 30 U/kg should not be exceeded.

Plasma levels of ADA more than twice the upper limit of 35 mcmol/hr/ml have occurred on occasion in several patients, and have been maintained for several weeks in one patient who received twice weekly injections (20 U/kg per dose). No adverse effects have been observed at these higher levels; there is no evidence that maintaining preinjection plasma ADA > 35 mcmol/hr/ml produces any additional clinical benefits.

Dose proportionality has not been established; closely monitor patients when the dosage is increased. Pegademase bovine is not recommended for IV administration.

Establish the optimal dosage and schedule of administration for each patient based on monitoring of plasma ADA activity levels (trough levels before maintenance injection), biochemical markers of ADA deficiency (primarily red cell deoxyadenosine triphosphate [dATP] content). Since improvement in immune function follows correction of metabolic abnormalities, maintenance dosage in individual patients should be aimed at achieving the following biochemical goals: 1) Maintain plasma ADA activity (trough levels before maintenance injection) in the range of 15 to 35 mcmol/hr/ml (assayed at 37°C [98.6°F]); and 2) decline in erythrocyte dATP to ≤ 0.005 to 0.015 mcmol/ml packed erythrocytes, or ≤ 1% of the total erythrocyte adenine nucleotide (ATP = dATP) content, with a normal ATP level, as measured in a pre-injection sample. In addition, continued monitoring of immune function and clinical status is essential in any patient with a primary immunodeficiency disease and should be continued in patients being treated with pegademase bovine.

➤*Admixture incompatibility:* Pegademase bovine should not be diluted nor mixed with any other drug prior to administration.

➤*Storage/Stability:* Refrigerate. Store between 2°C and 8°C (36°F and 46°F). Do not freeze. Pegademase bovine should not be stored at room temperature. This product should not be used if there are any indications that it may have been frozen.

Actions

➤*Pharmacology:* Pegademase bovine is a modified enzyme used for enzyme replacement therapy for the treatment of severe combined immunodeficiency disease (SCID) associated with a deficiency of adenosine deaminase. The drug will not benefit patients with immunodeficiency due to other causes. It is a conjugate of numerous strands of monomethoxypolyethylene glycol (PEG), covalently attached to the enzyme ADA. ADA, used in the manufacture of pegademase bovine, is derived from bovine intestine.

Pegademase bovine provides specific replacement of the deficient enzyme. In the absence of the enzyme ADA, the purine substrates adenosine, 2'-deoxyadenosine and their metabolites are toxic to lymphocytes. The direct action of pegademase bovine is the correction of these metabolic abnormalities. Improvement in immune function and diminished frequency of opportunistic infections only occurs after metabolic abnormalities are corrected. There is a lag between the correction of the metabolic abnormalities and improved immune function. This period of time is variable, from a few weeks to as long as 6 months. In contrast to the natural history of combined immunodeficiency disease due to ADA deficiency, a trend toward diminished frequency of opportunistic infections and fewer complications of infections has occurred in patients receiving pegademase bovine.

SCID associated with ADA deficiency is a rare, inherited and often fatal disease. In the absence of ADA enzyme, purine substrates adenosine and 2'-deoxyadenosine accumulate, causing metabolic abnormalities that are directly toxic to lymphocytes.

The immune deficiency can be cured by bone marrow transplantation. When a suitable bone marrow donor is unavailable or when bone marrow transplantation fails, non-selective replacement of the ADA enzyme has been provided by periodic irradiated red blood cell transfusions. However, transmission of viral infections and iron overload are serious risks, and relatively few ADA-deficient patients have benefited from chronic transfusion therapy.

In patients with ADA deficiency, rigorous adherence to a schedule of pegademase bovine can eliminate toxic metabolites of ADA deficiency and improve immune function. Carefully monitor by measuring the level of ADA activity in plasma. Monitoring the level of dATP in erythrocytes is also helpful in determining that the dose is adequate.

➤*Pharmacokinetics:* Pharmacokinetics and biochemical effects have been studied in six children ranging in age from 6 weeks to 12 years with SCID associated with ADA deficiency. After IM injection, peak plasma ADA activity levels were reached in 2 to 3 days. ADA plasma elimination half-life of was variable, even for the same child. Range was 3 to > 6 days. Following weekly injections of 15 U/kg, average trough level of ADA activity in plasma was between 20 and 25 mcmol/hr/ml.

The changes in red blood cell deoxyadenosine nucleotide (ie, dATP) and S-adenosylhomocysteine hydrolase (SAHase) have been evaluated. In patients with ADA deficiency, inadequate elimination of 2'-deoxyadenosine caused a marked elevation in dATP and a decrease in SAHase level in red blood cells. Prior to treatment with pegademase bovine, the levels of dATP in the red blood cells ranged from 0.056 to 0.899 mcmol/ml of erythrocytes. After 2 months of maintenance treatment, the levels decreased to 0.007 to 0.015 mcmol/ml. The normal value of dATP is below 0.001 mcmol/ml. In the same period of time, SAHase increased from pretreatment range of 0.09 to 0.22 nmol/hr/mg protein to 2.37 to 5.16 nmol/hr/mg protein. Normal value for SAHase is 4.18 ± 1.9 nmol/hr/mg protein.

Contraindications

There is no evidence to support the safety and efficacy of pegademase bovine as preparatory or support therapy for bone marrow transplantation. Since the drug is administered by IM injection, use with caution in patients with thrombocytopenia and do not use if thrombocytopenia is severe.

Warnings

➤*Product potency:* Product potency testing prior to distribution may not assure the initial and continuing potency of each new lot of pegademase bovine. Report any laboratory or clinical indication of a decrease in potency immediately by telephone to Enzon (732-980-4500).

➤*Pregnancy: Category C.* It is not known whether pegademase bovine can cause fetal harm when administered to a pregnant woman or can affect reproduction capacity. Give to a pregnant woman only if clearly needed.

➤*Lactation:* It is not known whether pegademase bovine is excreted in breast milk. Exercise caution when administering to a nursing woman.

Precautions

➤*Monitoring:*

Laboratory test monitoring – Monitor the treatment of SCID associated with ADA deficiency with pegademase bovine by measuring plasma ADA activity and red blood cell dATP levels.

Determine plasma ADA activity and red cell dATP prior to treatment. Once treatment has been initiated, a desirable range of plasma ADA activity (trough level before maintenance injection) should be 15 to 35 mcmol/hr/ml. This minimum trough level will ensure that plasma ADA activity from injection to injection is maintained above the level of total erythrocyte ADA activity in the blood of normal individuals.

Determine plasma ADA activity (pre-injection) every 1 to 2 weeks during the first 8 to 12 weeks of treatment in order to establish an effective dose. After 2 months of maintenance treatment, red cell dATP levels should decrease to a range of ≤ 0.005 to 0.015 mcmol/ml. The normal value of dATP is below 0.001 mcmol/ml. Once the level of dATP has fallen adequately, measure 2 to 4 times during the remainder of the first year and 2 to 3 times a year thereafter, assuming no interruption in therapy.

PEGADEMASE BOVINE

Between 3 and 9 months, determine plasma ADA twice a month, then monthly until after 18 to 24 months of treatment. In patients who have successfully been maintained on therapy for 2 years, continue to have plasma ADA measured every 2 to 4 months and red cell dATP measured twice yearly. More frequent monitoring would be necessary if therapy were interrupted or if an enhanced rate of clearance of plasma ADA activity develops.

Once effective ADA plasma levels have been established, should a patient's plasma ADA activity level fall below 10 mcmol/hr/ml (which cannot be attributed to improper dosing, sample handling or antibody development) then all patients receiving this lot of pegademase bovine will be required to have a blood sample for plasma ADA determination taken prior to their next injection. The index patient will require retesting for determination of plasma ADA activity prior to their next injection. If this value, as well as the value from one of the other patients from a different site, is < 10 mcmol/hr/ml, then the lot in use will be recalled and replaced with a new clinical lot by Enzon.

➤*Immunodeficiency:* Maintain appropriate care to protect immune-deficient patients until improvement in immune function has been documented. The degree of immune function improvement may vary from patient to patient and, therefore, each patient will require appropriate care consistent with immunologic status.

➤*Immune function:* Immune function, including the ability to produce antibodies, generally improves after 2 to 6 months of therapy, and matures over a longer period. Compared with the natural history of combined immunodeficiency disease due to ADA deficiency, a trend toward diminished frequency of opportunistic infections and fewer complications of infections has occurred in patients receiving pegademase bovine. However, the lag between the correction of the metabolic abnormalities and improved immune function with a trend toward diminished frequency of infections and complications of infection is variable, and has ranged from a few weeks to ≈ 6 months. Improvement in the general clinical status of the patient may be gradual (as evidenced by improvement in various clinical parameters) but should be apparent by the end of the first year of therapy.

A decline in immune function, with increased risk of opportunistic infections and complications of infection, will result from failure to maintain adequate levels of plasma ADA activity (whether due to the development of antibody, improper calculation of dosage, interruption of treatment or to improper storage with subsequent loss of activity). If a persistent decline in plasma ADA activity occurs, monitor immune function and clinical status closely and take precautions to minimize the risk of infection. If antibody to ADA or pegademase bovine is found to be the cause of a persistent fall in plasma ADA activity, then adjustment in the dosage and other measures may be taken to induce tolerance and restore adequate ADA activity.

➤*Antibody:* Antibody to pegademase bovine may develop in patients and may result in more rapid clearance of the drug. Suspect antibody to pegademase bovine if a persistent fall in pre-injection level of plasma ADA to < 10 mcmol/hr/ml occurs. If other causes for a decline in plasma ADA levels can be ruled out (eg, improper storage of vials [freezing or prolonged storage at temperatures> 4°C], or improper handling of plasma samples [eg, repeated freezing and thawing during transport to laboratory]), then perform a specific assay for antibody to ADA and pegademase bovine (ELISA, enzyme inhibition).

One of 12 patients showed an enhanced rate of clearance of plasma ADA activity after 5 months of therapy at 15 U/kg/week. Enhanced clearance was correlated with the appearance of an antibody that directly inhibited both unmodified ADA and pegademase bovine. Subsequently, the patient was treated with twice weekly IM injections at an increased dose of 20 U/kg, or a total weekly dose of 40 U/kg. No adverse effects were observed at the higher dose and effective levels of plasma ADA were restored. After 4 months, the patient returned to a weekly dosage schedule of 20 U/kg and effective plasma levels have been maintained.

Drug Interactions

➤*Vidarabine:* Vidarabine is a substrate for ADA and **2'-deoxycoformycin** is a potent inhibitor of ADA. Thus, the activities of these drugs and pegademase bovine could be substantially altered if they are used in combination with one another.

Adverse Reactions

Clinical experience is limited. The following adverse reactions have occurred: Headache (1 patient) and pain at the injection site (2 patients).

Overdosage

An intraperitoneal dose of 50,000 U/kg of pegademase bovine in mice resulted in weight loss up to 9%.

ALEFACEPT

| *Rx* | **Amevive** (Biogen Idec) | **Powder for injection, lyophilized:** 7.5 mg | 12.5 mg sucrose. Preservative-free. In dose pack 1s and 4s.[1] |
| | | 15 mg | 12.5 mg sucrose. Preservative-free. In dose pack 1s and 4s.[2] |

[1] In single-use vials with 10 mL single-use diluent (sterile water for injection) vial, syringe, winged infusion set, and needles.

[2] In single-use vials with 10 mL single-use diluent (sterile water for injection) vial, syringe, and needles.

Indications

➤*Plaque psoriasis:* For the treatment of adult patients with moderate to severe chronic plaque psoriasis who are candidates for systemic therapy or phototherapy.

Administration and Dosage

➤*Approved by the FDA:* January 31, 2003.

➤*Dosage regimen:* The recommended dose of alefacept is 7.5 mg given once weekly as an IV bolus or 15 mg given once weekly as an IM injection. The recommended regimen is a course of 12 weekly injections. Retreatment with an additional 12-week course may be initiated provided that CD4+ T lymphocyte counts are within the normal range and a minimum of a 12-week interval has passed since the previous course of treatment. Data on retreatment beyond 2 cycles are limited.

➤*Monitoring:* Monitor the CD4+ T lymphocyte counts of patients receiving alefacept weekly before initiating dosing and throughout the course of the 12-week dosing regimen. Withhold dosing if CD4+ T lymphocyte counts are below 250 cells/mcL. Discontinue the drug if the counts remain below 250 cells/mcL for 1 month.

➤*Reconstitution:* Reconstitute 15 mg alefacept lyophilized powder for IM administration with 0.6 mL of the supplied diluent (sterile water for injection); 0.5 mL of the reconstituted solution contains 15 mg alefacept.

Reconstitute 7.5 mg alefacept lyophilized powder for IV administration with 0.6 mL of the supplied diluent; 0.5 mL of the reconstituted solution contains 7.5 mg alefacept.

Do not add other medications to solutions containing alefacept. Do not reconstitute alefacept with other diluents. Do not filter reconstituted solution during preparation or administration.

Using the supplied syringe and one of the supplied needles, withdraw only 0.6 mL of the supplied diluent (sterile water for injection). Keeping the needle pointed at the sidewall of the vial, slowly inject the diluent into the vial of alefacept. Some foaming will occur, which is normal. To avoid excessive foaming, do not shake or vigorously agitate. Swirl the contents gently during dissolution. Generally, dissolution of alefacept takes less than 2 minutes. Use the solution as soon as possible after reconstitution.

The reconstituted solution should be clear and colorless to slightly yellow. Do not use the solution if it is discolored or cloudy or if undissolved material remains.

Following reconstitution, use the product immediately or within 4 hours if stored in the vial at 2° to 8°C (36° to 46°F). Discard alefacept not used within 4 hours of reconstitution.

➤*Administration:*

IM – For IM use, inject the full 0.5 mL of solution. Rotate injection sites so that a different site is used for each new injection. Give new injections at least 1 inch from an old site and never into areas where the skin is tender, bruised, red, or hard.

IV – For IV use, prepare 2 syringes with 3 mL normal saline for pre- and postadministration flush. Prime the winged infusion set with 3 mL saline and insert the set into the vein. Attach the alefacept-filled syringe to the infusion set and administer the solution over no more than 5 seconds. Flush the infusion set with 3 mL saline.

➤*Storage/Stability:* Store the dose tray containing alefacept lyophilized powder at controlled room temperature (15° to 30°C; 59° to 86°F). Protect from light. Retain in carton until time of use.

Following reconstitution, use the product immediately or within 4 hours if stored in the vial at 2° to 8°C (36° to 46°F). Discard alefacept not used within 4 hours of reconstitution.

Actions

➤*Pharmacology:* Alefacept is an immunosuppressive dimeric fusion protein that consists of the extracellular CD2-binding portion of the human leukocyte function antigen-3 (LFA-3) linked to the Fc (hinge, CH2 and CH3 domains) portion of human IgG1. Alefacept interferes with lymphocyte activation by specifically binding to the lymphocyte antigen, CD2, and inhibiting LFA-3/CD2 interaction. Activation of T lymphocytes involving the interaction beween LFA-3 on antigen-presenting cells and CD2 on T lymphocytes plays a role in the pathophysiology of chronic plaque psoriasis. The majority of T lymphocytes in psoriatic lesions are of the memory effector phenotype characterized by the presence of the CD45RO marker, express activation markers (eg, CD25, CD69) and release inflammatory cytokines, such as interferon γ.

Alefacept also causes a reduction in subsets of CD2+ T lymphocytes (primarily CD45RO+), presumably by bridging between CD2 on target lymphocytes and immunoglobulin Fc receptors on cytotoxic cells, such

as natural killer cells. Treatment with alefacept results in a reduction in circulating total CD4+ and CD8+ T lymphocyte counts. CD2 also is expressed at low levels on the surface of natural killer cells and certain bone marrow B lymphocytes. Therefore, the potential exists for alefacept to affect the activation and numbers of cells other than T lymphocytes. In clinical studies of alefacept, minor changes in the numbers of circulating cells other than T lymphocytes have been observed.

➤*Pharmacokinetics:* In patients with moderate to severe plaque psoriasis, following a 7.5 mg IV administration, the mean volume of distribution of alefacept was 94 mL/kg, the mean clearance was 0.25 mL/h/kg, and the mean elimination half-life was approximately 270 hours. Following an IM injection, bioavailability was 63%.

Pharmacodynamics – At doses tested in clinical trials, alefacept therapy resulted in a dose-dependent decrease in circulating total lymphocytes. The reduction predominantly affected the memory effector subset of the CD4+ and CD8+ T lymphocyte compartments, the predominant phenotype in psoriatic lesions. Circulating naive T lymphocyte and natural killer cell counts appeared to be only minimally susceptible to alefacept treatment, while circulating B lymphocyte counts appeared not to be affected by alefacept.

Contraindications

Hypersensitivity to alefacept or any of its components.

Warnings

➤*Lymphopenia:* Alefacept induces dose-dependent reductions in circulating CD4+ and CD8+ T lymphocyte counts.

Do not initiate a course of alefacept therapy in patients with a CD4+ T lymphoctye count below normal. Monitor the CD4+ T lymphocyte counts of patients receiving alefacept weekly throughout the course of the 12-week dosing regimen. Withhold dosing if CD4+ T lymphocyte counts are below 250 cells/mcL. Discontinue the drug if the counts remain below 250 cells/mcL for 1 month (see Administration and Dosage).

➤*Malignancies:* Alefacept may increase the risk of malignancies. Some patients who received alefacept in clinical studies developed malignancies. In preclinical studies, animals developed B cell hyperplasia, and 1 animal developed a lymphoma. Do not administer alefacept to patients with a history of systemic malignancy. Exercise caution when considering the use of alefacept in patients at high risk for malignancy. If a patient develops a malignancy, discontinue alefacept.

➤*Serious infections:* Alefacept is an immunosuppressive agent and, therefore, has the potential to increase the risk of infection and reactivate latent, chronic infections. Do not administer alefacept to patients with a clinically important infection. Exercise caution when considering the use of alefacept in patients with chronic infections or a history of recurrent infection. Monitor patients for signs and symptoms of infection during or after a course of alefacept. Closely monitor new infections. Discontinue alefacept if a patient develops a serious infection.

➤*Hypersensitivity reactions:* Hypersensitivity reactions (ie, urticaria, angioedema) were associated with the administration of alefacept. If an anaphylactic reaction or other serious allergic reaction occurs, immediately discontinue alefacept administration and initiate appropriate therapy.

➤*Carcinogenesis:* In a chronic toxicity study, cynomolgus monkeys were dosed weekly for 52 weeks with IV alefacept at 1 or 20 mg/kg/dose. One animal in the high-dose group developed a B-cell lymphoma that was detected after 28 weeks of dosing. Additional animals in both dose groups developed B-cell hyperplasia of the spleen and lymph nodes.

All animals in the study were positive for an endemic primate gamma-herpes virus also known as lymphocryptovirus (LCV). Latent LCV infection is generally asymptomatic but can lead to B-cell lymphomas when animals are immune suppressed.

In a separate study, baboons given 3 doses of alefacept at 1 mg/kg every 8 weeks were found to have centroblast proliferation in B-cell dependent areas in the germinal centers of the spleen following a 116-day washout period.

The role of alefacept in the development of the lymphoid malignancy and the hyperplasia observed in nonhuman primates and the relevance to humans is unknown. Immunodeficiency-associated lymphocyte disorders (plasmacytic hyperplasia, polymorphic proliferation, and B-cell lymphomas) occur in patients who have congenital or acquired immunodeficiencies including those resulting from immunosuppressive therapy.

➤*Elderly:* Because the incidence of infections and certain malignancies is higher in the elderly population, in general, use caution in treating the elderly.

ALEFACEPT

►*Pregnancy:* Category B. Because the effect of alefacept on pregnancy and fetal development, including immune system development, is not known, health care providers are encouraged to enroll patients currently taking alefacept who become pregnant into the manufacturer's pregnancy registry by calling (866) 263-8483.

Alefacept underwent transplacental passage and produced in utero exposure in developing monkeys. In utero, serum levels of exposure in these monkeys were 23% of maternal serum levels. No evidence of fetal toxicity including adverse effects on immune system development was observed in any of these animals.

There are no adequate and well-controlled studies in pregnant women. Because the risk to the development of the fetal immune system and postnatal immune function in humans is unknown, use alefacept during pregnancy only if clearly needed. If pregnancy occurs while taking alefacept, assess continued use of the drug.

►*Lactation:* It is not known whether alefacept is excreted in human milk. Because many drugs are excreted in human milk, and because there exists the potential for serious adverse reactions in nursing infants from alefacept, decide whether to discontinue nursing while taking the drug or to discontinue the use of the drug, taking into account the importance of the drug to the mother.

►*Children:* The safety and efficacy of alefacept in pediatric patients have not been studied. Alefacept is not indicated for pediatric patients.

Precautions

►*Monitoring:* Monitor CD4+ T lymphocyte counts weekly during the 12-week dosing period and use them to guide dosing. Patients should have normal CD4+ T lymphocyte counts prior to an initial or a subsequent course of treatment with alefacept. Withhold dosing if CD4+ T lymphocyte counts are below 250 cells/mcL. Discontinue alefacept if CD4+ T lymphocyte counts remain below 250 cells/mcL for 1 month.

►*Immunosuppression:* Patients receiving other immunosuppressive agents or phototherapy should not receive concurrent therapy with alefacept because of the possibility of excessive immunosuppression. The duration of the period following treatment with alefacept before one should consider starting another immunosuppressive therapy has not been evaluated.

►*Vaccinations:* The safety and efficacy of vaccines, specifically live or live-attenuated vaccines, administered to patients being treated with alefacept have not been studied. In a study of 46 patients with chronic plaque psoriasis, the ability to mount immunity to tetanus toxoid (recall antigen) and an experimental neo-antigen was preserved in those patients undergoing alefacept therapy.

►*Immunogenicity:* Approximately 3% of patients receiving alefacept developed low-titer antibodies to alefacept. No apparent correlation of antibody development and clinical response or adverse events was observed. The long-term immunogenicity of alefacept is unknown.

Drug Interactions

No formal interaction studies have been performed. The duration of the period following treatment with alefacept before one should consider starting another immunosuppressive therapy has not been evaluated.

Adverse Reactions

The most serious adverse reactions were lymphopenia, malignancies, serious infections requiring hospitalization, and hypersensitivity reactions (see Warnings).

Commonly observed adverse events seen in the first course of placebo-controlled clinical trials with at least a 2% higher incidence in the alefacept-treated patients compared with placebo-treated patients were the following: Pharyngitis, dizziness, increased cough, nausea, pruritus, myalgia, chills, injection site pain, injection site inflammation, accidental injury. The only adverse event that occurred at a 5% or higher incidence among alefacept-treated patients compared with placebo-treated patients was chills (1% placebo vs 6% alefacept), which occurred predominantly with IV administration.

The adverse reactions that most commonly resulted in clinical intervention were cardiovascular events, including coronary artery disorder and MI (less than 1%). These events were not observed in any of the 413 placebo-treated patients. The total number of patients hospitalized for cardiovascular events in the alefacept-treated group was 1.2%.

The most common events resulting in discontinuation of treatment with alefacept were the following: CD4+ T lymphocyte levels below 250 cells/mcL; headache, nausea (0.2%).

►*Hematologic/Lymphatic:* In the IM study (Study 2), 4% of patients temporarily discontinued treatment and no patients permanently discontinued treatment because of CD4+ T lymphocyte counts below the specified threshold of 250 cells/mcL. In Study 2, 10%, 28%, and 42% of patients had total lymphocyte, CD4+, and CD8+ T lymphocyte counts below normal, respectively. Twelve weeks after a course of therapy (12 weekly doses), 2%, 8%, and 21% of patients had total lymphocyte, CD4+, and CD8+ T lymphocyte cell counts below normal.

In the first course of the IV study (Study 1), 10% of patients temporarily discontinued treatment and 2% permanently discontinued treatment because of CD4+ T lymphocyte counts below the specified threshold of 250 cells/mcL. During the first course of Study 1, 22% of patients had total lymphocyte counts below normal, 48% had CD4+ T lymphocyte counts below normal, and 59% had CD8+ T lymphocyte counts below normal. The maximal effect on lymphocytes was observed within 6 to 8 weeks of initiation of treatment. Twelve weeks after a course of therapy (12 weekly doses), 4% of patients had total lymphocyte counts below normal, 19% had CD4+ T lymphocyte counts below normal, and 36% had CD8+ T lymphocyte counts below normal.

For patients receiving a second course of alefacept in Study 1, 17% of patients had total lymphocyte counts below normal, 44% had CD4+ T lymphocyte counts below normal, and 56% had CD8+ T lymphocyte counts below normal. Twelve weeks after completing dosing, 3% of patients had total lymphocyte counts below normal, 17% had CD4+ T lymphocyte counts below normal, and 35% had CD8+ T lymphocyte counts below normal (see Warnings).

►*Hepatic:* Rare cases (9) of transaminase elevations to 5 to 10 times the upper limit of normal were observed.

►*Hypersensitivity:* In clinical studies, 2 patients were reported to experience angioedema, one of whom was hospitalized. In the 24-week period constituting the first course of placebo-controlled studies, urticaria was reported in 6 (fewer than 1%) alefacept-treated patients vs 1 patient in the control group. Urticaria resulted in discontinuation of therapy in one of the alefacept-treated patients.

►*Local:* In the IM study (Study 2), 16% of alefacept-treated patients and 8% of placebo-treated patients reported injection site reactions. Reactions at the site of injection generally were mild, typically occurred on single occasions, and included the following: Pain (7%); inflammation, bleeding (4%); edema, nonspecific reaction (2%); mass (1%); skin hypersensitivity (less than 1%). In the clinical trials, a single case of injection site reaction led to the discontinuation of alefacept.

►*Miscellaneous:*

Malignancies – In the 24-week period constituting the first course of placebo-controlled studies, 13 malignancies were diagnosed in 11 alefacept-treated patients. The incidence of malignancies was 1.3% for alefacept-treated patients compared with 0.5% in the placebo group.

Among the 1357 patients who received alefacept, 25 patients were diagnosed with 35 treatment-emergent malignancies. The majority of these malignancies (23 cases) were basal (6) or squamous cell cancers (17) of the skin. Three cases of lymphoma were observed; one was classified as non-Hodgkin follicle-center cell lymphoma and two were classified as Hodgkin disease.

Infections – In the 24-week period constituting the first course of placebo-controlled studies, serious infections (infections requiring hospitalization) were seen at a rate of 0.9% in alefacept-treated patients and 0.2% in the placebo group. In patients receiving repeated courses of alefacept therapy, the rates of serious infections were 0.7% and 1.5% in the second and third course of therapy, respectively. Serious infections among 1357 alefacept-treated patients included necrotizing cellulitis, peritonsillar abscess, postoperative and burn wound infection, toxic shock, pneumonia, appendicitis, preseptal cellulitis, cholecystitis, gastroenteritis, and herpes simplex infection.

Overdosage

The highest dose tested in humans (0.75 mg/kg IV) was associated with chills, headache, arthralgia, and sinusitis within 1 day of dosing. Closely monitor patients who have been inadvertently administered an excess of the recommended dose for effects on total lymphocyte count and CD4+ T lymphocyte count.

Patient Information

Inform patients of the need for regular monitoring of white blood cell (lymphocyte) counts during therapy and that alefacept must be administered under the supervision of a physician. Inform patients that alefacept reduces lymphocyte counts, which could increase their chances of developing an infection or a malignancy. Advise patients to promptly inform their physician if they develop any signs of an infection or malignancy while undergoing a course of treatment with alefacept.

Advise female patients to notify their physicians if they become pregnant while taking alefacept (or within 8 weeks of discontinuing alefacept) and be advised of the existence of and encouraged to enroll in the pregnancy registry. Call (866) 263-8483 to enroll.

EFALIZUMAB

Rx	**Raptiva** (Genentech)	**Powder for injection, lyophilized:** 150 mg (designed to deliver 125 mg/1.25 mL)	Preservative-free. In single-use vials[1]. With 1 single-use, prefilled diluent syringe containing 1.3 mL sterile water for injection, two 25 gauge × ⅝ inch needles, and 2 alcohol prep pads.

[1] With 123.2 mg sucrose, 6.8 mg L-histidine hydrochloride monohydrate, and 4.3 mg L-histidine.

Indications

➤*Psoriasis:* For the treatment of adult patients (18 years of age and older) with chronic moderate to severe plaque psoriasis who are candidates for systemic therapy or phototherapy.

Administration and Dosage

➤*Approved by the FDA:* October 27, 2003.

➤*Dosage:* The recommended dose of efalizumab is a single 0.7 mg/kg SC conditioning dose followed by weekly SC doses of 1 mg/kg (maximum single dose not to exceed a total of 200 mg).

➤*Preparation for administration:* Administer efalizumab using the sterile, disposable syringe and needles provided. To prepare the efalizumab solution, slowly inject the 1.3 mL of sterile water for injection into the efalizumab vial using the provided prefilled diluent syringe. Swirl the vial with a gentle rotary motion to dissolve the product. Do not shake; shaking will cause foaming of the efalizumab solution. Generally, dissolution takes less than 5 minutes. Efalizumab is provided as a single-use vial and contains no antibacterial preservatives. Reconstitute immediately before use and use only once. If the reconstituted efalizumab is not used immediately, store the vial at room temperature and use within 8 hours. Do not add other medications to solutions containing efalizumab and do not reconstitute efalizumab with other diluents.

Administration – Sites for injection include thigh, abdomen, buttocks, or upper arm. Rotate injection sites. Following administration, discard any unused reconstituted efalizumab solution. If it is determined to be appropriate, patients may self-inject efalizumab after proper training in the preparation and injection technique and with medical follow-up. The safety and efficacy of efalizumab therapy beyond 1 year have not been established.

➤*Storage/Stability:* Do not use a vial beyond the expiration date stamped on the carton or vial label. Refrigerate efalizumab at 2° to 8°C (36° to 46°F). Protect the vial from exposure to light. Store in original carton until time of use.

Actions

➤*Pharmacology:* Efalizumab is an immunosuppressive, recombinant, humanized IgG1 kappa isotype monoclonal antibody that binds to human CD11a. Efalizumab binds to CD11a, the α subunit of leukocyte function antigen-1 (LFA-1) that is expressed on all leukocytes, and decreases cell surface expression of CD11a. Efalizumab inhibits the binding of LFA-1 to intercellular adhesion molecule-1 (ICAM-1), thereby inhibiting the adhesion of leukocytes to other cell types. Interaction between LFA-1 and ICAM-1 contributes to the initiation and maintenance of multiple processes, including activation of T lymphocytes, adhesion of T lymphocytes to endothelial cells, and migration of T lymphocytes to sites of inflammation, including psoriatic skin. Lymphocyte activation and trafficking to skin play a role in the pathophysiology of chronic plaque psoriasis. In psoriatic skin, ICAM-1 cell surface expression is upregulated on endothelium and keratinocytes. CD11a also is expressed on the surface of B lymphocytes, monocytes, neutrophils, natural killer cells, and other leukocytes. Therefore, the potential exists for efalizumab to affect the activation, adhesion, migration, and numbers of cells other than T lymphocytes.

At a dose of 1 mg/kg/week SC, efalizumab reduced expression of CD11a on circulating T lymphocytes to approximately 15% to 25% of predose values and reduced free CD11a binding sites to a mean of 5% or less of predose values. These pharmacodynamic effects were seen 1 to 2 days after the first dose and were maintained between weekly 1 mg/kg SC doses. Following discontinuation of efalizumab, CD11a expression returned to a mean of 74% of baseline at 5 weeks and stayed at comparable levels at 8 and 13 weeks. Following discontinuation of efalizumab, free CD11a binding sites returned to a mean of 86% of baseline at 8 weeks and stayed at comparable levels at 13 weeks.

In clinical trials, efalizumab treatment resulted in a mean increase in white blood cell (WBC) count of 34%, a doubling of mean lymphocyte counts, and an increase in eosinophil counts of 29% because of decreased leukocyte adhesion to blood vessel walls and decreased trafficking from the vascular compartment to tissues. At day 56 of 1 mg/kg/week efalizumab treatment, 32% of patients had a shift in total WBC from low or normal baseline value to above normal, 46% had a shift to above normal absolute lymphocyte counts, and 5% had a shift to above normal eosinophil counts. Following discontinuation of efalizumab treatment, the abnormal elevated lymphocyte counts took approximately 8 weeks to normalize among patients who had above normal lymphocyte counts. Plasma samples collected after first administration of 0.3 mg/kg IV efalizumab indicate that at 2 hours, TNF-α and IL-6 plasma levels were elevated 9- and 90-fold, respectively, compared with baseline. Plasma samples collected after first administration of 0.7 mg/kg SC efalizumab indicate that at 2 days, IL-6 levels were

elevated (10 pg/mL as compared with 5 pg/mL at baseline), whereas TNF-α was not detectable. In efalizumab-treated patients, the mean levels of C reactive protein increased from baseline by 67% and the mean levels of fibrinogen increased by 15%.

➤*Pharmacokinetics:*

Absorption/Distribution – In patients with moderate to severe plaque psoriasis, following an initial SC efalizumab dose of 0.7 mg/kg followed by 11 weekly SC doses of 1 mg/kg/week, serum concentrations reached steady state at 4 weeks with a mean trough concentration of approximately 9 mcg/mL (n = 26). After the last dose, the mean peak concentration was approximately 12 mcg/mL (n = 25). The mean estimated efalizumab SC bioavailability was 50%.

Metabolism/Excretion – Mean steady-state clearance was 24 mL/kg/day (range, 5 to 76 mL/kg/day, n = 25). Mean time to eliminate efalizumab after the last steady-state dose was 25 days (range, 13 to 35 days, n = 17).

Contraindications

Hypersensitivity to efalizumab or any of its components.

Warnings

➤*Infections:* Efalizumab is an immunosuppressive agent and has the potential to increase the risk of infection and reactivate latent, chronic infections. Do not administer efalizumab to patients with clinically important infections. Exercise caution when considering the use of efalizumab in patients with a chronic infection or history of recurrent infections. If a patient develops a serious infection, discontinue efalizumab. Monitor new infections developing during efalizumab treatment. During the first 12 weeks of controlled trials, serious infections occurred in 7 of 1620 (0.4%) efalizumab-treated patients compared with 1 of 715 (0.1%) placebo-treated patients (see Adverse Reactions). Serious infections requiring hospitalization included cellulitis, pneumonia, abscess, sepsis, bronchitis, gastroenteritis, aseptic meningitis, Legionnaire disease, and vertebral osteomyelitis (note some patients had more than 1 infection).

➤*Malignancies:* Many immunosuppressive agents have the potential to increase the risk of malignancy. The role of efalizumab in the development of malignancies is not known. Exercise caution when considering the use of efalizumab in patients at high risk for malignancy or with a history of malignancy. If a patient develops a malignancy, discontinue efalizumab.

➤*Thrombocytopenia:* Platelet counts at or below 52,000 cells/mcL were observed in 8 (0.3%) efalizumab-treated patients during clinical trials compared with none among the placebo-treated patients. Five of the 8 patients received a course of systemic steroids for thrombocytopenia. Thrombocytopenia resolved in the 7 patients receiving adequate follow-up (1 patient was lost to follow-up). Follow patients closely for signs and symptoms of thrombocytopenia. Assessment of platelet counts is recommended during treatment with efalizumab; discontinue efalizumab if thrombocytopenia develops.

➤*Worsening of psoriasis:* Worsening of psoriasis can occur during or after discontinuation of efalizumab. During clinical studies, 0.7% of efalizumab-treated patients had serious worsening of psoriasis during treatment or worsening past baseline after discontinuation of efalizumab. In some patients, these events took the form of psoriatic erythroderma or pustular psoriasis. Some patients required hospitalization and alternative antipsoriatic therapy to manage the psoriasis worsening. Closely observe patients, including those not responding to efalizumab treatment, following discontinuation of efalizumab and institute appropriate psoriasis treatment as necessary.

➤*Elderly:* Because the incidence of infections is higher in the elderly population, in general, use caution in treating the elderly.

➤*Pregnancy: Category C.* At 11 weeks of age, the offspring of female mice administered doses 3 to 30 times the equivalent of the recommended clinical dose exhibited a significant reduction in their ability to mount an antibody response, which showed evidence of partial reversibility by 25 weeks of age. It is not known whether efalizumab can cause fetal harm when administered to a pregnant woman or if efalizumab can affect reproduction capacity. Give to a pregnant woman only if clearly needed.

Pregnancy registry – Health care providers are encouraged to enroll patients who become pregnant while taking efalizumab (or within 6 weeks of discontinuing efalizumab) in the efalizumab Pregnancy Registry.

➤*Lactation:* It is not known whether efalizumab is excreted in human milk. An antimouse CD11a antibody was detected in milk samples of lactating mice exposed to antimouse CD11a antibody and the offspring of the exposed females exhibited significant reduction in antibody responses. Since maternal immunoglobulins are known to be present in

EFALIZUMAB

milk of lactating mothers and animal data suggest the potential for adverse effects in nursing infants from efalizumab, decide whether to discontinue nursing while taking the drug or to discontinue the use of the drug, taking into account the importance of the drug to the mother.

➤*Children:* The safety and efficacy of efalizumab in pediatric patients have not been studied.

Precautions

➤*Monitoring:* Assessment of platelet counts is recommended upon initiating and periodically while receiving efalizumab treatment. It is recommended that assessments become more frequent while initiating therapy (eg, monthly). Assessments may decrease in frequency with continued treatment (eg, every 3 months). Severe thrombocytopenia has been observed (see Warnings).

➤*Immunosuppression:* The safety and efficacy of efalizumab in combination with other immunosuppressive agents or phototherapy have not been evaluated. Patients receiving other immunosuppressive agents should not receive concurrent therapy with efalizumab because of the possibility of increased risk of infections and malignancies.

➤*Vaccinations:* The safety and efficacy of vaccines administered to patients being treated with efalizumab have not been studied. In a small clinical study with IV administered efalizumab, a single dose of 0.3 mg/kg given before primary immunization with a neoantigen decreased the secondary immune response, and a dose of 1 mg/kg almost completely ablated it. A dose of 0.3 mg/kg IV has comparable pharmacodynamic effects to the recommended dose of 1 mg/kg SC. Do not administer acellular, live, and live-attenuated vaccines during efalizumab treatment.

➤*First-dose reactions:* First-dose reactions including headache, fever, nausea, and vomiting are associated with efalizumab treatment and are dose-level related in incidence and severity. Therefore, a conditioning dose of 0.7 mg/kg is recommended to reduce the incidence and severity of reactions associated with initial dosing (see Administration and Dosage). One case of aseptic meningitis resulting in hospitalization has been observed in association with initial dosing (see Adverse Reactions).

Drug Interactions

➤*Immunosuppressive agents:* Do not use efalizumab with other immunosuppressive drugs (see Precautions).

➤*Live vaccines:* Do not administer acellular, live, and live-attenuated vaccines during efalizumab treatment (see Precautions).

➤*Drug/Lab test interactions:* Increases in lymphocyte counts related to the pharmacologic mechanism of action are frequently observed during efalizumab treatment (see Pharmacology).

Adverse Reactions

The most serious adverse reactions observed during treatment with efalizumab were serious infections, malignancies, thrombocytopenia, and psoriasis worsening and variants (see Warnings).

The most common adverse reactions associated with efalizumab were a first-dose reaction complex that included headache, chills, fever, nausea, and myalgia within 2 days following the first 2 injections. These reactions are dose-level related in incidence and severity and were largely mild to moderate in severity when a conditioning dose of 0.7 mg/kg was used as the first dose. In placebo-controlled trials, 29% of patients treated with efalizumab 1 mg/kg developed 1 or more of these symptoms following the first dose, compared with 15% of patients receiving placebo. After the third dose, 4% and 3% of patients receiving efalizumab 1 mg/kg and placebo, respectively, experienced these symptoms. Less than 1% of patients discontinued efalizumab treatment because of these adverse events. Other adverse events resulting in discontinuation of efalizumab treatment were psoriasis (0.6%), pain (0.4%), arthritis (0.4%), and arthralgia (0.3%).

The following table enumerates the adverse events occurring during controlled periods of the clinical trials where the frequency of the adverse events is at least 2% greater in the efalizumab-treated group than the placebo group.

Efalizumab Adverse Events (≥ 2)		
Adverse reaction	Efalizumab 1 mg/kg/week (n = 1213)	Placebo (n = 715)
Headache	32	22
Infection[1]	29	26
Chills	13	4
Nausea	11	7
Pain	10	5
Myalgia	8	5
Flu syndrome	7	4
Fever	7	3
Back pain	4	2
Acne	4	1

[1] Includes diagnosed infections and other nonspecific infections. Most common nonspecific infection was upper respiratory infection.

➤*Other adverse events:* Adverse events occurring at a rate between 1% and 2% greater in the efalizumab group compared with placebo were arthralgia, asthenia, peripheral edema, and psoriasis.

Infections – In the first 12 weeks of placebo-controlled studies, the proportion of patients with serious infection was 0.4% in the efalizumab-treated group (5 of these were hospitalized, 0.3%) and 0.1% in the placebo group (see Warnings). In the complete safety data from both controlled and uncontrolled studies, the overall incidence of hospitalization for infections was 1.6 per 100 patient-years for efalizumab-treated patients compared with 1.2 per 100 patient-years for placebo-treated patients. Including both controlled, uncontrolled, and follow-up study treatment periods, there were 27 serious infections in 2475 efalizumab-treated patients. These infections included cellulitis, pneumonia, abscess, sepsis, sinusitis, bronchitis, gastroenteritis, aseptic meningitis, Legionnaire disease, septic arthritis, and vertebral osteomyelitis. In controlled trials, the overall rate of infections in efalizumab-treated patients was 3% higher than in placebo-treated patients.

Malignancies – Among the 2762 psoriasis patients who received efalizumab at any dose (median duration 8 months), 31 patients were diagnosed with 37 malignancies (see Warnings). The overall incidence of malignancies of any kind was 1.8 per 100 patient-years for efalizumab-treated patients compared with 1.6 per 100 patients-years for placebo-treated patients. Malignancies observed in the efalizumab-treated patients included nonmelanoma skin cancer, noncutaneous solid tumors, Hodgkin and non-Hodgkin lymphoma, and malignant melanoma. The incidence of noncutaneous solid tumors (8 in 1790 patient-years) and malignant melanoma were within the range expected for the general population.

The majority of the malignancies were nonmelanoma skin cancers; 26 cases (13 basal, 13 squamous) in 20 patients (0.7% of 2762 efalizumab-treated patients). The incidence was comparable for efalizumab-treated and placebo-treated patients. However, the size of the placebo group and duration of follow-up were limited, and a difference in rates of nonmelanoma skin cancers cannot be excluded.

Thrombocytopenia – In the combined safety database of 2762 efalizumab-treated patients, there were 8 occurrences (0.3%) of thrombocytopenia of less than 52,000 cells/mcL reported (see Warnings). Three of the 8 patients were hospitalized for thrombocytopenia, including 1 patient with heavy uterine bleeding; all cases were consistent with an immune-mediated thrombocytopenia. Antiplatelet antibody was evaluated in 1 patient and was found to be positive. Each case resulted in discontinuation of efalizumab. Based on available platelet count measurements, the onset of platelet decline was between 8 and 12 weeks after the first dose of efalizumab in 5 of the patients. Onset was more delayed in 3 patients, occurring as late as 1 year in 1 patient. In these cases, the platelet count nadirs occurred between 12 and 72 weeks after the first dose of efalizumab.

Psoriasis – In the combined safety database from all studies, serious psoriasis adverse events occurred in 19 efalizumab-treated patients (0.7%) including hospitalization in 17 patients (see Warnings). Most of these events (14/19) occurred after discontinuation of study drug and occurred in both patients responding and not responding to efalizumab treatment. Serious adverse events of psoriasis included pustular, erythrodermic, and guttate subtypes. During the first 12 weeks of treatment within placebo-controlled studies, the rate of psoriasis adverse events (serious and nonserious) was 3.2% in the efalizumab-treated patients and 1.4% in the placebo-treated patients.

Hypersensitivity reactions – In the first 12 weeks of controlled clinical studies, the proportion of patients reporting at least 1 hypersensitivity reaction was 8% in the 1 mg/kg/week group and 7% of patients in the placebo group. Urticaria was observed in 1% of patients receiving efalizumab and 0.4% of patients receiving placebo during the initial 12-week treatment period. Other observed adverse events in patients receiving efalizumab that may be indicative of hypersensitivity included: Laryngospasm, angioedema, erythema multiforme, asthma, and allergic drug eruption. One patient was hospitalized with a serum sickness-like reaction.

Inflammatory/immune-mediated reactions – In the entire efalizumab clinical development program of 2762 efalizumab-treated patients, inflammatory, potentially immune-mediated adverse events resulting in hospitalization included inflammatory arthritis (12 cases, 0.4% of patients) and interstitial pneumonitis (2 cases). One case of each of the following serious adverse reactions was observed: Transverse myelitis, bronchiolitis obliterans, aseptic meningitis, idiopathic hepatitis, sialedenitis, and sensorineural hearing loss.

Lab test abnormalities – In efalizumab-treated patients, a mean elevation in alkaline phosphatase (5 units/L) was observed; 4% of efalizumab-treated patients experienced a shift to above normal values compared with 0.6% of placebo-treated patients. The clinical significance of this change is unknown. Higher numbers of efalizumab-treated patients experienced elevations above normal in 2 or more liver function tests than placebo (3.1% vs 1.5%). Other laboratory adverse reactions that were observed included thrombocytopenia, lymphocytosis (40%) (including 3 cases of transient atypical lymphocytosis), and leukocytosis (26%).

EFALIZUMAB

Immunogenicity – In patients evaluated for antibodies to efalizumab after efalizumab treatment ended, predominantly low-titer antibodies to efalizumab or other protein components of the efalizumab drug product were detected in 6.3% of patients. The long-term immunogenicity of efalizumab is unknown.

Overdosage

➤*Symptoms:* The maximum administered single dose was 10 mg/kg IV. This was administered to 1 patient, who subsequently was admitted to the hospital for severe vomiting.

➤*Treatment:* In case of overdose, it is recommended that the patient be monitored for 24 to 48 hours for any acute signs or symptoms of adverse reactions or effects and appropriate treatment instituted.

Patient Information

Refer patients to the efalizumab patient package insert.

Inform patients that their physician may monitor platelet counts during therapy. Advise patients to seek immediate medical attention if they develop any of the signs or symptoms associated with severe thrombocytopenia, such as easy bleeding from the gums, bruising, or petechiae.

Inform patients that efalizumab is an immunosuppressant and could increase their chances of developing an infection or a malignancy. Advise patients to promptly call the prescribing doctor's office if they develop any new signs of, or receive a new diagnosis of infection or malignancy while undergoing treatment with efalizumab.

Advise female patients to notify their physicians if they become pregnant while taking efalizumab (or within 6 weeks of discontinuing efalizumab). Advise female patients of the existence of and encourage them to enroll in the efalizumab Pregnancy Registry.

If a patient or caregiver is to administer efalizumab, instruct he/she regarding injection techniques and how to measure the correct dose to ensure proper administration of efalizumab. In addition, patients should have available materials for and be instructed in the proper disposal of needles and syringes. Caution patients against reuse of syringes and needles.

Advise patients not to change or stop treatment without first talking with their health care provider.

Advise patients not to take other medicines called immunosuppressives or to take treatments called phototherapy.

AZATHIOPRINE

Rx	Azasan (aaiPharma)	Tablets: 25 mg	Lactose. Yellow, oval, scored. In 100s.
Rx	Azathiprine (aaiPharma)	Tablets: 50 mg	In 100s.
Rx	Imuran (Prometheus)		(Imuran 50). Yellow to off-white, scored. In 100s and UD 100s.
Rx	Azasan (aaiPharma)		Lactose. Yellow, capsule shape, scored. In 100s.
Rx	Azasan (aaiPharma)	Tablets: 75 mg	Lactose. Yellow, triangular, scored. In 100s.
Rx	Azasan (aaiPharma)	Tablets: 100 mg	Lactose. Yellow, diamond shape, scored. In 100s.
Rx	Azathioprine Sodium (Various, eg, Bedford)	Injection: 100 mg (as sodium) per vial	In 20 ml vials.
Rx	Imuran (Prometheus)		In 20 ml vials.

WARNING

Chronic immunosuppression with azathioprine increases the risk of neoplasia. Physicians using this drug should be familiar with this risk as well as with the mutagenic potential to both men and women and with possible hematologic toxicities.

Indications

➤*Renal homotransplantation:* As an adjunct for the prevention of rejection in renal homotransplantation. Experience with > 16,000 transplants shows a 5-year patient survival rate of 35% to 55%, but this is dependent on donor and many other variables.

➤*Rheumatoid arthritis:* Indicated only in adult patients meeting criteria for classic or definite rheumatoid arthritis as specified by the American Rheumatism Association. Restrict use to patients with severe, active and erosive disease not responsive to conventional management. Continue rest, physiotherapy and salicylates while azathioprine is given, but it may be possible to reduce the dose of corticosteroids.

➤*Unlabeled uses:* Azathioprine has been used in the treatment of chronic ulcerative colitis; however, serious adverse effects may offset its limited value.

Azathioprine 2 to 3 mg/kg/day has been used for the treatment of generalized myasthenia gravis; however, adverse reactions may occur in > 35% of patients.

Azathioprine 2.5 mg/kg/day may be effective in controlling the progression of Behcet's syndrome, especially eye disease, the most serious manifestation.

Although controversial, low-dose azathioprine (75 to 100 mg) may be effective in treating Crohn's disease.

Administration and Dosage

➤*Renal homotransplantation:* The dose required to prevent rejection and minimize toxicity varies. Initial dose is usually 3 to 5 mg/kg/day, given as a single daily dose on the day of transplantation, and in a minority of cases, 1 to 3 days before transplantation. It is often initiated IV, with subsequent use of tablets (at the same dose level) after the postoperative period. Reserve IV administration for patients unable to tolerate oral medications. Maintenance levels are 1 to 3 mg/kg/day. Do not increase the dose to toxic levels because of threatened rejection. Discontinuation may be necessary for severe hematologic or other toxicity, even if homograft rejection may be a consequence.

Children – An initial dose of 3 to 5 mg/kg/day IV or orally followed by a maintenance dose of 1 to 3 mg/kg/day has been recommended.

➤*Rheumatoid arthritis:* Usually given daily. Initial dose is approximately 1 mg/kg (50 to 100 mg) given as a single dose or twice daily. The dose may be increased, beginning at 6 to 8 weeks and thereafter by steps at 4 week intervals, if there are no serious toxicities and if initial response is unsatisfactory. Use dose increments of 0.5 mg/kg/day, up to a maximum dose of 2.5 mg/kg/day.

Therapeutic response occurs after 6 to 8 weeks of treatment; an adequate trial should be a minimum of 12 weeks. Patients not improved after 12 weeks are refractory. Continue the drug in patients with clinical response, but monitor carefully, and attempt gradual dosage reduction to reduce risk of toxicity. Optimum duration of therapy has not been determined. Use the lowest effective dose for maintenance therapy; lower decrementally with changes of 0.5 mg/kg or approximately 25 mg/day every 4 weeks while other therapy is kept constant. Azathioprine can be discontinued abruptly, but delayed effects are possible.

➤*Renal function impairment:* Relatively oliguric patients, especially those with tubular necrosis in the immediate postcadaveric transplant period, may have delayed clearance of azathioprine or its metabolites. They may be particularly sensitive to this drug and may require lower doses.

➤*Use with allopurinol:* Reduce dose of azathioprine to approximately 25% to 33% of the usual dose.

➤*Parenteral administration:* For IV use only. Add 10 ml Sterile Water for Injection and swirl until a clear solution results; use within 24 hours. Further dilution into sterile saline or dextrose is usually made for infusion. The final volume depends on the infusion time; it is usually 30 to 60 minutes, but ranges from 5 minutes to 8 hours for the daily dose.

Actions

➤*Pharmacology:* Azathioprine, an imidazoyl derivative of 6-mercaptopurine (6-MP), has many biological effects similar to those of the parent compound.

Homograft survival – Although the use of azathioprine for inhibition of renal homograft rejection is well established, the mechanism(s) for this action are obscure. The drug suppresses cell-mediated hypersensitivities and alters antibody production. Suppression of T-cell effects, including ablation of T-cell suppression, depends on the temporal relationship to antigenic stimulus or engraftment. This agent has little effect on established graft rejections or secondary responses.

AZATHIOPRINE

Alterations in specific immune responses or immunologic functions in transplant recipients are difficult to relate specifically to immunosuppression by azathioprine. These patients have subnormal responses to vaccines, low numbers of T-cells and abnormal phagocytosis by peripheral blood cells, but their mitogenic responses, serum immunoglobulins and secondary antibody responses are usually normal.

Immunoinflammatory response – The severity of adjuvant arthritis is reduced by azathioprine. The mechanisms whereby it affects autoimmune diseases are not known. Azathioprine is immunosuppressive; delayed hypersensitivity and cellular cytotoxicity tests are suppressed to a greater degree than are antibody responses. In the rat model of adjuvant arthritis, azathioprine inhibits the lymph node hyperplasia that precedes the onset of the signs of the disease. Both the immunosuppressive and therapeutic effects in animal models are dose-related. Azathioprine is a slow-acting drug and effects may persist after the drug has been discontinued.

►*Pharmacokinetics:* Azathioprine is well absorbed following oral administration. Maximum serum radioactivity occurs at 1 to 2 hours after oral radioactive azathioprine and decays with a half-life of 5 hours. This is not an estimate of the half-life of azathioprine itself but is the decay rate for all radioactive metabolites of the drug. Because of extensive metabolism, only a fraction of the radioactivity is present as azathioprine. Usual doses produce blood levels of < 1 mcg/ml azathioprine and 6-MP. Blood levels are of little value for therapy since the magnitude and duration of clinical effects correlate with thiopurine nucleotide levels in tissues rather than with plasma drug levels. Azathioprine and 6-MP are 30% bound to serum proteins.

Azathioprine is cleaved in vivo to 6-MP. Both compounds are rapidly eliminated from blood and are oxidized or methylated in erythrocytes and liver; no azathioprine or 6-MP is detectable in urine after 8 hours. Conversion to inactive 6-thiouric acid by xanthine oxidase is an important degradative pathway. Proportions of metabolites are different in individual patients, and this presumably accounts for variable magnitude and duration of drug effects. Renal clearance is probably not important in predicting effectiveness or toxicity, although dose reduction is practiced in patients with poor renal function. Azathioprine and 6-MP are partially dialyzable.

Contraindications

Hypersensitivity to azathioprine; pregnancy in rheumatoid arthritis patients.

Warnings

►*Hematologic effects:* Severe leukopenia or thrombocytopenia, macrocytic anemia, severe bone marrow depression and selective erythrocyte aplasia may occur in patients on azathioprine. Hematologic toxicities are dose-related, may occur late in the course of therapy and may be more severe in renal transplant patients whose homograft is undergoing rejection. Perform complete blood counts, including platelet counts, weekly during the first month, twice monthly for the second and third months of treatment, then monthly or more frequently if dosage alterations or other therapy changes are necessary. Delayed hematologic suppression may occur. Prompt reduction in dosage or temporary withdrawal of the drug may be necessary if there is a rapid fall in, or persistently low leukocyte count or other evidence of bone marrow depression. Leukopenia does not correlate with therapeutic effect; do not increase the dose intentionally to lower the white blood cell count. Drugs that affect leukocyte production (eg, TMP-SMZ) may lead to exaggerated leukopenia when used concurrently with azathioprine.

►*Infections:* Serious infections are a constant hazard for patients on chronic immunosuppression, especially for homograft recipients. The incidence of infection in renal homotransplantation is 30 to 60 times that in rheumatoid arthritis. Fungal, viral, bacterial and protozoal infections may be fatal and should be treated vigorously. Infection may occur as a secondary manifestation of bone marrow suppression or leukopenia. Consider reduction of azathioprine dosage or use of other drugs.

►*GI toxicity:* A GI hypersensitivity reaction characterized by severe nausea and vomiting has been reported (12% of 676 rheumatoid arthritis patients). These symptoms may also be accompanied by diarrhea, rash, fever, malaise, myalgias, elevations in liver enzymes, and occasionally hypotension. Symptoms of GI toxicity most often develop within the first several weeks of therapy and are reversible upon discontinuation of the drug. The reaction can recur within hours after rechallenge with a single azathioprine dose. The frequency of gastric disturbance can be reduced by administration in divided doses or after meals. Vomiting with abdominal pain may occur rarely with a hypersensitivity pancreatitis. Diarrhea and steatorrhea have been reported (< 1%).

►*Hepatotoxicity:* Hepatotoxicity with elevated serum alkaline phosphatase and bilirubin may occur primarily in allograft recipients. This is generally reversible after interruption of azathioprine. Hepatotoxicity has been uncommon in rheumatoid arthritis patients (< 1%). Hepatotoxicity following transplantation most often occurs within 6 months of transplantation and is generally reversible after interruption of aza-

thioprine. A rare, but life-threatening hepatic veno-occlusive disease associated with chronic administration of the drug has occurred in transplant patients and in one patient with panuveitis. Periodically measure serum transaminases, alkaline phosphatase and bilirubin for early detection of hepatotoxicity. If hepatic veno-occlusive disease is suspected, permanently withdraw azathioprine.

►*Carcinogenesis:* Azathioprine is carcinogenic in animals and may increase the patient's risk of neoplasia. Renal transplant patients have an increased risk of malignancy, predominantly skin cancer and reticulum cell or lymphomatous tumors. The risk of posttransplant lymphomas may be increased in patients who receive aggressive treatment with immunosuppressive drugs. The degree of immunosuppression is determined not only by the immune suppression regimen but also by a number of other patient factors. The number of immunosuppressive agents may not necessarily increase the risk of posttransplant lymphomas. However, transplant patients who receive multiple immunosuppressive agents may be at risk for over-immunosuppression; therefore, maintain immunosuppressive drug therapy at the lowest effective levels. The precise risk of neoplasia due to azathioprine has not been defined, but the risk is lower for rheumatoid arthritis patients than for transplant recipients. However, acute myelogenous leukemia as well as solid tumors have occurred in patients with rheumatoid arthritis receiving azathioprine. Also, rheumatoid arthritis patients previously treated with alkylating agents (eg, cyclophosphamide, chlorambucil, melphalan) may have a prohibitive risk of neoplasia if treated with azathioprine.

►*Mutagenesis:* Azathioprine is mutagenic in animals and humans.

►*Fertility impairment:* Temporary depression in spermatogenesis and reduction in sperm viability and sperm count have occurred in mice at doses 10 times the therapeutic human dose. A reduced percentage of fertile matings occurred in animals receiving 5 mg/kg.

►*Pregnancy: Category D.* Azathioprine can cause fetal harm when administered to a pregnant woman. Whenever possible, avoid use of this drug in pregnant patients. Do not use for treatment of rheumatoid arthritis in pregnant women.

Limited immunologic and other abnormalities have occurred in a few infants born of renal allograft recipients on azathioprine. In one report, documented lymphopenia, diminished IgG and IgM levels, CMV infection and a decreased thymic shadow were noted in an infant born to a mother receiving 150 mg azathioprine and 30 mg prednisone daily throughout pregnancy. Most of the infants' features had normalized at 10 weeks old. Another case reported pancytopenia and severe immune deficiency in a premature infant whose mother received 125 mg azathioprine daily. One infant was born with preaxial polydactyly; another infant whose father received long-term azathioprine had a large myelomeningocele in the upper lumbar region, bilateral dislocated hips and bilateral talipes equinovarus.

Carefully weigh the benefits vs the risks of azathioprine therapy in women of reproductive potential. There are no adequate and well controlled studies in pregnant women. If this drug is used during pregnancy, or if the patient becomes pregnant while taking it, apprise the patient of the potential hazard to the fetus. Advise women of childbearing age to avoid becoming pregnant.

►*Lactation:* Use in nursing mothers is not recommended. The drug or its metabolites are transferred at low levels, both transplacentally and in breast milk. Because of potential tumorigenicity shown for azathioprine, decide whether to discontinue nursing or the drug, taking into account the importance of the drug to the mother.

►*Children:* Safety and efficacy in children have not been established. However, it has been used in children (see Administration and Dosage).

Drug Interactions

Azathioprine Drug Interactions			
Precipitant drug	Object drug*		Description
ACE inhibitors	Azathioprine	↑	Concurrent use may induce severe leukopenia.
Allopurinol	Azathioprine	↑	Allopurinol may increase the pharmacologic and toxic effects of azathioprine.
Methotrexate	Azathioprine	↑	Plasma levels of the 6-MP metabolite may be increased.
Azathioprine	Anticoagulants	↓	Azathioprine may decrease the action of the anticoagulants.
Azathioprine	Cyclosporine	↓	Cyclosporine plasma levels may be decreased.
Azathioprine	Nondepolarizing neuromuscular blockers	↓	Pharmacologic actions of the neuromuscular blockers may be decreased or reversed.

* ↑ = Object drug increased. ↓ = Object drug decreased.

Adverse Reactions

The principal and potentially serious toxic effects are hematologic and GI (see Warnings). The risks of secondary infection and neoplasia are

AZATHIOPRINE

also important. The frequency and severity of adverse reactions depend on the dose and duration, as well as on the patient's underlying disease or concomitant therapies. The incidence of hematologic toxicities and neoplasia encountered in groups of renal homograft recipients is significantly higher than that in rheumatoid arthritis patients.

Incidence of Hematologic Toxicities and Neoplasia with Azathioprine		
Toxicity	Renal homograft	Rheumatoid arthritis
Leukopenia		
Any degree	> 50%	28%
< 2500/mm^3	> 16%	5.3%
Infections	> 20%	< 1%
Neoplasia		†^{1}
Lymphoma	> 0.5%	
Others	> 2.8%	

^{1} 1.8 cases per 1000 patient years of follow-up (one study).

➤*Miscellaneous:* Skin rashes (≈ 2%); alopecia, fever, arthralgias, negative nitrogen balance (< 1%).

BASILIXIMAB

Rx	**Simulect** (Novartis)	**Powder for injection, lyophilized:** 20 mg	Preservative free. Sucrose, mannitol, potassium phosphate, sodium chloride. In single-use vials.

WARNING

Only physicians experienced in immunosuppression therapy and management of organ transplantation patients should prescribe basiliximab. The physician responsible for basiliximab administration should have complete information requisite for the follow-up of the patient. Manage patients receiving the drug in facilities equipped and staffed with adequate laboratory and supportive medical resources.

Indications

➤*Organ rejection, prophylaxis:* Prophylaxis of acute organ rejection in patients receiving renal transplantation when used as part of an immunosuppresive regimen that includes cyclosporine and corticosteroids.

Administration and Dosage

➤*Approved by the FDA:* May 12, 1998.

Basiliximab is used as part of an immunosuppressive regimen that includes cyclosporine and corticosteroids. Basiliximab is for central or peripheral IV administration only. Give reconstituted basiliximab either as a bolus injection or dilute to a volume of 50 mL with normal saline or 5% Dextrose and administer as an IV infusion over 20 to 30 minutes. Bolus administration may be associated with nausea, vomiting, and local reactions, including pain.

Only administer basiliximab once it has been determined that the patient will receive the graft and concomitant immunosuppression. Patients previously administered basiliximab should only be re-exposed to a subsequent course of therapy with extreme caution.

➤*Adult:* The recommended regimen is 2 doses of 20 mg each. Give the first 20 mg dose within 2 hours prior to transplantation surgery and the second 20 mg dose 4 days after transplantation. Withhold the second dose if complications such as severe hypersensitivity reactions to basiliximab or graft loss occur.

➤*Children / Adolescents:* In pediatric patients weighing < 35 kg, the recommended regimen is 2 doses of 10 mg each. Discard any remaining product after each dose. In pediatric patients weighing ≥ 35 kg, the recommended regimen is 2 doses of 20 mg each. Give the first dose within 2 hours prior to transplantation surgery and the second dose 4 days after transplantation. Withhold the second dose if complications such as severe hypersensitivity reactions to basiliximab or graft loss occur.

➤*Reconstitution:* To prepare the reconstituted solution, add 5 mL of Sterile Water for Injection to the vial containing the basiliximab powder. Shake the vial gently to dissolve the powder.

The reconstituted solution is isotonic and may be given either as a bolus injection or diluted to a volume of 50 mL with normal saline or 5% Dextrose for infusion. When mixing the solution, gently invert the bag to avoid foaming; do not shake.

After reconstitution, basiliximab should be a clear to opalescent, colorless solution. If particulate matter is present or the solution is colored, do not use.

Take care to assure sterility of the prepared solution because the drug product does not contain any antimicrobial preservatives or bacteriostatic agents.

➤*Admixture incompatibility:* No incompatibility between basiliximab and polyvinyl chloride bags or infusion sets has been observed. No data are available on the compatibility of basiliximab with other IV substances. Other drug substances should not be added or infused simultaneously through the same IV line.

➤*Storage / Stability:* Refrigerate lyophilized basiliximab at 2° to 8°C (36° to 46°F).

It is recommended that after reconstitution the solution be used immediately. If not used immediately, it can be stored at 2° to 8°C (36° to 46°F) for 24 hours or at room temperature for 4 hours. Discard the reconstituted solution if not used within 24 hours.

Actions

➤*Pharmacology:* Basiliximab, an interleukin-2 (IL-2) receptor antagonist, is a chimeric (murine/human) monoclonal antibody (IgG$_{1κ}$) produced by recombinant DNA technology that functions as an immunosuppressive agent, specifically binding to and blocking the IL-2 receptor α-chain (IL-2Rα, also known as CD25 antigen), which is selectively expressed on the surface of activated T-lymphocytes. This specific high-affinity binding of basiliximab to IL-2Rα competitively inhibits IL-2-mediated activation of lymphocytes, a critical pathway in the cellular immune response involved in allograft rejection.

While in the circulation, basiliximab impairs the response of the immune system to antigenic challenges. Whether the ability to respond to repeated or ongoing challenges with those antigens returns to normal after basiliximab is cleared is unknown.

Complete and consistent binding to IL-2Rα in adults is maintained as long as serum basiliximab levels exceed 0.2 mcg/mL. As concentrations fall below this threshold, the IL-2Rα sites are no longer fully bound, and the number of T-cells expressing unbound IL-2Rα returns to pretherapy values within 1 to 2 weeks. The relationship between serum concentration and receptor saturation was assessed in 13 pediatric patients and was similar to that characterized in adult renal transplantation patients. In vitro studies using human tissues indicate that basiliximab binds only to lymphocytes.

When added to a regimen of cyclosporine and corticosteroids, the mean duration of basiliximab saturation of IL-2Rα was 36 days. The duration of clinically relevant IL-2 receptor blockade after the recommended course of basiliximab is not known. No significant changes to circulating lymphocyte numbers or cell phenotypes were observed by flow cytometry.

➤*Pharmacokinetics:*

Adults – Peak mean serum concentration following IV infusion of 20 mg over 30 minutes is ≈ 7.1 mg/L. There is a dose-proportional increase in C$_{max}$ and AUC up to the highest tested single dose of 60 mg. The volume of distribution at steady state is ≈ 8.6 L. The extent and degree of distribution to various body compartments have not been fully studied. The terminal half-life is ≈ 7.2 days. Total body clearance is ≈ 41 mL/hr.

Children – The pharmacokinetics of basiliximab were assessed in 39 pediatric renal transplantation patients. In infants and children (1 to 11 years of age; n = 25), the distribution volume and clearance were reduced by ≈ 50% compared with adult renal transplantation patients. The volume of distribution at steady state was ≈ 4.8 L, half-life was ≈ 9.5 days and clearance was ≈ 17 mL/hr. In adolescents (12 to 16 years of age; n = 14) disposition was similar to that in adult renal transplantation patients. The volume of distribution at steady state was ≈ 7.8 L, half-life was ≈ 9.1 days, and clearance was ≈ 31 mL/hr.

Contraindications

Hypersensitivity to basiliximab or any component of the formulation.

Overdosage

Very large doses may lead to marrow hypoplasia, bleeding, infection and death. About 30% is bound to serum proteins, but ≈ 45% is removed by 8-hour hemodialysis. A single case of azathioprine overdosage has been reported in a renal transplant patient who ingested a single dose of 7500 mg. The immediate toxic reactions were nausea, vomiting and diarrhea, followed by mild leukopenia and mild abnormalities in liver function. The WBC count, AST and bilirubin returned to normal 6 days after the overdose.

Patient Information

If GI upset occurs, administer in divided doses or take with food.

Notify physician if any of the following occurs: Unusual bleeding or bruising, fever, sore throat, mouth sores, signs of infection, abdominal pain, pale stools or darkened urine. Inform patients of the necessity of periodic blood counts

May cause nausea, vomiting, skin rash, fever, arthralgias and diarrhea; notify physician if these persist or become bothersome.

Advise patients of the potential risks of therapy during pregnancy and breastfeeding.

BASILIXIMAB

Warnings

➤*Opportunistic infections/Lymphoproliferative disorders:* While neither the incidence of lymphoproliferative disorders nor of opportunistic infections was higher in basiliximab-treated patients than in placebo-treated patients, patients on immunosuppressive therapy are at increased risk for developing these complications and should be monitored accordingly.

➤*Infectious episodes:* Cytomegalovirus infection was reported in 15% of basiliximab-treated patients and 17% of placebo-treated patients receiving a dual or triple immunosuppression regimen. The rates of infections, serious infections, and infectious organisms were similar in the basiliximab and placebo treatment groups among dual and triple therapy-treated patients.

➤*Hypersensitivity reactions:* Severe acute (onset within 24 hours) hypersensitivity reactions, including anaphylaxis, have been observed on initial exposure to basiliximab or following re-exposure after several months. These reactions may include hypotension, tachycardia, cardiac failure, dyspnea, wheezing, bronchospasm, pulmonary edema, respiratory failure, urticaria, rash, pruritus, or sneezing. If a severe hypersensitivity reaction occurs, permanently discontinue therapy with basiliximab. Medications for the treatment of severe hypersensitivity reactions including anaphylaxis should be available for immediate use. Patients previously administered basiliximab should only be re-exposed to a subsequent course of therapy with extreme caution. The potential risks of such re-administration, specifically those associated with immunosuppression, are not known. Refer to Management of Acute Hypersensitivity Reactions.

➤*Elderly:* Controlled clinical studies of basiliximab have included a small number of patients ≥ 65 years of age (basiliximab, 28; placebo, 32). The adverse event profile in patients ≥ 65 years of age is not different from patients < 65 years of age, and no age-related dosing adjustment is required. Caution must be used in giving immunosuppressive drugs to elderly patients.

➤*Pregnancy:* Category B. There are no adequate and well-controlled studies in pregnant women. Because IgG molecules are known to cross the placental barrier and because IL-2 receptors may play an important role in development of the immune system, use in pregnant women only when the potential benefit justifies the potential risk to the fetus. Women of childbearing potential should use effective contraception before beginning basiliximab therapy, during therapy, and for 4 months after completion of therapy.

➤*Lactation:* It is not known whether basiliximab is excreted in breast milk. Because human antibodies are excreted in human milk and because of the potential for adverse reactions, decide whether to discontinue nursing or to discontinue the drug, taking into account the importance of the drug to the mother.

➤*Children:* No adequate and well-controlled studies have been completed in pediatric patients. In a safety and pharmacokinetic study, 41 pediatric patients (1 to 11 years of age [n = 27], 12 to 16 years of age [n = 14], median age 8.1 years) were treated with basiliximab via IV bolus injection in addition to standard immunosuppressive agents including cyclosporine, corticosteroids, azathioprine, and mycophenolate mofetil. The acute rejection rate at 6 months was comparable to that in adults in the triple therapy trials. The most frequently reported adverse events were hypertension, hypertrichosis, and rhinitis (49% each), urinary tract infections (46%), and fever (39%). Overall, the adverse event profile was consistent with general clinical experience in the pediatric renal transplantation population and with the profile in the controlled adult renal transplantation studies.

It is not known whether the immune response to vaccines, infection, and other antigenic stimuli administered or encountered during basiliximab therapy is impaired or whether such response will remain impaired after basiliximab therapy.

Precautions

➤*Immunosuppression:* It is not known whether basiliximab use will have a long-term effect on the ability of the immune system to respond to antigens first encountered during basiliximab-induced immunosuppression.

➤*Immunogenicity:* Of renal transplantation patients treated with basiliximab and tested for anti-idiotype antibodies, 4/339 developed an anti-idiotype antibody response, with no deleterious clinical effect upon the patient. In the US study, the incidence of human antimurine antibody (HAMA) in renal transplantation patients treated with basiliximab was 2/138 in patients not exposed to muromonab-CD3 and 4/34 in patients who subsequently received muromonab-CD3. The available clinical data on the use of muromonab-CD3 in patients previously treated with basiliximab suggest that subsequent use of muromonab-CD3 or other murine antilymphocytic antibody preparations is not precluded.

Adverse Reactions

Basiliximab did not appear to add to the background of adverse events seen in organ transplantation patients as a consequence of their underlying disease and the concurrent administration of immunosuppressants and other medications. Adverse events were reported by 96% of the patients in the placebo and basiliximab groups. Basiliximab did not increase the incidence of serious adverse events observed compared with placebo. The most frequently reported adverse events were GI disorders (69% basiliximab, 67% placebo).

➤*The following adverse events occurred in ≥ 10% of basiliximab-treated patients.:*
CNS – Headache; tremor; insomnia.

Dermatologic – Surgical wound complications; acne.

GI – Constipation; nausea; diarrhea; abdominal pain; vomiting; dyspepsia.

Metabolic/Nutritional – Hyperkalemia; hypokalemia; hyperglycemia; hyperuricemia; hypophosphatemia; hypercholesterolemia.

Respiratory – Dyspnea; upper respiratory tract infection.

Miscellaneous – Anemia; pain; peripheral edema; fever; viral infection; hypertension; urinary tract infection.

➤*The following adverse events were reported with an incidence of ≥ 3% and < 10% in patients treated with basiliximab.:*
Cardiovascular – Angina pectoris; cardiac failure; chest pain; abnormal heart sounds; aggravated hypertension; hypotension; arrhythmia; atrial fibrillation; tachycardia; vascular disorder.

CNS – Hypesthesia; neuropathy; paresthesia; dizziness; agitation; anxiety; depression.

Dermatologic – Cyst; herpes simplex; herpes zoster; hypertrichosis; pruritus; rash; skin disorder; skin ulceration.

GI – Enlarged abdomen; flatulence; GI disorder; gastroenteritis; GI hemorrhage; gum hyperplasia; melena; esophagitis; ulcerative stomatitis; moniliasis.

GU – Impotence, male; genital edema, male; albuminuria; bladder disorder; hematuria; frequent micturition; oliguria; abnormal renal function; renal tubular necrosis; surgery; ureteral disorder; urinary retention; dysuria; increased nonprotein nitrogen.

Hematologic – Hematoma; hemorrhage; purpura; thrombocytopenia; thrombosis; polycythemia; leukopenia.

Metabolic/Nutritional – Acidosis; hypertriglyceridemia; hypocalcemia; weight increase; dehydration; diabetes mellitus; fluid overload; hypercalcemia; hyperlipemia; hypoglycemia; hypoproteinemia; hypomagnesemia.

Musculoskeletal – Arthralgia; arthropathy; bone fracture; cramps; hernia; myalgia; back pain; leg pain.

Respiratory – Bronchitis; bronchospasm; abnormal chest sounds; coughing; pharyngitis; rhinitis; pneumonia; pulmonary disorder; pulmonary edema; sinusitis.

Special senses – Cataract; conjunctivitis; abnormal vision.

Miscellaneous – Accidental trauma; asthenia; dependent edema; leg edema; increased drug level; face edema; fatigue; infection; malaise; generalized edema; rigors; sepsis; increased glucocorticoids.

➤*Postmarketing experience:* Severe acute hypersensitivity reactions, including anaphylaxis characterized by hypotension, tachycardia, cardiac failure, dyspnea, wheezing, bronchospasm, pulmonary edema, respiratory failure, urticaria, rash, pruritus, or sneezing, as well as capillary leak syndrome and cytokine release syndrome, have been reported during postmarketing experience with basiliximab.

Overdosage

A maximum tolerated dose has not been determined in patients. In clinical studies, basiliximab has been administered to adult renal transplantation patients in single doses of ≤ 60 mg, or in divided doses over 3 to 5 days of ≤ 120 mg, without any associated serious adverse events. There has been one spontaneous report of a pediatric renal transplantation patient who received a single 20 mg dose (2.3 mg/kg) without adverse events.

Immunosuppressives

CYCLOSPORINE (Cyclosporin A)[1]

Rx	Gengraf (Abbott)	Capsules: 25 mg	12.8% alcohol, castor oil. (25 mg OR). White, oval. In UD 30s.
		100 mg	12.8% alcohol, castor oil. (100 mg OT). White, oval. In UD 30s.
Rx	Cyclosporine (Apotex, Eon Labs, Pliva)	Capsules, soft gelatin: 25 mg	Castor oil, sorbitol, alcohol. (0932). Clear, oblong. In UD 30s.
Rx	Neoral (Novartis)		11.9% dehydrated alcohol. (Neoral 25 mg). Blue-gray, oval. In UD 30s.
Rx	Sandimmune (Novartis)		Sorbitol, ≤ 12.7% dehydrated alcohol. (78/240). Pink, oblong. In UD 30s.
Rx	Cyclosporine (Apotex, Eon Labs, Pliva)	100 mg	Castor oil, sorbitol, alcohol. (0933). Clear, oblong. In UD 30s.
Rx	Neoral (Novartis)		11.9% dehydrated alcohol. (Neoral 100 mg). Blue-gray, oblong. In UD 30s.
Rx	Sandimmune (Novartis)		Sorbitol, ≤ 12.7% dehydrated alcohol. (78/241). Rose, oblong. In UD 30s.
Rx	Cyclosporine (Pliva)	Oral solution: 100 mg/mL	In 50 mL.
Rx	Neoral (Novartis)		11.9% dehydrated alcohol. In 50 mL.
Rx	Sandimmune (Novartis)		12.5% alcohol. In 50 mL with syringe.
Rx	Cyclosporine Injection (Bedford Labs)	Injection: 50 mg/mL	In 5 mL single-use vials.
Rx	Sandimmune (Novartis)		650 mg polyoxyethylated castor oil/mL and 32.9% alcohol. In 5 mL amps.

[1] Product tables do not imply bioequivalence (see page xi). Also refer to Bioequivalency (in Administration and Dosage).

WARNING

Only physicians experienced in the management of systemic immunosuppressive therapy for the indicated disease should prescribe cyclosporine. Patients receiving the drug should be managed in facilities equipped and staffed with adequate laboratory and supportive medical resources. The physician responsible for maintenance therapy should have complete information requisite for the follow-up of the patient.

Administer *Sandimmune* with adrenal corticosteroids but not with other immunosuppressive agents. Increased susceptibility to infection and other possible development of lymphoma may result from immunosuppression.

Neoral and *Gengraf* may increase the susceptibility to infection and the development of neoplasia. In kidney, liver, and heart transplant patients, *Gengraf* and *Neoral* may be administered with other immunosuppressive agents. Increased susceptibility to infection and the possible development of lymphoma and other neoplasms may result from the increase in the degree of immunosuppression in transplant patients.

The absorption of *Sandimmune* during chronic administration was found to be erratic. It is recommended that patients taking *Sandimmune* over a period of time be monitored at repeated intervals to avoid toxicity from high levels and possible organ rejection from low absorption. This is of special importance in liver transplants.

Sandimmune capsules and oral solution have decreased bioavailability in comparison with *Neoral* capsules, *Neoral* oral solution, and *Gengraf* capsules. *Gengraf* and *Neoral* are not bioequivalent to *Sandimmune* and cannot be used interchangeably without physician supervision. For given trough concentrations, cyclosporine exposure will be greater with *Neoral* and *Gengraf* than with *Sandimmune*. If a patient receiving exceptionally high doses of *Sandimmune* is converted to *Neoral* or *Gengraf*, exercise particular caution. Monitor cyclosporine blood levels in transplant and rheumatoid arthritis (RA) patients taking *Gengraf* and *Neoral* to minimize possible organ rejection due to high concentrations. Make dose adjustments in transplant patients to minimize possible organ rejection due to low concentrations. Comparison of blood concentrations in the published literature with blood concentrations obtained using current assays must be done with detailed knowledge of the assay methods employed.

Psoriasis patients previously treated with PUVA and to a lesser extent, methotrexate or other immunosuppressive agents, UVB, coal tar, or radiation therapy, are at an increased risk of developing skin malignancies when taking *Neoral* or *Gengraf*.

Cyclosporine, in recommended doses, can cause systemic hypertension and nephrotoxicity. The risk increases with increasing dose and duration of cyclosporine therapy. Renal dysfunction, including structural kidney damage, is a potential consequence of cyclosporine, and therefore, renal function must be monitored during therapy.

Indications

➤*Allogeneic transplants:* For prophylaxis of organ rejection in kidney, liver, and heart allogeneic transplants. *Gengraf* and *Neoral* have been used in combination with azathioprine and corticosteroids. *Sandimmune* always is to be used with adrenal corticosteroids. *Sandimmune* also may be used in the treatment of chronic rejection in patients previously treated with other immunosuppressive agents. Because of

the risk of anaphylaxis, reserve *Sandimmune* injection for patients who are unable to take the soft gelatin capsule or oral solution.

➤*Psoriasis: Neoral* and *Gengraf* are indicated for the treatment of adult, nonimmunocompromised patients with severe (ie, extensive and/or disabling), recalcitrant, plaque psoriasis who have failed to respond to at least 1 systemic therapy (eg, PUVA, retinoids, methotrexate) or in patients for whom other systemic therapies are contraindicated or cannot be tolerated. While rebound rarely occurs, most patients will experience relapse with *Neoral* or *Gengraf* as with other therapies upon cessation of treatment.

➤*RA: Neoral* and *Gengraf* are indicated for the treatment of patients with severe, active, RA where the disease has not adequately responded to methotrexate. *Neoral* and *Gengraf* can be used in combination with methotrexate in RA patients who do not respond adequately to methotrexate alone.

Administration and Dosage

➤*Bioequivalency: Sandimmune* capsules and oral solution have decreased bioavailability in comparison with *Neoral* capsules, *Neoral* oral solution, and *Gengraf* capsules. *Gengraf* and *Neoral* are not bioequivalent to *Sandimmune* and cannot be used interchangeably without physician supervision.

➤*Allogenic transplants:* In children, the same dose and dosing regimen may be used as in adults; although, in several studies, children have required and tolerated higher doses than those used in adults.

➤*Sandimmune, oral:* Give the initial dose of Sandimmune 4 to 12 hours prior to transplantation as a single dose of 15 mg/kg. Although a single daily dose of 14 to 18 mg/kg was used in most clinical trials, few centers continue to use the highest dose, most favoring the lower end of the scale. There is a trend towards use of even lower initial doses for renal transplantation in the ranges of 10 to 14 mg/kg/day. The initial single daily dose is continued postoperatively for 1 to 2 weeks and then tapered by 5% per week to a maintenance dose of 5 to 10 mg/kg/day. Some centers have successfully tapered the maintenance dose to as low as 3 mg/kg/day in selected renal transplant patients without an apparent rise in rejection rate.

➤*Sandimmune, parenteral:* For infusion only. *Sandimmune* injection is administered at one-third the oral dose. Give the initial dose 4 to 12 hours prior to transplantation as a single IV dose of 5 to 6 mg/kg/day. This single dose is continued postoperatively until the patient can tolerate oral therapy. Switch patients to oral therapy as soon as possible after surgery.

Immediately before use, dilute the IV concentrate 1 mL *Sandimmune* in 20 to 100 mL 0.9% sodium chloride injection or 5% dextrose injection and given in a slow IV infusion over approximately 2 to 6 hours. Discard diluted infusion solutions after 24 hours. The *Cremophor EL* (polyoxyethylated castor oil) contained in the concentrate for IV infusion can cause phthalate stripping from PVC.

➤*Neoral and Gengraf:* Always give the daily dosage of *Neoral* and *Gengraf* in 2 divided doses (bid) on a consistent schedule with regard to time of day and relation to meals.

➤*Newly transplanted patients:* Give the initial dose of *Neoral* and *Gengraf* 4 to 12 hours prior to transplantation or postoperatively. The initial dose of *Neoral* and *Gengraf* varies depending on the transplanted organ and the other immunosuppressive agents included in the immunosuppressive protocol. In newly transplanted patients, the initial oral dose of *Neoral* and *Gengraf* are the same as the initial dose of *Sandimmune*. The mean approximate initial doses were 9 mg/kg/day for renal transplant patients, 8 mg/kg/day for liver transplant patients, and 7 mg/kg/day for heart transplant patients. Total daily doses were

CYCLOSPORINE (Cyclosporin A)[1]

divided into equal daily doses. The *Neoral* and *Gengraf* dose is subsequently adjusted to achieve a predefined cyclosporine blood concentration. Using the same trough concentration target for *Neoral* and *Gengraf* as for *Sandimmune* results in greater cyclosporine exposure when *Neoral* and *Gengraf* are administered. Titrate dosing based on clinical assessments of rejection and tolerability. Lower *Neoral* and *Gengraf* doses may be sufficient as maintenance therapy.

➤*Conversion from Sandimmune:* In transplanted patients who are considered for conversion to *Neoral* or *Gengraf* from *Sandimmune*, start *Neoral* or *Gengraf* with the same daily dose as was previously used with *Sandimmune* (1:1 dose conversion). Subsequently, adjust the *Neoral* or *Gengraf* dose to attain the preconversion cyclosporine blood trough concentration. Using the same trough concentration target range for *Neoral* and *Gengraf* as for *Sandimmune* results in greater cyclosporine exposure when *Neoral* and *Gengraf* are administered. Patients with suspected poor absorption of *Sandimmune* require different dosing strategies. In some patients, the increase in blood trough concentration is more pronounced and may be of clinical significance.

Until the blood trough concentration attains the preconversion value, it is strongly recommended that the cyclosporine blood-trough concentration be monitored every 4 to 7 days after conversion to *Neoral* or *Gengraf*. In addition, monitor clinical safety parameters such as serum creatinine and blood pressure every 2 weeks during the first 2 months after conversion. If the blood trough concentrations are outside the desired range and/or if the clinical safety parameters worsen, adjust the dosage of *Neoral* or *Gengraf* accordingly.

➤*Poor Sandimmune absorption:* Patients with lower than expected cyclosporine blood trough concentrations in relation to the oral dose of *Sandimmune* may have poor or inconsistent absorption of cyclosporine from *Sandimmune*. After conversion to *Neoral* or *Gengraf*, patients tend to have higher cyclosporine concentrations. Due to the increase in bioavailability of cyclosporine following conversion to *Neoral* or *Gengraf*, the cyclosporine blood trough concentration may exceed the target range. Exercise particular caution when converting patients to *Neoral* or *Gengraf*; the cyclosporine blood trough concentration may exceed the target range. Exercise particular caution when converting patients to *Neoral* or *Gengraf* at doses greater than 10 mg/kg/day. Individually titrate the dose of *Neoral* or *Gengraf* based on cyclosporine trough concentrations, tolerability, and clinical response. In this population, measure the cyclosporine trough concentrations more frequently, at least twice a week (daily, if initial dose exceeds 10 mg/kg/day), until the concentration stabilizes within the desired range.

➤*Oral solution preparation:*
Sandimmune – To make *Sandimmune* oral solution more palatable, it may be diluted with milk, chocolate milk, or orange juice, preferably at room temperature. Instruct patients to stir well and drink at once, not allowing the solution to stand before drinking. It is best to use a glass container and rinse it with more diluent to ensure that the total dose is taken. Instruct patients to not rinse the dosage syringe with water or other cleaning agents either before or after use. If the dosage syringe requires cleaning, it must be completely dry before resuming use. Introduction of water into the product by any means will cause variation in dose. Patients should avoid switching diluents frequently. Administer *Sandimmune* soft gelatin capsules and oral solution on a consistent schedule with regard to time of day and relation to meals.

Neoral or *Gengraf* – It is recommended that *Neoral* and *Gengraf* be administered on a consistent schedule with regard to time of day and relation to meals. Grapefruit and grapefruit juice affect metabolism, increasing blood concentration of cyclosporine, and thus, should be avoided. To make *Neoral* more palatable, it should be diluted with orange or apple juice that is at room temperature. Instruct patients to not switch diluents frequently. The combination of *Neoral* solution with milk can be unpalatable. The effect of milk on the bioavailability of cyclosporine when administered as *Neoral* oral solution has not been evaluated. Instruct patients to remove the protective cover from dosing syringe supplied, and transfer the solution to a glass of orange or apple juice. Advise patients to stir well and drink at once, not allowing the diluted solution to stand before drinking. A glass container, not plastic, should be used. Tell patients to rinse the glass with more diluent to ensure that the total dose is consumed. After use, the outside of the dosing syringe should be dried with a clean towel and the protective cover should be replaced. The dosing syringe should not be rinsed with water or other cleaning agents. If the syringe requires cleaning, it must be completely dry before resuming use.

➤*Adjunct therapy:* Adjunct therapy with adrenal corticosteroids is recommended initially. Different tapering dosage schedules of prednisone appear to achieve similar results. A representative dosage schedule based on the patient's weight started with 2 mg/kg/day for the first 4 days tapered to 1 mg/kg/day by 1 week, 0.6 mg/kg/day by 2 weeks, 0.3 mg/kg/day by 1 month, and 0.15 mg/kg/day by 2 months and thereafter as a maintenance dose. Steroid doses may be further tapered on an individualized basis depending on status of patient and function of graft. Adjustments in dosage of prednisone must be made according to the clinical situation.

➤*Psoriasis:* The initial dose of *Neoral* or *Gengraf* should be 2.5 mg/kg/day. Take *Neoral* or *Gengraf* twice daily, as a divided (1.25 mg/kg BID) oral dose. Keep patients at that dose for at least 4 weeks, barring adverse events. Increase dosage at 2-week intervals if significant clinical improvement has not occurred by that time. Based on patient response, make dose increases of approximately 0.5 mg/kg/day to a maximum of 4 mg/kg/day.

Make dose decreases by 25% to 50% at any time to control adverse events, such as hypertension, serum creatinine elevations (greater than or equal to 25% above the patient's pretreatment level), or clinically significant laboratory abnormalities. If dose reduction is not effective in controlling abnormalities, or if the adverse event or abnormality is severe, discontinue *Neoral* or *Gengraf* therapy.

Patients generally show some improvement in the clinical manifestations of psoriasis in 2 weeks. Satisfactory control and stabilization of the disease may take 12 to 16 weeks to achieve. Discontinue treatment if satisfactory response cannot be achieved after 6 weeks at 4 mg/kg/day or the patient's maximum tolerated dose. Once a patient is adequately controlled and appears stable, lower the dose of *Neoral* or *Gengraf*. Doses below 2.5 mg/kg/day may also be equally effective.

Upon stopping treatment with cyclosporine, relapse will occur in approximately 6 weeks (50% of patients) to 16 weeks (75% of patients). In the majority of patients, rebound does not occur after cessation of treatment with cyclosporine. Continuous treatment for extended periods longer than 1 year is not recommended. Consider alteration with other forms of treatment in the long-term management of patients with life-long disease.

➤*RA:* The initial dose of *Neoral* or *Gengraf* is 2.5 mg/kg/day, taken twice daily as a divided (bid) oral dose. Salicylates, NSAIDS, and oral corticosteroids may be continued. Onset of action generally occurs between 4 and 8 weeks. If sufficient clinical benefit is seen and tolerability is good (including serum creatinine less than 30% above baseline), the dose may be increased by 0.5 to 0.75 mg/kg/day after 8 weeks and again after 12 weeks to a maximum of 4 mg/kg/day. If no benefit is seen by 16 weeks of therapy, discontinue *Neoral* or *Gengraf* therapy.

Make dose decreases by 25% to 50% at any time to control adverse events, such as hypertension, serum creatinine elevations (greater than or equal to 25% above the patient's pretreatment level), or clinically significant laboratory abnormalities. If dose reduction is not effective in controlling abnormalities, or if the adverse event or abnormality is severe, discontinue *Neoral* or *Gengraf*.

Use with methotrexate – Use the same initial dose and dosage range if *Neoral* or *Gengraf* is combined with the recommended dose of methotrexate. Most patients can be treated with *Neoral* or *Gengraf* doses of 3 mg/kg/day or less when combined with methotrexate doses of up to 15 mg/week.

➤*Storage/Stability:*
Sandimmune –
Capsules: Store at 25°C (77°F); excursions permitted to 15° to 30°C (59°F to 86°F).
Oral solution: Store in the original container at temperatures below 30°C (86°F). Do not store in the refrigerator. Protect from freezing. Once opened, the contents must be used within 2 months.
IV: Store at temperatures below 30°C (86°F) and protect from light.
Neoral –
Capsules: Store in the original unit-dose container at controlled room temperature 20° to 25°C (68° to 77°F).
Oral Solution: Store in the original container at controlled room temperature 20° to 25°C (68° to 77°F). Do not store in the refrigerator. Once opened, the contents must be used within 2 months. At temperatures below 20°C (68°F), the solution may gel; light flocculation or the formation of a light sediment also may occur. There is no impact on product performance or dosing using the syringe provided. Allow to warm to room temperature 25°C (77°F) to reverse these changes.
Gengraf –
Capsules: Store in the original unit-dose container at controlled room temperature 15° to 30°C (59° to 86°F).

Actions

➤*Pharmacology:* Cyclosporine is a potent immunosuppressive agent that in animals prolongs survival of allogenic transplants involving skin, kidney, liver, heart, pancreas, bone marrow, small intestine, and lung. Cyclosporine has been demonstrated to suppress some humoral immunity and to a greater extent, cell-mediated immune reactions such as allograft rejection, delayed hypersensitivity, experimental allergic encephalomyelitis, Freund's adjuvant arthritis, and graft vs host disease in many animal species for a variety of organs.

The effectiveness of cyclosporine results from specific and reversible inhibition of immunocompetent lymphocytes in the G_0 and G_1-phase of the cell cycle. T-lymphocytes are preferentially inhibited. The T-helper cell is the main target, although the T-suppressor cell also may be suppressed. Cyclosporine also inhibits lymphokine production and release including interleukin-2.

CYCLOSPORINE (Cyclosporin A)[1]

►*Pharmacokinetics:*
Absorption –

Select Pharmacokinetic Parameters of Cyclosporine Formulations				
	Absolute bioavailability (%)	T_{max} (hours)	C_{max} (ng/mL/mg of dose)	$t_{1/2}$ (hours)
Sandimmune	30[a]	3.5	≈ 1 (2.7 to 1.4)[b]	19 (range, 10 to 27)
Neoral	Not determined in adults	1.5 to 2	40% to 106% or greater[c]	8.4 (range, 5 to 18)
Gengraf	Not determined in adults	1.5 to 2	40% to 106% or greater[c]	8.4 (range, 5 to 18)

[a] Based upon the results in 2 patients.
[b] Blood levels for low to high doses, respectively.
[c] In renal transplant patients treated with *Neoral* and *Gengraf*, peak levels were 40% to 106% greater than those following *Sandimmune* administration.

The absorption of cyclosporine from the GI tract is incomplete and variable. The extent of absorption of cyclosporine is dependent on the individual patient, the patient population, and the formulation. Very little difference in absorption was observed when patients were administered *Gengraf* or *Neoral* with and without T-tube diversion of bile. For *Sandimmune*, C_{max} and area under the plasma or blood concentration-time curve (AUC) increase with administered dose; for blood, the relationship is curvilinear (parabolic) between 0 and 1400. The relationship between administered dose and exposure AUC is linear within the therapeutic dose range for *Neoral* and *Gengraf*. The intersubject variability of cyclosporine exposure (AUC) when *Gengraf*, *Neoral*, or *Sandimmune* is administered ranges from about 20% to 50% in renal transplant patients. This intersubject variability contributes to the need for individualization of the dosing regimen for optimal therapy. Intrasubject variability of AUC in renal transplant recipients was 9% to 21% for *Gengraf* and *Neoral* and 19% to 26% for *Sandimmune*. In the same studies, intrasubject variability of trough concentrations was 17% to 30% for *Gengraf* and *Neoral* and 16% to 38% for *Sandimmune*.

The dose normalized AUC in renal transplant patients taking *Gengraf* or *Neoral* 28 days after transplantation was 50% greater than in those patients administered *Sandimmune*. The increase in AUC is accompanied by an increase in peak blood cyclosporine concentration in the range of 40% to 106% in renal transplant patients and approximately 90% in liver transplant patients. AUC and C_{max} also are increased (*Gengraf* or *Neoral* relative to *Sandimmune*) in heart transplant patients, but data are very limited. Although the AUC and C_{max} values are higher with *Gengraf* and *Neoral* relative to *Sandimmune*, the pre-dose trough concentrations (dose-normalized) are similar between the formulations.

The administration of food with *Gengraf* or *Neoral* decreases the cyclosporine AUC and C_{max}. A high-fat meal (669 kcal, 45 g fat) consumed within one-half hour before *Gengraf* or *Neoral* administration decreased the AUC by 13% and C_{max} by 33%. The effects of a low-fat meal (667 kcal, 15 g fat) were similar.

Distribution – Cyclosporine is distributed largely outside the blood volume; approximately 33% to 47% is in plasma, 4% to 9% in lymphocytes, 5% to 12% in granulocytes, and 41% to 58% in erythrocytes. At high concentrations, the binding capacity of leukocytes and erythrocytes becomes saturated. In plasma, approximately 90% is bound to proteins, primarily lipoproteins. The steady-state volume of distribution during IV dosing has been reported as 3 to 5 L/kg in solid organ transplant recipients. In blood, the distribution is concentration dependent.

Blood level monitoring is useful in patient management (see Precautions).

Metabolism – Cyclosporine is extensively metabolized by the cytochrome P450 3A4 enzyme system in the liver and, to a lesser degree, in the GI tract and the kidney. At least 25 metabolites have been identified from human bile, feces, blood, and urine. The biological activity of the metabolites and their contributions to toxicity are considerably less than those of the parent compound. At steady-state following the oral administration of *Sandimmune*, the mean AUCs for blood concentrations of the major metabolites M1, M9, and M4N are about 70%, 21%, and 7.5% of the AUC for blood cyclosporine concentrations, respectively. Based on blood concentration data from stable renal transplant patients and bile concentration data from de novo liver transplant patients, the percentage of dose present as M1, M9, and M4N metabolites is similar when *Gengraf*, *Neoral*, or *Sandimmune* is administered.

Excretion – Only 0.1% of a dose is excreted unchanged in the urine. Excretion is primarily biliary with only 6% of the dose (parent drug and metabolites) excreted in urine. Neither dialysis nor renal failure alter cyclosporine clearance significantly.

Special populations –
  Children: Pharmacokinetic data in pediatric patients administered *Neoral*, *Gengraf*, or *Sandimmune* is very limited. In 15 renal transplant patients 3 to 16 years of age, cyclosporine whole blood clearance after IV administration of *Sandimmune* was approximately 10.6 mL/min/kg.

In a study of 7 renal transplant patients 2 to 16 years of age, the cyclosporine clearance ranged from 9.8 to 15.5 mL/min/kg. In 9 liver transplant patients 0.6 to 5.6 years of age, clearance was approximately 9.3 mL/min/kg.

In the pediatric population, *Neoral* and *Gengraf* also demonstrate an increased bioavailability as compared with *Sandimmune*. In 7 liver de novo transplant patients 1.4 to 10 years of age, the absolute bioavailability of *Neoral* and *Gengraf* was 43% (range, 30% to 68%) and for *Sandimmune*, in the same individuals, absolute bioavailability was 28% (range, 17% to 42%).

Contraindications

Hypersensitivity to polyoxyethylated castor oil (injection only; see Warnings and Administration and Dosage), cyclosporine, or any component of the products; *Gengraf* and *Neoral* in psoriasis or RA patients with abnormal renal function, uncontrolled hypertension, or malignancies; *Gengraf* and *Neoral* concomitantly with PUVA or UVB, methotrexate or other immunosuppressive agents, coal tar or radiation therapy in psoriasis patients.

Warnings

►*Elevated BUN and serum creatinine:* It is not unusual for serum creatinine and BUN levels to be elevated during cyclosporine therapy. These elevations in renal transplant patients do not necessarily indicate rejection, and each patient must be fully evaluated before dosage adjustment is indicated. These increases reflect a reduction in the glomerular filtration rate. Impaired renal function at any time requires close monitoring, and frequent dosage adjustments may be indicated. The frequency and severity of serum creatinine elevations increase with dose and duration of cyclosporine therapy. These elevations are likely to become more pronounced without dose reduction or discontinuation.

►*Nephrotoxicity:* Nephrotoxicity has been noted in 25% of cases of renal transplantation, 38% of cases of cardiac transplantation, and 37% of cases of liver transplantation. Mild nephrotoxicity was generally noted 2 to 3 months after transplant and consisted of an arrest in the fall of the preoperative elevations of BUN and creatinine at a range of 35 to 45 mg/dL and 2 to 2.5 mg/dL, respectively. These elevations are often responsive to dosage reductions. More overt nephrotoxicity was seen early after transplantation and was characterized by a rapidly rising BUN and creatinine. Because these events are similar to rejection episodes, care must be taken to differentiate between them. This form of toxicity is usually responsive to cyclosporine dosage reduction.

Although specific diagnostic criteria that reliably differentiate renal graft rejection from drug toxicity have not been found, a number of parameters have been significantly associated to one or the other. However, it should be noted that up to 20% of patients may have simultaneous nephrotoxicity and rejection.

A form of a cyclosporine-associated nephrotoxicity is characterized by serial deterioration in renal function and morphologic changes in the kidneys. From 5% to 15% of transplant patients who have received cyclosporine will fail to show a reduction in rising serum creatinine despite a decrease or discontinuation of cyclosporine therapy. Renal biopsies from these patients will demonstrate one or several of the following alterations: tubular vacuolization, tubular microcalcifications, peritubular capillary congestion, arteriolopathy, and a striped form of interstitial fibrosis with tubular atrophy. Though none of these morphologic changes are entirely specific, a diagnosis of cyclosporine-associated structural nephrotoxicity requires evidence of these findings. When considering the development of cyclosporine-associated nephropathy, it is noteworthy that several authors have reported an association between the appearance of interstitial fibrosis and higher cumulative doses or persistently high circulating trough levels of cyclosporine. This is particularly true during the first 6 posttransplant months when the dosage tends to be highest and when, in kidney recipients, the organ appears to be most vulnerable to the toxic effects of cyclosporine. Among other contributing factors to the development of interstitial fibrosis in these patients are prolonged perfusion time, warm ischemia time, as well as episodes of acute toxicity, and acute and chronic rejection. The reversibility of interstitial fibrosis and its correlation to renal function have not yet been determined. Reversibility of arteriopathy has been reported after stopping cyclosporine and lowering the dosage.

Cyclosporine nephropathy was detected in renal biopsies of 6 out of 60 (10%) RA patients after the average treatment duration of 19 months. Only 1 patient out of these 6 patients was treated with a dose of approximately 4 mg/kg/day. Serum creatinine improved in all but 1 patient after discontinuation of cyclosporine. The maximal creatinine increase appears to be a factor in predicting cyclosporine nephropathy.

Kidney biopsies from 86 psoriasis patients treated for a mean duration of 23 months with 1.2 to 7.6 mg/kg/day of cyclosporine showed evidence of cyclosporine nephropathy in 18/86 (21%) of the patients. The pathology consisted of renal tubular atrophy and interstitial fibrosis. On repeat biopsy of 13 of these patients maintained on various dosages of cyclosporine for a mean of 2 additional years, the number with cyclosporine induced nephropathy rose to 26/86 (30%). The majority of patients (19/26) were on a dose of greater than or equal to 5 mg/kg/day.

CYCLOSPORINE (Cyclosporin A)[1]

The patients were also on cyclosporine for greater than 15 months (18/26) and/or had a clinically significant increase for greater than 1 month (21/26). Creatinine levels returned to normal in 7 of 11 patients in whom cyclosporine therapy was discontinued.

Parameter	Diagnostic Criteria Differentiating Nephrotoxicity From Rejection	
	Nephrotoxicity	Rejection
History	• Donor > 50 years of age or hypotensive, • Prolonged kidney preservation, • Prolonged anastomosis time, • Concomitant nephrotoxic drugs	• Antidonor immune response, • Retransplant patient
Clinical	• Often > 6 weeks post-op, • Prolonged initial nonfunction (acute tubular necrosis)	• Often < 4 weeks post-op • Fever> 37.5°C, • Decrease in daily urine volume > 500 mL (or 50%), • Graft swelling and tenderness, • Weight gain > 0.5 kg
Laboratory	• CyA serum trough level > 200 ng/mL, • Gradual rise in Cr (< 0.15 mg/dL/day), • Cr plateau < 25% above baseline, • BUN/Cr ≥ 20	• CyA serum trough level < 150 ng/mL, • Rapid rise in Cr (> 0.3 mg/dL/day), • Cr> 25% above baseline, • BUN/Cr < 20
Biopsy	• Arteriolopathy (medial hypertrophy, hyalinosis, nodular deposits, intimal thickening, endothelial vacuolization, progressive scarring), • Tubular atrophy, isometric vacuolization, isolated calcifications, • Minimal edema, • Mild focal infiltrates, • Diffuse interstitial fibrosis, often striped form	• Endovasculitis (proliferation, intimal arteritis, necrosis, sclerosis), • Tubulitis with RBC and WBC casts, some irregular vacuolization, • Interstitial edema and hemorrhage, • Diffuse moderate to severe mono-nuclear infiltrates, • Glomerulitis (mononuclear cells)
Aspiration cytology	• CyA deposits in tubular and endothelial cells, • Fine isometric vacuolization of tubular cells	• Inflammatory infiltrate with mono-nuclear phagocytes, macro-phages, lymphoblastoid cells, and activated T-cells, • These strongly express HLA-DR antigens
Urine cytology	• Tubular cells with vacuolization and granularization	• Degenerative tubular cells, plasma cells and lymphocyturia > 20% of sediment
Manometry	• Intracapsular pressure < 40 mm Hg	• Intracapsular pressure > 40 mm Hg
Ultrasonography	• Unchanged graft cross sectional area	• Increase in graft cross sectional area, • AP diameter ≥ transverse diameter
Magnetic resonance imagery	• Normal appearance	• Loss of distinct corticomedullary junction, swelling image intensity of parachyma approaching that of psoas, loss of hilar fat
Radionuclide scan	• Normal or generally decreased perfusion, • Decrease in tubular function, • (^{131}I-hippuran) > decrease in perfusion (^{99m}Tc DTPA)	• Patchy arterial flow, • Decrease in perfusion > decrease in tubular function, • Increased uptake of indium 111 labeled platelets or Tc-99m in colloid
Therapy	• Responds to decreased cyclosporine	• Responds to increased steroids or antilymphocyte globulin

▶*Thrombocytopenia and microangiopathic hemolytic anemia:* Occasionally patients have developed a syndrome of thrombocytopenia and microangiopathic hemolytic anemia that may result in graft failure. The vasculopathy can occur in the absence of rejection and is accompanied by avid platelet consumption within the graft. Neither the pathogenesis nor the management of this syndrome is clear. Though resolution has occurred after reduction or discontinuation of cyclosporine and 1) administration of streptokinase and heparin or 2) plasmapheresis, this appears to depend upon early detection with Indium 111 platelet scans.

▶*Hyperkalemia:* Significant hyperkalemia (sometimes associated with hyperchloremic metabolic acidosis) and hyperuricemia have been seen occasionally in individual patients.

▶*Hepatotoxicity:* Hepatotoxicity has been noted in 4% of cases of renal transplantation, 7% of cases of cardiac transplantation, and 4% of cases of liver transplantation. This was usually noted during the first month of therapy when high doses of cyclosporine were used and consisted of elevations of hepatic enzymes and bilirubin. The chemistry elevations usually decreased with a reduction in dosage.

▶*Convulsions:* Convulsions have occurred in adult and pediatric patients receiving cyclosporine, particularly in combination with high-dose methylprednisolone.

▶*Encephalopathy:* Encephalopathy has been described in postmarketing reports and in the literature. Manifestations include impaired consciousness, convulsions, visual disturbances (including blindness), loss of motor function, movement disorders, and psychiatric disturbances. In many cases, changes in the white matter have been detected using imaging techniques and pathologic specimens. Predisposing factors such as hypertension, hypomagnesemia, hypocholesterolemia, high-dose corticosteroids, high cyclosporine blood concentrations, and graft vs host disease have been noted in many but not all of the reported cases. The changes in most cases have been reversible upon discontinuation of cyclosporine, and in some cases improvement was noted after reduction of dose. It appears that patients receiving liver transplants are more susceptible to encephalopathy than those receiving kidney transplants.

▶*Bioequivalency:* Because *Sandimmune* is not bioequivalent to *Neoral* or *Gengraf,* conversion from *Neoral* or *Gengraf* to *Sandimmune* using a 1:1 ratio (mg/kg/day) may result in lower cyclosporine blood concentration. Conversion from *Neoral* or *Gengraf* to *Sandimmune* should be made with increased blood concentration monitoring to avoid the potential of underdosing.

▶*Nephrotoxic drugs:* Care should be taken in using cyclosporine with nephrotoxic drugs (see Drug Interactions).

▶*Vaccination:* During treatment with cyclosporine, vaccination may be less effective; avoid the use of live attenuated vaccines.

▶*Glomerular capillary thrombosis:* Glomerular capillary thrombosis has been reported and may progress to graft failure. The pathologic changes resemble those seen in the hemolytic-uremic syndrome and include thrombosis of the renal microvasculature, with platelet-fibrin thrombi occluding glomerular capillaries and afferent arterioles, microangiopathic hemolytic anemia, thrombocytopenia, and decreased renal function. Similar findings have been observed when other immunosuppressives have been employed posttransplantation.

▶*Hypomagnesemia:* Hypomagnesemia has been reported in some, but not all, patients exhibiting convulsions while on cyclosporine therapy. Although magnesium-depletion studies in normal subjects suggest that hypomagnesemia is associated with neurologic disorders, multiple factors, including hypertension, high-dose methylprednisolone, hypocholesterolemia, and nephrotoxicity associated with high plasma concentrations of cyclosporine appear to be related to the neurological manifestations of cyclosporine toxicity.

▶*Hypersensitivity reactions:* Rarely (approximately 1 in 1000), patients receiving *Sandimmune* injection have experienced anaphylactic reactions. Although the exact cause of these reactions is unknown, it is believed to be due to the *Cremophor EL* (polyoxyethylated castor oil) used as the vehicle for the IV formulation. These reactions have consisted of flushing of the face and upper thorax, acute respiratory dis-

CYCLOSPORINE (Cyclosporin A)[1]

tress with dyspnea and wheezing, blood pressure changes, and tachycardia. One patient died after respiratory arrest and aspiration pneumonia. In some cases, the reaction subsided after the infusion stopped. Continually observe patients receiving *Sandimmune* injection for at least the first 30 minutes following the start of the infusion and at frequent intervals thereafter. If anaphylaxis occurs, stop the infusion. An aqueous solution of epinephrine 1:1000 should be available at the bedside as well as a source of oxygen. Anaphylactic reactions have not been reported with the capsules or oral solution, which lack *Cremophor EL* (polyoxyethylated castor oil). In fact, patients experiencing anaphylactic reactions have been treated subsequently with the capsules or oral solution without incident.

➤*Renal function impairment:* Renal function impairment requires close monitoring and possibly frequent dosage adjustment. In patients with persistent high elevations of BUN and creatinine unresponsive to dosage adjustments, consider switching to other immunosuppressive therapy. In the event of severe and unremitting rejection, when rescue therapy with pulse steroids and monoclonal antibodies fails to reverse the rejection episode, it is preferable to switch to alternative immunosuppressive therapy or allow the kidney transplant to be rejected and removed rather than increase the dosage to a very high level in an attempt to reverse the rejection.

➤*Carcinogenesis:* As in patients receiving other immunosuppressants, those patients receiving cyclosporine are at increased risk of development of lymphomas and other malignancies, particularly those of the skin. The increased risk appears related to the intensity and duration of immunosuppression rather than to the use of specific agents. Because of the danger of oversuppression of the immune system resulting in increased risk of infection or malignancy, use a treatment regimen containing multiple immunosuppressants with caution. Reduction or discontinuance of immunosuppression may cause the lesions to regress.

It is not clear whether the risk with cyclosporine is greater than that in RA patients or in RA patients on cytotoxic treatment for this indication. Five cases of lymphoma were detected: 4 in a survey of approximately 2,300 patients treated with cyclosporine for RA; and another case of lymphoma was reported in a clinical trial. Although other tumors (12 skin cancers, 24 solid tumors of diverse types, and 1 multiple myeloma) also were reported in this survey, epidemiologic analyses did not support a relationship to cyclosporine other than for malignant lymphomas.

Tumors were reported in 32 (2.2%) of 1439 psoriasis patients treated with cyclosporine worldwide from clinical trials. Additional tumors have been reported in 7 patients in cyclosporine postmarketing experience. Skin malignancies were reported in 16 (1.1%) of these patients; all but 2 of them had previously received PUVA therapy. Methotrexate was received by 7 patients. UVB and coal tar had been used by 2 and 3 patients, respectively. Seven patients had either a history of previous skin cancer or a potentially predisposing lesion was present prior to cyclosporine exposure. Of the 16 patients with skin cancer, 11 patients had 18 squamous cell carcinomas and 7 patients had 10 basal cell carcinomas.

There were 2 lymphoproliferative malignancies; 1 case of non-Hodgkin lymphoma that required chemotherapy, and 1 case of mycosis fungoides which regressed spontaneously upon discontinuation of cyclosporine. There were 4 cases of benign lymphocytic infiltration: 3 regressed spontaneously upon discontinuation of cyclosporine, while the fourth regressed despite continuation of the drug. The remainder of the malignancies, 13 cases (0.9%), involved various organs.

Do not treat patients for psoriasis concurrently with cyclosporine and PUVA or UVB, other radiation therapy, or other immunosuppressive agents because of the possibility of excessive immunosuppression and the subsequent risk of malignancies (see Contraindications).

Thoroughly evaluate patients before and during cyclosporine treatment for the development of malignancies. Moreover, use of cyclosporine therapy with other immunosuppressive agents may induce an excessive immunosuppression that is known to increase the risk of malignancy.

➤*Elderly:* In RA clinical trials with cyclosporine, 17.5% of patients were 65 years of age and older. These patients were more likely to develop systolic hypertension on therapy, and more likely to show serum creatinine rises greater than or equal to 50% above the baseline after 3 to 4 months of therapy. Monitor elderly patients with particular care, because decreases in renal function also occur with age. If patients are not properly monitored and dosages are not properly adjusted, cyclosporine therapy can cause structural kidney damage and persistent renal dysfunction.

➤*Pregnancy:* Category C. *Sandimmune* oral solution is embryotoxic and fetotoxic as indicated by increased pre- and postnatal mortality and reduced fetal weight together with related skeletal retardation in rats and rabbits when given in doses 2 to 5 times the human dose. There are no adequate and well-controlled studies in pregnant women. Use during pregnancy only if the potential benefit justifies the risk to the fetus.

The following data represent the reported outcomes of 116 pregnancies in women receiving cyclosporine during pregnancy, 90% of whom were transplant patients and most of whom received cyclosporine throughout the entire gestational period. The only consistent patterns of abnormality were premature birth (gestational period of 28 to 36 weeks) and low birth weight for gestational age. Sixteen fetal losses occurred. Most of the pregnancies (85 of 100) were complicated by disorders, including pre-eclampsia, eclampsia, premature labor, abruptio placentae, oligohydramnios, Rh incompatibility, and fetoplacental dysfunction. Preterm delivery occurred in 47%. Seven malformations were reported in 5 viable infants and in 2 cases of fetal loss. Twenty-eight percent of the infants were small for gestational age. Neonatal complications occurred in 27%. Therefore, weigh the risks and benefits of using cyclosporine during pregnancy.

Because of the possible disruption of maternal-fetal interaction, carefully weigh the risk/benefit ratio of using cyclosporine in psoriasis patients during pregnancy with seriously considering discontinuing cyclosporine.

➤*Lactation:* Cyclosporine is excreted in breast milk; avoid nursing.

➤*Children:* Although no adequate and well-controlled studies have been completed in children, patients as young as 6 months of age have received *Sandimmune* with no unusual adverse effects. Transplant recipients as young as 1 year of age have received *Neoral* or *Gengraf* with no unusual adverse effects.

The safety and efficacy of *Neoral* or *Gengraf* treatment in children with juvenile RA or psoriasis younger than 18 years of age have not been established.

Precautions

➤*Monitoring:*

Blood levels – Transplant centers have found blood concentration monitoring of cyclosporine to be an essential component of patient management. Of importance to blood concentration analysis are the type of assay used, the transplanted organ, and other immunosuppressant agents being administered. While no fixed relationship has been established, blood concentration monitoring may assist in the clinical evaluation of rejection and toxicity, dose adjustments, and the assessment of compliance.

Various assays have been used to measure blood concentrations of cyclosporine. HPLC is the standard reference, but the monoclonal antibody RIAs and the monoclonal antibody FPIA offer sensitivity, reproducibility, and convenience. Most clinicians base their monitoring on trough cyclosporine concentrations. Blood concentration monitoring is not a replacement for renal function monitoring or tissue biopsies.

Laboratory tests – Assess renal and liver functions repeatedly by measurement of BUN, serum creatinine, serum bilirubin, and liver enzymes. Also monitor serum lipids, magnesium, and potassium. Routinely monitor cyclosporine blood concentrations in transplant patients and periodically in RA patients.

Special monitoring for RA patients – Before initiating treatment, perform a careful physical exam, including blood pressure measurements (on at least 2 occasions) and 2 creatinine levels to estimate baseline. Evaluate blood pressure and serum creatinine every 2 weeks during the initial 3 months and then monthly if the patient is stable. It is advisable to monitor serum creatinine and blood pressure always after an increase of the dose of NSAIDs and after initiation of new NSAID therapy during *Neoral* or *Gengraf* treatment. If coadministered with methotrexate, CBC and liver function tests are recommended to be monitored monthly.

Special monitoring for psoriasis patients – Before initiating treatment, perform a careful dermatological and physical examination, including blood pressure measurements (on at least 2 occasions). Because *Neoral* and *Gengraf* are immunosuppressive agents, evaluate patients for the presence of occult infection on their first physical examination and for the presence of tumors initially, and throughout treatment with *Neoral* or *Gengraf*. Biopsy skin lesions are not typical for psoriasis before starting *Neoral* or *Gengraf*. Treat patients with malignant or premalignant changes of the skin with *Neoral* or *Gengraf* only after appropriate treatment of such lesions and if no other treatment option exists. Baseline laboratories include serum creatinine (on 2 occasions), BUN, CBC, serum magnesium, potassium, uric acid, and lipids.

Evaluate serum creatinine and BUN every 2 weeks during the initial 3 months of therapy and then monthly if the patient is stable. If the serum creatinine is greater than or equal to 25% above the patient's pretreatment level, repeat serum creatinine within 2 weeks. If the change in serum creatinine remains greater than or equal to 25% above baseline, reduce *Neoral* or *Gengraf* by 25% to 50%. Discontinue *Neoral* or *Gengraf* if reversibility (within 25% of baseline) of serum creatinine is not achievable after 2 dosage modifications.

Evaluate blood pressure every 2 weeks during the initial 3 months of therapy and then monthly if the patient is stable, or more frequently when dosage adjustments are made. Patients without a history of previous hypertension before initiation of treatment with *Neoral* or *Gengraf* should have the drug reduced by 25% to 50% if found to have sustained hypertension. If the patient continues to be hypertensive

Immunosuppressives

CYCLOSPORINE (Cyclosporin A)[1]

despite multiple reductions of *Neoral* or *Gengraf*, then discontinue *Neoral* or *Gengraf*. For patients treated with hypertension, before the initiation of *Neoral* or *Gengraf* therapy, discontinue their medication if a change in hypertension management is not effective or tolerable.

Also monitor CBC, uric acid, potassium, lipids, and magnesium every 2 weeks for the first 3 months of therapy, and then monthly if the patient is stable or more frequently when dosage adjustments are made. Reduce *Neoral* or *Gengraf* dosage by 25% to 50% for any abnormality of clinical concern. In controlled trials of cyclosporine in psoriasis patients, cyclosporine blood concentrations did not correlate well with either improvement or with side effects such as renal dysfunction.

➤*Hypertension:* Mild or moderate hypertension is encountered more frequently than severe hypertension and the incidence decreases over time. In recipients of kidney, liver, and heart allografts treated with cyclosporine, antihypertensive therapy may be required. However, because cyclosporine may cause hyperkalemia, do not use potassium-sparing diuretics. While calcium antagonists can be effective agents in treating cyclosporine-associated hypertension, they can interfere with cyclosporine metabolism.

➤*Malabsorption:* Patients with malabsorption may have difficulty achieving therapeutic levels with *Sandimmune* capsules or oral solution.

> **Drug Interactions**

➤*Nephrotoxic drugs:* Concomitant nonsteroidal anti-inflammatory drugs (NSAIDS), particularly in the setting of dehydration, may potentiate renal dysfunction. Other drugs that may potentiate renal dysfunction are antibiotics such as gentamycin, tobramycin, vancomycin, TMP-SMZ; antineoplastics such as melphalan; antifungals such as amphotericin B, ketoconazole; anti-inflammatory drugs such as diclofenac, naproxen, sulindac, colchicines; GI drugs such as cimetidine and ranitidine; and immunosuppressives such as tacrolimus.

➤*Cytochrome P450 system:* Cyclosporine is extensively metabolized by cytochrome P450 3A4. Monitoring of circulating cyclosporine concentrations and appropriate *Neoral* or *Gengraf* dosage adjustments are essential when these drugs are used concomitantly with other drugs that are inducers or inhibitors of this isoenzyme (eg, calcium channel blockers, glucocorticoids, anticonvulsants, protease inhibitors).

Cyclosporine Drug Interactions			
Precipitant Drug	Object Drug*		Description
Allopurinol	Cyclosporine	↑	Coadministration may increase cyclosporine concentrations.
Amiodarone	Cyclosporine	↑	Amiodarone may increase cyclosporine blood levels, possibly increasing the risk of nephrotoxicity.
Androgens (eg, danazol, methyl-testosterone)	Cyclosporine	↑	Increased cyclosporine blood concentrations and possible nephrotoxicity.
Anticonvulsants (eg, carbamazepine, phenytoin)	Cyclosporine	↓	Cyclosporine levels may be decreased, resulting in a reduction in the pharmacologic effects.
Azole antifungals (eg, fluconazole, ketoconazole)	Cyclosporine	↑	Cyclosporine levels and toxicity may increase 1 to 3 days after starting therapy and persist more than 1 week after stopping antifungal therapy.
Beta blockers (eg, carvedilol)	Cyclosporine	↑	Elevated cyclosporine concentrations with a risk of nephrotoxicity and neurotoxicity may occur.
Bosentan	Cyclosporine	↑↓	Trough concentrations of bosentan may be elevated, increasing the risk of adverse effects, while cyclosporine plasma levels may be decreased. Coadministration is contraindicated.
Cyclosporine	Bosentan		
Bromocriptine	Cyclosporine	↑	Coadministration may increase cyclosporine concentrations.
Calcium channel blockers (eg, nicardipine, diltiazem, verapamil)	Cyclosporine	↑	Increased cyclosporine levels with possible nephrotoxicity. However, administration of verapamil before cyclosporine may be nephroprotective. The interaction is typically observed within 7 days of starting verapamil and may abate within 1 week after discontinuation.
Colchicine	Cyclosporine	↑	Severe adverse clinical symptoms including GI, hepatic, renal, and neuromuscular toxicity may occur during concurrent administration.
Contraceptives, oral	Cyclosporine	↑	Severe hepatotoxicity and raised plasma-cyclosporine trough values have resulted with coadministration in one case.

Cyclosporine Drug Interactions			
Precipitant Drug	Object Drug*		Description
Corticosteroids	Cyclosporine	↑	Although this combination is therapeutically beneficial for organ transplants, toxicity may be enhanced.
Fluoroquinolones (eg, ciprofloxacin)	Cyclosporine	↑	Increased cyclosporine toxicity may occur.
Foscarnet	Cyclosporine	↑	The risk of renal failure may be increased.
Imipenem-cilastatin	Cyclosporine	↑	The CNS side effects of both agents may be increased.
Macrolide antibiotics	Cyclosporine	↑	Elevated cyclosporine levels, increasing the risk of nephrotoxicity and neurotoxicity, may occur.
Metoclopramide	Cyclosporine	↑	An increase in the immunosuppressive and toxic effects of cyclosporine may result with metoclopramide coadministration.
Nafcillin	Cyclosporine	↓	Coadministration may decrease cyclosporine concentrations.
Nefazodone	Cyclosporine	↑	Cyclosporine concentrations and toxicity may be increased.
Orlistat	Cyclosporine	↓	Whole blood cyclosporine concentrations may be decreased, possibly resulting in a decrease in the immunosuppressive action of cyclosporine.
Probucol	Cyclosporine	↓	Whole blood cyclosporine concentrations may be reduced, producing a decrease in clinical effect.
Rifamycins (rifampin and rifabutin)	Cyclosporine	↓	The immunosuppressive effect of cyclosporine may be reduced. This appears to occur as early as 2 days following the initiation of rifamycins and may persist for 1 to 3 weeks after their discontinuation.
Serotonin reuptake inhibitors (SSRIs) (eg, fluoxetine, sertraline)	Cyclosporine	↑	SSRIs may increase cyclosporine concentrations and toxicity.
St. John's wort	Cyclosporine	↓	Decreased cyclosporine levels and efficacy may occur with coadministration.
Sulfonamides (eg, TMP-SMZ)	Cyclosporine	↓	The action of cyclosporine may be reduced. Oral sulfonamides may increase the risk of nephrotoxicity.
Terbinafine	Cyclosporine	↓	Terbinafine may decrease cyclosporine concentrations.
Ticlopidine	Cyclosporine	↓	Cyclosporine whole blood concentrations may decrease, producing a decrease in pharmacologic effects.
Cyclosporine	Digoxin	↑	Elevated digoxin levels with toxicity may occur.
Cyclosporine	Etoposide	↑	Serum etoposide concentration may be elevated, resulting in increased toxicity.
Cyclosporine	HMG-CoA reductase inhibitors	↑	Severe myopathy or rhabdomyolysis may occur with coadministration.
Cyclosporine	Methotrexate	↑	Coadministration resulted in increased methotrexate AUC ≈ 30% and the AUC of its metabolite was decreased ≈ 80%.
Cyclosporine	Potassium-sparine diuretics	↑	Coadministration may lead to hyperkalemia. Avoid concomitant use.
Cyclosporine	Sirolimus	↑	Sirolimus plasma concentrations may be increased, resulting in increased toxicity. Administer sirolimus 4 hours after cyclosporine to prevent variations in sirolimus concentrations.

* ↑ = Object drug increased. ↓ = Object drug decreased.

➤*Drug/Food interactions:* Administration of food with *Gengraf* and *Neoral* decreases the AUC and C_{max} of cyclosporine. A high-fat meal (669 kcal, 45 g fat) consumed within 30 minutes of *Gengraf* and *Neoral* administration decreased the AUC by 13% and C_{max} by 33%. The

CYCLOSPORINE (Cyclosporin A)[1]

effects of a low-fat meal (667 kcal, 15 g fat) were similar. Unless patients have been instructed by a health care provider to take cyclosporine with grapefruit juice, caution them to avoid fluctuations in the ingestion of grapefruit juice while taking cyclosporine.

Adverse Reactions

▶*Most common:* The principal adverse reactions of cyclosporine therapy are renal dysfunction, tremor, hirsutism, hypertension, and gum hyperplasia. Hypertension, which is usually mild to moderate, may occur in approximately 50% of patients following renal transplantation and in most cardiac transplant patients.

Glomerular capillary thrombosis – Glomerular capillary thrombosis has been found in patients treated with cyclosporine and may progress to graft failure. The pathologic changes resemble those seen in the hemolytic-uremic syndrome and include thrombosis of the renal microvasculature, with platelet-fibrin thrombi occluding glomerular capillaries and afferent arterioles, microangiopathic hemolytic anemia, thrombocytopenia, and decreased renal function. Similar findings have been observed when other immunosuppressives have been employed posttransplantation.

Polyoxyethylated castor oil – *Cremophor EL* (polyoxyethylated castor oil) is known to cause hyperlipidemia and electrophoretic abnormalities of lipoproteins. These effects are reversible upon discontinuation of treatment but are usually not a reason to stop treatment.

Hypomagnesemia – Hypomagnesemia has been reported in some, but not all, patients exhibiting convulsions while on cyclosporine therapy. Although magnesium-depletion studies in normal subjects suggest that hypomagnesemia is associated with neurologic disorders, multiple factors, including hypertension, high dose methylprednisolone, hypocholesterolemia, and nephrotoxicity associated with high plasma concentrations of cyclosporine appear to be related to the neurological manifestations of cyclosporine toxicity.

Cyclosporine (*Sandimmune*) Adverse Reactions (%)

| Adverse reactions | Randomized kidney patients | | All *Sandimmune* patients (kidney, heart, liver transplants) (n = 892) |
	Sandimmune (n = 227)	Azathioprine (n = 228)	
Cardiovascular			
Flushing	< 1	0	≤ 4
Hypertension	26	18	13 - 53
CNS			
Confusion	≤ 2	—	—
Convulsions	3	1	1 - 5
Headache	2	< 1	2 - 15
Paresthesia	3	0	1 - 2
Tremor	12	0	21 - 55
Dermatologic			
Acne	6	8	1 - 2
Brittle fingernails	≤ 2	—	—
Hirsutism	21	< 1	21 - 45
GI			
Abdominal dis- comfort	< 1	0	≤ 7
Anorexia	≤ 2	—	—
Diarrhea	3	< 1	3 - 8
Gastritis	≤ 2	—	—
Gum hyperplasia	4	0	5 - 16
Nausea/vomiting	2	< 1	4 - 10
Peptic ulcer	≤ 2	—	—
Hematopoietic			
Anemia	≤ 2	—	—
Leukopenia	2	19	≤ 6
Lymphoma	< 1	0	1 - 6
Thrombocytopenia	≤ 2	—	—
Miscellaneous			
Allergic reaction	≤ 2	—	—
Conjunctivitis	≤ 2	—	—
Cramps	4	< 1	≤ 2
Edema	≤ 2	—	—
Fever	≤ 2	—	—
Gynecomastia	< 1	0	≤ 4
Hearing loss	≤ 2	—	—
Hepatotoxicity	< 1	< 1	4 - 7
Hiccoughs	≤ 2	—	—
Hyperglycemia	≤ 2	—	—
Muscle pain	≤ 2	—	—
Renal dysfunction	32	6	25 - 38
Sinusitis	< 1	0	3 - 7
Tinnitus	≤ 2	—	—

The following reactions occurred rarely: anxiety, chest pain, constipation, depression, hair breaking, hematuria, joint pain, lethargy, mouth sores, MI, night sweats, pancreatitis, pruritus, swallowing difficulty, tingling, upper GI bleeding, visual disturbance, weakness, weight loss.

Among 705 kidney transplant patients treated with *Sandimmune* in clinical trials, the reason for treatment discontinuation was renal toxicity (5.4%), infection (0.9%), lack of efficacy (1.4%), acute tubular necrosis (1%), lymphoproliferative disorders (0.3%), hypertension (0.3%), and other reasons (0.7%).

Infectious Complications in Randomized Renal Transplant Patients (%)

Complication	Cyclosporine (n = 227)	Azathioprine with steroids[a] (n = 228)
Abscess	4.4	5.3
Cytomegalovirus	4.8	12.3
Local fungal infections	7.5	9.6
Pneumonia	6.2	9.2
Septicemia	5.3	4.8
Systemic fungal infections	2.2	3.9
Urinary tract infections	21.1	20.2
Viral infections	15.9	18.4
Wound and skin infections	7	10.1

[a] Some patients also received antilymphocytic globulin.

▶*Sandimmune, Neoral, Gengraf:*

RA – The principal adverse reactions associated with the use of cyclosporine in RA are renal dysfunction, hypertension, headache, GI disturbances, and hirsutism/hypertrichosis.

In RA patients treated in clinical trials within the recommended dose range, cyclosporine was discontinued in 5.3% of patients because of hypertension and in 7% of patients because of increased creatinine. These changes are usually reversible with timely dose decreases or discontinuation. The frequency and severity of serum creatinine elevations increase with dose and duration of cyclosporine therapy. These elevations are likely to become more pronounced without dose reduction or discontinuation.

Neoral/Sandimmune RA Adverse Events (≥ 3%)

Adverse event	*Sandimmune*[a] (N = 269)	*Sandimmune* (N = 155)	Methotrexate + *Sandimmune* (N = 74)	*Neoral* (N = 143)
Cardiovascular				
Arrhythmia	2	5	5	2
Chest pain	4	5	1	6
Flushing	2	2	3	5
Hypertension	8	26	16	25
CNS				
Depression	3	6	3	1
Dizziness	8	6	7	8
Headache	17	23	22	25
Insomnia	4	1	1	3
Migraine	2	3	0	3
Paresthesia	8	7	8	11
Tremor	8	7	7	13
Dermatologic				
Alopecia	3	0	1	4
Bullous eruptions	1	0	4	1
Hypertrichosis	19	17	12	15
Rash	7	12	10	8
Skin ulceration	1	1	3	0
GI				
Abdominal pain	15	15	15	15
Anorexia	3	3	1	3
Diarrhea	12	12	18	13
Dyspepsia	12	12	10	8
Flatulence	5	5	5	4
GI disorder NOS[b]	0	2	1	4
Gingivitis	4	3	0	0
Gum hyperplasia	2	4	1	4
Nausea	23	14	24	18
Rectal hemorrhage	0	3	0	1
Stomatitis	7	5	16	6
Vomiting	9	8	14	6
GU				
Dysuria	0	0	11	1
Leukorrhea	1	0	4	1
Menstrual disorder	3	2	1	1
Micturition frequency	2	4	3	2
NPN, increased	0	19	12	18
UTI	0	3	5	3

CYCLOSPORINE (Cyclosporin A)[1]

Neoral/Sandimmune RA Adverse Events (≥ 3%)				
Adverse event	Sandimmune[a] (N = 269)	Sandimmune (N = 155)	Methotrexate + Sandimmune (N = 74)	Neoral (N = 143)
Lab test abnormalities				
Creatinine elevations ≥ 30%	43	39	55	48
Creatinine elevations ≥ 50%	24	18	26	18
Respiratory				
Bronchitis	1	3	1	1
Coughing	5	3	5	4
Dyspnea	5	1	3	1
Infection NOS	9	5	0	3
Pharyngitis	3	5	5	4
Pneumonia	1	0	4	1
Rhinitis	0	3	11	1
Sinusitis	4	4	8	3
Upper respiratory tract infection	0	14	23	13
Miscellaneous				
Accidental trauma	0	1	10	4
Edema NOS	5	14	12	10
Fatigue	6	3	8	3
Fever	2	3	0	2
Flu-like symptoms	< 1	6	1	3
Pain	6	9	10	13
Rigors	1	1	4	3
Ear disorder NOS	0	5	0	1
Purpura	3	4	1	2

[a] Includes patients in 2.5 mg/kg/day dose group only.
[b] NOS = not otherwise specified.

In addition, the following adverse events have been reported in 1% to less than 3% of the RA patients in the cyclosporine treatment group in controlled clinical trials.

Cardiovascular – Abnormal heart sounds, cardiac failure, MI, peripheral ischemia.

CNS – Anxiety, confusion, decreased libido, emotional lability, hypoesthesia, impaired concentration, increased libido, nervousness, neuropathy, paranoia, somnolence, vertigo.

Dermatologic – Abnormal pigmentation, angioedema, dermatitis, dry skin, eczema, nail disorder, pruritus, skin disorder, urticaria.

GI – Constipation, dysphagia, enanthema, eructation, esophagitis, gastric ulcer, gastritis, gastroenteritis, gingival bleeding, glossitis, peptic ulcer, salivary gland enlargement, tongue disorder, tooth disorder.

GU – Abnormal urine, breast pain, breast fibroadenosis, hematuria, increased BUN, micturition urgency, nocturia, polyuria, pyelonephritis, urinary incontinence, uterine hemorrhage.

Hematologic – Anemia, epistaxis, leucopenia, lymphadenopathy.

Metabolic/Nutritional – Diabetes mellitus, hyperkalemia, hyperuricemia, hypoglycemia, weight decrease, weight increase.

Musculoskeletal – Arthralgia, bone fracture, bursitis, joint dislocation, myalgia, stiffness, synovial cyst, tendon disorder.

Respiratory – Abnormal chest sounds, bronchospasm, tonsillitis.

Special senses – Abnormal vision, cataract, conjunctivitis, deafness, eye pain, taste perversion, tinnitus, vestibular disorder.

Miscellaneous – Abcess, allergy, asthenia, bacterial infection, bilirubinemia, carcinoma, cellulitis, dry mouth, folliculitis, fungal infection, goiter, herpes simplex, herpes zoster, hot flushes, increased sweating, malaise, moniliasis, overdose, procedure NOS, renal abscess, tumor NOS, viral infection.

Psoriasis – The principal adverse reactions associated with the use of cyclosporine in patients with psoriasis are renal dysfunction, headache, hypertension, hypertriglyceridemia, hirsutism/hypertrichosis, paresthesia or hyperesthesia, influenza-like symptoms, nausea/vomiting, diarrhea, abdominal discomfort, lethargy, and musculoskeletal or joint pain.

In psoriasis patients treated in US controlled trials within the recommended dose range, cyclosporine therapy was discontinued in 1% of patients because of hypertension and in 5.4% of patients because of increased creatinine. In the majority of cases, these changes were reversible after dose reduction or discontinuation of cyclosporine. There has been one reported death associated with the use of cyclosporine in psoriasis. A 27-year-old male developed renal deterioration and was continued on cyclosporine. He had progressive renal failure leading to death.

Frequency and severity of serum creatinine increases with dose and duration of cyclosporine therapy. These elevations are likely to become more pronounced and may result in irreversible renal damage without dose reduction or discontinuation.

Adverse Events Occurring in Psoriasis Patients (≥ 1%)		
Adverse reaction	Neoral (n = 182)	Sandimmune (n = 185)
Cardiovascular		
Chest pain	1 to < 3	1 to < 3
Hypertension	27.5	25.4
CNS		
Dizziness	1 to < 3	1 to < 3
Headache	15.9	14
Insomnia	1 to < 3	1 to < 3
Nervousness	1 to < 3	1 to < 3
Paresthesia	7.1	4.8
Vertigo	1 to < 3	1 to < 3
Dermatologic		
Acne	1 to < 3	1 to < 3
Dry skin	1 to < 3	1 to < 3
Folliculitis	1 to < 3	1 to < 3
Hypertrichosis	6.6	5.4
Keratosis	1 to < 3	1 to < 3
Pruritus	1 to < 3	1 to < 3
Rash	1 to < 3	1 to < 3
GI		
Abdominal pain	2.7	6
Abdominal distention	1 to < 3	1 to < 3
Constipation	1 to < 3	1 to < 3
Diarrhea	5	5.9
Dyspepsia	2.2	3.2
Gingival bleeding	1 to < 3	1 to < 3
Gum hyperplasia	3.8	6
Nausea	5.5	5.9
GU		
Increased creatinine	19.8	15.7
Micturition frequency	1 to < 3	1 to < 3
Hematologic		
White cell and RES	4.4	2.7
Platelet, bleeding, and clotting disorders	1 to < 3	1 to < 3
Red blood cell disorders	1 to < 3	1 to < 3
Respiratory		
Bronchospasm	5	4.9
Coughing	5	4.9
Dyspnea	5	4.9
Infection (viral, other)	1 to < 3	1 to < 3
Rhinitis	5	4.9
Upper respiratory tract infections	7.7	11.3
Miscellaneous		
Abnormal vision	1 to < 3	1 to < 3
Arthralgia	6	1.1
Fever	1 to < 3	1 to < 3
Flu-like symptoms	9.9	8.1
Flushes	1 to < 3	1 to < 3
Hot flushes	1 to < 3	1 to < 3
Hyperbilirubinemia	1 to < 3	1 to < 3
Increased appetite	1 to < 3	1 to < 3
Pain	4.4	3.2
Skin malignancies (squamous cell [0.9%], basal cell [0.4%] carcinomas)	1 to < 3	1 to < 3

Mild hypomagnesemia and hyperkalemia may occur but are asymptomatic. Increases in uric acid may occur and attacks of gout have been rarely reported. A minor dose-related hyperbilirubinemia has been observed in the absence of hepatocellular damage. Cyclosporine therapy may be associated with a modest increase of serum triglycerides and cholesterol. Elevations of triglycerides (greater than 750 mg/dL) occur in about 15% of psoriasis patients; elevations of cholesterol (greater than 300 mg/dL) are observed in less than 3% of psoriasis patients. Generally these laboratory abnormalities are reversible upon dose reduction or discontinuation of cyclosporine.

Overdosage

▶*Oral:* There is minimal experience with cyclosporine overdosage. Forced emesis can be of value up to 2 hours after administration of cyclosporine. Follow general supportive measures and symptomatic treatment in all cases of overdosage. Cyclosporine is not dialyzable to any great extent, nor is it cleared well by charcoal hemoperfusion.

Patient Information

Advise patients to take cyclosporine with food at the same time each day.

Advise patients to not eat grapefruit or drink grapefruit juice while taking this medicine.

CYCLOSPORINE (Cyclosporin A)[1]

Women who could become pregnant should use nonhormonal contraceptives (diaphragms, condoms) while taking cyclosporine.

Instruct patients to contact their health care provider if fever, sore throat, tiredness, unusual bleeding or bruising, urination, or yellow skin/eyes occurs.

An odor may be present upon opening the *Sandimmune* package. The odor will disappear shortly after opening and does not mean that there is anything wrong with the medicine.

Instruct patients to not take potassium supplements while taking cyclosporine.

Cyclosporine may increase skin cancer risk. Advise patients to avoid prolonged exposure to the sun and other UV light and to use sun-screens and wear protective clothing while taking this medicine. Patients who are being treated for psoriasis will need to have at least 2 careful skin and physical examinations, including blood pressure measurements, before starting cyclosporine.

Patients should avoid live vaccines (eg, measles, mumps, oral polio) while taking cyclosporine. The vaccination may be less effective.

Cyclosporine may increase risk of high blood pressure and abnormal kidney function.

Cyclosporine may affect blood sugar level in diabetic patients.

Instruct patients not to switch to another form of this medication without contacting a health care provider.

DACLIZUMAB

| *Rx* | **Zenapax** (Roche) | **Injection:** 25 mg/5 mL | Preservative-free. In single-use vials. |

WARNING

Only physicians experienced in immunosuppressive therapy and management of organ transplant patients should prescribe daclizumab. The physician responsible for daclizumab administration should have complete information requisite for the follow-up of the patient. Daclizumab should only be administered by health care personnel trained in the administration of the drug who have available adequate laboratory and supportive medical resources.

Indications

➤*Organ rejection, prophylaxis:* Prophylaxis of acute organ rejection in patients receiving renal transplants. It is used as part of an immunosuppressive regimen that includes cyclosporine and corticosteroids.

Administration and Dosage

➤*Approved by the FDA:* December 10, 1997.

The recommended dose for daclizumab in adults and children is 1 mg/kg IV used as part of an immunosuppressive regimen that includes cyclosporine and corticosteroids. Mix the calculated volume of daclizumab with 50 mL of sterile 0.9% sodium chloride solution, and administer via a peripheral or central vein over a 15-minute period.

The standard course of daclizumab therapy is 5 doses. Give the first dose no more than 24 hours before transplantation. Give the 4 remaining doses at intervals of 14 days.

➤*Instructions for administration:*
• Not for direct injection. Dilute the calculated volume in 50 mL of sterile 0.9% sodium chloride solution before administration. When mixing the solution, gently invert the bag in order to avoid foaming; do not shake.
• This product contains no antimicrobial preservative or bacteriostatic agents. Once the infusion is prepared, administer IV within 4 hours. If it must be held longer, refrigerate between 2° to 8°C (36° to 46°F) for up to 24 hours. After 24 hours, discard the prepared solution. Discard any unused portion of the drug.
• Do not add or infuse other drug substances simultaneously through the same IV line.

➤*Compatibility / Incompatibility:* No incompatibility has been observed between daclizumab and polyvinyl chloride, polyethylene bags, or infusion sets. Do not add or infuse other drug substances simultaneously through the same IV line.

➤*Storage / Stability:* Refrigerate vials at 2° to 8°C (36° to 46°F); do not shake or freeze. Protect undiluted solution against direct light. Diluted medication is stable for 24 hours at 4°C (39°F) or for 4 hours at room temperature.

Actions

➤*Pharmacology:* Daclizumab is an immunosuppressive, humanized IgG1 monoclonal antibody produced by recombinant DNA technology that binds specifically to the alpha subunit (Tac subunit) of the human high-affinity interleukin-2 (IL-2) receptor that is expressed on the surface of activated lymphocytes. Daclizumab is a composite of human (90%) and murine (10%) antibody sequences.

Daclizumab functions as an IL-2 receptor antagonist that binds with high affinity to the Tac subunit of the high affinity IL-2 receptor complex and inhibits IL-2 binding. Daclizumab binding is highly specific for Tac, which is expressed on activated but not resting lymphocytes. Daclizumab inhibits IL-2-mediated activation of lymphocytes, a critical pathway in the cellular immune response involved in allograft rejection.

At recommended doses, daclizumab saturates the Tac sub-unit of the IL-2 receptor for approximately 90 and 120 days posttransplant, respectively, in pediatric and adult patients; the duration of clinically significant IL-2 receptor blockade is not known. It is unknown if daclizumab-impaired immune responses to repeated or ongoing antigenic challenges return to normal after drug elimination.

➤*Pharmacokinetics:* In clinical trials involving renal allograft patients treated with a 1 mg/kg IV dose every 14 days for a total of 5 doses, peak serum concentrations rose between the first dose (21 ± 14 mcg/mL) and the fifth dose (32 ± 22 mcg/mL). The mean trough serum concentration before the fifth dose was 7.6 ± 4 mcg/mL. In vitro and in vivo data suggest that serum levels of 5 to 10 mcg/mL are necessary for saturation of the Tac subunit of the IL-2 receptors to block the responses of activated T-lymphocytes.

Population pharmacokinetic analysis gave the following values for a reference patient (white male, 45 years of age, with a body weight of 80 kg and no proteinuria): Systemic clearance = 15 mL/hr, volume of central compartment = 2.5 L, volume of peripheral compartment = 3.4 L. The estimated terminal elimination half-life for the reference patient was 20 days (480 hours), which is similar to the terminal elimination half-life for human IgG (18 to 23 days). Bayesian estimates of terminal elimination half-life ranged from 11 to 38 days for the 123 patients included in the population analysis.

The influence of body weight on systemic clearance supports the dosing of daclizumab on a mg/kg basis. For patients studied, this dosing maintained drug exposure within 30% of the reference exposure.

Special populations –
Children: Pharmacokinetic parameters were evaluated in 61 pediatric patients treated with a 1 mg/kg IV dose of daclizumab every 14 days for a total of 5 doses. Peak serum concentration (mean ± SD) rose between the first dose (16 ± 12 mcg/mL) and fifth dose (21 ± 14 mcg/mL). The mean trough serum concentration before the fifth dose was 5 ± 2.7 mcg/mL. Population pharmacokinetic analysis of the data using a 2-compartment open model gave the following values for a reference patient (white patient with a body weight of 29.7 kg): systemic clearance = 10 mL/hr, volume of central compartment = 2 L, volume of peripheral compartment = 1.4 L. The estimated terminal elimination half-life for the reference patient was 13 days (317 hours). For the patients studied, this dosing maintained drug exposure within 50% of the reference exposure. The estimated interpatient variability (percent coefficient of variation) in systemic clearance and central volume of distribution were 30% and 40%, respectively.

Contraindications

Hypersensitivity to daclizumab or to any components of this product.

Warnings

➤*Mortality:* The use of daclizumab as part of an immunosuppressive regimen including cyclosporine, mycophenolate mofetil, and corticosteroids may be associated with an increase in mortality. In a randomized, double-blind, placebo-controlled trial of daclizumab for the prevention of allograft rejection in 434 cardiac transplant recipients receiving concomitant cyclosporine, mycophenolate mofetil, and corticosteroids, mortality at 6 and 12 months was increased in those patients receiving daclizumab compared to those receiving placebo (7% vs 5%, respectively at 6 months; 10% vs 6% respectively at 12 months). Some, but not all, of the increase in mortality appeared related to a higher incidence of severe infections. Concomitant use of anti-lymphocyte, antibody therapy may also be a factor in some of the fatal infections.

➤*Benefit / Risk:* Administer under qualified medical supervision. Inform patients of the potential benefits of therapy and the risks associated with administration of immunosuppressive therapy.

➤*Lymphoproliferative disorders:* While the incidence of lymphoproliferative disorders and opportunistic infections in the limited clinical trial experience was no higher in daclizumab-treated patients compared with placebo-treated patients, patients on immunosuppressive therapy are at increased risk for developing lymphoproliferative disorders and opportunistic infections and should be monitored accordingly.

➤*Hypersensitivity reactions:* Severe, acute (onset within 24 hours) hypersensitivity reactions including anaphylaxis have been observed both on initial exposure to daclizumab and following re-exposure. These reactions may include hypotension, bronchospasm, wheezing, laryngeal edema, pulmonary edema, cyanosis hypoxia, respiratory arrest, cardiac arrhythmia, cardiac arrest, peripheral edema, loss of consciousness, fever, rash, urticaria, diaphoresis, pruritus, and/or injection site reactions. If a severe hypersensitivity reaction occurs, permanently discontinue therapy with daclizumab. Ensure that medications

DACLIZUMAB

for the treatment of severe hypersensitivity reactions including anaphylaxis are available for immediate use. Use caution if re-exposing patients previously administered daclizumab to a subsequent course of therapy. The potential risks of such readministration, specifically those associated with immunosuppression, are not known.

➤*Elderly:* Use caution in giving immunosuppressive drugs to elderly patients.

➤*Pregnancy: Category C.* It is not known whether daclizumab can cause fetal harm when administered to pregnant women or can affect reproductive capacity. In general, IgG molecules are known to cross the placental barrier. Do not use daclizumab in pregnant women unless the potential benefit justifies the potential risk to the fetus. Women of childbearing potential should use effective contraception before beginning daclizumab therapy, during therapy and for 4 months after completing daclizumab therapy.

➤*Lactation:* It is not known whether daclizumab is excreted in human milk. Because of the potential for adverse reactions, decide whether to discontinue nursing or discontinue the drug, taking into account the importance of the drug to the mother.

➤*Children:* The safety and efficacy of daclizumab have been established in pediatric patients from 11 months to 17 years of age.

Precautions

➤*Immune system effects:* It is not known whether daclizumab use will have a long-term effect on the ability of the immune system to respond to antigens first encountered during daclizumab-induced immunosuppression.

➤*Re-administration:* Re-administration of daclizumab after an initial course of therapy has not been studied in humans. The potential risks of such re-administration, specifically those associated with immunosuppression and/or the occurrence of anaphylaxis/anaphylactoid reactions, are not known.

➤*Immunogenicity:* Low titers of anti-idiotype antibodies to daclizumab were detected in the adult patients treated with daclizumab with an overall incidence of 14%. The incidence of anti-daclizumab antibodies observed in the pediatric patients was 34%. No antibodies that affected efficacy, safety, serum daclizumab levels or any other clinically related parameter were detected.

Adverse Reactions

➤*Adults:* Adverse events were reported by 95% of placebo-treated patients and 96% of daclizumab-treated patients (all received cyclosporine and corticosteroids). The proportion of patients prematurely withdrawn from the combined studies because of adverse events was 8.5% and 8.6% in the placebo and daclizumab groups, respectively.

The incidence and types of adverse events were similar in both groups. The most frequently reported adverse events were GI disorders, which were reported with equal frequency (placebo, 68% vs daclizumab, 67%). The following adverse events occurred in 2% or more of daclizumab-treated patients.

Cardiovascular – Aggravated hypertension, bleeding, hypertension, hypotension, tachycardia, thrombosis (5% or more).

CNS – Dizziness, headache, insomnia, tremor, (5% or more); anxiety, depression, prickly sensation (2% to less than 5%).

Dermatologic – Acne , impaired wound healing without infection (5% or more); hirsutism, increased sweating, night sweats, pruritus, rash (2% to less than 5%).

GI – Abdominal distension, abdominal pain, constipation, diarrhea, dyspepsia, epigastric pain (not food-related), nausea, pyrosis, vomiting (5% or more); flatulence, gastritis, hemorrhoids (2% to less than 5%).

GU – Dysuria, oliguria, renal tubular necrosis (5% or more); hydronephrosis, renal damage, renal insufficiency, urinary retention, urinary tract bleeding, urinary tract disorder (2% to less than 5%).

Metabolic/Nutritional – Edema, peripheral edema (5% or more); dehydration, diabetes mellitus, fluid overload (2% to less than 5%).

Hyperglycemia: A total of 32% of daclizumab-treated patients (16% for placebo) had high fasting blood-glucose values. Most of these high values occurred either on the first day post-transplant when patients received high doses of corticosteroids or in patients with diabetes.

Musculoskeletal – Back pain, musculoskeletal pain (5% or more); arthralgia, leg cramps, myalgia (2% to less than 5%).

Respiratory – Coughing, dyspnea, pulmonary edema (5% or more); abnormal breath sounds, atelectasis, congestion, hypoxia, pharyngitis, pleural effusion, rales, rhinitis (2% to less than 5%).

Miscellaneous – Chest pain, fatigue, fever, lymphocele, pain, post-traumatic pain (5% or more); blurred vision, generalized weakness, injection site reaction, shivering (2% to less than 5%).

Incidence of malignancies: One and 3 years post-transplant, the incidence of malignancies was 1.5% and 6.4%, respectively, in the daclizumab group (2.7% and 7.8%, respectively, for placebo). Addition of daclizumab did not increase the number of post-transplant lymphomas, which occurred with a frequency of ≤ 1.5% in both placebo-treated and daclizumab-treated groups.

Incidence of infectious episodes: In a large randomized study of daclizumab used for the prevention of allograft rejection in patients receiving cardiac allografts, more patients receiving daclizumab experienced severe or fatal infections after 12 months of therapy when compared with those receiving placebo (10% vs 7%, respectively). The risks of infection or death may be increased in patients receiving concomitant anti-lymphocyte antibody therapy (see Warnings).

The types of infections reported were similar in both groups. Cytomegalovirus infection was reported in 13% of the patients in the daclizumab group (16% for placebo). One exception was cellulitis and wound infections, which occurred in 8.4% of daclizumab-treated patients (4.1% for placebo). At 1 year post-transplant, 7 placebo patients and only 1 daclizumab-treated patient had died of an infection.

Children – The safety profile of daclizumab in pediatric transplant patients was shown to be comparable with that in adult transplant patients with the exception of the following adverse events, which occurred more frequently in pediatric patients (greater than 15% difference in incidence): diarrhea, post-operative pain, fever, vomiting, aggravated hypertension, pruritus, and infections of the upper respiratory tract and urinary tracts.

Postmarketing – Severe acute hypersensitivity reactions including anaphylaxis characterized by hypotension, bronchospasm, wheezing, laryngeal edema, pulmonary edema, cyanosis, hypoxia, respiratory arrest, cardiac arrhythmia, cardiac arrest, peripheral edema, loss of consciousness, fever, rash, urticaria, diaphoresis, pruritus, and/or injection site reactions, as well as cytokine release syndrome, have been reported during postmarketing experience with daclizumab. The relationship between these reactions and the development of antibodies to daclizumab is unknown.

Overdosage

Overdose with daclizumab has not been reported. A maximum tolerated dose has not been determined in patients. A dose of 1.5 mg/kg has been administered to bone marrow transplant recipients without any associated adverse events.

Patient Information

Tell your health care provider or pharmacist if any of the following occur: Serious allergic reactions (eg, rash, hives, difficulty breathing), chest pain, fast heartbeat, urinary tract bleeding, constipation, nausea, diarrhea, vomiting, stomach pain, swelling, tremors, headache, dizziness, difficulty urinating, pain, fever, tiredness, coughing, impaired wound healing without infection, urinary tract disorder, reaction at the injection site.

Advise women of childbearing potential to use effective birth control methods before beginning treatment with this medicine and to continue using birth control for 4 months after completing therapy.

This medicine may cause dizziness or blurred vision. Use caution while driving or performing other tasks requiring alertness, coordination, or physical dexterity.

GLATIRAMER ACETATE

Rx	**Copaxone** (Teva)	**Injection, premixed:** 20 mg/mL	40 mg mannitol. Preservative free. In single-use prefilled syringes.

Indications

➤*Relapsing-remitting multiple sclerosis (RR MS):* For the reduction of the frequency of relapses in patients with RR MS.

Administration and Dosage

The recommended dose is 20 mg/day injected SC. Sites for injection include arms, abdomen, hips, and thighs. Before injection, allow syringe to warm to room temperature (20 minutes). See the Glatiramer Acetate Patient Information booklet for Self-Injection Procedure.

➤*Storage/Stability:* Refrigerate at 2° to 8°C (36° to 46°F). However, excursions at room temperature 15° to 30°C (59° to 86°F) for up to 1 week are permitted.

Actions

➤*Pharmacology:* Glatiramer, for use in patients with MS, is a random synthetic copolymer of L-alanine, L-glutamic acid, L-lysine, and L-tyrosine.

The mechanism by which glatiramer exerts its effects in patients with MS is unknown. However, glatiramer is thought to act by modifying immune processes that are currently believed to be responsible for the pathogenesis of MS. This view of glatiramer derives from knowledge that it reduces the incidence and severity of experimental allergic encephalomyelitis (EAE), a condition induced in several animal species through immunization against CNS-derived material containing myelin and often used as an experimental animal model of MS.

GLATIRAMER ACETATE

➤**Pharmacokinetics:** Pharmacokinetic studies in humans have not been performed. However, it is assumed, based in part on the results of animal studies, that a substantial fraction of SC injection of glatiramer is hydrolyzed locally. Some fraction of injected material is presumed to enter the lymphatic circulation, enabling it to reach regional lymph nodes, and some may enter the systemic circulation intact.

Contraindications

Hypersensitivity to glatiramer acetate or mannitol.

Warnings

➤*Administration:* Administer SC, not IV.

➤*Immediate postinjection reaction:* A constellation of side effects including flushing, chest pain, palpitations, anxiety, dyspnea, laryngeal constriction, and urticaria immediately after injection has been reported (approximately 10%). Symptoms were invariably transient and self-limited and did not require specific treatment. In general, these symptoms have their onset several months after the initiation of treatment, although they may occur earlier in the course of treatment, and a given patient may experience 1 or several episodes of these symptoms.

Whether these episodes are mediated by an immunologic or nonimmunologic mechanism, or whether several similar episodes seen in a given patient have identical mechanisms is unknown.

➤*Chest pain:* Approximately 21% of glatiramer patients (compared with 11% of placebo patients) experienced at least 1 episode of what was described as transient chest pain. While some of these episodes occurred in the context of the immediate postinjection reaction, many did not. The temporal relationship of the chest pain to an injection of glatiramer was not always known, although the pain was transient (usually lasting only a few minutes), often unassociated with other symptoms, and appeared to have no important clinical sequelae. Some patients experienced more than 1 such episode, and episodes usually began at least 1 month after the initiation of treatment. The pathogenesis of this symptom is unknown.

➤*Pregnancy: Category B.* There are no adequate and well-controlled studies in pregnant women. Use glatiramer acetate during pregnancy only if clearly needed.

➤*Lactation:* It is not known whether glatiramer is excreted in breast milk. Exercise caution when administering to a nursing woman.

➤*Children:* Safety and efficacy have not been established in individuals younger than 18 years of age.

Precautions

➤*Immunosuppression:* Because glatiramer can modify immune response, consider the possibility that it could interfere with useful immune function. For example, treatment with glatiramer might interfere with the recognition of foreign antigens in a way that would undermine the body's defenses against infections and tumor surveillance. There is no evidence that it does so, but there has not been systematic evaluation of this risk as yet.

Although glatiramer is intended to minimize the autoimmune response to myelin, there is the possibility that continued alteration of cellular immunity caused by chronic treatment with glatiramer might result in untoward effects.

➤*Immunogenicity:* Glatiramer acetate-reactive antibodies are formed in practically all patients exposed to daily treatment with the recommended dose. Studies in animals have suggested that immune complexes are deposited in the renal glomeruli. In studies of patients given 20 mg glatiramer acetate SC every day for 2 years, serum IgG levels reached at least 3 times baseline values in 80% of patients by 3 months of initiation of treatment. By 12 months of treatment, however, 30% of patients still had IgG levels at least 3 times baseline values, and 90% had levels above baseline. The antibodies are exclusively of the IgG subtype and predominantly of the IgG-1 subtype. No IgE type antibodies could be detected in any of the 94 sera tested; nevertheless, anaphylaxis can be associated with the administration of most any foreign substance, and therefore, this risk cannot be excluded.

Adverse Reactions

The most common adverse reactions associated with discontinuation were: injection site reaction (6.5%), depression, dizziness, dyspnea, tachycardia, tremor, unintended pregnancy, urticaria, and vasodilation.

Glatiramer Adverse Reactions (%)		
Adverse reaction	Glatiramer (N = 201)	Placebo (N = 206)
Cardiovascular		
Chest pain	21	11
Migraine	5	2
Palpitations	17	8
Syncope	5	2
Tachycardia	5	4
Vasodilation	27	10

Glatiramer Adverse Reactions (%)		
Adverse reaction	Glatiramer (N = 201)	Placebo (N = 206)
CNS		
Agitation	4	2
Anxiety	23	19
Confusion	2	0
Foot drop	3	2
Hypertonia	22	18
Nervousness	2	1
Nystagmus	2	1
Speech disorder	2	1
Tremor	7	3
Vertigo	6	5
Dermatologic		
Erythema	4	2
Herpes simplex	4	3
Pruritus	18	13
Rash	18	15
Skin nodule	2	0
Sweating	15	10
Urticaria	4	2
GI		
Anorexia	8	7
Diarrhea	12	11
Gastroenteritis	3	1
GI disorder	5	4
Nausea	22	17
Vomiting	6	4
GU		
Dysmenorrhea	6	5
Urinary urgency	10	8
Vaginal mono-liasis	8	4
Hematologic		
Ecchymosis	8	6
Lymphadeno-pathy	12	6
Injection Site		
Erythema	66	19
Hemorrhage	5	3
Induration	13	0
Inflammation	49	11
Mass	27	10
Pain	73	38
Pruritus	40	6
Urticaria	5	0
Welt	11	2
Metabolic/Nutritional		
Edema	3	0
Peripheral edema	7	4
Weight gain	3	0
Respiratory		
Bronchitis	9	6
Dyspnea	19	7
Laryngismus	5	3
Rhinitis	14	13
Special senses		
Ear pain	7	6
Eye disorder	4	0
Miscellaneous		
Arthralgia	24	19
Asthenia	41	38
Back pain	16	15
Bacterial infection	5	4
Chills	4	1
Face edema	6	1
Fever	8	7
Flu syndrome	19	17
Infection	50	48
Neck pain	8	4
Cyst	2	0
Pain	28	25

➤*Cardiovascular:* Hypertension (greater than or equal to 1%); atrial fibrillation, bradycardia, fourth heart sound, hypotension, midsystolic click, postural hypotension, systolic murmur, varicose veins (0.1% to 1%).

Immunosuppressives

GLATIRAMER ACETATE

➤*CNS:* Abnormal gait, abnormal thinking, amnesia, depression, dizziness, dysesthesia, emotional lability, euphoria, hypesthesia, incoordination, insomnia, Lhermitte sign, paresthesia, sleep disorder, somnolence, twitching (greater than or equal to 2%); abnormal dreams, emotional lability, stupor (greater than or equal to 1%); aphasia, ataxia, circumoral paresthesia, coma, concentration disorder, convulsion, decreased libido, depersonalization, facial paralysis, hallucinations, hostility, hypokinesia, mania reaction, memory impairment, myoclonus, paranoid reaction, paraplegia, psychotic depression, transient stupor (0.1% to 1%).

➤*Dermatologic:* Acne, alopecia, nail disorder (greater than or equal to 2%); eczema, herpes zoster, pustular rash, skin atrophy, warts (greater than or equal to 1%); angioedema, benign skin neoplasm, contact dermatitis, dermatitis, dry skin, erythema nodosum, furunculosis, fungal dermatitis, maculopapular rash, pigmentation, psoriasis, skin carcinoma, skin hypertrophy, skin striae, vesiculobullous rash (0.1% to 1%).

➤*Endocrine:* Goiter, hyperthyroidism, hypothyroidism (0.1% to 1%).

➤*GI:* Abdominal pain, constipation, dry mouth, dyspepsia, dysphagia, fecal incontinence, flatulence, gastritis, gingivitis, nausea and vomiting, periodontal abscess (greater than or equal to 2%); bowel urgency, oral moniliasis, salivary gland enlargement, tooth caries, ulcerative stomatitis (greater than or equal to 1%); burning sensation on tongue, carcinoma, cholecystitis, colitis, dry mouth, duodenal ulcer, esophageal ulcer, esophagitis, gum hemorrhage, hepatomegaly, increased appetite, melena, mouth ulceration, pancreas disorder, pancreatitis, rectal hemorrhage, stomatitis, tenesmus, tongue discoloration (0.1% to 1%).

➤*GU:* Breast pain, cystitis, dysuria, metrorrhagia, urinary frequency, urinary incontinence, urinary retention, UTI, vaginitis (greater than or equal to 2%); amenorrhea, hematuria, impotence, menorrhagia, suspicious papanicolaou smear, vaginal hemorrhage (greater than or equal to 1%); abnormal sexual function, abortion, breast engorgement, breast enlargement, carcinoma in situ cervix, fibrocystic breast, flank pain (kidney), kidney calculus, nocturia, ovarian cyst, priapism, pyelonephritis, urethritis, vaginitis (0.1% to 1%).

➤*Hematologic/Lymphatic:* Anemia, cyanosis, eosinophilia, hematemesis, leukopenia, lymphedema, pancytopenia, splenomegaly (0.1% to 1%).

➤*Metabolic/Nutritional:* Abnormal healing, alcohol intolerance, Cushing syndrome, gout, weight loss, xanthoma (0.1% to 1%).

➤*Musculoskeletal:* Myalgia, myasthenia (greater than or equal to 2%); arthritis, bone pain, bursitis, muscle atrophy, muscle disorder, myopathy, osteomyelitis, tendon pain, tenosynovitis (0.1% to 1%).

➤*Respiratory:* Increased cough, laryngitis, pharyngitis, sinusitis (greater than or equal to 2%); hay fever, hyperventilation (greater than or equal to 1%); asthma, epistaxis, hypoventilation, pneumonia, voice alteration (0.1% to 1%).

➤*Special senses:* Abnormal vision, amblyopia, conjunctivitis, deafness, diplopia, eye pain, taste perversion, tinnitus (greater than or

equal to 2%); visual field defect (greater than or equal to 1%); dry eyes, cataract, corneal ulcer, mydriasis, optic neuritis, otitis externa, photophobia, ptosis, taste loss (0.1% to 1%).

➤*Miscellaneous:* Accidental injury, allergic rhinitis, headache, injection site ecchymosis, neck rigidity, malaise (greater than or equal to 2%); abscess, injection site atrophy, injection site edema, injection site hypersensitivity (greater than or equal to 1%); cellulitis, generalized edema, hernia, injection site abscess, injection site fibrosis, injection site hematoma, injection site hypertrophy, injection site melanosis, lipoma, moon face, photosensitivity reaction, serum sickness, suicide attempt (0.1% to 1%).

➤*Postmarketing:*

Cardiovascular – Angina pectoris, arrhythmia, cardiomegaly, cardiomyopathy, CHF, coronary occlusion, deep thrombophlebitis, MI, pericardial effusion, peripheral vascular disease, thrombosis.

CNS – Abnormal dreams, aphasia, brain edema, CNS neoplasm, cerebrovascular accident, convulsion, meningitis, myelitis, neuralgia.

EENT – Blindness, glaucoma.

GI – Cholelithiasis, cirrhosis of the liver, eructation, hemorrhage, hepatitis, liver damage, liver function abnormality, stomach ulcer, tongue edema.

GU – Bladder carcinoma, breast carcinoma, kidney failure, nephrosis, ovarian carcinoma, urine abnormality, urogenital neoplasm.

Hematologic/Lymphatic – Acute leukemia, lymphoma-like reaction, thrombocytopenia.

Metabolic/Nutritional – Hypercholesterolemia.

Musculoskeletal – Generalized spasm, rheumatoid arthritis.

Respiratory – Carcinoma of lung, pleural effusion, pulmonary embolus.

Miscellaneous – Allergic reaction, anaphylactoid reaction, enlarged abdomen, hydrocephalus, LE syndrome, sepsis.

Patient Information

Advise patients to inform physician if they are pregnant, planning to become pregnant, or become pregnant, or if they are nursing while taking this medication.

Advise patients to not stop taking the drug without consulting the physician.

Provide appropriate instructions on self-injection and safe needle disposal procedures.

Instruct patient on injection sites (eg, arm, abdomen, hips, thighs) and the importance of rotating each injection site.

Counsel patient about possible injection site reaction (eg, hives, skin rash, irritation, severe pain, flushing, chest tightness or pain), and advise the patient to report them to their physician immediately if symptoms do not go away.

MUROMONAB-CD3

| *Rx* | **Orthoclone OKT3** (Ortho Biotech) | **Injection:** 5 mg per 5 ml | With 1 mg polysorbate 80. In 5 ml amps. |

WARNING

Only physicians experienced in immunosuppressive therapy and management of renal transplant patients should use muromonab-CD3.

Anaphylactic or anaphylactoid reactions may occur following administration of any dose or course of muromonab-CD3. Serious and occasionally life-threatening systemic, cardiovascular and CNS reactions have been reported. These have included: Pulmonary edema, especially in patients with volume overload; shock; cardiovascular collapse; cardiac or respiratory arrest; seizures; coma. Hence, a patient being treated with muromonab-CD3 must be managed in a facility equipped and staffed for cardiopulmonary resuscitation.

Indications

➤*Renal allograft rejection:* Treatment of acute allograft rejection in renal transplant patients.

➤*Cardiac/Hepatic allograft rejection:* Treatment of steroid-resistant acute allograft rejection in cardiac and hepatic transplant patients.

Administration and Dosage

➤*Approved by the FDA:* 1986.

Administer as an IV bolus in < 1 minute. Do not give by IV infusion or in conjunction with other drug solutions.

➤*Renal allograft rejection, acute:* 5 mg/day for 10 to 14 days. Begin treatment once acute renal rejection is diagnosed.

➤*Cardiac/hepatic allograft rejection, steroid resistant:* 5 mg/day for 10 to 14 days. Begin treatment when it is determined that a rejec-

tion has not been reversed by an adequate course of corticosteroid therapy.

➤*Monitor:* Monitor patients closely for the first few doses. Methylprednisolone sodium succinate 8 mg/kg IV given 1 to 4 hours prior to muromonab-CD3 administration is strongly recommended to decrease the incidence of reactions to the first dose. Acetaminophen and antihistamines, given concomitantly, may reduce early reactions. Patient temperature should not exceed 37.8°C (100°F) prior to first administration.

➤*Other immune-suppressive drugs:* Reduce the dose of concomitant immunosuppressive drugs during muromonab-CD3 administration to the lowest level compatible with an effective therapeutic response. Resume maintenance immunosuppression ≈ 3 days prior to cessation of muromonab-CD3.

➤*Preparation of solution:* Draw solution into a syringe through a low protein-binding 0.2 or 0.22 micrometer (μm) filter.

➤*Admixture incompatibility:* Do not add or infuse other drugs simultaneously through the same IV line. If the same IV line is used for sequential infusion of several different drugs, flush with saline before and after infusion of muromonab-CD3.

➤*Storage/Stability:* Refrigerate at 2° to 8°C (36° to 46°F). Do not freeze or shake. Because this drug is a protein solution, it may develop a few fine translucent particles which do not affect its potency. Since no bacteriostatic agent is present in this product, use the amp immediately once opened and discard the unused portion.

Actions

➤*Pharmacology:* Muromonab-CD3 is a murine monoclonal antibody to the T3 (CD3) antigen of human T-cells that functions as an immunosuppressant. Muromonab-CD3 is for IV use only. The antibody is a biochemically purified IgG$_{2a}$ immunoglobulin. It reverses graft rejection, probably by blocking the T-cell function, which plays a major role in acute allograft rejection. The drug reacts with, and blocks the function

MUROMONAB-CD3

of, a molecule (CD3) in the membrane of human T-cells that is associated with the antigen recognition structure of T-cells and is essential for signal transduction. Muromonab-CD3 blocks all known T-cell functions and reacts with most peripheral T-cells in blood and in body tissues. Following termination of therapy, T-cell function usually returns to normal within 1 week.

A rapid concomitant decrease in the number of circulating CD2, CD3, CD4 and CD8 positive T-cells was observed within minutes after administration. This decrease in the number of CD3 positive T-cells results from the specific interaction between muromonab-CD3 and the CD3 antigen on the surface of all T-lymphocytes. T-cell activation results in the release of numerous cytokines/lymphokines, which are thought to be responsible for many of the acute clinical manifestations seen following muromonab-CD3 therapy (see Warnings).

Between days 2 and 7, increasing numbers of circulating CD4 and CD8 positive cells have been observed, although CD3 positive cells are not detectable. CD3 positive cells reappear rapidly and reach pretreatment levels within a week after therapy termination. Increasing numbers of CD3 positive cells have been observed in patients prior to termination of therapy, possibly caused by the development of neutralizing antibodies.

Antibodies have occurred (incidence of 21% for IgM, 86% for IgG and 29% for IgE). Mean time of appearance of IgG antibodies was 20 days. Early IgG antibodies occur towards the end of the second week of treatment in 3% of patients.

➤*Pharmacokinetics:* Serum levels are measured with an enzyme-linked immunosorbent assay (ELISA). During treatment with 5 mg/day for 14 days, mean serum trough levels rose over the first 3 days and then averaged 0.9 mcg/mL on days 3 to 14. Circulating serum levels ≥ 0.8 mcg/mL block the function of cytotoxic T-cells in vitro and in vivo.

➤*Clinical trials:*

Acute renal allograft rejection – In a controlled randomized clinical trial, muromonab-CD3 was significantly more effective than conventional high-dose steroid therapy in reversing acute renal allograft rejection. Patients undergoing acute rejection of cadaveric renal transplants were treated either with muromonab-CD3 daily for a mean of 14 days, with concomitant lowering of the dosage of azathioprine and maintenance steroids (62 patients), or with conventional high-dose steroids (60 patients). Muromonab-CD3 reversed 94% of the rejections compared with a 75% reversal rate obtained with conventional high-dose steroid treatment. The 1-year Kaplan-Meier (actuarial) estimates of graft survival rates for these patients who had acute rejection were 62% and 45% for muromonab-CD3 and steroid-treated patients, respectively; at 2 years, the rates were 56% and 42%, respectively. One- and 2-year patient survivals were not significantly different between the two groups (85% and 75% for muromonab-CD3-treated patients and 90% and 85% for steroid-treated patients).

In additional open clinical trials, the observed rate of reversal of acute renal allograft rejection was 92% for muromonab-CD3 therapy. The drug was also effective in reversing acute renal allograft rejections in 65% of cases where steroids and lymphocyte immune globulin preparations were contraindicated or were not successful (rescue).

Acute cardiac or hepatic allograft rejection – The rate of reversal in acute cardiac allograft rejection and in hepatic allograft rejection in patients unresponsive to treatment with steroids was 90% and 83%, respectively.

Contraindications

Hypersensitivity to this or any product of murine origin; anti-mouse antibody titers ≥ 1:1000; patients in fluid overload or uncompensated heart failure, as evidenced by chest x-ray or > 3% weight gain within the week prior to treatment; history of seizures or predisposition to seizures; pregnancy, breastfeeding (see Warnings).

Warnings

➤*Cytokine release syndrome (CRS):* Temporally associated with the administration of the first few doses of muromonab-CD3 (particularly, the first two to three doses), most patients have developed an acute clinical syndrome (CRS) that has been attributed to the release of cytokines by activated lymphocytes or monocytes. This clinical syndrome has ranged from a more frequently reported mild, self-limited, "flu-like" illness to a less frequently reported severe, life-threatening shock-like reaction, which may include serious cardiovascular and CNS manifestations. The syndrome typically begins approximately 30 to 60 minutes after administration of a dose (but may occur later) and may persist for several hours. The frequency and severity of this symptom complex is usually greatest with the first dose. With each successive dose, both the frequency and severity of the CRS tend to diminish. Increasing the amount of a dose or resuming treatment after a hiatus may result in a reappearance of the CRS.

Common clinical manifestations – High fever (often spiking, up to 107°F); chills/rigors; headache; tremor; nausea/vomiting; diarrhea; abdominal pain; malaise; muscle/joint aches and pains; generalized weakness. Less frequently reported adverse experiences include minor dermatologic reactions (eg, rash, pruritus) and a spectrum of often seri-

ous, occasionally fatal, cardiorespiratory and neuro-psychiatric adverse experiences.

Cardiorespiratory – Cardiorespiratory findings may include the following: Dyspnea; shortness of breath; bronchospasm/wheezing; tachypnea; respiratory arrest/failure/distress; cardiovascular collapse; cardiac arrest; angina/MI; chest pain/tightness; tachycardia (including ventricular); hypertension; hemodynamic instability; hypotension, including profound shock; heart failure; pulmonary edema (cardiogenic and non-cardiogenic); adult respiratory distress syndrome; hypoxemia; apnea; arrhythmias.

Pulmonary edema – In the initial renal rejection studies, potentially fatal, severe pulmonary edema, the most serious postdose reaction, occurred in 4.7% of the initial 107 patients. Fluid overload was present before treatment in all of these cases. However, it occurred in none of the subsequent 311 patients treated with first-dose volume/weight restrictions. In subsequent trials and in postmarketing experience, severe pulmonary edema has occurred in patients who appeared to be euvolemic. The pathogenesis of pulmonary edema may involve all or some of the following: Volume overload; increased pulmonary vascular permeability; reduced left ventricular compliance/contractility.

Serum creatinine – During the first 1 to 3 days of therapy, some patients have experienced an acute and transient decline in the glomerular filtration rate and diminished urine output with a resulting increase in the level of serum creatinine. Massive release of cytokines appears to lead to reversible renal function impairment or delayed renal allograft function. Similarly, transient elevations in hepatic transaminases have been reported following administration of the first few doses.

Fluid status – Prior to administration, assess the patient's volume (fluid) status carefully. It is imperative, especially prior to the first few doses, that there be no clinical evidence of volume overload or uncompensated heart failure, including a clear chest X-ray and weight restriction of ≤ 3% above the patient's minimum weight during the week prior to injection.

Prevention / Minimization of CRS – Manifestations of the CRS may be prevented or minimized by pretreatment with 8 mg/kg methylprednisolone (ie, high-dose steroids), given 1 to 4 hours prior to administration of the first dose of muromonab-CD3 and by closely following recommendations for dosage and treatment duration. If any of the more serious presentations of the CRS occur, intensive treatment including oxygen, IV fluids, corticosteroids, pressor amines, antihistamines, and intubation may be required.

➤*Neuropsychiatric events:* Seizures, encephalopathy, cerebral edema, aseptic meningitis, and headaches have occurred during therapy with muromonab-CD3, even following the first dose, resulting in part from T-cell activation and subsequent systemic release of cytokines.

Seizures – Seizures, some accompanied by loss of consciousness or cardiorespiratory arrest, or death, have occurred independently or in conjunction with any of the neurologic syndromes described below. Patients predisposed to seizures may include those with the following conditions: Acute tubular necrosis/uremia; fever; infection; a precipitous fall in serum calcium; fluid overload; hypertension; hypoglycemia, history of seizures and electrolyte imbalances; those who are taking a medication concomitantly that may, by itself, cause seizures. The number and regularity of seizure reports indicate that this hazard appears not to be rare. Anticipate convulsions clinically with appropriate patient monitoring.

Encephalopathy – Manifestations may include the following: Impaired cognition; confusion; obtundation; altered mental status; auditory/visual hallucinations; psychosis (delirium, paranoia); mood changes (eg, mania, agitation, combativeness); diffuse hypotonus; hyperreflexia; myoclonus; tremor; asterixis; involuntary movements; major motor seizures; lethargy/stupor/coma; diffuse weakness. Approximately one-third of patients with a diagnosis of encephalopathy may have had coexisting aseptic meningitis syndrome.

Cerebral edema – Cerebral edema and other signs of increased vascular permeability (eg, otitis media, nasal and ear stuffiness) have been seen in patients treated with muromonab-CD3 and may accompany some of the other neurologic manifestations.

Aseptic meningitis syndrome – The incidence of this syndrome was 6%. Fever (89%), headache (44%), meningismus (ie, neck stiffness; 14%) and photophobia (10%) were the most commonly reported symptoms; a combination of these 4 symptoms occurred in 5% of patients. Diagnosis is confirmed by CSF analysis demonstrating leukocytosis with pleocytosis, elevated protein and normal or decreased glucose, with negative viral, bacterial, and fungal cultures. In any immunosuppressed transplant patient with clinical findings suggesting meningitis, evaluate the possibility of infection. Approximately one-third of the patients with a diagnosis of aseptic meningitis had coexisting signs and symptoms of encephalopathy. Most patients with the aseptic meningitis syndrome had a benign course and recovered without any permanent sequelae during therapy or subsequent to its completion or discontinuation.

MUROMONAB-CD3

Headache – Headache is frequently seen after any of the first few doses and may occur in any of the aforementioned neurologic syndromes or by itself.

The following additional neurologic events have been reported occasionally: Irreversible blindness; impaired vision; quadri- or paraparesis/plegia; cerebrovascular accident (hemiparesis/-plegia); aphasia; transient ischemic attack; subarachnoid hemorrhage; palsy of the VI cranial nerve; hearing loss.

Signs or symptoms of encephalopathy, meningitis, seizures, and cerebral edema, with or without headache, have typically been reversible. Headache, aseptic meningitis, seizures, and less severe forms of encephalopathy resolved in most patients despite continued treatment. However, some events have been irreversible.

CNS adverse experiences – Patients who may be at greater risk for CNS adverse experiences include the following: Known or suspected CNS disorders (eg, history of seizure disorder); cerebrovascular disease (small or large vessel); conditions having associated neurologic problems (eg, head trauma, uremia); underlying vascular diseases; concomitant medication that may, by itself, affect the CNS.

➤*Infections:* Muromonab-CD3 is usually added to immunosuppressive therapeutic regimens, thereby augmenting the degree of immunosuppression. This increase in the total burden of immunosuppression may alter the spectrum of infections observed and increase the risk, the severity and the potential gravity (morbidity) of infectious complications. Approximately 1 to 6 months posttransplant, patients are at risk for viral infections (eg, cytomegalovirus, Epstein-Barr virus, herpes simplex virus), which produce serious systemic disease and also increase the overall state of immunosuppression. Multiple or intensive courses of any anti-T cell antibody preparation, including muromonab-CD3, which produce profound impairment of cell-mediated immunity, further increase the risk of (opportunistic) infection, especially with the herpes viruses and fungi. Anti-infective prophylaxis may reduce the morbidity associated with certain potential pathogens and should be considered for high-risk patients.

➤*Hypersensitivity reactions:* Serious and occasionally fatal, immediate (usually within 10 minutes) hypersensitivity (anaphylactic) reactions have occurred. Manifestations of anaphylaxis may appear similar to manifestations of the CRS. It may be impossible to determine the mechanism responsible for any systemic reaction(s). Reactions attributed to hypersensitivity have been reported less frequently than those attributed to cytokine release. Acute hypersensitivity reactions may be characterized by the following: Cardiovascular collapse; cardiorespiratory arrest; loss of consciousness; hypotension/shock; tachycardia; tingling; angioedema (including laryngeal, pharyngeal or facial edema); airway obstruction; bronchospasm; dyspnea; urticaria; pruritus.

Serious allergic events, including anaphylactic or anaphylactoid reactions, have been reported in patients re-exposed to muromonab-CD3 subsequent to their initial course of therapy. Pretreatment with antihistamines or steroids may not reliably prevent anaphylaxis in this setting. Weigh the possible allergic hazards of retreatment against expected therapeutic benefits and alternatives. If retreatment is employed, have epinephrine and other emergency life-support equipment available, and monitor the patient closely.

If hypersensitivity is suspected, discontinue the drug immediately and do not resume therapy or re-expose the patient to muromonab-CD3. Serious acute hypersensitivity reactions may require emergency treatment with 0.3 to 0.5 mL aqueous epinephrine (1:1000 dilution) SC and other resuscitative measures. Refer to Management of Acute Hypersensitivity Reactions.

➤*Carcinogenesis:* As a result of depressed cell-mediated immunity, organ transplant patients have an increased risk of developing malignancies. This risk is evidenced almost exclusively by the occurrence of lymphoproliferative disorders (LPD), lymphomas and skin cancers. Following the initiation of muromonab-CD3 therapy, continuously monitor patients for evidence of LPD. Vigilant surveillance is advised, as early detection with subsequent reduction of total immunosuppression may result in regression of some of these lymphoproliferative disorders.

Because the potential for the development of LPD is related to the duration and extent (intensity) of total immunosuppression, it is advisable to adhere to the recommended dosage and duration of muromonab-CD3 and other anti-T lymphocyte antibody preparations administered within a short period of time. If appropriate, reduce the dosage(s) of immunosuppressive drugs used concomitantly to the lowest level compatible with an effective therapeutic response.

➤*Pregnancy:* Category C. It is not known whether muromonab-CD3 can cause fetal harm when administered to a pregnant woman or can affect reproduction capacity. However, it is an IgG antibody and may cross the placenta. If this drug is used during pregnancy, or the patient becomes pregnant while taking this drug, apprise the patient of the potential hazard to the fetus.

➤*Lactation:* It is not known whether muromonab-CD3 is excreted in breast milk. Because of the potential for serious adverse reactions/oncogenesis, decide whether to discontinue nursing or to discontinue the drug, taking into account the importance of the drug to the mother.

➤*Children:* Safety and efficacy in children have not been established. Muromonab-CD3 has been used in infants/children, beginning with a dose of ≤ 5 mg. Based on immunologic monitoring, the dosage has been adjusted accordingly. Pediatric recipients may be significantly immunosuppressed for a prolonged period of time and therefore require close monitoring posttherapy for opportunistic infection, particularly varicella (VZV), which poses an infectious complication unique to this population. GI fluid loss secondary to diarrhea or vomiting resulting from the CRS may be significant when treating small children and may require parenteral hydration. It is unknown whether there may be significant long-term sequelae (eg, neurodevelopmental language difficulties in infants < 1 year of age) related to the occurrence of seizures, high fever, CNS infections, or aseptic meningitis following muromonab-CD3 treatment. In cases where administration would be deemed medically appropriate, more vigilant and frequent monitoring is required for children than in adults.

Precautions

➤*Monitoring:* Monitor the following tests prior to and during therapy:

Renal – BUN, serum creatinine;

Hepatic – Transaminases, alkaline phosphatase, bilirubin;

Hematopoietic – WBCs and differential, platelet count;

Chest X-ray – Within 24 hours before initiating treatment, which should be free of any evidence of heart failure or fluid overload.

Monitor one of the following immunologic tests during therapy:

Plasma levels determined by an ELISA (target levels should be ≥ 800 ng/mL); or

Quantitative T-lymphocyte surface phenotyping (CD3, CD4, CD8); target CD3 positive T-cells < 25 cells/mm[3].

Testing for human-mouse antibody titers is strongly recommended; a titer ≥ 1:1000 is a contraindication for use.

➤*Intravascular thrombosis:* As with other immunosuppressive therapies, arterial, or venous thrombosis of allografts and other vascular beds (eg, heart, lungs, brain, bowel) have been reported. Consider these findings when deciding to use muromonab-CD3 in patients with a history of thrombotic events or underlying vascular disease. Consider concomitant use of prophylactic anti-thrombotic interventions (eg, minidose heparin).

➤*Special risk:* Patients at risk for more serious complications of the CRS may include those with the following conditions: Unstable angina; recent MI or symptomatic ischemic heart disease; heart failure of any etiology; pulmonary edema of any etiology; any form of chronic obstructive pulmonary disease; intravascular volume overload or depletion of any etiology (eg, excessive dialysis, recent intensive diuresis, blood loss); cerebrovascular disease; patients with advanced symptomatic vascular disease or neuropathy; history of seizures; septic shock. Make efforts to correct or stabilize background conditions prior to the initiation of therapy.

Drug Interactions

➤*Indomethacin:* Encephalopathy and other CNS effects have occurred with concurrent use.

Adverse Reactions

Cytokine release syndrome – See Warnings. In trials, the majority of patients experienced pyrexia (90%), of which 19% were ≥ 40°C (104°F), and chills (59%). Other adverse experiences occurring in ≥ 8% during the first 2 days included the following: Dyspnea (21%); nausea, vomiting (19%); chest pain, diarrhea (14%); tremor, wheezing (13%); headache (11%); tachycardia (10%); rigor, hypertension (8%).

Infections – See Warnings.
Renal rejection trial: The most common infections during the first 45 days of therapy were due to herpes simplex (27%) and cytomegalovirus (CMV; 19%). Other severe and life-threatening infections were *Staphylococcus epidermidis* (4.8%), *Pneumocystis carinii* (3.1%), *Legionella, Cryptococcus, Serratia,* and gram-negative bacteria (1.6%).
Hepatic rejection trial: The most common infections during the first 45 days of treatment were CMV (15.7%), fungal infections (14.9%) and herpes simplex (7.5%). Other severe and life-threatening infections were gram-positive (9%), gram-negative (7.5%), viral (1.5%), *Legionella* (0.7%). In another hepatic rejection trial, incidence of fungal infections was 34% and of herpes simplex virus infections was 31%.
Cardiac rejection trial: The most common infections reported during the first 45 days of treatment were herpes simplex (5%), fungal (4%), and CMV (3%).

Neoplasia – See Warnings.

Neuropsychiatric – See Warnings.

➤*Hypersensitivity:* See Warnings.

➤*Other:*

Cardiovascular – Cardiac arrest; hypotension/shock; heart failure; cardiovascular collapse; angina/MI; tachycardia; bradycardia; hemodynamic instability; hypertension; left ventricular dysfunction; arrhythmias; chest pain/tightness.

MUROMONAB-CD3

Dermatologic – Rash; Stevens-Johnson syndrome; urticaria; pruritus; erythema; flushing; diaphoresis.

GI – Diarrhea; nausea/vomiting; abdominal pain; bowel infarction; GI hemorrhage.

Hepatic – Increases in transaminases (eg, AST, ALT); hepato/splenomegaly or hepatitis, usually secondary to viral infection or lymphoma.

Musculoskeletal – Arthralgia; arthritis; myalgia; stiffness/aches/pains.

Renal – Anuria/oliguria; delayed graft function; transient and reversible increases in BUN and serum creatinine; abnormal urinary cytology, including exfoliation of damaged lymphocytes, collecting duct cells and cellular casts.

Respiratory – Respiratory arrest; adult respiratory distress syndrome (ARDS); respiratory failure; pulmonary edema (cardiogenic or noncardiogenic); apnea; dyspnea; bronchospasm; wheezing; shortness of breath; hypoxemia; tachypnea/hyperventilation; abnormal chest sounds; pneumonia/pneumonitis.

Special senses – Blindness; blurred vision; diplopia; hearing loss; otitis media; tinnitus; vertigo; VI cranial nerve palsy; photophobia; conjunctivitis; nasal/ear stuffiness.

Miscellaneous – Pancytopenia; aplastic anemia; neutropenia; leukopenia; thrombocytopenia; lymphopenia; leukocytosis; lymphadenopathy; arterial and venous thrombosis of allografts and other vascular beds (eg, heart, lung, brain, bowel); disturbances of coagulation; fever (including spiking temperatures as high as 107°F); chills/rigors; flu-like syndrome; fatigue/malaise; generalized weakness; anorexia.

Overdosage

Symptoms of overdose may include hyperthermia, severe chills, myalgia, vomiting, diarrhea, edema, oliguria, pulmonary edema, and acute renal failure. A high incidence (5%) of microangiopathic hemolytic anemia/HUS syndrome in patients receiving 10 mg/day was also reported. In the event of acute overdosage, carefully observe the patient and give symptomatic and supportive treatment.

Patient Information

Advise patients of the signs and symptoms associated with the cytokine release syndrome, including the potentially serious nature of this symptom complex (eg, systemic, cardiovascular, neuro-psychiatric events).

Advise patients to seek medical attention at the first sign of skin rash, urticaria, rapid heartbeat, difficulty in swallowing and breathing, or any swelling that may suggest angioedema or other allergic reaction.

Patients should know how they might react before operating an automobile or machinery, or engaging in activities requiring mental alertness, coordination, or physical dexterity.

MYCOPHENOLATE MOFETIL

Rx	**CellCept** (Roche)	**Capsules:** 250 mg	(CellCept 250 Roche). Blue/brown. In 100s, 500s, and packages containing 12 bottles of 120s.
		Tablets: 500 mg	Alcohols. (CellCept 500 Roche). Lavender. Caplet-shaped. Film coated. In 100s and 500s.
Rx	**Myfortic** (Novartis)	**Tablets, extended-release:** 180 mg	Lactose. (C). Lime green. Film-coated. In 120s.
		360 mg	Lactose. (CT). Pale orange-red. Film-coated. In 120s.
Rx	**CellCept** (Roche)	**Powder for oral suspension:** 200 mg/mL (constituted)	Aspartame,[1] methylparaben, sorbitol. Mixed fruit flavor. In 225 mL.
		Powder for injection, lyophilized: 500 mg (as HCl)	Preservative free. In 20 mL vials.

[1] 0.56 mg/mL phenylalanine.

WARNING

Increased susceptibility to infection and the possible development of lymphoma may result from immunosuppression. Only physicians experienced in immunosuppressive therapy and management of renal, hepatic, or cardiac transplant patients should use mycophenolate. Manage patients receiving the drug in facilities equipped and staffed with adequate laboratory and supportive medical resources. The physician responsible for maintenance therapy should have complete information requisite for the follow-up of the patient.

Indications

➤*Allogeneic transplants:* For the prophylaxis of organ rejection in patients receiving allogeneic renal, hepatic, or cardiac transplants. Use mycophenolate concomitantly with cyclosporine and corticosteroids.

➤*Unlabeled uses:* Refractory uveitis (2 g/day alone or in combination with previous corticosteroid, cyclosporine, or tacrolimus therapy); second-line therapy for Churg-Strauss syndrome; in combination with prednisolone for the treatment of diffuse proliferative lupus nephritis.

Administration and Dosage

➤*Approved by the FDA:* May 9, 1995.

➤*Renal transplantation:* 1 g twice daily administered orally or IV (over 2 hrs) (daily dose of 2 g). Although a dose of 1.5 g twice daily was used in clinical trials and was shown to be safe and effective, no efficacy advantage could be established for renal transplant patients. Patients receiving 2 g/day demonstrate an overall better safety profile than patients receiving 3 g/day.

➤*Tablets, ER:*

Adults – 720 mg administered twice daily (1440 mg total daily dose) on an empty stomach, 1 hour before or 2 hours after food intake.

The mycophenolate mofetil ER tablets and mycophenolate mofetil tablets and capsules should not be used interchangeably without physician supervision because the rate of absorption following the administration of these two products is not equivalent.

Patients are to be instructed that mycophenolate mofetil ER tablets should not be crushed, chewed, or cut prior to ingesting. The ER tablets should be swallowed whole in order to maintain the integrity of the enteric coating.

Children – The recommended dose of mycophenolate mofetil ER in stable pediatric patients is 400 mg/m² body surface area (BSA) administered twice daily (up to a maximum dose of 720 mg administered twice daily). Patients with a BSA of 1.19 to 1.58 m² may be dosed either with three 180 mg ER tablets or one 180 mg ER tablet plus one 360 mg ER tablet twice daily (1080 mg daily dose). Patients with a BSA of more than 1.58 m² may be dosed either with four 180 mg ER tablets or two 360 mg ER tablets twice daily (1440 mg daily dose). Pediatric doses for patients with BSA more than 1.19 m² cannot be accurately administered using currently available formulations of ER tablets.

Elderly – The maximum recommended dose is 720 mg administered twice daily.

➤*Cardiac transplantation:* 1.5 g twice daily administered orally or IV (over ≥ 2 hours) (daily dose of 3 g) is recommended.

➤*Hepatic transplantation:* 1 g twice daily administered IV (over ≥ 2 hours) or 1.5 g twice daily orally (daily dose of 3 g) is recommended.

➤*Capsules, oral suspension, and tablets:* Give the initial oral dose as soon as possible following transplantation. Food has been shown to decrease mycophenolic acid (MPA) C_{max} by 40%. It is recommended that mycophenolate be administered on an empty stomach. However, in stable renal transplant patients, it may be administered with food if necessary.

If required, the oral suspension can be administered via a nasogastric tube with a minimum size of 8 French (minimum 1.7 mm interior diameter).

➤*IV administration:* Do not administer IV solution by rapid or bolus IV injection. Mycophenolate IV is recommended for patients unable to take capsules, oral suspension, or tablets. Administer ≤ 24 hours follow-

ing transplantation and for ≤ 14 days; switch patients to oral mycophenolate as soon as they can tolerate oral medication.

Following reconstitution, administer by slow IV infusion over a period of ≥ 2 hours by either peripheral or central vein.

➤*Preparation of oral suspension:* Tap the closed bottle several times to loosen the powder. Measure 94 mL of water in a graduated cylinder. Add ≈ ½ the total amount of water for constitution to the bottle and shake the closed bottle well for ≈ 1 minute. Add the remainder of water and shake the closed bottle well for ≈ 1 minute. Remove the child-resistant cap and push bottle adapter into neck of bottle. Close bottle with child-resistant cap tightly. This will assure the proper seating of the bottle adapter in the bottle and child-resistant status of the cap.

➤*Preparation of infusion solution (6 mg/mL):* Exercise caution in the handling and preparation of solutions of mycophenolate IV. Mycophenolate IV must be reconstituted and diluted to a concentration of 6 mg/mL using 5% Dextrose Injection. Mycophenolate IV is incompatible with other IV infusion solutions.

Mycophenolate IV does not contain an antibacterial preservative. If the infusion solution is not prepared immediately prior to administration, the commencement of administration of the infusion solution should be within 4 hours of reconstitution and dilution. Reconstitution and dilution of the product must be performed under aseptic conditions.

Reconstitute the contents of each vial with 14 mL of 5% Dextrose Injection. Gently shake the vial to dissolve the drug. The resulting solution is slightly yellow. Discard the vial if particulate matter or discoloration is observed.

For a 1 g dose, further dilute the contents of 2 reconstituted vials into 140 mL of 5% Dextrose Injection. For a 1.5 g dose, further dilute the contents of 3 reconstituted vials into 210 mL of 5% Dextrose Injection. The final concentration of both solutions is 6 mg/mL. Discard the infusion solution if particulate matter or discoloration is observed.

➤*Renal function impairment:* In renal transplant patients with severe chronic renal impairment (GFR < 25 mL/min/1.73 m²) outside of the immediate posttransplant period, avoid doses > 1 g administered twice daily; carefully observe these patients. No dose adjustments are needed in patients experiencing delayed graft function postoperatively. No data are available for cardiac or hepatic transplant patients with severe chronic renal impairment.

➤*Neutropenia:* If neutropenia develops (ANC < 1.3×10^3/mcL), interrupt dosing or reduce the dose, perform appropriate diagnostic tests, and appropriately manage the patient (see Warnings and Precautions).

➤*Handling/Disposal:* Because mycophenolate has demonstrated teratogenic effects in rats and rabbits, do not crush tablets, and do not open or crush the capsules. Avoid inhalation or direct contact with skin or mucous membranes of the powder contained in mycophenolate capsules, oral suspension, and injection (before or after constitution). If such contact occurs, wash thoroughly with soap and water; rinse eyes with plain water. Should a spill occur, wipe up using paper towels wetted with water to remove spilled powder or suspension.

➤*Admixture incompatibility:* Do not mix or administer mycophenolate IV concurrently via the same infusion catheter with other IV drugs or infusion admixtures.

➤*Storage/Stability:* Store at 25°C (77°F). Storage in a refrigerator at 2° to 8°C (36° to 46°F) is acceptable. Do not freeze. Discard any unused portion 60 days after constitution.

Extemporaneous oral liquid – A 100 mg/mL oral suspension prepared with the contents of mycophenolate mofetil capsules and a cherry-flavored vehicle was stable for 121 days when stored at 23° to 25°C (73° to 77°F) and 2° to 8°C (36° to 46°F) in amber PETG bottles.

Actions

➤*Pharmacology:* Mycophenolate mofetil (MMF) prolongs the survival of allogeneic transplants in animals (eg, kidney, heart, liver, intestine, limb, small bowel, pancreatic islets, and bone marrow). It also reverses ongoing acute rejection in the canine renal and rat cardiac allograft models, and inhibits proliferative arteriopathy in experimental models of aortic and heart allografts in rats, as well as in primate cardiac xenografts. Mycophenolate was used alone or with other immunosuppressive agents in these studies. The drug inhibits immunologically mediated inflammatory responses in animal models, inhibits

MYCOPHENOLATE MOFETIL

tumor development, and prolongs survival in murine tumor transplant models.

Mycophenolate is hydrolyzed to form MPA, a potent, selective, uncompetitive, and reversible inhibitor of inosine monophosphate dehydrogenase (IMPDH), which inhibits the de novo pathway of guanosine nucleotide synthesis without incorporation into DNA. Because T- and B-lymphocytes are critically dependent for their proliferation on de novo synthesis of purines whereas other cell types can use salvage pathways, MPA has potent cytostatic effects on lymphocytes. MPA inhibits proliferative responses of T- and B-lymphocytes to mitogenic and allospecific stimulation. Addition of guanosine or deoxyguanosine reverses the cytostatic effects of MPA on lymphocytes. MPA also suppresses antibody formation by B-lymphocytes. MPA prevents the glycosylation of lymphocyte and monocyte glycoproteins that are involved in intercellular adhesion to endothelial cells and may inhibit recruitment of leukocytes into sites of inflammation and graft rejection.

➤*Pharmacokinetics:*

Absorption/Distribution – Following oral and IV administration, mycophenolate undergoes rapid and complete metabolism to MPA, the active metabolite. Metabolism to MPA occurs presystemically after oral dosing. MPA is further metabolized to form the phenolic glucuronide of MPA (MPAG), which is not pharmacologically active. The parent drug, MMF, can be measured systemically during the IV infusion; however, shortly ($\approx$ 5 minutes) after the infusion is stopped or after oral administration, MMF concentration is below the limit of quantitation (0.4 mcg/mL). MPA C_{max} was decreased by 40% in the presence of food (see Drug Interactions). In 12 healthy volunteers, the mean absolute bioavailability of oral mycophenolate relative to IV mycophenolate (based on MPA AUC) was 94%. The AUC for MPA appears to increase in a dose-proportional fashion in renal transplant patients receiving multiple doses of mycophenolate up to a daily dose of 3 g.

In the early posttransplant period (< 40 days posttransplant), renal, cardiac, and hepatic transplant patients had mean MPA AUCs $\approx$ 20% to 41% lower and mean C_{max} $\approx$ 32% to 44% lower compared with the late transplant period (3 to 6 months posttransplant).

The mean apparent volume of distribution of MPA in 12 healthy volunteers is $\approx$ 3.6 and 4 L/kg following IV and oral administration, respectively. MPA, at clinically relevant concentrations, is 97% bound to plasma albumin. MPAG is 82% bound to plasma albumin at MPAG concentration ranges normally seen in stable renal transplant patients; however, at higher MPAG concentrations (observed in patients with renal impairment or delayed graft function), the binding of MPA may be reduced as a result of competition between MPAG and MPA for protein binding.

Metabolism – In addition to MPA, the following metabolites of the 2-hydroxyethyl-morpholine moiety are also recovered in urine following oral administration in healthy subjects: N-(2-carboxymethyl)-morpholine, N-(2-hydroxyethyl)-morpholine, and the N-oxide of N-(2-hydroxyethyl)-morpholine. Secondary peaks in plasma MPA concentration-time profile are usually observed 6 to 12 hours postdose. It appears that enterohepatic recirculation contributes to MPA plasma levels.

Excretion – Negligible amount of drug is excreted as MPA (< 1% of dose) in the urine. Oral administration resulted in complete recovery of the administered dose; 93% was recovered in the urine and 6% was recovered in feces. Most ($\approx$ 87%) of the administered dose is excreted in the urine as MPAG. MPA and MPAG are usually not removed by hemodialysis. However, at high MPAG plasma concentrations (> 100 mcg/mL), small amounts of MPAG are removed.

Mean apparent half-life and plasma clearance of MPA are $\approx$ 17.9 hours and $\approx$ 193 mL/min following oral administration and $\approx$ 16.6 hours and $\approx$ 177 mL/min following IV administration, respectively.

Mean Pharmacokinetic Parameters for MPA Following Mycophenolate Administration				
Parameter	Dose/ Route	T_{max} (hr)	C_{max} (mcg/mL)	AUC (mcg•hr/mL)
Healthy volunteers (n = 129) (single dose)	1 g/oral	$\approx$ 0.8	$\approx$ 24.5	$\approx$ 63.9 (n = 117)
Renal transplant patients				
Time after renal transplantation				
5 days (n = 31)	1 g bid/IV	$\approx$ 1.58	$\approx$ 12	$\approx$ 40.8[1]
6 days (n = 31)	1 g bid/oral	$\approx$ 1.33	$\approx$ 10.7	$\approx$ 32.9[1]
Early (< 40 days; n = 25)	1 g bid/oral	$\approx$ 1.31	$\approx$ 8.16	$\approx$ 27.3[1]
Early (< 40 days; n = 27)	1.5 g bid/oral	$\approx$ 1.21	$\approx$ 13.5	$\approx$ 38.4[1]
Late (> 3 months; n = 23)	1.5 g bid/oral	$\approx$ 0.9	$\approx$ 24.1	$\approx$ 65.3[1]
Cardiac transplant patients				
Time after cardiac transplantation				
Early (day before discharge)	1.5 g bid/oral	$\approx$ 1.8 (n = 11)	$\approx$ 11.5 (n = 11)	$\approx$ 43.3 (n = 9)[1]
Late (> 6 months)	1.5 g bid/oral	$\approx$ 1.1 (n = 52)	$\approx$ 20 (n = 52)	$\approx$ 54.1 (n = 49)[2]
Hepatic transplant patients				
Time after hepatic transplantation				
4 to 9 days (n = 22)	1 g bid/IV	$\approx$ 1.5	$\approx$ 17	$\approx$ 34[1]
Early (5 to 8 days) (n = 20)	1.5 g bid/oral	$\approx$ 1.15	$\approx$ 13.1	$\approx$ 29.2[1]
Late (> 6 months) (n = 6)	1.5 g bid/oral	$\approx$ 1.54	$\approx$ 19.3	$\approx$ 49.3[1]

Mean Pharmacokinetic Parameters for MPA Following Mycophenolate Administration				
Parameter	Dose/ Route	T_{max} (hr)	C_{max} (mcg/mL)	AUC (mcg•hr/mL)
Renal impairment (single dose) (GFR, mL/min/1.73 m^2)				
Healthy volunteers (GFR > 80; n = 6)	1 g/oral	$\approx$ 0.75	$\approx$ 25.3	$\approx$ 45[3]
Mild renal impairment (GFR 50 to 80; n = 6)	1 g/oral	$\approx$ 0.75	$\approx$ 26	$\approx$ 59.9[3]
Moderate renal impairment (GFR 25 to 49; n = 6)	1 g/oral	$\approx$ 0.75	$\approx$ 19	$\approx$ 52.9[3]
Severe renal impairment (GFR < 25; n = 7)	1 g/oral	$\approx$ 1	$\approx$ 16.3	$\approx$ 78.6[3]
Hepatic impairment (single dose)				
Healthy volunteers (n = 6)	1 g/oral	$\approx$ 0.63	$\approx$ 24.3	$\approx$ 29[4]
Alcoholic cirrhosis (n = 18)	1 g/oral	$\approx$ 0.85	$\approx$ 22.4	$\approx$ 29.8[4]

[1] Interdosing interval AUC_{0-12}.
[2] AUC_{0-12} values quoted are extrapolated from data from samples collected over 4 hours.
[3] Interdosing interval AUC_{0-96}.
[4] Interdosing interval AUC_{0-48}.

Renal insufficiency – In a single-dose study, plasma MPA AUCs observed in volunteers with severe chronic renal impairment (GFR < 25 mL/min/1.73 m^2) were $\approx$ 75% higher relative to those observed in healthy volunteers (GFR > 80). In addition, the single-dose plasma MPAG AUC was 3- to 6-fold higher in volunteers with severe renal impairment than in volunteers with mild renal impairment or healthy volunteers, consistent with the known renal elimination of MPAG.

In patients with delayed graft function posttransplant, mean MPA AUC_{0-12} was comparable to that seen in posttransplant patients without delayed graft function. Mean plasma MPAG AUC_{0-12} was 2- to 3-fold higher than in posttransplant patients without delayed graft function.

Hemodialysis usually does not remove MPA or MPAG. At high concentrations of MPAG (> 100 mcg/mL), hemodialysis removes only small amounts of MPAG.

Pediatrics –

Mean Pharmacokinetic Parameters for MPA Following Multiple Oral Doses of Mycophenolate in Pediatric Renal Transplant Patients 21 Days Posttransplant				
Age range	Dose	T_{max} (hr)	C_{max} (mcg/mL)	AUC_{0-12} (mcg•hr/mL)
$\geq$ 3 mo to < 6 yr (n = 4)	15 mg/kg bid	$\approx$ 1.25	$\approx$ 3.7	$\approx$ 13.6
$\geq$ 6 yr to < 12 yr (n = 4)	15 mg/kg bid	$\approx$ 0.5	$\approx$ 13.5	$\approx$ 23.4
$\geq$ 6 yr to < 12 yr (n = 5)	23 mg/kg bid	$\approx$ 1.46	$\approx$ 17	$\approx$ 40.1
$\geq$ 12 yr to 18 yr (n = 5)	15 mg/kg bid	$\approx$ 0.5	$\approx$ 13.2	$\approx$ 30
$\geq$ 12 yr to 18 yr (n = 5)	23 mg/kg bid	$\approx$ 1.32	$\approx$ 11.5	$\approx$ 31.1

➤*Clinical trials:* The safety and efficacy of mycophenolate in combination with corticosteroids and cyclosporine for the prevention of organ rejection were assessed in randomized, double-blind, multicenter trials in renal (3 trials), in cardiac (1 trial), and in hepatic (1 trial) transplant patients. Treatment failure was measured within the first 6 months. The following table summarizes the results of these studies.

Incidence of Organ Rejection and Patient Survival from Mycophenolate Studies for the Prevention of Organ Rejection (%)[1]				
	Mycophenolate		Azathioprine	Placebo
	2 g/day	3 g/day		
Renal transplants				
Transplant treatment failure[2]	30.3 to 38.2	31.3 to 38.8	47.6 to 50	56
Biopsy-proven rejection	17 to 19.8	13.8 to 17.5	35.5 to 38	46.4
Graft loss and patient death	8.5 to 11.7	10 to 11.5	11.5 to 13.6[3]	11.5 to 13.6[3]
Cardiac transplants				
Biopsy-proven rejection[4]	nd	32	35	nd
Retransplantation or patient death	nd	6.2	11.4	nd
	Mycophenolate[5]		Azathioprine[6]	
Hepatic transplants				
Biopsy-proven rejection[7]	38.5		47.7	
Retransplantation or patient death	14.7		14.6	

[1] Data pooled from several studies; not intended to be comparative.
[2] All treatment failures; biopsy-proven rejection or early termination for any reason.
[3] Cumulative incidence that includes those patients who received azathioprine and those who received placebo.
[4] With hemodynamic compromise.
[5] Patients received mycophenolate 1.5 g twice daily IV for up to 14 days followed by 1.5 g twice daily orally.
[6] Patients received azathioprine 1 to 2 mg/kg/day IV followed by 1 to 2 mg/kg/day orally.
[7] Rejection at 6 months (including death or retransplantation).
* nd = No data available.

MYCOPHENOLATE MOFETIL

Contraindications

Hypersensitivity to the drug, mycophenolic acid, or any component of the drug product; sensitivity to polysorbate 80 (Tween) (IV only).

Warnings

➤*Lymphomas/Malignancies:* Patients receiving immunosuppressive regimens involving combinations of drugs, including mycophenolate, as part of an immunosuppressive regimen are at increased risk of developing lymphomas and other malignancies, particularly of the skin. Lymphoproliferative disease or lymphoma developed in 0.4% to 1% of patients receiving mycophenolate (2 or 3 g) with other immunosuppressive agents in controlled clinical trials of renal, hepatic, and cardiac transplant patients. The risk appears to be related to the intensity and duration of immunosuppression rather than to the use of any specific agent. Oversuppression of the immune system can also increase susceptibility to infection, including opportunistic infections, fatal infections, and sepsis.

Instruct patients with increased risk for skin cancer to limit exposure to sunlight and UV light by wearing protective clothing and using a strong sunscreen.

➤*Neutropenia:* Up to 2% of renal transplant patients, up to 3.6% of hepatic transplant patients, and up to 2.8% of cardiac transplant patients receiving mycophenolate 3 g daily developed severe neutropenia (absolute neutrophil count [ANC] < 0.5 x 10^3/mcL). Monitor patients receiving mycophenolate for neutropenia (see Monitoring in Precautions). The development of neutropenia may be related to mycophenolate itself, concomitant medications, viral infections, or some combination of these causes. If neutropenia develops (ANC < 1.3 x 10^3/mcL), interrupt dosing or reduce the dose, perform appropriate diagnostic tests, and manage the patient appropriately (see Administration and Dosage). Neutropenia has been observed most frequently in the period from 31 to 180 days posttransplant in patients treated for prevention of renal, hepatic, and cardiac rejection.

➤*Renal function impairment:* Renal transplant subjects with severe chronic renal impairment (GFR < 25 mL/min/1.73 m²) who have received single doses of mycophenolate showed higher plasma MPA and MPAG AUCs relative to subjects with lesser degrees of renal impairment or to healthy volunteers (see Pharmacokinetics). Avoid mycophenolate doses > 1 g twice a day and carefully observe patients.

No data are available for cardiac or hepatic transplant patients with severe chronic renal impairment. Mycophenolate may be used for cardiac or hepatic transplant patients with severe chronic renal impairment if the potential benefits outweigh the potential risks.

➤*Mutagenesis:* The genotoxic potential of mycophenolate was determined in 5 assays. Mycophenolate was genotoxic in the mouse lymphoma/thymidine kinase assay and the in vivo mouse micronucleus assay. Mycophenolate was not genotoxic in the bacterial mutation assay, the yeast mitotic gene conversion, or the Chinese hamster ovary cell chromosomal aberration assay.

➤*Elderly:* Elderly patients, particularly those who are receiving mycophenolate as part of a combination immunosuppressive regimen, may be at increased risk of certain infections (including CMV tissue invasive disease) and possibly GI hemorrhage and pulmonary edema, compared with younger individuals.

➤*Pregnancy:* Category C. In teratology studies in rats and rabbits, fetal resorptions and malformations occurred in rats at 6 mg/kg/day and in rabbits at 90 mg/kg/day, in the absence of maternal toxicity. These levels are equivalent to 0.03 to 0.92 times the recommended clinical dose in renal transplant patients and 0.02 to 0.61 times the recommended clinical dose in cardiac transplant patients on a body surface area (BSA) basis. In a female fertility and reproduction study in rats, oral doses of 4.5 mg/kg/day (0.01 to 0.02 times the recommended clinical dose when corrected for BSA) caused malformations (principally of head and eyes) in first-generation offspring in the absence of maternal toxicity. Adverse effects on fetal development (including malformations) occurred when pregnant rats and rabbits were dosed during organogenesis. Responses occurred at doses lower than those associated with maternal toxicity, and at doses below the recommended clinical dose for renal or cardiac transplantation.

There are no adequate and well-controlled studies in pregnant women. Do not use in pregnant women unless the potential benefit justifies the potential risk to the fetus. Women of childbearing potential should have a negative serum or urine pregnancy test with a sensitivity of ≥ 50 mIU/mL ≤ 1 week prior to beginning therapy. Do not initiate mycophenolate therapy until a negative pregnancy test report is obtained.

Effective contraception must be used before beginning mycophenolate therapy, during therapy, and for 6 weeks following discontinuation of therapy, even when there has been a history of infertility, unless because of a hysterectomy. Two reliable forms of contraception must be used simultaneously unless abstinence is the chosen method. If pregnancy does occur during treatment, the physician and patient should discuss the desirability of continuing the pregnancy.

➤*Lactation:* Studies in rats treated with mycophenolate have shown mycophenolic acid to be excreted in milk. It is not known whether this drug is excreted in human breast milk. Because of the potential for serious adverse reactions in nursing infants from mycophenolate, decide whether to discontinue nursing or to discontinue the drug, taking into account the importance of the drug to the mother.

➤*Children:* Safety and efficacy have not been established.

Precautions

➤*Monitoring:* Perform CBCs weekly during the first month of treatment, twice monthly for the second and third months, then monthly through the first year.

➤*GI bleeding:* GI tract bleeding has been observed in ≈ 3% of renal transplants, 5.4% of hepatic transplants, and 1.7% of cardiac transplants treated with mycophenolate 3 g daily. GI perforations have rarely been observed. Most patients receiving mycophenolate also were receiving other drugs known to be associated with these complications. Because mycophenolate has been associated with an increased incidence of GI adverse events, including infrequent cases of GI tract ulceration, hemorrhage, and perforation, administer with caution in patients with active serious GI disease.

➤*Delayed renal graft function posttransplant:* In patients with delayed graft function posttransplant, mean MPA AUC was comparable, but MPAG AUC was 2- to 3-fold higher, compared with that seen in posttransplant patients without delayed graft function. In the 3 controlled studies of rejection prevention, 20% of patients had delayed graft function. Although patients with delayed graft function have a higher incidence of certain adverse events (eg, anemia, thrombocytopenia, hyperkalemia) than patients without delayed graft function, these events were not more frequent in patients receiving mycophenolate than azathioprine or placebo. No dose adjustment is recommended for these patients; however, carefully observe them.

➤*Rare hereditary deficiency:* On theoretical grounds, because mycophenolate is an inosine monophosphate dehydrogenase (IMPDH) inhibitor, avoid in patients with rare hereditary deficiency of hypoxanthine-guanine phosphoribosyl-transferase (HGPRT), such as Lesch-Nyhan and Kelley-Seegmiller syndrome.

➤*Phenylketonuria:* Mycophenolate oral suspension contains aspartame, a source of phenylalanine (0.56 mg phenylalanine/mL suspension). Therefore, take care if the oral suspension is administered to patients with phenylketonuria.

Drug Interactions

➤*Drugs that alter the GI flora:* Drugs that alter the GI flora may interact with mycophenolate by disrupting enterohepatic recirculation. Interference of MPAG hydrolysis may lead to less MPA available for absorption.

Mycophenolate Drug Interactions			
Precipitant drug	Object drug*		Description
Acyclovir Ganciclovir	Mycophenolate	↑	MPAG and acyclovir plasma AUCs were increased 10.6% and 21.9%, respectively. Because MPAG plasma concentrations are increased in the presence of renal impairment, as are acyclovir and ganciclovir concentrations, the potential exists for the 2 drugs to compete for tubular secretion, further increasing the concentrations of both drugs.
Mycophenolate	Acyclovir Ganciclovir		
Antacids	Mycophenolate	↓	Absorption of a single mycophenolate dose was decreased when coadministered with an aluminum/magnesium hydroxide antacid. The C_{max} and AUC for MPA were 33% and 17% lower, respectively, than when mycophenolate was given alone. Avoid simultaneous administration.
Azathioprine	Mycophenolate	↔	It is recommended to avoid concomitant use because of a lack of clinical studies.
Cholestyramine	Mycophenolate	↓	Following coadmistration, MPA AUC decreased ≈ 40%. Do not give with cholestyramine or agents that may interfere with enterohepatic recirculation.
Iron	Mycophenolate	↓	Following coadministration, mycophenolate absorption and MPA AUC were significantly decreased. Avoid concomitant administration.
Probenecid	Mycophenolate	↑	In animals, coadministration resulted in a 3-fold increase in plasma MPAG AUC and a 2-fold increase in plasma MPA AUC.
Salicylates	Mycophenolate	↑	Coadministration increased the free fraction of MPA.

MYCOPHENOLATE MOFETIL

Mycophenolate Drug Interactions			
Precipitant drug	Object drug*		Description
Mycophenolate	Live attenuated vaccines	↓	Coadministration may cause vaccinations to be less effective. Avoid if possible.
Mycophenolate	Oral contraceptives	↓	Coadministration of mycophenolate and oral contraceptives containing levonorgestrel produced a significant decrease in the levonorgestrel AUC by ≈ 15%. Mean serum levels of LH, FSH, and progesterone were not significantly affected. Administer with caution and consider additional birth control methods.
Mycophenolate	Phenytoin	↑	MPA decreased protein binding of phenytoin and may, therefore, increase free phenytoin levels.
Mycophenolate	Theophylline	↑	MPA decreased protein binding of theophylline and may, therefore, increase free theophylline levels.

* ↑ = Object drug increased. ↓ = Object drug decreased. ⟷ = Undetermined clinical effect.

▶ *Drug/Food interactions:* Food (27 g fat, 650 calories) had no effect on the extent of absorption (MPA AUC) of mycophenolate when administered at doses of 1.5 g twice daily to renal transplant patients. However, MPA C_{max} was decreased by 40% in the presence of food.

Adverse Reactions

The principal adverse reactions associated with mycophenolate include diarrhea, leukopenia, sepsis, and vomiting, and evidence of a higher frequency of certain types of infections.

Patients receiving mycophenolate 2 g/day had an overall better safety profile than did patients receiving 3 g/day. Sepsis, which was generally CMV viremia, was slightly more common in renal transplant patients treated with mycophenolate, compared with patients receiving azathioprine. The incidence of sepsis was comparable to mycophenolate and in azathioprine-treated patients in cardiac and hepatic studies. In the digestive system, diarrhea was increased in renal and cardiac transplant patients receiving mycophenolate compared with patients receiving azathioprine, but was comparable in hepatic transplant patients treated with mycophenolate or azathioprine. Severe neutropenia developed in up to 2% of renal transplant patients, up to 2.8% of cardiac transplant patients, and up to 3.6% of hepatic transplant patients receiving mycophenolate 3 g daily (see Warnings).

Mycophenolate Adverse Reactions in Renal, Cardiac, or Hepatic Allograft Rejection (%)[1]						
	Renal studies			Cardiac study		Hepatic study
Adverse reaction	Mycophenolate 2 g/day (n = 336)	Mycophenolate 3 g/day (n = 330)	Azathioprine 1 to 2 mg/kg/day or 100 to 150 mg/day (n = 326)	Mycophenolate 3 g/day (n = 289)	Azathioprine 1.5 to 3 mg/kg/day (n = 289)	Mycophenolate 3 g/day (n = 277)	Azathioprine 1 to 2 mg/kg/day (n = 287)
Cardiovascular							
Hypertension	32.4	28.2	32.2	77.5	72.3	62.1	59.6
Hypotension	-	-	-	32.5	36	18.4	20.9
Cardiovascular disorder	-	-	-	25.6	24.2	-	-
Tachycardia	-	-	-	20.1	18	22	15.7
Arrhythmia	-	-	-	19	18.7	-	-
Bradycardia	-	-	-	17.3	17.3	-	-
Pericardial effusion	-	-	-	15.9	13.5	-	-
Heart failure	-	-	-	11.8	8.7	-	-
CNS							
Headache	21.1	16.1	21.2	54.3	51.9	53.8	49.1
Tremor	11	11.8	12.3	24.2	23.9	33.9	35.5
Insomnia	8.9	11.8	10.4	40.8	37.7	52.3	47
Anxiety	-	-	-	28.4	23.9	19.5	17.8
Paresthesia	-	-	-	20.8	18	15.2	15.3
Hypertonia	-	-	-	15.6	14.5	-	-
Depression	-	-	-	15.6	12.5	17.3	16.7
Agitation	-	-	-	13.1	12.8	-	-
Somnolence	-	-	-	11.1	10.4	-	-
Confusion	-	-	-	13.5	7.6	17.3	18.8
Nervousness	-	-	-	11.4	9	10.1	10.5
Dizziness	5.7	11.2	11	28.7	27.7	16.2	14.3
Dermatologic							
Acne	10.1	9.7	6.4	12.1	9.3	-	-
Skin disorder	-	-	-	12.5	8.7	-	-
Pruritus	-	-	-	-	-	14.1	10.5
Sweating	-	-	-	-	-	10.8	10.1
Rash	-	-	-	22.1	18	17.7	18.5
GI							
Diarrhea	31	36.1	20.9	45.3	34.3	51.3	49.8
Abdominal pain	24.7	27.6	23	33.9	33.2	62.5	51.2
Constipation	22.9	18.5	22.4	41.2	37.7	37.9	38.3
Nausea	19.9	23.6	24.5	54	54.3	54.5	51.2
Dyspepsia	17.6	13.6	13.8	18.7	19.4	22.4	20.9
Vomiting	12.5	13.6	9.2	33.9	28.4	32.9	33.4
Nausea and vomiting	10.4	9.7	10.7	11.1	7.6	-	-
Flatulence	-	-	-	13.8	15.6	12.6	9.8
Abdomen, enlarged	-	-	-	-	-	18.8	17.8
Anorexia	-	-	-	-	-	25.3	17.1
Cholangitis	-	-	-	-	-	14.1	13.6
Hepatitis	-	-	-	-	-	13	16
Cholestatic jaundice	-	-	-	-	-	11.9	10.8
Oral moniliasis	10.1	12.1	11.3	11.4	11.8	10.1	10.1
GU							
Urinary tract infection	37.2	37	33.7	13.1	11.8	18.1	17.8
Hematuria	14	12.1	11.3	-	-	-	-
Kidney function, abnormal	-	-	-	21.8	26.3	25.6	28.9
Oliguria	-	-	-	14.2	12.8	17	20.6
Kidney tubular necrosis	6.3	10	5.8	-	-	-	-
Hemic/Lymphatic							
Anemia	25.6	25.8	23.6	42.9	43.9	43	53
Leukopenia	23.2	34.5	24.8	30.4	39.1	45.8	39
Thrombocytopenia	10.1	8.2	13.2	23.5	27	38.3	42.2
Hypochromic anemia	7.4	11.5	9.2	24.6	23.5	13.7	10.8

MYCOPHENOLATE MOFETIL

Mycophenolate Adverse Reactions in Renal, Cardiac, or Hepatic Allograft Rejection (%)[1]

Adverse reaction	Renal studies — Mycophenolate 2 g/day (n = 336)	Renal studies — Mycophenolate 3 g/day (n = 330)	Renal studies — Azathioprine 1 to 2 mg/kg/day or 100 to 150 mg/day (n = 326)	Cardiac study — Mycophenolate 3 g/day (n = 289)	Cardiac study — Azathioprine 1.5 to 3 mg/kg/day (n = 289)	Hepatic study — Mycophenolate 3 g/day (n = 277)	Hepatic study — Azathioprine 1 to 2 mg/kg/day (n = 287)
Ecchymosis	-	-	-	16.6	8	-	-
Leukocytosis	7.1	10.9	7.4	40.5	35.6	22.4	21.3
Metabolic/Nutritional							
Peripheral edema	28.6	27	28.2	64	53.3	48.4	47.7
Hypercholesteremia	12.8	8.5	11.3	41.2	38.4	-	-
Hypophosphatemia	12.5	15.8	11.7	-	-	-	-
Edema	12.2	11.8	13.5	26.6	25.6	14.4	9.1
Hypokalemia	10.1	10	8.3	31.8	25.6	28.2	28.2
Hyperglycemia	8.6	12.4	15	46.7	52.6	37.2	41.1
Liver function tests, abnormal	-	-	-	-	-	43.7	48.8
Creatinine, increased	-	-	-	39.4	36	24.9	19.2
BUN, increased	-	-	-	34.6	32.5	19.9	21.6
Lactic dehydrogenase, increased	-	-	-	23.2	17	10.1	12.9
Bilirubinemia	-	-	-	18	21.8	-	-
Hypervolemia	-	-	-	16.6	22.8	14.4	18.8
Generalized edema	-	-	-	18	20.1	-	-
Hyperuricemia	-	-	-	16.3	17.6	14.8	16
AST, increased	-	-	-	17.3	15.6	-	-
Hypomagnesemia	-	-	-	18.3	12.8	-	-
Acidosis	-	-	-	14.2	16.6	39	37.6
Weight gain	-	-	-	15.6	15.2	-	-
ALT, increased	-	-	-	15.6	12.5	-	-
Hyponatremia	-	-	-	11.4	11.8	-	-
Hyperlipemia	-	-	-	10.7	9.3	-	-
Hypocalcemia	-	-	-	-	-	30	30
Hypoproteinemia	-	-	-	-	-	13.4	13.9
Hypoglycemia	-	-	-	-	-	10.5	9.1
Healing, abnormal	-	-	-	-	-	10.5	8.7
Hyperkalemia	8.9	10.3	16.9	14.5	19.7	22	23.7
Musculoskeletal							
Leg cramps	-	-	-	16.6	15.6	-	-
Myasthenia	-	-	-	12.5	9.7	-	-
Myalgia	-	-	-	12.5	9.3	-	-
Respiratory							
Infection	22	23.9	19.6	37	35.3	15.9	19.9
Dyspnea	15.5	17.3	16.6	36.7	36.3	31	30.3
Cough, increased	15.5	13.3	15	31.1	25.6	15.9	12.5
Pharyngitis	9.5	11.2	8	18.3	13.5	14.1	12.5
Lung disorder	-	-	-	30.1	29.1	22	18.8
Sinusitis	-	-	-	26	19	11.2	9.8
Rhinitis	-	-	-	19	15.6	-	-
Pleural effusion	-	-	-	17	13.8	34.3	35.9
Asthma	-	-	-	11.1	11.4	-	-
Atelectasis	-	-	-	-	-	13	12.9
Pneumonia	-	-	-	10.7	10.4	13.7	11.5
Miscellaneous							
Pain	33	31.2	32.2	75.8	74.7	74	77.7
Fever	21.4	23.3	23.3	47.4	46.4	52.3	56.1
Sepsis	17.6	19.7	15.6	18.7	18.7	27.4	26.5
Infection	18.2	20.9	19.9	25.6	19.4	27.1	25.1
Asthenia	13.7	16.1	19.9	43.3	36.3	35.4	33.8
Chest pain	13.4	13.3	14.7	26.3	26	15.9	13.2
Back pain	11.6	12.1	14.1	34.6	28.4	46.6	47.4
Accidental injury	-	-	-	19	14.9	11.2	15
Chills	-	-	-	11.4	11.4	10.8	10.1
Ascites	-	-	-	-	-	24.2	22.6
Hernia	-	-	-	-	-	11.6	8.7
Amblyopia	-	-	-	14.9	6.6	-	-
Peritonitis	-	-	-	-	-	10.1	12.5

[1] Data are pooled from 3 separate studies and are not necessarily comparable.

Lymphoproliferative disease or lymphoma developed in 0.4% to 1% of patients receiving mycophenolate (2 or 3 g daily) with other immunosuppressive agents in controlled clinical trials of renal, cardiac, and hepatic transplant patients followed for ≥ 1 year. Nonmelanoma skin carcinomas occurred in 1.6% to 4.2% of patients, other types of malignancy in 0.7% to 2.1% of patients. Three-year safety data in renal and cardiac transplant patients did not reveal any unexpected changes in incidence of malignancy compared with the 1-year data.

In the 3 controlled studies for prevention of renal or cardiac rejection, similar rates of fatal infections/sepsis (< 2%) occurred in patients while receiving mycophenolate (2 or 3 g) or control therapy in combination with other immunosuppressive agents (see Warnings). In cardiac transplant patients, the overall incidence of opportunistic infections was ≈ 10% higher in patients treated with mycophenolate than in those receiving azathioprine, but this difference was not associated with excess mortality because of infection/sepsis among patients treated with mycophenolate.

Serious life-threatening infections such as meningitis and infectious endocarditis have been reported occasionally, and there is evidence of a higher frequency of certain types of serious infections such as tuberculosis and atypical mycobacterial infection.

MYCOPHENOLATE MOFETIL

	Viral and Fungal Infections in Prevention of Renal, Cardiac, or Hepatic Transplant Rejection with Mycophenolate (%)[1]						
	Renal studies			Cardiac study		Hepatic study	
Infection	Mycophenolate 2 g/day (n = 336)	Mycophenolate 3 g/day (n = 330)	Azathioprine 1 to 2 mg/kg/day or 100 to 150 mg/day (n = 326)	Mycophenolate 3 g/day (n = 289)	Azathioprine 1.5 to 3 mg/kg/day (n = 289)	Mycophenolate 3 g/day (n = 277)	Azathioprine 1 to 2 mg/kg/day (n = 287)
Herpes simplex	16.7	20	19	20.8	14.5	10.1	5.9
CMV							
Viremia/Syndrome	13.4	12.4	13.8	12.1	10	14.1	12.2
Tissue invasive disease	8.3	11.5	6.1	11.4	8.7	5.8	8
Herpes zoster	6	7.6	5.8	10.7	5.9	4.3	4.9
Cutaneous disease	6	7.3	5.5	10	5.5	4.3	4.9
Candida	17	17.3	18.1	18.7	17.6	22.4	24.4
Mucocutaneous	15.5	16.4	15.3	18	17.3	18.4	17.4

[1] Data pooled from 3 separate studies and are not necessarily comparable.

Other adverse reactions occurring in 3% to < 10% of patients, in combination with cyclosporine and corticosteroids, are as follows:

➤*Cardiovascular:* Angina pectoris; atrial fibrillation; palpitation; peripheral vascular disorder; postural hypotension; thrombosis; vasodilation; ventricular extrasystole; CHF; supraventricular tachycardia; ventricular tachycardia; atrial flutter; pulmonary hypertension; cardiac arrest; venous pressure increased; syncope; supraventricular extrasystoles; extrasystoles; pallor; vasospasm; arterial thrombosis.

➤*CNS:* Emotional lability; neuropathy; convulsions; hallucinations; abnormal thinking; vertigo; delirium; dry mouth; hypesthesia; psychosis.

➤*Dermatologic:* Alopecia; fungal dermatitis; hirsutism; benign skin neoplasm; skin hypertrophy; skin ulcer; hemorrhage; skin carcinoma; vesiculobullous rash.

➤*Endocrine:* Diabetes mellitus; parathyroid disorder; Cushing syndrome; hypothyroidism.

➤*GI:* Esophagitis; flatulence; gastritis; gastroenteritis; GI hemorrhage; gingivitis; gum hyperplasia; ileus; infection; mouth ulceration; rectal disorder; GI disorder; liver damage; dysphagia; jaundice; stomatitis; thirst; GI moniliasis; melena; stomach ulcer.

➤*GU:* Albuminuria; dysuria; hydronephrosis; impotence; pain; pyelonephritis; urinary frequency; nocturia; kidney failure; urine abnormality; urinary incontinence; prostatic disorder; urinary retention; urinary tract disorder; dysuria; acute kidney failure; scrotal edema.

➤*Hematologic:* Hemorrhage; ecchymosis; polycythemia; pancytopenia; increased prothrombin; increased thromboplastin; coagulation disorder; petechia; thrombosis (with IV).

➤*Metabolic/Nutritional:* Liver function tests abnormal; dehydration; weight gain/loss; hypercholesterolemia; hyponatremia; increased alkaline phosphatase, creatinine, gamma glutamyl transpeptidase, lactic dehydrogenase, AST, and ALT; hypercalcemia; hyperlipemia; hypocalcemia; hypoglycemia; hypoproteinemia; acidosis; hypoxia; alkalosis; hypochloremia.

➤*Musculoskeletal:* Arthralgia; joint disorder; osteoporosis.

➤*Respiratory:* Lung edema; hiccough; pneumothorax; increased sputum; epistaxis; apnea; voice alteration; pain; hemoptysis; neoplasm; respiratory acidosis; bronchitis; respiratory disorder; hyperventilation; respiratory moniliasis.

➤*Special senses:* Cataract; conjunctivitis; ear pain; deafness; ear disorder; tinnitus; abnormal vision; lacrimation disorder; eye hemorrhage.

➤*Miscellaneous:* Cyst; face edema; flu syndrome; malaise; pelvic pain; neck pain; cellulitis (with IV); phlebitis; abnormal healing; abscess; abnormal lab test; gout.

➤*Postmarketing:*

GI – Colitis (sometimes caused by CMV); pancreatitis.

Respiratory – Interstitial lung disorders, including fatal pulmonary fibrosis, have been reported rarely and should be considered in the differential diagnosis of pulmonary symptoms ranging from dyspnea to respiratory failure in post-transplant patients receiving mycophenolate.

Miscellaneous – Serious life-threatening infections such as meningitis and infectious endocarditis have been reported occasionally and there is evidence of a higher frequency of certain types of serious infections such as tuberculosis and atypical mycobacterial infection.

Overdosage

➤*Symptoms:* At doses of 4 or 5 g/day, there appears to be a higher rate, compared with the use of ≤ 3 g/day, of GI intolerance (eg, nausea, vomiting, diarrhea), and occasional hematologic abnormalities, principally neutropenia, leading to a need to reduce or discontinue dosing.

➤*Treatment:* MPA and MPAG usually are not removed by hemodialysis. However, at high MPAG plasma concentrations (> 100 mcg/mL), small amounts of MPAG are removed. By increasing excretion of the drug, MPA can be removed by bile acid sequestrants, such as cholestyramine.

Patient Information

Inform patients of the need for repeated appropriate laboratory tests while they are receiving mycophenolate.

Instruct patients with increased risk for skin cancer to limit exposure to sunlight and UV light by wearing protective clothing and using a strong sunscreen.

Give patients complete dosage instructions and inform them of the increased risk of lymphoproliferative disease and certain other malignancies.

Instruct patients to report immediately any evidence of infection, unexpected bruising, bleeding, or any other manifestation of bone marrow depression.

Inform women of childbearing potential of the possible risks during pregnancy; instruct them to use effective contraception before beginning therapy, during therapy, and for 6 weeks after mycophenolate has been stopped (see Pregnancy).

Immunosuppressives

TACROLIMUS (FK506)

Rx	Prograf (Fujisawa)	Capsules: 0.5 mg	Lactose. (0.5 mg 607). Light yellow, oblong. In 60s and 100s.
		1 mg	Lactose. (1 mg 617). White, oblong. In 100s and blister cards of 100s.
		5 mg	Lactose. (5 mg 657). Grayish/red, oblong. In 100s and blister cards of 100s.
		Injection: 5 mg/mL	In 1 mL amps.[1]

[1] Contains 200 mg/mL polyoxyl 60 hydrogenated castor oil (HCO-60) and 80% dehydrated alcohol.

Tacrolimus also is available as an ointment for use in mild to moderate atopic dermatitis. For complete prescribing information for the ointment, refer to the Dermatologics chapter.

WARNING

Increased susceptibility to infection and the possible development of lymphoma may result from immunosuppression. Only physicians experienced in immunosuppressive therapy and management of organ transplant patients should prescribe tacrolimus. Manage patients receiving the drug in facilities equipped and staffed with adequate laboratory and supportive medical resources. The physician responsible for maintenance therapy should have complete information necessary for the follow-up of the patient.

Indications

➤*Organ rejection prophylaxis:* Prophylaxis of organ rejection in patients receiving allogeneic liver or kidney transplants. It is recommended that tacrolimus be used concomitantly with adrenal corticosteroids. Because of the risk of anaphylaxis, reserve the injection for patients unable to take the capsules orally.

➤*Unlabeled uses:* Tacrolimus is being investigated for bone marrow, cardiac, pancreas, pancreatic island cell, small bowel, and lung transplantation. It may be beneficial for the treatment of autoimmune disease (ie, rheumatoid arthritis, inflammatory bowel disease) and severe recalcitrant psoriasis.

Administration and Dosage

➤*Approved by the FDA:* April 8, 1994 (1P,E classification).

➤*Injection:* Anaphylactic reactions have occurred with injectables containing castor oil derivatives. See Warnings.

For IV infusion only.

In patients unable to take the capsules, therapy may be initiated with the injection. Administer the initial dose no sooner than 6 hours after transplantation. The recommended starting dose is 0.03 to 0.05 mg/kg/day as a continuous IV infusion. Give adult patients doses at the lower end of the dosing range. Concomitant adrenal corticosteroid therapy is recommended early posttransplantation. Continue continuous IV infusion only until the patient can tolerate oral administration.

Preparation for administration – Tacrolimus must be diluted with 0.9% Sodium Chloride Injection or 5% Dextrose Injection to a concentration between 0.004 and 0.02 mg/mL prior to use.

➤*Oral:*

Summary of Initial Oral Dosage Recommendations and Typical Whole Blood Trough Concentrations

Patient population	Recommended initial oral dose[1]	Typical whole blood trough concentrations
Adult kidney transplant patients	0.2 mg/kg/day	Month 1 through 3: 7 to 20 ng/mL Month 4 through 12: 5 to 15 ng/mL
Adult liver transplant patients	0.1 to 0.15 mg/kg/day	Month 1 through 12: 5 to 20 ng/mL
Pediatric liver transplant patients	0.15 to 0.2 mg/kg/day	Month 1 through 12: 5 to 20 ng/mL

[1] 2 divided doses, every 12 hours.

Liver transplantation – Convert patients from IV to oral therapy as soon as oral therapy can be tolerated. This usually occurs within 2 to 3 days. Administer the initial dose no sooner than 6 hours after transplantation. Give the first dose of oral therapy 8 to 12 hours after discontinuing the IV infusion. The recommended starting oral dose is 0.1 to 0.15 mg/kg/day administered in 2 divided daily doses every 12 hours. Administer the initial dose no sooner than 6 hours after transplantation.

Titrate dosing based on clinical assessments of rejection and tolerability. Lower dosages may be sufficient as maintenance therapy. Adjunct therapy with adrenal corticosteroids is recommended early posttransplant.

Kidney transplantation – The recommended starting oral dose is 0.2 mg/kg/day administered every 12 hours in 2 divided doses. The initial dose of tacrolimus may be administered within 24 hours of transplantation, but should be delayed until renal function has recovered (as indicated for example by a serum creatinine of 4 mg/dL or less). Black

patients may require higher doses to achieve comparable blood concentrations.

The data in kidney transplant patients indicate that the black patients required a higher dose to attain comparable trough concentrations compared with Caucasian patients.

Trough Concentrations in Kidney Transplantation Patients

Time after transplant	Caucasian (n = 114)		Black (n = 56)	
	Dose (mg/kg)	Trough concentrations (ng/mL)	Dose (mg/kg)	Trough concentrations (ng/mL)
Day 7	0.18	12	0.23	10.9
Month 1	0.17	12.8	0.26	12.9
Month 6	0.14	11.8	0.24	11.5
Month 12	0.13	10.1	0.19	11

➤*Children:* Pediatric liver transplantation patients without pre-existing renal or hepatic dysfunction have required and tolerated higher doses than adults to achieve similar blood concentrations. Therefore, it is recommended that therapy be initiated in pediatric patients in the IV and oral dosing ranges of 0.03 to 0.05 mg/kg/day IV and 0.15 to 0.2 mg/kg/day oral. Dose adjustments may be required.

➤*Hepatic/Renal function impairment:* Because of the potential for nephrotoxicity, give patients with renal and hepatic impairment doses at the lowest value of the recommended IV and oral dosing ranges. Further reductions in dose below these ranges may be required. Therapy may need to be delayed by up to 48 hours or longer in patients with postoperative oliguria.

➤*Conversion from one immunosuppressive regimen to another:* Do not use tacrolimus simultaneously with cyclosporine. Discontinue either agent at least 24 hours before initiating the other. In the presence of elevated tacrolimus or cyclosporine concentrations, dosing with the other drug usually should be further delayed.

➤*Blood concentration monitoring:* Most study centers have found tacrolimus blood concentration monitoring helpful in patient management. While no fixed relationship has been established, such blood monitoring may assist in the clinical evaluation of rejection and toxicity, dose adjustments, and assessment of compliance.

Various assays have been used to measure blood concentrations of tacrolimus. Comparison of the concentrations in published literature to patient concentrations using current assays must be made with detailed knowledge of the assay methods employed.

Liver transplantation – US clinical trials show that tacrolimus whole blood concentrations, as measured by ELISA, were most variable during the first week post-transplantation. After this early period, median trough blood concentrations, measured at intervals from the second week to 1 year posttransplantation, ranged from 9.8 to 19.4 ng/mL.

Kidney transplantation – Data from the Phase III study indicates that trough concentrations of tacrolimus in whole blood were most variable during the first week of dosing. During the first 3 months, 80% of the patients maintained trough concentrations between 7 to 20 ng/mL, and then between 5 to 15 ng/mL, through 1 year.

➤*Storage/Stability:* Store capsules at 25°C (77°F); excursions permitted to 15° to 30°C (59° to 86°F). Store injection between 5° and 25°C, 41° and 77°F). Store diluted infusion solution in glass or polyethylene containers and discard after 24 hours. Do not store the diluted infusion solution in a PVC container because of decreased stability and the potential for extraction of phthalates.

Actions

➤*Pharmacology:* Tacrolimus, previously known as FK506, is a macrolide immunosuppressant produced by *Streptomyces tsukubaensis.* Tacrolimus prolongs the survival of the host and transplanted graft in animal transplant models of liver, kidney, heart, bone marrow, small bowel and pancreas, lung and trachea, skin, cornea, and limb.

In animals, tacrolimus suppresses some humoral immunity and, to a greater extent, cell-mediated reactions such as allograft rejection, delayed-type hypersensitivity, collagen-induced arthritis, experimental allergic encephalomyelitis, and graft vs host disease.

Tacrolimus inhibits T-lymphocyte activation, although the exact mechanism of action is not known. Evidence suggests that the drug binds to an intracellular protein, FKBP-12. A complex of tacrolimus-FKBP-12, calcium, calmodulin, and calcineurin is then formed, and the phosphatase activity of calcineurin is inhibited. This effect may prevent the generation of nuclear factor of activated T-cells (NF-AT), a nuclear component thought to initiate gene transcription for the formation of

TACROLIMUS (FK506)

lymphokines (interleukin-2, gamma interferon). The net result is the inhibition of T-lymphocyte activation (ie, immunosuppression).

➤*Pharmacokinetics:*

Absorption – Absorption of tacrolimus from the GI tract after oral administraton is variable. The absolute bioavailability of tacrolimus was about 17% in adult kidney transplant patients, about 22% in adult liver transplant patients, and about 18% in healthy volunteers. Tacrolimus maximum blood concentrations (C_{max}) and area under the curve (AUC) appeared to increase in a dose-proportional fashion in 18 fasted healthy volunteers receiving a single oral dose of 3, 7, and 10 mg.

In kidney transplant patients, tacrolimus trough concentrations from 3 to 30 ng/mL measured at 10 to 12 hours postdose (C_{min}) and in liver transplant patients over a concentration range of 10 to 60 ng/mL correlated well with the AUC.

Food effects: The rate and extent of tacrolimus absorption were greatest under fasted conditions. The rate and extent of tacrolimus absorption were greatest under fasted conditions. The presence and composition of food decreased the rate and extent of tacrolimus absorption. The effect was most pronounced with a high-fat meal (848 kcal, 46% fat): Mean AUC and C_{max} were decreased 37% and 77%, respectively; T_{max} was lengthened 5-fold. A high-carbohydrate meal (668 kcal, 85% carbohydrate) decreased mean AUC and mean C_{max} by 28% and 65%, respectively.

Distribution – The plasma protein binding of tacrolimus is approximately 99%. Tacrolimus is bound mainly to albumin and alpha-1-acid glycoprotein and has a high level of association with erythrocytes. The distribution of tacrolimus between whole blood and plasma depends on several factors, such as hematocrit, temperature at the time of plasma separation, drug concentration, and plasma protein concentration. In a US study, the ratio of whole blood concentration to plasma concentration averaged 35 (range, 12 to 67).

Metabolism – Tacrolimus is extensively metabolized by the mixed-function oxidase system, primarily the cytochrome P450 system (CYP3A). A metabolic pathway leading to the formation of 8 possible metabolites has been proposed. Demethylation and hydroxylation were identified as the primary mechanisms of biotransformation in vitro. The major metabolite identified is 13-demethyl tacrolimus.

Excretion – The mean clearance following IV administration of tacrolimus is 0.04, 0.083, and 0.053 L/hr/kg in healthy volunteers, adult kidney transplant patients, and adult liver transplant patients, respectively. Less than 1% of the dose administered is excreted unchanged in urine.

After IV administration, fecal elimination accounted for about 92.4% and the elimination half-life was about 48.1 hours, whereas it was about 43.5 hours based on tacrolimus concentrations. When administered orally, fecal elimination accounted for about 92.6%, urinary elimination accounted for about 2.3%, and the elimination half-life was about 31.9 hours, whereas it was about 48.4 hours based on tacrolimus concentrations. The pharmacokinetic parameters of tacrolimus have been determined following IV and oral administration in healthy volunteers, kidney transplant, and liver transplant patients.

Pharmacokinetic Parameters of Tacrolimus

Population	N	Route (dose)	C_{max} (ng/mL)	T_{max} (hr)	AUC (ng·hr/mL)	t½ (hr)	Clearance (L/hr/kg)	Vd (L/kg)
Healthy volunteers	8	IV (0.025 mg/kg/4 hr)	—	—	≈ 598[1]	≈ 34.2	≈ 0.04	≈ 1.91
	16	PO (5 mg)	≈ 29.7	≈ 1.6	≈ 243[2]	≈ 34.8	≈ 0.041[3]	≈ 1.94[3]
Kidney transplant patients	26	IV (0.02 mg/kg/12 hr)	—	—	≈ 294[4]	≈ 18.8	≈ 0.083	1.41
		PO (0.2 mg/kg/day)	≈ 19.2	3	≈ 203[4]	NA[5]	NA	NA
		PO (0.3 mg/kg/day)	≈ 24.2	1.5	≈ 288[4]	NA	NA	NA
Liver transplant patients	17	IV (0.05 mg/kg/12 hr)	—	—	≈ 3300[4]	≈ 11.7	≈ 0.053	≈ 0.85
		PO (0.3 mg/kg/day)	≈ 68.5	≈ 2.3	≈ 519[4]	NA	NA	NA

[1] AUC_{0-120}
[2] AUC_{0-72}
[3] Corrected for individual bioavailability.
[4] $AUC_{0-\infty}$
[5] NA = Not available
– = Not applicable

Special populations –

Children: Trough concentrations obtained from 31 children younger than 12 years of age showed that children need higher doses than adults to achieve similar trough concentrations (see Administration and Dosage).

Hepatic insufficiency: The mean clearance was substantially lower and half-life was prolonged in patients with severe hepatic dysfunction.

➤*Clinical trials:*

Liver transplant patients – The safety and efficacy of tacrolimus-based immunosuppression following orthotopic liver transplantation were assessed in 2 prospective, randomized, nonblinded multicenter studies. The active control groups were treated with a cyclosporine-based immunosuppressive regimen (CBIR). Both studies used concomitant adrenal corticosteroids as part of the immunosuppressive regimens. These studies were designed to evaluate whether the 2 regimens were therapeutically equivalent, with patient and graft survival at 12 months following transplantation as the primary endpoints. The tacrolimus-based immunosuppressive regimen was found to be equivalent to the cyclosporine-based immunosuppressive regimens.

One-year patient survival (CBIR and tacrolimus-based treatment groups combined) was 78% to 88%. The overall 1-year graft survival (CBIR and tacrolimus-based treatment groups combined) was 73% to 81%. Median time to convert from IV to oral tacrolimus dosing was 2 days.

Contraindications

Hypersensitivity to tacrolimus; hypersensitivity to HCO-60 polyoxyl 60 hydrogenated castor oil (used in vehicle for injection).

Warnings

➤*Insulin-dependent post-transplant diabetes mellitus (PTDM):* Insulin-dependent PTDM was reported in 20% of tacrolimus-treated kidney patients without pretransplant history of diabetes mellitus in the Phase III study. The median time to onset of PTDM was 68 days. Insulin dependence was reversible in 15% of these PTDM patients at 1 year and in 50% at 2 years post-transplant. Black and Hispanic kidney transplant patients were at an increased risk of development of PTDM.

Insulin-dependent PTDM was reported in 18% and 11% of tacrolimus-treated liver transplant patients and was reversible in 45% and 31% of these patients at 1 year post-transplant, in the US and European randomized studies, respectively. Hyperglycemia was associated with the use of tacrolimus in 47% and 33% of liver transplant recipients in the US and European randomized studies, respectively, and may require treatment.

➤*Nephrotoxicity:* Tacrolimus can cause neurotoxicity and nephrotoxicity, particularly when used in high doses. Nephrotoxicity has been noted in approximately 52% of kidney transplantation patients and in 36% to 40% of liver transplantation patients receiving the drug. More overt nephrotoxicity is seen early after transplantation, characterized by increasing serum creatinine and a decrease in urine output. Closely monitor patients with impaired renal function; the dosage may need to be reduced. In patients with persistent elevations of serum creatinine who are unresponsive to dosage adjustments, consider changing to another immunosuppressive therapy. Take care in using tacrolimus with other nephrotoxic drugs; in particular, to avoid excess nephrotoxicity, do not use simultaneously with cyclosporine. Discontinue tacrolimus or cyclosporine at least 24 hours prior to initiating the other. In the presence of elevated tacrolimus or cyclosporine concentrations, usually delay dosing with the other drug (see Drug Interactions).

➤*Hyperkalemia:* Mild to severe hyperkalemia that may require treatment has been noted in 31% of kidney transplant recipients and in 13% to 45% of liver transplant recipients treated with tacrolimus. Monitor serum potassium levels and do not use potassium-sparing diuretics therapy.

➤*Neurotoxicity:* Neurotoxicity, including tremor, headache, and other changes in motor function, mental status, and sensory function occurred in approximately 55% of liver transplant recipients. Tremor occurred more often in tacrolimus-treated kidney transplant patients (54%) compared with cyclosporine-treated patients. Tremor and headache have been associated with high whole-blood concentrations of tacrolimus and may respond to dosage adjustment. Seizures have occurred in adult and pediatric patients. Coma and delirium also have been associated with high plasma concentrations of tacrolimus.

➤*Lymphomas:* As with other immunosuppressants, patients receiving tacrolimus are at increased risk of developing lymphomas and other malignancies, particularly of the skin. The risk appears to be related to the intensity and duration of immunosuppression rather than to the use of any specific agent. A lymphoproliferative disorder (LPD) related to Epstein-Barr virus (EBV) infection has been reported in immunosuppressed organ transplant recipients. The risk of LPD appears greatest in young children who are at risk for primary EBV infection while immunosuppressed or who are switched to tacrolimus following long-term immunosuppressive therapy. Because of the danger of oversuppression of the immune system, which can increase susceptibility to infection, use combination immunosuppressant therapy with caution.

➤*Myocardial hypertrophy:* Myocardial hypertrophy has been reported in association with the administration of tacrolimus and is generally manifested by echocardiographically demonstrated concen-

TACROLIMUS (FK506)

tric increases in left ventricular posterior wall and interventricular septum thickness. Hypertrophy has been observed in infants, children, and adults. This condition appears reversible in most cases following dose reduction or discontinuance of therapy. In a group of 20 patients with pre- and post-treatment echocardiograms who showed evidence of myocardial hypertrophy, mean tacrolimus whole blood concentrations during the period prior to diagnosis of myocardial hypertrophy ranged from 11 to 53 ng/mL in infants, 4 to 46 ng/mL in children, and 11 to 24 ng/mL in adults.

➤*Hypersensitivity reactions:* A few patients receiving the injection have experienced anaphylactic reactions. Although the exact cause of these reactions is not known, other drugs with castor oil derivatives in the formulation have been associated with anaphylaxis in a small percentage of patients. Because of this potential risk of anaphylaxis, reserve the injection for patients who are unable to take capsules.

Continuously observe patients receiving the injection for at least the first 30 minutes following the start of the infusion and at frequent intervals thereafter. If signs or symptoms of anaphylaxis occur, stop the infusion. Have an aqueous solution of epinephrine available at the bedside as well as a source of oxygen. Refer to Management of Acute Hypersensitivity Reactions.

➤*Renal/Hepatic function impairment:* Use lower doses for patients with renal insufficiency (see Administration and Dosage).

The use of tacrolimus in liver transplant recipients experiencing post-transplant hepatic impairment may be associated with increased risk of developing renal insufficiency related to high whole-blood levels of tacrolimus. Monitor these patients closely and consider dosage adjustments. Use lower doses in these patients (see Administration and Dosage).

➤*Carcinogenesis:* An increased incidence of malignancy is a recognized complication of immunosuppression in recipients of organ transplants. The most common forms of neoplasms are non-Hodgkin's lymphomas and carcinomas of the skin. As with other immunosuppressive therapies, the risk of malignancies in tacrolimus recipients may be higher than in the healthy population. Lymphoproliferative disorders associated with Epstein-Barr virus infection have been seen. It has been reported that reduction or discontinuation of immunosuppression may cause the lesions to regress (see also Lymphomas).

➤*Fertility impairment:* Tacrolimus, given orally at 1 mg/kg (0.7 to 1.4 times the recommended clinical dose range of 0.1 to 0.2 mg/kg/day) to male and female rats prior to and during mating, as well as to dams during gestation and lactation, was associated with embryolethality and with adverse effects on female reproduction. Effects on female reproductive function (parturition) and embryolethal effects were indicated by a higher rate of pre-implantation loss and increased numbers of undelivered and nonviable pups. When given at 3.2 mg/kg, tacrolimus was associated with maternal and paternal toxicity, as well as reproductive toxicity including marked adverse effects on estrus cycles, parturition, pup viability, and pup malformations.

➤*Pregnancy: Category C.* In reproduction studies in rats and rabbits, adverse effects on the fetus were observed mainly at dose levels that were toxic to dams. Tacrolimus at oral doses of 0.32 and 1 mg/kg during organogenesis in rabbits was associated with maternal toxicity as well as an increase in incidence of abortions; these doses are equivalent to 0.5 to 1 times and 1.6 to 3.3 times the recommended clinical dose range (0.1 to 0.2 mg/kg). At the higher dose only, an increased incidence of malformations and developmental variations also was seen. Tacrolimus, at oral doses of 3.2 mg/kg during organogenesis in rats, was associated with maternal toxicity and caused an increase in late resorptions, decreased numbers of live births, and decreased pup weight and viability. Oral tacrolimus (1 and 3.2 mg/kg) to pregnant rats after organogenesis and during lactation was associated with reduced pup weights.

There are no adequate and well-controlled studies in pregnant women. Tacrolimus is transferred across the placenta. The use of tacrolimus during pregnancy has been associated with neonatal hyperkalemia and renal dysfunction. Use during pregnancy only if the potential benefit to the mother justifies potential risk to the fetus.

➤*Lactation:* Tacrolimus is excreted in breast milk; avoid nursing.

➤*Children:* Successful liver transplants have been performed in pediatric patients (up to 16 years of age) using tacrolimus. Pediatric patients generally require higher doses to maintain blood trough levels of tacrolimus similar to adult patients (see Administration and Dosage).

Precautions

➤*Monitoring:* Regularly assess serum creatinine, potassium, and fasting glucose. Perform routine monitoring of metabolic and hematologic systems as clinically warranted.

➤*Hypertension:* Hypertension is a common adverse effect of tacrolimus therapy. Mild or moderate hypertension is more frequently reported than severe hypertension. Antihypertensive therapy may be required; the control of blood pressure can be accomplished with any of the common antihypertensive agents. Because tacrolimus may cause hyperkalemia, avoid potassium-sparing diuretics. While calcium-

channel blocking agents can be effective in treating tacrolimus-associated hypertension, take care because interference with tacrolimus metabolism may require a dosage reduction (see Drug Interactions).

Drug Interactions

Tacrolimus Drug Interactions			
Precipitant drug		Object drug*	Description
Nephrotoxic agents (eg, Aminoglycosides,	amphotericin B, cisplatin, cyclosporine)	Tacrolimus ⬆	Because of the potential for additive or synergistic impairment of renal function, take care when administering tacrolimus with drugs that may be associated with renal dysfunction. Coadministration with cyclosporine resulted in additive/synergistic nephrotoxicity; tacrolimus blood levels also may be increased. Give the first tacrolimus dose no sooner than 24 hours after the last cyclosporine dose.
Bromocriptine Cimetidine Cisapride Chloramphenicol Danazol Ethinyl estradiol Methylprednisolone Metoclopromide Metronidazole Nefazodone Omeprazole Protease inhibitors Macrolide antibiotics (eg, clarithromycin, erythromycin, troleandomycin)	Calcium channel blockers (eg, diltiazem, nicardepine, nifedipine, verapamil) Antifungal Agents (eg, clotrimazole, fluconazole, itraconazole, ketoconazole, miconazole)	Tacrolimus ⬆	These agents may increase tacrolimus blood levels, increasing risk of toxicity.
Carbamazepine Fosphenytoin Phenobarbital Phenytoin	Antibiotics (eg, rifabutin, rifampin, rifapentine)	Tacrolimus ⬇	These agents may decrease tacrolimus blood levels.
St. John's wort		Tacrolimus ⬇	St. John's wort induces CYP3A4 and P-glycoprotein. Because tacrolimus is a substrate for CYP3A4, tacrolimus blood levels may decrease.
Tacrolimus		Mycophenolate mofetil ⬆	Mycophenolate trough plasma concentrations may be elevated, increasing risk of side effects.
Tacrolimus		Vaccines ⬇	Immunosuppressants may affect vaccination. Therefore, during treatment with tacrolimus, vaccination may be less effective. Avoid the use of live vaccines (eg, measles, mumps, rubella, oral polio, BCG, yellow fever, TY 21a typhoid).

* ⬆ = Object drug increased. ⬇ = Object drug decreased.

Because tacrolimus is metabolized mainly by the cytochrome P450 3A enzyme systems, substances known to inhibit these enzymes may affect the metabolism or increase bioavailability of tacrolimus with resultant increases or decreases in whole blood or plasma levels. Monitoring of blood levels and appropriate dosage adjustments are essential when such drugs are used concomitantly.

➤*Drug/Food interactions:* The rate and extent of tacrolimus absorption were greatest under fasted conditions. The presence and composition of food decreased both the rate and extent of tacrolimus absorption. The effect was most pronounced with a high-fat meal (848 kcal, 46% fat): Mean AUC and C_{max} were decreased 37% and 77%, respectively; T_{max} was lengthened 5-fold. A high-carbohydrate meal (668 kcal, 85% carbohydrate) decreased mean AUC and mean C_{max} by 28% and 65%, respectively.

Coadministered grapefuit juice has been reported to increase tacrolimus blood trough concentrations in liver transplant patients.

TACROLIMUS (FK506)

Adverse Reactions

Tacrolimus Adverse Reactions in Kidney and Liver Transplant Patients (%)[1]

Adverse reaction	Liver transplant patients		Kidney transplant patients	
	Tacrolimus (n = 514)	CBIR (n = 515)	Tacrolimus (n = 205)	CBIR (n = 207)
Cardiovascular				
Chest pain	—	—	19	13
Hypertension[2]	38-47	43-56	50	52
CNS				
Dizziness	—	—	19	16
Headache[2]	37-64	26-60	44	38
Insomnia	32-64	23-68	32	30
Paresthesia	17-40	17-30	23	16
Tremor[2]	48-56	32-46	54	34
GI				
Anorexia	7-34	5-24	—	—
Constipation	23-24	21-27	35	43
Diarrhea	37-72	27-47	44	41
Dyspepsia	—	—	28	20
LFT abnormal	6-36	5-30	—	—
Nausea	32-46	27-37	38	36
Vomiting	14-27	11-15	29	23
GU				
BUN increased[2]	12-30	9-22	—	—
Creatinine increased[2]	24-39	19-25	45	42
Kidney function abnormal[2]	36-40	23-27	—	—
Oliguria	18-19	12-15	—	—
Urinary tract infection	16-21	18-19	34	35
Hemic/Lymphatic				
Anemia	5-47	1-38	30	24
Leukocytosis	8-32	8-26	—	—
Leukopenia	—	—	15	17
Thrombocytopenia	14-24	19-20	—	—
Metabolic/Nutritional				
Diabetes mellitus[2]	—	—	24	9
Hyperglycemia[2]	33-47	22-38	22	16
Hyperkalemia[2]	13-45	9-26	31	32
Hyperlipemia	—	—	31	38
Hypokalemia	13-29	16-34	22	25
Hypomagnesemia	16-48	9-45	34	17
Hypophosphatemia	—	—	49	53
Respiratory				
Atelectasis	5-28	4-30	—	—
Cough increased	—	—	18	15
Dyspnea	5-29	4-23	22	18
Pleural effusion	30-36	32-35	—	—
Skin/Appendages				
Pruritus	15-36	7-20	15	7
Rash	10-24	4-19	17	12
Miscellaneous				
Abdominal pain	29-59	22-54	33	31
Arthralgia	—	—	25	24
Ascites	7-27	8-22	—	—
Asthenia	11-52	7-48	34	30
Back pain	17-30	17-29	24	20
Edema	—	—	18	19
Fever	19-48	22-56	29	29
Infection	—	—	45	49
Pain	24-63	22-57	32	30
Peripheral edema	12-26	14-26	36	48

[1] Data are pooled from separate US and European studies and are not necessarily comparable.
[2] See Precautions or Warnings.

Liver transplant patients – The principal adverse reactions of tacrolimus are tremor, headache, diarrhea, hypertension, nausea, and renal dysfunction. These occur with oral and IV administration and may respond to a reduction in dosing. Diarrhea was sometimes associated with other GI complaints such as nausea and vomiting.

Hyperkalemia, hypomagnesemia, and hyperuricemia have occurred. Hyperglycemia has been noted in many patients; some may require insulin therapy (see Warnings and Precautions).

Kidney transplant patients – The most common adverse reactions reported in kidney transplant patients were infection, tremor, hypertension, decreased renal function, constipation, diarrhea, headache, abdominal pain, and insomnia. The following adverse events were reported in more than 3% and less than 15% incidence in liver or kidney transplant recipients receiving tacrolimus.

➤*Cardiovascular:* Angina pectoris; chest pain; deep thrombophlebitis; abnormal ECG; hemorrhage; hypotension; postural hypotension; peripheral vascular disorder; phlebitis; tachycardia; thrombosis; vasodilation.

➤*CNS:* Abnormal dreams; agitation; amnesia; anxiety; confusion; convulsions; depression; dizziness; emotional lability; encephalopathy; hallucinations; hypertonia; incoordination; myoclonus; nervousness; neuropathy; psychosis; somnolence; thinking abnormal.

➤*Dermatologic:* Acne; alopecia; exfoliative dermatitis; fungal dermatitis; herpes simplex; hirsutism; skin discoloration; skin disorder; skin ulcer; sweating.

➤*Endocrine:* Cushing's syndrome; diabetes mellitus (see Warnings).

➤*GI:* Anorexia; cholangitis; cholestatic jaundice; dyspepsia; dysphasia; esophagitis; flatulence; gastritis; GI hemorrhage; GGT increase; GI perforation; hepatitis; ileus; increased appetite; jaundice; liver damage; liver function test abnormal; oral moniliasis; rectal disorder; stomatitis.

➤*GU:* Albuminuria; cystitis; dysuria; hematuria; hydronephrosis; kidney failure; kidney tubular necrosis; nocturia; pyuria; toxic nephropathy; oliguria; urinary frequency; urinary incontinence; vaginitis.

➤*Hematologic/Lymphatic:* Coagulation disorder; ecchymosis; hypochromic anemia; leukocytosis; leukopenia; polycythemia; prothrombin decreased; serum iron decreased; thrombocytopenia.

➤*Metabolic/Nutritional:* Acidosis; alkaline phosphatase increased; alkalosis; ALT increased; AST increased; bicarbonate decreased; bilirubinemia; BUN increased; dehydration; GGT increased; healing abnormal; hypercalcemia; hypercholesterolemia; hyperlipidemia; hyperphosphatemia; hyperuricemia; hypervolemia; hypocalcemia; hypoglycemia; hypophosphatemia; hyponatremia; hypoproteinemia; lactic dehydrogenase increase; weight gain.

➤*Musculoskeletal:* Arthralgia; cramps; generalized spasm; joint disorder; leg cramps; myalgia; myasthenia; osteoporosis.

➤*Respiratory:* Asthma; bronchitis; cough increased; lung disorder; pneumothorax; pulmonary edema; pharyngitis; pneumonia; respiratory disorder; rhinitis; sinusitis; voice alteration.

➤*Special senses:* Abnormal vision; amblyopia; ear pain; otitis media; tinnitus.

➤*Miscellaneous:* Abdomen enlarged; abscess; accidental injury; allergic reaction; cellulitis; chills; flu syndrome; generalized edema; hernia; peritonitis; photosensitivity reaction; sepsis.

There have been rare spontaneous reports of myocardial hypertrophy associated with clinically manifested ventricular dysfunction in patients receiving tacrolimus therapy.

Postmarketing – The following have been reported: Increased amylase including pancreatitis, hearing loss including deafness, leukoencephalopathy, thrombocytopenic purpura, hemolytic-uremic syndrome, acute renal failure, Stevens-Johnson syndrome, stomach ulcer, glycosuria, cardiac arrhythmia, gastroenteritis.

Overdosage

There is minimal experience with overdosage. Acute overdosages of up to 30 times the intended dose have been reported. Almost all cases have been asymptomatic and all patients recovered with no sequelae. In patients who have received inadvertent overdosage of tacrolimus, no adverse reactions different from those reported in patients receiving therapeutic doses have been described. Follow general supportive measures and systemic treatment in all cases of overdosage. Refer to General Management of Acute Overdosage. Based on the poor aqueous solubility and extensive erythrocyte and plasma protein binding, it is anticipated that tacrolimus is not dialyzable to any significant extent; there is no experience with charcoal hemoperfusion.

Patient Information

Inform patients of the need for repeated appropriate lab tests while they are receiving tacrolimus. Give patients complete dosage instructions, advise them of potential risks during pregnancy and inform them of the increased risk of neoplasia.

Inform patients that changes in dosage should not be undertaken without first consulting their physician.

Inform patients that tacrolimus can cause diabetes mellitus and advise them of the need to see their physician if they develop frequent urination or increased thirst or hunger.

Immunosuppressives

SIROLIMUS

Rx	**Rapamune** (Wyeth Laboratories)	**Tablets:** 1 mg	Sucrose, lactose. (RAPAMUNE 1 mg). White, triangular. In 100s and *Redipak* UD 100s.
		2 mg	Sucrose, lactose. (RAPAMUNE 2 mg) Yellow to beige, triangular. In 100s and *Redipak* 100s.
		Solution, oral: 1 mg/mL	Ethanol. In 60 mL fill with oral syringe adaptor.

WARNING

Increased susceptibility to infection and the possible development of lymphoma may result from immunosuppression. Only physicians experienced in immunosuppressive therapy and management of renal transplant patients should use sirolimus. Manage patients receiving the drug in facilities equipped and staffed with adequate laboratory and supportive medical resources. The physician responsible for maintenance therapy should have complete information needed for the follow-up of the patient.

Liver transplantation-excess mortality, graft loss, and hepatic artery thrombosis (HAT): The use of sirolimus in combination with tacrolimus was associated with excess mortality and graft loss in a study in de novo liver transplant recipients. Many of these patients had evidence of infection at or near the time of death.

In this and another study in de novo liver transplant recipients, the use of sirolimus in combination with cyclosporine or tacrolimus was associated with an increase in HAT; most cases of HAT occurred within 30 days post-transplantation and most led to graft loss or death.

Lung transplantation-bronchial anastomotic dehiscence: Cases of bronchial anastomotic dehiscence, most fatal, have been reported in de novo lung transplant patients when sirolimus has been used as part of an immunosuppressive regimen.

The safety and efficacy of sirolimus as immunosuppressive therapy have not been established in liver or lung transplant patients, and therefore, such use is not recommended.

Indications

►*Organ rejection prophylaxis:* Prophylaxis of organ rejection in patients receiving renal transplants. It is recommended that sirolimus be used initially in a regimen with cyclosporine and corticosteroids. In patients at low to moderate immunological risk, cyclosporine should be withdrawn 2 to 4 months after transplantation and sirolimus dose should be increased to reach recommended blood concentrations.

►*Unlabeled uses:* Treatment of psoriasis.

Administration and Dosage

►*Approved by the FDA:* September 15, 1999.

For oral administration only.

►*Concomitant use with cyclosporine and corticosteroids:* It is recommended that sirolimus be used initially in a regimen with cyclosporine and corticosteroids. It is recommended that sirolimus be taken 4 hours after cyclosporine. Cyclosporine withdrawal is recommended 2 to 4 months after transplantation in patients at low to moderate immunological risk.

►*Sirolimus and cyclosporine combination therapy:* Administer the initial dose as soon as possible after transplantation. For de novo transplant recipients, give a loading dose of sirolimus 3 times the maintenance dose. A daily maintenance dose of 2 mg is recommended for use in renal transplant patients, with a 6 mg loading dose. Although a 5 mg/day maintenance dose with a 15 mg loading dose was found to be safe and effective, no efficacy advantage over the 2 mg dose could be established for renal transplant patients.

►*Sirolimus following cyclosporine withdrawal:* Initially, patients considered for cyclosporine withdrawal should be receiving sirolimus and cyclosporine combination therapy. At 2 to 4 months following transplantation, progressively discontinue cyclosporine over 4 to 8 weeks and adjust the sirolimus dose to obtain whole blood trough concentrations within the range of 12 to 24 ng/mL. Therapeutic drug monitoring should not be the sole basis for adjusting sirolimus therapy. Careful attention should be made to clinical signs/symptoms, tissue biopsy, and laboratory parameters. The sirolimus dose will need to be approximately 4-fold higher to account for both the absence of the pharmacokinetic interaction (approximately 2-fold increase) and the augmented immunosuppressive requirement in the absence of cyclosporine (approximately 2-fold increase).

►*Dosage adjustment:* Frequent sirolimus dose adjustments based on non-steady-state sirolimus concentrations can lead to overdosing or underdosing because sirolimus has a long half-life. Once sirolimus maintenance dose is adjusted, retain patients on the new maintenance dose for at least 7 to 14 days before further dosage adjustment with concentration monitoring. In most patients dose adjustments can be based on simple proportion: new sirolimus dose = current dose × (target concentration/current concentration). Consider a loading dose in addition to a new maintenance dose when it is necessary to considerably increase sirolimus trough concentration: sirolimus loading dose =

3 × (new maintenance dose − current maintenance dose). The maximum sirolimus dose administered on any day should not exceed 40 mg. If an estimated daily dose exceeds 40 mg because of the addition of a loading dose, administer the loading dose over 2 days. Monitor sirolimus trough concentrations for at least 3 to 4 days after a loading dose(s).

►*Patients at least 13 years of age weighing less than 40 kg (88 lbs):* Adjust the initial dosage based on body surface area to 1 mg/m²/day. The loading dose should be 3 mg/m² in this population.

►*Administration:* To minimize the variability of exposure to sirolimus, take this drug consistently with or without food. Grapefruit juice reduces CYP3A4-mediated metabolism of sirolimus and must not be administered with sirolimus or used for dilution.

►*Oral solution:* Two mg of oral solution has been demonstrated to be clinically equivalent to 2 mg oral tablets, making them interchangeable on a milligram-to-milligram basis. However, it is not known if higher doses of oral solution are clinically equivalent to higher doses of tablets on a milligram-to-milligram basis. Patients receiving 2 mg/day oral solution demonstrated an overall better safety profile than did patients receiving 5 mg/day oral solution.

►*Hepatic function impairment:* Reduce the maintenance dose of sirolimus by approximately 33% in patients with hepatic function impairment. It is not necessary to modify the sirolimus loading dose.

►*Blood concentration monitoring:* Whole blood trough concentrations of sirolimus should be monitored in patients receiving concentration-controlled sirolimus. Monitor blood sirolimus levels in pediatric patients, in patients with hepatic function impairment, during coadministration of strong CYP3A4 and/or P-glyco-protein inducers and inhibitors, and/or if cyclosporine dosing is markedly reduced or discontinued. In controlled clinical trials with concomitant cyclosporine, mean sirolimus whole blood trough levels, as measured by immunoassay, were 9 ng/mL for the 2 mg/day treatment group, and 17 ng/mL for the 5 mg/day dose. Results from other assays may differ from those with an immunoassay.

In a controlled trial with cyclosporine withdrawal, the mean sirolimus whole blood trough concentrations during months 4 through 12 following transplantation, as measured by immunoassay, were 10.7 ng/mL in the concomitant sirolimus and cyclosporine treatment group and were 23.3 ng/mL in the cyclosporine withdrawal treatment group.

►*Instructions for dilution and administration of oral solution:*
Bottles – Use the amber oral dose syringe to withdraw the prescribed amount of sirolimus oral solution from the bottle. Empty the correct amount of sirolimus from the syringe into only a glass or plastic container holding at least 2 ounces (¼ cup, 60 mL) of water or orange juice. No other liquids, including grapefruit juice, should be used for dilution. Stir vigorously and drink at once. Refill the container with an additional volume (minimum of 4 ounces [½ cup, 120 mL]) of water or orange juice, stir vigorously, and drink at once.

Pouches – When using the pouch, squeeze the entire contents of the pouch into only a glass or plastic container holding at least 2 ounces (¼ cup, 60 mL) of water or orange juice. No other liquids, including grapefruit juice, should be used for dilution. Stir vigorously and drink at once. Refill the container with an additional volume (minimum of 4 ounces [½ cup, 120 mL]) of water or orange juice, stir vigorously, and drink at once.

►*Storage / Stability:*
Oral solution – Protect oral solution from light. Refrigerate at 2° to 8°C (36° to 46°F). Use the contents within 1 month once the bottle is opened. If necessary, the patient may store the bottles and pouches at room temperature up to 25°C (77°F) for a short period of time (eg, up to 24 hours for the pouches and not more than 15 days for the bottles).

An amber syringe and cap are provided for dosing and the product may be kept in the syringe for a maximum of 24 hours at room temperature up to 25°C (77°F) or refrigerated at 2° to 8°C (36° to 46°F). Discard the syringe after 1 use. After dilution, use the preparation immediately.

Sirolimus oral solution provided in bottles may develop a slight haze when refrigerated. If such a haze occurs, allow the product to stand at room temperature and shake gently until the haze disappears. The presence of this haze does not affect the quality of the product.

Tablets – Store tablets at 20° to 25°C (68° to 77°F). Use cartons to protect blister cards and strips from light. Dispense in a tight, light-resistant container.

Actions

►*Pharmacology:* Sirolimus, a macrolide immunosuppressive agent, inhibits T-lymphocyte activation and proliferation that occurs in response to antigenic and cytokine (interleukin [IL]-2, IL-4, and IL-15)

SIROLIMUS

stimulation and also inhibits antibody production. In cells, sirolimus binds to the immunophilin, FK binding protein-12 (FKBP-12), to generate an immunosuppressive complex. The sirolimus: FKBP-12 complex has no effect on calcineurin activity. This complex binds to and inhibits the activation of the mammalian target of rapamycin (mTOR), a key regulatory kinase. This inhibition suppresses cytokine-driven T-cell proliferation, inhibiting the progression from the G_1 to the S phase of the cell cycle. In some studies, the immunosuppressive effect of sirolimus lasted up to 6 months after discontinuation of therapy. This tolerization effect is alloantigen-specific.

In rodent models of autoimmune disease, sirolimus suppresses immune-mediated events associated with systemic lupus erythematosus, collagen-induced arthritis, autoimmune type 1 diabetes, autoimmune myocarditis, experimental allergic encephalomyelitis, graft-vs-host disease, and autoimmune uveoretinitis.

▶*Pharmacokinetics:*

Absorption – Sirolimus oral solution is rapidly absorbed following oral administration, with a mean time-to-peak concentration of approximately 1 hour after a single dose in healthy subjects and approximately 2 hours after multiple oral doses in renal transplant recipients. The systemic bioavailability of sirolimus oral solution was estimated to be approximately 14%.

The mean bioavailability of sirolimus after administration of the tablet is about 27% higher relative to the oral solution. Sirolimus tablets are not bioequivalent to the oral solution; however, clinical equivalence has been demonstrated at the 2 mg dose level.

Distribution – The mean volume of distribution is 12 ± 7.52 L/kg. Sirolimus is extensively bound (approximately 92%) to human plasma proteins. The binding of sirolimus was shown mainly to be associated with serum albumin (97%), α_1-acid glycoprotein, and lipoproteins. The mean blood-to-plasma ratio of sirolimus was 36 ± 17.9 in stable renal allograft recipients, indicating that sirolimus is extensively partitioned into formed blood elements.

Metabolism – Sirolimus is a substrate for both cytochrome P450 3A4 (CYP3A4) and P-glyco-protein. Sirolimus is extensively metabolized by O-demethylation and/or hydroxylation. Seven major metabolites, including hydroxy, demethyl, and hydroxydemethyl, are identifiable in whole blood. Some of these metabolites are also detectable in plasma, fecal, and urine samples. Glucuronide and sulfate conjugates are not present in any of the biologic matrices. Sirolimus is the major component in human whole blood and contributes to more than 90% of the immunosuppressive activity.

Excretion – After a single dose of sirolimus in healthy volunteers, 91% was recovered from the feces and 2.2% was excreted in urine.

Food effects – A high-fat meal alters the bioavailability of sirolimus (see Drug Interactions).

Special populations –
  Hepatic function impairment: Dosage adjustment is recommended for patients with mild to moderate hepatic impairment (see Administration and Dosage).

Sirolimus (15 mg) was administered as a single oral dose to 18 subjects with normal hepatic function and to 18 patients with Child-Pugh classification A or B hepatic impairment in which hepatic impairment was primary and not related to any underlying systemic disease. The hepatic impairment group had higher mean values for sirolimus AUC (61%) and half-life (43%) and had lower mean values for sirolimus oral dose clearance (CL/F/WT) (33%). The mean half-life increased from 79 ± 12 hours in subjects with normal hepatic function to 113 ± 41 hours in patients with impaired hepatic function. The pharmacokinetics of sirolimus in patients with severe hepatic dysfunction are unknown.

  Renal transplant patients: Pharmacokinetic parameters for sirolimus given daily in combination with cyclosporine and corticosteroids in renal transplant patients are summarized below.

Mean Sirolimus Pharmacokinetic Parameters in Renal Transplant Patients (Multiple Dose)[1]					
Dose	$C_{max, ss}$ (ng/mL)	$T_{max, ss}$ (h)	$AUC_{\tau, ss}$ (ng•h/mL)	CL/F/WT[2] (mL/h/kg)	C_{min} (ng/mL)
Oral solution:					
2 mg (n = 19)	12.2	3.01	158	182	8.9
5 mg (n = 23)	37.4	1.84	396	221	-
Tablets:					
2 mg (n = 13)	15	3.46	230	139	9.5

[1] Sirolimus administered 4 hours after cyclosporine oral solution or cyclosporine capsules.
[2] CL/F/WT = oral dose clearance.

Mean whole blood sirolimus trough concentrations for the 2 and 5 mg/day dose groups were approximately 8.6 ng/mL (n = 226) and 17.3 ng/mL (n = 219), respectively. Whole blood trough sirolimus concentrations were significantly correlated with $AUC_{\tau, ss}$. Upon repeated twice-daily administration without an initial loading dose in a multiple-dose study, the average trough concentration of sirolimus increases approximately 2- to 3-fold over the initial 6 days of therapy at which time steady state is reached. A loading dose of 3 times the main-

tenance dose will provide near-steady-state concentrations within 1 day in most patients. The mean terminal elimination half-life of sirolimus after multiple dosing in stable renal transplant patients was estimated to be 62 ± 16 hours.

Average sirolimus doses and sirolimus whole blood trough concentrations for tablets administered daily in combination with cyclosporine and following cyclosporine withdrawal, in combination with corticosteroids in renal transplant patients are summarized in the table below.

Mean Sirolimus C_{min} Concentrations[1] in Renal Transplant Patients after Tablet Administration (Multiple Dose)				
	Sirolimus with cyclosporine		Sirolimus following cyclosporine withdrawal	
Time	Sirolimus dose (mg/day)	C_{min} (ng/mL)	Sirolimus dose (mg/day)	C_{min} (ng/mL)
4 to 12 months	2.1	10.7	8.2	23.3
12 to 24 months	2	11.2	6.4	22.5

[1] Expressed by immunoassay and equivalence.

The withdrawal of cyclosporine and concurrent increases in sirolimus trough concentrations to steady-state required approximately 6 weeks. Larger sirolimus doses were required because of the absence of the inhibition of sirolimus metabolism and transport by cyclosporine and to achieve higher target concentrations during concentration-controlled administration following cyclosporine withdrawal.

  Pediatric: The table below summarizes pharmacokinetic data obtained in pediatric dialysis patients with chronically impaired renal function.

Mean Sirolimus Pharmacokinetic Parameters in Pediatric Patients with Stable Chronic Renal Failure Maintained on Hemodialysis or Peritoneal Dialysis (1, 3, 9, 15 mg/m² single dose)			
Age group (years)	t_{max} (h)	$t_{1/2}$ (h)	CL/F/WT (mL/h/kg)
5 to 11 (n = 9)	1.1	71	580
12 to 18 (n = 11)	0.79	55	450

  Elderly: Sirolimus trough concentration data in renal transplant patients older than 65 years of age were similar to those in the adult population from 18 to 65 years of age.
  Gender: Sirolimus oral dose clearance in males was 12% lower than that in females; male subjects had a significantly longer half-life than did female subjects (72.3 vs 61.3 hours). Dose adjustments are not recommended.

▶*Clinical trials:*

Oral solution – Two randomized, double-blind, multicenter, controlled studies compared 2 dose levels of sirolimus oral solution (2 and 5 mg once daily) with azathioprine (study 1) or placebo (study 2) when administered in combination with cyclosporine and corticosteroids. Sirolimus, at doses of 2 and 5 mg/day, significantly reduced the incidence of efficacy failure at 6 months following transplantation compared with azathioprine and placebo. The graft and patient survival rates at 1 year were similar in the sirolimus- and comparator-treated patients. The reduction in the incidence of first biopsy-confirmed acute rejection episodes in sirolimus-treated patients compared with the control groups included a reduction in all grades of rejection.

In study 1, efficacy failure was similar for sirolimus 2 mg/day and lower for sirolimus 5 mg/day compared with azathioprine in black patients. In study 2, which was not prospectively stratified by race, efficacy failure was similar for both sirolimus doses compared with placebo in black patients. The decision to use the higher dose of sirolimus in black patients must be weighed against the increased risk of dose-dependent adverse events that were observed with the 5 mg sirolimus dose (see Adverse Reactions).

In both studies, the mean glomerular filtration rate (GFR) at 12 and 24 months (study 1) and 12 and 36 months (study 2) was lower in patients treated with cyclosporine and sirolimus compared with those treated with cyclosporine and the respective azathioprine or placebo control. Within each treatment group in studies 1 and 2, mean GFR at 1 year post-transplant was lower in patients who experienced at least 1 episode of biopsy-proven acute rejection, compared with those who did not.

Contraindications

Hypersensitivity to sirolimus, its derivatives, or any component of the drug product.

Warnings

▶*Interstitial lung disease:* Cases of interstitial lung disease (including pneumonitis, and infrequently bronchiolitis obliterans organizing pneumonia [BOOP] and pulmonary fibrosis), some fatal, have occurred in patients receiving immunosuppressive regimens including sirolimus. In some cases, the interstitial lung disease has resolved upon discontinuation of sirolimus. The risk may be increased as the trough sirolimus concentration increases.

▶*High-risk patients:* The safety and efficacy of cyclosporine withdrawal in high-risk patients have not been adequately studied and it is therefore not recommended. This includes patients with Banff grade III acute rejection or vascular rejection prior to cyclosporine withdrawal,

SIROLIMUS

those who are dialysis-dependent, or with serum creatinine greater than 4.5 mg/dL, black patients, retransplants, multi-organ transplants, or patients with high panel of reactive antibodies.

►*Hepatic artery thrombosis:* In de novo liver transplant recipients, the use of sirolimus in combination with cyclosporine or tacrolimus was associated with an increase in hepatic artery thrombosis. Most cases occurred within 30 days post-transplantation and most led to graft loss or death. The safety and efficacy of sirolimus as immunosuppressive therapy have not been established in liver transplant patients; therefore, such use is not recommended (see Warning box).

►*Infection/Lymphoma/Other malignancies:* Increased susceptibility to infection and the possible development of lymphoma and other malignancies, particularly of the skin, may result from immunosuppression (see Adverse Reactions). Oversuppression of the immune system also can increase susceptibility to infection including opportunistic infections, fatal infections, and sepsis.

As usual for patients with increased risk for skin cancer, exposure to sunlight and UV light should be limited by wearing protective clothing and using a sunscreen with a high protection factor.

►*Lipids:* Increased serum cholesterol and triglycerides that required treatment occurred more frequently in patients treated with sirolimus compared with azathioprine or placebo controls.

In phase III clinical trials in de novo renal transplant recipients who began the study with normal, fasting, total serum cholesterol (fasting serum cholesterol less than 200 mg/dL), there was an increased incidence of patients who developed hypercholesterolemia (fasting serum cholesterol more than 240 mg/dL) in patients receiving both sirolimus 2 and 5 mg compared with azathioprine and placebo controls.

In phase III clinical trials in de novo renal transplant recipients who began the study with normal, fasting, total serum triglycerides (fasting serum triglycerides less than 200 mg/dL), there was an increased incidence of hypertriglyceridemia (fasting serum triglycerides more than 500 mg/dL) in patients receiving sirolimus 2 and 5 mg compared with azathioprine and placebo controls.

Treatment of new-onset hypercholesterolemia with lipid-lowering agents was required in 42% to 52% of patients enrolled in the sirolimus arms of the study compared with 16% of patients in the placebo arm and 22% of patients in the azathioprine arm.

During the prerandomization period of the cyclosporine withdrawal study, mean fasting serum cholesterol and triglyceride values rapidly increased, and peaked at 2 months with mean cholesterol values greater than 240 mg/dL and triglycerides greater than 250 mg/dL. After randomization, mean cholesterol and triglyceride values remained higher in the cyclosporine withdrawal arm compared with the sirolimus and cyclosporine combination.

Renal transplant patients have a higher prevalence of clinically significant hyperlipidemia. Accordingly, carefully consider the risk/benefit in patients with established hyperlipidemia before initiating an immunosuppressive regimen including sirolimus.

Monitor patients who are administered sirolimus for hyperlipidemia using laboratory tests. If hyperlipidemia is detected, initiate subsequent interventions such as diet, exercise, and lipid-lowering agents, as outlined by the National Cholesterol Education Program guidelines.

The coadministration of sirolimus and HMG-CoA reductase inhibitors and/or fibrates appeared to be well tolerated. Monitor all patients administered sirolimus with cyclosporine in conjunction with HMG-CoA reductase inhibitors for the development of rhabdomyolysis and other adverse effects.

►*Concurrent immunosuppressants:* Sirolimus has been administered concurrently with cyclosporine and corticosteroids. The efficacy and safety of the use of sirolimus in combination with other immunosuppressive agents have not been determined.

►*Renal function impairment:* Mean serum creatinine was increased and mean glomerular filtration rate was decreased in patients treated with sirolimus and cyclosporine compared with those treated with cyclosporine and placebo or azathioprine controls. Monitor renal function closely during the administration of sirolimus in combination with cyclosporine since long-term administration can be associated with deterioration of renal function. Consider appropriate adjustment of the immunosuppression regimen, including discontinuation of sirolimus and/or cyclosporine, in patients with elevated or increasing serum creatinine levels. Exercise caution when using agents that are known to impair renal function (eg, aminoglycosides, amphotericin B). In patients at low to moderate immunological risk, continuation of combination therapy with cyclosporine beyond 4 months following transplantation should only be considered when the benefits outweigh the risks of this combination for the individual patients.

►*Carcinogenesis:* In the 86-week female mouse study at dosages of 0, 12.5, 25, and 50/6 mg (dosage lowered from 50 to 6 mg/kg/day at week 31 because of infection secondary to immunosuppression), there was a statistically significant increase in malignant lymphoma at all dosages (approximately 16 to 135 times the clinical doses adjusted for body surface area) compared with controls. In the 104-week rat study at dosages of 0, 0.05, 0.1, and 0.2 mg/kg/day, there was a statistically significant increased incidence of testicular adenoma in the 0.2 mg/kg/day group (approximately 0.4 to 1 times the clinical doses adjusted for body surface area).

Fertility impairment – Reductions in testicular weights and histological lesions (eg, tubular atrophy and tubular giant cells) were observed in rats following dosages of 0.65 mg/kg (approximately 1 to 3 times the clinical doses adjusted for body surface area) and in a study with monkeys at 0.1 mg/kg (approximately 0.4 to 1 times the clinical doses adjusted for body surface area). Sperm counts were reduced in male rats following the administration of sirolimus for 13 weeks at a dosage of 6 mg/kg (approximately 12 to 32 times the clinical doses adjusted for body surface area), but showed improvement by 3 months after dosing was stopped.

►*Pregnancy:* Category C. Sirolimus was embryo- and fetotoxic in rats at dosages of 0.1 mg/kg and above (approximately 0.2 to 0.5 the clinical doses adjusted for body surface area). Embryo- and fetotoxicity was manifested as mortality and reduced fetal weights (with associated delays in skeletal ossification). However, no teratogenesis was evident. In combination with cyclosporine, rats had increased embryofetal mortality compared with sirolimus alone. There are no adequate and well-controlled studies in pregnant women. Effective contraception must be initiated before, during, and for 12 weeks after sirolimus therapy has been discontinued. Use during pregnancy only if the potential benefit outweighs the potential risk to the embryo or fetus.

►*Lactation:* Sirolimus is excreted in trace amounts in the milk of lactating rats. It is not known whether sirolimus is excreted in human milk. The pharmacokinetic and safety profiles of sirolimus in infants are not known. Because of the potential for adverse reactions in nursing infants from sirolimus, decide whether to discontinue nursing or to discontinue the drug, taking into account the importance of the drug to the mother.

►*Children:* The safety and efficacy of sirolimus in pediatric patients below 13 years of age have not been established.

Precautions

►*Monitoring:* Monitor whole blood sirolimus concentrations in patients receiving concentration-controlled sirolimus. Monitoring is also necessary in patients likely to have altered drug metabolism, in patients at least 13 years old who weigh less than 40 kg, in patients with hepatic impairment, and during concurrent administration of potent CYP3A4 inducers and inhibitors.

►*Lymphocele:* Lymphocele, a known surgical complication of renal transplantation, occurred significantly more often in a dose-related fashion in sirolimus-treated patients. Consider appropriate postoperative measures to minimize this complication.

►*Antimicrobial prophylaxis:* Cases of *Pneumocystis carinii* pneumonia have been reported in patients not receiving antimicrobial prophylaxis. Therefore, administer antimicrobial prophylaxis for *P. carinii* pneumonia for 1 year following transplantation. Cytomegalovirus (CMV) prophylaxis is recommended for 3 months after transplantation, particularly for patients at increased risk for CMV disease.

Drug Interactions

►*CYP450 system:* Sirolimus is extensively metabolized by the CYP3A4 isoenzyme in the gut wall and liver. Therefore, absorption and the subsequent elimination of systemically absorbed sirolimus may be influenced by drugs that affect this isoenzyme. Exercise care when concomitantly administering drugs metabolized by CYP3A4 with sirolimus.

Sirolimus Drug Interactions			
Precipitant drug	Object drug*		Description
Cyclosporine	Sirolimus	↑	Sirolimus plasma concentrations may be increased, resulting in increased toxicity. Administer sirolimus 4 hours after cyclosporine to prevent variations in sirolimus concentrations.

SIROLIMUS

Sirolimus Drug Interactions			
Precipitant drug	Object drug*		Description
CYP3A4 inhibitors such as: Bromocriptine Cimetidine Cisapride Clarithromycin Clotrimazole Danazol Erythromycin Fluconazole Itraconazole Metoclopramide Nicardipine Troleandomycin Verapamil Protease inhibitors (eg, ritonavir, indinavir)	Sirolimus	↑	Concomitant use may decrease the metabolism of sirolimus and increase sirolimus levels because of CYP3A4 inhibition.
CYP3A4 inducers such as: Carbamazepine Phenobarbital Phenytoin Rifabutin Rifapentine St. John's Wort	Sirolimus	↓	Concomitant use may increase metabolism of sirolimus decrease sirolimus levels because of CYP3A4 induction.
Diltiazem	Sirolimus	↑	Sirolimus C_{max}, T_{max}, and AUC were increased 1.4-, 1.3-, and 1.6-fold, respectively, following coadministration of sirolimus and diltiazem. If diltiazem is administered, monitor sirolimus; a dose adjustment may be necessary.
Azole antifungal agents	Sirolimus	↑	Plasma sirolimus concentrations may be elevated, increasing the risk of toxicity. Monitor sirolimus plasma concentrations and observe the patient for toxicity when starting or stopping an azole antifungal agent. Adjust the dose of sirolimus as needed.
Rifampin	Sirolimus	↓	Rifampin greatly increased sirolimus oral-dose clearance by 5.5-fold, which represents mean decreases in AUC and C_{max} of about 82% and 71%, respectively. Consider alternative therapeutic agents with less enzyme induction potential where rifampin is indicated.
Sirolimus	Vaccines	↓	Immunosuppressants may affect response to vaccination. Vaccination may be less effective in patients during treatment with sirolimus. Avoid live vaccines.

* ↑ = Object drug increased. ↓ = Object drug decreased.

▶ *Drug / Food interactions:* In 22 healthy volunteers, a high-fat meal (861.8 kcal, 54.9% fat) altered the bioavailability characteristics of sirolimus oral solution. Compared with fasting, a 34% decrease in the peak blood sirolimus concentration (C_{max}), a 3.5-fold increase in the time-to-peak concentration (T_{max}), and a 35% increase in total exposure (AUC) was observed. After administration of sirolimus tablets with a high-fat meal in 24 healthy volunteers, C_{max}, T_{max}, and AUC showed increases of 65%, 32%, and 23%, respectively. To minimize variability, take sirolimus oral solution and tablets consistently with or without food (see Administration and Dosage).

Grapefruit juice reduced CYP3A4-mediated metabolism of sirolimus and must not be used for dilution.

Adverse Reactions

▶ *Oral solution:* Patients maintained on 5 mg/day sirolimus oral solution, when compared with patients on 2 mg/day sirolimus oral solution, demonstrated an increased incidence of the following adverse events: anemia, leukopenia, thrombocytopenia, hypokalemia, hyperlipidemia, fever, diarrhea.

In general, adverse events related to the administration of sirolimus were dependent on dose/concentration.

	Sirolimus Oral Solution Adverse Reactions (≥ 20%)[1]					
	Sirolimus (2 mg/day)		Sirolimus (5 mg/day)		Azathioprine 2 to 3 mg/kg/day	Placebo
Adverse reaction	Study 1 (n = 281)	Study 2 (n = 218)	Study 1 (n = 269)	Study 2 (n = 208)	Study 1 (n = 160)	Study 2 (n = 124)
CNS						
Headache	23	34	27	34	21	31
Insomnia	14	13	22	14	18	8
Tremor	31	21	30	22	28	19
Dermatologic						
Acne	31	22	20	22	17	19
Rash	12	10	13	20	6	6
GI						
Constipation	28	36	34	38	37	31
Abdominal pain	28	29	30	36	29	30
Diarrhea	32	25	42	35	28	27
Dyspepsia	17	23	23	25	24	34
Nausea	31	25	36	31	39	29
Vomiting	21	19	25	25	31	21
Hemic/Lymphatic						
Anemia	27	23	37	33	29	21
Leukopenia	9	9	15	13	20	8
Thrombocytopenia	13	14	20	30	9	9
Metabolic/Nutritional						
Creatinine increase	35	39	37	40	28	38
Edema	24	20	16	18	23	15
Hypercholesterolemia	38	43	42	46	33	23
Hyperkalemia	15	17	12	14	24	27
Hyperlipidemia	38	45	44	57	28	23
Hypokalemia	17	11	21	17	11	9
Hypophosphatemia	20	15	23	19	20	19
Peripheral edema	60	54	64	58	58	48
Weight gain	21	11	15	8	19	15
Respiratory						
Dyspnea	22	24	28	30	23	30
Pharyngitis	17	16	16	21	17	22
Upper respiratory tract infection	20	26	24	23	13	23
Miscellaneous						
Asthenia	38	22	40	28	37	28
Back pain	16	23	26	22	23	20
Chest pain	16	18	19	24	16	19
Fever	27	23	33	34	33	35
Pain	24	33	29	29	30	25
Arthralgia	25	25	27	31	21	18
Urinary tract infection	20	26	23	33	31	26
Hypertension	43	45	39	49	29	48

[1] In any treatment group in prevention of acute renal rejection trials at least 12 months post-transplantation. Patients were additionally receiving cyclosporine and corticosteroids.

With longer term follow-up, the adverse event profile remained similar. Some new events became significantly different among the treatment groups. For events that occurred at a frequency of at least 20% by 24 months for study 1 and 36 months for study 2, only the incidence of edema became significantly higher in both sirolimus groups as compared with the control group. The incidence of headache became significantly more common in the 5 mg/day sirolimus group as compared with control therapy.

Infections – At 24 months for study 1, the following treatment-emergent infections were significantly different among the treatment groups: Bronchitis, herpes simplex, pneumonia, pyelonephritis, upper respiratory infections. In each instance, the incidence was highest in the 5 mg/day sirolimus group, lower in the 2 mg/day sirolimus group, and lowest in the azathioprine group. Except for upper respiratory tract infections in the 5 mg/day sirolimus cohort, the remainder of events occurred with a frequency of less than 20%.

At 36 months in study 2 only the incidence of treatment-emergent herpes simplex was significantly different among the treatment groups, being higher in the 5 mg/day sirolimus group than either of the other groups.

Malignancies – The table below summarizes the incidence of malignancies in the 2 controlled trials for the prevention of acute rejection. At 24 (study 1) and 36 months (study 2) there were no significant differences among treatment groups.

SIROLIMUS

Incidence of Malignancies with Sirolimus Oral Solution in Studies 1 (24 months) and 2 (36 months) Post-transplant (%)[1,2]						
	Sirolimus 2 mg/day		Sirolimus 5 mg/day		Azathioprine 2 to 3 mg/kg/day	Placebo
Malignancy	Study 1 (n = 284)	Study 2 (n = 227)	Study 1 (n = 274)	Study 2 (n = 219)	Study 1 (n = 161)	Study 2 (n = 130)
Lymphoma/ Lympho-proliferative disease	0.7	1.8	1.1	3.2	0.6	0.8
Skin carcinoma						
Any squamous cell[3]	0.4	2.7	2.2	0.9	3.8	3
Any basal cell[3]	0.7	2.2	1.5	1.8	2.5	5.3
Melanoma	0	0.4	0	1.4	0	0
Miscellaneous/ not specified	0	0	0	0	0	0.8
Total	1.1	4.4	3.3	4.1	4.3	7.7
Other malignancy	1.1	2.2	1.5	1.4	0.6	2.3

[1] Patients received cyclosporine and corticosteroids.
[2] Includes patients who prematurely discontinued treatment.
[3] Patients may be counted in more than 1 category.

The overall incidence of malignancy was higher in patients receiving sirolimus plus cyclosporine compared with patients who had cyclosporine withdrawn.

Incidence of Malignancies in Cyclosporine Withdrawal Study at 36 Months Post-transplant (%)[1,2]			
Malignancy	Nonrandomized (n = 95)	Sirolimus with cyclosporine therapy (n = 215)	Sirolimus following cyclosporine withdrawal (n = 215)
Lymphoma/Lympho-proliferative disease	1.1	1.4	0.5
Skin carcinoma			
Any squamous cell[3]	1.1	1.9	2.3
Any basal cell[3]	3.2	4.7	2.3
Melanoma	0	0.5	0
Miscellaneous/not specified	1.1	0.9	0
Total	4.2	6.5	3.7
Other malignancy	1.1	3.3	1.4

[1] Patients received cyclosporine and corticosteroids.
[2] Includes patients who prematurely discontinued treatment.
[3] Patients may be counted in more than 1 category.

Adverse events of at least 3% and less than 20% – Among the adverse events that were reported at a rate of at least 3% and less than 20%, the following were more prominent in patients on 5 mg/day sirolimus vs 2 mg/day sirolimus: Epistaxis, lymphocele, insomnia, thrombotic thrombocytopenic purpura (hemolytic-uremic syndrome), skin ulcer, increased LDH, hypotension, facial edema.

The following adverse events were reported with at least 3% and less than 20% incidence in patients in any sirolimus treatment group in the 2 controlled clinical trials for the prevention of acute rejection:

Cardiovascular: Atrial fibrillation; CHF; hemorrhage; hypervolemia; hypotension; palpitation; peripheral vascular disorder; postural hypotension; syncope; tachycardia; thrombophlebitis; thrombosis; vasodilation.

CNS: Anxiety; confusion; depression; dizziness; emotional lability; hypertonia; hypesthesia; hypotonia; insomnia; neuropathy; paresthesia; somnolence.

Dermatologic: Fungal dermatitis; hirsutism; pruritus; skin hypertrophy; skin ulcer; sweating.

GI: Anorexia; dysphagia; eructation; esophagitis; flatulence; gastritis; gastroenteritis; gingivitis; gum hyperplasia; ileus; mouth ulceration; oral moniliasis; stomatitis.

GU: Albuminuria; bladder pain; dysuria; hematuria; hydronephrosis; impotence; kidney pain; kidney tubular necrosis; nocturia; oliguria; pyelonephritis; pyuria; scrotal edema; testis disorder; toxic nephropathy; urinary frequency; urinary incontinence; urinary retention.

Endocrine: Cushing syndrome; diabetes mellitus; glycosuria.

Hematologic/Lymphatic: Ecchymosis; leukocytosis; lymphadenopathy; polycythemia; thrombotic thrombocytopenic purpura (hemolytic-uremic syndrome).

Metabolic/Nutritional: Acidosis; alkaline phosphatase increased; BUN increased; creatine phosphokinase increased; dehydration; abnormal healing; abnormal liver function tests; hypercalcemia; hyperglycemia; hyperphosphatemia; hypocalcemia; hypoglycemia; hypomagnesemia; hyponatremia; increased LDH; increased ALT; increased AST; weight loss.

Musculoskeletal: Arthrosis; bone necrosis; leg cramps; myalgia; osteoporosis; tetany.

Respiratory: Asthma; atelectasis; bronchitis; increased cough; epistaxis; hypoxia; lung edema; pleural effusion; pneumonia; rhinitis; sinusitis.

Special senses: Abnormal vision; cataract; conjunctivitis; deafness; ear pain; otitis media; tinnitus.

Miscellaneous: Abdomen enlarged; abscess; ascites; cellulitis; chills; face edema; flu syndrome; generalized edema; hernia; herpes zoster infection; lymphocele; malaise; pelvic pain; peritonitis; sepsis.

• *Less frequent adverse events* – Mycobacterial infections, Epstein-Barr virus infections, pancreatitis. There have been rare reports of pancytopenia.

Among the events that were reported at an incidence of at least 3% and less than 20% by 24 months for study 1 and 36 months for study 2, tachycardia and Cushing syndrome were reported significantly more commonly in both sirolimus groups as compared with control therapy. Events that were reported more commonly in the 5 mg/day sirolimus group than either the 2 mg/day sirolimus group and/or control group were the following: Abnormal healing, bone necrosis, chills, CHF, dysuria, hernia, hirsutism, urinary frequency, and lymphadenopathy.

► *Tablets:* The adverse events were similar with the oral solution and the tablets with the exception of acne and hypertonia, which occurred more frequently in the oral solution group, and tremor (particularly in black patients) and diabetes mellitus, which occurred more frequently in the tablet group.

Hispanic patients in the tablet group experienced hyperglycemia more frequently than Hispanic patients in the oral solution group. Menorrhagia, metrorrhagia, and polyuria occurred with an incidence of at least 3% and less than 20%.

► *Sirolimus following cyclosporine withdrawal:* Following randomization (at 3 months) patients who had cyclosporine eliminated from their therapy experienced significantly higher incidences of abnormal liver function tests (including increased AST and increased ALT), hypokalemia, thrombocytopenia, abnormal healing, ileus, and rectal disorder. Conversely, the incidence of hypertension, cyclosporine toxicity, increased creatinine, abnormal kidney function, toxic nephropathy, edema, hyperkalemia, hyperuricemia, and gum hyperplasia was significantly higher in patients who remained on cyclosporine than those who had cyclosporine withdrawn from therapy. Mean systolic and diastolic blood pressure improved significantly following cyclosporine withdrawal. The incidence of herpes zoster infection was significantly lower in patients receiving sirolimus following cyclosporine withdrawal compared with patients who continued to receive sirolimus and cyclosporine.

► *Interstitial lung disease:* Cases of interstitial lung disease (including pneumonitis, and infrequently BOOP and pulmonary fibrosis), some fatal, have occurred in patients receiving immunosuppressive regimens including sirolimus. In some cases, the interstitial lung disease has resolved upon discontinuation of sirolimus. The risk may be increased as the trough sirolimus concentration increases.

► *Miscellaneous:* Hepatotoxicity has been reported, including fatal hepatic necrosis with elevated sirolimus trough levels. Abnormal healing following transplant surgery has been reported, including fascial dehiscence and anastomotic disruption (eg, wound, vascular, airway, ureteral, biliary).

Overdosage

Reports of overdose with sirolimus have been received; however, experience has been limited. In general, the adverse effects of overdose are consistent with those listed in the Adverse Reactions section.

Follow general supportive measures in all cases of overdose. Based on the poor aqueous solubility and high erythrocyte and plasma protein binding of sirolimus, it is anticipated that sirolimus is not dialyzable to any significant extent. In mice and rats, the acute oral lethal dose was greater than 800 mg/kg.

Patient Information

Give patients complete dosage instructions (see Patient Instructions). Inform women of childbearing potential to use effective contraception prior to the initiation of sirolimus therapy, during therapy, and for 12 weeks after sirolimus therapy has been discontinued because of potential risk during pregnancy (see Warnings).

Tell patients that exposure to sunlight and UV light should be limited by wearing protective clothing and using a sunscreen with a high protection factor because of the increased risk for skin cancer.

INTERFERON ALFA-2a, RECOMBINANT (rIFN-A; IFLrA)

Rx	**Roferon-A** (Hoffman La-Roche)	**Prefilled syringes:** 3 million IU/syringe[1]	In 0.5 mL single-use, prefilled syringes. In 1s and 6s.
		6 million IU/syringe[1]	In 0.5 mL single-use, prefilled syringes. In 1s and 6s.
		9 million IU/syringe[1]	In 0.5 mL single-use, prefilled syringes. In 1s and 6s.

[1] With NaCl, polysorbate 80, benzyl alcohol, and ammonium acetate.

WARNING

Alpha interferons, including interferon alfa-2a, recombinant, cause or aggravate fatal or life-threatening neuropsychiatric, autoimmune, ischemic, and infectious disorders. Closely monitor patients with periodic clinical and laboratory evaluations. Withdraw patients with persistently severe or worsening signs or symptoms of these conditions from therapy. In many, but not all cases, these disorders resolve after stopping interferon alfa-2a, recombinant therapy (see Warnings and Adverse Reactions.

Indications

➤*Chronic hepatitis C:* In select patients 18 years of age and older.

➤*Hairy cell leukemia:* In select patients 18 years of age and older.

➤*AIDS-related Kaposi's sarcoma:* In select patients 18 years of age and older.

➤*Chronic myelogenous leukemia (CML):* In chronic phase, Philadelphia chromosome (Ph)-positive CML patients who are minimally pretreated (within 1 year of diagnosis).

➤*Unlabeled uses:* Bladder tumors, mycosis fungoides, essential thrombocythemia, non-Hodgkin's lymphoma, ovarian and cervical cancer, renal cell carcinoma, melanoma.

Administration and Dosage

➤*Approved by the FDA:* 1986.

The route of administration for the vial is SC or IM; the route of administration for the prefilled syringe is SC only. SC administration is suggested for, but not limited to, patients who are thrombocytopenic (platelet count less than 50,000/mm³) or who are at risk for bleeding.

➤*Chronic hepatitis C:* The recommended dosage is 3 million IU 3 times/week administered SC or IM for 12 months (48 to 52 weeks). As an alternative, patients may be treated with an induction dose of 6 million IU 3 times/week for the first 3 months (12 weeks) followed by 3 million IU 3 times/week for 9 months (36 weeks). Normalization of serum ALT generally occurs within a few weeks after initiation of treatment in responders. Approximately 90% of patients who respond to interferon alfa-2a do so within the first 3 months of treatment; however, patients responding to interferon alfa-2a with a reduction in ALT should complete 12 months of treatment. Patients who have no response to interferon alfa-2a within the first 3 months of therapy are not likely to respond with continued treatment; consider treatment discontinuation in these patients.

Patients who tolerate and partially or completely respond to therapy with interferon alfa-2a but relapse following its discontinuation may be retreated. Consider retreatment with either 3 million IU 3 times/week or with 6 million IU 3 times/week for 6 to 12 months.

Temporary dose reduction by 50% is recommended in patients who do not tolerate the prescribed dose. If adverse events resolve, treatment with the original prescribed dose can be re-initiated. In patients who cannot tolerate the reduced dose, cessation of therapy, at least temporarily, is recommended.

➤*Hairy cell leukemia:*

Induction dose – 3 million IU daily for 16 to 24 weeks, SC or IM.

Maintenance dose – 3 million IU 3 times/week. Dosage reduction by 50% or withholding of individual doses may be needed when severe adverse reactions occur. The use of doses more than 3 million IU is not recommended.

Patients with hairy cell leukemia have been treated for up to 24 consecutive months. The optimal duration of treatment for this disease has not been determined.

➤*AIDS-related Kaposi's sarcoma:*

Induction dose – 36 million IU daily for 10 to 12 weeks, administered IM or SC.

Maintenance dose – 36 million IU, 3 times/week. An escalating schedule of 3, 9, and 18 million IU daily for 3 days followed by 36 million IU daily for the remainder of the 10- to 12-week induction period also has produced equivalent therapeutic benefit with some amelioration of the acute toxicity in some patients.

If severe reactions occur, modify dosage (50% reduction) or temporarily discontinue therapy until the adverse reactions abate.

➤*CML:*

Chronic phase Ph-positive CML – Prior to initiation of therapy, make a diagnosis of Ph-positive CML in chronic phase by the appropriate peripheral blood, bone marrow, and other diagnostic testing. Regularly monitor hematologic parameters (eg, monthly). Because

significant cytogenic changes are not readily apparent until after hematologic response has occurred, and usually not until several months of therapy have elapsed, cytogenic monitoring may be performed at less frequent intervals. Achievement of complete cytogenic response has been observed up to 2 years following the start of interferon alfa-2a treatment.

Induction dose – 9 million IU daily administered SC or IM. Based on clinical experience, short-term tolerance may be improved by gradually increasing the dose of interferon alfa-2a over the first week of administration from 3 million IU daily for 3 days to 6 million IU daily for 3 days to the target dose of 9 million IU daily for the duration of the treatment period.

Maintenance – Optimal dose and duration of therapy have not been determined.

Even though the median time to achieve a complete hematologic response was 5 months in clinical studies, hematologic responses have been observed up to 18 months after starting treatment. Continue therapy until disease progression. If severe side effects occur, a treatment interruption or reduction in either the dose or the frequency of injections may be necessary to achieve the individual maximally tolerated dose.

Children – Limited data are available on the use of interferon alfa-2a in children with CML. In one report of 15 children with Ph-positive, adult-type CML, doses between 2.5 to 5 million IU/m²/day given IM were tolerated. In another study, severe adverse effects including death were noted in children with previously untreated Ph-negative juvenile CML who received interferon doses of 30 million IU/m²/day.

➤*Storage/Stability:* Refrigerate the injection solution and prefilled syringes at 2° to 8°C (36° to 46°F). Do not freeze; do not shake.

Actions

➤*Pharmacology:* Interferon alfa-2a is a sterile protein product manufactured by recombinant DNA technology that employs a genetically engineered *Escherichia coli* bacterium. Interferon alfa-2a is a highly purified protein containing 165 amino acids.

The mechanism by which interferons exert antitumor or antiviral activity is not clearly understood. However, direct antiproliferative action against tumor cells and modulation of the host immune response may play important roles.

Using human cells in culture, interferon alfa-2a has antiproliferative and immunomodulatory activities that are very similar to those of the mixture of interferon alfa subtypes produced by human leukocytes. In vivo, interferon alfa-2a inhibits the growth of several human tumors growing in immunocompromised mice.

➤*Pharmacokinetics:*

Absorption/Distribution – In healthy people, interferon alfa-2a exhibited an elimination half-life of 3.7 to 8.5 hours (mean, 5.1 hours), volume of distribution at steady state of 0.223 to 0.748 L/kg (mean, 0.4 L/kg) and a total body clearance of 2.14 to 3.62 mL/min/kg (mean, 2.79 mL/min/kg) after a 36 million IU (2.2 x 10⁸ pg) IV infusion. After IM and SC administrations of 36 million IU, peak serum concentrations ranged from 1500 to 2580 pg/mL (mean, 2020 pg/mL) at a mean time to peak of 3.8 hours and from 1250 to 2320 pg/mL (mean, 1730 pg/mL) at a mean time to peak of 7.3 hours, respectively. The serum concentrations of interferon alfa-2a reflected a large intersubject variation. Dose proportional increases in serum concentrations were observed after single doses up to 198 million IU. There were no changes in the distribution or elimination of interferon alfa-2a during twice daily (0.5 to 36 million IU), once daily (1 to 54 million IU) or 3 times weekly (1 to 136 million IU) dosing regimens up to 28 days of dosing. Multiple IM doses resulted in accumulation of 2 to 4 times the single dose serum concentrations. The apparent fraction of the dose absorbed after IM injection was greater than 80%.

Metabolism/Excretion – Alpha interferons are filtered through the glomeruli and undergo rapid proteolytic degradation during tubular reabsorption, rendering a negligible reappearance of intact alpha interferon in the systemic circulation, suggesting near-complete reabsorption of interferon alfa-2a catabolites. Liver metabolism and subsequent biliary excretion are minor pathways of elimination.

➤*Clinical trials:*

Hairy cell leukemia – During the first 1 to 2 months of treatment, significant depression of hematopoiesis was likely to occur. Subsequently, there was improvement in circulating blood cell counts.

Of the 75 patients evaluated for at least 16 weeks of therapy, 46 (61%) achieved complete or partial response. Twenty-one patients (28%) had a minor remission, 8 (11%) remained stable and none had worsening of disease. All patients who achieved either a complete or partial response had complete or partial normalization of all peripheral blood elements with a concomitant decrease in peripheral blood and bone marrow

INTERFERON ALFA-2a, RECOMBINANT (rIFN-A; IFLrA)

hairy cells. Responding patients also exhibited a marked reduction in red blood cell and platelet transfusion requirements, a decrease in infectious episodes, and improvement in performance status. The probability of survival for 2 years in patients receiving interferon alfa-2a (94%) was statistically increased compared with a historical control group (75%).

AIDS-related Kaposi's sarcoma – Doses of 3 to 54 million IU daily were evaluated in more than 350 patients. An additional 91 patients received interferon alfa-2a in combination with vinblastine. The best response rate associated with acceptable toxicity was observed when interferon alfa-2a was administered as a single agent at a dose of 36 million IU daily. The escalating regimen of 3 to 36 million IU provided equivalent therapeutic benefit with some amelioration of acute toxicity in some patients. Lower doses were less effective in inducing tumor regression and doses higher than 36 million IU daily were associated with unacceptable toxicity.

The likelihood of response to interferon alfa-2a varies with the clinical manifestations of human immunodeficiency virus (HIV) infection. Patients with prior opportunistic infection or B symptoms (eg, night sweats, weight loss greater than 10% of body weight or 15 lbs, fever greater than 100°F without identifiable source of infection) are unlikely to respond to treatment.

Patients who were otherwise asymptomatic, with no prior opportunistic infection and near-normal levels of CD4 lymphocytes, experienced higher response rates. Responding patients with a baseline CD4 lymphocyte count greater than 200 cells/mm^3 had a distinct survival advantage over both responding patients with a baseline CD4 lymphocyte count of 200 cells/mm^3 or less and nonresponding patients regardless of their baseline CD4 lymphocyte count.

The median time to response was 2.7 months. The median duration of response for patients achieving a partial or complete response was 6.3 and 20.7 months, respectively. Complete and partial responses lasting in excess of 3 years have been observed.

Contraindications

Hypersensitivity to alfa interferon or any component of the product.

Warnings

➤*Administration:* Administer interferon alfa-2a under the guidance of a qualified physician (see Administration and Dosage). Appropriate management of the therapy and its complication is possible only when adequate facilities are readily available.

➤*Depression / Suicidal behavior:* Depression and suicidal behavior including suicidal ideation, suicidal attempts, and suicides have been reported in association with treatment with alfa interferons, including interferon alfa-2a. Inform patients to be treated with interferon alfa-2a that depression and suicidal ideation may be side effects of treatment and advise them to report these side effects immediately to the prescribing physician. Patients receiving interferon alfa-2a therapy should receive close monitoring for the occurrence of depressive symptomatology. Consider cessation of treatment for patients experiencing depression. Although dose reduction or treatment cessation may lead to resolution of the depressive symptomatology, depression may persist and suicides have occurred after withdrawing therapy.

➤*GI hemorrhage:* Infrequently, severe or fatal GI hemorrhage has been reported in association with alfa interferon therapy.

➤*Special patient populations:* Use with caution in patients with severe renal or hepatic disease, seizure disorders, or compromised CNS function.

Administer with caution to patients with cardiac disease or with any history of cardiac illness. Acute, self-limited toxicities (ie, fever, chills) frequently associated with interferon alfa administration may exacerbate preexisting cardiac conditions. Rarely, MI has occurred.

➤*Autoimmune disease:* Do not treat patients with a history of autoimmune hepatitis or a history of autoimmune disease or immunosuppressed transplant recipients with interferon alfa-2a. Controlled studies of interferon alfa-2a therapy in patients with advanced cirrhosis and/or decompensated liver disease have not been performed. In chronic hepatitis C, initiation of alfa-interferon therapy, including interferon alfa-2a, has been reported to cause transient liver abnormalities, which in patients with poorly compensated liver disease can result in increased ascites, hepatic failure, or death.

Rare cases of autoimmune diseases including thrombocytopenia, vasculitis, Raynaud's phenomenon, rheumatoid arthritis, lupus erythematosus, and rhabdomyolysis have been observed in patients treated with alpha interferons. Closely monitor any patient developing an autoimmune disorder during treatment and, if appropriate, discontinue treatment.

➤*CNS reactions:* CNS reactions have occurred in a number of patients and included decreased mental status, dizziness, impaired memory, agitation, manic behavior, and psychotic reactions. More severe obtundation and coma have been rarely observed. Most of these were mild and reversible within a few days to 3 weeks upon dose reduc-

tion or drug discontinuation. Careful periodic neuropsychiatric monitoring of all patients is recommended.

➤*Leukopenia and elevation of hepatic enzymes:* Leukopenia and elevation of hepatic enzymes occurred frequently but were rarely dose-limiting. Thrombocytopenia occurred less frequently. Proteinuria and increased cells in urinary sediment also were seen infrequently.

➤*Bone marrow toxicity:* Alpha interferons suppress bone marrow function and may result in severe cytopenias including very rare events of aplastic anemia. It is advised that complete blood counts (CBC) be obtained pretreatment and monitored routinely during therapy. Discontinue alpha interferon therapy in patients who develop severe decreases in neutrophil (less than 0.5 × 10^9/L) or platelet counts (less than 25 × 10^9/L).

➤*Myelosuppression:* Exercise caution when administering interferon alfa-2a to patients with myelosuppression or when interferon alfa-2a is used in combination with other agents that are known to cause myelosuppression. Synergistic toxicity has been observed when interferon alfa-2a is administered in combination with zidovudine (AZT). The effects of interferon alfa-2a when combined with other drugs used in the treatment of AIDS-related disease are not known.

➤*Hyperglycemia:* Hyperglycemia has been observed rarely in patients treated with interferon alfa-2a. Symptomatic patients should have their blood glucose measured and followed-up accordingly. Patients with diabetes mellitus may require adjustment of their antidiabetic regimen.

➤*Visceral AIDS-related Kaposi's sarcoma:* Do not use interferon alfa-2a for the treatment of visceral AIDS-related Kaposi's sarcoma associated with rapidly progressive or life-threatening disease.

➤*Neutralizing antibodies:* Serum neutralizing activity, determined by a highly sensitive enzyme immunoassay, and a neutralization bioassay, was detected in approximately 25% of all patients who received interferon alfa-2a. Antibodies to human leukocyte interferon may occur spontaneously in certain clinical conditions (cancer, systemic lupus erythmatosus, herpes zoster) in patients who have never received exogenous interferon.

➤*Renal / Hepatic function impairment:* Dose-limiting hepatic or renal toxicities are unusual. Severe renal toxicities, sometimes requiring renal dialysis, have been reported.

➤*Pregnancy:* Category C. Safety in pregnancy has not been established. Use during pregnancy only if the potential benefit justifies the potential risk to the fetus. Fertile women should not receive interferon alfa-2a unless they are using effective contraception during therapy.

The injectable solution contains benzyl alcohol. The excipient benzyl alcohol can be transmitted via the placenta. The possibility of toxicity should be taken into account in premature infants after the administration of interferon alfa-2a solution for injection immediately prior to birth or Cesarean section.

➤*Lactation:* It is not known whether this drug is excreted in breast milk. Because of the potential for serious adverse reactions in nursing infants, decide whether to discontinue nursing or to discontinue the drug, taking into account the importance of the drug to the mother.

➤*Children:* Safety and efficacy in children below 18 years of age have not been established.

Use of interferon alfa-2a in children with Ph-positive adult-type CML is supported by evidence from adequate and well-controlled studies of interferon alfa-2a in adults with additional data from the literature on the use of alfa interferon in children with CML. A published report on 15 children with Ph-positive adult-type CML suggests a safety profile similar to that seen in adult CML; clinical responses were also observed.

The injectable solutions are not indicated for use in neonates or infants and should not be used by patients in that age group. There have been rare reports of death in neonates and infants associated with excessive exposure to benzyl alcohol.

Precautions

➤*Monitoring:* Prior to initiation of therapy, perform tests to quantitate peripheral blood hemoglobin, platelets, granulocytes, hairy cell, and bone marrow hairy cells. Monitor periodically (eg, monthly) during treatment to determine response to treatment. If a patient does not respond within 6 months, discontinue treatment. If a response occurs, continue treatment until no further improvement is observed and these laboratory parameters have been stable for about 3 months.

Perform periodic complete blood with differential platelet counts and clinical chemistry tests. Perform prior to therapy and at appropriate periods during therapy. Because responses of hairy cell leukemia, AIDS-related Kaposi's sarcoma, chronic hepatitis C, and CML are not generally observed for 1 to 3 months after initiation of treatment, very careful monitoring for severe depression of blood cell counts is warranted during the initial phase of treatment.

For patients being treated for chronic hepatitis C, serum ALT should be evaluated before therapy to establish baselines and repeated at week 2 and monthly thereafter following initiation of therapy for monitoring clinical response. Patients with neutrophil count less than 1500/mm^3,

INTERFERON ALFA-2a, RECOMBINANT (rIFN-A; IFLrA)

platelet count less than 75,000/mm³, hemoglobin less than 10 g/dL and creatinine greater than 1.5 mg/dL were excluded from several major chronic hepatitis C studies; patients with these laboratory abnormalities should be carefully monitored if treated with interferon alfa-2a.

Patients with pre-existing thyroid abnormalities may be treated if normal thyroid stimulating hormone (TSH) levels can be maintained by medication. Testing of TSH levels in these patients is recommended at baseline and every 3 months following initiation of therapy.

Cardiovascular – Those patients who have preexisting cardiac abnormalities or who are in advanced stages of cancer should have ECGs taken prior to and during the course of treatment.

►*Benzyl alcohol:* The injectable solutions contain benzyl alcohol and should not be used by patients with a known allergy to benzyl alcohol. This product is not indicated for use in neonates or infants and should not be used by patients in that age group. There have been rare reports of death in neonates and infants associated with excessive exposure to benzyl alcohol. There have been reports of permanent neuropsychiatric deficits and multiple system organ failure associated with benzyl alcohol in neonates and infants. The amount of benzyl alcohol at which toxicity or adverse effects may occur in neonates or infants is not known.

Drug Interactions

Interferon alfa-2a Drug Interactions		
Precipitant drug	Object drug*	Description
Interferon alfa-2a	Theophylline ↑	Reduced clearance of theophylline following coadministration has been reported.
Interferon alfa-2a	Neurotoxic, hematotoxic or cardiotoxic drugs ↑	Effects of previously or coadministered drugs may be increased by interferons.
Interferon alfa-2a	Interleukin-2 ↑	Potential risk of renal failure.
Interferon alfa-2a	CNS drugs ↔	Interactions could occur following coadministration of centrally acting drugs.

* ↑ = Object drug increased. ↔ = Undetermined clinical effect.

►*Other interactions:* Alfa-interferons may affect the oxidative metabolic process by reducing the activity of hepatic microsomal cytochrome enzymes in the P-450 group. Although the clinical relevance is still unclear, take into account when prescribing concomitant therapy with drugs metabolized by this route.

Adverse Reactions

The physician must evaluate the need and usefulness of the drug against the risk of adverse reactions. Most adverse reactions are reversible if detected early. If severe reactions occur, reduce dosage or discontinue the drug and take appropriate corrective measures according to the clinical judgment of the physician. Reinstitute interferon alfa-2a therapy with caution and with adequate consideration of the further need for the drug and alertness to possible recurrence of toxicity.

►*Chronic hepatitis C (most frequent adverse reactions associated with 3 million IU dose):*
CNS – Headache (52%); depression (16%); irritability (15%); insomnia (14%); dizziness (13%); paresthesia, confusion (7%); anxiety (5%); concentration impaired (4%); change in taste or smell, behavior disturbances (3%).

Dermatologic – Injections site reaction (29%); partial alopecia (19%); rash (8%); dry skin or pruritus (7%); hematoma (1%); psoriasis, cutaneous eruptions, eczema, seborrhea (less than 1%).

GI – Nausea/vomiting (33%); diarrhea (20%); anorexia (14%); abdominal pain (12%); flatulence, liver pain (3%); digestion impaired, gingival bleeding (2%).

Respiratory – Dryness or inflammation of oropharynx (6%); epistaxis (4%); rhinitis (3%); sinusitis (less than 1%).

Miscellaneous – Conjunctivitis (4%); menstrual irregularity (2%); arrhythmia (1%); visual acuity decreased (less than 1%).
Flu-like symptoms: Fatigue (58%); myalgia/arthralgia (51%); flu-like symptoms (33%); fever (28%); chills (23%); asthenia (6%); sweating (5%); leg cramps (3%); malaise (1%).
Other: Patients receiving 6 million IU 3 times/week experienced a higher incidence of severe psychiatric events (9%) than those receiving 3 million IU 3 times/week (6%) in 2 large US studies. In addition, more patients withdrew from these studies when receiving 6 million IU 3 times/week (11%) than when receiving 3 million IU 3 times/week (7%). Up to 50% of patients receiving 3 million IU or 6 million IU 3 times/week withdrawing from the study experienced depression or other psychiatric adverse events. At higher doses, anxiety, sleep disorders, and irritability were observed more frequently. An increased incidence of fatigue, myalgia/arthralgia, headache, fever, chills, alopecia, sleep disturbances and dry skin or pruritus was also generally observed during treatment with higher doses of interferon alfa-2a.

Generally there were fewer adverse events reported in the second 6 months of treatment than in the first 6 months for patients treated with 3 million IU 3 times/week. Patients tolerant of initial therapy with interferon alfa-2a generally tolerate retreatment at the same dose, but tend to experience more adverse reactions at higher doses.

Infrequent adverse events (greater than 1% but less than 3% incidence) included the following: Cold feeling, cough, muscle cramps, diaphoresis, dyspnea, eye pain, reactivation of herpes simplex, lethargy, edema, sexual dysfunction, shaking, skin lesions, stomatitis, tooth disorder, urinary tract infection, weakness in extremities.

►*Hairy cell leukemia:*
Cardiovascular – Chest pain, edema, hypertension (11%).

CNS – Dizziness (21%); depression (16%); paresthesia, numbness (12%); sleep disturbance, decreased mental status (10%); anxiety, lethargy, visual disturbance (6%); confusion (5%).

Dermatologic – Skin rash (44%); diaphoresis (22%); partial alopecia, dry skin (17%); pruritus (13%).

GI – Anorexia (43%); nausea/vomiting (39%); diarrhea (34%); throat irritation (21%).

Musculoskeletal – Joint or bone pain (25%); arthritis or polyarthritis (5%).

Respiratory – Coughing (16%); dyspnea, rhinorrhea (12%); pneumonia, sinusitis (11%).

Miscellaneous – Generalized pain (24%); back pain (16%).
Flu-like syndrome: Fever (92%); fatigue (86%); myalgia (71%); headache (64%); chills (64%); weight loss (33%); flu-like symptoms (16%).
Other: Gait disturbance, nervousness, syncope, vertigo, cardiac murmur, thrombophlebitis, hypotension (less than 5%); ecchymosis, epistaxis, bleeding gums, petechiae, urticaria, inflammation at injection site (rare).

►*AIDS-related Kaposi's sarcoma:*
CNS – Dizziness (40%); decreased mental status (17%); depression (16%); paresthesia, confusion (8%); diaphoresis (7%); sleep disturbance, visual disturbance (5%); numbness (3%).

Dermatologic – Partial alopecia (22%); rash (11%); dry skin or pruritus (5%).

GI – Anorexia (65%); nausea (51%); diarrhea (42%); emesis (17%); abdominal pain (15%).

Respiratory – Coughing (27%); dryness or inflammation of oropharynx (14%); dyspnea (11%); chest pain, rhinorrhea (4%).

Miscellaneous – Weight loss, taste perversion (25%); edema (9%); night sweats (8%); hypotension (4%).
Flu-like symptoms: Fatigue (95%); fever (74%); myalgia (69%); headache (66%); chills (41%); arthralgia (24%).
Other: Anxiety, nervousness, emotional lability, vertigo, forgetfulness, cardiac palpitations, arrhythmia, sinusitis, constipation, chest congestion, pneumonia, urticaria, flatulence (less than 3%); ataxia, seizures, cyanosis, gastric distress, bronchospasm, pain at injection site, earache, eye irritation, rhinitis (less than 1%); poor coordination, lethargy, muscle contractions, neuropathy, tremor, involuntary movements, syncope, aphasia, aphonia, dysarthria, amnesia, weakness, flushing of skin (less than 0.5%); cardiomyopathy (rare).

►*CML:*
CNS – Headache (44%); depression (28%); decreased mental status (16%); dizziness, sleep disturbances (11%); paresthesia (8%); involuntary movements (7%); visual disturbances (6%).

Dermatologic – Hair changes (including alopecia), skin rash (18%); sweating (15%); dry skin, pruritus (7%).

GI – Anorexia (48%); nausea, vomiting, diarrhea (37%).

Miscellaneous – Coughing (19%); dyspnea (8%); dysrhythmia (7%).
Flu-like syndrome: Fever (92%); asthenia, fatigue (88%); myalgia (68%); chills (63%); arthralgia/bone pain (47%); headache (44%).
Other: Chest pain, syncope, hypotension, impotence, alterations in taste or hearing, confusion, seizures, memory loss, disturbances of libido, bruising, coagulopathy (less than 4%); Coombs positive hemolytic anemia, aplastic anemia, hypothyroidism, cardiomyopathy, hypertriglyceridemia, bronchospasm (rare).

►*Other infrequent adverse events:* Pancreatitis, colitis, GI hemorrhage, stomatitis, thyroid dysfunction (including hypothyroidism and hyperthyroidism), diabetes (in some patients requiring insulin therapy), and pneumonitis (some cases responding to interferon cessation and corticosteroid therapy) (less than 5%); autoimmune diseases (eg, vasculitis, arthritis, hemolytic anemia, lupus erythematosus syndrome) (less than 3%); abdominal fullness, hypermotility, hepatitis, gait disturbance, hallucinations, encephalopathy, psychomotor retardation, coma, stroke, transient ischemic attacks, dysphasia, sedation, apathy, irritability, hyperactivity, claustrophobia, loss of libido, CHF, MI, Raynaud phenomenon, hot flashes, tachypnea, ischemic retinopathy, excessive salivation, and anaphylactic reactions (less than 1%).

INTERFERON ALFA-2a, RECOMBINANT (rIFN-A; IFLrA)

➤*Abnormal laboratory test values:*

	Chronic hepatitis C (3 million IU 3 times/week) (n = 203)	CML[1]		Hairy cell leukemia (n = 218)	AIDS-related Kaposi sarcoma (n = 241)
Abnormality		US study (n = 91)	Non-US study (n = 219)		
Leukopenia	1.5	20	3	45[2]	49
Neutropenia	10	22	0	68[2]	52
Thrombocytopenia	4.5	27	5	62[2]	35
Anemia (Hb)	0	15	4	31[2]	27
AST	NAP	5	1	9	46
Alkaline phosphatase	0	3	1	3	11
LDH	NAP	NA	NA	< 1	10
Proteinuria	0	NA	NA	10[3]	< 1

Significant Abnormal Laboratory Test Values (%)

NAP = not applicable.   NA = not assessed.
[1] Patients enrolled in the 2 clinical studies receiving at least 1 dose of interferon alfa-2a.
[2] In the majority of patients, initial hematologic laboratory test values were abnormal because of their underlying disease.
[3] Ten percent of the patients experienced a proteinuria of more than 1+ at least once.

Chronic hepatitis C: The incidence of neutropenia (WHO grades III or IV) was over twice as high in those treated with 6 million IU 3 times/week (21%) as those treated with 3 million IU 3 times/week (10%).

CML: In the 2 clinical studies, a severe or life-threatening anemia was seen in up to 15% of patients. A severe or life-threatening leukopenia and thrombocytopenia were observed in up to 20% and 27% of patients, respectively. Changes were usually reversible when therapy was discontinued. One case of aplastic anemia and one case of Coombs positive hemolytic anemia were seen in 310 patients treated with interferon alfa-2a in clinical studies. Severe cytopenias led to discontinuation of therapy in 4% of all interferon alfa-2a treated patients.

Transient increases in liver transaminases or alkaline phosphatase of any intensity were seen in up to 50% of patients during treatment with interferon alfa-2a. Only 5% of patients had a severe or life-threatening increase in AST. In the clinical studies, such abnormalities required termination of therapy in less than 1% of patients.

Hairy cell leukemia: Increases in serum phosphorus (1.6 mmol/L or more) and serum uric acid (9.1 mg/dL or more) were observed in 9% and 10% of patients, respectively. The increase in serum uric acid is likely to be related to underlying disease. Decreases in serum calcium (1.9 mmol/L or less) and serum phosphorus (0.9 mmol/L or less) were seen in 28% and 22% of patients, respectively.

Overdosage

There are no reports of overdosage, but repeated large doses of interferon can be associated with profound lethargy, fatigue, prostration, and coma. Such patients should be hospitalized for observation and appropriate supportive treatment given.

Patient Information

Patient package insert is available with product.

Thoroughly instruct patients in the importance of proper disposal procedures and caution them against reusing syringes and needles. If home use is prescribed, supply the patient with a puncture-resistant container for the disposal of used syringes and needles. Instruct patients to dispose of the full container according to directions provided by the physician.

Caution patients receiving high-dose alfa interferon against performing tasks that require complete mental alertness, such as operating machinery or driving a motor vehicle.

Inform patients treated with interferon alfa-2a that depression and suicidal ideation may be side effects of treatment and advise them to report these side effects immediately to the prescribing physician.

Warn patients not to change brands of interferon; changes in dosage may result.

Hydrate patients well, especially during initial treatment.

PEGINTERFERON ALFA-2a

Rx   **Pegasys** (Roche)   **Injection:** 180 mcg   In 1 mL single-use vials[a] and 0.5 mL prefilled syringes.[b] Available in vial[c] and prefilled syringe[d] monthly convenience packs.

[a] With 8 mg sodium chloride, 0.05 mg polysorbate 80, and 10 mg benzyl alcohol.
[b] With 4 mg sodium chloride, 0.025 mg polysorbate 80, and 5 mg benzyl alcohol.

[c] Contains 4 single-use vials, four 1 mL syringes with needles, and 8 alcohol swabs.
[d] Contains 4 single-use prefilled syringes, 4 needles, and 4 alcohol swabs.

WARNING

Alpha interferons, including peginterferon alfa-2a, may cause or aggravate fatal or life-threatening neuropsychiatric, autoimmune, ischemic, and infectious disorders. Closely monitor patients with periodic clinical and laboratory evaluations. Withdraw therapy in patients with persistently severe or worsening signs or symptoms of these conditions. In many, but not all cases, these disorders resolve after stopping peginterferon alfa-2a treatment (see Warnings and Adverse Reactions).

Use with ribavirin: Ribavirin may cause birth defects and/or death of the fetus. Take extreme care to avoid pregnancy in female patients and in female partners of male patients. Ribavirin causes hemolytic anemia. The anemia associated with ribavirin therapy may result in a worsening of cardiac disease. Ribavirin is genotoxic and mutagenic; consider it a potential carcinogen.

Indications

➤*Chronic hepatitis C virus (HCV):* Alone or in combination with ribavirin tablets for the treatment of adults with chronic HCV infection who have compensated liver disease and have not been treated previously with interferon alpha.

When used in combination with ribavirin, refer to the ribavirin monograph for additional prescribing information.

➤*Unlabeled uses:* Renal cell carcinoma.

Administration and Dosage

➤*Approved by the FDA:* October 17, 2002.

There are no safety and efficacy data on treatment for longer than 48 weeks. Consider discontinuing therapy after 12 to 24 weeks of therapy if the patient has failed to demonstrate an early virologic response.

Instruct patients to self-inject peginterferon alfa-2a only if the physician determines that it is appropriate, the patient agrees to medical follow-up as necessary, and training in proper injection technique has been provided.

➤*Monotherapy:* 180 mcg peginterferon alfa-2a once weekly for 48 weeks by SC administration in the abdomen or thigh.

➤*Peginterferon alfa-2a/Ribavirin tablet combination:* 180 mcg peginterferon alfa-2a once weekly. The recommended dose of ribavirin and duration for the peginterferon alfa-2a/ribavirin tablet combination therapy is based on viral genotype.

The daily dose of ribavirin tablets is 800 to 1200 mg administered orally in 2 divided doses. Individualize the dose depending on baseline disease characteristics (eg, genotype), response to therapy, and tolerability of the regimen.

Because ribavirin tablet absorption increases when administered with a meal, advise patients to take the tablet with food.

Peginterferon Alfa-2a/Ribavirin Tablet Combination Dosing Recommendations			
Genotype	Peginterferon alfa-2a dose	Ribavirin tablet dose	Duration
Genotype 1, 4	180 mcg	< 75 kg = 1000 mg	48 weeks
		≥ 75 kg = 1200 mg	48 weeks
Genotype 2, 3	180 mcg	800 mg	24 weeks

➤*Dose reduction:* When dose modification is required for moderate to severe adverse reactions (clinical or laboratory), initial dose reduction to 135 mcg generally is adequate. However, in some cases, dose reduction to 90 mcg may be needed. Following improvement of the adverse reaction, re-escalation of the dose may be considered. If intolerance persists after dose adjustment, discontinue therapy.

Hematologic toxicity –
Peginterferon alfa-2a:

Peginterferon Alfa-2a Hematological Dose Modification Guidelines		
Laboratory values	Peginterferon alfa-2a dose reduction	Discontinue peginterferon alfa-2a if:
ANC < 750/mm³	135 mcg	If ANC < 500/mm³, suspend treatment until ANC values return to more than 1000/mm³. Reinstitute at 90 mcg and monitor ANC
Platelet < 50,000/mm³	90 mcg	Platelet count < 25,000/mm³

PEGINTERFERON ALFA-2a

Ribavirin tablets:

Ribavirin Tablet Dosage Modification Guidelines		
Laboratory values	Reduce only ribavirin tablet dose to 600 mg/day[a] if:	Discontinue ribavirin tablet if:
Hemoglobin in patients with no cardiac disease	< 10 g/dL	< 8.5 g/dL
Hemoglobin in patients with history of stable cardiac disease	≥ 2 g/dL decrease in hemo-globin during any 4-week period treatment	< 12 g/dL despite 4 weeks at reduced dose.

[a] One 200 mg tablet in the morning and two 200 mg tablets in the evening.

Once the ribavirin tablet has been withheld because of a laboratory abnormality or clinical manifestation, an attempt may be made to restart the ribavirin tablet at 600 mg/day and further increase the dose to 800 mg/day depending upon the physician's judgment. However, it is not recommended that the ribavirin tablet be increased to the original dose (1000 or 1200 mg).

Psychiatric depression –

Guidelines for Modification or Discontinuation of Peginterferon alfa-2a and for Scheduling Visits for Patients with Depression					
Depression severity	Initial management (4 to 8 weeks)		Depression		
	Dose modification	Visit schedule	Remains stable	Improves	Worsens
Mild	No change	Evaluate once weekly by visit and/or phone	Continue weekly visit schedule	Resume normal visit schedule	(See moderate or severe depression.)
Moderate	Decrease peg-interferon alfa-2a dose to 135 mcg (in some cases dose reduction to 90 mcg may be needed)	Evaluate once weekly (office visit at least every other week)	Consider psychiatric consultation. Continue reduced dosing	If symptoms improve and are stable for 4 weeks, may resume normal visit schedule. Continue reduced dosing or return to normal dose.	(See severe depression.)
Severe	Discontinue peginterferon alfa-2a permanently	Obtain immediate psychiatric consultation	Psychiatric therapy necessary.		

Renal function impairment – In patients with end-stage renal disease requiring hemodialysis, dose reduction to 135 mcg peginterferon alfa-2a is recommended. Closely monitor for signs and symptoms of interferon toxicity. Do not administer ribavirin tablets in patients with creatinine clearance (Ccr) less than 50 mL/min.

Liver function impairment – In patients with progressive ALT increases above baseline values, reduce the dose of peginterferon alfa-2a to 135 mcg. Immediately discontinue therapy if ALT increases are progressive despite dose reduction or are accompanied by increased bilirubin or evidence of hepatic decompensation.

►*Storage/Stability:* Store in a refrigerator at 2° to 8°C (36° to 46°F). Do not freeze or shake. Protect from light. Vials and prefilled syringes are for single use only. Discard any unused portion.

Actions

►*Pharmacology:* Interferons bind to specific receptors on the cell surface, initiating intracellular signaling via a complex cascade of protein-protein interactions, which leads to rapid activation of gene transcription. Interferon-stimulated genes modulate many biological effects, including the inhibition of viral replication in infected cells, inhibition of cell proliferation, and immunomodulation. The clinical relevance of these in vitro activities is not known. Peginterferon alfa-2a stimulates the production of effector proteins such as serum neopterin and 2′,5′-oligoadenylate synthetase.

►*Pharmacokinetics:*

Absorption/Distribution – Maximal C_{max} occurs between 72 to 96 hours postdose. The C_{max} and AUC measurements of peginterferon alfa-2a increase in a dose-related manner. Week 48 mean trough concentrations (16 ng/mL; range, 4 to 28) at 168 hours postdose are approximately 2-fold higher than week 1 mean trough concentrations (8 ng/mL; range, 0 to 15). Steady-state serum levels are reached within 5 to 8 weeks of once-weekly dosing. The peak-to-trough ratio at week 48 is approximately 2.

Metabolism/Excretion – The mean systemic clearance in healthy patients given peginterferon alfa-2a was 94 mL/h. The mean terminal half-life after SC dosing in patients with chronic hepatitis C was 80 hours (range, 50 to 140 hours).

Special populations –

Elderly: The AUC was increased from 1295 to 1663 ng•h/mL in subjects older than 62 years of age taking 180 mcg peginterferon alfa-2a, but peak concentrations were similar (9 vs 10 ng/mL) in those older and younger than 62 years of age.

Renal function impairment: In patients with end-stage renal disease undergoing hemodialysis, there is a 25% to 45% reduction in peginterferon alfa-2a clearance (see Warnings).

►*Clinical trials:*

Monotherapy – The safety and efficacy of peginterferon alfa-2a for the treatment of HCV infection were assessed in 3 randomized, open-label, active-controlled clinical studies. All patients were adults with compensated liver disease, detectable HCV, and liver biopsy diagnosis of chronic hepatitis and previously were untreated with interferon. All patients received therapy by SC injection for 48 weeks and were followed for an additional 24 weeks to assess the durability of response. Response to treatment was defined in the protocol as undetectable HCV RNA and normalization of ALT on or after study week 68.

In study 1 (n = 630), patients received 3 million international units (MIU) interferon alfa-2a 3 times/week, 135 mcg peginterferon alfa-2a once/week, or 180 mcg peginterferon alfa-2a once/week. In study 2 (n = 526), patients received 6 MIU interferon alfa-2a 3 times/week for 12 weeks followed by 3 MIU 3 times/week for 36 weeks or 180 mcg peginterferon alfa-2a once/week. In study 3 (n = 269), patients received 3 MIU interferon alfa-2a 3 times/week, 90 mcg peginterferon alfa-2a once/week, or 180 mcg peginterferon alfa-2a once/week.

In all 3 studies, treatment with 180 mcg peginterferon alfa-2a resulted in significantly more patients who experienced a sustained response compared with treatment with interferon alfa-2a (see table below).

Combination therapy – The safety and efficacy of peginterferon alfa-2a in combination with ribavirin tablets for the treatment of HCV infection were assessed in 2 randomized, controlled clinical trials. All patients were adults with compensated liver disease, detectable HCV, and liver biopsy diagnosis of chronic hepatitis and previously were untreated with interferon.

Patients were randomized to receive one of the following: 180 mcg peginterferon alfa-2a SC once/week with an oral placebo; 180 mcg peginterferon alfa-2a once/week with 1000 mg (body weight less than 75 kg) or 1200 mg (body weight 75 kg or more) oral ribavirin tablets; 3 MIU interferon alfa-2b SC 3 times/week plus 1000 or 1200 mg oral ribavirin. All patients received 48 weeks of therapy followed by 24 weeks of treatment-free follow-up. Peginterferon alfa-2a in combination with ribavirin tablets resulted in a higher sustained virologic response (SVR) (defined as undetectable HCV RNA at the end of the 24-week treatment-free follow-up period) compared with peginterferon alfa-2a alone or interferon alfa-2b and ribavirin. In all treatment arms, patients with viral genotype 1, regardless of viral load, had a lower response rate.

Sustained Virologic Response to Combination Therapy (%)			
	Interferon alfa-2b + 1000 or 1200 mg ribavirin	Peginterferon alfa-2a + placebo	Peginterferon alfa-2a + 1000 or 1200 mg ribavirin tablets
All patients	44	29	53
Genotype 1	36	20	44
Genotypes 2-6	59	46	70

In the next study, all patients received 180 mcg peginterferon alfa-2a SC once/week and were randomized to treatment for either 24 or 48 weeks and to a ribavirin tablet dose of either 800 or 1000/1200 mg. Assignment to the 4 treatment arms was stratified by viral genotype and baseline HCV viral titer. Patients with genotype 1 and high viral titer (defined as more than 2×10^6 HCV RNA copies/mL serum) preferentially were assigned to treatment for 48 weeks.

Sustained Virologic Response as a Function of Genotype (%)				
	24 weeks treatment		48 weeks treatment	
	Peginterferon alfa-2a + ribavirin tablets 800 mg (N = 207)	Peginterferon alfa-2a + ribavirin tablets 1000 or 1200 mg[a] (N = 280)	Peginterferon alfa-2a + ribavirin tablets 800 mg (N = 361)	Peginterferon alfa-2a + ribavirin tablets 1000 or 1200 mg[a] (N = 436)
Genotype 1	29	41	40	51
Genotype 2-3	82	81	76	76

[a] 1000 mg for body weight less than 75 kg; 1200 mg for body weight 75 kg or more.

PEGINTERFERON ALFA-2a

Peginterferon Alfa-2a Sustained Response to Monotherapy Treatment						
	Study 1		Study 2		Study 3	
Protocol[a]	Interferon alfa-2a 3 MIU (N = 207)	Peginterferon alfa-2a 180 mcg (N = 208)	Interferon alfa-2a 6/3 MIU (N = 261)	Peginterferon alfa-2a 180 mcg (N = 265)	Interferon alfa-2a 3 MIU (N = 86)	Peginterferon alfa-2a 180 mcg (N = 87)
Combined virological and biologic sustained response	11	24	17	35	7	23
Sustained virological response	11	26	19	38	8	30

[a] See text for response definition.

Contraindications

►*Peginterferon alfa-2a:* In neonates and infants because it contains benzyl alcohol (see Warnings); hypersensitivity to peginterferon alfa-2a or any of its components; autoimmune hepatitis; hepatic decompensation (Child-Pugh class B and C) before or during treatment with peginterferon alfa-2a.

►*Peginterferon alfa-2a/Ribavirin tablets combination:* Known hypersensitivity to ribavirin tablets or to any component of the tablet; women who are pregnant; men whose female partners are pregnant; patients with hemoglobinopathies (eg, thalassemia major, sickle-cell anemia).

Warnings

►*Autoimmune disorders:* Development or exacerbation of autoimmune disorders, including hepatitis, idiopathic thrombocytopenic purpura, interstitial nephritis, myositis, psoriasis, rheumatoid arthritis, systemic lupus erythematosus, and thyroiditis have been reported in patients receiving alpha interferon. Use peginterferon alfa-2a with caution in patients with autoimmune disorders.

►*Hemolytic anemia:* The primary toxicity of ribavirin is hemolytic anemia. Hemoglobin less than 10 g/dL was observed in approximately 13% of patients treated with ribavirin tablet and peginterferon alfa-2a in clinical trials. Anemia associated with ribavirin tablets occurs within 1 to 2 weeks of initiation of therapy with maximum drop in hemoglobin observed during the first 8 weeks. Because the initial drop in hemoglobin may be significant, it is advised that hemoglobin or hematocrit be obtained pretreatment and at weeks 2 and 4 of therapy or more frequently, if clinically indicated.

►*Benzyl alcohol:* Peginterferon alfa-2a is contraindicated in neonates and infants because it contains benzyl alcohol. Benzyl alcohol is associated with an increased incidence of neurologic and other complications in neonates and infants that are sometimes fatal.

►*Bone marrow toxicity:* Peginterferon alfa-2a suppresses bone marrow function and may result in severe cytopenias. Ribavirin may potentiate the neutropenia and lymphopenia induced by alpha interferons including peginterferon alfa-2a. Alpha interferons very rarely may be associated with aplastic anemia. Obtain complete blood counts (CBCs) pretreatment and routinely monitor during therapy (see Precautions).

Use peginterferon alfa-2a and ribavirin tablets with caution in patients with baseline neutrophil counts under 1500 cells/mm^3, baseline platelet counts less than 90,000 cells/mm^3, or baseline hemoglobin less than 10 g/dL. Discontinue peginterferon alfa-2a therapy, at least temporarily, in patients who develop severe decreases in neutrophil and/or platelet counts (see Administration and Dosage).

►*Cardiovascular events:* Hypertension, supraventricular arrhythmias, chest pain, and MI have been observed in patients treated with peginterferon alfa-2a. Administer peginterferon alfa-2a with caution to patients with preexisting cardiac disease.

Fatal and nonfatal MIs have been reported in patients with anemia caused by ribavirin. Assess patients for underlying cardiac disease before initiation of ribavirin therapy. Administer electrocardiogram (ECG) before treating patients with preexisting cardiac disease, and appropriately monitor them during therapy. If there is any deterioration of cardiovascular status, suspend or discontinue therapy. Because cardiac disease may be worsened by drug-induced anemia, patients with a history of significant or unstable cardiac disease should not use ribavirin tablets.

►*Colitis:* Ulcerative and hemorrhagic/ischemic colitis, sometimes fatal, have been observed within 12 weeks of starting alpha interferon treatment. Abdominal pain, bloody diarrhea, and fever are the typical manifestations of colitis. Immediately discontinue peginterferon alfa-2a if these symptoms develop. The colitis usually resolves within 1 to 3 weeks of discontinuation of alpha interferon.

►*Endocrine disorders:* Peginterferon alfa-2a causes or aggravates hypothyroidism and hyperthyroidism. Hyperglycemia, hypoglycemia, and diabetes mellitus have developed in patients treated with peginterferon alfa-2a. Patients with these conditions at baseline who cannot be treated effectively by medication should not begin peginterferon alfa-2a therapy. Patients who develop these conditions during treatment and cannot be controlled with medication may require discontinuation of peginterferon alfa-2a therapy.

►*Hypersensitivity reactions:* Severe acute hypersensitivity reactions (eg, urticaria, angioedema, bronchoconstriction, anaphylaxis) rarely have been observed during alpha interferon and ribavirin therapy. If such reaction occurs, discontinue therapy with peginterferon alfa-2a and ribavirin tablets and immediately institute appropriate medical therapy.

►*Neuropsychiatric events:* Life-threatening or fatal neuropsychiatric reactions may manifest in patients receiving therapy with peginterferon alfa-2a. Depression, drug overdose, relapse of drug addiction, suicidal ideation, and suicide may occur in patients with and without previous psychiatric illness.

Use peginterferon alfa-2a with extreme caution in patients who report a history of depression. Neuropsychiatric adverse events observed with alpha interferon treatment include aggressive behavior, bipolar disorders, hallucinations, mania, and psychoses.

Physicians should monitor all patients for evidence of depression and other psychiatric symptoms. Advise patients to report any sign or symptom of depression or suicidal ideation to their prescribing physicians. In severe cases, immediately stop therapy and institute psychiatric intervention.

►*Infections:* Serious and severe bacterial infections, some fatal, have been observed in patients treated with alpha interferons including peginterferon alfa-2a. Some of the infections have been associated with neutropenia. Discontinue peginterferon alfa-2a in patients who develop severe infections and institute appropriate antibiotic therapy.

►*Ophthalmologic disorders:* Decrease or loss of vision, retinopathy (including macular edema, retinal artery or vein thrombosis), retinal hemorrhages and cotton wool spots, optic neuritis, and papilledema are induced or aggravated by treatment with peginterferon alfa-2a or other alpha interferons. All patients should receive an eye examination at baseline. Patients with preexisting ophthalmologic disorders (eg, diabetic or hypertensive retinopathy) should receive periodic ophthalmologic exams during interferon alpha treatment. Any patient who develops ocular symptoms should receive a prompt and complete eye examination. Discontinue peginterferon alfa-2a in patients who develop new or worsening ophthalmologic disorders.

►*Pancreatitis:* Pancreatitis, sometimes fatal, has occurred during alpha interferon and ribavirin treatment. Suspend peginterferon alfa-2a/ribavirin tablet treatment if symptoms or signs suggestive of pancreatitis are observed. Discontinue peginterferon alfa-2a and ribavirin tablets in patients diagnosed with pancreatitis.

►*Pulmonary disorders:* Dyspnea, pulmonary infiltrates, pneumonia, bronchiolitis obliterans, interstitial pneumonitis, and sarcoidosis, some resulting in respiratory failure and/or patient deaths, may be induced or aggravated by peginterferon alfa-2a or alpha interferon therapy. Discontinue treatment in patients who develop persistent or unexplained pulmonary infiltrates or pulmonary function impairment.

►*Renal function impairment:* A 25% to 45% higher exposure to peginterferon alfa-2a is seen in subjects undergoing hemodialysis. In patients with impaired renal function, closely monitor for signs and symptoms of interferon toxicity. Adjust doses of peginterferon alfa-2a accordingly. Use peginterferon alfa-2a with caution in patients with Ccr less than 50 mL/min (see Administration and Dosage).

►*Fertility impairment:* Peginterferon alfa-2a may impair fertility in women. Prolonged menstrual cycles and/or amenorrhea were observed in female cynomolgus monkeys given SC injections of 600 mcg/kg/dose (7200 mcg/m^2/dose) peginterferon alfa-2a every other day for 1 month, at approximately 180 times the recommended weekly human dose for a 60 kg person (based on body surface area). Menstrual cycle irregularities were accompanied by a decrease and a delay in peak 17β-estradiol and progesterone levels following administration of peginterferon alfa-2a to female monkeys. A return to normal menstrual rhythm followed cessation of treatment. Every-other-day dosing with 100 mcg/kg (1200 mcg/m^2) peginterferon alfa-2a (equivalent to approximately 30 times the recommended human dose) had no effects on cycle duration or reproductive hormone status.

►*Elderly:* Clinical studies of peginterferon alfa-2a alone or in combination with ribavirin tablets did not include sufficient numbers of subjects 65 years of age and older to determine whether they respond differently from younger subjects. Adverse reactions related to alpha interferons, such as CNS, cardiac, and systemic (eg, flu-like) effects

PEGINTERFERON ALFA-2a

may be more severe in the elderly; exercise caution in the use of peginterferon alfa-2a in this population. Peginterferon alfa-2a and ribavirin tablets are excreted by the kidney, and the risk of toxic reaction to this drug may be greater in patients with impaired renal function. Because elderly patients are more likely to have decreased renal function, take care in dose selection; it also may be useful to monitor renal function.

➤*Pregnancy:* Category C. Peginterferon alfa-2a has not been studied for its teratogenic effect. Nonpegylated interferon alfa-2a treatment of pregnant Rhesus monkeys at approximately 20 to 500 times the human weekly dose resulted in a statistically significant increase in abortions. No teratogenic effects were seen in the offspring delivered at term. Assume peginterferon alfa-2a also has abortifacient potential. There are no adequate and well-controlled studies of peginterferon alfa-2a in pregnant women. Peginterferon alfa-2a is to be used during pregnancy only if the potential benefit justifies the potential risk to the fetus. Peginterferon alfa-2a is recommended for use in women of childbearing potential only when they are using effective contraception during therapy.

Use with ribavirin – Category X. Ribavirin may cause birth defects and/or death of the exposed fetus. Take extreme care to avoid pregnancy in female patients and in female partners of male patients taking peginterferon alfa-2a and ribavirin tablet combination therapy. Ribavirin tablet therapy should not be started unless a report of a negative pregnancy test has been obtained immediately prior to initiation of therapy. Women of childbearing potential and men must use 2 forms of effective contraception during treatment and for at least 6 months after treatment has concluded. Perform routine monthly pregnancy tests during this time.

If pregnancy occurs in a patient or partner of a patient during treatment or during the 6 months after treatment cessation, such cases should be reported to the ribavirin tablet Pregnancy Registry at (800) 526-6367 (please refer to ribavirin monograph for additional information).

➤*Lactation:* It is not known whether peginterferon alfa-2a or ribavirin or its components are excreted in human milk. The effect of orally ingested peginterferon alfa-2a or ribavirin from breast milk on the nursing infant has not been evaluated. Because of the potential for adverse reactions from the drug in nursing infants, decide whether to discontinue nursing or discontinue the treatment.

➤*Children:* Safety and efficacy of peginterferon alfa-2a alone or in combination with ribavirin tablets in children younger than 18 years of age have not been established.

Peginterferon alfa-2a contains benzyl alcohol. Benzyl alcohol has been associated with an increased incidence of neurological and other complications in neonates and infants that are sometimes fatal.

Precautions

➤*Monitoring:* Before beginning peginterferon alfa-2a or peginterferon alfa-2a/ribavirin tablet combination therapy, standard hematological and biochemical laboratory tests are recommended for all patients. Perform pregnancy screening for women of childbearing potential. After initiation of therapy, perform hematological tests at 2 and 4 weeks and biochemical tests at 4 weeks. Periodically perform additional testing during therapy. In the clinical studies, the CBC (including hemoglobin level and white blood cell [WBC] and platelet counts) and chemistries (including liver function tests and uric acid) were measured at 1, 2, 4, 6, and 8, and then every 4 weeks, or more frequently if abnormalities were found. Thyroid-stimulating hormone (TSH) was measured every 12 weeks. Perform monthly pregnancy testing during combination therapy and for 6 months after discontinuing therapy.

Clinical study criteria – The entrance criteria used for the clinical studies of peginterferon alfa-2a may be considered as a guideline to acceptable baseline values for initiation of treatment:
- Platelet count 90,000 cells/mm^3 or more (as low as 75,000 cells/mm^3 in patients with cirrhosis or transition to cirrhosis).
- Exercise caution in initiating treatment in any patient with baseline risk of severe anemia (eg, spherocytosis, history of GI bleeding).
- ANC 1500 cells/mm^3 or more.
- Serum creatinine concentration less than 1.5 times the upper limit of normal.
- TSH and T$_4$ within normal limits or adequately controlled thyroid function.

➤*Immunogenicity:* Nine percent of patients treated with peginterferon alfa-2a with or without ribavirin tablets developed binding antibodies to interferon alfa-2a, as assessed by an ELISA assay. Three percent of patients receiving peginterferon alfa-2a with or without ribavirin tablets, developed low-titer neutralizing antibodies. The clinical and pathological significance of the appearance of serum neutralizing antibodies is unknown.

➤*HIV or HBV coinfections:* The safety and efficacy of peginterferon alfa-2a alone or in combination with ribavirin tablets for the treatment of hepatitis C have not been established in patients coinfected with HIV or HBV.

➤*Hepatitis C:* The safety and efficacy of peginterferon alfa-2a alone or in combination with ribavirin tablets for the treatment of hepatitis C in patients who have failed other alpha interferon treatments or who have received liver or other organ transplants have not been established.

➤*Lab test abnormalities:* Peginterferon alfa-2a treatment was associated with decreases in WBC, ANC, lymphocytes, and platelet counts, often starting within the first 2 weeks of treatment. Dose reduction is recommended in patients with hematologic abnormalities.

While fever commonly is caused by peginterferon alfa-2a therapy, other causes of persistent fever must be ruled out, particularly in patients with neutropenia.

Transient elevations in ALT (2- to 5-fold above baseline) were observed in some patients receiving peginterferon alfa-2a and were not associated with deterioration of other liver function tests. However, discontinue therapy when the increase in ALT levels is progressive, despite dose reduction, or is accompanied by increased bilirubin.

Drug Interactions

➤*Methadone:* In a study of HCV patients concomitantly receiving methadone, treatment with peginterferon alfa-2a once weekly for 4 weeks was associated with methadone levels that were 10% to 15% higher than at baseline. The clinical significance of this finding is unknown; however, monitor patients for signs and symptoms of methadone toxicity.

➤*Theophylline:* Treatment with once-weekly peginterferon alfa-2a for 4 weeks in healthy subjects was associated with inhibition of P450 1A2 and a 25% increase in theophylline AUC. Monitor theophylline serum levels and consider appropriate dose adjustments for patients given theophylline and peginterferon alfa-2a concurrently.

Adverse Reactions

The most common life-threatening or fatal events induced or aggravated by peginterferon alfa-2a and ribavirin tablets were depression, suicide, relapse of drug abuse/overdose, and bacterial infections; each occurred at a frequency of less than 1%. The most commonly reported adverse reactions were psychiatric reactions, including anxiety, depression, irritability, and flu-like symptoms such as fatigue, headache, myalgia, pyrexia, and rigors.

Overall, 11% of patients receiving 48 weeks of therapy with peginterferon alfa-2a either alone (7%) or in combination with ribavirin tablets (10%) discontinued therapy. The most common reasons for discontinuation of therapy were dermatologic, flu-like syndrome (eg, lethargy, fatigue, headache), GI, and psychiatric disorders.

The most common reason for dose modification in patients receiving combination therapy was for laboratory abnormalities including the following: Neutropenia (20%) and thrombocytopenia (4%) for peginterferon alfa-2a and anemia (22%) for ribavirin tablets.

Peginterferon alfa-2a dose was reduced in 12% of patients receiving 1000 to 1200 mg ribavirin tablets for 48 weeks and in 7% of patients receiving 800 mg ribavirin tablets for 24 weeks. Ribavirin tablet dose was reduced in 21% of patients receiving 1000 to 1200 mg ribavirin tablets for 48 weeks and 12% in patients receiving 800 mg ribavirin tablets for 24 weeks.

Peginterferon Alfa-2a Adverse Reactions in Hepatitis C Clinical Trials (Pooled Studies 1, 2, and 3 and Study 4) (≥ 5%)			
Adverse reaction	Peginterferon alfa-2a 180 mcg (48 weeks)[a] (N = 559)	Interferon alfa-2a[a,b] (N = 554)	Peginterferon alfa-2a 180 mcg + 1000 or 1200 mg ribavirin tablets (48 weeks)[c] (N = 451)	Interferon alfa-2b + 1000 or 1200 mg ribavirin capsules (48 weeks)[c] (N = 443)
CNS				
Concentration impairment	8	10	10	13
Depression	18	19	20	28
Dizziness	16	12	14	14
Headache	54	58	43	49
Insomnia	19	23	30	37
Irritability/Anxiety/ Nervousness	19	22	33	38
Memory impairment	5	4	6	5
Mood alteration	3	2	5	6
Dermatologic				
Alopecia	23	30	28	33
Dermatitis	8	3	16	13
Dry skin	4	3	10	13
Eczema	1	1	5	4
Pruritus	12	8	19	18
Rash	5	4	8	5
Sweating increased	6	7	6	5

PEGINTERFERON ALFA-2a

Peginterferon Alfa-2a Adverse Reactions in Hepatitis C Clinical Trials (Pooled Studies 1, 2, and 3 and Study 4) (≥ 5%)

Adverse reaction	Peginterferon alfa-2a 180 mcg (48 weeks)[a] (N = 559)	Interferon alfa-2a[a,b] (N = 554)	Peginterferon alfa-2a 180 mcg + 1000 or 1200 mg ribavirin tablets (48 weeks)[c] (N = 451)	Interferon alfa-2b + 1000 or 1200 mg ribavirin capsules (48 weeks)[c] (N = 443)
GI				
Abdominal pain	15	15	8	9
Anorexia	17	17	24	26
Diarrhea	16	16	11	10
Dry mouth	6	3	4	7
Dyspepsia	< 1	1	6	5
Nausea/Vomiting	24	33	25	29
Hematologic[d]				
Anemia	2	1	11	11
Lymphopenia	3	5	14	12
Neutropenia	21	8	27	8
Thrombocyto-penia	5	2	5	< 1
Musculoskeletal				
Arthralgia	28	29	22	23
Back pain	9	10	5	5
Myalgia	37	38	40	49
Respiratory				
Cough	4	3	10	7
Dyspnea	4	2	13	14
Dyspnea, exertional	< 1	< 1	4	7
Miscellaneous				
Fatigue/Asthenia	56	57	65	68
Hypothyroidism	3	2	4	5
Injection-site reaction	22	18	23	16
Overall resistance mechanism disorders	10	6	12	10
Pain	11	12	10	9
Pyrexia	37	41	41	55
Rigors	35	44	25	37
Vision blurred	4	2	5	2
Weight decrease	4	3	10	10

[a] Pooled studies 1, 2, and 3.
[b] Either 3 MIU or 6/3 MIU interferon alfa-2a.
[c] Study 4.
[d] Severe hematologic abnormalities.

The most common serious adverse event (3%) was bacterial infection (eg, sepsis, osteomyelitis, endocarditis, pyelonephritis, pneumonia). Serious adverse events occurring in less than 1% included the following: aggression, angina, anxiety, aplastic anemia, arrhythmia, autoimmune phenomena (eg, hyperthyroidism, hypothyroidism, rheumatoid arthritis, sarcoidosis, systemic lupus erythematosus), cerebral hemorrhage, cholangitis, colitis, coma, corneal ulcer, diabetes mellitus, drug abuse and overdose, fatty liver, GI bleeding, hepatic dysfunction, myositis, pancreatitis, peptic ulcer, peripheral neuropathy, psychosis, pulmonary embolism, suicidal ideation, and suicide.

►*Lab test abnormalities:*

Hemoglobin – The hemoglobin concentration decreased below 12 g/dL in 17% of monotherapy and 52% of combination therapy patients. Severe anemia (hemoglobin less than 10 g/dL) was encountered in 13% of patients receiving combination therapy and 2% of monotherapy recipients. Dose modification for anemia was required in 22% of ribavirin recipients treated for 48 weeks. Hemoglobin decreases in peginterferon alfa-2a monotherapy generally were mild and did not require dose modification.

Neutrophils – Decreases in neutrophil count below normal were observed in 95% of patients treated with peginterferon alfa-2a either alone or in combination with ribavirin tablets. Severe potentially life-threatening neutropenia (ANC less than 0.5×10^9/L) occurred in approximately 5% of patients receiving peginterferon alfa-2a alone or in combination with ribavirin tablets. Seventeen percent of patients receiving peginterferon alfa-2a monotherapy and 20% to 24% of patients receiving peginterferon alfa-2a/ribavirin tablet combination therapy required modification of interferon dosage for neutropenia. Two percent of patients required permanent reductions of peginterferon alfa-2a dosage and less than 1% required permanent discontinuation. Median neutrophil counts returned to pretreatment levels 4 weeks after cessation of therapy.

Lymphocytes – Decreases in lymphocyte count are induced by interferon alpha therapy. Lymphopenia was observed during monotherapy (86%) and combination therapy with peginterferon alfa-2a and ribavirin tablets (94%). Severe lymphopenia (less than 0.5×10^9/L) occurred in approximately 5% of monotherapy patients and 14% of combination peginterferon alfa-2a/ribavirin tablet therapy recipients. Dose adjustments were not required by protocol. Median lymphocyte counts return to pretreatment levels after 4 to 12 weeks of the cessation of therapy. The clinical significance of the lymphopenia is not known.

Platelets – Platelet counts decreased in 52% of patients treated with peginterferon alfa-2a alone (median drop 45% from baseline) and 33% of patients receiving combination with ribavirin tablets (median drop 30% from baseline). Median platelet counts return to pretreatment levels 4 weeks after the cessation of therapy.

Triglycerides – Triglyceride levels are elevated in patients receiving alfa interferon therapy and were elevated in the majority of patients participating in clinical studies receiving either peginterferon alfa-2a alone or in combination with ribavirin tablets. Random levels higher than 400 mg/dL were observed in approximately 20% of patients.

ALT elevations – Less than 1% of patients experienced marked elevations (5- to 10-fold above baseline) in ALT levels during treatment. These transaminase elevations were on occasion associated with hyperbilirubinemia and were managed by dose reduction or discontinuation of study treatment. Liver function test abnormalities generally were transient. One case was attributed to autoimmune hepatitis that persisted beyond study medication discontinuation.

Thyroid function – Peginterferon alfa-2a treatment alone or in combination with ribavirin tablets was associated with the development of abnormalities in thyroid laboratory values, some with associated clinical manifestations. Hypothyroidism or hyperthyroidism (requiring treatment, dose modification, or discontinuation) occurred in 4% and 1% of patients treated with peginterferon alfa-2a alone and 4% and 2% of patients treated with peginterferon alfa-2a and ribavirin tablets, respectively. Among the patients who developed thyroid abnormalities during peginterferon alfa-2a treatment, approximately 50% still had abnormalities during the follow-up period.

Overdosage

There is limited experience with overdosage. The maximum dose received by any patient was 7 times the intended dose of peginterferon alfa-2a (180 mcg/day for 7 days). There were no serious reactions attributed to overdosages. Weekly doses of up to 630 mcg have been administered to patients with cancer. Dose-limiting toxicities were fatigue, elevated liver enzymes, neutropenia, and thrombocytopenia. There is no specific antidote for peginterferon alfa-2a. Hemodialysis and peritoneal dialysis are not effective.

Patient Information

Direct patients receiving peginterferon alfa-2a alone or in combination with ribavirin tablets in the appropriate use, inform them of the benefits and risks associated with treatment, and refer them to the peginterferon alfa-2a or ribavirin tablets medication guide.

Caution patients who develop dizziness, confusion, somnolence, and fatigue to avoid driving or operating machinery.

If home use is prescribed, supply the patients with a puncture-resistant container for the disposal of used needles and syringes. Thoroughly instruct patients in the importance of proper disposal, and caution them against any reuse of any needles and syringes. Instruct patients to dispose the full container according to the directions provided by the physician.

Peginterferon alfa-2a and ribavirin tablet combination therapy must not be used by women who are pregnant or by men whose female partners are pregnant. Do not initiate ribavirin tablet therapy until a report of a negative pregnancy test has been obtained immediately before starting therapy. Advise female patients of childbearing potential and male patients with female partners of childbearing potential of the teratogenic/embryocidal risks, and instruct them to practice 2 forms of effective contraception during ribavirin tablet therapy and for 6 months posttherapy. Notify patients that routine monthly pregnancy tests will be performed during this time. Advise patients to immediately notify their physician in the event of a pregnancy.

If pregnancy does occur during treatment or during 6 months posttherapy, advise patients of the significant teratogenic risk of ribavirin therapy to the fetus. To monitor maternal-fetal outcomes of pregnant women exposed to ribavirin, the ribavirin tablet Pregnancy Registry has been established. Physicians and patients are strongly encouraged to register by calling (800) 526-6367.

Advise patients that laboratory evaluations are required before starting therapy and periodically thereafter. Instruct patients to remain well hydrated, especially during the initial stages of treatment.

Inform patients that it is not known if therapy with peginterferon alfa-2a alone or in combination with ribavirin will prevent transmission of HCV infection to others or prevent cirrhosis, liver failure, or liver cancer that might result from HCV infection.

PEGINTERFERON ALFA-2a

Advise patients to visually inspect the product for particles and discoloration before use and to return the medicine to their pharmacist if it contains particles or discolored matter.

Instruct patients to contact their health care provider if signs of a serious allergic reaction (eg, hives, tightness in the chest, difficulty breathing, swelling of the mouth, face, lips, or tongue), bloody stools, depression or thoughts of suicide, fever, increased pulse rate, nausea, stomach pain, vision problems, or vomiting occur while using this medicine.

INTERFERON ALFA-2b, RECOMBINANT (IFN-alpha 2; rIFN-α2; α-2-interferon)

Rx	Intron A[1] (Schering)	**Powder for injection:**[2] 5 million IU/vial	In vials with 1 mL diluent vial.[3]
		10 million IU/vial	In vials with 2 mL diluent vial.[3]
		18 million IU/vial	In vials with 5 mL diluent vial.[3]
		25 million IU/vial	In vials with 5 mL diluent vial.[3]
		50 million IU/vial	In vials with 1 mL diluent vial.[3]
		Injection:[4] 3 million IU/dose	In multidose pens (6 doses; 22.5 million IU/1.5 mL per pen) with needles.
		5 million IU/dose	In multidose pens (6 doses; 37.5 million IU/1.5 mL per pen) with needles.
		10 million IU/dose	In multidose pens (6 doses; 75 million IU/1.5 mL per pen) with needles.
		Solution for injection:[4] 3 million IU/vial	In vials, Pak-3 (6 vials, 6 syringes).
		5 million IU/vial	In vials, Pak-5 (6 vials, 6 syringes).
		10 million IU/vial	In vials, Pak-10 (6 vials, 6 syringes).
		18 million IU/vial	In multidose vials (22.8 million IU/3.8 mL per vial).
		25 million IU/vial	In multidose vials (32 million IU/3.2 mL per vial).

[1] Not all dosage forms and strengths are appropriate for some indications.
[2] Each milliliter includes 1 mg human albumin, 20 mg glycine, 2.3 mg sodium phosphate dibasic, 0.55 mg sodium phosphate monobasic.
[3] Diluent is bacteriostatic water for injection containing 0.9% benzyl alcohol as a preservative.

[4] Each milliliter contains 7.5 mg sodium chloride, 1.8 mg sodium phosphate dibasic, 1.3 mg sodium phosphate monobasic, 0.1 mg EDTA, 0.1 mg polysorbate 80, and 1.5 mg m-cresol as a preservative.

WARNING

Alpha interferons, including interferon alfa-2b, recombinant, cause or aggravate fatal or life-threatening neuropsychiatric, autoimmune, ischemic, and infectious disorders. Closely monitor patients with periodic clinical and laboratory evaluations. Withdraw patients with persistently severe or worsening signs or symptoms of these conditions from therapy. In many, but not all cases, these disorders resolve after stopping interferon alfa-2b, recombinant therapy. (See Warnings and Adverse Reactions.)

Indications

▶*Hairy-cell leukemia:* In patients 18 years of age or older with hairy-cell leukemia.

▶*Malignant melanoma:* Adjuvant to surgical treatment in patients 18 years of age or older with malignant melanoma who are free of disease but are at high risk for systemic recurrence within 56 days of surgery.

▶*Follicular lymphoma:* Initial treatment of clinically aggressive follicular non-Hodgkin lymphoma in conjunction with anthracycline-containing combination chemotherapy in patients 18 years of age or older.

▶*Condylomata acuminata:* Intralesional treatment of external genital or perianal warts in select patients 18 years of age or older.

▶*AIDS-related Kaposi sarcoma:* In select patients 18 years of age or older with AIDS-related Kaposi sarcoma.

▶*Chronic hepatitis C:* In patients 18 years of age or older with compensated liver disease who have a history of blood or blood product exposure and/or patients who are hepatitis C virus (HCV)-antibody-positive. (Interferon alfa-2b also is indicated for hepatitis C in combination with ribavirin capsules. Please refer to the interferon alfa-2b/ribavirin capsules combination monograph for more information.)

▶*Chronic hepatitis B:* In patients 1 year of age or older with compensated liver disease and hepatitis B virus (HBV) replication. Patients must be serum HBsAg-positive for at least 6 months and have HBV replication (serum HBeAg-positive) with elevated serum ALT.

▶*Unlabeled uses:* Alpha interferons have been used for a variety of conditions, a list of which follows. Clinical trials are currently in progress to further determine clinical efficacy, optimal dosage, and length of treatment.

Interferon Alfa Unlabeled Uses		
Neoplastic diseases		
Significant activity	Limited activity	No activity
Bladder tumors (local use for superficial tumors) Chronic myelogenous leukemia Cutaneous T-cell lymphoma Non-Hodgkin lymphoma Essential thrombocytosis Chronic granulocytic leukemia	Melanoma Multiple myeloma Acute leukemias Carcinoid tumor Hodgkin disease	

Interferon Alfa Unlabeled Uses		
Neoplastic diseases		
Significant activity	Limited activity	No activity
Viral infections		*Miscellaneous*
Cytomegaloviruses Herpes simplex	Papillomaviruses Rhinoviruses Varicella zoster HIV[1]	Behçet syndrome Hypereosinophilic syndrome Polycythemia vera treatment

[1] Interferons have anti-HIV activity and may be enhanced by foscarnet/zidovudine.

Administration and Dosage

Do not use interferon alfa-2b solution for injection IV; only powder for injection may be used IV.

▶*Hairy-cell leukemia:* 2 million IU/m², IM or SC 3 times/week for up to 6 months. Do not use the 50 million IU strength of the powder for injection for the treatment of hairy-cell leukemia. Higher doses are not recommended. Responding patients may benefit from continued treatment.

If severe adverse reactions develop, modify dosage (50% reduction) or temporarily discontinue therapy until reactions abate. Discontinue if intolerance persists or recurs following adequate dosage adjustment, or if disease progresses.

▶*Malignant melanoma:* 20 million IU/m² IV infusion on 5 consecutive days/week for 4 weeks. Maintenance dosage is 10 million IU/m² SC 3 times/week for 48 weeks. Interferon alfa-2b solution for injection is not recommended for the IV treatment of malignant melanoma.

Dose modification – Perform regular lab testing to monitor abnormalities for the purpose of dose modification. If adverse reactions develop during interferon alfa-2b treatment, particularly if granulocytes decrease to less than 500/mm³ or ALT/AST rises to more than 5 times the upper limit of normal (ULN), temporarily discontinue treatment until adverse reactions abate. Restart interferon alfa-2b at 50% of the previous dose. If intolerance persists, granulocytes decrease to less than 250/mm³, or ALT/AST rises to more than 10 times the ULN, discontinue interferon alfa-2b therapy.

▶*Follicular lymphoma:* 5 million IU SC 3 times/week for up to 18 months in conjunction with an anthracycline-containing chemotherapy regimen.

In published reports, the doses of myelosuppressive drugs were reduced 25% from those used in a full-dose CHOP regimen (cyclophosphamide, doxorubicin, vincristine, prednisone), and cycle length increased 33% (eg, from 21 to 28 days) when an alfa interferon was added to the regimen. The following dose modification guidelines for hematologic toxicity were used in the clinical trial: The chemotherapy regimen was delayed if the neutrophil count was less than 1500/mm³ or the platelet count was less than 75,000/mm³. Administration of interferon alfa-2b therapy was temporarily interrupted for a neutrophil count less than 1000/mm³, or a platelet count less than 50,000/mm³, or reduced by 50%

INTERFERON ALFA-2b, RECOMBINANT (IFN-alpha 2; rIFN-α2; α-2-interferon)

to 2.5 million IU 3 times/week for a neutrophil count of more than 1000/mm³ but less than 1500/mm³. Reinstitution of the initial interferon alfa-2b dose (5 million IU 3 times/week) was tolerated after resolution of hematologic toxicity (1500/mm³ or more).

Discontinue interferon alfa-2b therapy if AST exceeds more than 5 times the ULN or serum creatinine is more than 2 mg/dL.

▶*Condylomata acuminata:* Inject 1 million IU/lesion (either 0.1 mL of reconstituted 10 million IU or 0.1 mL of the 5 million IU, 10 million IU, or 25 million IU strengths of solution for injections, each having a final concentration of 10 million IU/mL) 3 times/week for 3 weeks on alternate days intralesionally. Use tuberculin or similar syringe and a 25- to 30-gauge needle. The needle should be directed at the center of the base of the wart and at an angle almost parallel to the plane of the skin, infiltrating the lesion and causing a small wheal. Do not go beneath the lesion too deeply or inject too superficially. As many as 5 lesions can be treated at one time. To reduce side effects, give in the evening with acetaminophen.

Maximum response usually occurs 4 to 8 weeks after therapy initiation. If results are not satisfactory after 12 to 16 weeks, a second course may be instituted. Patients with 6 to 10 condylomata may receive a second (sequential) course. Patients with more than 10 condylomata may receive additional sequences, depending on how many condylomata are present.

The 10 million IU vial of interferon alfa-2b powder for injection must be reconstituted with 1 mL of diluent (bacteriostatic water for injection). Do not reconstitute the 10 million IU vial of interferon alfa-2b powder for injection with more than 1 mL of diluent because the injection would be subpotent. Do not use the 5, 18, 25, or 50 million IU vials of interferon alfa-2b powder for injection for the treatment of condylomata acuminata because the resulting reconstituted solution would be hypertonic or an inappropriate concentration. Do not use the multidose pens and 3 million IU vial or the 18 million IU multidose vial of interferon alfa-2b solution for injection for the intralesional treatment of condylomata acuminata because the concentrations are inappropriate for such use.

▶*AIDS-related Kaposi sarcoma:* 30 million IU/m² 3 times/week administered SC or IM. Do not use the multidose pens and the 18 and 25 million IU multidose strengths of the interferon alfa-2b solution for injection for the treatment of AIDS-related Kaposi sarcoma because the concentrations are inappropriate. Maintain the selected dosage regimen unless the disease progresses rapidly or severe intolerance occurs. If severe adverse reactions develop, modify dosage (50% reduction) or temporarily discontinue therapy until adverse reactions abate. When patients initiate therapy at 30 million IU/m² 3 times/week, average dose tolerated at the end of 12 weeks of therapy is 110 million IU/week and 75 million IU/week at end of 24 weeks of therapy.

When disease stabilization or response to treatment occurs, continue treatment until there is no further evidence of tumor or until discontinuation is required by evidence of a severe opportunistic infection or adverse effect.

▶*Chronic hepatitis C:* 3 million IU 3 times/week SC or IM. In patients tolerating therapy with normalization of ALT at 16 weeks of treatment, extend therapy to 18 to 24 months at 3 million IU 3 times/week to improve the sustained response. Consider discontinuing therapy in non-responders after 16 weeks. If severe adverse reactions develop, modify the dose (50% reduction) or temporarily discontinue therapy until reactions abate. If intolerance persists after dose adjustment, discontinue therapy. See interferon alfa-2b recombinant and ribavirin combination therapy monograph when used in combination with ribavirin capsules.

▶*Chronic hepatitis B:*

Adults – 30 to 35 million IU/week SC or IM, as 5 million IU daily or 10 million IU 3 times/week for 16 weeks.

Pediatrics – 3 million IU/m² 3 times/week for the first week of therapy followed by dose escalation to 6 million IU/m² 3 times/week (maximum of 10 million IU 3 times/week) administered SC for a total therapy duration of 16 to 24 weeks.

If serious adverse reactions or lab abnormalities develop during therapy, decrease the dose by 50% or discontinue if appropriate until adverse reactions abate. If intolerance persists after dose adjustment, discontinue the drug.

Decreased white blood cell, granulocyte, or platelet counts – Use the following guidelines:

Interferon Alfa-2b Dose with Decreased White Blood Cell, Granulocyte, or Platelet Counts			
Granulocyte count	White blood cell count	Platelet count	Interferon alfa-2b dose
< 750/mm³	< 1500/mm³	< 50,000/mm³	Reduce by 50%
< 500/mm³	< 1000/mm³	< 25,000/mm³	Permanently discontinue

When white blood cell, platelet, or granulocyte counts return to normal or baseline values, therapy can be reinstituted at up to 100% of initial dose.

▶*Reconstitution or administration of powder for injection:* Inject appropriate amount of diluent (bacteriostatic water for injection) stated in chart below into vial. Swirl gently. The appropriate interferon alfa-2b dose should then be withdrawn and injected IM, SC, or intralesionally.

Interferon alfa-2b powder for injection is not indicated for use in infants and should not be used in pediatric patients in this age group because the provided diluent contains benzyl alcohol (see Warnings).

▶*Preparation and administration of interferon alfa-2b powder for injection for IV infusion:* Prepare the infusion solution immediately prior to use. Based on the desired dose, reconstitute the appropriate vial strength(s) of interferon alfa-2b powder for injection with the diluent provided. Then withdraw the appropriate dose and inject it into a 100 mL bag of 0.9% sodium chloride injection. The final concentration of interferon alfa-2b should not be less than 10 million IU/100 mL. Infuse the prepared solution over a 20-minute period.

Preparation of Interferon Alfa-2b Powder for Injection Based on Indication	
Vial strength	Amount of diluent
Hairy-cell leukemia	
5 million IU	1 mL
10 million IU	2 mL
25 million IU	5 mL
Malignant melanoma Induction:[1]	
5 million IU	1 mL
10 million IU	1 mL
18 million IU	1 mL
25 million IU	5 mL
50 million IU[2]	1 mL
Maintenance:	
5 million IU	1 mL
10 million IU	1 mL
18 million IU	1 mL
50 million IU[2]	1 mL
Follicular lymphoma	
5 million IU	1 mL
10 million IU	1 mL
25 million IU	5 mL
Condylomata acuminata	
10 million IU[3]	1 mL
AIDS-related Kaposi sarcoma	
50 million IU[2]	1 mL
Chronic hepatitis B	
5 million IU	1 mL
10 million IU	1 mL

[1] Based on the desired dose, the appropriate vial strengths should be reconstituted and administered IV.
[2] This vial size is to be used *only* for treatment of patients with AIDS-related Kaposi sarcoma or for patients with malignant melanoma.
[3] Reconstitute the 10 million IU vial with *only* 1 mL of the diluent to reach a final concentration of 10 million IU/mL for intralesional administration.

▶*Preparation and administration of solution for injection:* Multidose vials of interferon alfa-2b solution for injection do not require reconstitution prior to administration. Inject the appropriate interferon alfa-2b dose IM, SC, or intralesionally (5 and 10 million IU vials and 25 million IU multidose vials only).

Interferon Alfa-2b, Recombinant Solution for Injection					
	3 million IU	5 million IU	10 million IU	18 million IU multidose[1]	25 million IU multidose[2]
Chronic hepatitis B		X	X		X[3]
Chronic hepatitis C	X			X	
Hairy cell leukemia	X	X	X	X	X
Condylomata acuminata		X	X		X
Malignant melanoma	X[4]	X	X	X[4]	X[5]
Follicular lymphoma		X			X

[1] This is a multidose vial that contains a total of 22.8 million IU of interferon alfa-2b, recombinant per 3.8 mL in order to provide the delivery of six 0.5 mL doses, each containing 3 million IU of interferon alfa-2b, recombinant for injection (for a label strength of 18 million IU).
[2] This is a multidose vial that contains a total of 32 million IU of interferon alfa-2b, recombinant per 3.2 mL in order to provide the delivery of five 0.5 mL doses, each containing 5 million IU of interferon alfa-2b, recombinant for injection (for a label strength of 25 million IU).
[3] Use only for the 5 million IU daily regimen.
[4] Use only for dose reduction.
[5] Use only for maintenance treatment.

INTERFERON ALFA-2b, RECOMBINANT (IFN-alpha 2; rIFN-α2; α-2-interferon)

➤*Solution for injection in multidose pens:* The interferon alfa-2b solution for injection multidose pen contains a prefilled, multidose cartridge for SC administration. It is designed to deliver individual doses using a simple dial mechanism. The needles provided in the packaging should be used for the multidose pen only. A new needle is to be used each time a dose is delivered using the pen. To avoid the possible transmission of disease, each multidose pen is for single patient use only.

Interferon Alfa-2b, Recombinant Solution in Multidose Pens

	3 million IU/ 0.2 mL[1]	5 million IU/ 0.2 mL[2]	10 million IU/ 0.2 mL[3]
Chronic hepatitis B		X	X
Chronic hepatitis C	X		
Hairy cell leukemia	X	X	
Malignant melanoma			X
Follicular lymphoma		X	

[1] The 3 million IU multidose pen contains a total of 22.5 million IU of interferon alfa-2b per 1.5 mL in order to provide delivery of six 0.2 mL doses each containing 3 million IU (for a label strength of 18 million IU).

[2] The 5 million IU multidose pen contains a total of 37.5 million IU of interferon alfa-2b per 1.5 mL in order to provide delivery of six 0.2 mL doses each containing 5 million IU (for a label strength of 30 million IU).

[3] The 10 million IU multidose pen contains a total of 75 million IU of interferon alfa-2b per 1.5 mL in order to provide delivery of six 0.2 mL doses each containing 10 million IU (for a label strength of 80 million IU).

Do not use the 3 million IU vial and the 18 million IU multidose vial of interferon alfa-2b solution for injection for chronic hepatitis B or condylomata acuminata. Do not use the multidose pen for condylomata acuminata. Do not use the 10 million IU vial of interferon alfa-2b solution for injection for chronic hepatitis C. Do not use interferon alfa-2b solution for injection for AIDS-related Kaposi sarcoma because the concentrations are inappropriate. Interferon alfa-2b solution for injection is not recommended for IV administration and should not be used for the induction phase of malignant melanoma.

➤*Storage / Stability:*

Solution for injection – Store interferon alfa-2b solution between 2° and 8°C (36° and 46°F).

Multidose pens and vials: Interferon alfa-2b solution for injection multidose pens provided in strengths ranging from 18 to 80 million IU per pen is stable at 30°C (86°F) for up to 2 days. Interferon alfa-2b solution for injection provided in vials ranging from 3 to 25 million IU per vial is stable at 35°C (95°F) for up to 7 days and at 30°C (86°F) for up to 14 days. The solution is clear and colorless.

Powder for injection – Store interferon alfa-2b powder both before and after reconstitution between 2° to 8°C (36° to 46°F); the solution is stable for 1 month.

Actions

➤*Pharmacology:* Interferon alfa-2b is a protein produced by recombinant DNA techniques. It is obtained from a strain of *Escherichia coli* bearing a genetically engineered plasmid containing an interferon alfa-2b gene from human leukocytes.

The interferons are naturally occurring small protein molecules. They are produced and secreted by cells in response to viral infections or synthetic and biological inducers. Three major classes of interferons have been identified: Alpha, beta, and gamma.

Interferons exert their cellular activities by binding to specific membrane receptors on the cell surface. Once bound to the cell membrane, interferons initiate a complex sequence of intracellular events that includes the induction of certain enzymes. These events include inhibition of virus replication in virus-infected cells, suppression of cell proliferation, and such immunomodulating activities as enhancement of the phagocytic activity of macrophages and augmentation of the specific cytotoxicity of lymphocytes for target cells.

➤*Pharmacokinetics:*

Absorption / Distribution – Maximum serum concentrations obtained via SC and IM were approximately 18 to 116 IU/mL and occurred 3 to 12 hours after administration. Serum concentrations were below the detection limit by 16 hours after the injections.

After IV use, serum concentrations peaked (135 to 273 IU/mL) by the end of infusion, then declined at a slightly more rapid rate than after IM or SC administration, becoming undetectable 4 hours after infusion.

Metabolism / Excretion – Following IM/SC injections and IV administration, the elimination half-lives were approximately 2 to 3 hours. Interferon could not be detected in urine; the kidney may be the main site of interferon catabolism.

Contraindications

Hypersensitivity to interferon alfa-2b or any components of the product. Interferon alfa-2b and ribavirin must not be used by women who are pregnant or by men whose female partners are pregnant. Extreme care must be taken to avoid pregnancy in female patients and in female partners of patients taking combination interferon alfa-2b/ribavirin therapy. Patients with autoimmune hepatitis must not be treated with combination interferon alfa-2b/ribavirin therapy.

Warnings

➤*Hemolytic anemia:* Combination therapy containing interferon alfa-2b and ribavirin capsules was associated with hemolytic anemia. Hemoglobin less than 10 g/dL was observed in approximately 10% of patients in clinical trials. Anemia occurred within 1 to 2 weeks of initiation of ribavirin therapy. Interferon alfa-2b/ribavirin capsule combination therapy is not recommended in patients with severe renal impairment and should be used with caution in patients with moderate renal impairment.

➤*Thrombocytopenia:* Do not give IM to patients with platelet counts less than 50,000/mm[3]. Instead, give SC.

➤*50 million IU vial size:* This vial size is to be used only for treatment of patients with AIDS-related Kaposi sarcoma or for patients with malignant melanoma. The 50 million IU strength of interferon powder for injection is not to be used for the treatment of hairy-cell leukemia, condylomata acuminata, follicular lymphoma, chronic hepatitis C, or chronic hepatitis B.

➤*Condylomata acuminata:* Do not use 5, 18, 25, or 50 million IU vials of powder for injection or the 3 or 18 million IU multidose vials for intralesional treatment of condylomata acuminata because the dilution required for the intralesional use would result in a hypertonic solution or an inappropriate concentration.

➤*AIDS-related Kaposi sarcoma:* Do not use interferon alfa-2b solution for injection, multidose pens, or the 18 or 25 million IU multidose strengths; concentrations are inappropriate. Do not use in patients with rapidly progressive visceral disease. There may be synergistic adverse effects between interferon alfa-2b and zidovudine. Patients have had a higher incidence of neutropenia than that expected with zidovudine alone. Careful monitoring of the WBC count is indicated.

➤*Malignant melanoma:* Interferon solution for injection is not recommended for the IV treatment of malignant melanoma.

➤*Neuropsychiatric events:* Depression and suicidal behavior, including suicidal ideation, suicidal attempts, and completed suicides have been reported. Patients with a pre-existing psychiatric condition, especially depression, or a history of severe psychiatric disorder should not be treated with interferon alfa-2b. Discontinue therapy for any patient developing severe depression or other psychiatric disorders during treatment. Obtundation and coma also have been observed in some patients, usually elderly, treated at higher doses. These effects are usually rapidly reversible upon discontinuation of therapy; full resolution of symptoms has taken up to 3 weeks in a few severe episodes. Use concurrent narcotics, hypnotics, or sedatives with caution, and monitor patients closely until the adverse effects have resolved.

➤*Bone marrow toxicity:* Interferon alfa-2b therapy suppresses bone marrow function and may result in severe cytopenias, including very rare events of aplastic anemia. It is advised that complete blood counts (CBCs) be obtained pretreatment and monitored routinely during therapy. Discontinue interferon alfa-2b therapy in patients who develop severe decreases in neutrophil (less than 0.5×10^9/L) or platelet counts (less than 25×10^9/L).

➤*Thyroid abnormalities:* Infrequently, patients receiving interferon alfa-2b therapy developed thyroid abnormalities, either hypothyroid or hyperthyroid. Do not treat patients with pre-existing thyroid abnormalities whose thyroid function cannot be maintained in the normal range by medication. Prior to initiation of therapy, evaluate serum thyroid stimulating hormone (TSH). TSH levels must be within normal limits upon initiation; repeat TSH testing at 3 and 6 months. Patients developing symptoms consistent with possible thyroid dysfunction during the course of therapy should have their thyroid function evaluated and appropriate treatment instituted. Discontinue therapy for patients developing thyroid abnormalities during treatment whose thyroid function cannot be normalized by medication. Discontinuation of therapy has not always reversed thyroid dysfunction occurring during treatment.

➤*Fever / "Flu-like" symptoms:* Because of fever and other flu-like symptoms associated with this drug, use cautiously in patients with debilitating medical conditions, such as those patients with a history of pulmonary disease (eg, chronic obstructive pulmonary disease) or diabetes mellitus prone to ketoacidosis. Observe caution in coagulation disorders (eg, thrombophlebitis, pulmonary embolism) or severe myelosuppression.

While fever may be related to the flu-like syndrome reported commonly in patients treated with interferon, rule out other causes of persistent fever.

INTERFERON ALFA-2b, RECOMBINANT (IFN-alpha 2; rIFN-α2; α-2-interferon)

➤*Pulmonary disorders:* Pulmonary infiltrates, pneumonitis, and pneumonia, including fatality, have been observed. The etiologic explanation for these pulmonary findings has not been established. Take chest x-rays of any patient developing fever, cough, dyspnea, or other respiratory symptoms. If x-ray shows pulmonary infiltrates or if there is evidence of pulmonary function impairment, closely monitor the patient, and discontinue therapy if appropriate. While this has been reported more often in patients with chronic hepatitis C treated with interferon alfa, it also has been reported in patients with oncologic diseases treated with interferon alfa.

➤*Cardiovascular:* Use therapy cautiously in patients with a history of cardiovascular disease. Monitor those patients with a history of MI or previous or current arrhythmic disorder who require therapy. Cardiovascular adverse experiences, including hypotension, arrhythmia, or tachycardia of 150 bpm or more and, rarely, cardiomyopathy and MI, have been observed. Hypotension may occur during administration, or 2 days or less posttherapy, and may require supportive therapy, including fluid replacement to maintain intravascular volume. Supraventricular arrhythmias occurred rarely and appeared to be correlated with pre-existing conditions and prior therapy with cardiotoxic agents. These adverse experiences were controlled by modifying the dose or discontinuing treatment but may require specific additional therapy.

➤*Ophthalmologic disorders:* Decrease or loss of vision, retinopathy (including macular edema), retinal artery or vein thrombosis, retinal hemorrhages and cotton wool spots, optic neuritis, and papilledema may be induced or aggravated by treatment with interferon alfa-2b or other alpha interferons. All patients should receive an eye examination at baseline. Patients with pre-existing ophthalmologic disorders (eg, diabetic or hypertensive retinopathy) should receive periodic ophthalmologic exams during interferon alpha treatment. Any patient who develops ocular symptoms should receive a prompt and complete eye examination. Interferon alfa-2b treatment should be discontinued in patients who develop new or worsening ophthalmologic disorders.

A baseline ocular examination is recommended prior to treatment with interferon alfa-2b in patients with diabetes mellitus or hypertension because the retinal events may have to be differentiated from those seen with diabetic or hypertensive retinopathy.

➤*Hepatotoxicity:* Hepatotoxicity, including fatality, has been observed. Closely monitor any patient developing liver function abnormalities during treatment; discontinue treatment if appropriate.

➤*Autoimmune disorders:* Rare cases of autoimmune diseases, including thrombocytopenia, vasculitis, Raynaud phenomenon, rheumatoid arthritis, lupus erythematosus, and rhabdomyolysis have been observed in patients treated with alpha interferons. In very rare cases, the event resulted in fatality. Monitor any patient developing an autoimmune disorder during treatment. Discontinue treatment if appropriate.

➤*Hyperglycemia:* Diabetes mellitus and hyperglycemia have been observed rarely in patients treated with interferon alfa-2b. Symptomatic patients should have their blood glucose measured and followed up accordingly. Patients with diabetes mellitus may require adjustment of their antidiabetic regimen.

➤*Benzyl alcohol:* The powder for injection for interferon alfa-2b, when reconstituted with the provided diluent (bacteriostatic water for injection) contains benzyl alcohol and is not indicated for use in infants. There have been reports of death in infants associated with excessive exposure to benzyl alcohol.

➤*Hypersensitivity reactions:* Acute, serious hypersensitivity reactions (eg, urticaria, angioedema, bronchoconstriction, anaphylaxis) have been observed rarely in treated patients; if an acute reaction develops, discontinue the drug immediately, and institute appropriate medical therapy. Refer to Management of Acute Hypersensitivity Reactions. Transient rashes have occurred following injection but have not necessitated treatment interruption.

➤*Hepatic function impairment:* Do not treat patients with decompensated liver disease, autoimmune hepatitis, history of autoimmune disease, or immunosuppressed transplant recipients. In these patients, worsening liver disease, including jaundice, hepatic encephalopathy, hepatic failure, and death have occurred following therapy. Discontinue therapy for any patient developing signs and symptoms of liver failure.

➤*Fertility impairment:* Interferon may impair fertility. In nonhuman primates, abnormalities of the menstrual cycle have been observed. Decreases in serum estradiol and progesterone concentrations have occurred in women treated with human leukocyte interferon. Fertile women should not receive interferon alfa-2b unless they are using effective contraception. Use with caution in fertile men.

➤*Elderly:* In general, administer interferon alfa-2b therapy cautiously to elderly patients, reflecting the greater frequency of decreased hepatic, renal, bone marrow, and/or cardiac function and concomitant disease or other drug therapy. Interferon alfa-2b is known to be substantially excreted by the kidney and the risk of adverse reactions to interferon alfa-2b may be greater in patients with impaired renal function. Because elderly patients often have decreased renal function,

carefully monitor patients during treatment, and make dose adjustments based on symptoms and/or laboratory abnormalities.

In a database consisting of clinical study and postmarketing reports for various indications, cardiovascular adverse events and confusion were reported more frequently in elderly patients receiving interferon alfa-2b therapy compared with younger patients.

➤*Pregnancy: Category C.* Interferon alfa-2b has abortifacient effects in rhesus monkeys at 15 and 30 million IU/kg (estimated human equivalent of 5 and 10 million IU/kg, based on body surface area adjustment for a 60 kg adult). Therefore, use during pregnancy only if the potential benefit justifies the potential risk to the fetus.

Use with ribavirin – Category X. If interferon alfa-2b is used in combination therapy with ribavirin, instruct patients that this therapy must not be used by pregnant women or by men whose female partners are pregnant. Extreme caution must be taken to avoid pregnancy. Do not initiate therapy until a report of a negative pregnancy test is obtained. Refer to ribavirin monograph for additional information.

➤*Lactation:* It is not known if this drug is excreted in breast milk. Because of the potential for serious reactions in nursing infants, decide whether to discontinue nursing or to discontinue the drug, taking into account the importance of the drug to the mother.

➤*Children:* Safety and efficacy in children less than 18 years of age have not been established for indications other than chronic hepatitis B (in children 1 year of age and older).

Precautions

➤*Monitoring:* In addition to tests normally required for monitoring patients, the following are recommended for all patients on interferon therapy prior to beginning treatment and periodically thereafter: Standard hematologic tests, including hemoglobin with CBCs and differential, platelet counts, blood chemistries, electrolytes, TSH, and liver function tests. Patients with pre-existing cardiac abnormalities or in advanced stages of cancer should have ECGs taken before and during treatment.

Mild to moderate leukopenia and AST levels have been reported with intralesional administration of interferon alfa-2b; therefore, consider monitoring these laboratory parameters.

Baseline chest x-rays are suggested; repeat if clinically indicated.

For malignant melanoma patients, monitor differential WBC count and liver function tests weekly during the induction phase of therapy and monthly during the maintenance phase of therapy.

If increases in ALT occur during therapy for chronic hepatitis B, carefully monitor clinical symptomatology and liver function tests, including ALT, prothrombin time, alkaline phosphatase, albumin, and bilirubin.

➤*Triglycerides:* Elevated triglyceride levels have been observed in patients treated with interferon therapy. Manage elevated triglyceride levels as clinically appropriate. Hypertriglyceridemia may result in pancreatitis. Consider discontinuation of therapy for patients with persistently elevated triglycerides (more than 1000 mg/dL) associated with symptoms of potential pancreatitis, such as abdominal pain, nausea, or vomiting.

➤*Chronic hepatitis B:* Perform a liver biopsy to establish presence of chronic hepatitis and extent of liver damage. Establish that the patient has compensated liver disease. Before treatment, establish and consider the following criteria: No history of hepatic encephalopathy, variceal bleeding, ascites, or other signs of clinical decompensation; bilirubin normal; albumin stable and within normal limits; prothrombin time (PT) less than 3 seconds prolonged (adults), 2 seconds or less prolonged (pediatrics); WBC at least 4000/mm³; and platelets at least 100,000/mm³ (adults), at least 150,000/mm³ (pediatrics). Evaluate CBC and platelet counts, then repeat at weeks 1, 2, 4, 8, 12, and 16. Evaluate liver function tests, including serum ALT, albumin, and bilirubin at treatment weeks 1, 2, 4, 8, 12, and 16. Evaluate HBeAg, HBsAg, and ALT at the end of therapy and 3- and 6-month posttherapy.

ALT increase – A transient increase in ALT 2 times or more baseline (flare) can occur, generally 8 to 12 weeks after therapy initiation, and is more frequent in responders. Continue therapy unless signs and symptoms of hepatic failure occur. During the ALT flare, monitor clinical symptomatology and liver function tests (including ALT, PT, alkaline phosphatase, albumin, and bilirubin) at about 2-week intervals.

Chronic hepatitis B patients with evidence of decreasing hepatic synthetic functions (eg, decreasing albumin levels, prolongation of PT) may be at increased risk of clinical decompensation in association with a flare of aminotransferases.

➤*Chronic hepatitis C:* Perform a liver biopsy to establish diagnosis, and test for presence of antibody to HCV. Exclude patients with other causes of chronic hepatitis, including autoimmune hepatitis. Establish that the patient has compensated liver disease. Before treatment, establish and consider the following criteria: No history of hepatic encephalopathy, variceal bleeding, ascites, or other signs of clinical decompensation; bilirubin 2 mg/dL or less; albumin stable and within normal limits; PT less than 3 seconds prolonged; WBC 3000/mm³ or more; platelets 70,000/mm³ or more; serum creatinine normal or near

INTERFERON ALFA-2b, RECOMBINANT (IFN-alpha 2; rIFN-α2; α-2-interferon)

normal. Evaluate CBC and platelet counts, repeat at weeks 1 and 2 after therapy initiation, monthly thereafter. Evaluate ALT levels at about 3-month intervals.

▶*Psoriasis and sarcoidosis:* There have been reports of interferon exacerbating pre-existing psoriasis and sarcoidosis as well as development of new sarcoidosis; therefore, use therapy in these patients only if the potential benefit justifies the potential risk.

▶*Immunogenicity:* In interferon alfa-2b-treated patients tested for antibody activity in clinical trials, serum anti-interferon neutralizing antibodies were detected in 0% of patients with hairy-cell leukemia, 0.8% of patients treated intralesionally for condylomata acuminata, and 4% of patients with AIDS-related Kaposi sarcoma. Serum neutralizing antibodies have been detected in less than 3% of patients treated with higher interferon alfa-2b doses in malignancies other than hairy-cell leukemia or AIDS-related Kaposi sarcoma. The clinical significance of the appearance of serum anti-interferon neutralizing activity in these indications is not known.

Serum anti-interferon neutralizing antibodies were detected in 7% of patients either during treatment or after completing 12 to 48 weeks of treatment with 3 million IU 3 times/week of interferon alfa-2b therapy for chronic hepatitis C, in 13% of patients who received interferon alfa-2b therapy for chronic hepatitis B at 5 million IU/day for 4 months, and in 3% of patients treated at 10 million IU 3 times/week. Serum anti-interferon neutralizing antibodies were detected in 9% of pediatric patients who received interferon alfa-2b therapy for chronic hepatitis B and 6 million IU/m^2 3 times/week. The titers detected were low among all adult and pediatric patients with chronic hepatitis B or C with detectable serum neutralizing antibodies. The appearance of serum anti-interferon neutralizing activity did not appear to affect safety or efficacy.

▶*Photosensitivity:* Photosensitivity may occur; therefore, caution patients to take protective measures (eg, sunscreens, protective clothing) against exposure to ultraviolet light or sunlight until tolerance is determined.

Drug Interactions

Interferon Alfa-2b Drug Interactions			
Precipitant drug	Object drug*		Description
Interferon alfa-2b	Theophyllines	↑	Concomitant use significantly reduces theophylline clearance (33% to 81%), resulting in a 100% increase in serum theophylline levels.
Interferon alfa-2b	Zidovudine	↑	There may be synergistic adverse effects between interferon alfa-2b and zidovudine. Patients have had a higher incidence of neutropenia than that expected with zidovudine alone. Carefully monitor WBC count in myelosuppressed patients or those receiving myelosuppressive agents.

* ↑ = Object drug increased.

Adverse Reactions

Most adverse effects are mild to moderate in severity. Some are transient and most diminish with continued therapy. The most frequently reported adverse reactions are flu-like symptoms, particularly fever, headache, chills, myalgia, and fatigue. More severe toxicities are observed generally at higher doses and may be difficult for patients to tolerate. In addition, the following spontaneous adverse experiences have been reported during the marketing surveillance of interferon alfa-2b, recombinant, for injection: Nephrotic syndrome; pancreatitis; psychosis, including hallucinations; renal failure; and renal insufficiency. Vary rarely, interferon alfa-2b used alone or in combination with ribavirin capsules may be associated with aplastic anemia. Rarely sarcoidosis or exacerbation of sarcoidosis has been reported.

Malignant melanoma – The interferon alfa-2b dose was modified because of adverse events in 65% of the patients. Interferon alfa-2b therapy was discontinued because of adverse events in 8% of the patients during induction and 18% of the patients during maintenance. Adverse reactions classified as severe or life threatening (ECOG Toxicity Criteria grade 3 or 4) were recorded in 66% and 14% of interferon alfa-2b-treated patients, respectively. Severe adverse reactions recorded in more than 10% of interferon alfa-2b-treated patients included neutropenia/leukopenia (26%); fatigue (23%); fever (18%); myalgia, headache (17%); chills (16%); and increased AST (14%). Grade 4 fatigue was recorded in 4% and grade 4 depression was recorded in 2% of interferon alfa-2b-treated patients. No other grade 4 adverse event was reported in more than 2 interferon alfa-2b-treated patients. Lethal hepatotoxocity occurred in 2 interferon alfa-2b-treated early in the clinical trial. No subsequent lethal hepatotoxicities were observed with adequate monitoring of liver function tests.

Follicular lymphoma – Ninety-six percent of patients treated with CHVP (cyclophosphamide, doxorubicin, teniposide, prednisone) plus interferon alfa-2b therapy and 91% of patients treated with CHVP alone reported an adverse event of any severity. Asthenia, fever, neutropenia, increased hepatic enzymes, alopecia, headache, anorexia, flu-like symptoms, myalgia, dyspnea, thrombocytopenia, paresthesia, and polyuria occurred more frequently in the CHVP plus interferon alfa-2b-treated patients than in patients treated with CHVP alone. Adverse reactions classified as severe or life-threatening (World Health Organization [WHO] grade 3 or 4) recorded in more than 5% of CHVP plus interferon alfa-2b-treated patients included neutropenia (34%), asthenia, vomiting (10%). The incidence of neutropenic infection was 6% in CHVP plus interferon alfa-2b vs 2% in CHVP alone. One patient in each treatment group required hospitalization.

Twenty-eight percent of CHVP plus interferon alfa-2b-treated patients had a temporary modification/interruption of their interferon alfa-2b therapy but only 10% of patients permanently stopped interferon alfa-2b therapy because of toxicity. There were 4 deaths in the study; 2 patients committed suicide in the CHVP plus interferon alfa-2b arm and 2 patients in the CHVP arm had unwitnessed sudden death. Three patients with hepatitis B (one of whom also had alcoholic cirrhosis) developed hepatotoxicity leading to discontinuation of interferon alfa-2b. Other reasons for discontinuation included intolerable asthenia (4%), severe flu symptoms (1%), and 1 patient each with exacerbation of ankylosing spondylitis, psychosis, and decreased ejection fraction.

AIDS-related Kaposi sarcoma – In patients with AIDS-related Kaposi sarcoma, some type of adverse reaction occurred in 100% of the 74 patients treated with 30 million IU/m^2 3 times/week and in 97% of the 29 patients treated with 35 million IU/day.

Of these adverse reactions, those classified as severe (WHO grade 3 or 4) were reported in 27% to 55% of patients. Severe adverse reactions in the 30 million IU/m^2 3 times/week study included: Fatigue (20%); influenza-like symptoms (15%); anorexia (12%); dry mouth, headache (4%); confusion, fever, myalgia (3%); nausea, vomiting (1%). Severe adverse reactions for patients who received the 35 million IU QD included: Fever (24%); fatigue (17%); influenza-like symptoms, dyspnea (14%); headache (10%); pharyngitis (7%); ataxia, confusion, dysphagia, GI hemorrhage, abnormal hepatic function, increased AST, myalgia, cardiomyopathy, face edema, depression, emotional lability, suicide attempt, chest pain, and coughing (1 patient each). Overall, the incidence of severe toxicity was higher among patients who received the 35 million IU/day dose.

Chronic hepatitis C – Two studies of extended treatment (18 to 24 months) with interferon alfa-2b, recombinant for injection show that approximately 95% of all patients treated experience some type of adverse event and that patients treated for extended duration continue to experience adverse events throughout treatment. Most adverse events reported are mild to moderate in severity. However 19% of patients treated for 18 to 24 months experienced a serious adverse event compared with 7% of those treated for 6 months. Adverse events that occur or persist during extended treatment are similar in type and severity to those occurring during short-course therapy.

Of the patients achieving a complete response after 6 months of therapy, 15% subsequently discontinued interferon alfa-2b treatment during extended therapy because of adverse events, and 29% experienced severe adverse events (WHO grade 3 or 4) during extended therapy.

In patients using interferon alfa-2b/ribavirin capsule combination therapy, the primary toxicity observed was hemolytic anemia. Reductions in hemoglobin levels occurred within the first 1 to 2 weeks of therapy. Cardiac and pulmonary events associated with anemia occurred in approximately 10% of patients treated with interferon alfa-2b/ribavirin capsule combination therapy. See interferon alfa-2b/ribavirin capsule combination therapy package insert for additional information.

Chronic hepatitis B –

Adults: In patients with chronic hepatitis B, some type of adverse reaction occurred in 98% of the 101 patients treated at 5 million IU QD and 90% of the 78 patients treated at 10 million IU 3 times/week. Most of these adverse reactions were mild to moderate in severity, manageable, and reversible following the end of therapy.

Adverse reactions classified as severe (causing a significant interference with normal daily activities or clinical state) were reported in 21% to 44% of patients. The severe adverse reactions reported most frequently were the flu-like symptoms of fever (28%); fatigue (15%); headache (5%); myalgia, rigors (4%); and other severe flu-like symptoms (1% to 3%). Other severe adverse reactions occurring in more than one patient were alopecia (8%); anorexia (6%); depression, nausea (3%); and vomiting (2%).

To manage side effects, the dose was reduced or interferon alfa-2b therapy was interrupted in 25% to 38% of patients. Five percent of patients discontinued treatment because of adverse experiences.

Children: In pediatric patients, the most frequently reported adverse events were these commonly associated with interferon treatment: Flu-like symptoms (100%), GI system disorders (46%), and nausea/vomiting (40%). Neutropenia (13%) and thrombocytopenia (3%) also were reported. None of the adverse events were life-threatening. The majority were moderate to severe and resolved upon dose reduction or drug discontinuation.

INTERFERON ALFA-2b, RECOMBINANT (IFN-alpha 2; rIFN-α2; α-2-interferon)

	Interferon Alfa-2b Adverse Reactions Based on Indication (%)							
Adverse reaction	Malignant melanoma (n=143)	Follicular lymphoma (n = 135)	Hairy-cell leukemia (n = 145)	Condylomata acuminata (n = 352)	AIDS-related Kaposi sarcoma (n = 103)	Chronic hepatitis C (n = 183)	Chronic hepatitis B (adults) (n = 179)	Chronic hepatitis B (pediatrics) (n = 116)
Bone, joint, muscle								
Arthralgia	6	8	8	9	3	16	8-19	15
Back pain	—	15	19	6	1-3	—	—	15
Musculoskeletal pain	—	18	—	—	—	21	1-9	10
Myalgia	75	16	39	44	28-34	43	40-59	27
CNS								
Amnesia	*	1	< 5	—	14	—	—	—
Anxiety	1	9	5	< 1	1-3	5	2	3
Confusion	8	2	< 5	4	10-12	1	—	2
Decreased libido	1	1	< 5	—	—	1	1-5	—
Depression	40	9	6	3	9-28	19	6-17	4
Dizziness	23	—	12	9	7-24	9	10-13	8
Hypesthesia	—	1	< 5	1	10	—	—	—
Impaired concentration	—	1	—	< 1	3-14	3	5-8	3
Insomnia	5	4	—	< 1	3	12	6-11	8
Irritability	1	1	—	—	—	13	12-16	22
Nervousness	1	1	—	1	3	2	3	3
Paresthesia	13	13	6	1	3-21	5	3-6	< 1
Somnolence	1	2	< 5	3	3	33[1]	9-14	5
Dermatologic								
Alopecia	29	23	8	—	12-31	28	26-38	17
Dermatitis	1	—	8	—	—	2	1	—
Dry skin	1	3	9	—	9-10	4	3	< 1
Facial edema	—	1	—	< 1	10	< 1	1-3	< 1
Injection site inflammation	—	1	—	—	—	5	3	—
Rash	19	13	25	—	9-10	5	1-8	5
Pruritus	—	10	11	1	7	9	4-6	3
Flu-like symptoms								
Chills	54	—	46	45	—	—	—	—
Dry mouth	1	2	19	—	22-28	5	5-6	—
Fatigue	96	8	61	18	48-84	23	69-75	71
Fever	81	56	68	56	47-55	34	66-86	94
Flu-like symptoms	10	18	37	—	45-79	26	5	< 1
Headache	62	21	39	47	21-36	43	44-61	57
GI								
Abdominal pain	2	20	< 5	1	5-21	16	4-5	23
Anorexia	69	21	19	1	38-41	14	43-53	43
Constipation	1	14	< 1	—	1-10	4	5	2
Diarrhea	35	19	18	2	18-45	13	8-19	12
Dry mouth/thirst	1	—	19	—	22-28	5	5-6	—
Dyspepsia	—	2	—	2	4	7	3-8	3
Gingivitis	2[2]	7[2]	—	—	14	—	1	—
Loose stools	—	1	—	< 1	10	2	2	2
Nausea	66	24	21	17	21-28	19	33-50	18
Taste alteration	24	2	13	< 1	5-7	2	10	—
Vomiting	**	32	6	2	11-14	8	7-10	27
Respiratory								
Coughing	6	13	< 1	—	31	1	4	5
Dyspnea	15	14	< 1	—	1-34	3	5	—
Nasal congestion	1	7	—	1	10	< 1	4	—
Nonproductive coughing	2	7	—	—	14	0	1	—
Pharyngitis	2	8	< 5	1	1-31	3	1-7	7
Sinusitis	1	4	—	—	21	2	—	—
Miscellaneous								
Asthenia	—	63	7	—	11	40	5-15	5
Chest pain	2	8	< 1	< 1	1-28	4	4	—
Herpes simplex	1	2	—	1	3	1	5	—
Increased sweating	6	13	8	2	4-21	4	1	3
Malaise	6	—	—	14	5	13	6-9	3
Moniliasis	—	1	—	< 1	17	—	—	—
Pain (unspecified)	15	9	18	3	3	—	—	—
Rigors	2	7	—	—	14-30	16	38-42	30
Weight loss	3	13	< 1	< 1	3-5	10	2-5	3

* Amnesia was reported with confusion as a single term.
** Vomiting was reported with nausea as a single term.

[1] Predominantly lethargy.
[2] Includes stomatitis/mucositis.

INTERFERON ALFA-2b, RECOMBINANT (IFN-alpha 2; rIFN-α2; α-2-interferon)

Lab test	Malignant melanoma (n = 143)	Follicular lymphoma (n = 135)	Hairy-cell leukemia (n = 145)	Condylomata acuminata (n = 352)	AIDS-related Kaposi sarcoma (n = 54 to 142)	Chronic hepatitis C (n = 140 to 171)	Chronic hepatitis B (adults) (n = 178 to 197)	Chronic hepatitis B (pediatrics) (n = 113 to 115)
Interferon Alfa-2b Abnormal Laboratory Test Values Based on Indication (%)								
Hemoglobin	22	8	NA	—	1-15	26[1]	23-32[2]	17[3]
WBC count	*	—	NA	17	10-22	26[4]	34-68[4]	9[4]
Platelet count	15	13	NA	—	0-8	15[5]	5-12[5]	1[5]
Serum creatinine	3	2	0	—	—	6	0-3	3
Alkaline phosphatase	13	—	4	—	—	—	4-8	0
Lactate dehydrogenase	1	—	0	—	—	—	—	—
Serum urea nitrogen	12	4	0	—	—	—	0-2	2
AST	63	24	4	12	11-41	—	—	—
ALT	2	—	13	—	10-15	—	—	—
Granulocyte count								
Total	92	36	NA	—	31-39	45[6]	61-75[6]	70[6]
1000 to < 1500/mm³	66	—	—	—	—	32	30-32	43
750 to < 1000/mm³	—	21	—	—	—	10	18-24	18
500 to < 750/mm³	25	—	—	—	—	1	9-17	7
< 500/mm³	1	13	—	—	—	2	2-4	2

Dash (–) indicates not reported. NA = not applicable.
* WBC count was reported as neutropenia.
[1] Decrease of 2 g/dL or more; 20% 2 to less than 3 g/dL; 6% 3 g/dL or more.
[2] Decrease of 2 g/dL or more.
[3] Decrease of 2 g/dL or more; 14% 2 to less than 3 g/dL; 3% 3 g/dL or more.
[4] Decrease to less than 3000/mm³.
[5] Decrease to less than 70,000/mm³.
[6] Neutrophils plus bands.

➤*All indications (less than 5%):*

Cardiovascular – Angina, arrhythmia, atrial fibrillation, bradycardia, cardiac failure, cardiomegaly, cardiomyopathy, coronary artery disorder, extrasystoles, heart valve disorder, hematoma, hypertension (9% in chronic hepatitis C patients); hypotension, palpitations, postural hypotension, pulmonary embolism, Raynaud disease, tachycardia, thrombosis, varicose veins.

CNS – Abnormal coordination/dreaming/gait/thinking, aggravated depression, aggressive reaction, agitation (7% in chronic hepatitis B pediatric patients); alcohol intolerance, apathy, aphasia, ataxia, Bell palsy, CNS dysfunction, coma, convulsions, dysphonia, emotional lability, extrapyramidal disorder, feeling of ebriety, flushing, hearing disorder, hearing impairment, hot flashes, hyperesthesia, hyperkinesia, hypertonia, hypokinesia, impaired consciousness, labyrinthine disorder, manic depression, manic reaction, migraine, neuralgia, neuritis, neuropathy, neurosis, paresis, paroniria, parosmia, personality disorder, polyneuropathy, speech disorder, stroke, suicide attempt, syncope, tinnitus, tremor, vertigo, delirium, loss of consciousness, psychosis, suicidal ideation, twitching (8% in follicular lymphoma patients).

Dermatologic – Abnormal hair texture, acne, cellulitis, cyanosis of the hand, cold/clammy skin, dermatitis lichenoides, eczema, epidermal necrolysis, erythema, erythema nodosum, folliculitis, furunculosis, increased hair growth, lacrimal gland disorder, lacrimation, lipoma, maculopapular rash, melanosis, nail disorder, nonherpetic cold sores, pallor, peripheral ischemia, photosensitivity (see Precautions), pruritus genital, psoriasis, psoriasis aggravated, purpura (5% in chronic hepatitis C patients); erythematous rash, skin depigmentation, skin discoloration, urticaria, vitiligo, sebaceous cyst, skin nodule.

Injection site bleeding, pain, burning, and reaction (5% in chronic hepatitis B pediatrics patients); itching.

Endocrine – Aggravation of diabetes mellitus; gynecomastia; goiter; hyperglycemia; hyperthyroidism; hypertriglyceridemia; hypothyroidism; virilism.

GI – Abdominal ascites, abdominal distention, colitis, dysphagia, eructation, esophagitis, flatulence, gallstones, gastric ulcer, gastritis, gastroenteritis, GI disorder (7% in follicular lymphoma patients); GI hemorrhage; GI mucosal discoloration; gingival bleeding; gum hyperplasia; halitosis; hemorrhoids; increased appetite; increased salivation; intestinal disorder; melena; mouth ulceration; mucositis; oral hemorrhage; oral leukoplakia; rectal bleeding after stool; rectal hemorrhage; stomatitis; tongue disorder; tooth disorder; ulcerative stomatitis; taste loss.

GU – Amenorrhea (12% in follicular lymphoma patients); albumin/protein in urine, cystitis, dysuria, hematuria, incontinence, increased BUN, micturition disorder/frequency, nocturia, polyuria (10% in follicular lymphoma patients); renal insufficiency, urinary tract infection (5% in chronic hepatitis C patients); dysmenorrhea; impotence; leukorrhea; menorrhagia; menstrual irregularity; pelvic pain; penis disorder; sexual dysfunction; uterine bleeding; vaginal dryness; scrotal/penile edema.

Hematologic – Anemia, anemia hypochromic, granulocytopenia, hemolytic anemia, leukopenia, lymphocytosis, neutropenia (9% in chronic hepatitis C patients, 14% in chronic hepatitis B pediatric patients); thrombocytopenia (10% in chronic hepatitis C patients); bleeding (8% in malignant melanoma patients); thrombocytopenic purpura.

Hepatic – Abnormal hepatic function tests; biliary pain; bilirubinemia; hepatitis; increased lactate dehydrogenase; increased transaminases (ALT/AST) (elevated AST 63% in malignant melanoma patients, 24% in follicular lymphoma patients); jaundice, right upper quadrant pain (15% in chronic hepatitis C patients); and very rarely, hepatic encephalopathy, hepatic failure, and death.

Musculoskeletal – Arteritis; arthritis; arthritis aggravated; arthrosis; bone pain; bone disorder; carpal tunnel syndrome; leg cramps; muscle weakness; polyarteritis nodosa; tendinitis; hyporeflexia; muscle atrophy; rheumatoid arthritis; spondylitis.

Respiratory – Asthma, bronchitis (10% in follicular lymphoma patients); bronchospasm, cyanosis, epistaxis (7% in chronic hepatitis B pediatric patients); hemoptysis; hypoventilation; laryngitis; lung fibrosis; pleural effusion; orthopnea; pleural pain; pneumonia; pneumonitis; pneumothorax; rales; respiratory disorder; respiratory insufficiency; sneezing; wheezing; tonsillitis; tracheitis.

Special senses – Abnormal/Blurred vision; diplopia; dry eyes; eye pain; photophobia; nystagmus; earache.

Miscellaneous – Allergic reaction, cachexia, dehydration, edema, hypercalcemia, hyperglycemia, hypothermia, inflammation (nonspecific), lymphadenitis, lymphadenopathy, mastitis, periorbital edema, poor peripheral circulation, peripheral edema (6% in follicular lymphoma patients); chest pain substernal, hyperthermia, rhinitis, rhinorrhea (less than 5%); phlebitis superficial; thirst; weakness; weight increase; hernia.

Resistance mechanism disorders: Abscess, conjunctivitis, fungal/hemophilus/herpes zoster/bacterial/nonspecific infection (7% in follicular lymphoma patients); parasitic infection, otitis media, sepsis, stye, trichomonas, upper respiratory tract infection, viral infection (7% in chronic hepatitis C patients).

Overdosage

There is limited experience with overdosage. Postmarketing surveillance includes reports of patients receiving a single dose as great as 10 times the recommended dose. In general, the primary effects of an overdosage are consistent with the effects seen with therapeutic doses of interferon alfa-2b. Hepatic enzyme abnormalities, renal failure, hemorrhage, and MI have been reported with single administration overdoses and/or with longer durations of treatment than prescribed. Toxic effects after ingestion of interferon alfa-2b are not expected because interferons are poorly absorbed orally. There is no specific antidote for interferon alfa-2b. Hemodialysis and peritoneal dialysis are not considered effective for treatment of overdose.

Patient Information

A patient package insert is available with product.

May cause drowsiness or dizziness. Use caution while driving or performing other tasks requiring alertness, coordination, or physical dexterity.

Notify your doctor if hives, itching, tightness in the chest, cough, difficulty breathing, visual problems, wheezing, low blood pressure, or lightheadedness occurs.

Contraceptive measures are recommended during therapy with these drugs. Notify your doctor immediately if you suspect pregnancy.

Avoid prolonged exposure to sunlight. Photosensitivity may occur. Wear protective clothing and use sunscreens until tolerance is determined.

INTERFERON ALFA-2b, RECOMBINANT (IFN-alpha 2; rIFN-α2; α-2-interferon)

Do not change brands of interferon; changes in dosage may be necessary.

The most common adverse effects are flu-like symptoms, such as fever, headache, fatigue, anorexia, nausea, and vomiting. These appear to decrease in severity as treatment continues. Some of these flu-like symptoms may be minimized by bedtime doses. Use antipyretics to prevent or partially alleviate fever and headache. Another common adverse experience is thinning of the hair.

Patients should be well hydrated, especially during the initial stages of treatment.

If home use is prescribed, a puncture-resistant container for the disposal of used syringes and needles should be supplied. Thoroughly instruct patients in the importance of proper disposal and caution against any reuse of needles and syringes. Dispose of the full container according to the directions provided by the physician.

If interferon alfa-2b is used in combination therapy with ribavirin, this therapy must not be used by pregnant women or by men whose female partners are pregnant. Extreme caution must be taken to avoid pregnancy, and do not initiate therapy until a report of a negative pregnancy test is obtained.

PEGINTERFERON ALFA-2B

Rx	PEG-Intron[1] (Schering)	Powder for injection, lyophilized: 50 mcg/0.5 mL when reconstituted	In 2 mL vials[2] with 1 mL diluent vial, 2 syringes, and 2 alcohol swabs and *Redipen*[3] with 1 B-D needle and 2 alcohol swabs.
		80 mcg/0.5 mL when reconstituted	In 2 mL vials[2] with 1 mL diluent vial, 2 syringes, and 2 alcohol swabs and *Redipen*[3] with 1 B-D needle and 2 alcohol swabs.
		120 mcg/0.5 mL when reconstituted	In 2 mL vials[2] with 1 mL diluent vial, 2 syringes, and 2 alcohol swabs and *Redipen*[3] with 1 B-D needle and 2 alcohol swabs.
		150 mcg/0.5 mL when reconstituted	In 2 mL vials[2] with 1 mL diluent vial, 2 syringes, and 2 alcohol swabs and *Redipen*[3] with 1 B-D needle and 2 alcohol swabs.

[1] Effective October 22, 2001, *PEG-Intron* only will be made available through the *PEG-Intron* Access Assurance program. Pharmacists must obtain an order authorization number prior to placing an order with their wholesaler. To obtain this number, call (888) 437-2608 to provide the patient's Access Assurance ID# and the quantity to be dispensed (maximum 4 units). Patients without an Access Assurance ID# also may call this number to enroll. Next, contact the wholesaler and provide the authorization number and order information.

[2] Contains 1.11 mg dibasic and monobasic sodium phosphate, 0.074 mg polysorbate 80, and 59.2 mg sucrose.
[3] Contains 1.013 mg dibasic and monobasic sodium phosphate, 0.0675 mg polysorbate 80, and 54 mg sucrose.

WARNING

Alpha interferons, including peginterferon alfa-2b, may cause or aggravate fatal or life-threatening neuropsychiatric, autoimmune, ischemic, and infectious disorders. Closely monitor patients with periodic clinical and laboratory evaluations. Withdraw patients with persistently severe or worsening signs or symptoms of these conditions from therapy. In many, but not all cases, these disorders resolve after stopping peginterferon alfa-2b therapy (see Precautions, Adverse Reactions).

Ribavirin use: Ribavirin may cause birth defects and/or death of the unborn child. Take extreme care to avoid pregnancy in female patients and in female partners of male patients. Ribavirin causes hemolytic anemia. The anemia associated with ribavirin therapy may result in a worsening of cardiac disease. Ribavirin is genotoxic and mutagenic; consider it a potential carcinogen (see Ribavirin monograph for additional information and warnings).

Indications

➤*Chronic hepatitis C:* For use alone or in combination with ribavirin capsules for the treatment of chronic hepatitis C in patients with compensated liver disease who have not been previously treated with interferon alpha and are at least 18 years of age.

When used in combination with ribavirin, refer to ribavirin monograph for additional prescribing information.

➤*Unlabeled uses:* Treatment of renal cell carcinoma.

Administration and Dosage

➤*Approved by the FDA:* January 22, 2001.

There are no safety and efficacy data on treatment for longer than 1 year. Instruct patient to self-inject only if the physician determines that it is appropriate, the patient agrees to medical follow-up as necessary, and the patient receives training in proper injection technique.

➤*Monotherapy:* 1 mcg/kg/week subcutaneously for 1 year. Administer the dose on the same day of the week. Base initial dosing on the patient's weight as described in the following table.

Recommended Dosing of Peginterferon Alfa-2b

Redipen or vial strength to use (mcg/0.5 mL)	Body weight (kg)	Amount of peginterferon alfa-2b to administer (mcg)	Volume[1] of peginterferon alfa-2b to administer (mL)
50	≤ 45	40	0.4
	46 to 56	50	0.5
80	57 to 72	64	0.4
	73 to 88	80	0.5
120	89 to 106	96	0.4
	107 to 136	120	0.5
150	137 to 160	150	0.5

[1] When reconstituted as directed.

➤*Peginterferon alfa-2b/Ribavirin capsules combination therapy:* When administered in combination with ribavirin capsules, the recommended dose of peginterferon alfa-2b is 1.5 mcg/kg/week. The volume of peginterferon alfa-2b to be injected depends on the strength of peginterferon alfa-2b and the patient's body weight.

Recommended Peginterferon Alfa-2b Combination Therapy Dosing

Redipen or vial strength to use (mcg/0.5 mL)	Body weight (kg)	Amount of peginterferon alfa-2b to administer (mcg)	Volume[1] of peginterferon alfa-2b to administer (mL)
50	< 40	50	0.5
80	40 to 50	64	0.4
	51 to 60	80	0.5
120	61 to 75	96	0.4
	76 to 85	120	0.5
150	> 85	150	0.5

[1] When reconstituted as directed.

The recommended dose of ribavirin capsules is 800 mg/day in 2 divided doses; 2 capsules (400 mg) with breakfast and 2 capsules (400 mg) with dinner. Do not use ribavirin capsules in patients with Ccr less than 50 mL/min.

➤*Discontinuation:* It is recommended that patients receiving peginterferon alfa-2b alone or in combination with ribavirin be discontinued from therapy if hepatitis C virus (HCV) viral levels remain high after 6 months of therapy.

➤*Dose reduction:* If a serious adverse reaction develops during the course of treatment (see Warnings, Precautions), discontinue or modify the dosage of peginterferon alfa-2b and/or ribavirin capsules until the adverse reaction abates or decreases in severity. If persistent or recurrent serious adverse reactions develop despite adequate dosage adjustment, discontinue treatment. Decreases in hemoglobin, neutrophils, and platelets may require dose reduction or permanent discontinuation from therapy. For guidelines for dose modifications and discontinuation based on laboratory parameters, see the tables below. In the combination therapy trial, dose reductions occurred among 42% of patients receiving peginterferon alfa-2b 1.5 mcg/kg/ribavirin capsules 800 mg/day, including 57% of those patients 60 kg or less.

Guidelines for Modification or Discontinuation of Peginterferon Alfa-2b or Peginterferon Alfa-2b/Ribavirin Capsules and for Scheduling Visits for Patients with Depression

Depression severity[1]	Initial management (4 to 8 weeks)		Depression		
	Dose modification	Visit schedule	Remains stable	Improves	Worsens
Mild	No change.	Evaluate once/week by visit or phone.	Continue weekly visit schedule.	Resume normal visit schedule.	(See moderate or severe depression.)

PEGINTERFERON ALFA-2B

Guidelines for Modification or Discontinuation of Peginterferon Alfa-2b or Peginterferon Alfa-2b/Ribavirin Capsules and for Scheduling Visits for Patients with Depression

| Depression severity[1] | Initial management (4 to 8 weeks) | | Depression | | |
	Dose modification	Visit schedule	Remains stable	Improves	Worsens
Moderate	Decrease IFN dose 50%.	Evaluate once/week (office visit at least every other week).	Consider psychiatric consultation. Continue reduced dosing.	If symptoms improve and are stable for 4 weeks, may resume normal visit schedule. Continue reduced dosing or return to normal dose.	(See severe depression.)
Severe	Discontinue IFN/R permanently.	Obtain immediate psychiatric consultation.	Psychiatric therapy necessary.		

[1] See DSM-IV for definitions.

Guidelines for Dose Modification and Discontinuation of Peginterferon Alfa-2b or Peginterferon Alfa-2b/Ribavirin Capsules for Hematologic Toxicity

Laboratory values		Peginterferon alfa-2b	Ribavirin capsules
Hemoglobin[1]	< 10 g/dL	—	Decrease by 200 mg/day
	< 8.5 g/dL	Permanently discontinue	Permanently discontinue
WBC	< 1.5 × 10⁹/L	Reduce dose by 50%	—
	< 1 × 10⁹/L	Permanently discontinue	Permanently discontinue
Neutrophils	< 0.75 × 10⁹/L	Reduce dose by 50%	—
	< 0.5 × 10⁹/L	Permanently discontinue	Permanently discontinue
Platelets	< 80 × 10⁹/L	Reduce dose by 50%	—
	< 50 × 10⁹/L	Permanently discontinue	Permanently discontinue

[1] For patients with a history of stable cardiac disease receiving peginterferon alfa-2b in combination with ribavirin capsules, reduce the peginterferon alfa-2b dose by half and the ribavirin capsule dose by 200 mg/day if a more than 2 g/dL decrease in hemoglobin is observed during any 4-week period. Permanently discontinue peginterferon alfa-2b and ribavirin capsules if patient has hemoglobin levels less than 12 g/dL after this ribavirin dose reduction.

➤*Reconstitution:* Visually inspect the solution for particulate matter and discoloration prior to administration. The reconstituted solution should be clear and colorless. Do not use the solution if discolored or cloudy or if particulates are present. The prepared solution is to be injected subcutaneously.

Redipen – To reconstitute the lyophilized peginterferon alfa-2b in the *Redipen*, hold the *Redipen* upright (dose button down) and press the two halves of the pen together until there is an audible click. Gently invert the pen to mix the solution. Do not shake. Keeping the pen upright, attach the supplied needle and select the appropriate peginterferon alfa-2b dose by pulling back on the dosing button until the dark bands are visible and turning the button until the dark band is aligned with the correct dose. The *Redipen* is for single use only.

Vials – Reconstitute the peginterferon alfa-2b lyophilized product with only 0.7 mL of supplied diluent (sterile water for injection). The diluent vial is for single use only. Discard the remaining diluent. Do not add any other medication to solutions containing peginterferon alfa-2b, and do not reconstitute peginterferon alfa-2b with other diluents. Swirl gently to hasten complete dissolution of the powder.

➤*Storage/Stability:*
Redipen – Store at 2° to 8°C (36° to 46°F). After reconstitution, use the solution immediately, or it may be stored up to 24 hours at 2° to 8°C (36° to 46°F). The reconstituted solution contains no preservative and is clear and colorless. Do not freeze.

Vials – Store at 25°C (77°F); excursions permitted to 15° to 30°C (59° to 86°F). After reconstitution with supplied diluent, use the solution immediately, or it may be stored up to 24 hours at 2° to 8°C (36° to 46°F). The reconstituted solution contains no preservative and is clear and colorless. Do not freeze.

Actions

➤*Pharmacology:* The biological activity of peginterferon alfa-2b is derived from its interferon alfa-2b moiety. Interferons exert their cellular activities by binding to specific membrane receptors on the cell surface and initiating a complex sequence of intracellular events. These include the induction of certain enzymes, suppression of cell proliferation, immunomodulating activities, such as enhancement of the phagocytic activity of macrophages and augmentation of the specific cytotoxicity of lymphocytes for target cells, and inhibition of virus replication in virus-infected cells.

➤*Pharmacokinetics:*

Absorption/Distribution – Following a single subcutaneous dose of peginterferon alfa-2b, the mean absorption half-life ($t_{1/2}$ k_a) was 4.6 hours. Maximal serum concentrations (C_{max}) occur between 15 and 44 hours postdose and are sustained for up to 48 to 72 hours. The C_{max} and AUC measurements of peginterferon alfa-2b increase in a dose-related manner. After multiple dosing, there is an increase in bioavailability of peginterferon alfa-2b. Week 48 mean trough concentrations (320 pg/mL; range, 0, 2960) are approximately 3-fold higher than week 4 mean trough concentrations (94 pg/mL; range, 0, 416).

Metabolism/Excretion – The mean peginterferon alfa-2b elimination half-life is approximately 40 hours (range, 22 to 60 hours) in patients with HCV infection. The apparent clearance of peginterferon alfa-2b is estimated to be approximately 22 mL/h•kg. Renal elimination accounts for 30% of the clearance. Single-dose peginterferon alfa-2b pharmacokinetics following a 1 mcg/kg subcutaneous dose suggest the clearance of peginterferon alfa-2b is reduced by approximately 50% in patients with impaired renal function (Ccr less than 50 mL/min).

Pegylation of interferon alfa-2b produces a product (peginterferon alfa-2b) whose clearance is lower than that of nonpegylated interferon alfa-2b. When compared with interferon alfa-2b, peginterferon alfa-2b (1 mcg/kg) has an approximately 7-fold lower mean apparent clearance and a 5-fold greater mean half-life, permitting a reduced dosing frequency. At effective therapeutic doses, peginterferon alfa-2b has approximately 10-fold greater C_{max} and 50-fold greater AUC than interferon alfa-2b.

➤*Clinical trials:*

Monotherapy – A randomized study compared peginterferon alfa-2b treatment (0.5, 1, or 1.5 mcg/kg once weekly subcutaneous) with interferon alfa-2b treatment (3 million units 3 times/week subcutaneous) in 1219 adults with chronic hepatitis from HCV infection. The patients were not previously treated with interferon alfa and had compensated liver disease, detectable HCV RNA, elevated ALT, and liver histopathology consistent with chronic hepatitis. Patients were treated for 48 weeks and were followed for 24 weeks posttreatment. Of all patients, 70% were infected with HCV genotype 1 and 74% of all patients had high baseline levels of HCV RNA (more than 2 million copies/mL of serum), 2 factors known to predict poor response to treatment.

Response to treatment was defined as undetectable HCV RNA and normalization of ALT at 24 weeks posttreatment. The response rates to the 1 and 1.5 mcg/kg peginterferon alfa-2b doses were similar (approximately 24%) to each other and were both higher than the response rate to inteferon alfa-2b (12%).

Rates of Response to Treatment with Peginterferon Alfa-2b

	A Peginterferon alfa-2b 0.5 mcg/kg (n = 315)	B Peginterferon alfa-2b 1 mcg/kg (n = 298)	C Interferon alfa-2b 3 MIU 3 times/week (n = 307)	B – C (95% CI) Difference between peginterferon alfa-2b 1 mcg/kg and interferon alfa-2b
Treatment response (combined virologic response and ALT normalization)	17%	24%	12%	11 (5, 18)
Virologic response[1]	18%	25%	12%	12 (6, 19)
ALT normalization	24%	29%	18%	11 (5, 18)

[1] Serum HCV is measured by a research-based quantitative polymerase chain reaction assay by a central laboratory.

PEGINTERFERON ALFA-2B

Combination therapy – A randomized study compared treatment with 2 peginterferon alfa-2b/ribavirin capsules regimens (peginterferon alfa-2b 1.5 mcg/kg subcutaneous once weekly/ribavirin capsules 800 mg oral daily [in divided doses]; peginterferon alfa-2b 1.5 mcg/kg subcutaneous once weekly for 4 weeks then 0.5 mcg/kg subcutaneous once weekly for 44 weeks/ribavirin capsules 1000/1200 mg oral daily [in divided doses]) with interferon alfa-2b (3 million IU subcutaneous 3 times weekly/ribavirin capsules 1000/1200 mg oral daily [in divided doses]) in 1530 adults with chronic hepatitis C. Interferon-naive patients were treated for 48 weeks and followed for 24 weeks posttreatment. Eligible patients had compensated liver disease, detectable HCV RNA, elevated ALT, and liver histopathology consistent with chronic hepatitis.

Response to treatment was defined as undetectable HCV RNA at 24 weeks posttreatment. The response rate to the peginterferon alfa-2b 1.5 mcg/kg plus ribavirin 800 mg dose was higher than the response rate to interferon alfa-2b/ribavirin capsules (see table below). The response rate to peginterferon alfa-2b 1.5 → 0.5 mcg/kg/ribavirin capsules was essentially the same as the response to interferon alfa-2b/ribavirin capsules (data not shown).

Rates of Response to Peg-Interferon Alfa 2b/ Ribavirin vs Interferon Alfa-2b/Ribavirin Treatment (%)		
	Peginterferon alfa-2b 1.5 mcg/kg once/week ribavirin capsules 800 mg once/day	Interferon alfa-2b 3 MIU 3 times/week ribavirin capsules 1000/1200 mg once/day
Overall[1],[2] response	52	46
Genotype 1	41	33
Genotype 2-6	75	73

[1] Serum HCV RNA is measured with a research-based quantitative polymerase chain reaction assay by a central laboratory.
[2] Difference in overall treatment response (peginterferon alfa-2b/ribavirin capsules vs interferon alfa-2b/ribavirin capsules) is 6% with 95% confidence interval of (0.18, 11.63) adjusted for viral genotype and presence of cirrhosis at baseline.

Contraindications

➤*Peginterferon alfa-2b:* Hypersensitivity to peginterferon alfa-2b or any component of the product; autoimmune hepatitis; decompensated liver disease.

➤*Peginterferon alfa-2b/Ribavirin capsules combination:* Hypersensitivity to ribavirin capsules or any other component of the product; pregnant women; men whose female partners are pregnant; patients with hemoglobinopathies (eg, thalassemia major, sickle-cell anemia).

Warnings

➤*Neuropsychiatric events:* Life-threatening or fatal neuropsychiatric events, including suicide, suicidal and homicidal ideation, depression, relapse of drug addiction/overdose, and aggressive behavior have occurred in patients with and without a previous psychiatric disorder during peginterferon alfa-2b treatment and follow-up. Psychoses, hallucinations, bipolar disorders, and mania have been observed in patients treated with alpha interferons. Use peginterferon alfa-2b with extreme caution in patients with a history of psychiatric disorders. Advise patients to report immediately any symptoms of depression and/or suicidal ideation to their prescribing physicians. Physicians should monitor all patients for evidence of depression and other psychiatric symptoms. In severe cases, stop peginterferon alfa-2b immediately and institute psychiatric intervention.

➤*Bone marrow toxicity:* Peginterferon alfa-2b suppresses bone marrow function, sometimes resulting in severe cytopenias. Discontinue peginterferon alfa-2b in patients who develop severe decreases in neutrophil or platelet counts. Ribavirin may potentiate the neutropenia induced by interferon alpha. Very rarely, alpha interferons may be associated with aplastic anemia.

➤*Colitis:* Fatal and nonfatal ulcerative or hemorrhagic/ischemic colitis have been observed within 12 weeks of the start of alpha interferon treatment. Abdominal pain, bloody diarrhea, and fever are the typical manifestations. Immediately discontinue peginterferon alfa-2b in patients who develop these symptoms and signs. The colitis usually resolves within 1 to 3 weeks of discontinuation of alpha interferons.

➤*Pancreatitis:* Fatal and nonfatal pancreatitis have been observed in patients treated with alpha interferons. Suspend peginterferon alfa-2b therapy in patients with signs and symptoms suggestive of pancreatitis, and discontinue in patients diagnosed with pancreatitis.

➤*Pulmonary disorders:* Dyspnea, pulmonary infiltrates, pneumonia, bronchiolitis obliterans, interstitial pneumonitis, and sarcoidosis, some resulting in respiratory failure and/or patient deaths, may be induced or aggravated by peginterferon alfa-2b or alpha-interferon therapy. Recurrence of respiratory failure has been observed with interferon rechallenge. Suspend peginterferon alfa-2b combination treatment in patients who develop pulmonary infiltrates or pulmonary function impairment. Closely monitor patients who resume interferon treatment.

➤*Endocrine disorders:* Peginterferon alfa-2b causes or aggravates hypothyroidism and hyperthyroidism. Hyperglycemia has been observed in patients treated with peginterferon alfa-2b. Diabetes mellitus has been observed in patients treated with alpha interferons. Do not begin peginterferon alfa-2b therapy in patients with these conditions who cannot be effectively treated by medication. Do not continue peginterferon alfa-2b therapy in patients who develop these conditions during treatment and cannot be controlled with medication.

➤*Cardiovascular events:* Cardiovascular events, including hypotension, arrhythmia, tachycardia, cardiomyopathy, angina pectoris, and MI have been observed in patients treated with peginterferon alfa-2b. Use peginterferon alfa-2b cautiously in patients with cardiovascular disease. Closely monitor patients with a history of MI and arrhythmic disorder who require peginterferon alfa-2b therapy. Do not treat patients with a history of significant or unstable cardiac disease with peginterferon/ribavirin capsules combination therapy.

➤*Autoimmune disorders:* Development or exacerbation of autoimmune disorders (eg, thyroiditis, thrombocytopenia, rheumatoid arthritis, interstitial nephritis, systemic lupus erythematosus, psoriasis) has been observed in patients receiving peginterferon alfa-2b. Use peginterferon alfa-2b with caution in patients with autoimmune disorders.

➤*Ophthalmologic disorders:* Decrease or loss of vision, retinopathy (including macular edema), retinal artery or vein thrombosis, retinal hemorrhages and cotton wool spots, optic neuritis, and papilledema may be induced or aggravated by treatment with peginterferon alfa-2b or other alpha interferons. All patients should receive an eye examination at baseline. Patients with preexisting ophthalmologic disorders (eg, diabetic or hypertensive retinopathy) should receive periodic ophthalmologic exams during interferon alpha treatment. Any patient who develops ocular symptoms should receive a prompt and complete eye examination. Discontinue peginterferon alfa-2b treatment in patients who develop new or worsening ophthalmologic disorders.

➤*Anemia:* Ribavirin caused hemolytic anemia in 10% of peginterferon alfa-2b/ribavirin capsule-treated patients within 1 to 4 weeks of initiation of therapy. Obtain complete blood counts pretreatment and at weeks 2 and 4 of therapy or more frequently if clinically indicated. Anemia associated with ribavirin capsule therapy may result in a worsening of cardiac disease. Decrease in dosage or discontinuation of ribavirin capsules may be necessary.

➤*Hypersensitivity reactions:* Serious, acute hypersensitivity reactions (eg, urticaria, angioedema, bronchoconstriction, anaphylaxis) rarely have been observed during alpha interferon therapy. If such a reaction develops during treatment with peginterferon alfa-2b, discontinue treatment and immediately institute appropriate medical therapy. Transient rashes do not necessitate interruption of treatment.

➤*Renal function impairment:* Increases in serum creatinine levels have been observed in patients treated with interferons, including peginterferon alfa-2b therapy. Closely monitor patients with impairment of renal function for signs and symptoms of interferon toxicity, including increases in serum creatinine, and adjust doses of peginterferon alfa-2b accordingly. Use peginterferon alfa-2b with caution in patients with Ccr less than 50 mL/min. Do not use ribavirin in patients with Ccr less than 50 mL/min.

➤*Fertility impairment:* Irregular menstrual cycles were observed in female cynomolgus monkeys given subcutaneous injections of 4239 mcg/m^2 peginterferon alfa-2b every other day for 1 month (at approximately 345 times the recommended weekly human dose based on body surface area). These effects included transiently decreased serum levels of estradiol and progesterone, suggestive of anovulation. Normal menstrual cycles and serum hormone levels resumed in these animals 2 to 3 months following cessation of peginterferon alfa-2b treatment. Every other day dosing with 262 mcg/m^2 (approximately 21 times the recommended weekly human dose) had no effects on cycle duration or reproductive hormone status. The effects of peginterferon alfa-2b on male fertility have not been studied.

➤*Elderly:* In general, younger patients tend to respond better than older patients to interferon-based therapies. However, clinical studies of peginterferon alfa-2b alone or in combination with ribavirin capsules did not include sufficient numbers of subjects 65 years of age and older to determine whether they respond differently than younger subjects. Treatment with alpha interferons, including peginterferon alfa-2b, is associated with neuropsychiatric, cardiac, pulmonary, GI, and systemic (flu-like) adverse effects. Because these adverse reactions may be more severe in the elderly, exercise caution in the use of peginterferon alfa-2b in this population. This drug is known to be substantially excreted by the kidney. Because elderly patients are more likely to have decreased renal function, the risk of toxic reactions to this drug may be greater in patients with impaired renal function. Do not use ribavirin capsules in patients with Ccr less than 50 mL/min. When using peginterferon alfa-2b/ribavirin therapy, also refer to the ribavirin capsules medication guide.

➤*Pregnancy:* Category C. Assume that peginterferon alfa-2b has abortifacient potential. There are no adequate and well-controlled studies in pregnant women. Use during pregnancy only if the potential benefit justifies the potential risk to the fetus. Peginterferon alfa-2b is recommended for use in fertile women only when they are using effective contraception during the treatment period.

PEGINTERFERON ALFA-2B

If pregnancy occurs in a patient or partner of a patient during treatment with peginterferon alfa-2b and ribavirin capsules during the 6 months after treatment cessation, physicians should report such cases by calling (800) 727-7064.

Use with ribavirin – Category X. Ribavirin capsules may cause birth defects and/or death of the unborn child. Do not start ribavirin therapy until a report of a negative pregnancy test has been obtained immediately prior to planned initiation of therapy. Instruct patients to use at least 2 forms of contraception and have monthly pregnancy tests (see Warning Box and Contraindications; also see ribavirin prescribing information).

➤*Lactation:* It is not known whether the components of peginterferon alfa-2b are excreted in human milk. Because of the potential for adverse reactions from the drug in nursing infants, decide whether to discontinue nursing or discontinue the treatment, taking into account the importance of the product to the mother.

➤*Children:* Safety and efficacy in patients younger than 18 years of age have not been established.

Precautions

➤*Monitoring:* Patients on peginterferon alfa-2b or peginterferon alfa-2b/ribavirin capsules combination therapy should have hematology and blood chemistry testing before the start of treatment and then periodically thereafter. Measure HCV RNA at 6 months of treatment. Discontinue peginterferon alfa-2b or peginterferon alfa-2b/ribavirin capsules combination therapy in patients with persistent high viral levels. Administer an ECG to patients who have preexisting cardiac abnormalities before treatment with peginterferon alfa-2b/ribavirin capsules.

➤*Immunogenicity:* Approximately 2% of patients receiving peginterferon alfa-2b or interferon alfa-2b with or without ribavirin capsules developed low-titer (160 or less) neutralizing antibodies to peginterferon alfa-2b or interferon alfa-2b. The clinical and pathological significance of the appearance of serum neutralizing antibodies is unknown.

➤*HIV or HBV coinfections:* The safety and efficacy of peginterferon alfa-2b/ribavirin capsules for the treatment of patients with HCV coinfected with HIV or HBV have not been established.

➤*Organ transplants:* The safety and efficacy of peginterferon alfa-2b alone or in combination with ribavirin capsules for the treatment of hepatitis C in patients who have received liver or other organ transplants have not been studied. Preliminary data indicate that interferon alpha therapy may be associated with an increased rate of kidney graft rejection. Liver graft rejection also has been reported, but a causal association to interferon alpha therapy has not been established.

➤*Triglycerides:* Elevated triglyceride levels have been observed in patients treated with interferons, including peginterferon alfa-2b therapy. Manage elevated triglyceride levels as clinically appropriate. Hypertriglyceridemia may result in pancreatitis. Consider discontinuation of peginterferon alfa-2b therapy for patients with persistently elevated triglycerides (ie, triglycerides greater than 1000 mg/dL) associated with symptoms of potential pancreatitis, such as abdominal pain, nausea, or vomiting.

➤*Lab test abnormalities:* Peginterferon alfa-2b alone or in combination with ribavirin capsules may cause severe decreases in neutrophil and platelet counts and hematologic, endocrine (eg, thyroid-stimulating hormone [TSH]), and hepatic abnormalities. In 10% of patients treated with peginterferon alfa-2b, ALT levels rose 2- to 5-fold above baseline. The elevations were transient and were not associated with deterioration of other liver functions.

Adverse Reactions

Nearly all study patients in clinical trials experienced 1 or more adverse events. In the peginterferon alfa-2b monotherapy trial, the incidence of serious adverse events was similar (approximately 12%) in all treatment groups. In the peginterferon alfa-2b/ribavirin capsules trial, the incidence of serious adverse events was 17% in the peginterferon alfa-2b/ribavirin capsules groups compared with 14% in the interferon alfa-2b/ribavirin capsules group.

In many, but not all cases, adverse events resolved after dose reduction or discontinuation of therapy. Some patients experienced ongoing or new serious adverse events during the 6-month, follow-up period. In the peginterferon alfa-2b/ribavirin capsules trial, 13 patients experienced life-threatening psychiatric events (suicidal ideation or attempt) and 1 patient committed suicide.

There have been 5 patient deaths that occurred in clinical trials: 1 suicide in a patient receiving peginterferon alfa-2b monotherapy and 1 suicide in a patient receiving peginterferon alfa-2b/ribavirin capsules combination therapy; 2 deaths among patients receiving interferon alfa-2b monotherapy (1 murder/suicide and 1 sudden death); and 1 patient death in the interferon alfa-2b/ribavirin capsules group (motor vehicle accident).

Overall, 10% to 14% of patients receiving peginterferon alfa-2b, alone or in combination with ribavirin capsules, discontinued therapy compared with 6% treated with interferon alfa-2b alone and 13% treated with interferon alfa-2b in combination with ribavirin capsules. The most common reasons for discontinuation of therapy were related to psychiatric, systemic (eg, fatigue, headache), or GI adverse events.

In the combination therapy trial, dose reductions caused by adverse reactions occurred in 42% of patients receiving peginterferon alfa-2b (1.5 mcg/kg)/ribavirin capsules and in 34% of those receiving interferon alfa-2b/ribavirin capsules. The majority of patients (57%) weighing 60 kg or less receiving peginterferon alfa-2b (1.5 mcg/kg)/ribavirin capsules required dose reduction. Reduction of interferon was dose-related (peginterferon alfa-2b 1.5 mcg/kg greater than peginterferon alfa-2b 0.5 mcg/kg or interferon alfa-2b), 40%, 27%, 28%, respectively. Dose reduction for ribavirin capsules was similar across all 3 groups, 33% to 35%. The most common reasons for dose modifications were neutropenia (18%) or anemia (9%). Other common reasons included depression, fatigue, nausea, and thrombocytopenia.

In the peginterferon alfa-2b/ribavirin capsules combination trial, the most common adverse events were psychiatric, occurring among 77% of patients and included most commonly depression, irritability, and insomnia, each reported by approximately 30% to 40% of subjects in all treatment groups. Suicidal behavior (eg, ideation, attempts, suicides) occurred in 2% of all patients during treatment or during follow-up after treatment cessation.

Peginterferon alfa-2b induced fatigue or headache in approximately two thirds of patients and induced fever or rigors in approximately 50% of the patients. The severity of some of these systemic symptoms (eg, fever, headache) tended to decrease as treatment continued. The incidence tends to be higher with peginterferon alfa-2b than with interferon alfa-2b therapy alone or in combination with ribavirin capsules.

Application-site inflammation and reaction (eg, bruising, itchiness, irritation) occurred at approximately twice the incidence with peginterferon alfa-2b therapies (in up to 75% of patients) compared with interferon alfa-2b. However, injection-site pain was infrequent (2% to 3%) in all groups.

Other common adverse events in the peginterferon alfa-2b/ribavirin capsules group included alopecia (36%), anorexia (32%), arthralgia (34%), myalgia (56%), nausea (43%), pruritus (29%), and weight loss (29%).

In the peginterferon alfa-2b monotherapy trial, the incidence of severe adverse events was 13% in the interferon alfa-2b group and 17% in the peginterferon alfa-2b groups. In the peginterferon alfa-2b/ribavirin capsules combination therapy trial, the incidence of severe adverse events was 23% in the interferon alfa-2b/ribavirin capsules group and 31% to 34% in the peginterferon alfa-2b/ribavirin capsules groups. The incidence of life-threatening adverse events was 1% or less across all groups in the monotherapy and combination therapy trials.

Adverse events that occurred in the clinical trials at more than 5% incidence are provided in the table below by treatment group. Because of potential differences in ascertainment procedures, do not make adverse event rate comparisons across studies.

Peginterferon Alfa-2b Adverse Events Occurring in > 5% of Patients[1]			
	Study 1		Study 2
Adverse reaction	Peginterferon alfa-2b 1 mcg/kg (n = 297)	Interferon alfa-2b 3 MIU (n = 303)	Peginterferon alfa-2b (1.5 mcg/kg)/ ribavirin capsules (n = 511)	Interferon alfa-2b/ ribavirin capsules (n = 505)
CNS				
Agitation	2	2	8	5
Anxiety/ Emotional lability/ Irritability	28	34	47	47
Concentration impaired	10	8	17	21
Depression	29	25	31	34
Dizziness	12	10	21	17
Fatigue/ Asthenia	52	54	66	63
Headache	56	52	62	58
Insomnia	23	23	40	41
Nervousness	4	3	6	6
Dermatologic				
Alopecia	22	22	36	32
Dry skin	11	9	24	23
Flushing	6	3	4	3
Pruritus	12	8	29	28
Rash	6	7	24	23
Sweating increased	6	7	11	7
GI				
Abdominal pain	15	11	13	13
Anorexia	20	17	32	27
Constipation	1	3	5	5

PEGINTERFERON ALFA-2B

Peginterferon Alfa-2b Adverse Events Occurring in > 5% of Patients[1]				
	Study 1		Study 2	
Adverse reaction	Peginterferon alfa-2b 1 mcg/kg (n = 297)	Interferon alfa-2b 3 MIU (n = 303)	Peginterferon alfa-2b (1.5 mcg/kg)/ribavirin capsules (n = 511)	Interferon alfa-2b/ribavirin capsules (n = 505)
Diarrhea	18	16	22	17
Dry mouth	6	7	12	8
Dyspepsia	6	7	9	8
Nausea	26	20	43	33
Vomiting	7	6	14	12
Hematologic				
Anemia	0	0	12	17
Leukopenia	< 1	0	6	5
Neutropenia	6	2	26	14
Thrombocyto-penia	7	< 1	5	2
Musculoskeletal				
Arthralgia	23	27	34	28
Musculoskel-etal pain	28	22	21	19
Myalgia	54	53	56	50
Respiratory				
Coughing	8	5	23	16
Dyspnea	4	2	26	24
Pharyngitis	10	7	12	13
Rhinitis	2	2	8	6
Sinusitis	7	7	5	5
Miscellaneous				
Chest pain	6	4	8	7
Conjunctivitis	4	2	4	5
Fever	22	12	46	33
Hepatomegaly	6	5	4	4
Hypothyroid-ism	5	3	5	4
Infection, fungal	< 1	3	6	1
Infection, viral	11	10	12	12
Injection-site inflammation/reaction	47	20	75	49
Malaise	7	6	4	6
Menstrual disorder	4	3	7	6
Right upper quadrant pain	8	8	12	6
Rigors	23	19	48	41
Taste perver-sion	< 1	2	9	4
Vision blurred	2	3	5	6
Weight decrease	11	13	29	20

[1] Patients reporting 1 or more adverse event. A patient may have reported more than 1 adverse event within a body system/organ class category.

Many patients continued to experience adverse events several months after discontinuation of therapy. By the end of the 6-month follow-up period, the incidence of ongoing adverse events by body class in the peginterferon alfa-2b 1.5/ribavirin capsules group was 33% (psychiatric), 20% (musculoskeletal), and 10% (for endocrine and GI). In approximately 10% to 15% of patients, weight loss, fatigue, and headache had not resolved.

➤*Cardiovascular:* Angina, cardiomyopathy, MI, pericardial effusion, supraventricular arrhythmias, transient ischemic attack (1% or less).

➤*CNS:* Aggressive reaction, loss of consciousness, nerve palsy (facial, oculomotor), psychosis, relapse of drug addiction/overdose, severe depression, suicidal ideation, suicide attempt (1% or less).

➤*Dermatologic:* Aggravated psoriasis, injection-site necrosis, phototoxicity, urticaria, vasculitis (1% or less).

➤*Hematologic:* Autoimmune thrombocytopenia with or without purpura, neutropenia (1% or less).

➤*Metabolic:* Gout, hyperglycemia (1% or less).

➤*Respiratory:* Bronchiolitis obliterans, emphysema, pleural effusion (1% or less).

➤*Special senses:* Blindness, decreased visual acuity, optic neuritis, retinal artery or vein thrombosis, retinal ischemia (1% or less).

➤*Miscellaneous:* Gastroenteritis, hyperthyroidism, hypothyroidism, infection (eg, pneumonia, abscess, sepsis, cellulitis), interstitial nephritis, lupus-like syndrome, pancreatitis, rheumatoid arthritis, sarcoidosis (1% or less).

➤*Lab test abnormalities:*

Hemoglobin – Ribavirin capsules induced a decrease in hemoglobin levels in approximately two thirds of patients. Hemoglobin levels decreased to less than 11 g/dL in approximately 30% of patients. Severe anemia (less than 8 g/dL) occurred in less than 1% of patients. Dose modification was required in 9% and 13% of patients in the peginterferon alfa-2b/ribavirin capsule and interferon alfa-2b/ribavirin capsule groups, respectively. Hemoglobin levels become stable by treatment week 4 to 6 on average. Hemoglobin levels return to baseline between 4 and 12 weeks posttreatment. In the peginterferon alfa-2b monotherapy trial, hemoglobin decreases were generally mild and dose modifications were rarely necessary.

Neutrophils – Decreases in neutrophil counts were observed in a majority of patients treated with peginterferon alfa-2b alone (70%) or as combination therapy with ribavirin capsules (85%) and interferon alfa-2b/ribavarin capsules (60%). Severe and potentially life-threatening neutropenia (less than 0.5×10^9/L) occurred in 1% of patients treated with peginterferon alfa-2b monotherapy, 2% of patients treated with interferon alfa-2b/ribavirin capsules, and in 4% of patients treated with peginterferon alfa-2b/ribavirin capsules. Two percent of patients receiving peginterferon alfa-2b monotherapy and 18% of patients receiving peginterferon alfa-2b/ribavirin capsules required modification of interferon dosage. Few patients (1% or less) required permanent discontinuation of treatment. Neutrophil counts generally return to pretreatment levels within 4 weeks of cessation of therapy.

Platelets – Platelet counts decrease in approximately 20% of patients treated with peginterferon alfa-2b alone or with ribavirin capsules and in 6% of patients treated with interferon alfa-2b/ribavirin capsules. Severe decreases in platelet counts (less than 50,000/mm^3) occur in less than 1% of patients. Patients may require discontinuation or dose modification as a result of platelet decreases. In the peginterferon alfa-2b/ribavirin capsules combination therapy trial, 1% or 3% of patients required dose modification of interferon alfa-2b or peginterferon alfa-2b, respectively. Platelet counts generally returned to pretreatment levels within 4 weeks of the cessation of therapy.

Thyroid function – Development of TSH abnormalities, with and without clinical manifestations, are associated with interferon therapies. Clinically apparent thyroid disorders occur among patients treated with either interferon alfa-2b or peginterferon alfa-2b (with or without ribavirin capsules) at a similar incidence (5% for hypothyroidism and 3% for hyperthyroidism). Subjects developed new-onset TSH abnormalities while on treatment and during the follow-up period. At the end of the follow-up period, 7% of subjects still had abnormal TSH values.

Bilirubin and uric acid – In the peginterferon alfa-2b/ribavirin capsules trial, 10% to 14% of patients developed hyperbilirubinemia and 33% to 38% developed hyperuricemia in association with hemolysis. Six patients developed mild to moderate gout.

➤*Postmarketing:*

Cardiovascular – Cardiac ischemia.

CNS – Peripheral neuropathy, seizures, vertigo.

Dermatologic – Erythema multiforme, Stevens-Johnson syndrome, toxic epidermal necrolysis.

Metabolic – Renal failure, renal insufficiency.

Special senses – Hearing impairment, hearing loss.

Miscellaneous – Rhabdomyolysis, stomatitis.

Overdosage

There is limited experience with overdosage. In the clinical studies, a few patients accidentally received a dose greater than that prescribed. There were no instances in which a participant in the monotherapy or combination therapy trials received more than 10.5 times the intended dose of peginterferon alfa-2b. The maximum dose received by any patient was 3.45 mcg/kg weekly over a period of approximately 12 weeks. The maximum known overdosage of ribavirin capsules was an intentional ingestion of 10 g (fifty 200 mg capsules). There were no serious reactions attributed to these overdosages. In cases of overdosing, symptomatic treatment and close observation of the patient are recommended.

Patient Information

Direct patients receiving peginterferon alfa-2b alone or in combination with ribavirin capsules in its appropriate use, inform them of the benefits and risks associated with treatment, and refer them to the medication guide.

Advise patients to use a puncture-resistant container for the disposal of used syringes, needles, and the *Redipen*. Thoroughly instruct patients in the importance of proper disposal, and caution them against any reuse of needles, syringes, or the *Redipen*. Instruct patients to dispose of the full container in accordance with state and local laws.

Inform patients that there are no data evaluating whether peginterferon alfa-2b therapy will prevent transmission of HCV infection to oth-

PEGINTERFERON ALFA-2B

ers. Also, it is not known if treatment with peginterferon alfa-2b will cure hepatitis C or prevent cirrhosis, liver failure, or liver cancer that may be the result of infection with HCV.

Advise patients that laboratory evaluations are required before starting therapy and periodically thereafter. It is advised that patients be well-hydrated, especially during the initial stages of treatment. Flulike symptoms associated with administration of peginterferon alfa-2b may be minimized by bedtime administration or by use of antipyretics.

Inform patients that ribavirin may cause birth defects and/or death of the unborn child. Extreme care must be taken to avoid pregnancy in female patients and in female partners of male patients during treatment with combination peginterferon alfa-2b/ribavirin capsules therapy and for 6 months posttherapy. Do not initiate combination peginterferon alfa-2b/ribavirin capsule therapy until a report of a negative pregnancy test has been obtained immediately prior to initiation of therapy. It is recommended that patients undergo monthly pregnancy tests during therapy and for 6 months posttherapy.

INTERFERON ALFA-2b, RECOMBINANT AND RIBAVIRIN COMBINATION

Rx	Rebetron (Schering)	Injection/Capsules (combination packages): 3 million IU interferon alfa-2b, recombinant/0.5 mL and 200 mg ribavirin

Patients ≤ 75 kg:
Intron A (injection): In single-dose vials (6s), one 18 million IU multidose vial, or one 18 million IU multidose pen. *Rebetol* (capsules): (REBETOL 200 MG). White. In 70s.

Patients > 75 kg:
Intron A (injection): In single-dose vials (6s), one 18 million IU multidose vial, or one 18 million IU multidose pen. *Rebetol* (capsules): (REBETOL 200 MG). White. In 84s.

Dose reduction:
Intron A (injection): In single-dose vials (6s), one 18 million IU multidose vial, or one 18 million IU multidose pen. *Rebetol* (capsules): (REBETOL 200 MG). White. In 42s.

For complete prescribing information, refer to the individual interferon alfa-2b and ribavirin monographs.

WARNING

Combination ribavirin/interferon alfa-2b therapy is contraindicated in women who are pregnant and in the male partners of women who are pregnant. Extreme care must be taken to avoid pregnancy during therapy and for 6 months after completion of treatment in female patients, and in female partners of male patients who are taking combination ribavirin/interferon alfa-2b therapy. Women of childbearing potential and men must use 2 reliable forms of effective contraception during treatment and during the 6-month posttreatment follow-up period. Significant teratogenic or embryocidal effects have been demonstrated for ribavirin in all animal species studied. Ribavirin monotherapy is not effective for the treatment of chronic hepatitis C and should not be used for this indication. Alpha interferons, including interferon alfa-2b, cause or aggravate fatal or life-threatening neuropsychiatric, autoimmune, ischemic, and infectious disorders. Closely monitor patients with periodic clinical and laboratory elevations. Withdraw patients from therapy who have persistently severe or worsening signs or symptoms of these conditions. In many, but not all cases, these disorders resolve after stopping interferon alfa-2b therapy.

Indications

▶*Hepatitis C:* Treatment of chronic hepatitis C in patients with compensated liver disease previously untreated with alpha interferon or who have relapsed following alpha interferon therapy.

Ribavirin monotherapy is not effective for the treatment of chronic hepatitis C and should not be used for this indication.

Administration and Dosage

Administer interferon alfa-2b SC and ribavirin orally without regard to food. Hydrate patients well, especially during initial treatment stages.

Initiate combination therapy only after a negative pregnancy test has been obtained. Patients or partners of patients should report any pregnancy that occurs during treatment or within 6 months after treatment cessation to their physician immediately. Physicians are encouraged to report such cases by calling (800) 727-7064.

The recommended ribavirin dose depends on the patient's body weight. Administer doses of ribavirin and interferon alfa-2b according to the following table for 6 months (24 weeks). The safety and efficacy of the combination therapy has not been established for > 6 months of treatment.

Recommended Interferon Alfa-2b/Ribavirin Combination Dosing		
Body weight	Ribavirin	Interferon alfa-2b injection
≤ 75 kg	400 mg am PO 600 mg pm PO	3 million IU 3 times/week SC
> 75 kg	600 mg am PO 600 mg pm PO	

▶*Dose modifications:* If severe adverse reactions or laboratory abnormalities develop during combination therapy, modify the dose, or discontinue if appropriate, until the adverse reactions abate. If intolerance persists after dose adjustment, discontinue therapy.

For patients with a history of stable cardiovascular disease, a permanent dose reduction is required if the hemoglobin decreases by ≥ 2 g/dL during any 4-week period. In addition, for these cardiac history patients, if the hemoglobin remains < 12 g/dL after 4 weeks on a reduced dose, discontinue combination therapy.

It is recommended that patients whose hemoglobin level falls below 10 g/dL have their ribavirin dose reduced to 600 mg daily (200 mg am, 400 mg pm). Permanently discontinue treatment in patients whose hemoglobin level falls below 8.5 g/dL from combination therapy.

It is recommended that patients who experience moderate depression (persistent low mood, loss of interest, poor self image, or hopelessness) have their interferon alfa-2b dose temporarily reduced or be considered for medical therapy. Discontinue treatment in patients experiencing severe depression or suicidal ideation/attempt from combination therapy and follow closely with appropriate medical management.

Interferon Alfa-2b/Ribavirin Combination Dose Modification Guidelines		
Parameter	Dose reduction[1] ribavirin - 600 mg/day, interferon alfa-2b - 1.5 million IU 3 times/week	Permanent discontinuation of combination treatment
Hemoglobin	< 10 g/dL (reduce ribavirin) *Cardiac history patients only:* ≥ 2 g/dL decrease during any 4-week period during treatment (reduce ribavirin/ interferon alfa-2b)	< 8.5 g/dL *Cardiac history patients only:* < 12 g/dL after 4 weeks of dose reduction
White blood count	< 1.5 × 10^9/L (reduce interferon alfa-2b)	< 1 × 10^9/L
Neutrophil count	< 0.75 × 10^9/L (reduce interferon alfa-2b)	< 0.5 × 10^9/L
Platelet count	< 50 × 10^9/L (reduce interferon alfa-2b)	< 25 × 10^9/L

[1] Medication to be reduced in dose is shown in parentheses.

▶*Administration of interferon alfa-2b injection:* At the discretion of the physician, the patient may self-administer interferon alfa-2b.

Withdraw the appropriate dose from the vial or set on the multidose pen and inject SC. After administration, follow the procedure for proper disposal of syringes and needles.

Administration of Interferon Alfa-2b Injection		
Vial/Pen label strength	Fill volume	Concentration
3 million IU vial	0.5 mL	3 million IU/0.5 mL
18 million IU multidose vial[1]	3.8 mL	3 million IU/0.5 mL
18 million IU multidose pen[2]	1.5 mL	3 million IU/0.2 mL

[1] This is a multidose vial that contains 22.8 million IU of interferon alfa-2b/3.8 mL in order to provide the delivery of six 0.5 mL doses, each containing 3 million IU of interferon alfa-2b (for a label strength of 18 million IU).
[2] This is a multidose pen that contains a 22.5 million IU of interferon alfa-2b/1.5 mL in order to provide the delivery of six 0.2 mL doses, each containing 3 million IU of interferon alfa-2b (for a label strength of 18 million IU).

▶*Treatment duration:* The recommended duration of treatment for patients previously untreated with interferon is 24 to 48 weeks. Individualize the duration of treatment to the patient depending on baseline disease characteristics, response to therapy, and tolerability of the regimen. After 24 weeks of treatment, assess virologic response. Consider treatment discontinuation in any patient who has not achieved an HCV RNA below the limit of detection of the assay by 24 weeks. There are no safety and efficacy data on treatment for > 48 weeks in the previously untreated patient population.

In patients who relapse following interferon therapy, the recommended duration of treatment is 24 weeks. There are no safety and efficacy data on treatment for > 24 weeks in the relapsed patient population.

INTERFERON ALFA-2b, RECOMBINANT AND RIBAVIRIN COMBINATION

➤*Storage / Stability:* Interferon alfa-2b injection in vials is stable at 35°C (95°F) for ≤ 7 days and at 30°C (86°F) for ≤ 14 days; the multidose pen is stable at 30°C (86°F) for ≤ 2 days.

Refrigerate the combination package or the individual cartons between 2° and 8°C (36° and 46°F). The ribavirin carton may alternately be stored at 25°C (77°F).

Precautions

➤*Monitoring:* The following laboratory tests are recommended for all patients on combination therapy, prior to beginning treatment and then periodically thereafter: Standard hematologic tests including hemoglobin (pretreatment, week 2 and week 4 of therapy, and as clinically appropriate), complete and differential white blood cell counts, and platelet count; liver function tests and TSH; pregnancy including monthly monitoring for women of childbearing potential.

➤*Cardiac disease:* Administer therapy with caution to patients with preexisting cardiac disease. Assess patients before commencement of therapy and appropriately monitor them during therapy. If there is any deterioration of cardiovascular status, stop therapy.

➤*Renal function impairment:* Administer with caution in patients with Ccr < 50 mL/min.

Patient Information

Advise patients (male and female) to practice adequate contraception (2 reliable forms) during combination therapy and to notify the physician in the event of pregnancy.

Advise female patients of the need to perform a pregnancy test monthly during therapy and for 6 months post-therapy.

INTERFERON ALFACON-1

Rx	Infergen (InterMune)	Injection: 9 mcg	Preservative free. In 0.3 mL single-dose vials.
		15 mcg	Preservative free. In 0.5 mL single-dose vials.

For complete prescribing information on interferon-alfa 2a and -alfa 2b, refer to the individual monographs.

```
WARNING

Alpha interferons, including interferon alfacon-1, cause or aggra-
vate fatal or life-threatening neuropsychiatric, autoimmune, ische-
mic, and infectious disorders.

Monitor patients closely with periodic clinical and laboratory evalu-
ations. Withdraw patients with persistently severe or worsening
symptoms of these conditions from therapy. In many but not all
cases, these disorders resolve after stopping interferon alfacon-1
therapy.
```

Indications

➤*Hepatitis C infection, chronic:* For the treatment of chronic hepatitis C virus (HCV) infection in patients 18 years of age or older with compensated liver disease who have anti-HCV serum antibodies or the presence of HCV RNA.

Administration and Dosage

➤*Approved by the FDA:* October 6, 1997.

9 mcg subcutaneous as a single injection 3 times/week for 24 weeks. At least 48 hours should elapse between doses.

Patients who tolerated previous interferon therapy and did not respond or relapsed following its discontinuation may be subsequently treated with 15 mcg 3 times/week for 48 weeks.

➤*Dose reduction:* Withhold dosage temporarily if patients experience severe adverse reactions on interferon alfacon-1. If the adverse reaction does not become tolerable, discontinue therapy. Dose reduction to 7.5 mcg may be necessary following an intolerable adverse event. If adverse reactions continue to occur at reduced dosage, discontinue treatment or reduce dosage further. However, decreased efficacy may result from continued treatment at dosages less than 7.5 mcg.

➤*Storage / Stability:* Store refrigerated at 2° to 8°C (36° to 46°F). Do not freeze. Avoid vigorous shaking and exposure to direct sunlight.

Actions

➤*Pharmacology:* Interferons are a family of naturally occurring protein molecules that are produced and secreted by cells in response to viral infections or to various synthetic and biological inducers. All type-I interferons share common biological activities generated by binding of interferon to the cell-surface receptor, leading to the production of several interferon-stimulated gene products. Type-I interferons induce biologic responses, which include antiviral, antiproliferative, and immunomodulatory effects, regulation of cell surface major histocompatibility antigen (HLA class I and class II) expression and regulation of cytokine expression. Interferon alfacon-1 is a recombinant nonnaturally occurring type-I interferon with a molecular weight of 19,434 daltons.

The antiviral, antiproliferative, natural killer (NK) cell activation , and gene-induction activities of interferon alfacon-1 have been compared with other recombinant alpha interferons in in vitro assays and have demonstrated similar ranges of activity. Interferon alfacon-1 exhibited at least 5 times higher specific activity in vitro than Interferon alfa-2a and Interferon alfa-2b. Comparison of interferon alfacon-1 with a WHO international potency standard for recombinant alpha interferon (83/514) revealed that the specific activity of interferon alfacon-1 in both in vitro antiviral cytopathic effect assay and an antiproliferative assay was 1×10^9 U/mg.

➤*Pharmacokinetics:* Plasma levels after subcutaneous injection of 1, 3, or 9 mcg in healthy subjects were too low to be detected by enzyme-linked immunoabsorbent assay (ELISA) or by inhibition of viral cytopathic effect. However, analysis of interferon alfacon-1-induced cellular products 2′5′ oligoadenylate synthetase and β-2 microglobulin revealed a statistically significant dose-related increase in the AUC. Peak concentrations of these interferon-stimulated gene products were maximal at 24 to 36 hours after dosing.

➤*Clinical trials:* In a double-blind trial, 704 patients with chronic HCV infection previously untreated with alpha interferon were randomized to receive 3 or 9 mcg interferon alfacon-1 or 3 million IU interferon alpha-2b recombinant (IFN α2b). All patients received subcutaneous administrations 3 times/week for 24 weeks and were observed for an additional 24 weeks to assess sustained response determined by ALT normalization. Reduction of HCV RNA to less than 100 copies/mL was used as a secondary endpoint. The 9 mcg interferon alfacon-1 group demonstrated similar efficacy to the IFN α2b group at the end of 24 weeks (normalized ALT 39% vs 35% and HCV RNA negative 33% vs 25%, respectively) and at 48 weeks (normalized ALT 17% vs 17% and HCV RNA negative 9% vs 8%, respectively). Similar improvement in liver histology was observed in all groups; 3 and 9 mcg interferon alfacon-1 (63% and 68%) and IFN α2b (65%).

Contraindications

Hypersensitivity to alpha interferons, to products derived from *E. coli*, or to any component of the product.

Warnings

➤*Adverse events:* Treatment should be administered under the guidance of a qualified physician, and may lead to moderate-to-severe adverse experiences requiring dose reduction, temporary dose cessation, or discontinuation of further therapy.

Withdrawal from study because of adverse events occurred in 7% of patients initially treated with 9 mcg interferon alfacon-1 (including 4% because of psychiatric events). Withdrawal from study because of adverse events occurred in 5% of patients subsequently treated with 15 mcg interferon alfacon-1 for 24 weeks and 11% of patients subsequently treated with 15 mcg interferon alfacon-1 for 48 weeks.

➤*Cardiac disease:* Administer with caution to patients with preexisting cardiac disease. Hypertension and supraventricular arrhythmias, chest pain, and MI have been associated with alpha interferon therapies.

➤*Myelosuppression:* Alpha interferons suppress bone marrow function and may result in severe cytopenias including very rare events of aplastic anemia. Use cautiously in patients with abnormally low peripheral blood cell counts, patients who are chronically immunosuppressed, transplant patients, or patients receiving agents that are known to cause myelosuppression.

Decreases in mean platelet count of 16%, white blood cells of 19%, and absolute neutrophil count of 23%, compared with baseline, have been observed. Three percent of patients developed platelet values less than 50×10^9 cells/L and 2 patients developed decreases in ANC to levels below 500×10^6 cells/L. These events usually necessitated a dose reduction. These effects reversed during the post-treatment observation period.

Mean decreases from baseline up to 23% for WBCs and up to 27% for ANC were observed for patients subsequently treated with interferon alfacon-1. Two patients in the 24-week group experienced reversible reductions in ANC to less than 500×106 cells/L, which were not associated with infectious complications. No patients discontinued therapy as a result of hematologic toxicity in subsequent treatment trials.

➤*Psychiatric events:* Severe psychiatric events may manifest in patients receiving therapy with alpha interferon, including interferon alfacon-1. Depression, suicidal ideation, and suicide attempt may occur. The incidence of suicidal ideation was small (1%) for patients treated with 9 mcg interferon alfacon-1 compared with the overall incidence (55%) of psychiatric events. Use with caution in patients with a history of depression; monitor all patients for evidence of depression. Other prominent psychiatric adverse events may include nervousness, anxiety, emotional lability, abnormal thinking, agitation, or apathy. Discontinue in patients developing severe depression, suicidal ideation, or other severe psychiatric disorders.

INTERFERON ALFACON-1

➤*Hypersensitivity reactions:* Serious acute hypersensitivity reactions have occurred rarely following treatment with alpha interferons. Discontinue immediately if hypersensitivity reactions occur (eg, urticaria, angioedema, bronchoconstriction, anaphylaxis), and institute appropriate medical treatment.

➤*Hepatic function impairment:* Do not treat patients with decompensated hepatic disease with interferon alfacon-1; discontinue therapy in patients who develop symptoms of hepatic decompensation, such as jaundice, ascites, coagulopathy, or decreased serum albumin.

➤*Elderly:* Treatment with interferons, including interferon alfacon-1, is associated with psychiatric, cardiac, and systemic (flu-like) adverse effects. Because decreased hepatic, renal, or cardiac function, concomitant disease, and the use of other drug therapies in elderly patients may produce adverse reactions of greater severity, exercise caution in the administration of interferon alfacon-1 to this population.

➤*Pregnancy: Category C.* Interferon alfacon-1 has embryolethal or abortifacient effects in hamsters and monkeys at 135 and 9 to 81 times the human dose, respectively. There are no adequate and well-controlled studies in pregnant women. Do not use during pregnancy. If a patient becomes pregnant or plans to become pregnant while taking interferon alfacon-1, inform her of the potential hazards to the fetus. Advise men and women treated with interferon alfacon-1 to use effective contraception.

➤*Lactation:* It is not known whether interferon alfacon-1 is excreted in breast milk. Use caution if administered to a nursing woman.

➤*Children:* The safety and efficacy have not been established in patients younger than 18 years of age and is not recommended in this population.

Precautions

➤*Monitoring:* Laboratory tests are recommended for all patients on interferon alfacon-1 therapy, prior to beginning treatment (baseline), 2 weeks after initiation of therapy, and periodically thereafter during the 24 or 48 weeks of therapy. Following completion of therapy, monitor any abnormal test values periodically. The following are acceptable baseline values for initiation of treatment:

- Platelet counts (at least 75×10^9/L)
- Hemoglobin concentration (at least 100 g/L)
- ANC (at least 1500×10^6/L)
- Serum creatinine concentration (less than 180 mmol/L [less than 2 mg/dL]) or creatinine clearance (greater than 0.83 mL/second [greater than 50 mL/min])
- Serum albumin (at least 25 g/L)
- Bilirubin (within normal limits)
- TSH and T_4 (within normal limits)

Neutropenia, thrombocytopenia, hypertriglyceridemia, and thyroid disorders have been reported with administration of interferon alfacon-1 (see Adverse Reactions). Therefore, closely monitor these laboratory parameters.

Use cautiously in patients with abnormally low peripheral blood cell counts or in patients who are receiving agents that are known to cause myelosuppression. Mean decreases from baseline of 19% for WBCs and 23% for ANC have been observed with interferon alfacon-1 therapy. These effects reversed during the post-treatment observation period. In 2 interferon alfacon-1-treated patients in the phase 3 trial, decreases in ANC to levels below 500×10^6 cells/L were seen. In both cases, the ANC returned to clinically acceptable levels with reduction of the dose of interferon alfacon-1, and these transient decreases in neutrophils were not associated with infections.

Decreases in mean platelet count of 16% compared with baseline were seen by the end of treatment with 3% of patients developing values less than 50×10^9 cells/L, usually necessitating dose reduction. These decreases were reversed during the post-treatment observation period.

➤*Autoimmune disease:* Exacerbation of autoimmune disease has been reported in patients receiving type-I interferon therapy. Do not use in patients with autoimmune hepatitis. Use with caution in patients with other autoimmune disorders.

➤*Fever:* Fever may be related to the flu-like symptoms reported with interferon alfacon-1 therapy; rule out other possible causes when persistent fever occurs.

➤*Hemoglobin and hematocrit:* Treatment with interferon alfacon-1 was associated with gradual decreases in mean values for hemoglobin and hematocrit, which were 4% and 5% below baseline at the end of treatment, respectively. Decreases from baseline of at least 20% in hemoglobin or hematocrit were seen in up to 1% of patients.

➤*Ophthalmologic disorders:* Decrease or loss of vision, retinopathy including macular edema, retinal artery or vein thrombosis, retinal hemorrhages and cotton wool spots; optic neuritis, and papilledema are induced or aggravated by treatment with interferon alfacon-1 or other alpha interferons. All patients should receive an eye examination at baseline. Patients with preexisting ophthalmologic disorders (eg, diabetic or hypertensive retinopathy) should receive periodic ophthalmologic exams during interferon alpha treatment. Any patient who develops ocular symptoms should receive a prompt and complete eye

examination. Discontinue interferon alfacon-1 therapy in patients who develop new or worsening ophthalmologic disorders.

➤*Thyroid disorders:* Abnormal thyroid stimulating hormone (TSH) and free thyroxine (T_4) level with hypothyroidism occurred in 4% of patients administered 9 mcg interferon alfacon-1, and thyroid supplements were required in approximately two-thirds of those patients. Increases in TSH more than 7 mU/L were seen in 10% of patients treated with 9 mcg interferon alfacon-1. Thyroid supplements may be required.

➤*Triglycerides:* Mean values for serum triglyceride increased shortly after the start of interferon alfacon-1 therapy, with increases of 41% compared with baseline at the end of the treatment period. Seven percent of the patients developed values that were at least 3 times above pretreatment levels during treatment. This effect was promptly reversed after discontinuation of treatment.

Drug Interactions

Interferon Alfacon-1 Drug Interactions			
Precipitant Drug	Object Drug*		Description
Interferon alfacon-1	Myelosuppressive agents	↑	Use caution when administering with other agents known to cause myelosuppression.
Myelosuppressive agents	Interferon alfacon-1		
Interferon alfacon-1	Drugs metabolized by cytochrome P450	↔	Use caution when administering to patients who are receiving agents metabolized via cytochrome P450, and monitor closely for changes in therapeutic and/or toxic levels of these concomitant drugs.

* ↑ = Object drug increased. ↔ = Undetermined clinical effect.

Adverse Reactions

Interferon Alfacon-1 Adverse Reactions				
Adverse reaction	Interferon alfacon-1 9 mcg (n = 231)	Interferon alpha-2b (n = 236)	Interferon alfacon-1 15 mcg 24 weeks (n = 165)	Interferon alfacon-1 15 mcg 48 weeks (n = 168)
Cardiovascular				
Hypertension	5	3	2	4
Palpitation	3	6	5	2
CNS				
Amnesia	10	6	2	5
Confusion	4	6	4	5
Dizziness	22	25	18	25
Hyperesthesia	1	1	1	5
Hypertonia	7	10	6	6
Hypoesthesia	10	8	8	10
Insomnia	39	30	24	28
Paresthesia	13	10	9	9
Somnolence	4	8	6	7
Dermatologic				
Alopecia	14	25	10	13
Dry skin	6	5	2	5
Erythema	6	6	7	9
Pruritus	14	14	11	10
Rash	13	15	13	10
Wound	4	7	3	4
Endocrine disorders				
Thyroid test abnormal	9	5	4	6
Flu-like symptoms				
Arthralgia	51	44	43	46
Fatigue	69	67	65	71
Fever	61	45	58	55
Headache	82	83	78	80
Myalgia	58	56	51	55
Rigors	57	45	62	66
Sweating, increased	12	11	13	11
GI				
Abdominal pain	41	40	24	32
Anorexia	24	17	24	14
Constipation	9	6	5	6
Diarrhea	29	24	24	22
Dyspepsia	21	18	12	10
Flatulence	8	9	6	5
Gingivitis	2	3	1	5
Hemorrhoids	6	3	1	2
Nausea	40	36	30	36

INTERFERON ALFACON-1

Interferon Alfacon-1 Adverse Reactions				
Adverse reaction	Interferon alfacon-1 9 mcg (n = 231)	Interferon alpha-2b (n = 236)	Interferon alfacon-1 15 mcg 24 weeks (n = 165)	Interferon alfacon-1 15 mcg 48 weeks (n = 168)
Saliva decreased	6	7	4	1
Toothache	7	7	3	7
Ulcerative stomatitis	3	4	2	6
Vomiting	12	11	13	11
GU				
Breast mass	0	3	0	5
Breast pain	0	5	2	0
Dysmenorrhea	9	9	2	7
Genital moniliasis	2	6	2	0
Menorrhagia	3	0	2	5
Menstrual disorder	6	5	2	5
Vaginitis	8	2	5	5
Hematologic				
Anemia	2	3	2	6
Ecchymosis	6	4	4	2
Granulocytopenia	23	25	42	39
Leukopenia	15	13	19	28
Lymphadenopathy	6	8	4	4
Lymphocytosis	5	7	11	5
PT increased	3	5	1	0
Thrombocytopenia	19	16	18	18
Hepatic				
Hepatomegaly	3	5	5	2
Liver tender	5	3	6	2
Local				
Injection site ecchymosis	6	7	5	5
Injection site erythema	23	15	17	22
Injection site pain	9	3	8	11
Musculoskeletal				
Back pain	42	37	29	23
Limb pain	26	25	13	23
Musculoskeletal disorder	4	4	7	4
Neck pain	14	13	8	5
Skeletal pain	14	14	10	12
Psychiatric				
Agitation	6	6	4	4
Anxiety	19	18	9	14
Apathy	2	3	4	5
Depression	26	25	18	19
Emotional lability	12	11	6	3
Libido, decreased	5	5	5	4
Nervousness	31	29	16	22
Thinking abnormal	8	12	10	20
Respiratory				
Bronchitis	6	6	2	1
Cough	22	17	12	11
Dyspnea	7	12	8	7
Epistaxis	8	12	6	6
Pharyngitis	34	31	17	21
Respiratory tract congestion	12	7	4	9
Rhinitis	13	16	7	9
Sinusitis	17	22	12	16
Upper respiratory tract congestion	10	14	7	9
Upper respiraory tract infection	31	34	16	18

Interferon Alfacon-1 Adverse Reactions				
Adverse reaction	Interferon alfacon-1 9 mcg (n = 231)	Interferon alpha-2b (n = 236)	Interferon alfacon-1 15 mcg 24 weeks (n = 165)	Interferon alfacon-1 15 mcg 48 weeks (n = 168)
Special senses				
Conjunctivitis	8	8	4	6
Earache	5	7	5	5
Eye pain	5	6	4	2
Otitis	2	5	1	3
Taste perversion	3	6	3	5
Tinnitus	6	4	4	2
Vision abnormal	3	5	5	5
Miscellaneous				
Access pain	8	9	1	1
Allergic reaction	7	5	3	4
Asthenia	9	11	10	7
Body pain	54	45	62	66
Chest pain (non-cardiac)	13	14	5	9
Edema, peripheral	9	8	4	3
Flu-like symptoms, viral	15	11	8	8
Hot flushes	13	7	7	4
Hypertriglyceridemia	6	7	5	5
Infection	3	5	2	6
Malaise	11	10	2	5
Thyroid test, abnormal	9	5	4	6
Weight decrease	5	7	5	2

Flu-like symptoms (eg, headache, fatigue, fever, rigors, myalgia, sweating increased, arthralgia) were the most frequently reported treatment-related adverse reactions. The most common adverse event resulting in drug discontinuation was mild to moderate depression (26% of 9 mcg treatment group).

Overdosage

The maximum overdose reported is 150 mcg interferon alfacon-1 administered subcutaneously. The patient received 10 times the prescribed dosage for 3 days and experienced a mild increase in anorexia, chills, fever, and myalgia. Increases in ALT (15 to 127 IU/L), AST (15 to 164 IU/L), and LDH (183 to 281 IU/L) were also reported. These laboratory values returned to normal or to baseline within 30 days.

Patient Information

Inform patients of the possible development of depression prior to initiation of therapy. Patients should report any sign or symptom of depression immediately.

If home use is determined to be desirable by a physician, a health care professional should give instructions on appropriate. The patient must be instructed as to the proper dosage and administration. Fully review information included in the Medication Guide with the patient; it is not a disclosure of all, or possible, adverse effects. The most common adverse reactions occurring with interferon alfacon-1 therapy are flu-like symptoms including fatigue, fever, rigors, headache, arthralgia, myalgia, and increased sweating. Nonnarcotic analgesics and bedtime administration may be used to prevent or lessen some of these symptoms. Additionally, patients must be thoroughly instructed in the importance of proper disposal procedures and cautioned against the reuse of needles, syringes, or re-entry of the drug product. Inform the patient to use a puncture-resistant container for the disposal of used syringes and needles and to dispose according to the directions provided by the health care provider.

Warn patients not to change brands of interferon without medical consultation. Instruct patients not to reduce the dosage of interferon alfacon-1 prior to medical consultation.

Advise men and women treated with interferon alfacon-1 to use effective contraception.

INTERFERON ALFA-N3 (HUMAN LEUKOCYTE DERIVED)

Rx	**Alferon N** (Interferon Sciences, Inc.)	**Injection:** 5 million IU/ml	8 mg NaCl, 1.74 mg Na phosphate dibasic, 0.2 mg K phosphate monobasic, 0.2 mg KCl. In 1 ml vials.

Indications

➤*Condylomata acuminata:* Intralesional treatment of refractory or recurring external condylomata acuminata (venereal/genital warts) in patients ≥ 18 years of age.

Administration and Dosage

➤*Approved by the FDA:* 1989.

The physician should select patients for treatment with interferon alfa-n3 (human leukocyte derived) after consideration of a number of factors: Locations and sizes of the lesions, past treatment and response thereto, and the patient's ability to comply with the treatment regimen. Interferon alfa-n3 is particularly useful for patients who have not responded satisfactorily to other treatment modalities (eg, podophyllin resin, surgery, laser, cryotherapy).

There have been no studies with this product in adolescents. This product is not recommended for use in patients < 18 years of age.

The recommended dose of interferon alfa-n3 for the treatment of condylomata acuminata is 0.05 ml (250,000 IU) per wart. Administer interferon alfa-n3 twice weekly for up to 8 weeks. The maximum recommended dose per treatment session is 0.5 ml (2.5 million IU). Inject interferon alfa-n3 into the base of each wart, preferably using a 30-gauge needle. For large warts, inject interferon alfa-n3 at several points around the periphery of the wart, using a total dose of 0.05 ml/wart.

The minimum effective dose of interferon alfa-n3 for the treatment of condylomata acuminata has not been established. Moderate-to-severe adverse experiences may require modification of the dosage regimen or, in some cases, termination of therapy with interferon alfa-n3.

Genital warts usually begin to disappear after several weeks of treatment with interferon alfa-n3. Continue treatment for a maximum of 8 weeks. In clinical trials with interferon alfa-n3, many patients who had partial resolution of warts during treatment experienced further resolution of their warts after cessation of treatment. Of the patients who had complete resolution of warts due to treatment, half the patients had complete resolution of warts by the end of the treatment, and half had complete resolution of warts during the 3 months after cessation of treatment. Thus, it is recommended that no further therapy (interferon alfa-n3 or conventional therapy) be administered for 3 months after the initial 8-week course of treatment unless the warts enlarge or new warts appear. Studies to determine the safety and efficacy of a second course of treatment with interferon alfa-n3 have not been conducted.

Inspect parenteral drug products visually for particulate matter and discoloration prior to administration, whenever solution and container permit.

➤*Storage/Stability:* Store at 2° to 8°C (36° to 46°F). Do not freeze or shake.

Actions

➤*Pharmacology:* Interferons bind to specific membrane receptors on cell surfaces. Interferon alfa-n3 has been shown to bind to the same receptors as interferon alfa-2b. The receptors have a high degree of selectivity for the binding of human but not mouse interferon. This correlates with the high species specificity found in laboratory studies.

Binding of interferon to membrane receptors initiates a series of events including induction of protein synthesis. These actions are followed by a variety of cellular responses, including inhibition of virus replication and suppression of cell proliferation. Immunomodulation, including enhancement of phagocytosis by macrophages, augmentation of the cytotoxicity of lymphocytes, and enhancement of human leukocyte antigen expression occurs in response to exposure to interferons. One or more of these activities may contribute to the therapeutic effect of interferon.

Contraindications

Known hypersensitivity to human interferon alpha proteins or any component of the product; anaphylactic sensitivity to mouse immunoglobulin (IgG), egg protein, or neomycin.

Warnings

➤*Hypersensitivity reactions:* Acute, serious hypersensitivity reactions (eg, urticaria, angioedema, bronchoconstriction, anaphylaxis) have not been observed in patients receiving interferon alfa-n3. However, if such reactions develop, discontinue drug administration immediately and institute appropriate medical therapy.

➤*Fertility impairment:* In studies with adult females, interferon alpha has been shown to affect the menstrual cycle and decrease serum estradiol and progesterone levels.

Use interferon alfa-n3 (human leukocyte derived) with caution in fertile men. Caution fertile women to use effective contraception while being treated with interferon alfa-n3.

Changes in the menstrual cycle and abortions have been reported to occur in nonhuman primates given extremely high doses of recombinant interferon alpha. In these studies, *Macaca mulatta* (rhesus monkeys) were given interferon daily by IM injection. When given at daily IM doses 326 times the average intralesional dose of interferon alfa-n3 (120 times the maximum recommended dose), this recombinant interferon formulation produced menstrual cycle changes in the monkeys.

➤*Pregnancy: Category C.* Animal reproduction studies have not been conducted with interferon alfa-n3. It is also not known whether interferon alfa-n3 can cause fetal harm when administered to a pregnant woman or can affect reproductive capacity. Give interferon alfa-n3 to a pregnant woman only if clearly needed.

➤*Lactation:* It is not known whether interferon alfa-n3 is excreted in breast milk. Studies in mice have shown that mouse interferons are excreted in milk. Because many drugs are excreted in human breast milk and because of the potential for serious adverse reactions in nursing infants, make a decision whether to discontinue nursing or to not initiate drug treatment, taking into account the importance of the drug to the mother and the potential risks to the infant.

➤*Children:* Safety and efficacy have not been established in patients < 18 years of age.

Precautions

➤*Monitoring:* Because this product is made from human blood, it may carry a risk of transmitting infectious agents (eg, viruses, and theoretically, Creutzfeldt-Jakob disease [CJD] agents).

➤*Special risk:* Because of fever and other "flu-like" symptoms associated with interferon alfa-n3, use interferon alfa-n3 cautiously in patients with debilitating medical conditions such as cardiovascular disease (eg, unstable angina, uncontrolled CHF), severe pulmonary disease (eg, chronic obstructive pulmonary disease), or diabetes mellitus with ketoacidosis.

Use interferon alfa-n3 cautiously in patients with coagulation disorders (eg, thrombophlebitis, pulmonary embolism, hemophilia), severe myelosuppression, or seizure disorders.

➤*Lab test abnormalities:* Abnormalities were seen with statistically equivalent frequencies in the interferon alfa-n3 injection and placebo groups. None of the laboratory abnormalities were considered clinically significant. The abnormalities in the interferon alfa-n3-treated patients consisted primarily of decreased WBC (11%). Decreases also occurred in 4% of the placebo patients.

The number and percentage of patients with cancer who experienced a significant abnormal laboratory test value (values that changed from WHO Grades 0, 1, or 2 at baseline to WHO Grades 3 or 4 during or after treatment) at least once during the trials were the following: Hemoglobin level (7%); WBC count (3%); platelet count (3%); GGT (6%); AST (3%); alkaline phosphatase (8%); and total bilirubin (4%).

Adverse Reactions

➤*Adverse reactions in patients with condylomata acuminata:* A total of 104 patients with condylomata acuminata were treated with interferon alfa-n3 during a double-blind clinical trial. Adverse reactions were reported to be likely, unlikely, or not known to be related to interferon alfa-n3. Adverse reactions consisted primarily of "flu-like" symptoms (eg, myalgia, fever, headache), which were in most cases mild or moderate and transient and did not interfere with treatment.

The "flu-like" adverse reactions, consisting of fever, myalgias, or headache occurred primarily after the first treatment session and were reported by 30% of the patients. The frequency of "flu-like" adverse reactions abated with repeated dosing of interferon alfa-n3 so that the incidence due to interferon alfa-n3 and placebo were similar after 3 to 4 weeks of treatment (after 6 to 8 treatment sessions). "Flu-like" symptoms were relieved by administration of acetaminophen.

Adverse reactions were reported at least once during the course of treatment in the following percentages of patients in each treatment group.

Interferon Alfa-n3 Adverse Reactions (%)		
Adverse reaction	Interferon alfa-n3 (n = 104)	Placebo (n = 85)
CNS		
Headache	31	15
Dizziness	9	4
Insomnia	2	1
Depression	2	1
GI		
Nausea	4	7
Vomiting	3	0
Dyspepsia/Heartburn	3	1
Diarrhea	2	2

INTERFERON ALFA-N3 (HUMAN LEUKOCYTE DERIVED)

Interferon Alfa-n3 Adverse Reactions (%)		
Adverse reaction	Interferon alfa-n3 (n = 104)	Placebo (n = 85)
Musculoskeletal		
Myalgias	45	15
Arthralgia	5	1
Back pain	4	1
Miscellaneous		
Fever	40	19
Fatigue	14	6
Chills	14	2
Malaise	9	9
Generalized pruritus	2	0
Nose/Sinus drainage	2	2
Sweating	2	1
Vasovagal reaction	2	0

Most of the systemic adverse reactions were mild or moderate. Severe systemic adverse reactions were reported by 18% of interferon alfa-n3-treated patients and 13% of placebo-treated patients. Most of the severe systemic adverse reactions reported were "flu-like." Other severe systemic adverse reactions included back pain, insomnia, and sensitivity to allergens. Adverse reactions reported by 1% of patients treated with interferon alfa-n3 in the double-blind trial include the following: Left groin lymph node swelling, tongue hyperaesthesia, thirst, tingling of legs/feet, hot sensation on bottom of feet, strange taste in mouth, increased salivation, heat intolerance, visual disturbances, pharyngitis, sensitivity to allergens, muscle cramps, nosebleed, throat tightness, and papular rash on neck. Additional adverse reactions reported by 1% of patients treated with placebo include: Pharyngitis, oral pain, penile discharge, cold, knuckle stiffness, herpes outbreak, cough, disorientation, and weight/appetite loss.

Additional adverse reactions that occurred only in open clinical trials included the following: Herpes labialis, hot flashes, nervousness, decrease in concentration, dysuria, photosensitivity, and swollen lymph nodes. These reactions occurred in 1% of the patients. One patient with a history of epilepsy, who was not taking anticonvulsant medication, had a grand mal seizure while being treated with interferon alfa-n3; this seizure was judged to be unrelated to interferon alfa-n3 administration.

➤*Adverse reactions in cancer patients:* Thirty-one patients with cancer were treated with a maximum of 10 IM injections of interferon alfa-n3 in doses of 3, 9, or 15 million IU per treatment session. The occurrence of adverse reactions was judged to be unrelated to the dose of interferon alfa-n3.

The following adverse reactions were reported at least once (the percentage of patients experiencing the reaction is indicated in parentheses): Chills (87%); fever (81%); anorexia (68%); malaise (65%); nausea (48%); vomiting (29%); myalgias (16%); arthralgia, chest pains, soreness at injection site, sleepiness, headache (10%); diarrhea, fatigue, low blood pressure, sore mouth/stomatitis, blurred vision (6%).

Those adverse reactions that were each reported by only 1 patient treated with interferon alfa-n3 include the following: Stiff shoulders, flushed face, edema, dry mouth, mucositis, coughing, numbness, numbness in hands and fingers, pain on ocular rotation, shakes/shivers, ringing in ears, cramps, constipation, muscle soreness, confusion, lightheadedness, depression, upset stomach, and sweating. The following adverse reactions were reported as severe by ≥ 1 patient: Fever (55%); malaise (54%); anorexia, chills (45%); nausea (16%); myalgias (13%); vomiting (10%); fatigue, low blood pressure, chest pains, sore mouth/stomatitis (6%); headache, diarrhea, sleepiness, arthralgia, blurred vision, stiff shoulders, numbness, pain on ocular rotation, muscle soreness, confusion, light-headedness, depression, sweating (3%).

➤*Dermatologic:* The frequency of application site disorders (eg, itching, pain) for patients treated with interferon alfa-n3 was significantly less than that reported with placebo (12% vs 26%). No severe application site disorders were reported by patients treated with interferon alfa-n3, while 7% of placebo-treated patients reported severe disorders.

Patient Information

Inform patients of the early signs of hypersensitivity reactions including hives, generalized urticaria, tightness of the chest, wheezing, hypotension, and anaphylaxis. Advise patient to contact physician if these symptoms occur.

Inform patients being treated with interferon alfa-n3 of the benefits and risks associated with treatment. Caution patients not to change brands of interferon without medical consultation, as a change in dosage may occur.

INTERFERON GAMMA-1B

Rx	**Actimmune** (InterMune Pharm.)	**Injection:** 100 mcg (2 million IU)/0.5 ml	Preservative free. In single-dose vials.[1]

[1] With 20 mg mannitol, 0.36 mg sodium succinate, 0.05 mg polysorbate 20.

Indications

➤*Chronic granulomatous disease (CGD):* For reducing the frequency and severity of serious infections associated with chronic granulomatous disease.

➤*Osteopetrosis:* For delaying time to disease progression in patients with severe, malignant osteopetrosis.

Administration and Dosage

➤*Chronic granulomatous disease and severe, malignant osteopetrosis:* 50 mcg/m² (1 million IU/m²) for patients whose body surface area is > 0.5 m² and 1.5 mcg/kg/dose for patients whose body surface area is ≤ 0.5 m². Administer SC 3 times weekly (eg, Monday, Wednesday, Friday). The optimum sites of injection are the right and left deltoid and anterior thigh. Interferon gamma-1b can be administered by a physician, nurse, family member, or patient who is trained in the administration of SC injections.

The formulation does not contain a preservative. Discard the unused portion of any vial.

Safety and efficacy have not been established for interferon gamma-1b given in doses greater or less than the recommended dose of 50 mcg/m². The minimum effective dose has not been established.

If severe reactions occur, modify the dosage (50% reduction) or discontinue therapy until the adverse reaction abates.

Interferon gamma-1b may be administered using either sterilized glass or plastic disposable syringes.

➤*Storage/Stability:* Vials must be placed in a 2° to 8°C (36° to 46°F) refrigerator immediately upon receipt to ensure optimal retention of physical and biochemical integrity; do not freeze. Avoid excessive or vigorous agitation; do not shake. Do not leave an unentered vial at room temperature for a total time exceeding 12 hours prior to use. Discard and do not return vials exceeding this time period to the refrigerator.

Actions

➤*Pharmacology:* Interferon gamma-1b, a biologic response modifier, is a single-chain polypeptide containing 140 amino acids. Production of interferon gamma-1b is achieved by fermentation of a genetically engineered *Escherichia coli* bacterium containing the DNA that encodes for the human protein.

Interferons are a family of functionally related, species-specific proteins synthesized by eukaryotic cells in response to viruses and a variety of natural and synthetic stimuli. The most striking differences between interferon gamma and other classes of interferon concern the immunomodulatory properties of this molecule. While gamma, alpha, and beta interferons share certain properties, interferon gamma has potent phagocyte-activating effects not seen with other interferon preparations, including generation of toxic oxygen metabolites within phagocytes, which are capable of mediating the intracellular killing of microorganisms such as *Staphylococcus aureus, Toxoplasma gondii, Leishmania donovani, Listeria monocytogenes,* and *Mycobacterium avium* intracellulare.

Clinical studies in patients using interferon gamma have revealed a broad range of biological activities including the enhancement of the oxidative metabolism of tissue macrophages, enhancement of antibody-dependent cellular cytotoxicity, and natural killer cell activity. Additionally, effects of Fc receptor expression on monocytes and major histocompatibility antigen expression have been noted.

To the extent that interferon gamma is produced by antigen-stimulated T lymphocytes and regulates activity of immune cells, it is appropriate to characterize it as a lymphokine of the interleukin type. There is growing evidence that interferon gamma interacts functionally with other interleukin molecules such as interleukin-2, and that all interleukins form part of a complex, lymphokine regulatory network. For example, interferon gamma and interleukin-4 appear to reciprocally interact to regulate murine IgE levels; interferon gamma can suppress IgE levels and inhibit collagen production at the transcription level in human systems.

With respect to CGD, pilot clinical trials of the systemic administration of interferon gamma-1b in patients with CGD provided evidence for a treatment-related enhancement of phagocyte function including elevation of superoxide levels and improved killing of *Staphylococcus aureus.*

In severe, malignant osteopetrosis (another inherited disorder characterized by an osteoclast defect leading to bone overgrowth and deficient phagocyte oxidative metabolism), a treatment-related enhancement of superoxide production by phagocytes was observed in situ. Interferon gamma-1b was found to enhance osteoclast function in vitro.

➤*Pharmacokinetics:* Following single-dose administration of 100 mcg/m², interferon gamma is rapidly cleared after IV use (1.4 L/

Immunomodulators

INTERFERON GAMMA-1B

minute) and slowly absorbed after IM or SC injection. After IM or SC injection, the apparent fraction of dose absorbed was > 89%. The mean elimination half-life after IV administration was 38 minutes. The mean elimination half-lives for IM and SC dosing were 2.9 and 5.9 hours, respectively. Peak plasma concentrations occurred ≈ 4 hours (1.5 ng/ml) after IM dosing and 7 hours (0.6 ng/ml) after SC dosing. Multiple-dose SC pharmacokinetic studies were conducted in 38 healthy male subjects. There was no accumulation of drug after 12 consecutive daily injections of 100 mcg/m^2.

➤*Clinical trials:*

CGD – A randomized, double-blind, placebo-controlled study in patients (n = 128; 1 to 44 years of age) with CGD (an inherited disorder characterized by deficient phagocyte oxidative metabolism) was performed to determine whether SC interferon gamma-1b 3 times weekly could decrease the incidence of serious infectious episodes and improve existing infectious and inflammatory conditions. Most patients received prophylactic antibiotics. Serious infection was defined as a clinical event requiring hospitalization and the use of parenteral antibiotics. There was a 67% reduction in relative risk of serious infection in patients receiving interferon gamma-1b (n = 63) compared with placebo (n = 65). Additional supportive evidence of treatment benefit included a 2-fold reduction in the number of primary serious infections in the interferon gamma-1b group and the total number and rate of serious infections including recurrent events. Placebo patients required 3 times as many inpatient hospitalization days for treatment of clinical events compared with patients receiving interferon gamma-1b. The beneficial effect of therapy was observed throughout the entire study, in which the mean duration of administration was 8.9 months per patient.

Osteopetrosis – A controlled, randomized study in patients with severe, malignant osteopetrosis was conducted with interferon gamma-1b administered SC 3 times weekly. Sixteen patients were randomized to receive either interferon gamma-1b plus calcitriol (n = 11), or calcitriol alone (n = 5). The median time to disease progression was significantly delayed in the interferon gamma-1b plus calcitriol arm versus calcitriol alone. Based on the observed data, the median time to progression was ≥ 165 days versus a median of 65 days in calcitriol alone. In an analysis that combined data from a second study, 19 of 24 patients treated with interferon gamma-1b plus or minus calcitriol for ≥ 6 months had reduced trabecular bone volume compared with baseline.

Contraindications

Hypersensitivity to interferon gamma, *E. coli*-derived products, or any component of the product.

Warnings

➤*CNS disorders:* CNS adverse reactions including decreased mental status, gait disturbance, and dizziness have been observed, particularly in patients receiving doses > 250 mcg/m^2/day. Most of these abnormalities were mild and reversible within a few days upon dose reduction or discontinuation of therapy. Exercise caution in patients with seizure disorders and compromised CNS function.

➤*Cardiac disease:* Use with caution in preexisting cardiac disease, including symptoms of ischemia, CHF, or arrhythmia. No direct cardiotoxic effect has been demonstrated, but it is possible that acute and transient "flu-like" or constitutional symptoms such as fever and chills frequently associated with interferon gamma-1b administration at doses of ≥ 250 mcg/m^2/day may exacerbate preexisting conditions.

➤*Myelosuppression:* Exercise caution in patients with myelosuppression. Reversible neutropenia and elevation of hepatic enzymes can be dose-limiting at doses > 250 mcg/m^2/day. Thrombocytopenia and proteinuria have also occurred rarely.

➤*Hypersensitivity reactions:* Acute serious hypersensitivity reactions have not been observed in patients receiving interferon gamma-1b; however, if such an acute reaction develops, discontinue the drug immediately and institute appropriate medical therapy. Refer to Management of Acute Hypersensitivity Reactions. Transient cutaneous rashes have occurred in some patients following injection but have rarely necessitated treatment interruption.

➤*Fertility impairment:* Female monkeys treated with daily SC doses of 30 or 150 mcg/kg (≈ 20 and 100 times the human dose) exhibited irregular menstrual cycles or absence of cyclicity during treatment.

➤*Pregnancy: Category C.* Interferon gamma-1b has shown an increased incidence of abortions in primates when given in doses ≈ 100 times the human dose. There are no adequate and well-controlled studies in pregnant women. Use during pregnancy only if the potential benefit justifies the potential risk to the fetus. In addition, studies evaluating recombinant murine interferon gamma in pregnant mice revealed increased incidences of uterine bleeding and abortifacient activity and decreased neonatal viability at maternally toxic doses. The clinical significance of this observation with recombinant murine interferon gamma tested in a homologous system is uncertain.

➤*Lactation:* It is not known whether interferon gamma is excreted in breast milk. Because of the potential for serious adverse reactions in nursing infants, decide whether to discontinue nursing or to discontinue the drug, depending on the importance of the drug to the mother.

➤*Children:* Safety and efficacy in children < 1 year of age have not been established.

Precautions

➤*Monitoring:* In addition to tests normally required for monitoring patients with CGD and osteopetrosis, the following laboratory tests are recommended for all patients prior to beginning therapy and at 3-month intervals during treatment: Hematologic tests including complete blood counts and differential and platelet counts; blood chemistries including renal and liver function tests; urinalysis.

Drug Interactions

➤*CYP450:* Preclinical studies in rodents using species-specific interferon gamma have demonstrated a decrease in hepatic microsomal cytochrome P450 concentrations. This could potentially lead to a depression of the hepatic metabolism of certain drugs that utilize this degradative pathway.

➤*Myelosuppressive agents:* Exercise caution when administering interferon gamma-1b in combination with other potentially myelosuppressive agents (see Warnings).

Adverse Reactions

The following data on adverse reactions are based on the SC use of 50 mcg/m^2 interferon gamma-1b 3 times weekly in patients with CGD.

Similar safety data were observed in 34 patients with severe malignant osteopetrosis.

Interferon Gamma-1B Adverse Reactions (%)		
Adverse reaction	Interferon gamma-1b (n = 63)	Placebo (n = 65)
Fever	52	28
Headache	33	9
Rash	17	6
Chills	14	0
Injection site erythema or tenderness	14	2
Fatigue	14	11
Diarrhea	14	12
Vomiting	13	5
Nausea	10	2
Abdominal pain[1]	8	3
Myalgia	6	0
Depression[1]	3	0
Arthralgia	2	0
Back pain[1]	2	0

[1] May have been related to underlying disease.

Interferon gamma-1b has also been evaluated in additional disease states in studies in which patients have generally received higher doses (> 100 mcg/m^2/day) administered by IM injection or IV infusion. All of the previously described adverse reactions that occurred in patients with CGD have also been observed in patients receiving higher doses. Adverse reactions not observed in patients with CGD receiving doses < 100 mcg/m^2/day but seen rarely in patients receiving interferon gamma-1b in other studies include the following:

➤*Cardiovascular:* Hypotension; syncope; tachyarrhythmia; heart block; heart failure; MI.

➤*CNS:* Confusion; disorientation; gait disturbance; parkinsonian symptoms; seizure; hallucinations; transient ischemic attacks.

➤*GI:* Hepatic insufficiency; GI bleeding; pancreatitis.

➤*Hematologic:* Deep venous thrombosis; pulmonary embolism.

➤*Pulmonary:* Tachypnea; bronchospasm; interstitial pneumonitis.

➤*Metabolic:* Hyponatremia; hyperglycemia.

➤*Miscellaneous:* Exacerbation of dermatomyositis; reversible renal insufficiency.

Patient Information

Inform patients and/or their parents of the potential benefits and risks associated with treatment. If home use is determined to be desirable by the physician, give instructions on appropriate use, including a review of the contents of the Patient Information insert. This information is intended to aid in the safe and effective use of the medication; it is not a disclosure of all possible adverse or intended effects.

If home use is prescribed, supply the patients with a puncture resistant container for the disposal of used syringes and needles. Thoroughly instruct patients in the importance of proper disposal and caution against any reuse of needles and syringes. Dispose of the full container according to the directions provided by the physician.

The most common adverse experiences are "flu-like" or constitutional symptoms such as fever, headache, chills, myalgia, or fatigue that may decrease in severity as treatment continues. Some of the "flu-like" symptoms may be minimized by bedtime administration. Acetaminophen may be used to prevent or partially alleviate the fever and headache.

INTERFERON BETA

Indications

▶*Multiple sclerosis (MS):* Treatment of MS. See individual monographs for specific indications.

Actions

▶*Pharmacology:* **Interferon beta-1a** is a 166 amino acid glycoprotein. It is produced by mammalian cells (Chinese hamster ovary cells) into which the human interferon beta gene has been introduced. The amino acid sequence of interferon beta-1a is identical to that of natural human interferon beta. **Interferon beta-1b** is manufactured by bacterial fermentation of a strain of *Escherichia coli* that bears a genetically engineered plasmid containing the gene for human interferon beta$_{ser17}$. Interferon beta-1b is a purified protein that has 165 amino acids. It does not include the carbohydrate side chains found in the natural material.

Interferons are a family of naturally occurring proteins and glycoproteins that are produced by eukaryotic cells in response to viral infection and other biological inducers. Interferon beta is produced by various cell types including fibroblasts and macrophages. Three major classes of interferons have been identified: Alpha, beta, and gamma; they each have overlapping yet distinct biologic activities.

Interferon beta has antiviral, antiproliferative, and immunoregulatory activities. The mechanisms by which it exerts its actions in MS are not clearly understood. However, it is known that the binding of interferon beta to its receptors initiates a complex cascade of intracellular events that leads to the expression of numerous interferon-induced gene products and markers, including 2′,5′-oligoadenylate synthetase, beta 2-microglobulin, and neopterin, which may mediate some of the biological activities.

▶*Pharmacokinetics:*

Interferon beta-1a – Biological response markers (eg, neopterin and β_2-microglobulin) are induced by interferon beta-1a following parenteral doses of 15 to 75 mcg in healthy subjects and treated patients. Biological response marker levels increase within 12 hours of dosing and remain elevated for at least 4 days. Peak biological response marker levels are typically observed 48 hours after dosing.

	Interferon Beta-1a Pharmacokinetic Parameters[1]			
Route	Mean C_{max} (IU/mL)	T_{max} (h)	Mean AUC (IU•h/mL)	$t_{1/2}$ (h)
IM	4.9	3 to 15	65	10
SC[2]	5.1	16 (median)	294	69

[1] Data are pooled from different studies and are not necessarily comparable.
[2] Based on a single dose of 60 mcg.

Interferon beta-1b – Because serum concentrations of interferon beta-1b are low or not detectable following SC administration of up to 0.25 mg, pharmacokinetic information in patients with MS receiving the recommended dose is not available. Following single and multiple daily SC administrations of 0.5 mg (16 mIU) to healthy volunteers (n = 12), serum concentrations were generally less than 100 IU/mL. Peak serum concentrations occurred between 1 to 8 hours, with a mean peak serum concentration of 40 IU/mL. Bioavailability, based on a total dose of 0.5 mg given as 2 SC injections at different sites, was approximately 50%.

After IV administration (0.006 to 2 mg), similar pharmacokinetic profiles were obtained from healthy volunteers (n = 12) and from patients with diseases other than MS (n = 142). In patients receiving single IV doses up to 2 mg, increases in serum concentrations were dose-proportional. Mean serum clearance values ranged from 9.4 to 28.9 mL/min/kg and were independent of dose. Mean terminal elimination half-life values ranged from 8 minutes to 4.3 hours and mean steady-state volume of distribution values ranged from 0.25 to 2.88 L/kg. IV dosing 3 times/week for 2 weeks resulted in no accumulation of interferon beta-1b in the serum of patients. Pharmacokinetic parameters after single and multiple IV doses were comparable.

Following SC administration every other day, biologic response marker levels increased significantly above baseline 6 to 12 hours after the first dose. Peak biologic response marker levels usually occur between 40 and 124 hours after dosing and remain elevated for at least 7 days.

▶*Clinical trials:*

Interferon beta-1a – Patients with relapsing-remitting MS were randomized to treatment with 44 mcg *Rebif* 3 times/week via SC injection (n = 339) or 30 mcg *Avonex* weekly by IM injection (n = 338). Seventy-five percent and 62% of *Rebif* patients vs 63% and 52% of *Avonex*-treated patients were relapse-free at 24 and 48 weeks, respectively. Injection-site disorders, hepatic function disorders, and leukopenia were observed with greater frequency in the *Rebif* group vs the *Avonex* group.

Contraindications

Hypersensitivity to natural or recombinant interferon beta, human albumin, or any other component of the formulations.

Warnings

▶*Chronic progressive MS:* The safety and efficacy of interferon beta in chronic progressive MS have not been evaluated.

▶*Depression:* Use interferon beta with caution in patients with depression or other mood disorders, conditions that are common with MS. Depression and suicide have been reported in patients receiving interferon compounds. Depression, suicidal ideation, and suicidal attempts are known to occur at an increased frequency in patients receiving interferon compounds. Additionally, there have been postmarketing reports of depression, suicidal ideation, and/or development of new or worsening pre-existing psychiatric disorders, including psychosis. Some of these patients improved upon cessation of dosing.

Advise patients treated with interferon beta to immediately report any symptoms of depression or suicidal ideation. If a patient develops depression or other severe psychiatric symptoms, consider cessation of therapy.

▶*Injection-site necrosis (ISN):* ISN has been reported. Typically, ISN occurs within the first 4 months of therapy, although postmarketing reports have been received of ISN occurring over 1 year after initiation of therapy. Necrosis may occur at a single or multiple injection sites. The necrotic lesions are typically 3 cm or less in diameter, but larger areas have been reported. Generally, the necrosis has extended only to subcutaneous fat. However, there also are reports of necrosis extending to and including fascia overlaying muscle. In some lesions where biopsy results are available, vasculitis has been reported. For some lesions, debridement and, infrequently, skin grafting have been required.

As with any open lesion, it is important to avoid infection and, if it occurs, to treat the infection. Time to healing varied depending on the severity of the necrosis at the time of treatment. In most cases, healing was associated with scarring.

Some patients have experienced healing of necrotic skin lesions while **interferon beta-1b** therapy continued; others have not. Whether to discontinue therapy following a single site of necrosis is dependent on the extent of necrosis. For patients who continue therapy with interferon beta-1b after ISN has occurred, do not administer interferon beta-1b into the affected area until it is fully healed. If multiple lesions occur, discontinue therapy until healing occurs.

Periodically re-evaluate patient understanding and use of aseptic self-injection techniques, particularly if ISN has occurred.

▶*Anaphylaxis:* Anaphylaxis has been reported as a rare complication of interferon beta use. Other allergic reactions have included dyspnea, bronchospasm, tongue edema, orolingual edema, skin rash, and urticaria, and have ranged from mild to severe without a clear relationship to dose or duration of exposure. Several allergic reactions, some severe, have occurred after prolonged use.

▶*Decreased peripheral blood counts:* Decreased peripheral blood counts in all cell lines, including rare pancytopenia and thrombocytopenia, have been reported from postmarketing experience. Some cases of thrombocytopenia have had nadirs below 10,000/mcL. Some cases reoccur with rechallenge. Monitor patients for signs of these disorders.

▶*Albumin (human):* Some of these products contain albumin, a derivative of human blood. Based on effective donor screening and product manufacturing processes, it carries an extremely remote risk for transmission of viral diseases. A theoretical risk for transmission of Creutzfeldt-Jakob disease (CJD) also is considered extremely remote. No cases of transmission of viral diseases or CJD have been identified for albumin.

▶*Special risk patients:* Exercise caution when administering **interferon beta-1a** to patients with pre-existing seizure disorders. Seizures have been associated with the use of beta interferons. A relationship between occurrence of seizures and the use of interferon beta has not been established. Leukopenia and new or worsening thyroid abnormalities have developed in some patients treated with interferon beta. Regular monitoring for these conditions is recommended.

▶*Cardiac disease:* Closely monitor patients with cardiac disease, such as angina, CHF, or arrhythmia, for worsening of their clinical condition during initiation and continued treatment. While interferon beta does not have any known direct-acting cardiac toxicity, during the postmarketing period infrequent cases of CHF, cardiomyopathy, and cardiomyopathy with CHF have been reported in patients without known predisposition to these events and without other known etiologies being established. In rare cases, these events have been temporally related to the administration of interferon beta. In some of these instances, recurrence upon rechallenge was observed.

▶*Hepatic function impairment:* Severe liver dysfunction, leading to hepatic failure requiring liver transplantation, has been reported very rarely in patients taking interferon beta. Symptomatic hepatic dysfunction (including hepatitis), primarily presenting as jaundice, has been reported as a rare complication of use. Asymptomatic elevation of hepatic transaminases (particularly ALT) is common with interferon therapy. Initiate therapy with caution in patients with active liver disease, alcohol abuse, increased serum ALT (greater than 2.5 times the upper limit of normal [ULN]), or a history of significant liver disease.

INTERFERON BETA

Consider dose reduction if ALT rises above 5 times the ULN. The dose may be re-escalated gradually once the enzyme levels have normalized. Stop treatment if jaundice or other clinical symptoms of liver dysfunction appear.

➤*Fertility impairment:* Menstrual irregularities were observed in monkeys administered **interferon beta-1a** at a dose 100 times the recommended weekly human dose. Anovulation and decreased serum progesterone levels also were noted transiently in some animals. These effects were reversible after discontinuation of the drug.

➤*Pregnancy: Category C.* There are no adequate and well-controlled studies in pregnant women. Abortifacient activity has been shown in animals and 6 spontaneous abortions were reported in patients on interferon beta therapy during the clinical trials. If the patient becomes pregnant or plans to become pregnant while taking interferon beta, apprise the patient of the potential hazards to the fetus and recommend that the patient discontinue therapy.

➤*Lactation:* It is not known whether interferon beta is excreted in breast milk. Decide whether to discontinue nursing or discontinue the drug, taking into account the importance of the drug to the mother.

➤*Children:* Safety and efficacy in children younger than 18 years of age have not been established.

Precautions

➤*Monitoring:* In addition to the laboratory tests normally required for monitoring patients with MS, blood cell counts and liver function tests are recommended at baseline and regular intervals (1, 3, and 6 months) following introduction of interferon beta therapy and then periodically thereafter in the absence of clinical symptoms. Thyroid function tests are recommended every 6 months in patients with a history of thyroid dysfunction or as clinically indicated. Patients with myelosuppression may require more intensive monitoring of complete blood cell counts, with differential and platelet counts.

➤*Self-administration:* Instruct patients in injection techniques to ensure the safe self-administration of interferon beta. A patient information sheet is provided with the product.

➤*Flu-like symptoms complex:* Flu-like symptoms, including headache, fever, fatigue, rigors, chest pain, back pain, and myalgia, have been commonly reported with interferon beta therapy. Symptoms usually occur 4 hours after injection and subside within 24 hours. Acetaminophen or NSAIDs prior to and/or following injection may help to prevent or treat these symptoms.

➤*Autoimmune disorders:* Autoimmune disorders of multiple target organs have been reported postmarketing, including idiopathic thrombocytopenia, hyper- and hypothyroidism, and rare cases of autoimmune hepatitis. Monitor patients for signs of these disorders and implement appropriate treatment when observed.

➤*Hepatic injury:* Hepatic injury, including elevated serum hepatic enzyme levels and hepatitis, some of which have been severe, has been reported postmarketing. In some patients, a recurrence of elevated serum levels of hepatic enzymes has occurred upon rechallenge. In some cases, these events have occurred in the presence of other drugs associated with hepatic injury. The potential of additive effects from multiple drugs or other hepatotoxic agents (eg, alcohol) has not been determined. Monitor patients for signs of hepatic injury and exercise caution when interferons are used concomitantly with other drugs associated with hepatic injury.

➤*Immunogenicity:* As with all therapeutic proteins, there is a potential for immunogenicity. Antibodies to interferon beta have developed during therapy. The relationship between antibody formation and clinical safety or efficacy is unknown.

➤*Latex sensitivity:* Administer with caution to patients with a possible history of latex sensitivity; packaging may contain dry natural rubber.

➤*Photosensitivity:* Photosensitization (photoallergy or phototoxicity) may occur; therefore, caution patients to take protective measures (ie, sunscreens, protective clothing) against exposure to sunlight or ultraviolet light (eg, tanning beds) until tolerance is determined.

Drug Interactions

➤*Myelosuppressive agents:* Because of the potential of **interferon beta-1a** to cause neutropenia and lymphopenia, proper monitoring is required if administered concomitantly with myelosuppressive agents.

Adverse Reactions

The most serious adverse reactions associated with interferon beta therapy were depression, suicidal ideation, and ISN (see Warnings). The most commonly reported adverse reactions were asthenia, flu-like symptoms complex (see Precautions), headache, injection site reaction, lymphopenia (lymphocytes less than 1500/mm³), and pain. The most frequently reported adverse reactions resulting in clinical intervention (ie, discontinuation of therapy, adjustment in dosage, or the need for concomitant medication to treat an adverse reaction symptom) were asthenia, depression, flu-like symptoms complex, hypertonia, injection site reactions, increased liver enzymes, leukopenia, and myasthenia.

		Interferon Beta Adverse Reactions (%)[1]		
		Rebif		
Adverse reactions	Avonex (n = 351)	22 mcg 3 times/week (n = 189)	44 mcg 3 times/week (n = 184)	Interferon beta-1b (n = 1115)
Cardiovascular				
Hypertension	–	–	–	7
Migraine	5	–	–	–
Palpitations	–	–	–	4
Peripheral edema	–	–	–	15
Peripheral vascular disorder	–	–	–	6
Tachycardia	–	–	–	4
Vasodilation	2	–	–	8
CNS				
Anxiety	–	–	–	10
Asthenia	24	–	–	61
Convulsions	–	5	4	–
Depression	18	–	–	–
Dizziness	14	–	–	24
Fatigue	–	33	41	–
Headache	58	65	70	57
Incoordination	–	5	4	21
Nervousness	–	–	–	7
Hypertonia	–	7	6	50
Sleep difficulty	–	–	–	24
Somnolence	–	4	5	–
Dermatologic				
Alopecia	4	–	–	4
Rash (erythematous, maculopapular)	–	5-7	4-5	24
Skin disorder	–	–	–	12
Sweating	–	–	–	8
GI				
Abdominal pain	8	22	20	19
Constipation	–	–	–	20
Diarrhea	–	–	–	19
Dry mouth	–	1	5	–
Dyspepsia	–	–	–	14
Nausea	23	–	–	27
GU				
Dysmenorrhea[2]	–	–	–	7
Impotence[3]	–	–	–	9
Menorrhagia[2]	–	–	–	8
Metrorrhagia[2]	–	–	–	11
Prostatic disorder[3]	–	–	–	3
Urinary frequency	–	2	7	7
Urinary incontinence	–	4	2	–
Urinary urgency	–	–	–	13
Urine constituents, abnormal	3	–	–	–
UTI	17	–	–	–
Hemic/Lymphatic				
ANC < 1500/mm³	–	–	–	14
Anemia	4	3	5	–
Leukopenia	–	28	36	–
Lymphadenopathy	–	11	12	8
Lymphocytes < 1500/mm³	–	–	–	88
Thrombocytopenia	–	2	8	–
WBC < 3000/mm³	–	–	–	14
Hepatic				
ALT > 5 × baseline	–	20	27	10
AST > 5 × baseline	–	10	17	3
Bilirubinemia	–	3	2	–
Hepatic function abnormal	–	4	9	–
Musculoskeletal				
Arthralgia	9	–	–	31
Back pain	–	23	25	–
Myalgia	29	25	25	27

INTERFERON BETA

		Rebif		
Adverse reactions	Avonex (n = 351)	22 mcg 3 times/week (n = 189)	44 mcg 3 times/week (n = 184)	Interferon beta-1b (n = 1115)
Myasthenia	–	–	–	46
Skeletal pain	–	15	10	–
Respiratory				
Bronchitis	8	–	–	–
Dyspnea	–	–	–	7
Sinusitis	14	–	–	–
Upper respiratory tract infection	14	–	–	–
Special senses				
Eye disorder	4	–	–	–
Vision abnormal	–	7	13	–
Xerophthalmia	–	3	1	–
Miscellaneous				
Chest pain	5	6	8	11
Chills	19	–	–	25
Fever	20	25	28	36
Flu-like symptoms	49	56	59	60
Infection	7	–	–	–
ISN/inflammation/ecchymosis	6	1	3	5
Injection site reaction/pain	3-8	89	92	85
Leg cramps	–	–	–	4
Malaise	–	4	5	8
Pain	23	–	–	51
Rigors	–	6	13	–
Thyroid disorder	–	4	6	–
Toothache	3	–	–	–
Weight gain	–	–	–	7

Table title: **Interferon Beta Adverse Reactions (%)[1]**

[1] Data are pooled from separate studies and are not necessarily comparable.
[2] Premenopausal patients.
[3] Male patients
– = Not reported.

➤*Postmarketing:*
Interferon beta-1a –
  Cardiovascular: CHF, cardiomyopathy, cardiomyopathy with CHF.
  CNS: New or worsening psychiatric disorders, seizures in patients without history.
  GU: Menorrhagia, metrorrhagia.
  Hematologic: Decreased peripheral blood counts, including pancytopenia (rare); thrombocytopenia (some cases with nadirs below 10,000/mcL and have reoccurred upon rechallenge); idiopathic thrombocytopenia.

  Hepatic: Autoimmune hepatitis; hepatic injury, including elevated serum hepatic enzyme levels; hepatitis.
  Miscellaneous: Anaphylaxis, hyper- and hypothyroidism.
Interferon beta-1b –
  Cardiovascular: Cardiomyopathy, deep vein thrombosis, pulmonary embolism.
  CNS: Ataxia, confusion, convulsion, depersonalization, emotional lability, paresthesia.
  Dermatologic: Pruritus, skin discoloration, urticaria.
  Endocrine: Hypothyroidism, hyperthyroidism, thyroid dysfunction.
  GU: UTI, urosepsis.
  Hemic/Lymphatic: Anemia, thrombocytopenia.
  Metabolic/Nutritional: Gamma GT increase, hypocalcemia, hyperuricemia, triglyceride increase.
  Respiratory: Bronchospasm, pneumonia.
  Miscellaneous: Fatal capillary leak syndrome (may appear in patients with a pre-existing monoclonal gammopathy); hepatitis; pancreatitis; vomiting.

Patient Information

➤*Instruction on self-injection technique and procedures:* Instruct patients in the use of aseptic technique when administering interferon beta. Give appropriate instruction for reconstitution of the product and self-injection, including careful review of the patient information sheet that is provided. If possible, perform the first injection under the supervision of an appropriately qualified health care professional.

➤*Dosage schedule:* Caution patients not to change the dosage or the schedule of administration without medical consultation.

➤*Disposal:* Caution patients against the re-use of needles or syringes and instruct them in safe disposal procedures. Supply the patient with a puncture-resistant container for disposal of used needles/syringes along with instructions for safe disposal of containers.

➤*Injection site reactions:* Injection site reactions may occur at least one time during therapy. In general, these are transient and do not require discontinuation of therapy, but carefully assess the nature and severity of all reported reactions. Periodically re-evaluate patient understanding and use of aseptic self-injection technique and procedures.

Advise patients to promptly report any break in the skin, which may be associated with blue-black discoloration, swelling, or drainage of fluid from the injection site, prior to continuing interferon beta therapy.

➤*Flu-like symptoms:* Flu-like symptoms are common following initiation of therapy. Symptoms of flu syndrome are most prominent at the initiation of therapy and decrease in frequency with continued treatment. Concurrent use of analgesics and/or antipyretics may help ameliorate flu-like symptoms on treatment days.

➤*Depression/Suicide:* Caution patients to report depression or suicidal ideation.

➤*Abortifacient potential:* Advise patients about the abortifacient potential.

➤*Photosensitivity:* Advise patients to avoid prolonged exposure to sunlight or sunlamps; interferon beta may cause photosensitivity.

➤*Latex sensitivity:* Some of the packaging may contain latex; caution patients with a possible history of latex allergy.

INTERFERON BETA-1A

Rx	**Rebif** (Serono)	**Injection:** 22 mcg/0.5 mL	Preservative-free. In prefilled single-use syringes.[1] In 12s.
		44 mcg/0.5 mL (12 million IU)	Preservative-free. In prefilled single-use syringes.[2] In 1s, 3s, and 12s.
Rx	**Avonex** (Biogen Idec)	**Powder for injection, lyophilized:** 33 mcg (6.6 million IU [30 mcg/vial when reconstituted])	Preservative-free. In administration dose packs (single-use vial[3] with diluent [sterile water for injection], alcohol wipes, gauze pad, syringe, *Micro Pin* vial access pin, needle, and bandage).
		Prefilled syringe: 30 mcg/0.5 mL	Albumin-free. In administration dose packs (single-use syringe[4], needle, recloseable accessory pouch, alcohol wipes, gauze pads, and bandages).

[1] With 2 mg human albumin, 27.3 mg mannitol, 0.4 mg sodium acetate in water for injection.
[2] With 4 mg human albumin, 27.3 mg mannitol, 0.4 mg sodium acetate in water for injection.
[3] With 16.5 mg human albumin, 6.4 mg sodium chloride, 6.3 mg dibasic sodium phosphate, 1.3 mg monobasic sodium phosphate/vial.
[4] With 0.79 mg sodium acetate trihydrate, 0.25 mg glacial acetic acid, 15.8 mg arginine HCl, 0.025 mg polysorbate 20 in water for injection.

Indications

➤*Multiple sclerosis (MS):* For the treatment of relapsing forms of MS to slow the accumulation of physical disability and decrease the frequency of clinical exacerbations. Patients with MS in whom efficacy has been demonstrated include patients who have experienced a first clinical episode and have MRI features consistent with MS. Safety and efficacy in patients with chronic progressive MS have not been established.

Administration and Dosage

➤*Approved by the FDA:* May 17, 1996.

➤*Avonex:* 30 mcg IM once/week. *Avonex* is intended for use under the guidance and supervision of a physician. Patients may self-inject only if their physician determines that it is appropriate and with medical follow-up, as necessary, after proper training in IM injection technique. Sites for injection include the thigh or upper arm.

Do not substitute SC administration of *Avonex* for IM administration. SC and IM administration have been observed to have nonequivalent pharmacokinetic and pharmacodynamic parameters following administration to healthy volunteers.

Reconstitution of powder for injection – Use a sterile syringe and *Micro Pin* to inject 1.1 mL of the supplied diluent, sterile water for injection. Gently swirl to dissolve drug completely; do not shake. Withdraw 1 mL of reconstituted solution into a sterile syringe.

Vial and syringes are for single use only; discard any unused portion.

➤*Rebif:* 44 mcg SC 3 times/week. Administer, if possible, at the same time (preferably in the late afternoon or evening) on the same 3 days (eg, Monday, Wednesday, and Friday) at least 48 hours apart each week. Generally, start patients at 8.8 mcg SC 3 times/week and increase over a 4-week period to 44 mcg 3 times/week. A starter kit containing 22 mcg syringes is available for use in titrating the dose during the first 4 weeks of treatment. Following the administration of each

INTERFERON BETA-1A

dose, discard any residual product remaining in the syringe in a safe and proper manner.

Rebif Schedule for Patient Titration				
	Recommended titration (%)	Dose (mcg)	Volume (mL)	Syringe strength (per 0.5 mL) (mcg)
Weeks 1 to 2	20	8.8	0.2	22
Weeks 3 to 4	50	22	0.5	22
Weeks 5+	100	44	0.5	44

Leukopenia or elevated liver function tests may necessitate dose reductions of 20% to 50% until toxicity is resolved.

Rebif is intended for use under the guidance and supervision of a physician. It is recommended that physicians or qualified medical personnel train patients in the proper technique for self-administering SC injections using the prefilled syringe. Advise patients to rotate sites for SC injections. Concurrent use of analgesics or antipyretics may help ameliorate flu-like symptoms on treatment days.

➤*Storage / Stability:*

Avonex – Refrigerate lyophilized powder and prefilled syringes at 2° to 8°C (36° to 46°F). Do not expose to high temperatures. Do not freeze. Do not use beyond the expiration date. Protect from light.

   Powder for reconstitution: Should refrigeration be unavailable, store the powder at 25°C (77°F) for a period of up to 30 days. Following reconstitution, use as soon as possible (within 6 hours) stored at 2° to 8°C (36° to 46°F). Do not freeze reconstituted interferon beta-1a.

   Prefilled syringe: Once removed from the refrigerator, allow the prefilled syringe to warm to room temperature (approximately 30 minutes) and use it within 12 hours. Do not use external heat sources, such as hot water, to warm the prefilled syringe.

Rebif – Refrigerate at 2° to 8°C (36° to 46°F). Do not freeze. If a refrigerator is temporarily unavailable, store at or below 25°C (77°F) for up to 30 days away from heat and light. Do not use beyond the expiration date printed on the packages.

INTERFERON BETA-1B

Rx	**Betaseron** (Berlex)	**Powder for injection, lyophilized:** 0.3 mg	Preservative-free. In single-use 3 mL capacity vials with 1.2 mL prefilled syringe of diluent (sodium chloride 0.54%)[1], alcohol prep pads, and vial adaptor with attached needle for each drug vial. In blister unit 15s.

[1] With 15 mg human albumin, 15 mg mannitol/vial.

Indications

➤*Multiple sclerosis (MS):* For the treatment of relapsing forms of MS to reduce the frequency of clinical exacerbations.

Administration and Dosage

➤*Approved by the FDA:* July 23, 1993.

Interferon beta-1b is intended for use under the guidance and supervision of a physician. It is recommended that physicians or qualified medical personnel train patients in the proper technique for self-administering SC injections. Advise patients to rotate sites for SC injections. Concurrent use of analgesics and/or antipyretics may help ameliorate flu-like symptoms on treatment days.

➤*Dose:* 0.25 mg SC every other day. Sites for injection include arms, abdomen, hips, and thigh.

Generally, start patients at 0.0625 mg (0.25 mL) SC every other day, and increase over a 6-week period to 0.25 mg (1 mL) every other day.

Interferon Beta-1b Schedule for Dose Titration			
	Recommended titration (%)	Interferon beta-1b dose (mg)	Volume (mL)
Weeks 1 to 2	25	0.0625	0.25
Weeks 3 to 4	50	0.125	0.50

Interferon Beta-1b Schedule for Dose Titration			
	Recommended titration (%)	Interferon beta-1b dose (mg)	Volume (mL)
Weeks 5 to 6	75	0.1875	0.75
Weeks 7+	100	0.25	1

➤*Preparation of solution:* To reconstitute, attach the prefilled syringe containing the diluent to the interferon beta-1b vial using the vial adapter. Slowly inject 1.2 mL of diluent into the interferon beta-1b vial. Gently swirl the vial to dissolve the drug completely; do not shake. Foaming may occur during reconstitution or if the vial is swirled or shaken too vigorously. If foaming occurs, allow the vial to sit undisturbed until the foam settles. Keeping the syringe and vial adapter in place, turn the assembly over so that the vial is on top. Withdraw the appropriate dose of interferon beta-1b solution. Remove the vial from the vial adapter before injecting interferon beta-1b. One milliliter of reconstituted interferon beta-1b solution contains 0.25 mg interferon beta-1b.

➤*Storage / Stability:* The reconstituted product contains no preservatives. A vial is suitable for single use only; discard unused portions. Before reconstitution with diluent, store at room temperature 25°C (77°F), excursions permitted to 15° to 30°C (59° to 86°F). After reconstitution, if not used immediately, refrigerate the product and use within 3 hours. Avoid freezing.

ETANERCEPT

Rx	**Enbrel** (Amgen)	**Powder for Injection, lyophilized:** 25 mg	Preservative-free. 40 mg mannitol, 10 mg sucrose, 1.2 mg tromethamine. With syringe, needle, alcohol swabs, plunger, and diluent (1 mL sterile bacteriostatic water for injection contains 0.9% benzyl alcohol). Carton contains 4 dose trays. In multiple-use vials.

Indications

➤*Ankylosing spondylitis:* For reducing signs and symptoms in patients with active ankylosing spondylitis.

➤*Polyarticular-course juvenile rheumatoid arthritis (JRA):* For reducing signs and symptoms of moderately to severely active polyarticular-course JRA in patients who have had an inadequate response to 1 or more disease-modifying antirheumatic drugs (DMARD).

➤*Psoriatic arthritis:* For reducing signs and symptoms and inhibiting the progression of structural damage of active arthritis in patients with psoriatic arthritis. It can be used in combination with methotrexate in patients who do not respond adequately to methotrexate alone.

➤*Rheumatoid arthritis (RA):* For reduction in signs and symptoms, inhibiting the progression of structural damage, and improving physical function in moderately to severely active RA. It can be used in combination with methotrexate in patients who do not respond adequately to methotrexate alone.

➤*Unlabeled uses:* Treatment of Wegener granulomatosis (orphan drug status), psoriasis.

Administration and Dosage

➤*Approved by the FDA:* November 2, 1998.

➤*JRA (children 4 to 17 years of age):* 0.8 mg/kg/week (up to a maximum of 50 mg/week). The maximum dose that should be administered at a single injection site is 25 mg (1 mL). Therefore, for pediatric patients weighing more than 31 kg (68 lb), administer the total weekly dose as 2 SC injections either on the same day or 3 or 4 days apart. Administer the dose for pediatric patients weighing 31 kg (68 lb) or less as a single SC injection once weekly. Glucocorticoids, NSAIDs, or analgesics may be continued during treatment with etanercept. Concurrent use with methotrexate and higher doses of etanercept have not been studied in pediatric patients.

➤*RA, psoriatic arthritis, or ankylosing spondylitis (adults):* 50 mg/week given as two 25 mg SC injections at separate sites. Administer dose as two 25 mg injections given either on the same day or 3 or 4 days apart. Methotrexate, glucocorticoids, salicylates, nonsteroidal anti-inflammatory drugs (NSAIDs), or analgesics may be continued during treatment. Doses higher than 50 mg/week are not recommended.

➤*Preparation:* Reconstitute aseptically with 1 mL of the supplied sterile bacteriostatic water for injection (containing 0.9% benzyl alcohol) to yield a solution of 25 mg/mL etanercept. During reconstitution, inject the diluent slowly into the vial. Some foaming will occur; this is normal. To avoid excessive foaming, do not shake or vigorously agitate. Swirl the contents gently during dissolution. Generally, dissolution takes less than 10 minutes.

Withdraw the solution into the syringe, removing only the dose to be given from the vial. Some foam or bubbles may remain in the vial. Do not filter reconstituted solution during preparation or administration.

➤*Admixture incompatibilities:* Do not add other medications to solutions containing etanercept, and do not reconstitute with other diluents.

➤*Administration:* Etanercept is intended for use under the guidance and supervision of a physician. Patients may self-inject only if the physician determines that it is appropriate and if medical follow-up is provided, as necessary, after proper training in injection technique and how to measure the correct dose.

ETANERCEPT

Rotate injection sites (thigh, abdomen, or upper arm). Give new injections at least 1 inch from an old site and never into areas where the skin is tender, bruised, red, or hard.

➤*Storage / Stability:* Do not use a dose tray beyond the date stamped on the carton, dose tray label, vial label, or diluent syringe label. Store the dose tray containing etanercept (sterile powder) at 2° to 8°C (36° to 46°F). Do not freeze. Reconstituted solutions of etanercept prepared with the supplied bacteriostatic water for injection (0.9% benzyl alcohol) may be stored for up to 14 days if refrigerated at 2° to 8°C (36° to 46°F). Discard reconstituted solution after 14 days. Product stability and sterility cannot be assured after 14 days.

Actions

➤*Pharmacology:* Etanercept is a dimeric fusion protein consisting of the extracellular ligand-binding portion of the human 75 kd (p75) tumor necrosis factor receptor (TNFR) linked to the Fc portion of human IgG1. Etanercept binds specifically to tumor necrosis factor (TNF) and blocks its interaction with cell surface TNFRs. TNF is a naturally occurring cytokine that is involved in normal inflammatory and immune responses. It plays an important role in the inflammatory processes of RA, polyarticular-course JRA, and ankylosing spondylitis and the resulting joint pathology. Elevated levels of TNF are found in involved tissues and fluids of patients with RA, psoriatic arthritis, and ankylosing spondylitis.

Two distinct TNFRs, a 55 kd protein (p55) and a 75 kd protein (p75), exist naturally as monomeric molecules on cell surfaces and in soluble forms. Biological activity of TNF is dependent on binding to either cell surface TNFR.

Etanercept inhibits TNF activity in vitro and affects several animal models of inflammation, including murine collagen-induced arthritis. Etanercept inhibits binding of both TNFα and TNFβ (lymphotoxin alpha [LTα]) to cell surface TNFRs, rendering TNF biologically inactive. Cells expressing transmembrane TNF that bind etanercept are not lysed in vitro in the presence or absence of complement.

Etanercept also can modulate biological responses that are induced or regulated by TNF, including expression of adhesion molecules responsible for leukocyte migration, serum levels of cytokines (eg, IL-6), and serum levels of matrix metalloproteinase-3 (MMP-3 or stromelysin).

➤*Pharmacokinetics:*

Mean Pharmacokinetic Parameters for Etanercept in RA Patients (n = 25)				
	C_{max} (mcg/mL)	T_{max} (hr)	Clearance (mL/hr)	$t\frac{1}{2}$ (hr)
Single 25 mg SC injection	1.1	69	160	102

After 6 months of twice weekly 25 mg doses in these same RA patients, the mean C_{max} was approximately 2.4 mcg/mL (n = 23). Patients exhibited a 2- to 7-fold increase in peak serum concentrations and an approximate 4-fold increase in $AUC_{0-72 hr}$ (range, 1- to 17-fold) with repeated dosing. Serum concentration profiles at steady state appear comparable among patients with RA treated with 50 mg etanercept once weekly and those treated with 25 mg etanercept twice weekly. Serum concentrations in patients with RA have not been measured for periods of dosing that exceed 6 months.

Special populations –

Children: Pediatric patients 4 to 17 years of age with JRA were administered 0.4 mg/kg of etanercept twice weekly for up to 18 weeks. The mean serum concentration after repeated SC dosing was 2.1 mcg/mL (range, 0.7 to 4.3 mcg/mL). Limited data suggests that etanercept clearance is reduced slightly in children 4 to 8 years of age. Population analyses predict that administration of 0.8 mg/kg of etanercept once weekly will result in C_{max} 11% higher, and C_{min} 20% lower at steady state as compared with administration of 0.4 mg/kg of etanercept twice weekly.

➤*Clinical trials:* The efficacy of etanercept was compared with methotrexate in 424 patients with active RA. Patients were administered 25 mg etanercept SC twice a week or methotrexate 7.5 mg/week titrated to 20 mg/week for 12 months. Results are provided in the table below.

Response	ACR 20[1] (%)			ACR 50[2] (%)			ACR 70[3] (%)		
	Month 3	Month 6	Month 12	Month 3	Month 6	Month 12	Month 3	Month 6	Month 12
Etanercept (n = 207)	62	65	72	29	40	49	13[4]	21[4]	25
Methotrexate (n = 217)	56	58	65	24	32	43	7	14	22

[1] At least 20% improvement in the American College of Rheumatology response criteria.
[2] At least 50% improvement in the American College of Rheumatology response criteria.
[3] At least 70% improvement in the American College of Rheumatology response criteria.
[4] $P < 0.05$, etanercept vs methotrexate.

ACR response rates and improvement in all the individual ACR response criteria were maintained through 24 months of etanercept therapy.

In a 24-week study, 242 patients with active RA on methotrexate were randomized to receive either etanercept alone or etanercept and anakinra combination. The ACR 50 response rate was 31% for the combination and 41% for the etanercept alone group. Serious infections were increased in the combination etanercept-anakinra group vs the etanercept alone group.

Contraindications

Sepsis; hypersensitivity to etanercept or any of its components.

Warnings

➤*Serious infections:* In postmarketing reports, serious infections and sepsis, including fatalities, have been reported with the use of etanercept. Many of these serious infections have occurred in patients on concomitant immunosuppressive therapy that, in addition to their underlying disease, could predispose them to infections. Rare cases of tuberculosis (TB) have been observed in patients treated with TNF antagonists, including etanercept. Closely monitor patients who develop a new infection while undergoing treatment with etanercept. Discontinue administration of etanercept if a patient develops serious infection or sepsis. Do not initiate etanercept treatment in patients with active infections, including chronic or localized infections. Exercise caution when considering etanercept use in patients with a history of recurring infections or underlying conditions that may predispose them to infections (eg, advanced or poorly controlled diabetes; see Adverse Reactions).

In a 24-week study of concurrent etanercept and anakinra therapy, the rate of serious infections in the combination arm (7%) was higher than with etanercept alone (0%).

➤*Neurologic events:* Treatment with etanercept and other agents that inhibit TNF have been associated with rare cases of new onset or exacerbation of CNS demyelinating disorders, some presenting with mental status changes and some associated with permanent disability. Cases of transverse myelitis, optic neuritis, multiple sclerosis (MS), and new onset or exacerbation of seizure disorders have been observed in association with etanercept therapy. The causal relationship to etanercept therapy is unclear. However, while no clinical trials have been performed evaluating etanercept therapy in patients with MS, other TNF antagonists administered to patients with MS have been associated with increases in disease activity. Exercise caution in considering the use of etanercept in patients with preexisting or recent-onset CNS demyelinating disorders.

➤*Hematologic events:* Rare cases of pancytopenia including aplastic anemia, some fatal, have been reported in patients treated with etanercept. The causal relationship remains unclear. Although no high-risk group has been identified, exercise caution in patients being treated with etanercept who have a history of significant hematologic abnormalities. Advise all patients to seek immediate medical attention if they develop signs and symptoms suggestive of blood dyscrasias or infection (eg, persistent fever, bruising, bleeding, pallor) while on etanercept. If significant hematologic abnormalities are confirmed, consider discontinuation of etanercept therapy. Two percent of patients treated concurrently with etanercept and anakinra developed neutropenia (ANC less than 1×10^9/L). While neutropenic, 1 patient developed cellulitis which recovered with antibiotic therapy.

➤*Malignancies:* In the controlled portions of clinical trials of all the TNF-blocking agents, more cases of lymphoma have been observed among patients receiving the TNF blocker compared with control patients. During the controlled portions of etanercept trials, 1 lymphoma was observed among 2502 etanercept-treated patients vs 0 among 921 control patients (mean duration of controlled treatment approximately 6 months). In the controlled and open-label portions of clinical trials of etanercept in RA patients, 6 lymphomas were observed in 3389 patients over approximately 8000 patient-years of therapy. This is 2-fold higher than that expected in the general population. While patients with RA, particularly those with highly active disease, may be at a higher risk (up to several fold) for the development of lymphoma, the potential role of TNF-blocking therapy in the development of malignancies is not known.

Fifty-five malignancies other than lymphoma were observed. Of these, the most common malignancies were colon, breast, lung, and prostate, which were similar in type and number to what would be expected in the general population. Analysis of the cancer rates at 6-month intervals suggest constant rates over 3 years of observation.

➤*Heart failure:* There have been postmarketing reports of worsening of CHF, with and without identifiable precipitating factors, in patients taking etanercept. There also have been rare reports of new onset CHF, including CHF in patients without known preexisting cardiovascular disease. Some of these patients have been younger than 50 years of age. Exercise caution and monitor carefully when using etanercept in patients who also have heart failure.

➤*Hypersensitivity reactions:* Allergic reactions associated with etanercept during clinical trials have been reported in less than 2% of patients. Discontinue etanercept administration immediately and initiate appropriate therapy if an anaphylactic reaction or other serious allergic reaction occurs. Refer to Management of Acute Hypersensitivity Reactions.

ETANERCEPT

➤*Elderly:* A total of 197 RA patients 65 years of age or older have been studied in clinical trials. No overall differences in safety or effectiveness were observed between these patients and younger patients. However, because there is a higher incidence of infections in the elderly population in general, use caution in treating the elderly.

➤*Pregnancy: Category B.* There are no studies in pregnant women. Use during pregnancy only if clearly needed.

➤*Lactation:* It is not known whether etanercept is excreted in breast milk or absorbed systemically after ingestion. Because many drugs and immunoglobulins are excreted in breast milk and because of the potential for serious adverse reactions in nursing infants from etanercept, decide whether to discontinue breastfeeding or to discontinue the drug.

➤*Children:* Etanercept has not been studied in children younger than 4 years of age. Limited data suggest the clearance of etanercept is reduced slightly in children 4 to 8 years of age.

Precautions

➤*Immunogenicity:* Patients were tested at multiple timepoints for antibodies to etanercept. Antibodies, all nonneutralizing, were detected at least once in sera of less than 5% of adult RA, psoriatic arthritis, or ankylosing spondylitis patients. No apparent correlation of antibody development to clinical response or adverse events was observed. Results from the JRA patients were similar to those seen in adult RA patients treated with etanercept. The long-term immunogenicity of etanercept is unknown.

➤*Injection-site reactions:* In controlled trials, approximately 37% of patients developed injection site reactions. Reactions were mild to moderate (eg, erythema and/or itching, pain, swelling) and generally did not necessitate drug discontinuation. Injection site reactions generally occurred in the first month and subsequently decreased in frequency. The mean duration was 3 to 5 days; 7% experienced redness at a previous injection site when subsequent injections were given. In postmarketing experience, injection site bleeding and bruising also have been observed.

➤*Immunosuppression:* Anti-TNF therapies, including etanercept, affect host defenses against infections and malignancies (see Warnings) because TNF mediates inflammation and modulates cellular immune responses. In a study of 49 RA patients treated with etanercept, there was no evidence of depression of delayed-type hypersensitivity, depression of immunoglobulin levels, or change in enumeration of effector cell populations. The impact of treatment on the development and course of malignancies as well as active or chronic infections is not fully understood. Safety and efficacy in patients with immunosuppression or chronic infections have not been evaluated.

➤*Vaccinations:* Patients receiving etanercept may receive concurrent vaccinations, except for live vaccines. No data are available in patients receiving etanercept on the effects of vaccination or on the secondary transmission of infection by live vaccines.

It is recommended that JRA patients, if possible, be brought up to date with all immunizations in agreement with current immunization guidelines prior to initiating therapy. Two JRA patients developed varicella infection and signs and symptoms of aseptic meningitis, which resolved without sequelae. Patients with a significant exposure to varicella virus should temporarily discontinue etanercept and be considered for prophylactic treatment with varicella zoster immune globulin.

➤*Autoantibodies:* Treatment with etanercept may result in the formation of autoimmune antibodies, and, rarely, in the development of a lupus-like syndrome which may resolve following withdrawal of etanercept. If a patient develops symptoms and findings suggestive of a lupus-like syndrome following treatment with etanercept, discontinue treatment and carefully evaluate the patient. Patients had serum samples tested for autoantibodies at multiple timepoints. In studies 1 and 2, the percentage of patients who developed new positive ANA (greater than or equal to 1:40) was higher in etanercept-treated patients (11%) than in placebo-treated patients (5%). The percentage of patients who developed new positive anti-double stranded DNA antibodies was also higher by radioimmunoassay (15% etanercept vs 4% placebo) and by *Crithidia luciliae* assay (3% etanercept vs 0% placebo). The proportion of patients treated with etanercept who developed anticardiolipin antibodies was similarly increased compared with placebo-treated patients. In study 3, no pattern of increased autoantibody development was seen in etanercept patients compared with methotrexate patients. The impact of long-term treatment with etanercept on the development of autoimmune diseases is unknown. Rare adverse event reports have described patients with rheumatoid factor positive and/or erosive RA who have developed additional autoantibodies in conjunction with rash and other features suggesting a lupus-like syndrome.

➤*Benzyl alcohol:* Benzyl alcohol, a preservative contained in the diluent supplied, has been associated with a fatal "gasping syndrome" in premature infants.

Adverse Reactions

➤*RA/Psoriatic arthritis/Ankylosing spondylitis:* The following adverse events were reported in patients treated with etanercept compared with controls in placebo-controlled RA trials (including the combination methotrexate trial) and relevant events. Adverse events in the psoriatic arthritis and ankylosing spondylitis trials were similar to those reported in RA clinical trials.

Etanercept Adverse Reactions in RA Patients (%)[1]

Adverse reaction	Placebo-controlled		Active-controlled	
	Etanercept (n = 349)	Placebo (n = 152)[2]	Etanercept (n = 415)	Methotrexate (n = 217)
CNS				
Dizziness	7	5	8	11
Headache	17	13	24	27
Dermatologic				
Alopecia	1	1	6	12
Rash	5	3	14	23
GI				
Abdominal pain	5	3	10	10
Dyspepsia	4	1	11	10
Mouth ulcer	2	1	6	14
Nausea	9	10	15	29
Vomiting	3	-	5	8
Respiratory				
Cough	6	3	5	6
Pharyngitis	7	5	6	9
Respiratory disorder	5	1	N/A	N/A
Rhinitis	12	8	16	14
Sinusitis	3	2	5	3
Miscellaneous				
Asthenia	5	3	11	12
Infection	35	32	64	72
Injection site reaction	37	10	34	7
Non-upper respiratory tract infection[3]	38	32	51	60
Peripheral edema	2	3	8	4
Upper respiratory tract infection[3]	29	16	31	39

[1] Includes data from the 6-month study in which patients received concurrent methotrexate therapy.
[2] Duration of exposure for patients receiving placebo was less than the etanercept-treated patients.
[3] Includes data from 2 of the 3 placebo-controlled trials.

The following serious adverse events were observed in the etanercept 50 mg twice weekly arm: GI bleeding, normal pressure hydrocephalus, seizure, and stroke. No serious adverse events were observed in the 25 mg arm.

In controlled trials of RA and psoriatic arthritis, rates of serious adverse events were seen at a frequency of approximately 5% among etanercept- and control-treated patients. Among RA patients in placebo-controlled, active-controlled, and open-label trials of etanercept, malignancies and infections (see Warnings) were the most common serious adverse events observed.

Cardiovascular – Deep vein thrombosis; heart failure; hypertension; hypotension; MI; myocardial ischemia; thrombophlebitis.

CNS – Cerebral ischemia; depression; MS.

GI – Cholecystitis; GI hemorrhage; pancreatitis.

GU – Membranous glomerulonephropathy.

Musculoskeletal – Bursitis; polymyositis.

Respiratory – Dyspnea; pulmonary embolism.

Miscellaneous – Injection-site reactions (see Precautions); malignancies (see Warnings).

Infection: In controlled trials, there were no differences in rates of infection among RA, psoriatic arthritis, and ankylosing spondylitis patients treated with etanercept and those treated with placebo or methotrexate. The most common type of infection was upper respiratory tract infection, which occurred in approximately 20% among etanercept- and placebo-treated patients.

In placebo-controlled trials in RA, psoriatic arthritis, and ankylosing spondylitis, no increase in the incidence of serious infections was observed (approximately 1% in placebo- and etanercept-treated groups). In all RA clinical trials, serious infections experienced by patients have included: abdominal abscess, bronchitis, cellulitis, diar-

ETANERCEPT

rhea, foot abscess, leg ulcer, osteomyelitis, pneumonia, pyelonephritis, sepsis, septic arthritis, sinusitis, and wound infection. Serious infections, including sepsis and death, also have been reported during postmarketing etanercept use. Some have occurred within a few weeks after treatment initiation with etanercept. Many of the patients had underlying conditions (eg, diabetes, CHF, history of active or chronic infections) in addition to RA (see Warnings). In a clinical trial not specifically in RA patients, data suggest that etanercept treatment may increase mortality in patients with established sepsis.

In patients who received both etanercept and anakinra for up to 24 weeks, the incidence of serious infections was 7%. The most common infections consisted of bacterial pneumonia (4 cases) and cellulitis (4 cases). One patient with pulmonary fibrosis and pneumonia died because of respiratory failure.

In postmarketing experience, infections have been observed with various pathogens including viral, bacterial, fungal, and protozoal organisms. Infections have been noted in all organ systems and have been reported in patients receiving etanercept alone or in combination with immunosuppressive agents.

➤*JRA:* Adverse events in children were similar in frequency and type as those in adults. Differences from adults and other special considerations are discussed below.

Etanercept Adverse Reactions in Patients with JRA (%)	
Adverse reaction	Etanercept (n = 69)
GI	
Abdominal pain	19[1]
Nausea	9[2]
Vomiting	13[1]
Miscellaneous	
Headache	19[3]
Infection	62

[1] 0.74 events/patient year.
[2] 1 event/patient year.
[3] 1.7 events/patient year.

Severe adverse reactions reported in 69 JRA patients 4 to 17 years of age included cutaneous ulcer, depression/personality disorder, esophagitis/gastritis, gastroenteritis, group A streptococcal septic shock, soft tissue and postoperative wound infection, type I diabetes mellitus, and varicella (see Precautions).

Infection – Of 69 children with JRA, 43 (62%) experienced an infection while receiving etanercept during 3 months of study, and the frequency and severity of infections were similar in 58 patients completing 12 months of open-label extension therapy. The types of infections reported in JRA patients were generally mild and consistent with those commonly seen in outpatient pediatric populations. Two JRA patients developed varicella infection and signs and symptoms of aseptic meningitis which resolved without sequelae.

Postmarketing – Abscess with bacteremia, coagulopathy, cutaneous vasculitis, optic neuritis, pancytopenia, seizures, tuberculous arthritis, transaminase elevations, and urinary tract infection.

➤*Postmarketing:*

Cardiovascular – Chest pain; new onset of CHF; vasodilation (flushing).

CNS – Fatigue; paresthesias, seizures, stroke, and CNS events suggestive of MS or isolated demyelinating conditions such as transverse myelitis or optic neuritis (see Warnings).

Dermatologic – Cutaneous vasculitis; pruritus; SC nodules; urticaria.

GI – Altered sense of taste; anorexia; diarrhea; dry mouth; intestinal perforation.

Hematologic / Lymphatic – Adenopathy; anemia; aplastic anemia; leukopenia; neutropenia (see Warnings); pancytopenia; thrombocytopenia.

Musculoskeletal – Joint pain; lupus-like syndrome with manifestations including rash consistent with subacute or discoid lupus.

Ophthalmic – Dry eyes; ocular inflammation.

Respiratory – Dyspnea; interstitial lung disease; pulmonary disease; worsening of prior lung disorder.

Miscellaneous – Angioedema; fever; flu syndrome; generalized pain; weight gain.

Overdosage

The maximum tolerated dose of etanercept has not been established in humans. Toxicology studies have been performed in monkeys at doses up to 30 times the human dose with no evidence of dose-limiting toxicities. No dose-limiting toxicities have been observed during clinical trials. Single IV doses up to 60 mg/m^2 have been administered to healthy volunteers in an endotoxemia study without evidence of dose-limiting toxicities.

Patient Information

If the patient or caregiver is to administer etanercept, instruct him or her in injection techniques and how to measure the correct dose to ensure proper administration of etanercept. Have the patient/caregiver perform the first injection under the supervision of a qualified health care professional. Assess the ability of the patient's or caregiver's ability to inject SC. Instruct patients and caregivers in the technique and proper syringe and needle disposal. Caution against the reuse of these items. Use a puncture-resistant container for disposal of needles and syringes.

ANAKINRA

Rx	Kineret (Amgen)	Injection: 100 mg/0.67 mL	Preservative-free. Sodium chloride, EDTA. In 1 mL single-use prefilled syringe with 27-gauge needle.

Indications

➤*Rheumatoid arthritis (RA):* For the reduction in signs and symptoms of moderately to severely active RA in patients 18 years of age and older who have failed 1 or more disease-modifying antirheumatic drugs (DMARDs). Anakinra can be used alone or in combination with DMARDs other than tumor necrosis factor (TNF)-blocking agents.

Administration and Dosage

➤*Approved by the FDA:* November 14, 2001.

The recommended dose of anakinra is 100 mg/day administered daily by SC injection. Higher doses did not result in a higher response. Administer the dose at approximately the same time every day.

➤*Storage / Stability:* Do not use anakinra beyond the expiration date shown on the carton. Store anakinra in the refrigerator at 2° to 8°C (36° to 46°F). Do not freeze or shake. Protect from light.

Do not use the prefilled syringe if particulates or discoloration are observed. Discard any unused portions; anakinra is preservative free.

Actions

➤*Pharmacology:* Anakinra is a recombinant, nonglycosylated form of the human interleukin-1 receptor antagonist (IL-1Ra). Anakinra differs from native human IL-1Ra in that it has the addition of a single methionine residue at its amino terminus. Anakinra consists of 153 amino acids and has a molecular weight of 17.3 kilodaltons. It is produced by recombinant DNA technology using an *Escherichia coli* bacterial expression system.

Anakinra blocks the biologic activity of IL-1 by competitively inhibiting IL-1 binding to the interleukin-1 type I receptor (IL-1RI), which is expressed in a wide variety of tissues and organs.

IL-1 production is induced in response to inflammatory stimuli and mediates various physiologic responses including inflammatory and immunological responses. IL-1 has a broad range of activities, including cartilage degradation by its induction of the rapid loss of proteoglycans and stimulation of bone resorption. The levels of the naturally occurring IL-1Ra in synovium and synovial fluid from RA patients are not sufficient to compete with the elevated amount of locally produced IL-1.

➤*Pharmacokinetics:* The absolute bioavailability of anakinra after a 70 mg SC bolus injection in healthy subjects (n = 11) is 95%. In subjects with RA, maximum plasma concentrations of anakinra occurred 3 to 7 hours after SC administration of anakinra at clinically relevant doses (1 to 2 mg/kg; n = 18); the terminal half-life ranged from 4 to 6 hours. In RA patients, no unexpected accumulation of anakinra was observed after daily SC doses for up to 24 weeks. The estimated anakinra clearance increased with increasing Ccr and body weight.

Special populations –

Renal function impairment: The mean plasma clearance of anakinra decreased 70% to 75% in normal subjects with severe or end-stage renal disease (defined as Ccr less than 30 mL/min, as estimated from serum creatinine levels). No formal studies have been conducted examining the pharmacokinetics of anakinra administered SC in RA patients with renal impairment.

Contraindications

Known hypersensitivity to *E. coli*-derived proteins, anakinra, or any component of the product.

Warnings

➤*Infections:* Anakinra has been associated with an increased incidence of serious infections (2%) vs placebo (less than 1%). Discontinue administration of anakinra if a patient develops a serious infection. Do not initiate treatment with anakinra in patients with active infections. The safety and efficacy of anakinra in immunocompromised patients or in patients with chronic infections have not been evaluated. In a 24-week study of concurrent etanercept and anakinra therapy, the rate of serious infections in the combination arm (7%) was higher than with etanercept alone (0%). The combination of anakinra and etanercept did not result in higher ACR response rates compared to etanercept alone.

ANAKINRA

Coadministration of anakinra and etanercept has not demonstrated increased clinical benefit. Carefully monitor patients when considering initiation of anakinra therapy concurrently with etanercept therapy.

➤*Immunosuppression:* The impact of treatment with anakinra on active and/or chronic infections and the development of malignancies is unknown.

➤*Vaccinations:* No data are available on the effects of vaccination in patients receiving anakinra. Do not give live vaccines concurrently with anakinra. No data are available on the secondary transmission of infections by live vaccines in patients receiving anakinra. Because anakinra interferes with normal immune response mechanisms to new antigens such as vaccines, vaccination may not be effective in patients receiving anakinra.

➤*Hematologic events:* Patients receiving anakinra may experience a decrease in neutrophil counts. In the placebo-controlled studies, 8% of patients receiving anakinra had decreases in neutrophil counts of at least 1 World Health Organization (WHO) toxicity grade compared with 2% in the placebo control group. Nine anakinra-treated patients (0.4%) experienced neutropenia (ANC less than 1×10^9/L).

➤*Hypersensitivity reactions:* Hypersensitivity reactions associated with anakinra administration are rare. If a severe hypersensitivity reaction occurs, discontinue anakinra administration and initiate appropriate therapy.

➤*Renal function impairment:* This drug is known to be substantially excreted by the kidney; the risk of toxic reactions to this drug may be greater in patients with impaired renal function.

➤*Elderly:* Greater sensitivity of some older individuals cannot be ruled out. Because there is a higher incidence of infections in the elderly population in general, use caution in treating the elderly.

➤*Pregnancy: Category B.* Reproductive studies have been conducted with anakinra on rats and rabbits at doses up to 100 times the human dose and have revealed no evidence of impaired fertility or harm to the fetus. However, there are no adequate and well-controlled studies in pregnant women. Because animal reproduction studies are not always predictive of human response, use anakinra during pregnancy only if clearly needed.

➤*Lactation:* It is not known whether anakinra is secreted in human milk. Because many drugs are secreted in human milk, exercise caution if anakinra is administered to nursing women.

➤*Children:* The safety and efficacy of anakinra in patients with juvenile RA have not been established.

Precautions

➤*Monitoring:* Assess neutrophil counts prior to initiating anakinra treatment, while receiving anakinra monthly for 3 months, and quarterly for a period up to 1 year thereafter.

➤*Immunogenicity:* In 2 studies, 26% of patients tested positive for anti-anakinra antibodies at month 12 in a highly sensitive, anakinra-binding biosensor assay. Of the 1318 subjects with available data at week 12 or later, 1% were seropositive in a cell-based bioassay for antibodies capable of neutralizing the biologic effects of anakinra. Two of the 15 of these subjects were positive for neutralizing antibodies at more than 1 time point up to the week 52 visit and 4 were positive at week 52. No correlation between antibody development, clinical response, or adverse events was observed. The long-term immunogenicity of anakinra is unknown.

Adverse Reactions

Anakinra Adverse Reactions Occurring in ≥ 5% of RA Patients (%)		
Adverse reaction	Anakinra 100 mg/day (n = 1565)	Placebo (n = 733)
Injection-site reaction	71	29
Worsening of RA	19	29
Upper respiratory tract infection	14	17
Headache	12	9
Nausea	8	7
Diarrhea	7	5

Anakinra Adverse Reactions Occurring in ≥ 5% of RA Patients (%)		
Adverse reaction	Anakinra 100 mg/day (n = 1565)	Placebo (n = 733)
Sinusitis	7	7
Arthralgia	6	6
Influenza-like symptoms	6	6
Pain, abdominal	5	5

The most serious adverse reactions were serious infection and neutropenia, particularly when used in combination with TNF-blocking agents. The most common adverse reaction with anakinra is injection-site reactions (ISRs). These reactions were the most common reason for withdrawing from studies.

➤*Infections:* In 2 combined studies, the incidence of infection was 39% in the anakinra-treated patients and 37% in placebo-treated patients. The incidence of serious infections was 2% in anakinra-treated patients and 1% in placebo-treated patients over 6 months. The incidence of serious infection over 1 year was 3% in anakinra-treated patients and 2% in patients receiving placebo. These infections consisted primarily of bacterial events such as cellulitis, pneumonia, and bone and joint infections, rather than unusual, opportunistic, fungal, or viral infections. Patients with asthma appeared to be at higher risk of developing serious infections; anakinra 4% vs placebo 0%. Most patients continued on study drug after the infection resolved. There were no on-study deaths caused by serious infectious episodes in either study.

In 2 studies in which patients were receiving etanercept and anakinra for up to 24 weeks, the incidence of serious infections was 7%. The common infections consisted of bacterial pneumonia (4 cases) and cellulitis (4 cases). One patient with pulmonary fibrosis and pneumonia died because of respiratory failure.

➤*Hematologic:* In placebo-controlled studies with anakinra, treatment was associated with small reductions in the mean values for total white blood count, platelets, and ANC, and a small increase in the mean eosinophil differential percentage.

In all placebo-controlled studies, 8% of patients receiving anakinra had decreases in ANC of at least 1 WHO toxicity grade, compared with 2% of placebo patients. Nine anakinra-treated patients (0.4%) developed neutropenia (ANC less than 1×10^9/L). Additional patients treated with anakinra plus etanercept (2%) developed ANC less than 1×10^9/L. One neutropenic patient developed cellulitis and recovered with antibiotic therapy.

➤*Malignancies:* Twenty-three malignancies of various types were observed in 2730 RA patients treated in clinical trials with anakinra for up to 60 months. The observed rates and incidences were similar to those expected for the population studied.

➤*Injection-site reaction:* The most common and consistently reported treatment-related adverse event associated with anakinra is an ISR. The majority of ISRs were reported as mild. These typically lasted for 14 to 28 days and were characterized by: Erythema, ecchymosis, inflammation, and/or pain. In 2 studies, 71% of patients developed an ISR, which was typically reported within the first 4 weeks of therapy. The development of ISRs in patients who had not previously experienced ISRs was uncommon after the first month of therapy.

Overdosage

There have been no cases of overdose reported with anakinra in clinical trials of RA. In sepsis trials, no serious toxicities attributed to anakinra were seen when administered at mean calculated doses of up to 35 times those given to patients with RA over a 72-hour treatment period.

Patient Information

Instruct patients and their caregivers on the proper dosage and administration of anakinra. Provide all patients with the "Information for Patients and Caregivers" insert.

Inform patients of the signs and symptoms of allergic and other adverse drug reactions, and advise patients on appropriate actions. Thoroughly instruct patients and their caregivers on the importance of proper disposal and caution against the reuse of needles, syringes, and drug product. Have a puncture-resistance container available for the patient for the disposal of used syringes.

ADALIMUMAB

Rx **Humira** (Abbott)   **Injection:** 40 mg/0.8 mL   Preservative free. In 2 mL vials. With syringe and alcohol preps.

WARNING

Risk of infections: Cases of tuberculosis (frequently disseminated or extrapulmonary at clinical presentation) have been observed in patients receiving adalimumab.

Evaluate patients for latent tuberculosis infection with a tuberculin skin test. Initiate treatment of latent tuberculosis infection prior to therapy with adalimumab.

Indications

➤*Rheumatoid arthritis (RA):* For reducing signs and symptoms and inhibiting the progression of structural damage in adult patients with moderately to severely active RA who have had an inadequate response to one or more disease-modifying antirheumatic drugs (DMARDs). Adalimumab can be used alone or in combination with methotrexate (MTX) or other DMARDs.

Administration and Dosage

➤*Approved by the FDA:* December 31, 2002.

➤*Dose:* The recommended dose for adult patients with RA is 40 mg administered every other week as an SC injection. MTX, glucocorticoids, salicylates, nonsteroidal anti-inflammatory drugs (NSAIDs), analgesics, or other DMARDs may be continued during treatment with adalimumab. Some patients not taking concomitant MTX may derive additional benefit from increasing the dosing frequency of adalimumab to 40 mg every week.

➤*Self-administration:* Patients may self-inject adalimumab if their physician determines that it is appropriate and with medical follow-up, as necessary, after proper training in injection technique.

Rotate injection sites and never give injections into areas where the skin is tender, bruised, red, or hard.

➤*Storage/Stability:* Adalimumab does not contain preservatives; therefore, discard unused portions of drug remaining from the syringe or vial. Do not use beyond the expiration date on the container. Adalimumab must be refrigerated at 2° to 8°C (36° to 46°F). Do not freeze. Protect the vial and/or prefilled syringe from exposure to light. Store in original carton until time of administration.

Actions

➤*Pharmacology:* Adalimumab is a recombinant human IgG1 monoclonal antibody specific for human tumor necrosis factor (TNF). It binds specifically to TNF-alpha and blocks its interaction with the p55 and p75 cell surface TNF receptors. Adalimumab also lyses surface TNF expressing cells in vitro in the presence of complement. Adalimumab does not bind or inactivate lymphotoxin (TNF-beta). TNF is a naturally occurring cytokine that is involved in normal inflammatory and immune responses. Elevated levels of TNF are found in the synovial fluid of RA patients and play an important role in both the pathologic inflammation and the joint destruction that are hallmarks of RA.

Adalimumab also modulates biological responses that are induced or regulated by TNF, including changes in the levels of adhesion molecules responsible for leukocyte migration.

After treatment with adalimumab, a rapid decrease in levels of acute phase reactants of inflammation (C-reactive protein [CRP] and erythrocyte sedimentation rate [ESR]) and serum cytokines (IL-6) was observed compared with baseline in patients with RA. Serum levels of matrix metalloproteinases (MMP-1 and MMP-3) that produce tissue remodeling responsible for cartilage destruction were also decreased after adalimumab administration.

➤*Pharmacokinetics:*

Absorption/Distribution – The maximum serum concentration (C_{max}) and the time to reach maximum concentration (T_{max}) were approximately 4.7 mcg/mL and approximately 131 hours, respectively, following a single 40 mg SC dose of adalimumab to healthy adult subjects. The average absolute bioavailability of adalimumab estimated from 3 studies following a single 40 mg SC dose was 64%. The pharmacokinetics of adalimumab were linear over the dose range of 0.5 to 10 mg/kg following a single IV dose. Adalimumab mean steady-state trough concentrations of approximately 5 mcg/mL and 8 to 9 mcg/mL were observed with and without MTX, respectively. The serum adalimumab trough levels at steady state increased approximately proportionally with dose following 20, 40, and 80 mg every other week and every week SC dosing.

The single-dose pharmacokinetics of adalimumab were determined in several studies with IV doses ranging from 0.25 to 10 mg/kg. The distribution volume (V_{ss}) ranged from 4.7 to 6 L. Adalimumab concentrations in the synovial fluid from 5 RA patients ranged from 31% to 96% of those in serum.

Excretion – The systemic clearance of adalimumab is approximately 12 mL/h. The mean terminal half-life was approximately 2 weeks, ranging from 10 to 20 days across studies. In long-term studies with dosing more than 2 years, there was no evidence of changes in clearance over time.

Contraindications

Hypersensitivity to adalimumab or any of its components.

Warnings

➤*Infections:* Serious infections and sepsis, including fatalities, have been reported with the use of TNF blocking agents including adalimumab. Many of the serious infections have occurred in patients on concomitant immunosuppressive therapy that, in addition to their RA, could predispose them to infections. Tuberculosis and invasive opportunistic fungal infections have been observed in patients treated with TNF blocking agents, including adalimumab.

Do not initiate treatment with adalimumab in patients with active infections including chronic or localized infections. Closely monitor patients who develop a new infection while undergoing treatment with adalimumab. Discontinue adalimumab administration if a patient develops a serious infection. Physicians should exercise caution when considering the use of adalimumab in patients with a history of recurrent infection or underlying conditions that may predispose them to infections, or patients who have resided in regions where tuberculosis and histoplasmosis are endemic. Carefully consider the benefits and risks of adalimumab before initiation of therapy.

➤*Neurologic events:* Use of TNF blocking agents, including adalimumab, has been associated with rare cases of exacerbation of clinical symptoms and/or radiographic evidence of demyelinating disease. Exercise caution in considering the use of adalimumab in patients with pre-existing or recent-onset CNS demyelinating disorders.

➤*Malignancies:* Lymphomas have been observed in patients treated with TNF blocking agents including adalimumab. In clinical trials, patients treated with adalimumab had a higher incidence of lymphoma than the expected rate in the general population. While patients with RA, particularly those with highly active disease, may be at a higher risk (up to several fold) for the development of lymphoma, the role of TNF blockers in the development of malignancy is not known.

➤*Hypersensitivity reactions:* Allergic reactions have been observed in approximately 1% of patients receiving adalimumab. If an anaphylactic reaction or other serious allergic reaction occurs, immediately discontinue administration of adalimumab and initiate appropriate therapy.

➤*Elderly:* The frequency of serious infection and malignancy among adalimumab-treated subjects over 65 years of age was higher than for those under 65 years of age. Because there is a higher incidence of infections and malignancies in the elderly population in general, use caution when treating the elderly.

➤*Pregnancy: Category B.* An embryo-fetal perinatal developmental toxicity study has been performed in cynomolgus monkeys at dosages up to 100 mg/kg (266 times human AUC when given 40 mg SC with MTX every week or 373 times human AUC when given 40 mg SC without MTX) and has revealed no evidence of harm to the fetuses caused by adalimumab. There are, however, no adequate and well-controlled studies in pregnant women. Because animal reproduction and developmental studies are not always predictive of human response, use adalimumab during pregnancy only if clearly needed.

➤*Lactation:* It is not known whether adalimumab is excreted in human milk or absorbed systemically after ingestion. Because many drugs and immunoglobulins are excreted in human milk, and because of the potential for serious adverse reactions in nursing infants from adalimumab, decide whether to discontinue nursing or discontinue the drug, taking into account the importance of the drug to the mother.

➤*Children:* Safety and efficacy of adalimumab in pediatric patients have not been established.

Precautions

➤*Latex allergy:* The needle cover of the syringe contains dry rubber (latex), which should not be handled by people sensitive to this substance.

➤*Tuberculosis:* As observed with other TNF blocking agents, tuberculosis associated with the administration of adalimumab in clinical trials has been reported. While cases were observed at all doses, the incidence of tuberculosis reactivation was particularly increased at doses of adalimumab that were higher than the recommended dose. All patients recovered after standard antimicrobial therapy. No deaths caused by tuberculosis occurred during the clinical trials.

Before initiation of therapy with adalimumab, evaluate patients for active or latent tuberculosis infection with a tuberculin skin test. If latent infection is diagnosed, institute appropriate prophylaxis in accordance with the Centers for Disease Control and Prevention guidelines. Instruct patients to seek medical advice if signs/symptoms (eg, persistent cough, wasting/weight loss, low grade fever) suggestive of a tuberculosis infection occur.

ADALIMUMAB

▶*Immunosuppression:* The possibility exists for TNF blocking agents, including adalimumab, to affect host defenses against infections and malignancies since TNF mediates inflammation and modulates cellular immune responses. In a study of 64 patients with RA treated with adalimumab, there was no evidence of depression of delayed-type hypersensitivity, depression of immunoglobulin levels, or change in enumeration of effector T- and B-cells and NK-cells, monocyte/macrophages, and neutrophils. The impact of treatment with adalimumab on the development and course of malignancies, as well as active and/or chronic infections is not fully understood. The safety and efficacy of adalimumab in patients with immunosuppression have not been evaluated.

▶*Vaccinations:* No data are available on the effects of vaccination in patients receiving adalimumab. Live vaccines should not be given concurrently with adalimumab. No data are available on the secondary transmission of infection by live vaccines in patients receiving adalimumab.

▶*Immunogenicity:* Treatment with adalimumab may result in the formation of autoantibodies and, rarely, in the development of a lupus-like syndrome. If a patient develops symptoms suggestive of a lupus-like syndrome following treatment with adalimumab, discontinue treatment (see Adverse Reactions).

Drug Interactions

▶*Methotrexate:* MTX reduced adalimumab apparent clearance after single and multiple dosing by 29% and 44%, respectively. The data do not suggest the need for dose adjustment of adalimumab or MTX.

Adverse Reactions

The most serious adverse reactions were serious infections, neurologic events, and malignancies. The most common adverse reaction with adalimumab was injection site reactions. In placebo-controlled trials, 20% of patients treated with adalimumab developed injection site reactions (erythema and/or itching, hemorrhage, pain, or swelling), compared with 14% of patients receiving placebo. Most injection site reactions were described as mild and generally did not necessitate drug discontinuation.

The proportion of patients who discontinued treatment because of adverse events was 7% for patients taking adalimumab and 4% for placebo-treated patients. The most common adverse events leading to discontinuation of adalimumab were clinical flare reaction (0.7%), rash (0.3%), and pneumonia (0.3%).

▶*Infections:* In placebo-controlled trials, the rate of infection was 1 per patient-year in the adalimumab-treated patients and 0.9 per patient-year in the placebo-treated patients. The infections consisted primarily of upper respiratory tract infections, bronchitis, and urinary tract infections. Most patients continued on adalimumab after the infection resolved. The incidence of serious infections was 0.04 per patient year in adalimumab-treated patients and 0.02 per patient year in placebo-treated patients. Serious infections observed included pneumonia, septic arthritis, prosthetic and postsurgical infections, erysipelas, cellulitis, diverticulitis, and pyelonephritis.

Thirteen cases of tuberculosis, including miliary, lymphatic, peritoneal, and pulmonary were reported in clinical trials. Most of the cases of tuberculosis occurred within the first 8 months after initiation of therapy and may reflect recrudescence of latent disease. Six cases of invasive opportunistic infections caused by histoplasma, aspergillus, and nocardia were also reported in clinical trials (see Warnings).

▶*Malignancies:* Among 2468 RA patients treated in clinical trials with adalimumab for a median of 24 months, 48 malignancies of various types were observed, including 10 patients with lymphoma. The other malignancies observed during use of adalimumab were breast, colon-rectum, uterine-cervical, prostate, melanoma, gallbladder-bile ducts, and other carcinomas.

▶*Immunogenicity:* In the controlled trials, 12% of patients treated with adalimumab and 7% of placebo-treated patients that had negative baseline ANA titers developed positive titers at week 24. One patient out of 2334 treated with adalimumab developed clinical signs suggestive of new-onset lupus-like syndrome. The patient improved following discontinuation of therapy.

Patients in clinical studies were tested at multiple time points for antibodies to adalimumab during the 6 to 12 month period. Approximately 5% of adult RA patients receiving adalimumab developed low-titer antibodies to adalimumab at least once during treatment, which were neutralizing in vitro. Patients treated with concomitant MTX had a lower rate of antibody development than patients on adalimumab monotherapy (1% vs 12%). No apparent correlation of antibody development to adverse events was observed. With monotherapy, patients receiving every other week dosing may develop antibodies more frequently than those receiving weekly dosing. In patients receiving the recommended dosage of 40 mg every other week as monotherapy, the ACR 20 response was lower among antibody-positive patients than among antibody-negative patients. The long-term immunogenicity of adalimumab is unknown.

▶*Other adverse reactions:*

Adalimumab Adverse Reactions in RA Patients (%)		
Adverse reaction	Adalimumab 40 mg SC every other week (N = 705)	Placebo (N = 690)
GI		
Nausea	9	8
Abdominal pain	7	4
Respiratory		
Upper respiratory infection	17	13
Sinusitis	11	9
Flu syndrome	7	6
Miscellaneous		
Injection site pain	12	12
Headache	12	8
Rash	12	6
Accidental injury	10	8
Injection site reaction[1]	8	1
Back pain	6	4
Urinary tract infection	8	5
Hypertension	5	3
Lab test abnormalities[2]		
Lab test abnormal	8	7
Hypercholesterolemia	6	4
Hyperlipidemia	7	5
Hematuria	5	4
Alkaline phosphatase increased	5	3

[1] Does not include erythema and/or itching, hemorrhage, pain, or swelling.
[2] Lab test abnormalities were reported as adverse events in European trials.

Other infrequent serious adverse events occurring at an incidence of less than 5% in patients treated with adalimumab were the following:

Cardiovascular – Arrhythmia, atrial fibrillation, cardiovascular disorder, chest pain, CHF, coronary artery disorder, heart arrest, hypertensive encephalopathy, MI, palpitation, pericardial effusion, pericarditis, syncope, tachycardia, vascular disorder.

CNS – Confusion; multiple sclerosis; paresthesia; subdural hematoma; tremor.

Dermatologic – Cellulitis; erysipelas; herpes zoster.

GI – Cholecystitis; cholelithiasis; esophagitis; gastroenteritis; GI disorder; GI hemorrhage; hepatic necrosis; vomiting.

GU – Cystitis; kidney calculus; menstrual disorder; pyelonephritis.

Hematologic/Lymphatic – Agranulocytosis; granulocytopenia; leukopenia; lymphoma-like reaction; pancytopenia; polycythemia.

Metabolic/Nutritional – Dehydration; healing abnormal; ketosis; paraproteinemia; peripheral edema.

Musculoskeletal – Arthritis; bone disorder; bone fracture (not spontaneous); bone necrosis; joint disorder; muscle cramps; myasthenia; pyogenic arthritis; synovitis; tendon disorder.

Respiratory – Asthma; bronchospasm; dyspnea; lung disorder; lung function decreased; pleural effusion; pneumonia.

Miscellaneous – Fever; infection; pain in extremity; pelvic pain; sepsis; surgery; thorax pain; tuberculosis reactivated; lupus erythematosus syndrome; parathyroid disorder; adenoma, carcinomas such as breast, GI, skin, GU, and others; lymphoma; melanoma; cataract; leg thrombosis.

Overdosage

The maximum tolerated dose of adalimumab has not been established in humans. Multiple doses up to 10 mg/kg have been administered to patients in clinical trials without evidence of dose-limiting toxicities. In case of overdosage, it is recommended that the patient be monitored for any signs or symptoms of adverse reactions or effects and appropriate symptomatic treatment instituted immediately.

Patient Information

Perform the first injection under the supervision of a qualified health care professional. If patients or caregivers are to administer adalimumab, instruct them in injection techniques and assess their ability to inject SC to ensure the proper administration of adalimumab. A puncture-resistant container for disposal of needles and syringes should be used. Instruct patients or caregivers in the technique as well as proper syringe and needle disposal and caution them against reuse of these items.

There have been rare cases where patients taking adalimumab or other TNF-blocking agents have developed serious infections, including tuberculosis and infections caused by bacteria or fungi.

There have been rare cases of disorders that affect the nervous system of people taking adalimumab or other TNF blockers. Signs of a problem include the following: Numbness or tingling, vision problems, weakness in the legs, dizziness.

ADALIMUMAB

There have been very rare cases of certain kinds of cancer in patients taking adalimumab or other TNF blockers. People with more serious RA that have had the disease for a long time may have a higher-than-average risk of getting lymphoma, a cancer that affects the lymph system. Taking adalimumab or other TNF blockers may increase this risk.

Some patients have developed lupus-like symptoms that became better after their treatment was stopped. Advise patients who experience chest pains that do not go away, shortness of breath, joint pain, or a rash on their cheeks and arms that is sensitive to the sun to call their health care provider right away. Their health care provider may decide to stop treatment.

Advise patients to call their health care provider right away if they develop a severe rash, swollen face, or difficulty breathing while taking adalimumab.

Many patients experience a reaction where the injection was given. These reactions are usually mild and include redness, rash, swelling, itching, or bruising. Usually, the rash will go away within a few days. If the skin around the area where adalimumab was injected still hurts or is swollen, advise patients to try using a towel soaked with cold water on the injection site. Advise patients to call their health care provider right away if they have pain, redness, or swelling around the injection site that doesn't go away within a few days or gets worse. Other side effects are upper respiratory infections (sinus infections), headache, and nausea.

Advise patients that if they forget to take adalimumab when they are supposed to, they should inject the next dose right away and then take their next dose when their next scheduled dose is due.

THALIDOMIDE

Rx	Thalomid[a] (Celgene)	Capsules: 50 mg	(Celgene/50 mg). White, opaque. In blister pack 28s and 280s.
		100 mg	(Celgene/100 mg). Tan. In blister pack 28s and 140s.
		200 mg	(Celgene/200 mg). Blue. In blister pack 28s and 84s.

[a] Available only to be prescribed and dispensed under the terms of the S.T.E.P.S. Restricted Distribution Program.

WARNING

If thalidomide is taken during pregnancy, it can cause severe birth defects or death to an unborn baby. Thalidomide should never be used by women who are pregnant or who could become pregnant while taking the drug. Even a single dose (1 capsule [50, 100, 200 mg]) taken by a pregnant woman can cause severe birth defects. Because of this toxicity and in an effort to make the chance of fetal exposure to thalidomide as negligible as possible, thalidomide is approved for marketing only under a special restricted distribution program approved by the FDA. This program is called the "System for Thalidomide Education and Prescribing Safety (S.T.E.P.S.)." Under this restricted distribution program, only prescribers and pharmacists registered with the program are allowed to prescribe and dispense the product. In addition, patients must be advised of, agree to, and comply with the requirements of the S.T.E.P.S. program in order to receive the product.

Prescribers: Thalidomide may be prescribed only by licensed prescribers who are registered in the S.T.E.P.S. program and understand the risk of teratogenicity if thalidomide is used during pregnancy. The following major human fetal abnormalities related to thalidomide administration during pregnancy have been documented: Amelia (absence of limbs), phocomelia (short limbs), hypoplasticity of the bones, absence of bones, external ear abnormalities (including anotia, micro pinna, small or absent external auditory canals), facial palsy, eye abnormalities (anophthalmos, microphthalmos), and congenital heart defects. Alimentary tract, urinary tract, and genital malformations also have been documented. Mortality at or shortly after birth has been reported at about 40%. Effective contraception must be used for at least 1 month before beginning thalidomide therapy, during therapy, and for 1 month following discontinuation of therapy. Reliable contraception is indicated even where there has been a history of infertility, unless the patient has had a hysterectomy or has been postmenopausal for at least 24 months. Because thalidomide is present in the semen of patients receiving the drug, males receiving thalidomide must always use a latex condom during any sexual contact with women of childbearing potential even if he has undergone a successful vasectomy. Two reliable forms of contraception must be used simultaneously unless continuous abstinence from reproductive heterosexual sexual intercourse is the chosen method. Refer women of childbearing potential to a qualified provider of contraceptive methods, if needed. Sexually mature women who have not undergone a hysterectomy or who have not been postmenopausal for at least 24 consecutive months (ie, who have had menses at some time in the preceding 24 consecutive months) are considered to be women of childbearing potential. Before starting treatment, administer a pregnancy test (sensitivity of at least 50 mIU/mL) to women of childbearing potential. Perform the test within the 24 hours prior to beginning therapy. A prescription for thalidomide for a woman of childbearing potential must not be issued by the prescriber until a written report of a negative pregnancy test has been obtained by the prescriber. Once treatment has started, test for pregnancy weekly during the first month of use, then monthly thereafter in women with regular menstrual cycles. If menstrual cycles are irregular, test for pregnancy every 2 weeks. Perform pregnancy testing and counseling if a patient misses her period or if there is any abnormality in menstrual bleeding. If pregnancy occurs during thalidomide treatment, discontinue the drug immediately. Report any suspected fetal exposure to thalidomide to the FDA immediately via the MedWatch number at (800) FDA-1088 and also to the Celgene Corporation. Refer patient to an obstetrician/gynecologist experienced in reproductive toxicity for further evaluation and counseling.

WARNING (cont.)

➤*Female patients:* Thalidomide is contraindicated in women of childbearing potential unless alternative therapies are considered inappropriate and the patient meets ALL of the following conditions (ie, she is essentially unable to become pregnant while on thalidomide therapy):
- She understands and can reliably carry out instructions.
- She is capable of complying with the mandatory contraceptive measures, pregnancy testing, patient registration, and patient survey as described in the S.T.E.P.S. program.
- She has received both oral and written warnings of the hazards of taking thalidomide during pregnancy and of exposing a fetus to the drug.
- She has received both oral and written warnings of the risk of possible contraception failure and of the need to use 2 reliable forms of contraception simultaneously, unless continuous abstinence from reproductive heterosexual intercourse is the chosen method.
- She acknowledges, in writing, her understanding of these warnings and of the need for using 2 reliable methods of contraception for 1 month prior to starting thalidomide therapy, during thalidomide therapy, and for 1 month after stopping thalidomide therapy.
- She has had a negative pregnancy test with a sensitivity of at least 50 mIU/mL, within the 24 hours prior to beginning therapy.
- If the patient is between 12 and 18 years of age, her parent or legal guardian must have read this material and agreed to ensure compliance with the above.

➤*Male patients:* Thalidomide is contraindicated in sexually mature males unless the patient meets ALL of the following conditions:
- He understands and can reliably carry out instructions.
- He is capable of complying with the mandatory contraceptive measures that are appropriate for men, patient registration, and patient survey as described in the S.T.E.P.S. program.
- He has received both oral and written warnings of the hazards of taking thalidomide and exposing a fetus to the drug.
- He has received both oral and written warnings of the risk of possible contraception failure and of the need to use barrier contraception when having sexual intercourse with women of childbearing potential, even if he has undergone successful vasectomy.
- He acknowledges, in writing, his understanding of these warnings and of the need to use barrier contraception (latex condom), even if he has undergone successful vasectomy, when having sexual intercourse with women of childbearing potential.
- If the patient is between 12 and 18 years of age, his parent or legal guardian must have read this material and agreed to ensure compliance with the above.

Indications

➤*Erythema nodosum leprosum (ENL):*

Acute treatment – Acute treatment of the cutaneous manifestations of moderate to severe ENL. Not indicated as monotherapy for such ENL treatment in the presence of moderate to severe neuritis.

Maintenance therapy – Maintenance therapy for prevention and suppression of the cutaneous manifestations of ENL recurrence.

➤*Unlabeled uses:* Prostate cancer (in combination with docetaxel).

Orphan status – Clinical manifestations of mycobacterial infection caused by mycobacterium tuberculosis and non-tuberculous mycobacteria; Crohn disease; HIV-associated wasting syndrome; Kaposi sarcoma; lupus erythematosus, multiple myeloma; myelofibrosis with myeloid metaplasia, primary brain malignancies; treatment and maintenance of reactional lepromatous leprosy; treatment and prevention of graft vs

THALIDOMIDE

host disease; treatment and prevention of recurrent aphthous stomatitis and treatment and prevention of recurrent aphthous ulcer in severely, terminally immunocompromised patients.

Administration and Dosage

➤*Approved by the FDA:* July 16, 1998.

Thalidomide must only be administered in compliance with all of the terms outlined in the S.T.E.P.S. program. Thalidomide may only be prescribed by prescribers registered with the S.T.E.P.S. program and dispensed by pharmacists registered with the S.T.E.P.S. program.

Prescribing thalidomide to women of childbearing potential is contingent upon initial and continued confirmed negative results of pregnancy testing.

➤*Dosing:* Initiate dosing at 100 to 300 mg/day, once daily with water, preferably at bedtime and at least 1 hour after the evening meal. Start patients weighing less than 50 kg (110 lb) at the low end of the dose range.

In patients with a severe cutaneous ENL reaction, or in those who have previously required higher doses to control the reaction, thalidomide dosing may be initiated at higher doses, up to 400 mg/day once daily at bedtime or in divided doses with water at least 1 hour after meals.

In patients with moderate to severe neuritis associated with a severe ENL reaction, corticosteroids may be started concomitantly with thalidomide. Steroid usage can be tapered and discontinued when the neuritis has ameliorated.

Continue dosing with thalidomide until signs and symptoms of active reaction have subsided, usually at least 2 weeks. Patients may then be tapered off medication in 50 mg decrements every 2 to 4 weeks.

Maintain patients who have a documented history of requiring prolonged maintenance treatment to prevent the recurrence of cutaneous ENL or who flare during tapering on the minimum dose necessary to control the reaction. Attempt tapering of medication every 3 to 6 months, in decrements of 50 mg every 2 to 4 weeks.

➤*Dispensing instructions:* This product is only supplied to pharmacists registered with the S.T.E.P.S. program (see Warning Box). Pharmacists note: Before dispensing thalidomide, activate the authorization number on every prescription by calling the Celgene customer center at (888) 4-CELGENE (888-423-5436) and obtain a confirmation number. Write the confirmation number on the prescription. Accept a thalidomide prescription only if it has been issued within the previous 7 days (telephone prescriptions are not permitted). A new prescription is required for further dispensing. Dispense blister packs intact (capsules cannot be repackaged). Dispense subsequent prescriptions only if fewer than 7 days of therapy remain on the previous prescription.

➤*Storage/Stability:* Store at 25°C (77°F); excursions permitted to 15° to 30°C (59° to 86°F). Protect from light.

Actions

➤*Pharmacology:* Thalidomide is an immunomodulatory agent with a spectrum of activity that is not fully characterized. In patients with ENL, the mechanism of action is not fully understood.

Data suggest that the immunologic effects of this compound can vary substantially under different conditions, but may be related to suppression of excessive tumor necrosis factor-alpha (TNF-α) production and down-modulation of selected cell surface adhesion molecules involved in leukocyte migration. For example, administration of thalidomide has been reported to decrease circulating levels of TNF-α in patients with ENL; however, it also has been shown to increase plasma TNF-α levels in HIV-seropositive patients.

➤*Pharmacokinetics:*

Absorption/Distribution – The absolute bioavailability of oral thalidomide has not yet been characterized in human subjects because of its poor aqueous solubility. In studies of healthy volunteers and subjects with Hansen disease, the mean time to peak plasma concentrations (T_{max}) of thalidomide ranged from 2.9 to 5.7 hours, indicating that thalidomide is slowly absorbed from the GI tract. While the extent of absorption as measured by AUC is proportional to the dose in healthy subjects, the C_{max} increased in a less than proportional manner (see table below). This lack of C_{max} dose proportionality, coupled with the observed increase in T_{max} values, suggests that the poor solubility of thalidomide in aqueous media may be hindering the rate of absorption.

Various Thalidomide Pharmacokinetic Parameters (mean)				
Population/Single dose	AUC$_{0-\infty}$ (mcg•h/mL)	C$_{max}$ (mcg/mL)	T$_{max}$ (h)	Half-life (h)
Healthy subjects (n = 14)				
50 mg	4.9	0.62	2.9	5.52
200 mg	18.9	1.76	3.5	5.53
400 mg	36.4	2.82	4.3	7.29
Patients with Hansen disease (n = 6)				
400 mg	46.4	3.44	5.7	6.86

Coadministration of thalidomide with a high-fat meal causes minor (less than 10%) changes in the observed AUC and C_{max} values; however, it causes an increase in T_{max} to approximately 6 hours. The extent of plasma protein binding of thalidomide is unknown.

Metabolism – The exact metabolic route and fate of thalidomide is not known. Thalidomide does not appear to be hepatically metabolized to any large extent, but appears to undergo nonenzymatic hydrolysis in plasma to multiple metabolites. In a repeat dose study in which 200 mg was given to 10 healthy females for 18 days, thalidomide showed similar pharmacokinetic profiles on the first and last day of dosing. Thalidomide does not appear to induce or inhibit its own metabolism.

Excretion – As indicated in the table above, the mean elimination half-life ranges from approximately 5 to 7 hours after a single dose and is not altered by multiple dosing. Thalidomide has a renal clearance of 1.15 mL/min with less than 0.7% of the dose excreted in the urine as unchanged drug. Following a single dose, urinary levels of thalidomide were undetectable 48 hours after dosing. Although thalidomide is thought to be hydrolyzed to a number of metabolites, only a very small amount (0.02% of the administered dose) of 4-OH-thalidomide was identified in the urine of subjects 12 to 24 hours after dosing.

Contraindications

Pregnancy (*Category X;* see Warning Box and Warnings); hypersensitivity to the drug and its components.

Warnings

➤*Severe birth defects:* See Black Box Warnings.

➤*Drowsiness and somnolence:* Thalidomide frequently causes drowsiness and somnolence. Instruct patients to avoid situations where drowsiness may be a problem and not to take other medications that may cause drowsiness without adequate medical advice. Advise patients about the possible impairment of mental or physical abilities required for the performance of hazardous tasks, such as driving a car or operating other complex or dangerous machinery.

➤*Peripheral neuropathy:* Thalidomide is known to cause nerve damage that may be permanent. Peripheral neuropathy is a common, potentially severe, and irreversible side effect of treatment with thalidomide. Peripheral neuropathy generally occurs following chronic use over a period of months; however, reports following relatively short-term use also exist. The correlation with cumulative dose is unclear. Symptoms may occur some time after thalidomide treatment has been stopped and may resolve slowly or not at all. Few reports of neuropathy have arisen in the treatment of ENL despite long-term thalidomide treatment. However, the inability clinically to differentiate thalidomide neuropathy from the neuropathy often seen in Hansen disease makes it difficult to determine accurately the incidence of thalidomide-related neuropathy in ENL patients.

Examine patients at monthly intervals for the first 3 months of therapy to enable the clinician to detect early signs of neuropathy, which include numbness, tingling, or pain in the hands and feet. Evaluate patients periodically thereafter during treatment. Regularly counsel, question, and evaluate patients for signs or symptoms of peripheral neuropathy. Give consideration to electrophysiological testing, consisting of measurement of sensory nerve action potential amplitudes at baseline and thereafter every 6 months in an effort to detect asymptomatic neuropathy. If symptoms of drug-induced neuropathy develop, discontinue thalidomide immediately to limit further damage, if clinically appropriate. Usually reinitiate thalidomide treatment only if the neuropathy returns to baseline status.

Use medications known to be associated with neuropathy with caution in patients receiving thalidomide.

➤*Dizziness/Orthostatic hypotension:* Thalidomide may cause dizziness and orthostatic hypotension. Advise patients to sit upright for a few minutes prior to standing up from a recumbent position.

➤*Neutropenia:* Decreased white blood cell counts, including neutropenia, have been reported. Do not initiate treatment with an absolute neutrophil count (ANC) of less than 750/mm^3. Monitor white blood cell count and differential on an ongoing basis, especially in patients who may be more prone to neutropenia, such as patients who are HIV-seropositive. If ANC decreases to less than 750/mm^3 while on treatment, reevaluate the patient's medication regimen and, if the neutropenia persists, consider withholding thalidomide if clinically appropriate.

➤*HIV patients:* In a randomized, placebo-controlled trial of thalidomide in HIV-seropositive patients, plasma HIV RNA levels were found to increase. A similar trend was observed in a second study conducted in patients who were HIV-seropositive. The clinical significance of this increase is unknown. Both studies were conducted prior to availability of highly active antiretroviral therapy. Until the clinical significance of this finding in HIV-seropositive patients is further understood, measure viral load after the first and third months of treatment and every 3 months thereafter.

➤*Hansen disease patients:* Data suggest that these patients, relative to healthy subjects, may have an increased bioavailability of thalidomide. The increase is reflected in an increased AUC and in increased peak plasma levels. Clinical significance is unknown.

THALIDOMIDE

►*Thrombotic events:* Thrombotic events have been reported in patients treated with thalidomide. Patients with neoplastic and various inflammatory conditions being treated with thalidomide may have an increased incidence of pulmonary embolism, deep vein thrombophlebitis, thrombophlebitis, or thrombosis. It is not known if concomitant therapy with other medications, including anticancer agents, are a contributing factor.

►*Hypersensitivity reactions:* Hypersensitivity to thalidomide has been reported. Signs and symptoms have included the occurrence of erythematous macular rash, possibly associated with fever, tachycardia, and hypotension. May necessitate interruption of therapy if severe. If the reaction recurs when dosing is resumed, discontinue thalidomide. Refer to Management of Acute Hypersensitivity Reactions.

►*Pregnancy:* Category X. Because of its known human teratogenicity, even following a single dose, thalidomide is contraindicated in pregnant women and women capable of becoming pregnant (see Warning Box). When there is no alternative treatment, women of childbearing potential may be treated with thalidomide provided adequate precautions are taken to avoid pregnancy. Women must commit either to abstain continuously from heterosexual sexual intercourse or to use 2 methods of reliable birth control, including at least 1 highly effective method (eg, IUD, hormonal contraception, tubal ligation, partner's vasectomy) and 1 additional effective method (eg, latex condom, diaphragm, cervical cap), beginning 4 weeks prior to initiating treatment with thalidomide, during therapy, and continuing for 4 weeks following discontinuation of therapy. If hormonal or IUD contraception is medically contraindicated (see Drug Interactions), 2 other effective or highly effective methods may be used.

Have pregnancy testing (sensitivity of at least 50 mIU/mL) performed on women of childbearing potential who are being treated with thalidomide. Perform the test within the 24 hours before beginning thalidomide therapy, weekly during the first month of thalidomide therapy, then monthly thereafter in women with regular menstrual cycles or every 2 weeks in women with irregular menstrual cycles. Perform pregnancy testing and counseling if a patient misses her period or if there is any abnormality in menstrual bleeding. If pregnancy occurs during treatment, thalidomide must be immediately discontinued. Under these conditions, refer the patient to an obstetrician/gynecologist experienced in reproductive toxicity for further evaluation and counseling. Because thalidomide is present in the semen of males receiving the drug, males receiving thalidomide must always use a latex condom when engaging in sexual activity with women of childbearing potential.

Any suspected fetal exposure to thalidomide must be reported to the FDA via the MedWatch program at (800) FDA-1088 and also to the Celgene Corporation.

►*Lactation:* It is not known whether thalidomide is excreted in breast milk. Because of the potential for serious adverse reactions in nursing infants from thalidomide, decide whether to discontinue nursing or to discontinue the drug, taking into account the importance of the drug to the mother.

►*Children:* No pharmacokinetic data are available in subjects younger than 18 years of age. Safety and efficacy in patients younger than 12 years of age have not been established.

Precautions

►*Monitoring:* Have pregnancy testing (sensitivity of at least 50 mIU/mL) performed on women of childbearing potential. Perform the test within the 24 hours prior to beginning thalidomide therapy, weekly during the first month of use, then monthly thereafter in women with regular menstrual cycles or every 2 weeks in women with irregular menstrual cycles. Also perform pregnancy testing if a patient misses her period or if there is any abnormality in menstrual bleeding (see Warnings).

►*Exposure:* The only type of thalidomide exposure known to result in drug-associated birth defects are as a result of direct oral ingestion of thalidomide. Currently, no specific data are available regarding the cutaneous absorption or inhalation of thalidomide in women of childbearing potential and whether these exposures may result in any birth defects. Instruct patients not to handle extensively or open thalidomide capsules and to maintain storage of capsules in blister packs until ingestion. If there is contact with non-intact thalidomide capsules or the powder contents, wash the exposed area with soap and water.

Thalidomide has been shown to be present in the serum and semen of patients receiving thalidomide. If health care providers or other care givers are exposed to body fluids from patients receiving thalidomide, utilize appropriate precautions, such as wearing gloves to prevent the potential cutaneous exposure to thalidomide or wash the exposed area with soap and water.

►*Bradycardia:* Bradycardia in association with thalidomide use has been reported. There have been reports of cases of bradycardia requiring medical interventions. The clinical significance is unknown.

►*Serious dermatological reactions:* Serious dermatologic reactions, including Stevens-Johnson syndrome and toxic epidermal necrolysis, which may be fatal, have been reported. Discontinue thalidomide if a skin rash occurs and only resume following appropriate clinical evaluation. If the rash is exfoliative, purpuric, or bullous, or if Stevens-Johnson syndrome or toxic epidermal necrolysis is suspected, do not resume use of thalidomide.

►*Seizures:* Seizures, including grand mal convulsions, have been reported during postapproval use of thalidomide. During therapy with thalidomide, closely monitor patients with a history of seizures or with other risk factors for the development of seizures for clinical changes that could precipitate acute seizure activity.

►*Drug abuse and dependence:* Physical and psychological dependence has not been reported in patients taking thalidomide. However, as with other tranquilizers/hypnotics, thalidomide has been reported to create habituation to its soporific effects.

►*Photosensitivity:* Photosensitization (photoallergy or phototoxicity) may occur; therefore, caution patients to take protective measures (ie, sunscreens, protective clothing) against exposure to sunlight or ultraviolet light (eg, tanning beds) until tolerance is determined.

Drug Interactions

Thalidomide Drug Interactions			
Precipitant drug	Object drug*		Description
Thalidomide	Alcohol Barbiturates Chlorpromazine Reserpine	↑	Thalidomide may enhance sedative activity of these agents..
Thalidomide	Medication associated with peripheral neuropathy (eg, metronidazole, vincristine, isoniazid)	↑	Symptoms of peripheral neuropathy may be enhanced when thalidomide is taken with other medications known to cause peripheral neuropathy. Use caution when administering concomitantly.
Medication associated with peripheral neuropathy (eg, metronidazole, vincristine, isoniazid)	Thalidomide		

* ↑ = Object drug increased.

►*Drugs that interfere with hormonal contraceptives:* Concomitant use of carbamazepine, griseofulvin, HIV-protease inhibitors, modafinil, penicillins, rifabutin, rifampin, phenytoin, or certain herbal supplements such as St. John's wort with hormonal contraceptive agents may reduce the effectiveness of the contraception for up to 1 month after discontinuation of these concomitant therapies. Therefore, women requiring treatment with 1 or more of these drugs must use 2 other effective or highly effective methods of contraception or abstain from heterosexual sexual contact while taking thalidomide.

►*Drug/Food interactions:* Administration of thalidomide with a high-fat meal causes minor (less than 10%) changes in the observed AUC and C_{max} values; however, it causes an increase in T_{max} to approximately 6 hours.

Adverse Reactions

The most serious toxicity associated with thalidomide is its documented human teratogenicity (see Warnings). The risk of severe birth defects, primarily phocomelia or fetal death, is extremely high during the critical period of pregnancy. The critical period is estimated, depending on the source of information, to range from 35 to 50 days after the last menstrual period. The risk of other potentially severe birth defects outside this critical period is unknown but may be significant. Based on present knowledge, thalidomide must not be used at any time during pregnancy.

Because thalidomide is present in the semen of patients receiving the drug, males receiving thalidomide must always use a latex condom during any sexual contact with women of childbearing potential.

Thalidomide is associated with bradycardia, dizziness/orthostatic hypotension, drowsiness/somnolence, HIV viral load increase, hypersensitivity, neutropenia, and peripheral neuropathy (see Warnings and Precautions). Dizziness, rash, and somnolence are the most commonly observed adverse events associated with the use of thalidomide.

All adverse events listed in the following table were mild to moderate in severity, and none resulted in discontinuation. Events that were more frequent in the placebo-treated group are not included.

THALIDOMIDE

Thalidomide Adverse Reactions (%)				
	All ARs reported in ENL patients	ARs reported in ≥ 3 HIV-seropositive patients		
		Thalidomide		Placebo
Adverse reaction	50 to 300 mg/day (n = 24)	100 mg/day (n = 36)	200 mg/day (n = 32)	(n = 35)
CNS				
Agitation	0	0	9.4	0
Dizziness	4.2	19.4	18.7	0
Headache	12.5	16.7	18.7	11.4
Insomnia	0	0	9.4	5.7
Nervousness	0	2.8	9.4	0
Neuropathy	0	8.3	0	0
Paresthesia	0	5.6	15.6	11.4
Somnolence	37.5	36.1	37.5	11.4
Tremor	4.2	0	0	0
Vertigo	8.3	0	0	0
Dermatologic				
Acne	0	11.1	3.1	0
Dermatitis, fungal	4.2	5.6	9.4	0
Nail disorder	4.2	0	3.1	0
Pruritus	8.3	2.8	6.3	5.7
Rash	20.8	25	25	31.4
Rash, maculo-papular	4.2	16.7	18.7	5.7
Sweating	0	0	12.5	11.4
GI				
Abdominal pain	4.2	2.8	3.1	11.4
Anorexia	0	2.8	9.4	5.7
Constipation	4.2	2.8	9.4	0
Diarrhea	4.2	11.1	18.7	17.1
Dry mouth	0	8.3	9.4	5.7
Flatulence	0	8.3	0	5.7
Liver function tests (multiple abnormalities)	0	0	9.4	0
Nausea	4.2	0	12.5	2.9
Oral moniliasis	4.2	11.1	6.3	0
Tooth pain	4.2	0	0	0
GU				
Albuminuria	0	8.3	3.1	5.7
Hematuria	0	11.1	0	2.9
Impotence	8.3	2.8	0	0
Hematologic/ Lymphatic				
Anemia	0	5.6	12.5	8.6
Leukopenia	0	16.7	25	8.6
Lymphaden-opathy	0	5.6	12.5	8.6
Metabolic/ Endocrine				
AST increased	0	2.8	12.5	5.7
Edema, peripheral	4.2	8.3	3.1	0
Hyperlipemia	0	5.6	9.4	2.9
Respiratory				
Pharyngitis	4.2	8.3	6.3	5.7
Rhinitis	4.2	0	0	11.4
Sinusitis	4.2	8.3	3.1	5.7
Miscellaneous				
Accidental injury	4.2	5.6	0	2.9
Asthenia	8.3	5.6	21.9	2.9
Back pain	4.2	5.6	0	0
Chills	4.2	0	9.4	11.4
Facial edema	4.2	0	0	0
Fever	0	19.4	21.9	17.1
Infection	0	8.3	6.3	2.9
Malaise	8.3	0	0	0
Neck pain	4.2	0	0	0
Neck rigidity	4.2	0	0	0
Pain	8.3	0	3.1	5.7

Other adverse events observed in ENL patients – Thalidomide in doses no more than 400 mg/day has been administered investigationally in the US over a 19-year period in 1465 patients with ENL. The published literature describes the treatment of an additional 1678 patients. All reported events are included except those already listed in the previous table. Because of the fact that these data were collected from uncontrolled studies, the incidence rate cannot be determined.

➤*Cardiovascular:* Bradycardia; hypertension; hypotension; peripheral vascular disorder; tachycardia; vasodilation.

➤*CNS:* Abnormal thinking; agitation; amnesia; anxiety; causalgia; circumoral paresthesia; confusion; depression; euphoria; hyperesthesia; insomnia; nervousness; neuralgia; neuritis; neuropathy; paresthesia; peripheral neuritis; psychosis.

➤*Dermatologic:* Acne; alopecia; dry skin; eczematous rash; exfoliative dermatitis; ichthyosis; perifollicular thickening; photosensitivity; skin necrosis; seborrhea; sweating; urticaria; vesiculobullous rash.

➤*GI:* Anorexia; appetite increase/weight gain; dry mouth; dyspepsia; enlarged liver; eructation; flatulence; intestinal obstruction; vomiting.

➤*GU:* Hematuria; orchitis; proteinuria; pyuria; urinary frequency.

➤*Hematologic/Lymphatic:* Eosinophilia; ESR decrease; granulocytopenia; hypochromic anemia; leukemia; leukocytosis; leukopenia; MCV elevated; RBC abnormal; spleen palpable; thrombocytopenia.

➤*Lab test abnormalities:* ALT increased; BUN increased; creatinine increased; decreased creatinine clearance; electrolyte abnormalities; increased liver function tests; LDH increased; phosphorus decreased.

➤*Metabolic:* ADH inappropriate; alkaline phosphatase; amyloidosis; bilirubinemia; cyanosis; diabetes; edema; hyperglycemia; hyperkalemia; hyperuricemia; hypocalcemia; hypoproteinemia.

➤*Musculoskeletal:* Arthritis; bone tenderness; hypertonia; joint disorder; leg cramps; myalgia; myasthenia; periosteal disorder.

➤*Respiratory:* Cough; emphysema; epistaxis; pulmonary embolus; rales; upper respiratory tract infection; voice alteration.

➤*Special senses:* Amblyopia; deafness; dry eye; eye pain; tinnitus.

➤*Miscellaneous:* Abdomen enlarged; fever; upper extremity pain.

➤ *Other adverse events observed in HIV-seropositive patients:* In addition to controlled clinical trials, thalidomide has been used in uncontrolled studies in 145 patients.

Adverse reactions are as follows:

Cardiovascular – Angina pectoris; arrhythmia; atrial fibrillation; bradycardia; cerebral ischemia; cerebrovascular accident; CHF; deep thrombophlebitis; heart arrest; heart failure; hypertension; hypotension; MI; murmur; palpitation; pericarditis; peripheral vascular disorder; postural hypotension; syncope; tachycardia; thrombophlebitis; thrombosis.

CNS – Abnormal gait; ataxia; decreased libido; decreased reflexes; dementia; dysesthesia; dyskinesia; emotional lability; hostility; hypalgesia; hyperkinesia; incoordination; meningitis; neurologic disorder; tremor; vertigo.

Dermatologic – Angioedema; benign skin neoplasm; eczema; herpes simplex; incomplete Stevens-Johnson syndrome; nail disorder; photosensitivity reaction; pruritus; psoriasis; skin discoloration; skin disorder.

GI – Cholangitis; cholestatic jaundice; colitis; dyspepsia; dysphagia; esophagitis; gastroenteritis; GI disorder; GI hemorrhage; gum disorder; hepatitis; pancreatitis; parotid gland enlargement; periodontitis; stomatitis; tongue discoloration; tooth disorder.

Hematologic/Lymphatic – Aplastic anemia; macrocytic anemia; megaloblastic anemia; microcytic anemia.

Metabolic – Avitaminosis; bilirubinemia; dehydration; hypercholesteremia; hypoglycemia; increased alkaline phosphatase; increased lipase; increased serum creatinine; peripheral edema.

Musculoskeletal – Myalgia; myasthenia.

Respiratory – Apnea; bronchitis; lung disorder; lung edema; pneumonia (including *Pneumocystis carinii* pneumonia); rhinitis.

Special senses – Conjunctivitis; eye disorder; lacrimation disorder; retinitis; taste perversion.

Miscellaneous – AIDS; allergic reaction; ascites; cellulitis; chest pain; chills and fever; cyst; decreased CD4 count; facial edema; flu syndrome; hernia; hormone level altered; moniliasis; sarcoma; sepsis; viral infection.

Other adverse events in the published literature or reported from other sources – The following additional events have been identified either in the published literature or from spontaneous reports from other sources: Acute renal failure; amenorrhea; aphthous stomatitis; bile duct obstruction; carpal tunnel; chronic myelogenous leukemia; diplopia; dysesthesia; dyspnea; enuresis; erythema nodosum; erythroleukemia; foot drop; galactorrhea; gynecomastia; hangover effect; hypomagnesemia; hypothyroidism; lymphedema; lymphopenia; metrorrhagia; migraine; myxedema; nodular sclerosing Hodgkin disease; nystagmus; oliguria; pancytopenia; petechiae; purpura; Raynaud syndrome; stomach ulcer; suicide attempt.

➤*Postmarketing:*

Cardiovascular – Cardiac arrhythmias including atrial fibrillation; bradycardia; EKG abnormalities; sick sinus syndrome; tachycardia.

CNS – Changes in mental status or mood including depression and suicide attempts; disturbances in consciousness including lethargy, loss of consciousness, or stupor; seizures including grand mal convulsions; status epilepticus; syncope.

THALIDOMIDE

Hematologic / Lymphatic – Decreased white blood cell counts including neutropenia and febrile neutropenia; changes in prothrombin time.

Metabolic / Endocrine – Electrolyte imbalance including hypercalcemia and hypocalcemia; hyperkalemia and hypokalemia; hyponatremia; hypothyroidism; increased alkaline phosphatase.

Miscellaneous – Erythema multiforme; pleural effusion.

Overdosage

There have been 3 cases of overdose reported, all attempted suicides. There have been no reported fatalities in doses of at least 14.4 g, and all patients recovered without reported sequelae.

Patient Information

See Warning Box.

Instruct patients about the potential teratogenicity of thalidomide and the precautions that must be taken to preclude fetal exposure as per the S.T.E.P.S. program and boxed Warnings. Take thalidomide only as prescribed in compliance with all of the provisions of the S.T.E.P.S. Restricted Distribution Program.

Instruct patients not to extensively handle or open thalidomide capsules and to maintain storage of capsules in blister packs until ingestion.

Instruct patients not to share medication with anyone else.

Thalidomide frequently causes drowsiness and somnolence. Instruct patients to avoid situations where drowsiness may be a problem and not to take other medications that may cause drowsiness without adequate medical advice. Advise patients as to the possible impairment of mental or physical abilities required for the performance of hazardous tasks, such as driving a car or operating other complex machinery. Thalidomide may potentiate the somnolence caused by alcohol.

Thalidomide may cause photosensitivity (sensitivity to sunlight). Instruct patients to avoid prolonged exposure to the sun and other ultraviolet light. Instruct patients to use sunscreens and wear protective clothing until tolerance is determined.

Thalidomide can cause peripheral neuropathies that may be initially signaled by numbness, tingling, pain, or a burning sensation in the feet or hands. Instruct patients to report such occurrences to their prescriber immediately.

Thalidomide may cause dizziness and orthostatic hypotension. Instruct patients to sit upright for a few minutes prior to standing from a recumbent position.

Patients are not permitted to donate blood while taking thalidomide. In addition, instruct male patients not to donate sperm while taking thalidomide.

MITOXANTRONE HCl

| *Rx* | **Novantrone** (Serono) | **Injection:** 2 mg mitoxantrone free base/ml | Preservative free. In 10, 12.5, and 15 ml multi-dose vials.[1] |

[1] With 0.8% NaCl, 0.005% sodium acetate, and 0.046% acetic acid.

For complete prescribing information, see the Mitoxantrone monograph in the Antineoplastics chapter.

WARNING

Administer mitoxantrone for injection concentrate under the supervision of a physician experienced in the use of cytotoxic chemotherapy agents.

Give mitoxantrone slowly into a freely flowing IV infusion. Never give SC, IM, or intra-arterially. Severe local tissue damage may occur if there is extravasation during administration (see Adverse Reactions).

Not for intrathecal use. Severe injury with permanent sequelae can result from intrathecal administration (see Warnings).

Except for the treatment of acute nonlymphocytic leukemia, generally do not give mitoxantrone therapy to patients with baseline neutrophil counts less than 1500 cells/mm^3. In order to monitor the occurrence of bone marrow suppression, primarily neutropenia, which may be severe and result in infection, it is recommended that frequent peripheral blood cell counts be performed on all patients receiving mitoxantrone.

Myocardial toxicity, manifested in its most severe form by potentially fatal congestive heart failure (CHF), may occur either during therapy with mitoxantrone or months to years after termination of therapy. Mitoxantrone use has been associated with cardiotoxicity; this risk increases with cumulative dose. In cancer patients, the risk of symptomatic CHF was estimated to be 2.6% for patients receiving up to a cumulative dose of 140 mg/m^2. For this reason, monitor patients for evidence of cardiac toxicity and question them about symptoms of heart failure prior to initiation of treatment. Monitor patients with multiple sclerosis (MS) who reach a cumulative dose of 100 mg/m^2 for evidence of cardiac toxicity prior to each subsequent dose. Ordinarily, patients with MS should not receive a cumulative dose > 140 mg/m^2. Active or dormant cardiovascular disease, prior or concomitant radiotherapy to the mediastinal/pericardial area, previous therapy with other anthracyclines or anthracenediones, or concomitant use of other cardiotoxic drugs may increase the risk of cardiac toxicity. Cardiac toxicity with mitoxantrone may occur at lower cumulative doses whether or not cardiac risk factors are present (see Warnings and Administration and Dosage).

Secondary acute myelogenous leukemia (AML) has been reported in cancer patients treated with anthracyclines. Mitoxantrone is an anthracenedione, a related drug. Secondary AML has also been reported in cancer patients and multiple sclerosis patients who have been treated with mitoxantrone. The occurrence of refractory secondary leukemia is more common when anthracyclines are given in combination with DNA-damaging antineoplastic agents, when patients have been heavily pretreated with cytotoxic drugs, or when doses of anthracyclines have been escalated. The cumulative risk of developing treatment-related AML, in 1774 patients with breast cancer who received mitoxantrone concomitantly with other cytotoxic agents and radiotherapy, was estimated as 1.1% and 1.6% at 5 and 10 years, respectively (see Warnings).

Indications

➤*Multiple sclerosis:* For reducing neurologic disability or the frequency of clinical relapses in patients with secondary (chronic) progressive, progressive relapsing, or worsening relapsing-remitting MS (ie, patients whose neurologic status is significantly abnormal between relapses). Mitoxantrone is not indicated in the treatment of patients with primary progressive MS.

The clinical patterns of MS in the studies were characterized as follows: Secondary progressive and progressive relapsing disease were characterized by gradual increasing disability with or without superimposed clinical relapses, and worsening relapsing-remitting disease was characterized by clinical relapses resulting in a step-wise worsening of disability.

Administration and Dosage

➤*Approved by the FDA:* October 13, 2000.

➤*MS:* The recommended dosage of mitoxantrone is 12 mg/m^2 given as a short (approximately 5 to 15 minutes) IV infusion every 3 months.

Evaluation of left ventricular ejection fraction (LVEF) by echocardiogram or multiple-gated acquisition scanning (MUGA) is recommended prior to administration of the initial dose of mitoxantrone. Subsequent LVEF evaluations are recommended if signs or symptoms of CHF develop, and prior to all doses administered to patients who have received a cumulative dose of 100 mg/m^2 or more. Do not administer mitoxantrone to MS patients who have received a cumulative lifetime dose of 140 mg/m^2 or more, or those with either LVEF of less than 50% or a clinically significant reduction in LVEF.

Monitor complete blood counts, including platelets, prior to each course of mitoxantrone and in the event that signs or symptoms of infection develop. Mitoxantrone generally must not be administered to MS patients with neutrophil counts less than 1500 cells/mm^3. Monitor liver function tests prior to each course. Mitoxantrone therapy in MS patients with abnormal liver function tests is not recommended because mitoxantrone clearance is reduced by hepatic impairment and no laboratory measurement can predict drug clearance and dose adjustments.

Women with MS who are biologically capable of becoming pregnant, even if they are using birth control, should have a pregnancy test, and the results must be known before receiving each dose of mitoxantrone (see Warnings).

Therapeutic alternatives in the treatment of rheumatoid arthritis and related conditions include a diverse array of agents ranging from aspirin and similarly acting nonsteroidal anti-inflammatory agents (NSAIDs), to the slow-acting and possibly disease-modifying agents such as gold compounds and penicillamine. Because of their toxicity, the slow-acting agents are generally reserved for progressive disease unresponsive to more conservative therapy. Drugs and groups of drugs useful in the treatment of rheumatoid arthritis are listed below (refer to individual monographs).

➤*Anti-inflammatory Agents:*

Glucocorticoids – Glucocorticoids provide dramatic anti-inflammatory effects by inhibiting the initiation of inflammatory reactions. However, because of the consequences of prolonged therapy, use chronically only in patients with uncontrollable rheumatoid arthritis who fail to respond to other measures. Short-term therapy can be used in acute flares until other agents have a chance to act.

Salicylates – Aspirin, the most widely used NSAID, is generally considered the drug of first choice for rheumatoid arthritis. Adequate analgesia is usually achieved with 3 g/day of aspirin; 3 to 6 g/day are usually required for significant anti-inflammatory effects. At maximum doses, aspirin is as effective as any of the other NSAIDs. GI intolerance is the most common side effect. Other salicylate derivatives may offer the advantage of fewer GI complaints without interfering with platelet aggregation at recommended doses; however, when comparing anti-inflammatory agents, nonaspirin salicylates have not been proven as effective as aspirin.

NSAIDs – NSAIDs have essentially the same therapeutic benefits as aspirin. With the exception of indomethacin, the NSAIDs may offer the advantage of a lower incidence of GI side effects.

➤*Slow-acting antirheumatic agents:*

Hydroxychloroquine sulfate – Hydroxychloroquine sulfate, an antimalarial agent, may be effective in moderate to severe rheumatoid arthritis unresponsive to conventional treatment. Up to 6 months may be required for a clinical response. Side effects are frequent.

Gold compounds – Gold compounds are quite effective in the treatment of actively progressing rheumatoid arthritis. Prolonged therapy is required. Serious side effects may require discontinuation of therapy.

Penicillamine – Penicillamine is used in severe rheumatoid arthritis unresponsive to conventional therapy. Response to therapy is slow (2 to 3 months); adverse effects may be severe.

Azathioprine and cyclosporine – Azathioprine and cyclosporine are immunosuppressive agents used in the treatment of severe, active, and erosive disease not responsive to conventional therapy.

Methotrexate – Methotrexate is used in severe, active, classical, or definite rheumatoid arthritis unresponsive to other therapy.

Captopril – Captopril has been used investigationally to treat severe rheumatoid arthritis.

HYDROXYCHLOROQUINE SULFATE

Rx	**Hydroxychloroquine Sulfate** (Various, eg, Geneva, Mylan, Teva, Watson)	**Tablets:** 200 mg (equivalent to 155 mg base)	In 100s, 500s, and 1000s.
Rx	**Plaquenil** (Sanofi Synthelabo)		(PLAQUENIL). White to off-white. Film-coated. In 100s.

WARNING

Physicians should completely familiarize themselves with the complete contents of the package insert before prescribing hydroxychloroquine.

Indications

➤*Lupus erythematosus:* For the treatment of chronic discoid and systemic lupus erythematosus (SLE) in patients who have not responded satisfactorily to drugs with less potential for serious side effects.

➤*Malaria:* For the suppressive treatment and treatment of acute attacks of malaria caused by *Plasmodium vivax, P. malariae, P. ovale,* and susceptible strains of *P. falciparum.* Refer to the monograph in the Anti-infectives chapter for more information.

➤*Rheumatoid arthritis (RA):* For the treatment of acute or chronic RA in patients who have not responded satisfactorily to drugs with less potential for serious side effects.

Administration and Dosage

➤*Approved by the FDA:* April 18, 1955.

➤*Lupus erythematosus:* Initially, 400 mg once or twice daily in adults, continued for several weeks or months depending on response. For prolonged maintenance therapy, a smaller dose (200 to 400 mg daily) frequently will suffice. The incidence of retinopathy reportedly has been higher when the maintenance dose is exceeded.

➤*RA:*

Initial dosage – 400 to 600 mg daily, taken with a meal or a glass of milk. Side effects may require temporary reduction. Later (usually from 5 to 10 days), dose may be increased gradually to optimum response level, often without return of side effects.

Maintenance dosage – When a good response is obtained (usually in 4 to 12 weeks), reduce dosage by 50% and continue at a level of 200 to 400 mg daily. Incidence of retinopathy is higher when this dose is exceeded.

The compound is cumulative and requires several weeks to exert therapeutic effects; minor side effects may occur early. Maximum effects may not be obtained for several months. If objective improvement (reduced joint swelling, increased mobility) does not occur within 6 months, discontinue use. Safe use of hydroxychloroquine to treat juvenile rheumatoid arthritis (JRA) has not been established.

If relapse occurs after drug withdrawal, resume therapy or continue on an intermittent schedule if there are no ocular contraindications.

Corticosteroids and salicylates may be used with this compound; generally they can be decreased gradually or eliminated after hydroxychloroquine has been used for several weeks. When gradual reduction of steroid dosage is indicated, reduce (every 4 to 5 days) dose of cortisone by no more than 5 to 15 mg; hydrocortisone by 5 to 10 mg; prednisolone and prednisone by 1 to 2.5 mg; methylprednisolone and triamcinolone by 1 to 2 mg; or dexamethasone by 0.25 to 0.5 mg.

➤*Storage/Stability:* Store at room temperature, up to 30°C (86°F). Dispense in a tight, light-resistant container.

Actions

➤*Pharmacology:* Inhibition of heme polymerization appears crucial for antimalarial action. Hydroxychloroquine binds initially to heme and then prevents further heme polymerization by incorporating as hemequinoline complexes into growing heme polymer chains. It is unknown whether the accumulation of heme, heme-quinoline complexes, or both suffices to kill the parasites or if other actions of the antimalarial quinolones are required.

➤*Pharmacokinetics:*

Absorption/Distribution – Pharmacokinetics of hydroxychloroquine are similar to chloroquine. Both drugs are absorbed very rapidly and almost completely after oral administration. Hydroxychloroquine is distributed widely into body tissues and concentrates in the spleen, liver, kidney, melanin-containing tissues, lungs, and, to a lesser extent, the spinal cord and brain. It has a large apparent volume of distribution (more than 100 L/kg). It is bound approximately 60% to plasma proteins.

Metabolism/Excretion – Chloroquine is extensively metabolized in the liver. The renal clearance is approximately half of its total systemic clearance. Renal excretion is increased by acidification of the urine. The terminal half-life ranges from 30 to 60 days, and traces of the drug can be found in the urine for years after a therapeutic regimen.

Contraindications

Retinal or visual field changes attributable to any 4-aminoquinoline compound; hypersensitivity to 4-aminoquinoline compounds; long-term therapy in children.

Warnings

➤*Psoriasis:* Use in patients with psoriasis may precipitate a severe attack. Porphyria may be exacerbated. Do not use unless the benefit to the patient outweighs possible risks.

➤*Ophthalmic effects:* Irreversible retinal damage has been observed in some patients who had received long-term or high-dosage 4-aminoquinoline therapy for discoid and SLE or RA. Retinopathy has been reported to be dose-related. When prolonged therapy is contemplated, perform initial (baseline) and periodic (every 3 months) ophthalmologic examinations (including visual acuity, expert slit-lamp, funduscopic, and visual field tests). If there is any indication of abnormality in the visual acuity, visual field, or retinal macular areas (eg, pigmentary changes, loss of foveal reflex) or any visual symptoms (eg, light flashes or streaks) not fully explainable by difficulties of accommodation or corneal opacities, discontinue drug immediately and observe patient for possible progression (see Adverse Reactions).

Retinal changes – Retinal changes and visual disturbances may progress even after cessation of therapy.

Chloroquine retinopathy – Methods recommended for early diagnosis of "chloroquine retinopathy" consist of (1) funduscopic examination of macula for fine pigmentary disturbances or loss of the foveal reflex and (2) examination of central visual field with a small red test object for pericentral or paracentral scotoma or determination of retinal thresholds to red. Regard unexplained visual symptoms (eg, light flashes or streaks) as possible manifestations of retinopathy.

➤*Muscular weakness:* Examine patients on long-term therapy periodically, and test knee and ankle reflexes to detect evidence of muscular weakness. If weakness occurs, discontinue drug.

HYDROXYCHLOROQUINE SULFATE

➤*RA:* In RA, discontinue if objective improvement does not occur within 6 months. Safety for use in JRA has not been established.

➤*Renal / Hepatic function impairment:* Use with caution.

➤*Pregnancy:* According to *Drugs in Pregnancy and Lactation* by Briggs, the pregnancy risk factor is a *C*. The Centers for Disease Control and Prevention recommends use for prophylaxis in pregnant women who are traveling to areas with chloroquine-sensitive *P. falciparum* malaria.

Avoid use during pregnancy, except in the suppression of malaria when the benefit outweighs the possible hazard. Chloroquine administered IV to pregnant mice rapidly crossed the placenta, accumulated selectively in the melanin structures of the fetal eyes, and was retained in the ocular tissues for 5 months after the drug was eliminated from the rest of the body.

➤*Lactation:* The drug has been detected in breast milk from 2 mothers receiving 400 mg daily doses for SLE or RA.

➤*Children:* Children are especially sensitive to 4-aminoquinolines. A number of fatalities have been reported following ingestion of chloroquine in small doses (0.75 g or 1 g in one 3-year-old).

Safe use of the drug in the treatment of JRA and SLE has not been established.

Precautions

➤*Monitoring:* Perform periodic blood cell counts during prolonged therapy. If a severe blood disorder appears, consider discontinuation. Use caution in glucose-6-phosphate dehydrogenase (G-6-PD) deficiency.

➤*Hepatic disease:* Use with caution in patients with hepatic disease or in conjunction with hepatotoxic drugs.

➤*Alcoholism:* Use with caution in patients with alcoholism.

➤*Dermatologic reactions:* Dermatologic reactions may occur; exercise care when given to any patient receiving a drug with significant tendency to produce dermatitis.

➤*Toxic symptoms:* If serious toxic symptoms occur, administer ammonium chloride (8 g daily in divided doses for adults) 3 or 4 days a week for several months after therapy has been stopped; acidification of the urine increases renal excretion by 20% to 90%. Exercise caution in renal function impairment and/or metabolic acidosis.

Drug Interactions

Hydroxychloroquine Drug Interactions			
Precipitant drug	Object drug*		Description
Cimetidine	Aminoquino-lones (eg, hy-droxychloro-quine)	↑	The hydroxychloroquine dose may need to be lowered during coadministration because of increased pharmacologic effects of the hydroxychloroquine.
Aminoquino-lones (eg, hy-droxychloro-quine)	Beta-blockers (eg, metoprolol)	↑	Plasma concentrations and cardiovascular effects of certain beta-blockers may be increased. Carefully monitor patients when hydroxychloroquine is started or stopped with concomitant use of certain beta-blockers (eg, meto-prolol). Consider use of an alternative beta-blocker (eg, atenolol).
Aminoquino-lones (eg, hy-droxychloro-quine)	Cyclosporine	↑	Elevated cyclosporine concentrations may occur, increasing the risk of nephrotoxicity. Consider monitoring cyclosporine and serum creatinine levels. Adjust cyclosporine dose accordingly.
Aminoquino-lones (eg, hy-droxychloro-quine)	Digoxin	↑	Serum levels and actions of digoxin may be increased. Monitor for signs/symptoms of digoxin toxicity; reduce dosage if necessary.
Aminoquino-lones (eg, hy-droxychloro-quine)	Magnesium salts	↓	Oral magnesium salts may decrease the absorption and effect of hydroxychloroquine. The antacid activity of magnesium salts also may be reduced. Separate doses of each drug by 2 to 4 hours. It may be necessary to increase the hydroxychloroquine dose.
Aminoquino-lones (eg, hy-droxychloro-quine)	Mefloquine	↑	Coadministration may lead to an increased risk of seizures.

* ↑ = Object drug increased. ↓ = Object drug decreased.

Adverse Reactions

The following have occurred with 1 or more of the 4-aminoquinoline compounds.

➤*Cardiovascular:* Cardiomyopathy has been reported rarely with high daily doses of hydroxychloroquine.

➤*CNS:* Ataxia; convulsions; dizziness; emotional changes; headache; irritability; nerve deafness; nervousness; nightmares; nystagmus; psychosis; tinnitus; vertigo.

➤*Dermatologic:* Alopecia; bleaching of hair; photosensitivity; precipitation of nonlight-sensitive psoriasis; pruritus; skin and mucosal pigmentation; skin eruptions (urticarial, morbilliform, lichenoid, maculopapular, purpuric, erythema annulare centrifugum, Stevens-Johnson syndrome, acute generalized exanthematous pustulosis, and exfoliative dermatitis).

➤*GI:* Abdominal cramps; anorexia; diarrhea; nausea; vomiting. Isolated cases of abnormal liver function and fulminant hepatic failure.

➤*Hematologic:* Agranulocytosis; aplastic anemia; hemolysis in individuals with G-6-PD deficiency; leukopenia; thrombocytopenia.

➤*Musculoskeletal:* Skeletal muscle palsies, myopathy, or neuromyopathy leading to progressive weakness and atrophy of proximal muscle groups which may be associated with mild sensory changes, depression of tendon reflexes, and abnormal nerve conduction.

➤*Ophthalmic:*

Ciliary body – See Warnings. Disturbance of accommodation with blurred vision. This reaction is dose-related and reversible with cessation of therapy.

Cornea – Decreased corneal sensitivity; punctate to lineal opacities; transient edema. The corneal changes, with or without accompanying symptoms (eg, blurred vision, halos around lights, photophobia), are fairly common but reversible. Corneal deposits may appear as early as 3 weeks following initiation of therapy. The incidence of corneal changes and visual side effects appears to be considerably lower with hydroxychloroquine than with chloroquine.

Retina – Abnormal pigmentation (mild pigment stippling to a "bull's eye" appearance); atrophy; edema; elevated retinal threshold to red light in macular, paramacular, and peripheral retinal areas; increased macular recovery time following exposure to a bright light (photo-stress test); loss of foveal reflex.

Retinopathy – The most common visual symptoms attributed to retinopathy are: Reading and seeing difficulties (ie, words, letters, or parts of objects missing); photophobia; blurred distance vision; missing or blacked out areas in the central or peripheral visual field; light flashes and streaks. Retinopathy appears to be dose-related and has occurred within several months (rarely) to several years of daily therapy; a few cases have been reported several years after the drug was discontinued.

Patients with retinal changes may have visual symptoms or may be asymptomatic (with or without visual field changes). Rarely, scotomatous vision or field defects may occur without obvious retinal change. Retinopathy may progress even after the drug is discontinued. In a number of patients, early retinopathy (macular pigmentation sometimes with central field defects) diminished or regressed completely after therapy was discontinued. Paracentral scotoma to red targets ("premaculopathy") is indicative of early retinal dysfunction, which is usually reversible with cessation of therapy.

A small number of cases of retinal changes have occurred in patients who received only hydroxychloroquine. These usually consisted of alteration in retinal pigmentation that was detected on periodic ophthalmologic examination; visual field defects also were present in some. A case of delayed retinopathy has been reported with vision loss starting 1 year after the drug was discontinued.

Other fundus changes – Attenuation of retinal arterioles; fine granular pigmentary disturbances in the peripheral retina; optic disc pallor and atrophy; prominent choroidal patterns in advanced stage.

Visual field defects – Central scotoma with decreased visual acuity; field constriction (rare); pericentral or paracentral scotoma.

➤*Miscellaneous:* Weight loss; lassitude; exacerbation or precipitation of porphyria.

Overdosage

➤*Symptoms:* Toxic symptoms may occur within 30 minutes and consist of headache, drowsiness, visual disturbances, cardiovascular collapse, and convulsions, followed by sudden and early respiratory and cardiac arrest. Electrocardiogram may reveal atrial standstill, nodal rhythm, prolonged intraventricular conduction time, and progressive bradycardia leading to ventricular fibrillation and/or arrest. Rarely, these symptoms occur with lower doses in hypersensitive patients.

HYDROXYCHLOROQUINE SULFATE

►*Treatment:* Treatment is symptomatic and must be prompt, with immediate evacuation of the stomach by emesis or gastric lavage. Treatment includes usual supportive measures. Refer to General Management of Acute Overdosage. Activated charcoal, in a dose at least 5 times the estimated dose ingested, may inhibit further intestinal absorption if introduced by stomach tube after lavage within 30 minutes after ingestion. Control convulsions before attempting gastric lavage. If caused by cerebral stimulation, attempt cautious administration of an ultrashort-acting barbiturate; if caused by anoxia, correct with oxygen, artificial respiration, or, in shock with hypotension, use vasopressor therapy. Perform tracheal intubation or tracheostomy followed by gastric lavage if necessary. Exchange transfusions have been used to reduce the level of the drug in the blood. Closely observe, for at least 6 hours, patients surviving the acute phase who are asymptomatic. Fluids may be forced. Sufficient ammonium chloride (8 g daily in divided doses for adults) administered for a few days will acidify the urine and help promote urinary excretion.

Patient Information

May cause GI upset; instruct patients to take with food or milk.

Instruct patients to notify physician if any of the following occur: Blurring or other vision changes; ringing in the ears or hearing loss; fever; sore throat; unusual bleeding or bruising; unusual pigmentation (blue-black) of the skin; muscle weakness; bleaching or loss of hair; mood or mental changes.

Advise the patient to stop taking this medicine for RA if there is no improvement (reduced joint swelling, increased mobility) within 6 months.

If RA recurs after the medicine has been stopped, this medicine may be resumed or taken on a periodic basis if there are no existing vision problems.

This medicine may cause dizziness. Instruct patients to use caution while driving or performing other tasks requiring alertness, coordination, or physical dexterity.

Lab tests, including eye exams, may be required to monitor therapy. Instruct patients to be sure to keep appointments.

GOLD COMPOUNDS

WARNING

Signs of gold toxicity include the following: Fall in hemoglobin, leukopenia < 4000 WBC/mm^3, granulocytes < 1500/mm^3, platelets < 100,000 to 150,000/mm^3, proteinuria, hematuria, pruritus, rash, stomatitis or persistent diarrhea. Review recommended laboratory work results before instituting therapy and before each injection or written prescription for oral gold. See patient before each injection to determine presence or absence of adverse reactions; some of these can be severe or even fatal. Physicians planning to use gold compounds should be experienced with chrysotherapy and thoroughly familiar with both toxicity and benefits of gold.

Explain the possibility of adverse reactions to patients before starting therapy.

Advise patients to report promptly any toxicity symptoms (see Patient Information).

Indications

►*Rheumatoid arthritis:*

Parenteral – Active early rheumatoid arthritis, both adult and juvenile types (cases not adequately controlled by other anti-inflammatory agents or conservative measures). Use only as one part of therapy program; alone, it is not a complete treatment.

Oral – Management of adults with active classical or definite rheumatoid arthritis (ARA criteria) with insufficient therapeutic response to or intolerant of an adequate trial of full doses of one or more NSAIDs. Add **auranofin** to baseline program; include non-drug therapies.

►*Unlabeled uses:* Alternative or adjuvant to corticosteroids in treatment of pemphigus. For psoriatic arthritis in patients who do not tolerate or respond to NSAIDs.

Actions

►*Pharmacology:* Gold suppresses or prevents, but does not cure, arthritis and synovitis. It is taken up by macrophages, resulting in inhibition of phagocytosis and possibly, lysosomal enzyme activity. Gold decreases concentrations of rheumatoid factor and immunoglobulins. The exact mode of action in rheumatoid arthritis is unknown; however, gold compounds may decrease synovial inflammation and retard cartilage and bone destruction. No substantial evidence exists that gold induces remission of rheumatoid arthritis.

Therapeutic effects from gold compounds occur slowly. Early improvement, often limited to reduction in morning stiffness, may begin after 6 to 8 weeks of treatment with **gold sodium thiomalate**, but beneficial effects may not be observed until after months of therapy. Therapeutic effects from **auranofin** may be seen after 3 to 4 months of treatment, but in some patients, not before 6 months.

►*Pharmacokinetics:* Due to differences in administration routes (IM vs oral), dosage regimens (weekly vs daily), and actual quantity of gold administered to the patient, expect differences in the pharmacokinetic parameters of injectable and oral gold.

Parenteral gold compounds are water soluble. **Aurothioglucose** is an oily suspension; suspension results in delayed IM absorption. Both are similar in biologic and pharmacokinetic behavior.

After initial injection, serum levels of gold rise sharply and decline over the next week. Peak levels of aqueous preparations are higher and decline faster than oily preparations. After a standard weekly dose, considerable individual variation in levels of gold has been found. Small amounts are found in the serum for months after discontinuation.

Although parenteral gold is widely distributed in body tissues, highest concentrations occur in the reticuloendothelial system and in adrenal and renal cortices. Binding of gold to red blood cells from injectable gold compounds is lower compared with **auranofin**-derived gold. Blood to synovial fluid ratios are similar, ≈ 1.7:1, and synovial fluid levels are ≈ 50% of the blood concentrations. No correlation between blood-gold concentrations and safety or efficacy has been established.

Major pharmacokinetic differences are summarized in the table below:

				Pharmacokinetics of Auranofin and Injectable Gold Compounds				
Drug	Gold content (%)	Absorbed (%)	Time to peak (h)	Mean steady-state plasma levels (mcg/mL)	Protein binding (%)	Plasma half-life (days)	Excreted in urine (%)	Excreted in feces (%)
Auranofin	29	25 (15-33)	1-2	0.2-1	60	26 (21-31)	60[1]	85-95
Aurothioglucose	50	nd	4-6	1-5	95-99	3-27 (single dose) 14-40 (3rd dose)	70	30
Gold sodium thiomalate			2-6			up to 168 (11th dose)		

[1] 60% of the absorbed gold (15% of administered dose).   nd – No data.

Contraindications

►*Parenteral:* Hypersensitivity to any component; uncontrolled diabetes mellitus; severe debilitation; renal disease; hepatic dysfunction or history of infectious hepatitis; marked hypertension; uncontrolled CHF; systemic lupus erythematosus; agranulocytosis or hemorrhagic diathesis; blood dyscrasias; patients recently radiated; those with severe toxicity from previous exposure to gold or other heavy metals; urticaria; eczema; colitis; pregnancy (see Warnings).

►*Oral:* A history of any of the following gold-induced disorders: Anaphylactic reactions, necrotizing enterocolitis, pulmonary fibrosis, exfoliative dermatitis, bone marrow aplasia or other severe hematologic disorders; pregnancy (see Warnings).

Warnings

►*Active disease:* When cartilage and bone damage has already occurred, gold cannot reverse structural damage to joints caused by previous disease. The greatest potential benefit occurs in patients with active synovitis, particularly in its early stage.

►*Thrombocytopenia:* Thrombocytopenia has occurred in 1% to 3% of patients treated with **auranofin**, some of whom developed bleeding. It appears peripheral in origin and is usually reversible upon withdrawal. Onset is not related to duration of therapy; its course may be rapid. Monitor platelet counts at least monthly; however, if a precipitous decline in platelets or a platelet count < 100,000/mm^3 occurs or if signs and symptoms of thrombocytopenia (eg, purpura, ecchymoses or petechiae) occur, immediately withdraw auranofin and other therapies; obtain additional platelet counts. Do not reinstate auranofin unless thrombocytopenia resolves and studies show that it was not due to gold therapy.

►*Immediate effects:* Immediate effects following injection, or at any time during therapy include the following: anaphylactic shock, syncope, bradycardia, thickening of the tongue, difficulty swallowing or breathing, and angioneurotic edema. These effects may occur immediately after injection or as late as 10 minutes after injection. If such effects occur, discontinue treatment.

►*Renal / Hepatic function impairment:* Weigh the potential benefits of using **auranofin** in patients with progressive renal disease or significant hepatocellular disease against potential risks of gold toxicity on compromised organ systems and the difficulty in quickly detecting and correctly attributing the toxic effect.

►*Carcinogenesis:* Renal adenomas developed in rats receiving injectable gold at doses higher and more frequent than recommended human doses. Sarcomas at the injection site occurred in some rats.

Studies demonstrated a significant increase in the frequency of renal tubular cell karyomegaly and cytomegaly, renal adenoma, and malignant renal epithelial tumors in animals treated with **auranofin** and **gold sodium thiomalate**.

►*Elderly:* Tolerance to gold usually decreases with advancing age.

►*Pregnancy:* Category C. Gold crosses the placenta. The placenta showed gold deposits; smaller amounts were detected in fetal liver and kidneys.

Gold therapy is usually contraindicated in pregnant patients. Warn the patient about the hazards of becoming pregnant while on gold therapy. Rheumatoid arthritis frequently improves when a patient becomes pregnant. Do not superimpose the potential nephrotoxicity of gold on the increased renal burden which normally occurs in pregnancy. Discontinue therapy upon recognition of pregnancy, if possible. Consider slow excretion of gold and its persistence in body tissues after discontinuing treatment when a woman receiving gold plans to become pregnant.

Animals – **Gold sodium thiomalate** was teratogenic during the organogenic period in small animals when given in doses 140 to 175 times the usual human dose. **Auranofin** showed impaired food intake, decreased maternal and fetal weights, and increased resorptions, abortions, and congenital abnormalities, mainly abdominal defects (eg, gastroschisis, umbilical hernia).

There are no adequate, well controlled studies in pregnant women. Use only when benefits outweigh potential hazards to the fetus.

►*Lactation:* Injectable gold is excreted in breast milk. Following **auranofin** administration, gold is excreted in the milk of rodents; human data are not available. Trace amounts appear in the serum and red blood cells of nursing offspring. This may cause rashes, nephritis, hepatitis and hematologic aberrations in nursing infants. Decide whether to discontinue nursing or to discontinue parenteral gold, taking into account the importance of the drug to the mother. Nursing during auranofin therapy is not recommended. Consider the slow excretion and persistence of gold in the mother even after therapy is discontinued.

►*Children:* Safety and efficacy for use of **aurothioglucose** in children < 6 years of age have not been established. **Auranofin** is not recommended for use in children; safety and efficacy have not been established (however, see Administration and Dosage).

Precautions

►*Monitoring:* Before instituting treatment, rule out pregnancy; perform CBC with differential, platelet, hemoglobin, WBC and erythrocyte counts, urinalysis and renal and liver function tests. Perform urinalysis for protein and sediment changes prior to each injection. Perform CBC, including platelet estimation, before every second injection (every 2 weeks) throughout treatment. Purpura or ecchymoses always require a platelet count. Inquire regarding pruritus, rash, sore mouth, metallic taste and indigestion before each injection. Observe patient at least 15 minutes after each injection. For patients on auranofin, monitor CBC with differential, platelet count and urinalysis at least monthly.

Rapid reduction of hemoglobin, granulocytes < 1500/mm^3, leukopenia < 4000 WBC/mm^3, eosinophilia > 5%, platelets < 100,000 to 150,000/mm^3, albuminuria, hematuria, rash, dermatitis, pruritus, skin eruption, stomatitis, persistent diarrhea, jaundice or petechiae are signs of possible gold toxicity. Do not give additional therapy unless further studies show these abnormalities to be caused by conditions other than gold toxicity. Monitor patients with GI symptoms for GI bleeding (**auranofin**).

►*Proteinuria:*

Auranofin – Proteinuria has developed in 3% to 9% of auranofin patients. If clinically significant proteinuria or microscopic hematuria is found, immediately stop auranofin and other therapies with the potential to cause proteinuria or microscopic hematuria.

Aurothioglucose – Patients with HLA-D locus histocompatibility antigens DRw2 and DRw3 may have a genetic predisposition to develop certain toxic reactions, such as proteinuria, during treatment with gold or D–penicillamine. Use aurothioglucose with caution in patients with compromised cardiovascular or cerebral circulation.

►*Concomitant antirheumatic therapy:* Use of salicylates, NSAIDs and systemic corticosteroids may be continued when parenteral gold therapy is instituted. After improvement begins, slowly discontinue analgesics and NSAIDs as symptoms permit. Do not use penicillamine with gold salts.

►*Nonvasomotor postinjection reaction:* Arthralgia may occur for a day or two after injection; it usually subsides after the first few injections. The mechanism of the transient increase in rheumatic symptoms after gold injection is unknown. These reactions are usually mild, but occasionally may be so severe that treatment is stopped prematurely.

►*Special risk:* Control diabetes mellitus or CHF before gold therapy begins.

Extreme caution is indicated in patients with any of the following: History of blood dyscrasias such as agranulocytopenia or anemia caused by drug sensitivity; allergy or hypersensitivity to medications; skin rash; previous kidney or liver disease; marked hypertension; compromised cerebral or cardiovascular circulation.

Weigh the potential benefits of using auranofin in patients with inflammatory bowel disease, skin rash or history of bone marrow depression against potential risks of gold toxicity on compromised organ systems and the difficulty in quickly detecting and correctly attributing the toxic effect.

Drug Interactions

►*Phenytoin:* One report suggests coadministration with auranofin may increase phenytoin blood levels.

Adverse Reactions

Adverse reactions to gold therapy may occur during treatment or many months after discontinuation. Incidence of toxic reactions is apparently unrelated to gold plasma levels, but may relate to cumulative body content of gold. Higher than conventional dosages may increase occurrence and severity of toxicity. Adverse reactions are most frequent when cumulative dose is 400 to 800 mg (**gold sodium thiomalate**) or 300 to 500 mg (**aurothioglucose**). **Auranofin** appears to cause fewer adverse reactions than injectable gold; however, therapeutic efficacy may also be less.

Adverse Reactions of Oral vs Parenteral Gold (%)		
Adverse reaction	Auranofin (oral gold) (n = 445)	Injectable gold (n = 445)
Diarrhea	42.5	13
Rash	26	39
Stomatitis	13	18
Anemia	3.1	2.7
Elevated liver function tests	1.9	1.7
Leukopenia	1.3	2.2
Proteinuria	0.9	5.4
Thrombocytopenia	0.9	2.2
Pulmonary	0.2	0.2

►*Dermatologic:* Dermatitis is the most common reaction to **injectable gold** and second most common to **auranofin**. Any eruption, especially pruritic, is considered to be a reaction until proven otherwise. Rash, urticaria (auranofin, 1 to 3%) and angioedema (auranofin, < 0.1%) may occur. Pruritus (auranofin, 17%) often exists before dermatitis, and is a warning of reaction. Erythema, and occasionally more severe reactions, such as papular, vesicular and exfoliative dermatitis leading to alopecia and nail shedding, may occur. Chrysiasis (gray-to-blue pigmentation caused by gold deposits in tissues) has occurred, especially on photoexposed areas. Gold dermatitis may be aggravated by exposure to sunlight or an actinic rash may develop.

►*Renal:* Gold may produce a nephrotic syndrome or glomerulitis with proteinuria and hematuria; these are usually relatively mild and subside completely if recognized early and treatment is discontinued. They may become severe and chronic if treatment continues after onset. Acute renal failure secondary to acute tubular necrosis, acute nephritis or degeneration of proximal tubular epithelium may occur; perform regular urinalysis and discontinue treatment immediately if proteinuria or hematuria develop. Hematuria (1% to 3%) and proteinuria (3% to 9%) occur with **auranofin**.

►*Hematologic:*

Auranofin – Thrombocytopenia (with or without purpura), leukopenia, eosinophilia, anemia (1% to 3%); neutropenia (0.1% to 1%); agranulocytosis, pancytopenia, hypoplastic anemia, aplastic anemia, pure red cell aplasia (< 0.1%).

Granulocytopenia; panmyelopathy; hemorrhagic diathesis. Constantly monitor patients throughout treatment for blood dyscrasias of the formed elements of the blood (see Warnings and Precautions). Though rare, these reactions have potentially serious consequences. These reactions may occur separately or in combination at any time during treatment.

►*Hepatic:* Elevated liver enzymes (**auranofin** 1% to 3%), jaundice (auranofin < 0.1%) with or without cholestasis, hepatitis with jaundice, toxic hepatitis, intrahepatic cholestasis.

►*GI:*

Auranofin – Diarrhea/loose stools (50%), generally manageable by reducing the dose (eg, from 6 to 3 mg/day), and only 6% need permanent drug discontinuation; abdominal pain (14%); nausea (10%); anorexia, flatulence, dyspepsia (3% to 9%); constipation, dysgeusia (1% to 3%); GI bleeding, melena, positive stool for occult blood (0.1% to 1%); ulcerative enterocolitis (can be severe or fatal), dysphagia (< 0.1%).

Aurothioglucose – Nausea, vomiting, anorexia, abdominal cramps, ulcerative enterocolitis (can be severe or fatal), colitis (rare).

►*CNS:* Confusion; hallucinations; seizures.

►*Miscellaneous:* Iritis, corneal ulcers and gold deposits in ocular tissues (**gold sodium thiomalate**; rare). These include deposits in the lens or cornea unassociated clinically with eye disorders or visual impairment (**auranofin** incidence < 0.1%). Acute yellow atrophy; encephalitis; immunological destruction of the synovia; EEG abnormalities; peripheral neuropathy (auranofin < 0.1%) with and without fasciculations or neuritis; partial or complete hair loss (auranofin 1% to 3%); fever; headache (aurothioglucose rare); sensorimotor effects (including Guillain-Barre syndrome) and elevated spinal fluid protein have occurred (gold sodium thiomalate rare).

Mucous membranes – Stomatitis, the second most common adverse reaction with **injectable gold**, is also seen with **auranofin** (13%). It may be manifested by shallow ulcers on buccal membranes, on borders of tongue and on palate or in pharynx and may be the only adverse reaction or occur with dermatitis. Diffuse glossitis or gingivitis may develop. Metallic taste may precede these reactions. Careful oral hygiene is important. Inflammation of upper respiratory tract, pharyngitis, gastritis, colitis, tracheitis, vaginitis and rarely, conjunctivitis (auranofin 3% to 9%) have been reported. Glossitis (auranofin 1% to 3%), gingivitis (auranofin 0.1% to 1%) and thickening of the tongue have occurred.

Pulmonary – Pulmonary injury may be shown by gold bronchitis, interstitial pneumonitis (**auranofin** < 0.1%) or fibrosis, fever and partial or complete hair loss.

Nitritoid and allergic (parenteral) – Reactions of the "nitritoid type" may resemble anaphylactoid effects. Flushing, fainting, dizziness and sweating are most frequent. Other symptoms may include nausea, vomiting, malaise, headache and weakness.

Management of adverse reactions – Discontinue immediately if toxic reactions occur. Minor complications (ie, localized dermatitis, mild stomatitis, slight proteinuria) generally require no other therapy and resolve spontaneously with therapy suspension. For mild reactions, it may be sufficient to briefly stop use and then resume with smaller doses. Moderately severe skin and mucous membrane reactions often benefit from topical corticosteroids, oral antihistamines and anesthetic lotions.

If stomatitis or dermatitis become severe or more generalized, systemic corticosteroids (generally, 10 to 40 mg prednisone daily in divided doses) may provide symptomatic relief.

For serious renal, hematologic, pulmonary and enterocolitic complications, use high doses of systemic corticosteroids (40 to 100 mg prednisone daily in divided doses). The duration of corticosteroid treatment varies. Larger doses and a longer treatment period may be required than for dermatologic reactions. Often this treatment may be required for many months because of the slow elimination of gold from the body. Therapy may also be required for months when adverse effects are unusually severe or progressive.

In high-dose gold patients whose serious adverse reactions do not improve with high-dose corticosteroids, or who develop significant steroid-related adverse reactions, a chelating agent may be given to enhance gold excretion (eg, dimercaprol, penicillamine). Monitor patients given dimercaprol carefully; untoward reactions may occur. Corticosteroids and a chelating agent may be coadministered. Adjunctive use of an anabolic steroid with other drugs (eg, dimercaprol, penicillamine, corticosteroids) may contribute to recovery of bone marrow deficiency.

Do not reinstitute after severe or idiosyncratic reactions: After resolution of mild reactions, reduced doses may be given. If test dose of 5 mg is well tolerated, give progressively larger doses (5 to 10 mg increments) at weekly to monthly intervals until 25 to 50 mg is reached.

Overdosage

►Symptoms: Overdosage from too rapid increases in dosing are manifested by rapid appearance of toxic reactions, particularly renal damage (eg, hematuria, proteinuria), and hematologic effects (eg, thrombocytopenia, granulocytopenia). Other toxic effects include fever, nausea, vomiting, diarrhea and skin disorders (eg, papulovesicular lesions, urticaria and exfoliative dermatitis, all with severe pruritus).

Auranofin overdosage – Auranofin overdosage experience is limited. A 50-year-old female took 27 mg daily for 10 days and developed encephalopathy and peripheral neuropathy. Auranofin was discontinued, and she eventually recovered.

►Treatment: Promptly discontinue; give dimercaprol. Use specific supportive therapy for renal/hematologic complications. Refer to General Management of Acute Overdosage. Chelating agents are used with injectable gold; consider their use also for **auranofin** overdosage. In acute overdosage, immediately induce emesis or perform gastric lavage with supportive therapy.

Patient Information

Patient package insert is available with **auranofin**.

Notify physician of the following: Itching, rash, sore mouth, indigestion, metallic taste, easy bruising or nosebleed.

Increased joint pain may continue 1 or 2 days after an injection and usually subsides after the first few injections.

Chrysiasis (gray-to-blue pigmentation) may occur, especially on photo-exposed areas. Minimize exposure to sunlight or artificial ultraviolet light.

Observe careful oral hygiene in conjunction with therapy.

Warn women of childbearing potential of the risks of using gold therapy during pregnancy.

AURANOFIN (29% Gold)

Rx	Ridaura (SK-Beecham)	**Capsules:** 3 mg	(Ridaura SKF). Tan and brown. In 60s.

For complete prescribing information, refer to the Gold Compounds group monograph.

Administration and Dosage

►Adults: 6 mg daily, either as 3 mg twice daily or 6 mg once daily. Initiating dosages> 6 mg/day is not recommended; it is associated with increased incidence of diarrhea. If response is inadequate after 6 months, an increase to 9 mg/day (3 mg 3 times/day) may be tolerated. If response remains inadequate after 3 months of 9 mg/day, discontinue. Safety at doses > 9 mg/day has not been studied.

Transfer from injectable gold – Discontinue the injectable agent and start auranofin with 6 mg daily. At 6 months, control of disease activity of patients transferred to auranofin and those maintained on the injectable agent was not different.

►Children: The following doses have been recommended.

Initial – 0.1 mg/kg/day.

Maintenance – 0.15 mg/kg/day.

Maximum dose – 0.2 mg/kg/day.

AUROTHIOGLUCOSE (≈ 50% Gold)

Rx	Solganal (Schering)	**Injection Suspension:** 50 mg/ml[1]	In 10 ml vials.

[1] In sesame oil with 2% aluminum monostearate and 1 mg propylparaben.

For complete prescribing information, refer to the Gold Compounds group monograph.

Administration and Dosage

Administer only by IM injection, preferably intragluteally, using an 18-gauge, 1½ inch needle. For obese patients, an 18-gauge, 2 inch needle may be used.

►Adults:

Weekly injections – First dose, 10 mg; second and third doses, 25 mg; fourth and subsequent doses, 50 mg. Continue the 50 mg dose at weekly intervals until 0.8 to 1 g has been given. If the patient has improved and has no signs of toxicity, continue the 50 mg dose many months longer, at 3 to 4 week intervals. A weekly dose above 50 mg is usually unnecessary and contraindicated; tend toward lower dosage. A 25 mg dose may be the dose of choice. If no improvement is demonstrated after a total administration of 1 g, reevaluate the necessity of gold therapy.

►Children (6 to 12 years): One-fourth the adult dose, governed by body weight, not to exceed 25 mg per dose. Patient should remain recumbent ≈ 10 minutes after injection. Observe patient at least 15 minutes after each injection.

GOLD SODIUM THIOMALATE ($\approx$ 50% Gold)

Rx	**Aurolate** (Pasadena)	**Injection**: 50 mg/ml[1]	In 2 and 10 ml vials.
Rx	**Myochrysine** (Taylor)		In 2 and 10 ml vials.

[1] With 0.5% benzyl alcohol.

For complete prescribing information, refer to the Gold Compounds group monograph.

Administration and Dosage

Administer only by IM injection, preferably intragluteally. Have patient remain recumbent for $\approx$ 10 minutes after injection.

► *Adults:* For the average size adult, the following dosage schedule is recommended:

Weekly injections – First injection, 10 mg; second injection, 25 mg; third and subsequent injections, 25 to 50 mg until major clinical improvement or toxicity occurs, or until the cumulative dose reaches 1 g. If significant clinical improvement occurs before a cumulative dose of 1 g has been administered, the dose may be decreased or the interval between injections increased as with maintenance therapy.

Maintenance – 25 to 50 mg every other week for 2 to 20 weeks. If the clinical course remains stable, give 25 to 50 mg every third and subsequently every fourth week indefinitely. Some patients may require maintenance intervals of 1 to 3 weeks. Should arthritis exacerbate during maintenance, resume weekly injections temporarily until disease activity is suppressed.

Should a patient fail to improve during initial therapy (cumulative dose of 1 g), several options are available: Discontinue the drug, continue the same dose (25 to 50 mg) for $\approx$ 10 additional weeks or increase the dose by increments of 10 mg every 1 to 4 weeks, not to exceed 100 mg in a single injection.

If significant clinical improvement occurs using the second or third option, initiate the maintenance schedule described above. If there is no significant improvement or if toxicity occurs, discontinue therapy. The higher the individual dose, the greater the risk of toxicity. Base selection of these options on several factors, including the physician's experience with gold therapy, the course of the patient's condition, the choice of alternative treatments and patient availability for close supervision.

► *Children:* The pediatric dose is proportional to the adult dose on a weight basis. After the initial test dose of 10 mg, give 1 mg/kg, not to exceed 50 mg for a single injection. Otherwise, adult guidelines apply.

Other doses recommended are as follows: Initial, 0.25 mg/kg/dose (one dose); incremental dose increases of 0.25 mg/kg/dose may be used, increasing with each weekly dose; maintenance dose is 1 mg/kg/dose weekly for a total of 20 doses, then every 2 to 4 weeks, using the longest interval consistent with remission.

► *Storage / Stability:* Do not use if material has darkened. Color should not exceed pale yellow.

METHOTREXATE (Amethopterin; MTX)

Rx	**Methotrexate** (Various, eg, Major, Roxane, UDL)	**Tablets:** 2.5 mg (as sodium)	In 36s and 100s.
Rx	**Rheumatrex Dose Pack** (STADA Pharm)		(LL/M1). Yellow, scored. 4 cards, each w/ 2, 3, 4, 5 or 6 tablets, ie, 5, 7.5, 10, 12.5 or 15 mg/week.
Rx	**Trexall** (Barr)	**Tablets:** 5 mg	Lactose. (b 927/5). Green, oval, scored. Film-coated. In 30s, 60s, and 100s.
		7.5 mg	Lactose. (b 928/7 1/2). Blue, oval, scored. Film-coated. In 30s, 60s, and 100s.
		10 mg	Lactose. (b 929/10). Pink, oval, scored. Film-coated. In 30s, 60s, and 100s.
		15 mg	Lactose. (b 945/15). Purple, oval, scored. Film-coated. In 30s, 60s, and 100s.

This is an abbreviated monograph. For complete prescribing information and use of methotrexate as an antineoplastic agent, see Methotrexate Antimetabolite monograph in the Antineoplastics chapter.

WARNING

Severe reactions: Because of the possibility of severe toxic reactions, fully inform patient of the risks involved and assure constant supervision.

Deaths: Deaths have occurred with the use of methotrexate.

In rheumatoid arthritis treatment: Restrict use to patients with severe, recalcitrant, disabling disease, which is not adequately responsive to other forms of therapy, and only after established diagnosis and appropriate consultation.

Pregnancy: Fetal death or congenital anomalies have occurred; do not use in women of childbearing potential unless benefits outweigh possible risks. Pregnant rheumatoid arthritis patients should not receive methotrexate.

Periodic monitoring: Periodic monitoring for toxicity, including CBC with differential and platelet counts, and liver and renal function tests is mandatory. Periodic liver biopsies may be indicated in some situations. Monitor patients at increased risk for impaired methotrexate elimination (eg, renal dysfunction, pleural effusions or ascites) more frequently.

Liver: Methotrexate causes hepatotoxicity, fibrosis and cirrhosis, but generally only after prolonged use. Acutely, liver enzyme elevations are frequent, usually transient and asymptomatic, and also do not appear predictive of subsequent hepatic disease. Liver biopsy after sustained use often shows histologic changes, and fibrosis and cirrhosis have been reported; these latter lesions often are not preceded by symptoms or abnormal liver function tests. Periodic liver biopsies are usually recommended for patients under long-term treatment. Persistent abnormalities in liver function tests may precede appearance of fibrosis or cirrhosis in the rheumatoid arthritis population.

Methotrexate-induced lung disease: Methotrexate-induced lung disease, a potentially dangerous lesion, may occur acutely at any time during therapy and has been reported at doses as low as 7.5 mg/week. It is not always fully reversible. Pulmonary symptoms (especially a dry, nonproductive cough) may require treatment interruption and careful investigation.

Marked bone marrow depression: Marked bone marrow depression may occur, with resultant anemia, leukopenia or thrombocytopenia.

Unexpectedly severe (sometimes fatal) marrow suppression, aplastic anemia, and GI toxicity have been reported with coadministration of methotrexate (usually in high dosage) and some NSAIDs.

GI: Diarrhea and ulcerative stomatitis require interruption of therapy; hemorrhagic enteritis and death from intestinal perforation may occur.

Renal use: Use methotrexate in patients with impaired renal function with extreme caution, and at reduced dosages, because renal dysfunction will prolong elimination.

Severe skin reactions: Severe, occasionally fatal skin reactions have been reported following single or multiple doses of methotrexate. Reactions have occurred within days of oral methotrexate administration. Recovery has been reported with discontinuation of therapy.

Opportunistic infections: Potentially fatal opportunistic infections, especially *Pneumocystis carinii* pneumonia, may occur with methotrexate therapy.

Radiotherapy: Methotrexate given concomitantly with radiotherapy may increase the risk of soft tissue necrosis and osteonecrosis.

Indications

➤*Severe, active, classical or definite adult rheumatoid arthritis:* (ACR criteria) in selected adults who have had an insufficient therapeutic response to, or are intolerant of, an adequate trial of first line therapy including full dose NSAIDs.

➤*Polyarticular-course juvenile rheumatoid arthritis (JRA):* Methotrexate is indicated in the management of children with active polyarticular-course JRA who have had an insufficient therapeutic response to, or are intolerant of, an adequate trial of first-line therapy including full-dose NSAIDs.

Administration and Dosage

The patient should be fully informed of the risks involved and should be under constant supervision of the physician. Assessment of hematologic, hepatic, renal, and pulmonary function should be made by history, physical examination, and laboratory tests before beginning, periodically during, and before reinstituting methotrexate therapy. Appropriate steps should be taken to avoid conception during methotrexate therapy.

Weekly therapy may be instituted with the *Rheumatrex Dose Packs,* which are designed to provide doses over a range of 5 to 15 mg administered as a single weekly dose. The dose packs are not recommended for administration of methotrexate in weekly doses greater than 15 mg. All schedules should be continually tailored to the individual patient. An initial test dose may be given prior to the regular dosing schedule to detect any extreme sensitivity to adverse effects. Maximal myelosuppression usually occurs in 7 to 10 days.

➤*Adult RA:*

Starting dose – Single oral doses of 7.5 mg/week or divided oral dosages of 2.5 mg at 12 hour intervals for 3 doses given as a course once weekly.

Therapeutic response usually begins within 3 to 6 weeks and the patient may continue to improve for another 12 weeks or more.

➤*Polyarticular-course JRA:*

Starting dose – The recommended starting dose is 10 mg/m² given once weekly.

Therapeutic response usually begins within 3 to 6 weeks and the patient may continue to improve for another 12 weeks or more.

➤*Duration of therapy:* Optimal duration of therapy is unknown. Limited data from long-term studies in adults indicate that initial clinical improvement is maintained at least 2 years with continued therapy. When methotrexate is discontinued, the arthritis usually worsens within 3 to 6 weeks.

➤*Dose adjustment:* For either adult RA or polyarticular-course JRA, dosages may be adjusted gradually to achieve an optimal response. Limited experience shows a significant increase in the incidence and severity of serious toxic reactions, especially bone marrow suppression at doses greater than 20 mg/week in adults. Although there is experience with doses up to 30 mg/m²/week in children, there are too few published data to assess how doses over 20 mg/m²/week might affect the risk of serious toxicity in children. Experience does suggest, however, that children receiving 20 to 30 mg/m²/week (0.65 to 1 mg/kg/week) may have better absorption and fewer GI side effects if methotrexate is administered either IM or SC.

➤*Concomitant therapy:* Aspirin, NSAIDs, and/or low dose steroids may be continued, although the possibility of increased toxicity with concomitant use of NSAIDs including salicylates has not been fully explored. Steroids may be reduced gradually in patients who respond to methotrexate. Combined use of methotrexate with gold, penicillamine, hydroxychloroquine, sulfasalazine, or cytotoxic agents has not been studied and may increase the incidence of adverse effects. Note that the doses used in RA (7.5 to 15 mg/week) are somewhat lower than those used in psoriasis and that larger doses could lead to toxicity. Rest and physiotherapy as indicated should be continued.

➤*Storage/Stability:* Store at controlled room temperature (20° to 25°C; 68° to 77°F); excursions permitted to 15° to 30°C (59° to 86°F). Protect from light.

Actions

➤*Pharmacology:* The mechanism of action in rheumatoid arthritis is unknown; it may affect immune function. Two reports describe in vitro methotrexate inhibition of DNA precursor uptake by stimulated mononuclear cells and another (in animals) describes polyarthritis partial correction by methotrexate of spleen cell hyporesponsiveness and suppressed interleukin-2 production. Other laboratories, however, have been unable to demonstrate similar effects. Clarification of its effect on immune activity and its relation to rheumatoid immunopathogenesis await further studies.

In patients with rheumatoid arthritis, effects of methotrexate on articular swelling and tenderness can be seen as early as 3 to 6 weeks. Although methotrexate clearly ameliorates symptoms of inflammation (pain, swelling, stiffness), there is no evidence that it induces remission of rheumatoid arthritis nor has a beneficial effect been demonstrated on bone erosions and other radiologic changes which result in impaired joint use, functional disability and deformity.

METHOTREXATE (Amethopterin; MTX)

Most studies of methotrexate in patients with rheumatoid arthritis are relatively short term (3 to 6 months). Limited data from long-term studies indicate that an initial clinical improvement is maintained for at least 2 years with continued therapy.

Contraindications

Pregnant and nursing patients (see Warnings); alcoholism, alcoholic liver disease or other chronic liver disease; overt or laboratory evidence of immunodeficiency syndromes; pre-existing blood dyscrasias, such as bone marrow hypoplasia, leukopenia, thrombocytopenia or significant anemia; hypersensitivity to methotrexate.

Warnings

▶*Pregnancy: Category X.* Methotrexate can cause fetal death or teratogenic effects when administered to a pregnant woman and is contraindicated in pregnant patients with rheumatoid arthritis. Women of childbearing potential should not be started on methotrexate until pregnancy is excluded and should be fully counseled on the serious risk to the fetus should they become pregnant while undergoing treatment. Avoid pregnancy if either partner is receiving methotrexate: During and for a minimum of 3 months after therapy for male patients, and during and for at least one ovulatory cycle after therapy for female patients.

▶*Lactation:* Because of the potential for serious adverse reactions from methotrexate in breastfed infants, it is contraindicated in nursing mothers.

▶*Children:* Safety and efficacy in children have been established only in cancer chemotherapy and in polyarticular-course JRA.

Published clinical studies evaluating the use of methotrexate in children and adolescents 2 to 16 years of age with JRA demonstrated safety comparable to that observed in adults with RA.

Precautions

▶*Monitoring:* Monitor hematology at least monthly, and liver and renal function every 1 to 2 months during therapy. During initial or changing doses, or periods of increased risk of elevated methotrexate blood levels (eg, dehydration), more frequent monitoring may be indicated. Stop methotrexate immediately if there is a significant drop in blood counts.

Transient liver function test abnormalities are observed frequently after methotrexate administration and are usually not cause for modification of methotrexate therapy. Persistent liver function test abnormalities and/or depression of serum albumin may be indicators of serious liver toxicity and require evaluation.

▶*Weekly dose:* Physicians and pharmacists should emphasize that the dose is taken weekly. Mistaken daily use has led to fatal toxicity. Encourage patients to read the Patient Instructions in the Dose Pack. Do not write or refill prescriptions on a PRN basis.

Adverse Reactions

▶*Adult rheumatoid arthritis:* Elevated liver function tests (15%); nausea/vomiting (10%); thrombocytopenia (platelet count < 100,000/mm^3), stomatitis (3% to 10%); rash/pruritus/dermatitis, diarrhea, alopecia, leukopenia (WBC < 3000/mm^3), pancytopenia, dizziness (1% to 3%).

Other less common reactions included the following: Decreased hematocrit; headache; upper respiratory infection; anorexia; arthralgias; chest pain; coughing; dysuria; eye discomfort; epistaxis; fever; infection; sweating; tinnitus; vaginal discharge.

Almost all of these patients were on concomitant NSAIDs and some were also taking low dosages of corticosteroids.

▶*Polyarticular-course JRA:* Pediatric patients with JRA treated with oral, weekly doses of methotrexate (5 to 20 mg/m^2/week or 0.1 to 0.65 mg/kg/week) were as follows (virtually all patients were receiving concomitant NSAIDs, and some also were taking low doses of corticosteroids): Elevated liver function tests (14%); GI reactions (eg, nausea, vomiting, diarrhea) (11%); stomatitis, leukopenia (2%); headache (1.2%); alopecia (0.5%); dizziness, rash (0.2%).

SULFASALAZINE

Rx	**Sulfasalazine** (Various, eg, Mutual Pharm, Major, Watson)	**Tablets:** 500 mg	In 50s, 100s, 500s, and 1000s.
Rx	**Azulfidine** (Pharmacia & Upjohn)		(101 KPh). Gold, scored. In 100s, 300s, and UD 100s.
Rx	**Azulfidine EN-tabs** (Pharmacia & Upjohn)	**Tablets, delayed-release:** 500 mg	(102 KPh). Gold, elliptical. Enteric coated. In 100s and 300s.

Sulfasalazine is also indicated for use in ulcerative colitis. Refer to the monograph in the GI chapter.

Indications

▶*Ulcerative colitis:* For complete prescribing information, refer to the monograph in the GI chapter. In the treatment of mild-to-moderate ulcerative colitis, and as adjunctive therapy in severe ulcerative colitis; for the prolongation of the remission period between acute attacks of ulcerative colitis.

▶*Rheumatoid arthritis (RA; enteric-coated tablets):* In the treatment of patients with RA who have responded inadequately to salicylates or other nonsteroidal anti-inflammatory drugs (NSAIDs).

▶*Juvenile rheumatoid arthritis (JRA; enteric-coated tablets):* In the treatment of pediatric patients ≥ 6 years of age with polyarticular-course JRA who have responded inadequately to salicylates or other NSAIDs.

▶*Unlabeled uses:* Ankylosing spondylitis; Crohn's disease; psoriatic arthritis (2 g/day).

Administration and Dosage

Individualize dosage. Give the drug in evenly divided doses over each 24-hour period; intervals between nighttime doses should not exceed 8 hours, with administration after meals recommended when feasible. Swallow tablets whole; do not crush or chew. Experience suggests that with daily dosages of ≥ 4 g, the incidence of adverse effects tends to increase. Instruct patients receiving these dosages about the appearance of adverse effects, and carefully observe patients for these effects.

Some patients may be sensitive to treatment with sulfasalazine. Various desensitization-like regimens have been reported to be effective. These regimens suggest starting with a total daily dose of 50 to 250 mg initially, and doubling it every 4 to 7 days until the desired therapeutic level is achieved. If the symptoms of sensitivity recur, discontinue sulfasalazine. Do not attempt desensitization in patients who have a history of agranulocytosis, or who have experienced an anaphylactoid reaction while previously receiving sulfasalazine.

▶*Adult RA:* 2 g daily in 2 evenly divided doses. It is advisable to initiate therapy with a lower dosage (eg, 0.5 to 1 g daily) to reduce possible GI intolerance. A suggested dosing schedule is given below.

In RA, the effect of sulfasalazine delayed-release tablets can be assessed by the degree of improvement in the number and extent of actively inflamed joints.

Adult RA Sulfasalazine Dosing Schedule		
	Number of delayed-release tablets	
Week of treatment	Morning	Evening
1	—	1
2	1	1
3	1	2
4	2	2

A therapeutic response has been observed as early as 4 weeks after starting treatment, but treatment for 12 weeks may be required in some patients before clinical benefit is noted. Give consideration to increasing the daily dose to 3 g if the clinical response after 12 weeks is inadequate. Careful monitoring is recommended for doses > 2 g/day.

▶*JRA-polyarticular course:*

Children ≥ 6 years of age – 30 to 50 mg/kg of body weight daily in 2 evenly divided doses. Typically, the maximum dose is 2 g/day. To reduce possible GI intolerance, begin with a quarter to a third of the planned maintenance dose and increase weekly until reaching the maintenance dose at 1 month.

Desensitization – Some patients may be sensitive to treatment. These regimens suggest starting with a total daily dose of 50 to 250 mg initially, and doubling it every 4 to 7 days until the desired therapeutic level is achieved. Discontinue if the symptoms of sensitivity recur. Do not attempt desensitization in patients who have a history of agranulocytosis or who have experienced an anaphylactoid reaction while previously receiving sulfasalazine.

Actions

▶*Pharmacology:* The mode of action of sulfasalazine or its metabolites, 5-aminosalicyclic acid (5-ASA) and sulfapyridine (SP), is still under investigation, but may be related to the anti-inflammatory or immunomodulatory properties that have been observed in animals and in vitro, to its affinity for connective tissue, or to the relatively high concentration it reaches in serous fluids, the liver, and intestinal walls. In ulcerative colitis, clinical studies utilizing rectal administration of sulfasalazine, SP, and 5-ASA have indicated the major therapeutic action may reside in the 5-ASA moiety. The relative contribution of the parent drug and the major metabolites in RA is unknown.

SULFASALAZINE

▶*Pharmacokinetics:*

Absorption – The absolute bioavailability of orally administered sulfasalazine is < 15% for parent drug. In the intestine, sulfasalazine is metabolized by intestinal bacteria to SP and 5-ASA. Of the two, SP is relatively well absorbed from the colon and highly metabolized with an estimated bioavailability of 60%. 5-ASA is much less well absorbed with an estimated bioavailability of 10% to 30%. Detectable serum concentrations of sulfasalazine have been found in healthy subjects within 90 minutes after the dose. In comparison, peak plasma levels of both SP and 5-ASA occur ≈ 10 hours after dosing.

Distribution – Following IV injection, the calculated volume of distribution (Vd_{ss}) for sulfasalazine was ≈ 7.5 L. Sulfasalazine is highly bound to albumin (> 99.3%), while SP is only ≈ 70% bound to albumin. Acetylsulfapyridine (AcSP), the principal metabolite of SP, is ≈ 90% bound to plasma proteins.

Metabolism – The observed plasma half-life for IV sulfasalazine is 7.6 hours. The primary route of metabolism of SP is via acetylation to form AcSP. The rate of metabolism of SP to AcSP is dependent on acetylator phenotype. In fast acetylators, the mean plasma half-life of SP is 10.4 hours, while in slow acetylators it is 14.8 hours. SP can also be metabolized to 5-hydroxy-sulfapyridine (SPOH) and N-acetyl-5-hydroxy-sulfapyridine. 5-ASA is primarily metabolized in both the liver and intestine to N-acetyl-5-aminosalicylic acid via a non-acetylation-phenotype-dependent route. Because of low plasma levels produced by 5-ASA after oral administration, reliable estimates of plasma half-life are not possible.

Excretion – Absorbed SP and 5-ASA and their metabolites are primarily eliminated in the urine either as free metabolites or as glucuronide conjugates. The majority of 5-ASA stays within the colonic lumen and is excreted as 5-ASA and acetyl-5-ASA with the feces. The calculated clearance of sulfasalazine following IV administration was 1 L/hour. Renal clearance was estimated to account for 37% of total clearance.

Elderly – Elderly patients with RA showed a prolonged plasma half-life for sulfasalazine, SP, and their metabolites.

Fast / Slow acetylators – The metabolism of SP to AcSP is mediated by polymorphic enzymes such that two distinct populations of slow and fast metabolizers exist. Approximately 60% of the white population can be classified as belonging to the slow acetylator phenotype. These subjects will display a prolonged plasma half-life for SP (14.8 vs 10.4 hours) and an accumulation of higher plasma levels of SP than fast acetylators. Subjects who were slow acetylators of SP showed a higher incidence of adverse events.

Contraindications

Pediatric patients < 2 years of age; intestinal or urinary obstruction; porphyria; hypersensitivity to sulfasalazine, its metabolites, salicylates, or sulfonamides.

Warnings

▶*Porphyria:* Do not administer sulfonamides to patients with porphyria as these drugs have been reported to precipitate an acute attack.

▶*GI intolerance:* Sulfasalazine enteric-coated tablets are indicated in patients with ulcerative colitis who cannot take uncoated sulfasalazine tablets because of GI intolerance, and in whom there is evidence that this intolerance is not primarily the result of high blood levels of sulfapyridine and its metabolites (eg, patients experiencing nausea and vomiting with the first few doses of the drug, or patients in whom a reduction in dosage does not alleviate the adverse GI effects).

▶*Special risk patients:* The presence of clinical signs such as sore throat, fever, pallor, purpura, or jaundice may be indications of serious blood disorders. Use with caution in patients with severe allergy or bronchial asthma.

▶*Deaths:* Deaths associated with the administration of sulfasalazine have been reported from hypersensitivity reactions, agranulocytosis, aplastic anemia, other blood dyscrasias, renal and liver damage, irreversible neuromuscular and CNS changes, and fibrosing alveolitis. If toxic or hypersensitivity reactions occur, discontinue sulfasalazine immediately.

▶*Renal / Hepatic function impairment:* Only after critical appraisal should sulfasalazine be given to patients with hepatic or renal damage or blood dyscrasias.

▶*Carcinogenesis:* Sulfasalazine was tested at 84, 168 and 337.5 mg/kg/day doses in rats. A statistically significant increase in the incidence of urinary bladder transitional cell papillomas was observed in male rats. In female rats, two (4%) of the 337.5 mg/kg rats had transitional cell papilloma of the kidney. The increased incidence of neoplasms in the urinary bladder and kidney of rats was also associated with an increase in the renal calculi formation and hyperplasia of transitional cell epithelium. For the mouse study, sulfasalazine was tested at 675, 1350 and 2700 mg/kg/day. The incidence of hepatocellular adenoma or carcinoma in male and female mice was significantly greater than the control at all doses tested.

▶*Fertility impairment:* Oligospermia and infertility have been observed in men treated with sulfasalazine. Withdrawal of the drug appears to reverse these effects.

▶*Pregnancy: Category B.* There are no adequate and well-controlled studies in pregnant women. Use during pregnancy only if clearly needed.

A national survey evaluated the outcome of pregnancies associated with inflammatory bowel disease (IBD). In 186 pregnancies in women treated with sulfasalazine alone or sulfasalazine and concomitant steroid therapy, the incidence of fetal morbidity and mortality was comparable both to that of 245 untreated IBD pregnancies and to pregnancies in the general population.

A study of 1455 pregnancies associated with exposure to sulfonamides, including sulfasalazine, indicated that the group of drugs was not associated with fetal malformation. A review of the medical literature covering 1155 pregnancies in women with ulcerative colitis suggested that the outcome was similar to that expected in the general population.

Sulfasalazine and sulfapyridine pass the placental barrier. Although sulfapyridine has been shown to have poor bilirubin-displacing capacity, there is potential for kernicterus.

▶*Lactation:* Sulfonamides are excreted in breast milk. In newborns, they compete with bilirubin for binding sites on the plasma proteins and may cause kernicterus. Insignificant amounts of uncleaved sulfasalazine have been found in breast milk, whereas the sulfapyridine levels in breast milk are ≈ 30% to 60% of those in the maternal serum. Sulfapyridine has been shown to have a poor bilirubin-displacing capacity. Exercise caution.

▶*Children:* The safety and efficacy of sulfasalazine in pediatric patients < 2 years of age with ulcerative colitis have not been established. It has been reported that the frequency of adverse events in patients with systemic-course juvenile arthritis is high.

Precautions

▶*Monitoring:* Perform complete blood counts, including differential white cell count, and liver function tests before starting sulfasalazine and every second week during the first 3 months of therapy. During the second 3 months, perform the same tests once monthly and, thereafter, once every 3 months and as clinically indicated. Also perform urinalysis and an assessment of renal function periodically during treatment.

The determination of serum sulfapyridine levels may be useful because concentrations > 50 mcg/ml appear to be associated with an increased incidence of adverse reactions.

▶*RA:* RA rarely remits. Therefore, continued administration of sulfasalazine enteric-coated tablets as needed.

▶*Glucose-6-phosphate dehydrogenase deficiency:* Observe patients with glucose-6-phosphate dehydrogenase deficiency closely for signs of hemolytic anemia. This reaction is frequently dose-related.

▶*Undisintegrated tablets:* Isolated instances have occurred where sulfasalazine enteric-coated tablets have passed undisintegrated. If this is observed, discontinue the administration of the drug immediately.

▶*Adequate fluid intake:* Maintain adequate fluid intake in order to prevent crystalluria and stone formation.

Drug Interactions

Sulfasalazine Drug Interactions			
Precipitant drug	Object drug*		Description
Sulfasalazine	Digoxin	↓	Reduced absorption of digoxin has been reported when coadministered with sulfasalazine.
Sulfasalazine	Folic acid	↓	Reduced GI absorption of folic acid has been reported when coadministered with sulfasalazine. Periodically monitor patients taking sulfasalazine. If folate deficiency is noted, potential treatment measures include increasing dietary folate, giving sulfasalazine between meals, and administering additional folic acid or folinic acid.
Sulfonamides (eg, sulfasalazine)	Sulfonylureas (eg, glipizide)	↑	Sulfonamides may impair hepatic metabolism of sulfonylureas or alter plasma protein binding. Monitor blood glucose and decrease the sulfonylurea dose as necessary.

* ↑ = Object drug increased.   ↓ = Object drug decreased.

Adverse Reactions

The most common adverse reactions associated with sulfasalazine in ulcerative colitis are anorexia, headache, nausea, vomiting, gastric distress, and reversible oligospermia. These occur in ≈ 33% of patients. Less frequent adverse reactions are skin rash, pruritus, urticaria, fever, Heinz body anemia, hemolytic anemia, and cyanosis, which may occur at a frequency of ≤ 1 in 30 patients.

Similar adverse reactions are associated with use in adult RA, although there was a greater incidence of some reactions. In RA studies, the following common adverse reactions were noted: Nausea (19%); dyspep-

SULFASALAZINE

sia, rash (13%); headache (9%); abdominal pain, vomiting (8%); fever (5%); dizziness, stomatitis, pruritus, abnormal liver function tests (4%); leukopenia (3%); thrombocytopenia (1%). One report showed a 10% rate of immunoglobulin suppression, which was slowly reversible and rarely accompanied by clinical findings.

The following adverse reactions occur rarely ($\approx \leq 1$ in 1000 patients).

➤*CNS:* Transverse myelitis; convulsions; meningitis; transient lesions of the posterior spinal column; cauda equina syndrome; Guillain-Barré syndrome; peripheral neuropathy; mental depression; vertigo; hearing loss; insomnia; ataxia; hallucinations; tinnitus; drowsiness.

➤*GI:* Hepatitis; pancreatitis; bloody diarrhea; impaired folic acid absorption; impaired digoxin absorption; stomatitis; diarrhea; abdominal pains; neutropenic enterocolitis.

➤*Hematologic:* Aplastic anemia; agranulocytosis; leukopenia; megaloblastic (macrocytic) anemia; purpura; thrombocytopenia; hypoprothrombinemia; methemoglobinemia; congenital neutropenia; myelodysplastic syndrome.

➤*Hypersensitivity:* Erythema multiforme (Stevens-Johnson syndrome); exfoliative dermatitis; epidermal necrolysis (Lyell's syndrome) with corneal damage; anaphylaxis; serum sickness syndrome; pneumonitis with or without eosinophilia; vasculitis; fibrosing alveolitis; pleuritis; pericarditis with or without tamponade; allergic myocarditis; polyarteritis nodosa; lupus erythematosus-like syndrome; hepatitis and hepatic necrosis with or without immune complexes; fulminant hepatitis, sometimes leading to liver transplantation; parapsoriasis varioformis acuta (Mucha-Haberman syndrome); rhabdomyolysis; photosensitization; arthralgia; periorbital edema; conjunctival and scleral injection; alopecia.

➤*Renal:* Toxic nephrosis with oliguria and anuria; nephritis; nephrotic syndrome; hematuria; crystalluria; proteinuria; hemolytic-uremic syndrome.

➤*Miscellaneous:* Urine discoloration; skin discoloration.

Children – In general, the adverse reactions in JRA patients are similar to those seen in patients with adult RA except for a high frequency of serum sickness-like syndrome in systemic-course JRA.

Overdosage

➤*Symptoms:* Symptoms of overdosage may include nausea, vomiting, gastric distress, and abdominal pains. In more advanced cases, CNS symptoms (eg, drowsiness, convulsions) may be observed. Serum sulfapyridine concentrations may be used to monitor the progress of recovery from overdosage. Doses of regular sulfasalazine tablets of 16 g/day have been given to patients without mortality.

➤*Treatment:* Gastric lavage or emesis plus catharsis as indicated. Alkalinize urine. If kidney function is normal, force fluids. If anuria is present, restrict fluids and salt, and treat appropriately. Catheterization of the ureters may be indicated for complete renal blockage by crystals. The low molecular weight of sulfasalazine and its metabolites may facilitate their removal by dialysis. For agranulocytosis, discontinue the drug immediately, hospitalize the patient, and institute appropriate therapy.

Patient Information

If sore throat, fever, pallor, purpura, or jaundice occur, have patients contact their physician.

Instruct patients to take sulfasalazine in evenly divided doses, preferably after meals, and to swallow the tablets whole.

Advise patients that sulfasalazine may produce an orange-yellow discoloration of the urine or skin.

Instruct patients to drink plenty of water.

LEFLUNOMIDE

Rx	Arava (Hoechst Marion Roussel)	**Tablets:** 10 mg	Lactose. (ZBN). White. Film coated. In 30s and 100s.
		20 mg	Lactose, yellow ferric oxide. (ZBO). Light yellow, triangular. Film coated. In 30s and 100s.
		100 mg	Lactose. (ZBP). White. Film coated. In 3-count blister packs.

WARNING

Pregnancy must be excluded before the start of treatment with leflunomide. It is contraindicated in pregnant women, or women of childbearing potential who are not using reliable contraception (see Warnings). Pregnancy must be avoided during leflunomide treatment or prior to the completion of the drug elimination procedure after treatment.

Indications

➤*Rheumatoid arthritis (RA):* Treatment of active RA in adults to reduce signs and symptoms and to retard structural damage as evidenced by x-ray erosions and joint space narrowing.

Administration and Dosage

➤*Approved by the FDA:* September 10, 1998.

➤*RA:*

Loading dose – Initiate therapy with a single oral 100 mg/day dose for 3 days.

Maintenance therapy – 20 mg/day; doses > 20 mg/day are not recommended due to greater incidence of side effects. If dosing at 20 mg/day is not well tolerated clinically, the dose may be decreased to 10 mg/day.

Monitor liver enzymes; dose adjustments may be necessary (see Warnings, Hepatotoxicity). Due to the prolonged half-life of the active metabolite of leflunomide, observe patients carefully after dose reduction since it may take several weeks for metabolite levels to decline.

➤*Drug elimination procedure:* The following drug elimination procedure is recommended to achieve nondetectable plasma levels < 0.02 mg/L (0.02 mcg/ml) after stopping treatment with leflunomide:
1.) Administer cholestyramine 8 g 3 times daily for 11 days. (The 11 days do not need to be consecutive unless there is a need to lower the plasma level rapidly.)
2.) Verify plasma levels < 0.02 mg/L (0.02 mcg/ml) by 2 separate tests at least 14 days apart. If plasma levels are > 0.02 mg/L, consider additional cholestyramine treatment.

Without the drug elimination procedure, it may take ≤ 2 years to reach plasma M1 metabolite levels < 0.02 mg/L due to individual variation in drug clearance.

➤*Hepatotoxicity:* For confirmed ALT elevations > 2-fold ULN, dose reduction to 10 mg/day may allow continued administration of leflunomide. If elevations > 2 but ≤ 3-fold ULN persist despite dose reduction, liver biopsy is recommended if continued treatment is desired. If elevations > 3-fold ULN persist despite cholestyramine administration (see Overdosage) and dose reduction, discontinue and administer cholestyramine with close monitoring and retreatment with cholestyramine as indicated.

Actions

➤*Pharmacology:* Leflunomide, a pyrimidine synthesis inhibitor, is an isoxazole immunomodulatory agent that inhibits dihydroorotate dehydrogenase (an enzyme involved in de novo pyrimidine synthesis) and has antiproliferative activity. An anti-inflammatory effect has been demonstrated in vitro and in vivo.

➤*Pharmacokinetics:*

Absorption – Following oral administration, leflunomide is metabolized to an active metabolite (M1), which is responsible for essentially all of its activity in vivo. Relative to an oral solution, leflunomide tablets are 80% bioavailable.

Distribution – Peak levels of the active metabolite, M1, occurred between 6 to 12 hours after dosing. Due to the very long half-life of M1 ($\approx$ 2 weeks), a loading dose of 100 mg for 3 days was used in clinical studies to facilitate the rapid attainment of steady-state levels of M1. Without a loading dose, it is estimated that attainment of steady-state concentrations would require nearly 2 months of dosing. The resulting plasma concentrations following both loading doses and continued clinical dosing indicate that M1 plasma levels are dose-proportional.

Mean Pharmacokinetics Parameters for M1 After Administration of Leflunomide for 24 Days to Patients With Rheumatoid Arthritis (n = 54)			
Parameter	Maintenance (loading) dose		
	5 mg (50 mg)	10 mg (100 mg)	25 mg (250 mg)
C_{24} (Day 1) (mcg/ml)[1]	4	8.4	8.5
C_{24} (ss) (mcg/ml)[2]	8.8	18	63
$t_{1/2}$ (days)	15	14	18

[1] Concentration at 24 hours after loading dose.
[2] Concentration at 24 hours after maintenance doses at steady state.

M1 has a low volume of distribution (Vss = 0.13 L/kg) and is extensively bound (> 99.3%) to albumin in healthy subjects. The free fraction of M1 is slightly higher in patients with rheumatoid arthritis and approximately doubled in patients with chronic renal failure; the mechanism and significance of these increases are unknown.

Metabolism – Leflunomide is metabolized to one primary (M1) and many minor metabolites. Of these minor metabolites, only 4-trifluoromethylaniline (TFMA) is quantifiable, occurring at low levels in the plasma of some patients. The parent compound is rarely detectable in plasma. The specific site of leflunomide metabolism is unknown. In vivo and in vitro studies suggest a role for both the GI wall and the liver in drug metabolism. No specific enzyme has been identified as the primary route of metabolism for leflunomide; however, hepatic cytosolic and microsomal cellular fractions have been identified as sites of drug metabolism.

LEFLUNOMIDE

Excretion – The active metabolite M1 is eliminated by further metabolism, subsequent renal excretion, and direct biliary excretion. The primary urinary metabolites are leflunomide glucuronides and an oxanilic acid derivative of M1. The primary fecal metabolite was M1. Renal elimination is more significant over the first 96 hours, after which fecal elimination begins to predominate; ≈ 43% was eliminated in urine and 48% was eliminated in feces. In a study involving IV administration of M1, the clearance was estimated to be 31 ml/hr. Biliary recycling is a major contributor to the long elimination half-life of M1.

Special populations –

Smoking: A pharmacokinetic analysis indicated that smokers had a 38% increase in clearance; however, no difference in clinical efficacy was seen between smokers and nonsmokers.

Chronic renal insufficiency: In 6 patients with chronic renal insufficiency requiring either chronic ambulatory peritoneal dialysis (CAPD) or hemodialysis, neither had a significant impact on circulating levels of M1. The free fraction of M1 was almost doubled, but the mechanism of this increase is not known.

Hepatic insufficiency: Given the need to metabolize leflunomide into the active species, the role of the liver in drug elimination/recycling, and the possible risk of increased hepatic toxicity, the use of leflunomide in patients with hepatic insufficiency or positive hepatitis B or C serologies is not recommended.

➤*Clinical trials:* The efficacy of leflunomide in the treatment of RA was demonstrated in 3 controlled trials. All leflunomide patients used an initial loading dose of 100 mg/day for 3 days. Subjects with active RA of at least 6 months' duration received leflunomide 20 mg/day (n = 182), methotrexate (MTX) 7.5 mg/week increasing to 15 mg/week (n = 182), or placebo (n = 118). All patients received folate 1 mg twice daily. Treatment duration was 52 weeks. A second study treated subjects with active RA with leflunomide 20 mg/day (n = 133), sulfasalazine 2 g/day (n = 133), or placebo (n = 92). Treatment duration was 24 weeks. A third study treated subjects with active RA with leflunomide 20 mg/day (n = 501) or MTX at 7.5 mg/week increasing to 15 mg/week (n = 498). Folate supplementation was used in 10% of patients. Treatment duration was 52 weeks.

No consistent differences were demonstrated between leflunomide and MTX or between leflunomide and sulfasalazine. Leflunomide treatment effect was evident by 1 month, stabilized by 3 to 6 months, and continued throughout the course of treatment.

Contraindications

Hypersensitivity to leflunomide or any of the other components of leflunomide; pregnancy (see Warnings).

Warnings

➤*Hepatotoxicity:* In clinical trials, leflunomide treatment was associated with elevations of liver enzymes, primarily ALT and AST. In a significant number of patients, these effects were generally reversible. Most transaminase elevations were mild (≤ 2-fold ULN) and usually resolved while continuing treatment. Marked elevations (> 3-fold ULN) occurred infrequently and reversed with dose reduction or discontinuation of treatment. At minimum, perform ALT at baseline, and monitor initially at monthly intervals, then if stable, at intervals determined by the individual clinical situation. For guidelines for dose adjustment or discontinuation based on the severity and persistence of ALT elevation, refer to Administration and Dosage. Rare elevations of alkaline phosphatase and bilirubin have been observed.

➤*Concomitant therapy:* Aspirin, NSAIDs, or low-dose corticosteroids may be continued during treatment (see Drug Interactions). Concurrent use with other agents used for RA has not been adequately studied.

➤*Renal function impairment:* Single-dose studies in dialysis patients show a doubling of the free fraction of M1 in plasma. There is no clinical experience in the use of leflunomide in patients with renal impairment. In light of the fact that the kidney plays a role in drug elimination, and without adequate studies in subjects with renal insufficiency, use caution when leflunomide is administered to these patients.

➤*Hepatic function impairment:* Given the need to metabolize leflunomide into the active species, the role of the liver in drug elimination/recycling, and the possible risk of increased hepatic toxicity, the use of leflunomide in patients with hepatic insufficiency or positive hepatitis B or C serologies is not recommended.

➤*Carcinogenesis:* The risk of malignancy, particularly lymphoproliferative disorders, is increased with the use of some immunosuppression medications. There is a potential for immunosuppression with leflunomide. No apparent increase in the incidence of malignancies and lymphoproliferative disorders was reported in the trials.

Male mice in a 2-year bioassay exhibited an increased incidence in lymphoma at an oral dose of 15 mg/kg, the highest dose studied (1.7 times the human M1 exposure based on AUC). Female mice in the same study exhibited a dose-related increased incidence of bronchoalveolar adenomas and carcinomas combined beginning at 1.5 mg/kg (≈ 1/10 the human M1 exposure based on AUC).

4-trifluoromethylaniline (TFMA), a minor metabolite of leflunomide, was mutagenic in the Ames Assay and the HGPRT Gene Mutation Assay and was clastogenic in the in vitro Assay for Chromosome Aberrations in the Chinese Hamster Cells.

➤*Pregnancy: Category X.* Leflunomide can cause fetal harm when administered to a pregnant woman. When administered orally to rats during organogenesis at a dose of 15 mg/kg, leflunomide was teratogenic (most notably anophthalmia or microphthalmia and internal hydrocephalus). The systemic exposure of rats at this dose was ≈ 1/10 the human exposure level based on AUC. Under these exposure conditions, leflunomide also caused a decrease in the maternal body weight and an increase in embryolethality with a decrease in fetal body weight for surviving fetuses. In rabbits, oral treatment with 10 mg/kg during organogenesis resulted in fused, dysplastic sternebrae. The exposure level at this dose was essentially equivalent to the maximum human exposure level based on AUC.

When female rats were treated with 1.25 mg/kg of leflunomide beginning 14 days before mating and continuing until the end of lactation, the offspring exhibited marked (> 90%) decreases in postnatal survival. The systemic exposure level at 1.25 mg/kg was ≈ 1/100 the human exposure level based on AUC.

There are no adequate and well controlled studies evaluating leflunomide in pregnant women. However, based on animal studies, leflunomide may increase the risk of fetal death or teratogenic effects when administered to a pregnant woman. Women of childbearing potential must not be started on leflunomide until pregnancy is excluded and it has been confirmed that they are using reliable contraception. Before starting treatment, fully counsel patients on the potential for serious risk to the fetus. If this drug is used during pregnancy, or if the patient becomes pregnant while taking this drug, apprise the patient of the potential hazard to the fetus.

Advise patient that if there is any delay in onset of menses or any other reason to suspect pregnancy, they must notify the physician immediately for pregnancy testing, and if positive, the physician and patient must discuss the risk to the pregnancy. It is possible that rapidly lowering the blood level of the active metabolite by instituting the drug elimination procedure at the first delay of menses may decrease the risk to the fetus (see Administration and Dosage).

It is recommended that all women of childbearing potential who discontinue leflunomide and women receiving treatment who wish to become pregnant undergo the drug elimination procedure described in Administration and Dosage. This includes verification of M1 metabolite plasma levels < 0.02 mg/L (0.02 mcg/ml). Human plasma levels of the active metabolite (M1) < 0.02 mg/L (0.02 mcg/ml) are expected to have minimal risk based on available animal data.

To minimize any possible risk, men wishing to father a child should consider discontinuing leflunomide and taking cholestyramine 8 g 3 times daily for 11 days.

➤*Lactation:* Leflunomide should not be used by nursing mothers. It is not known whether it is excreted in breast milk. There is potential for serious adverse reactions in nursing infants from leflunomide. Therefore, decide whether to proceed with nursing or to initiate treatment, taking into account the importance of the drug to the mother.

➤*Children:* Safety and efficacy have not been studied. Use of leflunomide in patients < 18 years of age is not recommended.

Precautions

➤*Monitoring:* At minimum, perform ALT at baseline and monitor initially at monthly intervals, then if stable, at intervals determined by the individual clinical situation.

➤*Immunosuppression potential:* Although there is no clinical experience in the following patient populations, leflunomide is not recommended for patients with severe immunodeficiency, bone marrow dysplasia, or severe uncontrolled infections because of the theoretical potential for immunosuppression.

No clinical data are available on the efficacy and safety of vaccinations during leflunomide treatment. However, vaccination with live vaccines is not recommended. Consider the long half-life of leflunomide when contemplating administration of a live vaccine after stopping leflunomide.

➤*Lab test abnormalities:* Due to a specific effect on the brush border of the renal proximal tubule, leflunomide has a uricosuric effect. A separate effect of hypophosphatemia is seen in some patients. These effects have not been seen together nor have there been alterations in renal function.

Drug Interactions

Leflunomide Drug Interactions			
Precipitant drug	Object drug*		Description
Cholestyramine Charcoal	Leflunomide	↓	Coadministration resulted in a rapid and significant decrease in the active metabolite of leflunomide.
Rifampin	Leflunomide	↑	Following concomitant administration of a single dose of leflunomide to subjects receiving multiple doses of rifampin, M1 peak levels were increased (40%).

LEFLUNOMIDE

Leflunomide Drug Interactions

Precipitant drug	Object drug[*]		Description
Leflunomide	Hepatotoxic drugs	↑	Increased side effects may occur when leflunomide is given concomitantly with hepatotoxic substances. This is also to be considered when leflunomide treatment is followed by such drugs without a drug elimination procedure. Concomitant use of leflunomide with methotrexate resulted in a 2- to 3-fold elevation in liver enzymes in 5 of 30 patients. All elevations resolved, 2 with continuation of both drugs and 3 after discontinuation of leflunomide. A > 3-fold increase was seen in another 5 patients. All of these also resolved, 2 with continuation of both drugs and 3 after discontinuation of leflunomide. Three patients met "ACR criteria" for liver biopsy.
Leflunomide	NSAIDs	↑	In vitro, M1 caused an increase (13% to 50%) in the free fraction of diclofenac and ibuprofen. In vitro studies indicate that M1 inhibits cytochrome P450 2C9, which is responsible for the metabolism of many NSAIDs. The clinical significance of this finding is unknown.
Leflunomide	Tolbutamide	↔	In vitro, M1 caused increases (13% to 50%) in the free fraction of tolbutamide at concentrations in the clinical range. The clinical significance of this finding is unknown.

[*] ↑ = Object drug increased. ↓ = Object drug decreased. ↔ = Undetermined clinical effect.

Adverse Reactions

Leflunomide Adverse Reactions (≥ 3%)

	All RA studies	Placebo-controlled trials				Active-controlled trials	
	LEF[1] (n = 1339)	LEF (n = 315)	PL[2] (n = 210)	SSZ[3] (n = 133)	MTX[4] (n = 182)	LEF (n = 501)	MTX (n = 498)
Cardiovascular							
Hypertension[5]	10	9	4	4	3	10	4
Chest pain	2	4	2	2	4	1	2
CNS							
Dizziness	4	5	3	6	5	7	6
Headache	7	13	11	12	21	10	8
Paresthesia	2	3	1	1	2	4	3
Dermatologic							
Alopecia	10	9	1	6	6	17	10
Eczema	2	1	1	1	1	3	2
Pruritus	4	5	2	3	2	6	2
Rash	10	12	7	11	9	11	10
Dry skin	2	3	2	2	0	3	1
GI							
Anorexia	3	3	2	5	2	3	3
Diarrhea	17	27	12	10	20	22	10
Dyspepsia	5	10	10	9	13	6	7
Gastroenteritis	3	1	1	0	6	3	3
Abnormal liver enzymes	5	10	2	4	10	6	17
Nausea	9	13	11	19	18	13	18
GI/Abdominal pain	5	6	4	7	8	8	8
Mouth ulcer	3	5	4	3	10	3	6
Vomiting	3	5	4	4	3	3	3
Metabolic/ Nutritional							
Hypokalemia	1	3	1	1	1	1	< 1
Weight loss	4	2	1	2	0	2	2
Musculoskeletal							
Arthralgia	1	4	3	0	9	< 1	2
Leg cramps	1	4	2	2	6	0	0
Joint disorder	4	2	2	2	2	8	6
Synovitis	2	< 1	1	0	2	4	2
Tenosynovitis	3	2	0	1	2	5	1
Respiratory							
Bronchitis	7	5	2	4	7	8	7
Increased cough	3	4	5	3	6	5	7
Respiratory infection	15	21	21	20	32	27	25

Leflunomide Adverse Reactions (≥ 3%)

	All RA studies	Placebo-controlled trials				Active-controlled trials	
	LEF[1] (n = 1339)	LEF (n = 315)	PL[2] (n = 210)	SSZ[3] (n = 133)	MTX[4] (n = 182)	LEF (n = 501)	MTX (n = 498)
Pharyngitis	3	2	1	2	1	3	3
Pneumonia	2	3	0	0	1	2	2
Rhinitis	2	5	2	4	3	2	2
Sinusitis	2	5	5	0	10	1	1
Miscellaneous							
Allergic reaction	2	5	2	0	6	1	2
Asthenia	3	6	4	5	6	3	3
Flu syndrome	2	4	2	0	7	0	0
Infection	4	0	0	0	0	0	0
Injury accident	5	7	5	3	11	6	7
Pain	2	4	2	2	5	1	< 1
Abdominal pain	6	5	4	4	8	6	4
Back pain	5	6	3	4	9	8	7
Urinary tract infection	5	5	7	4	2	5	6

[1] Leflunomide.
[2] Placebo.
[3] Sulfasalazine.
[4] Methotrexate.
[5] Hypertension as a preexisting condition was over-represented in all leflunomide treatment groups in Phase III trials. Analysis of new onset hypertension revealed no difference among the treatment groups.

In addition, the following adverse events have been reported in 1% to < 3%:

➤*Cardiovascular:* Angina pectoris; migraine; palpitation; tachycardia; vasculitis; vasodilation; varicose vein.

➤*CNS:* Anxiety; depression; dry mouth; insomnia; neuralgia; neuritis; sleep disorder; sweat; vertigo.

➤*Dermatologic:* Acne; contact dermatitis; fungal dermatitis; hair discoloration; hematoma; herpes simplex; herpes zoster; nail disorder; skin nodule; subcutaneous nodule; maculopapular rash; skin disorder; skin discoloration; ulcer skin.

➤*Endocrine:* Diabetes mellitus; hyperthyroidism.

➤*GI:* Cholelithiasis; colitis; constipation; esophagitis; flatulence; gastritis; gingivitis; melena; oral moniliasis; pharyngitis; enlarged salivary gland; stomatitis (or aphthous stomatitis); tooth disorder.

➤*GU:* Albuminuria; cystitis; dysuria; hematuria; menstrual disorder; vaginal moniliasis; prostate disorder; urinary frequency.

➤*Hematologic / Lymphatic:* Anemia (including iron deficiency anemia); ecchymosis.

➤*Metabolic / Nutritional:* Creatine phosphokinase increase; peripheral edema; hyperglycemia; hyperlipidemia.

➤*Musculoskeletal:* Arthrosis; bursitis; muscle cramps; myalgia; bone necrosis; bone pain; tendon rupture.

➤*Respiratory:* Asthma; dyspnea; epistaxis; lung disorder.

➤*Special senses:* Blurred vision; cataract; conjunctivitis; eye disorder; taste perversion.

➤*Miscellaneous:* Abscess; cyst; fever; hernia; malaise; pain; neck pain; pelvic pain.

Other less common adverse events seen in clinical trials include the following: One case of anaphylactic reaction occurred in Phase II following rechallenge of drug after withdrawal due to rash (rare); urticaria; eosinophilia; transient thrombocytopenia (rare); and leukopenia (WBC < 2000/mm[3]; rare). A causal relationship of these events to leflunomide has not been established.

Overdosage

In the event of a significant overdose or toxicity, cholestyramine or charcoal administration is recommended to accelerate elimination. Oral cholestyramine given at a dose of 8 g 3 times a day for 24 hours to 3 healthy volunteers decreased plasma levels of M1 by ≈ 40% in 24 hours and by 49% to 65% in 48 hours.

Administration of activated charcoal (powder made into a suspension) orally or via nasogastric tube (50 g every 6 hours for 24 hours) has been shown to reduce plasma concentrations of the active metabolite, M1, by 37% in 24 hours and by 48% in 48 hours.

These drug elimination procedures may be repeated if clinically necessary.

Patient Information

Discuss the potential for increased risk of birth defects with female patients of childbearing potential. Advise women that they may be at increased risk of having a child with birth defects if they are pregnant while taking leflunomide, become pregnant while taking leflunomide, or do not wait to become pregnant until they have stopped taking leflunomide and followed the drug elimination procedure (see Warnings).

ANTIHISTAMINE-CONTAINING PREPARATIONS

otc	**Maximum Strength Bena-dryl 2%** (Parke-Davis)	**Cream:** 2% diphenhydramine HCl and parabens in a greaseless base	In 15 g.
		Spray, non-aerosol: 2% diphenhydramine HCl, 85% alcohol	In 60 ml.
otc	**Dermamycin** (Pfeiffer)	**Cream:** 2% diphenhydramine HCl, parabens, polyethylene glycol monostearate, propylene glycol	In 28.35 g.
		Spray: 2% diphenhydramine HCl, 1% menthol, alcohol, methylparaben	In 60 ml.
otc	**Maximum Strength Bena-dryl Itch Relief** (Pfeiffer)	**Cream:** 2% diphenhydramine HCl, 0.1% zinc acetate, parabens, aloe vera	In 14.2 g.
		Stick: 2% diphenhydramine HCl, 0.1% zinc acetate, 73.5% alcohol, aloe vera	In 14 ml.
otc	**Ziradryl** (Parke-Davis)	**Lotion:** 1% diphenhydramine HCl, 2% zinc oxide, 2% alcohol, camphor, parabens	In 180 ml.
otc	**Caladryl Clear** (Warner-Lambert)	**Lotion:** 1% diphenhydramine HCl, 2% zinc oxide, 2% alcohol, camphor, chlorophyllin sodium, parabens	In 180 ml.
otc	**Benadryl** (Parke-Davis)	**Cream:** 1% diphenhydramine HCl, parabens in a greaseless base	In 15 g.
		Spray, non-aerosol: 1% diphenhydramine HCl, 85% alcohol	In 60 ml.
otc	**Caladryl** (Parke-Davis)	**Cream:** 1% diphenhydramine HCl, 8% calamine, parabens, camphor	In 45 g.
		Lotion: 1% diphenhydramine HCl, 8% calamine, camphor, 2% alcohol	In 75 and 180 ml.
otc	**Di-Delamine** (Commerce)	**Gel and Spray, non-aerosol:** 1% diphenhydramine HCl, 0.5% tripelennamine HCl, 0.12% benzalkonium Cl, menthol, EDTA	**Gel:** In 37.5 g. **Spray:** In 120 ml.
otc	**Sting-Eze** (Wisconsin Pharm.)	**Concentrate:** Diphenhydramine HCl, camphor, phenol, benzocaine, eucalyptol	In 15 ml.
otc	**Medacote** (Dal-Med)	**Lotion:** 1% pyrilamine maleate, dimethyl polysiloxane, zinc oxide, menthol and camphor in a greaseless base	In 120 ml.
otc	**Derma-Pax** (Recsei Labs)	**Lotion:** 0.44% pyrilamine maleate, 0.06% chlorpheniramine, 1% benzyl alcohol, 35% isopropanol, chlo-robutanol	In 120 ml and pt.
otx	**Z-Xtra** (Magna)	**Lotion:** 2.07 mg pyrilamine maleate, 41.35 mg zinc oxide/mL. Benzocaine, apple blossom oil, silicone oil, lanolin oil, Wysteria oil, isopropanol, camphor, menthol, parabens	In 118 mL.
otc	**Calamycin** (Pfeiffer)	**Lotion:** Zinc oxide and 10% calamine, benzocaine, chloroxylenol, pyrilamine maleate, 2% isopropyl alcohol	In 120 ml.
otc	**Benadryl Itch Stopping Children's Formula** (Warner Wellcome)	**Gel:** 1% diphenhydramine HCl, 1% zinc acetate, camphor, parabens	In 118 g.
otc	**Benadryl Itch Stopping Maximum Strength** (Warner Wellcome)	**Gel:** 2% diphenhydramine HCl, 1% zinc acetate, camphor, parabens	In 118 g.
otc	**Dermarest** (Del)	**Gel:** 2% diphenhydramine HCl, 2% resorcinol, aloe vera gel, benzalkonium chloride, EDTA, menthol, methylparaben, propylene glycol	In 29.25 and 56.25 g.
otc	**Dermarest Plus** (Del)	**Gel:** 2% diphenhydramine HCl, 1% menthol, aloe vera gel, benzalkonium chloride, isopropyl alcohol, methylparaben, propylene glycol	In 15 and 30 g.
		Spray: 2% diphenhydramine HCl, 1% menthol, aloe vera gel, benzalkonium chloride, methylparaben, propylene glycol, SD alcohol 40, EDTA	In 15 and 30 g.
otc	**Clearly Cala-gel** (Tec Labs)	**Gel:** Diphenhydramine HCl, zinc acetate, menthol, EDTA	Clear. In 180 g.
otc	**Benadryl Itch Relief** (GlaxoWellcome)	**Spray:** 2% diphenhydramine HCl, 0.1% zinc acetate, 73.6% alcohol, aloe vera	In 59 ml.
otc	**Benadryl Itch Relief Children's** (GlaxoWellcome)	**Cream:** 1% diphenhydramine HCl, 0.1% zinc acetate, aloe vera, cetyl alcohol, parabens	In 14.2 g.
		Spray: 1% diphenhydramine HCl, 0.1% zinc acetate, 73.6% alcohol, aloe vera, povidone	In 59 ml.
otc	**Benadryl Itch Stopping Spray, Extra Strength** (Warner Lambert)	**Spray:** 2% diphenhydramine HCl, 0.1% zinc acetate, 73.5% v/v alcohol, glycerin, tromethamine	In 59 ml.
otc	**Benadryl Itch Stopping Spray, Original Strength** (Warner Lambert)	**Spray:** 1% diphenhydramine HCl, 0.1% zinc acetate, 73.6% v/v alcohol, glycerin, tromethamine	In 59 ml.

Indications

Temporary relief of itching due to minor skin disorders, ivy, sumac and oak poisoning, sunburn, insect bites (nonpoisonous) and stings.

Ingredients

Other ingredients used with the antihistamines include:

BENZOCAINE as a local anesthetic.

CHLOROXYLENOL, BENZALKONIUM CHLORIDE, EUCALYPTOL as bacteriostatic agents.

BENZYL ALCOHOL, CAMPHOR and *MENTHOL* for antipruritic effects.

CALAMINE and *ZINC OXIDE* as astringents.

DIMETHYL POLYSILOXANE as a skin protectant.

CHLOROPHYLLIN SODIUM promotes healing.

ISOPROPYL ALCOHOL as an antiseptic.

CHLOROBUTANOL for antipruritic and antiseptic effects.

Actions

➤*Pharmacology:* Topical antihistamines have some local anesthetic activity and are used to relieve itching. Some transdermal absorption may occur, but not in sufficient quantities to produce systemic side effects. They may cause local irritation and sensitization, especially with prolonged use. Refer to Antihistamine monograph in Respiratory Drugs chapter for further information on systemic antihistamines.

Warnings

➤*Do not apply:* To blistered, raw or oozing areas of the skin, or around the eyes or other mucous membranes (eg, nose, mouth).

Precautions

➤*For external use only:* Avoid contact with the eyes.

➤*Discontinue use:* If the condition persists, recurs after a few days or irritation develops.

➤*Avoid prolonged use:* For > 7 days or use on extensive skin areas.

DOXEPIN HCl

Rx	Zonalon (Bioglan)	**Cream:** 5%	Cetyl alcohol, petrolatum, benzyl alcohol, titanium dioxide. In 30 g.

For information on the systemic use of doxepin, refer to the individual monographs in the CNS Drugs chapter.

Indications

➤*Pruritus:* Short-term (up to 8 days) management of moderate pruritus in adults with the following forms of eczematous dermatitis: Atopic dermatitis; lichen simplex chronicus.

Administration and Dosage

➤*Approved by the FDA:* April 1, 1994.

Apply a thin film of cream 4 times each day with at least a 3 to 4 hour interval between applications. There are no data to establish the safety and efficacy when used for > 8 days. Chronic use beyond 8 days may result in higher systemic levels.

Drowsiness is significantly more common in patients applying doxepin cream to > 10% of body surface area. If excessive drowsiness occurs it may be necessary to do one or more of the following: Reduce the body surface area treated, reduce the number of applications per day, reduce the amount of cream applied or discontinue the drug. Occlusive dressings may increase the absorption of most topical drugs; therefore, occlusive dressings with doxepin cream should not be utilized.

Actions

➤*Pharmacology:* Doxepin cream, a dibenzoxepin tricyclic compound, is a topical antipruritic. The exact mechanism by which doxepin exerts its antipruritic effect is unknown. However, it does have potent H_1 and H_2 receptor blocking actions. Histamine-blocking drugs appear to compete at histamine receptor sites and inhibit the biological activation of histamine receptors. In addition, doxepin produces drowsiness in significant numbers of patients. Sedation may have an effect on certain pruritic symptoms.

➤*Pharmacokinetics:* In 19 pruritic eczema patients treated with doxepin cream, plasma doxepin concentrations ranged from nondetectable to 47 ng/ml from percutaneous absorption. Target therapeutic plasma levels of oral doxepin for the treatment of depression range from 30 to 150 ng/ml.

Once absorbed into the systemic circulation, doxepin undergoes hepatic metabolism that results in conversion to pharmacologically active desmethyldoxepin. Further glucuronidation results in urinary excretion of the parent drug and its metabolites. Desmethyldoxepin has a half-life that ranges from 28 to 52 hours and is not affected by multiple dosing. Plasma levels of both doxepin and desmethyldoxepin are highly variable and are poorly correlated with dosage. Renal disease, genetic factors, age and other medications affect the metabolism and subsequent elimination of doxepin.

Contraindications

Untreated narrow-angle glaucoma, tendency to urinary retention (since doxepin has an anticholinergic effect and because significant plasma levels are detectable after topical application); hypersensitivity to any components of the product.

Warnings

➤*For external use only:* Do not use ophthalmically, orally or intravaginally.

➤*Drowsiness:* This occurs in > 20% of patients treated with doxepin cream, especially in patients receiving treatment to > 10% of their body surface area. Warn patients of this possibility and caution them against driving a motor vehicle or operating hazardous machinery while being treated with doxepin cream. Also warn patients that the effects of alcoholic beverages can be potentiated when using doxepin cream. If excessive drowsiness occurs it may be necessary to reduce the number of applications, the amount of cream applied or the percentage of body surface area treated, or discontinue the drug.

➤*Pregnancy: Category B.* There are no adequate and well controlled studies in pregnant women. Use during pregnancy only if clearly needed.

➤*Lactation:* Doxepin is excreted in breast milk after oral administration. Significant systemic levels of doxepin are obtained after topical administration; therefore, it is possible that doxepin could be secreted in breast milk following topical administration. One case of apnea and drowsiness occurred in a nursing infant whose mother was taking an oral dosage form of doxepin. Because of the potential for serious adverse reactions in nursing infants, decide whether to discontinue nursing or to discontinue the drug, taking into account the importance of the drug to the mother.

➤*Children:* Safety and efficacy in children have not been established.

Drug Interactions

➤*Drugs metabolized by P450 2D6:* A subset (3% to 10%) of the population has reduced activity of certain drug metabolizing enzymes such as the cytochrome P450 isozyme P450 2D6. Such individuals are referred to as "poor metabolizers" and may have higher than expected plasma concentrations of tricyclic antidepressants (TCAs) when given usual doses. In addition, certain drugs that are metabolized by this isozyme may inhibit its activity, and thus may make normal metabolizers resemble poor metabolizers, leading to drug interactions. Concomitant use of TCAs with other drugs metabolized by cytochrome P450 2D6 may require lower doses than usually prescribed for either the TCA or the other drug. Therefore, coadministration of TCAs with other drugs that are metabolized by this isoenzyme should be approached with caution.

Since plasma levels of doxepin similar to therapeutic ranges for antidepressant use can be obtained following topical application of the cream, it would not be unexpected for the following drug interactions to be possible following topical application.

Topical Doxepin Drug Interactions			
Precipitant drug	Object drug[*]		Description
Alcohol	Doxepin	↑	Alcohol ingestion may exacerbate the potential sedative effects of doxepin cream.
Cimetidine	Doxepin	↑	Cimetidine produces clinically significant fluctuations in steady-state serum concentrations of various tricyclic antidepressants (TCAs). Serious anticholinergic symptoms have occurred with elevated TCA levels.
MAO inhibitors	Doxepin	↑	Serious side effects and even death have been reported following the concomitant use of MAOIs and other drugs chemically related to doxepin. Therefore, discontinue MAOIs at least 2 weeks prior to the initiation of treatment with doxepin cream.

[*] ↑ = Object drug increased.

Adverse Reactions

➤*Systemic:* The most common systemic effect was drowsiness (22%); ≈ 5% discontinued therapy. Other effects included: Dry mouth/lips, thirst, headache, fatigue, dizziness, emotional changes, taste changes (1% to 10%); nausea, anxiety, fever (< 1%).

➤*Local:* The most common local effect was burning or stinging at the application site (21%; ≈ 25% reported the reaction as "severe"); four patients withdrew from therapy. Other effects included: Pruritus or eczema exacerbation, dryness/tightness of skin, paresthesias, edema (1% to 10%); irritation, tingling, scaling, cracking (< 1%).

Overdosage

➤*Symptoms:*

Mild – Drowsiness, stupor, blurred vision, excessive dryness of mouth.

Severe – Respiratory depression, hypotension, coma, convulsions, cardiac arrhythmias, tachycardias, urinary retention (bladder atony), decreased GI motility (paralytic ileus), hyperthermia, hypothermia, hypertension, dilated pupils, hyperactive reflexes.

➤*Treatment:*

Mild – Observation and supportive therapy is all that is usually necessary. It may be necessary to reduce the percent of body surface area treated or the frequency of application or apply a thinner layer of cream.

Severe – Management consists of aggressive supportive therapy. Thoroughly wash the area covered with cream. Establish an adequate airway in comatose patients and use assisted ventilation if necessary. ECG monitoring may be required for several days because relapse after apparent recovery has been reported with oral doxepin. Treat arrhythmias with the appropriate antiarrhythmic agent. Many of the cardiovascular and CNS symptoms of TCA poisoning in adults may be reversed by the slow IV administration of 1 to 3 mg of physostigmine salicylate. Because physostigmine is rapidly metabolized, repeat the dosage as required. Convulsions may respond to standard anticonvulsant therapy; however, barbiturates may potentiate any respiratory depression. Dialysis and forced diuresis generally are not of value due to high tissue and protein binding of doxepin.

Patient Information

Caution patients about operating hazardous machinery, including automobiles, until they are reasonably certain that doxepin therapy does not adversely affect their ability to engage in such activities.

Do not use occlusive dressings since absorption may be increased.

Antibiotic Agents

GENTAMICIN SULFATE

Rx	Gentamicin (Various, eg, Fougera)	Ointment: 0.1% (as base)	May contain white petrolatum, parabens. In 15 g.
		Cream: 0.1% (as base)	May contain propylene glycol, parabens. In 15 g.

Indications

Gentamicin is a bactericidal agent that is not effective against viruses or fungi in skin infections.

➤*Primary skin infections:* Impetigo contagiosa, superficial folliculitis, ecthyma, furunculosis, sycosis barbae, and pyoderma gangrenosum.

Cream – Cream is recommended for wet, oozing primary infections.

➤*Secondary skin infections:* Infectious eczematoid dermatitis, pustular acne, pustular psoriasis, infected seborrheic dermatitis, infected contact dermatitis (including poison ivy), infected excoriations, and bacterial superinfections of fungal or viral infections.

Cream – Cream is used for greasy, secondary infections, such as pustular acne or infected seborrheic dermatitis.

Ointment – Ointment helps retain moisture and has been useful in infection on dry eczematous or psoriatic skin.

➤*Skin cysts:* Gentamycin is useful in the treatment of infected skin cysts and certain other skin abscesses when preceded by incision and drainage to permit adequate contact between the antibiotic and the infecting bacteria.

➤*Other infections:* Infected stasis and other skin ulcers, superficial burns, paronychia, infected insect bites and stings, lacerations and abrasions, and wounds from minor surgery.

Administration and Dosage

Apply 3 to 4 times daily to affected area. In cases of impetigo contagiosa, crusts should be removed before application. Cover treated area with gauze dressing if desired.

➤*Storage/Stability:* Store at controlled room temperature 15° to 30°C (59° to 86°F).

Actions

➤*Pharmacology:* Gentamicin sulfate is a wide spectrum bactericidal antibiotic that appears to inhibit protein synthesis and provides highly effective topical treatment in primary and secondary bacterial infections of the skin.

➤*Pharmacokinetics:* Systemic absorption of gentamicin has been reported with topical use through denuded skin, burns, and ulcers. More rapid absorption seems to occur with gentamicin cream compared with the ointment.

➤*Microbiology:* Bacteria susceptible to the action of gentamicin sulfate include Streptococci (group A beta-hemolytic, alpha hemolytic), *Staphylococcus aureus* (coagulase-positive, coagulase negative, and some penicillinase-producing strains), and the gram-negative bacteria, *Pseudomonas aeruginosa*, *Aerobacter aerogenes*, *Escherichia coli*, *Proteus vulgaris*, and *Klebsiella pneumoniae*.

Contraindications

History of sensitivity to any component of the product.

Warnings

➤*Pregnancy:* Category C. There are no adequate and well-controlled studies when using topical gentamicin in pregnant women. Use only when clearly needed and when the potential benefits outweigh the unknown potential hazards to the fetus.

➤*Lactation:* It is not known whether topical gentamicin is distributed through breast milk; although, parenteral gentamicin appears in breast milk. Consider discontinuing nursing or the drug, taking into account the importance of the drug to the mother.

➤*Children:* Gentamycin has been used successfully in infants older than 1 year of age.

Precautions

➤*Superinfection:* The use of topical antibiotics occasionally allows overgrowth of nonsusceptible organisms, including fungi. If this condition occurs, or if irritation, sensitization, or superinfection develops, treatment with gentamicin sulfate should be discontinued and appropriate therapy instituted.

Adverse Reactions

Irritation (erythema, pruritus); possible photosensitization.

Patient Information

For external use only. Avoid contact with the eyes.

Wash hands after applying medication to the affected area.

BACITRACIN

otc	Bacitracin (Various, eg, Fougera, Ivax, Rugby)	Ointment: 500 units/g	May contain mineral oil or white petrolatum. In 14, 28, 120, and 454 g and UD 144s.

Indications

As first aid to help prevent infection in minor cuts, wounds, scrapes, and burns.

Administration and Dosage

Clean the affected area. Apply a small amount of the antibiotic on the area 1 to 3 times/day. Do not use longer than 1 week unless directed by a physician. The affected area may be covered with a sterile bandage.

➤*Storage/Stability:* Store at 15° to 30°C (59° to 86°F).

Actions

➤*Pharmacology:* Bacitracin is believed to be bactericidal or bacteriostatic in action depending on the concentration of the drug and the susceptibility of the organism. Bacitracin inhibits cell-wall synthesis by preventing amino acids and nucleotides into the cell. Absorption is reported to be negligible following topical administration.

Contraindications

Known hypersensitivity to any of the ingredients; use in eyes.

Warnings

➤*Systemic therapy:* Deeper cutaneous infections may require systemic antibiotic therapy in addition to local treatment. Use caution when applying over large areas of the body for deep puncture wounds, animal bites, or serious burns.

➤*External use:* For external use only. Do not use in or near the eyes, nose, mouth, mucous membranes, or apply over large areas of the body.

➤*Pregnancy:* Category C. There are no adequate and well-controlled studies in pregnant women. Use during pregnancy only when clearly needed.

➤*Lactation:* It is not known whether bacitracin is excreted in breast milk. Use caution when applying on a breastfeeding woman.

Adverse Reactions

Rash; hypersensitivity reaction (rare).

Patient Information

Discontinue use of medication if a rash or other allergic reaction develops, or if condition persists or worsens.

For external use only. Do not use near eyes, nose, mouth, or mucous membranes.

Cleanse affected area prior to application of medicine.

Notify physician if condition worsens or if rash or irritation develops.

Not for prolonged use. Do not used for longer than 1 week unless directed by a physician.

AZELAIC ACID

Rx	Azelex (Allergan)	Cream: 20%	Glycerin, cetearyl alcohol, benzoic acid. In 30 and 50 g.
Rx	Finacea (Berlex Labs)	Gel: 15%	Benzoic acid, EDTA. In 30 g.

Indications

➤*Acne vulgaris (cream):* Topical treatment of mild to moderate inflammatory acne vulgaris.

➤*Rosacea (gel):* Topical treatment of inflammatory papules and pustules of mild to moderate rosacea. Safety and efficacy have not been studied beyond 12 weeks. Instruct patients to avoid spicy foods, thermally hot foods and drinks, alcoholic beverages, and to use only very mild soaps or soapless cleansing lotion for facial cleansing.

Administration and Dosage

After the skin is thoroughly washed and patted dry, gently but thoroughly massage a thin film of azelaic acid cream in to the affected areas twice daily, in the morning and evening. Wash the hands following application. The duration of use of azelaic acid can vary from person to person and depends on the severity of the acne. In the majority of patients with inflammatory lesions, improvement of the condition occurs within 4 weeks.

➤*Storage / Stability:* Protect from freezing. Store between 15° to 30°C (59° to 86°F).

Actions

➤*Pharmacology:* The exact mechanism of action of azelaic acid is not known. In vitro, azelaic acid possesses antimicrobial activity against *Propionibacterium acnes* and *Staphylococcus epidermidis*. The antimicrobial action may be attributable to inhibition of microbial cellular protein synthesis. A normalization of keratinization leading to an anticomedonal effect of azelaic acid may also contribute to its clinical activity. Evaluation of skin biopsies from human subjects treated with azelaic acid demonstrated a reduction in the thickness of the stratum corneum, a reduction in number and size of keratohyalin granules and a reduction in the amount and distribution of filaggrin (a protein component of keratohyalin) in epidermal layers. This is suggestive of the ability to decrease microcomedo formation.

➤*Pharmacokinetics:*

Cream – Following a single application to human skin in vitro, azelaic acid penetrates into the stratum corneum (approximately 3% to 5% of the applied dose) and other viable skin layers (up to 10% of the dose is found in the epidermis and dermis). Negligible cutaneous metabolism occurs after topical application. Approximately 4% of the topically applied azelaic acid is systemically absorbed. Azelaic acid is mainly excreted unchanged in the urine but undergoes some β-oxidation to shorter chain dicarboxylic acids. The observed half-lives in healthy subjects are approximately 45 minutes after oral dosing and 12 hours after topical dosing, indicating percutaneous absorption rate-limited kinetics.

Azelaic acid is a dietary constituent (whole grain cereals and animal products), and can be formed endogenously from longer-chain dicarboxylic acids, metabolism of oleic acid, and omega-oxidation of monocarboxylic acids. Endogenous plasma concentration (20 to 80 ng/mL) and daily urinary excretion (4 to 28 mg) of azelaic acid are highly dependent on dietary intake. After topical treatment, plasma concentration and urinary excretion are not significantly different from baseline levels.

Gel – The percutaneous absorption of azelaic acid after topical application could not be reliably determined. Mean plasma azelaic acid concentrations in rosacea patients treated twice daily for at least 8 weeks are in the range of 42 to 63.1 ng/mL. These values are within the maximum concentration range of 24 to 90.5 ng/mL observed in rosacea patients treated with vehicle only. This indicates that azelaic acid gel does not increase plasma azelaic acid concentration beyond the range derived from nutrition and endogenous metabolism. Azelaic acid is mainly excreted unchanged in the urine but undergoes some β-oxidation to shorter chain dicarboxylic acids.

Contraindications

Hypersensitivity to any component of the product.

Warnings

➤*For external dermatologic use only:* Not for ophthalmic, oral, or intravaginal use.

➤*Hypopigmentation:* There have been isolated reports of hypopigmentation after use of azelaic acid. Because azelaic acid has not been well studied in patients with dark complexions, monitor these patients for early signs of hypopigmentation.

➤*Pregnancy:* Category B. Embryotoxic effects were observed in rats receiving 2500 mg/kg/day of azelaic acid. Similar effects were observed in rabbits given 150 to 500 mg/kg/day and in monkeys given 500 mg/kg/day. The doses at which these effects were noted were all within toxic dose ranges for the dams. No teratogenic effects were observed. There are no adequate and well-controlled studies in pregnant women. Use during pregnancy only if clearly needed.

Gel – An oral peri- and postnatal developmental study was conducted in rats. Azelaic acid was administered from gestational day 15 through day 21 postpartum up to a dose level of 2500 mg/kg/day. Embryotoxicity was observed in rats at an oral dose that generated some maternal toxicity. In addition, slight disturbances in the postnatal development of fetuses was noted in rats at oral doses that generated some maternal toxicity (500 and 2500 mg/kg/day; 32 and 162 times the maximum recommended human dose based on body surface area). No effects on sexual maturation of the fetuses were noted in this study.

➤*Lactation:* In vitro, at an azelaic acid concentration of 25 mcg/mL, the milk/plasma distribution coefficient was 0.7 and the milk/buffer distribution was 1, indicating that passage of drug into breast milk may occur. Because less than 4% of a topically applied dose is systemically absorbed, the uptake of azelaic acid into breast milk is not expected to cause a significant change from baseline azelaic acid levels in the milk. However, exercise caution when administering to a nursing mother.

➤*Children:* Safety and efficacy in children younger than 12 years of age have not been established.

Precautions

➤*Sensitivity / Irritation:* If sensitivity or severe irritation develops, discontinue treatment and institute appropriate therapy.

Adverse Reactions

Cream – In clinical trials, adverse reactions were generally mild and transient and included: Pruritus, burning, stinging, tingling (1% to 5%); erythema, dryness, rash, peeling, irritation, contact dermatitis (less than 1%); worsening of asthma, vitiligo depigmentation, small depigmented spots, hypertrichosis, reddening (signs of keratosis pilaris), exacerbation of recurrent herpes labialis (rare); potential for allergic reactions.

Gel – In the vehicle-controlled clinical studies, treatment safety was monitored in patients who used azelaic acid gel, 15% or the gel vehicle, twice daily for 12 weeks.

Adverse Events in Rosacea Trials by Treatment Group and Maximum Intensity (≥ 1%)[1]						
	Azelaic acid gel, 15% (N = 333)			Vehicle (N = 331)		
Adverse reaction	Mild (n = 86) (26%)	Moderate (n = 44) (13%)	Severe (n = 20) (6%)	Mild (n = 49) (15%)	Moderate (n = 27) (8%)	Severe (n = 5) (2%)
Burning/stinging/ tingling	20	9	4	2	2	1
Pruritus	7	4	1	3	2	0
Scaling/dry skin/ xerosis	6	2	1	10	4	0
Erythema/irritation	2	2	0	2	1	1
Edema	1	1	0	1	0	0
Contact dermatitis	1	1	0	0	0	0
Acne	1	0	0	0	0	0
Seborrhea	1	0	0	0	0	0
Photosensitivity	0	0	0	1	0	0
Skin disease	0	0	0	0	1	0

[1] Subjects may have more than 1 cutaneous adverse event; thus, the sum of the frequencies of preferred terms may exceed the number of subjects with at least 1 cutaneous adverse event.

In patients using azelaic acid formulations, the following additional adverse experiences have been reported rarely: Worsening of asthma, vitiligo depigmentation, small depigmented spots, hypertrichosis, reddening (signs of keratosis pilaris), and exacerbation of recurrent herpes labialis.

Patient Information

Use for the full prescribed treatment period.

Avoid the use of occlusive dressings or wrappings.

Keep away from the mouth, eyes and other mucous membranes. If it does come in contact with the eyes, patients should wash their eyes with large amounts of water and consult a physician if eye irritation persists.

If patients have dark complexions, they should report abnormal changes in skin color to their physician (see Warnings).

Due in part to the low pH of azelaic acid, temporary skin irritation (eg, pruritus, burning, stinging) may occur when azelaic acid is applied to broken or inflamed skin, usually at the start of treatment. However, this irritation commonly subsides if treatment is continued. If it continues, apply only once a day or stop the treatment until these effects have subsided. If troublesome irritation persists, discontinue use and consult the physician (see Adverse Reactions).

Antibiotic Agents

AZELAIC ACID

Instruct patients to avoid spicy foods, thermally hot foods and drinks, alcoholic beverages, and to use only very mild soaps or soapless cleansing lotion for facial cleansing (gel only).

Avoid alcoholic cleansers, tinctures, astringents, abrasives and peeling agents (gel only).

Cosmetics may be applied after medication dries.

BENZOYL PEROXIDE

Rx	**Benzoyl Peroxide 2½ Wash** (Various, eg, Glades)	**Liquid:** 2.5%	In 237 mL.
Rx	**Benzac AC Wash 2½** (Galderma)		Glycerin, water based. In 240 mL.
Rx	**Triaz** (Medicis)	**Liquid:** 3%	Glycerin, petrolatum, lavender extract, menthol. In 170.3 and 340.2 g.
Rx	**Brevoxyl Creamy Wash** (Stiefel)	**Liquid:** 4%	Glycerin, castor oil, parabens, mineral oil. In 170 g.
Rx	**Benzac AC Wash 5** (Galderma)	**Liquid:** 5%	Glycerin, water based. In 240 mL.
Rx	**Benzac W Wash 5** (Galderma)		Water based. In 120 and 240 mL.
Rx	**Benzoyl Peroxide 5% Wash** (Various, eg, Glades)		In 118, 148, and 237 mL.
Rx	**Triaz** (Medicis)	**Liquid:** 6%	Glycerin, petrolatum, lavender extract, menthol. In 170.3 and 340.2 g.
Rx	**Brevoxyl Creamy Wash** (Stiefel)	**Liquid:** 8%	Glycerin, castor oil, parabens, mineral oil. In 170 g.
Rx	**Triaz** (Medicis)	**Liquid:** 9%	Glycerin, white petrolatum, zinc lactate, lavender extract, menthol. In 340.2 g.
Rx	**Benzac AC Wash 10** (Galderma)	**Liquid:** 10%	Glycerin, water based. In 240 mL.
Rx	**Benzac W Wash 10** (Galderma)		Water based. In 240 mL.
Rx	**Benzoyl Peroxide 10% Wash** (Various, eg, Glades)		In 148 and 237 mL.
otc	**Oxy Oil-Free Maximum Strength Acne Wash** (GlaxoSmithKline)		Parabens, diazolidinyl urea. In 237 mL.
otc	**PanOxyl** (Stiefel)	**Bar:** 5%	Soap-free. Cetostearyl alcohol, glycerin, castor oil, mineral oil. In 113 g.
otc	**PanOxyl** (Stiefel)	**Bar:** 10%	Soap free. Cetostearyl alcohol, glycerin, castor oil, mineral oil. In 113 g.
Rx	**Desquam-X 10** (Westwood Squibb)		Lactic acid, EDTA, sorbitol. In 106 g.
otc	**Neutrogena Clear Pore** (Neutrogena)	**Cleanser/Mask:** 3.5%	Glycerin, titanium dioxide, EDTA, menthol. In 125 mL.
Rx	**Brevoxyl 4 Cleansing** (Stiefel)	**Lotion:** 4%	Cetyl alcohol. In 297 g.
Rx[1]	**Benzoyl Peroxide** (Various, eg, Thames)	**Lotion:** 5%	In 30 mL.
Rx	**Brevoxyl 8 Cleansing** (Stiefel)	**Lotion:** 8%	Cetyl alcohol. In 297 g.
Rx[1]	**Benzoyl Peroxide** (Various, eg, Thames)	**Lotion:** 10%	In 30 mL.
otc	**Clearasil Maximum Strength Acne Treatment** (Boots Healthcare)	**Cream:** 10%	Parabens. Vanishing. In 18 g.
Rx[1]	**Benzoyl Peroxide** (Various, eg, Glades)	**Gel:** 2.5%	In 60 g.
Rx	**Benzac W 2½** (Galderma)		EDTA, water based. In 60 and 90g.
Rx	**Benzac AC 2½** (Galderma)		Glycerin, EDTA, water based. In 60 and 90 g.
Rx	**PanOxyl AQ 2½** (Stiefel)		EDTA, methylparaben, glycerin. In 57 and 113 g.
Rx	**Triaz** (Medicis)	**Gel:** 3%	Glycerin, zinc lactate, EDTA. In 42.5 g.
Rx	**Brevoxyl-4** (Stiefel)	**Gel:** 4%	Cetyl alcohol, stearyl alcohol. In 42.5 and 90 g.
Rx[1]	**Benzoyl Peroxide** (Various, eg, Glades)	**Gel:** 5%	In 60 and 90 g.
Rx	**Benzac AC 5** (Galderma)		Glycerin, EDTA, water based. In 60 and 90 g.
Rx	**Benzac 5** (Galderma)		12% alcohol. In 60 g.
Rx	**Benzac W 5** (Galderma)		EDTA, water based. In 60 and 90 g.
Rx	**Desquam-E 5** (Westwood Squibb)		EDTA, water based. In 42.5 g.
Rx	**Desquam-X 5** (Westwood Squibb)		EDTA, water based. In 42.5 and 85 g.
Rx	**PanOxyl 5** (Stiefel)		12% alcohol. In 56.7 and 113.4 g.
Rx	**PanOxyl AQ 5** (Stiefel)		Methylparaben, glycerin, EDTA. In 56.7 and 113.4 g.
Rx	**Triaz** (Medicis)	**Gel:** 6%	Glycerin, cetyl stearyl alcohol, zinc lactate, EDTA. In 42.5 g.
Rx	**Clinac BPO** (Ferndale)	**Gel:** 7%	EDTA. In 45 and 90 g.
Rx	**Brevoxyl-8** (Stiefel)	**Gel:** 8%	Cetyl alcohol, stearyl alcohol. In 42.5 and 90 g.
Rx	**Triaz** (Medicis)	**Gel:** 9%	Cetyl stearyl alcohol, glycolic acid, zinc lactate, EDTA. In 42.5 g.
Rx[1]	**Benzoyl Peroxide** (Various, eg, Glades)	**Gel:** 10%	In 60 and 90 g.
Rx	**Benzac AC 10** (Galderma)		Glycerin, EDTA, water based. In 60 and 90 g.
Rx	**Benzac 10** (Galderma)		12% alcohol. In 60 g.
Rx	**Benzac W 10** (Galderma)		Water based. In 60 and 90 g.
Rx	**Benzagel Wash** (Dermik)		14% alcohol. In 60 g.
Rx	**Desquam-E 10** (Westwood Squibb)		EDTA, water based. In 42.5 g.
Rx	**Desquam-X 10** (Westwood Squibb)		EDTA, water based. In 42.5 and 85 g.
Rx	**PanOxyl 10** (Stiefel)		20% alcohol. In 56.7 and 113.4 g.
Rx	**PanOxyl AQ 10** (Stiefel)		Methylparaben, EDTA, glycerin. In 56.7 and 113.4 g.

[1] Product available otc or Rx, depending on product labeling.

Indications

►*Acne:* Treatment of mild to moderate acne vulgaris.

May be used in more severe cases as an adjunct in therapeutic regimens including antibiotics, retinoic acid products, and sulfur/salicylic acid-containing preparations. Improvement of the treated condition depends on degree and type of acne, frequency of product use, and nature of other therapies.

Administration and Dosage

►*Cleansers:* Wash once or twice daily. Wet skin areas to be treated prior to administration. Rinse thoroughly and pat dry. Control amount of drying or peeling by modifying dose frequency or concentration. Adjust frequency of use to obtain the desired clinical response. Clinically visible improvement will normally occur by the third week of therapy. Maximum lesion reduction may be expected after approxi-

Antibiotic Agents

BENZOYL PEROXIDE

mately 8 to 12 weeks of drug use. Continuing use of the drug is normally required to maintain a satisfactory clinical response.

➤*Other doseforms:* Apply once or twice daily. After cleansing skin, smooth small amount over affected area. If bothersome dryness or peeling occurs, reduce dose frequency or drug concentration. If excessive stinging or burning occurs after any single application, remove with mild soap and water; resume use the next day.

➤*Storage/Stability:* Store at room temperature 15° to 30°C (59° to 86°F).

Actions

➤*Pharmacology:* The effectiveness of benzoyl peroxide in the treatment of acne vulgaris is primarily attributable to its antibacterial activity, especially with respect to *Propionibacterium acnes*, the predominant organism in sebaceous follicles and comedones. The antibacterial activity of this compound is presumably because of the release of active or free-radical oxygen capable of oxidizing bacterial proteins. In acne patients treated topically with benzoyl peroxide, resolution of the acne usually coincides with reduction in the levels of *P. acnes* and free fatty acids (FFA). Mild desquamation is another observed action of topically applied benzoyl peroxide and may also play a role in the drug's effectiveness in acne. Studies also indicate that topical benzoyl peroxide may exert a sebostatic effect with a resultant reduction of skin surface lipids.

➤*Pharmacokinetics:* Benzoyl peroxide is absorbed by the skin, where it is metabolized to benzoic acid and then excreted as benzoate in the urine.

Contraindications

Hypersensitivity to benzoyl peroxide or any components of the products. Cross-sensitivity may occur with benzoic acid derivatives (see Precautions).

Warnings

➤*Sun exposure:* When using this product, avoid unnecessary sun exposure and use a sunscreen.

➤*Carcinogenesis:* Based upon considerable evidence, benzoyl peroxide is not considered to be a carcinogen. However, in one study, using mice known to be highly susceptible to cancer, there was evidence for benzoyl peroxide as a tumor promoter. The clinical significance of this is unknown. Benzoyl peroxide has been found to be inactive as a mutagen in the Ames Salmonella and other assays, including the mouse dominant lethal assay. This assay is frequently used to assess the effect of substances on spermatogenesis.

➤*Pregnancy: Category C.* It is not known whether benzoyl peroxide can cause fetal harm when administered to a pregnant woman or can affect reproductive capacity. However, there are no available data on the effect of benzoyl peroxide on the later growth, development, and functional maturation of the unborn child. Use in pregnant women only if clearly needed.

➤*Lactation:* It is not known whether this drug is excreted in breast milk. Administer with caution to nursing mothers.

➤*Children:* Safety and efficacy in children younger than 12 years of age have not been established.

Precautions

➤*External use only:* Avoid contact with eyes, eyelids, lips, mucous membranes, and highly inflamed or damaged skin. If accidental contact occurs, rinse with water.

➤*Irritation:* If severe irritation develops, consult a doctor, discontinue use, and institute appropriate therapy. After the reaction clears, treatment may often be resumed with less frequent application.

➤*Bleaching effect:* Benzoyl peroxide is an oxidizing agent; it may bleach hair and colored fabric.

➤*Cross-sensitization:* With benzoic acid derivatives (eg, cinnamon, certain topical anesthetics), cross-sensitization may occur.

Drug Interactions

➤*Tretinoin:* Concomitant use may cause significant skin irritation.

Adverse Reactions

Excessive drying, manifested by marked peeling, erythema, possible edema, and allergic contact sensitization/dermatitis.

Overdosage

➤*Symptoms:* Excessive scaling, erythema, or edema.

➤*Treatment:* Discontinue use. If reaction is caused by excessive use and not allergy, cautiously reinstate at reduced dosage after signs and symptoms subside. To hasten resolution of adverse effects, use emollients, cool compresses, and/or topical corticosteroids.

Patient Information

Keep away from eyes, mouth, inside of nose and mucous membranes. If contact occurs, rinse with water.

May cause transitory feeling of warmth or slight stinging. Expect dryness and peeling; if excessive redness or discomfort occurs, decrease or discontinue use temporarily. If excessive irritation develops, discontinue use and contact a physician.

Avoid other sources of skin irritation (eg, sunlight, sun lamps, other topical acne medications) unless directed by a physician.

Avoid contact with hair or colored fabric; bleaching may occur.

Normal use of water-based cosmetics is permissible.

BENZOYL PEROXIDE COMBINATIONS

Rx	Sulfoxyl Regular (Stiefel)	Lotion: 5% benzoyl peroxide, 2% sulfur	Stearic acid, zinc laurate. In 59 mL.
Rx	Sulfoxyl Strong (Stiefel)	Lotion: 10% benzoyl peroxide, 5% sulfur	Stearic acid, zinc laurate. In 59 mL.
Rx	Duac (Stiefel)	Gel: 5% benzoyl peroxide, 1% clindamycin	EDTA, glycerin, methylparaben. In 45 g.
Rx	BenzaClin (Dermik)		In 25 g.
Rx	Erythromycin-Benzoyl Peroxide (Various, eg, Clay-Park)	Gel: 5% benzoyl peroxide, 3% erythromycin	In 23 and 46 g.
Rx	Benzamycin (Dermik)		20% alcohol. In 0.8, 23, and 46 g.
Rx	Benzamycin Pak (Dermik)		SD alcohol 40B. In 0.8 g pouches. In 60s.

Indications

➤*Acne vulgaris:* Topical treatment of acne vulgaris.

➤*Acne vulgaris, inflamed (Duac only):* Topical treatment of inflammatory acne vulgaris.

Administration and Dosage

➤*Sulfoxyl Lotion, regular and strong:* Apply the medication to the affected areas once a day during the first week, and then twice daily thereafter as tolerated. Adjust frequency of use to desired clinical response. Cleanse the affected areas with a nonmedicated soap prior to application. Improvement is typically seen by the third week of therapy. Maximum lesion reduction can be seen in approximately 8 to 12 weeks. Continue use of drug to maintain satisfactory response.

➤*Duac:* Apply once daily in the evening to the affected areas after the skin is thoroughly washed and patted dry.

➤*Benzamycin/Benzamycin Pak and BenzaClin:* Apply twice daily, morning and evening to affected areas after the skin is thoroughly washed and patted dry.

➤*Preparation of gel:*

Benzamycin Pak – Instruct patient to mix 2 separate components in foil pouch before applying this medication.

BenzaClin – Prior to dispensing, add purified water to the vial of powder (up to the mark) and shake until contents dissolve. Add this solution to the gel and stir until homogenous.

Benzamycin – Prior to dispensing, add ethyl alcohol (70%) to the vial of powder (up to the mark) and shake until contents dissolve. Add this solution to the gel and stir until homogenous.

➤*Storage/Stability:*

Sulfoxyl Lotion regular and strong – Store at room temperature 15° to 30°C (59° to 86°F). Shake well.

Duac – Before dispensing, store in a cold place preferably a refrigerator, between 2° to 8°C (36° to 46°F). Do not freeze. Once dispensed, store in room temperature up to 25°C (77°F) with a 2 month expiration date, discard any unused medication.

Benzamycin Pak – Store at room temperature 20° to 25°C (68° to 77°F). Keep away from heat and any open flame.

Benzamycin, BenzaClin – Prior to reconstitution store at room temperature 20° to 25°C (68° to 77°F). After reconstitution, store refrigerated at 2° to 8°C (36° to 46°F). Do not freeze. Following mixing, *BenzaClin* gel is good for 2 months. *Benzamycin* is good for 3 months; discard any unused medication after expiration date.

Actions

➤*Pharmacology:*

Benzoyl peroxide – Benzoyl peroxide is an antibacterial agent and has been shown to be effective against *Propionibacterium acnes*, an anaerobe found in sebaceous follicles and comedones. The antibacterial action of benzoyl peroxide is believed to be due to the release of active oxygen, it also has a keratolytic and desquamative effect, which may

BENZOYL PEROXIDE COMBINATIONS

also contribute to its efficacy. When benzoyl peroxide is applied to the skin, it is absorbed and converted to benzoic acid.

Erythromycin/Clindamycin – Erythromycin and clindamycin are antibiotics that reduce lesions of acne vulgaris in part due to the antibacterial activity; however, the exact mechanism is not fully known. Erythromycin and clindamycin act by inhibition of protein synthesis in susceptible organisms by reversibly binding to 50 S ribosomal subunits, thereby inhibiting translocation of aminoacyl transfer-RNA and inhibiting polypeptide synthesis. Antagonism has been demonstrated in vitro between erythromycin, lincomycin, chloramphenicol, and clindamycin.

➤*Pharmacokinetics:* Benzoyl peroxide has been shown to be absorbed by the skin where it is converted to benzoic acid. Less than 2% of the dose enters systemic circulation as benzoic acid. Mean systemic bioavailability of topical clindamycin is suggested to be less than 1%.

Drug resistance – There are reports of an increase of *Propionibacterium acnes* resistance to clindamycin in the treatment of acne. In patients with *P. acnes* resistant to clindamycin, the clindamycin component may provide no additional benefit beyond benzoyl peroxide alone.

Contraindications

History of hypersensitivity to erythromycin, clindamycin, benzoyl peroxide, sulfur, or to any of its components.

➤*Duac/BenzaClin:* Hypersensitivity to any of its components or to lincomycin; history of regional enteritis, ulcerative colitis, or antibiotic-associated colitis.

Warnings

➤*Colitis:* Orally and parenterally administered antibacterial agents, including erythromycin and clindamycin have been associated with severe colitis, which may result in patient death. Use of the topical formulation results in absorption of the antibiotic from the skin surface. Diarrhea, bloody diarrhea, and colitis (including pseudomembranous colitis) have been reported with topical and systemic use of antibiotics. The colitis is characterized by severe persistent diarrhea and severe abdominal cramps and may be associated with the passage of blood and mucus. Endoscopic examination may reveal pseudomembranous colitis, stool culture for *Clostridium difficile* and stool assay for *C. difficile* toxin may be helpful diagnostically. When severe diarrhea occurs, discontinue the drug and institute therapeutic measures. Diarrhea, colitis, and pseudomembranous colitis have been known to occur up to several weeks after cessation of oral and parenteral antibiotic therapy.

Mild cases of pseudomembranous colitis usually respond to drug discontinuation. In moderate to severe cases, consider management with fluids and electrolytes, protein supplementation and treatment with an antibacterial drug clinically effective against *C. difficile* colitis.

➤*Concomitant therapy:* Use concomitant topical acne therapy with caution because a possible cumulative irritancy effect may occur, especially with the use of peeling, desquamating, or abrasive agents. Clindamycin and erythromycin containing products should not be used in combination. In vitro studies have shown antagonism between these 2 antimicrobials. The clinical significance of this is not known.

➤*Carcinogenesis:* Benzoyl peroxide has been shown to be a tumor promoter and progression agent in a number of animal studies. The clinical significance of this is unknown. Benzoyl peroxide in acetone at doses of 5 to 10 mg administered twice per week induced skin tumors in transgenic mice in a study using 20 weeks of topical treatment.

➤*Mutagenesis:* Benzoyl peroxide has been found to cause DNA strand breaks in a variety of mammalian cell types, to be mutagenic in *Salmonella typhimurium* tests by some but not all investigators, and to cause sister chromatid exchanges in Chinese hamster ovary cells.

➤*Pregnancy: Category C.* There are no adequate and well-controlled trials in pregnant women. Use during pregnancy only if clearly needed.

➤*Lactation:* It is not known whether erythromycin, clindamycin, sulfur, or benzoyl peroxide is excreted in human milk after topical application. However, erythromycin and clindamycin is excreted in human milk following oral and parenteral administration. Because of the potential for serious adverse reactions in nursing infants, a decision should be made whether to discontinue nursing or to discontinue the drug, taking into account the importance of the drug to the mother.

➤*Children:* Safety and efficacy in children younger than 12 years of age have not been established.

Precautions

➤*Superinfection:* The use of antibiotic agents (especially prolonged or repeated therapy) may be associated with the overgrowth of nonsusceptible organisms including fungi. Such overgrowth may lead to a secondary infection. If this occurs, discontinue use and take appropriate measures.

➤*For external use:* Use externally only. Avoid contact with the eyes, nose, mouth, and mucous membranes. Benzoyl peroxide may cause bleaching when in contact with hair, fabrics, or carpeting.

Adverse Reactions

Topical Antibiotic and Benzoyl Peroxide Combination Adverse Reactions (%)[1]						
Adverse reaction	*BenzaClin* gel (N = 420)	*Benzamycin* gel	*Benzamycin Pak* gel (N = 236)	*Duac* gel (N = 397) (mild to moderate)	Erythromycin-benzoyl peroxide gel	*Sulfoxyl* lotion, *Regular* and *Strong*
Application site reaction	3	—	—	—	—	—
Blepharitis	—	—	1.7	—	—	—
Burning sensation	—	✔	2.5	5/< 1	✔	—
Dry skin	12	3	7.6	19/1	3	—
Erythema	1	✔	2.5	26/5	✔	5
Eye inflammation	—	✔	—	—	✔	—
Eye irritation	—	✔	—	—	✔	—
Face inflammation	—	✔	—	—	✔	—
Irritation	—	✔	—	—	✔	—
Itching	—	✔	—	—	✔	—
Nose inflammation	—	✔	—	—	✔	—
Oiliness	—	✔	—	—	✔	—
Peeling	2	✔	0.5	17/2	✔	5
Photosensitivity reaction (eg, sunburn, stinging with sun exposure)	1	—	1.3	—	—	—
Pruritus	2	—	1.7	—	—	—
Skin discoloration	—	✔	—	—	✔	—
Stinging	—	—	2.5	—	—	—
Tenderness	—	✔	—	—	✔	—
Urticarial reaction	—	3	—	—	3	—

[1] All events; data are pooled from separate studies and are not necessarily comparable.
— = not applicable   ✔ = Incidence not provided.

Patient Information

Benzoyl peroxide may bleach hair, fabrics, or carpets.

Patients should not use any other topical acne preparation unless otherwise directed by a physician.

This medication is to be used externally. Avoid eyes, nose, mouth, and mucous membranes.

Inform patients to mix the *Benzamycin Pak* prior to use. The medication is dispensed in a foil pouch containing medication in 2 separate compartments. Mix contents thoroughly in palm of hand prior to application.

Excessive or prolonged exposure to sunlight should be limited.

After application of medicine, be sure to wash hands.

BenzaClin should be stored in a refrigerator; discard any unused portion after 2 months. *Duac* should be stored at room temperature with a 2 month expiration. *Benzamycin* should be refrigerated and discarded after 3 months.

Antibiotic Agents

CLINDAMYCIN, TOPICAL

Rx	**Clindamycin Phosphate** (Various, eg, Fougera)	**Gel**: 1%	In 30 and 60 g.
Rx	**Cleocin T** (Pharmacia & Upjohn)		Methylparaben. In 30 and 60 g.
Rx	**Clindagel** (Galderma)		Methylparaben. In 7.5, 42, and 77 g.
Rx	**ClindaMax** (PharmaDerm)		Methylparaben. In 30 and 60 g.
Rx	**Clindamycin Phosphate** (Various, eg, Fougera)	**Lotion**: 1%	In 60 mL.
Rx	**Cleocin T** (Pharmacia & Upjohn)		2.5% cetostearyl alcohol, glycerin, 2.5% isostearyl alcohol, 0.3% methylparaben. In 60 mL.
Rx	**Clindamycin Phosphate** (Various, eg, Fougera, Morton Groves)	**Suspension, topical**: 1%	In 30 and 60 mL.
Rx	**Cleocin T** (Pharmacia & Upjohn)		50% isopropyl alcohol. In 30 and 60 mL and single-use pledget applicators.
Rx	**Clindets** (Stiefel Labs)		52% isopropyl alcohol. In 1 mL pledgets.
Rx	**ClindaMax Lotion** (PharmaDerm)	**Suspension, topical**: 1%	2.5% cetostearyl alcohol, glycerin, 2.5% isostearyl alcohol, 0.3% methylparaben. In 60 mL.

For information on the systemic and vaginal use of clindamycin, refer to the specific monographs in the Anti-infectives and Renal and Genitourinary chapters.

Indications
➤*Acne:* Treatment of acne vulgaris.

➤*Unlabeled uses:* Clindamycin lotion has been used in the treatment of rosacea.

Administration and Dosage
Apply a thin film to affected area once (*Clindagel*) or twice daily. More than 1 pledget may be used; however, use each pledget only once, then discard. Use enough to cover the entire affected area lightly.

➤*Lotion:* Shake well immediately before using.

➤*Pledget:* Remove from foil just before use. Discard after single use.

➤*Storage / Stability:* Store under controlled room temperature 20° to 25°C (68° to 77°F) excursions permitted between 15° to 30°C (59° to 86°F). Do not store in direct sunlight. Protect from freezing. Keep container tightly closed.

Actions
➤*Pharmacology:* Clindamycin demonstrates in vitro activity against isolates of *Propionibacterium acnes* which may account for its usefulness in acne. Free fatty acids on the skin surface decrease from approximately 14% to 2% following application. In vitro, clindamycin inhibits all *P. acnes* cultures tested.

➤*Pharmacokinetics:* Following multiple topical applications at a concentration equivalent to 10 mg/mL, very low levels (0 to 3 ng/mL) are present in the serum and less than 0.2% of the dose is recovered in urine as clindamycin. The mean concentration of activity in comedonal extracts from acne patients was 597 mcg/g (range, 0 to 1490).

In an open label, parallel group study of 24 patients with acne vulgaris, once-daily topical administration of approximately 3 to 12 g/day of clindamycin for 5 days resulted in peak plasma clindamycin concentrations that were less than 5.5 ng/mL. Following multiple applications of clindamycin, less than 0.04% of the total dose was excreted in the urine.

➤*Microbiology:* Although clindamycin phosphate is inactive in vitro, rapid in vitro hydrolysis converts this compound to clindamycin, which has antibacterial activity. Clindamycin inhibits bacteria protein synthesis at the ribosomal level by binding to the 50S ribosomal subunit and affecting the process of peptide chain initiation. In vitro studies indicated that clindamycin inhibited all tested *P. acnes* cultures at a minimum inhibitory concentration (MIC) of 0.4 mcg/mL. Cross-resistance has been demonstrated between clindamycin and erythromycin.

Contraindications
Hypersensitivity to clindamycin or lincomycin; history of regional enteritis, ulcerative colitis or antibiotic-associated colitis.

Warnings
➤*Colitis:* Diarrhea, bloody diarrhea, and colitis (including pseudomembranous colitis) have occurred with topical and systemic clindamycin. Symptoms can occur after a few days, weeks, or months after therapy initiation, but have also begun up to several weeks after cessation of therapy. Toxin(s) produced by *Clostridium difficile* is 1 primary cause of antibiotic-associated colitis, which is usually characterized by severe persistent diarrhea, severe abdominal cramps, and the passage of blood and mucus. When significant diarrhea occurs, stop the drug. Consider large bowel endoscopy in severe diarrhea.

Treatment – Vancomycin is effective in the treatment of antibiotic-associated pseudomembranous colitis produced by *C. difficile* (see individual monograph). The usual adult dosage is 500 mg to 2 g of vancomycin orally per day in 3 to 4 divided doses administered for 7 to 10 days. Cholestyramine or colestipol resins bind vancomycin in vitro. If both a resin and vancomycin are to be administered concurrently, it may be advisable to separate the time of administration of each drug.

Antiperistaltic agents such as opiates and diphenoxylate with atropine may prolong or worsen the condition.

➤*Pregnancy: Category B.* There are no adequate and well-controlled studies in pregnant women. Because animal reproduction studies are not always predictive of human response, use this drug during pregnancy only if clearly needed.

➤*Lactation:* It is not known whether topical clindamycin is excreted in breast milk, although oral and parenteral clindamycin appear in breast milk. Because of the potential for serious adverse reactions in nursing infants, discontinue nursing or discontinue the drug, taking into account the importance of the drug to the mother.

➤*Children:* Safety and efficacy in children younger than 12 years of age have not been established.

Precautions
➤*For external use only:* Avoid contact with the eyes. Clindamycin topical solution, suspension, and lotion have an alcohol base that will cause burning and irritation of the eye. In case of accidental contact with eyes, abraded skin or mucous membranes, bathe with copious amounts of cool tap water. Use caution when applying medication around the mouth.

➤*Atopic patients:* Prescribe with caution in atopic individuals.

Drug Interactions
➤*Erythromycin:* Antagonism has been demonstrated with clindamycin.

➤*Neuromuscular blocking agents:* Clindamycin has been shown to have neuromuscular blocking properties that may enhance the action of other neuromuscular blocking agents. Therefore, use with caution in patients receiving such agents.

Adverse Reactions
➤*Dermatologic:*

Clindamycin Dermatologic Adverse Events (%)			
Adverse reaction	Solution (n = 553)	Gel (N = 148)	Lotion (n = 160)
Burning	11	10	11
Itching	7	10	11
Burning/Itching	11	–[1]	–[1]
Dryness	19	23	18
Erythema	16	7	14
Oiliness/Oily skin	1	18	10[2]
Peeling	11	–[1]	7
Pruritus	NA[3]	0.6[4]	NA[3]

[1] Number not recorded.
[2] Out of 126 subjects.
[3] NA = not applicable.
[4] Incidence from a different study.

➤*GI:* Diarrhea, bloody diarrhea, abdominal pains and colitis (including pseudomembranous colitis); GI disturbance; gram-negative folliculitis.

Overdosage
Topical clindamycin can be absorbed enough to produce systemic effects.

Patient Information
This medicine is for external use only. Avoid contact with the eyes as burning or irritation can occur. If contact occurs with the eyes or sensitive surfaces (eg, scraped skin, mucous membranes) wash the area with cool tap water.

This medicine has an unpleasant taste. Use caution when applying this medicine around the mouth.

If severe diarrhea, stomach cramps/pain, or bloody stools occur, contact your doctor at once. This could be a symptom of a serious side effect requiring immediate medical attention. Do not treat diarrhea without consulting your doctor.

Antibiotic Agents

ERYTHROMYCIN, TOPICAL

Rx	Staticin (Westwood Squibb)	Solution: 1.5%	55% alcohol. In 60 mL with optional applicator.
Rx	Erythromycin (Various, eg, Morton Grove)	Solution: 2%	Contains alcohol. In 60 mL.
Rx	A/T/S (Medicis)		66% alcohol. In 60 mL.
Rx	Eryderm 2% (Abbott)		77% alcohol. In 60 mL with applicator.
Rx	T-Stat (Westwood Squibb)		71.2% alcohol. In pads (60s) and 60 mL with optional applicator.
Rx	A/T/S (Medicis)	Gel: 2%	92% alcohol. In 30 g.
Rx	Emgel (GlaxoSmithKline)		77% alcohol. In 27 and 50 g.
Rx	Erythromycin (Various, eg, Glades)		Contains alcohol. In 30 and 60 g.
Rx	Akne-Mycin (Healthpoint)	Ointment: 2%	Cetostearyl alcohol, petrolatum, mineral oil. In 25 g.
Rx	Ery Pads (Glades)	Pledgets: 2%	60.5% alcohol. In 60s.

For information on the systemic and ophthalmic use of erythromycin, refer to the specific monographs in the Anti-infectives and Ophthalmic chapters and the Antibiotics group monograph in this chapter.

Indications
➤*Acne:* Topical control of acne vulgaris.

Administration and Dosage
Apply sparingly morning and evening to affected areas. Before applying, thoroughly wash with warm water and soap, rinse and pat dry all areas to be treated. Apply with fingertips or applicator. Wash hands after use. If there is no improvement in 6 to 8 weeks or if condition worsens, consult a physician. Drying and peeling may be controlled by reducing the frequency of applications.

➤*Storage/Stability: Erygel, A/T/S* gel, *T-Stat, Staticin,* and *Emgel* should be stored between 15° and 25°C (59° to 77°F). Store *Akne-Mycin* below 27°C (80°F). The *A/T/S* solution and *Ery 2% Pads* should be stored at 15° to 30°C (59° to 86°F) and *Eryderm* should be stored below 30°C (86°F).

Actions
➤*Pharmacology:* Erythromycin is a bacteriostatic macrolide antibiotic, but may be bactericidal in high concentrations. Although the mechanism by which topical erythromycin acts in reducing inflammatory lesions of acne vulgaris is unknown, it is presumably due to its antibiotic action. Erythromycin acts by inhibition of protein synthesis in susceptible organisms by reversibly binding to 50 S ribosomal subunits, thereby inhibiting translocation of aminoacyl transfer-RNA and inhibiting polypeptide synthesis. Antagonism has been demonstrated in vitro between erythromycin, lincomycin, chloramphenicol, and clindamycin.

Contraindications
Hypersensitivity to erythromycin or to any component of these products.

Warnings
➤*Pseudomembranous colitis:* Pseudomembranous colitis has been reported with nearly all antibacterial agents, including erythromycin, and may range in severity from mild to life-threatening. Therefore, it is important to consider this diagnosis in patients who present with diarrhea subsequent to the administration of antibacterial agents.

Treatment with antibacterial agents alters the normal flora of the colon and may permit overgrowth of clostridia. Studies indicate that a toxin produced by *Clostridium difficile* is one primary cause of "antibiotic-associated colitis."

After the diagnosis of pseudomembranous colitis has been established, initiate therapeutic measures. Mild cases of pseudomembranous colitis usually respond to drug discontinuation alone. In moderate to severe cases, consider management with fluids and electrolytes, protein supplementation, and treatment with an antibacterial drug clinically effective against *C. difficile* colitis.

➤*Concomitant therapy:* Concomitant topical acne therapy should be used with caution because a possible cumulative irritancy effect may occur, especially with the use of peeling, desquamating, or abrasive agents. Clindamycin- and erythromycin-containing products should not be used in combination. In vitro studies have shown antagonism between these 2 antimicrobials. The clinical significance is not known.

➤*Pregnancy: Category B.* Safety for use during pregnancy has not been established. Use only when clearly needed and when the potential benefits outweigh potential hazards to the fetus. Erythromycin has been reported to cross the placental barrier in humans, but fetal plasma levels are low.

➤*Lactation:* It is not known whether erythromycin is excreted in human milk after topical application. However, erythromycin is excreted in human milk following oral and parenteral erythromycin administration. Therefore, exercise caution when erythromycin is administered to a nursing woman.

➤*Children:* Safety and efficacy in children have not been established.

Precautions
➤*For external use only:* Keep away from eyes, nose, mouth, and other mucous membranes.

➤*Superinfection:* Use of antibiotics (especially prolonged or repeated therapy) may result in bacterial or fungal overgrowth of nonsusceptible organisms. Such overgrowth may lead to a secondary infection. Discontinue use and take appropriate measures if superinfection occurs.

Adverse Reactions
Erythema; desquamation; burning sensation; eye irritation; tenderness; dryness; pruritus; oily skin; peeling; itching; contact sensitization; generalized urticarial reaction that required the use of systemic steroids (1 case).

Patient Information
Wash, rinse, and dry affected areas before application.

Keep away from the eyes, nose, mouth, and other mucous membranes.

Patients should not use any other topical acne medication unless directed by their physician.

Advise patients to wash hands after application of medicine.

METRONIDAZOLE

Rx	MetroLotion (Galderma)	Lotion: 0.75%	Benzyl alcohol, stearyl alcohol, glycerin, mineral oil. In 59 mL.
Rx	Metronidazole (Fougera)	Cream: 0.75%	Glycerin, benzyl alcohol, lactic acid. In 45 g.
Rx	MetroCream (Galderma)		Glycerin, benzyl alcohol. In 45 g.
Rx	Noritate (Dermik Labs)	Cream: 1%	Parabens, glycerin. In 30 g.
Rx	MetroGel (Galderma)	Gel: 0.75%	Parabens, EDTA. In 28.4 and 45 g.

For information on the systemic and vaginal use of metronidazole, refer to the individual monographs in the Anti-infectives and Renal and Genitourinary chapters.

Indications
➤*Rosacea:* Topical application in the treatment of inflammatory papules, pustules, and erythema of rosacea.

➤*Unlabeled uses:* Topical metronidazole has been used as a gel or 1% solution or suspension to treat infected decubitus ulcers; perioral dermatitis has been treated with topical metronidazole gel or cream.

Administration and Dosage
Apply and rub in a thin film once (1% cream) or twice daily, morning and evening, to entire affected areas after washing.

Cleanse areas to be treated before application of topical metronidazole. Patients may use cosmetics after application of topical metronidazole 5 minutes after allowing medication to dry.

➤*Storage/Stability:* Store at controlled room temperature, 15° to 30°C (59° to 86°F) for 0.75% cream and gel; and 20° to 25°C (68° to 77°F) for 0.75% lotion and 1% cream.

Actions
➤*Pharmacology:* Metronidazole is classified therapeutically as an antiprotozoal and antibacterial agent. The mechanisms by which topical metronidazole acts in reducing inflammatory lesions of acne rosacea are unknown, but may include an antibacterial or an anti-inflammatory effect.

➤*Pharmacokinetics:* Bioavailability studies on administration of 1 g topical metronidazole (7.5 mg metronidazole) to the faces of 10 rosacea patients showed a maximum serum concentration of 66 ng/mL. This is about 100 times less than concentrations afforded by a single 250 mg oral tablet. Three patients had no detectable serum concentrations of metronidazole. The mean dose of gel applied during clinical studies was 600 mg (4.5 mg metronidazole) per application. Therefore, under nor-

METRONIDAZOLE

mal usage levels, the formulation affords minimal serum concentrations. The time to peak plasma concentration (T_{max}) with detectable metronidazole was 8 to 12 hours after topical application.

Contraindications

History of hypersensitivity to metronidazole, parabens, or other ingredients.

Warnings

►*Carcinogenesis:* In several long-term studies in mice, oral doses of approximately 225 mg/m²/day or greater (approximately 37 times the human topical dose on a mg/m² basis) were associated with an increase in pulmonary tumors and lymphomas. Several long-term oral studies in the rat have shown statistically significant increases in mammary and hepatic tumors at doses more than 885 mg/m²/day (144 times the topical human dose).

In 1 study, using albino hairless mice, intraperitoneal administration of metronidazole at a dose of 45 mg/m²/day (approximately 7 times the human topical dose on a mg/m² basis) was associated with an increase in ultraviolet radiation-induced skin carcinogenesis. Neither dermal carcinogenicity nor photocarcinogenicity studies have been performed with any topical metronidazole.

►*Mutagenesis:* A dose-related increase in the frequency of micronuclei was observed in mice after intraperitoneal injections. An increase in chromosomal aberrations in peripheral blood lymphocytes was reported in patients with Crohn disease who were treated with 200 to 1200 mg/day of metronidazole for 1 to 24 months.

►*Pregnancy: Category B.* There has been no experience to date with the use of topical metronidazole in pregnant women. Metronidazole crosses the placental barrier and enters the fetal circulation rapidly. Since oral metronidazole is a carcinogen in some rodents, use during pregnancy only if clearly needed.

►*Lactation:* After oral administration, metronidazole is excreted in breast milk in concentrations similar to those in plasma. Even though metronidazole blood levels are significantly lower than those achieved after oral metronidazole, discontinue nursing or the drug, taking into account the importance of the drug to the mother.

►*Children:* Safety and efficacy in children have not been established.

Precautions

►*Conjunctivitis:* Conjunctivitis associated with topical use of metronidazole on the face has been reported.

►*For external use only:* Tearing of the eyes has occurred; avoid eye contact. If a reaction suggesting local irritation occurs, direct patients to use the medication less frequently, discontinue use temporarily, or discontinue use until further instructions.

►*Blood dyscrasia:* Metronidazole is a nitroimidazole; use with care in patients with evidence of, or history of, blood dyscrasia.

Drug Interactions

►*Anticoagulants:* Drug interactions are less likely with topical administration but should be kept in mind when topical metronidazole is prescribed for patients who are receiving anticoagulant treatment. Oral metronidazole may potentiate the anticoagulant effect of warfarin and coumarin resulting in a prolongation of prothrombin time.

Adverse Reactions

Topical Metronidazole Adverse Events (%)[1]				
Adverse reaction	0.75% cream	1% cream (N = 200)	0.75% lotion (N = 71)	0.75% gel
Acne	–	✔	–	–
Burning/stinging	–	–	1	✔
Conjunctivitis	–	✔	–	–
Constipation	–	✔	–	–
Contact dermatitis	–	–	3	–
Dryness	✔	✔	0	✔
Erythema	< 3	–	6	–
Eye irritation (eg, watering/tearing)	✔	✔	✔	✔
Headache	–	✔	–	–
Local allergic reaction	–	✔	3	–
Metallic taste	✔	–	✔	✔
Nausea	✔	✔	✔	✔
Paresthesia	–	✔	–	–
Pruritus	< 3	–	1	–
Rash	–	✔	–	–
Severe flare of comedonal acne	–	✔	–	–
Skin irritation	< 3	✔	✔	✔
Tingling/numbness of extremities	✔	✔	✔	✔
Transient redness	✔	–	✔	✔
Worsening of rosacea	< 3	✔	1	–

[1] All events; data are pooled from separate studies and are not necessarily comparable.
✔ = Incidence not provided.
– = not applicable.

Patient Information

For external use only. Avoid contact with the eyes.

Cleanse affected area(s) before applying the medication. Report any adverse reaction or irritation to your physician.

May apply cosmetics to face after medication is dry.

Antibiotic Agents

MUPIROCIN (Pseudomonic Acid A)

Rx	**Mupirocin** (Various, eg, Clay-Park, Teva)	**Ointment:** 2%	In a polyethylene glycol base. In 15, 22, and 30 g.
Rx	**Bactroban** (GlaxoSmithKline)	**Ointment:** 2% (20 mg/g)	Polyethylene glycol base. In 22 g.
Rx	**Centany** (OrthoNeutrogena)	**Ointment:** 2%	In a base containing castor oil and hard fat. In 15 and 30 g.
Rx	**Bactroban** (GlaxoSmithKline)	**Cream:** 2% mupirocin (2.15% as calcium)	Oil/water base. Benzyl alcohol, cetyl alcohol, stearyl alcohol. In 15 and 30 g.
Rx	**Bactroban Nasal** (GlaxoSmithKline)	**Ointment:** 2% mupirocin (2.15% as calcium)	Glycerin esters. In 1 g.

Indications

►*Topical ointment:* Impetigo caused by *Staphylococcus aureus*, beta-hemolytic streptococcus, and *Streptococcus pyogenes*.

►*Topical cream:* Treatment of secondarily infected traumatic skin lesions (up to 10 cm in length or 100 cm² in area) caused by susceptible strains of *S. aureus* and *S. pyogenes*.

►*Nasal:* Eradication of nasal colonization with methicillin-resistant *S. aureus* in adult patients and health care workers as part of a comprehensive infection control program to reduce infection risk among patients at high risk of methicillin-resistant *S. aureus* infection during institutional outbreaks of infections with this pathogen.

►*Unlabeled uses:* Topical mupirocin may be effective in treating diaper dermatitis caused by *Candida*.

Administration and Dosage

►*Topical ointment:* Apply a small amount to the affected area 3 times daily. The area may be covered with gauze dressing. Reevaluate those not showing a response in 3 to 5 days.

►*Topical cream:* Apply a small amount to the affected area 3 times daily for 10 days. The area may be covered with gauze dressing. Reevaluate those not showing a response in 3 to 5 days.

►*Nasal (12 years of age and older):* Divide approximately one half of the ointment from the single-use tube between the nostrils and apply twice daily (morning and evening) for 5 days.

After application, close nostrils by pressing together and releasing sides of the nose repeatedly for about 1 minute. The single-use tube will deliver a total of approximately 0.5 g of the ointment (approximately 0.25 g/nostril).

►*Storage/Stability:* Store the topical ointment between 20° and 25°C (68° to 77°F), and store the nasal ointment and topical cream at or below 25°C (77°F). Do not freeze the cream.

Actions

►*Pharmacology:* Mupirocin is an antibacterial agent produced by fermentation using the organism *Pseudomonas fluorescens*. Mupirocin is considered a topical antibacterial structurally unrelated to other agents, inhibits bacterial protein synthesis by reversibly and specifically binding to bacterial isoleucyl transfer-RNA synthetase. Mupirocin demonstrates no in vitro cross-resistance with other antimicrobials. However, when resistance does occur, it appears to result from the production of a modified isoleucyl-tRNA synthetase. High level plasmid-mediated resistance (MIC greater than 1024 mcg/mL) has been reported in some strains of *S. aureus* and coagulase negative staphylococci.

►*Pharmacokinetics:*

Absorption/Distribution –

Cream: Systemic absorption of mupirocin through human intact skin is minimal. Systemic absorption was studied following application of mupirocin cream 3 times/day for 5 days to various skin lesions (greater than 10 cm in length or 100 cm² in area) in 16 adults (29 to 60 years of age) and 10 children (3 to 12 years of age). Some systemic absorption was observed by detection of the metabolite, monic acid in urine. More frequent occurrence of percutaneous absorption in children (90%) was found compared with adults (44%). However, urinary concentrations in children and adults were within range. Mupirocin is highly protein bound (more than 97%), and the effect of wound secretions on the MICs of mupirocin has not been determined.

Ointment: Mupirocin ointment applied to the lower arm of healthy male subjects followed by occlusion for 24 hours showed no measurable systemic absorption (less than 1.1 ng mupirocin/mL of whole blood).

Nasal: Following single or repeated intranasal applications of 0.2 g of mupirocin nasal 3 times/day for 3 days to adults showed no evidence of systemic absorption. A study in neonates and premature infants indicated that, unlike adults, significant systemic absorption occurred following intranasal administration. Mupirocin nasal has not been adequately studied in children less than 12 years of age.

Metabolism/Excretion – Any mupirocin reaching the systemic circulation is rapidly metabolized, predominantly to inactive monic acid which is eliminated by renal excretion and demonstrates no antibacterial activity. The elimination half-life after IV administration was 20 to 40 minutes for mupirocin and 30 to 80 minutes for monic acid.

►*Microbiology:* The aerobic isolates of *Staphylococcus aureus* (including methicillin-resistant and β-lactamase producing strains), *S. epidermidis*, *S. saprophyticus*, and *Streptococcus pyogenes* are susceptible to mupirocin in vitro. Mupirocin also has been found to be active against certain gram-negative bacteria.

►*Clinical trials:* The efficacy of topical mupirocin cream for the treatment of secondarily infected traumatic skin lesions (eg, lacerations, sutured wounds and abrasions not more than 10 cm in length or 100 cm² in total area) was compared to that of oral cephalexin in 2 randomized clinical trials. Clinical efficacy rates at follow-up (adults and pediatric patients included) were 96.1% for mupirocin cream (n = 231) and 93.1% for oral cephalexin (n = 219). Pathogen eradication rates were 100% for both mupirocin cream and oral cephalexin.

Pediatrics – There were 93 pediatric patients 2 weeks to 16 years of age in the secondarily infected skin lesion studies. Patients were randomized to either 10 days of topical mupirocin cream 3 times/day or 10 days of oral cephalexin (250 mg 4 times/day for patients more than 40 kg or 25 mg/kg/day oral suspension in 4 divided doses for patients 40 kg or less). Clinical efficacy at follow-up (7 to 12 days post-therapy) was 97.7% for mupirocin cream and 93.9% for cephalexin. Only 1 adverse event (headache) was thought to be possibly or probably related to drug therapy in the mupirocin cream population (1.4%).

Contraindications

Hypersensitivity reactions to any components of the products.

Warnings

►*For external use only:* Avoid mucosal surfaces and contact with the eyes.

►*Pregnancy: Category B.* There are no adequate and well-controlled studies in pregnant women. Use during pregnancy only if clearly needed.

►*Lactation:* It is not known whether mupirocin is excreted in breast milk. Exercise caution when administering to a nursing woman.

►*Children:* Safety and efficacy of mupirocin ointment and cream have been established in children 2 months to 16 years of age.

Safety in children younger than 12 years of age has not been established for mupirocin nasal.

Precautions

►*Open wounds:* Polyethylene glycol can be absorbed from open wounds and damaged skin and is excreted by the kidney. Do not use if absorption of large quantities of polyethylene glycol is possible, especially if there is evidence of moderate or severe renal impairment.

►*Prophylaxis:* There are insufficient data at this time to recommend use of mupirocin nasal for general prophylaxis of any infection in any patient population or to establish that this product is safe and effective as part of an intervention program to prevent autoinfection of high-risk patients from their own nasal colonization.

►*Sensitivity reaction:* If a reaction suggesting sensitivity or chemical irritation occurs, discontinue treatment and institute appropriate alternative therapy.

►*Superinfection:* Prolonged use of antibiotics may result in overgrowth of nonsusceptible organisms, including fungi.

Drug Interactions

Do not use mupirocin nasal concurrently with any other nasal products.

Adverse Reactions

Topical ointment – Burning, stinging, or pain (1.5%); itching (1%); rash, nausea, erythema, dry skin, tenderness, swelling, contact dermatitis, and increased exudate (less than 1%); systemic reactions (rare).

Topical cream – Headache (1.7%); rash, nausea (1.1%); abdominal pain, burning at application site, cellulitis, dermatitis, dizziness, pruritus, secondary wound infection, and ulcerative stomatitis (less than 1%).

Secondarily infected eczema: Adverse events thought to be possibly or probably drug-related are as follows: Nausea (4.9%); headache and burning at application site (3.6%); pruritus (2.4%); 1 report each of abdominal pain, bleeding secondary to eczema, pain secondary to eczema, hives, dry skin, and rash.

Nasal – Headache (9%); rhinitis (6%); respiratory disorder including upper respiratory tract congestion (5%); pharyngitis (4%); taste perversion (3%); burning/stinging, cough (2%); pruritus (1%); blepharitis, diarrhea, dry mouth, ear pain, epistaxis, nausea, rash (< 1%).

Patient Information

This medication is for external use only. Avoid eyes and mucosal membranes.

Stop the medication and contact your doctor if irritation, severe itching or rash occurs.

If no improvement is seen within 3 to 5 days, contact your doctor.

Antibiotic Agents

MUPIROCIN (Pseudomonic Acid A)
The treated area may be covered by a gauze dressing.

➤*Nasal:* Press the sides of the nose together and gently massage after application to spread the ointment throughout the inside of the nostrils.

ANTIBIOTIC COMBINATIONS

Product and Distributor	Polymyxin B Sulfate (units/g)	Neomycin (mg/g)[1]	Bacitracin Zinc (units/g)	Other	How Supplied
otc **Lanabiotic Ointment** (Combe)	10,000	3.5	500	40 mg lidocaine	Aloe, lanolin, mineral oil, petrolatum. In 28 g.
otc **Tri-Biozene Ointment** (Reese)				10 mg pramoxine HCl/g	White petrolatum. In 15 g.
otc **Neosporin Plus Pain Relief Ointment** (Pfizer)					White petrolatum. In 15 and 30 g.
otc **Spectrocin Plus Ointment** (Numark Labs)					White petrolatum. In 28 g.
otc **Betadine First Aid Antibiotics Plus Moisturizer Ointment** (Purdue Frederick)			500		Cholesterolized ointment base. In 14 g.
otc **Double Antibiotic Ointment** (Fougera)					In ≈ 15 and ≈ 30 g, UD 0.9 g (144s).
otc **Polysporin Ointment** (Pfizer)					White petrolatum base. In ≈ 15 and ≈ 30 g.
otc **Polysporin Powder** (Pfizer)					Lactose base. In 10 g.
otc **Betadine Plus First Aid Antibiotics and Pain Reliever Ointment** (Purdue Frederick)				10 mg pramoxine HCl/g	Cholesterolized ointment base. In 14 g.
otc **Neosporin Plus Pain Relief Cream** (Pfizer)		3.5		10 mg pramoxine HCl/g	Methylparaben, mineral oil, white petrolatum. In 15 g.
otc **Neosporin Original Ointment** (Pfizer)	5000		400		Cocoa butter, cottonseed oil, olive oil, white petrolatum. In 14 and 28 g, UD 0.9 g (10s).
otc **Triple Antibiotic Ointment** (Various, eg, Alpharma)					In 15, 30, and 454 g.

[1] As base; equivalent to 5 mg neomycin sulfate.

Indications
Used as a first aid to help prevent skin infection and for the temporary relief of pain in minor cuts, wounds, scrapes, and burns.

Administration and Dosage
Clean the affected area. Apply a small amount of the antibiotic on the area 1 to 3 times/day. Do not use for longer than 1 week unless consulted by a physician. The affected area may be covered with a sterile bandage.

Actions
➤*Pharmacology:* The topical anti-infectives may be either bactericidal or bacteriostatic. Most inhibit protein synthesis. **Bacitracin** inhibits cell-wall synthesis.

Contraindications
Known sensitivity to any of the ingredients; use in the eyes.

Warnings
➤*Systemic therapy:* Deeper cutaneous infections may require systemic antibiotic therapy in addition to local treatment. Use caution when applying over large areas of the body for deep puncture wounds, animal bites, or serious burns.

➤*Neomycin toxicity:* Because of the potential nephrotoxicity and ototoxicity of neomycin, use with care in treating extensive burns, trophic ulceration, or other extensive conditions where absorption is possible. Do not apply more than once daily in burn cases where more than 20% of the body is affected. Especially if the patient has impaired renal function.

➤*External use:* For external use only. Do not use in or near the eyes, nose, mouth, mucous membranes, or apply over large areas of the body.

➤*Pregnancy:* Category C (bacitracin zinc/neomycin). There are no adequate and well-controlled studies in pregnant women. Use only when clearly needed and when the potential benefits outweigh the unknown potential hazards to the fetus. Ototoxicity is known to occur after oral, parenteral, and topical neomycin; however, it has not been reported to affect in utero exposure. Cranial nerve toxicity has been reported in the fetus following exposure to other aminoglycosides (eg, kanamycin, streptomycin) and may potentially occur with neomycin.

Category B (polymyxin B). There are no adequate and well-controlled studies in pregnant women. Use during pregnancy only if clearly needed.

➤*Lactation:* It is not known whether **bacitracin zinc**, **polymyxin B**, or **neomycin** are excreted in breast milk. Exercise caution when applying on a breastfeeding woman. Neomycin has been reported to be excreted into the milk of lactating cows and ewes after a single 10 mg/kg IM dose; also small amounts of other aminoglycosides (eg, gentamicin) are excreted into breast milk and absorbed by the nursing infant.

➤*Children:* Safety and efficacy in children younger than 2 years of age have not been established.

Precautions
➤*Neomycin hypersensitivity:* Chronic application of neomycin sulfate to inflamed skin of individuals with allergic contact dermatitis and chronic dermatoses (eg, chronic otitis externa, stasis dermatitis) increases the possibility of sensitization. Low grade reddening with swelling, dry scaling, itching, or a failure to heal are usually manifestations of this hypersensitivity. Discontinue use if these symptoms appear and avoid neomycin-containing products thereafter.

➤*Superinfection:* Prolonged use of antibiotics may result in overgrowth of nonsusceptible organisms, particularly fungi. Such overgrowth may lead to a secondary infection. Discontinue the drug and take appropriate measures if superinfection occurs.

Adverse Reactions
Bacitracin ointment – Allergic contact dermatitis has occurred.

Neomycin – Hypersensitivity (see Precautions); ototoxicity and nephrotoxicity have occurred (see Warnings).

Patient Information
Discontinue use of medication if rash or other allergic reaction develops or if condition persists or worsens.

For external use only. Cleanse affected area prior to application of medicine.

Notify physician if condition worsens or if rash or irritation develops.

Not for prolonged use. Do not use for longer than 1 week unless directed by a physician.

Antifungal Agents

BUTENAFINE HCl

otc	**Lotrimin Ultra** (Schering Plough)	**Cream:** 1% butenafine HCl	Benzyl alcohol, cetyl alcohol, glycerin, white petrolatum. In 12 and 24 g.
Rx	**Mentax** (Bertek)		Benzyl and cetyl alcohol, glycerin, white petrolatum. In 15 and 30 g.

Indications

➤*Dermatologic infections:* For the topical treatment of the following dermatologic infections: Tinea (pityriasis) versicolor caused by *Malassezia furfur* (formerly *Pityrosporum orbiculare*), interdigital tinea pedis (athlete's foot), tinea corporis (ringworm), and tinea cruris (jock itch) due to *Epidermophyton floccosum, Trichophyton mentagrophytes, Trichophyton rubrum,* and *Trichophyton tonsurans.* Butenafine cream was not studied in immunocompromised patients.

Administration and Dosage

➤*Approved by the FDA:* October 18, 1996.

Apply sufficient butenafine to cover the affected area and immediately surrounding skin. If a patient shows no clinical improvement after the treatment period, review the diagnosis and therapy.

➤*Tinea (pityriasis) versicolor, tinea corporis, or tinea cruris:* Apply butenafine once daily for 2 weeks.

➤*Interdigital tinea pedis:* Apply butenafine twice daily for 7 days or once daily for 4 weeks.

➤*Storage/Stability:* Store between 5° and 30°C (41° and 86°F).

Actions

➤*Pharmacology:* Butenafine is a benzylamine derivative with a mode of action similar to that of the allylamine class of antifungal drugs. Butenafine is hypothesized to act by inhibiting the epoxidation of squalene, thus blocking the biosynthesis of ergosterol, an essential component of fungal cell membranes. The benzylamine derivatives, like the allylamines, act at an earlier step in the ergosterol biosynthesis pathway than the azole class of antifungal drugs. Depending on the concentration of the drug and the fungal species tested, butenafine may be fungicidal in vitro.

➤*Pharmacokinetics:* Following once daily application for 14 days of 6 g of butenafine cream 1% to the dorsal skin (3000 cm^2), the mean maximum plasma concentration (C_{max}) of butenafine was about 1.4 ng/mL. The mean time to peak plasma concentration (T_{max}) was approximately 15 hours and the mean area under the plasma concentration-time curve ($AUC_{0-24\ h}$) was approximately 23.9 ng•h/mL. After once daily dosing to the arms, trunk, and groin areas (10,000 cm^2) for 14 days with 20 g of butenafine cream 1%, the mean C_{max} of butenafine was about 5 ng/mL, a mean T_{max} of about 6 hours, and the mean $AUC_{0-24\ h}$ was about 87.8 ng•h/mL. The total amount of butenafine absorbed through the skin into the systemic circulation has not been quantitated. The primary urine metabolite was formed through hydroxylation at the terminal t-butyl side chain.

➤*Microbiology:* Butenafine has been shown to be active against most strains of the following microorganisms, both in vitro and in clinical infections: *Malassezia furfur, Epidermophyton floccosum, Trichophyton mentagrophytes, T. rubrum,* and *T. tonsurans.*

Contraindications

Known or suspected sensitivity to butenafine or any of its components.

Warnings

➤*Irritation:* If irritation or sensitivity develops with the use of butenafine, discontinue treatment and institute appropriate therapy.

➤*For dermatologic use only:* Not for ophthalmic, oral, or intravaginal use.

➤*Allylamine antifungals:* Patients who are known to be sensitive to allylamine antifungals should use butenafine with caution, because it is possible that these drugs may be cross-reactive.

➤*Pregnancy: Category B.* There are no adequate and well-controlled studies of topically applied butenafine in pregnant women. Use during pregnancy only if clearly needed.

➤*Lactation:* It is not known if butenafine is excreted in breast milk. Exercise caution when administering to a nursing woman. Nursing mothers should avoid application of butenafine cream to the breast.

➤*Children:* Safety and efficacy in pediatric patients younger than 12 years of age have not been established.

Adverse Reactions

Burning/stinging, itching, and worsening of the condition (about 1%); contact dermatitis, erythema, irritation, and itching (less than 2%). No patient treated with butenafine discontinued treatment because of an adverse event.

In provocative testing in over 200 subjects, there was no evidence of allergic contact sensitization for either cream or vehicle base.

Patient Information

Use as directed by the physician. Wash hands after applying the medication to the affected area(s). Avoid contact with the eyes, nose, mouth, and other mucous membranes.

Butenafine is for external use only.

If the patient wishes to apply the medication after bathing, dry the affected area thoroughly before application.

Use the medication for the full treatment time recommended by the physician, even though symptoms may have improved. Notify the physician if the condition worsens or if there is no improvement.

Inform the physician if the area of application shows signs of increased irritation, redness, itching, burning, blistering, swelling, or oozing.

Avoid the use of occlusive dressings unless otherwise directed by the physician.

Do not use this medication for any disorder except that for which it is prescribed.

CICLOPIROX

Rx	**Loprox** (Medicis)	**Cream:** 0.77%	Water miscible base. 1% benzyl alcohol, cetyl alcohol, stearyl alcohol, myristyl alcohol, mineral oil. In 15, 30, and 90 g.
		Gel: 0.77%	Isopropyl alcohol. In 30, 45, and 100 g.
		Suspension, topical: 0.77%	Stearyl alcohol, cetyl alcohol, mineral oil, myristyl alcohol, benzyl alcohol, lactic acid. In 30 and 60 mL.
		Shampoo: 1%	In 120 mL.
Rx	**Penlac Nail Lacquer** (Dermik Labs.)	**Solution, topical:** 8%	Isopropyl alcohol. In 3.3 and 6.6 mL with brushes.

Indications

➤*Loprox:*

Cream and suspension – Tinea pedis (athlete's foot), tinea cruris (jock itch), and tinea corporis due to *Trichophyton rubrum, Trichophyton mentagrophytes, Epidermophyton floccosum,* and *Microsporum canis*; candidiasis (moniliasis) due to *Candida albicans*; and tinea (pityriasis) versicolor due to *Malassezia furfur.*

Gel – Interdigital tinea pedis and tinea corporis due to *T. rubrum, T. mentagrophytes,* or *E. floccosum.* For the topical treatment of seborrheic dermatitis of the scalp.

Shampoo – For the topical treatment of seborrheic dermatitis of the scalp.

➤*Penlac:* As a component of a comprehensive management program for the topical treatment in immunocompetent patients with mild-to-moderate onychomycosis of fingernails and toenails without lunula involvement caused by *T. rubrum.*

Administration and Dosage

➤*Loprox:* Gently massage cream, gel, or suspension into the affected and surrounding skin areas twice daily, morning, and evening. Clinical improvement usually occurs within the first week of treatment. Treat interdigital tinea pedis and tinea corporis for 4 weeks. If no improvement occurs after 4 weeks of treatment, reevaluate the diagnosis. Patients with tinea versicolor usually exhibit clinical and mycological clearing after 2 weeks of treatment.

Shampoo – Wet hair and apply approximately 1 teaspoon (5 mL) of the shampoo to the scalp. Up to 2 teaspoons (10 mL) may be used for long hair. Lather and leave on hair and scalp for 3 minutes. A timer may be used. Avoid contact with eyes. Rinse off. Repeat treatment twice weekly for 4 weeks, with a minimum of 3 days between applications.

Review the diagnosis if the patient with seborrheic dermatitis shows no clinical improvement after 4 weeks.

➤*Penlac:* Apply once daily (preferably at bedtime or 8 hours before washing) to all affected nails with the applicator brush provided. Apply evenly over the entire nail plate.

If possible, apply to the nail bed, hyponychium, and the undersurface of the nail plate when it is free of the nail bed (eg, onycholysis).

Do not remove product on a daily basis. Make daily applications over the previous coat and remove with alcohol every 7 days. Repeat this cycle throughout the duration of therapy.

CICLOPIROX

Use as a component of a comprehensive management program for ony-chomycosis. Removal of the unattached, infected nail, as frequently as monthly, by a health care professional, weekly trimming by the patient, and daily application of the medication are all integral parts of this therapy.

➤*Storage/Stability:*

Loprox cream, gel, and shampoo – Store between 15° and 30°C (59° and 86°F).

Loprox suspension – Store between 5° and 25°C (41° and 77°F).

Penlac – Store at controlled room temperature between 15° and 30°C (59° and 86°F). The product is flammable; keep away from heat and flame.

Actions

➤*Pharmacology:* Ciclopirox is a broad-spectrum, antifungal agent that inhibits the growth of pathogenic dermatophytes, yeasts, and *M. furfur*. It exhibits fungicidal activity in vitro against isolates of *T. rubrum, T. mentagrophytes, E. floccosum, M. canis,* and *C. albicans*. It also acts by chelation of polyvalent cations (Fe^{3+} or Al^{3+}) resulting in the inhibition of the metal-dependent enzymes that are responsible for the degradation of peroxides within the fungal cell.

➤*Pharmacokinetics:* An average of 1.3% of the dose was absorbed when a solution of ciclopirox in polyethylene glycol was applied topically, followed by occlusion for 6 hours. The half-life was 1.7 hours and excretion occurred via the kidney. Fecal excretion was negligible. Glucuronidation is the main metabolic pathway.

Studies in human cadaverous skin with ciclopirox cream showed 0.8% to 1.6% of the dose in stratum corneum 1.5 to 6 hours after application. Levels in the dermis were still 10 to 15 times above the minimum inhibitory concentrations. In other studies, ciclopirox penetrated into the hair and through the epidermis and hair follicles into the sebaceous glands and dermis, while a portion of the drug remained in the stratum corneum. Studies have indicated the therapeutic equivalence of cream and suspension formulations. Systemic absorption of ciclopirox was determined in 5 patients with dermatophytic onychomycoses after application of *Penlac* to all 20 digits and adjacent 5 mm of skin once daily for 6 months. In this study, ciclopirox serum levels ranged from 12 to 80 ng/mL. Based on urinary data, mean absorption of ciclopirox from the dosage form was less than 5% of the applied dose.

Application of 5 mL ciclopirox shampoo 1% twice weekly for 4 weeks, with an exposure time of 3 minutes per application, resulted in detectable serum concentrations in 6 of 18 patients. The serum concentrations measured throughout the dosing interval on days 1 and 29 ranged from 10.3 to 13.2 ng/mL. Total urinary excretion of ciclopirox was less than 0.5% of the administered dose.

Contraindications

Hypersensitivity to ciclopirox or any of its components.

Warnings

➤*For external use only:* Not for ophthalmic, oral, or intravaginal use. The topical solution nail lacquer is for use on nails and immediately adjacent skin only.

➤*Mutagenesis:* Chromosome aberration assays in V79 Chinese hamster lung fibroblasts, with and without metabolic activation, were positive (*Loprox* and *Penlac*). Cell transformation assays in BALB/c3T3 cell assays were positive (*Penlac* only).

➤*Pregnancy: Category B.* There are no adequate or well-controlled studies in pregnant women. Use during pregnancy only if clearly needed.

➤*Lactation:* It is not known whether this drug is excreted in breast milk. Exercise caution when administering to a breastfeeding woman.

➤*Children:* Safety and efficacy in children younger than 10 years of age have not been established (*Loprox* cream and suspension); safety and efficacy in children have not been established (*Penlac*); safety and efficacy in patients younger than 16 years of age have not been established (*Loprox* gel and shampoo).

Precautions

➤*Sensitivity:* If sensitivity or chemical irritation occurs, discontinue treatment and institute appropriate therapy.

➤*Insulin-dependent diabetes mellitus/diabetic neuropathy:* There is no relevant clinical experience in patients with insulin-dependent diabetes or who have diabetic neuropathy. Carefully weigh the risk of removal of the unattached, infected nail before prescribing to patients with a history of insulin-dependent diabetes mellitus or diabetic neuropathy.

➤*Immunosuppression:* There is no relevant clinical experience with patients who have a history of immunosuppression (eg, extensive, persistent, or unusual distribution of dermatomycoses, recent or recurring herpes zoster, or persistent herpes simplex), who are immunocompromised (eg, HIV-infected patients and transplant patients).

Drug Interactions

No studies have been conducted to determine whether ciclopirox might reduce the effectiveness of systemic antifungal agents for onychomycosis. Therefore, the concomitant use of the topical solution and systemic antifungal agents for onychomycosis is not recommended.

Adverse Reactions

➤*Loprox cream:* Pruritus at site of application, worsening of the clinical signs and symptoms, burning.

➤*Loprox gel:* Skin burning sensation upon application, which occurred in approximately 34% of seborrheic dermatitis patients and 7% of tinea pedis patients. Contact dermatitis and pruritus (1% to 5%); dry skin, acne, rash, alopecia, pain upon application, eye pain, and facial edema (less than 1%).

➤*Loprox topical suspension:* Pruritus, burning.

➤*Loprox shampoo:* Increased itching, application site reactions (eg, burning, erythema, itching) (1%); seborrhea, rash, headache, ventricular tachycardia, skin disorder.

➤*Penlac topical solution:* Periungual erythema and erythema of the proximal nail fold (5%); nail disorders (eg, shape change, irritation, ingrown toenail, discoloration), application site reactions and/or burning of the skin (1%); mild rash.

Patient Information

For external use only. Avoid contact with the eyes and mucous membranes.

➤*Loprox:* Use the medication for the full treatment time even though symptoms may have improved. Notify the physician if no improvement occurs after 4 weeks.

Inform physician if the area of application shows signs of increased irritation (eg, redness, itching, burning, blistering, swelling, oozing), which is indicative of possible sensitization.

Avoid the use of occlusive wrappings or dressings.

A transient burning/stinging sensation may be felt. This may occur in approximately 15% to 20% of cases when *Loprox* gel is used to treat seborrheic dermatitis of the scalp.

Loprox shampoo is for external use on the scalp only. Do not swallow.

Shake *Loprox* suspension vigorously before each use.

➤*Penlac:* Avoid contact with skin other than skin immediately surrounding the treated nail(s).

Avoid contact with the eyes and mucous membranes.

Removal of the unattached, infected nail, as frequently as monthly, by a health care professional is needed with use of this medication.

File away loose nail material and trim nails every 7 days after the solution is removed with alcohol.

Apply evenly over entire nail plate and 5 mm of surrounding skin. If possible, apply to the nail bed, hyponychium, and the under surface of the nail plate when it is free of the nail bed (eg, onycholysis). Contact with surrounding skin may produce mild, transient irritation (redness).

Inform health care provider if the area of application shows signs of increased irritation (eg, redness, itching, burning, blistering, swelling, oozing).

Up to 48 weeks of daily applications and professional removal, as frequently as monthly, of the unattached, infected nail are considered the full treatment to achieve a clear or almost clear nail. Six months of therapy with professional removal of the unattached, infected nail may be required before initial improvement of symptoms is noticed.

A completely clear nail may not be achieved with use of this medication. In clinical studies, less than 12% of patients were able to achieve either a clear or almost clear toenail.

Do not use nail polish or other nail cosmetic products on the treated nails.

Avoid use near heat or open flame; product is flammable.

Protect from light (eg, store the bottle in the carton after every use).

Patients should have detailed instructions regarding the use of *Penlac* as a component of a comprehensive management program for onychomycosis in order to achieve maximum benefit with the use of the product.

CLOTRIMAZOLE

otc/Rx[1]	**Clotrimazole** (Various, eg Taro)	**Cream:** 1%	1% benzyl alcohol, cetostearyl alcohol. Vanishing base. In 15, 30, 45, and 2 x 45 g tubes.
otc	**Cruex** (Novartis Consumer Health)		1% benzyl alcohol, cetostearyl alcohol. In 15 g.
otc	**Lotrimin AF** (Schering-Plough)		Benzyl alcohol, cetearyl alcohol. In 12 and 24 g.
otc	**Desenex** (Novartis Consumer Health)		1% benzyl alcohol, cetearyl alcohol. In 15 and 30 g.
otc	**Lotrimin AF** (Schering-Plough)	**Lotion:** 1%	Benzyl alcohol, cetearyl alcohol. In 20 mL.
otc/Rx[1]	**Clotrimazole** (Various, eg Taro)	**Solution, topical:** 1%	PEG 400. In 30 mL.
otc	**Lotrimin AF** (Schering-Plough)		PEG. In 10 mL.

[1] Products are available *OTC* or *Rx*, depending on product labeling.

For information on oral and vaginal clotrimazole, refer to individual monographs.

Indications

➤*OTC products:* Topical treatment of tinea pedis (athlete's foot), tinea cruris (jock itch), and tinea corporis (ringworm) due to *Trichophyton rubrum, Trichophyton mentagrophytes, Epidermophyton floccosum,* and *Microsporum canis.* For effective relief of the itching, cracking, burning, and discomfort that can accompany these conditions.

➤*Rx products:* Topical treatment of candidiasis due to *Candida albicans* and tinea versicolor due to *Malassezia furfur.*

Administration and Dosage

➤*OTC:* Clean skin with soap and water, and dry thoroughly. Apply a thin layer and gently massage over affected area morning and evening. For athlete's foot, pay special attention to spaces between toes. Wear well-fitting, ventilated shoes, and change shoes and socks at least once daily. For athlete's foot and ringworm, use daily for 4 weeks; for jock itch, use daily for 2 weeks. If condition persists longer, consult a physician or pharmacist. Not effective on scalp or nails.

➤*Rx:* Gently massage into affected and surrounding skin areas twice daily, morning, and evening. Clinical improvement, with relief of pruritus, usually occurs within the first week of treatment. If patient shows no clinical improvement after 4 weeks, re-evaluate the diagnosis.

Actions

➤*Pharmacology:* In studies of the mechanism of action, the minimum fungicidal concentration of clotrimazole caused leakage of intracellular phosphorus compounds into the ambient medium with concomitant breakdown of cellular nucleic acids and accelerated potassium efflux. Both of these events began rapidly and extensively after addition of the drug.

➤*Pharmacokinetics:* Clotrimazole appears to be minimally absorbed following topical and vaginal administration.

➤*Microbiology:* Clotrimazole, a broad-spectrum antifungal agent, inhibits growth of various pathogenic dermatophytes, yeasts, and *M. furfur.* Exhibits fungistatic and fungicidal activity in vitro against *T. rubrum, T. mentagrophytes, E. floccosum, M. canis,* and *Candida* sp., including *C. albicans.* Strains of fungi having natural resistance to clotrimazole are rare. No single-step or multiple-step resistance to clotrimazole has developed during successive passages of *C. albicans* and *T. mentagrophytes.* Slight, reversible resistance was noted in 3 isolates of *C. albicans* tested by 1 investigator. There is a single report that records the clinical emergence of a *C. albicans* strain with considerable resistance to flucytosine and miconazole, and with cross-resistance to clotrimazole; the strain remained sensitive to nystatin and amphotericin B.

Contraindications

Hypersensitivity to clotrimazole or any product component.

Warnings

➤*Pregnancy:* Category B. In clinical trials, vaginal use in pregnant women in their second and third trimesters has not been associated with ill effects. However, there are no adequate and well-controlled studies in pregnant women during the first trimester of pregnancy. Use only if clearly indicated during the first trimester.

➤*Lactation:* It is not known whether this drug is excreted in breast milk. Exercise caution when administering to a breastfeeding woman.

➤*Children:* Safety and efficacy in children have been established for clotrimazole when used as indicated and in the recommended dosage. Do not use in children younger than 2 years of age unless directed by a physician.

Precautions

➤*For external use only:* Avoid contact with the eyes.

➤*Development of irritation or sensitivity:* Discontinue use and institute appropriate therapy.

Adverse Reactions

Erythema; stinging; blistering; peeling; edema; pruritus; urticaria; burning; general skin irritation.

Patient Information

For external use only. Avoid contact with the eyes.

Apply after cleansing and drying affected area (unless directed otherwise).

If condition worsens or persists after the treatment period or if irritation occurs, discontinue use and notify physician.

Use the medication for the full treatment time even though the symptoms may have improved. Notify physician if there is no improvement after 4 weeks of treatment for tinea pedis, tinea corporis, cutaneous candidiasis, or tinea versicolor, or after 2 weeks for tinea cruris.

Inform the physician if the area of application shows signs of increased irritation (eg, redness, itching, burning, blistering, swelling, oozing) indicative of possible sensitization.

Avoid use of occlusive wrappings/dressings.

Avoid sources of infection or reinfection.

Not effective on scalp or nails.

ECONAZOLE NITRATE

Rx	**Econazole Nitrate** (Various, eg, Fougera, Taro)	**Cream:** 1%	In 15, 30, and 85 g.
Rx	**Spectazole** (Ortho Pharm. Corp.)		Water miscible base. Mineral oil. In 15, 30, and 85 g.

Indications

Treatment of tinea pedis (athlete's foot), tinea cruris (jock itch) and tinea corporis (ringworm) caused by *T. rubrum, T. mentagrophytes, T. tonsurans, M. canis, M. audouini, M. gypseum,* and *E. floccosum;* cutaneous candidiasis; tinea versicolor.

Administration and Dosage

➤*Tinea pedis, tinea cruris, tinea corporis, and tinea versicolor:* Apply sufficient quantity to cover affected areas once daily.

➤*Cutaneous candidiasis:* Apply to affected areas twice daily (morning and evening).

Early relief of symptoms is experienced by most patients, and clinical improvement may be seen fairly soon after treatment is begun. However, treat candidal infections and tinea cruris and corporis for 2 weeks and tinea pedis for 1 month to reduce the possibility of recurrence. If no clinical improvement occurs after the treatment period, reevaluate diagnosis. Patients with tinea versicolor usually exhibit clinical and mycological clearing after 2 weeks of treatment.

➤*Storage / Stability:* Store below 30°C (86°F).

Actions

➤*Pharmacokinetics:* After topical application to the skin, systemic absorption is extremely low. Although most of the applied drug remains on the skin surface, drug concentrations were found in the stratum corneum which exceeded the minimum inhibitory concentration for dermatophytes. Inhibitory concentrations were achieved in the epidermis and as deep as the middle region of the dermis. Less than 1% of the applied dose was recovered in the urine and feces.

➤*Microbiology:* In vitro and clinical studies revealed econazole nitrate's antifungal activity against the dermatophytes, *Trichophyton rubrum, T. mentagrophytes, T. tonsurans, Microsporum canis, M. audouini, M. gypseum,* and *Epidermophyton floccosum,* and against the yeasts, *Candida albicans* and *Malassezia furfur* (the organism responsible for tinea versicolor).

Contraindications

Hypersensitivity to econazole nitrate or any ingredients of the product.

Antifungal Agents

ECONAZOLE NITRATE

Warnings

➤*Ophthalmic:* Econazole nitrate is not for ophthalmic use.

➤*Pregnancy: Category C.* Fetotoxic or embryotoxic effects were observed in animal studies with oral doses 10 to 80 times the human dermal dose.

Do not use in the first trimester of pregnancy unless essential to the patient's welfare. Use during the second and third trimesters only if clearly needed.

➤*Lactation:* It is not known whether econazole is excreted in breast milk. Following oral administration to lactating rats, econazole and its metabolites were excreted in milk. Exercise caution when administering to a breastfeeding woman.

Precautions

➤*Sensitivity:* If sensitivity or chemical irritation occurs, discontinue use.

➤*For external use only:* Avoid contact with the eyes.

Adverse Reactions

➤*Local:* Burning, itching, stinging, erythema ($\approx$ 3%); pruritic rash (one case).

Patient Information

For external use only. Avoid contact with the eyes.

If condition worsens or persists after the treatment period or if irritation (burning, itching, stinging, redness) occurs, discontinue use and notify physician.

Use medication for the full treatment time even though symptoms may have improved. Notify physician if there is no improvement after 2 weeks (tinea cruris and corporis) or 4 weeks (tinea pedis).

GENTIAN VIOLET (Methylrosaniline Chloride; Crystal Violet)

otc	Gentian Violet (Various, eg, Humco)	Solution, topical: 1%	In 30 ml.
		2%	In 30 ml.

Indications

Topical anti-infective for external treatment of abrasions, minor cuts, surface injuries, and superficial fungus infections of the skin.

Administration and Dosage

Apply locally 1 to 2 times daily or as directed. Do not bandage.

Actions

➤*Pharmacology:* An antibacterial and antifungal dye. Active against some gram-positive bacteria especially *Staphylococcus* species. It inhibits the growth of *Candida, Cryptococcus, Epidermophyton,* and *Trichophyton*. Because of its staining properties and the availability of effective alternatives, gentian violet has generally been replaced in practice by other agents.

Warnings

➤*Pregnancy:* Use in pregnant women is not recommended.

Precautions

➤*For external or topical use only:* Avoid contact with the eyes; do not swallow.

➤*Irritation / Sensitivity:* May cause irritation or sensitivity reactions.

Patient Information

For external use only. Avoid contact with the eyes.

Gentian violet will stain skin and clothing.

Do not apply to an ulcerative lesion; may result in "tattooing" of the skin.

Discontinue use if irritation or sensitivity occurs.

SERTACONAZOLE NITRATE

Rx	Ertaczo (OrthoNeutrogena)	Cream: 2%	Lt. mineral oil, methylparaben. In 15 and 30 g tubes.

Indications

➤*Tinea pedis:* For the topical treatment of interdigital tinea pedis caused by *Trichophyton rubrum, Trichophyton mentagrophytes,* and *Epidermophyton floccosum* in immunocompetent patients 12 years of age and older.

Administration and Dosage

➤*Approved by the FDA:* December 10, 2003.

➤*Tinea pedis:* Apply twice daily for 4 weeks. Apply a sufficient amount of sertaconazole to cover the affected areas between the toes and the immediately surrounding healthy skin. If a patient shows no clinical improvement 2 weeks after the treatment period, review the diagnosis.

➤*Storage / Stability:* Store at 25°C (77°F); excursions permitted to 15° to 30°C (59° to 86°F).

Actions

➤*Pharmacology:* Sertaconazole is an antifungal that belongs to the imidazole class of antifungals. While the exact mechanism of action of this class of antifungals is not known, it is believed that they act primarily by inhibiting the cytochrome P450-dependent synthesis of ergosterol. Ergosterol is a key component of the cell membrane of fungi, and the lack of this component leads to fungal cell injury primarily by leakage of key constituents in the cytoplasm from the cell.

Sertaconazole has been shown to be active against isolates of the following microorganisms in clinical infections: *T. rubrum, T. mentagrophytes, E. floccosum.*

➤*Pharmacokinetics:* In a multiple-dose, pharmacokinetic study that included 5 male patients with interdigital tinea pedis (range of diseased area, 42 to 140 cm^2; mean, 93 cm^2), sertaconazole was topically applied every 12 hours for a total of 13 doses to the diseased skin (0.5 g sertaconazole/100 cm^2). Sertaconazole concentrations in plasma measured by serial blood sampling for 72 hours after the thirteenth dose were below the limit of quantitation (2.5 ng/mL) of the analytical method used.

Contraindications

Known or suspected hypersensitivity to sertaconazole or any of its components or to other imidazoles.

Warnings

➤*For external use only:* Sertaconazole is not indicated for ophthalmic, oral, or intravaginal use.

➤*Hypersensitivity reactions:* Exercise caution in patients known to be sensitive to imidazole antifungals, because cross-reactivity may occur.

➤*Pregnancy: Category C.* In an oral peripostnatal study in rats, a reduction in live birth indices and an increase in the number of stillborn pups was seen at 80 and 160 mg/kg/day. There are no adequate and well-controlled studies that have been conducted on topically applied sertaconazole in pregnant women. Use during pregnancy only if clearly needed.

➤*Lactation:* It is not known if sertaconazole is excreted in human milk. Exercise caution when prescribing sertaconazole to a nursing woman.

➤*Children:* Safety and efficacy have not been established in patients younger than 12 years of age.

Precautions

➤*Sensitivity:* If irritation or sensitivity develops with use of sertaconazole, discontinue treatment and institute appropriate therapy.

Adverse Reactions

➤*Dermatologic:* Application-site reaction, burning skin, contact dermatitis, dry skin, skin tenderness (2%).

➤*Postmarketing:* In non-US, postmarketing surveillance for sertaconazole, the following cutaneous adverse events were reported: Contact dermatitis, desquamation, erythema, hyperpigmentation, pruritus, vesiculation.

Patient Information

Instruct patients to wash hands after applying medication to the affected areas and to avoid contact with eyes, nose, mouth, and other mucous membranes. Sertaconazole is for external use only.

Instruct patients to thoroughly dry the affected areas before application if they wish to use sertaconazole after bathing.

Instruct patients to use medication for the full treatment time recommended by the physician, even though symptoms may have improved. Advise them to notify the physician if there is no improvement after the end of the prescribed treatment period, or sooner, if the condition worsens.

Advise patients to inform the physician if the area of application shows signs of increased irritation, redness, itching, burning, blistering, swelling, or oozing.

Instruct patients to avoid the use of occlusive dressings unless otherwise directed by the physician.

Advise patients not to use the medication for any disorder other than that for which it was prescribed.

KETOCONAZOLE

Rx	**Ketoconazole** (Teva)	**Cream:** 2% in an aqueous vehicle[1]	Cetyl alcohol, stearyl alcohol, sodium sulfite. In 15, 30, and 60 g.
Rx	**Nizoral** (McNeil)		In 15, 30, and 60 g.
otc	**Nizoral A-D** (McNeil Consumer)	**Shampoo:** 1%	In 207 ml.
Rx	**Ketoconazole** (Clay-Park)	**Shampoo:** 2%	In 118 mL.
Rx	**Nizoral** (McNeil)	**Shampoo:** 2% in an aqueous suspension	In 120 ml.

[1] With sodium sulfite.

For information on the systemic use of ketoconazole, refer to the individual monograph in the Anti-infectives chapter.

Indications

➤*Cream:* Tinea corporis (ringworm), tinea cruris (jock itch) and tinea pedis (athlete's foot) caused by *Trichophyton rubrum*, *T. mentagrophytes* and *E. floccosum*; tinea (pityriasis) versicolor caused by *P. orbiculare* (*M. furfur*); cutaneous candidiasis caused by *Candida* sp.; seborrheic dermatitis.

➤*Shampoo:* Reduction of scaling due to dandruff.

Administration and Dosage

➤*Cream:*

Cutaneous candidiasis, tinea corporis, tinea cruris and tinea (pityriasis) versicolor – Apply once daily to cover the affected and immediate surrounding area. Clinical improvement may be seen fairly soon after treatment is begun; however, treat candidal infections and tinea cruris and corporis for 2 weeks in order to reduce the possibility of recurrence. Patients with tinea versicolor usually require 2 weeks of treatment. Patients with tinea pedis require 6 weeks of treatment.

Seborrheic dermatitis – Apply to the affected area twice daily for 4 weeks or until clinical clearing.

If a patient shows no clinical improvement after the treatment period, redetermine the diagnosis.

➤*Shampoo:*

Dandruff – Moisten hair and scalp thoroughly with water. Apply sufficient shampoo to produce enough lather to wash scalp and hair and gently massage it over the entire scalp area for ≈ 1 minute. Rinse hair thoroughly with warm water. Repeat, leaving shampoo on scalp for an additional 3 minutes. After the second thorough rinse, dry hair with towel or warm air flow.

Shampoo twice a week for 4 weeks with at least 3 days between each shampooing, and then intermittently as needed to maintain control.

➤*Storage/Stability:* Do not store above room temperature (25°C; 77°F); protect from light.

Actions

➤*Pharmacology:* Ketoconazole is a broad spectrum antifungal agent. In vitro studies suggest it impairs ergosterol synthesis, which is a vital component of fungal cell membranes. The therapeutic effect in seborrheic dermatitis and dandruff may be due to reduction of *Pityrosporum ovale* (*Malassezia ovale*).

➤*Pharmacokinetics:* In animal and human studies, there were no detectable plasma levels following the use of the shampoo.

➤*Microbiology:* Ketoconazole inhibits the growth of the following common dermatophytes and yeasts by altering the permeability of the cell membrane. Dermatophytes: *Trichophyton rubrum*, *T. mentag-rophytes*, *T. tonsurans*, *Microsporum canis*, *M. audouini*, *M. gypseum* and *Epidermophyton floccosum*. Yeasts: *Candida albicans*, *C. tropicalis*, *P. ovale* (*M. ovale*); and *P. orbiculare* (*M. furfur*, the organism responsible for tinea versicolor). Development of resistance to the drug has not been reported.

➤*Clinical trials:* In a 4 week, double-blind, placebo controlled trial, the decrease in P ovale on the scalp was significantly greater with ketoconazole shampoo than with placebo and was comparable to selenium sulfide. Ketoconazole and selenium sulfide reduced the severity of adherent dandruff significantly more than placebo.

Contraindications

Hypersensitivity to any component of the product.

Warnings

➤*Pregnancy:* Category C. There are no adequate and well controlled studies in pregnant women. Use during pregnancy only if the potential benefits outweigh the potential hazards to the fetus.

➤*Lactation:* Safety for use in the nursing mother has not been established; however, exercise caution when applying on a nursing woman.

➤*Children:* Safety and efficacy in children have not been established.

Precautions

➤*For external use only:* Avoid contact with the eyes.

➤*Sensitivity:* Discontinue if sensitivity or chemical irritation occurs.

➤*Sulfite sensitivity:* The cream contains sulfites that may cause allergic-type reactions including anaphylactic symptoms and life-threatening or less severe asthmatic episodes in certain susceptible persons. The overall prevalence of sulfite sensitivity in the general population is unknown and probably low. It is seen more frequently in asthmatic or atopic nonasthmatic persons.

Adverse Reactions

Cream – Severe irritation, pruritus, stinging (≈ 5%); painful allergic reaction (one patient).

Shampoo – Increase in normal hair loss, irritation (< 1%); abnormal hair texture; scalp pustules; mild dryness of skin; itching; oiliness/dryness of hair and scalp.

Overdosage

➤*Shampoo:* In the event of ingestion, employ supportive measures, including gastric lavage with sodium bicarbonate. Refer to General Management of Acute Overdosage.

Patient Information

For external use only. Avoid contact with the eyes.

➤*Shampoo:* Removal of the curl from permanently waved hair may occur.

MICONAZOLE NITRATE

otc	**Tetterine** (S.S.S. Company)	**Ointment:** 2%	Petrolatum. In 28.4 g.
otc	**Miconazole Nitrate** (Taro)	**Cream:** 2%	Benzoic acid, mineral oil, apricot kernal oil. In 15 and 30 g.
otc	**Micatin** (Ortho)		Mineral oil. In 15 and 30 g.
Rx	**Monistat-Derm** (Ortho)		Water miscible, mineral oil base. In 15, 30 and 90 g.
otc	**Micatin** (Ortho)	**Powder:** 2%	In 90 g.
otc	**Lotrimin AF** (Schering-Plough)		Talc. In 90 g.
otc	**Zeasorb-AF** (Stiefel)		In 70 g.
otc	**Breezee Mist Antfungal** (Pedinol)		Isobutane, talc, aluminum chlorhydrate, cyclomenticone, isopropyl myristate, propylene carbonate, menthol
otc	**Lotrimin AF** (Schering-Plough)	**Spray Powder:** 2%	10% SD alcohol 40. In 100 g.
otc	**Micatin** (Ortho)		Alcohol. Available with and without deodorant. In 90 g.
otc	**Prescription Strength Desenex** (Ciba)		10% SD alcohol 40-B, aloe vera gel. In 90 ml.
otc	**Ting** (Heritage)		10% SD alcohol 40, aloe vera gel. In 85 g.
otc	**Micatin** (Ortho)	**Spray Liquid:** 2%	Alcohol. In 105 ml.
otc	**Lotrimin AF** (Schering-Plough)		17% SD alcohol 40. In 113 ml.
otc	**Prescription Strength Desenex** (Ciba)		15% SD alcohol 40-B. In 105 ml.
otc	**Fungoid Tincture** (Pedinol)	**Solution:** 2%	Alcohol. In 7.39 and 29.57 ml with brush applicator.

For information on vaginal miconazole, see the Miconazole Nitrate monograph in the Renal and Genitourinary chapter.

Indications

➤*Rx and otc:* Tinea pedis (athlete's foot), tinea cruris (jock itch) and tinea corporis (ringworm) caused by *T. rubrum*, *T. mentagrophytes* and *E. floccosum*.

➤*Rx only:* Cutaneous candidiasis (moniliasis); tinea versicolor.

Administration and Dosage

➤*Cream and lotion:* Cover affected areas twice daily, morning and evening (once daily in patients with tinea versicolor). Lotion is preferred in intertriginous areas; if cream is used, apply sparingly to avoid maceration effects.

➤*Powder:* Spray or sprinkle liberally over affected area morning and evening.

Early relief of symptoms (2 to 3 days) occurs in most patients; clinical improvement may be seen fairly soon after treatment. However, treat candida, tinea cruris and tinea corporis for 2 weeks, and tinea pedis for 1 month, to reduce chance of recurrence. If no clinical improvement after 1 month, reevaluate diagnosis. Patients with tinea versicolor usually exhibit clinical and mycological clearing in 2 weeks.

Actions

➤*Pharmacokinetics:* Miconazole alters cellular membrane permeability and interferes with mitochondrial and peroxisomal enzymes, resulting in intracellular necrosis. It inhibits growth of the common dermatophytes, *Trichophyton rubrum*, *T. mentagrophytes*, *Epidermophyton floccosum*, *Candida albicans* and the active organism in tinea versicolor, *Malassezia furfur*.

Precautions

➤*For external use only:* Avoid contact with the eyes.

➤*Sensitivity:* If a reaction occurs suggesting sensitivity or chemical irritation, discontinue use.

Adverse Reactions

Isolated reports of irritation, burning, maceration and allergic contact dermatitis.

Patient Information

For external use only.

If condition persists or worsens, or if irritation (burning, itching, stinging, redness) occurs, discontinue use and notify physician.

Use for full treatment time, even if symptoms improve. Notify physician if there is no improvement after 2 weeks (*Candida* infections, tinea cruris and corporis) or 4 weeks (tinea pedis).

NAFTIFINE HCl

Rx	**Naftin** (Allergan Herbert)	**Cream:** 1%	In 15, 30 and 60 g.
		Gel: 1%	In 20, 40 and 60 g.

Indications

Topical treatment of tinea pedis (athlete's foot), tinea cruris (jock itch) and tinea corporis (ringworm) caused by the organisms *T. rubrum*, *T. mentagrophytes*, *T. tonsurans†* and *E. floccosum*.

Administration and Dosage

Gently massage a sufficient quantity into the affected area and surrounding skin once a day with the cream, twice a day (morning and evening) with the gel. Wash hands after application.

If no clinical improvement is seen after 4 weeks of treatment, re-evaluate the patient.

Actions

➤*Pharmacology:* Naftifine, a broad spectrum antifungal agent, is a synthetic allylamine derivative. Although the exact mechanism of action against fungi is not known, naftifine appears to interfere with sterol biosynthesis by inhibiting the enzyme squalene 2,3-epoxidase. This inhibition of enzyme activity results in decreased amounts of sterols, especially ergosterol, and a corresponding accumulation of squalene in the cells.

➤*Pharmacokinetics:* Naftifine penetrates the stratum corneum to inhibit the growth of dermatophytes. Following a single topical application of 1% naftifine to the skin of healthy subjects, systemic absorption was ≈ 6% (cream) and ≤ 4.2% (gel). Naftifine or its metabolites are excreted via the urine and feces with a half-life of ≈ 2 to 3 days.

➤*Microbiology:* Naftifine exhibits fungicidal activity in vitro against a broad spectrum of organisms including *Trichophyton rubrum*, *T. mentagrophytes*, *T. tonsurans*, *Epidermophyton floccosum*, *Microsporum* *canis*, *M. audouini* and *M. gypseum*, and fungistatic activity against *Candida* sp., including *C. albicans*.

Contraindications

Hypersensitivity to naftifine or any component of the product.

Warnings

➤*Pregnancy:* Category B. There are no adequate studies in pregnant women. Use only when clearly needed and when potential benefits outweigh potential hazards to the fetus.

➤*Lactation:* It is not known whether naftifine is excreted in breast milk. Exercise caution when applying on a nursing woman.

➤*Children:* Safety and efficacy for use in children have not been established.

Precautions

➤*For external use only:* Avoid contact with the eyes.

➤*If irritation or sensitivity develops:* Discontinue treatment and institute appropriate therapy.

Adverse Reactions

➤*Local:*

Cream – Burning/stinging (6%); dryness (3%); erythema, itching, local irritation (2%).

Gel – Burning/stinging (5%); itching (1%); erythema, rash, tenderness (0.5%).

† Gel; efficacy studied in < 10 infections.

Antifungal Agents

NAFTIFINE HCl

Patient Information

Avoid the use of occlusive dressings or wrappings unless otherwise directed by the physician.

For external use only. Keep away from the eyes, nose, mouth and other mucous membranes.

NYSTATIN

Rx	Nystatin (Various, eg, Major, NMC)	Cream: 100,000 units per g	In 15 and 30 g.
Rx	Mycostatin (Westwood Squibb)		Aqueous vanishing cream base. In 15 and 30 g.
Rx	Nilstat (Lederle)		Aqueous vanishing cream base. In 15 and 240 g.
Rx	Nystatin (Various, eg, Goldline, Major, Moore, NMC)	Ointment: 100,000 units per g	In 15 and 30 g.
Rx	Mycostatin (Westwood Squibb)		Polyethylene and mineral oil gel base. In 15 and 30 g.
Rx	Nilstat (Lederle)		Light mineral oil and plastibase 50W. In 15 g.
Rx	Mycostatin (Westwood Squibb)	Powder: 100,000 units per g	Dispersed in talc. In 15 g.
Rx	Nystop (Paddock)		Dispersed in talc. In 15 and 30 g.

For further information, refer to the individual monographs in the Antifungal Agents, Mouth and Throat Products, and Vaginal Preparations sections.

Indications

Treatment of cutaneous or mucocutaneous mycotic infections caused by *Candida (Monilia) albicans* and other *Candida* species.

Administration and Dosage

Apply to affected areas 2 to 3 times daily, or as indicated, until healing is complete. For fungal infection of the feet caused by *Candida*, dust the powder freely on the feet as well as in shoes and socks. The cream is usually preferred in candidiasis involving intertriginous areas; very moist lesions, however, are best treated with powder.

Actions

➤*Pharmacology:* An antifungal antibiotic which is both fungistatic and fungicidal in vitro against a wide variety of yeasts and yeast-like fungi. It probably acts by binding to sterols in the cell membrane of the fungus with a resultant change in membrane permeability allowing leakage of intracellular components. It provides specific therapy for all localized forms of candidiasis, and cure is effected both clinically and mycologically in most localized cases. Symptomatic relief is rapid, often occurring within 24 to 72 hours after initiation of treatment.

Contraindications

Hypersensitivity to any component; not for ophthalmic use.

Precautions

➤*For external use only:* Avoid contact with the eyes.

➤*Hypersensitivity:* Should a hypersensitivity reaction occur, withdraw drug and take appropriate measures.

Adverse Reactions

Virtually nontoxic and nonsensitizing; well tolerated by all age groups including debilitated infants, even on prolonged administration. If irritation occurs, discontinue use.

Patient Information

For external use only. Avoid contact with the eyes.

Apply after cleansing affected area (unless directed otherwise).

If irritation occurs, discontinue use and notify physician.

OXICONAZOLE NITRATE

Rx	Oxistat (GlaxoWellcome)	Cream: 1%	White petrolatum, propylene glycol, stearyl alcohol NF, cetyl alcohol NF, 0.2% benzoic acid. In 15, 30 and 60 g tubes.
		Lotion: 1%	White petrolatum, propylene glycol, stearyl alcohol NF, cetyl alcohol NF, 0.2% benzoic acid. In 30 ml.

Indications

➤*Dermatomycosis:* For topical treatment of tinea pedis (athlete's foot), tinea cruris (jock itch) and tinea corporis (ringworm) caused by *Trichophyton rubrum*, *T. mentagrophytes* and *Epidermophyton floccosum* in adults and children.

➤*Cream only:* Topical treatment of tinea (pityriasis) versicolor caused by *Malassezia furfur* in adults and children.

Administration and Dosage

➤*Approved by the FDA:* August 18, 1997.

Shake well before using.

Apply cream or lotion to affected and immediately surrounding areas once or twice daily for tinea pedis, tinea corporis and tinea cruris. Apply cream only to affected areas once daily for tinea (pityriasis) versicolor. Treat tinea corporis, tinea cruris and tinea (pityriasis) versicolor for 2 weeks and tinea pedis for 1 month to reduce the possibility of recurrence. If a patient shows no clinical improvement after the treatment period, review the diagnosis.

➤*Children:* Cream is effective in pediatric patients for tinea corporis, tinea cruris, tinea pedis and tinea (pityriasis) versicolor; however, these indications rarely occur in children < 12 years of age.

➤*Note:* Tinea (pityriasis) versicolor may give rise to hyperpigmented or hypopigmented patches on the trunk that may extend to the neck, arms and upper thighs. Treatment may not immediately result in restoration of pigment to the affected sites. Normalization of pigment following successful therapy is variable and may take months, depending on individual skin type and incidental sun exposure. Although tinea (pityriasis) versicolor is not contagious, it may recur because the organism that causes the disease is part of the normal skin flora.

Actions

➤*Pharmacology:* Oxiconazole is a broad-spectrum antifungal for topical dermatologic use. The fungicidal activity of oxiconazole results primarily from the inhibition of ergosterol synthesis, which is needed for cellular membrane integrity. It has in vitro activity against a wide range of pathogenic fungi.

➤*Pharmacokinetics:* Five hours after application of 2.5 mg/cm² of oxiconazole cream, the concentration of oxiconazole nitrate in the epidermis, upper corium and deeper corium was 16.2, 3.64 and 1.29 mcmol, respectively. Systemic absorption of oxiconazole is low. Less than 0.3% of the applied dose was recovered in the urine of subjects up to 5 days after application.

➤*Microbiology:* Oxiconazole is active against most strains of the following organisms in vitro and in clinical infections: *Epidermophyton floccosum*, *Trichophyton rubrum*, *T. mentagrophytes* and *Malassezia furfur*.

Oxiconazole is active against the following microorganisms in vitro; however, clinical significance is unknown. Safety and efficacy in treating clinical infections caused by these organisms have not been established in adequate and well controlled trials: *T. tonsurans*, *T. violaceum*, *Microsporum canis*, *M. audouinii*, *M. gypseum* and *Candida albicans*.

Contraindications

Hypersensitivity to oxiconazole or any of the components of the product.

Warnings

➤*Fertility impairment:* At doses > 3 mg/kg/day in female rats and > 15 mg/kg/day in male rats, the following effects were observed: Reduction in the fertility parameters in males and females; reduction in the number of sperm in vaginal smears; extended estrous cycle; decrease in mating frequency.

➤*Pregnancy: Category B.* There are no adequate and well controlled studies in pregnant women. Use during pregnancy only if clearly needed.

➤*Lactation:* Because oxiconazole is excreted in breast milk, exercise caution when the drug is administered to a nursing woman.

Precautions

➤*Sensitivity:* If a reaction suggesting sensitivity or chemical irritation occurs with the use of oxiconazole nitrate, discontinue treatment and institute appropriate therapy.

➤*For external use only:* Avoid contact with the eyes or vagina.

Adverse Reactions

Pruritus (0.4% to 1.6%); burning (0.7% to 1.4%); stinging (0.1% to 0.7%); irritation, contact dermatitis, scaling, tingling, pain, dyshidrotic eczema (0.4%); folliculitis (0.3%); erythema (0.2%); papules, rash, nodules, maceration, fissure (0.1%).

OXICONAZOLE NITRATE

Patient Information

For external use only. Wash hands after applying the medication to the affected area(s). Avoid contact with the eyes, nose, mouth, vagina or other mucous membranes.

Use the medication for the full treatment time recommended, even though symptoms may have improved. Notify physician if the condition worsens or if there is no improvement after 2 to 4 weeks.

Inform the physician if the area of application shows signs of increased irritation, itching, burning, blistering, swelling or oozing.

Avoid the use of occlusive dressings unless otherwise directed.

Only use this medication for the disorder for which it was prescribed.

SULCONAZOLE NITRATE

Rx	Exelderm (Westwood Squibb)	Cream: 1%	In 15, 30 and 60 g tubes.
		Solution: 1%	In 30 ml.

Indications

Treatment of tinea pedis (athlete's foot; cream only), tinea cruris (jock itch) and tinea corporis (ringworm) caused by *T. rubrum, T. mentagrophytes, E. floccosum* and *M. canis*; tinea versicolor.

➤*Solution:* Efficacy has not been proven in tinea pedis (athlete's foot).

Administration and Dosage

Gently massage a small amount into the affected and surrounding skin areas once or twice daily, except in tinea pedis, where administration should be twice daily.

Early relief of symptoms is experienced by the majority of patients and clinical improvement may be seen fairly soon after treatment is begun. To reduce the possibility of recurrence, treat tinea cruris, tinea corporis and tinea versicolor for 3 weeks and tinea pedis for 4 weeks.

If significant clinical improvement is not seen after 4 to 6 weeks of treatment, consider an alternate diagnosis.

Actions

➤*Pharmacology:* Sulconazole nitrate, a broad-spectrum antifungal agent for topical use, is an imidazole derivative with antifungal and antiyeast activity. It inhibits growth of the common pathogenic dermatophytes including *Trichophyton rubrum* (cream only), *T. mentagrophytes, Epidermophyton floccosum* and *Microsporum canis*. It also inhibits the organism responsible for tinea versicolor, (*Malassezia furfur*), *Candida albicans* (cream only) and certain gram-positive bacteria.

A maximization test showed no evidence of irritation or contact sensitization. A modified Draize test showed no allergic contact dermatitis and a phototoxicity study showed no phototoxic or photoallergic reaction to sulconazole nitrate cream.

Contraindications

Hypersensitivity to any of the components of the product.

Warnings

➤*Pregnancy: Category C.* There are no adequate and well controlled studies in pregnant women. Use during pregnancy only if clearly needed. Sulconazole is embryotoxic in rats when given in doses 125 times the adult human dose. Sulconazole given orally to rats at a dose 125 times the human dose resulted in prolonged gestation and dystocia. Several females died during the perinatal period, most likely due to labor complications.

➤*Lactation:* Use with caution in nursing mothers since it is not known if sulconazole appears in breast milk.

➤*Children:* Safety and efficacy for use in children have not been established.

Precautions

➤*For external use only:* Avoid contact with the eyes.

➤*If irritation develops:* Discontinue the solution and institute appropriate therapy.

Adverse Reactions

➤*Local:* Itching, burning, stinging (3%); redness (1%).

Patient Information

Use only as directed.

For external use only. Avoid contact with the eyes.

TERBINAFINE HCl

otc	DesenexMax (Novartis)	Cream: 1%	Benzyl alcohol, stearyl alcohol, cetyl alcohol. In 24 g.
otc	Lamisil AT (Novartis)		With benzyl alcohol, cetyl alcohol and stearyl alcohol. In 15 and 30 g.
otc	Lamisil AT (Novartis)	Spray: 1%	Ethanol, propylene glycol. In 30 mL.

Indications

➤*Topical treatment of the following dermatologic infections:* Interdigital tinea pedis (athlete's foot), tinea cruris (jock itch) or tinea corporis (ringworm) due to *E. floccosum, T. mentagrophytes* or *T. rubrum.*

➤*Unlabeled uses:* Terbinafine is effective in the treatment of cutaneous candidiasis and pityriasis (tinea) versicolor.

Administration and Dosage

➤*Approved by the FDA:* December 30, 1992.

➤*Interdigital tinea pedis (athlete's foot):* Apply to cover the affected and immediate surrounding areas twice daily until clinical signs and symptoms are significantly improved. In many patients, this occurs by day 7. Duration should be for a minimum of 1 week and should not exceed 4 weeks.

Spray – Twice daily (morning and night) for 1 week or as directed by physician.

➤*Tinea cruris (jock itch) or tinea corporis (ringworm):* Apply to cover the affected and immediate surrounding areas once or twice daily until clinical signs and symptoms are significantly improved. In many patients, this occurs by day 7 of therapy. Therapy should be for a minimum of 1 week and should not exceed 4 weeks.

Spray – Once daily (morning and night) for 1 week or as directed by physician.

Many patients treated with shorter durations of therapy (1 to 2 weeks) continue to improve during the 2 to 4 weeks after drug therapy has been completed. As a consequence, patients should not be considered therapeutic failures until they have been observed for a period of 2 to 4 weeks off therapy.

If successful outcome is not achieved during the posttreatment observation period, review the diagnosis.

➤*Storage/Stability:* Store cream between 5° and 30°C (41° and 86°F).

Actions

➤*Pharmacology:* Terbinafine HCl is a synthetic allylamine derivative, which exerts its antifungal effect by inhibiting squalene epoxidase, a key enzyme in sterol biosynthesis in fungi. This action results in a deficiency in ergosterol and a corresponding accumulation of squalene within the fungal cell and causes fungal cell death.

➤*Pharmacokinetics:* Following a single application of 100 mcl (1 mg) to a 30 cm^2 area of the ventral forearm of six healthy subjects, the recovery in urine and feces averaged 3.5% of the administered dose.

In a study of 16 healthy subjects (eight of whose skin was artificially compromised by stripping the stratum corneum to the viable layer), single and multiple applications (average, 0.1 mg/cm^2 twice daily for 5 days) of terbinafine were made to various sites. Systemic absorption was highly variable. The maximum measured plasma concentration of terbinafine was 11.4 ng/ml, and the maximum measured plasma concentration of the demethylated metabolite was 11 ng/ml. In many patients, there were no detectable plasma levels of either parent compound or metabolite. Urinary excretion accounted for ≤ 9% of the topically applied dose; the majority excreted < 4%.

In a study of 10 patients with tinea cruris, once daily application for 7 days resulted in plasma concentrations of 0 to 11 ng/ml on day 7. Plasma concentrations of the metabolites of terbinafine ranged from 11 to 80 ng/ml in these patients.

Approximately 75% of cutaneously absorbed terbinafine is eliminated in the urine, predominantly as metabolites.

➤*Microbiology:* Terbinafine is active against most strains of the following organisms both in vitro and in clinical infections: *Epidermophy-*

TERBINAFINE HCl

ton floccosum; T. mentagrophytes; T. rubrum. Terbinafine exhibits satisfactory in vitro MICs against most strains of the following organisms; however, safety and efficacy of terbinafine in treating clinical infections due to these organisms have not been established: *Microsporum canis, gypseum* and *nanum; T. verrucosum.*

➤*Clinical trials:* In the following tables, the term "successful outcome" refers to those patients evaluated at a specific time point who had both negative mycological results (culture and KOH preparation) and a total clinical score of < 2 graded on a scale from 0 = absent to 3 = severe for each sign and symptom. Mean clinical scores at entry ranged from 8 to 11.

Terbinafine Therapy: Successful Outcomes for Tinea Pedis					
	1 week therapy			4 week therapy	
Therapy	At 1 week	At 4 weeks	At 6 weeks	At 4 weeks	At 6 weeks
Terbinafine	14%	51%	65%	71%	73%
Vehicle	6%	13%	12%	nd	nd
Active control	nd	nd	nd	63%	59%

nd = no data

Terbinafine Therapy: Successful Outcomes for Tinea Corporis/Cruris after 1 Week of Therapy			
Disease	Drug	At 1 week	At 4 weeks
Tinea corporis	Terbinafine	21%	83%
	Vehicle	0	31%
Tinea cruris	Terbinafine	43%	92%
	Vehicle	9%	25%

Contraindications

Hypersensitivity to terbinafine or any component of the product.

Warnings

➤*Diagnosis:* Confirm diagnosis of the disease either by direct microscopic examination of scrapings from infected tissue mounted in a solution of potassium hydroxide or by culture.

➤*For external use only:* Not for oral, ophthalmic or intravaginal use.

➤*Pregnancy:* Category B. There are no adequate and well controlled studies in pregnant women.

➤*Lactation:* After administering a single oral dose of 500 mg to two volunteers, the total dose of terbinafine secreted in breast milk during the 72 hour postdosing period was 0.65 mg in one person and 0.15 mg in the other. The total excretion of terbinafine in the breast milk was 0.13% and 0.03% of the administered dose, respectively. The concentrations of the one metabolite measured in breast milk of these two volunteers were below the detection limit of the assay used (150 ng/ml of milk).

Decide whether to discontinue nursing or the drug, taking into account the importance of the drug to the mother. Nursing mothers should not apply to the breast.

➤*Children:* Safety and efficacy in children < 12 years of age have not been established.

Precautions

➤*Irritation / Sensitivity:* If irritation or sensitivity develops, discontinue treatment and institute appropriate therapy.

Adverse Reactions

In clinical trials, 0.2% of patients discontinued therapy because of adverse events and 2.3% reported adverse reactions. These reactions included: Irritation (1%); burning (0.8%); itching, dryness (0.2%).

Overdosage

Acute overdosage with topical application is unlikely because of the limited absorption and would not be expected to lead to a life-threatening situation.

Overdosage in rats and mice by the oral and IV routes of drug administration has produced sedation, drowsiness, ataxia, dyspnea, exophthalmos and piloerection. The majority of deaths in animals occurred following oral administration of doses exceeding 3 g/kg or following 200 mg/kg administered IV. In rabbits, overdosage produced edema, erythema and scale formation following topical doses > 1.5 g/kg.

Patient Information

Use as directed; avoid contact with eyes, nose, mouth or other mucous membranes.

Use the medication for the recommended treatment time.

Inform the physician if the area of application shows signs of increased irritation or possible sensitization (redness, itching, burning, blistering, swelling or oozing).

Avoid the use of occlusive dressings unless otherwise directed.

TOLNAFTATE

otc	**Tolnaftate** (Various, eg, Fougera, Goldline, IDE, Moore, Parmed, NMC, Rugby, UDL)	**Cream:** 1%	In 15 g.
otc	**Absorbine Athlete's Foot Cream** (W.F. Young)		Parabens. In 21.3 g.
otc	**Genaspor** (Goldline)		In 15 g.
otc	**Tinactin** (Schering-Plough)		In 15 and 30 g.
otc	**Tinactin for Jock Itch** (Schering-Plough)		Petrolatum, mineral oil. In 15 g.
otc	**Ting** (Fisons)		In 15 g.
otc	**Tolnaftate** (Various, eg, Copley, Fougera, Goldline, Major, Moore, Parmed, Rugby)	**Solution:** 1%	In 10 ml.
otc	**Tinactin** (Schering-Plough)		In 10 ml.
otc	**Aftate for Athlete's Foot** (Schering-Plough)	**Gel:** 1%	In 15 g.
otc	**Aftate for Jock Itch** (Schering-Plough)		In 15 g.
otc	**Tolnaftate** (Various)	**Powder:** 1%	In 45 g.
otc	**Quinsana Plus** (Stephan)		Cornstarch, talc. In 90 g.
otc	**Tinactin** (Schering-Plough)		Cornstarch, talc. In 45 and 90 g.
otc	**Aftate for Athlete's Foot** (Schering-Plough)	**Spray Powder:** 1%	14% alcohol, talc. In 105 g.
otc	**Aftate for Jock Itch** (Schering-Plough)		14% alcohol. In 105 g.
otc	**Tinactin** (Schering-Plough)		14% alcohol, talc. **Deodorant:** In 100 g. **Regular:** In 100, 150 g.
otc	**Tinactin for Jock Itch** (Schering-Plough)		14% alcohol, talc. In 100 g.
otc	**Absorbine Footcare** (W.F. Young)	**Spray Liquid:** 1%	Acetone, chloroxylenol, menthol, wormwood oil. In 59.2 and 118.3 ml.
otc	**Aftate for Athlete's Foot** (Schering-Plough)		36% alcohol. In 120 ml.
otc	**Tinactin** (Schering-Plough)		36% alcohol. In 120 ml.

Indications

Treatment of tinea pedis (athlete's foot), cruris (jock itch) or corporis (ringworm) due to infection with *Trichophyton rubrum, T. mentagrophytes, T. tonsurans, Microsporum canis, M. audouini* and *Epidermophyton floccosum* and for tinea versicolor due to *Malassezia furfur.*

In onychomycosis, in chronic scalp infections in which fungi are numerous and widely distributed in skin and hair follicles, where kerion has formed and in fungus infections of palms and soles, use tolnaftate concurrently for adjunctive local benefit in these lesions.

➤*Powder and powder aerosol:* Also effective prophylactically against athlete's foot.

Administration and Dosage

Only small quantities are required. Treatment twice a day for 2 or 3 weeks is usually adequate, although 4 to 6 weeks may be required if the skin has thickened. Continue treatment to maintain remission.

The choice of vehicle is important for these products. Ointments, creams and liquids are used as primary therapy. In general, powders

Antifungal Agents

TOLNAFTATE

are used as adjunctive therapy, but they may be acceptable as primary therapy in very mild conditions.

Actions

➤*Pharmacology:* Effective in the treatment of superficial fungal infections of the skin.

Warnings

➤*Sensitization or irritation:* Discontinue treatment.

➤*Nail/Scalp infections:* Not recommended for these infections except as adjunctive therapy to systemic treatment.

➤*If symptoms do not improve:* After 10 days of use as recommended by the labeling and no improvement, discontinue use unless otherwise directed.

Precautions

➤*For external use only:* Keep out of eyes.

➤*Reevaluate patient:* If no improvement occurs after 4 weeks, reevaluate patient.

Adverse Reactions

A few cases of sensitization have been confirmed; mild irritation has occurred.

Patient Information

For external use only. Avoid contact with the eyes.

Cleanse skin with soap and water and dry thoroughly before applying product.

For athlete's foot, wear well-fitting, ventilated shoes; change shoes and socks at least once a day.

TRIACETIN (Glyceryl Triacetate)

Rx	**Fungoid Tincture** (Pedinol)	**Solution:** Triacetin, cetylpyridinium chloride, chloroxylenol, benzyl alcohol, acetone, benzalkonium chloride	In 30 ml and pt.
Rx	**Fungoid** (Pedinol)	**Solution:** Triacetin, PEG-8, cetylpyridinium chloride, chloroxylenol and benzalkonium chloride	In 15 ml.
Rx	**Fungoid Creme** (Pedinol)	**Cream:** Triacetin, cetylpyridinium chloride, chloroxylenol, mineral oil, lanolin, propylene glycol, parabens in a vanishing cream base	In 30 g.

Indications

Treatment of onychomycosis (nail fungus), tinea pedis (athlete's foot), tinea cruris (jock itch), tinea corporis (ringworm), monilial impetigo and dermatitis.

➤*Spray and tincture:* Only for treatment of onychomycosis.

Administration and Dosage

➤*Cream, solution:* Cleanse and dry affected areas. Gently massage sufficient amount into affected and surrounding skin areas 3 times daily. Clinical improvement usually occurs within the first week of therapy. If no clinical improvement occurs after 4 weeks of treatment, review the diagnosis.

➤*Tincture:* Cleanse and dry affected areas. Use brush to apply twice daily to affected areas of nail surface, beds, edges and under surface of the nail. Continued use may be necessary for several months before results are seen.

➤*Spray:* Shake well. Dry affected areas. Spray onto affected nails, holding actuator down 1 to 2 seconds.

Actions

➤*Pharmacology:* Triacetin, broad-spectrum antifungal and antimicrobial agent, inhibits growth of fungus, yeast and bacterial infections of skin, intertriginous areas and topical mycoses. Effective against the following organisms:

➤*Microbiology:*

Fungus, yeasts – *Aureobasidium mansonii* (*Cladosporium werneckii* and *mansonii*); *Alternaria solani*; *Aspergillus niger*; *Candida albicans*; *Epidermophyton floccosum*; *Microsporum audouinii, canis* and *gypseum*; *Penicillium chrysogenum*; *Piedraia hortae*; *Rhizopus (nigricans) arrhizus*; *(pastorianus) bayanus*; *Torula roseus* (*Candida* sp.); *Tricho-*

phyton mentagrophytes, and *rubrum, schoenleinii, tonsurans* and *violaceum*; *Trichosporon beigelii.*

Gram-positive – *Bacillus ammoniagenes* (*Brevibacterium ammoniagenes*), *cereus* (subsp. *mycoides*) and *subtilis*; *Staphylococcus aureus*; *Streptococcus faecalis.*

Gram-negative – *Enterobacter aerogenes*; *Escherichia coli*; *Pseudomonas aeruginosa*; *Proteus vulgaris.*

When used for onychomycosis, it facilitates removal of hyperkeratotic or mycotic tissue before debriding nail groove due to its apparent softening effect.

Contraindications

Sensitivity to any components of the products.

Precautions

➤*Irritation or sensitivity:* Discontinue treatment and notify physician.

➤*For external use only:* Not for ophthalmic use.

➤*Diabetics or patients with impaired blood circulation:* Use spray with caution.

Patient Information

For external use only. Avoid contact with the eyes.

Apply after cleansing affected area (unless directed otherwise).

Notify the physician if there is no improvement after 4 weeks of treatment (except when treating nail fungus, which may take several months).

Inform the physician if the area of application shows signs of increased irritation indicative of possible sensitization.

UNDECYLENIC ACID AND DERIVATIVES

otc	**Caldesene** (Fisons)	**Powder:** 10% calcium undecylenate	In 60 and 120 g.
otc	**Cruex** (Ciba Consumer)		Talc. In 45 g.
otc	**Cruex Aerosol** (Ciba Consumer)	**Powder:** 19% total undecylenate as undecylenic acid and zinc undecylenate	Menthol, talc. In 54, 105 and 165 g.
otc	**Desenex** (Ciba Consumer)	**Powder:** 25% total undecylenate as undecylenic acid and zinc undecylenate	Talc. In 45 g.
otc	**Phicon F** (T.E. Williams)	**Cream:** 8% undecylenic acid, 0.05% pramoxine HCl	In 60 g.
otc	**Breezee Mist Aerosol** (Pedinol)	**Powder:** Undecylenic acid, menthol and aluminum chlorhydrate	Talc. In 113 g.
Rx	**Blis-To-Sol** (Chattem)	**Powder:** 12% zinc undecylenate	Talc, zinc oxide. In 60 g.
Rx	**Pedi-Dri** (Pedinol)	**Powder:** Zinc undecylenate, aluminum chlorhydroxide, menthol and formaldehyde	Cornstarch. In 60 g.
otc	**Pedi-Pro** (Pedinol)	**Powder:** Zinc undecylenate, aluminum chlorhydroxide, menthol, chloroxylenol	Starch. In 60 g.
otc	**Cruex** (Ciba Consumer)	**Cream:** 20% total undecylenate as undecylenic acid and zinc undecylenate	Lanolin, parabens, white petrolatum. In 15 g.
otc	**Fungoid AF** (Pedinol)	**Solution:** 25% undecylenic acid	In 30 ml.
otc	**Gordochom** (Gordon)	**Solution:** 25% undecylenic acid and chloroxylenol in an oily base.	In 30 mL.
otc	**Desenex** (Ciba Consumer)	**Soap:** Undecylenic acid	In 97.5 g.

Indications

Antifungal and antibacterial agents for tinea pedis (athlete's foot), exclusive of the nails and hairy areas. Also recommended for the relief

and prevention of diaper rash, itching, burning and chafing, prickly heat, tinea cruris (jock itch), excessive perspiration and irritation in the groin area and bromhidrosis.

UNDECYLENIC ACID AND DERIVATIVES

Administration and Dosage

Cleanse and dry area well; smooth or spray on. Apply as needed or as directed.

The choice of vehicle is important for these products. Ointments, creams and liquids are used as primary therapy. In general, powders are used as adjunctive therapy, but they may be acceptable as primary therapy in very mild conditions.

Precautions

➤*For external use only:* Avoid inhaling and contact with the eyes or other mucous membranes. Patients with impaired circulation, including diabetics, should consult a physician before using. Do not use in children < 2 years old except on advice of physician.

ANTIFUNGAL COMBINATIONS

otc	**SteriNail** (Dr. Nordyke's Labs)	**Solution:** Undecylenic acid tolnaftate, propylene glycol, acetone, acetic acid, pripionic acid, benzyl alcohol, eucalyptol and benzyl acetate	In 30 ml. 3-step kit includes SteriScrub (28.35 g) and SteriBrush.
otc	**Blis-To-Sol** (Chattem)	**Liquid:** 1% tolnaftate	In 30 ml.
Rx	**Bensal HP** (7 Oaks Pharmaceutical Co.)	**Ointment:** 6% benzoic acid and 3% salicylic acid	Extract of oak bark. In 15 and 30 g tubes and 30 and 60 g jars.
otc	**Whitfield's** (Various, eg, Dixon-Shane, Fougera, Goldline, Lannett, Lilly, Moore, NMC, Rugby, URL)		In 30 g and 1 lb.
otc	**Blis-To-Sol** (Chattem)	**Powder:** 12% zinc undecylenate	Talc, zinc oxide. In 60 g.
Rx	**Versiclear** (Hope Pharmaceuticals)	**Lotion:** 25% sodium thiosulfate, 1% salicylic acid, 10% isopropyl alcohol, menthol, propylene glycol, EDTA and colloidal alumina	In 120 ml.
Rx	**Castellani Paint Modified** (Pedinol)	**Liquid:** Basic fuchsin, phenol, resorcinol and acetone	In 30 and 480 ml.
		Also available as a colorless solution with alcohol and without basic fuchsin.	In 30 and 480 ml.
otc	**Fungi-Nail** (Kramer)	**Liquid:** 1% resorcinol, 2% salicylic acid, 2% chloroxylenol, 0.5% benzocaine, 50% isopropyl alcohol	In 30 ml.

Ingredients

The principal active components of these formulations include:

➤*Antifungal agents:* UNDECYLENIC ACID (see individual monograph), SODIUM PROPIONATE, BENZOIC ACID, SODIUM THIOSULFATE.

➤*Other components include:*

SALICYLIC ACID – For its topical keratolytic action (see individual monograph).

BORIC ACID – As an astringent and antiseptic.

CHLOROXYLENOL – As an antiseptic.

BENZOCAINE – As an anesthetic (see individual monograph).

MENTHOL and PHENOL – For their antipruritic, anesthetic and antiseptic effects.

RESORCINOL – As an antipruritic and antiseptic.

CHLOROPHYLL DERIVATIVES – To promote healing, although there is no evidence to support this effect. These agents do have a deodorant action.

BASIC FUCHSIN – For its antifungal and antibacterial activity.

➤*Note:* The choice of vehicle is important for these products. Ointments, creams and liquids are used as primary therapy. In general, powders are used as adjunctive therapy, but they may be acceptable as primary therapy in very mild conditions.

Antiseptics and Germicides

BENZALKONIUM CHLORIDE (BAC)

otc	**Benzalkonium Chloride** (Various, eg, A-A Spectrum)	**Concentrate:** 17%	In 500 ml and 4 L.
otc	**Benza** (Century)	**Solution:** 1:750	In 60 and 120 ml.
otc	**Ony-Clear** (Pedinol Pharmacal)	**Solution, topical:** 1%	Urea. In 30 ml with brush-on applicator.
otc	**Zephiran** (Sanofi Winthrop)	**Solution, aqueous:** 1:750	In 240 ml and gal.
		Disinfectant concentrate: 17%	In 120 ml and gal.
		Tincture: 1:750	In gal.
		Tissue: 1:750. With chlorothymol, isopropyl alcohol and alcohol (20%)	In individual single use packets.
otc	**Mycocide NS** (Woodward)	**Solution:** Benzalkonium chloride, propylene glycol, diazolidinyl urea, methylparaben	In 30 ml.
otc	**no more germies towelettes** (Johnson & Johnson)	**Towelettes:** Benzalkonium chloride, aloe vera gel, EDTA, methylparaben, 15% SD alcohol 40.	In 24 individually wrapped towelettes.

Indications

➤*Aqueous solutions in appropriate dilutions:* Antisepsis of skin, mucous membranes and wounds; preoperative preparation of the skin; surgeons' hand and arm soaks; treatment of wounds; preservation of ophthalmic solutions; irrigations of the eye, body cavities, bladder and urethra; vaginal douching.

➤*Tinctures and sprays:* Preoperative preparation of the skin and treatment of minor skin wounds and abrasions.

Sterile storage of instruments and hospital utensils.

Administration and Dosage

Thoroughly rinse anionic detergents and soaps from the skin or other areas prior to use of solutions because they reduce the antibacterial activity of BAC.

➤*Incompatibilities:* The following are incompatible with BAC solutions: Iodine; silver nitrate; fluorescein; nitrates; peroxide; lanolin; potassium permanganate; aluminum; caramel; kaolin; pine oil; zinc sulfate; zinc oxide; yellow oxide of mercury.

➤*Recommended dilutions for specific applications of BAC solutions:*

Bladder retention lavage – 1:20,000 to 1:40,000 aqueous solution.

Bladder and urethral irrigation – 1:5000 to 1:20,000 aqueous solution.

Breast/nipple hygiene – 1:1000 to 1:2000 aqueous solution.

Catheters and other adsorbent articles – 1:500 aqueous solution (replenish frequently).

Deep infected wounds – 1:3000 to 1:20,000 aqueous solution.

Denuded skin and mucous membranes – 1:5000 to 1:10,000 aqueous solution.

Eye irrigation – 1:5000 to 1:10,000 aqueous solution.

Hospital disinfection – 1:750 aqueous solution.

Metallic instruments, ampuls and thermometers – 1:750 aqueous solution (replenish frequently).

Minor wounds/lacerations – 1:750 tincture or spray.

Oozing and open infections – 1:2000 to 1:5000 aqueous solution.

Postepisiotomy care – 1:5000 to 1:10,000 aqueous solution.

Preoperative disinfection of skin – 1:750 tincture, aqueous solution or spray.

Preservation of ophthalmic solutions – 1:5000 to 1:7500 aqueous solution.

Surgeons' hand and arm soaks – 1:750 aqueous solution.

Vaginal douche/irrigation – 1:2000 to 1:5000 aqueous solution.

Wet dressings – 1:5000 or less aqueous solution.

Preoperative prep – Perform preoperative periorbital skin or head prep only before the patient or eye is anesthetized.

➤*Prevention of rust:* To protect metal instruments stored in BAC solution, add crushed Anti-Rust Tablets (eg, Sanofi Winthrop, Lannett). Add 4 tablets/quart to the antiseptic solution. Change solution at least once a week. Not for storage of aluminum or zinc instruments, instruments with lenses fastened by cement (such as cystoscopes or optical instruments), lacquered catheters or some synthetic rubber goods.

Actions

➤*Pharmacology:* Benzalkonium chloride (BAC), a cationic surface-active agent, is also a rapidly acting anti-infective agent with a moderately long duration of action. It is active against bacteria and some viruses, fungi and protozoa. Bacterial spores are resistant. Solutions are bacteriostatic or bactericidal according to their concentration. The exact mechanism of bactericidal action is unknown, but may be due to enzyme inactivation. Solutions also have deodorant, wetting, detergent, keratolytic and emulsifying activity.

Contraindications

Use in occlusive dressings, casts and anal or vaginal packs because irritation or chemical burns may result.

Warnings

➤*Diluents:* Use Sterile Water for Injection as a diluent for aqueous solutions intended for deep wounds or for irrigation of body cavities. Otherwise, use freshly distilled water. Tap water containing metallic ions and organic matter may reduce antibacterial potency. Do not use resin deionized water since it may contain pathogenic bacteria.

➤*Storage:* Organic, inorganic and synthetic materials and surfaces may adsorb sufficient quantities to significantly reduce the antibacterial potency in solutions, resulting in serious contamination of solutions with viable pathogenic bacteria. Do not use corks to stopper bottles containing BAC solution. Do not store cotton, wool, rayon or other materials in solutions. Use sterile gauze sponges and fiber pledgets to apply solutions to the skin, and store in separate containers; immerse in BAC solutions immediately prior to application.

➤*Soaps:* BAC solutions are inactivated by soaps and anionic detergents; therefore, rinse thoroughly if these agents are employed prior to BAC use.

➤*Sterilization:* Do not rely upon antiseptic solutions to achieve complete sterilization; they do not destroy bacterial spores and certain viruses, including the etiologic agent of infectious hepatitis, and may not destroy *Mycobacterium tuberculosis* and other bacteria. In addition, when applied to the skin, BAC may form a film under which bacteria remain viable.

➤*Flammable solvents:* The tinted tincture and spray contain flammable solvents; do not use near an open flame or cautery.

➤*Eyes/Mucous membranes:* If solutions stronger than 1:3000 enter the eyes, irrigate immediately and repeatedly with water; obtain medical attention promptly. Do not use concentrations> 1:5000 on mucous membranes, except the vaginal mucosa (see recommended dilutions). Keep the tinted tincture and spray, which contain irritating organic solvents, away from the eyes or other mucous membranes.

Precautions

➤*Prolonged contact:* In preoperative antisepsis, do not prolong solution contact with the patient's skin. Avoid pooling of the solution on the operating table.

➤*Inflamed/Irritated tissues:* Solutions used must be more dilute than those used on normal tissues (see recommended dilutions).

➤*Corrosion of instruments:* To prevent corrosion of metal instruments, sodium nitrite (Anti-Rust Tablets) is added to the BAC solution. See Administration and Dosage.

Adverse Reactions

Solutions in concentrations normally used have low systemic and local toxicity and are generally well tolerated, although a rare individual may exhibit hypersensitivity.

Overdosage

➤*Symptoms:* Marked local GI tract irritation (eg, nausea, vomiting) may occur after ingestion. Signs of systemic toxicity include restlessness, apprehension, weakness, confusion, dyspnea, cyanosis, collapse, convulsions and coma. Death occurs as a result of respiratory muscle paralysis.

➤*Treatment:* Immediately administer several glasses of mild soap solution, milk or egg whites beaten in water. This may be followed by gastric lavage with a mild soap solution. Avoid alcohol as it promotes absorption.

To support respiration, clear airway and administer oxygen; employ artificial respiration if necessary. If convulsions occur, a short-acting parenteral barbiturate may be given with caution.

CHLORHEXIDINE GLUCONATE

otc	**BactoShield 2** (Amsco)	**Solution:** 2% with 4% isopropyl alcohol	In 960 ml.
otc	**Dyna-Hex 2 Skin Cleanser** (Western Medical)	**Liquid:** 2% with 4% isopropyl alcohol	In 120, 240, 480 and 960 ml and gal.
otc	**Betasept** (Purdue Frederick)	**Liquid:** 4% with 4% isopropyl alcohol	In 946 ml.
otc	**Dyna-Hex Skin Cleanser** (Western Medical)		In 120, 240 and 480 ml and gal.
otc	**Exidine Skin Cleanser** (Baxter Health Care)		In 120 and 240 ml, qt and gal.
otc	**Hibiclens Antiseptic/Anti-microbial Skin Cleanser** (Stuart)		In 120, 240, 480, and 960 ml.
otc	**Hibistat Germicidal Hand Rinse** (Stuart)	**Rinse:** 0.5% with 70% isopropanol and emollients	In 120 and 240 ml.
otc	**Hibistat Towelettes** (Stuart)	**Wipes:** 0.5% with 70% isopropanol	In 50s.
otc	**Hibiclens** (Stuart)	**Sponge/Brush:** 4% with 4% isopropyl alcohol	In unit-of-use 22 ml.
otc	**Bactoshield** (Amsco)	**Foam:** 4% with 4% isopropyl alcohol	In 180 ml aerosol.

Indications

Surgical scrub; skin cleanser; preoperative skin preparation; skin wound cleanser; preoperative showering and bathing (*Hibiclens* liquid).

➤*Hand rinse:* Health care personnel germicidal hand rinse; when hands are physically clean, but need degerming, and when routine handwashing is inconvenient or undesirable.

Chlorhexidine gluconate 0.12% is also indicated for the treatment of gingivitis. See monograph in the Mouth and Throat Products section.

➤*Unlabeled uses:* Chlorhexidine gluconate 4% skin cleanser twice daily appears effective in the treatment of acne vulgaris (significant reduction of papules plus pustules count).

Administration and Dosage

➤*Cleanser:*

Surgical scrub – Wet hands and forearms with warm water. Apply about 5 ml and scrub 3 minutes using a wet brush, paying particular attention to the nails, cuticles and interdigital spaces. Rinse thoroughly. Wash for an additional 3 minutes with 5 ml and rinse under running water. Dry thoroughly.

Preoperative skin preparation – Apply liberally to surgical site and swab for ≥ 2 minutes. Dry with sterile towel. Repeat for an additional 2 minutes and dry with sterile towel.

➤*Preoperative showering and whole-body bathing (Hibiclens liquid):* Instruct patient to wash the entire body, including the scalp, on two consecutive occasions immediately prior to surgery. Each procedure should consist of two consecutive thorough applications followed by thorough rinsing. If the patient's condition allows, showering is recommended for whole-body bathing. The recommended procedure is: Wet the body, including hair. Wash the hair using 25 ml and the body with another 25 ml. Rinse. Repeat. Rinse thoroughly after second application.

Hand wash – Wet hands with water. Apply about 5 ml into cupped hands and wash vigorously for 15 seconds. Rinse and dry thoroughly.

Skin wound and general skin cleanser – Thoroughly rinse affected area with water. Apply a sufficient amount to cover skin or wound area and wash gently. Rinse again thoroughly.

➤*Hand rinse/wipe:* Dispense about 5 ml into cupped hand or use one towelette and rub vigorously until dry (about 15 seconds), paying particular attention to nails and interdigital spaces. Rinse dries rapidly; no water or toweling are necessary.

➤*Sponge/Brush for surgical hand scrub:* Wet hands. Use nail cleaner under fingernails and to clean cuticles. Wet hands and forearms to the elbow with warm water. Wet sponge side of sponge/brush. Squeeze and pump immediately to work up adequate lather. Apply lather to hands and forearms using sponge side of the product. Start 3 minute scrub by using the brush side of the product to scrub *only* nails, cuticles and interdigital areas. Use sponge side for scrubbing hands and forearms (avoid using brush on these more sensitive areas). Rinse thoroughly with warm water. Scrub for an additional 3 minutes using sponge side only. To produce additional lather, add a small amount of water and pump the sponge. (While scrubbing, do not use excessive pressure to produce lather – a small amount of lather is all that is required to adequately cleanse skin.) Rinse and dry thoroughly, blotting hands and forearms with a soft sterile towel.

Actions

➤*Pharmacology:* Provides a persistent antimicrobial effect against a wide range of microorganisms, including gram-positive and gram-negative bacteria such as *Pseudomonas aeruginosa*.

Contraindications

Hypersensitivity to chlorhexidine gluconate or any component of the product.

Warnings

➤*Hypersensitivity reactions:* There have been several case reports of anaphylaxis following disinfection with 0.05% to 1% chlorhexidine. Symptoms included generalized urticaria, bronchospasm, cough, dyspnea, wheezing and malaise. Symptoms resolved following therapy with various agents including oxygen, aminophylline, epinephrine, corticosteroids or antihistamines. Refer to Management of Acute Hypersensitivity Reactions.

➤*Lactation:* In one case report, a mother sprayed chlorhexidine gluconate on her breasts to prevent mastitis. Her 2-day-old infant developed bradycardia episodes after breastfeeding; symptoms resolved when the chlorhexidine was discontinued.

Precautions

➤*For external use only:* Keep out of eyes, ears and mouth; if this accidentally occurs, rinse out promptly and thoroughly with water. Do not use as a preoperative skin preparation of the face or head (except *Hibiclens* liquid). Serious and permanent eye injury has occurred when it enters and remains in the eye during surgery (see Adverse Reactions).

➤*Meninges:* Avoid contact with meninges (see Adverse Reactions).

➤*Excessive heat:* Avoid exposing the drug to excessive heat (> 40°C; 104°F).

➤*Do not use:* For routine use on wounds involving more than the superficial layers of skin, or for repeated general skin cleansing of large body areas except in those patients whose underlying condition makes it necessary to reduce the bacterial population of the skin.

➤*Deafness:* May cause deafness when instilled in the middle ear. Take particular care in the presence of a perforated eardrum to prevent exposure of inner ear tissues.

Adverse Reactions

Irritation; dermatitis; photosensitivity (rare); deafness (see Precautions). Sensitization and generalized allergic reactions have occurred, especially in the genital areas. If adverse reactions occur, discontinue use immediately. If severe, contact physician.

Antiseptics and Germicides

GLUTARALDEHYDE

otc	Cidex[1] (J & J Medical)	Solution: 2%	In qt, gal and 2.5 gal.[3]
otc	Cidex Plus 28[2] (J & J Medical)	Solution: 3.2%	In qt, gal and 2.5 gal.[4]

[1] Activated dialdehyde is stable for 14 days after activation.
[2] Long-life activated dialdehyde is stable for 28 days after activation.

[3] Vial of activator contains solid sodium salts as buffer to adjust pH to 8.2 to 8.9.
[4] Vial of activator contains aqueous potassium salts as buffer to adjust pH to 7.2 to 7.8.

Indications

Germicidal agent for disinfection and sterilization of rigid and flexible fiberoptic endoscopes, plastic and rubber respiratory and anesthesia equipment, surgical and dental instruments and thermometers.

Actions

➤*Pharmacology:* Glutaraldehyde (pH 3 to 4) is a mildly acidic dialdehyde. Following alkalinization to a pH of 7.5 to 8.5 with sodium bicarbonate or aqueous potassium salt, it becomes a highly effective antimicrobial agent with potent bactericidal, tuberculocidal, fungicidal, sporicidal and virucidal activity. A high degree of effectiveness is retained even in the presence of organic material (eg, blood, tissue, mucus).

Precautions

➤*Avoid contact:* With eyes, skin and mucous membranes. If contact with skin or mucous membranes occurs, wash promptly with water. Should accidental contact with the eye occur, promptly irrigate with water and report to a physician.

➤*Fumes:* Solution fumes may be irritating to the respiratory tract, therefore keep solutions covered and use only in a well ventilated area.

➤*Directions:* To remove debris from equipment thoroughly brush clean with a mild detergent solution that does not contain an emollient; rinse and rough dry equipment prior to placement in the solution.

Place clean, dry instruments or equipment in perforated pail or tray and immerse in container of alkalinized glutaraldehyde solution. Cover container to minimize odor and prevent evaporation.

Disinfection – Follow specific label directions for immersion to destroy vegetative pathogens on inanimate surfaces. Rinse equipment thoroughly before use.

Sterilization – Immerse completely for a minimum of 10 hours to destroy resistant pathogenic spores. Use sterile technique to remove instruments from solution. Rinse thoroughly with sterile water. Carefully flush all lumens and cannulas. Dry prior to use.

Preparation of solution – Add activator to the solution. The activator contains a rust inhibitor; do not add any other such agent. Upon mixing, the colorless solution changes to a nonstaining green.

HEXACHLOROPHENE

Rx	pHisoHex (Winthrop Pharm.)	Liquid: 3%	Petrolatum, lanolin, PEG. In 150 ml, pt and gal and UD 8 ml (50s).

Indications

Surgical scrub and bacteriostatic skin cleanser; control of an outbreak of gram-positive infection when other procedures are unsuccessful.

Administration and Dosage

➤*Surgical wash or scrub:* As indicated.

➤*Bacteriostatic cleansing:* Wet hand with water and squeeze ≈ 5 ml into palm; add water; work up lather; apply to area to be cleansed. Rinse thoroughly after each washing.

➤*Infant care:* Do not use routinely for bathing infants (see Warnings). Use of baby skin products containing alcohol may decrease the antibacterial action.

➤*Storage/Stability:* Prolonged direct exposure to strong light may cause brownish surface discoloration, but this does not affect its action. Shaking disperses the color.

Actions

➤*Pharmacology:* Hexachlorophene is a bacteriostatic agent with activity against staphylococci and other gram-positive bacteria. Cumulative antibacterial action develops with repeated use.

Contraindications

Use on burned or denuded skin; as an occlusive dressing, wet pack or lotion; routine prophylactic total body bathing; as a vaginal pack or tampon or on any mucous membrane; sensitivity to any component; primary light sensitivity to halogenated phenol derivatives because of the possibility of cross sensitivity to hexachlorophene.

Warnings

➤*Rinse thoroughly after use:* Especially from sensitive areas (eg, scrotum, perineum).

➤*Rapid absorption:* This may occur with resultant toxic blood levels when applied to skin lesions such as ichthyosis congenita, the dermatitis of Letterer-Siwe's syndrome, or other generalized dermatological conditions. Application to burns has produced neurotoxicity and death.

➤*Cerebral irritability:* Discontinue promptly if signs and symptoms of cerebral irritability occur.

➤*Fertility impairment:* Topical exposure of neonatal rats to 3% hexachlorophene solution caused reduced fertility in 7-month-old males, due to inability to ejaculate.

➤*Pregnancy: Category C.* Placental transfer occurs in rats. There are no adequate and well controlled studies in pregnant women. Use during pregnancy only if the potential benefit justifies the risk to the fetus. Hexachlorophene is not recommended as an antiseptic lubricant for vaginal exams during labor because appreciable amounts have been detected in maternal and cord serum.

➤*Lactation:* It is not known whether this drug is excreted in breast milk. Decide whether to discontinue nursing or discontinue the drug, taking into account the importance of the drug to the mother.

➤*Children:* Infants, especially those who weigh < 1200 g and those with a gestational age of < 35 weeks, or those with dermatoses, are particularly susceptible to hexachlorophene absorption. Systemic toxicity may manifest as CNS stimulation (irritation), sometimes with convulsions.

Infants have developed dermatitis, irritability, generalized clonic muscular contractions and decerebrate rigidity following application of 6% hexachlorophene powder. Examination of brain stems revealed vacuolization. Moreover, histologic sections of premature infants who died of unrelated causes have shown a correlation between hexachlorophene baths and white matter brain lesions.

Precautions

➤*For external use only:* Avoid contact with the eyes. If contact occurs, rinse out promptly and thoroughly with water.

Adverse Reactions

Dermatitis; photosensitivity. Sensitivity to hexachlorophene is rare; however, persons who have developed photoallergy to similar compounds may also become sensitive to hexachlorophene.

Persons with highly sensitive skin may develop a reaction characterized by redness or mild scaling or dryness, especially when combined with mechanical factors such as excessive rubbing or exposure to heat or cold.

Overdosage

➤*Symptoms:* Ingestion of 30 to 120 ml has caused anorexia, vomiting, abdominal cramps, diarrhea, dehydration, convulsions, hypotension, shock and fatalities.

➤*Treatment:* If patients are seen early, evacuate the stomach by emesis or gastric lavage. Administer olive oil or vegetable oil (60 ml) to delay absorption, followed by a saline cathartic to hasten removal. Treatment is symptomatic and supportive; may give IV fluids (5% dextrose in physiologic saline solution) for dehydration. Correct electrolyte imbalance. If marked hypotension occurs, vasopressor therapy is indicated. Consider use of opiates if GI symptoms (eg, cramping, diarrhea) are severe.

Patient Information

For external use only.

Avoid getting suds in eyes; if this occurs, rinse promptly and thoroughly with water.

Rinse skin thoroughly after washing.

Do not use on burns or mucous membranes.

IODINE COMPOUNDS
IODINE

otc	**Iodine Topical** (Various, eg, AA–Spectrum)	**Solution:** 2% iodine and 2.4% sodium iodide in purified water	In 500 and 4000 ml.
otc¹	**Strong Iodine (Lugol's Solution)** (Various, eg, Lannett)	**Solution:** 5% iodine and 10% potassium iodide in water	In pt and gal.
otc	**Iodine Tincture** (Various, eg, Century, Lannett)	**Solution:** 2% iodine and 2.4% sodium iodide in 47% alcohol, purified water	In pt and gal.
otc	**Strong Iodine Tincture** (Various, eg, A-A Spectrum)	**Solution:** 7% iodine and 5% potassium iodide in 83% alcohol	In 500 and 4000 ml.

¹ Some of these products may be available *Rx*, depending on distributor discretion.

Indications

Iodine preparations are used externally for their broad microbicidal spectrum against bacteria, fungi, viruses, spores, protozoa and yeasts. Iodine may be used to disinfect intact skin preoperatively. Potassium iodide is added to increase the solubility of the iodine. Sodium iodide is present to stabilize the tincture and make it miscible with water in all proportions.

Contraindications

Hypersensitivity to iodine.

Warnings

➤*For external use only:* Avoid contact with the eyes and mucous membranes.

➤*Highly toxic if ingested:* Sodium thiosulfate is the most effective chemical antidote.

➤*Staining:* Iodine preparations stain skin and clothing.

➤*Occlusive dressings:* Do not use.

POVIDONE IODINE

otc	**Povidone-Iodine** (Various, eg, Humco, IDE, Major)	**Ointment:** 10%	In 30 g and lb.
		Solution: 10%	In pt and gal.
		Liquid	In pt.
otc	**Betadine** (Purdue Frederick)	**Aerosol:** 5%. Glycerin, dibasic sodium phosphate	In 88.7 ml.
		Gel (vaginal): 10%. Polyehtylene glycols.	In 18 and 90 g w/vaginal applicator.
		Ointment: 10%. Polyethylene glycols.	In 28 g tube, lb jar and 0.94 and 3.8 g packets.
		Skin cleanser, foam: 7.5%. Ammonium nonoxynol-4-sulfate, lauramide DEA	In 170 g.
		Solution: 10%. Citric acid, dibasic sodium phosphate, glycerin	In 15, 120 and 237 ml, pt, qt, gal and 30 ml packets.
		Solution, swab aid: 10%. Citric acid, dibasic sodium phosphate, glycerin	In 100s.
		Solution, swabsticks: 10%. Citric acid, dibasic sodium phosphate, glycerin	In packets of 1 (200s) or 3 (50s).
		Surgical scrub: 7.5%. Ammonium nonoxynol-4-sulfate, lauramide DEA	In pt with or without pump, qt, gal and 15 ml packets.
otc	**Betagen** (Goldline)	**Ointment:** 1/5 available iodine. PEG-8 and PEG-75	In 28.35 g and lb.
		Solution: 10%	In pt and gal.
		Surgical scrub: 7.5%	In pt.
otc	**Biodine Topical 1%** (Major)	**Solution:** 1% iodine	In pt and gal.
otc	**Etodine** (Fougera)	**Ointment:** 1% available iodine	In 30 g, lb and 0.94 g (144s).
otc	**Mallisol** (Hauck)	**Ointment**	In 1 g packets.
otc	**Minidyne** (Pedinol)	**Solution:** 10%. Citric acid and sodium phosphate dibasic	In 15 ml.
otc	**Polydine** (Century)	**Ointment**	In 30 and 120 g & lb.
		Scrub	In 30, 120 and 240 ml, pt and gal.
		Solution	In 30, 120 and 240 ml, pt and gal.
otc	**Povidine** (Various, eg, Barre-National, Moore, Rugby)	**Ointment:** 10%	In 28.4 g and lb.
		Solution: 10%	In pt and gal.
		Surgical scrub: 5.5	In pt and gal.

¹ Glycerin, sodium chloride, sodium hydroxide and sodium phosphate.

Indications

➤*Shampoo:* Temporary relief of scaling and itching due to dandruff.

Administration and Dosage

Unlike iodine tincture, treated areas may be bandaged.

➤*Shampoo:* Apply 2 tsp to hair and scalp; use warm water to lather. Rinse. Repeat application. Massage gently into scalp. Allow to remain on scalp for at least 5 minutes. Work up lather to a golden color, using warm water. Rinse scalp thoroughly. Repeat twice weekly until improvement is noted. Thereafter, shampoo weekly.

Actions

➤*Pharmacology:* Water-soluble complex of iodine with povidone. Povidone-iodine contains 9% to 12% available iodine. It retains the bactericidal activity of iodine but is less potent, therefore causes less irritation to skin and mucous membranes. In vitro, HIV appears to be completely inactivated by povidone-iodine preparations; further study is needed.

A broad-spectrum antimicrobial agent. Liberates free iodine.

Warnings

➤*Hypothyroidism:* A 6–week-old infant developed low serum total thyroxine concentration and high thyroid stimulating hormone concentration following maternal use of topical povidone-iodine during pregnancy and lactation. In one study, the use of povidone-iodine solution on very-low birthweight infants resulted in neonatal hypothyroidism. In contrast, women who used povidone-iodine douche daily for 14 days did not develop overt hypothyroidism; however, there was a significant increase in serum total iodine concetration and urine iodine excretion. Use with caution during pregnancy and lactation and in infants.

➤*Open wounds:* Avoid solutions containing a detergent if treating open wounds with povidone-iodine. The value of povidone-iodine on open wounds has not been established.

Precautions

➤*Shampoo:*

For external use only – Avoid contact with eyes.

Irritation / Inflammation – Discontinue if signs of irritation or inflammation develop.

MERCURY COMPOUNDS
THIMEROSAL (49% mercury)

otc	**Thimerosal** (Lannett)	**Solution:** 1:1000	Stainless. In pt and gal.
otc	**Mersol** (Century Pharm.)	**Tincture:** 1:1000 with 50% alcohol	In 120 ml, pt and gal.

Indications
➤*Tincture/Solution:* For antisepsis of the skin prior to surgery and for first aid treatment.

➤*Spray:* For cuts, scratches, wounds, lacerations and abrasions; as a pre- and postoperative antiseptic.

Administration and Dosage
Apply locally 1 to 3 times a day.

Actions
➤*Pharmacology:* An organomercurial antiseptic with sustained bacteriostatic and fungistatic activity against common pathogens.

Contraindications
Hypersensitivity to thimerosal.

Precautions
➤*For external use only:* Avoid contact with the eyes.

➤*Prolonged repeated applications:* Frequent or prolonged use or application to large areas may cause serious mercury poisoning.

➤*Incompatibilities:* Thimerosal is incompatible with strong acids, salts of heavy metals, potassium permanganate and iodine; do not use in combination with or immediately following their application.

➤*Discontinue:* If redness, swelling, pain, infection, rash or irritation persists or increases, discontinue and consult physician.

Adverse Reactions
Some individuals are hypersensitive to the thio or mercuri radicals. Symptoms include erythematous, papular and vesicular eruptions over the application area.

Overdosage
For ingestion of the tincture, consider alcohol and acetone content.

➤*Treatment:* Supportive therapy. Refer to General Management of Acute Overdosage.

OXYCHLOROSENE SODIUM

otc	**Clorpactin WCS-90** (Guardian)	**Powder for Solution:** 2 g sodium oxychlorosene	In 2 g bottles (5s).

Indications
Used for treating localized infections, particularly when resistant organisms are present; to remove necrotic debris in massive infections or from radiation necrosis; to counteract odorous discharges; as a preoperative and postoperative irrigant and for the cleansing and disinfection of fistulae, sinus tract, empyemas and wounds.

Administration and Dosage
Apply by irrigation, instillation, spray, soaks or wet compresses, preferably thoroughly cleansing with gravity flow irrigation or syringe to provide copious quantities of fresh solution to remove organic wastes and debris. Also for preoperative skin preparation and postoperative protection. Apply topically as the 0.4% solution in water or isotonic saline. Use dilutions of 0.1% to 0.2% in urology and ophthalmology.

Actions
➤*Pharmacology:* Oxychlorosene is a complex of the sodium salt of dodecylbenzenesulfonic acid and hypochlorous acid. Its action is markedly cidal, rapid and complete against both gram-negative and gram-positive bacteria, fungi, yeast, mold, viruses and spores.

Contraindications
Infection sites not exposed to direct contact with the solution; systemic use.

Precautions
➤*Bladder/Eye instillation:* Instillation of 0.2% solution, particularly into the bladder or into the eye, may cause severe discomfort. Pretreat the eye with a topical anesthetic. In the bladder, use a 0.1% concentration for the first treatment, instilling the solution to the capacity of the bladder without over-distention.

SILVER NITRATE

Rx	**Silver Nitrate** (Gordon Labs)	**Ointment:** 10%	Petrolatum base. In 30 g.
		Solution: 10%	In 30 ml.
		25%	In 30 ml.
		50%	In 30 ml.

For prevention of gonorrheal ophthalmia neonatorum, see monograph in Ophthalmic and Otic Agents.

Indications
To treat indolent wounds, destroy exuberant granulations, freshen the edges of ulcers and fissures, touch the bases of vesicular, bullous or aphthous lesions and provide styptic action.

➤*10% Ointment:*
Podiatry – To treat neurovascular helomas; to cauterize and destroy small nerve endings and blood vessels. It forms a protective covering after the removal of corns and calluses.

➤*10% Solution:* Impetigo vulgaris.
Podiatry – Helomas.

➤*25% Solution:* Pruritus.
Podiatry – Plantar warts.

➤*50% Solution:*
Podiatry – Plantar warts; granulation tissue; papillomatous growths; granuloma pyogenicum.

➤*Unlabeled uses:* Concentrations of 0.1% to 0.5% are used as wet dressings in burns and on lesions.

Administration and Dosage
➤*Ointment:* Apply in apertured pad on affected area for ≈ 5 days, as needed.

➤*Solution:* Apply a cotton applicator dipped in solution on the affected area or lesion 2 or 3 times a week for 2 or 3 weeks, as needed.

Actions
➤*Pharmacology:* Silver nitrate is a strong caustic and escharotic providing antiseptic, astringent, germicidal, local (epithelial) stimulant or caustic action externally.

The attachment of silver to a reactive group of a protein sharply decreases the protein's solubility; the protein's conformation may also be altered and denaturation may occur. Precipitation of the protein generally results. At low concentrations of silver, precipitation is confined to proteins in the interstices and an astringent action occurs. At high concentrations, membrane and intracellular structures are damaged and there is a casutic or corrosive effect.

Because silver ions attach so readily to the various groups of proteins, the ions are captured before they diffuse far into tissues. Precipitation of silver as silver chloride also limits extent of ion movement. Thus, local effects of silver are self-limiting and spread of damage occurs only when the dose overwhelms the capacity of tissues to fix the ion at the application site. Antiseptic effects of silver may derive in part from the reaction with bacterial and viral proteins.

Contraindications
Application on wounds, cuts or broken skin.

Warnings
➤*Skin discoloration:* Prolonged or frequent use may permanently discolor skin due to deposition of reduced silver. However, topical silver nitrate for local application to suppress granulation tissue apparently does not produce argyria.

➤*Staining of clothes:* Will stain clothing and linens.

➤*Electrolyte abnormalities:* If wet dressings are used over extensive areas or prolonged periods, electrolyte abnormalities can result. Sodium and chloride leach into the dressing and hyponatremia or hypochloremia can occur. Absorbed nitrate can cause methemoglobinemia.

Precautions
➤*Irritation:* Discontinue use if redness or irritation occurs.

➤*For external use only:* Avoid contact with the eyes.

SILVER NITRATE

Overdosage

➤*Symptoms:* The fatal dose of silver nitrate may be as low as 2 g. Oral intake of silver nitrate causes a local corrosive effect including pain and burning of mouth, salivation, vomiting, diarrhea progressing

to anuria, shock, coma, convulsions and death. Blackening of skin and mucous membranes occurs (sometimes permanent).

➤*Treatment:* Give NaCl in water, 10 g/L, to precipitate silver Cl. Follow with catharsis, including NaCl solution. Also attend to shock and methemoglobinemia if present.

If splashed in eyes, wash with copious amounts of water and see a physician.

SODIUM HYPOCHLORITE

| otc | Dakin's (Century Pharm.) | Solution: 0.25% | In pt. |
| | | 0.5% | In pt and gal. |

Indications

Applied topically to the skin as an antiseptic.

Actions

➤*Pharmacology:* Sodium hypochlorite has germicidal, deodorizing and bleaching properties. It is effective against vegetative bacteria and viruses, and also, to some degree, against spores and fungi.

Precautions

➤*Chemical burns:* May be produced; avoid skin or eye contact with this solution.

TRICLOSAN (Irgasan)

otc	Oxy ResiDon't (SK Beecham)	Liquid: 0.6%, diazolidinyl urea	In 240 ml
otc	no more germies (J & J)	Soap: 0.25%, PEG, EDTA	In 237 ml
otc	Septi-Soft (Calgon Vestal)	Solution: 0.25%. With glycerin, emollients	In 240 ml, qt, gal.
otc	Septisol (Calgon Vestal)		In 240 ml, qt, gal.
otc	Stridex Face Wash (Sterling Health)	Solution: 1% triclosan	Glycerin, EDTA. Alcohol free. In 237 ml.
otc	Clearasil Daily Face Wash (Procter & Gamble)	Liquid: 0.3% triclosan	Aloe vera gel, glycerin, EDTA. In 135 ml.

Indications

➤*Septi-Soft:* Skin cleanser. May use as hand/body wash, shampoo, bed or towel bath.

➤*Septisol:* Healthcare personnel handwash and skin degermer.

Administration and Dosage

Dispense a small amount (5 ml) on hands, rub thoroughly for 30 seconds, rinse thoroughly, dry.

➤*Septi-Soft:* May also be used as hand/body wash, shampoo, bed or towel bath.

Actions

➤*Pharmacology:* Triclosan, a bis-phenol disinfectant, is a bacteriostatic agent with activity against a wide range of gram-positive and gram-negative bacteria.

Contraindications

Use on burned or denuded skin or mucous membranes; routine prophylactic total body bathing.

➤*Septi-Soft:* Not a surgical scrub; do not use in preparation for surgery.

Precautions

For external use only. Avoid contact with the eyes.

MISCELLANEOUS ANTISEPTICS

otc	Stat·One Isopropyl Rubbing Alcohol (Continental)	Gel: 70% isopropyl rubbing alcohol	In 28.4 g.
otc	Stat·One Hydrogen Peroxide (Continental)	Gel: 3% hydrogen peroxide	In 28.4 g.
otc	Kleen-Handz (American Medical)	Solution: 62% SD alcohol	Aloe vera, purified water. In 60 ml.
otc	S.T. 37 (Menley & James)	Solution: 0.1% hexylresorcinol, 28% glycerin	In 165 and 360 ml.
otc	Mercurochrome (Humco)	Solution: 2% merbromin	In 30 mL.
otc	Tincture of Green Soap (Paddock)	Liquid: With 28% to 32% alcohol	In gal.
otc	Stat·One Hydrogen Peroxide (Continental)	Gel: 3% hydrogen peroxide	In 28.4 g.
otc	Stat·One Isopropyl Rubbing Alcohol (Continental)	Gel: 70% isopropyl rubbing alcohol	In 28.4 g.
otc	B.F.I. Antiseptic (Menley & James)	Powder: 16% bismuth-formic-iodide, zinc phenol sulfonate, potassium alum, bismuth subgallate, boric acid, menthol, eucalyptol, thymol	In 7.5, 37.5 and 240 g.
otc	Alco-Gel (Tweezerman)	Gel: 60% ethyl alcohol	In 60 and 480 g.

Antiviral Agents

ACYCLOVIR (Acycloguanosine)

Rx	Zovirax (Biovail)	Ointment: 5% (50 mg/g)	In a polyethylene glycol base. In 15 g tubes.
		Cream: 5% (50 mg/g)	Cetostearyl alcohol, mineral oil, in an aqueous cream base. In 2 g tubes.

For information on systemic acyclovir, refer to the monograph in the Anti-infectives chapter.

Indications

➤*Ointment:* Management of initial episodes of herpes genitalis and in limited non-life-threatening mucocutaneous herpes simplex virus infections in immunocompromised patients.

➤*Cream:* Treatment of recurrent herpes labialis (cold sores) in adults and adolescents (12 years of age and older).

Administration and Dosage

Initiate therapy as early as possible following onset of signs and symptoms.

➤*Ointment:* Apply sufficient quantity to adequately cover all lesions every 3 hours 6 times daily for 7 days. The dose size per application will vary depending upon the total lesion area; use approximately a one-half inch ribbon of ointment per 4 square inches of surface area. Use a finger cot or rubber glove when applying acyclovir to prevent autoinoculation of other body sites and transmission of infection to other people.

➤*Cream:* Apply 5 times/day for 4 days. For adolescents 12 years of age and older the dosage is the same as in adults.

➤*Storage/Stability:*

Ointment – Store at 15° to 25°C (59° to 77°F) in a dry place.

Cream – Store at or below 25°C (77°F); excursions permitted to 15° to 30°C (59° to 86°F).

Actions

➤*Pharmacology:* Acyclovir, a synthetic acyclic purine nucleoside analog, has in vitro inhibitory activity against herpes simplex types 1 and 2 (HSV-1, HSV-2), and varicella-zoster (VZV).

The inhibitory activity of acyclovir is highly selective due to its affinity for the enzyme thymidine kinase (TK) encoded by HSV and VZV. This viral enzyme converts acyclovir into acyclovir monophosphate, a nucleotide analog. The monophosphate is further converted into diphosphate by cellular guanylate kinase and into triphosphate by a number of cellular enzymes. In vitro, acyclovir triphosphate stops replication of herpes viral DNA. This is accomplished in 3 ways: 1) competitive inhibition of viral DNA polymerase; 2) incorporation into and termination of the growing viral DNA chain; and 3) inactivation of the viral DNA polymerase. The greater antiviral activity of acyclovir against HSV compared with VZV is due to its more efficient phosphorylation by the viral TK.

Drug resistance – Resistance of HSV and VZV to acyclovir can result from qualitative and quantitative changes in the viral TK and/or DNA polymerase. Clinical isolates of HSV and VZV with reduced susceptibility to acyclovir have been recovered from immunocompromised patients, especially with advanced HIV infection. While most of the acyclovir-resistant mutants isolated thus far from immunocompromised patients have been found to be TK-deficient mutants, other mutants involving the viral TK gene (TK partial and TK altered) and DNA polymerase have been isolated. TK-negative mutants may cause severe disease in infants and immunocompromised adults. Consider the possibility of viral resistance to acyclovir in patients who show poor clinical response during therapy.

➤*Pharmacokinetics:*

Ointment – Studies were performed with acyclovir ointment in immunocompromised adults at risk of developing mucocutaneous HSV infections or with localized VZV infections.

In 1 study with 16 inpatients the complete ointment or its vehicle were randomly administered in a dose of 1 cm strips (25 mg acyclovir) 4 times a day for 7 days to an intact skin surface area of 4.5 square inches. No local intolerance, systemic toxicity, or contact dermatitis were observed. In addition, no drug was detected in blood and urine by radioimmunoassay (sensitivity, 0.01 mcg/mL).

In another study with 11 patients, acyclovir was detected in the blood of 9 patients and in the urine of all patients tested. Acyclovir levels in plasma ranged from less than 0.01 to 0.28 mcg/mL in 8 patients with normal renal function and from less than 0.01 to 0.78 mcg/mL in 1 patient with impaired renal function. Acyclovir excreted in the urine ranged from less than 0.02% to 9.4% of the daily dose. Therefore, systemic absorption of acyclovir after topical application is minimal.

Cream – A study was performed with acyclovir cream in adult volunteers to evaluate the percutaneous absorption of acyclovir. The cream was applied to the backs of 6 male volunteers 5 times/day every 2 hours for 4 days. Plasma concentration of acyclovir was assayed 1 hour after the final application. Average daily urinary excretion of acyclovir was approximately 0.04% of the daily applied dose. Plasma acyclovir concentrations were below the limit of detection (0.01 mcM) in 5 subjects and barely detectable (0.014 mcM) in 1 subject. Systemic absorption of acyclovir from the cream is minimal in adults.

➤*Clinical trials:*

Ointment – In clinical trials of initial herpes genitalis, acyclovir decreased healing time and, in some cases, decreased duration of viral shedding and pain. Studies in immunocompromised patients with mainly herpes labialis showed decreased duration of viral shedding and slight decrease in pain duration. In contrast, studies of recurrent herpes genitalis and herpes labialis in nonimmunocompromised patients showed no clinical benefit; there was some decrease in duration of viral shedding.

Contraindications

Hypersensitivity or chemical intolerance to the components of the formulation.

Warnings

➤*For cutaneous use only:* Do not use in eyes, nose, or mouth.

➤*Pregnancy: Category B.* There are no adequate and well-controlled studies in pregnant women. Use during pregnancy only if the potential benefits outweigh the potential hazards to the fetus.

➤*Lactation:* It is not known whether this drug is excreted in breast milk. Exercise caution when administering to a breastfeeding mother.

Systemic exposure following topical administration is minimal. After oral administration of product, acyclovir concentrations have been documented in breast milk in 2 woman and ranged from 0.6 to 4.1 times the corresponding plasma levels. These concentrations would potentially expose the breastfeeding infant to a dose of acyclovir up to 0.3 mg/kg daily. Breastfeeding mothers who have active herpetic lesions near or on the breast should avoid breastfeeding.

➤*Children:* Safety and efficacy in pediatric patients less than 12 years of age have not been established.

Adverse Reactions

➤*Ointment:* Mild pain with transient burning/stinging (30%); pruritus (4%).

Post-marketing events – Edema and/or pain at application site; rash.

➤*Cream:* The most common were dry lips, desquamation, dryness of skin, cracked lips, burning skin, pruritus, flakiness of skin, and stinging on skin (less than 1%).

Post-marketing events – Angioedema, anaphylaxis, contact dermatitis, eczema, and application site reactions including inflammation.

Patient Information

Acyclovir is most effective when used early at the start of herpes simplex virus infection.

When applying ointment, use a finger cot or glove to prevent autoinoculation of other body sites.

For external use only, do not use in eyes, nose, or mouth.

Apply only to the affected area. Do not apply another type of skin product (eg, cosmetics, sunscreen, lip balm) to the area while using this medication.

These products will not prevent transmission of infection to others.

Acyclovir is not a cure for herpes simplex infections and it is of little benefit in treating recurrent attacks without signs or symptoms.

Wash hands with soap and water after application.

Transient burning, stinging, itching, and rash may occur when applied; notify physician if these symptoms become pronounced or persist.

PENCICLOVIR

Rx **Denavir** (Novartis) | **Cream:** 1% (10 mg/g) | Cetostearyl alcohol, mineral oil, white petrolatum. In 1.5 g tubes.

Indications

➤*Herpes labialis:* For the treatment of recurrent herpes labialis (cold sores) in adults.

Administration and Dosage

➤*Approved by the FDA:* September 24, 1996.

Apply penciclovir every 2 hours while awake for 4 days. Start treatment as early as possible (ie, during the prodrome or when lesions appear).

➤*Storage/Stability:* Store at controlled room temperature, 20° to 25°C (68° to 77°F).

Actions

➤*Pharmacology:* Penciclovir is an antiviral agent active against herpes viruses. It has in vitro inhibitory activity against herpes simplex virus types 1 (HSV-1) and 2 (HSV-2). In cells infected with HSV-1 or HSV-2, viral thymidine kinase phosphorylates penciclovir to a monophosphate form which, in turn, is converted to penciclovir triphosphate by cellular kinases. In vitro studies demonstrate that penciclovir triphosphate inhibits HSV polymerase competitively with deoxyguanosine triphosphate. Consequently, herpes viral DNA synthesis and replication are selectively inhibited.

Drug resistance – Penciclovir-resistant mutants of HSV can result from qualitative changes in viral thymidine kinase or DNA polymerase. The most commonly encountered acyclovir-resistant mutants that are deficient in viral thymidine kinase are also resistant to penciclovir.

➤*Pharmacokinetics:* Measurable penciclovir concentrations were not detected in plasma or urine of healthy male volunteers following single or repeat application of the 1% cream at a dose of 180 mg penciclovir daily (approximately 67 times the estimated usual clinical dose).

Contraindications

Hypersensitivity to the product or any of its components.

Warnings

➤*Carcinogenesis:* Two-year carcinogenicity studies were conducted with famciclovir (the oral prodrug of penciclovir) in rats and mice. An increase in the incidence of mammary adenocarcinoma was seen in female rats receiving 600 mg/kg/day (approximately 395 times the maximum theoretical human exposure to penciclovir following application of the topical product).

➤*Mutagenesis:* An increase in clastogenic responses was seen with penciclovir in mouse lymphoma cell assay (at doses at least 1000 mcg/mL). When tested in vivo, penciclovir caused an increase in micronuclei in mouse bone marrow following the IV administration of doses at least 500 mg/kg (at least 810 times the maximum human dose, based on body surface area conversion).

➤*Fertility impairment:* Testicular toxicity was observed in multiple animal species (rats and dogs) following repeated IV administration of penciclovir at doses approximately 1155 and 3255, respectively, times the human dose. Testicular changes seen in both species included atro-

phy of the seminiferous tubules and reductions in epididymal sperm counts and/or an increased incidence of sperm with abnormal morphology or reduced motility. Adverse testicular effects were related to an increasing dose or duration of exposure to penciclovir.

➤*Pregnancy: Category B.* No adverse effects on the course and outcome of pregnancy or on fetal development were noted in rats and rabbits following the IV administration of penciclovir at doses of 80 and 60 mg/kg/day, respectively. There are no adequate and well-controlled studies in pregnant women. Use during pregnancy only if clearly needed.

➤*Lactation:* There is no information on whether penciclovir is excreted in breast milk after topical administration. However, following oral administration of famciclovir (the oral prodrug of penciclovir) to lactating rats, penciclovir was excreted in breast milk at concentrations higher than those seen in the plasma. Therefore, decide whether to discontinue the drug or discontinue breastfeeding, taking into account the importance of the drug to the mother. There are no data on the safety of penciclovir in newborns.

➤*Children:* Safety and efficacy in pediatric patients have not been established.

Precautions

➤*Mucous membranes:* Use penciclovir on herpes labialis on the lips and face only. Because no data are available, application to human mucous membranes is not recommended. Take particular care to avoid application in or near the eyes because it may cause irritation.

➤*Immunocompromised patients:* Penciclovir's effect in immunocompromised patients has not been established.

Adverse Reactions

Penciclovir Adverse Reactions (%)		
Adverse reaction	Penciclovir (n = 1516)	Placebo (n = 1541)
Application site reaction	1.3	1.8
Hypesthesia/local anesthesia	0.9	1.4
Taste perversion	0.2	0.3
Pruritus	0.0	0.3
Pain	0.0	0.1
Rash (erythematous)	0.1	0.1
Allergic reaction	0.0	0.1
Headache	5.3	5.8
Mild erythema[1]	≈ 50	-

[1] A 5% penciclovir cream was applied.

Overdosage

Because penciclovir is poorly absorbed following oral administration, adverse reactions related to penciclovir ingestion are unlikely. There is no information on overdose.

BORIC ACID

otc	**Boric Acid** (Various, eg, Clay-Park, IDE, Major, Moore, Rugby, URL)	**Ointment:** 10%	In 30 and 60 g and lb.

Indications

A soothing application for chafed skin, abrasions, burns and other skin irritations.

Administration and Dosage

For external use only. Avoid contact with the eyes.

Apply directly to affected area once or twice daily.

Burn Preparations

MAFENIDE

Rx	Sulfamylon (Bertek)	Solution, topical: 5% mafenide (as acetate)	In 50 g packets for reconstitution.
Rx	Sulfamylon (Dow B. Hickam)	Cream: 85 mg (as acetate) per g	EDTA, cetyl alcohol, stearyl alcohol, parabens. sodium metabisulfite. In 37, 114 and 411 g.

Indications

➤*Burn treatment:* Adjunctive therapy of second and third degree burns.

Administration and Dosage

➤*Application:* Apply to the clean and debrided wound with a sterile gloved hand, once or twice daily, to a thickness of approximately $\frac{1}{16}$ inch; thicker application is not recommended. Cover the burned areas with mafenide at all times. Reapply to any areas from which it has been removed (eg, by patient activity). Dressings are usually not required, but if necessary, use only a thin layer of dressing.

➤*Bathing:* When feasible, bathe the patient daily to aid in debridement. A whirlpool bath is particularly helpful, but the patient may be bathed in bed or in a shower.

➤*Duration of therapy:* Continue treatment until healing is progressing well or until the site is ready for grafting. Do not withdraw mafenide while infection is still possible. However, if allergic manifestations occur, consider discontinuing treatment.

➤*Storage/Stability:* Avoid exposure to excessive heat (> 40°C; 104°F).

Actions

➤*Pharmacology:* Mafenide, a sulfonamide, is bacteriostatic against many gram-negative and gram-positive organisms, including *Pseudomonas aeruginosa* and certain strains of anaerobes. It is active in the presence of pus and serum; its activity is not altered by changes in the acidity of the environment.

Mafenide reduces the bacterial population present in the avascular tissues of second and third degree burns. This permits spontaneous healing of deep partial-thickness burns and prevents conversion of burn wounds from partial thickness to full thickness. However, delayed eschar separation has occurred in some cases.

➤*Pharmacokinetics:* Applied topically, mafenide diffuses through devascularized areas and is absorbed and rapidly metabolized to p-carboxybenzenesulfonamide which is cleared through the kidneys. The metabolite has no antibacterial activity but retains the ability to inhibit carbonic anhydrase.

Contraindications

Hypersensitivity to the drug. It is a not known whether there is cross-sensitivity to other sulfonamides.

Warnings

➤*Renal function impairment:* Use with caution in patients with acute renal failure.

➤*Pregnancy: Category C.* It is not known whether mafenide can cause fetal harm when administered to a pregnant woman or can affect reproduction capacity. Not recommended for the treatment of women of childbearing potential unless the burned area covers > 20% of the total body surface or benefit is greater than the possible risk to the fetus.

➤*Lactation:* It is not known whether mafenide is excreted in breast milk. Because of the potential for serious adverse reactions in nursing infants, decide whether to discontinue nursing or discontinue the drug, taking into account the importance of the drug to the mother.

➤*Children:* Use the same administration and dosage as for adults.

Precautions

➤*For external use only:* Avoid contact with eyes.

➤*Metabolic acidosis:* Mafenide and its metabolite inhibit carbonic anhydrase, which may result in metabolic acidosis, usually compensated by hyperventilation. In the presence of renal function impairment, high blood levels of mafenide and its metabolite may exaggerate the carbonic anhydrase inhibition. Therefore, close monitoring of acid-base balance is necessary, particularly in patients with extensive second degree or partial thickness burns and in those with pulmonary and renal dysfunction. Some burn patients treated with mafenide have also manifested an unexplained syndrome of marked hyperventilation with resulting respiratory alkalosis (slightly alkaline blood pH, low arterial pCO_2 and decreased total CO_2); change in arterial pO_2 is variable. The etiology and significance of these findings are unknown.

If acidosis occurs and becomes difficult to control, particularly in patients with pulmonary dysfunction, discontinuing therapy for 24 to 48 hours while continuing fluid therapy may aid in restoring acid-base balance.

➤*Superinfection:* Use may result in bacterial or fungal overgrowth of nonsusceptible organisms. Such overgrowth may lead to a secondary infection. Appropriate measures should be taken if superinfection occurs.

Fungal colonization in and below the eschar may occur concomitantly with reduction of bacterial growth in the burn wound. However, fungal dissemination through the infected burn wound is rare.

➤*Sulfite sensitivity:* Some of these products contain sulfites that may cause allergic-type reactions (including anaphylactic symptoms and life-threatening or less severe asthmatic episodes) in certain susceptible persons. The overall prevalence of sulfite sensitivity in the general population is unknown and probably low. It is seen more frequently in asthmatic or atopic nonasthmatic persons.

Adverse Reactions

It is difficult to distinguish a reaction to mafenide from the effect of a severe burn.

➤*Allergic:* Rash; itching; facial edema; swelling; hives; blisters; erythema; eosinophilia.

➤*Dermatologic:* Pain on application or a burning sensation (most frequent); excoriation of new skin, bleeding of skin (rare).

➤*Metabolic:* Acidosis; increase in serum chloride.

➤*Respiratory:* Tachypnea or hyperventilation; decrease in arterial pCO_2.

➤*Miscellaneous:* Bone marrow depression, acute attack of porphyria (one case each); fatal hemolytic anemia with disseminated intravascular coagulation, presumably related to a glucose-6-phosphate dehydrogenase deficiency; diarrhea due to accidental ingestion.

Patient Information

Notify physician if condition worsens, if irritation occurs or if hyperventilation occurs.

Bathe burned area daily; a whirlpool bath is particularly helpful.

Continue treatment until healing occurs or until site is ready for grafting.

NITROFURAZONE

Rx	Nitrofurazone (Various, eg, Clay-Park)	Topical Solution: 0.2%	In pt and gal.
Rx	Furacin (Roberts)		In 480 ml.
Rx	Nitrofurazone (Various, eg, Clay-Park)	Ointment (soluble): 0.2%	In 480 g.
Rx	Furacin Soluble Dressing (Roberts)		In a polyethylene glycol base. In 28, 56 and 454 g.
Rx	Furacin (Roberts)	Cream: 0.2%	Cetyl alcohol, mineral oil, parabens. Water-miscible base. In 28 g.

Indications

➤*Burn treatment:* Adjunctive therapy of patients with second and third degree burns when bacterial resistance to other agents is a real or potential problem.

➤*Skin grafting:* For use where bacterial contamination may cause graft rejection or donor site infection, particularly in hospitals with historical resistant bacteria epidemics.

Administration and Dosage

For the treatment of burns, apply directly to the lesion or place on gauze. Reapply once daily or every few days, depending on dressing technique. Flushing dressing with sterile saline facilitates removal.

➤*Storage/Stability:*

Cream – Avoid exposure to direct sunlight, excessive heat (> 40°C; 104°F), strong fluorescent lighting and alkaline materials.

Actions

➤*Pharmacology:* Nitrofurazone, a synthetic nitrofuran with a broad antibacterial spectrum, is bactericidal against a number of gram-negative and -positive bacteria commonly causing surface infections, including *Staphylococcus aureus, Streptococcus, Escherichia coli, Clostridium perfringens, Aerobacter aerogenes* and *Proteus* sp.

Contraindications

Hypersensitivity to nitrofurazone or any component of the product.

NITROFURAZONE

Warnings

➤*Minor burns/infections:* There is no evidence of effectiveness in treatment of minor burns or surface bacterial infections involving wounds, cutaneous ulcers or the various pyodermas.

➤*Renal function impairment:* Use the soluble burn dressing with caution in patients with known or suspected renal impairment. The polyethylene glycol present in the base can be absorbed through denuded skin and may not be excreted normally by a compromised kidney, leading to symptoms of progressive renal impairment including increased BUN, anion gap and metabolic acidosis.

➤*Pregnancy:* Category C. There are no adequate and well controlled studies in pregnant women. Use only when potential benefits outweigh risk to the fetus.

➤*Lactation:* It is not known whether this drug is excreted in breast milk. Decide whether to discontinue nursing or to discontinue the drug, taking into account the importance of the drug to the mother.

➤*Children:* Safety and efficacy have not been established.

Precautions

➤*For external use only:* Avoid contact with eyes.

➤*Superinfection:* Use may result in bacterial or fungal overgrowth of nonsusceptible organisms, including fungi and *Pseudomonas.* Such overgrowth may lead to a secondary infection. If this occurs, or if irritation, sensitization or superinfection develops, discontinue treatment and institute appropriate therapy.

Adverse Reactions

Varying degrees of contact dermatitis such as rash, pruritus and local edema ($\approx$1%). Treat allergic reactions symptomatically.

Patient Information

Notify physician if condition worsens or if rash or irritation occurs.

SILVER SULFADIAZINE

Rx	SSD Cream (Boots)	**Cream**: 10 mg per g in a water-miscible base[1]	Cetyl alcohol. In 25, 50, 85, 400 and 1000 g.
Rx	Silvadene (Hoescht Marion Roussel)		In 20, 50, 85, 400 and 1000 g.
Rx	Thermazene (Sherwood)		In 50, 400 and 1000 g.
Rx	SSD AF Cream (Boots)		In 50, 400 and 1000 g.

[1] Contains white petrolatum, stearyl alcohol, 0.3% methylparaben.

Indications

➤*Burn treatment:* As an adjunct for prevention and treatment of sepsis in second and third degree burns.

Administration and Dosage

➤*Application:* Apply under sterile conditions once or twice daily to a thickness of approximately $\frac{1}{16}$ inch to the clean and debrided wound. Cover the burn areas with silver sulfadiazine at all times. Whenever necessary, reapply the cream to any areas from which it has been removed by patient activity. Reapply immediately after hydrotherapy. Dressings are not required, but may be used if individual patient requirements make them necessary.

➤*Bathing:* When feasible, bathe patient daily to aid in debridement. A whirlpool bath is particularly helpful, but the patient may be bathed in bed or in a shower.

➤*Duration of therapy:* Continue treatment until satisfactory healing occurs or until the site is ready for grafting. Do not withdraw the drug while the possibility of infection remains, unless a significant adverse reaction occurs.

Actions

➤*Pharmacology:* Silver sulfadiazine acts only on the cell membrane and cell wall to produce its bactericidal effect. Silver is slowly released from the preparation in concentrations that are selectively toxic to bacteria. It is not a carbonic anhydrase inhibitor.

Reduction in bacterial growth after application of topical antibacterial agents has been reported to permit spontaneous healing of deep partial thickness burns by preventing conversion of the partial thickness to full thickness by sepsis. However, reduction in bacterial colonization has caused delayed separation, in some cases necessitating escharotomy in order to prevent contracture.

➤*Pharmacokinetics:* While ≤ 1% of the silver content is absorbed, up to 10% of the sulfadiazine may be absorbed. Serum concentrations of 10 to 20 mcg/ml have been reported when extensive areas were involved.

➤*Microbiology:* Silver sulfadiazine is bactericidal for many gram-negative and gram-positive bacteria and is effective against yeast. Silver sulfadiazine will inhibit bacteria resistant to other antimicrobial agents and is superior to sulfadiazine.

Organisms Generally Susceptible to Silver Sulfadiazine		
Pseudomonas aeruginosa	Proteus mirabilis	Staphylococcus epidermidis
Pseudomonas maltophilia	Morganella morganii	β-hemolytic streptococcus
Enterobacter species	Providencia rettgeri	Enterococcus species
Enterobacter cloacae	Proteus vulgaris	Candida albicans
Klebsiella species	Providencia species	Corynebacterium diphtheriae
Escherichia coli	Citrobacter species	
Serratia species	Acinetobacter calcoaceticus	Clostridium perfringens
	Staphylococcus aureus	

Contraindications

Hypersensitivity to the contents of the preparation; pregnant women at or near term, premature infants, infants ≤ 2 months old (sulfonamides may increase the possibility of kernicterus).

Warnings

➤*G-6-PD deficiency:* Use in glucose-6-phosphate dehydrogenase-deficient individuals may be hazardous, as hemolysis may occur.

➤*Fungal colonization:* Fungal colonization in and below the eschar may occur; however, incidence of fungal superinfection is low.

➤*Serum sulfonamide concentrations:* In the treatment of burn wounds involving extensive areas of the body, the serum sulfa concentration may approach adult therapeutic levels (8 to 12 mg/dl). Therefore, in these patients, monitor serum sulfa concentrations. Monitor renal function carefully and check the urine for sulfa crystals.

➤*Leukopenia (< 5000 WBC/mm³):* It has been reported which reverted to normal upon drug discontinuation or recovered spontaneously. Leukopenia associated with silver sulfadiazine administration is primarily characterized by decreased neutrophil count. Maximal WBC depression occurs within 2 to 4 days of initiation of therapy. Rebound to normal leukocyte levels follows onset within 2 to 3 days. Recovery is not influenced by continuation of silver sulfadiazine therapy. The incidence of leukopenia averages about 20%. An increased incidence of leukopenia has been reported in patients treated concurrently with cimetidine.

➤*Hypersensitivity reactions:* There is potential cross-sensitivity between silver sulfadiazine and other sulfonamides. If allergic reactions attributable to silver sulfadiazine occur, continuation of therapy must be weighed against the potential hazards of the particular allergic reaction. Refer to Management of Acute Hypersensitivity Reactions.

➤*Renal/Hepatic function impairment:* If hepatic or renal function becomes impaired and drug elimination decreases, accumulation may occur. Weigh discontinuation against the therapeutic benefit being achieved.

➤*Pregnancy:* Category B. There are no adequate and well controlled studies in pregnant women. Use during pregnancy only if clearly justified, especially in pregnant women approaching or at term.

➤*Lactation:* It is not known whether silver sulfadiazine cream is excreted in breast milk. However, sulfonamides are excreted in breast milk and all sulfonamide derivatives increase the possibility of kernicterus. Decide whether to discontinue nursing or to discontinue the drug, taking into acccount the importance of the drug to the mother.

➤*Children:* Safety and efficacy have not been established.

Precautions

➤*For external use only:* Avoid contact with eyes.

➤*Reduction in bacterial colonization:* This has caused delayed separation, in some cases necessitating escharotomy to prevent contracture.

➤*Absorption:* Silver sulfadiazine absorption varies depending upon the percent of the body surface area and the extent of the tissue damage. Although few have been reported, since significant quantities of sulfadiazine are absorbed, it is possible that any of the adverse reactions attributable to sulfonamides may occur (see monograph in Anti-Infectives chapter).

Drug Interactions

➤*Topical proteolytic enzymes:* Silver may inactivate such enzymes if these agents are used in conjunction with silver sulfadiazine.

➤*Drug/Lab test interactions:* Absorption of the propylene glycol vehicle, affecting serum osmolality, has occurred.

Adverse Reactions

Leukopenia (20%; see Warnings); skin necrosis, erythema multiforme, skin discoloration, burning sensation, rashes, interstitial nephritis (infrequent).

CHLOROXINE

Rx	**Capitrol** (Westwood Squibb)	**Shampoo:** 2%	In 120 ml.

Indications

Treatment of dandruff and mild to moderately severe seborrheic dermatitis of the scalp.

Administration and Dosage

Massage thoroughly into wet scalp. Allow lather to remain on scalp for 3 minutes; rinse. Repeat application and rinse. Two treatments per week are usually sufficient.

Actions

➤*Pharmacology:* A synthetic antibacterial compound; also has antifungal activity. Chloroxine reduces excess scaling in patients with scaling or seborrheic dermatitis.

Contraindications

Hypersensitivity to any of the ingredients. Do not use on acutely inflamed lesions.

Warnings

➤*Pregnancy: Category C.* Safety for use during pregnancy has not been established. Use only when clearly needed and when the potential benefits outweigh the potential hazards to the fetus.

➤*Lactation:* It is not known whether the drug is excreted in breast milk. Exercise caution when administering to a nursing woman.

➤*Children:* Safety and efficacy for use in children have not been established.

Precautions

➤*For external use only:* Avoid contact with eyes; if contact occurs, flush with cool water.

Adverse Reactions

Irritation and burning of the scalp and adjacent areas have occurred. Discoloration of light colored hair has occurred.

Patient Information

For external use only. Avoid contact with eyes.

If irritation, burning or rash occurs, discontinue use.

May discolor blond, gray or bleached hair.

Corticosteroids, Topical

Indications

▶*Relief of inflammatory and pruritic manifestations of corticosteroid-responsive dermatoses:* Some of the conditions in which topical corticosteroids have been proven effective include: Contact dermatitis, atopic dermatitis, nummular eczema, stasis eczema, asteatotic eczema, lichen planus, lichen simplex chronicus, insect and arthropod bite reactions, first- and second-degree localized burns and sunburns.

▶*Alternative/Adjunctive treatment:* Psoriasis, seborrheic dermatitis, severe diaper rash, disidrosis, nodular prurigo, chronic discoid lupus erythematosus, alopecia areata, lymphocytic infiltration of the skin, mycosis fungoides and familial benign pemphigus of Hailey-Hailey.

▶*Possibly effective in the following conditions:* Bullous pemphigoid, cutaneous mastocytosis, lichen sclerosus et atrophicus and vitiligo.

Topical corticosteroids relieve inflammatory symptoms associated with dermatophyte and yeast infections of the skin and may be used concomitantly with antifungal agents for initial treatment.

The use of topical corticosteroids in combination with antibiotics in secondary infected dermatoses remains controversial.

▶*Nonprescription hydrocortisone preparations:* Temporary relief of itching associated with minor skin irritations, inflammation and rashes due to eczema, insect bites, poison ivy, poison oak, poison sumac, soaps, detergents, cosmetics, jewelry, seborrheic dermatitis, psoriasis and external genital and anal itching.

Administration and Dosage

▶*Usual dose:* Apply sparingly to affected areas 2 to 4 times daily.

▶*General considerations:* Topical corticosteroids have a repository effect; with continuous use, one or two applications per day may be as effective as three or more. Many clinicians advise applying twice daily until clinical response is achieved, and then only as frequently as needed to control the condition.

Short term or intermittent therapy using high potency agents (eg, every other day, 3 to 4 consecutive days per week, or once per week) may be more effective and cause fewer adverse effects than continuous regimens using lower potency products.

Do not discontinue treatment abruptly. After long-term use or after using a potent agent, in order to prevent a rebound effect, switch to a less potent agent or alternate use of topical corticosteroids and emollient products.

Use low potency agents in children, on large areas, and on body sites especially prone to steroid damage such as the face, scrotum, axilla, flexures and skin folds. Reserve higher potency agents for areas and conditions resistant to treatment with milder agents; they may be alternated with milder agents.

Perform appropriate clinical and laboratory tests if a topical corticosteroid is used for long periods or over large areas of the body.

Treatment with very high potency topical corticosteroids should not exceed 2 consecutive weeks and the total dosage should not exceed 50 g per week because of the potential for these drugs to suppress the HPA axis.

▶*Occlusive dressing technique:*
1.) Soak the area in water or wash it well.
2.) While the skin is still moist, gently rub medication into the affected areas.
3.) Cover the area with a plastic wrap (eg, *Saran Wrap, Handi Wrap*). Alternatively, plastic gloves may be used for hands, plastic bags for feet, or a bathing cap for scalp.
4.) Seal edges with tape or bandage, ensuring that the wrap adheres closely to the skin.
5.) Leave in place overnight or at least 6 hours. Do not use for > 12 hours in a 24 hour period. Do not use this technique with very high potency topical corticosteroids.

Actions

▶*Pharmacology:* Topical corticosteroids are adrenocorticosteroid derivatives incorporated into a vehicle suitable for application to skin or external mucous membranes. Modifications of the essential 4-ring steroid structure such as hydroxylation, methylation, fluorination or esterification are often made to increase lipid solubility and potency and decrease mineralocorticoid effects.

The primary therapeutic effects of the topical corticosteroids are due to their anti-inflammatory activity which is non-specific (ie, they act against most causes of inflammation including mechanical, chemical, microbiological and immunological).

Topically applied corticosteroids diffuse across cell membranes to interact with cytoplasmic receptors located in both the dermal and intradermal cells. The intracellular effects are similar to those that occur with systemically administered corticosteroids.

At the cellular level, corticosteroids appear to induce phospholipase A_2 inhibitory proteins (lipocortins), thus depressing formation, release and activity of the endogenous mediators of inflammation such as prostaglandins, kinins, histamine, liposomal enzymes and the complement system.

When corticosteroids are applied to inflamed skin, they inhibit the migration of macrophages and leukocytes into the area by reversing vascular dilation and permeability. The clinical result is a decrease in edema, erythema and pruritus.

By suppressing DNA synthesis, topically applied corticosteroids have an antimitotic effect on epidermal cells. This property is useful in proliferative disorders such as psoriasis, but also can be demonstrated in normal skin.

▶*Pharmacokinetics:* The amount of corticosteroid absorbed from the skin depends on the intrinsic properties of the drug itself, the vehicle used, the duration of exposure and the surface area and condition of the skin to which it is applied. In general, absorption will be enhanced by increased skin temperature, hydration, application to inflamed or denuded skin, intertriginous areas (eg, eyelids, groin, axilla) or skin surfaces with a thin stratum corneum layer (eg, face, scrotum). Palms, soles and crusted surfaces are less permeable. Occlusive dressings greatly enhance skin penetration and, therefore, increase drug absorption.

Infants and children have a higher total body surface to body weight ratio that decreases with age. Therefore, proportionately more topically applied medications will be absorbed systemically in this population, putting them at a greater risk for systemic effects.

Following topical absorption, corticosteroids enter the systemic circulation and are metabolized and excreted via pathways described for systemically administered corticosteroids.

Vehicles – Ointments are more occlusive and are preferred for dry scaly lesions. Use creams on oozing lesions or in intertriginous areas where the occlusive effects of ointments may cause maceration and folliculitis. Creams are often preferred by patients for aesthetic reasons even though their water content makes them more drying than ointments. Gels, aerosols, lotions and solutions are useful on hairy areas. Urea enhances the penetration of hydrocortisone and selected steroids by hydrating the skin. As a general rule, ointments and gels are more potent than creams or lotions. However, optimized vehicles that have been formulated for some products have demonstrated equal potency in cream, gel and ointment forms. Steroid impregnated tapes are useful for occlusive therapy in small areas.

Occlusive dressings – Occlusive dressings such as a plastic wrap increase skin penetration approximately tenfold by increasing the moisture content of the stratum corneum. Occlusion can be beneficial in resistant cases but it may also lead to sweat retention and increased bacterial and fungal infections. Additionally, increased absorption of the corticosteroid may produce systemic side effects. Therefore, do not use occlusive dressings > 12 hours per day and when using very potent topical corticosteroids.

Relative potency – The relative potency of a product depends on several factors including the characteristics and concentration of the drug and the vehicle used. Vasoconstrictor assays are used to measure the relative potency of the commercially available products. The estimated relative potency of selected topical corticosteroid preparations is given in the following table. Ranking is based on vasoconstrictor assays of brand name products. In some cases, generic "equivalents" have less vasoconstrictive activity.

Relative Potency of Selected Topical Corticosteroid Products		
Drug	Dosage Form	Strength
I. *Very high potency*		
Augmented betamethasone dipropionate	Ointment	0.05%
Clobetasol propionate	Cream, Ointment	0.05%
Diflorasone diacetate	Ointment	0.05%
Halobetasol propionate	Cream, Ointment	0.05%
II. *High potency*		
Amcinonide	Cream, Lotion, Ointment	0.1%
Augmented betamethasone dipropionate	Cream	0.05%
Betamethasone dipropionate	Cream, Ointment	0.05%
Betamethasone valerate	Ointment	0.1%
Desoximetasone	Cream, Ointment	0.25%
	Gel	0.05%
Diflorasone diacetate	Cream, Ointment (emollient base)	0.05%
Fluocinolone acetonide	Cream	0.2%
Fluocinonide	Cream, Ointment, Gel	0.05%
Halcinonide	Cream, Ointment	0.1%
Triamcinolone acetonide	Cream, Ointment	0.5%

Relative Potency of Selected Topical Corticosteroid Products		
Drug	Dosage Form	Strength
III. *Medium potency*		
Betamethasone benzoate	Cream, Gel, Lotion	0.025%
Betamethasone dipropionate	Lotion	0.05%
Betamethasone valerate	Cream	0.1%
Clocortolone pivalate	Cream	0.1%
Desoximetasone	Cream	0.05%
Fluocinolone acetonide	Cream, Ointment	0.025%
Flurandrenolide	Cream, Ointment	0.025%
	Cream, Ointment, Lotion	0.05%
	Tape	4 mcg/cm²
Fluticasone propionate	Cream	0.05%
	Ointment	0.005%
Hydrocortisone butyrate	Ointment, Solution	0.1%
Hydrocortisone valerate	Cream, Ointment	0.2%
Mometasone furoate	Cream, Ointment, Lotion	0.1%
Triamcinolone acetonide	Cream, Ointment, Lotion	0.025%
	Cream, Ointment, Lotion	0.1%
IV. *Low potency*		
Aclometasone dipropionate	Cream, Ointment	0.05%
Desonide	Cream	0.05%
Dexamethasone	Aerosol	0.01%
	Aerosol	0.04%
Dexamethasone sodium phosphate	Cream	0.1%
Fluocinolone acetonide	Cream, Solution	0.01%
Hydrocortisone	Lotion	0.25%
	Cream, Ointment, Lotion, Aerosol	0.5%
	Cream, Ointment, Lotion, Solution	1%
	Cream, Ointment, Lotion	2.5%
Hydrocortisone acetate	Cream, Ointment	0.5%
	Cream, Ointment	1%

Contraindications

Hypersensitivity to any component; monotherapy in primary bacterial infections such as impetigo, paryonchia, erysipelas, cellulitis, angular cheilitis, erythrasma (clobetasol), treatment of rosacea, perioral dermatitis or acne; use on the face, groin or axilla (very high or high potency agents); ophthalmic use (prolonged ocular exposure may cause steroid-induced glaucoma and cataracts). When applied to the eyelids or skin near the eyes, the drug may enter the eyes.

Warnings

➤*Pregnancy:* Category C. Corticosteroids are teratogenic in animals when administered systemically at relatively low dosages. The more potent corticosteroids are teratogenic after dermal application in animals. There are no adequate and well controlled studies in pregnant women. Therefore, use during pregnancy only if the potential benefits outweigh the potential hazards to the fetus. In pregnant patients, do not use extensively; do not use in large amounts or for prolonged periods of time.

➤*Lactation:* It is not known whether topical corticosteroids could result in sufficient systemic absorption to produce detectable quantities in breast milk. Systemic corticosteroids are secreted into breast milk in quantities not likely to have a deleterious effect on the infant. Nevertheless, exercise caution when administering topical corticosteroids to a nursing mother.

➤*Children:* Children may be more susceptible to topical corticosteroid-induced hypothalamic-pituitary-adrenal (HPA) axis suppression and Cushing's syndrome than adults because of a larger skin surface area to body weight ratio.

HPA axis suppression, Cushing's syndrome and intracranial hypertension have occurred in children receiving topical corticosteroids. Manifestations of adrenal suppression include linear growth retardation, delayed weight gain, low plasma cortisol levels and absence of response to ACTH stimulation. Manifestations of intracranial hypertension include bulging fontanelles, headaches and bilateral papilledema.

Limit administration to the least amount compatible with effective therapy. Chronic corticosteroid therapy may interfere with the growth and development of children.

Do not use potent topical corticosteroids to treat diaper dermatoses in infants.

Safety and efficacy of augmented betamethasone dipropionate, clobetasol, fluticasone propionate, desoximetasone and halobetasol propionate are not established.

Precautions

➤*Systemic effects:* Systemic absorption of topical corticosteroids has produced reversible HPA axis suppression, Cushing's syndrome, hyperglycemia and glycosuria. Conditions that augment systemic absorption include the application of the more potent steroids, use over large surface areas, prolonged use and the addition of occlusive dressings.

Periodically evaluate patients for evidence of HPA axis suppression by using morning plasma cortisol, urinary free cortisol and ACTH stimulation tests. If HPA axis suppression is noted, attempt to withdraw the drug, reduce the frequency of application, substitute a less potent steroid or use a sequential approach with the occlusive technique. Also test for impairment of thermal homeostasis.

Recovery of HPA axis function and thermal homeostasis are generally prompt and complete upon discontinuation of the drug. Infrequently, signs and symptoms of steroid withdrawal may occur, requiring supplemental systemic corticosteroids.

Clobetasol suppresses the HPA axis at doses as low as 2 g per day.

Children – They may absorb proportionally larger amounts of topical corticosteroids and may be more susceptible to systemic toxicity (see Warnings).

As a general rule, little effect on the HPA axis will occur with use of a potent topical corticosteroid in amounts of < 50 g weekly for an adult and 15 g weekly for a small child, without occlusion. To cover the adult body one time requires 12 to 26 g.

For information regarding systemic corticosteroids, refer to the Adrenal Cortical Steroids, Glucocorticoids group monograph in the Endocrine and Metabolic Agents chapter.

➤*Local irritation:* If local irritation develops, discontinue use and institute appropriate therapy. Medications containing alcohol may produce dry skin or burning sensations/irritation in open lesions. Allergic contact dermatitis is usually diagnosed by observing failure to heal rather than noting clinical exacerbation as with most topical products not containing corticosteroids. Corroborate such an observation with diagnostic patch testing.

Skin atrophy – This is common and may be clinically significant in 3 to 4 weeks with potent preparations. Atrophy occurs most readily at sites where percutaneous absorption is high.

Take care when using periorbitally or in the genital area. Avoid use of high potency topical corticosteroids on the face and in intertriginous areas because of resulting striae.

➤*Psoriasis:* Do not use topical corticosteroids as sole therapy in widespread plaque psoriasis.

In rare instances, treatment (or withdrawal of treatment) of psoriasis with corticosteroids is thought to have provoked the pustular form of the disease.

➤*Atrophic changes:* Certain areas of the body, such as the face, groin and axillae, are more prone to atrophic changes than other areas of the body following treatment with corticosteroids. Frequent observation of the patient is important if these areas are to be treated.

➤*Infections:* In the presence of an infection, institute therapy with an antifungal or antibacterial agent. If a favorable response does not occur promptly, discontinue the corticosteroid until the infection has been controlled. Treating skin infections with topical corticosteroids can extensively worsen the infection.

➤*For external use only:* Avoid inhalation of aerosols, ingestion or contact with eyes.

➤*Vehicles:* Many topical corticosteroids are in specially formulated bases designed to maximize their release and potency. Mixing with other bases or vehicles may affect potency far beyond that normally expected from the dilution. Exercise caution before mixing; if necessary, contact the manufacturer to determine if there may be an incompatibility.

➤*Occlusive therapy:* Discontinue the use of occlusive dressings if infection develops, and institute appropriate antimicrobial therapy.

Occasionally, a patient may develop a sensitivity reaction to a particular occlusive dressing material or adhesive; a substitute material may be necessary.

Do not use occlusive dressings in **augmented betamethasone dipropionate**, **betamethasone dipropionate**, **clobetasol**, **halobetasol propionate** and **mometasone** treatment regimens.

Adverse Reactions

➤*Local:* Burning; itching; irritation; erythema; dryness; folliculitis; hypertrichosis; pruritus; acneiform eruptions; hypopigmentation; perioral dermatitis; allergic contact dermatitis; numbness of fingers; stinging and cracking/tightening of skin; maceration of the skin; secondary infection; skin atrophy; striae; miliaria; telangiectasia. These may occur more frequently with occlusive dressings.

Also, there have been reports of development of pustular psoriasis from chronic plaque psoriasis following reduction or discontinuation of potent topical corticosteroids.

Sensitivity to a particular dressing material or adhesive may occur occasionally.

Corticosteroids, Topical

▶**Systemic:** Systemic absorption of topical corticosteroids has produced reversible HPA axis suppression, manifestations of Cushing's syndrome, hyperglycemia and glycosuria (see Precautions). This is more likely to occur with occlusive dressings and with the more potent steroids. Patients with liver failure or children (see Warnings) may be at at higher risk. Lightheadedness and hives have been reported rarely.

Following prolonged application around the eyes, cataracts and glaucoma may develop. In diffusely atrophied skin, blood vessels may become visible on the skin surface; telangiectasia and purpura may occur at the site of trauma.

The risk of adverse reactions may be minimized by changing to a less potent agent, reducing the dosage or using intermittent therapy.

Overdosage

Topical corticosteroids can be absorbed in sufficient amounts to produce systemic effects (see Precautions).

Patient Information

Apply ointments, creams or gels sparingly in a light film; rub in gently. Washing or soaking the area before application may increase drug penetration.

To use a lotion, solution or gel on your scalp, part your hair, apply a small amount of the medicine on the affected area and rub it in gently.

Protect the area from washing, clothing, rubbing, etc until the lotion dries. You may wash your hair as usual but not right after applying the medicine.

To apply aerosols, shake well and spray on affected area holding container about 3 to 6 inches away. Spray for about 2 seconds to cover an area the size of your hand. Take care not to inhale the vapors. If you are spraying your face or near your face, cover your eyes.

Use only as directed. Do not put bandages, dressing, cosmetics or other skin products over the treated area unless directed by your physician.

Notify your physician if the condition being treated gets worse, or if burning, swelling or redness develop.

Avoid prolonged use around the eyes, in the genital and rectal areas, on the face, armpits and in skin creases unless directed by your physician. Avoid contact with the eyes.

If you forget a dose, apply it as soon as you remember and continue on your regular schedule. If it is almost time for the next application, wait and continue on your regular schedule. Do not apply double doses.

For parents of pediatric patients: Do not use tight-fitting diapers or plastic pants on a child treated in the diaper area; these garments may work like occlusive dressings and cause more of the drug to be absorbed into your child's body.

ALCLOMETASONE DIPROPIONATE

Rx	**Aclovate** (GlaxoWellcome)	**Ointment:** 0.05%	Hexylene glycol, white wax, propylene glycol stearate, white petrolatum. In 15 and 45 g.
		Cream: 0.05%	Hydrophilic, emollient base. Propylene glycol, white petrolatum, glyceryl stearate, PEG-100 stearate, chlorocresol. In 15 and 45 g.

Complete prescribing information begins in the Topical Corticosteroids group monograph.

AMCINONIDE

Rx	**Cyclocort** (Fujisawa)	**Ointment:** 0.1%	White petrolatum. 2% benzyl alcohol. In 15, 30 and 60 g.
Rx	**Amcinonide** (Taro)	**Cream:** 0.1%	In 15, 30, and 60 g.
Rx	**Cyclocort** (Fujisawa)		Hydrophilic base. 2% benzyl alcohol, glycerin. In 15, 30 and 60 g.
Rx	**Cyclocort** (Fujisawa)	**Lotion:** 0.1%	Hydrophilic base. 1% benzyl alcohol, glycerin. In 20 and 60 ml.

Complete prescribing information begins in the Topical Corticosteroids group monograph.

AUGMENTED BETAMETHASONE DIPROPIONATE

Rx	**Betamethasone Dipropionate, Augmented** (Various, eg, Alpharma, Fougera, Warrick)	**Ointment:** 0.05%	In an optimized vehicle. Propylene glycol, propylene glycol stearate, white wax, white petrolatum. In 15, 45, and 50 g.
Rx	**Diprolene** (Schering)		In an optimized vehicle. Propylene glycol, propylene glycol stearate, white wax, white petrolatum. In 15 and 45 g.
Rx	**Diprolene AF** (Schering)	**Cream:** 0.05%	Emollient base. Chlorocresol, propylene glycol, white petrolatum, white wax. In 15 and 45 g.
Rx	**Diprolene** (Schering)	**Gel:** 0.05%	Propylene glycol. In 15 and 45 g.
Rx	**Diprolene** (Schering)	**Lotion:** 0.05%	30% isopropyl alcohol, hydroxypropylcellulose, propylene glycol. In 30 and 60 ml.

Complete prescribing information begins in the Topical Corticosteroids group monograph.

BETAMETHASONE DIPROPIONATE

Rx	**Betamethasone Dipropionate** (Various, eg, NMC)	**Ointment:** 0.05%	In 15 and 45 g.
Rx	**Diprosone** (Schering)		Mineral oil, white petrolatum. In 15 and 45 g.
Rx	**Maxivate** (Westwood Squibb)		Mineral oil, white petrolatum.
Rx	**Betamethasone Dipropionate** (Various, eg, NMC, Schein)	**Cream:** 0.05%	In 15 and 45 g.
Rx	**Alphatrex** (Savage)		Hydrophilic. Mineral oil, white petrolatum, polyethylene glycol, chlorocresol. In 15 and 45 g.
Rx	**Diprosone** (Schering)		Hydrophilic, emollient. Mineral oil, white petrolatum, chlorocresol, propylene glycol. In 15 and 45 g.
Rx	**Maxivate** (Westwood Squibb)		Hydrophilic base. Mineral oil, white petrolatum, polyethylene glycol, chlorocresol. In 15 and 45 g.
Rx	**Teladar** (Dermol)		Mineral oil, white petrolatum, polyethylene glycol, 4 chloro-m-cresol, propylene glycol. In 15 and 45 g.
Rx	**Betamethasone Dipropionate** (Various, eg, Goldline, Major, Moore, Rugby)	**Lotion:** 0.05%	In 20 and 60 ml.
Rx	**Diprosone** (Schering)		46.8% alcohol. In 30 ml.
Rx	**Maxivate** (Westwood Squibb)		Isopropyl alcohol. In 60 ml.
Rx	**Diprosone** (Schering)	**Aerosol:** 0.1%	10% isopropyl alcohol, mineral oil. In 85 g.

Complete prescribing information begins in the Topical Corticosteroids group monograph.

BETAMETHASONE VALERATE

Rx	**Betamethasone Valerate** (Various, eg, Genetco, Goldline, Major, Taro)	**Ointment:** 0.1%	In 15 and 45 g.
Rx	**Psorion Cream** (ICN)	**Cream:** 0.05%	Mineral oil, white petrolatum, propylene glycol. In 15 and 45 g.
Rx	**Betamethasone Valerate** (Various, eg, Genetco, Major, Moore, Taro)	**Cream:** 0.1%	In 15 and 45 g.
Rx	**Beta-Val** (Lemmon)		Aqueous, vanishing base. Mineral oil, white petrolatum, 4-chloro-m-cresol. In 15 and 45 g.
Rx	**Betamethasone Valerate** (Various, eg, Moore)	**Lotion:** 0.1%	In 60 ml.
Rx	**Beta-Val** (Lemmon)		47.5% isopropyl alcohol. In 60 ml.
Rx	**Luxiq** (Connetics)	**Foam:** 1.2 mg/g	60.4% ethanol, cetyl alcohol, stearyl alcohol. In 100 g.
Rx	**Betamethasone Valerate** (Paddock)	**Powder for compounding**	In micronized 5 and 10 g.

Complete prescribing information begins in the Topical Corticosteroids group monograph.

CLOBETASOL PROPIONATE

Rx	**Clobetasol Propionate** (Various, eg, Copley, NMC Labs)	**Ointment:** 0.05%	In 15, 30, and 45 g.
Rx	**Temovate** (GlaxoWellcome)		White petrolatum, sorbitan sesquioleate. In 15, 30, and 45 g.
Rx	**Cormax** (Oclassen)		White petrolatum, sorbitan sesquioleate. In 15 and 45 g.
Rx	**Embeline** (Healthpoint)		White petrolatum. In 15, 30, 45, and 60 g.
Rx	**Clobetasol Propionate** (Various, eg, Copley, NMC Labs)	**Cream:** 0.05%	In 15, 30, and 45 g.
Rx	**Embeline** (Healthpoint)		White petrolatum, cetyl alcohol, stearyl alcohol, lanolin oil, parabens. In 15, 30, 45, and 60 g.
Rx	**Temovate** (GlaxoWellcome)		Chlorocresol. In 15, 30, and 45 g.
Rx	**Temovate Emollient** (Glaxo-Wellcome)		Emollient base. In 15, 30, and 60 g.
Rx	**Embeline E, 0.05%** (Healthpoint)		Cetostearyl alcohol. In 15, 30, and 60 g tubes.
Rx	**Clobex** (Galderma)	**Lotion:** 0.05%	Mineral oil. In 15, 30, 59, and 118 mL.
Rx	**Embeline** (Healthpoint)	**Scalp application:** 0.05%	40% isopropyl alcohol. In 25 and 50 mL.
Rx	**Temovate** (GlaxoWellcome)		39.3% isopropyl alcohol. In 25 and 50 ml.
Rx	**Clobetasol Propionate** (Various, eg, Fougera, Glades)	**Gel:** 0.05%	In 15, 30, and 60 g.
Rx	**Embeline** (Healthpoint)		In 15, 30, and 60 g.
Rx	**Temovate** (GlaxoWellcome)		In 15, 30, and 60 g.
Rx	**Olux** (Connetics)	**Foam:** 0.05%	60% ethanol, cetyl alcohol, stearyl alcohol. In 100g.
Rx	**Clobex** (Galderma)	**Shampoo:** 0.05%	Alcohol. In 118 mL.

Complete prescribing information begins in the Topical Corticosteroids group monograph.

CLOCORTOLONE PIVALATE

Rx	**Cloderm** (Hermal)	**Cream:** 0.1%	Water-washable, emollient base. White petrolatum, mineral oil, EDTA, parabens. In 15 and 45 g.

Complete prescribing information begins in the Topical Corticosteroids group monograph.

DESONIDE

Rx	**Desonide** (Various, eg, Copley, Goldline, Major, Moore, Rugby, Taro)	**Ointment:** 0.05%	In 15 and 60 g.
Rx	**DesOwen** (Owen/Galderma)		Mineral oil. In 15 and 60 g.
Rx	**Tridesilon** (Bayer)		White petrolatum. In 15 and 60 g.
Rx	**Desonide** (Taro)	**Cream:** 0.05%	Methylparaben, mineral oil, white petrolatum. In 15 and 60 g.
Rx	**DesOwen** (Owen/Galderma)		In 15 and 60 g.
Rx	**Tridesilon** (Bayer)		White petrolatum, glycerin, mineral oil, methylparaben. In 15 and 60 g.
Rx	**Desonide** (Various, eg, Fougera, Glades)	**Lotion:** 0.05%	May contain light mineral oil, cetyl alcohol, stearyl alcohol, parabens, EDTA. In 59 and 118 mL.
Rx	**DesOwen** (Owen/Galderma)		Light mineral oil, parabens, EDTA. In 60 and 120 ml.
Rx	**LoKara** (PharmaDerm)		Light mineral oil, cetyl alcohol, stearyl alcohol, parabens, EDTA. In 59 and 118 mL.

Complete prescribing information begins in the Topical Corticosteroids group monograph.

Corticosteroids, Topical

DESOXIMETASONE

Rx	**Topicort** (Taro)	**Ointment:** 0.25%	White petrolatum, sorbitan sesquioleate. In 15 and 60 g.
Rx	**Desoximetasone** (Various, eg, Taro)	**Cream:** 0.05%	Emollient base. White petrolatum, lanolin alcohols, mineral oil, EDTA. In 15 and 60 g.
Rx	**Topicort LP** (Taro)		Emollient. White petrolatum, mineral oil, lanolin alcohols, EDTA. In 15 and 60 g.
Rx	**Desoximetasone** (Various, eg, Taro)	**Cream:** 0.25%	Emollient base. White petrolatum, lanolin alcohols, mineral oil. In 15 and 60 g.
Rx	**Topicort** (Taro)		Emollient. White petrolatum, mineral oil, lanolin alcohols. In 15, 60, 120 g.
Rx	**Topicort** (Taro)	**Gel:** 0.05%	20% SD alcohol 40, EDTA, docusate sodium, trolamine. In 15 and 60 g.

Complete prescribing information begins in the Topical Corticosteroids group monograph.

DEXAMETHASONE

Rx	**Decaspray** (Merck)	**Aerosol:** 0.04%	In 25 g.

Complete prescribing information begins in the Topical Corticosteroids group monograph.

DEXAMETHASONE SODIUM PHOSPHATE

Rx	**Decadron Phosphate** (Merck)	**Cream:** 0.1%	Greaseless base. Mineral oil, EDTA, 0.15% methylparaben, 0.1% sorbic acid. In 15 and 30 g.

Complete prescribing information begins in the Topical Corticosteroids group monograph.

DIFLORASONE DIACETATE

Rx	**ApexiCon** (PharmaDerm)	**Ointment:** 0.05%	White petrolatum. In 30 and 60 g.
Rx	**Diflorasone Diacetate** (Taro)		In 15, 30, and 60 g tubes.
Rx	**Maxiflor** (Allergan)		Emollient, occlusive base. Lanolin alcohol, white petrolatum. In 15, 30 and 60 g.
Rx	**Psorcon E** (Dermik)		Emollient, occlusive base. Lanolin alcohol, white petrolatum. In 15, 30 and 60 g.
Rx	**ApexiCon E** (PharmaDerm)	**Cream:** 0.05%	Stearyl alcohol, mineral oil, cetyl alcohol. In 30 and 60 g.
Rx	**Diflorasone Diacetate** (Taro)		In 15, 30, and 60 g tubes.
Rx	**Florone** (Dermik)		Emulsified, hydrophilic base. Propylene glycol. In 30 and 60 g.
Rx	**Florone E** (Dermik)		Emollient, hydrophilic vanishing base. Mineral oil. In 15, 30 and 60 g.
Rx	**Maxiflor** (Allergan)		Emulsified, hydrophilic base. 15% propylene glycol. In 15, 30 and 60 g.
Rx	**Psorcon E** (Dermik)		Hydrophilic base. Stearyl alcohol, cetyl alcohol, mineral oil. In 15 and 30 g.

Complete prescribing information begins in the Topical Corticosteroids group monograph.

FLUOCINOLONE ACETONIDE

Rx	**Fluocinolone** (Various, eg, Fougera, Goldline, Moore)	**Ointment:** 0.025%	In 15 and 60 g.
Rx	**Flurosyn** (Rugby)		In 15 and 60 g.
Rx	**Synalar** (Syntex)		White petrolatum. In 15, 30 and 425 g.
Rx	**Fluocinolone** (Various, eg, Fougera, Geneva, Goldline, Major, Moore, NMC)	**Cream:** 0.01%	In 15 and 60 g.
Rx	**Flurosyn** (Rugby)		Washable. Parabens. In 15, 60, 425 g.
Rx	**Synalar** (Syntex)		Water-washable, aqueous base. Mineral oil, EDTA, parabens. In 30 and 425 g.
Rx	**Fluocinolone** (Various, eg, Fougera, Geneva, Goldline, Major, Moore)	**Cream:** 0.025%	In 15 and 60 g.
Rx	**Flurosyn** (Rugby)		Washable. Parabens. In 15, 60, 425 g.
Rx	**Synalar** (Syntex)		Water-washable, aqueous base. Mineral oil, EDTA, parabens. In 30, 60 and 425 g.
Rx	**Synalar-HP** (Syntex)	**Cream:** 0.2%	Water-washable, aqueous base. Mineral oil, parabens. In 12 g.
Rx	**Fluocinolone** (Various, eg, Fougera, Goldline, Major, Moore, Rugby)	**Solution:** 0.01%	In 20 and 60 ml.
Rx	**Synalar** (Syntex)		Water-washable base. In 20, 60 ml.
Rx	**Capex** (Galderma)	**Shampoo:** 0.01%	In 12 mg capsule with shampoo base to be mixed by pharmacist before dispensing. 5.48 mg dibasic calcium phosphate dihydrate. In 180 ml.
Rx	**Derma-Smoothe/FS** (Hill)	**Oil:** 0.01%	A blend of oils, including mineral oil and peanut oil. In 120 ml

Complete prescribing information begins in the Topical Corticosteroids group monograph.

FLUOCINONIDE

Rx	**Fluocinonide** (Various, eg, Goldline, Lemmon, Taro)	**Cream:** 0.05%	In 15, 30, 60 and 120 g.
Rx	**Fluocinonide "E" Cream** (Various, eg, Goldline, Taro, URL)		In 15, 30, 60 and 120 g.
Rx	**Fluonex** (ICN)		Greaseless, anhydrous, water-washable. In 15 and 30 g.
Rx	**Lidex** (Syntex)		Water-miscible, emollient, hydrophilic, anhydrous, greaseless. In 15, 30, 60 and 120 g.
Rx	**Lidex-E** (Syntex)		Water-washable, aqueous emollient base. Mineral oil. In 15, 30 and 60 g.
Rx	**Fluocinonide** (Various, eg, Lemmon, Rugby, Taro)	**Ointment:** 0.05%	In 15, 30 and 60 g.
Rx	**Lidex** (Syntex)		Occlusive, emollient. White petrolatum. In 15, 30, 60 and 120 g.
Rx	**Fluocinonide** (Various, eg, Fougera, Goldline, Lemmon, Major, Moore)	**Solution:** 0.05%	In 60 ml.
Rx	**Lidex** (Syntex)		35% alcohol. In 20 and 60 ml.
Rx	**Fluocinonide** (Various, eg, Fougera, Lemmon, Moore)	**Gel:** 0.05%	In 60 g.
Rx	**Lidex** (Syntex)		Water-miscible, greaseless. EDTA. In 15, 30, 60, and 120 g.

Complete prescribing information begins in the Topical Corticosteroids group monograph.

FLURANDRENOLIDE

Rx	**Cordran** (Oclassen)	**Ointment:** 0.05%	White petrolatum. In 15, 30 and 60 g.
Rx	**Cordran SP** (Oclassen)	**Cream:** 0.05%	Emulsified base. Mineral oil. In 15, 30 and 60 g.
Rx	**Flurandrenolide** (Various, eg, Barre-National)	**Lotion:** 0.05%	In 60 ml.
Rx	**Cordran** (Oclassen)		Oil-in-water base. Mineral oil, glycerin, menthol, benzyl alcohol. In 15 and 60 ml.
Rx	**Cordran** (Oclassen)	**Tape:** 4 mcg per square cm	In 24″ x 3″ and 80″ x 3″ rolls.

Complete prescribing information begins in the Topical Corticosteroids group monograph.

FLUTICASONE PROPIONATE

Rx	**Fluticasone Propionate** (Sandoz)	**Cream:** 0.05%	Cetostearyl alcohol, mineral oil. In 15, 30, and 60 g tubes.
	Cutivate (GlaxoWellcome)		Mineral oil base. Imidurea. In 15, 30 and 60 g.
Rx	**Fluticasone Propionate** (Fougera)	**Ointment:** 0.005%	In 15, 30, and 60 g tubes.
	Cutivate (GlaxoWellcome)		In 15 and 60 g.

Complete prescribing information begins in the Topical Corticosteroids group monograph.

HALCINONIDE

Rx	**Halog** (Princeton)	**Ointment:** 0.1%	Polyethylene and mineral oil gel base. In 15, 30, 60 and 240 g.
Rx	**Halog** (Princeton)	**Cream:** 0.025%	In 15 and 60 g.
Rx	**Halog** (Princeton)	**Cream:** 0.1%	Titanium dioxide. In 15, 30, 60 and 240 g.
Rx	**Halog-E** (Princeton)		Water-washable, greaseless, hydrophilic, vanishing, emollient. White petrolatum. In 15, 30 and 60 g.
Rx	**Halog** (Princeton)	**Solution:** 0.1%	EDTA. In 20 and 60 ml.

Complete prescribing information begins in the Topical Corticosteroids group monograph.

HALOBETASOL PROPIONATE

Rx	**Ultravate** (Westwood Squibb)	**Ointment:** 0.05%	Petrolatum. In 15 and 45 g.
		Cream: 0.05%	Glycerin, diazolidinyl urea. In 15 and 45 g.

Complete prescribing information begins in the Topical Corticosteroids group monograph.

HYDROCORTISONE

Rx[1]	**Hydrocortisone** (Various, eg, Carolina Medical, Fougera, Parmed, Rugby[2], URL)	**Ointment:** 0.5%	In 30 g.
otc	**Cortizone•5** (Thompson)		White petrolatum. In 30 g.
Rx[1]	**Hydrocortisone** (Various, eg, Carolina Medical[3], Fougera, Major, Parmed, Rugby, URL)	**Ointment:** 1%	In 20, 30 and 120 g and lb.
otc	**HydroSkin** (Rugby)		Mineral oil, white petrolatum base. In 28.4 g.
otc	**Cortizone•10** (Thompson)		White petrolatum. In 30 g.
Rx	**Hycort** (Everett)		White petrolatum and mineral oil base. In 30 g.
otc	**Tegrin-HC** (Block)		Mineral oil, white petrolatum. In 28 g.
Rx	**1% HC** (C & M)		Washable. Petrolatum base. In 15, 20, 30, 60, 120 and 240 g and lb.
Rx	**Hydrocortisone** (Various, eg, Major, Parmed, Rugby, URL)	**Ointment:** 2.5%	In 20 g.
Rx	**Hytone** (Dermik)		Emollient base. Mineral oil, white petrolatum. In 30 g.

HYDROCORTISONE

Rx[1]	**Hydrocortisone** (Various, eg, Fougera, Geneva, Major, Roberts Hauck, Rugby[2], URL)	**Cream:** 0.5%	In 15, 30 and 120 g and lb.
otc	**Cortizone for Kids** (Pfizer)		Parabens, cetearyl alcohol, glycerin, white petrolatum. In 14 g.
otc	**Cortizone•5** (Thompson)		Glycerin, mineral oil, white petrolatum, parabens. In 60 g.
otc	**Delcort** (Roberts Med)		In 1 g packets.
otc	**Dermolate** (Schering-Plough)		Greaseless, vanishing. Petrolatum, mineral oil, chlorocresol. In 15 and 30 g.
otc	**HydroTex** (Syosset)		In 30 and 60 g.
Rx[1]	**Hydrocortisone** (Various, eg, Fougera, Geneva, Goldline, Major, Moore, Parmed, Roberts Hauck, Rugby, URL[2])	**Cream:** 1%	In 20, 30 and 120 g and lb.
otc	**HydroSkin** (Rugby)		Mineral oil, lanolin alcohol, cetyl alcohol, parabens. In 113.4 g.
Rx	**Ala-Cort** (Del-Ray)		Glycerin. In 30 and 90 g.
otc	**Maximum Strength Bactine** (Miles Inc.)		Glycerin, lt. mineral oil, methylparaben, white petrolatum. In 30 g.
Rx	**Cort-Dome** (Miles Inc.)		Glycerin, white petrolatum, lt. mineral oil, methylparaben. In 30 g.
Rx	**Delcort** (Roberts Med)		In 1 g packets.
Rx	**Hi-Cor 1.0** (C & M)		Washable. Petrolatum, glycerin. In 15, 20, 30, 60, 120 & 240 g & lb.
Rx	**Hytone** (Dermik)		Water-washable. Cholesterol. In 30 and 120 g.
otc	**Procort** (Roberts)		In 30 g.
Rx	**Synacort** (Syntex)		Mineral oil. In 15, 30 and 60 g.
otc	**Maximum Strength KeriCort-10** (Bristol-Myers Squibb)		Parabens, cetyl alcohol, stearyl alcohol. In 56.7 g.
otc	**Cortaid Intensive Therapy** (Pharmacia & Upjohn)		Alcohol, parabens. In 56 g tubes.
otc	**Cortizone-10 Plus** (Pfizer Consumer)		Alcohol, aloe, glycerin, mineral oil, parabens, petrolatum. In 28 and 57 g.
Rx	**Hydrocortisone** (Various, eg, Geneva, Goldline, King, Major, Moore, NMC, Rugby, URL)	**Cream:** 2.5%	In 20 and 30 g and lb.
Rx	**Anusol-HC 2.5%** (Parke-Davis)		Water-washable. Benzyl alcohol, petrolatum, EDTA. In 30 g.
Rx	**Eldecort** (ICN)		Light mineral oil, propylene glycol, allantoin. In 15 and 30 g.
Rx	**Hi-Cor 2.5** (C & M)		Washable. Petrolatum, glycerin. In 15, 20, 30, 60, 120 & 240 g & lb.
Rx	**Hydrocort** (Parmed)		In 20 and 30 g and lb.
Rx	**Hytone** (Dermik)		Water-washable base. Cholesterol. In 30 and 60 g.
Rx	**Synacort** (Syntex)		Mineral oil. In 30 g.
Rx	**proctoCream•HC 2.5%** (Schwarz Pharma)		Glyceryl monostearate, glycerin, stearyl alcohol, benzyl alcohol. In 30 g tubes.
Rx	**Cetacort** (Owen/Galderma)	**Lotion:** 0.25%	Parabens. In 120 ml.
Rx[1]	**Hydrocortisone** (Various, eg, Goldline, Mericon, Parmed, Rugby, URL)	**Lotion:** 0.5%	In 30, 60 and 120 ml.
Rx	**Cetacort** (Owen/Galderma)		Parabens. In 60 ml.
otc[1]	**Hydrocortisone** (Various, eg, Geneva, Glades, Mericon)	**Lotion:** 1%	In 120 ml.
otc	**HydroSkin** (Rugby)		Cetyl alcohol, parabens. In 118 mL.
Rx	**Acticort 100** (Baker Cummins)		In 60 ml.
Rx	**Ala-Cort** (Del-Ray)		Light mineral oil, glycerin. In 118 ml.
Rx	**Hytone** (Dermik)		Cholesterol, triethanolamine. In 120 ml.
Rx	**LactiCare-HC** (Stiefel)		Light mineral oil, lactic acid. In 120 ml.
Rx	**Ala-Scalp** (Del-Ray)	**Lotion:** 2%	Isopropyl alcohol, benzalkonium chloride. In 30 ml.
Rx	**Hydrocortisone** (Glades)	**Lotion:** 2.5%	Stearyl alcohol, cetyl alcohol, light mineral oil. In 59 and 120 mL.
Rx	**Hytone** (Dermik)		Cholesterol, triethanolamine. In 60 ml.
Rx	**LactiCare-HC** (Stiefel)		Light mineral oil, lactic acid. In 60 ml.
otc	**Scalpicin** (Combe)	**Liquid:** 1%	Menthol, SD alcohol 40. In 45, 75 and 120 ml.
otc	**T/Scalp** (Neutrogena)		Greaseless. In 60 and 600 ml.
otc	**Extra Strength CortaGel** (Norstar)	**Gel:** 1%	Greaseless. EDTA. In 15 and 30 g.
Rx	**Alcortin** (Primus)	**Gel:** 2%	Alcohols, glycerin. In 2 g tubes.
Rx	**Penecort** (Allergan)	**Solution:** 1%	Alcohol, petrolatum, propylene glycol. In 30 and 60 ml.
Rx	**Texacort** (GenDerm)		Lipid free. 33% SD alcohol 40-2. In 30 ml.
otc	**Maximum Strength Cortaid** (Pharmacia & Upjohn)	**Pump Spray:** 1%	55% alcohol, glycerin, methylparaben. In 45 ml.
otc	**Procort** (Roberts)	**Spray:** 1%	In 45 ml.
otc	**Cortizone-10 Quickshot** (Pfizer Consumer)		Alcohols. In 44 mL.
otc	**Maximum Strength Cortaid Faststick** (Pharmacia & Upjohn)	**Stick, roll-on:** 1%	55% alcohol, glycerin, methylparaben. In 14 g.

[1] Products are available *otc* or *Rx* depending on product labeling.
[2] Also available with aloe.

[3] In *Absorbase* (a water-in-oil emulsion of cholesterolized petrolatum and purified water).

Complete prescribing information begins in the Topical Corticosteroids group monograph.

Corticosteroids, Topical

HYDROCORTISONE ACETATE

otc	**Lanacort-5** (Combe)	**Ointment:** 0.5%	Acetylated lanolin alcohols, aloe, petrolatum. In 15 g.
otc	**Corticaine** (UCB)	**Cream:** 0.5%	Greaseless. Glycerin, EDTA, menthol, parabens. In 30 g.
otc	**Cortaid with Aloe** (Pharmacia & Upjohn)		Aloe vera, parabens. In 15 and 30 g.
otc	**Cortef Feminine Itch** (Pharmacia & Upjohn)		Vanishing. Aloe vera, parabens. In 15 g.
otc	**Lanacort-5 Creme** (Combe)		Aloe, parabens. In 15 and 22.5 g.
otc	**Anusol HC-1** (Parke-Davis)	**Ointment:** 1%	Diazolidinyl urea, parabens, mineral oil, sorbitan sesquioleate, white petrolatum. In 21 g.
otc	**Maximum Strength Cortaid** (Pharmacia & Upjohn)		Mineral oil, parabens, cholesterol, white petrolatum. In 30 g.
otc	**Maximum Strength Hydrocortisone Acetate** (Clay-Park Labs)		Aloe extract, white petrolatum. In 28 g.
Rx[1]	**Hydrocortisone Acetate** (Various, eg, Thames)	**Cream:** 1%	Mineral oil, parabens. In 20, 30 and 120 g.
otc	**Gynecort Female Creme** (Combe)		Parabens, sorbitol, zinc pyrithione. In 15 g.
otc	**Lanacort 10 Creme** (Combe)		Parabens. In 15 and 30 g.
otc	**Maximum Strength Cortaid** (Pharmacia & Upjohn)		Parabens, glycerin, white petrolatum. In 15 g.
otc	**Maximum Strength Caldecort** (Ciba Self-Medication)		Cetostearyl alcohol, white petrolatum. In 14 g.

[1] Products are available *otc* or *Rx* depending on product labeling.

Complete prescribing information begins in the Topical Corticosteroids group monograph.

HYDROCORTISONE PROBUTATE

Rx	**Pandel** (Savage)	**Cream:** 0.1%	In 15 and 45 g.

Complete prescribing information begins in the Topical Corticosteroids group monograph.

Administration and Dosage

Apply a thin film to the affected area once or twice a day depending on the severity of the condition. Massage gently until the medication disappears. Use occlusive dressings only under the advice of a physician for the management of refractory lesions of psoriasis and other deep-seated dermatoses. Do not apply in the diaper area, as diapers or plastic pants may constitute occlusive dressings.

➤*Storage / Stability:* Store at controlled room temperature 15° to 30°C (59° to 86°F).

HYDROCORTISONE BUTYRATE

Rx	**Locoid** (Ferndale)	**Ointment:** 0.1%	Mineral oil. In 15 and 45 g.
		Cream: 0.1%	Alcohol, mineral oil, parabens, white petrolatum. In 15 and 45 g.
Rx	**Hydrocortisone Butyrate** (Taro)	**Solution:** 0.1%	50% isopropyl alcohol, glycerin. In 20 and 60 mL.
Rx	**Locoid** (Ferndale)		50% alcohol, glycerin. In 20 and 60 mL.

Complete prescribing information begins in the Topical Corticosteroids group monograph.

Administration and Dosage

➤*Cream and ointment:* Apply to the affected area as a thin film 2 or 3 times daily depending on the severity of the condition. Use occlusive dressings under the direction of a physician for the management of psoriasis or recalcitrant conditions. Do not use tight-fitting diapers or plastic pants on a child being treated in the diaper area, as these garments may constitute occlusive dressings. If an infection develops, discontinue occlusive dressings and institute appropriate antimicrobial therapy.

➤*Solution:* Apply to the affected area as a thin film 2 or 3 times daily depending on the severity of the condition. Use occlusive dressings only under the advice of a physician. Do not use tight-fitting diapers or plastic pants on a child being treated in the diaper area, as these garments may constitute occlusive dressing.

HYDROCORTISONE VALERATE

Rx	**Hydrocortisone Valerate** (Taro)	**Ointment:** 0.2%	Hydrophilic base. White petrolatum, alcohol, mineral oil. In 15, 45, and 60 g.
	Westcort (Westwood Squibb)		Hydrophilic base. White petrolatum, mineral oil. In 15, 45, and 60 g.
Rx	**Hydrocortisone Valerate** (Copley)	**Cream:** 0.2%	Hydrophlic base. White petrolatum, alcohol. In 15, 45, and 60 g.
	Westcort (Westwood Squibb)		Hydrophilic base. White petrolatum. In 15, 45, 60, and 120 g.

Complete prescribing information begin in the Topical Corticosteroids group monograph.

MOMETASONE FUROATE

Rx	**Elocon** (Schering)	**Ointment:** 0.1%	White petrolatum. In 15 and 45 g.
		Cream: 0.1%	White petrolatum. In 15 and 45 g.
		Lotion: 0.1%	40% isopropyl alcohol. In 27.5 and 55 ml.

Complete prescribing information begins in the Topical Corticosteroids group monograph.

PREDNICARBATE

Rx	**Dermatop E** (Dermik)	**Cream:** 0.1% prednicarbate	White petrolatum, mineral oil, EDTA, lanolin alcohols, cetostearyl alcohol, lactic acid. In 15 and 60 g.
		Ointment: 0.1% prednicarbate	White petrolatum, glycerin. In 15 and 60 g.

Complete prescribing information begins in the Topical Corticosteroids group monograph.

Corticosteroids, Topical

TRIAMCINOLONE ACETONIDE

Rx	Triamcinolone Acetonide (Various, eg, Fougera, Goldline, Moore, URL)	Ointment: 0.025%	In 15, 80 and 454 g.
Rx	Flutex (Syosset)		White petrolatum, mineral oil. In 28, 57 and 113 g.
Rx	Kenalog (Westwood Squibb)		In *Plastibase* (polyethylene, mineral oil gel base). In 15, 80 and 240 g.
Rx	Triamcinolone Acetonide (Various, eg, Fougera, Goldline, Moore, NMC, URL)	Ointment: 0.1%	In 15 and 80 g and lb.
Rx	Aristocort (Fujisawa)		White petrolatum. In 15, 60 and 240 g.
Rx	Aristocort A (Fujisawa)		White petrolatum. In 15 and 60 g.
Rx	Flutex (Syosset)		White petrolatum, mineral oil. In 28, 57 and 113 g.
Rx	Kenalog (Westwood Squibb)		In *Plastibase* (polyethylene, mineral oil gel base). In 15, 60, 80 and 240 g.
Rx	Triamcinolone Acetonide (Various, eg, URL)	Ointment: 0.5%	In 15 g.
Rx	Aristocort (Fujisawa)		White petrolatum base. In 15 and 240 g.
Rx	Flutex (Syosset)		White petrolatum, mineral oil. In 28, 57 and 113 g.
Rx	Kenalog (Westwood Squibb)		In *Plastibase* (polyethylene, mineral oil gel base). In 20 g.
Rx	Triamcinolone Acetonide (Various, eg, Goldline, Major, Moore, Schein, URL)	Cream: 0.025%	In 15, 80 and 454 g.
Rx	Aristocort (Fujisawa)		In 15 & 60 g & lb.
Rx	Aristocort A (Fujisawa)		Water-washable. 2% benzyl alcohol. In 15 & 60 g.
Rx	Flutex (Syosset)		Mineral oil, lanolin alcohol, sodium bisulfite. In 15, 30, 60, 120 and 240 g.
Rx	Kenalog (Westwood Squibb)		Vanishing base. White petrolatum. In 15, 80, 240 g.
Rx	Triamcinolone Acetonide (Various, eg, Fougera, Goldline)	Cream: 0.1%	In 15, 80 and 454 g.
Rx	Aristocort (Fujisawa)		In 15, 60 and 240 g and lb.
Rx	Aristocort A (Fujisawa)		Water-washable base. Glycerin, 2% benzyl alcohol. In 15, 60 and 240 g.
Rx	Delta-Tritex (Dermol)		In 30 and 80 g.
Rx	Flutex (Syosset)		Mineral oil, lanolin alcohol, sodium bisulfite. In 15, 30, 60, 120 and 240 g.
Rx	Kenalog (Westwood Squibb)		Vanishing base. White petrolatum. In 15, 60, 80 & 240 g.
Rx	Kenonel (Marnel)		In 20 g.
Rx	Triderm (Del-Rey)		Mineral oil. In 30 and 90 g.
Rx	Triamcinolone Acetonide (Various, eg, Fougera, Goldline, Moore, URL)	Cream: 0.5%	In 15 g.
Rx	Aristocort (Fujisawa)		In 15 and 240 g.
Rx	Aristocort A (Fujisawa)		Water-washable base. 2% benzyl alcohol. In 15 g.
Rx	Flutex (Syosset)		Mineral oil, lanolin alcohol, sodium bisulfite. In 15, 30, 60, 120 and 240 g.
Rx	Kenalog (Westwood Squibb)		Vanishing base. White petrolatum. In 20 g.
Rx	Triamcinolone Acetonide (Various, eg, Major, Morton Grove, Rugby)	Lotion: 0.025%	In 60 ml.
Rx	Kenalog (Westwood Squibb)		In 60 ml.
Rx	Triamcinolone Acetonide (Various, eg, Goldline, Morton Grove, Moore, PBI)	Lotion: 0.1%	In 60 ml.
Rx	Kenalog (Westwood Squibb)		In 15 and 60 ml.
Rx	Delta-Tritex (Dermol)	Ointment: 0.1%	In 30 g.
Rx	Kenalog (Westwood Squibb)	Aerosol: (2 sec. spray)	10.3% alcohol. In 23 and 63 g.

Complete prescribing information begins in the Topical Corticosteroids group monograph.

CORTICOSTEROID COMBINATIONS

	Product & Distributor	Hydrocortisone (%)	Clioquinol (%)	Pramoxine (%)	Other Content and How Supplied
Rx	**Hydrocortisone with Clioquinol Cream** (Various, eg, Moore, Rugby)	0.5	3		In 30 g.
Rx	**Ala-Quin Cream** (Del-Ray)				Glycerin. In 30 g.
Rx	**Hydrocortisone with Clioquinol Cream** (Various, eg, Goldline, Moore, Rugby, Schein, URL)	1	3		In 20, 30 and 300 g.
Rx	**Corque Cream** (Geneva)	1	3		In 20 g.
Rx	**Hysone Cream** (Roberts Med)	1	3		In 20 g tube.
Rx	**Hydrocortisone with Clioquinol Ointment** (Various, eg, Moore, Rugby)	1	3		In 20 and 30 g.
Rx	**1 + 1-F Creme** (Dunhall)	1	3	1	Mineral oil, lanolin alcohol, parabens. In 30 g.
Rx	**Analpram-HC Cream** (Ferndale)	1[1]		1	0.1% potassium sorbate, 0.1% sorbic acid. In 30 g.
Rx	**Enzone Cream** (UAD)				Hydrophilic. 0.1% K sorbate, 0.1% sorbic acid. In 30 g.
Rx	**Pramosone Cream** (Ferndale)				Hydrophilic base. 0.1% potassium sorbate, 0.1% sorbic acid. In 30, 60 and 120 g.
Rx	**ProctoCream-HC Cream** (Reed & Carnrick)				Hydrophilic base. Propylene glycol. In 30 g.
Rx	**Pramosone Ointment** (Ferndale)				Emollient base. White petrolatum. In 30 and 120 g.
Rx	**Pramosone Lotion** (Ferndale)				Hydrophilic. Glycerin, 0.1% potassium sorbate, 0.1% sorbic acid. In 60, 120, 240 ml.
Rx	**Epifoam Aerosol Foam** (Schwarz Pharma)				Parabens, propylene glycol. In 10 g.
Rx	**ProctoFoam-HC Aerosol Foam** (Reed & Carnrick)				Hydrophilic base. Parabens. In 10 g.
Rx	**Cortane-B Lotion** (Blansett)	1		1	0.1% chloroxylenol. Benzalkonium Cl. In 60 mL.
Rx	**Carmol HC Cream** (Doak)	1[1]			Water-washable, vanishing. 10% urea, sodium metabisulfite. In 30 and 120 g.
Rx	**Hydrocortison Iodoquinol 1% Cream** (Various, eg, Cypress, Glades)	1			1% iodoquinol. In 30 g.
Rx	**Vytone Cream** (Dermik)	1			Greaseless. 1% iodoquinol, propylene glycol. In 30 g.
Rx	**Novacort Gel** (Primus)	2		1	Alcohols, aloe, glycerin. In 29 g tubes.
Rx	**Analpram-HC Cream** (Ferndale)	2.5[1]		1	In 30 g.
Rx	**Pramosone Cream** (Ferndale)				Hydrophilic. 0.1% K sorbate, 0.1% sorbic acid. In 30, 120 g.
Rx	**Pramosone Ointment** (Ferndale)				Emollient base. White petrolatum. In 30 and 120 g.
Rx	**Pramosone Lotion** (Ferndale)				Hydrophilic. Glycerin, 0.1% potassium sorbate, 0.1% sorbic acid. In 60 and 120 ml.
Rx	**Zone-A Forte Lotion** (UAD)				Hydrophilic. Glycerin, triethanolamine, 0.1% K sorbate, 0.1% sorbic acid. In 60 ml.
Rx	**AnaMantle HC Cream** (Bradley)	0.5[1]			3% lidocaine HCl, cetyl alcohol, light mineral oil, parabens, glycerin, stearyl alcohol, petrolatum. In kits of 7 g tubes with single-use applicators (14s).
Rx	**Lida-Mantle-HC Cream** (Doak)	0.5[1]			3% lidocaine HCl, glycerin, parabens. In 30 g.
Rx	**LidaMantle HC Lotion** (Doak)				3% lidocaine HCl, cetyl alcohol, mineral oil, methylparaben, petrolatum. In 177 mL.
otc	**HC Derma-Pax Liquid** (Recsei)	0.5[1]			0.44% pyrilamine maleate, 0.06% chlorpheniramine maleate, 1% benzyl alcohol, 35% isopropanol, 25% chlorobutanol. In 60 and 120 ml.
otc	**Massengill Medicated Towelettes** (SK-Beecham)				Diazolidinyl urea, parabens, propylene glycol. In 10 and 16 softcloth towelettes.
Rx	**Vanoxide-HC Lotion** (Dermik)				Water-washable. 5% benzoyl peroxide, mineral oil, propylene glycol, EDTA, parabens. In 25 ml.

[1] Hydrocortisone acetate.

These products contain corticosteroids in combination with various other components. They are indicated for a variety of specific and non-specific dermatoses. For further information see individual monographs. Components of these formulations include:

Ingredients

➤*CORTICOSTEROID:* Used for their anti-inflammatory, antipruritic and vasoconstrictive effects.

➤*CLIOQUINOL, IODOQUINOL, TRIACETIN, CLOTRIMA-ZOLE, NYSTATIN, POLYMYXIN B SULFATE, BACITRACIN ZINC, CETYLPYRIDINIUM Cl and CHLOROXYLENOL:* Used for their antifungal, antibacterial and anti-eczematous effects.

➤*LIDOCAINE:* Used as a local anesthetic.

➤*UREA:* This is a mild keratolytic and hydrates dry skin.

➤*CHLORPHENIRAMINE:* This is an antihistamine.

➤*BENZOYL PEROXIDE:* Used for its peeling and drying effects.

Corticosteroids, Topical

CORTICOSTEROID AND ANTIBIOTIC COMBINATIONS

		Dosage form	Corticosteroid	Neomycin sulfate	Other	Base/ How Supplied
Rx	**Cortisporin** (GlaxoWellcome)	Cream	0.5% hydrocortisone acetate	0.5%	10,000 units polymyxin B sulfate per g; white, liquid petrolatum; 0.25% methylparaben	In 7.5 g.
Rx	**Myco-Biotic** II (Moore)		0.1% triamcinolone acetonide		Aqueous vanishing. 100,000 units nystatin per g, white petrolatum	In 15, 30 and 60 g and lb.
Rx	**Hydrocortisone-Neomycin** (Various)	Ointment	1% hydrocortisone	0.5%	White petrolatum, mineral oil	In 20 g.
Rx	**Cortisporin** (GlaxoWellcome)		1% hydrocortisone		400 units bacitracin zinc, white petrolatum, and 5000 units polymyxin B sulfate per g	In 15 g.

Consider the information for Topical Corticosteroids, Antibiotics and Antifungals when using these products (see individual monographs).

CORTICOSTEROID AND ANTIFUNGAL COMBINATIONS

		Dosage form	Corticosteroid	Antifungal	Base/How Supplied
Rx	**Clotrimazole and Betamethasone Dipropionate** (Fougera)	Cream	0.05% betamethasone (as dipropionate)	1% clotrimazole	Mineral oil, white petrolatum, cetearyl alcohol, benzyl alcohol. In 15 and 45 g.
Rx	**Lotrisone** (Schering)				Hydrophilic. Mineral oil, white petrolatum, benzyl alcohol. In 15 and 45 g.
Rx	**Nystatin-Triamcinolone Acetonide** (Various, eg, Fougera, Taro)		0.1% triamcinolone acetonide	100,000 units nystatin per g	In 15, 30 and 60 g and UD 1.5 g.
Rx	**Mycogen** II (Goldline)				In 15, 30, 60 and 120 g.
Rx	**Mycolog**-II (B-M Squibb)				Vanishing base. White petrolatum. In 15, 30, 60 and 120 g.
Rx	**Myconel** (Marnel)				In 20 g.
Rx	**Myco-Triacet** II (Lemmon)				Aqueous, vanishing base. White petrolatum, parabens. In 15, 30 and 60 g.
Rx	**Tri-Statin** II (Rugby)				Vanishing base. White petrolatum. In 15, 30 and 60 g.
Rx	**Nystatin-Triamcinolone Acetonide** (Various, eg, Fougera)	Ointment	0.1% triamcinolone acetonide	100,000 units nystatin per g	In 15, 30 and 60 g.
Rx	**Mycogen** II (Goldline)				In 15, 30 and 60 g.
Rx	**Mycolog**-II (B-M Squibb)				Mineral oil, gel base. In 15, 30, 60 and 120 g.
Rx	**Myco-Triacet** II (Lemmon)				Vanishing base. White petrolatum and mineral oil. In 15 and 30 g.

Consider the information given for Topical Corticosteroids and for Topical Antifungals when using these products.

In addition to the products described here, other products for treatment of psoriasis include: Coal tar; corticosteroids; salicylic acid. Refer to individual monographs.

ANTHRALIN (Dithranol)

Rx	**Anthra-Derm** (Dermik)	**Ointment:** 0.1%	In 42.5 g
		0.25%	In 42.5 g.
Rx	**Anthra-Derm** (Dermik)	**Ointment:** 0.5%	In 42.5 g.
		1%	In 42.5 g.
Rx	**Drithocreme** (Dermik)	**Cream:** 0.25%	White petrolatum, cetostearyl alcohol. In 50 g.
Rx	**Anthralin** (Rising Pharmaceuticals[1])	**Cream:** 1%	In 50 g.
Rx	**Psoriatec** (Sirius)		In 50 g.

[1] Rising Pharmaceuticals, Inc., 411 Sette Drive, Paramus, NJ 07652; 201-262-4200, fax 201-262-4284.

Indications

➤*Psoriasis:* Quiescent or chronic psoriasis.

Administration and Dosage

Generally, apply once a day or as directed. Anthralin is known to be a potential skin irritant. The irritant potential of anthralin is directly related to the strength being used and each patient's individual tolerance. Therefore, where the response to treatment has not previously been established, always commence treatment for at least 1 week using the lowest strength possible. Increase strengths when directed. Apply as directed and remove by washing or showering. The optimal period of contact will vary according to the strength used and the patient's response to treatment. Continue treatment until the skin is entirely clear (ie, when there is nothing to feel with fingers and the texture is normal).

➤*Skin application:* Apply sparingly only to the psoriatic lesions and rub gently and carefully into the skin until absorbed. It is most important to avoid applying an excessive quantity which may cause unnecessary soiling and staining of the clothing or bed linen. At the end of each treatment period, take a bath or shower to remove any surplus (cream may have become red/brown in color). The margins of the lesions may gradually become stained purple/brown as treatment progresses, but this will disappear after treatment cessation.

➤*Scalp application:* Comb the hair to remove scalar debris and, after suitably parting, rub the cream well into the lesions, taking care to prevent the cream from spreading onto the forehead. Keep away from the eyes. Take care to avoid application to uninvolved scalp margins. Remove any unintended residue which may be deposited behind the ears. At the end of each period of contact, wash the hair and scalp to remove any surplus (cream may have become red/brown in color).

Short-contact regimens have been used preferably for stable plaque-type psoriasis. Initial contact time is 0.1% to 2% for 15 to 20 minutes, followed by thorough removal of the anthralin with an appropriate solvent (soap or petrolatum) and application of an emollient. Short-contact therapy plus other treatments (eg, ultraviolet light, retinoids, topical steroids, psoralens plus UV light) may improve the response.

Actions

➤*Pharmacology:* Anthralin reduces the mitotic rate; in vitro evidence suggests that anthralin's antimitotic effect results from inhibition of DNA synthesis. Additionally, the chemically reducing properties of anthralin may upset oxidative metabolic processes, providing a further slowing down of epidermal mitosis.

Contraindications

Hypersensitivity to anthralin or any component of the product; use on the face; acutely or actively inflamed psoriatic eruptions.

Warnings

➤*For external use only:* Avoid contact with the eyes (severe conjunctivitis may occur) or mucous membranes. Anthralin should not normally be applied to intertriginous skin areas and high strengths should not be used on these sites. Do not apply to face or genitalia. Remove any unintended residue which may be deposited behind the ears. Avoid applying to the folds and creases of the skin. Discontinue use if a sensitivity reaction occurs or if excessive irritation develops on uninvolved skin areas. Wash hands thoroughly after using.

➤*Renal/Hepatic function impairment:* Although no renal or hepatic abnormalities have occurred with topical application, use caution in patients with renal disease and in those having extensive and prolonged applications. Perform periodic urine tests for albuminuria. Discontinue use if sensitivity reactions occur.

➤*Carcinogenesis:* In long-term studies with mice, anthralin demonstrated carcinogenic and tumorigenic activity.

➤*Pregnancy: Category C.* It is not known whether anthralin can cause fetal harm when administered to a pregnant woman or can affect reproduction capacity. Administer only if clearly needed.

➤*Lactation:* It is not known whether this drug is excreted in breast milk. Because of the potential for tumorigenicity in animal studies, discontinue nursing or the drug, taking into account the importance of the drug to the mother.

➤*Children:* Safety and efficacy have not been established.

Precautions

➤*Staining:* May stain fabrics, skin or hair; apply sparingly and carefully to psoriatic lesions only. To prevent the possibility of staining clothing or bed linen while gaining experience in using anthralin, it may be advisable to use protective dressings. To prevent the possibility of discoloration, especially when using higher strengths, always rinse the bath/shower with hot water immediately after washing/showering and then use a suitable cleanser to remove any deposit on the surface of the bath or shower. Contact with fabrics, plastics and other materials may cause staining and should be avoided.

Drug Interactions

➤*Corticosteroids, topical:* As long-term use of topical corticosteroids may destabilize psoriasis, and withdrawal may also give rise to a "rebound" phenomenon, allow an interval of at least 1 week between the discontinuance of such steroids and the commencement of therapy. Petrolatum or a suitably bland emollient may be applied during the intervening period.

Adverse Reactions

Very few instances of contact allergic reactions to anthralin have been reported. However, transient primary irritation of normal skin or uninvolved skin surrounding the treated lesions is more frequently seen and may occasionally be severe. Application must be restricted to the psoriatic lesions. If the initial treatment produces excessive soreness or if the lesions spread, reduce frequency of application and, in extreme cases, discontinue use and consult physician.

Some temporary discoloration of hair and fingernails may arise during the period of treatment but should be minimized by careful application. Anthralin may stain skin, hair or fabrics. Staining of fabrics may be permanent; avoid contact. See Precautions.

Patient Information

Patient instructions are available with products.

CALCIPOTRIENE

Rx	Dovonex (Westwood Squibb)	Ointment: 0.005%	In 30, 60 and 100 g.
		Cream: 0.005%	In 30, 60 and 100 g.
		Solution: 0.005%	Menthol. In 60 ml.

Indications

➤*Psoriasis:* Treatment of moderate plaque psoriasis.

Administration and Dosage

➤*Approved by the FDA:* December 29, 1993 (1S classification).

Apply a thin layer to the affected skin twice daily and rub in gently and completely. Safety and efficacy have been demonstrated in patients treated for 8 weeks.

Actions

➤*Pharmacology:* Calcipotriene is a synthetic vitamin D_3 analog for the treatment of moderate plaque psoriasis. In humans, the natural supply of vitamin D depends mainly on exposure to the ultraviolet rays of the sun for conversion of 7-dehydrocholesterol to vitamin D_3 (cholecalciferol) in the skin. After entering the bloodstream, it is metabolized in the liver and kidneys to its active form, the hormone calcitriol. Vitamin D_3 receptors, proteins that bind chemically to calcitriol, occur in many parts of the body, including the skin cells known as keratinocytes. The scaly red patches of psoriasis are caused by the abnormal growth and production of the keratinocytes. Calcipotriene regulates skin cell production and development.

➤*Pharmacokinetics:* Approximately 6% of an applied dose is absorbed systemically when the ointment is applied topically to psoriasis plaques or 5% when applied to normal skin; much of the absorbed active drug is converted to inactive metabolites within 24 hours of application.

Vitamin D and its metabolites are transported in the blood, bound to specific plasma proteins. The active form of the vitamin, 1,25-dihydroxy vitamin D_3 (calcitriol), is known to be recycled via the liver and excreted in the bile. Calcipotriene metabolism following systemic uptake is rapid, and occurs via a similar pathway to the natural hormone. The primary metabolites are much less potent than the parent compound. The systemic disposition of calcipotriene is expected to be similar to that of the naturally occurring vitamin.

➤*Clinical trials:* Patients treated with calcipotriene have demonstrated improvement usually beginning after 2 weeks of therapy. This improvement continued with approximately 70% of patients showing at least marked improvement after 8 weeks of therapy, but only approximately 10% showing complete clearing.

Contraindications

Hypersensitivity to any components of the preparation; patients with demonstrated hypercalcemia or evidence of vitamin D toxicity; use on the face.

Warnings

➤*Dermatoses:* The safety and efficacy of topical calcipotriene in dermatoses other than psoriasis have not been established.

➤*For external use only:* Not for ophthalmic, oral or intravaginal use.

➤*Elderly:* Of the total number of patients in clinical studies of calcipotriene ointment, approximately 12% were ≥ 65 years of age, while approximately 4% were ≥ 75. The results of an analysis of severity of skin-related adverse events showed a statistically significant difference for subjects > 65 years of age (more severe) compared to those < 65 (less severe).

➤*Pregnancy:* Category C. Doses of calcipotriene up to 36 mcg/kg/day in the rabbit did not result in teratogenic effects; however, increased maternal and fetal toxicity was observed at ≥ 12 mcg/kg/day. In the rat, oral doses of 54 mcg/kg/day resulted in a significantly higher incidence of skeletal abnormalities consisting primarily of enlarged fontanelles and extra ribs. The enlarged fontanelles is most likely due to calcipotriene's effect upon calcium metabolism. There is evidence that maternal calcitriol may enter the fetal circulation. There are no adequate and well controlled studies in pregnant women. Use during pregnancy only if the potential benefit justifies the potential risk to the fetus.

➤*Lactation:* It is not known whether calcipotriene is excreted in breast milk. Exercise caution when administering to a nursing woman.

➤*Children:* Safety and efficacy have not been established. Because of a higher ratio of skin surface area to body mass, children are at greater risk than adults of systemic adverse effects when they are treated with topical medication.

Precautions

➤*Irritation:* Use of calcipotriene may cause irritation of lesions and surrounding uninvolved skin. If irritation develops, discontinue the drug.

➤*Hypercalcemia:* Transient, rapidly reversible elevation of serum calcium has occurred with use of calcipotriene. If elevation in serum calcium occurs outside the normal range, discontinue treatment until normal calcium levels are restored.

Adverse Reactions

Burning, itching, skin irritation (≈ 10% to 15%); erythema, dry skin, peeling, rash, worsening of psoriasis (including development of facial/scalp psoriasis), dermatitis (1% to 10%); skin atrophy, hyperpigmentation, hypercalcemia, folliculitis (< 1%).

Overdosage

Topically applied calcipotriene can be absorbed in sufficient amounts to produce systemic effects. Elevated serum calcium has been observed with excessive use.

Patient Information

Use as directed. It is for external use only; avoid contact with the face or eyes. As with any topical medication, wash hands after application.

Do not use for any disorder other than that for which it was prescribed.

Patients should report any signs of local adverse reactions.

METHOTREXATE (Amethopterin; MTX)

Rx	Methotrexate (Various, eg, Major, Roxane, UDL)	Tablets: 2.5 mg	In 36s, 100s, and UD 20s.
Rx	Rheumatrex Dose Pack (STADA)		In 5, 7.5, 10, 12.5, and 15 mg/week dose packs.
Rx	Trexall (Barr)	Tablets: 5 mg	Lactose. (b 927/5). Green, oval, scored. Film-coated. In 30s, 60s, and 100s.
		7.5 mg	Lactose. (b 928/7 1/2). Blue, oval, scored. Film-coated. In 30s, 60s, and 100s.
		10 mg	Lactose. (b 929/10). Pink, oval, scored. Film-coated. In 30s, 60s, and 100s.
		15 mg	Lactose. (b 945/15). Purple, oval, scored. Film-coated. In 30s, 60s, and 100s.
Rx	Methotrexate sodium (Various, eg, Bedford Labs, APP[1])	Injection: 25 mg/mL (as base)	Preservative-free. In 2, 4, 8, 10, 20, and 40 mL single-use vials.
Rx	Methotrexate sodium (Various, eg, Xanodyne, APP)		In 2 and 10 mL vials[2].
Rx	Methotrexate LPF sodium (Xanodyne)		Preservative-free. In 2, 4, and 10 mL single-use vials[3].
Rx	Methotrexate sodium (Various, eg, Xanodyne, APP)	Powder for injection, lyophilized: 20 mg (as base)	Preservative-free. In single–use vials[4].
		Powder for injection, lyophilized: 1 g (as base)	Preservative-free. In single-use vials[4].

[1] The 2, 4, 8, 10, 20, and 40 mL solutions contain approximately 0.43, 0.86, 1.72, 2.15, 4.3, and 8.6 mEq of sodium per vial, respectively.
[2] Contains 0.9% benzyl alcohol as a preservative; must not be used for intrathecal or high dose therapy.

[3] The 2, 4, and 10 mL vials contain approximately 0.43, 0.86, and 2.15 mEq of sodium per vial, respectively.
[4] Approximately 0.14 mEq of sodium in 20 mg vial; 7 mEq of sodium in 1 g vial.

This is an abbreviated monograph. For complete prescribing information and use of methotrexate as an antineoplastic or immunomodulator agent, see monographs in the Antineoplastics and Biologicals and Immunologics chapters.

METHOTREXATE (Amethopterin; MTX)

WARNING

Due to the possibility of fatal or severe toxic reactions, inform patient of risks involved; keep under constant supervision. Deaths have occurred. Restrict use to severe, recalcitrant, disabling psoriasis not adequately responsive to other therapy when diagnosis is established by biopsy or after dermatologic consultation.

May produce marked bone marrow depression with resultant anemia, leukopenia or thrombocytopenia.

Methotrexate has caused fetal death or congenital anomalies. Therefore, it is not recommended for women of childbearing potential unless there is clear medical evidence that the benefits can be expected to outweigh the considered risks. Pregnant patients with psoriasis should not receive methotrexate.

Diarrhea and ulcerative stomatitis require interruption of therapy; otherwise, hemorrhagic enteritis and death from intestinal perforation may occur.

Periodic monitoring for toxicity, including CBC with differential and platelet counts, and liver and renal function tests is a mandatory part of methotrexate therapy. Periodic liver biopsies may be indicated in some situations. Monitor patients at increased risk for impaired methotrexate elimination (eg, renal dysfunction, pleural effusions, ascites) more frequently.

Methotrexate causes hepatotoxicity, fibrosis and cirrhosis, but generally only after prolonged use. Acutely, liver enzyme elevations are frequently seen, these are usually transient and asymptomatic and also do not appear predictive of subsequent hepatic disease. Liver biopsy after sustained use often shows histologic changes, and fibrosis and cirrhosis have been reported; these latter lesions often are not preceded by symptoms or abnormal liver function tests. For this reason, periodic liver biopsies are usually recommended for psoriatic patients who are under long-term treatment.

Methotrexate-induced lung disease is a potentially dangerous lesion, which may occur acutely at any time during therapy and which has been reported at doses as low as 7.5 mg per week. It is not always fully reversible. Pulmonary symptoms (especially a dry, nonproductive cough) may require interruption of treatment and careful investigation.

Use with extreme caution, and at reduced dosages, in patients with impaired renal function because renal dysfunction will prolong methotrexate elimination.

Unexpectedly severe (sometimes fatal) marrow suppression, aplastic anemia, and GI toxicity have occurred with coadministration of methotrexate (usually in high dosage) along with some nonsteroidal anti-inflammatory drugs.

Methotrexate formulations and diluents containing preservatives must not be used for intrathecal or high-dose methotrexate therapy.

Severe, occasionally fatal, skin reactions have been reported following single or multiple doses of methotrexate. Reactions have occurred within days of oral, intramuscular, intravenous, or intrathecal methotrexate administration. Recovery has been reported with discontinuation of therapy.

Potentially fatal opportunistic infections, especially *Pneumocystis carinii* pneumonia, may occur with methotrexate therapy.

Methotrexate given concomitantly with radiotherapy may increase the risk of soft tissue necrosis and osteonecrosis.

Indications

➤*Psoriasis:* For the symptomatic control of severe, recalcitrant, disabling psoriasis which is not adequately responsive to other therapy. Use only when the diagnosis has been established by biopsy or after dermatologic consultation. It is important to ensure that a psoriasis "flare" is not due to an undiagnosed concomitant disease affecting immune responses.

Methotrexate is also used as an antineoplastic agent and in the management of rheumatoid arthritis (see individual monographs).

Administration and Dosage

Fully inform the patient of the risks involved, and keep patient under constant supervision of the physician.

Assess hematologic, hepatic, renal and pulmonary function before beginning, periodically during, and before reinstituting therapy.

➤*Severe, recalcitrant, disabling psoriasis:* Individualize dosage. A test dose may be given prior to therapy to detect extreme sensitivity to adverse effects.

Weekly single oral, IM or IV dosage schedule – 10 to 25 mg/week until adequate response is achieved. Do not exceed 30 mg per week.

Divided oral dose schedule – 2.5 mg at 12 hour intervals for 3 doses. Do not exceed 30 mg per week.

Once optimal clinical response is achieved, reduce to lowest possible amount of drug with the longest possible rest period. Methotrexate may permit return to conventional topical therapy, which should be encouraged.

➤*Storage/Stability:* Store at controlled room temperature, 20° to 25°C (68° to 77°F); excursions permitted to 15° to 30°C (59° to 86°F). Protect from light.

Actions

➤*Pharmacology:* Methotrexate interferes with DNA synthesis, repair and cellular replication. Actively proliferating tissues are generally more sensitive to the effect of methotrexate. In psoriasis, the rate of production of epithelial cells in the skin is greatly increased over normal skin. This differential in proliferation rates is the basis for the use of this drug to control the psoriatic process.

Contraindications

Pregnant and nursing patients; alcoholism, alcoholic liver disease or other chronic liver disease; overt or laboratory evidence of immunodeficiency syndromes; pre-existing blood dyscrasias, such as bone marrow hypoplasia, leukopenia, thrombocytopenia or significant anemia; hypersensitivity to methotrexate.

Warnings

➤*Pregnancy:* Category X. Methotrexate can cause fetal death or teratogenic effects when administered to a pregnant woman and is contraindicated in pregnant patients with psoriasis. Do not start women of childbearing potential on methotrexate until pregnancy is excluded, and fully counsel them on the serious risk to the fetus should they become pregnant while undergoing treatment. Avoid pregnancy if either partner is receiving methotrexate: During and for a minimum of 3 months after therapy for male patients, and during and for at least one ovulatory cycle after therapy for female patients.

➤*Lactation:* Because of the potential for serious adverse reactions from methotrexate in breastfed infants, it is contraindicated in nursing mothers.

➤*Children:* Safety and efficacy in children have been established only in cancer chemotherapy and in polyarticular-course JRA.

Precautions

➤*Hematologic:* Methotrexate can suppress hematopoiesis and cause anemia, aplastic anemia, pancytopenia, leukopenia, neutropenia, and/or thrombocytopenia. Stop methotrexate immediately if there is a significant drop in blood counts.

➤*Hepatic:* Liver function tests, including serum albumin, should be performed periodically prior to dosing but are often normal in the face of developing fibrosis or cirrhosis. These lesions may be detectable only by biopsy. The usual recommendation is to obtain a liver biopsy at 1) pretherapy or shortly after initiation of therapy (2 to 4 months), 2) a total cumulative dose of 1.5 g, and 3) after each additional 1 to 1.5 grams. Moderate fibrosis or any cirrhosis normally leads to discontinuation of the drug; mild fibrosis normally suggests a repeat biopsy in 6 months. Milder histologic findings such as fatty change and low grade portal inflammation are relatively common pretherapy. Although these mild changes are usually not a reason to avoid or discontinue methotrexate therapy, use the drug with caution.

Adverse Reactions

There are 2 literature reports describing large series (n = 204, 248) of psoriasis patients treated with methotrexate. Dosages ranged up to 25 mg/week, and treatment was administered for up to 4 years. With the exception of alopecia, photosensitivity, and "burning of skin lesions" (each 3% to 10%), the adverse reaction rates in these reports were very similar to those in the rheumatoid arthritis studies. Rarely, painful plaque erosions may appear.

SELENIUM SULFIDE

otc	**Selenium Sulfide** (Various, eg, Rugby)	**Lotion/Shampoo:** 1%	In 210 mL.
otc	**Head & Shoulders Intensive Treatment** (Procter & Gamble)		In 400 mL.
otc	**Selsun Blue Medicated Treatment** (Chattem)		Menthol. In 325 mL.
Rx	**Selenium Sulfide** (Various, eg, Clay-Park)	**Lotion:** 2.5%	In 120 mL.
Rx	**Selsun** (Abbott)		In 120 mL.

Indications

Treatment of dandruff, seborrheic dermatitis of the scalp; tinea versicolor (2.5% only).

➤*Unlabeled uses:* Adjunctive therapy for tinea capitis.

Administration and Dosage

Shake well.

➤*Dandruff/seborrheic dermatitis:* Massage 5 to 10 mL into wet scalp. Allow to remain on scalp 2 to 3 minutes. Rinse thoroughly. Repeat application and rinse thoroughly. Wash hands after treatment.

Usually, 2 applications each week for 2 weeks will afford control. After this, it may be used at less frequent intervals-weekly, every 2 weeks or even every 3 or 4 weeks in some cases. Do not apply more frequently than required to maintain control.

➤*Tinea versicolor:* Apply to affected areas and lather with a small amount of water. Allow to remain on skin for 10 minutes; rinse body thoroughly. Repeat once a day for 7 days.

➤*Storage/Stability:* Store at controlled room temperature (15° to 30°C; 59° to 86°F). Keep tightly capped.

Actions

➤*Pharmacology:* Selenium sulfide appears to have a cytostatic effect on cells of the epidermis and follicular epithelium, thus reducing corneocyte production.

Contraindications

Allergy to any component of the product.

Warnings

➤*Pregnancy: Category C* (tinea versicolor). It is not known whether this drug can cause fetal harm or can affect reproduction capacity. Use only if clearly needed. Under ordinary circumstances, do not use for tinea versicolor in pregnant women.

➤*Children:* Safety and efficacy in infants have not been established.

Precautions

➤*Hypersensitivity:* Discontinue use if sensitivity reactions occur.

➤*Treatment of tinea versicolor:* Selenium sulfide may irritate the skin, especially in the genital area and in skin folds. Rinse these areas thoroughly after application.

➤*For external use only:* Avoid contact with the eyes.

➤*Acute inflammation/exudation:* Do not use when present; absorption may be increased.

Adverse Reactions

➤*Decreasing order of severity:*

Dermatologic – Skin irritation; greater than normal hair loss; hair discoloration (avoid or minimize by thorough rinsing after treatment); oiliness or dryness of hair and scalp.

Patient Information

For external use only. Avoid contact with the eyes. Do not use on acutely inflamed skin.

If irritation occurs, discontinue use. Thoroughly rinse after application.

If using on bleached, tinted, or permed hair, rinse hair for at least 5 minutes in cool running water after use.

May damage jewelry; remove before using.

Antiseborrheic Combinations

Ingredients

➤*SALICYLIC ACID and SULFUR (see individual monographs):* These are used for antiseborrheic and keratolytic/keratoplastic actions.

➤*TAR PREPARATIONS, PYRITHIONE ZINC (see individual monographs) and MYRISTYLTRIMETHYLAMMONIUM BROMIDE:* These are used for their antipruritic, antibacterial or antiseborrheic actions.

➤*MENTHOL:* This is used as an antipruritic.

➤*BENZALKONIUM CHLORIDE, ISOPROPYL ALCOHOL, PHENOL and MENTHOL:* These are used as antiseptics.
➤*IODOQUINOL and BENZYL ALCOHOL:* These are antimicrobial agents.

Precautions

➤*For external use only:* Avoid contact with eyes; in case of contact, flush with water.

If undue skin irritation develops or increases, discontinue use and consult physician. Preparations containing tar may temporarily discolor blond, bleached or tinted hair. Slight staining of clothing may also occur.

ANTISEBORRHEIC SHAMPOOS

otc	**Maximum Strength Meted** (GenDerm)	**Shampoo:** 5% sulfur and 3% salicylic acid	In 118 ml.
otc	**MG217 Medicated Tar-Free Shampoo** (Triton)		In 4 and 8 oz.
otc	**MG400** (Triton)	**Shampoo:** 3% salicylic acid, 5% colloidal sulfur in Guy-Base II.	In 240 ml and pt.
otc	**Scalpicin** (Combe)	**Shampoo:** 3% salicylic acid, menthol	SD alcohol 40. In 45 and 75 ml.
otc	**Sebex** (Rugby)	**Shampoo:** 2% sulfur and 2% salicylic acid	In 118 ml.
otc	**Sulfoam** (Doak)	**Shampoo:** 2% sulfur	In 237 ml.
otc	**P & S** (Baker Cummins)	**Shampoo:** 2% salicylic acid	In 120 ml.
otc	**Neutrogena T/Sal** (Triton)	**Shampoo:** 2% salicyclic acid, 2% solubilized coal tar extract	In 135 ml.
otc	**Ionil** (Owen/Galderma)	**Shampoo:** Salicylic acid, benzalkonium chloride, EDTA	In 120 and 240 ml, pt and qt.
otc	**X●Seb** (Baker Cummins)	**Shampoo:** 4% salicylic acid	In 120 ml.
otc	**Tarsum** (Summers)	**Shampoo/Gel:** 10% crude coal tar and 5% salicylic acid	In 120 and 240 ml.
otc	**X●Seb T** (Baker Cummins)	**Shampoo:** 10% coal tar solution, 4% salicylic acid	In 120 ml.
otc	**X●Seb T Plus** (Baker Cummins)	**Shampoo:** 10% coal tar solution, 3% salicylic acid and 1% menthol	In 120 ml.
otc	**Ionil T** (Owen/Galderma)	**Shampoo:** Coal tar solution, salicylic acid, benzalkonium chloride	In 120 and 240 ml, pt and qt.
otc	**Sebaquin** (Summers)	**Shampoo:** 3% iodoquinol, lanolin	In 120 ml.
otc	**X●Seb Plus** (Baker Cummins)	**Shampoo:** 1% pyrithione zinc and 2% salicylic acid	In 120 ml.

Complete prescribing information begins in the Antiseborrheic Combinations introduction.

MEDICATED HAIR DRESSINGS

Rx	**Sal-Oil-T** (Syosset)	**Solution:** 10% crude coal tar, 6% salicylic acid, vegetable oil	In 59.14 ml.
otc	**SLT Lotion** (C & M)	**Lotion:** 2% coal tar solution, 3% salicylic acid, 5% lactic acid, 65% isopropyl alcohol, 1.6% benzyl alcohol and benzalkonium chloride	In 129 ml.
otc	**Sebucare** (Westwood Squibb)	**Lotion:** 1.8% salicylic acid with 61% alcohol	In 120 ml.
otc	**P & S** (Baker Cummins)	**Liquid:** Phenol, mineral oil and glycerin	In 120 and 240 ml.

Complete prescribing information begins in the Antiseborrheic Combinations introduction.

ARNICA

otc	**Arnica** (Various, eg, Humco)	**Tincture:** 20%	In 30, 60, 120 ml, pt, gal.

Indications

Relief of pain from sprains and bruises; of doubtful value.

Administration and Dosage

Apply locally with massage 2 or 3 times daily.

Precautions

➤*For external use only:* Avoid getting into eyes or mucous membranes.

➤*Irritation:* Do not apply to irritated skin or if excessive irritation develops.

Adverse Reactions

Arnica is an irritant to mucous membranes; when ingested, it has produced severe gastroenteritis, nervous disturbances, tachycardia, bradycardia and collapse.

Arnica may cause dermatitis in sensitive persons.

ALUMINUM ACETATE SOLUTION (Burow's or Modified Burow's Solution)

otc	**Buro-Sol** (Doak)	**Powder:** 0.23% aluminum acetate	In 12 packets.
otc	**Burow's Solution** (Various, eg, Paddock)	Aluminum acetate solution	In 480 ml.
otc	**Bluboro Powder** (Allergan Herbert)	Aluminum sulfate and calcium acetate. One packet or tablet in a pint of water produces a modified 1:40 Burow's solution. Apply every 15 to 30 minutes for 4 to 8 hours.	**Powder packets:** 1.8 g. In 12s and 100s.
otc	**Boropak Powder** (Glenwood)		**Powder packets:** 2.4 g. In 12s and 100s.
otc	**Domeboro Powder and Tablets** (Miles)		**Effervescent tablets:** In 12s and 100s.
			Powder packets: In 12s and 100s.
otc	**Pedi-Boro Soak Paks** (Pedinol)		**Powder packets:** 2.7 g. In 12s and 100s.
otc	**Bite Rx** (International Lab. Tech. Corp.)[1]	**Solution:** 0.5% w/w aluminum acetate	Benzalkonium chloride. In 120 ml.

[1] (954) 893-1118

Indications

An astringent wet dressing for relief of inflammatory conditions of the skin, such as insect bites, poison ivy, swelling, allergy, bruises and athlete's foot.

Precautions

➤*Discontinue use:* If intolerance, irritation or extension of inflammatory condition being treated occurs. If symptoms persist > 7 days, discontinue use and consult physician.

➤*Do not use plastic:* Do not use plastic nor any other impervious material to prevent evaporation.

➤*For external use only:* Avoid contact with the eyes.

Drug Interactions

➤*Collagenase:* The enzyme activity of topical collagenase may be inhibited by aluminum acetate solution because of the metal ion and low pH. Cleanse the site of the solution with repeated washings of normal saline before applying the enzyme ointment.

HAMAMELIS WATER (Witch Hazel)

otc	**Witch Hazel** (Various, eg, Humco, Lannett)	**Liquid**	In 120 and 240 ml, pt and gal.
otc	**A•E•R** (Birchwood)	**Pads:** 50%. 12.5% glycerin, methylparaben, benzalkonium chloride.	In 40s.

Indications

Temporary relief of anal or vaginal irritation and itching, hemorrhoids, postepisiotomy discomfort and hemorrhoidectomy discomfort.

Administration and Dosage

Apply locally up to 6 times daily or after each bowel movement.

Actions

➤*Pharmacology:* Hamamelis water is a mild astringent prepared from twigs of *Hamamelis virginiana*; the distillate is then adjusted with an appropriate amount of alcohol.

Warnings

➤*Worsened conditions:* If condition worsens or does not improve within 7 days consult a physician.

➤*Bleeding:* In case of bleeding, consult physician promptly.

Precautions

➤*For external use only:* Avoid contact with eyes.

Anti-Acne

MEDICATED BAR CLEANSERS

otc	**Clearasil Antibacterial Soap** (Procter & Gamble)	**Bar:** Triclosan	In 92 g.
otc	**Oxy Medicated Soap** (SmithKline Beecham)	**Bar:** 1% triclosan, EDTA	In 97.5 g.
otc	**Stri-Dex Cleansing Bar** (Sterling Health)	**Bar:** 1% triclosan, lanolin alcohol, EDTA	In 105 g.
otc	**Salicylic Acid Cleansing** (Stiefel)	**Bar:** 2% salicylic acid, EDTA	In 113 g.
otc	**Sulfur Soap** (Stiefel)	**Bar:** 10% precipitated sulfur, EDTA	In 116 g.
otc	**Fostex Acne Medication Cleansing** (Westwood Squibb)	**Bar:** 2% salicylic acid, EDTA	In 106 g.
otc	**Salicylic Acid and Sulfur Soap** (Stiefel)	**Bar:** 10% precipitated sulfur, 3% salicylic acid, EDTA	In 116 g.
otc	**SAStid Soap** (Stiefel)	**Bar:** 10% precipitated sulfur, EDTA	In 116 g.
otc	**Aveeno Cleansing for Acne-Prone Skin** (Rydelle)	**Bar:** Salicylic acid, colloidal oatmeal, glycerin and titanium dioxide	Soap free. In 90 g.

ABRASIVE CLEANSERS

otc	**Pernox Lathering Abradant Scrub** (Westwood Squibb)	**Lotion:** Sulfur, salicylic acid	In 141 g.
otc	**Pernox Scrub for Oily Skin** (Westwood Squibb)	**Cleanser:** Sulfur, salicylic acid, EDTA	Regular or lemon scent. In 56 and 113 g.
otc	**Brasivol** (Stiefel)	**Cleanser:** Aluminum oxide particles in a surfactant cleansing base	In fine (153 g), medium (180 g) and rough (195 g) textures.
otc	**Ionax** (Galderma)	**Scrub:** Benzalkonium chloride, SD alcohol 40	Lemon scented. In 60 and 120 g.
otc	**Seba-Nil Cleansing Mask** (Galderma)	**Scrub:** SD alcohol-40, castor oil, methylparaben	In 105 g.
otc	**PROPApH Peel-off Acne Mask** (Del Pharm.)	**Mask:** 2% salicylic acid, polyvinyl alcohol, parabens, SD alcohol 40, vitamin E acetate	In 60 ml.

LIQUID CLEANSERS

otc	**Stridex Anti-Bacterial Foaming Wash** (Blistex)	1% triclosan, parabens, glycerin, meadow foam oil, peppermint oil, spearmint oil, aloe, menthol	In 177 ml.
otc	**Clearasil Medicated Deep Cleanser** (Procter & Gamble)	0.5% salicylic acid and 42% alcohol, menthol, EDTA, aloe vera gel, hydrogenated castor oil	In 229 ml.
otc	**Clearasil Acne-Fighting Pads** (Procter & Gamble)	2% salicylic acid, alcohol, EDTA, aloe	In 65s.
otc	**PROPApH Astringent Cleanser Maximum Strength** (Del)	**Liquid:** 2% salicylic acid, aloe vera gel, 55.1% SD alcohol 40-2	In 355 mL.
otc	**Clearasil Double Textured Pads** (Procter & Gamble)	**Regular Strength:** 2% salicylic acid, 40% alcohol, glycerin, aloe vera gel, disodium EDTA	In 32s and 40s.
		Maximum Strength: 2% salicylic acid, 40% alcohol, aloe vera gel, menthol, disodium EDTA	In 32s and 40s.
otc	**Stri-Dex Pads** (Sterling Health)	**Regular Strength:** 0.5% salicylic acid, 28% SD alcohol, citric acid, menthol	In 55s.
		Maximum Strength: 2% salicylic acid, 44% SD alcohol, citric acid, menthol	In 55s and 90s. Dual textured in 32s.
		Oil Fighting Formula: 2% salicylic acid, citric acid, menthol, 54% SD alcohol	In 55 Super Scrub pads.
		Sensitive Skin: 0.5% salicylic acid, citric acid, aloe vera gel, menthol, 28% SD alcohol	In 55s.
otc	**Oxy Medicated Cleanser and Pads** (SK-Beecham)	**Regular Strength Pads:** 0.5% salicylic acid, 40% alcohol, citric acid, menthol, propylene glycol	**Pads:** In 50s and 90s.
		Maximum Strength Pads: 2% salicylic acid, 50% alcohol, citric acid, menthol, propylene glycol	In 50s and 90s.
		Sensitive Skin Pads: 0.5% salicylic acid, 22% alcohol, disodium lauryl sulfosuccinate, menthol, trisodium EDTA	In 50s and 90s.
otc	**Ionax Astringent Cleanser** (Galderma)	Salicylic acid, EDTA, isopropyl alcohol	In 240 ml.
otc	**Drytex Lotion** (C & M)	Salicylic acid, 10% acetone, 40% isopropyl alcohol, tartrazine	In 240 ml.
otc	**Seba-Nil Oily Skin Cleanser** (Galderma)	SD alcohol 40, acetone	In 240 and 473 ml.
otc	**Tyrosum Cleanser** (Summers)	50% isopropanol, 10% acetone, 2% polysorbate 80	**Liquid:** In 120 ml and pt.
			Packets: In 24s and 50s.
otc	**Acno Cleanser** (Baker Cummins)	60% isopropyl alcohol, EDTA	In 240 ml.
Rx	**Xerac AC** (Person & Covey)	6.25% aluminum chloride-hexahydrate in 96% anhydrous ethyl alcohol	In 35 and 60 ml.
otc	**Exact** (Premier)	2% salicylic acid, propylene glycol, aloe vera gel, disodium EDTA, menthol, parabens, glycerin, diazolidinyl urea	In 118 ml.
otc	**Neutrogena Oil-free Acne Wash** (Neutrogena)	2% salicylic acid, EDTA, propylene glycol, tartrazine, aloe extract	In 180 ml.
otc	**Neutrogena Antiseptic Cleanser for Acne-Prone Skin** (Neutrogena)	Benzethonium chloride, butylene glycol, methylparaben, menthol, peppermint oil, eucalyptus oil, cornmint oil, rosemary oil, witch hazel extract, camphor	In 135 ml.
otc	**PROPApH Cleansing for Sensitive Skin** (Del Pharm.)	**Pads:** 0.5% salicylic acid, SD alcohol 40, EDTA, menthol, aloe vera gel	In 45s.
otc	**PROPApH Cleansing Maximum Strength** (Del Pharm)	**Pads:** 2% salicylic acid, SD alcohol 40, propylene glycol, EDTA, menthol, aloe vera gel	In 45s.
otc	**PROPApH Foaming Face Wash** (Del Pharm.)	2% salicylic acid, EDTA, menthol, aloe vera gel	Alcohol-, oil-, and soap-free. In 180 ml.
otc	**Oil of Olay Foaming Face Wash Liquid** (Procter & Gamble)	Potassium cocoyl hydrolyzed collagen, glycerin, EDTA	Regular and sensitive skin formulas: In 90 ml tubes and 210 ml pump.

SOAP FREE CLEANSERS

These products are recommended for patients with sensitive, dry or irritated skin, who may react adversely to common soap products. Some products may be useful for patients with atopic dermatitis, diaper dermatitis and other eczematous skin conditions. Therapeutic cleansers include "soap free" cleansers, which may be adjusted to a neutral pH and are less irritating to sensitive skin, and "modified" soap products, which may contain emollient components or may be adjusted to a neutral or slightly acidic pH.

otc	**Aquanil Cleanser** (Person & Covey)	**Lotion:** Lipid free. Glycerin, cetyl, stearyl and benzyl alcohol, sodium laureth sulfate, xanthan gum	In 240 and 480 ml.
otc	**Bacti-Cleanse** (Pedinol)	**Lotion:** Benzalkonium chloride, mineral oil, isopropyl palmitate, cetyl alcohol, glycerine, glyceryl stearate, PEG 100 stearate, dimethicone, diazolidinyl urea, parabens, DMDM hydantoin, EDTA	In 453.6 ml.
otc	**Derm-Cleanse** (Yers Pharm)	**Liquid:** Soap free. Sodium lauryl sulfate, mineral oil, propylene glycol, hydroxyethylcellulose, EDTA	In 240 ml.
otc	**Drytergent** (C & M)	**Liquid:** TEA-dodecylbenzenesulfonate, boric acid, lauramide DEA, propylene glycol, tartrazine	In 240 and 480 ml.
otc	**Duplex** (C & M)	**Liquid:** 15% sodium lauryl sulfate, lauramide DEA	In 480 ml.
otc	**Free & Clear** (Pharmaceutical Specialties)	**Shampoo:** Ammonium laureth sulfate, disodium cocamido MEA sulfosuccinate, cocamidopropyl hydroxysultaine, cocamide DEA, PEG-120 methyl glucose dioleate, EDTA, potassium sorbate, citric acid	Dye free. In 240 ml
otc	**Green Soap** (Paddock)	**Liquid:** Soybean oil, potassium salt, ethanol	For skin and hair. In 3780 ml.
otc	**Lowila Cake** (Westwood Squibb)	**Bar:** Soap free. Dextrin, sodium lauryl sulfoacetate, boric acid, urea, sorbitol, mineral oil, PEG-14 M, lactic acid, cellulose gum, DSS	In 112.5 g.
otc	**Cetaphil** (Galderma)	**Bar:** Soap-free. Petrolatum	In 127 g.
		Bar, antibacterial: Soap-free. Triclosan, petrolatum	In 127 g.
		Cleanser: Cetyl alcohol, stearyl alcohol, parabens	In 236 ml.
		Cream: Lipid free. Cetyl alcohol, stearyl alcohol, sodium lauryl sulfate, propylene glycol, parabens	In 480 g.
		Lotion: Cetyl alcohol, propylene glycol, sodium lauryl sulfate, stearyl alcohol, parabens	In 120, 240, 480 ml.
otc	**Ancet** (C & M)	**Liquid:** Sodium lauryl sulfate, lauramide DEA, propylene glycol, hydroxyethyl ethylcellulose, PCMX	In 240 ml.
otc	**Ceta** (C & M)	**Liquid:** Soap free. Propylene glycol, hydroxyethylcellulose, cetyl and cetearyl alcohols, sodium lauryl sulfate, parabens	In 240 ml.
otc	**pHisoDerm** (Chattem)	**Liquid:** Soap free. Sodium octoxynol-2 ethane sulfonate solution, petrolatum, octoxynol-3, mineral oil (with lanolin alcohol and oleyl alcohol), cocamide MEA, imidazolidinyl urea, sodium benzoate, tetrasodium EDTA and methylcellulose	Regular formula: Scented and unscented. In 150, 270, 480 ml and gal.
			Oily skin formula: In 150 and 480 ml.
otc	**pHisoDerm For Baby** (Chattem)	**Liquid:** Sodium octoxynol-2 ethane sulfonate solution, petrolatum, octoxynol-3, mineral oil (with lanolin alcohol and oleyl alcohol), cocamide MEA, imidazolidinyl urea, sodium benzoate, tetrasodium EDTA and methylcellulose. pH adjusted with hydrochloric acid.	In 150 and 270 ml.
otc	**Spectro-Jel** (Recsei)	**Gel:** Soap free. Iodo-methyl-cellulose, carboxypolymethylene, cetyl alcohol, sorbitan monooleate, fumed silica, triethanolamine stearate, glycol polysiloxane, propylene glycol, glycerine and 5% isopropyl alcohol	In 127.5 ml, pt and gal.
otc	**Lobana Body Shampoo** (Ulmer)	**Liquid:** Chloroxylenol in a mild sudsing base with conditioners and emollients	In 240 ml and gal.
otc	**Sulfoil** (C & M)	**Liquid:** Soap free. Neutral pH. Sulfonated castor oil	For skin and hair. In pt and gal.
otc	**Tersaseptic** (Doak)	**Shampoo/Liquid:** DEA-lauryl sulfate, lauramide DEA, propylene glycol, ethoxydiglycol, PEG-12 distearate, EDTA, triclosan, citric acid	In 475 ml.
otc	**Lobana Liquid Lather** (Ulmer)	**Body wash:** Sodium laureth sulfate, sodium lauroyl sarcosinate, sodium myristyl sarcosonate, lauramide DEA, linoleamide DEA, octyl hydroxystearate, polyquaternium 7, tetrasodium EDTA, quaternium 15, sodium chloride, citric acid	In 240 ml and gal.
otc	**Neutrogena Non-Drying Cleansing** (Neutrogena)	**Lotion:** Glycerin, caprylic/capric triglyceride, PEG-20 almond glycerides, cetyl recinoleate, isohexadecane, TEA-cocoyl glutamate, PEG-20 methyl glucose sesquistearate, methyl glucose sesquistearate, stearyl alcohol, cetyl alcohol, EDTA, dipotassium glycyrrhizate, stearyl glycyrrhetinate, bisabolol, parabens, acrylates/C 10-30 alkyl acrylate crosspolymer, triethanolamine, diazolidinyl urea	In 165 ml.
otc	**SFC** (Stiefel)	**Lotion:** Soap free. PEG-75, stearyl alcohol, sodium cocoyl isethionate, parabens	In 237 and 480 ml.

MODIFIED BAR SOAPS

otc	**pHisoDerm Cleansing Bar** (Chattem)	**Bar:** Sodium tallowate, sodium cocoate, petrolatum, glycerin, lanolin, sodium chloride, BHT, EDTA, titanium dioxide	Scented or unscented. In 99 g.
otc	**Oilatum Soap** (Stiefel)	**Bar:** Sodium tallowate, sodium cocoate, peanut oil, octyl hydroxystearate, lecithin, NaCl, PEG-14M, titanium dioxide, o-tolyl biguanide, EDTA, sodium borohydride, glyceryl oleate, corn oil, t-butyl hydroquinone, propylene glycol	Scented or unscented. In 120 and 240 g.
otc	**Neutrogena Dry Skin Soap** (Neutrogena Corp.)	**Bar:** TEA-stearate, triethanolamine, sodium tallowate, glycerin, sodium cocoate, sodium ricinoleate, TEA-oleate, laneth-10 acetate, cocamide DEA, nonoxynol 12, PEG-5 octanoate, tocopherol	Transparent. Scented or unscented. In 105 and 165 (scented only) g.
otc	**Neutrogena Oily Skin Soap** (Neutrogena Corp.)	**Bar:** TEA-stearate, triethanolamine, sodium tallowate, glycerin, sodium lauroyl sarcosinate, sodium cocoate, sodium ricinoleate, witch hazel, tocopherol	Transparent. Scented. In 105 g.
otc	**Neutrogena Soap** (Neutrogena Corp.)	**Bar:** TEA-stearate, triethanolamine, glycerin, sodium tallowate, sodium cocoate, sodium ricinoleate, TEA-oleate, cocamide DEA, tocopherol	Transparent. Scented or unscented. In 105 and 165 g.
otc	**Neutrogena Cleansing for Acne-Prone Skin** (Neutrogena Corp.)	**Bar:** TEA-stearate, triethanolamine, glycerin, sodium tallowate, sodium cocoate, TEA-oleate, sodium ricinoleate, acetylated lanolin alcohol, cocamide DEA, TEA lauryl sulfate, tocopherol	Transparent, nonmedicated. In 105 g.
otc	**Ambi 10** (Kiwi Brands)	**Bar:** Triclosan, sodium tallowate, PEG-20, titanium dioxide	In 99 g.
otc	**Alpha Keri Moisturizing Soap** (Bristol-Myers)	**Bar:** Sodium tallowate, sodium cocoate, mineral oil, lanolin oil, PEG-75, glycerin, titanium dioxide, sodium chloride, BHT, EDTA	Nondetergent, emollient. In 120 g.
otc	**Purpose Soap** (Johnson & Johnson)	**Bar:** Sodium tallowate, sodium cocoate, glycerin, NaCl, BHT, EDTA	In 108 and 180 g.
otc	**Nivea Moisturizing Creme Soap** (Beiersdorf)	**Bar:** Sodium tallowate, sodium cocoate, glycerin, petrolatum, titanium dioxide, NaCl, octyldodecanol, macadamia nut oil, aloe, sodium thiosulfate, lanolin alcohol, pentasodium pentetate, EDTA, BHT, beeswax	In 90 and 150 g.
otc	**Cuticura Medicated Soap** (DEP Corp.)	**Bar:** 1% triclocarban, sodium tallowate, sodium cocoate, glycerin, mineral oil, petrolatum, sodium chloride, tetrasodium EDTA, sodium bicarbonate, magnesium silicate and iron oxides	Phosphorus free. Emollient. Mildly antibacterial. In 97.5 and 142 g.
otc	**Formula 405** (Doak)	**Bar:** Sodium tallowate, sodium cocoate, Doak Additive A, PPG-20 methyl glucose ether, titanium dioxide, trochlorocarbanilide, pentasodium pentetate, EDTA	Fragrance free. In 100 g.

CAPSAICIN

otc	**Capsin** (Fleming)	**Lotion:** 0.025%	Benzyl alcohol, propylene glycol, denatured alcohol. In 59 ml.
otc	**Capsin** (Fleming)	**Lotion:** 0.075%	Benzyl alcohol, propylene glycol, denatured alcohol. In 59 ml.
otc	**Capsaicin** (Various, eg, Alpharma, Ferndale, Ivax)	**Cream:** 0.025%	In 45 and 60 g.
otc	**Pain Doctor** (Fougera)		25% methyl salicylate, 10% menthol, propylene glycol, parabens. In 60 g.
otc	**Zostrix** (Rodlen Labs[a])	**Cream:** 0.025% in an emollient base	In 45 and 90 g.
otc	**Zostrix-HP** (Rodlen Labs[a])	**Cream:** 0.075% in an emollient base	In 30 and 60 g.
otc	**Capsaicin** (Various, eg, Alpharma, Ferndale, Ivax)	**Cream:** 0.075%	In 60 g.
otc	**Rid·a·Pain·HP** (Pfeiffer)		Alcohols, parabens. In 45 g.
otc	**Dolorac** (GenDerm)	**Cream:** 0.25% in an emollient base	Benzyl alcohol and cetyl alcohol. In 28 g tubes.
otc	**R-Gel** (Healthline Labs)	**Gel:** 0.025%	EDTA. In 15 and 30 g.
otc	**Pain-X** (B.F. Ascher)	**Gel:** 0.05%	5% menthol, 4% camphor, alcohol, parabens. In 42.5 g.
otc	**No Pain-HP** (Young Again Products)	**Roll-on:** 0.075%	In 60 ml.

[a] Rodlen Laboratories, 100 Fairway Drive, Suite 134, Vernon Hills, IL 60061; (847) 362–8200.

Indications

Temporary relief of pain from rheumatoid arthritis, osteoarthritis and relief of neuralgias such as the pain following shingles (herpes zoster) or painful diabetic neuropathy.

➤*Unlabeled uses:* Capsaicin is being investigated for use in other disorders including psoriasis, vitiligo and intractable pruritus, as well as postmastectomy and postamputation neuroma (phantom limb syndrome), vulvar vestibulitis, apocrine chromhidrosis and reflex sympathetic dystrophy.

Administration and Dosage

➤*Adults and children ≥ 2 years of age:* Apply to affected area not more than 3 or 4 times daily. May cause transient burning on application. This is observed more frequently when application schedules of < 3 or 4 times daily are used. If applied with the fingers, wash hands immediately after application.

Actions

➤*Pharmacology:* Capsaicin is a natural chemical derived from plants of the solanaceae family. Although the precise mechanism of action is not fully understood, evidence suggests that the drug renders skin and joints insensitive to pain by depleting and preventing reaccumulation of substance P in peripheral sensory neurons. Substance P is thought to be the principle chemomediator of pain impulses from the periphery to the central nervous system.

Warnings

➤*For external use only:* Avoid getting in eyes or on broken or irritated skin. Use care when handling contact lenses following application of capsaicin; irritation and burning may occur following lens insertion. Washing hands or using gloves or an applicator may alleviate this problem.

➤*Bandage use:* Do not bandage tightly.

➤*Worsened condition:* If condition worsens or if symptoms persist 14 to 28 days, discontinue use and consult physician.

Adverse Reactions

Burning (≥ 30%; usually diminishes with repeated use); stinging; erythema; cough; respiratory irritation

Patient Information

For external use only. Avoid contact with the eyes. Use caution when handling contact lens following application; washing hands or using gloves or an applicator is recommended.

Do not bandage tightly.

If condition worsens or symptoms persist 14 to 28 days, contact a physician.

Chloroacetic Acids

Indications

➤*Dichloroacetic acid:* Verrucae (warts); calluses; hard and soft corns; xanthoma palpebrarum; seborrheic keratoses; ingrown nails; cysts and benign erosion of the cervix; endocervicitis; epistaxis.

➤*Monochloroacetic and trichloroacetic acid:* Removal of verrucae.

The CDC recommends trichloroacetic acid as an alternative regimen to cryotherapy for treatment of external genital/perianal warts and vaginal and anal warts.

Actions

➤*Pharmacology:* Rapidly penetrates and cauterizes skin, keratin and other tissues. Monochloroacetic acid is more deeply destructive than trichloroacetic acid.

Contraindications

Treatment of malignant or premalignant lesions; hypersensitivity to any component.

Warnings

➤*Cauterant properties:* These acids are powerful keratolytics and cauterants. Restrict use to areas where these effects are desired. May cause severe burning, inflammation or tenderness of skin.

➤*Cervical lesions:* A careful diagnosis and possibly a biopsy is required to rule out malignancy; treatment is contraindicated in the event of positive findings.

➤*Normal tissue:* Apply only to the lesion being treated. To prevent acid from spreading onto normal skin, apply petrolatum around the area to be treated. If any acid is spilled on normal tissue or if too much acid is applied, remove immediately and wash with water. Sodium bicarbonate may be applied as a local antidote.

DICHLOROACETIC ACID

Rx	Bichloracetic Acid (Glenwood)	**Liquid:** 10 ml	In treatment kit with 16 g petrolatum, applicators, acid receptacles, microdropper and holder.

Complete prescribing information begins in the Chloroacetic Acids group monograph.

Administration and Dosage

➤*Amount applied:* This varies with the nature of the lesion. Dense horny lesions (corns, warts, calluses, plantar warts) require repeated intensive treatment. Lesions of light density (pedunculated warts, xanthoma palpebrarum, soft corns, seborrheic keratoses, condyloma acuminata) receive lighter applications.

➤*Application technique:* This depends on the type of lesion. Treat dense growths by rubbing the acid into the lesion with a pointed wooden or cotton-tipped applicator; 3 or 4 treatments may be necessary. Lesions of light density should receive a lighter application at each visit. Usually 1 or 2 such treatments are sufficient.

Apply thin layer of petrolatum to normal tissue surrounding the lesion. Use microdropper to transfer some acid to small-stemmed acid recep-

tacle. The acid should not contact the microdropper's neoprene bulb. Use microdropper upright; fill no more than halfway. Moisten a sharpened applicator stick in acid and draw over flared lip to remove excess. There should never be a large excess drop on applicator.

When applying very small amounts, hold applicator level or with the point up so that a tiny fraction of one drop can be transferred to small lesions. To follow cauterization progress, observe change in color of treated area to gray-white, using a magnifying lens if necessary. It is sometimes advantageous to apply by rolling applicator over surface of lesion, using the point only at the edges. To avoid contamination, do not return any remaining acid from receptacle to bottle. Keep bottle tightly capped except when removing acid. Discard applicators after use.

See manufacturer's package insert for treatment of specific lesions.

MONOCHLOROACETIC ACID

Rx	Mono-Chlor (Gordon)	**Liquid:** 80%	In 15 ml.

Complete prescribing information begins in the Chloroacetic Acids group monograph.

Administration and Dosage

Remove callus tissue. Apply to verruca. Apply bandage and allow to remain in place for 5 to 6 days. Remove verruca tissue and reapply as needed. If crystallization of liquid occurs, place capped bottle in hot water to redissolve.

TRICHLOROACETIC ACID

Rx	Tri-Chlor (Gordon)	**Liquid:** 80%	In 15 ml.

Complete prescribing information begins in the Chloroacetic Acids group monograph.

Administration and Dosage

Debride callus tissue. Apply to verruca. Cover with bandage for 5 to 6 days. Remove verruca. Reapply as needed. If crystallization of liquid occurs, place capped bottle in hot water to redissolve.

PODOFILOX

Rx	**Condylox** (Oclassen)	**Topical Gel:** 0.5% podofilox	Alcohol. In 3.5 ml aluminum tubes.
Rx	**Podofilox** (Various, eg, Paddock, Watson)	**Topical Solution:** 0.5% podofilox	95% alcohol. In 3.5 mL.
Rx	**Condylox** (Oclassen)		Alcohol. In 3.5 ml bottles.

Indications

➤*Gel:* Topical treatment of anogenital warts (external genital and perianal warts). Not indicated in treatment of mucous membrane warts.

➤*Solution:* Topical treatment of external warts (*Condylomata acuminata*). Not indicated in the treatment of perianal or mucous membrane warts.

Administration and Dosage

➤*Solution:* Apply twice daily morning and evening (every 12 hours) to the warts with a cotton-tipped applicator supplied with the drug. Touch the drug-dampened applicator to the wart to be treated, applying the minimum amount of solution necessary to cover the lesion. Limit treatment to < 10 cm ^{2} of wart tissue and to ≤ 0.5 ml of the solution per day. There is no evidence to suggest that more frequent application will increase efficacy, but additional applications would be expected to increase the rate of local adverse reactions and systemic absorption. Allow the solution to dry before allowing the return of opposing skin surfaces to their normal positions. After each treatment, dispose of the used applicator and wash hands.

➤*Gel:* Apply twice daily to the warts with the applicator tip or finger. Minimize application on the surrounding normal tissue. Limit to ≤ 10 cm ^{2} of wart tissue and to ≤ 0.5 g of the gel per day. Allow the gel to dry before allowing the return of opposing skin surfaces to their normal positions. Instruct patients to wash their hands thoroughly before and after each application.

The prescriber should ensure that the patient is fully aware of the correct method of therapy and identify which specific warts should be treated. If there is incomplete response after 4 treatment weeks, consider alternate treatment. Safety and effectiveness of > 4 treatment weeks have not been established. Apply twice daily for 3 consecutive days, then withhold use for 4 consecutive days. This 1–week cycle of treatment may be repeated up to 4 times until there is no visible wart tissue.

➤*Storage/Stability:* Store at room temperature between 15° to 30°C (59° to 86°F). Avoid excessive heat. Do not freeze.

Actions

➤*Pharmacology:* Podofilox is a topical antimitotic drug which can be chemically synthesized or purified from the plant families *Coniferae* and *Berberidaceae* (eg, species of *Juniperus* and *Podophyllum*). Treatment of anogenital warts with podofilox results in necrosis of visible wart tissue. The exact mechanism of action is unknown. Condylomas, or genital warts, are caused by the human papillomavirus. In males the warts appear on the penis, anus and perineum; in females they are found on the vagina, cervix, perineum and anus. The number of warts increases in immunosuppressed patients and in those with AIDS and other immunologic deficiencies. Genital warts are epidemiologically associated with cervical carcinoma. Distinguishing between these conditions can be difficult. Obtain histopathologic confirmation if there is any doubt of the diagnosis.

➤*Pharmacokinetics:* In 52 patients, topical application of 0.05 ml of 0.5% podofilox solution to external genitalia did not result in detectable serum levels. Applications of 0.1 to 1.5 ml resulted in peak serum levels of 1 to 17 ng/ml 1 to 2 hours after application. The elimination half-life ranged from 1 to 4.5 hours. The drug did not accumulate after multiple treatments.

➤*Clinical trials:*

Solution – In double-blind clinical studies, patients were treated for 2 to 4 weeks and reevaluated at a 2 week follow-up examination. Although the number of patients and warts evaluated at each time period varied, the results among investigators were relatively consistent.

Patient Response to Podofilox Treatment[1]			
	Initially cleared	Recurred after clearing	Cleared at 2 week follow-up
Warts (n = 524)	79%	35%	60%
Patients (n = 70)	50%	60%	25%

[1] Cleared and clearing mean no visible wart tissue remained at the treated sites.

Gel – In 326 patients with anogenital warts, podofilox and its vehicle were applied in a double-blind fashion to comparable patient groups; 176 were treated with podofilox. Patients applied podofilox twice daily for 3 consecutive days followed by a 4–day rest period. At the end of 4 weeks, 38.4% of the patients had complete clearing of the wart tissue when treated with podofilox.

In another trial in 108 evaluable patients with anogenital warts, podofilox solution was compared with podofilox gel for efficacy. Patients applied podofilox gel twice daily for 3 consecutive days followed by a 4–day rest period. Similar clearance rates were observed. At the end of

4 weeks, 25.6% of the patients had complete clearing of the wart tissue when treated with podofilox gel.

Contraindications

Hypersensitivity or intolerance to any component of the formulation.

Warnings

➤*Diagnosis:* Correct diagnosis of the lesions to be treated is essential. Although anogenital warts have a characteristic appearance, obtain histopathologic confirmation if there is any doubt of the diagnosis. Differentiating warts from squamous cell carcinoma (so-called "Bowenoid papulosis") is of particular concern. Squamous cell carcinoma may also be associated with human papillomavirus but should not be treated with podofilox.

The gel is not indicated for treatment of mucous membrane warts; the solution is not indicated for perianal or mucous membrane warts.

➤*External use only:* Podofilox is intended for cutaneous use only. Avoid contact with the eyes. If eye contact occurs, immediately flush the eye with copious quantities of water and seek medical advice.

In mouse studies, crude podophyllum resin (containing podofilox) applied topically to the cervix produced changes resembling carcinoma in situ. These changes were reversible at 5 weeks after treatment cessation. In one report, epidermal carcinoma of the vagina and cervix was found in 1 of 18 mice after 120 applications of podophyllin (applied twice weekly over 15 months).

Results from the mouse micronucleus in vivo assay using podofilox 0.5% solution in concentrations up to 25 mg/kg indicate that podofilox should be considered a potential clastogen (a chemical that induces disruption and breakage of chromosomes).

➤*Pregnancy:* Category C. Podofilox is embryotoxic in rats when administered at ≈ 250 times the recommended maximum human dose systemically or ≈19 times the recommended maximum human dose intraperitoneally. There are no adequate and well controlled studies in pregnant women. Use in pregnancy only if the potential benefit justifies the potential risk to the fetus.

➤*Lactation:* It is not known whether this drug is excreted in breast milk. Decide whether to discontinue nursing or to discontinue the drug, taking into account the importance of the drug to the mother.

➤*Children:* Safety and efficacy in children have not been established.

Precautions

➤*Perianal/Mucous membrane warts:* Data are not available on the safe and effective use of this product for treatment of warts occurring on mucous membranes of the genital area (including the urethra, rectum and vagina). Data are not available on the safe and effective use of podofilox **solution** for treatment of warts occurring in the perianal area. Do not exceed the recommended method of application, frequency of application or duration of usage (see Administration and Dosage).

Adverse Reactions

In clinical trials, the following local adverse reactions occurred at some point during treatment. Reports of burning and pain were more frequent and of greater severity in women than in men treated with the solution. The severity of local adverse reactions in gel-treated patients were predominantly mild or moderate and did not increase during the treatment period; severe reactions were most frequent within the first 2 weeks of treatment.

Podofilox Adverse Reactions (%)		
Adverse Reaction	Solution	Gel
Burning	64-78	12-37
Pain	50-72	12-24
Inflammation	63-71	9-32
Erosion	67	9-27
Itching	50-65	8-32
Bleeding	N/A	1-19

Miscellaneous (< 5%) –

Solution: Pain with intercourse; insomnia; tingling; bleeding; tenderness; chafing; malodor; dizziness; scarring; vesicle formation; crusting edema; dryness/peeling; foreskin irretraction; hematuria; vomiting; ulceration.

Gel: Headache, stinging, and erythema; less commonly reported local adverse events included desquamation, scabbing, discoloration, tenderness, dryness, crusting, fissures, soreness, ulceration, swelling/edema, tingling, rash and blisters.

Overdosage

➤*Symptoms:* Topically applied podofilox may be absorbed systemically. Toxicity reported following systemic administration of podofilox in investigational use for cancer treatment included: Nausea; vomiting; fever; diarrhea; bone marrow depression; oral ulcers. Following 5 to 10

PODOFILOX

daily IV doses of 0.5 to 1 mg/kg/day, significant hematological toxicity occurred but was reversible. Other toxicities occurred at lower doses.

Toxicity reported following systemic administration of podophyllum resin included: Nausea; vomiting; fever; diarrhea; peripheral neuropathy; altered mental status; lethargy; coma; tachypnea; respiratory failure; leukocytosis; pancytosis; hematuria; renal failure; seizures.

➤*Treatment:* Topical overdosage treatment should include washing the skin free of any remaining drug and symptomatic and supportive therapy. Refer to General Management of Acute Overdosage.

Patient Information

Provide the patient with a Patient Information leaflet when a podofilox prescription is filled.

Use only as directed by the health care provider. Instruct patients to wash their hands thoroughly before and after each application. It is for external use only. Avoid contact with the eyes.

Advise patients not to use this medication for any disorder other than for which it was prescribed.

Patients should report any signs of adverse reactions to the health care provider.

If no improvement is observed after 4 weeks of treatment, discontinue the medication and consult the health care provider.

PODOPHYLLUM RESIN (Podophyllin)

Rx	**Podocon-25** (Paddock)	**Liquid:** 25% podophyllum resin in tincture of benzoin	In 15 ml.
Rx	**Podofin** (Syosset)		In 15 ml.

Indications

➤*Wart removal:* For the removal of soft genital (venereal) warts (condylomata acuminata) and other papillomas; for multiple superficial epitheliomatosis and keratoses.

The CDC recommends podophyllum resin as an alternative regimen to cryotherapy for the treatment of external genital/perianal warts, vaginal warts and urethral meatus warts (CDC 1989 Sexually Transmitted Diseases Treatment Guidelines. *Morbidity and Mortality Weekly Report* 1989 Sept 1;38(No.S-8):20-21).

Administration and Dosage

Podophyllum is to be applied only by a physician. It is not to be dispensed to the patient. Thoroughly cleanse affected area. Use applicator to apply sparingly to lesion. Avoid contact with healthy tissue. Allow to dry thoroughly. Treat only intact (non-bleeding) lesions. As podophyllum is a powerful caustic and severe irritant, it is recommended the first application be left in contact for only a short time (30 to 40 minutes) to determine patient's sensitivity. To avoid systemic absorption, use the minimum time of contact necessary to produce the desired result (1 to 4 hours, depending on condition of lesion and of patient), with the physician developing their own experience and technique. Do not treat large areas or numerous warts at once. After treatment time has elapsed, remove dried podophyllum resin thoroughly with alcohol or soap and water.

Actions

➤*Pharmacology:* Podophyllum resin is the powdered mixture of resins removed from the May apple or Mandrake (*Podophyllum peltatum* Linne'), a perennial plant of the northern and middle US. Podophyllum is a cytotoxic agent that has been used topically in the treatment of genital warts. It arrests mitosis in metaphase, an effect it shares with other cytotoxic agents such as the vinca alkaloids. The active agent is podophyllotoxin, whose concentration varies with the type of podophyllum resin used; American podophyllum typically has a reduced level of podophyllotoxin and normally contains one-fourth the amount of the Indian source.

Contraindications

Diabetics; patients using steroids or with poor blood circulation; use on bleeding warts, moles, birthmarks or unusual warts with hair growing from them; pregnancy, lactation (see Warnings).

Warnings

➤*For external use only:* Podophyllum is a powerful caustic and severe irritant. Keep away from the eyes; if eye contact occurs, flush with copious amounts of warm water and consult physician or poison control center immediately for advice.

➤*Physician use (application) only:* Podophyllum resin is to be applied only by a physician. It is not to be dispensed to the patient.

➤*Pregnancy:* There have been reports of complications associated with the topical use of podophyllum on condylomas of pregnant patients including birth defects, fetal death and stillbirth. Do not use on pregnant patients or patients who plan to become pregnant.

➤*Lactation:* It is not known whether podophyllum is excreted in breast milk following topical application. Do not use on nursing patients.

Precautions

➤*Inflamed / Irritated tissue:* Do not use if wart or surrounding tissue is inflamed or irritated. Do not use on bleeding warts, moles, birthmarks or unusual warts with hair growing from them.

Adverse Reactions

Paresthesia; polyneuritis; paralytic ileus; pyrexia; leukopenia; thrombocytopenia; nausea; vomiting; diarrhea; abdominal pain; confusion; dizziness; stupor; convulsions; coma; death.

Significant neuropathy and death are generally related to large amounts used for multiple and widespread lesions. Onset of neuropathy may occur within hours of application and duration may range from months to years with some neurologic deficit.

Patient Information

To be applied only by a physician.

For external use only. Avoid contact with eyes and healthy tissue.

METHIONINE

Rx	**M-Caps** (Pal-Pak)	**Capsules:** 200 mg	In 1000s.
Rx	**Uracid** (Wesley)		In 1000s.
Rx[1]	**Methionine** (Various, eg, Mason, Tyson & Assoc.)	**Tablets:** 500 mg	In 30s and 60s.
Rx	**Pedameth** (Forest)	**Liquid:** 75 mg per 5 ml	Fruit flavor. In pt.

[1] Products available *otc* or *Rx*, depending on product labeling.

Indications

Treatment of diaper rash in infants and for control of odor, dermatitis and ulceration caused by ammoniacal urine in incontinent adults.

Administration and Dosage

➤*Diaper rash caused by ammoniacal urine:* 75 mg in warm formula or other liquid, 3 or 4 times daily or 3 to 5 days. In severe cases or when the infant is > 1 year old it may be necessary to double the dosage the first two days of treatment.

➤*Control of odor in incontinent adults:* 200 to 500 mg, 3 or 4 times daily after meal.

Actions

➤*Pharmacology:* The acid-producing effect of methionine on urine pH creates an ammonia free urine.

Contraindications

A history of liver disease; large doses of methionine may exaggerate the toxemia of the disease.

Precautions

➤*Protein intake:* Excessive methionine added alone to the diet over extended periods may result in a less than normal weight gain in infants when protein intake is insufficient. Maintain adequate protein intake during therapy and do not exceed the recommended dosage.

Patient Information

Take with food, milk or other liquid.

DIAPER RASH PRODUCTS, TOPICAL

otc	**Diaper Rash** (Various, eg, Goldline, Rugby)	**Ointment:** Zinc oxide, cod liver oil, lanolin, methylparaben, petrolatum, talc	In 113 g.
otc	**A and D Medicated** (Schering-Plough)	**Ointment:** White petrolatum, zinc oxide, benzyl alcohol, cod liver oil, light mineral oil, propylparabens, vitamins A and D	In 113 g.
otc	**A+D Ointment with Zinc Oxide** (Schering-Plough)	**Ointment:** 1% dimethicone, 10% zinc oxide, aloe, benzyl alcohol, vitamins A and D, cod liver oil, light mineral oil, synthetic beeswax	In 81 g.
otc	**Bottom Better** (InnoVisions)	**Ointment:** 49% petrolatum, 15.5% lanolin, lanolin alcohols, EDTA, parabens	In 3.75 g packets (18).
otc	**Desitin** (Leeming)	**Ointment:** 40% zinc oxide, cod liver oil, talc, petrolatum, lanolin, methylparaben	In 30, 60, 120, 240 and 270 g.
otc	**Diaper Guard** (Del)	**Ointment:** 1% dimethicone, 66% white petrolatum, cocoa butter, parabens, vitamins A, D₃ and E, zinc oxide	In 49.6 and 99.2 g.
otc	**Diaparene Diaper Rash** (Lehn & Fink)	**Ointment:** Zinc oxide, petrolatum, parabens, imidazolidinyl urea	In 60 g.
otc	**Flanders Buttocks** (Flanders Inc.)	**Ointment:** Zinc oxide, castor oil, balsam peru	In 60 g.
otc	**Desitin Creamy** (Pfizer)	**Ointment:** 10% zinc oxide, mineral oil, white petrolatum, parabens	In 57 g.
otc	**Diaparene Baby** (Lehn & Fink)	**Cream:** Mineral oil, petrolatum, aloe, EDTA, diazolidinyl urea, parabens	In 60 g.
otc	**Amerigel** (Amerx Health Care Corp.)	**Lotion:** Glycerin, lemon oil, parabens, oak extract (oakin).	In 228 g.
otc	**Dyprotex** (Blistex)	**Pads:** 40% micronized zinc oxide, 37.6% petrolatum, 2.5% dimethicone, cod liver oil, aloe	In 3 pads (9 applications) and 8 pads (24 applications).
otc	**Diaparene Cornstarch Baby** (Lehn & Fink)	**Powder:** Corn starch, aloe	In 120, 270 and 420 g.
otc	**Mexsana Medicated** (Schering-Plough)	**Powder:** Kaolin, eucalyptus oil, camphor, corn starch, lemon oil, zinc oxide	In 90, 187.5 and 330 g.
otc	**Desitin with Zinc Oxide** (Pfizer)	**Powder:** 88.2% cornstarch, 10% zinc oxide	In 28 and 397 g.
otc	**Gold Bond Medicated Baby Powder** (Chattem)	**Powder:** Talc, zinc oxide	In 113 and 283 g.
otc	**Gold Bond Cornstarch Plus Medicated Baby Powder** (Chattem)	**Powder:** Cornstarch, zinc oxide, kaolin	In 113 and 283 g.
otc	**Gold Bond Triple Action Medicated Baby Powder** (Chattem)	**Powder:** 89% talc, 10% zinc oxide	In 113 and 283 g.

Indications

These products are intended for use in diaper rash or ammonia dermatitis.

Ingredients

The principal active components of these formulations include:

➤*EUCALYPTOL:* Antimicrobial agent. Minimizes bacterial proliferation.

➤*ZINC OXIDE:* For drying.

➤*CAMPHOR:* A local anesthetic. Relieves pain, itching and irritation.

➤*BALSAM PERU:* It is claimed to promote wound healing or tissue repair, but effectiveness has not been conclusively demonstrated.

➤*CALCIUM CARBONATE and KAOLIN:* Used for their moisture absorbing abilities.

➤*PROTECTANTS and LUBRICANTS:* To minimize chafing and irritation.

ALUMINUM CHLORIDE (HEXAHYDRATE)

Rx	**Aluminum Chloride (Hexahydrate)** (Glades)	**Solution:** 20% in 88.5% SD alcohol 40-2	In 37.5 mL bottle and 35 and 60 mL *Dab-O-Matic* applicator bottle.
Rx	**Drysol** (Person & Covey)	**Solution:** 20% in 93% SD alcohol 40	In 37.5 mL or 35 and 60 mL with *Dab-O-Matic* applicator.

Indications

An astringent used as an aid in the management of hyperhidrosis.

Administration and Dosage

Apply to the affected area once daily, only at bedtime. To help prevent irritation, completely dry area prior to application. Do not apply to broken, irritated, or recently shaved skin.

For maximum effect, cover the treated area with plastic wrap, held in place by a snug fitting T-shirt or body shirt, mitten, or sock. (Never hold plastic wrap in place with tape.) Wash the treated area the following morning. Excessive sweating may stop after ≥ 2 treatments. Thereafter, apply once or twice weekly or as needed.

Warnings

➤*For external use only:* Avoid contact with the eyes.

➤*Discontinue use:* If irritation or sensitization occurs, discontinue use.

➤*Metals / Fabrics:* Aluminum chloride (hexahydrate) may be harmful to certain metals and fabrics.

Adverse Reactions

Burning or prickling sensation may occur.

FORMALDEHYDE

Rx	**Formalyde-10** (Pedinol)	**Spray:** 10%	SD-40 alcohol. In 60 mL.
Rx	**Lazer Formalyde** (Pedinol)	**Solution:** 10%	In 90 mL.

Indications

Drying agent for pre- and post-surgical removal of warts or for Histofreezer treatment of warts where dryness is required. Safeguards against offensive odor and dries excessive moisture of feet.

Administration and Dosage

Apply once daily to affected areas as directed.

➤*Storage / Stability:* Store at controlled room temperature (15° to 30°C; 59° to 86°F).

Contraindications

Hypersensitivity to any ingredients of the product.

Precautions

➤*For external use only:* Avoid contact with and keep away from face, eyes, nose, and mucous membranes.

➤*Irritation / Sensitivity:* May be irritating and sensitizing to the skin of some patients; check skin for sensitivity prior to application. If redness or irritation persists, consult physician.

COLLAGENASE

| Rx | Collagenase Santyl (Ross) | Ointment: 250 units collagenase enzyme/g. | White petrolatum. In 15 and 30 g. |

Indications

For debriding chronic dermal ulcers and severely burned areas.

Administration and Dosage

Apply once daily (or more frequently if the dressing becomes soiled).

Prior to application, cleanse the lesion of debris and digested material by gently rubbing with a gauze pad saturated with normal saline solution or with the desired cleansing agent compatible with collagenase, followed by a normal saline solution rinse.

When infection is present, use an appropriate topical antibacterial powder. Apply to the lesion prior to the application of collagenase ointment. Should the infection not respond, discontinue therapy until remission of the infection occurs.

Apply ointment directly to wounds or to a sterile gauze pad and apply to wound and secure properly.

Cross-hatching thick eschar with a #10 blade allows collagenase more surface contact with necrotic debris. Remove as much loosened tissue debris as possible with forceps and scissors.

Remove all excess ointment each time dressing is changed.

Terminate use of the ointment when debridement of necrotic tissue is complete and granulation tissue is well established.

Actions

➤*Pharmacology:* Since collagen accounts for 75% of the dry weight of skin tissue, the ability of collagenase to digest collagen in the physiological pH and temperature range makes it effective in the removal of detritus. Collagenase thus contributes to the formation of granulation tissues and subsequent epithelialization of dermal ulcers and severely burned areas. Collagen in healthy tissue or in newly formed granulation tissue is not attacked.

Contraindications

Local or systemic hypersensitivity to collagenase.

Precautions

➤*For external use only:* Avoid contact with the eyes.

➤*Optimal pH range:* Optimal pH range for the enzyme is 6 to 8.

➤*Systemic bacterial infections:* Monitor debilitated patients for systemic bacterial infections because debriding enzymes may increase the risk of bacteremia.

➤*Slight transient erythema:* This has been noted occasionally in surrounding tissue, particularly when the ointment was not confined to the lesion. Therefore, apply carefully within the area of the lesion.

➤*Inhibition of enzymatic activity:* Enzymatic activity is inhibited by certain detergents and heavy metal ions, such as mercury and silver, that are used in some antiseptics. When such materials have been used, carefully cleanse the site by repeated washings with normal saline before ointment is applied. Avoid soaks containing metal ions or acidic solutions such as Burow's solution because of the metal ion and low pH. Cleansing materials such as hydrogen peroxide, Dakin's solution, or normal saline do not interfere with enzyme activity.

Adverse Reactions

No allergic sensitivity or toxic reactions have been noted in clinical investigations. However, 1 case of systemic manifestations of hypersensitivity to collagenase in a patient treated for > 1 year with a combination of collagenase and cortisone has been reported.

Overdosage

Action of the enzyme may be stopped by washing with povidone iodine.

ENZYME COMBINATIONS, TOPICAL

Rx	Granulderm (Qualitest)	Aerosol: 0.1 mg trypsin, 72.5 mg balsam peru and 650 mg castor oil per 0.82 mL.	In 113.4 g.
Rx	Granulex (Bertek)	Aerosol: 0.12 mg trypsin, 87 mg balsam peru, and 788 mg castor oil per g.	In 57 and 113 g.
Rx	Accuzyme (Healthpoint)	Ointment: 8.3×10^5 units papain and 100 mg urea per g in a hydrophilic ointment base; parabens, glycerin.	In 30 g.
Rx	Ethezyme 830 (Ethex)	Ointment: 8.3×10^5 units papain and 100 mg urea per g in a hydrophilic ointment base; EDTA, parabens, glycerin.	In 30 g.
Rx	Gladase (Glades)	Ointment: 8.3×10^5 units papain and 100 mg urea per g; parabens, glycerin.	In 30 g.
Rx	Papain-Urea Debriding (Cypress)	Ointment: 1.1×10^6 units papain and 10% urea per g in a hydrophilic ointment base; parabens, glycerin.	In 30 g.
Rx	Papain Urea Chlorophyllin (Cypress)	Ointment: 521,700 units papain, 10% urea, 0.5% chlorophyllin copper complex per g.	In 30 g.
Rx	Panafil (Healthpoint)	Ointment: ≥ 521,700 units papain, 10% urea, 0.5% chlorophyllin copper complex sodium per g in a hydrophilic base with propylene glycol, white petrolatum, stearyl alcohol, boric acid, chlorobutanol (anhydrous).	In 30 g tube and 1 lb jar.
Rx	Panafil (Healthpoint)	Spray: ≥ 521,700 units papain, 10% urea, 0.5% chlorophyllin copper complex sodium/g in a base with glycerin, cetearyl alcohol, mineral oil, parabens.	In 33 mL.

Indications

For debridement of necrotic tissue and liquefication of slough in acute and chronic lesions such as pressure ulcers, varicose and diabetic ulcers, burns, postoperative wounds, pilonidal cyst wounds, carbuncles, and miscellaneous traumatic or infected wounds.

Administration and Dosage

Apply medication once or twice daily.

Clean wound prior to application and at each redressing. For papain-containing products, avoid hydrogen peroxide solution because it may inactivate papain.

➤*Aerosols:* Shake well. Hold upright and ≈ 12 inches from the area to be treated.

Ingredients

➤*TRYPSIN and PAPAIN:* Used for the enzymatic debridement and promotion of normal healing, especially where healing is retarded by eschar, necrotic tissue, and debris.

➤*BALSAM OF PERU:* An effective capillary bed stimulant intended to improve circulation to the wound site. It may have a mildly antiseptic action.

➤*CASTOR OIL:* (Also refer to Laxative monograph in the Gastrointestinal Agents chapter). Used to improve epithelialization by reducing premature epithelial desiccation and cornification, and as protective cover.

➤*UREA:* (See monograph in Emollients section). An emollient and keratolytic.

➤*CHLOROPHYLL DERIVATIVES:* (See individual monograph). Adds healing action to the cleansing action of the proteolytic papain-urea combination. The basic wound-healing properties are promotion of healthy granulations, control of local inflammation, and reduction of wound odors.

Contraindications

Sensitivity to papain or any other components of these preparations.

Warnings

➤*Arterial clots:* Do not spray aerosol products on fresh arterial clots.

➤*For external use only:* Avoid contact with the eyes.

➤*Transient burning:* Transient burning may be experienced upon application.

➤*Papain:* Papain may be inactivated by the salts of heavy metals such as lead, silver, and mercury. Avoid contact with medications containing these metals.

Adverse Reactions

Generally well-tolerated and non-irritating. A transient burning sensation may be experienced by a small percentage of patients. Occasionally, the profuse exudate from enzymatic digestion may irritate the skin. In such cases, more frequent dressing changes will alleviate discomfort until exudate decreases.

IMIQUIMOD

Rx Aldara (3M Pharm)	**Cream:** 5%	Cetyl alcohol, stearyl alcohol, white petrolatum, benzyl alcohol, parabens. In single-use packets. In boxes of 12.

Indications

➤*Genital and perianal warts:* Treatment of external genital and perianal warts/condyloma acuminata in individuals 12 years of age and older.

➤*Unlabeled uses:* May be effective for the treatment of basal cell carcinoma.

Administration and Dosage

➤*Approved by the FDA:* February 27, 1997.

Apply imiquimod 3 times per week, prior to normal sleeping hours, and leave on the skin for 6 to 10 hours. Following the treatment period, remove cream by washing the treated area with mild soap and water. Examples of 3 times per week application schedules are Monday, Wednesday, Friday; or Tuesday, Thursday, Saturday. Continue imiquimod treatment until there is total clearance of the genital/perianal warts or for a maximum of 16 weeks. A rest period of several days may be taken if required by the patient's discomfort or severity of the local skin reaction. Treatment may resume once the reaction subsides.

Nonocclusive dressings such as cotton gauze or cotton underwear may be used in the management of skin reactions. Hand-washing before and after cream application is recommended. Imiquimod is packaged in single-use packets that contain sufficient cream to cover a wart area of up to 20 cm^2; avoid use of excessive amounts of cream. Instruct patients to apply imiquimod to external, genital, or perianal warts. Apply a thin layer to the wart area and rub in until the cream is no longer visible. Do not occlude the application site.

➤*Storage/Stability:* Store below 25°C (77°F). Avoid freezing.

Actions

➤*Pharmacology:* Imiquimod is an immune response modifier. The mechanism of action of imiquimod in treating genital/perianal warts is unknown. Imiquimod has no direct antiviral activity in cell culture. Mouse skin studies suggest that imiquimod induces cytokines, including interferon-alpha and others, in humans and animals. However, the clinical relevance of these findings is unknown.

➤*Pharmacokinetics:* Percutaneous absorption of imiquimod was minimal in a study involving 6 healthy subjects treated with a single topical application (5 mg) of radiolabeled imiquimod cream. Less than 0.9% of the dose was excreted in the urine and feces following topical application.

Contraindications

None known.

Warnings

➤*Other conditions:* Imiquimod has not been evaluated for the treatment of urethral, intravaginal, cervical, rectal, or intra-anal human papilloma viral disease and is not recommended for these conditions.

➤*Pregnancy: Category B.* There are no adequate and well-controlled studies in pregnant women. Imiquimod was not found to be teratogenic in rat or rabbit teratology studies.

➤*Lactation:* It is not known whether imiquimod is excreted in breast milk.

➤*Children:* Safety and efficacy in patients under 12 years of age have not been established.

Precautions

➤*Skin reactions:* The most frequently reported adverse reactions were local skin and application site reactions. These reactions were usually mild-to-moderate in intensity. These reactions were more frequent and more intense with daily application than with 3-times-a-week application. In the 3-times-a-week application clinical studies, 1.2% (4/327) of the patients discontinued because of local skin/application site reactions.

Local skin reactions such as erythema, erosion, excoriation/flaking, and edema are common. Should severe local skin reaction occur, remove the cream by washing the treatment area with mild soap and water. Treatment with imiquimod cream can be resumed after the skin reaction has subsided. There is no clinical experience with imiquimod cream therapy immediately following the treatment of genital/perianal warts with other cutaneously applied drugs; therefore, imiquimod cream administration is not recommended until genital/perianal tissue is

healed from any previous drug or surgical treatment. Imiquimod has the potential to exacerbate inflammatory conditions of the skin.

Adverse Reactions

Imiquimod Adverse Reactions (3 Times a Week Application) (%)

	Mild/moderate		Severe	
Adverse reaction	Females (n = 114)	Males (n = 156)	Females (n = 114)	Males (n = 156)
Erythema	61	54	4	4
Erosion	30	29	1	1
Excoriation/flaking	18	25	0	1
Edema	17	12	1	0
Induration	5	7	0	0
Ulceration	5	4	3	0
Scabbing	4	13	0	0
Vesicles	3	2	0	0

Imiquimod Adverse Reactions (3 times per week application) (%)

Adverse reaction	Females (n = 117)	Males (n = 156)
Local		
Itching	32	22
Burning	26	9
Pain	8	2
Soreness	3	0
Fungal infection[1]	11	2
Systemic reactions		
Headache	4	5
Influenza-like symptoms	3	1
Myalgia	1	1

[1] Incidences reported without regard to causality with imiquimod.

Females – Erythema (3%); ulceration (2%); edema (1%).

Males – Erosion (2%); erythema, edema, induration, excoriation/flaking (1%).

➤*Miscellaneous:* Other adverse reactions (> 1%) include: Application site disorders; wart site reactions (eg, burning, hypopigmentation, irritation, itching, pain, rash, sensitivity, soreness, stinging, tenderness); remote site reactions (eg, bleeding, burning, itching, pain, tenderness, tinea cruris); fatigue; fever; influenza-like symptoms; headache; diarrhea; myalgia.

Overdosage

Overdosage of imiquimod in humans is unlikely because of minimal percutaneous absorption. Animal studies reveal a rabbit dermal lethal imiquimod dose of greater than 1600 mg/m^2. Persistent topical overdosing of imiquimod could result in severe local skin reactions. The most clinically serious adverse event reported following multiple oral imiquimod doses of greater than 200 mg was hypotension that resolved following oral or IV fluid administration.

Patient Information

Imiquimod may weaken condoms and vaginal diaphragms. Therefore, concurrent use is not recommended.

This medication is for external use only. Avoid contact with eyes.

Do not occlude the treatment area with bandages or other covers or wraps.

Avoid sexual (genital, anal, oral) contact while the cream is on the skin.

Wash the treatment area with mild soap and water 6 to 10 hours following application of imiquimod.

Patients commonly experience local skin reactions such as erythema, erosion, excoriation/flaking and edema at the site of application or surrounding areas. Most skin reactions are mild-to-moderate. Severe skin reactions occur; promptly report severe reactions to the physician.

Uncircumcised males treating warts under the foreskin should retract the foreskin and clean the area daily.

Imiquimod is not a cure; new warts may develop during therapy.

TACROLIMUS

Rx	Protopic (Fujisawa)	Ointment: 0.03%	Mineral oil, white petrolatum. In 30 and 60 g.
		0.1%	Mineral oil, white petrolatum. In 30 and 60 g.

Tacrolimus is also available as a capsule for organ rejection prophylaxis; see Biological and Immunologic Agents chapter.

Indications

➤*Moderate to severe atopic dermatitis:* Tacrolimus ointment, both 0.03% and 0.1% for adults, and only 0.03% for children 2 to 15 years of age, is indicated for short-term and intermittent long-term therapy in the treatment of patients with moderate-to-severe atopic dermatitis in whom the use of alternative, conventional therapies are deemed inadvisable because of potential risks, or in the treatment of patients who are not adequately responsive to or are intolerant of alternative, conventional therapies.

Administration and Dosage

➤*Approved by the FDA:* December 8, 2000.

➤*Adults:*

0.03% and 0.1% – Apply a thin layer to the affected skin areas twice daily and rub in gently and completely. Continue treatment for 1 week after clearing of signs and symptoms of atopic dermatitis.

➤*Children:*

0.03% – Apply a thin layer to the affected skin areas twice daily and rub in gently and completely. Continue treatment for 1 week after clearing of signs and symptoms of atopic dermatitis.

The safety of tacrolimus ointment under occlusion, which may promote systemic exposure, has not been evaluated. Do not use tacrolimus ointment with occlusive dressings.

➤*Storage/Stability:* Store at room temperature 25°C (77°F); excursions permitted to 15° to 30°C (59° to 86°F).

Actions

➤*Pharmacology:* Tacrolimus is a macrolide immunosuppressant produced by *Streptomyces tsukubaensis.* The mechanism of action of tacrolimus in atopic dermatitis is not known. It has been demonstrated that tacrolimus inhibits T-lymphocyte activation by first binding to an intracellular protein, FKBP-12. A complex of tacrolimus-FKBP-12, calcium, calmodulin, and calcineurin is then formed and the phosphatase activity of calcineurin is inhibited. This effect has been shown to prevent the dephosphorylation and translocation of nuclear factor of activated T-cells (NF-AT), a nuclear component thought to initiate gene transcription for the formation of lymphokines (such as interleukin-2, gamma interferon). Tacrolimus also inhibits the transcription for genes that encode IL-3, IL-4, IL-5, GM-CSF, and TNF-α, all of which are involved in the early stages of T-cell activation. Additionally, tacrolimus has been shown to inhibit the release of pre-formed mediators from skin mast cells and basophils, and to downregulate the expression of $F_{CE}RI$ on Langerhans cells.

➤*Pharmacokinetics:*

Absorption/Distribution – In atopic dermatitis patients, tacrolimus is absorbed after topical application of 0.1% tacrolimus ointment. Peak tacrolimus blood concentrations ranged from undetectable to 20 ng/mL after single or multiple doses of 0.1% tacrolimus ointment, with 45 of the 49 patients having peak blood concentrations < 5 ng/mL.

There was no evidence based on blood concentrations that tacrolimus accumulates systemically upon intermittent topical application for periods of up to 1 year. The absolute bioavailability of topical tacrolimus is unknown. Using IV historical data for comparison, the bioavailability of tacrolimus in atopic dermatitis patients is < 0.5%. In adults with an average of 53% BSA treated, exposure of tacrolimus is ≈ 30-fold less than that seen with oral immunosuppressive doses in kidney and liver transplant patients.

Contraindications

A history of hypersensitivity to tacrolimus or any other component of the preparation.

Warnings

➤*Carcinogenesis:* A 104-week dermal carcinogenicity study was performed in mice with tacrolimus ointment at doses equivalent to 1.1 to 118 mg/kg/day tacrolimus. A statistically significant elevation in the incidence of pleomorphic lymphoma in high-dose male and female animals and in the incidence of undifferentiated lymphoma in high-dose female animals was noted in the mouse dermal carcinogenicity study. Lymphomas were noted in the mouse dermal carcinogenicity study at a daily dose of 3.5 mg/kg (0.1% tacrolimus ointment) (26 × MRHD based on AUC comparisons).

In a 52-week photocarcinogenicity study, the median time to onset of skin tumor formation was decreased in hairless mice following chronic topical dosing with concurrent exposure to UV radiation (40 weeks of treatment followed by 12 weeks of observation) with tacrolimus ointment at ≥ 0.1% tacrolimus.

➤*Pregnancy:* Category C. There are no adequate and well-controlled studies of topically administered tacrolimus in pregnant women. The experience with tacrolimus ointment when used by pregnant women is too limited to permit assessment of the safety of its use during pregnancy.

There are no adequate and well-controlled studies of systemically administered tacrolimus in pregnant women. Tacrolimus is transferred across the placenta. The use of systemically administered tacrolimus during pregnancy has been associated with neonatal hyperkalemia and renal dysfunction. Use tacrolimus ointment during pregnancy only if the potential benefit to the mother justifies the potential risk to the fetus.

➤*Lactation:* Although systemic absorption of tacrolimus following topical applications of tacrolimus ointment is minimal relative to systemic administration, it is known that tacrolimus is excreted in human milk. Because of the potential for serious adverse reactions in nursing infants from tacrolimus, a decision should be made whether to discontinue nursing or to discontinue the drug, taking into account the importance of the drug to the mother.

➤*Children:* Tacrolimus 0.03% ointment may be used in children ≥ 2 years of age.

Precautions

➤*Infected atopic dermatitis:* Studies have not evaluated the safety and efficacy of tacrolimus ointment in the treatment of clinically infected atopic dermatitis. Before commencing treatment with tacrolimus ointment, clear clinical infections at treatment sites.

➤*Viral infection:* While patients with atopic dermatitis are predisposed to superficial skin infections, including eczema herpeticum (Kaposi's varicelliform eruption), treatment with tacrolimus ointment may be associated with an increased risk of varicella zoster virus infection (chicken pox or shingles), herpes simplex virus infection, or eczema herpeticum. In the presence of these infections, evaluate the balance of risks and benefits associated with tacrolimus ointment.

➤*Lymphadenopathy:* In clinical studies, 33 cases of lymphadenopathy (0.8%) were reported and were usually related to infections (particularly of the skin) and noted to resolve upon appropriate antibiotic therapy. The majority had either a clear etiology or were known to resolve. Transplant patients receiving immunosuppressive regimens (eg, systemic tacrolimus) are at increased risk for developing lymphoma; therefore, patients who receive tacrolimus ointment and who develop lymphadenopathy should have the etiology of their lymphadenopathy investigated. In the absence of a clear etiology for the lymphadenopathy, or in the presence of acute infectious mononucleosis, consider discontinuation of tacrolimus ointment. Monitor patients who develop lymphadenopathy to ensure that the lymphadenopathy resolves.

➤*Phototoxicity:* The enhancement of ultraviolet carcinogenicity is not necessarily dependent on phototoxic mechanisms. Despite the absence of observed phototoxicity in humans (see Adverse Reactions), tacrolimus ointment shortened the time to skin tumor formation in animal photocarcinogenicity study (see Warnings). Therefore, it is prudent for patients to minimize or avoid natural or artificial sunlight exposure.

➤*Other skin disorders:* The use of tacrolimus ointment in patients with Netherton's syndrome is not recommended because of the potential for increased systemic absorption of tacrolimus. The safety of tacrolimus ointment has not been established in patients with generalized erythroderma.

Drug Interactions

Formal topical drug interaction studies with tacrolimus ointment have not been conducted. Based on its minimal extent of absorption, interactions of tacrolimus ointment with systemically administered drugs are unlikely to occur but cannot be ruled out. The concomitant administration of known CYP3A4 inhibitors in patients with widespread or erythrodermic disease should be done with caution. Some examples of such drugs are erythromycin, itraconazole, ketoconazole, fluconazole, calcium channel blockers, and cimetidine.

Adverse Reactions

The use of tacrolimus ointment may cause local symptoms such as skin burning (burning sensation, stinging, soreness) or pruritus. Localized symptoms are most common during the first few days of application and typically improve as the lesions of atopic dermatitis heal. With tacrolimus ointment 0.1%, 90% of the skin burning events had a duration between 2 minutes and 3 hours (median, 15 minutes). Of the pruritus events, 90% had a duration between 3 minutes and 10 hours (median, 20 minutes).

The following table depicts the adjusted incidence of adverse events pooled across the 3 identically designed 12-week studies for patients in 0.03% and 0.1% tacrolimus ointment treatment groups, and the unadjusted incidence of adverse events in two 1-year long-term safety studies, regardless of relationship to study drug.

TACROLIMUS

Incidence of Treatment-Emergent Adverse Events with Tacrolimus (%)

Adverse reaction	12-week, randomized, double-blind phase 3 studies; 12-week adjusted incidence rate			Open-label studies (up to 1 year) 0.1% tacrolimus ointment	
	Adults		Children	Adults (n = 316)	Children (n = 255)
	0.03% (n = 210)	0.1% (n = 209)	0.03% (n = 118)		
Dermatologic					
Skin burning[1]	46	58	43	47	26
Pruritus[1]	46	46	41	25	25
Skin erythema	25	28	12	12	9
Skin infection	12	5	10	11	11
Herpes simplex	4	4	0	12	5
Eczema herpeticum	1	1	2	2	0
Pustular rash	3	4	2	6	8
Folliculitis[1]	6	4	2	11	2
Urticaria	3	6	1	5	5
Maculopapular rash	2	2	0	4	3
Rash[1]	5	2	2	2	5
Fungal dermatitis	2	1	0	2	6
Acne[1]	4	7	0	2	4
Sunburn	2	1	0	4	4
Skin disorder	2	1	4	1	4
Vesiculobullous rash[1]	3	2	4	2	2
Skin tingling[1]	3	8	2	2	1
Dry skin	3	3	1	0	1
Benign skin neoplasm[2]	1	1	0	2	3
Contact dermatitis	3	3	4	1	1
Eczema	2	2	0	3	0
Exfoliative dermatitis	3	1	0	0	2
GI					
Diarrhea	3	4	5	4	6
Vomiting	1	1	6	1	5
Abdominal pain	1	1	3	1	5
Gastroenteritis	2	2	0	4	2
Nausea	3	2	1	1	2
Dyspepsia[1]	1	4	0	1	4
Respiratory					
Cough increased	1	1	18	3	15
Asthma	6	4	6	5	16
Pharyngitis	3	4	6	5	10
Rhinitis	3	2	6	5	5
Sinusitis[1]	4	2	3	3	7
Bronchitis	2	2	3	3	6
Pneumonia	1	1	0	1	2
Miscellaneous					
Flu-like symptoms[1]	23	31	28	22	35
Allergic reaction	12	6	4	22	15
Headache[1]	20	19	5	10	18
Fever	4	1	21	2	18
Infection	1	2	7	14	8
Accidental injury	3	6	6	4	12
Otitis media	0	1	12	1	7
Lack of drug effect	1	0	1	10	2
Alcohol intolerance[1]	3	7	0	6	0
Conjunctivitis	2	2	1	4	2
Pain	2	2	1	4	3
Lymphadenopathy	2	1	3	2	3

Incidence of Treatment-Emergent Adverse Events with Tacrolimus (%)

Adverse reaction	12-week, randomized, double-blind phase 3 studies; 12-week adjusted incidence rate			Open-label studies (up to 1 year) 0.1% tacrolimus ointment	
	Adults		Children	Adults (n = 316)	Children (n = 255)
	0.03% (n = 210)	0.1% (n = 209)	0.03% (n = 118)		
Face edema	2	1	1	3	1
Hyperesthesia[1]	3	7	0	3	0
Back pain[1]	2	2	1	3	1
Peripheral edema	4	3	0	2	1
Varicella zoster/ herpes zoster[1,3]	1	0	5	1	3
Asthenia	2	3	0	2	1
Insomnia	4	3	1	1	0
Dysmenorrhea	4	4	0	0	2
Periodontal abscess	0	1	0	3	0
Myalgia[1]	3	2	0	1	0
Cyst[1]	1	3	0	0	0

[1] May be reasonably associated with the use of this drug product.
[2] Generally, "warts."
[3] Four cases of chicken pox in the pediatric 12-week study; 1 case of "zoster of the lip" in the adult 12–week study; 7 cases of chicken pox and 1 case of shingles in the open-label pediatric study; 2 cases of herpes zoster in the open-label adult study.

Other adverse events that occurred at an incidence ≥ 1% in any clinical study include the following:

➤*Cardiovascular:* Angina pectoris, arrhythmia, cerebrovascular accident, hypertension, palpitations, peripheral vascular disorder, vasodilation.

➤*CNS:* Anxiety, depression, dizziness, migraine, neuritis, paresthesia, vertigo.

➤*Dermatologic:* Alopecia, cellulitis, ecchymosis, skin discoloration, sweating.

➤*GI:* Anorexia, constipation, gastritis.

➤*Lab test abnormalities:* Abnormal liver function tests, ALT or AST increased, bilirubinemia, creatinine increased, hyperglycemia, hypoglycemia, leukocytosis, leukopenia.

➤*Musculoskeletal:* Arthralgia, arthritis.

➤*Respiratory:* Dyspnea, hypoxia, laryngitis, lung disorder.

➤*Special senses:* Ear pain, eye disorder, eye pain, taste perversion.

➤*Miscellaneous:* Anaphylactoid reaction, angioedema, breast pain, cheilitis, chills, dehydration, edema, epistaxis, exacerbation of untreated area, furunculosis, hernia, malaise, neck pain, photosensitivity reaction, procedural complication, routine procedure, tooth disorder, unintended pregnancy, vaginal moniliasis.

Overdosage

Tacrolimus ointment is not for oral use. Oral ingestion of tacrolimus ointment may lead to adverse effects associated with systemic administration of tacrolimus. If oral ingestion occurs, seek medical advice.

Patient Information

Use tacrolimus ointment as directed by the physician. It is for external use only. As with any topical medication, patients or caregivers should wash hands after application if hands are not an area for treatment.

Minimize or avoid exposure to natural or artificial sunlight (tanning beds or UVA/B treatment) while using tacrolimus ointment.

Do not use this medication for any disorder other than that for which it was prescribed.

Patients should report any signs of adverse reactions to their physician.

Before applying tacrolimus ointment after a bath or shower, be sure the skin is completely dry.

PIMECROLIMUS

Rx **Elidel** (Novartis) **Cream:** 1% In 30 and 100 g tubes.

Indications

➤*Mild to moderate atopic dermatitis:* Short-term and intermittent long-term therapy in the treatment of mild to moderate atopic dermatitis in nonimmunocompromised patients ≥ 2 years of age in whom the use of alternative, conventional therapies is deemed inadvisable because of potential risks, or in the treatment of patients who are not adequately responsive to or intolerant of alternative, conventional therapies.

Administration and Dosage

➤*Approved by the FDA:* December 13, 2001.

Apply a thin layer of pimecrolimus to the affected skin twice daily and rub in gently and completely. Pimecrolimus may be used on all skin surfaces, including the head, neck, and intertriginous areas.

Use pimecrolimus twice daily for as long as signs and symptoms persist. Discontinue treatment if resolution of disease occurs. If symptoms persist beyond 6 weeks, reevaluate patient. Do not use pimecrolimus with occlusive dressings.

➤*Storage / Stability:* Store at 25°C (77°F); excursions permitted to 15°C to 30°C (59° to 86°F). Do not freeze.

Actions

➤*Pharmacology:* Pimecrolimus is the 33-epi-chloro-derivative of the macrolactam ascomycin. Its mechanism of action in atopic dermatitis is not known. It has been demonstrated that pimecrolimus binds with high affinity to macrophilin-12 (FKBP-12) and inhibits the calcium-dependent phosphatase, calcineurin. As a consequence, it inhibits T-cell activation by blocking the transcription of early cytokines. In particular, pimecrolimus inhibits at nanomolar concentrations interleukin-2

PIMECROLIMUS

and interferon gamma (Th1-type) and interleukin-4 and interleukin-10 (Th2-type) cytokine synthesis in human T-cells. In addition, pimecrolimus prevents the release of inflammatory cytokines and mediators from mast cells in vitro after stimulation by antigen/IgE.

▶*Pharmacokinetics:*

Absorption – In adult patients treated for atopic dermatitis (13% to 62% body surface area [BSA] involvement) for periods up to 1 year, pimecrolimus blood concentrations are routinely either at or below the limit of quantification of the assay (< 0.5 ng/mL). In those subjects with detectable blood levels, they are routinely < 2 ng/mL and show no sign of drug accumulation with time.

Distribution – In vitro studies of the protein binding of pimecrolimus indicate that it is 74% to 87% bound to plasma proteins.

Metabolism – Following the administration of a single oral dose of pimecrolimus, numerous circulating O-demethylation metabolites were seen. Studies with human liver microsomes indicate that pimecrolimus is metabolized in vitro by the CYP3A subfamily of metabolizing enzymes. No evidence of skin-mediated drug metabolism was identified.

Excretion – Following a single oral dose of pimecrolimus ≈ 81% was recovered, primarily in the feces (78.4%) as metabolites; < 1% found in the feces was caused by unchanged pimecrolimus.

Contraindications

A history of hypersensitivity to pimecrolimus or any of the components of the cream.

Warnings

▶*Carcinogenesis:* In a 2-year rat dermal carcinogenicity study using pimecrolimus, a statistically significant increase in the incidence of follicular cell adenoma of the thyroid was noted in low-, mid-, and high-dose male animals compared with vehicle and saline control male animals. Follicular cell adenoma of the thyroid was noted in the dermal rat carcinogenicity study at the lowest dose of 2 mg/kg/day (0.2% pimecrolimus cream; 1.5 times the maximum recommended human dose [MRHD] based on AUC comparisons). Lymphoproliferative changes (including lymphoma) were noted in a 13-week repeat-dose dermal toxicity study conducted in mice using pimecrolimus in an ethanolic solution at a dose of 25 mg/kg/day (47 times the MRHD based on AUC comparisons). The latency time to lymphoma formation was shortened to 8 weeks after dermal administration of pimecrolimus dissolved in ethanol at a dose of 100 mg/kg/day (179 to 217 times the MRHD based on AUC comparisons).

In a mouse oral (gavage) carcinogenicity study, a statistically significant increase in the incidence of lymphoma was noted in high-dose male and female animals compared with vehicle control male and female animals. Lymphomas were noted in the oral mouse carcinogenicity study at a dose of 45 mg/kg/day (258 to 340 times the MRHD based on AUC comparisons). In an oral (gavage) rat carcinogenicity study, a statistically significant increase in the incidence of benign thymoma was noted in 10 mg/kg/day pimecrolimus-treated male and female animals compared with vehicle control-treated male and female animals. In addition, a significant increase in the incidence of benign thymoma was noted in another oral (gavage) rat carcinogenicity study in 5 mg/kg/day pimecrolimus-treated male animals compared with vehicle control treated male animals.

▶*Fertility impairment:* An oral fertility and embryofetal developmental study in rats revealed estrus cycle disturbances, postimplantation loss and reduction in litter size at the 45 mg/kg/day dose (38 times the MRHD based on AUC comparisons).

▶*Pregnancy: Category C.* There are no adequate and well-controlled studies of topically administered pimecrolimus in pregnant women. Use this drug during pregnancy only if clearly needed. The experience with pimecrolimus when used by pregnant women is too limited to permit assessment of the safety of its use during pregnancy.

A combined oral fertility and embryofetal developmental study was conducted in rats and an oral embryofetal developmental study was conducted in rabbits. Pimecrolimus was administered during the period of organogenesis (2 weeks prior to mating until gestational day 16 in rats, gestational days 6 to 18 in rabbits) up to dose levels of 45 mg/kg/day in rats and 20 mg/kg/day in rabbits. In the absence of maternal toxicity, indicators of embryofetal toxicity (postimplantation loss and reduction in litter size) were noted at 45 mg/kg/day (38 times the MRHD based on AUC comparisons) in the oral fertility and embryofetal developmental study conducted in rats.

▶*Lactation:* It is not known whether this drug is excreted in human milk. Because of the potential for serious adverse reactions in nursing infants from pimecrolimus, decide whether to discontinue nursing or to discontinue the drug, taking into account the importance of the drug to the mother.

▶*Children:* Pimecrolimus may be used in pediatric patients ≥ 2 years of age.

Precautions

▶*Dermal infections:* Do not apply pimecrolimus should not be applied to areas of active cutaneous viral infections. Before commencing treatment with pimecrolimus, clear clinical infections at treatment sites.

While patients with atopic dermatitis are predisposed to superficial skin infections including eczema herpeticum (Kaposi's varicelliform eruption), treatment with pimecrolimus may be associated with an increased risk of varicella zoster virus infection (chicken pox or shingles), herpes simplex virus infection, or eczema herpeticum. In the presence of these skin infections, evaluate the balance of risks and benefits associated with pimecrolimus use.

▶*Lymphadenopathy:* In clinical studies, 14 cases of lymphadenopathy (0.9%) were reported while using pimecrolimus cream. These cases usually were related to infections and noted to resolve upon appropriate antibiotic therapy. Of these 14 cases, the majority had a clear etiology or were known to resolve. In the absence of a clear etiology or in the presence of acute infectious mononucleosis, consider discontinuation of pimecrolimus. Monitor patients who develop lymphadenopathy to ensure that the lymphadenopathy resolves.

▶*Other skin disorders:* In clinical studies, 15 cases of skin papilloma or warts (1%) were observed in patients using pimecrolimus cream. In cases where there is worsening of skin papillomas or they do not respond to conventional therapy, consider discontinuation of pimecrolimus until complete resolution of the warts is achieved. The use of pimecrolimus in patients with Netherton syndrome is not recommended because of the potential for increased systemic absorption of pimecrolimus.

▶*Phototoxicity:* The enhancement of ultraviolet carcinogenicity is not necessarily dependent on phototoxic mechanism. Despite the absence of observed phototoxicity in humans, pimecrolimus shortened the time to skin tumor formation in an animal photocarcinogenicity study. Therefore, it is prudent for patients to minimize or avoid natural or artificial sunlight exposure.

Drug Interactions

Potential interactions between pimecrolimus and other drugs, including immunizations, have not been systematically evaluated. Because of the very low blood levels of pimecrolimus detected in some patients after topical application, systemic drug interactions are not expected, but cannot be ruled out. Coadminister known CYP3A inhibitors (eg, erythromycin, itraconazole, ketoconazole, fluconazole, calcium channel blockers, cimetidine) with caution in patients with widespread or erythrodermic disease.

Adverse Reactions

The use of pimecrolimus may cause local symptoms such as skin burning. Localized symptoms are most common during the first few days of application and typically improve as the lesions of atopic dermatitis resolve. Most application site reactions started within 1 to 5 days, were mild to moderate in severity, and lasted no more than 5 days.

Treatment Emergent Adverse Events in Pimecrolimus Treatment Groups (≥ 1%)						
	Pediatric patients[1] vehicle-controlled (6 weeks)		Pediatric patients[1] open-label (20 weeks)	Pediatric patients[1] vehicle-controlled (1 year)		Adult active comparator (1 year)
Adverse event	Pimecrolimus (n = 267)	Vehicle (n = 136)	Pimecrolimus (n = 335)	Pimecrolimus (n = 272)	Vehicle (n = 75)	Pimecrolimus (n = 328)
≥ 1 adverse event	68.2	71.3	72	84.6	74.7	78
Dermatological						
Skin infection NOS	3	5.1	5.4	2.2	4	6.4
Impetigo	1.9	2.2	3.6	4	5.3	2.4
Folliculitis	1.1	0.7	0.9	2.2	4	6.1
Molluscum contagiosum	0.7	0	1.2	1.8	0	0
Skin papilloma	0.4	0	0.6	3.3	< 1	0
Herpes simplex dermatitis	0	0	0.3	1.5	0	0.6
Urticaria	1.1	0	0.3	0.4	< 1	0.9
Acne NOS	0	0.7	0.3	1.5	< 1	1.8
GI						
Gastroenteritis NOS	0	2.2	0.6	7.4	2.7	1.8
Abdominal pain, upper	4.1	4.4	3	5.5	6.7	0.3
Sore throat	3.4	3.7	5.4	8.1	5.3	3.7
Vomiting NOS	3	4.4	4.2	6.6	8	0.6
Diarrhea NOS	1.1	0.7	0.6	7.7	5.3	2.1
Nausea	0.4	2.2	1.2	4	6.7	1.8
Abdominal pain NOS	0.4	0.7	1.5	4.4	4	0.3
Toothache	0.4	0.7	0.6	2.6	1.3	0.6
Constipation	0.4	0	0.6	3.7	< 1	0
Loose stools	0	0.7	1.2	< 1	< 1	0

PIMECROLIMUS

Treatment Emergent Adverse Events in Pimecrolimus Treatment Groups (≥ 1%)						
	Pediatric patients[1] vehicle-controlled (6 weeks)		Pediatric patients[1] open-label (20 weeks)	Pediatric patients[1] vehicle-controlled (1 year)		Adult active comparator (1 year)
Adverse event	Pimecrolimus (n = 267)	Vehicle (n = 136)	Pimecrolimus (n = 335)	Pimecrolimus (n = 272)	Vehicle (n = 75)	Pimecrolimus (n = 328)
Musculoskeletal						
Back pain	0.4	1.5	0.3	< 1	0	1.8
Arthralgias	0	0	0.3	1.1	1.3	1.5
Respiratory						
Upper respiratory tract infection NOS	14.2	13.2	19.4	4.8	8	4.3
Nasopharyngitis	10.1	7.4	19.6	26.5	21.3	7.6
Sinusitis	1.1	0.7	3.3	2.2	1.3	0.6
Pneumonia NOS	1.1	0.7	1.5	0	1.3	0.3
Pharyngitis NOS	0.7	1.5	0.9	8.1	2.7	0.9
Pharyngitis streptococcal	0.7	1.5	3	0	< 1	0
Bronchitis NOS	0.4	2.2	1.2	10.7	8	2.4
Upper respiratory tract infection viral NOS	0.4	0	0.9	1.5	0	0.3
Bronchitis acute NOS	0	0	0	1.5	0	0
Cough	11.6	8.1	9.3	15.8	10.7	2.4
Nasal congestion	2.6	1.5	1.8	1.5	1.3	0.6
Rhinorrhea	1.9	0.7	0.9	0.4	1.3	0
Asthma aggravated	1.5	2.2	3.9	1.1	1.3	0
Sinus congestion	1.1	0.7	0.6	< 1	< 1	0.9
Rhinitis	0.4	0	1.5	4.4	6.7	2.1
Wheezing	0.4	0.7	1.2	0.7	< 1	0
Asthma NOS	0.7	0.7	3.3	3.7	2.7	2.4
Epistaxis	0	0.7	0	3.3	1.3	0.3
Dyspnea NOS	0	0	0	1.8	1.3	0.6
Special senses						
Ear infection NOS	2.2	1.5	5.7	3.3	1.3	0.6
Otitis media	2.2	0.7	3	2.9	5.3	0.6
Eye infection NOS	0	0	0	1.1	< 1	0.3
Conjunctivitis NEC	0.7	0.7	2.1	2.2	4	3
Earache	0.7	0.7	0	2.9	2.7	0

Treatment Emergent Adverse Events in Pimecrolimus Treatment Groups (≥ 1%)						
	Pediatric patients[1] vehicle-controlled (6 weeks)		Pediatric patients[1] open-label (20 weeks)	Pediatric patients[1] vehicle-controlled (1 year)		Adult active comparator (1 year)
Adverse event	Pimecrolimus (n = 267)	Vehicle (n = 136)	Pimecrolimus (n = 335)	Pimecrolimus (n = 272)	Vehicle (n = 75)	Pimecrolimus (n = 328)
Miscellaneous						
Influenza	3	0.7	6.6	13.2	4	9.8
Bacterial infection	1.5	2.2	1.2	1.1	0	1.8
Staphylococcal infection	0.4	3.7	2.1	0	< 1	0.9
Herpes simplex	0.4	0	1.2	3.3	2.7	4
Tonsillitis NOS	0.4	0	0.9	6.3	0	0.6
Viral infection NOS	0.7	0.7	0.3	6.6	1.3	0
Chickenpox	0.7	0	0.9	2.9	4	0.3
Tonsillitis acute NOS	0	0	0	2.6	0	0
Application site burning	10.4	12.5	1.5	8.5	6.7	25.9
Pyrexia	7.5	8.8	12.2	12.5	5.3	1.2
Application site reaction NOS	3	5.1	2.1	3.3	2.7	14.6
Application site irritation	3	5.9	0.9	0.4	4	6.4
Influenza-like illness	0.4	0	0.6	1.8	2.7	1.8
Application site erythema	0.4	0	0	2.2	0	2.1
Application site pruritus	1.1	1.5	0.6	1.8	0	5.5
Dysmenorrhea	1.1	0	1.5	1.1	1.3	1.2
Hypersensitivity NOS	4.1	4.4	4.8	5.1	1.3	3.4
Accident NOS	1.1	0.7	0.3	< 1	1.3	0
Laceration	0.7	0.7	1.5	< 1	< 1	0
Headache	13.9	8.8	11.3	25.4	16	7

[1] 2 to 17 years of age.
NOS = Not otherwise specified.

Overdosage

There has been no experience with pimecrolimus overdose. No incidents of accidental ingestion have been reported. If oral ingestion occurs, seek medical advice.

Patient Information

Pimecrolimus is for external use on the skin only. Wash hands after application if hands are not an area for treatment. Pimecrolimus may cause local reactions such as mild to moderate feeling of warmth or sensation of burning. See a physician if an application site reaction is severe or persists for > 1 week.

Minimize or avoid exposure to natural or artificial sunlight (tanning beds or UVA/B treatment) while using pimecrolimus.

Discontinue therapy after signs and symptoms of atopic dermatitis have resolved. Resume treatment at the first signs of recurrence.

Contact the physician if no improvement in the atopic dermatitis is seen following 6 weeks of treatment, or if at any time the condition worsens.

DICLOFENAC SODIUM

Rx	**Solaraze** (SkyePharma)	**Gel:** 3%[1]	Benzyl alcohol. In 25 and 50 g.

[1] 1 g contains 30 mg diclofenac sodium

For information on CNS and ophthalmic/otic uses of diclofenac sodium, refer to individual monographs.

Indications

➤*Actinic keratoses (AK):* For the topical treatment of AK. Sun avoidance is indicated during therapy.

Administration and Dosage

Apply gel to lesion areas twice daily. It is to be smoothed onto the affected skin gently. The amount needed depends upon the size of the lesion site. Assure that enough gel is applied to adequately cover each lesion. Normally, 0.5 g of gel is used on each 5 cm × 5 cm lesion site. The recommended duration of therapy is from 60 to 90 days. Complete healing of the lesion(s) or optimal therapeutic effect may not be evident for up to 30 days following cessation of therapy. Lesions that do not respond to therapy must be carefully reevaluated and management reconsidered.

➤*Storage/Stability:* Store at controlled room temperatures (15° to 30°C; 59° to 86°F). Protect from heat. Avoid freezing.

Actions

➤*Pharmacology:* The mechanism of action of diclofenac in the treatment of AK is unknown. The contribution to efficacy of individual components of the vehicle has not been established.

➤*Pharmacokinetics:*

Absorption – When diclofenac is applied topically, it is absorbed into the epidermis. In a study in patients with compromised skin (mainly atopic dermatitis and other dermatitic conditions) of the hands, arms, or face, ≈ 10% of the applied dose (2 g of 3% gel over 100 cm^2) of diclofenac was absorbed systemically in normal and compromised epidermis after 7 days, with 4 times daily applications.

After topical application of 2 g diclofenac 3 times daily for 6 days to the calf of the leg in healthy subjects, diclofenac could be detected in plasma. The systemic bioavailability after topical application of diclofenac is lower than after oral dosing.

Blood drawn at the end of treatment from 60 patients with AK lesions treated with topical diclofenac in 3 adequate and well-controlled clinical trials were assayed for diclofenac levels. Each patient was administered 0.5 g diclofenac gel twice a day for ≤ 105 days. There were ≤ three 5 cm × 5 cm treatment sites per patient on the face, forehead, hands, forearm, and scalp. Serum concentrations of diclofenac were on the average ≤ 20 ng/ml. These data indicate that systemic absorption of diclofenac in patients treated topically with diclofenac is much lower than that occurring after oral daily dosing of diclofenac sodium.

No information is available on the absorption of diclofenac when it is used under occlusion.

Distribution – Diclofenac binds tightly to serum albumin. Diclofenac's volume of distribution following oral administration is ≈ 550 ml/kg.

Metabolism – Biotransformation of diclofenac following oral administration involves conjugation at the carboxyl group of the side chain or single or multiple hydroxylations resulting in several phenolic metabolites, most of which are converted to glucuronide conjugates. Two of these phenolic metabolites are biologically active; however, to a much smaller extent than diclofenac. Metabolism following topical administration is thought to be similar to that after oral administration. The small amounts of diclofenac and its metabolites appearing in the plasma following topical administration makes the quantification of specific metabolites imprecise.

Excretion – Diclofenac and its metabolites are excreted mainly in the urine after oral dosing. Systemic clearance of diclofenac from plasma is ≈ 263 ml/min. The terminal plasma half-life is 1 to 2 hours. Four of the metabolites also have short terminal half-lives of 1 to 3 hours.

Contraindications

Patients with a known hypersensitivity to diclofenac, benzyl alcohol, polyethylene glycol monomethyl ether 350, or hyaluronate sodium.

Warnings

➤*Hypersensitivity reactions:* As with other NSAIDs, anaphylactoid reactions may occur in patients without prior exposure to diclofenac. Administer diclofenac with caution to patients with the aspirin triad. The triad typically occurs in asthmatic patients who experience rhinitis with or without nasal polyps, or who exhibit severe, potentially fatal bronchospasm after taking aspirin or other NSAIDs.

➤*Carcinogenesis:* A photocarcinogenicity study with ≤ 0.035% diclofenac in the vehicle gel was conducted in hairless mice at topical doses ≤ 2.8 mg/kg/day. Median tumor onset was earlier in the 0.035% group.

➤*Elderly:* Of the 211 subjects treated with diclofenac in controlled clinical studies, 143 subjects were ≥ 65 years of age. Of those 143 subjects, 55 subjects were ≥ 75 years of age. No overall differences in safety or effectiveness were observed between these subjects and younger subjects, and other reported clinical experience has not identified differences in responses between the elderly and younger patients, but greater sensitivity of some older individuals cannot be ruled out.

➤*Pregnancy: Category B.* The safety of diclofenac gel has not been established during pregnancy. However, reproductive studies performed with diclofenac alone at oral doses ≤ 20 mg/kg/day (15 times the estimated systemic human exposure) in mice, 10 mg/kg/day (15 times the estimated systemic human exposure) in rats, and 10 mg/kg/day (30 times the estimated systemic human exposure) in rabbits have revealed no evidence of teratogenicity despite the induction of maternal toxicity. In rats, maternally toxic doses were associated with dystocia, prolonged gestation, reduced fetal weights and growth, and reduced fetal survival.

Diclofenac has been shown to cross the placental barrier in mice and rats. However, there are no adequate and well-controlled studies in pregnant women. Because animal reproduction studies are not always predictive of human response, do not use during pregnancy unless the benefits to the mother justify the potential risk to the fetus. Because of the risk to the fetus resulting in premature closure of the ductus arteriosus, avoid diclofenac in late pregnancy.

The effects of diclofenac on labor and delivery in pregnant women are unknown. Because of the known effects of prostaglandin-inhibiting drugs on the fetal cardiovascular system (closure of ductus arteriosus), avoid use of diclofenac during late pregnancy. As with other NSAIDs, it is possible that diclofenac may inhibit uterine contractions and delay parturition.

➤*Lactation:* Because of the potential for serious adverse reactions in nursing infants from diclofenac, a decision should be made whether to discontinue nursing or to discontinue the drug, taking into account the importance of the drug to the mother.

➤*Children:* AK is not a condition seen within the pediatric population; do not use diclofenac gel in children.

Precautions

➤*Monitoring:* Do not allow gel to come in contact with the eyes. The safety of the concomitant use of sunscreens, cosmetics, or other topical medications and diclofenac is unknown.

➤*Special risk:* Use diclofenac gel with caution in patients with active GI ulceration or bleeding and severe renal or hepatic impairments. Do not apply to open skin wounds, infections, or exfoliative dermatitis.

Drug Interactions

Although the systemic absorption of diclofenac is low, minimize concomitant oral administration of other NSAIDs such as aspirin at anti-inflammatory/analgesic doses.

Adverse Reactions

Of the 423 patients evaluable for safety in adequate and well-controlled trials, 211 were treated with diclofenac and 212 were treated with vehicle gel. Eighty-seven percent of the diclofenac-treated patients and 84% of the vehicle-treated patients experienced ≥ 1 adverse reactions during the studies. The majority of these reactions were mild-to-moderate in severity and resolved upon discontinuation of therapy.

Of the 211 patients treated with diclofenac, 82% experienced adverse reactions involving skin and the application site compared to 75% of the vehicle-treated patients. Application site reactions were the most frequent adverse reactions in both groups. Contact dermatitis, rash, dry skin, and exfoliation (scaling) were significantly more prevalent in the diclofenac group than in the vehicle-treated patients.

Eighteen percent of diclofenac-treated patients and 4% of vehicle-treated patients discontinued from the clinical trials because of adverse reactions (whether considered related to treatment or not). These discontinuations were mainly caused by skin irritation or related cutaneous adverse reactions.

DICLOFENAC SODIUM

Adverse Reactions Reported During Diclofenac Phase 3 Clinical Trials for 60- and 90-day Treatments (%)				
	60-day treatment		90-day treatment	
Adverse reaction	Diclofenac (n = 48)	Gel vehicle (n = 49)	Diclofenac (n = 114)	Gel vehicle (n = 114)
Cardiovascular				
Chest pain	2	0	1	0
Hypertension	2	0	1	0
Phlebitis	0	2	0	0
CNS				
Anxiety	0	2	0	1
Dizziness	0	0	0	4
Hypokinesia	2	0	0	0
Headache	0	6	7	6
Migraine	0	2	1	0
Dermatologic				
Acne	0	2	0	1
Application site reaction	75	71	84	70
Acne	0	4	1	0
Alopecia	2	0	1	1
Contact dermatitis	19	4	33	4
Dry skin	27	12	25	17
Edema	4	0	3	0
Exfoliation	6	4	24	13
Hyperesthesia	0	0	3	1
Pain	15	22	26	30
Paresthesia	8	4	20	20
Photosensitivity reaction	0	2	3	0
Pruritus	31	59	52	45
Rash	35	20	46	17
Vesiculobullous rash	0	0	4	1
Contact dermatitis	2	0	0	0
Dry skin	0	4	3	0
Herpes simplex	0	2	0	0
Maculopapular rash	0	2	0	0
Pain	2	2	1	0
Pruritus	4	6	4	1
Rash	2	10	4	0
Skin carcinoma	0	6	2	2
Skin nodule	0	2	0	0
Skin ulcer	2	0	1	0
GI				
Abdominal pain	2	0	1	0
Constipation	0	0	0	2
Diarrhea	2	0	2	3
Dyspepsia	2	0	3	4
Lab test abnormalities				
Increased creatine phosphokinase	0	0	4	1
Increased creatinine	2	2	0	1
Hypercholesteremia	0	2	1	0
Hyperglycemia	0	2	1	0
AST increased	0	0	3	0
ALT increased	0	0	2	0
Musculoskeletal				
Back pain	4	0	2	2
Arthralgia	2	0	0	2
Arthrosis	2	0	0	0
Myalgia	2	0	3	1
Respiratory				
Asthma	2	0	0	0
Dyspnea	2	0	2	0
Pharyngitis	2	8	2	4
Pneumonia	2	0	0	1
Rhinitis	2	2	2	2
Sinusitis	0	0	2	0
Miscellaneous				
Accidental injury	0	0	4	2
Allergic reaction	0	0	1	3
Asthenia	0	0	2	0
Chills	0	2	0	0
Edema	0	2	0	0
Flu syndrome	10	6	1	4
Infection	4	6	4	5
Neck pain	0	0	2	0
Pain	2	0	2	2
Conjunctivitis	2	0	4	1
Eye pain	0	2	2	0
Hematuria	0	0	2	1
Procedure	0	0	0	3

DICLOFENAC SODIUM

▶*Dermatologic:* Skin hypertrophy, paresthesia, seborrhea, urticaria, application site reactions (skin carcinoma, hypertonia, skin hypertrophy lacrimation disorder, maculopapular rash, purpuric rash, vasodilation) (< 1%).

Overdosage

▶*Symptoms:* Because of the low systemic absorption of topically applied diclofenac gel, overdosage is unlikely.

▶*Treatment:* In the event of oral ingestion of diclofenac gel, resulting in significant systemic side effects, it is recommended that the stomach be emptied by vomiting or lavage. Forced diuresis may theoretically be beneficial because the drug is excreted in the urine. The effect of dialysis or hemoperfusion in the elimination of diclofenac (99% protein-bound) remains unproven. In addition to supportive measures, the use of oral activated charcoal may help to reduce the absorption of diclofenac. Give supportive and symptomatic treatment for complications such as renal failure, convulsions, GI irritation, and respiratory depression.

Patient Information

In clinical studies, localized dermal side effects such as contact dermatitis, exfoliation, dry skin, and rash were found in patients treated with diclofenac at a higher incidence than in those with placebo.

Patients should understand the importance of monitoring and follow-up evaluation, the signs and symptoms of dermal adverse reactions, and the possibility of irritant or allergic contact dermatitis. If severe dermal reactions occur, treatment with diclofenac may be interrupted until the condition subsides.

Avoid exposure to sunlight and the use of sunlamps.

Safety and efficacy of the use of diclofenac together with other dermal products, including cosmetics, sunscreens, and other topical medications on the area being treated have not been studied.

SALICYLIC ACID

otc	**Panscol** (Baker Cummins)	**Ointment:** 3%	In 90 g.
otc	**MG217 Sal-Acid Ointment** (Triton)	**Ointment:** 3% with vitamin E	In 2 oz.
otc	**Fostex** (Bristol Products)	**Cream:** 2% with etetic acid, stearyl alcohol	In 118 g.
Rx	**Salex** (Healthpoint)	**Cream:** 6%	Alcohols, glycerin, parabens. In 400 g bottles.
otc	**Panscol** (Baker Cummins)	**Lotion:** 3%	In 120 ml.
otc	**Fung-O** (S.S.S. Company)	**Liquid:** 17% salicylic acid, 2% alcohol and 68% ether	In 15 ml w/drop applicator.
otc	**Mosco** (Medtech)	**Liquid:** 17.6% in a flexible collodion base with 33% alcohol and 65.5% ether	In 10 ml.
otc	**Dr Scholl's Wart Remover Kit** (Schering-Plough)	**Liquid:** 17% in a flexible collodion with 17% alcohol, 52% ether, acetone	In 10 ml with brush and cushions.
otc	**Occlusal-HP** (GenDerm)	**Liquid:** 17% in a polyacrylic vehicle with isopropyl alcohol	In 10 ml with brush applicator.
otc	**Compound W** (Whitehall)	**Liquid:** 17% with collodion, 21.2% alcohol, 63.6% ether, camphor, castor oil, menthol	In 9 ml.
otc	**DuoFilm** (Schering-Plough)	**Liquid:** 17% in flexible collodion with 15.8% alcohol, castor oil, 42.6% ether	In 15 ml with brush applicator.
otc	**Maximum Strength Wart Remover** (Glades)	**Liquid:** 17% with 29% alcohol, castor oil in a flexible collodion	In 13.3 ml with applicator.
otc	**Off-Ezy Wart Remover Kit** (Del Pharm)	**Liquid:** 17% in collodion-like vehicle with 21% alcohol and 65% ether, acetone	In 13.5 ml with skin buffer and applicator.
otc	**Off-Ezy Corn & Callus Remover Kit** (Del Pharm)	**Liquid:** 17% in collodion-like vehicle with 21% alcohol and 65% ether, acetone	In 13.5 ml with callus smoother and corn cushions.
otc	**Wart-Off** (Pfizer)	**Liquid:** 17% in flexible collodion with 26.35% alcohol, propylene glycol dipelargonate	In 15 ml with applicator.
otc	**Salactic Film** (Pedinol)	**Liquid:** 17% in collodion-like vehicle	In 15 ml with brush applicator.
otc	**Gordofilm** (Gordon)	**Liquid:** 16.7% in flexible collodion	In 15 ml with brush applicator.
otc	**Freezone** (Whitehall)	**Liquid:** 13.6% in a collodion-like vehicle, 20.5% alcohol, 64.8% ether, castor oil	In 9 ml.
otc	**Dr Scholl's Corn/Callus Remover** (Schering-Plough)	**Liquid:** 12.6% in flexible collodion with 18% alcohol, 55% ether, acetone, hydrogenated vegetable oil	In 10 ml with 3 cushions.
otc	**Sal-Plant** (Pedinol)	**Gel:** 17% in collodion-like vehicle	In 14 g.
otc	**Compound W** (Whitehall)	**Gel:** 17% with 67.5% alcohol, camphor, castor oil, collodion, colloidal silicon dioxide, hydroxypropyl cellulose, hypophosphorous acid, polysorbate 80	In 7 g.
otc	**DuoPlant** (Schering-Plough)	**Gel:** 17% in flexible collodion with 57.6% alcohol, 16.42% ether, ethyl lactate, hydroxypropyl cellulose, polybutene	In 14.2 g.
otc	**Keralyt** (Summers)	**Gel:** 6%, 21% SD-40 alcohol	In 28.4 g.
otc	**Psor-a-set** (Hogil)	**Soap:** 2%	In 97.5 g.
otc	**DuoFilm** (Schering-Plough)	**Transdermal Patch:** 40% in a rubber-based vehicle	In 18s (containing 3 sizes).
otc	**Trans-Ver-Sal PlantarPatch** (Doak)	**Transdermal Patch:** 15% with karaya, PEG-300, propylene glycol, quaternium-15	20 mm patches in 25s with 25 securing tapes and one emery file.
otc	**Trans-Ver-Sal PediaPatch** (Doak)	**Transdermal Patch:** 15% in karaya gum base	In 6 mm (20s) with bandage tapes.
otc	**Trans-Ver-Sal AdultPatch** (Doak)	**Transdermal Patch:** 15% with karaya, PEG-300, propylene glycol, quaternium-15	6 or 12 mm patches in 40s with 42 securing tapes and one emery file.
otc	**Mediplast** (Beiersdorf)	**Plaster:** 40%	2″ x 3″ patches in 2s and 25s.
otc	**Dr Scholl's Advanced Pain Relief Corn Removers** (Schering-Plough)	**Disk:** 40% in a rubber-based vehicle	In 6s with cushions.
otc	**Dr Scholl's Callus Removers** (Schering-Plough)		In 4s with 6 pads and 4s with 4 pads (extra-thick).
otc	**Dr Scholl's Clear Away Plantar** (Schering-Plough)		In 24s with cushions.
otc	**Dr Scholl's Clear Away** (Schering-Plough)		In 18s with cover-up disks.
otc	**Dr Scholl's Corn Removers** (Schering-Plough)		In 9s (pads and disks) as regular, extra-thick, soft, small, waterproof and ultra-thin and 6s (pads and disks) as wrap-around.
otc	**Dr Scholl's Moisturizing Corn Remover Kit** (Schering-Plough)		In 6s with moisturizing cream and cushions.
otc	**Dr Scholl's Clear Away OneStep** (Schering-Plough)	**Strips:** 40% in a rubber-based vehicle	In 14s.
otc	**Dr Scholl's OneStep Corn Removers** (Schering-Plough)		In 6s.
otc	**Compound W for Kids** (Medtech)	**Pad:** 40% in a plaster vehicle	Lanolin, rubber. In 12s.

Indications

A topical aid in the removal of excessive keratin in hyperkeratotic skin disorders, including common and plantar warts, psoriasis, calluses and corns.

▶*Unlabeled uses:* The use of a 40% salicylic acid disk covered with an adhesive strip has been used to aid in the removal of inaccessible splinters in children.

Administration and Dosage

For specific instructions for use of these products, refer to individual product labeling.

Apply to affected area. May soak in warm water for 5 minutes prior to use to hydrate skin and enhance the effect. Remove any loose tissue with brush, wash cloth or emery board and dry thoroughly.

In general, for treatment of warts, improvement should occur in 1 to 2 weeks; maximum resolution may be expected after 4 to 6 weeks,

SALICYLIC ACID

although application for up to 12 weeks may be necessary. If skin irritation develops or there is no improvement after several weeks, contact a physician.

➤**Storage / Stability:** Some products are flammable; keep away from fire or flame. Keep bottle tightly capped and store at room temperature away from heat.

Actions

➤**Pharmacology:** Salicylic acid is the only *otc* product considered safe and effective by the FDA for use as a keratolytic for corns, calluses and warts. Salicylic acid produces desquamation of the horny layer of skin, while not affecting the structure of the viable epidermis, by dissolving intercellular cement substance. The keratolytic action causes the cornified epithelium to swell, soften, macerate and then desquamate.

Salicylic acid is keratolytic at concentrations of ≈ 2% to 6%. These concentrations are generally used for treatment of dandruff, seborrhea and psoriasis. Concentrations of 5% to 17% in collodion are safe and effective for the removal of common and plantar warts; up to 40% in plasters is used to remove warts, corns and calluses.

Salicylic acid preparations, alone or in combination, have also been used to treat dandruff, seborrheic dermatitis, acne, tinea infections and psoriasis.

➤**Pharmacokinetics:** In a study of the percutaneous absorption of salicylic acid in four patients with extensive active psoriasis, peak serum salicylate levels never exceeded 5 mg/dl even though > 60% of the applied salicylic acid was absorbed. Systemic toxic reactions are usually associated with much higher serum levels (30 to 40 mg/dl). Peak serum levels occurred within 5 hours of the topical application under occlusion.

The major urinary metabolites identified after topical administration differ from those after oral salicylate administration; those derived from percutaneous absorption contain more salicylate glucuronides (42%) and less salicyluric (52%) and salicylic acid (6%).

Contraindications

Sensitivity to salicylic acid; prolonged use, especially in infants, diabetics and patients with impaired circulation; use on moles, birthmarks or warts with hair growing from them, genital or facial warts or warts on mucous membranes, irritated skin or any area that is infected or reddened.

Warnings

➤**Salicylate toxicity:** Prolonged use over large areas, especially in young children and those patients with significant renal or hepatic impairment, could result in salicylism. Limit the area to be treated and be aware of signs of salicylate toxicity (eg, nausea, vomiting, dizziness, loss of hearing, tinnitus, lethargy, hyperpnea, diarrhea, psychic disturbances). In the event of salicylic acid toxicity, discontinue use.

Refer to the Salicylates monograph in the CNS Drugs chapter for additional information on the systemic effects of salicylates.

➤**Special risk patients:** Do not use if diabetic or poor blood circulation exists.

➤**Pregnancy:** Category C. There are no adequate and well controlled studies in pregnant women. Use during pregnancy only if the potential benefit justifies the potential risk to the fetus.

Precautions

➤**For external use only:** Avoid contact with eyes, mucous membranes and normal skin surrounding warts. If contact with eyes or mucous membranes occurs, immediately flush with water for 15 minutes. Avoid inhaling vapors.

Drug Interactions

Interactions have been reported with both topical and oral salicylates. Refer to the Salicylates monograph for a complete listing.

Adverse Reactions

Local irritation may occur from contact with normal skin surrounding the affected area. If irritation occurs, temporarily discontinue use and take care to apply only to wart site when treatment is resumed.

Patient Information

For external use only. Avoid contact with eyes, face, genitals, mucous membranes and normal skin surrounding warts.

Medication may cause reddening or scaling of skin when used on open skin lesions.

Contact with clothing, fabrics, plastics, wood, metal or other materials may cause damage; avoid contact.

SULFUR PREPARATIONS

otc	**Sulpho-Lac Acne Medication** (Doak)	**Cream:** 5% sulfur	27% zinc sulfate, 53% Vleminckx's solution base. Greaseless. In 28.35 and 50 g.
otc	**Acne Lotion 10** (C & M)	**Lotion:** 10% colloidal sulfur	22.5% isopropyl alcohol. Tinted. Aqueous. In 60 ml.
otc	**Liquimat** (Galderma)	**Lotion:** 4% sulfur	22% SD alcohol 40, cetyl alcohol. Assorted tints. In 45 ml.
otc	**Sulpho-Lac** (Doak)	**Soap:** 5% sulfur	In a coconut and tallow oil soap base. In 85 g.
otc	**Sulmasque** (C & M)	**Mask:** 6.4% sulfur	With 15% isopropyl alcohol, methylparaben. In 150 g.

Indications

➤**Acne:** An aid in the treatment of mild acne and oily skin.

Administration and Dosage

Apply a thin layer. Use 1 to 3 times daily. For best results, wash skin thoroughly with a mild cleanser prior to application.

Actions

➤**Pharmacology:** Sulfur, a keratolytic, provides peeling and drying actions. Although it may help to resolve comedones, it may also promote the development of new ones by increasing horny cell adhesion.

Precautions

For external use only. Avoid contact with eyes. Certain individuals may be sensitive to one or more components. If undue skin irritation develops or increases, discontinue use and consult physician.

➤**Concomitant treatment:** Using other topical acne medications at the same time or immediately following sulfur products may increase dryness or irritation of the skin. If this occurs, use only one medication unless otherwise directed.

Patient Information

Keep away from the eyes.

May cause irritation of the skin; discontinue use and notify physician if this occurs.

KERATOLYTIC AGENT COMBINATION

otc	**Gets-It** (Oakhurst)	**Liquid:** Salicylic acid, zinc chloride and collodion in ≈ 35% ether and ≈ 28% alcohol	In 12 ml.

ACNE PRODUCTS, COMBINATIONS

		Sulfur	Salicylic Acid	Resorcinol	Other Content	How Supplied
otc	**Finac Lotion** (C & M)		2%		22.5% isopropyl alcohol, propylene glycol, acetone	In 60 ml.
otc	**PROPApH Cleansing Lotion for Normal/Combination Skin** (Del)		0.5%		SD alcohol 40, menthol, EDTA	In 180 ml (lotion) and 45s (pads).
otc	**PROPApH Cleansing Pads** (Del)		0.5%		SD alcohol 40, EDTA, menthol	In 45s.
otc	**PROPApH Cleansing for Oily Skin Lotion** (Del)		0.6%		SD alcohol 40, EDTA, menthol	In 180 ml.
Rx	**Clenia Cream** (Upsher-Smith)	5%			10% sodium sulfacetamide, parabens, EDTA	In 28 g tubes.
Rx	**Clenia Foam** (Upsher-Smith)	5%			10% sodium sulfacetamide, parabens, EDTA	In 170 and 340 mg bottles.
Rx	**Rosac Cream** (Stiefel)	5%			10% sodium sulacetamide, benzyl alcohol, cetostearyl alcohol, EDTA	In 45 g.
Rx	**Sodium Sulfacetamide 10% and Sulfur 5%** (Glades)	5%			10% sodium sulfacetamide, cetyl alcohol, benzyl alcohol, EDTA	In 30 ml tube and 25 ml.
Rx	**Zetacet Topical Suspension** (Stiefel)	5%			10% sodium sulfacetamide, cetyl alcohol, benzyl alcohol, EDTA	In 30 g.
Rx	**Avar Cleanser** (Sirius)	5%			10% sodium sulfacetamide, cetyl alcohol, stearyl alcohol	In 226.8 g.
Rx	**Avar Gel** (Sirius)	5%			10% sodium sulfacetamide, EDTA, benzyl alcohol	In 45 g.
Rx	**Avar Green Gel** (Sirius)	5%			10% sodium sulfacetamide, EDTA, benzyl alcohol	For color correction. In 45 g.
Rx	**Plexion Cleanser** (Medicis)	5%			10% sodium sulfacetamide, cetyl alcohol, stearyl alcohol, EDTA, parabens	In 170 and 340 g.
Rx	**Plexion SCT Cream** (Medicis)	5%			10% sodium sulfacetamide, witch hazel, benzyl alcohol	In 120 g.
Rx	**Rosanil Cleanser** (Galderma)	5%			10% sodium sulfacetamide, EDTA, light mineral oil, parabens	In 170 g.
Rx	**Rosula Gel** (Doak)	5%			10% sodium sulfacetamide in a 10% urea vehicle	In 45 mL.
Rx	**Vanocin** (Stratus)	5%			10% sodium sulfacetamide, benzyl alcohol, cetyl alcohol, EDTA, parabens, stearyl alcohol	In 30 and 60 g.
Rx	**Sulfacet-R Lotion** (Dermik)	5%			10% sodium sulfacet amide, parabens	Tinted. In 25 ml.
Rx	**Nicosyn Lotion** (Sirius[1])	5%			10% sodium sulfacetamide, glycerin, cetyl alcohol, zinc oxide, benzyl alcohol, EDTA	In 45 g.
Rx	**Novacet Lotion** (Genderm)	5%			10% sodium sulfacetamide, cetyl alcohol, benzyl alcohol, EDTA, sodium thiosulfate	In 30 ml.
otc	**Acno Lotion** (Baker Cummins)	3%				Greaseless. In 120 ml.
otc	**Therac Lotion** (C & M)	10%[2]				In 60 ml.
otc	**Acnotex Lotion** (C & M)	8%	2%		20% isopropyl alcohol	In 60 ml.
otc	**Acnomel Cream** (Numark)	8%	2%		11% alcohol	In 28 g.
otc	**Adult Acnomel Cream** (Numark)	8%	2%		15% alcohol, propylene glycol	Tinted. In 28 g.
otc	**Medicated Acne Cleanser** (C & M)	4%	2%			In 129 g.
otc	**Sulforcin Lotion** (Galderma)	5%	2%		11.65% SD alcohol 40, methylparaben	In 120 ml.
otc	**Rezamid Lotion** (Summers)	5%	2%		28% alcohol	In 56.7 ml.
otc	**R/S Lotion** (Summers)					In 56.7 ml.
otc	**Clearasil Clearstick Maximum Strength** (Procter & Gamble)		2%		39% alcohol, menthol, EDTA	For regular and sensitive skin. In 35 ml.
otc	**Clearasil Double Clear Maximum Strength Pads** (Procter & Gamble)		2%		40% alcohol, witch hazel distillate, menthol	In 32s.
otc	**Fostex Acne Cleansing Cream** (Westwood Squibb)		2%		Stearyl alcohol, EDTA	In 118 g.
otc	**Oxy Night Watch Maximum Strength Lotion** (SK-Beecham)		2%		Cetyl alcohol, EDTA, parabens, stearyl alcohol	In 60 ml.

ACNE PRODUCTS, COMBINATIONS

	Sulfur	Salicylic Acid	Resorcinol	Other Content	How Supplied
otc **PROPApH Acne Maximum Strength Cream** (Del)		2%		Lanolin alcohol, cetearyl alcohol, EDTA, menthol, stearyl alcohol	In 19.5 g.
otc **Sal-Clens Acne Cleanser Gel** (C & M)		2%			In 240 g.
otc **Sebasorb Lotion** (Summers)		2%		10% attapulgite	In 45 ml.
otc **Stridex Clear Gel** (Sterling Health)		2%		9.3% SD alcohol	In 30 g.
otc **Clearasil Clearstick Regular Strength** (Procter & Gamble)		1.25%		39% alcohol, aloe vera gel, menthol, disodium EDTA	In 35 ml.
otc **Clearasil Double Clear Pads Regular Strength** (Procter & Gamble)		1.25%		40% alcohol, witch hazel distillate, menthol	In 32s.
otc **Oxy Night Watch Sensitive Skin Lotion** (SK-Beecham)		1%		Cetyl alcohol. EDTA, stearyl alcohol, parabens	In 60 ml.
otc **RA Lotion** (Medco Lab)			3%	43% alcohol	In 120, 240 and 480 ml.
otc **Clearasil Adult Care Cream** (Procter & Gamble)				Sulfur, resorcinol, 10% alcohol, parabens	In 17 g.
otc **Fostril Lotion** (Westwood Squibb)				Sulfur, zinc oxide, parabens, EDTA	In 28 ml.
Rx **Klaron** (Dermik)				10% sodium sulfacetamide, propylene glycol, polyethylene glycol 400, methylparaben, EDTA	In 59 ml.

[1] Sirius Laboratories, Inc., 100 Fairway Drive, Suite 130, Vernon Hills, IL 60061; (847) 968–2424. [2] As colloidal sulfur.

Ingredients

These products contain keratolytics and astringents to aid in removing keratin and to dry the skin. Many products also have hydroalcoholic or organic solvent bases to aid in removal of sebum. Individual components include:

➤*ANTIMICROBIAL:* Sodium thiosulfate and sodium sulfacetamide.

➤*ANTISEPTIC:* Ethanol, isopropyl alcohol, phenol, sulfur and acetone.

➤*KERATOLYTICS:* Salicylic acid, resorcinol and sulfur.

➤*PROTECTIVES and ADSORBANTS:* Zinc oxide.

Hydrocortisone-containing acne products are listed under Topical Corticosteroid Combinations.

In addition to the single entity products listed in this section, other products containing topical local anesthetics are listed in other sections, based on their specific uses. These include: Anorectal Preparations and Ophthalmic Local Anesthetics (see individual monographs).

Indications

Because of the diversity of uses of these products, the following is a general discussion. For information on specific applications of individual products, consult the manufacturer's package literature.

➤*Skin disorders:* For topical anesthesia in local skin disorders, including: Pruritus and pain due to minor burns, skin manifestations of systemic disease (eg, chickenpox), prickly heat, abrasions, sunburn, plant poisoning, insect bites, eczema; local analgesia on normal, intact skin (EMLA).

➤*Mucous membranes:* For local anesthesia of accessible mucous membranes, including: Oral, nasal and laryngeal mucous membranes; respiratory or urinary tracts. Also for the treatment of pruritus ani, pruritus vulvae and hemorrhoids.

Administration and Dosage

➤*Topical:* Apply to the affected area as needed. Ointments and creams can be applied to gauze or to a bandage prior to applying to the skin.

➤*Mucous membranes:* Dosage varies and depends upon the area to be anesthetized, vascularity of tissues, individual tolerance and technique of anesthesia. Administer the lowest dose possible that still provides adequate anesthesia. Apply to affected areas using the proper technique (see individual manufacturer inserts).

In debilitated, elderly patients or children, administer lower concentrations.

A combination of tetracaine 0.5%, epinephrine 1:2000 and cocaine 11.8% (also known as TAC) in a liquid topical formulation has been used for minor skin lacerations, especially of the face and scalp. Other preparations include cocaine 11.8% and epinephrine 1:1000, and lidocaine 4%, epinephrine 1:1000 and tetracaine 0.5%, both utilizing methylcellulose for a more viscous gel formulation. Use results in decreased pain on application, allowing for better compliance and tolerance of repair procedure. This may be beneficial in patients who cannot tolerate injection anesthesia or those who are difficult to control (eg, children). A commercial preparation of lidocaine and prilocaine (EMLA) was developed for a similar purpose (increased absorption in children) on intact skin. However, toxic effects are also more likely to occur in infants and children with all of these preparations.

The use of the lidocaine/prilocaine combination appears to be beneficial as a pretreatment in decreasing the pain of DPT vaccinations (and presumably other vaccinations) in infants. The cream is applied at the injection site with occlusive dressing for at least 60 minutes prior to the vaccination.

Actions

➤*Pharmacology:* Local anesthetics inhibit conduction of nerve impulses from sensory nerves. This action results from an alteration of the cell membrane permeability to ions. Although poorly absorbed through the intact epidermis (except for the lidocaine/prilocaine mixture; penetration and subsequent systemic absorption is enhanced over use of each agent alone), these agents are readily absorbed from mucous membranes. When skin permeability has been increased by abrasions or ulcers, the absorption and, subsequently, the efficacy of local anesthetics improves; however, the incidence of side effects also increases. Onset, depth and duration of dermal analgesia provided by the lidocaine/prilocin mixture depends primarily on duration of application.

Topical Local Anesthetics: Indications, Dose, Strength, Peak Effect and Duration						
Local anesthetics, topical	Indications		Maximum adult dose (mg)	Available or recommended strengths (%)	Peak[1] effect (minutes)	Duration[1] of effect (minutes)
	Skin	Mucous membrane				
Amides						
Dibucaine	✔		25	0.5-1	< 5	15-45
Lidocaine	✔	✔	†[2]	2-5	2-5	15-45
Esters						
Benzocaine	✔	✔		0.5-20	< 5	15-45
Butamben picrate	✔			1		
Cocaine		✔	50-200	4-10	1-5	30-60
Tetracaine	✔	✔	50	0.5-2	3-8	30-60
Miscellaneous						
Dyclonine		✔	100	0.5-1	< 10	< 60
Pramoxine	✔		200	1	3-5	
Lidocaine/Prilocaine	✔			2.5/2.5	60-120	60-120

[1] Based primarily on application to mucous membranes.

[2] Variable depending on doseform.

Contraindications

Hypersensitivity to any component of these products; ophthalmic use.

Warnings

➤*Systemic effects:* Use the lowest dose effective for anesthesia to avoid high plasma levels and serious adverse effects. Repeated doses of **lidocaine** and **dyclonine** may cause significant increases in blood levels with each repeated dose because of slow accumulation of the drug or its metabolites. Have resuscitative equipment available for immediate use. Lidocaine/prilocaine is not recommended for use on mucous membranes because of its much greater absorption through this area than through intact skin, potentially resulting in serious adverse effects.

➤*Methomoglobinemia:* **Benzoacaine**, **lidocaine** and **prilocaine** should not be used in those rare patients with congenital or idiopathic methemoglobinemia and in infants < 12 months of age who are receiving treatment with methemoglobin-inducing agents. Very young patients or patients with glucose-6–phosphate deficiencies are more susceptible to methemoglobinemia.

➤*Ototoxic effects:* **Lidocaine/prilocaine** has an ototoxic effect when instilled into the middle ear of animals, but not when used in the external auditory canal. Do not use this combination in any situation where penetration or migration beyond the tympanic membrane into the middle ear is possible.

➤*Hepatic function impairment:* Patients with severe hepatic disease, because of their inability to metabolize local anesthetics normally, are at greater risk of developing toxic plasma concentrations of lidocaine and prilocaine.

➤*Pregnancy: Category B* (lidocaine); *Category C* (benzocaine, cocaine, dyclonine, tetracaine). Safety for use during pregnancy has not been established. Use in women of childbearing potential, and particularly in early pregnancy, only when the potential benefits outweigh the potential hazards to the fetus.

➤*Lactation:* Lidocaine, and probably prilocaine, are excreted in breast milk. Exercise caution when administering any of these drugs to a nursing woman.

➤*Children:* Safety and efficacy of dyclonine and tetracaine have not been established in children < 12 years of age. Do not use benzocaine in infants < 1 year of age. Dosages in children should be reduced commensurate with age, body weight and physical condition.

Precautions

➤*For external or mucous membrane use only:* Do not use in the eyes.

➤*Minimal effective dose:* Reactions and complications are best averted by using the minimal effective dose. Not for prolonged use. Give debilitated or elderly patients, acutely ill patients and children dosages commensurate with their age, size and physical condition.

➤*Severe shock / heartblock:* Use **lidocaine** and **dyclonine** with caution.

➤*Traumatized mucosa:* Use cautiously in persons with known drug sensitivities or in patients with severely traumatized mucosa and sepsis in the region of the application. If irritation or rash occurs, discontinue treatment and institute appropriate therapy.

➤*Oral use:* Topical anesthetics may impair swallowing and enhance danger of aspiration. Do not ingest food for 1 hour after anesthetic use in mouth or throat. This is particularly important in children because of their frequency of eating.

➤*Tartrazine sensitivity:* Some of these products contain tartrazine, which may cause allergic-type reactions (including bronchial asthma) in susceptible individuals. Although the incidence of tartrazine sensitivity in the general population is low, it is frequently seen in patients who also have aspirin hypersensitivity. Specific products containing tartrazine are identified in the product listings.

➤*Sulfite sensitivity:* Some of these products contain sulfites which may cause allergic-type reactions including anaphylactic symptoms and life-threatening or less severe asthmatic episodes in certain susceptible persons. The overall prevalence of sulfite sensitivity in the general population is unknown and probably low. Sulfite sensitivity is seen more frequently in asthmatic or atopic non-asthmatic persons. Specific products containing sulfites are identified in the product listings.

Drug Interactions

➤*Class I antiarrhythmic agents:* Use with caution in patients receiving Class I antiarrhythmic drugs (such as tocainide and mexiletine) because the toxic effects are additive and potentially synergistic.

➤*Drug/Lab test interactions:* Dyclonine topical solutions should not be used in cystoscopic procedures folliwng intravenous pyelography because an iodine precipitate occurs which interferes with visualization.

Adverse Reactions

Adverse reactions are, in general, dose-related and may result from high plasma levels due to excessive dosage or rapid absorption, hypersensitivity, idiosyncrasy or diminished tolerance. (See Overdosage.)

➤*Hypersensitivity:* Cutaneous lesions; urticaria; edema; contact dermatitis; bronchospasm; shock; anaphylactoid reactions. The detection of sensitivity by skin testing is of doubtful value.

➤*Local:* Burning; stinging; tenderness; sloughing.

➤*Miscellaneous:* Urethritis with and without bleeding. In a few case reports, methemoglobinemia characterized by cyanosis has followed topical application of **benzocaine** or **lidocaine/prilocaine** and may be more common with prilocaine (see Warnings). Seizures in children have occurred from overuse of **oral lidocaine**.

Overdosage

➤*Symptoms:* Reactions due to overdosage (high plasma levels) are systemic and involve the CNS (convulsions) or the cardiovascular system (hypotension).

CNS – Reactions are excitatory or depressant, and may be characterized by: Nervousness; apprehension; euphoria; confusion; dizziness; lightheadedness; tinnitus; blurred vision; vomiting; sensations of heat, cold or numbness; twitching; tremors; drowsiness; convulsions; unconsciousness; respiratory depression or arrest. Excitatory reactions may be very brief or not occur at all; in this case, first sign of toxicity may be drowsiness, merging into unconsciousness and respiratory arrest.

Cardiovascular – Reactions are depressant, and may be characterized by: Hypotension; myocardial depression; bradycardia; cardiac arrest; cardiovascular collapse.

➤*Treatment:* Maintain airway and support ventilation. Cardiovascular support consists of vasopressors, preferably those that stimulate the myocardium, IV fluids and perhaps blood transfusions. Control convulsions by slow IV of 0.1 mg/kg diazepam or 10 to 50 mg succinylcholine, with continued use of oxygen. Refer to General Management of Acute Overdosage.

Methemoglobinemia – This may be treated with methylene blue 1%, 1 to 2 mg/kg IV over 10 minutes (refer to individual monograph).

Patient Information

Do not ingest food for 1 hour following use of oral topical anesthetic preparations in the mouth or throat. Topical anesthesia may impair swallowing, thus enhancing the danger of aspiration.

Numbness of the tongue or buccal mucosa may increase the danger of biting trauma. Do not eat or chew gum while the mouth or throat area is anesthetized.

When lidocaine/prilocaine is used, the patient should be aware that the production of dermal analgesia may be accompanied by the block of all senstions in the treated skin. For this reason, the patient should avoid inadvertent trauma to the treated area by scratching, rubbing, or exposure to extreme hot or cold temperatures until complete sensation has returned.

Amide Local Anesthetics

DIBUCAINE

otc	**Dibucaine** (Various, eg, IDE, Moore)	Ointment: 1%	In 30 g.
otc	**Nupercainal** (Ciba Consumer)		Acetone, sodium bisulfite, lanolin, mineral oil, white petrolatum. In 30 and 60 g.
otc	**Nupercainal** (Ciba Consumer)	Cream: 0.5%	Acetone, sodium bisulfite, glycerin. In 42.5 g.

Complete prescribing information begins in the Local Anesthetics, Topical group monograph.

LIDOCAINE HCl

otc	**Zilactin-L** (Zila)	**Liquid:** 2.5%	79.3% alcohol. In 10 ml.
Rx	**Numby Stuff** (Iomed)	**Solution, topical:** 2% For iontophoretic dermal delivery.	1:100,000 epinephrine/30 ml multiple-unit fliptop vial.
Rx	**LidoSite Topical System** (Vyteris)	**Patch:** 10% for iontophoretic delivery.	0.1% edpinephrine, EDTA, sodium metabisulfite. Topical system includes 1 **Lidosite** controller and 25 **Lidosite** patches.
Rx	**Lidocaine HCl** (Moore)	**Ointment:** 5%	In 50 g.
otc	**Solarcaine Aloe Extra Burn Relief** (Schering-Plough)	**Cream:** 0.5%	Aloe, lanolin oil, lanolin, camphor, propylparaben, eucalyptus oil, EDTA, menthol, tartrazine. In 120 g.
Rx	**LidaMantle** (Doak Dermatologics)	**Cream:** 3%	Cetyl alcohol, stearyl alcohol, glycerin, petrolatum, parabens, light mineral oil. In 28 and 85 g.
otc	**L-M-X4** (Ferndale)	**Cream:** 4% (40 mg/g)	Benzyl alcohol. In 5 and 30 g.
otc	**Solarcaine Aloe Extra Burn Relief** (Schering-Plough)	**Gel:** 0.5%	Aloe vera gel, glycerin, EDTA, isopropyl alcohol, menthol, diazolidinyl urea, tartrazine. In 120 and 240 g.
otc	**Burn-O-Jel** (S.S.S. Company)		Aloe vera gel, EDTA, glycerin, ethyl alcohol. In 85 g.
otc	**DermaFlex** (Zila)	**Gel:** 2.5%	79% alcohol. In 15 g.
otc	**Solarcaine Aloe Extra Burn Relief** (Schering-Plough)	**Spray:** 0.5%	Aloe vera gel, glycerin, EDTA, diaolidinyl urea, vitamin E, parabens. In 135 mg.
Rx	**Lidocaine HCl Topical**[1] (Various, eg, Moore, Roxane)	**Solution:** 4% For topical anesthesia of accessible mucous membranes of the oral and nasal cavities and proximal portions of the digestive tract.	In 50 ml.[1]
Rx	**Xylocaine** (Astra)		Parabens. In 50 ml.
Rx	**Lidocaine 2% Viscous**[2] (Various, eg, Moore, Roxane)	**Solution:** 2% For topical anesthesia of irritated or inflamed mucous membranes of the mouth and pharynx. Also used to reduce gagging during the taking of x-rays or dental impressions.	In 50 and 100 ml and UD 20 ml.[1,2,3]
Rx	**Xylocaine Viscous** (Astra)		Sodium carboxymethylcellulose, parabens, saccharin. In 100 and 450 ml.
Rx	**Anestacon** (PolyMedica)	**Jelly:** 2% For prevention and control of pain in procedures involving the male and female urethra, for topical treatment of painful urethritis and as an anesthetic lubricant for endotracheal intubation.	1% hydroxypropylmethylcellulose, 0.01% benzalkonium chloride. In 15 and 240 ml disposable units.
Rx	**Lidocaine HCl** (IMS)	**Jelly:** 2%	Preservative-free. In UD 5, 10, and 20 mL single-use vials. In 25s.
Rx	**Dentipatch** (Noven)	**Patch:** 23/2 cm² patch For production of mild topical anesthesia of accessible muous membranes of the mouth prior to superficial dental procedures.	Aspartame. In 50s or 100s.
		46.1/2 cm² patch For production of mild topical anesthesia of accessible mucous membranes of the mouth prior to superficial dental procedures.	Aspartame. In 50s and 100s.
Rx	**Lidoderm** (Endo)	**Patch:** 10 × 14 cm. 5% lidocaine. For relief of pain associated with postherpetic neuralgia	EDTA, glycerin, parabens, polyvinyl alcohol. In 5s.

[1] May contain parabens.
[2] May contain sodium carboxymethylcellulose.
[3] May contain saccharin.

Complete prescribing information begins in the Local Anesthetics, Topical group monograph.

Ester Local Anesthetics

BENZOCAINE

otc	**Americaine Anesthetic** (Fisons)	**Spray:** 20%	In 60 ml.
otc	**Boil-Ease** (Del)	**Ointment:** 20% with camphor, lanolin, eucalyptus oil, menthol, petrolatum, phenol	In 30 g.
otc	**Dermoplast** (Whitehall-Robins)	**Spray:** 20% with 0.5% menthol, methylparaben, aloe, lanolin	In 82.5 ml.
otc	**Lanacane** (Combe)	**Spray:** 20% with 0.1% benzethonium Cl, 36% ethanol, aloe extract	In 113 ml.
otc	**Solarcaine Medicated First Aid Spray** (Schering-Plough)	**Spray:** 20% with 0.13% triclosan, alcohol	In 90 ml.
otc	**Dermoplast** (Whitehall-Robins)	**Lotion:** 8% with 0.5% menthol, aloe, glycerin, parabens, lanolin	In 90 ml.
otc	**Solarcaine** (Schering-Plough)	**Aerosol:** 20% with 0.13% triclosan, 35% SD alcohol 40, tocopheryl acetate	In 90 and 120 ml.
otc	**Bicozene** (Sandoz)	**Cream:** 6% with 1.67% resorcinol, castor oil, glycerin	In 30 g.
otc	**Foille Plus** (Blistex)	**Aerosol:** 20% with 12% alcohol	In 105 ml.
otc	**Foille** (Blistex)	**Spray:** 5% with 0.63% chloroxylenol	In 97.5 ml.
otc	**Benzocaine** (Various, eg, IDE)	**Cream:** 5%	In 480 g.
otc	**Foille Medicated First Aid** (Blistex)	**Ointment:** 5% with 0.1% chloroxylenol, benzyl alcohol, EDTA in corn oil base	In 3.5 and 28 g.
		Aerosol: 5% with 0.6% chloroxylenol, benzyl alcohol in corn oil base	In 92 ml.
otc	**Chigger-Tox** (Scherer)	**Liquid:** Benzocaine with benzyl benzoate and green soap in an isopropanol base	In 30 ml.
otc	**Solarcaine** (Schering-Plough)	**Lotion:** Benzocaine with triclosan, mineral oil, alcohol, aloe extract, tocopheryl acetate, menthol, camphor, parabens, EDTA	In 120 ml.
otc	**Lanacane** (Combe)	**Cream:** 6% with 0.1% benzethonium Cl, aloe, parabens, castor oil, glycerin, isopropyl alcohol	In 28 and 56 g.
otc	**Maximum Strength Anbesol** (Whitehall)	**Liquid:** 20%	50% alcohol, saccharin. In 9 ml.
otc	**Hurricaine** (Beutlich)	**Gel:** 20%	60% alcohol, saccharin. In 7 g.
		Spray: 20% For oral and mucosal anesthesia to conrol pain and suppress the gag reflex.	Cherry flavor. In 60 ml.
Rx	**Americaine Anesthetic Lubricant** (Fisons)	**Gel:** 20% For use as a lubricant and anesthetic on intratracheal catheters and pharyngeal and nasal airways; on nasogastric and endoscopic tubes; urinary catheters; laryngoscopes; proctoscopes; sigmoidoscopes; vaginal specula.	0.1% benzethonium chloride. In 30 g and UD 2.5 g.
otc	**Orajel Mouth-Aid** (Del)	**Liquid:** 20%	0.1% cetylpyridinium Cl, 70% ethyl alcohol, tartrazine, saccharin. in 13.5 ml.
		Gel: 20%	0.02 benzalkonium Cl, 0.1% zinc Cl, EDTA, saccharin. In 5.6 and 10 g.

Complete prescribing information begins in the Local Anesthetics, Topical group monograph.

COCAINE

c-ii	**Cocaine HCl** (Roxane)	**Topical Solution:** 4%	In 10 ml multidose and UD 4 ml.
		10%	In 10 ml multidose and UD 4 ml.
c-ii	**Cocaine Viscous** (Roxane)	**Topical Solution:** 4%	In 10 ml multidose and UD 4 ml.
		10%	In 10 ml multidose bottles and UD 4 ml.
c-ii	**Cocaine HCl** (Mallinckrodt)	**Powder**	In 5 and 25 g.

Indications

Topical anesthesia for mucous membranes.

Administration and Dosage

Reduce dosages for children and for elderly and debilitated patients. Cocaine solution can be given by means of cotton applicators or packs, instilled into a cavity or as a spray.

For topical application (ear, nose, throat, bronchoscopy), concentrations of 1% to 4% are used. As a general guide, the maximum single dose should be 1 mg/kg. Concentrations > 4% are not advisable because of the potential for increased incidence and severity of systemic toxic reactions.

Actions

➤*Pharmacology:* Cocaine is an alkaloid derived from the plant *Erythroxylon coca*; chemically, it is benzoylmethylecgonine. Following local application, cocaine blocks the initiation or conduction of the nerve impulse and causes intense vasoconstriction. It not only lessens sensibility to pain and touch but, when applied to the nose or mouth, diminishes the acuity of taste and smell. Its most striking systemic effect is general CNS stimulation, manifested in descending order of frequency as euphoria, stimulation, reduced fatigue, loquacity, sexual stimulation, increased mental ability, alertness and increased sociality. As the dose is increased, tremors and tonic-clonic convulsions may occur. In addition, vomiting centers may also be stimulated. Central stimulation is soon followed by depression. The medullary centers are eventually depressed; death results from respiratory failure.

Small doses of cocaine may slow the heart as a result of central sympathetic stimulation, but after moderate doses, the heart rate increases. Although blood pressure may finally fall, there is at first a prominent rise in blood pressure due to sympathetically mediated tachycardia and vasoconstriction.

Cocaine is markedly pyrogenic. It increases muscular activity which augments heat production; vasoconstriction decreases heat loss. Cocaine may also have a direct action on central heat regulating centers.

Cocaine interferes with the uptake of norepinephrine and dopamine by the presynaptic adrenergic nerve terminals; therefore, it may produce sensitization to catecholamines, causing vasoconstriction and mydriasis.

➤*Pharmacokinetics:*

Absorption/Distribution – Cocaine is rapidly absorbed from all sites of application and absorption is enhanced in the presence of inflammation. When it is applied to mucous membranes, maximum local anesthesia occurs within 5 minutes. A 10% cocaine solution (1.5 mg/kg) applied to nasal mucosa yielded peak plasma levels in 15 to 60 minutes that declined over 3 to 5 hours. Peak effects occur in 2 to 5 minutes, persisting for 30 minutes. Absorption from mucous membranes may exceed the rate of metabolism and excretion.

Metabolism/Excretion – Cocaine is degraded in the liver to its principal metabolite, benzoylecgonine, which is then excreted in the urine. Cocaine is also metabolized by plasma cholinesterase. At therapeutic doses, < 20% is excreted unchanged in the urine. Half-life is approximately 1 to 2.5 hours.

COCAINE

For comparative data of cocaine with other local anesthetics, refer to the Topical Local Anesthetics group monograph.

Contraindications

Systemic use; hypersensitivity to cocaine; ophthalmologic anesthesia (see Warnings).

Warnings

➤**Dependence:** Although cocaine does not produce true physical dependence with definite withdrawal symptoms, continual exposure creates an excessively strong psychological dependence, and sometimes depression, as an indirect effect. Chronic use may cause progression from euphoria to paranoid psychosis; included may be perceptual changes (halo lights) and intense pruritus ("cocaine bugs"). This drug produces the highest degree of psychic dependence seen among recreationally abused drugs; thus, cocaine does produce an addictive syndrome.

"Crack" – This is a form of cocaine that is prepared with ammonia to alkalinize the solution and precipitate alkaloidal cocaine, thereby making it suitable for smoking. This form of cocaine is widely abused, highly addictive and potentially lethal.

Treatment of dependence – In addition to behavior modification and supportive psychotherapy, several agents may help decrease withdrawal symptoms associated with cocaine abuse or dependence, including: Amantadine; bromocriptine; desipramine; mazindol; carbamazepine.

➤**Systemic effects:** Concentrations > 4% are not advisable because of the potential for increasing the incidence and severity of systemic toxic reactions.

➤**Ophthalmic use:** Cocaine causes sloughing of the corneal epithelium, causing clouding, pitting and occasionally, ulceration of the cornea. Ophthalmic use is contraindicated.

➤**Elderly:** Because elderly patients with vascular disease may be sensitive to the vasoconstrictive effects of the drug and may have slowed cocaine metabolism, a lower dosage is recommended.

➤**Pregnancy:** *Category C.* Cocaine use/abuse can lead to major toxicity in the mother, fetus and neonate. Consider cocaine abuse by a pregant woman as possibly teratogenic. Cocaine causes placental vasoconstriction, decreasing blood flow to the fetus. An increase in uterine contractility has occurred. A study compared 23 women who used cocaine only (n = 12) or cocaine plus narcotics (n = 11) during pregnancy with a group of women who were on methadone (n = 15) and a control group (n = 15). There was a higher rate of spontaneous abortion in the cocaine group. In addition, infants exposed to cocaine had depression of interactive behavior and a poor organizational response to environmental stimuli. In one retrospective trial, pregnant women who used "crack" delivered infants who were more likely to have a birth weight and head circumference under the tenth percentile for their gestational age. Other fetal effects noted following maternal cocaine use include growth retardation, fetal distress, cerebrovascular accidents and congential anomalies. Abnormal mild neurobehavioral signs (eg, irritability, muscular rigidity, tremulousness) were also more prevalent after birth, and GI symptoms (eg, nausea, vomiting) have occurred.

Women who use cocaine during pregnancy are at significant risk for shorter gestations, premature delivery, spontaneous abortions, abruptio placentae and death. Use only when clearly needed.

➤**Lactation:** Safety for use in the nursing mother has not been established. In one report, benzoylecgonine was detected in breast milk for up to 36 hours after the mother's last dose. Cocaine and its metabolite have been found in the urine of an infant following breastfeeding. Several case reports indicated that infants exposed via breastfeeding may develop symptoms of cocaine toxicity (eg, irritability, tremulousness, increased startle responese).

Because of the potential for serious adverse reactions in nursing infants from cocaine, it is recommended that nursing be discontinued during cocaine use. Strongly discourage cocaine use during breastfeeding. The American Academy of Pediatrics considers cocaine to be contraindicated during breastfeeding.

➤**Children:** Safety and efficacy for use in children have not been established. See Lactation.

Convulsions have occurred in infants, who may be especially susceptible to cocaine-induced toxicity.

Precautions

➤**Limit administration:** Limit to office and surgical procedures. Safety and efficacy depends on proper dosage, correct technique, adequate precautions and readiness for emergencies.

➤**Traumatized mucosa:** Use with caution in patients with severely traumatized mucosa and sepsis in the region of the proposed application.

Adverse Reactions

➤**Cardiovascular:** Small doses of cocaine slow the heart rate; after moderate doses, the rate is increased due to central sympathetic stimulation. Hypertension, tachycardia, tachypnea and myocardial ischemia may occur.

➤**CNS:** Reactions are excitatory or depressant. Nervousness, restlessness, euphoria, excitement, tremors and tonic-clonic convulsions may result. Central stimulation is followed by depression, with death resulting from respiratory failure.

Overdosage

➤**Symptoms:** Toxicity may occur following ingestion, parenteral administration, inhalation or absorption from topical administration to mucous membranes. Initial symptoms of acute poisoning are anxiety, restlessness, excitability, hallucinations, tachycardia, dilated pupils, chills or fever, abdominal pain, nausea, vomiting, numbness and muscular spasm, followed by irregular respirations, convulsions, coma and circulatory failure. If acute poisoning ends in death, it occurs quickly, from minutes to a maximum of 3 hours.

Chronic poisoning may be similar, but long-term changes involve mental deterioration, weight loss, change of character and perhaps, perforated nasal septum from chronic sniffing of cocaine.

Fatal dose – 500 mg to 1.2 g orally. Severe toxic effects have occurred with doses as low as 20 mg.

➤**Treatment:** Maintain airway and respiration. If drug was ingested, attempt delay of absorption with activated charcoal, gastric lavage or emesis. Limit absorption from an injection site by tourniquet or ice pack. Control convulsions with diazepam (0.1 mg/kg orally or slow IV) or 2.5% thiopental sodium slowly IV; in severe cases, use pancuronium bromide or succinylcholine with mechanical ventilation. The drug of choice for tachycardia and other arrhythmias is propranolol (1 mg slowly IV, every 5 minutes, up to a dose of 5 to 8 mg) or lidocaine 1 mg/minute IV.

Maintain blood pressure with fluids (vasopressors are hazardous). For hypertensive reactions, give phentolamine, 5 mg slowly IV. Treat hyperthermia if it occurs.

Refer to General Management of Acute Overdosage. If the patient survives the first 3 hours after acute poisoning, recovery is likely.

TETRACAINE HCl

otc	**Cepacol Viractin** (J.B. Williams)	**Gel:** 2%	Parabens. In 7.1 g.
		Cream: 2%	Hydrochloric acid, methylparaben. In 7.1 g.

Complete prescribing information begins in the Local Anesthetics, Topical group monograph.

PRAMOXINE HCl

otc	**AmLactin AP** (Upsher-Smith)	**Cream:** 1%	12% lactic acid, light mineral oil, cetyl alcohol, glycerin, parabens. In 140 g.
otc	**Prax** (Ferndale)		Hydrophilic base with glycerin, cetyl alcohol, white petrolatum. In 30, 113.4 g and 1 lb.
otc	**Tronothane HCl** (Abbott)		Water miscible base with cetyl alcohol, glycerin, parabens. In 28.4 g.
otc	**Prax** (Ferndale)	**Lotion:** 1%	Hydrophilic base with mineral oil, cetyl alcohol, glycerin, lanolin, 0.1% potassium sorbate, 0.1% sorbic acid. In 15, 120 and 240 ml.
otc	**PrameGel** (Bioglan)	**Gel:** 1%	Emollient base with 0.5% menthol, benzyl alcohol, SD alcohol 40. In 118 g.
otc	**Itch-X** (Ascher & Co.)		10% benzyl alcohol, aloe vera gel, diazolidinyl urea, SD alcohol 40, parabens. In 35.4 g.
otc	**Itch-X** (Ascher & Co.)	**Spray:** 1%	10% benzyl alcohol, aloe vera gel, SD alcohol 40. In 60 ml.
otc	**Bactine Pain Relieving Cleansing** (Bayer)	**Wipes:** 1%	0.13% benzalkonium chloride, EDTA. In 16s.

Complete prescribing information begins in the Local Anesthetics, Topical group monograph.

LOCAL ANESTHETICS, TOPICAL COMBINATIONS

otc	**Detane** (Del)	**Gel:** 7.5% benzocaine, carbomer 940, PEG 400	In 15 g.
otc	**Sting-Kill** (Kiwi)	**Swabs:** 18.9% benzocaine, 0.9% menthol	In 0.5 & 14 ml.
Rx	**Cetacaine** (Cetylite)	14% benzocaine, 2% tetracaine HCl, 2% butamben and 0.5% benzalkonium chloride with 0.005% cetyl dimethyl ethyl ammonium bromide in a bland water soluble base	**Gel:** In 29 g.
			Liquid: In 56 ml.
			Ointment: In 37 g.
			Aerosol: In 56 g.
otc	**Aerocaine** (Aeroceuticals)	**Aerosol:** 13.6% benzocaine with 0.5% benzethonium Cl	In 15 and 75 ml.
otc	**Aerotherm** (Aeroceuticals)		In 150 ml.
otc	**Anbesol** (Whitehall)	**Liquid:** 6.3% benzocaine with 0.5% phenol, povidone-iodine, 70% alcohol, camphor, menthol	In 9.3 & 22.2 ml.
		Gel: 6.3% benzocaine, 0.5% phenol, 70% alcohol	In 7.5 g.
Rx	**EMLA** (Astra)	**Cream:** 2.5% lidocaine, 2.5% prilocaine	In 5 g with *Tegaderm* dressings and 30 g.
otc	**Vagisil** (Combe)	**Cream:** Benzocaine and resorcin with lanolin alcohol, parabens, trisodium HEDTA, mineral oil and sodium sulfite	In 30 and 60 g.
otc	**Unguentine Maximum Strength** (Lee)	**Cream:** 5% benzocaine, 2% resorcinol.	Alcohols, methylparaben, mineral oil. In 28.3 g.
otc	**Chiggerex** (Scherer)	**Ointment:** Benzocaine with camphor, menthol	In 50 g.
otc	**Skeeter Stik** (Triton)	**Liquid:** 4% lidocaine with 2% phenol in an isopropyl alcohol base	In 14 ml.
otc	**Bactine Pain Relieving Cleansing** (Bayer)	**Spray:** 2.5% lidocaine, 0.13% benzalkonium chloride, EDTA	In 150 mL.
otc	**Bactine Antiseptic Anesthetic** (Bayer)	2.5% lidocaine HCl, 0.13% benzalkonium chloride, EDTA, 3.17% alcohol	**Aerosol:** In 90 g.
			Spray: In 60, 120 and 480 ml.
otc	**Unguentine Plus** (Mentholatum)	**Cream:** 2% lidocaine HCl with 2% chloroxylenol and 0.5% phenol, parabens, mineral oil	In 30 g.
otc	**Medi-Quik** (Mentholatum)	**Aerosol:** Lidocaine HCl and benzalkonium chloride	In 90 ml.
		Spray: 2% lidocaine, 0.13% benzalkonium chloride, 0.2% camphor, benzyl alcohol	In 85 ml.
otc	**Dr. Scholl's Cracked Heel Relief** (Schering-Plough)	**Cream:** 2% lidocaine, 0.13% benzethonium Cl	Aloe. In 89 ml.
otc	**ProTech First-Aid Stik** (Triton)	**Liquid:** 2.5% lidocaine HCl, 10% povidone iodine	In 14 ml dab-on applicator.
otc	**TheraPatch Cold Sore** (LecTec)	**Patch:** 4% lidocaine HCl, 0.5% camphor, aloe vera, eucalyptus oil, glycerin	In 21s.
Rx	**EMLA Anesthetic** (Astra-Zeneca)	**Disc:** 1 g EMLA emulsion (2.5% lidocaine, 2.5% prilocaine). Contact surface ≈ 10 cm^2	In 2s and 10s.
otc	**Campho-Phenique Cold Sore Treatment and Scab Relief** (Bayer)	**Cream:** 1% pramoxine hydrochloride	30% petrolatum, alcohols, EDTA, glycerin, parabens, ureas. Mint flavor. In 6.5 g.

Refer to the general discussion of these products beginning in the Local Anesthetics, Topical group monograph.

MISCELLANEOUS TOPICAL ANESTHETICS

Rx	**Ethyl Chloride** (Gebauer)	**Spray:** Chloroethane **Indications:** Topical vapo-coolant to control pain associated with minor surgical procedures (eg, lancing boils, incision and drainage of small abscesses), athletic injuries, injections and for treatment of myofascial pain, restricted motion and muscle spasm	In 100 g metal tubes, 105 ml "Spra-Pak" and 120 ml bottles (fine, medium and coarse spray).
Rx	**Fluro-Ethyl** (Gebauer)	**Aerosol spray:** 25% ethyl chloride and 75% dichlorotetrafluoroethane **Indications:** Topical refrigerant anesthetic to control pain associated with minor surgical procedures, dermabrasion, injections, contusions and minor strains	In 270 ml.
Rx	**Fluori-Methane** (Gebauer)	**Spray:** 15% dichlorodifluoromethane and 85% trichloromonofluoromethane **Indications:** Vapo-coolant for topical application in management of myofascial pain, restricted motion and muscle spasm, and for control of pain associated with injections	In 105 ml glass bottles (fine or medium spray).
otc	**Aerofreeze** (Graham-Field)	**Spray:** Trichloromonofluoromethane and dichlorodifluoromethane **Indications:** Topical anesthesia for preinjection, skin planing, dermabrasion and minor surgical procedures; for treatment of strains, sprains and muscle spasms	In 240 ml.

Complete prescribing information begins in the Local Anesthetics, Topical group monograph.

MINOXIDIL

otc	**Rogaine** (Pharmacia & Upjohn)	**Solution: 2%**	In 60 ml bottle with multiple applicators.
otc	**Minoxidil Extra Strength for Men** (Apotex)	**Solution: 5%**	30% alcohol. In 60 mL bottles (1s and 2s).
otc	**Rogaine Extra Strength for Men** (Pharmacia & Upjohn)		Alcohol. In two 60 ml bottles w/ dropper and sprayer applicators.

Indications

Treatment of androgenetic alopecia, expressed in males as baldness of the vertex of the scalp and in females as diffuse hair loss or thinning of the frontoparietal areas. At least 4 months of twice daily applications are generally required before evidence of hair growth can be expected.

➤*Unlabeled uses:* Although further study is needed, topical minoxidil may be useful in the treatment of alopecia areata (a systemic disease in which patches of hair fall out over a period of a few days; any part of the body may be involved).

Administration and Dosage

Dry the hair and scalp prior to application. Apply 1 ml to the total affected areas of the scalp twice daily, once in the morning and at night. The total daily dosage should not exceed 2 ml. If finger tips are used to facilitate drug application, wash hands afterwards. Twice daily application for ≥ 4 months may be required before evidence of hair regrowth is observed. Onset and degree of hair regrowth may be variable among patients. If hair regrowth is realized, twice daily applications are necessary for additional and continued hair regrowth. Some anecdotal patient reports indicate that regrown hair and the balding process return to their untreated state 3 to 4 months following cessation of the drug.

➤*Other topical agents:* Do not use in conjunction with other topical agents including topical corticosteroids, retinoids and petrolatum or agents that are known to enhance cutaneous drug absorption.

Actions

➤*Pharmacology:* Minoxidil topical solution stimulates vertex hair growth in individuals with alopecia androgenetica, expressed in males as baldness of the vertex of the scalp and in females as diffuse hair loss or thinning of the frontoparietal areas. There is no effect in patients with predominantly frontal hair loss. The mechanism is not known, but like minoxidil, some other arterial dilating drugs also stimulate hair growth when given systemically.

In placebo controlled trials involving > 3500 male patients given topical minoxidil for 4 months (longer treatment was given after the placebo group was discontinued), and in > 300 female patients given topical minoxidil for 8 months, typical systemic effects of oral minoxidil (weight gain, edema, tachycardia, fall in blood pressure and their more serious consequences) did not occur more frequently in patients given topical minoxidil than in those given topical placebo.

To study the potential for systemic effects of topical minoxidil, three concentrations (1%, 2% and 5%) applied twice daily were compared to low oral doses (2.5 and 5 mg given once daily) and placebo in hypertensive patients in a double-blind controlled trial. The 5 mg oral dose had readily detectable effects, including a fall in diastolic pressure of about 5 mm Hg and an increase in heart rate of 7 bpm. No other group had a clear effect, although there was some evidence of a weak and inconsistent effect in the 2.5 mg oral, and possibly the 5% topical, treatments.

➤*Pharmacokinetics:* Topical minoxidil has poor absorption, averaging ≈ 1.4% (range 0.3% to 4.5%) from normal intact scalp, and about 2% in the hypertensive patients, whose scalps were shaved.

In a comparison of topical and oral absorption, peak serum levels of unchanged drug after 1 ml twice a day of 2% solution (the maximum recommended dose) averaged 5.8% (range, 1.4% to 12.7%) of the level observed after 2.5 mg orally twice a day. Similarly, in the hypertension study where patients had shaved scalps, mean concentrations after 1 ml twice a day of 2% topical solution (1.7 ng/ml) were 1/20 the concentrations seen after daily oral doses of 2.5 mg (32.8 ng/ml) or 5 mg (59.2 ng/ml). Blood levels obtained in the large controlled hair growth trials averaged < 2 ng/ml for the 2% solution (range, up to 30 ng/ml). If more than the recommended dose is applied to inflamed skin in an individual with relatively high absorption, blood levels with systemic effects might rarely be obtained.

Serum levels resulting from topical administration are governed by the drug's percutaneous absorption rate. Following cessation of topical dosing, ≈ 95% of systemically absorbed minoxidil is eliminated within 4 days.

➤*Clinical trials:*

Males – Three main parameters of efficacy were used: Hair counts in a 1 inch diameter circle on the vertex of the scalp; investigator evaluation of terminal hair regrowth; and patient evaluation of hair regrowth. At the end of 4 month placebo controlled portions of 12 month clinical studies (ie, baseline to month 4), topical minoxidil (20 mg/ml) demonstrated the following efficacy:

Hair counts: Topical minoxidil was significantly more effective than placebo in producing hair regrowth as assessed by hair counts. Patients using topical minoxidil had a mean increase from baseline of 72 nonvellus hairs in the 1 inch diameter circle compared with a mean increase of 39 nonvellus hairs in patients on placebo.

Investigator evaluation: Of patients on topical minoxidil, 8% demonstrated moderate to dense terminal hair regrowth compared with 4% on placebo. During the initial 4 months of treatment, however, very little regrowth of terminal hair can be expected. Although most patients did not demonstrate cosmetically significant hair regrowth, 26% of the patients showed minimal terminal hair regrowth using topical minoxidil compared with 16% of those using placebo.

Patient evaluation: 26% using topical minoxidil demonstrated moderate to dense hair regrowth compared with 11% using placebo.

Patients who continued on topical minoxidil during the remaining 8 months of the 12 month clinical studies (ie, the non-placebo controlled portion of the studies) continued to sustain a regrowth response. At the end of the 8 months, the following results were obtained:

Hair counts – Patients using topical minoxidil had a mean increase of 112 nonvellus hairs in the same 1 inch diameter circle as compared to month 4.

Investigator evaluation – 39% of the patients achieved moderate to dense terminal hair regrowth by month 12.

Patient evaluation – 48% felt they had achieved moderate to dense hair regrowth at month 12.

Trends in the data suggest that those patients who are older, who have been balding for a longer period of time, or who have a larger area of baldness, may do less well.

Females (18 to 45 years of age; 90% white) – In females with Ludwig grade I and II diffuse frontoparietal hair thinning, the main parameters of efficacy were: Nonvellus hair counts in a designated 1 cm² site on the frontoparietal areas of the scalp; investigator evaluation of hair regrowth; and patient evaluation of hair regrowth. Data demonstrate that 44% to 63% of women with androgenetic alopecia will have discernible growth of nonvellus hair when treated with minoxidil for 32 weeks vs 29% to 39% for vehicle control treated women.

Two 8 month placebo controlled studies produced the following results:

Hair counts – Minoxidil was significantly more effective than placebo in producing hair regrowth as assessed by hair counts in both studies. Patients using minoxidil had a mean increase from baseline of 22.7 and 33.2 nonvellus hairs, respectively, in the same 1 cm² site compared with a mean increase of 11 and 19.1 nonvellus hairs, respectively, in patients using placebo.

Investigator evaluation – Based on the investigators' evaluation, 63% (13% moderate and 50% minimal) and 44% (12% moderate and 32% minimal), respectively, of the patients using minoxidil in the two studies achieved hair regrowth at week 32, compared with 39% (6% moderate and 33% minimal) and 29% (5% moderate and 24% minimal), respectively, of those using placebo.

Patient evaluation – Based on the patients' self evaluation, 59% (19% moderate and 40% minimal) and 55% (1% dense, 24% moderate and 30% minimal), respectively, of the patients using minoxidil reported hair regrowth at week 32, compared with 40% (7% moderate and 33% minimal) and 41% (12% moderate and 29% minimal), respectively, of those using placebo.

Hair growth was defined as follows:

Investigator evaluation of growth – No visible new hair growth; minimal growth (definite growth but no substantial covering of thinning areas); moderate growth (new growth partially covering thinning areas, less dense than non-thinning areas; readily discernible); dense growth (full covering of thinning areas; hair density similar to non-thinning areas).

Patient evaluation of growth – No visible hair growth; minimal hair growth (barely discernible); moderate new hair growth (readily discernible); dense new hair growth.

Contraindications

Hypersensitivity to any component of the preparation.

Warnings

➤*Cardiac lesions:* Minoxidil produces several cardiac lesions in animals. The significance of these lesions for humans is not clear, as they have not been recognized in patients treated with oral minoxidil at systemically active doses (see the systemic Minoxidil monograph in the Antihypertensive Vasodilators section in the Cardiovascular chapter).

➤*Need for normal scalp:* The majority of clinical studies included only healthy patients with normal scalps and no cardiovascular disease. Before starting a patient on topical minoxidil, ascertain that the patient has a healthy, normal scalp. Local abrasion or dermatitis may increase absorption and, hence, increase the risk of side effects.

➤*Systemic effects:* Although extensive use has not revealed evidence that enough topical drug is absorbed to cause systemic effects, greater absorption because of misuse, individual variability or unusual sensitivity could lead to a systemic effect.

MINOXIDIL

As is the case with other topically applied drugs, decreased integrity of the epidermal barrier caused by inflammation or disease processes in the skin (eg, excoriations of the scalp, scalp psoriasis, severe sunburn) may increase percutaneous absorption. Also, do not use in conjunction with other topical agents (eg, corticosteroids, retinoids, petrolatum) or agents that are known to enhance cutaneous drug absorption.

➤*Heart disease:* Adverse effects might be especially serious in patients with a history of underlying heart disease. Be alert for tachycardia and fluid retention and watch for increased heart rate, weight gain, or other systemic effects.

➤*Pregnancy: Category C.* Adequate and well-controlled studies have not been conducted in pregnant women. Do not administer to a pregnant woman.

➤*Lactation:* Because of the potential for adverse effects in nursing infants from minoxidil absorption, do not apply on a nursing woman.

➤*Children:* Safety and efficacy in patients < 18 years of age have not been established.

Precautions

➤*Monitoring:* Give a history and physical examination to patients being considered for topical minoxidil. Advise of the potential risk; the patient and physician should decide that the benefits outweigh the risks.

Monitor patients ≥ 1 month after starting topical minoxidil and ≥ 6 months thereafter. If systemic effects occur, discontinue use.

➤*Alcohol base:* This product contains an alcohol base that will cause burning and irritation of the eyes. In the event of accidental contact with sensitive surfaces (eg, eyes, abraded skin, mucous membranes), bathe the area with large amounts of cool tap water.

➤*Avoid inhalation:* Avoid inhaling the spray mist.

➤*For topical use only:* Accidental ingestion could lead to adverse systemic effects.

Adverse Reactions

➤*Cardiovascular:* Edema, chest pain, blood pressure increases/decreases, palpitations, pulse rate increases/decreases (1.5%; placebo 1.6%).

➤*CNS:* Headache, dizziness, faintness, lightheadedness (3.4%; placebo 3.5%).

➤*Dermatologic:* Irritant dermatitis, allergic contact dermatitis (7.4%; placebo 5.4%); eczema; hypertrichosis; local erythema; pruritus; dry skin/scalp flaking; exacerbation of hair loss; alopecia.

➤*Endocrine:* Menstrual changes, breast symptoms (0.5%; placebo 0.5%).

➤*GI:* Diarrhea, nausea, vomiting (4.3%; placebo 6.6%).

➤*GU:* Urinary tract infections, renal calculi, urethritis, prostatitis, epididymitis, vaginitis, vulvitis, vaginal discharge, itching (0.9%; placebo 0.8% to 1.1%); sexual dysfunction.

➤*Hematologic:* Lymphadenopathy, thrombocytopenia, anemia (0.3%; placebo 0.6%).

➤*Hypersensitivity:* Non-specific allergic reactions, hives, allergic rhinitis, facial swelling, sensitivity (1.3%; placebo 1%).

➤*Metabolic:* Edema, weight gain (1.2%; placebo 1.3%).

➤*Musculoskeletal:* Fractures, back pain, tendinitis, aches and pains (2.6%; placebo 2.2%).

➤*Psychiatric:* Anxiety, depression, fatigue (0.4%; placebo 1%).

➤*Respiratory:* Bronchitis, upper respiratory tract infection, sinusitis (7.2%; placebo 8.6%).

➤*Special senses:* Conjunctivitis, ear infection, vertigo (1.2%; placebo 1.2%); visual disturbances, including decreased visual acuity.

Overdosage

➤*Topical:* Increased systemic absorption of minoxidil may potentially occur if more frequent or larger doses than directed are used or if the drug is applied to large surface areas of the body or areas other than the scalp. There are no known cases of minoxidil overdosage resulting from topical administration.

In a 14-day controlled clinical trial, 1 ml of 3% minoxidil solution was applied 8 times daily (6 times the recommended dose) to the scalp of 11 healthy male volunteers and to the chest of 11 other volunteers. No significant systemic effects were observed in these subjects when compared with a similar number of placebo-treated subjects.

➤*Systemic:* Because of the high concentration of minoxidil in the topical solution, accidental ingestion has the potential of producing systemic effects related to the pharmacologic action of the drug (5 ml contains 100 mg minoxidil, the maximum adult dose for oral minoxidil administration when used to treat hypertension).

➤*Symptoms:* Signs and symptoms of minoxidil overdosage would most likely be cardiovascular effects associated with fluid retention and tachycardia.

➤*Treatment:* Manage fluid retention with appropriate diuretic therapy. Control clinically significant tachycardia by administration of a β-adrenergic blocking agent. If encountered, control hypotension by IV administration of normal saline. Avoid sympathomimetic drugs, such as norepinephrine and epinephrine, because of their excessive cardiac-stimulating activity.

Patient Information

Evidence of hair growth usually will take ≥ 4 months.

First hair growth may be soft, downy, colorless hair that is barely visible. After further treatment, the new hair should be the same color and thickness as the other hair on the scalp.

If there is no response to treatment after a reasonable period of time (≥ 4 months), consult physician as to whether to discontinue use.

If treatment is stopped, new hair will probably be shed within a few months.

If 1 or 2 daily applications are missed, restart twice-daily application and return to the usual schedule. Do not attempt to make up for missed applications.

More frequent applications or use of larger doses (> 1 ml twice a day) will not speed up the process of hair growth and may increase the possibility of side effects.

Minoxidil topical solution contains alcohol, that could cause burning or irritation of the eyes, mucous membranes, or sensitive skin areas. If accidental contact occurs, bathe the area with large amounts of cool tap water. Consult physician if irritation persists.

Because absorption of minoxidil may be increased and the risk of side effects may become greater, apply only to the scalp; do not use on other parts of the body. Do not use if scalp becomes irritated or is sunburned; do not use along with other topical medications on the scalp.

EFLORNITHINE HCl

Rx **Vaniqa** (Women First HealthCare) | **Cream:** 13.9% (139 mg/g) of anhydrous eflornithine HCl as eflornithine HCl monohydrate (150 mg/g) | Parabens, cetearyl alcohol, mineral oil, stearyl alcohol. In 30 and 2 x 30 g tubes.

For information on IV use of eflornithine as an antiprotozoal, refer to the specific monograph in the Systemic Anti-Infectives chapter.

Indications

➤*Facial hair:* For the reduction of unwanted facial hair in women.

Administration and Dosage

➤*Approved by the FDA:* July 27, 2000.

For topical dermatological use only. Not for ophthalmic, oral, or intravaginal use.

Eflornithine HCl has only been studied on the face and adjacent involved areas under the chin of affected individuals. Limit usage to these areas of involvement.

Apply a thin layer of eflornithine HCl to affected areas of the face and adjacent involved areas under the chin and rub in thoroughly. Do not wash treated area for ≥ 4 hours. Use twice daily ≥ 8 hours apart or as directed by a physician. Continue to use hair removal techniques as needed in conjunction with eflornithine HCl. Apply eflornithine HCl ≥ 5 minutes after hair removal. Cosmetics or sunscreens may be applied over treated areas after cream has dried.

➤*Storage/Stability:* Store at 25°C (77°F); excursions permitted to 15° to 30°C (59° to 86°F). Do not freeze.

Actions

➤*Pharmacology:* It is postulated that topical eflornithine HCl irreversibly inhibits ornithine decarboxylase (ODC) activity in skin. This enzyme is necessary in the synthesis of polyamines. Animal data indicate that inhibition of ODC inhibits cell division and synthetic functions, which affect the rate of hair growth. Eflornithine HCl has been shown to retard the rate of hair growth in nonclinical and clinical studies.

➤*Pharmacokinetics:* The mean percutaneous absorption of eflornithine in women with unwanted facial hair is < 1% of the dose, following either single or multiple doses under conditions of clinical use that included shaving within 2 hours before dose application in addition to other forms of cutting, plucking, and tweezing to remove facial hair. Steady-state was reached within 4 days of twice-daily application. The apparent steady-state plasma $t_{1/2}$ of eflornithine was ≈ 8 hours. Following twice-daily application of 0.5 g of the cream (total dose, 1 g/day; 139 mg as anhydrous eflornithine HCl), under conditions of clinical use in women with unwanted facial hair (n = 10), the steady-state C_{max}, C_{trough}, and AUC_{12hr} were ≈ 10 ng/ml, 5 ng/ml, and 92 ng•hr/ml, respectively. At steady-state, the dose-normalized peak concentrations (C_{max}) and the extent of daily systemic exposure (AUC) of eflornithine following twice-daily application of 0.5 g of the cream (total dose, 1 g/day) is estimated to be ≈ 100- and 60-fold lower, respectively, when compared to 370 mg/day once-daily oral doses. This compound is not known to be metabolized and is primarily excreted unchanged in the urine.

Contraindications

History of sensitivity to any components of the preparation.

Warnings

Discontinue if hypersensitivity occurs.

➤*Pregnancy: Category C.* Although eflornithine HCl was not formally studied in pregnant patients, 22 pregnancies occurred during the trials. Nineteen of these pregnancies occurred while patients were using eflornithine HCl. Of the 19 pregnancies, there were 9 healthy infants, 4 spontaneous abortions, 5 induced/elective abortions, and 1 birth defect (Down's Syndrome to a 35-year-old). Because there are no adequate and well-controlled studies in pregnant women, weigh the risk/benefit ratio of using eflornithine HCl in women with unwanted facial hair who are pregnant carefully with serious consideration for either not implementing or discontinuing use of eflornithine HCl.

➤*Lactation:* It is not known whether eflornithine HCl is excreted in human milk. Exercise caution when eflornithine HCl is administered to a nursing woman.

➤*Children:* The safety and efficacy of eflornithine HCl have not been established in pediatric patients < 12 years of age.

Precautions

For external use only.

Transient stinging or burning may occur when applied to abraded or broken skin.

Drug Interactions

It is not known if eflornithine HCl has any interaction with other topically applied drug products.

➤*Drug/Lab test interactions:* In an open-labeled study, some patients showed an increase in their transaminases; however, the clinical significance of these findings is unknown.

Adverse Reactions

Adverse events reported for most body systems occurred at similar frequencies in eflornithine HCl and vehicle control groups. The most frequent adverse events related to treatment with eflornithine HCl were skin-related.

Adverse Events (> 1%) Associated with Use of Eflornithine HCl or its Vehicle			
	Vehicle-controlled studies		Vehicle-controlled and open-label studies
Adverse reaction	Eflornithine HCl (N = 393)	Vehicle (N = 201)	Eflornithine HCl (n = 1373)
CNS			
Headache	3.8	5	4
Dizziness	1.5	1.5	1.3
Vertigo	0.3	1	0.1
Dermatologic			
Acne	21.3	21.4	10.8
Pseudofolliculitis barbae	16.3	15.4	4.9
Stinging skin	7.9	2.5	4.1
Burning skin	4.3	2	3.5
Dry skin	1.8	3	3.3
Pruritus	3.8	4	3.1
Erythema	1.3	0	2.5
Tingling skin	3.6	1.5	2.2
Skin irritation	1	1	1.8
Rash	2.8	0	1.5
Alopecia	1.5	2.5	1.3
Folliculitis	0.5	0	1
Ingrown hair	0.3	2	0.9
Facial edema	0.3	3	0.7
GI			
Dyspepsia	2.5	2	1.9
Anorexia	1	2	0.7
Nausea	0.5	1	0.7
Miscellaneous			
Asthenia	0	1	0.3

Treatment-related skin adverse events that occurred in < 1% of the subjects treated with eflornithine HCl include the following: Bleeding skin, cheilitis, contact dermatitis, swelling of the lips, herpes simplex, numbness, and rosacea.

Adverse events were primarily mild in intensity and generally resolved without medical treatment or discontinuation of eflornithine HCl. Only 2% of subjects discontinued studies because of an adverse event related to use of eflornithine HCl.

➤*IV:* Use of an IV formulation of eflornithine HCl at high doses (400 mg/kg/day or ≈ 24 g/day) for the treatment of *Trypanosoma brucei gambiense* infection (African sleeping sickness) has been associated with adverse events and laboratory abnormalities. Adverse events in this setting have included hair loss, facial swelling, seizures, hearing impairment, stomach upset, loss of appetite, headache, weakness, and dizziness. A variety of hematological toxicities, including anemia, thrombocytopenia, and leukopenia also have been observed, but these were usually reversible upon discontinuation of treatment.

Overdosage

If very high topical doses (eg, multiple tubes per day) or oral ingestion are encountered (a 30 g tube contains 4.2 g of eflornithine HCl), monitor the patient and administer appropriate supportive measures as necessary.

Patient Information

This medication is not a depilatory, but rather appears to retard hair growth to improve the condition and the patient's appearance. Patients likely will need to continue using a hair removal method (eg, shaving, plucking) in conjunction with eflornithine HCl.

Onset of improvement was seen after as little as 4 to 8 weeks of treatment in the 24-week clinical trials. The condition may return to pretreatment levels 8 weeks after discontinuing treatment.

If skin irritation or intolerance develops, direct the patient to temporarily reduce the frequency of application (eg, once a day). If irritation continues, discontinue use of the product.

Instruct patients to refer to the Patient Information Leaflet for additional important information and instructions.

AMINOLEVULINIC ACID HCl

Rx　　Levulan Kerastick (DUSA)　　　　**Solution, topical:** 20% (354 mg aminolevulinic acid HCl)　　48% v/v ethanol, isopropyl alcohol. In 4s, 6s, and 12s. Applicator contains 2 glass ampules and an applicator tip. One ampule contains 1.5 ml solution vehicle, the other ampule contains 354 mg aminolevulinic acid HCl.

Indications

▶*Non-hyperkeratotic actinic keratoses (face/scalp):* For the treatment of non-hyperkeratotic actinic keratoses of the face or scalp.

▶*Unlabeled uses:* (In conjunction with a photodynamic therapy.) Barrett's esophagus; Bowen's disease; epidermodysplasia verruciformis; intraepithelial neoplasia of the lower genital tract; nevus sebaceus; mycosis fungoides; actinic cheilitis; premalignant epithelial lesions of the oral cavity; intraepithelial neoplasia and associated human papillomavirus of the uterine cervix; oral leukoplakia; multifocal superficial transitional cell carcinoma of the upper urinary tract; vulvar lichen sclerosus; advanced-stage esophageal cancer; non-melanoma skin malignancies of the eyelid; squamous cell carcinoma; Kaposi's sarcoma; xeroderma pigmentosum; aids in diagnosis of basal cell carcinomas.

Administration and Dosage

▶*Approved by the FDA:* December 3, 1999.

Aminolevulinic acid (ALA) topical solution is intended for direct application to individual lesions diagnosed as actinic keratoses and not to perilesional skin. This product is not intended for application by patients or unqualified medical personnel. Application should involve either scalp or face lesions, but not both simultaneously.

The recommended treatment frequency is: One application of the topical solution and 1 dose of illumination per treatment site per 8-week treatment session. Use each individual applicator for only 1 patient. Photodynamic therapy for actinic keratoses with the topical solution is a 2-stage process involving the following: Application of the product to the target lesions with ALA topical solution, followed 14 to 18 hours later by illumination with blue light using Blue Light Photodynamic Therapy Illuminator (BLU-U). The second visit for illumination must take place in the 14- to 18-hour window following application.

| Schedule for Aminolevulinic Acid and Blue Light Administration ||
Topical solution application	Time window for blue light illumination
6 am	8 pm to midnight
7 am	9 pm to 1 am
8 am	10 pm to 2 am
9 am	11 pm to 3 am
10 am	Midnight to 4 am
11 am	1 am to 5 am
12 am	2 am to 6 am
1 pm	3 am to 7 am
2 pm	4 am to 8 am
3 pm	5 am to 9 am
4 pm	6 am to 10 am
5 pm	7 am to 11 am
6 pm	8 am to noon
7 pm	9 am to 1 pm
8 pm	10 am to 2 pm
9 pm	11 am to 3 pm
10 pm	Noon to 4 pm

Treated lesions that have not completely resolved after 8 weeks may be treated a second time with ALA topical solution and photodynamic therapy. Patients did not receive follow-up past 12 weeks after the initial treatment, so the incidence of recurrence of treated lesions past 12 weeks and the role of further treatment is not known.

▶*Preparation:* Prepare the ALA topical solution as follows:
1.) Hold the applicator so that the applicator cap is pointing up.
2.) Crush the bottom ampule containing the solution vehicle by applying finger pressure to Position A on the cardboard sleeve.
3.) Crush the top ampule containing ALA powder by applying finger pressure to Position B on the cardboard sleeve. Continue crushing the applicator downward, applying finger pressure to Position A.
4.) Holding the applicator between the thumb and forefinger, point the applicator cap away from the face, shake the applicator gently for ≥ 3 minutes to completely dissolve the drug powder in the solution vehicle.

Following solution admixture, remove the cap from the applicator. Dab the dry applicator tip on a gauze pad until uniformly wet with solution.

▶*Application:* Clean and dry the actinic keratoses targeted for treatment prior to application of the topical solution. Apply the solution directly to the targeted lesions by dabbing gently with the wet applicator tip. Apply enough solution to uniformly wet the lesion surface, including the edges without excess running or dripping. Once the initial application has dried, apply again in the same manner. Use the topical solution immediately following preparation (dissolution) because of the instability of the activated product. If the solution application is not completed within 2 hours of activation, discard the applicator and use a new ALA topical solution.

Photosensitization of the treated lesions will take place over the next 14 to 18 hours. Do not wash the actinic keratoses during this time. Advise the patient to wear a wide-brimmed hat or other protective apparel to shade the treated actinic keratosis lesions from sunlight or other bright light sources until BLU-U treatment. Advise the patient to reduce light exposure if the sensations of stinging or burning are experienced.

If for any reason a patient cannot be given BLU-U treatment during the prescribed time after topical solution application, he or she may, nonetheless, experience sensations of stinging or burning if the photosensitized actinic keratoses are exposed to sunlight or prolonged or intense light at that time. Advise the patient to wear a wide-brimmed hat or other protective apparel to shade the treated actinic keratosis lesions from sunlight or other bright light sources ≥ 40 hours after the application of the topical solution. Advise the patient to reduce light exposure if the sensations of stinging or burning are experienced.

The effect of the topical solution on ocular tissues is unknown. It should not be applied to the periorbital area or allowed to contact ocular or mucosal surfaces.

▶*Administration of BLU-U treatment 14 to 18 hours after application of the topical solution:* At the visit for light illumination, gently rinse the actinic keratoses to be treated with water and pat dry. Photoactivation of actinic keratoses treated with ALA topical solution is accomplished with BLU-U illumination from the BLU-U. A 1000-second (16 minutes 40 seconds) exposure is required to provide a 10 J/cm² light dose. During light treatment, provide both patients and medical personnel with blue-blocking protective eyewear, as specified in the BLU-U operating instructions, to minimize ocular exposure. Please refer to the BLU-U operating instructions for further information on conducting the light treatment. Advise patients that transient stinging or burning at the target lesion sites occurs during the period of light exposure.

If blue light treatment with BLU-U therapy is interrupted or stopped for any reason, do not restart. Advise the patient to protect the treated lesions from exposure to sunlight or prolonged or intense light for ≥ 40 hours after application of the topical solution from the first visit.

▶*Patients with facial lesions:*
1.) The BLU-U is positioned so that the base is slightly above the patient's shoulder, parallel to the patient's face.
2.) The BLU-U is positioned around the patient's head so the entire surface area to be treated lies between 2 to 4 inches from the BLU-U surface: The patient's nose should be no closer than 2 inches from the surface; the patient's forehead and cheeks should be no further than 4 inches from the surface; the sides of the patient's face and ears should be no closer than 2 inches from the BLU-U surface.

A chin rest is available to provide support for the patient's head during treatment.

▶*Patients with scalp lesions:*
1.) The knobs on either side of the BLU-U are loosened and the BLU-U is rotated to a horizontal position.
2.) The BLU-U is positioned around the patient's head so the entire surface area to be treated lies between 2 to 4 inches from the BLU-U surface: The patient's scalp should be no closer than 2 inches from the surface; the patient's scalp should be no further than 4 inches from the surface; the sides of the patient's face and ears should be no closer than 2 inches from the BLU-U surface.

A chin rest is available to provide support for the patient's head during treatment.

ALA topical solution is not intended for use with any device other than the BLU-U Blue Light Photodynamic Illuminator. Use of the topical solution without subsequent BLU-U illumination is not recommended.

▶*Storage/Stability:* Store ALA at 25°C (77°F).

Actions

▶*Pharmacology:* The mechanism of ALA is the first step in the biochemical pathway resulting in heme synthesis. ALA is not a photosensitizer but rather a metabolic precursor of protoporphyrin IX (PpIX), which is a photosensitizer. The synthesis of ALA is normally tightly controlled by feedback inhibition of the enzyme, ALA synthetase, presumably by intracellular heme levels. ALA, when provided to the cell, bypasses this control point and results in the accumulation of PpIX, which is converted into heme by ferrochelatase through the addition of iron to the PpIX nucleus.

According to the presumed mechanism of action, photosensitization following application of ALA topical solution occurs through the metabolic conversion of ALA to PpIX, which accumulates in the skin to which ALA topical solution has been applied. When exposed to light of appropriate

AMINOLEVULINIC ACID HCl

wavelength and energy, the accumulated PpIX produces a photodynamic reaction, a cytotoxic process dependent upon the simultaneous presence of light and oxygen. The absorption of light results in an excited state of the porphyrin molecule, and subsequent spin transfer from PpIX to molecular oxygen generates singlet oxygen, which can further react to form superoxide and hydroxyl radicals. Photosensitization of actinic (solar) keratosis lesions using ALA, plus illumination with the BLU-U, is the basis for ALA photodynamic therapy (PDT).

➤*Pharmacokinetics:* In a human pharmacokinetic study (n=6) using a 128 mg dose of sterile IV ALA and oral ALA (equivalent to 100 mg ALA) in which plasma ALA and PpIX were measured, the mean half-life of ALA was ≈ 0.7 hr after the oral dose and ≈ 0.83 hr after the IV dose. The oral bioavailability of ALA was 50% to 60% with a mean C_{max} of ≈ 4.65 mcg/ml. PpIX concentrations were low and were detectable only in 42% of the plasma samples. PpIX concentrations in plasma were quite low relative to ALA plasma concentrations, and were below the level of detection (10 ng/ml) after 10 to 12 hours. ALA is not indicated for internal use.

ALA does not exhibit fluorescence, while PpIX has a high fluorescence yield. Time-dependent changes in surface fluorescence have been used to determine PpIX accumulation and clearance in actinic keratosis lesions and perilesional skin after application of ALA topical solution in 12 patients. Peak fluorescence intensity was reached in ≈ 11 hr in actinic keratoses and ≈ 12 hr in perilesional skin. The mean clearance half-life of fluorescence for lesions was ≈ 30 hr and ≈ 28 hr for perilesional skin. The fluorescence in perilesional skin was similar to that in actinic keratoses. Therefore, apply ALA topical solution only to the affected skin.

Contraindications

Cutaneous photosensitivity at wavelengths of 400 to 450 nm; porphyria or known allergies to porphyrins; sensitivity to any components of ALA topical solution.

Warnings

➤*Topical therapy:* ALA topical solution contains alcohol and is intended for topical use only. Do not apply to the eyes or to mucous membranes.

➤*Pregnancy:* Category C. It is not known whether ALA topical solution can cause fetal harm when administered to a pregnant woman or can affect reproductive capacity. Give to a pregnant woman only if clearly needed.

➤*Lactation:* The levels of ALA or its metabolites in the milk of subjects treated with ALA topical solution have not been measured. Exercise caution when administering ALA topical solution to a nursing woman.

Precautions

➤*Photosensitivity:* During the time period between the application and exposure to activating light from the BLU-U, the treatment site will become photosensitive. After application, patients should avoid exposure of the photosensitive treatment sites to sunlight or bright indoor light (eg, examination lamps, operating room lamps, tanning beds, lights at close proximity) during the period prior to blue light treatment. Exposure may result in a stinging or burning sensation and may cause erythema or edema of the lesions. Before exposure to sunlight, patients should, therefore, protect treated lesions from the sun by wearing a wide-brimmed hat or similar head covering of light-opaque material. Sunscreens will not protect against photosensitivity reactions caused by visible light. It has not been determined if perspiration can spread ALA topical solution outside the treatment site to the eye or surrounding skin.

Application to perilesional areas of photodamaged skin of the face or scalp may result in photosensitization. Upon exposure to activating light from the BLU-U, such photosensitized skin may produce a stinging or burning sensation and may become erythematous or edematous in a manner similar to that of actinic keratoses treated with ALA-PDT.

➤*Inherited or acquired coagulation defects:* ALA topical solution has not been tested on patients with inherited or acquired coagulation defects.

Drug Interactions

There have been no formal studies of the interaction of ALA topical solution with any other drugs. No drug-specific interactions were noted during any of the controlled clinical trials. However, it is possible that concomitant use of other known photosensitizing agents, such as griseofulvin, thiazide diuretics, sulfonylureas, phenothiazines, sulfonamides, and tetracyclines might increase the photosensitivity reaction of actinic keratoses treated with ALA topical solution.

Adverse Reactions

Post-Photodynamic Therapy (Including Aminolevulinic Acid HCl) Cutaneous Adverse Events (%)				
	Face		Scalp	
	Aminolevulinic acid HCl (n=139)		Aminolevulinic acid HCl (n=42)	
Adverse reaction	Mild/Moderate	Severe	Mild/Moderate	Severe
Scaling/Crusting	71	1	64	2
Pain	1	0	0	0
Tenderness	1	0	2	0
Itching	25	1	14	7
Edema	1	0	0	0
Ulceration	4	0	2	0
Bleeding/Hemorrhage	4	0	2	0
Hypo/Hyperpigmentation	22	22	36	36
Vesiculation	4	0	5	0
Pustules	4	0	0	0
Oozing	1	0	0	0
Dysesthesia	2	0	0	0
Scabbing	2	1	0	0
Erosion	14	1	2	0
Excoriation	1	0	0	0
Wheal/Flare	7	1	2	0
Skin disorder NOS	5	0	12	0

Overdosage

In the unlikely event that the drug is ingested, monitoring and supportive care are recommended. Advise the patient to avoid incidental exposure to intense light sources for ≥ 40 hours. The consequences of exceeding the recommended topical dosage are unknown.

Patient Information

➤*Photodynamic therapy for actinic keratoses:* The first step in ALA-PDT for actinic keratoses is application of the ALA topical solution to actinic keratoses located on the patient's face or scalp. After the solution is applied to the actinic keratoses in the doctor's office, the patient will be told to return the next day. During this time, the actinic keratoses will become sensitive to light (photosensitive). Take care to keep the treated actinic keratoses dry and out of bright light. After the solution is applied, it is important for the patient to wear light-protective clothing, such as a wide-brimmed hat, when exposed to sunlight or sources of light. Fourteen to 18 hours after application, the patient will return to the doctor's office to receive blue light treatment, which is the second and final step in the treatment. Prior to blue light treatment, the actinic keratoses will be rinsed with tap water. The patient will be given goggles to wear as eye protection during the blue light treatment. The blue light is of low intensity and will not heat the skin. However, during the light treatment, which lasts ≈ 17 minutes, the patient will experience sensations of tingling, stinging, prickling, or burning of the treated lesions. These feelings of discomfort should improve at the end of the light treatment. Following treatment, the actinic keratoses and, to some degree, the surrounding skin, will redden, and swelling and scaling may also occur. However, these lesion changes are temporary and should completely resolve by 4 weeks after treatment.

➤*Photosensitivity:* After the solution is applied to the actinic keratoses in the doctor's office, the patient should avoid exposure of the photosensitive actinic keratoses to sunlight or bright indoor light (eg, from examination lamps, operating room lamps, tanning beds, lights at close proximity) during the period prior to blue light treatment. If the patient feels stinging or burning on the actinic keratoses, reduce exposure to light. Before going into sunlight, the patient should protect treated lesions from the sun by wearing a wide-brimmed hat or similar head covering of light-opaque material. Sunscreens will not protect the patient against photosensitivity reactions.

If for any reason the patient cannot return for blue light treatment during the prescribed period after application of ALA topical solution (14 to 18 hours), the patient should call the doctor. The patient also should continue to avoid exposure of the photosensitized lesions to sunlight or prolonged or intense light for ≥ 40 hours. If stinging or burning is noted, reduce exposure to light.

WARNING

Methoxsalen with ultraviolet (UV) radiation is to be used only by physicians with competence in diagnosis and treatment of psoriasis and vitiligo, and with special training and experience in photochemotherapy. Constantly supervise such therapy. For psoriasis, restrict photochemotherapy to patients with severe, recalcitrant, disabling psoriasis not adequately responsive to other therapies, and only when diagnosis is supported by biopsy. Because of possible ocular damage, skin aging, and skin cancer (including melanoma), inform patient of risks.

For specific warnings, precautions, indications, and instructions related to photopheresis, consult the *UVAR Photopheresis System* operator's manual before using *Uvadex*.

These are potent drugs, capable of producing severe burns if improperly used. Read entire monograph before prescribing or dispensing these medications.

Never dispense methoxsalen lotion to a patient. The lotion should be applied only by a physician under controlled conditions for light exposure and subsequent light shielding.

Caution: Do not use *Oxsoralen-Ultra* interchangeably with *8-MOP* without retitration of the patient. This new dosage form of methoxsalen exhibits significantly greater bioavailability and earlier photosensitization onset time than previous dosage forms. Treat patients in accordance with dosimetry specifically recommended for this product. Determine minimum phototoxic dose (MPD) and phototoxic peak time after drug administration prior to onset of photochemotherapy with this dosage form.

Indications

➤*Oxsoralen-Ultra, 8-MOP:* Symptomatic control of severe recalcitrant disabling psoriasis not responsive to other therapy when the diagnosis has been supported by biopsy. Administer only in conjunction with a schedule of controlled doses of long wave UV radiation.

➤*Oxsoralen (lotion), 8-MOP, trioxsalen:* With long wave UV radiation for repigmentation of idiopathic vitiligo.

➤*8-MOP, Uvadex:* For extracorporeal administration with long wave UV radiation of white blood cells (photopheresis) and the *UVAR Photopheresis System* in the palliative treatment of the skin manifestations of cutaneous T-cell lymphoma (CTCL) that is unresponsive to other forms of treatment. Refer to the *UVAR Photopheresis System* operator's manual for specific warnings, precautions, indications, and instructions related to photopheresis.

➤*Trioxsalen:* For increasing tolerance to sunlight and for enhancing pigmentation.

Actions

➤*Pharmacology:* Normal skin pigmentation is due to melanin formed by the oxidation of tyrosine to DOPA (dihydroxyphenylalanine). Melanin must be activated by radiant energy in the form of UV light, preferably between 290 and 380 nm. The combination treatment regimen of psoralen (P) and UV radiation of 320 to 400 nm wavelength (UVA) is known by the acronym PUVA. Skin reactivity to UVA radiation is markedly enhanced by the ingestion of methoxsalen.

Oral **methoxsalen** reaches the skin via the blood, and UVA penetrates well into the skin. If sufficient cell injury occurs in the skin, an inflammatory reaction occurs. The most obvious manifestation of this reaction is delayed erythema, which may not begin for several hours and peaks at 48 to 72 hours. The inflammation is followed over several days to weeks by repair, which is manifested by increased melanization of the epidermis and thickening of the stratum corneum.

The exact mechanism of action of psoralens in the process of melanogenesis is not known. The action of these drugs depends upon the presence of functional melanocytes and their proliferation (mitotic activation) by the photoactivated psoralen. One belief is that exposure of methoxsalen-treated patients to UV light thickens the stratum corneum, induces an inflammatory reaction, and increases the amount of melanin in exposed areas. The exact mechanism of action of methoxsalen with the epidermal melanocytes and keratinocytes is not known.

Methoxsalen acts as a photosensitizer; subsequent exposure to UVA can lead to cell injury. In the treatment of psoriasis, the mechanism is assumed to be DNA photodamage and resulting decrease in cell proliferation, but other vascular, leukocyte, or cell regulatory mechanisms may also be involved. The best known biochemical reaction of methoxsalen is with DNA. Methoxsalen, upon photoactivation, conjugates and forms covalent bonds with DNA, which leads to the formation of both monofunctional (addition to a single strand of DNA) and bifunctional (cross-linking of psoralen to both strands of DNA) adducts. Reactions with proteins have also been described.

➤*Pharmacokinetics:* Oral psoralen is > 95% absorbed from the GI tract. Concomitant administration with food increases peak serum concentrations.

Oxsoralen-Ultra Capsules – Oxsoralen-Ultra Capsules reach peak drug levels in 0.5 to 4 hours (mean, 1.8 hours) when given with

8 ounces of milk. Maximum bioavailability of *8-MOP* is reached in 1.5 to 3 hours (mean, 2 hours) and may last up to 8 hours. Detectable methoxsalen levels were observed up to 12 hours post-dose. Half-life is ≈ 2 hours. Photosensitivity studies demonstrate a short peak photosensitivity time of 1.5 to 2.1 hours for *Oxsoralen-Ultra Capsules*.

Methoxsalen is reversibly bound to serum albumin and is preferentially taken up by epidermal cells. It is rapidly metabolized. Accumulation does not occur during continuous use; metabolism occurs in hepatic microsomal enzymes. Approximately 95% is excreted in urine within 24 hours; 4% to 10% is excreted in feces.

Trioxsalen possesses greater activity than methoxsalen, yet its median lethal dose is 6 times that of methoxsalen.

Contraindications

Idiosyncratic reactions to psoralen compounds; melanoma or a history of melanoma; invasive squamous cell carcinomas; aphakia (increased risk of retinal damage because of the absence of lenses); patients possessing a specific history of a light-sensitive disease state; diseases associated with photosensitivity including porphyria, acute lupus erythematosus, porphyria cutanea tarda, erythropoietic protoporphyria, variegate porphyria, xeroderma pigmentosum, leukoderma of infectious origin, and in albinism; concomitant use with any preparation having internal or external photosensitizing capacity.

➤*Oral trioxsalen and methoxsalen lotion:* Children ≤ 12 years of age.

Warnings

➤*Skin burning:* Serious burns from either UVA or sunlight (even through window glass) can result if recommended drug dosage or exposure schedules are exceeded or protective covering or sunscreens are not used. The blistering of the skin sometimes encountered after UV exposure generally heals without complication or scarring. Suitable covering of the area of application or a topical sunblock should follow the therapeutic UVA exposure.

➤*Cataracts:* Exposure to large doses of UVA light causes cataracts in animals. Oral methoxsalen exacerbates this toxicity. Serum methoxsalen concentrations are substantially lower after extracorporeal methoxsalen treatment than after oral methoxsalen treatment. The concentration of methoxsalen in the lens is proportional to the serum level. If the lens is exposed to UVA during the presence of methoxsalen in the lens, photochemical action may lead to irreversible binding of methoxsalen to proteins and the DNA components of the lens. However, if the lens is shielded from UVA, the methoxsalen will diffuse out of the lens in a 24-hour period. Emphatically instruct patients to wear UVA-absorbing, wraparound sunglasses for the 24 hours following ingestion of methoxsalen, whether exposed to direct or indirect sunlight in the open, or through window glass.

Among patients using proper eye protection, there is no evidence for a significantly increased risk of cataracts in association with PUVA therapy. Of 1380 patients, 35 have developed cataracts in the 5 years since their first PUVA treatment, an incidence comparable to that expected in a population of this size and age distribution. No relationship between PUVA dose and cataract risk has been noted.

➤*Actinic degeneration:* Exposure to sunlight or UV radiation may prematurely age skin.

➤*Cardiac disease:* Do not treat patients with cardiac disease or who may be unable to tolerate prolonged standing or exposure to heat stress in a vertical UVA chamber.

➤*UVA dosage:* Total cumulative safe UVA dosage over long periods of time is not established.

Do not increase the dosage of **trioxsalen** and exposure time. To prevent harmful effects, instruct patient to adhere to prescribed dosage schedule and procedure.

➤*Hepatic function impairment:* Because hepatic biotransformation is necessary for drug urinary excretion, treat patients with hepatic insufficiency with caution.

➤*Carcinogenesis:* In a prospective study of 1380 patients given PUVA therapy for psoriasis, 237 patients developed 1422 cutaneous squamous cell cancers. This appears greatest among patients who are fair-skinned or who had pre-PUVA exposure to prolonged tar and UVB treatment, ionizing radiation, or arsenic.

A study in 690 patients for up to 4 years showed no increase in risk of nonmelanoma skin cancer. However, patients had significantly less PUVA exposure. There is no evidence of an increased risk of melanoma in PUVA patients, but there is a need for continued evaluation of melanoma risk in these patients.

In a study in Indian patients treated for 4 years for vitiligo, 12% developed keratoses, but not cancer, in the depigmented, vitiliginous areas.

➤*Pregnancy:* Category C. It is not known whether psoralens can cause fetal harm when administered to a pregnant woman or can affect reproduction capacity. Use only if clearly needed.

Category D (Uvadex only). Methoxsalen may cause fetal harm when given to a pregnant woman. Doses of 80 to 160 mg/kg/day given during organogenesis caused significant fetal toxicity in rats. The lowest of these doses, 80 mg/kg/day, is over 4000 times greater than a single dose of methoxsalen on a mg/m² basis. Fetal toxicity was associated with significant maternal weight loss, anorexia, and increased relative liver weight. Signs of fetal toxicity included increased fetal mortality, increased resorptions, late fetal death, fewer fetuses per litter, and decreased fetal weight. Methoxsalen caused an increase in skeletal malformation and variations at doses of ≥ 80 mg/kg/day. There are no adequate and well-controlled studies of methoxsalen in pregnant women. If methoxsalen is used during pregnancy, or if the patient becomes pregnant while receiving methoxsalen, apprise the patient of the potential hazard to the fetus. Advise women of childbearing potential to avoid becoming pregnant.

➤*Lactation:* It is not known whether these agents are excreted in breast milk. Exercise caution when administering to a nursing woman.

➤*Children:* Safety of **methoxsalen** use has not been established. Potential hazards include possible carcinogenicity and cataractogenicity, and probable actinic degeneration. Oral **trioxsalen** and **methoxsalen** lotion are contraindicated in children ≤ 12 years of age.

Precautions

➤*Monitoring:* Perform the following before therapy: CBC (hemoglobin or hematocrit; WBC, and if abnormal, a differential count), antinuclear antibodies, liver and renal function tests (creatinine or blood urea nitrogen), and ophthalmologic examination; retest in 6 to 12 months and conduct additional tests at more extended time periods as indicated. Conduct ophthalmologic examinations yearly after the start of therapy.

➤*Basal cell carcinoma:* Diligently observe and treat patients exhibiting multiple basal cell carcinomas or having a history of basal cell carcinomas.

➤*Vitiligo therapy:* Do not increase the dosage of methoxsalen above 0.6 mg/kg; overdosage may result in serious burning of the skin. Protect eyes and skin from sun.

➤*Furocoumarin-containing foods:* No clinical reports or tests verify that more severe reactions may result from concomitant ingestion of furocoumarin-containing foods, but warn the patient that eating limes, figs, parsley, parsnips, mustard, carrots, and celery might be dangerous.

➤*PUVA erythema/sunburn differences:* PUVA-induced inflammation differs from sunburn or UVB phototherapy in several ways. The percent transmission of UVB varies between 0% to 34% through skin, whereas UVA varies between 1% to 80% transmission; thus, UVA is transmitted to a larger percent through the skin. The in situ depth of photochemistry is deeper within the tissue because UVA is transmitted further into the skin. The DNA lesions induced by PUVA are very different from UV-induced thymine dimers and may lead to a DNA crosslink. The DNA lesion may be more problematic to the cell because cross-links are more lethal and psoralen-DNA photoproducts may be "new" or unfamiliar substrates for DNA repair enzymes. DNA synthesis is also suppressed longer after PUVA. The time course of delayed erythema is different with PUVA and may not involve the usual mediators seen in sunburn. PUVA-induced redness may be just beginning at 24 hours, when UVB erythema has already passed its peak. The erythema dose-response curve is also steeper for PUVA. Compared to equally erythemogenic doses of UVB, the histologic alterations induced by PUVA show more dermal vessel damage and longer duration of epidermal and dermal abnormalities.

Exercise special care in treating patients who are receiving concomitant therapy (either topically or systemically) with known photosensitizing agents such as **anthralin**, **coal tar** or **coal tar derivatives**, **griseofulvin**, **phenothiazines**, **nalidixic acid**, **halogenated salicylanilides** (bacteriostatic soaps), **sulfonamides**, **tetracyclines**, **thiazides**, and certain organic staining dyes such as **methylene blue**, **toluidine blue**, **rose bengal**, and **methyl orange**.

Adverse Reactions

Severe burns and blisters can result from excessive sunlight or sunlamp UV exposure.

Basal cell epitheliomas have been removed from exposed and unexposed areas.

Nausea is common (10%).

Other effects of **methoxsalen** include the following: Nervousness; insomnia; psychological depression; edema; dizziness; headache; malaise; hypopigmentation; vesiculation and bullae formation; nonspecific rash; herpes simplex; miliaria; urticaria; folliculitis; GI disturbances; cutaneous tenderness; leg cramps; hypotension; extension of psoriasis and depression; gastric discomfort.

➤*Combined methoxsalen/UVA therapy:*

Pruritus (≈ 10%): Alleviate with frequent application of bland emollients or other topical agents; severe pruritus may require systemic treatment. If pruritus is unresponsive, shield pruritic areas from further UVA exposure until the condition resolves. If intractable pruritus is generalized, discontinue UVA treatment until pruritus disappears.

Erythema: Mild, transient erythema 24 to 48 hours after PUVA therapy is expected; it indicates a therapeutic interaction between methoxsalen and UVA. Shield any area showing moderate erythema

during subsequent UVA exposures until the erythema has resolved. Erythema greater than Grade 2, which appears within 24 hours after UVA treatment may signal a potentially severe burn. Erythema may worsen progressively over the next 24 hours since peak erythemal reaction characteristically occurs 48 hours or later after methoxsalen ingestion. Protect the patient from further UVA exposures and sunlight; monitor closely.

Uvadex: Side effects of photopheresis (*Uvadex* used with the *UVAR Photopheresis System*) were primarily related to hypotension secondary to changes in extracorporeal volume (> 1%). In one study, 6 serious cardiovascular adverse experiences were reported in 5 patients (10%). Five of these 6 events were not related to photopheresis and did not interfere with the scheduled photopheresis treatments. One patient (2%) with ischemic heart disease had an arrhythmia after the first day of photopheresis, but this resolved by the next day. Six infections were also reported in 5 patients. Two of the 6 events were Hickman catheter infections in 1 patient, which did not interrupt the scheduled photopheresis. The other 4 infections were not related to photopheresis and did not interfere with scheduled treatments.

Overdosage

Induce emesis within the first 2 to 3 hours after ingestion of methoxsalen, since maximum blood levels are reached by this time. Follow accepted procedures for treatment of severe burns. Keep the individual in a darkened room for ≥ 24 hours or until cutaneous reactions subside. There are no known reports of overdosage with extracorporeal administration of methoxsalen.

This does not apply to topical use. In the unlikely event that the lotion is ingested, follow standard procedures for poisoning, including gastric lavage. Protection from UVA or daylight for hours or days would also be necessary.

Patient Information

Use **topical methoxsalen** only on small, well-defined lesions that can be protected by clothing or sunscreen (≥ SPF 15) from subsequent exposure to radiant energy. If used to treat vitiligo of face or hands, keep the treated area protected from light by use of protective clothing or sunscreens. The area of application may be highly photosensitive for several days and may result in severe burns if exposed to additional UV or sunlight.

➤*Before methoxsalen ingestion:* Do not sunbathe during the 24 hours prior to methoxsalen ingestion and UV exposure. Sunburn may prevent an accurate evaluation of the patient's response to photochemotherapy.

➤*After methoxsalen ingestion:* Wear UVA-absorbing wraparound sunglasses during daylight for 24 hours to prevent cataracts (see Warnings). The protective eyewear must prevent entry of stray radiation to the eyes, including that which may enter from the sides of the eyewear. Visual discrimination should be permitted by the eyewear for patient well-being and comfort.

Avoid sun exposure, even through window glass or cloud cover, for ≥ 8 hours after methoxsalen ingestion. If sun exposure cannot be avoided, wear protective devices such as a hat and gloves, or apply sunscreens that filter out UVA radiation (eg, sunscreens with SPF ≥ 15). Apply sunscreens to all areas that might be exposed to the sun (including lips). Do not apply sunscreens to areas affected by psoriasis until after treatment in the UVA chamber.

➤*Before PUVA therapy:* Certain other medicines can make the patient more sensitive to the combination drug and light treatment. In addition, certain other medical conditions can be aggravated by this treatment. Before starting treatment, the patient should be sure to tell his/her physician if experiencing any of the following: Severe reaction to *Oxsoralen-Ultra*; recent or planned x-ray treatment; history of skin cancer, eye problems such as cataracts or loss of the lens of the eyes, liver problems, heart or blood pressure problems, any medical condition that requires the patient to stay out of the sun such as lupus erythematosus; or are taking any drugs (either prescription or nonprescription).

Some drugs can increase the patient's sensitivity to UV light either from the sun or man-made sources. Examples of such drugs include major tranquilizers, sulfa drugs for the treatment of infection or diabetes, tetracycline, antibiotics, griseofulvin products, thiazide-containing diuretics (blood pressure or water elimination drugs), and certain antibacterial or deodorant soaps.

➤*During PUVA therapy:* Wear total UVA-absorbing/blocking goggles mechanically designed to give maximal ocular protection. Failure to do so may increase the risk of cataract formation. A radiometer can verify elimination of UVA transmission through the goggles.

Protect abdominal skin, breasts, genitalia, and other sensitive areas for approximately one-third of the initial exposure time until tanning occurs. Unless affected by disease, shield male genitalia.

➤*After combined methoxsalen/UVA therapy:* Wear UVA-absorbing wraparound sunglasses during the daylight for 24 hrs after therapy. Do not sunbathe for 48 hrs after therapy. Erythema or burning because of photochemotherapy and sunburn are additive.

Psoralens

➤*PUVA therapy risks:* Premature skin aging may result from prolonged PUVA therapy, especially in those individuals who tan poorly. This problem is similar to excessive exposure to sunlight. There is an increased risk of developing non-fatal skin cancer. This risk is greater for individuals who fall into the following categories: Fair skin that burns rather than tans; prior treatment with x-rays, grenz rays, or arsenic; prior coal tar and UVB treatment.

Even though the physician will be examining the patient, the patient should routinely and completely examine himself/herself for small growths on his/her skin or skin sores that will not heal. Immediately report such observations to the physician.

Minimize or avoid nausea by taking the drug with milk or food, or by dividing into 2 doses, taken 30 minutes apart.

Do not exceed prescribed dosage or exposure time.

Avoid furocoumarin-containing foods (eg, limes, figs, parsley, parsnips, mustard, carrots, celery).

METHOXSALEN (8-Methoxypsoralen, 8-MOP), ORAL

Rx	8-MOP (ICN Pharmaceuticals)	**Capsules:** 10 mg	In 50s.
Rx	Oxsoralen-Ultra (ICN Pharmaceuticals)	**Capsules, soft gelatin:** 10 mg	(ICN 650). Green. In 50s.

For complete prescribing information, refer to the Psoralens group monograph.

WARNING

Methoxsalen should be used only by physicians who have special competence in the diagnosis and treatment of psoriasis and vitiligo and who have special training and experience in photochemotherapy. Constantly supervise psoralen and UV radiation therapy. For the treatment of patients with psoriasis, restrict photochemotherapy to patients with severe, recalcitrant, disabling psoriasis that is not adequately responsive to other forms of therapy, and only when the diagnosis is certain. Because of the possibilities of ocular damage, aging of the skin, and skin cancer (including melanoma), fully inform the patient of the risks inherent in this therapy. When methoxsalen is used in combination with photopheresis, refer to the *UVAR Photopheresis System* operator's manual for specific warnings, cautions, indications, and instructions related to photopheresis.

Oxsoralen-Ultra: Exhibits significantly greater bioavailability and earlier photosensitization onset time than previous forms. Determine the minimum phototoxic dose and phototoxic peak time after drug administration prior to onset of photochemotherapy with this dosage form.

8-MOP: May not be interchanged with *Oxsoralen-Ultra* capsules without retitration of the patient.

Indications

➤*Psoriasis:* For the symptomatic control of severe, recalcitrant, disabling psoriasis not responsive to other therapy when the diagnosis has been supported by biopsy. Administer only in conjunction with a schedule of controlled doses of long wave UV radiation.

➤*Vitiligo (8-MOP only):* With long wave UV radiation for repigmentation of idiopathic vitiligo.

➤*Cutaneous T-cell lymphoma (8-MOP only):* With long wave UV radiation of white blood cells (photopheresis) with the *UVAR Photopheresis System* in the palliative treatment of skin manifestations of cutaneous T-cell lymphoma (CTCL) in people who have not been responsive to other forms of treatment. Refer to the *UVAR Photopheresis System* operator's manual for specific warnings, precautions, indications, and instructions related to photopheresis.

Administration and Dosage

➤*Vitiligo (8-MOP):* 20 mg daily in 1 dose with milk or food, taken 2 to 4 hours before UV exposure. Therapy should be on alternate days, and never on consecutive days.

Limit exposure time to sunlight according to the following table:

	Basic skin color		
Suggested Sun Exposure Guide with Methoxsalen Use			
Exposure	Light	Medium	Dark
Initial exposure	15 min	20 min	25 min
Second exposure	20 min	25 min	30 min
Third exposure	25 min	30 min	35 min
Fourth exposure	30 min	35 min	40 min
Subsequent exposure	Gradually increase exposure based on erythema and tenderness of amelanotic skin.		

➤*Psoriasis:*

Initial therapy – Take dose 2 hours before UVA exposure with food or milk (*Oxsoralen-Ultra*-take 1.5 to 2 hours before UVA exposure with low-fat food or milk), according to the following table:

Methoxsalen Dosing	
Patient weight (kg)	Dose (mg)
< 30	10
30 - 50	20
51 - 65	30
66 - 80	40
81 - 90	50
91 - 115	60
> 115	70

Weight change – If the patient's weight changes during treatment and falls into an adjacent weight range/dose category, no dose change is usually required. If a weight change is sufficiently great enough to modify the dose, then adjust UVA exposure.

Doses/week – Determine the number of doses per week of methoxsalen capsules by the patient's schedule of UVA exposures. Never give treatments more often than once every other day because the full extent of phototoxic reactions may not be evident until 48 hours after each exposure.

Dosage increase – If there is no response or only minimal response after 15 treatments, increase dosage by 10 mg (a one-time increase). Continue this increased dosage for the remainder of the course of treatment, but do not exceed it.

Refer to the *UVAR Photopheresis System* for further details.

For UVA source specifications and PUVA protocols, see manufacturer information.

➤*Storage/Stability:* Store at 25°C (77°F); excursions permitted to 15° to 30°C (59° to 86°F).

METHOXSALEN (8-Methoxypsoralen), SOLUTION

Rx	Uvadex (Therakos)	Solution: 20 mcg/mL	Alcohol (0.05 mL). In 10 mL vials.

For complete prescribing information, refer to the Psoralens group monograph.

WARNING

Methoxsalen should be used only by physicians who have special competence in the diagnosis and treatment of cutaneous T-cell lymphoma and have special training and experience in the *UVAR* or *UVAR XTS Photopheresis System*. Consult the *UVAR Photopheresis System* operator's manual before using this product.

Indications

➤*Cutaneous T-cell lymphoma:* For extracorporeal administration with the *UVAR Photopheresis System* in the palliative treatment of skin manifestations of cutaneous T-cell lymphoma (CTCL) that is unresponsive to other forms of treatment.

Administration and Dosage

➤*Normal treatment schedule:* Give methoxsalen on 2 consecutive days every 4 weeks for a minimum of 7 treatment cycles (6 months). The total dose of methoxsalen used with the *UVAR Photopheresis System* in conjunction with *Uvadex* is substantially lower (approximately 200 times) than that used with oral administration.

➤*Accelerated treatment schedule:* If the assessment of the patient during the fourth treatment cycle (approximately 3 months) reveals an increased skin score from the baseline score, the frequency of treatment may be increased to 2 consecutive treatments every 2 weeks. If a 25% improvement in the skin score is attained after 4 consecutive weeks, the regular treatment schedule may resume. Patients who are maintained in the accelerated treatment schedule may receive a maximum of 20 cycles. There is no clinical evidence to show that treatment with methoxsalen for more than 6 months or using a different schedule provides additional benefit. In a study, 15 of the 17 responses were seen within 6 months of treatment, and only 2 patients responded to treatment after 6 months.

➤*Instruction for administration:* Each methoxsalen treatment involves collection of leukocytes, photoactivation, and reinfusion of photoactivated cells. During each photopheresis treatment performed with the *UVAR system*, 10 mL (200 mcg) of methoxsalen is injected directly into the photoactivation bag during the first buffy coat collection cycle. At the end of 6 cycles, a total of 740 mL (240 mL of buffy coat, 300 mL of plasma, and 200 mL of normal saline priming fluid) is collected and mixed with the 200 mcg of methoxsalen present in the photoactivation bag. After photoactivation, the cells are reinfused. Consult the *UVAR Photopheresis System* operator's manual before using this product.

During treatments with the *UVAR XTS System*, the dosage of methoxsalen for each treatment will be calculated according to the treatment volume (displayed on the XTS display panel). The prescribed amount of methoxsalen will be injected into the recirculation bag prior to the Photoactivation Phase using the following formula:

Treatment Volume $\times$ 0.017 = mL of methoxsalen for each treatment.

➤*Storage/Stability:* Store between 15° and 30°C (59° and 86°F).

METHOXSALEN (8–Methoxypsoralen, 8–MOP), TOPICAL

Rx	Oxsoralen (ICN Pharmaceuticals, Inc.)	Lotion: 1% (10 mg/mL)	Acetone. Alcohol (71%). In 30 mL.

For complete prescribing information, refer to the Psoralens group monograph.

WARNING

Methoxsalen lotion is a potent drug capable of producing severe burns if improperly used. Apply only by a physician under controlled conditions for light exposure and subsequent light shielding. This preparation should never be dispensed to a patient.

Indications

➤*Vitiligo:* Repigmenting agent in vitiligo, used in conjunction with controlled doses of UVA (320 to 400 nm) or sunlight.

Administration and Dosage

Apply lotion to a small, well-defined, vitiliginous lesion, then expose this area to UVA light. Initial exposure time must not exceed one half the minimal erythema dose.

Regulate treatment intervals by erythema response (once a week or less, depending on the results).

Pigmentation may begin after a few weeks; significant repigmentation may take up to 6 to 9 months. Periodic treatment may be needed to retain the new pigment.

Essentially, idiopathic vitiligo is reversible, but not equally in every patient. Individualize treatment. Repigmentation varies in completeness, time of onset, and duration; it occurs more rapidly on fleshy regions such as the face, abdomen, and buttocks, and less rapidly over bony areas such as the dorsum of the hands and feet.

Protect the hands and fingers of the person applying the medication with gloves or finger cots to avoid photosensitization and possible burns.

➤*Storage/Stability:* Store at 25°C (77°F); excursions permitted to 15° to 30°C (59° to 88°F).

Patient Information

Instruct patient to keep the treated areas protected from light by use of protective clothing or sunscreening agents. The area of application may be highly photosensitive for several days and may result in severe burn injury if exposed to additional UV or sunlight.

Tar-Containing Preparations

TAR DERIVATIVES, SHAMPOOS

otc	**DHS Tar** (Person & Covey)	**Shampoo:** 0.5% coal tar	**Liquid:** In 120, 240 & 480 mL.
			Gel: In 240 g.
otc	**Zetar** (Dermik)	**Shampoo:** 1% coal tar	In 177 mL.
otc	**Doak Tar** (Doak)	**Shampoo:** 1.2% coal tar	Isopropyl alcohol. In 237 mL.
otc	**Ionil T Plus** (Healthpoint)	**Shampoo:** 2% coal tar	In 120 and 240 mL.
otc	**Neutrogena T/Gel Original** (Neutrogena Corp.)	**Shampoo:** 2% coal tar extract	In 132, 255, 480 mL.
otc	**Pentrax** (Medicis)	**Shampoo:** 5% coal tar	In 236 mL.
otc	**Creamy Tar** (Genesis)	**Shampoo:** 6.65% coal tar solution, 0.67% crude coal tar (2% coal tar)	In 240 mL.
otc	**MG 217 Medicated Tar** (Triton)	**Shampoo:** 15% coal tar solution (3% coal tar)	In 120 and 240 mL.
otc	**Polytar** (Stiefel)	**Shampoo:** 4.5% polytar (coal tar solution, solubilized crude coal tar equivalent to 0.5% coal tar).	Lanolin. In 177 and 355 mL.

Indications

For treatment of scalp psoriasis, seborrheic dermatitis, dandruff, cradle-cap, and other oily, itchy conditions of the body and scalp.

Administration and Dosage

Refer to specific product labeling. Rub shampoo liberally into wet hair and scalp. Leave on for several minutes. Rinse thoroughly. Repeat and rinse. Depending on product, use from once daily to at least twice a week or as directed by a physician. For severe scalp problems, use daily.

Actions

➤*Pharmacology:* Tar derivatives have antiseptic, antibacterial, and antiseborrheic properties and loosen and soften scales and crusts.

Contraindications

Acute inflammation; open or infected lesions.

Warnings

➤*Carcinogenesis:* High concentrations of some chemicals in coal tar may cause cancer. However, concentrations of 0.5% to 5% appear to be safe.

➤*Children:* Use on children less than 2 years of age only as directed by a physician.

Precautions

➤*For external use only:* Avoid contact with eyes. If contact occurs, rinse eyes thoroughly with water. Do not use in or around the rectum or in the genital or groin area.

➤*Irritation:* Discontinue if irritation develops and contact a physician. In rare instances, temporary discoloration of blond, bleached, or tinted hair may occur.

➤*If condition worsens or does not improve:* After regular use as directed, if excessive dryness or any undesirable effect occurs, discontinue use and contact physician.

➤*Other treatment:* Do not use this product with other forms of psoriasis therapy, such as ultraviolet radiation or prescription drugs, unless directed to do so by a physician.

➤*Photosensitivity:* Use caution in exposing skin to sunlight after application. It may increase sunburn for up to 24 hours after application.

Adverse Reactions

Minor dermatologic side effects include rash or burning sensation. Photosensitivity may occur. May discolor skin.

Patient Information

For external use only. Avoid contact with the eyes.

Use caution in the sunlight after applying; it may increase the tendency to sunburn up to 24 hours after application.

Do not use for prolonged periods without consulting physician.

If condition covers a large part of the body, consult a physician before using.

TAR-CONTAINING PRODUCTS, BATH PREPARATIONS

otc	**Balnetar** (Westwood Squibb)	**Liquid:** 2.5% coal tar in mineral oil, lanolin oil	In 221 mL.
otc	**Cutar Emulsion** (Summers)	**Liquid:** 7.5% LCD (1.5% coal tar) in mineral oil, lanolin alcohols extract, parabens	In 177 mL and 1 gal.
otc	**Doak Tar Oil** (Doak)	**Oil:** 2% doak tar distillate (equivalent to 0.8% coal tar), mineral oil	In 237 mL.

Indications

These products contain tar derivatives, which have keratoplastic, antieczematous, and antipruritic effects. They are used as adjuncts in a wide range of pruritic dermatoses including psoriasis and seborrheic dermatitis.

Administration and Dosage

➤*Directions:* Add to bath water. Soak 10 to 20 minutes and then pat dry.

Contraindications

Hypersensitivity to any ingredient of the product.

Warnings

➤*Carcinogenesis:* High concentrations of some chemicals in coal tar may cause cancer. However, concentrations of 0.5% to 5% appear to be safe.

Precautions

➤*For external use only:* Avoid contact with the eyes. If contact occurs, rinse with water and contact physician.

➤*Use caution:* To avoid slipping in the bathtub.

➤*Staining:* May occur on plastic or fiberglass tubs.

➤*Irritation:* If irritation persists, discontinue use. Coal tar may cause allergic irritation.

➤*Application considerations:* Do not apply to acutely inflamed or broken skin or to the genital or rectal areas.

➤*Photosensitivity:* Coal tar is photosensitizing; for 24 hours after use, avoid exposure to direct sunlight or sunlamps.

Adverse Reactions

Dermatitis; allergic sensitization; folliculitis; photosensitization (see Precautions).

Patient Information

Keep this and all other drugs out of the reach of children. In case of accidental ingestion, seek professional assistance or contact a Poison Control Center immediately.

Discontinue use and consult with physician if condition worsens or does not improve after regular use, covers a large area of the body, or causes irritation or allergic reaction.

Discontinue use and consult with physician if used for a prolonged period of time.

TAR-CONTAINING PRODUCTS, MISCELLANEOUS

otc	**Medotar** (Medco)	**Ointment:** 1% coal tar	Octoxynol-5, zinc oxide, white petrolatum. In 454 g.
otc	**Taraphilic** (Medco)	**Ointment:** 1% coal tar distillate	Stearyl alcohol, petrolatum, parabens. In 454 g.
otc	**MG217 Medicated Tar** (Triton)	**Ointment:** 10% coal tar solution USP (equivalent to 2% coal tar)	Petrolatum, cetyl alcohol. In 107 g.
otc	**Fototar** (ICN Pharm)	**Cream:** coal tar extract (equivalent to 2% coal tar)	Emollient moisturizing base. In 85 and 454 g.
otc	**MG217 Medicated Tar Lotion** (Triton)	**Lotion:** 5% coal tar solution (equivalent to 1% coal tar)	Moisturizing base. Cetyl alcohol, mineral oil. In 120 mL.
otc	**Oxipor VHC** (Medtech)	**Lotion:** 25% coal tar solution (equivalent to 5% coal tar)	79% alcohol. In 56 mL.
otc	**Estar** (Westwood Squibb)	**Gel:** Coal tar extract (equivalent to 5% coal tar)	Benzyl alcohol, 15.6% SD alcohol 40. In 85 g.
otc	**PsoriGel** (Healthpoint)	**Gel:** 7.5% coal tar solution	28.3% alcohol. In 113 g.
otc	**Packer's Pine Tar** (GenDerm)	**Soap:** Pine tar, pine oil	Soap base. In 99 g.
otc	**Polytar** (Stiefel)	**Soap:** 2.5% coal tar solution (equivalent to 0.5% coal tar)	Glycerin, ethyl alcohol, peanut oil. In 113 g.

Indications

For the relief and control of itching, irritation, and skin flaking associated with psoriasis and seborrheic dermatitis.

Administration and Dosage

Refer to specific product labeling. Depending on product, use from 1 to 4 times/day.

Contraindications

Hypersensitivity to any ingredient in the product.

Warnings

➤*Carcinogenesis:* High concentrations of some chemicals in coal tar may cause cancer. However, concentrations of 0.5% to 5% appear to be safe.

Precautions

➤*For external use only:* Avoid contact with the eyes. If contact occurs, rinse eyes thoroughly with water and contact physician.

➤*Application considerations:* Do not apply preparations to acutely inflamed or broken skin or to the genital or rectal areas except on the advice of a physician.

➤*Discoloration/Staining:* Staining of clothing may occur which is normally removed by standard laundry methods. Use on the scalp may cause temporary staining of light colored hair.

➤*Other treatment:* Do not use with other forms of psoriasis therapy (eg, ultraviolet radiation, drug therapy) unless directed to do so by a physician.

➤*Flammable:* Some coal tar products are extremely flammable. Keep away from fire and flame.

➤*Photosensitivity:* Avoid exposure to sunlight for up to 24 hours as it may increase tendency to sunburn. Do not use on patients who have a disease characterized by photosensitivity (eg, lupus erythematosus, sunlight allergy).

Patient Information

Do not use for prolonged periods without consulting physician.

If condition worsens or does not improve after regular use, consult physician.

If condition covers a large part of the body, consult physician before using.

DIHYDROXYACETONE

otc	**Chromelin Complexion Blender** (Summers)	**Suspension:** 5%	Isopropyl alcohol, propylene glycol. In 30 mL.

Indications

➤*Idiopathic vitiligo:* Used to darken light or unpigmented areas of skin affected by vitiligo, scars, and other causes.

Administration and Dosage

Use applicator top to apply evenly to areas of skin to be darkened. Allow to remain on the skin at least 3 hours before washing. The first effects appear in about 6 hours after initial application. To achieve a darker color, repeat application instructions once or twice in 24 hours, more often if darker color is desired. The coloration will last 3 to 10 days with gradual and even fading. To prevent darkening of skin surrounding treated areas, take a damp tissue and gently wipe off any dihydroxyacetone (DHA) that has overlapped onto normally pigmented skin. Maintenance applications of once a day or every other day should be sufficient.

Actions

➤*Pharmacology:* The mechanism of action is not fully understood; however, DHA may involve a reaction (similar to that caused by sun exposure) with amino acids in the stratum corneum of the skin to produce a brownish color. As the concentration of the drug increases, so does the pigmentation.

Precautions

➤*For external use only:* Avoid contact with hair, eyes, eyelids, abraded skin, and clothes.

➤*Sun exposure:* Use sunscreen before exposing treated areas to the sun.

Adverse Reactions

Rashes with erythema and allergic dermatitis; skin irritation or sensitivity (rare).

Patient Information

Use sunscreen before exposing treated skin to the sun.

Use applicator to evenly apply to affected areas to be treated; to prevent darkening of skin in surrounding areas, take a damp cloth to wipe off excess.

Do not wash the treated area for 3 hours after application.

First application takes about 6 hours to develop color.

Cosmetics may be applied on treated areas.

May stain clothing; let treated areas dry.

HYDROQUINONE

otc	**Eldopaque** (ICN)	**Cream:** 2%	With sunblock. In 14.2 and 28.4 g.
otc	**Esoterica Facial** (Medicis)		Octyl dimethyl PABA, benzophenone, stearyl alcohol, sodium bisulfite, parabens, EDTA. In 90 g.
otc	**Esoterica Regular** (Medicis)		Light mineral oil, stearyl alcohol, parabens, sodium bisulfite, EDTA. In 90 g.
otc	**Esoterica Sunscreen** (Medicis)		3.3% padimate O, 2.5% oxybenzone, mineral oil, parabens, sodium bisulfite, EDTA. In 85 g.
otc	**Solaquin** (ICN)		With sunscreens. In 28.4 g.
Rx	**Hydroquinone** (Various, eg, Ethex, Glades)	**Cream:** 4%	May contain EDTA, parabens, mineral oil, sodium metabisulfite. In 28.35 g.
Rx	**Hydroquinone with Sunscreen** (Various, eg, Ethex, Glades)		May contain padimate O, dioxybenzone, oxybenzone, octyl methoxycinnamate, octyl dimethyl-p-aminobenzoate, cetearyl alcohol, vitamin E, parabens, mineral oil, cetearyl alcohol, stearyl alcohol, lactic acid, EDTA, sodium metabisulfite. In 28.35 g.
Rx	**Claripel** (Stiefel)		Cetostearyl alcohol, EDTA, parabens, octyl methoxycinnamate, avobenzone, oxybenzone, sodium metabisulfite, stearyl alcohol, glycerin. In 45 g.
Rx	**Eldopaque Forte** (ICN)		In a sunblock base. Talc, light mineral oil, EDTA, sodium metabisulfite. In 28.4 g.
Rx	**Eldoquin-Forte** (ICN)		In a vanishing base. Light mineral oil, propylparaben, sodium metabisulfite. In 28.4 g.
Rx	**EpiQuin Micro** (SkinMedica)		Vitamins A, E, and C, cetyl alcohol, benzyl alcohol, EDTA, glycerin, methylparaben, sodium metabisulfite. In 30 g.
Rx	**Glyquin** (ICN)		In a vanishing base. Padimate O, oxybenzone, octyl methoxycinnamate, methylparaben. SPF 15. In 28 g.
Rx	**Glyquin-XM** (ICN)		In a vanishing base. Octocrylene, oxybenzone, avobenzone, vitamin E, methylparaben, EDTA. SPF 15. In 28 g.
Rx	**Solaquin Forte** (ICN)		In a vanishing base. Dioxybenzone, padimate O, oxybenzone, EDTA, sodium metabisulfite, cetearyl alcohol, stearyl alcohol, lactic acid. In 28.4 g.
Rx	**Lustra** (Medicis)		Glycerin, alcohol, cetyl alcohol, cetearyl alcohol, benzyl alcohol, sodium metabisulfite, EDTA. In 28.4 g.
Rx	**Lustra-AF** (Medicis)		Glycerin, alcohol, cetyl alcohol, cetearyl alcohol, benzyl alcohol, sodium metabisulfite, EDTA, octyl methoxycinnamate, avobenzone. In 28.4 g.
Rx	**Nuquin HP** (Stratus)		Octyl methoxycinnamate, glycerin, cetyl alcohol, cetostearyl alcohol, stearyl alcohol, sodium metabisulfite. In 14.2, 28.4, and 56.7 g.
Rx	**Melquin HP** (Stratus)		In a vanishing base. Mineral oil, petrolatum, cetostearyl alcohol, glycerin, sodium metabisulfite. In 14.2 and 28.4 g.
Rx	**Melpaque HP** (Stratus)		In a sunblocking base. Mineral oil, parabens, EDTA, sodium metabisulfite, talc. Tinted. In 14.2 and 28.4 g.
Rx	**Hydroquinone** (Glades)	**Solution:** 3%	SD alcohol 40-B, isopropyl alcohol. In 29 mL with applicator.
otc	**NeoStrata Skin Lightening** (NeoStrata)	**Gel:** 2%	Denatured alcohol. sodium bisulfite, EDTA. In 4.8 g.
Rx	**Hydroquinone** (Glades)	**Gel:** 3%	Hydroalcoholic base. Padimate O, dioxybenzone, EDTA, sodium metabisulfite. In 30 g.
Rx	**Hydroquinone** (Glades)	**Gel:** 4%	Hydroalcoholic base. Padimate O, dioxybenzone, alcohol, EDTA, sodium metabisulfite. In 28.35 g.
Rx	**Solaquin Forte** (ICN)		Hydroalcoholic base. Padimate O, dioxybenzone, EDTA, alcohol, sodium metabisulfite. In 28.4 g.
Rx	**Aclaro** (Harmony)	**Emulsion:** 4%	Alcohols, EDTA. In 50 mL spray bottles.

Indications

For the gradual bleaching of hyperpigmented skin conditions (eg, freckles, senile lentigines, age spots, chloasma, and melasma) and other forms of melanin hyperpigmentation. Hydroquinone is also indicated for the gradual treatment of ultraviolet-induced dyschromia and discoloration resulting from the use of oral contraceptives, pregnancy, hormone replacement therapy, or skin trauma.

Administration and Dosage

Apply to affected skin twice daily. Rub in well. Use morning and before bedtime or as directed by physician.

Not recommended for children 12 years of age and younger.

➤*Storage/Stability:* Store at controlled room temperature (15° to 30°C; 59° to 86°F). Slight darkening of *Nuquin HP* and *Melpaque HP* is normal and does not affect potency of the product.

HYDROQUINONE

Actions

►*Pharmacology:* Hydroquinone depigments hyperpigmented skin by inhibiting the enzymatic oxidation of tyrosine and suppressing other melanocyte metabolic processes.

Exposure to sunlight or UV light will cause repigmentation; prevent by using sunblocking agents. In addition to hydroquinone, some products contain sunscreens (eg, octocrylene, octyl methoxycinnamate, padimate O, avobenzone, octyl dimethyl PABA, dioxybenzone, oxybenzone).

Contraindications

Hypersensitivity to hydroquinone or any other ingredients of the products.

Warnings

►*Use as directed:* Hydroquinone is a depigmenting agent that may produce unwanted cosmetic effects if not used as directed. The physician should become familiar with the contents of the prescribing information before prescribing or dispensing this medication.

►*Sunscreen use:* Sunscreen use is an essential aspect of hydroquinone therapy because minimal sun exposure sustains melanocytic activity. Therefore, avoid sun exposure by using a sunscreen, a sun block, or protective clothing to prevent repigmentation. Some products provide the necessary sun protection during therapy.

►*Sensitivity testing:* Test for skin sensitivity before using. Apply small amount to unbroken skin and check in 24 hours. If vesicle formation, itching, or excessive inflammation occurs, do not use. Minor redness is not a contraindication. Limit treatment to relatively small areas of the body at one time.

►*Discontinue use:* If no bleaching or lightening effect is noted after 2 months (3 months, topical solution and 2% cream) of use, discontinue treatment.

►*Pregnancy: Category C.* Safety for use during pregnancy has not been established. It is not known whether hydroquinone can cause fetal harm when used topically on a pregnant woman or affect reproductive capacity. It is also not known to what degree, if any, systemic absorption occurs. Use only if clearly needed.

►*Lactation:* It is not known whether topical hydroquinone is absorbed or excreted in breast milk. Caution is advised when used by a nursing mother.

►*Children:* Safety and efficacy in children 12 years of age and younger have not been established.

Precautions

Hydroquinone is formulated for use as a treatment for dyschromia and should not be used for sunburn prevention.

►*Lips:* A bitter taste and anesthetic effect may occur if applied to lips.

►*For external use only:* If rash or irritation develops, discontinue treatment. Do not use near eyes.

►*Blue-black darkening:* Rarely, a gradual blue-black darkening of the skin may occur, in which case use of hydroquinone should be discontinued and a physician contacted immediately.

►*Concomitant topical products:* Inform patient not to use these products in combination with externally applied products containing resorcinol, phenol, or salicylic acid unless directed by physician.

►*Sulfite sensitivity:* Some of these products contain sulfites which may cause allergic-type reactions (eg, hives, itching, wheezing, anaphylaxis) in certain susceptible persons. Although the overall prevalence of sulfite sensitivity in the general population is probably low, it is seen more frequently in asthmatics or atopic nonasthmatics.

Adverse Reactions

No systemic reactions have been reported. Occasional cutaneous hypersensitivity (localized contact dermatitis) may occur, in which case the medication should be discontinued and the physician notified immediately.

Dryness and fissuring of paranasal and infraorbital areas, erythema, and stinging (topical solution).

Overdosage

There have been no systemic reactions from the use of topical hydroquinone. However, limit treatment to relatively small areas of the body at one time, since some patients experience a transient skin reddening and a mild burning sensation. This does not preclude treatment.

Patient Information

For external use only. Avoid contact with the eyes. In case of accidental contact with eyes, inform patient to rinse thoroughly with water and contact physician.

Protection from the sun (eg, sunscreens, clothing) is an essential aspect of therapy.

Inform patient not to use on irritated, denuded, or damaged skin.

Inform patient to discontinue use and consult physician if rash or irritation develops.

MONOBENZONE

| *Rx* | **Benoquin** (ICN) | **Cream:** 20%[1] | Cetyl alcohol, propylene glycol. In 35.4 g. |

[1] In a water washable base.

Indications

►*Idiopathic vitiligo:* For treatment of final depigmentation in extensive vitiligo.

Monobenzone is a potent depigmenting agent, not a mild cosmetic bleach. Do not use except for indication.

Administration and Dosage

Apply and rub into the pigmented areas to be treated 2 or 3 times/day. Depigmentation is usually observed after 1 to 4 months of therapy. If satisfactory results have not been obtained within 4 months, discontinue treatment. When the desired degree of depigmentation is obtained, apply only as often as needed to maintain (usually only 2 times/week).

►*Storage / Stability:* Store at 25°C (77°F).

Actions

►*Pharmacology:* Monobenzone is the monobenzyl ether of hydroquinone whose mechanism of action is not fully understood. The topical application of monobenzone increases the excretion of melanin from the melanocytes. Monobenzone may cause destruction of melanocytes and permanent depigmentation. This effect is erratic and may take 1 to 4 months to occur while existing melanin is lost with normal sloughing of the stratum corneum. Hyperpigmented skin appears to fade more rapidly than does normal skin and exposure to sunlight reduces the depigmenting effect of the drug. The histology of the skin after depigmentation with topical monobenzone is the same as that seen in vitiligo; the epidermis is normal except for the absence of identifiable melanocytes.

Contraindications

Freckling; hyperpigmentation because of photosensitization following use of certain perfumes or following inflammation of the skin; melasma (chloasma) of pregnancy; cafe-au-lait spots; pigmented nevi; malignant melanoma; pigment resulting from pigments other than melanin, including bile, silver, and artificial pigments; hypersensitivity to monobenzone or any ingredients of the product.

Warnings

►*Skin sensitivity:* Following therapy with monobenzone, the skin will be sensitive for the rest of the patient's life. Use sunscreens during exposure.

►*Discontinue use:* Discontinue use when irritation, a burning sensation, or dermatitis occur.

►*For external use only:* Avoid contact with eyes, hair, and abraded skin.

►*Pregnancy: Category C.* It is not known whether the drug can cause fetal harm when used topically on a pregnant woman. Use only when clearly needed.

►*Lactation:* It is not known whether monobenzone is absorbed or excreted in breast milk. Use with caution in nursing mothers.

►*Children:* Safety and efficacy in children younger than 12 years of age have not been established.

Adverse Reactions

►*Dermatologic:* Mild, transient skin irritation and sensitization, including erythematous and eczematous reactions. Discontinue use if irritation, a burning sensation, or dermatitis occur. Areas of normal skin distant to the site of monobenzone application have frequently become depigmented. In addition, irregular, excessive, unsightly, and permanent depigmentation has frequently occurred.

Patient Information

Inform patient that depigmentation in areas of normal skin distant to the site of application may become irregular, excessive, unsightly, and frequently permanent.

Use sunscreens during sun exposure.

For external use only, avoid contact with the eyes and abraded skin.

Discontinue use and contact physician if irritation, a burning sensation, or dermatitis occurs.

PIGMENT AGENT COMBINATIONS

Rx	**Tri-Luma** (Galderma)	**Cream:** 0.01% fluocinolone acetonide, 4% hydroquinone, 0.05% tretinoin	Cetyl alcohol, glycerin, parabens, sodium metabisulfite, stearyl alcohol. In 30 g.
Rx	**Solage** (Galderma)	**Topical solution:** 2% mequinol, 0.01% tretinoin	Ethyl alcohol, EDTA. In 30 mL.

Indications

➤*Tri-Luma:* Short-term treatment of moderate to severe melasma of the face, in the presence of measures for sun avoidance, including the use of sunscreens.

➤*Solage:* Treatment of solar lentigines as an adjunct to a comprehensive skin care and sun avoidance program. Efficacy of daily use longer than 24 weeks has not been established.

Administration and Dosage

➤*Tri-Luma:* Apply once daily at night. Apply at least 30 minutes before bedtime. Gently wash the face and neck with a mild cleanser. Rinse and pat the skin dry. Apply a thin film of the cream to the hyperpigmented areas of melasma including about ½ inch of healthy-appearing skin surrounding each lesion. Rub lightly and uniformly into the skin. Do not use occlusive dressing. During the day, use a sunscreen of SPF 30 and wear protective clothing. Avoid sunlight exposure. Patients may use moisturizers and/or cosmetics during the day.

➤*Solage:* Apply to the solar lentigines using the applicator tip while avoiding application to the surrounding skin. Use twice daily, morning and evening, at least 8 hours apart. Patients should not shower or bathe the treatment area for at least 6 hours after application.

➤*Storage/Stability:* Store at controlled room temperature (20° to 25°C; 68° to 77°F).

Tri-Luma – Keep tightly closed. Protect from freezing.

Solage – Protect from light by continuing to store in the carton after opening.

Actions

➤*Pharmacology:*

Tri-Luma – One of the components is hydroquinone, a depigmenting agent, which may interrupt 1 or more steps in the tyrosine-tyrosinase pathway of melanin synthesis. However, the mechanism of action of the active ingredients in the treatment of melasma is unknown.

Solage – The mechanism of action of mequinol is unknown. Although mequinol is a substrate for the enzyme tyrosinase and acts as a competitive inhibitor of the formation of melanin precursors, the clinical significance of these findings is unknown. The mechanism of action of tretinoin as a depigmenting agent also is unknown.

➤*Pharmacokinetics:*

Tri-Luma – Percutaneous absorption of unchanged tretinoin, hydroquinone, and fluocinolone acetonide into the systemic circulation of 2 groups of healthy volunteers (n = 59) was found to be minimal following 8 weeks of daily application of 1 or 6 g.

Solage – The percutaneous absorption of tretinoin and the systemic exposure to tretinoin and mequinol were assessed in healthy subjects (n = 8) following 2 weeks of twice daily topical treatment with *Solage*. Approximately 0.8 mL was applied to a 400 cm^2 area of the back, corresponding to a dose of 37.3 mcg/cm^2 for mequinol and 0.23 mcg/cm^2 for tretinoin. The percutaneous absorption of tretinoin was approximately 4.4%, and systemic concentrations did not increase over endogenous levels. The mean C_{max} for mequinol was 9.92 ng/mL and the T_{max} was 2 hours.

Contraindications

Hypersensitivity, allergy or intolerance to the product or any of its components; pregnancy or use in women of childbearing potential (*Solage* only).

Warnings

➤*Hydroquinone:* Hydroquinone (contained in *Tri-Luma*) may produce exogenous ochronosis, a gradual blue-black darkening of the skin, whose occurrence should prompt discontinuation of therapy. The majority of patients developing this condition are black, but it may also occur in Caucasians and Hispanics.

➤*Eczema:* Tretinoin has been reported to cause severe irritation on eczematous skin and should be used only with utmost caution in patients with this condition.

➤*Irritation:*

Solage – *Solage* may cause skin irritation, erythema, burning, stinging or tingling, peeling, and pruritus. If the degree of such local irritation warrants, patients should be directed to use less medication, decrease the frequency of application, discontinue use temporarily, or discontinue use altogether.

Tri-Luma – *Tri-Luma* contains hydroquinone and tretinoin that may cause mild to moderate irritation. Local irritation such as skin reddening, peeling, mild burning sensation, dryness, and pruritus may be expected at the site of application. Transient skin reddening or mild burning sensation does not preclude treatment. If a reaction suggests hypersensitivity or chemical irritation, discontinue the medication.

➤*Vitiligo: Solage* should be used with caution by patients with a history or family history of vitiligo.

➤*Adrenal suppression: Tri-Luma* contains the corticosteroid fluocinolone acetonide. Systemic absorption of topical corticosteroids can produce reversible hypothalamic-pituitary-adrenal (HPA) axis suppression with the potential for glucocorticosteroid insufficiency after withdrawal of treatment. Manifestations of Cushing syndrome, hyperglycemia, and glucosuria can also be produced by systemic absorption of topical corticosteroid while on treatment. If HPA axis suppression is noted, the use of *Tri-Luma* should be discontinued. Recovery of HPA axis function generally occurs upon discontinuation of topical corticosteroids.

➤*Hypersensitivity reactions:* Cutaneous hypersensitivity to the active ingredients of *Tri-Luma* has been reported in the literature. In a patch test study to determine sensitization potential in 221 healthy volunteers, 3 volunteers developed sensitivity reactions to *Tri-Luma* or its components.

➤*Carcinogenesis:*

Tri-Luma – Studies of hydroquinone in animals have demonstrated some evidence of carcinogenicity. The carcinogenic potential of hydroquinone in humans is unknown. Studies in hairless albino mice suggest that concurrent exposure to tretinoin may enhance the tumorigenic potential of carcinogenic doses of UVB and UVA light from a solar simulator. Published studies have demonstrated that hydroquinone is a mutagen and a clastogen.

Solage – In a photocarcinogenicity study in mice administered *Solage*, median time to onset of tumors decreased.

➤*Pregnancy: Category C (Tri-Luma), Category X (Solage).*

Tri-Luma – *Tri-Luma* contains the teratogen tretinoin, which may cause embryofetal death, altered fetal growth, congenital malformations, and potential neurologic deficits. There are no adequate and well-controlled studies in pregnant women. *Tri-Luma* should be used during pregnancy only if the potential benefit justifies the potential risk to the fetus.

Solage – The combination of mequinol and tretinoin may cause fetal harm when administered to a pregnant woman. Due to the known effects of these active ingredients, *Solage* should not be used in women of childbearing potential. No adequate or well-controlled trials have been conducted with *Solage* in pregnant women.

➤*Lactation:* Corticosteroids (contained in *Tri-Luma*), when systemically administered, appear in human milk. It is not known if the other ingredients in *Tri-Luma* or *Solage* are excreted in human milk. Exercise caution when administering to a nursing woman.

➤*Children:* Safety and efficacy in pediatric patients have not been established. *Solage* should not be used on children.

Precautions

➤*Weather extremes:* Weather extremes such as wind or cold may be more irritating to patients using *Solage.*

➤*Photosensitivity: Solage* should not be administered if the patient is also taking drugs known to be photosensitizers (eg, thiazides, tetracyclines, fluoroquinolones, phenothiazines, sulfonamides) because of the possibility of augmented phototoxicity. Because of heightened burning susceptibility, exposure to sunlight (including sunlamps) to treated areas should be avoided or minimized. Patients must be advised to use protective clothing and comply with a comprehensive sun avoidance program. Patients with sunburn should be advised not to use *Solage* until fully recovered. Patients who may have considerable sun exposure because of their occupation and those patients with inherent sensitivity to sunlight should exercise particular caution.

➤*Sulfite sensitivity: Tri-Luma* contains sodium metabisulfite, which may cause allergic-type reactions, including anaphylactic symptoms and life-threatening/less severe asthmatic episodes in susceptible people. The overall prevalence in the general population is unknown and probably low. It is seen more frequently in asthmatic or atopic nonasthmatic people.

Drug Interactions

➤*Topical preparations:* Concomitant topical products with a strong skin drying effect, products with high concentrations of alcohol, astringents, spices or lime, medicated soaps or shampoos, permanent wave solutions, electrolysis, hair depilatories or waxes, or other preparations that might dry or irritate the skin should be used with caution in patients being treated with *Solage* because they may increase irritation.

➤*Photosensitizers:* Avoid drugs known to be photosensitizers (eg, thiazides, tetracyclines, fluoroquinolones, phenothiazines, sulfonamides) because of the possibility of augmented phototoxicity.

PIGMENT AGENT COMBINATIONS

Adverse Reactions

➤*Tri-Luma:* The most frequently reported events were erythema, desquamation, burning, dryness, and pruritus at the site of application. The majority of these events were mild to moderate in severity.

Tri-Luma Adverse Reactions (≥ 1% of Patients; n = 161)	
Adverse reaction	Incidence
Erythema	41
Desquamation	38
Burning	18
Dryness	14
Pruritus	11
Acne	5
Paresthesia	3
Telangiectasia	3
Hyperesthesia	2
Pigmentary changes	2
Irritation	2
Papules	1
Acne-like rash	1
Rosacea	1
Dry mouth	1
Rash	1
Vesicles	1

The following local adverse reactions have been reported infrequently with topical corticosteroids. They may occur more frequently with the use of occlusive dressings, especially with higher potency corticosteroids. These reactions are listed in an approximate decreasing order of occurrence: Burning, itching, irritation, dryness, folliculitis, acneiform eruptions, hypopigmentation, perioral dermatitis, allergic contact dermatitis, secondary infection, skin atrophy, striae, miliaria.

Tri-Luma contains hydroquinone, which may produce exogenous ochronosis, a gradual blue-black darkening of the skin, whose occurrence should prompt discontinuation of therapy.

Cutaneous hypersensitivity to the active ingredients of *Tri-Luma* has been reported in the literature. In a patch test study to determine sensitization potential in 221 healthy volunteers, 3 volunteers developed sensitivity reactions to *Tri-Luma* or its components.

➤*Solage:* The most frequent adverse reactions were erythema (49%); burning, stinging, or tingling (26%); desquamation (14%); pruritus (12%); skin irritation (5%).

Some patients experienced temporary hypopigmentation of treated lesions (5%) or of the skin surrounding treated lesions (7%); 89% had resolution of hypopigmentation upon discontinuation of treatment to the lesion, and/or re-instruction on proper application to the lesion only. Another 8% of patients with hypopigmentation events had resolution within 120 days after the end of treatment, and 2.8% had persistence of hypopigmentation beyond 120 days. Approximately 6% of patients discontinued study participation with *Solage* because of adverse reactions.

These discontinuations were due primarily to skin redness (erythema) or related cutaneous adverse reactions.

Solage Adverse Events (> 1%)	
Adverse event	Incidence
Erythema	44.6
Burning/Stinging/Tingling	21.9
Desquamation	12.6
Pruritus	11
Skin irritation	7.3
Halo hypopigmentation	6.2
Hypopigmentation	4.1
Dry skin	3.1
Rash	2.5
Crusting	2.4
Rash vesicular bullae	2.1
Dermatitis	2

Overdosage

If applied excessively, no more rapid or better results will be obtained and marked redness, peeling, discomfort, or hypopigmentation may occur. Oral ingestion of *Solage* may lead to the same adverse effects as those associated with excessive oral intake of vitamin A (hypervitaminosis A). If oral ingestion occurs, the patient should be monitored, and appropriate supportive measures administered as necessary. The maximal no-effect level for oral administration of *Solage* in rats was 5 mL/kg (30 mg/m^2). Clinical signs observed were attributed to the high alcohol content (77%) of the drug formulation.

Patient Information

Solage should not be used in women of childbearing potential or in pregnant women.

Exposure to sunlight, sunlamp, or UV light should be avoided. Patients who are consistently exposed to sunlight or skin irritants either through their work environment or habits should exercise particular caution. Sunscreen and protective covering (such as the use of a hat) over the treated areas should be used.

Sunscreen use is an essential aspect of melasma therapy, as even minimal sunlight sustains melanocytic activity.

Weather extremes such as heat or cold may be irritating to patients. Because of the drying effect of *Tri-Luma*, a moisturizer may be applied to the face in the morning after washing.

Application should be kept away from the eyes, nose, or angles of the mouth because the mucosa is much more sensitive than the skin to the irritant effect. If local irritation persists or becomes severe, application of the medication should be discontinued and the health care provider consulted. Allergic contact dermatitis, blistering, crusting, and severe burning or swelling of the skin, and irritation of the mucous membranes of the eyes, nose, and mouth require medical attention. If the medication is applied excessively, marked redness, peeling, or discomfort may occur.

POISON IVY TREATMENT PRODUCTS

otc	**Maximum Strength Ivarest** (Blistex)	**Cream:** 14% calamine and 2% diphenhydramine HCl[1]	Lanolin oil, petrolatum, propylene glycol. In 56 g.
otc	**Zanfel** (Zanfel Labs)	**Cream:** Polyethylene granules, nonoxynol-9, disodium EDTA, triethanolamine	In 30 g.
otc	**Calamine** (Various, eg, Goldline, Major, Moore)	**Lotion:** 6.97% calamine, 6.97% zinc oxide	Glycerin. In 118, 240, and 480 mL.
otc	**Phenolated Calamine** (Humco)	**Lotion:** Calamine, zinc oxide	Glycerin, 1% liquefied phenol. In 177 mL.
otc	**Caladryl** (Pfizer)	**Lotion:** 8% calamine, 1% pramoxine HCl	Alcohol, camphor, diazolidinyl urea, parabens. In 177 mL.
otc	**Ivy Super Dry** (Ivy Corp)	**Liquid:** 2% zinc acetate, 10% benzyl alcohol, 35% isopropanol, menthol, camphor	Glycerin, parabens. In 177 mL.
otc	**Ivy-Dry** (Ivy Corp)	**Lotion:** 2% zinc acetate, 12.5% isopropanol	Glycerin, methylparaben. In 118 mL.
otc	**Caladryl Clear** (Pfizer)	**Lotion:** 1% pramoxine HCl, 0.1% zinc acetate	Alcohol, camphor, diazolidinyl urea, parabens. In 177 mL.
otc	**Anti-Itch Gel** (Band-Aid)	**Gel:** 0.45% camphor	37% SD alcohol 23 A. In 60 g.
otc	**Itch Relief Gel Spritz** (Band-Aid)	**Spray:** 0.5% camphor	Benzyl alcohol, glycerin, SD alcohol 40 B (43%). In 56 g.
otc	**Ivy Soothe** (Enviroderm)	**Cream:** 1% hydrocortisone	Parabens, cetyl alcohol, glycerin, white petrolatum. In 28 g.

[1] Do not use with other products that contain diphenhydramine.

For other products used for relief of symptoms associated with contact dermatoses, see also: Antihistamine-Containing Preparations, Topical; Local Anesthetics, Topical; Corticosteroids, Topical.

Indications

For the relief of itching, pain, and discomfort of ivy, oak, and sumac poisoning. Some products are also recommended for insect bites and other minor skin irritations.

Administration and Dosage

Please refer to individual product labeling for specific information. Apply to affected area 3 to 4 times daily as needed.

Shake calamine lotions well before using.

Ingredients

The principal active components of these products include:

➤*Antimicrobial:* Benzyl alcohol.

➤*Antiseptic:* Phenol, isopropyl alcohol, benzalkonium chloride, camphor, menthol, zinc oxide.

➤*Protectants/Astringents:* Calamine, zinc oxide.

➤*Local anesthetics/Analgesics:* Benzocaine, camphor, pramoxine, menthol, phenylcarbinol (benzyl alcohol), methyl salicylate.

➤*Antipruritics:* Benzyl alcohol, camphor.

➤*Antihistamines:* Diphenhydramine.

Precautions

➤*For external use only:* Do not use in the eyes. If the condition for which these preparations are used persists or recurs, or if rash, irritation or sensitivity develops, discontinue use and consult physician.

➤*Irritation:* Do not use on blistered or broken skin.

➤*Application considerations:* Do not use on large areas of the body.

➤*Children:* Most of these products are not recommended for use on children younger than 2 years of age.

Ivy Super Dry is not recommended for use in children younger than 6 years of age.

➤*Sulfite sensitivity:* Some of these products contain sulfites that may cause allergic-type reactions, including anaphylactic symptoms and life-threatening/less severe asthmatic episodes in susceptible persons. The overall prevalence in the general population is unknown and probably low. It is seen more frequently in asthmatic or atopic nonasthmatic persons.

POISON IVY PREVENTATIVES

otc	Tecnu Outdoor Skin Cleanser (Tec Labs)	**Lotion:** Deodorized mineral spirits, propylene glycol, octylphenoxy-polyethoxyethanol, mixed fatty acid soap	In 118 and 355 mL.
otc	Ivy Stat (Tec Labs)	**Gel:** 1% hydrocortisone	Propylene glycol, menthol, SD alcohol 40-B. In 89 mL.
otc	Ivy Block (EnviroDerm)	**Lotion:** 5% bentoquatam	Benzyl alcohol, methylparaben, SDA 40 denatured alcohol. In 118 mL.
otc	Ivy Cleanse (EnviroDerm)	**Wipes:** Isopropyl and cetyl alcohol	In packet of 12 individually wrapped towelettes.

Indications

➤*Poison ivy, oak, and sumac:* For the removal of the toxic oils that cause rash and itching of poison ivy, oak, and sumac from affected skin; and to stop the irritant from spreading.

Administration and Dosage

Please refer to individual product labeling for more specific information.

➤*Tecnu:* Use within the first few hours after exposure or as soon as the rash appears. Use before smoking, going to the bathroom, and at day's end to minimize spreading oils.

Before rash has started – Apply to exposed, dry skin within 2 to 8 hours after exposure to poison plant. Rub vigorously for 2 minutes to remove oils. If hypersensitive, wash entire body. Rinse skin clean with cool running water or wipe off with a cloth; repeat.

As soon as rash appears – Rub on affected skin and surrounding areas or to entire body for best results for 2 minutes. Avoid breaking skin. Rinse off with cool running water to remove cleanser and oils. If itching persists, reapply and rinse in a very warm shower (not a bath). Towel dry gently. Repeat as needed and before bedtime.

To clean clothing and equipment – Saturate contaminated, dry clothing. Let soak for several minutes. Launder clothing by itself as usual with detergent and hot water. Wipe off equipment and tools with a clean cloth saturated with the cleanser. Then wipe off or rinse with running water. Clean hands with cleanser after handling contaminated items.

➤*Ivy Block (6 years of age and older):* Shake well before use. Apply 15 minutes before risk of exposure. Avoid intentional contact with poison ivy, oak, and sumac. Remove with soap and water after risk of exposure. Apply every 4 hours for continued protection or sooner if needed.

➤*IvyStat (2 years of age and older):*
Step 1 – Cleanse affected skin with exfoliate. Rub gently for 15 to 30 seconds. Rinse off with running water and towel dry gently. Repeat as needed and before bedtime.

Step 2 – Apply 1% hydrocortisone gel and rub thoroughly into skin 3 to 4 times/day as needed. If itching recurs, repeat steps 1 and 2.

➤*Ivy Cleanse:* Immediately wipe exposed skin areas with towelette; discard. Avoid contaminating cleansed areas. Clean hands with fresh towelette.

Precautions

➤*Irritation:* Do not apply to deep puncture wounds, burns, or oozing areas of skin. May irritate sensitive skin.

➤*For external use only:* Do not use in eyes or near other mucous membranes.

➤*Hydrocortisone:* Do not use within 3 days of using hydrocortisone ointments on affected areas.

➤*Colorfastness:* May cause colorfastness when used on clothing. Check for colorfastness of fabric first by testing a corner of the fabric.

Adverse Reactions

➤*Dermatologic:* Rash; may irritate sensitive skin.

Patient Information

Advise patient to discontinue use and consult doctor if symptoms persist for more than 7 days or if redness, irritation, increased itching, or infection occurs.

Advise patient that this product is for external use only.

Advise patient to launder clothing and decontaminate exposed pets, tools, etc.

FLUOROURACIL

Rx	Carac (Dermik)	Cream: 0.5%	Glycerin, parabens. In 30 g.
Rx	Fluoroplex (Allergan)	Cream: 1%	Benzyl alcohol, emulsifying wax, and mineral oil. In 30 g.
Rx	Efudex (ICN Pharmaceuticals)	Cream: 5%	Parabens in a white petrolatum base. In 25 g.
Rx	Fluoroplex (Allergan)	Solution: 1%	In 30 mL dropper bottle.
Rx	Fluorouracil (Taro)	Solution: 2%	In 10 mL.
Rx	Efudex (ICN Pharmaceuticals)		EDTA, and parabens. In 10 mL dropper bottle.
Rx	Fluorouracil (Taro)	Solution: 5%	In 10 mL.
Rx	Efudex (ICN Pharmaceuticals)		EDTA, and parabens. In 10 mL dropper bottle.

For information on the systemic use of fluorouracil, refer to the monograph in the Antineoplastics chapter.

Indications

➤*Multiple actinic or solar keratoses:* For the topical treatment of multiple actinic or solar keratoses. The 0.5% cream is only indicated for the face and anterior scalp areas.

➤*Superficial basal cell carcinomas:* The 5% strength is useful in the treatment of superficial basal cell carcinoma when conventional methods are impractical (ie, multiple lesions, difficult treatment sites). Establish diagnosis prior to treatment.

Administration and Dosage

➤*Multiple actinic or solar keratoses:* Apply twice daily to cover lesions. Apply preferably with a nonmetal applicator or suitable glove. If applied with fingers, wash hands immediately afterward. Continue until inflammatory response reaches erosion, necrosis, and ulceration stage, then discontinue use. Usual duration of therapy is from 2 to 6 weeks. Complete healing may not be evident for 1 to 2 months following cessation. Increasing the frequency of application and a longer period of administration may be required on areas other than the head and neck.

Carac – Using fingertips, apply once/day to cover lesions with a thin film. Do not apply near eyes, nostrils, or mouth. Apply 10 minutes after thoroughly washing, rinsing, and drying the entire area. Immediately after application, wash hands thoroughly. Continued treatment up to 4 weeks results in greater lesion reduction. Local irritation is not markedly increased by extending treatment from 2 to 4 weeks, and is generally resolved within 2 weeks of cessation of treatment.

➤*Superficial basal cell carcinomas:* Only the 5% strength is recommended. Apply twice daily in an amount sufficient to cover the lesions. Continue treatment for at least 3 to 6 weeks. Therapy may be required for as long as 10 to 12 weeks.

➤*Storage/Stability:* Store at 25°C (77°F); excursions permitted to 15° to 30°C (59° to 86°F).

Actions

➤*Pharmacology:* There is evidence that the metabolism of fluorouracil in the anabolic pathway blocks the methylation reaction of deoxyuridylic acid to thymidylic acid. Fluorouracil appears to inhibit the synthesis of deoxyribonucleic acid (DNA); to a lesser extent, ribonucleic acid (RNA) is inhibited. These effects are most marked on rapidly growing cells that take up fluorouracil at a rapid pace.

When applied to keratotic skin, a response occurs with the following sequence: Erythema, usually followed by scaling, tenderness, erosion, ulceration, necrosis, and re-epithelization. When the inflammatory reaction reaches the erosion, ulceration, and necrosis stages, terminate the use of the drug should be. Responses may sometimes occur in areas that appear clinically normal. These may be sites of subclinical actinic (solar) keratosis that the medication is affecting.

➤*Pharmacokinetics:* Fluorouracil is not significantly absorbed (approximately 6%).

Contraindications

Hypersensitivity to any component; in women who are pregnant or who may become pregnant (see Warnings); dihydropyrimidine dehydrogenase (DPD) enzyme deficiency (*Carac* only).

Warnings

➤*Occlusive dressings:* May increase the incidence of inflammatory reactions in the adjacent normal skin. A porous gauze dressing may be applied for cosmetic reasons without increase in reaction.

➤*Inflammation:* There is a possibility of increased absorption through ulcerated or inflamed skin.

➤*Photosensitivity:* Avoid prolonged exposure to UV rays while under treatment with fluorouracil because the intensity of the reaction may be increased.

➤*Mucous membranes:* Avoid application to mucous membranes because of the possibility of local inflammation and ulceration. Cases of miscarriage and a birth defect (ventricular septal defect) have been reported when applied to mucous membrane areas during pregnancy.

➤*DPD deficiency:* Do not use *Carac* in patients with DPD enzyme deficiency. A large percentage of fluorouracil is catabolized by the enzyme DPD. DPD enzyme deficiency can result in shunting of fluorouracil to the anabolic pathway, leading to cytotoxic activity and potential toxicities. Rarely, life-threatening toxicities such as stomatitis, diarrhea, neutropenia, and neurotoxicity have been reported with IV administration of fluorouracil in patients with DPD enzyme deficiency.

A case of life-threatening systemic toxicity has been reported with the topical use of fluorouracil 5% in a patient with DPD enzyme deficiency. Symptoms included severe abdominal pain, bloody diarrhea, vomiting, fever, and chills. Physical examination revealed stomatitis, erythematous skin rash, neutropenia, thrombocytopenia, inflammation of the esophagus, stomach, and small bowel. Although this case was observed with 5% fluorouracil cream, it is unknown whether patients with profound DPD enzyme deficiency would develop systemic toxicity with lower concentrations of topically applied fluorouracil.

➤*Hypersensitivity reactions:* The potential for a delayed hypersensitivity reaction to fluorouracil exists. Patch testing to prove hypersensitivity may be inconclusive.

➤*Mutagenesis:* In vitro and in vivo studies of fluorouracil have shown positive effects for mutagenicity.

➤*Fertility impairment:* In vitro and in vivo studies of fluorouracil have shown positive effects for fertility impairment.

➤*Pregnancy: Category X.* Fluorouracil may cause fetal harm when administered to a pregnant woman. In animal studies, parenteral fluorouracil is both teratogenic and embryolethal. The drug is contraindicated in women who are or who may become pregnant. If fluorouracil is used during pregnancy, or if the patient becomes pregnant while taking this drug, apprise her of the potential hazard to the fetus.

No adequate and well-controlled studies have been conducted in pregnant women with either topical or parenteral forms of fluorouracil. One birth defect (cleft lip and palate) has been reported in the newborn of a patient using fluorouracil as recommended. One birth defect (ventricular septal defect) and cases of miscarriage have been reported when fluorouracil was applied to mucous membrane areas. Multiple birth defects have been reported in the fetus of a patient treated with IV fluorouracil.

➤*Lactation:* It is not known whether this drug is excreted in breast milk. Because there is some systemic absorption of the drug after topical administration, mothers should not breastfeed while receiving this drug.

➤*Children:* Safety and efficacy have not been established.

Precautions

➤*Biopsies:* To rule out the presence of a frank neoplasm, biopsy those areas failing to respond to treatment or recurring after treatment. Perform follow-up biopsies as indicated in the management of superficial basal cell carcinoma.

Adverse Reactions

➤*Local:* Burning; crusting; allergic contact dermatitis; erosions; erythema; hyperpigmentation; irritation; pain; pruritus; scarring; rash; soreness; ulceration; inflammation; photosensitivity; leukocytosis.

➤*Infrequent:* Although a causal relationship is remote, the following adverse reactions have been reported infrequently:

CNS – Emotional upset; insomnia; irritability.

GI – Metallic taste; stomatitis.

Hematologic – Eosinophilia; thrombocytopenia; toxic granulation.

Dermatologic – Alopecia; blistering; bullous pemphigoid; discomfort; ichthyosis; scaling; suppuration; swelling; telangiectasia; tenderness; urticaria; skin rash.

Special senses – Conjunctival reaction; corneal reaction; lacrimation; nasal irritation.

Miscellaneous – Herpes simplex.

FLUOROURACIL

Carac Adverse Reactions (%)					
Adverse reaction	Week 1 (n = 85)	Week 2 (n = 87)	Week 4 (n = 85)	All active treatments (n = 257)	Vehicle (n = 127)
Dermatologic					
Application-site reaction	91.8	95.4	96.5	94.6	65.4
Burning	60	80.5	83.5	74.7	22
Dryness	69.4	87.4	92.9	83.3	47.2
Edema	14.1	32.2	60	35.4	4.7
Erosion	24.7	43.7	63.5	44	13.4
Erythema	89.4	94.3	96.5	93.4	59.8
Irritation	1.2	0	2.4	1.2	0
Pain	30.6	39.1	61.2	43.6	5.5
Miscellaneous					
Allergy	0	2.3	1.2	1.2	1.6
Common cold	4.7	0	2.4	2.3	2.4
Headache	3.5	2.3	3.5	3.1	2.4
Eye irritation	5.9	3.4	7.1	5.4	2.4
Sinusitis	4.7	0	0	1.6	1.6

Overdosage

Ordinarily topical overdosage will not cause acute problems. If fluorouracil accidently comes in contact with the eye, flush the eye with water or normal saline. If fluorouracil is accidentally ingested, induce emesis and gastric lavage. Administer symptomatic and supportive care as needed.

Patient Information

Avoid prolonged exposure to UV rays or other forms of UV irradiation while under treatment; intensity of reaction may be increased.

Avoid contact with eyes, nose, and mouth.

If applied with fingers, wash hands immediately afterward. Apply with care near the eyes, nose, and mouth.

Reaction in the treated areas may be unsightly during therapy and, in some cases, for several weeks following cessation of therapy.

Inform physician if able to become pregnant; physician may advise about birth control.

Do not use fluorouracil if pregnant, planning on becoming pregnant, or if breastfeeding.

PYRITHIONE ZINC

otc	**Dermazinc** (Dermalogix)	**Shampoo:** 0.25%	Parabens. In 240 mL.
otc	**Zincon** (Medtech)	**Shampoo:** 1%	Propylene glycol. In 118 and 240 mL.
otc	**Head & Shoulders** (Procter & Gamble)		Cetyl and benzyl alcohol. In "normal to oily" and "normal to dry" formulas. In 200, 400, and 750 mL.
otc	**Head & Shoulders Dry Scalp** (Procter & Gamble)		Cetyl and benzyl alcohol. In regular and conditioning formulas. In 200, 400, 750, and 1000 mL.
otc	**DHS Zinc** (Person & Covey)	**Shampoo:** 2%	In 240 and 360 mL.
otc	**Denorex Everyday Dandruff** (Medtech)		Propylene glycol, menthol. In 118 and 240 mL.
otc	**ZNP Bar** (Stiefel)	**Soap:**[1] 2%	Cetostearyl alcohol. In 119 g.

[1] Also contains corn starch, glycerin, hydrogenated castor oil, and mineral oil.

Indications

For control of dandruff and seborrheic dermatitis of the face, body, and scalp. Relieves the itching and scalp flaring associated with dandruff. Also relieves the itching, irritation, and skin flaking associated with seborrheic dermatitis.

Administration and Dosage

➤*Shampoo:* Apply shampoo; lather, rinse, and repeat. Use at least twice weekly for best results.

➤*Soap:* Use on affected areas in place of your regular soap. Work up a rich lather using warm water and massage into affected areas; rinse well, then repeat. Use twice a week for best results. May be used as a shampoo.

Actions

➤*Pharmacology:* Pyrithione zinc, a cytostatic agent, reduces cell turnover rate. Its action is thought to be due to a nonspecific toxicity for epidermal cells. The compound strongly binds to hair and external skin layers.

Warnings

➤*Children:* Do not use on children under 2 years of age, unless directed by a physician (*Zincon*).

Precautions

➤*For external use only:* Keep out of eyes; if contact occurs, rinse thoroughly with water.

Adverse Reactions

Irritation of skin (rare).

Patient Information

Avoid contact with eyes; rinse with water thoroughly if contact occurs.

If condition worsens, or does not improve after regular use, consult a physician.

ADAPALENE

| *Rx* | **Differin** (Galderma) | **Solution:** 0.1% | 30% alcohol, PEG-400. In 30 mL glass bottles with applicator and 60 unit-of-use pledgets. |

Indications

➤*Acne vulgaris:* Topical treatment of acne vulgaris.

Administration and Dosage

➤*Approved by the FDA:* May 31, 1996.

Apply once a day to affected areas after washing in the evening before bedtime. Apply a thin film, avoiding eyes, lips, and mucous membranes.

During the early weeks of therapy, an apparent exacerbation of acne may occur. This is because of the action of the medication on previously unseen lesions and should not be considered a reason to discontinue therapy. Therapeutic results should be noticed after 8 to 12 weeks of treatment.

➤*Storage/Stability:* Store at controlled room temperature 20° to 25°C (68° to 77°F). Keep bottle tightly closed and store upright. Protect from freezing.

Actions

➤*Pharmacology:* Adapalene is a retinoid-like compound and acts on retinoid receptors. It is a modulator of cellular differentiation, keratinization and inflammatory processes, all of which represent important features in the pathology of acne vulgaris.

Adapalene binds to specific retinoic acid nuclear receptors but does not bind to the cytosolic receptor protein. Although the exact mode of action of adapalene is unknown, it is suggested that topical adapalene may normalize the differentiation of follicular epithelial cells resulting in decreased microcomedone formation.

➤*Pharmacokinetics:*

Absorption –

Gel/Solution: Absorption of adapalene gel or solution through human skin is low. Only trace amounts (less than 0.25 ng/mL) of parent substance have been found in the plasma of acne patients following chronic topical application of adapalene.

Cream: Absorption of adapalene from the cream through human skin is low. In a pharmacokinetic study with 6 acne patients treated once daily for 5 days with 2 g of adapalene cream applied to 1000 cm² of acne involved skin, there were no quantifiable amounts (limit of quantification = 0.35 ng/mL) of adapalene in the plasma samples from any patient.

Excretion – Excretion appears to be primarily by the biliary route.

Contraindications

Hypersensitivity to adapalene or any of the components in the vehicle.

Warnings

➤*Hypersensitivity reactions:* Discontinue use of adapalene if hypersensitivity or chemical irritation occurs.

➤*Pregnancy: Category C.* No teratogenic effects were seen in rats at oral doses of adapalene 0.15 to 5 mg/kg/day, up to 120 times the maximal daily human topical dose. However, adapalene administered orally at doses of greater than or equal to 25 mg/kg (100 times the recommended topical human dose [MRHD] for rats and 200 times the MRHD for rabbits) has been shown to be teratogenic. There are no adequate and well-controlled studies in pregnant women. Use adapalene during pregnancy only if the potential benefit justifies the potential risk to the fetus.

➤*Lactation:* It is not known whether this drug is excreted in breast milk. Exercise caution when administering adapalene to a nursing mother.

➤*Children:* Safety and effectiveness in pediatric patients below the age of 12 years have not been established.

Precautions

➤*For external use only:* Avoid contact with the eyes, lips, angles of the nose, and other mucous membranes. Do not apply to cuts, abrasions, eczematous skin, or sunburned skin. As with other retinoids, avoid the use of "waxing" as a depilatory method on skin treated with adapalene.

➤*Local adverse reactions:* Certain cutaneous signs and symptoms such as erythema, dryness, scaling, burning, or pruritus may occur during treatment. These are most likely to occur during the first 2 to 4 weeks, are mostly mild to moderate in intensity, and will usually lessen with continued use of the medication. Depending upon the severity of adverse events, instruct patients to reduce the frequency of application or discontinue use.

➤*Photosensitivity:* Advise patients with sunburn not to use the product until fully recovered. Minimize exposure to sunlight, including sunlamps, during the use of adapalene. Warn patients who normally experience high levels of sun exposure and those with inherent sensitivity to sun, to exercise caution. Use of sunscreen products and protective clothing over treated areas is recommended when exposure cannot be avoided. Weather extremes, such as wind or cold, also may be irritating to patients under treatment with adapalene.

Drug Interactions

➤*Local irritants:* As adapalene has the potential to produce local irritation in some patients, concomitant use of other potentially irritating topical products (medicated or abrasive soaps and cleansers; soaps and cosmetics that have a strong drying effect; products with high concentrations of alcohol, astringents, spices, or lime) should be approached with caution. Exercise particular caution in using preparations containing sulfur, resorcinol, or salicylic acid in combination with adapalene. If these preparations have been used, it is advisable not to start therapy with adapalene until the effects of such preparations in the skin have subsided.

Adverse Reactions

➤*Gel/Solution:*

Dermatologic – Erythema, scaling, dryness, pruritus, burning (gel, 10% to 40%; solution, 30% to 60%); pruritus or burning immediately after application (gel, approximately 20%; solution, approximately 30%); skin irritation, burning/stinging, erythema, sunburn, acne flares (approximately 1% or less).

These adverse reactions are most commonly seen during the first month of therapy and decrease in frequency and severity thereafter. All adverse effects with use of adapalene during clinical trials were reversible upon discontinuation of therapy.

➤*Cream:*

Dermatologic –

Adapalene Cream Local Adverse Reactions (N = 285) (%)				
Adverse reaction	None	Mild	Moderate	Severe
Erythema	52	38	10	< 1
Scaling	58	35	6	< 1
Dryness	48	42	9	< 1
Pruritus (persistent)	74	21	4	< 1
Burning/Stinging (persistent)	71	24	4	< 1

Other reported local cutaneous adverse events in patients who used adapalene cream once daily included the following: Sunburn (2%), skin discomfort/burning and stinging (1%), and skin irritation (1%). Events occurring in fewer than 1% of patients treated with adapalene cream included the following: Acne flare, dermatitis and contact dermatitis, eyelid edema, conjunctivitis, erythema, pruritus, skin discoloration, rash, eczema.

Overdosage

Adapalene is intended for cutaneous use only. If the medication is applied excessively, no more rapid or better results will be obtained and marked redness, peeling, or discomfort may occur. The acute oral toxicity of adapalene in mice and rats is greater than 10 mL/kg. Chronic ingestion of the drug may lead to the same side effects as those associated with excessive oral intake of vitamin A.

Patient Information

Adapalene cream is for external use only. Avoid contact with the eyes, lips, angles of the nose, and mucous membranes. Exposure of the eye to this medication may result in reactions such as swelling, conjunctivitis, and eye irritation. Do not apply this medication to cuts, abrasions, or eczematous or sunburned skin.

Cleanse area with a mild or soapless cleanser before applying this medication.

Moisturizers may be used if necessary; however, avoid products containing alpha hydroxy or glycolic acids.

Do not perform wax epilation on treated skin because of the potential for skin erosions.

During the early weeks of therapy, an apparent exacerbation of acne may occur. This is due to the action of this medication on previously unseen lesions and should not be considered a reason to discontinue therapy. Overall clinical benefit may be noticed after 2 weeks of therapy, but at least 8 weeks are required to obtain consistent beneficial effects.

TRETINOIN (trans-Retinoic Acid; Vitamin A Acid)

Rx	Renova (Ortho Dermatological)	Cream: 0.02%	Parabens, benzyl alcohol, cetyl alcohol, stearyl alcohol, EDTA. In 40 g.
Rx	Tretinoin (Alpharma, Spear Dermatology)	Cream: 0.025%	May contain stearyl alcohol. In 20 and 45 g.
Rx	Avita (Bertek)		Stearyl alcohol. In 20 and 45 g.
Rx	Retin-A (Ortho)		Hydrophilic vehicle. In 20 and 45 g.
Rx	Tretinoin (Spear Dermatology)	Cream: 0.05%	Stearyl alcohol. In 20 and 45 g.
Rx	Renova (Ortho Dermatological)		Methylparaben, stearyl alcohol, EDTA. In 20, 40, and 60 g.
Rx	Retin-A (Ortho)		Hydrophilic vehicle. In 20 and 45 g.
Rx	Tretinoin (Spear Dermatology)	Cream: 0.1%	Stearyl alcohol. In 20 and 45 g.
Rx	Retin-A (Ortho)		Stearyl alcohol. In 20 and 45 g.
Rx	Tretinoin (Spear Dermatology)	Gel: 0.01%	Alcohol. In 15 and 45 g.
Rx	Retin-A (Ortho)		90% alcohol. In 15 and 45 g.
Rx	Tretinoin (Spear Dermatology)	Gel: 0.025%	Alcohol. In 15 and 45 g.
Rx	Avita (Bertek)		83% ethanol. In 20 and 45 g.
Rx	Retin-A (Ortho)		90% alcohol. In 15 and 45 g.
Rx	Retin-A Micro (Ortho)	Gel: 0.04%	Glycerin, EDTA, propylene glycol, benzyl alcohol. In 20 and 45 g.
Rx	Retin-A Micro (Ortho)	Gel: 0.1%	Glycerin, EDTA, propylene glycol, benzyl alcohol. In 20 and 45 g.
Rx	Retin-A (Ortho)	Liquid: 0.05%	55% alcohol. In 28 mL.

Indications

➤*Acne (except Renova):* Topical treatment of acne vulgaris.

➤*Renova:*

Dermatologic conditions –

0.02% cream: Adjunctive agent for use in the mitigation (palliation) of fine wrinkles in patients who use comprehensive skin care and sun avoidance programs.

0.05% cream: Adjunctive agent for use in the mitigation (palliation) of fine wrinkles, mottled hyperpigmentation, and tactile roughness of facial skin in patients who do not achieve such palliation using comprehensive skin care and sun avoidance programs alone.

➤*Unlabeled uses:* Tretinoin has been used to treat hyperpigmentation of photoaged skin, postinflammatory hyperpigmentation, melasma, and facial actinic keratoses.

Administration and Dosage

➤*Acne treatment:* Apply once a day before bedtime or in the evening. Cover the entire affected area lightly.

Closely monitor alterations of vehicle, drug concentration, or dose frequency. During the early weeks of therapy, an apparent exacerbation of inflammatory lesions may occur due to the action of the medication on deep, previously undetected lesions; this is not a reason to discontinue therapy.

Therapeutic results should be seen after 2 to 3 weeks, but may not be optimal until after 6 weeks. Once lesions have responded satisfactorily, maintain therapy with less frequent applications or other dosage forms.

Patients may use cosmetics, but thoroughly cleanse area to be treated before applying medication.

➤*Liquid:* Apply with fingertip, gauze pad, or cotton swab. Do not oversaturate gauze or cotton to the extent that liquid will run into unaffected areas.

➤*Gel:* Excessive application results in "pilling" of the gel, which minimizes the likelihood of overapplication by the patient.

➤*Renova:* Gently wash face with a mild soap, pat the skin dry, and wait 20 to 30 minutes before applying. Apply tretinoin to the face once a day in the evening, using only enough to cover the entire affected area lightly. Apply a pea-sized amount of cream to cover the entire face. Take caution to avoid contact with eyes, ears, nostrils, and mouth.

For best results, do not apply another skin care product or cosmetic for at least 1 hour after applying tretinoin.

Do not wash face for at least 1 hour after applying tretinoin.

Application of tretinoin may cause a transitory feeling of warmth or slight stinging.

Mitigation (palliation) of fine facial wrinkling, mottled hyperpigmentation, and tactile roughness may occur gradually over the course of therapy. Up to 6 months of therapy may be required before the effects are seen. Most of the improvement noted with tretinoin is seen during the first 24 weeks of therapy. Thereafter, therapy primarily maintains the improvement noticed during the first 24 weeks.

Patients treated with tretinoin may use cosmetics, but the areas to be treated should be cleansed thoroughly before the medication is applied.

➤*Storage/Stability:* Store between 15° and 30°C (59° and 86°F). Do not freeze.

Actions

➤*Pharmacology:* Tretinoin is a retinoid metabolite of vitamin A. Although the exact mode of action of tretinoin is unknown, current evidence suggests that topical tretinoin decreases cohesiveness of follicular epithelial cells with decreased microcomedo formation. Additionally, tretinoin stimulates mitotic activity and increases turnover of follicular epithelial cells, causing extrusion of the comedones.

➤*Pharmacokinetics:* The transdermal absorption of tretinoin from various topical formulations ranged from 1% to 31% of applied dose, depending on whether it was applied to healthy skin or dermatitic skin.

In vitro and in vivo pharmacokinetic studies with tretinoin cream and gel indicated that less than 0.3% of the topically applied dose is bioavailable. Circulating plasma levels of tretinoin are only slightly elevated above those found in healthy normal controls. Estimates of in vivo bioavailability of *Retin-A Micro* following single and multiple daily applications, for a period of 28 days with the 0.1% gel, were approximately 0.82% and 1.41%, respectively. When percutaneous absorption of *Renova* was assessed in healthy male subjects (n = 14) after a single application, as well as after repeated daily applications for 28 days, the absorption of tretinoin was less than 2% and endogenous concentrations of tretinoin and its major metabolites were unaltered.

Contraindications

Hypersensitivity to any component of the product; discontinue if hypersensitivity to any ingredient is noted.

Warnings

➤*For external use only:* Keep tretinoin away from the eyes, mouth, angles of the nose, and mucous membranes.

➤*Renova:*

Mitigating effects – Tretinoin has shown no mitigating effects on significant signs of chronic sun exposure (eg, coarse or deep wrinkling, skin yellowing, lentigines, telangiectasia, skin laxity, keratinocytic atypia, melanocytic atypia, dermal elastosis).

Tretinoin 0.02% cream has shown no mitigating effects on tactile roughness or mottled hyperpigmentation.

Tretinoin does not eliminate wrinkles, repair sun damaged skin, reverse photoaging, or restore a more youthful or younger dermal histologic pattern.

Many patients achieve desired palliative effect on fine wrinkling, mottled hyperpigmentation, and tactile roughness of facial skin with the use of comprehensive skin care and sun avoidance programs including sunscreens, protective clothing, and nonprescription emollient creams.

Long-term use – Tretinoin is a dermal irritant, and the results of continued irritation of the skin for greater than 48 weeks are not known. There is evidence of atypical changes in melanocytes and keratinocytes and of increased dermal elastosis in some patients treated with tretinoin 0.05% for longer than 52 weeks.

➤*Pregnancy:* Category C. Oral tretinoin is teratogenic. There are no adequate and well-controlled studies in pregnant women. Use during pregnancy only if the potential benefit justifies the potential risk. Do not use *Renova* and *Avita* during pregnancy.

Topical tretinoin in animal teratogenicity tests has generated equivocal results. There is evidence of teratogenicity (shortened or kinked tail) of topical tretinoin in Wistar rats at doses greater than 1 mg/kg/day (200 times the recommended human topical clinical dose) Anomalies

TRETINOIN (trans-Retinoic Acid; Vitamin A Acid)

(humerus: short 13%, bent 6%; os parietal incompletely ossified 14%) also have been reported in rats when 10 mg/kg/day was dermally applied.

There are other reports in New Zealand White rabbits with doses of approximately 80 times the recommended human topical clinical dose of an increased incidence of domed head and hydrocephaly, typical of retinoid-induced fetal malformations in this species.

In contrast, several well-controlled animal studies have shown that dermally applied tretinoin was not teratogenic at doses of 100 and 200 times the recommended human topical clinical dose in rats and rabbits, respectively.

Dermal tretinoin has been shown to be fetotoxic in rabbits when administered in doses 100 times the recommended topical human clinical dose.

Thirty cases of temporally associated congenital malformations have been reported during 2 decades of clinical use of another formulation of topical tretinoin (acne preparation). Although no definite pattern of teratogenicity and no causal association has been established from these cases, 5 of the reports describe the rare birth defect category holoprosencephaly (defects associated with incomplete midline development of the forebrain). The significance of these spontaneous reports in terms of risk to the fetus is unknown.

➤*Lactation:* It is not known whether this drug is excreted in breast milk. Exercise caution when tretinoin is administered to a nursing mother.

➤*Children:*

Renova – Safety and efficacy in patients less than 18 years of age have not been established.

Precautions

➤*Irritation:* Tretinoin may induce severe local erythema, pruritus, burning, stinging, and peeling at the application site. If the degree of local irritation warrants, use medication less frequently or discontinue use temporarily or completely. Tretinoin may cause severe irritation to eczematous skin; use with caution in patients with this condition.

➤*Photosensitivity:* It is advisable to "rest" a patient's skin until effects of keratolytic agents subside before beginning tretinoin. Minimize exposure to sunlight and sunlamps, and advise patients with sunburn not to use tretinoin until fully recovered because of heightened susceptibility to sunlight as a result of tretinoin use. Patients who undergo considerable sun exposure due to occupation and those with inherent sun sensitivity should exercise particular caution. Use sunscreen products and wear protective clothing over treated areas. Weather extremes, such as wind and cold, also may irritate treated areas.

Drug Interactions

➤*Sulfur, resorcinol, benzoyl peroxide, or salicylic acid:* Cautiously use concomitant topical medications because of possible interactions with tretinoin. Significant skin irritation may result. It also is advisable to "rest" a patient's skin until the effects of such preparations subside before use of tretinoin is begun.

➤*Topical preparations:* Cautiously use medicated or abrasive soaps and cleansers, soaps and cosmetics that have a strong drying effect, and products with high concentrations of alcohol, astringents, spices, or lime, permanent wave solutions, electrolysis, hair depilatories or waxes, and products that may irritate the skin in patients being treated with tretinoin because they may increase irritation.

➤*Photosensitizers:* Do not use tretinoin if the patient also is taking drugs known to be photosensitizers (eg, thiazides, tetracyclines, fluoro-quinolones, phenothiazines, sulfonamides) because of the possibility of augmented phototoxicity.

Adverse Reactions

Almost all patients reported 1 or more local reactions such as peeling, dry skin, burning, stinging, erythema, and pruritus during therapy with tretinoin.

Sensitive skin may become excessively red, edematous, blistered, or crusted. If these effects occur, discontinue medication until skin integrity is restored or adjust to a tolerable level. True contact allergy is rare.

Temporary hyperpigmentation or hypopigmentation has been reported with repeated application. Some individuals have a heightened susceptibility to sunlight while under treatment.

All adverse effects have been reversible upon discontinuation.

Overdosage

Application of larger amounts of medication than recommended will not lead to more rapid or better results, and marked redness, peeling, or discomfort may occur. Oral ingestion of tretinoin may lead to the same side effects as those associated with excessive oral intake of vitamin A.

Patient Information

Apply once daily before bedtime or as directed by your physician. Wash with a mild soap and dry skin gently. Wait 20 to 30 minutes before applying medication; it is important for skin to be completely dry in order to minimize possible irritation.

Keep away from eyes, mouth, angles of the nose, and mucous membranes.

Avoid excessive exposure to sunlight and sunlamps. Wear an effective sunscreen any time you are outside. For extended sun exposure, wear protective clothing, like a hat. If you do become sunburned, stop therapy with tretinoin until skin has recovered.

Application may cause a transitory feeling of warmth and slight stinging. The skin of certain sensitive individuals may become excessively red, swollen, blistered, or crusted. If you are experiencing severe or persistent irritation, discontinue the use of tretinoin and consult your physician.

Avoid preparations that may dry or irritate your skin. These preparations may include certain astringents, toiletries containing alcohol, spices, or lime, or certain medicated soaps, shampoos, and hair permanent solutions.

Weather extremes, such as wind or cold, may be more irritating to patients using tretinoin-containing products.

Normal use of cosmetics is permissible.

➤*Renova:* Apply only as an adjunct to a comprehensive skin care and sun avoidance program. Apply a moisturizing sunscreen with a minimum SPF of 15 every morning when being treated with tretinoin. Avoid direct sun exposure as much as possible and totally avoid sunlamps while using tretinoin. Do not use if sunburned or if eczema or other chronic skin conditions exist. Do not use if inherently sensitive to sunlight or if also taking other drugs that increase sensitivity to sunlight.

Do not use if pregnant, attempting to become pregnant, or at high risk of pregnancy.

A majority of patients will lose most mitigating effects on fine wrinkles, mottled hyperpigmentation, and tactile roughness of facial skin with discontinuation of a comprehensive skin care and sun avoidance program including tretinoin; however, the safety and efficacy of tretinoin daily use for greater than 48 weeks have not been established.

ISOTRETINOIN (13-cis-Retinoic Acid)

Rx	**Accutane** (Roche)	**Capsules:**[1] 10 mg	(ACCUTANE 10 ROCHE). Light pink. In UD 10s.	
		20 mg	(ACCUTANE 20 ROCHE). Maroon. In UD 10s.	
		40 mg	(ACCUTANE 40 ROCHE). Yellow. In UD 10s.	
Rx	**Amnesteem** (Bertek)	**Capsules:** 10 mg	(I10). Reddish brown. In 30s and 100s.	
Rx	**Claravis** (Barr Laboratories)		(BARR 934). Lt. gray. In blister pack 30s and 100s.	
Rx	**Amnesteem** (Bertek)	**Capsules:** 20 mg	(I20). Reddish brown and cream. In 30s and 100s.	
Rx	**Claravis** (Barr Laboratories)		(BARR 935). Brown-orange. In blister pack 30s and 100s.	
Rx	**Amnesteem** (Bertek)	**Capsules:** 40 mg	(I40). Orange brown. In 30s and 100s.	
Rx	**Claravis** (Barr Laboratories)		(BARR 936). Lt. orange. In blister pack 30s and 100s.	
Rx	**Sotret** (Ranbaxy)	**Capsules, soft gel:** 10 mg	(5R). Parabens. Lt. Pink. In 30s and 100s.	
		20 mg	(6R). Parabens. Maroon. In 30s and 100s.	
		30 mg	(8R). Parabens. Golden yellow. In 30s and 100s.	
		40 mg	(7R). Parabens. Yellow. In 30s and 100s.	

[1] Capsule contains suspension of drug in soybean oil; also contains parabens and EDTA.

WARNING

Isotretinoin must not be used by females who are pregnant. Although not every fetus exposed to isotretinoin has resulted in a deformed child, there is an extremely high risk that a deformed infant can result if pregnancy occurs while taking isotretinoin in any amount even for short periods of time. Potentially any fetus exposed during pregnancy can be affected. Presently, there are no accurate means of determining, after isotretinoin exposure, which fetus has been affected and which fetus has not been affected.

Major human fetal abnormalities related to isotretinoin administration in females have been documented. There is an increased risk of spontaneous abortion. In addition, premature births have been reported.

Documented external abnormalities include the following: Skull abnormality; ear abnormalities (including anotia, micropinna, small or absent external auditory canals); eye abnormalities (including microphthalmia); facial dysmorphia; cleft palate. Documented internal abnormalities include the following: CNS abnormalities (including cerebral abnormalities, cerebellar malformation, hydrocephalus, microcephaly, cranial nerve deficit); cardiovascular abnormalities; thymus gland abnormality; parathyroid hormone deficiency. In some cases death has occurred with certain of the abnormalities previously noted.

Cases of IQ scores less than 85 with or without obvious CNS abnormalities also have been reported.

Isotretinoin is contraindicated in females of childbearing potential unless the patient meets all of the following conditions:
• Must not be pregnant or breastfeeding,
• Must be capable of complying with mandatory contraceptive measures required for isotretinoin therapy and understand behaviors associated with an increased risk of pregnancy, and
• Must be reliable in understanding and carrying out instructions.

Accutane must be prescribed under the System to Manage Accutane-Related Teratogenicity (SMART). The prescriber must obtain a supply of yellow self-adhesive *Accutane* qualification stickers. To obtain these stickers: 1) Read the booklet entitled *SMART Guide to Best Practices*; 2) sign and return the completed SMART letter of understanding containing the prescriber checklist; and 3) use the yellow self-adhesive *Accutane* qualification sticker. *Accutane* should not be prescribed or dispensed to any patient (male or female) without a yellow self-adhesive *Accutane* qualification sticker.

►*Female patients:* For female patients, the yellow self-adhesive *Accutane* qualification sticker signifies that she understands the following:
• Must have had 2 negative urine or serum pregnancy tests with a sensitivity of at least 25 mIU/mL before receiving the initial isotretinoin prescription. The first test (a screening test) is obtained by the prescriber when the decision is made to pursue qualification of the patient for isotretinoin. The second pregnancy test (a confirmation test) should be done during the first 5 days of the menstrual period immediately preceding the beginning of isotretinoin therapy. For patients with amenorrhea, the second test should be done at least 11 days after the last act of unprotected sexual intercourse (without using 2 effective forms of contraception). Each month of therapy, the patient must have a negative result from a urine or serum pregnancy test. A pregnancy test must be repeated every month prior to the female patient receiving each prescription. The manufacturer will make available urine pregnancy test kits for female isotretinoin patients for the initial, second, and monthly testing during therapy.
• Must have selected and have committed to using 2 forms of effective contraception simultaneously, at least 1 of which must be a primary form, unless absolute abstinence is the chosen method, or

WARNING (cont.)

the patient has undergone a hysterectomy. Patients must use 2 forms of effective contraception for at least 1 month prior to initiation of isotretinoin therapy, during isotretinoin therapy, and for 1 month after discontinuing isotretinoin therapy. Counseling about contraception and behaviors associated with an increased risk of pregnancy must be repeated on a monthly basis.

Effective forms of contraception include both primary and secondary forms of contraception. Primary forms of contraception include: Tubal ligation, partner's vasectomy, intrauterine devices, birth control pills, and injectable/implantable/insertable hormonal birth control products. Secondary forms of contraception include diaphragms, latex condoms, and cervical caps; each must be used with a spermicide.

Any birth control method can fail. Therefore, it is critically important that women of childbearing potential use 2 effective forms of contraception simultaneously. A drug interaction that decreases effectiveness of hormonal contraceptives has not been entirely ruled out for isotretinoin. Although hormonal contraceptives are highly effective, there have been reports of pregnancy from women who have used oral contraceptives, as well as injectable/implantable contraceptive products. These reports occurred while these patients were taking isotretinoin. These reports are more frequent for women who use only a single method of contraception. Patients must receive written warnings about the rates of possible contraception failure (included in patient education kits).

Prescribers are advised to consult the package insert of any medication administered concomitantly with hormonal contraceptives, because some medications may decrease the effectiveness of these birth control products. Patients should be prospectively cautioned not to self-medicate with the herbal supplement St. John's wort because a possible interaction has been suggested with hormonal contraceptives based on reports of breakthrough bleeding while on oral contraceptives shortly after starting St. John's wort. Pregnancies have been reported by users of combined hormonal contraceptives who also used some form of St. John's wort.
• Must have signed a patient information/consent form that contains warnings about the risk of potential birth defects if the fetus is exposed to isotretinoin.
• Must have been informed of the purpose and importance of participating in the *Accutane* survey and have been given the opportunity to enroll.

The yellow self-adhesive *Accutane* qualification sticker documents that the female patient is qualified and includes the date of qualification, patient gender, cut-off date for filling the prescription, and up to a 30-day supply limit with no refills.

If a pregnancy does occur during treatment with isotretinoin, the prescriber and patient should discuss the desirability of continuing the pregnancy. Prescribers are strongly encouraged to report all cases of pregnancy to Roche at (800) 526-6367 where a Roche pregnancy prevention program specialist will be available to discuss Roche pregnancy information, or prescribers may contact the FDA MedWatch program at (800) FDA-1088.

Isotretinoin should be prescribed only by prescribers who have demonstrated special competence in the diagnosis and treatment of severe recalcitrant nodular acne, are experienced in the use of systemic retinoids, have read the *SMART Guide to Best Practices*, signed and returned the completed SMART letter of understanding, and obtained yellow self-adhesive *Accutane* qualification stickers. Do not prescribe or dispense *Accutane* without a yellow self-adhesive *Accutane* qualification sticker.

ISOTRETINOIN (13-cis-Retinoic Acid)

WARNING (cont.)

➤*Male patients:* These yellow self-adhesive *Accutane* qualification stickers also should be used for male patients.

➤*Information for pharmacists:* Isotretinoin must only be dispensed as follows:

• In no more than 30-day supply.
• Only on presentation of an *Accutane* prescription with a yellow self-adhesive *Accutane* qualification sticker.
• Prescription written within the previous 7 days.
• Refills require a new prescription with a yellow self-adhesive *Accutane* qualification sticker.
• No telephone or computerized prescriptions are permitted.

An *Accutane* medication guide must be given to the patient each time isotretinoin is dispensed, as required by law. This guide is an important part of the risk management program for the patient.

Indications

➤*Severe recalcitrant nodular acne:* Nodules are inflammatory lesions with a diameter of 5 mm or greater. The nodules may become suppurative or hemorrhagic. "Severe," by definition, means "many" as opposed to "few or several" nodules.

Adverse effects are significant; reserve treatment for patients unresponsive to conventional therapy, including systemic antibiotics. In addition, isotretinoin is indicated only for those females who are not pregnant, because isotretinoin can cause severe birth defects. A single course of therapy for 15 to 20 weeks has resulted in complete, prolonged remission in many patients. If a second course is needed, do not initiate therapy until at least 8 weeks after completion of the first course. Patients may continue to improve while not receiving the drug. The optimal interval before retreatment has not been defined for patients who have not completed skeletal growth.

➤*Unlabeled uses:* Low-dose isotretinoin has been shown to be effective in the treatment of rosacea. It also has been shown to be temporarily effective in the treatment of cornification disorders, such as ichthyoses, keratodermas, Papillon-Lefevre syndrome, and Darier's disease. Various forms of folliculitis and neoplastic disorders (including sebaceous hyperplasia, recurrent condylomata acuminata, and cutaneous T-cell lymphoma) also have been shown to be responsive to isotretinoin. Successful treatment of recurrent malignant gliomas and spinal cord astrocytoma with isotretinoin also has been shown.

Administration and Dosage

➤*Approved by the FDA:* May 7, 1982.

Individualize dosage. Adjust the dose according to side effects and disease response.

➤*Recommended course of therapy:* The recommended dose is 0.5 to 1 mg/kg/day divided into 2 doses for 15 to 20 weeks. Administer isotretinoin with food. Adult patients whose disease is very severe with scarring or is primarily manifested on the trunk may require up to the maximum recommended dose, 2 mg/kg/day, as tolerated. Failure to take isotretinoin with food will signifcantly decrease absorption. Before upward dose adjustments are made, question patients about their compliance with food instructions. The safety of once-daily dosing with isotretinoin has not been established. Once-daily dosing is not recommended. If the total nodule count decreases by more than 70% prior to completing 15 to 20 weeks of treatment, the drug may be discontinued. After 2 months or more off therapy, and if warranted by persistent or recurring severe nodular acne, a second course of therapy may be initiated.

In studies comparing 0.1, 0.5, and 1 mg/kg/day, all doses provided initial clearing of disease, but there was a greater need for retreatment with the lower doses.

Isotretinoin Dosing by Body Weight				
Body weight		Total mg/day		
kg	lbs	0.5 mg/kg	1 mg/kg	2 mg/kg[1]
40	88	20	40	80
50	110	25	50	100
60	132	30	60	120
70	154	35	70	140
80	176	40	80	160
90	198	45	90	180
100	220	50	100	200

[1] The recommended dosage range is 0.5 to 1 mg/kg/day.

➤*Storage/Stability:* Store at controlled room temperature (15° to 30°C; 59° to 86°F). Protect from light.

Actions

➤*Pharmacology:* Isotretinoin is a retinoid that, when administered in pharmacologic dosages of 0.5 to 1 mg/kg/day, inhibits sebaceous gland function and keratinization. The exact mechanism of action of isotretinoin is unknown.

Clinical improvement in nodular acne occurs in association with a reduction in sebum secretion. The decrease in sebum secretion is temporary, is related to the dose and duration of treatment with isotretinoin, and reflects a reduction in sebaceous gland size and an inhibition of sebaceous gland differentiation.

➤*Pharmacokinetics:*

Absorption – Because of its high lipophilicity, oral absorption of isotretinoin is enhanced when given with a high-fat meal. In a crossover study, 74 healthy adult subjects received a single 80 mg oral dose (two 40 mg capsules) of isotretinoin under fasted and fed conditions. Peak plasma concentration (C_{max}) and the total exposure (AUC) of isotretinoin were more than doubled following a standardized high-fat meal when compared with isotretinoin given under fasted conditions. The observed elimination half-life was unchanged. This lack of change in half-life suggests that food increases the bioavailability of isotretinoin without altering its disposition. The time to peak concentration (T_{max}) also was increased with food and may be related to a longer absorption phase. Therefore, isotretinoin always should be taken with food.

Pharmacokinetic Parameters of Isotretinoin Mean (%CV), N = 74				
Isotretinoin 2 × 40 mg capsules	$AUC_{(0-\infty)}$ (ng•hr/mL)	C_{max} (ng/mL)	T_{max} (hr)	$t_{1/2}$ (hr)
Fed[1]	10,004 (22%)	862 (22%)	5.3 (77%)	21 (39%)
Fasted	3703 (46%)	301 (63%)	3.2 (56%)	21 (30%)

[1] Eating a standardized high-fat meal.

Distribution – Isotretinoin is more than 99.9% bound to plasma proteins, primarily albumin.

Metabolism – Following oral administration of isotretinoin, at least 3 metabolites have been identified in human plasma: 4-*oxo*-isotretinoin, retinoic acid (tretinoin), and 4-*oxo*-retinoic acid (4-*oxo*-tretinoin). Retinoic acid and 13-*cis*-retinoic acid are geometric isomers and show reversible interconversion. The administration of one isomer will give rise to the other. Isotretinoin also is irreversibly oxidized to 4-*oxo*-isotretinoin, which forms its geometric isomer 4-*oxo*-tretinoin.

After a single 80 mg oral dose of isotretinoin to 74 healthy adult subjects, concurrent administration of food increased the extent of formation of all metabolites in plasma when compared with the extent of formation under fasted conditions.

All of these metabolites possess retinoid activity that is in some in vitro models more than that of the parent isotretinoin. However, the clinical significance of these models is unknown. After multiple oral dose administration of isotretinoin to adult cystic acne patients (18 years of age and older), the exposure of patients to 4-*oxo*-isotretinoin at steady state under fasted and fed conditions was approximately 3.4 times higher than that of isotretinoin. In vitro studies indicated that the primary P450 isoforms involved in isotretinoin metabolism are 2C8, 2C9, 3A4, and 2B6. Isotretinoin and its metabolites are further metabolized into conjugates, which are then excreted in urine and feces.

Excretion – Following oral administration of an 80 mg dose of ^{14}C-isotretinoin as a liquid suspension, ^{14}C-activity in blood declined with a half-life of 90 hours. The metabolites of isotretinoin and any conjugates are ultimately excreted in the feces and urine in relatively equal amounts (total of 65% to 83%). After a single 80 mg oral dose of isotretinoin to 74 healthy adult subjects under fed conditions, the mean elimination half-lives of isotretinoin and 4-*oxo*-isotretinoin were approximately 21 and 24 hours, respectively. After single and multiple doses, the observed accumulation ratios of isotretinoin ranged from 0.9 to 5.43 in patients with cystic acne.

Contraindications

Pregnancy (see Warning Box); hypersensitivity to this medication or any of its components; hypersensitivity to parabens (used as a preservative in the formulation).

Warnings

➤*Psychiatric disorders:* Isotretinoin may cause depression, psychosis, and rarely, suicidal ideation, suicide attempts, suicide, and aggressive or violent behavior. Discontinuation of isotretinoin therapy may be insufficient; further evaluation may be necessary. No mechanism of action has been established for these events.

➤*Pseudotumor cerebri (benign intracranial hypertension):* Isotretinoin use has been associated with a number of cases of pseudotumor cerebri, some of which involved concomitant use of tetracyclines. Therefore, avoid concomitant treatment with tetracyclines. Early signs and symptoms include papilledema, headache, nausea, vomiting, and visual disturbances. Screen patients with these symptoms for papilledema; if present, discontinue drug immediately and consult a neurologist.

➤*Pancreatitis:* Acute pancreatitis has been reported in patients with elevated or normal serum triglyceride levels. In rare instances, fatal hemorrhagic pancreatitis has been reported. Stop isotretinoin if hypertriglyceridemia cannot be controlled at an acceptable level or if symptoms of pancreatitis occur.

ISOTRETINOIN (13-cis-Retinoic Acid)

➤*Visual impairment:* Carefully monitor visual problems. If visual difficulties occur, discontinue the drug and have an ophthalmological examination.

Corneal opacities – These have appeared in patients receiving isotretinoin for acne and more frequently in patients on higher dosages for keratinization disorders. Corneal opacities have either completely resolved or were resolving at follow-up 6 to 7 weeks after discontinuation.

Decreased night vision – Decreased night vision has occurred during therapy and in some cases persisted after therapy was discontinued. Because the onset in some patients was sudden, advise patients of this potential problem and warn them to be cautious when driving or operating any vehicle at night.

➤*Inflammatory bowel disease:* Inflammatory bowel disease, including regional ileitis, has been associated with isotretinoin in patients without a history of intestinal disorders. In some instances, symptoms have been reported to persist after isotretinoin therapy has been stopped. Discontinue treatment immediately if abdominal pain, rectal bleeding, or severe diarrhea occurs.

➤*Hypertriglyceridemia:* Hypertriglyceridemia in excess of 800 mg/dL occurred in approximately 25% of patients; approximately 15% developed a decrease in high density lipoproteins (HDL) and approximately 7% showed an increase in cholesterol levels. Perform blood lipid determinations before isotretinoin is given and then at intervals until the lipid response to isotretinoin is established, which usually occurs within 4 weeks.

These effects are reversible after cessation of therapy. Patients who are at high risk of developing hypertriglyceridemia include those with diabetes, obesity, increased alcohol intake, a lipid metabolism disorder, and a familial history.

Reduction of weight, dietary fat intake, alcohol intake, and dose may reverse the effects on serum triglycerides, allowing patients to continue therapy.

➤*Musculoskeletal effects:* In a clinical trial (N = 217) of a single course of therapy for isotretinoin, 7.9% of patients had decreases in lumbar spine bone mineral density greater than 4%, and 10.6% of patients had decreases in total hip bone mineral density greater than 5%.

Spontaneous reports of osteoporosis, osteopenia, bone fractures, and delayed healing of bone fractures have been seen in the isotretinoin population. While causality to isotretinoin has not been established, an effect cannot be ruled out. Physicians should use caution when prescribing isotretinoin to patients with a genetic predisposition for age-related osteoporosis, a history of childhood osteoporosis conditions, osteomalacia, or other disorders of bone metabolism. This would include patients diagnosed with anorexia nervosa and those who are on chronic drug therapy that causes drug-induced osteoporosis/osteomalacia and/or affects vitamin D metabolism, such as systemic corticosteroids and any anticonvulsants.

There are spontaneous reports of premature epiphyseal closure in acne patients receiving recommended doses of isotretinoin.

In clinical trials for disorders of keratinization, a high prevalence of skeletal hyperostosis was noted with a mean dose of 2.24 mg/kg/day.

Minimal skeletal hyperostosis and calcification of ligaments and tendons has been observed by x-ray in prospective studies of nodular acne patients treated with a single course of therapy at recommended doses. The skeletal effects of multiple isotretinoin treatment courses for acne are unknown.

➤*Hepatotoxicity:* Clinical hepatitis possibly or probably related to isotretinoin therapy has been reported. Additionally, mild to moderate elevations of liver enzymes have been seen in approximately 15% of patients, some of whom normalized with dosage reduction or continued administration of the drug. If normalization does not readily occur, or if hepatitis is suspected, stop the drug and further investigate etiology.

➤*Hearing impairment:* Impaired hearing has been reported in patients taking isotretinoin; in some cases, the hearing impairment has been reported to persist after therapy has been discontinued. Mechanisms and causality for this event have not been established. Patients who experience tinnitus or hearing impairment should discontinue isotretinoin treatment and be referred to specialized care for further evaluation.

➤*Hormonal contraceptives:* Microdosed progesterone preparations (minipills) may be an inadequate method of contraception during isotretinoin therapy. Although other hormonal contraceptives are highly effective, there have been reports of pregnancy from women who have used combined oral contraceptives, as well as injectable/implantable contraceptive products. These reports are more frequent for women who use only a single method of contraception. It is not known if hormonal contraceptives differ in their effectiveness when used with isotretinoin. Therefore, it is critically important that women of childbearing potential use 2 effective forms of contraception simultaneously, at least 1 of which must be a primary form, unless absolute abstinence is the chosen method, or the patient has undergone a hysterectomy (see Warning Box).

➤*Hypersensitivity reactions:* Anaphylactic reactions and other allergic reactions have been reported. Cutaneous allergic reactions and serious cases of allergic vasculitis, often with purpura (bruises and red patches), of the extremities and extracutaneous involvement (including renal) have been reported. Severe allergic reaction necessitates discontinuation of therapy and appropriate medical management.

➤*Carcinogenesis:* In male and female Fischer 344 rats given oral isotretinoin at dosages of 8 or 32 mg/kg/day (1.3 to 5.3 times the recommended clinical dose of 1 mg/kg/day, respectively, after normalization for total body surface area) for more than 18 months, there was a dose-related increased incidence of pheochromocytoma relative to controls. The incidence of adrenal medullary hyperplasia also was increased at the higher dosage in both sexes.

➤*Pregnancy:* Category X (see Warning Box).

➤*Lactation:* It is not known whether this drug is excreted in breast milk. Because of the potential for adverse effects, do not give to a nursing mother.

➤*Children:* The use of isotretinoin in pediatric patients less than 12 years of age has not been studied. Carefully consider isotretinoin use in pediatric patients 12 to 17 years of age, especially for those patients in whom a known metabolic or structural bone disease exists.

Precautions

➤*Monitoring:*

Pregnancy test – Female patients of childbearing potential must have negative results from 2 urine or serum pregnancy tests with a sensitivity of at least 25 mIU/mL before receiving the initial isotretinoin prescription. The first test is obtained by the prescriber when the decision is made to pursue qualification of the patient for isotretinoin (a screening test). Perform the second pregnancy test (a confirmation test) during the first 5 days of the menstrual period immediately preceding the beginning of isotretinoin therapy. For patients with amenorrhea, the second test should be done at least 11 days after the last act of unprotected sexual intercourse (without using 2 effective forms of contraception).

Each month of therapy, the patient must have a negative result from a urine or serum pregnancy test. Repeat the pregnancy test each month prior to the female patient receiving each prescription.

Lipids – Obtain pretreatment and follow-up blood lipids under fasting conditions. After consumption of alcohol, at least 36 hours should elapse before these determinations are made. It is recommended that these tests be performed at weekly or biweekly intervals until the lipid response to isotretinoin is established. The incidence of hypertriglyceridemia is 1 patient in 4 on isotretinoin therapy.

Liver function tests – Because elevations of liver enzymes have been observed during clinical trials and hepatitis has been reported, perform pretreatment and follow-up liver function tests at weekly or biweekly intervals until the response to isotretinoin has been established.

➤*Exacerbation of acne (transient):* Transient exacerbation of acne has occurred, generally during the initial therapy period.

➤*Contact lens:* Tolerance may decrease.

➤*Diabetes:* Certain patients have experienced problems in the control of their blood sugar. In addition, new cases of diabetes have been diagnosed during therapy, although no causal relationship has been established.

➤*Blood donation:* Because of isotretinoin's teratogenic potential, patients receiving the drug should not donate blood for transfusion during treatment and for 1 month after discontinuing therapy.

➤*Neutropenia/Agranulocytosis:* Neutropenia and rare cases of agranulocytosis have been reported. Discontinue isotretinoin if clinically significant decreases in white cell counts occur.

➤*Photosensitivity:* Photosensitization (photoallergy or phototoxicity) may occur; caution patients to take protective measures (eg, sunscreens, protective clothing) against exposure to ultraviolet light or sunlight until tolerance is determined.

Drug Interactions

➤*Vitamin A:* To avoid additive toxic effects, do not take concomitantly with isotretinoin.

➤*Tetracyclines:* Avoid concomitant treatment with isotretinoin and tetracyclines. Isotretinoin use has been associated with a number of cases of pseudotumor cerebri (benign intracranial hypertension), some of which involved concomitant use of tetracyclines.

Adverse Reactions

Most adverse reactions are reversible upon discontinuation; however, some have persisted after cessation of therapy. Many are similar to those described in patients taking high doses of vitamin A (dryness of the skin and mucous membranes, eg, of the lips, nasal passage, and eyes).

➤*Cardiovascular:* Palpitation; tachycardia; vascular thrombotic disease.

ISOTRETINOIN (13-cis-Retinoic Acid)

➤*CNS:* Fatigue; headache; pseudotumor cerebri, including headache, visual disturbances, and papilledema; dizziness; drowsiness; insomnia; lethargy; malaise; nervousness; paresthesias; seizures; stroke; syncope; weakness; suicidal ideation; suicide attempts; suicide; psychosis; emotional instability; aggression; violent behaviors. Depression has occurred and has subsided with discontinuation of therapy and recurred upon reinstitution.

➤*Dermatologic:* Acne fulminans; alopecia (which persists in some cases); bruising; cheilitis (dry lips); dry skin; eruptive xanthomas; flushing; fragility of skin; hair abnormalities; hirsutism; hyperpigmentation and hypopigmentation; infections (including disseminated herpes simplex); nail dystrophy; paronychia; peeling of palms and soles; photoallergic/photosensitizing reactions; pruritus; pyogenic granuloma; rash (including facial erythema, seborrhea, and eczema); sunburn susceptibility increased; sweating; urticaria; abnormal wound healing (delayed healing or exuberant granulation tissue with crusting).

➤*GI:* Dry mouth; nausea; nonspecific GI symptoms; inflammatory bowel disease; bleeding and inflammation of the gums; hepatitis; pancreatitis; colitis; ileitis; esophagitis/esophageal ulceration.

➤*GU:* White cells in urine; proteinuria; microscopic or gross hematuria; nonspecific urogenital findings; abnormal menses; glomerulonephritis.

➤*Hypersensitivity:* Allergic reactions; systemic hypersensitivity.

➤*Musculoskeletal:* Mild to moderate musculoskeletal symptoms, including arthralgia, that occasionally require drug discontinuation and rarely persist after discontinuation (16%); skeletal hyperostosis (see Warnings); calcification of tendons and ligaments; premature epiphyseal closure; arthritis; tendonitis; other bone abnormalities; decreases in bone mineral density; back pain; rhabdomyolysis (rare postmarketing reports).

➤*Ophthalmic:* Conjunctivitis; optic neuritis; photophobia; eyelid inflammation; corneal opacities (see Warnings); cataracts; visual disturbances; color vision disorder; keratitis; dry eyes; decreased night vision that may persist.

➤*Respiratory:* Bronchospasms, with or without a history of asthma; respiratory infections; voice alterations.

➤*Miscellaneous:* Epistaxis; dry nose or mouth; transient chest pain (rarely persists after discontinuation); vasculitis (including Wegener granulomatosis); anemia; lymphadenopathy; edema; tinnitus; hearing impairment; weight loss.

➤*Lab test abnormalities:* Hypertriglyceridemia; elevated sedimentation rate; decreased red blood cell parameters and white blood cell counts, including severe neutropenia and rare reports of agranulocyto- sis; elevated platelet counts; decrease in serum HDL levels; elevations of serum cholesterol; increased alkaline phosphatase, AST, ALT, GGTP, and LDH; increased fasting blood sugar; hyperuricemia; thrombocytopenia; elevated CPK levels in patients who undergo vigorous physical activity.

Overdosage

Overdosage has been associated with vomiting, facial flushing, cheilosis, abdominal pain, headache, dizziness, and ataxia. All symptoms quickly resolved without apparent residual effects.

Patient Information

Patient information leaflet available with product.

Prior to use, have patients complete a consent form included with package insert.

Take with food. To decrease the risk of esophageal irritation, swallow the capsules with a full glass of liquid. Do not take vitamin supplements containing vitamin A.

Instruct females of childbearing potential that they must not be pregnant when isotretinoin therapy is initiated, and that they should use 2 forms of effective contraception 1 month before starting isotretinoin, while taking isotretinoin, and for 1 month after isotretinoin has been stopped. They also should sign a consent form prior to beginning isotretinoin therapy. Female patients should be seen by their prescribers monthly and have a urine or serum pregnancy test performed each month during treatment to confirm negative pregnancy status before another isotretinoin prescription is written (see Contraindications and Warnings). Notify physician immediately if pregnancy is suspected.

A transient exacerbation of acne may occur during the initial period of therapy.

May cause photosensitivity; avoid prolonged exposure to sunlight or UV rays.

Immediately report depression, visual disturbances, abdominal pain, rectal bleeding, severe diarrhea, difficulty in controlling blood sugar, and decreased tolerance to contact lens wear to physician.

Do not donate blood during therapy or for 1 month after stopping therapy because the blood might be given to a pregnant woman whose fetus must not be exposed to isotretinoin.

Do not share isotretinoin with anyone else because of the risk of birth defects and other serious adverse events.

Avoid wax epilation and skin resurfacing procedures (eg, dermabrasion, laser) during therapy and for at least 6 months thereafter because of the possibility of scarring.

ACITRETIN

Rx	Soriatane (Roche)	Capsules[1]: 10 mg	(SORIATANE 10 ROCHE). Brown/white. In 30s.
		25 mg	(SORIATANE 25 ROCHE). Brown/yellow. In 30s.

[1] Capsule shells contain gelatin, iron oxide, titanium dioxide, and may also contain benzyl alcohol.

WARNING

Pregnancy: Acitretin must not be used by females who are pregnant, or who intend to become pregnant during therapy, or at any time for at least 3 years following discontinuation of therapy. Acitretin also must not be used by females who may not use reliable contraception while undergoing treatment or for at least 3 years following discontinuation of treatment. Acitretin is a metabolite of etretinate and major human fetal abnormalities have been reported with the administration of etretinate and acitretin. Potentially, any fetus exposed can be affected.

Clinical evidence has shown that concurrent ingestion of acitretin and ethanol has been associated with the formation of etretinate, which has a longer elimination half-life than acitretin. Because the longer elimination half-life of etretinate would increase the duration of teratogenic potential for female patients, ethanol must not be ingested by female patients either during treatment with acitretin or for 2 months after cessation of therapy. This allows for elimination of acitretin, thus removing the substrate for transesterification to etretinate. The mechanism of the metabolic process for conversion of acitretin to etretinate has not been fully defined. It is not known whether substances other than ethanol are associated with transesterification.

Acitretin has been shown to be embryotoxic and teratogenic in rabbits, mice, and rats at doses approximately 0.2, 0.3, and 3 times the maximum recommended therapeutic dose, respectively.

Major human fetal abnormalities associated with acitretin administration have been reported, including meningomyelocele; meningoencephalocele; multiple synostoses; facial dysmorphia; syndactylies; absence of terminal phalanges; malformations of hip, ankle, and forearm; low set ears; high palate; decreased cranial volume; cardiovascular malformation; and alterations of the skull and cervical vertebrae.

Acitretin should be prescribed only by those who have special competence in the diagnosis and treatment of severe psoriasis, are experienced in the use of systemic retinoids, and understand the risk of teratogenicity.

➤*Female patients:* Consider only for women with severe psoriasis unresponsive to other therapies or whose clinical condition contraindicates the use of other treatments.

Females of reproductive potential must not be given acitretin until pregnancy is excluded. Acitretin is contraindicated in females of reproductive potential unless the patient meets all of the following conditions:

- Must have had 2 negative urine or serum pregnancy tests with a sensitivity of at least 25 mIU/mL. The first test (a screening test) is obtained by the prescriber when the decision is made to pursue acitretin therapy. The second pregnancy test (a confirmation test) should be done during the first 5 days of the menstrual period immediately preceding the beginning of acitretin therapy. For patients with amenorrhea, the second test should be done at least 11 days after the last act of unprotected sexual intercourse (without using 2 effective forms of contraception [birth control] simultaneously). Timing of pregnancy testing throughout the treatment course should be monthly or individualized based on the prescriber's clinical judgement.

- Must have selected and have committed to use 2 effective forms of contraception (birth control) simultaneously, at least 1 of which must be a primary form, unless absolute abstinence is the chosen method, or the patient has undergone a hysterectomy or is clearly postmenopausal.

- Must use 2 effective forms of contraception (birth control) simultaneously for at least 1 month prior to initiation of acitretin therapy, during acitretin therapy, and for at least 3 years after discontinuing acitretin therapy.

Effective forms of contraception include both primary and secondary forms of contraception. Primary forms of contraception include the following: Tubal ligation, partner's vasectomy, intrauterine devices, birth control pills, and injectable/implantable/insertable/topical hormonal birth control products. Secondary forms of contraception include diaphragms, latex condoms, and cervical caps; each secondary form must be used with a spermicide.

WARNING (cont.)

It has not been established if there is a pharmacokinetic interaction between acitretin and combined oral contraceptives. However, it has been established that acitretin interferes with the contraceptive effect of microdosed progestin preparations. Microdosed "minipill" progestin preparations are not recommended for use with acitretin. It is not known whether other progestational contraceptives, such as implants and injectables, are adequate methods of contraception during acitretin therapy.

If pregnancy does occur during acitretin therapy or at any time for at least 3 years following discontinuation of acitretin therapy, the prescriber and patient should discuss the possible effects on the pregnancy. The risk of severe fetal malformations is well established when systemic retinoids are taken during pregnancy. Pregnancy must also be prevented after stopping acitretin therapy. The duration of posttherapy contraception to achieve adequate elimination cannot be calculated precisely. It is strongly recommended that contraception be continued for at least 3 years after stopping acitretin treatment.

- Severe birth defects have been reported where conception occurred during the time interval when the patient was being treated with acitretin and/or etretinate. In addition, severe birth defects have also been reported when conception occurred after the mother completed therapy.

➤*Male patients:* Samples of seminal fluid from 3 male patients treated with acitretin and 6 male patients treated with etretinate have been assayed for the presence of acitretin. The maximum concentration of acitretin observed in the seminal fluid of these men was 12.5 ng/mL. Assuming an ejaculate volume of 10 mL, the amount of drug transferred in semen would be 125 ng, which is 1/200,000 of a single 25 mg capsule. Thus, it appears that residual acitretin in seminal fluid poses little, if any, risk to a fetus while a male patient is taking the drug or after it is discontinued (see Warnings under Pregnancy).

➤*Hepatotoxicity:* Clinical hepatotoxicity, hepatitis, and hepatitis related deaths have been reported in patients taking acitretin (see Warnings).

➤*Patient consent form:* Female patients must have signed a Patient Agreement/Informed Consent Form that contains warnings about the risk of potential birth defects if the fetus is exposed to acitretin, about contraceptive failure, and about the fact that they must not ingest beverages or products containing ethanol while taking acitretin and for 2 months after acitretin treatment has been discontinued.

➤*Blood donation:* Male and female patients should not donate blood during and for at least 3 years following the completion of acitretin therapy because women of childbearing potential must not receive blood from patients being treated with acitretin.

➤*Medication guide:* An acitretin medication guide must be given to the patient each time acitretin is dispensed, as required by law.

Indications

➤*Psoriasis:* Treatment of severe psoriasis.

➤*Unlabeled uses:* Darier disease, palmoplantar pustulosis, lichen planus, lamellar ichthyosis in children, nonbullous and bullous ichthyosiform erythroderma, Sjögren-Larsson syndrome, lichen sclerosus et atrophicus of the vulva, palmoplantar lichen nitidus, cutaneous T-cell lymphoma (CTCL).

Administration and Dosage

➤*Approved by the FDA:* October 28, 1997.

Individualization of dosage is required to achieve sufficient therapeutic response while minimizing side effects. Initiate acitretin therapy at 25 to 50 mg/day given as a single dose with the main meal. Maintenance doses of 25 to 50 mg/day may be given after response to initial treatment. Females who have taken etretinate must continue to follow the contraceptive recommendations for etretinate.

➤*Relapse:* Most patients experience relapse of psoriasis after discontinuing therapy. Subsequent courses, when clinically indicated, have produced efficacy results similar to the initial course of therapy. Relapses may be treated as outlined for initial therapy.

➤*Concomitant use with phototherapy:* When acitretin is used with phototherapy, decrease the phototherapy dose, dependent on the patient's individual response.

➤*Information for the pharmacists:* A *Soriatane* Medication Guide must be given to the patient each time *Soriatane* is dispensed, as required by law.

ACITRETIN

►*Storage / Stability:* Store between 15° and 25°C (59° and 77°F). Protect from light. Avoid exposure to high temperatures and humidity after the bottle is opened.

Actions

►*Pharmacology:* Acitretin, a retinoid, is a metabolite of etretinate and is related to both retinoic acid and retinol (vitamin A). The mechanism of action is unknown. However, acitretin is thought to exert its therapeutic effect by modulating the following pathogenic processes: Keratinocyte differentiation, keratinocyte hyperpoliferation, and tissue infiltration by inflammatory cells.

►*Pharmacokinetics:*

Absorption / Distribution – Oral absorption is optimal when given with food and is approximately 72% (range, 47% to 109%). Maximum plasma concentrations after a single 50 mg dose range from 196 to 728 ng/mL (mean, 416 ng/mL) and are achieved in 2 to 5 hours (mean, 2.7 hours). Following multiple-dose administration, steady-state concentrations of acitretin and cis-acitretin are achieved within approximately 3 weeks. Acitretin is more than 99.9% bound to plasma proteins, primarily albumin.

Metabolism / Excretion – Acitretin undergoes extensive metabolism and interconversion by simple isomerization to its 13-cis form (cis-acitretin). The formation of cis-acitretin relative to parent compound is not altered by dose or fed/fast conditions. Both parent compound and isomer are further metabolized into chain-shortened breakdown products and conjugates which are excreted in the feces (34% to 54%) and urine (16% to 53%). The terminal elimination half-life following multiple-dose administration is 49 hours (range, 33 to 96 hours), and that of cis-acitretin under the same conditions is 63 hours (range, 28 to 157 hours).

Ethanol – Etretinate (a retinoid with a much longer half-life) can be formed with concurrent ingestion of acitretin and ethanol. In a 2-way crossover study, all 10 subjects formed etretinate with concurrent ingestion of a single 100 mg dose of acitretin during a 3-hour period of ethanol ingestion (total ethanol, approximately 1.4 g/kg body weight). A mean peak etretinate concentration of 59 ng/mL (range, 22 to 105 ng/mL) was observed, and extrapolation of AUC values indicated that the formation of etretinate in this study was comparable to a single 5 mg oral dose of etretinate. There was no detectable formation of etretinate when a single 100 mg oral dose of acitretin was administered without concurrent ethanol ingestion, although the formation of etretinate without concurrent ethanol ingestion cannot be excluded. Of 93 psoriatic patients on acitretin therapy (10 to 80 mg/day), 16% had measurable etretinate levels (more than 5 ng/mL). In one study the apparent mean terminal half-life after 6 months of therapy was approximately 120 days (range, 84 to 168 days). The long half-life appears to be due to storage of etretinate in adipose tissue.

Special populations –

Psoriasis: In patients with psoriasis, mean steady-state trough concentrations of acitretin increased in a dose-proportional manner with dosages ranging from 10 to 50 mg/day. Acitretin plasma concentrations were nonmeasurable (less than 4 ng/mL) in all patients 3 weeks after cessation of therapy.

Elderly: A 2-fold increase in acitretin plasma concentrations was seen in elderly subjects, although the elimination half-life did not change.

Renal function impairment: Plasma concentrations of acitretin were significantly (59.3%) lower in end-stage renal failure subjects when compared with age-matched controls, following single 50 mg oral doses. Acitretin was not removed by hemodialysis.

Contraindications

Pregnancy (see Warning Box); severe hepatic or renal function impairment; chronic abnormally elevated blood lipid values (see Warning Box); concomitant use with methotrexate or tetracyclines; hypersensitivity to the preparation (acitretin or excipients) or to other retinoids.

Warnings

►*Psychiatric symptoms:* Depression and/or other psychiatric symptoms such as aggressive feelings or thoughts of self-harm have been reported. These events, including self-injurious behavior, have been reported in patients taking other systemically administered retinoids, as well as in patients taking acitretin. Because other factors may have contributed to these events, it is not known if they are related to acitretin. Counsel patients to stop taking acitretin and notify their prescriber immediately if they experience psychiatric symptoms.

►*Pancreatitis:* Lipid elevations occur in 25% to 50% of patients treated with acitretin. Triglyceride increases sufficient to be associated with pancreatitis are much less common, although fatal fulminant pancreatitis has been reported. There have been rare reports of pancreatitis during acitretin therapy in the absence of hypertriglyceridemia.

►*Hepatotoxicity:* Treatment with acitretin has been shown to cause hepatotoxicity. In clinical trials, 2 patients had clinical jaundice with elevated serum bilirubin and transaminases considered related to acitretin treatment. Liver function test results in these patients returned to normal after acitretin was discontinued. Two patients developed biopsy-confirmed toxic hepatitis. A second biopsy in 1 of these patients revealed nodule formation suggestive of cirrhosis. One developed a 3-fold increase of transaminases. A liver biopsy of this patient showed mild lobular disarray, multifocal hepatocyte loss, and mild triaditis of the portal tracts compatible with acute reversible hepatic injury. The patient's transaminase levels returned to normal 2 months after acitretin was discontinued.

In another study, a comparison of liver biopsy findings before and after therapy revealed 58% of patients showed no change, 25% improved, and 17% patients had a worsening of their liver biopsy status. For 6 patients, the classification changed from class 0 (no pathology) to class 1 (normal fatty infiltration; nuclear variability and portal inflammation; both mild); for 7 patients the change from class 1 to class 2 (fatty infiltration, nuclear variability, portal inflammation, and focal necrosis; all moderate to severe); and for 1 patient, the change was from class 2 to class 3b (fibrosis; moderate to severe). No correlation could be found between liver function test result abnormalities and the change in liver biopsy status, and no cumulative dose relationship was found.

Elevations of AST, ALT, GGT, or LDH have occurred in approximately 1 in 3 patients treated with acitretin. Treatment was discontinued in 3.8% due to elevated liver function test results. If hepatotoxicity is suspected during treatment with acitretin, discontinue the drug and further investigate the etiology.

Ten patients had clinical or histologic hepatitis considered to be possibly or probably related to etretinate treatment. There have been reports of hepatitis-related deaths worldwide; a few of these patients had received etretinate for a month or less before presenting with hepatic symptoms or signs.

►*Lipids:* Perform blood lipid determinations before acitretin is administered and again at intervals of 1 to 2 weeks until the lipid response to the drug is established, usually within 4 to 8 weeks. In patients receiving acitretin during clinical trials, 66% and 33% experienced elevation in triglycerides and cholesterol, respectively. Decreased high density lipoproteins (HDL) occurred in 40%. These effects of acitretin were generally reversible upon cessation of therapy.

Patients with an increased tendency to develop hypertriglyceridemia included those with diabetes mellitus, obesity, increased alcohol intake, or a familial history of these conditions. Because of the risk of hypertriglyceridemia, serum lipids must be more closely monitored in high-risk patients and during long-term treatment.

Hypertriglyceridemia and lowered HDL may increase a patient's cardiovascular risk status. Although no causal relationship has been established, there have been postmarketing reports of acute MI or thromboembolic events in patients on acitretin therapy. In addition, elevation of serum triglycerides to more than 800 mg/dL has been associated with fatal fulminant pancreatitis. Therefore, use dietary modifications, reduction in acitretin dose, or drug therapy to control significant elevations of triglycerides.

►*Pseudotumor cerebri:* Acitretin and other oral retinoids have been associated with cases of pseudotumor cerebri (benign intracranial hypertension). Some of these events involved concomitant use of isotretinoin and tetracyclines. However, the event seen in a single acitretin patient was not associated with tetracycline use. Early signs and symptoms include papilledema, headache, nausea, vomiting, and visual disturbances. Examine patients with these signs and symptoms for papilledema and, if present, discontinue acitretin immediately and refer for neurological evaluation and care. Since both acitretin and tetracyclines can cause increased intracranial pressure, their combined use is contraindicated.

►*Ophthalmologic effects:* The eyes and vision of 329 patients treated with acitretin were examined by ophthalmologists. The findings included dry eyes (23%), irritation of eyes (9%) and brow and lash loss (5%). The following were reported in less than 5% of patients: Bell Palsy, blepharitis or crusting of lids, blurred vision, conjunctivitis, corneal epithelial abnormality, cortical cataract, decreased night vision, diplopia, itchy eyes or eyelids, nuclear cataract, pannus, papilledema, photophobia, posterior subcapsular cataract, recurrent sties, and subepithelial corneal lesions.

Any patient treated with acitretin who is experiencing visual difficulties should discontinue the drug and undergo ophthalmologic evaluation.

►*Hyperostosis:* In adults receiving long-term treatment with acitretin, perform appropriate examinations periodically in view of possible ossification abnormalities. Because the frequency and severity of iatrogenic bony abnormality in adults is low, periodic radiography is only warranted in the presence of symptoms or long-term use of acitretin. If such disorders arise, the continuation of therapy should be discussed with the patient on the basis of a careful risk/benefit analysis. In clinical trials with acitretin, patients were prospectively evaluated for evidence of development or change in bony abnormalities of the vertebral column, knees, and ankles.

Vertebral results – Of 380 patients treated with acitretin, 15% had preexisting abnormalities of the spine which showed new changes or progression of preexisting findings. Changes included degenerative spurs, anterior bridging of spinal vertebrae, diffuse idiopathic skeletal hyperostosis, ligament calcification, and narrowing and destruction of a

ACITRETIN

cervical disc space. De novo changes (formation of small spurs) were seen in 3 patients after 1.5 to 2.5 years.

Skeletal appendicular results – Six of 128 patients treated with acitretin showed abnormalities in the knees and ankles before treatment that progressed during treatment. In 5 patients, these changes involved the formation of additional spurs or the enlargement of existing spurs. The sixth patient had degenerative joint disease that worsened. No patients developed spurs de novo.

➤*Diabetes:* Certain patients receiving retinoids have experienced problems in the control of their blood sugar. In addition, new cases of diabetes have been diagnosed during retinoid therapy, including diabetic ketoacidosis. Monitor blood sugar very carefully.

➤*Elderly:* In general, dose selection for an elderly patient should be cautious, usually starting at the low end of the dosing range, reflecting the greater frequency of decreased hepatic, renal, or cardiac function, and of concomitant disease or other drug therapy. A 2-fold increase in acitretin plasma concentrations was seen in healthy elderly subjects compared with young subjects, although the elimination half–life did not change.

➤*Pregnancy:* Category X (see Warning Box). There have been 318 prospectively reported cases involving pregnancies and the use of etretinate, acitretin, or both. In 238 of these cases, the conception occurred after the last dose of etretinate (103 cases), acitretin (126), or both (9). Fetal outcome remained unknown in approximately 50% of these cases, of which 62 were terminated and 14 were spontaneous abortions. Fetal outcome is known for the other 118 cases and 15 of the outcomes were abnormal (including cases of absent hand/wrist, clubfoot, GI malformation, hypocalcemia, hypotonia, limb malformation, neonatal apnea/anemia, neonatal ichthyosis, placental disorder/death, undescended testicle, and 5 cases of premature birth). In the 126 prospectively reported cases where conception occurred after the last dose of acitretin only, 43 cases involved conception at least 1 year but less than 2 years after the last dose. There were 3 reports of abnormal outcomes out of these 43 cases (involving limb malformation, GI tract malformations, and premature birth).

There is also a total of 35 retrospectively reported cases where conception occurred at least 1 year after the last dose of etretinate, acitretin, or both. From these cases there are 3 reports of birth defects when the conception occurred at least 1 year but less than 2 years after the last dose of acitretin (including heart malformations, Turner Syndrome, and unspecified congenital malformations) and 4 reports of birth defects when conception occurred at least 2 years after the last dose of acitretin (including foot malformation, cardiac malformations [2 cases] and unspecified neonatal and infancy disorder). There were 3 additional abnormal outcomes in cases where conception occurred at least 2 years after the last dose of etretinate (including chromosome disorder, forearm aplasia, and stillbirth).

Male patients – There have been 25 cases of reported conception when the male partner was taking acitretin. The pregnancy outcome is known in 13 of these 25 cases. Of these, 9 reports were retrospective and 4 were prospective (meaning the pregnancy was reported prior to knowledge of the outcome).

Pregnancy Outcomes of Paternal Acitretin Therapy

Timing of paternal acitretin treatment relative to conception	Delivery of healthy neonate	Spontaneous abortion	Induced abortion	Total
At time of conception	5[1]	5	1	11
Discontinued ≈ 4 weeks prior	0	0	1[2]	1
Discontinued ≈ 6 to 8 months prior	0	1	0	1

[1] Four of 5 cases were prospective.
[2] With malformation pattern not typical of retinoid embryopathy (bilateral cystic hygromas of neck, hypoplasia of lungs bilateral, pulmonary atresia, VSD with overriding truncus arteriosus).

➤*Lactation:* Etretinate is excreted in the milk of rats. There is 1 prospective case report where acitretin is reported to be excreted in human milk. Therefore, mothers should not receive acitretin prior to or during breastfeeding because of the potential for serious adverse reactions in breastfeeding infants.

➤*Children:* No clinical studies have been conducted in pediatric patients. Safety and efficacy have not been established. Ossification of interosseous ligaments and tendons of the extremities, skeletal hyperostoses, decreases in bone mineral density, and premature epiphyseal closure have been reported with other systemic retinoids. While it is not known that these occurrences are more severe or more frequent in children, there is concern in pediatric patients because of the implications for growth potential.

Precautions

➤*Monitoring:* Perform blood lipid determinations before acitretin is administered and again at intervals of 1 to 2 weeks until the lipid response to the drug is established, usually within 4 to 8 weeks. It is recommended that AST, ALT, and LPH tests be performed prior to intiation of acitretin therapy at 1- to 2-week intervals until stable and thereafter at intervals as clinically indicated.

➤*Phototherapy:* Significantly lower doses of phototherapy are required when acitretin is used because acitretin-induced effects on the stratum corneum can increase the risk of erythema.

➤*Night vision:* Decreased night vision has been reported with acitretin therapy. Advise patients of this potential problem and warn them to be cautious when driving or operating any vehicle at night. Carefully monitor visual problems.

➤*Contact lenses:* A decreased tolerance to contact lenses during the treatment period and sometimes after treatment has stopped has been reported.

➤*Blood donation:* Acitretin can cause birth defects and women of childbearing potential must not receive blood from patients being treated with acitretin. Do not donate blood during and for at least 3 years following therapy.

➤*Worsening symptoms:* Worsening of psoriasis is sometimes seen during the initial treatment period. Advise patients that they may have to wait 2 to 3 months before they get the full benefit of acitretin, although some patients may achieve significant improvements within the first 8 weeks of treatment.

➤*Photosensitivity:* Photosensitization may occur; therefore, caution patients to avoid the use of sun lamps and excessive exposure to sunlight (nonmedical UV exposure) because the effects of UV light are enhanced by retinoids.

Drug Interactions

Acitretin Drug Interactions

Precipitant drug	Object drug[*]		Description
Acitretin	Glyburide	⟷	Possible potentiation of blood glucose lowering effect of glyburide in 3 of 7 subjects. Careful supervision is recommended.
Acitretin	Methotrexate	↑	Increased risk of hepatitis with combined use. Concomitant use is contraindicated.
Acitretin	Oral contraceptives (progestin only)	↓	It has been established that acitretin interferes with the contraceptive effect of microdosed progestin "minipill" preparations. It is not known if there is an interaction with combined oral contraceptives.
Acitretin	Phenytoin	↑	The protein binding of phenytoin may be decreased.
Ethanol	Acitretin	↑	Etretinate formation has occurred with concomitant ingestion of alcohol and acitretin. Etretinate has a much longer half-life than acitretin (≈ 120 days) which appears to be a result of storage in adipose tissue (see Pharmacokinetics).
Acitretin	Tetracyclines	↑	Concomitant use is contraindicated due to the increased risk for increased intracranial pressure.
Tetracyclines	Acitretin		
Acitretin	Vitamin A and oral retinoids	↑	Avoid coadministration because of the increased risk of hypervitaminosis A.
Vitamin A and oral retinoids	Acitretin		

[*] ↑ = Object drug increased. ↓ = Object drug decreased. ⟷ = Undetermined clinical effect.

ACITRETIN

Adverse Reactions

Hypervitaminosis A produces a wide spectrum of signs and symptoms primarily of the mucocutaneous, musculoskeletal, hepatic, neuropsychiatric, and CNS. Many of the clinical adverse reactions reported to date with acitretin administration resemble those of the hypervitaminosis A syndrome.

Acitretin Adverse Reactions (%)	
Adverse reaction	Acitretin (n = 525)
CNS	
Rigors	10 to 25
Headache	1 to 10
Pain	1 to 10
Depression	1 to 10
Insomnia	1 to 10
Somnolence	1 to 10
Fatigue	1 to 10
Dermatologic	
Alopecia	50 to 75
Skin peeling	50 to 75
Dry skin	25 to 50
Nail disorder	25 to 50
Pruritus	25 to 50
Erythematous rash	10 to 25
Hyperesthesia	10 to 25
Paresthesia	10 to 25
Paronychia	10 to 25
Skin atrophy	10 to 25
Sticky skin	10 to 25
Abnormal skin odor	1 to 10
Abnormal hair texture	1 to 10
Bullous eruption	1 to 10
Cold/clammy skin	1 to 10
Dermatitis	1 to 10
Increased sweating	1 to 10
Infection	1 to 10
Psoriasiform rash	1 to 10
Purpura	1 to 10
Pyogenic granuloma	1 to 10
Rash	1 to 10
Seborrhea	1 to 10
Skin fissures	1 to 10
Skin ulceration	1 to 10
Sunburn	1 to 10
GI	
Abdominal pain	1 to 10
Diarrhea	1 to 10
Nausea	1 to 10
Tongue disorder	1 to 10
Anorexia	1 to 10
Increased appetite	1 to 10
Mucous membranes	
Cheilitis	> 75
Rhinitis	25 to 50
Dry mouth	10 to 25
Epistaxis	10 to 25
Gingival bleeding	1 to 10
Gingivitis	1 to 10
Increased saliva	1 to 10
Stomatitis	1 to 10
Thirst	1 to 10
Ulcerative stomatitis	1 to 10
Musculoskeletal	
Arthralgia	10 to 25
Spinal hyperostosis	10 to 25
Arthritis	1 to 10
Arthrosis	1 to 10
Back pain	1 to 10
Hypertonia	1 to 10
Myalgia	1 to 10
Osteodynia	1 to 10
Peripheral joint hyperostosis	1 to 10
Special senses	
Earache	1 to 10
Taste perversion	1 to 10
Xerophthalmia	10 to 25
Abnormal/blurred vision	1 to 10
Blepharitis	1 to 10

Acitretin Adverse Reactions (%)	
Adverse reaction	Acitretin (n = 525)
Conjunctivitis/irritation	1 to 10
Corneal epithelial abnormality	1 to 10
Decreased night vision/blindness	1 to 10
Eye abnormality	1 to 10
Eye pain	1 to 10
Photophobia	1 to 10
Tinnitus	1 to 10
Miscellaneous	
Edema	1 to 10
Hot flashes	1 to 10
Flushing	1 to 10
Sinusitis	1 to 10

Abnormal Laboratory Test Results				
Body system	50% to 75%	25% to 50%	10% to 25%	1% to 10%
Electrolytes			*Increased:* Phosphorus Potassium Sodium *Increased and decreased:* Magnesium	*Decreased:* Phosphorus Potassium Sodium *Increased and decreased:* Calcium Chloride
Hematologic		*Increased:* Reticulo cytes	*Decreased:* Hematocrit Hemoglobin WBC *Increased:* Haptoglobin Neutrophils WBC	*Increased:* Bands Basophils Eosinophils Hematocrit Hemoglobin Lympho cytes Moncytes *Decreased:* Haptoglobin Lympho cytes Neutrophils Reticulo cytes *Increased or decreased:* Platelets RBC
Hepatic		*Increased:* Choles terol LDH AST ALT *Decreased:* HDL choles terol	*Increased:* Alkaline phospha tase Direct biliru bin GGTP	*Increased:* Globulin Total biliru bin Total protein *Increased and decreased:* Serum albu min
Miscellaneous	*Increased:* Triglycerides	*Increased:* CPK Fasting blood sugar	*Decreased:* Fasting blood sugar High occult blood	*Increased and decreased:* Iron
Renal			*Increased:* Uric acid	*Increased:* BUN Creatinine
Urinary		WBC in urine	Acetonuria Hematuria RBC in urine	Glycosuria Proteinuria

▶*Adverse reactions less than 1%:*

Cardiovascular – Chest pain, cyanosis, increased bleeding time, intermittent claudication, peripheral ischemia.

CNS – Malaise, dizziness, abnormal gait, migraine, neuritis, pseudotumor cerebri (intracranial hypertension), anxiety, dysphonia, nervousness.

Dermatologic – Acne, cyst, eczema, fungal infection, furunculosis, hair discoloration, herpes simplex, hyperkeratosis, hypertrichosis, hypoesthesia, impaired healing, photosensitivity reaction, psoriasis aggravated, scleroderma, skin nodule, skin hypertrophy, skin disorder, skin irritation, sweat gland disorder, urticaria, verrucae.

GI – Altered saliva, anal disorder, gum hyperplasia, constipation, dyspepsia, esophagitis, gastritis, gastroenteritis, glossitis, hemorrhoids, melena, tenesmus, tongue ulceration, weight increase.

GU – Libido decreased, atrophic vaginitis, leukorrhea, abnormal urine, dysuria, penis disorder.

Hepatic – Abnormal hepatic function, hepatitis, jaundice.

Musculoskeletal – Muscle weakness, bone disorder, olecranon bursitis, spinal hyperostosis (new lesions), tendonitis.

Respiratory – Coughing, increased sputum, laryngitis, pharyngitis.

Special senses – Ceruminosis, deafness, taste loss, otitis media, otitis externa, abnormal lacrimation, chalazion, conjunctival hemorrhage, corneal ulceration, diplopia, ectropion, itchy eyes/lids, papilledema, recurrent sties, subepithelial corneal lesions.

Miscellaneous – Alcohol intolerance, fever, hemorrhage, influenza-like symptoms, moniliasis, breast pain.

ACITRETIN

➤*Postmarketing:*

Cardiovascular – Acute MI, thromboembolism, stroke.

CNS – Myopathy with peripheral neuropathy (both conditions improved with discontinuation of the drug). Aggressive feelings and/or suicidal thoughts. These events, including self-injurious behavior, have been reported in patients taking other systemically administered retinoids, as well as in patients taking acitretin. Since other factors may have contributed to these events, it is not known if they are related to acitretin.

Dermatologic – Thinning of the skin, skin fragility, and scaling may occur all over the body, particularly on the palms and soles; nail fragility is frequently observed.

GU – Vulvo vaginitis due to *Candida albicans.*

Overdosage

In the event of acute overdosage, acitretin must be withdrawn at once. Symptoms of overdose are identical to acute hypervitaminosis A (eg, headache, vertigo). One overdose has been reported. A male 32 years of age took a 525 mg single dose. He vomited several hours later but experienced no other ill effects. The acute oral toxicity (LD_{50}) of acitretin in both mice and rats was greater than 4000 mg/kg.

All female patients of childbearing potential who have taken an overdose of acitretin must have a pregnancy test at the time of overdose. They also must be counseled as per the boxed Contraindications, Warnings, and Precautions sections regarding birth defects and contraceptive use for at least 3 years' duration after the overdose.

Patient Information

Females of reproductive potential must not be pregnant when acitretin therapy is initiated and should use 2 forms of effective contraception for at least 1 month prior to and during acitretin therapy. The risk of severe fetal malformation is well established when systemic retinoids are taken during pregnancy. Pregnancy also must be prevented after stopping therapy; the duration of posttherapy contraception to achieve adequate elimination cannot be calculated precisely. It is strongly recommended that contraception be continued for at least 3 years after stopping treatment with acitretin.

Advise females of reproductive potential that they must not ingest beverages or products containing ethanol while taking acitretin and for

2 months after acitretin treatment has been discontinued. This allows for elimination of the acitretin, which can be converted to etretinate in the presence of alcohol.

Advise female patients that certain methods of birth control can fail, including tubal ligation and microdosed progestin "minipill" preparations.

Because of the relationship of acitretin to vitamin A, advise patients against taking vitamin A supplements in excess of minimum recommended daily allowances to avoid possible additive toxic effects.

Advise patients that a transient worsening of psoriasis is sometimes seen during the initial treatment period.

Advise patients that the full benefit of acitretin may not be seen for 2 to 3 months.

Advise patients that they may experience decreased tolerance to contact lenses during the treatment period and sometimes after treatment has stopped.

It is recommended that patients (male and female) do not donate blood during and for 3 years following acitretin therapy.

Patients should avoid the use of sunlamps and excessive exposure to sunlight because the effects of UV light are enhanced by retinoid therapy.

Advise patients that they must not give their acitretin to any other person.

May cause photosensitivity (sensitivity to sunlight). Avoid prolonged exposure to the sun and other ultraviolet light. Use sunscreens and wear protective clothing until tolerance is determined.

Female patients must sign a consent form prior to beginning acitretin therapy.

Instruct patients to read the Medication Guide supplied as required by law when acitretin is dispensed.

Decreased night vision has been reported with acitretin therapy. Advise patients of this potential problem, and warn them to be cautious when driving or operating any vehicle at night. Carefully monitor visual problems.

Advise diabetic patients that some have experienced problems with blood sugar control. Monitor carefully.

ALITRETINOIN

Rx	**Panretin** (Ligand)	**Gel:** 0.1%	Dehydrated alcohol. In 60 g tubes.

Indications

➤*Kaposi's sarcoma (KS) cutaneous lesions:* Topical treatment of cutaneous lesions in patients with AIDS-related KS.

Administration and Dosage

➤*Approved by the FDA:* February 2, 1999.

Do not use occlusive dressings with alitretinoin gel.

Initially apply 2 times/day to cutaneous KS lesions. The application frequency can be gradually increased to 3 or 4 times/day, according to individual lesion tolerance. If application site toxicity occurs, the application frequency can be reduced. If severe irritation occurs, application of drug can be discontinued for a few days until the symptoms subside.

Apply sufficient gel to cover the lesion with a generous coating. Allow the gel to dry for 3 to 5 minutes before covering with clothing. Because unaffected skin may become irritated, avoid application of the gel to healthy skin surrounding the lesions. In addition, do not apply the gel on or near mucosal surfaces of the body.

A response of KS lesions may be seen as soon as 2 weeks after initiation of therapy, but most patients require longer application. With continued application, further benefit may be attained. Some patients have required over 14 weeks to respond. In clinical trials, alitretinoin gel was applied for up to 96 weeks. Continue alitretinoin gel as long as the patient is deriving benefit.

Actions

➤*Pharmacology:* Alitretinoin (9-cis-retinoic acid) is a naturally occurring endogenous retinoid that binds to and activates all known intracellular retinoid receptor subtypes (RARα, RARβ, RARγ, RXRα, RXRβ, and RXRγ). Once activated, these receptors function as transcription factors that regulate the expression of genes that control the process of cellular differentiation and proliferation in healthy and neoplastic cells. Alitretinoin inhibits the growth of KS cells in vitro.

➤*Pharmacokinetics:* There is indirect evidence that absorption of 9-cis-retinoic acid is not extensive. Plasma concentrations were evaluated during clinical studies in patients with cutaneous lesions of AIDS-related KS after repeated multiple daily dose application of alitretinoin gel for up to 60 weeks. The range of 9-cis-retinoic acid plasma concentrations in these patients was similar to the range of circulating, naturally occurring 9-cis-retinoic acid plasma concentrations in untreated healthy volunteers.

Although there are no detectable plasma concentrations of 9-cis-retinoic acid metabolites after topical application of alitretinoin gel, in vitro studies indicate that the drug is metabolized to 4-hydroxy-9-cis-retinoic acid and 4-oxo-9-cis-retinoic acid by CYP 2C9, 3A4, 1A1, and 1A2 enzymes. In vivo, 4-oxo-9-cis-retinoic acid is the major circulating metabolite following oral administration of 9-cis-retinoic acid.

Contraindications

Hypersensitivity to retinoids or to any of the ingredients of the product; when systemic anti-KS therapy is required (eg, more than 10 new KS lesions in the prior month, symptomatic lymphedema, symptomatic pulmonary KS, symptomatic visceral involvement).

Warnings

➤*Systemic therapy:* Alitretinoin gel is not a systemic therapy; therefore, it cannot treat visceral KS, nor prevent the development of new KS lesions where it has not been applied. Alitretinoin is not indicated when systemic anti-KS therapy is required (see Contraindications). There is no experience to date using alitretinoin gel with systemic anti-KS treatment.

➤*Elderly:* Inadequate information is available to assess safety and efficacy in patients 65 years of age and older.

➤*Pregnancy: Category D.* Alitretinoin gel could cause fetal harm if significant absorption were to occur in a pregnant woman. 9-cis-retinoic-acid is teratogenic in rabbits and mice. An increased incidence of fused sternebrae, and limb and craniofacial defects occurred in rabbits given oral doses of 0.5 mg/kg/day (about 5 times the estimated daily human topical dose on a mg/m² basis) during the period of organogenesis. Oral 9-cis-retinoic acid also was embryocidal, as indicated by early resorptions and postimplantation loss when it was given to rabbits during the period of organogenesis at doses of 1.5 mg/kg/day and to rats at doses of 5 mg/kg/day. It is not known whether topical alitretinoin gel can modulate endogenous 9-cis-retinoic acid levels in a pregnant woman nor whether systemic exposure is increased by application to ulcerated lesions or by duration of treatment. There are no adequate and well-controlled studies in pregnant women. If alitretinoin gel is used during pregnancy, or if the patient becomes pregnant while taking the drug, apprise the patient of the potential hazard to the fetus. Advise women of childbearing potential to avoid becoming pregnant.

➤*Lactation:* It is not known whether alitretinoin or its metabolites are excreted in breast milk. Because of the potential for adverse reactions from alitretinoin gel in nursing infants, mothers should discontinue nursing prior to using the drug.

ALITRETINOIN

▶*Children:* Safety and efficacy in children have not been established.

Precautions

▶*Response:* In the clinical trials, responses were seen as early as 2 weeks; however, most patients required 4 to 8 weeks of treatment, and some patients did not experience significant improvement until 14 weeks or more of treatment. The cumulative percentage of patients who achieved a response was less than 1% at 2 weeks, 10% at 4 weeks, and 28% at 8 weeks.

▶*Cutaneous T-cell lymphoma:* Alitretinoin gel is indicated for topical treatment of KS. Patients with cutaneous T-cell lymphoma were less tolerant of topical alitretinoin gel; 5 of 7 patients had 6 episodes of treatment-limiting toxicities (grade 3 dermal irritation) with alitretinoin gel (0.01% or 0.05%).

▶*Photosensitivity:* Retinoids as a class have been associated with photosensitivity. There were no reports of photosensitivity associated with the use of alitretinoin gel in clinical studies. Nonetheless, because in vitro data indicate that 9-cis-retinoic acid may have a weak photosensitizing effect, advise patients to minimize exposure of treated areas to sunlight and sunlamps during the use of alitretinoin gel.

Drug Interactions

▶*DEET:* Do not use products that contain DEET (N,N-diethyl-m-toluamide), a common component of insect repellent products, while using alitretinoin gel. Animal toxicology studies showed increased DEET toxicity when DEET was included as part of the formulation.

Adverse Reactions

Adverse events associated with the use of alitretinoin gel in patients with AIDS-related KS occurred almost exclusively at the site of application. The dermal toxicity begins as erythema; with continued application, erythema may increase and edema may develop. Dermal toxicity may become treatment-limiting, with intense erythema, edema, and vesiculation. Adverse events are usually mild to moderate in severity; they led to withdrawal from the study in only 7% of the patients. Severe local (application site) skin adverse events occurred in about 10% of patients in the US study (vs 0% in the control group).

Alitretinoin Application Site Reactions (≥ 5%)				
	Study 1		Study 2	
Adverse reaction	Alitretinoin gel (n = 134)	Vehicle gel (n = 134)	Alitretinoin gel (n = 36)	Vehicle gel (n = 46)
Rash (eg, erythema, scaling, irritation, redness, rash, dermatitis)	77	11	25	4
Pain (eg, burning, pain)	34	7	0	4
Pruritus (eg, itching)	11	4	8	4
Exfoliative dermatitis (eg, flaking, peeling, desquamation, exfoliation)	9	2	3	0
Skin disorder (eg, excoriation, cracking, scabbing, crusting, drainage, eschar, fissure, oozing)	8	1	0	0
Paresthesia (eg, stinging, tingling)	3	0	22	7
Edema (eg, swelling, inflammation)	8	3	3	0

Overdosage

Systemic toxicity following acute overdosage with topical application of alitretinoin gel is unlikely because of limited systemic plasma levels observed with normal therapeutic doses. There is no specific antidote for overdosage.

Patient Information

Advise patients against applying gel on or near mucosal surfaces of the body such as eyes, nostrils, mouth, lips, vagina, tip of the penis, rectum, or anus.

Advise patients against using insect repellents containing DEET or other products containing DEET while using alitretinoin.

Instruct patients to keep out of reach of children.

Product contains alcohol; keep away from open flame.

Do not administer to patients who are pregnant or breastfeeding. Instruct patients to take precautions to avoid becoming pregnant while using altretinoin. If the patient is pregnant, thinking of becoming pregnant, or breastfeeding, advise them to speak with their health care provider for more information.

Inform patients that KS lesions can appear and affect other parts of their body, including internal organs (eg, lungs and intestines). Advise patients to regularly consult their health care provider about the status of their KS disease, especially if they note changes.

Alitretinoin does not treat lung or intestinal KS.

Alitretinoin does not prevent the appearance of new KS lesions or the increased growth of KS lesions not treated with alitretinoin.

Alitretinoin does not treat extremity swelling associated with KS.

Instruct patients to avoid applying the gel to areas of healthy skin around a KS lesion. Exposure of healthy skin to alitretinoin may cause unnecessary irritation or redness.

Instruct patients to avoid showering, bathing, or swimming for at least 3 hours after any application, if possible.

Instruct patients to avoid covering the KS lesions treated with gel with any bandage or material other than loose clothing.

Instruct patients to avoid prolonged exposure of the treated area to sunlight or other ultraviolet light (eg, tanning lamps).

Instruct patients to avoid the use of other topical products on treated KS lesions. Mineral oil may be used between alitretinoin applications in order to help prevent excessive dryness or itching. Mineral oil should not be applied for at least 2 hours before or after the application of alitretinoin.

Instruct patients to avoid scratching the treated areas.

Instruct patients to always use the cap to close the tube tightly after each use.

TAZAROTENE

Rx	Tazorac (Allergan)	Cream: 0.05%	1% benzyl alcohol, EDTA, medium chain triglycerides, mineral oil. In 15, 30, and 60 g.
Rx	Avage (Allergan)	Cream: 0.1%	1% benzyl alcohol, EDTA, medium chain triglycerides, mineral oil. In 15 and 30 g.
Rx	Tazorac (Allergan)		1% benzyl alcohol, EDTA, medium chain triglycerides, mineral oil. In 15, 30, and 60 g.
Rx	Tazorac (Allergan)	Gel: 0.05%	1% benzyl alcohol, EDTA. In 30 and 100 g.
		0.1%	1% benzyl alcohol, EDTA. In 30 and 100 g.

Indications

➤*Tazorac cream:*

Acne – Topical treatment of patients with acne vulgaris (0.1% only).

Psoriasis – Topical treatment of patients with plaque psoriasis.

➤*Tazorac Gel:*

Acne – Topical treatment of patients with facial acne vulgaris of mild to moderate severity (0.1% only).

Psoriasis – Topical treatment of patients with stable plaque psoriasis of up to 20% body surface area involvement.

The efficacy of tazarotene in the treatment of acne previously treated with other retinoids or resistant to oral antibiotics has not been established.

➤*Avage:*

Wrinkling, hyper- and hypopigmentation, lentigines – As an adjunctive agent in the mitigation (palliation) of facial fine wrinkling, facial mottled hyper- and hypopigmentation, and benign facial lentigines in patients who use comprehensive skin care and sunlight avoidance programs. This product does not eliminate or prevent wrinkles, repair sun-damaged skin, reverse photoaging, or restore more youthful or younger skin.

• *Avage* has not demonstrated a mitigating effect on significant signs of chronic sunlight exposure such as coarse or deep wrinkling, tactile roughness, telangiectasia, skin laxity, keratinocytic atypia, melanocytic atypia, or dermal elastosis.

• *Avage* should be used under medical supervision as an adjunct to a comprehensive skin care and sunlight avoidance program that includes the use of effective sunscreens (minimum SPF 15) and protective clothing.

• Neither the safety nor the effectiveness of *Avage* for the prevention or treatment of actinic keratoses, skin neoplasms, or lentigo maligna has been established.

• Neither the safety nor the efficacy of using *Avage* daily for greater than 52 weeks has been established, and daily use beyond 52 weeks has not been systematically and histologically investigated in adequate and well-controlled trials.

Administration and Dosage

➤*Approved by the FDA:* June 13, 1997.

For topical use only. Not for ophthalmic, oral, or intravaginal use.

Application may cause excessive irritation in the skin of certain sensitive individuals. In cases where it has been necessary to temporarily discontinue therapy or where the dosing has been reduced to a lower concentration (in patients with psoriasis) or to an interval the patient can tolerate, therapy can be resumed, or the drug concentration or frequency of application can be increased as the patient becomes able to tolerate the treatment. Closely monitor frequency of application by careful observation of the clinical therapeutic response and skin tolerance. Efficacy has not been established for less than once daily dosing frequencies.

➤*Acne:* Cleanse the face gently. After the skin is dry, apply a thin film of tazarotene (2 mg/cm^2) once a day in the evening to the skin where acne lesions appear. Use enough to cover the entire affected area. Tazarotene was investigated for up to 12 weeks during clinical trials for acne.

➤*Psoriasis:* Apply tazarotene once a day in the evening to psoriatic lesions, using enough (2 mg/cm^2) to cover only the lesion with a thin film. The gel should cover no more than 20% of body surface area. If a bath or shower is taken prior to application, dry the skin before applying. If emollients are used, apply them at least 1 hour before *Tazorac* cream. Because unaffected skin may be more susceptible to irritation, carefully avoid application of tazarotene to these areas. It is recommended that treatment start with the 0.05% cream with strength increase to 0.1% if tolerated and medically indicated. Tazarotene gel was investigated for up to 12 months during clinical trials for psoriasis.

➤*Wrinkling, hyper- and hypopigmentation, lentigines:* Apply a pea-sized amount once a day at bedtime to lightly cover the entire face including the eyelids if desired. Facial moisturizers may be used as frequently as desired. Remove any makeup before applying the cream to the face. If the face is washed or a bath or shower is taken prior to application, the skin should be dry before applying the cream. If emollients or moisturizers are used, they can be applied before or after application of tazarotene cream, ensuring that the first cream or lotion has absorbed into the skin and has dried completely. Closely monitor frequency of application by careful observation of the clinical therapeutic response and skin tolerance. If the frequency of dosing is reduced, it

should be noted that efficacy at a reduced frequency of application has not been established. The duration of the mitigating effects on facial fine wrinkling, mottled hypo- and hyperpigmentation, and benign facial lentigines following discontinuation has not been studied.

➤*Storage/Stability:*

Tazorac and Avage creams – Store at 25°C (77°F). Excursions permitted from -5° to 30°C (23° to 86°F).

Gel – Store at 25°C (77°F). Excursions permitted from 15° to 30°C (59° to 86°F).

Actions

➤*Pharmacology:* Tazarotene is a retinoid prodrug that is converted to its active form, tazarotenic acid, by rapid de-esterification in most biological systems. Tazarotenic acid binds to all 3 members of the retinoic acid receptor (RAR) family (RARα, RARβ and RARγ), but shows relative selectivity for RARβ and RARγ and may modify gene expression. The clinical significance of these findings is unknown.

The mechanism of tazarotene action is not defined. Tazarotene inhibited corneocyte accumulation in rhino mouse skin and cross-linked envelope formation in cultured human keratinocytes. Topical tazarotene blocks induction of mouse epidermal ornithine decarboxylase (ODC) activity, which is associated with cell proliferation and hyperplasia. In cell culture and in vitro models of skin, tazarotene suppresses expression of MRP8, a marker of inflammation present in the epidermis of psoriasis subjects at high levels. In human keratinocyte cultures, it inhibits cornified envelope formation, whose build-up is an element of psoriatic scale. Tazarotene also induces the expression of a gene that may be a growth suppressor in human keratinocytes and that may inhibit epidermal hyperproliferation in treated plaques. The clinical significance of these findings is unknown.

➤*Pharmacokinetics:*

Absorption/Distribution – Following topical application, tazarotene undergoes esterase hydrolysis to form its active metabolite, tazarotinic acid. Little parent compound can be detected in the plasma. Tazarotenic acid is highly bound to plasma proteins (more than 99%).

Cream: In a multiple dose study with a once-daily dose for 14 consecutive days in 9 psoriatic patients, measured doses of tazarotene 0.1% cream were applied to involved skin without occlusion. The C_{max} of tazarotenic acid was 2.31 ng/mL occurring 8 hours after the final dose, and the AUC_{0-24h} was 31.2 ng•h/mL on day 15 in the 5 patients who were administered clinical doses of 2 mg cream/cm^2.

Tazarotene cream 0.1% was applied once daily to the face (N = 8) or to 15% of body surface area (N = 10) of female patients with moderate to severe acne vulgaris. The mean C_{max} and AUC values of tazarotenic acid peaked at day 15 for both dosing groups during a 29-day treatment period. Mean C_{max} and AUC_{0-24h} values of tazarotenic acid from patients in the 15% body surface area dosing group were more than 10 times higher than those from patients in the face-only dosing group. In the face-only group, the C_{max} and AUC_{0-24h} of tazarotenic acid on day 15 were 0.1 ng/mL and 1.54 ng•h/mL, respectively, whereas in the 15% body surface area dosing group, the C_{max} and AUC_{0-24h} of tazarotenic acid on day 15 were 1.2 ng/mL and 17.01 ng•h/mL, respectively. The steady state pharmacokinetics of tazarotenic acid had been reached by day 8 in the face-only and by day 15 in the 15% body surface area dosing groups.

Tazarotene cream 0.1% was topically applied once daily to the face or to 15% of body surface area over 4 weeks in patients with fine wrinkling and mottled hyperpigmentation. In the "face-only" dosing group, the maximum average C_{max} and AUC_{0-24h} values of tazarotenic acid occurred on day 15 with C_{max} and AUC_{0-24h} of tazarotenic acid being 0.236 ng/mL and 2.44 ng•h/mL, respectively. The mean C_{max} and AUC_{0-24h} values of tazarotenic acid from patients in the 15% body surface area dosing group were approximately 10 times higher than those from patients in the face-only dosing group. The single highest C_{max} throughout the study period was 3.43 ng/mL on day 29 from patients in the 15% body surface area dosing group.

Gel: Studies following a single, topical dose of tazarotene determined that systemic absorption of the total dose was less than 1% without occlusion in psoriatic patients and approximately 5% under occlusion in healthy patients. Another study found the C_{max} and AUC for the 0.1% gel to be 40% higher than the 0.05% gel. Systemic absorption of 2 mg/cm^2 doses of 0.1% gel applied topically without occlusion was less than 1% after 7 days of therapy when applied to 20% of the total body surface area (BSA) of healthy patients and was about 15% after 14 days when applied to approximately 13% of total BSA in psoriatic patients. The results of these in vivo studies refer to the active metabolite only.

TAZAROTENE

An in vitro percutaneous absorption study indicated that about 4% to 5% of the applied dose was in the stratum corneum (tazarotene:metabolite, 5:1) and 2% to 4% was in the viable epidermis-dermis layer (tazarotene:metabolite, 2:1) 24 hours after topical application of the gel.

Metabolism/Excretion – The half-life of the metabolite following topical application of tazarotene is approximately 18 hours and is similar among healthy and psoriatic patients. The parent drug and metabolite are further metabolized and eliminated through urinary and fecal pathways.

Contraindications

Pregnancy (see Warnings); hypersensitivity to any components of the product.

Warnings

➤*Carcinogenesis:* In evaluation of photocarcinogenicity, median time to onset of tumors was decreased and the number of tumors increased in hairless mice following chronic topical dosing with intercurrent exposure to ultraviolet radiation at tazarotene concentrations of 0.001%, 0.005%, and 0.01% for up to 40 weeks.

➤*Fertility impairment:* There was a significant decrease in the number of estrous stages and an increase in developmental effects at oral doses up to 2 mg/kg/day. That dose produced an AUC_{0-24h} that was 6.7 times the maximum AUC_{0-24h} in patients treated with 2 mg/cm^2 of tazarotene cream 0.1% over 15% body surface area for signs of fine wrinkling and mottled hyperpigmentation.

➤*Pregnancy: Category X.* In rabbits, topical tazarotene caused retinoid malformations, including spina bifida, hydrocephaly, and heart anomalies.

As with other retinoids, when tazarotene was given orally to experimental animals, developmental delays were seen in rats, and teratogenic effects and postimplantation loss were observed in rats and rabbits at doses producing 2.1 and 52 times, respectively, the maximum AUC_{0-24h} in patients treated with 2 mg/cm^2 of tazarotene cream 0.1% over 15% body surface area for fine wrinkling and mottled hyperpigmentation.

In a study of the effect of oral tazarotene on fertility and early embryonic development in rats, decreased number of implantation sites, decreased litter size, decreased number of live fetuses, and decreased fetal body weights, all classic developmental effects of retinoids, were observed when female rats were administered 2 mg/kg/day from 15 days before mating through gestation day 7. A low incidence of retinoid-related malformations at that dose were reported to be related to treatment. That dose produced an AUC_{0-24h} that was 6.7 times the maximum AUC_{0-24h} in patients treated with 2 mg/cm^2 of tazarotene cream 0.1% over 15% body surface area for signs of fine wrinkling and mottled hyperpigmentation.

Tazarotene is contraindicated in women who are or may become pregnant. If this drug is used during pregnancy or if the patient becomes pregnant while taking this drug, discontinue treatment and apprise the patient of the potential hazard to the fetus. Warn women of childbearing potential of the potential risk and to use adequate birth-control measures when using tazarotene. Consider the possibility that a woman of childbearing potential is pregnant at the time of institution of therapy. Obtain a negative result for a pregnancy test having a sensitivity down to at least 50 mIU/mL for human chorionic gonadotropin (hCG) within 2 weeks prior to tazarotene therapy, which should begin during a normal menstrual period.

➤*Lactation:* Tazarotene is excreted in breast milk of rats. It is not known whether this drug is excreted in human milk. Exercise caution when tazarotene is administered to a nursing woman.

➤*Children:*

Tazorac cream – Safety and efficacy have not been established in patients under 18 years of age with psoriasis or in patients under 12 years of age with acne.

Avage – Safety and efficacy have not been established in patients under 17 years of age with facial fine wrinkling, facial mottled hypo- and hyperpigmentation, and benign facial lentigines.

Gel – Safety and efficacy have not been established in children less than 12 years of age.

Precautions

➤*For external use only:* Apply only to the affected areas. Avoid contact with eyes, eyelids (*Tazorac* only), and mouth. If contact with the eyes occurs, rinse thoroughly with water. The safety of use of tazarotene gel over more than 20% of body surface area has not been established in psoriasis or acne.

➤*Eczematous skin:* Do not use retinoids on eczematous skin, as they may cause severe irritation.

➤*Dermatologic medications and cosmetics:* Avoid those medications and cosmetics that have a strong drying effect. It also is advisable to "rest" a patient's skin until the effects of such preparations subside before use of tazarotene is begun.

➤*Photosensitizers (eg, thiazides, tetracyclines, fluoroquinolones, phenothiazines, sulfonamides):* Administer with caution if the patient is also taking drugs known to be photosensitizers because of the increased possibility of augmented photosensitivity.

➤*Discontinue:* If pruritus, burning, skin redness, or peeling is excessive, discontinue until the integrity of the skin is restored, or reduce the dosing to an interval the patient can tolerate. However, efficacy at reduced frequency of application has not been established. Alternatively, patients with psoriasis who are being treated with *Tazorac* 1% cream can be switched to the lower concentration (0.05%).

➤*Weather extremes:* Wind or cold may be more irritating to patients using tazarotene.

➤*Lentigo maligna:* Some facial pigmented lesions are not lentigines, but rather lentigo maligna, a type of melanoma. Facial pigmented lesions of concern should be carefully assessed by a qualified physician (eg, dermatologist) before application of *Avage.* Do not treat lentigo maligna with *Avage.*

➤*Photosensitivity:* Photosensitization (photoallergy or phototoxicity) may occur; therefore, caution patients to take protective measures (ie, sunscreens, protective clothing) against exposure to sunlight or ultraviolet light (eg, tanning beds) until tolerance is determined.

Because of heightened burning susceptibility, avoid exposure to sunlight (including sunlamps) unless deemed medically necessary; in such cases, minimize exposure during the use of tazarotene. Warn patients to use sunscreens (minimum SPF 15) and protective clothing when using tazarotene. Advise patients with sunburn not to use tazarotene until fully recovered. Patients who may have considerable sun exposure because of their occupation and those patients with inherent sensitivity to sunlight should exercise particular caution when using tazarotene.

In human dermal safety studies, tazarotene did not induce allergic contact sensitization, phototoxicity, or photoallergy.

Adverse Reactions

The most frequent adverse events with tazarotene are limited to the skin and include the following:

➤*Gel:*

Acne: Desquamation, burning/stinging, dry skin, erythema, pruritus (10% to 30%); irritation, skin pain, fissuring, localized edema, skin discoloration (1% to 10%).

Psoriasis: Pruritus, burning/stinging, erythema, worsening of psoriasis, irritation, skin pain (10% to 30%); rash, desquamation, irritant contact dermatitis, skin inflammation, fissuring, bleeding, dry skin (1% to 10%). In general, the incidence of adverse events with 0.05% gel was 2% to 5% lower than that seen with 0.1% gel.

Increases in psoriasis worsening and sun-induced erythema were noted in some patients over months 4 to 12, as compared with the first 3 months of a 1-year study.

➤*Tazorac cream:*

Acne: Desquamation, dry skin, erythema, burning sensation (10% to 30%); pruritus, irritation, face pain, stinging (1% to 5%).

Psoriasis: Pruritus, erythema, burning (10% to 23%); irritation, desquamation, stinging, contact dermatitis, dermatitis, eczema, worsening of psoriasis, skin pain, rash, hypertriglyceridemia, dry skin, skin inflammation, peripheral edema (more than 1% to less than 10%).

Tazorac 0.1% cream was associated with a somewhat greater degree of local irritation than the 0.05% cream. In general, the rates of irritation adverse events reported during psoriasis studies with 0.1% cream were 1% to 4% higher than those reported for the 0.05% cream.

➤*Avage cream:* Desquamation (40%); erythema (34%); burning sensation (26%); dry skin (16%); skin irritation, pruritus (10%); irritant contact dermatitis (8%); stinging, acne (3%); cheilitis (1%). A few patients reported adverse events at week 0; however, for patients who were treated with *Avage,* the highest number of new reports for each adverse event was at week 2. When combining data from the 2 pivotal studies, 5.3% of patients in the tazarotene group and 0.9% of patients in the vehicle group discontinued because of adverse events. Overall, 3.5% of patients in the tazarotene group and 2.8% of patients in the vehicle group reported adverse events (including edema, irritation, and inflammation) directly related to the eye or eyelid. The majority of these conditions were mild.

Overdosage

➤*Symptoms:* Excessive topical use of tazarotene may lead to marked redness, peeling, or discomfort.

Oral ingestion of the drug may lead to the same adverse effects as those associated with excessive oral intake of vitamin A (hypervitaminosis A) or other retinoids.

➤*Treatment:* If oral ingestion occurs, monitor the patient and administer appropriate supportive measures as necessary. Refer to General Management of Acute Overdosage.

TAZAROTENE

Patient Information

Do not use tazarotene if you are pregnant, plan to become pregnant, or may become pregnant because of the potential harm to the unborn child. Talk with your doctor about effective birth control if you are a woman who is able to become pregnant. If you become pregnant while using tazarotene, contact your physician immediately.

Do not use tazarotene if you have a sunburn, eczema, or other continuing skin conditions.

Do not use tazarotene if you are sensitive to sunlight.

For best results, if emollients or moisturizers are used, they can be applied before or after tazarotene cream, ensuring that the first cream or lotion has absorbed into the skin and dried completely.

Avoid sunlight and other medicines that may increase your sensitivity to sunlight. Avoidance of excessive sun exposure and the use of sunscreens with protective measures (hat, visor) are recommended. In the morning, apply a moisturizing sunscreen SPF 15 or greater.

Refer to patient package insert for additional patient information.

➤*Avage:* Apply only a small, pea-sized amount (about ¼ inch or 5 mm diameter) of *Avage* to your face at one time.

Avage does not remove or prevent wrinkles or repair sun-damaged skin.

➤*Tazorac:* Apply a thin film to your psoriasis areas once a day in the evening.

Usually your acne will begin to improve in about 4 weeks. Continue to use *Tazorac* for up to 12 weeks as directed by your doctor.

BEXAROTENE

Rx **Targretin** (Ligand Pharmaceuticals) | **Gel:** 1% | Dehydrated alcohol. In 60 g.

Bexarotene is also available as a soft gelatin capsule for the treatment of cutaneous T-cell lymphoma (CTCL). Refer to the Antineoplastic Agents chapter.

Indications

➤*Cutaneous T-cell lymphoma (CTCL) lesions:* For the topical treatment of cutaneous lesions in patients with CTCL (Stage IA and IB) who have refractory or persistent disease after other therapies or who have not tolerated other therapies.

Administration and Dosage

➤*Approved by the FDA:* June 28, 2000.

Initially apply once every other day for the first week. Increase the application frequency at weekly intervals to once daily, then twice daily, then 3 times daily, and finally 4 times daily according to individual lesion tolerance. Generally, patients were able to maintain a dosing frequency of 2 to 4 times/day. Most responses were seen at dosing frequencies of ≥ 2 times/day. If application site toxicity occurs, the application frequency can be reduced. Should severe irritation occur, application of drug can be temporarily discontinued for a few days until the symptoms subside.

Apply sufficient gel to cover the lesion with a generous coating. Allow the gel to dry before covering with clothing. Because unaffected skin may become irritated, avoid application of the gel to normal skin surrounding the lesions. In addition, do not apply the gel near mucosal surfaces of the body.

A response may be seen as soon as 4 weeks after initiation of therapy but most patients require longer application. With continued application, further benefit may be attained. The longest onset time for the first response among the responders was 392 days. In clinical trials, bexarotene gel was applied for up to 172 weeks.

Continue bexarotene gel as long as the patient is deriving benefit.

Do not use occlusive dressings with bexarotene gel.

Bexarotene gel is a topical therapy and is not intended for systemic use. It has not been studied in combination with other CTCL therapies.

➤*Storage/Stability:* Store at 15° to 30°C (59° to 86°F). Avoid exposing to high temperatures and humidity after the tube is opened. Protect from light.

Actions

➤*Pharmacology:* Bexarotene selectively binds and activates retinoid X receptor subtypes (RXRα, RXRβ, RXRγ). RXRs can form heterodimers with various receptor partners, such as retinoic acid receptors (RARs), vitamin D receptor, thyroid receptor, and peroxisome proliferator activator receptors (PPARs). Once activated, these receptors function as transcription factors that regulate the expression of genes that control cellular differentiation and proliferation. Bexarotene inhibits the growth in vitro of some tumor cell lines of hematopoietic and squamous cell origin. It also induces tumor regression in vivo in some animal models. The exact mechanism of action of bexarotene in the treatment of CTCL is unknown.

➤*Pharmacokinetics:*

Absorption/Distribution – Sporadically observed and generally low plasma bexarotene concentrations indicate that, in patients receiving doses of low-to-moderate intensity, there is a low potential for significant plasma concentrations following repeated application of the gel. Bexarotene is highly bound (> 99%) to plasma proteins. The plasma proteins to which bexarotene binds have not been elucidated, and the ability of bexarotene to displace drugs bound to plasma proteins and the ability of drugs to displace bexarotene binding have not been studied. The uptake of bexarotene by organs or tissues has not been evaluated.

Metabolism – Four bexarotene metabolites have been identified in plasma following oral administration of bexarotene: 6- and 7-hydroxy-bexarotene and 6- and 7-oxo-bexarotene. In vitro studies suggest that cytochrome P450 3A4 is the major cytochrome P450 responsible for formation of the oxidative metabolites and that the oxidative metabolites may be glucuronidated. The oxidative metabolites are active in in vitro assays of retinoid receptor activation, but the relative contribution of the parent and any metabolites to the efficacy and safety of bexarotene gel is unknown.

Excretion – The renal elimination of bexarotene and its metabolites was examined in patients with Type 2 diabetes mellitus following oral administration of bexarotene. Neither bexarotene nor its metabolites were excreted in urine in appreciable amounts.

Contraindications

Pregnancy; known hypersensitivity to bexarotene or other components of the product.

Warnings

➤*Hypersensitivity reactions:* Use bexarotene with caution in patients with a known hypersensitivity to other retinoids. No clinical instances of cross-reactivity have been noted.

➤*Renal function impairment:* Urinary elimination of bexarotene and its known metabolites is a minor excretory pathway for bexarotene (< 1% of an orally administered dose), but because renal insufficiency can result in significant protein binding changes, and bexarotene is > 99% protein bound, pharmacokinetics may be altered in patients with renal insufficiency.

➤*Hepatic function impairment:* Because < 1% of the dose of oral bexarotene is excreted in the urine unchanged and there is in vitro evidence of extensive hepatic contribution to bexarotene elimination, hepatic impairment would be expected to lead to greatly decreased clearance.

➤*Mutagenesis:* Bexarotene was not mutagenic to bacteria (Ames assay) or mammalian cells (mouse lymphoma assay). Bexarotene was not clastogenic in vivo (micronucleus test in mice).

➤*Fertility impairment:* No formal fertility studies were conducted with bexarotene. Bexarotene caused testicular degeneration when oral doses of 1.5 mg/kg/day were given to dogs for 91 days.

➤*Elderly:* No overall differences in safety were observed between patients ≥ 65 years of age and younger patients, but greater sensitivity of some older individuals to bexarotene cannot be ruled out. Responses to bexarotene gel were observed across all age group decades, without preference for any individual age group decade.

➤*Pregnancy: Category X.* Bexarotene may cause fetal harm when administered to a pregnant woman. It must not be given to a pregnant woman or a woman who intends to become pregnant. If a woman becomes pregnant while taking bexarotene, bexarotene must be stopped immediately and the woman given appropriate counseling.

Advise women of childbearing potential to avoid becoming pregnant when bexarotene is used. Consider the possibility that a woman of childbearing potential is pregnant at the time therapy is instituted. A negative pregnancy test (eg, serum beta-human chorionic gonadotropin, beta-HCG) with a sensitivity of ≥ 50 mIU/L should be obtained within 1 week prior to bexarotene therapy, and the pregnancy test must be repeated at monthly intervals while the patient remains on bexarotene. Effective contraception must be used for 1 month prior to the initiation of therapy, during therapy, and for ≥ 1 month following discontinuation of therapy; it is recommended that 2 reliable forms of contraception be used simultaneously unless abstinence is the chosen method. Male patients with sexual partners who are pregnant, possibly pregnant, or who could become pregnant must use condoms during sexual intercourse while applying bexarotene gel and for ≥ 1 month after the last dose of drug. Initiate the gel on the second or third day of a normal menstrual period. Do not give more than a 1-month supply of gel to the patient so that the results of pregnancy testing can be assessed and counseling regarding avoidance of pregnancy and birth defects can be reinforced.

➤*Lactation:* It is not known whether bexarotene is excreted in human milk. Because many drugs are excreted in human milk and because of the potential for serious adverse reactions in nursing infants from bexarotene, a decision should be made whether to discontinue nursing or to discontinue the drug, taking into account the importance of the drug to the mother.

➤*Children:* Safety and efficacy in pediatric patients have not been established.

Precautions

➤*Photosensitivity:* Retinoids as a class have been associated with photosensitivity. In vitro assays indicate that bexarotene is a potential photosensitizing agent. There were no reports of photosensitivity in patients in the clinical studies. Advise patients to minimize exposure to sunlight and artificial ultraviolet light during the use of bexarotene.

Drug Interactions

➤*Cytochrome P450 3A4:* Bexarotene oxidative metabolites appear to be formed through cytochrome P450 3A4. Drugs that affect levels or activity of cytochrome P450 3A4 may potentially affect the disposition of bexarotene.

Bexarotene Drug Interactions			
Precipitant drug	Object drug*		Description
CYP450 inhibitors (eg, ketoconazole, itraconazole, erythromycin, grapefruit juice)	Bexarotene	↑	Concomitant ketoconazole, itraconazole, erythromycin, and grapefruit juice could increase bexarotene plasma concentrations.

BEXAROTENE

Bexarotene Drug Interactions			
Precipitant drug	Object drug*		Description
Gemfibrozil	Bexarotene	↑	Based on data that gemfibrozil increases bexarotene concentrations following oral bexarotene administration, concomitant gemfibrozil could increase bexarotene plasma concentrations. However, because of the low systemic exposure to bexarotene after low to moderately intense gel regimens, increases that occur are unlikely to be of sufficient magnitude to result in adverse effects.
Bexarotene	DEET (N,N-diethyl-m-toluamide)	↑	Do not concurrently use products that contain DEET, a common component of insect repellent products. An animal toxicology study showed increased DEET toxicity when DEET was included as part of the formulation.
Bexarotene	Vitamin A	↑	In clinical studies, patients were advised to limit vitamin A intake to ≤ 15,000 IU/day. Because of the relationship of bexarotene to vitamin A, advise patients to limit vitamin A supplements to avoid potential additive toxic effects.
Vitamin A	Bexarotene	↑	

* ↑ = Object drug increased.

Adverse Reactions

The most common adverse events reported with an incidence at the application site of ≥ 10% in patients with CTCL were rash, pruritus, skin disorder, and pain.

Adverse events leading to dose reduction or study drug discontinuation in ≥ 2 patients were rash, contact dermatitis, and pruritus.

Of the 98% who experienced any adverse event, most experienced events categorized as mild (18%) or moderate (54%). There were 24% who experienced ≥ 1 moderately severe adverse event. The most common moderately severe events were rash (14%) and pruritus (6%). Only 2% experienced a severe adverse event (rash).

Adverse Events[1] for All Application Frequencies of Bexarotene Gel in the Multicenter CTCL Study (≥ 5%)		
	All adverse reactions n = 50	Application site adverse reactions n = 50
Dermatological		
Contact dermatitis[2]	14	8
Exfoliative dermatitis	6	0
Pruritus[3]	36	18
Rash[4]	72	56
Maculopapular rash	6	0
Skin disorder (NOS)[5]	26	18
Sweating	6	0

Adverse Events[1] for All Application Frequencies of Bexarotene Gel in the Multicenter CTCL Study (≥ 5%)		
	All adverse reactions n = 50	Application site adverse reactions n = 50
Hemic/Lymphatic		
Leukopenia	6	0
Lymphadenopathy	6	0
WBC abnormal	6	0
Respiratory		
Cough increased	6	0
Pharyngitis	6	0
Miscellaneous		
Asthenia	6	0
Edema	10	0
Headache	14	0
Hyperlipemia	10	0
Infection	18	0
Paresthesia	6	6
Pain	30	18
Peripheral edema	6	0

[1] Regardless of association with treatment.
[2] Contact dermititis, irritant contact dermatitis, irritant dermatitis.
[3] Pruritus, itching, itching of lesion.
[4] Erythema, scaling, irritation, redness, rash, dermatitis.
[5] Skin inflammation, excoriation, sticky or tacky sensation; NOS = not otherwise specified.

Overdosage

Systemic toxicity following acute overdosage with topical application of bexarotene gel is unlikely because of low systemic plasma levels observed with normal therapeutic doses. There is no specific antidote for overdosage.

There has been no experience with acute overdose of bexarotene gel in humans. Treat any overdose with bexarotene gel with supportive care for the signs and symptoms exhibited by the patient.

Patient Information

Advise women of childbearing potential to avoid becoming pregnant when bexarotene is used. A negative pregnancy test (eg, serum beta-human chorionic gonadotropin, beta-HCG) with a sensitivity of ≥ 50 mIU/L should be obtained within 1 week prior to bexarotene therapy, and the pregnancy test must be repeated at monthly intervals while the patient remains on bexarotene. Effective contraception must be used for 1 month prior to the initiation of therapy, during therapy, and for ≥ 1 month following discontinuation of therapy; it is recommended that 2 reliable forms of contraception be used simultaneously unless abstinence is the chosen method.

Advise patients to limit vitamin A supplements.

May cause photosensitivity; avoid prolonged exposure to sunlight or UV rays.

CROTAMITON

Rx	Eurax (Bristol-Myers Squibb)	Cream: 10%	Vanishing base. Cetyl alcohol. In 60 g.
		Lotion: 10%	Emollient base. Cetyl alcohol. In 60 and 454 g.

Indications

Eradication of scabies (*Sarcoptes scabiei*) and symptomatic treatment of pruritic skin.

Administration and Dosage

Shake well before using.

➤*Scabies:* Thoroughly massage into the skin of the whole body from the chin down, paying particular attention to all folds and creases. A second application is advisable 24 hours later. Change clothing and bed linen the next morning. Take a cleansing bath 48 hours after the last application.

➤*Pruritus:* Massage gently into affected areas until medication is completely absorbed. Repeat as necessary.

➤*Storage/Stability:* Store at room temperature, 20° to 25°C (68° to 77°F).

Actions

➤*Pharmacology:* Scabicidal and antipruritic; the mechanisms of action are not known.

Contraindications

Do not administer to patients who develop a sensitivity to or are allergic to crotamiton or who manifest a primary irritation response.

Warnings

➤*For external use only:* Do not apply to acutely inflamed skin, raw weeping surfaces, eyes, or mouth. Defer use until acute inflammation has subsided.

➤*Irritation/Sensitization:* If severe irritation or sensitization develops, discontinue use.

➤*Pregnancy: Category C.* It is not known whether crotamiton can cause fetal harm when applied topically to a pregnant woman or if it can affect reproduction capacity. Use on a pregnant woman only if clearly needed.

➤*Children:* Safety and efficacy for use in children have not been established.

Adverse Reactions

Allergic sensitivity or primary irritation reactions may occur.

Overdosage

➤*Symptoms:* Signs of ingestion include burning sensation in mouth, irritation of the buccal, esophageal, and gastric mucosa, nausea, vomiting, and abdominal pain. Acute toxicity (after accidental oral administration in children): Highest known doses ingested–cream, 2 g (1½ years of age); lotion, 30 mL (2 years of age). A death was reported, but cause was not confirmed.

➤*Treatment:* There is no specific antidote. General measures to eliminate the drug and reduce its absorption, combined with symptomatic treatment, are recommended. Refer to General Management of Acute Overdosage.

Patient Information

Patient instructions available with product.

Shake well before using.

Patients with scabies should take a routine bath or shower before applying the medicated cream or lotion to the skin; a second application is advisable 24 hours later.

Change clothing and bed linen the next day. Contaminated clothing and bed linen may be dry cleaned or washed in the hot cycle of the washing machine.

For external use only. Keep away from the eyes and mucous membranes (eg, nose, mouth); do not apply to inflamed skin.

Discontinue use and notify physician if irritation or sensitization occurs.

LINDANE (Gamma Benzene Hexachloride)

Rx	Lindane (Various, eg, Alpharma, Major)	Lotion: 1%	In 30 and 59 mL, and pharmacy-size only pint.
		Shampoo: 1%	In 30 and 59 mL, and pharmacy-size only pint.

WARNING

Only use lindane in patients who cannot tolerate or have failed first-line treatment with safer medications for the treatment of scabies.

Neurologic toxicity: Seizures and deaths have been reported following lindane use with repeat or prolonged application, but also in rare cases following a single application used according to directions. Exercise caution when using lindane in infants, children, the elderly, and individuals with other skin conditions (eg, atopic dermatitis, psoriasis) and in those who weigh less than 110 lbs (50 kg) as they may be at risk of serious neurotoxicity.

Contraindications: Lindane is contraindicated in premature infants and individuals with known uncontrolled seizure disorders.

Proper use: Instruct patients on the proper use of lindane, the amount to apply, how long to leave it on, and avoiding retreatment. Inform patients that itching occurs after the successful killing of scabies and is not necessarily an indication for retreatment with lindane.

Indications

➤*Lotion:* For the treatment of scabies (*Sarcoptes scabiei*) only in patients who cannot tolerate or who have failed other treatments.

➤*Shampoo:* For the treatment of head lice (*Pediculosis humanis capitis*), crab lice (*Pthirus pubis*), and their ova only in patients who cannot tolerate or who have failed other treatments.

Administration and Dosage

All patients must be provided a medication guide each time lindane is dispensed.

Washing of all recently worn clothing, underwear, pajamas, sheets, pillows, and towels is very important. Do not administer orally. Instruct caregivers to wear gloves or wash hands immediately after applying the lotion or shampoo. Inform patient that itching occurs after the successful killing of scabies or lice and it is not necessarily an indication for retreatment with lindane. Lindane does not prevent infestation or reinfestation and should not be used to ward off a possible infestation.

➤*Scabies (lotion):* Apply a thin layer of lotion over all skin (ie, entire trunk, extremities, soles of feet, underneath finger nails) from the neck down. Wash hands immediately or use gloves when applying lindane. One ounce (30 mL) is sufficient for an average adult. Do not prescribe more than 2 ounces (60 mL) for larger adults. Apply once and wash off

in 8 to 12 hours. Do not retreat unless instructed to do so by a physician; 1 application of lindane is generally successful. Do not cover areas where medication is applied. Treat sexual contacts concurrently.

Patient may bathe prior to application; however, wait at least 1 hour after bathing before applying lindane to skin. Wet and warm skin may increase absorption, leading to toxicity (eg, seizures).

➤*Head lice/crab lice (shampoo):* Apply shampoo directly to dry hair without adding water. Work thoroughly into the hair and allow to remain in place for 4 minutes only. Give special attention to the fine hairs along the neck. After 4 minutes, add small quantities of water to hair until a good lather forms. Immediately rinse all lather away. Towel briskly and then remove nits with nit comb or tweezers. Do not cover the hair with shower cap or towel. Avoid unnecessary contact of lather with other body surfaces. Do not prescribe more than 2 ounces (60 mL) for larger adults. Do not retreat or use as a routine shampoo. Treat sexual contacts concurrently.

Actions

➤*Pharmacology:* An ectoparasiticide and ovicide effective against *Sarcoptes scabiei* (scabies). Parasiticidal action is exerted direct absorbtion into the parasites and their ova.

➤*Pharmacokinetics:* Approximately 10% systemic absorption of a lindane acetone solution was reported when applied to the forearm of human subjects and left in place for 24 hours. A blood level of 290 ng/mL was associated with convulsions following the accidental ingestion of a lindane-containing product. It was found that the greatest peak blood level of 64 ng/mL occurred 6 hours after total body application of lindane in 1 of 8 nonscabietic pediatric patients. The half-life in blood was determined to be approximately 18 hours. Data available suggest that lindane has a rapid distribution phase followed by a longer β-elimination phase.

Contraindications

Premature neonates, because their skin may be more permeable than that of full-term infants and their liver enzymes may not be sufficiently developed; patients with known seizure disorders; hypersensitivity to lindane or any component of the products; crusted (Norwegian) scabies and other skin conditions (eg, atopic dermatitis, psoriasis) that may increase systemic absorption.

Warnings

➤*Absorption:* Simultaneous application of creams, ointments, or oils may enhance absorption.

LINDANE (Gamma Benzene Hexachloride)

➤*Neurotoxicity:* Seizures and deaths have been reported following lindane use with repeat or prolonged application, but also in rare cases following a single application. Infants, children, the elderly, individuals with other skin conditions, and those who weigh less than 110 lbs (50 kg) may be at greater risk of serious neurotoxicity. Give careful consideration before prescribing lindane to patients with conditions that may increase the risk of seizure, such as HIV infection, history of head trauma or a prior seizure, CNS tumor, the presence of severe hepatic cirrhosis, excessive use of alcohol, abrupt withdrawal from alcohol or sedatives, as well as concomitant use of medications known to lower seizure threshold.

➤*Deaths:* Serious outcomes such as hospitalization and disability or death has occurred. In approximately 20% of the total reported cases, lindane was reported to have been used according to the labeled directions. Of these cases, 13 deaths were reported, many cases of which were remote from the time of actual lindane use. Lindane toxicity, verified by autopsy, was the cause of 1 infant's death and was the cause of death reported for an adult who ingested it orally in a successful suicide. The direct causes of death for the other cases were attributed to reasons other than lindane. Most of these adverse events occurred with lindane lotion.

➤*Fertility impairment:* The number of spermatids in the testes of rats 2 weeks after oral administration of a single dose of 30 mg/kg body weight (12 times the estimated human exposure) was significantly reduced compared with the control rats.

➤*Elderly:* There have been no studies of lindane in the elderly. There are 4 postmarketing reports of deaths in elderly patients who were treated for scabies with lindane. Two patients died within 24 hours of lindane application, and the third patient died 41 days after application of lindane, having suffered a seizure on the day of death. A fourth patient died of an unreported cause of death on the same day that lindane treatment for scabies was administered.

➤*Pregnancy: Category C.* Give lindane to pregnant women only if clearly needed. There are no adequate and well-controlled studies in pregnant women. There are no known maternal or fetal health risks if the scabies is not treated. Lindane is lipophilic and may accumulate in the placenta. There has been a single case report of a stillborn infant following multiple maternal exposures to lindane during pregnancy. The relationship of the maternal exposures to the fetal outcome is unknown.

Animal data suggest that lindane exposure of the fetus may increase the likelihood of neurologic developmental abnormalities. The immature central nervous system (as in the fetus) may have increased susceptibility to the effects of the drug.

When rats received lindane in the diet from day 6 of gestation through day 10 of lactation, reduced pup survival, decreased pup weight and decreased weight gains during lactation, increased motor activity, and decreased motor activity habituation were seen in pups at 5.6 mg/kg. An increased number of stillborn pups was seen at 8 mg/kg, and increased pup mortality was seen at 5.6 mg/kg.

➤*Lactation:* Lindane is lipophilic and is present in human breast milk, but exact quantities are not known. There may be a risk of toxicity if lindane is ingested from breast milk, or from skin absorption from mother to baby in the course of breastfeeding when lindane is applied topically to the chest area. Advise nursing mothers who require treatment with lindane of the potential risks. Counsel them to avoid large areas of skin-to-skin contact with the infant while lindane is applied, as well as to interrupt breastfeeding, with expression and discarding of milk, for at least 24 hours following use.

➤*Children:* Animal data demonstrated increased risk of adverse events in the young across species. Pediatric patients have a higher surface to volume ratio and may be at risk of greater systemic exposure when lindane is applied to the body. Infants and children may be at an even higher risk due to immaturity of organ systems such as skin and liver. Use lindane with extreme caution in patients who weigh less than approximately 110 lbs (50 kg) and especially in infants.

Precautions

➤*For external use only:* Avoid contact with eyes; if this occurs, immediately flush eyes with water.

➤*Oils:* Oils may enhance absorption of lindane. Avoid using oil treatment, oil-based hair dressings, or conditioners before and after applying lindane.

Drug Interactions

Use lindane with caution with drugs that lower seizure threshold. These drugs may include the following: Antipsychotics, antidepressants, theophylline, cyclosporine, mycophenolate mofetil, tacrolimus capsules, penicillins, imipenem, quinolone antibiotics, chloroquine sulfate, pyrimethamine, isoniazid, meperidine, radiographic contrast agents, centrally active anticholinesterases, methocarbamol.

Adverse Reactions

Lindane has been reported to cause CNS stimulation ranging from dizziness to seizures. Although seizures were almost always associated with ingestion or misuse of the product (to include repeat treatment), seizures and deaths have been reported when lindane was used according to directions. Irritant dermatitis from contact with this product has also been reported.

➤*Postmarketing experience:* Alopecia, dermatitis, headache, pain, paresthesia, pruritus, and urticaria. The relationship of some of these events to lindane therapy is unknown.

Overdosage

➤*Symptoms:* Overdosage or oral ingestion can cause CNS excitation and, if taken in sufficient quantities, seizures may occur. A blood level of 290 ng/mL was associated with convulsions following the accidental ingestion of a lindane-containing product.

➤*Treatment:* If accidental ingestion occurs, institute prompt gastric emptying. However, because oils favor absorption, give saline cathartics for intestinal evacuation rather than oil laxatives. If CNS manifestations occur, administer pentobarbital, phenobarbital, or diazepam. Refer to General Management of Acute Overdosage.

Patient Information

The skin should be clean and without any other lotion, cream, or oil on it. Oils can make lindane go through the skin faster and possibly increase the risk of neurotoxicity (eg, seizures).

Wait at least 1 hour after bathing or showering before putting lindane on the skin.

Wet or warm skin can make lindane go through skin faster; make sure skin is dry and cool before application.

Put lotion under fingernails after trimming the fingernails short, because scabies are very likely to remain there. A toothbrush can be used to apply the lotion under the fingernails. Immediately after use, wrap the toothbrush in paper and throw away.

Use only a single application, applied as a very thin layer over all skin from the neck down.

Do not use any covering over the applied lindane that does not breathe (eg, diapers with plastic lining, plastic clothes, tight clothes, or blankets).

Wash the lindane completely off after 8 to 12 hours. Never leave lindane on the skin for more than 12 hours. Warm, but not hot water can be used.

Wash all recently worn clothing, underwear, pajamas, used sheets, pillow cases, and towels in very hot water or dry-clean.

The patient may still itch after using lindane, even after all the scabies (insects) are dead.

For external use only (oral ingestion can lead to serious CNS toxicity). Do not apply to face. Avoid eyes; if there is contact, flush well with water for several minutes. Avoid unnecessary skin contact or contact with mucous membranes (eg, nose, mouth). Wear rubber gloves, particularly when applying to more than 1 person.

Notify physician if condition worsens or if itching, redness, swelling, burning, or skin rash occurs.

Avoid use on open cuts and extensive excoriations.

Treat sexual contacts simultaneously.

Lindane does not prevent infestation or reinfestation and should not be used to ward off a possible infestation.

A lindane medication guide must be given to the patient each time lindane is dispensed.

MALATHION

Rx	Ovide (Medicis)	Lotion: 0.5%[1]	In 59 mL.

[1] In a vehicle of 78% isopropyl alcohol, terpineol, dipentene, and pine needle oil.

Indications

Treatment of head lice (*Pediculus humanus capitis*) and their ova of the scalp hair.

Administration and Dosage

Because the potential for transdermal absorption of malathion is not known at this time, strict adherence to the dosing instructions regarding its use in children, method of application, duration of exposure, and frequency of application is required.

Apply lotion on dry hair in an amount just sufficient to thoroughly wet the hair and scalp. Pay particular attention to the back of the head and neck while applying the lotion. Wash hands after applying to scalp. Allow hair to dry naturally; use no heat and leave uncovered. After 8 to 12 hours, wash the hair with a nonmedicated shampoo. Rinse and use a fine-toothed nit comb to remove dead lice and eggs. If required, repeat with second application in 7 to 9 days.

Further treatment is generally not necessary. Evaluate other family members to determine if infested; if so, treat.

➤*Storage/Stability:* Store at controlled room temperature, 20° to 25°C (68° to 77°F).

Actions

➤*Pharmacology:* Malathion is an organophosphate pediculicide lotion for topical application to the hair and scalp. Malathion acts via cholinesterase inhibition and exerts both lousicidal and ovicidal actions in vitro. This activity is selective to insects because malathion is rapidly hydrolyzed and detoxified in mammals.

➤*Pharmacokinetics:* Malathion in an acetone vehicle is absorbed through human skin only to the extent of 8% of the applied dose. However, percutaneous absorption from the *Ovide* lotion formulation has not been studied and the parameters of distribution and excretion after absorption are not known.

Contraindications

Neonates and infants because their scalps are more permeable and may have increased absorption of malathion; sensitivity to malathion or any components of the product.

Warnings

➤*Pregnancy: Category B.* Use during pregnancy only if clearly needed.

➤*Lactation:* It is not known whether malathion is excreted in breast milk. However, because malathion is transdermally absorbed to the extent of 8% of the applied dose, exercise caution when using on a nursing mother.

➤*Children:* Safety and efficacy in children younger than 6 years of age have not been established. Strict adherence to the dosing instructions regarding its use in children, method of application, duration of exposure, and frequency of application is required.

Precautions

➤*Contains flammable alcohol:* The lotion and wet hair should not be exposed to open flame or electric heat, including hair dryers and electric curlers. Do not smoke while applying lotion or while hair is wet. Allow hair to dry naturally and uncovered after application.

➤*For external use only:* Avoid contact with the eyes; if accidentally placed in the eye, flush immediately with water.

➤*Carbamate or organophosphate-type insecticides/pesticides:* Inadvertent transdermal absorption of malathion has occurred from its agricultural use. In such cases, acute toxicity was manifested by excessive cholinergic activity (ie, increased sweating, salivary and gastric secretion, GI and uterine motility, and bradycardia).

Adverse Reactions

Irritation of the skin and scalp has occurred. Accidental contact with the eyes can result in mild conjunctivitis. It is not known if malathion has the potential to cause contact allergic sensitization.

Overdosage

➤*Symptoms:* Malathion, although a weaker cholinesterase inhibitor than some other organophosphates, may be expected to exhibit the same symptoms of cholinesterase depletion after accidental ingestion orally. If accidentally swallowed, vomiting should be induced promptly or the stomach lavaged with 5% sodium bicarbonate solution. Severe respiratory distress is the major and most serious symptom of organophosphate poisoning requiring artificial respiration, and atropine may be needed to counteract the symptoms of cholinesterase depletion. Repeat analyses of serum and RBC cholinesterase may assist in establishing the diagnosis and formulating a long-range prognosis.

Inadvertent transdermal absorption of malathion has occurred from its agricultural use. In such cases, acute toxicity was manifested by excessive cholinergic activity (ie, increased sweating, salivary and gastric secretion, GI and uterine motility, and bradycardia).

Patient Information

For external use only (serious toxicity may occur if ingested). Avoid contact with the eyes.

Contact your physician before using malathion if you are pregnant or nursing.

If skin irritation occurs, wash scalp and hair immediately. If the irritation clears, malathion may be reapplied. If irritation recurs, consult a physician.

Slight stinging sensations may be produced when using malathion.

Allow hair to dry naturally and to remain uncovered. Shampoo hair after 8 to 12 hours, again paying attention to the back of the head and neck while shampooing.

Rinse hair and use a fine-toothed (nit) comb to remove dead lice and eggs.

If lice are still present after 7 to 9 days, repeat with a second application of malathion.

Further treatment is generally not necessary. A physician should evaluate other family members to determine if infested.

See patient instructions available with the product.

PERMETHRIN

Rx	Permethrin (Various, eg, Clay-Park)	Cream: 5%	In 60 g tubes.
Rx	Elimite (Allergen)		Lanolin alcohols, coconut oil, mineral oil. In 60 g tubes.
Rx	Acticin (Bertek)		Coconut oil, lanolin alcohols, light mineral oil. In 60 g tubes.
otc	Permethrin (Various, eg, Alpharma)	Lotion: 1%	In 60 mL with comb.
otc	Nix Creme Rinse (Pfizer)	Liquid (cream rinse): 1%	20% isopropyl alcohol, cetyl alcohol, parabens. In 60 mL with comb.

Indications

➤*Cream:* For the treatment of scabies (*Sarcoptes scabiei*) infestation.

➤*Lotion/Cream rinse:* For the treatment of head lice (*Pediculus humanus capitis*) and its nits (eggs).

➤*Liquid:* For the treatment of infestation with *Pediculus humanus var. capitis* (the head louse) and its nits (eggs). Treatment for recurrences is required in less than 1% of patients since the ovicidal activity may be supplemented by residual persistence in the hair. If live lice are observed 7 or more days following the initial application, give a second application.

➤*Unlabeled uses:* Permethrin appears to be effective for the topical treatment of papulopustular rosacea.

Administration and Dosage

➤*Scabies (cream):* Thoroughly massage cream into the skin from the head to the soles of the feet. Scabies rarely infest the scalp of adults, although the hairline, neck, temple, and forehead may be infested in infants and geriatric patients. Remove the cream by washing (shower or bath) after 8 to 14 hours. Treat infants on the scalp, temple, and forehead. One application is generally curative. Usually 30 g is sufficient for an average adult.

Patients often experience pruritus after treatment. This is rarely a sign of treatment failure and is not an indication for retreatment. Demonstrable living mites after 14 days indicate that retreatment is necessary.

➤*Head lice (lotion/cream rinse):* Apply to hair after washing with shampoo; rinse with water and towel dry. Apply a sufficient amount to saturate hair and scalp (especially behind the ears and nape of neck). Leave on hair for no longer than 10 minutes, then rinse with water. A single application is generally sufficient; however, if lice are observed within 7 days after application, apply a second treatment. Remove any remaining nits with the nit comb provided.

➤*Storage/Stability:* Store at 15° to 25°C (59° to 77°F).

Actions

➤*Pharmacology:* Permethrin is a pyrethroid active against lice, ticks, mites, and fleas. It acts on the parasites' nerve cell membranes to dis-

PERMETHRIN

rupt the sodium channel current, resulting in delayed repolarization and paralysis of the pests.

➤*Pharmacokinetics:* Permethrin is rapidly metabolized by ester hydrolysis to inactive metabolites that are excreted primarily in the urine. Although the amount of permethrin absorbed after a single application of the 5% cream has not been determined precisely, preliminary data suggest it is 2% or less of the amount applied. Residual persistence is detectable on the hair for at least 10 days following a single application.

Contraindications

Hypersensitivity to any synthetic pyrethroid or pyrethrin, or to any component of the product. If hypersensitivity develops, discontinue use.

Warnings

➤*Carcinogenesis:* Species-specific increases in pulmonary adenomas, a common benign tumor of mice, were seen in the mouse studies. In 1 study, incidence of pulmonary alveolar-cell carcinomas and benign liver adenomas increased only in female mice when permethrin was given in their food at a concentration of 5000 ppm.

➤*Pregnancy: Category B.* There are no adequate and well-controlled studies in pregnant women. Use during pregnancy only if clearly needed.

➤*Lactation:* It is not known whether this drug is excreted in breast milk. Because of the evidence for tumorigenic potential of permethrin in animal studies, consider discontinuing nursing temporarily or withholding the drug while the mother is nursing.

➤*Children:* Safety and efficacy for use in children younger than 2 months of age have not been established.

Precautions

➤*For external use only:* Do not use near eyes, mucous membranes (ie, nose, mouth, vagina), or ingest orally. If infestation of eyelashes or eyebrows occurs, consult physician.

➤*Asthmatics:* Permethrin may cause breathing difficulties or exacerbate asthmatic episodes.

➤*Pruritus, erythema, and edema:* These often accompany scabies and head lice infestation. Treatment with permethrin may temporarily exacerbate these conditions.

Adverse Reactions

The most frequent adverse reaction is pruritus. Usually a consequence of scabies or head lice infestation itself, it may be temporarily aggravated following treatment.

➤*Cream:* Mild transient burning/stinging (10%); itching (7%); tingling, numbness, erythema, or rash (2% or less).

Postmarketing reactions – Headache, fever, dizziness, abdominal pain, diarrhea, nausea, vomiting (5%); seizure (rare).

➤*Lotion / Cream rinse:* Itching, redness, swelling of scalp.

Overdosage

If ingested, perform gastric lavage and employ general supportive measures. Excessive topical use may result in increased irritation and erythema.

Patient Information

For external use only. Avoid contact with the mucous membranes (eg, nose, mouth, vagina). May be irritating to the eyes. Avoid contact with the eyes; flush with water immediately if eye contact with the drug occurs.

Itching, redness, or swelling of the scalp may occur; notify physician if irritation persists.

Patient instructions and information are available with the product. Do not exceed the prescribed dosage.

Inform patients that they may still experience pruritus after treatment. This is rarely a sign of treatment failure or an indication for retreatment.

Inform patients on the importance of washing in hot water all personal articles susceptible to infestation (eg, sheets, pillows, clothing, combs, brushes). It is recommended to thoroughly vacuum rooms.

MISCELLANEOUS PEDICULICIDES

otc	**Tisit**[1] (Pfeiffer)	**Lotion:** 0.3% pyrethrins, 2% piperonyl butoxide	In 59 and 118 mL.
otc	**Tisit** (Pfeiffer)	**Gel:** 0.3% pyrethrins, 3% piperonyl butoxide	In 30 mL.
otc	**A-200** (Hogil)	**Shampoo:** 0.33% pyrethrins, 4% piperonyl butoxide	In 59 and 118 mL with comb, and in 118 mL kits containing comb and lice control spray.
otc	**Pronto** (Del)		Benzyl alcohol, decyl alcohol, isopropyl alcohol. In 60 and 120 mL with comb.
otc	**Pyrinyl Plus** (Rugby)		Benzyl alcohol. In 59 mL.
otc	**RID** (Bayer)		SD alcohol. In 60, 120, and 240 mL, and 120 mL kits containing gel, comb, and lice control spray.
otc	**Tisit** (Pfeiffer)		In 59 and 118 mL with comb.
otc	**Lice Treatment** (Goldline)		Benzyl alcohol. In 59 and 118 mL with comb.
otc	**RID** (Bayer)	**Mousse:** 0.33% pyrethrins, 4% piperonyl butoxide	Cetearyl alcohol, SD alcohol, isobutane. In 165 mL with comb.

[1] Contains petroleum distillate and piperonyl butoxide equivalent to 1.6% ether.

Indications

Treatment of infestations of head lice, body lice, and pubic (crab) lice and their eggs.

Administration and Dosage

Administration and dosage varies. Refer to individual package inserts for information.

Contraindications

Hypersensitivity to ingredients; ragweed sensitized persons (pyrethrins and permethrins).

Precautions

➤*For external use only:* Harmful if swallowed or inhaled. May be irritating to the eyes and mucous membranes (eg, nose, mouth, vagina). In case of contact with eyes, flush with water. Discontinue use and notify physician if irritation or infection occurs.

➤*Infestation of eyelashes or eyebrows:* Do not use in these areas; consult physician.

➤*Reinfestation:* To prevent reinfestation, sterilize or treat all brushes/combs, towels, clothing, and bedding concurrently. It is recommended that all rooms inhabited by infected patients be thoroughly vacuumed. A second treatment may need to be repeated in 7 to 10 days to kill any newly hatched lice.

➤*Pubic lice:* May be transmitted by sexual contact. Treat sexual partners simultaneously.

BECAPLERMIN

| *Rx* | **Regranex** (Johnson & Johnson Wound Management) | **Gel:** 100 mcg | Parabens. In 2, 7.5 and 15 g multi-use tubes. |

Indications

>*Diabetic neuropathic ulcers:* Treatment of lower-extremity diabetic neuropathic ulcers that extend into the subcutaneous tissue or beyond and have an adequate blood supply. To be used as an adjunct to, and not a substitute for, good ulcer care practices including initial sharp debridement, pressure relief and infection control.

Administration and Dosage

>*Approved by the FDA:* December 16, 1997.

The amount of becaplermin gel to be applied will vary depending on the size of the ulcer area. To calculate the length of gel to apply to the ulcer, measure the greatest length of the ulcer by the greatest width of the ulcer in either inches or centimeters. To calculate the length of gel, refer to the following table:

Formula to Calculate Daily Application Length of Becaplermin		
Unit of measure	Tube size (g)	Formula
Inches	15 or 7.5	length × width × 0.6
	2	length × width × 1.3
Centimeters	15 or 7.5	length × width ÷ 4
	2	length × width ÷ 2

>*Inches:* Each square inch of ulcer surface will require ≈ ⅔ inch length of gel squeezed from a 7.5 or 15 g tube or ≈ 1⅓ inch length of the gel from a 2 g tube. For example, if the ulcer measures 1 inch by 2 inches, then use a 1¼ inch length of gel for a 7.5 or 15 g tube (1 × 2 × 0.6 = 1¼) and 2¾ inch gel length for a 2 g tube (1 × 2 × 1.3 = 2¾).

>*Centimeters:* Each square centimeter of ulcer surface will require ≈ 0.25 cm length of gel squeezed from a 7.5 or 15 g tube or ≈ 0.5 cm length of gel from a 2 g tube. For example, if the ulcer measures 4 cm by 2 cm, then use a 2 cm length of gel for a 7.5 or 15 g tube [(4 × 2) ÷ 4 = 2] and a 4 cm length of gel for a 2 g tube [(4 × 2) ÷ 2 = 4].

>*Application procedure:* Apply once daily to the ulcer(s) until complete healing has occurred. Recalculate the amount of gel to be applied at weekly or biweekly intervals depending on the rate of change in ulcer area. Reassess continued treatment if the ulcer does not decrease in size by ≈ 30% after 10 weeks or has not completely healed by 20 weeks. Excess application has not been shown to be beneficial.

Squeeze the calculated length of gel on to a clean measuring surface (eg, wax paper) and transfer to the ulcer using an application aid (eg, clean cotton swab, tongue depressor). Spread gel over the entire ulcer area to yield a thin continuous layer ≈ ¹⁄₁₆ of an inch thickness. Cover the site(s) of application with a saline-moistened dressing and leave in place for ≈ 12 hours. Remove the dressing and rinse ulcer with saline or water to remove residual gel and cover again with a second moist dressing (without gel) for the remainder of the day.

>*Storage / Stability:* Store in the refrigerator. Do not freeze.

Actions

>*Pharmacology:* Becaplermin is a recombinant human platelet-derived growth factor (rhPDGF-BB) for topical administration. Becaplermin is produced by recombinant DNA technology by insertion of the gene for the B chain of platelet-derived growth factor (PDGF) into the yeast, *Saccharomyces cerevisiae*. Becaplermin has biological activity similar to that of endogenous platelet-derived growth factor, which includes promoting the chemotactic recruitment and proliferation of cells involved in wound repair and enhancing the formation of granulation tissue.

>*Pharmacokinetics:* Ten patients with Stage III or IV lower-extremity diabetic ulcers received topical applications of becaplermin gel 0.01% at the dose range of 0.32 to 2.95 mcg/kg (7 mcg/cm²) daily for 14 days. Six patients had non-quantifiable PDGF levels at baseline, and throughout the study, two patients had PDGF levels at baseline that did not increase substantially, and two patients had PDGF levels that increased sporadically above their baseline values during the 14-day study period.

Systemic bioavailability of becaplermin was < 3% in rats with full thickness wounds receiving single or multiple (5 days) topical application of 127 mcg/kg (20.1 mcg/cm² of wound area) of becaplermin.

>*Clinical trials:* The effects of becaplermin on the incidence of and time to complete healing in lower-extremity diabetic ulcers were assessed in four randomized controlled studies. In the four trials, 95% of the ulcers measured in area ≤ 10 cm² and the median ulcer size at baseline ranged from 1.4 to 3.5 cm². Becaplermin gel 0.003% or 0.01% or placebo gel was applied once a day and covered with a saline moist-

ened dressing. Patients were treated until complete healing or for a period of up to 20 weeks and were considered a treatment failure if their ulcer did not show an ≈ 30% reduction in inital ulcer area after 8 to 10 weeks of therapy.

In study 1 (n = 118), the incidence of complete ulcer closure for becaplermin 0.003% (n = 61) was 48% vs 25% for placebo.

In study 2 (n = 382), the incidence of complete ulcer closure for becaplermin 0.01% (n = 123) was 50% vs 36% for becaplermin 0.003% (n = 132) and 35% for placebo (n = 127). Only becaplermin 0.01% was significantly different from placebo.

The primary goal of study 3 (n = 172) was to assess the safety of vehicle gel (placebo; n = 70) compared with good ulcer care alone (n = 68). The study included a small (n = 34) becaplermin 0.01% arm. Incidences of complete ulcer closure were 44% for becaplermin, 36% for placebo and 22% for good ulcer care alone.

In study 4 (n = 250), the incidences of complete ulcer closure in the becaplermin 0.01% arm (n = 128; 36%) and good ulcer care alone (n = 122; 32%) were not statistically different.

In a 3-month follow-up period where no standardized regimen of preventative care was used, the incidence of ulcer recurrence was ≈ 30% in all treatment groups, demonstrating that the durability of ulcer closure was comparable.

Contraindications

Hypersensitivity to any component of this product (eg, parabens); neoplasm(s) at the site of application.

Warnings

>*Other wounds:* Becaplermin is a non-sterile, low-bioburden, preserved product; do not use in wounds that close by primary intention.

The efficacy of becaplermin for the treatment of diabetic neuropathic ulcers that do not extend through the dermis into subcutaneous tissue (Stage I or II, IAET staging classification) or ischemic diabetic ulcers has not been evaluated.

>*Pregnancy: Category C.* It is not known whether becaplermin can cause fetal harm when administered to a pregnant woman or can affect reproductive capacity. Give to pregnant women only if clearly needed.

>*Lactation:* It is not known whether becaplermin is excreted in breast milk. Exercise caution when becaplermin is administered to nursing women.

>*Children:* Safety and efficacy in children < 16 years of age have not been established.

Precautions

>*For external use only:*

>*Application site reaction:* If application site reactions occur, consider the possibility of sensitization or irritation caused by parabens or m-cresol.

>*Exposed areas:* The effects of becaplermin on exposed joints, tendons, ligaments and bone have not been established. In preclinical studies, rats injected at the metatarsals with 3 or 10 mcg/site (≈ 60 or 200 mcg/kg) of becaplermin every other day for 13 days displayed histological changes indicative of accelerated bone remodeling consisting of periosteal hyperplasia and subperiosteal bone resorption and exostosis. The soft tissue adjacent to the injection site had fibroplasia with accompanying mononuclear cell infiltration reflective of the ability of PDGF to stimulate connective tissue growth.

Adverse Reactions

Patients receiving becaplermin, placebo and good ulcer care alone had a similar incidence of ulcer-related adverse events such as infection, cellulitis or osteomyelitis. However, erythematous rashes occurred in 2% of patients treated with becaplermin and placebo, and none in patients receiving good ulcer care alone.

Patient Information

Advise patients to wash hands thoroughly before applying becaplermin.

Do not allow the tip of the tube to come into contact with the ulcer or any other surface; recap the tube tightly after each use.

Apply only once a day in a carefully measured quantity (see Administration and Dosage). Spread the measured quantity of gel evenly over the ulcerated area to yield a thin continuous layer of ≈ ¹⁄₁₆ of an inch thickness. Adjust the measured length of the gel to be squeezed from the tube according to the size of the ulcer. Use a cotton swab, tongue depressor or other application aid to apply becaplermin.

CHLOROPHYLL DERIVATIVES

| *otc* | **Chloresium**
(Rystan) | **Ointment:** 0.5% chlorophyllin copper complex in a hydrophilic base | In 30 and 120 g and lb. |
| | | **Solution:** 0.2% chlorophyllin copper complex in isotonic saline | In 240 and 960 ml. |

Indications

Arteriosclerotic, diabetic and varicose ulcers; trophic decubitus ulcers and chronic ulcers of nonspecific origin; malignant lesions (where deodorization is desired); traumatic injuries; skin grafting and skin defects; thermal, chemical and irradiation injuries; a wide variety of dermatoses.

Administration and Dosage

➤*Ointment:* Apply generously and cover with gauze, linen or other appropriate dressing. For best results, do not change dressings more often than every 48 to 72 hours.

➤*Solution:* Apply full strength as continuous wet dressing, or instill directly into sinus tracts, fistulae, deep ulcers or cavities.

Actions

➤*Pharmacology:* Aids wound healing by helping to produce a clean, granulating wound base for epithelialization or skin grafting. It also soothes inflamed, painful tissues and controls wound odor, even in malignant lesions. This is a true deodorizing, not a masking, action.

Adverse Reactions

Sensitivity reactions (rare); itching; irritation.

DEXTRANOMER

| *otc* | **Debrisan**
(Johnson & Johnson) | **Beads** | In 25, 60 and 120 g containers and 4 g packets (in 7s and 14s). |
| | | **Paste** | Premixed, sterile. In 10 g packets (6s). |

Indications

For use in cleaning wet ulcers and wounds such as venous stasis ulcers, decubitus ulcers, infected traumatic and surgical wounds and infected burns.

Administration and Dosage

➤*Application:* Debride and clean the wound (dextranomer is not an enzyme and will not debride). Leave cleansed area moist. Apply to at least a thickness of ¼ inch to achieve desired suction effects. Cover area with a dry dressing and close on all sides.

➤*Removal:* When saturated, dextranomer changes colors and should be removed. Removal should be as complete as possible and is best achieved by irrigation. Vigorous irrigation (ie, soaking or whirlpool) may be necessary to remove patches that adhere to the wound surface.

➤*Paste:* May be needed for hard to reach areas or irregular body surfaces.

Mix beads with glycerin either on the dry dressing or in a receptacle or use premixed paste. Do not mix with any substance but glycerin. (See package insert for complete procedure.) Dress wound in the usual manner. Mix a fresh paste for each application. Do not reuse.

➤*Reapply:* Dextranomer beads or paste should be reapplied every 12 hours or more frequently if necessary. Reduce number of applications as exudate diminishes. Discontinue applications when the area is free of exudate and edema, or when a healthy granulation base is present. Consult physician if condition worsens or persists beyond 14 to 21 days.

Actions

➤*Pharmacology:* Dextranomer's ability to remove exudates rapidly and continuously from the surface of the wound results in a reduction of inflammation and edema. In vitro evidence suggests that the suction forces created by the drug may remove bacteria and inflammatory exudates from the surface of the wound.

Dextranomer is a hydrophilic dextran polymer in the form of tiny beads or paste. The hydrophilic beads absorb approximately 4 ml of fluid per 1 g of beads. The beads swell to approximately 4 times their original size. This swelling causes significant suction forces and capillary action in the spaces between the beads. This action continues as long as unsaturated beads or paste are in proximity to the wound.

When applied to the surface of wet ulcers or wounds, dextranomer removes various exudates and particles that impede tissue repair. Low molecular weight components of wound exudates are drawn up within the beads or paste, while higher molecular weight components (plasma proteins and fibrinogen) are found between the swollen beads. Removal of these latter components (particularly fibrin and fibrinogen) retards eschar formation.

Precautions

➤*For external use only:* Avoid contact with the eyes.

➤*Wound packing:* When treating cratered decubitus ulcers, do not pack wound tightly. Allow for expansion of beads. Maceration of surrounding skin may result if occlusive dressings are used.

➤*Removal of dextranomer:* Do not use dextranomer in deep fistulas, sinus tracts or any body cavity where complete removal is not assured.

Remove the beads or paste once they are saturated. This avoids encrustation which makes removal more difficult. All dextranomer must be removed before any surgical procedures to close the wound (ie, graft or flap).

➤*Edema reduction:* Wounds may appear larger during the first few days of treatment due to reduction of edema.

➤*Dry wounds:* Not effective in cleansing dry wounds.

➤*Complete healing:* Not all wounds require treatment with dextranomer to complete healing. When the wound is no longer wet and a healthy granulation base is established, discontinue dextranomer.

➤*Treatment of the underlying condition:* This (eg, venous or arterial flow, pressure) should proceed concurrently with the use of dextranomer.

Adverse Reactions

Upon application or removal of beads, transitory pain, bleeding, blistering and erythema have occurred. Severe infections have been associated with administration in both diabetic and immunosuppressed patients.

Patient Information

For external use only. Avoid contact with the eyes.

DEXPANTHENOL

otc	**Panthoderm** (Jones Medical)	**Cream:** 2% in a water miscible base	In 30 and 60 g.

Indications

Relieves itching and aids healing of skin in mild eczemas and dermatoses; itching skin, minor wounds, stings, bites, poison ivy, poison oak (dry stage) and minor skin irritations. Also used in infants and children for diaper rash, chafing and mild skin irritations.

Administration and Dosage

For external use only. Avoid contact with the eyes.

Apply to affected areas once or twice daily.

UREA (Carbamide)

otc	**Aquacare** (Menley & James)	**Cream:** 10%	Petrolatum, glycerin, lanolin oil, mineral oil, lanolin alcohol, benzyl alcohol. In 75 g.
otc	**Carmol 20** (Doak)	**Cream:** 20%	Nonlipid vanishing cream base. In 90 g and lb.
otc	**Gormel Creme** (Gordon)		Mineral oil, parabens. In 75, 120 g, lb.
otc	**Lanaphilic** (Medco)		Petrolatum, lanolin oil, PPG, lactic acid, parabens. In lb.
otc	**Ureacin-20** (Pedinol)		Lactic acid, glycerin, mineral oil, parabens, EDTA. In 75 g.
Rx	**Urea** (Hi-Tech)	**Cream:** 40%	Mineral oil, petrolatum, cetyl alcohol. In 28.35 and 198.6 g.
Rx	**Carmol 40** (Doak)		Mineral oil, petrolatum, cetyl alcohol. In 28.35 and 85 g.
Rx	**Gordon's Urea 40%** (Gordon)		Petrolatum base. In 30 g.
Rx	**Vanamide** (Dermik)		Light mineral oil, cetyl alcohol, petrolatum. In 85 and 199 g.
Rx	**Keralac** (Doak)	**Cream:** 50%	Cetyl alcohol, EDTA, lactic acid. In 142 and 255 g.
otc	**Aquacare** (Menley & James)	**Lotion:** 10%	Mineral oil, petrolatum, parabens. In 240 ml.
otc	**Carmol 10** (Doak)		In 180 ml.
otc	**Ureacin-10** (Pedinol)		EDTA, parabens, lactic acid. In 240 ml.
otc	**Ultra Mide 25** (Baker Cummins)	**Lotion:** 25%	Mineral oil, glycerin, lanolin, EDTA. In 240 ml.
Rx	**Keralac** (Doak)	**Lotion:** 35%	Cetyl alcohol, EDTA, lactic acid. In 207 and 325 ml.
Rx	**Urea** (Hi-Tech)	**Lotion:** 40%	Mineral oil, petrolatum, cetyl alcohol. In 236.6 mL.
Rx	**Carmol 40** (Doak)	**Gel:** 40%	Glycerin, EDTA. In 15 mL.
Rx	**Keralac** (Doak)	**Gel:** 50%	EDTA, lactic acid. In 18 mL.
Rx	**Umecta** (Harmony)	**Emulsion:** 40%	Helianthus annuus oil, EDTA. In 240 mL.

Indications

Promote hydration, remove excess keratin in dry skin and hyperkeratotic conditions.

➤*40% urea:* Treatment of nail destruction and dissolution. It removes dystrophic and potentially disabling nails without local anesthesia and surgery.

Administration and Dosage

For external use only. Avoid contact with the eyes.

Apply 2 to 4 times daily to affected area or as directed. Rub in completely.

➤*40% urea:* Cover surrounding surfaces. Generously apply directly to the diseased nail surface and cover with plastic film, wrap and anchor with adhesive tape. Cover with a "finger" cut from plastic or vinyl glove and anchor with more tape. Keep completely dry. Remove treated nails in either 3, 7 or 14 days. Nail bed usually hardens in 12 to 36 hours when left open to the air.

VITAMIN E, TOPICAL

otc	**Vitamin E** (Various, eg, Nature's Bounty)	**Cream**	In 60 g.
otc	**Vitec** (Pharmaceutical Specialities)	**Cream:** dl-alpha tocopheryl acetate in a vanishing cream base, cetearyl alcohol, sorbitol, propylene glycol, simethicone, glyceryl monostearate, PEG monostearate	In 120 g.
otc	**Vite E Creme** (Gordon)	**Cream:** 50 mg dl-alpha tocopheryl acetate per g	In lb.
otc	**Vitamin E** (Various, eg, Nature's Bounty)	**Lotion**	In 120 ml.
otc	**Coppertone Aloe Aftersun Lotion** (Schering-Plough)	**Lotion:** Vitamin E, aloe, glyceryl, lanolin, paraben, EDTA, jojoba oil, cocoa butter, mineral oil	In 473 ml.
otc	**Vitamin E** (Various, eg, Mission, Nature's Bounty)	**Oil**	In 30 and 60 ml.[1]

[1] May or may not contain aloe.

Indications

Temporary relief of minor skin disorders such as diaper rash, burns, sunburn and chapped or dry skin.

Administration and Dosage

For external use only. Avoid contact with the eyes.

Apply a thin layer over affected area.

VITAMINS A, D and E, TOPICAL

otc	**Vitamin A & D** (Various, eg, Goldline, Rugby)	**Ointment**	In 60 g and lb.
otc	**A and D** (Schering-Plough)	**Ointment:** Fish liver oil, cholecalciferol, lanolin, petrolatum, mineral oil	In 45, 120, 480 g, 75 g pump dispenser.
otc	**Caldesene** (Fisons)	**Ointment:** Cod liver oil (vitamins A and D), 15% zinc oxide, lanolin oil, 54% petrolatum, parabens, talc	In 37.5 g.
otc	**Comfortine** (Dermik)	**Ointment:** Vitamins A and D, lanolin, zinc oxide, chloroxylenol, iron oxides, lanolin alcohol, mineral oil, triethanolamine, vegetable oil	In 45 and 120 g.
otc	**Desitin** (Pfizer)	**Ointment:** Cod liver oil (vit A & D), 40% zinc oxide, talc, petrolatum-lanolin base	In 30, 60, 120, 240, 270 g.
otc	**Lobana Peri-Garde** (Ulmer)	**Ointment:** Vitamins A, D and E and chloroxylenol in an emollient base	In 240 g.
otc	**Clocream** (Roberts)	**Cream:** Cod liver oil (vitamins A and D), cholecalciferol, vitamin A palmitate, cottonseed oil, glycerin, parabens, mineral oil	Vanishing base. In 30 g.
otc	**Lazer Creme** (Pedinol)	**Cream:** Vitamins A (3333.3 units/g) and E (116.67 units/g)	In 60 g.
otc	**Lobana Derm-Ade** (Ulmer)	**Cream:** Vitamins A, D and E, moisturizers, emollients, silicone	Vanishing base. In 270 g.
otc	**Retinol** (Nature's Bounty)	**Cream:** 100,000 IU vitamin A, glycol stearate, mineral oil, propylene glycol, lanolin oil, propylene glycol stearate SE, lanolin alcohol, retinol, parabens, EDTA	In 60 g.

VITAMINS A, D and E, TOPICAL

otc	**Retinol-A** (Young Again Products)	**Cream:** 300,000 IU vitamin A palmitate per 30 g.	In 60 g.
otc	**Aloe Grande** (Gordon)	**Lotion:** Vitamins A (3333.3 units/g) and E (50 units/g), petrolatum, mineral oil, sodium lauryl sulfate, oleic acid, parabens, triethanolamine, aloe	In 240 ml.
otc	**Coppertone Cool Beads** (Schering-Plough)	**Lotion:** Vitamins A and E, aloe vera, glycol, EDTA, lactose	In 340 g.

Indications

For temporary relief of discomfort due to minor burns, sunburn, windburn, abrasions, chapped or chafed skin and other minor non-infected skin irritations including diaper rash and irritations associated with ileostomy and colostomy skin drainage.

Warnings

➤*For external use only:* Avoid contact with the eyes.

➤*Worsened condition:* If the condition for which these preparations is used worsens or does not improve within 7 days, consult a physician.

Administration and Dosage

Apply locally to affected skin with gentle massage.

EMOLLIENTS, MISCELLANEOUS

otc	**Balmex** (Block)	**Ointment:** 11.3% zinc oxide, aloe vera gel, parabens, mineral oil	In 30, 60, 120 and 454 g.
otc	**Allercreme Ultra Emollient** (Carme)	**Cream:** Mineral oil, petrolatum, lanolin, lanolin alcohol, lanolin oil, glycerin, glyceryl stearate, PEG-100 stearate, squalane, parabens	Unscented. In 60 g.
otc	**AmLactin** (Upsher-Smith)	**Cream:** 12% ammonium lactate	In 140, 225 and 400g.
Rx	**LAC-Lotion** (Paddock)	**Cream:** 12% ammonium lactate (12% lactic acid neutralized with ammonium hydroxide), light mineral oil, cetyl alcohol, parabens, glycerin	In 225 and 400 g.
otc	**AquaBalm** (Quintessa[1])	**Cream:** Petrolatum, methyl glucate dioleate, propylene glycol, DMDM hydantoin, iodopropynyl butylcarbamate	Fragrance-free. In 114 g.
otc	**Aveeno Moisturizing** (Rydelle)	**Cream:** 1% colloidal oatmeal, glycerin, petrolatum, dimethicone, phenylcarbinol	In 120 g.
otc	**Catrix Correction** (Donell DerMedex)	**Cream:** Dipentaerythrityl, hexacaprylate/hexacaprate, sesame oil, *Catrix* (bovine derived complex mucopolysaccharide), ceteareth-20, glycerin, caprylic/capric triglyceride, glycereth-7, dimethicone, xanthan gum, tocopheryl linoleate, alanine, glycine, urea, EDTA, imidazolidinyl urea, parabens, phenoxyethanol, orange oil, cardamon oil, titanium dioxide	In 36.9 g.
otc	**Complex 15 Face** (Schering-Plough)	**Cream:** Caprylic/capric triglyceride, squalane, glycerin, glyceryl stearate, lecithin, PEG-50 stearate, propylene glycol, dimethicone, diazolidinyl urea, carbomer-934P, EDTA	In 75 g.
otc	**Complex 15 Hand & Body** (Schering-Plough)	**Cream:** Mineral oil, glycerin, squalane, caprylic/capric triglyceride, glycol stearate, PEG-50, carboxylic acid sterol ester, glyceryl stearate, lecithin, dimethicone, diazolidinyl urea, carbomer-934, EDTA	In 120 g.
otc	**Curel Moisturizing** (Bausch & Lomb)	**Cream:** Glycerin, petrolatum, dimethicone, parabens	In 90 g.
otc	**Cutemol** (Summers)	**Cream:** Allantoin, mineral oil, acetylated lanolin, lanolin alcohols extract, mineral wax, beeswax, sorbitan sesquioleate, parabens	In 60 and 240 g.
otc	**DML Forte** (Person & Covey)	**Cream:** Petrolatum, PPG-2 myristyl ether propionate, glyceryl stearate, glycerin, simethicone, benzyl alcohol, silica, EDTA, sodium carbomer 1342	In 113 g.
otc	**Hydrisinol** (Pedinol)	**Cream:** Sulfonated hydrogenated castor oil, hydrogenated vegetable oil	In 120 g and lb.
otc	**Keri Creme** (Westwood Squibb)	**Cream:** Mineral oil, lanolin alcohol, talc, sorbitol, ceresin, propylene glycol, magnesium stearate, glyceryl oleate, parabens	In 75 g.
otc	**Kinerase** (ICN Pharm.)	**Cream:** 0.1% N[6]-furfuryladenine, stearic acid, cetyl alcohol, safflower oil, stearyl alcohol, aloe vera, parabens	In 40 and 80 g tubes.
otc	**Kinerase Intensive Eye Cream** (ICN Pharm)	**Cream:** 0.125% kinetin, safflower seed oil, cetyl alcohol, urea, parabens	In 20 g.
otc	**Lanolor** (Westwood Squibb)	**Cream:** Lanolin oil, glyceryl stearates, propylene glycol, sodium lauryl sulfate, simethicone, polyoxyl 40 stearate, cetyl esters wax, methylparaben	In 60 and 240 g.
otc	**Lubriderm** (Warner-Lambert)	**Cream:** Mineral oil, petrolatum, lanolin, lanolin alcohol, lanolin oil, glycerin, glyceryl stearate, PEG-100 stearate, sorbitan laurate, parabens	Scented and unscented. In 81 g.
otc	**Neutrogena Norwegian Formula Hand** (Neutrogena)	**Cream:** Glycerin, sodium cetearyl sulfate, sodium sulfate, parabens	Scented and unscented. In 56.7 g.
Rx	**Lactinol-E Creme** (Pedinol)	**Cream:** 10% lactic acid, 3500 IU/30 g vitamin E	In 56.7
otc	**Lactrex 12%** (SDR Pharmaceuticals[2])	**Cream:** 12% lactic acid, petrolatum, EDTA	In 184 g.
otc	**Lady Esther** (Menley & James)	**Cream:** Mineral oil	In 120 g
otc	**Nouriva Repair** (Ferndale)	**Cream:** Petrolatum, parafin, mineral oil, sorbitan oleate, carnauba wax, ceramide 3, cholesterol, glycerin, oleic acid, palmitic acid, acrylates/C 10-30 albyl acrylate crosspolymer, tromethamine	In 30 g.
otc	**Nutraderm** (Owen/Galderma)	**Cream:** Mineral oil, sorbitan stearate, stearyl alcohol, sorbitol, citric acid, cetyl esters wax, sodium lauryl sulfate, dimethicone, parabens, diazolidinyl urea	In 90, 240 and 480 g.
otc	**Pacquin Medicated** (Pfizer)	**Cream:** Dimethicone, glycerin, cetyl alcohol, parabens	In 227 g.
otc	**Pacquin Dry Skin** (Pfizer)	**Cream:** Glycerin, cetyl alcohol, parabens	In 227 g.
otc	**Pacquin Plus** (Pfizer)	**Cream:** Glycerin, lanolin, cetyl alcohol, parabens	In 227 g.
otc	**Pacquin Plus with Aloe** (Pfizer)	**Cream:** Aloe vera gel, mineral oil, petrolatum, synthetic beeswax, cetyl alcohol, lanolin, dimethicone, stearic acid, methylparaben	In 227 g.
otc	**Pacquin Skin Cream with Aloe** (Pfizer)	**Cream:** Aloe vera gel, mineral oil, petrolatum, synthetic beeswax, cetyl alcohol, methylparaben	In 227 g.
otc	**Penecare** (Reed & Carnrick)	**Cream:** Lactic acid, mineral oil, imidurea	In 120 g.
otc	**Pedi-Vit-A Creme** (Pedinol)	**Cream:** 100,000 units vitamin A/30 g	In 60 g.
otc	**Pen·Kera** (B.F. Ascher)	**Cream:** Glycerin, mineral oil, sorbitan stearate, urea, wheat germ glycerides, carbomer 940, triethanolamine, DMDM hydantoin, diazolidinyl urea	Dye and fragrance free. In 237 ml.

EMOLLIENTS, MISCELLANEOUS

otc	**Phicon** (T.E. Williams)	**Cream:** 250 IU vitamin A and 66.7 IU E per g, aloe vera, 5% pramoxine HCl	In 60 g.
otc	**Polysorb Hydrate** (Fougera)	**Cream:** Sorbitan sesquioleate in a wax and petrolatum base	In 56.7 g and lb.
otc	**Pretty Feet and Hands** (B.F. Ascher)	**Cream:** Mineral oil, glyceryl stearate, stearyl alcohol, cetyl alcohol, aloe vera gel, parabens	In 88.7 ml.
otc	**Penecare** (Reed & Carnrick)	**Lotion:** Lactic acid, imidurea	In 240 ml.
otc	**Allercreme Skin** (Carme)	**Lotion:** Mineral oil, sorbitol, triethanolamine, parabens	In 240 ml.
otc	**Aloe Vesta** (ConvaTec)	**Lotion:** 3% dimethicone	Alcohols, aloe, glycerin, petrolatum. In 60 mL.
otc	**AmLactin** (Upsher-Smith)	**Lotion:** 12% ammonium lactate, parabens, light mineral oil	In 225 and 400 g.
otc	**Aquanil** (Person & Covey)	**Lotion:** Glycerin, benzyl alcohol, sodium laureth sulfate, stearyl alcohol, xanthan gum	In 240 and 480 ml.
otc	**Aveeno** (Rydelle)	**Lotion:** 1% colloidal oatmeal, glycerin, phenylcarbinol, petrolatum, dimethicone, benzyl alcohol	In 240 ml.
otc	**Balmex Emollient** (Macsil)	**Lotion:** Lanolin oil, silicone, Balsam Peru, glycerol monostearate	In 180 ml.
otc	**Complex 15 Hand & Body** (Schering-Plough)	**Lotion:** Caprylic/capric triglyceride, PEG-50 stearate, squalane, carboxylic acid sterol ester, diazolidinyl urea, glycerin, glyceryl stearate, lecithin, dimethicone, glycol stearate, carbomer-934P, EDTA	Unscented. In 30 ml.
otc	**Corn Huskers** (Warner-Lambert)	**Lotion:** 6.7% glycerin, 5.7% SD alcohol 40, algin, guar gum, methylparaben	In 120 and 210 ml.
otc	**Dermasil** (Unilever)	**Lotion:** Dimethicone, mineral oil, glycerin, sunflower seed oil, borage seed oil, cetyl alcohol, lanolin alcohol, sweet almond oil, rose extract, sandalwood oil, EDTA, parabens	In 472 ml.
otc	**Derma Viva** (Rugby)	**Lotion:** Mineral oil, glyceryl stearate, laureth-4, lanolin oil, PEG-100 stearate, PEG-40 stearate, PEG-4 dilaurate, trolamine, DSS, parabens	In 237 ml.
otc	**DML** (Person & Covey)	**Lotion:** Petrolatum, glycerin, dimethicone, benzyl alcohol, volatile silicone, glyceryl stearate, palmitic acid, carbomer 941, xanthan gum	Unscented. In 240 and 480 ml.
otc	**Emollia** (Gordon Labs)	**Lotion:** Mineral oil, propylene glycol, white wax, sodium lauryl sulfate, oleic acid, parabens	In 120 and 240 ml and gal.
otc	**Epilyt** (Stiefel)	**Lotion concentrate:** Propylene glycol, glycerin, oleic acid, lactic acid	In 118 ml.
otc	**Esotérica Dry Skin Treatment** (SK-Beecham)	**Lotion:** Propylene glycol, dicaprylate/dicaprate, mineral oil, glyceryl stearate, cetyl esters wax, hydrolyzed animal protein, dimethicone, TEA-carbomer-941, parabens	In 37.5 ml.
otc	**Eucerin Moisturizing** (Beiersdorf)	**Lotion:** Mineral oil, PEG-40 sorbitan peroleate, lanolin acid glycerin ester, sorbitol, propylene glycol, cetyl palmitate, lanolin alcohol	Unscented. In 52.5, 120 and 240 ml, pt and gal.
otc	**Hydrisea** (Pedinol)	**Lotion:** 8% Dead Sea salts concentrate, NaCl, MgCl, KCl, CaCl, mineral oil, propylene glycol, sorbitan stearate, glyceryl stearate, PEG-75 lanolin, EDTA, imidazolidinyl urea, tartrazine, parabens	In 120 ml.
otc	**Hydrisinol** (Pedinol)	**Lotion:** Sulfonated castor oil, hydrogenated vegetable oil, propylene glycol stearate SE, mineral oil, lanolin, lanolin alcohol, sesame oil, sunflower oil, aloe, triethanolamine, sorbitan stearate, parabens, hydroxyethyl cellulose	In 240 ml.
otc	**Keri** (Westwood Squibb)	**Lotion:** Mineral oil, lanolin oil, propylene glycol, glyceryl stearate, PEG–100 stearate, PEG–40 stearate, PEG-4 dilaurate, laureth–4, carbomer-934, triethanolamine, docusate sodium, parabens	Scented and unscented. In 195, 390 and 600 ml.
otc	**Keri Light** (Westwood Squibb)	**Lotion:** Glycerin, stearyl alcohol, ceteareth–20, cetearyl octanoate, stearyl heptanoate, squalane, parabens, carbomer-934	In 195 and 390 ml.
otc	**Kinerase** (ICN)	**Lotion:** 0.1% N^6-furfuryladenine glycerin, stearyl alcohol, safflower oil, cetyl alcohol, aloe, parabens, corn oil	In 53 and 112 ml.
Rx	**Lac-Hydrin** (Westwood Squibb)	**Lotion:** 12% ammonium lactate (12% lactic acid neutralized with ammonium hydroxide), light mineral oil, cetyl alcohol, parabens	In 150 and 360 ml.
otc	**Lac-Hydrin Five** (Westwood Squibb)	**Lotion:** Lactic acid, glycerin, petrolatum, squalane, steareth-2, PCE-21-stearyl ether, propylene glycol dioctanoate, dimethicone, cetyl palmitate, diazolidinyl urea	Unscented. In 120 and 240 ml.
otc	**LactiCare** (Stiefel)	**Lotion:** Lactic acid, mineral oil, sodium hydroxide, glyceryl stearate, PEG-100 stearate, carbomer-940, DMDM hydantoin	In 222 and 345 ml.
otc	**Lobana Body** (Ulmer)	**Lotion:** Mineral oil, triethanolamine stearate, lanolin, propylene glycol and parabens	In 120 and 240 ml and gal.
otc	**Lubriderm** (Warner-Lambert)	**Lotion:** Mineral oil, petrolatum, sorbitol, lanolin, lanolin alcohol, triethanolamine and parabens	Scented and unscented. In 75, 120, 240, 360, 480 ml.
otc	**Neutrogena Body** (Neutrogena)	**Lotion:** Glyceryl stearate, PEG–100 stearate, imidazolidinyl urea, carbomer-954, parabens, sodium lauryl sulfate, triethanolamine	Scented and unscented. In 240 ml.
otc	**Nivea After Tan** (Beiersdorf)	**Lotion:** SD alcohol 40B, mineral oil, PEG-40 castor oil, glyceryl stearate, parabens, aloe extract, lanolin alcohol, imidazolidinyl urea, phenoxyethanol, triethanolamine, chamomile extract, carbomer, simethicone	In 120 ml.
otc	**Nivea Moisturizing Extra Enriched** (Beiersdorf)	**Lotion:** Mineral oil, PEG-40 sorbitan peroleate, glycerin, polyglyceryl-3 diisostearate, petrolatum, glyceryl lanolate, lanolin alcohol, phenoxyethanol	In 120, 240 and 360 ml.
otc	**Nutraderm** (Owen/Galderma)	**Lotion:** Mineral oil, sorbitan stearate, stearyl alcohol, sodium lauryl sulfate, carbomer 940, diazolidinyl urea, parabens, triethanolamine	In 240 and 480 ml.
otc	**Shepard's Cream** (Dermik)	**Lotion:** Glycerin, sesame oil, vegetable oil, SD alcohol 40-B, propylene glycol, ethoxydiglycol, triethanolamine, glyceryl stearate, simethicone, monoglyceride citrate, parabens	Unscented. In 240 and 480 ml.
otc	**Sofenol 5** (C & M)	**Lotion:** Glycerin, petrolatum, allantoin, dimethicone, soluble collagen, PEG-40-stearate, carbomer 940, kaolin	Unscented. In 240 ml.
otc	**Therapeutic Bath** (Goldline)	**Lotion:** Mineral oil, glyceryl stearate, PEG-100 stearate, propylene glycol, PEG-40 stearate, laureth-4, PEG-4 dilaurate, lanolin oil, parabens, carbomer 934, trolamine, DSS	In 236 ml.
otc	**Ultra Derm** (Baker Cummins)	**Lotion:** Mineral oil, petrolatum, lanolin oil, glycerin, propylene glycol, glyceryl stearate, PEG–50 stearate, propylene glycol stearate SE, sorbitan laurate, potassium sorbate, phosphoric acid, EDTA	In 240 ml.
otc	**Vaseline Intensive Care** (Unilever)	**Lotion:** Ethylhexyl p-methoxycinnamate, (SPF5). Glycerin, sunflower seed oil, cetyl alcohol, corn oil, methylparaben, EDTA	In 325 ml.
otc	**Wibi** (Owen/Galderma)	**Lotion:** Glycerin, SD alcohol 40, PEG-4, PEG–6-32 stearate, PEG–6-32, carbomer–940, PEG–75, parabens, triethanolamine, menthol	In 240 and 480 ml.
otc	**Wondra** (Richardson-Vicks)	**Lotion:** Petrolatum, lanolin acid, glycerin, EDTA, hydrogenated vegetable glycerides phosphate, carbomer, dimethicone, imidazolidinyl urea, EDTA, titanium dioxide, parabens	Scented and unscented. In 300 ml.
otc	**Xeroderm** (Dermol)	**Lotion:** Mineral oil, acetylate lanolin alcohol, cetyl alcohol, glycerin, triethanolamine, parabens, imidazolidinyl urea	In 267 ml.

EMOLLIENTS, MISCELLANEOUS

otc	**Collastin Oil Free Moisturizer** (Dermol)	**Lotion:** Solluble collagen, hydrolyzed elastin	In 60 ml.
otc	**Eucerin Plus** (Beiersdorf)	**Lotion:** Mineral oil, hydrogenated castor oil, 5% sodium lactate, 5% urea, glycerin, lanolin alcohol	In 177 ml.
Rx	**Lactinol** (Pedinol)	**Lotion:** 10% lactic acid	In 237 ml.
otc	**Hawaiian Tropic Cool Aloe With I.C.E.** (Tanning Research)	**Gel:** Lidocaine, menthol, aloe, SD alcohol 40, diazolidinyl urea, EDTA, vitamins A and E, tartrazine	In 360 g.
otc	**Coppertone Aloe Vera Gel** (Schering-Plough)	**Gel:** Aloe vera, glycerin, parabens, EDTA	Alcohol free. In 454 g.
otc	**Neutrogena Body** (Neutrogena)	**Oil:** Sesame oil, PEG-40 sorbitan peroleate	In 240 ml.
otc	**Nivea Skin** (Beiersdorf)	**Oil:** Mineral oil, lanolin, petrolatum, glyceryl lanolate, lanolin alcohol	In 240 ml.
otc	**Eucerin Itch-Relief Moisturizing Spray** (Beiersdorf)	**Spray:** 0.15% menthol, glycerin, mineral oil, cetyl alcohol, *Oenothera biennis* (evening primrose oil)	In 200 mL.
otc	**Sardoettes** (Schering-Plough)	**Towelettes:** Mineral oil, tocopherol, beta-carotene	In 25s.

[1] Quintessa Corporation, PO Box 808, Lancaster, CA 93584; (661) 940–5600. [2] SDR Pharmaceuticals, Inc., Andover, NJ 07821; (973) 786–7996.

Indications

These preparations lubricate and moisturize the skin, counteracting dryness and itching.

EMOLLIENT BATH PREPARATIONS

otc	**ActiBath Effervescent Tablets** (Jergens)	20% colloidal oatmeal	In 4s.
otc	**Aveeno Shave Gel** (Rydelle)	Oatmeal flour	In 210 g.
otc	**Nutra·Soothe** (Pertussin)	Colloidal oatmeal, light mineral oil	In individual oil (9) & oatmeal powder packets (9).
otc	**Nutraderm Bath Oil** (Owen/Galderma)	Mineral oil, lanolin oil, PEG-4 dilaurate, benzophenone-3, butylparaben	In 240 ml.
otc	**Sardo Bath & Shower Oil** (Schering-Plough)	Mineral oil, tocopherol	In 112.5 ml.
otc	**Ultra Derm Bath Oil** (Baker Cummins)	Mineral oil, lanolin oil, octoxynol–3	In 240 ml.
otc	**Alpha Keri Therapeutic Bath Oil** (Westwood)	Mineral oil, lanolin oil, PEG-4 dilaurate, benzophenone-3	In 120 and 240 ml and pt.
otc	**Therapeutic Bath Oil** (Goldline)		In 473 ml.
otc	**LubraSol Bath Oil** (Pharmaceutical Specialties)	Mineral oil, lanolin oil, PEG-200 dilaurate, oxybenzone	In 240 ml.
otc	**Domol Bath & Shower Oil** (Miles)	Di-isopropyl sebacate, mineral oil	In 240 ml.
otc	**Lubriderm Bath Oil** (Warner-Lambert)	Mineral oil, PPG-15, stearyl ether oleth-2, nonoxynol-5	In 480 ml.
otc	**Cameo Oil** (Medco)	Mineral oil, PEG-8 dioleate, lanolin oil	Unscented. In 240, 480 and 960 ml.
otc	**RoBathol Bath Oil** (Pharmaceutical Specialties)	Cottonseed oil and alkyl aryl polyether alcohol	Lanolin free. Dye free. In 240 ml, pt and gal.
otc	**Esoterica Soap** (Medicis)	Sodium tallowate, sodium cocoate, mineral oil, acacia, sodium cocoyl isethionate, lauramide DEA, potassium oleate, titanium dioxide, pentasodium pentetate, tetra sodium etidronate	In 85 g.
otc	**Dermasil Lotion** (Chesebrough-Ponds)	Glycerin, dimethicone, sunflower seed oil, petrolatum, borage seed oil, vitamin E acetate, vitamin A palmitate, vitamin D_3, corn oil, EDTA, methylparaben.	In 120 and 240 ml.
otc	**Aveeno Shower & Bath Oil** (Rydelle)	5% colloidal oatmeal, mineral oil, glyceryl stearate, PEG 100 stearate, laureth-4, benzyl alcohol, silica benzaldehyde	In 240 ml.

Indications

These products contain colloidal solids and various oils which act as emollients. They are recommended for relief of minor skin irritations and pruritus associated with common dermatoses and dry skin conditions.

Precautions

▶*For external use only:* Avoid contact with the eyes; if this occurs, flush with clear water.

Use caution – To avoid slipping in tub when using bath oils.

Do not use – On acutely inflamed areas.

ZINC OXIDE

otc	Dr. Smith's Adult Care (Beta Dermaceuticals)[1]	Ointment: 10%	Petrolatum, lanolin, mineral oil, olive oil. In 85 g.
otc	Dr. Smith's Diaper Ointment (Beta Dermaceuticals)[1]		Petrolatum, lanolin, mineral oil, olive oil. In 85 g.
otc	Zinc Oxide (Various, eg, Moore, Paddock, Rugby)	Ointment: 20%	In 30 and 60 g and lb.
otc	Borofax Skin Protectant (Warner-Wellcome)	Ointment: 15%. 68.6% petrolatum, lanolin, mineral oil	In 50 g.

[1] Beta Dermaceuticals, PO Box 691106, San Antonio, TX 78269–1106; (210) 349–9326, (800) 434–BETA (2382), fax (210) 349–9363; http://www.beta-derm.com.

Indications

Minor skin irritations, burns, abrasions, chafed skin and diaper rash.

Administration and Dosage

For external use only. Avoid contact with the eyes.
Apply to affected areas as required.

PROTECTANTS, MISCELLANEOUS

otc	Hydropel (C & M)	Ointment: 30% silicone, 10% hydrophobic starch derivative, petrolatum	In 60 g and lb.
otc	Silicone No. 2 (C & M)	Ointment: 10% silicone in petrolatum, hydrophobic starch derivative, methylparaben	In 30 and 480 g.
otc	White Cloverine Salve (Medtech)	Ointment: 97% white petrolatum, rectified turpentine oil, white wax	In 30 g.
otc	Kerodex (Whitehall)	Cream: #51-Bentonite, calcium carbonate, cellulose gum, chloroxylenol, glycerin, iron oxides, isopropyl alcohol, kaolin, parabens, petrolatum, sodium lauryl sulfate, spermaceti. Nongreasy invisible barrier for dry or oily work	In 113 g.
		Cream: #71-Calcium carbonate, cetrimonium bromide, iron oxide, isopropyl alcohol, kaolin, parabens, mineral oil, paraffin, petrolatum, sodium hexametaphosphate, sodium lauryl sulfate, zinc oxide. Nongreasy invisible water repellent barrier for wet work	In 113 g.
otc	BlisterGard (Medtech)	Liquid: 6.7% alcohol, pyroxylin solution, oil of cloves, 8-hydroxyquinoline	In 30 ml.
otc	New-Skin (Medtech)		In 10 and 30 ml bottle and 3.5 ml tube.
otc	Skin Shield (Del)	Liquid: 0.75% dyclonine HCl, 0.2% benzethonium chloride, acetone, castor oil, 10% SD alcohol 40. Waterproof.	In 13.3 ml.
otc	New-Skin Antiseptic (Medtech)	Spray Liquid: Pyroxylin solution, acetone ACS, oil of cloves, 8-hydroxyquinoline, 4.2% alcohol	In 28.5 g.
otc	Aerozoin (Graham Field)	Spray: 30% tincture of benzoin compound, 44.8% isopropyl alcohol	In 105 ml.
otc	Benzoin (Various, eg, Humco, Lannett)	Tincture	In 60 and 120 ml, pt and gal.
otc	Benzoin Compound (Various, eg, Century, Humco, Lannett, Paddock, Purepac)	Tincture: Benzoin, aloe, storax, tolu balsam, 74% to 80% alcohol	In 30, 60 and 120 ml, pt and gal.
otc	TinBen (Ferndale)	Tincture: Benzoin, 75% to 83% alcohol	In 120 ml.
otc	TinCoBen (Ferndale)	Tincture: Benzoin, aloe, tolu balsam, storax, 77% alcohol	In 120 ml.
otc	Pro-Q (CollaGenex)	Foam: Dimethicone, glycerin, parabens	In 75 and 161 mL.

Indications

To protect skin against contact irritants.

Contraindications

Do not use silicone on wet, exudative lesions or inflamed or abraded skin.

SUNSCREENS

		SPF		
otc	**Hawaiian Tropic Baby Faces Sunblock** (Tanning Research)	30+	**Lotion**: Titanium dioxide, octyl methoxycinnamate, octocrylene, benzophenone-3, octyl salicylate	PABA free. Waterproof. In 120 ml.
otc	**SolBar PF** (Person & Covey)	30+	**Cream**: Oxybenzone, octyl methoxycinnamate, octocrylene	PABA free. Waterproof. In 120 g.
otc	**Coppertone Sport** (Schering-Plough)	30+	**Lotion**: Ethylhexyl, p-methoxycinnamate, oxybenzone, 2-ethylhexyl salicylate, homosalate. Parabens, aloe	PABA free. Waterproof. In 118 ml.
otc	**Hawaiian Tropic Sunblock** (Tanning Research)	30+	**Lotion**: Titanium dioxide, octyl methoxycinnamate, benzophenone-3, octyl salicylate, octocrylene	PABA free. Waterproof. In 120 and 300 ml.
otc	**Coppertone Moisturizing Sunblock** (Schering-Plough)	30+	**Lotion**: Ethylhexyl p-methoxycinnamate, 2-ethylhexyl salicylate, octocrylene, oxybenzone	PABA free. Waterproof. In 120 and 300 ml.
otc	**Coppertone Shade Sunblock** (Schering-Plough)	30+	**Lotion**: Ethylhexyl p-methoxycinnamate, 2-ethylhexyl salicylate, oxybenzone, homosalate. Sorbitol, benzyl alcohol, aloe, vitamin E, parabens, jojoba oil, EDTA, phenethyl alcohol	PABA free. Waterproof. In 118 ml.
otc	**Coppertone Water Babies** (Schering-Plough)	30+	**Lotion**: Ethylhexyl p-methoxycinnamate, 2-ethylhexyl salicylate, oxybenzone, homosalate. Alcohol, aloe, parabens	PABA free. Waterproof. In 118 ml.
otc	**Water Babies UVA/UVB Sunblock** (Schering-Plough)	30+	**Lotion**: Ethylhexyl p-methoxycinnamate, 2-ethylhexyl salicylate, octocrylene, oxybenzone	PABA free. Waterproof. In 120 ml.
otc	**Hawaiian Tropic Just For Kids Sunblock** (Tanning Research)	30+	**Lotion**: Octyl methoxycinnamate, benzophenone-3, octyl salicylate, octocrylene, titanium dioxide	PABA free. Waterproof, all day protection. In 88.7 ml.
otc	**Coppertone Kids** (Schering-Plough)	30+	**Lotion**: Ethylhexyl p-methoxycinnamate, 2-ethylhexyl salicylate, oxybenzone, homosalate. Sorbitol, benzyl alcohol, aloe, jojoba oil, parabens	PABA free. Waterproof. In 237 ml.
otc	**Vaseline Intensive Care Blockout** (Chesebrough Ponds)	30+	**Lotion**: Padimate, ethylhexyl p-methoxycinnamate, oxybenzone, 2-ethylhexyl salicylate, titanium dioxide	Waterproof. In 120 ml.
otc	**Bullfrog Sunblock** (Chattem)	30+	**Gel**: Benzophenone-3, octocrylene, octyl methoxycinnamate. Aloe, vitamin E, isostearyl alcohol	PABA free. Waterproof, all day protection. In 120 g.
otc	**Hawaiian Tropic Baby Faces Sunblock** (Tanning Research)	30+	**Lotion**: Octyl methoxycinnamate, benzophenone-3, octyl salicylate, titanium dioxide, octocrylene	PABA free. Waterproof, all day protection. In 60, 120 and 300 ml.
otc	**Hawaiian Tropic Sunblock** (Tanning Research)	30+	**Lotion**: Homosalate, octyl methoxycinnamate, benzophenone-3, menthyl anthranilate, octyl salicylate	PABA free. Waterproof, all day protection. In 120 ml.
otc	**Coppertone Oil Free** (Schering-Plough)	30	**Lotion**: Ethylhexyl p-methoxycinnamate, oxybenzone, 2-ethylhexyl salicylate, homosalate. Parabens, EDTA, glyceryl	PABA free. Waterproof. In 118 ml.
otc	**Coppertone Water Babies** (Schering-Plough)	30	**Lotion**: Ethylhexyl p-methoxycinnamate, oxybenzone, 2-ethylhexyl salicylate, homosalate. Glyceryl, alcohol, parabens	PABA free. Waterproof. In 118 ml.
otc	**Neutrogena No-Stick Sunscreen** (Neutrogena)	30	**Cream**: 7.5% octyl methoxycinnamate, 15% homosalate, 6% benzophenone-3, 5% octyl salicylate	EDTA, parabens, diazolidinyl urea. In 118 g.
otc	**Ti-Screen** (Pedinol)	30	**Lotion**: 7.5% octyl methoxycinnamate, 6% oxybenzone, 5% octyl salicylate, 7.5% octocrylene	PABA free. Waterproof. In 120 ml.
otc	**PreSun Active** (Bristol-Myers)	30	**Gel**: Octyl methoxycinnamate, oxybenzone, octyl salicylate. 69% SD alcohol 40	PABA free. Waterproof, non-greasy. In 120 ml.
otc	**PreSun Ultra** (Westwood Squibb)	30	**Lotion**: 7.5% octyl methoxycinnamate, 5% octyl salicylate, 3% oxybenzone, 3% avobenzone	In 120 ml.
otc	**PreSun Ultra** (Westwood Squibb)	30	**Gel**: 7.5% octyl methoxycinnamate, 5% octyl salicylate, 3% oxybenzone, 3% avobenzone	In 120 ml.
otc	**Sundown Sunblock** (Johnson & Johnson)	30	**Lotion**: Octyl methoxycinnamate, octyl salicylate, oxybenzone, titanium dioxide	PABA free. Waterproof, non-greasy. In 120 ml.
otc	**Bain de Soleil All Day for Kids** (Procter & Gamble)	30	**Lotion**: Ethylhexyl p-methoxycinnamate, 2-ethylhexyl 2-cyano-3, 3-diphenylacrylate, oxybenzone, titanium dioxide. Stearyl alcohol, vitamin E, EDTA	PABA free. Waterproof. In 120 ml.
otc	**Bain de Soleil All Day Waterproof Sunblock** (Procter & Gamble)	30	**Lotion**: Ethylhexyl p-methoxycinnamate, 2-ethylhexyl 2-cyano-3, 3-diphenylacrylate, oxybenzone, titanium dioxide. Stearyl alcohol, vitamin E, EDTA	PABA free. Waterproof, non-greasy, all day protection. In 120 ml.
otc	**Coppertone Moisturizing Sunblock** (Schering-Plough)	30	**Lotion**: Ethylhexyl p-methoxycinnamate, oxybenzone, 2-ethylhexyl salicylate, homosalate	PABA free. Waterproof. In 120 and 240 ml.
otc	**Coppertone Sport** (Schering-Plough)	30	**Lotion**: Ethylhexyl p-methoxycinnamate, oxybenzone, 2-ethylhexyl salicylate	PABA free. Waterproof. In 120 ml.
otc	**Shade Sunblock** (Schering-Plough)	30	**Stick**: Ethylhexyl p-methoxycinnamate, oxybenzone, 2-ethylhexyl salicylate, homosalate	Waterproof. In 18 g.
otc	**Shade Sunblock** (Schering-Plough)	30	**Lotion**: Ethylhexyl p-methoxycinnamate, 2-ethylhexyl salicylate, homosalate, oxybenzone	Waterproof. In 120 ml.
otc	**Shade Sunblock** (Schering-Plough)	30	**Gel**: Ethylhexyl p-methoxycinnamate, homosalate, oxybenzone. 73% SD alcohol 40	Waterproof. Oil free. In 120 g.
otc	**Water Babies UVA/UVB Sunblock** (Schering-Plough)	30	**Lotion**: Ethylhexyl p-methoxycinnamate, 2-ethylhexyl salicylate, homosalate, oxybenzone	PABA free. Waterproof. In 120 and 240 ml.
otc	**Hawaiian Tropic Just For Kids Sunblock** (Tanning Research)	30	**Lotion**: Homosalate, octyl methoxycinnamate, benzophenone-3, menthyl anthranilate, octyl salicylate	PABA free. Waterproof, all day protection. In 88.7 ml.
otc	**Hawaiian Tropic Sport Sunblock** (Tanning Research)	30	**Lotion**: Octyl methoxycinnamate, octocrylene, benzophenone-3, octyl salicylate, titanium dioxide	PABA free. Waterproof, all day protection. In 88.7 ml.
otc	**SolBar PF** (Person & Covey)	30	**Liquid**: 10% octocrylene, 7.5% octyl methoxycinnamate, 6% oxybenzone. 77% SD alcohol 40	PABA free. In 114 ml.
otc	**Bain de Soleil SPF 30 + Color** (Procter & Gamble)	30	**Lotion**: Octocrylene, octyl methoxycinnamate, oxybenzone. Mineral oil, cetyl alcohol, EDTA	Waterproof. In 118 ml.
otc	**Coppertone Kids Sunblock** (Schering-Plough)	30	**Lotion**: Octocrylene, ethylhexyl p-methoxycinnamate, oxybenzone, 2-ethylhexyl salicylate	PABA free. Waterproof. In 120 and 240 ml.
otc	**Tréo** (Biopharm Lab)	30	**Lotion**: Octocrylene, octyl methoxycinnamate, benzophenone-3, octyl salicylate. Isostearyl alcohol, diazolidinyl urea, propylparabens. Also contains 0.05% citronella oil as an insect repellent	PABA free. Waterproof. In 118 ml.
otc	**Coppertone Kids Spray 'n Splash** (Schering-Plough)	30	**Spray**: Ethylhexyl p-methoxycinnamate, oxybenzone, 2-ethylhexyl salicylate, homosalate. Parabens, EDTA	PABA free. Waterproof. In 236 ml.
otc	**Coppertone To Go Sunblock** (Schering-Plough)	30	**Spray**: Ethylhexyl p-methoxycinnamate, oxybenzone, 2-ethylhexyl salicylate, homosalate. Alcohol	PABA free. Waterproof. In 112 ml.

SUNSCREENS

		SPF		
otc	**Coppertone Sport Sunblock Spray** (Schering-Plough)	30	**Spray:** Ethylhexyl p-methoxycinnamate, oxybenzone, 2-ethylhexyl salicylate, homosalate. Alcohol	PABA free. Waterproof. In 112 ml.
otc	**Coppertone Moisturizing Sunblock** (Schering-Plough)	25	**Lotion:** Ethylhexyl p-methoxycinnamate, oxybenzone, 2-ethylhexyl salicylate, homosalate	PABA free, Waterproof. In 120 ml.
otc	**Vaseline Intensive Care Moisturizing Sunblock** (Chesebrough Ponds)	25	**Lotion:** Ethylhexyl p-methoxycinnamate, oxybenzone, 2-ethylhexyl salicylate. Glycerin, aloe vera gel, C12-15 alkyl benzoate, cetyl alcohol, petrolatum, vitamin E, parabens, EDTA	PABA free. In 118 ml.
otc	**Neutrogena Sunblock Stick** (Neutrogena)	25	**Stick:** Octyl methoxycinnamate, benzophenone-3, octyl salicylate. Castor oil, cetearyl alcohol, propylparaben, shea butter	PABA free. Waterproof. In 12.6 g.
otc	**PreSun Moisturizing Sunscreen with Keri** (Bristol-Myers)	25	**Lotion:** Octyl methoxycinnamate, oxybenzone, octyl salicylate. Petrolatum, cetyl alcohol, diazolidinyl urea	Waterproof. In 120 ml.
otc	**PreSun for Kids Spray Mist** (Bristol-Myers)	23	Waterproof. In 105 ml.	
otc	**Eucerin Dry Skin Care Daily Facial** (Beiersdorf)	20	**Lotion:** Ethylhexyl p-methoxycinnamate, titanium dioxide, 2-phenylbenzimidazole-5-sulfonic acid, 2-ethylhexyl salicylate. Mineral oil, cetearyl alcohol, castor oil, lanolin alcohol, EDTA	In 120 ml.
otc	**Hawaiian Tropic Baby Faces** (Tanning Research)	20	**Gel:** Octyl methoxycinnamate, octocrylene, benzophenone-3, menthyl anthranilate	PABA free. Waterproof. In 120 g.
otc	**Bullfrog Sunblock** (Chattem)	18	**Gel:** Octocrylene, benzophenone-3, octyl methoxycinnamate. Isostearyl alcohol, vitamin E, aloe	PABA free. Waterproof, all day protection. In 120 g.
otc	**Bullfrog** (Chattem)	18	**Stick:** Benzophenone-3, octyl methoxycinnamate. Isostearyl alcohol, aloe, hydrogenated vegetable oil, vitamin E	Waterproof. In 16.5 g.
otc	**Bullfrog Extra Moisturizing Gel** (Chattem)	18	**Gel:** Benzophenone-3, octocrylene, octyl methoxycinnamate. Vitamin E, aloe	PABA free. Waterproof, all day protection. In 90 g.
otc	**Bullfrog Sport Lotion** (Chattem)	18	**Lotion:** Benzophenone-3, octocrylene, octyl methoxycinnamate, octyl salicylate, titanium dioxide. Diazolidinyl urea, EDTA, parabens, vitamin E, aloe	Waterproof, all day protection. In 120 ml.
otc	**Bullfrog for Kids** (Chattem)	18	**Gel:** Octocrylene, octyl methoxycinnamate, octyl salicylate. Vitamin E, aloe, C12-15 alcohols benzoate	Waterproof, non-greasy, all day protection. In 60 g.
otc	**Neutrogena Chemical-Free Sunblocker** (Neutrogena)	17	**Lotion:** Titanium dioxide. Parabens, diazolidinyl urea, shea butter	PABA free. In 120 ml.
otc	**SUNPRuF 17** (C & M)	17	**Gel:** 7.8% octyl methoxycinnamate, 5.2% octyl salicylate	Oil free, water-resistant. In 120 g.
otc	**TI·Screen Sunless** (Pedinol)	17	**Creme:** 7.5% octyl methoxycinnamate, 3% benzophenone-3. Mineral oil, alcohols, PEG-100, parabens	In 118 ml.
otc	**TI·Baby Natural** (Pedinol)	16	**Lotion:** 5% titanium dioxide	PABA free. Waterproof. In 120 ml.
otc	**TI·Screen Natural** (Pedinol)	16	**Lotion:** 5% titanium dioxide	PABA free. Waterproof. In 120 ml.
otc	**Hawaiian Tropic 15 Plus Sunblock** (Tanning Research)	15+	**Lotion:** Menthyl anthranilate, octyl methoxycinnamate, benzophenone-3	PABA free. Waterproof, all day protection. In 7.5, 15, 60, 120, 240 and 300 ml.
otc	**Hawaiian Tropic 15 Plus** (Tanning Research)	15+	**Gel:** Octyl methoxycinnamate, octocrylene, benzophenone-3, menthyl anthranilate	PABA free. Waterproof, all day protection. In 120 g.
otc	**TI·Screen** (Pedinol)	15+	**Lotion:** 7.5% ethylhexyl p-methoxycinnamate, 5% oxybenzone	PABA free. Water resistant. In 120 ml.
otc	**TI·Lite** (Pedinol)	15	**Cream:** 7.5% ethylhexyl p-methoxycinnamate, 2% titanium dioxide. Cetyl alcohol, phenethyl alcohol, parabens, EDTA	In 60 g.
otc	**Aquaderm** (Baker Cummins)	15	**Cream:** 7.5% octyl methoxycinnamate, 6% oxybenzone	In 105 g.
otc	**SolBar PF Sunscreen** (Person & Covey)	15	**Liquid:** 7.5% octyl methoxycinnamate, 5% oxybenzone. 76% SD alcohol 40	PABA free. In 120 ml.
otc	**SUNPRuF 15** (C & M)	15	**Lotion:** 7.5% octyl methoxycinnamate, 5% benzophenone-3	PABA free. Water-resistant. In 240 ml.
otc	**Bain de Soleil SPF 15 + Color** (Procter & Gamble)	15	**Lotion:** Octyl methoxycinnamate, octocrylene, oxybenzone. Mineral oil, cetyl alcohol, EDTA	Waterproof. In 118 ml.
otc	**Catrix Correction** (Donell DerMedex)	15	**Cream:** Octyl methoxycinnamate, menthyl anthranilate, benzophenone 3, titanium dioxide. Sesame oil, cetearyl alcohol, urea, EDTA, imidazolidinyl urea, parabens	PABA free. In 39 g.
otc	**Oil of Olay Daily UV Protectant** (Procter & Gamble)	15	**Cream:** Octyl methoxycinnamate, titanium dioxide. Phenylbenzimidazole sulfonic acid, glycerin, cetyl alcohol, imidazolidinyl urea, parabens, EDTA, castor oil	Scented or unscented. In 51 g.
otc	**Bain de Soleil All Day Waterproof Sunblock** (Procter & Gamble)	15	**Lotion:** Ethylhexyl p-methoxycinnamate, 2-ethylhexyl 2-cyano-3, 3-diphenylacrylate, oxybenzone, titanium dioxide. Stearyl alcohol, vitamin E, EDTA	PABA free. Waterproof, non-greasy, all day protection. In 120 ml.
otc	**Coppertone Sport** (Schering-Plough)	15	**Lotion:** Ethylhexyl p-methoxycinnamate, oxybenzone	PABA free. Waterproof. In 120 ml.
otc	**Shade Sunblock** (Schering-Plough)	15	**Gel:** Ethylhexyl p-methoxycinnamate, oxybenzone. 75% SD alcohol 40	Waterproof. Oil free. In 120 g.
otc	**Vaseline Intensive Care Sport Sunblock** (Chesebrough Ponds)	15	**Lotion:** Ethylhexyl p-methoxycinnamate, oxybenzone, C12-15 alkyl benzoate. Aloe vera gel, vitamin E, EDTA	PABA free. Waterproof, non-greasy. In 118 ml.
otc	**Coppertone Kids Sunblock** (Schering-Plough)	15	**Lotion:** Ethylhexyl p-methoxycinnamate, oxybenzone, 2-ethylhexyl salicylate, homosalate	PABA free. Waterproof. In 120 and 240 ml.
otc	**Coppertone Moisturizing Sunblock** (Schering-Plough)	15	**Lotion:** Ethylhexyl p-methoxycinnamate, oxybenzone	PABA free. Waterproof. In 120, 240 and 300 ml.
otc	**Faces Only Moisturizing Sunblock by Coppertone** (Schering-Plough)	15	**Lotion:** Ethylhexyl p-methoxycinnamate, oxybenzone	PABA free. In 55.5 ml.
otc	**Oil of Olay Daily UV Protectant** (Procter & Gamble)	15	**Lotion:** Ethylhexyl p-methoxycinnamate, 2-phenylbenzimidazole-5-sulfonic acid, titanium dioxide. Cetyl alcohol, imidazolidinyl urea, parabens, EDTA, castor oil, tartrazine	PABA free. Greaseless. Scented or unscented. In 105 and 157.7 ml.
otc	**Vaseline Intensive Care Ultra Violet Daily Defense** (Chesebrough Ponds)	15	**Lotion:** Ethylhexyl p-methoxycinnamate, oxybenzone. Vitamin E, cetyl alcohol, acetylated lanolin alcohol, parabens, EDTA	PABA free. Non-greasy. In 120 and 300 ml.
otc	**Hawaiian Tropic Sport Sunblock** (Tanning Research)	15	**Lotion:** Octyl methoxycinnamate, benzophenone-3, octocrylene	PABA free. Waterproof, all day protection. In 88.7 ml.

SUNSCREENS

		SPF		
otc	**Neutrogena Intensified Day Moisture** (Neutrogena)	15	**Cream:** Octyl methoxycinnamate, 2-phenylbenzimidazole sulfonic acid, titanium dioxide. Cetyl alcohol, diazolidinyl urea, parabens, EDTA	PABA free. In 67.5 g.
otc	**Ray Block** (Del Ray)	15	**Lotion:** 5% octyl dimethyl PABA, 3% benzophenone-3. SD alcohol	In 118.3 ml.
otc	**Solex A15 Clear Lotion** (Dermol)	15	**Lotion:** 5% octyl dimethyl PABA, 33% benzophenone. SD alcohol	Non-oily. In 120 ml.
otc	**Johnson's Baby Sunblock** (Johnson & Johnson)	15	**Lotion:** Titanium dioxide. Hydrogenated castor oil, EDTA, hydroxylated lanolin, zinc oxide, mineral oil	PABA free. Waterproof. In 120 ml.
otc	**Total Eclipse Oily and Acne Prone Skin Sunscreen** (Triangle Labs)	15	**Lotion:** Padimate O, oxybenzone, glyceryl PABA. 77% alcohol	In 120 ml.
otc	**Total Eclipse Moisturizing** (Triangle Labs)	15	**Lotion:** Padimate O, oxybenzone, octyl salicylate	In 120 ml.
otc	**Shade UVAGuard** (Schering-Plough)	15	**Lotion:** 7.5% octyl methoxycinnamate, 3% avobenzone, 3% oxybenzone	Waterproof. In 120 ml.
otc	**SolBar Plus 15** (Person & Covey)	15	**Cream:** 4% oxybenzone, 2% dioxybenzone, 6% octyl dimethyl PABA	In 113 g.
otc	**PreSun Moisturizing Sunscreen with Keri** (Bristol-Myers)	15	**Lotion:** Octyl dimethyl PABA, oxybenzone. Cetyl alcohol, diazolidinyl urea	Waterproof. In 120 ml.
otc	**SolBar PF** (Person & Covey)	15	**Cream:** 7.5% octyl methoxycinnamate, 5% oxybenzone	PABA free. In 222 g.
otc	**Sundown Sunblock** (Johnson & Johnson)	15	**Lotion:** Octyl methoxycinnamate, oxybenzone, octyl salicylate, titanium dioxide	PABA free. Waterproof, non-greasy. In 120 ml.
otc	**Water Babies UVA/UVB Sunblock** (Schering-Plough)	15	**Lotion:** Ethylhexyl p-methoxycinnamate, oxybenzone	PABA free. Waterproof. In 120 ml.
otc	**DML Facial Moisturizer** (Person & Covey)	15	**Cream:** 8% octyl methoxycinnamate, 4% oxybenzone. Benzyl alcohol, petrolatum, EDTA	In 45 g.
otc	**Hawaiian Tropic Self Tanning Sunblock** (Tanning Research)	15	**Cream:** Octyl methoxycinnamate, benzophenone-3. Aloe, cetyl alcohol, stearyl alcohol, cocoa butter, parabens, vitamin E	PABA free. In 93.75 ml.
otc	**Nivea Sun** (Beiersdorf)	15	**Lotion:** Octyl methoxycinnamate, octyl salicylate, benzophenone-3, 2-phenylbenzimidazole-5-sulfonic acid	PABA free. Waterproof. In 120 ml.
otc	**Neutrogena Moisture** (Neutrogena)	15	**Lotion:** Octyl methoxycinnamate, benzophenone-3. Parabens, diazolidinyl urea	PABA free. In sheer tint and untinted. In 120 ml.
otc	**Neutrogena Sunblock** (Neutrogena)	15	**Cream:** Octyl methoxycinnamate, octyl salicylate, menthyl anthranilate, titanium dioxide. Mineral oil, propylparaben	PABA free. Waterproof. In 67.5 g.
otc	**Tréo** (Biopharm Lab)	15	**Lotion:** Octocrylene, octyl methoxycinnamate, benzophenone-3, octyl salicylate. Isostearyl alcohol, diazolidinyl urea, propylparabens. Also contains 0.05% citronella oil as an insect repellent	PABA free. Waterproof. In 118 ml.
otc	**Coppertone Oil Free** (Schering-Plough)	15	**Lotion:** Ethylhexyl p-methoxycinnamate, oxybenzone. Aloe, parabens, EDTA	PABA free. Waterproof. In 118 and 237 ml.
otc	**Coppertone Sport Sunblock Spray** (Schering-Plough)	15	**Spray:** Ethylhexyl p-methoxycinnamate, 2-ethylhexyl salicylate, homosalate, oxybenzone. Alcohol	PABA free. Waterproof. In 112 ml.
otc	**Hawaiian Tropic 10 Plus** (Tanning Research)	10+	**Lotion:** Octyl methoxycinnamate, benzophenone-3, menthyl anthranilate	PABA free. Waterproof, all day protection. In 120 ml.
otc	**Original Eclipse Sunscreen** (Triangle Labs)	10	**Lotion:** Padimate O, glyceryl PABA	In 120 ml.
otc	**Scar Cream Maximum Strength** (Clay-Park Labs)	10	**Cream:** 7.5% octyl methoxycinnamate, 5% octyl salicylate.	Alcohols, mineral oil, parabens, urea. In 28 g.
otc	**Hawaiian Tropic 8 Plus** (Tanning Research)	8+	**Gel:** Octyl methoxycinnamate, benzophenone-3, menthyl anthranilate	PABA free. Waterproof, all day protection. In 120 g.
otc	**Vaseline Intensive Care No Burn No Bite** (Chesebrough Ponds)	8	**Lotion:** Ethylhexyl p-methoxycinnamate, oxybenzone	PABA free. Waterproof. In 180 ml.
otc	**Ti-Screen** (Pedinol)	8	**Lotion:** 6% ethylhexyl p-methoxycinnamate, 2% oxybenzone	PABA free. Water resistant. In 120 ml.
otc	**Bain de Soleil All Day Waterproof Sunfilter** (Procter & Gamble)	8	**Lotion:** 2-ethylhexyl 2-cyano-3, 3-diphenylacrylate, ethylhexyl p-methoxycinnamate, titanium dioxide. Stearyl alcohol, vitamin E, EDTA	PABA free. Waterproof, non-greasy, all day protection. In 120 ml.
otc	**Coppertone Moisturizing Sunscreen** (Schering-Plough)	8	**Lotion:** Ethylhexyl p-methoxycinnamate, oxybenzone	PABA free. Waterproof. In 120 and 240 ml.
otc	**Coppertone Oil Free** (Schering-Plough)	8	**Lotion:** Ethylhexyl p-methoxycinnamate, oxybenzone. Aloe, parabens, vitamin E, EDTA	PABA free. Waterproof. In 118 ml.
otc	**Coppertone Sport** (Schering-Plough)	8	**Lotion:** Ethylhexyl p-methoxycinnamate, oxybenzone	PABA free. Waterproof. In 120 ml.
otc	**Bain de Soleil SPF 8 + Color** (Procter & Gamble)	8	**Lotion:** Octyl methoxycinnamate, octocrylene. Mineral oil, cetyl alcohol, EDTA	Waterproof. In 118 ml.
otc	**Neutrogena Glow Sunless Tanning** (Neutrogena)	8	**Lotion:** Octyl methoxycinnamate. Cetyl alcohol, diazolidinyl urea, parabens, EDTA	PABA free. In 120 ml.
otc	**Neutrogena Sunblock** (Neutrogena)	8	**Cream:** Octyl methoxycinnamate, menthyl anthranilate, titanium dioxide. Mineral oil	PABA free. Waterproof. In 67.5 g.
otc	**Sundown Sunscreen** (Johnson & Johnson)	8	**Lotion:** Octyl methoxycinnamate, octyl salicylate, oxybenzone, titanium dioxide	PABA free. Waterproof. In 120 ml.
otc	**Tréo** (Biopharm Lab)	8	**Lotion:** Octocrylene, octyl methoxycinnamate, benzophenone-3, octyl salicylate. Isostearyl alcohol, diazolidinyl urea, propylparabens. Also contains 0.05% citronella oil as an insect repellent	PABA free. Waterproof. In 118 ml.
otc	**Hawaiian Tropic Protective Tanning** (Tanning Research)	6	**Lotion:** Titanium dioxide	PABA free. Waterproof. In 240 ml.
otc	**Coppertone Moisturizing Sunscreen** (Schering-Plough)	6	**Lotion:** Ethylhexyl p-methoxycinnamate, oxybenzone	PABA free. Waterproof. In 120 ml.
otc	**Faces Only Clear Sunscreen by Coppertone** (Schering-Plough)	6	**Gel:** Ethylhexyl p-methoxycinnamate, oxybenzone	PABA free. In 55.5 g.
otc	**Hawaiian Tropic Protective Tanning Dry** (Tanning Research)	6	**Oil:** 2-ethylhexyl p-methoxycinnamate, homosalate, menthyl anthranilate	Waterproof. In 180 ml.
			Gel: Phenylbenzimidazole, sulfonic acid, benzophenone-4	In 180 g.
otc	**Neutrogena Moisture** (Neutrogena)	5	**Lotion:** Octyl methoxycinnamate. Petrolatum, cetyl alcohol, parabens, diazolidinyl urea, EDTA, cetyl alcohol	PABA free. In 60 and 120 ml.

SUNSCREENS

		SPF		
otc	**Bain de Soleil Mega Tan** (Procter & Gamble)	4	**Lotion:** Ethylhexyl p-methoxycinnamate, 2-ethylhexyl salicylate. Lanolin, cocoa butter, palm oil, aloe, DMDM hydantoin, xanthan gum, shea butter, EDTA	Waterproof. In 120 ml.
otc	**Bain de Soleil Orange Gelée** (Procter & Gamble)	4	**Gel:** Ethylhexyl p-methoxycinnamate, 2-ethylhexyl salicylate	PABA free. In 93.75 g.
otc	**Bain de Soleil Tropical Deluxe** (Procter & Gamble)	4	**Lotion:** Ethylhexyl p-methoxycinnamate, 2-ethylhexyl salicylate. Cetyl alcohol, EDTA	PABA free. Waterproof. In 240 ml.
otc	**Coppertone Moisturizing Suntan** (Schering-Plough)	4	**Lotion:** Ethylhexyl p-methoxycinnamate, oxybenzone	PABA free. Waterproof. In 120 and 240 ml.
otc	**Hawaiian Tropic Dark Tanning with Sunscreen** (Tanning Research)	4	**Oil:** Ethylhexyl p-methoxycinnamate, octyl dimethyl PABA	Waterproof. In 240 ml.
			Gel: Phenylbenzimidazole, sulfonic acid	PABA free. In 240 g.
otc	**Tropical Blend Dark Tanning** (Schering-Plough)	4	**Lotion:** Ethylhexyl p-methoxycinnamate, oxybenzone	Waterproof. In 240 ml.
			Oil: Padimate O, oxybenzone	Waterproof. In 240 ml.
otc	**Coppertone Sport** (Schering-Plough)	4	**Lotion:** Ethylhexyl p-methoxycinnamate, oxybenzone	PABA free. Waterproof. In 120 ml.
otc	**Coppertone Tan Magnifier Suntan** (Schering-Plough)	4	**Lotion:** Ethylhexyl p-methoxycinnamate	PABA free. In 120 ml.
			Gel: 2-phenylbenzimidazole-5-sulfonic acid	PABA free. In 120 g.
otc	**Bain de Soleil All Day** (Procter & Gamble)	4	**Lotion:** 2-ethylhexyl 2-cyano-3, 3-diphenylacrylate, ethylhexyl p-methoxycinnamate, titanium dioxide. Stearyl alcohol, vitamin E, EDTA	PABA free. Waterproof. In 120 ml.
otc	**Tropical Blend Dry Oil** (Schering-Plough)	4	**Oil:** Homosalate, oxybenzone	Non-greasy. In 180 ml.
otc	**Tropical Blend Tan Magnifier** (Schering-Plough)	4	**Oil:** Triethanolmine salicylate	Waterproof. In 240 ml.
otc	**Coppertone Gold Dark Tanning Oil** (Schering Plough)	4	**Spray:** Homosalate, oxybenzone. Aloe, vitamin E, mineral oil, paraben	In 236 ml.
otc	**Coppertone Gold Dark Tanning Exotic Oil** (Schering-Plough)	*	**Spray:** Homosalate. Mineral oil, coconut oil, olive oil, macadamia nut oil, cocoa butter, vitamin E, lanolin oil, sweet almond oil, jojoba oil, aloe	In 236 ml.
otc	**Q.T. Quick Tanning Suntan by Coppertone** (Schering-Plough)	2	**Lotion:** Ethylhexyl p-methoxycinnamate, dihydroxyacetone	PABA free. In 120 ml.
otc	**Coppertone Moisturizing Suntan** (Schering-Plough)	2	**Oil:** Homosalate	PABA free. Waterproof. In 120 ml.
otc	**Tropical Blend Dark Tanning** (Schering-Plough)	2	**Lotion/Oil:** Homosalate	Waterproof. In 240 ml.
otc	**Tropical Blend Dry Oil** (Schering-Plough)	2	**Oil:** Homosalate	Non-greasy. In 180 ml.
otc	**Hawaiian Tropic Dark Tanning** (Tanning Research)	2	**Gel:** Phenylbenzimidazole sulfonic acid	In 240 ml.
			Oil: 2-ethylhexyl methoxycinnamate, octyl dimethyl PABA	Waterproof. In 240 ml.
otc	**Coppertone Tan Magnifier Suntan** (Schering-Plough)	2	**Oil:** Triethanolamine salicylate	PABA free. In 120 ml.
otc	**Tropical Blend Tan Magnifier** (Schering-Plough)	2	**Oil:** Triethanolamine salicylate	Waterproof. In 240 ml.
otc	**Coppertone Gold Tan Magnifier Oil** (Schering-Plough)	2	**Oil:** Triethanolamine salicylate. Glycerin, aloe, lanolin oil, cocoa butter, macadamia nut oil, olive oil, sweet almond oil, vitamin E, jojoba oil, coconut oil, parabens	In 236 ml.
otc	**Coppertone Gold Dark Tanning Sandproof Dry Oil** (Schering-Plough)	2	**Spray:** Homosalate. Aloe, vitamin E, mineral oil, paraben	In 236 ml.
otc	**A-Fil** (GenDerm)	*	**Cream:** 5% menthyl anthranilate, 5% titanium dioxide	In 45 g.
otc	**RVPaque** (ICN)	*	**Cream:** Red petrolatum, zinc oxide, cinoxate	Water resistant. Greaseless. Tinted. In 15 and 37.5 g.
otc	**Coppertone Sunless Tanner Spray** (Schering-Plough)	*	**Spray, non-aerosol:** Aloe vera, vitamin E, glycerin	In 118 ml.
otc	**Hawaiian Tropic 45 Plus Sunblock Lip Balm** (Tanning Research)	30+	**Lip balm:** Octyl methoxycinnamate, benzophenone-3, octyl salicylate, titanium dioxide, menthyl anthranilate	PABA free. Waterproof. Tropical, mint and cherry flavors. In 4.2 g.
otc	**Herpecin-L** (Chattem)	30+ / 30	**Lip balm:** 7.5% octyl methoxycycinnamate, 6% oxybenzone, 5% octyl salicylate, 1% dimethicone. Beeswax, petrolatum, zinc oxide	In 2.8 g.
otc	**Blistex Ultra Protection** (Blistex)	30	**Lip balm:** Octyl methoxycinnamate, oxybenzone, octyl salicylate, menthyl anthranilate, homosalate, dimethicone	PABA free. Water resistant. In 4.2 g.
otc	**Coppertone Little Licks** (Schering-Plough)	30	**Lip balm:** Ethylhexyl p-methoxycinnamate, oxybenzone, 2-ethylhexyl salicylate. Paraben, aloe, saccharin	Waterproof. Cherry flavor. In 4.2 g.
otc	**Water Babies Little Licks by Coppertone** (Schering-Plough)	30	**Lip Balm:** Ethylhexyl p-methoxycinnamate, oxybenzone, 2-ethylhexyl salicylate	PABA free. Waterproof. In 4.5 g.
otc	**Stay Moist Lip Conditioner** (Stanback)	15+	**Lip balm:** Padimate O, oxybenzone. Aloe vera, vitamin E	Tropical fruit flavor. In 4.8 g.
otc	**Ti-Screen** (Pedinol)	15+	**Lip balm:** 7.5% ethylhexyl p-methoxycinnamate, 5% oxybenzone. Petrolatum	PABA free. In 4.5 g.
otc	**Catrix Lip Saver** (Donell DerMedex)	15	**Lip Balm:** Allantoin, ethylhexyl p-methoxycinnamate, oxybenzone. Mineral oil, castor oil, petrolatum, vitamin E, propylparaben	PABA free. In 4.5 g.
otc	**ChapStick Sunblock 15 Petroleum Jelly Plus** (Robins)	15	**Ointment:** 89% white petrolatum, 7% padimate O, 3% oxybenzone. Aloe, lanolin	In 10 g.
otc	**Chapstick Sunblock 15** (Robins)	15	**Lip balm:** 7% padimate O, 3% oxybenzone. 0.5% cetyl alcohol, 44% petrolatums, 0.5% lanolin, 0.5% isopropyl myristate, parabens, mineral oil, titanium dioxide	In 4.25 g.
otc	**Eclipse Lip and Face Protectant** (Triangle Labs)	15	**Stick:** Padimate O, oxybenzone	In 4.5 g.
otc	**Neutrogena Lip Moisturizer** (Neutrogena)	15	**Lip balm:** Octyl methoxycinnamate, benzophenone-3. Corn oil, castor oil, mineral oil, lanolin oil, petrolatum, lanolin, stearyl alcohol	PABA free. In 4.5 g.

SUNSCREENS

		SPF		
otc	**Daily Conditioning Treatment** (Blistex)	15	**Lip balm:** 7.5% padimate O, 3.5% oxybenzone, cetyl alcohol, aloe, cocoa butter, lanolin, vitamins A and E, petrolatum	In 7 g.
otc	**Blistex** (Blistex)	10	**Lip balm:** 6.6% padimate O, 2.5% oxybenzone. 2% dimethicone, cocoa butter, lanolin, parabens, mineral oil, petrolatum	Regular, mint, berry flavors. In 4.5 g.

Indications

Sunburn prevention. Overexposure to the sun may cause premature skin aging and skin cancer. The liberal and regular use of these products may help reduce the occurrence of these harmful effects.

For persons with conditions such as systemic lupus erythematosus, solar urticaria, erythropoietic protoporphyria or those taking photosensitizing drugs. Following is a partial list of drugs that may cause photosensitivity:

Antihistamines (eg, cyproheptadine, diphenhydramine)
Anti-infectives (eg, tetracyclines, nalidixic acid, sulfonamides)
Antineoplastic agents (eg, fluorouracil, methotrexate, procarbazine)
Antipsychotic agents (eg, phenothiazines, haloperidol)
Diuretics (eg, thiazides, acetazolamide, amiloride)
Hypoglycemic agents (eg, sulfonylureas)
Nonsteroidal anti-inflammatory drugs (eg, phenylbutazone, ketoprofen, naproxen)
Miscellaneous (eg, bergamot oils, etc, used in cosmetics; coal tar; psoralens; amiodarone; oral contraceptives; quinidine; disopyramide; gold salts; isotretinoin; captopril; carbamazepine)

Administration and Dosage

Apply liberally to all exposed areas (2 mg/cm^2 is recommended) at least 30 minutes prior to sun exposure (up to 2 hours for aminobenzoic acid and its esters) to allow for penetration and binding to the skin. Reapply after swimming or excessive sweating.

▶*Children:* Do not use sunscreens on infants < 6 months old. Do not use SPFs as low as 2 or 3 on children < 2 years of age.

▶*Sun protection factor (SPF):* Sunscreen products include SPF ratings. This factor indicates the amount of increased resistance to sunburning the product provides, relative to unprotected skin. The SPF value is based on a numerical index designed to tell how much protection from the sun a product will provide. The SPF value is defined as the ratio of the amount of energy required to produce a minimal erythema dose (MED) or minimal sunburn through a film of a sunscreen drug product to the amount of energy required to produce the same MED without any treatment. (Example: Using a product with an SPF value of 6 would permit 6 times as much sun exposure.) Base product selection on the patient's history of response to sun exposure.

Recommended Sunscreen Product Guide[1]		
Skin type	Patient characteristics[2]	Suggested product SPF
I	Always burns easily; rarely tans	20 to 30
II	Always burns easily; tans minimally	12 to < 20
III	Burns moderately; tans gradually	8 to < 12
IV	Burns minimally; always tans well	4 to < 8
V	Rarely burns; tans profusely	2 to < 4
VI[3]	Never burns; deeply pigmented (insensitive)	None indicated

[1] Based on the FDA's tentative final monograph (TFM) for sunscreen products.
[2] Based on first 45 to 60 minutes sun exposure after winter season or no sun exposure.
[3] This skin type not included in TFM.

▶*Waterproof formulas:* Maintain sunburn protection after being in the water up to 80 minutes.

▶*Water resistant formulas:* Maintain sunburn protection after being in the water up to 40 minutes.

Sweat resistant formulas – Maintain protection after ≤ 30 minutes of continuous heavy perspiration.

SPFs > 15 were not recommended by the 1978 FDA advisory panel on sunscreens. However, the agency issued a tentative final monograph on this product class in May 1993, and is proposing an upper limit for SPF values of 30. Scientific evidence shows a point of diminishing returns at levels > SPF 30; any benefits that might be derived from using sunscreens with SPFs > 30 are negligible. An SPF of at least 15 for most individuals is recommended by the Skin Cancer Foundation.

In addition to the products listed on the following pages, there are other sunscreens available from various cosmetic manufacturers.

Actions

▶*Pharmacology:* Sunscreens provide either a chemical or a physical barrier to sunlight. These agents help to prevent sunburn, actinic keratosis, premature aging, photosensitivity reactions, and to reduce incidences of skin cancer. Chemical sunscreens act by absorbing ultraviolet (UV) radiation in the medium wavelength range of 290 to 320 nm (UVB range). This is the spectrum of UV radiation primarily responsible for sunburning and inducing skin cancer. UVA may augment the carcinogenic effects of UVB. Long wavelength UV radiation in the 320 to 400 nm (UVA range) can cause tanning and is responsible for most photosensitivity reactions that occur with many drugs, plants, soaps and cosmetics; it is also a major risk factor for serious skin damage. UVA irradiation can exceed that of UVB by 10 to 1000 fold. UVA deeply penetrates into the dermis; UVB is primarily absorbed in the epidermis. There has been discussion of dividing UVA into UVA I (340 to 400 nm) and UVA II (320 to 340 nm); besides UVB, UVA II may cause the most skin damage. Physical sunscreens reflect or scatter light in both the visible and UV spectrum (290 to 700 nm), preventing penetration of the skin.

UV radiation in the 200 to 290 nm band is known as UVC; although little reaches the earth from the sun, some artificial sources emit UVC. UVC is thought to cause some erythema of the skin.

Sunscreen effectiveness is dependent on UV absorption spectrum, concentration, vehicle and ability to withstand swimming or sweating.

Sunscreen Ingredients			
	Sunscreens	UV spectrum (nm)	Concentrations (%)
Chemical	*Benzophenones*	UVA and UVB	
	Oxybenzone	270-350	2-6
	Dioxybenzone	260-380[1]	3
	PABA and PABA esters	UVB	
	p-aminobenzoic acid	260-313	5-15
	Ethyl dihydroxy propyl PABA	280-330	1-5
	Padimate O (octyl dimethyl PABA)	290-315	1.4-8
	Glyceryl PABA	264-315	2-3
	Cinnamates	UVB[2]	
	Cinoxate	270-328	1-3
	Ethylhexyl p-methoxycinnamate	290-320	2-7.5
	Octocrylene	250-360	7-10
	Octyl methoxycinnamate	290-320	—
	Salicylates	UVB[3]	
	Ethylhexyl salicylate	280-320	3-5
	Homosalate	295-315	4-15
	Octyl salicylate	280-320	3-5
	Miscellaneous	UVB	
	Menthyl anthranilate	260-380[4]	3.5-5
	Digalloyl trioleate	270-320	2-5
	Avobenzone (butyl-methoxy-dibenzoylmethane; Parsol 1789)	UVA 320-400	3
Physical	Titanium dioxide	290-700	2-25
	Red petrolatum	290-365[5]	30-100
	Zinc oxide	290-700	—

[1] Values available when used in combination with other screens.
[2] Some UVA spectrum.
[3] Primarily UVB, but has about ⅓ the absorbency of PABA.
[4] Values are for concentrations higher than normally found in nonprescription drugs.
[5] At 334 nm, 16% UV radiation is transmitted; at 365 nm, 58% is transmitted.

Precautions

▶*Sensitivity:* Avoid prolonged exposure to sun and to tanning lamps. Sun-sensitive persons particularly should exercise caution. If irritation or sensitization occurs, discontinue use.

Do not use sunscreens containing PABA or its derivatives if sensitive to benzocaine, procaine, sulfonamides, thiazides, PABA or PABA esters.

▶*For external use only:* Avoid contact with eyes.

▶*Vehicle:* Do not use sunscreens in highly alcoholic vehicles on eczematous or inflamed skin.

▶*PABA:* May cause a permanent yellow stain on clothing.

▶*Vitamin D deficiency:* May occur in elderly patients; sunscreens that block UV-B may block cutaneous vitamin D synthesis.

▶*UV exposure:* The amount of UV exposure is influenced by many factors (eg, time of day, season, latitude, altitude, atmospheric conditions). UVB radiation is strongest between 10 am and 2 pm; UVA is relatively constant. Each 1000 foot increase in altitude adds 4% to UV light intensity. Reflectance from water depends on the angle of exposure, with almost 100% when the sun is directly overhead. Fresh snow reflects approximately 85% to 100% of UV light, and sand reflects 20% to 25%.

Adverse Reactions

Contact dermatitis may develop with PABA or its esters (especially glyceryl PABA), benzophenones and cinnamates. Physical sunscreens are occlusive; miliaria or folliculitis may occur.

SUNSCREENS

Patient Information

Follow directions on product container concerning frequency of application; reapply after swimming or sweating. Reapplication does not extend the protection period.

➤*For external use only:* Do not swallow. Avoid contact with the eyes.

Discontinue use if signs of irritation or rash appear.

PABA may permanently stain clothing yellow.

Wear protective eye coverings or sunglasses; UV light can cause corneal damage.

OINTMENT AND LOTION BASES

otc	**Lanaphilic** (Medco)	**Ointment:** Stearyl alcohol, white petrolatum, isopropyl palmitate, lanolin oil, propylene glycol, sorbitol, sodium lauryl sulfate, parabens	In lb.
otc	**Lanaphilic w/Urea 10%** (Medco)	**Ointment:** Urea, stearyl alcohol, white petrolatum, isopropyl palmitate, lanolin oil, sorbitol, propylene glycol, sodium lauryl sulfate, lactic acid, parabens	In lb.
otc	**Petrolatum** (Carolina Medical)	**Ointment:** Petrolatum, mineral oil, ceresin wax, woolwax alcohol	In 430 g.
otc	**Absorbase** (Carolina Medical)	**Ointment:** Petrolatum, mineral oil, ceresin wax, woolwax alcohol, potassium sorbate	Unscented. In 114 and 454 g.
otc	**Hydrophilic** (Rugby)	**Ointment:** White petrolatum, stearyl alcohol, propylene glycol, sodium lauryl sulfate, parabens	In 454 g.
otc	**Aquabase** (Paddock)	**Ointment:** Petrolatum, mineral oil, mineral wax, woolwax alcohol, sorbitan sesquioleate	Unscented. Dye free. In 454 g.
otc	**Aquaphilic** (Medco)	**Ointment:** Stearyl alcohol, white petrolatum, isopropyl palmitate, sorbitol, propylene glycol, sodium lauryl sulfate, parabens	In lb.
otc	**Aquaphilic w/Carbamide 10% and 20%** (Medco)	**Ointment:** Urea, stearyl alcohol, white petrolatum, isopropyl palmitate, propylene glycol, sorbitol, sodium lauryl sulfate, lactic acid, parabens	In lb.
otc	**Aquaphor Healing Ointment** (Beiersdorf)	**Ointment:** Petrolatum, mineral oil, lanolin, alcohol, panthenol, glycerin.	In 10 and 50 g tubes and 99 and 396 g jars.
otc	**Polyethylene Glycol** (Medco)	**Ointment:** Water soluble greaseless base with PEG-8 and PEG-75	In lb.
otc	**Solumol** (C & M)	**Ointment:** Petrolatum, mineral oil, cetearyl alcohol, sodium lauryl sulfate, glycerin, propylene glycol	In lb.
otc	**Unibase** (Warner Chilcott)	**Ointment:** Nongreasy, water removable base with white petrolatum, glycerin, sodium lauryl sulfate, propylparaben. Will absorb 30% of its weight in water	In lb.
otc	**Acid Mantle** (Doak)	**Cream:** Water, cetearyl alcohol, sodium lauryl sulfate, sodium cetearyl sulfate, glycerin, petrolatum, synthetic beeswax, mineral oil, methylparaben, aluminum sulfate, calcium acetate, white potato dextrin	In 120 g.
otc	**Velvachol** (Owen/Galderma)	**Cream:** Water miscible vehicle containing petrolatum, mineral oil, stearyl alcohol, sodium lauryl sulfate, cholesterol, parabens	In lb.
otc	**Dermabase** (Paddock)	**Cream:** Mineral oil, petrolatum, cetostearyl alcohol, propylene glycol, sodium lauryl sulfate, isopropyl palmitate, imidazolidinyl urea, parabens	In 454 g.
otc	**Dermovan** (Owen/Galderma)	**Cream:** Nonionic, water miscible vanishing cream vehicle containing glyceryl stearate, stearamidoethyl diethylamine, glycerin, mineral oil, cetyl esters, parabens	In lb.
otc	**Hydrocream Base** (Paddock)	**Cream:** Petrolatum, mineral oil, mineral wax, woolwax alcohol, cholesterol, imidazolidinyl urea, parabens	In 454 g.
otc	**Eucerin** (Beiersdorf)	**Cream:** Petrolatum, mineral oil, mineral wax, woolwax alcohol	In 60, 120, 240 and 480 g.
otc	**Hydrocerin** (Geritrex[1])	**Cream:** Petrolatum, mineral oil, lanolin alcohol, parabens	In 120 g.
otc	**Vanicream** (Pharmaceutical Specialties)	**Cream:** White petrolatum, cetearyl alcohol, ceteareth-20, sorbitol solution, propylene glycol, simethicone, glyceryl monostearate, polyethylene glycol monostearate	In 120 g and lb.
otc	**Nutraderm** (Owen/Galderma)	**Lotion:** Mineral oil, sorbitan stearate, stearyl alcohol, sodium lauryl sulfate, cetyl alcohol, carbomer-940, parabens, triethanolamine	In 240 and 480 ml.
otc	**Hydrocerin** (Geritrex[1])	**Lotion:** Mineral oil, lanolin alcohol, parabens	In 473 mL.
otc	**Vehicle/N** (Neutrogena)	**Solution:** 45% SD alcohol 40, laureth-4, propylene glycol, 4% isopropyl alcohol	In 50 ml with applicator.
otc	**Vehicle/N Mild** (Neutrogena)	**Solution:** 37.5% SD alcohol 40, laureth-4, 5% isopropyl alcohol	In 50 ml with applicator.
otc	**Solvent-G** (Syosset)	**Liquid:** 55% SD alcohol 40B, laureth-4, isopropyl alcohol, propylene glycol	In 50 ml.

[1] Geritrex Corp., 144 Kingsbridge Road East, Mt. Vernon, NY 10550; 914-668-4003, fax 914-668-4047.

Indications

►*Uses:* These products are used as bases for incorporation of various active ingredients in extemporaneously compounded dermatological prescriptions.

Indications

These products are used for relief of pain of muscular aches, neuralgia, rheumatism, arthritis, sprains and like conditions, when skin is intact.

Ingredients

Individual components include:

➤*COUNTERIRRITANTS:* Cajuput oil, camphor, capsicum preparations (capsicum oleoresin, capsaicin), eucalyptus oil, menthol, methyl nicotinate, methyl salicylate, mustard oil, wormwood oil.

➤*ANTISEPTICS:* Chloroxylenol, thymol.

➤*ANALGESIC:* Trolamine salicylate.

Contraindications

Allergy to components of any formulation or to salicylates.

Warnings

➤*For external use only:* Avoid contact with eyes and mucous membranes.

Precautions

➤*Apply to affected parts only:* Do not apply to irritated skin; if excessive irritation develops, discontinue use. If pain persists for more than 7 to 10 days, or if redness is present, or in conditions affecting children < 10 years of age, consult a physician.

➤*Heat therapy:* Do not use an external source of heat (eg, heating pad) with these agents since irritation or burning of the skin may occur.

➤*Protective covering:* Applying a tight bandage or wrap over these agents is not recommended since increased absorption may occur.

Drug Interactions

➤*Anticoagulants:* An enhanced anticoagulant effect (eg, increased prothrombin time) occurred in several patients receiving an anticoagulant and using topical methylsalicylate concurrently.

Adverse Reactions

If applied to large skin areas, salicylate side effects may occur, such as tinnitus, nausea or vomiting. Toxic if ingested.

Counterirritants may cause local irritation, especially in patients with sensitive skin.

GELS, CREAMS AND OINTMENTS

otc	**Aspercreme Cream** (Chattem)	10% trolamine salicylate	In 37.5, 90 and 150 g.
otc	**Flex-Power Performance Sports** (Flex-Power)		Cetyl alcohol, EDTA, parabens, glycerols, stearyl alcohol, sodium metabisulfite. Citrus light and clean scents. In 120 g.
otc	**Mobisyl Creme** (Ascher)		In 35.4, 100 and 227 g.
otc	**Myoflex Creme** (Fisons)		In 60, 120 and 240 g and lb.
otc	**Sportscreme** (Chattem)		In 37.5 and 90 g.
otc	**Panalgesic Cream** (E.C. Robins/Poythress)	35% methyl salicylate, 4% menthol	In 120 g.
otc	**Icy Hot Cream** (Chattem)	30% methyl salicylate, 10% menthol, carbomer, cetyl esters wax, emulsifying wax, trolamine	In 37.5 and 90 g.
otc	**ArthriCare Triple-Medicated Gel** (Commerce)	30% methyl salicylate, 1.25% menthol, 0.7% methyl nicotinate, isopropyl alcohol, propylene glycol, hydroxypropylmethylcellulose, DSS	In 90 g.
otc	**Musterole Deep Strength Rub** (Schering-Plough)	30% methyl salicylate, 0.5% methyl nicotinate and 3% menthol	In 37 and 90 g.
otc	**Ben-Gay Ultra Strength Cream** (Pfizer)	30% methyl salicylate, 10% menthol, 4% camphor, EDTA, glyceryl stearate SE, anhydrous lanolin, polysorbate 80, potassium carbomer and stearate, triethanolamine carbomer and stearate	In 35 g.
otc	**Arthritis Formula Ben-Gay** (Pfizer)	30% methyl salicylate, 8% menthol, glyceryl stearate SE, anhydrous lanolin, polysorbate 85, potassium stearate, sorbitan tristearate, xanthan gum	In 35 g.
otc	**Exocaine Plus Rub** (Commerce Drug)	30% methyl salicylate	In 39 and 120 g.
otc	**Icy Hot Stick** (Chattem)	30% methyl salicylate, 10% menthol, ceresin, cyclomethicone, hydrogenated castor oil, microcrystalline wax, paraffin, PEG-150 distearate, propylene glycol	In 52.5 g.
otc	**Icy Hot Balm** (Chattem)	29% methyl salicylate, 7.6% menthol, paraffin, white petrolatum	In 105 g.
otc	**Exocaine Medicated Rub** (Commerce)	25% methyl salicylate, clove oil, eucalyptus oil, lanolin, cetyl alcohol, glycerin, glyceryl, menthol, parabens	In 120 g.
otc	**Improved Analgesic Ointment** (Rugby)	18.3% methyl salicylate, 16% menthol	In 36, 85 and 454 g.
otc	**Ben-Gay Original Ointment** (Pfizer)	18.3% methyl salicylate, 16% menthol, anhydrous lanolin, microcrystalline wax, synthetic bees wax	In 35 and 90 g.
otc	**Pain Bust·RII** (Continental)	17% methyl salicylate, 12% menthol	In 90 g.
otc	**Arthritis Hot Creme** (Chattem)	15% methyl salicylate, 10% menthol, glyceryl stearate, carbomer 934, lanolin, PEG-100 stearate, propylene glycol, trolamine, parabens	In 90 g.
otc	**Icy Hot Arthritis Therapy Gel** (Chattem)	0.025% capsaicin, parabens, aloe vera, alcohol, wax, soybean oil	In 70.8 g.
otc	**Deep-Down Rub** (SK-Beecham)	15% methyl salicylate, 5% menthol, 0.5% camphor, 40.5% SD alcohol	In 37.5 and 90 g.
otc	**Minit-Rub** (Bristol-Myers)	15% methyl salicylate, 3.5% menthol, 2.3% camphor, anhydrous lanolin	In 45 and 90 g.
otc	**Thera-gesic Cream** (Mission)	15% methyl salicylate, menthol, dimethylpolysiloxane, glycerin, carbopol, triethanolamine, parabens	In 90 and 150 g.
otc	**Ziks Cream** (Nodum)	12% methyl salicylate, 1% menthol, 0.025% capsaicin, cetyl alcohol	In 60 g.
otc	**Gordogesic Creme** (Gordon)	10% methyl salicylate, propylene glycol, mineral oil, white wax, triethanolamine, parabens	In 75 g and lb.
otc	**Methagual** (Gordon)	8% methyl salicylate, 2% guaiacol, petrolatum, white wax, parabens	In 60 g and lb.
otc	**Blue Gel Muscular Pain Reliever** (Rugby)	Menthol	In 240 g.
otc	**Eucalyptamint Maximum Strength Ointment** (Ciba)	16% menthol, lanolin, eucalyptus oil	In 60 ml.
otc	**Flexall Ultra Plus** (Chattem)	16% menthol, 10% methyl salicylate, 3.1% camphor in aloe vera gel base, eucalyptus oil, glycerin, peppermint oil, alcohol	In 70.8 g.
otc	**Maximum Strength Flexall 454** (Chattem)	16% menthol, aloe vera gel, eucalyptus oil, methyl salicylate, peppermint oil, SD alcohol 38-B, thyme oil	In 90 g.

GELS, CREAMS AND OINTMENTS

otc	**Bayer Muscle and Joint Cream** (Bayer)	10% menthol, 4% camphor, 30% methyl salicylate, EDTA, glyceryl, lanolin, stearyl alcohol	In 56 and 114 g
otc	**Ben Gay SPA Cream** (Pfizer)	10% menthol	In 57 g.
otc	**Eucalyptamint Gel** (Ciba Consumer)	8% menthol, eucalyptus oil, SD 3A alcohol	In 60 g.
otc	**Wonder Ice Gel** (Pedinol)	5.25% menthol	In 113 and 473 g.
otc	**Double Ice ArthriCare Gel** (Commerce)	4% menthol, 3.1% camphor, aloe vera gel, carbomer 940, dioctylsodium sulfosuccinate, isopropyl alcohol, propylene glycol, triethanolamine	In 90 g.
otc	**Absorbine Power Gel** (W.F. Young)	4% menthol	In 88 g.
otc	**Pain Gel Plus** (Mentholatum Co.)	4% menthol, aloe, vitamin E	In 57 g.
otc	**Vanishing Scent Ben-Gay** (Pfizer)	2.5% menthol, alcohol, camphor	In 120 g.
otc	**Odor Free ArthriCare Rub** (Commerce)	1.25% menthol, 0.25% methyl nicotinate, 0.025% capsaicin, aloe vera gel, carbomer 940, DMDM hydantoin, emulsifying wax, glyceryl stearate SE, isopropyl alcohol, myristyl propionate, propylparaben, triethanolamine	In 90 g.
otc	**Soltice Quick-Rub** (Chattem)	Methyl salicylate, camphor, menthol, eucalyptus oil, glycerin, oleic acid	In 40 and 112 g.
otc	**Dermal-Rub Balm** (Hauck)	Methyl salicylate, camphor, racemic menthol, cajuput oil	In 30 g and lb.
otc	**Analgesic Balm** (Various, eg, URL)	Methyl salicylate, menthol	In 30 and 454 g.
otc	**Argesic Cream** (Econo Med)	Methyl salicylate, triethanolamine	Vanishing base. In 60 g.
otc	**TheraFlu Vapor Stick Cough & Muscle Aches** (Novartis)	4.8% camphor, 2.6% menthol, cetyl alcohol, eucalyptus oil, parabens	In 51 g.
otc	**Vicks VapoRub Cream** (Richardson-Vicks)	4.7% camphor, 2.6% menthol, 1.2% eucalyptus oil, cedarleaf oil, EDTA, glycerin, imidazolidinyl urea, cetyl and stearyl alcohols, parabens, nutmeg oil, titanium dioxide, spirits of turpentine	In 45, 60, 90 and 180 g.
otc	**Methalgen Cream** (Alra)	Camphor, menthol, methyl salicylate, oil of mustard	In 60 and 480 g.
otc	**Therapeutic Mineral Ice Exercise Formula Gel** (Bristol-Myers)	4% menthol, ammonium hydroxide, carbomer 934P or 934, cupric sulfate, isopropyl alcohol, thymol	In 90 g.
otc	**Ben-Gay Vanishing Scent Gel** (Pfizer)	3% menthol, benzophenone-4, camphor, diazolidinyl urea, EDTA, isopropyl alcohol, potassium carbomer 940	In 35 g.
otc	**Sportscreme Ice Gel** (Thompson)	2% menthol, carbomer 934, styrene/acrylate copolymer, triethanolamine, 38% SD alcohol 40	In 227 g.
otc	**Therapeutic Mineral Ice Gel** (Bristol-Myers)	2% menthol, ammonium hydroxide, carbomer 934, cupric sulfate, isopropyl alcohol, thymol	In 105, 240 and 480 g.
otc	**Flex-all 454 Gel** (Chattem)	Menthol in an aloe vera gel, methyl salicylate, alcohol, allantoin, boric acid, carbomer 940, diazolidinyl urea, iodine, polysorbate 60, propylene glycol, potassium iodide, triethanolamine, eucalyptus oil, glycerin, parabens	In 60, 120 and 240 g.
otc	**Eucalyptamint** (Ciba Consumer)	**Gel:** 8% menthol	

LIQUIDS

otc	**Extra Strength Absorbine Jr. Liquid** (W.F. Young)	4% menthol	In 59 and 118 ml.

LOTIONS AND LINIMENTS

otc	**Aspercreme Rub Lotion** (Thompson)	10% trolamine salicylate, cetyl alcohol, glyceryl stearate, lanolin, parabens, potassium phosphate, propylene glycol, sodium lauryl sulfate, stearic acid	In 180 ml.
otc	**Panalgesic Gold Liniment** (ECR Pharm)	55% methyl salicylate, 3.1% camphor, 1.25% menthol, 18.6% emollient oils, 22% alcohol	In 120 ml.
otc	**Gordobalm** (Gordon)	Menthol, camphor, methyl salicylate, 16% isopropyl alcohol, tragacanth, thymol, acetone, eucalyptus oil, tartrazine	In 120 ml and gal.
otc	**Heet Liniment** (Whitehall)	15% methyl salicylate, 3.6% camphor, capsicum oleoresin (as 0.025% capsaicin), acetone, 70% alcohol	In 68.5 and 150 ml.
otc	**Banalg Hospital Strength Lotion** (Forest)	14% methyl salicylate, 3% menthol	In 60 ml.
otc	**Banalg Lotion** (Forest)	4.9% methyl salicylate, 2% camphor, 1% menthol	In 60 and 480 ml.
otc	**Extra Strength Absorbine Jr.** (W.F. Young)	4% natural menthol	In 60 ml.
otc	**Absorbine Jr. Liniment** (W.F. Young)	1.27% menthol, plant extracts of calendula, echinacea and wormwood, iodine, potassium iodide, thymol, acetone, chloroxylenol	In 60 and 120 ml.
otc	**Arth-Rx Topical Analgesic Lotion** (Phillips Gulf)	0.5% methyl nicotinate, 0.025% capsaicin, aloe vera gel, extracts of arnica, rue, chamomile, boswellia	In 90 ml roll-on applicator.
otc	**Yager's Liniment** (Oakhurst Company)	3.1% camphor, 8.3% turpentine, clove oil	In 120 and 240 ml.

SPRAYS

otc	**Sports Spray** (Mentholatum)	35% methyl salicylate, 10% menthol, 5% camphor, 58% alcohol	In 85 g.

PATCHES

otc	**BENGAY** (Pfizer)	**Patch:** 1.4% menthol	Glycerin. In regular and large sizes. In 1s.

TOPICAL COMBINATIONS, MISCELLANEOUS

otc	**Boyol Salve** (Pfeiffer)	**Salve:** 10% ichthammol, benzocaine, lanolin, petrolatum	In 30 g.
otc	**Wonderful Dream** (Wonderful Dream Salve Corp.)	**Salve:** Phenyl mercury nitrate 1:5000, oil of tar, turpentine, olive oil, linseed oil, posin, burgundy pitch, camphor, beeswax, mutton tallow	In 34 g.
otc	**Dr. Dermi-Heal** (Quality)	**Ointment:** 1% allantoin, zinc oxide, Balsam Peru, castor oil, petrolatum *For relief of diaper rash, chafing, minor burns, bed sores, external vaginal itching and irritation, ostomy irritation and heat rash.*	In 75 g.
otc	**Saratoga** (Blair)	**Ointment:** Zinc oxide, boric acid, eucalyptol, acetylated lanolin alcohols, white petrolatum, white beeswax *For temporary relief of itching and minor skin irritations, chapped and chafed skin, diaper rash, bed sores, mild burns.*	In 28 and 60 g.
otc	**Unguentine** (Mentholatum)	**Ointment:** 1% phenol, petrolatum, oleostearine, zinc oxide, eucalyptus oil, thyme oil *For pain relief in minor burns.*	In 30 g.
otc	**Amerigel** (Amerx Health Care Corp.)	**Ointment:** Meadowsweet extract, oakbark extract, polyethylene glycol 400, polyethylene glycol 3350, zinc acetate. *For stage I-IV pressure ulcers, stasis ulcers, diabetic skin ulcers, post-surgical incisions, 1st and 2nd degree burns, cuts, and abrasions.*	In 28.3 g.
otc	**Ostiderm** (Pedinol)	**Lotion:** Aluminum sulfate, zinc oxide *For foot odor/excessive moisture.*	In 42.5 ml.
		Roll-On: Aluminum chlorohydrate, camphor, alcohol, EDTA, diazolidinyl urea, *Safeguards against offensive odor and dries excessive moisture of the feet.*	In 88.7 ml.
otc	**Sarna Anti-Itch** (Stiefel)	**Lotion:** 0.5% camphor, 0.5% menthol, carbomer 940, DMDM hydantoin, glyceryl stearate, PEG-8 stearate, PEG-100 stearate, petrolatum *For relief of dry, itching skin, sunburn, poison ivy and poison oak.*	In 222 ml.
otc	**Schamberg's** (C & M)	**Lotion:** Zinc oxide, 0.15% menthol, 1% phenol, peanut oil and lime water *For the temporary relief of itching.*	In 480 ml.
otc	**Soothaderm** (Pharmakon)	**Lotion:** 2.07 mg pyrilamine maleate, 2.08 mg benzocaine and 41.35 mg zinc oxide per ml, simethicone, parabens, propylene glycol, camphor, menthol *For relief of itching due to chickenpox, diaper rash, insect bites, poison ivy/oak, prickly heat and sunburn.*	In 118 ml.
otc	**Florida Sunburn Relief** (Pharmacel)	**Lotion:** 3% benzyl alcohol, 0.4% phenol, 0.2% camphor, 0.15% menthol *For relief of pain due to sunburn.*	In 60 ml.
otc	**Outgro** (Whitehall)	**Solution:** 25% tannic acid, 5% chlorobutanol, 83% isopropyl alcohol *For temporary pain relief of ingrown toenails.*	In 9.3 ml.
otc	**Stypto-Caine** (Pedinol)	**Solution:** 250 mg aluminum chloride, 2.5 mg tetracaine HCl, 1 mg oxyquinoline sulfate per g with glycerin *To stop bleeding in minor cuts.*	In 59 ml.
otc	**Campho-Phenique** (Sterling Health)	**Liquid:** 10.8% camphor, 4.7% phenol, eucalyptus oil, light mineral oil *To relieve pain and combat infections.*	In 22.5, 45 and 120 ml.
otc	**Oxyzal Wet Dressing** (Gordon)	**Liquid:** Oxyquinoline sulfate, benzalkonium Cl 1:2000 *For minor infections.*	In 30, 120 and 480 ml.
otc	**Campho-Phenique** (Sterling Health)	**Gel:** 4.7% phenol, 10.8% camphor, colloidal silicon dioxide, eucalyptus oil, glycerin, light mineral oil *Pain relief in cold sores, fever blisters, cuts, scrapes, burns and insect bites.*	In 6.9 and 15 g.
otc	**Topic** (Syntex)	**Gel:** 5% benzyl alcohol, camphor, menthol, 30% isopropyl alcohol *For temporary relief of itching from poison oak/ivy, insect bites, eczema, minor skin allergies and heat rash.*	In 60 g.
otc	**Mederma** (Merz)	**Gel:** Water (purified), PEG-4, onion (allium cepa) extract, xanthan gum, allantoin, fragrance, methylparaben, sorbic acid. *Helps scars appear softer and smoother.*	In 50g.
otc	**Aluminum Paste** (Paddock)	**Ointment:** 10% metallic aluminum *An occlusive skin protectant.*	White petrolatum base. In lb.
otc	**Sarna Anti-Itch** (Stiefel)	**Foam:** 0.5% camphor, 0.5% menthol, carbomer 940, DMDM hydantoin, glyceryl stearate, PEG-8 and PEG-100 stearate, petrolatum *For relief of dry, itching skin.*	In 99 g.
otc	**ProTech First-Aid Stik** (Triton)	**Liquid:** 10% povidone-iodine, 2.5% lidocaine HCl *For cleaning and pain relief of cuts, scrapes and burns.*	In 14 ml.
otc	**Proderm Topical** (Dow B. Hickam)	**Dressing:** 650 mg castor oil and 72.5 mg Balsam Peru per 0.82 ml *For prevention and management of decubitus ulcers.*	In 113.4 g.
otc	**Dome-Paste** (Miles)	**Wound dressing:** Zinc oxide, calamine, gelatin *For conditions of extremities (eg, varicose ulcers) requiring protection.*	3″ by 10 yd or 4″ by 10 yd bandages.
otc	**Columbia Antiseptic Powder** (F.C. Sturtevant[1])	**Powder:** Zinc oxide, talc, carbolic acid, boric acid.	In 30 and 420 g.
Rx	**Scarlet Red Ointment Dressings** (Sherwood Medical)	**Wound dressings:** 5% scarlet red, lanolin, olive oil and petrolatum in fine mesh absorbent gauze *For epithelialization of donor sites, burns and wounds.*	In 5″ x 9″ strips.

[1] The F.C. Sturtevant Company, P.O. Box 607, Bronxville, NY 10708; 914-337-5131, 888-871-5661; fax 914-337-5309; http://www.columbiapowder.com

Ingredients

Principal active ingredients of these formulations include:

➤**BORIC ACID, OXYQUINOLINE and BENZALKONIUM Cl:** Used as antiseptics.

➤**ZINC OXIDE and ALUMINUM:** Provide astringent and topical protectant actions.

➤**CAMPHOR, EUCALYPTOL, MENTHOL and PHENOL:** Used as antipruritics, mild local anesthetics and counterirritants.

➤**BENZOCAINE and LIDOCAINE:** Local anesthetics.

➤**PYRILAMINE MALEATE:** An antihistamine.

➤**CASTOR OIL (RICINUS OIL), GLYCERIN and MINERAL OIL:** Used as emollients.

➤**BENZYL ALCOHOL:** Used as an antipruritic.

➤**BISMUTH SUBNITRATE:** Used as a skin protectant.

➤**BALSAM PERU:** Used to stimulate tissue growth.

➤**BIEBRICH SCARLET RED:** Used to promote wound healing.

➤**ICHTHAMMOL:** Used as an anti-infective.

FLEXIBLE HYDROACTIVE DRESSINGS AND GRANULES

otc	**IntraSite** (Smith & Nephew)	**Gel:** 2% graft T starch copolymer, 78% water, 20% propylene glycol. Sterile amorphous hydrogel dressing	In UD 25 g (10s).
otc	**Shur-Clens** (Calgon Vestal)	**Solution:** 20% poloxamer 188	In UD 100 and 200 ml.
otc	**FlexiGel Strands** (Smith-Nephew)	**Absorbent wound dressing**	Single-use absorbent matrix. 6 g unit. In 10s.
otc	**DuoDerm** (ConvaTec)	**Dressings, sterile:** 4″ x 4″, 6″ x 8″, 8″ x 8″ and 8″ x 12″	In 3s (8″ x 12″ only), 5s and 20s
		Dressing, adhesive border: 4″ x 4″ 8″ x 8″	In 5s. In 3s.
		Granules, sterile: 5 g per tube	In 5s.
		Paste, sterile	In 30 g tube.
otc	**DuoDerm CGF** (ConvaTec)	**Control gel formula dressing, sterile:** 4″ x 4″, 6″ x 6″, 8″ x 8″	In 5s.
		Control gel formula border dressing, sterile: 2.5″ x 2.5″, 4″ x 4″, 6″ x 6″, 4″ x 5″, 6″ x 7″ with adhesive borders	In 5s.
otc	**DuoDerm Extra Thin** (ConvaTec)	**Control gel formula dressing, extra thin, sterile:** 4″ x 4″, 6″ x 6″	In 10s.
otc	**Sorbsan** (Dow B. Hickam)	**Pads, sterile:** Calcium alginate fiber 2″ x 2″, 3″ x 3″, 4″ x 4″ and 4″ x 8″	In 1s.
		Wound packing fibers, sterile: Calcium alginate fiber. 12″ (2 g)	In 1s.

Indications

➤*Dressings:* For the local management of: Dermal ulcers; pressure ulcers; leg ulcers; superficial wounds (eg, minor abrasions, donor sites, second-degree burns); protective dressings; postoperative wounds.

➤*Granules:* For use in the local management of exudating dermal ulcers in association with the dressings.

➤*Paste:* For use in association with *DuoDerm* dressings for local management of exudating dermal ulcers.

Administration and Dosage

Clean and prepare the wound site before application. See package labeling for wound management and application/removal instructions for the dressing and granules. Dressings are designed to remain in place from 1 to 7 days.

Actions

➤*Pharmacology:* The dressings interact with wound exudate producing a soft moist gel at the wound surface enabling removal of the dressing with little or no damage to newly formed tissues. They are designed to remain in place from 1 to 7 days.

Contraindications

Dermal ulcers involving muscle, tendon or bone; ulcers resulting from infection, such as tuberculosis, syphilis and deep fungal infections; lesions in patients with active vasculitis, such as periarteritis nodosa, systemic lupus erythematosus and cryoglobulinemia; third-degree burns; clinically infected wounds.

Precautions

➤*Excess exudate:* In the presence of excess exudate, the ability of the dressings to remain in place with less frequent leakage may be improved by applying the granules directly into the wound site. Used in this way, with the dressings, the granules may reduce the frequency of dressing change.

➤*Odor:* Wounds often have a characteristic disagreeable odor. The odor usually disappears following wound cleansing.

➤*Wound deterioration:* When using any occlusive dressing, the wound will increase in size and depth during the initial phase as the necrotic debris is cleaned away.

➤*Infection:* If clinical infection develops, discontinue DuoDerm and institute appropriate treatment. Restart *DuoDerm* when the infection has been eradicated.

PHYSIOLOGICAL IRRIGATING SOLUTIONS

Rx	**0.45% Sodium Chloride Irrigation** (Abbott)	**Solution:** 450 mg sodium chloride per 100 ml	In 250 and 500 ml and 1, 1.5, 2 and 3 L.
Rx	**0.9% Sodium Chloride Irrigation** (Abbott)	**Solution:** 900 mg sodium chloride per 100 ml	In 100, 250 and 500 ml and 1, 1.5, 2 and 3 L.
Rx	**Ringer's Irrigation** (Various, eg, McGaw)	**Solution:** 860 mg sodium chloride, 30 mg potassium chloride, 33 mg calcium chloride per 100 ml	In 1 L.
Rx	**Tis-U-Sol** (Baxter)	**Solution:** 800 mg NaCl, 40 mg KCl, 20 mg magnesium sulfate, 8.75 mg dibasic sodium phosphate heptahydrate and 6.25 mg monobasic potassium phosphate per 100 ml	In 1 L.
Rx	**Lactated Ringer's Irrigation** (Abbott)	**Solution:** 600 mg sodium chloride, 310 mg sodium lactate, anhydrous, 30 mg potassium chloride, 20 mg calcium chloride, dihydrate per 100 ml	In 300 ml.
Rx	**Physiolyte** (American McGaw)	**Solution:** 530 mg NaCl, 370 mg sodium acetate, 500 mg sodium gluconate, 37 mg KCl and 30 mg magnesium Cl per 100 ml	In 1 L.
Rx	**PhysioSol** (Abbott)	**Solution:** 526 mg NaCl, 222 mg sodium acetate, 502 mg sodium gluconate, 37 mg KCl and 30 mg magnesium chloride hexahydrate per 100 ml	In 250 and 500 ml and 1 L.
Rx	**Cytosol** (Cytosol Ophthalmics)	**Solution:** 48 mg calcium chloride, 30 mg magnesium chloride, 75 mg potassium chloride, 390 mg sodium acetate, 640 mg sodium chloride, 170 mg sodium citrate per 100 ml	In 200 and 500 ml.
Rx	**Saf-Clens** (Calgon Vestal)	**Spray:** Meroxapol 105, NaCl, potassium sorbate NF, DMDM hydantoin	In 177 ml.

Indications

For general irrigation, washing and rinsing purposes which permit use of a sterile, nonpyrogenic electrolyte solution.

Administration and Dosage

The dose depends on the capacity or surface area of the structure to be irrigated and the nature of the procedure. When used as a vehicle for other drugs, follow manufacturer's recommendations.

➤*Storage/Stability:* Avoid excessive heat. Do not freeze. Store at 25°C (77°F); however, brief exposure to 40°C (104°F) does not cause adverse effects.

Contraindications

Irrigation during electrosurgical procedures.

Warnings

➤*For irrigation only:* Not for injection.

➤*Absorption:* Irrigating fluids enter the systemic circulation in relatively large volumes and must be regarded as a systemic drug. Absorption of large amounts can cause fluid or solute overloading resulting in dilution of serum electrolyte concentrations, overhydration, congested states or pulmonary edema.

➤*Dilutional states:* The risk of dilutional states is inversely proportional to the electrolyte concentrations of administered parenteral solutions. The risk of solute overload causing congested states with peripheral and pulmonary edema is directly proportional to the electrolyte concentrations of such solutions.

➤*Do not heat:* Do not heat to > 66°C (> 150°F).

➤*Pregnancy: Category C.* It is not known whether these solutions can cause fetal harm when administered to a pregnant woman or can affect reproduction capacity. Give to a pregnant woman only if clearly needed.

Precautions

➤*Continuous irrigation:* Observe caution when solution is used for continuous irrigation or allowed to "dwell" inside body cavities because of possible absorption into the blood stream and circulatory overload.

➤*Aseptic technique:* This is essential for irrigation of body cavities, wounds and urethral catheters or for wetting dressings that come in contact with body tissues.

➤*Accidental contamination:* Careless technique may transmit infection.

➤*Containers:* When used as a "pour" irrigation, do not allow any part of the contents to contact the surface below the outer protected thread area of the semi-rigid wide mouth container. When used via irrigation equipment, attach the administration set promptly. Discard unused portions and use a fresh container for the start-up of each cycle or repeat procedure. For repeated irrigations of urethral catheters, use a separate container for each patient.

➤*Displaced catheters/drainage tubes:* This can lead to irrigation or infiltration of unintended structures or cavities.

➤*Additives:* May be incompatible. When introducing additives, use aseptic technique, mix thoroughly and do not store.

➤*Tissue distention/disruption:* Excessive volume or pressure during irrigation of closed cavities may cause undue distention or disruption of tissues.

Adverse Reactions

Should any adverse reaction occur, discontinue the irrigant, evaluate the patient, institute appropriate countermeasures and save the remainder of the fluid for examination.

Overdosage

In overhydration or solute overload, reevaluate and institute corrective measures.

►*General Considerations in Topical Ophthalmic Drug Therapy:* Proper administration is essential to optimal therapeutic response. In many instances, health professionals may be too casual when instructing patients on proper use of ophthalmics. The administration technique used often determines drug safety and efficacy.

• The normal eye retains ≈ 10 mcL of fluid (adjusted for blinking). The average dropper delivers 25 to 50 mcL/drop. The value of more than one drop is questionable.

• Minimize systemic absorption of ophthalmic drops by compressing lacrimal sac for 3 to 5 minutes after instillation. This retards passage of drops via nasolacrimal duct into areas of potential absorption such as nasal and pharyngeal mucosa.

• Because of rapid lacrimal drainage and limited eye capacity, if multiple drop therapy is indicated, the best interval between drops is 5 minutes. This ensures that the first drop is not flushed away by the second or that the second is not diluted by the first.

• Topical anesthesia will increase the bioavailability of ophthalmic agents by decreasing the blink reflex and the production and turnover of tears.

• Factors that may increase absorption from ophthalmics include lax eyelids of some patients, usually the elderly, which creates a greater reservoir for retention of drops, and hyperemic or diseased eyes.

• Eyecup use is discouraged due to risk of contamination.

• Ophthalmic suspensions mix with tears less rapidly and remain in the cul-de-sac longer than solutions.

• Ophthalmic ointments maintain contact between the drug and ocular tissues by slowing the clearance rate to as little as 0.5% per minute. Ophthalmic ointments provide maximum contact between drug and external ocular tissues.

• Ophthalmic ointments may impede delivery of other ophthalmic drugs to the affected side by serving as a barrier to contact.

• Ointments may blur vision during the waking hours. Use with caution in conditions where visual clarity is critical (eg, operating motor equipment, reading) or use at bedtime.

• Monitor expiration dates closely. Do not use outdated medication.

• Solutions and ointments are frequently misused. Do not assume that patients know how to maximize safe and effective use of these agents. Combine appropriate patient education and counseling with prescribing and dispensing of ophthalmics.

Topical application is the most common route of administration for ophthalmic drugs. Advantages include convenience, simplicity, noninvasive nature and the ability of the patient to self-administer. Because of blood and aqueous losses of drug, topical medications do not typically penetrate in useful concentrations to posterior ocular structures and therefore are of no therapeutic benefit for diseases of retina, optic nerve and other posterior segment structures.

►*Ingredients:* The following inactive agents may be present in ophthalmic products:

PRESERVATIVES – Preservatives destroy or inhibit multiplication of microorganisms introduced into the product by accident and are as follows:

Benzalkonium Cl, benzethonium Cl, cetylpyridinium Cl, chlorobutanol, EDTA, mercurial preservatives (phenylmercuric nitrate, phenyl mercuric acetate, thimerosal), methyl/propylparabens, phenylethyl alcohol, sodium benzoate, sodium propionate, sorbic acid.

VISCOSITY-INCREASING AGENTS – Viscosity-increasing agents slow drainage of the product from the eye, thus increasing retention time of the active drug. Increased bioavailability may result. Viscosity-increasing agents are as follows:

Carboxymethylcellulose sodium, dextran 70, gelatin, glycerin, hydroxyethylcellulose, hydroxypropyl methylcellulose, methylcellulose, PEG, poloxamer 407, polysorbate 80, propylene glycol, polyvinyl alcohol, polyvinylpyrrolidone (povidone).

ANTIOXIDANTS – Antioxidants prevent or delay deterioration of products by oxygen in the air and are as follows:

EDTA, sodium bisulfite, sodium metabisulfite, sodium thiosulfate, thiourea.

WETTING AGENTS – Wetting agents reduce surface tension, allowing drug solution to spread over eye and are as follows:

Polysorbate 20 and 80, poloxamer 282, tyloxapol.

BUFFERS – Buffers help maintain ophthalmic products in the range of pH 6 to 8, which is the comfortable range for ophthalmic instillation and are as follows:

Acetic acid, boric acid, phosphoric acid, potassium bicarbonate, potassium borate and tetraborate, potassium carbonate, potassium citrate, potassium phosphates, sodium acetate, sodium bicarbonate, sodium biphosphate, sodium borate, sodium carbonate, sodium citrate, sodium hydroxide, sodium phosphate, hydrochloric acid.

TONICITY AGENTS – Tonicity agents help the ophthalmic product solutions to be isotonic with natural tears. Products in the sodium chloride equivalence range of 0.9% ± 0.2% are considered isotonic and will help prevent ocular pain and tissue damage. A range of 0.6% to 1.8% is usually comfortable for ophthalmic use. Tonicity agents are as follows:

Buffers, dextran 40 and 70, dextrose, glycerin, potassium Cl, propylene glycol, sodium Cl.

►*Packaging Standards:* To help reduce confusion in labeling and identification of various topical ocular medications, drug packaging standards have been proposed. When fully implemented by the ophthalmic drug industry, the standard colors for drug labels and bottle caps will include the following:

Ophthalmic Drug Packaging Standards	
Therapeutic class	Proposed color
Beta blockers	Yellow, blue or both
Mydriatics and cycloplegics	Red
Miotics	Green
Nonsteroidal anti-inflammatory agents	Grey
Anti-infectives	Brown, tan

►*Medications:*

Solutions and suspensions – Most topical ocular preparations are commercially available as solutions or suspensions that are applied directly to the eye from the bottle, which serves as the eye dropper. Avoid touching the dropper tip to the eye because this can lead to contamination of the medication and may also cause ocular injury. Resuspend suspensions (notably, many ocular steroids) by shaking to provide an accurate dosage of drug.

Recommended procedures for administration of solutions or suspensions –

• Wash hands thoroughly before administration.

• Tilt head backward or lie down and gaze upward.

• Gently grasp lower eyelid below eyelashes and pull the eyelid away from the eye to form a pouch.

• Place dropper directly over eye. Avoid contact of the dropper with the eye, finger or any surface.

• Look upward just before applying a drop.

• After instilling the drop, look downward for several seconds.

• Release the lid slowly and close eyes gently.

• With eyes closed, apply gentle pressure with fingers to the inside corner of eye for 3 to 5 min. This retards drainage of solution from intended solution.

• Do not rub the eye or squeeze the eyelid. Minimize blinking.

• Do not rinse the dropper.

• Do not use eye drops that have changed color or contain a precipitate.

• If more than one type of ophthalmic drop is used, wait ≥ 5 minutes before administering the second agent.

• When the instillation of eye drops is difficult (eg, pediatric patients, adults with particularly strong blink reflex), the close-eye method may be used. This involves lying down, placing the prescribed number of drops on the eyelid in the inner corner of the eye, then opening eye so that drops will fall into the eye by gravity.

Ointments – The primary purpose for an ophthalmic ointment vehicle is to prolong drug contact time with the external ocular surface. This is particularly useful for treating children, who may "cry out" topically applied solutions, and for medicating ocular injuries, such as corneal abrasions, when the eye is to be patched. Administer solutions before ointments. Ointments preclude entry of subsequent drops.

Recommended procedures for administration of ointments –

• Wash hands thoroughly before administration.

• Holding the ointment tube in the hand for a few minutes will warm the ointment and facilitate flow.

• When opening the ointment tube for the first time, squeeze out and discard the first 0.25 inch of ointment as it may be too dry.

• Tilt head backward or lie down and gaze upward.

• Gently pull down the lower eyelid to form a pouch.

• Place 0.25 to 0.5 inch of ointment with a sweeping motion inside the lower eyelid by squeezing the tube gently and slowly release the eyelid.

• Close the eye for 1 to 2 minutes and roll the eyeball in all directions.

• Temporary blurring of vision may occur. Avoid activities requiring visual acuity until blurring clears.

• Remove excessive ointment around the eye or ointment tube tip with a tissue.

• If using more than one kind of ointment, wait about 10 minutes before applying the second drug.

Gels – Ophthalmic gels are similar in viscosity and clinical usage to ophthalmic ointments. Pilocarpine (*Pilopine HS*) is currently the only ophthalmic preparation available in gel form, and it is intended to serve as a "sustained-release" pilocarpine, requiring only once-daily administration (at bedtime).

Sprays – Although not commercially available, some practitioners use mydriatics or cycloplegics, alone or in combination, administered as a spray to the eye to dilate the pupil or for cycloplegic examination. This is most often used for pediatric patients, and the solution is administered using a sterile perfume atomizer.

Lid scrubs – Commercially available eyelid cleansers or antibiotic solutions or ointments can be applied directly to the lid margin for the treatment of noninfectious blepharitis. This is best accomplished by applying the medication to the end of a cotton-tipped applicator and then scrubbing the eyelid margin several times daily. The gauze pads supplied with commercially available eyelid cleansers are also convenient.

►*Devices:*

Contact lenses – Soft contact lenses can absorb water-soluble drugs and release them over prolonged periods of time. This has the clinical advantage of promoting sustained-release solutions or suspensions that would otherwise be removed quickly from the external ocular tissues. Soft contact lenses as delivery devices are most often used in the management of dry eye disorders, but the technique is occasionally used for the treatment of ocular infections, including corneal ulcers.

Corneal shields – A non-cross-linked, homogenized, porcine scleral collagen shield is available (*Bio-Cor Fyodoror Collagen Corneal Shield*). This is placed as a bandage on the cornea following surgery or injury, protecting and lubricating the cornea. Topical antibiotics have been used with the shield to promote healing of corneal ulcers.

Cotton pledgets – Small pieces of cotton can be saturated with ophthalmic solutions and placed in the conjunctival sac. These devices allow a prolonged ocular contact time with solutions that are normally administered topically into the eye. The clinical use of pledgets is usually reserved for mydriatic solutions such as cocaine or phenylephrine.

This drug delivery method promotes maximum mydriasis in an attempt to break posterior synechiae or to dilate sluggish pupils.

Filter paper strips – Sodium fluorescein and rose bengal dyes are commercially available as drug-impregnated filter paper strips. The strips help ensure sterility of sodium fluorescein which, when prepared in solution, can become easily contaminated with Pseudomonas aeruginosa. These dyes are used diagnostically to disclose corneal injuries, infections such as herpes simplex, and dry eye disorders.

Artificial tear inserts – A rod-shaped pellet of hydroxypropyl cellulose without preservative (*Lacrisert*), is inserted into the inferior conjunctival sac with a specially designed applicator. Following placement, the device releases the nonmedicated polymer to the eye for up to 24 hours. The device is designed as a sustained-release artificial tear for the treatment of dry eye disorders.

Membrane-bound inserts – A membrane-controlled drug delivery system (*Ocusert*) delivers a constant quantity of pilocarpine to the eye for up to 1 week. Placed onto the bulbar conjunctiva under the upper or lower eyelid, it is a useful substitute for pilocarpine drops or gel in glaucoma patients who cannot comply with more frequent instillation or in those with ocular or visual side effects from pilocarpine solutions.

Glaucoma is a condition of the eye in which an elevation of the intraocular pressure (IOP) leads to progressive cupping and atrophy of the optic nerve head, deterioration of the visual fields, and, ultimately, blindness. Primary open-angle glaucoma is the most common type of glaucoma. Angle-closure glaucoma and congenital glaucoma are treated primarily by surgical methods, although short-term drug therapy is used to decrease IOP prior to surgery.

Drugs used in the therapy of primary open-angle glaucoma include a variety of agents with different mechanisms of action. The therapeutic goal in treating glaucoma is reducing the elevated IOP, a major risk factor in the pathogenesis of glaucomatous visual field loss. The higher the level of IOP, the greater the likelihood of glaucomatous visual field loss and optic nerve damage. Reduction of IOP may be accomplished by: 1) Decreasing the rate of production of aqueous humor, or 2) increasing the rate of outflow (drainage) of aqueous humor from the anterior chamber of the eye.

The 6 groups of agents used in therapy of primary open-angle glaucoma are listed in the table, which summarizes their mechanism of decreasing IOP, effects on pupil size and ciliary muscle, and duration of action.

Agents for Glaucoma

Drug	Strength	Duration (h)	Decrease aqueous production	Increase aqueous outflow	Effect on pupil	Effect on ciliary muscle
Sympathomimetics						
Apraclonidine[1]	0.5%-1%	7-12	+++	NR	NR	NR
Epinephrine	0.1%-2%	12	+	++	mydriasis	NR
Dipivefrin	0.1%	12	+	++	mydriasis	NR
Brimonidine	0.2%	12	++	++	NR	NR
Beta blockers						
Betaxolol	0.25%-0.5%	12	+++	NR	NR	NR
Carteolol	1%	12	+++	nd	NR	NR
Levobunolol	0.25%-0.5%	12-24	+++	NR	NR	NR
Metipranolol	0.3%	12-24	+++	+	NR	NR
Timolol	0.25%-0.5%	12-24	+++	+	NR	NR
Miotics, direct-acting						
Acetylcholine[2]	1%	10-20 min	NR	+++	miosis	accommodation
Carbachol[2]	0.75%-3%	6-8	NR	+++	miosis	accommodation
Pilocarpine[3]	0.25%-10%	4-8	NR	+++	miosis	accommodation
Miotics, cholinesterase inhibitors						
Physostigmine	0.25%-0.5%	12-36	NR	+++	miosis	accommodation
Demecarium	0.125%-0.25%	days/wk	NR	+++	miosis	accommodation
Echothiophate	0.03%-0.25%	days/wk	NR	+++	miosis	accommodation
Carbonic anhydrase inhibitors						
Dichlorphenamide[4]	50 mg	6-12	+++	NR	NR	NR
Acetazolamide[4]	125-500 mg	8-12	+++	NR	NR	NR
Methazolamide[4]	25-50 mg	10-18	+++	NR	NR	NR
Dorzolamide[5]	2%	≈ 8	+++	NR	NR	NR
Prostaglandin analog						
Latanoprost	.005%	24	NR	+++	NR	NR

* +++ = significant activity   ++ = moderate activity   + = some activity   NR = no activity reported   nd = No data available
[1] 1% used only to decrease IOP in surgery.
[2] Intraocular administration only for miosis during surgery; carbachol also available as a topical agent.
[3] Also available as a gel and an insert; the duration of these doseforms is longer (18 to 24 hours and 1 week, respectively) than the solution.
[4] Systemic agents; for detailed information, see group monograph in Cardiovascular section.
[5] Topical ophthalmic agent.

➤ *Sympathomimetic agents:* Sympathomimetic agents (adrenergic agonists) have both α and β activity (apraclonidine is a relatively selective alpha adrenergic agonist). They lower IOP mainly by increasing outflow and reducing production of aqueous humor. Epinephrine is used as an adjunct to miotic or beta-blocker therapy; however, it is also used as primary therapy, especially in young patients or patients with cataracts. The combination of a miotic and a sympathomimetic will have additive effects in lowering IOP.

Dipivefrin HCl is a prodrug that is metabolized to epinephrine in vivo. The IOP-lowering and intraocular effects are qualitatively and quantitatively similar to epinephrine; however, extraocularly, dipivefrin may be better tolerated and have a lower incidence of adverse effects.

➤ *Beta-adrenergic blocking agents:* Beta-adrenergic blocking agents may be used alone or in conjunction with other agents. They may be more effective than either pilocarpine or epinephrine alone and have the advantage of not affecting either pupil size or accommodation. They lower IOP by decreasing the rate of aqueous production.

➤ *Miotics (direct-acting):* Direct-acting miotics were considered the first step in glaucoma therapy. They have now yielded to the beta-blockers. Pilocarpine is a useful adjunctive agent that is additive to the beta-blockers, carbonic anhydrase inhibitors, or sympathomimetics. Dosage and frequency of administration must be individualized. Patients with darkly pigmented irides may require higher strengths of pilocarpine.

➤ *Miotics (cholinesterase inhibitors):* Cholinesterase inhibitor miotics include both reversible/short-acting (eg, physostigmine) and irreversible/long-acting (eg, echothiophate) agents that enhance the effects of endogenous acetylcholine by inactivation of the enzyme acetylcholinesterase. These agents are more potent and longer-acting than the direct-acting cholinergic agents. Side effects and systemic toxicity are more common and of greater significance. Using a direct-acting cholinergic and a cholinesterase inhibitor provides no improvement in response.

➤ *Carbonic anhydrase inhibitors:* Carbonic anhydrase inhibitors are administered systemically, except for the topical agent dorzolamide. IOP is lowered by suppressing the secretion of aqueous humor (inflow). Systemic carbonic anhydrase inhibitors are used as adjunctive therapy and do not replace topical therapy.

➤ *Hyperosmotic agents:* Hyperosmotic agents (mannitol, urea, glycerin, and isosorbide) are administered systemically and are useful in lowering IOP in acute situations. These agents lower IOP by creating an osmotic gradient between the ocular fluids and plasma. They are not for chronic use.

➤ *Prostaglandin analogs:* Prostaglandin analogs increase uveoscleral outflow through a new mechanism of action, selective prostenoid receptor agonism. Latanoprost, currently the only agent available in this class, can be used concomitantly with other topical ophthalmic drug products to reduce IOP.

Alpha Adrenergic Agonist

BRIMONIDINE TARTRATE

Rx	**Brimonidine Tartrate** (Various, eg, Bausch & Lomb, Falcon)	**Solution**: 0.2%	In 5, 10, 15 mL.
Rx	**Alphagan** (Allergan)	**Solution**: 0.2%[1]	In 5, 10, and 15 mL bottles.
Rx	**Alphagan P** (Allergan)	**Solution**: 0.15%[2]	In 5, 10, and 15 mL bottles.

[1] With 0.05 mg benzalkonium chloride; polyvinyl alcohol; sodium chloride; sodium citrate; hydrochloric acid and/or sodium hydroxide may be added to adjust pH.

[2] With 0.005% *Purite*; boric acid; potassium chloride; sodium borate; sodium chloride; hydrochloric acid and/or sodium hydroxide to adjust pH.

Refer to Topical Ophthalmic Drugs introduction for more complete information.

Indications

➤*Intraocular pressure (IOP):* Lowering IOP in patients with open-angle glaucoma or ocular hypertension.

Administration and Dosage

➤*Dose:* The recommended dose is 1 drop of brimonidine in the affected eye(s) 3 times daily, approximately 8 hours apart.

➤*Concomitant therapy:* May be used concomitantly with other topical ophthalmic drug products to lower intraocular pressure. If more than 1 topical ophthalmic product is being used, administer the products at least 5 minutes apart.

➤*Storage/Stability:* Store between 15° to 25°C (59° to 77°F).

Actions

➤*Pharmacology:* Brimonidine is an alpha-2 adrenergic receptor agonist. It has a peak ocular hypotensive effect occurring at 2 hours post-dosing. Fluorophotometric studies in animals and humans suggest that brimonidine has a dual mechanism of action by reducing aqueous humor production and increasing uveoscleral outflow.

➤*Pharmacokinetics:* After ocular administration of a 0.1% or 0.2% solution, plasma concentrations peaked within 0.5 to 2.5 hours and declined with a systemic half-life of approximately 2 hours.

Systemic metabolism of brimonidine is extensive. It is metabolized primarily by the liver. Urinary excretion is the major route of elimination of the drug and its metabolites. Approximately 87% of an orally administered radioactive dose was eliminated within 120 hours, with 74% found in the urine.

➤*Clinical trials:* In comparative clinical studies with timolol 0.5% lasting up to 1 year, the IOP-lowering effect of brimonidine was approximately 4 to 6 mm Hg compared with approximately 6 mm Hg for timolol. In these studies, both patient groups were dosed twice daily. Eight percent of subjects were discontinued from studies because of inadequately controlled IOP, which occurred in 30% of patients during the first month of therapy. Approximately 20% were discontinued because of adverse experiences.

Contraindications

Hypersensitivity to brimonidine or any component of this medication; patients receiving monoamine oxidase inhibitor (MAOI) therapy.

Warnings

➤*Soft contact lenses:* The preservative in brimonidine, benzalkonium chloride, may be absorbed by soft contact lenses. Instruct patients wearing soft contact lenses to wait at least 15 minutes after instilling brimonidine to insert soft contact lenses.

➤*Renal/Hepatic function impairment:* Brimonidine has not been studied in patients with hepatic or renal impairment; use caution when treating such patients.

➤*Pregnancy:* Category B. There are no adequate and well-controlled studies of brimonidine in pregnant women. However, in animal studies, brimonidine crossed the placenta and entered into the fetal circulation to a limited extent. Use brimonidine during pregnancy only if the potential benefit to the mother justifies the potential risk to the fetus.

➤*Lactation:* It is not known whether brimonidine is excreted in human breast milk. In animal studies brimonidine was excreted in breast milk. Decide whether to discontinue nursing or to discontinue the drug, taking into account the importance of the drug to the mother.

➤*Children:* Safety and effectiveness have not been studied in pediatric patients under 2 years of age. Brimonidine is not recommended for use in pediatric patients under 2 years of age.

Precautions

➤*Cardiovascular disease:* Although brimonidine had minimal effect on blood pressure of patients in clinical studies, exercise caution in treating patients with severe cardiovascular disease.

➤*Use with caution:* Use caution in patients with depression, cerebral or coronary insufficiency, Raynaud's phenomenon, orthostatic hypotension, or thromboangiitis obliterans.

➤*Loss of effect:* Loss of effect in some patients may occur. The IOP-lowering efficacy observed with brimonidine during the first month of therapy may not always reflect the long-term level of IOP reduction. Therefore, routinely monitor IOP.

Drug Interactions

Brimonidine Drug Interactions			
Precipitant Drug	Object Drug[*]		Description
Brimonidine	Beta blockers, antihypertensives, cardiac glycosides	↑	Because alpha-agonists, as a class, may reduce pulse and blood pressure, use caution with concomitant drugs such as beta-blockers (ophthalmic and systemic), antihypertensives, and/or cardiac glycosides.
Brimonidine	CNS depressants (eg, alcohol, barbiturates, opiates, sedatives or anesthetics)	↑	Consider the possibility of an additive or potentiating effect with CNS depressants.
Brimonidine	MAOIs	↑	Coadministration is contraindicated.
Tricyclic antidepressants	Brimonidine	↓	Tricyclic antidepressants can affect the metabolism and uptake of circulating amines.

[*] ↑ = Object drug increased. ↓ = Object drug decreased.

Adverse Reactions

The following adverse events were reported (approximate percentages):

➤*Cardiovascular:*

0.2% solution – Hypertension, palpitations/arrhythmias, syncope (less than 3%).

0.15% solution – Hypertension (5% to 9%).

➤*CNS:*

0.2% solution – Somnolence (50% to 83% in patients 2 to 6 years of age); headache, fatigue/drowsiness (10% to 30%); dizziness, asthenia (3% to 9%); insomnia, depression, anxiety (less than 3%).

0.15% solution – Asthenia, dizziness, headache (1% to 4%); insomnia, somnolence (less than 1%).

➤*GI:*

0.2% solution – Oral dryness (10% to 30%); GI symptoms (3% to 9%); abnormal taste (less than 3%).

0.15% solution – Oral dryness (5% to 9%); dyspepsia (1% to 4%); taste perversion (less than 1%).

➤*Respiratory:*

0.2% solution – Upper respiratory symptoms (3% to 9%); nasal dryness (less than 3%).

0.15% solution – Bronchitis, cough, dyspnea, pharyngitis, rhinitis, sinus infection, sinusitis (1% to 4%); nasal dryness (less than 1%).

➤*Special senses:*

0.2% solution – Ocular hyperemia, burning/stinging, blurring, foreign body sensation, conjunctival follicles, ocular allergic reactions, ocular pruritus (10% to 30%); corneal staining/erosion, photophobia, eyelid erythema, ocular ache/pain, ocular dryness, tearing, eyelid edema, conjunctival edema, blepharitis, ocular irritation, conjunctival blanching, abnormal vision (3% to 9%); lid crusting, conjunctival hemorrhage, conjunctival discharge (less than 3%).

0.15% solution – Allergic conjunctivitis, conjunctival hyperemia, eye pruritus (10% to 20%); burning sensation, conjunctival folliculosis, visual disturbance (5% to 9%); blepharitis, conjunctival edema, conjunctival hemorrhage, conjunctivitis, epiphora, eye discharge, eye dryness, eye irritation, eye pain, eyelid edema, eyelid erythema, follicular conjunctivitis, foreign body sensation, photophobia, stinging, superficial punctate keratopathy, visual field defect, vitreous floaters, worsened visual acuity (1% to 4%); corneal erosion (less than 1%).

➤*Miscellaneous:*

0.2% solution – Muscular pain (3% to 9%).

0.15% solution – Allergic reaction, rash, flu syndrome (1% to 4%).

➤*Postmarketing:* Bradycardia; hypotension; iritis; miosis; skin reactions (eg, erythema, eyelid pruritus, rash, vasodilation); tachycardia. Apnea, bradycardia, hypotension, hypothermia, hypotonia, and somnolence have been reported in infants receiving brimonidine.

Alpha Adrenergic Agonist

BRIMONIDINE TARTRATE

Overdosage

No information is available on overdosage in humans. Treatment of an oral overdose includes supportive and symptomatic therapy; maintain a patent airway.

Patient Information

Instruct patients wearing soft contact lenses to wait at least 15 minutes after instilling brimonidine to insert soft contact lenses.

As with other drugs in this class, brimonidine may cause fatigue or drowsiness in some patients. Caution patients who engage in hazardous activities of the potential for a decrease in mental alertness.

APRACLONIDINE HCl

Rx	**Iopidine** (Alcon)	**Solution: 1%**	0.01% benzalkonium chloride. In 0.1 mL (2s).
		Solution: 0.5%	0.01% benzalkonium chloride. In 5 mL and 10 mL *Drop-Tainers*.

Refer to Topical Ophthalmic Drugs introduction for more complete information.

Indications

➤*1% solution:* To control or prevent post-surgical elevations in IOP that occur in patients after argon laser trabeculoplasty or iridotomy.

➤*0.5% solution:* Short-term adjunctive therapy in patients on maximally tolerated medical therapy who require additional IOP reduction.

Administration and Dosage

➤*0.5% solution:* Instill one to two drops in the affected eye(s) 3 times daily. Since apraclonidine 0.5% will be used with other ocular glaucoma therapies, use an approximate 5 minute interval between instillation of each medication to prevent washout of the previous dose. Not for injection into the eye.

➤*1% solution:* Instill 1 drop in scheduled operative eye 1 hour before initiating anterior segment laser surgery. Instill second drop into same eye immediately upon completion of surgery.

➤*Storage/Stability:* Store at room temperature. Protect from light and freezing (0.5%).

Actions

➤*Pharmacology:* Apraclonidine has the action of reducing elevated, as well as normal, intraocular pressure (IOP) whether accompanied by glaucoma or not. Apraclonidine is a relatively selective α-adrenergic agonist that does not have significant membrane stabilizing (local anesthetic) activity. When instilled into the eyes, apraclonidine reduces IOP and has minimal effect on cardiovascular parameters.

Optic nerve head damage and visual field loss may result from an acute elevation in IOP that can occur after argon laser surgical procedures. The higher the peak or spike of IOP, the greater the likelihood of visual field loss and optic nerve damage, especially in patients with previously compromised optic nerves. The onset of action is usually within 1 hour and the maximum IOP reduction occurs 3 to 5 hours after application of a single dose. Apraclonidine's mechanism of action is not completely established, although its predominant action may be related to a reduction of aqueous formation via stimulation of the alpha-adrenergic system.

➤*Pharmacokinetics:* Topical use of apraclonidine 0.5% leads to systemic absorption. Studies of apraclonidine ophthalmic solution dosed 1 drop 3 times daily in both eyes for 10 days in healthy volunteers yielded mean peak and trough concentrations of 0.9 and 0.5 ng/mL, respectively. The half-life of apraclonidine 0.5% was calculated to be 8 hours.

➤*Clinical trials:* The clinical utility of apraclonidine 0.5% is most apparent for those glaucoma patients on maximally tolerated medical therapy (ie, patients were using combinations of a topical beta blocker, sympathomimetics, parasympathomimetics and oral carbonic anhydrase inhibitors). Patients with advanced glaucoma and uncontrolled IOP scheduled to undergo laser trabeculoplasty or trabeculectomy surgery were enrolled in a study to determine whether apraclonidine dosed 3 times daily could delay the need for surgery for ≤ 3 months. Apraclonidine treatment resulted in a significantly greater percentage of treatment successes compared with patients treated with placebo.

Contraindications

Hypersensitivity to any component of this medication or to clonidine; concurrent monoamine oxidase inhibitor therapy (see Drug Interactions).

Warnings

➤*Concomitant therapy:* The addition of apraclonidine 0.5% to patients already using two aqueous suppressing drugs (eg, beta-blocker plus carbonic anhydrase inhibitor) as part of their maximally tolerated medical therapy may not provide additional benefit. This is because apraclonidine is an aqueous suppressing drug and the addition of a third aqueous suppressant may not significantly reduce IOP.

➤*Tachyphylaxis:* The IOP lowering efficacy of apraclonidine 0.5% diminishes over time in some patients. This loss of effect, or tachyphylaxis, appears to be an individual occurrence with a variable time of onset and should be closely monitored. The benefit for most patients is < 1 month.

➤*Hypersensitivity reactions:* Apraclonidine can lead to an allergic-like reaction characterized wholly or in part by the symptoms of hyperemia, pruritus, discomfort, tearing, foreign body sensation and edema of the lids and conjunctiva. If ocular allergic-like symptoms occur, discontinue therapy. Refer to Management of Acute Hypersensitivity Reactions.

➤*Renal/Hepatic function impairment:* Although the topical use of apraclonidine has not been studied in renal failure patients, structurally related clonidine undergoes a significant increase in half-life in patients with severe renal impairment. Close monitoring of cardiovascular parameters in patients with impaired renal function is advised if they are candidates for topical apraclonidine therapy. Close monitoring of cardiovascular parameters in patients with impaired liver function is also advised as the systemic dosage form of clonidine is partly metabolized in the liver.

➤*Pregnancy:* Category C. Apraclonidine has an embryocidal affect in rabbits when given in an oral dose of 3 mg/kg (60 times the maximum recommended human dose). There are no adequate and well controlled studies in pregnant women. Use during pregnancy only if the potential benefit justifies the potential risk to the fetus.

➤*Lactation:* It is not known if topically applied apraclonidine is excreted in breast milk. Exercise caution when apraclonidine is administered to a nursing woman. Consider discontinuing nursing for the day on which apraclonidine is used.

➤*Children:* Safety and efficacy for use in children have not been established.

Precautions

➤*Monitoring:* Glaucoma patients on maximally tolerated medical therapy who are treated with apraclonidine 0.5% to delay surgery should have their visual fields monitored periodically. Discontinue treatment if IOP rises significantly.

➤*IOP reduction:* Since apraclonidine is a potent depressor of IOP, closely monitor patients who develop exaggerated reductions in IOP. An unpredictable decrease of IOP control in some patients and incidence of ocular allergic responses and systemic side effects may limit the utility of apraclonidine 0.5%. However, patients on maximally tolerated medical therapy may still benefit from the additional IOP reduction provided by the short-term use of apraclonidine 0.5%.

➤*Cardiovascular disease:* Acute administration of apraclonidine has had minimal effect on heart rate or blood pressure; however, observe caution in treating patients with severe cardiovascular disease, including hypertension.

Use apraclonidine 0.5% with caution in patients with coronary insufficiency, recent myocardial infarction, cerebrovascular disease, chronic renal failure, Raynaud's disease or thromboangiitis obliterans.

➤*Depression:* Caution and monitor depressed patients since apraclonidine has been infrequently associated with depression.

➤*Vasovagal attack:* Consider the possibility of a vasovagal attack occurring during laser surgery; use caution in patients with a history of such episodes.

➤*Corneal changes:* Topical ocular administration of apraclonidine 1.5% to rabbits 3 times daily for 1 month resulted in sporadic and transient instances of minimal corneal cloudiness. No corneal changes were observed in humans given at least one dose of apraclonidine 1%.

Drug Interactions

Apraclonidine Drug Interactions			
Precipitant drug	Object drug*		Description
Apraclonidine	Cardiovascular agents	↓	Since apraclonidine may reduce pulse and blood pressure, caution in using cardiovascular drugs is advised. Patients using cardiovascular drugs concurrently with apraclonidine 0.5% should have pulse and blood pressures frequently monitored.
Apraclonidine	MAO inhibitors	↑	Apraclonidine should not be used in patients receiving MAO inhibitors (see Contraindications).

* ↑ = Object drug increased.　↓ = Object drug decreased.

Alpha Adrenergic Agonist

APRACLONIDINE HCl

Adverse Reactions

In clinical studies the overall discontinuation rate related to apraclonidine was 15%. The most commonly reported events leading to discontinuation included (in decreasing order of frequency): Hyperemia; pruritus; tearing; discomfort; lid edema; dry mouth; foreign body sensation.

The following adverse effects were reported with the use of apraclonidine in laser surgery: Upper lid elevation (1.3%); conjunctival blanching (0.4%); mydriasis (0.4%).

The following additional adverse effects were reported:

➤*Cardiovascular:*

1% solution – Bradycardia; vasovagal attack; palpitations; orthostatic episode.

0.5% solution – Asthenia (< 3%); peripheral edema, arrhythmia (< 1%). Although there are no reports of bradycardia, consider the possibility.

➤*CNS:*

1% solution – Insomnia; dream disturbances; irritability; decreased libido; headache; paresthesia.

0.5% solution – Headache (< 3%); somnolence, dizziness, nervousness, depression, insomnia, paresthesia (< 1%).

➤*GI:*

1% solution – Abdominal pain; diarrhea; stomach discomfort; emesis; dry mouth.

0.5% solution – Dry mouth (2%); constipation, nausea (< 1%).

➤*Hypersensitivity:* Use can lead to an allergic-like reaction (see Warnings).

➤*Ophthalmic:*

1% solution – Conjunctival blanching; upper lid elevation; mydriasis; burning; discomfort; foreign body sensation; dryness; itching; hypotony; blurred or dimmed vision; allergic response; conjunctival microhemorrhage.

0.5% solution – Hyperemia (13%); pruritus (10%); discomfort (6%); tearing (4%); lid edema, blurred vision, foreign body sensation, dry eye, conjunctivitis, discharge, blanching (< 3%); lid margin crusting, conjunctival follicles, conjunctival edema, edema, abnormal vision, pain, lid disorder, keratitis, blepharitis, photophobia, corneal staining, lid erythema, blepharoconjunctivitis, irritation, corneal erosion, corneal infiltrate, keratopathy, lid scales, lid retraction (< 1%).

➤*Respiratory:*

0.5% solution – Dry nose (2%); rhinitis, dyspnea, pharyngitis, asthma (< 1%).

➤*Miscellaneous:*

1% solution – Taste abnormalities; nasal burning or dryness; head cold sensation; chest heaviness or burning; clammy or sweaty palms; body heat sensation; shortness of breath; increased pharyngeal secretion; extremity pain or numbness; fatigue; pruritus not associated with rash.

0.5% solution – Taste perversion (3%); contact dermatitis, dermatitis, chest pain, abnormal coordination, malaise, facial edema (< 1%); myalgia, parosmia (0.2%)

Patient Information

Do not touch dropper tip to any surface as this may contaminate the contents.

Apraclonidine can cause dizziness and somnolence. Patients who engage in hazardous activities requiring mental alertness should be warned of the potential for a decrease in mental alertness, physical dexterity or coordination while using apraclonidine.

EPINEPHRINE

Rx	**Epinephrine HCl** (Novartis Ophthalmic)	**Solution:** 0.1%	In 1 mL *Dropperettes* (12s).[1]
Rx	**Epifrin** (Allergan)	**Solution:** 0.5% (as base)	In 15 mL dropper bottles.[2]
Rx	**Epifrin** (Allergan)	**Solution:** 1% (as base)	In 15 mL dropper bottles.[2]
Rx	**Glaucon** (Alcon)	**Solution:** 1%	In 10 mL *Drop-Tainers.*[3]
Rx	**Epifrin** (Allergan)	**Solution:** 2% (as base)	In 15 mL dropper bottles.[2]
Rx	**Glaucon** (Alcon)	**Solution:** 2%	In 10 mL *Drop-Tainers.*[3]

[1] With 0.5% chlorobutanol and sodium bisulfite.
[2] With benzalkonium chloride, sodium metabisulfite, EDTA and hydrochloric acid.
[3] With 0.01% benzalkonium chloride, sodium metabisulfite, EDTA, sodium chloride, hydrochloric acid and sodium hydroxide.

Refer to Topical Ophthalmic Drugs introduction for more complete information.

Indications

➤*Glaucoma:* Management of open-angle (chronic simple) glaucoma; may be used in combination with miotics, beta blockers, hyperosmotic agents or carbonic anhydrase inhibitors.

Administration and Dosage

Instill 1 drop into affected eye(s) once or twice daily. Determine frequency of instillation by tonometry.

More frequent instillation than 1 drop twice daily does not usually elicit any further improvement in therapeutic response.

When used in conjunction with miotics, instill the miotic first.

➤*Storage/Stability:* Store at 2° to 24°C (36° to 75°F). Keep container tightly sealed. Protect solution from light; store in cool place. Do not freeze. Discard if solution becomes discolored or contains a precipitate.

Actions

➤*Pharmacology:* Epinephrine, a direct-acting sympathomimetic agent, acts on α and β receptors. Therefore, topical application causes conjunctival decongestion (vasoconstriction), transient mydriasis (pupillary dilation) and reduction in intraocular pressure (IOP). It is believed IOP reduction is primarily due to reduced aqueous production and increased aqueous outflow. The duration of decrease in IOP is 12 to 24 hours.

Epinephrine is available as hydrochloride and borate salts. These preparations are therapeutically equal when given in equivalent doses of epinephrine base.

Contraindications

Hypersensitivity to epinephrine or any component of the formulation; narrow- or shallow-angle (angle Y closure) glaucoma; aphakia; patients with a narrow angle but no glaucoma; if the nature of the glaucoma is not clearly established. Do not use while wearing soft contact lenses; discoloration of lenses may occur.

Warnings

For ophthalmic use only. Not for injection or intraocular use.

➤*Gonioscopy:* Because pupil dilation may precipitate an acute attack of narrow-angle glaucoma, evaluate anterior chamber angle by gonioscopy prior to beginning therapy.

➤*Anesthesia:* Discontinue use prior to general anesthesia with anesthetics that sensitize the myocardium to sympathomimetics (eg, cyclopropane, halothane).

➤*Aphakic patients:* Maculopathy with associated decrease in visual acuity may occur in the aphakic eye; if this occurs, promptly discontinue use.

➤*Elderly:* Use with caution.

➤*Pregnancy: Category C.* Safety for use during pregnancy has not been established. Use only when clearly needed.

➤*Lactation:* It is not known whether this drug is excreted in breast milk. Exercise caution when administering to a nursing woman.

➤*Children:* Safety and efficacy for use in children have not been established.

Precautions

➤*Instillation discomfort:* Epinephrine is relatively uncomfortable upon instillation. Discomfort lessens as concentration of epinephrine decreases.

➤*Potentially hazardous tasks:* Epinephrine may cause temporarily blurred or unstable vision after instillation; observe caution while driving, operating machinery or performing other tasks requiring coordination or physical dexterity.

➤*Special risk:* Use with caution in the presence of or history of: Hypertension; diabetes; hyperthyroidism; heart disease; cerebral arteriosclerosis; bronchial asthma.

➤*Sulfite sensitivity:* Some of these products contain sulfites that may cause allergic-type reactions (eg, hives, itching, wheezing, anaphylaxis) in certain susceptible persons. Although the overall prevalence of sulfite sensitivity in the general population is probably low, it is seen more frequently in asthmatics or atopic nonasthmatics.

Drug Interactions

Consider interactions that occur with systemic use of epinephrine (see Epinephrine monograph in the Vasopressors Used in Shock section).

Adverse Reactions

➤*Local:* Transient stinging and burning; eye pain/ache; browache; headache; allergic lid reaction; conjunctival hyperemia; conjunctival or corneal pigmentation, ocular irritation (hypersensitivity), localized adrenochrome deposits in conjunctiva and cornea (prolonged use); reversible cystoid macular edema may result from use in aphakic patients.

➤*Systemic:* Headache; palpitations; tachycardia; extrasystoles; cardiac arrhythmia; hypertension; faintness.

Overdosage

If ocular overdosage occurs, flush eye(s) with water or normal saline.

Patient Information

To avoid contamination, do not touch tip of container to any surface. Replace cap after using.

Do not use if solution is brown or contains a precipitate.

Do not use while wearing soft contact lenses.

Transitory stinging may occur upon initial instillation. Headache or browache may occur.

Patients should immediately report any decrease in visual acuity.

EPINEPHRYL BORATE

Rx	**Epinal** (Alcon)	**Solution:** 0.5%	In 7.5 mL.[1]
		1%	In 7.5 mL.[1]

[1] With 0.01% benzalkonium chloride, ascorbic acid, acetylcysteine, boric acid and sodium carbonate.

DIPIVEFRIN HCl (Dipivalyl epinephrine)

Rx	**Dipivefrin HCl** (Various, eg, Falcon)	**Solution:** 0.1%	In 5, 10 and 15 mL.
Rx	**Propine** (Allergan)		In 5, 10 & 15 mL C Cap Compliance Cap B.I.D.[1]

[1] With 0.005% benzalkonium chloride, sodium chloride, EDTA and hydrochloric acid.

Refer to Topical Ophthalmic Drugs introduction for more complete information.

Indications

➤*Glaucoma:* Initial therapy or as an adjunct with other antiglaucoma agents for the control of IOP in chronic open-angle glaucoma.

Administration and Dosage

➤*Initial glaucoma therapy:* Instill 1 drop into the eye(s) every 12 hours.

➤*Replacement therapy:* When transferring patients to dipivefrin from antiglaucoma agents other than epinephrine, continue the previous medication the first day and add 1 drop of dipivefrin in affected eye(s) every 12 hours. The next day, discontinue the other agent and continue with dipivefrin. Monitor with tonometry.

When transferring patients from conventional epinephrine therapy, discontinue the epinephrine and institute the dipivefrin regimen. Monitor with tonometry.

➤*Concomitant therapy:* When patients receiving other antiglaucoma agents require additional therapy, add 1 drop of dipivefrin every 12 hours.

Actions

➤*Pharmacology:* Dipivefrin is a prodrug of epinephrine formed by diesterification of epinephrine and pivalic acid, enhancing its lipophilic character and, consequently, penetration into anterior chamber. Dipivefrin, converted to epinephrine in the eye by enzymatic hydrolysis, appears to act by decreasing aqueous production and enhancing outflow facility. It has the same therapeutic effects as epinephrine with fewer local and systemic side effects.

Dipivefrin does not produce the miosis or accommodative spasm that cholinergic agents produce. The blurred vision and night blindness often associated with miotic agents do not occur with dipivefrin. In patients with cataracts the inability to see around lenticular opacities caused by constricted pupil is avoided.

➤*Pharmacokinetics:* The onset of action with 1 drop occurs about 30 minutes after treatment, with maximum effect seen at about 1 hour.

➤*Clinical trials:* In patients with a history of epinephrine intolerance, only 3% of dipivefrin-treated patients exhibited intolerance, while 55% treated with epinephrine again developed an intolerance. Response to dipivefrin twice daily is less than that to 2% epinephrine twice daily and comparable to 2% pilocarpine 4 times daily. Patients using dipivefrin twice daily had mean IOP reductions ranging from 20% to 24%.

Contraindications

Hypersensitivity to dipivefrin or any formulation component; narrow-angles (any dilation of pupil may predispose patient to an attack of angle-closure glaucoma).

Warnings

➤*Pregnancy: Category B.* There are no adequate and well controlled studies in pregnant women. Use only when clearly needed.

➤*Lactation:* It is not known whether this drug is excreted in breast milk. Use caution in nursing mothers.

➤*Children:* Safety and efficacy for use in children have not been established.

Precautions

➤*Aphakic patients:* Macular edema occurs in up to 30% of aphakic patients treated with epinephrine. Discontinuation generally results in reversal of the maculopathy.

Adverse Reactions

➤*Cardiovascular:* Tachycardia, arrhythmias, hypertension (reported with epinephrine).

➤*Local:* Burning and stinging (6%); conjunctival injection (6.5%); follicular conjunctivitis, mydriasis, allergic reactions (infrequent). Epinephrine therapy can lead to adrenochrome deposits in the conjunctiva and cornea.

Dipivefrin 0.1% is less irritating than 1% epinephrine HCl. Only 1.8% of dipivefrin patients reported discomfort due to photophobia, glare or light sensitivity.

Patient Information

Slight stinging or burning on initial instillation may occur.

Do not try to "catch up" on missed doses by applying more than one dose at a time.

DAPIPRAZOLE HCl

Rx	**Rēv-Eyes** (Storz/Lederle)	**Powder, lyophilized:** 25 mg (0.5% solution when reconstituted)	In vial with 5 mL diluent and dropper.[1]

[1] With 2% mannitol, 0.4% hydroxypropyl methylcellulose, 0.01% EDTA, 0.01% benzalkonium chloride and sodium chloride.

Refer to Topical Ophthalmic Drugs introduction for more complete information.

Indications

➤*Mydriasis:* Treatment of iatrogenically induced mydriasis produced by adrenergic (phenylephrine) or parasympatholytic (tropicamide) agents.

Administration and Dosage

Instill 2 drops into the conjunctiva of each eye followed 5 minutes later by an additional 2 drops. Administer after the ophthalmic examination to reverse the diagnostic mydriasis.

Shake container for several minutes to ensure mixing.

➤*Storage/Stability:* Store at room temperature 15° to 30°C (59° to 86°F) for 21 days after reconstitution.

Actions

➤*Pharmacology:* Dapiprazole acts through blocking the alpha-adrenergic receptors in smooth muscle and produces miosis through an effect on the dilator muscle of the iris.

The drug does not have any significant activity on ciliary muscle contraction and, therefore, does not induce a significant change in the anterior chamber depth or the thickness of the lens.

Dapiprazole has demonstrated safe and rapid reversal of mydriasis produced by phenylephrine and, to a lesser degree, tropicamide. In patients with decreased accommodative amplitude due to treatment with tropicamide, the miotic effect of dapiprazole may partially increase the accommodative amplitude.

Eye color affects the rate of pupillary constriction. In individuals with brown irides, the rate of pupillary constriction may be slightly slower than in individuals with blue or green irides. Eye color does not appear to affect the final pupil size.

Dapiprazole does not significantly alter intraocular pressure (IOP) in normotensive eyes or in eyes with elevated IOP.

Contraindications

When constriction is undesirable, such as acute iritis; hypersensitivity to any component of this preparation.

Warnings

➤*For topical ophthalmic use only.:* Not for injection.

➤*Frequency of use:* Do not use in the same patient more frequently than once a week.

➤*IOP reduction:* Not indicated for the reduction of IOP or in the treatment of open-angle glaucoma.

➤*Vision reduction:* May cause difficulty in dark adaptation and may reduce field of vision. Patients should exercise caution in night driving or when performing other activities in poor illumination.

➤*Pregnancy: Category B.* There are no adequate and well controlled studies in pregnant women. Use during pregnancy only when clearly needed and when potential benefits outweigh the potential hazards to the fetus.

➤*Lactation:* It is not known whether this drug is excreted in breast milk. Exercise caution when dapiprazole is administered to a nursing woman.

➤*Children:* Safety and efficacy for use in children have not been established.

Adverse Reactions

Conjunctival injection lasting 20 minutes (> 80%); burning on instillation (≈ 50%); ptosis, lid erythema, lid edema, chemosis, itching, punctate keratitis, corneal edema, browache, photophobia, headaches (10% to 40%); dryness of the eye, tearing, blurring of vision (less frequent).

Patient Information

May cause difficulty in dark adaptation and may reduce field of vision. Exercise caution when driving at night or performing other activities in poor illumination.

To avoid contamination, do not touch tip of container to any surface.

Do not use in the same patient more frequently than once a week.

Discard any solution that is not clear and colorless.

Beta-Adrenergic Blocking Agents

Refer to the general discussion of these products in the Topical Ophthalmic Introduction for more complete information.

Indications

►*Glaucoma:* Lowering intraocular pressure (IOP) in patients with chronic open-angle glaucoma.

For specific approved indications, refer to individual drug monographs.

Administration and Dosage

►*Concomitant therapy:* If IOP is not controlled with these agents, institute concomitant pilocarpine, other miotics, dipivefrin or systemic carbonic anhydrase inhibitors.

Use of epinephrine with topical β-blockers is controversial. Some reports indicate initial effectiveness of the combination decreases over time (see Drug Interactions).

►*Monitoring:* The IOP-lowering response to betaxolol and timolol may require a few weeks to stabilize.

Because of diurnal IOP variations in individual patients, satisfactory response to once-a-day therapy is best determined by measuring IOP at different times during the day.

Actions

►*Pharmacology:* Timolol, levobunolol, carteolol and metipranolol are noncardioselective (β_1 and β_2) β-blockers; betaxolol and levobetaxolol are cardioselective (β_1) β-blockers. Topical β-blockers do not have significant membrane-stabilizing (local anesthetic) actions or intrinsic sympathomimetic activity. They reduce elevated and normal IOP, with or without glaucoma.

The exact mechanism of ocular antihypertensive action is not established, but it appears to be a reduction of aqueous production. However, some studies show a slight increase in outflow facility with timolol and metipranolol.

These agents reduce IOP with little or no effect on pupil size or accommodation. Blurred vision and night blindness often associated with miotics are not associated with these agents. The inability to see around lenticular opacities when the pupil is constricted is avoided. These agents may be absorbed systemically (see Warnings).

►*Pharmacokinetics:*

Pharmacokinetics of Ophthalmic β-Adrenergic Blocking Agents				
Drug	β-receptor selectivity	Onset (min)	Maximum effect (hr)	Duration (hr)
Carteolol	β_1 and β_2	nd[1]	2	12
Betaxolol	β_1	≤ 30	2	12
Levobunolol	β_1 and β_2	< 60	2 to 6	≤ 24
Metipranolol	β_1 and β_2	≤ 30	≈ 2	24
Timolol	β_1 and β_2	≤ 30	1 to 2	≤ 24
Levobetaxolol	β_1	≤ 30	2	≈ 12

[1] nd = No data

►*Clinical trials:*

Timolol – In controlled studies of untreated IOP of ≥ 22 mmHg, timolol 0.25% or 0.5% bid caused greater IOP reduction than 1%, 2%, 3%, or 4% pilocarpine solution 4 times daily or 0.5%, 1%, or 2% epinephrine HCl solution twice daily. In comparative studies, mean IOP reduction was 31% to 33% with timolol, 22% with pilocarpine, and 28% with epinephrine.

Timolol, generally well tolerated, produces fewer and less severe side effects than pilocarpine or epinephrine.

Betaxolol – Betaxolol ophthalmic was compared to ophthalmic timolol and placebo in patients with reactive airway disease. Betaxolol had no significant effect on pulmonary function as measured by Forced Expiratory Volume (FEV_1), Forced Vital Capacity (FVC) and FEV_1/VC. Also, action of isoproterenol was not inhibited. Timolol significantly decreased these pulmonary functions. No evidence of cardiovascular β-blockade during exercise was observed with betaxolol. Mean arterial blood pressure was not affected by any treatment; however, timolol significantly decreased mean heart rate. Betaxolol reduces mean IOP 25% from baseline. In controlled studies, the magnitude and duration of the ocular hypotensive effects of betaxolol and timolol were clinically equivalent.

Clinical observation of glaucoma patients treated with betaxolol solution for up to 3 years shows that the IOP-lowering effect is well maintained.

Betaxolol has been successfully used in glaucoma patients who have undergone laser trabeculoplasty and have needed long-term antihypertensive therapy. The drug is well tolerated in glaucoma patients with hard or soft contact lenses and in aphakic patients.

Levobunolol – In controlled clinical studies of ≈ 2 years duration, intraocular pressure was well-controlled in ≈ 80% of subjects treated with levobunolol 0.5% twice daily. The mean IOP decrease from baseline was between 6.87 mmHg and 7.81 mmHg.

Metipranolol – Metipranolol reduced the average intraocular pressure approximately 20% to 26% in controlled studies of patients with IOP > 24 mmHg at baseline. Clinical studies in patients with glaucoma treated ≤ 2 years indicate that an intraocular pressure lowering effect is maintained.

Carteolol – Carteolol produced a median percent IOP reduction of 22% to 25% when given twice daily in clinical trials ranging from 1.5 to 3 months.

Contraindications

Bronchial asthma, a history of bronchial asthma or severe chronic obstructive pulmonary disease; sinus bradycardia; second-degree and third-degree AV block; overt cardiac failure; cardiogenic shock; hypersensitivity to any component of the products.

Warnings

►*Systemic absorption:* These agents may be absorbed systemically. The same adverse reactions found with systemic β-blockers (see group monograph in Cardiovascular section) may occur with topical use. For example, severe respiratory reactions and cardiac reactions, including death due to bronchospasm in asthmatics, and rarely, death associated with cardiac failure, have been reported with topical β-blockers.

►*Cardiovascular:* Timolol may decrease resting and maximal exercise heart rate even in healthy subjects.

Cardiac failure – Sympathetic stimulation may be essential for circulation support in diminished myocardial contractility; its inhibition by β-receptor blockade may precipitate more severe failure.

In patients without history of cardiac failure, continued depression of myocardium with β-blockers may lead to cardiac failure. Discontinue at the first sign or symptom of cardiac failure.

►*Non-allergic bronchospasm:* Patients with a history of chronic bronchitis, emphysema, etc, should receive β-blockers with caution; they may block bronchodilation produced by catecholamine stimulation of β_2-receptors.

►*Major surgery:* Withdrawing β-blockers before major surgery is controversial. Beta-receptor blockade impairs the heart's ability to respond to β-adrenergically mediated reflex stimuli. This may augment the risk of general anesthesia. Some patients on β-blockers have had protracted severe hypotension during anesthesia. Difficulty restarting and maintaining heartbeat has been reported. In elective surgery, gradual withdrawal of β-blockers may be appropriate.

The effects of β-blocking agents may be reversed by β-agonists such as isoproterenol, dopamine, dobutamine, or levarterenol.

►*Diabetes mellitus:* Administer with caution to patients subject to spontaneous hypoglycemia or to diabetic patients (especially labile diabetics). Beta-blocking agents may mask signs and symptoms of acute hypoglycemia.

►*Thyroid:* Beta-adrenergic blocking agents may mask clinical signs of hyperthyroidism (eg, tachycardia). Manage patients suspected of developing thyrotoxicosis carefully to avoid abrupt withdrawal of β-blockers, which might precipitate thyroid storm.

►*Cerebrovascular insufficiency:* Because of potential effects of β-blockers on blood pressure and pulse, use with caution in patients with cerebrovascular insufficiency. If signs or symptoms suggesting reduced cerebral blood flow develop, consider alternative therapy.

►*Carcinogenesis:* In female mice receiving oral metipranolol doses of 5, 50 and 100 mg/kg/day, the low dose had an increased number of pulmonary adenomas.

►*Pregnancy: Category C.* There have been no adequate and well controlled studies in pregnant women. Use during pregnancy only if the potential benefits outweigh potential hazards to the fetus.

Carteolol – Increased resorptions and decreased fetal weights occurred in rabbits and rats at maternal doses ≈ 1052 and 5264 times the maximum human dose, respectively. A dose-related increase in wavy ribs was noted in the developing rat fetus when pregnant rats received doses ≈ 212 times the maximum human dose.

Betaxolol – In oral studies with rats and rabbits, evidence of post-implantation loss was seen at dose levels above 12 mg/kg and 128 mg/kg, respectively. Betaxolol was not teratogenic, however, and there were no other adverse effects on reproduction at subtoxic dose levels.

Levobunolol – Fetotoxicity was observed in rabbits at doses 200 and 700 times the glaucoma dose.

Metipranolol – Increased fetal resorption, fetal death and delayed development occurred in rabbits receiving 50 mg/kg orally during organogenesis.

Timolol – Doses of 1000 mg/kg/day (142,000 times the maximum recommended human ophthalmic dose) were maternotoxic in mice and resulted in increased fetal resorptions. Increased fetal resorptions were also seen in rabbits at 14,000 times the systemic exposure following the maximum recommended human ophthalmic dose, in this case without apparent maternotoxicity.

Levobetaxolol – There was evidence of drug-related postimplantation loss in rabbits with levobetaxolol at 12 mg/kg/day and sternebrae malformations at 4 mg/kg/day. No other adverse effects on reproduction were noted at subtoxic dose levels.

➤*Lactation:* It is not known whether betaxolol, levobunolol or metipranolol are excreted in breast milk. Systemic β-blockers and topical and ophthalmic timolol maleate are excreted in milk. Carteolol is excreted in breast milk of animals. Exercise caution when administering to a nursing mother.

Because of the potential for serious adverse reactions from timolol in nursing infants, decide whether to discontinue nursing or discontinue the drug taking into account the importance of the drug to the mother.

➤*Children:* Safety and efficacy for use in children have not been established.

Precautions

➤*Angle-closure glaucoma:* The immediate objective is to reopen the angle, requiring constriction of the pupil with a miotic. These agents have little or no effect on the pupil. When they are used to reduce elevated IOP in angle-closure glaucoma, use with a miotic.

➤*Muscle weakness:* Beta-blockade may potentiate muscle weakness consistent with certain myasthenic symptoms (eg, diplopia, ptosis, generalized weakness). Timolol has increased muscle weakness in some patients with myasthenic symptoms or myasthenia gravis.

➤*Long-term therapy:* In long-term studies (2 and 3 years), no significant differences in mean IOP were observed after initial stabilization.

➤*Sulfite sensitivity:* Some of these products contain sulfites which may cause allergic-type reactions (eg, hives, itching, wheezing, anaphylaxis) in certain susceptible persons. Although the overall prevalence of sulfite sensitivity in the general population is probably low, it is seen more frequently in asthmatics or atopic nonasthmatics.

Drug Interactions

Ophthalmic Beta Blocker Drug Interactions			
Precipitant drug	Object drug*		Description
Beta blockers, ophthalmic	Beta blockers, oral	↑	Use topical beta blockers with caution because of the potential for additive effects on systemic and ophthalmic beta-blockade.
Beta blockers, ophthalmic	Calcium antagonists	↑	Possible cases of hypotension, left ventricular failure, and atrioventricular conduction disturbances may occur from coadministration of timolol maleate and calcium antagonists. Avoid use in patients with impaired cardiac function.
Beta blockers, ophthalmic	Catecholamine-depleting drugs (eg, reserpine)	↑	Use of reserpine with ophthalmic beta blockers can cause additive effects and the production of hypotension or marked bradycardia, which may result in syncope, vertigo, or postural hypotension. Close observation is recommended.
Catecholamine-depleting drugs (eg, reserpine)	Beta blockers, ophthalmic		
Beta blockers, ophthalmic	Digitalis	↑	Coadministration of ophthalmic beta blockers with digitalis and calcium antagonists may have additive effects in prolonging atrioventricular conduction time.
Digitalis	Beta blockers, ophthalmic		
Quinidine	Beta blockers, ophthalmic	↑	Decreased heart rate has been reported during combined treatment with timolol maleate and quinidine, possibly because quinidine inhibits the metabolism of timolol maleate via the P450 enzyme, CYP2D6.
Beta blockers	Phenothiazine compounds	↑	Potential additive hypotensive effects due to mutual inhibition of metabolism.

* ↑ = Object drug increased.

Other drugs that may interact with systemic β-adrenergic blocking agents may also interact with ophthalmic agents. For further information, refer to the β-blocker group monograph in the Cardiovasculars chapter.

Adverse Reactions

➤*The following have occurred with ophthalmic* β₁ *and* β₂ *(nonselective) blockers:*

Cardiovascular – Arrhythmia; syncope; heart block; cerebral vascular accident; cerebral ischemia; congestive heart failure; palpitation.

CNS – Headache; depression.

Dermatologic – Hypersensitivity, including localized and generalized rash.

Endocrine – Masked symptoms of hypoglycemia in insulin-dependent diabetics (see Warnings).

GI – Nausea.

Ophthalmic – Keratitis; blepharoptosis; visual disturbances including refractive changes (due to withdrawal of miotic therapy in some cases); diplopia; ptosis.

Respiratory – Bronchospasm (predominantly in patients with preexisting bronchospastic disease); respiratory failure.

➤*Carteolol:*

Ophthalmic – Transient irritation, burning, tearing, conjunctival hyperemia, edema (≈ 25%); blurred/cloudy vision; photophobia; decreased night vision; ptosis; blepharoconjunctivitis; abnormal corneal staining; corneal sensitivity.

Systemic – Bradycardia; decreased blood pressure; arrhythmia; heart palpitation; dyspnea; asthenia; headache; dizziness; insomnia; sinusitis; taste perversion.

➤*Betaxolol:*

Cardiovascular – Bradycardia; heart block; CHF.

CNS – Dizziness; vertigo; headaches; depression; lethargy; increase in signs and symptoms of myasthenia gravis.

Ophthalmic – Brief discomfort (25%); occasional tearing (5%). Rare: Decreased corneal sensitivity; erythema; itching; corneal punctate staining; keratitis, anisocoria; photophobia; edema.

Pulmonary – Pulmonary distress characterized by dyspnea, bronchospasm, thickened bronchial secretions, asthma, and respiratory failure.

Miscellaneous – Taste and smell perversions; hives; toxic epidermal necrolysis; hair loss; glossitis; insomnia.

➤*Metipranolol:*

Ophthalmic – Transient local discomfort; conjunctivitis; eyelid dermatitis; blepharitis; blurred vision; tearing; browache; abnormal vision; photophobia; edema; uveitis.

Systemic – Allergic reaction; headache; asthenia; hypertension; MI; atrial fibrillation; angina; palpitation; bradycardia; nausea; rhinitis; dyspnea; epistaxis; bronchitis; coughing; dizziness; anxiety; depression; somnolence; nervousness; arthritis; myalgia; rash.

➤*Levobetaxolol:*

Cardiovascular – Bradycardia, heart block, hypertension, hypotension, tachycardia, vascular anomaly (< 2%).

CNS – Anxiety, dizziness, hypertonia, vertigo (< 2%).

Dermatologic – Alopecia, dermatitis, psoriasis (< 2%).

Endocrine – Diabetes, hypothyroidism (< 2%).

GI – Constipation, dyspepsia (< 2%).

GU – Breast abscess, cystitis (< 2%).

Metabolic/Nutritional – Gout, hypercholesteremia, hyperlipidemia (< 2%).

Musculoskeletal – Arthritis, tendonitis (< 2%).

Ophthalmic – Transient ocular discomfort upon instillation (11%); transient blurred vision (≈ 2%); cataracts, vitreous disorders (< 2%).

Pulmonary – Pulmonary distress characterized by bronchitis, dyspnea, pharyngitis, pneumonia, rhinitis, and sinusitis (< 2%).

Special senses – Ear pain, otitis media, taste perversion, tinnitus (< 2%).

Miscellaneous – Accidental injury, headache, infection (< 2%).

➤*Levobunolol:*

Cardiovascular – Effects may resemble timolol.

CNS – Ataxia, dizziness, headache, lethargy (rare).

Dermatologic – Urticaria, pruritus (rare).

Ophthalmic – Transient burning/stinging (≤ 33%); blepharoconjunctivitis (≤ 5%); iridocyclitis (rare); decreased corneal sensitivity.

➤*Timolol:*

Cardiovascular – Bradycardia; arrhythmia; hypotension; syncope; heart block; cerebral vascular accident; cerebral ischemia; heart failure; palpitation; cardiac arrest.

CNS – Dizziness; depression; fatigue; lethargy; hallucinations; confusion.

Ophthalmic – Ocular irritation including conjunctivitis; blepharitis; keratitis; blepharoptosis; decreased corneal sensitivity; visual disturbances including refractive changes; diplopia; ptosis.

Respiratory – Bronchospasm (mainly in patients with preexisting bronchospastic disease); respiratory failure; dyspnea.

Miscellaneous – Aggravation of myasthenia gravis; alopecia; nausea; localized and generalized rash; urticaria; impotence; decreased libido; masked symptoms of hypoglycemia in diabetics; diarrhea.

➤*Systemic* β-*adrenergic blocker-associated reactions:* Consider potential effects with ophthalmic use (see Warnings).

Beta-Adrenergic Blocking Agents

Overdosage

If ocular overdosage occurs, flush eye(s) with water or normal saline. If accidentally ingested, efforts to decrease further absorption may be appropriate (gastric lavage).

The most common signs and symptoms of overdosage from systemic β-blockers are bradycardia, hypotension, bronchospasm and acute cardiac failure. If these occur, discontinue therapy and initiate appropriate supportive therapy.

Patient Information

Transient stinging/discomfort is relatively common; notify physician if severe.

Do not touch dropper tip to any surface; do not use with contact lenses in eyes.

LEVOBUNOLOL HCl

Rx	**Levobunolol** (Various, eg, Bausch & Lomb)	**Solution:** 0.25%	In 5 and 10 mL.
Rx	**Betagan Liquifilm** (Allergan)		In 5 and 10 mL dropper bottles with B.I.D. *C Cap.*[1]
Rx	**Levobunolol** (Various, eg, Bausch & Lomb, Falcon)	**Solution:** 0.5%	In 5, 10, and 15 mL.
Rx	**Betagan Liquifilm** (Allergan)		In 2 mL bottles with standard cap and 5, 10, and 15 mL with B.I.D. and Q.D. *C Cap.*[1]

[1] With 1.4% polyvinyl alcohol; 0.004% benzalkonium chloride; sodium metabisulfite; EDTA; sodium phosphate, dibasic; potassium phosphate, monobasic; NaCl; hydrochloric acid; sodium hydroxide.

For complete prescribing information, refer to the Beta-Adrenergic Blocking Agents group monograph.

Indications

➤*Elevated IOP:* Lowering IOP in chronic open-angle glaucoma or ocular hypertension.

Administration and Dosage

➤*Usual dose:*

0.5% solution – 1 to 2 drops in the affected eye(s) once a day.

0.25% solution – 1 to 2 drops in the affected eye(s) twice daily.

In patients with more severe or uncontrolled glaucoma, the 0.5% solution can be administered twice a day. As with any new medication, carefully monitor patients.

Dosages > 1 drop of 0.5% levobunolol twice daily are not generally more effective. If IOP is not at a satisfactory level on this regimen, concomitant therapy can be instituted. Do not administer ≥ 2 topical ophthalmic beta-adrenergic blocking agents simultaneously.

BETAXOLOL HCl

Rx	**Betaxolol HCl** (Various, Akorn, Falcon)	**Solution:** 5.6 mg (equiv. to 5 mg base) per mL (0.5%)	In 2.5, 5, 10, and 15 mL.
Rx	**Betoptic** (Alcon)		In 2.5, 5, 10, and 15 mL *Drop-Tainer* dispensers.[1]
Rx	**Betoptic S** (Alcon)	**Suspension:** 2.8 mg (equiv. to 2.5 mg base) per mL (0.25%)	In 2.5, 5, 10, and 15 mL *Drop-Tainer* dispensers.[2]

[1] With 0.01% benzalkonium chloride, NaCl, hydrochloric acid and/or sodium hydroxide, EDTA.

[2] With 0.01% benzalkonium chloride, mannitol, poly sulfonic acid, hydrochloric acid or sodium hydroxide, EDTA.

For complete prescribing information, refer to the Beta-Adrenergic Blocking Agents group monograph.

Indications

➤*Elevated IOP:* Lowering IOP; ocular hypertension; chronic open-angle glaucoma.

Administration and Dosage

➤*Usual dose:* Instill 1 to 2 drops in the affected eye(s) twice daily. Consider concomitant therapy if IOP is not at a satisfactory level.

➤*Replacement therapy (single agent):* Continue the agent already used and add 1 drop of betaxolol twice daily. The following day, discontinue the previous agent and continue betaxolol. Monitor with tonometry.

➤*Replacement therapy (multiple agents):* When transferring from several concomitant antiglaucoma agents, individualize dosage. Adjust 1 agent at a time at intervals of ≥ 1 week. One may continue the agents being used and add 1 drop betaxolol twice daily. The next day, discontinue another agent. Decrease or discontinue remaining antiglaucoma agents according to patient response.

➤*Storage/Stability:* Store at room temperature. Shake suspension well.

METIPRANOLOL HCl

Rx	**Metipranolol** (Falcon)	**Solution:** 0.3%	In 5 and 10 mL.[1]
Rx	**OptiPranolol** (Bausch & Lomb)		In 5 and 10 mL dropper bottles.[2]

[1] With 0.004% benzalkonium chloride, povidone, hydrochloric acid, NaCl,EDTA.

[2] With 0.004% benzalkonium chloride, glycerin, povidone, hydrochloric acid, NaCl, sodium hydroxide and/or hydrochloric acid, EDTA.

For complete prescribing information, refer to the Beta-Adrenergic Blocking Agents group monograph.

Indications

➤*Elevated IOP:* Treatment of elevated IOP in patients with ocular hypertension or open-angle glaucoma.

Administration and Dosage

➤*Usual dose:* Instill 1 drop in the affected eye(s) twice a day. If the patient's IOP is not at a satisfactory level on this regimen, more frequent administration or a larger dose is not known to be of benefit. Concomitant therapy to lower IOP may be used.

CARTEOLOL HCl

Rx	**Carteolol HCl** (Various, eg, Akorn, Falcon)	**Solution:** 1%	In 5, 10, and 15 mL.
Rx	**Ocupress** (Novartis Pharmaceuticals)		In 5, 10, and 15 mL dispenser bottles.[1]

[1] With 0.005% benzalkonium chloride; NaCl; sodium phosphate, dibasic and monobasic.

For complete prescribing information, refer to the Beta-Adrenergic Blocking Agents group monograph.

Indications

➤*Elevated IOP:* Lowering of IOP in chronic open-angle glaucoma and intraocular hypertension.

Administration and Dosage

➤*Usual dose:* Instill 1 drop in affected eye(s) twice daily. If the patient's IOP is not at a satisfactory level on this regimen, concomitant therapy can be instituted.

Beta-Adrenergic Blocking Agents

TIMOLOL

Rx	**Timolol Maleate** (Various, eg, Akorn, Bausch & Lomb, Falcon, Fougera)	**Solution:** 0.25%	In 2.5, 5, 10, and 15 mL.
Rx	**Betimol**[1] (Novartis Ophthalmic)		In 2.5, 5, 10, and 15 mL.[2]
Rx	**Timoptic**[3] (Merck)		Preservative free. In UD 60s *Ocudose*.[4]
Rx	**Timoptic**[3] (Merck)		In 2.5, 5, 10, and 15 mL *Ocumeters*.[5]
Rx	**Timolol Maleate** (Various, eg, Akorn, Bausch & Lomb, Falcon, Fougera)	**Solution:** 0.5%	In 2.5, 5, 10, and 15 mL.
Rx	**Betimol**[1] (Novartis Ophthalmics)		In 2.5, 5, 10, and 15 mL.[2]
Rx	**Istolol**[1] (Bausch & Lomb)		In 5 mL.[4]
Rx	**Timoptic**[3] (Merck)		Preservative free. In UD 60s *Ocudose*.[5]
Rx	**Timoptic**[3] (Merck)		In 2.5, 5, 10, and 15 mL *Ocumeters*.[6]
Rx	**Timolol Maleate** (Falcon)	**Solution, gel-forming:** 0.25%	In 2.5 and 5 mL.[7]
Rx	**Timoptic-XE**[3] (Merck)		In 2.5 and 5 mL *Ocumeters*.[7]
Rx	**Timolol Maleate** (Falcon)	**Solution, gel-forming:** 0.5%	In 2.5 and 5 mL.[7]
Rx	**Timoptic-XE**[3] (Merck)		In 2.5 and 5 mL *Ocumeters*.[7]

[1] As hemihydrate.
[2] With 0.01% benzalkonium chloride and monosodium and disodium phosphate dihydrate.
[3] As maleate.
[4] With 0.005% benzalkonium chloride, monobasic sodium phosphate monohydrate, 0.47% potassium sorbate, and sodium hydroxide.
[5] Preservative free; use immediately after opening; discard remaining contents. With monobasic and dibasic sodium phosphate and sodium hydroxide.
[6] With 0.01% benzalkonium chloride, sodium hydroxide, and monobasic and dibasic sodium phosphate.
[7] With 0.012% benzododecinium bromide.

For complete prescribing information, refer to the Beta-Adrenergic Blocking Agents group monograph.

Indications

➤*Elevated IOP:* Treatment of elevated IOP in open-angle glaucoma, ocular hypertension.

Administration and Dosage

➤*Solution:*

Initial therapy – Instill 1 drop of 0.25% or 0.5% in the affected eye(s) twice daily (once daily *Istalol* only in the morning). If clinical response is not adequate, change the dosage to 1 drop of 0.5% solution in the affected eye(s) twice a day. If the IOP is maintained at satisfactory levels, change the dosage to 1 drop in the affected eye(s) once a day. Consider concomitant therapy if IOP is not at a satisfactory level. The concomitant use of 2 topical β-blocking agents is not recommended.

Replacement therapy (single agent) – When a patient is transferred from another ophthalmic β-adrenergic blocker, discontinue that agent after proper dosing on 1 day, and start treatment the next day with 1 drop of 0.25% timolol in the affected eye(s) twice daily. Increase to 1 drop of 0.5% twice a day if response is inadequate.

When changing from an agent other than an ophthalmic β-blocker, on the first day, continue with the agent being used, and add 1 drop 0.25% timolol twice daily. The next day, discontinue the previously used agent completely, and continue with timolol. If a higher dosage is required, substitute 1 drop 0.5% in the affected eye(s) twice daily.

Replacement therapy (multiple agents) – When transferring from several concomitantly administered agents, individualize dosage. If any of the agents is an ophthalmic β-blocker, discontinue it before starting timolol. Adjust 1 agent at a time, at intervals of ≥ 1 week. Continue the agents being used and add 1 drop of 0.25% twice a day. The next day, discontinue one of the other agents. Decrease or discontinue remaining agents according to patient response. If a higher dosage is required, use 1 drop of 0.5% twice daily.

➤*Gel:* Invert the closed container and shake once before each use; it is not necessary to shake it more than once. Administer other ophthalmics ≥ 10 minutes before the gel. Dose is 1 drop (0.25% or 0.5%) once daily. Dosages > 1 drop of 0.5% per day have not been studied. Consider concomitant therapy if IOP is not at a satisfactory level. When patients are switched from timolol solution twice daily to the gel once daily, the ocular hypotensive effect has remained consistent.

Because the pressure-lowering response may require a few weeks to stabilize, determine IOP after ≈ 4 weeks of treatment.

LEVOBETAXOLOL HCl

Rx	**Betaxon** (Alcon)	**Suspension, ophthalmic:** 0.5% as base (5.6 mg/mL)	0.01% benzalkonium chloride, EDTA, hydrochloric acid, boric acid. In 5, 10, and 15 mL *Drop-tainers*.

For complete prescribing information, refer to the Beta-Adrenergic Blocking Agents group monograph.

Indications

➤*Intraocular pressure:* For lowering intraocular pressure in patients with chronic open-angle glaucoma or ocular hypertension.

Administration and Dosage

➤*Approved by the FDA:* February 24, 2000.

➤*Recommended dose:* The recommended dose is 1 drop in the affected eye(s) twice daily. In some patients, the intraocular pressure lowering responses may require a few weeks to stabilize.

As with any new medication, careful monitoring of patients is advised. The concomitant use of 2 topical beta-adrenergic agents is not recommended.

➤*Storage/Stability:* Store upright 39° to 77°F (4° to 25°C). Protect from light. Shake well before using.

Refer to the Topical Ophthalmic Drugs introduction and Agents for Glaucoma introduction for a general discussion of these products. For information on the oral use of pilocarpine, refer to the monograph in the Mouth and Throat Products section.

Indications

➤*Carbachol, topical; pilocarpine:*
Glaucoma – To decrease elevated IOP in glaucoma.

➤*Acetylcholine; carbachol, intraocular:*
Miosis – To induce miosis during surgery.

See individual monographs for specific indications.

Actions

➤*Pharmacology:* The direct-acting miotics are parasympathomimetic (cholinergic) drugs which duplicate the muscarinic effects of acetylcholine. When applied topically, these drugs produce pupillary constriction, stimulate the ciliary muscles and increase aqueous humor outflow facility. Miosis, produced through contraction of the iris sphincter, causes increased tension on the scleral spur (reducing outflow resistance) and opening of the trabecular meshwork spaces facilitating outflow. With the increase in outflow facility, there is a decrease in intraocular pressure (IOP). Topical ophthalmic instillation of acetylcholine causes no discernible response as cholinesterase destroys the molecule more rapidly than it can penetrate the cornea; therefore, acetylcholine is only used intraocularly.

Miosis Induction of Direct-Acting Miotics

Miotic	Onset	Peak	Duration
Acetylcholine, intraocular	seconds	—	10 min
Carbachol			
Intraocular	seconds	2 to 5 min	1 to 2 days
Topical	10 to 20 min	—	4 to 8 hours
Pilocarpine, topical	10 to 30 min	—	4 to 8 hours

Contraindications

Hypersensitivity to any component of the formulation; where constriction is undesirable (eg, acute iritis, acute or anterior uveitis, some forms of secondary glaucoma, pupillary block glaucoma, acute inflammatory disease of the anterior chamber).

Warnings

➤*Corneal abrasion:* Use carbachol with caution in the presence of corneal abrasion to avoid excessive penetration.

➤*Pregnancy: Category C* (carbachol, pilocarpine). Safety for use during pregnancy has not been established. Use only when clearly needed.

➤*Lactation:* It is not known whether these drugs are excreted in breast milk; exercise caution when administering to a nursing woman.

➤*Children:* Safety and efficacy for use in children have not been established.

Precautions

➤*Systemic reactions:* Caution is advised in patients with acute cardiac failure, bronchial asthma, peptic ulcer, hyperthyroidism, GI spasm, urinary tract obstruction, Parkinson's disease, recent MI, hypertension or hypotension.

➤*Retinal detachment:* Retinal detachment has been caused by miotics in susceptible individuals, in individuals with preexisting retinal disease or in those who are predisposed to retinal tears. Fundus examination is advised for all patients prior to initiation of therapy.

➤*Miosis:* Miosis usually causes difficulty in dark adaptation. Advise patients to use caution while night driving or performing hazardous tasks in poor light.

➤*Angle-closure:* Although withdrawal of the peripheral iris from the anterior chamber angle by miosis may reduce the tendency for narrow-angle closure, miotics can occasionally precipitate angle closure by increasing resistance to aqueous flow from posterior to anterior chamber.

➤*Pilocarpine ocular system (Ocusert):* Carefully consider and evaluate patients with acute infectious conjunctivitis or keratitis prior to use.

Drug Interactions

➤*Nonsteroidal anti-inflammatory agents (NSAIDs), topical:* Although studies with acetylcholine chloride or carbachol revealed no interference, and there is no known pharmacological basis for an interaction, there have been reports that these drugs have been ineffective when used in patients treated with topical NSAIDs.

Adverse Reactions

➤*Acetylcholine:*
Ophthalmic – Corneal edema; clouding; decompensation.

Systemic – Bradycardia; hypotension; flushing; breathing difficulties; sweating.

➤*Carbachol:*
Ophthalmic – Transient stinging and burning; corneal clouding; persistent bullous keratopathy; postoperative iritis following cataract extraction with intraocular use; retinal detachment; transient ciliary and conjunctival injection; ciliary spasm with resultant temporary decrease of visual acuity.

Systemic – Headache; salivation; GI cramps; vomiting; diarrhea; asthma; syncope; cardiac arrhythmia; flushing; sweating; epigastric distress; tightness in bladder; hypotension; frequent urge to urinate.

➤*Pilocarpine:*
Ophthalmic – Transient stinging and burning; tearing; ciliary spasm; conjunctival vascular congestion; temporal, peri- or supra-orbital headache; superficial keratitis; induced myopia (especially in younger individuals who have recently started administration); blurred vision; poor dark adaptation; reduced visual acuity in poor illumination in older individuals and in individuals with lens opacity. A subtle corneal granularity has occurred with pilocarpine gel. Lens opacity (prolonged use), retinal detachment (rare; see Precautions).

Systemic – Hypertension, tachycardia, bronchiolar spasm, pulmonary edema, salivation, sweating, nausea, vomiting, diarrhea (rare).

Pilocarpine ocular system (Ocusert): Conjunctival irritation, including mild erythema with or without a slight increase in mucus secretion with first use. These symptoms tend to lessen or disappear after the first week of therapy. Ciliary spasm may occur with pilocarpine usage but is not a contraindication to continued therapy unless the induced myopia is debilitating to the patient. Rarely, a sudden increase in pilocarpine effects has been reported during use.

Irritation from pilocarpine has been infrequently encountered and may require cessation of therapy. True allergic reactions are uncommon, but require discontinuation of therapy. Corneal abrasion and visual impairment have been reported.

Overdosage

Should accidental overdosage in the eye(s) occur, flush with water.

➤*Treatment:* Treatment includes usual supportive measures. Refer to General Management of Acute Overdosage. Observe patients for signs of toxicity (eg, salivation, lacrimation, sweating, nausea, vomiting, diarrhea). If these occur, anticholinergics (atropine) may be necessary. Bronchial constriction may be a problem in asthmatic patients.

Patient Information

May sting upon instillation, especially first few doses.

May cause headache, browache and decreased night vision. Use caution while night driving or performing hazardous tasks in poor light.

To avoid contamination, do not touch tip of container to any surface. Replace cap after using. Keep bottle tightly closed when not in use. Discard solution after expiration date.

ACETYLCHOLINE CHLORIDE, INTRAOCULAR

Rx	**Miochol-E** (Novartis Pharmaceuticals)	**Solution:** 1:100 acetylcholine chloride when reconstituted	In 2 mL dual chamber univial (lower chamber 20 mg lyophilized acetylcholine chloride and 56 mg mannitol; upper chamber 2 mL electrolyte diluent[1] and sterile water for injection).

[1] Sodium chloride, potassium chloride, magnesium chloride hexahydrate, calcium chloride dihydrate.

For complete prescribing information, refer to the Miotics, Direct-Acting group monograph.

Indications

➤*Miosis:* To produce complete miosis in seconds after delivery of the lens in cataract surgery. In penetrating keratoplasty, iridectomy and other anterior segment surgery where rapid, complete miosis may be required.

Administration and Dosage

Instill the solution into the anterior chamber before or after securing one or more sutures. The pupil is rapidly constricted and the peripheral iris drawn away from the angle of the anterior chamber if there are no mechanical hindrances. Any anatomical hindrance to miosis may require surgery to permit desired effect of drug.

In cataract surgery, use only after delivery of the lens.

➤*Solution:* 0.5 to 2 mL produces satisfactory miosis. Solution need not be flushed from the chamber after miosis occurs. Since acetylcholine has a short duration of action, pilocarpine may be applied topically before dressing to maintain miosis.

➤*Preparation of solution:* The aqueous solution of acetylcholine chloride is unstable. Prepare solution immediately before use. Do not use solution which is not clear and colorless. Discard any solution that has not been used. Do not gas sterilize.

➤*Storage/Stability:* Store at room temperature 15° to 30°C (59° to 86°F). Do not freeze.

CARBACHOL, INTRAOCULAR

Rx	**Carbastat** (Novartis Ophthalmics)	**Solution:** 0.01%	In 1.5 mL vials.[1]
Rx	**Miostat** (Alcon)		In 1.5 mL vials.[1]

[1] With 0.64% sodium chloride, 0.075% potassium chloride, 0.048% calcium chloride dihydrate, 0.03% magnesium chloride hexahydrate, 0.39% sodium acetate trihydrate, 0.17% sodium citrate dihydrate, sodium hydroxide, hydrochloric acid.

For complete prescribing information, refer to the Miotics, Direct-Acting group monograph.

Indications

➤*Miosis:* Intraocular use for miosis during surgery.

Administration and Dosage

For single-dose intraocular use only. Discard unused portion.

Open under aseptic conditions only.

Gently instill no more than 0.5 mL into the anterior chamber before or after securing sutures. Miosis is usually maximal 2 to 5 minutes after application.

➤*Storage/Stability:* Store at room temperature 15° to 30°C (59° to 86°F).

CARBACHOL, TOPICAL

Rx	**Isopto Carbachol** (Alcon)	**Solution:** 0.75%	In 15 and 30 mL *Drop-Tainers.*[1]
		1.5%	In 15 and 30 mL *Drop-Tainers.*[1]
		2.25%	In 15 mL *Drop-Tainers.*[1]
Rx	**Isopto Carbachol** (Alcon)	3%	In 15 and 30 mL *Drop-Tainers.*[1]
Rx	**Carboptic** (Optopics)		In 15 mL.[2]

[1] With 0.005% benzalkonium chloride, 1% hydroxypropyl methylcellulose, sodium chloride, boric acid and sodium borate.

[2] With benzalkonium chloride, polyvinyl alcohol and sodium phosphate dibasic and monobasic.

For complete prescribing information, refer to the Miotics, Direct-Acting group monograph.

Indications

➤*Glaucoma:* For lowering intraocular pressure in the treatment of glaucoma.

Administration and Dosage

Instill 2 drops into eye(s) up to 3 times daily.

➤*Storage/Stability:* Store at 8° to 27°C (46° to 80°F).

PILOCARPINE HCl

Rx	**Isopto Carpine** (Alcon)	**Solution:** 0.25%	In 15 mL.[1]
Rx	**Pilocarpine HCl** (Various, eg, Rugby)	**Solution:** 0.5%	In 15 and 30 mL.
Rx	**Isopto Carpine** (Alcon)		In 15 and 30 mL.[1]
Rx	**Pilocar** (Novartis Ophthalmics)		In 15 mL.[2]
Rx	**Pilocarpine HCl** (Various, eg, Alcon, Goldline, Rugby)	**Solution:** 1%	In 2, 15 and 30 mL and UD 1 mL.
Rx	**Akarpine** (Akorn)		In 15 mL.
Rx	**Isopto Carpine** (Alcon)		In 15 and 30 mL.[1]
Rx	**Pilocar** (Novartis Ophthalmics)		In 15 mL and 1 mL dropperettes.[2]
Rx	**Pilocarpine HCl** (Various eg, Alcon, Goldline, Rugby)	**Solution:** 2%	In 2, 15, and 30 mL.
Rx	**Akarpine** (Akorn)		In 15 mL dropper bottles.
Rx	**Isopto Carpine** (Alcon)		In 15 and 30 mL.[1]
Rx	**Pilocar** (Novartis Ophthalmics)		In 15 mL, twin-pack (2 × 15 mL) and 12 × 1 mL dropperettes.[2]
Rx	**Isopto Carpine** (Alcon)	**Solution:** 3%	In 15 mL and 30 mL.[1]
Rx	**Pilocarpine HCl** (Various, eg, Alcon, Goldline, Rugby)	**Solution:** 4%	In 2, 15 and 30 mL.
Rx	**Akarpine** (Akorn)		In 15 mL dropper bottles.
Rx	**Isopto carpine** (Alcon)		In 15 and 30 mL.[1]
Rx	**Pilocar** (Novartis Ophthalmics)		In 15 mL, twin-pack (2 × 15 mL) and 12 × 1 mL dropperettes.[2]
Rx	**Isopto Carpine** (Alcon)	**Solution:** 5%	In 15 mL.[1]
Rx	**Pilocarpine HCl** (Various, eg, Rugby)	**Solution:** 6%	In 15 mL.
Rx	**Isopto Carpine** (Alcon)		In 15 and 30 mL.[1]
Rx	**Pilocar** (Novartis Ophthalmics)		In 15 mL.[3]
Rx	**Pilocarpine HCl** (Alcon)	**Solution:** 8%	In 2 mL.
Rx	**Isopto Carpine** (Alcon)		In 15 mL.
Rx	**Isopto Carpine** (Alcon)	**Solution:** 10%	In 15 mL.[1]
Rx	**Pilopine HS** (Alcon)	**Gel:** 4%	In 3.5 g.[6]

[1] With 0.5% hydroxypropyl methylcellulose and 0.01% benzalkonium chloride.
[2] With dydroxypropyl methylcellulose, benzalkonium chloride and EDTA.
[3] With polyvinyl alcohol, benzalkonium chloride and EDTA.

[4] With 0.004% benzalkonium chloride, EDTA, povidone, PEG and hydroxyethyl cellulose.
[5] With dydroxypropyl methylcellulose, 0.01% benzalkonium chloride and EDTA.
[6] With 0.008% benzalkonium chloride, carbopol 940 and EDTA.

For complete prescribing information, refer to the Miotics, Direct-Acting group monograph.

Indications

➤*Chronic simple glaucoma:* Chronic simple glaucoma, especially open-angle glaucoma. Patients may be maintained on pilocarpine as long as intraocular pressure (IOP) is controlled and there is no deterioration in the visual fields.

Chronic angle-closure glaucoma.

➤*Acute (angle-dose) glaucoma:* Alone, or in combination with other miotics, β-adrendergic blocking agents, epinephrine, carbonic anhydrase inhibitors or hyperosmotic agents to decrease IOP prior to surgery.

Pre- and postoperative intraocular tension.

➤*Mydriasis:* Mydriasis caused by mydriatic or cycloplegic agents.

Administration and Dosage

➤*Solution:*

Initial – 1 or 2 drops 3 to 4 times a daily. The frequency of instillation and the concentration are determined by patient response. Individuals with heavily pigmented irides may require higher strengths.

➤*Gel:* Apply a 0.5 inch ribbon in the lower conjunctival sac of affected eye(s) once daily at bedtime. If other glaucoma medication is also used at bedtime, use drops at least 5 minutes before the gel.

➤*Storage/Stability:* Do not freeze. Store at room temperature.

PILOCARPINE OCULAR THERAPEUTIC SYSTEM

Rx	Ocusert Pilo-20 (Alza)	**Ocular Therapeutic System:** Releases 20 mcg pilocarpine per hour for 1 week	In packs of 8 individ. sterile systems.

For complete prescribing information, refer to the Miotics, Direct-Acting group monograph.

Indications

➤*IOP reduction:* Control of elevated IOP in pilocarpine-responsive patients.

Administration and Dosage

➤*Damaged or deformed systems:* Do not place or retain in the eye. Remove and replace systems believed to be associated with an unexpected increase in drug action.

➤*Initiation of therapy:* There is no direct correlation between the strength of *Ocusert* used and the strength of pilocarpine eyedrop solutions required to achieve a given level of pressure lowering. It has been estimated that *Ocusert* 20 mcg is roughly equal to 0.5% or 1% drops and 40 mcg is roughly equal to 2% or 3% drops. *Ocusert* reduces the amount of drug necessary to achieve adequate medical control; therefore, therapy may be started with the 20 mcg system, regardless of the strength of pilocarpine solution the patient previously required. Because of the patient's age, family history and disease status or progression, however, therapy may be started with the 40 mcg system. The patient should return during the first week of therapy for evaluation of IOP, and as often thereafter as deemed necessary.

If pressure is satisfactorily reduced with the 20 mcg system, the patient should continue its use, replacing each unit every 7 days. If IOP reduction greater than that achieved by 20 mcg is needed, transfer the patient to the 40 mcg system. If necessary, concurrently use epinephrine, a β-blocker or carbonic anhydrase inhibitor; *Ocusert*'s release rate is not influenced by other ophthalmic preparations.

➤*Placement and removal of the system:* The system is placed in and removed from the eye by the patient. Since pilocarpine-induced myopia may occur during the first several hours of therapy, place the system into the conjunctival cul-de-sac at bedtime. By morning, the myopia is at a stable level (≤ 0.5 diopters).

In those patients in whom retention is a problem, superior cul-de-sac placement is often more desirable. The unit can be manipulated from lower to upper conjunctival cul-de-sac by gentle digital massage through the eyelid. If possible, move the unit before sleep to the upper conjunctival cul-de-sac for best retention. Should the unit slip out during sleep, its ocular hypotensive effect after loss continues for a period comparable to that following instillation of eyedrops.

Ocusert has been used concomitantly with various ophthalmic medications.

➤*Storage / Stability:* Refrigerate at 2° to 8°C (36° to 46°F).

Actions

➤*Pharmacology:* An elliptical unit designed for continuous release of pilocarpine following placement in the cul-de-sac of the eye. Pilocarpine is released from the system as soon as it is placed in contact with the conjunctival surfaces.

➤*Pharmacokinetics: Ocusert* initially releases the drug at 3 times the rated value in the first hours and declines to the rated value in approximately 6 hours. A total of 0.3 to 0.7 mg pilocarpine is released during this initial 6 hour period (one drop of 2% pilocarpine ophthalmic solution contains 1 mg pilocarpine). During the remainder of the 7 day period, the release rate is within ± 20% of the rated value.

Ocular hypotensive effect is fully developed within 1.5 to 2 hours after placement in cul-de-sac. A satisfactory ocular hypotensive response is maintained around the clock. IOP reduction for the entire week is achieved with the system from either 3.4 or 6.7 mg pilocarpine (20 or 40 mcg/hr times 24 hrs/day times 7 days, respectively), vs 28 mg given as a 2% ophthalmic solution 4 times daily.

During the first several hours after insertion, induced myopia may occur. In contrast to fluctuating and high levels of induced myopia typical of pilocarpine use, the amount of induced myopia with *Ocusert* decreases after the first several hours to a low baseline level (≤ 0.5 diopters), which persists for the therapeutic life of the system. Pilocarpine-induced miosis approximately parallels induced myopia.

Patient Information

Patient package insert is available with the product.

Wash hands with soap and water before touching or manipulating the system. If a displaced system contacts unclean surfaces, rinse with cool tap water before replacing. Discard contaminated systems and replace with a fresh unit.

Check for the presence of the system before retiring at night and upon arising.

Refer to the general discussion of these products in the Topical Oph-thalmics Introduction.

Indications

➤*Glaucoma:* Therapy of open-angle glaucoma.

For other specific indications, refer to the individual monographs.

Actions

➤*Pharmacology:* These indirect-acting agents inhibit the enzyme cholinesterase, potentiating the action of acetylcholine on the parasym-pathomimetic end organs. Topical application to the eye produces intense miosis and muscle contraction. Intraocular pressure (IOP) is reduced by a decreased resistance to aqueous outflow.

Cholinesterase inhibitors are subdivided into reversible and irrevers-ible agents. Reversible agents (eg, physostigmine, demecarium) quickly combine with cholinesterase; the resulting complex is slowly hydro-lyzed and the inhibited enzyme is regenerated. The demecarium-en-zyme complex is hydrolyzed more slowly than the physostigmine complex; therefore, its duration of action is longer.

Irreversible agents (eg, echothiophate) also bind to cholinesterase; how-ever, the resulting covalent bond is not hydrolyzed. Therefore, cholin-esterase is not regenerated. More cholinesterase must be synthesized or supplied from depots elsewhere in the body before ophthalmic action dependent on cholinesterase returns. Echothiophate will depress both plasma and erythrocyte cholinesterase levels in most patients after a few weeks of eyedrop therapy.

These effects are accompanied by increased capillary permeability of the ciliary body and iris, increased permeability of the blood-aqueous barrier and vasodilation. Myopia may be induced or, if present, may be augmented by the increased refractive power of the lens that results from the accommodative effect of the drug. Demecarium indirectly pro-duces some of the muscarinic and nicotinic effects of acetylcholine as quantities of the latter accumulate.

Cholinesterase-Inhibiting Miotics					
	Miosis		IOP reduction		
Miotics	Onset (min)	Duration	Onset (hrs)	Peak (hrs)	Duration
Reversible					
Physostigmine	20 to 30	12 to 36 hrs	—	2 to 6	12 to 36 hrs
Demecarium	15 to 60	3 to 10 days	—	24	7 to 28 days
Irreversible					
Echothiophate	10 to 30	1 to 4 weeks	4 to 8	24	7 to 28 days

Contraindications

Hypersensitivity to cholinesterase inhibitors or any component of the formulation; active uveal inflammation or any inflammatory disease of the iris or ciliary body; glaucoma associated with iridocyclitis.

➤*Demecarium:* Pregnancy.

➤*Echothiophate:* Most cases of angle-closure glaucoma (due to the possibility of increasing angle-block).

Warnings

➤*Myasthenia gravis:* Because of possible additive adverse effects, administer demecarium and echothiophate only with extreme caution to patients with myasthenia gravis who are receiving systemic anticho-linesterase therapy. Conversely, exercise extreme caution in the use of anticholinesterase drugs for the treatment of myasthenia gravis patients who are already undergoing topical therapy with cholinester-ase inhibitors.

➤*Surgery:* In patients receiving cholinesterase inhibitors, administer succinylcholine with extreme caution before and during general anes-thesia (see Drug Interactions). Use prior to ophthalmic surgery only as a considered risk because of the possible occurrence of hyphema.

➤*Pregnancy: Category X* (demecarium). Contraindicated in women who are or who may become pregnant. If this drug is used during preg-nancy, or if the patient becomes pregnant while taking this drug, apprise the patient of the potential hazard to the fetus.

Category C (physostigmine, echothiophate). Safety for use during preg-nancy has not been established. Use only when clearly needed and when the potential benefits outweigh the potential hazards to the fetus.

➤*Lactation:* It is not known whether these drugs are excreted in breast milk. Exercise caution when administering to a nursing woman. Because of the potential for serious adverse reactions in nursing infants, decide whether to discontinue nursing or the drug, taking into account the importance of the drug to the mother.

➤*Children:* The occurrence of iris cysts is more frequent in children (see Precautions). Exercise extreme caution in children receiving deme-carium who may require general anesthesia. Safety and efficacy for use of physostigmine have not been established.

Precautions

➤*Concomitant therapy:* Cholinesterase inhibitors may be used in combination with adrenergic agents, β-blockers, carbonic anhydrase inhibitors or hyperosmotic agents.

➤*Narrow angle glaucoma:* Use with caution in patients with chronic angle-closure (narrow-angle) glaucoma or in patients with nar-row angles, because of the possibility of producing pupillary block and increasing angle blockage.

➤*Ophthalmic ointments:* Ophthalmic ointments may retard corneal healing.

➤*Miosis:* Miosis usually causes difficulty in dark adaptation. Use cau-tion while driving at night or performing hazardous tasks in poor light.

➤*Gonioscopy:* Use only when shorter-acting miotics have proved inadequate. Gonioscopy is recommended prior to use of medication. Routine examination (eg, slit-lamp) to detect lens opacities should accompany therapy.

➤*Concomitant ocular conditions:* When an intraocular inflamma-tory process is present, breakdown of the blood-aqueous barrier from anticholinesterase therapy requires abstention from, or cautious use of, these drugs. Use with great caution where there is a history of quies-cent uveitis. After long-term use, blood vessel dilation and resultant greater permeability increase possibility of hyphema during or prior to ophthalmic surgery. Discontinue 3 to 4 weeks before surgery.

➤*Systemic effects:* Repeated administration may cause depression of the concentration of cholinesterase in the serum and erythrocytes, with resultant systemic effects. Discontinue if salivation, urinary inconti-nence, diarrhea, profuse sweating, muscle weakness, respiratory diffi-culties, shock or cardiac irregularities occur.

Although systemic effects are infrequent, use digital compression of the nasolacrimal ducts for 1 to 2 minutes after instillation to minimize drainage into the nasopharyngeal area.

➤*Iris cysts:* Iris cysts may form, enlarge and obscure vision (more fre-quent in children). The iris cyst usually shrinks upon discontinuance of the miotic, or following reduction in strength of the drops or frequency of instillation. Rarely, the cyst may rupture or break free into the aque-ous humor. Frequent examination for this occurrence is advised.

➤*Special risk:* Use caution in patients with marked vagotonia, bron-chial asthma, spastic GI disturbances, peptic ulcer, pronounced brady-cardia/hypotension, recent MI, epilepsy, parkinsonism and other disorders that may respond adversely to vagotonic effects. Temporarily discontinue if cardiac irregularities occur.

➤*Sulfite sensitivity:* Some of these products contain sulfites which may cause allergic-type reactions (eg, hives, itching, wheezing, anaphy-laxis) in certain susceptible persons. Although the overall prevalence of sulfite sensitivity in the general population is probably low, it is seen more frequently in asthmatics or atopic nonasthmatics.

Drug Interactions

Ophthalmic Cholinesterase Inhibitor Drug Interactions			
Precipitant drug	Object drug*		Description
Carbamate/ Or-ganophosphate insecticides, pes-ticides	Cholinesterase inhibitors	↑	Warn persons on cholinesterase inhibitors who are exposed to these substances (eg, gardeners, organophosphate plant or ware-house workers, farmers) of sys-temic effects possible from absorption through respiratory tract or skin. Advise use of respi-ratory masks, frequent washing and clothing changes.
Succinylcholine	Cholinesterase inhibitors	↑	Use extreme caution before or during general anesthesia to patients on cholinesterase inhibi-tors because of possible respira-tory and cardiovascular collapse.
Anticholinester-ases, systemic	Cholinesterase inhibitors	↑	Additive effects are possible; coadminister topical cholinester-ase inhibitors cautiously, regard-less of which therapy is added (see Warnings).

* ↑ = Object drug increased

Adverse Reactions

➤*Ophthalmic:* Iris cysts (see Precautions); burning; lacrimation; lid muscle twitching; conjunctival and ciliary redness; browache; head-ache; activation of latent iritis or uveitis; induced myopia with visual blurring; retinal detatchment; lens opacities (see Precautions); con-juntival thickening and destruction of nasolacrimal canals (prolonged use).

Paradoxical increase in IOP by pupillary block may follow instillation. Alleviate with pupil-dilating medication.

➤*Systemic:* Nausea; vomiting; abdominal cramps; diarrhea; urinary incontinence; fainting sweating; salivation; difficulty in breathing; cardiac irregularities.

Overdosage

➤*Treatment:* If systemic effects occur, give parenteral atropine sulfate (IV if necessary):

Adults – 0.4 to 0.6 mg.

Infants and children up to 12 years – 0.01 mg/kg repeated every 2 hours as needed until the desired effect is obtained, or adverse effects of atropine preclude further usage. The maximum single dose should not exceed 0.4 mg.

Much larger atropine doses for anticholinesterase intoxication in adults have been used. Initially, 2 to 6 mg followed by 2 mg every hour or more often, as long as muscarinic effects continue. Consider the greater possibility of atropinization with large doses, particularly in sensitive individuals.

Pralidoxime chloride (see Antidotes) has been useful in treating systemic effects due to cholinesterase inhibitors. However, use in addition to, not as a substitute for, atropine.

A short-acting barbiturate is indicated for convulsions not relieved by atropine. Promptly treat marked weakness or paralysis of respiratory muscles by maintaining a clear airway and by artificial respiration.

Patient Information

Local irritation and headache may occur at initiation of therapy.

Notify physician if abdominal cramps, diarrhea or excessive salivation occurs.

Wash hands immediately after administration.

Use caution while driving at night or performing hazardous tasks in poor light.

DEMECARIUM BROMIDE

Rx	Humorsol (Merck)	Solution: 0.125%	In 5 mL *Ocumeters.*[1]
		0.25%	In 5 mL *Ocumeters.*[1]

[1] With 1:5000 benzalkonium chloride and sodium chloride.

For complete prescribing information, refer to the Miotics, Cholinesterase Inhibitors group monograph.

Indications

➤*Glaucoma:* Treatment of open-angle glaucoma (use only when shorter-acting miotics have proved inadequate).

➤*Aqueous outflow:* Conditions affecting aqueous outflow (eg, synechial formation) that are amenable to miotic therapy.

➤*Iridectomy:* Following iridectomy procedure.

➤*Accommodative esotripia:* Treatment of accomodative esotripia (accomodative convergent stabismus).

Administration and Dosage

Do not use more often than directed. Caution is necessary to avoid overdosage. Individualize dosage to obtain maximal therapeutic effect.

Closely observe the patient during the initial period. If the response is not adequate within the first 24 hours, consider other measures. Keep frequency of use to a minimum in all patients, especially children, to reduce chance of iris cyst development.

➤*Glaucoma:*

Initial – Instill 1 or 2 drops into eye(s). A decrease in IOP should occur within a few hours. During this period, keep patient under supervision and perform tonometric examinations at least hourly for 3 or 4 hours to make sure no immediate rise in pressure occurs.

Usual dose – Instill 1 or 2 drops twice a week to 1 or 2 drops twice a day. The 0.125% strength used twice daily usually results in smooth control of the physiologic diurnal variation in IOP.

➤*Strabismus:* Essentially equal visual acuity of both eyes is a prerequisite to successful treatment.

Diagnosis – For initial evaluation, use as a diagnostic aid to determine if an accommodative factor exists. This is especially useful preoperatively in young children and in patients with normal hypermetropic refractive errors. Instill 1 drop daily for 2 weeks, then 1 drop every 2 days for 2 to 3 weeks. If the eyes become straighter, an accommodative factor is demonstrated. This technique may supplement or complement standard testing with atropine and trial with glasses for the accommodative factor.

Therapy – In esotropia uncomplicated by amblyopia or anisometropia, instill not more than 1 drop at a time in both eyes every day for 2 to 3 weeks; too severe a degree of miosis may interfere with vision. Then reduce dosage to 1 drop every other day for 3 to 4 weeks and reevaluate the patient's status. Continue with a dosage of 1 drop every 2 days to 1 drop twice a week (the latter dosage may be maintained for several months). Evaluate the patient's condition every 4 to 12 weeks. If improvement continues, reduce to 1 drop once a week and eventually to a trial without medication. However discontinue therapy after 4 months if control of the condition still requires 1 drop every 2 days.

➤*Storage / Stability:* Do not freeze. Protect from heat.

ECHOTHIOPHATE IODIDE

Rx	Phospholine Iodide (Wyeth-Ayerst)	Powder for Reconstitution: 6.25 mg to make 0.125%	With 5 mL diluent.[1]

[1] With potassium acetate, 0.55% chlorobutanol and 1.2% mannitol.

For complete prescribing information, refer to the Miotics, Cholinesterase Inhibitors group monograph.

Indications

➤*Glaucoma:* Chronic open-angle glaucoma; subacute or chronic angle-closure glaucoma after iridectomy or where surgery is refused or contraindicated; certain nonuveitic secondary types of glaucoma, especially glaucoma following cataract surgery.

➤*Accomodative esotropia:* Concomitant esotropias with a significant accommodative component.

Administration and Dosage

Tolerance may develop after prolonged use; a rest period restores response to the drug.

➤*Glaucoma:* Two doses per day are preferred to maintain a smooth diurnal tension curve, although 1 dose/day or every other day has been used with satisfactory results. It is unnecessary and undesirable to exceed a schedule of twice a day. Instill the daily dose or 1 of the 2 daily doses just before bedtime to avoid inconvenience due to miosis.

Early chronic simple glaucoma – Instill a 0.03% solution just before retiring and in the morning in cases not controlled with pilocarpine. Control during the night and early morning hours may then be obtained. Change therapy if IOP fails to remain at an acceptable level.

Advanced chronic simple glaucoma and glaucoma secondary to cataract surgery – Instill 0.03% solution twice daily, as above. When transferring a patient to echothiophate because of unsatisfactory control with other miotics, one of the higher strengths will be

needed. In this case, a brief trial with 0.03% solution will be advantageous because higher strengths will then be more easily tolerated.

➤*Concomitant therapy:* May be coadministered with epinephrine, a carbonic anhydrase inhibitor or both.

➤*Accommodative esotropia:*

Diagnosis – Instill 1 drop of 0.125% solution once a day into both eyes at bedtime for 2 or 3 weeks. If the esotropia is accommodative, a favorable response may begin within a few hours.

Treatment – Use lowest concentration and frequency which gives satisfactory results. After initial period of treatment for diagnostic purposes, reduce schedule to 0.125% every other day or 0.06% every day. Dosages can often be gradually lowered as treatment progresses. The 0.03% strength has proven effective in some cases. The maximum recommended dose is 0.125% once a day, although more intensive therapy has been used for short periods.

Duration of treatment – In diagnosis, only a short period is required and little time will be lost in instituting other procedures if the esotropia proves to be unresponsive. In therapy, there is no definite limit if the drug is well tolerated. However, if the eyedrops, with or without eyeglasses, are gradually withdrawn after a year or two and deviation recurs, consider surgery.

➤*Storage / Stability:* Store at room temperature 15° to 30°C (59° to 86°F). After reconstitution, keep eye drops in refrigerator to obtain maximum useful life of 6 months. Use within 1 month if stored at room temperature.

Refer to the Topical Ophthalmic Drugs introduction for more complete information.

Indications

➤*Elevated intraocular pressure (IOP):* Treatment of elevated IOP in patients with ocular hypertension or open-angle glaucoma.

Actions

➤*Pharmacology:* Dorzolamide and brinzolamide are carbonic anhydrase inhibitors for ophthalmic use. Carbonic anhydrase (CA) is an enzyme found in many tissues of the body, including the eye. It catalyzes the reversible reaction involving the hydration of carbon dioxide and the dehydration of carbonic acid. In humans, CA exists as a number of isoenzymes, the most active being CA-II, found primarily in red blood cells (RBCs), but also in other tissues. Inhibition of CA in the ciliary processes of the eye decreases aqueous humor secretion, presumably by slowing the formation of bicarbonate ions with subsequent reduction in sodium and fluid transport. The result is a reduction in intraocular pressure (IOP). Dorzolamide and brinzolamide reduce elevated IOP by inhibiting CA-II. Elevated IOP is a major risk factor in the pathogenesis of optic nerve damage and glaucomatous visual field loss.

➤*Pharmacokinetics:* When topically applied, dorzolamide and brinzolamide reach the systemic circulation and accumulate in RBCs during chronic dosing as a result of binding to CA-II. Extensive distribution into RBCs yields a long half-life, ≈ 3.5 to 4 months. The parent drugs form a single N-desethyl metabolite that inhibits CA-II less potently than the parent drug, but also inhibits CA-I. The metabolite also accumulates in RBCs, where it binds primarily to CA-I. Plasma concentrations of parent and metabolite are generally below the assay limit of quantitation. Plasma protein binding is moderate (≈ 33%) for dorzolamide and ≈ 60% for brinzolamide. These agents are primarily excreted unchanged in the urine, and the metabolite also is excreted in urine.

Contraindications

Hypersensitivity to any component of these products.

Warnings

➤*Systemic effects:* Dorzolamide and brinzolamide are sulfonamides and, although administered topically, are absorbed systemically. Therefore, the same types of adverse reactions attributable to systemic sulfonamides may occur with topical administration of these agents (refer to the systemic Sulfonamides monograph in the Anti-Infectives chapter). Fatalities have occurred, although rarely, because of severe reactions to sulfonamides including Stevens-Johnson syndrome, toxic epidermal necrolysis, fulminant hepatic necrosis, agranulocytosis, aplastic anemia, and other blood dyscrasias. Sensitization may recur when a sulfonamide is readministered regardless of the route of administration. If signs of serious reactions or hypersensitivity occur, discontinue the use of this preparation.

➤*Renal/Hepatic function impairment:* These agents have not been studied in patients with severe renal impairment (Ccr < 30 mL/min). However, because dorzolamide, brinzolamide, and their metabolites are excreted predominantly by the kidney, these agents are not recommended in such patients.

Dorzolamide and brinzolamide have not been studied in patients with hepatic impairment and should be used with caution in such patients.

➤*Carcinogenesis:* In a 2-year study of dorzolamide administered orally to male and female Sprague-Dawley rats, urinary bladder papillomas were seen in male rats in the highest dosage group of 20 mg/kg/day (250 times the recommended human ophthalmic dose); papillomas were not seen in rats given oral doses equivalent to ≈ 12 times the recommended dose. The increased incidence of urinary bladder papillomas is a class effect of CA inhibitors in rats.

➤*Elderly:* Of all the patients in dorzolamide clinical studies, 44% were ≥ 65 years of age, and 10% were ≥ 75 years of age. No overall differences in efficacy or safety were observed between these patients and younger patients, but greater sensitivity of some older individuals to the product cannot be ruled out.

➤*Pregnancy:* Category C. Maternal toxicity and a significant increase in the number of fetal variations (eg, malformations of the vertebral bodies) was seen in animals at doses > 20 times the recommended human ophthalmic dose. These malformations occurred at doses that caused metabolic acidosis with decreased body weight gain in dams and decreased fetal weights. There are no adequate and well controlled studies in pregnant women. Use during pregnancy only if the potential benefit justifies the risk to the fetus.

➤*Lactation:* In lactating rats, decreases in body weight gain were seen in offspring with these agents at oral doses > 94 times the recommended human ophthalmic dose. A slight delay in postnatal development (incisor eruption, vaginal canalization, and eye openings), secondary to lower fetal body weight, also was noted with dorzolamide.

It is not known whether this drug is excreted in breast milk. Because of the potential for serious adverse reactions in nursing infants, decide whether to discontinue nursing or to discontinue the drug, taking into account the importance of the drug to the mother.

➤*Children:* Safety and efficacy in children have not been established.

Precautions

➤*Corneal endothelium effects:* Carbonic anhydrase activity has been observed in both the cytoplasm and around the plasma membranes of the corneal endothelium. The effect of continued administration of dorzolamide or brinzolamide on the corneal endothelium has not been fully evaluated.

➤*Acute angle-closure glaucoma:* The management of patients with acute angle-closure glaucoma requires therapeutic interventions in addition to ocular hypotensive agents. Dorzolamide and brinzolamide have not been studied in patients with acute angle-closure glaucoma.

➤*Ocular effects:* Local ocular adverse effects, primarily conjunctivitis and lid reactions, were reported with chronic administration of dorzolamide. Many of these reactions had the clinical appearance and course of an allergic-type reaction that resolved upon discontinuation of drug therapy. If such reactions are observed, discontinue the drug and evaluate the patient before considering restarting the drug.

➤*Concomitant oral CA inhibitors:* There is a potential for an additive effect on the known systemic effects of CA inhibition in patients receiving an oral CA inhibitor and dorzolamide or brinzolamide. Concomitant administration of ophthalmic and oral CA inhibitors is not recommended.

➤*Bacterial keratitis:* There have been reports of bacterial keratitis associated with the use of topical ophthalmic products in multiple-dose containers. These containers had been inadvertently contaminated by patients who, in most cases, had a concurrent corneal disease or a disruption of the ocular epithelial surface. Serious damage to the eye and subsequent loss of vision may result from using contaminated solutions.

➤*Contact lenses:* The preservative used in these products, benzalkonium chloride, may be absorbed by soft contact lenses. Do not administer these agents while wearing soft contact lenses; reinsert lenses ≥ 15 minutes after drug administration.

Drug Interactions

Although acid-base and electrolyte disturbances were not reported in the clinical trials with dorzolamide and brinzolamide, these disturbances have been reported with oral CA inhibitors and have, in some instances, resulted in drug interactions (eg, toxicity associated with high-dose salicylate therapy). Therefore, consider the potential for such drug interactions in patients receiving either of these agents.

Adverse Reactions

➤*Dorzolamide:*

Miscellaneous – Ocular burning, stinging or discomfort immediately following administration (≈ 33%); bitter taste following administration (≈ 25%); superficial punctate keratitis (10% to 15%); signs and symptoms of ocular allergic reaction (≈ 10%); blurred vision, tearing, dryness, photophobia (≈ 1% to 5%); headache, nausea, asthenia/fatigue (infrequent); skin rashes, urolithiasis, iridocyclitis (rare).

➤*Brinzolamide:*

Miscellaneous – Blurred vision, bitter, sour, or unusual taste (≈ 5% to 10%); blepharitis, dermatitis, dry eye, foreign body sensation, headache, hyperemia, ocular discharge, ocular discomfort, ocular keratitis, ocular pain, ocular pruritus, rhinitis (1% to 5%); allergic reactions, alopecia, chest pain, conjunctivitis, diarrhea, diplopia, dizziness, dry mouth, dyspnea, dyspepsia, eye fatigue, hypertonia, keratoconjunctivitis, keratopathy, kidney pain, lid margin crusting or sticky sensation, nausea, pharyngitis, tearing, urticaria (< 1%).

Overdosage

Electrolyte imbalance, development of an acidotic state and possible CNS effects may occur. Monitor serum electrolyte levels (particularly potassium) and blood pH levels. Significant lethality was observed in female rats and mice after single oral doses of 1927 and 1320 mg/kg of dorzolamide, respectively.

Patient Information

Dorzolamide and brinzolamide are sulfonamides and, although administered topically, are absorbed systemically. Therefore, the same types of adverse reactions that are attributable to systemic sulfonamides may occur with topical administration. Advise patients that if serious or unusual reactions or signs of hypersensitivity occur, they should discontinue use of the product and consult their physician.

Vision may be temporarily blurred. Instruct patients to exercise care in operating machinery or driving a motor vehicle.

Advise patients that if they develop any ocular reactions, particularly conjunctivitis and lid reactions, they should discontinue medication use and seek their physician's advice.

Instruct patients to avoid allowing the tip of the dispensing container to contact the eye or surrounding structures. Ocular solutions, if handled improperly or if the tip of the dispensing container contacts the eye or surrounding structures, can become contaminated by common bacteria known to cause ocular infections. Serious damage to the eye and subsequent loss of vision may result from using contaminated solutions.

Advise patients that if they develop an intercurrent ocular condition (eg, trauma, ocular surgery, infection), they should immediately seek their physician's advice concerning the continued use of the present multidose container.

If more than one topical ophthalmic drug is being used, administer the drugs at least 10 minutes apart.

DORZOLAMIDE HYDROCHLORIDE

| *Rx* | **Trusopt** (Merck) | **Solution:** 2% (as base) | In 5 and 10 mL *Ocumeters*.[1] |

[1] With 0.0075% benzalkonium chloride, hydroxyethylcellulose, sodium hydroxide, and mannitol.

For complete prescribing information, refer to the Carbonic Anhydrase Inhibitors group monograph.

Indications

➤*Elevated intraocular pressure (IOP):* Treatment of elevated IOP in patients with ocular hypertension or open-angle glaucoma.

Administration and Dosage

➤*Approved by the FDA:* December 9, 1994.

➤*Dosage:* One drop in the affected eye(s) 3 times daily.

➤*Concomitant therapy:* Dorzolamide may be used concomitantly with other topical ophthalmic drug products to lower intraocular pressure. If more than one ophthalmic drug is being used, administer the drugs at least 10 minutes apart.

➤*Storage/Stability:* Store at 15° to 30°C (59° to 86°F). Protect from light.

BRINZOLAMIDE

| *Rx* | **Azopt** (Alcon) | **Suspension:** 1% | In 2.5, 5, 10, and 15 mL *Drop-Tainers*.[1] |

[1] With 0.01% benzalkonium chloride, mannitol, carbomer 974P, tyloxapol, sodium chloride, hydrochloric acid and/or sodium hydroxide, and EDTA.

For complete prescribing information, refer to the Carbonic Anhydrase Inhibitors group monograph.

Indications

➤*Elevated intraocular pressure (IOP):* Treatment of elevated IOP in patients with ocular hypertension or open-angle glaucoma.

Administration and Dosage

➤*Approved by the FDA:* April 3, 1998.

➤*Dosage:* One drop in the affected eye(s) 3 times daily.

➤*Concomitant therapy:* Brinzolamide may be used concomitantly with other topical ophthalmic drug products to lower intraocular pressure. If more than one topical ophthalmic drug is being used, administer the drugs at least 10 minutes apart.

➤*Storage/Stability:* Store at 4° to 30°C (39° to 86°F). Shake well.

LATANOPROST

Rx	Xalatan (Pfizer)	Solution: 0.005%	0.02% benzalkonium chloride, sodium chloride. In 2.5 mL fill dropper bottles.

Refer to the Topical Ophthalmic Drugs introduction for more complete information.

Indications

➤*Elevated intraocular pressure (IOP):* For reduction of elevated IOP in patients with open-angle glaucoma and ocular hypertension.

Administration and Dosage

➤*Approved by the FDA:* June 5, 1996.

The recommended dosage is 1 drop (1.5 mcg) in the affected eye(s) once daily in the evening. Do not exceed once-daily dosage because it has been shown that more frequent administration may decrease the IOP-lowering effect. Reduction of the IOP starts approximately 3 to 4 hours after administration, and the maximum effect is reached after 8 to 12 hours.

Latanoprost may be used concomitantly with other topical ophthalmic drug products to lower IOP. If more than one topical ophthalmic drug is being used, administer the drugs at least 5 minutes apart.

➤*Storage / Stability:* Protect from light. Refrigerate unopened bottle at 2° to 8°C (36° to 46°F). Once opened, the container may be stored at room temperature up to 25°C (77°F) for 6 weeks.

Actions

➤*Pharmacology:* Latanoprost is a prostaglandin $F_{2\alpha}$ analog that is believed to reduce the IOP by increasing the outflow of aqueous humor.

➤*Pharmacokinetics:*

Absorption – Latanoprost is absorbed through the cornea where the isopropyl ester prodrug is hydrolyzed to the biologically active acid. Peak concentration in the aqueous humor is reached approximately 2 hours after topical administration.

Distribution – The distribution volume is approximately 0.16 L/kg. The acid of latanoprost could be measured in aqueous humor during the first 4 hours and in plasma only during the first hour after local administration.

Metabolism – The active acid of latanoprost reaching systemic circulation is primarily metabolized by the liver to the 1,2-dinor and 1,2,3,4-tetranor metabolites via fatty acid β-oxidation.

Excretion – The elimination of the acid of latanoprost from human plasma was rapid (half-life was 17 min) after both IV and topical administration. Systemic clearance is approximately 7 mL/min/kg. Following hepatic β-oxidation, the metabolites are mainly eliminated via the kidneys. Approximately 88% to 98% of the administered dose is recovered in the urine after topical and IV dosing, respectively.

➤*Clinical trials:* Patients with mean baseline IOP of 24 to 25 mm Hg who were treated for 6 months in multicenter, randomized, controlled trials demonstrated 6 to 8 mm Hg reductions in IOP. This IOP reduction with 0.005% latanoprost dosed once daily was equivalent to the effect of 0.5% timolol dosed twice daily.

Contraindications

Hypersensitivity to any component of this product.

Warnings

➤*Eye pigment changes:* Latanoprost ophthalmic solution has been reported to cause changes to pigmented tissues. The most frequently reported changes have been increased pigmentation of the iris, periorbital tissue (eyelid) and eyelashes, and growth of eyelashes. Pigmentation is expected to increase as long as latanoprost is administered. After discontinuation of latanoprost, pigmentation of the iris is likely to be permanent while pigmentation of the periorbital tissue and eyelash changes have been reported to be reversible in some patients. Patients who receive treatment should be informed of the possibility of increased pigmentation. The effects of increased pigmentation beyond 5 years are not known.

The eye color change is due to increased melanin content in the stromal melanocytes of the iris rather than to an increase in the number of melanocytes. This change may not be noticeable for several months to years. Typically, the brown pigmentation around the pupil spreads concentrically towards the periphery of the iris and the entire iris or parts of the iris become more brownish. Neither nevi nor freckles of the iris appear to be affected by treatment. While treatment with latanoprost can be continued in patients who develop noticeably increased iris pigmentation, these patients should be examined regularly.

The increase in brown iris pigment has not shown to progress further upon discontinuation of treatment, but the resultant color change may be permanent.

Eyelid skin darkening, which may be reversible, has been reported in association with the use of latanoprost.

Latanoprost may gradually change eyelashes and vellus hair in the treated eye; these changes include increased length, thickness, pigmen-

tation, the number of lashes or hairs, and misdirected growth of eyelashes. Eyelash changes are usually reversible upon discontinuation of treatment.

➤*Pregnancy: Category C.* In rabbits, 4 out of 16 dams had no viable fetuses at a dose that was approximately 80 times the maximum human dose, and the highest nonembryocidal dose in rabbits was approximately 15 times the maximum human dose. There are no adequate and well controlled studies in pregnant women. Use during pregnancy only if the potential benefit justifies the potential risk to the fetus.

➤*Lactation:* It is not known whether this drug or its metabolites are excreted in breast milk. Exercise caution when administering latanoprost to a nursing woman.

➤*Children:* Safety and efficacy have not been established.

Precautions

➤*Intraocular inflammation:* Use latanoprost with caution in patients with a history of intraocular inflammation (iritis/uveitis). Generally, do not use latanoprost in patients with active intraocular inflammation.

➤*Macular edema:* Macular edema, including cystoid macular edema, has been reported during treatment with latanoprost. These reports have mainly occurred in aphakic patients, in pseudophakic patients with a torn posterior lens capsule, or in patients with known risk factors for macular edema. Use latanoprost with caution in patients who do not have an intact posterior capsule or who have known risk factors for macular edema.

➤*Bacterial keratitis:* There have been reports of bacterial keratitis associated with the use of multiple-dose containers of topical ophthalmic products. These containers had been inadvertently contaminated by patients who, in most cases, had a concurrent corneal disease or a disruption of the ocular epithelial surface.

➤*Contact lenses:* Do not administer latanoprost while wearing contact lenses. They may be reinserted 15 minutes after administration.

Drug Interactions

In vitro studies have shown that precipitation occurs when eye drops containing thimerosal are mixed with latanoprost. If such drugs are used, administer with an interval of at least 5 minutes between applications.

Adverse Reactions

➤*Local:* The ocular adverse events and ocular signs and symptoms reported in 5% to 15% of the patients on latanoprost in the three 6-month controlled trials were blurred vision, burning and stinging, conjunctival hyperemia, foreign body sensation, itching, increased pigmentation of the iris, and punctate epithelial keratopathy. Local conjunctival hyperemia was observed; however, less than 1% of the latanoprost-treated patients required discontinuation of therapy because of intolerance to conjunctival hyperemia. Also reported were dry eye, excessive tearing, eye pain, lid crusting, lid edema, lid erythema, lid discomfort/pain, photophobia (1% to 4%); conjunctivitis, diplopia, discharge from the eye (less than 1%); retinal artery embolus, retinal detachment, vitreous hemorrhage from diabetic retinopathy (rare).

The following also occurred: Eyelash changes (increased length, thickness, pigmentation, and number of lashes); eyelid skin darkening; intraocular inflammation (iritis/uveitis); iris pigmentation changes; and macular edema, including cystoid macular edema (see Warnings).

➤*Systemic:* The most common systemic adverse events seen with latanoprost were upper respiratory tract infection/cold/flu (4%); pain in muscle/joint/back, chest pain/angina pectoris, rash/allergic skin reaction (1% to 2%).

➤*Post-marketing:* The events that have been chosen for inclusion because of their seriousness, frequency of reporting, possible causal connection to latanoprost, or a combination of these factors, include: Asthma and exacerbation of asthma; corneal edema and erosions; dyspnea; eyelash and vellus hair changes (increased length, thickness, pigmentation, and number); eyelid skin darkening; herpes keratitis; intraocular inflammation (iritis/uveitis); keratitis; macular edema, including cystoid macular edema; misdirected eyelashes sometimes resulting in eye irritation; and toxic epidermal necrolysis.

Overdosage

➤*Symptoms:* Apart from ocular irritation and conjunctival or episcleral hyperemia, the ocular effects of latanoprost administered at high doses are not known. IV administration of large doses of latanoprost in monkeys has been associated with transient bronchoconstriction; however, in 11 patients with bronchial asthma treated with latanoprost, bronchoconstriction was not induced. IV infusions of up to 3 mcg/kg in healthy volunteers produced mean plasma concentrations 200 times higher than during clinical treatment, and no adverse reactions were observed. IV dosages of 5.5 to 10 mcg/kg caused abdominal

LATANOPROST

pain, dizziness, fatigue, hot flushes, nausea, and sweating.

➤*Treatment:* If overdosage occurs, treatment should be symptomatic.

Patient Information

Inform patients of the potential for increased brown pigmentation of the iris that may be permanent. Inform patients about the possibility of eyelid skin darkening, which may be reversible after discontinuation of latanoprost.

Inform patients of the possibility of eyelash and vellus hair changes in the treated eye during treatment with latanoprost. These changes may result in a disparity between eyes in length, thickness, pigmentation, number of eyelashes or vellus hair, and/or direction of eyelash growth. Eyelash changes are usually reversible upon discontinuation of treatment.

Advise patients that if they develop an intercurrent ocular condition (eg, trauma, infection) or have ocular surgery, they should immediately seek their physician's advice concerning the continued use of the multiple-dose container.

Advise patients to avoid allowing the tip of the dispensing container to contact the eye or surrounding structures because this could cause the tip to become contaminated by common bacteria known to cause ocular infections. Serious damage to the eye and subsequent loss of vision may result from using contaminated solutions.

Advise patients that if they develop any ocular reactions, particularly conjunctivitis and lid reactions, they should immediately seek their physician's advice.

Latanoprost contains benzalkonium chloride, which may be absorbed by contact lenses. Remove contact lenses prior to administration of the solution. Lenses may be reinserted 15 minutes following latanoprost administration.

If more than one topical ophthalmic drug is being used, administer the drugs at least 5 minutes apart.

TRAVOPROST

Rx	**Travatan** (Alcon)	**Solution:** 0.004%	0.015% benzalkonium chloride/mL, EDTA. In 2.5 mL *Drop-Tainers*.

Indications

➤*Elevated intraocular pressure (IOP):* For the reduction of IOP in patients with open-angle glaucoma or ocular hypertension who are intolerant of other IOP-lowering medications or insufficiently responsive (failed to achieve target IOP determined after multiple measurements over time) to another IOP-lowering medication. Travoprost has not been evaluated for the treatment of angle closure, inflammatory, or neovascular glaucoma.

Administration and Dosage

➤*Approved by the FDA:* March 16, 2001.

The recommended dosage is 1 drop in the affected eye(s) once daily in the evening. The dosage of travoprost should not exceed once daily because it has been shown that more frequent administration may decrease the IOP-lowering effect.

Reduction of IOP starts ≈ 2 hours after administration, and the maximum effect is reached after 12 hours.

Travoprost may be used concomitantly with other topical ophthalmic drugs to lower IOP. If more than 1 topical ophthalmic drug is being used, the drugs should be administered at least 5 minutes apart.

➤*Storage/Stability:* Store between 2° to 25°C (36° to 77°F). Discard the container within 6 weeks of removing it from the sealed pouch.

Actions

➤*Pharmacology:* Travoprost is a synthetic prostaglandin $F_{2\alpha}$ analog. Travoprost free acid is a selective FP prostanoid receptor agonist, which is believed to reduce IOP by increasing uveoscleral outflow. The exact mechanism of action is unknown at this time.

➤*Pharmacokinetics:*

Absorption – Travoprost is absorbed through the cornea. In humans, peak plasma concentrations of travoprost free acid (≤ 25 pg/mL) were reached within 30 minutes following topical ocular administration and was rapidly eliminated.

Metabolism – Travoprost, an isopropyl ester prodrug, is hydrolyzed by esterases in the cornea to its biologically active free acid.

Excretion – Elimination of travoprost free acid from human plasma is rapid. Plasma levels are below the limit of quantitation (< 10 pg/mL) within 1 hour following ocular instillation.

➤*Clinical trials:* In clinical studies, patients with open-angle glaucoma or ocular hypertension and baseline pressure of 25 to 27 mmHg who were treated with travoprost dosed once daily in the evening demonstrated 7 to 8 mmHg reductions in intraocular pressure. In subgroup analyses of these studies, mean IOP reduction in black patients was up to 1.8 mmHg greater than in non-black patients. It is not known at this time whether this difference is attributed to race or to heavily pigmented irides.

In a multi-center, randomized, controlled trial, patients with mean baseline IOP of 24 to 26 mmHg on timolol 0.5% twice daily were treated with travoprost 0.004% dosed every day adjunctively to timolol 0.5% twice daily demonstrate 6 to 7 mmHg reductions in IOP.

Contraindications

Known hypersensitivity to travoprost, benzalkonium chloride, or any other ingredients of the product. Travoprost may interfere with the maintenance of pregnancy and should not be used by women during pregnancy or by women attempting to become pregnant.

Warnings

➤*Ocular changes:* Travoprost has been reported to cause changes to pigmented tissues. The most frequently reported changes have been increased pigmentation of the iris and periorbital tissue (eyelid) and increased pigmentation and growth of eyelashes. These changes may be permanent.

Travoprost may gradually change eye color, increasing the amount of brown pigmentation in the iris by increasing the number of melanosomes (pigment granules) in melanocytes. This change may not be noticeable for months to years. Iris pigmentation changes may be more noticeable in patients with mixed color irides (ie, blue-brown, grey-brown, yellow-brown, and green-brown); however, it also has been observed in patients with brown eyes. The color change is believed to be due to increased melanin content in the stromal melanocytes of the iris. The exact mechanism of action is unknown at this time. Typically, the brown pigmentation around the pupil spreads concentrically towards the periphery in affected eyes, but the entire iris or parts of it may become more brownish. Until more information about increased brown pigmentation is available, examine patients regularly and, depending on the situation, treatment may be stopped if increased pigmentation ensues. The long-term effects on the melanocytes and the consequences of potential injury to the melanocytes or deposition of pigment granules to other areas of the eye are currently unknown. The change in iris color occurs slowly and may not be noticeable for months to years. Inform patients of the possibility of iris color change.

Eyelid skin darkening has been reported in association with the use of travoprost.

Travoprost may gradually change eyelashes in the treated eye; these changes include increased length, thickness, pigmentation, or number of lashes. Inform patients who are expected to receive treatment in only 1 eye about the potential for increased brown pigmentation of the iris, periorbital, or eyelid tissue, and eyelashes in the treated eye and thus heterochromia between the eyes. Advise them of the potential for a disparity between the eyes in length, thickness, or number of eyelashes.

➤*Mutagenesis:* Travoprost was not mutagenic in the Ames test, mouse micronucleus test, and rat chromosome assay. A slight increase in the mutant frequency was observed in 1 of 2 mouse lymphoma assays in the presence of rat S-9 activation enzymes.

➤*Fertility impairment:* Travoprost did not affect mating or fertility indices in male or female rats at SC doses up to 10 mcg/kg/day (250 times the maximum recommended human ocular dose of 0.04 mcg/kg/day on a mcg/kg basis [MRHOD]). At 10 mcg/kg/day, the mean number of corpora lutea was reduced, and the post-implantation losses were increased. These effects were not observed at 3 mcg/kg/day (75 times the MRHOD).

➤*Pregnancy:* Category C. Because prostaglandins are biologically active and may be absorbed through the skin, women who are pregnant or attempting to become pregnant should exercise appropriate precautions to avoid direct exposure to the contents of the bottle. In case of accidental contact with the contents of the bottle, thoroughly cleanse the exposed area with soap and water immediately.

Travoprost was teratogenic in rats, at an IV dose up to 10 mcg/kg/day (250 times the MRHOD), evidenced by an increase in the incidence of skeletal malformations as well as external and visceral malformations, such as fused sternebrae, domed head, and hydrocephaly. Travoprost produced an increase in post-implantation losses and a decrease in fetal viability in rats at IV doses > 3 mcg/kg/day (75 times the MRHOD) and in mice at SC doses > 0.3 mcg/kg/day (7.5 times the MRHOD).

In the offspring of female rats that received travoprost SC from day 7 of pregnancy to lactation day 21 at the doses of ≥ 0.12 mcg/kg/day (3 times the MRHOD), the incidence of postnatal mortality was increased, and neonatal body weight gain was decreased. Neonatal development was also affected, evidenced by delayed eye opening, pinna detachment, and preputial separation, and by decreased motor activity.

No adequate and well-controlled studies have been performed in pregnant women. Travoprost may interfere with the maintenance of preg-

TRAVOPROST

nancy and should not be used by women during pregnancy or by women attempting to become pregnant.

➤*Lactation:* A study in lactating rats demonstrated that radiolabeled travoprost or its metabolites were excreted in milk. It is not known whether this drug or its metabolites are excreted in human milk. Because many drugs are excreted in human milk, exercise caution when travoprost is administered to a nursing woman.

➤*Children:* Safety and efficacy in pediatric patients have not been established.

Precautions

➤*Bacterial keratitis:* There have been reports of bacterial keratitis associated with the use of multiple-dose containers of topical ophthalmic products. These containers had been inadvertently contaminated by patients, who, in most cases, had a concurrent corneal disease or a disruption of the epithelial surface (see Patient Information).

➤*Active intraocular inflammation:* Use travoprost with caution in patients with active intraocular inflammation (iritis/uveitis).

➤*Macular edema:* Macular edema, including cystoid macular edema, has been reported during treatment with prostaglandin $F_{2\alpha}$ analogs. These reports have mainly occurred in aphakic patients, pseudophakic patients with a torn posterior lens capsule, or in patients with known risk factors for macular edema. Use travoprost with caution in these patients.

➤*Contact lenses:* Travoprost should not be administered while wearing contact lenses.

Advise patients that travoprost contains benzalkonium chloride, which may be absorbed by the contact lenses. Contact lenses should be removed prior to the administration of the solution. Lenses may be reinserted 15 minutes following administration of travoprost.

Adverse Reactions

➤*Ophthalmic:* The most common ocular adverse event observed in controlled clinical studies with travoprost was ocular hyperemia, which was reported in 35% to 50% of patients. Approximately 3% of patients discontinued therapy due to conjunctival hyperemia.

Ocular adverse events reported at an incidence of 5% to 10% included decreased visual acuity, eye discomfort, foreign body sensation, pain, and pruritus.

Ocular adverse events reported at an incidence of 1% to 4% included abnormal vision, blepharitis, blurred vision, cataract, cells, conjunctivitis, dry eye, eye disorder, flare, iris discoloration, keratitis, lid margin crusting, photophobia, subconjunctival hemorrhage, and tearing.

➤*Systemic:* Nonocular adverse events reported at a rate of 1% to 5% were the following: Accidental injury, angina pectoris, anxiety, arthritis, back pain, bradycardia, bronchitis, chest pain, cold syndrome, depression, dyspepsia, GI disorder, headache, hypercholesterolemia, hypertension, hypotension, infection, pain, prostate disorder, sinusitis, urinary incontinence, and urinary tract infection.

Patient Information

Instruct patients to avoid allowing the tip of the dispensing container to contact the eye or surrounding structures because this could cause the tip to become contaminated by common bacteria known to cause ocular infections. Serious damage to the eye and subsequent loss of vision may result from using contaminated solutions.

Advise patients that if they develop an intercurrent ocular condition (eg, trauma, infection) or have ocular surgery, they should immediately seek their physician's advice concerning the continued use of the multidose container.

Advise patients that if they develop any ocular reactions, particularly conjunctivitis and lid reactions, they should immediately seek their physician's advice.

If more than 1 topical ophthalmic drug is being used, administer the drugs at least 5 minutes apart.

BIMATOPROST

Rx	Lumigan (Allergan)	Solution: 0.03%	0.05 mg benzalkonium chloride/mL. In 2.5 and 5 mL.

Indications

➤*Elevated intraocular pressure (IOP):* For the reduction of elevated IOP in patients with open angle glaucoma or ocular hypertension who are intolerant of other IOP-lowering medications or insufficiently responsive (failed to achieve target IOP determined after multiple measurements over time) to another IOP-lowering medication. Bimatoprost has not been evaluated for the treatment of angle closure, inflammatory, or neovascular glaucoma.

Administration and Dosage

➤*Approved by the FDA:* March 16, 2001.

The recommended dosage is 1 drop in the affected eye(s) once daily in the evening. The dosage should not exceed once daily because it has been shown that more frequent administration may decrease the IOP-lowering effect.

Reduction of IOP starts ≈ 4 hours after the first administration with maximum effect reached within ≈ 8 to 12 hours.

Bimatoprost may be used concomitantly with other topical ophthalmic drug products to lower IOP. If more than 1 topical ophthalmic drug is being used, the drugs should be administered at least 5 minutes apart.

➤*Storage / Stability:* Bimatoprost should be stored in the original container at 15° to 25°C (59° to 77°F).

Actions

➤*Pharmacology:* Bimatoprost is a prostamide, a synthetic structural analog of prostaglandin with ocular hypotensive activity. It selectively mimics the effects of naturally occurring substances, prostamides. Bimatoprost is believed to lower IOP in humans by increasing outflow of aqueous humor through the trabecular meshwork and uveoscleral routes. Elevated IOP presents a major risk factor for glaucomatous field loss. The higher the level of IOP, the greater the likelihood of optic nerve damage and visual field loss.

➤*Pharmacokinetics:*

Absorption – After 1 drop of bimatoprost ophthalmic solution 0.03% was administered once daily to both eyes of 15 healthy subjects for 2 weeks, blood concentrations peaked within 10 minutes after dosing and were below the lower limit of detection (0.025 ng/mL) in most subjects within 1.5 hours after dosing. Mean C_{max} and $AUC_{0-24\ hr}$ values were similar on days 7 and 14 at ≈ 0.08 ng/mL and 0.09 ng•hr/mL, respectively, indicating that steady state was reached during the first week of ocular dosing. There was no significant systemic drug accumulation over time.

Distribution – Bimatoprost is moderately distributed into body tissues with a steady-state volume of distribution of 0.67 L/kg. In human blood, bimatoprost resides mainly in the plasma. Approximately 12% of bimatoprost remains unbound in human plasma.

Metabolism – Bimatoprost is the major circulating species in the blood once it reaches the systemic circulation following ocular dosing. Bimatoprost then undergoes oxidation, N-deethylation and glucuronidation to form a diverse variety of metabolites.

Excretion – Following an IV dose of radiolabeled bimatoprost (3.12 mcg/kg) to 6 healthy subjects, the maximum blood concentration of unchanged drug was 12.2 ng/mL and decreased rapidly with an elimination half-life of ≈ 45 minutes. The total blood clearance of bimatoprost was 1.5 L/hr/kg. Up to 67% of the administered dose was excreted in the urine while 25% of the dose was recovered in the feces.

➤*Clinical trials:* In clinical studies of patients with open angle glaucoma or ocular hypertension with a mean baseline IOP of 26 mmHg, the IOP-lowering effect of bimatoprost 0.03% once daily (in the evening) was 7 to 8 mmHg.

Contraindications

Hypersensitivity to bimatoprost or any other ingredient of this product.

Warnings

➤*Ocular changes:* Bimatoprost has been reported to cause changes to pigmented tissues. These reports include increased pigmentation and growth of eyelashes and increased pigmentation of the iris and periorbital tissue (eyelid). These changes may be permanent.

Bimatoprost may gradually change eye color, increasing the amount of brown pigment in the iris by increasing the number of melanosomes (pigment granules) in melanocytes. Typically, the brown pigmentation around the pupil is expected to spread concentrically towards the periphery in affected eyes, but the entire iris or parts of it may also become more brownish. Until more information about increased brown pigmentation is available, examine patients regularly and, depending on the clinical situation, treatment may be stopped if increased pigmentation ensues. The increase in brown iris pigment is not expected to progress further upon discontinuation of treatment, but the resultant color change may be permanent. Neither nevi nor freckles of the iris are expected to be affected by treatment. The long-term effects on the melanocytes and the consequences of potential injury to the melanocytes or deposion of pigment granules to other areas of the eye are currently unknown. The change in iris color occurs slowly and may not be noticeable for several months to years. Inform patients of the possibility of iris color change.

Eyelid skin darkening has been reported in association with the use of bimatoprost.

Bimatoprost may gradually change eyelashes; these changes include increased length, thickness, pigmentation, and number of lashes.

BIMATOPROST

Inform patients who are expected to receive treatment in only 1 eye about the potential for increased brown pigmentation of the iris, periorbital tissue, and eyelashes in the treated eye and thus, heterochromia between the eyes. Advise them of the potential for a disparity between the eyes in length, thickness, or number of eyelashes.

➤*Pregnancy: Category C.* In embryo/fetal developmental studies in pregnant mice and rats, abortion was observed at oral doses of bimatoprost that achieved at least 33 or 97 times, respectively, the intended human exposure based on blood AUC levels.

At doses 41 times the intended human exposure based on blood AUC levels, the gestation length was reduced in the dams, the incidence of dead fetuses, late resorptions, peri- and postnatal pup mortality was increased, and pup body weights were reduced.

There are no adequate and well-controlled studies of bimatoprost administration in pregnant women. Because animal reproductive studies are not always predictive of human response, bimatoprost should be administered during pregnancy only if the potential benefit justifies the potential risk to the fetus.

➤*Lactation:* It is not known whether bimatoprost is excreted in human milk, although in animal studies, bimatoprost has been shown to be excreted in breast milk. Because many drugs are excreted in human milk, exercise caution when bimatoprost is administered to a nursing woman.

➤*Children:* Safety and efficacy in pediatric patients have not been established.

Precautions

➤*Bacterial keratits:* There have been reports of bacterial keratitis associated with the use of multiple-dose containers of topical ophthalmic products. These containers had been inadvertently contaminated by patients who, in most cases, had a concurrent corneal disease or a disruption of the ocular epithelial surface (see Patient Information).

➤*Active intraocular inflammation:* Use bimatoprost with caution in patients with active intraocular inflammation (eg, uveitis).

➤*Macular edema:* Macular edema, including cystoid macular edema, has been reported during treatment with bimatoprost ophthalmic solution. Use bimatoprost with caution in aphakic patients, in pseudophakic patients with a torn posterior lens capsule, or in patients with known risk factors for macular edema.

➤*Contact lenses:* Do not administer bimatoprost while wearing contact lenses. Remove contact lenses prior to instillation of bimatoprost; lenses may be reinserted 15 minutes after bimatoprost administration. Advise patients that bimatoprost contains benzalkonium chloride, which may be absorbed by soft contact lenses.

Adverse Reactions

In clinical trials, the most frequent events associated with the use of bimatoprost occurring in ≈ 15% to 45% of patients, in descending order of incidence, included conjunctival hyperemia, growth of eyelashes, and ocular pruritus. Approximately 3% of patients discontinued therapy due to conjunctival hyperemia.

➤*Ophthalmic:* Adverse events that occurred in ≈ 3% to 10% of patients, in descending order or incidence, included the following: Ocular dryness, visual disturbances, ocular burning, foreign body sensation, eye pain, pigmentation of the periocular skin, blepharitis, cataract, superficial punctate keratitis, eyelid erythema, ocular irritation, and eyelash darkening. The following ocular adverse events reported in ≈ 1% to 3% of patients, in descending order of incidence, included the following: Eye discharge, tearing, photophobia, allergic conjunctivitis, asthenopia, increases in iris pigmentation, and conjunctival edema. In < 1% of patients, intraocular inflammation was reported as iritis.

➤*Systemic:* Systemic adverse events reported in ≈ 10% of patients were infections (primarily colds and upper respiratory tract infections). The following systemic adverse events reported in ≈ 1% to 5% of patients, in descending order of incidence, included headaches, abnormal liver function tests, asthenia, and hirsutism.

Overdosage

No information is available on overdosage in humans. If overdose with bimatoprost occurs, treatment should be symptomatic.

In oral (by gavage) mouse and rat studies, doses up to 100 mg/kg/day did not produce any toxicity. This dose expressed as mg/m^2 is at least 70 times higher than the accidental dose of one bottle of bimatoprost for a 10 kg child.

Patient Information

Inform patients that bimatoprost has been reported to cause increased growth and darkening of eyelashes and darkening of the skin around the eye in some patients. These changes may be permanent.

Some patients may slowly develop darkening of the iris, which may be permanent.

When only 1 eye is treated, there is a potential for a cosmetic difference between the eyes in eyelash length, darkness or thickness, or color changes of the eyelid skin or iris.

Avoid allowing the tip of the dispensing container to contact the eye, surrounding structures, fingers, or any other surface in order to avoid contamination of the solution by common bacteria known to cause ocular infections. Serious damage to the eye and subsequent loss of vision may result from using contaminated solutions.

If patients develop an intercurrent ocular condition (eg, trauma or infection) or have ocular surgery, they should immediately seek their physician's advice concerning the continued use of the multidose container.

If patients develop any ocular reactions, particularly conjunctivitis and eyelid reactions, they should immediately seek their physician's advice.

Remove contact lenses prior to instillation of bimatoprost; lenses may be reinserted 15 minutes after bimatoprost administration. Advise patients that bimatoprost contains benzalkonium chloride, which may be absorbed by soft contact lenses.

If more than 1 topical ophthalmic drug is being used, administer the drugs at least 5 minutes apart.

UNOPROSTONE ISOPROPYL

| *Rx* | **Rescula** (Novartis Pharmaceuticals) | **Solution:** 0.15% | 0.015% benzalkonium chloride/mL, EDTA, sodium hydroxide, hydrochloric acid. In 5 mL. |

Indications

➤*Elevated intraocular pressure (IOP):* For the lowering of IOP in patients with open-angle glaucoma or ocular hypertension who are intolerant of other IOP-lowering medications or insufficiently responsive (failed to achieve target IOP determined after multiple measurements over time) to another IOP-lowering medication.

Administration and Dosage

➤*Approved by the FDA:* August 3, 2000.

The recommended dosage is 1 drop in the affected eye(s) twice daily. Unoprostone may be used concomitantly with other topical ophthalmic drug products to lower IOP. If 2 drugs are used, administer ≥ 5 minutes apart.

➤*Storage/Stability:* Store between 2° to 25°C (36° to 77°F).

Actions

➤*Pharmacology:* Unoprostone is a prostaglandin F$_{2\alpha}$ analog that is believed to reduce elevated IOP by increasing the outflow of aqueous humor, but the exact mechanism is unknown at this time.

➤*Pharmacokinetics:*

Absorption – Unoprostone is absorbed through the cornea and conjunctival epithelium, where it is hydrolyzed by esterases to unoprostone-free acid.

The systemic exposure of its metabolite unoprostone-free acid was minimal following the ocular administration.

Excretion – Elimination of unoprostone-free acid from human plasma is rapid, with a half-life of 14 minutes. Plasma levels of unoprostone-free acid dropped below the lower limit of quantitation (< 0.25 ng/mL) 1 hour following ocular instillation. The metabolites are excreted predominately in urine.

➤*Clinical trials:* In patients with mean baseline IOP of 23 mmHg, unoprostone lowers IOP by ≈ 3 to 4 mmHg throughout the day. Unoprostone appears to lower IOP without affecting cardiovascular or pulmonary function.

Contraindications

Known hypersensitivity to unoprostone isopropyl, benzalkonium chloride, or any other ingredients in this product.

Warnings

➤*Ocular changes:* Unoprostone has been reported to cause changes in pigmented tissue. These changes may be permanent.

It may gradually change eye color, increasing the amount of brown pigment in the iris. The long-term effects and the consequences of potential injury to the eye are currently unknown. The change in iris color occurs slowly and may not be noticeable for months to several years. Inform patients of the possibility of iris color change.

➤*Carcinogenesis:* Unoprostone was not carcinogenic in rats administered oral doses up to 12 mg/kg/day for up to 2 years (≈ 580- and 240-fold the recommended human dose).

➤*Pregnancy: Category C.* There are no adequate and well-controlled studies in pregnant women. Because animal studies are not always predictive of human response, use unoprostone during pregnancy only if the potential benefit justifies the potential risk to the fetus.

UNOPROSTONE ISOPROPYL

➤*Lactation:* It is not known whether topical ocular administration could result in sufficient systemic absorption to produce detectable quantities in breast milk. Nevertheless, exercise caution when unoprostone is administered to a nursing mother.

➤*Children:* Safety and efficacy in pediatric patients have not been established.

Precautions

➤*Bacterial keratitis:* There have been reports of bacterial keratitis associated with the use of multiple-dose containers of topical ophthalmic products. These containers had been inadvertently contaminated by patients who, in most cases, had a concurrent corneal disease or a disruption of the ocular epithelial surface.

➤*Active intraocular inflammation:* Use unoprostone with caution in patients with active intraocular inflammation (eg, uveitis).

➤*Contact lenses:* Unoprostone should not be administered while wearing contact lenses.

Advise patients that unoprostone contains benzalkonium chloride, which may be adsorbed by contact lenses. Contact lenses should be removed prior to administration of the solution. Lenses may be reinserted 15 minutes following administration of unoprostone.

Adverse Reactions

➤*Ophthalmic:* The most common ocular adverse events were burning/stinging, burning/stinging upon drug instillation, dry eyes, itching, increased length of eyelashes, and injection. These were reported in ≈ 10% to 25% of patients. Approximately 10% to 14% of patients were observed to have an increase in the length of eyelashes (≥ 1 mm) at 12 months, while 7% of patients were observed to have a decrease in the length of eyelashes.

Ocular adverse events occurring in ≈ 5% to 10% of patients were abnormal vision, eyelid disorder, foreign body sensation, and lacrimation disorder.

Ocular adverse events occurring in ≈ 1% to 5% of patients were blepharitis, cataract, conjunctivitis, corneal lesion, discharge from the eye, eye hemorrhage, eye pain, keratitis, irritation, photophobia, and vitreous disorder.

Other ocular adverse events reported in < 1% of patients were acute elevated IOP, color blindness, corneal deposits, corneal edema, corneal opacity, diplopia, hyperpigmentation of the eyelid, increased number of eyelashes, iris hyperpigmentation, iritis, optic atrophy, ptosis, retinal hemorrhage, and visual field defect.

➤*Systemic:* Flu syndrome (≈ 6%); accidental injury, allergic reaction, back pain, bronchitis, cough increased, diabetes mellitus, dizziness, headache, hypertension, insomnia, pharyngitis, pain, rhinitis, sinusitis (1% to 5%).

Overdosage

There is no published information available regarding overdosage with unoprostone. The risk of adverse effects caused by accidental oral ingestion is very low since the amount of active ingredient in each bottle is limited (7.5 mg in a 5 mL vial). Accidental ingestion of a vial by a child with 30 kg body weight will amount to 0.25 mg/kg body weight.

If overdosage does occur, treatment should be symptomatic.

Patient Information

Instruct patients to avoid allowing the tip of the dispensing container to contact the eye or surrounding structures because this could cause the tip to become contaminated by common bacteria known to cause ocular infections. Serious damage to the eye and subsequent loss of vision may result from using contaminated solutions.

Advise patients that if they develop an intercurrent ocular condition (eg, trauma, infection) or have ocular surgery, they should immediately seek their physician's advice concerning the continued use of the multidose container.

Advise patients that if they develop any ocular reactions, particularly conjunctivitis and eyelid reactions, they should immediately seek their physician's advice.

If more than 1 topical ophthalmic drug is being used, administer the drugs at least 5 minutes apart.

Combinations

PILOCARPINE AND EPINEPHRINE

Rx	P₁E₁ (Alcon)	**Solution:** 1% pilocarpine HCl, 1% epinephrine bitartrate	In 15 mL *Drop-Tainers*.[1]
Rx	P₂E₁ (Alcon)	**Solution:** 2% pilocarpine HCl, 1% epinephrine bitartrate	In 15 mL *Drop-Tainers*.[1]
Rx	P₄E₁ (Alcon)	**Solution:** 4% pilocarpine HCl, 1% epinephrine bitartrate	In 15 mL *Drop-Tainers*.[1]
Rx	P₆E₁ (Alcon)	**Solution:** 6% pilocarpine HCl, 1% epinephrine bitartrate+	In 15 mL *Drop-Tainers*.[1]

[1] With 0.01% benzalkonium chloride, methylcellulose, EDTA, chlorobutanol, polyethylene glycol and sodium bisulfite.

Also refer to the general discussion of Miotics, Cholinesterase Inhibitors.

Indications

➤*Glaucoma:* Therapy of open-angle glaucoma.

For other specific indications, refer to the individual monographs.

Administration and Dosage

Instill 1 or 2 drops into the eye(s) 1 to 4 times daily. Determine concentration and frequency of instillation by severity of the glaucoma and by patient response.

Individuals with heavily pigmented irides may require larger doses.

➤*Storage/Stability:* Store at 8° to 30°C (46° to 86°F). Keep tightly closed. Do not use solution if it is brown or contains a precipitate. Protect from light and heat.

Ingredients

PILOCARPINE lowers IOP by a direct cholinergic action that improves outflow facility on chronic administration (see Agents for Glaucoma: Miotics, Direct-Acting).

EPINEPHRINE reduces IOP by increasing outflow facility (see Agents for Glaucoma, Sympathomimetics).

The combination of pilocarpine and epinephrine provides additive effects in lowering IOP; opposing actions on the pupil may prevent marked miosis or mydriasis. These fixed combinations do not permit the flexibility necessary to adjust the dosage of each agent.

DORZOLAMIDE HCl AND TIMOLOL MALEATE

Rx	Cosopt (Merck)	**Solution:** 2% dorzolamide, 0.5% timolol	In 5 and 10 mL *Ocumeters*.[1]

[1] With 0.0075% benzalkonium chloride and mannitol.

Refer to the general discussion of Carbonic Anhydrase Inhibitors and Beta-adrenergic Blocking Agents.

Indications

➤*Elevated intraocular pressure (IOP):* Treatment of elevated IOP in patients with ocular hypertension or open-angle glaucoma.

Administration and Dosage

Instill one drop into the affected eye(s) two times daily. If more than one topical ophthalmic drug is being used, the drugs should be administered at least 10 minutes apart.

➤*Storage/Stability:* Store between 15° and 25°C (59° to 77°F). Protect from light.

Ingredients

DORZOLAMIDE is a carbonic anhydrase inhibitor that lowers IOP by decreasing aqueous humor secretion. It presumably slows bicarbonate ion formation with subsequent reduction in sodium and fluid transport.

TIMOLOL is a non-selective beta-adrenergic receptor blocker that decreases IOP by decreasing aqueous humor secretion and may slightly increase outflow facility.

The combined effect of these two agents administered together twice a day results in additional intraocular pressure reduction compared with either component administered alone, but the reduction is not as much as when dorzolamide 3 times a day and timolol 2 times a day are administered concomitantly.

Refer to the Topical Ophthalmic Drugs introduction for more complete information.

Indications

➤*Flurbiprofen, suprofen:* Inhibition of intraoperative miosis.

➤*Diclofenac:* Treatment of postoperative inflammation following cataract extraction.

➤*Ketorolac:* Relief of ocular itching caused by seasonal allergic conjunctivitis. Treatment of postoperative inflammation following cataract extraction.

➤*Unlabeled uses:*

Flurbiprofen – Topical treatment of cystoid macular edema, inflammation after cataract or glaucoma laser surgery and uveitis syndromes.

Actions

➤*Pharmacology:* Flurbiprofen, suprofen, diclofenac and ketorolac are NSAIDs available as ophthalmic solutions. Flurbiprofen and suprofen are phenylalkanoic acids, diclofenac is a phenylacetic acid and ketorolac tromethamine is a member of the pyrrolo-pyrrolle group; they have analgesic, antipyretic and anti-inflammatory activity. Their mechanism of action is believed to be through inhibition of the cyclo-oxygenase enzyme that is essential in the biosynthesis of prostaglandins.

In animals, prostaglandins are mediators of certain kinds of intraocular inflammation. Prostaglandins produce disruption of the blood-aqueous humor barrier, vasodilation, increased vascular permeability, leukocytosis and increased intraocular pressure (IOP). These agents have no significant effect on IOP.

Prostaglandins also appear to play a role in the miotic response produced during ocular surgery by constricting the iris sphincter independently of cholinergic mechanisms. These agents inhibit the miosis induced during the course of cataract surgery.

Contraindications

Hypersensitivity to the drugs or any component of the products.

➤*Flurbiprofen, suprofen:* Epithelial herpes simplex keratitis (dendritic keratitis).

➤*Diclofenac, ketorolac:* Patients wearing soft contact lenses (see Precautions).

Warnings

➤*Cross-sensitivity:* The potential for cross-sensitivity to acetylsalicylic acid and other NSAIDs exists. Use caution when treating individuals who have previously exhibited sensitivities to these drugs.

➤*Bleeding tendencies:* Systemic absorption occurs with drugs applied ocularly. With some NSAIDs, there exists the potential for increased bleeding time caused by interference with thrombocyte aggregation. There have been reports that ocularly applied NSAIDs may cause increased bleeding of ocular tissues (including hyphemas) in conjunction with ocular surgery. Use with caution in surgical patients with known bleeding tendencies or in patients taking drugs known to cause bleeding (eg, anticoagulants).

➤*Flank pain/Renal function impairment:* Use of oral suprofen has been associated with a syndrome of acute flank pain and generally reversible renal insufficiency, which may present as acute uric acid nephropathy. This syndrome occurs in $\approx$ 1 in 3500 patients and has been reported with as few as one to two doses of a 200 mg capsule.

➤*Pregnancy:* Category C (flurbiprofen, ketorolac, suprofen); Category B (diclofenac). **Flurbiprofen** is embryocidal, delays parturition, prolongs gestation, reduces weight and slightly retards fetal growth in rats at daily oral doses of $\geq$ 0.4 mg/kg ($\approx$ 185 times the human daily topical dose).

Oral doses of **ketorolac** at 1.5 mg/kg (8.8 mg/m^2), which was half of the human oral exposure, administered after gestation day 17 caused dystocia and higher pup mortality in rats.

Oral doses of **suprofen** of up to 200 mg/kg/day in animals resulted in an increased incidence of fetal resorption associated with maternal toxicity. There was an increase in still-births and a decrease in postnatal survival in pregnant rats treated with $\geq$2.5 mg/kg/day.

Oral **diclofenac** in mice and rats crosses the placental barrier. In rats, maternally toxic doses were associated with dystocia, prolonged gestation and reduced fetal weights, growth and survival.

There are no adequate and well controlled studies in pregnant women. Use during pregnancy only if the potential benefits outweigh the potential hazards to the fetus.

➤*Lactation:* It is not known whether **flurbiprofen** is excreted in breast milk. Because of the potential for serious adverse reactions in nursing infants, decide whether to discontinue nursing or to discontinue the drug, taking into account the importance of the drug to the mother.

Suprofen is excreted in breast milk after a single oral dose. Based on measurements of plasma and milk levels in women taking oral suprofen, the milk concentration is $\approx$ 1% of the plasma level. Because systemic absorption may occur from topical ocular administration, consider discontinuing nursing while on suprofen; its safety in human neonates has not been established.

Exercise caution while **ketorolac** is administered to a nursing woman.

➤*Children:* Safety and efficacy for use in children have not been established.

Precautions

➤*Wound healing:* may be delayed with the use of flurbiprofen.

➤*Contact lenses:* Patients wearing hydrogel soft contact lenses who have used diclofenac concurrently have experienced ocular irritation manifested by redness and burning.

Drug Interactions

➤*Acetylcholine chloride and carbachol:* Although clinical and animal studies revealed no interference, and there is no known pharmacological basis for an interaction, both of these drugs have reportedly been ineffective when used in patients treated with flurbiprofen or suprofen.

Adverse Reactions

Most frequent – Transient burning and stinging upon instillation (diclofenac 15%, ketorolac $\approx$ 40%); other minor symptoms of ocular irritation.

Suprofen: Discomfort; itching; redness; allergy, iritis, pain, chemosis, photophobia, irritation, punctate epithelial staining (< 0.5%).

Diclofenac: Keratitis (28%, although most cases occurred in cataract studies prior to drug therapy); elevated IOP (15%, although most cases occurred post-surgery and prior to drug therapy); anterior chamber reaction; ocular allergy; nausea, vomiting (1%); viral infections ($\leq$ 1%).

Ketorolac: Ocular irritation; allergic reactions; superficial keratitis; superficial ocular infections; eye dryness; corneal infiltrates; corneal ulcer; blurry vision.

Flurbiprofen – Increased bleeding tendency of ocular tissues in conjunction with ocular surgery.

Overdosage

Overdosage will not ordinarily cause acute problems. If accidentally ingested, drink fluids to dilute.

FLURBIPROFEN SODIUM

Rx	**Ocufen** (Allergan)	**Solution** : 0.03%	In 2.5 mL dropper bottles.[1]
Rx	**Flurbiprofen Sodium Ophthalmic** (Various, eg, Bausch & Lomb)		In 2.5 mL.[1]

[1] With 1.4% polyvinyl alcohol, 0.005% thimerosal and EDTA.

Complete prescribing information begins in the Ophthalmic NSAIDs group monograph.

Indications

Inhibition of intraoperative miosis.

➤*Unlabeled uses:* Topical treatment of cystoid macular edema, inflammation after cataract or glaucoma laser surgery and uveitis syndromes.

Administration and Dosage

➤*Inhibition of intraoperative miosis:* Instill 1 drop approximately every 30 minutes, beginning 2 hours before surgery (total of 4 drops).

SUPROFEN

Rx	**Profenal** (Alcon)	Solution: 1%	In 2.5 mL *Drop-Tainers.*[1]

[1] With 0.005% thimerosal, 2% caffeine and EDTA.

Complete prescribing information begins in the Ophthalmic NSAIDs group monograph.

Indications

Inhibition of intraoperative miosis.

Administration and Dosage

➤*Inhibition of intraoperative miosis:* On the day of surgery, instill 2 drops into the conjunctival sac at 3, 2 and 1 hour(s) prior to surgery. On the day preceding surgery, 2 drops may be instilled into the conjunctival sac every 4 hours while awake.

DICLOFENAC SODIUM

Rx	**Voltaren** (Novartis Pharmaceuticals)	Solution: 0.1%	In 2.5 and 5 mL dropper bottles.[1]

[1] With 1 mg/mL EDTA, boric acid, polyoxyl 35 castor oil, 2 mg/mL sorbic acid and tromethamine.

Complete prescribing information begins in the Ophthalmic NSAIDs group monograph.

Indications

Treatment of postoperative inflammation following cataract extraction and for the temporary relief of pain and photophobia following corneal refractive surgery.

Administration and Dosage

➤*Following cataract surgery:* Instill 1 drop to the affected eye 4 times/day beginning 24 hours after cataract surgery and continuing throughout the first 2 weeks of the postoperative period.

➤*Corneal refractive surgery:* Instill 1 or 2 drops within 1 hour prior to surgery. Apply 1 to 2 drops within 15 minutes after surgery to affected eye(s) and continue 4 times/day for up to 3 days.

➤*Storage/Stability:* Store at 15° to 25°C (59° to 77°F). Dispense in original, unopened container only.

KETOROLAC TROMETHAMINE

Rx	**Acular** (Allergan)	Solution : 0.5%	In 3, 5, and 10 mL dropper bottles.[1]
Rx	**Acular LS** (Allergan)	Solution: 0.4%	In 5 mL dropper bottles.[2]

[1] With 0.01% benzalkonium Cl, 0.1% EDTA and octoxynol 40.   [2] With 0.015% EDTA, 0.006% benzalkonium chloride.

Complete prescribing information begins in the Ophthalmic NSAIDs group monograph.

Indications

➤*Acular:* Relief of ocular itching caused by seasonal allergic conjunctivitis. Treatment of postoperative inflammation following cataract extraction.

➤*Acular LS:* Reduction of ocular pain and burning/stinging following corneal refractive surgery.

Administration and Dosage

➤*Acular:*

Ocular itching – Administer 1 drop (0.25 mg) 4 times/day.

Following cataract extraction – Apply 1 drop to the affected eye(s) 4 times/day beginning 24 hours after cataract surgery and continuing through the first 2 weeks of the postoperative period.

➤*Acular LS:* 1 drop 4 times daily in the operated eye as needed for pain and burning/stinging for up to 4 days following corneal refractive surgery.

Refer to the Topical Ophthalmics introduction for complete information on administration and use.

Indications

➤*Inflammatory conditions:* For the treatment of steroid-responsive inflammatory conditions of the palpebral and bulbar conjunctiva, cornea, lid, sclera and anterior segment of the globe, such as: Allergic conjunctivitis; acne rosacea; superficial punctate keratitis; herpes zoster keratitis; iritis; cyclitis; selected infective conjunctivitis; vernal conjunctivitis; episcleritis; epinephrine sensitivity; and anterior uveitis.

Ocular surgery – For treatment of postoperative inflammation following ocular surgery.

➤*Corneal injury:* For corneal injury from chemical, radiation or thermal burns or penetration of foreign bodies.

See individual monographs for specific indications and administration and dosage.

Administration and Dosage

Treatment duration varies with type of lesion and may extend from a few days to several weeks, depending on therapeutic response. If signs and symptoms fail to improve after 2 days, the patients should be re-evaluated. Relapse may occur if therapy is reduced too rapidly; taper over several days. Relapses, more common in chronic active lesions than in self-limited conditions, usually respond to retreatment.

Actions

➤*Pharmacology:* Topical corticosteroids exert an anti-inflammatory action. Aspects of the inflammatory process such as edema, fibrin deposition, capillary dilation, leukocyte migration, capillary proliferation, deposition of collagen, scar formation and fibroblastic proliferation are suppressed. Steroids inhibit inflammatory response to inciting agents of mechanical, chemical or immunological nature. Topical corticosteroids are effective in acute inflammatory conditions of the conjunctiva, sclera, cornea, lids, iris and anterior segment of the globe; and in ocular allergic conditions. In ocular disease, route of administration depends on site and extent of disorder.

The mechanism of the anti-inflammatory action is thought to be potentiation of epinephrine vasoconstriction, stabilization of lysosomal membranes, retardation of macrophage movement, prevention of kinin release, inhibition of lymphocyte and neutrophil function, inhibition of prostaglandin synthesis and, in prolonged use, decrease of antibody production.

Inhibiting fibroblastic proliferation may prevent symblepharon formation in chemical and thermal burns. Decreased scarring with clearer corneas after topical corticosteroids is a result of inhibiting fibroblastic proliferation and vascularization.

Contraindications

Acute epithelial herpes simplex keratitis (dendritic keratitis); fungal diseases of ocular structures; vaccinia, varicella and most other viral diseases of the cornea and conjunctiva; ocular tuberculosis; hypersensitivity; after uncomplicated removal of a superficial corneal foreign body; mycobacterial eye infection; acute, purulent, untreated eye infections that may be masked or enhanced by the presence of steroids (see Warnings).

➤*Medrysone:* Medrysone is not for use in iritis and uveitis; its efficacy has not been demonstrated.

Warnings

➤*Moderate-to-severe inflammation:* Use higher strengths for moderate-to-severe inflammations. In difficult cases of anterior segment eye disease, systemic therapy may be required. When deeper ocular structures are involved, use systemic therapy.

➤*Ocular damage:* Prolonged use may result in glaucoma, elevated IOP, optic nerve damage, defects in visual acuity and fields of vision, posterior subcapsular cataract formation or secondary ocular infections from pathogens liberated from ocular tissues. Check IOP and lens frequently if used for ≥ 10 days. In diseases that cause thinning of cornea or sclera, perforation has occurred with topical steroids.

➤*Cataract surgery:* The use of steroids after cataract surgery may delay healing and increase the incidence of bleb formation.

➤*Mustard gas keratitis or Sjögren's keratoconjunctivitis:* Topical steroids are not effective.

➤*Infections:* Prolonged use may result in secondary ocular infections caused by suppression of host response. Acute, purulent, untreated eye infections may be masked or the activity enhanced by steroids. Fungal infections of the cornea have been reported with long-term local steroid applications. Therefore, suspect fungal invasion in any persistent corneal ulceration where a steroid has been used or is being used. Take fungal cultures when appropriate.

Stromal herpes simplex keratitis treatment with steroid medication requires great caution; frequent slit-lamp microscopy is mandatory.

➤*Pregnancy: Category C.* There are no adequate and well controlled studies in pregnant women. Use only when clearly needed and when potential benefits outweigh potential hazards.

➤*Lactation:* Topically applied steroids are absorbed systemically. It is not known if sufficient systemic absorption occurs to produce detectable quantities in breast milk. Therefore, because of the potential for serious adverse reactions in nursing infants, decide whether to discontinue nursing or discontinue the drug, taking into account the importance of the drug to the mother.

➤*Children:* Safety and efficacy have not been established.

Fluorometholone – Safety and efficacy in children < 2 years of age have not been established.

Precautions

➤*Bacterial keratitis:* Bacterial keratitis associated with the use of multiple-dose containers of topical ophthalmic products has been reported. Containers had been inadvertently contaminated by patients who, in most cases, had a concurrent corneal disease or a disruption of the ocular epithelial surface. Serious damage to the eye and subsequent loss of vision may result from using contaminated preparations.

➤*Benzalkonium chloride:* Benzalkonium chloride is a preservative used in some of these products that may be absorbed by soft contact lenses. Patients wearing soft contact lenses should wait ≥ 15 minutes after instilling products containing this preservative before inserting their lenses.

➤*Sulfite sensitivity:* Some of these products contain sulfites that may cause allergic-type reactions (eg, hives, itching, wheezing, anaphylaxis) in certain susceptible people. Although the overall prevalence of sulfite sensitivity in the general population is probably low, it is seen more frequently in asthmatics or in atopic nonasthmatic people. Specific products containing sulfites are identified in the product listings.

Adverse Reactions

Glaucoma (elevated IOP) with optic nerve damage, loss of visual acuity and field defects; posterior subcapsular cataract formation; delayed wound healing; secondary ocular infection from pathogens, including herpes simplex and fungi liberated from ocular tissues; acute uveitis; perforation of globe where there is corneal or scleral thinning; exacerbation of viral, bacterial and fungal corneal infections; transient stinging or burning; chemosis; dry eyes; epiphora; photophobia; keratitis; conjunctivitis; corneal ulcers; mydriasis; ptosis; blurred vision, discharge, discomfort, ocular pain, foreign body sensation, hyperemia, pruritus (rimexolone). Rarely, filtering blebs have been reported with steroid use after cataract surgery.

➤*Systemic:* Systemic side effects may occur with extensive use (eg, hypercorticoidism) (see Adrenocortical Steroids group monograph in the Endocrine and Metabolic Agents chapter).

Patient Information

Medical supervision during therapy is recommended.

Instruct patients that use of contaminated ocular solutions can cause ocular infections and serious damage to the eye with subsequent loss of vision. To avoid contamination, do not touch applicator tip to any surface. Replace cap after using.

If improvement in the condition being treated does not occur within 2 days, or if pain, redness, itching or swelling of the eye occurs, discontinue medication and notify the physician. Take care not to discontinue prematurely.

Advise patients to immediately seek physician's advice concerning continued use of the present multidose container if they develop an intercurrent ocular condition (eg, trauma, ocular surgery, infection).

Benzalkonium chloride is absorbed by contact lenses. Do not administer medications containing benzalkonium chloride while wearing soft contact lenses. Instruct patients to wait ≥ 15 minutes after instilling medication before inserting their lenses.

FLUOROMETHOLONE

Rx	**Fluor-Op** (Novartis Ophthalmics)	**Suspension:** 0.1%	In 3, 5, 10 and 15 mL.[1]
Rx	**FML** (Allergan)		In 5 and 10 mL.[2]
Rx	**Fluorometholone Ophthalmic Suspension** (Various, eg, Falcon)		In 5, 10 and 15 mL.[1]
Rx	**Flarex** (Alcon)	**Suspension:** 0.1% fluorometholone acetate	In 2.5, 5 and 10 mL Drop-Tainers.[3]
Rx	**FML Forte** (Allergan)	**Suspension:** 0.25%	In 2, 5, 10 and 15 mL.[4]
Rx	**FML S.O.P.** (Allergan)	**Ointment:** 0.1%	In 3.5 g.[5]

[1] With 0.004% benzalkonium chloride, EDTA, polysorbate 80 and 1.4% polyvinyl alcohol.
[2] With 0.004% benzlkonium chloride, EDTA, polysorbate 80 and polyvinyl alcohol.
[3] With 0.01% benzalkonium chloride, EDTA, hydroxyethylcellulose and tyloxapol.

[4] With 0.005% benzalkonium chloride, EDTA, polysorbate 80 and 1.4% polyvinyl alcohol.
[5] With 0.0008% phenylmercuric acetate, white petrolatum, mineral oil and lanolin alcohol.

Complete prescribing information begins in the Ophthalmic Corticosteroids group monograph.

Indications

➤*Inflammatory conditions:* For steroid-responsive inflammation of the palpebral and bulbar conjunctiva, cornea and anterior segment of the globe.

Administration and Dosage

Consult a physician if there is no improvement after 2 days. Do not discontinue therapy prematurely. In chronic conditions, withdraw treatment by gradually decreasing the frequency of applications.

➤*Suspension:* Shake well before using. Instill 1 to 2 drops into the conjunctival sac(s) 2 to 4 times daily. During the initial 24 to 48 hours, the dosage may be increased to 2 drops every 2 hours.

➤*Ointment:* Apply a small amount (≈ ½ inch ribbon) of ointment to the conjunctival sac 1 to 3 times daily. During the first 24 to 48 hours, the dosing frequency may be increased to one application every 4 hours.

MEDRYSONE

Rx	**HMS** (Allergan)	**Suspension:** 1%	In 5 and 10 mL.[1]

[1] With 0.004% benzalkonium chloride, EDTA, 1.4% polyvinyl alcohol and hydroxypropyl methyl-cellulose.

Complete prescribing information begins in the Ophthalmic Corticosteroids group monograph.

Indications

➤*Inflammatory conditions:* For the treatment of allergic conjunctivitis, vernal conjunctivitis, episcleritis and ephinephrine sensitivity.

Administration and Dosage

Shake well before using. Instill 1 drop into the conjunctival sac up to every 4 hours.

PREDNISOLONE

Rx	**Pred Mild** (Allergan)	**Suspension:** 0.12% prednisolone acetate	In 5 and 10 mL.[1]
Rx	**Econopred** (Alcon)	**Suspension:** 0.125% prednisolone acetate	In 5 and 10 mL *Drop-Tainers.*[2]
Rx	**Econopred Plus** (Alcon)	**Suspension:** 1% prednisolone acetate	In 5 and 10 mL *Drop-Tainers.*[2]
Rx	**Pred Forte** (Allergan)		In 1, 5, 10 and 15 mL.[1]
Rx	**Prednisolone Acetate Ophthalmic** (Falcon)		In 10 and 15 mL.[2]
Rx	**Prednisolone Sodium Phosphate** (Various, eg, Schein)	**Solution:** 0.125% prednisolone sodium phosphate	In 5, 10 and 15 mL.
Rx	**AK-Pred** (Akorn)		In 5 and 10 mL.[3]
Rx	**Inflamase Mild** (Novartis Ophthalmics)		In 5 and 10 mL.[3]
Rx	**Prednisolone Sodium Phosphate** (Various, eg, Bausch & Lomb, Schein)	**Solution:** 1% prednisolone sodium phosphate	In 5, 10 and 15 mL.
Rx	**AK-Pred** (Akorn)		In 5, 10 and 15 mL.[3]
Rx	**Inflamase Forte** (Novartis Pharmaceuticals)		In 5, 10 and 15 mL.[3]

[1] With benzalkonium chloride, EDTA, polysorbate 80, hydroxypropyl methylcellulose and sodium bisulfite.
[2] With 0.01% benzalkonium chloride, EDTA, polysorbate 80, hydroxypropyl methylcellulose and glycerin.

[3] With 0.01% benzalkonium chloride and EDTA.

Complete prescribing information begins in the Ophthalmic Corticosteroids group monograph.

Indications

➤*Inflammatory conditions:* For the treatment of steroid-responsive inflammatory conditions of the palpebral and bulbar conjunctiva, cornea and anterior segment of the globe, such as allergic conjunctivitis, acne rosacea, superficial punctate keratitis, herpes zoster keratitis, iritis, cyclitis, selected infective conjunctivitis when the inherent hazard of steroid use is accepted to obtain an advisable diminution in edema and inflammation.

Mild-to-moderate – For the treatment of mild-to-moderate noninfectious allergic and inflammatory disorders of the lid, conjunctiva, cornea and sclera (including chemical and thermal burns).

Moderate-to-severe – Use higher strengths for moderate-to-severe inflammations. In difficult cases of anterior segment eye disease, systemic therapy may be required. When deeper ocular structures are involved, use systemic therapy.

➤*Corneal injury:* Corneal injury from chemical, radiation or thermal burns or penetration of foreign bodies.

Administration and Dosage

➤*Solutions:* Depending on the severity of inflammation, instill 1 or 2 drops of solution into the conjunctival sac up to every hour during the day and every 2 hours during the night as necessary as initial therapy.

When a favorable response is observed, reduce dosage to 1 drop every 4 hours. Further reduction in dosage to 1 drop 3 to 4 times daily may suffice to control symptoms.

➤*Suspensions:* Shake well before using. Instill 1 to 2 drops into the conjunctival sac 2 to 4 times daily. During the initial 24 to 48 hours, the dosing frequency may be increased if necessary.

In cases of bacterial infections, concomitant use of anti-infective agents is mandatory.

If signs and symptoms do not improve after 2 days, re-evaluate the patient.

Dosing may be reduced, but advise patients not to discontinue therapy prematurely. In chronic conditions, withdraw treatment by gradually decreasing the frequency of applications.

DEXAMETHASONE

Rx	**Dexamethasone Sodium Phosphate** (Various, eg, Bausch & Lomb, Schein, Zenith Goldline)	**Solution:** 0.1% dexamethasone phosphate (as sodium phosphate)	In 5 mL.
Rx	**Decadron Phosphate** (Merck)		In 5 mL *Ocumeters.*[1]
Rx	**Maxidex** (Alcon)	**Suspension:** 0.1% dexamethasone	In 5 and 15 mL *Drop-Tainers.*[2]
Rx	**Dexamethasone Sodium Phosphate** (Various, eg, Zenith Goldline)	**Ointment:** 0.05% dexamethasone phosphate (as sodium phosphate)	In 3.5 g.

[1] With polysorbate 80, EDTA, 0.1% sodium bisulfite, 0.25% phenylethanol, 0.02% benzalkonium chloride.

[2] With 0.01% benzalkonium chloride, EDTA, 0.5% hydroxypropylmethylcellulose, polysorbate 80.

[3] With lanolin anhydrous, parabens, PEG-400, white petrolatum and mineral oil.

[4] With white petrolatum and mineral oil.

Complete prescribing information begins in the Ophthalmic Corticosteroids group monograph.

Indications

➤*Inflammatory conditions:* Treatment of steroid-responsive inflammatory conditions of the palpebral and bulbar conjunctiva, cornea and anterior segment of the globe, such as allergic conjunctivitis, acne rosacea, superficial punctate keratitis, herpes zoster iritis, selected infective conjunctivitis when the inherent hazard of steroid use is accepted to obtain advisable edema and inflammation diminution.

➤*Corneal injury:* Corneal injury from chemical, radiation or thermal burns or penetration of foreign bodies.

Administration and Dosage

➤*Solutions:* Instill 1 to 2 drops into the conjunctival sac every hour during the day and every 2 hours during the night as initial therapy.

When a favorable response is observed, reduce dosage to 1 drop every 4 hours. Further reduction in dosage to 1 drop 3 or 4 times daily may suffice to control symptoms.

➤*Suspension:* Shake well before using. Instill 1 or 2 drops in the conjunctival sac(s). In severe disease, drops may be used hourly, being tapered to discontinuation as inflammation subsides. In mild disease, drops may be used ≤ 4 to 6 times daily.

➤*Ointment:* Apply a thin coating of ointment 3 to 4 times a day. When a favorable response is observed, reduce the number of daily applications to twice daily and later to once daily as a maintenance dose if this is sufficient to control symptoms.

The ointment is particularly convenient when an eye pad is used. It may also be the preparation of choice for patients in whom therapeutic benefit depends on prolonged contact of the active ingredients with ocular tissues.

RIMEXOLONE

Rx	**Vexol** (Alcon)	**Suspension:** 1%	In 2.5, 5 and 10 mL *Drop-Tainers.*[1]

[1] With 0.01% benzalkonium chloride, polysorbate 80 and EDTA.

Complete prescribing information begins in the Ophthalmic Corticosteroids group monograph.

Indications

➤*Inflammatory conditons:* Treatment of anterior uveitis.

Ocular surgery – Treatment of postoperative inflammation after ocular surgery.

Administration and Dosage

Shake well before using.

➤*Postoperative inflammation:* Apply 1 to 2 drops into the conjunctival sac of the affected eye(s) 4 times daily begining 24 hours after surgery and continuing throughout the first 2 weeks of the postoperative period.

➤*Anterior uveitis:* Apply 1 to 2 drops into the conjunctival sac of the affected eye every hour during waking hours for the first week, 1 drop every 2 hours during waking hours of the second week, and then taper until uveitis is resolved.

LOTEPREDNOL ETABONATE

Rx	**Lotemax** (Bausch & Lomb)	**Suspension:** 0.5%	In 2.5, 5, 10 and 15 mL.[1]
Rx	**Alrex** (Bausch & Lomb)	**Suspension:** 0.2%	In 5 and 10 mL.[1]

[1] With 0.01% benzalkonium chloride and EDTA.

Complete prescribing information begins in the Ophthalmic Corticosteroids group monograph.

Indications

➤*0.2% suspension:*

Inflammatory conditions – For the temporary relief of the signs and symptoms of seasonal allergic conjunctivitis.

➤*0.5% suspension:*

Inflammatory conditions – For the treatment of steroid-responsive inflammatory conditions of the palpebral and bulbar conjunctiva, cornea and anterior segment of the globe such as allergic conjunctivitis, acne rosacea, superficial punctate keratitis, herpes zoster keratitis, iritis, cyclitis, selected infective conjunctivitis, when the inherent hazard of steroid use is accepted to obtain an advisable dimunition in edema and inflammation.

Ocular surgery – Treatment of postoperative inflammation following ocular surgery.

Administration and Dosage

➤*Approved by the FDA:* March 9, 1998.

Shake well before using.

➤*0.2% suspension:* Instill 1 drop into the affected eye(s) 4 times daily.

➤*0.5% suspension:*

Steroid responsive disease – Apply 1 to 2 drops into the conjunctival sac of the affected eye(s) 4 times daily. During the initial treatment within the first week, the dosing may be increased up to 1 drop every hour. Advise patients not to discontinue therapy prematurely. If signs and symptoms fail to improve after 2 days, re-evaluate the patient.

Postoperative inflammation – Apply 1 to 2 drops into the conjunctival sac of the operated eye(s) 4 times daily beginning 24 hours after surgery and continuing throughout the first 2 weeks of the postoperative period.

PEMIROLAST POTASSIUM

Rx	Alamast (Santen)	Solution, ophthalmic: 0.1% (1 mg/mL)	0.005% lauralkonium chloride, glycerin, dibasic and monobasic sodium phosphate, phosphoric acid, and/or sodium hydroxide. In 10 mL.

Indications

➤*Allergic conjunctivitis:* For the prevention of eye itching caused by allergic conjunctivitis.

Administration and Dosage

➤*Approved by the FDA:* September 24, 1999.

➤*Allergic conjunctivitis:* 1 to 2 drops in each affected eye 4 times daily.

Symptomatic response to therapy (decreased itching) may be evident within a few days, but frequently requires longer treatment (up to 4 weeks).

➤*Storage/Stability:* Store at 15° to 25°C (59° to 77°F).

Actions

➤*Pharmacology:* Pemirolast potassium is a mast cell stabilizer that inhibits the in vivo Type I immediate hypersensitivity reaction.

In vitro and in vivo studies have demonstrated that pemirolast potassium inhibits the antigen-induced release of inflammatory mediators (eg, histamine, leukotriene C_4, D_4, E_4) from human mast cells.

In addition, pemirolast potassium inhibits the chemotaxis of eosinophils into ocular tissue and blocks the release of mediators from human eosinophils.

Although the precise mechanism of action is unknown, the drug has been reported to prevent calcium influx into mast cells upon antigen stimulation.

➤*Pharmacokinetics:* Topical ocular administration of 1 to 2 drops of pemirolast potassium ophthalmic solution in each eye 4 times daily in 16 healthy volunteers for 2 weeks resulted in detectable concentrations in the plasma. The mean peak plasma level of ≈ 4.7 ng/mL occurred at ≈ 0.42 hours and the mean $t_{1/2}$ was ≈ 4.5 hours. When a single 10 mg pemirolast potassium dose was taken orally, a peak plasma concentration of 0.723 mcg/mL was reached.

Following topical administration, ≈ 10% to 15% of the dose was excreted unchanged in the urine.

Contraindications

Hypersensitivity to any of the ingredients.

Warnings

For topical ophthalmic use only. Not for injection or oral use.

➤*Pregnancy: Category C.* Pemirolast potassium caused an increased incidence of thymic remnant in the neck, interventricular septal defect, fetuses with wavy rib, splitting of thoracic vertebral body, and reduced numbers of ossified sternebrae, sacral and caudal vertebrae, and metatarsi when rats were given oral doses ≥ 250 mg/kg (≈ 20,000 fold the human dose at 2 drops/eye, 40 mcL/drop, 4 times daily for a 50 kg adult) during organogenesis. Increased incidence of dilation of renal pelvis/ureter in the fetuses and neonates was also noted when rats were given an oral dose of 400 mg/kg pemirolast potassium (≈ 30,000 fold the human dose). Pemirolast potassium was not teratogenic in rabbits given oral doses ≤ 150 mg/kg (≈ 12,000 fold the human dose) during the same time period. There are no adequate and well-controlled studies in pregnant women. Because animal reproductive studies are not always predictive of human response, use during pregnancy only if the benefit outweighs the risk.

Pemirolast potassium produced increased pre- and postimplantation losses, reduced embryo/fetal and neonatal survival, decreased neonatal body weight, and delayed neonatal development in rats receiving an oral dose at 400 mg/kg (≈ 30,000 fold the human dose). Pemirolast potassium also caused a reduction in the number of corpus lutea, the number of implantations, and number of live fetuses in the F_1 generation in rats when F_0 dams were given oral dosages ≥ 250 mg/kg (≈ 20,000 fold the human dose) during late gestation and the lactation period.

➤*Lactation:* Pemirolast potassium is excreted in the milk of lactating rats at concentrations higher than those in plasma. It is not known whether pemirolast potassium is excreted in human breast milk; exercise caution when pemirolast ophthalmic solution is administered to a nursing woman.

➤*Children:* Safety and efficacy in pediatric patients < 3 years of age have not been established.

Precautions

➤*Contact lens:* Do not wear contact lens if eye is red. Do not use to treat contact lens-related irritation. The preservative in pemirolast potassium, lauralkonium chloride, may be absorbed by soft contact lenses. Instruct patients who wear soft contact lenses and whose eyes are not red to wait ≥ 10 minutes after instilling pemirolast potassium before they insert their contact lenses.

Adverse Reactions

In clinical studies lasting ≤ 17 weeks with pemirolast potassium ophthalmic solution, headache, rhinitis, and cold/flu symptoms were reported (10% to 25%). The occurrence of these side effects was generally mild. Some of these events were similar to the underlying ocular disease being studied.

➤*Ophthalmic:* Burning, dry eye, foreign body sensation, ocular discomfort (< 5%).

➤*Miscellaneous:* Allergy, back pain, bronchitis, cough, dysmenorrhea, fever, sinusitis, sneezing/nasal congestion (< 5%).

Overdosage

No accounts of pemirolast potassium ophthalmic solution overdose were reported following topical ocular application.

Oral ingestion of the contents of a 10 mL bottle would be equivalent to 10 mg of pemirolast potassium.

Patient Information

For topical ophthalmic use only. Not for injection or oral use.

To prevent contaminating the dropper tip and solution, do not touch the eyelids or surrounding areas with the dropper tip. Keep the bottle tightly closed when not in use.

Advise patients not to wear contact lens if their eye is red. Instruct patients who wear soft contact lenses and whose eyes are not red to wait ≥ 10 minutes after instilling pemirolast potassium before they insert their contact lenses.

NEDOCROMIL SODIUM

Rx	Alocril (Allergan)	Solution, ophthalmic: 2% (20 mg/mL)	0.01% benzalkonium Cl, 0.5% NaCl, 0.05% EDTA. In 5 mL w/ dropper tip.

Indications

➤*Allergic conjunctivitis:* For the treatment of itching associated with allergic conjunctivitis.

Administration and Dosage

➤*Approved by the FDA:* December 15, 1999.

1 or 2 drops in each eye twice a day. Use at regular intervals.

Continue treatment throughout the period of exposure (ie, until the pollen season is over or until exposure to the offending allergen is terminated), even when symptoms are absent.

➤*Storage/Stability:* Store between 2° to 25°C (36° to 77°F). Keep tightly closed and out of the reach of children.

Actions

➤*Pharmacology:* Nedocromil sodium is a mast cell stabilizer. It inhibits the release of mediators from cells involved in hypersensitivity reactions. Decreased chemotaxis and decreased activation of eosinophils have also been demonstrated.

In vitro studies with adult human bronchoalveolar cells showed that nedocromil sodium inhibits histamine release from a population of mast cells as belonging to the mucosal subtype and beta-glucuronidase release from macrophages.

➤*Pharmacokinetics:* Nedocromil sodium exhibits low systemic absorption, with < 4% of the total dose systemically absorbed following multiple dosing. Absorption is mainly through the nasolacrimal duct rather than through the conjunctiva. It is not metabolized and is eliminated primarily unchanged in urine (70%) and feces (30%).

Contraindications

Hypersensitivity to nedocromil sodium or to any of the other ingredients.

Warnings

➤*Pregnancy: Category B.* Reproduction studies performed in mice, rats, and rabbits using an SC dose of 100 mg/kg/day (> 1600 times the maximum recommended human daily ocular dose on a mg/kg basis) revealed no evidence of teratogenicity or harm to the fetus caused by nedocromil sodium. However there are no adequate and well-controlled studies in pregnant women. Because animal reproduction studies are not always predictive of human response, use nedocromil sodium during pregnancy only if clearly needed.

➤*Lactation:* After IV administration to lactating rats, nedocromil was excreted in milk. It is not known whether this drug is excreted in human milk. Exercise caution when nedocromil sodium is administered to nursing women.

➤*Children:* Safety and efficacy in children < 3 years of age have not been established.

NEDOCROMIL SODIUM

Adverse Reactions

The most frequently reported adverse experience was headache ($\approx$ 40%). Ocular burning, irritation and stinging, unpleasant taste, nasal congestion (10% to 30%); asthma, conjunctivitis, eye redness, photophobia, rhinitis (1% to 10%).

Patient Information

Advise patients to follow the instructions listed on the Information for Patients sheet.

Instruct patients to refrain from wearing contact lenses while exhibiting the signs and symptoms of allergic conjunctivitis.

LODOXAMIDE TROMETHAMINE

Rx	**Alomide** (Alcon)	Solution: 0.1%	In 10 mL *Drop-Tainers*.

Indications

Treatment of the ocular disorders referred to by the terms vernal keratoconjunctivitis, vernal conjunctivitis and vernal keratitis.

Administration and Dosage

➤*Approved by the FDA:* September 23, 1993.

➤*Adults and children > 2 years of age:* Instill 1 to 2 drops in each affected eye 4 times daily for up to 3 months.

Actions

➤*Pharmacology:* Lodoxamide is a mast cell stabilizer that inhibits, in vivo, the Type I immediate hypersensitivity reaction. Lodoxamide therapy inhibits the increases in cutaneous vascular permeability that are associated with reagin or IgE and antigen-mediated reactions. In vitro, lodoxamide stabilizes rodent mast cells and prevent mast cell inflammatory mediators (ie, SRS-A, slow-reacting substances of anaphylaxis, also known as the peptidoleukotrienes) and inhibits eosinophil chemotaxis. Although lodoxamide's precise mechanism of action is unknown, the drug may prevent calcium influx into mast cells upon antigen stimulation.

Lodoxamide has no intrinsic vasoconstrictor, antihistaminic, cyclooxygenase inhibition or other anti-inflammatory activity.

➤*Pharmacokinetics:* The disposition of lodoxamide was studied in six healthy adult volunteers receiving a 3 mg oral dose. Urinary excretion was the major route of elimination. The elimination half-life was 8.5 hours in urine. In a study in 12 healthy adult volunteers, topical administration of one drop in each eye 4 times per day for 10 days did not result in any measurable lodoxamide plasma levels at a detection limit of 2.5 ng/mL.

Contraindications

Hypersensitivity to any component of this product.

Warnings

For ophthalmic use only. Not for injection.

➤*Contact lenses:* As with all ophthalmic preparations containing benzalkonium chloride, instruct patients not to wear soft contact lenses during treatment with lodoxamide.

➤*Pregnancy: Category B.* There are no adequate and well controlled studies in pregnant women. Use during pregnancy only if clearly needed.

➤*Lactation:* It is not known whether lodoxamide is excreted in breast milk. Exercise caution when administering to a nursing woman.

➤*Children:* Safety and efficacy in children < 2 years of age have not been established.

Precautions

➤*Burning / Stinging:* Patients may experience a transient burning or stinging upon instillation of lodoxamide. Should these symptoms persist, advise the patient to contact their physician.

Adverse Reactions

➤*Ophthalmic:* Transient burning, stinging or discomfort upon instillation ($\approx$ 15%); ocular itching/pruritus, blurred vision, dry eye, tearing/discharge, hyperemia, crystalline deposits, foreign body sensation (1% to 5%); corneal erosion/ulcer, scales on lid/lash, eye pain, ocular edema/swelling, ocular warming sensation, ocular fatigue, chemosis, corneal abrasion, anterior chamber cells, keratopathy/keratitis, blepharitis, allergy, sticky sensation, epitheliopathy (< 1%).

➤*Systemic:* Headache (1.5%); heat sensation, dizziness, somnolence, nausea, stomach discomfort, sneezing, dry nose, rash (< 1%).

Overdosage

Overdose of an oral preparation of 120 to 180 mg resulted in a temporary sensation of warmth, profuse sweating, diarrhea, lightheadedness and a feeling of stomach distension; no permanent adverse effects were observed. Side effects reported following oral administration of 0.1 to 10 mg included a feeling of warmth or flushing, headache, dizziness, fatigue, sweating, nausea, loose stools and urinary frequency/urgency. Consider emesis in the event of accidental ingestion.

CROMOLYN SODIUM

Rx	**Crolom** (Dura)	Solution: 4%	In 2.5 and 10 mL bottles with controlled drop tip.
Rx	**Cromolyn Sodium Ophthalmic Solution** (Akorn)		In 10 mL with controlled dropper tip.
Rx	**Cromolyn Sodium Ophthalmic Solution** (Falcon)		In 10 and 15 mL.
Rx	**Cromolyn Sodium Ophthalmic** (Teva)		In 10 mL.

Indications

➤*Conjunctivitis:* Treatment of vernal keratoconjunctivitis, vernal conjunctivitis and vernal keratitis.

Administration and Dosage

Instill 1 or 2 drops in each eye 4 to 6 times a day at regular intervals. One drop contains approximately 1.6 mg cromolyn sodium.

Actions

➤*Pharmacology:* In vitro and in vivo animal studies have shown that cromolyn inhibits the degranulation of sensitized mast cells that occurs after exposure to specific antigens. Cromolyn acts by inhibiting the release of histamine and SRS-A (slow-reacting substance of anaphylaxis) from the mast cell.

Another activity demonstrated in vitro is the capacity of cromolyn to inhibit the degranulation of non-sensitized rat mast cells by phospholipase A and the subsequent release of chemical mediators. In another study, cromolyn did not inhibit the enzymatic activity of released phospholipase A on its specific substrate.

Cromolyn has no intrinsic vasoconstrictor, antihistaminic or anti-inflammatory activity.

➤*Pharmacokinetics:* Cromolyn is poorly absorbed. When multiple doses of cromolyn ophthalmic solution are instilled into normal rabbit eyes, < 0.07% of the dose is absorbed into the systemic circulation (presumably by way of the eye, nasal passages, buccal cavity and GI tract). Trace amounts (< 0.01%) of the dose penetrate into the aqueous humor, and clearance from this chamber is virtually complete within 24 hours after treatment is stopped.

In healthy volunteers, analysis of drug excretion indicates that approximately 0.03% of cromolyn is absorbed following administration to the eye.

Contraindications

Hypersensitivity to cromolyn or to any of the other ingredients.

Warnings

➤*Stinging / Burning:* Patients may experience a transient stinging or burning sensation following instillation of cromolyn.

➤*Duration / Frequency of therapy:* The recommended frequency of administration should not be exceeded. Symptomatic response to therapy (decreased itching, tearing, redness and discharge) is usually evident within a few days, but longer treatment for up to 6 weeks is sometimes required. Once symptomatic improvement has been established, continue therapy for as long as needed to sustain improvement.

➤*Contact lens use:* As with all ophthalmic preparations containing benzalkonium chloride, users of soft (hydrophilic) contact lenses should refrain from wearing lenses while under treatment with cromolyn ophthalmic solution. Wear can be resumed within a few hours after discontinuation of the drug.

➤*Concomitant therapy:* If required, corticosteroids may be used concomitantly with cromolyn ophthalmic solution.

➤*Pregnancy: Category B.* In animals receiving parenteral cromolyn, adverse fetal effects (increased resorption and decreased fetal weight) were noted only at the very high parenteral doses that produced maternal toxicity. There are no adequate and well controlled studies in pregnant women. Use during pregnancy only if clearly needed.

➤*Lactation:* It is not known whether this drug is excreted in breast milk. Exercise caution when cromolyn is administered to a nursing woman.

➤*Children:* Safety and efficacy in children < 4 years of age have not been established.

CROMOLYN SODIUM

Adverse Reactions

The most frequently reported adverse reaction is transient ocular stinging or burning upon instillation. Other adverse reactions (infrequent) include: Conjunctival injection; watery eyes; itchy eyes; dryness around the eye; puffy eyes; eye irritation; styes.

Patient Information

Advise patients that the effect of cromolyn therapy is dependent on its administration at regular intervals, as directed.

Do not wear soft contact lenses while using cromolyn.

Refer to the Topical Ophthalmic Drugs introduction for more complete information.

Indications

Refer to individual product listings for specific indications.

Actions

➤*Pharmacology:* The effects of sympathomimetic agents on the eye include: Pupil dilation, increase in outflow of aqueous humor and vasoconstriction (α-adrenergic effects); relaxation of the ciliary muscle and a decrease in the formation of aqueous humor (β-adrenergic effects). Hydroxyamphetamine dilates the pupil, probably by stimulating the dilator muscles of the iris.

Strong (α) vasoconstriction preparations (phenylephrine 2.5% and 10%; hydroxyamphetamine) cause vasoconstriction and pupillary dilation for diagnostic eye exams, during surgery and to prevent synechiae formation in uveitis. Weak sympathomimetic solutions (phenylephrine 0.12%; naphazoline; tetrahydrozoline) are used as ophthalmic decongestants (vasoconstriction of conjunctival blood vessels) for symptomatic relief of minor eye irritations. Epinephrine is used for open-angle glaucoma and is not included in this monograph (see Epinephrine monograph in the Agents for Glaucoma section).

Ophthalmic Vasoconstrictors/Mydriatics			
Vasoconstrictor/ Mydriatic	Duration of action (hr)	Available concentration	Prescription status
Hydroxyamphetamine	few hours	1%	Rx
Naphazoline	3 to 4	0.012%	otc
		0.02%	otc
		0.03%	otc
		0.1%	Rx
Oxymetazoline	4 to 6	0.025%	otc
Phenylephrine	0.5 to 1.5	0.12%	otc
	—	2.5%	Rx
	—	10%	Rx
Tetrahydrozoline	1 to 4	0.05%	otc

Contraindications

Hypersensitivity to any of these agents; narrow-angle glaucoma or anatomically narrow (occludable) angle and no glaucoma; prior to peripheral iridectomy in eyes capable of angle closure because mydriatic action may precipitate angle block.

➤*Phenylephrine 10%:* Patients with insulin-dependent diabetes; hypertensive patients; generalized arteriosclerosis; aneurysms; preexisting cardiovascular diseases; infants, small children with low body weight; elderly patients.

Warnings

➤*Anesthetics:* Discontinue prior to use of anesthetics which sensitize the myocardium to sympathomimetics (eg, cyclopropane, halothane).

Local anesthetics can increase absorption of topically applied drugs; exercise caution when applying prior to use of phenylephrine. However, use of a local anesthetic prior to phenylephrine 2.5% or 10% may help prevent pain.

➤*Overuse:* Overuse may produce increased redness of the eye.

➤*Pregnancy: Category C.* Safety for use during pregnancy is not established. Use only if clearly needed and if the potential benefits outweigh potential hazards to the fetus.

➤*Lactation:* Safety for use during breastfeeding has not been established. Use caution when administering to a nursing woman.

➤*Children:* Safety and efficacy have not been established. Phenylephrine 10% is contraindicated in infants.

Precautions

➤*Special risk patients:* Use with caution in the presence of hypertension, diabetes, hyperthyroidism, cardiovascular abnormalities, arteriosclerosis.

➤*Narrow-angle glaucoma:* Ordinarily, any mydriatic is contraindicated in patients with glaucoma. However, when temporary pupil dilation may free adhesions, or when vasoconstriction of intrinsic vessels may lower intraocular tension, these advantages may temporarily outweigh danger from coincident pupil dilation.

➤*Rebound congestion:* Rebound congestion may occur with frequent or extended use of ophthalmic vasoconstrictors. This may be of importance when there is retinal detachment or prior to cataract surgery. Rebound miosis has occurred in older persons 1 day after receiving phenylephrine; reinstillation produced a reduction in mydriasis.

➤*Systemic absorption:* Exceeding recommended dosages of these agents or applying **phenylephrine** 2.5% to 10% solutions to the instrumented, traumatized, diseased or postsurgical eye or adnexa, or to patients with suppressed lacrimation, as during anesthesia, may result in the absorption of sufficient quantities to produce a systemic vasopressor response.

➤*Pigment floaters:* Older individuals may develop transient pigment floaters in the aqueous humor 30 to 45 minutes after instillation of phenylephrine. The appearance may be similar to anterior uveitis or to a microscopic hyphema.

➤*Potentially hazardous tasks:* **Phenylephrine** may cause temporary blurred or unstable vision; observe caution while driving or performing other hazardous tasks.

➤*Sulfite sensitivity:* Some of these products contain sulfites that may cause allergic-type reactions (eg, hives, itching, wheezing, anaphylaxis) in certain susceptible persons. Although the overall prevalence of sulfite sensitivity in the general population is probably low, it is seen more frequently in asthmatics or in atopic nonasthmatic persons.

Drug Interactions

Ophthalmic Sympathomimetic Drug Interactions			
Precipitant drug	Object drug*		Description
Anesthetics	Ophthalmic sympatho-mimetics	↑	Cautiously use anesthetics that sensitize the myocardium to sympathomimetics (eg, cyclopropane, halothane). Local anesthetics can increase absorption of topical drugs; exercise caution when applying prior to use of phenylephrine.
Beta blockers	Ophthalmic sympatho-mimetics	↑	Systemic side effects may occur more readily in patients taking these drugs.
MAOIs	Ophthalmic sympatho-mimetics	↑	When given with, or up to 21 days after MAOIs, exaggerated adrenergic effects may result. Supervise and adjust dosage carefully.

* ↑ = Object drug increased.

Also consider drug interactions that may occur with systemic use of the sympathomimetics (see Vasopressors Used for Shock).

Adverse Reactions

➤*Ophthalmic:* Transitory stinging on initial instillation; blurring of vision; mydriasis; increased redness; irritation; discomfort; blurring; punctate keratitis; lacrimation; increased IOP.

Phenylephrine – Phenylephrine may cause rebound miosis and decreased mydriatic response to therapy in older persons.

➤*Cardiovascular:* Palpitation; tachycardia; cardiac arrhythmia; hypertension; ventricular arrhythmias (ie, premature ventricular contractions); reflex bradycardia; coronary occlusion; pulmonary embolism; subarachnoid hemorrhage; myocardial infarction; stroke; death associated with cardiac reactions. Headache or browache may occur.

Phenylephrine 10% – Significant elevation of blood pressure is rare but can occur after conjunctival instillation. Exercise caution with elderly patients and children of low body weight. Carefully monitor the blood pressure of these patients. (See Warnings and Contraindications.) There have been rare reports of the development of serious cardiovascular reactions, including ventricular arrhythmias and myocardial infarctions. These episodes, some fatal, have usually occurred in elderly patients with preexisting cardiovascular diseases.

➤*Miscellaneous:* Headache; blanching; tremor; trembling; sweating; dizziness; nausea; nervousness; drowsiness; weakness; hyperglycemia.

Overdosage

➤*Hydroxyamphetamine:* If ocular overdosage occurs, dilute pilocarpine (1%) may be administered. If accidentally ingested, sedation is indicated. Further treatment is symptomatic.

Patient Information

Do not use beyond 48 to 72 hours without consulting a physician.

If irritation, blurring or redness persists, or if severe eye pain, headache, vision changes, floating spots, dizziness, decrease in body temperature, drowsiness, acute eye redness or pain with light exposure occur, discontinue use and consult a physician.

Do not use if you have glaucoma except under the advice of a physician.

Refer to the Topical Ophthalmic Introduction for more complete information.

➤*Potentially hazardous tasks:* Phenylephrine may cause temporary blurred or unstable vision; observe caution while driving or performing other hazardous tasks.

TETRAHYDROZOLINE HCl

otc	**Tetrahydrozoline HCl** (Various, eg, Moore, Rugby, Steris)	**Solution:** 0.05%	In 15 and 30 mL.
otc	**Collyrium Fresh** (Wyeth-Ayerst)		In 15 mL.[1]
otc	**Geneye** (Goldline)		In 15 mL.[3]
otc	**Geneye Extra** (Goldline)		In 15 mL.[4]
otc	**Murine Plus** (Ross)		In 15 and 30 mL.[5]
otc	**Optigene 3** (Pfeiffer)		In 15 mL.[3]
otc	**Tetrasine** (Optopics)		In 15 and 22.5 mL.
otc	**Tetrasine Extra** (Optopics)		In 15 mL.[4]

[1] With 0.01% benzalkonium chloride and EDTA.
[2] With 0.01% benzalkonium chloride and 0.1% EDTA.
[3] With benzalkonium chloride and EDTA.

[4] With 1% polyethylene glycol 400, benzalkonium chloride and EDTA.
[5] With 0.013% benzalkonium chloride, 0.1% EDTA and 1% PEG-400.

For complete prescribing information, refer to the Vasoconstrictors/Mydriatics group monograph.

Indications

➤*Redness:* For relief of redness of the eye due to minor irritations.

➤*Burning/irritation:* For temporary relief of burning and irritation due to dryness of the eye or discomfort due to minor irritations or to exposure to wind or sun.

Administration and Dosage

Instill 1 or 2 drops into eye(s) up to 4 times a day.

➤*Storage/Stability:* Do not use if solution changes color or becomes cloudy.

PHENYLEPHRINE HCl

otc	**Prefrin Liquifilm** (Allergan)	**Solution:** 0.12%	In 20 mL.[2]
otc	**Relief** (Allergan)		Preservative free. In UD 0.3 mL.[3]
Rx	**Phenylephrine HCl** (Various)	**Solution:** 2.5%	In 15 mL.
Rx	**AK-Dilate** (Akorn)		In 2 and 15 mL.[4]
Rx	**Mydfrin 2.5%** (Alcon)		In 3 and 5 mL *Drop-Tainers*.[5]
Rx	**Neo-Synephrine** (Sanofi Winthrop)		In 15 mL.[6]
Rx	**Phenylephrine HCl** (Various, eg, Iolab, Steris)	**Solution:** 10%	In 2 and 5 mL.
Rx	**AK-Dilate** (Akorn)		In 2 and 5 mL.[4]
Rx	**Neo-Synephrine** (Sanofi Winthrop)		In 5 mL.[7]
Rx	**Neo-Synephrine Viscous** (Sanofi Winthrop)		In 5 mL.[8]

[1] With 0.005% benzalkonium chloride, 1.4% polyvinyl alcohol and EDTA.
[2] With 1.4% polyvinyl alcohol, 0.004% benzalkonium chloride and EDTA.
[3] With 1.4% polyvinyl alcohol and EDTA.
[4] With benzalkonium chloride.

[5] With 0.01% benzalkonium chloride, EDTA and sodium bisulfite.
[6] With 1:7500 benzalkonium chloride.
[7] With 1:10,000 benzalkonium chloride.
[8] With 1:10,000 benzalkonium chloride and methylcellulose.

For complete prescribing information, refer to the Vasoconstrictors/Mydriatics group monograph.

Indications

➤*2.5% and 10% solutions:* Decongestant and vasoconstrictor and for pupil dilation in uveitis (posterior synechiae), open-angle glaucoma, refraction without cycloplegia, prior to surgery, ophthalmoscopic examination, diagnostic procedures (funduscopy).

➤*0.12% solution:* A decongestant to provide relief of minor eye irritations.

Administration and Dosage

➤*Vasoconstrictors and pupil dilation:* Apply a drop of topical anesthetic. Follow in a few minutes by 1 drop of the 2.5% or 10% phenylephrine. The anesthetic prevents stinging and consequent dilution of solution by lacrimation. It may be necessary to repeat the instillation after 1 hour, again preceded by a topical anesthetic.

➤*Uveitis:* The formation of synechiae may be prevented by using the 2.5% or 10% solution and atropine to produce wide dilation of the pupil. However, the vasoconstrictor effect of phenylephrine may be antagonistic to the increase of local blood flow in uveal infection.

To free recently formed posterior synechiae, instill 1 drop of the 2.5% or 10% solution to the upper surface of the cornea. Continue treatment the following day, if necessary. In the interim, apply hot compresses for 5 or 10 minutes, 3 times daily using 1 drop of 1% or 2% solution of atropine sulfate and before and after each series of compresses.

➤*Glaucoma:* Instill 1 drop of 10% solution on the upper surface of the cornea as often as necessary. The 2.5% and 10% solutions may be used in conjunction with miotics in patients with open-angle glaucoma. Phenylephrine reduces the difficulties experienced by the patient because of the small field produced by miosis, and permits and often supports the effect of the miotic in lowering the IOP in open-angle glaucoma. Hence, there may be marked improvement in visual acuity after using phenylephrine with miotic drugs.

➤*Surgery:* When a short-acting mydriatic is needed for wide dilation of the pupil before intraocular surgery, the 2.5% or 10% solution may be instilled from 30 to 60 minutes before the operation.

➤*Refraction:* Prior to determination of refractive errors, the 2.5% solution may be used effectively with homatropine HBr, atropine sulfate, cyclopentolate, tropicamide HCl or a combination of homatropine and cocaine HCl.

Adults – Place 1 drop of the preferred cycloplegic in each eye; follow in 5 minutes with 1 drop phenylephrine 2.5% solution and in 10 minutes with another drop of the cycloplegic. In 50 to 60 minutes, the eyes are ready for refraction.

Since adequate cycloplegia is achieved at different time intervals after the necessary number of drops, different cycloplegics will require different waiting periods.

Children – Place 1 drop of atropine sulfate 1% in each eye; follow in 10 to 15 minutes with 1 drop of phenylephrine 2.5% solution and in 5 to 10 minutes with a second drop of atropine sulfate 1%. In 1 to 2 hours, the eyes are ready for refraction.

For a "one application method", combine 2.5% phenylephrine solution with a cycloplegic to elicit synergistic action. The additive effect varies depending on the patient. Therefore, when using a "one application method", it may be desirable to increase the concentration of the cycloplegic.

➤*Ophthalmoscopic examination:* Place 1 drop of 2.5% phenylephrine solution in each eye. Sufficient mydriasis is produced in 15 to 30 minutes and lasts 1 to 3 hours.

➤*Diagnostic procedures:* Heavily pigmented irides may require larger doses in all the following procedures.

Provocative test for angle block in patients with glaucoma – The 2.5% solution may be used as a provocative test when latent increased IOP is suspected. Measure tension before application and again after dilation. A 3 to 5 mm Hg rise in pressure suggests the presence of angle block in patients with glaucoma; however, failure to obtain such a rise does not preclude the presence of glaucoma from other causes.

Shadow test (retinoscopy) – When dilation of the pupil without cycloplegic action is desired, the 2.5% solution may be used alone.

Blanching test – Instill 1 to 2 drops of the 2.5% solution in the injected eye. After 5 minutes, examine for perilimbal blanching. If blanching occurs, the congestion is superficial and probably does not indicate iritis.

➤*Minor eye irritations:* Instill 1 or 2 drops of the 0.12% solution in eye(s) up to 4 times daily as needed.

➤*Storage/Stability:* Prolonged exposure to air or strong light may cause oxidation and discoloration. Do not use if solution changes color, becomes cloudy or contains a precipitate.

OXYMETAZOLINE HCl

otc	**OcuClear** (Schering-Plough)	**Solution:** 0.025%	In 30 mL.[1]
otc	**Visine L.R.** (Pfizer)		In 15 and 30 mL.[1]

[1] With 0.01% benzalkonium chloride and 0.1% EDTA.

For complete prescribing information, refer to the Vasoconstrictors/ Mydriatics group monograph.

Indications

➤*Redness:* For relief of redness of the eye due to minor eye irritations.

Administration and Dosage

➤*Adults and children ≥ 6 years of age:* Instill 1 or 2 drops in the affected eye(s) every 6 hours.

➤*Storage / Stability:* Do not use if solution changes color or becomes cloudy.

NAPHAZOLINE HCl

otc	**20/20 Eye Drops** (S.S.S. Company)	**Drops:** 0.012%	In 15 mL.[2]
otc	**All Clear** (Bausch & Lomb)	**Solution:** 0.012%	In 15 mL.[11]
otc	**Allerest Eye Drops** (Novartis Ophthalmic)		In 15 mL.[1]
otc	**Clear Eyes** (Ross)		In 15 and 30 mL.[2]
otc	**Clear Eyes ACR** (Ross)		In 15 and 30 mL.[3]
otc	**Naphcon** (Alcon)		In 15 mL.[5]
otc	**VasoClear** (Novartis Ophthalmics)	**Solution:** 0.02%	In 15 mL.[7]
otc	**All Clear AR** (Bausch & Lomb)	**Solution:** 0.03%	In 15 mL.[9]
otc	**Comfort Eye Drops** (Pilkington/Barnes Hind)		In 15 mL.[8]
otc	**Maximum Strength Allergy Drops** (Bausch & Lomb)		In 15 mL.[9]
Rx	**Naphazoline HCl** (Various, eg, Goldline)	**Solution:** 0.1%	In 15 mL.
Rx	**AK-Con** (Akorn)		In 15 mL.[5]
Rx	**Albalon** (Allergan)		In 15 mL.[10]
Rx	**Nafazair** (Bausch & Lomb)		In 15 mL.[5]
Rx	**Naphcon Forte** (Alcon)		In 15 mL *Drop-Tainers.*[5]

[1] With benzalkonium chloride, EDTA.
[2] With benzalkonium chloride, EDTA, 0.2% glycerin.
[3] With benzalkonium chloride, EDTA, 0.25% zinc sulfate, 0.2% glycerin.
[4] With 0.0067% benzalkonium chloride, 0.02% EDTA, hydroxyethylcellulose, povidone.
[5] With 0.01% benzalkonium chloride, EDTA.
[6] With 0.2% PEG-300, 0.01% benzalkonium chloride.

[7] With 0.01% benzalkonium chloride, 0.25% polyvinyl alcohol, 1% PEG-400, EDTA.
[8] With 0.005% benzalkonium chloride and 0.02% EDTA.
[9] With 0.01% benzalkonium chloride, 0.5% hydroxypropyl methylcellulose and EDTA.
[10] With 0.004% benzalkonium chloride, EDTA, 1.4% polyvinyl alcohol.
[11] With 0.2% PEG 300, 0.01% benzalkonium chloride, EDTA.

For complete prescribing information, refer to the Vasoconstrictors/ Mydriatics group monograph.

Indications

➤*Redness:* To soothe, refresh and remove redness due to minor eye irritations such as smoke, smog, sunglare, wearing contact lenses, allergies or swimming.

Administration and Dosage

Instill 1 or 2 drops into the conjunctival sac of affected eye(s) every 3 to 4 hours, up to 4 times daily.

➤*Storage / Stability:* Do not use if solution changes color or becomes cloudy.

OLOPATADINE HCl

| *Rx*   **Patanol** (Alcon) | **Solution:** 0.1% | Benzalkonium chloride. In 5 mL *Drop-Tainer* dispenser. |

Indications
➤*Allergic conjunctivitis:* For temporary prevention of itching of the eye due to allergic conjunctivitis.

Administration and Dosage
The recommended dose is 1 to 2 drops in each affected eye 2 times per day at an interval of 6 to 8 hours.

➤*Storage / Stability:* Store at 39° to 86°F (4° to 30°C).

Actions
➤*Pharmacology:* Olopatadine is an inhibitor of histamine release from the mast cell and a relatively selective histamine H_1-antagonist that inhibits the in vivo and in vitro type 1 immediate hypersensitivity reaction. Olopatadine is devoid of effects on alpha-adrenergic, dopamine, muscarinic type 1 and 2, and serotonin receptors.

➤*Pharmacokinetics:* Olopatadine has low systemic exposure. Plasma concentrations are generally below the quantitation limit of the assay (< 0.5 ng/mL). Samples in which olopatadine is quantifiable are typically found within 2 hours of dosing and range from 0.5 to 1.3 ng/mL. The half-life in plasma is ≈ 3 hours, and elimination is predominantly through renal excretion. Approximately 60% to 70% of the dose is recovered in the urine as parent drug. Two metabolites, the mono-desmethyl and the N-oxide, were detected at low concentrations in the urine.

Contraindications
Hypersensitivity to any component of this product.

Warnings
➤*Pregnancy: Category C.* Olopatadine was not found to be teratogenic in rats and rabbits. There are no adequate and well controlled studies in pregnant women. Use this drug in pregnant women only if the potential benefit to the mother justifies the potential risk to the embryo or fetus.

➤*Lactation:* Olopatadine has been identified in the milk of nursing rats following oral administration. It is not known whether topical ocular administration could result in sufficient systemic absorption to produce detectable quantities in breast milk. Exercise caution when olopatadine is administered to a nursing mother.

➤*Children:* Safety and effectiveness in pediatric patients < 3 years old have not been established.

Precautions
➤*For topical use only.:* Not for injection. Do not instill olopatadine while wearing contact lenses.

Adverse Reactions
➤*Ophthalmic:* Burning or stinging, dry eye, foreign body sensation, hyperemia, keratitis, lid edema, pruritus (< 5%).

➤*Miscellaneous:* Headache (7%); asthenia, cold syndrome, pharyngitis, rhinitis, sinusitis, taste perversion (< 5%).

Patient Information
To prevent contaminating the dropper tip and solution, do not touch the eyelids and surrounding areas with the dropper tip of the bottle.

Keep bottle tightly closed when not in use.

EMEDASTINE DIFUMARATE

| *Rx*   **Emadine** (Alcon) | **Solution:** 0.05% | Benzalkonium chloride. In 5 mL. |

Indications
➤*Allergic Conjunctivitis:* Temporary relief of the signs and symptoms of allergic conjunctivitis.

Administration and Dosage
➤*Approved by the FDA:* December 29, 1997.

One drop in the affected eye(s) up to four times a day.

➤*Storage / Stability:* Store at 4° to 30°C (39° to 86°F).

Actions
➤*Pharmacology:* Emedastine is a relatively selective, histamine H_1 antagonist for ophthalmic use. In vivo studies have shown concentration-dependent inhibition of histamine-stimulated vascular permeability in the conjunctiva following topical ocular administration. Emedastine appears to be devoid of effects on adrenergic, dopaminergic and serotonin receptors.

➤*Pharmacokinetics:* Following topical administration, emedastine has low systemic exposure. In a study involving 10 healthy volunteers dosed bilaterally twice daily for 15 days with emedastine, plasma concentrations of the parent compound were generally below the quantitation limit of the assay (< 0.3 ng/mL). Samples in which emedastine was quantifiable ranged from 0.3 to 0.49 ng/mL. The elimination plasma half-life of oral emedastine was 3 to 4 hours. Approximately 44% of the oral dose is recovered in the urine over 24 hours with only 3.6% of the dose excreted as parent drug. Two primary metabolites, 5– and 6–hydroxyemedastine, are excreted in the urine as both free and conjugated forms. The 5'-oxoanalogs of 5– and 6–hydroxyemedastine and the N-oxide are also formed as minor metabolites.

➤*Clinical trials:* Patients with allergic conjunctivitis were treated with emedastine for 6 weeks. The results demonstrated that emedastine provides relief of the signs and symptoms of allergic conjunctivitis. In conjunctival antigen challenge studies, in which subjects were challenged with antigen both initially and ≤ 4 hours after dosing, emedastine was demonstrated to be significantly more effective than placebo in preventing ocular itching associated with allergic conjunctivitis.

Contraindications
Hypersensitivity to emedastine difumarate or any product components.

Warnings
➤*Topical (ophthalmic) use only:* Not for injection or oral use.

➤*Pregnancy: Category B.* At 70,000 times the maximum recommended ocular human use level, emedastine difumarate increased the incidence of external, visceral and skeletal anomalies in rats. There are no adequate and well controlled studies in pregnant women. Use this drug during pregnancy only if clearly needed.

➤*Lactation:* Oral emedastine has been identified in rat milk. It is not known whether topical ocular administration could result in sufficient systemic absorption to produce detectable quantities in breast milk. Exercise caution when administering to a breastfeeding woman.

➤*Children:* Safety and efficacy in children < 3 years old have not been established.

Adverse Reactions
In controlled clinical studies of emedastine lasting 42 days, the most frequent adverse reaction was headache (11%). The following adverse reactions were reported in < 5% of patients: Abnormal dreams; asthenia; bad taste; blurred vision; burning or stinging; corneal infiltrates; corneal staining; dermatitis; discomfort; dry eyes; foreign body sensation; hyperemia; keratitis; pruritus; rhinitis; sinusitis; tearing. Some of these events were similar to the underlying disease being studied.

Overdosage
Somnolence and malaise have been reported following daily oral administration. Oral ingestion of the contents of a 15 mL container of emedastine would be equivalent to 7.5 mg. In case of overdosage, treatment is symptomatic and supportive. Refer to General Management of Acute Overdosage.

Patient Information
To prevent contaminating the dropper tip and solution, take care not to touch the eyelids or surrounding areas with the dropper tip of the bottle. Keep the bottle tightly closed when not in use. Do not use if the solution has become discolored.

Advise patients not to wear contact lenses if their eyes are red. Do not use emedastine to treat contact lens-related irritation. The preservative in emedastine, benzalkonium chloride, may be absorbed by soft contact lenses. Instruct patients who wear soft contact lenses and whose eyes are not red to wait at least 10 minutes after instilling emedastine before inserting contact lenses.

AZELASTINE HCl

| *Rx* | **Optivar** (MedPointe Healthcare[1]) | **Solution:** 0.5 mg/mL (equiv. to 0.457 mg azelastine base) | 0.125 mg benzalkonium chloride, EDTA dihydrate, hydroxypropylmethylcellulose, sodium hydroxide. In 10 mL containers with 6 mL solution with dropper. |

[1] MedPointe Healthcare Inc., 265 Davidson Avenue, Suite 300, Somerset, NJ 08873–4120; (732) 564–2200; http://www.medpointeinc.com.

For more information, see Azelastine HCl in the Antihistamines group monograph.

Indications

➤*Allergic conjunctivitis:* For the treatment of itching of the eye associated with allergic conjunctivitis.

Administration and Dosage

Instill 1 drop into each affected eye twice daily.

➤*Storage/Stability:* Store upright between 2° and 25°C (36° and 77°F).

Actions

➤*Pharmacology:* Azelastine is a relatively selective histamine H_1 antagonist and an inhibitor of the release of other mediators from cells (eg, mast cells) involved in the allergic response. Decreased chemotaxis and activation of eosinophils also has been demonstrated.

➤*Pharmacokinetics:*

Absorption/Distribution – Absorption of azelastine following ocular administration was relatively low. A study in symptomatic patients receiving 1 drop of azelastine in each eye 2 to 4 times/day (0.06 to 0.12 mg azelastine) demonstrated plasma concentrations of azelastine to generally be between 0.02 to 0.25 ng/mL after 56 days of treatment. Three of 19 patients had quantifiable amounts of N-desmethylazelastine that ranged from 0.25 to 0.87 ng/mL at day 56. Steady-state volume of distribution was 14.5 L/kg.

Metabolism/Excretion – Based on IV and oral administration, the elimination half-life and plasma clearance were 22 hours and 0.5 L/hr/kg, respectively. Approximately 75% of an oral dose of azelastine was excreted in the feces with < 10% as unchanged azelastine. Azelastine is oxidatively metabolized to the principal metabolite, N-desmethylazelastine, by the cytochrome P450 enzyme system. In vitro studies in human plasma indicate that the plasma protein binding of azelastine and N-desmethylazelastine are ≈ 88% and 97%, respectively.

Contraindications

Known or suspected hypersensitivity to any of its components.

Warnings

For topical ophthalmic use only; not for injection or oral use.

➤*Pregnancy:* Category C. Azelastine has been shown to be embryotoxic, fetotoxic, and teratogenic (external and skeletal abnormalities) in mice at an oral dose of 68.6 mg/kg/day (57,000 times the recommended ocular human use level). At an oral dose of 30 mg/kg/day (25,000 times the recommended ocular human use level), delayed ossification (undeveloped metacarpus) and the incidence of 14th rib were increased in rats. At 68.6 mg/kg/day azelastine caused resorption and fetotoxic effects in rats. The relevance to humans of these skeletal findings noted at only high drug exposure levels is unknown.

There are no adequate and well-controlled studies in pregnant women. Use azelastine during pregnancy only if the potential benefit justifies the potential risk to the fetus.

➤*Lactation:* It is not known whether azelastine is excreted in breast milk. Because many drugs are excreted in breast milk, exercise caution when administering to a nursing woman.

➤*Children:* Safety and efficacy in pediatric patients < 3 years of age have not been established.

Adverse Reactions

In controlled, multiple-dose studies where patients were treated for up to 56 days, the most frequently reported adverse reactions were transient eye burning/stinging (≈ 30%), headaches (≈ 15%), and bitter taste (≈ 10%). The severity of these events was generally mild.

The following events were reported in 1% to 10% of patients: Asthma, conjunctivitis, dyspnea, eye pain, fatigue, influenza-like symptoms, pharyngitis, pruritus, rhinitis, and temporary blurring. Some of these events were similar to the underlying disease being studied.

Patient Information

To prevent contaminating the dropper tip and solution, advise patients to take care not to touch any surface, the eyelids, or surrounding areas with the dropper tip of the bottle. Keep bottle tightly closed when not in use. This product is sterile when packaged.

Advise patients not to wear a contact lens if their eye is red. Do not use azelastine to treat contact lens-related irritation. The preservative, benzalkonium chloride, may be absorbed by soft contact lenses. Instruct patients who wear soft contact lenses and whose eyes are not red to wait at least 10 minutes after instilling azelastine before they insert their contact lenses.

LEVOCABASTINE HCl

| *Rx* | **Livostin** (Novartis Pharmaceuticals) | **Ophthalmic suspension:** 0.05% | With 0.15 mg benzalkonium chloride, propylene glycol, EDTA. In 2.5, 5, and 10 mL dropper bottles. |

Indications

➤*Allergic conjunctivitis:* For the temporary relief of th e signs and symptoms of seasonal allergic conjunctivitis.

Administration and Dosage

Shake well before using.

The usual dose is 1 drop instilled in affected eyes 4 times daily. Treatment may be continued for up to 2 weeks.

➤*Storage/Stability:* Keep tightly closed when not in use. Do not use if the suspension has discolored. Store at controlled room temperature of 15° to 30°C (59° to 86°F). Protect from freezing.

Actions

➤*Pharmacology:* Levocabastine is a potent, selective histamine H_1-receptor antagonist for topical ophthalmic use. Antigen challenge studies performed 2 and 4 hours after initial drug instaillation indicated activity was maintained for at least 2 hours.

➤*Pharmacokinetics:* After instillation in the eye, levocabastine is systemically absorbed. However, the amount of systemically absorbed levocabstine after therapeutic ocular doses is low (mean plasma concentrations in the range of 1 to 2 ng/mL).

➤*Clinical trials:* Levocabastine instilled 4 times/day was significantly more effective than its vehicle in reducing ocular itching associated with seasonal allergic conjunctivitis.

Contraindications

Hypersensitivity to any components of the product; while soft contact lenses are being worn.

Warnings

➤*For ophthalmic use only:* Not for injection.

In female mise, levocabastine doses of 5000 and 21,500 times the maximum recommended ocular human use level resulted in an increased incidence of pituitary gland adenoma and mammary gland adenocarcinoma possibly produced by increased prolactin levels. The clinical relevance of this finding is unknown with regard to the interspecies differences in prolactin physiology and the very low plasma concentrations of levocabastine following ocular administration.

➤*Pregnancy:* Category C. Levocabastine is teratogenic (polydactyly) in rats when given in doses 16,500 times the maximum recommended human ocular dose. Teratogenicity (polydactyly, hydrocephaly, brachygnathia), embryotoxicity and maternal toxicity were observed in rats at 66,000 times the maximum recommended ocular human dose. There are no adequate and well-controlled studies in pregnant women. Use during pregnancy only if the potential benefit justifies the potential risk to the fetus.

➤*Lactation:* Based on determinations of levocabastine in breast milk after ophthalmic administration of the drug ot one nursing woman, it was calculated that the daily dose of levocabastine in the infant was ≈ 0.5 mcg.

➤*Children:* Safety and efficacy in children < 12 years of age have not been established.

Adverse Reactions

Mild, transient stinging and burning (15%); headache (5%); visual disturbances, dry mouth, fatigue, pharyngitis, eyepain/dryness, somnolence, red dyds, lacrimation/discharge, cough, nausea, rash/erythema, eyelid edema, dyspnea (1% to 3%).

Patient Information

Shake well before using.

To prevent contaminating the dropper tip and suspension, take care not to touch the eyelids or surrounding areas with the dropper tip of the bottle.

Keep bottle tightly closed when not in use. Do not use if the suspension has discolored. Store at controlled room temperature. Protect from freezing.

KETOTIFEN FUMARATE

Rx	**Zaditor** (Novartis Pharmaceuticals)	Solution: 0.025%	In 5 mL and 7.5 mL.[1]

[1] With glycerol, sodium hydroxide/hydrochloric acid, purified water, and benzalkonium chloride 0.01% as a preservative.

Indications

➤*Conjunctivitis:* Temporary prevention of itching of the eye due to allergic conjunctivitis.

Administration and Dosage

➤*Approved by the FDA:* July 2, 1999.

The recommended dose is one drop in the affected eye(s) every 8 to 12 hours.

Actions

➤*Pharmacology:* Ketotifen is a relatively selective, non-competitive histamine antagonist (H_1 receptor) and mast cell stabilizer. Ketotifen inhibits the release of mediators from cells involved in hypersensitivity reactions. Decreased chemotaxis and activation of eosinophils has also been demonstrated. The action of ketotifen occurs rapidly with an effect seen within minutes after administration.

Contraindications

Hypersensitivity to any component of this product.

Warnings

➤*Ophthalmic use:* For topical ophthalmic use only. Not for injection or oral use.

➤*Fertility impairment:* Treatment of male rats with oral doses of ketotifen ≥ 10 mg/kg/day orally [6,667 times the maximum recommended human ocular dose (MRHOD) of 0.0015 mg/kg/day on a mg/kg basis] for 70 days prior to mating resulted in mortality and a decrease in fertility.

➤*Pregnancy: Category C.* Oral treatment of pregnant rabbits during organogenesis with 45 mg/kg/day of ketotifen (30,000 the MRHOD) resulted in an increased incidence of retarded ossification of the sternebrae. The offspring of the rats that received ketotifen orally from day 15 of pregnancy to day 21 post partum at 50 mg/kg/day (33,333 times the MRHOD), a maternally toxic treatment protocol, the incidence of postnatal mortality was slightly increased, and body weight gain during the first 4 days post partum was slightly decreased.

There are no adequate and well controlled studies in pregnant women. Use during pregnancy only if the potential benefits outweigh the potential hazards to the fetus.

➤*Lactation:* Ketotifen has been identified in milk in rats following oral administration. It is not known whether topical ocular administration could result in sufficient systemic absorption to produce detectable quantities in breast milk. Nevertheless, exercise caution when ketotifen is administered to a nursing mother.

➤*Children:* Safety and efficacy in pediatric patients < 3 years of age have not been established.

Adverse Reactions

Conjunctival injection, headaches, rhinitis (10% to 25%). The occurrence of these side effects were generally mild. Some of these events were similar to the underlying ocular disease being studied.

➤*Ophthalmic:* Burning or stinging, conjunctivitis, discharge, dry eyes, eye pain, eyelid disorder, itching, keratitis, lacrimation disorder, mydriasis, photophobia (< 5%).

➤*Miscellaneous:* Allergic reactions, rash, flu syndrome, pharyngitis (< 5%).

Overdosage

Oral ingestion of the contents of a 5 mL bottle would be equivalent to 1.725 mg of ketotifen. Clinical results have shown no serious signs or symptoms after the ingestion of up to 20 mg of ketotifen.

Patient Information

To prevent contaminating the dropper tip and solution, take care not to touch the eyelids or surrounding areas with the dropper tip of the bottle. Keep the bottle tightly closed when not in use.

Advise patients not to wear contact lenses if their eyes are red. Do not use ketotifen to treat contact lens-related irritation. The preservative in ketotifen, benzalkonium chloride, may be absorbed by soft contact lenses. Instruct patients who wear soft contact lenses and whose eyes are not red to wait ≥ 10 minutes after instilling ketotifen before they insert their contact lenses.

EPINASTINE HCl

Rx	**Elestat** (Allergan)	Solution, ophthalmic: 0.05%	0.01% benzalkonium chloride, EDTA. In 8 and 15 mL.

Indications

➤*Allergic conjunctivitis:* For the prevention of itching associated with allergic conjunctivitis.

Administration and Dosage

➤*Approved by the FDA:* October 16, 2003.

The recommended dosage is 1 drop in each eye twice a day.

Continue treatment throughout the period of exposure (ie, until the pollen season is over or until exposure to the offending allergen is terminated), even when symptoms are absent.

➤*Storage/Stability:* Store at 15° to 25°C (59° to 77°F). Keep bottle tightly closed.

Actions

➤*Pharmacology:* Epinastine is a topically active, direct H_1-receptor antagonist and an inhibitor of the release of histamine from the mast cell. Epinastine is selective for the histamine H_1-receptor and has affinity for the histamine H_2-receptor. Epinastine also possesses affinity for the alpha-1, alpha-2, and 5-HT_2-receptors. Epinastine does not penetrate the blood/brain barrier, and, therefore, is not expected to induce side effects of the CNS.

➤*Pharmacokinetics:*

Absorption/Distribution – Fourteen subjects with allergic conjunctivitis received 1 drop of epinastine in each eye twice daily for 7 days. On day 7, average maximum epinastine plasma concentrations of approximately 0.04 ng/mL were reached after about 2 hours, indicating low systemic exposure. While these concentrations represented an increase over those seen following a single dose, the day 1 and day 7 AUC values were unchanged indicating that there is no increase in systemic absorption with multiple dosing. Epinastine is 64% bound to plasma proteins.

Metabolism/Excretion – The total systemic clearance is approximately 56 L/h and the terminal plasma elimination half-life is about 12 hours. Epinastine is mainly excreted unchanged. About 55% of an IV dose is recovered unchanged in the urine with about 30% in feces. Less than 10% is metabolized. The renal elimination is mainly via active tubular secretion.

Contraindications

Hypersensitivity to epinastine or to any of the other ingredients.

Warnings

Epinastine is for topical ophthalmic use only and not for injection or oral use.

➤*Pregnancy: Category C.* There are no adequate and well-controlled studies in pregnant women. Only use epinastine ophthalmic solution during pregnancy if the potential benefit justifies the potential risk to the fetus.

➤*Lactation:* A study in lactating rats revealed excretion of epinastine into the breast milk. It is not known whether this drug is excreted in human milk. Exercise caution when administering epinastine ophthalmic solution to a nursing woman.

➤*Children:* Safety and efficacy in pediatric patients younger than 3 years of age have not been established.

Adverse Reactions

The most frequently reported ocular adverse events occurring in approximately 1% to 10% of patients were burning sensation in the eye, folliculosis, hyperemia, and pruritus.

The most frequently reported nonocular adverse events were infection (cold symptoms and upper respiratory infections), seen in approximately 10% of patients, and headache, rhinitis, sinusitis, increased cough, and pharyngitis seen in approximately 1% to 3% of patients.

Some of these events were similar to the underlying disease being studied.

Patient Information

Advise patients not to wear a contact lens if their eye is red. Do not use epinastine to treat contact lens-related irritation. The preservative in epinastine, benzalkonium chloride, may be absorbed by soft contact lenses. Remove contact lenses prior to instillation; they may be reinserted after 10 minutes following epinastine administration.

Instruct patients to avoid allowing the tip of the dispensing container to contact the eye, surrounding structures, fingers, or any other surface in order to avoid contamination of the solution by common bacteria known to cause ocular infections. Serious damage to the eye and subsequent loss of vision may result from using contaminated solutions.

The bottle should be kept tightly closed when not in use.

OPHTHALMIC DECONGESTANT/ANTIHISTAMINE COMBINATIONS

	Product & Distributor	Decongestant	Antihistamine	How Supplied
otc	**Zincfrin Solution** (Alcon)	phenylephrine HCl 0.12%		In 15 and 30 mL *Drop-Tainers.*[1]
otc	**Clear Eyes ACR Solution** (Ross)	naphazoline HCl 0.012%		In 15 and 30 mL.[2]
otc	**VasoClear A Solution** (Novartis Ophthalmics)	naphazoline HCl 0.02%		In 15 mL.[3]
otc	**Naphazoline HCl & Pheniramine Maleate Solution** (Various, eg, Moore)	naphazoline HCl 0.025%	pheniramine maleate 0.3%	In 15 mL.
otc	**Naphazoline Plus Solution** (Parmed)			In 15 mL.[4]
otc	**Naphcon-A Solution** (Alcon)			In 15 mL *Drop-Tainers.*[4]
otc	**Opcon-A Solution** (Bausch & Lomb)	naphazoline HCl 0.027%	pheniramine maleate 0.315%	In 15 mL.[5]
otc	**Naphazoline HCl & Antazoline Phosphate Sodium** (Various, eg, Moore, Steris)	naphazoline HCl 0.05%	antazoline phosphate 0.5%	In 5 and 15 mL.
otc	**Visine Allergy Relief** (Pfizer)	tetrahydrozoline HCl 0.05%		In 15 and 30 mL.[6]
otc	**Geneye AC Allergy Formula** (Goldline)			In 15 mL.[7]

[1] With 0.01% benzalkonium Cl, polysorbate 80, 0.25% zinc sulfate.
[2] With 0.2% glycerin, benzalkonium Cl, EDTA, boric acid, 0.25% zinc sulfate.
[3] With 0.005% benzalkonium Cl, EDTA, 0.25% polyvinyl alcohol, PEG-400, 0.25% zinc sulfate.
[4] With 0.01% benzalkonium Cl, EDTA.

[5] With 0.5% hydroxypropyl methylcellulose, 0.01% benzalkonium CL, 0.1% EDTA, boric acid.
[6] With 0.01% benzalkonium Cl, 0.1% EDTA, 0.25% zinc sulfate.
[7] With 0.01% benzalkonium Cl, EDTA, 0.25% zinc sulfate.

Indications

►*Itching/Redness:* Temporary relief of the minor eye symptoms of itching and redness caused by pollen, animal hair, etc.

Administration and Dosage

Recommendations vary. Refer to manufacturer package insert for instructions.

Ingredients

►*In these combinations: PHENYLEPHRINE HCL, NAPHA-ZOLINE HCL* and *TETRAHYDROZOLINE* have decongestant actions. See individual monographs for further information.

HYDROXYPROPYLMETHYLCELLULOSE and *POLYVINYL ALCO-HOL* increase the viscosity of the solution, thereby increasing contact time.

ZINC SULFATE is an astringent.

PHENIRAMINE MALEATE and *ANTAZOLINE* are antihistamines.

Warnings

►*Antihistamines:* Topical antihistamines are potential sensitizers and may produce a local sensitivity reaction. Because they may produce angle closure, use with caution in persons with a narrow angle or a history of glaucoma.

Refer to the Topical Ophthalmic Drugs introduction for more complete information.

Indications

►*Mydriasis/Cycloplegia:* For cycloplegic refraction and for dilating the pupil in inflammatory conditions of the iris and uveal tract. See individual monographs for specific indications.

Actions

►*Pharmacology:* Anticholinergic agents block the responses of the sphincter muscle of the iris and the muscle of the ciliary body to cholinergic stimulation, producing pupillary dilation (mydriasis) and paralysis of accommodation (cycloplegia).

Cycloplegic Mydriatics					
	Mydriasis		Cycloplegia		
Drug	Peak (min)	Recovery (days)	Peak (min)	Recovery (days)	Solution available
Atropine	30 - 40	7 - 10	60 - 180	6 - 12	0.5% - 2%
Homatropine	40 - 60	1 - 3	30 - 60	1 - 3	2% - 5%
Scopolamine	20 - 30	3 - 7	30 - 60	3 - 7	0.25%
Cyclopentolate	30 - 60	1	25 - 75	.25 - 1	0.5% - 2%
Tropicamide	20 - 40	0.25	20 - 35	< 0.25	0.5% - 1%

Contraindications

Primary glaucoma or a tendency toward glaucoma (eg, narrow anterior chamber angle); hypersensitivity to belladonna alkaloids or any component of the products; adhesions (synechiae) between the iris and the lens; children who have previously had a severe systemic reaction to atropine.

Warnings

For topical ophthalmic use only. Not for injection.

►*Glaucoma:* Determine the intraocular tension and the depth of the angle of the anterior chamber before and during use to avoid glaucoma attacks.

►*Elderly:* Use these products with caution in the elderly and others where increased IOP may be encountered.

►*Pregnancy: Category C* (atropine, homatropine). Safety for use during pregnancy has not been established. Give to a pregnant woman only if clearly needed.

►*Lactation:* Atropine and homatropine may be detectable, in very small amounts, in breast milk. Although this is controversial, according to the American Academy of Pediatrics, these agents are compatible with breastfeeding. It is not known if cyclopentolate is excreted in breast milk. Exercise caution when administering to a nursing woman.

►*Children:* Excessive use in children and in certain susceptible individuals may product systemic toxic symptoms. Use with extreme caution in infants and small children.

Tropicamide and cyclopentolate may cause CNS disturbances, which may be dangerous in infants and children. Keep in mind the possibility of occurrence of psychotic reaction and behavioral disturbance due to hypersensitivity to anticholinergic drugs. Use with extreme caution. Increased susceptibility to cyclopentolate has been reported in infants, young children and in children with spastic paralysis or brain damage. Feeding intolerance may follow ophthalmic use of this product in neonates. It is recommended that feeding be withheld for 4 hours after examination. Do not use in concentrations > 0.5% in small infants.

Precautions

►*Systemic effects:* Avoid excessive systemic absorption by compressing the lacrimal sac by digital pressure for 1 to 3 minutes after instillation.

►*Down's syndrome/children with brain damage:* Use cycloplegics with caution. These patients may demonstrate a hyperreactive response to topical atropine.

►*Hazardous tasks:* May produce drowsiness, blurred vision or sensitivity to light (due to dilated pupils); observe caution while driving or performing other tasks requiring alertness, coordination or physical dexterity.

►*Sulfite sensitivity:* Some of these products contain sulfites which may cause allergic-type reactions (eg, hives, itching, wheezing, anaphylaxis) in certain susceptible persons. Although the overall prevalence of sulfite sensitivity in the general population is probably low, it is seen more frequently in asthmatics or in atopic nonasthmatic persons. Specific products containing sulfites are identified in the product listings.

Adverse Reactions

►*Local:* Increased intraocular pressure; transient stinging/burning; irritation with prolonged use (eg, allergic lid reactions, hyperemia, follicular conjunctivitis, blepharoconjunctivitis, vascular congestion, edema, exudate, eczematoid dermatitis).

►*Systemic:* Dryness of the mouth and skin; blurred vision; photophobia with or without corneal staining; tachycardia; headache; parasympathetic stimulation; somnolence; visual hallucinations.

Other toxic manifestations of anticholinergic drugs include: Skin rash; abdominal distention in infants; unusual drowsiness; hyperpyrexia; vasodilation; urinary retention; diminished GI motility; decreased secretion in salivary and sweat glands, pharynx, bronchii and nasal passages. Severe manifestations of toxicity include: Coma; medullary paralysis; death. Severe reactions are manifested by hypotension with progressive respiratory depression.

Cyclopentolate and tropicamide have been associated with psychotic reactions and behavioral disturbances in children. CNS disturbances have occurred in children on tropicamide. Ataxia, incoherent speech, restlessness, hallucinations, hyperactivity, seizures, disorientation as to time and place, and failure to recognize people have occurred with cyclopentolate.

Overdosage

►*Ocular:* If ocular overdosage occurs, flush eye(s) with water or normal saline. Use of a topical miotic may be required. If accidentally ingested, induce emesis or gastric lavage.

►*Systemic:* If symptoms develop (see Adverse Reactions), patients usually recover spontaneously when the drug is discontinued. In cases of severe toxicity, give physostigmine salicylate (see individual monograph). Have atropine (1 mg) available for immediate injection if physostigmine causes bradycardia, convulsions or bronchoconstriction.

►*Cyclopentolate toxicity:* Cyclopentolate toxicity may cause exaggerated symptoms (see Adverse Reactions). When administration of the drug product is discontinued, the patient usually recovers spontaneously. In case of severe manifestation of toxicity, the antidote of choice is physostigmine salicylate.

Children – Slowly inject 0.5 mg physostigmine salicylate IV. If toxic symptoms persist and no cholinergic symptoms are produced, repeat at 5 minute intervals to a maximum cumulative dose of 2 mg.

Adults and adolescents – Slowly inject 2 mg physostigmine salicylate IV. A second dose of 1 to 2 mg may be given after 20 minutes if no reversal of toxic manifestations has occurred.

Patient Information

To avoid contamination, do not touch dropper tip to any surface. Replace cap after using.

May cause blurred vision. Do not drive or engage in any hazardous activities while the pupils are dilated.

May cause sensitivity to light. Protect eyes in bright illumination during dilation.

Keep out of the reach of children. These drugs should not be taken orally. Wash your own hands and the child's following administration.

If eye pain occurs, discontinue use and consult physician immediately.

Refer to the Topical Ophthalmics Introduction for more complete information on administration and use.

ATROPINE SULFATE

Rx	**Atropine Sulfate Ophthalmic** (Various, eg, Bausch & Lomb, Goldline)	**Ointment:** 1%	In 3.5 and UD 1 g.
Rx	**Isopto Atropine** (Alcon)	**Solution:** 0.5%	In 5 mL *Drop-Tainers*.[1]
Rx	**Atropine Sulfate** (Various, eg, Alcon)	**Solution:** 1%	In 2, 5 and 15 mL and UD 1 mL.
Rx	**Atropine-1** (Optopics)		In 2, 5 and 15 mL.
Rx	**Isopto Atropine** (Alcon)		In 5 and 15 mL *Drop-Tainers*.[1]
Rx	**Atropine Sulfate** (Alcon)	**Solution:** 2%	In 2 mL.

[1] With 0.01% benzalkonium chloride, 0.5% hydroxypropyl methylcellulose and boric acid.
[2] With 0.01% benzalkonium chloride, hydroxypropyl methylcellulose and boric acid.
[3] With benzalkonium chloride, EDTA and boric acid.

For complete prescribing information, refer to the Cycloplegic Mydriatics group monograph.

> **Indications**

➤*Mydriasis/Cycloplegia:* For cycloplegic refraction or pupil dilation in acute inflammatory conditions of iris and uveal tract.

> **Administration and Dosage**

➤*Solution:*
Adults –
 Uveitis: Instill 1 or 2 drops into the eye(s) up to 4 times daily.
 Refraction: Instill 1 or 2 drops of 1% solution into eye(s) 1 hour before refracting.

Children –
 Uveitis: Instill 1 or 2 drops of 0.5% solution into the eye(s) up to 3 times daily.
 Refraction: Instill 1 or 2 drops of 0.5% solution into the eye(s) twice daily for 1 to 3 days before examination.
➤*Ointment:* Apply a small amount in the conjunctival sac up to 3 times daily.

Compress the lacrimal sac by digital pressure for several minutes after instillation.

Individuals with heavily pigmented irides may require larger doses.

➤*Storage/Stability:* Keep from heat.

SCOPOLAMINE HBr (Hyoscine HBr)

Rx	**Isopto Hyoscine** (Alcon)	**Solution:** 0.25%	In 5 and 15 mL *Drop-Tainers*.[1]

[1] With 0.01% benzalkonium chloride and 0.5% hydroxypropyl methylcellulose.

For complete prescribing information, refer to the Cycloplegic Mydriatics group monograph.

> **Indications**

➤*Mydriasis/Cycloplegia:* For cycloplegia and mydriasis in diagnostic procedures.
➤*Iridocyclitis:* For preoperative and postoperative states in the treatment of iridocyclitis.

> **Administration and Dosage**

➤*Uveitis:* Instill 1 or 2 drops into the eye(s) up to 4 times daily.

➤*Refraction:* Instill 1 or 2 drops into the eye(s) 1 hour before refracting.

Compress the lacrimal sac by digital pressure for several minutes after instillation.

➤*Storage/Stability:* Protect from light. Store at 8° to 27°C (46° to 80°F).

HOMATROPINE HBr

Rx	**Isopto Homatropine** (Alcon)	**Solution:** 2%	In 5 and 15 mL *Drop-Tainers*.[1]
Rx	**Homatropine HBr** (Various, eg, Alcon, Novartis Ophthalmics)	**Solution:** 5%	In 1, 2 and 5 mL.
Rx	**Isopto Homatropine** (Alcon)		In 5 and 15 mL *Drop-Tainers*.[1]

[1] With 0.01% benzalkonium chloride, 0.5% hydroxypropylmethylcellulose and polysorbate 80.

For complete prescribing information, refer to the Cycloplegic Mydriatics group monograph.

> **Indications**

➤*Mydriasis/Cycloplegia:* A moderately long-acting mydriatic and cycloplegic for refraction, and in the treatment of inflammatory conditions of the uveal tract. For preoperative and postoperative states when mydriasis is required.
➤*Lens opacity:* As an optical aid in some cases of axial lens opacities.

> **Administration and Dosage**

➤*Uveitis:* Instill 1 or 2 drops into the eye(s) up to every 3 to 4 hours.

➤*Refraction:* Instill 1 or 2 drops into the eye(s); repeat in 5 to 10 minutes if necessary.

Individuals with heavily pigmented irides may require larger doses.

➤*Children:* Use only the 2% strength.

Compress the lacrimal sac by digital pressure for several minutes after instillation.

➤*Storage/Stability:* Store at 8° to 24°C (46° to 75°F).

TROPICAMIDE

Rx	**Tropicamide** (Various, eg, Bausch & Lomb)	**Solution:** 0.5%	In 2 and 15 mL.
Rx	**Mydriacyl** (Alcon)		In 15 mL *Drop-Tainers*.[1]
Rx	**Tropicacyl** (Akorn)		In 15 mL.[2]
Rx	**Tropicamide** (Various, eg, Bausch & Lomb)	**Solution:** 1%	In 15 mL.
Rx	**Mydriacyl** (Alcon)		In 3 and 15 mL *Drop-Tainers*.[1]
Rx	**Tropicacyl** (Akorn)		In 2 and 15 mL.[2]

[1] With 0.01% benzalkonium chloride and EDTA.
[2] With 0.1% benzalkonium chloride and EDTA.

For complete prescribing information, refer to the Cycloplegic Mydriatics group monograph.

> **Indications**

➤*Mydriasis/Cycloplegia:* For mydriasis and cycloplegia for diagnostic purposes.

> **Administration and Dosage**

➤*Refraction:* Instill 1 or 2 drops of 1% solution into the eye(s); repeat in 5 minutes. If patients is not seen within 20 to 30 minutes, instill an additional drop to prolong mydriatic effect.

➤*Examination of fundus:* Instill 1 or 2 drops of 0.5% solution 15 to 20 minutes prior to examination. Compress the lacrimal sac by digital pressure for several minutes after instillation to avoid excessive absorption.

Individuals with heavily pigmented irides may require larger doses.

➤*Storage/Stability:* Store away from heat. Do not refrigerate.

CYCLOPENTOLATE HCl

Rx	Cyclogyl (Alcon)	Solution: 0.5%	In 2, 5 and 15 mL *Drop-Tainers.*[1]
Rx	Cyclopentolate HCl (Various, eg, Steris)	Solution: 1%	In 2, 5 and 15 mL.
Rx	AK-Pentolate (Akorn)		In 1 and 15 mL.[1]
Rx	Cyclogyl (Alcon)		In 2, 5 and 15 mL.[1]
Rx	Pentolair (Bausch & Lomb)		In 2 and 15 mL squeeze bottles.[2]
Rx	Cyclogyl (Alcon)	Solution: 2%	In 2, 5 and 15 mL *Drop-Tainers.*[1]

[1] With 0.01% benzalkonium chloride, EDTA and boric acid.

[2] With 0.01% benzalkonium chloride and EDTA.

For complete prescribing information, refer to the Cycloplegic Mydriatics group monograph.

Indications

➤*Mydriasis / Cycloplegia:* For mydriasis and cycloplegia in diagnostic procedures.

Administration and Dosage

➤*Adults:* Instill 1 or 2 drops of 0.5%, 1% or 2% solution into eye(s). Repeat in 5 to 10 minutes, if necessary. Complete recovery usually occurs in 24 hours.

➤*Children:* Instill 1 or 2 drops of 0.5%, 1% or 2% solution into eye(s).

Repeat in 5 to 10 minutes, if necessary, with a second application of 0.5% or 1% solution.

➤*Small infants:* Instill 1 drop of 0.5% solution into eye(s). Observe patient closely for at least 30 minutes following instillation.

Compress the lacrimal sac by digital pressure for several minutes after instillation.

Individuals with heavily pigmented irides may require higher strengths.

➤*Storage / Stability:* Store at 8° to 27°C (46° to 80°F).

MYDRIATIC COMBINATIONS

Rx	Cyclomydril (Alcon)	Solution: 0.2% cyclopentolate HCl/1% phenylephrine HCl.	In 2 and 5 mL *Drop-Tainers.*[1]
Rx	Murocoll-2 (Bausch & Lomb)	Drops: 0.3% scopolamine HBr/10% phenylephrine HCl.	In 5 mL.[2]

[1] With 0.01% benzalkonium chloride, EDTA and boric acid.

[2] With 0.01% benzalkonium chloride, sodium metabisulfite and EDTA.

These combinations induce mydriasis that is considerably greater than that of either drug alone. See individual monographs for complete prescribing information.

Indications

➤*Cyclomydril:* Production of mydriasis.

➤*Murocoll-2:* For mydriasis, cycloplegia and to break posterior synechiae in iritis.

Administration and Dosage

➤*Cyclomydril:* Instill 1 drop into each eye every 5 to 10 minutes, not to exceed 3 times.

➤*Murocoll-2:*

Mydriasis – 1 or 2 drops into eye(s); repeat in 5 minutes, if necessary.

Postoperatively – 1 or 2 drops into the eye(s) 3 or 4 times daily.

Refer to the Topical Ophthalmic Drugs introduction for more complete information.

Indications

➤*Ocular infections:* Treatment of superficial ocular infections involving the conjunctiva or cornea (eg, conjunctivitis, keratitis, keratoconjunctivitis, corneal ulcers, blepharitis, blepharoconjunctivitis, acute meibomianitis and dacryocystitis) due to strains of microorganisms susceptible to antibiotics.

➤*Erythromycin:* Prophylaxis of ophthalmia neonatorum due to Neisseria gonorrhoeae or Chlamydia trachomatis.

➤*Chloramphenicol:* Use only in those serious infections for which less potentially dangerous drugs are ineffective or contraindicated (see Warnings).

For a list of microorganisms usually susceptible to these agents, refer to systemic monographs in the Anti-infectives chapter.

		Miscellaneous							Quinolones			Aminoglycosides			Sulfonamides	
Organism/Infection		Bacitracin	Gramicidin	Polymyxin B	Erythromycin	Chloramphenicol	Trimethoprim	Oxytetracycline	Norfloxacin	Ciprofloxacin	Ofloxacin	Neomycin	Gentamicin	Tobramycin	Sodium Sulfacetamide	Sulfisoxazole
Gram-Positive	Staphylococcus sp.	✓	✓						✓	✓	✓		✓	✓		
	S. aureus	✓	✓		✓	✓	✓		✓	✓	✓	✓	✓[1]	✓	✓	✓
	Streptococcus sp.	✓	✓							✓	✓			✓	✓	✓
	S. pneumoniae	✓	✓		✓	✓							✓[1]	✓	✓	✓
	α-hemolytic streptococci (viridans group)				✓										✓	✓
	β-hemolytic streptococci	✓											✓[1]	✓		
	S. pyogenes	✓			✓		✓			✓	✓		✓		✓	✓
	Corynebacterium sp.	✓	✓		✓							✓	✓	✓		
Gram-Negative	Escherichia coli			✓		✓	✓	✓		✓	✓	✓	✓	✓	✓	✓
	Haemophilus aegyptius					✓	✓		✓				✓	✓	✓	✓
	H. ducreyi					✓		✓		✓			✓	✓		
	H. influenzae or parainfluenzae			✓	✓	✓		✓	✓	✓	✓		✓	✓		
	Klebsiella sp					✓			✓	✓	✓				✓	✓
	K. pneumoniae			✓			✓		✓	✓	✓		✓	✓		
	Neisseria sp	✓			✓					✓		✓	✓	✓		
	N. gonorrhoeae	✓			✓[2]				✓	✓	✓		✓		✓	
	Proteus sp.						✓		✓	✓	✓	✓	✓	✓	✓	✓
	Acinetobacter calcoaceticus								✓	✓	✓		✓	✓		
	Enterobacter aerogenes			✓		✓		✓	✓	✓	✓	✓	✓	✓		
	Enterobacter sp.					✓			✓	✓	✓	✓	✓	✓	✓	✓
	Serratia marcescens						✓		✓	✓	✓		✓	✓		
	Moraxella sp.					✓				✓			✓	✓		
	Chlamydia trachomatis				✓[2]					✓	✓				✓	✓
	Pasteurella tularensis							✓								
	Pseudomonas aeruginosa			✓					✓	✓	✓		✓[1]	✓		
	Bartonella bacilliformis							✓								
	Bacteroides sp.							✓								
	Vibrio sp					✓			✓	✓	✓		✓	✓		
	Providencia sp.									✓	✓					

[1] Increasing resistance has been seen.
[2] For prophylaxis.

Administration and Dosage

Administration and dosage varies for the individual products. Refer to the individual manufacturer inserts.

Contraindications

Hypersensitivity to any component of these products; epithelial herpes simplex keratitis (dendritic keratitis); vaccinia; varicella; mycobacterial infections of the eye; fungal diseases of the ocular structure; use of steroid combinations after uncomplicated removal of a corneal foreign body.

Warnings

➤*Sensitization:* Sensitization from the topical use of an antibiotic may contraindicate the drug's later systemic use in serious infections. For this reason, topical preparations containing antibiotics not ordinarily administered systemically are preferable.

Products with neomycin sulfate may cause cutaneous/conjunctival sensitization.

➤*Cross-sensitivity:* Allergic cross-reactions may occur that could prevent future use of any or all of these antibiotics: Kanamycin, neomycin, paromomycin, streptomycin, and possibly, gentamicin.

➤*Hematopoietic toxicity:* Hematopoietic toxicity has occurred occasionally with the systemic use of **chloramphenicol** and rarely with topical administration. It is generally a dose-related toxic effect on bone marrow, and is usually reversible on cessation of therapy. Rare cases of aplastic anemia, bone marrow hypoplasia and death have been reported with prolonged (months to years) or frequent intermittent (over months and years) use of ocular chloramphenicol.

➤*Corneal healing:* Ophthalmic ointments may retard corneal epithelial healing.

➤*Pregnancy:* Category B (erythromycin, tobramycin), Category C (gentamicin, ciprofloxacin, norfloxacin, ofloxacin, polymyxin B). Safety for use during pregnancy has not been established. Use only when clearly needed and when the potential benefits outweigh the potential hazards to the fetus.

➤*Lactation:* It is not known whether **ciprofloxacin, norfloxacin** or **ofloxacin** appears in breast milk following ophthalmic use. Exercise caution when administering **ciprofloxacin** to a nursing mother. Because of the potential for adverse reactions in nursing infants from **norfloxacin, ofloxacin, chloramphenicol** and **tobramycin,** decide whether to discontinue nursing or discontinue the drug, taking into account the importance of the drug to the mother.

➤*Children:* **Tobramycin** is safe and effective in children. Safety and efficacy of **fluoroquinolones** in infants < 1 year of age, and **polymyxin B/trimethoprim** in infants < 2 months have not been established.

Precautions

➤*Monitoring:* Perform culture and susceptibility testing during treatment.

➤*Systemic antibiotics:* In all except very superficial infections, supplement the topical use of antibiotics with appropriate systemic medication. Systemic aminoglycoside antibiotics require monitoring the total serum concentration (peak and trough).

➤*Crystalline precipitate:* A white crystalline precipitate located in the superficial portion of the corneal defect was observed in ≈ 17% of patients on **ciprofloxacin**. Onset was within 1 to 7 days after starting therapy. The precipitate resolved in most patients within 2 weeks, and did not preclude continued use nor adversely affect the clinical course or outcome.

➤*Superinfection:* Do not use topical antibiotics in deep-seated ocular infections or in those that are likely to become systemic. Use of antibiotics (especially prolonged or repeated therapy) may result in bacterial or fungal overgrowth of nonsusceptible organisms. Such overgrowth may lead to a secondary infection. Take appropriate measures if superinfection occurs.

➤*Sulfite sensitivity:* Some of these products contain sulfites which may cause allergic-type reactions (eg, hives, itching, wheezing, anaphylaxis) in certain susceptible persons. Although the overall prevalence of sulfite sensitivity in the general population is probably low, it is seen more frequently in asthmatics or in atopic nonasthmatic persons. Specific products containing sulfites are identified in the product listings.

Adverse Reactions

Sensitivity reactions such as transient irritation, burning, stinging, itching, inflammation, angioneurotic edema, urticaria, vesicular and maculopapular dermatitis have occurred in some patients.

➤*Chloramphenicol:* Hematological events (including aplastic anemia) have been reported (see Warnings).

➤*Fluoroquinolones:* White crystalline precipitates; lid margin crusting; crystals/scales; foreign body sensation; conjunctival hyperemia; bad/bitter taste in mouth; corneal staining; keratopathy/keratitis; allergic reactions; lid edema; tearing; photophobia; corneal infiltrates; nausea; decreased vision; chemosis.

➤*Aminoglycosides:* Localized ocular toxicity and hypersensitivity, lid itching, lid swelling and conjunctival erythema (< 3% with tobramycin); bacterial/fungal corneal ulcers; nonspecific conjunctivitis; conjunctival epithelial defects; conjunctival hyperemia (gentamicin). Similar reactions may occur with the topical use of other aminoglycoside antibiotics.

Overdosage

➤*Symptoms:* Symptoms of tobramycin overdose include punctate keratitis, erythema, increased lacrimation, edema and lid itching. These may be similar to adverse reactions.

➤*Treatment:* A topical overdose of **ciprofloxacin** may be flushed from the eyes with warm tap water.

Patient Information

Tilt head back, place medication in conjunctival sac and close eyes. Apply light finger pressure on lacrimal sac for 1 minute following instillation.

May cause temporary blurring of vision or stinging following administration. Notify physician if stinging, burning or itching becomes pronounced or if redness, irritation, swelling, decreasing vision or pain persists or worsens.

To avoid contamination, do not touch tip of container to any surface. Replace cap after using.

In general, patients being treated for bacterial conjunctivitis should not wear contact lenses; however, if the physician considers contact lens use appropriate, wait at least 15 minutes after using any solutions containing benzalkonium chloride before inserting the lens, as it may be absorbed by the lens.

➤*Quinolones:* Discontinue use and notify physician at the first sign of a skin rash or other allergic reaction.

CHLORAMPHENICOL

Rx	**Chloramphenicol** (Various, eg, Goldline,Schein)	**Solution**[1]: 5 mg/mL	In 7.5 and 15 mL.
Rx	**Chloramphenicol** (Various, eg, Schein)	**Ointment**: 10 mg/g	In 3.5 g.
Rx	**Chloroptic S.O.P.** (Allergan)		In 3.5 g.[6]
Rx	**Chloromycetin** (Parke-Davis)	**Powder for solution**: 25 mg/vial.	Preservative free. In 15 mL with diluent.

[1] Refrigerate until dispensed.
[2] With 0.5% chlorobutanol, boric acid, sodium borate, hydroxypropyl methylcellulose, sodium hydroxide and hydrochloric acid.
[3] With 0.5% chlorobutanol, PEG-300, polyoxyl 40 stearate and sodium hydroxide or hydrochloric acid.
[4] With white petrolatum, mineral oil and polysorbate 60.
[5] With liquid petrolatum and polyethylene base.
[6] With 0.5% chlorobutanol, white petrolatum, mineral oil, polyoxyl 40 stearate, petrolatum (and) lanolin alcohol and PEG-300.

Complete prescribing information begins in the Ophthalmic Antibiotics group monograph.

Indications

➤*Ocular infections:* Treatment of superficial ocular infections involving the conjunctiva or cornea (eg, conjunctivitis, keratitis, keratoconjunctivitis, corneal ulcers, blepharitis, blepharoconjunctivitis, acute meibomianitis and dacryocystitis) due to strains of microorganisms susceptible to antibiotics.

➤*Chloramphenicol:* Use only in those serious infections for which less potentially dangerous drugs are ineffective or contraindicated (see Warnings).

For a list of microorganisms usually susceptible to these agents, refer to systemic monographs in the Anti-infectives chapter.

Administration and Dosage

Administration and dosage varies for the individual products. Refer to the individual manufacturer inserts.

ERYTHROMYCIN

Rx	**Erythromycin** (Various, eg, Akorn,Bausch & Lomb, Fougera,Goldline,Rugby)	**Ointment**: 0.5%	In 3.5 g.
Rx	**Ilotycin** (Dista)		In 3.5 g.[1]

[1] With white petrolatum and mineral oil.

Complete prescribing information begins in the Opthalmic Antibiotics group monograph.

Indications

➤*Ocular infections:* Treatment of superficial ocular infections involving the conjunctiva or cornea (eg, conjunctivitis, keratitis, keratoconjunctivitis, corneal ulcers, blepharitis, blepharoconjunctivitis, acute meibomianitis and dacryocystitis) due to strains of microorganisms susceptible to antibiotics.

➤*Erythromycin:* Prophylaxis of ophthalmia neonatorum due to *Neisseria gonorrhoeae* or *Chlamydia trachomatis.*

For a list of microorganisms usually susceptible to these agents, refer to systemic monographs in the Anti-infectives chapter.

Administration and Dosage

Administration and dosage varies for the individual products. Refer to the individual manufacturer inserts.

GENTAMICIN SULFATE

Rx	**Gentamicin Ophthalmic** (Various, eg, Bausch & Lomb, Goldline, Rugby, Schein)	**Solution**: 3 mg/mL	In 5 and 15 mL.
Rx	**Garamycin** (Schering)		In 5 mL dropper bottles.[1]
Rx	**Genoptic** (Allergan)		In 1 and 5 mL dropper bottles.[2]
Rx	**Gentacidin** (Novartis Ophthalmics)		In 5 mL dropper bottles.[1]
Rx	**Garamycin** (Schering)	**Ointment**: 3 mg/g	In 3.5 g.[3]
Rx	**Genoptic S.O.P.** (Allergan)		In 3.5 g.[3]
Rx	**Gentak** (Akorn)		In 3.5 g.[3]

[1] With 0.1 mg/mL benzalkonium chloride, sodium phosphate and NaCl.
[2] With benzalkonium chloride, 1.4% polyvinyl alcohol, EDTA, sodium phosphate dibasic, NaCl and hydrochloric acid or sodium hydroxide.
[3] With white petrolatum and parabens.

Complete prescribing information begins in the Ophthalmic Antibiotics group monograph.

Indications

➤*Ocular infections:* Treatment of superficial ocular infections involving the conjunctiva or cornea (eg, conjunctivitis, keratitis, keratocon-

GENTAMICIN SULFATE

junctivitis, corneal ulcers, blepharitis, blepharoconjunctivitis, acute meibomianitis and dacryocystitis) due to strains of microorganisms susceptible to antibiotics.

For a list of microorganisms usually susceptible to these agents, refer to systemic monographs in the Anti-infectives chapter.

Administration and Dosage

Administration and dosage varies for the individual products. Refer to the individual manufacturer inserts.

TOBRAMYCIN

Rx	**Tobramycin** (Various, eg, Bausch & Lomb)	**Solution:** 0.3% tobramycin	In 5 mL bottle.[1]
Rx	**AKTob** (Akorn)		In 5 mL.[2]
Rx	**Defy** (Akorn)		In 5 mL.
Rx	**Tobrex** (Alcon)		In 5 mL Drop-Tainers.[3]
Rx	**Tobrex** (Alcon)	**Ointment:** 3 mg tobramycin per g	In 3.5 g.[4]

[1] With 0.01% benzalkonium Cl and boric acid.
[2] With 0.01% benzalkonium chloride, boric acid and sodium sulfate.
[3] With 0.01% benzalkonium chloride, tyloxapol and boric acid.
[4] With white petrolatum, mineral oil and 0.5% chlorobutanol.

Complete prescribing information begins in the Opthalmic Antibiotics group monograph.

Indications

➤*Ocular infections:* Treatment of superficial ocular infections involving the conjunctiva or cornea (eg, conjunctivitis, keratitis, keratoconjunctivitis, corneal ulcers, blepharitis, blepharoconjunctivitis, acute meibomianitis and dacryocystitis) due to strains of microorganisms susceptible to antibiotics.

For a list of microorganisms usually susceptible to these agents, refer to systemic monographs in the Anti-infectives chapter.

Administration and Dosage

Administration and dosage varies for the individual products. Refer to the individual manufacturer inserts.

POLYMYXIN B SULFATE

Rx	**Polymyxin B Sulfate Sterile** (Roerig)	**Powder for solution:** 500,000 units	In 20 mL vials.

Complete prescribing information begins in the Opthalmic Antibiotics group monograph.

Indications

➤*Ocular infections:* Treatment of superficial ocular infections involving the conjunctiva or cornea (eg, conjunctivitis, keratitis, keratoconjunctivitis, corneal ulcers, blepharitis, blepharoconjunctivitis, acute meibomianitis and dacryocystitis) due to strains of microorganisms susceptible to antibiotics.

For a list of microorganisms usually susceptible to these agents, refer to systemic monographs in the Anti-infectives chapter.

Administration and Dosage

Administration and dosage varies for the individual products. Refer to the individual manufacturer inserts.

BACITRACIN

Rx	**Bacitracin** (Various, eg, Goldline, Major, Schein, URL)	**Ointment:** 500 units/g	In 3.5 and 3.75 g.
Rx	**AK-Tracin** (Akorn)		Preservative free. In 3.5 g.[1]

[1] With white petrolatum and mineral oil.

Complete prescribing information begins in the Ophthalmic Antibiotics group monograph.

Indications

➤*Ocular infections:* Treatment of superficial ocular infections involving the conjunctiva or cornea (eg, conjunctivitis, keratitis, keratoconjunctivitis, corneal ulcers, blepharitis, blepharoconjunctivitis, acute meibomianitis and dacryocystitis) due to strains of microorganisms susceptible to antibiotics.

For a list of microorganisms usually susceptible to these agents, refer to systemic monographs in the Anti-infectives chapter.

Administration and Dosage

Administration and dosage varies for the individual products. Refer to the individual manufacturer inserts.

CIPROFLOXACIN

Rx	**Ciprofloxacin** (Various, eg, Bausch & Lomb, Novax)	**Solution:** 3.5 mg/mL (equivalent to 3 mg base)	In 2.5, 5, and 10 mL dropper bottles.[a]
Rx	**Ciloxan** (Alcon)		In 2.5 and 5 mL *Drop-Tainers.*[b]
Rx	**Ciloxan** (Alcon)	**Ointment:** 3.33 mg/g (equivalent to 3 mg base)	Mineral oil, white petrolatum. In 3.5 g.

[a] With 0.006% benzalkonium chloride, mannitol, and EDTA.
[b] With 0.006% benzalkonium chloride, 4.6% mannitol, and 0.05% EDTA.

Complete prescribing information begins in the Opthalmic Antibiotics group monograph.

Indications

➤*Ocular infections:* Treatment of superficial ocular infections involving the conjunctiva or cornea (eg, conjunctivitis, keratitis, keratoconjunctivitis, corneal ulcers, blepharitis, blepharoconjunctivitis, acute meibomianitis and dacryocystitis) due to strains of microorganisms susceptible to antibiotics.

For a list of microorganisms usually susceptible to these agents, refer to systemic monographs in the Anti-infectives chapter.

Administration and Dosage

Administration and dosage varies for the individual products. Refer to the individual manufacturer inserts.

GATIFLOXACIN

Rx	**Zymar** (Allergan)	**Solution:** 0.3% (3 mg/mL)	In 2.5 and 5 mL dropper bottles.[1]

[1] With 0.005% benzalkonium chloride and EDTA.

Complete prescribing information begins in the Ophthalmic Antibiotics group monograph.

Indications

Treatment of bacterial conjunctivitis caused by susceptible strains of the following organisms listed below:

➤*Gram positive bacteria: Cornyebacterium propinquum*†, *Staphylococcus aureus, S. epidermidis, Streptococcus mitis*†, *S. pneumoniae.*

➤*Gram negative bacteria: Haemophilus influenzae.*

Administration and Dosage

➤*Approved by the FDA:* March 28, 2003.

➤*Days 1 and 2:* Instill 1 drop in affected eye(s) every 2 hours while awake, up to 8 times/day.

➤*Days 3 through 7:* Instill 1 drop up to 4 times/day while awake.

➤*Storage:* Store between 15° to 25°C (59° to 77°F). Protect from freezing.

† Efficacy for this organism was studied in fewer than 10 infections.

MOXIFLOXACIN HCl

| *Rx* | **Vigamox** (Alcon) | **Solution:** 0.5% (5 mg/mL) | In 3 mL *Drop-Tainer.*[1] |

[1] With boric acid, sodium chloride, and purified water.

Complete prescribing information begins in the Ophthalmic Antibiotics group monograph.

Indications

➤*Conjunctivitis:*

Gram-positive bacteria – *Corynebacterium* species†, *Micrococcus luteus*†, *Staphylococcus aureus*, *S. epidermidis*, *S. haemolyticus*, *S. hominis*, *S. warneri*†, *Streptococcus pneumoniae*, *Streptococcus* viridans group.

Gram negative bacteria – *Acinetobacter lwoffii*†, *Haemophilus influenzae*, *H. parainfluenzae*†.

Other microorganisms – *Chlamydia trachomatis.*

Administration and Dosage

➤*Approved by the FDA:* April 15, 2003.

➤*Adults and children at least 1 year of age:* Instill 1 drop in the affected eye 3 times a day for 7 days.

➤*Storage/Stability:* Store at 2° to 25°C (36° to 77°F).

OFLOXACIN

| *Rx* | **Ocuflox** (Allergan) | **Solution:** 0.3% (3 mg/mL) | In 1, 5, and 10 mL.[1] |

[1] With 0.005% benzalkonium chloride.

Complete prescribing information begins in the Ophthalmic Antibiotics group monograph.

Indications

Treatment of infections caused by susceptible strains of the following bacteria in the conditions listed below:

➤*Conjunctivitis:*

Gram positive bacteria – *Staphylococcus aureus*, *S. epidermidis*, *Streptococcus pneumoniae.*

Gram negative bacteria – *Enterobacter cloacae*, *Haemophilus influenzae*, *Proteus mirabilis*, *Pseudomonas aeruginosa.*

➤*Corneal ulcers:*

Gram positive bacteria – *S. aureus*, *S. epidermidis*, *S. pneumoniae.*

Gram negative bacteria – *P aeruginosa*, *S. marcescens* (efficacy for this organism was studied in < 10 infections).

Anaerobic species – *Propionibacterium acnes.*

Administration and Dosage

➤*Bacterial conjunctivitis:*

Days 1 and 2 – 1 to 2 drops every 2 to 4 hours in the affected eye(s).

Days 3 through 7 – 1 to 2 drops 4 times daily.

➤*Bacterial corneal ulcer:*

Days 1 and 2 – 1 to 2 drops into the affected eye every 30 minutes while awake. Awaken at ≈ 4 and 6 hours after retiring and instill 1 to 2 drops.

Days 3 through 7 to 9 – Instill 1 to 2 drops hourly while awake.

Days 7 to 9 through treatment completion – Instill 1 to 2 drops 4 times daily.

LEVOFLOXACIN

| *Rx* | **Quixin** (Santen) | **Solution:** 0.5% (5 mg/mL) | In 2.5 and 5 mL.[1] |
| *Rx* | **Iquix** (Santen) | **Solution:** 1.5% (15 mg/mL) | In 5 mL. |

[1] With 0.005% benzalkonium chloride.

Complete prescribing information begins in the Ophthalmic Antibiotics group monograph.

Indications

➤*Quixin:*

Conjunctivitis – Treatment of bacterial conjunctivitis caused by susceptible strains of the following organisms:

Gram-positive bacteria: Corynebacterium species (efficacy for this organism was studied in < 10 infections), *Staphylococcus aureus* (methicillin-susceptible strains only), *Staphylococcus epidermidis* (methicillin-susceptible strains only), *Streptococcus pneumoniae*, *Streptococcus* (Groups C/F and G), Viridans group streptococci.

Gram-negative bacteria: Acinetobacter lwoffii (efficacy for this organism was studied in < 10 infections), *Haemophilus influenzae*, *Pseudomonas aeruginosa* (Iquix only), *Serratia marcescens* (efficacy for this organism was studied in < 10 infections).

➤*Iquix:*

Corneal ulcer – Treatment of corneal ulcer caused by susceptible strains of the following organisms:

Gram-positive bacteria: Corynebacterium species (efficacy for this organism was studied in < 10 infections), *S. aureus* (methicillin-suscep-tible strains only), *S. epidermidis* (methicillin-susceptible strains only), *S. pneumoniae*, *S.* (Groups C/F and G), Viridans group streptococci.

Gram-negative bacteria: Pseudomonas aeruginosa, *Serratia marcescens* (efficacy for this organism was studied in < 10 infections).

Administration and Dosage

➤*Approved by the FDA:* August 2000.

➤*Quixin:*

Days 1 and 2 – Instill 1 to 2 drops in the affected eye(s) every 2 hours while awake, up to 8 times per day.

Days 3 through 7 – Instill 1 to 2 drops in the affected eye(s) every 4 hours while awake, up to 4 times per day.

➤*Iquix:*

Days 1 through 3 – Instill 1 to 2 drops in the affected eye(s) every 30 minutes to 2 hours while awake and approximately 4 and 6 hours after retiring.

Day 4 through treatment completion – Instill 1 to 2 drops in the affected eye(s) every 1 to 4 hours while awake.

---

† Efficacy for this organism was studied in fewer than 10 infections.

Refer to Topical Ophthalmic Drugs introduction for more complete information.

Indications

➤*Ocular infections:* For conjunctivitis, corneal ulcer and other superficial ocular infections due to susceptible microorganisms.

➤*Trachoma:* As an adjunct to systemic sulfonamide therapy in the treatment of trachoma.

Administration and Dosage

Usual duration of treatment is 7 to 10 days.

➤*Solutions:*

Conjunctivitis or other superficial ocular infections – Instill 1 to 2 drops into the lower conjunctival sac(s) every 1 to 4 hours initially according to severity of infection. Dosages may be tapered by increasing the time interval between doses as the condition responds.

Trachoma – 2 drops every 2 hours. Concomitant systemic sulfonamide therapy is indicated.

Storage/Stability – Protect from light. On long standing, solutions will darken in color and should be discarded.

➤*Ointments:* Apply a small amount (0.5 inch) into the lower conjunctival sac(s) 3 to 4 times daily and at bedtime. Dosages may be tapered by increasing the time interval between doses as the condition responds. Or apply 0.5 to 1 inch into the conjunctival sac(s) at night in conjunction with the use of drops during the day, or before an eye is patched.

Storage/Stability – Store away from heat.

Actions

➤*Pharmacology:* Sulfonamides are bacteriostatic against a wide range of susceptible gram-positive and gram-negative microorganisms. Through competition with para-aminobenzoic acid (PABA), they restrict synthesis of folic acid which bacteria require for growth. For complete information, refer to the systemic sulfonamides monograph in the Anti-infectives chapter.

➤*Pharmacokinetics:* Sulfonamides do not appear to be appreciably absorbed from mucous membranes.

➤*Microbiology:* Topically applied sulfonamides are considered active against susceptible strains of the following common bacterial eye pathogens: *Escherichia coli, Staphylococcus aureus, Streptococcus pneumoniae, Streptococcus* (viridans group), *Haemophilus influenzae, Klebsiella* sp and *Enterobacter* sp.

Topically applied sulfonamides do not provide adequate coverage against *Neisseria* sp, *Serratia marcescens* and *Pseudomonas aeruginosa.* A significant percentage of staphylococcal isolates are completely resistant to sulfa drugs.

Contraindications

Hypersensitivity to sulfonamides or any component of the product; infants < 2 months of age; in epithelial herpes simplex keratitis (dendritic keratitis), vaccinia, varicella and many other viral diseases of the cornea and conjunctiva; mycobacterial infection or fungal diseases of the ocular structures; after uncomplicated removal of a corneal foreign body (steroid combinations).

Warnings

➤*Staphylococcus species:* A significant percentage of isolates are resistant to sulfa drugs.

➤*Hypersensitivity reactions:* Severe sensitivity reactions have been identified in individuals with no prior history of sulfonamide hypersensitivity (see Adverse Reactions).

➤*Pregnancy: Category C.* Safety for use during pregnancy has not been established. Use only when clearly needed and when potential benefits outweigh potential hazards to the fetus.

➤*Lactation:* Systemic sulfonamides are excreted in breast milk.

➤*Children:* Safety and efficacy not established. Contraindicated in infants < 2 months old.

Precautions

For topical ophthalmic use only. Not for injection.

➤*Epithelial healing:* Ophthalmic ointments may retard corneal wound healing.

➤*Sensitization:* Sensitization may occur when a sulfonamide is readministered, regardless of route. Cross-sensitivity between different sulfonamides may occur. If signs of sensitivity or other untoward reactions occur, discontinue use of the preparation.

➤*PABA:* PABA present in purulent exudates inactivates sulfonamides.

➤*Dry eye:* Use with caution in patients with severe dry eye.

➤*Superinfection:* Use of antibiotics (especially prolonged or repeated therapy) may result in bacterial or fungal overgrowth of nonsusceptible organisms. Such overgrowth may lead to a secondary infection. Take appropriate measures if this occurs.

➤*Sulfite sensitivity:* May cause allergic-type reactions (eg, hives, itching, wheezing, anaphylaxis) in certain susceptible persons. Although overall prevalence in the general population is probably low, it is more common in asthmatics or in atopic nonasthmatics. Specific products containing sulfites are identified in product listings.

Drug Interactions

Silver preparations are incompatible with these solutions.

Adverse Reactions

Headache; local irritation; itching; periorbital edema, burning and transient stinging; bacterial and fungal corneal ulcers. As with all sulfonamide preparations, severe sensitivity reactions include rare occurrences of Stevens-Johnson syndrome, exfoliative dermatitis, toxic epidermal necrolysis, photosensitivity, fever, skin rash, GI disturbance and bone marrow depression; fatalities have occurred.

Patient Information

For topical use only.

To avoid contamination, do not touch tip of container to any surface.

Keep bottle tightly closed when not in use. Do not use if solution has darkened.

Notify physician if improvement is not seen after several days, if condition worsens, or if pain, increased redness, itching or swelling of the eye occurs or persists for > 48 hours. Do not discontinue use without consulting physician.

SULFISOXAZOLE DIOLAMINE

| *Rx* | **Gantrisin** (Roche) | **Solution:** 4% | With 1:100,000 phenylmercuric nitrate. In 15 mL with dropper. |

Complete prescribing information is found in the Sulfonamides group monograph.

Indications

➤*Ocular infections:* For conjunctivitis, corneal ulcer and other superficial ocular infections due to susceptible microorganisms.

➤*Trachoma:* As an adjunct to systemic sulfonamide therapy in the treatment of trachoma.

Administration and Dosage

Usual duration of treatment is 7 to 10 days.

➤*Solutions:*

Conjunctivitis or other superficial ocular infections – Instill 1 to 2 drops into the lower conjunctival sac(s) every 1 to 4 hours initially according to severity of infection. Dosages may be tapered by increasing the time interval between doses as the condition responds.

Trachoma – 2 drops every 2 hours. Concomitant systemic sulfonamide therapy is indicated.

➤*Storage/Stability:* Protect from light. On long standing, solutions will darken in color and should be discarded.

Sulfonamides

SULFACETAMIDE SODIUM

Rx	Sulster (Akorn)	**Solution:** 1%	In 5 and 10 mL.
Rx	**Sulfacetamide Sodium** (Various, eg, Bausch & Lomb, Fougera, Goldline, Moore, Optopics, Rugby, Steris, URL)	**Solution:** 10%	In 15 mL.
Rx	**AK-Sulf** (Akorn)		In 2, 5 and 15 mL.[1]
Rx	**Bleph-10** (Allergan)		In 2.5, 5 and 15 mL.[2]
Rx	**Ocusulf-10** (Optopics)		In 2, 5 and 15 mL.[3]
Rx	**Storz Sulf** (Lederle)		In 15 mL.
Rx	**Sulfacetamide Sodium** (Various, eg, Schein, Steris)	**Solution:** 30%	In 15 mL.
Rx	**Sodium Sulfacetamide** (Various, eg, Moore, URL)	**Ointment:** 10%	In 3.5 g
Rx	**AK-Sulf** (Akorn)		In 3.5 g.[5]
Rx	**Cetamide** (Alcon)		In 3.5 g.[7]

[1] 3.1 mg sodium thiosulfate pentahydrate, 5 mg methylcellulose, 0.5 mg methylparaben and 0.1 mg propylparaben per mL.
[2] With 1.4% polyvinyl alcohol, 0.005% benzalkonium chloride, polysorbate 80, sodium thiosulfate and EDTA.
[3] With parabens, 1.4% polyvinyl alcohol and sodium thiosulfate.
[4] With 1.5 mg sodium thiosulfate pentahydrate, 0.5 mg methylparaben and 0.1 mg propylparaben per mL.

[5] With 0.5 mg methylparaben, 0.1 mg propylparaben, 0.25 mg benzalkonium chloride and petrolatum base per g.
[6] With 0.0008% phenylmercuric acetate, white petrolatum, mineral oil, petrolatum and lanolin alcohol.
[7] With 0.05% methylparaben, 0.01% propylparaben, white petrolatum, anhydrous liquid lanolin and mineral oil.

Complete prescribing information begins in the Sulfonamides group monograph.

Indications

➤*Ocular infections:* For conjunctivitis, corneal ulcer and other superficial ocular infections due to susceptible microorganisms.

➤*Trachoma:* As an adjunct to systemic sulfonamide therapy in the treatment of trachoma.

Administration and Dosage

Usual duration of treatment is 7 to 10 days.

➤*Solutions:*

Conjunctivitis or other superficial ocular infections – Instill 1 to 2 drops into the lower conjunctival sac(s) every 1 to 4 hours initially according to severity of infection. Dosages may be tapered by increasing the time interval between doses as the condition responds.

Trachoma – 2 drops every 2 hours. Concomitant systemic sulfonamide therapy is indicated.

Storage/Stability – Protect from light. On long standing, solutions will darken in color and should be discarded.

➤*Ointments:* Apply a small amount (0.5 inch) into the lower conjunctival sac(s) 3 to 4 times daily and at bedtime. Dosages may be tapered by increasing the time interval between doses as the condition responds. Or apply 0.5 to 1 inch into the conjunctival sac(s) at night in conjunction with the use of drops during the day, or before an eye is patched.

Storage/Stability – Store away from heat.

COMBINATION ANTIBIOTIC PRODUCTS

	Product and Distributor	Polymyxin B Sulfate (units/g or mL)	Neomycin (mg/g or mL)	Bacitracin Zinc (units/g)	Other Antibiotics	How Supplied
Rx	**Neomycin and Polymyxin B Sulfates and Bacitracin Zinc Ophthalmic Ointment** (Various, eg, Bausch & Lomb, Fougera)	10,000	3.5[1]	400		White petrolatum, mineral oil. In 3.5 g.
Rx	**Neosporin Ophthalmic Ointment** (Monarch)					White petrolatum. In 3.5 g.
Rx	**Neomycin and Polymyxin B Sulfates and Gramicidin Ophthalmic Solution** (Various, eg, Bausch & Lomb, URL, Zenith Goldline)	10,000	1.75		0.025 mg/mL gramicidin	Sodium chloride, 0.5% alcohol, propylene glycol, hydrochloric acid, 0.001% thimerosal, poloxamer 188, ammonium hydroxide. In 10 mL.
Rx	**Neosporin Ophthalmic Solution** (Monarch)					Alcohol 0.5%, 0.001% thimerosal, propylene glycol, sodium chloride. In 10 mL *Drop Dose.*
Rx	**Bacitracin Zinc and Polymyxin B Sulfate Ophthalmic Ointment** (Bausch & Lomb)	10,000		500		White petrolatum, mineral oil. In 3.5 g.
Rx	**AK-Poly-Bac Ophthalmic Ointment** (Akorn)					White petrolatum, mineral oil. In 3.5 g.
Rx	**Polysporin Ophthalmic Ointment** (Monarch)					White petrolatum. In 3.5 g.
Rx	**Terramycin w/Polymyxin B Sulfate Ophthalmic Ointment** (Roerig)	10,000			5 mg/g oxytetracycline HCl	White and liquid petrolatum. In 3.5 g.
Rx	**Terak with Polymyxin B Sulfate Ophthalmic Ointment** (Akorn)					White and liquid petrolatum. In 3.5 g.
Rx	**Trimethoprim Sulfate and Polymyxin B Sulfate Ophthalmic Solution** (Various, eg, Bausch and Lomb, Falcon)	10,000			1 mg/mL trimethoprim sulfate	In 10 mL.
Rx	**Polytrim Ophthalmic Solution** (Allergan)					0.04 mg/mL benzalkonium chloride, sodium chloride, sodium hydroxide. In 5 and 10 mL.

[1] Equivalent to 5 g neomycin sulfate.

Complete prescribing information begins in the Ophthalmic Antibiotics group monograph.

STEROID ANTIBIOTIC COMBINATIONS

STEROID AND ANTIBIOTIC SOLUTIONS AND SUSPENSIONS

	Product & Distributor	Steroid	Antibiotic	Other Content	How Supplied
Rx	Cortisporin Ophthalmic Suspension (Monarch)	1% hydrocortisone	Neomycin sulfate equivalent to 0.35% neomycin base and 10,000 units/mL polymyxin B sulfate	0.001% thimerosal, cetyl alcohol, glyceryl monostearate, mineral oil, propylene glycol	In 7.5 mL *Drop Dose.*
Rx	Poly-Pred Liquifilm Ophthalmic Suspension (Allergan)	0.5% prednisolone acetate	Neomycin sulfate equivalent to 0.35% neomycin base and 10,000 units/mL polymyxin B sulfate	1.4% polyvinyl alcohol, 0.001% thimerosal, polysorbate 80, propylene glycol, sodium acetate	In 5 and 10 mL.
Rx	Pred-G Ophthalmic Suspension (Allergan)	1% prednisolone acetate	Gentamicin sulfate equivalent to 0.3% gentamicin base	0.005% benzalkonium chloride, 1.4% polyvinyl alcohol, EDTA, hydrochloric acid, hydroxypropyl methylcellulose, NaCl, polysorbate 80, sodium citrate dihydrate, sodium hydroxide	In 2, 5 and 10 mL.
Rx	NeoDecadron Ophthalmic Solution (Merck)	0.1% dexamethasone phosphate (as dexamethasone sodium phosphate)	Neomycin sulfate equivalent to 0.35% neomycin base	0.02% benzalkonium chloride, EDTA, hydrochloric acid, 0.1% sodium bisulfite, polysorbate 80, sodium borate, sodium citrate	In 5 mL *Ocumeters.*
Rx	Neo-Dexameth Ophthalmic Solution (Major)	0.1% dexamethasone phosphate	Neomycin sulfate equivalent to 0.35% neomycin base	0.01% benzalkonium chloride, EDTA, hydrochloric acid, polysorbate 80, sodium bisulfite, sodium borate, sodium citrate	In 5 mL.
Rx	TobraDex Ophthalmic Suspension (Alcon)	0.1% dexamethasone	0.3% tobramycin	0.01% benzalkonium chloride, EDTA, hydroxyethyl cellulose, NaCl, sodium hydroxide, tyloxapol	In 2.5, 5 and 10 mL *Drop-Tainers.*
Rx	Neomycin and Polymyxin B Sulfates and Dexamethasone Ophthalmic Suspension (Various, eg, Falcon)	0.1% dexamethasone	Neomycin sulfate equivalent to 0.35% neomycin base and 10,000 units/mL polymyxin B sulfate	0.004% benzalkonium chloride, 0.5% hydroxypropyl methylcellulose, hydrochloric acid, NaCl, polysorbate 20, sodium hydroxide	In 5 mL.
Rx	Maxitrol Ophthalmic Suspension (Alcon)				In 5 mL *Drop-Tainers.*

Indications

➤ *Inflammatory conditions:* For steroid-responsive inflammatory ocular conditions in which a corticosteroid is indicated and in which superficial bacterial infection or risk of infection exists.

For inflammatory conditions of the palpebral and bulbar conjunctiva, cornea and anterior segment of the globe in which the inherent risk of corticosteroid use in certain infective conjunctivitides is accepted to obtain a diminution in edema and inflammation. For chronic anterior uveitis and corneal injury from chemical, radiation or thermal burns, or penetration of foreign bodies.

The use of a combination drug with an anti-infective component is indicated when the risk of infection is high or when there is an expectation that potentially dangerous numbers of bacteria will be present in the eye.

Administration and Dosage

Store suspensions upright and shake well before using.
➤ *Dexacidin:* Taper to discontinuation as inflammation subsides.
➤ *Poly-Pred:* Reduce dose frequency as inflammation is brought under control.
➤ *Pred-G:* Do not discontinue prematurely.
Do not prescribe > 20 mL initially; do not refill without further evaluation.
For complete dosage instructions, see individual manufacturer inserts.

2198

STEROID ANTIBIOTIC COMBINATIONS

STEROID AND ANTIBIOTIC OINTMENTS

	Product & Distributor	Steroid (per g)	Antibiotic (per g)	Other Content	How Supplied
Rx	**Ophthocort** (Parke-Davis)	0.5% hydrocortisone acetate	1% chloramphenicol, 10,000 units polymyxin B (as sulfate)	Liquid petrolatum, polyethylene	Preservative free. In 3.5 g.
Rx	**Bacitracin Zinc/Neomycin Sulfate/Polymyxin B Sulfate/Hydrocortisone** (Various, eg, Fougera)	1% hydrocortisone	Neomycin sulfate equivalent to 0.35% neomycin base, 400 units bacitracin zinc, 10,000 units polymyxin B sulfate		In 3.5 g.
Rx	**Cortisporin** (Glaxo Wellcome)			White petrolatum	
Rx	**Pred-G S.O.P.** (Allergan)	0.6% prednisolone acetate	Gentamicin sulfate equivalent to 0.3% gentamicin base	0.5% chlorobutanol, white petrolatum, mineral oil, petrolatum, lanolin alcohol	In 3.5 g.
Rx	**Neomycin/Polymyxin B Sulfate/Dexamethasone** (Various, eg, Fougera, Rugby)	0.1% dexamethasone	Neomycin sulfate equivalent to 0.35% neomycin base, 10,000 units polymyxin B sulfate		In 3.5 g.
Rx	**AK-Trol** (Akorn)			White petrolatum, lanolin oil, mineral oil, parabens	In 3.5 g.

Indications

► *Inflammatory conditions:* For steroid-responsive inflammatory ocular conditions in which a corticosteroid is indicated and in which bacterial infection or risk of infection exists. For inflammatory conditions of the palpebral and bulbar conjunctiva, cornea and anterior segment of the globe in which the inherent risk of steroid use in certain infective conjunctivitis is accepted to obtain a diminution in edema and inflammation. For chronic anterior uveitis and corneal injury from chemical, radiation or thermal burns, or penetration of foreign bodies.

Administration and Dosage

Apply ointment to the affected eye(s) every 3 or 4 hours, depending on the severity of the condition.

Do not prescribe > 8 g initially, and the prescription should not be refilled until further evaluation. For complete dosage instructions, see individual manufacturer inserts.

STEROID ANTIBIOTIC COMBINATIONS

Steroid Sulfonamide Combinations

STEROID AND SULFONAMIDE COMBINATIONS, SUSPENSIONS AND SOLUTIONS

	Product & Distributor	Steroid	Sulfonamide	Other Content	How Supplied
Rx	FML-S Suspension (Allergan)	0.1% fluorometholone	10% sodium sulfacetamide	EDTA, 1.4% polyvinyl alcohol, 0.006% benzalkonium chloride, polysorbate 80, povidone, sodium thiosulfate and sodium chloride	In 5 and 10 mL.
Rx	Blephamide Suspension (Allergan)	0.2% prednisolone acetate	10% sodium sulfacetamide	EDTA, 1.4% polyvinyl alcohol, polysorbate 80, sodium thiosulfate, benzalkonium chloride	In 2.5, 5 and 10 mL.
Rx	Metimyd Suspension (Schering)	0.5% prednisolone acetate	10% sodium sulfacetamide	0.5% phenylethyl alcohol, 0.025% benzalkonium chloride, sodium thiosulfate, EDTA, tyloxapol	In 5 mL.
Rx	Sulfacetamide Sodium and Prednisolone Sodium Phosphate (Schein)	0.25% prednisolone sodium phosphate	10% sodium sulfacetamide	0.01% mg thimerosal, EDTA, boric acid	In 5 and 10 mL.
Rx	Sulster Solution (Akorn)			0.01% thimerosal, EDTA	In 5 and 10 mL.
Rx	Vasocidin Solution (Novartis)			EDTA, 0.01% thimerosal, poloxamer 407	In 5 and 10 mL.

The information for steroid preparations and sulfonamide preparations must be considered when using these products. See individual monographs.

Indications

▶*Inflammation/Infection:* For corticosteroid-responsive inflammatory ocular conditions for which a corticosteroid is indicated and where superficial bacterial ocular infection or a risk of infection exists.

Administration and Dosage

▶*Solutions/Suspensions:* Instill 1 to 3 drops into the conjunctival sac(s) every 1 to 4 hours during the day and at bedtime until a favorable response is obtained.

Do not prescribe > 20 mL initially or refill prescription without further evaluation.

For complete dosage instructions, see individual manufacturer inserts.

Storage/Stability – Protect from light. Do not freeze. Shake well before using. Do not use if solution or suspension has darkened. Clumping may occur on long standing at high temperatures.

▶*Ointments:* Apply a small amount (≈ ½ inch ribbon) into the conjunctival sac(s) 3 or 4 times daily and once at bedtime (or once or twice at night) until a favorable response is obtained.

Do not prescribe > 8 g initially, and the prescription should not be refilled without further evaluation.

For complete dosage instructions, see individual manufacturer inserts.

Storage/Stability – Keep tightly closed. Store away from heat.

STEROID AND SULFONAMIDE COMBINATIONS, OINTMENTS

	Product & Distributor	Steroid	Sulfonamide	Other Content	How Supplied
Rx	Blephamide (Allergan)	0.2% prednisolone acetate	10% sodium sulfacetamide	0.0008% phenylmercuric acetate, mineral oil, white petrolatum, lanolin alcohol	In 3.5 g.

POVIDONE IODINE

| *Rx* | **Betadine 5% Sterile Ophthalmic Prep Solution** (Alcon) | **Solution:** 5% povidone iodine | In 50 mL.[1] |

[1] Glycerin, sodium chloride, sodium hydroxide and sodium phosphate.

Indications

➤*Ophthalmic preoperative prep:* Used prior to eye surgery to prep the periocular region (lids, brow and cheek) and irrigate the ocular surface (cornea, conjunctiva and palpebral fornices).

Administration and Dosage

Transfer solution to a sterile prep cup. Apply to lashes and lid margins with sterile applicator, repeat once. Apply to lids, brow and cheek with sterile applicator, repeat 3 times. Irrigate cornea, conjunctiva and palpebral fornices with solution and leave in for 2 minutes; flush with sterile saline solution.

Actions

➤*Pharmacology:* Povidone iodine has broad-spectrum antimicrobial action.

Contraindications

Hypersensitivity to iodine.

Warnings

➤*For external use only:* Not for intraocular injection or irrigation.

➤*Pregnancy: Category C.* Safety for use during pregnancy has not been established. Use only when clearly needed.

➤*Lactation:* Because of the potential for adverse reactions in nursing infants, decide whether to discontinue nursing or discontinue the drug, taking into account the importance of the drug to the mother.

➤*Children:* Safety and efficacy have not been established.

Precautions

➤*Thyroid disorders:* Use caution in patients with thyroid disorders due to the possibility of iodine absorption.

Adverse Reactions

Local sensitivity has been exhibited by some individuals.

SILVER NITRATE

| *Rx* | **Silver Nitrate** (Lilly) | **Solution:** 1% | With acetic acid and sodium acetate. In 100s (wax ampules). |

Indications

➤*Ophthlamic neonatorum:* Prevention of gonorrheal ophthalmia neonatorum.

Administration and Dosage

Immediately after birth, clean the eyelids with steril absorbent cotton or gauze and sterile water. Use a separate pledget for each eye; wash unopened lids from the nose outward until free of blood, mucus or meconium. Next, separate the lids and instill 2 drops of 1% solutions. Elevate lids away from the eyeball so that a lake of silver nitrate may lie for ≥ 30 seconds between them, contacting the entire conjunctival sac.

The American Academy of Pediatrics has endorsed a statement from the Committee on Ophthalmia Neonatorum of the National Society for the prevention of Blindness, which does not recommend irrigation of the eyes following instillation of the silver nitrate.

➤*Storage / Stability:* Do not freeze. Do not use when cold. Protect from light.

Actions

➤*Pharmacology:* Silver nitrate ophthalmic solution is an anti-infective. In weak solutions, it is used as a germicide and astringent to mucous membranes. The germicidal action is due to precipitation of bacterial proteins by liberated silver ions.

Contraindications

Hypersensitivity to any component of the formulation.

Warnings

➤*Neonatal chlamydial conjunctivitis:* Silver nitrate has not been effective for the prevention of neonatal chlamydial conjunctivitis.

➤*Cauterization of cornea:* A 1% solution is considered optimal. Use with caution, since cauterization of the cornea and blindness may result, especially with repeated applications.

➤*Caustic / Irritant:* Silver nitrate is caustic and irritating to the skin and mucous membranes.

Precautions

➤*Staining:* Handle solutions carefully because they tend to stain skin and utensils. Stains may be removed from linen by applications of iodine tincture followed by sodium thiosulfate solution.

Drug Interactions

➤*Sulfonamide:* Sulfonamide preparations are incompatible with silver preparations.

Adverse Reactions

A mild chemical conjunctivitis should result from a properly performed Credé prophylaxis using silver nitrate. A more severe chemical conjunctivitis occurs in ≤ 20% of cases.

Overdosage

When ingested, silver nitrate is highly toxic to the GI tract and CNS. Swallowing can cause severe gastroenteritis that may be fatal. Sodium chloride may be used by gastric lavage to remove the chemical.

When a solution of ≥ 2% silver nitrate concentration is used in the eye, conjunctivits may be produced. Irrigate the eye with an isotonic solution of sodium chloride after solutions of silver nitrate stronger than 1% are instilled.

NATAMYCIN

Rx **Natacyn** (Alcon)	**Suspension:** 5%	With 0.02% benzalkonium chloride. In 15 mL.

Indications

➤*Fungal blepharitis, conjunctivitis and keratitis:* Fungal blepharitis, conjunctivitis, and keratitis caused by susceptible organisms. Natamycin is the initial drug of choice in Fusarium solani keratitis.

Administration and Dosage

➤*Fungal keratitis:* Instill 1 drop into the conjunctival sac at 1 or 2 hour intervals. The frequency of application can usually be reduced to 1 drop 6 to 8 times daily after the first 3 to 4 days. Generally, continue therapy for 14 to 21 days, or until there is resolution of active fungal keratitis. In many cases, it may help to reduce the dosage gradually at 4 to 7 day intervals to ensure that the organism has been eliminated.

➤*Fungal blepharitis and conjunctivitis:* 4 to 6 daily applications may be sufficient.

➤*Storage/Stability:* Store at room temperature 8° to 24°C (46° to 75°F) or refrigerate at 2° to 8°C (36° to 46°F). Do not freeze. Avoid exposure to light and excessive heat. Shake well before each use.

Actions

➤*Pharmacology:* Natamycin, a tetraene polyene antibiotic, is derived from Streptomyces natalensis. It possesses in vitro activity against a variety of yeast and filamentous fungi, including *Candida*, *Aspergillus*, *Cephalosporium*, *Fusarium* and *Penicillium*. The mechanism of action appears to be through binding of the molecule to the fungal cell membrane. The polyenesterol complex alters membrane permeability, depleting essential cellular constituents. Although activity against fungi is dose-related, natamycin is predominantly fungicidal. It is not effective in vitro against gram-negative or -positive bacteria.

➤*Pharmacokinetics:* Topical administration appears to produce effective concentrations within the corneal stroma, but not in intraocular fluid. Absorption from the GI tract is very poor. Systemic absorption should not occur after topical administration.

Contraindications

Hypersensitivity to any component of the formulation.

Warnings

➤*Pregnancy:* Catagory C. Safety for use during pregnancy has not been established. Use only when clearly needed and when potential benefits outweigh potential hazards to the fetus.

➤*Lactation:* It is not known if natamycin is excreted in breast milk. Use with caution in nursing women.

➤*Children:* Safety and efficacy have not been established

Precautions

For topical use only. Not for injection.

➤*Fungal endophthalmitis:* The effectiveness of topical natamycin as a single agent in fungal endophthalmitis has not been established.

➤*Resistance:* Failure of keratitis to improve following 7 to 10 days of administration suggests that the infection may be caused by a microorganism not susceptible to natamycin. Base continuation of therapy on clinical reevaluation and additional laboratory studies.

➤*Toxicity:* Adherence of the suspension to areas of epithelial ulceration or retention in the fornices occurs regularly. Should suspicion of drug toxicity occur, discontinue the drug.

➤*Diagnosis/Monitoring:* Determine initial and sustained therapy of fungal keratitis by the clinical diagnosis (laboratory diagnosis by smear and culture of corneal scrapings) and by response to the drug. Whenever possible, determine the in vitro activity of natamycin against the responsible fungus. Monitor tolerance to natamycin at least twice weekly.

Adverse Reactions

One case of conjunctival chemosis and hyperemia, thought to be allergic in nature, was reported.

Patient Information

Refer to the Topical Ophthalmics introduction.

The topical ophthalmic antiviral preparations appear to interfere with viral reproduction by altering DNA synthesis. Idoxuridine, vidarabine and trifluridine are effective treatment for herpes simplex infections of the conjunctiva and cornea. Ganciclovir is indicated for use in immuno-compromised patients with cytomegalovirus (CMV) retinitis and for prevention of CMV retinitis in transplant patients. Foscarnet is indicated for use only in AIDS patients with CMV retinitis.

Agents for Ophthalmic Conditions			
Indications	Generic name	Trade name (manufacturer)	Preparations
Cytomegalovirus (CMV) retinitis	Foscarnet sodium[1]	*Foscavir* (Astra)	Solution for Injection
	Ganciclovir sodium[1]	*Cytovene* (Syntex)	Reconstituted powder Capsules 250 mg
Herpes simplex types 1 and 2; idoxu-ridine-resistant herpes	Vidarabine	*Vira-A* (Parke-Davis)	Ointment 3%

Agents for Ophthalmic Conditions			
Indications	Generic name	Trade name (manufacturer)	Preparations
Herpes simplex types 1 and 2; idoxu-ridine hypersensi-tivity; vidarabine-resistant keratitis	Trifluridine	*Viroptic* (Burroughs Wellcome)	Solution 1%

[1] Refer to specific monograph in the Antivirals section.

Viral infection, especially epidemic keratoconjunctivitis (EKC), is more often associated with a follicular conjunctivitis, a serous conjunctival discharge and preuricular lymphadenopathy. The exceptionally conta-gious organism causing EKC is not susceptible to antiviral therapy at this time.

VIDARABINE (Adenine Arabinoside; Ara-A)

Rx   **Vira-A** (Monarch)   **Ointment:** 3% vidarabine monohydrate (equivalent to 2.8% vidarabine)   Liquid petrolatum base. In 3.5 g.

Refer to the Topical Ophthalmics introduction for more complete infor-mation.

Indications

➤*Acute keratoconjunctivitis and recurrent epithelial keratitis:* Acute keratoconjunctivitis and recurrent epithelial keratitis caused by herpes simplex virus types 1 and 2.

➤*Superficial keratitis:* Superficial keratitis caused by herpes sim-plex virus that has not responded to topical idoxuridine, or when toxic or hypersensitivity reactions to idoxuridine have occurred.

Administration and Dosage

Administer ≈ 0.5 inch of ointment into the lower conjunctival sac(s) 5 times/day at 3-hour intervals.

If there are no signs of improvement after 7 days, or if complete re-epi-thelialization has not occurred in 21 days, consider other forms of therapy. Some severe cases may require longer treatment. After re-epi-thelialization has occurred, treat for an additional 7 days at a reduced dosage (such as twice daily) to prevent recurrence.

➤*Concomitant therapy:* Topical corticosteroids have been adminis-tered concurrently with vidarabine without an increase in adverse reactions, although their advantages and disadvantages must be con-sidered (see Warnings).

Actions

➤*Pharmacology:* The antiviral mechanism of action has not been established. Vidarabine appears to interfere with the early steps of viral DNA synthesis. It is rapidly deaminated to arabinosylhypoxan-thine (Ara-Hx), the principal metabolite. Ara-Hx possesses less in vitro antiviral activity than vidarabine. In contrast to topical idoxuridine, vidarabine demonstrated less cellular toxicity in regenerating corneal epithelium of rabbits.

➤*Pharmacokinetics:*

Absorption – Systemic absorption is not expected to occur following ocular administration and swallowing lacrimal secretions. In labora-tory animals, vidarabine is rapidly deaminated in the GI tract to Ara-Hx.

Distribution – Because of its low solubility, trace amounts of both vidarabine and Ara-Hx can be detected in the aqueous humor only if there is an epithelial defect in the cornea. If the cornea is normal, only trace amounts of Ara-Hx can be recovered from the aqueous humor.

➤*Microbiology:* Vidarabine possesses antiviral activity against her-pes simplex types 1 and 2, varicella-zoster, and vaccinia viruses. Except for rhabdovirus and oncornavirus, it does not display in vitro antiviral activity against other RNA or DNA viruses, including adenovirus.

Contraindications

Hypersensitivity to vidarabine.

Warnings

➤*Efficacy in other conditions:* Vidarabine is not effective against RNA virus; adenoviral ocular infections; bacterial, fungal, or chla-mydial infections of the cornea; or nonviral trophic ulcers. Effectiveness against stromal keratitis and uveitis caused by herpes simplex virus has not been established.

➤*Corticosteroids:* Corticosteroids alone are normally contraindicated in herpes simplex virus eye infections. If vidarabine is coadministered with topical corticosteroid therapy, consider corticosteroid-induced ocu-lar side effects such as glaucoma or cataract formation and progression of bacterial or viral infection.

➤*Temporary visual haze:* A temporary visual haze may be produced with vidarabine.

➤*Carcinogenesis:* In female mice treated with IM vidarabine, there was an increase in liver tumor incidence; some male mice developed kidney neoplasia.

In rats, intestinal, testicular, and thyroid neoplasia occurred with greater frequency among the vidarabine-treated animals.

➤*Mutagenesis:* In vitro, vidarabine can be incorporated into mamma-lian DNA and can induce mutation. In vivo studies have not been con-clusive; however, vidarabine may be capable of producing mutagenic effects in male germ cells.

Vidarabine has caused chromosome breaks and gaps when added to human leukocytes in vitro. While the significance is not fully under-stood, there is a well known correlation between the ability of various agents to produce such effects and their ability to produce heritable genetic damage.

➤*Pregnancy: Category C.* A 10% ointment applied to 10% of the body surface during organogenesis induced fetal abnormalities in rabbits. The possibility of embryonic or fetal damage in pregnant women is remote. The topical ophthalmic dose is small, and the drug is relatively insoluble. Its ocular penetration is very low. However, a safe dose for a human embryo or fetus has not been established, and there are no adequate and well controlled studies in pregnant women. Therefore, use only if the potential benefit outweighs the potential risk to the fetus.

➤*Lactation:* It is not known whether vidarabine is excreted in breast milk. Excretion of vidarabine in breast milk is unlikely because the drug is rapidly deaminated in the GI tract. However, it is still recom-mended that either nursing or the drug be discontinued, taking into account the importance of the drug to the mother.

Precautions

➤*Viral resistance:* Viral resistance to vidarabine has not been observed, although this possibility exists.

Adverse Reactions

Lacrimation; foreign body sensation; conjunctival infection; burning; irritation; superficial punctate keratitis; pain; photophobia; punctal occlusion; sensitivity.

Uveitis, stromal edema, secondary glaucoma, trophic defects, corneal vascularization, and hyphema have occurred but may be disease-related.

Overdosage

The rapid deamination to Ara-Hx should preclude any difficulty. No untoward effects should result from ingestion of the entire contents of a tube. Overdosage by ocular instillation is unlikely because excess is quickly expelled from conjunctival sac. Avoid frequent administration.

Patient Information

May cause sensitivity to bright light; this may be minimized by wear-ing sunglasses.

Notify physician if improvement is not seen after 7 days, if condition or pain worsens, decrease in vision, burning or irritation of the eye occurs. Do not discontinue use without consulting a physician.

TRIFLURIDINE (Trifluorothymidine)

Rx	Trifluridine (Falcon)	Solution: 1%	In aqueous solution with NaCl, 0.001% thimerosal. In 7.5 mL.
Rx	Viroptic (Monarch)		In aqueous solution with NaCl and 0.001% thimerosal. In 7.5 mL Drop-Dose.

Refer to the Topical Ophthalmics introduction for more complete information.

Indications

➤*Keratoconjunctivitis / Keratitis:* Treatment of primary keratoconjunctivitis and recurrent epithelial keratitis caused by herpes simplex virus types 1 and 2.

➤*Epithelial keratitis:* Epithelial keratitis that has not responded clinically to topical idoxuridine, when ocular toxicity or hypersensitivity to idoxuridine has occurred, and in a small number of patients resistant to topical vidarabine.

Administration and Dosage

➤*Adults and children > 6 years:* Instill 1 drop onto the cornea of the affected eye(s) every 2 hours while awake for a maximum daily dosage of 9 drops until the corneal ulcer has completely re-epithelialized. Following re-epithelialization, treat for an additional 7 days with 1 drop every 4 hours while awake for a minimum daily dosage of 5 drops. If there are no signs of improvement after 7 days, or if complete re-epithelialization has not occurred after 14 days, consider other forms of therapy. Avoid continuous use for periods > 21 days because of potential ocular toxicity.

➤*Storage / Stability:* Store under refrigeration, 2° to 8°C (36° to 46°F).

Actions

➤*Pharmacology:* Trifluridine is a fluorinated pyrimidine nucleoside with activity against herpes simplex virus types 1 and 2 and vaccinia virus. Some strains of adenovirus are also inhibited in vitro. Trifluridine interferes with DNA synthesis in cultured mammalian cells. However, its antiviral mechanism of action is not completely known.

➤*Pharmacokinetics:*

Absorption – Intraocular penetration occurs after topical instillation. Decreased corneal integrity or stromal or uveal inflammation may enhance the penetration into the aqueous humor. Systemic absorption appears negligible.

Contraindications

Hypersensitivity reactions or chemical intolerance to trifluridine.

Warnings

➤*Efficacy in other conditions:* The clinical efficacy in the treatment of stromal keratitis and uveitis due to herpes simplex or ophthalmic infections caused by vaccinia virus and adenovirus has not been established by well controlled clinical trials. Trifluridine is not effective against bacterial, fungal, or chlamydial infections of the cornea or nonviral trophic lesions. Trifluridine has not been shown to be effective in the prophylaxis of herpes simplex virus keratoconjunctivitis and epithelial keratitis.

➤*Mutagenesis:* Trifluridine has exerted mutagenic, DNA-damaging, and cell-transforming activities in various standard in vitro test systems. Although the significance of these test results is not clear or fully understood, it is possible that mutagenic agents may cause genetic damage in humans.

➤*Pregnancy: Category C.* In animal studies, fetal toxicity consisting of delayed ossification of portions of the skeleton occurred at dose levels of 2.5 and 5 mg/kg/day. In addition, both doses produced fetal death and resorption. There are no adequate and well controlled studies in pregnant women. Use during pregnancy only if the potential benefit justifies the risk to the fetus.

➤*Lactation:* It is unlikely that trifluridine is excreted in breast milk after ophthalmic instillation because of the relatively small dosage (≤ 5 mg/day), its dilution in body fluids, and its extremely short half-life (≈ 12 minutes). However, do not prescribe for nursing mothers unless the potential benefits outweigh the potential risks.

➤*Children:* Safety and efficacy in children < 6 years of age have not been established.

Precautions

➤*Viral resistance:* Viral resistance, although documented in vitro, has not been reported following multiple exposure to trifluridine; this possibility may exist.

Adverse Reactions

The most frequent adverse reactions reported are mild, transient burning or stinging upon instillation (4.6%) and palpebral edema (2.8%). Other adverse reactions in decreasing order of reported frequency were as follows: Superficial punctate keratopathy; epithelial keratopathy; hypersensitivity reaction; stromal edema; irritation; keratitis sicca; hyperemia; increased intraocular pressure.

Overdosage

Overdosage by ocular instillation is unlikely because any excess solution is quickly expelled from the conjunctival sac. No adverse effects are likely to result from ingestion of the entire contents of a bottle. Single IV doses of 1.5 to 30 mg/kg/day in children and adults with neoplastic disease produce reversible bone marrow depression as the only potentially serious toxic effect and only after 3 to 5 courses of therapy.

Patient Information

Transient stinging may occur upon installation.

Notify physician if improvement is not seen after 7 days, if condition worsens, or if irritation occurs. Do not discontinue use without consulting a physician.

GANCICLOVIR

Rx	Vitrasert (Bausch & Lomb Surgical)	Implant: 4.5 mg	In individual unit boxes.

Indications

Treatment of CMV retinitis in patients with acquired immunodeficiency syndrome (AIDS).

Administration and Dosage

Each implant contains a minimum of 4.5 mg of ganciclovir, and is designed to release the drug over a 5 to 8 month period of time. Following depletion of ganciclovir from the insert, as evidenced by progression of retinitis, the implant may be removed and replaced.

➤*Handling and disposal:* Caution should be exercised in handling of the implant in order to avoid damage to the polymer coating on the implant, which may result in an increased rate of drug release from the implant. Thus, the implant should be handled only by the suture tab. Aseptic technique should be maintained at all times prior to and during the surgical implantation procedure. Because the insert contains ganciclovir, which shares some of the properties of anti-tumor agents (i.e., carcinogenicity and mutagenicity), consideration should be given to handling and disposal of the implant according to guidelines issued for antineoplastic drugs.

➤*Storage / Stability:* Store at room temperature, 16° to 30°C (59° to 86°F).

FOMIVIRSEN SODIUM

Rx	Vitravene (Novartis Ophthalmics)	Injection (as sodium): 6.6 mg/mL	Preservative-free. In 0.25 mL single-use vials.[1]

[1] With sodium bicarbonate, NaCl, and sodium carbonate.

Indications

➤*Cytomegalovirus (CMV) retinitis, treatment:* Local treatment of CMV retinitis in patients with acquired immunodeficiency syndrome (AIDS) who are intolerant of, or have a contraindication to, other treatments for CMV retinitis or who were insufficiently responsive to previous treatments for CMV retinitis.

Administration and Dosage

➤*Approved by the FDA:* August 26, 1998.

This product is intended for intravitreal injection only.

➤*Treatment:* The recommended induction dose is 330 mcg (0.05 mL) as a single intravi-treal injection every other week for 2 doses followed by maintenance doses of 330 mcg (0.05 mL) once every 4 weeks. For patients whose disease progresses on fomivirsen during maintenance,

an attempt at reinduction at the same dose may result in resumed disease control.

For unacceptable inflammation in the face of controlled CMV retinitis, it is worthwhile interrupting therapy until inflammation decreases and therapy can resume.

➤*Intravitreal injection instructions:* Fomivirsen sodium is administered by intravitreal injection (0.05 mL/eye) into the affected eye following application of standard topical or local anesthetics and antimicrobials using a 30-gauge needle on a low-volume (eg, tuberculin) syringe. The following steps should be used:

• Attach a 5 micron filter needle to the injection syringe for solution withdrawal (to further guard against the introduction of stopper particulate), and withdraw ≈ 0.15 mL through the filter needle.

• Remove filter needle and attach a 30-gauge needle to syringe containing fomivirsen sodium.

FOMIVIRSEN SODIUM

- Stabilize globe with cotton tip applicator and insert needle fully through an area 3.5 to 4 mm posterior to the limbus (avoiding the horizontal meridian) aiming toward the center of the globe, keeping fingers off the plunger until the needle has been completely inserted.
- Deliver the injection volume (0.05 mL) by injecting slowly. Roll cotton tip applicator over injection site as needle is withdrawn to reduce loss of eye fluid.

➤*Post-injection monitoring instructions:* Monitor light perception and optic nerve head perfusion. If not completely perfused by 7 to 10 minutes, perform anterior chamber paracentesis with a 30-gauge needle on a plungerless tuberculin syringe at the slit lamp.

➤*Storage/Stability:* Store between 2° to 25°C (35° to 77°F). Protect from excessive heat and light.

Actions

➤*Pharmacology:* Fomivirsen is a phosphorothioate oligonucleotide that inhibits human cytomegalovirus (CMV) replication through an antisense mechanism. The nucleotide sequence of fomivirsen is complementary to a sequence in mRNA transcripts of the major immediate early region 2 (IE2) of CMV. This region of mRNA encodes several proteins responsible for regulation of viral gene expression that are essential for production of infectious CMV. Binding of fomivirsen to the target mRNA results in inhibition of IE2 protein synthesis, subsequently inhibiting replication.

Cross-resistance – The antisense mechanism of action and molecular target of fomivirsen are different from that of other inhibitors of CMV replication, which function by inhibiting the viral DNA polymerase. Fomivirsen was equally potent against 21 independent clinical CMV isolates, including several that were resistant to ganciclovir, foscarnet, or cidofovir. Isolates which are resistant to fomivirsen may be sensitive to ganciclovir, foscarnet, or cidofovir.

➤*Pharmacokinetics:*
Ocular kinetics – Fomivirsen is cleared from the vitreous in rabbits over the course of 7 to 10 days by a combination of tissue distribution and metabolism, with metabolism as the primary route of elimination from the eye. Fomivirsen is metabolized by exonucleases in a process yielding shortened oligonucleotides and mononucleotide metabolites. Mononucleotide metabolites are further catabolized similar to endogenous nucleotides and are excreted as low molecular weight metabolites. Animal studies indicate a small amount is eliminated in urine (16%) or feces (3%) as low molecular weight metabolites.

Fomivirsen ocular concentrations were greatest in the retina and iris. It was detectable in retina within hours after injection, and concentrations increased over 3 to 5 days.

Systemic exposure – Systemic exposure to fomivirsen following single or repeated intravitreal injections in animals was below limits of quantitation. However, there were isolated instances when fomivirsen's metabolites were observed in liver, kidney, and plasma at a concentration near the level of detection.

Protein binding – In animal studies, analysis of vitreous samples indicate that ≈ 40% of fomivirsen is bound to proteins.

Contraindications

Hypersensitivity to any component of this preparation.

Warnings

➤*Route of administration:* Fomivirsen is for intravitreal injection (ophthalmic) use only.

➤*Systemic CMV disease:* CMV retinitis may be associated with CMV disease elsewhere in the body. Fomivirsen intravitreal injection provides localized therapy limited to the treated eye and does not provide treatment for systemic CMV disease. Monitor patients for extraocular CMV disease or disease in the contralateral eye.

➤*Previous CMV therapy:* Fomivirsen is not recommended for use in patients who have recently (2 to 4 weeks) been treated with either IV or intravitreal cidofovir because of the risk of exaggerated ocular inflammation.

➤*CMV retinitis diagnosis:* The diagnosis and evaluation of CMV retinitis is ophthalmologic and should be made by comprehensive retinal examination including indirect ophthalmoscopy. Consider other conditions in the differential diagnosis of CMV retinitis include ocular infections caused by syphilis, candidiasis, toxoplasmosis, histoplasmosis, herpes simplex virus, and varicella-zoster virus, as well as retinal scars and cotton wool spots, any of which may produce a retinal appearance similar to CMV. For this reason, it is essential that a physician familiar with a retinal presentation of these conditions establish the diagnosis of CMV retinitis.

➤*Pregnancy: Category C.* It is not known whether fomivirsen sodium can cause fetal harm when administered to a pregnant woman or can affect reproduction capacity. There are no adequate and well controlled studies in pregnant women. Use during pregnancy only if the potential benefit justifies the potential risk to the fetus.

➤*Lactation:* It is not known whether fomivirsen sodium is excreted in breast milk. Because of the potential for serious adverse reactions in nursing infants from fomivirsen, decide whether to discontinue nursing or to discontinue the drug, taking into account the importance of the drug to the mother.

➤*Children:* Safety and efficacy have not been established.

Precautions

➤*Monitoring:* Patients receiving fomivirsen should have regular ophthalmologic follow-up examinations. CMV may exist as a systemic disease in addition to CMV retinitis. Therefore, monitor patients for extraocular CMV infections (eg, pneumonitis, colitis) and retinitis in the opposite eye, if only 1 infected eye is being treated.

➤*Ocular inflammations:* Uveitis including iritis and vitritis has been reported in ≈ 25% of patients. Inflammatory reactions are more common during induction dosing. Topical corticosteroids have been useful in the management of inflammatory changes; patients may be able to continue to receive intravitreal injections of fomivirsen after the inflammation has resolved.

➤*Increased intraocular pressure (IOP):* IOP has been commonly reported and is usually a transient event; in most cases, pressure returns to the normal range without any treatment or with temporary use of topical medications. Monitor IOP at each visit and manage IOP elevations, if sustained, with medications to lower IOP.

Adverse Reactions

The most frequently observed adverse experiences have been cases of ocular inflammation (uveitis) including iritis and vitritis. Ocular inflammation has been reported to occur in ≈ 25% of patients (see Precautions).

➤*Ophthalmic:* Abnormal vision, anterior chamber inflammation, blurred vision, cataract, conjunctival hemorrhage, decreased visual acuity, desaturation of color vision, eye pain, floaters, increased intraocular pressure, photophobia, retinal detachment, retinal edema, retinal hemorrhage, retinal pigment changes, uveitis, vitritis (5% to 20%); application site reaction, conjunctival hyperemia, conjunctivitis, corneal edema, decreased peripheral vision, eye irritation, hypotony, keratic precipitates, optic neuritis, photopsia, retinal vascular disease, visual field defect, vitreous hemorrhage, vitreous opacity (2% to 5%).

➤*Systemic:* Abdominal pain, anemia, asthenia, diarrhea, fever, headache, infection, nausea, pneumonia, rash, sepsis, sinusitis, systemic CMV, vomiting (5% to 20%); abnormal liver function, abnormal thinking, allergic reactions, anorexia, back pain, bronchitis, cachexia, catheter infection, chest pain, decreased weight, dehydration, depression, dizziness, dyspnea, flu syndrome, increased cough, increased GGTP, kidney failure, lymphoma-like reaction, neuropathy, neutropenia, oral monilia, pain, pancreatitis, sweating, thrombocytopenia (2% to 5%).

Overdosage

In clinical trials, 1 patient with advanced CMV retinitis unresponsive to other antiviral treatments was accidentally dosed once bilaterally with 990 mcg per eye. Anterior chamber paracentesis was performed bilaterally and vision was retained.

Patient Information

Fomivirsen intravitreal injection is not a cure for CMV retinitis, and some immunocompromised patients may continue to experience progression of retinitis during and following treatment. Advise patients receiving fomivirsen to have regular ophthalmologic follow-up examinations. Patients may also experience other manifestations of CMV disease despite fomivirsen therapy.

Fomivirsen treats only the eye(s) in which it has been injected. CMV may exist as a systemic disease, in addition to CMV retinitis. Therefore, monitor patients for extraocular CMV infections (eg, pneumonitis, colitis) and retinitis in the opposite eye, if only 1 infected eye is being treated.

HIV-infected patients should continue antiretroviral therapy as otherwise indicated.

CYCLOSPORINE OPHTHALMIC EMULSION

| *Rx* | **Restasis** (Allergan) | **Emulsion, ophthalmic:** 0.05%[1] | Preservative-free. In 0.4 mL single-use vials. |

[1] With glycerin, castor oil, and polysorbate 80.

Indications

➤*Tear production:* To increase tear production in patients whose tear production is presumed to be suppressed because of ocular inflammation associated with keratoconjunctivitis sicca.

Administration and Dosage

➤*Approved by the FDA:* December 23, 2002.

For ophthalmic use only.

Invert the unit dose vial a few times to obtain a uniform, white, opaque emulsion before using. Instill 1 drop twice daily in each eye approximately 12 hours apart. Cyclosporine ophthalmic emulsion can be used concomitantly with artificial tears, allowing a 15-minute interval between products. Discard vial immediately after use.

➤*Storage/Stability:* Store at 15° to 25°C (59° to 77°F). Keep out of reach of children.

Actions

➤*Pharmacology:* Cyclosporine ophthalmic emulsion contains a topical immunomodulator with anti-inflammatory effects. Cyclosporine is an immunosuppressive agent when administered systemically. In patients whose tear production is presumed to be suppressed because of ocular inflammation associated with keratoconjunctivitis sicca, cyclosporine emulsion is thought to act as a partial immunomodulator. The exact mechanism of action is not known.

➤*Pharmacokinetics:* Blood cyclosporin A concentrations were measured using a specific high pressure liquid chromatography-mass spectrometry assay. Blood concentrations of cyclosporine in all the samples collected after topical administration of cyclosporine ophthalmic emulsion twice daily in humans for up to 12 months were below the quantitation limit of 0.1 ng/mL. There was no detectable drug accumulation in blood during 12 months of treatment with cyclosporine ophthalmic emulsion.

Contraindications

Active ocular infections; known or suspected hypersensitivity to any of the ingredients in the formulation.

Warnings

➤*Herpes keratitis:* Cyclosporine ophthalmic emulsion has not been studied in patients with a history of herpes keratitis.

➤*Carcinogenesis:* Systemic carcinogenicity studies were carried out in male and female mice and rats. In the 78-week oral (diet) mouse study, at doses of 1, 4, and 16 mg/kg/day, evidence of a statistically significant trend was found for lymphocytic lymphomas in females and the incidence of hepatocellular carcinomas in mid-dose males significantly exceeded the control value.

In the 24-month oral (diet) rat study conducted at 0.5, 2, and 8 mg/kg/day, pancreatic islet cell adenomas significantly exceeded the control rate in the low-dose level. The hepatocellular carcinomas and pancreatic islet cell adenomas were not dose-related. The low doses in mice and rats are approximately 1000 and 500 times greater, respectively, than the daily human dose of 1 drop (28 mcL) of cyclosporine ophthalmic emulsion twice daily into each eye of a 60 kg person (0.001 mg/kg/day), assuming that the entire dose is absorbed.

➤*Pregnancy: Category C.* Adverse effects were seen in reproduction studies in rats and rabbits only at dose levels toxic to dams. At toxic doses (rats at 30 mg/kg/day and rabbits at 100 mg/kg/day), cyclosporine oral solution was embryo- and fetotoxic as indicated by increased pre- and postnatal mortality and reduced fetal weight together with related skeletal retardations. These doses are 30,000 and 100,000 times greater, respectively, than the daily human dose of 1 drop (28 mcL) of cyclosporine ophthalmic emulsion twice daily into each eye of a 60 kg person (0.001 mg/kg/day), assuming that the entire dose is absorbed. No evidence of embryolethal toxicity was observed in rats or rabbits receiving cyclosporine at oral doses up to 17 or 30 mg/kg/day, respectively, during organogenesis. These doses in rats and rabbits are approximately 17,000 and 30,000 times greater, respectively, than the daily human dose.

Offspring of rats receiving a 45 mg/kg/day oral dose of cyclosporine from day 15 of pregnancy until day 21 postpartum, a maternally toxic level, exhibited an increase in postnatal mortality. This dose is 45,000 times greater than the daily human topical dose, 0.001 mg/kg/day, assuming that the entire dose is absorbed. No adverse events were observed at oral doses up to 15 mg/kg/day (15,000 times greater than the daily human dose).

There are no adequate and well-controlled studies in pregnant women. Administer cyclosporine ophthalmic emulsion to a pregnant woman only if clearly needed.

➤*Lactation:* Cyclosporine is known to be excreted in human milk following systemic administration, but excretion in human milk after topical treatment has not been investigated. Although blood concentrations are undetectable after topical administration of cyclosporine ophthalmic emulsion, exercise caution when it is administered to a nursing woman.

➤*Children:* Safety and efficacy have not been established in pediatric patients below 16 years of age.

Precautions

➤*Contact lenses:* Do not administer cyclosporine ophthalmic emulsion while wearing contact lenses. Patients with decreased tear production typically should not wear contact lenses. If contact lenses are worn, remove them prior to the administration of the emulsion. Lenses may be reinserted 15 minutes following administration.

Adverse Reactions

➤*Ophthalmic:* Ocular burning (17%); visual disturbance (most often blurring), conjunctival hyperemia, discharge, epiphora, eye pain, foreign body sensation, pruritus, stinging (1% to 5%).

Patient Information

The emulsion from 1 individual single-use vial is to be used immediately after opening for administration to one or both eyes; discard the remaining contents immediately after administration.

Do not allow the tip of the vial to touch the eye or any surface, as this may contaminate the emulsion.

Do not administer cyclosporine ophthalmic emulsion while wearing contact lenses. Patients with decreased tear production typically should not wear contact lenses. If contact lenses are worn, remove them prior to the administration of the emulsion. Lenses may be reinserted 15 minutes following administration.

VERTEPORFIN

Rx　**Visudyne** (QLT PhotoTherapeutics/Novartis Oph-　　**Lyophilized cake for injection:** 15 mg (reconsti-　Egg phosphatidylglycerol. In single-use vials.
　　thalmics)　　　　　　　　　　　　　　　　tuted to 2 mg/mL)

Indications

➤*Predominantly classic subfoveal choroidal neovascularization (CNV):* Treatment of predominantly classic subfoveal CNV caused by age-related macular degeneration, pathologic myopia, or presumed ocular histoplasmosis.

➤*Unlabeled uses:* Treatment of psoriasis, psoriatic arthritis, rheumatoid arthritis, nonmelanoma skin cancers, circumscribed choroidal hemangioma.

Administration and Dosage

➤*Approved by the FDA:* April 12, 2000.

Intended for IV use only.

A course of verteporfin therapy is a 2-step process requiring administration of both drug and light. The first step is the IV infusion of verteporfin. The second step is the activation of verteporfin with light from a nonthermal diode laser.

Re-evaluate patients every 3 months; if choroidal neovascular leakage is detected on fluorescein angiography, repeat therapy.

➤*Reconstitution:* Reconstitute each vial of verteporfin with 7 mL of sterile water for injection to provide 7.5 mL containing 2 mg/mL. Reconstituted verteporfin must be protected from light and used within 4 hours. Inspect visually for particulate matter and discoloration prior to administration. Reconstituted verteporfin is an opaque dark-green solution.

➤*Verteporfin administration:* The volume of reconstituted verteporfin required to achieve the desired dose of 6 mg/m^2 body surface area (BSA) is withdrawn from the vial and diluted with 5% dextrose for injection to a total infusion volume of 30 mL. The full infusion volume is administered IV over 10 minutes at a rate of 3 mL/min using an appropriate syringe pump and in-line filter. Clinical studies were conducted using a standard infusion line filter of 1.2 microns.

Take precautions to prevent extravasation at the injection site. If extravasation occurs, protect the site from light (see Precautions).

➤*Light administration:* Initiate 689 nm wavelength laser light delivery to the patient 15 minutes after the start of the 10-minute infusion with verteporfin.

Photoactivation of verteporfin is controlled by the total light dose delivered. In the treatment of CNV, the recommended light dose is 50 J/cm^2 of neovascular lesion administered at an intensity of 600 mW/cm^2. This dose is administered over 83 seconds.

Light dose, light intensity, ophthalmic lens magnification factor, and zoom-lens setting are important parameters for the appropriate delivery of light to the predetermined treatment spot. Follow the laser system manuals for procedure set up and operation.

The laser system must deliver a stable power output at a wavelength of 689 ± 3 nm. Light is delivered to the retina as a single circular spot via a fiber optic and a slit lamp, using a suitable ophthalmic magnification lens.

➤*Concurrent bilateral treatment:* The controlled trials only allowed the treatment of 1 eye per patient. In patients who present with eligible lesions in both eyes, evaluate the potential benefits and risks of treating both eyes concurrently. If the patient has already received previous verteporfin therapy in 1 eye with an acceptable safety profile, both eyes can be treated concurrently after a single administration of verteporfin. Treat the more aggressive lesion first at 15 minutes after the start of infusion. Immediately at the end of light application to the first eye, adjust the laser settings to introduce the treatment parameters for the second eye, with the same light dose and intensity as for the first eye, starting no later than 20 minutes from the start of infusion.

In patients who present for the first time with eligible lesions in both eyes without prior verteporfin therapy, it is prudent to treat only 1 eye (the most aggressive lesion) at the first course. One week after the first course, if no significant safety issues are identified, the second eye can be treated using the same treatment regimen after a second verteporfin infusion. Approximately 3 months later, both eyes can be evaluated and concurrent treatment following a new verteporfin infusion can be started if both lesions still show evidence of leakage.

➤*Safety and handling:* Wipe up spills of verteporfin with a damp cloth. Avoid skin and eye contact because of the potential for photosensitivity reactions upon exposure to light. Use of rubber gloves and eye protection is recommended. Dispose of all materials properly.

Because of the potential to induce photosensitivity reactions, it is important to avoid contact with the eyes and skin during preparation and administration of verteporfin. Any exposed person must be protected from bright light.

➤*Storage/Stability:* Store verteporfin between 20° and 25°C (68° and 77°F). Reconstituted verteporfin must be protected from light and used within 4 hours.

Actions

➤*Pharmacology:* Verteporfin is a light-activated drug used in photodynamic therapy. Therapy consists of a 2-stage process requiring administration of both verteporfin for injection and nonthermal red light.

Verteporfin is transported in the plasma primarily by lipoproteins. Once it is activated by light in the presence of oxygen, highly reactive, short-lived singlet oxygen and reactive oxygen radicals are generated. Light activation of verteporfin results in local damage to neovascular endothelium, resulting in vessel occlusion. Damaged endothelium is known to release procoagulant and vasoactive factors through the lipooxygenase (leukotriene) and cyclo-oxygenase (eicosanoids such as thromboxane) pathways, resulting in platelet aggregation, fibrin clot formation, and vasoconstriction. Verteporfin appears to preferentially accumulate in neovasculature, including choroidal neovasculature. However, animal models indicate that the drug also is present in the retina. Therefore, there may be collateral damage to retinal structures following photoactivation, including retinal pigmented epithelium and outer nuclear layer of the retina. The temporary occlusion of CNV following verteporfin therapy has been confirmed in humans by fluorescein angiography.

➤*Pharmacokinetics:* Following IV infusion, verteporfin exhibits a biexponential elimination with a half-life of approximately 5 to 6 hours. The extent of exposure and the maximal plasma concentration are proportional to the dose between 6 and 20 mg/m^2.

Verteporfin is metabolized to a small extent to its diacid metabolite by liver and plasma esterases. NADPH-dependent liver enzyme systems (including the CYP450 isozymes) do not appear to play a role in the metabolism of verteporfin. Elimination is by the fecal route with less than 0.01% of the dose recovered in urine.

Special populations –

　Hepatic function impairment: In a study of patients with mild hepatic insufficiency (defined as having 2 abnormal hepatic function tests at enrollment), AUC and C$_{max}$ were not significantly different from the control group; however, half-life was significantly increased by approximately 20%.

Contraindications

Patients with porphyria or hypersensitivity to any component of this preparation.

Warnings

➤*Photosensitivity:* Following injection with verteporfin, avoid exposure of skin or eyes to direct sunlight or bright indoor light for 5 days. In the event of extravasation during infusion, the extravasation area must be thoroughly protected from direct light until the swelling and discoloration have faded to prevent the occurrence of a local burn, which could be severe. If emergency surgery is necessary within 48 hours after treatment, protect as much of the internal tissue as possible from intense light.

➤*Ocular changes:* Do not retreat patients who experience severe decrease of vision of 4 lines or more within 1 week after treatment, at least until their vision completely recovers to pretreatment levels and the potential benefits and risks of subsequent treatment are carefully considered by the treating physician.

➤*Lasers:* Use of incompatible lasers that do not provide the required characteristics of light for the photoactivation of verteporfin could result in incomplete treatment caused by partial photoactivation of verteporfin, overtreatment caused by overactivation of verteporfin, or damage to surrounding normal tissue.

➤*Hepatic function impairment:* Carefully consider use in patients with moderate to severe hepatic impairment or biliary obstruction because there is no clinical experience with verteporfin.

➤*Mutagenesis:* Photodynamic therapy (PDT) as a class has been reported to result in DNA damage, including DNA strand breaks, alkali-labile sites, DNA degradation, and DNA-protein cross links that may result in chromosomal aberrations, sister chromatid exchanges (SCE), and mutations. In addition, other photodynamic therapeutic agents increase the incidence of SCE in Chinese hamster ovary (CHO) cells irradiated with visible light and in Chinese hamster lung fibroblasts irradiated with near-UV light, increased mutations and DNA-protein cross-linking in mouse L5178 cells, and increased DNA strand breaks in malignant human cervical carcinoma cells but not in normal cells. Verteporfin was not evaluated in these latter systems. It is not known how the potential for DNA damage with PDT agents translates into human risk.

➤*Elderly:* Approximately 90% of the patients treated with verteporfin in the clinical efficacy trials were over 65 years of age. A reduced treatment effect was seen with increasing age.

➤*Pregnancy: Category C.* There are no adequate and well-controlled studies in pregnant women. Use during pregnancy only if the benefit justifies the potential risk to the fetus.

VERTEPORFIN

Rat fetuses of dams administered verteporfin for IV injection at greater than or equal to 10 mg/kg/day during organogenesis (approximately 40-fold human exposure at 6 mg/m² based on AUC_∞ in female rats) exhibited an increase in the incidence of anophthalmia/microphthalmia. Rat fetuses of dams administered 25 mg/kg/day (approximately 125-fold human exposure at 6 mg/m² based on AUC_∞ in female rats) had an increased incidence of wavy ribs and anophthalmia/microphthalmia.

In pregnant rabbits, a decrease in body weight gain and food consumption was observed in animals that received verteporfin for IV injection at greater than or equal to 10 mg/kg/day during organogenesis. The no-observed-adverse-effect level for maternal toxicity was 3 mg/kg/day (approximately 7-fold human exposure at 6 mg/m² based on BSA). There were no teratogenic effects observed in rabbits at doses up to 10 mg/kg/day.

➤*Lactation:* It is not known whether verteporfin is excreted in breast milk. Use caution when verteporfin is administered to a nursing woman.

➤*Children:* Safety and efficacy have not been established.

Precautions

➤*Extravasation:* Standard precautions to avoid extravasation include the following:

- Establish a free-flowing IV line before starting verteporfin infusion and carefully monitor the line.
- Because of the possible fragility of vein walls of some elderly patients, use the largest arm vein possible, preferably antecubital.
- Avoid small veins in the back of the hand.

If extravasation does occur, stop the infusion immediately and apply cold compresses.

➤*Anesthetized patients:* There are no clinical data related to the use of verteporfin in anesthetized patients. At a greater than 10-fold higher dose given by bolus injection to sedated or anesthetized pigs, verteporfin caused severe hemodynamic effects, including death, probably as a result of complement activation. These effects were diminished or abolished by pretreatment with an antihistamine and they were not seen in conscious unsedated pigs. Verteporfin resulted in a concentration-dependent increase in complement activation in human blood in vitro. At 10 mcg/mL (approximately 5 times the expected plasma concentration in human patients), there was mild to moderate complement activation. At greater than or equal to 100 mcg/mL, there was significant complement activation. Signs (eg, chest pain, syncope, dyspnea, flushing) consistent with complement activation have been observed in less than 1% of patients administered verteporfin. Supervise patients during verteporfin infusion.

Drug Interactions

Based on the mechanism of action of verteporfin, many drugs used concomitantly could influence the effect of verteporfin therapy. Calcium channel blockers, polymyxin B, or radiation therapy could enhance the rate of verteporfin uptake by the vascular endothelium. Photosensitizing agents could increase the potential for skin photosensitivity reactions. Compounds that quench active oxygen species or scavenge radicals (eg, dimethyl sulfoxide, beta-carotene, ethanol, formate, mannitol) would be expected to decrease verteporfin activity. Drugs that decrease clotting, vasoconstriction, or platelet aggregation (eg, thromboxane A_2 inhibitors) also could decrease the efficacy of verteporfin therapy.

Adverse Reactions

Severe vision decrease, equivalent of 4 lines or more within 7 days after treatment has been reported in 1% to 5% of patients. Partial recovery of vision was observed in some patients. Photosensitivity reactions occurred in the form of sunburn following exposure to sunlight. The higher incidence of back pain in the verteporfin group occurred primarily during infusion.

The most frequently reported adverse events to verteporfin therapy are injection site reactions (including extravasation and rashes) and visual disturbances (including blurred vision, decreased visual acuity, and visual field defects). These events occurred in approximately 10% to 30% of patients. The following events were reported more frequently with verteporfin therapy than with placebo therapy and occurred in 1% to 10% of patients:

➤*Cardiovascular:* Atrial fibrillation; hypertension; peripheral vascular disorder; varicose veins.

➤*CNS:* Hypesthesia; sleep disorder; vertigo.

➤*GI:* Constipation; GI cancers; nausea.

➤*Hematologic/Lymphatic:* Anemia; decreased WBC count; increased WBC count.

➤*Metabolic/Nutritional:* Albuminuria; increased creatinine.

➤*Musculoskeletal:* Arthralgia; arthrosis; myasthenia.

➤*Ophthalmic:* Blepharitis; cataracts; conjunctivitis/conjunctival injection; lacrimation disorder; diplopia; dry eyes; ocular itching; severe vision loss with or without subretinal or vitreous hemorrhage.

➤*Respiratory:* Cough; pharyngitis; pneumonia.

➤*Miscellaneous:* Asthenia; back pain (primarily during infusion); eczema; elevated liver function tests; fever; flu syndrome; photosensitivity reactions; prostatic disorder; decreased hearing.

➤*Postmarketing:* The following adverse events have occurred at low incidence (less than 1%) during clinical trials or have been reported during the use of verteporfin in clinical practice where these events were reported voluntarily from a population of unknown size and frequency of occurrence cannot be determined precisely.

Ophthalmic – Retinal detachment (nonrhegmatogenous); retinal or choroidal vessel nonperfusion.

Miscellaneous – Chest pain and other musculoskeletal pain during infusion; hypersensitivity reactions (which can be severe); syncope; severe allergic reactions with dyspnea and flushing; vasovagal reactions.

Overdosage

➤*Symptoms:* Overdosage of drug or light in the treated eye may result in nonperfusion of normal retinal vessels with the possibility of a severe decrease in vision that could be permanent. An overdose of drug also will result in the prolongation of the period during which the patient remains photosensitive to bright light.

➤*Treatment:* Extend the photosensitivity precautions for a time proportional to the overdose.

Patient Information

Advise patients who receive verteporfin that they will become temporarily photosensitive after the infusion. Tell patients to wear a wrist band to remind them to avoid direct sunlight for 5 days. During that period, advise patients to avoid exposure of unprotected skin, eyes, or other body organs to direct sunlight or bright indoor light. Sources of bright light include, but are not limited to, tanning salons, bright halogen lighting, and high power lighting used in surgical operating rooms and dental offices. Prolonged exposure to light from light-emitting medical devices (eg, pulse oximeters) also should be avoided for 5 days following verteporfin administration.

Instruct patients to protect all parts of their skin and eyes by wearing protective clothing and dark sunglasses if they must go outdoors in daylight during the first 5 days after treatment. UV sunscreens are not effective in protecting against photosensitivity reactions because photoactivation of the residual drug in the skin can be caused by visible light.

Encourage patients to expose their skin to ambient indoor light and not stay in the dark, as it will help inactivate the drug in the skin through a process called photobleaching.

OCULAR LUBRICANTS

otc	**Akwa Tears** (Akorn)	**Ointment:** White petrolatum, mineral oil, lanolin	Preservative free. In 3.5 g.
otc	**Dry Eyes** (Bausch & Lomb)		Preservative free. In 3.5 g.
otc	**Artificial Tears** (Rugby)	**Ointment:** White petrolatum, anhydrous liquid lano-lin, mineral oil	In 3.5 g.
otc	**Duratears Naturale** (Alcon)		Preservative free. In 3.5 g.
otc	**HypoTears** (Novartis Ophthalmics)	**Ointment:** White petrolatum, light mineral oil	Preservative and lanolin free. In 3.5 g.
otc	**Puralube** (Fougera)		In 3.5 g.
otc	**Tears Renewed** (Akorn)		Preservative and lanolin free. In 3.5 g.
otc	**Stye** (Del Pharm)	**Ointment:** 55% white petrolatum, 32% mineral oil, boric acid, stearic acid, wheat germ oil	In 3.5 g.
otc	**Lacri-Lube NP** (Allergan)	**Ointment:** 55.5% white petrolatum, 42.5% mineral oil, 2% petrolatum/lanolin alcohol	Preservative free. In 0.7 g (UD 24s).
otc	**Lacri-Lube S.O.P.** (Allergan)	**Ointment:** 56.8% white petrolatum, 42.5% mineral oil, chlorobutanol, lanolin alcohols	In 3.5 and 7 g.
otc	**Preservative Free Moisture Eyes PM** (Bausch & Lomb)	**Ointment:** 80% white petrolatum, 20% mineral oil.	Preservative free. In 3.5 g.
otc	**Refresh PM** (Allergan)	**Ointment:** 56.8% white petrolatum, 41.5% mineral oil, lanolin alcohols, sodium chloride	Preservative free. In 3.5 g.

Refer to the Topical Ophthalmics introduction for more complete information.

Indications

➤*Ophthalmic lubrication:* Protection and lubrication of the eye.

Administration and Dosage

Pull down the lower lid of affected eye(s) and apply a small amount (0.25 inch) of ointment to the inside of the eyelid.

➤*Storage / Stability:* Store at room temperature 15° to 30°C (59° to 86°F). Store away from heat.

Actions

➤*Pharmacology:* These products serve as lubricants and emollients.

Contraindications

Hypersensitivity to any component of the products.

Patient Information

Do not touch tube tip to any surface since this may contaminate the product.

Do not use with contact lenses.

If eye pain, vision changes or continued redness or irritation occurs, or if the condition worsens or persists for > 72 hours, discontinue use and contact a physician.

TYLOXAPOL

otc	**Enuclene** (Alcon)	**Solution:** 0.25%	0.02% benzalkonium Cl. In 15 mL *Drop-Tainers.*

Indications

➤*Cleaner / Lubricant:* To lubricate, clean and wet artificial eyes to increase wearing comfort.

Administration and Dosage

Use drops just as ordinary eye drops are used. With the artificial eye in place, apply 1 or 2 drops 3 or 4 times daily. The artificial eye may be removed periodically if advised by your physician, and 2 or 3 drops applied to remove oily or mucous materials. The artificial eye is then rubbed between the fingers and rinsed with tap water. Then 1 or 2 drops may be applied to the artificial eye, either prior to or after reinsertion.

➤*Storage / Stability:* Store at 8° to 27°C (46° to 80°F).

Actions

➤*Pharmacology:* The cleaning/lubricant solution is a sterile, buffered isotonic solution formulated for artificial eye wearers. It contains the antibacterial agent benzalkonium chloride to kill most germs that are commonly found in the eye socket of artificial eye wearers. Tyloxapol, a detergent, liquifies the solid matter so that it is less irritating. Benzalkonium chloride, in addition to its germ-killing action, aids tyloxapol in wetting the artificial eye so it is completely covered.

Contraindications

Hypersensitivity to any component of the formulation.

Patient Information

If irritation persists or increases, discontinue use and consult your physician. Keep container tightly closed. Keep out of the reach of children.

To avoid contamination, do not touch dropper tip to any surface. Replace cap after using.

ARTIFICIAL TEAR SOLUTIONS

otc	**20/20 Tears** (S.S.S. Co.)	**Drops:** 1.4% PVA, NaCl, KCl, 0.05% EDTA, 0.01% benzalkonium Cl.	In 0.5 fl oz.
otc	**OptiZen** (InnoZen)	**Drops:** 0.5% polysorbate 80.	EDTA, NaCl, sodium phosphate, sorbic acid. In 10 mL.
otc	**TheraTears** (Advanced Vision Research)	**Gel:** 1% carboxymethylcellulose sodium, KCl, sodium bicarbonate, NaCl, sodium phosphate.	In UD 28s.
otc	**Akwa Tears** (Akorn)	**Solution:** 0.01% benzalkonium Cl, 1.4% polyvinyl alcohol, sodium phosphate, EDTA, NaCl	In 15 mL.
otc	**Artificial Tears** (Various, eg, Rugby, Steris, URL)	**Solution:** 0.01% benzalkonium chloride. May also contain EDTA, NaCl, polyvinyl alcohol, hydroxypropyl methylcellulose	In 15 and 30 mL.
otc	**Computer Eye Drops** (Bausch & Lomb)	**Solution:** 0.01% benzalkonium chloride, 1% glycerin, NaCl, boric acid, EDTA	In 15 mL.
otc	**AquaSite** (Novartis Ophthalmics)	**Solution:** 0.2% PEG-400, 0.1% dextran 70, polycarbophil, NaCl, EDTA, sodium hydroxide	Preservative free. In 24 × 1 single dose and 15 mL multidose.
otc	**Artificial Tears Plus** (Various)	**Solution:** 1.4% polyvinyl alcohol, 0.6% povidone, 0.5% chlorobutanol, NaCl	In 15 mL.
otc	**Bion Tears** (Alcon)	**Solution:** 0.1% dextran 70, 0.3% hydroxypropyl methylcellulose 2910, NaCl, KCl, sodium bicarbonate	Preservative free. In single-use 0.45 mL containers (28s).
otc	**Celluvisc** (Allergan)	**Solution:** 1% carboxymethylcellulose, NaCl, KCl, sodium lactate	Preservative free. In 0.3 mL (UD 30s).
otc	**Comfort Tears** (Allergan)	**Solution:** Hydroxyethylcellulose, 0.005% benzalkonium chloride, 0.02% EDTA	In 15 mL.
otc	**Dry Eyes** (Bausch & Lomb)	**Solution:** 1.4% polyvinyl alcohol, 0.01% benzalkonium chloride, sodium phosphate, EDTA, NaCl	In 15 mL.
otc	**GenTeal** (Novartis Ophthalmics)	**Drops:** 0.3% hydroxypropyl methylcellulose, boric acid, phosphone acid, sodium chloride, sodium perborate.	In 15 and 25 mL.
otc	**HypoTears** (Novartis Ophthalmics)	**Solution:** 1% polyvinyl alcohol, PEG-400, 1% dextrose, 0.01% benzalkonium Cl, EDTA	In 15 and 30 mL.
otc	**HypoTears PF** (Novartis Ophthalmics)	**Solution:** 1% polyvinyl alcohol, PEG-400, 1% dextrose, EDTA	Preservative free. In 0.6 mL (30s).
otc	**Isopto Plain** (Alcon)	**Solution:** 0.5% hydroxypropyl methylcellulose 2910, 0.01% benzalkonium chloride, NaCl, sodium phosphate, sodium citrate	In 15 mL Drop-Tainers.
otc	**Isopto Tears** (Alcon)		In 15 and 30 mL.
otc	**Just Tears** (Blairex)	**Solution:** Benzalkonium chloride, EDTA, 1.4% polyvinyl alcohol, NaCl, KCl	In 15 mL.
otc	**Liquifilm Tears** (Allergan)	**Solution:** 1.4% polyvinyl alcohol, 0.5% chlorobutanol, NaCl	In 15 and 30 mL.
otc	**Murine** (Ross)	**Solution:** 0.5% polyvinyl alcohol, 0.6% povidone, benzalkonium chloride, dextrose, EDTA, NaCl, sodium bicarbonate, sodium phosphate	In 15 and 30 mL.
otc	**Murocel** (Bausch & Lomb)	**Solution:** 1% methylcellulose, propylene glycol, NaCl, 0.046% methylparaben, 0.02% propylparaben, boric acid, sodium borate	In 15 mL.
otc	**Nu-Tears** (Optopics)	**Solution:** 1.4% polyvinyl alcohol, EDTA, sodium chloride, benzalkonium chloride, KCl	In 15 mL.
otc	**Nu-Tears** II (Optopics)	**Solution:** 1% polyvinyl alcohol, 1% PEG-400, EDTA, benzalkonium chloride	In 15 mL.
otc	**Preservative Free Moisture Eyes** (Bausch & Lomb)	**Solution:** 0.95% propylene glycol, boric acid, NaCl, KCl, sodium borate, edetate disodium	Preservative free. In 0.6 mL (UD 32s).
otc	**Puralube Tears** (Fougera)	**Solution:** 1% polyvinyl alcohol, 1% PEG 400, EDTA, benzalkonium Cl	In 15 mL.
otc	**Refresh** (Allergan)	**Solution:** 1.4% polyvinyl alcohol, 0.6% povidone, NaCl	Preservative free. In 0.3 mL (UD 30s, 50s).
otc	**Refresh Plus** (Allergan)	**Solution:** 0.5% carboxymethylcellulose sodium, KCl, NaCl	Preservative free. In 0.3 mL single-use containers (30s and 50s).
otc	**Refresh Tears** (Allergan)	**Solution:** 0.5% carboxymethylcellulose sodium	In 15 mL dropper bottles.
otc	**OcuCoat** (Storz Ophthalmics)	**Solution:** 0.1% dextran 70, 0.8% hydroxypropyl methylcellulose, sodium phosphate, KCl, NaCl, 0.01% benzalkonium chloride, dextrose	In 15 mL.
otc	**OcuCoat PF** (Storz Ophthalmics)	**Solution:** 0.1% dextran 70, 0.8% hydroxypropyl methylcellulose, sodium phosphate, KCl, NaCl, dextrose	Preservative free. In 0.5 mL single-dose containers (28s).
otc	**TearGard** (Lee)	**Solution:** 0.25% sorbic acid, 0.1% EDTA, hydroxyethylcellulose	Thimerosal free. In 15 mL.
otc	**Teargen** (Zenith Goldline)	**Solution:** 0.01% benzalkonium Cl, EDTA, NaCl, polyvinyl alcohol	In 15 mL.
otc	**Teargen II** (Zenith Goldline	**Solution:** 4 mg hydroxypropyl methylcellulose, 0.01% benzalkonium chloride, EDTA, KCl, NaCl, hydrochloric acid, sodium hydroxide.	In 15 mL.
otc	**Tearisol** (Novartis Ophthalmics)	**Solution:** 0.5% hydroxypropyl methylcellulose, 0.01% benzalkonium chloride, EDTA, boric acid, KCl	In 15 mL.
otc	**Tears Naturale** (Alcon)	**Solution:** 0.1% dextran 70, 0.01% benzalkonium chloride, 0.3% hydroxypropyl methylcellulose, NaCl, EDTA, hydrochloric acid, sodium hydroxide, KCl	In 15 and 30 mL.
otc	**Tears Naturale Free** (Alcon)	**Solution:** 0.3% hydroxypropyl methylcellulose 2910, 0.1% dextran 70, NaCl, KCl, sodium borate	Preservative free. In 0.6 mL single-use containers.
otc	**Tears Naturale** II (Alcon)	**Solution:** 0.1% dextran 70, 0.3% hydroxypropyl methylcellulose 2910, 0.001% polyquaternium-1, NaCl, KCl, sodium borate	In 15 and 30 mL Drop-Tainers.
otc	**Tears Plus** (Allergan)	**Solution:** 1.4% polyvinyl alcohol, NaCl, 0.6% povidone, 0.5% chlorobutanol	In 15 and 30 mL.
otc	**Tears Renewed** (Akorn)	**Solution:** 0.01% benzalkonium chloride, EDTA, 0.1% dextran 70, NaCl, 0.3% hydroxypropyl methylcellulose 2906	In 2, 15 and 30 mL.
otc	**Ultra Tears** (Alcon)	**Solution:** 1% hydroxypropyl methylcellulose 2910, 0.01% benzalkonium chloride, NaCl	In 15 mL.
otc	**Viva-Drops** (Vision Pharm)	**Solution:** Polysorbate 80, sodium chloride, EDTA, retinyl palmitate, mannitol, sodium citrate, pyruvate	Preservative free. In 10 and 15 mL.

ARTIFICIAL TEAR SOLUTIONS

Indications

➤*Ophthalmic lubricants:* These products offer tear-like lubrication for the relief of dry eyes and eye irritation associated with deficient tear production. Also used as ocular lubricants for artificial eyes.

Administration and Dosage

Instill 1 to 2 drops into eye(s) 3 or 4 times daily, as needed.

Actions

➤*Pharmacology:* These products contain balanced amounts of salts to maintain ocular tonicity (0.9% NaCl equivalent), buffers to adjust pH, viscosity agents to prolong eye contact time, and preservatives for sterility. See the Topical Ophthalmics introduction for a description and listing of these ingredients.

Patient Information

Do not touch the tip of the container or dropper to any surface. Close container immediately after use.

If headache, eye pain, vision changes, continued redness or irritation occurs, or if condition worsens or persists for > 3 days, discontinue use and consult a physician.

May cause mild stinging or temporary blurred vision.

Some of these products should not be used with soft contact lenses.

ARTIFICIAL TEAR INSERT

Rx	**Lacrisert** (Merck)	**Insert:** 5 mg hydroxpropyl cellulose	Preservative free. In 60s with applicator.

Indications

➤*Dry eye syndromes, moderate to severe:* Keratoconjunctivityis sicca (especially in patients who remain symptomatic after an adequate trial of artivicial tear solutions); exposure keratitis; decreased corneal sensitivity; recurrent corneal erosions.

Administration and Dosage

Once daily, inserted into inferior cul-de-sac beneath the base of the tarsus, not in apposition to the cornea nor beneath the eyelid at the level of the tarsal plate. Individual patients may require twice-daily use for optimal results.

If not properly positioned, the insert will be expelled into the interpalpebral fissure, and may cause symptoms of a foreign body.

Occasionally, the insert is inadvertently expelled from the eye, especially in patients with shallow conjunctival fornices. Caution the patient against rubbing the eyelid(s), especially upon awakening, so as not to dislodge or expel the insert. If required, another insert may be used. If transient blurred vision develops, the patient may want to remove the insert a few hours after insertion to avoid this.

Actions

➤*Pharmacology:* The hydroxypropyl cellulose insert acts to stabilize and thicken the precorneal tear film and prolong tear film breakup time, which is usually accelerated in patients with dry eye states. The insert also acts to lubricate and protect the eye.

Signs and symptoms resulting from moderate to severe dry eye syndromes, such as conjunctival hyperemia, corneal and conjunctival staining with rose bengal, exudation, itching, burning, foreign body sensation, smarting, photophobia, dryness and blurred or cloudy vision are reduced. Progressive visual deterioration may be retarded, halted or sometimes reversed.

➤*Pharmacokinetics:* Hydroxypropyl cellulose is a physiologically inert substance. Dissolution studies in rabbits showed that the inserts became softer within 1 hour after they were placed in the conjunctival sac. Most dissolved completely in 14 to 18 hours; with a single exception, all had disappeared by 24 hours after insertion. Similar dissolution of inserts was observed during prolonged use (up to 54 weeks).

➤*Clinical trials:* In a multicenter crossover study, the 5 mg insert administered into the inferior cul-de-sac once a day during the waking hours was compared to artificial tears used ≥ 4 times daily. There was a prolongation of tear film breakup time and a decrease in foreign body sensation associated with dry eye syndrome in patients during treatment with inserts as compared to artificial tears. Improvement was greater in most patients who used the inserts.

Contraindications

Hypersensitivity to hydroxypropyl cellulose.

Adverse Reactions

The following have occurred, but in most instances were mild and transient: Transient blurring of vision; ocular discomfort or irritation; matting or stickiness of eyelashes; ohotophobia; hypersensitivity; edema of the eyelids; hyperemia.

Patient Information

May produce transient blurring of vision; exercise caution while operating hazardous machinery or driving a motor vehicle.

If improperly placed in the inferior cul-de-sac, corneal abrasion may result. Patient should practice insertion and removal in physician's office until proficiency is achieved.

Illustrated instructions are included in each package.

If symptoms worsen, remove insert and notify physician.

PUNCTAL PLUGS

| Rx | **Herrick Lacrimal Plug** (Lacrimedics) | **Plug:** Silicone plug | In 0.3 and 0.5 mm sizes (packs of 2 plugs). |
| Rx | **Punctum Plug** (Eagle Vision) | | In 0.5, 0.6, 0.7 and 0.8 mm sizes (packs of 2 plugs). Contains one inserter tool. |

Indications

➤*Keratitis sicca (dry eye):* Treatment of symptoms of dry eye (eg, redness, burning, reflex tearing, itching, foreign body sensation); after eye surgery to prevent complications due to dry eye; to enhance the efficacy of ocular medications; for patients experiencing dry eye-related contact lens problems.

Administration and Dosage

Plugs must be inserted by a physician or doctor of optometry.

Actions

➤*Pharmacology:* These flexible silicone plugs partially block the puncta and horizontal canaliculus and eliminate tear loss by this route.

Contraindications

Hypersensitivity to silicone; eye infection.

Precautions

➤*Injection path:* If injecting an anesthetic agent in the region of the canaliculus, maintain approximately a 5 mm distance between the injection path and the angular vessels.

➤*Dilation:* Do not dilate punctal opening > 1.2 mm.

➤*Irritation:* If irritation caused by plug insertion persists longer than several days, reexamine the patient and consider plug removal.

Patient Information

Do not press fingers on or near the eyelid. Use a cotton-tipped swab to remove "sleep" from the corner of eyes.

Do not attempt to replace a plug that has fallen out.

Relief may not occur immediately after insertion; some discomfort and tearing may occur for a few days.

COLLAGEN IMPLANTS

| Rx | **Collagen Implant** (Lacrimedics) | **Implant:** Collagen implant | In 0.2, 0.3, 0.4, 0.5 and 0.6 mm sizes (72s). |
| Rx | **Temporary Punctal/Canalicular Collagen Implant** (Eagle Vision) | | In 0.2, 0.3, 0.4, 0.5 and 0.6 mm sizes (72s). |

Indications

➤*Dry eyes:* For the relief of dry eyes and secondary abnormalities such as conjunctivitis, corneal ulcer, pterygium, blepharitis, keratitis, red lid margins, recurrent chalazion, recurrent corneal erosion, filamentary keratitis and other noninfectious external eye diseases; to enhance the effect of ocular medications; treatment of symptoms of dry eye (eg, redness, burning, reflex tearing, itching, foreign body sensation); after eye surgery to prevent complications; for patients experiencing dry eye-related contact lens problems.

Administration and Dosage

Implants must be inserted by a physician or doctor of optometry. Placement of implants in all four canaliculi is recommended to prevent a false negative response.

Actions

➤*Pharmacology:* These absorbable implants partially block the puncta and horizontal canaliculus, eliminating tear loss by this route.

Contraindications

Tearing secondary to chronic dacryocystitis with mucopurulent discharge; allergy to bovine collagen; inflammation of eyelid; epiphoria.

Patient Information

Relief may not occur immediately after insertion.

No removal is necessary; implants dissolve within 7 to 10 days.

Reexamination is usually required within 14 days.

Successful treatment may indicate a need for permanent treatment (eg, nondissolvable silicone plugs).

SODIUM CHLORIDE, HYPERTONIC

otc	**Adsorbonac** (Alcon)	**Solution:** 2%	In 15 mL.[1]
otc	**Muro 128** (Bausch & Lomb)		In 15 mL.[2]
otc	**Adsorbonac** (Alcon)	**Solution:** 5%	In 15 mL.[1]
otc	**AK-NaCl** (Akorn)		In 15 mL.[3]
otc	**Muro 128** (Bausch & Lomb)		In 15 and 30 mL.[4]
otc	**AK-NaCl** (Akorn)	**Ointment:** 5%	Preservative free. In 3.5 g.[5]
otc	**Muro 128** (Bausch & Lomb)		In 3.5 g single and twin packs.[6]

[1] With povidone, hydroxyethylcellulose 2910, PEG-90M, poloxamer 188, 0.004% thimerosal, EDTA.
[2] With hydroxypropyl methylcellulose 2906, 0.046% methylparaben, 0.02% propylparaben, propylene glycol, boric acid.
[3] With hydroxypropyl methylcellulose, propylene glycol, 0.023% methylparaben, 0.01% propylparaben, boric acid.

[4] Boric acid, hydroxypropyl methylcellulose 2910, propylene glycol, 0.023% methylparaben, 0.01% propylparaben.
[5] With mineral oil, white petrolatum, lanolin oil.
[6] With mineral oil, white petrolatum, lanolin.

Indications
➤*Corneal edema:* Temporary relief.

Administration and Dosage
➤*Solution:* Instill 1 or 2 drops in affected eye(s) every 3 or 4 hours, or as directed.

➤*Ointment:* Pull down lower eyelid of the affected eye(s) and apply a small amount ($\approx$ ¼ inch) of ointment to the inside of the affected eye(s) every 3 or 4 hours, or as directed.

➤*Storage/Stability:* Store at 8° to 30°C (46° to 86°F). Keep tightly closed. Protect from light.

Actions
➤*Pharmacology:* A hypertonic (hyperosmolar) solution exerts an osmotic gradient greater than that present in the body tissues and fluids, so that water is drawn from the body tissues and fluids across semipermeable membranes. Applied topically to the eye, a hypertonicity agent creates an osmotic gradient which draws water out of the cornea.

Contraindications
Hypersensitivity to any component of the product.

Adverse Reactions
May cause temporary burning and irritation upon instillation.

Patient Information
To avoid contamination, do not touch tip of container to any surface. Replace cap after using.

Do not use this product except under the advice and supervision of a physician. If you experience eye pain, changes in vision, continued redness or irritation of the eye or if the condition worsens or persists, discontinue use and consult a physician.

Product may cause temporary burning and irritation when instilled into the eye.

If solution changes color or becomes cloudy, do not use.

➤*Contact lens guidelines:* Inadequate cleaning can lead to lens discoloration and lens surface buildup of protein, lipids, minerals and other environmental contaminants, which can contribute to giant papillary conjunctivitis (GPC), superficial punctate keratitis (SPK) and corneal abrasion. Irregular contact lens disinfection can cause severe ocular infection.

Contact Lens Guidelines

- Proper contact lens care will increase success and decrease complications.
- Cleaning does not disinfect lenses.
- Disinfecting does not clean lenses.
- Enzyme solutions are not a substitute for disinfection.
- Wash and rinse hands thoroughly before handling contact lenses.
- Do not insert contact lenses if eyes are red or irritated. If eyes become painful or vision worsens while wearing lenses, remove lenses and consult an eye-care practitioner immediately.
- Do not wear contact lenses while sleeping unless they have been prescribed for extended wear.
- For soft lens care, use only products designed for soft lenses.
- For rigid lens care, use only products designed for rigid lenses.
- Do not change or substitute products from a different manufacturer without consulting a doctor.
- Do not use non-sterile, home-prepared saline solutions unless recommended by your eye-care practitioner.
- Always follow label directions or doctor's recommendations.
- Do not store lenses in tap water.
- After removal, lenses must be cleaned, rinsed and disinfected before wearing again.
- Lenses that are stored > 12 hours may again require cleaning, rinsing and disinfection; consult package insert or eye care practitioner.
- Never use saliva to wet contact lenses.
- Keep lens care products out of the reach of children.
- Do not instill topical medications while contact lenses are being worn unless directed by a doctor.
- Do not get cosmetic lotions, creams or sprays in your eyes or on lenses. It is best to put on lenses before putting on makeup and remove them before removing makeup. Water-based cosmetics are less likely to damage lenses than oil-based products.
- Schedule and keep follow-up appointments with your eye-care practitioner (approximately every 6 to 12 months or as recommended).
- Contact lenses wear out with time and should be replaced regularly. Throw away disposable lenses after the recommended wearing period.
- Check with your eye-care practitioner regarding wearing lenses during sports activities.

➤*Contact lens materials:* Three types of contact lenses are manufactured: Hard, rigid gas permeable and soft.

➤*Hard contact lenses:* Hard contact lenses are made from polymethylmethacrylate (PMMA). PMMA does not transmit the oxygen needed for normal corneal integrity. Hard contact lenses have caused chronic corneal edema, corneal distortion, edematous corneal formations, spectacle blur, polymegathism and corneal abrasions. Because of these ocular complications, hard lenses are seldom the lens of choice for a new contact lens patient. Less than 1% of the contact lens population wear hard contact lenses.

➤*Rigid gas permeable lenses:* Approximately 20% of contact lens patients wear rigid gas permeable (RGP) lenses. These lenses are oxygen permeable; therefore, the RGP patient does not have the severe physiological complications of the hard lens patient. Several lens polymers with a high degree of oxygen permeability have been approved by the FDA for extended wear. RGP lenses provide the patient with good vision, durability and easy care.

➤*Soft contact lenses:* Soft contact lenses are made of hydroxyethylmethacrylate (HEMA), a plastic compound. The first soft lens was marketed in the US in 1971. Today, most soft lenses manufactured from HEMA contain 30% to 50% water.

Daily wear soft contact lenses are designed to be worn all day (12 to 14 hours), but must be removed nightly to be cleaned and disinfected. Extended wear soft lenses can be worn for ≥ 24 hours. The FDA and most eye care practitioners recommend a maximum wearing period of 7 days. The lenses must then be removed overnight for cleaning and disinfection. The major advantage of extended wear lenses is convenience. Daily wear soft lenses provide the same level of comfort and vision as extended wear soft lenses. The popularity of extended wear soft lenses has decreased due to the increased risk of infection.

➤*Disposable soft lenses:* Disposable soft lenses are designed to eliminate the complications of lens deposits by planned lens replacement. Lens deposits can interfere with vision, cause corneal irritation and contribute to ocular infection. In addition, disposable lenses offer the patient the convenience of reduced lens care.

Disposable lenses are approved for daily wear and extended wear. It is recommended that the lenses be discarded after a specified length of time; the physician will prescribe the replacement schedule for each patient. If a disposable lens is not discarded immediately after lens removal, it should be cleaned with a surfactant cleaner and stored in a disinfection solution.

➤*Contact Lens Care Products:* Products for use with contact lenses possess the same general characteristics of all ophthalmic products (eg,

sterile, isotonic, free of particulate matter). Additionally, product formulations contain various components to achieve specific goals of contact lens care.

Although all contact lenses serve similar functions in correcting visual defects, each distinct type of lens material requires a unique lens care program. In selecting appropriate lens care solutions, it is essential to correctly identify the type of lens the patient is using.

➤*Hard and rigid gas permeable lenses:* Similar lens care is used for the hard and RGP lenses. Products include *wetting/soaking/disinfecting solutions*, cleaning agents and rewetting solutions.

When a rigid contact lens is removed from the eye, it may be covered with lipids, proteins, eye makeup and other debris. After removal, immediately clean the lens with a *surfactant cleaner*. Improper cleaning can contribute to a lens surface buildup that can interfere with vision and potentially cause corneal irritation.

Soak rigid lenses overnight in a *wetting/soaking/disinfecting solution*. This solution has four major functions:
1.) To enhance the lens surface wettability
2.) To maintain the lens hydration similar to that achieved during daily contact lens wear
3.) To disinfect the lens
4.) To act as a mechanical buffer between the lens and the cornea

It is not uncommon for a rigid lens patient to experience dryness after several hours of wear. This is especially true with RGP lens patients because of the hydrophobic nature of the lens material. *Rewetting drops* can provide temporary relief by rinsing some debris off the lens surface and rewetting the eye and the lens.

Many clinicians recommend the weekly use of an enzyme (papain) cleaner with RGP lenses. This weekly cleaning process is very effective in removing protein deposits from the lens surface. A protein film on an RGP lens can decrease vision and cause giant papillary conjunctivitis.

➤*Soft contact lenses:* Soft contact lens care systems are designed to clean, disinfect and rewet the lenses. The first step is cleaning. Cleaning the lens gently in the palm of the hand with a *daily surfactant cleaner* will remove fresh lipids, oils and other debris. Clean soft lenses thoroughly with a surfactant cleaner each time a lens is removed. After cleaning the lens, thoroughly rinse with a soft lens *rinsing/storage solution*. All *rinsing/storage solutions* contain 0.9% saline. Some are available with no preservatives in unit-dose vials or aerosol containers. Other saline solutions contain preservatives to decrease microorganism growth. Discourage use of saline made with salt tablets because of risk of contamination and infection (see Precautions).

Enzymatic cleaners – Enzymatic cleaners are generally used on a weekly basis. They more effectively remove protein deposits than surfactant cleaners because they contain proteolytic enzymes (papain, pancreatin or subtilisin). Most enzymes are dissolved directly in saline, but the subtilisin enzyme tablet can be dissolved in a hydrogen peroxide disinfection solution.

Disinfection – Disinfection is the most important step in soft lens care. Disinfection is achieved by using a thermal (heat) or chemical (cold) system.

Thermal disinfection: was the first system approved for soft contact lenses. A heat unit designed for soft lenses is used for 10 min at 80°C (176°F). This procedure will kill most microorganisms that are dangerous to the eye. Recently, Acanthamoeba keratitis has become a concern to many clinicians. Heat disinfection is the most effective procedure to successfully kill Acanthamoeba; however, heat disinfection cannot be used with all soft lens material. Also, continued use of heat can shorten soft lens life.

Chemical disinfection: The original chemical soft lens disinfection systems used thimerosal with either chlorhexidine or a quaternary ammonium compound. These systems had a high incidence of sensitivity reactions. Various hydrogen peroxide care systems are currently available in the US. Most systems require two steps to achieve disinfection and hydrogen peroxide neutralization; one other system combines disinfection and neutralization in a single step. Hydrogen peroxide (3%) is very effective and can be used with all soft lens polymers. However, hydrogen peroxide care systems can be complex and expensive. Do not substitute generic peroxide solutions for solutions formulated for contact lenses. They may be contaminated with heavy metals, have different concentrations of hydrogen peroxide or use stabilizers that may discolor soft lenses.

The two newest chemical soft lens care systems introduced into the US marketplace include *Opti-Free* by Alcon and *ReNu* by Bausch & Lomb. Polyquad (polyquaternium-1) and Dymed (polyammopropylbiguamide) are the disinfection agents utilized in these care systems. Both are simple to use and may therefore increase patient compliance. These two chemical systems have become the care system of choice for the majority of soft lens patients.

Recommended Disinfection Times For Soft Lenses by Product			
System	Manufacturer	Disinfection time (minimum)	Neutralization time (minimum)
AOSEPT	Novartis Ophthalmics	6 hrs[1]	6 hrs[1]
Disinfecting Solution	Bausch & Lomb	4 hrs	none
Flex-Care	Alcon	4 hrs	none

Recommended Disinfection Times For Soft Lenses by Product			
System	Manufacturer	Disinfection time (minimum)	Neutralization time (minimum)
MiraSept System	Alcon	10 min	10 min
Opti-Free	Alcon	4 hrs	none
Opti-Soft	Alcon	4 hrs	none
ReNu Multi-Purpose	Bausch & Lomb	4 hrs	none
Soft Mate Consept	Pilkington Barnes Hind	10 min	10 min

[1] One-step method: Disinfection and neutralization occur together for a total of 6 hours.

Soft lens rewetting solutions – Soft lens rewetting solutions permit the lubrication of the soft lens while it is on the eye. Most patients find these rewetting drops minimally effective in reducing the symptoms of dryness. Maximum relief can be achieved by removing the lens, cleaning it with a daily surfactant cleaner and thoroughly rinsing it with a rinsing/storage saline solution.

➤*Precautions:*

Acanthamoeba keratitis – Soft contact lens wearers who use homemade saline solution are at risk of developing Acanthamoebakeratitis, a serious and painful corneal infection that may cause blindness or impaired vision. Homemade saline solutions (nonsterile) may be used during thermal disinfection but NOT after.

Drug interference with contact lens use – Systemic medications may affect the physiology of the cornea, lids and tear system. In addition, many drugs may discolor soft contact lenses. Pharmacists and eye-care practitioners should be aware of the interaction of systemic medications and contact lenses.

Drug Interference With Contact Lens Use		
Drug	RGP/Hard/Soft Lens	Action
Anticholinergics	RGP, hard, soft	Tear volume decreased
Antihistamines, sympathomimetics	RGP, hard, soft	Tear volume decreased, blink rate decreased
Chlorthalidone	RGP, hard, soft	Causes lid or corneal edema
Clomiphene	RGP, hard, soft	Causes lid or corneal edema
Diuretics, thiazide	RGP, hard, soft	Tear volume decreased
Dopamine	soft	Discoloration of contact lenses
Epinephrine, topical	soft	Discoloration of contact lenses
Fluorescein, topical	soft	Lens absorbs the yellow dye
Hypnotics, sedatives, muscle relaxants	RGP, hard, soft	Blink rate decreased
Iodine groups	soft	Discoloration of contact lenses

Drug Interference With Contact Lens Use		
Drug	RGP/Hard/Soft Lens	Action
Nitrofurantoin	soft	Discoloration of contact lenses
Oral contraceptives	RGP, hard, soft	Increased stickiness of mucus; corneal lid edema due to fluid retention properties of estrogens
Phenazopyridine	soft	Discoloration of contact lenses
Phenolphthalein	soft	Discoloration of contact lenses
Phenylephrine	soft	Discoloration of contact lenses
Primidone	RGP, hard, soft	Causes lid or corneal edema
Rifampin	soft	Lens absorbs drug, causing orange discoloration
Sulfasalazine	soft	Yellow staining
Tetracycline	soft	Discoloration of contact lenses
Tricyclic antidepressants	RGP, hard, soft	Tear volume decreased

Products are listed on the following pages and are grouped as follows:

Contact Lens Solutions	
Type of lens	Type of solution
Hard	Wetting Cleaning Cleaning/Soaking Wetting/Soaking Cleaning/Soaking/Wetting Rewetting
RGP	Disinfecting/Wetting/Soaking Cleaning Enzymatic Cleaners Cleaning/Disinfecting/Soaking Rewetting
Soft	Rinsing/Storage Chemical Disinfection Surfactant Cleaning Enzymatic Cleaners Rewetting

Hard (PMMA) Contact Lens Products

Refer to the general discussion of these products in the Contact Lens Products monograph.

Actions

➤*Pharmacology:* Conventional hard lenses are made of a rigid hydrophobic polymer, polymethylmethacrylate (PMMA). For optimum comfort, these lenses require care with separate wetting, cleaning and soaking solutions. Refer to the general discussion of these products in the Contact Lens Products monograph.

WETTING SOLUTIONS, HARD LENSES

otc	**Liquifilm Wetting** (Allergan)	**Solution:** 0.004% benzalkonium chloride, EDTA, hydroxypropyl methylcellulose, NaCl, KCl, polyvinyl alcohol	In 60 mL.
otc	**Sereine** (Optikem)	**Solution:** Buffered. 0.1% EDTA, 0.01% benzalkonium chloride	In 60 and 120 mL.
otc	**Wetting Solution** (Pilkington Barnes Hind)	**Solution:** Polyvinyl alcohol, 0.004% benzalkonium chloride, 0.02% EDTA	In 60 mL.

Actions

➤*Pharmacology:* Wetting solutions contain surfactants to facilitate hydration of the hydrophobic hard lens surface. These solutions include methylcellulose and derivatives, polyvinyl alcohol, povidone, some newer polymers, preservatives and buffers. These agents increase solution viscosity and act as a physical cushioning agent between lens and cornea.

WETTING/SOAKING SOLUTIONS, HARD LENSES

otc	**Sereine** (Optikem)	**Solution:** Buffered, isotonic. 0.1% EDTA, 0.01% benzalkonium chloride	In 120 mL.
otc	**Soac-Lens** (Alcon)	**Solution:** Buffered. 0.004% thimerosal, 0.1% EDTA, wetting agents	In 118 mL.
otc	**Wet-N-Soak Plus** (Allergan)	**Solution:** Buffered, isotonic. 0.003% benzalkonium chloride, polyvinyl alcohol, EDTA	In 120 and 180 mL.

Hard (PMMA) Contact Lens Products

REWETTING SOLUTIONS, HARD LENSES

otc	**20/20 Lubricating and Rewetting Solution** (S.S.S. Co.)	**Drops:** 1.4% PVA, NaCl, KCl, 0.05% EDTA, 0.01% benzalkonium Cl.	In 0.5 fl oz.
otc	**Adapettes** (Alcon)	**Solution:** Buffered, isotonic. Povidone and other water-soluble polymers, sorbic acid, EDTA	Thimerosal free. In 15 mL.
otc	**Clerz 2** (Alcon)	**Solution:** Isotonic. Hydroxyethylcellulose, poloxamer 407, NaCl, KCl, sodium borate, boric acid, sorbic acid, EDTA	Thimerosal free. In 5, 15 and 30 mL.
otc	**Lens Lubricant** (Bausch & Lomb)	**Solution:** Buffered, isotonic. 0.004% thimerosal, 0.1% EDTA, povidone, polyoxyethylene	In 15 mL.
otc	**Opti-Tears** (Alcon)	**Solution:** Isotonic. 0.1% EDTA, 0.001% polyquaternium-1, dextran, NaCl, KCl, hydroxymethylcellulose	Thimerosal and sorbic acid free. In 15 mL.
otc	**Lens Drops** (Novartis Ophthalmics)	**Solution:** Buffered, isotonic. NaCl, carbamide, poloxamer 407, 0.2% EDTA, 0.15% sorbic acid.	Thimerosal free. In 15 mL.

Actions

▶*Pharmacology:* Rewetting solutions are intended for use directly in the eye in conjunction with a contact lens. These products improve wearing time by rehydrating the lens, which may become dry and contaminated during wear, although more benefit is obtained by actually removing and rewetting the lens. The principle components of these solutions are wetting agents.

CLEANING SOLUTIONS, HARD LENSES

otc	**LC-65** (Allergan)	**Solution:** Buffered. 0.001% thimerosal, EDTA	In 15 and 60 mL.
otc	**Opti-Clean** (Alcon)	**Solution:** Buffered, isotonic. Tween 21, hydroxyethylcellulose, polymeric cleaners, 0.004% thimerosal, 0.1% EDTA	In 12 and 20 mL.
otc	**Opti-Clean II** (Alcon)	**Solution:** Buffered, isotonic. Tween 21, polymeric cleaners, 0.1% EDTA, 0.001% polyquaternium-1	Thimerosal free. In 12 and 20 mL.
otc	**Resolve/GP** (Allergan)	**Solution:** Buffered. Cocoamphocarboxyglycinate, sodium lauryl sulfate, hexylene glycol, alkyl ether sulfate, fatty acid amide surfactants	Preservative free. In 30 mL.
otc	**Sereine** (Optikem)	**Solution:** Cocoamphodiacetate and glycols, 0.1% EDTA, 0.01% benzalkonium chloride	In 60 mL.
otc	**Titan** (Pilkington Barnes Hind)	**Solution:** Buffered. Nonionic cleaning agents, 2% EDTA, 0.13% potassium sorbate	In 30 mL.

Actions

▶*Pharmacology:* Cleaning solutions contain surfactant cleaners to facilitate removal of oleaginous, proteinaceous and other types of debris from the lens surface. To adequately clean, physically rub lens in the palm of the hand or between thumb and finger with solution for about 20 seconds and rinse with water or sterile saline solution.

CLEANING AND SOAKING SOLUTIONS, HARD LENSES

otc	**Clean-N-Soak** (Allergan)	**Solution:** Buffered. Surfactant cleaning agent with 0.004% phenylmercuric nitrate	In 120 mL.

CLEANING/SOAKING/WETTING SOLUTIONS, HARD LENSES

otc	**Total** (Allergan)	**Solution:** Buffered, isotonic. Polyvinyl alcohol, benzalkonium chloride, EDTA	In 60 and 120 mL.

Rigid Gas Permeable Contact Lens Products

Refer to the general discussion of these products in Contact Lens Products monograph.

Actions

▶*Pharmacology:*

Gas permeable hard lenses – Silicone/acrylate and fluoropolymers are used in rigid gas permeable (RGP) contact lenses. Lens care regimens include the use of a surfactant cleaner, enzyme cleaner and storage in a chemical disinfecting solution. Advise patients to follow the lens care protocol provided by the lens manufacturer or the instructions of their doctor.

DISINFECTING/WETTING/SOAKING SOLUTIONS, RGP LENSES

otc	**Boston Advance Comfort Formula** (Polymer Tech)	**Solution:** Buffered, slightly hypertonic. 0.00015% polyaminopropyl biguanide, 0.05% EDTA, cationic cellulose derivative polymer (wetting agent)	In 120 mL.
otc	**Boston Conditioning Solution** (Polymer Tech)	**Solution:** Buffered, slightly hypertonic, low viscosity. 0.05% EDTA, 0.006% chlorhexidine gluconate, cationic cellulose derivative polymer as wetting agent	In 120 mL.
otc	**Flex-Care Especially for Sensitive Eyes** (Alcon)	**Solution:** Buffered, isotonic. 0.1% EDTA, 0.005% chlorhexidine gluconate, NaCl, sodium borate, boric acid	Thimerosal free. In 118, 237 and 355 mL.
otc	**Stay-Wet 3** (Sherman)	**Solution:** 0.02% sodium bisulfite, 0.1% benzyl alcohol, 0.05% sorbic acid, 0.1% EDTA, sodium and potassium chloride salts containing polyvinyl pyrrolidone, polyvinyl alcohol, hydroxyethylcellulose	Thimerosal free. In 30 mL.
otc	**Stay-Wet 4** (Sherman)	**Solution:** 0.15% benzyl alcohol, 0.1% EDTA, NaCl, KCl, polyvinyl alcohol, hydroxyethyl cellulose	Thimerosal free. In 30 mL.
otc	**Wetting and Soaking Solution** (Bausch & Lomb)	**Solution:** Buffered, hypertonic. 0.006% chlorhexidine gluconate, 0.05% EDTA, cationic cellulose derivative polymer	Thimerosal free. In 118 mL.
otc	**Wet-N-Soak Plus** (Allergan)	**Solution:** Buffered, isotonic. 0.003% benzalkonium chloride, polyvinyl alcohol, EDTA	In 120 and 180 mL.

CLEANING SOLUTIONS, RGP LENSES

otc	**Boston Advance Cleaner** (Polymer Tech)	**Solution:** Concentrated homogenous surfactant. Alkyl ether sulfate, ethoxylated alkyl phenol, tri-quaternary cocoa-based phospholipid, silica gel	In 30 mL.
otc	**Boston Cleaner** (Polymer Tech)	**Solution:** Concentrated homogenous surfactant. Alkyl ether sulfate, silica gel, titanium dioxide	In 30 mL.
otc	**Concentrated Cleaner** (Bausch & Lomb)	**Solution:** Surfactant solution with alkyl ether sulfate and silica gel	Preservative free. In 30 mL.
otc	**Gas Permeable Daily Cleaner** (Pilkington Barnes Hind)	**Solution:** 0.13% potassium sorbate, 2% EDTA, ethoxylated polyoxypropylene glycol, tris (hydroxymethyl) amino methane, hydroxyethylcellulose	Thimerosal free. In 30 mL.
otc	**LC-65** (Allergan)	**Solution:** Buffered cleaning agent. 0.001% thimerosal and EDTA	In 15 and 60 mL.
otc	**Opti-Clean** (Alcon)	**Solution:** Buffered, isotonic. 0.004% thimerosal, 0.1% EDTA, Tween 21, hydroxyethylcellulose, *Microclens* polymeric cleaners	In 12 and 20 mL.
otc	**Opti-Clean II Especially for Sensitive Eyes** (Alcon)	**Solution:** Buffered, isotonic. 0.1% EDTA, 0.001% polyquaternium-1, *Microclens* polymeric cleaners, Tween 21	Thimerosal free. In 12 and 20 mL.
otc	**Resolve/GP** (Allergan)	**Solution:** Buffered. Cocoamphocarboxyglycinate, sodium lauryl sulfate, hexylene glycol, alkyl ether sulfate, fatty acid amide surfactants	Preservative free. In 30 mL.

ENZYMATIC CLEANERS, RGP LENSES

otc	**Boston One Step Liquid Enzymatic Cleaner** (Polymer Tech)	**Solution:** Proteolytic enzyme (subtilisin).	Preservative free. Contains glycerol. In 2.4 mL.
otc	**Opti-Zyme Enzymatic Cleaner Especially for Sensitive Eyes** (Alcon)	**Tablets:** Highly purified pork pancreatin. *To make solution for soaking, dilute in preserved saline or sterile unpreserved saline solution*	Preservative free. In 8s, 24s, 36s and 56s.
otc	**ProFree/GP Weekly Enzymatic Cleaner** (Allergan)	**Tablets:** Papain, NaCl, sodium carbonate, sodium borate, EDTA	In 16s and 24s with vials.

CLEANING/DISINFECTING/SOAKING SOLUTIONS, RGP LENSES

otc	**de • STAT 3** (Sherman)	**Solution:** 0.1% benzyl alcohol, 0.5% EDTA, lauryl sulfate salt of imidazoline, octylphenoxypolyethoxyethanol	Thimerosal free. In 118 mL.
otc	**de • STAT 4** (Sherman)	**Solution:** 0.3% benzyl alcohol, 0.5% EDTA, lauryl sulfate salt of imidazoline, octylphenoxypolyethoxyethanol	Thimerosal free. In 118 mL.
otc	**Boston Simplicity Multi-Action** (Polymer Technology)	**Solution:** PEO sorbitan monolaurate, silicone glycol copolymer, cellulosic viscosifier, derivatized PEG, 0.003% chlorhexidine gluconate, 0.0005% polyaminopropyl biguanide, 0.05% EDTA	In 60, 90, and 120 mL.

REWETTING SOLUTIONS, RGP LENSES

otc	**Boston Rewetting Drops** (Polymer Tech)	**Solution:** Buffered, slightly hypertonic. 0.006% chlorhexidine gluconate, 0.05% EDTA, cationic cellulose derivative polymer as wetting agent	In 10 mL.
otc	**Boston Simplicity** (Polymer Tech)	**Solution:** Buffered, slightly hypertonic. 0.003% chlorhexidine gluconate, 0.0005% polyaminopropyl gidunanide, 0.05% EDTA, PEO sorbitan monolaurate, betaine surfactant, silicone glycol copolymer, derivatized polyethylene glycol, cellulosic viscosifier.	In 120 mL.
otc	**Wet-N-Soak** (Allergan)	**Solution:** Borate buffered, isotonic. 0.006% WSCP, hydroxyethylcellulose	In 15 mL.

Soft (Hydrogel) Contact Lens Products

Refer to the general discussion of these products in the Contact Lens Products monograph.

> ### WARNING
> Do NOT use conventional (hard) lens solutions on soft contact lenses. Use caution in product selection. Not all products are intended for use on all types of soft lenses.

Actions

➤*Pharmacology:* Soft (hydrogel) contact lenses are made of hydrophilic polymers. Hydrogel lenses must be maintained in a hydrated state in physiological saline to prevent them from becoming brittle. Hydrogel lenses will absorb many substances; therefore, use only solutions specifically formulated for hydrogel lenses. In addition, these lenses must be disinfected either by heating in saline solution or by soaking in a chemical solution. Heating a lens in solutions used for chemical disinfection only may cause the lens to become opaque.

Soft lens solutions are especially formulated to be compatible with, and to meet the particular needs of, soft contact lenses. Of particular importance to soft lens care is the need for thorough cleaning to remove deposits which coat and may discolor the lens, especially when subjected to asepticizing by heating.

RINSING/STORAGE SOLUTIONS, SOFT CONTACT LENSES

Actions

➤*Pharmacology:* Use these solutions for rinsing and storage of hydrogel lenses in conjunction with heat disinfection. Prepared saline solutions may contain chelating agents (EDTA) which prevent calcium deposits from forming. Thimerosal-free preserved saline solutions may be used by patients sensitive to thimerosal or mercury-containing compounds. Preservative-free solutions are for patients intolerant to preservatives. Salt tablets are available to make saline solution; however, these solutions are nonsterile and contain no preservatives; use only with heat disinfection methods. Because cases of *Acanthamoebakeratitis* (a serious eye infection) have occurred in patients using homemade saline solutions, the use of salt tablets for soft contact lens storage/rinsing solution is not recommended.

PRESERVED SALINE SOLUTIONS, SOFT CONTACT LENSES

otc	**Alcon Saline Especially for Sensitive Eyes** (Alcon)	**Solution:** Buffered, isotonic. NaCl, borate buffer system, sorbic acid, EDTA	Thimerosal free. In 360 mL.
otc	**BarnesHind Saline for Sensitive Eyes** (Pilkington Barnes Hind)	**Solution:** Isotonic. 0.13% potassium sorbate, 0.025% EDTA	In 360 mL (2s).
otc	**MiraSept Step 2** (Alcon)	**Solution:** Boric acid, sodium borate, NaCl, EDTA, sodium pyruvate.	In 120 mL.
otc	**Opti-Soft** (Alcon)	**Solution:** Buffered, isotonic. 0.1% EDTA, 0.001% polyquaternium-1, NaCl, borate buffer system. For lenses with ≤ 45% water content	Thimerosal free. In 355 mL.
otc	**ReNu** (Bausch & Lomb)	**Solution:** Buffered, isotonic. 0.00003% polyaminopropyl biguanide, NaCl, boric acid, EDTA	In 355 mL.
otc	**Saline** (Bausch & Lomb)	**Solution:** Buffered, isotonic. 0.001% thimerosal, boric acid, NaCl, EDTA	In 355 mL.
otc	**Sensitive Eyes** (Bausch & Lomb)	**Solution:** Buffered, isotonic. 0.1% sorbic acid, 0.025% EDTA, NaCl, boric acid, sodium borate	Thimerosal free. In 118, 237 and 355 mL.
otc	**Sensitive Eyes Plus** (Bausch & Lomb)	**Solution:** Boric acid, sodium borate, KCl, NaCl, 0.00003% polyaminopropyl biguanide, 0.025% EDTA	In 118 and 355 mL.
otc	**SoftWear** (Novartis Ophthalmics)	**Solution:** Isotonic, NaCl, boric acid, sodium borate, sodium perborate (generating up to 0.006% hydrogen peroxide stabilized with phosphonic acid)	Thimerosal free. In 120, 240 and 360 mL.
otc	**Your Choice Sterile Preserved Saline Solution** (Amcon)	**Solution:** Isotonic. 0.1% sorbic acid, boric buffer, EDTA, NaCl	In 60 and 360 mL.

PRESERVATIVE FREE SALINE SOLUTIONS, SOFT CONTACT LENSES

otc	**Blairex Sterile Saline** (Blairex)	**Solution:** Buffered, isotonic. NaCl, boric acid, sodium borate	In 90, 240 and 360 mL aerosol.
otc	**Unisol Plus** (Alcon)		In 240 and 360 mL aerosol.
otc	**Your Choice Non-Preserved Saline Solution** (Amcon)		In 360 mL.
otc	**Novartis Ophthalmic Vision Saline** (Novartis Ophthalmics)	**Solution:** Buffered, isotonic. NaCl, boric acid, sodium borate	In 240 and 360 mL aerosol.
otc	**Lens Plus Sterile Saline** (Allergan)	**Solution:** Buffered, isotonic. NaCl, boric acid, nitrogen	In 90, 240 and 360 mL aerosol.
otc	**Oxysept 2** (Allergan)	**Solution:** Buffered, isotonic. NaCl, catalytic neutralizing agent, EDTA, mono-and dibasic sodium phosphates	In 15 mL single-use containers (25s).

SALT TABLETS FOR NORMAL SALINE, SOFT CONTACT LENSES

otc	**Marlin Salt System** (Marlin)	**Tablets:** 250 mg NaCl	In 200s with 27.7 mL bottle.

Actions

➤*Pharmacology:* Reconstitute tablets in container provided with distilled, deionized or purified water; do not use mineral or tap water. These solutions are not sterile and are intended only for use in conjunction with heat disinfection regimens. Use only as a rinse prior to heat disinfection and as storage during heat disinfection. Not for use as a rinse after disinfection (eg, before lens placement in the eye). Not for use in the eye. See Precautions in the Contact Lens Products monograph.

Soft (Hydrogel) Contact Lens Products

SURFACTANT CLEANING SOLUTIONS, SOFT CONTACT LENSES

otc	**DURAcare** II (Blairex)	**Solution:** Buffered, hypertonic. 0.1% sodium bisulfite, 0.1% sorbic acid, 0.25% EDTA, salt buffers, ethylene/propylene oxide, octylphenoxypolyethoxyethanol, lauryl sulfate salt of imidazoline	Thimerosal free. In 30 mL.
otc	**LC-65** (Allergan)	**Solution:** Buffered. 0.001% thimerosal, EDTA	In 15 and 60 mL.
otc	**Novartis Ophthalmic Vision Cleaner for Sensitive Eyes** (Novartis Ophthalmics)	**Solution:** Cocoamphorcarboxyglycinate, sodium lauryl sulfate, hexylene glycol, 0.1% sorbic acid, 0.2% EDTA	In 15 mL.
otc	**Lens Plus Daily Cleaner** (Allergan)	**Solution:** Buffered. Cocoamphocarboxyglycinate, sodium lauryl sulfate, hexylene glycol, NaCl, sodium phosphate	Preservative free. In 15 and 30 mL.
otc	**MiraFlow Extra Strength** (Novartis Ophthalmics)	**Solution:** 15.7% isopropyl alcohol, poloxamer 407, amphoteric 10	Thimerosal free. In 12 and 20 mL.
otc	**Opti-Clean** (Alcon)	**Solution:** Buffered, isotonic. 0.004% thimerosal, 0.1% EDTA, Tween 21, hydroxyethyl cellulose, *Microclens* polymeric cleaners	In 12 and 20 mL.
otc	**Opti-Clean** II (Alcon)	**Solution:** Buffered, isotonic. 0.1% EDTA, 0.001% polyquaternium-1, *Microclens* polymeric cleaners, *Tween 21*	Thimerosal free. In 12 and 20 mL.
otc	**Opti-Free** (Alcon)	**Solution:** Buffered, isotonic. 0.01% EDTA, 0.001% polyquaternium-1, *Microclens* polymeric cleaners, *Tween 21*	Thimerosal free. In 12 and 20 mL.
otc	**Pliagel** (Alcon)	**Solution:** 0.25% sorbic acid, 0.5% EDTA, NaCl, KCl, poloxamer 407	In 25 mL.
otc	**Sensitive Eyes Daily Cleaner** (Bausch & Lomb)	**Solution:** Buffered, isotonic. 0.25% sorbic acid, 0.5% EDTA, NaCl, hydroxypropyl methylcellulose, poloxamine, sodium borate	In 20 mL.
otc	**Sensitive Eyes Saline/ Cleaning** (Bausch & Lomb)	**Solution:** Buffered, isotonic. 0.15% sorbic acid, 0.1% EDTA, boric acid, poloxamine, sodium borate, NaCl	In 237 mL.

> **Indications**

Cleaning solutions are used for daily prophylactic cleaning to prevent the accumulation of proteinaceous (mucus) deposits and to remove other debris.

ENZYMATIC CLEANERS, SOFT CONTACT LENSES

otc	**Allergan Enzymatic** (Allergan)	**Tablets:** Papain, NaCl, sodium carbonate, sodium borate, EDTA. *To make solution for soaking, dilute in sterile saline.*	In 12s, 24s, 36s and 48s.
otc	**Enzymatic Cleaner for Extended Wear** (Alcon)	**Tablets:** Highly purified pork pancreatin. *To make solution for soaking, dilute in preserved saline or sterile unpreserved saline.*	In 12s.
otc	**Opti-zyme Enzymatic Cleaner Especially for Sensitive Eyes** (Alcon)		Preservative free. In 8s, 24s, 36s and 56s.
otc	**Vision Care Enzymatic Cleaner** (Alcon)		In 24s.
otc	**Opti-Free** (Alcon)	**Tablets:** Highly purified pork pancreatin. *To make solution for soaking, dilute in Opti-Free disinfecting solution.*	In 6s, 12s and 18s.
otc	**ReNu Effervescent Enzymatic Cleaner** (Bausch & Lomb)	**Tablets:** Subtilisin, polyethylene glycol, sodium carbonate, NaCl, tartaric acid. *To make solution for soaking, dilute in preserved saline or sterile unpreserved saline solution.*	In 10s, 20s and 30s.
otc	**ReNu Thermal Enzymatic Cleaner** (Bausch & Lomb)	**Tablets:** Subtilisin, sodium carbonate, NaCl, boric acid. *To make solution for heat disinfection directly in lens carrying case.*	In 16s.
otc	**Ultrazyme Enzymatic Cleaner** (Allergan)	**Tablets:** Effervescing, buffering and tableting agents. Subtilisin A. *To make solution for soaking, dilute in 3% hydrogen peroxide disinfecting solution.*	In 5s, 10s, 15s and 20s.
otc	**Complete Weekly Enzymatic Cleaner** (Allergan)	**Tablets:** Effervescing, buffering and tableting agents. Subtilisin A. *To make solution for soaking, dilute in sterile saline.*	In 8s.

> **Actions**

▶*Pharmacology:* Enzymatic cleaning, by soaking in a solution prepared from enzyme tablets, is recommended once weekly to remove protein and other lens deposits.

REWETTING SOLUTIONS, SOFT CONTACT LENSES

otc	**20/20 Lubricating and Rewetting Solution** (S.S.S. Co.)	**Drops:** 1.4% PVA, NaCl, KCl, 0.05% EDTA, 0.01% benzalkonium Cl.	In 0.5 fl oz.
otc	**Clerz Plus** (Alcon)	**Drops:** Buffered, isotonic, citrate buffer, NaCl, 0.05% EDTA, 0.001% polyquaternium-1, PEG-11	In 5, 8, and 10 mL.
otc	**Blairex Lens Lubricant** (Blairex)	**Solution:** Isotonic. 0.25% sorbic acid, 0.1% EDTA, borate buffer, NaCl, hydroxypropyl methylcellulose, glycerin	Thimerosal free. In 15 mL.
otc	**Clerz 2** (Alcon)	**Solution:** Isotonic. NaCl, KCl, hydroxyethylcellulose, poloxamer 407, sodium borate, boric acid, sorbic acid, EDTA	Thimerosal free. In 5 (2s), 15 and 30 mL.
otc	**Lens Lubricant** (Bausch & Lomb)	**Solution:** Buffered, isotonic. 0.004% thimerosal, 0.1% EDTA, povidone, polyoxyethylene	In 15 mL.
otc	**Lens Plus Rewetting Drops** (Allergan)	**Solution:** Buffered, isotonic. NaCl, boric acid	Preservative free. In 0.35 mL (30s).
otc	**Opti-Tears** (Alcon)	**Solution:** Isotonic. 0.1% EDTA, 0.001% polyquaternium-1, dextran, NaCl, KCl, hydroxypropyl methylcellulose	Thimerosal free. In 15 mL.
otc	**Opti-Free** (Alcon)	**Solution:** Isotonic. Citrate buffer, NaCl, 0.05% EDTA, 0.001% polyquaternium-1	In 10 and 20 mL.
otc	**Opti-One** (Alcon)		In 10 mL.
otc	**Sensitive Eyes Drops** (Bausch & Lomb)	**Solution:** Buffered. 0.1% sorbic acid, 0.025% EDTA, NaCl, boric acid, sodium borate	In 30 mL.

Soft (Hydrogel) Contact Lens Products

REWETTING SOLUTIONS, SOFT CONTACT LENSES

otc	**Lens Drops** (Novartis Ophthalmics)	**Solution:** Buffered, isotonic. NaCl, borate buffer, poloxamer 407, 0.2% EDTA, 0.15% sorbic acid, carbamide	In 15 mL.
otc	**Complete** (Allergan)	**Solution:** Buffered, isotonic. NaCl, 0.0001% polyhexamethylene biguanide, tromethamine, tyloxapol, EDTA	In 15 mL.

Actions

➤*Pharmacology:* May be used directly in the eye to rehydrate and improve comfort of hydrogel lenses.

CHEMICAL DISINFECTION SYSTEMS

Actions

➤*Pharmacology:* Chemical disinfection is an alternative to heat. Two-solution systems use separate disinfecting and rinsing solutions. One-solution systems use the same solution for rinsing and storage.

Warnings

➤*Heat disinfection:* Lenses must NOT be disinfected by heating when using these solutions.

HYDROGEN PEROXIDE-CONTAINING SYSTEMS, SOFT LENSES

otc	**MiraSept** (Alcon)	**Disinfecting Solution:** 3% hydrogen peroxide, sodium stannate, sodium nitrate	In 120 mL.
		Rinse and Neutralizer: Isotonic. Boric acid, sodium borate, NaCl, sodium pyruvate, EDTA	In 120 mL (2s).
otc	**Oxysept** (Allergan)	**Disinfecting Solution:** 3% hydrogen peroxide, sodium stannate, sodium nitrate, phosphate buffer	In 240 and 360 mL.
		Neutralizer Tablets: Catalase, buffering agents	In 12s (with *Oxy-Tab* cup) and 36s.
otc	**Ultra-Care** (Allergan)	**Disinfecting Solution:** 3% hydrogen peroxide, sodium stannate, sodium nitrate, phosphate buffer	In 120 and 360 mL.
		Neutralizer Tablets: Catalase, hydroxypropyl methylcellulose, buffering agents	In 12s and 36s with cup.
otc	**Quick CARE** (Novartis Ophthalmics)	**Disinfecting Solution:** Isopropanol, NaCl, polyoxypropylenepolyoxy ethylene block copolymer, disodium lauroamphodiacetate	In 15 mL.
		Rinse and Neutralizer: Isotonic. Sodium borate, boric acid, sodium perborate (generating up to 0.006% hydrogen peroxide), phosphonic acid	In 360 mL.
otc	**AOSEPT** (Novartis Ophthalmics)	**Disinfecting Solution:** 3% hydrogen peroxide, 0.85% NaCl, phosphonic acid, phosphate buffers	In 120, 240 and 360 mL.
		AODISC Neutralizer: Platinum-coated tablet	Tablet good for 100 uses or 3 months of daily use.[1]

[1] For use only with the AOSEPT system.

NON-HYDROGEN PEROXIDE-CONTAINING SYSTEMS, SOFT LENSES

otc	**Disinfecting Solution** (Bausch & Lomb)	**Solution:** Buffered, isotonic. 0.005% chlorhexidine, 0.1% EDTA, 0.001% thimerosal, NaCl, sodium borate, boric acid	In 355 mL.
otc	**Flex-Care Especially for Sensitive Eyes** (Alcon)	**Solution:** Buffered, isotonic. 0.1% EDTA, 0.005% chlorhexidine gluconate, NaCl, sodium borate, boric acid	In 360 mL.
otc	**Opti-Free** (Alcon)	**Solution:** Isotonic. 0.05% EDTA, 0.001% polyquaternium-1, citrate buffer, NaCl	Thimerosal free. In 118, 237 and 355 mL.
otc	**Opti-One Multi-Purpose** (Alcon)	**Solution:** Buffered, isotonic. 0.05% EDTA, 0.001% polyquaternium-1, sodium chloride, NaCl	In 118, 237, 355 and 473mL.
otc	**Complete All-In-One Solution** (Allergan)	**Solution:** Buffered, isotonic. NaCl, 0.0001% polyhexamethylene biguanide, EDTA	In 60, 120 and 360 mL.
otc	**ReNu Multi-Purpose** (Bausch & Lomb)	**Solution:** Isotonic. 0.00005% polyaminopropyl biguanide, 0.01% EDTA, NaCl, sodium borate, boric acid, poloxamine	In 118, 237 and 355 mL.

Refer to the Topical Ophthalmic Drugs introduction for more complete information.

Indications

Corneal anesthesia of short duration (eg, tonometry, gonioscopy, removal of corneal foreign bodies and sutures); short corneal and conjunctival procedures; cataract surgery; conjunctival and corneal scraping for diagnostic purposes; paracentesis of the anterior chamber.

Ophthalmic Uses of Local Anesthetics	
Route	Use
Injectable	Facial nerve block
	Retrobulbar anesthesia
	Eyelid infiltration
Topical	Gonioscopy
	Tonometry
	Fundus contact lens biomicroscopy
	Evaluation of corneal abrasions
	Forced duction testing
	Schirmer tear testing
	Electroretinography
	Lacrimal dilation and irrigation
	Contact lens fitting
	Superficial foreign body removal
	Minor surgery of conjunctiva
	Suture removal
	Corneal epithelial debridement

Actions

➤*Pharmacology:* Local anesthetics stabilize the neuronal membrane so the neuron is less permeable to ions. This prevents the initiation and transmission of nerve impulses, thereby producing the local anesthetic action.

Studies indicate that local anesthetics influence permeability of the nerve cell membrane by limiting sodium ion permeability by closing the pores through which the ions migrate in the lipid layer of the nerve cell membrane. This limitation prevents the fundamental change necessary for the generation of the action potential.

➤*Pharmacokinetics:* Tetracaine and proparacaine are approximately equally potent. They have a rapid onset of anesthesia beginning within 13 to 30 seconds following instillation; the duration of action is 15 to 20 minutes.

Contraindications

Hypersensitivity to similar drugs (ester-type local anesthetics), para-aminobenzoic acid or its derivatives or to any other ingredient in these preparations; prolonged use, especially for self-medication (not recommended).

Warnings

➤*For topical ophthalmic use only.:* Prolonged use may diminish duration of anesthesia, retard wound healing and cause corneal epithelial erosions(see Adverse Reactions).

➤*Systemic toxicity:* Systemic toxicity is rare with topical ophthalmic application of local anesthetics. It usually occurs as CNS stimulation followed by CNS and cardiovascular depression.

➤*Protection of the eye:* Protection of the eye from irritating chemicals, foreign bodies and rubbing during the period of anesthesia is very important. Thoroughly rinse tonometers soaked in sterilizing or detergent solutions with sterile distilled water before use. Advise the patient to avoid touching the eye until anesthesia has worn off. Because the "blink" reflex is temporarily eliminated, it is advised that the eye be covered with a patch following instillation.

➤*Pregnancy: Category C.* Safety for use during pregnancy has not been established. Use only when clearly needed and when potential benefits outweigh potential hazards to the fetus.

➤*Lactation:* Safety for use during lactation has not been established. Use only when clearly needed and when potential benefits outweigh potential hazards to the infant.

➤*Children:* Safety and efficacy for use in children have not been established.

Precautions

➤*Tolerance:* varies with the status of the patient; give debilitated, elderly or acutely ill patients doses commensurate with their weight, age and physical status.

➤*Reduced plasma esterase:* Use caution in patients with abnormal or reduced levels of plasma esterases.

➤*Special risk patients:* Use cautiously and sparingly in patients with known allergies, cardiac disease or hyperthyroidism.

Adverse Reactions

Prolonged ophthalmic use of topical anesthetics has been associated with corneal epithelial erosions, retardation or prevention of healing of corneal erosions and reports of severe keratitis and permanent corneal opacification with accompanying visual loss and scarring or corneal perforation. Inadvertent damage may be done to the anesthetized cornea and conjunctiva by rubbing an eye to which topical anesthetics have been applied.

➤*Tetracaine:* Transient stinging, burning and conjunctival redness may occur. A rare, severe, immediate type allergic corneal reaction has been reported characterized by acute diffuse epithelial keratitis with filament formation and sloughing of large areas of necrotic epithelium, diffuse stromal edema, descemetitis and iritis.

Rarely, local reactions including lacrimation, photophobia and chemosis have occurred.

➤*Proparacaine:* Local or systemic sensitivity occurs occasionally. At recommended concentration and dosage, proparacaine usually produces little or no initial irritation, stinging, burning, conjunctival redness, lacrimation or increased winking. However, some local irritation and stinging may occur several hours after instillation.

Rarely, a severe, immediate-type, hyperallergic corneal reaction may occur, which includes acute, intense and diffuse epithelial keratitis, a gray, ground-glass appearance, sloughing of large areas of necrotic epithelium, corneal filaments and, sometimes, iritis with descemetitis. Pupillary dilation or cycloplegic effects have been observed rarely.

Allergic contact dermatitis with drying and fissuring of the fingertips and softening and erosion of the corneal epithelium and conjunctival congestion and hemorrhage have been reported.

Patient Information

Avoid touching or rubbing the eye until the anesthesia has worn off because inadvertent damage may be done to the anesthetized cornea and conjunctiva.

To avoid contamination, do not touch dropper tip to any surface. Replace cap after using.

Do not use if discolored, cloudy or if it contains a precipitate. Protect from light.

Refer to the Topical Ophthalmics introduction for more complete information.

TETRACAINE

Rx	**Tetracaine HCl** (Various, eg, Alcon, Iolab, Optopics, Schein)	**Solution:** 0.5%	In 1, 2 and 15 mL.

[1] With 0.4% chlorobutanol and 0.75% sodium chloride.

Complete prescribing information begins in the Local Anesthetics, Topical group monograph.

Administration and Dosage

➤*Solution:* Instill 1 or 2 drops. Not for prolonged use.

➤*Storage/Stability:* Store at 8° to 27°C (46° to 80°F). Protect from light.

PROPARACAINE HCl

Rx	**Proparacaine HCl** (Various, eg, Moore, Raway, Rugby)	**Solution:** 0.5%	In 2, 15 mL and UD 1 mL.
Rx	**Alcaine** (Alcon)		In 15 mL *Drop-Tainers.*[1, 2]
Rx	**Ophthaine** (Apothecon)		In 15 mL.[3, 4]
Rx	**Ophthetic** (Allergan)		In 15 mL.[4, 5]

[1] With glycerin and 0.01% benzalkonium Cl.
[2] Refrigerate after opening.
[3] With glycerin, 0.2% chlorobutanol and benzalkonium Cl.

[4] Refrigerate.
[5] With 0.01% benzalkonium Cl, glycerin and sodium Cl.

Complete prescribing information begins in the Local Anesthetics, Topical group monograph.

Administration and Dosage

➤*Deep anesthesia as in cataract extraction:* 1 drop every 5 to 10 minutes for 5 to 7 doses.

➤*Removal of sutures:* Instill 1 or 2 drops 2 or 3 minutes before removal of sutures.

➤*Removal of foreign bodies:* Instill 1 or 2 drops prior to operating.

➤*Tonometry:* Instill 1 or 2 drops immediately before measurement.

➤*Storage/Stability:* Store at 8° to 24°C (46° to 75°F). Protect from light.

MISCELLANEOUS LOCAL ANESTHETIC COMBINATIONS

Rx	**Fluoracaine** (Akorn)	**Solution:** 0.5% proparacaine HCl and 0.25% fluorescein sodium	In 5 mL.[1, 2]
Rx	**Fluorescein Sodium with Proparacaine HCl** (Pasadena)		In 5 mL with dropper.[3]
Rx	**Fluress** (Pilkington Barnes Hind)	**Solution:** 0.4% benoxinate HCl and 0.25% fluorescein sodium	In 5 mL with dropper.[4]
Rx	**Flurate** (Bausch & Lomb)		In 5 mL with dropper.[5]

[1] Refrigerate.
[2] With glycerin, povidone, polysorbate 80 and 0.01% thimerosal.
[3] With povidone, glycerin, EDTA and 0.01% thimerosal.

[4] With povidone, boric acid and 1% chlorobutanol.
[5] 1% chlorobutnol, povidone.

Complete prescribing information begins in the Local Anesthetics, Topical group monograph.

Indications

For procedures in which a topical ophthalmic anesthetic agent in conjunction with a disclosing agent is indicated: Corneal anesthesia of short duration (eg, tonometry, gonioscopy, removal of corneal foreign bodies); short corneal and conjunctival procedures.

Administration and Dosage

➤*Removal of foreign bodies or sutures; tonometry:* 1 to 2 drops (in single instillations) in each eye before operating.

➤*Deep ophthalmic anesthesia:*

Proparacaine/fluorescein – Instill 1 drop in each eye every 5 to 10 minutes for 5 to 7 doses. Use of an eye patch is recommended.

Benoxinate/fluorescein – Instill 2 drops into each eye at 90 second intervals for 3 instillations.

➤*Storage/Stability:* Protect from light.

In addition to the following products, the ophthalmic vasoconstrictors, cycloplegic mydriatics and topical local anesthetics are used in diagnostic procedures (see individual monographs).

➤*Vasoconstrictors/Mydriatics:* With α-sympathomimetic activity cause dilation of the pupil and are used to facilitate ophthalmoscopic examination and other diagnostic procedures.

➤*Cycloplegic Mydriatics:* Cycloplegic Mydriatics (anticholinergics) cause both dilation of the pupil and paralysis of accommodation. These agents are used to facilitate refraction.

➤*Local Anesthetics:* Used to facilitate gonioscopy, tonometry and other procedures.

FLUORESCEIN SODIUM

Rx	AK-Fluor (Akorn)	Injection: 10%	In 5 mL amps and vials.
Rx	Fluorescite (Alcon)		In 5 mL amps with syringes.
Rx	AK-Fluor (Akorn)	Injection: 25%	In 2 mL amps and vials.
Rx	Fluorescite (Alcon)		In 2 mL amps.
Rx	Fluorescein Sodium (Various, eg, Alcon)	Solution: 2%	In 1, 2 and 15 mL.
otc	Ful-Glo (Sola/Barnes-Hind)	Strips: 0.6 mg	In 300s.
otc	Fluorets (Akorn)	Strips: 1 mg	In 100s.

Indications

➤*Topical:* In fitting contact lenses; in applanation tonometry; diagnosis and detection of corneal stippling, abrasions, ulcerations, herpetic lesions, foreign bodies (not epithelialized), contact lens pressure points; making lacrimal drainage test; wound leakage tests (Seidel Test).

➤*Injection:* Diagnostic aid in ophthalmic angiography, including examination of the fundus; evaluation of the iris vasculature; distinction between viable and nonviable tissue; observation of the aqueous flow; differential diagnosis of malignant and nonmalignant tumors; determination of circulation time and adequacy.

Administration and Dosage

➤*Topical:* To detect foreign bodies and corneal abrasions, instill 1 or 2 drops of 2% solution; allow a few seconds for staining. Wash out excess with sterile irrigating solution.

➤*Strips:* Moisten strip with sterile water. Place moistened strip at the fornix in the lower cul-de-sac close to the punctum. For best results, patient should close lid tightly over strip until desired amount of staining is obtained. The patient should blink several times after application.

Applanation tonometry strips – Anesthetize the eyes. Retract upper lid and touch tip of strip moistened with saline or ocular irrigating solution (eg, *Blinx*) to the bulbar conjunctiva on the temporal side until an adequate amount of stain is available for a clearly defined endpoint reading.

➤*Injection:* Inject the contents of the ampule or pre-filled syringe rapidly into the antecubital vein *after taking precautions to avoid extravasation*. A syringe, filled with fluorescein, is attached to transparent tubing and a 25-gauge scalp vein needle for injection. Insert the needle and draw blood to the hub of the syringe so that a *small* air bubble separates the blood in the tubing from the fluorescein. With the room lights on, slowly inject the blood back into the vein while watching the skin over the needle tip. If the needle has extravasated, the patient's blood will bulge the skin, and the injection should be stopped before any fluorescein is injected. When assured that extravasation has not occurred, the room light may be turned off and the fluorescein injection completed. Luminescence appears in the retina and choroidal vessels in 9 to 15 seconds and can be observed by standard viewing equipment.

If potential allergy is suspected, an intradermal skin test may be performed prior to IV administration (ie, 0.05 mL injected intradermally to be evaluated 30 to 60 minutes following injection).

In patients with inaccessible veins where early phases of an angiogram are not necessary, such as cystoid macular edema, 1 g fluorescein has been given orally. Ten to 15 minutes are usually required before evidence of dye appears in the fundus.

Adults – 500 to 750 mg injected rapidly into the antecubital vein.

Children – 7.5 mg/kg (3.5 mg/lb) injected rapidly into the antecubital vein.

Have 0.1% epinephrine IM or IV, an antihistamine, soluble steroid, aminophylline IV and oxygen available.

➤*Storage/Stability:* Store at 8° to 30°C (46° to 86°F). Do not use if solution contains a precipitate. Discard any unused solution. Keep out of the reach of children.

Actions

➤*Pharmacology:* Sodium fluorescein, a yellow water-soluble dibasic acid xanthine dye, produces an intense green fluorescent color in alkaline (pH > 5) solution. Fluorescein demonstrates defects of corneal epithelium. It does not stain tissues, but is a useful indicator dye. Normal precorneal tear film will appear yellow or orange. The intact corneal epithelium resists fluorescein penetration and is not colored. Any break in the epithelial barrier permits rapid penetration. Whether resulting from trauma, infection or other causes, epithelial corneal defects appear bright green and are easily seen. If epithelial loss is extensive, topical fluorescein penetrates into the aqueous humor and is readily visible biomicroscopically as a green flare.

Contraindications

Hypersensitivity to fluorescein or any other component of the product; do not use with soft contact lenses (lenses may become discolored).

➤*Topical:* Not for injection. Do not use in intraocular surgery.

Warnings

➤*Topical (drops):* Discontinue if sensitivity develops. May stain soft contact lenses. Do not touch dropper tip to any surface, as this may contaminate the solution.

➤*Extravasation:* Avoid extravasation during injection. The high pH can result in severe local tissue damage. Complications have occurred from extravasation: Sloughing of skin, superficial phlebitis, SC granuloma and toxic neuritis along the median curve in the antecubital area. Extravasation can cause severe pain in the arm for several hours. When significant extravasation occurs, discontinue injection and use conservative measures to treat damaged tissue and relieve pain (see Warnings).

➤*Hypersensitivity reactions:* Exercise caution when administering to patients with a history of hypersensitivity, allergies or asthma. If signs of sensitivity develop, discontinue use.

➤*Pregnancy: Category C.* Avoid parenteral fluorescein angiography during pregnancy, especially in first trimester. There are no reports of fetal complications during pregnancy.

➤*Lactation:* Fluorescein is excreted in breast milk. Use caution when administering to a nursing woman.

➤*Children:* Safety and efficacy for use in children have not been established.

Adverse Reactions

Injection – Nausea; headache; GI distress; vomiting; syncope; hypotension and other symptoms and signs of hypersensitivity; cardiac arrest; basilar artery ischemia; thrombophlebitis at injection site; severe shock; convulsions; death (rare); temporary yellowish skin discoloration. Hives, itching, bronchospasm, anaphylaxis, pyrexia, transient dyspnea, angioneurotic edema and slight dizziness may occur. A strong taste may develop with use. Urine becomes bright yellow. Skin discoloration fades in 6 to 12 hours; urine fluorescence in 24 to 36 hours. Extravasation at injection site causes intense pain at the site and dull aching pain in the injected arm (see Warnings).

Patient Information

May cause strong taste with use.

May cause temporary yellowish discoloration of the skin. Urine will turn bright yellow. Discoloration of skin fades in 6 to 12 hours; urine in 24 to 36 hours.

Soft contact lenses may become stained. Do not wear lenses while fluorescein is being used. Whenever fluorescein is used, flush the eyes with sterile normal saline solution and wait at least 1 hour before replacing the lenses.

FLUOREXON

otc	**Fluoresoft-0.35%** (Various, eg, Amcon, Con-cise Lens, Eye Care and Cure, Holles, Ocusoft)	**Solution:** 0.35%	Preservative-free. In 0.35 mL ampules. In 20s.

Indications

►*Applanation tonometry:* For conducting the applanation tonometry procedure without removing the lens.

►*Contact lens fitting aid:* For the assessment of proper fitting characteristics of hydrogel lenses. For quickly and accurately locating the optic zone in aphakic or low-plus lenses.

For the evaluation of corneal integrity of patients wearing hydrogel contact lenses. In many instances, arcuate staining will show definite correlation with the edge of the optic zone, indicating improper bearing surfaces.

►*Tear break-up time test:* For use in place of sodium fluorescein when conducting the tear breakup time test.

►*Toric lenses:* For locating the lathe-cut index markings (toric lenses). Use as directed for fitting contact lenses.

Administration and Dosage

Place 1 drop on the concave surface of the lens and place the lens immediately on the eye. Alternately, place 1 or 2 drops in the lower cul-de-sac and have the patient blink several times.

As the dye passes under the lens, observe a central dark zone of 6 to 9 mm in diameter (ie, a limbal fluorescent ring about 2 mm wide) that forms after each blink. If such staining pattern cannot be observed immediately, slide the lens upward by gently pushing it with a finger, causing the dye to penetrate under the lens as it slides back into normal position. Additional drops may be used if the fluorescence starts to dissipate after prolonged examination. When the examination is completed, rinse the eye and lens with saline. The lens may be reinserted immediately, as opposed to the long waiting period required after the use of fluorescein.

Begin the examination immediately after instillation of fluorexon drops. The material tends to dissipate readily with the tear flow, leading to a progressive reduction in fluorescence. Prolonged examination may require sequential application of drops.

►*Applanation tonometry:* After seating the patient at the slit lamp and either removing the contact lens or displacing it to the side, instill a drop of proparacaine or similar topical anesthetic, followed 1 to 2 minutes later by a drop of fluorexon. Take the reading immediately after, followed by rinsing out the eye and replacing the contact lens.

►*Storage/Stability:* Store below 24°C (75°F). Avoid direct sunlight. For one-time use only; discard ampule after use.

Actions

►*Pharmacology:* Fluorexon is a large molecular weight fluorescent solution for use as a diagnostic and fitting aid for patients with hydrogel contact lenses. Fluorexon is used, with or without lens in place (when fluorescein is contraindicated), most commonly to avoid staining lenses. It may be used for soft and hard lenses.

Contraindications

Hypersensitivity to sodium fluorescein.

Warnings

►*Contact lenses:* When used with lenses of greater than 55% hydration, some color may remain on lens. Remove by washing repeatedly with washing solution approved for the lens. Rinse with saline or water. Any residual coloring will wash out with the tear flow when the lens is reinserted in the eye. With highly hydrated lenses, the amount of coloring picked up will vary with exposure. Avoid unnecessary delays in examination procedure.

Precautions

►*Hydrogen peroxide:* Do not use hydrogen peroxide solutions to clean or sterilize lenses until all traces of fluorexon are removed because this oxidizing agent can bind fluorexon molecules to the lens.

ROSE BENGAL

otc	**Rose Bengal** (Barnes-Hind)	**Strips:** 1.3 mg per strip	In 100s.
otc	**Rosets** (Akorn)		In 100s.

Indications

►*Suspected corneal/conjunctival damage:* A diagnostic agent in routine ocular examinations or when superficial corneal or conjunctival tissue damage is suspected. Effective aid for diagnosis of keratitis, keratoconjunctivitis sicca, corrosions or abrasions, and for the detection of foreign bodies.

Administration and Dosage

Thoroughly saturate tip of strip with 2 or 3 drops of sterile ophthalmic solution. Touch bulbar conjunctiva or lower fornix with moistened strip. The patient should blink several times after application.

Actions

►*Pharmacology:* Rose bengal is an iodine derivative of fluorescein and stains dead or degenerated epithelial cells (corneal and conjunctival) and the mucus of the precorneal tear film.

Contraindications

Hypersensitivity to rose bengal or any component of the formulation.

Precautions

►*Irritation:* The solution may be irritating.

►*Staining:* Rose bengal can stain eyelids, cheeks, fingers, and clothing in a concentration-dependent manner. Keeping the amount of dye at a minimum and irrigating the eye can help circumvent this problem.

Adverse Reactions

►*Ophthalmic:* Irritation and discomfort.

INDOCYANINE GREEN

Rx	**IC-Green** (Akorn)	**Powder for Injection:** 25 mg	In vials with 10 mL amps of aqueous solvent. In 6s.

Indications

►*Angiography:* For ophthalmic angiography.

►*In vivo diagnostics:* For determining cardiac output, hepatic function, and liver blood flow (see In Vivo Diagnostic Aids).

Administration and Dosage

►*Administer IV:* Use 40 mg dye in 2 mL of aqueous solvent. Immediately follow the injected dye bolus with a 5 mL bolus of normal saline. This injection regimen is designed to provide delivery of a spatially limited dye bolus of optimal concentration to the choroidal vasculature following IV injection.

►*Compatibility:* Use only the aqueous solvent (pH, 5.5 to 6.5) provided, which is especially prepared sterile water for injection, to dissolve indocyanine green. There have been reports of incompatibility with some commercially available water for injection products.

►*Storage/Stability:* Indocyanine green is unstable in aqueous solution and must be used within 10 hours. However, the dye is stable in plasma and whole blood so that samples obtained in discontinuous sampling techniques may be read hours later. Use sterile techniques in handling the dye solution and in the performance of the dilution curves.

Indocyanine green powder may cling to the vial or lump together because it is freeze-dried in the vials. *This is not because of the presence of water.*

Actions

►*Pharmacology:* Indocyanine green is a sterile, water soluble, tricarbocyanine dye with a peak spectral absorption at 800 to 810 nm in blood or blood plasma. Indocyanine green contains no more than 5% sodium iodide.

Indocyanine green permits recording of indicator-dilution curves for both diagnostic and research purposes independently of fluctuations in oxygen saturation. In the performance of dye dilution curves, a known amount of dye is usually injected as a single bolus as rapidly as possible via a cardiac catheter into selected sites in the vascular system. A recording instrument (oximeter or densitometer) is attached to a needle or catheter for sampling of the blood-dye mixture from a systemic arterial sampling site.

The peak absorption and emission of indocyanine green lie in a region (800 to 850 nm) where transmission of energy by the pigment epithelium is more efficient than in the region of visible light energy. Because indocyanine green is also nearly 98% bound to blood protein, excessive dye extravasation does not take place in the highly fenestrated choroidal vasculature. It is, therefore, useful in absorption and fluorescence infrared angiography of the choroidal vasculature when using appropriate filters and film in a fundus camera.

►*Pharmacokinetics:* Following IV injection, indocyanine green is rapidly bound to plasma protein, of which albumin is the principle carrier (95%). Indocyanine green undergoes no significant extrahepatic or enterohepatic circulation; simultaneous arterial and venous blood esti-

INDOCYANINE GREEN

mations have shown negligible renal, peripheral, lung, or cerebrospinal uptake of the dye. Indocyanine green is taken up from the plasma almost exclusively by the hepatic parenchymal cells and is secreted entirely into the bile. After biliary obstruction, the dye appears in the hepatic lymph, independently of the bile, suggesting that the biliary mucosa is sufficiently intact to prevent diffusion of the dye, though allowing diffusion of bilirubin. These characteristics make indocyanine green a helpful index of hepatic function.

Contraindications

Use with caution in patients who have a history of allergy to iodides.

Warnings

➤*Hypersensitivity reactions:* Two anaphylactic deaths have been reported following indocyanine green administration during cardiac catheterization. One of these was in a patient with a history of sensitivity to penicillin and sulfa drugs.

➤*Pregnancy: Category C.* It is not known whether indocyanine green can cause fetal harm when administered to a pregnant woman or can affect reproduction capacity. Give to a pregnant woman only if clearly indicated.

➤*Lactation:* It is not known whether this drug is excreted in breast milk. Exercise caution when indocyanine green is administered to a nursing woman.

Precautions

➤*Plasma fractional disappearance:* Plasma fractional disappearance rate at the recommended 0.5 mg/kg dose has been reported to be significantly greater in women than in men; however, there was no significant difference in the calculated value for clearance.

➤*Radioactive iodine uptake studies:* Do not perform for at least a week following the use of indocyanine green.

Drug Interactions

➤*Drug/Lab test interactions:* Heparin preparations containing sodium bisulfite reduce the absorption peak of indocyanine green in blood. Do not use heparin as an anticoagulant for the collection of samples for analysis.

Adverse Reactions

➤*Hypersensitivity:* Anaphylactic or urticarial reactions have been reported in patients without history of allergy to iodides. If such reactions occur, treat with appropriate agents (eg, epinephrine, antihistamines, corticosteroids).

TEAR TEST STRIPS

otc	**Sno-Strips** (Akorn)	**Strips:** Sterile tear flow test strips	In 100s.
Rx	**Schirmer Tear Test** (Various, eg, Alcon)	**Strips:** Sterile tear flow test strips	In 250s.

Indications

➤*Schirmer Tear Test:*

Test I – To diagnose dry eye syndrome, to evaluate lacrimal gland function in contact lens wearers, to check tear production prior to eyelid surgery and prior to corneal transplantation and cataract surgery.

Test II – To assess the adequacy of reflex lacrimation.

➤*Sno-Strips:* To assess tear secretion.

Administration and Dosage

Perform test on eye before any topical medication (especially anesthetic) is administered or other procedures are carried out (eg, manipulation of eyelids).

➤*Schirmer Tear Tests:* Strips are placed at the junction of the middle and temporal one third of the eyelid margin. To avoid increased reflex lacrimation and pain, do not touch the cornea. After 5 minutes, remove the strips and measure the length of the moistened area. A value of less than 5 mm is very suggestive of a true dry eye state.

For the Schirmer II Tear Test, insert the strips in the usual manner. Gently irritate the nasal mucosa with a cotton-tip applicator to provoke reflex lacrimation. Remove the strips after 5 minutes. A value of less than 10 mm suggests that the patient is unable to produce reflex lacrimation and has demonstrated reflex secretion failure.

➤*Sno-Strips:* Apply to lower temporal lid margin of eye. The distance between the notch and shoulder of strip is 10 mm, which should be wetted in approximately 3 minutes. Repeat if greater than 5 minutes; greater than 10 minutes indicates reduced tear secretion.

SODIUM HYALURONATE

Rx	**Healon** (Kabi Pharmacia)	Injection:10 mg/mL[1]	In 0.4, 0.55, 0.85 and 2 mL disp. syringes.
Rx	**Amvisc** (Chiron)	Injection: 12 mg/mL[2]	In 0.5 or 0.8 mL disp. syringe.
Rx	**Coease** (Advance Medical)		In 0.5 or 0.8 mL disposable syringes.
Rx	**Shellgel** (Cytosol Ophthalmics)		In 0.8 mL disposable syringes.
Rx	**Healon GV** (Kabi Pharmacia)	Injection: 14 mg/mL[1]	In 0.55 and 0.85 mL disp. syringes.
Rx	**Amvisc Plus** (Bausch & Lomb)	Injection: 16 mg/mL[2]	In 0.5 or 8 mL disp. syringe.
Rx	**AMO Vitrax** (Allergan)	Injection: 30 mg/mL[3]	In 0.65 mL disp. syringe.

[1] With 8.5 mg NaCl per mL.
[2] With 9 mg NaCl per mL.

[3] With 3.2 mg NaCl, 0.75 mg KCl, 0.48 mg calcium chloride, 0.3 mg magnesium chloride, 3.9 mg sodium acetate and 1.7 mg sodium citrate per mL.

Indications

➤*Surgical aid:* As a surgical aid in cataract extraction (intra- and extra-capsular), intraocular lens implantation (IOL), corneal transplant, glaucoma filtration, retinal attachment surgery and posterior segment surgery to gently separate, maneuver and hold tissues.

To maintain a deep anterior chamber in surgical procedures in the anterior segment of the eye, allowing for efficient manipulation with less trauma to the corneal endothelium and other surrounding tissues.

To push back the vitreous face and prevent formation of a postoperative flat chamber.

To create a clear field of vision, facilitating intra- and postoperative inspection of the retina and photocoagulation.

➤*Unlabeled uses:* Sodium hyaluronate has been used in the treatment of refractory dry eye syndrome.

Administration and Dosage

➤*Cataract surgery - IOL implantation:* Slowly introduce a sufficient amount (using cannula or needle) into anterior chamber. Inject either before or after delivery of lens. Injection before lens delivery protects corneal endothelium from possible damage from removal of the cataractous lens. May use to coat surgical instruments and the IOL prior to insertion. May inject additional amounts during surgery to replace any of the drug lost.

➤*Glaucoma filtration surgery:* In conjunction with the performance of the trabeculectomy, inject slowly and carefully through a corneal paracentesis to reconstitute the anterior chamber. Further injection can be continued to allow it to extrude into the subconjunctival filtration site through and around the sutured outer scleral flap.

➤*Corneal transplant surgery:* After removal of the corneal button, fill the anterior chamber with the drug. Then, suture the donor graft in place. An additional amount may be injected to replace the lost amount as a result of surgical manipulation.

Sodium hyaluronate has also been used in the anterior chamber of the donor eye prior to trepanation to protect the corneal endothelial cells of the graft.

➤*Retinal attachment surgery:* Slowly introduce into the vitreous cavity. The injection may be directed to separate membranes from retina for safe excision and release of traction. Also serves to maneuver tissues into desired position (eg, to gently push back a detached retina or unroll a retinal flap); aids in holding retina against the sclera for reattachment.

➤*Storage: Amvisc/Amvisc Plus, Healon/Healon GV:* Store at 2° to 8°C (36° to 46°F).

AMO Vitrax – Store at room temperature (15° to 30°C; 59° to 86°F). Do not freeze. Protect from light.

Actions

➤*Pharmacology:* Sodium hyaluronate and sodium chondroitin sulfate are widely distributed in extracellular matrix of connective tissues.

They are found in synovial fluid, skin, umbilical cord and vitreous and aqueous humor. The cornea is the ocular tissue having the greatest concentration of sodium chondroitin sulfate; the vitreous and aqueous humor contain the greatest concentration of sodium hyaluronate.

This preparation is a specific fraction of sodium hyaluronate developed for use in anterior segment and vitreous procedures as a viscoelastic agent. It has high molecular weight, is nonantigenic, does not cause inflammatory or foreign body reactions and has a high viscosity. The 1% solution is transparent and remains in the anterior chamber for < 6 days. It protects corneal endothelial cells and other ocular structures. It does not interfere with epithelialization and normal wound healing.

Warnings

➤*Hypersensitivity reactions:* Because this preparation is extracted from avian tissues and contains minute amounts of protein, risks of hypersensitivity may exist.

Precautions

➤*For intraocular use:* Use only if solution is clear.

➤*Postoperative intraocular pressure (IOP):* Postoperative intraocular pressure (IOP) may be elevated as a result of preexisting glaucoma, compromised outflow and by operative procedures and sequelae, including enzymatic zonulysis, absence of an iridectomy, trauma to filtration structures and by blood and lenticular remnants in the anterior chamber. Because the exact role of these factors is difficult to predict in any individual case, the following precautions are recommended:

Anterior chamber – Do not overfill the anterior chamber (except in glaucoma surgery). (See Administration and Dosage.)

Monitoring – Carefully monitor IOP, especially during the immediate postoperative period. Treat significant increases appropriately.

Posterior segment surgery – In posterior segment surgery, in aphakic diabetics, exercise special care to avoid using large amounts of the drug.

Remove some of the preparation by irrigation or aspiration at the close of surgery (except in glaucoma surgery). (See Administration and Dosage.)

Avoid trapping air bubbles behind the drug.

➤*Cloudiness/precipitate:* Reports indicate that the drug may become cloudy or form a slight precipitate after instillation. The clinical significance is not known because the majority do not indicate any harmful effects on ocular tissues. Be aware of this phenomenon and remove cloudy or precipitated material by irrigation or aspiration. In vitro studies suggest that this phenomenon may be related to interactions with certain concomitantly administered ophthalmic medications.

Adverse Reactions

Although well tolerated, a transient postoperative increase of IOP has been reported (see Precautions).

Other reactions that have occurred include postoperative inflammatory reactions (iritis, hypopyon); corneal edema; corneal decompensation.

SODIUM HYALURONATE AND CHONDROITIN SULFATE

Rx	**Viscoat** (Alcon)	**Solution:** ≤ 40 mg sodium chondroitin sulfate, 30 mg sodium hyaluronate per mL	0.45 mg sodium dihydrogen phosphate hydrate, 2 mg disodium hydrogen phosphate, 4.3 mg sodium chloride per mL. In 0.5 mL disposable syringes.

Refer to the Sodium Hyaluronate monograph for more complete information.

Indications

➤*Surgical aid:* A surgical aid in anterior segment procedures including cataract extraction and intraocular lens implantation.

Administration and Dosage

Carefully introduce (using a 27-gauge cannula) into the anterior chamber. May inject prior to or following delivery of the crystalline lens. Instillation prior to lens delivery provides additional protection to cor-

neal endothelium, protecting it from possible damage arising from surgical instrumentation. May also be used to coat intraocular lens and tips of surgical instruments prior to implantation surgery. May inject additional solution during anterior segment surgery to fully maintain the chamber or to replace solution lost during surgery. At the end of surgery, remove solution by thoroughly irrigating the eye with a balanced salt solution. Alternatively, the solution may be left in the eye when used as directed.

➤*Storage/Stability:* Store at 2° to 8°C (36° to 46°F). Do not freeze.

SODIUM HYALURONATE AND FLUORESCEIN SODIUM

Rx	Healon Yellow (Pharmacia)	Solution: 10 mg sodium hyaluronate, 0.005 mg fluorescein sodium per mL	8.5 mg NaCl, 0.28 mg disodium hydrogen phosphate dihydrate, 0.04 mg sodium dihydrogen phosphate hydrate per mL. In 0.55 or 0.85 mL disposable syringes with cannula.

Refer to the Sodium Hyaluronate and Fluorescein Sodium monographs for more complete information.

Indications

➤*Surgical aid:* A surgical aid in anterior segment procedures including cataract extraction, intraocular lens (IOL) implantation and corneal transplant surgery. The fluorescein sodium facilitates visualization of the product during the surgical procedure.

Administration and Dosage

➤*Cataract surgery/IOL implantation:* Carefully introduce (using a 27–gauge cannula) into the anterior chamber. May inject prior to or following delivery of the lens. Instillation prior to lens delivery provides additional protection to corneal endothelium, protecting it from possible damage arising from removal of the cataractous lens. May also be used to coat the intraocular lens and surgical instruments prior to insertion. May inject additional solution during surgery to replace solution lost during surgical manipulation. Remove solution by irrigation or aspiration at the close of surgery.

➤*Corneal transplant surgery:* After removal of the corneal button, fill the anterior chamber with the solution. Then, suture the donor graft in place. May inject additional solution to replace solution lost during surgical manipulation. Remove solution by irrigation or aspiration at the close of surgery.

➤*Storage/Stability:* Store at 2° to 8°C (36° to 46°F). Allow to attain room temperature (approximately 30 min) prior to use. Do not freeze. Protect from light.

Precautions

➤*IOP:* Do not overfill the anterior segment as it may result in increased intraocular pressure, glaucoma or other ocular damage.

HYDROXYPROPYL METHYLCELLULOSE

Rx	OcuCoat (Storz)	Solution: 2%	In a balanced salt solution. In 1 mL syringe with cannula.
otc	Gonak (Akorn)	Solution: 2.5%	In 15 mL.[1]
otc	Goniosol (Novartis Ophthalmics)		In 15 mL.[1]

[1] With 0.01% benzalkonium chloride and EDTA.

Indications

➤*Surgical aid:*

2% solution – An ophthalmic surgical aid in anterior segment surgical procedures including cataract extraction and intraocular lens implantation.

2.5% solution – For professional use in gonioscopic examinations.

Administration and Dosage

➤*Anterior segment surgery:* Carefully introduce into the anterior chamber using a 20-gauge or smaller cannula. The 2% solution may be used prior to or following delivery of the crystalline lens. Injection of 2% solution prior to lens delivery will provide additional protection to the corneal endothelium and other ocular tissues.

The 2% solution may also be used to coat an intraocular lens and tips of surgical instruments prior to implantation surgery. May inject during anterior segment surgery to fully maintain the chamber, or to replace fluid lost during the surgical procedure. Remove solution from the anterior chamber at the end of surgery.

➤*Gonioscopic examinations:* Fill gonioscopic prism with 2.5% solution, as necessary.

➤*Storage/Stability:* If this solution dries on optical surfaces, let them stand in cool water before cleansing. If solution changes color or becomes cloudy, do not use. Not for use with hot laser treatment as solution clouding will occur.

To avoid contamination, do not touch tip of container to any surface. Replace cap after using. Keep container tightly closed. Store at room temperature 15° to 30°C (59° to 86°F). Avoid excessive heat over 60°C (140°F). Protect from light.

Actions

➤*Pharmacology:* Hydroxypropyl methylcellulose is an isotonic, non-pyrogenic viscoelastic solution with a high molecular weight (> 80,000 daltons). It maintains a deep chamber during anterior segment surgery and allows for more efficient manipulation with less trauma to the corneal endothelium and other ocular tissues. The viscoelasticity helps the vitreous face to be pushed back, preventing formation of a postoperative flat chamber. It is also used as a demulcent agent.

Precautions

➤*Intraocular pressure (IOP):* Transient increased IOP may occur following surgery because of preexisting glaucoma or due to the surgery itself. If the postoperative IOP increases above expected values, administer appropriate therapy.

Adverse Reactions

Although well tolerated, a transient, postoperative increase in IOP has been reported (see Precautions). Other reactions that have occurred include postoperative inflammatory reactions (iritis, hypopyon), corneal edema and corneal decompensation.

HYDROXYETHYLCELLULOSE

Rx	Gonioscopic (Alcon)	Solution: Hydroxyethylcellulose	0.004% thimerosal, 0.1% EDTA. In 15 mL Drop-Tainers.

Indications

➤*Gonioscopic bonding:* For use in bonding gonioscopic prisms to the eye.

Administration and Dosage

➤*Storage/Stability:* Store at room temperature 15° to 30°C (59° to 86°F).

BOTULINUM TOXIN TYPE A

Rx	Botox (Allergan)	Powder for Injection (vacuum dried): 100 units of vacuum-dried Clostridium botulinum toxin type A neurotoxin complex[1]	Preservative free. 0.5 mg albumin (human), 0.9 mg sodium chloride. In single-use vials.

[1] One unit corresponds to the calculated median lethal intraperitoneal dose (LD_{50}) in mice.

For more information, refer to the Botulinum Toxin monographs in the CNS chapter.

Indications

➤*Strabismus and blepharospasm:* Treatment of strabismus and blepharospasm associated with dystonia, including benign essential blepharospasm or VII nerve disorders in patients ≥ 12 years of age.

➤*Unlabeled uses:* Treatment of hemifacial spasms, spasmodic torticollis (ie, clonic twisting of the head), oromandibular dystonia, spasmodic dysphonia (laryngeal dystonia), and for other dystonias (eg, writer's cramp, focal task-specific dystonias). Botulinum toxin is being assessed in the treatment of head and neck tremor unresponsive to pharmacologic therapy. Designated an orphan drug for the treatment of dynamic muscle contracture in pediatric cerebral palsy patients.

Other reported uses of botulinum toxin type A include the following: Acquired nystagmus, oscillopsia, tremor, tics, detrusor sphincter dyssynergia, achalasia, anismus/vaginismus, cosmesis, hyperhidrosis, myofacial pain, temporomandibular joint dysfunction, cervicogenic headache, and spasticity.

Admistration and Dosage

➤*Approved by the FDA:* December 1989.

➤*Strabismus:* Botulinum toxin type A is intended for injection into extraocular muscles utilizing the electrical activity recorded from the tip of the injection needle as a guide to placement within the target muscle. Do not attempt injection without surgical exposure or electromyographic guidance. Physicians should be familiar with electromyographic technique.

To prepare the eye for botulinum toxin type A injection, give several drops of a local anesthetic and an ocular decongestant several minutes prior to injection.

➤*Note:* The volume of botulinum toxin type A injected for treatment of strabismus should be between 0.05 to 0.15 mL per muscle.

The initial listed doses of the diluted botulinum toxin type A (see Dilution table) typically create paralysis of injected muscles beginning 1 to 2 days after injection and increasing in intensity during the first week. The paralysis lasts for 2 to 6 weeks and gradually resolves over a similar time period. Overcorrections lasting > 6 months have been rare. About one half of patients will require subsequent doses because of inadequate paralytic response of the muscle to the initial dose, because mechanical factors such as large deviations or restrictions, or because of the lack of binocular motor fusion to stabilize the alignment.

1.) Initial doses in units (U). Use the lower listed doses for treatment

BOTULINUM TOXIN TYPE A

of small deviations. Use the larger doses only for large deviations.

- a.) For vertical muscles, and for horizontal strabismus of < 20 prism diopters: 1.25 to 2.5 U in any one muscle.
- b.) For horizontal strabismus of 20 to 50 prism diopters: 2.5 to 5 U in any one muscle.
- c.) For persistent VI nerve palsy of ≥ 1 month duration: 1.25 to 2.5 U in the medial rectus muscle.

2.) Subsequent doses for residual or recurrent strabismus.

- a.) Re-examine patients 7 to 14 days after each injection to assess the effect of that dose.
- b.) Patients experiencing adequate paralysis of the target muscle who require subsequent injections should receive a dose comparable to the initial dose.
- c.) Subsequent doses for patients experiencing incomplete paralysis of the target muscle may be increased up to 2-fold the previously administered dose.
- d.) Do not administer subsequent injections until the effects of the previous dose have dissipated as evidenced by substantial function in the injected and adjacent muscles.
- e.) Maximum recommended dose as a single injection for any one muscle is 25 U.

➤*Blepharospasm:* Diluted botulinum toxin type A (see Dilution table) is injected using a sterile, 27- to 30-gauge needle without electromyographic guidance. Initially, 1.25 to 2.5 U (0.05 to 0.1 mL volume at each site) injected into the medial and lateral pre-tarsal orbicularis oculi of the upper lid and into the lateral pre-tarsal orbicularis oculi of the lower lid is the initial recommended dose. Avoiding injection near the levator palpebrae superioris may reduce the complication of ptosis. Avoiding medial lower lid injections, and thereby reducing diffusion into the inferior oblique, may reduce the complication of diplopia. Ecchymosis occurs easily in the soft eyelid tissues. This can be prevented by applying pressure at the injection site immediately after the injection.

In general, the initial effect of the injections is seen within 3 days and reaches a peak at 1 to 2 weeks post-treatment. Each treatment lasts ≈ 3 months, following which the procedure can be repeated. At repeat treatment sessions, the dose may be increased up to 2-fold if the response from the initial treatment is considered insufficient (usually defined as an effect that does not last > 2 months). However, there appears to be little benefit obtainable from injecting > 5 U per site. Some tolerance may be found when botulinum toxin type A is used in treating blepharospasm if treatments are given any more frequently than every 3 months, and it is rare for the effect to be permanent.

The cumulative dose of botulinum toxin type A in a 30-day period should not exceed 200 U.

➤*Dilution technique:* To reconstitute vacuum-dried botulinum toxin type A, use sterile normal saline without a preservative; 0.9% Sodium Chloride Injection is the recommended diluent. Draw up the proper amount of diluent in the appropriate size syringe, and slowly inject the diluent into the vial. Because botulinum toxin type A is denatured by bubbling or similar violent agitation, inject the diluent into the vial gently. Discard the vial if a vacuum does not pull the diluent into the vial. Gently mix botulinum toxin type A with the saline by rotating the vial. Record the date and time of reconstitution on the space on the label. Administer within 4 hours after reconstitution.

The use of 1 vial for > 1 patient is not recommended because the product and diluent do not contain a preservative.

Botulinum Toxin Type A Dilution	
Diluent added (0.9% Sodium Chloride Injection)	Resulting dose (U/0.1 mL)
1 mL	10 U
2 mL	5 U
4 mL	2.5 U
8 mL	1.25 U

➤*Note:* These dilutions are calculated for an injection volume of 0.1 mL. A decrease or increase in the botulinum toxin type A dose is also possible by administering a smaller or larger injection volume – from 0.05 mL (50% decrease in dose) to 0.15 mL (50% increase in dose).

The method for performing the potency assay is specific to Allergan's botulinum toxin type A. Because of specific details of this assay such as the vehicle, dilution scheme, and laboratory protocols for the various potency assays, units of biological activity of botulinum toxin type A cannot be compared to nor converted into units of any other botulinum toxin or any toxin assessed with any other specific assay method.

➤*Preparation:* An injection of botulinum toxin type A is prepared by drawing into an appropriately sized sterile syringe an amount of the properly diluted toxin (see Dilution table) slightly greater than the intended dose. Air bubbles in the syringe barrel are expelled and the syringe is attached to an appropriate injection needle. Confirm patency of the needle. Injection volume in excess of the intended dose is expelled through the needle into an appropriate waste container to assure patency of the needle and to confirm that there is no syringe-needle leakage. Use a new, sterile needle and syringe to enter the vial on each occasion for dilution or removal of botulinum toxin type A.

➤*Storage/Stability:* Store the vacuum-dried product in a freezer at or below -5°C (23°F). Administer within 4 hours after the vial is removed from the freezer and reconstituted. During these 4 hours, store reconstituted botulinum toxin type A in a refrigerator (2° to 8°C; 36° to 46°F). Reconstituted botulinum toxin type A should be clear, colorless, and free of particulate matter.

Actions

➤*Pharmacology:* Botulinum toxin neurotoxin complex is a sterile, lyophilized form of purified botulinum toxin type A, produced from a fermentation of the Hall strain of *Clostridium botulinum* type A grown in a medium containing casein hydrolysate and yeast extract. Botulinum toxin type A blocks neuromuscular conduction by binding to receptor sites on motor nerve terminals, entering the nerve terminals, and inhibiting the release of acetylcholine. This inhibition occurs as the neurotoxin cleaves SNAP-25, a protein integral to the successful docking and release of acetylcholine from vesicles situated within nerve endings. When injected IM at therapeutic doses, botulinum toxin type A produces a partial chemical denervation of the muscle, resulting in a localized reduction in muscle activity. In addition, the muscle may atrophy, axonal sprouting may occur, and extrajunctional acetylcholine receptors may develop, thus, slowly reversing muscle denervation produced by botulinum toxin type A.

The paralytic effect of botulinum toxin type A on injected muscles is useful in reducing the excessive, abnormal contractions associated with blepharospasm. When used for the treatment of strabismus, the administration of botulinum toxin type A may affect muscle pairs by inducing an atrophic lengthening of the injected muscle and a corresponding shortening of the muscle's antagonist.

➤*Clinical trials:*
Blepharospasm – In 1 study, botulinum toxin type A was evaluated in 27 patients with essential blepharospasm; 26 had previously undergone drug treatment utilizing benztropine mesylate, clonazepam, or baclofen without adequate clinical results. Three of these patients then underwent muscle stripping surgery, still without an adequate outcome. Upon using botulinum toxin, 25 of the 27 patients reported improvement within 48 hours. One of the other patients was later controlled with a higher dosage. The remaining patient reported only mild improvement and remained functionally impaired.

Patients with blepharospasm (n = 1684) evaluated in an open-label trial showed clinical improvement lasting an average of 12.5 weeks prior to need for retreatment.

Strabismus – Patients with strabismus (n = 677) treated with ≥ 1 injection of botulinum toxin type A were evaluated in an open-label trial; 55% were improved to an alignment of ≤ 10 prism diopters when evaluated ≥ 6 months following injection. These results are consistent with results from additional open-label trials.

Contraindications

Presence of infection at the proposed injection site(s); hypersensitivity to any ingredient in the formulation.

Warnings

➤*Strabismus:* The efficacy of botulinum toxin type A in deviations > 50 prism diopters, in restrictive strabismus, in Duane's syndrome with lateral rectus weakness, and in secondary strabismus caused by prior surgical over-recession of the antagonist has not been established. Botulinum toxin type A is ineffective in chronic paralytic strabismus, except to reduce antagonist contracture when used in conjunction with surgical repair.

➤*Neuropathic disorders:* Individuals with peripheral motor neuropathic diseases (eg, amyotrophic lateral sclerosis, motor neuropathy) or neuromuscular junctional disorders (eg, myasthenia gravis, Lambert-Eaton syndrome) should only receivie botulinum toxin type A with caution. Patients with neuromuscular disorders may be at increased risk of clinically significant systemic effects, including severe dysphagia and respiratory compromise, from typical doses of botulinum toxin type A. Published medical literature has reported rare cases of administration of a botulinum toxin to patients with known or unrecognized neuromuscular disorders where the patients have shown extreme sensitivity to the systemic effects of typical clincal doses. In some of these cases, dysphagia has lasted several months and required placement of a gastric feeding tube.

➤*Dysphagia:* Dysphagia is a commonly reported adverse event all botulinum toxins following for treatment of cervical dystonia. In these patients, there are reports of rare cases of dysphagia severe enough to warrant the insertion of a gastric feeding tube. There are also rare case reports where subsequent to the finding of dysphagia, a patient developed aspiration pneumonia and died.

➤*Albumin:* This product contains albumin, a derivative of human blood. Based on effective donor screening and product manufacturing processes, it carries an extremely remote risk for transmission of viral diseases. A theoretical risk for transmission of Creutzfeldt-Jakob disease (CJD) is considered extremely remote. No cases of transmission of viral diseases or CJD have ever been identified with albumin.

➤*Dosage, systemic toxicity:* Do not exceed the recommended dosages and frequencies of administration. Risks resulting from administration at higher dosages are not known. If accidental injection or oral inges-

BOTULINUM TOXIN TYPE A

tion occurs, medically supervise the person for several days on an outpatient basis for signs or symptoms of systemic weakness or muscle paralysis.

➤*Hypersensitivity reactions:* As with all biologic products, have epinephrine and other precautions available if an anaphylactic reaction occurs. Refer to General Management of Acute Hypersensitivity Reactions.

➤*Elderly:* In general, be cautious in dose selection for an elderly patient' usually starting at the low end of the dosing range, reflecting the greater frequency of decreased hepatic, renal, or cardiac function, and of concomitant disease or other drug therapy.

➤*Pregnancy: Category C.* When pregnant mice and rats were injected IM during the period of organogenesis, the developmental NOEL of botulinum toxin type A was 4 U/kg. Higher doses (8 or 16 U/kg) were associated with reductions in fetal body weights or delayed ossification which may be reversible.

In a range-finding study in rabbits, daily injection of 0.125 U/kg/day (days 6 to 18 of gestation) and 2 U/kg (days 6 and 13 of gestation) produced severe maternal toxicity, abortions, or fetal malformations. Higher doses resulted in death of the dams. The rabbit appears to be a very sensitive species to botulinum toxin type A.

There are no adequate and well-controlled studies of botulinum toxin type A in pregnant women. Because animal reproductive studies are not always predictive of human response, administer this product during pregnancy only if the potential benefit justifies the potential risk to the fetus. If this drug is used during pregnancy, or if the patient becomes pregnant while taking this drug, apprise the patient of the potential risks, including abortion or fetal malformations, which have been observed in rabbits.

➤*Lactation:* It is not known whether this drug is excreted in breast milk. Exercise caution when botulinum toxin type A is administered to a nursing woman.

➤*Children:* Safety and efficacy in children < 12 years of age have not been established for blepharospasm or strabismus.

Precautions

➤*Safe and effective use:* Safe and effective use of botulinum toxin type A depends upon proper storage of the product, selection of the correct dose and proper reconstitution, and administration techniques. Physicians administering botulinum toxin type A must understand the relevant neuromuscular and orbital anatomy, and any alterations to the anatomy due to prior surgical procedures and standard electromyographic techniques.

➤*Injection site:* Use caution when botulinum toxin type A treatment is used in the presence of inflammation at the proposed injection site(s) or when excessive weakness or atrophy is present in the target muscle(s).

➤*Retrobulbar hemorrhages:* During the administration of botulinum toxin type A for the treatment of strabismus, retrobulbar hemorrhages sufficient to compromise retinal circulation have occurred from needle penetrations into the orbit. Have appropriate instruments accessible to decompress the orbit. Ocular (globe) penetrations by needles have also occurred. An ophthalmoscope to diagnose this condition should be available. Inducing paralysis in ≥ 1 extraocular muscles may produce spatial disorientation, double vision, or past pointing. Covering the affected eye may alleviate these symptoms.

➤*Blepharospasm:* Reduced blinking from botulinum toxin type A injection of the orbicularis muscle can lead to corneal exposure, persistent epithelial defect, and corneal ulceration, especially in patients with VII nerve disorders. One case of corneal perforation in an aphakic eye requiring corneal grafting has occurred because of this effect. Carefully test corneal sensation in eyes previously operated upon, avoid injection into the lower lid area to avoid ectropion, and vigorously treat any epithelial defect. This may require protective drops, ointment, therapeutic soft contact lenses, or closure of the eye by patching or other means.

➤*Antibodies:* Formation of neutralizing antibodies to botulinum toxin type A may reduce the effectiveness of therapy by inactivating the biological activity of the toxin. The rate of formation of neutralizing antibodies in patients receiving botulinum toxin type A has not been well established. The results from some studies suggest that botulinum toxin type A injections at more frequent intervals or at higher doses may lead to greater incidence of antibody formation. The potential for antibody formation may be minimized by injecting with the lowest effective dose given at the longest feasible intervals between injections. Keep the dose of botulinum toxin type A for strabismus and blepharospasm as low as possible.

Drug Interactions

➤*Aminoglycosides:* The effect of botulinum toxin may be potentiated by aminoglycoside antibiotics or any other drug that interferes with neuromuscular transmission. Exercise caution when botulinum toxin type A is used in patients taking these drugs.

The effect of administering different botulinum neurotoxin serotypes at the same time or within several months of each other is unknown. Excessive neuromuscular weakness may be exacerbated by administra-

tion of another botulinum toxin prior to the resolution of the effects of a previously administered botulinum toxin.

Adverse Reactions

In general, adverse events occur within the first week following injection of botulinum toxin type A and, while generally transient, may have a duration of several months.

➤*Cardiovascular:* There have been rare reports of adverse events involving the cardiovascular system, including arrhythmia and MI, some with fatal outcomes. Some of these patients had risk factors including cardiovascular disease. The exact relationship of these events to the botulinum toxin injection has not been established.

➤*Local:* Localized pain, tenderness, or bruising may be associated with the injection. Local weakness of the injected muscle(s) represents the expected pharmacological action of botulinum toxin. However, weakness of adjacent muscles may also occur due to spread of toxin.

➤*Ophthalmic:*

Strabismus – Inducing paralysis in ≥ 1 extraocular muscle may produce spatial disorientation, double vision, or past-pointing. Covering the affected eye may alleviate these symptoms. Extraocular muscles adjacent to the injection site are often affected, causing ptosis or vertical deviation, especially with higher doses. Side effects in 2058 adults who received 3650 injections for horizontal strabismus included ptosis (15.7%) and vertical deviation (16.9%). The incidence of ptosis was much less after inferior rectus injection (0.9%) and much greater after superior rectus injection (37.7%).

Side effects persisting for > 6 months in an enlarged series of 5587 injections of horizontal muscles in 3104 patients included ptosis (0.3%) and vertical deviation > 2 prism diopters (2.1%).

In these patients, the injection procedure itself caused 9 scleral perforations. A vitreous hemorrhage occurred and later cleared in 1 case. No retinal detachment or visual loss occurred in any case; 16 retrobulbar hemorrhages occurred without visual loss. Decompression of the orbit after 5 minutes was done to restore retinal circulation in 1 case. Five eyes had pupillary change consistent with ciliary ganglion damage (Adies pupil).

One patient developed anterior segment ischemia after receiving botulinum toxin type A injection into the medial rectus muscle under direct visualization for esotropia.

Blepharospasm – In a study of blepharospasm patients who received an average dose per eye of 33 U (injected at 3 to 5 sites), the most frequently reported treatment-related adverse reactions were ptosis (20.8%), superficial punctate keratitis (6.3%), and eye dryness (6.3%).

In this study, the rate for ptosis in the current botulinum toxin type A treated group (20.8% of patients) was significantly higher than the original treated group (4% of patients). All of these events were mild or moderate exept for 1 case of ptosis which was rated severe.

Other events reported in prior clinical studies in decreasing order of incidence include the following: Irritation, tearing, lagophthalmos, photophobia, ectropion, keratitis, diplopia, and entropion, diffuse skin rash and local swelling of the eyelid skin lasting for several days following eyelid injection.

In 2 cases of VII nerve disorder (1 case of an aphakic eye), reduced blinking from botulinum toxin type A injection of the orbicularis muscle led to serious corneal exposure, persistent epithelial defect, and corneal ulceration. Perforation occurred in the aphakic eye and required corneal grafting.

There was a report of acute angle closure glaucoma 1 day after receiving an injection of botulinum toxin for blepharospasm, with recovery 4 months later after laser iridotomy and trabeculectomy. Focal facial paralysis, syncope, and exacerbation of myasthenia gravis have also been reported after treatment of blepharospasm.

➤*Miscellaneous:* There have been rare spontaneous reports of death, sometimes associated with dysphagia, pneumonia, or other significant debility after treatment with botulinum toxin.

Postmarketing – The following events have been reported since the drug has been marketed and a causal relationship to the botulinum toxin injection is unknown: Skin rash (including erythema multiforme, urticaria, and psoriasiform eruption), pruritus, and allergic reaction.

Overdosage

➤*Symptoms:* Signs and symptoms of overdose are not apparent immediately post injection. If accidental injection or oral ingestion occur, the medically supervise the person for up to several weeks for signs or symptoms of systemic weakness or muscle paralysis.

➤*Treatment:* An antitoxin is available in the event of immediate knowledge of an overdose or misinjection. In the event of overdosage or injection into the wrong muscle, additional information may be obtained by contacting Allergan Pharmaceuticals at (800) 433-8871 from 8 am to 4 pm Pacific Time, or at (714) 246-5954 for a recorded message at other times. The antitoxin will not reverse any botulinum toxin induced muscle weakness effects already apparent by the time of antitoxin administration.

BOTULINUM TOXIN TYPE A

Patient Information

As with any treatment with the potential to allow previously sedentary patients to resume activities, caution these patients to resume activity slowly and carefully following administration.

Advise patients or caregivers to seek immediate medical attention if swallowing, speech, or respiratory disorders arise.

POLYDIMETHYLSILOXANE (Silicone Oil)

| Rx | **AdatoSil 5000** (Escalon Ophthalmics) | **Injection:** Polydimethylsiloxane oil | In single-use 10 and 15 mL vials. |

Indications

➤*Retinal detachments:* Prolonged retinal tamponade in selected cases of complicated retinal detachments where other interventions are not appropriate for patient management. Complicated retinal detachments or recurrent retinal detachments occur most commonly in eyes with proliferative vitreoretinopathy (PVR), proliferative diabetic retinopathy (PDR), cytomegalovirus (CMV) retinitis, giant tears and following perforating injuries.

For primary use in detachments due to AIDS-related CMV retinitis and other viral infections.

Administration and Dosage

➤*Approved by the FDA:* November 7, 1994.

Polydimethylsiloxane can be used in conjunction with or following standard retinal surgical procedures including scleral buckle surgery, vitrectomy, membrane peeling and retinotomy or relaxing retinectomy.

Avoid introduction of air bubbles into the oil by careful withdrawal or decanting of the oil into the syringe. The oil can be injected into the vitreous from the syringe via a single use cannulated infusion line or syringe needle. Subretinal fluid can be drained with a flute needle concurrent with polydimethylsiloxane infusion. The vitreous space can be filled with the oil to between 80% and 100% while exchanging for fluid or air, taking necessary precautions to avoid high intraocular pressure from developing during the exchange. Because the polydimethylsiloxane is less dense than the eye aqueous fluid, a basal iridectomy at the 6 o'clock meridian (Ando iridectomy) is recommended to minimize oil induced pupillary block and early angle-closure glaucoma. Upon choice of the physician, it may be desirable to have the patient assume a face-down posture during the first 24 hours following surgery.

Monitor the patient closely for development of glaucoma, cataract and keratopathy complications and schedule for follow-up reexamination at regular intervals.

It is recommended that polydimethylsiloxane be removed at an appropriate interval within 1 year following instillation if the retina is stable, attached and without significant remnants of proliferation. Although there is insufficient clinical evidence to support justification for longer term tamponade, whether or not the oil should be removed in patients at high risk for redetachment or the development of phthisis and shrinkage due to hypotony must be determined individually by the physician. In order to minimize the number of invasive traumatic experiences for patients with AIDS and CMV retinitis at high risk for redetachment and who have a shortened expected lifespan, avoid silicone oil removal procedures if the patient concurs.

Polydimethylsiloxane can be removed from the posterior chamber by withdrawal with a normal 10 mL syringe and a wide bore 1 mm cannula. By repeated oil-fluid exchange most of the remaining small silicone oil droplets can subsequently be mobilized and removed from the eye. Alternatively, oil may be passively removed by infusion of an appropriate aqueous solution under the oil bubble, while allowing the oil to effuse out of a sclerotomy incision, or limbal incision in aphakic patients.

As there is a possible correlation between the migration of polydimethylsiloxane into the anterior chamber and the appearance of corneal changes such as edema, hazing or opacification, Descemet folds or decompensation, perform regular monitoring of the patient's corneal status and take early corrective action if necessary, including extraction of the oil from the anterior chamber. Large bubbles or droplets of oil in the anterior chamber can be removed manually by syringe. Further standard practice for medical treatment of the keratopathy is recommended.

Temporary pressure increases > 3 weeks after surgery that can normalize either spontaneously or that can be corrected by surgical treatment are those in which the polydimethylsiloxane causes a mechanical blockage of the pupil or inferior iridectomy or causes chamber angle closure by forcing its way anteriorly. In these situations some of the oil may be withdrawn to relieve the mechanical force of the oil interface. Presence of polydimethylsiloxane droplets in the anterior chamber may also cause a chronic outflow obstruction of the trabecular meshwork. In such situations elevated intraocular pressure can be managed with anti-glaucoma medication in the majority of outflow obstruction patients.

➤*Admixture incompatibility:* Do not admix with any other substances prior to injection.

➤*Storage/Stability:* Store at room or cool temperature (8° to 24°C; 46° to 75°F). Polydimethylsiloxane is supplied in a sterile vial intended for single use only and contains no preservative. Do not resterilize. Discard unused portions. Product should be discarded following expiration date.

Actions

➤*Pharmacology:* Polydimethylsiloxane, an oil that is injected into the vitreous space of the eye, is used as a prolonged retinal tamponade in select cases of retinal detachment.

➤*Clinical trials:*

Anatomic reattachment rates – Successful reattachment of the retina occurred in 64% to 75% of the patients who were treated with polydimethylsiloxane. This rate varied depending on the specific etiology of the disease and the severity of the condition. In AIDS CMV retinitis patients receiving silicone oil as a primary means for reattaching the retina, attachment rates were as high as 90% within an average 6 month follow up period.

Visual acuity outcomes – From 45% to 70% of patients showed improvements in visual acuity at 6 months. In about 15% to 26% of patients, visual acuity did not change and in about 15% to 30%, worsening of visual acuity occurred. Deterioration of visual acuity in treated patients appeared to be related to redetachment of the retina, further progression of retinal disease, or to keratopathy and cataract complications. In AIDS CMV retinitis patients, improvement or maintenance of visual acuity was documented in 57% of the patients within an average 6 month follow-up period. In AIDS patients, further decline in visual acuity was seen due to continuing progression of retinal and optic nerve disease and development of oil related cataracts in 33% of patients within 4 to 5 months of oil instillation.

Contraindications

Pseudophakic patients with silicone intraocular lens (silicone oil can chemically interact and opacify silicone elastomers).

Warnings

➤*Cataract:* Approximately 50% to 70% of phakic patients developed a cataract within 12 months of oil instillation. Approximately 33% of phakic AIDS CMV retinitis patients developed some degree of cataract within an average 4 to 5 month time frame from oil instillation.

➤*Anterior chamber oil migration:* In 17% to 20% of patients, oil emulsification or migration into the anterior chamber was observed. Migration into the anterior chamber occurred in both phakic and aphakic patients.

➤*Keratopathy:* From 8% to 20% of patients developed keratopathy (0.6%, AIDS patients). This complication occurred most frequently in aphakic patients (18% to 21%) and in the patients in whom oil had migrated into the anterior chamber (30%); the keratopathy in these cases was attributed to prolonged physical contact between the corneal endothelium and the silicone oil.

➤*Glaucoma:* Approximately 19% to 20% (0.06%, AIDS patients) of patients developed a persistent elevation in intraocular pressure (> 23 to 25 mm Hg). The neovascular glaucoma rate was about 8%. Moderate temporary postoperative increases occurred within the first 3 weeks of treatment. Thereafter, secondary ocular hypertension occurred by several mechanisms. Glaucoma complications occurred in approximately 30% of patients in which anterior chamber oil is noted. Patients with proliferative diabetic retinopathy were at highest risk for development of glaucoma following silicone oil instillation into the vitreous space.

Precautions

➤*Long-term use:* The safety and efficacy of long-term use have not been established.

Adverse Reactions

Most common – The most common adverse reactions include: Cataract (50% to 70%); anterior chamber oil migration (17% to 20%); keratopathy (8% to 20%); glaucoma (19% to 20%). See Warnings.

➤*Miscellaneous:* Other adverse reactions ranked by frequency of occurrence: Redetachment, optic nerve atrophy, rubeosis iritis, temporary IOP increase, macular pucker, vitreous hemorrhage, phthisis, traction detachment, angle block (> 2%); subretinal strands, retinal rupture, endophthalmitis, subretinal silicone oil, choroidal detachment, aniridia, PVR reproliferation, cystoid macular edema, enucleation (< 2%).

The otic preparations on the following pages are divided into groups as follows:

Steroid and Antibiotic Combinations
Miscellaneous Preparations
Antibiotics

➤*Patient Information:* For use in the ear only. Avoid contact with the eyes.

Notify physician if burning or itching occurs or if condition persists.

Perforated tympanic membrane is considered a contraindication to the use of any medication in the external ear canal.

Proper use of ear drops –
• Wash hands thoroughly.
• Avoid touching the dropper to the ear or any other surface. For accuracy and to avoid contamination, have another person insert the ear drops when possible.
• Hold container in the hand for a few minutes to warm to near body temperature if it has been refrigerated.
• If the drops are in a suspension form, shake well for 10 seconds before using.

• Lie on your side or tilt the affected ear up for ease of administration.To allow the drops to run in:
   Adults-Hold the earlobe up and back.
   Children-Hold the earlobe down and back.
• Instill the prescribed number of drops in the ear.
• Do not insert the dropper into the ear.
• Keep the ear tilted for about 2 minutes, or insert a soft cotton plug, whichever is recommended.

Products used to soften, loosen and remove earwax –
• Do not use if ear drainage, discharge, pain, irritation or rash occurs.
• If you become dizzy, consult a physician.
• Do not use if injury or perforation of the ear drum exists or after ear surgery unless directed otherwise.
• Do not use for > 4 days; if excessive earwax remains after use of this product, consult a physician.
• Any wax remaining after treatment may be removed by gently flushing with warm water using a soft rubber bulb ear syringe.

Steroid and Antibiotic Combinations

Refer also to Patient Information in the Otic Product Preparations introduction for instructions on the use of these products.

Indications

Treatment of superficial bacterial infections of the external auditory canal.

➤*Suspension:* Also used to treat infections of mastoidectomy and fenestration cavities.

Administration and Dosage

The usual adult dose is 4 drops instilled 3 or 4 times daily.

Actions

➤*Pharmacology:*
In these combinations –
  HYDROCORTISONE: Hydrocortisone is used for its antiallergic, antipruritic and anti-inflammatory effects.
  ANTIBIOTICS: Antibiotics are used for their antibacterial actions.

Contraindications

Hypersensitivity to any component.

Precautions

➤*Superinfection:* Prolonged treatment may result in overgrowth of nonsusceptible organisms and fungi (eg, herpes simplex, vaccinia, varicella).

STEROID AND ANTIBIOTIC COMBINATIONS, SOLUTIONS

Rx	**Antibiotic Ear Solution** (Various, eg, Geneva)	**Solution:** 1% hydrocortisone, 5 mg neomycin sulfate[1], 10,000 units polymyxin B	In 10 mL.
Rx	**AntibiOtic** (Parnell)		In 10 mL.[2]
Rx	**Cortisporin Otic** (Glaxo Wellcome)		In 10 mL with dropper.[3]
Rx	**Ear-Eze** (Hyrex)		In 10 mL with dropper.[2]
Rx	**LazerSporin-C** (Pedinol)		In 10 mL with dropper.
Rx	**Otosporin** (Calmic)		In 10 mL with dropper.

[1] 5 mg neomycin sulfate is equivalent to 3.5 mg neomycin base.
[2] With propylene glycol, glycerin and potassium metabisulfite.
[3] With cupric sulfate, propylene glycol, glycerin and potassium metabisulfite.

Complete prescribing information begins in the Steroid and Antibiotic Combinations monograph.

STEROID AND ANTIBIOTIC COMBINATIONS, SUSPENSIONS

Rx	**Antibiotic Ear Suspension** (Various, eg, Geneva)	**Suspension:** 1% hydrocortisone, 5 mg neomycin sulfate[1], 10,000 units polymyxin B	In 10 mL with dropper.
Rx	**Cortisporin Otic** (Glaxo Wellcome)		In 10 mL with dropper.[2]
Rx	**Octicair** (Bausch & Lomb)		In 10 mL with dropper.[3]
Rx	**Pediotic** (Glaxo Wellcome)		In 7.5 mL with dropper.[4]
Rx	**Neomycin/Polymyxin B Sulfates/Hydrocortisone Otic** (Steris)		In 10 mL with dropper.[2]
Rx	**Coly-Mycin S Otic** (Parke-Davis)	**Suspension:** 1% hydrocortisone, 4.71 neomycin sulfate[5]	With 3 mg colistin (as sulfate) and 0.05% thonzonium Br/mL. In 5 and 10 mL with dropper.[6]
Rx	**Cortisporin-TC Otic** (Monarch)	**Suspension:** 1% hydrocortisone, 3.3 mg neomycin sulfate	With 3 mg colistin (as sulfate) and 0.5 mg thonzonium bromide. In 10 mL with dropper
Rx	**Cipro HC Otic** (Bayer)	**Suspension:** 2 mg ciprofloxacin, 10 mg hydrocortisone/mL	Benzyl alcohol. In 10 mL.
Rx	**Ciprodex** (Alcon)	**Suspension:** 0.3% ciprofloxacin, 0.1% dexamethasone	Benzalkonium chloride, boric acid, EDTA. In 5 and 7.5 mL *Drop-Tainer*.

[1] 5 mg neomycin sulfate is equivalent to 3.5 mg neomycin base.
[2] With cetyl alcohol, propylene glycol, polysorbate 80 and thimerosal.
[3] With cetyl alcohol, polyoxyl 40 stearate, polysorbate 80, propylene glycol, sulfuric acid and benzalkonium Cl.
[4] With thimerosal, cetyl alcohol, glyceryl monostearate, mineral oil, polyoxyl 40 stearate and propylene glycol.
[5] 4.71 mg neomycin sulfate is equivalent to 3.3 mg neomycin base.
[6] With polysorbate 80, acetic acid, sodium acetate and thimerosal.

Complete prescribing information begins in the Steroid and Antibiotic Combinations group monograph.

MISCELLANEOUS OTIC PREPARATIONS

Rx	**VoSoL HC Otic** (Wallace)	**Solution:** 1% hydrocortisone, 2% acetic acid, 3% propylene glycol diacetate, 0.015% sodium acetate and 0.02% benzethonium chloride *Dose:* Insert saturated wick into ear; leave in for 24 hours, keeping moist with 3 to 5 drops every 4 to 6 hours. Keep moist for 24 hours. Remove wick and instill 5 drops 3 or 4 times daily	With 0.05% citric acid. In 10 mL with dropper.
Rx	**Acetasol HC** (Barre-National)		With 0.2% citric acid. In 10 mL with dropper.
otc	**EarSol-HC** (Parnell)	**Solution:** 1% hydrocortisone, 44% alcohol, propylene glycol, *Dermprotective Factor* yerba santa, benzyl benzoate *Dose:* Insert 4 to 6 drops into ear ≤ 3 to 4 times/day	In 30 mL.
Rx	**Cortic** (Everett)	**Drops:** 1% hydrocortisone, 1% pramoxine HCl, 0.1% chloroxylenol, 3% propylene glycol diacetate and benzalkonium chloride *Dose:* Insert saturated wick into ear; leave in for 24 hours, keeping moist with 3 to 5 drops every 4 to 6 hours. Remove wick and instill 5 drops 3 or 4 times daily	In 10 mL.
Rx	**Cortic-ND** (Everett)	**Drops:** 1% hydrocortisone, 1% pramoxine HCl, 0.1% chloroxylenol, and benzalkonium chloride *Dose:* Adults - 4 to 5 drops into affected ear tid or qid; infants and small children - 3 drops.	In 15 mL.
Rx	**Cortane-B Aqueous** (Blansett)	**Drops:** 1% hydrocortisone, 1% pramoxine HCl, 0.1% chloroxylenol *Dose:* 4 to 5 drops into affected ear tid or qid; infants and small children - 3 drops.	In 15 mL.
Rx	**Cortane-B Otic** (Blansett)	**Drops:** 1% hydrocortisone, 1% pramoxine HCl, 0.1% chloroxylenol *Dose:* 4 to 5 drops into affected ear tid or qid; infants and small children - 3 drops.	In 10 mL.
Rx	**Oti-Med** (Hyrex)	**Drops:** 0.1% chloroxylenol, 1% pramoxine HCl, 1% hydrocortisone, propylene glycol, benzalkonium Cl *Dose:* Adults - Instill 4 to 5 drops into affected ear 3 or 4 times daily. Children and infants - Instill 3 drops into affected ear 3 or 4 times daily.	In 10 mL vials.
Rx	**Tri-Otic** (Pharmics)	**Drops:** 0.1% chloroxylenol, 1% pramoxine HCl; 1% hydrocortisone	In 10 mL vials.
Rx	**Allergen Ear Drops** (Goldline)	**Solution:** 1.4% benzocaine, 5.4% antipyrine, glycerin *Dose:* Fill ear canal with 2 to 4 drops; insert saturated cotton pledget. Repeat 3 or 4 times daily, or up to once every 1 to 2 hours	In 15 mL with dropper.[1]
Rx	**Antipyrine and Benzocaine Otic** (URL)		In 15 mL with dropper.
Rx	**Auroto Otic** (Barre-National)		In 15 mL with dropper.[1]
Rx	**Auroguard Otic** (SDA)	**Solution:** 1.4% benzocaine, 5.4% antipyrine, glycerin, oxyquinoline sulfate *Dose:* Instill 2 to 4 drops into affected ear. Moisten cotton pledget with solution and gently insert into ear canal. Repeat 3 or 4 times daily.	In 15 mL.
Rx	**Americaine Otic** (Fisons)	**Solution:** 20% benzocaine, 0.1% benzethonium chloride, 1% glycerin, PEG 300 *Dose:* Instill 4 or 5 drops. Insert cotton pledget. Repeat every 1 to 2 hours	In 15 mL with dropper.
Rx	**Otocain** (Abana)		In 15 mL.
Rx	**Cresylate** (Recsei)	**Solution:** 25% m-cresyl acetate, 25% isopropanol, 1% chlorobutanol, 1% benzyl alcohol, 5% castor oil, propylene glycol *Dose:* 2 to 4 drops as required	In 15 mL with dropper and pt.
Rx	**Acetic Acid Otic** (Various, eg, Rugby)	**Solution:** 2% acetic acid with 3% propylene glycol diacetate, 0.02% benzethonium chloride, 0.015% sodium acetate *Dose:* Insert saturated wick; keep moist 24 hours. Remove wick and instill 5 drops 3 or 4 times daily	In 15 mL.
Rx	**Acetasol** (Barre)		In 15 mL.
Rx	**VoSoL Otic** (Wallace)		In 15 and 30 mL dropper bottles.
Rx	**Acetic Acid 2% and Aluminum Acetate Otic Solution** (Bausch & Lomb)	**Solution:** 2% acetic acid in aluminum acetate solution *Dose:* Insert saturated wick; keep moist for 24 hours. Instill 4 to 6 drops every 2 to 3 hours	In 60 mL.
Rx	**Burow's Otic** (Rugby)		In 60 mL.
Rx	**Otic Domeboro** (Bayer)		In 60 mL with dropper.
Rx	**Borofair Otic** (Major)	**Solution:** 2% acetic acid, aluminum acetate	In 60 mL.
Rx	**Cerumenex Drops** (Purdue Frederick)	**Solution:** 10% triethanolamine polypeptide oleate-condensate, 0.5% chlorobutanol, propylene glycol *Dose:* Fill ear canal. Insert cotton plug, allow to remain 15 to 30 minutes. Flush ear	In 6 and 12 mL with dropper.
Rx	**Zoto-HC** (Horizon)	**Drops:** 1 mg chloroxylenol, 10 mg pramoxine HCl, 10 mg hydrocortisone, 3% propylene glycol diacetate, benzalkonium chloride. *Dose:* Instill 4 to 5 drops into affected ear 3 or 4 times daily	In 10 mL plastic dropper vials.
Rx	**Otomar-HC** (Marnel)	**Solution:** 1 mg chloroxylenol, 10 mg hydrocortisone, 10 mg pramoxine HCl per mL. *Dose:* Instill 5 drops into affected ear 3 or 4 times daily.	In 10 mL plastic dropper vials.
otc	**Auro-Dri** (Commerce)	**Solution:** 2.75% boric acid, isopropyl alcohol *Dose:* Instill 3 to 8 drops in each ear	In 30 mL with dropper.
otc	**Dri/Ear** (Pfeiffer)		In 30 mL.
otc	**Ear-Dry** (Scherer)		In 30 mL w/ dropper.
otc	**Star-Otic** (Stellar)	**Solution:** Nonaqueous acetic acid, Burow's solution, boric acid, propylene glycol *Dose:* Instill 2 to 3 drops before and after swimming or showering	In 15 mL with dropper.
otc	**Debrox** (Marion Merrell Dow)	**Drops:** 6.5% carbamide peroxide, glycerin, propylene glycol, sodium stannate *Dose:* Instill 5 to 10 drops twice daily for up to 4 days	In 30 mL with dropper.
otc	**Murine Ear** (Ross)	**Drops:** 6.5% carbamide peroxide, 6.3% alcohol, glycerin, polysorbate 20 *Dose:* Instill 5 to 10 drops twice daily for up to 4 days	In 15 mL.
otc	**Auro Ear Drops** (Commerce)	**Solution:** 6.5% carbamide peroxide in an anhydrous glycerine base *Dose:* Instill 5 to 10 drops twice daily for up to 4 days	In 15 mL.
otc	**E·R·O Ear** (Scherer)	**Drops** 6.5% carbamide peroxide, anhydrous glycerin *Dose:* Instill 5 to 10 drops twice daily for up to 4 days	In 15 mL.
otc	**Mollifene Ear Wax Removing Formula** (Pfeiffer)		With propylene glycol and sodium stannate. In 15 mL with dropper.
otc	**Swim-Ear** (Fougera)	**Liquid:** 95% isopropyl alcohol, 5% anhydrous glycerin *Dose:* Instill 4 or 5 drops in affected ear after swimming, showering or bathing	In 30 mL.

[1] With oxyquinoline sulfate.

MISCELLANEOUS OTIC PREPARATIONS

Indications

➤*In these combinations:*

HYDROCORTISONE and DESONIDE – Hydrocortisone and desonide are steroids used for their anti-inflammatory and antipruritic effects.

PHENYLEPHRINE – Phenylephrine is a vasoconstrictor which may be a decongestant.

ACETIC ACID, M-CRESYL ACETATE, BORIC ACID, BENZALKONIUM CHLORIDE, BENZETHONIUM CHLORIDE and ALUMINUM ACETATE (BUROW'S SOLUTION) – Acetic acid, M-cresyl acetate, boric acid, benzalkonium chloride, benzethonium chloride and aluminum acetate (Burow's Solution) provide antibacterial or antifungal action.

CARBAMIDE PEROXIDE and TRIETHANOLAMINE – Carbamide peroxide and triethanolamine emulsify and disperse ear wax.

GLYCERIN – Glycerin is a solvent and vehicle; it has emollient, hygroscopic and humectant properties.

BENZOCAINE – Benzocaine is a local anesthetic.

ANTIPYRINE – Antipyrine is an analgesic.

OFLOXACIN

Rx	**Ofloxacin** (Various, eg, Allergan, Apotex, Bausch & Lomb, Falcon)	**Solution:** 0.3% (3 mg/mL)	In 5 and 10 mL dropper bottles.[a]
Rx	**Floxin Otic** (Daiichi)		In 5 and 10 mL dropper bottles.[b]

[a] With 0.005% benzalkonium chloride.   [b] With 0.0025% benzalkonium chloride, 0.9% sodium chloride.

Indications

Ofloxacin is indicated for the treatment of infections caused by susceptible strains of the designated microorganisms in the specific conditions listed below.

➤*Otitis externa:* In adults and pediatric patients 1 year of age and older caused by *Staphylococcus aureus* and *Pseudomonas aeruginosa.*

➤*Chronic suppurative otitis media:* In patients 12 years of age and older with perforated tympanic membranes caused by *S. aureus, Proteus mirabilis,* and *P. aeruginosa.*

➤*Acute otitis media:* In pediatric patients 1 year of age and older with tympanostomy tubes caused by *S. aureus, Streptococcus pneumoniae, Haemophilus influenzae, Moraxella catarrhalis,* and *P. aeruginosa.*

Administration and Dosage

➤*Approved by the FDA:* December 16, 1997.

Prior to administration, warm the solution by holding the bottle in the hand for 1 or 2 minutes to avoid dizziness that may result from the instillation of a cold solution.

For otic administration only. Not for ophthalmic use or injection.

➤*Otitis externa:* The recommended dosage regimen for the treatment of otitis externa is the following:

Pediatric patients 1 to 12 years of age – 5 drops (0.25 mL; 0.75 mg ofloxacin) instilled into the affected ear twice daily for 10 days.

12 years of age and older – 10 drops (0.5 mL; 1.5 mg ofloxacin) instilled into the affected ear twice daily for 10 days.

Have the patient lie with the affected ear upward, and then instill the drops. This position should be maintained for 5 minutes to facilitate penetration of the drops into the ear canal. Repeat if necessary for the opposite ear.

➤*Acute otitis media in pediatric patients with tympanostomy tubes:* The recommended dosage regimen for the treatment of acute otitis media in pediatric patients from 1 to 12 years of age with tympanostomy tubes is 5 drops (0.25 mL; 0.75 mg ofloxacin) instilled into the affected ear twice daily for 10 days.

Have the patient lie with the affected ear upward, and then instill the drops. Pump the tragus 4 times by pushing inward to facilitate penetration of the drops into the middle ear. This position should be maintained for 5 minutes. Repeat if necessary for the opposite ear.

➤*Chronic suppurative otitis media with perforated tympanic membranes:* The recommended dosage regimen for the treatment of chronic suppurative otitis media with perforated tympanic membranes in patients 12 years of age and older is 10 drops (0.5 mL; 1.5 mg ofloxacin) instilled into the affected ear twice daily for 14 days. The patient should lie with the affected ear upward before instilling the drops. The tragus should then be pumped 4 times by pushing inward to facilitate penetration into the middle ear. This position should be maintained for 5 minutes. Repeat if necessary for the opposite ear.

➤*Storage/Stability:* Store at 15° to 25°C (59° to 77°F).

Actions

➤*Pharmacology:* Ofloxacin has in vitro activity against a wide range of gram-negative and gram-positive microorganisms. Ofloxacin exerts its antibacterial activity by inhibiting DNA gyrase, a bacterial topoisomerase. DNA gyrase is an essential enzyme that controls DNA topology and assists in DNA replication, repair, deactivation, and transcription.

➤*Pharmacokinetics:* In 2 single-dose studies, mean ofloxacin serum concentrations were low in adult patients with tympanostomy tubes, with and without otorrhea, after otic administration of a 0.3% solution (4.1 ng/mL [n = 3] and 5.4 ng/mL [n = 5], respectively). In adults with perforated tympanic membranes, the maximum serum drug level of ofloxacin detected was 10 ng/mL after administration of a 0.3% solution. Ofloxacin was detectable in the middle ear mucosa of some adult subjects with perforated tympanic membranes. The variability of ofloxacin concentration in middle ear mucosa was high, ranging from 1.2 to 602 mcg/g after otic administration of a 0.3% solution. Ofloxacin was present in high concentrations in otorrhea (389 to 2850 mcg/g, n = 13) 30 minutes after otic administration of a 0.3% solution in subjects with chronic suppurative otitis media and perforated tympanic membranes.

Cross-resistance – Cross-resistance has been observed between ofloxacin and other fluoroquinolones.

Contraindications

History of hypersensitivity to ofloxacin, to other quinolones, or to any of the components in this medication.

Warnings

➤*Hypersensitivity reactions:* Serious and occasionally fatal hypersensitivity (anaphylactic) reactions, some following the first dose, have been reported in patients receiving systemic quinolones, including ofloxacin. Some reactions were accompanied by cardiovascular collapse, loss of consciousness, angioedema (including laryngeal, pharyngeal, or facial edema), airway obstruction, dyspnea, urticaria, and itching. If an allergic reaction to ofloxacin is suspected, stop the drug. Serious acute hypersensitivity reactions may require immediate emergency treatment. Administer oxygen and airway management, including intubation, as clinically indicated.

➤*Mutagenesis:* Ofloxacin was positive in the rat hepatocyte UDS assay and in the mouse lymphoma assay.

➤*Pregnancy: Category C.* Ofloxacin has been shown to have an embryocidal effect in rats at a dose of 810 mg/kg/day and in rabbits at 160 mg/kg/day. These dosages resulted in decreased fetal body weights and increased fetal mortality in rats and rabbits, respectively. Minor fetal skeletal variations were reported in rats receiving doses of 810 mg/kg/day. There are no adequate and well-controlled studies in pregnant women. Ofloxacin otic should be used during pregnancy only if the potential benefit justifies the risk to the fetus.

➤*Lactation:* In nursing women, a single 200 mg oral dose resulted in concentrations of ofloxacin in milk that were similar to those found in plasma. It is not known whether ofloxacin otic is excreted in human milk. Because of the potential for serious adverse reactions from ofloxacin in nursing infants, decide whether to discontinue nursing or to discontinue the drug, taking into account the importance of the drug to the mother.

➤*Children:* Safety and effectiveness in infants below 1 year of age have not been established.

Precautions

➤*Superinfection:* As with other anti-infective preparations, prolonged use may result in overgrowth of nonsusceptible organisms, including fungi. If the infection has not improved after 1 week, obtain cultures to guide further treatment. If otorrhea persists after a full course of therapy or if 2 or more episodes of otorrhea occur within 6 months, further evaluation is recommended to exclude an underlying condition such as cholesteatoma, foreign body, or a tumor.

Adverse Reactions

➤*Patients with otitis externa:* The following treatment-related adverse events occurred in 1% or more of the subjects with intact tympanic membranes: Pruritus (4%); application site reaction (3%); dizziness, earache, vertigo (1%).

The following treatment-related adverse events were each reported in a single subject: Dermatitis, eczema, erythematous rash, follicular rash, rash, hypesthesia, tinnitus, dyspepsia, hot flushes, flushing, and otorrhagia.

➤*Subjects with acute otitis media with tympanostomy tubes and subjects with chronic suppurative otitis media with perforated tympanic membranes:* The following treatment-related adverse events occurred in 1% or more of the subjects with nonintact tympanic membranes: Taste perversion (7%); earache, pruritus, paresthesia, rash, dizziness (1%).

Other treatment-related adverse reactions: Diarrhea, otorrhagia (0.6%); dry mouth, vertigo (0.5%); headache, tinnitus, fever, nausea, vomiting (0.3%). The following treatment-related adverse events were each reported in a single subject: Application site reaction, otitis externa, urticaria, abdominal pain, dysesthesia, hyperkinesia, halitosis, inflammation, pain, insomnia, coughing, pharyngitis, rhinitis, sinusitis, and tachycardia.

Patient Information

Avoid contaminating the applicator tip with material from the fingers or other sources. This precaution is necessary if the sterility of the drops is to be preserved. Immediately discontinue use and contact your physician at the first sign of a rash or allergic reaction.

Prior to administration, warm the solution by holding the bottle in the hand for 1 or 2 minutes to avoid dizziness, which may result from the instillation of a cold solution.

The chemotherapeutic agents include a wide range of compounds that work by various mechanisms. Although development has been directed toward agents capable of selective actions on neoplastic tissues, those presently available manifest significant toxicity on normal tissues as a major complication of therapy. Thoroughly consider the risks vs benefits of therapy when using these agents.

Because of the complexities and dangers in cancer chemotherapy, use should be restricted to, or under the direct supervision of, physicians experienced in its use. In addition to drug therapy, surgical excision and radiation therapy also are employed when appropriate.

➤*Handling of cytotoxic agents:* Most antineoplastics are toxic compounds known to be carcinogenic, mutagenic, or teratogenic. Direct contact may cause irritation of the skin, eyes, and mucous membranes. Safe and aseptic handling of parenteral chemotherapeutic drugs by medical personnel involved in preparation and administration of these agents is mandatory. Potential risks from repeated contact with parenteral antineoplastics can be controlled by a combination of specific containment equipment and proper work techniques. The NIH Division of Safety brochure outlines recommendations for safe handling of these agents.

➤*Mechanisms of action:* The mechanism of action by which these agents suppress proliferation of neoplasms is not fully understood. Generally, they affect ≥ 1 stages of cell growth or replication. Those more active at 1 specific phase of cellular growth are referred to as *cell cycle specific* agents; those that are active on both proliferating and resting cells are *cell cycle nonspecific* agents. The selectivity of cytotoxic agents inversely follows cell cycle specificity. Rapidly dividing normal tissues including bone marrow, blood components, hair follicles, and mucous membranes of the GI tract may also experience major adverse effects.

➤*Alkylating agents:* These agents form highly reactive carbonium ions that react with essential cellular components, thereby altering normal biological function. Alkylating agents replace hydrogen atoms with an alkyl radical causing cross-linking and abnormal base pairing in deoxyribonucleic acid (DNA) molecules. They also react with sulfhydryl, phosphate, and amine groups resulting in multiple lesions in both dividing and nondividing cells. The resultant defective DNA molecules are unable to carry out normal cellular reproductive functions. Examples of alkylating agents include the following:

busulfan
carboplatin
carmustine
chlorambucil
cisplatin
cyclophosphamide
dacarbazine
estramustine
ifosfamide
lomustine
mechlorethamine
melphalan
pipobroman
streptozocin
thiotepa
uracil mustard

➤*Antimetabolites:* Antimetabolites include a diverse group of compounds that interfere with various metabolic processes, thereby disrupting normal cellular functions. These agents may act by 2 general mechanisms: By incorporating the drug, rather than a normal cellular constituent, into an essential chemical compound; or by inhibiting a key enzyme from functioning normally. Their primary benefit is the ability to disrupt nucleic acid synthesis. These agents work only on dividing cells during the S phase of nucleic acid synthesis and are most effective on rapidly proliferating neoplasms. Examples of antimetabolites include the following:

cytarabine
floxuridine
5-fluorouracil
fludarabine
gemcitabine
hydroxyurea
mercaptopurine
methotrexate
thioguanine

➤*Hormones:* These have been used to treat several types of neoplasms. Hormonal therapy interferes at the cellular membrane level with growth stimulatory receptor proteins. The mechanism of action, however, is still unclear. Adrenocortical steroids are used primarily for their suppressant effect on lymphocytes in leukemias and lymphomas and as a component in many combination regimens. The counterbalancing effect of androgens, estrogens, and progestins has been used to advantage in the therapy of malignancies of tissues dependent upon these sex-related hormones (eg, tumors of the breast, endometrium, prostate). These agents have the advantage of greater specificity for tissues responsive to their effects, thus inhibiting proliferation without a direct cytotoxic action.

Examples of hormone agents include the following:
aminoglutethimide
anastrozole
bicalutamide
diethylstilbestrol
estramustine
flutamide
goserelin
leuprolide
medroxyprogesterone
megestrol
mitotane
polyestradiol
tamoxifen
testolactone

➤*Antibiotic:* Antibiotic-type agents, unlike their anti-infective relatives, are capable of disrupting cellular functions of host (mammalian) tissues. Their primary mechanisms of action are to inhibit DNA-dependent RNA synthesis and to delay or inhibit mitosis. The antibiotics are cell cycle nonspecific. Examples of antineoplastic antibiotics include the following:
bleomycin
dactinomycin
daunorubicin
doxorubicin
idarubicin
mitomycin
mitoxantrone
pentostatin
plicamycin.

➤*Mitotic inhibitors:* Mitotic inhibitor mechanisms that are not fully understood. Podophyllotoxin derivatives inhibit DNA synthesis at specific phases of the cell cycle. Vinca alkaloids bind to tubulin, the subunits of the microtubules that form the mitotic spindle. This complex inhibits microtubule assembly, causing metaphase arrest. In contrast, paclitaxel enhances the polymerization of tubulin and induces the production of stable, nonfunctional microtubules, thus inhibiting cell replication. Podophyllotoxin derivatives include etoposide and teniposide. Vinca alkaloids include vinblastine, vincristine, and vinorelbine. A new class of agents called taxanes includes paclitaxel and docetaxel.

➤*Radiopharmaceuticals:* Radiopharmaceuticals exert direct toxic effects on exposed tissue via radiation emission. Primary activity is against metastatic disease. Examples include strontium-89, sodium iodide I 131, and chromic phosphate P 32.

➤*Biological response modifiers:* Biological response modifiers have complex antineoplastic, antiviral, and immunomodulating activities. It is believed that the antitumor activity of interferons is a result of a direct antiproliferative action against tumor cells and modulation of the host immune response. Examples of biological agents include the following:
aldesleukin (human interleukin-2)
interferon alfa-2a (recombinant DNA)
interferon alfa-2b (recombinant DNA)
interferon alfa-n3 (human leukocyte)
interferon gamma-1B (recombinant DNA)

➤*Miscellaneous:* Metabolism of altretamine is required for cytotoxicity, although the mechanisms are not clear. Asparaginase is an enzyme that inhibits protein synthesis of malignant cells by inhibiting asparagine, which is required for protein synthesis. Intravesical BCG is a suspension of *Mycobacterium bovis* that promotes a local inflammatory reaction in the urinary bladder and reduces cancerous lesions. Cladribine inhibits DNA synthesis and repair through a complex mechanism. Levamisole is an immunomodulator with complex effects. Procarbazine produces toxic metabolites, which induce chromosomal breakage. Tretinoin is a retinoid related to retinol (vitamin A), which induces cytodifferentiation. Porfimer is a photosensitivity agent. Topotecan and irinotecan are topoisomerase I inhibitors.

➤*Extravasation:* This occurs when IV fluid and medication leak into interstitial tissue. Damage resulting from extravasation of certain antineoplastic agents can range from painful erythematous swelling to full-thickness injury with deep necrotic lesions requiring surgical debridement and skin grafting.

Prevention of extravasation injury – This is based on careful, accurate IV drug administration. Avoid areas of previous irradiation and extremities with poor venous circulation for IV cannula placement. Dilute drugs properly and give at an appropriate rate.

Treatment – Treatment of extravasation includes immediate discontinuation of infusion and appropriate antidote administration. Goals of treatment are palliation and prevention of severe tissue damage. For further information regarding the instillation of a specific antidote, refer to individual product monographs. Consider surgical evaluation if an open wound occurs. Some practitioners recommend leaving the IV cannula in place to aspirate some of the chemotherapeutic agent and administering an antidote to the injured site. Others recommend immediate removal of the cannula and administration of the antidote by intradermal or SC injections. Immediate removal of the cannula followed by application of ice has also been recommended for all agents except etoposide, vinblastine, and vincristine (warm compresses are recommended for these agents). Apply the ice for 15 to 20 minutes every 4 to 6 hours for the first 72 hours. Elevate the affected area.

Hydrocortisone sodium succinate or dexamethasone sodium phosphate have been used on the extravasated site for their anti-inflammatory activity. However, these agents as well as other drugs (sodium bicarbonate, DMSO) are unproven for antidote use. Specific antidotes that are recommended include sodium thiosulfate for mechlorethamine and hyaluronidase for vincristine and vinblastine.

Drugs associated with severe local necrosis (vesicants) include the following –

dacarbazine
dactinomycin
daunorubicin
doxorubicin
epirubicin
idarubicin
mechlorethamine
mitomycin
streptozocin
vinblastine
vincristine
vinorelbine

➤*Nausea and vomiting:* These may be the most prominent adverse reactions of cancer chemotherapy from the patient's perspective. In clinical trials, 17% to 98% of patients reported emesis. At least 30% of patients experience acute emesis despite antiemetic therapy. Uncontrolled emesis may cause serious complications, including dehydration, malnutrition, metabolic disorders, esophageal injury, and aspiration. In addition, the patient's quality of life may be reduced significantly. Prevention and management of nausea and vomiting is an important aspect of cancer treatment.

Antineoplastics can be categorized according to their emetogenic potential based on the frequency of emesis. Level 1 is the least emetogenic, while Level 5 is the most emetogenic. Combining antineoplastic agents may increase the overall risk for emesis. For example, a combination of drugs with the risks factors of 2 + 2 + 2 may give a combined emetogenic risk of Level 3 (or 2 + 2 + 3 = 4 and 3 + 3 + 3 = 5).

Emetogenic Potential of Antineoplastics		
Level	Frequency of emesis	Chemotherapetuic agent
1	< 10%	Bleomycin Busulfan (oral, < 4 mg/kg/day) Chlorambucil (oral) Cladribine Doxorubicin, liposomal Estramustine Floxuridine Fludarabine Hyroxyurea	Inteferon alfa Melphalan (oral) Mercaptopurine Methotrexate $\leq$ 50 mg/m^2 Pentostatin Thioguanine (oral) Tretinoin Vinblastine Vincristine Vinorelbine
2	10% to 30%	Asparaginase Cytarabine (< 1000 mg/m^2) Daunorubicin, liposomal Docetaxel Doxorubicin HCl (< 20 mg/m^2) Etoposide Fluorouracil (< 1000 mg/m^2) Denileukin diftitox	Gemcitabine Methotrexate (50 to 250 mg/m^2) Mitomycin Paclitaxel Pegaspargase Teniposide Thiotepa Topotecan
3	30% to 60%	Aldesleukin Altretamine (oral) Capecitabine (oral) Cyclophosphamide ($\leq$ 750 mg/m^2) Cyclophosphamide (oral) Dactinomycin ($\leq$ 1.5 mg/m^2) Daunorubicin ($\leq$ 50 mg/m^2)	Doxorubicin HCl (20 to 60 mg/m^2) Epirubicin Idarubicin Ifosfamide ($\leq$ 1500 mg/m^2) Methotrexate (250 to 1000 mg/m^2) Mitoxantrone (< 15 mg/m^2) Temozolomide
4	60% to 90%	Carboplatin Carmustine ($\leq$ 250 mg/m^2) Cisplatin (< 50 mg/m^2) Cyclophosphamide (750 to 1500 mg/m^2) Cytarabine ($\geq$ 1000 mg/m^2) Dactinomycin (> 1.5 mg/m^2) Daunorubicin (> 50 mg/m^2)	Doxorubicin HCl (> 60 mg/m^2) Irinotecan Lomustine ($\leq$ 60 mg/m^2) Melphalan (IV) Methotrexate ($\geq$ 1000 mg/m^2) Mitoxantrone ($\geq$ 15 mg/m^2) Procarbazine
5	> 90%	Carmustine (> 250 mg/m^2) Cisplatin ($\geq$ 50 mg/m^2) Cyclophosphamide (> 1500 mg/m^2) Dacarbazine	Ifosfamide (> 1500 mg/m^2) Lomustine (> 60 mg/m^2) Mechlorethamine Streptozocin

The incidence of emesis with these and other agents varies greatly among individuals. Dose, schedule, concomitant therapy, other medical complications, and psychologic parameters may affect the incidence, as well.

Prevention and treatment – Prevention and treatment of nausea and vomiting should include measures such as dietary adjustment, restriction of activity, and positive support. However, if pharmacologic management is necessary, several agents or groups of agents may prove useful. Some drugs that have been used with varying degrees of success, either alone or in combination, include 5-HT$_3$ receptor antagonists (such as ondansetron, dolasetron, and granisetron), phenothiazines, butyrophenones, cannabinoids, corticosteroids, antihistamines, benzodiazepines, metoclopramide, and scopolamine.

Combinations of antineoplastic agents are frequently superior to single drug therapy in the management of many diseases, leading to higher response rates and increased duration of remissions. Using agents that work by differing mechanisms may improve antineoplastic efficacy. Neoplastic cells that acquire rapid resistance to a single agent by random mutation develop resistance less rapidly when treated with a combination of agents.

Selection of agents for combination chemotherapeutic regimens is based on mechanism of drug action, cell-cycle specificity of action, responsiveness to dosage schedules, and drug toxicity.

Many lists of chemotherapy regimens have been published; most sort the regimens by the malignancy treated. Acronyms and abbreviations used to describe chemotherapy regimens can be a source of confusion and inaccuracy. Practitioners should be cautious for several reasons, including the following: 1) a given acronym may refer to several different regimens, 2) different acronyms may be used for the same regimen, 3) abbreviations are frequently cited inconsistently in the literature, and 4) inaccuracies have been propagated in the literature when regimens were cited incorrectly. Referring to a regimen by an acronym or abbreviation may cause misunderstandings and misinterpretations, with potentially serious consequences. Whenever possible, acronyms and abbreviations should not be used to order drug regimens for patients. Use of abbreviations sacrifices clarity.

As a guide, a number of commonly used combination chemotherapeutic regimens are listed below. **Note:** CI = continuous IV infusion.

5 + 2

Use:	Acute myelocytic leukemia (AML; reinduction). *Cycle:* 7 days. Regimen given once after an induction regimen has been used.
Regimen:	Cytarabine 100-200 mg/m² /day CI, days 1 through 5 *with* Daunorubicin 45 mg/m² IV, days 1 and 2 *or* Mitoxantrone 12 mg/m² IV, days 1 and 2

7 + 3

Use:	Acute myelocytic leukemia (AML; induction). *Cycle:* 7 days. Give 1 cycle only.
Regimen:	Cytarabine 100-200 mg/m² /day CI, days 1 through 7 *with* Daunorubicin 30 or 45 mg/m² IV, days 1 through 3 *or* Idarubicin 12 mg/m² IV, days 1 through 3 *or* Mitoxantrone 12 mg/m² IV, days 1 through 3

7 + 3 + 7

Use:	Acute myelogenous leukemia (AML induction - adults). *Cycle:* 21 days. Give 1 cycle. If patient has persistent leukemia at day 21, give 1 to 2 additional cycles.
Regimen:	Cytarabine 100 mg/m² /day CI, days 1 through 7 Daunorubicin 50 mg/m² /day IV, days 1 through 3 Etoposide 75 mg/m² /day IV, days 1 through 7

"8 in 1"

Use:	Brain tumors (pediatrics). *Cycle:* 14 days
Regimen:	Methylprednisolone 300 mg/m² /dose PO every 6 hours for 3 doses, day 1, starting at hour 0 Vincristine 1.5 mg/m² (2 mg maximum dose) IV, day 1, hour 0 Lomustine 100 mg/m² /day PO, day 1, hour 0 Procarbazine 75 mg/m² /day PO, day 1, hour 1 Hydroxyurea 3000 mg/m² /day PO, day 1, hour 2 Cisplatin 90 mg/m² IV, day 1, begin hour 3 (6-hour infusion) Cytarabine 300 mg/m² IV, day 1, hour 9 Dacarbazine 150 mg/m² IV, day 1, hour 12

ABV

Use:	Kaposi's sarcoma. *Cycle:* 28 days
Regimen:	Doxorubicin 40 mg/m² IV, day 1 Bleomycin 15 units IV, days 1 and 15 Vinblastine 6 mg/m² IV, day 1
Use:	Kaposi's sarcoma. *Cycle:* 28 days
Regimen:	Doxorubicin 10 mg/m² IV, days 1 and 15 Bleomycin 15 units IV, days 1 and 15 Vincristine 1 mg IV, days 1 and 15

ABVD

Use:	Lymphoma (Hodgkin's). *Cycle:* 28 days
Regimen:	Doxorubicin 25 mg/m² IV, days 1 and 15 Bleomycin 10 units/m² IV, days 1 and 15 Vinblastine 6 mg/m² IV, days 1 and 15 *with* Dacarbazine 375 mg/m² IV, days 1 and 15 *or* Dacarbazine 150 mg/m² IV, days 1 through 5

AC

Use:	Breast cancer. *Cycle:* 21 days
Regimen:	Doxorubicin 60 mg/m² IV, day 1 Cyclophosphamide 600 mg/m² IV, day 1
Use:	Sarcoma (bony). *Cycle:* 21 to 28 days
Regimen:	Doxorubicin 30 mg/m² /day CI, days 1 through 3 Cisplatin 100 mg/m² IV, day 4
Use:	Neuroblastoma (pediatrics). *Cycle:* 21 to 28 days
Regimen:	Cyclophosphamide 150 mg/m² /day PO, days 1 through 7 Doxorubicin 35 mg/m² IV, day 8

AC/Paclitaxel, Sequential

Use:	Breast cancer. *Cycle:* 21 days
Regimen:	Give 4 cycles of AC regimen for breast cancer *followed by* Paclitaxel 175 mg/m² IV, day 1 for 4 cycles

ACE (CAE)

Use:	Lung cancer (small cell). *Cycle:* 21 to 28 days
Regimen:	Cyclophosphamide 1000 mg/m² IV, day 1 Doxorubicin 45 mg/m² IV, day 1 Etoposide 50 mg/m² IV, days 1 through 5

ACe

Use:	Breast cancer. *Cycle:* 21 to 28 days
Regimen:	Cyclophosphamide 200 mg/m² /day PO, days 3 through 6 Doxorubicin 40 mg/m² IV, day 1

AD

Use:	Sarcoma (soft tissue). *Cycle:* 21 days
Regimen:	Doxorubicin 45-60 mg/m² IV, day 1 Dacarbazine 200-250 mg/m² IV, days 1 through 5

AP

Use:	Ovarian, endometrial cancer. *Cycle:* 21 to 28 days
Regimen:	Doxorubicin 50-60 mg/m² IV, day 1 Cisplatin 50-60 mg/m² IV, day 1

ARAC-DNR

Use:	Acute myelocytic leukemia (AML).
Regimen:	Cytarabine 100 mg/m² /day CI, days 1 through 7 Daunorubicin 30 or 45 mg/m² IV, days 1 through 3 If leukemia is persistent, additional doses are given: Cytarabine on days 1 through 5, daunorubicin on days 1 and 2

B-CAVe

Use:	Lymphoma (Hodgkin's). *Cycle:* 28 days
Regimen:	Bleomycin 5 units/m² IV on days 1, 28, and 35 Lomustine 100 mg/m² /day PO on day 1 Doxorubicin 60 mg/m² IV on day 1 Vinblastine 5 mg/m² IV on day 1

BCVPP

Use:	Lymphoma (Hodgkin's). *Cycle:* 28 days
Regimen:	Carmustine 100 mg/m² IV, day 1 Cyclophosphamide 600 mg/m² IV, day 1 Vinblastine 5 mg/m² IV, day 1 Procarbazine 50 mg/m² /day PO, day 1 Procarbazine 100 mg/m² /day PO, days 2 through 10 Prednisone 60 mg/m² /day PO, days 1 through 10

BEACOPP

Use:	Lymphoma (Hodgkin's). *Cycle:* 21 days
Regimen:	Bleomycin 10 units/m² IV, day 8 Etoposide 100 mg/m² IV, days 1 through 3 Doxorubicin 25 mg/m² IV, day 1 Cyclophosphamide 650 mg/m² IV, day 1 Vincristine 1.4 mg/m² (2 mg maximum dose) IV, day 1 Procarbazine 100 mg/m² /day PO, days 1 through 7 Prednisone 40 mg/m² /day PO, days 1 through 14 Filgrastim 300-480 mcg/day SC, starting on day 8, give for at least 3 days or until leukocytes exceed 2000 cells/mm³ for 3 days

BEP

Use:	Testicular cancer, germ cell tumors. *Cycle:* 21 days
Regimen:	Bleomycin 30 units IV, days 2, 9, and 16 Etoposide 100 mg/m² IV, days 1 through 5 Cisplatin 20 mg/m² IV, days 1 through 5

Bicalutamide + LHRH-A

Use:	Prostate cancer. *Cycle:* Ongoing
Regimen:	Bicalutamide 50 mg PO daily *with* Goserelin acetate 3.6 mg/dose implant SC every 28 days *or* Leuprolide depot 7.5 mg/dose IM every 28 days

BIP

Use:	Cervical cancer. *Cycle:* 21 days
Regimen:	Bleomycin 30 units/day CI, day 1 Cisplatin 50 mg/m² IV, day 2 Ifosfamide 5000 mg/m²/day CI, day 2 Mesna 6000 mg/m²/cycle CI over 36 hours, day 2 (start with ifosfamide)

BOMP

Use:	Cervical cancer. *Cycle:* 6 weeks
Regimen:	Bleomycin 10 units IM, days 1, 8, 15, 22, 29, and 36 Vincristine 1 mg/m² (2 mg maximum dose) IV, days 1, 8, 22, and 29 Cisplatin 50 mg/m² IV, days 1 and 22 Mitomycin 10 mg/m² IV, day 1

CA

Use:	Acute myelocytic leukemia (AML; induction - pediatrics). *Cycle:* 7 days. Give 2 cycles. If patient has persistent blasts at day 15, give a third cycle.
Regimen:	Cytarabine 3000 mg/m²/dose IV every 12 hours for 4 doses, days 1 and 2 Asparaginase 6000 units/m² IM, at hour 42

CABO

Use:	Head and neck cancer. *Cycle:* 21 days
Regimen:	Cisplatin 50 mg/m² IV, day 4 Methotrexate 40 mg/m² IV, days 1 and 15 Bleomycin 10 units/dose IV, days 1, 8, and 15 Vincristine 2 mg/dose IV, days 1, 8, and 15

CAE - see ACE

CAF

Use:	Breast cancer. *Cycle:* 28 days
Regimen:	Cyclophosphamide 100 mg/m²/day PO, days 1 through 14 Doxorubicin 30 mg/m² IV, days 1 and 8 Fluorouracil 500 mg/m² IV, days 1 and 8
Use:	Breast cancer. *Cycle:* 21 days
Regimen:	Cyclophosphamide 500 mg/m² IV, day 1 Doxorubicin 50 mg/m² IV, day 1 Fluorouracil 500 mg/m² IV, day 1

CAL-G

Use:	Acute lymphocytic leukemia (ALL induction - adult). *Cycle:* 4 weeks. Give 1 cycle only.
Regimen:	Cyclophosphamide 1200 mg/m² IV, day 1 Daunorubicin 45 mg/m² IV, days 1 through 3 Vincristine 2 mg IV, days 1, 8, 15, and 22 Prednisone 60 mg/m²/day PO or IV, days 1 through 21 *with* Asparaginase 6000 units/m²/day SC, days 5, 8, 11, 15, 18, and 22

CAMP

Use:	Lung cancer (non-small cell). *Cycle:* 28 days
Regimen:	Cyclophosphamide 300 mg/m²/day IV, days 1 and 8 Doxorubicin 20 mg/m² IV, days 1 and 8 Methotrexate 15 mg/m² IV, days 1 and 8 Procarbazine 100 mg/m²/day PO, days 1 through 10

CAP

Use:	Lung cancer (non-small cell). *Cycle:* 28 days
Regimen:	Cyclophosphamide 400 mg/m² IV, day 1 Doxorubicin 40 mg/m² IV, day 1 Cisplatin 60 mg/m² IV, day 1

Carbo-Tax

Use:	Ovarian cancer. *Cycle:* 21 days
Regimen:	Paclitaxel 175 mg/m² IV over 3 hours, day 1 Carboplatin IV dose by Calvert equation to AUC 7.5, day 1 (after paclitaxel) *or* Paclitaxel 185 mg/m² IV over 3 hours, day 1 Carboplatin IV dose by Calvert equation to AUC 6, day 1 (after paclitaxel)

CaT

Use:	Adenocarcinoma (unknown primary), lung cancer (non-small cell), ovarian cancer. *Cycle:* 21 days
Regimen:	Carboplatin IV dose by Calvert equation to AUC 7.5, day 1 or 2 (give after paclitaxel infusion) *with* Paclitaxel 175 mg/m² IV, day 1 *or* Paclitaxel 135 mg/m²/day CI over 24 hours, on day 1

CAV/EP

Use:	Lung cancer (small cell). *Cycle:* 42 days for 3 cycles
Regimen:	Cyclophosphamide 1000 mg/m² IV, day 1 Doxorubicin 50 mg/m² IV, day 1 Vincristine 1.2 mg/m² IV, day 1 Etoposide 100 mg/m²/day IV, days 22 and 23 and 24 Cisplatin 25 mg/m²/day IV, days 22 and 23 and 24

CAV (VAC)

Use:	Lung cancer (small cell). *Cycle:* 21 days
Regimen:	Cyclophosphamide 1000 mg/m² IV, day 1 Doxorubicin 40-50 mg/m² IV, day 1 Vincristine 1-1.4 mg/m² (2 mg maximum dose) IV, day 1

CAVE

Use:	Lung cancer (small cell). *Cycle:* 21 days
Regimen:	**Add to CAV**: Etoposide 100 mg/m² IV, days 2 through 4

CA-VP16

Use:	Lung cancer (small cell). *Cycle:* 21 days
Regimen:	Cyclophosphamide 1000 mg/m² IV, day 1 Doxorubicin 45 mg/m² IV, day 1 Etoposide 80 mg/m²/day, days 1 through 3

CC

Uses:	Ovarian cancer. *Cycle:* 28 days
Regimen:	Cyclophosphamide 600 mg/m² IV, day 1 Carboplatin 300-350 mg/m² IV, day 1

CDB

Use:	Melanoma. *Cycle:* 21 days
Regimen:	Cisplatin 25 mg/m²/day IV, days 1 through 3 Dacarbazine 220 mg/m² IV, days 1 through 3 Carmustine 150 mg/m² IV, day 1 of odd-numbered cycles only (eg, cycle 1, 3, 5)

CDDP/VP-16

Use:	Brain tumors (pediatrics). *Cycle:* 21 days
Regimen:	Cisplatin 90 mg/m² IV, day 1 Etoposide 150 mg/m² IV, days 3 and 4

CDE

Use:	Lymphoma (HIV-related, non-Hodgkins - adult). *Cycle:* 28 days
Regimen:	Cyclophosphamide 200 mg/m²/day CI, days 1 through 4 Doxorubicin 12.5 mg/m²/day CI, days 1 through 4 Etoposide 60 mg/m²/day CI, days 1 through 4 Filgrastim 5 mcg/kg/day SC starting on day 6, at least 24 hours after the end of the CIs, and ending when the absolute neutrophil count (ANC) is at least 10,000 cells/mm³

CEF

Use:	Breast cancer. *Cycle:* 28 days
Regimen:	Cyclophosphamide 75 mg/m²/day PO, days 1 through 14 Epirubicin 60 mg/m² IV, days 1 and 8 Fluorouracil 500 mg/m² IV, days 1 and 8 Cotrimoxazole 2 tablets PO twice daily, days 1 through 28

CEPP(B)

Use:	Lymphoma (non-Hodgkin's). *Cycle:* 28 days
Regimen:	Cyclophosphamide 600-650 mg/m² IV, days 1 and 8 Etoposide 70-85 mg/m² IV, days 1 through 3 Prednisone 60 mg/m²/day PO, days 1 through 10 *may or may not give with* Bleomycin 15 units/m² IV, days 1 and 15

CEV

Use:	Lung cancer (small cell). *Cycle:* 21 days
Regimen:	Cyclophosphamide 1000 mg/m² IV, day 1 Etoposide 50 mg/m² IV, day 1 Etoposide 100 mg/m²/day PO, days 2 through 5 Vincristine 1.4 mg/m² (2 mg maximum dose) IV, day 1

CF

Use:	Adenocarcinoma, head and neck cancer. *Cycle:* 21 to 28 days
Regimen:	Cisplatin 100 mg/m² IV, day 1 Fluorouracil 1000 mg/m²/day CI, days 1 through 4 or days 1 through 5
Use:	Head and neck cancer. *Cycle:* 21 to 28 days
Regimen:	Carboplatin 400 mg/m² IV, day 1 Fluorouracil 1000 mg/m²/day CI, days 1 through 4 or days 1 through 5

CFM - see CNF

CHAMOCA (Modified Bagshawe)

Use:	Gestational trophoblastic neoplasm. *Cycle*: At least 18 days, as toxicity permits
Regimen:	Hydroxyurea 500 mg/dose PO every 6 hours for 4 doses, day 1 (start at 6 am) Dactinomycin 0.2 mg IV, days 1 through 3 (give at 7 pm) Dactinomycin 0.5 mg IV, days 4 and 5 (give at 7 pm) Cyclophosphamide 500 mg/m² IV, days 3 and 8 (give at 7 pm) Vincristine 1 mg/m² IV (2 mg maximum dose), day 2 (give at 7 am) Methotrexate 100 mg/m² IV push, day 2 (give at 7 pm) Methotrexate 200 mg/m² IV over 12 hours, day 2 (give after IV push dose) Leucovorin 14 mg/dose IM every 6 hours for 6 doses, days 3 through 5 (begin at 7 pm on day 3) Doxorubicin 30 mg/m² IV, day 8 (give at 7 pm)

CHAP

Use:	Ovarian cancer. *Cycle*: 28 days
Regimen:	Cyclophosphamide 150 mg/m²/day PO, days 2 through 8 *or* Cyclophosphamide 400 mg/m²/day IV, day 1 *with* Altretamine 150 mg/m²/day PO, days 2 through 8 Doxorubicin 30 mg/m² IV, day 1 Cisplatin 50-60 mg/m² IV, day 1

ChlVPP

Use:	Lymphoma (Hodgkin's). *Cycle*: 28 days
Regimen:	Chlorambucil 6 mg/m²/day (10 mg/day maximum dose) PO, days 1 through 14 Vinblastine 6 mg/m² (10 mg/day maximum dose) IV, days 1 and 8 Procarbazine 100 mg/m²/day (150 mg/day maximum dose) PO, days 1 through 14 Prednisone 40-50 mg/day PO, days 1 through 14* *Note: Prednisolone is recommended in the British literature. In the US, prednisone is the preferred corticosteroid. The doses of these 2 corticosteroids are equivalent (ie, prednisone 40 mg PO = prednisolone 40 mg PO).

ChlVPP/EVA

Use:	Lymphoma (Hodgkin's). *Cycle*: 28 days
Regimen:	**See ChlVPP, except:** Chlorambucil, Procarbazine, and Prednisone* days 1 through 7 and Vinblastine day 1 only *with* Etoposide 200 mg/m² IV, day 8 Vincristine 2 mg IV, day 8 Doxorubicin 50 mg/m² IV, day 8 *Note: Prednisolone is recommended in the British literature. In the US, prednisone is the preferred corticosteroid. The doses of these 2 corticosteroids are equivalent (ie, prednisone 40 mg PO = prednisolone 40 mg PO).

CHOP

Use:	Lymphoma (non-Hodgkin's), HIV-related lymphoma. *Cycle*: 21 to 28 days
Regimen:	Cyclophosphamide 750 mg/m² IV, day 1 Doxorubicin 50 mg/m² IV, day 1 Vincristine 1.4 mg/m² (2 mg maximum dose) IV, day 1 Prednisone 100 mg/day PO, days 1 through 5

CHOP-BLEO

Use:	Lymphoma (non-Hodgkin's). *Cycle*: 21 to 28 days
Regimen:	**Add to CHOP:** Bleomycin 15 units/day IV, days 1 through 5

CISCA

Use:	Bladder cancer. *Cycle*: 21 to 28 days
Regimen:	Cyclophosphamide 650 mg/m² IV, day 1 Doxorubicin 50 mg/m² IV, day 1 Cisplatin 100 mg/m² IV, day 2

CISCA II /VB IV

Use:	Germ cell tumors. *Cycle*: Individualized based on duration of myelosuppression
Regimen:	Cyclophosphamide 500 mg/m² IV, days 1 and 2 Doxorubicin 40-45 mg/m² IV, days 1 and 2 Cisplatin 100-120 mg/m² IV, day 3 *alternating with* Vinblastine 3 mg/m²/day CI, days 1 through 5 Bleomycin 30 units/day CI, days 1 through 5

Cisplatin-Docetaxel

Use:	Bladder cancer. *Cycle*: Every 7 days for 8 weeks
Regimen:	Cisplatin 30 mg/m² IV, day 1 Docetaxel 40 mg/m² IV, day 4

Cisplatin-Fluorouracil

Use:	Cervical cancer. *Cycle*: 21 days
Regimen:	Cisplatin 75 mg/m² IV, day 1 *followed by* Fluorouracil 1000 mg/m²/day CI, for 96 hours total *Used in conjunction with* Radiation therapy
Use:	Cervical cancer. *Cycle*: 28 days
Regimen:	Cisplatin 50 mg/m² IV, day 1 starting 4 hours *before* external beam radiotherapy. Fluorouracil 1000 mg/m²/day CI, days 2 through 5

Cisplatin-Vinorelbine

Use:	Cervical cancer. *Cycle*: 21 days
Regimen:	Cisplatin 80 mg/m² IV, day 1 Vinorelbine 25 mg/m² IV, days 1 and 8

CLD-BOMP

Use:	Cervical cancer. *Cycle*: 21 days
Regimen:	Bleomycin 5 units/day CI, days 1 through 7 Cisplatin 10 mg/m² IV, days 1 through 7 Vincristine 0.7 mg/m² IV, day 7 Mitomycin 7 mg/m² IV, day 7

CMF

Use:	Breast cancer. *Cycle*: 28 days
Regimen:	Methotrexate 40-60 mg/m² IV, days 1 and 8 Fluorouracil 600 mg/m² IV, days 1 and 8 *with* Cyclophosphamide 100 mg/m²/day PO, days 1 through 14 *or* Cyclophosphamide 750 mg/m² IV, day 1

CMF-IV

Use:	Breast cancer. *Cycle*: 21 days
Regimen:	Cyclophosphamide 600 mg/m² IV, day 1 Methotrexate 40 mg/m² IV, day 1 Fluorouracil 600 mg/m² IV, day 1

CMFP

Use:	Breast cancer. *Cycle*: 28 days
Regimen:	Cyclophosphamide 100 mg/m²/day PO, days 1 through 14 Methotrexate 30-40 mg/m²/day IV, days 1 and 8 Fluorouracil 400-600 mg/m²/day IV, days 1 and 8 Prednisone 40 mg/m²/day PO, days 1 through 14

CMFVP

Use:	Breast cancer. *Cycle*: 28 days
Regimen:	Cyclophosphamide 400 mg/m² IV, day 1 Methotrexate 30 mg/m² IV, days 1 and 8 Fluorouracil 400 mg/m² IV, days 1 and 8 Vincristine 1 mg IV, days 1 and 8 Prednisone 80 mg/day PO, days 1 through 7

C-MOPP - see COPP

CMV

Use:	Bladder cancer. *Cycle*: 21 days
Regimen:	Cisplatin 100 mg/m² IV, day 2 (at least 12 hours after methotrexate) Methotrexate 30 mg/m² IV, days 1 and 8 Vinblastine 4 mg/m² IV, days 1 and 8

CNF

Use:	Breast cancer. *Cycle*: 21 days
Regimen:	Cyclophosphamide 500 mg/m² IV, day 1 Mitoxantrone 10 mg/m² IV, day 1 Fluorouracil 500 mg/m² IV, day 1

CNOP

Use:	Lymphoma (non-Hodgkin's). *Cycle*: 21 to 28 days
Regimen:	Cyclophosphamide 750 mg/m² IV, day 1 Mitoxantrone 12 mg/m² IV, day 1 Vincristine 1.4 mg/m² (2 mg maximum dose) IV, day 1 Prednisone 50 mg/m²/day PO, days 1 through 5

COB

Use:	Head and neck cancer. *Cycle*: 21 days
Regimen:	Cisplatin 100 mg/m² IV, day 1 Vincristine 1 mg IV, days 2 and 5 Bleomycin 30 units/day CI, days 2 through 5

CODE

Use: Lung cancer (small cell). *Cycle*: 9 week regimen

Regimen: Cisplatin 25 mg/m² IV, every week for 9 weeks
Vincristine 1 mg/m² (2 mg maximum dose) IV weekly, weeks 1, 2, 4, 6, and 8
Doxorubicin 40 mg/m² IV weekly, weeks 1, 3, 5, 7, and 9
Etoposide 80 mg/m² IV day 1 of weeks 1, 3, 5, 7, and 9
Etoposide 80 mg/m²/day PO, days 2 and 3 of weeks 1, 3, 5, 7, and 9
used in conjunction with
Prednisone 50 mg PO daily for 5 weeks, alternate days until chemotherapy completion, then taper over 2 weeks

COMLA

Use: Lymphoma (non-Hodgkin's). *Cycle*: 78-85 days

Regimen: Cyclophosphamide 1500 mg/m² IV, day 1
Vincristine 1.4 mg/m² (2 mg maximum dose) IV, days 1, 8, and 15
Methotrexate 120 mg/m² IV, days 22, 29, 36, 43, 50, 57, 64, and 71
Leucovorin 25 mg/m²/dose PO every 6 hours for 4 doses, beginning 24 hours after each methotrexate dose
Cytarabine 300 mg/m² IV, days 22, 29, 36, 43, 50, 57, 64, and 71

COMP

Use: Lymphoma (Hodgkin's - pediatrics). *Cycle*: 28 days

Regimen: Cyclophosphamide 1200 mg/m² IV, day 1
Vincristine 2 mg/m² (2 mg maximum dose) IV, days 3, 10, 17, and 24
Methotrexate 300 mg/m² IV, day 12
Prednisone 60 mg/m²/day (60 mg/day maximum) PO in 4 divided doses, days 3 through 30, then taper for 7 days

Cooper Regimen

Use: Breast cancer. *Cycle*: 36 weeks

Regimen: Cyclophosphamide 2 mg/kg/day PO, weeks 1 through 36
Methotrexate 0.7 mg/kg IV weekly, weeks 1 through 8
Methotrexate 0.7 mg/kg IV every other week, weeks 10, 12, 14, 16, 18, 20, 22, 24, 26, 28, 30, 32, 34, and 36
Fluorouracil 12 mg/kg IV weekly, weeks 1 through 8
Fluorouracil 12 mg/kg IV every other week, weeks 10, 12, 14, 16, 18, 20, 22, 24, 26, 28, 30, 32, 34, and 36
Vincristine 0.035 mg/kg IV (2 mg maximum dose) weekly, weeks 1 through 5
Vincristine 0.035 mg/kg IV monthly, weeks 8, 12, 16, 20, 24, 28, 32, and 36
Prednisone 0.75 mg/kg/day PO, days 1 through 10, then taper off over next 40 days

COP

Use: Lymphoma (non-Hodgkin's). *Cycle*: 14 to 28 days

Regimen: Cyclophosphamide 800-1000 mg/m² IV, day 1
Vincristine 2 mg IV, day 1
Prednisone 60 mg/m²/day (or 100 mg/day) PO, days 1 through 5, then taper off over next 3 days

COPE

Use: Lung cancer (small cell). *Cycle*: 21 days

Regimen: Cyclophosphamide 750 mg/m² IV, day 1
Vincristine 2 mg/cycle IV, day 14
Cisplatin 50 mg/m² IV, day 2
Etoposide 100 mg/m² IV, days 1 through 3

COPE (Baby Brain I)

Use: Brain tumors (pediatrics). *Cycle*: 28 days, alternate cycles AABAAB

Regimen: **Cycle A:**
Vincristine 0.065 mg/kg (1.5 mg maximum dose) IV, days 1 and 8
Cyclophosphamide 65 mg/kg IV, day 1
Cycle B: Cisplatin 4 mg/kg IV, day 1
Etoposide 6.5 mg/kg IV, days 3 and 4

COPP (C-MOPP)

Use: Lymphoma (non-Hodgkin's or Hodgkin's). *Cycle*: 28 days

Regimen: Cyclophosphamide 450-650 mg/m² IV, days 1 and 8
Vincristine 1.4-2 mg/m² (2 mg maximum dose) IV, days 1 and 8
Procarbazine 100 mg/m²/day PO, days 1 through 14
Prednisone 40 mg/m²/day PO, cycles 1 and 4,* days 1 through 14
*Note: Some clinicians give prednisone with every cycle of COPP. The original clinical trials gave prednisone only with the first and fourth cycles.

CP

Use: Chronic lymphocytic leukemia (CLL). *Cycle*: 14 days

Regimen: Chlorambucil 30 mg/m²/day PO, day 1
Prednisone 80 mg/day PO, days 1 through 5

Use: Ovarian cancer. *Cycle*: 21 to 28 days

Regimen: Cyclophosphamide 600-1000 mg/m² IV, day 1
Cisplatin 60-80 mg/m² IV, day 1

CT

Use: Ovarian cancer. *Cycle*: 21 days

Regimen: Cisplatin 75 mg/m² IV, day 2 (given after paclitaxel)
Paclitaxel 135 mg/m²/day CI, day 1

CVD

Use: Malignant melanoma. *Cycle*: 21 days

Regimen: Cisplatin 20 mg/m² IV, days 2 through 5
Vinblastine 1.6 mg/m² IV, days 1 through 5
Dacarbazine 800 mg/m² IV, day 1

CVD + IL-2I

Use: Malignant melanoma. *Cycle*: 21 days

Regimen: Cisplatin 20 mg/m² IV, days 1 through 4
Vinblastine 1.6 mg/m² IV, days 1 through 4
Dacarbazine 800 mg/m² IV, day 1
Aldesleukin 9 million units/m²/day CI, days 1 through 4
Interferon alfa 5 million units/m²/day SC, days 1 through 5, 7, 9, 11, and 13

CVI (VIC)

Use: Lung cancer (non-small cell). *Cycle*: 28 days

Regimen: Carboplatin 300-350 mg/m² IV, day 1
Etoposide 60-100 mg/m² IV, days 1, 3, and 5
Ifosfamide 1500 mg/m² IV, days 1, 3, and 5
Mesna 400 mg/m² IV before ifosfamide given, days 1, 3, and 5
Mesna 1600 mg/m²/day CI, days 1, 3, and 5 (give after mesna bolus)

CVP

Use: Lymphoma (non-Hodgkin's), chronic lymphocytic leukemia (CLL). *Cycle*: 21 days

Regimen: Cyclophosphamide 300-400 mg/m²/day PO, days 1 through 5
Vincristine 1.4 mg/m² (2 mg maximum dose) IV, day 1
Prednisone 100 mg/m²/day PO, days 1 through 5

CVPP

Use: Lymphoma (Hodgkin's). *Cycle*: 28 days

Regimen: Lomustine 75 mg/m²/day PO, day 1
Vinblastine 4 mg/m² IV, days 1 and 8
Procarbazine 100 mg/m²/day PO, days 1 through 14
Prednisone 40 mg/m²/day PO, cycles 1 and 4, days 1 through 14

CYVADIC

Use: Sarcoma (bony or soft tissue). *Cycle*: 21 days

Regimen: Cyclophosphamide 500 mg/m² IV, day 1
Vincristine 1 mg/m² (2 mg maximum dose) IV, days 1 and 5
Doxorubicin 50 mg/m² IV, day 1
Dacarbazine 250 mg/m² IV, days 1 through 5

DA

Use: Acute myelocytic leukemia (AML; induction - pediatrics).

Regimen: Daunorubicin 45-60 mg/m² IV, days 1 through 3
Cytarabine 100 mg/m²/day CI, days 1 through 7

DAT

Use: Acute myelocytic leukemia (AML; induction - pediatrics). *Cycle*: 14 to 21 days

Regimen: Daunorubicin 60 mg/m²/day CI, days 5 through 7
Cytarabine 100 mg/m² IV every 12 hours, days 1 through 7
Thioguanine 100 mg/m²/day PO, every 12 hours, day 1 through 7

DAV

Use: Acute myelocytic leukemia (AML; induction - pediatrics). *Cycle*: Give a single cycle.

Regimen: Daunorubicin 60 mg/m² IV, days 3 through 5
Cytarabine 100 mg/m²/day CI, days 1 through 2
Cytarabine 100 mg/m²/dose IV every 12 hours for 12 doses, days 3 through 8
Etoposide 150 mg/m²/day IV, days 6 through 8

DCT

Use: Acute myelocytic leukemia (AML; adult induction). *Cycle*: 7 days. Give once. May be given a second time based on individual response. Time between cycles not specified.

Regimen: Daunorubicin 40 mg/m² IV, days 1 through 3
Cytarabine 100 mg/m²/dose IV every 12 hours, days 1 through 7
Thioguanine 100 mg/m²/dose PO every 12 hours, days 1 through 7

DHAP

Use: Lymphoma (non-Hodgkin's). *Cycle*: 21 to 28 days

Regimen: Cisplatin 100 mg/m²/day CI, day 1
Cytarabine 2000 mg/m² IV every 12 hours for 2 doses (total dose, 4000 mg/m²), day 2
Dexamethasone 40 mg/day PO or IV, days 1 through 4

DI

Use:	Sarcoma (soft-tissue). *Cycle*: 21 days
Regimen:	Doxorubicin 50 mg/m²/day IV, day 1 Ifosfamide 5000 mg/m²/day CI, day 1 (after doxorubicin given) Mesna 600 mg/m² IV bolus before ifosfamide infusion Mesna 2500 mg/m²/day CI over 36 hours

Docetaxel-Cisplatin

Use:	Lung cancer (non-small cell). *Cycle*: 21 days
Regimen:	Docetaxel 75 mg/m² IV, day 1 Cisplatin 75 mg/m² IV, day 1 (after docetaxel)

Dox ➡ CMF, Sequential

Use:	Breast cancer. *Cycle*: 21 days
Regimen:	Doxorubicin 75 mg/m² IV, day 1 for 4 cycles *followed by* CMF-IV for 8 cycles

DTIC/Tamoxifen

Use:	Malignant melanoma. *Cycle*: 21 days
Regimen:	Dacarbazine 250 mg/m² IV, days 1 through 5 Tamoxifen 20 mg/m²/day PO, days 1 through 5

DVP

Use:	Acute lymphocytic leukemia (ALL; induction - pediatric). *Cycle*: 35 days. Give a single cycle.
Regimen:	Daunorubicin 25 mg/m² IV, days 1, 8, and 15 Vincristine 1.5 mg/m² (2 mg maximum dose) IV, days 1, 8, 15, and 22 Prednisone 60 mg/m²/day PO, days 1 through 28 then taper over next 14 days *used in conjunction with* intrathecal chemotherapy

EAP

Use:	Gastric, small bowel cancer. *Cycle*: 21 to 28 days
Regimen:	Etoposide 100-120 mg/m² IV, days 4 through 6 Doxorubicin 20 mg/m² IV, days 1 and 7 Cisplatin 40 mg/m² IV, days 2 and 8

EC

Use:	Lung cancer. *Cycle*: 21 to 28 days
Regimen:	Etoposide 100-120 mg/m² IV, days 1 through 3 Carboplatin 300-350 mg/m² IV, day 1 *or* Carboplatin IV dose by Calvert equation to AUC 6, day 1

EFP

Use:	Gastric, small bowel cancer. *Cycle*: 21 to 28 days
Regimen:	Etoposide 80-100 mg/m² IV, days 1, 3, and 5 Fluorouracil 800-900 mg/m²/day CI, days 1 through 5 Cisplatin 20 mg/m² IV, days 1 through 5

ELF

Use:	Gastric cancer. *Cycle*: 21 to 28 days
Regimen:	Etoposide 120 mg/m² IV, days 1 through 3 Leucovorin 300 mg/m² IV, days 1 through 3 Fluorouracil 500 mg/m² IV, days 1 through 3 (after leucovorin)

EMA 86

Use:	Acute myelocytic leukemia (AML; adult induction). *Cycle*: Give a single cycle.
Regimen:	Mitoxantrone 12 mg/m² IV, days 1 through 3 Etoposide 200 mg/m²/day CI, days 8 through 10 Cytarabine 500 mg/m²/day CI, days 1 through 3 and days 8 through 10

EP

Use:	Testicular cancer. *Cycle*: 21 days
Regimen:	Etoposide 100 mg/m² IV, days 1 through 5 Cisplatin 20 mg/m² IV, days 1 through 5
Use:	Lung cancer, adenocarcinoma. *Cycle*: 21 to 28 days
Regimen:	Etoposide 80-120 mg/m² IV, days 1 through 3 Cisplatin 80-100 mg/m² IV, day 1

ESHAP

Use:	Lymphoma (non-Hodgkin's). *Cycle*: 21 to 28 days
Regimen:	Methylprednisolone 250-500 mg/day IV, days 1 through 4 or 1 through 5 Etoposide 40-60 mg/m² IV, days 1 through 4 Cytarabine 2000 mg/m² IV, day 5 (after etoposide and cisplatin finished) Cisplatin 25 mg/m²/day CI, days 1 through 4

Estramustine/Vinblastine

Use:	Prostate cancer. *Cycle*: 8 weeks
Regimen:	Estramustine 10 mg/kg/day PO given in 3 divided doses, days 1 through 42 Vinblastine 4 mg/m² IV weekly, weeks 1 through 6

EVA

Use:	Lymphoma (Hodgkin's). *Cycle*: 28 days
Regimen:	Etoposide 100 mg/m² IV, days 1 through 3 Vinblastine 6 mg/m² IV, day 1 Doxorubicin 50 mg/m² IV, day 1

FAC

Use:	Breast cancer. *Cycle*: 21 to 28 days
Regimen:	Fluorouracil 500 mg/m² IV, days 1 and 8 Doxorubicin 50 mg/m² IV, day 1 Cyclophosphamide 500 mg/m² IV, day 1

FAM

Use:	Adenocarcinoma, gastric cancer. *Cycle*: 8 weeks
Regimen:	Fluorouracil 600 mg/m²/day IV, days 1, 8, 29, and 36 Doxorubicin 30 mg/m²/day IV, days 1 and 29 Mitomycin 10 mg/m² IV, day 1

FAMTX

Use:	Gastric cancer. *Cycle*: 28 days
Regimen:	Methotrexate 1500 mg/m² IV, day 1 Fluorouracil 1500 mg/m² IV, day 1 (give after methotrexate given) Leucovorin 15 mg/m²/dose PO every 6 hours for 8 doses (start 24 hours after methotrexate); increase dose to 30 mg/m²/dose PO every 6 hours for 16 doses if 24-hour methotrexate level at least 2.5 mol/L Doxorubicin 30 mg/m² IV, day 15

FAP

Use:	Gastric cancer. *Cycle*: 5 weeks
Regimen:	Fluorouracil 300 mg/m² IV, days 1 through 5 Doxorubicin 40 mg/m² IV, day 1 Cisplatin 60 mg/m² IV, day 1

F-CL (FU/LV)

Use:	Colorectal cancer. *Cycle*: 4 to 8 weeks
Regimen:	Fluorouracil 600 mg/m² IV, weekly for 6 weeks (after starting leucovorin), then 2-week rest period Leucovorin 500 mg/m² IV, weekly for 6 weeks, then 2-week rest period *or* Fluorouracil 370-425 mg/m² IV, days 1 through 5 (after starting leucovorin) Leucovorin 20 mg/m² IV, days 1 through 5

FEC

Use:	Breast cancer. *Cycle*: 21 days
Regimen:	Fluorouracil 500 mg/m² IV, day 1 Cyclophosphamide 500 mg/m² IV, day 1 Epirubicin 100 mg/m² IV, day 1

FED

Use:	Lung cancer (non-small cell). *Cycle*: 21 days
Regimen:	Fluorouracil 960 mg/m²/day CI, days 2 through 4 Etoposide 80 mg/m² IV, days 2 through 4 Cisplatin 100 mg/m² IV, day 1

FL

Use:	Prostate cancer. *Cycle*: Ongoing
Regimen:	Flutamide 250 mg/dose PO every 8 hours *with* Leuprolide acetate 1 mg SC daily *or* Leuprolide depot 7.5 mg IM/dose, every 28 days *or* Leuprolide depot 22.5 mg IM/dose, every 3 months

Fle

Use:	Colorectal cancer. *Cycle*: 1 year
Regimen:	Fluorouracil 450 mg/m² IV, days 1 through 5 Fluorouracil 450 mg/m² IV weekly, weeks 5 through 52 Levamisole 50 mg/dose PO every 8 hours, days 1 through 3 of every other week for 1 year

FNC - see CNF

FU/LV - see F-CL

FU/LV/CPT-11

Use:	Metastatic colorectal cancer.* Cycle: 42 days
Regimen:	Fluorouracil 500 mg/m² IV, days 1, 8, 15, and 22 Leucovorin 20 mg/m² IV, days 1, 8, 15, and 22 Irinotecan 125 mg/m² IV, days 1, 8, 15, and 22 *Note: A recent study analysis found an increased risk of early deaths (within 60 days of initiating treatment) with use of this regimen. Specific risk factors that may have contributed to death were not identified. Intensive patient monitoring and dosage modification is recommended to reduce the risk of severe adverse effects.

FUP

Use:	Gastric cancer. Cycle: 28 days
Regimen:	Fluorouracil 1000 mg/m²/day CI, days 1 through 5 Cisplatin 100 mg/m² IV, day 2

FZ

Use:	Prostate cancer. Cycle: Ongoing
Regimen:	Flutamide 250 mg/dose PO every 8 hours with Goserelin acetate 3.6 mg/dose implant SC every 28 days or Goserelin acetate 10.8 mg/dose implant SC every 12 weeks

Gemcitabine-Carboplatin

Use:	Lung cancer (non-small cell). Cycle: 28 days
Regimen:	Gemcitabine 1000 mg/m² or 1100 mg/m² IV, days 1 and 8 Carboplatin IV dose by Calvert equation to AUC 5, day 8

Gemcitabine-Cis

Use:	Lung cancer (non-small cell). Cycle: 28 days
Regimen:	Gemcitabine 1000-1200 mg/m² IV, days 1, 8, and 15 Cisplatin 100 mg/m²/cycle IV, day 1, 2, or 15

Gemcitabine-Cisplatin

Use:	Metastatic bladder cancer. Cycle: 28 days up to 6 cycles
Regimen:	Gemcitabine 1000 mg/m² IV, days 1, 8, and 15 Cisplatin 70 mg/m² IV, day 2

Gemcitabine-Vinorelbine

Use:	Lung cancer (non-small cell). Cycle: 21 days up to 6 cycles
Regimen:	Gemcitabine 1200 mg/m² IV, days 1 and 8 Vinorelbine 30 mg/m² IV, days 1 and 8
Use:	Lung cancer (non-small cell). Cycle: 28 days up to 6 cycles
Regimen:	Gemcitabine 800 mg/m² or 1000 mg/m² IV, days 1, 8, and 15 Vinorelbine 20 mg/m² IV, days 1, 8, and 15

HDMTX

Use:	Sarcoma (bony). Cycle: 1 to 4 weeks
Regimen:	Methotrexate 8000-12,000 mg/m² (20,000 mg maximum dose) IV, day 1 Leucovorin 15 mg/m²/dose PO or IV every 6 hours for 10 doses, beginning 20 to 30 hours after beginning of methotrexate infusion

Hexa-CAF

Use:	Ovarian cancer. Cycle: 28 days
Regimen:	Altretamine 150 mg/m²/day PO, days 1 through 14 Cyclophosphamide 100-150 mg/m²/day PO, days 1 through 14 Methotrexate 40 mg/m² IV, days 1 and 8 Fluorouracil 600 mg/m² IV, days 1 and 8

Hi-C DAZE

Use:	Acute myelogenous leukemia (AML induction - pediatrics). Cycle: Give a single cycle.
Regimen:	Daunorubicin 30 mg/m² IV, days 1 through 3 Cytarabine 3000 mg/m²/dose IV every 12 hours, days 1 through 4 (total of 8 doses) Etoposide 200 mg/m² IV, days 1 through 3 and days 6 through 8 5-azacytidine* 150 mg/m² IV, days 3 through 5 and days 8 through 10 *Note: 5-azacytidine is an investigational Group C drug. Although it is not currently marketed in the US, the product may be obtained from the NCI.

ICE - see MICE

ICE Protocol - see Idarubicin, Cytarabine, Etoposide

ICE-T

Use:	Breast cancer, sarcoma, lung cancer (non-small cell). Cycle: 28 days
Regimen:	Ifosfamide 1250 mg/m² IV, days 1 through 3 Carboplatin 300 mg/m² IV, day 1 Etoposide 80 mg/m² IV, days 1 through 3 Paclitaxel 175 mg/m² IV, day 4 with Mesna 20% of ifosfamide dose IV before, then mesna 40% of ifosfamide dose PO given 4 and 8 hours after ifosfamide or Mesna 1250 mg/m² IV, days 1 through 3

IDA-based BF 12 - see Idarubicin, Cytarabine, Etoposide

Idarubicin, Cytarabine, Etoposide (ICE Protocol)

Use:	Acute myelogenous leukemia (AML induction - adults). Cycle: Give a single cycle
Regimen:	Idarubicin 6 mg/m² IV, days 1 through 5 Cytarabine 600 mg/m² IV, days 1 through 5 Etoposide 150 mg/m² IV, days 1 through 3

Idarubicin, Cytarabine, Etoposide (IDA-based BF 12)

Use:	Acute myelogenous leukemia (AML induction - adults). Cycle: Usually 1 cycle used. A second cycle may be considered for patients with partial response. Time between cycles not specified.
Regimen:	Idarubicin 5 mg/m² IV, days 1 through 5 Cytarabine 2000 mg/m²/dose IV every 12 hours, days 1 through 5 (total of 10 doses) Etoposide 100 mg/m² IV, days 1 through 5

IDMTX/6-MP

Use:	Acute lymphocytic leukemia (ALL; consolidation - pediatrics). Cycle: 2 weeks, up to 12 cycles
Regimen:	**Week 1:** Methotrexate 200 mg/m² IV bolus, day 1 Mercaptopurine 200 mg/m² IV bolus, day 1 then Methotrexate 800 mg/m²/day CI, day 1 Mercaptopurine 800 mg/m² IV over 8 hours, day 1 Leucovorin 5 mg/m²/dose PO or IV every 6 hours for 5-13 doses, beginning 24 hours after methotrexate infusion finished. **Week 2:** Methotrexate 20 mg/m² IM day 8 Mercaptopurine 50 mg/m² PO, days 8 through 14

IE

Use:	Sarcoma (soft-tissue). Cycle: 21 days
Regimen:	Ifosfamide 1800 mg/m² IV, days 1 through 5 Etoposide 100 mg/m² IV, days 1 through 5 with Mesna 1800 mg/m² IV, days 1 through 5 or Mesna 20% of ifosfamide dose prior to, then 4 and 8 hours after ifosfamide

IfoVP

Use:	Sarcoma (osteosarcoma - pediatrics). Cycle: 21 days
Regimen:	Ifosfamide 1800 mg/m² IV, days 1 through 5 Etoposide 100 mg/m² IV, days 1 through 5 Mesna 1800 mg/m² IV, days 1 through 5

Interleukin 2-Interferon alfa 2

Use:	Renal cell carcinoma. Cycle: 56 days
Regimen:	Aldesleukin 20 million units/m²/dose SC 3 times weekly, weeks 1 and 4 Aldesleukin 5 million units/m²/dose SC 3 times weekly, weeks 2, 3, 5, and 6 Interferon alfa 6 million units/m²/dose SC once weekly, weeks 1 and 4 Interferon alfa 6 million units/m²/dose SC 3 times weekly, weeks 2, 3, 5, and 6

IPA

Use:	Hepatoblastoma (pediatrics). Cycle: 21 days
Regimen:	Ifosfamide 500 mg/m² IV bolus, day 1 Ifosfamide 1000 mg/m²/day CI, days 1 through 3 Cisplatin 20 mg/m² IV, days 4 through 8 Doxorubicin 30 mg/m²/day CI, days 9 and 10

Linker Protocol

Use: Acute lymphocytic leukemia (ALL; induction and consolidation).

Regimen: **Remission induction.** Give 1 cycle only.
Daunorubicin 50 mg/m² IV, days 1 through 3
Vincristine 2 mg IV, days 1, 8, 15, and 22
Prednisone 60 mg/m²/day PO, days 1 through 28
Asparaginase 6000 units/m² IM, days 17 through 28
If residual leukemia in marrow on day 14:
Daunorubicin 50 mg/m² IV, day 15
If residual leukemia in marrow on day 28:
Daunorubicin 50 mg/m² IV, days 29 and 30
Vincristine 2 mg IV, days 29 and 36
Prednisone 60 mg/m²/day PO, days 29 through 42
Asparaginase 6000 units/m² IM, days 29 through 35
Consolidation therapy. *Cycle:* 28 days
Treatment A (cycles 1, 3, 5, and 7)
Daunorubicin 50 mg/m² IV, days 1 and 2
Vincristine 2 mg IV, days 1 and 8
Prednisone 60 mg/m²/day PO, days 1 through 14
Asparaginase 12,000 units/m² IM, days 2, 4, 7, 9, 11, and 14
Treatment B (cycles 2, 4, 6, and 8)
Teniposide 165 mg/m² IV, days 1, 4, 8, and 11
Cytarabine 300 mg/m² IV, days 1, 4, 8, and 11
Treatment C (cycle 9)
Methotrexate 690 mg/m² IV over 42 hours
Leucovorin 15 mg/m² IV every 6 hours for 12 doses (start at end of methotrexate infusion)

M-2

Use: Multiple myeloma. *Cycle:* 5 weeks

Regimen: Vincristine 0.03 mg/kg (2 mg maximum dose) IV, day 1
Carmustine 0.5 mg/kg IV, day 1
Cyclophosphamide 10 mg/kg IV, day 1
Prednisone 1 mg/kg/day PO, days 1 through 7, tapered over next 14 days
with
Melphalan 0.25 mg/kg/day PO, days 1 through 4
or
Melphalan 0.1 mg/kg/day PO, days 1 through 7 or days 1 through 10

MAC III

Use: Gestational trophoblastic neoplasm (high-risk). *Cycle:* 21 days

Regimen: Methotrexate 1 mg/kg IM, days 1, 3, 5, and 7
Leucovorin 0.1 mg/kg IM, days 2, 4, 6, and 8 (give 24 hours after each methotrexate dose)
Dactinomycin 0.012 mg/kg IV, days 1 through 5
Cyclophosphamide 3 mg/kg IV, days 1 through 5

MACC

Use: Lung cancer (non-small cell). *Cycle:* 21 days

Regimen: Methotrexate 30-40 mg/m² IV, day 1
Doxorubicin 30-40 mg/m² IV, day 1 (total cumulative dose 550 mg/m²)
Cyclophosphamide 400 mg/m² IV, day 1
Lomustine 30 mg/m²/day PO, day 1

MACOP-B

Use: Lymphoma, (non-Hodgkin's). *Cycle:* Give only a single cycle

Regimen: Methotrexate 400 mg/m² IV weekly, weeks 2, 6, and 10
Leucovorin 15 mg/dose PO every 6 hours for 6 doses, begin 24 hours after each methotrexate dose
Doxorubicin 50 mg/m² IV weekly, weeks 1, 3, 5, 7, 9, and 11
Cyclophosphamide 350 mg/m² IV weekly, weeks 1, 3, 5, 7, 9, and 11
Vincristine 1.4 mg/m² (2 mg maximum dose) IV weekly, weeks 2, 4, 6, 8, 10, and 12
Bleomycin 10 units/m² IV weekly, weeks 4, 8, and 12
Prednisone 75 mg/day PO for 12 weeks, tapered over last 2 weeks

MAID

Use: Sarcoma (soft-tissue, bony). *Cycle:* 21 days

Regimen: Mesna 2500 mg/m²/day CI, days 1 through 4
Doxorubicin 15 mg/m²/day CI, days 1 through 4
Ifosfamide 2000 mg/m²/day CI, days 1 through 3
Dacarbazine 250 mg/m²/day CI, days 1 through 4

m-BACOD

Use: Lymphoma (non-Hodgkin's). *Cycle:* 21 days

Regimen: Bleomycin 4 units/m² IV, day 1
Doxorubicin 45 mg/m² IV, day 1
Cyclophosphamide 600 mg/m² IV, day 1
Vincristine 1 mg/m² (2 mg maximum dose) IV, day 1
Dexamethasone 6 mg/m²/day PO, days 1 through 5
Methotrexate 200 mg/m² IV, days 8 and 15
Leucovorin 10 mg/m²/dose PO every 6 hours for 8 doses, begin 24 hours after each methotrexate dose

m-BACOD (Reduced Dose)

Use: Lymphoma (non-Hodgkins) associated with HIV infection. *Cycle:* 21 days

Regimen: Methotrexate 200 mg/m² IV, day 15
Bleomycin 4 units/m² IV, day 1
Doxorubicin 25 mg/m² IV, day 1
Cyclophosphamide 300 mg/m² IV, day 1
Vincristine 1.4 mg/m² (2 mg maximum dose) IV, day 1
Dexamethasone 3 mg/m²/day PO, days 1 through 5

M-BACOD

Use: Lymphoma (non-Hodgkin's). *Cycle:* 21 days

Regimen: Bleomycin 4 units/m² IV, day 1
Doxorubicin 45 mg/m² IV, day 1
Cyclophosphamide 600 mg/m² IV, day 1
Vincristine 1 mg/m² (2 mg maximum dose) IV, day 1
Dexamethasone 6 mg/m²/day PO, days 1 through 5
Methotrexate 3000 mg/m² IV, day 15
Leucovorin 10 mg/m²/dose PO every 6 hours for 8 doses, begin 24 hours after each methotrexate dose

MBC

Use: Head and neck cancer. *Cycle:* 21 days

Regimen: Methotrexate 40 mg/m² IV, days 1 and 14
Bleomycin 10 units/m² IM or IV, days 1, 7, and 14
Cisplatin 50 mg/m² IV, day 4

MC

Use: Acute myelocytic leukemia (AML; adult induction). *Cycle:* Give a single cycle

Regimen: Mitoxantrone 12 mg/m² IV, days 1 through 3
Cytarabine 100-200 mg/m²/day CI or IV, days 1 through 7

MF

Use: Breast cancer. *Cycle:* 28 days

Regimen: Methotrexate 100 mg/m² IV, days 1 and 8
Fluorouracil 600 mg/m² IV, days 1 and 8, given 1 hour after methotrexate
Leucovorin 10 mg/m²/dose IV or PO every 6 hours for 6 doses, starting 24 hours after methotrexate

MICE (ICE)

Use: Sarcoma (adults, osteosarcoma - pediatrics), lung cancer. *Cycle:* 21 to 28 days

Regimen: Ifosfamide 1250-1500 mg/m² IV, days 1 through 3
Carboplatin 300-635 mg/m² IV, day 1 or 3
Etoposide 80-100 mg/m² IV, days 1 through 3
with
Mesna 1250 mg/m² IV, days 1 through 3
or
Mesna 20% of ifosfamide dose IV before, 4 hours after, and 8 hours after each ifosfamide infusion.

MINE

Use: Lymphoma (non-Hodgkin's). *Cycle:* 21 days

Regimen: Mesna 1330 mg/m² IV, days 1 through 3, given with ifosfamide
Mesna 500 mg/dose PO, 4 hours after ifosfamide, days 1 through 3
Ifosfamide 1330 mg/m² IV, days 1 through 3
Mitoxantrone 8 mg/m² IV, day 1
Etoposide 65 mg/m² IV, days 1 through 3

MINE-ESHAP

Use: Lymphoma (non-Hodgkin's). *Cycle:* 21 days

Regimen: Give MINE for 6 cycles, then give ESHAP for 3 to 6 cycles

mini-BEAM

Use: Lymphoma (Hodgkin's). *Cycle:* 4 to 6 weeks

Regimen: Carmustine 60 mg/m² IV, day 1
Etoposide 75 mg/m² IV, days 2 through 5
Cytarabine 100 mg/m²/dose IV every 12 hours for 8 doses, days 2 through 5
Melphalan 30 mg/m² IV, day 6

MOBP

Use: Cervical cancer. *Cycle:* 6 weeks

Regimen: Bleomycin 30 units/day CI, days 1 through 4
Vincristine 0.5 mg/m² IV, days 1 and 4
Cisplatin 50 mg/m² IV, days 1 and 22
Mitomycin 10 mg/m² IV, day 2

MOP

Use: Brain tumors (pediatrics). *Cycle:* 28 days.

Regimen: Mechlorethamine 6 mg/m² IV, days 1 and 8
Vincristine 1.5 mg/m² (2 mg maximum dose) IV, days 1 and 8
Procarbazine 100 mg/m²/day PO, days 1 through 14

MOPP

Use:	Lymphoma (Hodgkin's). *Cycle*: 28 days
Regimen:	Mechlorethamine 6 mg/m² IV, days 1 and 8 Vincristine 1.4 mg/m² (2 mg maximum dose) IV, days 1 and 8 Procarbazine 100 mg/m²/day PO, days 1 through 14 Prednisone 40 mg/m²/day PO, cycles 1 and 4,* days 1 through 14 *Note: Some clinicians give prednisone with every cycle of MOPP. The original clinical trials gave prednisone only with the first and fourth cycles.
Use:	Brain cancer (medulloblastoma). *Cycle*: 28 days
Regimen:	Mechlorethamine 3 mg/m² IV, days 1 and 8 Vincristine 1.4 mg/m² (2 mg maximum dose) IV, days 1 and 8 Prednisone 40 mg/m²/day PO, days 1 through 10 Procarbazine 50 mg PO, day 1 Procarbazine 100 mg PO, day 2 Procarbazine 100 mg/m²/day PO, days 3 through 10

MOPP/ABV

Use:	Lymphoma (Hodgkin's). *Cycle*: 28 days
Regimen:	Mechlorethamine 6 mg/m² IV, day 1 Vincristine 1.4 mg/m² (2 mg maximum dose) IV, day 1 Procarbazine 100 mg/m²/day PO, days 1 through 7 Prednisone 40 mg/m²/day PO, days 1 through 14 Doxorubicin 35 mg/m² IV, day 8 Bleomycin 10 units/m² IV, day 8 Vinblastine 6 mg/m² IV, day 8

MOPP/ABVD

Use:	Lymphoma (Hodgkin's). *Cycle*: 28 days
Regimen:	Alternate MOPP and ABVD regimens every month

MP

Use:	Multiple myeloma. *Cycle*: 21 to 28 days
Regimen:	Melphalan 8 mg/m²/day PO, days 1 through 4 Prednisone 60 mg/m²/day PO, days 1 through 4
Use:	Prostate cancer. *Cycle*: 21 days
Regimen:	Mitoxantrone 12 mg/m² IV, day 1 Prednisone 5 mg/dose PO twice daily

MTX/6-MP

Use:	Acute lymphocytic leukemia (ALL; continuation - pediatrics). *Cycle*: Ongoing, weeks 25 through 130
Regimen:	Methotrexate 20 mg/m² IM weekly Mercaptopurine 50 mg/m²/day PO *used in conjunction with* intrathecal therapy once every 12 weeks

MTX/6-MP/VP

Use:	Acute lymphocytic leukemia (ALL; continuation - pediatrics). *Cycle*: Ongoing, 2 to 3 years
Regimen:	Methotrexate 20 mg/m²/dose PO weekly Mercaptopurine 75 mg/m²/day PO Vincristine 1.5 mg/m² IV once monthly Prednisone 40 mg/m²/day PO for 5 days each month

MTX-CDDPAdr

Use:	Osteosarcoma (pediatrics). *Cycle*: 28 days
Regimen:	Methotrexate 12,000 mg/m² IV, days 1 and 8 Leucovorin 20 mg/m²/dose IV every 3 hours for 8 doses then give PO every 6 hours for 8 doses (begin 16 hours after end of methotrexate infusion) Cisplatin 75 mg/m² IV, day 15 of cycles 1 through 7 Cisplatin 120 mg/m² IV, day 15 of cycles 8 through 10 Doxorubicin 25 mg/m² IV, days 15 through 17 of cycles 1 through 7

MV

Use:	Breast cancer. *Cycle*: 6 to 8 weeks
Regimen:	Mitomycin 20 mg/m² IV, day 1 Vinblastine 0.15 mg/kg IV, days 1 and 21
Use:	Acute myelocytic leukemia (AML; induction). *Cycle*: Give 1 cycle. Second cycle may be considered if complete response not achieved.
Regimen:	Mitoxantrone 10 mg/m² IV, days 1 through 5 Etoposide 100 mg/m² IV, days 1 through 5

M-VAC

Use:	Bladder cancer. *Cycle*: 28 days
Regimen:	Methotrexate 30 mg/m² IV, days 1, 15, and 22 Vinblastine 3 mg/m² IV, days 2, 15, and 22 Doxorubicin 30 mg/m² IV, day 2 Cisplatin 70 mg/m² IV, day 2

MVP

Use:	Lung cancer (non-small cell). *Cycle*: 6 weeks
Regimen:	Mitomycin 8 mg/m² IV, day 1 Vinblastine 6 mg/m² IV, days 1 and 22 Cisplatin 50 mg/m² IV, days 1 and 22

MVPP

Use:	Lymphoma (Hodgkin's). *Cycle*: 4 to 6 weeks
Regimen:	Mechlorethamine 6 mg/m² IV, days 1 and 8 Vinblastine 4 mg/m² IV, days 1 and 8 Procarbazine 100 mg/m²/day PO, days 1 through 14 Prednisone 40 mg/m²/day PO, cycles 1 and 4,* days 1 through 14 *Note: Some clinicians give prednisone with every cycle of MVPP. The original clinical trials gave prednisone only with the first and fourth cycles.

NFL

Use:	Breast cancer. *Cycle*: 21 days
Regimen:	Mitoxantrone 12 mg/m² IV, day 1 Fluorouracil 350 mg/m² IV, days 1 through 3 after leucovorin Leucovorin 300 mg IV, days 1 through 3 *or* Mitoxantrone 10 mg/m² IV, day 1 Fluorouracil 1000 mg/m² CI, days 1 through 3 after leucovorin Leucovorin 100 mg/m² IV, days 1 through 3

NOVP

Use:	Lymphoma (Hodgkin's). *Cycle*: 21 days
Regimen:	Mitoxantrone 10 mg/m² IV, day 1 Vinblastine 6 mg/m² IV, day 1 Prednisone 100 mg/day PO, days 1 through 5 Vincristine 1.4 mg/m² (2 mg maximum dose) IV, day 8

OPA

Use:	Lymphoma (Hodgkin's - pediatrics). *Cycle*: 15 days. Up to 2 cycles used. Time between cycles not specified.
Regimen:	Vincristine 1.5 mg/m² (2 mg maximum dose) IV, days 1, 8, and 15 Prednisone 60 mg/m²/day PO in 3 divided doses, days 1 through 15 Doxorubicin 40 mg/m² IV, days 1 and 15

OPPA

Use:	Lymphoma (Hodgkin's - pediatrics). *Cycle*: 15 days. Up to 2 cycles used. Time between cycles not specified.
Regimen:	**Add to OPA**: Procarbazine 100 mg/m²/day PO in 2-3 divided doses, days 1 through 15

PAC

Use:	Ovarian, endometrial cancer. *Cycle*: 28 days
Regimen:	Cisplatin 50 mg/m² IV, day 1 Doxorubicin 50 mg/m² IV, day 1 Cyclophosphamide 500 mg/m² IV, day 1

PAC-I (Indiana Protocol)

Use:	Ovarian cancer. *Cycle*: 21 days
Regimen:	Cisplatin 50 mg/m² IV, day 1 (total cumulative dose 300 mg/m²) Doxorubicin 50 mg/m² IV, day 1 Cyclophosphamide 750 mg/m² IV, day 1

PA-CI

Use:	Hepatoblastoma (pediatrics). *Cycle*: 21 days
Regimen:	Cisplatin 90 mg/m² IV, day 1 Doxorubicin 20 mg/m² CI, days 2 through 5

Paclitaxel-Carboplatin-Etoposide

Use:	Adenocarcinoma (unknown primary), lung cancer (small cell). *Cycle*: 21 days
Regimen:	Paclitaxel 200 mg/m²/day IV, day 1 Carboplatin IV dose by Calvert equation to AUC 6, day 1 (give after paclitaxel) Etoposide 50 mg/day PO alternated with 100 mg/day PO, days 1 through 10

Paclitaxel-Vinorelbine

Use:	Breast cancer. *Cycle*: 28 days
Regimen:	Paclitaxel 135 mg/m² IV, day 1 (after vinorelbine infusion) Vinorelbine 30 mg/m² IV, days 1 and 8

PC

Use: Lung cancer (non-small cell). *Cycle:* 21 days

Regimen: Paclitaxel 135 mg/m²/day CI, day 1
Carboplatin IV dose by Calvert equation to AUC 7.5, day 2 (after paclitaxel)

Use: Lung cancer (non-small cell). *Cycle:* 21 days

Regimen: Paclitaxel 175 mg/m² IV, day 1
Cisplatin 80 mg/m² IV, day 1 after paclitaxel

Use: Bladder cancer. *Cycle:* 21 days

Regimen: Paclitaxel 200 or 225 mg/m²/day IV, day 1
Carboplatin IV dose by Calvert equation to AUC 5-6, day 1 (after paclitaxel)

PCV

Use: Brain tumor. *Cycle:* 6 to 8 weeks

Regimen: Lomustine 110 mg/m²/day PO, day 1
Procarbazine 60 mg/m²/day PO, days 8 through 21
Vincristine 1.4 mg/m² (2 mg maximum dose) IV, days 8 and 29

PE

Use: Prostate cancer. *Cycle:* 21 days

Regimen: Paclitaxel 30 mg/m²/day CI, days 1 through 4
Estramustine 600 mg/m²/day PO given in 2-3 divided doses (start 24 hours before first paclitaxel infusion)

PFL

Use: Head and neck, gastric cancer. *Cycle:* 28 days

Regimen: Cisplatin 25 mg/m²/day CI, days 1 through 5
Fluorouracil 800 mg/m²/day CI, days 2 through 6
Leucovorin 500 mg/m²/day CI, days 1 through 6

Use: Head and neck, gastric cancer. *Cycle:* 21 days

Regimen: Cisplatin 100 mg/m² IV, day 1
Fluorouracil 600-1000 mg/m²/day CI, days 1 through 5
Leucovorin 50 mg/m²/dose PO every 4-6 hours, days 1 through 6

POC

Use: Brain tumors (pediatrics). *Cycle:* 6 weeks

Regimen: Prednisone 40 mg/m²/day PO, days 1 through 14
Vincristine 1.5 mg/m² (2 mg maximum dose), days 1, 8, and 15
Lomustine 100 mg/m²/day PO, day 1

ProMACE

Use: Lymphoma (non-Hodgkin's). *Cycle:* 28 days

Regimen: Prednisone 60 mg/m²/day PO, days 1 through 14
Methotrexate 750 mg/m² IV, day 14
Leucovorin 50 mg/m²/dose IV every 6 hours for 5 doses, day 15 (start 24 hours after methotrexate)
Doxorubicin 25 mg/m² IV, days 1 and 8
Cyclophosphamide 650 mg/m² IV, days 1 and 8
Etoposide 120 mg/m² IV, days 1 and 8

ProMACE/cytaBOM

Use: Lymphoma (non-Hodgkin's). *Cycle:* 21 days

Regimen: Prednisone 60 mg/m²/day PO, days 1 through 14
Doxorubicin 25 mg/m² IV, day 1
Cyclophosphamide 650 mg/m² IV, day 1
Etoposide 120 mg/m² IV, day 1
Cytarabine 300 mg/m² IV, day 8
Bleomycin 5 units/m² IV, day 8
Vincristine 1.4 mg/m² (2 mg maximum dose) IV, day 8
Methotrexate 120 mg/m² IV, day 8
Leucovorin 25 mg/m²/dose PO every 6 hours for 4 doses (start 24 hours after methotrexate dose)
Cotrimoxazole DS 2 tablets PO twice daily, days 1 through 28

ProMACE/MOPP

Use: Lymphoma (non-Hodgkin's). *Cycle:* 28 days

Regimen: Prednisone 60 mg/m²/day PO, days 1 through 14
Doxorubicin 25 mg/m² IV, day 1
Cyclophosphamide 650 mg/m² IV, day 1
Etoposide 120 mg/m² IV, day 1
Mechlorethamine 6 mg/m² IV, day 8
Vincristine 1.4 mg/m² (2 mg maximum dose) IV, day 8
Procarbazine 100 mg/m²/day PO, days 8 through 14
Methotrexate 500 mg/m² IV, day 15
Leucovorin 50 mg/m²/dose PO every 6 hours for 4 doses (start 24 hours after methotrexate dose)

Pt/VM

Use: Neuroblastoma (pediatrics). *Cycle:* 21 to 28 days

Regimen: Cisplatin 90 mg/m² IV, day 1
Teniposide 100 mg/m² IV, day 3

PVA

Use: Acute lymphocytic leukemia (ALL; induction - pediatrics). *Cycle:* 28 days. Give a single cycle.

Regimen: Prednisone 40 mg/m²/day (60 mg maximum dose) PO, given in 3 divided doses, days 1 through 28
Vincristine 1.5 mg/m² (2 mg maximum dose) IV, days 1, 8, 15, and 22
with
Asparaginase 6000 units/m²/dose IM, 3 times weekly for 2 weeks (ie, days 2, 5, 7, 9, 12, and 14)
or
Asparaginase 6000 units/m²/dose IM, days 2, 5, 8, 12, 15, and 19
used in conjunction with
intrathecal therapy, day 1

PVB

Use: Testicular cancer, adenocarcinoma. *Cycle:* 21 days

Regimen: Cisplatin 20 mg/m² IV, days 1 through 5
Vinblastine 0.15 mg/kg IV, days 1 and 2
Bleomycin 30 units IV, days 2, 9, and 16

PVDA

Use: Acute lymphocytic leukemia (ALL; induction - pediatrics). *Cycle:* 28 days. Give a single cycle.

Regimen: Prednisone 40 mg/m²/day PO, days 1 through 28
Vincristine 1.5 mg/m² (2 mg maximum dose) IV, days 1, 8, 15, and 22
Daunorubicin 25 mg/m² IV, days 1, 8, 15, and 22
Asparaginase 10,000 units/m² IM, days 2, 4, 6, 9, 11, 13, 16, 18, and 20 (ie, 3 times weekly for 12 doses)
used in conjunction with
intrathecal therapy

Sequential AC/Paclitaxel - see AC/Paclitaxel, Sequential

Sequential Dox ➡ CMF - see Dox ➡ CMF, Sequential

SMF

Use: Pancreatic cancer. *Cycle:* 8 weeks

Regimen: Streptozocin 1000 mg/m² IV, days 1, 8, 29, and 36
Mitomycin 10 mg/m² IV, day 1
Fluorouracil 600 mg/m² IV, days 1, 8, 29, and 36

Stanford V

Use: Lymphoma (Hodgkin's). *Cycle:* 28 days

Regimen: Mechlorethamine 6 mg/m² IV, day 1
Doxorubicin 25 mg/m² IV, days 1 and 15
Vinblastine 6 mg/m² IV, days 1 and 15
Vincristine 1.4 mg/m² (2 mg maximum dose) IV, days 8 and 22
Bleomycin 5 units/m² IV, days 8 and 22
Etoposide 60 mg/m² IV, days 15 and 16
Prednisone 40 mg/m²/day PO, every other day continually for 10 weeks, then taper off by 10 mg every other day for next 14 days

TAD

Use: Acute myelocytic leukemia (AML; adult induction). *Cycle:* 21 days. Give 1 cycle only.

Regimen: Daunorubicin 60 mg/m² IV, days 3 through 5
Cytarabine 100 mg/m²/day CI, days 1 and 2
Cytarabine 100 mg/m² IV every 12 hours, days 3 through 8
Thioguanine 100 mg/m²/dose PO every 12 hours, days 3 through 9

Tamoxifen-Epirubicin

Use: Breast cancer. *Cycle:* 28 days for epirubicin for 6 cycles. Tamoxifen therapy continuous for 4 years.

Regimen: Tamoxifen 20 mg PO daily, continuously
Epirubicin 50 mg/m² IV, on days 1 and 8

TCF

Use: Esophageal cancer. *Cycle:* 28 days

Regimen: Paclitaxel 175 mg/m² IV, day 1
Cisplatin 20 mg/m² IV, days 1 through 5 (give after paclitaxel)
Fluorouracil 750 mg/m²/day, CI days 1 through 5

TIP

Use: Head and neck, esophageal cancer. *Cycle:* 21 to 28 days

Regimen: Paclitaxel 175 mg/m² IV, day 1
Ifosfamide 1000 mg/m² IV, days 1 through 3
Mesna 400 mg/m² IV pre-ifosfamide, days 1 through 3
Mesna 200 mg/m² IV given 4 hours after ifosfamide, days 1 through 3
Cisplatin 60 mg/m² IV, day 1 (give after paclitaxel infusion)

TIT

Use:	Acute lymphocytic leukemia (CNS prophylaxis - pediatrics).

Regimen:	Doses are based on patient's age. Give during weeks 1, 2, 3, 7, 13, 19, and 25 of intensification and every 12 weeks during maintenance.
	Age 1-2 years:
	  Methotrexate 8 mg intrathecal
	  Cytarabine 16 mg intrathecal
	  Hydrocortisone 8 mg intrathecal
	Age 2-3 years:
	  Methotrexate 10 mg intrathecal
	  Cytarabine 20 mg intrathecal
	  Hydrocortisone 10 mg intrathecal
	Age 3-9 years:
	  Methotrexate 12 mg intrathecal
	  Cytarabine 24 mg intrathecal
	  Hydrocortisone 12 mg intrathecal
	Age 9 years and older:
	  Methotrexate 15 mg intrathecal
	  Cytarabine 30 mg intrathecal
	  Hydrocortisone 15 mg intrathecal

Topo/CTX

Use:	Sarcomas (bony and soft-tissue - pediatrics). *Cycle*: 21 days
Regimen:	Cyclophosphamide 250 mg/m^2 IV, days 1 through 5 Topotecan 0.75 mg/m^2 IV, days 1 through 5 after cyclophosphamide Mesna 150 mg/m^2/dose IV before and 3 hours after each cyclophosphamide dose, days 1 through 5

Trastuzumab-Paclitaxel

Use:	Breast cancer. *Cycle*: 21 days for at least 6 cycles
Regimen:	Paclitaxel 175 mg/m^2/dose IV, day 1 Trastuzumab 4 mg/kg IV, day 1 first cycle only (loading dose) Trastuzumab 2 mg/kg IV weekly, days 1, 8, and 15, except for day 1 of first cycle.

VAB-6

Use:	Testicular cancer. *Cycle*: 21 to 28 days
Regimen:	Cyclophosphamide 600 mg/m^2 IV, day 1 Dactinomycin 1 mg/m^2 IV, day 1 Vinblastine 4 mg/m^2 IV, day 1 Cisplatin 120 mg/m^2 IV, day 4 Bleomycin 30 units IV push, day 1 (omit from cycle 3) *then* Bleomycin 20 units/m^2/day CI, days 1 through 3 (omit from cycle 3)

VAC Pediatric

Use:	Sarcoma (pediatrics). *Cycle*: 21 days
Regimen:	Vincristine 2 mg/m^2 IV (2 mg maximum dose), day 1 Dactinomycin 1 mg/m^2 IV, day 1 Cyclophosphamide 600 mg/m^2 IV, day 1

VAC Pulse

Use:	Sarcomas.
Regimen:	Vincristine 2 mg/m^2 (2 mg maximum dose) IV weekly, for 12 weeks Dactinomycin 0.015 mg/kg/day (0.5 mg/day maximum dose) CI, days 1 through 5, every 3 months for 5 courses Cyclophosphamide 10 mg/kg/day IV or PO, days 1 through 7, every 6 weeks

VAC Standard

Use:	Sarcomas.
Regimen:	Vincristine 2 mg/m^2 (2 mg maximum dose) IV weekly, for 12 weeks Dactinomycin 0.015 mg/kg/day (0.5 mg/day maximum dose) CI, days 1 through 5, every 3 months for 5 courses Cyclophosphamide 2.5 mg/kg/day PO, daily for 2 years

VACAdr

Use:	Sarcoma (bony and soft-tissue - pediatrics).
Regimen:	Vincristine 1.5 mg/m^2 (2 mg maximum dose) IV, days 1, 8, 15, 22, 29, and 36 Cyclophosphamide 500 mg/m^2 IV, days 1, 8, 15, 22, 29, and 36 Doxorubicin 60 mg/m^2 IV, day 36 *followed by 6 week rest period, then* Dactinomycin 0.015 mg/kg/day IV, days 1 through 5 Vincristine 1.5 mg/m^2 (2 mg maximum dose) IV, days 14, 21, 28, 35, and 42 Cyclophosphamide 500 mg/m^2 IV, days 14, 21, 28, 35, and 42 Doxorubicin 60 mg/m^2 IV, day 42 (give on day of final vincristine and cyclophosphamide doses)

VAD

Use:	Multiple myeloma. *Cycle*: 3 to 4 weeks
Regimen:	Vincristine 0.4 mg/day (dose is not in mg/m^2) CI, days 1 through 4 Doxorubicin 9 mg/m^2/day CI, days 1 through 4 Dexamethasone 40 mg/day PO, days 1 through 4, days 9 through 12, and days 17 through 20 *Note: After completing the first 2 cycles of VAD, some clinicians give dexamethasone only on days 1 through 4 of each cycle to reduce the risk of infection. Antibiotic prophylaxis with cotrimoxazole also has been used for this purpose.
Use:	Acute lymphocytic leukemia. *Cycle*: 24 to 28 days
Regimen:	Vincristine 0.4 mg/day (dose is not in mg/m^2) CI, days 1 through 4 Doxorubicin 9-12 mg/m^2/day CI, days 1 through 4 Dexamethasone 40 mg/day PO, days 1 through 4, days 9 through 12, and days 17 through 20
Use:	Wilm's tumor (pediatrics). *Cycle*: 1 year. Give 1 cycle only.
Regimen 1:	Vincristine 1.5 mg/m^2 (2 mg maximum dose) IV, weekly for first 10-11 weeks then every 3 weeks for 15 more weeks *with* Dactinomycin 1.5 mg/m^2 IV every 6 weeks, starting week 1 for 9 doses Doxorubicin 40 mg/m^2 IV every 6 weeks for 26 weeks, starting week 4, for 9 doses
Regimen 2:	Vincristine 1.5 mg/m^2 (2 mg maximum dose) IV, given every 6 weeks for 6 to 15 months Dactinomycin 0.015 mg/kg/day IV for 5 doses, given every 6 weeks for 6 to 15 months *or* Dactinomycin 0.06 mg/kg IV, given every 6 weeks for 6 to 15 months *may or may not give with* Doxorubicin 60 mg/m^2 IV, given every 6 weeks for 6 to 15 months

VATH

Use:	Breast cancer. *Cycle*: 21 days
Regimen:	Vinblastine 4.5 mg/m^2 IV, day 1 Doxorubicin 45 mg/m^2 IV, day 1 Thiotepa 12 mg/m^2 IV, day 1 Fluoxymesterone 30 mg/day PO in 3 divided doses, throughout entire course

VBAP

Use:	Multiple myeloma. *Cycle*: 21 days
Regimen:	Vincristine 1 mg/m^2 (2 mg maximum dose) IV, day 1 Carmustine 30 mg/m^2 IV, day 1 Doxorubicin 30 mg/m^2 IV, day 1 Prednisone 60 mg/m^2/day PO, days 1 through 4

VBCMP

Use:	Multiple myeloma. *Cycle*: 35 days
Regimen:	Vincristine 1.2 mg/m^2 (2 mg maximum dose) IV, day 1 Carmustine 20 mg/m^2 IV, day 1 Melphalan 8 mg/m^2/day PO, days 1 through 4 Cyclophosphamide 400 mg/m^2 IV, day 1 Prednisone 40 mg/m^2/day PO, days 1 through 7 of all cycles *with* Prednisone 20 mg/m^2/day PO, days 8 through 14 of first 3 cycles only

VC

Use:	Lung cancer (non-small cell).
Regimen:	Vinorelbine 30 mg/m^2 IV, weekly Cisplatin 120 mg/m^2 IV, days 1 and 29, then give 1 dose every 6 weeks

VCAP

Use:	Multiple myeloma. *Cycle*: 21 days
Regimen:	Vincristine 1 mg/m^2 (2 mg maximum dose) IV, day 1 Cyclophosphamide 125 mg/m^2/day PO, days 1 through 4 Doxorubicin 30 mg/m^2 IV, day 1 Prednisone 60 mg/m^2/day PO, days 1 through 4

VCMP - see VMCP

VD

Use:	Breast cancer. *Cycle*: 21 days
Regimen:	Vinorelbine 25 mg/m^2 IV, days 1 and 8 Doxorubicin 50 mg/m^2 IV, day 1

VelP

Use:	Genitourinary cancer, testicular cancer. *Cycle*: 21 days
Regimen:	Vinblastine 0.11 mg/kg IV, days 1 and 2 Cisplatin 20 mg/m^2 IV, days 1 through 5 Ifosfamide 1200 mg/m^2 IV, days 1 through 5 Mesna 1200 mg/m^2/day CI, days 1 through 5

VIC - see CVI

Vinorelbine-Cisplatin

Use:	Lung cancer (non-small cell). *Cycle*: 42 days
Regimen:	Vinorelbine 30 mg/m^2 IV, weekly Cisplatin 120 mg/m^2 IV, days 1 and 29 for first cycle; then day 1 of subsequent cycles

Vinorelbine-Doxorubicin

Use:	Breast cancer. *Cycle*: 21 days
Regimen:	Vinorelbine 25 mg/m^2 IV, days 1 and 8 Doxorubicin 50 mg/m^2 IV, day 1

Vinorelbine-Gemcitabine

Use:	Lung cancer (non-small cell). *Cycle*: 28 days
Regimen:	Vinorelbine 20 mg/m^2 IV, days 1, 8, and 15 Gemcitabine 800 mg/m^2 IV, days 1, 8, and 15

VIP

Use:	Genitourinary cancer, testicular cancer. *Cycle*: 21 days
Regimen:	Etoposide 75 mg/m^2 IV, days 1 through 5 Cisplatin 20 mg/m^2 IV, days 1 through 5 Ifosfamide 1200 mg/m^2 IV, days 1 through 5 Mesna 1200 mg/m^2/day CI, days 1 through 5

Use:	Lung cancer (small cell). *Cycle*: 21 to 28 days
Regimen:	Ifosfamide 1200 mg/m^2 IV, days 1 through 4 Cisplatin 20 mg/m^2 IV, days 1 through 4 Mesna 120-300 mg/m^2 IV, day 1 (give before ifosfamide started) Mesna 1200 mg/m^2/day CI, days 1 through 4 (after mesna bolus given) *with* Etoposide 37.5 mg/m^2/day PO, days 1 through 14 *or* Etoposide 75 mg/m^2/day IV, days 1 through 4

Use:	Lung cancer (non-small cell). *Cycle*: 28 days
Regimen:	Ifosfamide 1000-1200 mg/m^2 IV, days 1 through 3 Cisplatin 100 mg/m^2 IV, days 1 and 8 Etoposide 60-75 mg/m^2 IV, days 1 through 3 *with* Mesna 300 mg/m^2/dose IV every 4 hours, days 1 through 4 *or* Mesna 20% of ifosfamide dose IV before, 4 and 8 hours after ifosfamide

VM

Use:	Breast cancer. *Cycle*: 6 to 8 weeks
Regimen:	Mitomycin 10 mg/m^2 IV, days 1 and 28 for 2 cycles, then day 1 only Vinblastine 5 mg/m^2 IV, days 1, 14, 28, and 42 for 2 cycles, then days 1 and 21 only

VMCP

Use:	Multiple myeloma. *Cycle*: 21 days
Regimen:	Vincristine 1 mg/m^2 (2 mg maximum dose) IV, day 1 Melphalan 6 mg/m^2/day PO, days 1 through 4 Cyclophosphamide 125 mg/m^2/day PO, days 1 through 4 Prednisone 60 mg/m^2/day PO, days 1 through 4

VP

Use:	Lung cancer (small cell). *Cycle*: 21 days
Regimen:	Etoposide 100 mg/m^2/day IV, days 1 through 4 Cisplatin 20 mg/m^2 IV, days 1 through 4

V-TAD

Use:	Acute myelocytic leukemia (AML; induction). *Cycle*: 7 days. Give 1 cycle. Up to 3 cycles have been given, but time between cycles is not specified.
Regimen:	Etoposide 50 mg/m^2 IV, days 1 through 3 Thioguanine 75 mg/m^2/dose PO every 12 hours, days 1 through 5 Daunorubicin 20 mg/m^2 IV, days 1 and 2 Cytarabine 75 mg/m^2/day CI, days 1 through 5

➤*NCI INVESTIGATIONAL AGENTS:* For further information, contact Pharmaceutical Management Branch, National Cancer Institute, Executive Plaza North, Room 804, 6130 Executive Blvd., Rockville, MD 20892, (301) 496-5725.

CHLORAMBUCIL

| *Rx* | **Leukeran** (GlaxoSmithKline) | **Tablets:** 2 mg | (GX EG3 L). Brown. Film coated. In 50s. |

WARNING

Chlorambucil can severely suppress bone marrow function; is carcinogenic in humans; is probably mutagenic and teratogenic in humans; produces human infertility. (See Warnings).

Indications

➤*Leukemia/Lymphomas:* For the treatment of chronic lymphocytic leukemia, malignant lymphomas including lymphosarcoma, giant follicular lymphoma, and Hodgkin disease. It is not a curative in any of these disorders, but it may produce clinically useful palliation.

➤*Unlabeled uses:* Chlorambucil has shown activity in other malignancies such as ovarian and testicular carcinoma, non-Hodgkin lymphoma, and Waldenström macroglobulinemia.

Administration and Dosage

➤*Approved by the FDA:* March 18, 1957.

➤*Initial and short courses of therapy:* Usual dose is 0.1 to 0.2 mg/kg/day for 3 to 6 weeks as required (average, 4 to 10 mg/day). The entire daily dose may be given at one time. Carefully adjust to response of the patient and immediately reduce if there is an abrupt fall in the WBC count. Patients with Hodgkin disease usually require 0.2 mg/kg/day; patients with other lymphomas or chronic lymphocytic leukemia usually require only 0.1 mg/kg/day. When lymphocytic infiltration of bone marrow is present or bone marrow is hypoplastic, do not exceed 0.1 mg/kg/day (average, 6 mg/day).

An alternate schedule for the treatment of chronic lymphocytic leukemia using intermittent, biweekly, or monthly pulse doses of chlorambucil consists of an initial single dose of 0.4 mg/kg. Doses are increased by 0.1 mg/kg until control of lymphocytosis or toxicity is observed. Subsequent doses are modified to produce mild hematologic toxicity. The response rate of chronic lymphocytic leukemia to biweekly or monthly administration is similar to or better than that reported with daily administration, and hematologic toxicity is less than or equal to that encountered using daily chlorambucil.

Radiation and cytotoxic drugs render the bone marrow more vulnerable to damage. Therefore, use chlorambucil with particular caution within 4 weeks of a full course of radiation therapy or chemotherapy. However, small doses of palliative radiation over isolated foci remote from the bone marrow will not usually depress neutrophil and platelet count; chlorambucil may be given in the customary dosage.

Short courses of treatment are safer than continuous maintenance therapy, although both methods have been effective. It must be recognized that continuous therapy may give the appearance of "maintenance" in patients who are actually in remission and have no immediate need for further drug. It may be desirable to withdraw drug after maximal control has been achieved because intermittent therapy reinstituted at time of relapse may be as effective as continuous treatment.

➤*Maintenance therapy:* Do not exceed 0.1 mg/kg/day; may be as low as 0.03 mg/kg/day (usually 2 to 4 mg/day or less depending on blood counts).

➤*Storage/Stability:* Store in refrigerator at 2° to 8°C (36° to 46°F).

Actions

➤*Pharmacology:* Chlorambucil is a bifunctional alkylating agent of the nitrogen mustard type. A cell cycle nonspecific drug, chlorambucil interacts with cellular DNA to produce a cytotoxic cross-linkage.

➤*Pharmacokinetics:*

Absorption/Distribution – Chlorambucil is rapidly and completely absorbed from the GI tract following oral administration. Peak plasma levels of chlorambucil are reached in 1 hour.

Chlorambucil and its metabolites are extensively bound to plasma and tissue proteins. In vitro, it is 99% bound to plasma proteins, specifically albumin.

Metabolism/Excretion – Chlorambucil is extensively metabolized in the liver, primarily to phenylacetic acid mustard, which has antineoplastic activity. Chlorambucil and its major metabolite spontaneously degrade in vivo, forming monohydroxy and dihydroxy derivatives. Approximately 15% to 60% of the dose appears in the urine after 24 hours; less than 1% is in the form of chlorambucil or phenylacetic acid mustard. The terminal elimination half-life is approximately 1.5 hours.

Contraindications

Resistance to the agent; hypersensitivity. There may be cross-hypersensitivity (skin rash) between chlorambucil and other alkylating agents.

Warnings

➤*Seizures:* Rare, focal and/or generalized seizures have occurred in adults and children at therapeutic daily doses, pulse dosing regimens, and in acute overdosage.

Children with nephrotic syndrome and patients receiving high pulse doses of the drug may have an increased risk of seizures. Exercise caution when administering chlorambucil to patients with a history of seizure disorders, head trauma, or to patients receiving other potentially epileptogenic drugs.

➤*Bone marrow damage:* Observe patients carefully to avoid life-threatening damage to the bone marrow.

Many patients develop a slowly progressive lymphopenia during treatment. The lymphocyte count usually rapidly returns to normal levels upon completion of drug therapy. Most patients have some neutropenia after the third week of treatment that may continue for up to 10 days after the last dose. Subsequently, the neutrophil count usually rapidly returns to normal. Severe neutropenia appears to be dose-related and usually occurs only in patients who have received a total dose of 6.5 mg/kg or more in one course of therapy with continuous dosing. About one fourth of all patients receiving the continuous dose schedule and one third of those receiving this dosage in 8 weeks or fewer may be expected to develop severe neutropenia.

It is not necessary to discontinue chlorambucil at the first evidence of a fall in neutrophil count. Decreases may continue for 10 days after the last dose is given. As the total dose approaches 6.5 mg/kg, irreversible bone marrow damage may occur. Decrease dosage if leukocyte or platelet counts fall below normal values; discontinue if more severe depression occurs. Persistently low neutrophil and platelet counts or peripheral lymphocytosis suggest bone marrow infiltration. If confirmed by bone marrow examination, do not exceed a daily dosage of 0.1 mg/kg.

➤*Carcinogenesis:* Because of its carcinogenic properties, do not give to patients with conditions other than chronic lymphatic leukemia or malignant lymphomas. Convulsions, infertility, leukemia, and secondary malignancies are observed when chlorambucil is used in the therapy of malignant and nonmalignant diseases.

There are reports of acute leukemia arising in patients with both malignant and nonmalignant diseases following chlorambucil treatment. Patients often received additional chemotherapeutic agents or radiation therapy. Risk of leukemogenesis apparently increases with both chronicity of treatment and with large cumulative doses. However, it is impossible to define a cumulative dose below which there is no risk of inducing secondary malignancy. Weigh the potential benefits of therapy against the risk of inducing a secondary malignancy.

➤*Mutagenesis:* Chlorambucil has caused chromatid or chromosome damage in humans. Reversible and permanent sterility have occurred in both sexes.

➤*Fertility impairment:* A high incidence of sterility occurs when chlorambucil is administered to prepubertal and pubertal males. Prolonged or permanent azoospermia also has occurred in adult males. While most reports of gonadal dysfunction secondary to chlorambucil are related to males, the induction of amenorrhea in females with alkylating agents is well documented, and chlorambucil can produce amenorrhea. Autopsy studies of the ovaries from women with malignant lymphoma treated with combination chemotherapy including chlorambucil show varying degrees of fibrosis, vasculitis, and depletion of primordial follicles.

➤*Pregnancy:* Category D. Chlorambucil can cause fetal harm when administered to a pregnant woman. Unilateral renal agenesis has been observed in two offspring whose mothers received chlorambucil during the first trimester. Urogenital malformations, including absence of a kidney, were found in fetuses of rats given chlorambucil. There are no adequate and well-controlled studies in pregnant women. If this drug is used during pregnancy or if the patient becomes pregnant while taking this drug, apprise her of the potential hazard to the fetus. Advise women of childbearing potential to avoid becoming pregnant.

➤*Lactation:* It is not known whether this drug is excreted in breast milk. Because of the potential for serious adverse reactions in breastfeeding infants, decide whether to discontinue breastfeeding or to discontinue the drug, taking into account the importance of the drug to the mother.

➤*Children:* Safety and efficacy in children have not been established.

Precautions

➤*Monitoring:* Determine weekly hemoglobin levels, total and differential leukocyte counts, and quantitative platelet counts. Also, during the first 3 to 6 weeks of therapy, perform white blood cell (WBC) counts 3 to 4 days after each of the weekly complete blood counts. It is dangerous to allow a patient to go more than 2 weeks without hematological and clinical examinations.

➤*Radiation and chemotherapy:* Do not give at full dosage before 4 weeks after a full course of radiation therapy or chemotherapy because of the vulnerability of the bone marrow to damage under these conditions. If the pretherapy leukocyte or platelet counts are depressed from bone marrow disease process prior to institution of therapy, institute treatment at a reduced dosage.

CHLORAMBUCIL

Adverse Reactions

➤*CNS:* Tremors, muscular twitching, myoclonia, confusion, agitation, ataxia, flaccid paresis, hallucinations (rare; resolved upon discontinuation); seizures (see Warnings).

➤*Dermatologic:* Allergic reactions such as urticaria and angioneurotic edema have occurred following initial or subsequent dosing. Skin hypersensitivity (including rare reports of skin rash progressing to erythema multiforme, toxic epidermal necrolysis or Stevens-Johnson syndrome). Promptly discontinue in patients who develop skin reactions.

➤*GI:* Nausea, vomiting, diarrhea, oral ulceration (infrequent).

➤*GU:* Infertility; prolonged or permanent azoospermia; amenorrhea (see Warnings).

➤*Hematologic:* The most common side effect is bone marrow suppression. Although bone marrow suppression frequently occurs, it is usually reversible if the drug is withdrawn early enough. However, irreversible bone marrow failure has been reported (see Warnings).

➤*Pulmonary:* Pulmonary fibrosis; interstitial pneumonia.

➤*Miscellaneous:* Drug fever; hepatotoxicity and jaundice; peripheral neuropathy; sterile cystitis; leukemia; secondary malignancies.

Overdosage

➤*Symptoms:* Reversible pancytopenia was the main finding. Neurological toxicity ranging from agitated behavior and ataxia to multiple grand mal seizures has also occurred.

➤*Treatment:* As there is no known antidote, closely monitor the blood picture and institute general supportive measures, together with appropriate blood transfusions if necessary. Chlorambucil is not dialyzable. Refer to General Management of Acute Overdosage.

Patient Information

Inform patients that the major toxicities of chlorambucil are related to hypersensitivity, drug fever, myelosuppression, hepatotoxicity, infertility, seizures, GI toxicity, and secondary malignancies.

Advise patient to notify a physician of bleeding, fever, nausea, vomiting, skin rash, persistent cough, seizures, amenorrhea, unusual lumps or masses, or yellow discoloration of the skin or eyes.

Advise women of childbearing potential to avoid becoming pregnant.

Inform patient to store under refrigeration

CYCLOPHOSPHAMIDE

Rx	Cyclophosphamide (Gensia Sicor)	**Tablets:** 25 mg	Lactose. (54 639). Lt. blue. In 100s and UD 100s.
Rx	Cytoxan (Mead Johnson Oncology)		Lactose. White with blue flecks. In 100s.
Rx	Cyclophosphamide (Gensia Sicor)	**Tablets:** 50 mg	Lactose. (54 980). Lt. blue. In 100s and UD 100s.
Rx	Cytoxan (Mead Johnson Oncology)		Lactose. White with blue flecks. In 100s and 1000s.
Rx	Cytoxan Lyophilized (Mead Johnson Oncology)	**Powder for Injection:** 75 mg mannitol/100 mg cyclophosphamide	In 100, 200, 500 mg and 1 and 2 g vials.
Rx	Neosar (Gensia Sicor)	**Powder for Injection:** 82 mg sodium bicarbonate/100 mg cyclophosphamide	In 100, 200 and 500 mg and 1 and 2 g vials.

Indications

Frequently used concurrently or sequentially with other antineoplastics. The following malignancies are often susceptible to cyclophosphamide treatment:

➤*Malignant disease:* Malignant lymphomas (Stages III and IV, Ann Arbor Staging System): Hodgkin's disease; lymphocytic lymphoma (nodular or diffuse); mixed-cell type lymphoma; histiocytic lymphoma; Burkitt's lymphoma; multiple myeloma; neuroblastoma (disseminated disease); adenocarcinoma of the ovary; retinoblastoma; carcinoma of the breast.

➤*Leukemias:* Chronic lymphocytic leukemia; chronic granulocytic leukemia (usually ineffective in acute blastic crisis); acute myelogenous and monocytic leukemia; acute lymphoblastic (stem-cell) leukemia in children (given during remission, cyclophosphamide is effective in prolonging remission duration).

➤*Mycosis fungoides:* Advanced disease.

➤*Nonmalignant disease:*
Biopsy proven "minimal change" nephrotic syndrome in children – Cyclophosphamide is useful in carefully selected cases but should not be used as primary therapy. In children whose disease fails to respond adequately to appropriate corticosteroid therapy or in whom the corticosteroid therapy produces or threatens to produce intolerable side effects, cyclophosphamide may induce a remission. Cyclophosphamide is not indicated for the nephrotic syndrome in adults or for any other renal disease.

➤*Unlabeled uses:* Variety of severe rheumatologic conditions: Wegener's granulomatosis, other steroid-resistant vasculitides and in some cases of severe progressive rheumatoid arthritis and systemic lupus erythematosus. Toxicity is limiting.

Cyclophosphamide (total dose 1 to 12 g) has been used to halt the progression of multiple sclerosis or decrease the frequency and duration of episodes. It has also been used in the treatment of polyarteritis nodosa using an initial dose of 2 mg/kg/day orally or 4 mg/kg/day IV. Cyclophosphamide (500 mg over 1 hour every 1 to 3 weeks), alone or in combination with corticosteroids, may be useful in the treatment of polymyositis.

Possible treatment for severe neuropsychiatric systemic lupus erythematosus (NPSLE).

Administration and Dosage

➤*Malignant diseases (adults and children):*
IV – When used as the only oncolytic drug therapy, the initial IV dose for patients with no hematologic deficiency is 40 to 50 mg/kg, usually given in divided doses over 2 to 5 days. Other IV regimens include 10 to 15 mg/kg every 7 to 10 days or 3 to 5 mg/kg twice weekly.

Oral – Usual range of 1 to 5 mg/kg/day for initial and maintenance dosing.

When cyclophosphamide is included in combined cytotoxic regimens, it may be necessary to reduce the dose of cyclophosphamide as well as that of the other drugs.

Dosages must be adjusted in accord with evidence of antitumor activity or leukopenia. The total leukocyte count is a good, objective guide for regulating dosage.

➤*Nonmalignant diseases:*
Biopsy proven "minimal change" nephrotic syndrome in children – An oral dose of 2.5 to 3 mg/kg daily for a period of 60 to 90 days is recommended. In males, the incidence of oligospermia and azoospermia increases if the duration of treatment exceeds 60 days. Treatment beyond 90 days increases the probability of sterility. Corticosteroid therapy may be tapered and discontinued during the course of cyclophosphamide therapy. See Precautions section concerning hematologic monitoring.

➤*Preparation of parenteral solution:* Add Sterile Water for Injection to the vial and shake to dissolve. Use the quantity of diluent shown in the following table to reconstitute the product.

Reconstitution of Cyclophosphamide	
	Quantity of diluent (ml)
Vial strength	Powder for Injection
100 mg	5
200 mg	10
500 mg	25
1 g	50
2 g	100

Prepared solutions may be injected IV, IM, intraperitoneally or intrapleurally, or they may be infused IV in 5% Dextrose Injection or 5% Dextrose and 0.9% Sodium Chloride Injection, 5% Dextrose and Ringer's Injection, Lactated Ringer's Injection, 0.45% Sodium Chloride Injection or ⅙ molar Sodium Lactate Injection.

➤*Preparation of oral solution:* Dissolve injectable cyclophosphamide in Aromatic Elixir; store under refrigeration in glass containers and use within 14 days.

➤*Storage/Stability:* Use solutions prepared with Bacteriostatic Water for Injection (paraben preserved) within 24 hours if stored at room temperature or within 6 days if stored under refrigeration. If cyclophosphamide is not prepared with Bacteriostatic Water for Injection use the solution promptly (preferably within 6 hours). Cyclophosphamide does not contain an antimicrobial agent; take care to ensure the sterility of prepared solutions.

CYCLOPHOSPHAMIDE

Actions

➤*Pharmacology:* Cyclophosphamide is an alkylating agent chemically related to the nitrogen mustards.

Cyclophosphamide is first hydroxylated by hepatic microsomal (P450 mixed-function oxidase) enzymes to the intermediate metabolites 4-hydroxycyclophosphamide and aldophosphamide. These are oxidized to the active antineoplastic alkylating compounds acrolein and phosphoramide mustard. The mechanism of action of the active metabolites is thought to involve cross-linking of DNA, which interferes with growth of susceptible neoplasms and normal tissues. It has not been demonstrated that any single metabolite is responsible for either the therapeutic or toxic effects of cyclophosphamide.

➤*Pharmacokinetics:*

Absorption / Distribution – Cyclophosphamide is well absorbed after oral administration with a bioavailability> 75%. Several cytotoxic and noncytotoxic metabolites have been identified in urine and in plasma. Concentrations of metabolites reach a maximum in plasma 2 to 3 hours after an IV dose. Plasma protein binding of unchanged drug is low, but some metabolites are > 60% bound.

Metabolism / Excretion – The drug is activated and inactivated to alkylating and nonalkylating metabolites respectively, by the P450 system in the liver. It is eliminated primarily in the form of metabolites; 5% to 25% of a dose is excreted as unchanged cyclophosphamide which has an elimination half-life of 3 to 12 hours. Although elevated levels of metabolites have occurred in patients with renal failure, increased clinical toxicity has not been demonstrated.

Contraindications

Previous hypersensitivity to the drug; continued use in severely depressed bone marrow function.

Warnings

➤*Hematologic:* Leukopenia is an expected effect and is used as a guide to dosage. Leukopenia of < 2000 cells/mm^3 develops commonly in patients treated with an initial loading dose of the drug, and less frequently in patients maintained on smaller doses. The degree of neutropenia is particularly important because it correlates with a reduction in resistance to infections. Thrombocytopenia or anemia develop occasionally. These effects are usually reversible when therapy is interrupted. Recovery from leukopenia usually begins in 7 to 10 days after cessation of therapy.

➤*Cardiac toxicity:* Although a few instances of cardiac dysfunction have occurred following use of recommended doses of cyclophosphamide, no causal relationship has been established. Cardiotoxicity has been observed in some patients receiving high doses of cyclophosphamide ranging from 120 to 270 mg/kg administered over a period of a few days, usually as a portion of an intensive antineoplastic multidrug regimen or in conjunction with transplantation procedures. In a few instances with high doses of cyclophosphamide, severe, and sometimes fatal, congestive heart failure has occurred within a few days after the first cyclophosphamide dose. Histopathologic examination has primarily shown hemorrhagic myocarditis.

No residual cardiac abnormalities as evidenced by electrocardiogram or echocardiogram appear to be present in the patients surviving episodes of apparent cardiac toxicity associated with high doses of cyclophosphamide.

➤*Adrenalectomy patients:* Adjustment of the doses of both replacement steroids and cyclophosphamide may be necessary for the adrenalectomized patient.

➤*Wound healing:* Cyclophosphamide may interfere with normal wound healing.

➤*GU:* Acute hemorrhagic cystitis occurs in 7% to 12% of patients, although some report an occurrence of up to 40%. Hemorrhagic cystitis can be severe, even fatal, and is probably caused by urinary metabolites. Nonhemorrhagic cystitis and bladder fibrosis have also been reported. Ample fluid intake and frequent voiding help to prevent cystitis, but when it occurs, it is usually necessary to interrupt therapy. Hematuria usually resolves spontaneously within a few days after therapy is discontinued, but may persist. In protracted cases, medical or surgical supportive treatment may be required.

A formalin (37% formaldehyde solution diluted to a 1% solution) bladder instillation has successfully controlled the cystitis. Complications may occur with the 10% solution; there appears to be no additional value in using > 4% solutions. The use of mesna has reduced the incidence of cyclophosphamide-induced cystitis (see individual monograph).

Treatment with cyclophosphamide may cause significant suppression of immune responses. Serious, sometimes fatal, infections may develop in severely immunosuppressed patients. Cyclophosphamide treatment may not be indicated, should be interrupted or the dose reduced in patients who have or who develop viral, bacterial, fungal, protozoan or helminthic infections.

➤*Hypersensitivity reactions:* Hypersensitivity reactions (type I) have occurred, mediated through increased B-cell activity and production of IgE. Refer to Management of Acute Hypersensitivity Reactions.

Rare instances of anaphylactic reaction including one death have occurred. One instance of possible cross sensitivity with other alkylating agents has occurred.

➤*Renal / Hepatic function impairment:* Use cautiously. Patients with compromised renal function may show some measurable changes in pharmacokinetic parameters of cyclophosphamide metabolism, but there is no evidence indicating a need for modified dosage in these patients.

➤*Carcinogenesis:* Secondary neoplasia has developed with cyclophosphamide alone or with other antineoplastic drugs or radiation therapy. These most frequently have been urinary bladder, myeloproliferative and lymphoproliferative malignancies. Secondary malignancies have developed most frequently in patients with primary myeloproliferative and lymphoproliferative malignancies and nonmalignant diseases in which immune processes are pathologically involved. In some cases, the secondary malignancy was detected several years after drug discontinuance. Secondary urinary bladder malignancies generally have occurred in patients who previously developed hemorrhagic cystitis. One case of carcinoma of the renal pelvis occurred with long-term therapy for cerebral vasculitis. Consider the possibility of secondary malignancy in any benefit-to-risk assessment for use of the drug.

➤*Fertility impairment:* Cyclophosphamide interferes with oogenesis and spermatogenesis. It may cause sterility in both sexes. Development of sterility appears to depend on the dose, duration of therapy, and the state of gonadal function at the time of treatment. Cyclophosphamide-induced sterility may be irreversible in some patients.

Amenorrhea associated with decreased estrogen and increased gonadotropin secretion develops in a significant proportion of women treated with cyclophosphamide. Affected patients generally resume regular menses within a few months after cessation of therapy. Girls treated during prepubescence generally develop secondary sexual characteristics normally and have regular menses. Ovarian fibrosis with apparently complete loss of germ cells after prolonged cyclophosphamide treatment in late prepubescence has occurred. Girls treated with cyclophosphamide during prepubescence subsequently have conceived.

Men treated with cyclophosphamide may develop oligospermia or azoospermia associated with increased gonadotropin but normal testosterone secretion. Sexual potency and libido are unimpaired in these patients. Boys treated during prepubescence develop secondary sexual characteristics normally, but may have oligospermia or azoospermia and increased gonadotropin secretion. Some degree of testicular atrophy may occur. Cyclophosphamide-induced azoospermia is reversible in some patients, though the reversibility may not occur for several years after cessation of therapy. Men temporarily rendered sterile by cyclophosphamide have subsequently fathered normal children.

➤*Pregnancy: Category D.* Both normal and malformed newborns have been reported following the use of cyclophosphamide in pregnancy. Malformations have included limb abnormalities (missing fingers and toes), cardiac anomalies and hernias. In addition, 40% of infants exposed to anticancer drugs (timing of exposure not considered) were of low birth weight. However, use of cyclophosphamide in the second and third trimesters does not seem to place the infant at risk for congenital defects; this does not include the possibility of physical and mental growth abnormalities.

Also, *paternal* use of combination chemotherapy, including cyclophosphamide prior to conception, has been associated with cardiac and limb abnormalities in an infant.

If this drug is used during pregnancy, or if the patient becomes pregnant while taking this drug, apprise the patient of the potential hazard to the fetus. Advise women of childbearing potential to avoid becoming pregnant.

➤*Lactation:* Cyclophosphamide is excreted in breast milk. Because of the potential for serious adverse reactions and the potential for tumorigenicity decide whether to discontinue breastfeeding or to discontinue the drug, taking into account the importance of the drug to the mother.

➤*Children:* See Administration and Dosage.

Precautions

➤*Monitoring:* During treatment, monitor the patient's hematologic profile (particularly neutrophils and platelets) regularly to determine the degree of hematopoietic suppression. Examine urine regularly for red cells which may precede hemorrhagic cystitis.

➤*Immunosuppression:* Treatment with cyclophosphamide may cause significant suppression of immune responses. Serious, sometimes fatal infections may develop in severely immunosuppressed patients. Treatment may not be indicated or be interrupted or the dose reduced in patients who have or who develop viral, bacterial, fungal, protozoan or helminthic infections.

➤*Renal effects:* A syndrome of inappropriate antidiuretic hormone (SIADH) has occurred with IV doses > 50 mg/kg. It is both a limitation to and consequence of fluid loading. Hemorrhagic ureteritis and renal

CYCLOPHOSPHAMIDE

tubular necrosis have occurred. Such lesions usually resolve following cessation of therapy.

➤*Special risk:* Give cautiously to patients with: Leukopenia; thrombocytopenia; tumor cell infiltration of bone marrow; previous radiation therapy; previous cytotoxic therapy.

Drug Interactions

Cyclophosphamide Drug Interactions			
Precipitant drug	Object drug*		Description
Allopurinol	Cyclophospha-mide	↑	The myelosuppressive effects of cyclophosphamide may be enhanced, possibly increasing the risk of bleeding or infection.
Chloramphenicol	Cyclophospha-mide	↓	Cyclophosphamide half-life may increase and metabolite concentrations may be decreased.
Phenobarbital	Cyclophospha-mide	↓	The rate of metabolism and the leukopenic activity of cyclophosphamide reportedly are increased by chronic administration of high doses of phenobarbital.
Thiazide diuretics	Cyclophospha-mide[1]	↑	Antineoplastic-induced leukopenia may be prolonged.
Cyclophospha-mide	Anticoagulants	↑	Anticoagulant effect is increased.
Cyclophospha-mide[1]	Digoxin	↓	Digoxin serum levels may be reduced.
Cyclophospha-mide	Doxorubicin	↑	Doxorubicin-induced cardiotoxicity is potentiated.
Cyclophospha-mide	Quinolone	↓	The antimicrobial effects of quinolones may be decreased.
Cyclophospha-mide	Succinylcholine	↑	Neuromuscular blockade may be prolonged, because of inhibition of cholinesterase activity.

* ↑ = Object drug increased. ↓ = Object drug decreased.
[1] Cyclophosphamide used in combination with other antineoplastics.

Adverse Reactions

➤*Cardiovascular:* Cardiotoxicity (hemorrhagic cardiac necrosis, transmural hemorrhages, coronary artery vasculitis) (See Warnings).

➤*Dermatologic:* Alopecia (frequent); regrowth of hair can be expected, although it may be of a different color or texture; skin rash (occasionally); pigmentation of the skin and changes in nails.

➤*GI:* Anorexia; nausea; vomiting; diarrhea; stomatitis; abdominal discomfort or pain; hemorrhagic colitis; oral mucosal ulceration.

➤*GU:* Acute hemorrhagic cystitis; amenorrhea, oligospermia, azoospermia, sterility (see Warnings); urinary bladder fibrosis; hematuria; hemorrhagic ureteritis; renal tubular necrosis.

➤*Hematologic:* Leukopenia, thrombocytopenia, anemia (see Warnings).

➤*Pulmonary:* Interstitial pulmonary fibrosis.

➤*Miscellaneous:* Secondary neoplasia; anaphylactic reactions; infections (see Warnings); jaundice; interference with normal wound healing; interstitial pulmonary fibrosis with prolonged high dosage.

Overdosage

No specific antidote for cyclophosphamide is known. Use general supportive measures. Cyclophosphamide and its metabolites are dialyzable although there are probably quantitative differences depending upon the dialysis system being used. Refer to General Management of Acute Overdosage. Cyclophosphamide and its metabolites are dialyzable.

Patient Information

Take tablets preferably on an empty stomach. If GI upset is severe, take with food.

Notify your doctor of unusual bleeding or bruising, fever, chills, sore throat, cough, shortness of breath, seizures, lack of menstrual flow, unusual lumps or masses, flank or stomach pain, joint pain, sores in the mouth or on the lips, or yellow discoloration of the skin or eyes.

Contraceptive measures are recommended during therapy for both men and women.

IFOSFAMIDE

Rx	**Ifosfamide** (American Pharmaceutical Partners)	**Powder for Injection:** 1 g	In single-dose vials.
Rx	**Ifex** (Mead Johnson Oncology)		In single-dose vials.[1]
Rx	**Ifosfamide** (American Pharmaceutical Partners)	**Powder for Injection:** 3 g	In single-dose vials.
Rx	**Ifex** (Mead Johnson Oncology)		In single-dose vials.[2]

[1] Includes 200 mg amps *Mesnex* (mesna).

[2] Includes 400 mg amps *Mesnex* (mesna).

WARNING

Urotoxic side effects, especially hemorrhagic cystitis, as well as CNS toxicities such as confusion and coma have been associated with ifosfamide. When they occur, they may require cessation of ifosfamide therapy (see Warnings).

Severe myelosuppression has occurred (see Warnings).

Indications

➤*Germ cell testicular cancer:* In combination with certain other approved antineoplastics for third-line chemotherapy of germ cell testicular cancer.

Ordinarily used in combination with a prophylactic agent for hemorrhagic cystitis, such as mesna (see individual monograph).

➤*Unlabeled uses:* Ifosfamide has shown activity in lung, breast, ovarian, pancreatic and gastric cancer, sarcomas, acute leukemias (except AML) and malignant lymphomas. Further studies are needed with ifosfamide alone and with other agents.

Administration and Dosage

Administer IV at a dose of 1.2 g/m^2/day for 5 consecutive days. Repeat every 3 weeks or after recovery from hematologic toxicity (platelets ≥ 100,000/mm^3, WBC ≥ 4000/mm^3). To prevent bladder toxicity, give with extensive hydration consisting of ≥ 2 L of oral or IV fluid per day. Use a protector, such as mesna, to prevent hemorrhagic cystitis. Administer ifosfamide as slow IV infusion lasting ≥ 30 minutes. Ifosfamide has been used in a small number of patients with compromised hepatic or renal function.

➤*Preparation:* Add Sterile Water for Injection or Bacteriostatic Water for Injection (benzyl alcohol or parabens preserved) to the vial and shake to dissolve. Use the quantity of diluent shown below to reconstitute the product:

Reconstitution of Ifosfamide		
Dosage strength	Quantity of diluent	Final concentration
1 g	20 ml	50 mg/ml
3 g	60 ml	50 mg/ml

➤*Storage/Stability:* Solutions of ifosfamide may be diluted further to concentrations of 0.6 to 20 mg/ml in the following fluids: 5% Dextrose Injection; 0.9% Sodium Chloride Injection; Lactated Ringer's Injection; Sterile Water for Injection. Such admixtures, when stored in large volume parenteral glass bottles, Viaflex bags or *PAB* bags, are physically and chemically stable for ≥ 1 week at 30°C (86°F) or 6 weeks at 5°C (41°F).

Because essentially identical stability results were obtained for Sterile Water admixtures as for the other admixtures, the use of large volume parenteral glass bottles, Viaflex bags or *PAB* bags that contain intermediate concentrations or mixtures of excipients (eg, 2.5% Dextrose Injection, 0.45% Sodium Chloride Injection or 5% Dextrose and 0.9% Sodium Chloride Injection) is also acceptable.

Refrigerate dilutions not prepared by constitution with Bacteriostatic Water for Injection (benzyl alcohol or parabens preserved), and use within 6 hours.

May store dry powder at room temperature. Avoid storage > 40°C (104°F).

Actions

➤*Pharmacology:* Ifosfamide is a chemotherapeutic agent chemically related to the nitrogen mustards and a synthetic analog of cyclophosphamide. Ifosfamide requires metabolic activation by microsomal liver enzymes to produce biologically active metabolites. Activation occurs by hydroxylation to form the unstable intermediate 4-hydroxyifosfamide. This metabolite rapidly degrades to the stable urinary metabolite 4-ketoifosfamide. Formation of the stable urinary metabolite, 4-carboxyifosfamide also occurs. These urinary metabolites are not cytotoxic. Ifosphoramide and acrolein are also found. Enzymatic oxidation of the chloroethyl side chains and subsequent dealkylation produces the major urinary metabolites, dechloroethyl ifosfamide and dechloroethyl

IFOSFAMIDE

cyclophosphamide. The alkylated metabolites of ifosfamide interact with DNA.

➤*Pharmacokinetics:*

Absorption / Distribution – Ifosfamide exhibits dose-dependent pharmacokinetics. Small quantities (nmole/ml) of ifosfamide mustard and 4-hydroxyifosfamide are detectable in plasma.

Metabolism / Excretion – At single doses of 3.8 to 5 g/m², the plasma concentrations decay biphasically, and the mean terminal elimination half-life is ≈ 15 hours. At doses of 1.6 to 2.4 g/m²/day, the plasma decay is monoexponential, and the terminal elimination half-life is ≈ 7 hours. Ifosfamide is extensively metabolized, and the metabolic pathways appear to be saturated at high doses. Metabolism of ifosfamide is required for the generation of the biologically active species and while metabolism is extensive, it varies among patients. After administration of doses of 5 g/m², 70% to 86% of the dose was recovered in the urine, with about 61% of the dose excreted as parent compound. At doses of 1.6 to 2.4 g/m², only 12% to 18% of the dose was excreted in the urine as unchanged drug within 72 hours.

➤*Clinical trials:* In one study, 50 fully evaluable patients with germ cell testicular cancer were given ifosfamide and cisplatin and either vinblastine or etoposide after failing (47 of 50) at least two prior chemotherapy regimens consisting of cisplatin/vinblastine/bleomycin (PVB), cisplatin/vinblastine/actinomycin D/bleomycin/cyclophosphamide (VAB6) or the combination of cisplatin and etoposide. Patients were selected for remaining cisplatin sensitivity because they had previously responded to a cisplatin-containing regimen and had not progressed while on the regimen or within 3 weeks of stopping it. Patients served as their own control based on the premise that long-term complete responses could not be achieved by retreatment with a regimen to which they had previously responded and subsequently relapsed.

Ten of 50 patients were still alive 2 to 5 years after treatment. Four of the 10 long-term survivors were rendered free of cancer by surgical resection after the ifosfamide regimen; median survival for the entire group of 50 patients was 53 weeks.

Contraindications

Continued use in patients with severely depressed bone marrow function (see Warnings and Precautions); hypersensitivity to ifosfamide.

Warnings

➤*Urotoxic side effects:* Urotoxic side effects, especially hemorrhagic cystitis, have been frequently associated with ifosfamide. Obtain a urinalysis prior to each dose. If microscopic hematuria (> 10 RBCs per high power field) is present, then withhold subsequent administration until complete resolution. Use ifosfamide with a protector, such as mesna, to prevent hemorrhagic cystitis.

➤*Myelosuppression:* When given in combination with other chemotherapeutic agents, severe myelosuppression is frequent. In studies, this was dose-related and dose-limiting. It consisted mainly of leukopenia and, to a lesser extent, thrombocytopenia. A WBC count < 3000/mm³ is expected in 50% of patients given ifosfamide alone at 1.2 g/m²/day for 5 consecutive days. At this dose level, thrombocytopenia (platelets < 100,000/mm³) occurred in ≈ 20% of patients. At higher dosages, leukopenia was almost universal; at total dosages of 10 to 12 g/m²/cycle, half of the patients had a WBC count < 1000/mm³ and 8% had platelet counts < 50,000/mm³. Myelosuppression is usually reversible, and treatment can be given every 3 to 4 weeks. When used in combination with other myelosuppressive agents, dose adjustments may be necessary. Patients who experience severe myelosuppression are potentially at increased risk for infection.

Close hematologic monitoring is recommended. Obtain a WBC count, platelet count and hemoglobin prior to each administration and at appropriate intervals. Unless clinically essential, do not administer to patients with a WBC count < 2000/mm³ or a platelet count < 50,000/mm³.

➤*Neurologic manifestations:* Neurologic manifestations consisting of somnolence, confusion, hallucinations and in some instances, coma, have occurred. The occurrence of these symptoms requires discontinuing ifosfamide therapy. The symptoms have usually been reversible; maintain supportive therapy until their complete resolution.

➤*Hematuria:* At doses of 1.2 g/m²/day for 5 consecutive days without a protector, microscopic hematuria is expected in ≈ 50% of the patients and gross hematuria in ≈ 8% of patients. Dose fractionation, vigorous hydration and a protector (eg, mesna) can significantly reduce hematuria incidence, especially gross hematuria, associated with hemorrhagic cystitis. At 1.2 g/m²/day for 5 consecutive days, leukopenia, if it occurs, is usually mild to moderate.

➤*Renal function impairment:* Use with caution. Clinical signs (eg, elevation in BUN or serum creatinine or decrease in creatinine clearance) were usually transient and most likely related to tubular damage.

➤*Carcinogenesis:* Ifosfamide is carcinogenic in rats, with female rats showing a significant incidence of leiomyosarcomas and mammary fibroadenomas. The mutagenic potential is documented in bacterial systems in vitro and mammalian cells in vivo. In vivo, ifosfamide has induced mutagenic effects in mice and *Drosophila melanogaster* germ cells and has induced a significant increase in dominant lethal mutations in male mice as well as recessive sex-linked lethal mutations in *Drosophila.*

Ifosfamide has caused resorptions, fetal anomalies, embryolethality and embryotoxicity in various rodent species in doses ranging from 18 to 88 mg/m².

➤*Pregnancy: Category D.* Animal studies indicate that the drug can cause gene mutations and chromosomal damage in vivo. Embryotoxic and teratogenic effects have been observed in mice, rats and rabbits at doses 0.05 to 0.075 times the human dose. Ifosfamide can cause fetal damage when administered to a pregnant woman. If ifosfamide is used during pregnancy or if the patient becomes pregnant while taking this drug, apprise the patient of the potential hazard to the fetus.

➤*Lactation:* Ifosfamide is excreted in breast milk. Because of the potential for serious adverse events and the tumorigenicity shown in animal studies, discontinue nursing or the drug, taking into account the importance of the drug to the mother.

➤*Children:* Safety and efficacy in children have not been established.

Precautions

➤*Monitoring:* During treatment, monitor the patient's hematologic profile (particularly neutrophils and platelets) regularly to determine the degree of hematopoietic suppression. Examine regularly for red cells that may precede hemorrhagic cystitis. Closely monitor serum and urine chemistries including phosphorus, potassium, alkaline phosphatase and other appropriate laboratory studies. Administer appropriate replacement therapy as indicated.

➤*Compromised bone marrow reserve:* Administer cautiously to patients with compromised bone marrow reserve, as indicated by: Leukopenia, granulocytopenia, extensive bone marrow metastases, prior therapy with radiation or other cytotoxic agents.

➤*Wound healing:* Ifosfamide may interfere with normal wound healing.

Adverse Reactions

➤*CNS:* Somnolence, confusion, depressive psychosis, hallucinations (12%); dizziness, disorientation, cranial nerve dysfunction, seizures, coma (less frequent); encephalopathy (rare). CNS toxicity incidence may be higher with altered renal function.

➤*GI:* Nausea and vomiting (58%); anorexia, diarrhea, constipation (< 1%).

➤*GU:* Hematuria (6% to 92%, see Warnings); hemorrhagic cystitis; dysuria; urinary frequency; metabolic acidosis (31%); proteinuria and acidosis (rare); renal tubular acidosis that progressed into chronic renal failure (one episode).

➤*Miscellaneous:* Alopecia (≈ 83%); myelosuppression (50%); infection (8%); liver dysfunction (3%); phlebitis (2%); fever of unknown origin (1%); allergic reactions, cardiotoxicity, coagulopathy, dermatitis, fatigue, hypertension, hypotension, malaise, polyneuropathy, pulmonary symptoms, salivation, stomatitis (< 1%); acute pancreatitis (rare).

➤*Lab test abnormalities:* Increases in liver enzymes or bilirubin (3%).

Overdosage

No specific antidote for ifosfamide is known. Management includes general supportive measures to sustain patient through any toxicity that might occur. Refer to General Management of Acute Overdosage.

Patient Information

Notify physician of unusual bleeding/bruising, fever, chills, sore throat, cough, shortness of breath, seizures, lack of menstrual flow, unusual lumps or masses, flank, stomach or joint pain, sores in mouth or on lips, yellow discoloration of skin or eyes.

Contraceptive measures are recommended during therapy for men and women.

MECHLORETHAMINE HCl (Nitrogen Mustard; HN₂)

| Rx | **Mustargen** (Merck) | **Powder for Injection:** 10 mg | In sets of 4 vials. |

WARNING

Administer mechlorethamine only under the supervision of a physician experienced in the use of cancer chemotherapeutic agents.

This drug is highly toxic and the powder and solution must be handled and administered with care. Inhalation of dust or vapors and contact with skin or mucous membranes, especially those of the eyes, must be avoided. Avoid exposure during pregnancy. Because of the toxic properties of mechlorethamine (eg, corrosivity, carcinogenicity, mutagenicity, teratogenicity), review special handling procedures prior to handling and follow diligently.

Extravasation of the drug into subcutaneous tissues results in painful inflammation. The area usually becomes indurated; sloughing may occur. If leakage of drug is obvious, promptly infiltrate the area with sterile isotonic sodium thiosulfate (⅙ molar), and apply an ice compress for 6 to 12 hours. For a ⅙ molar solution of sodium thiosulfate, use 4.14 g sodium thiosulfate per 100 mL sterile water for injection or 2.64 g anhydrous sodium thiosulfate per 100 mL, or dilute 4 mL sodium thiosulfate injection (10%) with 6 mL sterile water for injection.

Indications

➤*Bronchogenic carcinoma (IV only):* For palliative treatment of bronchogenic carcinoma.

➤*Leukemia/Lymphomas (IV only):* For palliative treatment of Hodgkin disease (Stages III and IV), lymphosarcoma, chronic myelocytic, or chronic lymphocytic leukemia.

➤*Metastatic carcinoma:* For palliative treatment of metastatic carcinoma resulting in effusion when administered intrapleurally, intraperitoneally, or intrapericardially.

➤*Mycosis fungoides (IV only):* For palliative treatment of mycosis fungoides.

➤*Polycythemia vera (IV only):* For palliative treatment of polycythemia vera.

➤*Unlabeled uses:* A topical mechlorethamine solution has been used to treat patients with mycosis fungoides.

Administration and Dosage

➤*Approved by the FDA:* March 15, 1949.

➤*IV:* Individualize dosage. Give a total dose of 0.4 mg/kg for each course, either as a single dose or in divided doses of 0.1 to 0.2 mg/kg/day. Base dosage on ideal dry body weight. Administration at night is preferred in case sedation for side effects is required.

Do not give subsequent courses until the patient has recovered hematologically from the previous course; determine by repeated studies of the peripheral blood elements. It is possible to give repeated courses of mechlorethamine as early as 3 weeks after treatment.

The margin of safety is narrow; exercise considerable care with dosage.

Administration – It is preferable to inject into the rubber or plastic tubing of a flowing IV infusion set. This reduces the possibility of severe extravasation reactions or high drug concentration; it also minimizes a chemical reaction between the drug and the solution. The rate of injection is not critical provided it is completed within a few minutes.

➤*Intracavitary administration:* Intracavitary administration has been used with varying success for the control of pleural, peritoneal, and pericardial effusions caused by malignant cells.

Consult product labeling for details of intracavitary administration. The technique and dose used by any of these routes varies. The usual dose is 0.4 mg/kg, although 0.2 mg/kg (or 10 to 20 mg) has been used intrapericardially.

➤*Special handling:* This drug is highly toxic; the powder and solution must be handled and administered with care. Inhalation of dust or vapors and contact with skin or mucous membranes, especially those of the eyes, must be avoided. Wear appropriate protective equipment when handling mechlorethamine. Should accidental eye contact occur, immediately institute copious irrigation for at least 15 minutes with water, normal saline, or a balanced salt ophthalmic irrigating solution, followed by prompt ophthalmologic consultation. Should accidental skin contact occur, the affected part must be irrigated immediately with copious amounts of water for at least 15 minutes while removing contaminated clothing and shoes, followed by 2% sodium thiosulfate solution. Seek medical attention immediately. Destroy contaminated clothing.

➤*Preparation of solution:* Each vial contains 10 mg mechlorethamine HCl triturated with 100 mg sodium chloride. In neutral or alkaline aqueous solution, it undergoes rapid chemical transformation and is highly unstable. Prepare solutions immediately before each injection because they will decompose on standing.

Do not use if the solution is discolored or if droplets of water are visible within the vial prior to reconstitution.

Reconstitute with 10 mL of sterile water for injection or sodium chloride injection. The resultant solution contains 1 mg/mL mechlorethamine HCl.

➤*Decontamination:* To clean rubber gloves, tubing, glassware, etc, after administration, soak them in an aqueous solution containing equal volumes of sodium thiosulfate (5%) and sodium bicarbonate (5%) for 45 minutes. Excess reagents and reaction products are washed away easily with water. Neutralize any unused injection solution by mixing with an equal volume of sodium thiosulfate/sodium bicarbonate solution. Allow the mixture to stand for 45 minutes. Treat contaminated vials in the same way with sodium thiosulfate/sodium bicarbonate solution before disposal.

➤*Storage/Stability:* Store at controlled room temperature 15° to 30°C (59° to 86°F). Protect from light and humidity. Prepare immediately before use.

Actions

➤*Pharmacology:* Mechlorethamine, an antineoplastic nitrogen mustard also known as HN₂, is a nitrogen analog of sulfur mustard. It is a biologic alkylating agent that has a cytotoxic action of inhibiting rapidly proliferating cells.

➤*Pharmacokinetics:* In water or body fluids, mechlorethamine undergoes rapid chemical transformation and combines with water or reactive compounds so the active drug is no longer present within a few minutes.

Contraindications

Patients with infectious disease; previous anaphylactic reactions to the drug.

Warnings

➤*Extravasation:* Extravasation of the drug into subcutaneous tissues results in a painful inflammation. The area usually becomes indurated and sloughing may occur (see Warning Box).

➤*Special handling:* Animal studies show mechlorethamine to be corrosive to skin and eyes, a powerful vesicant, irritating to the mucous membranes of the respiratory tract, and highly toxic by the oral route. It also has been shown to be carcinogenic, mutagenic, and teratogenic. Because of the drug's toxic properties, appropriate precautions, including the use of appropriate safety equipment are recommended for the preparation of mechlorethamine for parenteral administration. Avoid exposure during pregnancy (see Administration and Dosage).

➤*Inoperable neoplasms or terminal stage:* Balance the potential risk and discomfort from use in patients with inoperable neoplasms or in the terminal stage of the disease against the limited gain obtainable. Routine use in cases of widely disseminated neoplasms is discouraged.

➤*Hematologic:* The usual course of treatment (total dose, 0.4 mg/kg) produces lymphocytopenia within 24 hours after the first injection; significant granulocytopenia occurs within 6 to 8 days and lasts for 10 days to 3 weeks. Agranulocytosis is infrequent and recovery from leukopenia is usually complete within 2 weeks of the maximum reduction. Thrombocytopenia is variable, but the time course of appearance and recovery of reduced platelet count generally parallels the sequence of granulocyte levels. Severe thrombocytopenia may lead to bleeding from the gums and GI tract, petechiae, and small subcutaneous hemorrhages; these symptoms appear transient and, in most cases, disappear with return to a normal platelet count. However, a severe and uncontrollable hematopoietic depression occasionally may follow the usual dose, particularly in patients with widespread disease and debility and in patients previously treated with other antineoplastic agents or x-ray. Persistent pancytopenia has been reported. In rare instances, hemorrhagic complications may be caused by hyperheparinemia. Erythrocyte and hemoglobin levels may decline, but rarely significantly, during the first 2 weeks after therapy. Depression of the hematopoietic system may occur up to 50 days after starting therapy.

The use of mechlorethamine in patients with leukopenia, thrombocytopenia, and anemia, caused by invasion of the bone marrow by tumor, carries a greater risk. In such patients a good response to treatment with disappearance of the tumor from the bone marrow may be associated with improvement of bone marrow function. However, in the absence of a good response or in patients who have been previously treated with chemotherapeutic agents, hematopoiesis may be further compromised, and leukopenia, thrombocytopenia, and anemia may become more severe and lead to death.

➤*Chronic lymphatic leukemia:* Drug toxicity, especially sensitivity to bone marrow failure, appears to be more common in chronic lymphatic leukemia than in other conditions; administer in this condition with great caution, if at all.

➤*Tumors:* Tumors of bone and nervous tissue respond poorly to therapy. Results are unpredictable in disseminated and malignant tumors of different types.

MECHLORETHAMINE HCl (Nitrogen Mustard; HN₂)

➤*Amyloidosis:* Nitrogen mustard therapy may contribute to extensive and rapid development of amyloidosis; use only if foci of acute and chronic suppurative inflammation are absent.

➤*Herpes zoster:* Herpes zoster, common with lymphomas, may first appear after therapy is instituted and may be precipitated by treatment. Discontinue further treatment during the acute phase of this illness to avoid progression to generalized herpes zoster.

➤*Hypersensitivity reactions:* Hypersensitivity reactions, including anaphylaxis, have occurred. Refer to Management of Acute Hypersensitivity Reactions.

➤*Carcinogenesis:* Therapy with alkylating agents such as mechlorethamine may be associated with an increased incidence of a second malignant tumor, especially when it is combined with other antineoplastic agents or radiation therapy.

➤*Mutagenesis:* Various chromosomal abnormalities have been reported in association with nitrogen mustard therapy.

➤*Fertility impairment:* Impaired spermatogenesis, azoospermia, and total germinal aplasia have occurred in male patients, especially those receiving combination therapy. Spermatogenesis may return in patients in remission, but this may occur several years after chemotherapy has been discontinued. Warn patients of the potential risks to their reproductive capacity.

➤*Pregnancy: Category D.* Mechlorethamine can cause fetal harm when administered to a pregnant woman. Mechlorethamine has been shown to produce fetal malformations in the rat and ferret when given as single SC injections of 1 mg/kg (2 to 3 times the maximum recommended human dose). There are no adequate and well-controlled studies in pregnant women. If this drug is used during pregnancy or if the patient becomes pregnant while taking this drug, apprise her of the potential hazard to the fetus. Advise women of childbearing potential to avoid becoming pregnant.

➤*Lactation:* It is not known whether this drug is excreted in human milk. Because of the potential for serious adverse reactions from nitrogen mustards in breastfeeding infants, decide whether to discontinue breastfeeding or to discontinue the drug, taking into account the importance of the drug to the mother.

➤*Children:* Safety and efficacy in children have not been established by well-controlled studies. Use in children has been limited. Nitrogen mustards have been used in Hodgkin disease (Stages III and IV) in combination with other oncolytic agents (MOPP schedule). The MOPP chemotherapy combination includes mechlorethamine, vincristine, procarbazine, and prednisone or prednisolone.

Precautions

➤*Monitoring:* Many renal, hepatic, and bone marrow function abnormalities occur in patients with neoplastic disease who receive mechlorethamine. Check renal, hepatic, and bone marrow functions frequently.

➤*Local toxicity:* Thrombosis and thrombophlebitis may result from direct contact of the drug with the intima of the injected vein. Avoid high concentration and prolonged contact with the drug, especially in cases of elevated pressure in the antebrachial vein (ie, in mediastinal tumor compression from severe vena cava syndrome).

➤*Concomitant therapy:* Hematopoietic function is characteristically depressed by x-ray therapy or other chemotherapy in alternating courses. Do not give mechlorethamine following x-ray or x-ray subsequent to the drug until bone marrow function has recovered. In particular, irradiation of such areas as the sternum, ribs, and vertebrae shortly after a nitrogen mustard course may lead to hematologic complications.

➤*Immunosuppression:* Immunosuppressive activity has occurred with mechlorethamine. Use may predispose the patient to bacterial, viral, or fungal infection.

➤*Hyperuricemia:* Hyperuricemia may develop during therapy with mechlorethamine. The problem of urate precipitation may develop during therapy, particularly in the treatment of lymphomas; institute adequate methods to control hyperuricemia and maintain adequate fluid intake before treatment.

➤*Intracavitary administration:* Pain rarely occurs with intrapleural use; it is common with intraperitoneal injection and is often associated with nausea, vomiting, and diarrhea of 2 to 3 days duration. Transient cardiac irregularities may occur with intrapericardial injection. Death, possibly accelerated by nitrogen mustard, has occurred following intracavitary use. Although absorption by the intracavitary route is probably not complete because of its rapid deactivation by body fluids, the systemic effect is unpredictable. The acute side effects such as nausea and vomiting are usually mild. Bone marrow depression is generally milder than when the drug is given IV. Avoid use by the intracavitary route when other agents that may suppress bone marrow function are being used systemically.

➤*GI effects:* Nausea and vomiting usually begin 1 to 3 hours after administration. Vomiting may disappear in the first 8 hours; nausea may persist for 24 hours. Nausea and vomiting may be so severe as to precipitate vascular accidents in patients with a hemorrhagic tendency. Premedication with antiemetics and sedatives may be beneficial. Anorexia, diarrhea, and weakness may occur.

Adverse Reactions

➤*Dermatologic:* Alopecia (infrequent); erythema multiforme; herpes zoster (see Warnings). Occasionally, a maculopapular skin eruption occurs, but this may be idiosyncratic and does not necessarily recur with subsequent courses of the drug.

➤*GI:* Anorexia; diarrhea; nausea, vomiting (see Precautions); .

➤*GU:* Azoospermia, total germinal aplasia, impaired spermatogenesis (see Warnings); temporary or permanent amenorrhea; delayed menses; oligomenorrhea.

➤*Hematologic:* Agranulocytosis, granulocytopenia, hematopoietic depression, hyperheparinemia, lymphocytopenia, thrombocytopenia (see Warnings); hemolytic anemia (rare); persistent pancytopenia.

➤*Local:* Extravasation (see Warning Box); thrombosis; thrombophlebitis.

➤*Special senses:* Diminished hearing, tinnitus, vertigo, (infrequent).

➤*Miscellaneous:* Chromosomal abnormalities; hypersensitivity (including anaphylaxis); hyperuricemia (see Precautions); jaundice, vertigo (infrequent).

Overdosage

With total doses exceeding 0.4 mg/kg for a single course, severe leukopenia, anemia, thrombocytopenia, and hemorrhagic diathesis with subsequent delayed bleeding may develop. Death may follow. The only treatment for excessive dosage appears to be repeated blood product transfusions, antibiotic treatment of complicating infections, and general supportive measures.

Patient Information

Inform patients that this medicine can reduce the body's ability to fight infection and to report any signs of infection (eg, fever, chills, sore throat) to a doctor or health care provider.

Instruct patients that if accidental contact with the eyes or skin occurs, rinse with water for at least 15 minutes and seek medical attention.

Advise patients to talk with a health care provider at once if the injection site becomes red, swollen, or tender.

Warn patients of the potential risks to their reproductive capacity.

Advise women of childbearing potential to avoid becoming pregnant.

MELPHALAN (L-PAM; L-Phenylalanine Mustard; L-Sarcolysin)

Rx	Alkeran (Celgene)	Tablets: 2 mg	(GX EH3 A). Lactose. White. Film-coated. In amber glass bottles. In 50s.
		Powder for Injection, lyophilized: 50 mg	In single-use vials[1] with 10 mL vial of sterile diluent.[2]

[1] With 20 mg povidone.

[2] Water for injection with 0.2 g sodium citrate, 6 mL propylene glycol and 0.52 mL ethanol.

WARNING

Administer melphalan under the supervision of a qualified physician experienced in the use of cancer chemotherapeutic agents. Severe bone marrow suppression with resulting infection or bleeding may occur. Controlled trials comparing IV with oral melphalan have shown more myelosuppression with the IV formulation. Hypersensitivity reactions, including anaphylaxis, have occurred in approximately 2% of patients who received the IV formulation. Melphalan is leukemogenic in humans. It produces chromosomal aberrations in vitro and in vivo; therefore, it is potentially mutagenic in humans.

Indications

➤*Epithelial ovarian cancer (tablets only):* For the palliative treatment of nonresectable epithelial carcinoma of the ovary.

➤*Multiple myeloma:* For the palliative treatment of multiple myeloma. Use the IV formulation in patients for whom oral therapy is not appropriate.

➤*Unlabeled uses:* Melphalan also has been used for the treatment of breast cancer, testicular cancer, and bone marrow transplantation.

Administration and Dosage

➤*Epithelial ovarian cancer:* 0.2 mg/kg/day orally for 5 days as a single course. Repeat courses every 4 to 5 weeks depending on hematologic tolerance.

➤*Multiple myeloma:*

Oral – The usual dose is 6 mg/day. May give entire daily dose at one time. Adjust the dose, as required, on the basis of weekly blood counts. After 2 to 3 weeks of treatment, discontinue drug for up to 4 weeks, and carefully monitor blood count. When WBC and platelet counts are rising, institute a maintenance dose of 2 mg/day. Because of patient-to-patient variations in melphalan plasma levels following oral use, some recommend a cautious dosage increase until myelosuppression is observed to ensure therapeutic drug levels have been reached.

Renal function impairment: In patients with moderate to severe renal impairment, pharmacokinetic data does not justify an absolute recommendation on dosage reduction, but it may be prudent to use a reduced dose initially.

Alternative regimens: Initial course of 10 mg/day for 7 to 10 days. Maximal suppression of the leukocyte and platelet counts occurs within 3 to 5 weeks and recovery within 4 to 8 weeks. Institute maintenance therapy with 2 mg/day when the WBC count is greater than 4000 cells/mcL and the platelet count is greater than 100,000 cells/mcL. Adjust dosage to between 1 and 3 mg/day depending on hematological response. Maintain a significant degree of bone marrow depression to keep the leukocyte count in the range of 3000 to 3500 cells/mcL.

Other investigators start treatment with 0.15 mg/kg/day for 7 days, followed by a rest period of at least 2 weeks (up to 5 to 6 weeks). Begin maintenance therapy at 0.05 mg/kg/day or less when the WBC and platelet counts are rising; adjust according to the blood count. About one third to one half of patients with multiple myeloma show a favorable response to oral administration of the drug. In one study, melphalan in combination with prednisone significantly improved the percentage of patients with multiple myeloma who achieved palliation. One regimen is to administer melphalan at 0.25 mg/kg/day for 4 consecutive days (or 0.2 mg/kg/day for 5 consecutive days) for a total dose of 1 mg/kg/course. These 4- to 5-day courses are then repeated every 4 to 6 weeks if the granulocyte and platelet counts have returned to normal.

Response may be very gradual over many months; it is important to give repeated courses or continuous therapy because improvement may continue slowly over many months and the maximum benefit may be missed if treatment is abandoned too soon.

IV – The usual dose is 16 mg/m^2. Administer as a single infusion over 15 to 20 minutes. Give at 2-week intervals for 4 doses, then, after adequate recovery from toxicity, at 4-week intervals. Experience suggests that repeated courses should be given because improvement may continue slowly over many months, and the maximum benefit may be missed if treatment is abandoned prematurely. Consider dose adjustment on the basis of blood cell counts at the nadir and day of treatment.

Renal function impairment: Consider reduction of up to 50% in patients with renal insufficiency (BUN 30 mg/dL or greater).

Preparation for IV administration: Exercise caution in handling and preparing the solution of melphalan HCl for injection. Skin reactions associated with accidental exposure may occur. The use of gloves is recommended. If the solution contacts the skin or mucosa, immediately wash the skin or mucosa thoroughly with soap and water.

1.) Reconstitute by rapidly injecting 10 mL of the supplied diluent into the vial and immediately shake vigorously until a clear solution is obtained. This provides a 5 mg/mL solution.
2.) Immediately dilute the dose to be administered in 0.9% sodium chloride injection to a concentration not greater than 0.45 mg/mL.
3.) Administer the diluted product over a minimum of 15 minutes.
4.) Complete administration within 60 minutes of reconstitution.

Keep the time between reconstitution/dilution and administration to a minimum because reconstituted and diluted solutions are unstable. Over as short a time as 30 minutes, a citrate derivative of melphalan has been detected in reconstituted material from the reaction of melphalan with the sterile diluent. Upon further dilution with saline, nearly 1% label strength of melphalan hydrolyzes every 10 minutes.

➤*Storage / Stability:*

Tablets – Refrigerate at 2° to 8°C (36° to 46°F). Protect from light. Dispense in glass.

IV – Store at 15° to 30°C (59° to 86°F). Protect from light. A precipitate forms if the reconstituted solution is stored at 5°C (41°F). Do not refrigerate the reconstituted product.

Actions

➤*Pharmacology:* Melphalan is a phenylalanine derivative of nitrogen mustard and is a bifunctional, alkylating agent of the bischloroethylamine type. Its cytotoxicity appears to be related to the extent of its interstrand cross-linking with DNA, probably by binding at the N^7 position of guanine. Like other bifunctional alkylating agents, it is active against both resting and rapidly dividing tumor cells.

➤*Pharmacokinetics:*

Absorption / Distribution – Plasma melphalan levels vary after oral dosing with respect to the time of first detectable levels (0 to 6 hours) and to the peak concentrations achieved (range, 70 to 4000 ng/mL), depending on dose. These results may be because of incomplete intestinal absorption, a variable first-pass hepatic metabolism, or to rapid hydrolysis. Mean AUCs after an oral dose of 0.6 mg/kg were 61% (range, 25% to 89%) of those of the same IV dose. In a separate study in 18 patients given single oral doses of 0.2 to 0.25 mg/kg of melphalan, the mean C_{max} and AUC, when dose adjusted to 14 mg, were 212 ng/mL and 498 ng•h/mL, respectively. Following injection, mean peak plasma levels were 1.2 and 2.8 ng/mL after 10 and 20 mg/m^2 doses, respectively. The steady-state volume of distribution is 0.5 L/kg. Penetration into cerebrospinal fluid is low. Plasma protein binding of melphalan ranges from 60% to 90%, with approximately 30% being covalently (irreversibly) bound. Melphalan binds primarily to albumin with alpha$_1$-acid glycoprotein, accounting for approximately 20% of plasma binding.

Metabolism / Excretion – Plasma half-life after oral dosing is approximately 90 minutes. Following injection, drug plasma concentrations decline rapidly in a bi-exponential manner, with distribution phase and terminal elimination phase half-lives of approximately 10 and 75 minutes, respectively. Total body clearance is approximately 7 to 9 mL/min/kg. Melphalan is eliminated from plasma primarily by chemical hydrolysis to monohydroxy and dihydroxy melphalan; no other metabolites have been seen. The contribution of renal elimination to melphalan clearance appears to be low; one pharmacokinetic study showed a significant positive correlation between the elimination rate constant for melphalan and renal function and a significant negative correlation between renal function and the area under the plasma melphalan concentration/time curve.

Contraindications

Hypersensitivity to melphalan; demonstrated prior resistance to the drug.

Warnings

➤*Bone marrow suppression:* As with other nitrogen mustard drugs, excessive dosage will produce marked bone marrow suppression, which is the most significant toxicity associated with melphalan in most patients. Therefore, perform the following tests at the start of therapy and prior to each subsequent dose: Platelet count, hemoglobin, WBC count and differential. Thrombocytopenia and/or leukopenia are indications to withhold further therapy until the blood counts have sufficiently recovered. Frequent blood counts are essential to determine optimal dosage and to avoid toxicity. Discontinue the drug or decrease the dosage upon evidence of bone marrow suppression. Consider dose adjustment on the basis of blood counts at the nadir and day of treatments.

➤*Hypersensitivity reactions:* Hypersensitivity reactions, including anaphylaxis, have occurred with oral and injection. Acute hypersensitivity reactions, including anaphylaxis, occurred in 2.4% of patients on

MELPHALAN (L-PAM; L-Phenylalanine Mustard; L-Sarcolysin)

IV melphalan. These were characterized by bronchospasm, dyspnea, edema, hypotension, pruritus, tachycardia, and urticaria. These usually occur after multiple courses. Treatment is symptomatic. Terminate melphalan immediately; follow with volume expanders, pressor agents, corticosteroids, or antihistamines. If a hypersensitivity reaction occurs, do not readminister melphalan. Refer to Management of Acute Hypersensitivity Reactions.

➤*Renal function impairment:*

IV – Consider dose reduction in patients with renal insufficiency receiving IV melphalan. In one trial, increased bone marrow suppression was seen in patients with BUN levels 30 mg/dL or more. A 50% reduction in IV dose decreased incidence of severe bone marrow suppression in the latter portion of this study.

Oral – Whether routine dosage reductions are needed in patients with renal insufficiency is unknown; only a small amount of a dose appears as parent drug in urine of patients with normal renal function. Closely observe patients with azotemia to make dosage reductions, if required, at the earliest possible time.

➤*Carcinogenesis:* Secondary malignancies, including acute nonlymphocytic leukemia, myeloproliferative syndrome, and carcinoma, occurred in cancer patients following therapy with alkylating agents (including melphalan). Some patients also received other chemotherapeutic agents or radiation therapy. Precise quantitation of the risk of acute leukemia, myeloproliferative syndrome, or carcinoma is not possible. Published reports of leukemia in patients who have received melphalan (and other alkylating agents) suggest that the risk of leukemogenesis increases with chronicity of treatment and with cumulative dose. In one study, the 10-year cumulative risk of developing acute leukemia or myeloproliferative syndrome after melphalan therapy was 19.5% for cumulative doses ranging from 730 to 9652 mg. In this same study, as well as in an additional study, the 10-year cumulative risk of developing acute leukemia or myeloproliferative syndrome after melphalan therapy was less than 2% for cumulative doses under 600 mg. This does not mean that there is a cumulative dose below which there is no risk of the induction of secondary malignancy. The potential benefits from melphalan therapy must be weighed on an individual basis against the possible risk of the induction of a second malignancy.

Adequate and well-controlled carcinogenicity studies have not been conducted in animals. However, intraperitoneal administration of melphalan in rats (5.4 to 10.8 mg/m^2) and in mice (2.25 to 4.5 mg/m^2) 3 times/week for 6 months followed by 12 months of postdose observation produced peritoneal sarcoma and lung tumors, respectively.

➤*Mutagenesis:* Melphalan has been shown to cause chromatid or chromosome damage in humans. IM administration of melphalan at 6 and 60 mg/m^2 produced structural aberrations of the chromatid and chromosomes in bone marrow cells of Wistar rats.

➤*Fertility impairment:* Suppression of ovarian function may occur in premenopausal women, resulting in amenorrhea in many patients. Reversible and irreversible testicular suppression has also occurred.

➤*Elderly:* In general, use caution in dose selection for elderly patients.

➤*Pregnancy: Category D.* Melphalan may cause fetal harm when administered to a pregnant woman. Melphalan was embryolethal and teratogenic in rats following oral (6 to 18 mg/m^2/day for 10 days) and intraperitoneal (18 mg/m^2) administration. Malformations resulting from melphalan included alterations of the brain (underdevelopment, deformation, meningocele, encephalocele) and eye (anophthalmia, microphthalmos), reduction of the mandible and tail, as well as hepatocele (exomphaly). There are no adequate and well-controlled studies in pregnant women. If this drug is used during pregnancy, or if the patient becomes pregnant while taking it, apprise her of the potential hazard to the fetus. Advise women of childbearing potential to avoid becoming pregnant.

➤*Lactation:* It is not known whether this drug is excreted in breast milk. Melphalan is expected to be excreted into breast milk because of the relatively low molecular weight. Do not give to nursing mothers.

➤*Children:* Safety and efficacy in children have not been established.

Precautions

➤*Monitoring:* Perform periodic CBCs with differential during the course of treatment. Obtain at least one determination prior to each dose. Observe patients closely for consequences of bone marrow suppression, which include severe infections, bleeding, and symptomatic anemia (see Warnings).

➤*Prior radiation and chemotherapy:* Use with extreme caution in patients whose bone marrow reserve may have been compromised by prior irradiation or chemotherapy or whose marrow function is recovering from previous cytotoxic therapy.

Drug Interactions

Melphalan Drug Interactions			
Precipitant drug	Object drug*		Description
Cisplatin	Melphalan	↑	Cisplatin may affect melphalan kinetics by inducing renal dysfunction and subsequently altering melphalan clearance.
Nalidixic acid	Melphalan	↑	Incidence of severe hemorrhagic necrotic enterocolitis has been reported to increase in pediatric patients.
Melphalan	Carmustine	↑	Carmustine lung toxicity threshold may be reduced.
Melphalan	Cyclosporine	↑	An increase in the toxicity of cyclosporine, particularly nephrotoxicity, has been observed following coadministration.

*↑ = Object drug increased.

Adverse Reactions

➤*Dermatologic:* Alopecia, skin hypersensitivity, skin necrosis (rarely requiring skin grafting), skin ulceration at injection site.

➤*GI:* Diarrhea, oral ulceration, nausea, vomiting, (infrequent); hepatic veno-occlusive disease and other hepatic disorders ranging from abnormal liver function tests to clinical manifestations, such as hepatitis and jaundice, have been reported.

➤*Miscellaneous:* Allergic reaction, bone marrow suppression, hemolytic anemia, interstitial pneumonitis, pulmonary fibrosis, vasculitis. White blood cell count and platelet count nadirs usually occur 2 to 3 weeks after treatment with recovery in 4 to 5 weeks after treatment. Irreversible bone marrow failure has been reported (see Warnings). Acute hypersensitivity reactions including anaphylaxis were reported in 2.5% of 425 patients receiving melphalan for injection for myeloma (see Warnings).

Overdosage

➤*Symptoms:* Overdoses resulting in death have occurred. Overdoses, including doses up to 290 mg/m^2 (IV) and 50 mg/day for 16 days (oral), have produced the following symptoms: Cholinomimetic effects; convulsions; decreased consciousness; elevations in liver enzymes and veno-occlusive disease (infrequent); muscular paralysis; severe mucositis, stomatitis, colitis, diarrhea, and hemorrhage of the GI tract at high doses (greater than 100 mg/m^2 IV); severe nausea and vomiting; ulceration of the mouth. Significant hyponatremia caused by an associated inappropriate secretion of ADH syndrome; nephrotoxicity and adult respiratory distress syndrome (rare). The principal toxic effect is bone marrow suppression. A pediatric patient survived a 254 mg/m^2 overdose treated with standard supportive care.

➤*Treatment:* Closely follow hematologic parameters for 3 to 6 weeks. An uncontrolled study suggests that administration of autologous bone marrow or hematopoietic growth factors (eg, sargramostim, filgrastim) may shorten the period of pancytopenia. Institute general supportive measures together with appropriate blood transfusions and antibiotics as deemed necessary. This drug is not removed from plasma to any significant degree by hemodialysis or hemoperfusion.

Patient Information

Inform patients that the major toxicities are related to myelosuppression, hypersensitivity, GI toxicity, pulmonary toxicity, infertility, and secondary malignancies. Do not take without close medical supervision.

Notify physician of unusual bleeding, fever, persistent cough, skin rash, vasculitis, amenorrhea, nausea, vomiting, weight loss, or unusual lumps or masses.

Inform patients to refrigerate tablets and keep them in the glass bottle.

Contraceptive measures are recommended during therapy. Advise women of childbearing potential to avoid becoming pregnant.

ESTRAMUSTINE PHOSPHATE SODIUM

| Rx | Emcyt (Pharmacia) | Capsules: 140 mg (as estramustine phosphate) | White. In 100s. |

Indications

Palliative treatment of metastatic and/or progressive carcinoma of the prostate.

Administration and Dosage

➤*Recommended daily dosage:* 14 mg/kg/day (ie, one 140 mg capsule for each 10 kg or 22 lb) given in 3 or 4 divided doses (dosage range, 10 to 16 mg/kg/day).

Take with water at least 1 hour before or 2 hours after meals.

Milk, milk products, and calcium-rich foods or drugs (such as calcium-containing antacids) must not be taken simultaneously with estramustine phosphate sodium.

Treat for 30 to 90 days before assessing the possible benefits of continued therapy. Continue therapy as long as response is favorable. Some patients have been maintained on therapy for more than 3 years at doses ranging from 10 to 16 mg/kg/day.

➤*Storage/Stability:* Refrigerate at 2° to 8°C (36° to 46°F). Capsules may be left out of the refrigerator for 24 to 48 hours without affecting potency.

Actions

➤*Pharmacology:* Estramustine phosphate combines estradiol and nornitrogen mustard by a carbamate link. The molecule is phosphorylated to make it water soluble. The intent of the molecule design was for the estradiol portion to facilitate the uptake of the alkylating agent into the hormone-sensitive prostate cancer cells. However, it was determined that estramustine does not function in vivo as an alkylating agent and not all of its effects can be attributed to the estrogenic hormones. Estramustine has been shown to have weaker estrogenic effects than estradiol. It has been called an antimicrotubule agent because it covalently binds to microtubule-associated proteins, thereby inhibiting microtubule assembly and eventually causing their disassembly.

➤*Pharmacokinetics:*

Absorption/Distribution – After oral administration, estramustine is well absorbed with a bioavailability of at least 75%. Estramustine phosphate is readily dephosphorylated during absorption, and the major metabolites in plasma are estramustine, the estrone analog, estradiol, and estrone.

Prolonged treatment produces elevated total plasma concentrations of estradiol that are within ranges similar to the elevated estradiol levels found in prostatic cancer patients given conventional estradiol therapy. Estrogenic effects, as demonstrated by changes in circulating levels of steroids and pituitary hormones, are similar in patients treated with either estramustine phosphate or conventional estradiol.

Metabolism/Excretion – Estramustine is found in the body mainly as estromustine (17-keto analog).

The metabolic urinary patterns of estradiol and the estradiol moiety of estramustine phosphate are very similar, although the metabolites derived from estramustine phosphate are excreted at a slower rate. The nornitrogen mustard and estradiol metabolites are excreted independently into the bile, feces, and urine.

Contraindications

Hypersensitivity to estradiol or nitrogen mustard.

Active thrombophlebitis or thromboembolic disorders, except where the actual tumor mass is the cause of the thromboembolic phenomenon and the benefits of therapy outweigh the risks.

Warnings

➤*Thrombosis:* The risk of thrombosis, including fatal and nonfatal myocardial infarction, increases in men receiving estrogens for prostatic cancer. Use with caution in patients with a history of thrombophlebitis, thrombosis or thromboembolic disorders, especially if they were associated with estrogen therapy. Use with caution in patients with cerebral vascular or coronary artery disease.

➤*Glucose tolerance:* Tolerance to glucose may be decreased; observe diabetic patients receiving this drug.

➤*Elevated blood pressure:* Blood pressure elevation may occur; monitor blood pressure periodically during therapy.

➤*Hypersensitivity reactions:* Allergic reactions and angioedema at times involving the airway have been reported.

➤*Hepatic function impairment:* Estramustine may be poorly metabolized in patients with impaired liver function. Administer with caution.

➤*Carcinogenesis:* Long-term continuous administration of estrogens in certain animal species increases frequency of carcinomas of the breast and liver. Compounds structurally similar are carcinogenic in mice.

➤*Mutagenesis:* Although testing by the Ames method failed to demonstrate mutagenicity for estramustine, both estradiol and nitrogen mustard are mutagenic. For this reason, and because some patients who had been impotent while on estrogen therapy have regained potency while taking the drug, advise use of contraceptive measures.

Precautions

➤*Fluid retention:* Exacerbation of pre-existing or incipient peripheral edema or congestive heart disease may occur in some patients. Other conditions potentially influenced by fluid retention, such as epilepsy, migraine, or renal dysfunction, require careful observation.

➤*Calcium/Phosphorus metabolism:* Calcium/Phosphorus metabolism may be influenced by estramustine; use with caution in patients with metabolic bone diseases associated with hypercalcemia or in patients with renal insufficiency.

➤*Gynecomastia/Impotence:* Gynecomastia and impotence are known estrogenic effects.

➤*Lab test abnormalities:* Certain endocrine and liver function tests may be affected by estrogen-containing drugs. Estramustine phosphate sodium may depress testosterone levels. Abnormalities of hepatic enzymes and of bilirubin have occurred. Perform such tests at appropriate intervals during therapy and repeat after the drug has been withdrawn for 2 months.

Drug Interactions

➤*Drug/Food interactions:* Milk, milk products, and calcium-rich foods or drugs may impair the absorption of estramustine phosphate sodium.

Adverse Reactions

Estramustine Phosphate Sodium Adverse Reactions		
Adverse reactions	Estramustine phosphate sodium (11.5 to 15.9 mg/kg/day) (n = 93)	Diethylstilbestrol (3 mg/day) (n = 93)
Cardiovascular		
Cardiac arrest	0	2
Cerebrovascular accident	2	0
MI	3	1
Thrombophlebitis	3	7
Pulmonary emboli	2	5
CHF	3	2
CNS		
Lethargy alone	4	3
Depression	0	2
Emotional lability	2	0
Insomnia	3	0
Headache	1	1
Anxiety	1	0
Dermatologic		
Rash	1	4
Pruritus	2	2
Dry skin	2	0
Pigment changes	0	3
Easy bruising	3	0
Flushing	1	0
Night sweats	0	1
Fingertip (peeling skin)	1	0
Thinning hair	1	1
GI		
Nausea	15	8
Diarrhea	12	11
Minor GI upset	11	6
Anorexia	4	3
Flatulence	2	0
Vomiting	1	1
GI bleeding	1	0
Burning throat	1	0
Thirst	1	0
GU		
Breast tenderness	66	64
Breast enlargement		
Mild	60	54
Moderate	10	16
Marked	0	5
Respiratory		
Dyspnea	11	3
Upper respiratory discharge	1	1
Hoarseness	1	0

ESTRAMUSTINE PHOSPHATE SODIUM

Estramustine Phosphate Sodium Adverse Reactions		
Adverse reactions	Estramustine phosphate sodium (11.5 to 15.9 mg/kg/day) (n = 93)	Diethylstilbestrol (3 mg/day) (n = 93)
Special senses		
Pain in eyes	0	1
Tearing of eyes	1	1
Tinnitus	0	1
Laboratory test abnormalities		
Hematologic		
Leukopenia	4	2
Thrombopenia	1	2
Hepatic		
Bilirubin alone	1	5
Bilirubin and LDH	0	1
Bilirubin and AST	2	1
Bilirubin, LDH, AST	2	0
LDH and/or AST	31	28

Estramustine Phosphate Sodium Adverse Reactions		
Adverse reactions	Estramustine phosphate sodium (11.5 to 15.9 mg/kg/day) (n = 93)	Diethylstilbestrol (3 mg/day) (n = 93)
Miscellaneous		
Hypercalcemia (transient)	0	1
Leg cramps	8	11
Edema	19	17
Chest pain	1	1
Hot flashes	0	1

Overdosage

Although there has been no experience with overdosage, it may produce pronounced manifestations of the adverse reactions. In the event of overdosage, evacuate gastric contents by gastric lavage and initiate symptomatic therapy. Monitor hematologic and hepatic parameters for at least 6 weeks after overdosage.

Patient Information

Because of the possibility of mutagenic effects, use contraceptive measures.

Take with water at least 1 hour before or 2 hours after meals.

Milk, milk products, and calcium-rich foods or drugs (such as calcium-containing antacids) must not be taken simultaneously with estramustine phosphate sodium.

CARMUSTINE (BCNU)

| Rx | BiCNU (Bristol Labs Oncology) | Powder for Injection, lyophilized: 100 mg | Preservative-free. In single-dose vials with 3 mL sterile diluent. |
| Rx | Gliadel (Guilford Pharm.) | Wafer: 7.7 mg | Preservative-free. In single-dose treatment box with 8 individually pouched wafers. |

WARNING

Because delayed bone marrow suppression is the major toxic effect of injectable carmustine, monitor complete blood counts weekly for at least 6 weeks after a dose. Do not give repeat doses more frequently than every 6 weeks. Bone marrow toxicity is cumulative; therefore, adjust dosage on the basis of nadir blood counts from prior dose (see dosage adjustment table under Administration and Dosage).

Bone marrow suppression, notably thrombocytopenia and leukopenia, which may contribute to bleeding and overwhelming infections in an already compromised patient, is the most common and severe of the toxic effects of injectable carmustine.

Pulmonary toxicity from injectable carmustine appears to be dose-related. Patients receiving greater than 1400 mg/m^2 cumulative dose are at significantly higher risk than those receiving less.

Delayed pulmonary toxicity can occur years after treatment and can result in death, particularly in patients treated in childhood.

Indications

➤*Injection:* Palliative therapy as a single agent or combined with other approved chemotherapeutic agents in the following:

Brain tumors – Glioblastoma, brainstem glioma, medulloblastoma, astrocytoma, ependymoma and metastatic brain tumors.

Multiple myeloma – In combination with prednisone.

Hodgkin disease and non-Hodgkin lymphomas – As secondary therapy in combination with other approved drugs in patients who relapse with, or who fail to respond to, primary therapy.

➤*Wafer:* As an adjunct to surgery and radiation in newly diagnosed high-grade malignant glioma patients; in recurrent glioblastoma multiforme patients as an adjunct to surgery.

➤*Unlabeled uses:* Topical carmustine has been shown to be effective in the treatment of primary cutaneous T-cell lymphoma (ie, mycosis fungoides and Sezary syndrome). Carmustine, alone or in combination therapy, has also shown some benefit in the management of malignant melanoma.

Administration and Dosage

➤*Wafer:* It is recommended that 8 wafers be placed in the resection cavity if the size and shape of cavity allows. Should the size and shape not accommodate 8 wafers, the maximum number of wafers as allowed should be used to cover as much of the resection cavity as possible. Slight overlapping of the wafer is acceptable. Wafers broken in half may be used, but discard wafers broken in more than 2 pieces. Oxidized regenerated cellulose may be placed over the wafers to secure them against the cavity surface. After placement of the wafers, the resection cavity should be irrigated and the dura closed in a water-tight fashion.

➤*Injection:* As a single agent in previously untreated patients, 150 to 200 mg/m^2 IV every 6 weeks given as a single dose or divided daily injections (eg, 75 to 100 mg/m^2 on 2 successive days).

When used in combination with other myelosuppressive drugs or in patients in whom bone marrow reserve is depleted, adjust doses accordingly.

Do not give a repeat course until circulating blood elements have returned to acceptable levels (platelets above 100,000/mm^3; leukocytes above 4000/mm^3). Adequate number of neutrophils should be present on a peripheral blood smear. Monitor blood counts weekly; do not give repeat courses before 6 weeks because of delayed and cumulative toxicity.

The following schedule is suggested as a guide to dosage adjustment based on the patient's hematologic response to the previous dose:

Suggested Carmustine Dose Following Initial Dose		
Nadir after prior dose		Prior dose to be given (%)
Leukocytes/mm^3	Platelets/mm^3	
> 4000	> 100,000	100
3000-3999	75,000-99,999	100
2000-2999	25,000-74,999	70
< 2000	< 25,000	50

➤*Preparation/Handling:*

Wafer – Use of double gloves is recommended because exposure to carmustine can cause severe burning and hyperpigmentation of the skin. Use surgical instruments dedicated to the handling of the wafers for implantation. Deliver the aluminum foil laminate pouches containing the wafer to the operating room and leave unopened until ready to implant the wafers.

Injection – Accidental contact of reconstituted carmustine injection with the skin has caused transient hyperpigmentation of the affected areas. The use of gloves is recommended. Dissolve with 3 mL of the supplied sterile diluent (dehydrated alcohol injection), then add 27 mL of sterile water for injection to the alcohol solution. The resulting solution contains 3.3 mg/mL carmustine in 10% ethanol.

Reconstitution as recommended results in a clear colorless to yellowish solution that may be further diluted with 5% dextrose for injection.

Administer the reconstituted solution by IV drip. Shorter infusion times than 1 to 2 hours may produce intense pain and burning at the injection site.

The lyophilized dosage formulation contains no preservatives and is not intended as a multiple dose vial.

➤*Storage/Stability:*

Wafer – Unopened foil pouches may be kept at ambient room temperature for a maximum of 6 hours at a time. Store at or below -20°C (-4°F).

Injection – Store unopened vials of the dry powder in a refrigerator (2° to 8°C; 36° to 46°F). The recommended storage of unopened vials provides a stable product for 2 years. After reconstitution as recommended, carmustine is stable for 8 hours at room temperature (25°C; 77°F). Protect from light.

Vials reconstituted as directed and further diluted to a concentration of 0.2 mg/mL in 5% dextrose injection are stable for 8 hours at room temperature (25°C; 77°F). Protect from light.

Only use glass containers.

Carmustine has a low melting point (30.5° to 32°C; about 87° to 90°F). Exposure of the drug to this temperature or above will cause it to liquefy and appear as an oil film on the bottom of the vials. This is a sign of decomposition; discard the vial. If there is a question of adequate refrigeration upon receipt of this product, immediately inspect the larger vial in each individual carton. Hold the vial to a bright light for inspection. The carmustine will appear as a very small amount of dry flakes or dry congealed mass. If this is evident, the carmustine is suitable for use; refrigerate immediately.

Actions

➤*Pharmacology:* Carmustine alkylates deoxyribonucleic acid (DNA) and ribonucleic acid (RNA) and also inhibits several enzymes by carbamoylation of amino acids in proteins. Carmustine is not cross resistant with other alkylators. Antineoplastic and toxic activities may be caused by metabolites.

➤*Pharmacokinetics:*

Injection – Because of the high lipid solubility and the lack of ionization at physiological pH, carmustine crosses the blood-brain barrier effectively. Levels of radioactivity in the CSF are at least 50% of those in plasma.

Following IV administration, it is rapidly degraded, with no intact drug detectable after 15 minutes. Following an IV infusion of carmustine at doses ranging from 30 to 170 mg/m^2, the average terminal half-life, clearance and steady-state volume of distribution were 22 minutes, 56 mL/min/kg, and 3.25 L/kg, respectively. Approximately 60% to 70% of the total dose is excreted in the urine in 96 hours, and 10% is expired as CO_2. The fate of the remainder is undetermined.

Wafer – Wafers are biodegradable in the human brain when implanted into the cavity after tumor resection. The carmustine released from the wafer diffuses into the surrounding brain tissue. The rate of biodegradation is variable from patient to patient. A wafer remnant may be observed on brain imaging scans or at re-operation even though extensive degradation of all components has occurred. The absorption, distribution, metabolism, and excretion of the copolymer in humans is unknown.

Contraindications

Hypersensitivity to carmustine or to any components of the wafer formulation.

Warnings

➤*Hematologic:* The most frequent and serious toxic effect of injectable carmustine is delayed myelosuppression, which usually occurs 4 to 6 weeks after administration and is dose related (see Warning Box). Thrombocytopenia occurs at about 4 weeks postadministration and persists for 1 to 2 weeks. Leukopenia occurs at 5 to 6 weeks after a dose and persists for 1 to 2 weeks. Thrombocytopenia is generally more severe than leukopenia; however, both may have dose-limiting toxicities. Carmustine injection may produce cumulative myelosuppression, manifested by more depressed indices or longer duration of suppression after repeated doses. Anemia is less frequent and less severe. The occurrence of acute leukemia and bone marrow dysplasias have been reported in patients following long-term nitrosourea therapy.

CARMUSTINE (BCNU)

➤*Renal toxicity:* Decrease in kidney size, progressive azotemia, and renal failure have occurred in patients who received large cumulative doses of injectable carmustine after prolonged therapy; kidney damage was occasionally reported in patients receiving lower total doses.

➤*Hepatic toxicity:* Reversible hepatic toxicity, manifested by increased transaminase, alkaline phosphatase, and bilirubin levels, has occurred in a small percentage of patients using injectable carmustine.

➤*Pulmonary toxicity:* Pulmonary infiltrates and/or fibrosis have occurred with injectable carmustine from 9 days to 43 months after treatment with carmustine injection and related nitrosoureas. Most of these patients were receiving prolonged therapy with total doses of injection greater than 1400 mg/m². However, there have been reports of pulmonary fibrosis in patients receiving lower total doses. Other risk factors include past history of lung disease and duration of treatment. Cases of fatal pulmonary toxicity have been reported.

Additionally, delayed-onset pulmonary fibrosis, occurring up to 17 years after treatment, has been reported in a long-term study with 17 patients who received carmustine injection in childhood and early adolescence (1 to 16 years of age) in cumulative doses ranging from 770 to 1800 mg/m² combined with cranial radiotherapy for intracranial tumors. Chest x-rays demonstrated pulmonary hypoplasia with upper zone contraction. Thoracic CT scans have demonstrated an unusual pattern of upper zone fibrosis. There was some late reduction of pulmonary function in all long-term survivors. This form of lung fibrosis may be slowly progressive and has resulted in death in some cases. In this long-term study, 8 of 17 died of delayed pulmonary lung fibrosis, including all those initially treated (5 of 17) at less than 5 years of age.

➤*Ocular:* Carmustine administration through an intra-arterial intra-carotid route is investigational and has been associated with ocular toxicity.

➤*Brain herniation:* Cases of intracerebral mass effect unresponsive to corticosteroids have been described in patients treated with the wafer, including one case leading to brain herniation.

➤*Seizures:* In the initial surgery trial, the incidence of seizures was 33.3% in patients receiving carmustine wafer and 37.5% in patients receiving placebo. Grand mal seizures occurred in 5% of wafer-treated patients and 4.2% of placebo-treated patients. The incidence of seizures within the first 5 days after wafer implantation was 2.5% in the wafer group and 4.2% in the placebo group. The time from surgery to the onset of the first postoperative seizure did not differ between the wafer and placebo-treated patients.

In the surgery for recurrent disease trial, the incidence of postoperative seizures was the same for the wafer treatment group and placebo (19%). Of the 22 patients, 54% of wafer-treated patients and 9% of placebo patients experienced the first new or worsened seizure within the first 5 postoperative days; the median time to onset was 3.5 days and 61 days, respectively.

➤*Brain edema:* Brain edema was noted in 22.5% of patients treated with the wafer and in 19.2% of placebo patients. Development of brain edema with mass effect (caused by tumor recurrence, intracranial infection, or necrosis) may necessitate re-operation and, in some cases, removal of the wafer or its remnants.

➤*Intracranial infection:* In the initial surgery trial, the incidence of brain abscess or meningitis was 5% in patients treated with carmustine wafer and 6% in patients receiving placebo. In the recurrent setting, the incidence of brain abscess or meningitis was 4% in patients treated with the wafer and 1% in patients receiving placebo.

➤*Obstructive hydrocephalus:* Avoid communication between the surgical resection cavity and the ventricular system to prevent the wafers from migrating into the ventricular system and causing obstructive hydrocephalus. If a communication exists larger than the diameter of a wafer, close it prior to wafer implantation.

➤*Carcinogenesis:* Carmustine injection is carcinogenic in rats and mice, producing a marked increase in tumor incidence in doses approximating those employed clinically. Nitrosourea therapy does have carcinogenic potential in humans. There were increases in tumor incidence in all treated animals, predominantly SC and lung neoplasms. Long-term use of nitrosoureas has been reported to be associated with the development of secondary malignancies.

➤*Mutagenesis:* Carmustine was mutagenic in vitro (Ames assay, human lymphoblast HGPRT assay) and clastogenic both in vitro (V79 hamster cell micronucleus assay) and in vivo (SCE assay in rodent brain tumors, mouse bone marrow micronucleus assay).

➤*Fertility impairment:* Carmustine injection affects fertility in male rats at doses somewhat higher than the human dose. Carmustine caused testicular degeneration at intraperitoneal doses of 8 mg/kg/week for 8 weeks (about 1.3 times the recommended human dose on a mg/m² basis) in male rats.

➤*Pregnancy: Category D.* Carmustine is embryotoxic and teratogenic in rats and embryotoxic in rabbits at dose levels equivalent to the human dose. Carmustine may cause fetal harm when administered to a pregnant woman. There are no adequate and well-controlled studies in pregnant women. If this drug is used during pregnancy, or if the patient becomes pregnant while taking this drug, advise her of the potential hazard to the fetus. Advise women of childbearing potential to avoid becoming pregnant.

➤*Lactation:* It is not known whether this drug is excreted in breast milk. Because of the potential for serious adverse reactions in breast-feeding infants from carmustine, discontinue nursing.

➤*Children:* Safety and efficacy for use in children have not been established. Delayed-onset pulmonary fibrosis occurring up to 17 years after treatment, has been reported in a long-term study of patients who received carmustine injection in childhood and early adolescence (1 to 16 years of age). Eight out of the 17 patients (47%) who survived childhood brain tumors, including all of the 5 patients initially treated at less than 5 years of age, died of pulmonary fibrosis. Therefore, the risks and benefits of carmustine injection therapy must be carefully considered, because of the extremely high risk of pulmonary toxicity (see Adverse Reactions).

Precautions

➤*Monitoring:*

Injection – Because of delayed bone marrow suppression, monitor blood counts weekly for at least 6 weeks after a dose.

Conduct baseline pulmonary function studies and frequent pulmonary function tests during treatment. Patients with a baseline less than 70% of predicted Forced Vital Capacity (FVC) or Carbon Monoxide Diffusing Capacity (DL$_{co}$) are at particular risk. Monitor liver and renal function tests periodically.

Wafer – Monitor patients undergoing craniotomy for malignant glioma and implantation of the wafer closely for known complications of craniotomy, including seizures, intracranial infections, abnormal wound healing, and brain edema.

Computed tomography and magnetic resonance imaging of the head may demonstrate enhancement in the brain tissue surrounding the resection cavity after implantation of carmustine wafers. This enhancement may represent edema and inflammation caused by the wafer or tumor progression.

➤*Healing abnormalities:* The following healing abnormalities have been reported in clinical trials of carmustine wafer: Wound dehiscence, delayed wound healing, subdural, subgaleal, or wound effusions, and cerebrospinal fluid lead. In the initial surgery trial, healing abnormalities occurred in 15.8% of carmustine wafer-treated patients and in 11.7% of placebo recipients. Cerebrospinal fluid leaks occurred in 5% of carmustine wafer recipients and 0.8% of those given placebo. During surgery, obtain a water-tight dural closure to minimize the risk of cerebrospinal fluid leak.

In the surgery for recurrent disease trial, the incidence of healing abnormalities was 14% in carmustine-wafer treated patients and 5% in patients receiving placebo wafers.

➤*GI:* Nausea and vomiting after IV administration have been noted frequently. This dose-related toxicity appears within 2 hours of dosing and lasts 4 to 6 hours. Prior administration of antiemetics is effective in diminishing or preventing these side effects.

Drug Interactions

Carmustine Drug Interactions			
Precipitant drug	Object drug*		Description
Cimetidine	Carmustine	↑	Cimetidine may enhance the myelosuppressive effects of carmustine, possibly to the point of toxicity. Avoid if possible.
Carmustine	Digoxin	↓	Digoxin serum levels may be reduced, and its actions may be decreased by a combination chemotherapy regimen including carmustine.
Carmustine	Phenytoin	↓	Phenytoin serum concentrations may be decreased by a combination chemotherapy regimen including carmustine.

* ↑ = Object drug increased. ↓ = Object drug decreased.

Adverse Reactions

➤*Injection:*

Pulmonary – Pulmonary toxicity appears to be dose related. Patients receiving greater than 1400 mg/m² cumulative dose are at significantly higher risk than those receiving less. Additionally, delayed-onset pulmonary fibrosis occurring up to 17 years after treatment has been reported in patients receiving carmustine in childhood and early adolescence (see Warnings).

GI – Nausea and vomiting are noted frequently. Toxicity appears within 2 hours of dosing, usually lasting 4 to 6 hours, and is dose related (see Precautions).

CARMUSTINE (BCNU)

Hematologic – Delayed myelosuppression is the major toxicity. It usually occurs 4 to 6 weeks after drug administration and is dose related (see Warnings).

Hepatic – A reversible type of hepatic toxicity, manifested by increased transaminase, alkaline phosphatase, and bilirubin levels, has been reported in a small percentage of patients.

Renal – Progressive azotemia, decrease in kidney size, and renal failure have been reported in patients who received large cumulative doses after prolonged therapy. Kidney damage has also been reported (see Warnings).

Miscellaneous – Accidental contact with skin has caused burning and hyperpigmentation of the affected areas.

Rapid IV infusion may produce intensive flushing of the skin and suffusion of the conjunctiva within 2 hours, lasting about 4 hours. Rapid infusion is also associated with burning at the site of injection, although true thrombosis is rare.

Neuroretinitis, chest pain, headache, allergic reaction, hypotension, and tachycardia also have been reported.

➤*Wafer:*

Adverse Events Observed in Patients Receiving Carmustine Wafer at Initial Surgery (≥ 5%)		
Adverse reaction	Carmustine wafer (N = 120)	Placebo (N = 120)
Cardiovascular		
Deep thrombophlebitis	10	9
Pulmonary embolus	8	8
Hemorrhage	7	6
CNS		
Headache	28	37
Hemiplegia	41	44
Convulsion	33	38
Confusion	23	21
Brain edema	23	19
Aphasia	18	18
Depression	16	10
Somnolence	11	15
Speech disorder	11	8
Amnesia	9	10
Intracranial hypertension	9	2
Personality disorder	8	8
Anxiety	7	4
Facial paralysis	7	4
Neuropathy	7	10
Ataxia	6	4
Hypesthesia	6	5
Paresthesia	6	8
Thinking abnormal	6	8
Abnormal gait	5	5
Dizziness	5	9
Grand mal convulsion	5	4
Hallucinations	5	3
Insomnia	5	6
Tremor	5	7
Coma	4	5
Incoordination	3	7
Hypokinesia	2	7
Endocrine system		
Diabetes mellitus	5	4
Cushing syndrome	3	5
Alopecia	10	12
GI		
Nausea	22	17
Vomiting	21	16
Constipation	19	12
Abdominal pain	8	2
Diarrhea	5	4
Liver function tests abnormal	1	5
GU		
Urinary tract infection	8	11
Urinary incontinence	8	8
Metabolic/Nutritional disorders		
Healing abnormal	16	12
Peripheral edema	9	9

Adverse Events Observed in Patients Receiving Carmustine Wafer at Initial Surgery (≥ 5%)		
Adverse reaction	Carmustine wafer (N = 120)	Placebo (N = 120)
Respiratory		
Pneumonia	8	8
Dyspnea	3	7
Special senses		
Conjunctival edema	7	7
Abnormal vision	6	6
Visual field defect	5	7
Eye disorder	3	5
Diplopia	1	5
Miscellaneous		
Aggravation reaction[1]	82	79
Asthenia	22	15
Infection	18	20
Fever	18	18
Pain	13	15
Rash	12	11
Back pain	7	3
Face edema	6	5
Abscess	5	3
Accidental injury	5	7
Chest pain	5	0
Allergic reaction	2	5
Myasthenia	4	5

[1] Adverse events coded to "aggravation reaction" were usually events involving tumor/disease progression or general deterioration of condition (eg, condition/health/Karnofsky/neurological/physical deterioration).

Adverse Reactions: Carmustine Wafer vs Placebo for Recurrent Disease (≥ 4%)		
Adverse reaction	Wafer with carmustine (n=110; %)	Wafer without carmustine (n=112; %)
CNS		
Convulsion	19	19
Hemiplegia	19	20
Headache	15	13
Somnolence	14	11
Confusion	10	8
Aphasia	9	11
Stupor	6	6
Brain edema	4	1
Intracranial hypertension	4	6
Meningitis or abscess	4	1
Miscellaneous		
Urinary tract infection	21	17
Healing abnormal	14	5
Fever	12	8
Nausea and vomiting	8	6
Pain	7	1
Rash	5	4

Cardiovascular – Hypertension (3%); hypotension (1%).

CNS – Seizures, brain edema (see Warnings); hydrocephalus, depression (3%); abnormal thinking, ataxia, dizziness, insomnia, monoplegia (2%); coma, amnesia, diplopia, paranoid reaction (1%); cerebral hemorrhage and cerebral infarct (less than 1%).

GI – Diarrhea, constipation (2%); dysphagia, GI hemorrhage, fecal incontinence (1%).

Hematologic / Lymphatic – Thrombocytopenia, leukocytosis (1%).

Metabolic / Nutritional – Hyponatremia, hyperglycemia (3%); hypokalemia (1%).

Respiratory – Infection (2%); aspiration pneumonia (1%).

Special senses – Visual field defect (2%); eye pain (1%).

Miscellaneous – Healing abnormalities, intracranial infection (see Warnings and Precautions); peripheral edema, neck pain, rash, urinary incontinence (2%); accidental injury, back pain, allergic reaction, asthenia, chest pain, sepsis (1%).

Overdosage

No proven antidotes have been established for carmustine overdosage.

Patient Information

Contraceptive measures are recommended during therapy.

Nitrosoureas

LOMUSTINE (CCNU)

Rx	**CeeNU**	**Capsules:** 10 mg	Mannitol. Two-tone white. In 20s.
	(Bristol Labs Oncology)	40 mg	Mannitol. White/green. In 20s.
		100 mg	Mannitol. Two-tone green. In 20s.

Dose Pack: Two 100 mg capsules, two 40 mg capsules and two 10 mg capsules.

WARNING

Bone marrow suppression, notably thrombocytopenia and leukopenia, which may contribute to bleeding and overwhelming infections in an already compromised patient, is the most common and severe of the toxic effects of lomustine.

Because the major toxicity is delayed bone marrow suppression, monitor blood counts weekly for ≥ 6 weeks after a dose. At the recommended dosage, do not give courses of lomustine more frequently than every 6 weeks.

Bone marrow toxicity is cumulative. Consider dosage adjustments on the basis of nadir blood counts from prior dosage (see Administration and Dosage and Warnings).

Indications

As a single agent in addition to other treatment modalities, or in established combination therapy with other agents in the following:

➤ *Brain tumors:* Both primary and metastatic in patients who have already received appropriate surgical or radiotherapeutic procedures.

➤ *Hodgkin's disease:* Secondary therapy in combination with other drugs in patients who relapse while on primary therapy, or who fail to respond to primary therapy.

Administration and Dosage

➤*Adults and children:* 130 mg/m² as a single oral dose every 6 weeks. In compromised bone marrow function, reduce dose to 100 mg/m² every 6 weeks. Do not give a repeat course until circulating blood elements have returned to acceptable levels (platelets > 100,000/mm³; leukocytes > 4000/mm³). Monitor blood counts weekly and do not give repeat courses before 6 weeks; hematologic toxicity is delayed and cumulative.

Adjust doses subsequent to the initial dose according to the hematologic response of the patient to the preceding dose as follows:

Suggested Lomustine Dose Following Initial Dose		
Nadir after prior dose		Prior dose to be given (%)
Leukocytes/mm³	Platelets/mm³	
> 4000	> 100,000	100
3000-3999	75,000-99,999	100
2000-2999	25,000-74,999	70
< 2000	< 25,000	50

➤*Concomitant therapy:* With other myelosuppressive drugs, adjust dosage accordingly.

➤*Storage / Stability:* Avoid excessive heat (over 40°C; 104°F).

Actions

➤*Pharmacology:* Lomustine acts as an alkylating agent, but like other nitrosoureas, it may also inhibit several key enzymatic processes. Its mechanism of action involves the inhibition of both DNA and RNA synthesis through DNA alkylation. Lomustine has been shown to affect a number of cellular processes including RNA, protein synthesis, and the processing of ribosomal and nucleoplasmic messenger RNA; DNA base component structure; the rate of DNA synthesis and DNA polymerase activity. It is cell cycle nonspecific.

➤*Pharmacokinetics:*

Absorption – The lipid soluble nitrosoureas are rapidly and completely absorbed when given orally; appearance in plasma occurs ≈ 10 minutes postadministration and peak levels of metabolites appear in ≈ 3 hours.

Distribution – The lipid solubility of lomustine results in extensive tissue distribution. Blood-brain penetration is good; cerebrospinal fluid levels of 15% to 50% of those in plasma have been noted.

Metabolism – Lomustine is rapidly degraded, apparently in the liver, to several cytotoxic metabolites. The serum half-life of the metabolites ranges from 16 hours to 2 days. Tissue levels are comparable with plasma levels at 15 minutes after IV administration.

Excretion – About half of the dose is excreted in the form of degradation products within 24 hours. Small amounts are excreted via the feces and lungs.

Contraindications

Hypersensitivity to lomustine.

Warnings

➤*Hematologic:* The most frequent and most serious toxicity is delayed myelosuppression. It usually occurs 4 to 6 weeks after drug administration and is dose related. Thrombocytopenia occurs ≈ 4 weeks after a dose and persists for 1 to 2 weeks. Leukopenia occurs ≈ 5 to 6 weeks after a dose and persists for 1 to 2 weeks. About 65% of patients develop white blood cell (WBC) counts < 5000/mm³, and 36% of patients develop WBC counts < 3000/mm³. Thrombocytopenia is generally more severe than leukopenia; however, both may be dose-limiting toxicities. Anemia also occurs, but is less frequent and less severe than thrombocytopenia or leukopenia. Cumulative myelosuppression may occur, manifested by more depressed indices or longer duration of suppression after repeated doses.

➤*Hepatic toxicity:* A reversible type of hepatic toxicity, manifested by increased transaminase, alkaline phosphatase, and bilirubin levels, has occurred in a small percentage of patients.

➤*Renal toxicity:* Decrease in kidney size, progressive azotemia, and renal failure have occurred in patients who received large cumulative doses after prolonged therapy. Kidney damage has occurred occasionally in patients receiving lower total doses.

➤*Pulmonary toxicity:* Pulmonary toxicity characterized by pulmonary infiltrates or fibrosis occurs rarely and appears to be dose related. Onset of toxicity has occurred after an interval of ≥ 6 months from start of therapy with cumulative doses usually > 1100 mg/m². There is one report of pulmonary toxicity at a cumulative dose of 600 mg.

Delayed-onset pulmonary fibrosis occurring ≤ 15 years after treatment has been reported in patients who received related nitrosoureas in childhood and early adolescence combined with cranial radiotherapy for intracranial tumors.

➤*Carcinogenesis:* Carcinogenic in rats and mice in approximately clinical doses. Acute leukemia and bone marrow dysplasias have occurred after long-term nitrosourea therapy.

➤*Fertility impairment:* There have been reports of persistent testicular damage causing infertility.

➤*Pregnancy: Category D.* Lomustine can cause fetal harm when administered to a pregnant woman. There are no adequate and well-controlled studies in pregnant women. Advise patient of the potential hazard to the fetus if she becomes pregnant while taking lomustine. Advise women of childbearing potential to avoid becoming pregnant while on lomustine.

➤*Lactation:* It is not known whether lomustine is excreted in breast milk. Because of the potential for serious adverse reactions, decide whether to discontinue breastfeeding or to discontinue the drug, taking into account the importance of the drug to the mother.

➤*Children:* See Administration and Dosage.

Precautions

➤*Monitoring:* Major toxicity is delayed bone marrow suppression; monitor blood counts weekly for 6 weeks after a dose. Monitor liver and renal function periodically.

Also conduct baseline pulmonary function studies during treatment. Patients with a baseline < 70% of the predicted Forced Vital Capacity (FVC) or Carbon Monoxide Diffusing Capacity (DL$_{CO}$) are particularly at risk.

➤*GI:* Nausea and vomiting may occur 3 to 6 hours after an oral dose and usually last < 24 hours. Antiemetics prior to dosing may diminish and sometimes prevent these effects. May also be reduced by administration to fasting patients.

Adverse Reactions

Most adverse reactions are reversible if detected early. When adverse reactions occur, reduce dosage or discontinue the drug and take appropriate corrective measures.

➤*GI:* Nausea, vomiting (see Precautions); sore mouth, lips and throat; bleeding.

➤*Hematologic:* Delayed myelosuppression, leukopenia, anemia (see Warnings).

➤*Renal:* Decrease in kidney size, progressive azotemia, renal failure (see Warnings).

➤*Miscellaneous:* Alopecia; stomatitis (infrequent); disorientation, lethargy, ataxia, dysarthria (the relationship to medication is unclear); hepatic toxicity, pulmonary toxicity, pulmonary fibrosis (see Warnings).

LOMUSTINE (CCNU)

Secondary malignancies – Long-term use of nitrosoureas may be associated with development of secondary malignancies (see Warnings).

Overdosage

There are no proven antidotes for lomustine overdosage. Refer to General Management of Acute Overdosage.

Patient Information

Notify physician if fever, chills, sore throat, unusual bleeding or bruising, shortness of breath, dry cough, swelling of feet or lower legs, yellowing of eyes and skin, confusion, sores on the mouth or lips or unusual tiredness occurs.

Medication may cause loss of appetite, nausea and vomiting; hair loss, skin rash or itching (infrequent); notify physician if these reactions become pronounced.

Take on an empty stomach to reduce nausea.

Avoid alcohol for short periods after taking a dose of lomustine.

Contraceptive measures are recommended during therapy.

STREPTOZOCIN

| Rx | Zanosar (Gensia Sicor) | Powder for Injection: 1 g (100 mg/ml) | In vials. |

WARNING

A patient need not be hospitalized but should have access to a facility with laboratory and supportive resources sufficient to monitor drug tolerance and to protect and maintain a patient compromised by drug toxicity. Renal toxicity is dose-related and cumulative and may be severe or fatal. Other major toxicities are nausea and vomiting, which may be severe and, at times, treatment limiting. In addition, liver dysfunction, diarrhea and hematological changes have been observed.

Judge the possible benefit against the known toxic effects of this drug.

Indications

➤*Metastatic islet cell carcinoma of the pancreas:* Metastatic islet cell carcinoma of the pancreas (functional and nonfunctional carcinomas). Because of its inherent renal toxicity, limit therapy with this drug to patients with symptomatic or progressive metastatic disease.

Administration and Dosage

Administer IV. Intra-arterial administration is not recommended because adverse renal effects may be evoked more rapidly.

➤*Dosage schedules:* The following two different dosage schedules have been used successfully. The ideal duration of maintenance therapy has not been established for either schedule:

Daily schedule – 500 mg/m^2 of body surface area (BSA) for 5 consecutive days every 6 weeks until maximum benefit or until treatment limiting toxicity is observed. Dosage increases are not recommended.

Weekly schedule – Initial dose is 1000 mg/m^2 BSA at weekly intervals for the first 2 courses (weeks). In subsequent courses, increase drug doses in patients who have not achieved a therapeutic response and have not experienced significant toxicity with the previous course of treatment. However, do not exceed a single dose of 1500 mg/m^2 BSA, because a greater dose may cause azotemia. On this schedule, the median time to onset of response is ≈ 17 days and the median time to maximum response is ≈ 35 days. The median total dose to onset of response is ≈ 2000 mg/m^2 BSA and the median total dose to maximum response is ≈ 4000 mg/m^2 BSA.

For patients with functional tumors, serial monitoring of fasting insulin levels allows a determination of biochemical response to therapy. For patients with either functional or nonfunctional tumors, response to therapy can be determined by measurable reductions of tumor size (reduction of organomegaly, masses or lymph nodes).

➤*Reconstitute:* with 9.5 ml of Dextrose Injection or 0.9% Sodium Chloride Injection. The resulting pale gold solution contains 100 mg/ml streptozocin. Where more dilute infusion solutions are desirable, further dilution in the above vehicles is recommended.

➤*Storage/Stability:* The total storage time for reconstituted streptozocin is 12 hours. This product contains no preservatives and is not intended as a multiple dose vial. Refrigerate unopened vials at 2° to 8°C (35° to 46°F) and protect from light.

Actions

➤*Pharmacology:* Streptozocin is a naturally occurring nitrosourea that contains a glucose moiety not present in the other compounds. The glucose moiety is believed to contribute to reduced myelotoxicity, specificity for pancreatic islet cells and the drug's much slower reactivity toward DNA compared with other nitrosoureas.

Streptozocin inhibits DNA synthesis without significantly affecting RNA or protein synthesis in bacterial and mammalian cells. The biochemical mechanism leading to mammalian cell death has not been established but is at least partially caused by DNA alkylation causing intrastrand crosslinks; streptozocin inhibits cell proliferation at a considerably lower level than that needed to inhibit precursor incorporation into DNA or to inhibit several of the enzymes involved in DNA synthesis. The drug is cell cycle nonspecific.

➤*Pharmacokinetics:* After rapid IV injection, unchanged drug is rapidly cleared from the plasma (half-life, 35 minutes). Two hours after administration, metabolites are detected in spinal fluid in equivalent concentration to plasma. Metabolites persist in plasma over 24 hours and concentrate in the liver and kidney. Approximately 60% to 72% of an administered dose can be detected in the urine within 4 hours; 10% to 20% as parent drug. Most excretion is completed in 24 hours.

Warnings

➤*Hematologic:* Hematologic toxicity has been rare, most often involving mild decreases in hematocrit. However, fatal hematologic toxicity with substantial reductions in leukocyte and platelet counts has been observed.

➤*GI:* Nausea and vomiting usually begins 1 to 4 hours after administration and lasts 24 hours; occasionally requiring discontinuation of drug therapy.

➤*Hypoglycemia:* Mild to moderate abnormalities of glucose tolerance have generally been reversible, but insulin shock with hypoglycemia has occurred.

➤*Hydration:* Because of renal toxicity, keep the patient well hydrated. Increase fluid intake for sore lips, mouth or throat, diarrhea or jaundice.

➤*Renal toxicity:* Renal toxicity occurs in up to ⅔ of all patients treated with streptozocin, as evidenced by azotemia, anuria, hypophosphatemia, glycosuria and renal tubular acidosis. *Such toxicity is dose-related and cumulative and may be severe or fatal.* Monitor renal function before and after each course of therapy. Obtain serial urinalysis, BUN, plasma creatinine, serum electrolytes and creatinine clearance prior to, at least weekly during, and for 4 weeks after drug administration. Serial urinalysis is particularly important for the early detection of proteinuria; quantitate with a 24 hour collection when proteinuria is detected. Mild proteinuria is one of the first signs of renal toxicity and may herald further deterioration of renal function. Reduce the dose or discontinue treatment in the presence of significant renal toxicity. In patients with preexisting renal disease, judge potential benefit of streptozocin against known risk of serious renal damage.

Do not use in combination or concomitantly with other potential nephrotoxins.

➤*Carcinogenesis:* When administered parenterally, streptozocin induces renal tumors in rats, and liver and other tumors in hamsters. Stomach and pancreatic tumors were observed in rats treated orally with streptozocin.

➤*Mutagenesis:* Streptozocin is mutagenic in mammalian cells.

➤*Fertility impairment:* It has also been carcinogenic in mice and has adversely affected fertility in rats.

➤*Pregnancy:* Category C. Streptozocin is teratogenic in rats and has abortifacient effects in rabbits. There are no studies in pregnant women. Use during pregnancy only if the potential benefit outweighs the potential risks.

➤*Lactation:* It is not known whether streptozocin is excreted in breast milk. Because of the potential for serious adverse reactions in breastfeeding infants, discontinue breastfeeding in patients receiving streptozocin.

Precautions

➤*Monitoring:* Closely monitor for evidence of renal (see Warnings), hepatic and hematopoietic toxicity. Perform complete blood counts and liver function tests at least weekly. Dosage adjustments or discontinuance of the drug may be indicated, depending upon the degree of toxicity.

➤*Topical exposure:* When exposed dermally, some rats developed benign tumors at the site of application. Consequently, streptozocin may pose a carcinogenic hazard following topical exposure if not properly handled.

STREPTOZOCIN

Adverse Reactions

➤*CNS:* Confusion, lethargy and depression have occurred with a 5 day continuous infusion regimen that may have facilitated these effects.

➤*GI:* Nausea, vomiting (> 90%; see Warnings); diarrhea; sore mouth, lips and throat; bleeding; duodenal ulcer.

➤*Hepatic:* Chemical liver dysfunction (≈ 25%); hepatic toxicity characterized by elevated liver enzymes (AST and LDH); hypoalbuminemia; jaundice.

➤*Miscellaneous:* Nephrogenic diabetes insipidus (two cases: One had spontaneous recovery; the second responded to indomethacin); hematological toxicity (rare); glucose intolerance (see Warnings).

Overdosage

No specific antidote for streptozocin is known. Refer to General Management of Acute Overdosage.

Triazenes

DACARBAZINE (DTIC; Imidazole Carboxamide)

Rx	Dacarbazine (Various, eg, American Pharmaceutical Partners, Bedford, Mayne, Gensia Sicor)	Powder for injection: 100 mg	May contain mannitol. In vials.
Rx	DTIC-Dome (Bayer)		May contain mannitol. In vials.
Rx	Dacarbazine (Various, eg, American Pharmaceutical Partners, Bedford, Mayne, Gensia Sicor)	Powder for injection: 200 mg	May contain mannitol. In vials.
Rx	DTIC-Dome (Bayer)		May contain mannitol. In vials.

WARNING

It is recommended that dacarbazine be administered under the supervision of a qualified physician experienced in the use of cancer chemotherapeutic agents.

Hemopoietic depression is the most common toxicity with dacarbazine (see Warnings).

Hepatic necrosis has been reported (see Warnings).

Studies have demonstrated this agent to have a carcinogenic and teratogenic effect when used in animals.

In treatment of each patient, the physician must carefully weigh the possibility of achieving therapeutic benefit against the risk of toxicity.

Indications

►*Metastatic malignant melanoma:* For treatment of metastatic malignant melanoma.

►*Hodgkin disease:* For second-line therapy in Hodgkin disease in combination with other agents.

►*Unlabeled uses:* In combination with cyclophosphamide and vincristine for malignant pheochromocytoma; in combination with other agents for the treatment of advanced metastatic soft tissue sarcoma; alone or in combination with other agents for the management of Kaposi sarcoma.

Administration and Dosage

►*Approved by the FDA:* 1975.

Administer IV only. Extravasation of the drug subcutaneously during IV administration may result in tissue damage and severe pain.

►*Malignant melanoma:* 2 to 4.5 mg/kg/day IV for 10 days. May repeat at 4-week intervals.

Alternatively, administer 250 mg/m²/day IV for 5 days. May repeat every 3 weeks.

►*Hodgkin disease:* 150 mg/m²/day for 5 days, in combination with other effective drugs. May repeat every 4 weeks.

Alternatively, administer 375 mg/m² on day 1, in combination with other effective drugs. Repeat every 15 days.

►*Preparation of the solution:* Reconstitute the 100 mg vials with 9.9 mL and the 200 mg vials with 19.7 mL of sterile water for injection. The resulting solution contains 10 mg/mL of dacarbazine with a pH of 3 to 4. The reconstituted solution may be further diluted with 5% dextrose injection or sodium chloride injection and administered as an IV infusion.

►*Storage/Stability:* Store vials in refrigerator 2° to 8°C (36° to 46°F). Protect from light. After reconstitution, store the solution in the vial at 4°C (39.2°F) up to 72 hours or at normal room conditions (temperature and light) up to 8 hours. If the reconstituted solution is further diluted in 5% dextrose injection or sodium chloride injection, store the resulting solution at 4°C (39.2°F) up to 24 hours or at normal room conditions up to 8 hours.

Actions

►*Pharmacology:* The exact mechanism of action is unknown. There is some evidence for activity via three mechanisms: action as an alkylating agent; inhibition of DNA synthesis by acting as a purine analog; interaction with sulfhydryl groups in proteins.

►*Pharmacokinetics:*

Absorption/Distribution – After IV administration of dacarbazine, the volume of distribution exceeds total body water content, suggesting tissue localization most likely in the liver. At therapeutic concentrations, the drug is not appreciably bound to plasma protein.

Metabolism/Excretion – Plasma disappearance is biphasic with an initial half-life of 19 minutes and a terminal half-life of 5 hours. In a patient with renal and hepatic dysfunction, half-lives increase to 55 minutes and 7.2 hours.

An average of 40% dacarbazine is excreted unchanged in the urine in 6 hours. Dacarbazine is subject to renal tubular secretion rather than glomerular filtration. Besides unchanged dacarbazine, 5-aminoimidazole-4 carboxamide (AIC) is a major metabolite in the urine.

Contraindications

Hypersensitivity to dacarbazine.

Warnings

►*Hemopoietic depression:* Hemopoietic depression is the most common toxicity and involves primarily the leukocytes and platelets, although anemia sometimes occurs. Leukopenia and thrombocytopenia may be severe enough to cause death. Possible bone marrow depression requires careful monitoring of WBC, RBC, and platelet levels. Hemopoietic toxicity may warrant temporary suspension or cessation of therapy.

►*Hepatotoxicity:* Hepatotoxicity, accompanied by hepatic vein thrombosis and hepatocellular necrosis resulting in death has been reported in approximately 0.01% of patients treated. This toxicity has been observed mostly when dacarbazine was coadministered with other antineoplastics, but it has also been reported with dacarbazine alone.

►*Hypersensitivity reactions:* Anaphylaxis can occur following the administration of dacarbazine.

►*Carcinogenesis:* Angiosarcomas of the spleen and proliferative endocardial lesions, including fibrosarcomas and sarcomas, were induced in small animals after administration.

►*Pregnancy: Category C.* Teratogenicity has been demonstrated in animals given 7 to 20 times the human dose. There are no adequate and well-controlled studies in pregnant women. Use during pregnancy only if the potential benefit justifies the potential risk to the fetus.

►*Lactation:* It is not known whether this drug is excreted in breast milk. Because of the potential for tumorigenicity, decide whether to discontinue nursing or to discontinue the drug, taking into account the importance of the drug to the mother.

Adverse Reactions

►*Dermatologic:* Erythematous and urticarial rashes (infrequent); alopecia; facial flushing. Photosensitivity reactions may occur rarely.

►*GI:* Anorexia, nausea, and vomiting occur in more than 90% of patients with the initial few doses. The vomiting lasts 1 to 12 hours and is incompletely and unpredictably palliated with phenobarbital and/or prochlorperazine. Rarely, intractable nausea and vomiting have necessitated discontinuation of therapy. Diarrhea occurs rarely. Restricting the patient's oral intake of food for 4 to 6 hours prior to treatment may be beneficial. Rapid tolerance to these symptoms suggests that a CNS mechanism may be involved; symptoms usually subside after the first 1 or 2 days.

►*Lab test abnormalities:* There have been few reports of significant liver or renal function test abnormalities.

►*Miscellaneous:* Facial paresthesia; a flu-like syndrome of fever up to 39°C (102.2°F), myalgia, and malaise have been reported. Symptoms usually occur after large single doses, may last for several days, and may occur with successive treatments.

Overdosage

Give supportive treatment and monitor blood cell counts.

Patient Information

Advise patients of common side effects, which include the following: increased risk of infection or bleeding for 21 to 25 days after therapy; nausea, vomiting, or loss of appetite for 1 to 2 days after each dose (restricting food intake for 4 to 6 hours before treatment may help); reversible hair loss.

BUSULFAN

Rx	Myleran (GlaxoSmithKline)	Tablets: 2 mg	Lactose. (GX EF3 M). White. Film coated. In 25s.
Rx	Busulfex (ESP Pharma)	Injection: 6 mg/ml	In 10 ml single-use amps with syringe filters.

WARNING

Busulfan is a potent cytotoxic drug that causes profound myelosuppression at the recommended dosage. Do not use unless a diagnosis of chronic myelogenous leukemia has been adequately established and the responsible physician is knowledgeable in assessing response to chemotherapy, experienced in allogeneic hematopoietic stem-cell transplantation, the use of cancer chemotherapeutic drugs, and the management of patients with severe pancytopenia. Appropriate management of therapy and complications is only possible when adequate diagnostic and treatment facilities are readily available (see Warnings).

Busulfan can induce severe bone marrow hypoplasia. Reduce or discontinue dosage immediately at the first sign of any unusual depression of bone marrow function as reflected by an abnormal decrease in any of the formed elements of the blood. Perform a bone marrow examination if bone marrow status is uncertain (see Warnings).

Indications

➤*Tablets:*

Palliative treatment of chronic myelogenous leukemia (myeloid, myelocytic, granulocytic) – Approximately 90% of adults with previously untreated chronic myelogenous leukemia (CML) will obtain hematologic remission with regression or stabilization of organomegaly following busulfan. It is superior to splenic irradiation with respect to survival times and maintenance of hemoglobin levels and equivalent to irradiation at controlling splenomegaly.

Busulfan is less effective in patients with CML who lack the Philadelphia (Ph[1]) chromosome. Juvenile CML, typically occurring in young children and associated with the absence of a Philadelphia chromosome, responds poorly to busulfan. The drug is of no benefit if the disease has entered a "blastic" phase.

➤*Injection:* For use in combination with cyclophosphamide as a conditioning regimen prior to allogeneic hematopoietic progenitor cell transplantation for CML.

Administration and Dosage

➤*Tablets:*

Remission induction – 4 to 8 mg/day total dose. Dosing on a weight basis is the same for children and adults, ≈ 60 mcg/kg or 1.8 mg/m^2 daily. Because the rate at which the leukocyte count falls is dose-related, reserve daily doses exceeding 4 mg/day for patients with the most compelling symptoms; the greater the total daily dose, the greater the possibility of inducing bone marrow aplasia.

A decrease in the leukocyte count is not usually seen during the first 10 to 15 days of treatment; the leukocyte count may actually increase during this period and should not be interpreted as drug resistance, nor should the dose be increased. Because the leukocyte count may continue to fall for > 1 month after discontinuing the drug, discontinue busulfan before the total leukocyte count falls into the normal range. When the total leukocyte count has declined to ≈ 15,000/mcl, withdraw the drug.

With a constant dose of busulfan, the total leukocyte count declines exponentially; a weekly plot of the leukocyte count on semilogarithmic graph paper aids in predicting the time when therapy should be discontinued. A normal leukocyte count is usually achieved in 12 to 20 weeks with the recommended dose of busulfan.

Maintenance therapy – During remission, examine the patient monthly and resume treatment with the induction dosage when total leukocyte count reaches ≈ 50,000/mcl. When remission is < 3 months, maintenance therapy of 1 to 3 mg/day may keep the hematological status under control and prevent rapid relapse.

➤*Injection:* Administer IV via a central venous catheter as a 2-hour infusion every 6 hours for 4 consecutive days for a total of 16 doses. Premedicate all patients with phenytoin because busulfan is known to cross the blood-brain barrier and induce seizures. In cases where other anticonvulsants must be used, monitor plasma busulfan exposure (see Drug Interactions). Administer antiemetics prior to the first dose of busulfan and continue on a fixed schedule through administration of busulfan.

The usual adult dose of busulfan as a component of a conditioning regimen prior to bone marrow or peripheral blood progenitor cell replacement support is 0.8 mg/kg of ideal body weight or actual body weight, whichever is lower, administered every 6 hours for 4 days (a total of 16 doses). For obese or severely obese patients, administer busulfan based on adjusted ideal body weight. Cyclophosphamide in combination with busulfan is given on each of 2 days as 1-hour infusion at a dose of 60 mg/kg beginning on BMT day −3, 6 hours following the 16th busulfan dose.

➤*Preparation and administration precautions:* As with other cytotoxic compounds, exercise caution in handling and preparing the solution of busulfan. Skin reactions may occur with accidental exposure. The use of gloves is recommended. If busulfan or diluted busulfan solution contacts the skin or mucosa, wash the skin or mucosa thoroughly with water.

➤*Administration preparation:* Busulfan must be diluted prior to use with either 0.9% Sodium Chloride Injection, USP (normal saline) or 5% Dextrose Injection, USP (D5W). The diluent quantity should be 10 times the volume of busulfan, ensuring that the final concentration of busulfan is approximately ≥ 0.5 mg/ml. Calculation of the dose for a 70 kg patient would be performed as follows: (70 kg) × (0.8 mg/kg) ÷ (6 mg/ml) = 9.3 ml busulfan (56 mg total dose).

To prepare the final solution for infusion, add 9.3 ml of busulfan to 93 ml of diluent (normal saline or D5W) as calculated: (9.3 ml busulfan) × (10) = 93 ml of either diluent plus the 9.3 ml of busulfan to yield a final busulfan concentration of 0.54 mg/ml (9.3 ml × 6 mg/ml ÷ 102.3 ml = 0.54 mg/ml).

All transfer procedures require strict adherence to aseptic techniques, preferably employing a vertical laminar flow safety hood while wearing gloves and protective clothing. Using sterile transfer techniques, break off the top of the ampule. Using a syringe fitted with a needle and the 5 micron nylon filter provided, remove the calculated volume of busulfan from the ampule. Remove the needle and filter, replace with a new needle, and dispense the contents of the syringe into an IV bag (or syringe) that already contains the calculated amount of either normal saline or D5W, making sure that the drug flows into and through the solution. Do not put the busulfan into an IV bag that does not contain normal saline or D5W. Always add the busulfan to the diluent, not the diluent to the busulfan. Mix thoroughly by inverting several times.

Use infusion pumps to administer the diluted busulfan solution. Set the flow rate of the pump to deliver the entire prescribed busulfan dose over 2 hours. Prior to and following each infusion, flush the catheter line with ≈ 5 ml of 0.9% Sodium Chloride Injection, USP or 5% Dextrose Injection, USP. Do not infuse concomitantly with another IV solution of unknown compatibility. Warning: Rapid infusion of busulfan has not been tested and is not recommended.

➤*Storage / Stability:*

Injection – Store unopened ampules under refrigerated conditions between 2° and 8°C (36° to 46°F).

Busulfan diluted in 0.9% Sodium Chloride Injection, USP or 5% Dextrose Injection, USP is stable at room temperature (25°C; 73°F) for up to 8 hours, but the infusion must be completed within that time. Busulfan diluted in 0.9% Sodium Chloride Injection, USP is stable at refrigerated conditions (2° to 8°C; 36° to 46°F) for up to 12 hours, but the infusion must be completed within that time.

Use of filters other than the specific type included in this package with each ampule is not recommended.

Actions

➤*Pharmacology:* An alkylsulfonate, busulfan's predominant effect is against cells of the granulocytic series. Although a polyfunctional alkylating agent, it appears to interact with cellular thiol groups. Little cross-linking of nucleoproteins is observed. The drug is cell cycle-phase nonspecific.

While this chemical reactivity is relatively nonspecific, alkylation of the DNA is felt to be an important biological mechanism for its cytotoxic effect.

The biochemical basis for acquired resistance to busulfan is speculative; altered transport of busulfan into the cell and increased intracellular inactivation before it reaches DNA are possibilities. Resistance to these compounds may reflect an acquired ability of the cell to repair alkylation damage more effectively.

➤*Pharmacokinetics:*

Absorption / Distribution – Busulfan is well absorbed following oral administration. There is a lag period of 0.6 to 2 hours prior to detection in blood. It is well distributed into the spinal fluid with a CSF:plasma ratio of 1.3:1; distribution into saliva is equivalent to that of plasma. Plasma protein binding is ≈ 32.4%.

Metabolism / Excretion – The plasma elimination half-life is 2.5 hours and is similar for CSF. The drug appears to be extensively metabolized and renally excreted with little unchanged drug (≈ 30%, injection) found in the urine. The clearance of busulfan is more rapid in children than in adults.

Injection: Busulfan is predominantly metabolized by conjugation with glutathione, spontaneously and by glutathione S-transferase (GST) catalysis. This conjugate undergoes further extensive oxidative metabolism in the liver.

BUSULFAN

Contraindications

➤*Tablets:* Do not use unless a diagnosis of chronic myelogenous leukemia has been adequately established and the responsible physician is knowledgeable in assessing chemotherapy response.

Patients whose disease has demonstrated prior resistance to this drug without a diagnosis of CML.

Busulfan is of no value in chronic lymphocytic leukemia, acute leukemia, or in the "blastic crisis" of CML.

➤*Injection:* Hypersensitivity to any of its components.

Warnings

➤*Hematopoietic toxicity:* The most frequent and serious side effect is bone marrow failure (which may or may not be anatomically hypoplastic), resulting in severe pancytopenia that may be more prolonged than that induced with other alkylating agents. The usual cause is the failure to stop administration of the drug soon enough; individual idiosyncrasy appears unimportant. Use with extreme caution in patients whose bone marrow reserve may be compromised by or recovering from prior irradiation or chemotherapy, or whose marrow function is recovering from previous cytotoxic therapy. Although recovery from busulfan-induced pancytopenia may take from 1 month to 2 years, it is potentially reversible; vigorously support the patient through any period of severe pancytopenia.

The most consistent dose-related toxicity is bone marrow suppression. This may be manifested by neutropenia, anemia, leukopenia, thrombocytopenia, or any combination of these. Instruct patients to report promptly the development of fever, sore throat, signs of local infection, bleeding from any site, or symptoms suggestive of anemia. Any of these findings may indicate busulfan toxicity or transformation of the disease to an acute "blastic" form. Because busulfan may have a delayed effect, it is important to withdraw the medication temporarily at the first sign of an abnormally large or exceptionally rapid fall in any of the formed elements of the blood.

Evaluate the hemoglobin or hematocrit, white blood cell (WBC) count, differential count, and platelet count weekly. If the cause of fluctuation in the formed element of the peripheral blood is obscure, bone marrow examination may be useful. Individualize therapy based not only on the absolute hematologic values, but also on the rapidity with which changes are occurring. The dosage of busulfan may need to be reduced if the agent is combined with other myelosuppressive drugs. Occasionally, patients may be unusually sensitive to busulfan administered at standard dosage and suffer neutropenia or thrombocytopenia after relatively short exposure to the drug. Do not use busulfan where facilities for complete blood counts, including quantitative platelet counts, are not available at weekly (or more frequent) intervals. Never allow patients to take the drug without supervision.

Busulfan may cause additive myelosuppression when used with other myelosuppressive agents.

➤*Adrenal insufficiency:* A clinical syndrome closely resembling adrenal insufficiency and characterized by weakness, severe fatigue, anorexia, weight loss, nausea, vomiting, and melanoderma has developed after prolonged therapy. The symptoms have sometimes been reversible when busulfan was withdrawn. Adrenal responsiveness to exogenously administered adrenocorticotropic hormone (ACTH) is usually normal. However, pituitary function testing with metyrapone revealed a blunted urinary 17-hydroxycorticosteroid excretion in 2 patients. Following the discontinuation of busulfan (which was associated with clinical improvement), rechallenge with metyrapone revealed normal pituitary-adrenal function.

Hyperuricemia and hyperuricosuria – May occur in patients with chronic myelogenous leukemia. Additional rapid destruction of granulocytes may accompany chemotherapy and increase the urate pool. Minimize adverse effects by increased hydration, urine alkalization, and the prophylactic administration of allopurinol.

➤*Pulmonary effects:* A rare but important complication of busulfan therapy is the development of bronchopulmonary dysplasia with pulmonary fibrosis. Symptoms have occurred within 8 months to 10 years after initiation of therapy (the average duration of therapy being 4 years). Histologic findings associated with "busulfan lung" mimic those seen following pulmonary irradiation. Clinically, patients report the insidious onset of cough, dyspnea, and low-grade fever. Pulmonary function studies reveal diminished diffusion capacity and decreased pulmonary compliance. Exclude more common conditions (such as opportunistic infections or leukemic infiltration of the lungs). If sputum cultures, virologic studies, and exfoliative cytology fail to establish an etiology for the pulmonary infiltrates, lung biopsy may be necessary.

Treatment is unsatisfactory; most patients have died within 6 months after diagnosis. There is no specific therapy other than the immediate discontinuation of busulfan. Corticosteroid administration has been suggested, but the results have not been impressive or uniformly successful.

➤*Seizures:* Seizures have been reported in patients receiving high oral doses of busulfan at doses producing plasma drug levels similar to those achieved following the recommended dosage of phenytoin. Exercise caution when administering the recommended (injection) or high doses of busulfan to patients with a history of seizure disorder, head trauma, or receiving other potentially epileptogenic drugs. Initiate anticonvulsant prophylactic therapy prior to busulfan treatment.

➤*Cellular dysplasia:* Busulfan may cause cellular dysplasia in many organs in addition to the lung. Giant hyperchromatic nuclei have been reported in the lymph nodes, pancreas, thyroid, adrenal glands, bone marrow, and liver. This cytologic dysplasia may be severe enough to cause difficulty in interpretation of exfoliative cytologic examinations from the lung, bladder, breast, and the uterine cervix.

➤*Hepatic function impairment:* Current literature suggests that high busulfan doses may be associated with an increased risk of developing hepatic veno-occulsive disease (VOD). Patients who are at an increased risk of developing hepatic VOD with the recommended busulfan dose and regimen include those who have received prior radiation therapy, $\geq$ 3 cycles of chemotherapy, or a prior progenitor cell transplant. Hepatic VOD, which may be life-threatening, has been reported following the investigational use of high doses of busulfan in combination with cyclophosphamide or other chemotherapeutic agents prior to bone marrow transplantation. Possible risk factors include the following: Total busulfan dose > 16 mg/kg based on ideal body weight and concurrent use of multiple alkylating agents. A clear cause-and-effect relationship with busulfan has not been demonstrated.

➤*Carcinogenesis:* Malignant tumors have occurred in patients on busulfan therapy; this drug may be a human carcinogen. Four cases of acute leukemia occurred among 243 patients treated with busulfan for 5 to 8 years as adjuvant chemotherapy following surgical resection of bronchogenic carcinoma. Busulfan is mutagenic in mice and possibly in humans. Chromosome aberrations have been reported in cells from patients receiving busulfan.

➤*Fertility impairment:* Ovarian suppression and amenorrhea with menopausal symptoms commonly occur during busulfan therapy in premenopausal patients. There have been clinical reports of sterility, azoospermia, and testicular atrophy in males. The IV administration of busulfan (48 mg/kg given as biweekly doses of 12 mg/kg, or 30% of the total busulfan dose on a mg/m^2 basis) has been shown to increase the incidence of thymic and ovarian tumors in mice.

The solvent, dimethylacetamide (DMA), may also impair fertility. A DMA daily dose of 0.45 g/kg/day given to rats for 9 days (equivalent to 44% of the daily dose of DMA contained in the recommended dose of busulfan on a mg/m^2 basis) significantly decreased spermatogenesis in rats. A single SC dose of 2.2 g/kg (27% of the total DMA dose contained in busulfan on a mg/m^2 basis) 4 days after insemination terminated pregnancy in 100% of tested hamsters.

➤*Pregnancy: Category D.*

Tablets – Although healthy children have been born after busulfan treatment during pregnancy, 1 malformed baby was delivered by a mother treated with busulfan. During this pregnancy, the mother received x-ray therapy early in the first trimester, mercaptopurine until the third month, then busulfan until delivery.

There are reports of small infants born to mothers who received busulfan during pregnancy, in particular, during the third trimester. In 1 case, an infant had mild anemia and neutropenia at birth after busulfan was administered to the mother from the eighth week of pregnancy to term.

Injection – Busulfan produced teratogenic changes in the offspring of mice, rats, and rabbits when given during gestation. Malformations and anomalies included significant alterations in the musculoskeletal system, body weight gain, and size. In pregnant rats, busulfan produced sterility in male and female offspring due to the absence of germinal cells in the testes and ovaries. The solvent, DMA, may also cause fetal harm when administered to a pregnant woman. In rats, DMA doses of 400 mg/kg/day ($\approx$ 40% of the daily dose of DMA in the busulfan dose on a mg/m^2 basis) given during organogenesis caused significant developmental anomalies. The most striking abnormalities included anasarca, cleft palate, vertebral anomalies, rib anomalies, and serious heart vessel anomalies.

Busulfan may cause fetal harm when administered to a pregnant woman. There are no adequate and well-controlled studies of either busulfan or DMA in pregnant women. If this drug is used during pregnancy or if the patient becomes pregnant while taking this drug, apprise her of the potential hazard to the fetus. Advise women of childbearing potential to avoid becoming pregnant.

➤*Lactation:* It is not known whether this drug is excreted in breast milk. Because of the potential for tumorigenicity, decide whether to discontinue nursing or to discontinue the drug, taking into account the importance of the drug to the mother.

➤*Children:*

Injection – Safety and efficacy of busulfan in children have not been established. Busulfan clearance has been demonstrated to be higher in children than in adults. This has necessitated the development of alternative dosing regimens for oral busulfan in this population. Studies are underway to define the pharmacokinetics of busulfan in children. Cur-

BUSULFAN

rently the recommended dose of busulfan in children has not been defined.

See Administration and Dosage.

Precautions

➤*Monitoring:* Monitor patients for signs of local or systemic infection or bleeding. Frequently evaluate their hematologic status. Periodic measurement of serum transaminases, alkaline phosphatase, and bilirubin is indicated for early detection of hepatotoxicity. It is recommended that evaluation of the hemoglobin or hematocrit, total white blood cell count, complete blood count, including differential count and quantitative platelet count, be obtained weekly (daily for injection) while the patient is on busulfan therapy, and until engraftment has been demonstrated. Evaluate serum transaminase, alkaline phosphatase, and bilirubin daily through transplant day 28 to detect hepatotoxicity, which may herald the onset of hepatic VOD. In cases where the cause of fluctuation in the formed elements of the peripheral blood is obscure, bone marrow examination may be useful for evaluation of marrow status. Do not use busulfan where facilities for complete blood counts, including quantitative platelet counts, are not available at weekly (or more frequent) intervals.

➤*Cardiovascular:* Cardiac tamponade, which was often fatal, has been reported in a small number of pediatric patients with thalassemia (2% in one series) who received high doses of busulfan and cyclophosphamide as the preparatory regimen for bone marrow transplantation and hematopoietic progenitor cell transplantation. Abdominal pain and vomiting preceded the tamponade in most patients.

Drug Interactions

Busulfan Drug Interactions			
Precipitant drug	Object drug*		Description
Acetaminophen	Busulfan	↑	Because busulfan is eliminated from the body via conjugation with glutathione, use of acetaminophen prior to (< 72 hours) or concurrently with busulfan may result in reduced busulfan clearance based on the known property of acetaminophen to decrease glutathione levels in the blood and tissues.
Cyclophospha-mide	Busulfan	↑	Cardiac tamponade, which was often fatal, has been reported in a small number of patients with thalassemia (2% in one series) who received high doses of busulfan and cyclophosphamide (see Precautions).
Itraconazole	Busulfan	↓	Itraconazole decreases busulfan clearance by up to 25% and may produce AUCs > 1500 mcM•min in some patients.
Phenytoin	Busulfan	↑	Phenytoin increases the clearance of busulfan by ≥ 15%, possibly caused by the induction of glutathione-S-transferase.
Thioguanine	Busulfan	↑	In one study, ≈ 3.6% of patients receiving continuous (6 to 45 months) concomitant therapy for treatment of CML had esophageal varices associated with abnormal liver function tests. Liver biopsies performed in 33% of these patients all showed evidence of nodular regenerative hyperplasia. Use with caution in long-term continuous therapy.

* ↑ = Object drug increased. ↓ = Object drug decreased.

Adverse Reactions

➤*Tablets:*

Dermatologic – Hyperpigmentation (5% to 10%, particularly in those with a dark complexion); urticaria; erythema multiforme; erythema nodosum; alopecia; porphyria cutanea tarda; excessive dryness and fragility of the skin with anhidrosis; dryness of the oral mucous membranes; cheilosis.

Hematologic – See Warnings.

Hepatic – Esophageal varices have been reported in patients receiving continuous busulfan and thioguanine therapy for treatment of chronic myelogenous leukemia (oral).

Hepatic VOD is a recognized potential complication of conditioning therapy prior to transplant. It has been observed in patients receiving higher than recommended doses of busulfan.

Metabolic – Adrenal insufficiency, hyperuricemia, hyperuricosuria (see Warnings).

Pulmonary – Interstitial pulmonary fibrosis (see Warnings).

Miscellaneous – Cataracts (0% to 10%) occurred only after prolonged administration of the drug. Gynecomastia, cholestatic jaundice, myasthenia gravis (a clear cause-and-effect relationship has not been demonstrated); endocardial fibrosis (see Precautions); seizures; sterility (80% to 100%; see Warnings).

Endocardial fibrosis: One case of endocardial fibrosis has been reported in a 79-year-old woman who received a total dose of 7200 mg busulfan over a period of 9 years for the management of chronic myelogenous leukemia (oral).

➤*Injection:*

Clinical Significant Busulfan Adverse Reactions (%)[1]	
Adverse reaction	Incidence (%)
Cardiovascular	
Tachycardia	44
Hypertension	36
Thrombosis	33
Vasodilation	25
Hypotension	11
Arrhythmia	5
Cardiomegaly	5
Atrial fibrillation	2
ECG abnormality	2
Heart block	2
Left-sided heart failure	2
Pericardial effusion	2
Ventricular extrasystoles	2
CNS	
Insomnia	84
Anxiety	72
Dizziness	30
Depression	23
Confusion	11
Lethargy	7
Hallucinations	5
Agitation	2
Delirium	2
Encephalopathy	2
Seizure	2
Somnolence	2
Cerebral hemorrhage/coma	1
Dermatologic	
Rash	57
Pruritus	28
Alopecia	17
Vesiculobullous rash	10
Vesicular rash	10
Maculopapular rash	8
Acne	7
Exfoliative dermatitis	5
Erythema nodosum	2
GI	
Nausea	98
Stomatitis (mucositis)	97
Vomiting	95
Anorexia	85
Diarrhea	84
Abdominal pain	72
Dyspepsia	44
Constipation	38
Dry mouth	26
Rectal disorder	25
Rectal discomfort	24
Abdominal enlargement	23
Jaundice	12
Hepatomegaly	6
Hematemesis	2
Pancreatitis	2
Metabolic/Nutritional	
Hypomagnesemia	77
Hyperglycemia	66
Hypokalemia	64
Hypercalcemia	49
Hyperbilirubinemia	49
Edema	36
ALT elevation	31
Creatinine increased	21
Hypophosphatemia	17
Oliguria	15

BUSULFAN

| Clinical Significant Busulfan Adverse Reactions (%)[1] ||
Adverse reaction	Incidence (%)
Alkaline phosphatase increased	15
Hematuria	8
Dysuria	7
Hemorrhagic cystitis	7
BUN increased	5
Hyponatremia	2
Respiratory	
Rhinitis	44
Lung disorder	34
Cough	28
Epistaxis	25
Dyspnea	25
Pharyngitis	18
Hiccup	18
Asthma	8
Alveolar hemorrhage	5
Hemoptysis	3
Pleural effusion	3
Sinusitis	3
Atelectasis	2
Hypoxia	2
Miscellaneous	
Fever	80
Edema	79
Headache	69
Asthenia	51
Infection	51
Chills	46
Pain	44
Allergic reaction	26
Chest pain	26
Inflammation at injection site	25
Back pain	23
Myalgia	16
Injection site pain	15
Arthralgia	13
Pneumonia	5
Ear disorder	3

[1] All events regardless of severity (toxicity grades 1 to 4).

Hematologic – The most frequent, serious, toxic effect of busulfan is myelosuppression resulting in leukopenia, thrombocytopenia, and anemia. Myelosuppression is most frequently the result of a failure to discontinue dosage in the face of an undetected decrease in leukocyte or platelet counts. At the indicated dose and schedule, busulfan produced profound myelosuppression in 100% of patients. Following hematopoietic progenitor cell infusion, recovery of neutrophil counts to ≥ 500 cells/mm^3 occurred at median day 13 when prophylactic granulocyte colony-stimulating factor (G-CSF) was administered to the majority of participants in the study. The median number of platelet transfusions per patient in the study was 6, and the median number of red blood cell transfusions in the study was 4. Prolonged prothrombin time was reported in 1 patient (2%).

Miscellaneous –

Graft-vs-host disease: Graft-vs-host disease (GVHD) developed in 18% (11/61) of patients receiving allogeneic transplants; it was severe in 3%, and mild or moderate in 15%. There were 3 (5%) deaths attributed to GVHD.

Death: There were 2 deaths through bone marrow transplant (BMT) day +28 in the allogeneic transplant setting. There were an additional 6 deaths BMT day +29 through BMT day +100 in the allogeneic transplant setting.

Overdosage

►*Tablets:* Oral LD-50 single doses in mice are 120 mg/kg. Two distinct types of toxic responses are seen at median lethal doses given intraperitoneally. Within hours, there are signs of stimulation of the CNS with convulsions and death on the first day. With doses at the LD-50, there is also delayed death because of bone marrow damage. The principal toxic effect is on the bone marrow. Survival after a single 140 mg dose has been reported in an 18 kg, 4-year-old child, but hematologic toxicity is likely to be more profound with chronic overdosage.

Closely monitor hematologic status and institute vigorous supportive measures if necessary. Induce vomiting or gastric lavage, and follow by administration of charcoal if ingestion is recent. It is not known whether busulfan is dialyzable. There is no known antidote to busulfan. Refer to General Management of Acute Overdosage.

►*Injection:* There is no known antidote to busulfan other than hematopoietic progenitor cell transplantation. In the absence of hematopoietic progenitor cell transplantation, the recommended dosage for busulfan would constitute an overdose of busulfan. The principal toxic effect is profound bone marrow hypoplasia/aplasia and pancytopenia but the CNS, liver, lungs, and GI tract may be affected. Closely monitor the hematologic status and institute vigorous supportive measures as medically indicated. Inadvertent administration of a greater than normal dose of oral busulfan (2.1 mg/kg; total dose of 23.3 mg/kg) occurred in a 2-year-old child prior to a scheduled bone marrow transplant without sequelae. An acute dose of 2.4 g was fatal in a 10-year-old boy. There is 1 report that busulfan is dialyzable; thus, consider dialysis in the case of overdose. Busulfan is metabolized by conjugation with glutathione; thus, administration of glutathione may be considered.

Patient Information

Inform patients beginning therapy with busulfan of the importance of having periodic blood counts.

Do not take the drug without medical supervision.

Notify physician if unusual bleeding or bruising, fever, persistent cough, congestion, shortness of breath, flank, stomach or joint pain, abrupt weakness, unusual fatigue, anorexia, or weight loss occurs.

Tell patient that diffuse pulmonary fibrosis is an infrequent but serious and potentially life-threatening complication of long-term busulfan therapy.

Inform patients that some toxicities to busulfan include infertility, amenorrhea, skin hyperpigmentation, drug hypersensitivity, dryness of the mucous membranes, and cataract formation (rare).

Medication may cause darkening of skin, diarrhea, dizziness, fatigue, appetite loss, mental confusion, nausea, vomiting, and melanoderma that could be associated with a syndrome resembling adrenal insufficiency; notify physician if these become pronounced.

Take medication at the same time each day.

Extra fluid intake may be recommended.

Contraceptive measures are recommended during therapy.

If nausea or vomiting occurs, take the drug on an empty stomach.

Explain the increased risk of a second malignancy to the patient.

ALTRETAMINE (Hexamethylmelamine)

Rx	**Hexalen** (MGI Pharma)	**Capsules:** 50 mg	Lactose. (USB001 Hexalen 50 mg). Clear. In 100s.

WARNING

Administer only under the supervision of a physician experienced in the use of antineoplastic agents.

Monitor peripheral blood counts at least monthly, prior to the initiation of each course of altretamine therapy and as clinically indicated (see Adverse Reactions).

Because of the possibility of altretamine-related neurotoxicity, perform neurologic examination regularly during administration (see Adverse Reactions).

Indications

For use as a single agent in the palliative treatment of patients with persistent or recurrent ovarian cancer following first-line therapy with a cisplatin- or alkylating agent-based combination.

Administration and Dosage

Altretamine is administered orally. Calculate doses on the basis of body surface area.

Altretamine may be administered either for 14 or 21 consecutive days in a 28 day cycle at a dose of 260 mg/m^2/day. Give the total daily dose as 4 divided oral doses after meals and at bedtime.

Temporarily discontinue altretamine (for ≥ 14 days) and subsequently restart at 200 mg/m^2/day for any of the following situations: GI intolerance unresponsive to symptomatic measures; WBC < 2000/mm^3 or granulocyte count < 1000/mm^3; platelet count < 75,000/mm^3; progressive neurotoxicity.

If neurologic symptoms fail to stabilize on the reduced dose schedule, discontinue altretamine indefinitely.

Actions

➤*Pharmacology:* Altretamine, formerly known as hexamethylmelamine, is a synthetic cytotoxic antineoplastic s-triazine derivative. The precise mechanism by which altretamine exerts its cytotoxic effect is unknown, although a number of theoretical possibilities have been studied. Structurally, altretamine resembles the alkylating agent triethylenemelamine, yet in vitro tests for alkylating activity of altretamine and its metabolites have been negative. Altretamine is efficacious for certain ovarian tumors resistant to classical alkylating agents. Metabolism of altretamine is a requirement for cytotoxicity. Synthetic monohydroxymethylmelamines and products of altretamine metabolism in vitro and in vivo can form covalent adducts with tissue macromolecules including DNA, but the relevance of these reactions to antitumor activity is unknown.

➤*Pharmacokinetics:* Altretamine is well absorbed following oral administration, but undergoes rapid and extensive demethylation in the liver, producing variations in altretamine plasma levels. The principal metabolites are pentamethylmelamine and tetramethylmelamine. After oral administration to 11 patients with advanced ovarian cancer in doses of 120 to 300 mg/m^2, peak plasma levels were reached between 0.5 and 3 hours, varying from 0.2 to 20.8 mg/L. Half-life of the β-phase of elimination ranged from 4.7 to 10.2 hours. Altretamine and metabolites show binding to plasma proteins. The free fractions of altretamine, pentamethylmelamine and tetramethylmelamine are 6%, 25% and 50%, respectively.

Following oral administration of 4 mg/kg, urinary recovery was 61% at 24 hours and 90% at 72 hours. Human urinary metabolites were N-demethylated homologues of altretamine with < 1% unmetabolized altretamine excreted at 24 hours. After intraperitoneal administration to mice, tissue distribution was rapid in all organs, reaching a maximum at 30 minutes. The excretory organs (liver and kidney) and the small intestine showed high concentrations, whereas relatively low concentrations were found in other organs, including the brain.

➤*Clinical trials:* In two studies in patients with persistent or recurrent ovarian cancer following first-line treatment with cisplatin or alkylating agent-based combinations, altretamine was administered as a single agent for 14 or 21 days of a 28 day cycle. In the 51 patients with measurable or evaluable disease, there were 6 clinical complete responses, 1 pathologic complete response, and 2 partial responses for an overall response rate of 18%. The duration of these responses ranged from 2 months in a patient with a palpable pelvic mass to 36 months in a patient who achieved a pathologic complete response. In some patients, tumor regression was associated with improvement in symptoms and performance status.

Contraindications

Hypersensitivity to altretamine.

Pre-existing severe bone marrow depression or severe neurologic toxicity; however, altretamine has been administered safely to patients heavily pretreated with cisplatin or alkylating agents including patients with pre-existing cisplatin neuropathies. Careful monitoring of neurologic function in these patients is essential.

Warnings

➤*Neurotoxicity:* Altretamine causes mild to moderate neurotoxicity. Peripheral neuropathy and CNS symptoms (eg, mood disorders, disorders of consciousness, ataxia, dizziness, vertigo) have occurred. They are more likely to occur in patients receiving continuous high-dose daily altretamine than moderate-dose altretamine administered on an intermittent schedule. Neurologic toxicity appears to be reversible when therapy is discontinued. It has been suggested that the incidence and severity of neurotoxicity may be decreased by concomitant administration of pyridoxine, but this remains unproven. Perform a neurologic examination prior to the initiation of each course of therapy.

➤*Hematologic:* Altretamine causes mild to moderate dose-related myelosuppression. Leukopenia < 3000 WBC/mm^3 occurred in < 15% of patients on a variety of intermittent or continuous dose regimens; < 1% had leukopenia < 1000 WBC/mm^3. Thrombocytopenia < 50,000 platelets/mm^3 was seen in < 10% of patients. When given in doses of 8 to 12 mg/kg/day over a 21 day course, nadirs of leukocyte and platelet counts were reached by 3 to 4 weeks, and normal counts were regained by 6 weeks. With continuous administration at doses of 6 to 8 mg/kg/day, nadirs are reached in 6 to 8 weeks (median). Monitor peripheral blood counts prior to the initiation of each course of therapy, monthly, and as clinically indicated. Adjust the dose as necessary (see Administration and Dosage).

➤*Carcinogenesis:* Drugs with similar mechanisms of action are carcinogenic.

➤*Mutagenesis:* Altretamine was weakly mutagenic when tested in strain TA100 of *Salmonella typhimurium.*

➤*Fertility impairment:* Altretamine administered to female rats 14 days prior to breeding through the gestation period had no adverse effect on fertility, but it decreased postnatal survival at 120 mg/m^2/day and was embryocidal at 240 mg/m^2/day. Administration of 120 mg/m^2/day to male rats for 60 days prior to mating resulted in testicular atrophy, reduced fertility and a possible dominant lethal mutagenic effect. Male rats treated with 450 mg/m^2/day for 10 days had decreased spermatogenesis and atrophy of testes, seminal vesicles and ventral prostate.

➤*Pregnancy:* Category D. Altretamine is embryotoxic and teratogenic in rats and rabbits when given at doses 2 and 10 times the human dose, and it may cause fetal damage when administered to a pregnant woman. If altretamine is used during pregnancy, or if the patient becomes pregnant while taking the drug, apprise the patient of the potential hazard to the fetus. Advise women to avoid becoming pregnant.

➤*Lactation:* It is not known whether altretamine is excreted in breast milk. Because there is a possibility of toxicity in nursing infants secondary to altretamine treatment of the mother, it is recommended that breastfeeding be discontinued if the mother is treated with altretamine.

➤*Children:* Safety and efficacy in children have not been established.

Precautions

➤*Nausea and vomiting:* With continuous high-dose daily altretamine, nausea and vomiting of gradual onset occur frequently. In most instances, these symptoms are controllable with antiemetics; at times, however, the severity requires dose reduction or, rarely, discontinuation of therapy. In some instances, a tolerance of these symptoms develops after several weeks of therapy. The incidence and severity of nausea and vomiting are reduced with moderate-dose administration of altretamine. In two clinical studies of single-agent altretamine using a moderate, intermittent dose and schedule, only 1 patient (1%) discontinued altretamine due to severe nausea and vomiting.

Drug Interactions

Altretamine Drug Interactions			
Precipitant drug	Object drug*		Description
Cimetidine	Altretamine	↑	Cimetidine, an inhibitor of microsomal drug metabolism, increased altretamine's half-life and toxicity in a rat model.
Altretamine	Monoamine oxidase inhibitors	↑	Monoamine oxidase inhibitors and concurrent altretamine may cause severe orthostatic hypotension. Four patients, all > 60 years of age, experienced symptomatic hypotension after 4 to 7 days of concomitant therapy.

Adverse Reactions

The most common adverse reactions are: Nausea and vomiting (see Precautions); peripheral neuropathy, CNS symptoms and myelosuppression (see Warnings).

ALTRETAMINE (Hexamethylmelamine)

Data in the following table are based on the experience of 76 patients with ovarian cancer previously treated with a cisplatin-based combination regimen who received single-agent altretamine. In one study, altretamine 260 mg/m^2/day was administered for 14 days of a 28 day cycle. In another study, altretamine 6 to 8 mg/kg/day was administered for 21 days of a 28 day cycle.

Altretamine Adverse Reactions in Previously Treated Ovarian Cancer Patients (n = 76)

Adverse reaction	Incidence (%)
GI	
Nausea and vomiting	
Mild to moderate	32
Severe	1
Increased alkaline phosphatase	9
Hematologic	
Leukopenia	
WBC 2000 to 2999/mm^3	4
WBC < 2000/mm^3	1
Thrombocytopenia	
Platelets 75,000 to 99,000/mm^3	6
Platelets < 75,000/mm^3	3
Anemia	
Mild	20

Altretamine Adverse Reactions in Previously Treated Ovarian Cancer Patients (n = 76)

Adverse reaction	Incidence (%)
Moderate to severe	13
Neurologic	
Peripheral sensory neuropathy	
Mild	22
Moderate to severe	9
Anorexia and fatigue	1
Seizures	1
Renal	
Serum creatinine 1.6 to 3.75 mg/dl	7
BUN	
25-40 mg/dl	5
41-60 mg/dl	3
Greater than 60 mg/dl	1

Additional adverse reaction information is available from 13 single-agent altretamine studies (total of 1014 patients). The treated patients had a variety of tumors and many were heavily pretreated with other chemotherapies; most of these trials utilized high, continuous daily doses of altretamine (6 to 12 mg/kg/day). In general, adverse reaction experiences were similar in the two trials described above. Additional toxicities not reported in the above table included hepatic toxicity, skin rash, pruritus and alopecia, each occurring in < 1% of patients.

THIOTEPA (Triethylenethiophosphoramide; TSPA; TESPA)

Rx	Thiotepa (Bedford)	Powder for Injection, lyophilized: 15 mg	In single-dose vials.
Rx	Thioplex (Amgen)		In vials.

Indications

➤*Carcinomas:* Adenocarcinoma of the breast or ovary.

Controlling intracavitary effusions secondary to diffuse or localized neoplastic disease of various serosal cavities.

Treatment of superficial papillary carcinoma of the urinary bladder.

➤*Lymphomas:* While now largely superseded by other treatments, this drug has been effective against lymphomas, such as lymphosarcoma and Hodgkin's disease.

Administration and Dosage

Do not administer orally because GI absorption is variable.

Individualize dosage. A slow response may be deceptive and may lead to unwarranted frequency of administration with subsequent toxicity. After maximum benefit is obtained by initial therapy, continue with maintenance therapy (1- to 4-week intervals). In order to sustain optimal effect, do not give maintenance doses more frequently than weekly to preserve correlation between dose and blood counts.

➤*Initial and maintenance doses:* Usually, the higher dose in the given range is administered initially. Adjust the maintenance dose weekly based on pretreatment control blood counts and subsequent blood counts.

➤*IV administration:* 0.3 to 0.4 mg/kg at 1- to 4-week intervals by rapid administration.

➤*Intracavitary administration:* Administer 0.6 to 0.8 mg/kg through the same tubing used to remove fluid from the cavity.

➤*Intravesical administration:* Dehydrate patients with papillary carcinoma of the bladder for 8 to 12 hours prior to treatment. Then instill 60 mg in 30 to 60 ml of sodium chloride injection into the bladder by catheter. For maximum effect, retain the solution for 2 hours. If the patient finds it impossible to retain 60 ml for 2 hours, give the dose in a volume of 30 ml. If desired, the patient may be repositioned every 15 minutes for maximum area contact. The usual course of treatment is once a week for 4 weeks. Repeat if necessary, but give second and third courses with caution because bone marrow depression may be increased. Deaths have occurred after intravesical use caused by bone marrow depression from systemically absorbed drug.

➤*Reconstitution:* Reconstitute with Sterile Water for Injection.

Withdrawable Quantities and Concentration of Thiotepa

Label claim (mg/vial)	Actual content (mg/vial)	Amount of diluent to be added (ml)	≈ Withdrawable volume (ml)	≈ Withdrawable amount (mg/vial)	≈ Reconstituted concentration (mg/ml)
15	15.6	1.5	1.4	14.7	10.4

The reconstituted solution is hypotonic and should be further diluted with Sodium Chloride Injection before use. In order to eliminate haze, filter solutions through a 0.22 micron filter prior to administration. Filtering does not alter potency. Do not use solutions that remain opaque or precipitate after filtration.

➤*Storage/Stability:* Store the powder in the refrigerator at 2° to 8°C (36° to 46°F). Protect from light. When reconstituted with Sterile Water for Injection, store in a refrigerator and use within 8 hours. Use reconstituted solutions further diluted with Sodium Chloride Injection immediately.

Actions

➤*Pharmacology:* Thiotepa is a cell cycle nonspecific alkylating agent related to nitrogen mustard. Its radiomimetic action is believed to occur through the release of ethylenimine radicals, which disrupt the bonds of deoxyribonucleic acid (DNA). The drug has no apparent differential affinity for neoplasms.

➤*Pharmacokinetics:* TEPA, which possesses cytotoxic activity, appears to be the major metabolite of thiotepa found in the serum and urine. Urinary excretion of thiotepa and metabolites was 63% in a 34-year-old patient with metastatic carcinoma of the cecum who received a dose of 0.3 mg/kg IV. Thiotepa and TEPA in urine each account for < 2% of the dose.

Thiotepa pharmacokinetics are essentially the same in children as in adults at conventional doses.

Select IV Thiotepa Pharmacokinetics

Parameters	Thiotepa		TEPA	
	60 mg	80 mg	60 mg	80 mg
Peak serum concentration (ng/ml)	1331	1828	273	353
Elimination half-life (hr)	2.4	2.3	17.6	15.7
AUC (ng/hr/ml)	2832	4127	4789	7452
Total body clearance (ml/min)	446	419	-	-

Contraindications

Hypersensitivity to thiotepa; existing hepatic, renal or bone marrow damage (see Warnings).

Warnings

➤*Hematopoietic toxicity:* This drug is highly toxic to the hematopoietic system. A rapidly falling white blood cell (WBC) or platelet count indicates a need to discontinue or reduce dosage. Perform weekly blood and platelet counts during therapy and for ≥ 3 weeks after therapy discontinuation.

The most serious complication of excessive therapy or sensitivity is bone marrow depression, causing leukopenia, thrombocytopenia and anemia. Death from septicemia and hemorrhage has occurred as a result of hematopoietic depression.

The most reliable guide to toxicity is the WBC count; if this falls to ≤ 3000/mm^3, discontinue use. If the platelet count falls to 150,000/mm^3, discontinue therapy. Red blood cell (RBC) count is a less accurate indicator of toxicity.

Death has occurred after intravesical administration. This was caused by bone marrow depression from systemically absorbed drug.

➤*Hypersensitivity reactions:* Allergic reactions have occurred (see Adverse Reactions). Refer to Management of Acute Hypersensitivity Reactions.

THIOTEPA (Triethylenethiophosphoramide; TSPA; TESPA)

➤*Renal/Hepatic function impairment:* If the benefits outweigh the potential risks, use in low doses and monitor hepatic and renal function.

➤*Carcinogenesis:* Like many alkylating agents, this drug has been shown to be carcinogenic.

➤*Mutagenesis:* Thiotepa is mutagenic. In vitro, it causes chromatid-type chromosomal aberrations. The frequency of induced aberrations increases with the patient's age.

➤*Fertility impairment:* Thiotepa impaired fertility in male mice at oral or IP doses ≥ 0.7 mg/kg (≈ 12–fold less than the maximum recommended human therapeutic dose). Thiotepa (0.5 mg) inhibited implantation in female rats when instilled into the uterine cavity. Thiotepa interfered with spermatogenesis in male mice at IP doses ≥ 0.5 mg/kg.

➤*Pregnancy: Category D.* Thiotepa can cause fetal harm when administered to a pregnant woman. Thiotepa given by the IP route was teratogenic in mice and rats at doses ≥ 1 and 3 mg/kg, respectively (≈ 8-fold less than and ≈ equal to the maximum recommended human therapeutic dose [0.8 mg/kg]) and lethal to rabbit fetuses at a dose of 3 mg/kg.

Use effective contraception during therapy if either the patient or partner is of childbearing potential. There are no adequate and well controlled studies in pregnant women. If thiotepa is used during pregnancy, or if pregnancy occurs during therapy, apprise the patient and partner of the potential hazard to the fetus.

➤*Lactation:* It is not known whether thiotepa is excreted in breast milk. Because of the potential for tumorigenicity in animals, decide whether to discontinue breastfeeding or to discontinue the drug, taking into account the importance of the drug to the mother.

➤*Children:* Safety and efficacy have not been established.

Precautions

➤*Monitoring:* Because of hematopoietic toxicity, perform weekly blood and platelet counts during therapy and for ≥ 3 weeks after therapy discontinuation.

➤*Concomitant therapy:* Do not combine therapeutic modalities having the same mechanism of action. Thiotepa combined with other alkylating agents, such as nitrogen mustard or cyclophosphamide, or with irradiation, would intensify toxicity rather than enhance therapeutic response. If these agents must follow each other, it is important that recovery from the first, as indicated by WBC count, be complete before therapy with the second agent is instituted.

➤*Lymphomas:* Thiotepa is now largely superseded by other treatments.

Drug Interactions

➤*Neuromuscular blocking agents:* Coadministration of thiotepa and **pancuronium** resulted in prolonged muscular paralysis and respiratory depression.

Avoid other drugs that are known to produce bone-marrow depression.

Adverse Reactions

➤*CNS:* Dizziness; headache; blurred vision.

➤*Dermatologic:* Contact dermatitis; pain at injection site; alopecia; dermatitis; skin depigmentation (following topical use).

➤*GI:* Nausea; vomiting; abdominal pain; anorexia.

➤*GU:* Dysuria; urinary retention; chemical or hemorrhagic cystitis (rare, following intravesical but not parenteral use); amenorrhea; interference with spermatogenesis (see Warnings).

➤*Hypersensitivity:* Allergic reactions have occurred (eg, rash, urticaria, laryngeal edema, asthma, anaphylactic shock, wheezing).

➤*Miscellaneous:* Conjunctivitis; fatigue; weakness; febrile reaction and discharge from a subcutaneous lesion (result of tumor tissue breakdown); hematopoietic toxicity (see Warnings).

Overdosage

Hematopoietic toxicity can occur, manifested by a decrease in the white cell count or platelets. RBC count is a less accurate indicator of toxicity. Bleeding manifestations may develop. The patient may become more vulnerable to infection and less able to combat such infection. Dosages within and minimally above the recommended therapeutic doses have been associated with potentially life-threatening hematopoietic toxicity. Thiotepa has a toxic effect on the hematopoietic system that is dose-related. Thiotepa is dialyzable. There is no known antidote for thiotepa overdosage. Transfusions of whole blood or platelets have proven beneficial for hematopoietic toxicity.

Patient Information

Notify the physician in the case of any sign of bleeding (epistaxis, easy bruising, change in color of urine, black stool) or infection (fever, chills).

Notify the physician if patient or partner may be pregnant. Use effective contraception during thiotepa therapy if either the patient or the partner is of childbearing potential.

METHOTREXATE (Amethopterin; MTX)

Rx	**Methotrexate** (Various, eg, Major, Roxane, UDL)	**Tablets:** 2.5 mg	In 36s, 100s, and UD 20s.
Rx	**Rheumatrex Dose Pack** (STADA)		(LLM1). Yellow, scored. In 5, 7.5, 10, 12.5, and 15 mg/week dose packs.
Rx	**Trexall** (Barr)	**Tablets:** 5 mg	Lactose. (b 927/5). Green, oval, scored. Film-coated. In 30s, 60s, and 100s.
		7.5	Lactose (b 928/7½). Blue, oval, scored. Film-coated. In 30s, 60s, and 100s.
		10 mg	Lactose. (b 929/10). Pink, oval, scored. Film-coated. In 30s, 60s, and 100s.
		15 mg	Lactose. (b 945/15). Purple, oval, scored. Film-coated. In 30s, 60s, and 100s.
Rx	**Methotrexate Sodium** (Various, eg, American Pharmaceutical Partners[1], Bedford Labs)	**Injection:** 25 mg/mL (as base)	Preservative free. In 2, 4, 8, 10, 20, and 40 mL single-use vials.
Rx	**Methotrexate Sodium** (Various, eg, American Pharmaceutical Partners, Xanodyne)		In 2 and 10 mL vials.[2]
Rx	**Methotrexate LPF Sodium** (Xanodyne)		Preservative free. In 2, 4, and 10 mL single-use vials.[3]
Rx	**Methotrexate Sodium** (Various, eg, American Pharmaceutical Partners, Xanodyne)	**Powder for Injection, lyophilized:** 20 mg (as base)	Preservative free. In single-use vials.[4]
		1 g (as base)	Preservative free. In single-use vials.[4]

[1] The 2, 4, 8, 10, 20, and 40 mL solutions contain approximately 0.43, 0.86, 1.72, 2.15, 4.3, and 8.6 mEq sodium per vial, respectively.

[2] Contains 0.9% benzyl alcohol as a preservative; must not be used for intrathecal or high dose therapy.

[3] The 2, 4, and 10 mL vials contain approximately 0.43, 0.86, and 2.15 mEq sodium per vial, respectively.

[4] Approximately 0.14 mEq sodium in the 20 mg vial; 7 mEq sodium in the 1 g vial.

For complete prescribing information regarding methotrexate's use in arthritis, refer to the abbreviated monograph in the Biological and Immunological agents chapter. For complete prescribing information regarding methotrexate's use in psoriasis, refer to the abbreviated monograph in the Dermatologics chapter.

WARNING

The high dose regimens recommended for osteosarcoma require meticulous care.

Deaths: Use methotrexate only in life-threatening neoplastic diseases, or in patients with psoriasis or rheumatoid arthritis (RA) with severe, recalcitrant, disabling disease that is not adequately responsive to other forms of therapy. Deaths have occurred with the use of methotrexate in malignancy, psoriasis, and RA. Closely monitor patients for bone marrow, liver, lung, and kidney toxicities.

Marked bone marrow depression may occur with resultant anemia, leukopenia, or thrombocytopenia.

Unexpectedly severe (sometimes fatal) bone marrow suppression, aplastic anemia, and GI toxicity have occurred with coadministration of methotrexate (usually in high dosage) along with some NSAIDs (see Precautions, Drug Interactions).

Monitoring: Periodic monitoring for toxicity, including CBC with differential and platelet counts, and liver and renal function testing is mandatory. Periodic liver biopsies may be indicated in some situations. Monitor patients at increased risk for impaired methotrexate elimination (eg, renal dysfunction, pleural effusions, ascites) more frequently (see Precautions).

Liver: Methotrexate causes hepatotoxicity, fibrosis, and cirrhosis, but generally only after prolonged use. Acutely, liver enzyme elevations are frequent, usually transient and asymptomatic, and also do not appear predictive of subsequent hepatic disease. Liver biopsy after sustained use often shows histologic changes, and fibrosis and cirrhosis have occurred; these latter lesions often are not preceded by symptoms or abnormal liver function tests (see Precautions). For this reason, periodic liver biopsies are usually recommended for psoriatic patients who are under long-term treatment. Persistent abnormalities in liver function tests may precede appearance of fibrosis or cirrhosis in the RA population.

Methotrexate-induced lung disease: Methotrexate-induced lung disease is a potentially dangerous lesion that may occur acutely at any time during therapy and has occurred at doses as low as 7.5 mg/week. It is not always fully reversible. Pulmonary symptoms (especially a dry, nonproductive cough) may require interruption of treatment and careful investigation.

Pregnancy: Fetal death and/or congenital anomalies have occurred; do not use in women of childbearing potential unless benefits outweigh possible risks. Pregnant women with psoriasis or RA should not receive methotrexate (see Contraindications).

Renal use: Use methotrexate in patients with impaired renal function with extreme caution, and at reduced dosages, because renal dysfunction will prolong elimination.

WARNING (cont.)

GI: Diarrhea and ulcerative stomatitis require interruption of therapy; hemorrhagic enteritis and death from intestinal perforation may occur.

Diluents: Do not use methotrexate formulations and diluents containing preservatives for intrathecal or experimental high dose MTX therapy.

Malignant lymphomas: Malignant lymphomas, which may regress following withdrawal of methotrexate, may occur in patients receiving low-dose methotrexate and, thus, may not require cytotoxic treatment. Discontinue methotrexate first and, if the lymphoma does not regress, appropriate treatment should be instituted.

Tumor lysis syndrome: Like other cytotoxic drugs, methotrexate may induce tumor lysis syndrome in patients with rapidly growing tumors.

Skin reactions: Severe, occasionally fatal skin reactions have been reported following single or multiple doses of methotrexate. Reactions have occurred within days of oral, IM, IV, or intrathecal methotrexate administration. Recovery has been reported with discontinuation of therapy.

Potentially fatal opportunistic infections: Potentially fatal opportunistic infections, especially *Pneumocystis carinii* pneumonia, may occur with methotrexate therapy.

Radiotherapy: Methotrexate given concomitantly with radiotherapy may increase the risk of soft tissue necrosis and osteonecrosis.

Severe reactions: Because of the possibility of severe toxic reactions (which can be fatal), fully inform patients of the risks involved and assure constant supervision.

Indications

➤*Antineoplastic chemotherapy:* Treatment of gestational choriocarcinoma, chorioadenoma destruens, and hydatidiform mole.

Methotrexate alone or in combination with other anticancer agents for treatment of breast cancer, epidermoid cancers of the head and neck, advanced mycosis fungoides (cutaneous T-cell lymphoma) and lung cancer, particularly squamous cell and small cell types; in combination therapy in the treatment of advanced-stage non-Hodgkin lymphomas.

Methotrexate in high doses followed by leucovorin rescue in combination with other chemotherapeutic agents is effective in prolonging relapse-free survival in patients with nonmetastatic osteosarcoma who have undergone surgical resection or amputation for the primary tumor.

➤*Acute lymphocytic leukemia:* Treatment and prophylaxis of meningeal leukemia and maintenance therapy in combination with other chemotherapeutic agents.

➤*Psoriasis:* Symptomatic control of severe, recalcitrant, disabling psoriasis that is not adequately responsive to other forms of therapy (see specific monograph in the Dermatologics Agents chapter).

➤*Rheumatoid arthritis (RA):* Management of selected adults with severe, active RA (ACR criteria), or children with active polyarticular-course juvenile rheumatoid arthritis (JRA) who have had an insufficient therapeutic response to, or are intolerant of, an adequate trial of

METHOTREXATE (Amethopterin; MTX)

first-line therapy including full dose NSAIDs (see specific monograph in the Biological and Immunological Agents chapter).

➤*Unlabeled uses:* Used as maintenance regimen for Wegener granulomatosis; dermatomyositis; relapsing-remitting multiple sclerosis; myositis; ulcerative colitis; refractory Crohn disease; uveitis; systemic lupus erythematosus; psoriatic arthritis.

Administration and Dosage

Oral administration is often preferred when low doses are being administered. Methotrexate preparations may be given IM, IV, intra-arterially or intrathecally, however, the preserved formulation contains benzyl alcohol and must not be used for intrathecal or high-dose therapy.

Consider procedures for proper handling and disposal of anticancer drugs.

➤*Intrathecal use:* Reconstitute immediately prior to use. Use preservative-free medium such as 0.9% sodium chloride injection. Concentration should be 1 mg/mL.

➤*Reconstitution:* Reconstitute immediately prior to use.

Reconstitute methotrexate sodium with an appropriate sterile, preservative free medium such as 5% dextrose solution or sodium chloride injection. Reconstitute the 20 mg vial to a concentration no greater than 25 mg/mL. The 1 g vial should be reconstituted with 19.4 mL to a concentration of 50 mg/mL. When high doses of methotrexate are administered by IV infusion, the total dose is diluted in 5% dextrose solution.

➤*Dilution:* Methotrexate sodium injection isotonic liquid contains a preservative.

If desired, the solution may be further diluted with a compatible medium such as sodium chloride injection.

Methotrexate LPF Sodium isotonic liquid preservative-free is for single use only.

If desired, the solution may be further diluted immediately prior to use with an appropriate sterile, preservative-free medium such as 5% dextrose solution or sodium chloride injection.

➤*Choriocarcinoma and similar trophoblastic diseases:* Administer 15 to 30 mg orally or IM daily for a 5 day course. Repeat courses 3 to 5 times, as required, with rest periods of 1 or more weeks between courses, until any toxic symptoms subside. Evaluate the effectiveness of therapy by 24 hour quantitative analysis of urinary chorionic gonadotropin hormone (hCG), which should return to normal or less than 50 IU/24 hr usually after the third or fourth course and is usually followed by a complete resolution of measurable lesions in 4 to 6 weeks. One to 2 courses of methotrexate after normalization of hCG is usually recommended. Careful clinical assessment is essential before each course. Cyclic combination therapy with other antitumor drugs may be useful.

Since hydatidiform mole may precede choriocarcinoma, prophylaxis chemotherapy with methotrexate has been recommended. Chorioadenoma destruens is an invasive form of hydatidiform mole. Administer methotrexate in doses similar to those for choriocarcinoma.

➤*Leukemia:* Acute lymphatic (lymphoblastic) leukemia in children and young adolescents is most responsive. In young adults and older patients, clinical remission is more difficult to obtain and early relapse is more common.

When used for induction, methotrexate in doses of 3.3 mg/m^2, in combination with prednisone 60 mg/m^2 given daily, produced remission in 50% of patients, usually within 4 to 6 weeks. Corticosteroid therapy, in combination with other antileukemic drugs or in cyclic combinations with methotrexate included, has appeared to produce rapid and effective remissions. Methotrexate in combination with other agents is the drug of choice for maintenance of remissions. When remission is achieved and supportive care has produced general clinical improvement, initiate maintenance therapy as follows: Give methotrexate orally or IM 2 times weekly in total weekly doses of 30 mg/m^2 or 2.5 mg/kg IV every 14 days. If relapse occurs, repeat initial induction regimen.

➤*Meningeal leukemia:* Dilute preservative-free methotrexate to a concentration of 1 mg/mL with a sterile, preservative-free medium such as 0.9% sodium chloride injection. May administer at intervals of 2 to 5 days, and repeat until the cell count of the CSF returns to normal, then give 1 additional dose. Administration at intervals of less than 1 week may result in increased subacute toxicity. For prophylaxis against meningeal leukemia, the dosage is the same as for treatment, except for the intervals of administration.

CSF volume is dependent on age and not body surface area (BSA). The CSF is at 40% of the adult volume at birth and reaches adult volume in several years.

Intrathecal methotrexate 12 mg/m^2 (max, 15 mg) has resulted in low CSF methotrexate concentrations and reduced efficacy in children, and high concentrations and neurotoxicity in adults. The following dosage regimen is based on age instead of BSA and appears to result in more consistent CSF methotrexate concentrations and less neurotoxicity:

Intrathecal Methotrexate Dose Based on Age	
Age (years)	Dose (mg)
< 1	6
1	8
2	10
≥ 3	12

Because the CSF volume and turnover may decrease with age, a dose reduction may be indicated in elderly patients.

➤*Lymphomas (Burkitt Tumor, Stages I and II):* 10 to 25 mg/day orally for 4 to 8 days. In Stage III, give methotrexate concomitantly with other antitumor agents. Treatment in all stages generally consists of several courses with 7 to 10 day rest periods. Lymphosarcomas in Stage III may respond to combined drug therapy with methotrexate given in doses of 0.625 to 2.5 mg/kg/day.

➤*Mycosis fungoides (cutaneous T-cell lymphoma):* Methotrexate therapy produces clinical responses in 50% of cases. Dosage in early stages is usually 5 to 50 mg once weekly. Dose reduction or cessation is guided by patient response and hematologic monitoring. Methotrexate has also been administered twice weekly in doses ranging from 15 to 37.5 mg in patients who have responded poorly to weekly therapy. Combination chemotherapy regimens that include IV methotrexate administered at higher doses with leucovorin rescue have been utilized in advanced stages of the disease.

➤*Osteosarcoma:* Effective therapy requires several cytotoxic chemotherapeutic agents. In addition to high-dose methotrexate with leucovorin rescue, these agents may include doxorubicin, cisplatin, and the combination of bleomycin, cyclophosphamide, and dactinomycin (BCD) in the doses and schedule shown in the table below. The starting dose for high dose methotrexate treatment is 12 g/m^2. If this dose is not sufficient to produce a peak serum concentration of 1000 micromolar (10^{-3} mol/L) at the end of the methotrexate infusion, the dose may be increased to 15 g/m^2 in subsequent treatments. If the patient is vomiting or is unable to tolerate oral medication, give leucovorin IV or IM at the same dose and schedule.

Chemotherapy Regimens for Osteosarcoma		
Drug[1]	Dose[1]	Treatment week after surgery
Methotrexate	12 g/m^2 IV as 4 hour infusion (starting dose)	4, 5, 6, 7, 11, 12, 15, 16, 29, 30, 44, 45
Leucovorin	15 mg orally every 6 hours for 10 doses starting at 24 hours after start of methotrexate infusion	
Doxorubicin[2] as a single drug	30 mg/m^2/day IV × 3 days	8, 17
Doxorubicin[2] Cisplatin[2]	50 mg/m^2 IV 100 mg/m^2 IV	20, 23, 33, 36 20, 23, 33, 36
Bleomycin[2] Cyclophosphamide[2] Dactinomycin[2]	15 units/m^2 IV × 2 days 600 mg/m^2 IV × 2 days 0.6 mg/m^{2}IV × 2 days	2, 13, 26, 39, 42 2, 13, 26, 39, 42 2, 13, 26, 39, 42

[1] Link MP, et al. The effect of adjuvant chemotherapy on relapse-free survival in patients with osteosarcoma of the extremity. *N Engl J Med* 1986;314:1600-1606.

[2] See each respective monograph for more complete information. Dosage modifications may be necessary because of drug-induced toxicity.

When administering high doses of methotrexate, closely observe the following guidelines.

➤*Guidelines for methotrexate therapy with leucovorin rescue:* Delay methotrexate administration until recovery if:
• the WBC count is less than 1500/mm^3
• the neutrophil count is less than 200/mm^3
• the platelet count is less than 75,000/mm^3

• the serum bilirubin level is more than 1.2 mg/dL
• the ALT level is more than 450 U
• mucositis is present, until there is evidence of healing
• persistent pleural effusion is present; drain dry prior to infusion.

Adequate renal function must be documented – Serum creatinine must be normal, and creatinine clearance must be greater than 60 mL/min, before initiation of therapy.

METHOTREXATE (Amethopterin; MTX)

Serum creatinine must be measured prior to each subsequent course of therapy. If serum creatinine has increased 50% or more compared to a prior value, the creatinine clearance must be measured and documented to be greater than 60 mL/min (even if serum creatinine is still within the normal range).

Patients must be well hydrated and must be treated with sodium bicarbonate for urinary alkalinization.

Administer 1000 mL/m^2 of IV fluid over 6 hours prior to initiation of the methotrexate infusion. Continue hydration at 125 mL/m^2/hr (3 L/m^2/day) during methotrexate infusion, and for 2 days after the infusion has been completed.

Alkalinize urine to maintain pH above 7 during methotrexate infusion and leucovorin calcium therapy by giving sodium bicarbonate orally or by incorporation into a separate IV solution.

Repeat serum creatinine and serum methotrexate 24 hours after starting methotrexate and at least once daily until the level is below 5 × 10^{-8} mol/L (0.05 micromolar).

Guidelines for leucovorin calcium dosage based upon serum methotrexate levels (see table below):

Leucovorin Rescue Schedules Following Treatment with Higher Doses of Methotrexate		
Clinical situation	Laboratory findings	Leucovorin dosage and duration
Normal methotrexate elimination	Serum methotrexate level ≈ 10 micromolar at 24 hrs after administration, 1 micromolar at 48 hrs, and < 0.2 micromolar at 72 hrs	15 mg PO, IM, or IV q 6 hrs for 60 hrs (10 doses starting at 24 hrs after start of methotrexate infusion)
Delayed late methotrexate elimination	Serum methotrexate level remaining > 0.2 micromolar at 72 hrs, and > 0.05 micromolar at 96 hrs after administration	Continue 15 mg PO, IM, or IV q 6 hrs, until methotrexate level is < 0.05 micromolar
Delayed early methotrexate elimination and/or evidence of acute renal injury	Serum methotrexate level of ≥ 50 micromolar at 24 hrs, or ≥ 5 micromolar at 48 hrs after administration; or a ≥ 100% increase in serum creatinine level at 24 hours after methotrexate administration (eg, an increase from 0.5 mg/dL to a level of ≥ 1 mg/dL)	150 mg IV q 3 hrs, until methotrexate level is < 1 micromolar; then 15 mg IV q 3 hrs until methotrexate level is < 0.05 micromolar

Patients who experience delayed early methotrexate elimination are likely to develop nonreversible oliguric renal failure. In addition to appropriate leucovorin therapy, these patients require continuing hydration and urinary alkalinization, and close monitoring of fluid and electrolyte status until serum methotrexate level has fallen to below 0.05 micromolar and the renal failure has resolved.

Some patients will have abnormalities in methotrexate elimination, or abnormalities in renal function following methotrexate administration that are significant but less severe than those described in the table; they may or may not be associated with significant clinical toxicity. If significant clinical toxicity is observed, extend leucovorin rescue for an additional 24 hours (total 14 doses over 84 hours) in subsequent courses of therapy. Consider the possibility that the patient is taking other medications which interact with methotrexate when laboratory abnormalities or clinical toxicities are observed.

➤*RA and polyarticular-course JRA:* Refer to the monograph in the Antirheumatic section of the Biological and Immunologic Agents chapter for dosing information.

➤*Psoriasis:* Refer to the monograph in the Antipsoriatics section of the Dermatologicals chapter for dosing information.

➤*Storage/Stability:* Store at controlled room temperature (20° to 25°C; 68° to 77°F); excursions permitted to 15° to 30°C (59° to 86°F). Protect from light. Methotrexate sodium injection, isotonic liquid contains a preservative. Storage for 24 hours at a temperature of 21° to 25°C results in a product that is within 90% of label potency.

Actions

➤*Pharmacology:* Methotrexate competitively inhibits dihydrofolic acid reductase. Dihydrofolates must be reduced to tetrahydrofolates by this enzyme before they can be utilized as carriers of one-carbon groups in the synthesis of purine nucleotides and thymidylate. Therefore, methotrexate interferes with DNA synthesis, repair, and cellular replication.

Actively proliferating tissues such as malignant cells, bone marrow, fetal cells, buccal and intestinal mucosa, and cells of the urinary bladder are generally more sensitive to this effect of methotrexate. Cellular proliferation in malignant tissue is greater than in most normal tissue; thus, methotrexate may impair malignant growth without irreversibly damaging normal tissues.

The original rationale for high-dose methotrexate therapy was based on the concept of selective rescue of normal tissues by leucovorin. More recent evidence suggests that high-dose methotrexate may also overcome methotrexate resistance caused by impaired active transport, decreased affinity of dihydrofolic acid reductase for methotrexate, increased levels of dihydrofolic acid reductase resulting from gene amplification, or decreased polyglutamation of methotrexate. The actual mechanism of action is unknown.

➤*Pharmacokinetics:*

Absorption/Distribution – In adults, oral absorption appears to be dose-dependent. After oral doses of 30 mg/m^2 or less, methotrexate is generally well absorbed with a mean bioavailability of about 60%. The absorption of doses greater than 80 mg/m^2 is significantly less, possibly due to a saturation effect. Peak serum levels are usually reached in 1 to 2 hours. In leukemic children, oral absorption reportedly varies widely (23% to 95%). A 20-fold difference between highest and lowest peak levels was reported. Significant interindividual variability was also noted in time to peak concentration and fraction of dose absorbed. Food delayed absorption and reduced peak concentration.

After injection, the drug is generally completely absorbed, and peak serum levels are seen in 30 to 60 minutes. Following oral administration of methotrexate in doses of 6.4 to 11.2 mg/m^2/week in pediatric patients with JRA, mean serum concentrations were approximately 0.59 micromolar at 1 hour, 0.44 micromolar at 2 hours, and 0.29 micromolar at 3 hours. After IV administration, the initial volume of distribution is approximately 0.18 L/kg (18% of body weight) and steady-state volume of distribution is approximately 0.4 to 0.8 L/kg (40% to 80% of body weight). Methotrexate competes with reduced folates for active transport across cell membranes by means of a single carrier-mediated active transport process. At serum concentrations greater than 100 micromolar, passive diffusion becomes a major pathway by which effective intracellular concentrations can be achieved. Approximately 50% of the absorbed drug is bound to serum protein. Methotrexate does not penetrate the blood-cerebrospinal fluid barrier in therapeutic amounts. High CSF drug concentrations may be attained by direct intrathecal administration.

Metabolism/Excretion – After absorption, methotrexate undergoes hepatic and intracellular metabolism to polyglutamated forms which can be converted back to methotrexate by hydrolase enzymes. These polyglutamates act as inhibitors of dihydrofolate reductase and thymidylate synthetase. Small amounts of methotrexate polyglutamates may remain in tissues for extended periods. The retention and prolonged drug action of these active metabolite(s) vary among different cells, tissues, and tumors. A small amount of metabolism to 7-hydroxymethotrexate may occur at doses commonly prescribed. Accumulation of this metabolite may become significant at the high doses used in osteogenic sarcoma. The aqueous solubility of 7-hydroxymethotrexate is threefold to fivefold lower than the parent compound. Methotrexate is partially metabolized by intestinal flora after oral administration.

The terminal half-life is approximately 3 to 10 hours for patients receiving treatment for psoriasis, RA, or low-dose antineoplastic therapy (less than 30 mg/m^2). For patients on high doses, the terminal half-life is 8 to 15 hours. In pediatric patients receiving methotrexate for acute lymphocytic leukemia (6.3 to 30 mg/m^2), or for JRA (3.75 to 26.2 mg/m^2), the terminal half-life has been reported to range from 0.7 to 5.8 hours or 0.9 to 2.3 hours, respectively.

Renal excretion is the primary route of elimination and is dependent upon dosage and route of administration. With IV administration, 80% to 90% of the administered dose is excreted unchanged in the urine within 24 hours. There is limited biliary excretion of 10% or less. Enterohepatic recirculation of methotrexate has been proposed. Renal excretion occurs by glomerular filtration and active tubular secretion. Impaired renal function, as well as concurrent use of drugs such as weak organic acids that also undergo tubular secretion, can markedly increase serum levels. Excellent correlation has been reported between methotrexate clearance and endogenous creatinine clearance.

Clearance rates vary widely and are generally decreased at higher doses. Delayed drug clearance is one of the major factors responsible for toxicity because the toxicity for normal tissues appears more dependent upon the duration of exposure to the drug rather than the peak level achieved. When a patient has delayed drug elimination due to compro-

METHOTREXATE (Amethopterin; MTX)

mised renal function or other causes, methotrexate serum concentrations may remain elevated for prolonged periods.

The potential for toxicity from high-dose regimens or delayed excretion is reduced by leucovorin calcium during the final phase of methotrexate plasma elimination. Guidelines for monitoring serum methotrexate levels, and for adjustment of leucovorin dosing to reduce the risk of toxicity, are provided in Administration and Dosage.

Contraindications

Hypersensitivity to the drug.

Patients with psoriasis or RA with alcoholism, alcoholic liver disease, or other chronic liver disease should not receive methotrexate. Patients with psoriasis or RA who have overt or laboratory evidence of immunodeficiency syndromes should not receive methotrexate.

Patients with psoriasis or RA who have pre-existing blood dyscrasias (eg, bone marrow hypoplasia, leukopenia, thrombocytopenia, significant anemia) should not receive methotrexate.

➤*Pregnancy:* Methotrexate can cause fetal death or teratogenic effects when administered to a pregnant woman. Methotrexate is contraindicated in pregnant women with psoriasis or RA and should be used in the treatment of neoplastic diseases only when the potential benefit outweighs the risk to the fetus. Women of childbearing potential should not be started on methotrexate until pregnancy is excluded and should be fully counseled on the serious risk to the fetus should they become pregnant while undergoing treatment. Pregnancy should be avoided if either partner is receiving methotrexate; during and for a minimum of 3 months after therapy for male patients, and during and for at least 1 ovulatory cycle after therapy for female patients.

Lactation – Because of the potential for serious adverse reactions from methotrexate in breastfed infants, it is contraindicated in nursing mothers.

Warnings

➤*Toxic effects:* Toxic effects, potentially serious, may be related in frequency and severity to dose or frequency of administration, but have been seen at all doses. These effects can occur at any time during therapy; follow patients closely. Most adverse reactions are reversible if detected early. When reactions occur, reduce dosage or discontinue drug and take appropriate corrective measures; this could include use of leucovorin calcium. Use caution if therapy is reinstituted. Consider further need for the drug and possibility of recurrence of toxicity.

➤*Renal function impairment:* Methotrexate is excreted principally by the kidneys. Its use in impaired renal function may result in accumulation of toxic amounts or additional renal damage. Determine the patient's renal status prior to and during therapy. Exercise caution should significant renal impairment occur. Reduce or discontinue drug dosage until renal function improves or is restored. The potential for toxicity from high dose regimens or delayed excretion is reduced by the administration of leucovorin calcium during the final phase of methotrexate plasma elimination.

➤*Carcinogenesis:* Non-Hodgkin lymphoma and other tumors have been reported in patients receiving low-dose oral methotrexate. However, there have been instances of malignant lymphoma arising during treatment with low-dose oral methotrexate that have regressed completely following withdrawal of methotrexate without requiring active antilymphoma treatment.

➤*Mutagenesis:* Although there is evidence that the drug causes chromosomal damage to animal somatic cells and human bone marrow cells, the clinical significance remains uncertain. Weigh the benefits against this potential risk before using methotrexate alone or in combination with other drugs, especially in children or young adults.

➤*Fertility impairment:* Impairment of fertility, oligospermia, and menstrual dysfunction in humans has been reported during and for a short period after cessation of therapy.

➤*Elderly:* Clinical pharmacology has not been well studied in these patients. Due to diminished hepatic and renal function and decreased folate stores in this population, consider relatively low doses. Closely monitor for early signs of toxicity.

Since decline in renal function may be associated with increases in adverse events and serum creatinine measurements may overestimate renal function in the elderly, more accurate methods (ie, creatinine clearance) should be considered. Elderly patients should be closely monitored for early signs of hepatic, bone marrow, and renal toxicity. Postmarketing experience suggests that the occurrence of bone marrow suppression, thrombocytopenia, and pneumonitis may increase with age.

➤*Pregnancy:* Category X. Methotrexate has caused fetal death or teratogenic effects when administered to pregnant women. Use in the treatment of neoplastic disease only when the benefits outweigh risks to the fetus. Women of childbearing potential should not receive methotrexate until pregnancy is excluded and they should be fully counseled on the serious risk to the fetus should they become pregnant while undergoing treatment. Avoid pregnancy if either partner is receiving methotrexate, during and for a minimum of 3 months after therapy for

males, and during and for at least one ovulatory cycle after therapy for females. Do not administer to pregnant psoriatic or RA patients.

➤*Lactation:* Contraindicated in nursing mothers. Methotrexate is excreted in breast milk in low concentrations with a milk:plasma ratio of 0.08:1. Decide whether to discontinue nursing, or to discontinue the drug, taking into account the importance of the drug to the mother.

➤*Children:* Safety and efficacy in children have not been established, other than in cancer chemotherapy and in polyarticular-course JRA.

Published clinical studies evaluating the use of methotrexate in children and adolescents (ie, patients 2 to 16 years of age) with JRA demonstrated safety comparable to that observed in adults with RA.

Precautions

➤*Monitoring:* Baseline assessment should include complete blood count with differential and platelet counts; hepatic enzymes; renal function tests; and chest x-ray. During therapy of RA and psoriasis, monitoring of these parameters is recommended: Hematology at least monthly, renal function and liver function every 1 to 2 months. More frequent monitoring is usually indicated during antineoplastic therapy. During initial or changing doses, or during periods of increased risk of elevated methotrexate blood levels (eg, dehydration), more frequent monitoring may be indicated. Pulmonary function tests may be useful if methotrexate-induced lung disease is suspected, especially if baseline measurements are available. Appropriate steps should be taken to avoid conception during methotrexate therapy.

Hepatic – A relationship between abnormal liver function tests and fibrosis or cirrhosis of the liver has not been established. Transient liver function test abnormalities are observed frequently after methotrexate administration and are usually not cause for modification of methotrexate therapy. Persistent liver function test abnormalities or depression of serum albumin may indicate serious liver toxicity; they require evaluation.

RA: Liver function tests should be performed at baseline and at 4 to 8 week intervals in patients receiving methotrexate for RA. Pretreatment liver biopsy should be performed for patients with a history of excessive alcohol consumption, persistently abnormal baseline liver function test values, or chronic hepatitis B or C infection. During therapy, liver biopsy should be performed if there are persistent liver function test abnormalities or there is a decrease in serum albumin below the normal range (in the setting of well-controlled RA).

➤*Intrathecal therapy:* Large doses may cause convulsions. Untoward side effects may occur with any intrathecal injection and are commonly neurological. Intrathecal methotrexate appears significantly in systemic circulation and may cause systemic toxicity; therefore, adjust systemic antileukemic therapy appropriately. Focal leukemic involvement of the CNS may not respond to intrathecal chemotherapy and is best treated with radiotherapy.

➤*Intrathecal use:* Methotrexate formulations and diluents containing preservatives must not be used for intrathecal or high dose methotrexate therapy

➤*Organ system toxicity:*

GI – If vomiting, diarrhea, or stomatitis occur, which may result in dehydration, discontinue methotrexate until recovery occurs. Use with extreme caution in the presence of peptic ulcer disease or ulcerative colitis.

Hematologic – Methotrexate can suppress hematopoiesis and cause anemia, aplastic anemia, pancytopenia, leukopenia, neutropenia and/or thrombocytopenia. Use with caution, if at all, in patients with malignancy and preexisting hematopoietic impairment. In controlled clinical trials in RA (n = 128), leukopenia (WBC less than 3000/mm^3) was seen in 2 patients, thrombocytopenia (platelets less than 100,000/mm^3) in 6 patients, and pancytopenia in 2 patients.

In psoriasis and RA, methotrexate should be stopped immediately if there is a significant drop in blood counts. In the treatment of neoplastic diseases, continue methotrexate only if potential benefit warrants risk of severe myelosuppression. Evaluate those with profound granulocytopenia and fever immediately; they usually require parenteral broad-spectrum antibiotics.

Hepatic – Methotrexate has the potential for acute (elevated transaminases) and chronic (fibrosis and cirrhosis) hepatotoxicity. Chronic toxicity is potentially fatal; it generally occurs after prolonged use (generally 2 years or more) and after a total dose of at least 1.5 g. An accurate incidence rate is undetermined; the rate of progression and reversibility of lesions is not known. Special caution is indicated in the presence of preexisting liver damage or impaired hepatic function.

Periodically perform liver function tests, including serum albumin, prior to dosing. They are often normal in the face of developing fibrosis or cirrhosis. These lesions may be detectable only by biopsy.

Psoriasis: In psoriasis, liver function tests, including serum albumin, should be performed periodically prior to dosing but are often normal in the face of developing fibrosis or cirrhosis. These lesions may be detectable only by biopsy. The usual recommendation is to obtain a liver biopsy at 1) pretherapy or shortly after initiation of therapy (2 to 4 months), 2) a total cumulative dose of 1.5 g, and 3) after each additional 1 to 1.5 g. Moderate fibrosis or any cirrhosis normally leads to

METHOTREXATE (Amethopterin; MTX)

discontinuation of the drug; mild fibrosis normally suggests a repeat biopsy in 6 months. Milder histologic findings such as fatty change and low grade portal inflammation are relatively common pretherapy. Although these mild changes are usually not a reason to avoid or discontinue methotrexate therapy, use the drug with caution.

RA: In RA, first use of methotrexate and duration of therapy have been reported as risk factors for hepatotoxicity; other risk factors similar to those observed in psoriasis may be present in RA but have not been confirmed to date. Persistent abnormalities in liver function tests may precede appearance of fibrosis or cirrhosis in this population. There is a combined reported experience in 217 RA patients with liver biopsies both before and during treatment (after a cumulative dose of at least 1.5 g) and in 714 patients with a biopsy only during treatment. There are 64 (7%) cases of fibrosis and 1 (0.1%) case of cirrhosis. Of the 64 cases of fibrosis, 60 were deemed mild. The reticulin stain is more sensitive for early fibrosis and its use may increase these figures. It is unknown whether even longer use will increase these risks.

Infection or immunologic states – Use with extreme caution in the presence of active infection; usually contraindicated in patients with overt or laboratory evidence of immunodeficiency syndromes. Hypogammaglobulinemia occurs rarely.

Potentially fatal opportunistic infections, especially *P. carinii* pneumonia may occur with methotrexate therapy. When a patient presents with pulmonary symptoms, the possibility of *P. carinii* pneumonia should be considered.

Neurologic – There have been reports of leukoencephalopathy following IV administration of methotrexate to patients who have had craniospinal irradiation. Serious neurotoxicity, frequently manifested as generalized or focal seizures, has been reported with unexpectedly increased frequency among pediatric patients with acute lymphoblastic leukemia who were treated with intermediate-dose IV methotrexate ($1 g/m^2$). Symptomatic patients were commonly noted to have leukoencephalopathy and/or microangiopathic calcifications on diagnostic imaging studies. Chronic leukoencephalopathy has also occurred in patients who received repeated doses of high-dose methotrexate with leucovorin rescue even without cranial irradiation. Discontinuation of methotrexate does not always result in complete recovery.

A transient acute neurologic syndrome has been observed in patients treated with high dosage regimens. Manifestations of this stroke-like encephalopathy may include confusion, hemiparesis, transient blindness, seizures, and coma. The exact cause is unknown.

Intrathecal use: After intrathecal use of methotrexate, the CNS toxicity that may occur can be classified as follows: Acute chemical arachnoiditis manifested by headache, back pain, nuchal rigidity, and fever; subacute myelopathy characterized by paraparesis/paraplegia associated with involvement with 1 or more spinal nerve roots; chronic leukoencephalopathy manifested by confusion, irritability, somnolence, ataxia, dementia, seizures, and coma. This condition can be progressive and even fatal.

Pulmonary – Pulmonary symptoms (especially a dry, nonproductive cough) or a nonspecific pneumonitis occurring during therapy indicate a potentially dangerous lesion and require interruption of treatment and careful investigation. The typical patient presents with fever, cough, dyspnea, hypoxemia, and an infiltrate on chest x-ray; infection (including pneumonia) needs to be excluded. This lesion can occur at all dosages.

Renal – Methotrexate may cause renal damage that may lead to acute renal failure. High doses used in the treatment of osteosarcoma may cause renal damage leading to acute renal failure. Nephrotoxicity is due primarily to the precipitation of methotrexate and 7-hydroxymethotrexate in the renal tubules. Close attention to renal function including adequate hydration, urine alkalinization and measurement of serum methotrexate and creatinine levels are essential for safe administration.

Skin – Severe, occasionally fatal dermatologic reactions including toxic epidermal necrolysis, Stevens-Johnson syndrome, exfoliative dermatitis, skin necrosis, and erythema multiforme, have been reported in children and adults within days of oral, IM, IV, or intrathecal methotrexate administration. Reactions were noted after single or multiple, low, intermediate, or high doses of methotrexate in patients with neoplastic and nonneoplastic diseases.

➤*Vaccines:* Immunization may be ineffective when given during methotrexate therapy. Immunization with live virus vaccines is generally not recommended. Disseminated vaccinia infections after smallpox immunization have occurred in patients receiving methotrexate.

➤*Debility:* Use with extreme caution in the presence of debility.

➤*Pleural effusions or ascites:* Methotrexate exits slowly from third space compartments (eg, pleural effusions or ascites). This results in a prolonged terminal plasma half-life and unexpected toxicity. In patients with significant third space accumulations, evacuate the fluid before treatment and monitor plasma methotrexate levels.

➤*Psoriasis lesions:* Lesions of psoriasis may be aggravated by concomitant exposure to ultraviolet radiation. Radiation dermatitis and sunburn may be "recalled" by the use of methotrexate.

➤*Folate deficiency:* Folate deficiency states may increase methotrexate toxicity.

➤*Benzyl alcohol:* Methotrexate sodium for injection contains the preservative benzyl alcohol and is not recommended for use in neonates. There have been reports of fatal gasping syndrome in neonates (children younger than 1 month of age) following the administration of IV solutions containing the preservative benzyl alcohol. Symptoms include a striking onset of gasping respiration, hypotension, bradycardia, and cardiovascular collapse.

Drug Interactions

Methotrexate Drug Interactions			
Precipitant drug	Object drug*		Description
Aminoglycosides, oral	Methotrexate	↓	The antitumorigenic actions of methotrexate may be decreased, but not predictably. Consider parenteral methotrexate if oral aminoglycosides are being coadministered.
Charcoal	Methotrexate	↓	Charcoal can reduce absorption of methotrexate and remove it from systemic circulation. Depending on the clinical situation, this will reduce the effectiveness or toxicity of methotrexate.
Chloramphenicol	Methotrexate	↓	Oral chloramphenicol may decrease intestinal absorption of methotrexate or interfere with the enterohepatic circulation by inhibiting bowel flora and suppressing metabolism of the drug by bacteria.
Folic acid	Methotrexate	↓	Vitamin preparations containing folic acid or its derivatives may decrease responses to systemically administered methotrexate.
NSAIDs	Methotrexate	↑	Concomitant administration of some NSAIDs with high dose methotrexate has been reported to elevate and prolong serum methotrexate levels, resulting in deaths from severe hematologic and GI toxicity. NSAIDs may reduce tubular secretion of methotrexate and enhance toxicity. Monitor renal impairment that could predispose to methotrexate toxicity, for signs of methotrexate toxicity, and methotrexate levels if indicated.
Penicillins	Methotrexate	↑	Serum methotrexate concentrations may be elevated, increasing the risk of toxicity. Monitor for methotrexate toxicity and measure methotrexate concentrations twice a week for at least the first 2 weeks. If a broad-spectrum antibiotic is needed, ceftazidime may be less likely to interact.
Probenecid	Methotrexate	↑	Methotrexate plasma levels, therapeutic effects, and toxicity may be enhanced. Monitor methotrexate concentrations and adjust dose accordingly.
Salicylates	Methotrexate	↑	Increased toxic effects of methotrexate may occur. Salicylates may reduce tubular secretion of methotrexate and enhance toxicity. Consider monitoring methotrexate levels.
Sulfonamides	Methotrexate	↑	Sulfonamides may increase the risk of methotrexate-induced bone marrow suppression. Methotrexate may predispose patients to trimethoprim-sulfamethoxazole (TMP-SMZ)-induced megaloblastic anemia. Closely monitor patients for signs of hematologic toxicity.
Methotrexate	Sulfonamides		
Tetracyclines	Methotrexate	↑	Methotrexate concentrations may be elevated, increasing the risk of toxicity (eg, bone marrow suppression). If tetracyclines cannot be avoided in patients receiving high-dose methotrexate, closely monitor methotrexate plasma concentrations and patients for signs and symptoms of toxicity.

METHOTREXATE (Amethopterin; MTX)

Methotrexate Drug Interactions			
Precipitant drug	Object drug*		Description
Trimethoprim	Methotrexate	↑	Trimethoprim may increase the risk of methotrexate-induced bone marrow suppression and megaloblastic anemia. If this drug combination cannot be avoided, closely monitor for signs of hematologic toxicity.
Methotrexate	Digoxin	↓	Serum levels of digoxin may be reduced and actions may be decreased. Monitor patient for signs of reduction in pharmacologic effect of digoxin and increase digoxin dose if necessary. Serum level monitoring may facilitate tailoring dosage.
Methotrexate	Phenytoin	↓	Serum concentrations of phenytoin may be decreased, resulting in a loss of therapeutic effect. Monitor phenytoin serum levels and adjust the phenytoin dosage appropriately. IV phenytoin may be useful.
Methotrexate	Theophylline	↑	Methotrexate may decrease the clearance of theophylline. Theophylline levels should be monitored when used concomitantly with methotrexate.
Methotrexate	Thiopurines (eg, azathioprine)	↑	The actions of thiopurines may be enhanced. Reduced thiopurine dosage may be used during coadministration with methotrexate.

* ↑ = Object drug increased. ↓ = Object drug decreased.

➤*Drug/Food interactions:* Food may delay the absorption and reduce the peak concentration of methotrexate.

Adverse Reactions

The incidence and severity of acute side effects are generally related to dose and dosing frequency. See also Precautions section under "Organ System Toxicity."

The most common adverse reactions are: Ulcerative stomatitis; leukopenia; nausea; abdominal distress; malaise; fatigue; chills; fever; dizziness; decreased resistance to infection.

➤*Cardiovascular:* Pericarditis, pericardial effusion, hypotension, and thromboembolic events (including arterial thrombosis, cerebral thrombosis, deep vein thrombosis, retinal vein thrombosis, thrombophlebitis, and pulmonary embolus).

➤*CNS:* Headaches; drowsiness; blurred vision; aphasia; hemiparesis; paresis; convulsions; transient blindness; speech impairment, including dysarthria. Following low doses, there have been occasional reports of transient subtle cognitive dysfunction, mood alteration, unusual cranial sensations, leukoencephalopathy, or encephalopathy.

After intrathecal use, the CNS toxicity that may occur can be classified as follows:

1.) Acute chemical arachnoiditis (headache, back pain, nuchal rigidity, fever);
2.) subacute myelopathy (paraparesis/paraplegia with involvement of spinal nerve roots);
3.) chronic leukoencephalopathy (confusion, irritability, somnolence, ataxia, dementia, seizures, and coma).

➤*Dermatologic:* Erythematous rashes; pruritus; urticaria; photosensitivity; pigmentary changes; alopecia; ecchymosis; telangiectasia; acne; furunculosis; erythema multiforme; toxic epidermal necrolysis; Stevens-Johnson syndrome; skin necrosis; skin ulceration; exfoliative dermatitis; photosensitivity; "burning of skin lesions"; rash; plaque erosions (rare).

➤*GI:* Gingivitis; stomatitis; pharyngitis; anorexia; nausea; vomiting; diarrhea; hematemesis; melena; GI ulceration and bleeding; enteritis; pancreatitis.

➤*GU:* Renal failure; azotemia; cystitis; hematuria; severe nephropathy; defective oogenesis or spermatogenesis; transient oligospermia; menstrual dysfunction and vaginal discharge; infertility; abortion; fetal defects; gynecomastia; dysuria; vaginal discharge.

➤*Hematologic:* Bone marrow depression; leukopenia; thrombocytopenia; suppressed hematopoiesis causing anemia; aplastic anemia; pancytopenia; neutropenia; decreased hematocrit; lymphadenopathy and lymphoproliferative disorders (including reversible); hypogammaglobulinemia (rare).

➤*Hepatic:* Hepatotoxicity; acute hepatitis; chronic fibrosis; cirrhosis; decrease in serum albumin; liver enzyme elevations.

➤*Musculoskeletal:* Stress fracture, arthralgias, chest pain.

➤*Pulmonary:* Chronic interstitial obstructive pulmonary disease has occasionally occurred; deaths from respiratory fibrosis, respiratory failure, and interstitial pneumonitis have been reported. Upper respiratory infections, coughing, and epistaxis have occurred.

➤*Special senses:* Conjunctivitis; serious visual changes of unknown etiology; eye discomfort; tinnitus.

➤*Miscellaneous:* Rare reactions related to the use of methotrexate include arthralgia/myalgia, diabetes, osteoporosis and sudden death. Cases of anaphylactoid reactions have occurred; nodulosis; vasculitis; loss of libido/impotence; reversible lymphomas; tumor lysis syndrome; soft tissue necrosis; osteonecrosis; sweating.

Infection – The following also occurred. Infections, pneumonia, sepsis, nocardiosis, histoplasmosis, cryptococcosis, herpes zoster, herpes simplex hepatitis, and disseminated herpes simplex. There have been case reports of sometimes fatal opportunistic infections. *Pneumocystis carinii* pneumonia was the most common infection.

Overdosage

➤*Symptoms:* Reports of oral overdose often indicate accidental daily administration instead of weekly (single or divided doses). Symptoms commonly reported following oral overdose include those symptoms and signs reported at pharmacologic doses, particularly hematologic and GI reaction. For example, leukopenia, thrombocytopenia, anemia, pancytopenia, bone marrow suppression, mucositis, stomatitis, oral ulceration, nausea, vomiting, GI ulceration, and GI bleeding. In some cases, no symptoms were reported. There have been reports of death following overdose. In these cases, events such as sepsis or septic shock, renal failure, and aplastic anemia were also reported.

Symptoms of intrathecal overdose are generally CNS symptoms, including headache, nausea and vomiting, seizure or convulsion, and acute toxic encephalopathy. In some cases, no symptoms were reported. There have been reports of death following intrathecal overdose. In these cases, cerebellar herniation associated with increased intracranial pressure and acute toxic encephalopathy have also been reported.

➤*Treatment:* Leucovorin (citrovorum factor) is used to diminish the toxicity and counteract the effect of inadvertent overdosages of methotrexate. Administer leucovorin as promptly as possible. As the time interval between administration and leucovorin rescue increases, leucovorin's effectiveness in counteracting toxicity diminishes. Monitoring of the serum methotrexate concentration is essential in determining the optimal dose and duration of leucovorin treatment.

In cases of massive overdosage, hydration and urinary alkalinization may be necessary to prevent the precipitation of methotrexate and its metabolites in the renal tubules. Neither hemodialysis nor peritoneal dialysis improves methotrexate elimination. Effective clearance of methotrexate has been reported with acute intermittent hemodialysis using a high-flux dialyzer.

Accidental intrathecal overdosage may require intensive systemic support, high-dose systemic leucovorin, alkaline diuresis and rapid CSF drainage, and ventriculolumbar perfusion.

In postmarketing experience, overdose with methotrexate has generally occurred with oral and intrathecal administration, although IV and IM overdose have also been reported.

Patient Information

Avoid alcohol, salicylates, and prolonged exposure to sunlight or sunlamps (particularly patients with psoriasis).

Use contraceptive measures during and for at least 3 months (males) or 1 ovulatory cycle (females) after cessation of therapy. The risk of effects on reproduction should be discussed with both males and females on methotrexate.

Notify physician if any of the following occurs: Diarrhea; abdominal pain; black stools; fever and chills; sore throat; sores in or around the mouth; cough; yellow discoloration of the skin or eyes; swelling of the feet or legs; joint pain. May cause nausea, vomiting, loss of appetite, hair loss, skin rash, fever, or dizziness. Notify the physician if these effects persist.

Inform patients of the early signs of toxicity, of the need to see their physician promptly if they occur, and the need for close follow-up, including laboratory tests to monitor toxicity.

PEMETREXED

Rx	**Alimta** (Eli Lilly)	**Powder for injection, lyophilized:** 500 mg	500 mg mannitol. In single-use vials.

Indications

▶*Malignant pleural mesothelioma:* In combination with cisplatin for the treatment of patients with malignant pleural mesothelioma whose disease is unresectable or who are otherwise not candidates for curative surgery.

▶*Unlabeled uses:* Refractory non-small cell lung cancer.

Administration and Dosage

▶*Approved by the FDA:* February 5, 2004.

For IV infusion only.

▶*Dosing schedule:*

Pemetrexed Dosing Schedule for 21-Day Cycle

	Drug	Dose	Frequency
Chemo-therapy	Pemetrexed	500 mg/m^2 infused over 10 minutes	Day 1
	Cisplatin	75 mg/m^2 infused over 2 h	Day 1 – Begin approximately 30 minutes after the end of the pemetrexed infusion.
Premed-ication	Folic acid	350 to 1000 mcg by mouth	Daily – Begin 1 week prior to treatment, continuing throughout treatment and 21 days after the last pemetrexed dose (see Warnings).
	Vitamin B$_{12}$	1000 mcg IM	Every 3 cycles – Begin 1 week prior to treatment, continuing throughout treatment every 3 cycles thereafter[a] (see Warnings).
	Dexamethasone	4 mg twice daily by mouth	3 days – Administer the day before, the day of, and the day after treatment to help prevent skin rash (see Precautions).

[a] Subsequent injections may be given the same day as pemetrexed.

▶*Combination use with cisplatin:* Ensure patients receive consistent hydration with local practice prior to and/or after receiving cisplatin. See cisplatin package insert for more information.

▶*Dosage adjustment:*

Hematologic toxicities – Base dose adjustments at the start of a subsequent cycle on nadir hematologic counts or maximum nonhematologic toxicity from the preceding cycle of therapy. Treatment may be delayed to allow sufficient time for recovery. Do not have patients begin a new cycle of treatment unless the ANC is 1500 cells/mm^3 or more, the platelet count is 100,000 cells/mm^3 or more, and creatinine clearance (Ccr) is 45 mL/min or more. Upon recovery, retreat patients using the guidelines in the following table.

Dose Reduction for Pemetrexed and Cisplatin in Patients with Hematologic Toxicities

Nadir ANC < 500/mm^3 and nadir platelets ≥ 50,000/mm^3	75% of previous dose (both drugs)
Nadir platelets < 50,000/mm^3 regardless of nadir ANC	50% of previous dose (both drugs)

Nonhematologic toxicities – If patients develop nonhematologic toxicities (excluding neurotoxicity) of grade 3 (except grade 3 transaminase elevations) or more, withhold pemetrexed until it resolves to less than or equal to the patient's pretherapy value. Resume treatment according to the guidelines in the following table.

Dose Reduction for Pemetrexed and Cisplatin in Patients with Nonhematologic Toxicities[a,b]

	Pemetrexed dose (mg/m^2)	Cisplatin dose (mg/m^2)
Any grade 3[c] or 4 toxicities except mucositis	75% of previous dose	75% of previous dose
Any diarrhea requiring hospitalization	75% of previous dose	75% of previous dose
Grade 3 or 4 mucositis	50% of previous dose	100% of previous dose

[a] NCI Common Toxicity Criteria (CTC).
[b] Excluding neurotoxicity.
[c] Except grade 3 transaminase elevations.

Neurotoxicity – In the event of neurotoxicity, the recommended dose adjustments for pemetrexed and cisplatin are described in the following table. Discontinue therapy in patients if grade 3 or 4 neurotoxicity is experienced.

Dose Reduction for Pemetrexed and Cisplatin in Patients with Neurotoxicity

CTC grade	Pemetrexed dose (mg/m^2)	Cisplatin dose (mg/m^2)
0 to 1	100% of previous dose	100% of previous dose
2	100% of previous dose	50% of previous dose

Discontinue pemetrexed therapy if a patient experiences any hematologic or nonhematologic grade 3 or 4 toxicity after 2 dose reductions (except grade 3 transaminase elevations), or discontinue immediately if grade 3 or 4 neurotoxicity is observed.

Renal function impairment – In clinical studies, patients with Ccr 45 mL/min or more required no dose adjustments other than those recommended for all patients. Insufficient numbers of patients with Ccr below 45 mL/min have been treated to make dosage recommendations for this group of patients. Therefore, do not administer pemetrexed to patients whose Ccr is less than 45 mL/min.

Concomitant use with NSAIDS – Exercise caution when administering pemetrexed concurrently with nonsteroidal anti-inflammatory drugs (NSAIDs) to patients whose Ccr is less than 80 mL/min.

Hepatic function impairment – Pemetrexed is not extensively metabolized by the liver. Dose adjustments based on hepatic impairment experienced during treatment with pemetrexed are provided in the nonhematologic dose reduction table above.

▶*Preparation and administration:* If a solution of pemetrexed contacts the skin, wash the skin immediately and thoroughly with soap and water. If pemetrexed contacts the mucous membranes, flush thoroughly with water.

Calculate the dose and the number of pemetrexed vials needed. Each vial contains 500 mg pemetrexed. The vial contains an excess of pemetrexed to facilitate delivery of label amount.

Reconstitute 500 mg vials with 20 mL 0.9% sodium chloride injection (preservative-free) to give a solution containing 25 mg/mL pemetrexed. Gently swirl each vial until the powder is completely dissolved. The resulting solution is clear and ranges in color from colorless to yellow or green-yellow without adversely affecting product quality. The pH of the reconstituted pemetrexed solution is between 6.6 and 7.8. Further dilution is required.

Further dilute the appropriate volume of reconstituted pemetrexed solution to 100 mL with 0.9% sodium chloride injection (preservative-free), and administer as an IV infusion over 10 minutes.

▶*Admixture incompatibilities:* Reconstitution and further dilution prior to IV infusion is only recommended with 0.9% sodium chloride injection (preservative-free). Pemetrexed is physically incompatible with diluents containing calcium, including lactated Ringer's injection and Ringer's injection; therefore, do not use these diluents. Coadministration of pemetrexed with other drugs and diluents has not been studied, and, therefore, is not recommended.

▶*Storage / Stability:* Store at 25°C (77°F); excursions permitted to 15° to 30°C (59° to 86°F). Chemical and physical stability of reconstituted and infusion solutions of pemetrexed were demonstrated for up to 24 hours following initial reconstitution when stored under refrigeration at 2° to 8°C (36° to 46°F) or at 25°C (77°F); excursions permitted to 15° to 30°C (59° to 86°F). When prepared as directed, reconstituted and infusion solutions of pemetrexed contain no antimicrobial preservatives. Discard unused portion. Pemetrexed is not light sensitive.

Actions

▶*Pharmacology:* Pemetrexed is an antifolate antineoplastic agent that exerts its action by disrupting folate-dependent metabolic processes essential for cell replication. In vitro studies have shown that pemetrexed inhibits thymidylate synthase (TS), dihydrofolate reductase (DHFR), and glycinamide ribonucleotide formyltransferase (GARFT), all folate-dependent enzymes involved in the de novo biosynthesis of thymidine and purine nucleotides. Pemetrexed is transported into cells by the reduced folate carrier and membrane folate binding protein transport systems. Once in the cell, pemetrexed is converted to polyglutamate forms by the enzyme folyl polyglutamate synthase. The polyglutamate forms are retained in cells and are inhibitors of TS and GARFT. Polyglutamation is a time- and concentration-dependent process that occurs in tumor cells and, to a lesser extent, in normal tissues. Polyglutamated metabolites have an increased intracellular half life, resulting in prolonged drug action in malignant cells.

Preclinical studies have shown that pemetrexed inhibits the in vitro growth of mesothelioma cell lines (MSTO-211H, NCI-H2052). Studies with the MSTO-211H mesothelioma cell line showed synergistic effects when pemetrexed was combined concurrently with cisplatin. It was also observed that lower ANC nadirs occurred in patients with elevated baseline cystathionine or homocysteine concentrations. The levels of these substances can be reduced by folic acid and vitamin B$_{12}$ supplementation. There is no cumulative effect of pemetrexed exposure on ANC nadir over multiple treatment cycles.

PEMETREXED

➤*Pharmacokinetics:*

Absorption/Distribution – The pharmacokinetics of pemetrexed administered as a single agent in doses ranging from 0.2 to 838 mg/m^2 infused over a 10-minute period have been evaluated in 426 cancer patients with a variety of solid tumors. Pemetrexed AUC and C_{max} increase proportionally with dose. The pharmacokinetics of pemetrexed do not change over multiple treatment cycles. Pemetrexed has a steady-state volume of distribution of 16.1 L. In vitro studies indicate that pemetrexed is approximately 81% bound to plasma proteins. Binding is not affected by degree of renal impairment.

Metabolism/Excretion – Pemetrexed is not metabolized to an appreciable extent and is primarily eliminated in the urine, with 70% to 90% of the dose recovered unchanged within the first 24 hours following administration. The total systemic clearance of pemetrexed is 91.8 mL/min and the elimination half life of pemetrexed is 3.5 hours in patients with normal renal function (Ccr 90 mL/min).

Special populations –

Renal function impairment: Pharmacokinetic analyses of pemetrexed included 127 patients with reduced renal function. Plasma clearance of pemetrexed in the presence of cisplatin decreases as renal function decreases with increase in systemic exposure. Patients with Ccr of 45, 50, and 80 mL/min had 65%, 54%, and 13% increases, respectively, in pemetrexed AUC compared with patients with Ccr 100 mL/min (see Warnings and Administration and Dosage).

Contraindications

History of severe hypersensitivity reaction to pemetrexed or to any other ingredient used in the formulation.

Warnings

➤*Bone marrow suppression:* Pemetrexed can suppress bone marrow function manifested by neutropenia, thrombocytopenia, and anemia (see Adverse Reactions); myelosuppression is usually the dose-limiting toxicity. Dose reductions for subsequent cycles are based on nadir ANC, platelet count, and maximum nonhematologic toxicity seen in the previous cycle (see Administration and Dosage).

➤*Folate and vitamin B$_{12}$ supplementation:* Instruct patients treated with pemetrexed to take folic acid and vitamin B$_{12}$ as a prophylactic measure to reduce treatment-related hematologic and GI toxicity (see Administration and Dosage). In clinical studies, less overall toxicity and reductions in grade 3/4 hematologic and nonhematologic toxicities such as neutropenia, febrile neutropenia, and infection with grade 3/4 neutropenia were reported when pretreatment with folic acid and vitamin B$_{12}$ was administered. In clinical trials, the folic acid dose studied ranged from 350 to 1000 mcg, and the vitamin B$_{12}$ dose was 1000 mcg. The most commonly used dose of oral folic acid in clinical trials was 400 mcg.

➤*Renal function impairment:* Pemetrexed is primarily eliminated unchanged by renal excretion. No dosage adjustment is needed in patients with Ccr 45 mL/min or more. Insufficient numbers of patients have been studied with Ccr less than 45 mL/min to give a dose recommendation; therefore, do not administer pemetrexed to patients with Ccr less than 45 mL/min (see Administration and Dosage). One patient with severe renal impairment (Ccr 19 mL/min) who did not receive folic acid and vitamin B$_{12}$ died of drug-related toxicity following administration of pemetrexed alone.

➤*Hepatic function impairment:* Patients with bilirubin greater than 1.5 times the upper limit of normal (ULN) were excluded from clinical trials of pemetrexed. Patients with transaminases greater than 3 times the ULN were routinely excluded from clinical trials if they had no evidence of hepatic metastases. Patients with transaminase from 3 to 5 times the ULN were included in the clinical trial of pemetrexed if they had hepatic metastases. Dose adjustments based on hepatic impairment experienced during treatment with pemetrexed are provided in Administration and Dosage.

➤*Fertility impairment:* Pemetrexed administered at IV doses of 0.1 mg/kg/day or greater to male mice (approximately 1/1666 the recommended human dose on a mg/m^2 basis) resulted in reduced fertility, hypospermia, and testicular atrophy.

➤*Elderly:* For fully supplemented patients treated with pemetrexed plus cisplatin, the incidence of CTC grade 3/4 fatigue, leukopenia, neutropenia, and thrombocytopenia were greater in patients 65 years of age and older compared with patients younger than 65 years of age.

➤*Pregnancy: Category D.* Pemetrexed may cause fetal harm when administered to pregnant women. Pemetrexed was fetotoxic and teratogenic in mice at IV doses of 0.2 mg/kg (0.6 mg/m^2) or 5 mg/kg (15 mg/m^2) when given on gestation days 6 through 15. Pemetrexed caused fetal malformations (incomplete ossification of talus and skull bone) at 0.2 mg/kg (approximately 1/833 the recommended IV human dose on a mg/m^2 basis), and cleft palate at 5 mg/kg (approximately 1/33 the recommended IV human dose on a mg/m^2 basis). Embryotoxicity was characterized by increased embryo-fetal deaths and reduced litter sizes. There are no studies of pemetrexed in pregnant women. Advise patients to avoid becoming pregnant. If pemetrexed is used during pregnancy or if the patient becomes pregnant while taking pemetrexed, apprise the patient of the potential hazard to the fetus.

➤*Lactation:* It is not known whether pemetrexed or its metabolites are excreted in human milk. Because many drugs are excreted in human milk and because of the potential for serious adverse reactions in nursing infants from pemetrexed, it is recommended that nursing be discontinued if the mother is treated with pemetrexed.

➤*Children:* The safety and efficacy of pemetrexed in pediatric patients have not been established.

Precautions

➤*Monitoring:* Perform complete blood counts, including platelet counts and periodic chemistry tests, on all patients receiving pemetrexed. Monitor patients for nadir and recovery, which were tested in the clinical study before each dose and on days 8 and 15 of each cycle. Do not have patients begin a new cycle of treatment unless the ANC is 1500 cells/mm^3 or more, the platelet count is 100,000 cells/mm^3 or more, and Ccr is 45 mL/min or more.

➤*General:* Administer pemetrexed under the supervision of a qualified physician experienced in the use of antineoplastic agents. Appropriate management of complications is possible only when adequate diagnostic and treatment facilities are readily available. Treatment-related adverse events of pemetrexed seen in clinical trials have been reversible.

➤*Cutaneous reaction:* Skin rash has been reported more frequently in patients not pretreated with a corticosteroid in clinical trials. Pretreatment with dexamethasone (or equivalent) reduces the incidence and severity of cutaneous reaction (see Administration and Dosage).

➤*Extravasation risk:* Pemetrexed is not a vesicant. There is no specific antidote for extravasation of pemetrexed. To date, there have been few reported cases of pemetrexed extravasation that were not assessed as serious by the investigator. Manage pemetrexed extravasation with local standard practice for extravasation as with other nonvesicants.

➤*Pleural effusions or ascites:* The effect of third space fluid, such as pleural effusion and ascites, on pemetrexed is unknown. In patients with clinically significant third space fluid, give consideration to draining the effusion prior to pemetrexed administration.

Drug Interactions

Pemetrexed Drug Interactions			
Precipitant drug	Object drug*		Description
NSAIDs (ie, ibuprofen)	Pemetrexed	↑	Use caution when administering ibuprofen concurrently with pemetrexed to patients with mild to moderate renal insufficiency (Ccr from 45 to 79 mL/min), and avoid giving NSAIDs with short elimination half lives 2 days before, the day of, and 2 days following pemetrexed administration. Interrupt dosing in all patients taking NSAIDs with long elimination half lives for at least 5 days before, the day of, and 2 days following pemetrexed administration. If coadministration of an NSAID is necessary, closely monitor patients for toxicity, especially myelosuppression, renal, and GI toxicity.
Nephrotoxic agents	Pemetrexed	↑	Coadministration of nephrotoxic drugs could result in delayed clearance of pemetrexed. Coadministration of substances that also are tubularly secreted (eg, probenecid) could potentially result in delayed clearance of pemetrexed.

↑ = Object drug increased. ↓ = Object drug decreased.

Adverse Reactions

Adverse effects more common in the pemetrexed group than in the cisplatin-alone group were primarily hematologic effects, fever and infection, stomatitis/pharyngitis, and rash/desquamation.

Pemetrexed/Cisplatin Adverse Reactions in ≥ 5% of Patients with Malignant Pleural Mesothelioma[a] (CTC Grades)						
	All reported adverse events regardless of causality					
	Pemetrexed/Cisplatin (N = 168)			Cisplatin (N = 163)		
Adverse reaction	All grades	Grade 3	Grade 4	All grades	Grade 3	Grade 4
CNS						
Mood alteration/depression	14	1	0	9	1	0
Neuropathy/sensory	17	0	0	15	1	0

PEMETREXED

Pemetrexed/Cisplatin Adverse Reactions in ≥ 5% of Patients with Malignant Pleural Mesothelioma[a] (CTC Grades)

	All reported adverse events regardless of causality					
	Pemetrexed/Cisplatin (N = 168)			Cisplatin (N = 163)		
Adverse reaction	All grades	Grade 3	Grade 4	All grades	Grade 3	Grade 4
GI						
Anorexia	35	2	0	25	1	0
Constipation	44	2	1	39	1	0
Dehydration	7	3	1	1	1	0
Diarrhea without colostomy	26	4	0	16	1	0
Dysphagia/ esophagitis/ odynophagia	6	1	0	6	0	0
Nausea	84	11	1	79	6	0
Stomatitis/pharyngitis	28	2	0	9	0	0
Vomiting	58	10	1	52	4	1
Hematologic						
Anemia	33	5	1	14	0	0
Febrile neutropenia	1	1	0	1	0	0
Leukopenia	55	14	2	20	1	0
Neutropenia	58	19	5	16	3	1
Thrombocytopenia	27	4	1	10	0	0
Renal						
Creatinine elevation	16	1	0	12	1	0
Renal failure	2	0	1	1	0	0
Miscellaneous						
Allergic reaction/ hypersensitivity	2	0	0	1	0	0
Chest pain	40	8	1	30	5	1
Dyspnea	66	10	1	62	5	2
Fatigue	80	17	0	74	12	1
Fever	17	0	0	9	0	0
Infection without neutropenia	11	1	1	4	0	0
Infection with grade 3 or 4 neutropenia	6	1	0	4	0	0
Infection/febrile neutropenia, other	3	1	0	2	0	0
Other constitutional symptoms	11	2	1	8	1	1
Rash/desquamation	22	1	0	9	0	0
Thrombosis/embolism	7	4	2	4	3	1

[a] Patients received daily folic acid and vitamin B_{12} supplementation.

Adverse Events Comparing Fully Supplemented[a] vs Never Supplemented[b] Patients in the Pemetrexed/Cisplatin Arm (%)

Adverse event regardless of causality[c]	Fully supplemented[a] patients (N = 168)	Never supplemented[b] patients (N = 32)
Cardiovascular		
Hypertension	11	3
Thrombosis/embolism	6	3
GI		
Anorexia[c]	2	9
Diarrhea without colostomy[c]	4	9
Nausea[c]	12	31
Vomiting[c]	11	34
Hematologic		
Febrile neutropenia[c]	1	9
Infection with grade 3/4 neutropenia[c]	1	6
Neutropenia[c]	24	38
Thrombocytopenia[c]	5	9

Adverse Events Comparing Fully Supplemented[a] vs Never Supplemented[b] Patients in the Pemetrexed/Cisplatin Arm (%)

Adverse event regardless of causality[c]	Fully supplemented[a] patients (N = 168)	Never supplemented[b] patients (N = 32)
Miscellaneous		
Chest pain	8	6
Dehydration[c]	4	9
Fatigue[c]	17	25
Fever[c]	0	6

[a] Patients received daily folic acid and vitamin B_{12} supplementation.
[b] Patients never received vitamin supplementation.
[c] Grade 3/4 adverse events.

Gender – An increased incidence of rash in men (24%) compared with women (16%) was seen in patients receiving pemetrexed.

Overdosage

➤*Symptoms:* There have been few cases of pemetrexed overdose. Reported toxicities included neutropenia, anemia, thrombocytopenia, mucositis, and rash. Anticipated complications of overdose include bone marrow suppression as manifested by neutropenia, thrombocytopenia, and anemia. In addition, infection with or without fever, diarrhea, and mucositis may be seen.

➤*Treatment:* If an overdose occurs, institute general supportive measures as deemed necessary by the treating physician. In clinical trials, leucovorin was permitted for CTC grade 4 leukopenia lasting at least 3 days, CTC grade 4 neutropenia lasting at least 3 days, and immediately for CTC grade 4 thrombocytopenia, bleeding associated with grade 3 thrombocytopenia, or grade 3 or 4 mucositis. The following IV doses and schedules of leucovorin were recommended for IV use: 100 mg/m^2 IV once followed by 50 mg/m^2 leucovorin IV every 6 hours for 8 days. The ability of pemetrexed to be dialyzed is unknown.

Patient Information

It is not known if pemetrexed passes into breast milk. Instruct patients to stop breastfeeding once they start treatment with pemetrexed.

Advise patients to avoid becoming pregnant. If pemetrexed is used during pregnancy or if the patient becomes pregnant while taking pemetrexed, apprise the patient of the potential hazard to the fetus.

Instruct patients to notify their physician if they are taking other medicines, including prescription and nonprescription medicines, vitamins, and herbal supplements. Pemetrexed and other medicines may affect each other, causing serious side effects. Advise patients to tell their physician if they are taking NSAIDS for pain or swelling. Notify patients that there are many NSAID medications and to ask their physician or pharmacist if they are unsure whether any of their medications are NSAIDS.

Advise patients that their physician will prescribe a corticosteroid to take for 3 days during treatment with pemetrexed. Notify patients that corticosteroids lower their chances for getting skin reactions from pemetrexed.

Inform patients that it is very important to take folic acid and vitamin B_{12} during treatment with pemetrexed to lower the chances of harmful side effects. Instruct patients to start taking 350 to 1000 mcg folic acid every day for at least 5 of the 7 days before the first dose of pemetrexed, and to keep taking folic acid every day during the time they are getting treatment and for 21 days after their last treatment. Folic acid can be found OTC and in many multivitamin pills. Instruct patients to ask their physician if they are not sure how to choose a folic acid product. Notify patients that their physician will give them vitamin B_{12} injections while they are getting treatment with pemetrexed; the first injection will be given during the week before their first dose of pemetrexed and then approximately every 9 weeks during treatment.

Advise patients that they will have regular blood tests before and during pemetrexed treatment and that their physician may adjust their dose of pemetrexed or delay treatment based on the results of their blood tests and on their general condition.

The most common side effects of pemetrexed when taken with cisplatin are stomach upset, including nausea, vomiting, and diarrhea, low blood cell counts, tiredness, mouth, throat, or lip sores, loss of appetite, and rash.

CAPECITABINE

Rx	Xeloda (Roche)	Tablets: 150 mg	Lactose. (Xeloda 150). Light peach, oblong. Film-coated. In 60s and 120s.
		500 mg	Lactose. (Xeloda 500). Peach, oblong. Film-coated. In 120s and 240s.

WARNING

Warfarin interaction: Patients receiving capecitabine and oral coumarin-derivative anticoagulant therapy should have their anticoagulant response (INR or prothrombin time [PT]) monitored frequently in order to adjust the anticoagulant dose accordingly. A clinically important capecitabine-warfarin drug interaction was demonstrated in a clinical pharmacology trial. Altered coagulation parameters or bleeding, including death, have been reported in patients taking capecitabine concomitantly with coumarin-derivative anticoagulants such as warfarin and phenprocoumon. Postmarketing reports have shown clinically significant increases in PT and INR in patients who were stabilized on anticoagulants at the time capecitabine was introduced. These events occurred within several days and up to several months after initiating capecitabine therapy and, in a few cases, within 1 month after stopping capecitabine. These events occurred in patients with and without liver metastases. Age > 60 years and a diagnosis of cancer independently predispose patients to an increased risk of coagulopathy.

Indications

➤*Colorectal cancer:* First-line treatment in patients with metastatic colorectal carcinoma when treatment with fluoropyrimidine therapy alone is preferred. Combination chemotherapy has shown a survival benefit compared with 5-fluorouracil (5-FU)/leucovorin (LV) alone. A survival benefit over 5-FU/LV has not been demonstrated with capecitabine monotherapy. Use of capecitabine instead of 5-FU/LV in combinations has not been adequately studied to assure safety or preservation of the survival advantage.

➤*Breast cancer combination therapy:* Capecitabine in combination with docetaxel is indicated for the treatment of patients with metastatic breast cancer after failure of prior anthracycline-containing chemotherapy.

➤*Breast cancer monotherapy:* For the treatment of patients with metastatic breast cancer resistant to both paclitaxel and an anthracycline-containing chemotherapy regimen or resistant to paclitaxel and for whom further anthracycline therapy is not indicated (eg, patients who have received cumulative doses of 400 mg/m² of doxorubicin or doxorubicin equivalents). Resistance is defined as progressive disease while on treatment, with or without an initial response, or relapse within 6 months of completing treatment with an anthracycline-containing adjuvant regimen.

Administration and Dosage

➤*Approved by the FDA:* April 30, 1998.

The recommended dose of capecitabine is 1250 mg/m² administered orally twice daily (morning and evening; equivalent to 2500 mg/m² total daily dose) for 2 weeks followed by a 1-week rest period given as 3-week cycles. Swallow capecitabine tablets with water within 30 minutes after a meal. In combination with docetaxel, the recommended dose of capecitabine is 1250 mg/m² twice daily for 2 weeks followed by a 1-week rest period, combined with docetaxel at 75 mg/m² as a 1-hour IV infusion every 3 weeks. Premedication, according to the docetaxel labeling, should be started prior to docetaxel administration for patients receiving the capecitabine plus docetaxel combination. The following table displays the total daily dose by body surface area and the number of tablets to be taken at each dose.

Capecitabine Dose Calculation According to Body Surface Area			
Dose level 1250 mg/m² twice daily		Number of tablets per dose (morning and evening)[1]	
Surface area (m²)	Total daily dose (mg)	150 mg	500 mg
≤ 1.25	3000	0	3
1.26 to 1.37	3300	1	3
1.38 to 1.51	3600	2	3
1.52 to 1.65	4000	0	4
1.66 to 1.77	4300	1	4
1.78 to 1.91	4600	2	4
1.92 to 2.05	5000	0	5
2.06 to 2.17	5300	1	5
≥ 2.18	5600	2	5

[1] Total daily dose divided by 2 to allow equal morning and evening doses.

➤*Dose modification guidelines:* Carefully monitor patients for toxicity. Toxicity caused by capecitabine administration may be managed by symptomatic treatment, dose interruptions, and adjustment of dose. Once the dose has been reduced, it should not be increased at a later time. See the following tables for recommendations.

Capecitabine combination therapy with docetaxel –

Capecitabine in Combination with Docetaxel Dose Reduction Schedule			
Toxicity NCIC grades[1]	Grade 2	Grade 3	Grade 4
First appearance	Grade 2 occurring during the 14 days of capecitabine treatment: Interrupt capecitabine treatment until resolved to grade 0 to 1. Treatment may be resumed during the cycle at the same dose of capecitabine. Doses of capecitabine missed during a treatment cycle are not to be replaced. Implement prophylaxis for toxicities where possible. Grade 2 persisting at the time the next capecitabine/docetaxel treatment is due: Delay treatment until resolved to grade 0 to 1, then continue at 100% of the original capecitabine and docetaxel dose. Implement prophylaxis for toxicities where possible.	Grade 3 occurring during the 14 days of capecitabine treatment: Interrupt the capecitabine treatment until resolved to grade 0 to 1. Treatment may be resumed during the cycle at 75% of the capecitabine dose. Doses of capecitabine missed during a treatment cycle are not to be replaced. Implement prophylaxis for toxicities where possible. Grade 3 persisting at the time the next capecitabine/docetaxel treatment is due: Delay treatment until resolved to grade 0 to 1. For patients developing grade 3 toxicity at any time during the treatment cycle, upon resolution to grade 0 to 1, continue subsequent treatment cycles at 75% of the original capecitabine dose and at 55 mg/m² of docetaxel. Implement prophylaxis for toxicities where possible.	Discontinue treatment unless treating physician considers it to be in the best interest of the patient to continue with capecitabine at 50% of original dose.

CAPECITABINE

Capecitabine in Combination with Docetaxel Dose Reduction Schedule			
Toxicity NCIC grades[1]	Grade 2	Grade 3	Grade 4
Second appearance of same toxicity	Grade 2 occurring during the 14 days of capecitabine treatment: Interrupt capecitabine treatment until resolved to grade 0 to 1. Treatment may be resumed during the cycle at 75% of original capecitabine dose. Doses of capecitabine missed during a treatment cycle are not to be replaced. Implement prophylaxis for toxicities where possible. Grade 2 persisting at the time the next capecitabine/docetaxel treatment is due: Delay treatment until resolved to grade 0 to 1. For patients developing second occurrence of grade 2 toxicity at any time during the treatment cycle, upon resolution to grade 0 to 1, continue subsequent treatment cycles at 75% of the original capecitabine dose and at 55 mg/m^2 of docetaxel. Implement prophylaxis for toxicities where possible.	Grade 3 occurring during the 14 days of capecitabine treatment: Interrupt the capecitabine treatment until resolved to grade 0 to 1. Treatment may be resumed during the cycle at 50% of the capecitabine dose. Doses of capecitabine missed during a treatment cycle are not to be replaced. Implement prophylaxis for toxicities where possible. Grade 3 persisting at the time the next capecitabine/docetaxel treatment is due: Delay treatment until resolved to grade 0 to 1. For patients developing grade 3 toxicity at any time during the treatment cycle, upon resolution to grade 0 to 1, continue subsequent treatment cycles at 50% of the original capecitabine dose and discontinue docetaxel. Implement prophylaxis for toxicities where possible.	Discontinue treatment.
Third appearance of same toxicity	Grade 2 occurring during the 14 days of capecitabine treatment: Interrupt capecitabine treatment until resolved to grade 0 to 1. Treatment may be resumed during the cycle at 50% of the original capecitabine dose. Doses of capecitabine missed during a treatment cycle are not to be replaced. Implement prophylaxis for toxicities where possible. Grade 2 persisting at the time the next capecitabine/docetaxel treatment is due: Delay treatment until resolved to grade 0 to 1. For patients developing third occurrence of grade 2 toxicity at any time during the treatment cycle, upon resolution to grade 0 to 1, continue subsequent treatment cycles at 50% of the original capecitabine dose and discontinue docetaxel. Implement prophylaxis for toxicities where possible.	Discontinue treatment.	
Fourth appearance of same toxicity	Discontinue treatment.		

[1] National Cancer Institute of Canada (NCIC) Common Toxicity Criteria were used except for the hand-and-foot syndrome (see Precautions).

Capecitabine monotherapy –

Recommended Dose Modifications of Capecitabine		
Toxicity NCIC Grades[1]	During a course of therapy	Dose adjustment for next cycle (% of starting dose)
Grade 1	Maintain dose level	Maintain dose level
Grade 2		
1st appearance	Interrupt until resolved to grade 0 to 1	100
2nd appearance	Interrupt until resolved to grade 0 to 1	75
3rd appearance	Interrupt until resolved to grade 0 to 1	50
4th appearance	Discontinue treatment permanently	
Grade 3		
1st appearance	Interrupt until resolved to grade 0 to 1	75
2nd appearance	Interrupt until resolved to grade 0 to 1	50
3rd appearance	Discontinue treatment permanently	
Grade 4		
1st appearance	Discontinue permanently or If physician deems it to be in the patient's best interest to continue, interrupt until resolved to grade 0 to 1	50

[1] National Cancer Institute of Canada Common Toxicity Criteria were used except for the hand-and-foot syndrome (see Precautions).

Dosage modifications are not recommended for grade 1 events. Interrupt therapy upon the occurrence of a grade 2 or 3 adverse experience. Once the adverse event has resolved or decreased in intensity to grade 1, capecitabine therapy may be restarted at full dose or as adjusted according to the above table. If a grade 4 experience occurs, discontinue or interrupt therapy until resolved or decreased to grade 1 and restart therapy at 50% of the original dose. Doses of capecitabine omitted for toxicity are not replaced or restored; instead the patient should resume the planned treatment cycles.

➤*Adjustment of starting dose in special populations:*
Hepatic function impairment – In patients with mild-to-moderate hepatic dysfunction caused by liver metastases, no starting dose adjustment is necessary; however, carefully monitor patients. Patients with severe hepatic dysfunction have not been studied.

Renal function impairment – No adjustment to the starting dose of capecitabine is recommended in patients with mild renal impairment (Ccr 51 to 80 mL/min [Cockroft and Gault]). In patients with moderate renal impairment (baseline Ccr 30 to 50 mL/min), a dose reduction to 75% of the capecitabine starting dose when used as monotherapy or in combination with docetaxel (from 1250 mg/m^2 to 950 mg/m^2 twice daily) is recommended. Subsequent dose adjustment is recommended as outlined in the above table if a patient develops a grade 2 to 4 adverse event.

➤*Storage/Stability:* Store at 25°C (77°F); excursions permitted to 15° to 30°C (59° to 86°F). Keep tightly closed.

Actions

➤*Pharmacology:* Capecitabine is a fluoropyrimidine carbamate with antineoplastic activity. It is an oral systemic prodrug of 5'-deoxy-5-fluorouridine (5'-DFUR) that is enzymatically converted to 5-FU. Capecitabine is relatively noncytotoxic in vitro.

Both healthy and tumor cells metabolize 5-FU to 5-fluoro-2-deoxyuridine monophosphate (FdUMP) and 5-fluorouridine triphosphate (FUTP). These metabolites cause cell injury by 2 different mechanisms. First, FdUMP and the folate cofactor, N$^{5-10}$-methylenetetrahydrofolate, bind to thymidylate synthase (TS) to form a covalently bound ternary complex. This binding inhibits the formation of thymidylate from 2'-deoxyuridylate. Thymidylate is the necessary precursor of thymidine triphosphate, which is essential for the synthesis of DNA, so that a deficiency of this compound can inhibit cell division. Second, nuclear transcriptional enzymes can mistakenly incorporate FUTP in place of uridine triphosphate (UTP) during the synthesis of RNA. This metabolic error can interfere with RNA processing and protein synthesis.

➤*Pharmacokinetics:*
Absorption/Distribution – Capecitabine is readily absorbed from the GI tract. Capecitabine reaches peak blood levels in approximately 1.5 hours (T$_{max}$) with peak 5-FU levels occurring slightly later, at 2 hours. Food reduces the rate and extent of absorption of capecitabine with mean C$_{max}$ and AUC decreased by 60% and 35%, respectively. The

CAPECITABINE

C_{max} and AUC of 5-FU are also reduced by food by 43% and 21%, respectively. Food delayed T_{max} of both parent and 5-FU by 1.5 hours.

The pharmacokinetics of capecitabine and its metabolite, 5′-deoxy-5-fluorocytidine (5′-DFCR) were dose-proportional; however, the increases in the AUCs of 5′-DFUR and 5-FU were greater than proportional to the increase in dose and the AUC of 5-FU was 34% higher on day 14 than on day 1. Plasma protein binding of capecitabine and its metabolites is less than 60% and is not concentration-dependent. Capecitabine was primarily bound to human albumin (approximately 35%).

Metabolism/Excretion – Capecitabine is extensively metabolized enzymatically to 5-FU. In the liver, a 60 kDa carboxylesterase hydrolyzes much of the compound to 5′-DFCR. Cytidine deaminase, an enzyme found in most tissues, including tumors, subsequently converts 5′-DFCR to 5′-DFUR. The enzyme, thymidine phosphorylase, then hydrolyzes 5′-DFUR to the active drug 5-FU. Many tissues throughout the body express thymidine phosphorylase. Some human carcinomas express this enzyme in higher concentrations than surrounding normal tissues. The enzyme dihydropyrimidine dehydrogenase hydrogenates 5-FU, the product of capecitabine metabolism, to the much less toxic 5-fluoro-5,6-dihydro-fluorouracil (FUH₂). Dihydropyrimidinase cleaves to the pyrimidine ring to yield 5-fluoro-ureido-propionic acid (FUPA). Finally, β-ureido-propionase cleaves to FUPA to α-fluoro-β-alanine (FBAL), which is cleared in the urine. The elimination half-life of both parent capecitabine and 5-FU was approximately 45 minutes.

Capecitabine and its metabolites are predominantly excreted in urine; 95.5% of administered capecitabine dose is recovered in urine. Fecal excretion is minimal (2.6%). The major metabolite excreted in urine is FBAL, which represents 57% of the administered dose. About 3% of the administered dose is excreted in urine as unchanged drug.

Special populations –

Hepatic function impairment: Both AUC and C_{max} of capecitabine increased by 60% in patients with hepatic dysfunction who received a single 1255 mg/m² dose compared with patients with normal hepatic function (n = 14). The AUC and C_{max} of 5-FU were not affected (see Warnings).

Renal function impairment: Following oral administration of 1250 mg/m² capecitabine twice/day, patients with moderate (creatinine clearance [Ccr] 30 to 50 mL/min) and severe (Ccr less than 30 mL/min) renal impairment showed 85% and 258% higher systemic exposure to FBAL on day 1 compared to normal renal function patients (Ccr greater than 80 mL/min). Systemic exposure to 5′-DFUR was 42% and 71% greater in moderately and severely renal impaired patients, respectively, than in normal patients. Systemic exposure to capecitabine was about 25% greater in both moderately and severely renal impaired patients.

Race: Following oral administration of 825 mg/m² capecitabine twice/day for 14 days, Japanese patients (n = 18) had about 36% lower C_{max} and 24% lower AUC for capecitabine than Caucasian patients (n = 22). Japanese patients also had about 25% lower C_{max} and 34% lower AUC for FBAL than Caucasian patients.

➤*Clinical trials:*

Colorectal carcinoma – Data from 2 open-label, multicenter, randomized, controlled clinical trials involving 1207 patients support the use of capecitabine in the first-line treatment of patients with metastatic colorectal carcinoma. The 2 clinical studies were identical in design and were conducted in 120 centers in different countries. Study 1 was conducted in the US, Canada, Mexico, and Brazil; study 2 was conducted in Europe, Israel, Australia, New Zealand, and Taiwan. Altogether, in both trials, 603 patients were randomized to treatment with capecitabine at a dose of 1250 mg/m² twice daily for 2 weeks followed by a 1-week rest period and given as 3-week cycles; 604 patients were randomized to treatment with 5-FU and leucovorin (20 mg/m² leucovorin IV followed by 425 mg/m² IV bolus 5-FU, on days 1 to 5, every 28 days). Overall survival, time to progression, and response rate (complete plus partial responses) were assessed. Capecitabine was superior to 5-FU/LV for objective response rate in studies 1 and 2.

Efficacy of Capecitabine vs 5-FU/LV in Colorectal Cancer				
	Study 1		Study 2	
Parameter	Capecitabine (n = 302)	5-FU/LV (n = 303)	Capecitabine (n = 301)	5-FU/LV (n = 301)
Overall response rate (95% CI)	21% (16% to 26%)	11% (8% to 15%)	21% (16% to 26%)	14% (10% to 18%)
p-value	0.0014		0.027	
Median time to progression (95% CI)	128 days (120 to 136)	131 days (105 to 153)	137 days (128 to 165)	131 days (102 to 156)
Median survival (95% CI)	380 days (321 to 434)	407 days (366 to 446)	404 days (367 to 452)	369 days (338 to 430)

Breast cancer combination therapy – Capecitabine in combination with docetaxel was assessed in an open-label, multicenter, randomized trial in 75 centers in Europe, North America, South America, Asia, and Australia. A total of 511 patients with metastatic breast cancer resistant to or recurring during or after an anthracycline-containing

therapy, or relapsing during or recurring within 2 years of completing an anthracycline-containing adjuvant therapy were enrolled. Patients (n = 255) were randomized to receive capecitabine 1250 mg/m² twice daily for 14 days followed by 1 week without treatment and docetaxel 75 mg/m² as a 1-hour IV infusion administered in 3-week cycles. In the monotherapy arm, 256 patients received docetaxel 100 mg/m² as a 1-hour IV infusion administered in 3-week cycles. Capecitabine in combination with docetaxel resulted in statistically significant improvement in time to disease progression, overall survival and objected response rate compared to monotherapy with docetaxel, as shown in the following table.

Efficacy of Capecitabine and Docetaxel Combination vs Docetaxel Monotherapy			
Efficacy parameter	Combination therapy	Monotherapy	p-value
Median time to disease progression (95% CI)	186 days (165 to 198)	128 days (105 to 136)	0.0001
Median overall survival (95% CI)	442 days (375 to 497)	352 (298 to 387)	0.0126
Response rate	32%	22%	0.009

Contraindications

Hypersensitivity to 5-FU, capecitabine, or to any of its components; severe renal impairment (Ccr below 30 mL/min); dihydropyrimidine dehydrogenase (DPD) deficiency.

Warnings

➤*Dihydropyrimidine dehydrogenase deficiency:* Rarely, unexpected, severe toxicity (eg, stomatitis, diarrhea, neutropenia, and neurotoxicity) associated with 5-fluorouracil has been attributed to a deficiency of dihydropyrimidine dehydrogenase (DPD) activity. A link between decreased levels of DPD and increased, potentially fatal toxic effects of 5-fluorouracil therefore cannot be excluded.

➤*Diarrhea:* Capecitabine can induce diarrhea, sometimes severe. Carefully monitor patients with severe diarrhea and give fluid and electrolyte replacement therapy if they become dehydrated. The median time to first occurrence of grade 2 through 4 diarrhea was 34 days (range, 1 to 369 days). NCIC defines grade 2 diarrhea as an increase of 4 to 6 stools/day or nocturnal stools, grade 3 diarrhea as an increase of 7 to 9 stools/day or incontinence and malabsorption, and grade 4 diarrhea as an increase of ≥ 10 stools/day, grossly bloody diarrhea, or the need for parenteral support. If grade 2, 3, or 4 diarrhea occurs, immediately interrupt administration of capecitabine until the diarrhea resolves or decreases in intensity to grade 1. The median duration of grade 3 to 4 diarrhea was 5 days. Following a recurrence of grade 2 diarrhea or occurrence of any grade 3 or 4 diarrhea, decrease subsequent doses of capecitabine (see Administration and Dosage). Standard antidiarrheal treatments (eg, loperamide) are recommended.

Necrotizing enterocolitis (typhlitis) has been reported.

➤*Renal function impairment:* Patients with moderate renal impairment at baseline require dose reduction (see Administration and Dosage). Carefully monitor patients with mild and moderate renal impairment at baseline for adverse events. Prompt interruption of therapy with subsequent dose adjustments is recommended if a patient develops a grade 2 to 4 adverse event as outlined in Administration and Dosage.

➤*Hepatic function impairment:* Carefully monitor patients with mild-to-moderate hepatic dysfunction caused by liver metastases when capecitabine is administered (see Pharmacokinetics). The effect of severe hepatic dysfunction on the disposition of capecitabine is not known.

➤*Mutagenesis:* Capecitabine was clastogenic in vitro to human peripheral blood lymphocytes, but not clastogenic in vivo to mouse bone marrow (micronucleus test). Fluorouracil causes mutations in bacteria and yeast. Fluorouracil also causes chromosomal abnormalities in the mouse micronucleus test in vivo.

➤*Fertility impairment:* In studies of fertility and general reproductive performance in mice, oral capecitabine doses of 760 mg/kg/day disturbed estrus and consequently caused a decrease in fertility. In pregnant mice, no fetuses survived this dose. The disturbance in estrus was reversible. In males, this dose caused degenerative changes in the testes, including decreases in the number of spermatocytes and spermatids. In separate pharmacokinetic studies, this dose in mice produced 5′-DFUR AUC values ≈ 0.7 times the corresponding values in patients administered the recommended daily dose.

➤*Elderly:* Patients 80 years of age and older may experience a greater incidence of grade 3 or 4 adverse events.

➤*Pregnancy:* Category D. Capecitabine may cause fetal harm when given to a pregnant woman. Capecitabine at doses of 198 mg/kg/day during organogenesis caused malformations and embryo death in mice. Malformations in mice included cleft palate, anophthalmia, microphthalmia, oligodactyly, polydactyly, syndactyly, kinky tail, and dilation of cerebral ventricles. At doses of 90 mg/kg/day, capecitabine given to

CAPECITABINE

pregnant monkeys during organogenesis caused fetal death.

There are no adequate and well-controlled studies in pregnant women using capecitabine. If the drug is used during pregnancy, or if the patient becomes pregnant while receiving this drug, apprise the patient of the potential hazard to the fetus. Advise women of childbearing potential to avoid becoming pregnant while receiving treatment with capecitabine.

➤*Lactation:* Because of the potential for serious adverse reactions in nursing infants, it is recommended that nursing be discontinued when receiving capecitabine therapy.

➤*Children:* Safety and efficacy in patients under 18 years of age have not been established.

Precautions

Patients receiving therapy with capecitabine should be monitored by a physician experienced in the use of cancer chemotherapeutic agents. Most adverse events are reversible and do not need to result in discontinuation, although doses may need to be withheld or reduced (see Administration and Dosage).

➤*Hand-and-foot syndrome:* Hand-and-foot syndrome (palmar-plantar erythrodysesthesia or chemotherapy-induced acral erythema) is a cutaneous toxicity (median time to onset of 79 days; range, 11 to 360 days) with a severity range of grades 1 to 3. Grade 1 is characterized by any of the following: Numbness, dysesthesia/paresthesia, tingling, painless swelling or erythema of the hands or feet, or discomfort that does not disrupt normal activities.

Grade 2 hand-and-foot syndrome is defined as painful erythema and swelling of the hands or feet or discomfort affecting the patient's activities of daily living. Grade 3 hand-and-foot syndrome is defined as moist desquamation, ulceration, blistering, or severe pain of the hands or feet or severe discomfort that causes the patient to be unable to work or perform activities of daily living. If grade 2 or 3 hand-and-foot syndrome occurs, interrupt administration of capecitabine until the event resolves or decreases in intensity to grade 1. Following grade 3 hand-and-foot syndrome, decrease subsequent doses of capecitabine (see Administration and Dosage).

➤*Cardiotoxicity:* The cardiotoxicity observed with capecitabine includes MI/ischemia, angina, dysrhythmias, cardiac arrest, cardiac failure, sudden death, ECG changes, and cardiomyopathy. These adverse events may be more common in patients with a history of coronary artery disease.

➤*Hyperbilirubinemia:* The median time to onset for grade 3 or 4 hyperbilirubinemia in the colorectal cancer population was 64 days and median total bilirubin increased from 8 mcm/L at baseline to 13 mcm/L during treatment with capecitabine. Of the 136 colorectal cancer patients with grade 3 or 4 hyperbilirubinemia, 49 patients had grade 3 or 4 hyperbilirubinemia as their last measured value, of which 46 had liver metastases at baseline.

If drug-related grade 2 to 4 elevations in bilirubin occur, immediately interrupt administration of capecitabine until the hyperbilirubinemia resolves or decreases in intensity to grade 1 (see Administration and Dosage). NCIC grade 2 hyperbilirubinemia is defined as $1.5 \times$ normal, grade 3 hyperbilirubinemia as 1.5 to $3 \times$ normal, and grade 4 hyperbilirubinemia as $> 3 \times$ normal.

➤*Hematologic effects:* In 875 patients with either metastatic breast or colorectal cancer who received a dose of 1250 mg/m² administered twice daily as monotherapy for 2 weeks followed by a 1-week rest period, 3.2%, 1.7%, and 2.4% of patients had grade 3 or 4 neutropenia, thrombocytopenia, or decreases in hemoglobin, respectively. In 251 patients with metastatic breast cancer who received a dose of capecitabine in combination with docetaxel, 68% had grade 3 or 4 neutropenia, 2.8% had grade 3 or 4 thrombocytopenia, and 9.6% had grade 3 or 4 anemia.

Drug Interactions

Capecitabine Drug Interactions			
Precipitant drug	Object drug*		Description
Capecitabine	Phenytoin	↑	Carefully monitor phenytoin levels in patients taking capecitabine. The phenytoin dose may need to be reduced. The mechanism of interaction is presumed to be inhibition of the CYP2C9 isoenzyme by capecitabine or its metabolites.
Capecitabine	Warfarin	↑	Altered coagulation parameters or bleeding have been reported in patients taking capecitabine concomitantly with warfarin. Monitor patients regularly for prothrombin time (PT) or International Normalized Ratio (INR) alterations and adjust anticoagulant dose as necessary.

Capecitabine Drug Interactions			
Precipitant drug	Object drug*		Description
Antacids	Capecitabine	↑	When 20 mL of an aluminum hydroxide- and magnesium hydroxide-containing antacid was administered immediately after capecitabine, AUC and C_{max} increased by 16% and 35%, respectively, for capecitabine and by 18% and 22%, respectively, for 5'-DFCR.
Leucovorin	Capecitabine	↑	The concentration of 5-FU is increased and its toxicity may be enhanced by leucovorin. Deaths from severe enterocolitis, diarrhea, and dehydration have been reported in elderly patients receiving weekly leucovorin and fluorouracil.

*↑ = Object drug increased.

➤*Drug/Food interactions:* Food reduced the rate and extent of absorption of capecitabine with mean C_{max} and AUC decreased by 60% and 35%, respectively. The C_{max} and AUC of 5-FU were also reduced by food by 43% and 21%, respectively. Food delayed T_{max} of both parent and 5-FU by 1.5 hours. In all clinical trials, patients were instructed to administer capecitabine within 30 minutes after a meal. Because current safety and efficacy data are based upon administration with food, it is recommended that capecitabine be administered with food.

Adverse Reactions

➤*Colorectal cancer:* The following table shows the adverse events occurring in at least 5% of patients from pooling the 2 phase III trials in colorectal cancer. Rates are rounded to the nearest whole number. A total of 596 patients with metastatic colorectal cancer were treated with 1250 mg/m² twice a day of capecitabine administered for 2 weeks followed by a 1-week rest period, and 593 patients were administered 5-FU and leucovorin in the Mayo regimen (20 mg/m² leucovorin IV followed by 425 mg/m² IV bolus 5-FU, on days 1 through 5 every 28 days). In the pooled colorectal database, the median duration of treatment was 139 days for capecitabine-treated patients and 140 days for 5-FU/LV-treated patients. A total of 13% and 11% of capecitabine and 5-FU/LV-treated patients, respectively, discontinued treatment because of adverse events/intercurrent illness. A total of 82 deaths from all causes occurred either on study or within 28 days of receiving study drug: 8.4% of patients randomized to capecitabine and 5.4% randomized to 5-FU/LV.

Phase III Colorectal Trials with Capecitabine vs 5-FU/LV Related or Unrelated to Treatment (%)						
	Capecitabine (n = 596)			5-FU/LV (n = 593)		
Adverse reaction	Total	Grade 3	Grade 4	Total	Grade 3	Grade 4
Number of patients with > 1 adverse event	96	52	9	94	45	9
CNS						
Peripheral sensory neuropathy	10	-	-	4	-	-
Headache	10	1	-	7	-	-
Dizziness, excluding vertigo	8	< 1	-	8	< 1	-
Insomnia	7	-	-	7	-	-
Taste disturbance	6	1	-	11	< 1	1
Mood alteration	5	-	-	6	< 1	-
Depression	5	-	-	4	< 1	-
Dermatologic						
Hand-and-foot syndrome	54	17	NA	6	1	NA
Dermatitis	27	1	-	26	-	-
Skin discoloration	7	< 1	-	5	-	-
Alopecia	6	-	-	21	< 1	-
GI						
Diarrhea	55	13	2	61	10	2
Nausea	43	4	-	51	3	< 1
Vomiting	27	4	< 1	30	4	< 1
Stomatitis	25	2	< 1	62	14	1
Abdominal pain	35	9	< 1	31	5	-
Constipation	14	1	< 1	17	1	-
GI motility disorder	10	< 1	-	7	< 1	-
Oral discomfort	10	-	-	10	-	-
Upper GI inflammatory disorders	8	< 1	-	10	1	-
GI hemorrhage	6	1	< 1	3	-	-
Ileus	6	4	1	5	2	1

CAPECITABINE

Phase III Colorectal Trials with Capecitabine vs 5-FU/LV Related or Unrelated to Treatment (%)

Adverse reaction	Capecitabine (n = 596)			5-FU/LV (n = 593)		
	Total	Grade 3	Grade 4	Total	Grade 3	Grade 4
Respiratory						
Dyspnea	14	1	-	10	< 1	1
Cough	7	< 1	1	8	-	-
Pharyngeal disorder	5	-	-	5	-	-
Epistaxis	3	< 1	-	6	-	-
Sore throat	2	-	-	6	-	-
Miscellaneous						
Anemia	80	2	< 1	79	1	< 1
Hyperbilirubinemia	48	18	5	17	3	3
Fatigue/Weakness	42	4	-	46	4	-
Appetite decreased	26	3	< 1	31	2	< 1
Pyrexia	18	1	-	21	2	-
Edema	15	1	-	9	1	-
Neutropenia	13	1	2	46	8	13
Eye irritation	13	-	-	10	< 1	-
Pain	12	1	-	10	1	-
Back pain	10	2	-	9	< 1	-
Venous thrombosis	8	3	< 1	6	2	-
Arthralgia	8	1	-	6	1	-
Dehydration	7	2	< 1	8	3	1
Chest pain	6	1	-	6	1	< 1
Viral infections	5	< 1	-	5	< 1	-
Vision abnormal	5	-	-	2	-	-

►*Breast cancer combination therapy:* The following data are shown for the combination study with capecitabine and docetaxel in patients with metastatic breast cancer. In the capecitabine and docetaxel combination arm, the treatment was capecitabine administered orally 1250 mg/m² twice daily as intermittent therapy (2 weeks of treatment followed by 1 week without treatment) for at least 6 weeks and docetaxel administered as a 1-hour IV infusion at a dose of 75 mg/m² on the first day of each 3-week cycle for at least 6 weeks. In the monotherapy arm, docetaxel was administered as a 1-hour IV infusion at a dose of 100 mg/m² on the first day of each 3-week cycle for at least 6 weeks. The mean duration of treatment was 129 days in the combination arm and 98 days in the monotherapy arm. A total of 26% of patients in the combination arm and 19% in the monotherapy arm withdrew from the study because of adverse events. The percentage of patients requiring dose reductions because of adverse events were 65% in the combination arm and 36% in the monotherapy arm. The percentage of patients requiring treatment interruptions because of adverse events in the combination arm was 79%. Treatment interruptions were part of the dose modification scheme for the combination therapy arm, but not for the docetaxel monotherapy-treated patients.

Incidence of Adverse Events Considered Related or Unrelated to Treatment in Capecitabine and Docetaxel Combination vs Docetaxel Monotherapy Study (%)

Adverse reaction	Capecitabine 1250 mg/m² BID with docetaxel 75 mg/m²/3 weeks (n = 251)			Docetaxel 100 mg/m²/ 3 weeks (n = 255)		
	Total	Grade 3	Grade 4	Total	Grade 3	Grade 4
Number of patients with ≥ 1 adverse event	99	76.5	29.1	97	57.6	31.8
CNS						
Taste disturbance	16	< 1	-	14	< 1	-
Headache	15	3	-	15	2	-
Paresthesia	12	< 1	-	16	1	-
Dizziness	12	-	-	8	< 1	-
Insomnia	8	-	-	10	< 1	-
Peripheral neuropathy	6	-	-	10	1	-
Depression	5	-	-	5	1	-
Hypesthesia	4	< 1	-	8	< 1	-
Dermatologic						
Hand-and-foot syndrome	63	24	NA	8	1	NA
Alopecia	41	6	-	42	7	-
Nail disorder	14	2	-	15	-	-
Erythematous rash	9	< 1	-	5	-	-
Dermatitis	8	-	-	11	1	-
Nail discoloration	6	-	-	4	< 1	-
Onycholysis	5	1	-	5	1	-
Pruritus	4	-	-	5	-	-

Incidence of Adverse Events Considered Related or Unrelated to Treatment in Capecitabine and Docetaxel Combination vs Docetaxel Monotherapy Study (%)

Adverse reaction	Capecitabine 1250 mg/m² BID with docetaxel 75 mg/m²/3 weeks (n = 251)			Docetaxel 100 mg/m²/ 3 weeks (n = 255)		
	Total	Grade 3	Grade 4	Total	Grade 3	Grade 4
GI						
Diarrhea	67	14	< 1	48	5	< 1
Stomatitis	67	17	< 1	43	5	-
Nausea	45	7	-	36	2	-
Vomiting	35	4	1	24	2	-
Abdominal pain	30	< 3	< 1	24	2	-
Constipation	20	2	-	18	-	-
Dyspepsia	14	-	-	8	1	-
Dry mouth	6	< 1	-	5	-	-
Infection						
Oral candidiasis	7	< 1	-	8	< 1	-
Urinary tract infection	6	< 1	-	4	-	-
Upper respiratory tract	4	-	-	5	1	-
Laboratory test abnormalities						
Leukopenia	91	37	24	88	42	33
Neutropenia/ Granulocytopenia	86	20	49	87	10	66
Thrombocytopenia	41	2	1	23	1	2
Lymphocytopenia	99	48	41	98	44	40
Anemia	80	7	3	83	5	< 1
Hyperbilirubinemia	20	7	2	6	2	2
Metabolic						
Anorexia	13	1	-	11	< 1	-
Appetite decreased	10	-	-	5	-	-
Dehydration	10	2	-	7	< 1	< 1
Weight decreased	7	-	-	5	-	-
Musculoskeletal						
Arthralgia	15	2	-	24	3	-
Myalgia	15	2	-	25	2	-
Back pain	12	< 1	-	11	3	-
Bone pain	8	< 1	-	10	2	-
Ocular						
Lacrimation increased	12	-	-	7	< 1	-
Conjunctivitis	5	-	-	4	-	-
Eye irritation	5	-	-	1	-	-
Respiratory						
Dyspnea	14	2	< 1	16	2	-
Cough	13	1	-	22	< 1	-
Sore throat	12	2	-	11	< 1	-
Epistaxis	7	< 1	-	6	-	-
Rhinorrhea	5	-	-	3	-	-
Pleural effusion	2	1	-	7	4	-
Miscellaneous						
Edema	33	< 2	-	34	< 3	1
Pyrexia	28	2	-	34	2	-
Asthenia	26	4	< 1	25	6	-
Fatigue	22	4	-	27	6	-
Neutropenic fever	16	3	13	21	5	16
Weakness	16	2	-	11	2	-
Pain in limb	13	< 1	-	13	2	-
Lethargy	7	-	-	6	2	-
Pain	7	< 1	-	5	1	-
Flushing	5	-	-	5	-	-
Influenza-like illness	5	-	-	5	-	-
Chest pain (noncardiac)	4	< 1	-	6	2	-
Lymphedema	3	< 1	-	5	1	-

Below are clinically relevant adverse events in less than 5% of patients in the overall clinical trial safety database of 251 patients reported as related to the administration of capecitabine in combination with docetaxel and that were clinically at least remotely relevant. In parentheses is the incidence of grade 3 and 4 occurrences of each adverse event. It is anticipated that the same types of adverse events observed in the capecitabine monotherapy studies may be observed in patients treated with the combination of capecitabine plus docetaxel.

CNS – Syncope (1.2%); taste loss (0.8%); ataxia, polyneuropathy, migraine (0.39%).

GI – Hemorrhagic diarrhea (0.8%); ileus, necrotizing enterocolitis, esophageal ulcer (0.39%).

CAPECITABINE

Cardiovascular – Hypotension (1.2%); postural hypotension (0.8%); venous phlebitis and thrombophlebitis, supraventricular tachycardia (0.39%).

Hepatic – Jaundice, abnormal liver function tests, hepatic failure, hepatic coma, hepatotoxicity (0.39%).

Miscellaneous – Neutropenia sepsis (2.39%); hypersensitivity (1.2%); agranulocytosis, sepsis, bronchopneumonia, PT decreased, renal failure (0.39%).

➤*Breast cancer monotherapy:* The following data are shown for the study in stage IV breast cancer patients who received a dose of 1250 mg/m² administered twice daily for 2 weeks followed by a 1-week rest period. The mean duration of treatment was 114 days. A total of 8% of patients discontinued treatment because of adverse events/intercurrent illness.

Adverse Events Considered Remotely, Possibly, or Probably Related to Capecitabine Treatment in the Single Arm Trial in Stage IV Breast Cancer			
	Phase II trial in stage IV breast cancer (n = 162)		
Adverse reaction	Total	Grade 3	Grade 4
CNS			
Paresthesia	21	1	-
Headache	9	1	-
Dizziness	8	-	-
Insomnia	8	-	-
Dermatologic			
Hand-and-foot syndrome	57	11	NA
Dermatitis	37	1	-
Nail disorder	7	-	-
GI			
Diarrhea	57	12	3
Nausea	53	4	-
Vomiting	37	4	-
Stomatitis	24	7	-
Abdominal pain	20	4	-
Constipation	15	1	-
Dyspepsia	8	-	-
Hematologic			
Lymphopenia	94	44	15
Anemia	72	3	1
Neutropenia	26	2	2
Thrombocytopenia	24	3	1
Miscellaneous			
Fatigue	41	8	-
Anorexia	23	3	-
Hyperbilirubinemia	22	9	2
Eye irritation	15	-	-
Pyrexia	12	1	-
Edema	9	1	-
Myalgia	9	-	-
Dehydration	7	4	1
Pain in limb	6	1	-

➤*Monotherapy:* Below are clinically relevant adverse events in less than 5% of patients in the overall clinical trial safety database of 875 patients (phase III colorectal studies – 596 patients, phase II colorectal study — 34 patients, phase 2 breast cancer studies — 245 patients) reported as related to the administration of capecitabine and that were clinically at least remotely relevant. In parentheses is the incidence of grade 3 or 4 occurrences of each adverse event.

Cardiovascular – Hypotension, pulmonary embolism (0.2%); cerebrovascular accident, hypertension, myocarditis, tachycardia (0.1%); atrial fibrillation, bradycardia, extrasystoles, pericardial effusion, ventricular extrasystoles.

CNS – Ataxia (0.5%); loss of consciousness (0.2%); confusion, encephalopathy (0.1%); abnormal coordination, depression, dysarthria, dysphasia, impaired balance, insomnia, sedation, tremor; vertigo.

Dermatologic – Radiation recall syndrome (0.2%); nail disorder, photosensitivity reaction, sweating increased (0.1%); pruritus, skin ulceration.

GI – Ileus (0.3%); ascites, gastric ulcer, gastroenteritis (0.1%); abdominal distension, dysphagia, proctalgia, thirst, toxic dilation of intestine.

Hematologic / Lymphatic – Idiopathic thrombocytopenia purpura (1%); leukopenia (0.2%); bone marrow depression, coagulation disorder, lymphedema, pancytopenia (0.1%); hemorrhage.

Hepatic – Cholestatic hepatitis, hepatic fibrosis, hepatitis (0.1%); abnormal liver function tests.

Metabolic – Cachexia (0.4%); hypertriglyceridemia (0.1%); edema, hypokalemia, hypomagnesemia, increased weight.

Musculoskeletal – Arthritis, bone pain, (0.1%); muscle weakness, myalgia.

Respiratory – Asthma, bronchitis, bronchopneumonia, pneumonia (0.2%); cough, epistaxis, respiratory distress (0.1%); dyspnea, hemoptysis.

Miscellaneous – Laryngitis (1%); renal impairment (0.6%); sepsis (0.3%); chest pain, fungal infections (including candidiasis) (0.2%); drug hypersensitivity, fibrosis, pain (0.1%); chest mass, collapse, conjunctivitis, difficulty in walking, hoarseness, hot flushes, influenza-like illness, irritability, keratoconjunctivitis.

Postmarketing – Hepatic failure.

Overdosage

Manifestations of acute overdose would be nausea, vomiting, diarrhea, GI irritation and bleeding, and bone marrow depression. Medical management of overdose should include customary supportive medical interventions aimed at correcting the presenting clinical manifestations. Refer to General Management of Acute Overdosage. Although no clinical experience has been reported, dialysis may be of benefit in reducing circulating concentrations of 5′-DFUR, a low-molecular weight metabolite of the parent compound.

Patient Information

Inform patients and patients' caregivers of the expected adverse effects of capecitabine, particularly nausea, vomiting, diarrhea, and hand-and-foot syndrome; patient-specific dose adaptations during therapy are expected and necessary (see Administration and Dosage). Encourage patients to recognize the common grade 2 toxicities associated with capecitabine treatment.

➤*Diarrhea:* Instruct patients experiencing grade 2 or greater diarrhea (an increase of 4 to 6 stools/day or nocturnal stools) to stop taking capecitabine immediately. Standard antidiarrheal treatments (eg, loperamide) are recommended.

➤*Nausea:* Instruct patients experiencing grade 2 or greater nausea (food intake significantly decreased but able to eat intermittently) to stop taking capecitabine immediately. Initiation of symptomatic treatment is recommended.

➤*Vomiting:* Instruct patients experiencing grade 2 or greater vomiting (2 to 5 episodes in a 24-hour period) to stop taking capecitabine immediately. Initiation of symptomatic treatment is recommended.

➤*Hand-and-foot syndrome:* Instruct patients experiencing grade 2 or greater hand-and-foot syndrome (painful erythema and swelling of the hands or feet or discomfort affecting the patients' activities of daily living) to stop taking capecitabine immediately.

➤*Stomatitis:* Instruct patients experiencing grade 2 or greater stomatitis (painful erythema, edema, or ulcers of the mouth or tongue, but able to eat) to stop taking capecitabine immediately. Initiation of symptomatic treatment is recommended (see Administration and Dosage).

➤*Fever and neutropenia:* Instruct patients who develop a fever of 100.5°F (38°C) or greater or other evidence of potential infection to call their physician.

CYTARABINE

WARNING

Conventional cytarabine: Only physicians experienced in chemotherapy should use cytarabine. For induction therapy, treat patients in a facility with laboratory and supportive resources sufficient to monitor drug tolerance, and protect and maintain a patient compromised by drug toxicity. The main toxic effect is bone marrow suppression with leukopenia, thrombocytopenia, and anemia. Less serious toxicity includes nausea, vomiting, diarrhea, abdominal pain, oral ulceration, and hepatic dysfunction. The physician must weigh possible benefit to the patient against known toxic effects of this drug in considering the advisability of cytarabine therapy.

Liposomal cytarabine: Administer liposomal cytarabine only under the supervision of a qualified physician experienced in the use of intrathecal cancer chemotherapeutic agents. Appropriate management of complications is possible only when adequate diagnostic and treatment facilities are readily available. In all clinical studies, chemical arachnoiditis, a syndrome manifested primarily by nausea, vomiting, headache, and fever was a common adverse event. If left untreated, chemical arachnoiditis may be fatal. The incidence and severity of chemical arachnoiditis can be reduced by coadministration of dexamethasone (see Warnings). Treat patients receiving liposomal cytarabine with dexamethasone to mitigate the symptoms of chemical arachnoiditis (see Administration and Dosage).

Indications

➤*Conventional cytarabine:* Induction and maintenance of remission in acute non–lymphocytic leukemia of adults and children. It has also been useful in the treatment of other leukemias, such as acute lymphocytic leukemia (ALL) and chronic myelocytic leukemia (blast phase).

Acute myelocytic leukemia (AML) – Response rates are higher in children than in adults with similar treatment schedules.

Acute lymphocytic leukemia (adults and children) – Cytarabine has been used alone or in combination for remission induction; however, combinations containing other antineoplastic agents are more effective.

Meningeal leukemia – Intrathecal administration is indicated in the prophylaxis and treatment of meningeal leukemia. Dosage schedule is usually governed by type and severity of CNS manifestations and response to previous therapy. Focal leukemic involvement of the CNS may not respond to intrathecal cytarabine and may be better treated with radiotherapy.

➤*Liposomal cytarabine:* For the intrathecal treatment of lymphomatous meningitis. This indication is based on demonstration of increased complete response rate compared to unencapsulated cytarabine. There are no controlled trials that demonstrate a clinical benefit resulting from this treatment, such as improvement in disease-related symptoms, increased time to disease progression, or increased survival.

Actions

➤*Pharmacology:* Cytarabine is available as conventional (cytosine arabinoside; ara-C) and liposomal formulations. Cytarabine exhibits cell-phase specificity, primarily killing cells undergoing deoxyribonucleic acid (DNA) synthesis (S-phase) and under certain conditions, blocking the progression of cells from the G_1-phase to the S-phase. Intracellularly, cytarabine is converted into cytarabine-5′-triphosphate (ara-CTP), which is the active metabolite. Although the mechanism of action is not completely understood, it appears that cytarabine inhibits DNA polymerase. Incorporation of cytarabine into DNA and ribonucleic acid (RNA) may also contribute to cytarabine cytotoxicity. Chromosomal damage has been produced, and malignant transformation of rodent cells in culture has been reported. Deoxycytidine prevents or delays (but does not reverse) the cytotoxic activity.

Cell culture studies have shown that cytarabine has an antiviral effect. However, efficacy against herpes zoster or smallpox could not be demonstrated in controlled clinical trials.

Cellular resistance and sensitivity – Cytarabine is metabolized by deoxycytidine kinase and other nucleotide kinases to the nucleotide triphosphate, an effective inhibitor of DNA polymerase; it is inactivated by a pyrimidine nucleoside deaminase, which converts it to the nontoxic uracil derivative. It appears that the balance of kinase and deaminase levels may be an important factor in determining sensitivity or resistance of the cell to cytarabine.

➤*Pharmacokinetics:* **Conventional cytarabine** is rapidly metabolized and is not effective orally. Less than 20% of the oral dose is absorbed form the GI tract. After SC or IM use, peak plasma levels are achieved in ≈ 20 to 60 minutes and are considerably lower than after IV use.

The pharmacokinetics of **liposomal cytarabine** administered intrathecally to patients at 50 mg every 2 weeks is currently under investigation. However, preliminary analysis of the pharmacokinetic data show that following liposomal cytarabine intrathecal administration in patients, in either the lumbar sac or by intraventricular reservoir, peak levels of free cytarabine were observed within 5 hours in the ventricle

and lumbar sac. These peak levels were followed by a biphasic elimination profile with a terminal phase half-life of 100 to 263 hours over a dose range of 12.5 mg to 75 mg.

Following rapid IV injection, the disappearance from plasma is biphasic; the distributive phase half-life is ≈ 10 minutes, and the elimination phase half-life is ≈ 1 to 3 hours. Cytarabine is eliminated by enzymatic deamination to nontoxic uracil arabinoside (ara-U). Within 24 hours, ≈ 80% of a dose is recovered in the urine, ≈ 90% of which is ara-U.

Relatively constant plasma levels can be achieved by continuous IV infusion.

Cerebrospinal fluid (CSF) levels of cytarabine are lower than plasma levels after single IV injection. However, in 1 patient in whom CSF levels were examined after 2 hours of constant IV infusion, levels approached 40% of the steady-state plasma level. With intrathecal administration of free cytarabine, CSF levels declined with a first-order half-life of ≈ 2 hours. Because CSF levels of deaminase are low, little conversion to ara-U was observed.

Immunosuppressive action – Cytarabine may obliterate immune responses with little or no accompanying toxicity. Suppression of antibody responses to E. coli-VI antigen and tetanus toxoid have been demonstrated. This suppression was obtained during primary and secondary antibody responses. Following 5 days of therapy, the immune response is suppressed as indicated by the following parameters: Macrophage ingress into skin windows; circulating antibody response following primary antigenic stimulation; lymphocyte blastogenesis with phytohemagglutinin. A few days after termination of therapy there was a rapid return to normal.

Cytarabine also suppresses cell-mediated immune responses such as delayed hypersensitivity skin reaction to dinitrochlorobenzene. However, it had no effect on already-established delayed hypersensitivity reactions.

Contraindications

Hypersensitivity to cytarabine; active meningeal infection (**liposomal cytarabine**).

Warnings

➤*Chemical arachnoiditis:* Administer **liposomal cytarabine** only under the supervision of a qualified physician experienced in the use of cancer chemotherapeutic agents. Appropriate management of complications is possible only when adequate diagnostic and treatment facilities are readily available. Chemical arachnoiditis, a syndrome manifested primarily by nausea, vomiting, headache, and fever, has been a common adverse event in all studies. If left untreated, chemical arachnoiditis may be fatal. The incidence and severity of chemical arachnoiditis can be reduced by coadministration of dexamethasone. Treat patients receiving liposomal cytarabine concurrently with dexamethasone to mitigate the symptoms of chemical arachnoiditis (see Administration and Dosage).

➤*Death:* During clinical studies, 2 deaths related to **liposomal cytarabine** were reported. One patient died after developing encephalopathy 36 hours after an intraventricular dose of 125 mg. This patient was receiving concurrent whole-brain irradiation and had previously received systemic chemotherapy with cyclophosphamide, doxorubicin, and fluorouracil, as well as intraventricular methotrexate. The other patient received liposomal cytarabine 50 mg by the intraventricular route and developed focal seizures progressing to status epilepticus. This patient died ≈ 8 weeks after the last dose of study medication. The death of 1 additional patient was considered "possibly" related to liposomal cytarabine. He was 63 years of age with extensive lymphoma involving the nasopharynx, brain, and meninges with multiple neurologic deficits and died of apparent disease progression 4 days after his second dose of liposomal cytarabine.

➤*Neurotoxicity:* Blockage to CSF flow may result in increased free cytarabine concentations in the CSF and an increased risk of neurotoxicity. Enhanced neurotoxicity has been associated with concurrent use of intrathecal cytarabine and other cytotoxic agents administered intrathecally.

➤*Myelosuppression/Hematologic:* Because cytarabine is a bone marrow suppressant, anemia, leukopenia, thrombocytopenia, megaloblastosis, and reduced reticulocytes can be expected. The severity of these reactions is dose- and schedule-dependent. Expect cellular changes in the morphology of bone marrow and peripheral smears. Start therapy cautiously in patients with preexisting drug-induced bone marrow suppression. Keep patients under close medical supervision and, during induction therapy, perform leukocyte and platelet counts daily. Perform bone marrow examinations frequently after blasts have disappeared from the peripheral blood. Have facilities available for management of bone marrow suppression complications, possibly fatal (infection resulting from granulocytopenia and other impaired body defenses, and hemorrhage secondary to thrombocytopenia).

Following a 5-day constant infusion or acute injections of 50 to 600 mg/m^2, white cell depression follows a biphasic course. Regardless of initial count, dosage level or schedule, there is an initial fall starting the first 24 hours with a nadir at days 7 to 9. A brief rise follows, which peaks

CYTARABINE

around day 12. A second and deeper fall reaches nadir at days 15 to 24, then there is rapid rise to above baseline in the next 10 days. Platelet depression is noticeable at 5 days with a peak depression occurring between days 12 to 15. A rapid rise to above baseline occurs in the next 10 days.

Although significant systemic exposure to free cytarabine following intrathecal treatment is not expected, some effect on bone marrow function cannot be excluded. Accordingly, careful monitoring of the hematopoietic system is advised.

➤*Experimental doses:* Severe and sometimes fatal CNS, GI, and pulmonary toxicity (different from that seen with conventional cytarabine regimens) have occurred. These reactions include reversible corneal toxicity and hemorrhagic conjunctivitis, which may be prevented or diminished by prophylaxis with local corticosteroid eye drops; cerebral and cerebellar dysfunction including personality changes, dysarthria, ataxia, confusion, somnolence, and coma, usually reversible; severe GI ulceration, including pneumatosis cystoides intestinalis leading to peritonitis; sepsis and liver abscess; pulmonary edema; liver damage with increased hyperbilirubinemia; bowel necrosis; and necrotizing colitis. Rarely, severe skin rash leading to desquamation may occur. Complete alopecia is more common with experimental high-dose therapy than with standard cytarabine treatment programs. If experimental high-dose therapy is used, do not use a diluent containing benzyl alcohol.

Cardiomyopathy with subsequent death has occurred following experimental high-dose therapy with cytarabine in combination with cyclophosphamide when used for bone marrow transplant preparation.

A syndrome of sudden respiratory distress, rapidly progressing to pulmonary edema and radiographically pronounced cardiomegaly, has been reported following experimental high-dose therapy with cytarabine used for the treatment of relapsed leukemia from 1 institution in 16 of 72 patients. The outcome of this syndrome can be fatal.

Ten patients treated with experimental intermediate doses of cytarabine (1 g/m^2) with and without other chemotherapeutic agents (meta-AMSA, daunorubicin, etoposide) at various dose regimens developed a diffuse interstitial pneumonitis without clear cause that it may be related to cytarabine.

➤*Benzyl alcohol:* Benzyl alcohol is contained in the diluent for some **conventional cytarabine** products. Benzyl alcohol has been reported to be associated with a fatal "gasping syndrome" in premature infants. Do not use conventional cytarabine injection with benzyl alcohol intrathecally.

➤*Hypersensitivity reactions:* Cases of anaphylaxis have occurred resulting in acute cardiopulmonary arrest which required resuscitation. This occurred immediately after IV administration. Anaphylactic reactions following IV administration of free cytarabine have been reported. Refer to Management of Acute Hypersensitivity Reactions.

➤*Renal/Hepatic function impairment:* The liver detoxifies much of an administered dose. In particular, patients with renal or hepatic function impairment may have a higher likelihood of CNS toxicity after high-dose cytarabine. Use the drug with caution and possibly at reduced doses in patients with poor liver or kidney function.

➤*Pregnancy:* Category D. Cytarabine can cause fetal harm when administered to a pregnant woman. There are no adequate and well-controlled studies in pregnant women. If cytarabine is used during pregnancy, or if the patient becomes pregnant while taking cytarabine, apprise the patient of the potential risk to the fetus. Advise women of childbearing potential to avoid becoming pregnant.

The potential for abnormalities exists, particularly during the first trimester. Inform patient of potential risk to the fetus and advisability of pregnancy continuation. There is a lesser risk if therapy is initiated during the second or third trimester. Healthy infants have been delivered to patients treated in all 3 trimesters of pregnancy; however, follow-up of such infants is advisable.

In 32 reported cases where cytarabine was given during pregnancy, either alone or in combination with other cytotoxic agents, 18 healthy infants were delivered. Four infants had first trimester exposure, and 5 were premature or of low birth weight. Twelve of the 18 healthy infants were followed up at ages ranging from 6 weeks to 7 years, and showed no abnormalities. One apparently healthy infant died of gastroenteritis at 90 days. Two cases of congenital abnormalities have been reported, one with upper and lower distal limb defects and the other with extremity and ear deformities. Both of these cases had first trimester exposure.

There were 7 infants with various problems in the neonatal period, which included: Pancytopenia; transient depression of WBC, hematocrit, or platelets; electrolyte abnormalities; transient eosinophilia; increased IgM levels and hyperpyrexia possibly due to sepsis (1 case). Six of the 7 infants were also premature. The child with pancytopenia died of sepsis at 21 days.

Therapeutic abortions were done in 5 cases. Four fetuses were grossly normal, but one had an enlarged spleen and another showed Trisomy C chromosomal abnormality in the chorionic tissue. The concern for fetal

harm following intrathecal liposomal cytarabine administration is low because systemic exposure to cytarabine is negligible.

➤*Lactation:* It is not known whether this drug is excreted in breast milk. Because of the potential for serious adverse reactions in nursing infants from cytarabine, decide whether to discontinue nursing or discontinue the drug, taking into account the importance of the drug to the mother.

➤*Children:* Safety and efficacy of **liposomal cytarabine** in pediatric patients have not been established. **Conventional cytarabine** is indicated for use in children.

Precautions

➤*Monitoring:* Monitor patients closely. Frequent platelet and leukocyte counts and bone marrow examinations are mandatory. Suspend or modify therapy when drug-induced marrow depression results in a platelet count < $50,000/\text{mm}^3$ or a polymorphonuclear granulocyte count < $1000/\text{mm}^3$. Counts of formed elements in the peripheral blood may continue to fall after the drug is stopped and reach lowest values after drug-free intervals of 12 to 24 days. Restart therapy when definite signs of marrow recovery appear (on successive bone marrow studies). Patients whose drug is withheld until "normal" peripheral blood values are attained may escape from control.

Perform periodic checks of bone marrow, liver, and kidney functions.

➤*Rapid administration:* When large IV doses are given rapidly, patients are frequently nauseated and may vomit for several hours postinjection. This tends to be less severe when the drug is infused.

➤*Toxicity:* **Liposomal cytarabine** may produce serious toxicity (see boxed Warning). Treat all patients receiving liposomal cytarabine concurrently with dexamethasone to mitigate the symptoms of chemical arachnoiditis (see Administration and Dosage). Toxic effects may be related to a single dose or to cumulative administration. Because toxic effects can occur at any time during therapy (although they are most likely within 5 days of drug administration), monitor patients receiving intrathecal therapy with liposomal cytarabine continuously for the development of neurotoxicity. If patients develop neurotoxicity, reduce subsequent doses of liposomal cytarabine, and discontinue if toxicity persists.

When cytarabine is administered both intrathecally and IV within a few days, there is an increased risk of spinal cord toxicity; however, in serious life-threatening disease, concurrent use of IV and intrathecal cytarabine is left to the discretion of the treating physician.

➤*Neoplastic meningitis:* Some patients with neoplastic meningitis receiving treatment with **liposomal cytarabine** may require concurrent radiation or systemic therapy with other chemotherapeutic agents; this may increase the rate of adverse events.

➤*CSF elevations:* Transient elevations in CSF protein and white blood cells have been observed in patients following **liposomal cytarabine** administration and have also been noted after intrathecal treatment with methotrexate or cytarabine.

➤*Hyperuricemia:* Hyperuricemia may be induced because of rapid lysis of neoplastic cells. Monitor patient's blood uric acid level; use supportive and pharmacologic measures as necessary.

➤*Acute pancreatitis:* Acute pancreatitis has occurred in a patient receiving cytarabine by continuous infusion and in patients being treated with cytarabine who have had prior treatment with L-asparaginase. There is evidence that this may be schedule-dependent.

Two other cases of pancreatitis have occurred following experimental doses of cytarabine and numerous other drugs. Cytarabine could have been the causative agent.

➤*Peripheral motor and sensory neuropathies:* Peripheral motor and sensory neuropathies have occurred in 2 patients with adult acute non-lymphocytic leukemia after consolidation with high-dose cytarabine, daunorubicin, and asparaginase. Observe patients on high-dose cytarabine for neuropathy because dose schedule alterations may be needed to avoid irreversible neurologic disorders.

➤*Intrathecal use:* Intrathecal cytarabine may cause systemic toxicity; carefully monitor the hematopoietic system. Modification of other antileukemia therapy may be necessary. Major toxicity is rare. The most frequent reactions after intrathecal administration are nausea, vomiting, and fever; these reactions are mild and self-limiting. Paraplegia and neurotoxicity have occurred. Necrotizing leukoencephalopathy occurred in 5 children who had also been treated with intrathecal methotrexate and hydrocortisone and CNS radiation. Blindness occurred in 2 patients in remission whose treatment had consisted of combination systemic chemotherapy, prophylactic CNS radiation, and intrathecal cytarabine. Focal leukemic involvement of the CNS may not respond to intrathecal cytarabine and may be better treated with radiotherapy.

Intrathecal administration of free cytarabine may cause myelopathy and other neurologic toxicity and can rarely lead to a permanent neurologic deficit. Administration of intrathecal cytarabine in combination with other chemotherapeutic agents or with cranial/spinal irradiation may increase this risk of neurotoxicity.

CYTARABINE

If used intrathecally, do not use a diluent with benzyl alcohol. Two patients with childhood acute myelogenous leukemia who received intrathecal and IV cytarabine at conventional doses (in addition to a number of other coadministered drugs) developed delayed progressive ascending paralysis resulting in death in 1 patient.

➤*Infection:* Viral, bacterial, fungal, parasitic, or saprophytic infections in any location in the body may be associated with the use of cytarabrine alone or in combination with other immunosuppressive agents following immunosuppressant doses that affect cellular or humoral immunity. These infections may be mild, but can be severe and sometimes fatal.

Drug Interactions

Cytarabine Drug Interactions			
Precipitant drug	Object drug*		Description
Cytarabine	Digoxin	↓	Combination chemotherapy (including cytarabine) may decrease digoxin absorption even several days after stopping chemotherapy. Digoxin capsules and digitoxin do not appear to be affected.
Cytarabine	Gentamicin	↓	An in vitro interaction between gentamicin and cytarabine showed a cytarabine-related antagonism for the susceptibility of K. pneumoniae strains. This study suggests that in patients on cytarabine being treated with gentamicin for a K. pneumoniae infection, the lack of a prompt therapeutic response may indicate the need for reevaluation of antibacterial therapy.

* ↓ = Object drug decreased.

➤*Drug/Lab test interactions:* Because **liposomal cytarabine**particles are similar in size and appearance to white blood cells, take care in interpreting CSF examinations following liposomal cytarabine administration.

Adverse Reactions

➤*Conventional cytarabine:*
Cytarabine (ara-C) syndrome: A cytarabine syndrome characterized by fever, myalgia, bone pain, occasional chest pain, maculopapular rash, conjunctivitis, and malaise has been described. It usually occurs 6 to 12 hours following drug administration. Corticosteroids have been beneficial in treating or preventing this syndrome. If the symptoms are treatable, consider use of corticosteroids as well as continuation of cytarabine therapy.

Most frequent: Anorexia; nausea and vomiting (following rapid IV injection); diarrhea; oral and anal inflammation or ulceration; hepatic dysfunction; fever; rash; thrombophlebitis; bleeding (all sites).

Less frequent: Sepsis; pneumonia; cellulitis at injection site; skin ulceration; urinary retention; renal dysfunction; neuritis or neural toxicity; sore throat; esophageal ulceration; esophagitis; chest pain; pericarditis; bowel necrosis; abdominal pain; pancreatitis; freckling; jaundice; conjunctivitis (may occur with rash); dizziness; alopecia; anaphylaxis (see Warnings); allergic edema; pruritus; shortness of breath; urticaria; headache.

Experimental doses – Severe and sometimes fatal CNS, GI, and pulmonary toxicity (different from that seen with conventional therapy regimens of cytarabine) have occurred. Cardiomyopathy and a syndrome of sudden respiratory distress are other possibly fatal reactions to experimental doses of cytarabine (see Warnings).

➤*Liposomal cytarabine:* Arachnoiditis is an expected and well-documented side effect of neoplastic meningitis and intrathecal chemotherapy (see Warnings). For clinical studies of liposomal cytarabine, chemical arachnoiditis was defined as the occurrence of any 1 of the symptoms of neck rigidity, neck pain, meningism, or any 2 of the symptoms of nausea, vomiting, headache, fever, back pain, or CSF pleocytosis; the grade assigned to an episode of chemical arachnoiditis was the highest severity grade of its component symptoms. Because most of the adverse events reported in the trials were transient episodes associated with drug exposure, the incidence of these events is best expressed by drug cycle. A cycle of treatment for all treatment groups was defined as the 14-day period between liposomal cytarabine doses. The duration of

reported symptoms was from 1 to 5 days. Although it was sometimes difficult to distinguish between drug-related chemical arachnoiditis, infectious meningitis, or disease progression, > 90% of the chemical arachnoiditis cases reported occurred within 48 hours of the administration of intrathecal drug, indicating a drug etiology.

In the early study, chemical arachnoiditis was observed in 100% of cycles without dexamethasone prophylaxis; with concurrent administration of dexamethasone, chemical arachnoiditis was observed in 33% of cycles. Treat patients receiving cytarabine concurrently with dexamethasone to mitigate the symptoms of chemical arachnoiditis.

Comparison of Cytarabine (Liposomal vs Conventional) Adverse Reactions (≥ 10%)[1]				
	All adverse events		Grade 3 or 4 adverse events	
Adverse reaction	Liposomal (n = 74)[2]	Conventional (n = 45)[2]	Liposomal (n = 74)[2]	Conventional (n = 45)[2]
CNS				
Abnormal gait	4	11	1	2
Confusion	14	7	4	2
Somnolence	12	11	4	2
GI				
Constipation	7	11	0	0
Nausea[3]	11	16	0	4
Vomiting[3]	12	18	3	2
Hematologic				
Anemia	1	13	1	4
Neutropenia	9	11	8	11
Thrombocytopenia	8	16	5	11
Miscellaneous	53	60	18	22
Asthenia	19	33	5	9
Back pain[3]	7	11	0	2
Fever[3]	11	24	4	0
Headache[3]	28	9	5	2
Pain	11	20	3	0
Peripheral edema	7	11	0	0
Special senses	16	18	1	2
Urinary incontinence	3	11	0	0

[1] Patients with lymphomatous meningitis receiving liposomal or conventional cytarabine in the randomized study, by cycle.
[2] Number of cycles.
[3] Components of chemical arachnoiditis.

Overdosage

➤*Conventional cytarabine:* There is no antidote for cytarabine overdosage. Doses of 4.5 g/m^2 by IV infusion over 1 hour every 12 hours for 12 doses has caused an unacceptable increase in irreversible CNS toxicity and death.

Single doses as high as 3 g/m^2 have been administered by rapid IV infusion without apparent toxicity.

➤*Liposomal cytarabine:* No overdosages with liposomal cytarabine have been reported. An overdose with liposomal cytarabine may be associated with severe chemical arachnoiditis including encephalopathy.

In an early uncontrolled study without dexamethasone prophylaxis, single doses up to 125 mg were administered. One patient at the 125 mg dose level died of encephalopathy 36 hours after receiving an intraventricular dose of liposomal cytarabine (see Warnings). This patient, however, was also receiving concomitant whole brain irradiation and had previously received intraventricular methotrexate.

There is no antidote for overdose of intrathecal liposomal cytarabine or unencapsulated cytarabine released from liposomal cytarabine. Exchange of CSF with isotonic saline has been carried out in a case of intrathecal overdose of free cytarabine, and such a procedure may be considered in the case of liposomal cytarabine overdose. Direct management of overdose at maintaining vital functions.

Patient Information

Inform patients about the expected adverse events of headache, nausea, vomiting, and fever, and about the early signs and symptoms of neurotoxicity. Emphasize the importance of concurrent dexamethasone administration at the initiation of each cycle of **liposomal cytarabine**treatment. Instruct patients to seek medical attention if signs or symptoms of neurotoxicity develop, or if oral dexamethasone is not well tolerated.

CYTARABINE, CONVENTIONAL

Rx	**Tarabine PFS** (Adria)	**Injection:** 20 mg/ml	Preservative free. In 5 ml single vials and 50 ml bulk package vials.
Rx	**Cytarabine** (Mayne)		In 5 ml single- and multi-[1] dose vials and preservative free 50 ml flip-top vial (pharmacy bulk package).
Rx	**Cytarabine** (Various, eg, Bedford, Gensia)	**Powder for Injection:** 100 mg	In vials.
Rx	**Cytosar-U** (Gensia Sicor)		In multidose vials.
Rx	**Cytarabine** (Various, eg, Gensia)	**Powder for Injection:** 500 mg	In vials.
Rx	**Cytosar-U** (Gensia Sicor)		In multidose vials.
Rx	**Cytarabine** (Various, eg, Bedford, Gensia)	**Powder for Injection:** 1 g	In vials.
Rx	**Cytosar-U** (Gensia Sicor)		In multidose vials.
Rx	**Cytarabine** (Various, eg, Gensia)	**Powder for Injection:** 2 g	In vials.
Rx	**Cytosar-U** (Gensia Sicor)		In multidose vials.

[1] With 0.9% benzyl alcohol.

For complete prescribing information, refer to the Cytarabine group monograph.

Indications

➤*Conventional cytarabine:* Induction and maintenance of remission in acute non–lymphocytic leukemia of adults and children. It has also been useful in the treatment of other leukemias, such as acute lymphocytic leukemia (ALL) and chronic myelocytic leukemia (blast phase).

Acute myelocytic leukemia (AML) – Response rates are higher in children than in adults with similar treatment schedules.

Acute lymphocytic leukemia (adults and children) – Cytarabine has been used alone or in combination for remission induction; however, combinations containing other antineoplastic agents are more effective.

Meningeal leukemia – Intrathecal administration is indicated in the prophylaxis and treatment of meningeal leukemia. Dosage schedule is usually governed by type and severity of CNS manifestations and response to previous therapy. Focal leukemic involvement of the CNS may not respond to intrathecal cytarabine and may be better treated with radiotherapy.

Administration and Dosage

➤*Conventional cytarabine:* Cytarabine is not active orally; give SC or intrathecally or by IV infusion or injection. The purpose of the pharmacy bulk package is for the preparation of IV infusions. Thrombophlebitis has occurred at the injection or infusion site and, rarely, pain and inflammation occur at SC injection sites. The drug is generally well tolerated.

Patients can tolerate higher total doses when the drug is given by rapid IV injection as compared with slow infusion because of the drug's rapid inactivation and brief exposure of susceptible normal and neoplastic cells to significant levels after rapid injection. There is no distinct clinical advantage demonstrated for either.

Acute non-lymphocytic leukemia – In combination with other anticancer drugs, give 100 mg/m^2/day by continuous IV infusion (days 1 to 7) or 100 mg/m^2 IV every 12 hours (days 1 to 7).

Acute lymphocytic leukemia – Consult the literature for current recommendations.

Refractory acute leukemia – High-dose cytarabine 3 g/m^2 IV over 2 hours every 12 hours for 4 to 12 doses (repeated at 2- to 3-week intervals) has been used. Remission rates in 1 study were similar for patients with AML and ALL. Therapies using 4 to 6 doses every

2 weeks or 9 doses every 3 weeks appear equally effective and less toxic.

Meningeal leukemia (intrathecal use) – Dosage schedule is usually governed by type and severity of CNS manifestations and response to previous therapy.

Doses range from 5 to 75 mg/m^2 once daily for 4 days to once every 4 days. The most common dose is 30 mg/m^2 every 4 days until CSF findings are normal, followed by 1 additional treatment.

Do not use cytarabine injection that contains benzyl alcohol intrathecally.

Preparation of solutions –

	Preparation of Cytarabine Solutions	
Vial size	Amount of Bacteriostatic Water 0.9% to be added	Resultant solution
100 mg	5 ml	20 mg/ml
500 mg	10 ml	50 mg/ml
1 g	10 ml	100 mg/ml
2 g	20 ml	100 mg/ml

If used intrathecally, do not use a diluent containing benzyl alcohol. Reconstitute with autologous spinal fluid or preservative-free 0.9% Sodium Chloride for Injection; use immediately. The pharmacy bulk package is not intended to be used for the preparation of intrathecal doses.

When cytarabine is administered both intrathecally and IV within a few days, there is an increased risk of spinal cord toxicity; however, in serious life-threatening disease, concurrent use of IV and intrathecal cytarabine is left to the discretion of the treating physician.

Many investigators prefer to use a special diluent for intrathecal use that is physiologically similar to spinal fluid (Elliott's B Solution).

➤*Storage / Stability:*

Conventional cytarabine – Store reconstituted solutions at controlled room temperature 15° to 30°C (59° to 86°F) for 48 hours. Discard if a slight haze develops. When repackaged in glass or plastic, maximum stability appears to be provided by glass stored at 5°C (41°F); however, storage of cytarabine in plastic disposable syringes stored at 5°C is an acceptable alternative.

Chemical stability in infusion solutions: When the reconstituted cytarabine was added to Sterile Water for Injection, 5% Dextrose Injection, or Sodium Chloride Injection, 93% to 99% of the cytarabine was present after 192 hours of storage at room temperature.

CYTARABINE, LIPOSOMAL

Rx	**DepoCyt** (Enzon)	**Injection:** 10 mg/ml (liposomal)[1]	Preservative free. In 5 ml vials.

[1] In Sodium Chloride 0.9% w/v in Water for Injection.

For complete prescribing information, refer to the Cytarabine group monograph.

Indications

➤*Liposomal cytarabine:* For the intrathecal treatment of lymphomatous meningitis. This indication is based on demonstration of increased complete response rate compared to unencapsulated cytarabine. There are no controlled trials that demonstrate a clinical benefit resulting from this treatment, such as improvement in disease-related symptoms, increased time to disease progression, or increased survival.

Administration and Dosage

➤*Liposomal cytarabine:*

Preparation – Liposomal cytarabine is a cytotoxic anticancer drug; as with other potentially toxic compounds, use caution in handling the drug. The use of gloves is recommended. If liposomal cytarabine suspension contacts the skin, wash immediately with soap and water. If it contacts mucous membranes, flush thoroughly with water. Liposomal cytarabine particles are more dense than the diluent and have a tendency to settle with time. Allow vials of liposomal cytarabine to warm to room temperature and gently agitate or invert the vials to resuspend the particles immediately prior to withdrawal from the vial. Avoid aggressive agitation. No further reconstitution or dilution is required.

Administration – Withdraw liposomal cytarabine from the vial immediately before administration. Liposomal cytarabine is a single-use vial and does not contain any preservative; use within 4 hours of withdrawal from the vial. Discard unused portions of each vial properly. Do not save any unused portions for later administration. Do not mix liposomal cytarabine with any other medications.

Do not use in-line filters when administering liposomal cytarabine. Liposomal cytarabine is administered directly into the CSF via an intraventricular reservoir or by direct injection into the lumbar sac. Inject slowly over a period of 1 to 5 minutes. Following drug administration by lumbar puncture, instruct the patient to lie flat for 1 hour. Observe patients for immediate toxic reactions.

Start patients on dexamethasone 4 mg twice a day either PO or IV for 5 days beginning on the day of liposomal cytarabine injection.

Administer only by the intrathecal route.

Further dilution is not recommended.

Dosing regimen – For the treatment of lymphomatous meningitis, 50 mg is recommended to be given according to the following schedule:

Induction therapy: 50 mg administered intrathecally (intraventricular or lumbar puncture) every 14 days for 2 doses (weeks 1 and 3).

Consolidation therapy: 50 mg administered intrathecally (intraventricular or lumbar puncture) every 14 days for 3 doses (weeks 5, 7, and

CYTARABINE, LIPOSOMAL

9) followed by 1 additional dose at week 13.

Maintenance: 50 mg administered intrathecally (intraventricular or lumbar puncture) every 28 days for 4 doses (weeks 17, 21, 25, and 29).

If drug-related neurotoxicity develops, reduce the dose to 25 mg. If it persists, discontinue treatment.

FLUOROURACIL AND FLOXURIDINE

Indications

See individual product listings.

Actions

➤*Pharmacology:* There is evidence that the metabolism of fluorouracil in the anabolic pathway blocks the methylation reaction of deoxyuridylic acid to thymidylic acid. In this manner, fluorouracil interferes with the synthesis of deoxyribonucleic acid (DNA) and to a lesser extent inhibits the formation of ribonucleic acid (RNA). Since DNA and RNA are essential for cell division and growth, the effect of fluorouracil may be to create a thymine deficiency provoking unbalanced growth and death of the cell. DNA and RNA deprivation most affect those cells that grow rapidly and take up fluorouracil at a more rapid pace.

➤*Pharmacokinetics:* Following IV injection, fluorouracil distributes into tumors, intestinal mucosa, bone marrow, liver, and other body tissues. In spite of its limited lipid solubility, fluorouracil diffuses readily across the blood-brain barrier and distributes into CSF and brain tissue.

The parent drug is excreted unchanged (7% to 20%) in the urine in 6 hours; of this, > 90% is excreted in the first hour. The remaining percentage is metabolized, primarily in the liver. The catabolic metabolism of fluorouracil results in inactive degradation products (eg, CO_2, urea, α-fluoro-β-alanine). The inactive metabolites are excreted in the urine over the next 3 to 4 hours. Approximately 90% is excreted in expired CO_2. Following IV use, 90% of the dose is accounted for during the first 24 hours; the mean half-life of elimination from plasma is $\approx$ 16 minutes (range, 8 to 20 minutes) and is dose-dependent. No intact drug can be detected in the plasma 3 hours after an IV injection.

Floxuridine is rapidly catabolized to 5-fluorouracil. Thus, the same toxic and antimetabolic effects as 5-fluorouracil occur.

Contraindications

Poor nutritional status; depressed bone marrow function; potentially serious infections; hypersensitivity to fluorouracil.

Warnings

Hospitalize patients during initial course because of possible severe toxic reactions.

Use with extreme caution in poor-risk patients who have had high-dose pelvic irradiation or previous use of alkylating agents, who have widespread involvement of bone marrow by metastatic tumors, or impaired hepatic or renal function. These drugs are not intended as adjuvants to surgery.

➤*Combination therapy:* Any form of therapy which adds to the stress of the patient, interferes with nutrition or depresses bone marrow function will increase toxicity.

➤*Mutagenesis:* A positive effect was observed in the micronucleus test on bone marrow cells of the mouse, and fluorouracil at very high concentrations produced chromosomal breaks in hamster fibroblasts in vitro.

➤*Fertility impairment:* Intraperitoneal doses of 125 or 250 mg/kg induce chromosomal aberrations and changes in chromosomal organization of spermatogonia in rats. Spermatogonial differentiation was also inhibited by fluorouracil, resulting in transient infertility. In female rats, intraperitoneal fluorouracil 25 or 50 mg/kg/week for 3 weeks during the pre-ovulatory phase of oogenesis, significantly reduced the incidence of fertile matings, delayed pre- and postimplantation embryo development, increased preimplantation lethality incidence, and induced chromosomal anomalies in these embryos.

➤*Pregnancy: Category D* (fluorouracil). Fluorouracil crosses the placenta and enters into fetal circulation in the rat, resulting in increased resorptions and embryolethality. In monkeys, maternal doses > 40 mg/kg resulted in abortion of all embryos exposed to fluorouracil. Compounds which inhibit DNA, RNA, and protein synthesis might be expected to have adverse effects on peri- and postnatal development.

Fluorouracil may cause fetal harm when administered to a pregnant woman; it is teratogenic and mutagenic in laboratory animals. Malformations included cleft palates, skeletal defects, and deformed appendages, paws, and tails. Teratogenic dosages in animals are 1 to 3 times the maximum recommended human therapeutic dose. There are no adequate and well controlled studies in pregnant women. Advise women of childbearing potential to avoid pregnancy. If the drug is used during pregnancy, or if the patient becomes pregnant while taking the drug, tell her of the potential hazard to the fetus. Do not use during pregnancy (particularly in the first trimester) unless the potential benefit justifies the potential risk to the fetus.

➤*Storage/Stability:*

Liposomal cytarabine – Refrigerate at 2° to 8°C (36° to 46°F). Protect from freezing, and avoid aggressive agitation.

➤*Lactation:* It is not known whether fluorouracil is excreted in breast milk. Because fluorouracil inhibits DNA, RNA and protein synthesis, do not nurse while using it.

➤*Children:* Safety and efficacy of fluorouracil in children have not been established.

Precautions

Discontinue if signs of toxicity occur: Stomatitis or esophagopharyngitis (at first visible sign); rapidly falling WBC count; leukopenia (WBC < 3500/mm³); intractable vomiting; diarrhea or frequent bowel movements; GI ulceration and bleeding; thrombocytopenia (platelets < 100,000/mm³); hemorrhage.

These are highly toxic drugs with a narrow margin of safety. Therapeutic response is unlikely to occur without some toxicity. Inform patients of toxic effects, particularly oral manifestations. Measure WBC count with differential before each dose. Severe hematological toxicity, GI hemorrhage and death may result, despite meticulous patient selection and dosage adjustment. Although severe toxicity and fatalities are more likely in poor-risk patients, these effects may occur in patients in relatively good condition.

➤*Angina:* Coronary vasospasm with episodes of angina may occur in patients receiving fluorouracil. The angina appears to occur $\approx$ 6 hours (range, minutes to 7 days) after the third dose (range, 1 to 13 doses). Patients with preexisting coronary artery disease may be at increased risk. Nitrates or morphine appear effective in relieving the pain; pretreatment with a calcium channel blocker may also be successful.

Drug Interactions

➤*Leucovorin calcium:* Leucovorin calcium may enhance the toxicity of fluorouracil.

➤*Drug/Lab test interactions:* Elevations in **alkaline phosphatase, serum transaminase, serum bilirubin** and **lactic dehydrogenase** may occur.

Adverse Reactions

➤*Cardiovascular:* Myocardial ischemia; angina (see Precautions).

➤*CNS:* Lethargy, malaise, weakness, acute cerebellar syndrome (may persist following discontinuation of treatment); headache.

➤*Dermatologic:* Alopecia; dermatitis, often as a pruritic maculopapular rash on the extremities or trunk (usually reversible and responsive to symptomatic treatment); nonspecific skin toxicity; photosensitivity as manifested by erythema or increased skin pigmentation; nail changes including loss of nails; dry skin; fissuring; vein pigmentation.

➤*GI:* Stomatitis and esophagopharyngitis (which may lead to sloughing and ulceration), diarrhea, anorexia, nausea, vomiting, enteritis (common); cramps; duodenal ulcer; watery stools; duodenitis; gastritis; glossitis; pharyngitis; possible intra- and extrahepatic biliary sclerosis; acalculus cholecystitis; GI ulceration; bleeding.

➤*Hematologic:* Leukopenia; thrombocytopenia; pancytopenia; agranulocytosis; anemia; thrombophlebitis. Low WBC counts are usually observed between days 9 and 14 after the first course of treatment. The count usually normalizes by day 30.

➤*Hypersensitivity:* Anaphylaxis; generalized allergic reactions.

➤*Lab test abnormalities:* BSP; prothrombin; total proteins; sedimentation rate; thrombocytopenia.

➤*Ophthalmic:* Photophobia; lacrimation; decreased vision; nystagmus; diplopia; lacrimal duct stenosis; visual changes.

➤*Psychiatric:* Disorientation; confusion; euphoria.

➤*Miscellaneous:* Fever; epistaxis.

Regional arterial infusion complications – Arterial aneurysm; arterial ischemia; arterial thrombosis; bleeding at catheter site; catheter blocked, displaced or leaking; embolism; fibromyositis; abscesses; infection at catheter site; thrombophlebitis.

Overdosage

The possibility of overdosage with fluorouracil is unlikely in view of the mode of administration. Nevertheless, the anticipated manifestations would be nausea, vomiting, diarrhea, GI ulceration and bleeding, bone marrow depression (including thrombocytopenia, leukopenia and agranulocytosis). No specific antidotal therapy exists. Patients who have been exposed to an overdose of fluorouracil should be monitored hematologically for at least 4 weeks. Should abnormalities appear, utilize appropriate therapy.

FLUOROURACIL AND FLOXURIDINE

Patient Information

Transient alopecia may occur with fluorouracil; alert the patient to this possibility.

Contraceptive measures are recommended for men and women during therapy.

Notify doctor if chills, nausea, vomiting, unusual bleeding or bruising, yellowing of skin or eyes, abdominal pain, flank or joint pain, or swelling of feet or legs occurs.

May cause diarrhea, fever and weakness. Notify doctor if these become pronounced.

Drink plenty of liquids while taking this drug.

FLUOROURACIL (5-Fluorouracil; 5-FU)

Rx	Fluorouracil (Various, eg, American Pharmaceutical Partners)	Injection: 50 mg/ml	In 10, 20, and 100 ml vials and 10 ml amps.
Rx	Adrucil (Gensia Sicor)		In 10, 50, and 100 ml vials.

For complete prescribing information, refer to the Fluorouracil and Floxuridine group monograph.

Indications

Palliative management of colon, rectum, breast, stomach, and pancreas carcinoma.

Also used in combination with levamisole (see individual monograph) after surgical resection in patients with Dukes' stage C colon cancer.

In patients with metastatic colorectal carcinoma, IV leucovorin 200 mg/m^2/day for 5 days followed by fluorouracil 370 mg/m^2/day for 5 days and repeated every 28 days significantly increased response rate, decreased time to disease progression, and prolonged overall survival compared with fluorouracil alone.

Administration and Dosage

Give IV; avoid extravasation. No dilution required. Individualize dosage based on actual weight. Use lean body weight (dry weight) if patient is obese or has had spurious weight gain due to edema, ascites, or other abnormal fluid retention.

Although not FDA approved, fluorouracil has been administered orally in < 5% of patients when more acceptable methods are not possible. Absorption is erratic, and plasma concentrations are variable. If given orally, mix with water only.

➤*Initial dosage:* 12 mg/kg IV once daily for 4 days. Do not exceed 800 mg/day. If no toxicity is observed, give 6 mg/kg on days 6, 8, 10, and 12. No therapy is given on days 5, 7, 9, or 11. Discontinue at end of day 12, even with no apparent toxicity.

Poor-risk patients or those not in an adequate nutritional state receive 6 mg/kg/day for 3 days. If no toxicity is observed, give 3 mg/kg on days 5, 7, and 9. Give no therapy on days 4, 6, or 8. Do not exceed 400 mg/day.

A sequence of injections on either schedule constitutes a "course of therapy."

Discontinue therapy promptly when any signs of toxicity appear.

➤*Maintenance therapy:* Where toxicity has not been a problem, continue therapy using either of the following schedules: (1) Repeat dosage of first course every 30 days after last day of previous course; (2) when toxic signs from the initial course of therapy have subsided, administer a maintenance dose of 10 to 15 mg/kg/week as a single dose. Do not exceed 1 g/week. Use reduced doses for poor-risk patients. Consider the patient's reaction to the previous course, and adjust dosage accordingly. Some patients have received from 9 to 45 courses over 12 to 60 months.

➤*Storage/Stability:* Solution may discolor during storage; potency and safety are not adversely affected. Store at room temperature (15° to 30°C [59° to 86°F]) and protect from light. If precipitate forms due to exposure to low temperatures, heat to 60°C (140°F) with vigorous shaking; cool to body temperature before using.

FLOXURIDINE

Rx	Floxuridine (Bedford)	Powder for Injection, lyophilized: 500 mg	In 5 ml vials.
Rx	FUDR (Roche)		In 5 ml vials.

For complete prescribing information, refer to the Fluorouracil and Floxuridine group monograph.

Indications

Palliative management of GI adenocarcinoma metastatic to the liver, given by continuous regional intra-arterial infusion in selected patients considered incurable by surgery or other means. Patients with disease extending beyond an area capable of infusion via a single artery should, except in unusual circumstances, be considered for systemic therapy with other agents.

Administration and Dosage

➤*For intra-arterial infusion only:* Continuous arterial infusion of 0.1 to 0.6 mg/kg/day. The higher dose ranges (0.4 to 0.6 mg) are usually employed for hepatic artery infusion because the liver metabolizes the drug, thus reducing the potential for systemic toxicity. Administer until adverse reactions appear. When side effects have subsided, resume therapy. Maintain therapy as long as response continues. Use an infusion pump to overcome pressure in large arteries and to ensure a uniform infusion rate.

➤*Storage/Stability:*

Powder for injection – Reconstitute with 5 ml sterile water. Refrigerate reconstituted vials at 2° to 8°C (36° to 46°F) for ≤ 2 weeks.

GEMCITABINE HCl

Rx	Gemzar (Eli Lilly)	Powder for Injection, lyophilized: 20 mg/ml	Mannitol. In 10 and 50 ml vials.

Indications

➤*Pancreatic cancer:* First-line treatment for patients with locally advanced (nonresectable Stage II or Stage III) or metastatic (Stage IV) adenocarcinoma of the pancreas. Gemcitabine is indicated for patients previously treated with 5–FU.

➤*Non-small cell lung cancer:* In combination with cisplatin for the first-line treatment of patients with inoperable, locally advanced (Stage IIIA or IIIB) or metastatic (Stage IV) non-small cell lung cancer.

Administration and Dosage

➤*Approved by the FDA:* May 2, 1996.

IV use only. Gemcitabine may be administered on an outpatient basis.

➤*Pancreatic cancer:*

Single-agent use for adults – Administer IV at a dose of 1000 mg/m^2 over 30 minutes once weekly for up to 7 weeks (or until toxicity necessitates reducing or holding a dose), followed by 1 week of rest from treatment. Infuse subsequent cycles once weekly for 3 consecutive weeks out of every 4 weeks.

Dose modifications: Dosage adjustment is based on the degree of hematologic toxicity experienced by the patient. Monitor patient prior to each dose with a complete blood count (CBC) (see Gemcitabine Dosage Reduction Guidelines table). Patients who complete an entire 7-week initial cycle of gemcitabine therapy may have the dose for subsequent cycles increased by 25% (to 1250 mg/m^2), provided that the absolute granulocyte count (AGC) and platelet nadirs exceed 1500 × 10^6/L and 100,000 × 10^6/L, respectively, and if nonhematologic toxicity

has not been greater than World Health Organization Grade 1. If patients tolerate the subsequent course at a dose of 1250 mg/m^2, the dose for the next cycle can be increased by 20% to 1500 mg/m^2, provided that the ACG and platelet nadirs exceed 1500 × 10^6/L and 100,000 × 10^6/L, respectively, and again, if nonhematologic toxicity has not been greater than WHO Grade 1.

➤*Non-small cell lung cancer:*

Combination use – Two schedules have been investigated and the optimum schedule has not been determined. With the 4-week schedule, administer gemcitabine IV at a dose of 1000 mg/m^2 over 30 minutes on days 1, 8, and 15 of each 28-day cycle. Administer cisplatin IV at 100 mg/m^2 on day 1 after the infusion of gemcitabine. With the 3-week schedule, administer gemcitabine IV at a dose of 1250 mg/m^2 over 30 minutes on days 1 and 8 of each 21-day cycle. Administer cisplatin IV at a dose of 100 mg/m^2 after the infusion of gemcitabine on day 1.

Dose modifications: Dosage adjustment is based on the degree of hematologic toxicity experienced by the patient. Monitor patient prior to each dose with a complete blood count (CBC) (see Gemcitabine Dosage Reduction Guidelines table). For severe (grade 3 or 4) non-hematological toxicity, except alopecia and nausea/vomiting, hold or decrease gemcitabine plus cisplatin by 50%, depending on the judgment of the treating physician. During combination therapy with cisplatin, carefully monitor serum creatinine, serum potassium, serum calcium, and serum magnesium (grade 3/4 serum creatinine toxicity for gemcitabine plus cisplatin was 5% vs 2% for cisplatin alone).

GEMCITABINE HCl

Gemcitabine Dosage Reduction Guidelines			
Absolute granulocyte count ($\times 10^6$/L)		Platelet count ($\times 10^6$/L)	% of full dose
≥ 1000	and	≥ 100,000	100
500 to 999	or	50,000 to 99,000	75
< 500	or	< 50,000	hold

➤*Dilution:* Diluent for reconstitution of gemcitabine is 0.9% Sodium Chloride Injection without preservatives. Because of solubility considerations, the maximum concentration for gemcitabine upon reconstitution is 40 mg/ml. Avoid reconstitution at concentrations > 40 mg/ml; incomplete dissolution may result.

➤*Reconstitution:* To reconstitute, add 5 ml of 0.9% Sodium Chloride Injection to the 200 mg vial or 25 ml of 0.9% Sodium Chloride Injection to the 1 g vial. Shake to dissolve. These dilutions each yield a gemcitabine concentration of ≈ 40 mg/ml. The appropriate amount of drug may be administered as prepared by further diluting with 0.9% Sodium Chloride Injection to concentrations as low as 0.1 mg/ml.

➤*Storage/Stability:* Do not refrigerate solutions of reconstituted gemcitabine, as crystallization may occur. Store at controlled room temperature 20° to 25°C (68° to 77°F). Gemcitabine solutions are stable for 24 hours at controlled room temperature.

Actions

➤*Pharmacology:* Gemcitabine is a nucleoside analog that exhibits antitumor activity. It exhibits cell phase specificity, primarily killing cells undergoing DNA synthesis in the S-phase. It also blocks the progression of cells through the G1/S-phase boundary. The cytotoxic effect is attributed to its active metabolites, diphosphate (dFdCDP) and triphosphate nucleosides. First, gemcitabine diphosphate inhibits ribonucleotide reductase, which catalyzes the reactions that generate the deoxynucleoside triphosphates for DNA synthesis. Inhibition of this enzyme causes a reduction in the concentrations of deoxynucleotides, including dCTP. Second, gemcitabine triphosphate competes with dCTP for incorporation into DNA. After the gemcitabine nucleotide is incorporated into DNA, only 1 additional nucleotide is added to the growing DNA strands causing inhibition of further DNA synthesis. DNA polymerase epsilon is unable to remove the gemcitabine nucleotide and repair the growing DNA strands (masked chain termination).

➤*Pharmacokinetics:*

Absorption/Distribution – Patients receiving gemcitabine 1000 mg/m^2 once weekly generally demonstrate C_{max} values of 10 to 40 mg/L and achieve steady state after 15 to 30 minutes, during the 30-minute infusion protocol. Plasma protein binding of gemcitabine is negligible. A volume of distribution of 50 L/m^2 indicated that it is not extensively distributed into tissues following short infusions (< 70 minutes). For long infusions, the volume of distribution is 370 L/m^2, reflecting slow equilibration within the tissue compartment.

Metabolism/Excretion – It is metabolized intracellularly to the active diphosphate and triphosphate nucleosides. Clearance and elimination half-life is affected by gender and age, but this does not require dosing adjustments. Half-life ranges from 32 to 94 minutes for short infusions and 245 to 638 minutes for long infusions. The terminal phase half-life for the triphosphate metabolite from mononuclear cells ranges from 1.7 to 19.4 hours. A small amount (< 10%) of gemcitabine is excreted unchanged in the urine.

➤*Clinical trials:*

Pancreatic cancer – Patients with locally advanced or metastatic pancreatic cancer received gemcitabine 1000 mg/m^2 over 30 minutes once-weekly for up to 7 weeks (or until toxicity), followed by 1 week of rest, then subsequent cycles of once-weekly injections for 3 consecutive weeks in 2 trials. The first trial demonstrated that the gemcitabine-treated patients had statistically significant increases in clinical benefit response, survival, and time to progressive disease compared with 5-FU administered 600 mg/m^2 IV weekly. The second trial, involving patients previously treated with 5-FU or a 5-FU-containing regimen, showed a clinical benefit response rate of 27% and a median survival of 3.9 months.

Non-small cell lung cancer – Gemcitabine 1000 mg/m^2 on days 1, 8, and 15 with cisplatin 100 mg/m^2 on day 1 of a 28-day cycle was compared with single-agent cisplatin 100 mg/m^2 on day 1 of a 28-day cycle. Increased median survival time, median time to disease progression, and the objective response rate were statistically significant with gemcitabine plus cisplatin vs cisplatin alone. A second trial randomized patients to either gemcitabine 1250 mg/m^2 on days 1 and 8 plus cisplatin 100 mg/m^2 on day 1 of a 21-day cycle or to etoposide 100 mg/m^2 on days 1, 2, and 3 plus cisplatin 100 mg/m^2 on day 1 of a 21-day cycle. There was no statistically significant difference in survival between study groups. However, greater median time to disease progression and objective response rate were statistically significant in the gemcitabine plus cisplatin arm. Both studies demonstrated no difference in quality of life between the 2 treatment arms.

Contraindications

Known hypersensitivity to the drug.

Warnings

➤*Infusion time/frequency:* Infusion time > 60 minutes and more-frequent-than-weekly dosing have been shown to increase toxicity.

➤*Myelosuppression:* Bone marrow suppression as manifested by leukopenia, thrombocytopenia, and anemia, and myelosuppression is usually the dose-limiting toxicity. Monitor patients during therapy.

➤*Fever:* The overall incidence of fever was 41%. This is in contrast to the incidence of infection (16%) and indicates that gemcitabine may cause fever in the absence of clinical infection. Fever was frequently associated with other flu-like symptoms and was usually mild and clinically manageable.

➤*Rash:* Rash was reported in 30% of patients. The rash was typically a macular or finely granular maculopapular pruritic eruption of mild-to-moderate severity involving the trunk and extremities. Pruritus was reported in 13% of patients.

➤*Gender:* Older women were more likely not to proceed to a subsequent cycle and to experience grade 3/4 neutropenia and thrombocytopenia.

➤*Renal/Hepatic function impairment:* Use with caution in patients with preexisting renal impairment or hepatic insufficiency. Gemcitabine has not been studied in patients with significant renal or hepatic impairment.

Hepatic – Gemcitabine was associated with transient elevations of serum transaminases in ≈ 70% of patients, but there was no evidence of increasing hepatic toxicity with either longer duration of exposure to gemcitabine or with greater total cumulative dose.

Renal – Mild proteinuria and hematuria were commonly reported. Hemolytic uremic syndrome (HUS) with gemcitabine therapy or immediately post-therapy has been reported in 0.25% of patients. Consider the diagnosis of HUS if the patient develops anemia with evidence of microangiopathic hemolysis as indicated by elevated bilirubin, LDH, reticulocytosis, severe thrombocytopenia, and evidence of renal failure; discontinue therapy immediately if suspected. Renal failure may not be reversible even with discontinuation of therapy, and dialysis may be required.

➤*Elderly:* Gemcitabine clearance is affected by age. However, there is no evidence that unusual dose adjustments are necessary in patients > 65 years of age; in general, adverse reaction rates were similar in patients above and below 65 years of age. Grade 3/4 thrombocytopenia was more common in the elderly.

➤*Pregnancy: Category D.* Gemcitabine can cause fetal harm when administered to a pregnant woman. There are no studies of gemcitabine in pregnant women. If gemcitabine is used during pregnancy, or if the patient becomes pregnant while taking gemcitabine, inform the patient of the potential hazard to the fetus.

➤*Lactation:* It is not known whether gemcitabine or its metabolites are excreted in breast milk. Because of the potential for serious adverse reactions from gemcitabine in nursing infants, warn the mother and decide whether to discontinue nursing or the drug, taking into account the importance of the drug to the mother and the potential risk to the infant.

➤*Children:* Safety and efficacy have not been established.

Precautions

➤*Monitoring:* Monitor patients prior to each dose with a complete blood count (CBC), including differential and platelet count. Consider suspending or modifying therapy when marrow suppression is detected (see Administration and Dosage).

Hepatic and renal – Perform laboratory evaluations of renal and hepatic function prior to initiation of therapy and periodically thereafter.

Adverse Reactions

Myelosuppression is the principal dose-limiting factor with gemcitabine therapy.

GEMCITABINE HCl

Gemcitabine Adverse Reactions (%)					
	All patients (n = 699 to 974)	Pancreatic cancer patients (n = 161 to 241)	Discontinuations (n = 979)	Gemcitabine vs 5-FU	
				Gemcitabine (n = 58 to 63)	5-FU (n = 61 to 63)
Laboratory					
Hematologic					
Anemia	68	73	< 1	65	45
Leukopenia	62	64	< 1	71	15
Neutropenia	63	61		62	18
Thrombocytopenia	24	36	< 1	47	15
Hepatic			< 1		
ALT	68	72		72	38
AST	67	78		72	52
Alkaline phosphatase	55	77		71	64
Bilirubin	13	26		16	25
Renal			< 1		
Proteinuria	45	32		10	2
Hematuria	35	23		13	0
BUN	16	15		8	10
Creatinine	8	6		2	0
Non-laboratory					
Nausea and vomiting	69	71	< 1	64	58
Pain	48	42	< 1	10	7
Fever	41	38	< 1	30	16
Rash	30	28	< 1	24	13
Dyspnea	23	10	< 1	6	3
Constipation	23	31	0	10	11
Diarrhea	19	30	0	24	31
Hemorrhage	17	4	< 1	0	2
Infection	16	10	< 1	8	3
Alopecia	15	16	0	18	16
Stomatitis	11	10	< 1	14	15
Somnolence	11	11	< 1	5	7
Paresthesias	10	10	0	2	2

➤*Cardiovascular:* Two percent of patients discontinued therapy because of cardiovascular events such as myocardial infarction, cerebrovascular accident, arrhythmia, and hypertension. Many of these patients had a history of cardiovascular disease.

➤*CNS:* Mild paresthesias (10%); severe paresthesias (< 1%).

➤*Dermatologic:* Rash (30%; see Warnings); hair loss, usually minimal (15%).

➤*GI:* Nausea and vomiting (69%); transient elevations of serum transaminases (≈ 70%; see Warnings); diarrhea (19%); stomatitis (11%).

➤*Hematologic:* Red blood cell transfusions (19%); petechiae or mild blood loss (hemorrhage) (16%); sepsis, platelet transfusions (< 1%).

➤*Pulmonary:* Dyspnea (23%); severe dyspnea (3%); dyspnea may be due to an underlying disease such as lung cancer (40%) or pulmonary manifestations of other malignancies. Dyspnea was occasionally accompanied by bronchospasm (< 2 %); parenchymal lung toxicity consistent with drug-induced pneumonitis (rare); discontinuation of therapy because of pulmonary edema of unknown etiology (rare).

➤*Renal:* Mild proteinuria, hematuria, hemolytic uremic syndrome (see Warnings).

➤*Miscellaneous:* Peripheral edema (20%); "flu syndrome" (19%; including fever [41%; see Warnings]; asthenia, anorexia, headache, cough, chills, myalgia [common]; insomnia, rhinitis, sweating, malaise [infrequent]; < 1% discontinued because of flu-like symptoms); infections (16%); edema (13%); injection site related events (4%; there were no reports of injection site necrosis as gemcitabine is not a vesicant); bronchospasm (< 2%); sepsis (< 1%), generalized edema (< 1% [< 1% of patients discontinued because of edema]); anaphylactoid reaction (rare).

Overdosage

There is no known antidote for overdoses of gemcitabine. Myelosuppression, paresthesias, and severe rash were the principal toxicities seen when a single dose as high as 5700 mg/m^2 was infused IV over 30 minutes every 2 weeks.

➤*Treatment:* In the event of suspected overdose, monitor the patient with appropriate blood counts and provide supportive therapy, as necessary. Refer to General Management of Acute Overdosage.

Purine Analogs and Related Agents

CLADRIBINE (2-chlorodeoxyadenosine; CdA)

Rx	Cladribine (Bedford)	Solution for Injection: 1 mg/ml	9 mg NaCl/ml. In 10 ml fill in a 20 ml single-use vial.
Rx	Leustatin (Ortho Biotech)		Preservative free. In 10 ml or 10 ml fill in 20 ml single-use vials.

WARNING

Administer under the supervision of a qualified physician experienced in the use of antineoplastic therapy. Anticipate suppression of bone marrow function. This is usually reversible and appears to be dose-dependent. High doses (4 to 9 times the recommended dose for hairy cell leukemia) in conjunction with cyclophosphamide and total body irradiation as preparation for bone marrow transplantation, have been associated with severe, irreversible, neurologic toxicity (paraparesis/quadriparesis) or acute renal insufficiency in 45% of patients treated for 7 to 14 days.

Indications

➤*Hairy cell leukemia (HCL):* Treatment of active HCL as defined by clinically significant anemia, neutropenia, thrombocytopenia or disease-related symptoms.

➤*Unlabeled uses:* Cladribine (generally 0.1 mg/kg/day for 7 days) appears to be beneficial in the following conditions: Advanced cutaneous T-cell lymphomas; chronic lymphocytic leukemia; non-Hodgkin's lymphomas; acute myeloid leukemia; autoimmune hemolytic anemia; mycosis fungoides or the Sezary syndrome.

Administration and Dosage

➤*Approved by the FDA:* February 26, 1993.

➤*Usual dose:* The recommended dose and schedule for active HCL is a single course given by continuous infusion for 7 consecutive days at a dose of 0.09 mg/kg/day. Deviations from this dosage regimen are not advised. Consider delaying or discontinuing the drug if neurotoxicity or renal toxicity occurs (see Warnings).

Specific risk factors predisposing to increased toxicity from cladribine have not been defined. In view of the known toxicities of agents of this class, it would be prudent to proceed carefully in patients with known or suspected renal insufficiency or severe bone marrow impairment of any etiology. Monitor patients closely for hematologic and non-hematologic toxicity. (See Warnings and Precautions.)

➤*Preparation/Administration of IV solutions:* Cladribine must be diluted with the designated diluent prior to administration. Since the drug product does not contain any antimicrobial preservative or bacteriostatic agent, aseptic technique and proper environmental precautions must be observed in preparation of solutions.

Preparation of a single daily dose – Add the calculated dose (0.09 mg/kg or 0.09 ml/kg) to an infusion bag containing 500 ml 0.9% Sodium Chloride Injection, USP. Infuse continuously over 24 hours. Repeat daily for a total of 7 consecutive days. The use of 5% dextrose as a diluent is not recommended because of increased degradation of cladribine. Admixtures of cladribine are chemically and physically stable for at least 24 hours at room temperature under normal room fluorescent light in Baxter Viaflex PVC infusion containers. Since limited compatibility data are available, adherence to the recommended diluents and infusion systems is advised.

Preparation of Single Daily Cladribine Doses			
Method	Dose	Recommended diluent	Quantity of diluent
24 hour infusion	1 (day) × 0.09 mg/kg	0.9% sodium chloride	500 ml

Preparation of a 7 day infusion – Only prepare the 7 day infusion solution with Bacteriostatic 0.9% Sodium Chloride Injection, USP (0.9% benzyl alcohol preserved). In order to minimize the risk of microbial contamination, pass both cladribine and the diluent through a sterile 0.22 micron disposable hydrophilic syringe filter as each solution is being introduced into the infusion reservoir. First add the calculated dose of cladribine (7 days x 0.09 mg/kg or ml/kg) to the infusion reservoir through the sterile filter, then add a calculated amount of Bacteriostatic 0.9% Sodium Chloride Injection (also through the filter) to bring the total volume of the solution to 100 ml. After completing solution preparation, clamp off the line, disconnect and discard the filter. Aseptically aspirate air bubbles from the reservoir as necessary using the syringe and a dry second sterile filter or a sterile vent filter assembly. Reclamp the line and discard the syringe and filter assembly. Infuse continuously over 7 days. Solutions prepared with Bacteriostatic Sodium Chloride Injection for individuals weighing > 85 kg may have reduced preservative effectiveness due to greater dilution of the benzyl alcohol preservative. Admixtures for the 7 day infusion have demonstrated acceptable chemical and physical stability for at least 7 days in Pharmacia *Deltec* medication cassettes.

Preparation of 7 Day Cladribine Infusion			
Method	Dose	Recommended diluent	Quantity of diluent
7 day infusion method	7 days x 0.09 mg/kg	Bacteriostatic 0.9% Sodium Chloride	qs to 100 ml

➤*IV admixture incompatibility:* Since limited compatibility data are available, adherence to the recommended diluents and infusion systems is advised. Solutions containing cladribine should not be mixed with other IV drugs or additives or infused simultaneously via a common IV line, since compatibility testing has not been performed. Do not use preparations containing benzyl alcohol in neonates (see Warnings).

➤*Handling and disposal:* The use of disposable gloves and protective garments is recommended. If cladribine injection contacts the skin or mucous membranes, wash the involved surface immediately with copious amounts of water.

➤*Storage/Stability:* Refrigerate unopened vials (2° to 8°C; 36° to 46°F); protect from light. When stored in refrigerated conditions and protected from light, unopened vials are stable until the expiration date indicated on the package. Freezing does not adversely affect the solution. However, a precipitate may form during the exposure of cladribine to low temperatures; it may be resolubilized by allowing the solution to warm naturally to room temperature and by shaking vigorously. Do not heat or microwave. Once thawed, the vial is stable until expiration date if refrigerated. Do not refreeze. Once diluted, administer solutions containing cladribine injection promptly or store in the refrigerator for no more than 8 hours prior to administration. Vials of cladribine are for single use only. Discard any unused portion in an appropriate manner.

Actions

➤*Pharmacology:* Cladribine is a synthetic antineoplastic agent for continuous IV infusion. The selective toxicity of cladribine towards certain normal and malignant lymphocyte and monocyte populations is based on the relative activities of deoxycytidine kinase, deoxynucleotidase and adenosine deaminase. In cells with a high ratio of deoxycytidine kinase to deoxynucleotidase, cladribine, a purine nucleoside analog, passively crosses the cell membrane. It is phosphorylated by deoxycytidine kinase to 2-chloro-2'deoxy-β-D-adenosine mono-phosphate (2-CdAMP). Since cladribine is resistant to deamination by adenosine deaminase and there is little deoxynucleotide deaminase in lymphocytes and monocytes, 2-CdAMP accumulates intracellularly and is subsequently converted into the active triphosphate deoxynucleotide, 2-CdATP. It is postulated that cells with high deoxycytidine kinase and low deoxynucleotidase activities will be selectively killed by cladribine as toxic deoxynucleotides accumulate intracellularly.

Cells containing high concentrations of deoxynucleotides are unable to properly repair single-strand DNA breaks. The broken ends of DNA activate the enzyme poly (ADP-ribose) polymerase resulting in NAD and ATP depletion and disruption of cellular metabolism. There is also evidence that 2-CdATP is incorporated into the DNA of dividing cells, resulting in impairment of DNA synthesis. Thus, cladribine can be distinguished from other chemotherapeutic agents affecting purine metabolism in that it is cytotoxic to both actively dividing and quiescent lymphocytes and monocytes, inhibiting both DNA synthesis and repair.

➤*Pharmacokinetics:* Seventeen patients with hairy cell leukemia (HCL) and normal renal function were treated for 7 days with the recommended treatment regimen (0.09 mg/kg/day) by continuous IV infusion. The mean steady-state serum concentration was estimated to be 5.7 ng/ml with an estimated systemic clearance of 663.5 ml/hr/kg. Accumulation over the 7 day treatment period was not noted. In HCL patients, there does not appear to be a relationship between serum concentrations and ultimate clinical outcome.

Eight patients with hematologic malignancies received a 2 hour infusion (0.12 mg/kg). The mean end-of-infusion plasma concentration was 48 ± 19 ng/ml. For five of these patients, the disappearance of cladribine could be described by either a biphasic or triphasic decline. For patients with normal renal function, the mean terminal half-life was 5.4 hours. Mean values for clearance and steady-state volume of distribution were 978 ± 422 ml/hr/kg and 4.5 ± 2.8 L/kg, respectively. Cladribine is bound approximately 20% to plasma proteins.

In rats, approximately 41% to 44% of cladribine was recovered in the urine in the first 6 hours from 1 mg/kg bolus or infusion. Only small amounts were recovered after 6 hours; ≤ 1% was excreted in the feces following a bolus dose.

➤*Clinical trials:* Two single-center open label studies were conducted in patients with HCL with evidence of active disease requiring therapy. In one study, 89 patients were treated with a single course of cladribine (0.09 mg/kg/day) given by continuous IV infusion for 7 days. In a second study, 35 patients were treated with a 7 day continuous IV infusion at a comparable dose of 3.6 mg/m²/day.

CLADRIBINE (2-chlorodeoxyadenosine; CdA)

A complete response (CR) required clearing of the peripheral blood and bone marrow of hairy cells and recovery of the hemoglobin to 12 g/dl, platelet count to 100×10^9/L, and absolute neutrophil count to 1500×10^6/L. A good partial response (GPR) required the same hematologic parameters as a complete response, and that < 5% of hairy cells remain in the bone marrow. A partial response (PR) required that hairy cells in the bone marrow be decreased by at least 50% from baseline and the same response for hematologic parameters as for complete response. A pathologic relapse was defined as an increase in bone marrow hairy cells to 25% of pretreatment levels. A clinical relapse was defined as the recurrence of cytopenias, specifically, decreases in hemoglobin $\geq$ 2 g/dl, ANC $\geq$ 25% or platelet counts $\geq$ 50,000.

Response Rates to Cladribine Treatment in Patients with Hairy Cell Leukemia

Patient population	CR[1]	Overall[2]
Evaluable patients (n = 106)	66%	88%
Intent-to-treat population (n = 123)	54%	89%

[1] Complete response.
[2] Complete + good partial + partial responses.

In these studies, 60% of the patients had not received prior chemotherapy for HCL or had undergone splenectomy as the only prior treatment and were receiving cladribine as a first-line treatment. The remaining 40% of patients received cladribine as a second-line treatment, having been previously treated with other agents, including interferon alfa or pentostatin. The overall response rate for patients without prior chemotherapy was 92% compared with 84% for previously treated patients. Cladribine is active in previously treated patients; however, retrospective analysis suggests that the overall response rate is decreased in patients previously treated with splenectomy or pentostatin and in patients refractory to interferon alfa.

Overall Response Rates[1] To Cladribine Treatment in Patients with Hairy Cell Leukemia

	Overall response (n = 123)	NR[2]+ relapse
No prior chemotherapy	92%	6 + 4 (14%)
Any prior chemotherapy	84%	8 + 3 (22%)
Previous splenectomy	78%	9 + 1 (24%)
Previous interferon	83%	8 + 3 (23%)
Interferon refractory	55%	5 + 2 (64%)
Previous pentostatin	50%	3 + 1 (66%)

[1] CR + GPR + PR.
[2] No response.

After a reversible decline, normalization of peripheral blood counts (hemoglobin > 12 g/dl, platelets > 100×10^9/L, absolute neutrophil count [ANC] > 1500×10^6/L) was achieved by 92% of evaluable patients. The median time to normalization of peripheral counts was 9 weeks from the start of treatment (range, 2 to 72). With normalization of platelet count and hemoglobin, requirements for platelet and RBC transfusions were abolished after months 1 and 2, respectively, in those patients with complete response. Platelet recovery may be delayed in a minority of patients with severe baseline thrombocytopenia. Corresponding to normalization of ANC, a trend toward a reduced incidence of infection was seen after the third month, when compared to the months immediately preceding the therapy.

Time to Normalization of Peripheral Blood Counts Following Cladribine in HCL Patients

Parameter	Median time to normalization of count[1]
Platelet count	2 weeks
Absolute neutrophil count	5 weeks
Hemoglobin	8 weeks
ANC, hemoglobin and platelet count	9 weeks

[1] Day 1 = First day of infusion.

For patients achieving a complete response, the median time to response (absence of hairy cells in bone marrow and peripheral blood together with normalization of peripheral blood parameters), measured from treatment start, was $\approx$ 4 months. Since bone marrow aspiration and biopsy were frequently not performed at the time of peripheral blood normalization, the median time to complete response may actually be shorter than that which was recorded. At the time of data cut-off, the median duration of complete response was > 8 months and ranged to 25 + months. Among 93 responding patients, seven had evi-

dence of disease progression at the time of the data cut-off. In four of these patients, disease was limited to the bone marrow without peripheral blood abnormalities (pathologic progression), while in three patients there were also peripheral blood abnormalities (clinical progression). Seven patients who did not respond to a first course received a second course of therapy. In the five patients who had adequate follow-up, additional courses did not appear to improve their overall response.

Contraindications

Hypersensitivity to the drug or any of its components.

Warnings

➤*Bone marrow suppression:* Severe bone marrow suppression, including neutropenia, anemia and thrombocytopenia, has been commonly observed in patients treated with cladribine, especially at high doses. At initiation of treatment, most patients in the clinical studies had hematologic impairment as a manifestation of active HCL. Following treatment, further hematologic impairment occurred before recovery of peripheral blood counts began. During the first 2 weeks after treatment initiation, mean platelet count, ANC and hemoglobin concentration declined and subsequently increased with normalization of mean counts by day 12, week 5 and week 8, respectively. The myelosuppressive effects were most notable during the first month following treatment. Forty-four percent of patients received transfusions with RBCs and 14% received transfusions with platelets during month 1. Careful hematologic monitoring, especially during the first 4 to 8 weeks after treatment, is recommended.

➤*Nephrotoxicity/Neurotoxicity:* In a study using high-dose cladribine (4 to 9 times the recommended dose for HCL) as part of a bone marrow transplant conditioning regimen, which also included high-dose cyclophosphamide and total body irradiation, acute nephrotoxicity and delayed onset neurotoxicity were observed. Thirty-one poor-risk patients with drug-resistant acute leukemia in relapse (29 cases) or non-Hodgkin's lymphoma (two cases) received cladribine for 7 to 14 days prior to bone marrow transplantation. During infusion, eight patients experienced GI symptoms. While the bone marrow was initially cleared of all hematopoietic elements, including tumor cells, leukemia eventually recurred in all treated patients. Within 7 to 13 days after starting treatment, six patients (19%) developed manifestations of renal dysfunction (eg, acidosis, anuria, elevated serum creatinine) and five required dialysis. Several of these patients were also being treated with other medications having known nephrotoxic potential. Renal dysfunction was reversible in two of these patients. In the four patients whose renal function had not recovered at the time of death, autopsies were performed; in two of these, evidence of tubular damage was noted. Eleven patients (35%) experienced delayed onset neurologic toxicity. In the majority, this was characterized by progressive irreversible motor weakness (paraparesis/quadriparesis) of the upper or lower extremities, first noted 35 to 84 days after starting high-dose therapy. Non-invasive testing (electromyography and nerve conduction studies) was consistent with demyelinating disease.

In patients with HCL treated with the recommended treatment regimen (0.09 mg/kg/day for 7 consecutive days), there have been no reports of similar nephro- or neurologic toxicities. Mild neurologic toxicities, specifically paresthesias and dizziness, have been reported rarely.

➤*Fever:* Fever 37.8°C ($\geq$100°F) was associated with the use of cladribine in $\approx$ 66% of patients in the first month of therapy. Virtually all patients were treated empirically with parenteral antibiotics. Overall, 47% of patients had fever in the setting of neutropenia (ANC $\leq$ 1000), including 32% with severe neutropenia (ANC $\leq$ 500). Since the majority of fevers occurred in neutropenic patients, closely monitor patients during the first month of treatment and initiate empiric antibiotics as clinically indicated. Although 69% of patients developed fevers, < 33% of febrile events were associated with documented infection. Given the known myelosuppressive effects of cladribine, carefully evaluate the risks and benefits of administering this drug to patients with active infections.

➤*Death:* Of the 196 HCL patients entered in the trials, there were eight deaths following treatment. Of these, six were of infectious etiology (including three pneumonias), and 2 occurred in the first month following therapy. Of the eight deaths, six occurred in previously treated patients who were refractory to interferon alfa.

➤*Benzyl alcohol:* Benzyl alcohol, a constituent of the recommended diluent for the 7 day infusion solution, has been associated with a fatal "gasping syndrome" in premature infants.

➤*Renal function impairment:* The kidney has not been established as the pathway of excretion for cladribine. There are inadequate data on dosing of patients with renal or hepatic insufficiency. Development of acute renal insufficiency in some patients receiving high doses of cladribine has been described. Until more information is available, use caution when administering the drug to patients with known or suspected renal or hepatic insufficiency.

➤*Mutagenesis:* As expected for compounds in this class, the actions of cladribine yield DNA damage. In mammalian cells in culture, cladribine caused an imbalance of intracellular deoxyribonucleotide triphos-

CLADRIBINE (2-chlorodeoxyadenosine; CdA)

phate pools. This imbalance results in the inhibition of DNA synthesis and DNA repair, yielding DNA strand breaks and subsequently cell death. Inhibition of thymidine incorporation into human lymphoblastic cells was 90% at concentrations of 0.3 mcM. Cladribine was also incorporated into DNA of these cells.

➤*Fertility impairment:* When administered IV to Cynomolgus monkeys, cladribine caused suppression of rapidly generating cells, including testicular cells. The effect on human fertility is unknown.

➤*Pregnancy: Category D.* Cladribine is teratogenic in mice and rabbits and consequently has the potential to cause fetal harm when administered to a pregnant woman. A significant increase in fetal variations was observed in mice receiving 1.5 mg/kg/day, and increased resorptions, reduced litter size and increased fetal malformations were observed when mice received 3 mg/kg/day. Fetal death and malformations were observed in rabbits that received 3 mg/kg/day.

Although there is no evidence of teratogenicity in humans due to cladribine, other drugs that inhibit DNA synthesis (eg, methotrexate) are teratogenic in humans. Cladribine is embryotoxic in mice when given in doses equivalent to the recommended dose. If cladribine is used during pregnancy, or if the patient becomes pregnant while taking this drug, apprise the patient of the potential hazard to the fetus. Advise women of childbearing age to avoid becoming pregnant. Use during pregnancy only if the potential benefit justifies the potential risk to the fetus.

➤*Lactation:* It is not known whether this drug is excreted in breast milk. Because of the potential for serious adverse reactions in nursing infants, decide whether to discontinue nursing or discontinue the drug, taking into account the importance of the drug to the mother.

➤*Children:* Safety and efficacy in children have not been established. In a Phase I study involving patients 1 to 21 years old with relapsed acute leukemia, cladribine was given by continuous IV infusion in doses ranging from 3 to 10.7 mg/m²/day for 5 days (one-half to twice the dose recommended in HCL). In this study, the dose-limiting toxicity was severe myelosuppression with profound neutropenia and thrombocytopenia. At the highest dose (10.7 mg/m²/day), three of seven patients developed irreversible myelosuppression and fatal systemic bacterial or fungal infections. No unique toxicities were noted in this study.

Precautions

➤*Monitoring:* Cladribine is a potent antineoplastic agent with potentially significant toxic side effects. Administer only under the supervision of a physician experienced with the use of cancer chemotherapeutic agents. Closely observe patients undergoing therapy for signs of hematologic and non-hematologic toxicity. Periodic assessment of peripheral blood counts, particularly during the first 4 to 8 weeks post-treatment, is recommended to detect the development of anemia, neutropenia and thrombocytopenia and for early detection of any potential sequelae (eg, infection, bleeding). As with other potent chemotherapeutic agents, monitor renal and hepatic function, especially in patients with underlying kidney or liver dysfunction.

During and following treatment, monitor the patient's hematologic profile regularly to determine the degree of hematopoietic suppression. In the clinical studies, following reversible declines in all cell counts, the mean platelet count reached 100 x 10⁹/L by day 12, the mean ANC reached 1500 x 10⁶/L by week 5 and the mean hemoglobin reached 12 g/dl by week 8. After peripheral counts have normalized, perform bone marrow aspiration and biopsy to confirm response to treatment. Investigate febrile events with appropriate laboratory and radiologic studies. Perform periodic assessment of renal and hepatic function as clinically indicated.

➤*Hyperuricemia/Tumor lysis syndrome:* While hyperuricemia and tumor lysis syndrome is always possible in patients with large tumor burdens, patients in these studies were treated empirically with allopurinol and no episodes of tumor lysis were reported.

➤*Administration:* Cladribine must be diluted in designated IV solutions prior to administration (see Administration and Dosage).

Adverse Reactions

In month 1 of the HCL clinical trials, the following occurred: Severe neutropenia (70%); fever (69%); infection (28%). Other adverse experiences reported frequently during the first 14 days after initiating treatment included: Fatigue (45%); nausea (28%); rash (27%); headache (22%); injection site reactions (19%). Most non-hematologic adverse experiences were mild to moderate in severity.

➤*Cardiovascular:* Edema, tachycardia (6%).

➤*CNS:* Headache (22%); dizziness (9%); insomnia (7%).

➤*Dermatologic:* Rash (27%); injection site reactions (19%); pruritus, pain, erythema (6%).

➤*GI:* Nausea (28%); decreased appetite (17%); vomiting (13%); diarrhea (10%); constipation (9%); abdominal pain (6%).

➤*Hematologic/Lymphatic:* Purpura (10%); petechiae (8%); epistaxis (5%).

➤*Musculoskeletal:* Myalgia (7%); arthralgia (5%).

➤*Respiratory:* Abnormal breath sounds (11%); cough (10%); abnormal chest sounds (9%); shortness of breath (7%).

➤*Miscellaneous:* Fever (69%); fatigue (45%); chills, asthenia, diaphoresis (9%); malaise (7%); trunk pain (6%).

IV administration – Injection site infections (redness, swelling, pain; 9%); thrombosis, phlebitis (2%); broken catheter (1%). These appear to be related to the infusion procedure or indwelling catheter rather than the medication or the vehicle.

From day 15 to the last follow-up visit, the only events reported by> 5% of patients were: Fatigue (11%); rash (10%); headache, cough (7%); malaise (5%).

Myelosuppression – Myelosuppression was frequently observed during the first month after starting treatment. Neutropenia (ANC < 500 × 10⁶/L) was noted in 70% of patients, compared with 26% in whom it was present initially. Severe anemia (hemoglobin < 8.5 g/dl) developed in 37% of patients, compared with 10% initially and thrombocytopenia (platelets < 20 × 10⁹/L) developed in 12% of patients, compared to 4% in whom it was noted initially.

Infection – During the first month, 28% exhibited documented evidence of infection. Serious infections (eg, septicemia, pneumonia) were reported in 6% of all patients; the remainder were mild or moderate. Several deaths were attributable to infection or complications related to the underlying disease. During the second month, the overall rate of documented infection was 6%; these infections were mild to moderate and no severe systemic infections were seen. After the third month, the monthly incidence of infection was either less than or equal to that of the months immediately preceding therapy.

Fever – During the first month, 11% of patients experienced severe fever (≥ 40° C; 104° F). Documented infections were noted in < 33% of febrile episodes. Of the 196 patients studied, 19 were noted to have a documented infection in the month prior to treatment. In the month following treatment, there were 54 episodes of documented infection: 42% were bacterial, 20% were viral and 20% were fungal. Seven of 8 documented episodes of herpes zoster occurred during the month following treatment. Fourteen of 16 episodes of documented fungal infections occurred in the first 2 months following treatment. Virtually all of these patients were treated empirically with antibiotics.

CD4 count suppression – Analysis of lymphocyte subsets indicates that treatment with cladribine is associated with prolonged depression of the CD4 counts. Prior to treatment, the mean CD4 count was 766/mcl. The mean CD4 count nadir, which occurred 4 to 6 months following treatment, was 272/mcl. Fifteen months after treatment, mean CD4 counts remained < 500/mcl. CD8 counts behaved similarly, though increasing counts were observed after 9 months. There were no associated opportunistic infections reported during this time.

Bone marrow hypocellularity – Another event of unknown clinical significance includes the observation of prolonged bone marrow hypocellularity. Bone marrow cellularity of < 35% was noted after 4 months in 34% of patients treated in two trials. This hypocellularity was noted 2.8 years later. It is not known whether the hypocellularity is the result of disease-related marrow fibrosis or if it is the result of cladribine toxicity. There was no apparent clinical effect on the peripheral blood counts.

Rash – The vast majority of rashes were mild and occurred in patients who were receiving or had recently been treated with other medications (eg, allopurinol, antibiotics) known to cause rash.

Nausea – Most episodes of nausea were mild, not accompanied by vomiting, and did not require treatment with antiemetics. In patients requiring antiemetics, nausea was easily controlled, most frequently with chlorpromazine.

Other adverse reactions reported during the first 2 weeks following treatment initiation by > 5% of patients included:

Overdosage

➤*Symptoms:* High doses of cladribine have been associated with: Irreversible neurologic toxicity (paraparesis/quadriparesis), acute nephrotoxicity, severe bone marrow suppression resulting in neutropenia, anemia and thrombocytopenia (see Warnings). There is no known specific antidote.

➤*Treatment:* Treatment of overdosage consists of discontinuation of cladribine, careful observation and appropriate supportive measures. Refer to General Management of Acute Overdosage. It is not known whether the drug can be removed from the circulation by dialysis or hemofiltration.

FLUDARABINE PHOSPHATE

Rx	Fludara (Berlex)	Powder for Injection, lyophilized: 50 mg[1]	In single-dose vials.

[1] With 50 mg mannitol and sodium hydroxide.

WARNING

Administer fludarabine under the supervision of a qualified physician experienced in the use of antineoplastic therapy. Fludarabine can severely suppress bone marrow function. When used at high doses in dose-ranging studies in patients with acute leukemia, fludarabine was associated with severe neurologic effects, including blindness, coma, and death. This severe CNS toxicity occurred in 36% of patients treated with doses approximately 4 times greater (96 mg/m^2/day for 5 to 7 days) than the recommended dose. Similar severe CNS toxicity has rarely occurred (0.2% or less) in patients treated at doses in the range of the dose recommended for chronic lymphocytic leukemia (see Warnings).

Instances of life-threatening and sometimes fatal autoimmune hemolytic anemia have been reported to occur after 1 or more cycles of treatment with fludarabine. Evaluate and closely monitor patients undergoing treatment with fludarabine for hemolysis.

In a clinical investigation using fludarabine in combination with pentostatin (deoxycoformycin) for the treatment of refractory chronic lymphocytic leukemia (CLL), there was an unacceptably high incidence of fatal pulmonary toxicity. Therefore, the use of fludarabine in combination with pentostatin is not recommended.

Indications

➤*CLL:* Treatment of patients with B-cell CLL who have not responded to or whose disease has progressed during treatment with at least 1 standard alkylating agent-containing regimen.

The safety and efficacy in previously untreated or nonrefractory patients with CLL have not been established.

➤*Unlabeled uses:* Fludarabine may also be useful in the treatment of non-Hodgkin lymphoma; may be used in combination therapy for the treatment of primary resistant or relapsing acute myelogenous leukemia (AML), acute lymphoblastic leukemia (ALL), and secondary AML.

Administration and Dosage

➤*Approved by the FDA:* April 22, 1991.

➤*Usual dose:* 25 mg/m^2 administered IV over a period of approximately 30 minutes daily for 5 consecutive days. Commence each 5 day course of treatment every 28 days. Dosage may be decreased or delayed based on evidence of hematologic or nonhematologic toxicity. Consider delaying or discontinuing the drug if neurotoxicity occurs.

A number of clinical settings may predispose to increased toxicity including advanced age, renal insufficiency, and bone marrow impairment. Monitor such patients closely for excessive toxicity and modify the dose accordingly.

Duration – The optimal duration of treatment has not been clearly established. It is recommended that 3 additional cycles be administered following the achievement of a maximal response and then discontinue the drug.

Renal function impairment – Patients with moderate renal function impairment (creatinine clearance 30 to 70 mL/min/1.73 m^2) should have a 20% dose reduction of fludarabine. Fludarabine should not be administered to patients with severely impaired renal function (creatinine clearance less than 30 mL/min/1.73 m^2).

Preparation of solution – When reconstituted with 2 mL of sterile water for injection, the solid cake should fully dissolve in 15 seconds or less; each mL of the resulting solution will contain 25 mg fludarabine phosphate, 25 mg mannitol, and sodium hydroxide. In clinical studies, the product has been diluted in 100 or 125 mL of 5% dextrose injection or 0.9% sodium chloride.

➤*Storage/Stability:* Store under refrigeration, between 2° to 8°C (36° to 46°F). Reconstituted fludarabine contains no antimicrobial preservative; use within 8 hours of reconstitution.

Actions

➤*Pharmacology:* Fludarabine is a fluorinated nucleotide analog of the antiviral agent vidarabine that is relatively resistant to deamination by adenosine deaminase. Fludarabine is rapidly dephosphorylated to 2-fluoro-ara-A and then phosphorylated intracellularly by deoxycytidine kinase to the active triphosphate, 2-fluoro-ara-ATP. This metabolite appears to act by inhibiting DNA polymerase alpha, ribonucleotide reductase, and DNA primase, thus inhibiting DNA synthesis. The mechanism of action of this antimetabolite is not completely characterized and may be multifaceted.

➤*Pharmacokinetics:*

Absorption/Distribution – Fludarabine is rapidly converted to the active metabolite, 2-fluoro-ara-A, within minutes after IV infusion. Consequently, clinical pharmacology studies have focused on 2-fluoro-ara-A pharmacokinetics. After 5 daily doses of 25 mg/m^2/day to cancer patients infused over 30 minutes, 2-fluoro-ara-A concentrations showed

a moderate accumulation and an approximate increase in plasma trough levels by a factor of approximately 2. In vitro, plasma protein binding of fludarabine ranged between 19% and 29%. A correlation was noted between the degree of absolute granulocyte count nadir and increased area under the concentration time curve (AUC).

Metabolism/Excretion – The terminal half-life of 2-fluoro-ara-A is approximately 20 hours. The total body clearance of the metabolite 2-fluoro-ara-A correlates with the creatinine clearance, indicating the importance of the renal excretion pathway. Renal clearance represents approximately 40% of the total body clearance.

➤*Clinical trials:* Two single-arm, open-label studies have been conducted in patients with CLL refractory to at least 1 prior standard alkylating agent-containing regimen.

Fludarabine Efficacy in Refractory CLL Patients		
	Studies	
Parameter	MDAH[1] (n = 48)	SWOG[2] (n = 31)
Overall objective response	48%	32%
Complete response	13%	13%
Partial response	35%	19%
Median time to response	7 weeks (range, 1 to 68)	21 weeks (range, 1 to 53)
Median duration of disease control	91 weeks	65 weeks
Median survival	43 weeks	52 weeks

[1] M.D. Anderson Cancer Center. Dosage: 22 to 40 mg/m^2/day for 5 days every 28 days.
[2] Southwest Oncology Group. Dosage: 15 to 25 mg/m^2/day for 5 days every 28 days.

The ability of fludarabine to induce a significant rate of response in refractory patients suggests minimal cross-resistance with commonly used anti-CLL agents.

Rai stage improved to stage 2 or better in 7 of 12 MDAH responders (58%) and in 5 of 7 SWOG responders (71%) who were stage 3 or 4 at baseline. In the combined studies, mean hemoglobin concentration improved from 9 g/dL at baseline to 11.8 g/dL at the time of response in a subgroup of anemic patients. Similarly, average platelet count improved from 63,500/mm^3 to 103,300/mm^3 at the time of response in a subgroup of patients who were thrombocytopenic at baseline.

Contraindications

Hypersensitivity to this drug or its components.

Warnings

➤*Dose-dependent toxicity:* There are clear dose-dependent toxic effects seen with fludarabine. Dose levels approximately 4 times greater (96 mg/m^2/day for 5 to 7 days) than those recommended for CLL (25 mg/m^2/day for 5 days) were associated with a syndrome characterized by delayed blindness, coma, and death. Symptoms appeared from 21 to 60 days following the last dose. Thirteen of 36 patients (36%) who received high doses (96 mg/m^2/day for 5 to 7 days) developed this severe neurotoxicity. This syndrome has been reported rarely in patients treated with doses in the range of the recommended CLL dose of 25 mg/m^2/day for 5 days every 28 days. The effect of chronic administration on the CNS is unknown; however, patients have received the recommended dose for up to 15 courses of therapy.

➤*Hematologic effects:* Severe bone marrow suppression, notably anemia, thrombocytopenia, and neutropenia, has occurred in patients treated with fludarabine. In solid tumor patients, the median time to nadir counts was 13 days (range, 3 to 25 days) for granulocytes and 16 days (range, 2 to 32 days) for platelets. Most patients had hematologic impairment at baseline either as a result of disease or as a result of prior myelosuppressive therapy. Cumulative myelosuppression may be seen. While chemotherapy-induced myelosuppression is often reversible, administration of fludarabine requires careful hematologic monitoring.

Several instances of trilineage bone marrow hypoplasia or aplasia resulting in pancytopenia, sometimes resulting in death, have been reported. The duration of clinically significant cytopenia in the reported cases has ranged from approximately 2 months to approximately 1 year. These episodes have occurred in previously treated or untreated patients. Life-threatening and sometimes fatal autoimmune hemolytic anemia have been reported to occur after 1 or more cycles of treatment with fludarabine. in patients with or without a previous history of autoimmune hemolytic anemia or a positive Coombs' test and who may or may not be in remission from their disease. Steroids may or may not be effective in controlling these hemolytic episodes. The majority of patients rechallenged with fludarabine developed a recurrence in the hemolytic process.

➤*Pulmonary toxicity:* In a clinical investigation using fludarabine in combination with pentostatin (deoxycoformycin) for the treatment of refractory CLL, there was an unacceptably high incidence of fatal pulmonary toxicity. Therefore, the use of fludarabine in combination with pentostatin is not recommended.

FLUDARABINE PHOSPHATE

➤*Fatalities:* Of the 133 CLL patients in the 2 trials, there were 29 fatalities during study. Approximately 50% of the fatalities were caused by infection and 25% caused by progressive disease.

➤*Renal function impairment:* Administer cautiously. The total body clearance of 2-fluoro-ara-A is directly correlated with serum creatinine, suggesting renal elimination of the compound. Reduce the fludarabine dose 20% in patients with moderate impairment of renal function and monitor closely. Fludarabine is not recommended for patients with severely impaired renal function.

➤*Mutagenesis:* Chromosomal aberrations were seen in an in vitro assay. Fludarabine also was determined to increase sister chromatid exchanges in vitro.

➤*Fertility impairment:* Studies in mice, rats, and dogs have demonstrated dose-related adverse effects on the male reproductive system. Observations consisted of a decrease in mean testicular weights in mice and rats with a trend toward decreased testicular weights in dogs and degeneration and necrosis of spermatogenic epithelium of the testes in mice, rats, and dogs.

➤*Pregnancy: Category D.* Fludarabine may cause fetal harm when administered to a pregnant woman. Fludarabine was teratogenic in rats and rabbits. At 10 and 30 mg/kg/day in rats, there was an increased incidence of various skeletal malformations; dose-related teratogenic effects manifested by external deformities and skeletal malformations were observed in rabbits at 5 and 8 mg/kg/day. There are no adequate and well-controlled studies in pregnant women. If fludarabine is used during pregnancy or if the patient becomes pregnant while taking this drug, apprise her of the potential hazard to the fetus. Advise women of childbearing potential to avoid becoming pregnant.

➤*Lactation:* It is not known whether this drug is excreted in breast milk. Decide whether to discontinue nursing or to discontinue the drug, taking into account the importance of the drug to the mother.

➤*Children:* Safety and efficacy have not been established. Fludarabine was evaluated in 62 pediatric patients (median, 10 years of age) with refractory acute leukemia (45 patients) or solid tumors (17 patients). The fludarabine regimen tested for pediatric ALL patients was a loading bolus of 10.5 mg/m²/day followed by a continuous infusion of 30.5 mg/m²/day for 5 days. In 12 pediatric patients with solid tumors, dose-limiting myelosuppression was observed with a loading dose of 8 mg/m²/day followed by a continuous infusion of 23.5 mg/m²/day for 5 days. The maximum tolerated dose was a loading dose of 7 mg/m²/day followed by a continuous infusion of 20 mg/m²/day for 5 days. Treatment toxicity included bone marrow suppression. Platelet counts appeared to be more sensitive to the effects of fludarabine than hemoglobin and white blood cell counts. Other adverse events included fever, chills, asthenia, rash, nausea, vomiting, diarrhea, and infection.

Precautions

➤*Monitoring:* During treatment, monitor the patient's hematologic profile (particularly neutrophils and platelets) regularly to determine the degree of hematopoietic suppression. Evaluate and closely monitor for hemolysis.

➤*Hematologic toxicity:* Fludarabine is a potent antineoplastic with potentially significant toxic side effects. Closely observe patients for signs of hematologic and nonhematologic toxicity. Periodic assessment of peripheral blood counts is recommended to detect the development of anemia, neutropenia, and thrombocytopenia.

➤*Tumor lysis syndrome:* Tumor lysis syndrome associated with fludarabine treatment has occurred in CLL patients with large tumor burdens. Because fludarabine can induce a response as early as the first week of treatment, take precautions in patients at risk of developing this complication.

Drug Interactions

The use of fludarabine in combination with pentostatin is not recommended because of the risk of severe pulmonary toxicity.

Adverse Reactions

Fludarabine Adverse Reactions in the MDAH and SWOG Studies (%)		
Adverse reaction	MDAH (n = 101)	SWOG (n = 32)
Cardiovascular		
Aneurysm	1	0
Angina	0	6
Arrhythmia	0	3
Cerebrovascular accident	0	3
CHF	0	3
Deep venous thrombosis	1	3
Edema	8	19
Myocardial infarction	0	3
Phlebitis	1	3
Supraventricular tachycardia	0	3
Transient ischemic attack	1	0

Fludarabine Adverse Reactions in the MDAH and SWOG Studies (%)		
Adverse reaction	MDAH (n = 101)	SWOG (n = 32)
CNS		
Cerebellar syndrome	1	0
Depression	1	0
Fatigue	10	38
Headache	3	0
Impaired mentation	1	0
Paresthesia	4	12
Sleep disorder	1	3
Weakness	9	65
Dermatologic		
Alopecia	0	3
Pruritus	1	3
Rash	15	15
Seborrhea	1	0
GI		
Anorexia	7	34
Cholelithiasis	0	3
Constipation	1	3
Diarrhea	15	13
Dysphagia	1	0
Esophagitis	3	0
GI bleeding	3	13
Liver failure	1	0
Mucositis	2	0
Nausea/Vomiting	36	31
Stomatitis	9	0
GU		
Abnormal renal function test	1	0
Dysuria	4	3
Hematuria	2	3
Hesitancy	0	3
Proteinuria	1	0
Renal failure	1	0
Urinary infection	2	15
Musculoskeletal		
Arthralgia	1	0
Myalgia	4	16
Osteoporosis	2	0
Respiratory		
Allergic pneumonitis	0	6
Bronchitis	1	0
Cough	10	44
Dyspnea	9	22
Epistaxis	1	0
Hemoptysis	1	6
Hypoxia	1	0
Pharyngitis	0	9
Pneumonia	16	22
Sinusitis	5	0
Upper respiratory tract infection	2	16
Miscellaneous		
Abnormal liver function test	1	3
Anaphylaxis	1	0
Chills	11	19
Dehydration	1	0
Diaphoresis	1	13
Fever	60	69
Hearing loss	2	6
Hemorrhage	1	0
Hyperglycemia	1	6
Infection	33	44
Malaise	8	6
Pain	20	22
Tumor lysis syndrome	1	0
Visual disturbance	3	15

The most common adverse events include: anorexia; chills; fatigue; fever; infection; malaise; myelosuppression (anemia, neutropenia, thrombocytopenia); nausea; vomiting; weakness. Serious opportunistic infections occurred in CLL patients treated with fludarabine. Frequently reported, clearly drug-related adverse events appear below.

➤*Cardiovascular:* Edema (frequent); pericardial effusion (1 patient).

➤*CNS:* Agitation, coma (have occurred at the recommended dose), confusion, objective weakness, peripheral neuropathy, visual disturbances, wrist-drop (1 case).

FLUDARABINE PHOSPHATE

➤*Dermatologic:* Skin toxicity, consisting primarily of skin rashes.

➤*GI:* Anorexia, diarrhea, GI bleeding, nausea, stomatitis, vomiting.

➤*GU:* Rare cases of hemorrhagic cystitis.

➤*Hematologic:* Hematologic events (neutropenia, thrombocytopenia, anemia) were reported in the majority of CLL patients (see Warnings). During treatment of 133 patients with CLL, the absolute neutrophil count decreased to less than 500/mm^3 in 59% of patients, hemoglobin decreased from pretreatment values by at least 2 g in 60%, and platelet count decreased from pretreatment values by at least 50% in 55% of patients. Myelosuppression may be severe, cumulative, and affect multiple cell lines. Bone marrow fibrosis occurred in 1 CLL patient. Trilineage bone marrow hypoplasia or aplasia resulting in pancytopenia, sometimes resulting in death, have been reported. Life-threatening and sometimes fatal autoimmune hemolytic anemia have been reported.

➤*Metabolic:* Tumor lysis syndrome, which may include hematuria, hyperkalemia, hyperphosphatemia, hyperuricemia, hypocalcemia, metabolic acidosis, renal failure, urate crystalluria. The onset of this syndrome may be heralded by flank pain and hematuria (see Precautions).

➤*Pulmonary:* Pneumonia (16% to 22%; a frequent manifestation of infection in CLL patients); pulmonary hypersensitivity reactions characterized by cough, dyspnea, and interstitial pulmonary infiltrate.

Postmarketing – Cases of severe pulmonary toxicity have been observed, which resulted in ARDS, respiratory distress, pulmonary hemorrhage, pulmonary fibrosis, and respiratory failure. After an infectious origin has been excluded, some patients experienced symptom improvement with corticosteroids.

Overdosage

High doses are associated with an irreversible CNS toxicity characterized by delayed blindness, coma, and death (see Warnings). High doses are also associated with severe thrombocytopenia and neutropenia caused by bone marrow suppression. There is no known specific antidote for fludarabine overdosage. Treatment consists of drug discontinuation and supportive therapy. Refer to General Management of Acute Overdosage.

MERCAPTOPURINE (6-Mercaptopurine; 6-MP)

Rx	**Purinethol** (GlaxoSmithKline)	**Tablets:** 50 mg	(Purinethol O4A). Off-white, scored. In 25s and 250s.

Indications

For remission induction and maintenance therapy of acute lymphatic leukemia. Response to mercaptopurine depends upon the subclassification of acute lymphatic leukemia (ALL) and age of patient (child or adult).

➤*Acute lymphatic (lymphocytic, lymphoblastic) leukemia:* Given as a single agent, mercaptopurine induces complete remission in ≈ 25% of children and 10% of adults. Reliance upon mercaptopurine alone is not justified for initial remission induction of ALL since combination chemotherapy with vincristine, prednisone and L-asparaginase more frequently induces complete remission induction than mercaptopurine alone or in combination. The induced complete remission in acute lymphatic leukemia is so brief without use of maintenance therapy that some form of drug therapy is considered essential. Mercaptopurine, as a single agent, can significantly prolong complete remission duration; however, combination therapy has produced remission longer than mercaptopurine alone.

➤*Acute myelogenous (and acute myelomonocytic) leukemia:* As a single agent, mercaptopurine will induce complete remission in approximately 10% of children and adults. These results are inferior to those achieved with combination chemotherapy.

Administration and Dosage

➤*Induction therapy:* Individualize dosage.

Usual initial dose is 2.5 mg/kg/day (100 to 200 mg in the average adult and 50 mg in an average 5-year-old). Children with acute leukemia tolerate this dose without difficulty in most cases. Continue daily for several weeks or more. If, after 4 weeks on this dosage there is no clinical improvement and no definite evidence of leukocyte or platelet depression, increase dosage up to 5 mg/kg/day.

A dosage of 2.5 mg/kg/day may result in a rapid fall in leukocyte count within 1 to 2 weeks in some adults with ALL and high total leukocyte counts.

Daily dosage may be given at one time. Calculate to the closest multiple of 25 mg.

Monitor the leukocyte count closely; because the drug may have a delayed action, discontinue treatment at the first sign of an abnormally large or rapid fall in leukocyte count or platelet count. If the leukocyte count or platelet count subsequently remains constant for 2 or 3 days, or rises, resume treatment.

➤*Maintenance therapy:* If complete hematologic remission is obtained with mercaptopurine alone or in combination with other agents, maintenance therapy is essential. Maintenance doses vary from patient to patient. Usual daily dose - 1.5 to 2.5 mg/kg/day as a single dose. In children with acute lymphatic leukemia in remission, superior results have been obtained when mercaptopurine has been combined with other agents (most frequently with methotrexate) for remission maintenance. Mercaptopurine should rarely be relied upon as a single agent for maintenance of remissions induced in acute leukemia.

Actions

➤*Pharmacology:* Mercaptopurine (6-MP) competes with hypoxanthine and guanine for the enzyme hypoxanthine-guanine phosphoribosyltransferase and is converted to thioinosinic acid (TIMP). This intracellular nucleotide inhibits several reactions involving inosinic acid (IMP). In addition, 6-methylthioinosinate (MTIMP) is formed by the methylation of TIMP. Both TIMP and MTIMP inhibit *de novo* purine ribonucleotide synthesis. Radiolabeled 6-MP may be recovered from deoxyribonucleic acid (DNA) in the form of deoxythioguanosine. Some mercaptopurine is converted to nucleotide derivatives of 6-thioguanine.

Animal tumors resistant to mercaptopurine often have lost the ability to convert mercaptopurine to TIMP. Resistance may be acquired by other means as well, particularly in human leukemias. It is not known which biochemical effects of mercaptopurine and its metabolites are directly or predominantly responsible for cell death.

➤*Pharmacokinetics:*

Absorption / Distribution – The absorption of oral mercaptopurine is incomplete and variable, averaging 50%. Recent reports using a more sensitive assay indicate bioavailability may be less (range from 5% to 37%). There is negligible entry of mercaptopurine into cerebrospinal fluid. Plasma protein binding averages 19% over the concentration range 10 to 50 mcg/ml.

Metabolism / Excretion – There are two major pathways for hepatic drug metabolism: Methylation of the sulfhydryl group and oxidation by the enzyme xanthine oxidase. Allopurinol inhibits xanthine oxidase and retards catabolism of mercaptopurine and its active metabolites. Plasma half-life averages 21 and 47 minutes in children and adults, respectively. Metabolites appear in urine within 2 hours. After 24 hours, > 50% of a dose is recovered in urine as intact drug and metabolites.

Contraindications

Prior resistance to this drug. There is usually complete cross-resistance between mercaptopurine and thioguanine.

Mercaptopurine is not effective for prophylaxis or treatment of CNS leukemia, chronic lymphatic leukemia, the lymphomas (including Hodgkin's disease) or solid tumors.

Warnings

➤*Bone marrow toxicity:* The most consistent dose-related toxicity is bone marrow suppression. It may be manifested by anemia, leukopenia or thrombocytopenia. This may also indicate progression of the underlying disease. Patients should report any fever, sore throat, signs of local infection, bleeding from any site or symptoms suggestive of anemia. Since mercaptopurine may have a delayed effect, withdraw medication temporarily at the first sign of an abnormally large fall in any formed blood elements. Toxic effects are often unavoidable during the induction phase of adult acute leukemia if remission induction is to be successful. Whether these effects demand modifying or ceasing dosage depends upon both the response of the underlying disease and availability of supportive facilities. Life-threatening infections and bleeding have occurred as a result of granulocytopenia and thrombocytopenia. Supportive therapy with platelet transfusions for bleeding, and antibiotics and granulocyte transfusions for sepsis, may be required.

The induction of complete remission of acute lymphatic leukemia frequently is associated with marrow hypoplasia. Maintenance of remission generally involves multiple drug regimens whose component agents cause myelosuppression. Anemia, leukopenia and thrombocytopenia are frequently observed. Dosages and schedules are adjusted to prevent life-threatening cytopenias.

If it is not the intent to induce bone marrow hypoplasia, discontinue the drug temporarily at the first evidence of any abnormally large fall in white blood cell (WBC) count, platelet count or hemoglobin concentration. With severe depression of the formed elements of the blood due to mercaptopurine, the bone marrow may appear hypoplastic or normocellular on aspiration or biopsy.

Evaluate hemoglobin or hematocrit, total WBC, differential counts and platelet counts weekly during therapy. Where the cause of fluctuation in the formed elements in the peripheral blood is obscure, bone marrow examination may help evaluate marrow status. Base the decision to continue mercaptopurine on the absolute hematologic values and the rate at which changes occur in these values, particularly during the induction phase of acute leukemia. Perform complete blood counts more frequently than once a week to evaluate therapeutic effect. Dosage may

MERCAPTOPURINE (6-Mercaptopurine; 6-MP)

need to be reduced when combined with other drugs whose primary or secondary toxicity is myelosuppression.

▶*Hepatotoxicity:* Hepatotoxicity occurs with greatest frequency when doses of 2.5 mg/kg/day are exceeded. Deaths have occurred from hepatic necrosis. The histologic pattern includes both intrahepatic cholestasis and parenchymal cell necrosis, either of which may predominate. It is not clear how much hepatic damage is due to direct toxicity from the drug and how much may be due to a hypersensitivity reaction.

Published reports cite widely varying incidences of overt hepatotoxicity. In patients with various neoplastic diseases, mercaptopurine was given orally in doses ranging from 2.5 to 5 mg/kg without any hepatotoxicity. No definite clinical evidence of liver damage could be ascribed to the drug, although an occasional case of serum hepatitis occurred in patients receiving 6-MP who previously had transfusions. In smaller cohorts of adult and pediatric leukemic patients, the incidence of hepatotoxicity ranged from 0% to 6%. In one report, jaundice occurred more frequently (40%), especially when doses exceeded 2.5 mg/kg.

Usually, clinically detectable jaundice appears early in treatment (1 to 2 months), but has occurred from 1 week to 8 years after the start of treatment. In some patients, jaundice cleared following drug withdrawal and reappeared with reintroduction.

Monitoring – Monitoring of serum transaminase, alkaline phosphatase and bilirubin levels may allow early detection of hepatotoxicity. Monitor weekly when beginning therapy and monthly thereafter. More frequent liver function tests may be advisable in patients receiving other hepatotoxic drugs or with known preexisting liver disease. Approach all combination therapy involving mercaptopurine with caution. Use of mercaptopurine with doxorubicin was hepatotoxic in 19 of 20 patients undergoing remission induction therapy for leukemia resistant to previous therapy.

Hepatotoxicity has been associated with anorexia, jaundice, diarrhea and ascites. Hepatic encephalopathy has occurred. The onset of clinical jaundice, hepatomegaly or anorexia with tenderness in the right hypochondrium are immediate indications for withholding mercaptopurine until the exact etiology can be identified. Upon any evidence of deterioration in liver function, toxic hepatitis or biliary stasis, promptly discontinue drug and search for an etiology of hepatotoxicity.

▶*Immunosuppression:* This may be manifested by decreased cellular hypersensitivities and impaired allograft rejection. Immunity to infectious agents or vaccines will be subnormal. The degree of immunosuppression depends on antigen dose and temporal relationship to drug. Carefully consider with regard to intercurrent infections and risk of subsequent neoplasia.

▶*Renal function impairment:* Start with smaller doses due to the possibility of slower drug elimination and a greater cumulative effect.

▶*Carcinogenesis:* Mercaptopurine causes chromosomal aberrations in humans. Carcinogenic potential exists in humans, but risk is unknown.

▶*Pregnancy: Category D.* Mercaptopurine can cause fetal harm when administered to a pregnant woman. Women receiving the drug in the first trimester of pregnancy have an increased incidence of abortion; the risk of malformation in offspring surviving first trimester exposure is not known. In a series of 28 women receiving mercaptopurine after the first trimester, three mothers died undelivered, one delivered a stillborn child and one aborted; there were no cases of macroscopically abnormal fetuses. Use during pregnancy, especially the first trimester, only if the benefit justifies the risk to the fetus. The drug's effect on fertility is unknown. There are no adequate and well controlled studies in pregnant women. Inform patient of potential hazard to the fetus. Advise women of childbearing potential to avoid pregnancy.

▶*Lactation:* It is not known whether mercaptopurine is excreted in breast milk. Because of potential for serious adverse reactions in nursing infants, decide whether to discontinue nursing or the drug, taking into account the drug's importance to the mother.

Precautions

▶*Pancreatitis:* An increased risk of pancreatitis may be associated with the investigational use of mercaptopurine in inflammatory bowel disease.

Drug Interactions

Mercaptopurine Drug Interactions			
Precipitant drug	Object drug*		Description
Allopurinol	Mercaptopurine	↑	When administered concomitantly with mercaptopurine, reduce mercaptopurine to ⅓ to ¼ the usual dose. Failure to observe this dosage reduction will delay catabolism of mercaptopurine and increase likelihood of severe toxicity.
Trimethroprim-sulfamethoxazole			When coadministered with mercaptopurine, enhanced marrow suppression has occurred.

* ↑ = Object drug increased.

Adverse Reactions

▶*Dermatologic:* Dermatologic reactions can occur as a consequence of disease; however, mercaptopurine may cause skin rashes and hyperpigmentation.

▶*GI:* GI ulceration has occurred. Nausea, vomiting and anorexia are uncommon during initial administration. Mild diarrhea and sprue-like symptoms have been noted, but it is difficult to attribute these to the medication.

▶*Miscellaneous:*

Bone marrow toxicity and hepatotoxicity – See Warnings.

Oral lesions – These are rare and resemble thrush rather than antifolic ulcerations.

Hyperuricemia – This occurs as a consequence of rapid cell lysis accompanying the antineoplastic effect. Minimize adverse effects by increasing hydration, urine alkalinization and the prophylactic administration of allopurinol (see Drug Interactions).

Drug fever – This has occurred rarely with mercaptopurine. Exclude the more common causes of pyrexia, such as sepsis, in patients with acute leukemia.

Overdosage

Discontinue the drug immediately when toxicity develops. If a patient is seen immediately following overdosage of the drug, induced emesis may be useful.

Signs and symptoms of overdosage may be immediate (anorexia, nausea, vomiting, diarrhea) or delayed (myelosuppression, liver dysfunction and gastroenteritis). Dialysis cannot be expected to clear mercaptopurine. Hemodialysis is of marginal use due to the rapid intracellular incorporation of mercaptopurine into active metabolites with long persistence. There is no known pharmacologic antagonist.

Patient Information

Contraceptive measures are recommended during therapy for men and women.

Notify physician if fever, sore throat, chills, nausea, vomiting, unusual bleeding or bruising, yellow discoloration of the skin or eyes, abdominal pain, flank or joint pain, swelling of the feet or legs, or symptoms suggestive of anemia occurs.

May cause diarrhea, fever and weakness; notify physician if these become pronounced.

Maintain adequate fluid intake.

PENTOSTATIN (2'-deoxycoformycin; DCF)

Rx   **Nipent** (Super Gen)   **Powder for Injection:** 10 mg/vial[1]   In single dose vials.

[1] With 50 mg mannitol per vial.

> ### WARNING
>
> Administer under the supervision of a physician qualified and experienced in the use of cancer chemotherapeutic agents. The use of higher doses than those specified is not recommended. Dose-limiting severe renal, liver, pulmonary and CNS toxicities occurred in Phase I studies that used pentostatin at higher doses than recommended (20 to 50 mg/m^2 in divided doses over 5 days).
>
> In a clinical investigation in patients with refractory chronic lymphocytic leukemia using pentostatin at the recommended dose in combination with fludarabine phosphate, four of six patients had severe or fatal pulmonary toxicity. The use of pentostatin in combination with fludarabine phosphate is not recommended.

Indications

Single agent for adult patients with alpha-interferon-refractory hairy cell leukemia, defined as progressive disease after a minimum of 3 months of alpha-interferon treatment or no response after a minimum of 6 months of alpha-interferon.

Administration and Dosage

Hydrate with 500 to 1000 ml of 5% Dextrose in 0.5 Normal Saline or equivalent before pentostatin administration. Administer an additional 500 ml of 5% Dextrose or equivalent after pentostatin is given.

➤*Alpha-interferon-refractory hairy cell leukemia:* 4 mg/m^2 every other week. Pentostatin may be administered IV by bolus injection or diluted in a larger volume and given over 20 to 30 minutes. (See Preparation of IV Solution.)

Higher doses are not recommended.

No extravasation injuries were reported in clinical studies.

➤*Duration/Response:* The optimal duration of treatment has not been determined. In the absence of major toxicity and with observed continuing improvement, treat the patient until a complete response has been achieved. Although not established, the administration of two additional doses has been recommended following the achievement of a complete response.

Assess all patients receiving pentostatin at 6 months for response to treatment. If the patient has not achieved a complete or partial response, discontinue treatment.

If the patient has achieved a partial response, continue treatment in an effort to achieve a complete response. At any time that a complete response is achieved thereafter, two additional doses of pentostatin are recommended; then stop treatment. If the best response to treatment at the end of 12 months is a partial response, stop treatment with pentostatin.

➤*Therapy/Dose discontinuation:* Withholding or discontinuing individual doses may be needed when severe adverse reactions occur. Withhold drug treatment in patients with severe rash, and withhold or discontinue in patients showing evidence of CNS toxicity.

Withhold treatment in patients with active infection occurring during the treatment; may resume treatment when the infection is controlled.

Patients who have elevated serum creatinine should have their dose withheld and a Ccr determined. There are insufficient data to recommend a starting or a subsequent dose for patients with impaired renal function (Ccr < 60 ml/min).

➤*Renal function impairment:* Treat patients only when potential benefit justifies potential risk. Two patients with impaired renal function (Ccr 50 to 60 ml/min) achieved complete response without unusual adverse events when treated with 2 mg/m^2.

➤*Hematologic effects:* No dosage reduction is recommended at the start of therapy in patients with anemia, neutropenia or thrombocytopenia. In addition, dosage reductions are not recommended during treatment in patients with anemia and thrombocytopenia if patients can be otherwise supported hematologically. Temporarily withhold pentostatin if the absolute neutrophil count falls below 200 cells/mm^3 during treatment in a patient who had an initial neutrophil count > 500 cells/mm^3; treatment may be resumed when the count returns to predose levels.

➤*Preparation of IV solution:*
1.) Follow procedures for proper handling and disposal of anticancer drugs. Treat spills and wastes with 5% sodium hypochlorite solution prior to disposal.
2.) Protective clothing including polyethylene gloves must be worn.
3.) Transfer 5 ml Sterile Water for Injection, USP to the vial containing pentostatin and mix thoroughly to obtain complete dissolution of a solution yielding 2 mg/ml.

4.) Pentostatin may be given IV by bolus injection or diluted in a larger volume (25 to 50 ml) with 5% Dextrose Injection, USP or 0.9% Sodium Chloride Injection, USP. Dilution of the entire contents of a reconstituted vial with 25 or 50 ml provides a pentostatin concentration of 0.33 or 0.18 mg/ml, respectively, for the diluted solutions.
5.) Pentostatin solution, when diluted for infusion with 5% Dextrose Injection, USP or 0.9% Sodium Chloride Injection, USP does not interact with PVC infusion containers or administration sets at concentrations of 0.18 to 0.33 mg/ml.

➤*Storage/Stability:* Pentostatin vials are stable when stored at refrigerated temperatures (2° to 8°C; 36° to 46°F) for the period stated on the package. Vials reconstituted or reconstituted and further diluted as directed may be stored at room temperature and ambient light; however, use within 8 hours because pentostatin contains no preservatives.

Actions

➤*Pharmacology:* Pentostatin is a potent transition state inhibitor of the enzyme adenosine deaminase (ADA) and is isolated from fermentation cultures of Streptomyces antibioticus. The greatest activity of ADA is found in cells of the lymphoid system with T-cells having higher activity than B-cells and T-cell malignancies having higher ADA activity than B-cell malignancies. Pentostatin inhibition of ADA, particularly in the presence of adenosine or deoxyadenosine, leads to cytotoxicity due to elevated intracellular levels of d;ATP which can block DNA synthesis through inhibition of ribonucleotide reductase. Pentostatin can also inhibit RNA synthesis as well as cause increased DNA damage. In addition to elevated dATP, these mechanisms may contribute to the overall cytotoxic effect of pentostatin. However, the precise mechanism of pentostatin's antitumor effect in hairy cell leukemia is not known.

➤*Pharmacokinetics:* In rats pentostatin concentrations were highest in the kidneys with very little CNS penetration.

In man, following a single dose of 4 mg/m^2 pentostatin infused over 5 minutes, the distribution half-life was 11 minutes, the mean terminal half-life was 5.7 hours, the mean plasma clearance was 68 ml/min/m^2, and ≈ 90% of the dose was excreted in the urine as unchanged pentostatin or metabolites as measured by adenosine deaminase inhibitory activity. The plasma protein binding of pentostatin is low, ≈ 4%.

A positive correlation was observed between pentostatin clearance and creatinine clearance (Ccr) in patients with Ccr values ranging from 60 to 130 ml/min. Pentostatin half-life in patients with renal impairment (Ccr < 50 ml/min) was 18 hours, which was much longer than that observed in patients with normal renal function (Ccr > 60 ml/min), which was about 6 hours.

➤*Clinical trials:* Patients with hairy cell leukemia (n = 133) previously treated with alpha-interferon were treated with pentostatin in five clinical studies. Forty-four of these patients were refractory to alpha-interferon and were evaluable for response to pentostatin. Pentostatin was administered at a dose of 4 mg/m^2 every other week for 3 months; responding patients received 3 additional months (M.D. Anderson Hospital study). Another group of patients received 4 mg/m^2 pentostatin every other week for 3 months; responding patients were treated monthly for up to 9 additional months (Cancer and Leukemia Group B study; CALGB). A complete response required clearing of the peripheral blood and bone marrow of hairy cells, normalization of organomegaly and lymphadenopathy, and recovery of the hemoglobin to at least 12 g/dl, platelet count to at least 100,000/mm^3 and granulocyte count to at least 1500/mm^3. A partial response required that the percentage of hairy cells in the blood and bone marrow decrease by > 50%, enlarged organs and lymph nodes had to decrease by > 50%, and hematologic parameters had to meet the same criteria as for a complete response. For those patients who were clearly refractory to alpha-interferon, the complete response rate was 58% and the partial response rate was 28% giving a total response rate (complete plus partial responses) of 86%. Median time to achieve a response was 4.7 months (range, 2.9 to 24.1 months). Duration of response ranged from 1.4 to 35.1+ months in the CALGB study (median > 7.7 months) and from 1.3+ to 31.2+ months for the M.D. Anderson study (median > 15.2 months). Median duration of follow-up ranged from 3.9 months in the CALGB study to 19.3 months in the M.D. Anderson study. Only 4 of 20 and 2 of 13 responding patients had relapsed, respectively.

Responding patients with abnormal peripheral blood counts at the start of therapy showed increases in their hemoglobin, granulocyte count and platelet count in response to treatment with pentostatin.

Contraindications

Hypersensitivity to pentostatin.

Warnings

➤*Myelosuppression:* Patients with hairy cell leukemia may experience myelosuppression, primarily during the first few courses of treatment. Patients with infections prior to pentostatin treatment have in some cases developed worsening of their condition leading to death,

PENTOSTATIN (2'-deoxycoformycin; DCF)

whereas others have achieved complete response. Treat patients with infection only when the potential benefit justifies the potential risk to the patient. Attempt to control the infection before treatment is initiated or resumed.

In progressive hairy cell leukemia, initial courses of pentostatin were associated with worsening of neutropenia. Therefore, frequent monitoring of complete blood counts during this time is necessary. If severe neutropenia continues beyond initial cycles, evaluate for disease status, including a bone marrow examination.

➤*Renal toxicity:* Renal toxicity was observed at higher doses in early studies; however, in patients treated at the recommended dose, elevations in serum creatinine were usually minor and reversible. Some patients who began treatment with normal renal function had evidence of mild to moderate toxicity at a final assessment.

➤*Rashes:* Rashes, occasionally severe, were commonly reported and may worsen with continued treatment. Withholding of treatment may be required.

➤*Mutagenesis:* Pentostatin was nonmutagenic when tested with various Salmonella typhimurium strains; however, when tested with strain TA-100, a repeatable statistically significant response trend was observed with and without metabolic activation. Formulated pentostatin was clastogenic in the in vivo mouse bone marrow micronucleus assay at 20, 120 and 240 mg/kg.

➤*Fertility impairment:* In a 5 day IV toxicity study in dogs, mild seminiferous tubular degeneration was observed with doses of 1 and 4 mg/kg. The possible adverse effects on fertility in humans have not been determined.

➤*Pregnancy: Category D.* Pentostatin can cause fetal harm when administered to a pregnant woman. Pentostatin was administered IV to pregnant rats on days 6 through 15 of gestation; drug-related maternal toxicity occurred at doses of 0.1 and 0.75 mg/kg/day (0.6 and 4.5 mg/m^2). Teratogenic effects were observed at 0.75 mg/kg/day manifested by increased incidence of various skeletal malformations. In another study, fetal malformations that occurred were an omphalocele at 0.05 mg/kg (0.3 mg/m^2), gastroschisis at 0.75 and 1 mg/kg/day (4.5 and 6 mg/m^2), and a flexure defect of the hind limbs at 0.75 mg/kg/day (4.5 mg/m^2). Pentostatin was also teratogenic in mice when administered as a single 2 mg/kg (6 mg/m^2) intraperitoneal injection on day 7 of gestation. Pentostatin was not teratogenic in rabbits when administered IV on days 6 through 18 of gestation; however, maternal toxicity, abortions, early deliveries and deaths occurred in all drug-treated groups. There are no adequate and well controlled studies in pregnant women. If pentostatin is used during pregnancy, or if the patient becomes pregnant while taking this drug, apprise her of the potential hazard to the fetus. Advise women of childbearing potential to avoid becoming pregnant while taking this drug.

➤*Lactation:* It is not known whether pentostatin is excreted in breast milk. Decide whether to discontinue nursing or discontinue the drug, taking into account the importance of the drug to the mother.

➤*Children:* Safety and efficacy in children or adolescents have not been established.

Precautions

➤*Monitoring:* Therapy with pentostatin requires regular patient observation and monitoring of hematologic parameters and blood chemistry values. If severe adverse reactions occur, withhold the drug and take appropriate corrective measures.

Prior to initiating therapy, assess renal function with a serum creatinine or a Ccr assay. Perform complete blood counts and serum creatinine before each dose and at other appropriate periods during therapy. Severe neutropenia has been observed following the early courses of treatment; therefore, frequent monitoring of complete blood counts is recommended during this time. If hematologic parameters do not improve with subsequent courses, evaluate patients for disease status, including a bone marrow examination. Perform periodic monitoring of the peripheral blood for hairy cells to assess the response to treatment. In addition, bone marrow aspirates and biopsies may be required at 2 to 3 month intervals to assess response to treatment.

➤*CNS toxicity:* Withhold or discontinue therapy in those with evidence of CNS toxicity.

Drug Interactions

➤*Allopurinol:* Allopurinol and pentostatin are both associated with skin rashes. Based on clinical studies in 25 refractory patients, combined use did not appear to produce a higher incidence of skin rashes than observed with pentostatin alone. One patient experienced a hypersensitivity vasculitis that resulted in death. It was unclear whether this adverse event and subsequent death resulted from the drug combination.

➤*Fludarabine:* Concurrent use with pentostatin is not recommended because it may be associated with an increased risk of fatal pulmonary toxicity (see Warning Box).

➤*Vidarabine:* Pentostatin enhances the effects of vidarabine. The combined use may result in an increase in adverse reactions associated

with each drug. The therapeutic benefit of the drug combination has not been established.

Adverse Reactions

Pentostatin Adverse Reactions (%)	
Adverse reaction	Incidence
Cardiovascular	
Arrhythmia	3-10
Abnormal ECG	3-10
Thrombophlebitis	3-10
Hemorrhage	3-10
CNS	
Headache	13
Neurologic, CNS	11
Anxiety	3-10
Confusion	3-10
Depression	3-10
Dizziness	3-10
Insomnia	3-10
Nervousness	3-10
Paresthesia	3-10
Somnolence	3-10
Abnormal thinking	3-10
Dermatologic	
Rash	26
Skin disorder	17
Eczema	3-10
Dry skin	3-10
Herpes simplex/zoster	3-10
Maculopapular rash	3-10
Vesiculobullous rash	3-10
Pruritus	3-10
Seborrhea	3-10
Skin discoloration	3-10
Sweating	3-10
GI	
Nausea/Vomiting	22-53
Anorexia	16
Diarrhea	15
Constipation	3-10
Flatulence	3-10
Stomatitis	3-10
GU	
Genitourinary disorder	15
Hematuria	3-10
Dysuria	3-10
Increased BUN	3-10
Increased creatinine	3-10
Hematologic/Lymphatic	
Leukopenia	60
Anemia	35
Thrombocytopenia	32
Ecchymosis	3-10
Lymphadenopathy	3-10
Petechia	3-10
Metabolic/Nutritional	
Weight loss	3-10
Peripheral edema	3-10
Increased LDH	3-10
Hepatic	
Hepatic disorder/elevated liver function tests	19
Respiratory	
Cough	17
Upper respiratory tract infection	16
Lung disorder	12
Bronchitis	3-10
Dyspnea	3-10
Epistaxis	3-10
Lung edema	3-10
Pneumonia	3-10
Pharyngitis	3-10
Rhinitis	3-10
Sinusitis	3-10
Musculoskeletal	
Myalgia	11
Arthralgia	3-10

Purine Analogs and Related Agents

PENTOSTATIN (2'-deoxycoformycin; DCF)

Pentostatin Adverse Reactions (%)	
Adverse reaction	Incidence
Special senses	
Abnormal vision	3-10
Conjunctivitis	3-10
Ear pain	3-10
Eye pain	3-10
Miscellaneous	
Fever	42
Infection	36
Fatigue	29
Pain	20
Allergic reaction	11
Chills	11
Death	3-10
Sepsis	3-10
Chest pain	3-10
Abdominal pain	3-10
Back pain	3-10
Flu syndrome	3-10
Asthenia	3-10
Malaise	3-10
Neoplasm	3-10

The adverse events listed in the preceding table were reported during clinical studies with pentostatin in patients with hairy cell leukemia who were refractory to alpha-interferon therapy. Most patients experienced an adverse event. The drug association is uncertain since the adverse reactions may be associated with the disease itself (eg, fever, infection, anemia), but other events, such as the GI symptoms, hematologic suppression, rashes and abnormal liver function tests, can in many cases be attributed to the drug. Most adverse events that were assessed for severity were either mild (52%) or moderate (26%) and diminished in frequency with continued therapy; 11% of patients withdrew from treatment due to an adverse event.

The remaining adverse events occurred in < 3% of patients; their relationship to pentostatin is uncertain: Abscess; enlarged abdomen; ascites; cellulitis; cyst; face edema; fibrosis; granuloma; hernia; injection-site hemorrhage or inflammation; moniliasis; neck rigidity; pelvic pain; photosensitivity reaction; anaphylactoid reaction; immune system disorder; mucous membrane disorder; neck pain.

➤*Cardiovascular:* Aortic stenosis; arterial anomaly; cardiomegaly; congestive heart failure; cardiac arrest; flushing; hypertension; myocardial infarct; palpitation; shock; varicose vein.

➤*CNS:* Agitation; amnesia; apathy; ataxia; CNS depression; coma; convulsions; abnormal dreams; depersonalization; emotional lability; facial paralysis; abnormal gait; hyperesthesia; hypesthesia; hypertonia; incoordination; decreased libido; neuropathy; postural dizziness; decreased reflexes; stupor; tremor; vertigo.

➤*Dermatologic:* Acne; alopecia; contact dermatitis; exfoliative dermatitis; fungal dermatitis; psoriasis; benign skin neoplasm; subcutaneous nodule; skin hypertrophy; urticaria.

➤*GI:* Colitis; dysphagia; eructation; gastritis; GI hemorrhage; gum hemorrhage; hepatitis; hepatomegaly; intestinal obstruction; jaundice; leukoplakia; melena; periodontal abscess; proctitis; abnormal stools; dyspepsia; esophagitis; gingivitis; hepatic failure; mouth disorder.

➤*Hematologic/Lymphatic:* Abnormal erythrocytes; leukocytosis; pancytopenia; purpura; splenomegaly; eosinophilia; hematologic disorder; hemolysis; lymphoma-like reaction; thrombocythemia.

➤*Metabolic/Nutritional:* Acidosis; increased creatine phosphokinase; dehydration; diabetes mellitus; increased gamma globulins; gout; abnormal healing; hypocholesterolemia; weight gain; hyponatremia.

➤*Musculoskeletal:* Arthritis; bone pain; osteomyelitis; pathological fracture.

➤*Respiratory:* Asthma; atelectasis; hemoptysis; hyperventilation; hypoventilation; laryngitis; larynx edema; lung fibrosis; pleural effusion; pneumothorax; pulmonary embolus; increased sputum.

➤*Special senses:* Blepharitis; cataract; deafness; diplopia; exophthalmos; lacrimation disorder; optic neuritis; otitis media; parosmia; retinal detachment; taste perversion; tinnitus. One patient developed unilateral uveitis with vision loss.

➤*GU:* Albuminuria; fibrocystic breast; glycosuria; gynecomastia; hydronephrosis; kidney failure; oliguria; polyuria; pyuria; toxic nephropathy; urinary frequency/retention/urgency; urinary tract infection; impaired urination; urolithiasis; vaginitis.

➤*Lab test abnormalities:* Liver function test elevations occurred during treatment and were generally reversible.

Overdosage

➤*Symptoms:* Pentostatin administered at higher doses than recommended (20 to 50 mg/m^2 in divided doses over 5 days) was associated with deaths due to severe renal, hepatic, pulmonary and CNS toxicity.

➤*Treatment:* Management would include general supportive measures through any period of toxicity that occurs. Refer to General Management of Acute Overdosage.

THIOGUANINE (TG; 6-Thioguanine)

Rx	**Tabloid** (GlaxoSmithKline)	**Tablets:** 40 mg	Lactose. (Wellcome U3B). Greenish yellow, scored. In 25s.

WARNING

Thioguanine is a potent drug. Do not use unless a diagnosis of acute nonlymphocytic leukemia has been adequately established and the responsible physician is knowledgeable in assessing response to chemotherapy.

Indications

➤*Acute nonlymphocytic leukemias:* For the remission induction, consolidation, and maintenance therapy of acute nonlymphocytic leukemias. Response depends upon the age of the patient (younger patients faring better than older) and previous treatment. Reliance upon thioguanine alone is seldom justified for initial remission induction of acute nonlymphocytic leukemias because combination chemotherapy including thioguanine results in more frequent remission induction and longer duration of remission than thioguanine alone.

Thioguanine is not effective in chronic lymphocytic leukemia, Hodgkin lymphoma, multiple myeloma, or solid tumors. Although thioguanine is one of several agents with activity in the treatment of the chronic phase of chronic myelogenous leukemia, more objective responses are observed with busulfan; therefore, busulfan is usually regarded as the preferred drug.

➤*Unlabeled uses:* Possible second-line treatment for Crohn disease.

Administration and Dosage

Individualize dosage.

➤*Initial dosage for children and adults:* Approximately 2 mg/kg/day orally. If after 4 weeks there is no clinical improvement and no leukocyte or platelet depression, the dosage may be cautiously increased to 3 mg/kg/day. The total daily dose may be given at one time.

➤*Combination therapy:* Of 163 children with previously untreated acute nonlymphocytic leukemia, 96 (59%) obtained complete remission with a multiple-drug protocol including thioguanine, prednisone, cytarabine, cyclophosphamide, and vincristine. Remission was maintained with daily thioguanine, 4 day pulses of cytarabine and cyclo-phosphamide, and a single dose of vincristine every 28 days. The median duration of remission was 11.5 months. Of previously untreated adults with acute nonlymphocytic leukemias, 53% attained remission following use of the combination of thioguanine and cytarabine. A median duration of remission of 8.8 months was achieved with the multiple-drug maintenance that included thioguanine.

➤*Concomitant therapy:* In contrast to mercaptopurine or azathioprine, the dosage of thioguanine does not need to be reduced during coadministration of allopurinol.

➤*Storage/Stability:* Store at 15° to 25°C (59° to 77°F) in a dry place.

Actions

➤*Pharmacology:* Thioguanine, an analog of the nucleic acid constituent guanine, is closely related structurally and functionally to 6-mercaptopurine.

Thioguanine competes with hypoxanthine and guanine for the enzyme hypoxanthine-guanine phosphoribosyltransferase (HGPRTase) and is converted to 6-thioguanylic acid (TGMP). TGMP interferes at several points with the synthesis of guanine nucleotides. It inhibits de novo purine biosynthesis by inhibiting glutamine-5-phosphoribosylpyrophosphate amidotransferase. Thioguanine nucleotides are incorporated into both RNA and DNA by phosphodiester linkages and incorporation of such fraudulent bases may contribute to the cytotoxicity of thioguanine.

Thioguanine has multiple metabolic effects. Its tumor inhibitory properties may be because of one or more of its effects on feedback inhibition of de novo purine synthesis, inhibition of purine nucleotide interconversions, or incorporation into DNA and RNA. The net consequence of its actions is a sequential blockade of the synthesis and utilization of the purine nucleotides.

Resistance may result from the loss of HGPRTase activity (inability to convert thioguanine to TGMP) or increased catabolism of TGMP by a nonspecific phosphatase. Although variable, cross-resistance with mercaptopurine usually occurs.

THIOGUANINE (TG; 6-Thioguanine)

➤*Pharmacokinetics:*

Absorption/Distribution – Oral absorption averages 30% (14% to 46%). Following oral administration of ^{35}S-6-thioguanine, total plasma radioactivity reached a maximum at 8 hours and declined slowly thereafter.

Intravenous administration of ^{35}S-6-thioguanine disclosed a median plasma half-life of 80 minutes (25 to 240 minutes) when the compound was given in single doses of 65 to 300 mg/m^2. There was no correlation between the plasma half-life and the dose. Thioguanine does not appear to reach therapeutic concentrations in the CSF.

Metabolism/Excretion – The catabolism of thioguanine and its metabolites is complex. Only trace quantities of parent drug are excreted in the urine. However, a methylated metabolite, 2-amino-6-methylthiopurine (MTG), appeared very early, rose to a maximum 6 to 8 hours after drug administration, and was still being excreted after 12 to 22 hours. Radiolabeled sulfate appeared somewhat later than MTG, but was the principal metabolite after 8 hours. Thiouric acid and some unidentified products were found in the urine in small amounts.

Contraindications

Prior resistance to this drug. There is usually complete cross-resistance between mercaptopurine and thioguanine.

Warnings

➤*Bone marrow suppression:* The most consistent dose-related toxicity is bone marrow suppression. This may be manifested by anemia, leukopenia, thrombocytopenia, or any combination of these. Any one of these findings may also reflect progression of the underlying disease. Since thioguanine may have a delayed effect, it is important to withdraw the medication temporarily at the first sign of an abnormally large fall in any of the formed elements of the blood.

There are individuals with an inherited deficiency of the enzyme thiopurine methyltransferase (TPMT) who may be unusually sensitive to the myelosuppressive effects of mercaptopurine and prone to developing rapid bone marrow suppression following the initiation of treatment. This problem could be exacerbated by coadministration with drugs that inhibit TPMT (eg, olsalazine, mesalazine, sulfasalazine).

Frequently evaluate hemoglobin concentration or hematocrit, total white blood cell (WBC) and differential counts and quantitative platelet count during therapy. Where the cause of fluctuation in the formed elements in the peripheral blood is obscure, bone marrow examination may help evaluate marrow status. Base the decision to change thioguanine dosage on the absolute and rate of change of hematologic values. During the induction phase of acute leukemia, perform CBCs more frequently to evaluate therapeutic effect. The thioguanine dosage may need to be reduced when combined with other myelosuppressive drugs.

Myelosuppression is often unavoidable during the induction phase of adult acute nonlymphocytic leukemia if remission response is to be successful. Whether this demands modification or cessation of dosage depends upon both the response of the underlying disease and availability of supportive facilities. Life-threatening infections and bleeding have occurred as a result of thioguanine-induced granulocytopenia and thrombocytopenia.

➤*Carcinogenesis:* Thioguanine is potentially mutagenic and carcinogenic; consider risk of carcinogenesis when administering thioguanine.

➤*Elderly:* In general, dose selection for an elderly patient should be cautious, usually starting at the low end of the dosing range, reflecting the greater frequency of decreased hepatic, renal, or cardiac function, and of concomitant disease or other drug therapy.

➤*Pregnancy: Category D.* Drugs such as thioguanine are potential mutagens and teratogens. Thioguanine may cause fetal harm when administered to a pregnant woman. Thioguanine is teratogenic in rats at doses 5 times the human dose. When given to the rat on the fourth and fifth days of gestation, 13% of surviving placentas did not contain fetuses; 19% of offspring were malformed or stunted. Malformations included generalized edema, cranial defects and general skeletal hypoplasia, hydrocephalus, ventral hernia, situs inversus, and incomplete limb development. There are no adequate and well-controlled studies in pregnant women. Inform patient of the potential hazard to the fetus. Advise women of childbearing potential to avoid becoming pregnant.

➤*Lactation:* It is not known whether this drug is excreted in breast milk. Because of the potential for tumorigenicity, decide whether to discontinue nursing or to discontinue the drug, taking into account the importance of the drug to the mother.

Precautions

➤*Monitoring:* Monitor liver function tests (serum transaminases, alkaline phosphatase, bilirubin) at weekly intervals when first beginning therapy and at monthly intervals thereafter. More frequent liver function tests may be advisable in patients with pre-existing liver disease or who are receiving other hepatotoxic drugs. Instruct patients to immediately discontinue thioguanine if clinical jaundice is detected. If deterioration in liver function studies during thioguanine therapy occurs, promptly discontinue treatment and search for an explanation of the hepatotoxicity.

Frequently evaluate hemoglobin concentration or hematocrit, total white blood cell (WBC) and differential counts and quantitative platelet count during therapy.

➤*Hepatotoxicity:* Jaundice has occurred. Among these were two adult males and four children with acute myelogenous leukemia, and an adult male with acute lymphocytic leukemia who developed veno-occlusive hepatic disease while receiving chemotherapy. Six patients had received cytarabine prior to treatment with thioguanine, and some were receiving other chemotherapy in addition to thioguanine when they became symptomatic. Withhold thioguanine if there is evidence of toxic hepatitis or biliary stasis, clinical jaundice, hepatomegaly, or anorexia with tenderness in the right hypochondrium. Initiate appropriate clinical and laboratory investigations to establish the etiology of the hepatic dysfunction.

➤*Hyperuricemia:* Hyperuricemia frequently occurs as a consequence of rapid cell lysis accompanying the antineoplastic effect. Minimize adverse effects by increasing hydration, urine alkalinization, and the prophylactic administration of allopurinol. Unlike mercaptopurine and azathioprine, thioguanine may be continued in the usual dosage when allopurinol is used concurrently to inhibit uric acid formation.

Drug Interactions

➤*Busulfan:* After concomitant chronic busulfan and thioguanine therapy, esophageal varices associated with abnormal liver function tests and evidence of nodular regenerative hyperplasia were reported. Use long-term concomitant therapy with caution.

➤*Aminosalicylate derivatives (ie, olsalazine, sulfasalazine, mesalazine):* Aminosalicylate derivatives may inhibit the TPMT enzyme, therefore, use with caution when administering with thioguanine (see Warnings).

Adverse Reactions

➤*GI:* Nausea, vomiting, anorexia, and stomatitis may occur. Intestinal necrosis and perforation have also occurred in patients who received multiple-drug chemotherapy including thioguanine.

➤*GU:* Hyperuricemia frequently occurs as a consequence of rapid cell lysis accompanying the antineoplastic effect.

➤*Hepatic:* Liver enzyme and other liver function studies are occasionally abnormal. If jaundice, hepatomegaly, or anorexia with tenderness in the right hypochrondrium occurs, withhold thioguanine until the exact etiology can be determined. There have been reports of veno-occlusive liver disease occurring in patients who received combination chemotherapy including thioguanine. Esophageal varices have been reported in patients receiving continuous busulfan and thioguanine therapy for treatment of chronic myelogenous leukemia.

➤*Hematologic:* Myelosuppression is the most frequent adverse reaction to thioguanine. Induction of complete remission of acute myelogenous leukemia usually requires combination chemotherapy in dosages that produce marrow hypoplasia. Since consolidation and maintenance of remission are also affected by multiple-drug regimens whose component agents cause myelosuppression, pancytopenia is observed in nearly all patients. Dosages and schedules must be adjusted to prevent life-threatening cytopenias whenever these adverse reactions are observed (see Warnings).

Overdosage

➤*Symptoms:* Signs and symptoms of overdosage may be immediate (nausea, vomiting, malaise, hypotension, diaphoresis) or delayed (myelosuppression and azotemia). Hemodialysis is of marginal use because of the rapid intracellular incorporation of active thioguanine metabolites with long persistence. Symptoms of overdosage may occur after a single dose of as little as 2 to 3 mg/kg thioguanine. As much as 35 mg/kg has been given in a single oral dose with reversible myelosuppression observed. There is no known pharmacologic antagonist of thioguanine.

➤*Treatment:* Immediately discontinue if unintended toxicity occurs during treatment. Severe hematologic toxicity may require supportive therapy with platelet transfusions for bleeding, and granulocyte transfusions and antibiotics if sepsis is documented.

If a patient is seen immediately following an acute overdosage, induced emesis may be useful.

Patient Information

Advise patient to notify physician if fever, chills, nausea, vomiting, sore throat, unusual bleeding or bruising, yellow discoloration of the skin or eyes, swelling of the feet or legs, or abdominal, joint, or flank pain occurs.

May cause diarrhea, fever, and weakness. Advise patient to notify physician if these become pronounced.

Inform patient to drink plenty of liquids while taking this drug.

Contraceptive measures are recommended during therapy for men and women.

Purine Analogs and Related Agents

ALLOPURINOL

Rx	**Allopurinol** (Various, eg, Boots, Geneva, Major, Mylan, Parmed, Vangard)	**Tablets**: 100 mg	In 100s, 500s, 1000s, and UD 100s.
Rx	**Zyloprim** (GlaxoWellcome)		Lactose. (Zyloprim 100). White, scored. In 100s.
Rx	**Allopurinol** (Various, eg, Boots, Geneva, Major, Mylan, Parmed, Vangard)	**Tablets**: 300 mg	In 100s, 500s, 1000s, and UD 100s.
Rx	**Zyloprim** (GlaxoWellcome)		Lactose. (Zyloprim 300). Peach, scored. In 100s and 500s.
Rx	**Aloprim** (Nabi)	**Power for injection, lyophilized**: 500 mg	Preservative free. In 30 ml vials with rubber stoppers.

For more complete prescribing information on tablets, see the Allopurinol monograph in the Agents for Gout section.

Indications

➤*Injection:* For the management of patients with leukemia, lymphoma, and solid tumor malignancies who are receiving cancer therapy that causes elevations of serum and urinary uric acid levels and who cannot tolerate oral therapy.

➤*Tablets:* Management of patients with leukemia, lymphoma, and malignancies receiving therapy that causes elevations of serum and urinary uric acid. Discontinue allopurinol when the potential for overproduction of uric acid is no longer present. For more complete prescribing information on tablets, see the Allopurinol monograph in the Agents for Gout section.

Administration and Dosage

➤*Injection:*

Children and adults – The dosage of allopurinol sodium for injection to lower serum uric acid to normal or near-normal varies according to disease severity. The amount and frequency of dosage for maintaining the serum uric acid just within the normal range is best determined by using the serum uric acid level as an index. In adults, doses > 600 mg/day did not appear to be more effective. The recommended daily dose of allopurinol sodium for injection is as follows:

Recommended Daily Dose	
Adult	200 to 400 mg/m^2/day Maximum 600 mg/day
Child	Starting dose 200 mg/m^2/day

Hydration – A fluid intake sufficient to yield a daily urinary output of ≥ 2 L in adults and the maintenance of a neutral or, preferably, slightly alkaline urine is desirable.

Impaired renal function – Reduce the dose of allopurinol sodium for injection in patients with impaired renal function to avoid accumulation of allopurinol and its metabolites:

Recommended Daily Dose for Impaired Renal Function	
Ccr	Recommended daily dose
10 to 20 ml/min	200 mg/day
3 to 10 ml/min	100 mg/day
< 3 ml/min	100 mg/day at extended intervals

Administration – In adults and children, the daily dose can be given as a single infusion or in equally divided infusions at 6-, 8-, or 12-hour intervals at the recommended final concentration of ≤ 6 mg/ml (see Preparation of Solution. The rate of infusion depends on the volume of infusate. Whenever possible, initiate therapy with allopurinol sodium for injection 24 to 48 hours before the start of chemotherapy known to cause tumor lysis (including adrenocorticosteroids). Do not mix allopurinol sodium for injection with or administer through the same IV port with agents that are incompatible in solution with allopurinol sodium for injection (see IV incompatibilities).

Preparation of solution – Allopurinol sodium for injection must be reconstituted and diluted. Dissolve the contents of each 30 ml vial with 25 ml of Sterile Water for Injection. Reconstitution yields a clear, almost colorless solution with no more than a slight opalescence. This concentration solution has a pH of 11.1 to 11.8. Dilute it to the desired concentration with 0.9% Sodium Chloride Injection or 5% Dextrose for Injection. Do not use sodium bicarbonate-containing solutions. A final concentration of ≤ 6 mg/ml is recommended. Begin administration within 10 hours after reconstitution.

IV incompatibilities: Drugs that are physically incompatible in a solution with allopurinol sodium for injection include the following:
- Amikacin sulfate
- Amphotericin B
- Carmustine
- Cefotaxime sodium
- Chlorpromazine HCl
- Cimetidine HCl
- Clindamycin phosphate
- Cytarabine
- Dacarbazine
- Daunorubicin HCl
- Diphenhydramine HCl
- Doxorubicin HCl
- Doxycycline hyclate
- Droperidol
- Floxuridine
- Gentamicin sulfate
- Haloperidol lactate
- Hydroxyzine HCl
- Idarubicin HCl
- Imipenem-cilastatin sodium
- Mechlorethamine HCl
- Meperidine HCl
- Metoclopramide HCl
- Methylprednisolone sodium succinate
- Minocycline HCl
- Nalbuphine HCl
- Netilmicin sulfate
- Ondansetron HCl
- Prochlorperazine edisylate
- Promethazine HCl
- Sodium bicarbonate
- Streptozocin
- Tobramycin sulfate
- Vinorelbine tartrate

➤*Tablets:*
Prevention of uric acid nephropathy during vigorous therapy of neoplastic disease – 600 to 800 mg daily for 2 to 3 days with a high fluid intake. (For more complete prescribing information on tablets, see the Allopurinol monograph in the Agents for Gout section.)

➤*Storage/Stability:*
Powder for injection – Store unreconstituted powder at 25°C (77°F). Excursions permitted to 15° to 30°C (59° to 86°F). Store the reconstituted solution at 20° to 25°C (68° to 77°F). Do not refrigerate the reconstituted and/or diluted product.

Tablets – Store at 15° to 25°C (59° to 77°F) in a dry place, and protect from light.

Actions

➤*Pharmacology:* Allopurinol acts on purine catabolism without disrupting the biosynthesis of purines. It reduces the production of uric acid by inhibiting the biochemical reactions immediately preceding its formation. The degree of this decrease is dose-dependent.

Allopurinol is a structural analog of the natural purine base, hypoxanthine. It is an inhibitor of xanthine oxidase, the enzyme responsible for the conversion of hypoxanthine to xanthine and of xanthine to uric acid, the end product of purine metabolism in humans. Allopurinol is metabolized to the corresponding xanthine analog, oxypurinol (alloxanthine), which also is an inhibitor of xanthine oxidase.

Reutilization of both hypoxanthine and xanthine for nucleotide and nucleic acid synthesis is markedly enhanced when their oxidations are inhibited by allopurinol and oxypurinol. However, this reutilization does not disrupt normal nucleic acid anabolism because feedback inhibition is an integral part of purine biosynthesis. As a result of xanthine oxidase inhibition, the serum concentration of hypoxanthine plus xanthine in patients receiving allopurinol for treatment of hyperuricemia is usually in the range of 0.3 to 0.4 mg/dl compared with a normal level of ≈ 0.15 mg/dl. A maximum of 0.9 mg/dl of these oxypurines has been reported when the serum urate was lowered to < 2 mg/dl by high doses of allopurinol. These values are far below the saturation levels, at which point their precipitation would be expected to occur (> 7 mg/dl).

The renal clearance of hypoxanthine and xanthine is ≥ 10 times greater than that of uric acid. The increased xanthine and hypoxanthine in the urine have not been accompanied by problems of nephrolithiasis. There are isolated case reports of xanthine crystalluria in patients who were treated with oral allopurinol. The action of oral allopurinol differs from that of uricosuric agents, which lower the serum uric acid level by increasing urinary excretion of uric acid. Allopurinol reduces both the serum and urinary uric acid levels by inhibiting the formation of uric acid. The use of allopurinol to block the formation of urates avoids the hazard of increased renal excretion of uric acid posed by uricosuric drugs.

➤*Pharmacokinetics:* Following IV administration in 6 healthy male and female subjects, allopurinol was rapidly eliminated from the systemic circulation primarily via oxidative metabolism to oxypurinol,

ALLOPURINOL

with no detectable plasma concentration of allopurinol after 5 hours post-dosing. Approximately 12% of the allopurinol IV dose was excreted unchanged, 76% excreted as oxypurinol, and the remaining dose excreted as riboside conjugates in the urine. The rapid conversion of allopurinol to oxypurinol was not significantly different after repeated allopurinol dosing. Oxypurinol was present in systemic circulation in much higher concentrations and for a much longer period than allopurinol; thus, it is generally believed the pharmacological action of allopurinol is mediated via oxypurinol. Oxypurinol was primarily eliminated unchanged in urine by glomerular filtration and tubular reabsorption, with a net renal clearance of $\approx$ 30 ml/min.

To compare the pharmacokinetics of allopurinol and oxypurinol between IV and oral administration of allopurinol sodium for injection, a well-controlled, 4-way crossover study was conducted in 16 healthy male volunteers. Allopurinol sodium for injection was administered via an IV infusion over 30 minutes. Pharmacokinetic parameter estimates of allopurinol (mean $\pm$ S.D.) following single IV and oral administration of allopurinol sodium for injection are summarized as follows:

Administration of Allopurinol Sodium for Injection				
Allopurinol parameters	100 mg IV	300 mg IV	100 mg PO (n = 7)	300 mg PO
C_{max} (mcg/ml)	1.58	5.12	0.53	1.35
T_{max} (hr)	0.5	0.5	1	1.67
$T_{1/2}$ (hr)	1	1.21	0.98	1.32
$AUC_{0-\infty}$ (hr•mcg/ml)	1.99	7.1	1.03	3.69
CL (ml/min/kg)	12.2	9.94		
V_{ss} (L/kg)	0.84	0.87		
$F_{absolute}$ (%)[1]			48.8	52.7

[1] Absolute bioavailability.

Oxypurinol was measurable in the plasma within 10 to 15 minutes following the administration of allopurinol sodium for injection. Pharmacokinetic parameter estimates of oxypurinol following IV and oral administration of allopurinol sodium for injection are shown below:

Administration of Allopurinol Sodium for Injection				
Oxypurinol parameters	100 mg IV	300 mg IV	100 mg PO	300 mg PO
C_{max} (mcg/ml)	2.2	6.18	2.36	6.36
T_{max} (hr)	3.89	4.16	3.1	4.13
$T_{1/2}$ (hr)	24.1	23.5	24.9	23.7
$AUC_{0-\infty}$ (hr•mcg/ml)	80	231	83	245
$F_{relative}$ (%)[1]			107	108

[1] Relative bioavailability.

In general, the ratio of the area under the plasma concentration vs time curve ($AUC_{0-\infty}$) between oxypurinol and allopurinol was in the magnitude of 30 to 40. The C_{max} and $AUC_{0-\infty}$ for both allopurinol and oxypurinol following IV administration of allopurinol sodium for injection were dose-proportional in the dose range of 100 to 300 mg. The half-life of allopurinol and oxypurinol was not influenced by the route of allopurinol sodium for injection administration. Oral and IV administration of allopurinol sodium for injection at equal doses produced nearly superimposable oxypurinol plasma concentration vs time profiles, and the relative bioavailability of oxypurinol, ($F_{relative}$) was $\approx$ 100%. Thus, the pharmacokinetics and plasma profiles of oxypurinol, the major pharmacological components derived from allopurinol, are similar after IV and oral administration of allopurinol sodium for injection.

➤ Clinical trials: A compassionate plea trial was conducted from 1977 through 1989 in which 718 evaluable patients with malignancies requiring treatment with cytotoxic chemotherapy, but who were unable to ingest or retain oral medication, received IV allopurinol sodium for injection in the US. Of these patients, 411 had established hyperuricemia and 307 had normal serum urate levels at the time that treatment was initiated. Normal serum uric acid levels were achieved in 68% (reduction of serum uric acid was documented in 93%) of the former and were maintained throughout chemotherapy in 97% of the latter. Because of the study design, it was not possible to assess the impact of the treatment upon the clinical outcome of the patient groups.

Contraindications

Patients who previously have developed a severe reaction to allopurinol.

Warnings

➤ Hepatic function impairment: A few cases of reversible clinical hepatotoxicity have been noted in patients taking oral allopurinol, and in some patients asymptomatic rises in serum alkaline phosphatase or serum transaminase have been observed. If anorexia, weight loss, or pruritus develop in patients on allopurinol, include an evaluation of liver function as part of their diagnostic workup. In patients with pre-existing liver disease, periodic liver function tests are recommended during the early stages of therapy.

➤ Renal function impairment: The occurrence of hypersensitivity reactions to allopurinol may be increased in patients with decreased renal function receiving thiazides and allopurinol concurrently. Administer such combinations with caution in patients with decreased renal function.

➤ Hypersensitivity reactions: Discontinue allopurinol at the first appearance of skin rash or other signs that may indicate an allergic reaction. In some instances with oral allopurinol, a skin rash may be followed by more severe hypersensitivity reactions such as exfoliative, urticarial, and purpuric lesions as well as Stevens-Johnson syndrome (erythema multiforme exudativum), and/or generalized vasculitis, irreversible hepatotoxicity and, on rare occasions, death.

Because of the occasional occurrence of drowsiness, alert patients to the need for caution when engaging in activities where alertness is mandatory.

In patients receiving mercaptopurine or azathioprine, the concomitant administration of 300 to 600 mg of allopurinol sodium for injection per day will require a reduction in dose to approximately one-third to one-fourth of the usual dose of mercaptopurine or azathioprine. Adjust subsequent doses of mercaptopurine or azathioprine on the basis of therapeutic response and the appearance of toxic effects (see Drug Interactions).

➤ Elderly: Clinical studies of allopurinol sodium for injection did not include sufficient numbers of patients $\geq$ 65 years of age to determine whether they respond differently than younger patients. Other reported clinical experience has not identified differences in responses between the elderly and younger patients. In general, start at the low end of the dosing range when selecting a dose for the elderly.

➤ Pregnancy: Category C. There is a published report in pregnant mice that single intraperitoneal doses of 50 or 100 mg/kg ($\approx$ ⅓ or ¾ the human dose on a mg/m^2 basis) of allopurinol on gestation days 10 or 13 produced significant increases in fetal deaths and teratogenic effects (cleft palate, harelip, and digital defects). It is uncertain whether these findings represented a fetal effect or an effect secondary to maternal toxicity. There are, however, no adequate or well-controlled studies in pregnant women. Because animal reproduction studies are not always predictive of human response, use this drug during pregnancy only if the potential benefit justifies the potential risk to the fetus. Experience with allopurinol during human pregnancy has been limited partly because women of reproductive age rarely require treatment with allopurinol. Two unpublished reports and one published paper describe women giving birth to normal offspring after receiving oral allopurinol during pregnancy. There have been no pregnancies reported in patients receiving allopurinol sodium for injection, but it is assumed that the same risks would apply.

➤ Lactation: Allopurinol and oxypurinol have been found in the milk of a mother who was receiving allopurinol. Because the effect of allopurinol on the nursing infant is unknown, exercise caution when allopurinol is administered to a nursing woman.

➤ Children: Clinical data are available on $\approx$ 200 children treated with allopurinol sodium for injection. The efficacy and safety profile observed in this patient population were similar to that observed in adults (see Indications and Administration and Dosage).

Precautions

➤ Fluid intake: A fluid intake sufficient to yield a daily urinary output of $\geq$ 2 L in adults and the maintenance of a neutral or, preferably, slightly alkaline urine are desirable to 1) avoid the theoretical possibility of formation of xanthine calculi under the influence of allopurinol therapy and 2) help prevent renal precipitation of urates in patients receiving concomitant uricosuric agents.

A few patients with preexisting renal disease or poor urate clearance have shown a rise in BUN during allopurinol administration, although a decrease in BUN has also been observed. In patients with hyperuricemia due to malignancy, the vast majority of changes in renal function are attributable to the underlying malignancy rather than to therapy with allopurinol. Concurrent conditions such as multiple myeloma and congestive myocardial disease were present among those patients whose renal function deteriorated after allopurinol was begun. Renal failure is rarely associated with hypersensitivity reactions to allopurinol.

Patients with decreased renal function require lower doses of allopurinol. Observe patients carefully during the early stages of allopurinol administration so that the dosage can be appropriately adjusted for renal function.

In patients with severely impaired renal function or decreased urate clearance, the half-life of oxypurinol in the plasma is greatly prolonged. Treat patients with the lowest effective dose, in order to minimize possible side effects. The appropriate dose of allopurinol sodium for injection for patients with a creatinine clearance $\leq$ 10 ml/min is 100 mg per day. For patients with a creatinine clearance between 10 and 20 ml/min, a dose of 200 mg per day is recommended. With extreme renal impairment (creatinine clearance < 3 ml/min), the interval between doses may also need to be extended.

ALLOPURINOL

Bone marrow suppression has been reported in patients receiving allopurinol; however, most of these patients were receiving concomitant medications with the known potential to cause such an effect. The suppression has occurred from as early as 6 weeks to as long as 6 years after the initiation of allopurinol therapy.

➤*Lab test abnormalities:* The correct dosage and schedule for maintaining the serum uric acid within the normal range is best determined by using the serum uric acid as an index. In patients with pre-existing liver disease, periodic liver function tests are recommended during the early stages of therapy (see Warnings). Allopurinol and its primary active metabolite, oxypurinol, are eliminated by the kidneys; therefore, changes in renal function have a profound effect on dosage. In patients with decreased renal function, or who have concurrent illnesses that can affect renal function such as hypertension and diabetes mellitus, periodic laboratory parameters of renal function, particularly BUN and serum creatinine or creatinine clearance, should be performed and the patient's allopurinol dosage reassessed. Assess prothrombin time periodically in patients receiving dicumarol who are given allopurinol.

Drug Interactions

The following interactions were observed in some patients undergoing treatment with oral allopurinol. Although the pattern of use for oral allopurinol includes longer term therapy, particularly for gout and renal calculi, the experience gained may be relevant.

Allopurinol Drug Interactions			
Precipitant drug	Object drug*		Description
Uricosuric agents	Allopurinol	↑	Because the excretion of oxypurinol is similar to that of urate, uricosuric agents, which increase the excretion of urate, are also likely to increase the excretion of oxypurinol. As a result, the concomitant administration of uricosuric agents decreases the inhibition of xanthine oxidase by oxypurinol and increases the urinary excretion of uric acid.
Allopurinol	Ampicillin/ Amoxicillin	↑	An increase in the frequency of skin rash has been reported among patients receiving ampicillin or amoxicillin concurrently with allopurinol compared with patients who are not receiving both drugs. The cause of this reaction has not been established.
Allopurinol	Chlorpropamide	↑	The half-life of chlorpropamide in the plasma may be prolonged by allopurinol, because allopurinol and chlorpropamide may compete for excretion in the renal tubule. The risk of hypoglycemia secondary to this mechanism may be increased if allopurinol and chlorpropamide are given concomitantly in the presence of renal insufficiency.
Allopurinol	Cyclosporine	↑	Reports indicate that cyclosporine levels may be increased during concomitant treatment with allopurinol sodium for injection. Monitor cyclosporine levels, and adjust cyclosporine dosage when these drugs are co-administered.
Allopurinol	Cytotoxic agents	↑	Enhanced bone marrow suppression by cyclophosphamide and other cytotoxic agents has been reported among patients with neoplastic disease, except leukemia, in the presence of allopurinol. However, in a well-controlled study of patients with lymphoma on combination therapy, allopurinol did not increase the marrow toxicity of patients treated with cyclophosphamide, doxorubicin, bleomycin, procarbazine, or mechlorethamine.
Allopurinol	Dicumarol	↑	It has been reported that allopurinol prolongs the half-life of the anticoagulant, dicumarol. Consequently, reassess prothrombin time periodically in patients receiving both drugs. The clinical basis of this drug interaction has not been established.

Allopurinol Drug Interactions			
Precipitant drug	Object drug*		Description
Allopurinol	Mercaptopurine/ Azathioprine	↑	Allopurinol inhibits the enzymatic oxidation of mercaptopurine and azathioprine to 6-thiouric acid (inactive). This results in increased levels of the active drug. Therefore, the concomitant administration of 300 to 600 mg of oral allopurinol per day will require a reduction in dose to approximately one-third to one-fourth of the usual dose of mercaptopurine or azathioprine. Make subsequent adjustment of doses of mercaptopurine or azathioprine on the basis of therapeutic response and the appearance of toxic effects.

* ↑ = Object drug increased.

Adverse Reactions

In an uncontrolled, compassionate plea protocol, 125 of 1378 patients reported a total of 301 adverse reactions while receiving allopurinol sodium for injection. Most of the patients had advanced malignancies or serious underlying diseases and were taking multiple concomitant medications. Side effects directly attributable to allopurinol sodium for injection were reported in 19 patients. Fifteen of these adverse experiences were allergic in nature (rash, eosinophilia, local injection site reaction). One adverse experience of severe diarrhea and one indicidence of nausea were also reported as being possibly attributable to allopurinol sodium for injection. Two patients had serious adverse experiences (decreased renal function and generalized seizure) reported as being possibly attributable to allopurinol sodium for injection.

A listing of the adverse reactions regardless of causality reported from clinical trials follows:

➤*Cardiovascular:* Bradycardia, cardiorespiratory arrest, cardiovascular disorder, decreased venous pressure, ECG abnormality, flushing, headache, heart failure, hemorrhage, hypertension, hypotension, pulmonary embolus, septic shock, stroke, thrombophlebitis, ventricular fibrillation (< 1%).

➤*CNS:* Agitation, cerebral infarction, coma, dystonia, mental status changes, myoclonus, paralysis, seizure, status epilepticus, tremor, twitching (< 1%).

➤*Dermatologic:* Rash (1.5%); local injection site reaction, pruritus, urticaria (< 1%).

➤*GI:* Nausea (1.3%); vomiting (1.2%); diarrhea, GI bleeding, splenomegaly, hepatomegaly, intestinal obstruction, flatulence, constipation, proctitis (< 1%).

➤*GU:* Renal failure/insufficiency (1.2%); hematuria, increased creatinine, kidney function abnormality, oliguria, urinary tract infection (< 1%).

➤*Hematologic:* Anemia, bone marrow suppression, disseminated intravascular coagulation, ecchymosis, eosinophilia, leukopenia, marrow aplasia, neutropenia, pancytopenia, thrombocytopenia (< 1%).

➤*Hepatic:* Hepatomegaly, hyperbilirubinemia, liver failure, jaundice (< 1%).

➤*Metabolic:* Edema, electrolyte abnormality, glycosuria, hypercalcemia, hyperglycemia, hyperkalemia, hypernatremia, hyperphosphatemia, hyperuricemia, hypocalcemia, hypokalemia, hypomagnesemia, hyponatremia, lactic acidosis, metabolic acidosis, water intoxication (< 1%).

➤*Respiratory:* Apnea, ARDS, respiratory failure/insufficiency, increased respiration rate (< 1%).

➤*Miscellaneous:* Alopecia, blast crisis, cellulitis, chills, diaphoresis, enlarged abdomen, fever, hypervolemia, hypotonia, infection, mucositis/pharyngitis, pain, sepsis, tumor lysis syndrome, arthralgia (<1%).

The most frequent adverse reaction to oral allopurinol is skin rash. Skin reactions can be severe and sometimes fatal. Therefore, discontinue treatment with allopurinol sodium for injection immediately if a rash develops (see Warnings). For further details on hypersensitivity reactions to treatment with oral allopurinol, refer to the package insert for allopurinol tablets.

Overdosage

Massive overdosing or acute poisoning by allopurinol sodium for injection has not been reported. In mice, the minimal lethal dose is 45 mg/kg given IV or 500 mg/kg orally ($\approx$ $\frac{1}{3}$ or 4 times the usual human dose on a mg/m^2 basis). Hypoactivity was observed with these doses. In rats, the minimum lethal dose is 100 mg/kg IV and 5000 mg/kg orally ($\approx$ 1.5 and 75 times the usual human dose on a mg/m^2 basis). In the management of overdosage, there is no specific antidote for allopurinol sodium for injection. There has been no clinical experience in the management of a patient who has taken massive amounts of allopurinol. Both allopurinol and oxypurinol are dialyzable; however, the usefulness of hemodialysis or peritoneal dialysis in the management of an overdose of allopurinol sodium for injection is unknown.

RASBURICASE

Rx   **Elitek** (Sanofi-Synthelabo)   **Powder for injection, lyophilized:** 1.5 mg/vial   10.6 mg mannitol. In single-use vials with 1 mL amps of diluent.

WARNING

Anaphylaxis: Rasburicase may cause hypersensitivity reactions, including anaphylaxis. Immediately and permanently discontinue rasburicase in any patient developing clinical evidence of a serious hypersensitivity reaction (see Warnings).

Hemolysis: Rasburicase administered to patients with glucose-6-phosphate dehydrogenase (G6PD) deficiency can cause severe hemolysis. Immediately and permanently discontinue rasburicase administration in any patient developing hemolysis. It is recommended that patients at higher risk for G6PD deficiency (eg, patients of African or Mediterranean ancestry) be screened prior to starting rasburicase therapy (see Warnings).

Methemoglobinemia: Rasburicase use has been associated with methemoglobinemia. Immediately and permanently discontinue rasburicase administration in any patient identified as having developed methemoglobinemia (see Warnings).

Interference with uric acid measurements: Rasburicase will cause enzymatic degradation of the uric acid within blood samples left at room temperature, resulting in spuriously low uric acid levels. To ensure accurate measurements, blood must be collected into pre-chilled tubes containing heparin anticoagulant and immediately immersed and maintained in an ice water bath; plasma samples must be assayed within 4 hours of sample collection (see Precautions).

Indications

For the initial management of plasma uric acid levels in pediatric patients with leukemia, lymphoma, and solid tumor malignancies who are receiving anticancer therapy expected to result in tumor lysis and subsequent elevation of plasma uric acid.

Administration and Dosage

➤*Approved by the FDA:* July 12, 2002.

➤*Dose:* The recommended dose and schedule of rasburicase is 0.15 or 0.2 mg/kg as a single daily dose for 5 days. Because the safety and effectiveness of other schedules have not been established, dosing beyond 5 days or administration of more than 1 course of rasburicase is not recommended. Initiate chemotherapy 4 to 24 hours after the first dose of rasburicase. Do not administer as a bolus infusion. Rasburicase should be administered as an IV infusion over 30 minutes.

➤*Reconstitution:* Determine the number of vials of rasburicase needed to achieve the proper dosage, based on the individual patient's weight and the dose per kilogram. Rasburicase must be reconstituted in the diluent provided. Add 1 mL of the provided reconstitution solution (diluent) to each vial of rasburicase and mix by swirling very gently. Do not shake or vortex. Visually inspect parenteral drug products for particulate matter and discoloration prior to administration, and discard if particulate matter is visible or if product is discolored.

➤*Dilution and administration:* Remove the predetermined dose of rasburicase from the reconstituted vials and inject into an infusion bag continuing the appropriate volume of 0.9% sterile Sodium Chloride, to achieve a final total volume of 50 mL. This final solution for injection is to be infused over 30 minutes. Do not use filters for the infusion.

The reconstituted rasburicase contains no preservatives and must be administered within 24 hours of reconstitution. The reconstituted or diluted solution can be stored up to 24 hours at 2° to 8°C (36° to 46°F). Discard any unused product.

Infuse rasburicase through a different line than that used for the infusion of other concomitant medications. If use of a separate line is not possible, flush the line with at least 15 mL of saline solution prior to and after infusion with rasburicase.

➤*Storage/Stability:* Store the lyophilized drug product and the diluent for reconstitution at 2° to 8°C (36° to 46°F). Do not freeze. Protect from light. The reconstituted rasburicase contains no preservatives and must be administered within 24 hours of reconstitution. The reconstituted or diluted solution can be stored up to 24 hours at 2° to 8°C (36° to 46°F). Discard any unused product.

Actions

➤*Pharmacology:* Rasburicase is a recombinant urate-oxidase enzyme produced by a genetically modified *Saccharomyces cerevisiae* strain. In humans, uric acid is the final step in the catabolic pathway of purines. Rasburicase catalyzes enzymatic oxidation of uric acid into an inactive and soluble metabolite (allantoin). Rasburicase is only active at the end of the purine catabolic pathway.

➤*Pharmacokinetics:* Pharmacokinetics of rasburicase were evaluated in 2 studies that enrolled patients with lymphoid leukemia (B- and T-cell), non-Hodgkin's lymphoma (including Burkitt's lymphoma), or acute myelogenous leukemia. Rasburicase exposure, as measured by AUC_{0-24hr} and C_{max}, tended to increase linearly with doses over a lim-

ited dose range (0.15 to 0.2 mg/kg). The overall elimination half-life was 18 hours. No accumulation of rasburicase was observed between days 1 and 5 of dosing. Rasburicase mean volume of distribution was 110 to 127 mL/kg in pediatric patients. There are insufficient data to characterize pharmacokinetics in adult patients.

➤*Clinical trials:* A randomized, open-label, controlled study was conducted at 6 institutions in which 52 pediatric patients were randomized to receive rasburicase (n = 27) or allopurinol (n = 25). The dose of allopurinol varied according to local institutional practice. Rasburicase was administered as an IV infusion over 30 minutes once (n = 26) or twice (n = 1) daily at a dose of 0.2 mg/kg/dose (total daily dose 0.2 to 0.4 mg/kg/day). Initiation of dosing was permitted at any time between 4 to 48 hours before the start of antitumor therapy and could be continued for 5 to 7 days after initiation of antitumor therapy.

The uric acid AUC_{0-96hr} was significantly lower in the rasburicase group (128 ± s.e. 14 mg•hr/dL) as compared to the allopurinol group (328 ± s.e. 26 mg•hr/dL). All but 1 patient in the rasburicase arm had a reduction and maintenance of uric acid levels to within or below the normal range during the treatment. The incidence of renal dysfunction was similar in the 2 study arms; 1 patient in the allopurinol arm developed acute renal failure.

Contraindications

In individuals deficient in G6PD (see Warnings and Warning Box); known history of anaphylaxis or hypersensitivity reactions, hemolytic reactions, or methemoglobinemia reactions to rasburicase or any of the excipients.

Warnings

➤*Anaphylaxis:* The safety and efficacy of rasburicase have been established only for a single course of treatment once daily for 5 days (see Administration and Dosage).

Rasburicase may cause severe allergic reactions, including anaphylaxis. Signs and symptoms of these reactions include chest pain, dyspnea, hypotension, and urticaria. Immediately and permanently discontinue rasburicase administration in any patient developing clinical evidence of a serious hypersensitivity reaction.

➤*Hemolysis:* Rasburicase is contraindicated in patients with G6PD deficiency because hydrogen peroxide is one of the major by-products of the conversion of uric acid to allantoin. In clinical studies, 2 patients developed severe hemolytic reactions (National Cancer Institute Common Toxicity Criteria [NCI CTC] grade 3 and 4) within 2 to 4 days of starting rasburicase. G6PD deficiency subsequently was identified in one of these patients. Immediately and permanently discontinue rasburicase administration in any patient developing hemolysis, and initiate appropriate patient monitoring and support measures (eg, transfusion support). It is recommended that patients at higher risk for G6PD deficiency (eg, patients of African or Mediterranean ancestry) be screened prior to starting rasburicase therapy.

➤*Methemoglobinemia:* In clinical studies, methemoglobinemia has been reported in 2 patients receiving rasburicase. Both patients developed serious hypoxemia requiring intervention with the appropriate medical support measures. It is not known whether patients with deficiency of cytochrome b_5 reductase (formerly known as methemoglobin reductase) or of other enzymes with antioxidant activity are at increased risk for methemoglobinemia or hemolytic anemia. Immediately and permanently discontinue rasburicase administration in any patient identified as having developed methemoglobinemia, and implement appropriate monitoring and support measures (eg, transfusion support, methylene blue administration).

➤*Pregnancy: Category C.* Animal reproduction studies have not been conducted with rasburicase. It also is not known whether rasburicase can cause fetal harm when administered to a pregnant woman or can affect reproduction capacity. Give rasburicase to a pregnant woman only if clearly needed.

➤*Lactation:* It is not known whether this drug is excreted in human milk. Because many drugs are excreted in human milk and because of the potential for serious adverse reactions in nursing infants, decide whether to discontinue nursing or discontinue the drug, taking into account the importance of the drug to the mother.

➤*Children:* The safety and efficacy of rasburicase was studied in 246 pediatric patients ranging from 1 month to 17 years of age. Children less than 2 years of age had a higher mean uric acid AUC_{0-96hr} than those 2 to 17 years of age (150 ± s.e. 16 mg•hr/dL vs 108 ± s.e. 4 mg•hr/dL, respectively). In addition, the data suggest that children less than 2 years of age had a lower rate of success at achieving maintenance uric acid concentration by 48 hours (83% [95% CI of 62 to 95] vs 93% [95% CI of 89 to 95], respectively). Children less than 2 years of age also experienced more toxicity. The following adverse events were observed more frequently in children less than 2 years of age compared with those ages 2 to 17 years, respectively: Vomiting (75% vs 55%), diarrhea (63% vs 20%), fever (50% vs 38%), and rash (38% vs 10%).

RASBURICASE

Precautions

➤*Hydration:* Patients on rasburicase should receive IV hydration according to standard medical practice for the management of plasma uric acid in patients at risk for tumor lysis syndrome.

➤*Immunogenicity:* Rasburicase is immunogenic in healthy volunteers, and can elicit antibodies that inhibit the activity of rasburicase in vitro.

In a study of 28 healthy volunteers, the incidence of antibody responses to either a single dose or to 5 daily doses was assessed. Binding antibodies to rasburicase were detected by ELISA in 61% volunteers and neutralizing antibodies were detected in 64% volunteers. Time to detection of antibodies ranged from 1 to 6 weeks after rasburicase exposure. In 2 subjects with extended follow-up, antibodies persisted for 333 and 494 days.

The incidence of antibody responses in patients with hematologic malignancy has not been adequately assessed. In clinical trials of patients with hematologic malignancies 24 of the 218 patients tested (11%) developed antibodies by day 28 following rasburicase administration. However, this is not a reliable estimate of the true incidence of antibody responses in patients with hematologic malignancies because the data from the healthy volunteer study indicate that antibody may not be detectable until some time point beyond day 28.

The incidence of antibody responses detected is highly dependent on the sensitivity and specificity of the assay, which have not been fully evaluated. Additionally, the observed incidence of antibody positivity in an assay may be influenced by several factors, including serum sampling, timing, methodology, concomitant medications, and underlying disease. For these reasons, comparison of the incidence of antibodies to rasburicase with the incidence of antibodies to other products may be misleading.

Drug Interactions

No studies of interactions with other drugs have been conducted in humans.

➤*Drug/Lab test interactions:* At room temperature, rasburicase causes enzymatic degradation of the uric acid in blood/plasma/serum samples, potentially resulting in spuriously low plasma uric acid assay readings. The following special sample handling procedure must be followed to avoid ex vivo uric acid degradation.

Uric acid must be analyzed in plasma. Blood must be collected into prechilled tubes containing heparin anticoagulant. Samples must be immediately immersed in an ice water bath. Plasma samples must be prepared by centrifugation in a precooled centrifuge (4°C; 39°F). Finally, the plasma must be maintained in an ice water bath and analyzed for uric acid within 4 hours of collection.

Adverse Reactions

Among 703 patients for whom serious adverse reactions were assessed, the most serious adverse reactions caused by rasburicase were allergic reactions including anaphylaxis (less than 1%), rash (1%), hemolysis (less than 1%), and methemoglobinemia (less than 1%). The commonly observed serious adverse reactions were fever (5%), neutropenia with fever (4%), respiratory distress (3%), sepsis (3%), neutropenia (2%), and mucositis (2%). The following additional serious adverse reactions were observed in 1% or fewer of patients regardless of causality: Acute renal failure, arrhythmia, cardiac failure, cardiac arrest, cellulitis, cerebrovascular disorder, chest pain, convulsions, cyanosis, diarrhea, dehydration, hot flushes, ileus, infection, intestinal obstruction, hemorrhage, MI, paresthesia, pancytopenia, pneumonia, pulmonary edema, pulmonary hypertension, retinal hemorrhage, rigors, thrombosis, and thrombophlebitis.

Among the 347 patients for whom all adverse reactions regardless of severity were assessed, the most frequently observed adverse reactions (incidence at least 10%) were vomiting (50%), fever (46%), nausea (27%), headache (26%), abdominal pain (20%), constipation (20%), diarrhea (20%), mucositis (15%), and rash (13%). In 1 active control study, the following adverse events occurred more frequently in rasburicase-treated subjects than allopurinol-treated subjects: Vomiting, fever, nausea, diarrhea, and headache. Although the incidence of rash was similar in the 2 arms, severe rash (NCI CTC, Grade 3 or 4) was reported only in 1 rasburicase-treated patient.

Overdosage

No cases of overdosage with rasburicase have been reported. The maximum dose of rasburicase that has been administered as a single dose is 0.2 mg/kg; the maximum daily dose that has been administered is 0.4 mg/kg/day. According to the mechanism of action of rasburicase, an overdose will lead to low or undetectable plasma uric acid concentration, which has no known clinical consequences. Patients suspected of receiving an overdose should be monitored, and general supportive measures should be initiated as no specific antidote for rasburicase has been identified.

VINBLASTINE SULFATE (VLB)

Rx	Vinblastine Sulfate (Various, eg, Cetus, VHA Supply)	Powder for injection: 10 mg	In vials.
Rx	Velban (Lilly)		In vials.
Rx	Vinblastine Sulfate (Various, eg, Quad)	Injection: 1 mg/ml	In 10 and 25 ml vials.[1]

[1] With 0.9% benzyl alcohol.

WARNING

It is extremely important the needle be properly positioned in the vein before this product is injected. If leakage into surrounding tissue should occur during IV administration of vinblastine sulfate, it may cause considerable irritation. Immediately discontinue the injection, and introduce any remaining portion of the dose into another vein. Local injection of hyaluronidase and the application of moderate heat to the area of leakage will help disperse the drug and may minimize the discomfort and the possibility of cellulitis.

Fatal if given intrathecally. For IV use only.

See Warnings for the treatment of patients given intrathecal vinblastine sulfate injection.

Indications

Palliative treatment of the following:

▶*Frequently responsive malignancies:* Generalized Hodgkin's disease (stages III and IV, Ann Arbor modification of Rye staging system), lymphocytic lymphoma (nodular and diffuse, poorly and well differentiated); histiocytic lymphoma; mycosis fungoides (advanced stages); advanced testicular carcinoma; Kaposi's sarcoma and Letterer-Siwe disease (histiocytosis X).

▶*Less frequently responsive malignancies:* Choriocarcinoma resistant to other chemotherapy; breast cancer unresponsive to endocrine surgery and hormonal therapy.

▶*Multiple drug protocols:* Vinblastine, effective as a single agent, is usually administered with other antineoplastics. Combination therapy enhances therapeutic effect without additive toxicity when agents with different dose-limiting toxicities and mechanisms of action are selected.

▶*Hodgkin's disease:* Vinblastine used as a single agent; advanced Hodgkin's disease also has been successfully treated with multiple-drug regimens that included vinblastine.

▶*Advanced testicular germinal-cell cancers (embryonal carcinoma, teratocarcinoma, and choriocarcinoma):* Advanced testicular germinal-cell cancers are sensitive to vinblastine alone, but better clinical results are achieved with combination therapy. Vinblastine enhances the effect of bleomycin if given 6 to 8 hours prior to bleomycin administration; this schedule permits more cells to be arrested during metaphase, the stage in which bleomycin is active.

Administration and Dosage

Leukopenic responses vary following therapy. For this reason, do not administer drug more than once weekly. Initiate therapy for adults with a single IV dose of 3.7 mg/m² of body surface. Thereafter, measure WBC counts to determine patient's sensitivity. A 50% dose reduction is recommended for patients having a direct serum bilirubin value > 3 mg/dlL. Because metabolism and excretion are primarily hepatic, no modification is recommended for patients with impaired renal function.

Incremental Vinblastine Dosage (Weekly Intervals)		
	Adult dose (mg/m²)	Pediatric dose (mg/m²)
First dose	3.7	2.5
Second dose	5.5	3.75
Third dose	7.4	5
Fourth dose	9.25	6.25
Fifth dose	11.1	7.5

Use the same increments until a maximum dose not exceeding 18.5 mg/m² for adults and 12.5 mg/m² for children is reached. Do not increase dose after WBC count is reduced to ≈ 3000 cells/mm³. For most adults the weekly dosage range is 5.5 to 7.4 mg/m².

▶*Maintenance therapy:* When the dose produces the above degree of leukopenia, administer a dose one increment smaller at weekly intervals for maintenance. Even though 7 days have elapsed, do not give the next dose until the WBC count has returned to at least 4000/mm³. In some cases, oncolytic activity may be encountered before leukopenic effect but do not increase the size of subsequent doses.

Duration of maintenance therapy varies according to the disease and the combination of antineoplastics used. Prolonged chemotherapy for maintaining remission involves several risks: Life-threatening infections, sterility, secondary cancers through suppression of immune surveillance. In some disorders, survival following complete remission may not be as prolonged as that achieved with shorter periods of maintenance therapy. Conversely, failure to provide maintenance therapy may

lead to unnecessary relapse; complete remission in patients with testicular cancer, unless maintained for at least 2 years, often results in early relapse.

▶*IV:* Inject into either the tubing of a running IV infusion or directly into a vein over 1 minute. To prevent cellulitis or phlebitis, secure the needle within the vein so that no solution extravasates. To further minimize extravasation, rinse syringe and needle with venous blood before withdrawal of needle. Do not dilute the dose in large volumes of diluent (ie, 100 to 250 mL) or give IV for prolonged periods (≥ 30 min), because this often results in vein irritation and increases the chance of extravasation.

Because of the enhanced possibility of thrombosis, do not inject solution into an extremity in which circulation is impaired or potentially impaired by conditions such as compressing or invading neoplasm, phlebitis, or varicosity.

▶*Powder for injection:*

Preparation of solution – Add 10 mL of Bacteriostatic Sodium Chloride Injection (preserved with phenol or benzyl alcohol) to the vial for a concentration of 1 mg/mL. The drug dissolves instantly to give a clear solution. A preservative-containing solvent is unnecessary if unused portions are discarded immediately.

Compatibility – Do not dilute with solvents that raise or lower the pH of the resulting solution from between 3.5 and 5. Make solutions with either Normal Saline or 0.9% Sodium Chloride Injection (each with or without preservative) and do not combine in the same container with any other chemical.

▶*Storage/Stability:* After reconstitution and removal of a portion from the vial, refrigerate the remainder for 28 days without loss of potency. Refrigerate unopened vials at 2° to 8°C (36° to 46°F).

Actions

▶*Pharmacology:* Vinblastine sulfate, an alkaloid extracted from Vinca rosea Linn, interferes with metabolic pathways of amino acids leading from glutamic acid to the citric acid cycle and urea. Studies have demonstrated a stathmokinetic effect and various atypical mitotic figures. However, therapeutic responses are not fully explained by the cytologic changes, because these changes are sometimes observed clinically and experimentally in the absence of any oncolytic effects.

Vinblastine has an effect on cell energy production required for mitosis and interferes with nucleic acid synthesis. In vitro, the drug arrests growing cells in metaphase.

Reversal of the antitumor effect by glutamic acid or tryptophan has occurred.

▶*Pharmacokinetics:*

Absorption/Distribution – Similar to vincristine, vinblastine undergoes rapid distribution and extensive tissue binding following IV injection. Vinblastine also localizes in platelets and leukocyte fractions of whole blood.

Metabolism/Excretion – Vinblastine is partially metabolized to deacetyl vinblastine, which is more active than the parent drug. Plasma decline follows a triphasic pattern. The initial, middle, and terminal half-lives are 3.7 minutes, 1.6 hours and 24.8 hours, respectively. Toxicity may be increased if liver disease is present.

Vinblastine is metabolized by the hepatic P450 3A cytochromes, and the major route of excretion may be through the biliary system.

Contraindications

Leukopenia; presence of bacterial infection (infections must be under control prior to initiating therapy); significant granulocytopenia unless it is a result of the disease being treated.

Warnings

▶*This product is for IV use only:* The intrathecal administration of vinblastine has resulted in death. Label syringes containing this product "Vinblastine Sulfate for Intravenous Use Only."

Extemporaneously prepared syringes containing this product must be packaged in an overwrap that is labeled "Do Not Remove Covering Until Moment of Injection. Fatal if Given Intrathecally. For Intravenous Use Only."

The following treatment successfully arrested progressive paralysis in a single patient mistakenly given the related vinca alkaloid, vincristine sulfate, intrathecally. If vinblastine is mistakenly administered intrathecally, this treatment is recommended and should be initiated immediately after the intrathecal injection.

1.) Remove as much spinal fluid as can be safely done through the lumbar access.

VINBLASTINE SULFATE (VLB)

2.) Insert a catheter in a lateral cerebral ventricle for the purpose of flushing the subarachnoid space from above with removal through a lumbar access.

3.) Initiate flushing through the cerebral catheter with Lactated Ringer's Solution infused at the rate of 150 ml/hr.

4.) As soon as fresh frozen plasma becomes available, infuse 25 ml diluted in 1L of Lactated Ringer's Solution through the cerebral ventricular catheter at the rate of 75 ml/hr with removal through the lumbar access. The rate of infusion should be adjusted to maintain a protein level in the spinal fluid of 150 mg/dl.

5.) Administer 10 g of glutamic acid IV over 24 hours followed by 500 mg 3 times daily by mouth for 1 month or until neurological dysfunction stabilizes. The role of glutamic acid in this treatment is not certain and may not be essential.

The use of this treatment has not been reported following intrathecal vinblastine.

➤*Hematologic effects:* Leukopenia is expected; leukocyte count is an important guide to therapy. In general, the larger the dose, the more profound and longer lasting the leukopenia will be. If the WBC count returns to normal after drug-induced leukopenia, the white cell-producing mechanism is not permanently depressed. Usually, WBC count has completely returned to normal after virtual disappearance of white cells from peripheral blood. The nadir in WBC count occurs 5 to 10 days after the last dose of drug is given. Recovery of the WBC count is fairly rapid and usually complete within 7 to 14 days. With smaller doses employed for maintenance therapy, leukopenia may not occur.

Although the thrombocyte count ordinarily is not significantly lowered by therapy, recently impaired bone marrow by prior therapy with radiation or with other oncolytic drugs may show thrombocytopenia (< 200,000 platelets/mm³). When other chemotherapy or radiation has not been previously employed, thrombocytopenia is rare, even when vinblastine may be causing significant leukopenia. Rapid recovery (within a few days) from thrombocytopenia is the rule.

The effect on red blood cell count and hemoglobin is usually insignificant in the absence of other therapy; however, patients with malignant disease may exhibit anemia in the absence of any therapy.

If leukopenia (< 2000 WBC/mm³) occurs following a dose of this drug, carefully watch the patient for evidence of infection until a safe WBC count has returned.

When cachexia or ulcerated skin surface occurs, a more profound leukopenic response may occur; avoid use in older persons suffering from these conditions.

In patients with malignant cell infiltration of bone marrow, leukocyte and platelet counts have sometimes fallen precipitously after moderate doses, making further use of the drug inadvisable.

Leukopenia (granulocytopenia) may reach dangerously low levels following use of the higher recommended doses. Follow recommended dosage technique. Stomatitis and neurologic toxicity, although not common or permanent, can be disabling.

➤*Hepatic function impairment:* Toxicity may be enhanced in the presence of hepatic insufficiency. A dose reduction is recommended (see Administration and Dosage).

➤*Fertility impairment:* Aspermia has been reported. Amenorrhea has occurred in some patients treated with a combination of an alkylating agent, procarbazine, prednisone and vinblastine. Its occurrence was related to the total dose of these agents. Recovery of menses was frequent. The same combination of drugs given to male patients produced azoospermia; if spermatogenesis did return, it was not likely to do so with less than 2 years of unmaintained remission.

➤*Pregnancy:* Category D. Information is very limited. Animal studies suggest teratogenicity may occur. Animals given the drug early in pregnancy suffered resorption of the conceptus; surviving fetuses demonstrated gross deformities. There are no adequate and well controlled studies in pregnant women, but the drug can cause fetal harm. If the drug is used during pregnancy, or if the patient becomes pregnant while receiving this drug, apprise her of the potential hazard to the fetus. Advise women of childbearing potential to avoid becoming pregnant.

➤*Lactation:* It is not known whether this drug is excreted in breast milk. Because of the potential for serious adverse reactions in nursing infants, decide whether to discontinue nursing or to discontinue the drug, taking into account the importance of the drug to the mother.

Precautions

➤*Long-term use:* Using small amounts of drug daily for long periods is not advised, even though the resulting total weekly dose may be similar to that recommended. Strict adherence to the recommended dosage schedule is very important. When amounts equal to several times the recommended weekly dosage were given in 7 daily installments for long periods, convulsions, severe and permanent CNS damage and death occurred.

➤*Avoid eye contamination:* Severe irritation or corneal ulceration (if the drug was delivered under pressure) may result. Thoroughly wash the eye with water immediately.

➤*Pulmonary reactions:* Acute shortness of breath and severe bronchospasm have occurred following use of vinca alkaloids. These reactions occur most frequently when the vinca alkaloid is used with mitomycin. Onset may be within minutes or several hours after the vinca is injected and may occur up to 2 weeks after the dose of mitomycin. (See Drug Interactions.)

➤*Benzyl alcohol:* Benzyl alcohol, contained in some of these products as a preservative, has been associated with a fatal "gasping syndrome" in premature infants.

Drug Interactions

Vinblastine Drug Interactions			
Precipitant drug	Object drug*		Description
Vinblastine	Mitomycin	↑	Acute shortness of breath and severe bronchospasm have occurred following use of vinca alkaloids in patients who had previously or simultaneously received mitomycin. Onset may be within minutes or several hours after the vinca alkaloid is injected and may occur up to 2 weeks after the dose of mitomycin.
Vinblastine	Phenytoin	↓	Combination chemotherapy (including vinblastine) may reduce phenytoin plasma levels and increase seizure activity. Adjust the dosage based on serial blood level monitoring.
Erythromycin	Vinblastine	↑	May cause toxicity of vinblastine. Severe myalgia, neutropenia and constipation have been reported.
Agents that inhibit the cytochrome P450 pathway	Vinblastine	↑	Vinblastine is metabolized by the P450 3A enzyme. Use caution when coadministering drugs that inhibit P450 enzymes.

* ↑ = Object drug increased. ↓ = Object drug decreased.

Adverse Reactions

Incidence of adverse reactions is dose-related. Except for epilation, leukopenia and neurologic side effects, adverse reactions have not usually persisted for longer than 24 hours. Neurologic side effects are not common; when they occur, they often last for more than 24 hours. Leukopenia, the most common adverse reaction, is usually the dose-limiting factor.

➤*Cardiovascular:* Hypertension. Cases of unexpected myocardial infarction and cerebrovascular accidents have occurred in patients undergoing combination chemotherapy with vinblastine, bleomycin and cisplatin.

➤*CNS:* Numbness of digits; paresthesias; peripheral neuritis; mental depression; loss of deep tendon reflexes; headache; convulsions.

➤*Dermatologic:* Alopecia is common. Total epilation infrequently develops. In some cases, hair regrows during maintenance therapy. A single case of light sensitivity has been associated with this drug.

➤*GI:* Nausea and vomiting (may be controlled by antiemetics); pharyngitis; vesiculation of the mouth; ileus; diarrhea; constipation; anorexia; abdominal pain; rectal bleeding; hemorrhagic enterocolitis; bleeding from an old peptic ulcer.

➤*Hematologic:* Leukopenia (granulocytopenia), anemia, thrombocytopenia (myelosuppression). See Warnings.

➤*Miscellaneous:* Malaise; weakness; dizziness; pain in tumor site; bone and jaw pain. The syndrome of inappropriate secretion of antidiuretic hormone has occurred with higher than recommended doses.

Extravasation during IV injection may lead to cellulitis and phlebitis; sloughing may occur (see Administration and Dosage).

There are isolated reports of Raynaud's phenomenon occurring in patients with testicular carcinoma treated with bleomycin, cisplatin and vinblastine sulfate. It is unknown whether the cause was the disease, the drugs or a combination of these.

Overdosage

➤*Symptoms:* Side effects are dose-related. After an overdose, expected exaggerated effects. In addition, neurotoxicity similar to that with vincristine may occur.

➤*Treatment:* Supportive care should include prevention of side effects that result from the syndrome of inappropriate secretion of antidiuretic hormone (ie, restriction of the volume of daily fluid intake to that of the urine output plus insensible loss and perhaps use of a diuretic affecting the function of the loop of Henle and the distal tubule); administration of an anticonvulsant; prevention of ileus; monitoring the cardiovascular system; and determining daily blood counts for guidance in transfusion requirements and assessing the risk of infection. The major effect of excessive doses will be myelosuppression, which may be life-threatening. There is no information regarding the effectiveness of dialysis nor

VINBLASTINE SULFATE (VLB)

of cholestyramine for the treatment of overdosage.

In the dry state, the drug is irregularly and unpredictably absorbed from the GI tract following oral administration. Absorption of the solution has not been studied. If vinblastine is swallowed, oral activated charcoal in a water slurry may be given along with a cathartic. The use of cholestyramine in this situation has not been reported.

Patient Information

Immediately report sore throat, fever, chills or sore mouth to the physician.

The following may occur: Alopecia, jaw pain, pain in the organs containing tumor tissue, nausea and vomiting. Scalp hair will regrow to its pretreatment extent, even with continued treatment. Report any other serious medical event to the physician.

Avoid constipation.

VINCRISTINE SULFATE (VCR; LCR)

Rx	**Vincristine Sulfate** (Various, eg, Quad, VHA Supply)	**Injection:** 1 mg/ml	In 1, 2 and 5 ml vials.
Rx	**Vincasar PFS** (Gensia Sicor)		In 1, 2, 5 ml flip-top vials.[1]

[1] With 100 mg mannitol. Refrigerate.

WARNING

It is extremely important that the IV needle or catheter be properly positioned before injection. Leakage into surrounding tissue may cause considerable irritation.

This preparation is for IV use only. Intrathecal use usually results in death.

Indications

➤*Acute leukemia:* For acute leukemia.

➤*Combination therapy:* Combination therapy in Hodgkin's disease, non-Hodgkin's malignant lymphomas (lymphocytic, mixed-cell, histiocytic, undifferentiated, nodular and diffuse types), rhabdomyosarcoma, neuroblastoma and Wilms' tumor.

➤*Unlabeled uses:* Vincristine has been used in the treatment of idiopathic thrombocytopenic purpura, Kaposi's sarcoma, breast cancer and bladder cancer.

Administration and Dosage

Cautiously calculate and administer dose; overdosage may be serious or fatal.

Administer IV only, at weekly intervals. Inject solution either directly into a vein or into the tubing of a running IV infusion. Injection may be completed in about 1 minute.

➤*Adults:* 1.4 mg/m².

➤*Children:* 2 mg/m². For children weighing ≤ 10 kg or having a body surface area < 1 m², give 0.05 mg/kg once a week.

➤*Hepatic function impairment:* A 50% reduction in the dose is recommended for patients having a direct serum bilirubin value > 3 mg/dl.

➤*Extravasation:* Properly position needle in vein before injecting. Leakage into surrounding tissue may cause considerable irritation. Discontinue immediately; finish dose in another vein. Locally inject hyaluronidase; apply moderate heat to the area to disperse drug and minimize discomfort and possibility of cellulitis.

➤*Compatibility:* Do not dilute in solutions that raise or lower the pH outside the range of 3.5 to 5.5. Do not mix with anything other than normal saline or glucose in water.

Consider procedures for proper handling and disposal of anticancer drugs.

Actions

➤*Pharmacology:* Vincristine sulfate is an alkaloid obtained from the periwinkle (Vinca rosea Linn). Mode of action is unknown. In vitro, it arrests mitotic division at metaphase. Antineoplastic effects are related to interference with intracellular tubulin function. It reversibly binds to microtubule and spindle proteins in the S phase.

➤*Pharmacokinetics:*

Absorption / Distribution – Within 15 to 30 minutes following IV administration,> 90% of the drug is distributed from blood into tissue where it remains tightly, but not irreversibly, bound. Penetration across the blood-brain barrier is poor.

Metabolism / Excretion – Studies in cancer patients show a triphasic serum decay pattern following rapid IV injection. Initial, middle and terminal half-lives are 5 min, 2.3 hrs and 85 hrs, respectively; the range of the terminal half-life is 19 to 155 hrs. The liver is the major excretory organ; ≈ 80% of a dose appears in feces and 10% to 20% in urine. Hepatic dysfunction may alter elimination kinetics and augment toxicity.

Combination cancer chemotherapy – Combination cancer chemotherapy involves simultaneous use of several agents. Generally, each agent has a unique toxicity and mechanism so that therapeutic enhancement occurs without additive toxicity. It is rarely possible to achieve equally good results with single agent treatment. Vincristine is often chosen as part of polychemotherapy because of lack of significant bone marrow suppression (at recommended doses) and of unique clinical toxicity (neuropathy). See Administration and Dosage for possible increased toxicity when used in combination therapy.

Contraindications

Do not give to patients with demyelinating form of Charcot-Marie-Tooth syndrome.

Warnings

➤*Administer IV only:* Administer IV only; intrathecal administration is uniformly fatal.

➤*Hypersensitivity reactions:* Hypersensitivity temporally related to vincristine therapy, has occurred. Refer to Management of Acute Hypersensitivity Reactions. See Adverse Reactions.

➤*Carcinogenesis:* Patients who received vincristine with anticancer drugs known to be carcinogenic have developed secondary malignancies. Vincristine's contributing role in this development has not been determined.

➤*Fertility impairment:* Laboratory tests failed to conclusively demonstrate mutagenicity. Reports of both males and females who received multiple agent chemotherapy that included vincristine indicate azoospermia and amenorrhea can occur in postpubertal patients. Recovery occurred many months after chemotherapy completion in some. It is much less likely to cause permanent azoospermia and amenorrhea in prepubertal patients.

➤*Pregnancy: Category D.* Vincristine can cause fetal harm when administered to a pregnant woman. In several animal species, it induces teratogenic effects and embryolethality with doses that are nontoxic to the mother. There are no adequate and well controlled studies in pregnant women. If this drug is used during pregnancy or if the patient becomes pregnant while receiving it, apprise her of the potential hazard to the fetus. Advise women of childbearing potential to avoid becoming pregnant.

➤*Lactation:* It is not known whether this drug is excreted in breast milk. Because of the potential for serious adverse reactions in nursing infants, decide whether to discontinue nursing or the drug, taking into account importance of the drug to the mother.

Precautions

➤*Monitoring:* Dose-limiting clinical toxicity is manifested as neurotoxicity; clinical evaluation (history, physical examination) is necessary to detect need for dosage modification. Following vincristine, some patients may have a fall in WBC or platelet counts, particularly when previous therapy or the disease has reduced bone marrow function. Perform complete blood count before each dose. Acute serum uric acid elevation may occur during induction of remission in acute leukemia; thus determine such levels frequently during the first 3 to 4 treatment weeks or take appropriate measures to prevent uric acid nephropathy.

➤*Acute uric acid nephropathy:* Acute uric acid nephropathy has occurred.

➤*CNS leukemia:* CNS leukemia has occurred in patients undergoing otherwise successful therapy with vincristine. If CNS leukemia is diagnosed, additional agents may be required, since this drug does not adequately cross the blood-brain barrier.

➤*Leukopenia or complicating infection:* In the presence of these conditions, administration of the next dose warrants careful consideration.

➤*Neuromuscular disease:* Pay particular attention to dosage and neurological side effects if administered to patients with preexisting neuromuscular disease or when other neurotoxic drugs are used.

➤*Eye contamination:* Eye contamination should be avoided with concentrations used clinically. If accidental contamination occurs, severe irritation (or, if drug was delivered under pressure, even corneal ulceration) may result. Wash eyes immediately and thoroughly.

➤*Pulmonary reactions:* Acute shortness of breath and severe bronchospasm have followed administration of vinca alkaloids, most frequently when the drug was used with mitomycin-C. The onset may be within minutes or several hours after the vinca is injected and may occur up to 2 weeks following the dose of mitomycin.

➤*Concomitant radiation therapy:* Do not give to patients receiving radiation therapy through ports that include the liver.

VINCRISTINE SULFATE (VCR; LCR)

Drug Interactions

Vincristine Drug Interactions			
Precipitant drug	Object drug*		Description
Vincristine	Digoxin	↓	Combination chemotherapy (including vincristine) may decrease digoxin plasma levels and renal excretion.
L-asparaginase	Vincristine	↑	Administering L-asparaginase first may reduce hepatic clearance of vincristine. Give vincristine 12 to 24 hrs before L-asparaginase to minimize toxicity.
Mitomycin	Vincristine	↑	Acute pulmonary reactions may occur (see Precautions).
Vincristine	Phenytoin	↓	Combination chemotherapy (including vincristine) may reduce phenytoin plasma levels, requiring increased dosage to maintain therapeutic plasma levels.

* ↑ = Object drug increased. ↓ = Object drug decreased.

Adverse Reactions

Adverse reactions are generally reversible and dose-related. With single weekly doses, leukopenia, neuritic pain, and constipation may occur and are usually of short duration (ie, < 7 days). When dosage is reduced, reactions may lessen or disappear. They seem to increase when the drug is given in divided doses. Other adverse reactions, such as hair loss, sensory loss, paresthesia, difficulty in walking, slapping gait, loss of deep tendon reflexes, and muscle wasting may persist for at least as long as therapy is continued. Generalized sensorimotor dysfunction may become progressively more severe with continued treatment. Neuromuscular difficulties usually disappear by the sixth week after treatment is discontinued, but they may persist for prolonged periods in some patients. Hair regrowth may occur while maintenance therapy continues.

SIADH – The syndrome of inappropriate antidiuretic hormone secretion (SIADH), including high urinary sodium excretion in the presence of hyponatremia, occurs rarely. Renal or adrenal disease, hypotension, dehydration, azotemia, and clinical edema are absent. With fluid deprivation, hyponatremia and renal sodium loss improve.

➤*CNS:* Loss of deep-tendon reflexes, ataxia, footdrop, and paralysis have been seen with continued use. Cranial nerve manifestations, including isolated paresis or paralysis of muscles may occur; extraocular and laryngeal muscles are most commonly involved. Severe pain may occur in the jaw, pharynx, parotid gland, bones, back, and limbs. Myalgias have occurred. Reduced intestinal motility results in constipation. Convulsions, often with hypertension, have occurred in a few patients. Convulsions followed by coma have been seen in children. Frequently, there is a sequence in the development of neuropathy: Initially, sensory impairment and paresthesias, then neuritic pain may appear and later, motor difficulties. Neurotoxicity is dose-related and cumulative to where therapy must be stopped after a cumulative dose of 30 to 50 mg. It is reversible upon discontinuation, but recovery may take several months.

In one study, the administration of glutamic acid (500 mg 3 times daily) decreased the neurotoxicity induced by vincristine.

➤*GI:* Oral ulceration; abdominal cramps; nausea; vomiting; diarrhea; anorexia; intestinal necrosis or perforation.

Constipation – Constipation may take the form of upper colon impaction, and, on examination, the rectum may be empty. Colicky abdominal pain may accompany an empty rectum. A flat film of the abdomen demonstrates this condition. Cases respond to high enemas and laxatives. Use routine prophylaxis for constipation.

Paralytic ileus – Paralytic ileus that mimics the "surgical abdomen" may occur, particularly in young children. The ileus will reverse itself upon temporary discontinuation of vincristine and with symptomatic care.

➤*GU:* Polyuria; dysuria; urinary retention due to bladder atony. Discontinue other drugs known to cause urinary retention (particularly in the elderly), if possible, for the first few days following administration.

➤*Hematologic:* Serious bone marrow depression (usually not dose-limiting); anemia; leukopenia; thrombocytopenia. Thrombocytopenia, if present when therapy is begun, may improve before the appearance of marrow remission.

➤*Hypersensitivity:* Rare cases of allergic type reactions, such as anaphylaxis, rash and edema, that are temporally related to vincristine therapy have occurred in patients receiving vincristine as a part of multi-drug chemotherapy regimens (see Warnings).

➤*Ophthalmic:* Optic atrophy with blindness; transient cortical blindness; ptosis; diplopia; photophobia.

➤*Pulmonary:* Acute shortness of breath, severe bronchospasm (see Precautions).

➤*Miscellaneous:* Hyper- or hypotension; weight loss; fever; alopecia; rash; headache.

Overdosage

➤*Symptoms:* Side effects are dose-related. After an overdose, expect exaggerated side effects. In children < 13 years of age, death has occurred after doses 10 times those recommended; severe symptoms may occur with 3 to 4 mg/m². Adults may experience severe symptoms after single doses ≥ 3 mg/m².

➤*Treatment:* Supportive care should include prevention of side effects resulting from SIADH (eg, fluid intake restriction; perhaps a diuretic affecting function of Henle's loop and distal tubule); phenobarbital (anticonvulsant); enemas or cathartics to prevent ileus (in some instances, GI tract decompression may be necessary); monitor cardiovascular system; determine daily blood counts to guide transfusion requirements.

Folinic acid, 100 mg IV every 3 hours for 24 hours, then every 6 hours for at least 48 hours, may help treat overdose. Folinic acid does not eliminate the need for supportive measures.

Most of an IV dose is excreted into the bile after rapid tissue binding. Hemodialysis is not likely to be helpful. Patients with liver disease sufficient to decrease biliary excretion may experience increased severity of side effects.

VINORELBINE TARTRATE

Rx	Vinorelbine Tartrate (GensiaSicor)	Injection: 10 mg/ml	In 1 and 5 mL vials.
Rx	Navelbine (GlaxoSmithKline)		Preservative free. In 1 and 5 mL single-use vials.

WARNING

Administer vinorelbine under the supervision of a physician experienced in the use of cancer chemotherapeutic agents. This product is for IV use only. Intrathecal administration of other vinca alkaloids has resulted in death. Label syringes containing this product, "Warning: Vinorelbine for IV use only. Fatal if given intrathecally."

Severe granulocytopenia resulting in increased susceptibility to infection may occur. Granulocyte counts should be ≥ 1000 cells/mm³ prior to the administration of vinorelbine. Adjust dosage according to complete blood counts with differentials obtained on the day of treatment.

It is extremely important that the IV needle or catheter be properly positioned before vinorelbine is injected. Improper administration of vinorelbine may result in extravasation causing local tissue necrosis or thrombophlebitis (see Administration and Dosage).

Indications

➤*Non-small cell lung cancer (NSCLC):* Single agent or in combination with cisplatin for the first-line treatment of ambulatory patients with unresectable, advanced NSCLC. In patients with Stage IV NSCLC, vinorelbine is indicated as a single agent or in combination with cisplatin. In Stage III NSCLC, vinorelbine is indicated in combination with cisplatin.

➤*Unlabeled uses:* Metastatic breast cancer; carcinoma of the uterine cervix; desmoid tumors and fibromatosis; advanced Kaposi's sarcoma.

Administration and Dosage

➤*Approved by the FDA:* December 23, 1994.

The usual initial dose is 30 mg/m² administered weekly. The recommended method of administration is an IV injection over 6 to 10 minutes. In controlled trials, single-agent vinorelbine was given weekly until progression or dose-limiting toxicity. Vinorelbine was used at the same dose in combination with 120 mg/m² of cisplatin, given on days 1 and 29, then every 6 weeks.

➤*Hematologic toxicity:* Granulocyte counts should be ≥ 1000 cells/mm³ prior to the administration of vinorelbine. Base dosage adjustments on granulocyte counts obtained on the day of treatment as follows:

Vinorelbine Dose Adjustments Based on Granulocyte Counts	
Granulocytes (cells/mm³) on days of treatment	Dose (mg/m²)
≥ 1500	30
1000 to 1499	15

VINORELBINE TARTRATE

Vinorelbine Dose Adjustments Based on Granulocyte Counts	
Granulocytes (cells/mm³) on days of treatment	Dose (mg/m²)
< 1000	Do not administer. Repeat granulocyte count in 1 week. If 3 consecutive weekly doses are held because granulocyte count is < 1000 cells/mm³, discontinue vinorelbine.
Note: For patients who, during treatment, have experienced fever or sepsis while granulocytopenic or had 2 consecutive weekly doses held due to granulocytopenia, subsequent doses of vinorelbine should be: 22.5 mg/m² for granulocytes ≥ 1500 cells/mm³ 11.25 mg/m² for granulocytes 1000 to 1499 cells/mm³	

➤*Hepatic function impairment:* Administer with caution to patients with hepatic insufficiency. In patients who develop hyperbilirubinemia during treatment with vinorelbine, adjust the dose for total bilirubin as follows:

Vinorelbine Dose Modification Based on Total Bilirubin	
Total bilirubin (mg/dl)	Dose (mg/m²)
≤ 2	30
2.1 - 3	15
> 3	7.5

➤*Concurrent hematologic toxicity and hepatic insufficiency:* In patients with both hematologic toxicity and hepatic insufficiency, administer the lower of the doses determined from the previous tables.

➤*Administration precautions:* Administer vinorelbine IV. It is extremely important that the IV needle or catheter be properly positioned before any vinorelbine is injected. Leakage into surrounding tissue during IV administration may cause considerable irritation, local tissue necrosis, or thrombophlebitis. If extravasation occurs, discontinue the injection immediately and introduce any remaining portion of the dose into another vein. Since there are no established guidelines for the treatment of extravasation injuries with vinorelbine, institutional guidelines may be used. *The ONS Chemotherapy Guidelines* provide additional recommendations for the prevention of extravasation injuries. (ONS Clinical Practice Committee. Cancer Chemotherapy Guidelines: Recommendations for the management of vesicant extravasation, hypersensitivity, and anaphylaxis. Pittsburgh, PA: Oncology Nursing Society;1992:1-4.)

As with other toxic compounds, exercise caution in handling and preparing the solution of vinorelbine. Skin reactions may occur with accidental exposure. The use of gloves is recommended. If the solution of vinorelbine contacts the skin or mucosa, immediately wash the skin or mucosa thoroughly with soap and water. Severe irritation of the eye has been reported with accidental contamination of the eye with another vinca alkaloid. If this happens with vinorelbine, flush the eye with water immediately and thoroughly. Use procedures for proper handling and disposal of anticancer drugs.

➤*Preparation for administration:* Dilute vinorelbine in a syringe or IV bag using one of the recommended solutions. Administer the diluted vinorelbine over 6 to 10 minutes into the side port of a free-flowing IV closest to the IV bag followed by flushing with ≥ 75 to 125 ml of one of the solutions. Diluted vinorelbine may be used for up to 24 hours under normal room light when stored in polypropylene syringes or polyvinyl chloride bags at 5° to 30°C (41° to 86°F).

Syringe – Dilute the calculated dose of vinorelbine to a concentration between 1.5 and 3 mg/ml. The following solutions may be used for dilution: 5% Dextrose Injection; 0.9% Sodium Chloride Injection.

IV bag – Dilute the calculated dose of vinorelbine to a concentration between 0.5 and 2 mg/ml. The following solutions may be used for dilution: 5% Dextrose Injection; 0.45% or 0.9% Sodium Chloride Injection; 5% Dextrose and 0.45% Sodium Chloride Injection; Ringer's Injection; Lactated Ringer's Injection.

➤*Storage/Stability:* Unopened vials of vinorelbine are stable until the date indicated on the package when stored under refrigeration at 2° to 8°C (36° to 46°F) and protected from light in the carton. Unopened vials of vinorelbine are stable at temperatures up to 25°C (77°F) for up to 72 hours. Protect from light. Do not freeze. If particulate matter is seen, do not administer.

Actions

➤*Pharmacology:* Vinorelbine is a semi-synthetic vinca alkaloid with antitumor activity that interferes with microtubule assembly. The vinca alkaloids are structurally similar compounds comprised of 2 multi-ringed units, vindoline and catharanthine. Unlike other vinca alkaloids, the catharanthine unit is the site of structural modification for vinorelbine. The antitumor activity of vinorelbine is thought to be due primarily to inhibition of mitosis at metaphase through its inter-

action with tubulin. Like other vinca alkaloids, vinorelbine may also interfere with the following: 1) amino acid, cyclic AMP, and glutathione metabolism, 2) calmodulin-dependent Ca⁺⁺-transport ATPase activity, 3) cellular respiration, and 4) nucleic acid and lipid biosynthesis. In intact tectal plates from mouse embryos, vinorelbine, vincristine, and vinblastine inhibited mitotic microtubule formation at the same concentration (2 mcM), inducing a blockade of cells at metaphase. Vincristine produced depolymerization of axonal microtubules at 5 mcM, but vinblastine and vinorelbine did not have this effect until concentrations of 30 mcM and 40 mcM, respectively. These data suggest relative selectivity of vinorelbine for mitotic microtubules.

➤*Pharmacokinetics:* Following IV administration, vinorelbine concentration in plasma decays in a triphasic manner. The initial rapid decline primarily represents distribution of the drug to peripheral compartments followed by metabolism and excretion of the drug during subsequent phases. The prolonged terminal phase is due to relatively slow efflux of vinorelbine from peripheral compartments. The terminal phase half-life averages 27.7 to 43.6 hours and the mean plasma clearance ranges from 0.97 to 1.26 L/hr/kg. Steady-state volume of distribution values range from 25.4 to 40.1 L/kg.

Vinorelbine demonstrated high binding to human platelets and lymphocytes. The binding to plasma constituents in cancer patients ranged from 79.6% to 91.2%. Vinorelbine binding was not altered in the presence of cisplatin, 5-fluorouracil, or doxorubicin.

Vinorelbine undergoes substantial hepatic elimination, with large amounts recovered in feces. Two metabolites of vinorelbine have been identified in human blood, plasma, and urine; vinorelbine N-oxide and deacetylvinorelbine. Deacetylvinorelbine has been demonstrated to be the primary metabolite of vinorelbine in humans, and has shown to possess antitumor activity similar to vinorelbine. Therapeutic doses of vinorelbine (30 mg/m²) yield very small, if any, quantifiable levels of either metabolite in blood or urine. The metabolism of vinca alkaloids has been shown to be mediated by hepatic cytochrome P450 isoenzymes in the CYP3A subfamily. This metabolic pathway may be impaired in patients with hepatic dysfunction or who are taking concomitant potent inhibitors of these isoenzymes (see Precautions). The effects of renal or hepatic dysfunction on the disposition of vinorelbine have not been assessed, but based on experience with other anticancer vinca alkaloids, dose adjustments are recommended for patients with impaired hepatic function (see Administration and Dosage).

Approximately 18% of an administered dose was recovered in urine and 46% in feces; ≈ 10.9% of a 30 mg/m² IV dose was excreted unchanged in the urine.

➤*Clinical trials:* Patients (n = 612) were randomized to treatment with single-agent vinorelbine (30 mg/m²/week), vinorelbine (30 mg/m²/week) plus cisplatin (120 mg/m² days 1 and 29, then every 6 weeks), and vindesine (3 mg/m²/week for 7 weeks, then every other week) plus cisplatin (120 mg/m² days 1 and 29, then every 6 weeks). Vinorelbine plus cisplatin produced longer survival times than vindesine plus cisplatin (median survival 40 weeks vs 32 weeks). The median survival time for patients receiving single-agent vinorelbine was similar to that of vinorelbine plus cisplatin (31 vs 32 weeks). The 1-year survival rates were 35% for vinorelbine plus cisplatin, 27% for vindesine plus cisplatin, and 30% for single-agent vinorelbine. The overall objective response rate (all partial responses) was significantly higher with vinorelbine plus cisplatin (28%) than with vindesine plus cisplatin (19%) and with single-agent vinorelbine (14%). The response rates for vindesine plus cisplatin and single-agent vinorelbine were not significantly different. Significantly fewer incidences of nausea, vomiting, alopecia, and neurotoxicity were observed in patients receiving single-agent vinorelbine compared to vindesine and cisplatin.

In another study, patients were treated with vinorelbine (n = 143; 30 mg/m²) weekly or 5-fluorouracil (5-FU; n = 68; 425 mg/m² IV bolus) plus leucovorin (LV; 20 mg/m² IV bolus) daily for 5 days every 4 weeks. Vinorelbine showed improved survival time compared to 5-FU/LV. The median survival time for patients receiving vinorelbine was 30 weeks and for those receiving 5-FU/LV was 22 weeks. The 1-year survival rates were 24% for vinorelbine and 16% for the 5-FU/LV group. The median survival time with 5-FU/LV was similar to, or slightly better than, that usually observed in untreated patients with advanced NSCLC, suggesting that the difference was not related to some unknown detrimental effect of 5-FU/LV therapy. The response rates (all partial responses) for vinorelbine and 5-FU/LV were 12% and 3%, respectively. Quality of life was not adversely affected by vinorelbine when compared to control.

Contraindications

Pretreatment granulocyte counts < 1000 cells/mm³ (see Warnings).

Warnings

➤*Interstitial pulmonary changes:* Reported cases of interstitial pulmonary changes and ARDS, most of which were fatal, occurred in patients treated with single-agent vinorelbine. The mean time to onset of these symptoms after vinorelbine administration was 1 week (range, 3 to 8 days). Promptly evaluate patients with alterations in their baseline pulmonary symptoms or with new onset of dyspnea, cough, hypoxia, or other symptoms.

VINORELBINE TARTRATE

►*GI:* Vinorelbine has been reported to cause severe constipation (eg, grade 3 to 4), paralytic ileus, intestinal obstruction, necrosis, and perforation. Some events have been fatal.

►*Granulocytopenia:* Frequently monitor patients treated with vinorelbine for myelosuppression both during and after therapy. Granulocytopenia is dose-limiting. Granulocyte nadirs occur between 7 and 10 days after dosing with granulocyte count recovery usually within the following 7 to 14 days. Perform complete blood counts with differentials and review results prior to giving each dose. Do not administer to patients with granulocyte counts < 1000 cells/mm³. Carefully monitor patients developing severe granulocytopenia for evidence of infection or fever. See Administration and Dosage for recommended dose adjustments for granulocytopenia.

Prophylactic hematologic growth factors have not been routinely used with vinorelbine. If medically necessary, growth factors may be administered at recommended doses no earlier than 24 hours after the administration of cytotoxic chemotherapy. Growth factors should not be given within 24 hours before the administration of chemotherapy.

►*Hepatic function impairment:* There is no evidence that the toxicity of vinorelbine is enhanced in patients with elevated liver enzymes. However, exercise caution when administering vinorelbine to patients with severe hepatic injury or impairment (see Administration and Dosage).

►*Carcinogenesis:* In vivo, vinorelbine affects chromosome number and possibly structure.

Biweekly administration for 13 or 26 weeks in rats at 2.1 and 7.2 mg/m² (approximately one-fifteenth and one-fourth the human dose) resulted in decreased spermatogenesis and prostate/seminal vesicle secretion.

►*Elderly:* In patients ≥ 65 years of age, no overall differences in effectiveness or safety were observed between these patients and younger patients. However, greater sensitivity of some older individuals cannot be ruled out.

►*Pregnancy:* Category D. Vinorelbine may cause fetal harm if administered to a pregnant woman. A single dose of vinorelbine was embryo- or fetotoxic in mice and rabbits at doses of 9 mg/m² and 5.5 mg/m², respectively (one-third and one-sixth the human dose). At nonmaternotoxic doses, fetal weight was reduced and ossification was delayed. There have been no studies in pregnant women. If vinorelbine is used during pregnancy, or if the patient becomes pregnant while receiving this drug, apprise the patient of the potential hazard to the fetus. Advise women of childbearing potential to avoid becoming pregnant during therapy with vinorelbine.

►*Lactation:* It is not known whether the drug is excreted in breast milk. Because of the potential for serious adverse reactions in nursing infants from vinorelbine, discontinue nursing in women who are receiving vinorelbine therapy.

►*Children:* Safety and efficacy in children have not been established.

Precautions

►*Monitoring:* Since dose-limiting clinical toxicity is the result of depression of the white blood cell count, it is imperative that complete blood counts with differentials be obtained and reviewed on the day of treatment prior to each dose of vinorelbine (see Warnings).

Monitor patients with a history of or with preexisting neuropathy, regardless of etiology, for new or worsening signs and symptoms of neuropathy while receiving vinorelbine.

►*Prior radiation therapy:* Administration of vinorelbine to patients with prior radiation therapy may result in radiation recall reactions (see Adverse Reactions).

►*Bone marrow:* Use with extreme caution in patients whose bone marrow reserve may have been compromised by prior irradiation or chemotherapy or whose marrow function is recovering from the effects of previous chemotherapy.

►*Bronchospasm:* Acute shortness of breath and severe bronchospasm have been reported infrequently following the administration of vinorelbine and other vinca alkaloids, most commonly when the vinca alkaloid was used in combination with mitomycin. These adverse reactions may require treatment with supplemental oxygen, bronchodilators or corticosteroids, particularly when there is preexisting pulmonary dysfunction.

►*Eye contact:* Avoid contamination of the eye with concentrations of vinorelbine used clinically. Severe irritation of the eye has been reported with accidental exposure to another vinca alkaloid. If exposure occurs, immediately flush the eye(s) with water.

Drug Interactions

►*P450 isoenzymes:* Exercise caution in patients concurrently taking drugs known to inhibit drug metabolism by hepatic cytochrome P450 isoenzymes in the CYP3A subfamily, or in patients with hepatic dysfunction. Concurrent administration of vinorelbine tartrate with an inhibitor of this metabolic pathway may cause an earlier onset or an increased severity of side effects.

►*Prior or concomitant radiation therapy:* Administration of vinorelbine to patients with prior or concomitant radiation therapy may result in radiosensitizing effects.

Vinorelbine Drug Interactions			
Precipitant drug	Object drug*		Description
Cisplatin	Vinorelbine	↑	Although the pharmacokinetics of vinorelbine are not influenced by the concurrent administration of cisplatin, the incidence of granulocytopenia with vinorelbine used in combination with cisplatin is significantly higher than with single-agent vinorelbine.
Mitomycin	Vinorelbine	↑	Acute pulmonary reactions have been reported with vinorelbine and other anticancer vinca alkaloids used in conjunction with mitomycin.
Paclitaxel	Vinorelbine	↑	Monitor for signs and symptoms of neuropathy for patients who receive vinorelbine and paclitaxel, either concomitantly or sequentially.

* ↑ = Object drug increased.

Adverse Reactions

Most drug-related adverse reactions are reversible. If severe adverse reactions occur, reduce dosage or discontinue and take appropriate corrective measures. Reinstitution of therapy with vinorelbine should be carried out with caution and alertness as to possible recurrence of toxicity.

Vinorelbine (Single-Agent Use) Adverse Reactions (%)[1]						
	All grades		Grade 3		Grade 4	
Adverse reaction	All patients (n = 365)	NSCLC (n = 143)	All patients	NSCLC	All patients	NSCLC
Bone marrow						
Granulocytopenia (cells/mm³)						
< 2000	90	80	-	-	-	-
< 500	36	29	-	-	-	-
Leukopenia (cells/mm³)						
< 4000	92	81	-	-	-	-
< 1000	15	12	-	-	-	-
Thrombocytopenia (cells/mm³)						
< 100,000	5	4	-	-	-	-
< 50,000	1	1	-	-	-	-
Anemia (g/dl)						
< 11	83	77	-	-	-	-
< 8	9	1	-	-	-	-
Hospitalizations due to granulocytopenic complications	9	8	-	-	-	-

VINORELBINE TARTRATE

	Vinorelbine (Single-Agent Use) Adverse Reactions (%)[1]					
	All grades		Grade 3		Grade 4	
Adverse reaction	All patients (n = 365)	NSCLC (n = 143)	All patients	NSCLC	All patients	NSCLC
Lab test abnormalities						
Total bilirubin elevation (n = 351)	13	9	4	3	3	2
AST elevation (n = 346)	67	54	5	2	1	1
GI						
Nausea	44	34	2	1	0	0
Vomiting	20	15	2	1	0	0
Constipation	35	29	3	2	0	0
Diarrhea	17	13	1	1	0	0
Miscellaneous						
Asthenia	36	27	7	5	0	0
Injection site reactions	28	38	2	5	0	0
Injection site pain	16	13	2	1	0	0
Phlebitis	7	10	< 1	1	0	0
Peripheral neuropathy[2]	25	20	1	1	< 1	0
Dyspnea	7	3	2	2	1	0
Alopecia	12	12	≤ 1	1	0	0

[1] Grade based on modified criteria from the National Cancer Institute. Patients with NSCLC had not received prior chemotherapy; the majority of the remaining patients had received prior chemotherapy.

[2] Incidence of paresthesia plus hypesthesia.

➤*Cardiovascular:* Chest pain (5%); hypertension; hypotension; vasodilation; tachycardia; pulmonary edema. Most reports of chest pain were in patients who had either a history of cardiovascular disease or tumor within the chest. There have been rare reports of MI.

➤*CNS:* Mild-to-moderate peripheral neuropathy manifested by paresthesia and hypesthesia were the most frequently reported neurologic toxicities. Loss of deep tendon reflexes (< 5%); development of severe peripheral neuropathy (1%; generally reversible).

Peripheral neurotoxicities such as, but not limited to, muscle weakness and disturbance of gait, have been observed in patients with and without prior symptoms. There may be increased potential for neurotoxicity in patients with preexisting neuropathy, regardless of etiology, who receive vinorelbine. Vestibular and auditory deficits have been observed with vinorelbine, usually when used in combination with cisplatin.

➤*Dermatologic:* Alopecia (12%; was usually mild); injection site reactions, including localized rash and urticaria, blister formation, and skin sloughing (some may be delayed in appearance).

Like other anticancer vinca alkaloids, vinorelbine is a moderate vesicant. Injection site reactions, including erythema, pain at injection site and vein discoloration occurred in approximately one-third of patients; 5% were severe. Chemical phlebitis along the vein proximal to the site of injection was reported in 10% of patients.

➤*GI:* Mild or moderate nausea (34%); severe nausea (< 2%). Prophylactic antiemetics were not routine in patients treated with single-agent vinorelbine. Due to the low incidence of severe nausea and vomiting with single-agent vinorelbine, the use of serotonin antagonists is generally not required. Constipation (29%); vomiting, diarrhea, anorexia, stomatitis (< 20%; usually mild or moderate); paralytic ileus (1%); dysphagia; mucositis.

➤*Hematologic:* Granulocytopenia was the major dose-limiting toxicity; it was generally reversible and not cumulative over time. Granulocyte nadirs occurred 7 to 10 days after the dose, with granulocyte recovery usually within the following 7 to 14 days. Granulocytopenia resulted in hospitalizations for fever or sepsis in 8% of patients; septic deaths occurred in ≈ 1% of patients. Prophylactic hematologic growth factors have not been routinely used with vinorelbine. If medically necessary, growth factors may be administered at recommended doses no earlier than 24 hours after the administration of cytotoxic chemotherapy. Do not administer growth factors in the period 24 hours before the administration of chemotherapy.

Grade 3 or 4 anemia occurred in 1%, although blood products were administered to 18% of patients who received vinorelbine; grade 3 or 4 thrombocytopenia has occurred in 1% of patients.

Thromboembolic events (eg, pulmonary embolus, deep vein thrombosis) have been reported primarily in seriously ill and debilitated patients with known predisposing risk factors for these events.

➤*Hepatic:* Transient liver enzyme elevations occurred without clinical symptoms.

➤*Pulmonary:* Pneumonia; shortness of breath (3%; severe in 2%; see Precautions). Interstitial pulmonary changes were documented in a few patients.

➤*Miscellaneous:* Fatigue (27%), usually mild or moderate but tended to increase with cumulative dosing; jaw pain, myalgia, arthralgia, rash (< 5%); hemorrhagic cystitis, syndrome of inappropriate ADH secretion (< 1%); systemic allergic reactions (eg, anaphylaxis, pruritus, urticaria, angioedema); flushing; radiation recall events (eg, dermatitis, esophagitis); headache with and without other musculoskeletal aches and pains; pain in tumor-containing tissue; back pain; abdominal pain; electrolyte abnormalities, including hyponatremia with or without syndrome of inappropriate ADH secretion have been reported in seriously ill and debilitated patients.

Combination use – In a randomized study, 206 patients received treatment with vinorelbine plus cisplatin and 206 patients received single-agent vinorelbine. The incidence of severe nausea and vomiting was 30% for vinorelbine/cisplatin compared to < 2% for single-agent vinorelbine. Cisplatin did not appear to increase the incidence of neurotoxicity observed with single-agent vinorelbine. However, myelosuppression, specifically Grade 3 and 4 granulocytopenia, was greater with the combination of vinorelbine/cisplatin (79%) than with single-agent vinorelbine (53%). The incidence of fever and infection may be increased with the combination.

Monitor patients with prior exposure to paclitaxel who have demonstrated neuropathy for new or worsening neuropathy. Monitor patients who have experienced neuropathy with previous drug regimens for symptoms of neuropathy while receiving vinorelbine. Vinorelbine may result in radiosensitizing effects with prior or concomitant radiation therapy.

Overdosage

There is no known antidote for overdoses of vinorelbine. Overdoses involving quantities up to 10 times the recommended dose (30 mg/m^2) have been reported. The toxicities described were consistent with those listed in the adverse reactions section including paralytic ileus, stomatitis, and esophagitis. Bone marrow aplasia, sepsis, and paresis have also been reported. Fatalities have occurred following overdose of vinorelbine. If overdosage occurs, institute general supportive measures together with appropriate blood transfusions, growth factors, and antibiotics as deemed necessary by the physician. Refer to General Management of Acute Overdosage.

Patient Information

Inform patients that the major acute toxicities of vinorelbine are related to bone marrow toxicity, specifically granulocytopenia with increased susceptibility to infection. Advise them to report fever or chills immediately.

Advise women of childbearing potential to avoid pregnancy during treatment.

Advise patients to contact their physician if they experience increased shortness of breath, cough, or other new pulmonary symptoms, or if they experience symptoms of abdominal pain or constipation.

Taxoids

PACLITAXEL

Rx	**Taxol** (Bristol-Myers Squibb)	**Injection:** 6 mg/ml	In 5, 16.7, and 50 ml multi-dose vials.[1]
Rx	**Onxol** (Zenith-Goldline)		In 5, 25, and 50 ml multi-dose vials.[2]

[1] With 527 mg/ml polyoxyethylated castor oil (*Cremophor EL*) and 49.7% dehydrated alcohol.

[2] With 527 mg/ml polyoxyl 35 castor oil and 49.7% dehydrated alcohol.

WARNING

Administer under the supervision of a physician experienced in the use of cancer chemotherapeutic agents. Appropriate management of complications is possible only when adequate diagnostic and treatment facilities are readily available.

Anaphylaxis and severe hypersensitivity reactions characterized by dyspnea and hypotension requiring treatment, angioedema, and generalized urticaria have occurred in 2% to 4% of patients. Fatal reactions have occurred despite premedication. Pretreat patients receiving paclitaxel with corticosteroids, diphenhydramine, and H_2 antagonists to prevent these reactions (see Administration and Dosage). Do not rechallenge patients who experience severe hypersensitivity reactions to paclitaxel with the drug.

Do not give paclitaxel therapy to patients with solid tumors when the baseline neutrophil counts are < 1500 cells/mm^3. Do not give to patients with AIDS-related Kaposi's sarcoma if the baseline count is < 1000 cells/mm^3. In order to monitor the occurrence of bone marrow suppression, primarily neutropenia, which may be severe and result in infection, perform frequent peripheral blood cell counts on all patients receiving paclitaxel.

Indications

➤*Taxol:*

Ovarian cancer – Treatment of advanced carcinoma of the ovary as first-line and subsequent therapy. As first-line therapy, paclitaxel is indicated in combination with cisplatin.

Breast cancer – Adjuvant treatment of node-positive breast cancer administered sequentially to standard doxorubicin-containing combination chemotherapy. Treatment of breast cancer after failure of combination chemotherapy for metastatic disease or relapse within 6 months of adjuvant chemotherapy. Prior therapy should have included an anthracycline unless clinically contraindicated.

Non-small cell lung cancer (NSCLC) – First-line treatment of NSCLC in combination with cisplatin in patients who are not candidates for potentially curative surgery or radiation therapy.

AIDS-related Kaposi's sarcoma – As second-line treatment.

➤*Onxol:*

Ovarian cancer – Treatment of advanced carcinoma of the ovary as subsequent therapy.

Breast cancer – Treatment of breast cancer after failure of combination chemotherapy for metastatic disease or relapse within 6 months of adjuvant chemotherapy. Prior therapy should have included an anthracycline unless clinically contraindicated.

➤*Unlabeled uses:* Paclitaxel, alone or in combination with other chemotherapy agents, is being investigated for use in the following conditions: Advanced head and neck cancer, small-cell lung cancer, adenocarcinoma of the upper GI tract, hormone-refractory prostate cancer, non-Hodgkin's lymphoma, transitional cell carcinoma of the urothelium, pancreatic cancer, and polycystic kidney disease.

Administration and Dosage

➤*Approved by the FDA:* December 29, 1992.

➤*Recommended dose:*

Ovarian cancer – Either 175 mg/m^2 administered IV over 3 hours every 3 weeks or 135 mg/m^2 administered IV over 24 hours every 3 weeks, followed by cisplatin at a dose of 75 mg/m^2, in previously untreated patients with carcinoma of the ovary (*Taxol* only).

135 mg/m^2 or 175 mg/m^2 administered IV over 3 hours every 3 weeks in patients previously treated with chemotherapy for carcinoma of the ovary. Optimal regimen is not yet clear.

Breast cancer – 175 mg/m^2 IV over 3 hours every 3 weeks for 4 courses administered sequentially to doxorubicin-containing combination chemotherapy for the adjuvant treatment of node-positive breast cancer (*Taxol* only).

175 mg/m^2 IV over 3 hours every 3 weeks after failure of initial chemotherapy for metastatic disease or relapse within 6 months of adjuvant chemotherapy.

NSCLC – 135 mg/m^2 administered IV over 24 hours followed by 75 mg/m^2 cisplatin every 3 weeks.

AIDS-related Kaposi's sarcoma – 135 mg/m^2 given IV over 3 hours every 3 weeks or 100 mg/m^2 IV over 3 hours every 2 weeks (dose-intensity, 45 to 50 mg/m^2/week). In 2 clinical trials evaluating these schedules, the former schedule (135 mg/m^2 every 3 weeks) was more toxic than the latter. In addition, all patients with low performance status were treated with the latter schedule (100 mg/m^2 every 2 weeks).

Based upon the immunosuppression in patients with advanced HIV disease, the following modifications are recommended in these patients:

1.) Reduce the dose of dexamethasone as 1 of the 3 premedication drugs to 10 mg orally (instead of 20 mg orally);
2.) Initiate or repeat treatment with paclitaxel only if neutrophil count is ≥ 1000 cells/mm^3;
3.) Reduce the dose of subsequent courses of paclitaxel by 20% for patients who experience severe neutropenia (neutrophil count < 500 cells/mm^3 for ≥ 1 week);
4.) Initiate concomitant hematopoietic growth factor (G-CSF) as clinically indicated.

Do not repeat courses of paclitaxel until the neutrophil count is ≥ 1500 cells/mm^3 and the platelet count is ≥ 100,000 cells/mm^3. Do not give to patients with AIDS-related Kaposi's sarcoma if baseline or subsequent neutrophil count is < 1000 cells/mm^3. Reduce dosage by 20% for subsequent courses in patients who experience severe neutropenia (neutrophils < 500 cells/mm^3 for ≥ 1 week) or severe peripheral neuropathy during therapy. The incidence and severity of neurotoxicity and hematologic toxicity increase with dose, especially > 190 mg/m^2.

➤*Premedication regimen:* Premedicate patients prior to administration in order to prevent severe hypersensitivity reactions. Such premedication may consist of 20 mg oral dexamethasone administered ≈ 12 and 6 hours before paclitaxel, 50 mg diphenhydramine IV (or its equivalent) 30 to 60 minutes prior to paclitaxel, and 300 mg cimetidine, 20 mg famotidine, or 50 mg ranitidine IV 30 to 60 minutes before paclitaxel. Reduce the dose of dexamethasone to 10 mg orally in patients with Kaposi's sarcoma.

➤*Preparation:* Paclitaxel is a cytotoxic anticancer drug. As with other potentially toxic compounds, exercise caution in handling the drug; use gloves. If paclitaxel solution contacts the skin, wash the skin immediately and thoroughly with soap and water. Following topical exposure, adverse events have included tingling, burning, and redness. If paclitaxel contacts mucous membranes, thoroughly flush the membranes with water. Upon inhalation, dyspnea, chest pain, burning eyes, sore throat, and nausea have been reported.

Prior to infusion, dilute paclitaxel concentrate in 0.9% Sodium Chloride Injection, USP; 5% Dextrose Injection, USP; 5% Dextrose and 0.9% Sodium Chloride Injection, USP; or 5% Dextrose in Ringer's Injection to a final concentration of 0.3 to 1.2 mg/ml. The solutions are physically and chemically stable for ≤ 27 hours at ambient temperature (≈ 25°C; 77°F) and room lighting conditions. Inspect parenteral drug products visually for particulate matter and discoloration prior to administration whenever solution and container permit.

Upon preparation, solutions may show haziness, which is attributed to the formulation vehicle. No significant losses in potency have been noted following simulated delivery of the solution through IV tubing containing an in-line (0.22 micron) filter.

Administer through an in-line filter with a microporous membrane ≤ 0.22 microns. Use of filter devices such as *Ivex-2* filters, which incorporate short inlet and outlet PVC-coated tubing, has not resulted in significant leaching of DEHP (di-[2-ethylhexyl]phthalate).

Do not use the *Chemo Dispensing Pin* device or similar devices with spikes with paclitaxel vials because they can cause the stopper to collapse, resulting in the loss of sterile integrity of the drug solution.

➤*Admixture compatibility:* One study indicates compatibility in 5% Dextrose Injection, USP or normal saline at 0.1 and 1 mg/ml concentrations, at 4°, 22°, or 32°C (39.2°, 71.6°, or 89.6°F) for 3 days. Small, needlelike crystals form after 3 days.

Another study showed admixtures of 0.3 and 1.2 mg/ml paclitaxel with 2 mg/ml carboplatin in normal saline injection or 5% Dextrose Injection, USP were stable for at least 24 hours at 4°, 23°, and 32°C (39.2°, 71.6°, or 89.6°F). Paclitaxel 0.2 mg/ml mixed with 0.2 mg/ml cisplatin in normal saline injection showed unacceptable cisplatin loss in 24 hours. Utility time of paclitaxel mixed with carboplatin or cisplatin is limited due to paclitaxel microcrystalline precipitation and decomposition of carboplatin and cisplatin.

Paclitaxel 0.3 or 1.2 mg/ml combined with 200 mcg/ml doxorubicin in normal saline injection or 5% Dextrose Injection, USP was found to be stable for at least 24 hours at temperatures of 4°, 23°, and 32°C (39.2°, 71.6°, or 89.6°F). Microcrystalline precipitation of paclitaxel developed within 3 days.

➤*PVC equipment:* Contact of the undiluted concentrate with plasticized polyvinyl chloride equipment or devices used to prepare solutions for infusion is not recommended. To minimize patient exposure to the plasticizer DEHP (di-[2-ethylhexyl]phthalate), that may be leached from PVC infusion bags or sets, store diluted paclitaxel solutions in bottles (glass, polypropylene) or plastic bags (polypropylene, polyolefin), and administer through polyethylene-lined administration sets.

PACLITAXEL

➤*Storage / Stability:* Unopened vials of paclitaxel for injection concentrate are stable until the date indicated on the package when stored between 20° to 25°C (68° to 77°F) in the original package. Neither freezing nor refrigeration adversely affect the stability of the product. Upon refrigeration, components in the vial may precipitate but will redissolve upon reaching room temperature with little or no agitation. There is no impact on product quality. Discard the vial if the solution remains cloudy or if an insoluble precipitate is noted. Retain in the original package to protect from light. Solutions for infusion prepared as recommended are stable at ambient temperature (25°C; 77°F) and lighting conditions for ≤ 27 hours.

Actions

➤*Pharmacology:* Paclitaxel is a natural product, a taxane, with antitumor activity. It is a novel antimicrotubule agent that promotes the assembly of microtubules from tubulin dimers and stabilizes microtubules by preventing depolymerization. This stability inhibits the normal dynamic reorganization of the microtubule network that is essential for vital interphase and mitotic cellular functions. In addition, paclitaxel induces abnormal arrays or "bundles" of microtubules throughout the cell cycle and multiple esters of microtubules during mitosis, further disrupting cell function.

➤*Pharmacokinetics:*

Absorption – With a 24-hour infusion, a 30% increase in dose increased the C_{max} by 87%; with a 3-hour infusion, a 30% dose increase resulted in a 68% increase in C_{max}.

Distribution – The mean steady-state volume of distribution with the 24-hour infusion ranges from 227 to 688 L/m^2. The drug is 89% to 98% protein bound. Major plasma proteins involved are α_1-acid glycoprotein, albumin, and lipoproteins.

Metabolism – Paclitaxel is metabolized primarily to 6α-hydroxypaclitaxel by the cytochrome P450 isozyme CYP2C8 and to 2 minor metabolites, 3′-p-hydroxypaclitaxel and 6α, 3′-p-dihydroxypaclitaxel, by CYP3A4.

Excretion – Following IV administration, the drug exhibits a biphasic decline in plasma concentrations. The initial rapid decline represents distribution to the peripheral compartment and significant elimination of the drug. The later phase is caused, in part, by a relatively slow efflux of paclitaxel from the peripheral compartment. Following 3- and 24-hour infusions at dosing levels of 135 and 175 mg/m^2, mean terminal half-life ranges from 13.1 to 52.7 hours, respectively, and mean values for total body clearance range from 12.2 to 23.8 $L/hr/m^2$, respectively.

The disposition of paclitaxel has not been fully elucidated. After IV administration of 15 to 275 mg/m^2 doses as 1-, 6-, or 24-hour infusions, mean values for cumulative urinary recovery of unchanged drug range from 1.3% to 12.6% of the dose, indicating extensive non-renal clearance.

Contraindications

Hypersensitivity reactions to paclitaxel or other drugs formulated in *Cremophor EL* (polyoxyethylated castor oil; see Warnings) or polyoxyl 35 castor oil; patients with solid tumors who have baseline neutrophil count of < 1500 cells/mm^3 or in patients with AIDS-related Kaposi's sarcoma with baseline neutrophil counts of < 1000 cells/mm^3 (see Warnings).

Warnings

➤*Bone marrow suppression:* Bone marrow suppression (primarily neutropenia) is dose-dependent and is the major dose-limiting toxicity. Neutropenia is generally rapidly reversible. Neutrophil nadirs occurred at a median of 11 days. Do not administer to patients with baseline neutrophil counts of < 1500 cells/mm^3. Institute frequent monitoring of blood counts during treatment. Do not retreat with subsequent cycles of paclitaxel until neutrophils recover to a level of > 1500 cells/mm^3 and platelets recover to a level > 100,000 cells/mm^3. Do not give to patients with AIDS-related Kaposi's sarcoma if the baseline or subsequent neutrophil count is < 1000 cells/mm^3.

➤*Cardiac effects:* Severe conduction abnormalities have been documented in < 1% of patients during therapy, sometimes requiring a pacemaker. If patients develop significant conduction abnormalities during administration, administer appropriate therapy and perform continuous cardiac monitoring during subsequent therapy.

➤*Hypersensitivity reactions:* Do not use in patients with a history of severe hypersensitivity reactions to products containing *Cremophor EL* (polyoxyethylated castor oil). Pretreat patients with corticosteroids, diphenhydramine, and H$_2$ antagonists before administering paclitaxel to avoid the occurrence of severe hypersensitivity reactions. Fatal reactions have occurred despite premedication. Severe hypersensitivity reactions characterized by dyspnea and hypotension requiring treatment, angioedema, and generalized urticaria have occurred in 2% to 4% of patients, usually within 2 to 3 minutes and nearly always within 10 minutes, and require immediate discontinuation of paclitaxel and aggressive symptomatic therapy. Refer to Management of Acute Hypersensitivity Reactions. Do not rechallenge patients who experience severe hypersensitivity reactions to paclitaxel. Patients with a history

of allergic reactions to bee-stings may have an increased risk for a hypersensitivity reaction with paclitaxel. Minor symptoms such as flushing, skin reactions, dyspnea, hypotension, or tachycardia do not require interruption of therapy.

➤*Hepatic function impairment:* There is evidence that the toxicity of paclitaxel is enhanced in patients with elevated liver enzymes. Therefore, exercise caution when administering to patients with moderate-to-severe hepatic impairment and consider dose adjustments.

➤*Mutagenesis:* Paclitaxel is clastogenic in vitro (chromosome aberrations in human lymphocytes) and in vivo mammalian test systems (micronucleus test in mice).

➤*Fertility impairment:* Paclitaxel has caused low fertility and fetal toxicity in rats at a dose ≥ 1 mg/kg/day (≈ 0.04 the daily maximum recommended human dose on a mg/m^2 basis).

➤*Pregnancy: Category D.* Paclitaxel may cause fetal harm when administered to a pregnant woman. It is embryo- and fetotoxic in rats and rabbits and decreases fertility in rats. There are no adequate and well-controlled studies in pregnant women. If paclitaxel is used during pregnancy or if the patient becomes pregnant while receiving this drug, apprise the patient of the potential hazard. Advise women of childbearing potential to avoid becoming pregnant during therapy with paclitaxel.

➤*Lactation:* It is not known whether the drug is excreted in breast milk. Because of the potential for serious adverse reactions in nursing infants, discontinue nursing when receiving paclitaxel therapy.

➤*Children:* Safety and efficacy of paclitaxel in children have not been established. In investigations, CNS toxicity has been observed in these patients. This may be caused by high (350 to 420 mg/m^2) ethanol content of the formulation, rapid infusions (3 hours), or concomitant use of antihistamines. More data is needed.

Precautions

➤*Cardiovascular:* Hypotension, hypertension, and bradycardia have been observed during paclitaxel administration but generally do not require treatment. Occasionally, initial or recurrent hypertension requires interruption or discontinuation of paclitaxel. Frequently monitor vital signs, particularly during the first hour of infusion. Continuous cardiac monitoring is not required except for patients with serious conduction abnormalities (see Warnings and Adverse Reactions).

➤*CNS:* Although peripheral neuropathy (glove-and-stocking distribution) occurs frequently, the development of severe symptomatology is unusual and requires a dose reduction of 20% for all subsequent courses of paclitaxel. Also, consider that the formulation contains significant amounts of dehydrated alcohol (see Adverse Reactions).

➤*PVC equipment:* Contact of the undiluted concentrate of paclitaxel with plasticized PVC equipment or devices used to prepare solutions for infusion is not recommended (see Administration and Dosage).

➤*Injection site reaction:* Injection site reactions, including reactions secondary to extravasation, were usually mild and consisted of erythema, tenderness, skin discoloration, or swelling at the injection site. These reactions have been observed more frequently with 24-hour infusions than with 3-hour infusions. Recurrence of skin reactions at a site of previous extravasation following administration of paclitaxel at a different site (ie, "recall") has been reported rarely.

Rare reports of more severe events such as phlebitis, cellulitis, induration, skin exfoliation, necrosis, and fibrosis have been received as a part of the continuing surveillance of paclitaxel safety. In some cases, the onset of the injection site reaction either occurred during a prolonged infusion or was delayed by a week to 10 days.

Drug Interactions

➤*P450 system:* The metabolism of paclitaxel is catalyzed by cytochrome P450 isoenzymes CYP2C8 and CYP3A4. Exercise caution when administering paclitaxel concomitantly with known substrates or inhibitors of CYP2C8 and CYP3A4.

Paclitaxel Drug Interactions			
Precipitant drug	Object drug*		Description
Cisplatin	Paclitaxel	↑	In a Phase I trial using escalating doses of paclitaxel (110 to 200 mg/m^2) and cisplatin (50 or 75 mg/m^2) given as sequential infusions, myelosuppression was more profound when paclitaxel was given after cisplatin than with paclitaxel before cisplatin. Data demonstrated a decrease in paclitaxel clearance of ≈ 33% when paclitaxel was administered following cisplatin.
Cyclosporin Doxorubicin Felodipine Ketoconazole Valspodar Troleandomycin	Paclitaxel	↑	Metabolism of paclitaxel may be decreased through the inhibition of CYP3A4 by any of these drugs.

PACLITAXEL

Paclitaxel Drug Interactions			
Precipitant drug	Object drug*		Description
Diazepam Doxorubicin Felodipine 17α-ethinylestra-diol Ketoconazole Midazolam Retinoic acid	Paclitaxel	↑	Metabolism of paclitaxel may be decreased through the inhibition of CYP2C8 by any of these drugs.
Paclitaxel	Doxorubicin	↑	Doxorubicin and its active metabolite doxorubicinol may be increased when coadministered. Reports in the literature suggest that plasma levels of doxorubicin (and its active metabolite doxorubicinol) may be increased when paclitaxel and doxorubicin are used in combination.
Phenobarbital Carbamazepine	Paclitaxel	↓	Concomitant administration of either of these drugs may induce the metabolism of paclitaxel through the cytochrome CYP3A4 isoenzyme.

* ↑ = Object drug increased. ↓ = Object drug decreased.

Adverse Reactions

Data in the following table are based on 493 patients with ovarian carcinoma and 319 with breast carcinoma enrolled in 10 studies who received single-agent paclitaxel; 275 patients were treated with paclitaxel doses ranging from 135 to 300 mg/m^2 administered over 24 hours (in 4 of these studies, G-CSF was administered as hematopoietic support), 301 patients were treated in the randomized Phase 3 ovarian carcinoma study, which compared 2 doses (135 or 175 mg/m^2) and 2 schedules (3 or 24 hours) of paclitaxel, and 236 patients with breast carcinoma received paclitaxel (135 or 175 mg/m^2) administered over 3 hours in a controlled study.

Paclitaxel Adverse Reactions (%)[1]					
Adverse reaction	Paclitaxel (n = 812)[2]	Paclitaxel[3] 135 mg/m^2 (n = 195)[4]	Paclitaxel[5] 250 mg/m^2 (n = 197)[4]	Paclitaxel[6] 135 mg/m^2 (n = 29)[7]	Paclitaxel[8] 100 mg/m^2 (n = 56)[7]
Cardiovascular					
Abnormal ECG (all patients)	23	—	—	—	—
Abnormal ECG (patients with normal baseline)	14	—	—	—	—
Bradycardia	3	—	—	3	—
Hypotension	12	—	—	17	9
Syncope	1	—	—	—	—
Rhythm abnormalities	1	—	—	—	—
Hypertension	1	—	—	—	—
Venous thrombosis	1	—	—	—	—
Any symptoms	—	33	39	—	—
Severe symptoms[9]	—	13	12	—	—
CNS					
Peripheral neuropathy					
Any symptoms	60	—	—	79	46
Severe symptoms[9]	3	—	—	10	2
Neuromotor toxicity					
Any symptoms	—	37	47	—	—
Severe symptoms[9]	—	6	12	—	—
Neurosensory toxicity					
Any symptoms	—	48	61	—	—
Severe symptoms[9]	—	13	28	—	—
GI					
Diarrhea	38	—	—	90	73
Mucositis					
Any symptoms	31	18	28	45	20
Severe symptoms	—	1	4	—	—
Nausea and vomiting	—	—	—	69	70
Any symptoms	52	85	87	—	—
Severe symptoms[9]	—	27	29	—	—
Hematologic					
Anemia					
< normal	—	94	96	—	—
< 11 g/dl	78	—	—	86	73
< 8 g/dl	16	22	19	34	25
Bleeding	14	—	—	—	—
Leukopenia					
< 4000/mm^3	90	—	—	—	—
< 1000/mm^3	17	—	—	—	—
Neutropenia					
< 2000/mm^3	90	89	86	100	95
< 500/mm^3	52	74	65	76	35
Platelet transfusions	2	—	—	—	—

Paclitaxel Adverse Reactions (%)[1]					
Adverse reaction	Paclitaxel (n = 812)[2]	Paclitaxel[3] 135 mg/m^2 (n = 195)[4]	Paclitaxel[5] 250 mg/m^2 (n = 197)[4]	Paclitaxel[6] 135 mg/m^2 (n = 29)[7]	Paclitaxel[8] 100 mg/m^2 (n = 56)[7]
Red cell transfusions	25	—	—	—	—
Thrombocytopenia					
< normal	—	48	68	—	—
< 100,000/mm^3	20	—	—	52	27
< 50,000/mm^3	7	6	12	17	5
Febrile neutropenia	—	—	—	55	9
Hepatic					
Alkaline phosphatase increased	22	—	—	—	—
AST increased	19	—	—	—	—
Bilirubin increased	7	—	—	—	—
Hypersensitivity[10]					
All	41	16	27	14	9
Severe[9]	< 2	1	4	—	—
Flushing	28	—	—	—	—
Rash	12	—	—	—	—
Hypotension	4	—	—	—	—
Dyspnea	2	—	—	—	—
Tachycardia	2	—	—	—	—
Hypertension	1	—	—	—	—
Musculoskeletal					
Myalgia/arthralgia					
Any symptoms	60	21	42	93	48
Severe symptoms[9]	8	3	11	14	16
Opportunistic infections					
Any	30	38	31	76	54
Candidiasis, esophageal	—	—	—	7	9
Cryptosporidiosis	—	—	—	7	7
Cryptococcal meningitis	—	—	—	3	2
Cytomegalovirus	—	—	—	45	27
Herpes simplex	—	—	—	38	11
Leukoencephalopathy	—	—	—	—	2
M. avium-intracellulare	—	—	—	24	4
Pneumocystis carinii	—	—	—	14	21
Renal					
Creatinine increased					
All	—	—	—	34	18
Severe[9]	—	—	—	7	5
Miscellaneous					
Fever	12	—	—	—	—
Discontinuation due to drug toxicity	—	—	—	7	16
Injection site reactions	13	—	—	—	—
Alopecia	87	—	—	—	—
Nail changes	2	—	—	—	—
Edema	21	—	—	—	—

[1] Data are pooled from separate studies and are not necessarily comparable.
[2] Pooled analysis of patients with solid tumors (493 with ovarian carcinoma and 319 with breast carcinoma) receiving single-agent paclitaxel. Worst course analysis.
[3] As a 24-hour infusion with cisplatin 75 mg/m^2.
[4] Patients with NSCLC receiving paclitaxel (24-hour infusion) as first-line therapy. Worst course analysis.
[5] As a 24-hour infusion with G-CSF support; cisplatin dose is 75 mg/m^2.
[6] Administered as a 3-hour infusion every 3 weeks.
[7] Patients with AIDS-related Kaposi's sarcoma. Worst course analysis.
[8] Administered as a 3-hour infusion every 2 weeks.
[9] Severe events defined as at least grade III toxicity.
[10] All patients received premedication.

► *Cardiovascular:*

Hypotension/Bradycardia – Hypotension during the first 3 hours of infusion occurred in 12% of patients and 3% of courses administered. Bradycardia during the first 3 hours of infusion occurred in 3% of patients and 1% of courses. Neither dose nor schedule had an effect on the frequency of hypotension and bradycardia. These vital sign changes most often caused no symptoms and required neither specific therapy nor treatment discontinuation. The frequency of hypotension and bradycardia were not influenced by prior anthracycline therapy.

Cardiovascular events – Significant cardiovascular events occurred in ≈ 1% of patients. These events included syncope, rhythm abnormalities, hypertension, and venous thrombosis. One of the patients with syncope treated with 175 mg/m^2 > 24 hours had progressive hypotension and died. The arrhythmias included asymptomatic ventricular tachycardia, bigeminy, and complete AV block requiring pacemaker placement. Among patients with NSCLC treated with paclitaxel in combination with cisplatin in the Phase 3 study, significant cardiovascular events occured in 12% to 13%. This apparent increase in cardiovascular events is possibly because an increase in cardiovascular risk factors in patients with lung cancer.

ECG abnormalities – ECG abnormalities were common among patients at baseline. ECG abnormalities on study did not usually result

PACLITAXEL

in symptoms, were not dose-limiting, and required no intervention. ECG abnormalities were noted in 23% of patients. Among patients with a normal ECG prior to study entry, 14% of patients developed an abnormal tracing while on study. The most frequently reported ECG modifications were non-specific repolarization abnormalities, sinus bradycardia, sinus tachycardia, and premature beats. Among patients with normal ECG at baseline, prior therapy with anthracyclines did not influence the frequency of ECG abnormalities.

Rarely reported – Rarely reported are MI, CHF (notably after anthracyclines), atrial fibrillation, and supraventricular tachycardia.

➤*CNS:* The frequency and severity of neurologic manifestations were dose-dependent but not influenced by infusion duration. Peripheral neuropathy was observed in 60% of patients (3% severe) and in 52% of the patients without preexisting neuropathy (2% severe).

The frequency of peripheral neuropathy increased with cumulative dose. Neurologic symptoms were observed in 27% of the patients after the first course of treatment and in 34% to 51% from course 2 through 10.

Peripheral neuropathy was the cause of discontinuation in 1% of patients. Sensory symptoms have usually improved or resolved within several months of discontinuation. The incidence of neurologic symptoms did not increase in the subset of patients previously treated with cisplatin. Preexisting neuropathies resulting from prior therapies are not a contraindication for therapy. In patients with NSCLC, administration of paclitaxel followed by cisplatin resulted in greater incidence of severe neurotoxicity compared with the incidence in patients with ovarian or breast cancer treated with single-agent paclitaxel. Severe neurosensory symptoms were noted in 13% of NSCLC patients receiving 135 mg/m^2 paclitaxel by a 24-hour infusion followed by 75 mg/m^2 cisplatin; and 8% of NSCLC patients receiving cisplatin/etoposide.

Other serious neurologic events following administration have been rare (< 1%) and have included grand mal seizures, syncope, ataxia, neuroencephalopathy, and autonomic neuropathy resulting in paralytic ileus. Optic nerve and visual disturbances (scintillating scotoma) have been reported; usually reversible but rarely persistent optic nerve damage is reported. Postmarketing reports of ototoxicity (hearing loss and tinnitus) have also been reported.

➤*GI:* Nausea/vomiting (52%), diarrhea (38%), and mucositis (31%) have occurred. These manifestations were usually mild to moderate. Mucositis was schedule-dependent and occurred more frequently with the 24-hour than 3-hour infusion. Rates were higher in the AIDS-related Kaposi's sarcoma groups. Rare reports of intestinal obstruction, intestinal perforation, pancreatitis, dehydration, and ischemic colitis have occurred. Rare reports of neutropenic enterocolitis (typhlitis), despite the coadministration of G-CSF, were observed in patients treated with paclitaxel alone and in combination with other chemotherapeutic agents.

➤*Hematologic:* Bone marrow suppression was the major dose-limiting toxicity. Neutropenia, the most important hematologic toxicity, was dose- and schedule-dependent and was generally rapidly reversible. Among patients treated with a 3-hour infusion, neutrophil counts declined < 500 cells/mm^3 in 14% of the patients treated with a dose of 135 mg/m^2 compared with 27% at a dose of 175 mg/m^2. Severe neutropenia (< 500/mm^3) was more frequent with the 24-hour than 3-hour infusion; infusion duration had a greater impact on myelosuppression than dose. Neutropenia did not appear to increase with cumulative exposure and did not appear to be more frequent nor more severe for patients previously treated with radiation therapy.

Fever – Fever was frequent (12% of all treatment courses). Infectious episodes occurred in 30% of patients and 9% of courses; these episodes were fatal in 1% of patients and included sepsis, pneumonia, and peritonitis. Infectious episodes were reported in 20% to 26% of the patients given either a 135 or 175 mg/m^2 dose by a 3-hour infusion. Urinary tract infections and upper respiratory tract infections were the most frequently reported infectious complications.

In the immunosuppressed patient population with advanced HIV disease and poor-risk AIDS-related Kaposi's sarcoma, 61% of the patients reported ≥ 1 opportunistic infection. The use of supportive therapy, including G-CSF, is recommended for patients who have experienced severe neutropenia.

Thrombocytopenia – Thrombocytopenia was uncommon and almost never severe (< 50,000/mm^3); 20% of the patients experienced a drop in their platelet count to < 100,000 cells/mm^3 at least once while on treatment; 7% had a platelet count < 50,000 cells/mm^3 at the time of their worst nadir. Among the 812 patients, bleeding episodes were reported in 4% of courses and by 14% of patients, but most of the hemorrhagic episodes were localized and the frequency of these events was unrelated to the dose and schedule. Bleeding episodes were reported in 10% of the patients receiving either the 135 or 175 mg/m^2 dose given by a 3-hour infusion; no patients treated with the 3-hour infusion received platelet transfusions. In the adjuvant breast carcinoma trial, the incidence of severe thrombocytopenia and platelet transfusions increased with higher doses of doxorubicin.

Anemia – Anemia (Hgb < 11 g/dl) was observed in 78% of patients and was severe (Hgb < 8 g/dl) in 16% of cases. No consistent relationship between dose or schedule and the frequency of anemia was observed. Among patients with normal baseline hemoglobin, 69% became anemic on study but only 7% had severe anemia. Red cell transfusions were required in 25% of patients and in 12% of those with normal baseline hemoglobin levels.

➤*Hepatic:* No relationship was observed between liver function abnormalities and either dose or schedule of administration. Among patients with normal baseline liver function, 7%, 22%, and 19% had elevations in bilirubin, alkaline phosphatase, and AST, respectively. Prolonged exposure was not associated with cumulative hepatic toxicity. Hepatic necrosis/encephalopathy leading to death have occurred (rare).

➤*Hypersensitivity:* The frequency and severity were not affected by the dose or schedule. Hypersensitivity reactions were observed in 20% of courses and in 41% of patients. These reactions were severe in < 2% of the patients and 1% of the courses. No severe reactions were observed after course 3, and severe symptoms occurred generally within the first hour of infusion. The most frequent symptoms observed during these severe reactions were dyspnea, flushing, chest pain, and tachycardia (see Warnings).

Minor hypersensitivity reactions consisted mostly of flushing (28%); rash (12%); hypotension (4%); dyspnea, tachycardia (2%); hypertension (1%). The frequency of hypersensitivity reactions remained relatively stable during the entire treatment period. Chills and back pain have been reported rarely.

➤*Local:* Injection site reactions, including reactions secondary to extravasation, were usually mild and consisted of erythema, tenderness, skin discoloration, or swelling at the injection site. These reactions have been observed more frequently with 24-hour infusions than with 3-hour infusions. A specific treatment for extravasation reactions is unknown at this time. Rare reports of more severe events such as phlebitis, skin exfoliation, necrosis, fibrosis, induration, and cellulitis have occurred. "Recall" skin reactions have also been reported. Always closely monitor the injection site for extravasation. The onset of injection site reactions may develop during a prolonged infusion or ≤ 7 to 10 days later.

➤*Musculoskeletal:* There was no consistent relationship between dose or schedule and the frequency or severity of arthralgia/myalgia; 60% of patients treated experienced arthralgia/myalgia; 8% experienced severe symptoms. The symptoms were usually transient, occurred 2 or 3 days after administration and resolved within a few days. The frequency and severity of musculoskeletal symptoms remained unchanged throughout the treatment period.

➤*Renal:* Among the patients treated for Kaposi's sarcoma with paclitaxel, 5 patients had renal toxicity of grade III or IV severity. One patient with suspected HIV nephropathy of grade IV severity had to discontinue therapy, the other 4 patients had renal insufficiency with reversible elevations of serum creatinine.

➤*Respiratory:* Reports of interstitial pneumonia, lung fibrosis, and pulmonary embolism are rare. Rare reports of radiation pneumonitis have been received in patients receiving concurrent radiotherapy.

➤*Miscellaneous:* Alopecia was observed in almost all (87%) of the patients, usually within 13 to 21 days after doses of ≥ 135 mg/m^2; many patients have complete body hair loss. Transient skin changes caused by paclitaxel-related hypersensitivity reactions have been observed, but no other skin toxicities were significantly associated with administration. Nail changes (changes in pigmentation or discoloration of nail bed) were uncommon (2%). Edema was reported in 21% of patients (17% of those without baseline edema); only 1% had severe edema and none of these patients required treatment discontinuation. Edema was most commonly focal and disease-related. Edema was observed in 5% of courses for patients with normal baseline and did not increase with time on study. Rare reports of skin abnormalities related to radiation recall have occurred as well as maculopapular rash, pruritus, Stevens-Johnson syndrome, and toxic epidermal necrolysis. Reports of asthenia and malaise have been received as a part of the continuing surveillance of paclitaxel safety. In the Phase 3 trial of paclitaxel 135 mg/m^2 over 24 hours in combination with cisplatin as first-line therapy of ovarian cancer, asthenia was reported in 17% of the patients, significantly greater than the 10% incidence observed in the control arm of cyclophosphamide/cisplatin.

Overdosage

➤*Accidental exposure:* Upon inhalation, dyspnea, chest pain, burning eyes, sore throat, and nausea have been reported. Following topical exposure, events have included tingling, burning, and redness.

➤*Symptoms:* The primary anticipated complications of overdosage would consist of bone marrow suppression, peripheral neurotoxicity, and mucositis. Rare reports of radiation pneumonitis have been received in patients receiving concurrent radiotherapy. Overdoses in pediatric patients may be associated with ethanol toxicity.

➤*Treatment:* There is no known antidote for paclitaxel overdosage.

DOCETAXEL

Rx	**Taxotere** (Aventis)	**Injection:** 20 mg/0.5 mL	Polysorbate 80.[1] In single-dose vials with 1.5 mL diluent.[2]
		80 mg/2 mL	Polysorbate 80.[1] In single-dose vials with 6 mL diluent.[2]

[1] Polysorbate 80 1040 mg/mL.

[2] Contains 13% ethanol in water for injection.

WARNING

Administer docetaxel under the supervision of a qualified physician experienced in the use of antineoplastic agents. Appropriate management of complications is possible only when adequate diagnostic and treatment facilities are readily available.

The incidence of treatment-related mortality associated with docetaxel is increased in patients with abnormal liver function, patients receiving higher doses, and in patients with nonsmall cell lung carcinoma and a history of prior treatment with platinum-based chemotherapy who receive docetaxel as a single agent at a dose of 100 mg/m^2.

In general, do not give docetaxel to patients with bilirubin greater than the upper limit of normal (ULN) or to patients with AST and/or ALT over 1.5 × ULN concomitant with alkaline phosphatase (AP) over 2.5 × ULN. Patients with elevations of bilirubin or abnormalities of transaminases concurrent with alkaline phosphatase are at increased risk for the development of grade 4 neutropenia, febrile neutropenia, infections, severe thrombocytopenia, severe stomatitis, severe skin toxicity, and toxic death. Patients with isolated elevations of transaminases greater than 1.5 × ULN also had a higher rate of febrile neutropenia grade 4 but did not have an increased incidence of toxic death. Obtain and review bilirubin, AST or ALT, and alkaline phosphatase values prior to each cycle of docetaxel therapy.

Do not give to patients with a neutrophil count less than 1500 cells/mm^3. Perform frequent blood cell counts on all patients receiving docetaxel to monitor the occurrence of neutropenia, which may be severe and result in infection.

Severe hypersensitivity reactions characterized by hypotension and/or bronchospasm or generalized rash/erythema occurred in 2.2% of patients who received the recommended 3-day dexamethasone premedication. Hypersensitivity reactions requiring discontinuation of the docetaxel infusion were reported in 5 patients who did not receive premedication. These reactions resolved after discontinuation of the infusion and the administration of appropriate therapy. Do not give docetaxel to patients who have a history of severe hypersensitivity reactions to docetaxel or other drugs formulated with polysorbate 80.

Severe fluid retention occurred in 6.5% of patients despite use of a 3-day dexamethasone premedication regimen. It was characterized by 1 or more of the following events: Poorly tolerated peripheral edema, generalized edema, pleural effusion requiring urgent drainage, dyspnea at rest, cardiac tamponade, or pronounced abdominal distention (because of ascites).

Indications

▶*Breast cancer:* For the treatment of patients with locally advanced or metastatic breast cancer after failure of prior chemotherapy.

▶*Nonsmall cell lung cancer (NSCLC):* As a single agent for the treatment of patients with locally advanced or metastatic NSCLC after failure of prior platinum-based chemotherapy. Also in combination with cisplatin for the treatment of patients with unresectable locally advanced or metastatic nonsmall cell lung cancer who have not previously received chemotherapy for this condition.

▶*Unlabeled uses:* Gastric cancer, head and neck cancer, ovarian cancer, prostate cancer, and urothelial cancer.

Administration and Dosage

▶*Approved by the FDA:* May 14, 1996.

▶*Breast cancer:* 60 to 100 mg/m^2 administered IV over 1 hour every 3 weeks.

Adjust dose from 100 to 75 mg/m^2 in patients who are dosed initially at 100 mg/m^2 and who experience either febrile neutropenia, neutrophils fewer than 500 cells/mm^3 for more than 1 week or severe or cumulative cutaneous reactions, during docetaxel therapy. If the patient continues to experience these reactions, either decrease the dosage from 75 to 55 mg/m^2 or discontinue treatment. Patients who are dosed initially at 60 mg/m^2 and do not experience febrile neutropenia, neutrophils fewer than 500 cells/mm^3 for more than 1 week, severe or cumulative cutaneous reactions, or severe peripheral neuropathy may tolerate higher doses. Discontinue docetaxel treatment entirely if patients develop at least grade 3 peripheral neuropathy.

▶*NSCLC:*

After failure of prior platinum-base chemotherapy – Docetaxel was evaluated as monotherapy and the recommended dose is 75 mg/m^2 administered IV over 1 hour every 3 weeks. A dose of 100 mg/m^2 in patients previously treated with chemotherapy was associated with increased hematologic toxicity, infection, and treatment-related mortality in randomized, controlled trials.

Withhold treatment in patients who are dosed initially at 75 mg/m^2 and who experience either febrile neutropenia, neutrophils fewer than 500 cells/mm^3 for more than 1 week, severe or cumulative cutaneous reactions, or other grade 3 and 4 nonhematological toxicities during docetaxel treatment until resolution of the toxicity and then resume at 55 mg/m^2. Discontinue docetaxel treatment entirely if patients develop at least grade 3 peripheral neuropathy.

Chemotherapy naive patients – Docetaxel was evaluated in combination with cisplatin. Administer docetaxel 75 mg/m^2 IV over 1 hour immediately followed by cisplatin 75 mg/m^2 over 30 to 60 minutes every 3 weeks.

For patients who are dosed initially at docetaxel 75 mg/m^2 in combination with cisplatin, and whose nadir of platelet count during the previous course of therapy is less than 25,000 cells/mm^3, in patients who experience febrile neutropenia, and in patients with serious nonhematologic toxicities, the docetaxel dosage in subsequent cycles should be reduced to 65 mg/m^2. In patients who require a further dose reduction, a dose of 50 mg/m^2 is recommended. For cisplatin dosage adjustments, see manufacturer's prescribing information.

▶*Premedication regimen:* Premedicate patients with oral corticosteroids, such as dexamethasone 16 mg/day (eg, 8 mg twice daily), for 3 days starting 1 day prior to docetaxel administration to reduce the incidence and severity of fluid retention as well as the severity of hypersensitivity reactions (see Warnings).

▶*Preparation of solution:* Docetaxel is a cytotoxic anticancer drug, and as with other potentially toxic compounds, exercise caution when handling and preparing docetaxel solutions. The use of gloves is recommended. If docetaxel concentrate, initial diluted solution, or final dilution for infusion comes into contact with the skin, immediately and thoroughly wash with soap and water. If docetaxel concentrate, initial diluted solution, or final dilution for infusion comes into contact with mucosa, immediately and thoroughly wash with water. Docetaxel for injection concentrate requires 2 dilutions prior to administration. Dilute with 0.9% sodium chloride injection or 5% dextrose injection.

Preparation of the initial diluted solution

1.) Allow the vials and diluent to stand at room temperature for approximately 5 minutes.
2.) Aseptically withdraw the entire contents of the appropriate diluent vial into a syringe by partially inverting the vial, and transfer it to the appropriate vial of docetaxel for injection concentrate. If the procedure is followed as described, an initial diluted solution of 10 mg docetaxel/mL will result.
3.) Mix the initial diluted solution by repeated inversions for at least 45 seconds to assure full mixture of the concentrate and diluent. Do not shake.
4.) The initial diluted solution (10 mg/mL) should be clear; however, there may be some foam on top of the solution because of the polysorbate 80. Allow the solution to stand for a few minutes to allow any foam to dissipate. It is not required that all foam dissipate prior to continuing the preparation process. The initial diluted solution may be used immediately or stored either in the refrigerator or at room temperature for a maximum of 8 hours.

Preparation of the final dilution for infusion

1.) Aseptically withdraw the required amount of initial diluted docetaxel solution (10 mg/mL) with a calibrated syringe and inject into a 250 mL infusion bag or bottle of 0.9% sodium chloride solution or 5% dextrose solution to produce a final concentration of 0.3 to 0.74 mg/mL. If a dose greater than 200 mg is required, use a larger volume of the infusion vehicle so that a concentration of 0.74 mg/mL docetaxel is not exceeded.
2.) Thoroughly mix the infusion by manual rotation.
3.) If the docetaxel initial solution or final dilution for infusion is not clear or appears to have precipitation, these should be discarded.

PVC equipment – Contact of the docetaxel concentrate with plasticized PVC equipment or devices used to prepare solutions for infusion is not recommended. In order to minimize patient exposure to the plasticizer DEHP (di-2-ethyl-hexyl phthalate), which may be leached from PVC infusion bags or sets, store the final docetaxel dilution for infusion in bottles (glass, polypropylene) or plastic bags (polypropylene, polyolefin) and administer through polyethylene-lined administration sets.

▶*Storage/Stability:* Store between 2° and 25°C (36° and 77°F). Retain in the original package to protect from bright light. Freezing does not adversely affect the product. Docetaxel infusion solution, if stored between 2° and 25°C (36° and 77°F) is stable for 4 hours. Fully prepared docetaxel infusion solution (in either 0.9% sodium chloride

DOCETAXEL

solution or 5% dextrose solution) should be used within 4 hours (including the 1-hour IV administration).

Actions

➤*Pharmacology:* Docetaxel is an antineoplastic agent belonging to the taxoid family. It is prepared by semisynthesis beginning with a precursor extracted from the renewable needle biomass of the yew plant. It acts by disrupting cells' microtubular network that is essential for mitotic and interphase cellular functions. Docetaxel binds to free tubulin and promotes the assembly of tubulin into stable microtubules while simultaneously inhibiting their disassembly. This leads to the production of microtubule bundles without normal function and to the stabilization of microtubules, which results in the inhibition of mitosis in cells. Docetaxel's binding to microtubules does not alter the number of protofilaments in the bound microtubules, a feature that differs from most spindle poisons currently in clinical use.

➤*Pharmacokinetics:*

Absorption – The area under the curve (AUC) is dose-proportional following doses of 70 to 115 mg/m^2 with infusion times of 1 to 2 hours.

Distribution – Mean value for steady-state volume of distribution is 113 L. In vitro studies showed that docetaxel is about 94% protein bound, mainly to α_1-acid glycoprotein, albumin, and lipoproteins. In 3 cancer patients, the in vitro binding to plasma proteins was found to be approximately 97%. Dexamethasone does not affect the protein binding of docetaxel.

Metabolism – In vitro drug interaction studies revealed that docetaxel is metabolized by the CYP3A4 isoenzyme.

Excretion – Docetaxel's pharmacokinetic profile is consistent with a 3-compartment pharmacokinetic model, with half-lives for the α, β, and γ phases of 4 minutes, 36 minutes, and 11.1 hours, respectively. The initial rapid decline represents distribution to the peripheral compartments and the late (terminal) phase is due, in part, to a relatively slow efflux of docetaxel from the peripheral compartment. Mean value for total body clearance was 21 L/h/m^2. In 3 cancer patients, docetaxel was eliminated in the urine and feces following oxidative metabolism of tert-butyl ester group, but fecal excretion was the main elimination route. Within 7 days, urinary and fecal excretion accounted for approximately 6% and 75% of the administered radioactivity, respectively. About 80% of the radioactivity recovered in feces is excreted during the first 48 hours as 1 major and 3 minor metabolites with less than 8% of unchanged drug.

Special populations –

Hepatic function impairment: In patients with clinical chemistry data suggestive of mild to moderate liver function impairment (AST and/or ALT over 1.5 × ULN concomitant with alkaline phosphatase over 2.5 × ULN), total body clearance was lowered by an average of 27%, resulting in a 38% increase in systemic exposure (AUC). However, this average includes a substantial range, and there is, at present, no measurement that would allow recommendation for dose adjustment in such patients. Patients with combined abnormalities of transaminase and alkaline phosphatase should, in general, not be treated with docetaxel.

Contraindications

History of severe hypersensitivity reactions to docetaxel or to other drugs formulated with polysorbate 80; neutrophil counts of less than 1500 cells/mm^3.

Warnings

➤*Toxic deaths:*

Breast cancer – Docetaxel administered as 100 mg/m^2 was associated with deaths considered possibly or probably related to treatment in 2% of metastatic breast cancer patients, both previously treated and untreated, with normal liver function and in 11.5% of patients with various tumor types who had abnormal baseline liver function (AST and/or ALT over 1.5 × ULN together with AP over 2.5 × ULN). Among patients dosed at 60 mg/m^2, mortality related to treatment occurred in 0.6% of patients with normal liver function and in 3 of 7 patients with abnormal liver function. Approximately half of these deaths occurred during the first cycle. Sepsis accounted for the majority of deaths.

NSCLC – Docetaxel administered at a dose of 100 mg/m^2 in patients with locally advanced or metastatic NSCLC who had a history of prior platinum-based chemotherapy was associated with increased treatment-related mortality (14% and 5% in 2 randomized, controlled studies). There were 2.8% treatment-related deaths among the 176 patients treated at the 75 mg/m^2 dose in the randomized trials. Among patients who experienced treatment-related mortality at the 75 mg/m^2 dose level, 3 of 5 patients had a performance status (PS) of 2 at study entry.

➤*Fluid retention:* Severe fluid retention has occurred following docetaxel therapy. Premedicate patients with oral corticosteroids prior to docetaxel to reduce the severity of fluid retention (see Administration and Dosing and Boxed Warning). Closely monitor patients with pre-existing effusions from the first dose for the possible exacerbation of the effusions.

When fluid retention occurs, peripheral edema usually starts in the lower extremities and may become generalized with a median weight gain of 2 kg. Among 92 breast cancer patients premedicated with 3-day corticosteroids, moderate fluid retention occurred in 27.2% and severe fluid retention in 6.5%. The median cumulative dose to onset of moderate or severe fluid retention was 819 mg/m^2. 9.8% of patients discontinued treatment because of fluid retention: 4 patients discontinued with severe fluid retention; the remaining 5 had mild or moderate fluid retention. The median cumulative dose to treatment discontinuation because of fluid retention was 1021 mg/m^2. Fluid retention was completely, but sometimes slowly reversible with a median of 16 weeks from the last infusion of docetaxel to resolution (range 0 to 42+ weeks). Patients developing peripheral edema may be treated with standard measures (eg, salt restriction, oral diuretics).

➤*Hematologic:* Neutropenia (less than 2000 neutrophils/mm^3) occurs in virtually all patients given 60 to 100 mg/m^2 of docetaxel, and grade 4 neutropenia (less than 500 cells/mm^3) occurs in 85% of patients given 100 mg/m^2 and 75% of patients given 60 mg/m^2. Frequent monitoring of blood counts is essential so that dose may be adjusted. Do not administer to patients with neutrophils less than 1500 cells/mm^3. Febrile neutropenia occurred in about 12% of patients given 100 mg/m^2 but was very uncommon in patients given 60 mg/m^2. Hematologic responses, febrile reactions and infections, and rates of septic death for different regimens are dose-related. Three breast cancer patients with severe liver impairment (bilirubin more than 1.7 × ULN) developed fatal GI bleeding associated with severe drug-induced thrombocytopenia.

➤*Dermatologic:* Reversible cutaneous reactions characterized by a rash including localized eruptions, mainly on the feet and/or hands, but also on the arms, face, or thorax, usually associated with pruritus, have been observed. Eruptions generally occurred within 1 week after infusion, recovered before the next infusion, and were not disabling.

Localized erythema of the extremities with edema followed by desquamation has been observed. In case of severe skin toxicity, an adjustment in dosage is recommended.

Severe nail disorders were characterized by hypo- or hyperpigmentation and occasionally by onycholysis (in 0.8% of patients with solid tumors) and pain.

➤*Hypersensitivity reactions:* Observe patients closely for hypersensitivity reactions, especially during the first and second infusions. Severe hypersensitivity reactions characterized by hypotension and/or bronchospasm, or generalized rash/erythema occurred in 2.2% of the 92 patients premedicated with 3-day corticosteroids. Hypersensitivity reactions requiring discontinuation of docetaxel infusion were reported in 5 of 1260 patients with various tumor types who did not receive premedication, but in 0 of 92 patients premedicated with 3-day corticosteroids. Do not rechallenge patients with a history of severe hypersensitivity reactions to docetaxel. Hypersensitivity reactions may occur within a few minutes following initiation of docetaxel infusion. If minor reactions, such as flushing or localized skin reactions occur, interruption of therapy is not required. However, more severe reactions require immediate discontinuation of docetaxel and aggressive therapy. Premedicate all patients with an oral corticosteroid prior to the initiation of docetaxel infusion (see Warning Box).

➤*Hepatic function impairment:* Do not give docetaxel to patients with bilirubin greater than ULN. Also, do not administer docetaxel to patients with AST and/or ALT more than 1.5 × ULN concomitant with alkaline phosphatase more than 2.5 × ULN (see Warning Box).

➤*Mutagenesis:* Docetaxel has been shown to be clastogenic in the in vitro chromosome aberration test in CHO-K$_1$ cells and in the in vivo micronucleus test in the mouse, but it did not induce mutagenicity in the Ames test or the CHO/HGPRT gene mutation assays.

➤*Fertility impairment:* Docetaxel produced no impairment of fertility in rats when administered in multiple IV doses of up to 0.3 mg/kg (about 1/50 the recommended human dose on a mg/m^2 basis), but decreased testicular weights were reported. This correlates with findings of a 10-cycle toxicity study (dosing once every 21 days for 6 months) in rats and dogs in which testicular atrophy or degeneration was observed at IV doses of 5 mg/kg in rats and 0.375 mg/kg in dogs (about 1/3 and 1/15 the recommended human dose on a mg/m^2 basis, respectively). An increased frequency of dosing in rats produced similar effects at lower dose levels.

➤*Elderly:* In patients 65 years of age or older treated with docetaxel plus cisplatin, diarrhea (55%), peripheral edema (39%), and stomatitis (28%) were observed more frequently than in the vinorelbine plus cisplatin group (diarrhea 24%, peripheral edema 20%, stomatitis 20%). Patients treated with docetaxel plus cisplatin who were 65 years of age or older were more likely to experience diarrhea (55%), infections (42%), peripheral edema (39%), and stomatitis (28%) compared to patients younger than 65 years of age administered the same treatment (43%, 31%, 31%, and 21%, respectively).

Taxoids

DOCETAXEL

In general, dose selection for an elderly patient should be made with caution, reflecting the greater frequency of decreased hepatic, renal, or cardiac function and of concomitant disease or other drug therapy in elderly patients.

When docetaxel was combined with carboplatin for the treatment of chemotherapy-naive, advanced nonsmall cell lung carcinoma, patients 65 years of age and older (28%) experienced higher frequency of infection compared to similar patients treated with docetaxel plus cisplatin, and a higher frequency of diarrhea, infection, and peripheral edema than elderly patients treated with vinorelbine plus cisplatin.

➤*Pregnancy: Category D.* Docetaxel can cause fetal harm when administered to pregnant women. Studies in rats and rabbits at doses of 0.3 and 0.03 mg/kg/day or greater, respectively (about 1/50 and 1/300 the daily maximum recommended human dose on a mg/m² basis), administered during the period of organogenesis, have shown that docetaxel is embryotoxic and fetotoxic (characterized by intrauterine mortality, increased resorption, reduced fetal weight, and fetal ossification delay). The doses indicated above also caused maternal toxicity. There are no adequate and well-controlled studies in pregnant women using docetaxel. If docetaxel is used during pregnancy or if the patient becomes pregnant while receiving this drug, apprise the patient of the potential hazard to the fetus or potential risk for loss of the pregnancy. Advise women of childbearing potential to avoid becoming pregnant during therapy.

➤*Lactation:* It is not known whether docetaxel is excreted in breast milk. Because of the potential for serious adverse reactions in nursing infants from docetaxel, have the mother discontinue nursing prior to taking the drug.

➤*Children:* Safety and efficacy in children less than 16 years of age have not been established.

Precautions

➤*Monitoring:* Perform frequent peripheral blood cell counts on all patients to monitor the occurrence of myelotoxicity (see Warnings).

Do not retreat with subsequent cycles of docetaxel until neutrophils recover to a level of more than 1500 cells/mm³ and platelets recover to a level of more than 100,000 cells/mm³.

A 25% reduction in the docetaxel dose is recommended during subsequent cycles following severe neutropenia (fewer than 500 cells/mm³) lasting 7 days or more, febrile neutropenia, or a grade 4 infection in a docetaxel cycle.

Obtain bilirubin, AST or ALT, and alkaline phosphatase values prior to each cycle of docetaxel therapy.

➤*Neurologic:* Severe neurosensory symptoms (eg, paresthesia, dysesthesia, pain) were observed in 5.5% of metastatic breast cancer patients and resulted in treatment discontinuation in 6.1%. When these symptoms occur, dosage must be adjusted. If symptoms persist, discontinue treatment. Patients who experienced neurotoxicity in clinical trials and for whom follow-up information on the complete resolution of the event was available had spontaneous reversal of symptoms with a median of 9 weeks from onset (range, 0 to 106 weeks). Severe peripheral motor neuropathy mainly manifested as distal extremity weakness occurred in 4.4%.

➤*Asthenia:* Severe asthenia has been reported in 14.9% of metastatic breast cancer patients but has led to treatment discontinuation in only 1.8%. Fatigue and weakness may last from a few days to several weeks and may be associated with deterioration of performance status in patients with progressive disease.

Drug Interactions

➤*CYP450 system:* In vitro studies have shown that the metabolism of docetaxel may be modified by concomitant administration of compounds that induce, inhibit, or are metabolized by cytochrome P450 3A4, such as cyclosporine, ketoconazole, erythromycin, and troleandomycin. Exercise caution with these drugs when treating patients receiving docetaxel, as there is a potential for a significant interaction. Based on in vitro findings, it is likely that CYP3A4 inhibitors and/or substrates may lead to substantial increases in docetaxel blood concentrations.

Adverse Reactions

The adverse reactions are described for docetaxel 100 mg/m², the maximum dose approved for breast cancer, and 75 mg/m², the dose approved for advanced NSCLC after prior platinum-based chemotherapy and in combination with cisplatin for treatment of patients with nonsmall cell lung carcinoma who have not previously received chemotherapy for this condition.

Docetaxel Adverse Reactions (%)[1]								
				Nonsmall cell lung cancer patients				
	Patients with various tumor types[2]		Breast cancer patients	Previously treated with platinum-based chemotherapy			Chemotherapy-naive[3]	
							Docetaxel 75 mg/m² + cisplatin 75 mg/m² (n = 406)	Vinorelbine 25 mg/m² + cisplatin 100 mg/m² (n = 396)
Adverse reaction	Normal LFTs[4,5] at baseline (n = 2045)	Elevated LFTs[5,6] at baseline (n = 61)	Normal LFTs[4,5] at baseline (n = 965)	Docetaxel[4] 75 mg/m² (n = 176)	Best supportive care[4] (n = 49)	Vinorelbine/ Ifosamide[4] (n = 119)		
Dermatologic[7]								
Cutaneous								
any	47.6	54.1	47	19.9	6.1	16.8	16	14
grade 3/4	—	—	—	0.6	2	0.8	< 1	1
severe	4.8	9.8	5.2	—	—	—	—	—
Nail changes								
any	30.6	23	40.5	11.4	0	1.7	14	< 1
severe	2.5	4.9	3.7	1.1	0	0	< 1	0
GI								
Anorexia								
any	—	—	—	—	—	—	42	40
severe or life-threatening	—	—	—	—	—	—	5	5
Diarrhea	38.7	32.8	42.6	—	—	—	—	—
any	—	—	—	22.7	6.1	11.8	47	25
grade 3/4	—	—	—	2.8	0	4.2	7	3
severe	4.7	4.9	5.5	—	—	—	—	—
Nausea	38.8	37.7	42.1	—	—	—	—	—
any	—	—	—	33.5	30.6	31.1	72	76
grade 3/4	—	—	—	5.1	4.1	7.6	10	17
Stomatitis								
any	41.7	49.2	51.7	26.1	6.1	7.6	24	21
grade 3/4	—	—	—	1.7	0	0.8	2	1
severe	5.5	13	7.4	—	—	—	—	—
Vomiting	22.3	23	23.4	—	—	—	—	—
any	—	—	—	21.6	26.5	21.8	55	61
grade 3/4	—	—	—	2.8	2	5.9	8	16
Hematologic[7]								
Anemia								
hemoglobin < 11 g/dL	90.4	91.8	93.6	—	—	—	—	—
hemoglobin < 8 g/dL	8.8	31.1	7.7	—	—	—	—	—
any	—	—	—	9.1	55.1	90.8	89	94
grade 3/4	—	—	—	9.1	12.2	14.3	7	25
Febrile neutropenia[8]	11	26.2	12.3	6.3	NA[7,9]	0.8	5	5
Leukopenia								

DOCETAXEL

Docetaxel Adverse Reactions (%)[1]							
	Patients with various tumor types[2]		Breast cancer patients	Nonsmall cell lung cancer patients				
				Previously treated with platinum-based chemotherapy			Chemotherapy-naive[3]	
Adverse reaction	Normal LFTs[4,5] at baseline (n = 2045)	Elevated LFTs[5,6] at baseline (n = 61)	Normal LFTs[4,5] at baseline (n = 965)	Docetaxel[4] 75 mg/m² (n = 176)	Best supportive care[4] (n = 49)	Vinorelbine/ Ifosamide[4] (n = 119)	Docetaxel 75 mg/m² + cisplatin 75 mg/m² (n = 406)	Vinorelbine 25 mg/m² + cisplatin 100 mg/m² (n = 396)
< 4000 cells/mm³	95.6	98.3	98.6	—	—	—	—	—
< 1000 cells/mm³	31.6	46.6	43.7	—	—	—	—	—
any	—	—	—	83.5	6.1	89.1	—	—
grade 3/4	—	—	—	49.4	0	42.9	—	—
Neutropenia								
< 2000 cells/mm³	95.5	96.4	98.5	—	—	—	—	—
< 500 cells/mm³	75.4	87.5	85.9	—	—	—	—	—
any	—	—	—	84.1	14.3	83.2	91	90
grade 3/4	—	—	—	65.3	12.2	57.1	74	78
Thrombocytopenia								
< 100,000 cells/mm³	8	24.6	9.2	—	—	—	—	—
any	—	—	—	8	0	7.6	15	15
grade 3/4	—	—	—	2.8	0	1.7	3	4
Musculoskeletal								
Arthralgia	9.2	6.6	8.2	—	—	—	—	—
any	—	—	—	3.4	2	1.7	—	—
severe	—	—	—	0	0	0.8	—	—
Myalgia								
any	18.9	16.4	21.1	6.3	0	2.5	18	12
severe	1.5	1.6	1.8	0	0	0	< 1	< 1
Miscellanous								
Alopecia	75.8	62.3	74.2	56.3	34.7	49.6	—	—
any	—	—	—	—	—	—	75	42
grade 3	—	—	—	—	—	—	< 1	0
Asthenia								
any	61.8	52.5	66.3	52.8	57.1	53.8	74	75
severe	12.8	24.6	14.9	18.2	38.8	22.7	12[10]	14[10]
Fever in absence of infection								
any	31.2	41	35.1	—	—	—	33	29
severe	2.1	8.2	2.2	—	—	—	—	—
grade 3/4	—	—	—	—	—	—	< 1	1
Infections								
any	21.6	32.8	22.2	33.5	28.6	30.3	35	37
grade 3/4	—	—	—	10.2	6.1	9.2	8	8
severe	6.1	16.4	6.4	—	—	—	—	—
Infusion site reactions	4.4	3.3	4	—	—	—	—	—
Neurosensory[9]								
any	49.3	34.4	58.3	23.3	14.3	28.6	47	42
grade 3/4	—	—	—	1.7	6.1	5	4	4
severe	4.3	0	5.5	—	—	—	—	—
Neuromotor								
any	—	—	—	15.9	8.2	10.1	19	17
grade 3/4	—	—	—	4.5	6.1	3.4	3	6
Nonseptic death	0.6	6.6	0.6	—	—	—	—	—
Peripheral edema								
any	—	—	—	—	—	—	34	18
severe or life-threatening	—	—	—	—	—	—	< 1	< 1
Pleural effusion								
any	—	—	—	—	—	—	23	22
severe or life-threatening	—	—	—	—	—	—	2	2
Pulmonary								
any	—	—	—	40.9	49	45.4	—	—
grade 3/4	—	—	—	21	28.6	18.5	—	—
Septic death	1.6	4.9	1.4	—	—	—	—	—
Taste perversion								
any	—	—	—	5.7	0	0	—	—
severe	—	—	—	0.6	0	0	—	—
Treatment-related mortality	—	—	—	2.8	NA[11]	3.4	—	—
Weight gain								
any	—	—	—	—	—	—	15	9
severe or life-threatening	—	—	—	—	—	—	< 1	< 1

[1] Data are pooled from separate studies and are not necessarily comparable.
[2] Docetaxel 100 mg/m².
[3] In advanced unresectable or metastatic NSCLC.
[4] Normal baseline LFTs: Transaminases ≤ 1.5 times ULN or alkaline phosphatase ≤ 2.5 times ULN or isolated elevations of transaminases or alkaline phosphatase up to 5 times ULN.
[5] Liver function tests.
[6] Elevated baseline LFTs: AST and/or ALT > 1.5 times ULN concurrent with alkaline phosphatase > 2.5 times ULN.
[7] See Warnings.
[8] Febrile neutropenia: ANC grade 4 with fever > 38°C with IV antibiotics and/or hospitalization.
[9] See Precautions.
[10] Severe or life-threatening event.
[11] Not applicable.

Taxoids

DOCETAXEL

	Docetaxel Adverse Reactions (%)[1]							
	Patients with various tumor types[2]		Breast cancer patients	Nonsmall cell lung cancer patients				
				Previously treated with platinum-based chemotherapy			Chemotherapy-naive	
Adverse reactions	Normal LFTs[3],[4] at baseline	Elevated LFTs[4],[5] at baseline	Normal LFTs[3],[4] at baseline	Docetaxel[3] 75 mg/m² (n = 176)	Best supportive care[3] (n = 49)	Vinorelbine/ ifosamide[3] (n = 119)	Docetaxel 75 mg/m² + cisplatin 75 mg/m² (n = 406)	Vinorelbine 25 mg/m² + cisplatin 100 mg/m² (n = 396)
Fluid retention[6] any/severe	—	—	—	33.5/2.8	ND[7]/ND[7]	22.7/3.4	54/2[8]	42/2[8]
Fluid retention[6] w/3-day premedication any/severe	64.1/6.5 (n = 92)	66.7/33.3 (n = 3)	64.1/6.5 (n = 92)	—	—	—	—	—
Fluid retention[6] regardless of premedication any/severe	47/6.9 (n = 2045)	39.3/8.2 (n = 61)	59.7/8.9 (n = 965)	—	—	—	—	—
Hypersensitivity reaction any/grade 3/4	—	—	—	5.7/2.8	0/0	0.8/0	12/3	4/< 1
Hypersensitivity reaction[6] w/3-day premedication any/severe	15.2/2.2 (n = 92)	33.3/0 (n = 3)	15.2/2.2 (n = 92)	—	—	—	—	—
Hypersensitivity reaction[3] regardless of premedication any/severe	21/4.2 (n = 2045)	19.7/9.8 (n = 61)	17.6/2.6 (n = 965)	—	—	—	—	—

[1] Data are pooled from separate studies and are not necessarily comparable.
[2] Docetaxel 100 mg/m².
[3] Normal baseline LFTs: Transaminases ≤ 1.5 times ULN or alkaline phosphatase ≤ 2.5 times ULN or isolated elevations of transaminases or alkaline phosphatase up to 5 times ULN.
[4] Liver function tests.
[5] Elevated baseline LFTs: AST and/or ALT > 1.5 times ULN concurrent with alkaline phosphatase > 2.5 times ULN.
[6] See Warnings.
[7] Not Done.
[8] Severe or life-threatening event.

►*Cardiovascular:* Hypotension (2.8% with solid tumors, 1.2% required treatment); heart failure, sinus tachycardia, atrial flutter, dysrhythmia, unstable angina, pulmonary edema, hypertension (rare). 8.1% of metastatic breast cancer patients receiving docetaxel 100 mg/m² in a randomized trial and who had serial left ventricular ejection fractions assessed developed deterioration of LVEF by 10% or more associated with a drop below the institutional lower limit or normal.

►*Infusion site reactions:* Hyperpigmentation, inflammation, redness or dryness of the skin, phlebitis, extravasation, swelling of the vein (mild).

►*CNS:* Severe neurosensory symptoms (paresthesia, dysesthesia, pain) were observed in 5.5% of metastatic breast cancer patients, and resulted in treatment discontinuation in 6.1%. When these symptoms occur, dosage must be adjusted. If symptoms persist, discontinue treatment (see Precautions).

►*Dermatologic:* Reversible cutaneous reactions characterized by a rash including localized eruptions, mainly on the feet and/or hands, but also on the arms, face, or thorax, usually associated with pruritus, have been observed. Eruptions generally occurred within 1 week after infusion, recovered before the next infusion, and were not disabling.

Severe nail disorders were characterized by hypo- or hyperpigmentation and occasionally by onycholysis (in 0.8% of patients with solid tumors) and pain.

►*GI:* GI reactions (nausea and/or vomiting and/or diarrhea) were generally mild to moderate. Severe reactions occurred in 3% to 5% of patients with solid tumors and to a similar extent among metastatic breast cancer patients. The incidence of severe reactions was 1% or less for the 92 breast cancer patients premedicated with 3-day corticosteroids.

Severe stomatitis occurred in 5.5% of patients with solid tumors, in 7.4% of patients with metastatic breast cancer, and in 1.1% of the 92 breast cancer patients premedicated with 3-day corticosteroids.

►*Hematologic:* Reversible marrow suppression was the major dose-limiting toxicity of docetaxel. The median time to nadir was 7 days, while the median duration of severe neutropenia (fewer than 500 cells/mm³) was 7 days. Among 2045 patients with solid tumors and normal baseline LFTs, severe neutropenia occurred in 75.4% and lasted for more than 7 days in 2.9% of cycles.

Febrile neutropenia (fewer than 500 cells/mm³ with fever greater than 38°C with IV antibiotics and/or hospitalization) occurred in 11% of patients with solid tumors, in 12.3% of patients with metastatic breast cancer, and in 9.8% of 92 breast cancer patients premedicated with 3-day corticosteroids. Severe infectious episodes occurred in 6.1% of patients with solid tumors, in 6.4% of patients with metastatic breast cancer, and in 5.4% of 92 breast cancer patients premedicated with 3-day corticosteroids.

Thrombocytopenia (fewer than 100,000 cells/mm³) associated with fatal GI hemorrhage has been reported.

►*Hypersensitivity:* Minor events, including flushing, rash with or without pruritus, chest tightness, back pain, dyspnea, drug fever, or chills have been reported and resolved after discontinuing the infusion and appropriate therapy (see Warning Box and Warnings).

►*Metabolic:* Severe fluid retention occurred in 6.5% of patients despite use of a 3-day dexamethasone premedication regimen. It was characterized by one or more of the following events: Poorly tolerated peripheral edema, generalized edema, pleural effusion requiring urgent drainage, dyspnea at rest, cardiac tamponade, or pronounced abdominal distension (due to ascites).

When fluid retention occurs, peripheral edema usually starts in the lower extremities and may become generalized with a median weight gain of 2 kg.

►*Lab test abnormalities:* Increased ALT, AST, and alkaline phosphatase. In patients with normal LFTs at baseline, bilirubin values greater than the ULN occurred in 8.9% of patients. Increases in ALT or AST greater than 1.5 times the ULN or alkaline phosphatase greater than 2.5 times ULN were observed in 18.9% and 7.3% of patients, respectively. While on docetaxel, increases in ALT and/or AST greater than 1.5 times ULN concomitant with alkaline phosphatase greater than 2.5 times ULN occurred in 4.3% of patients with normal LFTs at baseline. Whether or not these changes were related to the drug or underlying disease has not been established (see Warnings).

►*Postmarketing:*

Cardiovascular – Atrial fibrillation, deep vein thrombosis, ECG abnormalities, thrombophlebitis, pulmonary embolism, syncope, tachycardia, MI.

CNS – Confusion, rare cases of seizures or transient loss of consciousness have been observed, sometimes appearing during the infusion of the drug.

Dermatologic – Bullous eruption (eg, erythema multiforme, Stevens-Johnson syndrome) (rare). Multiple factors may have contributed to the development of these effects.

GI – Abdominal pain, anorexia, constipation, duodenal ulcer, esophagitis, GI hemorrhage, GI perforation, ischemic colitis, colitis, intestinal obstruction, ileus, neutropenic enterocolitis, and dehydration as a consequence to GI events have been reported.

Ophthalmic – Conjunctivitis, lacrimation or lacrimation with or without conjunctivitis. Excessive tearing that may be attributable to lacrimal duct obstruction has been reported.

Respiratory – Dyspnea, acute pulmonary edema, acute respiratory distress syndrome, interstitial pneumonia. Pulmonary fibrosis has been reported rarely.

DOCETAXEL

Miscellaneous – Bleeding episodes; chest pain; diffuse pain; hepatitis (rare); radiation recall phenomenon; renal insufficiency.

Overdosage

➤*Symptoms:* Anticipated complications of overdosage include bone marrow suppression, peripheral neurotoxicity, and mucositis. In 2 overdose reports in which 1 patient received 150 mg/m² and the other received 200 mg/m² as 1-hour infusions, both patients experienced severe neutropenia, mild asthenia, cutaneous reactions, and mild paresthesia and recovered without incident.

In mice, lethality was observed following single IV doses that were 154 mg/kg or more (about 4.5 times the recommended human dose in a mg/m² basis); neurotoxicity associated with paralysis, nonextension of hind limbs, and myelin degeneration was observed in mice at 48 mg/kg (about 1.5 times the recommended human dose on a mg/m² basis). In male and female rats, lethality was observed at a dose of 20 mg/kg (comparable to the recommended human dose on a mg/m² basis) and was associated with abnormal mitosis and necrosis of multiple organs.

➤*Treatment:* There is no known antidote for docetaxel overdosage. In case of overdosage, keep patient in a specialized unit where vital functions may be closely monitored. Administer therapeutic G-CSF as soon as possible after discovery of overdose. Take other appropriate symptomatic measures as needed.

Patient Information

Side effects associated with docetaxel may include low white blood cell count, hair loss, fatigue, fluid retention, numbness, mouth irritation, cutaneous changes, nausea, and diarrhea.

Your doctor may prescribe other medications, including a corticosteroid such as dexamethasone, which is used to help avoid or lessen some of the side effects of treatment.

If you have a fever over 100°F, be sure to call your doctor immediately. Other symptoms of infection, such as sore throat, cough, or a burning sensation while urinating also should be reported.

If you feel a warm sensation, tightness in your chest, difficulty in breathing, or itching during or shortly after treatment, tell your doctor immediately.

Let your doctor know if you have any signs of fluid retention (eg, swelling of your feet or hands or increased weight).

If you feel prolonged fatigue during the course of your treatment, tell your doctor.

People receiving docetaxel may develop a red, blotchy rash. This usually occurs on the feet and hands, but may also appear on the arms, face, or body. If it occurs, the rash generally appears within the week after docetaxel treatment and usually disappears after a week or two. Tell your doctor if this occurs.

Some patients receiving docetaxel experience numbness, tingling, or burning sensations in their fingers and/or toes.

Changes in the color of your nails may occur. Occasionally, nails become soft and tender. In rare cases, nails may fall off.

WARNING

Severe myelosuppression: Severe myelosuppression with resulting infection or bleeding may occur.

Hypersensitivity reactions: Hypersensitivity reactions, including anaphylaxis-like symptoms, may occur with initial dosing or at repeated exposure to teniposide. Epinephrine, with or without corticosteroids and antihistamines, has been used to alleviate symptoms.

Indications

➤*Etoposide:*

Refractory testicular tumors – Refractory testicular tumors in combination with other chemotherapeutic agents in patients who have received surgery, chemotherapy and radiotherapy. Adequate data on the use of oral etoposide are not available.

Small cell lung cancer – Small cell lung cancer in combination with other agents as first line treatment.

➤*Teniposide:* In combination with other approved anticancer agents for induction therapy in patients with refractory childhood acute lymphoblastic leukemia (ALL). Available under a Treatment IND since 1988 for relapsed or refractory ALL.

➤*Unlabeled uses:*

Etoposide – Etoposide has been used alone or in combination in acute nonlymphocytic leukemias (monocytic), Hodgkin's disease, non-Hodgkin's lymphomas, Kaposi's sarcoma and neuroblastoma. Other tumors with a response rate of 5% to 20% to etoposide as a single agent include: Choriocarcinoma; rhabdomyosarcoma; hepatocellular carcinoma; epithelial ovarian, non-small and small cell lung, testicular, gastric, endometrial and breast cancers; acute lymphocytic leukemia; soft tissue sarcoma.

Actions

➤*Pharmacology:* These drugs are semisynthetic derivatives of podophyllotoxin.

Etoposide – Its main effect appears to be at the G_2 portion of the cell cycle. Two dose-dependent responses occur: At high concentrations ($\geq$ 10 mcg/ml), lysis of cells entering mitosis is seen; at low concentrations (0.3 to 10 mcg/ml), cells are inhibited from entering prophase. The predominant macromolecular effect appears to be DNA synthesis inhibition.

Teniposide – Teniposide is a phase-specific cytotoxic drug, acting in the late S or early G_2 phase of the cell cycle, thus preventing cells from entering mitosis. Teniposide causes dose-dependent single- and double-stranded breaks in DNA and DNA:protein cross-links. The mechanism of action appears to be related to the inhibition of type II topoisomerase activity since teniposide does not intercalate into DNA or bind strongly to DNA. The cytotoxic effects of teniposide are related to the relative number of double-stranded DNA breaks produced in cells, which are a reflection of the stabilization of a topoisomerase II-DNA intermediate. Teniposide has a broad spectrum of in vivo antitumor activity against murine tumors, including hematologic malignancies and various solid tumors. Notably, it is active against sublines of certain murine leukemias with acquired resistance to cisplatin, doxorubicin, amsacrine, daunorubicin, mitoxantrone or vincristine.

➤*Pharmacokinetics:*

Absorption / Distribution –

Various Pharmacokinetic Parameters for Etoposide and Teniposide

Parameter	Etoposide	Teniposide
Total body clearance (ml/min)	33-48	10.3
Terminal half-life (hrs)	4-11	5
Volume of distribution (L)	18-29	3-11 (children) 8-44 (adults)
Protein binding (%)	97	> 99
Elimination	Renal (35%) and nonrenal (ie, mostly metabolism, $\leq$ 6% bile)	Renal (44%) and fecal ($\leq$ 10%)
Excreted unchanged in urine (%)	< 50	4-12

Etoposide: The mean oral bioavailability is approximately 50% (range, 25% to 75%). There is no evidence of a first-pass effect for etoposide. On IV administration, the disposition of etoposide is a biphasic process with a distribution half-life of about 1.5 hours. The areas under the plasma concentration-time curves (AUC) and maximum plasma concentration (C_{max}) values increase linearly with dose. Etoposide does not accumulate in the plasma following daily administration of 100 mg/m² for 4 to 5 days. After either IV infusion or oral administration, C_{max} and AUC values exhibit marked intra- and intersubject variability. These values for oral etoposide consistently fall in the same range as the C_{max} and AUC values for an IV dose of half the size of the oral dose.

Although detectable in CSF and intracerebral tumors, the concentrations are lower than in extracerebral tumors and plasma. Concentra-

tions are higher in normal lung than in lung metastases and are similar in primary tumors and normal tissues of the myometrium. An inverse relationship between plasma albumin levels and renal clearance is found in children.

Metabolism / Excretion – The major urinary metabolite is the hydroxy acid. Glucuronide or sulfate conjugates of etoposide are excreted in human urine and represent 5% to 22% of the dose.

In adults, total body clearance is correlated with creatinine clearance, serum albumin concentration and nonrenal clearance. In children, elevated serum ALT levels are associated with reduced drug total body clearance. Prior use of cisplatin may also result in a decrease of etoposide total body clearance in children. The pharmacokinetic characteristics of teniposide differ from those of etoposide. Teniposide is more extensively bound to plasma proteins and its cellular uptake is greater. Teniposide also has a lower systemic clearance, a longer elimination half-life and is excreted in the urine as parent drug to a lesser extent than etoposide.

Teniposide – Plasma drug levels decline biexponentially following IV infusion in children. In adults, plasma levels increase linearly with dose. Drug accumulation did not occur after daily administration for 3 days. In children, C_{max} after infusions of 137 to 203 mg/m² over a period of 1 to 2 hours exceeded 40 mcg/ml; by 20 to 24 hours after infusion plasma levels were generally < 2 mcg/ml.

The blood-brain barrier appears to limit diffusion of teniposide into the brain, although in a study in patients with brain tumors, CSF levels were higher than in patients without brain tumors.

➤*Clinical trials:*

Teniposide – Nine children with acute lymphocytic leukemia (ALL) failing induction therapy with a cytarabine-containing regimen were treated with teniposide plus cytarabine. Three of these patients were induced into complete remission with durations of remission of 30 weeks, 59 weeks and 13 years. In another study, 16 children with ALL refractory to vincristine/prednisone-containing regimens were treated with teniposide plus vincristine and prednisone. Three patients were induced into complete remission with durations of remission of 5.5, 37 and 73 weeks.

Contraindications

Hypersensitivity to etoposide, teniposide or *Cremophor EL* (polyoxyethylated castor oil, present in the teniposide preparation).

Warnings

➤*Myelosuppression:* Observe patients for myelosuppression during and after therapy. Dose-limiting bone marrow suppression is the most significant toxicity.

Laboratory studies – Perform at the start of therapy and prior to each subsequent dose: Platelet count, hemoglobin, white blood cell count and differential. A platelet count < 50,000/mm³ or an absolute neutrophil count < 500/mm³ is an indication to withhold further therapy until the blood counts have sufficiently recovered.

➤*Anaphylaxis:* Anaphylaxis manifested by chills, fever, tachycardia, bronchospasm, dyspnea, facial flushing, hypertension or hypotension may occur (etoposide, 0.7% to 2%; teniposide, $\approx$ 5%). The reactions usually respond to cessation of infusion and institution of appropriate therapy. Refer to Management of Acute Hypersensitivity Reactions.

This reaction may occur with the first dose of teniposide and may be life threatening if not treated promptly with antihistamines, corticosteroids, epinephrine, IV fluids and other supportive measures as clinically indicated. The exact cause of these reactions is unknown; they may be due to the polyoxyethylated castor oil component of the vehicle or to teniposide itself. The incidence appears to be increased in patients with brain tumors and neuroblastoma. Patients who have experienced prior hypersensitivity reactions to teniposide are at risk for recurrence of symptoms and should only be retreated if the antileukemic benefit already demonstrated clearly outweighs the risk of a probable hypersensitivity reaction for that patient. When a decision is made to retreat a patient, pretreat with corticosteroids and antihistamines and carefully observe during and after the infusion. To date, there is no evidence to suggest cross-sensitization between teniposide and etoposide.

➤*Hypotension:* Administer by slow IV infusion (30 to 60 minutes or longer) since hypotension may occur with rapid IV injection. With teniposide, it may also be due to a direct effect of the polyoxyethylated castor oil component. If hypotension occurs, stop infusion and give fluids or other supportive therapy, as appropriate. When restarting infusion, use a slower rate.

➤*Benzyl alcohol:* Teniposide contains benzyl alcohol, which has been associated with a fatal "gasping" syndrome in premature infants.

➤*CNS depression:* Acute CNS depression and hypotension have occurred in patients receiving investigational infusions of high-dose teniposide who were pretreated with antiemetic drugs. The depressant effects of the antiemetic agents and the alcohol content of the teniposide formulation may place patients receiving higher than recommended doses at risk for CNS depression.

➤*Down's syndrome patients:* Patients with both Down's syndrome and leukemia may be especially sensitive to myelosuppressive chemotherapy; therefore, reduce initial dosing with teniposide in these patients. It is suggested that the first course be given at half the usual dose. Subsequent courses may be administered at higher dosages depending on the degree of myelosuppression and mucositis encountered in earlier courses in an individual patient.

➤*Hepatic function impairment:* There appears to be some association between an increase in serum alkaline phosphatase or gamma glutamyl-transpeptidase and a decrease in plasma clearance of teniposide. Therefore, exercise caution if teniposide is administered to patients with hepatic dysfunction. In children, elevated serum ALT levels are associated with reduced drug total body clearance of etoposide.

➤*Carcinogenesis:* These agents are possible carcinogens. Mutagenic and genotoxic potential has been established in mammalian cells.

Children with ALL in remission who received maintenance therapy with teniposide at weekly or twice weekly doses (plus other chemotherapeutic agents) had a relative risk of developing secondary acute nonlymphocytic leukemia (ANLL) approximately 12 times that of patients treated according to other less intensive schedules. A short course of teniposide for remission-induction or consolidation therapy was not associated with an increased risk of secondary ANLL, but the number of patients assessed was small. The potential benefit must be weighed on a case by case basis against the potential risk of the induction of a secondary leukemia.

➤*Pregnancy: Category D.* Etoposide and teniposide may cause fetal harm. They are teratogenic and embryotoxic in animals. There are no adequate and well controlled studies in pregnant women. If used during pregnancy, or if the patient becomes pregnant while receiving this drug, apprise her of the potential hazard to the fetus. Advise women of childbearing potential to avoid becoming pregnant.

➤*Lactation:* It is not known whether this drug is excreted in breast milk. Because of the potential for serious adverse reactions in nursing infants, decide whether to discontinue nursing or the drug, accounting for the importance of the drug to the mother.

➤*Children:* Safety and efficacy for use of etoposide in children have not been established. Teniposide is indicated for use in children.

Precautions

➤*Monitoring:* In addition to hematologic tests, carefully monitor renal and hepatic function tests prior to and during therapy.

Drug Interactions

Etoposide/Teniposide Drug Interactions

Precipitant drug	Object drug*		Description
Etoposide	Warfarin	↑	Prolongation of the prothrombin time may occur.
Teniposide	Methotrexate	↑	Plasma clearance of methotrexate may be slightly increased. In vitro, increased intracellular levels were observed.
Sodium salicylate Sulfamethizole Tolbutamide	Teniposide	↑	Teniposide was displaced from protein-binding sites by these agents to a small but significant extent. Because of the extremely high binding of teniposide to plasma proteins, these small decreases in binding could cause substantial increases in free drug levels, resulting in potentiation of toxicity.

* ↑ = Object drug increased.

Adverse Reactions

Most adverse reactions are reversible if detected early. If severe reactions occur, reduce or discontinue dosage and institute corrective measures. Reinstitute therapy with caution, consider further need for the drug and be alert to recurrence of toxicity.

Etoposide/Teniposide Adverse Reactions (%)

Adverse reaction	Etoposide	Teniposide
Cardiovascular		
Hypotension[1]	1-2	2
Hypertension	✔[3]	—[4]
Dermatologic		
Alopecia (reversible)[2]	≤ 66	9
Rash	✔	3
Pigmentation	✔	—
Pruritus	✔	—
Radiation recall dermatitis	one report	—
GI		
Mucositis	—	76
Nausea/Vomiting	31-43	29
Anorexia	10-13	—
Diarrhea	1-13	33
Abdominal pain	≤ 2	—
Stomatitis	1-6	—
Hepatic dysfunction/toxicity	≤ 3	< 1
Dysphagia	✔	—
Constipation	✔	—
Hematologic		
Myelosuppression, nonspecified	✔	75
Leukopenia (WBC/mm³)		
< 4000	60-91	—
< 3000	—	89
< 1000	3-17	—
Neutropenia (ANC/mm³)		
< 2000	—	95
Thrombocytopenia (platelets/mm³)		
< 100,000	22-41	85
< 50,000	1-20	—
Anemia	≤ 33	88
Miscellaneous		
Hypersensitivity/Anaphylactic reactions[1]	0.7-2 (< 1 oral)	≈ 5
Peripheral neurotoxicity	1-2	< 1
Aftertaste	✔	—
Fever	✔	3
Transient cortical blindness	✔	—
Infection	—	12
Bleeding	—	5
Renal dysfunction	—	< 1
Metabolic abnormalities	—	< 1

[1] See Warnings.
[2] Sometimes progressing to total baldness.
[3] ✔ = Adverse reaction observed, incidence not reported.
[4] — = Adverse reaction not reported.

Overdosage

➤*Symptoms:* The anticipated complications of overdosage are secondary to bone marrow suppression.

➤*Treatment:* There is no known antidote for overdosage. Treatment should consist of supportive care including blood products and antibiotics as indicated.

Patient Information

Contraceptive measures are recommended during treatment.

Notify physician of any of these: Fever; chills; rapid heartbeat; difficult breathing.

Podophyllotoxin Derivatives

ETOPOSIDE (VP-16-213)

Rx	VePesid (Bristol-Myers Oncology)	Capsules: 50 mg	Sorbitol. (Bristol 3091). Pink. In blisterpack 20s.
Rx	Etoposide (Various, eg, Pharmachemie B.V.)	Injection: 20 mg/ml	In 5, 12.5 and 25 ml vials.[1]
Rx	VePesid (Bristol-Myers Oncology)		In 5 ml vials.[2]
Rx	Toposar (Gensia Sicor)		In 5, 10 and 25 ml.[3]
Rx	Etopophos (Bristol-Myers Oncology)	Powder for Injection, lyophilized: 100 mg	In single dose vials.

[1] May contain alcohol, benzyl alcohol, 80 mg polysorbate 80, polyethylene glycol or citric acid.

[2] With 30 mg/ml benzyl alcohol, 80 mg polysorbate 80, 650 mg polyethylene glycol 300, 30.5% alcohol.

[3] With 30 mg/ml benzyl alcohol, 30.5% alcohol.

For complete prescribing information, refer to the Podophyllotoxin Derivatives group monograph.

Administration and Dosage

➤*Approved by the FDA:* 1983.

Modify the dosage, by either route, to account for the myelosuppressive effects of other drugs in combination, the effects of prior x–ray therapy or chemotherapy which may have compromised bone marrow reserve.

Administer solution over 30 to 60 minutes or longer. Do not give by rapid IV injection.

➤*Testicular cancer:*

Parenteral – Usual dose is 50 to 100 mg/m^2/day on days 1 to 5 to 100 mg/m^2/day on days 1, 3 and 5.

➤*Small cell lung cancer:*

Parenteral – 35 mg/m^2/day for 4 days to 50 mg/m^2/day for 5 days. Courses are repeated at 3- to 4-week intervals after recovery from toxicity.

Oral – 2 times the IV dose rounded to the nearest 50 mg.

➤*Preparation for IV administration:* Dilute with either 5% Dextrose Injection or 0.9% Sodium Chloride Injection to give a final concentration of 0.2 or 0.4 mg/ml.

Plastic devices made of acrylic or ABS have cracked and leaked when used with undiluted etoposide. This has not been reported with diluted solutions.

➤*Handling:* Skin reactions may occur with accidental exposure. Use gloves. If solution contacts the skin or mucosa, immediately wash the area thoroughly with soap and water.

➤*Storage/Stability:* Unopened vials are stable for 2 years at room temperature (25°C; 77°F). Diluted solutions (concentration of 0.2 or 0.4 mg/ml) are stable for 96 and 48 hours, respectively, at room temperature under normal room fluorescent light in both glass and plastic containers. Capsules must be stored at 2° to 8°C (36° to 46°F). Stable for 2 years under refrigeration, 3 months at room temperature. Do not freeze.

TENIPOSIDE (VM-26)

Rx	Vumon (Bristol-Myers Oncology)	Injection:[1] 50 mg (10 mg/ml)	In 5 ml amps.[2]

[1] Must be diluted prior to administration.

[2] With 30 mg benzyl alcohol and 500 mg *Cremophor EL* (polyoxyethylated castor oil) per ml, with 42.7% dehydrated alcohol.

For complete prescribing information, refer to the Podophyllotoxin Derivatives group monograph.

Administration and Dosage

➤*Approved by the FDA:* July 14, 1992.

Teniposide must be administered as an IV infusion. Take care to ensure that the IV catheter or needle is in the proper position and functional prior to infusion. Improper administration may result in extravasation causing local tissue necrosis or thrombophlebitis. In some instances, occlusion of central venous access devices has occurred during 24-hour infusion at a concentration of 0.1 to 0.2 mg/ml. Frequent observation during these infusions is necessary to minimize this risk.

➤*Administration:* Administer over ≥ 30 to 60 minutes. Do not give by rapid IV injection. Hypotension has been reported following rapid IV administration.

In one study, childhood acute lymphoblastic leukemia (ALL) patients failing induction therapy with a cytarabine-containing regimen were treated with the combination of teniposide 165 mg/m^2 and cytarabine 300 mg/m^2 IV twice weekly for 8 to 9 doses. In another study, patients with childhood ALL refractory to vincristine/prednisone-containing regimens were treated with the combination of teniposide 250 mg/m^2 and vincristine 1.5 mg/m^2 IV weekly for 4 to 8 weeks and prednisone 40 mg/m^2 orally for 28 days.

➤*Hepatic/Renal function impairment:* Adequate data in patients with hepatic or renal insufficiency are lacking, but dose adjustments may be necessary for patients with significant renal or hepatic impairment.

➤*Down's syndrome patients:* Reduce initial dosing; give the first course at half the usual dose (see Warnings).

➤*Preparation for IV administration:* Teniposide must be diluted with either 5% Dextrose Injection, USP, or 0.9% Sodium Chloride Injection, USP, to give final teniposide concentrations of 0.1, 0.2, 0.4, or 1 mg/ml.

Contact of undiluted teniposide with plastic equipment or devices used to prepare solutions for infusion may result in softening or cracking and possible drug product leakage. This effect has not been reported with diluted solutions.

In order to prevent extraction of the plasticizer DEHP, prepare and administer solutions in non-DEHP-containing LVP containers such as glass or polyolefin plastic bags or containers. The use of PVC containers is not recommended.

Lipid administration sets or low DEHP-containing nitroglycerin sets will keep patients' exposure to DEHP at low levels and are suitable for use. The diluted solutions are chemically and physically compatible with the recommended IV administration sets and LVP containers for up to 24 hours at ambient room temperature and lighting conditions.

Teniposide is a cytotoxic anticancer drug; use caution in handling and preparing the solution. Skin reactions associated with accidental exposure may occur. The use of gloves is recommended. If teniposide solution contacts the skin, immediately wash the skin thoroughly with soap and water. If the drug contacts mucous membranes, flush thoroughly with water.

➤*Admixture incompatibilities:* Heparin solution can cause precipitation of teniposide; therefore, flush the administration apparatus thoroughly with 5% Dextrose Injection or 0.9% Sodium Chloride Injection, USP, before and after administration of teniposide. Because of the potential for precipitation, compatibility with other drugs, infusion materials, or IV pumps cannot be assured.

➤*Storage/Stability:* Unopened amps are stable until the date indicated on the package when stored under refrigeration (2° to 8°C; 36° to 46°F) in the original package (to protect from light). Freezing does not adversely affect the product. Reconstituted solutions are stable at room temperature for up to 24 hours after preparation. Administer 1 mg/ml solutions within 4 hours of preparation to reduce the potential for precipitation. Refrigeration of solutions is not recommended. Stability and use times are identical in glass and plastic containers.

Although solutions are chemically stable under the conditions indicated, precipitation of teniposide may occur at the recommended concentrations, especially if the diluted solution is subjected to more agitation than is recommended to prepare the drug solution for parenteral administration. In addition, minimize storage time prior to administration and take care to avoid contact of the diluted solution with other drugs or fluids. Precipitation has been reported during 24-hour infusions of teniposide concentrations of 0.1 to 0.2 mg/ml, resulting in occlusion of central venous access catheters in several patients.

DAUNORUBICIN HCl

Rx	**Daunorubicin HCl for Injection** (Various, eg, Abbott, Bedford)	**Injection:** 5 mg/ml (equivalent to 5.34 mg daunorubicin HCl)[1]	Preservative-free. In 4 and 10 ml single-use vials.
Rx	**Daunorubicin HCl** (Various, eg, Abbott, Gensia Sicor)	**Powder for Injection, lyophilized:** 21.4 mg (equivalent to 20 mg daunorubicin)	100 mg mannitol. In 10 ml single-dose vials.
Rx	**Cerubidine** (Bedford)		100 mg mannitol. In single-dose vials.
Rx	**Daunorubicin HCl** (Various, eg, Abbott, Gensia Sicor)	**Powder for Injection, lyophilized:** 53.5 mg (equivalent to 50 mg daunorubicin)	250 mg mannitol. In 20 ml single-dose vials.

[1] 9 mg NaCl.

WARNING

Give daunorubicin into a rapidly flowing IV infusion. Do not administer IM or SC. Severe local tissue necrosis will result if extravasation occurs.

Myocardial toxicity, in its most severe form, as potentially fatal congestive heart failure, may occur when total cumulative dosage exceeds 400 to 550 mg/m^2 in adults, 300 mg/m^2 in children > 2 years of age, or 10 mg/kg in children < 2 years of age. This may occur during therapy or several months to years after therapy.

It is recommended that daunorubicin be administered only by physicians who are experienced in leukemia chemotherapy and in facilities with laboratory and supportive resources adequate to monitor drug tolerance and protect and maintain a patient compromised by drug toxicity.

The physician and institution must be capable of responding rapidly and completely to severe hemorrhagic conditions or overwhelming infection.

Severe myelosuppression occurs when used in therapeutic doses; this may lead to infection or hemorrhage.

Reduce dosage in patients with impaired hepatic or renal function.

Indications

➤*Leukemia:* In combination with other approved anticancer drugs, for remission induction in acute nonlymphocytic leukemia (myelogenous, monocytic, erythroid) of adults and for remission induction in acute lymphocytic leukemia of children and adults.

Administration and Dosage

For IV use only.

To eradicate the leukemic cells and induce a complete remission, a profound suppression of bone marrow is usually required. Evaluation of both the peripheral blood and bone marrow are mandatory in the formulation of treatment plans.

➤*Adult acute nonlymphocytic leukemia:* Representative dose schedules and combination for remission induction include the following.

Patients < 60 years of age – Daunorubicin 45 mg/m^2/day IV on days 1, 2, and 3 of the first course and on days 1 and 2 of subsequent courses and cytosine arabinoside 100 mg/m^2/day IV infusion daily for 7 days for the first course and for 5 days for subsequent courses.

Patients ≥ 60 years of age – Daunorubicin 30 mg/m^2/day IV on days 1, 2, and 3 of the first course and on days 1 and 2 of subsequent courses and cytosine arabinoside 100 mg/m^2/day IV infusion daily for 7 days for the first course and for 5 days for subsequent courses. This daunorubicin dose reduction is based on a single study and may not be appropriate if optimal supportive care is available.

Attaining a normal appearing bone marrow may require ≤ 3 courses of induction therapy. Evaluate bone marrow following recovery from the previous induction course to determine the need for a further course of induction treatment.

➤*Pediatric acute lymphocytic leukemia:* Representative dose schedules and combination for remission induction include the following.

Daunorubicin 25 mg/m^2 IV on day 1 every week, vincristine 1.5 mg/m^2 IV on day 1 every week, oral prednisone 40 mg/m^2/day. Generally, complete remission will be obtained with 4 courses of therapy; however, if after 4 courses the patient is in partial remission, an additional 1 or, if necessary, 2 courses may be given in an effort to obtain a complete remission.

In children < 2 years of age or < 0.5 m^2 body surface area, calculate dosage on the basis of weight (mg/kg) instead of body surface area.

➤*Adult acute lymphocytic leukemia:* Representative dose schedules and combination for the approved indication of remission induction include the following.

Daunorubicin 45 mg/m^2/day IV on days 1, 2, and 3 and vincristine 2 mg IV on days 1, 8, and 15; prednisone 40 mg/m^2/day orally on days 1 through 22, then tapered between days 22 to 29; L-asparaginase 500 IU/kg/day × 10 days IV on days 22 through 32.

➤*Hepatic or renal function impairment:* Reduce dosage.

Daunorubicin HCl Dosage in Hepatic or Renal Function Impairment (%)		
Serum bilirubin	Serum creatinine	Dose reduction
1.2 to 3.0 mg	—	25
> 3 mg	—	50
—	> 3 mg	50

➤*Preparation / Storage of solution:* Reconstitute vial contents with 4 ml Sterile Water for Injection to prepare a solution of 5 mg of daunorubicin activity per ml. Withdraw the desired dose into a syringe containing 10 to 15 ml of normal saline; inject into the tubing or sidearm of a rapidly flowing IV infusion of 5% glucose or normal saline solution.

➤*IV admixture compatibilities / incompatibilities:* Do not mix with other drugs or heparin.

➤*Storage / Stability:* Store unopened vials in refrigerator, 2° to 8°C (36° to 46°F). Store prepared solution for infusion at room temperature, 15° to 30°C (59° to 86°F) for ≤ 24 hours. Contains no preservative. Discard unused portion. Protect from light.

Actions

➤*Pharmacology:* Daunorubicin has antimitotic and cytotoxic activity through a number of proposed mechanisms of action. It forms complexes with DNA by intercalation between base pairs. It inhibits topoisomerase II activity by stabilizing the DNA-topoisomerase II complex, preventing the religation portion of the ligation-religation reaction that topoisomerase II catalyzes. Single-strand and double-strand DNA breaks result. Daunorubicin may also inhibit polymerase activity, affect regulation of gene expression, and produce free radical damage to DNA.

➤*Pharmacokinetics:*

Absorption / Distribution – Following IV injection, daunorubicin undergoes rapid tissue uptake and concentration. It does not cross the blood-brain barrier. Plasma and tissue protein binding is rapid and extensive; highest concentrations occur in the spleen, kidneys, liver, lungs, and heart.

Metabolism / Excretion – Daunorubicin is extensively metabolized in the liver and other tissues, mainly by cytoplasmic aldo-keto reductases, producing daunorubicinol, the major metabolite, which has antineoplastic activity. Approximately 40% of the drug in the plasma is present as daunorubicinol within 30 minutes and 60% in 4 hours after a dose of daunorubicin. Further metabolism via reduction cleavage of the glycosidic bond, 4-O demethylation and conjugation with both sulfate and glucuronide have been demonstrated. Terminal half-lives for daunorubicin and daunorubicinol are 18.5 and 26.7 hours, respectively. About 25% is eliminated in active form by urinary excretion and 40% by biliary excretion.

Special populations –

Elderly: Cardiotoxicity may be more frequent in the elderly. Use caution in patients who have inadequate bone marrow reserves due to old age. In addition, elderly patients are more likely to have age-related renal function impairment, which may require reduction of dosage in patients receiving daunorubicin (see Administration and Dosage).

Pediatric patients: Cardiotoxicity may be more frequent and occur at lower cumulative doses in children.

Renal and hepatic function impairment: Reduce doses of daunorubicin in patients with hepatic and renal impairment (see Administration and Dosage).

Contraindications

Hypersensitivity to daunorubicin or any component of the product.

Warnings

➤*Previous cumulative dose:* Do not use in patients who have previously received the recommended maximum cumulative dose of either doxorubicin or daunorubicin.

➤*Bone marrow suppression:* Bone marrow suppression will occur in all patients given a therapeutic dose of this drug. Do not start therapy in patients with preexisting drug-induced bone marrow suppression unless the benefit from such treatment warrants the risk. Persistent, severe myelosuppression may result in superinfection or hemorrhage.

➤*Cardiotoxicity:* Preexisting heart disease or previous doxorubicin therapy are cofactors of increased risk of cardiotoxicity; weigh benefit-to-risk ratio before starting therapy. Give attention to the drug's potential cardiac toxicity, particularly in infants and children.

In adults, at total cumulative doses < 550 mg/m^2, acute CHF is seldom encountered. However, rare instances of pericarditis-myocarditis, not

DAUNORUBICIN HCl

dose-related, have occurred. At cumulative doses > 550 mg/m², there is an increased incidence of CHF. This limit appears lower (400 mg/m²) in patients receiving radiation therapy that encompassed the heart. In infants and children, there is a greater susceptibility to anthracycline-induced cardiotoxicity compared with adults, which is more clearly dose-related. However, there is little risk for children > 2 years of age below a cumulative dose of 300 mg/m² or in children < 2 years of age (or < 0.5 m² body surface area) below a cumulative dose of 10 mg/kg. Furthermore, the total dose given to children and adults should take into account any previous or concomitant therapy with other potentially cardiotoxic agents or related compounds such as doxorubicin.

There is no reliable method for predicting patients who will develop acute CHF; certain ECG changes and a decrease in the systolic injection fraction from pretreatment baseline may aid in recognizing those patients at greatest risk. A decrease of ≥ 30% in limb lead QRS voltage has been associated with significant risk of drug-induced cardiomyopathy. Perform an ECG or determine systolic ejection fraction before each course. If one or the other of these predictive parameters occurs, weigh the benefit of continued therapy against the risk of producing cardiac damage.

➤*Secondary leukemias:* There have been reports of secondary leukemias in patients exposed to topoisomerase II inhibitors when used in combination with other antineoplastic agents or radiation therapy.

➤*Extravasation at injection site:* Extravasation at injection site can cause severe local tissue necrosis. Stop the injection immediately. For management see the Antineoplastics Introduction

➤*Renal / Hepatic function impairment:* Hepatic and renal function impairment can enhance toxicity; assess hepatic and renal function prior to therapy.

➤*Carcinogenesis:* Daunorubicin injected SC into mice caused fibrosarcomas to develop at the injection site. In male rats administered daunorubicin 3 times weekly for 6 months at 1/70 the recommended human dose on a body surface area basis, peritoneal sarcomas were found at 18 months. A single IV dose of daunorubicin administered to rats at 1.6-fold the recommended human dose on a body surface basis caused mammary adenocarcinomas to appear at 1 year.

➤*Mutagenesis:* Daunorubicin was mutagenic in vitro (Ames assay, V79 hamster cell assay), and clastogenic in vitro (CCRFCEM human lymphoblasts) and in vivo (SCE assay in mouse bone marrow) tests.

➤*Fertility impairment:* In male dogs, at a daily dose of 0.25 mg/kg administered IV, testicular atrophy was noted at autopsy. Histologic examination revealed total aplasia of the spermatocyte series in the seminiferous tubules with complete aspermatogenesis.

➤*Pregnancy: Category D.* Due to its teratogenic potential, daunorubicin can cause fetal harm if administered to a pregnant woman. An increased incidence of fetal abnormalities (parieto-occipital cranioschisis, umbilical hernias, or rachischisis) and abortions occurred in rabbits at doses of 0.05 mg/kg/day or ≈ 1/100 of the highest recommended human dose on a body-surface-area basis. Decreases in fetal birth weight and postdelivery growth rate were observed in mice. There are no adequate and well-controlled studies in pregnant women. Advise women of childbearing potential to avoid becoming pregnant.

➤*Lactation:* It is not known whether this drug is excreted in breast milk. Due to the potential for serious adverse reactions in nursing infants from daunorubicin, advise mothers to discontinue nursing during daunorubicin therapy.

Precautions

➤*Monitoring:* Observe patient closely and monitor chemical and laboratory tests extensively. Evaluate cardiac, renal, and hepatic function prior to each course of treatment.

➤*Urine discoloration:* Urine discoloration (red) may occur transiently; advise patient appropriately.

➤*Infections:* Control any systemic infection before beginning therapy.

➤*Lab test abnormalities:* Hyperuricemia may be induced secondary to rapid lysis of leukemic cells. As a precaution, administer allopurinol prior to initiating antileukemic therapy. Monitor serum uric acid levels; initiate therapy if hyperuricemia develops.

Drug Interactions

Daunorubicin HCl Drug Interactions			
Precipitant drug	Object drug*		Description
Cyclophospha-mide	Daunorubicin	↑	Cyclophosphamide used concurrently with daunorubicin may result in increased cardiotoxicity.
Myelosuppressive agents	Daunorubicin	↑	Dosage reduction of daunorubicin may be required when used concurrently with other myelosuppressive agents.
Hepatotoxic medications (eg, methotrexate)	Daunorubicin	↑	Hepatotoxic medications, such as high-dose methotrexate, may impair liver function and increase the risk of toxicity.

* ↑ = Object drug increased.

Adverse Reactions

Dose-limiting toxicity includes myelosuppression and cardiotoxicity (see Warnings).

➤*Dermatologic:* Reversible alopecia; rash; contact dermatitis; urticaria.

➤*GI:* Acute nausea and vomiting (usually mild). Antiemetic therapy may help. Mucositis may occur 3 to 7 days after administration. Diarrhea and abdominal pain occur occasionally.

➤*Local:* If extravasation occurs, tissue necrolysis, severe cellulitis, thrombophlebitis, or painful induration can result at the site.

➤*Miscellaneous:* Rarely, anaphylactoid reactions, fever, and chills can occur. Hyperuricemia may occur, especially in patients with leukemia; monitor serum uric levels.

DAUNORUBICIN CITRATE LIPOSOMAL

Rx	**DaunoXome** (Gilead Sciences)	**Injection:** 2 mg/mL (equivalent to 50 mg daunorubicin base)	In single-use vials and single-unit packs.

WARNING

Monitor cardiac function regularly in patients receiving liposomal daunorubicin because of the potential risk for cardiac toxicity and congestive heart failure (CHF). Cardiac monitoring is especially advised in those patients who have received prior anthracyclines, have had preexisting cardiac disease, or who have had prior radiotherapy encompassing the heart. Severe myelosuppression may occur.

Administer liposomal daunorubicin only under the supervision of a physician who is experienced in the use of cancer chemotherapeutic agents.

Reduce dosage in patients with impaired hepatic function (see Administration and Dosage).

A triad of back pain, flushing, and chest tightness has been reported in 13.8% of the patients (16/116) treated with liposomal daunorubicin in the phase 3 clinical trial, and in 2.7% of treatment cycles (27/994). This triad generally occurs during the first 5 minutes of the infusion, subsides with interruption of the infusion, and generally does not recur if the infusion is then resumed at a slower rate.

Indications

➤*Advanced HIV-associated Kaposi sarcoma:* As first-line cytotoxic therapy for advanced HIV-associated Kaposi sarcoma.

Administration and Dosage

➤*Approved by the FDA:* April 8, 1996.

Administer IV over a 60-minute period at a dose of 40 mg/m², with doses repeated every 2 weeks. Continue treatment until there is evidence of progressive disease (eg, based on best response achieved; new visceral sites of involvement or progression of visceral disease; development of 10 or more new cutaneous lesions or a 25% increase in the number of lesions compared with baseline; a change in the character of at least 25% of all previously counted flat lesions to raised; increase in surface area of the indicator lesions) or until other intercurrent complications of HIV disease preclude continuation of therapy.

Repeat blood counts prior to each dose and withhold therapy if the absolute granulocyte count is less than 750 cells/mm³.

➤*Hepatic or renal function impairment:* Reduce dosage.

Liposomal Daunorubicin Dosage in Hepatic or Renal Function Impairment		
Serum bilirubin	Serum creatinine	Recommended dose
1.2 to 3 mg/dL	—	¾ normal dose
> 3 mg/dL	> 3 mg/dL	½ normal dose

➤*Preparation:* Dilute liposomal daunorubicin 1:1 with 5% dextrose injection before administration. Do not use an in-line filter for IV infusion. Do not mix liposomal daunorubicin with other drugs.

The recommended concentration after dilution is 1 mg daunorubicin/mL of solution.

➤*Storage / Stability:* Refrigerate at 2° to 8°C (36° to 46°F). If not used immediately, store reconstituted solution for a maximum of 6 hours under refrigeration. Do not freeze. Protect from light.

DAUNORUBICIN CITRATE LIPOSOMAL

Actions

➤*Pharmacology:* Liposomal daunorubicin contains an aqueous solution of the citrate salt of daunorubicin encapsulated within lipid vesicles (liposomes) composed of a lipid bilayer of distearoylphosphatidylcholine and cholesterol (2:1 molar ratio). Daunorubicin is an anthracycline antibiotic with antineoplastic activity originally obtained from *Streptomyces peucetius*. It may also be isolated from *Streptomyces coeruleorubidus*. Daunorubicin has a 4-ring anthracycline moiety linked by a glycosidic bond to daunosamine, an amino sugar.

Liposomal daunorubicin is a liposomal preparation of daunorubicin formulated to maximize the selectivity of daunorubicin for solid tumors in situ. In the circulation, the liposomal daunorubicin formulation helps to protect the entrapped daunorubicin from chemical and enzymatic degradation, minimizes protein binding, and generally decreases uptake by normal (nonreticuloendothelial system) tissues. The specific mechanism by which liposomal daunorubicin is able to deliver daunorubicin to solid tumors in situ is not known. However, it is believed to be a function of increased permeability of the tumor neovasculature to some particles in the size range of liposomal daunorubicin. Once within the tumor environment, daunorubicin is released over time, enabling it to exert its antineoplastic activity.

➤*Pharmacokinetics:*
Absorption/Distribution –

Liposomal Daunorubicin Pharmacokinetic Parameters		
Parameters (units)	Daunorubicin citrate liposomal (n = 30)	Conventional daunorubicin (n = 4)
Plasma clearance (mL/min)	17.3 ± 6.1	236 ± 181[1]
Volume of distribution (L)	6.4 ± 1.5	1006 ± 622
Distribution half-life (h)	4.41 ± 2.33	0.77 ± 0.3
Elimination half-life (h)	4.4 (apparent)	55.4 ± 13.7

[1] Calculated.

The plasma pharmacokinetics of liposomal daunorubicin differ significantly from conventional daunorubicin HCl. The differences in the volume of distribution and clearance result in a higher daunorubicin exposure (in terms of AUC) from liposomal daunorubicin than with conventional daunorubicin HCl. The apparent elimination half-life of liposomal daunorubicin is far shorter than that of daunorubicin HCl, and probably represents a distribution half-life. Preclinical biodistribution data in animals suggest that liposomal daunorubicin crosses the normal blood-brain barrier, however, it is unknown if this occurs in humans.

Metabolism – Daunorubicinol, the major active metabolite of daunorubicin, was detected at low levels in the plasma.

➤*Clinical trials:* In advanced, HIV-related Kaposi sarcoma, 2 treatment regimens were compared as first-line cytotoxic therapy: Liposomal daunorubicin 40 mg/m^2 and ABV (doxorubicin 10 mg/m^2, bleomycin 15 U, and vincristine 1 mg). Twenty of 33 ABV patients and 11 of 27 liposomal daunorubicin patients responded to therapy by criteria more stringent than flattening of lesions (ie, shrinkage of lesions and/or reduction in the number of lesions). Photographic evidence of tumor response to liposomal daunorubicin and ABV was comparable across all anatomic sites (eg, face, oral cavity, trunk, legs, feet).

First-Line Cytotoxic Therapy for Advanced Kaposi Sarcoma		
	Daunorubicin citrate liposomal (n = 116)	ABV (n = 111)
Response rate	23%[1]	30%
Duration of response, median	110 days[2]	113 days
Time to progression, median	92 days[3]	105 days
Survival	342 days[4]	291 days

[1] The 95% confidence interval for difference in the response rates (ABV/liposomal daunorubicin) was −5%, 18%.
[2] The hazard ratio (ABV/liposomal daunorubicin) for duration of response 0.8, and the 95% confidence intervals were 0.44, 1.46.
[3] The hazard ratio (ABV/liposomal daunorubicin) for time to progression was 0.78, and the 95% confidence intervals were 0.57, 1.07.
[4] The hazard ratio (ABV/liposomal daunorubicin) for mortality was 1.29, and the 95% confidence intervals were 0.92, 1.79.

Contraindications

Hypersensitivity reaction to previous doses of liposomal daunorubicin or to any of its constituents.

Warnings

➤*Myelosuppression:* The primary toxicity of liposomal daunorubicin is myelosuppression, especially of the granulocytic series, which may be severe and associated with fever and may result in infection. Effects on the platelets and erythroid series are much less marked. Careful hematologic monitoring is required. Because patients with HIV infection are immunocompromised, carefully observe patients for evidence of intercurrent or opportunistic infections.

➤*Potential cardiac toxicity:* Give special attention to the potential cardiac toxicity of liposomal daunorubicin. Although there is no reliable means of predicting CHF, cardiomyopathy induced by anthracyclines is usually associated with a decrease of the left ventricular ejection fraction (LVEF). Evaluate cardiac function in each patient by means of a history and physical examination before each course of liposomal daunorubicin, and perform determination of LVEF at total cumulative doses of liposomal daunorubicin 320 mg/m^2 and every 160 mg/m^2 thereafter.

Patients who have received prior therapy with anthracyclines (doxorubicin greater than 300 mg/m^2 or equivalent), have preexisting cardiac disease, or have received previous radiotherapy encompassing the heart may be less "cardiac" tolerant to treatment with liposomal daunorubicin. Therefore, monitor LVEF at cumulative liposomal daunorubicin doses prior to therapy and every 160 mg/m^2 of liposomal daunorubicin.

In patients with Kaposi sarcoma, CHF has been reported in 1 patient at a cumulative dose of 340 mg/m^2 of liposomal daunorubicin. In 8 Kaposi sarcoma patients, LVEF decreases were reported at cumulative doses ranging from 200 to 2100 mg/m^2 (median dose 320 mg/m^2) of liposomal daunorubicin. In clinical studies in malignancies other than Kaposi sarcoma treated with doses of liposomal daunorubicin greater than the recommended dose of 40 mg/m^2, CHF has been reported at a cumulative dose as low as 200 mg/m^2 of liposomal daunorubicin; 7 patients have been reported with LVEF decreases. The proportion of patients at risk for cardiotoxicity is unknown because the denominator is uncertain since there were several instances of missing repeat cardiac evaluations.

➤*Back pain, flushing, and chest tightness:* A triad of back pain, flushing, and chest tightness have been reported (see Black Box Warning). This combination of symptoms appears to be related to the lipid component of liposomal daunorubicin, as a similar set of signs and symptoms has been observed with other liposomal products not containing daunorubicin.

➤*Extravasation at injection site:* Conventional daunorubicin has been associated with local tissue necrosis at the site of drug extravasation. Although grade 3 to 4 injection-site inflammation was reported in 2 patients treated with liposomal daunorubicin, no instances of local tissue necrosis were observed with extravasation. Take care to ensure there is no extravasation of the drug when liposomal daunorubicin is administered.

➤*Hepatic function impairment:* Reduce dosage in patients with impaired hepatic function (see Administration and Dosage).

➤*Carcinogenesis:* A high incidence of mammary tumors was observed approximately 120 days after a single IV dose of 12.5 mg/kg daunorubicin in rats (approximately 2 times the human dose on a mg/m^2 basis).

➤*Mutagenesis:* Daunorubicin was mutagenic in in vitro tests and clastogenic in in vitro and in vivo tests.

➤*Fertility impairment:* Daunorubicin IV doses of 0.25 mg/kg/day (approximately 8 times the human dose on a mg/m^2 basis) in male dogs caused testicular atrophy and total aplasia of spermatocytes in the seminiferous tubules.

➤*Elderly:* Safety and efficacy in the elderly have not been established.

➤*Pregnancy: Category D.* Liposomal daunorubicin can cause fetal harm when administered to a pregnant woman. If liposomal daunorubicin is used during pregnancy or if the patient becomes pregnant while taking liposomal daunorubicin, warn the patient of the potential hazard to the fetus.

➤*Children:* Safety and efficacy in children have not been established.

Adverse Reactions

Adverse Reactions of Liposomal Daunorubicin Compared with ABV (%)				
	Liposomal daunorubicin (n = 116)		ABV (n = 111)	
Adverse reaction	Mild/Moderate	Severe	Mild/Moderate	Severe
CNS				
Depression	7	3	6	-
Dizziness	8	-	9	-
Fatigue	43	6	44	7
Headache	22	3	23	2
Insomnia	6	-	14	-
Malaise	9	1	11	1
Neuropathy	12	1	38	3
Dermatologic				
Alopecia	8	-	36	-
Pruritus	7	-	14	-

DAUNORUBICIN CITRATE LIPOSOMAL

Adverse Reactions of Liposomal Daunorubicin Compared with ABV (%)

Adverse reaction	Liposomal daunorubicin (n = 116)		ABV (n = 111)	
	Mild/Moderate	Severe	Mild/Moderate	Severe
GI				
Abdominal pain	20	3	23	4
Anorexia	21	2	26	2
Constipation	7	-	18	-
Diarrhea	34	4	29	6
Nausea	51	3	45	5
Stomatitis	9	1	8	-
Vomiting	20	3	26	2
Musculoskeletal				
Arthralgia	7	-	6	-
Back pain	16	-	8	-
Myalgia	7	-	12	-
Rigors	19	-	23	-
Respiratory				
Cough	26	2	19	-
Dyspnea	23	3	17	3
Rhinitis	12	-	6	-
Sinusitis	8	-	5	1
Miscellaneous				
Abnormal vision	3	2	3	-
Allergic reaction	21	3	19	2
Chest pain	9	1	7	-
Edema	9	2	8	1
Fever	42	5	49	5
Influenza-like symptoms	5	-	5	-
Sweating, increased	12	2	12	-
Tenesmus	4	1	1	-

Summary of Important Safety Data (Liposomal Daunorubicin vs ABV)

	Daunorubicin citrate liposomal (n = 116)	ABV (n = 111)
Neutropenia (less than 1000 cells/mm^3)	36%	35%
Neutropenia (less than 500 cells/mm^3)	15%	5%
Opportunistic infections/illnesses	40%	27%
Median time to first opportunistic infections/illnesses	214 days	412 days[2]
Number of cases with absolute reduction in ejection fraction of 20% to 25%	3	1

Summary of Important Safety Data (Liposomal Daunorubicin vs ABV)

	Daunorubicin citrate liposomal (n = 116)	ABV (n = 111)
Number of cases removed from therapy because of cardiac causes[1]	2	0
Alopecia (all grades)	8%	36%[3]
Neuropathy (all grades)	13%	41%[3]

[1] The denominator is uncertain because there were several instances of missing repeat cardiac evaluations.
[2] $P = 0.21$.
[3] $P < 0.001$.

➤*Other adverse events (5% or less):*

Cardiovascular – Angina pectoris; atrial fibrillation; cardiac arrest; hot flushes; hypertension; myocardial infarction; palpitation; pericardial effusion; pericardial tamponade; pulmonary hypertension; sinus tachycardia; supraventricular tachycardia; syncope; tachycardia; ventricular extrasystoles.

CNS – Abnormal gait; abnormal thinking; amnesia; anxiety; ataxia; confusion; convulsions; emotional lability; hallucinations; hyperkinesia; hypertonia; meningitis; somnolence; tremors.

Dermatologic – Dry skin; folliculitis; seborrhea.

GI – Dry mouth; dysphagia; gastritis; GI hemorrhage; gingival bleeding; hemorrhoids; hepatomegaly; increased appetite; melena; tooth caries.

GU – Dysuria; nocturia; polyuria.

Respiratory – Hemoptysis; hiccups; increased sputum; pulmonary infiltration.

Special senses – Conjunctivitis; deafness; earache; eye pain; taste perversion; tinnitus.

Miscellaneous – Dehydration; injection-site inflammation; lymphadenopathy; splenomegaly; thirst.

Overdosage

Symptoms of acute overdosage are increased severities of the observed dose-limiting toxicities of therapeutic doses, myelosuppression (especially granulocytopenia), fatigue, nausea, and vomiting.

Patient Information

Advise patients that this medicine will be prepared and administered by a health care provider in a medical setting.

Advise patients that lab tests will be required to monitor therapy. Instruct patients to be sure to keep appointments.

Advise patients not to take any over-the-counter or prescription medications or dietary supplements without talking with their health care provider.

Advise patients to avoid becoming pregnant during therapy.

DOXORUBICIN, CONVENTIONAL

Rx	Doxorubicin HCl (Bedford Labs)	**Powder for Injection (lyophilized):** 10 mg	50 mg lactose. In single-dose flip-top vials.
Rx	Adriamycin RDF (Pharmacia & Upjohn)		In single-dose vials.[2] *Rapid dissolution formula.*
Rx	Doxorubicin HCl (Bedford Labs)	**Powder for Injection (lyophilized):** 20 mg	100 mg lactose. In single-dose flip-top vials.
Rx	Adriamycin RDF (Pharmacia & Upjohn)		In single-dose vials.[2] *Rapid dissolution formula.*
Rx	Doxorubicin HCl (Bedford Labs)	**Powder for Injection (lyophilized):** 50 mg	250 mg lactose. In single-dose flip-top vials.
Rx	Adriamycin RDF (Pharmacia & Upjohn)		In single-dose vials.[2] *Rapid dissolution formula.*
Rx	Adriamycin RDF (Pharmacia & Upjohn)	**Powder for Injection (lyophilized):** 150 mg[1]	In single-dose vials.[2] *Rapid dissolution formula.*
Rx	Doxorubicin HCl (Bedford Labs)	**Injection, aqueous:** 2 mg/ml	0.9% NaCl, hydrochloric acid. In 5, 10, 25, and 100 ml vials.
Rx	Adriamycin PFS (Pharmacia & Upjohn)	**Injection:** 2 mg/ml	Preservative-free. In 5, 10, 25, and 37.5 ml single-dose vials and 100 ml multi-dose vials.

[1] Multiple-dose vial.

[2] With methylparaben and 50, 100, 250, and 750 mg lactose, respectively.

Note: The following monograph pertains to the conventional form of doxorubicin only. For complete prescribing information for the liposomal form of doxorubicin, refer to the Doxorubicin, Liposomal monograph.

DOXORUBICIN, CONVENTIONAL

WARNING

Severe local tissue necrosis will result if extravasation occurs. Do not give IM or SC.

Myocardial toxicity manifested in its most severe form by potentially fatal CHF may occur either during therapy or months to years after termination of therapy. The risk of developing CHF increases rapidly with increasing total cumulative doses of doxorubicin in excess of 450 mg/m². This toxicity may occur at lower cumulative doses in patients with prior mediastinal irradiation or on concurrent cyclophosphamide therapy or with preexisting heart disease. Pediatric patients are at increased risk for developing delayed cardiotoxicity.

Reduce dosage in patients with impaired hepatic function (see Administration and Dosage).

Severe myelosuppression may occur.

Administer doxorubicin only under the supervision of a physician who is experienced in the use of cancer chemotherapeutic agents.

Indications

➤*Disseminated neoplastic conditions:* To produce regression in disseminated neoplastic conditions such as the following: Acute lymphoblastic leukemia, acute myeloblastic leukemia, Wilms' tumor, neuroblastoma, soft tissue and bone sarcomas, breast carcinoma, ovarian carcinoma, transitional cell bladder carcinoma, thyroid carcinoma, Hodgkin's and non-Hodgkin's lymphomas, bronchogenic carcinoma (the small-cell histologic type is the most responsive), and gastric carcinoma.

Administration and Dosage

➤*Approved by the FDA:* May 20, 1985.

For IV use only.

With IV administration of doxorubicin, extravasation may occur with or without an accompanying burning or stinging sensation, even if blood returns well on aspiration of the infusion needle. If any signs or symptoms of extravasation have occurred, immediately terminate the injection or infusion and restart in another vein. If extravasation is suspected, intermittent application of ice to the site for 15 minutes 4 times/day x 3 days may be helpful. The benefit of local administration of drugs has not been clearly established. Because of the progressive nature of extravasation reactions, close observation and plastic surgery consultation is recommended. Blistering, ulceration, and persistent pain are indications for wide excision surgery, followed by split-thickness skin grafting.

➤*Recommended dosage schedule:* 60 to 75 mg/m² as a single IV injection administered at 21-day intervals. Give the lower dose to patients with inadequate marrow reserves because of old age, prior therapy, or neoplastic marrow infiltration.

➤*Dosage in patients with elevated bilirubin:* Serum bilirubin 1.2 to 3 mg/dl, reduce the normal dose by 50%; 3.1 to 5 mg/dl, reduce the normal dose by 75%.

➤*IV infusion:* Administer slowly into the tubing of a freely running IV infusion of NaCl Injection or 5% Dextrose Injection. Attach the tubing to a butterfly needle inserted into a large vein. Avoid veins over joints or in extremities with compromised venous or lymphatic drainage. Rate depends on size of vein and dosage; however, administer in not less than 3 to 5 minutes. Local erythematous streaking along the vein as well as facial flushing may indicate too rapid administration.

Extravasation – A burning or stinging sensation may indicate perivenous infiltration. Immediately terminate the infusion and restart in another vein; perivenous infiltration may occur painlessly (see Warnings).

➤*Preparation / Storage of solution:*

Conventional doxorubicin – Dilute the 10 mg vial with 5 ml, the 20 mg vial with 10 ml, the 50 mg vial with 25 ml, and the 150 mg vial with 75 ml of 0.9% NaCl for a final concentration of 2 mg/ml. Bacteriostatic diluents are not recommended.

➤*IV compatibilities / incompatibilities:* Incompatible with heparin, fluorouracil, cephalothin, and dexamethasone sodium phosphate; a precipitate will form. A color change in doxorubicin from red to blue-purple, which denotes decomposition, occurs with aminophylline and 5-fluorouracil. Until specific data are available, do not mix doxorubicin with other drugs. One study reported that a solution of doxorubicin and vinblastine in 0.9% Sodium Chloride is compatible and relatively stable for ≥ 5 days.

➤*Storage / Stability:* After adding the diluent, shake the vial and allow the contents to dissolve. The reconstituted solution is stable for 7 days at room temperature and under normal room light (100 footcandles) and 15 days under refrigeration (2° to 8°C; 36° to 46°F). Protect from sunlight. Discard any of the unused solution from the 10, 20, and 50 mg single-dose vials. Discard unused solutions of the multiple-dose vial remaining beyond the recommended storage times.

Actions

➤*Pharmacology:* Doxorubicin is a cytotoxic anthracycline antibiotic isolated from cultures of *Streptomyces peucetius* var. *caesius*. The cytotoxic effect of doxorubicin on malignant cells and its toxic effects on various organs are thought to be related to nucleotide base intercalation and cell membrane lipid-binding activities of doxorubicin. Intercalation inhibits nucleotide replication and action of DNA and RNA polymerases. The interaction of doxorubicin with topoisomerase II to form DNA-cleavable complexes appears to be an important mechanism of doxorubicin cytocidal activity. Doxorubicin cellular membrane binding may affect a variety of cellular functions. Enzymatic electron reduction of doxorubicin by a variety of oxidases, reductases, and dehydrogenases generate highly reactive species including the hydroxyl free radical OH•. Free radical formation has been implicated in doxorubicin cardiotoxicity by means of CU (II) and Fe (III) reduction at the cellular level. Cells treated with doxorubicin have been shown to manifest the characteristic morphologic changes associated with apoptosis or programmed cell death. Doxorubicin-induced apoptosis may be an integral component of the cellular mechanism of action relating to therapeutic effects, toxicities, or both.

➤*Pharmacokinetics:*

Absorption / Distribution – The drug is rapidly distributed in body tissues with ≈ 75% binding to plasma proteins, principally albumin. In the blood, the free doxorubicin fraction is dependent on the patient's hematocrit, with greater free drug available in patients with a reduced hematocrit. Also, drug levels in various tissues are roughly proportional to the DNA content of the specific tissue. The volume of distribution is ≈ 28 L/kg. Human tissues with high drug concentrations include: Liver, lymph nodes, muscle, bone marrow, fat, and skin. The drug does not distribute into the CNS system and experimental efforts to increase CNS uptake by osmotic disruption produced significant neurotoxicity.

Metabolism / Excretion – Plasma disappearance follows a triphasic pattern with mean half-lives of ≈ 12 minutes, 3.3 hours, and ≈ 30 to 40 hours. Doxorubicin binding to DNA is believed to explain the prolonged terminal half-life. Doxorubicin is metabolized by carbonyl reduction to the active alcohol, doxorubicinol, and inactive aglycones. Other inactive metabolites have been identified in urine and bile.

Liver function impairment, as reflected by elevated serum bilirubin, results in slower excretion and increased retention and accumulation of drug and metabolites in plasma and tissues. Other liver function abnormalities are not predictive. Urinary excretion accounts for ≈ 4% to 5% of the dose in 5 days. Biliary excretion is the major excretion route; 40% to 50% is recovered in bile or feces in 7 days.

Contraindications

Do not initiate therapy in patients with marked myelosuppression induced by previous treatment with other antitumor agents or by radiotherapy.

A history of hypersensitivity reactions to conventional or liposomal doxorubicin or their components.

Previous treatment with complete cumulative doses of doxorubicin, daunorubicin, idarubicin, or other anthracyclines and anthracenes.

Warnings

➤*Non-responsive neoplastic conditions:* Malignant melanoma, kidney carcinoma, large bowel carcinoma, brain tumors, and metastases to the CNS are not significantly responsive to doxorubicin therapy.

➤*Myelosuppression:* The most common dose-limiting toxicity in the short term is myelosuppression. It is primarily of leukocytes and requires careful monitoring. With the recommended dosage schedule, leukopenia is usually transient, reaching its nadir 10 to 14 days after treatment, with recovery usually by the 21st day. Expect white blood cell counts as low as 1000/mm³ during treatment. Hematologic toxicity may require dose reduction, suspension, or delay of therapy. Persistent, severe myelosuppression may result in superinfection or hemorrhage.

➤*Necrotizing colitis:* Necrotizing colitis manifested by typhlitis (cecal inflammation), bloody stools, and severe and sometimes fatal infections have occurred with doxorubicin given by IV push daily for 3 days with cytarabine continuous infusion daily for ≥ 7 days.

➤*Cardiac toxicity:* Cardiac toxicity must be given special attention. Irreversible myocardial toxicity, manifested in its most severe form by life-threatening or fatal CHF, may occur either during therapy or months to years after termination of therapy. Although uncommon, acute left ventricular failure has occurred, particularly in patients who have received total dosage exceeding the recommended limit of 550 mg/m². Dose-related incidences range from ≤ 2% at total doses of 300 mg/m², 3% to 5% at total dose of 400 mg/m², 5% to 8% at a total dose of 450 mg/m², and 6% to 20% at a dose of 500 mg/m² given at a schedule of a bolus injection once every 3 weeks. This limit appears to be lower (400 mg/m²) in patients who received radiotherapy to the mediastinal area. Take into account the total dose of drug of any previous or concomitant therapy with other potentially cardiotoxic agents such as cyclophosphamide or daunorubicin. Cardiomyopathy or CHF may occur several weeks after drug discontinuation and is often unresponsive to

DOXORUBICIN, CONVENTIONAL

medical or physical therapy.

The elderly, very young, and those with preexisting hypertension or cardiac disease are at increased risk for cardiac toxicity.

Early diagnosis of drug-induced heart failure is essential for successful treatment with digitalis, diuretics, after load reducers such as angiotensin I converting enzyme (ACE) inhibitors, low-salt diet, and bed rest. Severe cardiac toxicity may occur precipitously without antecedent ECG changes. A baseline cardiac evaluation with an ECG, left ventricular ejection fraction (LVEF), and an echocardiogram (ECHO) or multigated radionuclide scans (MUGA) is recommended, especially in patients with risk factors for increased cardiac toxicity (preexisting heart disease, mediastinal irradiation, or concurrent cyclophosphamide therapy). Obtain subsequent evaluation at a cumulative dose of doxorubicin of ≥ 400 mg/m^2 and periodically thereafter during the course of therapy. Pediatric patients are at increased risk for developing delayed cardiotoxicity following doxorubicin administration; therefore, a follow-up cardiac evaluation is recommended periodically to monitor for this delayed cardiotoxicity.

Transient ECG changes (eg, T-wave flattening, ST depression, arrhythmias) lasting up to 2 weeks after a dose are not indications for therapy suspension. Doxorubicin cardiomyopathy is associated with persistent reduction in voltage of the QRS wave, prolongation of the systolic time interval, and reduction of ejection fraction. None of these tests have consistently identified patients approaching their maximally tolerated cumulative dose. If test results indicate cardiac function change, carefully evaluate benefit of continued therapy against risk of producing irreversible cardiac damage. In adults, a 10% decline in LVEF to below the lower limit of normal or an absolute LVEF of 45%, or a 20% decline in LVEF at any level is indicative of deterioration in cardiac function. In pediatric patients, deterioration in cardiac function during or after the completion of therapy with doxorubicin is indicated by a drop in fractional shortening (FS) by an absolute value of ≥ 10 percentile units or $< 29\%$, and a decline in LVEF of 10 percentile units or an LVEF $\leq 55\%$. In general, if test results indicate deterioration in cardiac function associated with doxorubicin, weigh the benefit of continued therapy against the risk of producing irreversible cardiac damage. Acute life-threatening arrhythmias occurred during or within a few hours of use. Preliminary evidence suggests cardiotoxicity may be reduced and total dosage safely increased by giving the drug on a weekly schedule or as a prolonged (48 to 96 hours) continuous infusion.

Dexrazoxane, a cardioprotective agent, may be effective in preventing doxorubicin-induced cardiotoxicity (see individual monograph).

➤*Extravasation:* Extravasation at injection site with or without a stinging or burning sensation may occur, even if blood returns well on aspiration of the infusion needle. If any signs of extravasation occur, terminate the infusion immediately and restart in another vein. For management, see the Antineoplastic Introduction.

The application of ice over the site of extravasation for ≈ 30 minutes may be helpful in alleviating the local reaction. Do not give IM or SC.

➤*Infusion reactions:* Infusion reactions appear to occur with the first infusion and do not appear to occur with later infusions if not present initially. In most patients, these reactions resolve over the course of several hours to a day once the infusion is terminated. In some patients, the reaction resolves by slowing the rate of infusion.

➤*Mucositis:* Mucositis may occur 5 to 10 days after administration, leading to ulceration, and represent a site or origin for severe infections. Incidence and severity of mucositis is greater with the 3 successive daily dosage regimen. Ulceration and necrosis of the colon, especially the cecum, may occur leading to bleeding or severe infections that can be fatal. This reaction has occurred in patients with acute nonlymphocytic leukemia treated with 3 days of doxorubicin plus cytarabine.

➤*Hepatic function impairment:* Doxorubicin is excreted primarily via the hepatobiliary route and toxicity is enhanced by hepatic impairment. Prior to dosing, evaluate hepatic function using clinical laboratory tests such as AST, ALT, alkaline phosphatase, and bilirubin.

➤*Carcinogenesis:* Doxorubicin and related compounds have mutagenic and carcinogenic properties in experimental models.

➤*Pregnancy: Category D.* Safety for use during pregnancy is not established. Use only when the potential benefits outweigh the potential hazards to the fetus. Doxorubicin is embryotoxic and teratogenic in rats and embryotoxic and abortifacient in rabbits. Doxorubicin has been given during pregnancy without adverse fetal effect and has been detected in fetal tissue; however, its effect on the human fetus is unknown.

➤*Lactation:* Doxorubicin was excreted in the milk of 1 lactating patient, with peak milk concentration at 24 hours after treatment being ≈ 4.4-fold greater than the corresponding plasma concentration. Doxorubicin was detectable in the milk up to 72 hours after therapy with 70 mg/m^2 of doxorubicin given as a 15-minute IV infusion and 100 mg/m^2 of cisplatin as a 26-hour IV infusion. The peak concentration of doxorubicinol in milk at 24 hours was 0.2 mcM and AUC up to 24 hours was 16.5 mcM/hr while the AUC for doxorubicin was 9.9 mcM/hr. Because of the potential for serious adverse reactions in nursing infants from doxorubicin, mothers should be advised to discontinue nursing during doxorubicin therapy.

➤*Children:* Pediatric patients are at increased risk for developing delayed cardiotoxicity. Perform follow-up cardiac evaluations periodically to monitor for this delayed cardiotoxicity (see Warnings). The risk of CHF and other acute manifestations of doxorubicin cardiotoxicity in pediatric patients may be as much or lower than in adults. Pediatric patients appear to be at particular risk for developing delayed cardiac toxicity in that doxorubicin-induced cardiomyopathy impairs myocardial growth as pediatric patients mature, subsequently leading to possible development of CHF during early adulthood. As many as 40% of pediatric patients may have subclinical cardiac dysfunction and 5% to 10% of pediatric patients may develop CHF on long-term follow-up. This late cardiac toxicity may be related to the dose of doxorubicin. The longer the length of follow-up the greater the increase in the detection rate. Doxorubicin, as a component of intensive chemotherapy regimens administered to pediatric patients, may contribute to prepubertal growth failure. It may also contribute to gonadal impairment, which is usually temporary.

Precautions

➤*Monitoring:* Initial treatment requires close patient observation and extensive laboratory monitoring. Hospitalize patients at least during the first phase of treatment. Initial treatment with doxorubicin requires observation of the patient and periodic monitoring of complete blood counts, hepatic function tests, and radionuclide left ventricular ejection fraction (see Warnings).

➤*Hyperuricemia:* Hyperuricemia may be induced by doxorubicin secondary to rapid lysis of neoplastic cells (tumor-lysis syndrome). Monitor patient's blood uric acid level.

➤*Urine discoloration:* Doxorubicin imparts a red color to the urine for 1 to 2 days after administration; advise patients to expect this during active therapy.

➤*Live vaccines:* Administration of live vaccines to immunosuppressed patients including those undergoing cytotoxic chemotherapy may be hazardous.

Drug Interactions

Doxorubicin Drug Interactions			
Precipitant drug	Object drug*		Description
Cyclosporine	Doxorubicin	↑	The addition of cyclosporine to doxorubicin may result in increases in AUC for doxorubicin and doxorubicinol possibly because of a decrease in clearance of parent drug and a decrease in metabolism of doxorubicinol. Literature reports suggest that adding cyclosporine to doxorubicin results in more profound and prolonged hemotologic toxicity than doxorubicin alone. Coma or seizures have also been described.
Paclitaxel	Doxorubicin	↑	Two published studies report that initial administration of paclitaxel infused over 24 hours followed by doxorubicin administered over 48 hours resulted in a significant decrease in doxorubicin clearance with more profound neutropenic and stomatitis episodes than the reverse sequence of administration.
Phenobarbital	Doxorubicin	↓	Phenobarbital increases doxorubicin elimination.
Progesterone	Doxorubicin	↑	In a published study, progesterone was given IV to patients with advanced malignancies (ECOG PS < 2) at high doses (up to 10 g over 24 hours) concomitantly with a fixed doxorubicin dose (60 mg/m^2) via bolus. Enhanced doxorubicin-induced neutropenia and thrombocytopenia were observed.
Streptozocin	Doxorubicin	↑	Streptozocin may inhibit hepatic metabolism of doxorubicin.
Verapamil	Doxorubicin	↑	A study of the effects of verapamil on the acute toxicity of doxorubicin in mice revealed higher initial peak concentrations of doxorubicin in the heart with a higher incidence and severity of degenerative changes in cardiac tissue resulting in shorter survival.

DOXORUBICIN, CONVENTIONAL

Doxorubicin Drug Interactions			
Precipitant drug	Object drug*		Description
Doxorubicin	Actinomycin-D	↑	Pediatric patients receiving concomitant doxorubicin and actinomycin-D have manifested acute "recall" pneumonitis at variable times after local radiation therapy.
Doxorubicin	Cyclophosphamide Mercaptopurine	↑	Exacerbation of cyclophosphamide-induced hemorrhagic cystitis and enhancement of 6-mercaptopurine have occurred.
Doxorubicin	Digoxin	↓	Serum levels may be decreased by combination chemotherapy (including doxorubicin). Digitoxin and digoxin capsules do not appear to be affected.
Doxorubicin	Phenytoin	↓	Phenytoin levels may be decreased by doxorubicin.
Doxorubicin	Radiation		Radiation-induced toxicity to the myocardium, mucosa, skin, and liver have been increased by doxorubicin administration.

* ↑ = Object drug increased. ↓ = Object drug decreased.

Adverse Reactions

➤*Cardiovascular:* Myocardial toxicity manifested in its most severe form by potentially fatal CHF may occur either during therapy or months to years after termination of doxorubicin therapy (see Warning Box and Warnings).

➤*CNS:* Peripheral neurotoxicity in the form of local-regional sensory or motor disturbances have been reported in patients treated intra-arterially with doxorubicin mostly in combination with cisplatin. Seizures were reported in 1 patient receiving a very high dose of doxorubicin (2 to 3 times the approved dosage) in combination with high-dose cyclophosphamide.

DOXORUBICIN, LIPOSOMAL

Rx	**Doxil** (Sequus)	**Injection:** 20 mg (liposomal)	Sucrose. In 10 ml single-use vials.

Note: The following monograph pertains to the liposomal form of doxorubicin only. For conventional prescribing information, refer to the Doxorubicin, Conventional monograph.

WARNING

Serious irreversible myocardial toxicity with delayed CHF often unresponsive to supportive therapy may occur as total dosage of liposomal doxorubicin approaches 550 mg/m^2. Prior use of other anthracyclines or anthracenediones will reduce the total dose of doxorubicin HCl that can be given without cardiac toxicity. Cardiac toxicity also may occur at lower cumulative doses in patients with prior mediastinal irradiation or who are receiving concurrent cyclophosphamide therapy.

Administer liposomal doxorubicin to patients with a history of cardiovascular disease only when the benefit outweighs the risk to the patient.

Accidental substitution of liposomal doxorubicin for conventional doxorubicin has resulted in severe side effects. Liposomal doxorubicin exhibits unique pharmacokinetic properties compared with conventional doxorubicin. **Do not substitute** on a mg per mg basis.

Administer liposomal doxorubicin only under the supervision of a physician who is experienced in the use of cancer chemotherapeutic agents.

Acute infusion-associated reactions (flushing, shortness of breath, facial swelling, headache, chills, back pain, tightness in the chest or throat, and hypotension) have occurred in ≈ 7% of patients treated with liposomal doxorubicin. In most patients, these reactions resolve over the course of several hours to a day once the infusion is terminated. In some patients, the reaction resolves by slowing the infusion rate.

Reduce dosage in patients with impaired hepatic function (see Administration and Dosage).

Severe myelosuppression may occur.

Indications

➤*Kaposi's sarcoma (KS):* Treatment of AIDS-related KS in patients with disease that has progressed on prior combination chemotherapy or in patients who are intolerant to such therapy.

Administration and Dosage

➤*Approved by the FDA:* November 17, 1995.

➤*Dermatologic:* Reversible complete alopecia, hyperpigmentation of nailbeds and dermal creases (primarily in children), onycholysis, recall of skin reaction due to prior radiotherapy.

➤*GI:* Acute nausea and vomiting may be severe and may be alleviated by antiemetic therapy. Mucositis (stomatitis and esophagitis; see Warnings); anorexia, diarrhea (occasionally).

➤*Hematologic:* The occurrence of secondary acute myeloid leukemia with or without a preleukemic phase has been reported rarely in patients concurrently treated with doxorubicin in association with DNA-damaging antineoplastic agents. Such cases could have a short (1 to 3 years) latency period. Pediatric patients are also at risk of developing secondary acute myeloid leukemia.

➤*Hypersensitivity:* Fever, chills, urticaria, anaphylaxis, lincomycin cross-sensitivity.

➤*Local:* Severe cellulitis, vesication, and tissue necrosis occur if drug is extravasated (see Warnings). Erythematous streaking along the vein next to the injection site has occurred.

➤*Ophthalmic:* Conjunctivitis and lacrimation (rare).

➤*Miscellaneous:*

Infection – Opportunistic infections occurred in 50.4% of patients, most commonly candidiasis (23.5%), cytomegalovirus (20.1%), herpes simplex (10.5%), Pneumocystis carinii pneumonia (9.2%), and mycobacterium avium (8.4%).

Vascular – Phlebosclerosis, especially when small veins or a single vein is used for repeated administration; facial flushing may occur if injection is too rapid.

Overdosage

Acute overdosage enhances the toxic effects of mucositis, leukopenia, pancytopenia, and thrombocytopenia. Treat the severely myelosuppressed patient with hospitalization, antibiotics, platelet transfusions, and symptomatic treatment of mucositis. Consider the use of hemopoietic growth factor (G-CSF, GM-CSF).

Chronic overdosage with cumulative doses > 550 mg/m^2 increases the risk of cardiomyopathy and resultant CHF. Vigorously manage CHF with digitalis preparations and diuretics. Use of afterload reducers such as ace inhibitors is recommended.

➤*Recommended dosage schedule:* Administer IV at a dose of 20 mg/m^2 (conventional doxorubicin equivalent) over 30 minutes, once every 3 weeks, for as long as the patient responds satisfactorily and tolerates treatment.

Do not administer as a bolus injection or an undiluted solution. Rapid infusion may increase the risk of infusion-related reactions.

➤*Alternative dose schedules:*

Liposomal Doxorubicin Dosing in Palmar-Plantar Erythrodysesthesia			
Toxicity grade	Symptoms	Weeks since last dose	
		3	4
0	No symptoms	Redose at 3-week interval	Redose at 3-week interval
1	Mild erythema, swelling, or desquamation not interfering with daily activities	Redose unless patient has experienced a previous grade 3 or 4 skin toxicity, in which case, wait an additional week.	Redose at 25% dose reduction; return to 3-week interval.
2	Erythema, desquamation, or swelling interfering with, but not precluding, normal physical activities; small blisters or ulcerations < 2 cm in diameter	Wait an additional week.	Redose at 50% dose reduction; return to 3-week interval.
3	Blistering, ulceration, or swelling interfering with walking or normal daily activities; cannot wear regular clothing	Wait an additional week.	Discontinue liposomal doxorubicin.
4	Diffuse or local process causing infectious complications, or a bedridden state or hospitalization		

DOXORUBICIN, LIPOSOMAL

Liposomal Doxorubicin Dosing in Hematological Toxicity			
Grade	ANC (cells/mm^3)	Platelets (cells/mm^3)	Modification
1	1500-1900	75,000-150,000	None
2	1000-< 1500	50,000-< 75,000	None
3	500-999	25,000-< 50,000	Wait until ANC is ≥ 1000 or platelets are ≥ 50,000, then redose at 25% dose reduction.
4	< 500	< 25,000	Wait until ANC is ≥ 1000 or platelets are ≥ 50,000, then redose at 50% dose reduction.

Liposomal Doxorubicin Dosing in Stomatitis		
Grade	Symptoms	Modification
1	Painless ulcers, erythema, or mild soreness	None
2	Painful erythema, edema, or ulcers, but can eat	Wait 1 week, and if symptoms improve, redose at 100% dose.
3	Painful erythema, edema, or ulcers, and cannot eat	Wait 1 week, and if symptoms improve, redose at 25% dose reduction.
4	Requires parenteral or enteral support	Wait 1 week, and if symptoms improve, redose at 50% dose reduction.

➤ *Patients with impaired hepatic function:* Limited clinical experience exists in treating hepatically impaired patients with liposomal doxorubicin. Therefore, based on experience with conventional doxorubicin, it is recommended that liposomal doxorubicin dosage be reduced if the bilirubin is elevated as follows: Serum bilirubin 1.2 to 3 mg/dl, give 50% of the normal dose; > 3 mg/dl, give 25% of the normal dose.

➤ *Preparation / Storage of solution:* Dilute the appropriate dose of liposomal doxorubicin, up to a maximum of 90 mg, in 250 ml of 5% Dextrose Injection, USP, prior to administration. Do not use with in-line filters.

➤ *IV compatibilities / incompatibilities:* Do not mix with other drugs. Do not use with any diluent other than 5% Dextrose Injection. Do not use any bacteriostatic agent, such as benzyl alcohol. Liposomal doxorubicin is not a clear solution but a translucent, red liposomal dispersion.

➤ *Storage / Stability:* Refrigerate diluted liposomal doxorubicin at 2° to 8°C (36° to 46°F), and administer within 24 hours. Avoid freezing. Prolonged freezing may adversely affect liposomal drug products; however, short-term freezing (< 1 month) does not appear to have a deleterious effect on liposomal doxorubicin.

Actions

➤ *Pharmacology:* Doxorubicin is a cytotoxic anthracycline antibiotic isolated from cultures of *Streptomyces peucetius* var. *caesius*. Liposomal doxorubicin is encapsulated in long-circulating liposomes. Liposomes are microscopic vesicles composed of a phospholipid bilayer that are capable of encapsulating active drugs. The liposomes of liposomal doxorubicin are formulated with surface-bound methoxypolyethylene glycol (MPEG), a process often referred to as pegylation, to protect liposomes from detection by the mononuclear phagocyte system (MPS) and to increase blood circulation time.

The liposomes have a half-life of ≈ 55 hours in humans. They are stable in blood, and direct measurement of liposomal doxorubicin shows that ≥ 90% of the drug (the assay used cannot quantify < 5% to 10% free doxorubicin) remains liposome-encapsulated during circulation.

It is hypothesized that because of their small size (ca. 100 nm) and persistence in the circulation to pegylated doxorubicin, liposomes are able to penetrate the altered and often compromised vasculature of tumors. This hypothesis is supported by studies using colloidal gold-containing liposomes, which can be visualized microscopically. Evidence of penetration of the liposomes from blood vessels and their entry and accumulation in tumors have been seen in mice with C-26 colon carcinoma tumors and in transgenic mice with Kaposi's sarcoma-like lesions. Once the liposomes distribute to the tissue compartment, the encapsulated doxorubicin becomes available. The exact mechanism of release is not understood.

Liposomal encapsulation can substantially affect a drug's functional properties relative to those of the unencapsulated drug. In addition, different liposomal products with a common active ingredient may vary from one another in the chemical composition and physical form. Such differences may affect functional properties of these drug products.

➤ *Pharmacokinetics:*
Absorption / Distribution – In contrast to original doxorubicin, the steady-state volume of distribution of liposomal doxorubicin indicates that it is confined mostly to the vascular fluid volume. Plasma protein binding has not been determined.

Metabolism / Excretion – Doxorubicinol, the major metabolite of doxorubicin, was detected at very low levels (range, 0.8 to 26.2 ng/ml) in the plasma of patients who received 10 or 20 mg/m^2 liposomal doxorubicin.

The plasma clearance of liposomal doxorubicin was slow, with a mean clearance value of 0.041 L/hr/m^2. This is in contrast to original doxorubicin.

Because of its slower clearance, the area under the curve (AUC) of liposomal doxorubicin, primarily representing the circulation of liposome-encapsulated doxorubicin, is ≈ 2 to 3 orders of magnitude larger than the AUC for a similar dose of conventional doxorubicin as reported. The plasma pharmacokinetics of liposomal doxorubicin were evaluated in 42 patients with AIDS-related KS who received single doses of 10 or 20 mg/m^2 administered by a 30-minute infusion. Twenty-three of these patients received single doses of both 10 and 20 mg/m^2 with a 3-week wash-out period between doses. The pharmacokinetic parameter values of liposomal doxorubicin, given for total doxorubicin (most liposomally bound), are presented in the following table.

Pharmacokinetic Parameters of Liposomal HCl Doxorubicin in AIDS Patients with Kaposi's Sarcoma[1]		
	Dose	
Parameter (units)	10 mg/m^2	20 mg/m^2
Peak plasma concentration (mcg/ml)	4.12	8.34
Plasma clearance (L/hr/m^2)	0.056	0.041
Steady-state volume of distribution (L/m^2)	2.83	2.72
AUC (mcg/ml•hr)	277	590
First phase (λ_1) half-life (hr)	4.7	5.2
Second phase (λ_2) half-life (hr)	52.3	55

[1] n = 23

Liposomal doxorubicin displayed linear pharmacokinetics. Disposition occurred in 2 phases after liposomal doxorubicin administration, with a relatively short first phase (≈ 5 hours) and a prolonged second phase (≈ 55 hours) that accounted for the majority of the AUC.

Contraindications

A history of hypersensitivity reactions to conventional or liposomal doxorubicin or their components.

Warnings

➤ *Myelosuppression:* The majority of experience with liposomal doxorubicin has been in AIDS-KS patients who present with baseline myelosuppression because of such factors as their HIV disease or numerous concomitant medications. In this population, myelosuppression appears to be the dose-limiting adverse event. Leukopenia is the most common adverse event (≈ 60%) experienced in this population; anemia (≈ 20%) and thrombocytopenia (≈ 10%) can also be expected.

Because of the potential for bone marrow suppression, monitor white blood cell and platelet counts and Hgb/Hct. With the recommended dosage schedule, leukopenia is usually transient. Hematologic toxicity may require dose reduction or suspension or delay of liposomal doxorubicin therapy. Persistent severe myelosuppression may result in superinfection or hemorrhage.

Patients treated with liposomal doxorubicin may require G-CSF (or GM-CSF) to support their blood counts (see Adverse Reactions).

➤ *Cardiac toxicity:* Experience with liposomal doxorubicin is limited in evaluating cardiac risk. Therefore, observe warnings related to the use of conventional doxorubicin. The long-term cardiac effects of liposomal doxorubicin in patients relative to the conventional doxorubicin have not been adequately evaluated.

Give special attention to cardiac toxicity. Although uncommon, acute left ventricular failure has occurred, particularly in patients who have received total dosage exceeding the recommended limit of 550 mg/m^2. This limit appears to be lower (400 mg/m^2) in patients who received radiotherapy to the mediastinal area. Take into account the total dose of drug of any previous or concomitant therapy with other potentially cardiotoxic agents such as cyclophosphamide or daunorubicin. Cardiomyopathy or CHF may occur several weeks after drug discontinuation and is often unresponsive to medical or physical therapy.

Early diagnosis of drug-induced heart failure is essential for successful treatment with digitalis, diuretics, after load reducers such as angiotensin I converting enzyme (ACE) inhibitors, low-salt diet, and bed rest. Severe cardiac toxicity may occur precipitously without antecedent ECG changes. A baseline cardiac evaluation with an ECG, left ventricular ejection fraction (LVEF), and an echocardiogram (ECHO) or

DOXORUBICIN, LIPOSOMAL

multigated radionuclide (MUGA) scans, is recommended especially in patients with risk factors for increased cardiac toxicity (preexisting heart disease, mediastinal irradiation, or concurrent cyclophosphamide therapy). Obtain subsequent evaluation at a cumulative dose of doxorubicin of ≥ 400 mg/m² and periodically thereafter during the course of therapy. Pediatric patients are at increased risk for developing delayed cardiotoxicity following doxorubicin administration; therefore, a follow-up cardiac evaluation is recommended periodically to monitor for this delayed cardiotoxicity.

Transient ECG changes (eg, T-wave flattening, ST depression, arrhythmias) lasting up to 2 weeks after a dose are not indications for therapy suspension. Doxorubicin cardiomyopathy is associated with persistent reduction in voltage of the QRS wave, prolongation of the systolic time interval, and reduction of ejection fraction. None of these tests have consistently identified patients approaching their maximally tolerated cumulative dose. If test results indicate cardiac function change, carefully evaluate benefit of continued therapy against risk of producing irreversible cardiac damage. In adults, a 10% decline in LVEF to below the lower limit of normal, an absolute LVEF of 45%, or a 20% decline in LVEF at any level is indicative of deterioration in cardiac function. In pediatric patients, deterioration in cardiac function during or after the completion of therapy with doxorubicin is indicated by a drop in fractional shortening (FS) by an absolute value of ≥ 10 percentile units or < 29% and a decline in LVEF of 10 percentile units or an LVEF ≤ 55%. In general, if test results indicate deterioration in cardiac function associated with doxorubicin, weigh the benefit of continued therapy against the risk of producing irreversible cardiac damage. Preliminary evidence suggests cardiotoxicity may be reduced and total dosage safely increased by giving the drug on a weekly schedule or as a prolonged (48 to 96 hours) continuous infusion.

Dexrazoxane, a cardioprotective agent, may be effective in preventing doxorubicin-induced cardiotoxicity (see individual monograph).

➤*Extravasation:* Extravasation at injection site with or without a stinging or burning sensation may occur, even if blood returns well on aspiration of the infusion needle. Consider liposomal doxorubicin an irritant. If any signs of extravasation occur, terminate the infusion immediately and restart in another vein. For management, see the Antineoplastic Introduction.

The application of ice over the site of extravasation for ≈ 30 minutes may be helpful in alleviating the local reaction. Do not give IM or SC.

➤*Infusion reactions:* Infusion reactions appear to occur with the first infusion and do not appear to occur with later infusions if not present initially. In most patients, these reactions resolve over the course of several hours to a day once the infusion is terminated. In some patients, the reaction resolves by slowing the rate of infusion. Similar reactions have not been reported with conventional doxorubicin, and they presumably represent a reaction to liposomal doxorubicin or one of its surface components.

Many patients were able to tolerate further infusions without complications; however, 6 patients were terminated from therapy because of an infusion reaction to liposomal doxorubicin.

➤*Palmar-plantar erythrodysesthesia:* Among 705 patients with AIDS-related KS treated with liposomal doxorubicin, 24 (3.4%) developed palmar-plantar skin eruptions characterized by swelling, pain, erythema, and desquamation of the skin on the hands and feet. The syndrome was generally seen after ≥ 6 weeks of treatment but may occur earlier. The incidence of this reaction may be higher when liposomal doxorubicin is administered at doses that are higher or at intervals that are shorter than those recommended. In most patients, the reaction is mild and resolves in 1 to 2 weeks so that prolonged delay of therapy need not occur. However, the reaction can be severe and debilitating in some patients and may require discontinuation of treatment.

➤*Mucositis:* Mucositis may occur 5 to 10 days after administration with doxorubicin, leading to ulceration, and represents a site or origin for severe infections.

➤*Radiation therapy:* Recall of skin reaction because of prior radiotherapy has occurred with administration of liposomal doxorubicin.

➤*Hepatic function impairment:* Doxorubicin is excreted primarily via the hepatobiliary route, and toxicity is enhanced by hepatic impairment. Prior to dosing, evaluate hepatic function using clinical laboratory tests such as AST, ALT, alkaline phosphatase, and bilirubin. Reduction of liposomal doxorubicin dose is recommended (see Administration and Dosage).

➤*Carcinogenesis:* Doxorubicin and related compounds have mutagenic and carcinogenic properties in experimental models.

➤*Pregnancy: Category D.* Safety for use during pregnancy is not established. Use only when the potential benefits outweigh the potential hazards to the fetus. Liposomal doxorubicin is embryotoxic at doses of 1 mg/kg/day (≈ 33% of the recommended human dose on a mg/m² basis) in rats. Liposomal doxorubicin is embryotoxic and abortifacient at 0.5 mg/kg/day (≈ 25% the recommended human dose on a mg/m² basis) in rabbits. Embryotoxicity was characterized by increased embryo-fetal deaths and reduced live litter sizes.

➤*Lactation:* It is not known whether liposomal doxorubicin is excreted in breast milk. Because many drugs are excreted in human milk and because of the potential for serious adverse reactions in nursing infants from liposomal doxorubicin, mothers should discontinue nursing prior to taking this drug.

➤*Children:* Safety and efficacy has not been established with liposomal doxorubicin.

Precautions

➤*Monitoring:* Initial treatment requires close patient observation and extensive laboratory monitoring. Obtain a CBC, including platelet counts, frequently and at a minimum prior to each dose.

➤*Live vaccines:* Administration of live vaccines to immunosuppressed patients including those undergoing cytotoxic chemotherapy may be hazardous.

Drug Interactions

Liposomal doxorubicin may interact with drugs known to interact with conventional doxorubicin.

Conventional Doxorubicin Drug Interactions			
Precipitant drug	Object drug*		Description
Cyclosporine	Doxorubicin	↑	The addition of cyclosporine to doxorubicin may result in increases in AUC for both doxorubicin and doxorubicinol, possibly because of a decrease in clearance of parent drug and a decrease in metabolism of doxorubicinol. Literature reports suggest that adding cyclosporine to doxorubicin results in more profound and prolonged hemotologic toxicity than doxorubicin alone. Coma or seizures have also been described.
Paclitaxel	Doxorubicin	↑	Two published studies report that initial administration of paclitaxel infused over 24 hours followed by doxorubicin administered over 48 hours resulted in a significant decrease in doxorubicin clearance with more profound neutropenic and stomatitis episodes than the reverse sequence of administration.
Phenobarbital	Doxorubicin	↓	Phenobarbital increases doxorubicin elimination.
Progesterone	Doxorubicin	↑	In a published study, progesterone was given IV to patients with advanced malignancies (ECOG PS < 2) at high doses (up to 10 g over 24 hours) concomitantly with a fixed doxorubicin dose (60 mg/m²) via bolus. Enhanced doxorubicin-induced neutropenia and thrombocytopenia were observed.
Streptozocin	Doxorubicin	↑	Streptozocin may inhibit hepatic metabolism of doxorubicin.
Verapamil	Doxorubicin	↑	A study of the effects of verapamil on the acute toxicity of doxorubicin in mice revealed higher initial peak concentrations of doxorubicin in the heart with a higher incidence and severity of degenerative changes in cardiac tissue resulting in a shorter survival.
Doxorubicin	Actinomycin-D	↑	Pediatric patients receiving concomitant doxorubicin and actinomycin-D have manifested acute recall pneumonitis at variable times after local radiation therapy.
Doxorubicin	Cyclophosphamide Mercaptopurine	↑	Exacerbation of cyclophosphamide-induced hemorrhagic cystitis and enhancement of 6-mercaptopurine have occurred.
Doxorubicin	Digoxin	↓	Serum levels may be decreased by combination chemotherapy (including doxorubicin). Digitoxin and digoxin capsules do not appear to affected.
Doxorubicin	Phenytoin	↓	Phenytoin levels may be decreased by doxorubicin.
Doxorubicin	Radiation	↑	Radiation-induced toxicity to the myocardium, mucosa, skin, and liver have been increased by doxorubicin administration.

*↑ = Object drug increased. ↓ = Object drug decreased.

DOXORUBICIN, LIPOSOMAL

Adverse Reactions

Eighty-three percent of the patients reported adverse events that were considered to be possibly or probably related to treatment with liposomal doxorubicin. These adverse events are provided below. Adverse reactions only infrequently (5%) led to discontinuation of treatment. Those that did so included bone marrow suppression, cardiac adverse events, infusion-related reactions, toxoplasmosis, palmar-plantar erythrodysethesia, pneumonia, cough/dyspnea, fatigue, optic neuritis, progression of a non-KS tumor, allergy to penicillin, and unspecified reasons.

Liposomal Doxorubicin Adverse Reactions (≥ 5%) (%)		
Adverse reactions	Refractory or intolerant AIDS-KS patients (n = 77)	Total AIDS-KS patients (n = 705)
Number of patients reporting adverse events	74	83.1
Alkaline phosphatase increase	1.3	7.8
Alopecia	9.1	8.9
Anemia	6.5	19.4
Asthenia	6.5	9.9
Diarrhea	5.2	7.8
Fever	7.8	9.1
Hypochromic anemia	5.2	9.8
Nausea	18.2	16.9
Neutropenia (ANC < 1000/mm³)	44.2	49.9
Oral moniliasis	1.3	5.5
Stomatitis	5.2	6.8
Thrombocytopenia	6.5	9.2
Vomiting	7.8	7.8

➤*Incidence 1% to 5% (possibly or probably related):*
Cardiovascular – Chest pain; hypotension; tachycardia.

Dermatologic – Herpes simplex; rash; itching.

GI – Mouth ulceration; glossitis; constipation; aphthous stomatitis; anorexia; dysphagia; abdominal pain.

Hematologic – Hemolysis; increased prothrombin time.

Metabolic/Nutritional – ALT increase; weight loss; hypocalcemia; hyperbilirubinemia; hyperglycemia.

Miscellaneous – Headache; back pain; infection; allergic reaction; chills; dyspnea; albuminuria; pneumonia; retinitis; emotional lability; dizziness; somnolence.

➤*Cardiovascular:* Sixty-eight (9.6%) patients experienced cardiac-related adverse events. In 30 patients (4.3%), the event was thought to be possibly or probably related to liposomal doxorubicin. Nine cases of possibly or probably related cardiomyopathy and CHF were reported. Seven (1%) of the possibly or probably related cardiac events were severe. These severe events included arrhythmia (nonspecific), cardiomyopathy, heart failure, pericardial effusion, and tachycardia. Three patients discontinued the study because of cardiac events.

➤*Dermatologic:* Three patients (0.4%) discontinued liposomal doxorubicin because of palmar-plantar erythrodysesthesia (see Warnings).

➤*Hematologic:*

Infection – Opportunistic infections occurred in 50.4% of patients, most commonly candidiasis (23.5%), cytomegalovirus (20.1%), herpes simplex (10.5%), *Pneumocystis carinii* pneumonia (9.2%), and mycobacterium avium (8.4%).

Neutropenia (< 1000 neutrophils/mm³) occurred in 49% of patients treated with liposomal doxorubicin in a study with 13% of patients having ≥ 1 episode of ANC < 500 cell/mm³. Sepsis occurred in 5% of patients; in 0.7% of patients, the event was considered possibly or probably related to liposomal doxorubicin. Ten patients developed sepsis in the setting of neutropenia. Eleven patients (1.6%) discontinued study because of bone marrow suppression or neutropenia.

➤*Hypersensitivity:* Fever, chills, urticaria, anaphylaxis, lincomycin cross-sensitivity (doxorubicin).

➤*Miscellaneous:*

Infusion reactions – Acute infusion-associated reactions characterized by flushing, shortness of breath, facial swelling, headache, chills, back pain, tightness in the chest and throat, and hypotension have occurred in ≈ 6.8% of patients treated with liposomal doxorubicin (see Warnings).

Radiation therapy – Recall of skin reaction because of prior radiotherapy has occurred with liposomal doxorubicin administration.

Overdosage

Acute overdosage enhances the toxic effects of mucositis, leukopenia, and thrombocytopenia. Treat the severely myelosuppressed patient with hospitalization, antibiotics, platelet and granulocyte transfusions, and symptomatic treatment of mucositis. Consider the use of hemopoietic growth factor (G-CSF, GM-CSF).

Chronic overdosage with cumulative doses > 550 mg/m² increases the risk of cardiomyopathy and resultant CHF. Vigorously manage CHF with digitalis preparations and diuretics. Use of afterload reducers such as ACE inhibitors is recommended.

EPIRUBICIN HCl

Rx	Ellence (Pharmacia & Upjohn)	Injection: 2 mg/mL	Preservative-free. In 25 and 100 mL single-use vials.

WARNING

Severe local tissue necrosis will occur if there is extravasation during administration (see Precautions). Epirubicin must not be given by the IM or SC route.

Myocardial toxicity, manifested in its most severe form by potentially fatal CHF, may occur either during therapy with epirubicin or months to years after termination of therapy. The probability of developing clinically evident CHF is estimated as approximately 0.9% at a cumulative dose of 550 mg/m^2, 1.6% at 700 mg/m^2, and 3.3% at 900 mg/m^2. In the adjuvant treatment of breast cancer, the maximum cumulative dose used in clinical trials was 720 mg/m^2. The risk of developing CHF increases rapidly with increasing total cumulative doses of epirubicin in excess of 900 mg/m^2; exceed this cumulative dose with extreme caution. Active or dormant cardiovascular disease, prior or concomitant radiotherapy to the mediastinal/pericardial area, previous therapy with other anthracyclines or anthracenediones, or concomitant use of other cardiotoxic drugs may increase the risk of cardiac toxicity. Cardiac toxicity with epirubicin may occur at lower cumulative doses whether or not cardiac risk factors are present.

Secondary acute myelogenous leukemia (AML) has been reported in patients with breast cancer treated with anthracyclines, including epirubicin. The occurrence of refractory secondary leukemia is more common when such drugs are given in combination with DNA-damaging antineoplastic agents, when patients have been heavily pretreated with cytotoxic drugs, or when doses of anthracyclines have been escalated. In 3844 patients with breast cancer who received adjuvant treatment with epirubicin-containing regimens, the cumulative risk of developing treatment-related AML was estimated at 0.2% at 3 years and 0.8% at 5 years.

Reduce dosage in patients with impaired hepatic function (see Administration and Dosage).

Severe myelosuppression may occur.

Administer epirubicin only under the supervision of a physician who is experienced in the use of cancer chemotherapeutic agents.

Indications

➤*Breast cancer:* As a component of adjuvant therapy in patients with evidence of axillary node tumor involvement following resection of primary breast cancer.

➤*Unlabeled uses:* Epirubicin has been used in combination with other chemotherapeutic agents for the treatment of various forms of cancer such as advanced esophageal cancer (epirubicin plus cisplatin and 5-fluorouracil).

Administration and Dosage

➤*Approved by the FDA:* September 16, 1999.

Epirubicin injection is administered to patients by IV infusion and is given in repeated 3- to 4-week cycles. The total dose of epirubicin may be given on day 1 of each cycle or divided equally and given on days 1 and 8 of each cycle.

➤*Starting doses:* 100 to 120 mg/m^2. The following regimens were used in the trials supporting the use of epirubicin as a component of adjuvant therapy in patients with axillary node-positive breast cancer.

Regimens Including Epirubicin as Adjuvant Therapy in Axillary Node-Positive Patients

FEC-100		CEF-120	
5-Fluorouracil	500 mg/m^2	Cyclophosphamide	75 mg/m^2 oral on days 1 to 14
Epirubicin	100 mg/m^2	Epirubicin	60 mg/m^2 IV on days 1 and 8
Cyclophosphamide	500 mg/m^2	5-Fluorouracil	500 mg/m^2 IV on days 1 and 8
All drugs administered IV on day 1 and repeated every 21 days for 6 cycles		Repeated every 28 day for 6 cycles	

Patients administered the 120 mg/m^2 regimen of epirubicin also received prophylactic antibiotic therapy with trimethoprim-sulfamethoxazole or a fluoroquinolone.

➤*Bone marrow dysfunction:* Consider administration of lower starting doses (eg, 75 to 90 mg/m^2) for heavily pretreated patients, patients with preexisting bone marrow depression, or in the presence of neoplastic bone marrow infiltration.

➤*Hepatic function impairment:* Definitive recommendations regarding use of epirubicin in patients with hepatic dysfunction are not available because patients with hepatic abnormalities were excluded from participation in adjuvant trials of FEC-100/CEF-120 therapy. In patients with elevated serum AST or serum total bilirubin concentra-

tions, the following dose reductions were recommended in clinical trials, although few patients experienced hepatic impairment:
• Bilirubin 1.2 to 3 mg/dL or AST 2 to 4 times upper limit of normal (ULN), give one-half of recommended starting dose
• Bilirubin more than 3 mg/dL or AST more than 4 times ULN, give one-fourth of recommended starting dose

➤*Renal function impairment:* While no specific dose recommendation can be made based on the limited available data in patients with renal impairment, consider lower doses in patients with severe renal impairment (serum creatinine more than 5 mg/dL).

➤*Dosage adjustments:* Make dosage adjustments after the first treatment cycle based on hematologic and nonhematologic toxicities.

Epirubicin Dosage Adjustments

Initial dose	Toxicity	Dosage adjustment
100 mg/m^2 on day 1 of each cycle	Nadir platelet counts < 50,000 mm^3, ANC < 250 mm^3, neutropenic fever, or Grade 3/4 nonhematologic toxicity	*Day 1 of next cycle:* Reduce dose to 75% of day 1 dose. Delay next cycle until platelet counts are ≥ 100,000 mm^3, ANC ≥ 1500 mm^3, and nonhematologic toxicities have recovered to ≤ Grade 1.
60 mg/m^2 on days 1 and 8 of each cycle	*Day 8:* Platelet counts 75,000 to 100,000 mm^3 and ANC 1000 to 1499 mm^3.	*Day 8 dose:* Reduce to 75% of day 1 dose.
	Day 8: Platelet counts < 75,000 mm^3, ANC < 1000 mm^3, or Grade 3/4 nonhematologic toxicity.	*Day 8 dose:* Omit dose.

➤*Preparation and administration precautions:*
Protective measures – Take the following protective measures when handling epirubicin:
• Train personnel in appropriate techniques for reconstitution and handling.
• Exclude pregnant staff from working with this drug.
• Personnel handling epirubicin should wear protective clothing (eg, goggles, gowns, disposable gloves, masks).
• Designate an area for syringe preparation (preferably under a laminar flow system), with the work surface protected by disposable, plastic-backed, absorbent paper.
• Place all items used for reconstitution, administration, or cleaning (including gloves) in high-risk, waste-disposal bags for high temperature incineration.

Treat spillage or leakage with dilute sodium hypochlorite (1% available chlorine) solution, preferably by soaking, and then water. Place all contaminated and cleaning materials in high-risk, waste-disposal bags for incineration. Treat accidental contact with the skin or eyes immediately by copious lavage with water, soap and water, or sodium bicarbonate solution. Do not abrade the skin by using a scrub brush. Seek medical attention.

Admixture incompatibilities – Avoid prolonged contact with any solution of any alkaline pH as it will result in hydrolysis of the drug. Do not mix epirubicin with heparin or fluorouracil because of chemical incompatibility that may lead to precipitation.

Epirubicin can be used in combination with other antitumor agents, but it is recommended that it not be mixed with other drugs in the same syringe.

➤*Preparation of infusion solution:* Epirubicin is provided as a preservative-free, ready-to-use solution.

It is recommended that epirubicin be administered into the tubing of a freely flowing IV infusion (0.9% sodium chloride or 5% glucose solution) over a period of 3 to 20 minutes, depending on dosage and volume of the infusion solution. This technique is intended to minimize the risk of thrombosis or perivenous extravasation, which could lead to severe cellulitis, vesication, or tissue necrosis. A direct push injection is not recommended because of the risk of extravasation, which may occur even in the presence of adequate blood return upon needle aspiration. Venous sclerosis may result from injection into small vessels or repeated injections into the same vein (see Precautions). Use epirubicin within 24 hours of first penetration of the rubber stopper. Discard any unused solution.

➤*Storage/Stability:* Store refrigerated between 2° to 8°C (36° to 46°F). Do not freeze. Protect from light. Discard unused portion.

Actions

➤*Pharmacology:* Although anthracyclines can interfere with a number of biochemical and biological functions within eukaryotic cells, the precise mechanisms of epirubicin's cytotoxic and/or antiproliferative properties have not been completely elucidated.

EPIRUBICIN HCl

Epirubicin forms a complex with DNA by intercalation of its planar rings between nucleotide base pairs with consequent inhibition of nucleic acid (DNA and RNA) and protein synthesis. Such intercalation triggers DNA cleavage by topoisomerase II, resulting in cytocidal activity. Epirubicin also inhibits DNA helicase activity, preventing the enzymatic separation of double-stranded DNA and interfering with replication and transcription. Epirubicin also is involved in oxidation/reduction reactions by generating cytotoxic free radicals.

Epirubicin is cytotoxic in vitro to a variety of established murine and human cell lines and primary cultures of human tumors. It also is active in vivo against a variety of murine tumors and human xenografts in athymic mice, including breast tumors.

➤*Pharmacokinetics:*

Distribution – Following IV administration, epirubicin is rapidly and widely distributed into the tissues. Binding of epirubicin to plasma proteins, predominantly albumin, is approximately 77% and is not affected by drug concentration. Epirubicin also appears to concentrate in red blood cells; whole blood concentrations are approximately twice those of plasma.

Metabolism – Epirubicin is extensively and rapidly metabolized by the liver and also is metabolized by other organs and cells, including red blood cells. Four main metabolic routes have been identified: Reduction of the C-13 keto-group with the formation of the 13(S)-dihydro derivative, epirubicinol; conjugation of both the unchanged drug and epirubicinol with glucuronic acid; loss of the amino sugar moiety through a hydrolytic process with the formation of the doxorubicin and doxorubicinol aglycones; loss of the amino sugar moiety through a redox process with the formation of the 7-deoxy-doxorubicin aglycone and 7-deoxy-doxorubicinol aglycone. Epirubicinol has in vitro cytotoxic activity one-tenth of epirubicin. As plasma levels of epirubicinol are lower than those of the unchanged drug, they are unlikely to reach in vivo concentrations sufficient for cytotoxicity. No significant activity or toxicity has been reported for the other metabolites.

Excretion – Epirubicin and its major metabolites are eliminated through biliary excretion and, to a lesser extent, by urinary excretion. Mass-balance data from 1 patient found approximately 60% of the total dose in feces (34%) and urine (27%). These data are consistent with those from 3 patients with extrahepatic obstruction and percutaneous drainage, in whom approximately 35% and 20% of the administered dose were recovered as epirubicin or its major metabolites in bile and urine, respectively, in the 4 days after treatment. The plasma concentration declined in a triphasic manner with mean half-lives for the alpha, beta, and gamma phases of approximately 3 minutes, 2.5 hours, and 33 hours, respectively. Epirubicin pharmacokinetics are linear over the dose range of 60 to 150 mg/m^2 and plasma clearance is not affected by the duration of infusion or administration schedule. Pharmacokinetic parameters for epirubicin following 6- to 10-minute, single-dose IV infusions of epirubicin at doses of 60 to 150 mg/m^2 in patients with solid tumors are shown in the following table.

Mean Epirubicin Pharmacokinetic Parameters in Patients[a] with Solid Tumors

Doses[b] (mg/m^2)	C_{max} (mcg/mL)[c]	AUC (mcg•h/mL)	Terminal $t_{1/2}$ (h)	CL (L/h)	Vss (L/kg)
60	5.7	1.6	35.3	65	21
75	5.3	1.7	32.1	83	27
120	9	3.4	33.7	65	23
150	9.3	4.2	31.1	69	21

[a] Advanced solid tumor cancers, primarily of the lung.
[b] 6 patients/dose level.
[c] At the end of 6- to 10-minute infusion.

Special populations –

Age: A population analysis of plasma data from 36 cancer patients (13 males and 23 females, 20 to 73 years of age) showed that age affects plasma clearance of epirubicin in female patients. The predicted plasma clearance for a female patient of 70 years of age was approximately 35% lower than that for a female patient 25 years of age. An insufficient number of males older than 50 years of age were included in the study to draw conclusions about age-related alterations in clearance in males. Although a lower epirubicin starting dose does not appear necessary in elderly female patients and was not used in clinical trials, take particular care in monitoring toxicity when epirubicin is administered to female patients older than 70 years of age.

Hepatic function impairment: Epirubicin is eliminated by hepatic metabolism and biliary excretion, and clearance is reduced in patients with hepatic dysfunction. In a study of the effect of hepatic dysfunction, patients with solid tumors were classified into 3 groups. Patients in Group 1 (n = 22) had serum AST levels above the ULN (median: 93 IU/L) and normal serum bilirubin levels (median: 0.5 mg/dL) and were given epirubicin doses of 12.5 to 90 mg/m^2. Patients in Group 2 had alterations in both serum AST (median: 175 IU/L) and bilirubin levels (median: 2.7 mg/dL) and were treated with an epirubicin dose of 25 mg/m^2 (n = 8). Their pharmacokinetics were compared with those patients with normal serum AST and bilirubin values who received epirubicin doses of 12.5 to 120 mg/m^2. The median plasma clearance of

epirubicin was decreased compared with patients with normal hepatic function by approximately 30% in patients in Group 1 and by 50% in patients in Group 2. Patients with more severe hepatic impairment have not been evaluated.

Renal function impairment: No significant alterations in the pharmacokinetics of epirubicin or its major metabolite, epirubicinol, have been observed in patients with serum creatinine 5 mg/dL or more. A 50% reduction in plasma clearance was reported in 4 patients with serum creatinine at least 5 mg/dL. Patients on dialysis have not been studied.

Contraindications

Baseline neutrophil count less than 1500 $cells/mm^3$; severe myocardial insufficiency or recent MI; severe arrhythmias; previous treatment with anthracyclines up to the maximum cumulative dose; hypersensitivity to epirubicin, other anthracyclines, or anthracenediones; severe hepatic dysfunction (see Warnings).

Warnings

➤*Hematologic:* A dose-dependent, reversible leukopenia and/or neutropenia is the predominant manifestation of hematologic toxicity associated with epirubicin and represents the most common acute dose-limiting toxicity of this drug. In most cases, the white blood cell (WBC) nadir is reached 10 to 14 days from drug administration. Leukopenia/neutropenia is usually transient, with the WBC and neutrophil counts generally returning to normal values by day 21 after drug administration. As with other cytotoxic agents, epirubicin at the recommended dose in combination with cyclophosphamide and fluorouracil can produce severe leukopenia and neutropenia. Severe thrombocytopenia and anemia also may occur. Clinical consequences of severe myelosuppression include fever, infection, septicemia, septic shock, hemorrhage, tissue hypoxia, symptomatic anemia, or death. If myelosuppressive complications occur, appropriate supportive measures (eg, IV antibiotics, colony-stimulating factors, transfusions) may be required. Myelosuppression requires careful monitoring. Assess total and differential WBC, RBC, and platelet counts before and during each cycle of therapy with epirubicin.

➤*Cardiac:* Cardiotoxicity is a known risk of anthracycline treatment. Anthracycline-induced cardiac toxicity may be manifested by early (acute) or late (delayed) events. Early cardiac toxicity of epirubicin consists mainly of sinus tachycardia and/or ECG abnormalities, such as nonspecific ST-T wave changes, but tachyarrhythmias, including premature ventricular contractions and ventricular tachycardia, bradycardia, as well as atrioventricular and bundle-branch block also have been reported. These effects do not usually predict subsequent development of delayed cardiotoxicity, are rarely of clinical importance, and are generally not considered an indication for the suspension of epirubicin treatment. Delayed cardiac toxicity results from a characteristic cardiomyopathy that is manifested by reduced left ventricular ejection function (LVEF) and/or signs and symptoms of CHF, such as tachycardia, dyspnea, pulmonary edema, dependent edema, hepatomegaly, ascites, pleural effusion, and gallop rhythm. Life-threatening CHF is the most severe form of anthracycline-induced cardiomyopathy. This toxicity appears to be dependent on the cumulative dose of epirubicin and represents the cumulative dose-limiting toxicity of the drug. If it occurs, delayed cardiotoxicity usually develops late in the course of therapy with epirubicin or within 2 to 3 months after completion of treatment, but later events (several months to years after treatment termination) have been reported.

The estimated risk of epirubicin-treated patients clinically evident CHF was 0.9% at a cumulative dose of 550 mg/m^2, 1.6% at 700 mg/m^2, and 3.3% at 900 mg/m^2. The risk of developing CHF in the absence of other cardiac risk factors increased steeply after an epirubicin cumulative dose of 900 mg/m^2.

Given the risk of cardiomyopathy, exceed a cumulative dose of 900 mg/m^2 epirubicin only with extreme caution. Risk factors (active or dormant cardiovascular disease, prior or concomitant radiotherapy to the mediastinal/pericardial area, previous therapy with other anthracyclines or anthracenediones, concomitant use of other drugs with the ability to suppress cardiac contractility) may increase the risk of cardiac toxicity. Although not formally tested, it is probable that the toxicity of epirubicin and other anthracyclines or anthracenediones is additive. Concomitant use of epirubicin with other cardioactive compounds that could cause heart failure (eg, calcium channel blockers), requires close monitoring of cardiac function throughout treatment. Cardiac toxicity with epirubicin may occur at lower cumulative doses whether or not cardiac risk factors are present.

Monitoring for potential cardiotoxicity is important (see Precautions).

➤*Secondary leukemia:* The occurrence of secondary AML, with or without a preleukemic phase, has been reported in patients treated with anthracyclines. Secondary leukemia is more common when such drugs are given in combination with DNA-damaging antineoplastic agents, when patients have been heavily pretreated with cytotoxic drugs, or when doses of the anthracyclines have been escalated. These leukemias can have a short 1- to 3-year latency period. An analysis of 3844 patients who received adjuvant treatment with epirubicin in controlled clinical trials showed a cumulative risk of secondary AML of approximately 0.2% at 3 years and approximately 0.8% at 5 years.

EPIRUBICIN HCl

►*Tumor lysis syndrome:* As with other cytotoxic agents, epirubicin may induce hyperuricemia as a consequence of the extensive purine catabolism that accompanies drug-induced rapid lysis of highly chemosensitive neoplastic cells (tumor lysis syndrome). Other metabolic abnormalities may also occur. While not generally a problem in patients with breast cancer, physicians should consider the potential for tumor-lysis syndrome in potentially susceptible patients and consider monitoring serum uric acid, potassium, calcium, phosphate, and creatinine immediately after initial chemotherapy administration. Hydration, urine alkalinization, and prophylaxis with allopurinol to prevent hyperuricemia may minimize potential complications of tumor-lysis syndrome.

►*Renal function impairment:* Assess serum creatinine before and during therapy. Dosage adjustment is necessary in patients with serum creatinine more than 5 mg/dL (see Administration and Dosage). Patients undergoing dialysis have not been studied.

►*Hepatic function impairment:* The major route of elimination of epirubicin is the hepatobiliary system. Evaluate serum total bilirubin and AST levels before and during treatment with epirubicin. Patients with elevated bilirubin or AST may experience slower clearance of drug with an increase in overall toxicity. Lower doses are recommended in these patients (see Administration and Dosage). Patients with severe hepatic impairment have not been evaluated; therefore, do not use epirubicin in this patient population.

►*Carcinogenesis:* Treatment-related AML has been reported in women treated with epirubicin-based adjuvant chemotherapy regimens. IV administration of a single 3.6 mg/kg dose to female rats (approximately 0.2 times the maximum recommended human dose [MRHD] on a body surface area basis) approximately doubled the incidence of mammary tumors (primarily fibroadenomas) observed at 1 year. Administration of 0.5 mg/kg epirubicin IV to rats every 3 weeks for 10 doses increased the incidence of SC fibromas in males over an 18-month observation period. In addition, SC administration of 0.75 or 1 mg/kg/day to newborn rats for 4 days on both the first and tenth day after birth for a total of 8 doses increased the incidence of animals with tumors compared to controls during a 24-month observation period.

Epirubicin is mutagenic, clastogenic, and carcinogenic in animals.

►*Mutagenesis:* Although experimental data are not available, epirubicin could induce chromosomal damage in human spermatozoa because of its genotoxic potential. Advise men undergoing treatment with epirubicin to use effective contraceptive methods. Epirubicin may cause irreversible amenorrhea (premature menopause) in premenopausal women.

►*Fertility impairment:* In fertility studies in rats, males were given epirubicin daily for 9 weeks and mated with females that were given epirubicin daily for 2 weeks prior to mating and through day 7 of gestation. When 0.3 mg/kg/day (approximately 0.015 times the MRHD on a body surface area basis) was administered to both sexes, no pregnancies resulted. No effects on mating behavior of fertility were observed at 0.1 mg/kg/day, but male rats had atrophy of the testes and epididymis and reduced spermatogenesis. The 0.1 mg/kg/day dose also caused embryolethality. An increased incidence of fetal growth retardation was observed in these studies at 0.03 mg/kg/day. Multiple daily doses of epirubicin to rabbits and dogs also caused atrophy of male reproductive organs. Single 20.5 and 12 mg/kg doses of IV epirubicin caused testicular atrophy in mice and rats, respectively. A single dose of 16.7 mg/kg epirubicin caused uterine atrophy in rats.

►*Elderly:* Although a lower starting dose of epirubicin was not used in trials in elderly female patients, take particular care in monitoring toxicity when epirubicin is administered to female patients 70 years of age and older.

►*Pregnancy: Category D.* Epirubicin may cause fetal harm when administered to a pregnant woman. Administration of 0.8 mg/kg/day IV of epirubicin to rats (approximately 0.04 times the single MRHD on a body surface area basis) during days 5 to 15 of gestation was embryotoxic (increased resorptions and postimplantation loss) and caused fetal growth retardation (decreased body weight), but was not teratogenic up to this dose. Administration of 2 mg/kg/day IV of epirubicin to rats on days 9 and 10 of gestation was embryotoxic (increased late resorptions, postimplantation losses, and dead fetuses; and decreased live fetuses), retarded fetal growth (decreased body weight), and caused decreased placental weight. This dose also was teratogenic, causing numerous external (anal atresia, misshapen tail, abnormal genital tubercle), visceral (primarily GI, urinary, and cardiovascular systems), and skeletal (deformed long bones and girdles, rib abnormalities, irregular spinal ossification) malformations. Administration of IV epirubicin to rabbits at doses up to 0.2 mg/kg/day during days 6 to 18 of gestation was not embryotoxic or teratogenic, but a maternally toxic dose of 0.32 mg/kg/day increased abortions and delayed ossification. Administration of a maternally toxic IV dose of 1 mg/kg/day epirubicin to rabbits on days 10 to 12 of gestation induced abortion, but no other signs of embryofetal toxicity or teratogenicity were observed.

There are no adequate and well-controlled studies in pregnant women. Two pregnancies have been reported in women taking epirubicin. A woman 34 years of age and 28 weeks pregnant at her diagnosis of breast cancer was treated with cyclophosphamide and epirubicin every 3 weeks for 3 cycles. She received the last dose at 34 weeks of pregnancy and delivered a healthy baby at 35 weeks. Another woman 34 years of age with breast cancer metastatic to the liver was randomized to FEC-50 but was removed from the study because of pregnancy. She experienced a spontaneous abortion. If epirubicin is used during pregnancy, or if the patient becomes pregnant while taking this drug, apprise the patient of the potential hazard to the fetus. Advise women of childbearing potential to avoid becoming pregnant.

►*Lactation:* Epirubicin was excreted into the milk of rats treated with 0.5 mg/kg/day of epirubicin during peri- and postnatal periods. It is not known whether epirubicin is excreted in human breast milk. Because many drugs, including other anthracyclines, are excreted in human milk and because of the potential for serious adverse reactions in nursing infants from epirubicin, advise mothers to discontinue nursing prior to taking this drug.

►*Children:* The safety and efficacy of epirubicin in pediatric patients have not been established. Pediatric patients may be at greater risk for anthracycline-induced acute manifestations of cardiotoxicity and for chronic CHF.

Precautions

►*Monitoring:* Administer epirubicin injection only under the supervision of qualified physicians experienced in the use of cytotoxic therapy. Precede initial treatment with epirubicin with a careful baseline assessment of blood counts, serum levels of total bilirubin, AST, and creatinine, and cardiac function as measured by LVEF. Carefully monitor patients during treatment for possible clinical complications caused by myelosuppression. Assess blood counts, including absolute neutrophil counts, and liver function before and during each cycle of therapy with epirubicin. Perform repeated evaluations of LVEF during therapy. Supportive care may be necessary for the treatment of severe neutropenia and severe infectious complications.

Monitoring for potential cardiotoxicity is also important, especially with greater cumulative exposure to epirubicin. Although endomyocardial biopsy is recognized as the most sensitive diagnostic tool to detect anthracycline-induced cardiomyopathy, this invasive examination is not practically performed on a routine basis. Electrocardiogram (ECG) changes such as dysrhythmias, a reduction of the electrocardiographic wave (QRS) voltage, or a prolongation beyond normal limits of the systolic time interval may be indicative of anthracycline-induced cardiomyopathy, but ECG is not a sensitive or specific method for following anthracycline-related cardiotoxicity. The risk of serious cardiac impairment may be decreased through regular monitoring of LVEF during the course of treatment with prompt discontinuation of epirubicin at the first sign of impaired function. The preferred method for repeated assessment of cardiac function is evaluation of LVEF measured by multi-gated radionuclide angiography (MUGA) or echocardiography (ECHO). A baseline cardiac evaluation with an ECG and a MUGA scan or an ECHO is recommended, especially in patients with risk factors for increased cardiac toxicity. Perform repeated MUGA or ECHO determinations of LVEF, particularly with higher, cumulative anthracycline doses. The technique used for assessment should be consistent through follow-up. In patients with risk factors, particularly prior anthracycline or anthracenedione use, the monitoring of cardiac function must be particularly strict and the risk-benefit of continuing treatment with epirubicin in patients with impaired cardiac function must be carefully evaluated.

►*Injection-site reactions:* Epirubicin injection is administered by IV infusion. Venous sclerosis may result from an injection into a small vessel or from repeated injections into the same vein. Extravasation of epirubicin during the infusion may cause local pain, severe tissue lesions (vesication, severe cellulitis), and necrosis. It is recommended that epirubicin be slowly administered into the tubing of a freely running IV infusion, usually between 3 and 20 minutes depending upon dosage and volume of the infusion solution. If possible, avoid veins over joints or in extremities with compromised venous or lymphatic drainage. A burning or stinging sensation may be indicative of perivenous infiltration; immediately terminate the infusion and restart in another vein. Perivenous infiltration may occur without causing pain.

Facial flushing, as well as local erythematous streaking along the vein, may be indicative of excessively rapid administration. It may precede local phlebitis or thrombophlebitis.

As with other cytotoxic agents, thrombophlebitis and thromboembolic phenomena including pulmonary embolism (in some cases fatal) have been coincidentally reported with the use of epirubicin.

►*Prophylactic antibiotics:* Patients administered the 120 mg/m² regimen of epirubicin as a component of combination chemotherapy should also receive prophylactic antibiotic therapy with trimethoprim-sulfamethoxazole or a fluoroquinolone.

►*Antiemetics:* Epirubicin is emetogenic. Antiemetics may reduce nausea and vomiting; consider prophylactic use of antiemetics before administration of epirubicin, particularly when given in conjunction with other emetogenic drugs.

►*Inflammatory recall reaction:* As with other anthracyclines, administration of epirubicin after previous radiation therapy may

EPIRUBICIN HCl

induce an inflammatory recall reaction at the site of irradiation.

➤*Radiation therapy:* There are few data regarding the coadministration of radiation therapy and epirubicin. In adjuvant trials of epirubicin-containing CEF-120 or FEC-100 chemotherapies, breast irradiation was delayed until after chemotherapy was completed. This practice resulted in no apparent increase in local breast cancer recurrence relative to published accounts in the literature. A small number of patients received epirubicin-based chemotherapy concomitantly with radiation therapy but had chemotherapy interrupted in order to avoid potential overlapping toxicities. It is likely that use of epirubicin with radiotherapy may sensitize tissues to the cytotoxic actions of irradiation. Administration of epirubicin after previous radiation therapy may induce an inflammatory recall reaction at the site of the irradiation.

➤*Concurrent cytotoxic therapy:* Epirubicin when used in combination with other cytotoxic drugs may show on-treatment additive toxicity, especially hematologic and GI effects.

Drug Interactions

➤*Cimetidine:* Cimetidine increased the AUC of epirubicin by 50%. Stop cimetidine treatment during treatment with epirubicin.

➤*Cardioactive compounds:* Concomitant use of epirubicin with other cardioactive compounds that could cause heart failure (eg, calcium channel blockers) requires close monitoring of cardiac function throughout treatment.

Adverse Reactions

Epirubicin Adverse Reactions in Patients with Early Breast Cancer (%)						
	FEC-100/CEF-120[a] (n = 620)		FEC-50[a] (n = 280)		CMF[a] (n = 360)	
Adverse reaction	Grades 1-4	Grades 3/4	Grades 1-4	Grades 3/4	Grades 1-4	Grades 3/4
Dermatologic						
Alopecia	95.5	56.6	69.6	19.3	84.4	6.7
Local toxicity	19.5	0.3	2.5	0.4	8.1	0
Rash/Itch	8.9	0.3	1.4	0	14.2	0
Skin changes	4.7	0	0.7	0	7.2	0
Endocrine						
Amenorrhea	71.8	0	69.3	0	67.7	0
Hot flashes	38.9	4	5.4	0	69.1	6.4
GI						
Anorexia	2.9	0	1.8	0	5.8	0.3
Diarrhea	24.8	0.8	7.1	0	50.7	2.8
Mucositis	58.5	8.9	9.3	0	52.9	1.9
Nausea/Vomiting	92.4	25	83.2	22.1	85	6.4
Hematologic						
Anemia	72.2	5.8	12.9	0	70.9	0.9
Leukopenia	80.3	58.6	49.6	1.5	98.1	60.3
Neutropenia	80.3	67.2	53.9	10.5	95.8	78.1
Thrombocytopenia	48.8	5.4	4.6	0	51.4	3.6
Infection						
Febrile neutropenia	NA[b]	6.1	0	0	NA[b]	1.1
Infection	21.5	1.6	15	0	25.9	0.6
Miscellaneous						
Conjunctivitis/ Keratitis	14.8	0	1.1	0	38.4	0
Fever	5.2	0	1.4	0	4.5	0
Lethargy	45.8	1.9	1.1	0	72.7	0.3

[a] FEC and CEF = cyclophosphamide + epirubicin + fluorouracil; CMF = cyclophosphamide + methotrexate + fluorouracil.
[b] NA = not available.

Grade 1 or 2 changes in transaminase levels were observed but were more frequently seen with CMF than with CEF.

The following delayed adverse reactions were noted in the FEC-100/CEF-120, FEC-50, and CMF patients, respectively: Asymptomatic drops in LVEF (1.8%, 1.4%, and 0.8%); CHF (1.5%, 0.4%, and 0.3%); AML (0.8%, 0%, and 0.3%). Two cases of acute lymphocytic leukemia (ALL) also were observed in patients receiving epirubicin. However, an association between anthracyclines such as epirubicin and ALL has not been clearly established.

➤*Dermatologic:* Alopecia occurs frequently, but is usually reversible with hair regrowth occurring within 2 to 3 months from the termination of therapy. Flushes, hypersensitivity to irradiated skin (radiation-recall reaction), photosensitivity, skin and nail hyperpigmentation have been observed.

➤*Hypersensitivity:* Urticaria and anaphylaxis have been reported in patients treated with epirubicin; signs and symptoms of these reactions may vary from skin rash and pruritus to fever, chills, and shock.

➤*GI:* A dose-dependent mucositis (mainly oral stomatitis, less often esophagitis) may occur in patients treated with epirubicin. Clinical manifestations of mucositis may include bleeding, erosions, erythema, infections, a pain or burning sensation, or ulcerations. Mucositis generally appears early after drug administration and, if severe, may progress over a few days to mucosal ulcerations; most patients recover from this adverse event by the third week of therapy. Hyperpigmentation of the oral mucosa may also occur.

Nausea, vomiting, and occasionally diarrhea and abdominal pain can also occur. Severe vomiting and diarrhea may produce dehydration. Antiemetics may reduce nausea and vomiting; consider prophylactic use of antiemetics before therapy (see Precautions).

➤*Miscellaneous:* See Warnings for cardiovascular, hematologic, and secondary leukemia. See Precautions for injection-site reactions.

Overdosage

➤*Symptoms:* A man 36 years of age with non-Hodgkin lymphoma received a daily 95 mg/m^2 dose of epirubicin injection for 5 consecutive days. Five days later, he developed bone marrow aplasia, grade 4 mucositis, and GI bleeding. No signs of acute cardiac toxicity were observed. He was treated with antibiotics, colony-stimulating factors, and antifungal agents and recovered completely. A woman 63 years of age with breast cancer and liver metastasis received a single 320 mg/m^2 dose of epirubicin. She was hospitalized with hyperthermia and developed multiple organ failure (respiratory and renal), with lactic acidosis, increased lactate dehydrogenase, and anuria. Death occurred within 24 hours after administration of epirubicin. Additional instances of administration of doses higher than recommended have been reported at doses ranging from 150 to 250 mg/m^2. The observed adverse events in these patients were qualitatively similar to known toxicities of epirubicin. Most of the patients recovered with appropriate supportive care.

➤*Treatment:* If an overdose occurs, provide supportive treatment including antibiotic therapy, blood and platelet transfusions, colony-stimulating factors, and intensive care as needed until the recovery of toxicities. Delayed CHF has been observed months after anthracycline administration. Patients must be observed carefully over time for signs of CHF and provided with appropriate supportive therapy. Refer to General Management of Acute Overdosage.

Patient Information

Inform patients of the expected adverse effects of epirubicin, including GI symptoms (eg, nausea, vomiting, diarrhea, stomatitis) and potential neutropenic complications.

Advise patients to consult their physician if vomiting, dehydration, fever, evidence of infection, symptoms of CHF, or injection-site pain occurs following therapy with epirubicin.

Advise women of childbearing potential to avoid becoming pregnant.

Inform patients that they will almost certainly develop alopecia.

Advise patients that their urine may appear red for 1 to 2 days after administration of epirubicin and that they should not be alarmed.

Patients should understand that there is a risk of irreversible myocardial damage associated with treatment with epirubicin, as well as a risk of treatment-related leukemia.

Because epirubicin may induce chromosomal damage in sperm, men undergoing treatment with epirubicin should use effective contraceptive methods.

Women treated with epirubicin may develop irreversible amenorrhea or premature menopause.

IDARUBICIN HCl

Rx	Idarubicin HCl (GensiaSicor)	Injection: 1 mg/mL	Preservative-free. In 5, 10, and 20 mL single-use vials.
Rx	Idamycin PFS (Pfizer)		Preservative-free. In 5, 10, and 20 mL single-use vials.

WARNING

Give idarubicin (IDR) slowly into a freely flowing IV infusion; never give IM or SC. Severe local tissue necrosis can occur if there is extravasation during administration.

Idarubicin can cause myocardial toxicity leading to congestive heart failure (CHF). Cardiac toxicity is more common in patients who have received prior anthracyclines or who have pre-existing cardiac disease.

Severe myelosuppression occurs when idarubicin is used at therapeutic doses.

Administer idarubicin only under the supervision of a physician who is experienced in leukemia chemotherapy and in facilities with laboratory and supportive resources adequate to monitor drug tolerance and protect and maintain a patient compromised by drug toxicity. The physician and institution must be capable of responding rapidly and completely to severe hemorrhagic conditions and/or overwhelming infection.

Reduce dosage in patients with impaired hepatic or renal function (see Administration and Dosage).

Indications

▶*Acute myeloid leukemia (AML):* In combination with other approved antileukemic drugs for the treatment of AML in adults. This includes French-American-British (FAB) classifications M1 through M7.

Administration and Dosage

▶*Approved by the FDA:* September 27, 1990.

▶*Induction therapy in adult patients with AML:* 12 mg/m²/day for 3 days by slow (10 to 15 minutes) IV injection in combination with cytarabine. The cytarabine may be given as 100 mg/m²/day by continuous infusion for 7 days or as cytarabine 25 mg/m² IV bolus followed by cytarabine 200 mg/m²/day for 5 days continuous infusion. In patients with unequivocal evidence of leukemia after the first induction course, a second course may be administered. Delay administration of the second course in patients who experience severe mucositis until recovery from this toxicity has occurred; a dose reduction of 25% is recommended.

▶*Renal/Hepatic function impairment:* In patients with hepatic and/or renal impairment, consider a dose reduction of idarubicin. Do not administer if the bilirubin level is more than 5 mg/dL (see Warnings).

▶*Administration:* Administer slowly (over 10 to 15 minutes) into the tubing of a freely running IV infusion of 0.9% sodium chloride injection or 5% dextrose injection. Attach the tubing to a butterfly needle or other suitable device and insert into a large vein.

▶*Extravasation:* Extravasation of idarubicin can cause severe local tissue necrosis. Extravasation may occur with or without an accompanying stinging or burning sensation even if blood returns well on aspiration of the infusion needle. If signs or symptoms of extravasation occur, terminate the injection or infusion immediately and restart in another vein.

Care in the administration of idarubicin will reduce the chance of perivenous infiltration. It may also decrease the chance of local reactions such as urticaria and erythematous streaking. If it is known or suspected that SC extravasation has occurred, it is recommended that intermittent ice packs (½ hour immediately, then ½ hour 4 times/day for 3 days) be placed over the area of extravasation and that the affected extremity be elevated. Because of the progressive nature of extravasation reactions, frequently examine the area of injection and obtain plastic surgery consultation early if there is any sign of a local reaction such as pain, erythema, edema, or vesication. If ulceration begins or there is severe persistent pain at the site of extravasation, consider early wide excision of the involved area.

▶*IV incompatibility:* Unless specific compatibility data are available, do not mix idarubicin with other drugs. Precipitation occurs with heparin. Prolonged contact with any solution of an alkaline pH will result in degradation of the drug.

▶*Storage/Stability:* Store preservative-free solutions under refrigeration (2° to 8°C; 36° to 46°F), and protect from light. Retain in carton until time of use.

Actions

▶*Pharmacology:* Idarubicin HCl is a semi-synthetic antineoplastic anthracycline for IV use; it is a DNA-intercalating analog of daunorubicin, which has an inhibitory effect on nucleic acid synthesis and interacts with the enzyme topoisomerase II. The compound has a high lipophilicity, which results in an increased rate of cellular uptake compared with other anthracyclines.

▶*Pharmacokinetics:*

Absorption/Distribution – Following IV administration of 10 to 12 mg/m²/day for 3 to 4 days (as a single agent or combined with cytarabine) to adult leukemia patients with normal renal and hepatic function, there is a rapid distributive phase with a very high volume of distribution presumably reflecting extensive tissue binding.

Peak cellular idarubicin concentrations are reached a few minutes after injection. Idarubicin and idarubicinol (the primary metabolite) concentrations in nucleated blood and bone marrow cells are more than 100 times the plasma concentrations.

The percentages of idarubicin and idarubicinol bound to human plasma proteins averaged 97% and 94%, respectively. The binding is concentration-independent.

Metabolism/Excretion – The plasma clearance is twice the expected hepatic plasma flow, indicating extensive extrahepatic metabolism. The drug is eliminated predominantly by biliary and to a lesser extent by renal excretion, mostly in the form of the primary metabolite, idarubicinol.

The estimated mean terminal half-life is 22 hours (range, 4 to 48 hours) when used as a single agent and 20 hours (range, 7 to 38 hours) when used in combination with cytarabine. The elimination of idarubicinol is considerably slower, with an estimated mean terminal half-life of more than 45 hours; hence, its plasma levels are sustained for more than 8 days. As idarubicinol has cytotoxic activity, it presumably contributes to the effects of idarubicin.

The extent of drug and metabolite accumulation predicted in leukemia patients for days 2 and 3 of dosing is 1.7- and 2.3-fold, respectively, and suggests no change in kinetics following a 3-day regimen.

Idarubicin disappearance rates in plasma and cells were comparable with a terminal half-life of about 15 hours. The terminal half-life of idarubicinol in cells was approximately 72 hours.

Special populations –

Hepatic/Renal function impairment: In patients with moderate or severe hepatic dysfunction, the metabolism of idarubicin may be impaired and lead to higher systemic drug levels. The disposition of idarubicin may be also affected by renal impairment. Therefore, consider a dose reduction in patients with hepatic and/or renal impairment (see Warnings and Administration and Dosage).

Children: Idarubicin studies in pediatric leukemia patients, at doses of 4.2 to 13.3 mg/m²/day for 3 days, suggest dose-independent kinetics. There is no difference between the half-lives of the drug following daily for 3 days or weekly for 3 weeks administration.

Cerebrospinal fluid (CSF) levels of idarubicin and idarubicinol were measured in pediatric leukemia patients. Idarubicin was detected in 2 of 21 CSF samples (0.14 and 1.57 ng/mL), while idarubicinol was detected in 20 of these 21 CSF samples obtained 18 to 30 hours after dosing (mean = 0.51 ng/mL; range, 0.22 to 1.05 ng/mL). The clinical relevance of these findings is unknown.

▶*Clinical trials:* Four prospective randomized studies have been conducted to compare the safety and efficacy of IDR to that of daunorubicin (DNR), each in combination with cytarabine as induction therapy in previously untreated adult patients with AML. These data are summarized in the following table and demonstrate significantly greater complete remission rates and significantly longer overall survival for the IDR regimen in 2 of the studies.

Efficacy of Idarubicin vs Daunorubicin in AML						
	Induction[1] regimen dose in mg/m² daily × 3 days		Complete remission rate		Median survival (days)	
Studies	IDR	DNR	IDR	DNR	IDR	DNR
Age ≤ 60 years	12[2]	50[2]	51/65[3] (78%)	38/65 (58%)	508[3]	435
Age ≥ 15 years	12[4]	45[4]	76/111[3] (69%)	65/119 (55%)	328	277
Age ≥ 18 years	13[4]	45[4]	68/101 (67%)	66/113 (58%)	393[3]	281
Age ≥ 55 years[5]	12[4]	45[4]	49/124 (40%)	49/125 (39%)	87	169

[1] Patients who had persistent leukemia after the first induction course received a second course.
[2] Cytarabine 25 mg/m² bolus IV followed by 200 mg/m² daily × 5 days by continuous infusion.
[3] Overall $P < 0.05$, unadjusted for prognostic factors or multiple endpoints.
[4] Cytarabine 100 mg/m² daily × 7 days by continuous infusion.
[5] Non-US study.

IDARUBICIN HCl

The following consolidation regimens were used in US controlled trials. Patients received the same anthracycline for consolidation as was used for induction.

Studies 1 and 3 – Studies 1 and 3 utilized 2 courses of consolidation therapy consisting of IDR 12 or 13 mg/m^2/day for 2 days, respectively (or DNR 50 or 45 mg/m^2/day for 2 days), and cytarabine, either 25 mg/m^2 by IV bolus followed by 200 mg/m^2/day by continuous infusion for 4 days (study 1), or 100 mg/m^2/day for 5 days by continuous infusion (study 3). A rest period of 4 to 6 weeks is recommended prior to initiation of consolidation and between the courses; hematologic recovery is mandatory prior to initiation of each consolidation course.

Study 2 – Study 2 utilized 3 consolidation courses, administered at intervals of 21 days or upon hematologic recovery. Each course consisted of IDR 15 mg/m^2 IV for 1 dose (or DNR 50 mg/m^2 IV for 1 dose), cytarabine 100 mg/m^2 every 12 hours for 10 doses and 6-thioguanine 100 mg/m^2 orally for 10 doses. If severe myelosuppression occurred, subsequent courses were given with a 25% reduction in the doses of all drugs. This study also included 4 courses of maintenance therapy (2 days of the same anthracycline that was used in induction and 5 days of cytarabine).

Toxicities and duration of aplasia were similar during induction except for an increase in mucositis on the IDR arm in 1 study. During consolidation, duration of aplasia on the IDR arm was longer in all 3 studies and mucositis was more frequent in 2 studies. During consolidation, transfusion requirements were higher on the IDR arm in the 2 studies in which they were tabulated, and patients on the IDR arm in study 3 spent more days on IV antibiotics (study 3 used a higher dose of IDR).

The benefit of consolidation and maintenance therapy in prolonging the duration of remission and survival is not proven.

Intensive maintenance with IDR is not recommended in view of the considerable toxicity (including deaths in remission) experienced by patients during the maintenance phase of study 2.

Warnings

➤*Administration:* Administer idarubicin under the supervision of a physician who is experienced in leukemia chemotherapy.

➤*Bone marrow suppression:* Idarubicin is a potent bone marrow suppressant. Do not give to patients with pre-existing bone marrow suppression induced by previous drug therapy or radiotherapy unless the benefit warrants the risk.

➤*Severe myelosuppression:* Severe myelosuppression will occur in all patients given a therapeutic dose of this agent for induction, consolidation, or maintenance. Careful hematologic monitoring is required. Deaths due to infection and/or bleeding have occurred during severe myelosuppression. Facilities with laboratory and supportive resources adequate to monitor drug tolerability and protect and maintain a patient compromised by drug toxicity should be available. It must be possible to treat rapidly and completely a severe hemorrhagic condition and/or a severe infection.

➤*Cardiotoxicity:* Pre-existing heart disease and previous therapy with anthracyclines at high cumulative doses or other potentially cardiotoxic agents are cofactors for increased risk of idarubicin-induced cardiac toxicity; weigh the benefit to risk ratio of idarubicin therapy in such patients before starting treatment.

Myocardial toxicity, as manifested by potentially fatal CHF, acute life-threatening arrhythmias, or other cardiomyopathies may occur following therapy with idarubicin. Appropriate therapeutic measures for the management of CHF and/or arrhythmias are indicated.

Carefully monitor cardiac function during treatment in order to minimize the risk of cardiac toxicity of the type described for other anthracycline compounds. The risk of such myocardial toxicity may be higher following concomitant or previous radiation to the mediastinal-pericardial area or in patients with anemia, bone marrow depression, infections, leukemic pericarditis, and/or myocarditis. While there are no reliable means for predicting CHF, cardiomyopathy induced by anthracyclines is usually associated with a decrease of the left ventricular ejection fraction (LVEF) from pretreatment baseline values.

➤*Renal/Hepatic function impairment:* Renal and hepatic function impairment can affect the disposition of idarubicin. Evaluate liver and kidney function with conventional clinical laboratory tests (using serum bilirubin and serum creatinine as indicators) prior to and during treatment. Consider dose reduction if the bilirubin or creatinine levels are above the normal range (see Administration and Dosage).

➤*Carcinogenesis:* Idarubicin and related compounds have mutagenic and carcinogenic properties when tested in experimental models (including bacterial systems and mammalian cells in culture and female Sprague-Dawley rats).

In male dogs given 1.8 mg/m^2/day idarubicin (3 times per week for 13 weeks times the human dose]), testicular atrophy was observed with inhibition of spermatogenesis and sperm maturation, and few or no mature sperm. Effects were not readily reversible after an 8-week recovery period.

➤*Elderly:* Patients older than 60 years of age who were undergoing induction therapy experienced CHF, serious arrhythmias, chest pain, myocardial infarction, and asymptomatic declines in LVEF more frequently than younger patients.

➤*Pregnancy: Category D.* Idarubicin was embryotoxic and teratogenic in the rat at a dose of 1.2 mg/m^2/day or one-tenth the human dose, which was nontoxic to dams. Idarubicin was embryotoxic but not teratogenic in the rabbit, even at a dose of 2.4 mg/m^2/day or two-tenths the human dose, which was toxic to dams. There has been 1 report of a fetal fatality after maternal exposure to idarubicin during the second trimester. There is no conclusive information about idarubicin adversely affecting human fertility or causing teratogenesis. There are no adequate and well-controlled studies in pregnant women. If idarubicin is to be used during pregnancy, or if the patient becomes pregnant during therapy, apprise the patient of the potential hazard to the fetus. Advise women of childbearing potential to avoid pregnancy.

➤*Lactation:* It is not known whether this drug is excreted in breast milk. Because of the potential for serious adverse reactions in nursing infants from idarubicin, mothers should discontinue nursing prior to taking this drug.

➤*Children:* Safety and efficacy in children have not been established.

Precautions

➤*Monitoring:* Therapy with idarubicin requires close observation of the patient and careful laboratory monitoring. Frequent complete blood counts and monitoring of hepatic and renal function tests are recommended.

➤*Hyperuricemia:* Hyperuricemia secondary to rapid lysis of leukemic cells may be induced. Take appropriate measures to prevent hyperuricemia and to control any systemic infection before beginning therapy.

➤*Administer slowly:* Administer slowly (over 10 to 15 minutes) into the tubing of a freely running IV infusion of 0.9% sodium chloride injection or 5% dextrose injection. Attach the tubing to a butterfly needle or other suitable device and insert into a large vein.

➤*Extravasation:* Extravasation of idarubicin can cause severe local tissue necrosis. Extravasation may occur with or without an accompanying stinging or burning sensation even if blood returns well on aspiration of the infusion needle. If signs or symptoms of extravasation occur, terminate the injection or infusion immediately and restart in another vein.

Care in the administration of idarubicin will reduce the chance of perivenous infiltration. It may also decrease the chance of local reactions such as urticaria and erythematous streaking. If it is known or suspected that SC extravasation has occurred, it is recommended that intermittent ice packs (½ hour immediately, then ½ hour 4 times/day for 3 days) be placed over the area of extravasation and that the affected extremity be elevated. Because of the progressive nature of extravasation reactions, frequently examine the area of injection and obtain plastic surgery consultation early if there is any sign of a local reaction such as pain, erythema, edema, or vesication. If ulceration begins or there is severe persistent pain at the site of extravasation, consider early wide excision of the involved area.

Adverse Reactions

The table below lists the adverse experiences reported in one US study and is representative of the experiences in other studies.

Adverse Reactions: Idarubicin vs Daunorubicin (%)		
Adverse Reactions	Idarubicin (n = 110)	Daunorubicin (n = 118)
Infection	95	97
Nausea and vomiting	82	80
Hair loss	77	72
Abdominal cramps/Diarrhea	73	68
Hemorrhage	63	65
Mucositis	50	55
Dermatologic	46	40
Mental status	41	34
Pulmonary-clinical	39	39
Fever	26	28
Headache	20	24
Cardiac-clinical	16	24
Neurologic-peripheral nerves	7	9
Seizure	4	5
Cerebellar	4	4
Pulmonary allergy	2	4

The duration of aplasia and incidence of mucositis were greater on the IDR arm than the DNR arm, especially during consolidation in some US controlled trials (see Clinical trials).

The following information reflects experience based on US controlled clinical trials.

IDARUBICIN HCl

➤*Cardiovascular:* CHF (frequently attributed to fluid overload), serious arrhythmias including atrial fibrillation, chest pain, MI, and asymptomatic declines in LVEF have occurred in patients undergoing induction therapy for AML. Myocardial insufficiency and arrhythmias were usually reversible and occurred in the setting of sepsis, anemia, and aggressive IV fluid administration. Events were reported more frequently in patients older than 60 years of age and in those with pre-existing cardiac disease (see Warnings).

➤*Dermatologic:* Alopecia occurred frequently, and dermatologic reactions including generalized rash, urticaria, and a bullous erythrodermatous rash of the palms and soles have occurred. The dermatologic reactions were usually attributed to concomitant antibiotic therapy. Local reactions including hives at the injection site have occurred. Recall of skin reaction due to prior radiotherapy has occurred with idarubicin administration.

➤*GI:* Nausea and/or vomiting, mucositis, abdominal pain, and diarrhea occurred frequently but were severe in less than 5% of patients. Severe enterocolitis with perforation has occurred rarely. The risk of perforation may be increased by instrumental intervention. Consider the possibility of perforation in patients who develop severe abdominal pain, and take appropriate steps for diagnosis and management.

Hepatic and renal – Changes in hepatic and renal function tests have been observed. These changes were usually transient and occurred in the setting of sepsis and while patients were receiving potentially hepatotoxic and nephrotoxic antibiotics and antifungal agents. Severe changes in renal function occurred in no more than 1% of patients, while severe changes in hepatic function occurred in fewer than 5% of patients.

Myelosuppression – Severe myelosuppression is the major toxicity associated with idarubicin therapy, but this effect of the drug is required in order to eradicate the leukemic clone. During the period of myelosuppression, patients are at risk of developing infection and bleeding, which may be life-threatening or fatal (see Warnings).

Overdosage

There is no known antidote. Two cases of fatal overdosage in patients receiving therapy for AML have occurred. The doses were 135 mg/m^2 over 3 days and 45 mg/m^2 of idarubicin and 90 mg/m^2 of daunorubicin over 3 days.

It is anticipated that overdosage with idarubicin will result in severe and prolonged myelosuppression and possibly in increased severity of GI toxicity. Adequate supportive care including platelet transfusions, antibiotics, and symptomatic treatment of mucositis is required. The effect of acute overdose on cardiac function is not fully known, but severe arrhythmia occurred in 1 of the 2 patients exposed. It is anticipated that very high doses of idarubicin may cause acute cardiac toxicity and may be associated with a higher incidence of delayed cardiac failure.

The profound multicompartment behavior, extensive extravascular distribution, and tissue binding, coupled with the low unbound fraction available in the plasma pool, make it unlikely that therapeutic efficacy or toxicity would be altered by conventional peritoneal or hemodialysis.

BLEOMYCIN SULFATE (BLM)

Rx	**Bleomycin** (Various, eg, Bedford Laboratories, Gensia Sicor)	**Powder for injection:** 15 units[1]	In vials.
		30 units[1]	In vials.
Rx	**Blenoxane** (Bristol-Myers Oncology)	**Powder for injection:** 15 units[1]	In vials.
		30 units[1]	In vials.

[1] A unit of bleomycin is equal to the formerly used milligram activity.

WARNING

Administer bleomycin under the supervision of a qualified physician experienced in the use of cancer chemotherapeutic agents. Appropriate management of therapy and complications is possible only when adequate diagnostic and treatment facilities are readily available.

Pulmonary fibrosis is the most severe toxicity. It is most frequently seen as pneumonitis, which occasionally progresses to pulmonary fibrosis. Incidence is higher in elderly patients and in those receiving greater than 400 units total dose, but pulmonary toxicity has occurred in young patients and those treated with low doses (see Warnings).

A severe idiosyncratic reaction consisting of hypotension, mental confusion, fever, chills, and wheezing has occurred in approximately 1% of lymphoma patients.

Indications

Palliative treatment in the following neoplasms as either a single agent or in combination with other chemotherapeutic agents:

➤*Lymphomas:* For the treatment of Hodgkin and non-Hodgkin lymphomas.

➤*Malignant pleural effusion:* Effective as a sclerosing agent for the treatment of malignant pleural effusion and prevention of recurrent pleural effusions.

➤*Squamous cell carcinoma:* For the treatment of head and neck squamous cell carcinoma including mouth, tongue, tonsil, nasopharynx, oropharynx, sinus, palate, lip, buccal mucosa, gingiva, epiglottis, skin, and larynx. Response is poorer in patients with head and neck cancer previously irradiated. Bleomycin is also indicated in carcinoma of the penis, cervix, and vulva.

➤*Testicular carcinoma:* For the treatment of embryonal cell, choriocarcinoma, and teratocarcinoma testicular carcinomas.

➤*Unlabeled uses:* Mycosis fungoides, osteosarcoma, AIDS-related Kaposi sarcoma. Has been used in children for palliative treatment of lymphomas, testicular carcinoma, germ cell tumors, and sclerosis of pleural effusions.

Administration and Dosage

➤*Approved by the FDA:* July 31, 1973.

Administer IM, IV, SC, or intrapleurally.

Because of the possibility of anaphylactoid reaction, treat lymphoma patients with no more than 2 units for the first 2 doses. If no acute reaction occurs, follow the regular dosage schedule.

Pulmonary toxicity of bleomycin appears dose-related with a striking increase when total dose is greater than 400 units. Give total doses greater than 400 units with great caution. When bleomycin is used in combination with other antineoplastic agents, pulmonary toxicities may occur at lower doses.

➤*Squamous cell carcinoma, non-Hodgkin lymphoma, testicular carcinoma:* 0.25 to 0.5 units/kg (10 to 20 units/m^2) IV, IM, or SC once or twice weekly.

Improvement of testicular tumors is prompt (less than or equal to 2 weeks). If no improvement is seen by this time, it is unlikely to occur. Squamous cell cancers respond more slowly, sometimes requiring 3 weeks for improvement.

➤*Hodgkin disease:* 0.25 to 0.5 units/kg (10 to 20 units/m^2) IV, IM, or SC once or twice weekly. After a 50% response, give a maintenance dose of 1 unit daily or 5 units per week IV or IM. Improvement of Hodgkin disease is prompt (less than or equal to 2 weeks).

➤*Malignant pleural effusion:* Sixty units administered as a single-dose bolus intrapleural injection. Sixty units of bleomycin are dissolved in 50 to 100 mL 0.9% NaCl for injection and administered through a thoracostomy tube following drainage of excess pleural fluid and confirmation of complete lung expansion. Ensure that the amount of drainage from the chest tube is as minimal as possible prior to installation of bleomycin. The thoracostomy tube is clamped after bleomycin instillation. The patient is moved from the supine to the left and right lateral positions several times during the next 4 hours. The clamp is then removed and suction reestablished (see Precautions).

➤*Preparation of solutions:*

IM or SC – Reconstitute the 15 unit vial with 1 to 5 mL or the 30 unit vial with 2 to 10 mL sterile water for injection, 0.9% NaCl for injection, or bacteriostatic water for injection.

IV solution – Dissolve contents of the 15 or 30 unit vial with 5 or 10 mL, respectively, of 0.9% NaCl for injection; administer slowly over 10 minutes.

Intrapleural – Dissolve 60 units of bleomycin in 50 to 100 mL of 0.9% NaCl for injection.

➤*Storage/Stability:* Bleomycin demonstrates a loss of potency. Do not reconstitute or dilute with 5% dextrose in water or other dextrose-containing diluents.

Bleomycin is stable for 24 hours at room temperature in 0.9% NaCl injection. Store the powder under refrigeration (2° to 8°C; 36° to 46°F).

Actions

➤*Pharmacology:* Bleomycin sulfate is a mixture of cytotoxic glycopeptide antibiotics isolated from a strain of *Streptomyces verticillus.* The exact mechanism of action is unknown; however, the main mode of action appears to be inhibition of DNA synthesis with lesser inhibition of RNA and protein synthesis.

When administered intrapleurally for the treatment of malignant pleural effusion, bleomycin acts as a sclerosing agent.

➤*Pharmacokinetics:*

Absorption/Distribution – Bleomycin plasma concentrations suggest a systemic absorption of approximately 45% following intrapleural administration. In mice, high concentrations of bleomycin are found in the skin, lungs, kidneys, peritoneum, and lymphatics. Tumor cells of the skin and lungs have high concentrations of bleomycin in contrast to the low concentrations in hematopoietic tissue. The low concentrations of bleomycin in bone marrow may be related to high levels of bleomycin degradative enzymes in that tissue.

Excretion – 60% to 70% of an administered dose is recovered in the urine as active bleomycin. In patients with a creatinine clearance of greater than 35 mL/min, the plasma terminal elimination half-life is approximately 115 minutes.

Special populations –

Renal function impairment: At Ccr less than 35 mL/min, the plasma terminal elimination half-life increases exponentially as the creatinine clearance decreases. It was reported that patients with moderately severe renal failure excreted less than 20% of the dose in the urine. This result would suggest that severe renal impairment could lead to accumulation of the drug in blood.

➤*Clinical trials:* The safety and efficacy of 60 units bleomycin and 1 g tetracycline as treatment for malignant pleural effusion were evaluated in a multicenter, randomized trial. Overall survival did not differ between the 60 units bleomycin (n = 44) and tetracycline (n = 41) groups. Of patients evaluated within 30 days of instillation, the recurrence rate was 36% (10/28) with bleomycin and 67% (18/27) with tetracycline (*P* = 0.023). Toxicity was similar between groups.

Contraindications

Hypersensitivity or idiosyncratic reaction to bleomycin sulfate (see Warnings).

Warnings

➤*Idiosyncratic reactions:* Idiosyncratic reactions similar to anaphylaxis have been reported in approximately 1% of lymphoma patients. These reactions (eg, hypotension, confusion, fever, chills, wheezing) may be immediate or delayed for several hours and usually occur after the first or second dose; careful and frequent monitoring is essential during and after therapy. Refer to Management of Acute Hypersensitivity Reactions.

➤*Skin toxicity:* Skin toxicity, a relatively late manifestation, appears to be related to the cumulative dose; it usually develops in the second and third week of treatment after administration of 150 to 200 units of the drug (see Adverse Reactions).

➤*Pulmonary toxicities:* Pulmonary toxicities, the most serious side effect, occur in 10% of treated patients. In approximately 1%, the drug-induced nonspecific pneumonitis progresses to pulmonary fibrosis and death. Although this is age- and dose-related, it is unpredictable. It is more common in patients older than 70 years of age and in those receiving more than 400 units total dose. However, pulmonary toxicity has been seen in young patients receiving low doses.

BLEOMYCIN SULFATE (BLM)

Identifying pulmonary toxicity is extremely difficult because of lack of specificity of the clinical syndrome. The earliest symptom is dyspnea; the earliest sign is fine rales.

Radiographically, the pneumonitis produces nonspecific patchy opacities, usually of the lower lung field. Pulmonary function tests show a decrease in total lung volume and vital capacity. These changes do not predict fibrosis development.

The nonspecific microscopic tissue changes include bronchiolar squamous metaplasia, reactive macrophages, atypical alveolar epithelial cells, fibrinous edema, and interstitial fibrosis. The acute stage may involve capillary changes and subsequent fibrinous exudation into alveoli, producing a change similar to hyaline membrane formation and progressing to a diffuse interstitial fibrosis resembling the Hamman-Rich syndrome.

Because of bleomycin's sensitization of lung tissue, patients are at greater risk of developing pulmonary toxicity when oxygen is given in surgery. Long exposure to very high oxygen concentrations is a known cause of lung damage; however, after bleomycin administration, lung damage can occur at concentrations usually considered safe. Suggested preventive measures are to maintain inspired oxygen fraction (FI O_2) at concentrations approximating that of room air (25%) during surgery and the postoperative period and to carefully monitor fluid replacement, focusing more on colloid administration rather than crystalloid.

Sudden onset of an acute chest pain syndrome suggestive of pleuropericarditis has occurred rarely during bleomycin sulfate infusions. Evaluate each patient individually, but further courses of bleomycin do not appear to be contraindicated.

➤*Renal/Hepatic function impairment:* At Ccr less than 35 mL/min, the plasma terminal elimination half-life increases exponentially as the creatinine clearance decreases. Renal or hepatic toxicity, beginning as a deterioration in renal or liver function tests, has occurred infrequently. These toxicities may occur at any time.

➤*Carcinogenesis:* Bleomycin has caused an increased incidence of nodular hyperplasia, fibrosarcomas, and various renal tumors in rats.

➤*Mutagenesis:* Bleomycin has been shown to be mutagenic in vitro and in vivo.

➤*Pregnancy: Category D.* Bleomycin can cause fetal harm when administered to a pregnant woman. There have been no studies in pregnant women. If bleomycin is used during pregnancy, or if the patient becomes pregnant while receiving this drug, apprise the patient of the potential hazard to the fetus. Advise women of childbearing age to avoid becoming pregnant during therapy.

It has been shown to be teratogenic in rats. Administration of intraperitoneal doses of 1.5 mg/kg/day to rats (about 1.6 times the recommended human dose on a unit/m² basis) on days 6 through 15 of gestation caused skeletal malformations, shortened innominate artery, and hydroureter. Bleomycin is an abortifacient but is not teratogenic in rabbits, at IV doses of 1.2 mg/kg/day (about 2.4 times the recommended human dose on a unit/m² basis) given on gestation days 6 through 18.

➤*Lactation:* It is not known whether this drug is excreted in breast milk. Because of the potential for serious adverse reactions in breastfeeding infants, it is recommended that breastfeeding be discontinued by women receiving therapy.

➤*Children:* Safety and efficacy of bleomycin have not been established.

Precautions

➤*Monitoring:* Frequent roentgenograms are recommended.

Take chest x-rays every 1 to 2 weeks to monitor the onset of pulmonary toxicity. If changes are noted, discontinue treatment until it is determined if they are drug related. Sequential measurements of the pulmonary diffusion capacity for carbon monoxide (DL_{co}) may indicate subclinical pulmonary toxicity. Monitor the DL_{co} monthly; discontinue the drug when the DL_{co} falls below 30% to 35% of the pretreatment value. Because of bleomycin's sensitization of lung tissue, patients are at greater risk of developing pulmonary toxicity when oxygen is given in surgery. Long exposure to very high oxygen concentrations is a known cause of lung damage; however, after bleomycin administration, lung damage can occur at concentrations usually considered safe. Suggested preventive measures are to maintain FI O_2 at concentrations approximating that of room air (25%) during surgery and the postoperative period and to carefully monitor fluid replacement, focusing more on colloid administration rather than crystalloid.

➤*Chest tube drainage:* It is generally accepted that chest tube drainage must be less than 100 mL in a 24-hour period prior to sclerosis. However, bleomycin instillation may be appropriate when drainage is between 100 and 300 mL under clinical conditions that necessitate sclerosis therapy. Clamp thoracostomy tube after bleomycin therapy. Move patient from supine to the left and right lateral positions several times during the next 4 hours, then remove clamp and reestablish suction.

Drug Interactions

Bleomycin Drug Interactions			
Precipitant drug	Object drug*		Description
Bleomycin	Digoxin	↓	Digoxin serum levels may be decreased by combination chemotherapy (including bleomycin). Digoxin capsules do not appear to be affected. Monitor patients for signs of reduction in pharmacologic effect (eg, deteriorating heart failure). Increase digoxin dose if necessary; serum level monitoring may facilitate tailoring dosage.
Bleomycin	Phenytoin	↓	Phenytoin serum concentrations may be decreased by combination chemotherapy. Monitor serum phenytoin levels and adjust the phenytoin dosage appropriately. IV phenytoin may be useful.
Oxygen	Bleomycin	↑	Risk for pulmonary toxicity is increased (see Warnings).
Bleomycin	Oxygen		

* ↑ = Object drug increased. ↓ = Object drug decreased.

Adverse Reactions

➤*Pulmonary:* Pneumonitis, pulmonary fibrosis (see Warnings).

➤*Idiosyncratic reactions:* In approximately 1% of the lymphoma patients treated with bleomycin, an idiosyncratic reaction, similar to clinical anaphylaxis, has been reported. The reaction may be immediate or delayed for several hours and usually occurs after the first or second dose. It consists of chills, fever, hypotension, mental confusion, and wheezing. Treatment is symptomatic including antihistamines, corticosteroids, pressor agents, and volume expansion.

➤*Integument and mucous membranes:* Alopecia, erythema, hyperkeratosis, hyperpigmentation, nail changes, pruritus, rash, skin tenderness, stomatitis, striae, vesiculation (approximately 50%). Drug therapy was stopped in 2% of patients because of these toxicities (see Warnings).

➤*Intrapleural administration:* Pulmonary adverse events that may be related to the intrapleural administration of bleomycin have been reported rarely.

Intrapleural administration of bleomycin has occasionally been associated with local pain. Hypotension possibly requiring symptomatic treatment has been reported infrequently. Death has been very rarely reported in association with bleomycin pleurodesis in these very seriously ill patients.

➤*Miscellaneous:* Chills, fever, vomiting (frequent); anorexia, weight loss (common, may persist long after termination of the drug); pain at tumor site, phlebitis, and other local reactions (infrequent).

➤*Combination therapy:* Vascular toxicities coincident with the use of bleomycin in combination with other antineoplastics occur rarely. The events are clinically heterogeneous and may include cerebral arteritis, cerebrovascular accident, MI, or thrombotic microangiopathy. There also are reports of Raynaud phenomenon with bleomycin with vinblastine with or without cisplatin or, in a few cases, bleomycin as a single agent. It is currently unknown if the cause of Raynaud phenomenon in these cases is the disease, underlying vascular compromise, bleomycin, vinblastine, hypomagnesemia, or a combination of any of these factors.

Sudden onset of an acute chest pain syndrome suggestive of pleuropericarditis has occurred rarely during bleomycin sulfate infusions. Evaluate each patient individually, but further courses of bleomycin do not appear to be contraindicated.

➤*Postmarketing:* Malaise, scleroderma-like skin changes.

Patient Information

Inform patient that this medicine will be prepared and administered by a health care provider in a health care facility.

Advise patient to contact a health care provider immediately if any of the following side effects occur: Chest pain, chills, confusion, fever, wheezing.

Advise patient to stop smoking or smoke less while taking bleomycin; coughing, wheezing, and shortness of breath may be worse if they smoke cigars, cigarettes, or pipe tobacco.

Advise patient not to take any other OTC or prescription medications or dietary supplements without consulting the health care provider.

Advise patients with other medical conditions to consult the health care provider before taking bleomycin.

Inform patients to keep appointments and that lab tests will be required to monitor therapy.

DACTINOMYCIN (Actinomycin D; ACT)

Rx	Cosmegen (Merck)	Powder for Injection, lyophilized: 0.5 mg	In vials.[1]

[1] With 20 mg mannitol.

> **WARNING**
>
> Dactinomycin is extremely corrosive to soft tissue. If extravasation occurs during IV use, severe damage to soft tissues will occur. In at least one instance, this has led to contracture of the arms.

Indications

➤*Wilms' tumor:* Combinations with vincristine, radiotherapy and surgery.

➤*Rhabdomyosarcoma:* Combinations with vincristine, cyclophosphamide and doxorubicin.

➤*Metastatic and nonmetastatic choriocarcinoma:* Combination with methotrexate.

➤*Nonseminomatous testicular carcinoma:* For the treatment of nonseminomatous testicular carcinoma.

➤*Ewing's sarcoma:* Palliative treatment alone, with other antineoplastics or x-ray.

Nonmetastatic Ewing's – Cyclosphosphamide and radiotherapy.

➤*Sarcoma botryoides:* Palliative treatment alone, with other antineoplastics or radiotherapy.

➤*Radiation therapy:* Radiation therapy effects may be potentiated by dactinomycin; the converse also appears likely. Dactinomycin may be tried in radiosensitive tumors not responding to x-ray therapy. Objective improvement in tumor size and activity may be observed when lower, better tolerated doses of both types of therapy are employed.

➤*Perfusion technique:* Dactinomycin alone or with other antineoplastics has been given by the isolation-perfusion technique, either as palliative treatment or as an adjunct to tumor resection; some tumors resistant to chemotherapy and radiation therapy may respond. Neoplasms in which dactinomycin has been tried using this technique include various types of sarcoma, carcinoma and adenocarcinoma. This technique offers advantages, provided drug leakage into the general circulation is minimal. By this technique the drug is in continuous contact with the tumor for the duration of treatment. The dose may be increased well over that used by the systemic route, usually without added toxicity.

Administration and Dosage

Toxic reactions are frequent and may limit the amount of drug that may be given. Severity of toxicity varies and is only partly dependent on dose. Administer the drug in short courses.

➤*IV:* Individualize dosage. Do not exceed 15 mcg/kg or 400 to 600 mcg/m² daily IV for 5 days. Calculate the dosage for obese or edematous patients on the basis of surface area in an effort to relate dosage to lean body mass.

Adults – 0.5 mg/day IV for a maximum of 5 days.

Children – 0.015 mg/kg/day IV for 5 days. Alternative schedule is a total dosage of 2.5 mg/m² IV over 1 week.

In both adults and children, administer a second course after at least 3 weeks, provided all signs of toxicity have disappeared.

➤*Isolation-perfusion technique:* 0.05 mg/kg for lower extremity or pelvis; 0.035 mg/kg for upper extremity. Use lower doses in obese patients, or when previous therapy has been employed. Complications are related to amount of drug that escapes into systemic circulation.

Use "two-needle technique" if given directly into the vein without use of an infusion. Reconstitute and withdraw dose from vial with one sterile needle. Use another needle for direct injection into vein.

➤*Preparation of solution:* Reconstitute by adding 1.1 ml Sterile Water for Injection (without preservative). The resulting solution contains approximately 0.5 mg/ml. Add directly to infusion solutions of 5% Dextrose or Sodium Chloride Injection or to the tubing of a running IV infusion. Although chemically stable after reconstitution, the product does not contain a preservative; discard any unused portion. Use of water that contains preservatives (benzyl alcohol or parabens) to reconstitute the drug for injection results in precipitate formation.

Partial removal of dactinomycin from IV solutions by cellulose ester membrane filters used in some IV in-line filters has been reported.

➤*Storage/Stability:* Protect from light.

Actions

➤*Pharmacology:* Dactinomycin is the principal component of the mixture of actinomycins produced by *Streptomyces parvullus*. Dactinomycin exerts an inhibitory effect on gram-positive and gram-negative bacteria and on some fungi. However, its toxic properties preclude its use as an antibiotic in treating infectious diseases.

Dactinomycin anchors into a purine-pyrimidine (DNA) base pair by intercalation, inhibiting messenger RNA synthesis. Although maximal cell-kill is noted in G_1 phase, the cytotoxic action is primarily cell cycle nonspecific. Actively proliferating cells are more sensitive.

➤*Pharmacokinetics:* Very little active drug can be detected in circulating blood 2 minutes after IV injection. It concentrates in nucleated cells and does not cross the blood-brain barrier. Dactinomycin is minimally metabolized. Plasma half-life is ≈ 36 hours.

Contraindications

If given at or about the time of infection with chicken pox or herpes zoster, a severe generalized disease may occur, which could result in death.

Warnings

➤*Radiation:* With combined dactinomycin-radiation therapy, the normal skin, as well as the buccal and pharyngeal mucosa, show early erythema. A smaller than usual x-ray dose, when given with dactinomycin, causes erythema and vesiculation which progress more rapidly through the tanning and desquamation stages. Healing may occur in 4 to 6 weeks rather than 2 to 3 months. Erythema from previous x-ray therapy may be reactivated by dactinomycin alone, even when irradiation occurred many months earlier, and especially when the interval between the two forms of therapy is brief. When the nasopharynx is irradiated, the combination may produce severe oropharyngeal mucositis. Severe reactions may appear if high doses are used or if the patient is particularly sensitive to such combined therapy.

Increased incidence of GI toxicity and marrow suppression has occurred when dactinomycin was given with x-ray therapy. Use particular caution in the first 2 months after irradiation for the treatment of right-sided Wilms' tumor, since hepatomegaly and elevated AST levels have been noted.

Reports indicate an increased incidence of second primary tumors following treatment with radiation and dactinomycin.

➤*Carcinogenesis:* The International Agency on Research on Cancer has judged that dactinomycin is a positive carcinogen in animals. Local sarcomas were produced in mice and rats after repeated SC or intraperitoneal injection. Mesenchymal tumors occurred in male rats given intraperitoneal injections of 0.05 mg/kg, 2 to 5 times per week for 18 weeks. The first tumor appeared at 23 weeks.

➤*Mutagenesis:* Dactinomycin has been mutagenic in a number of test systems in vitro and in vivo including human fibroblasts and leukocytes, and HELA cells. DNA damage and cytogenetic effects have been demonstrated in the mouse and the rat.

➤*Pregnancy: Category C.* The drug has caused malformations and embryotoxicity in the rat, rabbit and hamster in doses 3 to 7 times the maximum recommended human dose. There are no adequate and well controlled studies in pregnant women. Safety for use during pregnancy has not been established. Use only when clearly needed and when potential benefits outweigh potential hazards to the fetus.

➤*Lactation:* It is not known whether this drug is excreted in breast milk. Because of the potential for serious adverse reactions in nursing infants decide whether to discontinue nursing or to discontinue the drug, taking into account the importance of the drug to the mother.

Infants – Do not give to infants < 6 to 12 months of age because of greater frequency of toxic effects.

Precautions

Reactions may involve any body tissue; anaphylactoid reactions may occur.

➤*Nausea and vomiting:* Nausea and vomiting due to dactinomycin necessitates intermittent administration. Observe the patient daily for toxic side effects when multiple chemotherapy is used; a full course of therapy occasionally is not tolerated. If stomatitis, diarrhea or severe hematopoietic depression appear, discontinue use until the patient has recovered.

➤*Renal, hepatic and bone marrow function:* Many abnormalities have occurred.

➤*This drug is highly toxic:* Handle and administer both powder and solution with care. Avoid inhalation of dust or vapors and contact with skin or mucous membranes, especially those of the eyes. Should accidental eye contact occur, immediately institute copious irrigation with water, followed by prompt ophthalmologic consultation. Should accidental skin contact occur, immediately irrigate the affected part with copious amounts of water for at least 15 minutes.

➤*Extravasation:* Dactinomycin is extremely corrosive. Extravasation during IV administration causes severe damage to soft tissues. This has led to contracture of the arms in at least one instance. If extravasation occurs, immediately discontinue the infusion. Apply cold compresses to the area. Local infiltration with an injectable corticosteroid may lessen the local reaction. Dilute the drug by infusing saline injection through the line into the infiltrated area.

Drug Interactions

➤*Drug/Lab test interactions:* Dactinomycin may interfere with bioassay procedures for the determination of antibacterial drug levels.

DACTINOMYCIN (Actinomycin D; ACT)

Adverse Reactions

Toxic effects usually do not become apparent until 2 to 4 days after a course of therapy and may not be maximal before 1 to 2 weeks. Adverse reactions are usually reversible with discontinuation of therapy.

➤*Dermatologic:* Alopecia; skin eruptions; acne; flare-up of erythema; increased pigmentation of previously irradiated skin.

➤*GI:* Cheilitis; dysphagia; esophagitis; ulcerative stomatitis; pharyngitis; anorexia; abdominal pain; diarrhea; GI ulceration; proctitis; liver toxicity (including ascites, hepatomegaly, hepatitis and liver function test abnormalities). Alleviate nausea and vomiting occurring during the first few hours after use by giving antiemetics.

➤*Hematologic:* Anemia (including aplastic anemia); agranulocytosis; leukopenia; thrombocytopenia; pancytopenia; reticulopenia. Perform platelet and white cell counts daily. If either count markedly decreases, withhold drug until marrow recovery occurs; this often takes up to 3 weeks.

➤*Miscellaneous:* Malaise; fatigue; lethargy; fever; myalgia; hypocalcemia; death.

Perfusion technique – Complications may consist of hematopoietic depression, absorption of toxic products from massive destruction of neoplastic tissue, increased susceptibility to infection, impaired wound healing and superficial ulceration of the gastric mucosa. Other side effects may include edema of the extremity involved, damage to soft tissues of the perfused area and (potentially) venous thrombosis.

MITOMYCIN (Mitomycin-C; MTC)

| Rx | Mutamycin (Bristol-Myers Oncology) | Powder for Injection: 5, 20 and 40 mg | 10, 40 and 80 mg mannitol, respectively. In vials. |

WARNING

Bone marrow suppression: Bone marrow suppression, notably thrombocytopenia and leukopenia, which may contribute to overwhelming infection in an already compromised patient, is the most common and severe toxic effect (see Warnings and Adverse Reactions).

Hemolytic uremic syndrome: Hemolytic uremic syndrome, a serious syndrome of microangiopathic hemolytic anemia, thrombocytopenia and irreversible renal failure has occurred (see Warnings).

Indications

Therapy of disseminated adenocarcinoma of stomach or pancreas with other chemotherapeutic agents, and as palliative treatment when other modalities fail.

➤*Unlabeled uses:* Mitomycin has been given by the intravesical route for the management of superficial bladder cancer. Mitomycin as an ophthalmic solution appears beneficial as an adjunct to surgical excision in primary or recurrent pterygia.

Administration and Dosage

Give IV only. If extravasation occurs, cellulitis, ulceration and sloughing may result.

After hematological recovery (see dosage adjustment guide) from previous chemotherapy use 20 mg/m^2 IV as a single dose at 6 to 8 week intervals.

Because of cumulative myelosuppression, reevaluate patients after each course of therapy; reduce dose if patient experiences any toxicity. Doses> 20 mg/m^2 are not more effective, and are more toxic than lower doses. Do not repeat dosage until leukocyte count has returned to 4000/mm^3 and platelet count to 100,000/mm^3. If disease continues to progress after two courses, discontinue; chances of response are minimal. When used with other myelosuppressives, adjust dosage appropriately.

Dosage Adjustment for Mitomycin		
Nadir after prior dose per mm^3		% of prior dose to be given
Leukocytes	Platelets	
> 4000	> 100,000	100
3000-3999	75,000-99,999	100
2000-2999	25,000-74,999	70
< 2000	< 25,000	50

➤*Preparation of solution:* Reconstitute 5, 20 or 40 mg vial with 10, 40 or 80 ml Sterile Water for Injection, respectively. If product does not dissolve immediately, allow to stand at room temperature until solution is obtained.

➤*Storage/Stability:* Avoid excessive heat (> 40°C). Reconstituted with Sterile Water for Injection to 0.5 mg/ml, solution is stable for 14 days under refrigeration, 7 days at room temp.

Diluted in various IV fluids at room temperature to a concentration of 20 to 40 mcg/ml, stability is as follows: 5% Dextrose Injection, 3 hours; 0.9% NaCl Injection, 12 hours; Sodium Lactate Injection, 24 hours.

The combination of mitomycin (5 to 15 mg) and heparin (1000 to 10,000 units) in 30 ml of 0.9% NaCl Injection is stable for 48 hours at room temperature.

Actions

➤*Pharmacology:* Mitomycin is an antibiotic with antitumor activity isolated from *Streptomyces caespitosus.* It selectively inhibits the synthesis of deoxyribonucleic acid (DNA). The guanine and cytosine content correlates with the degree of mitomycin-induced cross-linking. At high concentrations, cellular ribonucleic acid (RNA) and protein synthesis are also suppressed.

➤*Pharmacokinetics:*

Absorption/Distribution – IV mitomycin is rapidly cleared from the serum. Maximal serum concentrations were 2.4 mcg/ml after IV injection of 30 mg; 1.7 mcg/ml after a 20 mg dose, and 0.52 mcg/ml after 10 mg. Serum half-life after a 30 mg bolus injection is 17 minutes.

Metabolism/Excretion – Clearance is effected primarily by hepatic metabolism, but metabolism occurs in other tissues as well. Clearance rate is inversely proportional to maximal serum concentration due to saturation of degradative pathways. About 10% of a dose is excreted unchanged in urine. Because of saturable metabolic pathways, the percent excreted in urine increases with increasing dose.

Contraindications

Primary therapy as a single agent; to replace surgery or radiotherapy; hypersensitivity or idiosyncratic reaction to mitomycin; patients with thrombocytopenia, coagulation disorder or an increase in bleeding tendency due to other causes.

Warnings

➤*Bone marrow suppression:* Bone marrow suppression, particularly thrombocytopenia and leukopenia, occurring in 64% of patients, is the most serious toxicity and is cumulative. Thrombocytopenia or leukopenia may occur any time within 8 weeks (average 4 weeks) of therapy; recovery after therapy is within 10 weeks. About 25% of the patients did not recover.

Perform the following during and for at least 8 weeks following therapy: Platelet count, WBC, differential and hemoglobin. A platelet count < 100,000/mm^3 or a WBC < 4000/mm^3, or a progressive decline in either, is an indication to interrupt therapy. Observe patients frequently during and after therapy. Advise patients of potential toxicity, particularly bone marrow suppression. Deaths have occurred due to septicemia as a result of leukopenia.

➤*Renal function impairment:* Observe patients for evidence of renal toxicity. Do not give to patients with a serum creatinine > 1.7 mg/dl.

➤*Carcinogenesis:* At doses approximating the recommended clinical dose in man, mitomycin produces a 50% to 100% increase in tumor incidence in rats and mice.

➤*Pregnancy:* Safety for use during pregnancy has not been established. Teratological changes have been noted in animal studies.

Precautions

➤*Adult respiratory distress syndrome:* A few cases have occurred in patients receiving mitomycin in combination with other chemotherapy and maintained at FIO$_2$ concentrations> 50% perioperatively. Exercise caution to use only enough oxygen to provide adequate arterial saturation since oxygen itself is toxic to the lungs. Pay careful attention to fluid balance; avoid overhydration.

Drug Interactions

➤*Vinca alkaloids:* Acute shortness of breath and severe bronchospasm have occurred following use of vinca alkaloids in patients who had previously or simultaneously received mitomycin. Onset of this acute respiratory distress occurs within minutes to hours after the vinca alkaloid injection. Total number of doses for each drug varies considerably. Bronchodilators, steroids or oxygen produce symptomatic relief.

Adverse Reactions

Bone marrow toxicity: (64%) – Thrombocytopenia and leukopenia (see Warnings).

➤*Integument and mucous membrane: (4%):* Cellulitis at injection site is occasionally severe; stomatitis; alopecia. Rashes occur rarely.

Extravasation: The most important dermatological problem with this drug is necrosis and consequent tissue sloughing if the drug is extravasated during injection, which may occur with or without stinging or burning and even if there is adequate blood return when the needle is aspirated. Delayed erythema or ulceration may occur either at or distant from injection site, weeks to months after use, even when no evidence of extravasation was seen during use. For management, see Antineoplastics Introduction.

➤*Renal:* 2% of 1281 patients had a significant rise in serum creatinine. There was no correlation between total dose or duration of therapy and degree of renal impairment.

Pulmonary toxicity – Infrequent, but can be severe or life-threatening. Dyspnea with nonproductive cough and radiographic evidence of

MITOMYCIN (Mitomycin-C; MTC)

pulmonary infiltrates may indicate pulmonary toxicity. If other etiologies are eliminated, discontinue therapy. Steroids have been used to treat this toxicity, but therapeutic value is not determined. Adult respiratory distress syndrome may also occur (see Precautions).

Hemolytic uremic syndrome (HUS) – This serious complication of chemotherapy, consisting primarily of microangiopathic hemolytic anemia (hematocrit ≤ 25%), thrombocytopenia (≤ 100,000/mm³) and irreversible renal failure (serum creatinine ≥ 16 mg/dl) has occurred in patients receiving mitomycin. Microangiopathic hemolysis with fragmented red blood cells on peripheral blood smears has occurred in 98% of patients with the syndrome. Other less frequent complications may include: Pulmonary edema (65%); neurologic abnormalities (16%); hypertension. Exacerbation of the symptoms associated with HUS has occurred in some patients receiving blood product transfusions. A high mortality rate (52%) has been associated with HUS.

The syndrome may occur at any time during therapy with mitomycin as a single agent or in combination with other cytotoxic drugs. Closely monitor patients receiving ≥ 60 mg for unexplained anemia with fragmented cells on peripheral blood smear, thrombocytopenia and decreased renal function.

Acute side effects (14%) – Fever; anorexia; nausea; vomiting.

➤*Miscellaneous:* Headache; blurred vision; confusion; drowsiness; syncope; fatigue; edema; thrombophlebitis; hematemesis; diarrhea; pain. These did not appear to be dose-related and were not unequivocally drug-related.

TESTOLACTONE

c-iii　**Teslac** (Bristol-Myers Squibb)　**Tablets:** 50 mg　Lactose. (690). White, biconvex. In 100s.

This is an abbreviated monograph. For complete information on Androgens, see the group monograph in the Endocrine/Metabolic chapter.

Indications

Adjunctive therapy in the palliative treatment of advanced disseminated breast carcinoma in postmenopausal women when hormonal therapy is indicated.

Premenopausal women with disseminated breast carcinoma in whom ovarian function has been subsequently terminated.

Administration and Dosage

Administer 250 mg 4 times daily. To evaluate response, continue therapy for a minimum of 3 months, unless there is active disease progression.

Actions

➤*Pharmacology:* The precise mechanism by which testolactone produces a clinical antineoplastic effect is unknown. Testolactone's principal action appears to be inhibition of steroid aromatase activity and consequent reduction in estrone synthesis from adrenal androstenedione, the major source of estrogen in postmenopausal women. Based on in vitro studies, the aromatase inhibition may be noncompetitive and irreversible. This phenomenon may account for the persistence of testolactone's effect on estrogen synthesis after drug withdrawal.

Testolactone is effective in 15% of patients with advanced or disseminated mammary cancer.

Testolactone is well absorbed from the GI tract. It is metabolized to several derivatives in the liver, all of which preserve the lactone D-ring. These metabolites, as well as some unmetabolized drug, are excreted in the urine. Additional pharmacokinetic data in humans are unavailable.

Contraindications

Carcinoma of the male breast; hypersensitivity to the drug.

Warnings

➤*Pregnancy: Category C.* Testolactone is intended for use in postmenopausal women and is not indicated for use during pregnancy.

➤*Lactation:* It is not known whether this drug is excreted in breast milk. Decide whether to discontinue nursing or to discontinue the drug, taking into account the importance of the drug to the mother.

➤*Children:* Safety and efficacy have not been established.

Precautions

➤*Monitoring:* Routinely monitor plasma calcium levels in any patient receiving therapy for mammary cancer, particularly during periods of active remission of bony metastases. If hypercalcemia occurs, institute appropriate measures.

The usual precautions pertaining to use of androgens apply (see the Androgen group monograph in the Endocrine/Metabolic chapter).

Consult the physician regarding missed doses.

Drug Interactions

➤*Anticoagulants, oral:* Pharmacologic effects may be increased by testolactone; monitor and adjust the anticoagulant dose accordingly.

➤*Drug/Lab test interactions:* Physiologic effects of testolactone may result in decreased estradiol concentrations with radioimmunoassays for estradiol, increased plasma calcium concentrations and increased 24 hour urinary excretion of creatine and 17-ketosteroids.

Adverse Reactions

➤*CNS:* Paresthesia.

➤*GI:* Glossitis; anorexia; nausea; vomiting.

➤*Miscellaneous:* Maculopapular erythema; aches and edema of the extremities; alopecia; nail growth disturbances (rare); increase in blood pressure.

Patient Information

Notify physician if numbness or tingling of fingers, toes, or face occurs.

Contraceptive measures are recommended during treatment.

Medication may cause diarrhea, loss of appetite, nausea, vomiting, loss of hair, swelling or redness of the tongue; notify physician if these become pronounced.

BICALUTAMIDE

Rx	**Casodex** (AstraZeneca)	**Tablets:** 50 mg	Lactose. (CDX50 Casodex). White. Film-coated. In 30s, 100s, and UD 30s.

Indications

➤*Prostate cancer:* For use in combination therapy with a luteinizing hormone-releasing hormone (LHRH) analog for the treatment of Stage D_2 metastatic carcinoma of the prostate.

Administration and Dosage

➤*Approved by the FDA:* October 4, 1995.

The recommended dose for bicalutamide therapy in combination with an LHRH analog is one 50 mg tablet once daily (morning or evening), with or without food. It is recommended that bicalutamide be taken at the same time each day. Start bicalutamide treatment at the same time as treatment with an LHRH analog.

➤*Storage/Stability:* Store at controlled room temperature 20° to 25°C (68° to 77°F).

Actions

➤*Pharmacology:* Bicalutamide is a nonsteroidal antiandrogen. It competitively inhibits the action of androgens by binding to cytosol androgen receptors in the target tissue. Prostatic carcinoma is known to be androgen-sensitive and responds to treatment that counteracts the effect of androgen or removes the source of androgen.

In clinical trials with bicalutamide as a single agent for prostate cancer, rises in serum testosterone and estradiol have been noted. When bicalutamide is combined with LHRH analog therapy, bicalutamide does not affect the suppression of serum testosterone induced by the LHRH analog.

➤*Pharmacokinetics:*

Absorption/Distribution – Bicalutamide is well-absorbed following oral administration, although the absolute bioavailability is unknown. Coadministration with food has no clinically significant effect on rate or extent of absorption. Bicalutamide is highly protein-bound (96%).

Metabolism/Excretion – Bicalutamide undergoes stereospecific metabolism. The S-(inactive) isomer is metabolized primarily by glucuronidation. The R-(active) isomer also undergoes glucuronidation but is predominantly oxidized to an inactive metabolite followed by glucuronidation. Both the parent and metabolite glucuronides are eliminated in the urine and feces. The S-enantiomer is rapidly cleared relative to the R-enantiomer, with the R-enantiomer accounting for ≈ 99% of total steady-state plasma levels. In healthy males, apparent oral clearance of the active enantiomer is 0.32 L/hr, peak concentration (single-dose) is 0.77 mcg/mL, time to peak concentration (single-dose) is 31.3 hours, and half-life is 5.8 days. Mean steady-state concentration of the active enantiomer in patients with prostate cancer is 8.9 mcg/mL.

➤*Clinical trials:* In a large multicenter, double-blind, controlled clinical trial, 813 patients with previously untreated advanced prostate cancer were randomized to receive bicalutamide 50 mg once daily (404 patients) or flutamide 250 mg (409 patients) 3 times per day, each in combination with LHRH analogs (either goserelin acetate implant or leuprolide acetate depot). After a median follow-up of 160 weeks was reached, 52.7% of patients treated with bicalutamide-LHRH analog therapy and 57.5% of patients treated with flutamide-LHRH analog therapy had died.

Contraindications

Hypersensitivity to the drug or any of the components of the product; pregnancy (see Warnings).

Warnings

➤*Hepatotoxicity:* Rare cases of death or hospitalization because of severe liver injury have been reported postmarketing in association with the use of bicalutamide. Hepatotoxicity in these reports generally occurred within the first 3 to 4 months of treatment. Hepatitis or marked increases in liver enzymes leading to drug discontinuation occurred in ≈ 1% of bicalutamide patients in controlled clinical trials.

Measure serum transaminase levels prior to starting treatment with bicalutamide, at regular intervals for the first 4 months of treatment, and periodically thereafter. If clinical symptoms or signs suggestive of liver dysfunction occur (eg, nausea, vomiting, abdominal pain, fatigue, anorexia, "flu-like" symptoms, dark urine, jaundice, right upper quadrant tenderness), measure the serum transaminases immediately, in particular the serum ALT. If at any time a patient has jaundice, or their ALT rises above 2 times the upper limit of normal, immediately discontinue bicalutamide, with close follow-up of liver function.

➤*Gynecomastia/Breast pain:* In clinical trials with bicalutamide as a single agent for prostate cancer, gynecomastia and breast pain were reported in up to 38% and 39% of patients, respectively.

➤*Women:* Bicalutamide has no indication for women and should not be used in this population, particularly for nonserious or non-life-threatening conditions.

➤*Hepatic function impairment:* Use bicalutamide with caution in patients with moderate-to-severe hepatic impairment. Bicalutamide is extensively metabolized by the liver. The half-life of the R-enantiomer was increased ≈ 76% (5.9 and 10.4 days for normal and impaired patients, respectively) in patients with severe liver disease (n = 4). Limited data in subjects with severe hepatic impairment suggest that excretion of bicalutamide may be delayed and could lead to further accumulation. Consider periodic liver function tests for hepatic impaired patients on long-term therapy (see Hepatotoxicity). No dosage adjustment is necessary for patients with mild-to-moderate hepatic impairment.

➤*Carcinogenesis:* Two-year oral carcinogenicity studies were conducted in male and female rats and mice. A variety of tumor target organ effects were identified and were attributed to the antiandrogenicity of bicalutamide, namely, testicular benign interstitial (Leydig) cell tumors in male rats and uterine adenocarcinoma in female rats. There is no evidence of Leydig cell hyperplasia in humans; uterine tumors are not relevant to the indicated patient population. A small increase in the incidence of hepatocellular carcinoma in male mice and an increased incidence of benign thyroid follicular cell adenomas in rats were recorded.

➤*Fertility impairment:* Administration of bicalutamide may lead to inhibition of spermatogenesis. In male rats the precoital interval and time to successful mating were increased in the first pairing, but no effects on fertility following successful mating were seen. These effects were reversed by 7 weeks after the end of an 11-week period of dosing. Administration of bicalutamide to pregnant females resulted in feminization of the male offspring, leading to hypospadias at all dose levels. Affected male offspring were also impotent.

➤*Pregnancy: Category X.* Bicalutamide may cause fetal harm when administered to pregnant women. The male offspring of rats receiving doses of ≥ 10 mg/kg/day (plasma drug concentrations in rats equal to ≈ ⅔ human therapeutic concentrations) were observed to have reduced anogenital distance and hypospadias in reproductive toxicology studies. These pharmacological effects have been observed with other antiandrogens. Bicalutamide is contraindicated in women who are or may become pregnant. If this drug is used during pregnancy, or if the patient becomes pregnant while taking this drug, apprise the patient of the potential hazard to the fetus.

➤*Lactation:* Bicalutamide is not indicated for use in women. It is not known whether this drug is excreted in breast milk. Exercise caution when administering to a nursing woman.

➤*Children:* Safety and efficacy in children have not been established. Because of the mechanism of action and the indication, bicalutamide has not been studied in pediatric subjects.

Precautions

➤*Monitoring:* Regular assessments of serum Prostate Specific Antigen (PSA) may be helpful in monitoring the patient's response. If PSA levels rise during therapy, evaluate the patient for clinical progression. For patients who have objective progression of disease together with an elevated PSA, consider a treatment-free period of antiandrogens while continuing the LHRH analog.

Measure serum transaminase levels prior to starting treatment with bicalutamide, at regular intervals for the first 4 months of treatment, and periodically thereafter (see Hepatotoxicity).

Drug Interactions

➤*Anticoagulants:* In vitro bicalutamide can displace coumarin anticoagulants (eg, warfarin), from their protein-binding sites. It is recommended that if bicalutamide is started in patients already receiving coumarin anticoagulants, closely monitor prothrombin times and adjust the anticoagulant dose if necessary.

Adverse Reactions

In patients with advanced prostate cancer treated with bicalutamide in combination with an LHRH analog, the most frequent adverse reaction was hot flashes (53%).

Adverse Reactions: Bicalutamide vs Flutamide (%)		
Adverse reaction	Bicalutamide + LHRH analog (n = 401)	Flutamide + LHRH analog (n = 407)
Cardiovascular		
Hot flashes	53	53
Hypertension	8	7
CNS		
Dizziness	10	9
Paresthesia	8	10
Insomnia	7	10
Anxiety	5	2
Depression	4	8

Antiandrogens

BICALUTAMIDE

Adverse Reactions: Bicalutamide vs Flutamide (%)		
Adverse reaction	Bicalutamide + LHRH analog (n = 401)	Flutamide + LHRH analog (n = 407)
Dermatologic		
Rash	9	7
Sweating	6	5
GI		
Constipation	22	17
Nausea	15	14
Diarrhea	12	26
Increased liver enzyme test[1]	7	11
Vomiting	6	8
Dyspepsia	7	6
Flatulence	6	5
Anorexia	6	7
GU		
Nocturia	12	14
Hematuria	12	6
Urinary tract infection	9	9
Impotence	7	9
Gynecomastia	9	7
Urinary incontinence	4	8
Breast pain	6	4
Urinary frequency	6	7
Urinary retention	5	3
Urination impaired	5	4
Metabolic/Nutritional		
Peripheral edema	13	10
Hyperglycemia	6	7
Weight loss	7	10
Alkaline phosphatase increased	5	6
Weight gain	5	4
Musculoskeletal		
Bone pain	9	11
Myasthenia	7	5
Arthritis	5	7
Pathological fracture	4	8
Respiratory		
Dyspnea	13	8
Cough increased	8	6
Pharyngitis	8	6
Bronchitis	6	3
Pneumonia	4	5
Rhinitis	4	5
Miscellaneous		
Pain (general)	35	31
Back pain	25	26
Asthenia	22	21
Pelvic pain	21	17

Adverse Reactions: Bicalutamide vs Flutamide (%)		
Adverse reaction	Bicalutamide + LHRH analog (n = 401)	Flutamide + LHRH analog (n = 407)
Infection	18	14
Abdominal pain	11	11
Anemia[2]	11	13
Chest pain	8	8
Flu syndrome	7	7
Headache	7	7

[1] Increased liver enzyme test includes increases in AST, ALT, or both.
[2] Anemia includes anemia and hypochromic and iron deficiency anemia.

Other adverse reactions (≥ 2% to < 5%) reported in the bicalutamide-LHRH analog treatment group are listed below in order of decreasing frequency within each body system.

➤*Cardiovascular:* Angina pectoris; CHF; myocardial infarct; cardiac arrest; coronary artery disorder; syncope.

➤*CNS:* Hypertonia; confusion; somnolence; libido decreased; neuropathy; nervousness.

➤*Dermatologic:* Dry skin; alopecia; pruritus; herpes zoster; skin carcinoma; skin disorder.

➤*GI:* Melena; rectal hemorrhage; dry mouth; dysphagia; GI disorder; periodontal abscess; GI carcinoma.

➤*GU:* Dysuria; urinary urgency; hydronephrosis; urinary tract disorder;

➤*Lab test abnormalities:* Elevated AST, ALT, bilirubin, BUN, and creatinine and decreased hemoglobin and white cell count have been reported in both bicalutamide-LHRH analog treated and flutamide-LHRH analog treated patients.

➤*Metabolic/Nutritional:* Edema; BUN increased; creatinine increased; dehydration; gout; hypercholesterolemia.

➤*Musculoskeletal:* Myalgia; leg cramps.

➤*Respiratory:* Lung disorder; asthma; epistaxis; sinusitis.

➤*Miscellaneous:* Neoplasm; neck pain; fever; chills; sepsis; hernia; cyst; cataract specified.

➤*Postmarketing:*

Miscellaneous – Rare cases of interstitial pneumonitis and pulmonary fibrosis have been reported.

Overdosage

Long-term clinical trials have been conducted with dosages of ≤ 200 mg daily, and these dosages have been well tolerated. A single dose of bicalutamide that results in symptoms of an overdose considered life-threatening has not been established. There is no specific antidote; treatment of an overdose should be symptomatic.

In the management of an overdose with bicalutamide, vomiting may be induced if the patient is alert. Remember that, in this patient population, multiple drugs may have been taken. Dialysis is not likely to be helpful because bicalutamide is highly protein bound and is extensively metabolized. General supportive care, including frequent monitoring of vital signs and close observation of the patient, is indicated.

Patient Information

Inform patients that therapy with bicalutamide and the LHRH analog should be initiated at the same time, and that they should not interrupt or stop taking these medications without consulting their physician.

FLUTAMIDE

Rx	**Flutamide** (Eon, Ivax, Zenith Goldline)	**Capsules:** 125 mg	May contain lactose. In 100s, 180s, 500s, and UD 100s.
Rx	**Eulexin** (Schering-Plough)		Lactose, parabens, EDTA. (Schering 525). Brown. In 180s, 500s, and UD 100s.

WARNING

Hepatic injury: There have been postmarketing reports of hospitalization and rarely death from liver failure in patients taking flutamide. Evidence of hepatic injury included elevated serum transaminase levels, jaundice, hepatic encephalopathy, and death related to acute hepatic failure. The hepatic injury was reversible after discontinuation of therapy in some patients. Approximately half of the reported cases occurred within the initial 3 months of treatment with flutamide.

Measure serum transaminase levels prior to starting treatment with flutamide. Flutamide is not recommended in patients whose ALT values exceed twice the upper limit or normal. Serum transaminase levels should then be measured monthly for the first 4 months of therapy, and periodically thereafter. Also obtain liver function tests at the first signs and symptoms suggestive of liver dysfunction (eg, nausea, vomiting, abdominal pain, fatigue, anorexia, "flu-like" symptoms, hyperbilirubinuria, jaundice, right upper quadrant tenderness). If at any time a patient has jaundice, or their ALT rises > 2 times the upper limit of normal, immediately discontinue flutamide, with close follow-up of liver function tests until resolution.

Indications

➤*Prostatic carcinoma:* For use in combination with luteinizing hormone-releasing hormone (LHRH) agonists for the management of locally confined Stage B$_2$-C and Stage D$_2$ metastatic carcinoma of the prostate.

➤*Unlabeled uses:* Treatment of hirsutism in women (250 mg/day).

Administration and Dosage

➤*Approved by the FDA:* January 27, 1989.

➤*Usual dose:* Two capsules 3 times a day at 8-hour intervals for a total daily dosage of 750 mg.

➤*Stage B$_2$-C prostatic carcinoma:* Treatment with flutamide capsules and goserelin acetate implant should start 8 weeks prior to initiating radiation therapy and continue during radiation therapy.

➤*Stage D$_2$ metastatic carcinoma:* To achieve benefit from treatment, initiate flutamide capsules with the LHRH agonist and continue until progression.

➤*Storage / Stability:* Store between 2° and 30°C (36° and 86°F). Protect unit dose packages from excessive moisture.

Actions

➤*Pharmacology:* Flutamide, a nonsteroidal agent, demonstrates potent antiandrogenic effects in animal studies. It exerts its antiandrogenic action by inhibiting androgen uptake or by inhibiting nuclear binding of androgen in target tissues or both. Prostatic carcinoma is androgen-sensitive and responds to treatment that counteracts the effect of androgen or removes the source of androgen (eg, castration). Elevations of plasma testosterone and estradiol levels have been noted following flutamide administration.

➤*Pharmacokinetics:*

Absorption / Distribution – Flutamide is rapidly and completely absorbed. The alpha-hydroxylate metabolite reaches maximum plasma levels in ≈ 2 hours, indicating that it is rapidly formed from flutamide. The plasma half-life for this metabolite is ≈ 6 hours. Flutamide and alpha-hydroxylate approach steady-state plasma levels (based on pharmacokinetic simulations) after the fourth dose. The half-life of alpha-hydroxylate in elderly volunteers after a single dose is ≈ 8 hours and at steady state is 9.6 hours. Flutamide is 94% to 96% bound to plasma proteins at steady-state plasma concentrations of 24 to 78 ng/mL. Alpha-hydroxylate at steady-state plasma concentrations of 1556 to 2284 ng/mL is 92% to 94% bound to plasma proteins.

Metabolism / Excretion – Flutamide is rapidly and extensively metabolized. At least 6 metabolites have been identified in plasma. The major plasma metabolite is a biologically active alpha-hydroxylate derivative that accounts for 23% of the dose in plasma 1 hour after drug administration. Flutamide and its metabolites are excreted mainly in the urine with only 4.2% of a single dose excreted in the feces over 72 hours.

Special risk patients –

Renal function impairment: In patients with creatinine clearance of < 29 mL/min, the half-life of the active metabolite was slightly prolonged. Flutamide and its active metabolite were not well dialyzed. Dose adjustment in patients with chronic renal insufficiency is not warranted.

➤*Clinical trials:*

Stage B$_2$-C prostatic carcinoma – In 1 trial (n = 466), administration of flutamide (250 mg 3 times daily) and goserelin acetate (3.6 mg depot) prior to and during radiation was associated with a significantly lower rate of local failure compared with radiation alone (16% vs 33% at 4 years). The combination therapy also resulted in a trend toward reduction in the incidence of distant metastases (27% vs 36% at 4 years). Median disease-free survival was significantly increased in patients who received complete hormonal therapy combined with radiation, as compared to those patients who received radiation alone (4.4 vs 2.6 years). Inclusion of normal PSA level as a criterion for disease-free survival also resulted in significantly increased median disease-free survival in patients receiving the combination therapy (2.7 vs 1.5 years).

Stage D$_2$ metastatic carcinoma – To study the effects of combination therapy, 617 patients (311 leuprolide + flutamide; 306 leuprolide + placebo) with previously untreated advanced prostatic carcinoma were enrolled in a large multicenter, controlled clinical trial.

Median survival had been reached 3.5 years after the study was initiated. The median actuarial survival time is 34.9 months for patients treated with leuprolide and flutamide vs 27.9 months for patients treated with leuprolide alone (a 25% improvement in overall survival time with flutamide therapy). Analysis of progression-free survival showed a 2.6 month improvement in patients who received leuprolide plus flutamide (a 19% increment over leuprolide and placebo).

Contraindications

Hypersensitivity to flutamide or any component of the preparation. Flutamide is contraindicated in patients with severe hepatic impairment (evaluate baseline hepatic enzymes prior to treatment).

Warnings

➤*Aniline exposure:* One metabolite of flutamide is 4-nitro-3-fluoromethylaniline. Several toxicities consistent with aniline exposure including methemoglobinemia, hemolytic anemia, and cholestatic jaundice occurred after flutamide administration. In patients susceptible to aniline toxicity (eg, people with glucose-6-phosphate dehydrogenase deficiency, hemoglobin M disease, smokers), monitoring of methemoglobin levels should be considered.

➤*Hepatotoxicity:* There have been postmarketing reports of hospitalization and rarely death from liver failure in patients taking flutamide. Evidence of hepatic injury included elevated serum transaminase levels, jaundice, hepatic encephalopathy, and death related to acute hepatic failure. The hepatic injury was reversible after discontinuation of therapy in some patients. Approximately half of the reported cases occurred within the initial 3 months of treatment with flutamide (see Warning Box).

➤*Women:* Flutamide is for use only in men. This product has no indication for women, and should not be used in this population, particularly for nonserious or non-life-threatening conditions.

➤*Carcinogenesis:* In a 1-year dietary study in male rats, interstitial cell adenomas of the testes were present in 49% to 75% of all treated rats (daily doses of 10, 30, and 50 mg/kg/day were administered). In a 2-year carcinogenicity study in male rats, daily administration of flutamide at these same doses produced testicular interstitial cell adenomas in 91% to 95% of all treated rats. There are likewise reports of malignant breast neoplasms in men treated with flutamide.

➤*Fertility impairment:* Reduced sperm counts were observed during a 6-week study of flutamide monotherapy in healthy volunteers. Male rats treated with 150 mg/kg/day (30 times the minimum effective antiandrogenic dose) failed to mate; mating behavior returned to normal after dosing was stopped. Conception rates were decreased in all dosing groups. Suppression of spermatogenesis was observed in rats dosed for 52 weeks at ≈ 3, 8, or 17 times the human dose and in dogs dosed for 78 weeks at 1.4, 2.3, and 3.7 times the human dose.

➤*Pregnancy: Category D.* Flutamide may cause fetal harm when administered to a pregnant woman. There was decreased 24-hour survival in the offspring of rats treated with flutamide at doses of 30, 100, or 200 mg/kg/day (≈ 3, 9, and 19 times the human dose) during pregnancy. A slight increase in minor variations in development of the sternebra and vertebra was seen in the fetuses of rats at the 2 higher doses. Feminization of the males also occurred at the 2 higher dose levels. There was a decreased survival rate in the offspring of rabbits receiving the highest dose (15 mg/kg/day), equal to 1.4 times the human dose.

Precautions

➤*Monitoring:* Measure serum transaminase levels prior to starting treatment with flutamide. Serum transaminase levels should then be measured monthly for the first 4 months of therapy, and periodically thereafter. Also obtain liver function tests at the first signs and symp-

FLUTAMIDE

toms suggestive of liver dysfunction (eg, nausea, vomiting, abdominal pain, fatigue, anorexia, "flu-like" symptoms, hyperbilirubinuria, jaundice, right upper quadrant tenderness). If at any time a patient has jaundice, or their ALT rises > 2 times the upper limit of normal, immediately discontinue flutamide, with close follow-up of liver function tests until resolution.

Monitor methemoglobin levels in patients susceptible to aniline toxicity (eg, people with glucose-6-phosphate dehydrogenase deficiency or hemoglobin M disease as well as patients who smoke).

Regular assessment of serum prostate specific antigen (PSA) may be helpful in monitoring the patient's response. If PSA levels rise significantly and consistently during flutamide therapy, evaluate the patients for clinical progression. For patients who have objective progression of disease together with an elevated PSA, a treatment period free of antiandrogen while continuing the LHRH analog may be considered.

➤*Gynecomastia:* In clinical trials, gynecomastia occurred in 9% of patients receiving flutamide together with medical castration.

➤*Urine discoloration:* The urine was noted to change to an amber or yellow-green appearance that can be attributed to the flutamide or its metabolites.

➤*Photosensitivity:* Photosensitization (photoallergy or phototoxicity) may occur; therefore, caution patients to take protective measures (eg, sunscreens, protective clothing) against exposure to sunlight or ultraviolet light (eg, tanning beds) until tolerance is determined.

Drug Interactions

➤*Warfarin:* Increases in prothrombin time have been noted in patients receiving long-term warfarin therapy after flutamide was initiated. Therefore, close monitoring of prothrombin time is recommended and adjustments of the anticoagulant dose may be necessary when flutamide is given concomitantly with warfarin.

Adverse Reactions

Stage B_2-C carcinoma –

Flutamide Adverse Reactions During Radiation Therapy (%)				
	Goserelin acetate implant + flutamide + radiation (n = 231)		Radiation only (n = 235)	
Adverse reaction	Acute radiation (≤ 90 days)	Late radiation (> 90 days)	Acute radiation (≤ 90 days)	Late radiation (> 90 days)
Diarrhea	-	36	-	40
Cystitis	-	16	-	16
Rectal bleeding	-	14	-	20
Proctitis	-	8	-	8
Hematuria	-	7	-	12
Rectum/Large bowel	80	-	76	-
Bladder	58	-	60	-
Skin	37	-	37	-

Additional adverse event data was collected for the combination therapy with radiation group over both the hormonal treatment and hormonal treatment plus radiation phases of the study. Adverse experiences occurring in > 5% of patients in this group, over both parts of the study, were hot flashes (46%); diarrhea (40%); nausea (9%); skin rash (8%).

Stage D_2 metastatic carcinoma –

Flutamide Adverse Reactions in Stage D₂ Metastatic Carcinoma (%)		
Adverse reaction	Flutamide + LHRH agonist (n = 294)	Placebo + LHRH agonist (n = 285)
Hot flashes	61	57
Loss of libido	36	31

Flutamide Adverse Reactions in Stage D₂ Metastatic Carcinoma (%)		
Adverse reaction	Flutamide + LHRH agonist (n = 294)	Placebo + LHRH agonist (n = 285)
Impotence	33	29
Diarrhea	12	4
Nausea/Vomiting	11	10
Gynecomastia	9	11
Other	7	9
Other GI	6	4

The only notable difference was the higher incidence of diarrhea in the flutamide + LHRH agonist group (12%), which was severe in 5%, as opposed to the placebo + LHRH agonist (4%), which was severe in < 1%.

The following adverse reactions occurred during treatment with flutamide + LHRH agonist.

➤*CNS:* Drowsiness, confusion, depression, anxiety, nervousness (1%).

➤*GI:* Anorexia (4%); other GI disorders (6%).

➤*Hematologic:* Anemia (6%); leukopenia (3%); thrombocytopenia (1%).

➤*Lab test abnormalities:* Laboratory abnormalities including elevated AST, ALT, bilirubin, SGGT, BUN, and serum creatinine.

➤*Miscellaneous:* Edema (4%); injection site irritation, rash (3%); genitourinary and neuromuscular symptoms (2%); hypertension (1%); hepatitis, jaundice, pulmonary symptoms (< 1%).

➤*Postmarketing:*

Miscellaneous – The following spontaneous adverse experiences have occurred during the marketing of flutamide: Hemolytic anemia, macrocytic anemia, methemoglobinemia, sulfhemoglobinemia, photosensitivity reactions (including erythema, ulceration, bullous eruptions, and epidermal necrolysis) and urine discoloration (see Precautions); cholestatic jaundice, hepatic encephalopathy, hepatic necrosis (see Warnings). The hepatic conditions were often reversible after discontinuing therapy; however, there have been reports of death following severe hepatic injury associated with use of flutamide. Malignant breast neoplasms have occurred rarely in male patients.

Overdosage

➤*Symptoms:* In animals, signs of overdose included the following: Hypoactivity; piloerection; slow respiration; ataxia; lacrimation; anorexia; tranquilization; emesis; methemoglobinemia.

Clinical trials have been conducted with flutamide in doses ≤ 1500 mg/day for periods ≤ 36 weeks with no serious adverse effects reported. Adverse reactions reported included gynecomastia, breast tenderness, and some increases in AST. The single dose of flutamide ordinarily associated with symptoms of overdose or considered to be life-threatening has not been established.

➤*Treatment:* Because flutamide is highly protein bound, hemodialysis may not be of any use. If it does not occur spontaneously, induce vomiting if the patient is alert. Use general supportive care, including frequent monitoring of the vital signs and close observation of the patient. Refer to General Management of Acute Overdosage.

Patient Information

Inform patients that flutamide and the drug used for medical castration should be administered concomitantly, and that they should not interrupt their dosing or stop taking these medications without consulting their physician.

Inform patients there may be a change in urine color.

May cause photosensitivity. Avoid prolonged exposure to the sun and other ultraviolet light. Use sunscreens and wear protective clothing until tolerance is determined.

NILUTAMIDE

Rx	**Nilandron** (Aventis)	**Tablets:** 50 mg	Lactose. (168). White, biconvex. In 90s.
		150 mg	Lactose. (168D). White, biconvex. In 30s.

WARNING

Interstitial pneumonitis: Interstitial pneumonitis has been reported in 2% of patients in controlled clinical trials in patients exposed to nilutamide. A small study in Japanese subjects showed that 8 of 47 (17%) developed interstitial pneumonitis. Reports of interstitial changes including pulmonary fibrosis that led to hospitalization and death have been rarely reported postmarketing. Symptoms included exertional dyspnea, cough, chest pain, and fever. X-rays showed interstitial or alveolo-interstitial changes, and pulmonary function tests revealed a restrictive pattern with decreased DL_{CO}. Most cases occurred within the first 3 months of treatment with nilutamide and most reversed with discontinuation of therapy.

Perform a routine chest x-ray prior to initiating treatment with nilutamide. Baseline pulmonary function tests may be considered. Instruct patients to report any new or worsening shortness of breath that they experience while on nilutamide. If symptoms occur, discontinue nilutamide immediately until it can be determined if the symptoms are drug-related.

Indications

➤*Metastatic prostate cancer:* For use in combination with surgical castration for the treatment of metastatic prostate cancer (Stage D_2).

For maximum benefit, nilutamide treatment must begin on the same day as or the day after surgical castration.

Administration and Dosage

➤*Approved by the FDA:* September 19, 1996.

300 mg once daily for 30 days followed thereafter by 150 mg once daily. Nilutamide tablets can be taken with or without food.

➤*Storage/Stability:* Store at 25°C (77°F). Excursions permitted between 15° and 30°C (59° and 86°F). Protect from light.

Actions

➤*Pharmacology:* Nilutamide is nonsteroidal with antiandrogen activity. In animal studies, nilutamide has demonstrated antiandrogenic activity without other hormonal (estrogen, progesterone, mineralocorticoid, and glucocorticoid) effects. In vitro, nilutamide blocks the effects of testosterone at the androgen receptor level. In vivo, nilutamide interacts with the androgen receptor and prevents the normal androgenic response.

➤*Pharmacokinetics:*

Absorption – Analysis of blood, urine, and feces samples following a single oral 150 mg dose of [^{14}C]-nilutamide in patients with metastatic prostate cancer showed that the drug is rapidly and completely absorbed and that it yields high and persistent plasma concentrations.

Distribution – After absorption of the drug, there is a detectable distribution phase with moderate binding of the drug to plasma proteins and low binding to erythrocytes. The binding is nonsaturable except in the case of alpha-1-glycoprotein, which makes a minor contribution to the total concentration of proteins in the plasma. The results of binding studies do not indicate any effects that would cause nonlinear pharmacokinetics.

Metabolism – Nilutamide is extensively metabolized and < 2% of the drug is excreted unchanged in the urine after 5 days. Five metabolites have been isolated from human urine. Two metabolites display an asymmetric center, due to oxidation of a methyl group, resulting in the formation of D- and L-isomers. One of the metabolites was shown, in vitro, to possess 25% to 50% of the pharmacological activity of the parent drug, and the D-isomer of the active metabolite showed equal or greater potency compared with the L-isomer. However, the pharmacokinetics and pharmacodynamics of the metabolites have not been fully investigated.

Excretion – The majority (62%) of orally administered [^{14}C]-nilutamide is eliminated in the urine during the first 120 hours after a single 150 mg dose. Fecal elimination is negligible, ranging from 1.4% to 7% of the dose after 4 to 5 days. Excretion of radioactivity in urine likely continues beyond 5 days. The mean elimination half-life of nilutamide determined in studies in which subjects received a single dose of 100 to 300 mg ranged from 38 to 59.1 hours with most values between 41 and 49 hours. The elimination of ≥ 1 metabolite is generally longer than that of unchanged nilutamide (59 to 126 hours). During multiple dosing of 3 × 50 mg twice a day, steady-state was reached within 2 to 4 weeks for most patients, and mean steady-state AUC_{0-12} was 110% higher than the $AUC_{0-\infty}$ obtained from the first dose of 3 × 50 mg.

These data and in vitro metabolism data suggest that, upon multiple dosing, metabolic enzyme inhibition may occur for this drug.

Contraindications

Severe hepatic impairment; severe respiratory insufficiency; hypersensitivity to nilutamide or any component of this preparation.

Warnings

➤*Hepatitis:* Rare cases of death or hospitalization because of severe liver injury have been reported postmarketing in association with the use of nilutamide. Hepatotoxicity in these reports generally occurred within the first 3 to 4 months of treatment. Hepatitis or marked increases in liver enzymes leading to drug discontinuation occurred in 1% of nilutamide patients in controlled clinical trials.

Measure serum transaminase levels prior to starting treatment with nilutamide and at regular intervals for the first 4 months of treatment, and periodically thereafter. Obtain liver function tests at the first sign or symptoms suggestive of liver dysfunction (eg, nausea, vomiting, abdominal pain, fatigue, anorexia, "flu-like" symptoms, dark urine, jaundice, right upper quadrant tenderness). If at any time, a patient has jaundice or their ALT rises above 2 times the upper limit of normal, nilutamide should be immediately discontinued with close follow-up of liver function tests until resolution.

➤*Aplastic anemia:* Foreign postmarketing surveillance has revealed isolated cases of aplastic anemia in which a causal relationship with nilutamide could not be ascertained.

➤*Women:* Nilutamide has no indication for women, and should not be used in this population, particularly for nonserious or non-life-threatening conditions.

➤*Carcinogenesis:* Administration of nilutamide to rats for 18 months at doses of 0, 5, 15, or 45 mg/kg/day produced benign Leydig cell tumors in 35% of the high-dose male rats. The increased incidence of Leydig cell tumors is secondary to elevated luteinizing hormone (LH) concentrations resulting from loss of feedback inhibition at the pituitary. Elevated LH and testosterone concentrations are not observed in castrated men receiving nilutamide. Nilutamide had no effect on the incidence, size, or time of onset of any spontaneous tumor in rats.

➤*Pregnancy:* Category C. Animal reproduction studies have not been conducted with nilutamide. It is also not known whether nilutamide can cause fetal harm when administered to a pregnant woman or can affect reproductive capacity. Give nilutamide to a pregnant woman only if clearly needed.

➤*Children:* Safety and efficacy in pediatric patients have not been established.

Precautions

➤*Delay in adaptation to the dark:* Thirteen percent to 57% of patients receiving nilutamide reported a delay in adaptation to the dark, ranging from seconds to a few minutes, when passing from a lighted area to a dark area. This effect sometimes does not abate as drug treatment is continued. Caution patients who experience this effect about driving at night or through tunnels. This effect can be alleviated by wearing tinted glasses.

Drug Interactions

In vitro, nilutamide has been shown to inhibit the activity of liver cytochrome P450 isoenzymes and, therefore, may reduce the metabolism of compounds requiring these systems. Drugs with a low therapeutic margin, such as vitamin K antagonists, phenytoin, and theophylline, could have a delayed elimination and increases in their serum half-life leading to a toxic level. The dosage of these drugs or others with a similar metabolism may need to be modified if they are administered concomitantly with nilutamide. For example, when vitamin K antagonists are administered concomitantly with nilutamide, carefully monitor prothrombin time and, if necessary, reduce the dosage of vitamin K antagonists.

Adverse Reactions

Adverse Reactions for Nilutamide + Leuprolide vs Nilutamide + Surgical Castration[1] (> 5%)		
Adverse experience	Nilutamide + leuprolide (n = 209)	Nilutamide + surgical castration (n = 225)
CNS		
Insomnia	16.3	—
Headache	13.9	—
Dizziness	10	7.1
Depression	8.6	—
Hypesthesia	5.3	—
Dermatologic		
Sweating	6.2	—
Alopecia	5.7	—
Dry skin	5.3	—
Rash	5.3	—

NILUTAMIDE

Adverse Reactions for Nilutamide + Leuprolide vs Nilutamide + Surgical Castration[1] (> 5%)		
Adverse experience	Nilutamide + leuprolide (n = 209)	Nilutamide + surgical castration (n = 225)
Endocrine		
Hot flushes	66.5	28.4
Impotence	11	—
Libido decrease	11	—
GI		
Nausea	23.9	9.8
Constipation	19.6	7.1
Anorexia	11	—
Abdominal pain	10	—
Dyspepsia	6.7	—
Vomiting	5.7	—
GU		
Testicular atrophy	16.3	—
Gynecomastia	10.5	—
Urinary tract infection	8.6	8
Hematuria	8.1	—
Urinary tract disorder	7.2	—
Nocturia	6.7	—
Metabolic/Nutritional		
Increased AST	12.9	8
Peripheral edema	12.4	—
Increased ALT	9.1	7.6
Respiratory		
Dyspnea	10.5	6.2
Upper respiratory tract infection	8.1	—
Pneumonia	5.3	—
Special senses		
Impaired adaptation to dark	56.9	12.9
Chromatopsia	8.6	—
Impaired adaptation to light	7.7	—
Abnormal vision	6.2	6.7
Miscellaneous		
Pain	26.8	—
Asthenia	19.1	—
Back pain	11.5	—
Hypertension	9.1	5.3
Anemia	7.2	—
Chest pain	7.2	—
Flu syndrome	7.2	—
Bone pain	6.2	—
Fever	5.3	—

[1] Data are pooled from 2 separate studies and are not necessarily comparable.

Some frequently occurring adverse experiences reported during one nilutamide + leuprolide study (eg, hot flushes, impotence, decreased libido) are known to be associated with low serum androgen levels and are known to occur with medical or surgical castration alone. Notable was the higher incidence of visual disturbances (variously described as impaired adaptation to darkness, abnormal vision, and colored vision), which led to treatment discontinuation in 1% to 2% of patients.

Interstitial pneumonitis occurred in 1 (< 1%) patient receiving nilutamide in combination with surgical castration, in 7 patients (3%) receiving nilutamide in combination with leuprolide, and 1 patient receiving placebo in combination with leuprolide. Overall, it has been reported in 2% of patients receiving nilutamide. This included a report of interstitial pneumonitis in 8 of 47 patients (17%) in a small study performed in Japan.

The following adverse experiences were reported in 2% to 5% of patients treated with nilutamide in combination with leuprolide or orchiectomy.

➤*Cardiovascular:* Heart failure (3%); angina, syncope (2%).

➤*CNS:* Paresthesia (3%); nervousness (2%).

➤*GI:* Diarrhea, dry mouth, GI disorder, GI hemorrhage, melena (2%).

➤*Lab test abnormalities:* Hyperglycemia (4%); alkaline phosphatase increased, leukopenia (3%); increased haptoglobin, BUN, and creatinine (2%).

➤*Metabolic/Nutritional:* Alcohol intolerance (5%); edema, weight loss (2%).

➤*Respiratory:* Lung disorder (4%); cough increased, interstitial lung disease, rhinitis (2%).

➤*Special senses:* Cataract, photophobia (2%).

➤*Miscellaneous:* Malaise, pruritus, arthritis (2%).

Overdosage

One case of massive overdosage has been published. A 79-year-old man attempted suicide by ingesting 13 g of nilutamide (ie, 43 times the maximum recommended dose). Despite immediate gastric lavage and oral administration of activated charcoal, plasma nilutamide levels peaked at 6 times the normal range 2 hours after ingestion. There were no clinical signs or symptoms or changes in parameters such as transaminases or chest x-ray. Maintenance treatment (150 mg/day) was resumed 30 days later.

In repeated-dose tolerance studies, doses of 600 mg/day and 900 mg/day were administered to 9 and 4 patients, respectively. The ingestion of these doses was associated with GI disorders, including nausea and vomiting, malaise, headache, and dizziness. In addition, a transient elevation in hepatic enzyme levels was noted in 1 patient.

Because nilutamide is protein bound, dialysis may not be useful as treatment for overdose. As in the management of overdosage with any drug, bear in mind that multiple agents may have been taken. General supportive care, including frequent monitoring of the vital signs and close observation of the patient, is indicated (refer to Management of Acute Overdose).

Patient Information

Inform patients that nilutamide tablets should be started on the day of, or the day after, surgical castration. Also inform them that they should not interrupt their dosing of nilutamide or stop taking the medication without consulting their physician.

Because of the possibility of interstitial pneumonitis, tell patients to report immediately any dyspnea or aggravation of preexisting dyspnea.

Because of the possibility of hepatitis, tell patients to consult with their physician should nausea, vomiting, abdominal pain, or jaundice occur.

Because of the possibility of an intolerance to alcohol (facial flushes, malaise, hypotension) following ingestion of nilutamide, it is recommended that intake of alcoholic beverages be avoided by patients who experience this reaction. This effect has been reported in ≈ 5% of patients treated with nilutamide.

Caution patients about the potential for a delayed adaptation to the dark. This is especially important when driving at night or through tunnels. This effect can be alleviated by the wearing of tinted glasses.

MEGESTROL ACETATE

Rx	**Megestrol Acetate** (Various, eg, Barr, Par, Roxane, UDL)	**Tablets:** 20 mg	In 20s, 100s, 500s, and UD 100s.
Rx	**Megestrol Acetate** (Various, eg, Barr, Major, Par, Roxane, UDL, Zenith Goldline)	**Tablets:** 40 mg	In 100s, 250s, 500s, UD 25s, and UD 100s.
Rx	**Megace** (Bristol-Myers Oncology/Immunology)		Light blue, scored. In 250s and 500s.

Megestrol acetate is also available as a suspension for appetite enhancement in AIDS patients; refer to the monograph in the Endocrine and Metabolic Agents chapter. For complete prescribing information, see the Progestins group monograph in the Endocrine/Metabolic chapter.

WARNING

Use of megestrol is not recommended during the first 4 months of pregnancy.

Indications

➤*Breast or endometrial carcinoma:* Palliative treatment of advanced carcinoma of the breast or endometrium (ie, recurrent, inoperable or metastatic disease). Do not use in place of surgery, radiation, or chemotherapy.

➤*Appetite enhancement in AIDS patients (suspension only):* Treatment of anorexia, cachexia, or an unexplained significant weight loss in patients with a diagnosis of acquired immunodeficiency syndrome (AIDS). (Refer to the monograph in the Endocrine and Metabolic Agents chapter).

Administration and Dosage

➤*Breast cancer:* 160 mg/day (40 mg 4 times daily).

➤*Endometrial carcinoma:* 40 to 320 mg/day in divided doses.

At least 2 months of continuous treatment is adequate for determining efficacy.

Actions

➤*Pharmacology:* The exact mechanism by which megestrol acetate produces its antineoplastic effects is unknown. An antiluteinizing effect mediated via the pituitary has been postulated. Evidence also suggests a local effect as a result of the marked changes from direct instillation of progestational agents into the endometrial cavity.

Contraindications

As a diagnostic test for pregnancy.

Warnings

The use of megestrol acetate in other types of neoplastic disease is not recommended.

➤*Pregnancy:* The use of progestational agents during the first 4 months of pregnancy is not recommended. Reports suggest an association between intrauterine exposure to female sex hormones and congenital anomalies.

If the patient is exposed to megestrol acetate during the first 4 months of pregnancy or becomes pregnant while taking this drug, apprise her of the potential risks to the fetus.

Precautions

Use with caution in patients with a history of thrombophlebitis.

Adverse Reactions

Weight gain – Weight gain is a frequent side effect of megestrol acetate. This effect has been associated with increased appetite, not necessarily with fluid retention.

Thromboembolic phenomena – Thromboembolic phenomena, including thrombophlebitis and pulmonary embolism, have occurred rarely.

➤*Miscellaneous:* Nausea/vomiting; edema; breakthrough bleeding; dyspnea; tumor flare (with or without hypercalcemia); hyperglycemia; alopecia; carpal tunnel syndrome; rash.

No serious side effects resulted from megestrol acetate studies using doses as high as 800 mg/day.

Patient Information

Medication may cause back or abdominal pain, headache, nausea, vomiting, or breast tenderness; notify physician if these effects become pronounced.

Contraceptive measures are recommended during therapy.

MEDROXYPROGESTERONE ACETATE

Rx	**Depo-Provera** (Pharmacia)	**Injection:** 400 mg/ml[1]	In 2.5 and 10 ml vials and 1 ml U-ject.

[1] With polyethylene glycol 3350, sodium sulfate anhydrous, myristyl-gamma-picolinium Cl.

For complete information, see the Progestins group monograph in the Endocrine/Metabolic chapter.

WARNING

Use is not recommended during the first 4 months of pregnancy.

Indications

➤*Endometrial or renal carcinoma:* Adjunctive therapy and palliative treatment of inoperable, recurrent, and metastatic endometrial carcinoma or renal carcinoma.

➤*Unlabeled uses:* Depot medroxyprogesterone acetate has been used as a long-acting contraceptive (150 mg IM every 3 months or 450 mg every 6 months) and in the treatment of advanced breast cancer.

Administration and Dosage

For IM administration only.

➤*Endometrial or renal carcinoma:* Initially, 400 to 1000 mg IM per week. If improvement occurs within a few weeks or months and the disease appears stabilized, it may be possible to maintain improvement with as little as 400 mg/month.

Actions

➤*Pharmacology:* When administered parenterally in recommended doses to women with adequate endogenous estrogen, it transforms proliferative endometrium into secretory endometrium. Medroxyprogesterone inhibits (in the usual dose range) the secretion of pituitary gonadotropin which, in turn, prevents follicular maturation and ovulation.

Contraindications

Thrombophlebitis, thromboembolic disorders, stroke, or history of these conditions; breast carcinoma; undiagnosed vaginal bleeding; missed abortion; sensitivity to medroxyprogesterone acetate; as a diagnostic test for pregnancy.

Warnings

➤*Hepatic function impairment:* Upon earliest manifestations of impaired liver function, discontinue the drug and re-evaluate the patient's status.

➤*Pregnancy:* The use of progestational agents during the first 4 months of pregnancy is not recommended. Several reports suggest an association between intrauterine exposure to female sex hormones and congenital anomalies. The risk of hypospadias, 5 to 8 per 1000 male births in the general population, may be approximately doubled with exposure to progestational agents. There are insufficient data to quantify the risk to exposed female fetuses, but because some of these drugs induce mild virilization of the external genitalia of the female fetus, and because of the increased association of hypospadias in the male fetus, it is prudent to avoid the use of these drugs during the first trimester of pregnancy.

If the patient is exposed to medroxyprogesterone acetate during the first 4 months of pregnancy or if she becomes pregnant while taking this drug, apprise her of the potential risks to the fetus.

➤*Lactation:* Medroxyprogesterone does not adversely affect lactation; if breastfeeding is desired, it may be used safely. Milk production and duration of lactation may be increased if given in the puerperium.

Adverse Reactions

Following repeated injections, amenorrhea and infertility may persist for up to 18 months and occasionally longer.

In a few instances there have been undesirable sequelae at the site of injection, such as residual lump, change in color of skin, or sterile abscess.

➤*CNS:* Nervousness; insomnia; somnolence; fatigue; dizziness; headache (rare).

➤*Dermatologic:* Angioneurotic edema; pruritus; urticaria; generalized rash; acne; alopecia; hirsutism.

➤*GI:* Nausea (rare); jaundice, including neonatal jaundice.

➤*Miscellaneous:* Hyperpyrexia (rare); anaphylaxis; thrombophlebitis; pulmonary embolism.

Antiestrogens

TAMOXIFEN CITRATE

Rx	Tamoxifen Citrate (Various, eg, Barr, Ivax, Mylan, Roxane, Teva)	Tablets: 10 mg (as base)	In 60s, 180s, 500s, 1000s, and UD 100s.
Rx	Nolvadex (AstraZeneca)		(NOLVADEX 600). White. In 60s.
Rx	Tamoxifen Citrate (Various, eg, Barr, Ivax, Mylan, Roxane, Teva)	Tablets: 20 mg (as base)	In 30s, 90s, 100s, 500s, 1000s, and UD 100s.
Rx	Nolvadex (AstraZeneca)		(NOLVADEX 604). White. In 30s.

WARNING

Women with ductal carcinoma in situ (DCIS) and women at high risk for breast cancer: Serious and life-threatening events associated with tamoxifen in the risk reduction setting (women at high risk for cancer and women with DCIS) include uterine malignancies, stroke, and pulmonary embolism. Incidence rates for these events were estimated from the NSABP P-1 trial. Uterine malignancies consist of both endometrial adenocarcinoma (incidence rate per 1000 women-years of 2.2 for tamoxifen vs 0.71 for placebo) and uterine sarcoma (incidence rate per 1000 women-years of 0.17 for tamoxifen vs 0 for placebo) (updated long-term follow-up data [median length of follow-up is 6.9 years] from NSABP P-1 study). For stroke, the incidence rate per 1000 women-years was 1.43 for tamoxifen vs 1 for placebo. For pulmonary embolism, the incidence rate per 1000 women-years was 0.75 for tamoxifen vs 0.25 for placebo.

Some of the strokes, pulmonary emboli, and uterine malignancies were fatal.

Health care providers should discuss the potential benefits vs the potential risks of these serious events with women at high risk of breast cancer and women with DCIS considering tamoxifen to reduce their risk of developing breast cancer.

The benefits of tamoxifen outweigh its risks in women already diagnosed with breast cancer.

Indications

➤*Breast cancer:*

Adjuvant therapy – For treatment of axillary node-negative breast cancer in women following total mastectomy or segmental mastectomy, axillary dissection, and breast irradiation.

For treatment of node-positive breast cancer in postmenopausal women following total mastectomy or segmental mastectomy, axillary dissection, and breast irradiation. In some tamoxifen adjuvant studies, most of the benefit to date has been in the subgroup with 4 or more positive axillary nodes.

The estrogen and progesterone receptor values may help predict whether adjuvant tamoxifen therapy is likely to be beneficial.

Tamoxifen reduces the occurrence of contralateral breast cancer in patients receiving adjuvant tamoxifen therapy for breast cancer.

Current data from clinical trials support 5 years of adjuvant tamoxifen therapy for patients with breast cancer.

Advanced disease therapy – Effective in the treatment of metastatic breast cancer in women and men. In premenopausal women with metastatic breast cancer, tamoxifen is an alternative to oophorectomy or ovarian irradiation. Women with estrogen receptor-positive tumors are most likely to benefit.

➤*Reduction in breast cancer incidence in high-risk women:* To reduce the incidence of breast cancer in women at high risk for breast cancer. "High risk" is defined as women at least 35 years of age with a 5-year predicted risk of breast cancer of at least 1.67%, as calculated by the Gail Model. Examples of combinations of factors predicting a 5-year risk of at least 1.67% are as follows:

Age 35 years or older and any of the following combination of factors – One first-degree relative with a history of breast cancer, 2 or more benign biopsies, and a history of a breast biopsy showing atypical hyperplasia; or at least 2 first-degree relatives with a history of breast cancer and a personal history of at least 1 breast biopsy; or lobular carcinoma in situ (LCIS).

Age 40 years or older and any of the following combination of factors – One first-degree relative with a history of breast cancer, 2 or more benign biopsies, age at first live birth 25 years or older, and age of menarche 11 years or younger; or at least 2 first-degree relatives with a history of breast cancer and age at first live birth 19 years or younger; or 1 first-degree relative with a history of breast cancer and a personal history of a breast biopsy showing atypical hyperplasia.

Age 45 years or older and any of the following combination of factors – At least 2 first-degree relatives with history of breast cancer and age at first live birth 24 years or younger; or 1 first-degree relative with a history of breast cancer with a personal history of a benign breast biopsy age at menarche 11 years or younger, and age at first live birth 20 years or older.

Age 50 years or older and any of the following combination of factors – At least 2 first-degree relatives with a history of breast cancer; or history of 1 breast biopsy showing atypical hyperplasia, age at

first live birth 30 years or older, and age at menarche 11 years or younger; or history of at least 2 breast biopsies with a history of atypical hyperplasia and age at first live birth 30 years or older.

Age 55 years or older and any of the following combination of factors – One first-degree relative with a history of breast cancer with a personal history of a benign breast biopsy and age at menarche 11 years or younger; or history of at least 2 breast biopsies with a history of atypical hyperplasia and age at first live birth 20 years or older.

Age 60 years or older – Five-year predicted risk of breast cancer at least 1.67%, as calculated by the Gail Model.

For women whose risk factors are not described above, the Gail Model is necessary to estimate absolute breast cancer risk. Health care professionals can obtain a Gail Model Risk Assessment Tool by calling (800) 544-2007.

After an assessment of the risk of developing breast cancer, base the decision regarding therapy with tamoxifen for the reduction in breast cancer incidence on an individual assessment of the benefits and risks of tamoxifen therapy. In trials, tamoxifen treatment lowered the risk of developing breast cancer during the follow-up period of the trial but did not eliminate breast cancer risk.

➤*DCIS:* In women with DCIS, following breast surgery and radiation, tamoxifen is indicated to reduce the risk of invasive breast cancer. Base the decision regarding therapy with tamoxifen for the reduction in breast cancer incidence upon an individual assessment of the benefits and risks of tamoxifen therapy.

➤*Unlabeled uses:* Ovulation stimulation in specially selected anovulatory women desiring pregnancy, mainly those with amenorrhea or oligomenorrhea who were previously taking oral contraceptives.

Management and treatment of some types of mastalgia (eg, cyclical); malignant carcinoid tumor and carcinoid syndrome; migraine associated with menstruation; metastatic malignant melanoma; male infertility (oligozoospermia); McCune-Albright syndrome in female pediatric patients (in combination with other agents).

Administration and Dosage

➤*Approved by the FDA:* December 10, 1985.

➤*Breast cancer patients:* 20 to 40 mg/day. Give doses greater than 20 mg/day in divided doses (morning and evening).

Some studies have used dosages of 10 mg 2 or 3 times/day for 2 years, and 10 mg twice daily for 5 years or more. The reduction in recurrence and mortality was greater in those studies that used the drug for about 5 years than in those that used it for a shorter period. There was no indication that doses greater than 20 mg/day were more effective. Current data from clinical trials support 5 years of adjuvant tamoxifen therapy for patients with breast cancer.

➤*Reduction in breast cancer incidence in high-risk women:* 20 mg/day for 5 years. There are no data to support the use of tamoxifen other than for 5 years.

For sexually active women of childbearing potential, initiate tamoxifen therapy during menstruation. In women with menstrual irregularity, a negative B-hCG immediately prior to the initiation of therapy is sufficient.

➤*DCIS:* 20 mg/day for 5 years.

➤*Storage/Stability:* Store at controlled room temperature, 20° to 25°C (68° to 77°F). Dispense in a well-closed, light-resistant container.

Actions

➤*Pharmacology:* Tamoxifen is a nonsteroidal agent with potent antiestrogenic properties, likely because of its ability to compete with estrogen for binding sites in target tissues such as the breast. Tamoxifen also may produce weak estrogenic and estrogenic-like activity at some sites.

➤*Pharmacokinetics:*

Absorption/Distribution – Following a single oral dose of 20 mg tamoxifen, an average peak plasma concentration of 40 ng/mL (range, 35 to 45 ng/mL) occurred approximately 5 hours after dosing. The decline in plasma concentrations of tamoxifen is biphasic. The average peak plasma concentration of N-desmethyl tamoxifen is 15 ng/mL (range, 10 to 20 ng/mL). Chronic administration of 10 mg tamoxifen given twice daily for 3 months results in average steady-state plasma concentrations of 120 ng/mL (range, 67 to 183 ng/mL) for tamoxifen and 336 ng/mL (range, 148 to 654 ng/mL) for N-desmethyl tamoxifen. The average steady-state plasma concentrations of tamoxifen and N-desmethyl tamoxifen after administration of 20 mg tamoxi-

TAMOXIFEN CITRATE

fen once daily for 3 months are 122 ng/mL (range, 71 to 183 ng/mL) and 353 ng/mL (range, 152 to 706 ng/mL), respectively. After initiation of therapy, steady-state concentrations for tamoxifen are achieved in about 4 weeks and steady-state concentrations for N-desmethyl tamoxifen are achieved in about 8 weeks.

Metabolism/Excretion – Tamoxifen is extensively metabolized after oral administration. N-desmethyl tamoxifen is the major metabolite found in patients' plasma. The biological activity of N-desmethyl tamoxifen appears to be similar to tamoxifen. 4-Hydroxytamoxifen and a side chain primary alcohol derivative of tamoxifen have been identified as minor metabolites in plasma. Tamoxifen is a substrate of cytochrome P450 3A, 2C9, and 2D6 and an inhibitor of P-glycoprotein. Studies in women receiving 20 mg of ^{14}C tamoxifen have shown that approximately 65% of the administered dose was excreted from the body over 2 weeks with fecal excretion as the primary route of elimination. The drug was excreted mainly as polar conjugates, with unchanged drug and unconjugated metabolites accounting for less than 30% of the total fecal radioactivity. Tamoxifen has a terminal elimination half-life of about 5 to 7 days and its N-desmethyl tamoxifen metabolite appears to have a half-life of approximately 14 days.

Special populations –

Children: In pediatric patients, an average steady-state peak plasma concentration ($C_{ss,\ max}$) and AUC were of 187 ng/mL and 4110 ng•h/mL, respectively, and $C_{ss,\ max}$ occurred approximately 8 hours after dosing. Clearance (CL/F) as body weight adjusted in female pediatric patients was approximately 2.3-fold higher than in female breast cancer patients. In the youngest cohort of female pediatric patients (2 to 6 years of age), CL/F was 2.6-fold higher; in the oldest cohort (7 to 10.9 years of age), CL/F was approximately 1.9-fold higher.

➤*Clinical trials:*

Adjuvant breast cancer – The Early Breast Cancer Trialists' Collaborative Group (EBCTCG) conducted worldwide overviews of systemic adjuvant therapy for early breast cancer in 1985, 1990, and again in 1995. In 1998, 10-year outcome data were reported for 36,689 women in 55 randomized trials of adjuvant tamoxifen using doses of 20 to 40 mg/day for 1 to 5+ years. Twenty-five percent of patients received 1 year or less of trial treatment, 52% received 2 years, and 23% received about 5 years. Forty-eight percent of tumors were estrogen-receptor (ER)-positive (greater than 10 fmol/mg), 21% were ER-poor (less than 10 fmol/mg), and 31% were ER-unknown. Among 29,441 patients with ER-positive or -unknown breast cancer, 58% were entered into trials comparing tamoxifen with no adjuvant therapy and 42% were entered into trials comparing tamoxifen in combination with chemotherapy vs the same chemotherapy alone. Among these patients, 54% had node-positive disease and 46% had node-negative disease.

Among women with ER-positive or unknown breast cancer and positive nodes who received about 5 years of treatment, overall survival at 10 years was 61.4% for tamoxifen vs 50.5% for control (logrank 2p < 0.00001). The recurrence-free rate at 10 years was 59.7% for tamoxifen vs 44.5% for control (logrank 2p < 0.00001). Among women with ER-positive or unknown breast cancer and negative nodes who received about 5 years of treatment, overall survival at 10 years was 78.9% for tamoxifen vs 73.3% for control (logrank 2p < 0.00001). The recurrence-free rate at 10 years was 79.2% for tamoxifen vs 64.3% for control (logrank 2p < 0.00001).

The effect of the scheduled duration of tamoxifen may be described as follows: In women with ER-positive or unknown breast cancer receiving 1 year or less, 2 years, or about 5 years of tamoxifen, the proportional reductions in mortality were 12%, 17%, and 26%, respectively (trend significant at 2p < 0.003). The corresponding reductions in breast cancer recurrence were 21%, 29%, and 47% (trend significant at 2p < 0.00001).

Benefit is less clear for women with ER-poor breast cancer in whom the proportional reduction in recurrence was 10% (2p = 0.007) for all durations taken together, or 9% (2p = 0.02) if contralateral breast cancers are excluded. The corresponding reduction in mortality was 6% (NS). The effects of about 5 years of tamoxifen on recurrence and mortality were similar regardless of age and concurrent chemotherapy. There was no indication that doses greater than 20 mg/day were more effective.

Duration of therapy – In the EBCTCG 1995 overview, the reduction in recurrence and mortality was greater in those studies that used tamoxifen for about 5 years than in those that used tamoxifen for a shorter period of therapy.

Node positive (individual studies) – Two studies (Hubay and NSABP B-09) demonstrated an improved disease-free survival following radical or modified radical mastectomy in postmenopausal women or women 50 years of age or older with surgically curable breast cancer with positive axillary nodes when tamoxifen was added to adjuvant cytotoxic chemotherapy. In the Hubay study, tamoxifen was added to "low-dose" CMF (cyclophosphamide, methotrexate, and fluorouracil). In the NSABP B-09 study, tamoxifen was added to melphalan (L-phenylalanine mustard [P]) and fluorouracil (F).

In the Hubay study, patients with a positive (more than 3 fmol) estrogen receptor were more likely to benefit. In the NSABP B-09 study in

women 50 to 59 years of age, only women with both estrogen and progesterone receptor levels 10 fmol or greater clearly benefited, while there was a nonstatistically significant trend toward adverse effect in women with both estrogen and progesterone receptor levels less than 10 fmol. In women 60 to 70 years of age, there was a trend toward a beneficial effect of tamoxifen without any clear relationship to estrogen or progesterone receptor status.

Three prospective studies (ECOG-1178, Toronto, NATO) using tamoxifen adjuvantly as a single agent demonstrated an improved disease-free survival following total mastectomy and axillary dissection for postmenopausal women with positive axillary nodes compared with placebo/no treatment controls. The NATO study also demonstrated an overall survival benefit.

Contraindications

Hypersensitivity to the drug or any ingredients; women who require concomitant coumarin-type anticoagulant therapy, women with a history of deep vein thrombosis or pulmonary embolus (reduction in breast cancer incidence and DCIS indications).

Warnings

➤*Thromboembolic effects:* There is evidence of an increased incidence of thromboembolic events, including deep vein thrombosis and pulmonary embolism (PE), during tamoxifen therapy. When tamoxifen is administered with chemotherapy, there may be a further increase in the incidence of thromboembolic effects. Consider the risks and benefits of tamoxifen carefully in women with a history of thromboembolic events. Data from 1 trial showed that participants receiving tamoxifen without a history of PE had a statistically significant increase in PE. Three of the PE incidences, all in the tamoxifen arm, were fatal. Among women receiving tamoxifen, the events appeared between 2 and 60 months from the start of treatment.

➤*Uterus-endometrial cancer and uterine sarcoma:* An increased incidence of uterine malignancies has been reported in association with tamoxifen treatment. The underlying mechanism is unknown, but may be related to the estrogen-like effect of tamoxifen. Most uterine malignancies seen in association with tamoxifen are classified as adenocarcinoma of the endometrium. However, rare uterine sarcomas, including malignant mixed mullerian tumors, also have been reported. Uterine sarcoma is generally associated with a higher FIGO stage (III/IV) at diagnosis, poorer prognosis, and shorter survival. Uterine sarcoma has been reported to occur more frequently among long-term users (at least 2 years) of tamoxifen than nonusers. Some of the uterine malignancies (endometrial carcinoma or uterine sarcoma) have been fatal.

In an updated review of long-term data (median length of total follow-up is 6.9 years, including blinded follow-up), endometrial adenocarcinoma was reported in 53 women randomized to tamoxifen and 17 women randomized to placebo. Uterine sarcomas were reported in 4 women randomized to tamoxifen and no patients randomized to placebo. A similar increased incidence in endometrial adenocarcinoma and uterine sarcoma was observed among women receiving tamoxifen in 5 other NSABP clinical trials.

➤*Ocular disturbances:* Ocular disturbances, including corneal changes, cataracts, the need for cataract surgery, decrement in color vision perception, retinal vein thrombosis, and retinopathy have occurred with tamoxifen use.

In the NSABP P-1 trial, an increased risk of borderline significance of developing cataracts among those women without cataracts at baseline (540 for tamoxifen, 483 for placebo; RR = 1.13, 95% CI: 1 to 1.28) was observed. Among these same women, tamoxifen was associated with an increased risk of having cataract surgery (101 for tamoxifen, 63 for placebo; RR = 1.62, 95% CI: 1.17 to 2.25). Among all women in the trial (with or without cataracts at baseline), tamoxifen was associated with an increased risk of having cataract surgery (201 for tamoxifen, 129 for placebo; RR = 1.51, 95% CI: 1.21 to 1.89). Eye examinations were not required during the study.

➤*Disease of bone:* Increased bone pain, tumor pain, and local disease flare are sometimes associated with a good tumor response shortly after starting tamoxifen, and generally subside rapidly. Patients with increased bone pain may require additional analgesics. Lesion size may increase suddenly in soft tissue disease, sometimes with new lesions, or with erythema in or around the lesion.

➤*Hypercalcemia:* Hypercalcemia has occurred in some breast cancer patients with bone metastases within a few weeks of starting therapy with tamoxifen. If hypercalcemia occurs, institute appropriate measures and, if severe, discontinue use.

➤*Hepatic effects:* Tamoxifen has been associated with changes in liver enzyme levels and, on rare occasions, a spectrum of more severe liver abnormalities including fatty liver, cholestasis, hepatitis, and hepatic necrosis. A few of these serious cases included fatalities. In most cases the relationship to tamoxifen was uncertain; however, some positive rechallenges and dechallenges have been reported. Perform periodic liver function tests.

➤*Carcinogenesis:* A study in rats revealed hepatocellular carcinomas at doses of 5 to 35 mg/kg/day for up to 2 years; incidence was significantly higher using doses of 20 or 35 mg/kg/day (69%) vs 5 mg/kg/day

TAMOXIFEN CITRATE

(14%). Also, in a trial using 40 mg/day for 2 to 5 years in humans, 3 cases of liver cancer were reported vs 1 case in the control group.

Granulosa-cell ovarian tumors and interstitial-cell testicular tumors were found in mice.

Uterine-endometrial changes and cancer – An increased frequency of endometrial changes including hyperplasia and polyps have been reported with tamoxifen. The incidence and pattern suggest that the underlying mechanism is related to the estrogenic properties.

➤*Mutagenesis:* Increased levels of DNA adducts were observed by ^{32}P postlabeling in DNA from rat liver and cultured human lymphocytes. Tamoxifen also has been found to increase levels of micronucleus formation in vitro in human lymphoblastoid cell line (MCL-5). Based on these findings, tamoxifen is genotoxic in rodent and human MCL-5 cells.

➤*Fertility impairment:* Fertility in female rats decreased following 0.04 mg/kg/day for 2 weeks prior to mating through day 7 of pregnancy.

➤*Pregnancy: Category D.* Tamoxifen may cause fetal harm when administered to a pregnant woman. Advise patients not to become pregnant while taking tamoxifen or within 2 months of discontinuing tamoxifen and to use barrier or nonhormonal contraceptive measures. Effects on reproductive functions are expected from the antiestrogenic properties of the drug. In reproductive studies in rats at dose levels equal to or below the human dose, nonteratogenic developmental skeletal changes were seen and were found to be reversible. In fertility and teratology studies in rats and rabbits using doses at or below those in humans, a lower incidence of embryo implantation and a higher incidence of fetal death or retarded in utero growth were observed, with slower learning behavior in some rat pups.

In rodent models of fetal reproductive tract development, tamoxifen (at doses 0.002- to 2.4-fold the human maximum recommended dose on a mg/m^2 basis) caused changes in both sexes that are similar to those caused by estradiol, ethinyl estradiol, and diethylstilbestrol. Although the clinical relevance of these changes is unknown, some of these changes, especially vaginal adenosis, are similar to those seen in young women exposed to diethylstilbestrol in utero and who have a 1 in 1000 risk of developing clear-cell adenocarcinoma of the vagina or cervix. To date, in utero exposure to tamoxifen has not been shown to cause vaginal adenosis or clear-cell adenocarcinoma of the vagina or cervix in young women. However, only a small number of young women have been exposed to tamoxifen in utero, and a smaller number have been followed long enough (to 15 to 20 years of age) to determine whether vaginal or cervical neoplasia could occur as a result of this exposure.

There are no adequate and well-controlled studies in pregnant women. Spontaneous abortions, birth defects, fetal deaths, and vaginal bleeding have occurred. If this drug is used during pregnancy or if the patient becomes pregnant while taking this drug or within about 2 months of discontinuing therapy, apprise her of the potential hazard to the fetus, including potential long-term risk of a DES-like syndrome.

➤*Lactation:* It is not known whether this drug is excreted in breast milk. Because there is potential for serious adverse reactions in nursing infants, decide whether to discontinue nursing or discontinue the drug. Because tamoxifen has been shown to inhibit lactation and because of the adverse effects noted in newborn animals and human adults given the drug directly, the drug should be considered contraindicated during nursing.

➤*Children:* The safety and efficacy of tamoxifen for girls 2 to 10 years of age with McCune-Albright syndrome and precocious puberty have not been studied beyond 1 year of treatment. The long-term effects of tamoxifen therapy for girls have not been established.

Precautions

➤*Monitoring:* Perform periodic complete blood counts, including platelet counts and liver function tests. Perform a breast examination, mammogram, and gynecologic examination prior to the initiation of therapy for women taking tamoxifen to reduce the incidence of breast cancer. Repeat these studies at regular intervals while on therapy.

➤*Leukopenia/Thrombocytopenia:* Leukopenia has been observed, sometimes in association with anemia or thrombocytopenia. Decreases in platelet counts (usually to 50,000 to 100,000/mm^3, infrequently lower) have occurred in patients taking tamoxifen for breast cancer. In patients with significant thrombocytopenia, rare hemorrhagic episodes have occurred, but it is uncertain if these episodes are because of tamoxifen therapy. There have been rare reports of neutropenia and pancytopenia, sometimes severe.

➤*Hyperlipidemias:* Hyperlipidemias have occurred infrequently. Periodic monitoring of plasma triglycerides and cholesterol may be indicated in patients with pre-existing hyperlipidemias.

Drug Interactions

Tamoxifen Drug Interactions			
Precipitant drug	Object drug*		Description
Aminoglutethimide	Tamoxifen	↓	Aminoglutethimide reduces tamoxifen and N-desmethyl tamoxifen plasma concentrations.
Bromocriptine	Tamoxifen	↑	Bromocriptine may elevate serum tamoxifen and N-desmethyl tamoxifen levels.
Cytotoxic agents	Tamoxifen	↑	The risk of thromboembolic events increases with coadministration.
Erythromycin Cyclosporin Nifedipine Diltiazem	Tamoxifen	↔	These agents have been shown to competitively inhibit the formation of N-desmethyl tamoxifen. The clinical significance of this is unknown.
Medroxyprogesterone	Tamoxifen	↓	Medroxyprogesterone reduces plasma concentrations of N-desmethyl tamoxifen (metabolite) but not tamoxifen.
Phenobarbital	Tamoxifen	↓	One patient receiving tamoxifen with concomitant phenobarbital exhibited a steady-state serum level of tamoxifen lower than that observed for other patients (ie, 26 ng/mL vs mean value of 122 ng/mL). The clinical significance of this is unknown.
Rifamycins	Tamoxifen	↓	Plasma concentrations of tamoxifen may be reduced. Rifampin reduced tamoxifen AUC and C$_{max}$ by 86% and 55%, respectively. It may be necessary to increase the tamoxifen dose during coadministration.
Tamoxifen	Anticoagulants	↑	The hypoprothrombinemic effect may be increased by concurrent tamoxifen. Carefully monitor prothrombin time.
Tamoxifen	Letrozole	↓	Tamoxifen reduced plasma letrozole concentrations by 37% when these drugs were coadministered.

* ↑ = Object drug increased. ↓ = Object drug decreased. ↔ = Undetermined clinical effect.

➤*Drug/Lab test interactions:* T$_4$ elevations occurred in a few postmenopausal patients but were not accompanied by clinical hyperthyroidism. An increase in thyroid-binding globulin in postmenopausal women on tamoxifen may explain T$_4$ elevations during treatment. Variations in the karyopyknotic index on vaginal smears and various degrees of estrogen effect on Pap smears have been infrequently seen in postmenopausal patients.

Adverse Reactions

Adverse reactions to tamoxifen are relatively mild and rarely require discontinuation of therapy.

Females –

Most frequent: Hot flashes.

Less frequent: Vaginal bleeding; vaginal discharge; menstrual irregularities; skin rash; headaches. Usually not severe enough to require dosage reduction or discontinuation.

Infrequent: Hypercalcemia; peripheral edema; food distaste; pruritus vulvae; depression; dizziness; lightheadedness; headache; hair thinning or partial loss; vaginal dryness.

Rare: Erythema multiforme; Stevens-Johnson syndrome; bullous pemphigoid; interstitial pneumonitis; hypersensitivity reactions, including angioedema; elevations of serum triglyceride levels, sometimes with pancreatitis.

Ovarian cysts have been observed in a small number of premenopausal patients with advanced breast cancer who have been treated with tamoxifen. There also have been reports of endometriosis and uterine fibroids.

Changes in liver enzyme levels have been associated with tamoxifen therapy (see Warnings).

TAMOXIFEN CITRATE
Adjuvant breast cancer –

Tamoxifen Adverse Reactions: 5-Year Therapy (%)		
Adverse reaction	Tamoxifen (n = 1422)	Placebo (n = 1437)
Hot flashes	64	48
Fluid retention	32	30
Vaginal discharge	30	15
Nausea	26	24
Irregular menses	25	19
Weight loss (> 5%)	23	18
Skin changes	19	15
Increased AST	5	3
Increased bilirubin	2	1
Increased creatinine	2	1
Thrombocytopenia (platelets < 100,000/mm^3)	2	1
Deep vein thrombosis[1]	0.8	0.2
Pulmonary embolism[1]	0.5	0.2
Superficial phlebitis[1]	0.4	0

[1] Two of the patients treated with tamoxifen who had thrombotic events died.

Premenopausal women with metastatic breast cancer –

Tamoxifen vs Ovarian Ablation (%)		
Adverse reaction	Tamoxifen (n = 104)	Ovarian ablation (n = 100)
Flush	33	46
Amenorrhea	16	69
Altered menses	13	5
Oligomenorrhea	9	1
Bone pain	6	6
Menstrual disorder	6	4
Nausea	5	4
Coughing	4	1
Edema	4	1
Fatigue	4	1
Musculoskeletal pain	3	0
Pain	3	4
Ovarian cyst(s)	3	2
Depression	2	2
Abdominal cramps	1	2
Anorexia	1	2

Reduction in breast cancer incidence – In the NSABP P-1 trial for reduction in breast cancer incidence in high-risk women, there was an increase in 6 serious adverse effects in the tamoxifen group: Endometrial cancer (33 cases in tamoxifen-treated patients vs 14 in placebo-treated patients), pulmonary embolism (18 cases tamoxifen vs 6 placebo), deep vein thrombosis (30 cases tamoxifen vs 19 placebo), stroke (34 cases tamoxifen vs 24 placebo), cataract formation (540 cases tamoxifen vs 483 placebo), and cataract surgery (101 cases tamoxifen vs 63 placebo).

The following table presents the adverse events observed in the NSABP P-1 by treatment arm. Only adverse events more common on tamoxifen than placebo are shown.

Adverse Reactions in NSABP P-1 Trial (%)		
Adverse reaction	Tamoxifen (n = 6681)	Placebo (n = 6707)
Hot flashes	80	68
Vaginal discharges	55	35
Vaginal bleeding	23	22
Mood changes	11.6	10.8
Infection/Sepsis	6	5.1
Alopecia	5.2	4.4
Constipation	4.4	3.2
Skin abnormality	5.6	4.7
Allergy	2.5	2.1
Platelets decreased	0.7	0.3

In the NSABP P-1 trial, 15% and 9.7% of participants receiving tamoxifen and placebo therapy, respectively, withdrew from the trial for medical reasons. The following are the medical reasons for withdrawing from tamoxifen therapy, respectively: Hot flashes (3.1% vs 1.5%) and vaginal discharge (0.5% vs 0.1%). In the NSABP P-1 trial 8.7% and 9.6% of participants receiving tamoxifen and placebo therapy, respectively withdrew for nonmedical reasons. In the NSABP P-1 trial, hot flashes of any severity occurred in 68% of women on placebo and in 80% of women on tamoxifen. Severe hot flashes occurred in 28% of women on placebo and 45% of women on tamoxifen. Vaginal discharge occurred in 35% and 55% of women on placebo and tamoxifen respectively; and was severe in 4.5% and 12.3%, respectively. There was no difference in the incidence of vaginal bleeding between treatment arms.

McCune-Albright syndrome – Mean uterine volume increased after 6 months of treatment and doubled at the end of the 1-year study. A causal relationship has not been established (see Warnings).

Males – Tamoxifen is well tolerated in males with breast cancer. The safety profile appears to be similar to that in females. Loss of libido and impotence have resulted in discontinuation of therapy. Also, in oligospermic males treated with tamoxifen, luteinizing hormone (LH), follicle-stimulating hormone (FSH), testosterone, and estrogen levels were elevated.

Overdosage

➤*Symptoms:* In animals, respiratory difficulties and convulsions occurred at high doses. In advanced metastatic cancer patients receiving loading doses of greater than 400 mg/m^2, followed by maintenance doses of 150 mg/m^2 twice daily, acute neurotoxicity manifested by tremor, hyperreflexia, unsteady gait, and dizziness was noted. Symptoms occurred within 3 to 5 days of beginning therapy and cleared within 2 to 5 days after stopping therapy. One patient experienced a seizure several days after discontinuation and after neurotoxic symptoms had resolved. The causal relationship to tamoxifen therapy is unknown. Prolongation of the QT interval also was noted in patients given doses higher than 250 mg/m^2 loading dose followed by maintenance treatment of 80 mg/m^2 twice daily. Minimal loading dose and maintenance doses given at which neurological symptoms and QT changes occurred were at least 6-fold higher than the maximum recommended dose.

➤*Treatment:* No specific treatment for overdosage is known; treatment must be symptomatic. Refer to General Management of Acute Overdosage.

Patient Information

Advise patients that tamoxifen reduces the incidence of breast cancer but may not eliminate risk. Instruct patients on the benefits of tamoxifen vs the risk.

Women with DCIS treated with lumpectomy and radiation therapy who are considering tamoxifen to reduce the incidence of a second breast cancer event should assess the risks and benefits of therapy because treatment with tamoxifen decreased the incidence of invasive breast cancer but has not been shown to affect survival.

Advise women who are receiving or who have previously received tamoxifen to have regular gynecologic examinations and promptly inform their physician of menstrual irregularities, abnormal vaginal bleeding, change in vaginal discharge, or pelvic pain or pressure.

Women who are pregnant or who plan to become pregnant should not take tamoxifen to reduce her risk of breast cancer. Effective nonhormonal contraception must be used by all premenopausal women taking tamoxifen and for approximately 2 months after discontinuing therapy if they are sexually active. Tamoxifen does not cause infertility, even in the presence of menstrual irregularity. For sexually active women of childbearing potential, initiate tamoxifen therapy during menstruation. In women with menstrual irregularity, a negative B-hCG immediately prior to the initiation of therapy is sufficient.

Notify physician of pain/swelling/tenderness of legs, unexplained shortness of breath, changes in vision, new breast lumps, vaginal bleeding, or gynecologic symptoms (eg, menstrual irregularities, changes in vaginal discharge, pelvic pain or pressure).

TOREMIFENE CITRATE

Rx	**Fareston** (Shire)	**Tablets:** 60 mg	Lactose. (TO 60). White. In 30s and 100s.

Indications

➤*Breast cancer:* Treatment of metastatic breast cancer in postmenopausal women with estrogen-receptor (ER)-positive or ER-unknown tumors.

Administration and Dosage

➤*Approved by the FDA:* May 30, 1997.

Dosage is 60 mg once daily, generally continued until disease progression is observed.

Actions

➤*Pharmacology:* Toremifene is a nonsteroidal triphenylethylene derivative (antiestrogen) differing from tamoxifene only by the addition of a chlorine atom. Toremifene binds to estrogen receptors and may exert estrogenic, antiestrogenic, or both activities, depending on duration of treatment, gender, target organ, or endpoint selected. In general, however, nonsteroidal triphenylethylene derivatives are predominantly antiestrogenic in rats and humans and estrogenic in mice. In rats, toremifene causes regression of established dimethylbenzanthracene (DMBA)-induced mammary tumors. The antitumor effect of toremifene in breast cancer is believed to be mainly because of its antiestrogenic effects (eg, its ability to compete with estrogen for binding sites in the cancer), blocking the growth-stimulating effects of estrogen in the tumor. Toremifene's antiestrogenic effect causes a decrease in the estradiol-induced vaginal cornification index in some postmenopausal women. Its estrogenic activity can decrease serum gonadotropin concentrations (FSH and LH).

➤*Pharmacokinetics:*

Absorption/Distribution – Toremifene is well absorbed and absorption is not influenced by food. Peak plasma concentrations are obtained within 3 hours. Toremifene displays linear pharmacokinetics after single oral doses of 10 to 680 mg. Steady-state concentrations were reached in ≈ 4 to 6 weeks. Toremifene has an apparent Vd of 580 L and binds extensively (> 99.5%) to serum proteins, mainly to albumin. The plasma concentration time profile of toremifene declines biexponentially after absorption with a mean distribution half-life of ≈ 4 hours.

Metabolism/Excretion – Toremifene is extensively metabolized, principally by CYP3A4 to N-demethyltoremifene, which also is antiestrogenic but with weak in vivo antitumor potency. Serum concentrations of N-demethyltoremifene are 2 to 4 times higher than toremifene at steady state. Elimination half-lives of major metabolites, N-demethyltoremifene and (deaminohydroxy) toremifene were 6 and 4 days, respectively. Mean total clearance of toremifene was ≈ 5 L/h. Toremifene is eliminated as metabolites predominantly in the feces, with ≈ 10% excreted in the urine during a 1-week period. Elimination of toremifene is slow, in part because of enterohepatic circulation. Elimination half-life is ≈ 5 days.

Special populations –

Hepatic insufficiency: The mean elimination half-life of toremifene was increased by < 2-fold in patients with hepatic impairment (cirrhosis or fibrosis). The pharmacokinetics of N-demethyltoremifene were unchanged in these patients.

Elderly: Increases in the elimination half-life (4.2 vs 7.2 days) and the volume of distribution (457 vs 627 L) of toremifene were observed in elderly females without any change in clearance or AUC.

➤*Clinical trials:* Three prospective, randomized, controlled clinical studies were conducted to evaluate the efficacy of toremifene in the treatment of breast cancer in postmenopausal women. Patients were randomized to parallel groups receiving 60 mg toremifene (TOR60) or 20 mg tamoxifen (TAM20) in the North American study or 40 mg tamoxifen (TAM40) in the Eastern European and Nordic studies. The North American and Eastern European studies also included high-dose toremifene arms of 200 and 240 mg daily, respectively, which were not superior to lower dose groups. The studies included postmenopausal women with ER-positive or ER-unknown metastatic breast cancer. The patients had ≥ 1 measurable or evaluable lesion. The median treatment duration was 5 months (range, 4.2 to 6.3 months).

Response to Toremifene vs Tamoxifen

	North American		Eastern European		Nordic	
	TOR60 (n = 221)	TAM20 (n = 215)	TOR60 (n = 157)	TAM40 (n = 149)	TOR60 (n = 214)	TAM40 (n = 201)
Responses[1]						
CR + PR	14 + 33	11 + 30	7 + 25	3 + 28	19 + 48	19 + 56
RR (CR +PR)%	21.3	19.1	20.4	20.8	31.3	37.3
Time to progression (TTP)						
Median (mo)	5.6	5.8	4.9	5	7.3	10.2
Survival (S)						
Median (mo)	33.6	34	25.4	23.4	33	38.7

[1] CR = complete response. PR = partial reponse. RR = response rate.

Contraindications

Hypersensitivity to the drug.

Warnings

➤*Hypercalcemia and tumor flare:* As with other antiestrogens, hypercalcemia and tumor flare have been reported in some breast cancer patients with bone metastases during the first weeks of treatment. Tumor flare is a syndrome of diffuse musculoskeletal pain and erythema with increased size of tumor lesions that later regress. It is often accompanied by hypercalcemia. Tumor flare does not imply treatment failure or represent tumor progression. Institute appropriate measures if hypercalcemia occurs, and if severe, discontinue treatment. Drugs that decrease renal calcium excretion (eg, thiazide diuretics) may increase the risk of hypercalcemia in patients receiving toremifene.

➤*Tumorigenicity:* Endometrial hyperplasia has occurred. Some patients treated with toremifene have developed endometrial cancer, but circumstances (eg, short duration of treatment, prior antiestrogen treatment or premalignant conditions) make it difficult to establish the role of toremifene. In general, patients with preexisting endometrial hyperplasia should not be given long-term toremifene treatment. Endometrial hyperplasia of the uterus was observed in monkeys following 52 weeks of treatment at ≥ 1 mg/kg and in dogs following 16 weeks of treatment at ≥ 3 mg/kg with toremifene (about ¼ and 1.4 times, respectively, the daily maximum recommended human dose on a mg/m^2 basis).

➤*Carcinogenesis:* Studies in mice at doses of 1 to 30 mg/kg/day (about 1/15 to 2 times the daily maximum recommended human dose on a mg/m^2 basis) for ≤ 2 years revealed increased incidence of ovarian and testicular tumors, and increased osteoma and osteosarcoma. The significance of the mouse findings is uncertain because of the different role of estrogens in mice and the estrogenic effects of toremifene in mice.

Toremifene is clastogenic in vitro (chromosomal aberrations and micronuclei formation in human lymphoblastoid MCL-5 cells) and in vivo (chromosomal aberrations in rat hepatocytes).

➤*Fertility impairment:* Toremifene produced impairment of fertility and conception in male and female rats at doses ≥ 25 and 0.14 mg/kg/day, respectively (about 3.5 times and 1/50 the daily maximum recommended human dose on a mg/m^2 basis). At these doses, sperm counts, fertility index and conception rates were reduced in males with atrophy of seminal vesicles and prostate. In females, fertility and reproductive indices were markedly reduced with increased pre- and postimplantation loss. In addition, offspring of treated rats exhibited depressed reproductive indices. Toremifene produced ovarian atrophy in dogs administered doses ≥ 3 mg/kg/day (about 1.5 times the daily maximum recommended human dose on a mg/m^2 basis) for 16 weeks. Cystic ovaries and reduction in endometrial stromal cellularity were observed in monkeys at doses ≥ 1 mg/kg/day (about ¼ the daily maximum recommended human dose on a mg/m^2 basis) for 52 weeks.

➤*Elderly:* The median ages in the three controlled studies ranged from 60 to 66 years. No significant age-related differences in toremifene were noted.

➤*Pregnancy: Category D.* Toremifene may cause fetal harm when administered to a pregnant woman. Studies in rats at doses ≥ 1 mg/kg/day (about ¼ the daily maximum recommended human dose on a mg/m^2 basis) administered during the period of organogenesis, have shown that toremifene is embryotoxic and fetotoxic, as indicated by intrauterine mortality, increased resorption, reduced fetal weight and fetal anomalies, including malformations of limbs, incomplete ossification, misshapen bones, ribs/spine anomalies, hydroureter, hydronephrosis, testicular displacement and subcutaneous edema. Fetal anomalies may have been a consequence of maternal toxicity. Toremifene crosses the placenta and accumulates in the rodent fetus. In rodent models of fetal reproductive tract development, toremifene inhibited uterine development in female pups similar to diethylstilbestrol (DES) and tamoxifen.

Embryotoxicity and fetotoxicity were observed in rabbits at doses ≥ 1.25 and 2.5 mg/kg/day, respectively (about ⅓ and ⅔ times the daily maximum recommended human dose on a mg/m^2 basis); fetal anomalies included incomplete ossification and anencephaly.

There are no studies in pregnant women. If toremifene is used during pregnancy, or if the patient becomes pregnant while receiving this drug, apprise the patient of the potential hazard to the fetus or potential risk for loss of the pregnancy.

➤*Lactation:* Toremifene is excreted in the milk of lactating rats. It is not known whether this drug is excreted in human breast milk.

➤*Children:* There is no indication for use of toremifene in pediatric patients.

Precautions

➤*Monitoring:* Obtain periodic complete blood counts, calcium levels and liver function tests. Closely monitor patients with bone metastases for hypercalcemia during the first weeks of treatment (see Warnings).

TOREMIFENE CITRATE

Leukopenia and thrombocytopenia have been reported rarely; monitor leukocyte and platelet counts when using toremifene.

➤*Thromboembolic disease:* Patients with a history of thromboembolic disease should generally not be treated with toremifene.

Drug Interactions

➤*Anticoagulants:* There is a known interaction between antiestrogenic compounds of the triphenylethylene derivative class and coumarin-type anticoagulants (eg, warfarin), leading to an increased prothrombin time. When concomitant use of anticoagulants with toremifene is necessary, careful monitoring of the prothrombin time is recommended.

Cytochrome P450 3A4 enzyme inducers, such as phenobarbital, phenytoin and carbamazepine, increase the rate of toremifene metabolism, lowering the steady-state concentration in serum. Metabolism of toremifene may be inhibited by drugs known to inhibit CYP3A4 to 6 enzymes. Examples of such drugs are ketoconazole and similar antimycotics as well as erythromycin and similar macrolides. Patients on anticonvulsants (phenobarbital, clonazepam, phenytoin and carbamazepine) showed a 2–fold increase in clearance and a decrease in elimination half-life of toremifene.

Adverse Reactions

Adverse drug reactions are principally caused by the antiestrogenic hormonal actions of toremifene and typically occur at the beginning of treatment.

Toremifene Adverse Reactions in the North American Study (%)

Adverse reaction	TOR60 (n = 221)	TAM20 (n = 215)
Hot flashes	35	30
Sweating	20	17
Nausea	14	15
Vaginal discharge	13	16
Dizziness	9	7
Edema	5	5
Vomiting	4	2
Vaginal bleeding	2	4

Approximately 1% of patients receiving toremifene (n = 592) in the three controlled studies discontinued treatment as a result of adverse events (nausea and vomiting, fatigue, thrombophlebitis, depression, lethargy, anorexia, ischemic attack, arthritis, pulmonary embolism and myocardial infarction).

Toremifene Adverse Reactions: Toremifene vs Tamoxifen (%)

Adverse reaction	North American TOR60 (n = 221)	North American TAM20 (n = 215)	Eastern European TOR60 (n = 157)	Eastern European TAM40 (n = 149)	Nordic TOR60 (n = 214)	Nordic TAM40 (n = 201)
Cardiovascular						
Cardiac failure	2	< 1	-	< 1	1	1.5
Myocardial infarction	1	1.5	< 1	1	-	< 1
Arrhythmia	-	-	-	-	1.5	< 1
Angina pectoris	-	-	< 1	-	< 1	1
Ophthalmic						
Cataracts	10	7.5	-	-	-	3
Dry eyes	9	7.5	-	-	-	-
Abnormal visual fields	4	5	-	-	-	< 1
Corneal keratopathy	2	1	-	-	-	-
Glaucoma	1.5	1	< 1	-	-	< 1
Abnormal vision/ diplopia	-	-	-	-	1.5	-

Toremifene Adverse Reactions: Toremifene vs Tamoxifen (%)

Adverse reaction	North American TOR60 (n = 221)	North American TAM20 (n = 215)	Eastern European TOR60 (n = 157)	Eastern European TAM40 (n = 149)	Nordic TOR60 (n = 214)	Nordic TAM40 (n = 201)
Thrombo-embolic						
Pulmonary embolism	2	1	< 1	-	-	< 1
Thrombo-phlebitis	-	1	< 1	< 1	2	1.5
Thrombosis	-	< 1	< 1	-	1.5	2
CVA/TIA	< 1	-	-	< 1	2	2
Elevated liver tests[1]						
AST	5	2	19	15	15	17
Alkaline phosphatase	19	11	10	9	8	15
Bilirubin	1.5	2	1	< 1	1	1.5
Miscellaneous						
Hyper-calcemia	3	3	< 1	-	-	-

[1] Elevated defined as: North American Study: AST > 100 IU/L; alkaline phosphatase > 200 IU/L; bilirubin > 2 mg/dl. Eastern European/Nordic Studies: AST, alkaline phosphatase, and bilirubin: WHO Grade 1 (1.25 times the upper limit of normal).

Other adverse events of unclear causal relationship to toremifene included leukopenia and thrombocytopenia, skin discoloration or dermatitis, constipation, dyspnea, paresis, tremor, vertigo, pruritus, anorexia, reversible corneal opacity (corneal verticulata), asthenia, alopecia, depression, jaundice, and rigors.

In the 200 and 240 mg toremifene dose arms, the incidence of AST elevation and nausea was higher. Approximately 4% of patients were withdrawn for toxicity from the high-dose toremifene treatment arms. Reasons for withdrawal included hypercalcemia, abnormal liver function tests, 1 case each of toxic hepatitis, depression, dizziness, incoordination, ataxia, blurred vision, diffuse dermatitis, and a constellation of symptoms consisting of nausea, sweating, and tremor.

Overdosage

➤*Symptoms:* Lethality was observed in rats following single oral doses that were ≥ 1000 mg/kg (≈ 150 times the recommended human dose on a mg/m² basis) and was associated with gastric atony/dilation leading to interference with digestion and adrenal enlargement.

Vertigo, headache, and dizziness were observed in healthy volunteers at a daily dose of 680 mg for 5 days. The symptoms occurred in 2 of the 5 subjects during the third day of treatment and disappeared within 2 days of discontinuation of the drug. No immediate concomitant changes in any measured clinical chemistry parameters were found. In a study of postmenopausal breast cancer patients, toremifene 400 mg/m²/day caused dose-limiting nausea, vomiting, and dizziness, as well as reversible hallucinations and ataxia in 1 patient.

Theoretically, overdose may be manifested as an increase of antiestrogenic effects, such as hot flashes; estrogenic effects such as vaginal bleeding; or nervous system disorders such as vertigo, dizziness, ataxia, and nausea.

➤*Treatment:* No specific antidote exists and treatment is symptomatic. Refer to General Management of Acute Overdosage.

Patient Information

Vaginal bleeding has been reported in patients using toremifene. Inform patients about this reaction and instruct them to contact their physician if such bleeding occurs.

Inform patients with bone metastases of typical signs/symptoms of hypercalcemia; instruct them to contact their physician if such signs or symptoms occur.

FULVESTRANT

Rx	**Faslodex** (AstraZeneca)	**Injection:** 50 mg/mL	Alcohol, benzyl alcohol, castor oil. In 5 mL or two 2.5 mL prefilled syringes.

Indications

➤*Breast cancer:* Treatment of hormone receptor-positive metastatic breast cancer in postmenopausal women with disease progression following antiestrogen therapy.

Administration and Dosage

➤*Approved by the FDA:* April 25, 2002.

➤*Adults:* The recommended dose is 250 mg to be administered IM into the buttock at intervals of 1 month as a single 5 mL injection or 2 concurrent 2.5 mL injections. Administer the injection slowly.

➤*Storage/Stability:* Store in a refrigerator 2° to 8°C (36° to 46°F) in original container.

Actions

➤*Pharmacology:* Many breast cancers have estrogen receptors (ERs) and the growth of these tumors can be stimulated by estrogen. Fulvestrant is an estrogen receptor antagonist that binds to the estrogen receptor in a competitive manner with affinity comparable with that of estradiol. Fulvestrant downregulates the ER protein in human breast cancer cells.

In a clinical study in postmenopausal women with primary breast cancer treated with single doses of fulvestrant 15 to 22 days prior to sur-

FULVESTRANT

gery, there was evidence of increasing downregulation of ER with increasing dose. This was associated with a dose-related decrease in the expression of the progesterone receptor, an estrogen-regulated protein. These effects on the ER pathway also were associated with a decrease in Ki67 labeling index, a marker of cell proliferation.

In vitro studies demonstrated that fulvestrant is a reversible inhibitor of the growth of tamoxifen-resistant, as well as estrogen-sensitive human breast cancer (MCF-7) cell lines.

In in vivo studies in immature rats and ovariectomized monkeys, fulvestrant blocked the uterotrophic action of estradiol. In postmenopausal women, the absence of changes in plasma concentrations of follicle-stimulating hormone (FSH) and luteinizing hormone (LH) in response to fulvestrant treatment (250 mg monthly) suggests no peripheral steroidal effects.

➤*Pharmacokinetics:*

Absorption/Distribution – Following IV administration, fulvestrant is rapidly cleared at a rate approximating hepatic blood flow (about 10.5 mL plasma/min/kg). After an IM injection, plasma concentrations are maximal at about 7 days and are maintained over a period of at least 1 month, with trough concentration about ⅓ of C_{max}. The apparent half-life was about 40 days. After administration of 250 mg fulvestrant IM every month, plasma levels approach steady state after 3 to 6 doses, with an average 2.5-fold increase in plasma AUC compared with single dose AUC and trough levels about equal to the single dose C_{max} (see table).

Fulvestrant Pharmacokinetic Parameters in Postmenopausal Advanced Breast Cancer Patients After a 250 mg IM Dose (Mean ± SD)

	C_{max} (ng/mL)	C_{min} (ng/mL)	AUC (ng·d/mL)	$t_{1/2}$ (days)	CL (mL/min)
Single dose	8.5 ± 5.4	2.6 ± 1.1	131 ± 62	40 ± 11	690 ± 226
Multiple-dose steady state	15.8 ± 2.4	7.4 ± 1.7	328 ± 48		

Fulvestrant was subject to extensive and rapid distribution. The apparent volume of distribution at steady state was approximately 3 to 5 L/kg. This suggests that distribution is largely extravascular. Fulvestrant was highly (99%) bound to plasma proteins; VLDL, LDL, and HDL lipoprotein fractions appear to be the major binding components. The role of sex hormone-binding globulin, if any, could not be determined.

Metabolism/Excretion – Biotransformation and disposition of fulvestrant in humans have been determined following IM and IV administration of ^{14}C-labeled fulvestrant. Metabolism of fulvestrant appears to involve combinations of a number of possible biotransformation pathways analogous to those of endogenous steroids, including oxidation, aromatic hydroxylation, conjugation with glucuronic acid and/or sulphate at the 2, 3, and 17 positions of the steroid nucleus, and oxidation of the side chain sulphoxide. Identified metabolites are less active or exhibit similar activity to fulvestrant in antiestrogen models. Studies using human liver preparations and recombinant human enzymes indicate that cytochrome P-450 3A4 (CYP 3A4) is the only P-450 isoenzyme involved in the oxidation of fulvestrant; however, the relative contribution of P-450 and non-P-450 routes in vivo is unknown.

Fulvestrant was rapidly cleared by the hepatobiliary route with excretion primarily via the feces (approximately 90%). Renal elimination was negligible (less than 1%).

➤*Clinical trials:* Efficacy of fulvestrant was established by comparison to the selective aromatase inhibitor anastrozole in 2 randomized, controlled clinical trials (one conducted in North America, the other in Europe) in postmenopausal women with locally advanced or metastatic breast cancer. All patients had progressed after previous therapy with an antiestrogen or progestin for breast cancer in the adjuvant or advanced disease setting. The majority of patients in these trials had ER+ and/or PgR+ tumors. Patients who had ER-/PgR- or unknown disease must have shown prior response to endocrine therapy.

In both trials, eligible patients with measurable and/or evaluable disease were randomized to receive either fulvestrant 250 mg IM once/month (28 days ± 3 days) or anastrozole 1 mg orally once daily. All patients were assessed monthly for the first 3 months and every 3 months thereafter. Patients on the fulvestrant arm of the North American trial received 2 separate injections (two 2.5 mL), whereas fulvestrant patients received a single injection (one 5 mL) in the European trial. In both trials, patients were initially randomized to a 125 mg/month dose as well, but interim analysis showed a very low response rate and low dose groups were dropped.

Results of the trials, after a minimum follow-up duration of 14.6 months, are summarized in the following table. The effectiveness of fulvestrant 250 mg was determined by comparing response rates (RR) and time to progression (TTP) results to anastrozole 1 mg, the active control. With respect to response rate, the 2 studies ruled out (by one-sided 97.7% confidence limit) inferiority of fulvestrant to anastrozole of 6.3% and 1.4%.

Fulvestrant vs Anastrozole Efficacy Results

End point	North American trial		European trial	
	Fulvestrant 250 mg (n = 206)	Anastrozole 1 mg (n = 194)	Fulvestrant 250 mg (n = 222)	Anastrozole 1 mg (n = 229)
Objective tumor response				
Number (%) of subjects with CR[1] + PR[2]	35 (17)	33 (17)	45 (20.3)	34 (14.9)
% Difference in tumor				
Response rate (FAS[3]-ANA[4])	0		5.4	
2-sided 95.4% CI[5]	(-6.3, 8.9)		(-1.44, 14.8)	
Stable disease for ≥ 24 weeks (%)	26.7	19.1	24.3	30.1
Time to progression (TTP)				
Median TTP (days)	165	103	166	156
Hazard ratio (FAS/ANA)	0.9		1	
2-sided 95.4% CI	(0.7 to 1.1)		(0.8 to 1.26)	
Survival time				
Died n (%)	109 (52.9)	92 (47.4)	125 (56.3)	130 (56.8)
Median survival (days)	837	901	803	742
Hazard ratio	1.1		1	
2-sided 95% CI	(0.8, 1.5)		(0.8, 1.3)	

[1] CR = complete response.
[2] PR = partial response.
[3] FAS = *Faslodex.*
[4] ANA = anastrozole.
[5] CI = confidence interval.

Contraindications

Pregnancy; hypersensitivity to the drug or to any of its components.

Warnings

➤*Hepatic function impairment:* Safety and efficacy have not been evaluated in patients with moderate to severe hepatic impairment (see Pharmacology and Administration and Dosage).

➤*Carcinogenesis:* A 2-year carcinogenesis study was conducted in female and male rats at IM doses of 15 mg/kg/30 days, 10 mg/rat/30 days and 10 mg/rat/15 days. These doses correspond to approximately 1-, 3-, and 5-fold (in females) and 1.3-, 1.3-, and 1.6-fold (in males) the systemic exposure ($AUC_{0-30\ days}$) achieved in women receiving the recommended dose of 250 mg/month. An increased incidence of benign ovarian granulosa cell tumors and testicular Leydig cell tumors was evident in females dosed at 10 mg/rat/15 days and males dosed at 15 mg/rat/30 days, respectively. Induction of such tumors is consistent with the pharmacology-related endocrine feedback alterations in gonadotropin levels caused by an antiestrogen.

➤*Fertility impairment:* In female rats, fulvestrant administered at doses of 0.01 mg/kg/day or greater (approximately one-hundredth of the human recommended dose based on body surface area [BSA], for 2 weeks prior to and for 1 week following mating, caused a reduction in fertility and embryonic survival. Restoration of female fertility to values similar to controls was evident following a 29-day withdrawal period after dosing at 2 mg/kg/day (twice the human dose based on BSA). The effects of fulvestrant on the fertility of female rats appear to be consistent with its antiestrogenic activity. The potential effects of fulvestrant on the fertility of male animals were not studied, but in a 6-month toxicology study, male rats treated with IM doses of 15 mg/rat/30 days, 10 mg/rat/30 days, or 10 mg/rat/15 days fulvestrant showed a loss of spermatozoa from the seminiferous tubules, seminiferous tubular atrophy, and degenerative changes in the epididymides. Changes in the testes and epididymides had not recovered 20 weeks after cessation of dosing. These fulvestrant doses correspond to approximately 2-, 3-, and 3-fold the systemic exposure ($AUC_{0-30\ days}$) achieved in women.

➤*Pregnancy: Category D.* Advise women of childbearing potential not to become pregnant while receiving fulvestrant. Fulvestrant can cause fetal harm when administered to a pregnant woman and has been shown to cross the placenta following single IM doses in rats and rabbits. In studies of the pregnant rat, IM doses of fulvestrant 100 times lower than the maximum recommended human dose (based on BSA), caused an increased incidence of fetal abnormalities and death. Similarly, rabbits failed to maintain pregnancy and the fetuses showed an increased incidence of skeletal variations when fulvestrant was administered at 50% of the recommended human dose (based on BSA).

There are no studies in pregnant women using fulvestrant. If fulvestrant is used during pregnancy or if the patient becomes pregnant while receiving this drug, apprise the patient of the potential hazard to the fetus or potential risk for loss of the pregnancy.

Before starting treatment with fulvestrant, pregnancy must be excluded.

FULVESTRANT

►*Lactation:* Fulvestrant is found in rat milk at levels significantly higher (approximately 12-fold) than plasma after administration of 2 mg/kg. Drug exposure in rodent pups from fulvestrant-treated lactating dams was estimated as 10% of the administered dose. It is not known if fulvestrant is excreted in human milk. Because many drugs are excreted in human milk, and because of the potential for serious adverse reactions from fulvestrant in nursing infants, a decision should be made whether to discontinue nursing or to discontinue the drug, taking into account the importance of the drug to the mother.

►*Children:* The safety and efficacy of fulvestrant in pediatric patients have not been established.

Drug Interactions

There are no known drug interactions. Fulvestrant does not significantly inhibit any of the major CYP isoenzymes.

Fulvestrant is metabolized by CYP 3A4 in vitro. Clinical studies of the effect of strong CYP 3A4 inhibitors on the pharmacokinetics of fulvestrant have not been performed.

Adverse Reactions

The most commonly reported adverse experiences in the fulvestrant and anastrozole treatment groups, regardless of the investigator's assessment of causality, were the following: GI symptoms (including nausea, vomiting, constipation, diarrhea, abdominal pain), headache, back pain, vasodilation (hot flushes), and pharyngitis.

Injection site reactions with mild transient pain and inflammation were seen with fulvestrant and occurred in 7% of patients (1% of treatments) given the single 5 mL injection (European trial) and in 27% of patients (4.6% of treatments) given the two 2.5 mL injections (North American trial).

Adverse Events: Fulvestrant vs Anastrozole (≥ 5%)[1]		
Adverse event[2]	Fulvestrant 250 mg IM once monthly (n = 423)	Anastrozole 1 mg PO daily (n = 423)
CNS	34.3	33.8
Headache	15.4	16.8
Dizziness	6.9	6.6
Insomnia	6.9	8.5
Paresthesia	6.4	7.6
Depression	5.7	6.9
Anxiety	5	3.8
Dermatologic	22.2	23.4
Rash	7.3	8
Sweating	5	5.2
GI	51.5	48
Nausea	26	25.3
Vomiting	13	11.8
Constipation	12.5	10.6
Diarrhea	12.3	12.8
Abdominal pain	11.8	11.6
Anorexia	9	10.9

Adverse Events: Fulvestrant vs Anastrozole (≥ 5%)[1]		
Adverse event[2]	Fulvestrant 250 mg IM once monthly (n = 423)	Anastrozole 1 mg PO daily (n = 423)
Musculoskeletal	25.5	27.9
Bone pain	15.8	13.7
Arthritis	2.8	6.1
Respiratory	38.5	33.6
Pharyngitis	16.1	11.6
Dyspnea	14.9	12.3
Cough increased	10.4	10.4
Miscellaneous		
Asthenia	22.7	27
Pain	18.9	20.3
Vasodilation	17.7	17.3
Back pain	14.4	13.2
Injection site pain[3]	10.9	6.6
Pelvic pain	9.9	9
Peripheral edema	9	10.2
Chest pain	7.1	5
Flu syndrome	7.1	6.4
Fever	6.4	6.4
Urinary tract infection	6.1	3.5
Accidental injury	4.5	5.7
Anemia	4.5	5

[1] Data combined from the North American and European trials.
[2] A patient may have more than 1 adverse event.
[3] All patients on fulvestrant received injections, but only those anastrozole patients who were in the North American study received placebo injections.

Other adverse events reported as drug-related and seen infrequently (less than 1%) include thromboembolic phenomena, myalgia, vertigo, and leukopenia.

Vaginal bleeding has been reported infrequently (less than 1%), mainly in patients during the first 6 weeks after changing from existing hormonal therapy to treatment with fulvestrant. If bleeding persists, consider further evaluation.

Overdosage

Animal studies have shown no effects other than those related directly or indirectly to antiestrogen activity with IM doses of fulvestrant higher than the recommended human dose. There is no clinical experience with overdosage in humans. No adverse effects were seen in healthy male and female volunteers who received IV fulvestrant, which resulted in peak plasma concentrations at the end of the infusion that were approximately 10 to 15 times those seen after IM injection.

LEUPROLIDE ACETATE

Rx	**Leuprolide Acetate Injection** (Various, eg, Bedford Laboratories)	**Injection:** 5 mg/ml	In 2.8 ml multiple-dose vials.[1]
Rx	**Lupron** (TAP Pharm)		In 2.8 ml multiple-dose vials.[1]
Rx	**Lupron for Pediatric Use** (TAP Pharm)		In 2.8 ml multiple-dose vials.[1]
Rx	**Eligard** (Sanofi-Synthelabo	**Powder for Injection, lyophilized:** 7.5 mg	In single-use kits with a 2-syringe mixing system and 20-gauge, ½ inch needle.
Rx	**Eligard 22.5 mg** (Sanofi-Synthelabo	**Injection:** 22.5 mg	In single-use kits with a 2-syringe mixing system and 20-gauge, ½ inch needle.
Rx	**Eligard** (Sanofi-Synthelabo	**Injection:** 30 mg	In single-use kit with 2-syringe mixing system and syringe containing *Atrigel*.
Rx	**Lupron Depot** (TAP Pharm)	**Microspheres for Injection, lyophilized:**[2] 3.75 mg	Mannitol. Preservative free. In single kits, multi-packs, and prefilled dual-chamber syringe.
		7.5 mg	Mannitol. Preservative free. In single kits, multi-packs, and prefilled dual-chamber syringe.
Rx	**Lupron Depot-Ped** (TAP Pharm)	**Microspheres for Injection, lyophilized:**[2] 7.5 mg	Mannitol. Preservative free. In single-dose kit and pre-filled dual-chamber syringe.
		11.25 mg	Mannitol. Preservative free. In single-dose kit and pre-filled dual-chamber syringe.
		15 mg	Mannitol. Preservative free. In single-dose kit and pre-filled dual-chamber syringe.
Rx	**Lupron Depot - 3 Month** (TAP Pharm)	**Microspheres for Injection, lyophilized:**[2] 11.25 mg	Mannitol. Preservative free. In single-use kit containing 11.25 mg vial leuprolide with 1.5 ml diluent and in pre-filled dual-chamber syringes.
		22.5 mg	Mannitol. Preservative free. In single-use kit containing 22.5 mg vial leuprolide with 1.5 ml diluent and in pre-filled dual-chamber syringes.
Rx	**Lupron Depot - 4 Month** (TAP Pharm)	**Microspheres for Injection, lyophilized:**[2] 30 mg	Mannitol. Preservative free. In single-use kit containing 30 mg vial leuprolide with 1.5 ml diluent and in pre-filled dual-chamber syringes.
Rx	**Viadur** (ALZA Corporation)	**Implant:** 72 mg	In single-dose kit.

[1] With 9 mg/ml benzyl alcohol as preservative and sodium chloride.

[2] Listed as total dose; vials are combined to provide proper strength.

Indications

➤*Advanced prostatic cancer (injection, implant, or depot 7.5, 22.5, and 30 mg):* Palliative treatment of advanced prostatic cancer that offers an alternative when orchiectomy or estrogen administration are not indicated or are unacceptable to the patient.

➤*Endometriosis (depot 3.75 and 11.25 mg):* Management of endometriosis, including pain relief and reduction of endometriotic lesions. Experience is limited to women ≥ 18 years of age treated for ≤ 6 months.

➤*Uterine leiomyomata (fibroids) (depot 3.75 and 11.25 mg):* Concomitantly with iron therapy for the preoperative hematologic improvement of patients with anemia caused by uterine leiomyomata. Experience with leuprolide depot in females has been limited to women ≥ 18 years of age and treated for ≤ 6 months.

➤*Central precocious puberty (CPP) (pediatric injection or Depot-Ped):* Treatment of children with CPP.

Administration and Dosage

➤*Depot:* Because of different release characteristics, a fractional dose of the 3-month or 4-month depot formulation is not equivalent to the same dose of the monthly formulation and should not be given.Do not use needles smaller than 22-gauge. Reconstitute only with diluent provided.

➤*Injection:* Vary the injection site periodically. Use the syringes provided in the kit; if alternate syringes are needed, use insulin syringes.

➤*Advanced prostate cancer:*

Injection – 1 mg SC daily.

Depot – 7.5 mg IM monthly, 22.5 mg IM every 3 months (84 days), 30 mg IM every 4 months (16 weeks).

Implant – One implant every 12 months.

➤*Endometriosis (depot only):* 3.75 mg IM monthly or 11.25 mg IM every 3 months.

Recommended duration is 6 months. Retreatment cannot be recommended since safety data are not available. If the symptoms of endometriosis recur after a course of therapy and further treatment is contemplated, it is recommended that bone density be assessed before retreatment begins to ensure that values are within normal limits.

➤*Uterine leiomyomata (depot only):* 3.75 mg IM monthly or one 11.25 mg IM injection with concomitant iron therapy.

11.25 mg is indicated only for women for whom 3 months of hormonal suppression is deemed necessary.

The clinician may wish to consider a 1-month trial period of iron alone, because some patients may respond to iron alone.

Recommended duration of therapy is ≤ 3 months. The symptoms associated with uterine leiomyomata will recur following discontinuation of

therapy. If additional treatment is contemplated, assess bone density prior to initiation of therapy to ensure that values are within normal limits.

➤*CPP:* Individualize dosage based on a mg/kg ratio of drug to body weight. Younger children require higher doses on a mg/kg basis.

Injection – May be administered by a patient/parent or health care professional. Recommended starting dose is 50 mcg/kg/day as a single SC injection. If total downregulation is not achieved, titrate upward by 10 mcg/kg/day, which will be considered the maintenance dose.

Depot-Ped (7.5, 11.25, and 15 mg) – Must be administered under physician supervision. Recommended starting dose is 0.3 mg/kg/ 4 weeks (minimum, 7.5 mg) as a single IM injection. Determine the starting dose as follows:

Leuprolide Depot Starting Dose for CPP	
Weight (kg)	Dose (mg)
≤ 25	7.5
> 25 to 37.5	11.25
> 37.5	15

If total downregulation is not achieved, titrate upward in 3.75 mg increments every 4 weeks, which will be considered the maintenance dose.

Injection / Depot – After 1 to 2 months of initiating therapy or changing doses, monitor with a GnRH stimulation test, sex steroids, and Tanner staging to confirm downregulation. Monitor measurements of bone age for advancement every 6 to 12 months. Titrate the dose upwards until no progression of the condition is noted either clinically or by lab parameters. The first dose to result in adequate downregulation can probably be maintained for duration of therapy in most children. However, there are insufficient data to guide dosage adjustment as patients move into higher weight categories. Verify adequate downregulation in patients whose weight has increased significantly while on therapy. Vary the injection site periodically. Consider discontinuation of therapy before 11 years of age in females and before 12 years of age in males.

➤*Depot preparation:*

Single use kit – For a single IM injection, reconstitute the lyophilized microspheres with diluent provided. Using a 22-gauge needle, withdraw appropriate amount of diluent from amp (1 or 1.5 ml); inject into vial. Shake well to obtain uniform suspension. It will appear milky. Withdraw entire contents into syringe and inject immediately.

Prefilled dual-chamber syringe – To prepare for injection, screw the white plunger into the end stopper until the stopper begins to turn. Remove and discard the tab around the base of the needle. Holding the syringe upright, release the diluent by slowly pushing the plunger until the first stopper is at the blue line in the middle of the barrel. Gently shake the syringe to thoroughly mix the particles to form a uniform suspension. The suspension will appear milky. If the microspheres (par-

LEUPROLIDE ACETATE

ticles) adhere to the stopper, tap the syringe against your finger. Remove the needle guard and advance the plunger to expel air from the syringe. Inject the entire contents of the syringe IM as you would for a normal injection. The suspension settles very quickly following reconstitution; therefore, it is preferable to mix and use immediately. Reshake suspension if settling occurs.

►*Storage/Stability:*

Injection – Store below room temperature (25°C; 77°F). Avoid freezing. Protect from light; store vial in carton until use.

Depot – May be stored at room temperature; protect from freezing. The suspension is stable for 24 hours following reconstitution; however, since the product does not contain a preservative, discard if not used immediately.

Implant – Store at 25°C (77°F); excursions permitted to 15° to 30°C (59° to 86°F).

Actions

►*Pharmacology:* Leuprolide, a luteinizing hormone-releasing hormone (LH-RH) agonist, is a synthetic nonapeptide analog of naturally occurring gonadotropin-releasing hormone (GnRH) possessing greater potency than the natural hormone. It inhibits gonadotropin secretion when given continuously and in therapeutic doses. After initial stimulation, chronic administration of leuprolide suppresses ovarian and testicular steroidogenesis, which is reversible upon discontinuation.

Leuprolide initially increases circulating levels of luteinizing hormone (LH) and follicle stimulating hormone (FSH), leading to a transient increase in gonadal steroids (testosterone and dihydrotestosterone in males; estrone and estradiol in premenopausal females). However, continuous daily administration results in decreased LH and FSH in all patients. In males, testosterone is reduced to castrate levels. In premenopausal females, estrogens are reduced to postmenopausal levels. These decreases occur within 2 to 4 weeks after initiation. Castrate levels of testosterone in prostatic cancer have been seen for ≤ 5 years. Leuprolide also inhibits growth of certain hormone-dependent tumors and atrophy of the reproductive organs.

CPP – In children with CPP, stimulated and basal gonadotropins are reduced to prepubertal levels. Testosterone and estradiol are reduced to prepubertal levels in males and females, respectively. Reduction of gonadotropins will allow for normal physical and psychological growth and development. Natural maturation occurs when gonadotropins return to pubertal levels following discontinuation of leuprolide acetate.

The following physiologic effects have been noted with the chronic administration of leuprolide acetate in this patient population:

Skeletal growth – A measurable increase in body length can be noted because the epiphyseal plates will not close prematurely;

Organ growth – Reproductive organs will return to a prepubertal state;

Menses – If present, will cease.

►*Pharmacokinetics:*

Absorption –

Depot: Mean peak plasma levels of ≈ 7, 20, 36.3, 48.9, and 59.3 ng/ml occurred at 4 hours and declined to 0.3, 0.36, 0.23, 0.67, and 0.44 ng/ml by week 4 after single injections of the 3.75, 7.5, 11.25, 22.5, and 30 mg depot formulations, respectively. After an initial burst, leuprolide release declined rapidly to provide steady-state plasma levels throughout the monthly, 3-, or 4-month dosing interval.

Implant: After insertion of leuprolide implant, mean serum leuprolide concentrations were 16.9 ng/ml at 4 hours and 2.4 ng/ml at 24 hours.

Mean serum leuprolide concentrations were maintained at ≈ 0.9 ng/ml for 12 months.

Distribution –

Depot and implant: The mean steady-state volume of distribution of leuprolide following 1 mg IV bolus administration to healthy volunteers was 27 L. In vitro binding to human plasma proteins ranged from 43% to 49%.

Metabolism –

Depot: Systemic clearance following a 1 mg IV bolus of leuprolide was 7.6 L/hr with a terminal half-life of ≈ 3 hours based on a 2 compartment mode.

Excretion –

Depot: Following administration of the 3.75 mg depot, < 5% of the dose was recovered.

►*Clinical trials:*

Advanced prostatic cancer – In a controlled study comparing leuprolide injection 1 mg/day SC with diethylstilbestrol (DES) 3 mg/day, the survival rate for the 2 groups was comparable after 2 years of treatment. The objective response to treatment was also similar for the 2 groups. The safety and efficacy of monthly leuprolide depot did not differ from that of the SC injection.

In clinical studies with the 3-month 22.5 mg and 4-month 30 mg depot formulations, mean serum testosterone was suppressed to castrate levels within ≤ 30 days in ≈ 95% of patients. Approximately 85% of patients had no tumor progression during the first 24 weeks of treatment with the 3-month depot and at week 16 with the 4-month formulation. A change in serum prostate-specific antigen (PSA) to within normal range (≤ 4 ng/ml) occurred in 63% and 50% of patients treated with 3- and 4-month depot, respectively.

Following the initial insertion in patients receiving 1 implant, mean serum testosterone concentrations increased from 422 ng/dl at baseline to 690 ng/dl on day 3, then decreased to below baseline by week 2. Serum testosterone decreased below the 50 ng/dl castrate threshold by week 4 in 99%. Once serum testosterone suppression was achieved, testosterone remained suppressed below the castrate threshold for the duration of the treatment phase.

Most patients (n = 118) had a new implant inserted for a second year of therapy following removal of the first implant(s). No patient experienced a clinically significant increase in serum testosterone (acute-on-chronic phenomenon) upon removal of the original implant(s) and insertion of a new implant. Suppression of serum testosterone was maintained in all patients through the 2-month follow-up period following removal of the first implant(s) and insertion of a new implant.

Endometriosis – Leuprolide depot 3.75 mg monthly for 6 months was comparable with danazol 800 mg/day in relieving clinical symptoms (eg, pelvic pain, dysmenorrhea, dyspareunia, pelvic tenderness, induration) and in reducing the size of endometrial implants.

Hormone replacement therapy: Clinical studies suggest that the addition of hormonal replacement therapy (estrogen or progestin) to leuprolide is effective in reducing loss of bone mineral density which occurs with leuprolide, without compromising the efficacy of leuprolide in relieving symptoms of endometriosis. The optimal drug/dose is not established.

Uterine leiomyomata (fibroids) – Administration of leuprolide depot 3.75 mg for 3 or 6 months decreased uterine and fibroid volume, thus allowing for relief of clinical signs and symptoms (eg, abdominal bloating, pelvic pain, pressure). Excessive vaginal bleeding (eg, menorrhagia, menometrorrhagia) decreased (in 1 study, 80% of the patients experienced relief), resulting in improvement in hematologic parameters.

Following administration of the 3-month 11.25 mg depot, the onset of estradiol suppression was observed for individual subjects between day 4 and week 4 after dosing. Serum estradiol was suppressed to ≤ 20 pg/ml in all subjects within 4 weeks and remained suppressed (≤ 40 pg/ml) in 80% of subjects until the end of the 12-week dosing interval.

The 3-month 11.25 mg depot produced similar pharmacodynamic effects in terms of hormonal and menstrual suppression to those achieved with monthly injections of 3.75 mg during the controlled clinical trials for the management of endometriosis and the anemia caused by uterine fibroids.

Contraindications

Pregnancy, lactation (see Warnings); hypersensitivity to GnRH, GnRH agonist analogs, or product excipients (a report of an anaphylactic reaction to synthetic GnRH (*Factrel*) has been reported in the medical literature); undiagnosed abnormal vaginal bleeding. The 30 mg depot formulation is contraindicated in women. The implant is contraindicated in women and children.

Warnings

►*Worsening of signs and symptoms:*

Prostatic cancer – There are isolated cases of worsening of signs and symptoms during the first few weeks of treatment with LH-RH analogs. Isolated cases of ureteral obstruction and spinal cord compression have been observed, which may contribute to paralysis with or without fatal complications. For patients at risk, consider initiating therapy with daily leuprolide injections for the first 2 weeks to facilitate withdrawal of treatment if necessary. Worsening of symptoms may manifest as an increase in bone pain, which can be treated symptomatically. In a few cases, a temporary worsening of existing hematuria and urinary tract obstruction occurred during the first week. Temporary weakness and paresthesia of the lower limbs have occurred; observe patients with metastatic vertebral lesions or urinary tract obstruction closely during the first few weeks of therapy.

CPP – During the early phase of therapy, gonadotropins and sex steroids rise above baseline because of the natural stimulatory effect of the drug. Therefore, an increase in clinical signs and symptoms may be observed. Noncompliance with drug regimen or inadequate dosing may result in inadequate control of the pubertal process. The consequences of poor control include the return of pubertal signs such as menses, breast development, and testicular growth. The long-term consequences of inadequate control of gonadal steroid secretion are unknown, but may include a further compromise of adult stature.

►*Hypersensitivity reactions:* Anaphylaxis has occurred with synthetic GnRH. Patients allergic to benzyl alcohol, a component of the leuprolide injection vehicle, may display symptoms of local hypersensitivity in the form of erythema and induration at the injection site. Leuprolide depot is preservative free.

LEUPROLIDE ACETATE

►*Carcinogenesis:* In rats, a dose-related increase in benign pituitary hyperplasia and benign pituitary adenomas was noted after 2 years with high daily doses. A significant, but not dose-related, increase of pancreatic islet cell adenomas in females and of testicular interstitial cell adenomas in males (highest incidence in the low dose group) was also observed.

Patients have been treated with leuprolide acetate for ≤ 3 years with doses ≤ 10 mg/day and for 2 years with doses ≤ 20 mg/day without demonstrable pituitary abnormalities.

Studies with leuprolide and similar analogs have shown full reversibility of fertility suppression when the drug is stopped after continuous use for up to 24 weeks.

►*Pregnancy:* Category X. Leuprolide is contraindicated in women who are or may become pregnant while receiving the drug. Major fetal abnormalities were observed in animal studies, including increased fetal mortality and decreased fetal weights. The effects on fetal mortality are logical consequences of the alterations in hormonal levels brought about by this drug. Therefore, the possibility exists that spontaneous abortion may occur if the drug is given during pregnancy.

Before starting therapy, pregnancy must be excluded. When used at the recommended dose and dosing interval, leuprolide depot usually inhibits ovulation and stops menstruation; however, contraception is not ensured (see Patient Information).

►*Lactation:* It is not known whether leuprolide is excreted in human breast milk. Do not use while nursing.

►*Children:* Although no clinical studies have been completed in children to assess the full reversibility of fertility suppression, animal studies with leuprolide acetate and other GnRH analogs have shown functional recovery.

Precautions

►*Monitoring:*

Prostatic cancer – Monitor response by measuring serum levels of testosterone, prostatic acid phosphatase, and PSA levels. In the majority of patients, testosterone levels increased above baseline during the first week, declining thereafter to baseline levels or below by the end of the second week. Castrate levels were reached within 2 to 4 weeks and were maintained for as long as drug administration was maintained. Occasional transient increases in acid phosphatase levels may occur early in treatment. By the fourth week, the elevated levels usually decreased to values at or near baseline.

X-rays do not affect leuprolide implant functionality. The implant is radio-opaque and is well visualized on X-rays.

The titanium alloy reservoir of the implant is nonferromagnetic and is not affected by MRI. Slight image distortion around the implant may occur during MRI procedures.

Endometriosis/Uterine leiomyomata – During the early phase of therapy, sex steroids temporarily rise above baseline because of the physiologic effect of the drug. Therefore, an increase in clinical signs and symptoms may occur during the initial days of therapy, but these will dissipate with continued therapy. The patient should notify her physician if regular menstruation persists beyond the second month.

CPP – Monitor response with leuprolide 1 to 2 months after the start of therapy with a GnRH stimulation test, sex steroid levels, and Tanner staging to confirm downregulation. Measurement of bone age for advancement should be done every 6 to 12 months.

Sex steroids may increase or rise above prepubertal levels if the dose is inadequate. Once a therapeutic dose has been established, gonadotropin and sex steroid levels will decline to prepubertal levels.

►*CPP, selection for use:* Select children for treatment of CPP based on the following criteria: 1) Clinical diagnosis of CPP (idiopathic or neurogenic) with onset of secondary sexual characteristics earlier than 8 years of age in females and 9 years of age in males; 2) confirmed diagnosis by a pubertal response to a GnRH stimulation test, bone age advanced 1 year beyond chronological age; 3) baseline evaluation including height, weight, sex steroid levels, adrenal steroid level to exclude congenital adrenal hyperplasia, beta human chorionic gonadotropin level to rule out a chorionic gonadotropin secreting tumor, pelvic/adrenal/testicular ultrasound to rule out a steroid secreting tumor, and computed tomography of the head to rule out intracranial tumor.

►*Uterine leiomyomata:* The clinician may want to consider a 1-month trial period on iron alone as some patients will respond to iron alone. Leuprolide may be added if the response to iron alone is considered inadequate. Recommended therapy duration with leuprolide is ≤ 3 months.

Patients Achieving Hemoglobin ≥ 12 g/dl: Leuprolide with Iron vs Iron Alone (%)			
Treatment	Week 4	Week 8	Week 12
Leuprolide 3.75 mg with iron	40	71	75
Iron alone	17	39	49

►*Bone density changes:* The induced hypoestrogen state results in a small loss in bone density over the course of treatment, some of which may not be reversible. For a period of ≤ 6 months, this bone loss should not be important. In patients with major risk factors for decreased bone mineral content (eg, chronic alcohol or tobacco use, strong family history of osteoporosis, chronic use of drugs that can reduce bone mass [eg, anticonvulsants, corticosteroids]), leuprolide may pose additional risk; weigh the risks and benefits before starting therapy. Repeated courses of therapy beyond 6 months are not recommended, particularly in patients with major risk factors for loss of bone mineral content.

Drug Interactions

►*Drug/Lab test interactions:* Since leuprolide suppresses the pituitary-gonadal system, diagnostic tests of pituitary gonadotropic and gonadal functions during treatment and up to 12 weeks after discontinuing leuprolide depot or implant may be misleading.

Adverse Reactions

	Leuprolide Acetate Adverse Reactions (%)[1]								
	Prostatic cancer					Endo-metriosis[2]	CPP		Uterine leiomyo-mata
Adverse reaction	Leupro-lide injection (n = 98)	Leupro-lide depot (7.5 mg) (n = 56)	Leupro-lide depot (22.5 mg) (n = 94)	Leupro-lide depot (30 mg) (n = 49)[3]	Leupro-lide implant (n = 131)	Leupro-lide depot (3.75 mg) (n = 166)	Leupro-lide Depot-Ped (n = 395)	Leupro-lide for Pedi-atric Use (n = 395)	Leupro-lide depot (3.75 mg) (n = 166)
Cardiovascular									
ECG changes/ischemia	19.4	—	—	—	—	—	—	—	—
High blood pressure	8.2	—	< 5	—	—	—	—	—	—
Murmur	3.1	—	—	—	—	—	—	—	—
Edema	12.2	12.5	< 5	8.2	< 2-3.1	7	< 2	< 2	5.4
CNS									
Depression/emotional lability	< 5	—	< 5	—	5.3	22	< 2	< 2	10.8
Insomnia/sleep disorders	7.1	< 5	8.5	< 5	< 2	< 5	—	—	< 5
Pain	13.3	7.1	26.6	32.7	< 2	19	2	2	8.4
Headache	7.1	—	6.4	10.2	4.6	32	< 2	< 2	25.9
Dizziness/lightheadedness	5.1	—	6.4	6.1	< 2	11	—	—	< 5
Nervousness	< 5	—	< 5	—	—	5	< 2	< 2	< 5
Paresthesias	< 5	< 5	< 5	8.2	< 2	7	—	—	< 5
Endocrine[4]									
Impotence/↓libido	4.1	5.4	< 5	< 5	2.3	11	—	—	< 5
Gynecomastia/breast tenderness/changes	7.1	< 5	< 5	—	3.1-6.9	6	< 2	< 2	< 5
Hot flashes/sweats	55	58.9	58.5	46.9	67.9/5.3	84	—	—	72.9

Gonadotropin-Releasing Hormone Analog

LEUPROLIDE ACETATE

	Leuprolide Acetate Adverse Reactions (%)[1]								
	Prostatic cancer					Endo-metriosis[2]	CPP		Uterine leiomyo-mata
Adverse reaction	Leupro-lide injection (n = 98)	Leupro-lide depot (7.5 mg) (n = 56)	Leupro-lide depot (22.5 mg) (n = 94)	Leupro-lide depot (30 mg) (n = 49)[3]	Leupro-lide implant (n = 131)	Leupro-lide depot (3.75 mg) (n = 166)	Leupro-lide *Depot-Ped* (n = 395)	Leupro-lide for Pedi-atric Use (n = 395)	Leupro-lide depot (3.75 mg) (n = 166)
GI									
GI disturbances	< 5	—	16	10.2	—	7	—	—	< 5
Anorexia	6.1	< 5	< 5	< 5	—	—	—	—	—
Constipation	7.1	—	—	< 2	—	—	—	—	—
Diarrhea	< 5	—	—	2.3	—	—	—	—	< 5
Nausea/vomiting	5.1	5.4	—	—	< 2	13	< 2	< 2	< 5
GU									
↓ testicular size/atrophy	7.1	5.4	20.2	< 5	3.8	—	—	—	—
Vaginitis/bleeding/discharge	—	—	—	—	—	28	2	2	11.4
Urinary frequency/urgency/disorders	6.1	< 5	14.9	10.2	3.8	—	< 2	< 2	—
Urinary tract infection	3.1	—	—	< 5	< 2	—	—	—	—
Nocturia	—	—	—	—	3.8	—	—	—	—
Hematuria	6.1	< 5	—	—	—	—	—	—	—
Musculoskeletal									
Joint disorder/pain	< 5	—	11.7	16.3	—	8	—	—	7.8
Myalgia	3.1	< 5	—	8.2	—	1	—	—	< 5
Bone pain	5.1	< 5	—	< 2	—	—	—	—	—
Neuromuscular disorders	—	—	9.6	6.1	—	7	—	—	< 5
Miscellaneous									
Dyspnea	2	5.4	—	—	2.3	—	—	—	—
Weight gain/loss	—	< 5	—	< 5	2.3	13	< 2	< 2	< 5
Anemia	5.1	—	< 5	—	2.3	—	—	—	—
Dermatitis/skin reactions/acne/seborrhea	5.1	< 5	8.5	12.2	—	10	2	2	< 5
Rash (including erythema multiforme)	—	—	—	—	< 2	—	2	2	—
Ecchymosis	< 5	—	—	—	4.6	—	—	—	—
Asthenia	10.2	5.4	7.4	12.2	7.6	3	—	—	8.4
Respiratory disorder	5	—	6.4	8.2	—	—	—	—	—
Flu syndrome	—	—	—	12.2	—	—	—	—	—
Dehydration	—	—	< 5	8.2	—	—	—	—	—
Alopecia	< 5	—	—	—	2.3	< 5	< 2	< 2	—
Injection site reaction	—	—	13.8	8.2	—	< 5	5	5	< 5

[1] Data are pooled from several separate studies and are not necessarily comparable.
[2] Percentages approximate.
[3] Nonorchiectomized patients.
[4] Physiologic effect of decreased testosterone.

►*Leuprolide injection and depot (< 5%):*
Cardiovascular – Angina, cardiac arrhythmia; vasodilation (< 2% in CPP).

CNS – Memory disorder, syncope, personality disorder, somnolence (< 2% in CPP); anxiety.

Dermatologic – Hair growth; hair loss, skin striae (< 2% in CPP).

GI – Taste disorders/perversion; dysphagia, gingivitis, GI bleeding (< 2% in CPP).

GU – Testicular pain, dysuria; incontinence, cervix disorder (< 2% in CPP).

Lab test abnormalities – Increased calcium; increased BUN (≥ 5% in 22.5 mg depot).

Miscellaneous – Ophthalmologic disorder/abnormal vision, diabetes, chills, fever; infection, body odor, epistaxis, accelerated sexual maturity (< 2% in CPP).

►*Leuprolide depot (< 5%):*
Cardiovascular – Tachycardia; bradycardia; heart failure; varicose vein; palpitations; hypertension; atrial fibrillation; deep thrombophlebitis; hypotension.

CNS – Delusions; hypesthesia; confusion; abnormal thinking; amnesia; convulsion; dementia; depression.

GI – Duodenal ulcer; dry mouth; appetite changes; thirst; eructation; GI hemorrhage; gum hemorrhage; hepatomegaly; intestinal obstruction; periodontal abscess.

GU – Penis disorder; testes disorder; bladder carcinoma; epididymitis; prostate disorder.

Lab test abnormalities – LDH (> 2 N) (19.6%); AST (> 2 N) (7.1%); alkaline phosphatase (> 1.5 N) (7.1%); increased uric acid (7.5 mg depot); hyperglycemia, hyperlipidemia (total cholesterol, LDL cholesterol, triglycerides), hyperphosphatemia, abnormal liver function tests, increased PT, increased PTT, decreased platelets, decreased potassium, increased glucose, increased WBC (≥ 5%, 22.5 mg and 30 mg depot); decreased bicarbonate, decreased hemoglobin/hematocrit/RBC,

decreased HDL cholesterol, eosinophilia, increased phosphorus, leukopenia, thrombocytopenia, uricaciduria (≥ 5%, 30 mg depot).

Endometriosis: In clinical trials, AST was > 2 × the ULN in 1 patient. There was no other clinical or laboratory evidence of abnormal liver function.

Uterine leiomyomata: Post-treatment transaminase levels were ≥ 2 × the baseline value and ULN in 5 (3%) patients. None of the laboratory increases were associated with clinical symptoms.

Respiratory – Rhinitis; pharyngitis; pleural effusion; asthma; bronchitis; hiccough; lung disorder; sinusitis; voice alteration; hypoxia.

Miscellaneous – Conjunctivitis; nail disorder; hair disorder; enlarged abdomen; lymphedema; amblyopia; dry eyes; lymphadenopathy; menstrual disorder; androgen-like effects; abscess; accidental injury; allergic reaction; cyst; hernia; neck pain; neoplasm; abnormal healing; leg cramps; pathological fracture; ptosis; herpes zoster; melanosis; hard nodule in throat; tinnitus; lactation.

►*Leuprolide implant (< 2%):*
CNS – Amnesia; anxiety.

Dermatologic – Pruritus; rash; hirsutism.

GU – Prostatic disorder; dysuria; urinary incontinence; urinary retention.

Miscellaneous – Chills; abdominal pain; malaise; dry mucous membranes; iron deficiency; anemia; arthritis.

►*Leuprolide injection (< 5%):*
Cardiovascular – MI; pulmonary emboli; CHF; phlebitis/thrombosis; pulmonary infiltrates.

CNS – Lethargy; mood swings; numbness; blackouts; fatigue; peripheral neuropathy.

Dermatologic – Carcinoma of skin/ear; dry skin; itching; pigmentation; skin lesions.

GI – GI bleeding; peptic ulcer; rectal polyps.

GU – Bladder spasms; urinary obstruction.

LEUPROLIDE ACETATE

Respiratory – Cough; pleural rub; pulmonary fibrosis; pneumonia.

Miscellaneous – Thyroid enlargement; hypoglycemia; increased creatinine; inflammation; swelling (temporal bone); blurred vision.

➤*Postmarketing experience (injection and depot):* During postmarketing surveillance with other dosage forms and in the same or different populations, the following adverse events were reported:

Like other drugs in this class, mood swings, including depression, have been reported as a physiologic effect of decreased sex steroids. There have been very rare reports of suicidal ideation and attempt. Many, but not all, of these patients had a history of depression or other psychiatric illness. Patients should be counseled on the possibility of worsening of depression.

Symptoms consistent with an anaphylactoid or asthmatic process have been reported. Rash, urticaria, and photosensitivity reactions have also been reported.

Localized reactions including induration and abscess have been reported at the site of injection.

Symptoms consistent with fibromyalgia (eg, joint and muscle pain, headaches, sleep disorders, GI distress, shortness of breath) have been reported individually and collectively.

Cardiovascular – Hypotension; transient ischemic attack/stroke; pulmonary embolism; pulmonary infiltrates.

CNS – Hearing disorder; peripheral neuropathy; spinal fracture/paralysis.

GU – Penile swelling; prostate pain.

Hematologic / Lymphatic – Decreased WBC; hemoptysis.

Musculoskeletal – Ankylosing spondylosis; pelvic fibrosis; tenosynovitis-like symptoms.

Miscellaneous – Hypoproteinemia; hard nodule in throat; weight gain; increased uric acid; hair growth; libido increase; hepatic dysfunction; respiratory disorders.

Overdosage

In rats, SC administration of 250 to 500 times the recommended human dose (125 to 250 times the pediatric dose) resulted in dyspnea, decreased activity, and local irritation at the injection site.

In clinical trials using daily SC leuprolide acetate in patients with prostate cancer, doses as high as 20 mg/day for up to 2 years caused no adverse effects differing from those observed with the 1 mg/day dose.

Patient Information

Patient package insert is available with each injection kit. Patient information for injection and depot is available at 1-800-622-2011; patient information for implant is available at 1-877-VIADUR or http://www.viadur.com.

Do not discontinue medication except on advice of physician.

➤*Prostatic cancer:* May cause increased bone pain and increased difficulty in urinating during the first few weeks of treatment. May cause hot flashes, injection site irritation (eg, burning, itching, swelling), and may cause or aggravate nerve symptoms; notify physician if these become pronounced.

➤*CPP:* Prior to starting therapy the parent or guardian must be aware of the importance of continuous therapy. Adherence to 4 week drug administration schedules must be accepted if therapy is to be successful.

During the first 2 months of therapy, a female may experience menses or spotting. If bleeding continues beyond the second month, notify the physician.

Report any irritation at the injection site to the physician immediately.

Report any unusual signs or symptoms to the physician.

➤*Endometriosis / Uterine leiomyomata:* Effective doses of leuprolide depot should stop menstruation; notify physician if it persists. Successive missed doses may cause breakthrough bleeding or ovulation with the potential for conception. Nonhormonal methods of birth control should be used during treatment. Do not use if pregnant or breastfeeding, allergic to any ingredients of product, or in the presence of undiagnosed abnormal vaginal bleeding. Adverse reactions associated with hypoestrogenism include the following: Hot flashes, headaches, emotional lability, decreased libido, acne, myalgia, decreased breast size, vaginal dryness. Estrogen levels return to normal after treatment discontinuation (see Bone Density Changes in Precautions).

GOSERELIN ACETATE

Rx	**Zoladex** (AstraZeneca)	**Implant:** 3.6 mg	In preloaded syringes (16-gauge needle).
		10.8 mg	In preloaded syringes (14-gauge needle).

Indications

➤*Prostatic carcinoma:* Palliative treatment of advanced carcinoma of the prostate. Goserelin offers an alternative treatment of prostatic cancer when orchiectomy or estrogen administration are either not indicated or unacceptable to the patient.

➤*Stage B₂-C prostatic carcinoma (10.8 mg only):* For use in combination with flutamide for the management of locally confined T2b-T4 (Stage B₂–C) carcinoma of the prostate. Treatment with goserelin and flutamide should start 8 weeks prior to initiating radiation therapy and continue during radiation therapy.

➤*Endometriosis (3.6 mg only):* Management of endometriosis, including pain relief and reduction of endometriotic lesions for the duration of therapy.

➤*Advanced breast cancer (3.6 mg only):* Palliative treatment of advanced breast cancer in pre- and perimenopausal women. Estrogen and progesterone receptor values may help predict whether goserelin therapy is likely to be beneficial.

➤*Endometrial thinning (3.6 mg only):* Endometrial-thinning agent prior to endometrial ablation for dysfunctional uterine bleeding.

Administration and Dosage

➤*Monthly (3.6 mg) implant:* Administer SC every 28 days into the upper abdominal wall. Local anesthesia may be used prior to injection. While a delay of a few days is permissible, attempt to adhere to the 28-day schedule.

➤*3-month (10.8 mg) implant:* Administer SC every 12 weeks into the upper abdominal wall. Local aneshthesia may be used prior to injection. While a delay of a few days is permissible, attempt to adhere to the 12–week schedule.

➤*Prostatic carcinoma / Breast carcinoma:* Intended for long-term administration unless clinically inappropriate.

➤*Endometriosis:* Recommended duration is 6 months. There are no clinical data on the effect of treatment of benign gynecological conditions with goserelin for periods > 6 months. Retreatment cannot be recommended because safety data are not available. If symptoms recur after a course of therapy and further treatment is contemplated, consider monitoring bone mineral density.

➤*Endometrial thinning:* For use as an endometrial-thinning agent prior to endometrial ablation, the dosing recommendation is 1 or 2 depots (with each depot given 4 weeks apart). When 1 depot is administered, surgery should be performed at 4 weeks. When 2 depots are administered, surgery should be performed within 2 to 4 weeks following administration of the second depot.

➤*Stage B₂-C prostatic carcinoma:* When goserelin is given in combination with radiotherapy and flutamide for patients with Stage T2b-T4 (Stage B₂–C) prostatic carcinoma, start treatment 8 weeks prior to initiating radiotherapy and continue during radiation therapy. Utilize treatment regimen using one goserelin 3.6 mg depot, followed in 28 days by one 10.8 mg depot.

➤*Removal of goserelin:* In the unlikely event of the need to surgically remove goserelin, it can be localized by ultrasound.

Actions

➤*Pharmacology:* Goserelin acetate is a synthetic decapeptide analog of luteinizing hormone-releasing hormone (LHRH or GnRH). It acts as a potent inhibitor of pituitary gonadotropin secretion when administered in the biodegradable formulation. Following initial administration in males, the drug causes an initial increase in serum luteinizing hormone (LH) and follicle-stimulating hormone (FSH) values with subsequent increases in serum levels of testosterone. Chronic administration leads to sustained suppression of pituitary gonadotropins; testosterone serum levels consequently fall into the range normally seen in surgically castrated men at ≈ 2 to 4 weeks after initiation of therapy. This leads to accessory sex organ regression. In clinical trials with follow-up of > 2 years, suppression of serum testosterone to castrate levels has been maintained for the duration of therapy.

In females, a similar down-regulation of the pituitary gland by chronic exposure to goserelin leads to suppression of gonadotropin secretion, a decrease in serum estradiol to levels consistent with the postmenopausal state, and would be expected to lead to a reduction in ovarian size and function, reduction in the size of the uterus and mammary gland, and a regression of sex hormone-responsive tumors, if present. Serum estradiol is suppressed to levels similar to those observed in postmenopausal women ≤ 3 weeks following initial administration; however, after this suppression was attained, isolated estradiol elevations were seen in 10% of patients in the clinical trials. Serum LH and FSH are suppressed to follicular phase levels ≤ 4 weeks after initial administration and are usually maintained in that range with contin-

GOSERELIN ACETATE

ued use of goserelin. In ≤ 5% of women treated with goserelin, FSH and LH levels may not be suppressed to follicular phase levels on day 28 post-treatment with use of a single 3.6 mg depot injection. In certain individuals, suppression of these hormones to such levels may not be achieved with goserelin. Estradiol, LH, and FSH levels return to pre-treatment values ≤ 12 weeks following the last implant administration in most cases.

➤*Pharmacokinetics:*

Absorption/Distribution – Absorption is rapid, but the pharmacokinetics of goserelin are determined by the release of drug from the depot.

Goserelin 3.6 mg implant is absorbed at a much slower rate initially for the first 8 days with peak serum concentrations achieved 12 to 15 days for males (8 to 22 days for females) after SC administration and a more rapid and continuous release for the remainder of the 28-day dosing period. Despite the change in the releasing rate of goserelin, administration every 28 days resulted in testosterone levels that were suppressed to and maintained in the range normally seen in surgically castrated men. For the 10.8 mg depot, mean concentrations increase to a peak of ≈ 8 ng/ml within the first 24 hours and then decline rapidly until day 4. Thereafter, mean concentrations remain relatively stable until the end of the treatment period.

The apparent volumes of distribution are 44.1 and 20.3 L for males and females, respectively. The plasma protein-binding of goserelin is low (27%).

Metabolism/Excretion – Clearance of goserelin following SC administration of the solution formulation is very rapid and occurs via a combination of hepatic metabolism and urinary excretion. More than 90% of an SC solution formulation dose is excreted in urine. Approximately 20% of the dose in urine is accounted for by unchanged goserelin. The total body clearance of goserelin was significantly greater (163.9 vs 110.5 ml/min) in females compared with males.

Renal function impairment – Male subjects with impaired renal function (creatinine clearance < 20 ml/min) had a serum elimination half-life of 12.1 hours compared with 4.2 hours for subjects with normal renal function. However, no dosage adjustment is required.

Body weight – A decline of ≈ 1% to 2.5% in the AUC after administration of a 10.8 mg depot was observed with a kg increase in body weight. Monitor testosterone levels closely in obese patients who have not responded clinically.

➤*Clinical trials:*

Prostatic carcinoma –

3.6 mg implant: In controlled studies of patients with advanced prostatic cancer comparing goserelin with orchiectomy, the long-term endocrine responses and objective responses were similar between the treatments. Additionally, duration of survival was similar between the treatments in a major comparative trial.

10.8 mg implant: In studies with advanced prostatic cancer, the 10.8 mg implant produced a similar effect in terms of suppression of serum testosterone to that achieved with the 3.6 mg implant. Clinical outcome similar to that produced with the use of goserelin 3.6 mg implant administered every 28 days is predicted with the 10.8 mg implant administered every 12 weeks.

Endometriosis – In controlled clinical studies using the 3.6 mg formulation every 28 days for 6 months, goserelin was as effective as danazol in relieving clinical symptoms (eg, dysmenorrhea, dyspareunia, pelvic pain) and signs (eg, pelvic tenderness, pelvic induration) of endometriosis and decreasing the size of endometrial lesions as determined by laparoscopy. The clinical significance of a decrease in endometriotic lesions is unknown at this time; goserelin led to amenorrhea in 80% to 92% of treated women ≤ 8 weeks after initial administration. Menses usually resumed ≤ 8 weeks following completion of therapy. Within 4 weeks following initial administration, clinical symptoms were significantly reduced and were reduced by ≈84% at the end of treatment.

Contraindications

Pregnancy, lactation, nondiagnosed vaginal bleeding (see Warnings); hypersensitivity to LHRH, LHRH-agonist analogs, or any component of the product.

Warnings

➤*Increased testosterone/estrogen:* Initially, goserelin, like other LHRH agonists, transiently increases serum levels of testosterone in men with prostate cancer or estrogen in women with breast cancer. Transient worsening of symptoms or the occurrence of additional signs and symptoms of prostatic or breast cancer may occasionally develop during the first few weeks of treatment. Some patients may experience a temporary increase in bone pain, which can be managed symptomatically.

As with other LHRH agonists, isolated cases of exacerbation of disease symptoms, either ureteral obstruction or spinal cord compression, have been observed in prostate cancer patients. Monitor closely during the first month of therapy. If spinal cord compression or renal impairment develops, institute standard treatment for these complications; in extreme cases, consider an immediate orchiectomy.

➤*Use in females:* The 10.8 mg implant is not indicated in women as the data are insufficient to support reliable suppression of serum estradiol.

➤*Hypercalcemia:* Hypercalcemia has occurred in some prostate and breast cancer patients with bone metastases after starting goserelin treatment. If hypercalcemia occurs, initiate appropriate treatment.

➤*Lipids:* In a controlled trial in women, 3.6 mg goserelin resulted in a minor but statistically significant effect on serum lipids. In patients treated for endometriosis, at 6 months following therapy initiation, goserelin increased LDL and HDL cholesterol by 21.3 and 2.7 mg/dl, respectively (vs 33.3 mg/dl increase and 21.3 mg/dl decrease with danazol). Triglycerides increased by 8 mg/dl with goserelin vs an 8.9 mg/dl decrease with danazol.

In endometriosis treatment, goserelin increased total cholesterol and LDL cholesterol during 6 months of treatment. However, goserelin resulted in HDL cholesterol levels that were significantly higher relative to danazol therapy. At the end of 6 months of treatment, HDL cholesterol fractions (HDL_2 and HDL_3) were decreased by 13.5 and 7.7 mg/dl, respectively, for danazol-treated patients compared with treatment increases of 1.9 and 0.8 mg/dl, respectively, for goserelin-treated patients.

➤*Hormone replacement therapy:* Clinical studies suggest the addition of hormone replacement therapy (estrogens or progestins) to goserelin may decrease the occurrence of vasomotor symptoms and vaginal dryness associated with hypoestrogenism without compromising the efficacy of goserelin in relieving pelvic symptoms. The optimal drugs, dose, and duration of treatment have not been established.

➤*Bone mineral density changes:* After 6 months of treatment, 109 female patients treated with goserelin showed an average 4.3% decrease of vertebral trabecular bone mineral density (BMD) compared with pretreatment values. Patients (n = 66) were assessed for BMD loss 6 months after the completion of the 6-month therapy. Data from these patients showed an average 2.4% BMD loss compared with pretreatment values. Data from 28 patients at 12 months post-therapy showed an average decrease of 2.5% in BMD compared with pretreatment values. These data suggest a possibility of partial reversibility.

In patients with a history of treatment that may have resulted in BMD loss or in patients with major risk factors for decreased BMD such as chronic alcohol abuse or tobacco abuse, significant family history of osteoporosis, or chronic use of drugs that can reduce bone density such as anticonvulsants or corticosteroids, therapy may pose an additional risk. In these patients the risks and benefits must be weighed carefully before therapy is instituted.

➤*Antibody formation:* Among 115 goserelin-treated patients tested for development of binding to goserelin following treatment with goserelin, 1 patient showed low titer-binding to goserelin. On further testing of this patient's plasma obtained after treatment, her goserelin binding component was not found to be precipitated with rabbit anti-human immunoglobulin polyvalent sera. These findings suggest the possiblity of antibody formation.

➤*Vaginal bleeding:* During the first 2 months of goserelin use, some women experience vaginal bleeding of variable duration and intensity. In all likelihood, the bleeding represents estrogen withdrawal bleeding and is expected to stop spontaneously.

➤*Carcinogenesis:* Animal studies resulted in an increased incidence of pituitary adenomas at doses of ≈ 3 to 9 times the recommended human dose after 1 year SC administration. There was also an increased incidence of histiocytic sarcoma of the vertebral column and femur at ≈ 70 times the recommended human dose following 2 years SC administration.

➤*Fertility impairment:* Administration of goserelin led to gonadal suppression at 30 to 60 times the recommended monthly dose in male and female rats as a result of its endocrine action. Except for the testes, almost complete histologic reversal of effects in males and females was observed several weeks after dosing was stopped; however, fertility and general reproductive performance were reduced in those that became pregnant after the drug was discontinued.

➤*Pregnancy:* Category D (breast cancer); Category X (endometriosis; endometrial thinning).Studies in both rats and rabbits at doses 2 times the maximum recommended dose given during organogenesis have confirmed that this drug will increase pregnancy loss in a dose-related manner.

Before starting treatment with goserelin, pregnancy must be excluded. Safe use of goserelin during pregnancy has not been established; goserelin can cause fetal harm when administered to a pregnant woman. Do not use in women who are or who may become pregnant while receiving the drug. If goserelin is used during pregnancy or if pregnancy occurs while taking this drug, apprise the patient of the potential hazard to the fetus or potential risk for loss of the pregnancy caused by possible hormonal imbalance as a result of the expected pharmacologic action of goserelin treatment. Advise women of childbearing potential to avoid becoming pregnant. Effective nonhormonal contraception must be used by all premenopausal women during

GOSERELIN ACETATE

goserelin therapy and for 12 weeks following discontinuation of therapy. There are no adequate and well controlled studies in pregnant women using goserelin.

When used every 28 days, goserelin usually inhibits ovulation and stops menstruation. Contraception is not ensured. Following the last goserelin injection, nonhormonal methods of contraception must be continued until the return of menses or for ≥ 12 weeks.

➤*Lactation:* It is not known if goserelin is excreted in breast milk. Because of the potential for serious adverse reactions in nursing infants from goserelin, discontinue the drug prior to breastfeeding.

➤*Children:* Safety and efficacy have not been established. Goserelin use for endometriosis has been limited to women who are ≥ 18 years old and have been treated for 6 months.

Drug Interactions

➤*Drug/Lab test interactions:* Goserelin suppresses the pituitary-gonadal system. Therefore, diagnostic tests of pituitary-gonadotropic and gonadal functions conducted during treatment and until resumption of menses may show misleading results. Normal function is usually restored within 12 weeks of treatment discontinuation.

Adverse Reactions

Goserelin Adverse Reactions in Males (%)		
Adverse reaction	Goserelin 3.6 mg (n = 242)	Orchiectomy (n = 254)
CNS		
Lethargy	8	4
Dizziness	5	4
Insomnia	5	1
GI		
Anorexia	5	2
Nausea	5	2
GU		
Sexual dysfunction	21	15
Decreased erections	18	16
Lower urinary tract symptoms	13	8
Miscellaneous		
Hot flashes	62[1]	53
Pain (may have worsened in the first 30 days)	8[2]	3
Edema	7	8
Upper respiratory tract infection	7	2
Rash	6	1
Sweating	6	4
Chronic obstructive pulmonary disease	5	3
CHF	5	1

[1] 64% with 10.8 mg (n = 157)
[2] 14% with 10.8 mg (n = 157)

Adverse Reactions in Endometriosis: Goserelin vs Danazol (%)		
Adverse reaction	Goserelin (n = 411)	Danazol (n = 207)
CNS		
Headache	75	63
Emotional lability	60	56
Depression	54	48
Asthenia	11	13
Insomnia	11	4
Dizziness	6	4
Nervousness	3	5
Dermatologic		
Sweating	45	30
Acne	42	55
Seborrhea	26	52
Hirsutism	7	15
Hair disorders	4	11
Pruritus	2	6
GI		
Nausea	8	14
Abdominal pain	7	7
Pharyngitis	5	2
Increased appetite	2	5
GU		
Vaginitis	75	43
Libido decreased	61	44
Pelvic symptoms	18	23

Adverse Reactions in Endometriosis: Goserelin vs Danazol (%)		
Adverse reaction	Goserelin (n = 411)	Danazol (n = 207)
Dyspareunia	14	5
Libido increased	12	19
Breast pain	7	4
Miscellaneous		
Hot flashes	96	67
Breast atrophy	33	42
Peripheral edema	21	34
Breast enlargement	18	15
Pain	17	16
Infection	13	11
Back pain	7	13
Application site reaction	6	-
Flu syndrome	5	5
Voice alterations	3	8
Myalgia	3	11
Weight gain	3	23
Leg cramps	2	6
Hypertonia	1	10

Goserelin Adverse Reactions in Endometrial Thinning (%)		
Adverse reaction	Goserelin 3.6 mg (n = 180)	Placebo (n = 177)
Cardiovascular		
Vasodilation	57	18
Migraine	7	4
Hypertension	6	2
CNS		
Nervousness	5	3
Depression	3	7
GU		
Dysmenorrhea	7	9
Uterine hemorrhage	6	4
Vulvovaginitis	5	1
Menorrhagia	4	5
Vaginitis	1	6
Respiratory		
Pharyngitis	6	9
Sinusitis	3	6
Miscellaneous		
Headache	32	22
Sweating	16	5
Abdominal pain	11	10
Pelvic pain	9	6
Nausea	5	6
Back pain	4	7

➤*Males:* Goserelin is generally well tolerated; withdrawal from treatment was rare. As seen with other hormonal therapies, the most commonly observed adverse events were caused by the expected physiological effects from decreased testosterone levels, including hot flashes, sexual dysfunction, and decreased erections.

Cardiovascular – Cerebrovascular accident (> 1% to < 5%); arrhythmia, hypertension, MI, peripheral vascular disorder, chest pain (> 1% to < 5% in 3.6 mg); angina pectoris, cerebral ischemia, heart failure, pulmonary embolus, varicose veins (> 1% to < 5% in 10.8 mg).

CNS – Asthenia (5% in 10.8 mg); anxiety, depression (> 1% to < 5% in 3.6 mg); headache (> 1% to < 5% in both).

GI – Diarrhea (> 1% to < 5%); constipation, diarrhea, ulcer, vomiting (> 1% to < 5% in 3.6 mg); hematemesis (> 1% to < 5% in 10.8 mg).

GU – Gynecomastia (8% in 10.8 mg); renal insufficiency, urinary obstruction, urinary tract infection (> 1% to < 5% in 3.6 mg); bladder neoplasm, breast pain, hematuria, impotence, urinary frequency/incontinence, urinary tract disorder, impaired urination, urinary tract infection (> 1% to < 5% in 10.8 mg).

Metabolic/Nutritional – Gout, hyperglycemia, weight increase (> 1% to < 5% in 3.6 mg); diabetes mellitus (> 1% to < 5% in 10.8 mg).

Miscellaneous – Pelvic/bone pain (6% in 10.8 mg; see Warnings); anemia (> 1% to < 5%); chills, fever, breast swelling/tenderness (> 1% to < 5% in 3.6 mg); abdominal/back pain, flu syndrome, sepsis, aggravation reaction, herpes simplex, pruritus; injection site reaction (< 1% in 3.6 mg); hypersensitivity (rare).

➤*Females (3.6 mg implant only):*
Cardiovascular – Hemorrhage, hypertension, migraine, palpitations, tachycardia (≥ 1%).

GOSERELIN ACETATE

CNS – Anxiety, paresthesia, somnolence, abnormal thinking (≥ 1%).

Dermatologic – Alopecia, dry skin, rash, skin discoloration (≥ 1%).

GI – Anorexia, constipation, diarrhea, dry mouth, dyspepsia, flatulence (≥ 1%).

GU – Dysmenorrhea, urinary frequency, urinary tract infection, vaginal hemorrhage (see Warnings).

Lab test abnormalities – Elevation of liver enzymes (AST, ALT; < 1%) with no other evidence of abnormal liver function; changes in serum lipids (see Warnings).

Musculoskeletal – Arthralgia, joint disorder (≥ 1%); bone mineral density changes (see Warnings).

Respiratory – Bronchitis, cough increased, epistaxis, rhinitis, sinusitis (≥ 1%).

Special senses – Amblyopia, dry eyes (≥ 1%).

Miscellaneous – Allergic reaction, chest pain, fever, malaise, edema, ecchymosis (≥ 1%); acne; hair disorders; osteoporosis; voice alterations; hypersensitivity (rare; see Warnings).

➤*Advanced breast cancer (goserelin [n = 57] vs oophorectomy [n = 55], respectively):* Hot flashes (70% vs 47%), tumor flare (23% vs 4%), nausea (11% vs 7%), edema (5% vs 0%), malaise/fatigue/lethargy (5% vs 2%), vomiting (4% vs 7%).

Overdosage

There is no experience with overdosage. If overdosage occurs, manage symptomatically. Refer to General Management of Acute Overdosage.

Patient Information

➤*Females (3.6 mg only):* Because menstruation should stop with effective doses of goserelin, the patient should notify her physician if regular menstruation persists. Patients missing 1 or more successive doses may experience breakthrough menstrual bleeding, and some patients may have delayed return to menses. The patient may rarely experience persistent amenorrhea.

Use of goserelin in pregnancy is contraindicated in women being treated for endometriosis or endometrial thinning. Therefore, use a nonhormonal method of contraception during treatment. Advise patients that if they miss ≥ 1 successive doses, breakthrough menstrual bleeding or ovulation may occur with the potential for conception. If a patient becomes pregnant during treatment, discontinue treatment and advise the patient of the possible risks (see Warnings).

Adverse events occurring most frequently are associated with hypoestrogenism. The most frequently reported are hot flashes (flushes), headache, vaginal dryness, emotional lability, change in libido, depression, sweating and change in breast size.

Treatment induces a hypoestrogenic state that results in a loss of bone mineral density over the course of treatment, some of which may not be reversible.

➤*Males:* Carefully consider the use of goserelin in patients at particular risk of developing ureteral obstruction or spinal cord compression, and monitor the patients closely during the first month of therapy. Patients with ureteral obstruction or spinal cord compression should have appropriate treatment prior to initiation of goserelin.

TRIPTORELIN PAMOATE

Rx	**Trelstar Depot** (Pharmacia)	**Microgranules for injection, lyophilized:** Equivalent to 3.75 mg triptorelin peptide base	Mannitol. In single-dose vials.
Rx	**Trelstar LA** (Pharmacia)	**Microgranules for injection, lyophilized:** Equivalent to 11.25 mg triptorelin peptide base	Mannitol. In single-dose vials.

Indications

➤*Advanced prostate cancer:* Palliative treatment of advanced prostate cancer. Triptorelin pamoate offers an alternative treatment for prostate cancer when orchiectomy or estrogen administration are not indicated or unacceptable to the patient.

Administration and Dosage

➤*Approved by the FDA:* June 15, 2000.

For IM use only. Administration must be under the supervision of a physician.

➤*Trelstar Depot:* The recommended dose is 3.75 mg incorporated in a depot formulation and is administered every 28 days as a single IM injection. Alternate injection site periodically.

Preparation for administration –
1.) Using a syringe fitted with a sterile 20-gauge needle, withdraw 2 mL sterile water for injection. Do not use other diluents. Inject into vial.
2.) Shake well to thoroughly disperse particles to obtain a uniform suspension. The suspension will appear milky.
3.) Withdraw vial content into the syringe and inject the reconstituted suspension immediately.

➤*Trelstar LA:* The recommended dose is 11.25 mg incorporated in a long acting formulation administered every 84 days as a single IM injection administered in either buttock. Alternate injection site periodically.

Preparation for administration –
1.) Using a syringe fitted with a sterile 20-gauge needle, withdraw 2 mL sterile water for injection. Do not use other diluents. Inject into vial.
2.) Shake well to thoroughly disperse particles to obtain a uniform suspension. The suspension will appear milky.
3.) Slowly withdraw the entire contents into the syringe.
4.) Inject the patient in either buttock with the contents of the syringe.

➤*Renal / Hepatic function impairment:* Patients with renal or hepatic impairment showed 2- to 4-fold higher exposure than young, healthy males. The clinical consequences of this increase, as well as the potential need for dose adjustment, is unknown.

➤*Storage / Stability:* Store at 20° to 25°C (77°F); excursions permitted to 15° to 30°C (59° to 86°F). Discard the suspension if not used immediately after reconstitution. Do not freeze long-acting triptorelin.

Actions

➤*Pharmacology:* Triptorelin is a synthetic decapeptide agonist analog of luteinizing hormone releasing hormone (LHRH or GnRH) with greater potency than the naturally occurring LHRH. It is a potent inhibitor of gonadotropin secretion when given continuously and in therapeutic doses. Following the first administration, there is a transient surge in circulating levels of luteinizing hormone (LH), follicle-stimulating hormone (FSH), testosterone, and estradiol. After chronic and continuous administration, usually 2 to 4 weeks after initiation of therapy, a sustained decrease in LH and FSH secretion and marked reduction of testicular and ovarian steroidogenesis is observed. In men, a reduction of serum testosterone concentration to a level typically seen in surgically castrated men is obtained. Consequently, the result is that tissues and functions that depend on these hormones for maintenance become quiescent. These effects usually are reversible after cessation of therapy.

Trelstar Depot – Following a single IM triptorelin injection to healthy, male volunteers, serum testosterone levels first increased, peaking on day 4, and declined thereafter to low levels by week 4. Similar testosterone profiles were observed in patients with advanced prostate cancer when injected with triptorelin. In healthy volunteers, testosterone serum levels returned to near baseline by week 8.

Trelstar LA – Following a single IM injection to men with advanced prostate cancer, serum testosterone levels first increased, peaking on days 2 to 3, and declined thereafter to low levels by weeks 3 to 4.

➤*Pharmacokinetics:*

Absorption – Triptorelin is not active when given orally.

Trelstar Depot: IM injection of the depot formulation provides plasma concentrations of triptorelin over a period of 1 month. The pharmacokinetic parameters following a single IM injection of 3.75 mg to 20 healthy, male volunteers are listed in the following table. The plasma concentrations declined to 0.084 ng/mL at 4 weeks.

Trelstar LA: The pharmacokinetic parameters following a single IM injection of 11.25 mg long acting triptorelin to 13 patients with prostate cancer are listed in the table below. Triptorelin did not accumulate over 9 months of treatment.

Pharmacokinetic Parameters Following IM Administration of Triptorelin

	Dose (mg)	C_{max} (mean) (ng/mL)	T_{max} (h)	AUC (h•ng/mL)	F (%)[1] (28 days)
Trelstar Depot	3.75 mg	≈ 28.43	1 to 3	≈ 223.15[2]	83
Trelstar LA	11.25	≈ 38.5	≈ 2.9[3]	≈ 2268[4]	-

[1] Computed as the mean AUC of the study divided by the mean AUC of healthy volunteers corrected for dose where AUC = 36.1 h•ng/mL and 500 mcg IV bolus dose of triptorelin was administered.
[2] Mean AUC from 0 to 28 days.
[3] Mean from 1 to 85 days.
[4] Mean AUC from 1 to 85 days.

Distribution – The volume of distribution following an IV bolus dose of 0.5 mg was 30 to 33 L in healthy, male volunteers. There is no evidence that triptorelin, at clinically relevant concentrations, binds to plasma proteins.

Metabolism – The metabolism of triptorelin in humans is unknown but is unlikely to involve hepatic microsomal enzymes (cytochrome P450). Thus far, no metabolites of triptorelin have been identified. Pharmacokinetic data suggest that C-terminal fragments produced by tissue degradation are completely degraded in the tissues, rapidly

Gonadotropin-Releasing Hormone Analog

TRIPTORELIN PAMOATE
degraded in plasma, or cleared by the kidneys.

Excretion – Triptorelin is eliminated by the liver and kidneys. Results of pharmacokinetic investigations conducted in healthy men indicate that after IV bolus administration, triptorelin is distributed and eliminated according to a 3-compartment model and corresponding half-lives are approximately 6 minutes, 45 minutes, and 3 hours. Following IV administration of 0.5 mg triptorelin peptide to 6 healthy, male volunteers with a creatinine clearance (Ccr) of 149.9 mL/min, 41.7% of the dose was excreted in urine as intact peptide with a total triptorelin clearance of 212 mL/min. This percentage increased to 62.3% in patients with liver disease who have a lower Ccr (89.9 mL/min). It also has been observed that the nonrenal clearance of triptorelin (patient anuric, Ccr = 0) was 76.2 mL/min, thus indicating that the nonrenal elimination of triptorelin is mainly dependent on the liver (see Special Populations).

Special populations –
Renal and hepatic function impairment: After an IV injection of 0.5 mg triptorelin peptide, renal insufficiency led to a decrease in total triptorelin clearance proportional to the decrease in Ccr, an increase in volume of distribution, and consequently an increase in elimination half-life (see following table). The decrease in triptorelin clearance was more pronounced in subjects with liver insufficiency, but the half-life was prolonged similarly in subjects with renal insufficiency since the volume of distribution was only minimally increased.

Pharmacokinetic Parameters (Mean) of Triptorelin in Healthy Volunteers and Special Populations						
Group	C_{max} (ng/mL)	AUC_{inf} (h•ng/mL)	Cl_p[1] (mL/min)	Cl_{renal} (mL/min)	$T_{\frac{1}{2}}$ (h)	Ccr (mL/min)
6 healthy males	≈ 48.2	≈ 36.1	≈ 211.9	≈ 90.6	≈ 2.81	≈ 149.9
6 males with moderate renal impairment	≈ 45.6	≈ 69.9	≈ 120	≈ 23.3	≈ 6.56	≈ 39.7
6 males with severe renal impairment	≈ 46.5	≈ 88	≈ 88.6	≈ 4.3	≈ 7.65	≈ 8.9
6 males with liver disease	≈ 54.1	≈ 131.9	≈ 57.8	≈ 35.9	≈ 7.58	≈ 89.9

[1] Plasma clearance.

Contraindications
Hypersensitivity to triptorelin or any other component of the product, other LHRH agonists, or LHRH (3 postmarketing reports of anaphylactic shock and 7 postmarketing reports of angioedema related to triptorelin administration have been reported since 1986; see Warnings); pregnancy.

Warnings
➤*Worsening of signs and symptoms:* Initially, triptorelin, like other LHRH agonists, causes a transient increase in serum testosterone levels. As a result, isolated cases of worsening of signs and symptoms of prostate cancer during the first weeks of treatment have been reported with LHRH agonists. Patients may experience worsening of symptoms or onset of new symptoms, including bone pain, neuropathy, hematuria, or urethral or bladder outlet obstruction. Cases of spinal cord compression, which may contribute to paralysis with or without fatal complications, have been reported with LHRH agonists.

If spinal cord compression or renal impairment develops, institute standard treatment of these complications and in extreme cases consider an immediate orchiectomy.

➤*Women:* Triptorelin has not been studied in women and is not indicated for use in women.

➤*Hypersensitivity reactions:* Do not administer to individuals who are hypersensitive to triptorelin, other LHRH agonists, or LHRH. Rare reports of anaphylactic shock and angioedema related to triptorelin administration have been reported. In the event of a reaction, immediately discontinue therapy with long-acting triptorelin and administer the appropriate supportive and symptomatic care. Refer to Management of Acute Hypersensitivity Reactions.

➤*Carcinogenesis:* In rats, doses of 120, 600, and 3000 mcg/kg given every 28 days (approximately 0.3, 2, and 8 times the recommended human therapeutic dose based on body surface area) resulted in increased mortality with a drug treatment period of 13 to 19 months. The incidence of benign and malignant pituitary tumors and histiosarcomas were increased in a dose-related manner.

➤*Pregnancy: Category X.* Triptorelin is contraindicated in women who are or may become pregnant while receiving the drug. Studies in pregnant rats administered triptorelin at doses of 2, 10, and 100 mcg/kg/day (approximately equivalent to 0.2, 0.8, and 8 times the recommended human therapeutic dose based on body surface area) during the period of organogenesis displayed maternal toxicity and embryotoxicity, but no fetotoxicity or teratogenicity. If this drug is used during pregnancy or if the patient becomes pregnant while taking this drug, inform the patient of the potential hazard to the fetus.

➤*Lactation:* It is not known whether triptorelin is excreted in breast milk. Do not use during nursing.

➤*Children:* Triptorelin is not indicated for use in pediatric patients.

Precautions
➤*Monitoring:* Monitor response by measuring serum levels of testosterone and prostate-specific antigen. Measure testosterone levels immediately prior to or immediately after dosing.

Closely observe patients with metastatic vertebral lesions and/or upper or lower urinary tract obstruction during the first few weeks of therapy (see Warnings).

Drug Interactions
No pharmacokinetic drug interaction studies have been conducted with triptorelin. In the absence of relevant data and as a precaution, do not prescribe hyperprolactinemic drugs concomitantly with triptorelin because hyperprolactinemia reduces the number of pituitary GnRH receptors.

➤*Drug/Lab test interactions:* Chronic or continuous administration of triptorelin in therapeutic doses results in suppression of the pituitary-gonadal axis. Diagnostic tests of the pituitary-gonadal function conducted during treatment and after cessation of therapy may therefore be misleading.

Adverse Reactions
In the majority of patients, testosterone levels increased above baseline during the first week following the initial injection, declining thereafter to baseline levels or below by the end of the second week of treatment. The transient increase in testosterone levels may be associated with temporary worsening of disease signs and symptoms, including bone pain, hematuria, and bladder outlet obstruction. Isolated cases of spinal cord compression with weakness or paralysis of the lower extremities have occurred (see Warnings).

In a controlled, comparative clinical trial, the following adverse reactions were reported to have a possible or probable relationship as reported by the treating physician in 1% or more of the patients receiving triptorelin. Often, causality is difficult to assess in patients with metastatic prostate cancer. Reactions considered not drug-related or unlikely to be related are excluded.

Triptorelin Adverse Reactions (%)		
Adverse reaction	Trelstar Depot (n = 140)	Trelstar LA (n = 174)
Cardiovascular		
Hypertension	3.6	4
Chest pain	–	1.7
CNS		
Headache	5	6.9
Fatigue	2.1	2.3
Insomnia	2.1	1.7
Dizziness	1.4	2.9
Emotional lability	1.4	–
Asthenia	–	1.1
Dermatologic		
Rash	-	1.7
Pruritus	1.4	-
GI		
Nausea	–	2.9
Vomiting	2.1	–
Anorexia	–	1.7
Constipation	–	1.7
Dyspepsia	–	1.7
Diarrhea	1.4	1.1
Abdominal pain	–	1.1
GU		
Impotence[1]	7.1	2.3
Dysuria	–	4.6
Urinary retention	1.4	1.1
Breast pain	–	2.3
Decreased libido[1]	–	2.3
Gynecomastia	–	1.7
Urinary tract infection	1.4	–
Musculoskeletal		
Skeletal pain	12.1	13.2
Arthralgia	–	2.3
Leg cramps	-	1.7
Myalgia	–	1.1
Respiratory		
Coughing	–	1.7
Dyspnea	–	1.1
Pharyngitis	–	1.1

TRIPTORELIN PAMOATE

Triptorelin Adverse Reactions (%)		
Adverse reaction	Trelstar Depot (n = 140)	Trelstar LA (n = 174)
Miscellaneous		
Hot flushes[1]	58.6	73
Leg edema	–	6.3
Injection site pain	3.6	4
Leg pain	2.1	5.2
Back pain	–	2.9
Pain	2.1	3.4
Dependent edema	–	2.3
Increased alkaline phosphatase	–	1.7
Anemia	1.4	–
Abnormal hepatic function	–	1.1
Conjunctivitis	–	1.1
Eye pain	–	1.1

Triptorelin Adverse Reactions (%)		
Adverse reaction	Trelstar Depot (n = 140)	Trelstar LA (n = 174)
Peripheral edema	–	1.1

[1] Expected pharmacologic consequences of testosterone suppression.

➤*Lab value changes (Trelstar LA):* The following abnormalities in lab values not present at baseline were observed in 10% or more of patients: Decreased hemoglobin and RBC count; increased glucose, BUN, AST, ALT, and alkaline phosphatase. The relationship of these changes to drug treatment is difficult to assess in this population.

Overdosage

The pharmacological properties of triptorelin and its mode of administration make accidental or intentional overdosage unlikely. There were no reported overdoses in clinical trials. In single-dose toxicity studies in mice and rats, the SC LD_{50} of triptorelin was 400 mg/kg in mice and 250 mg/kg in rats, approximately 7000 and 4000 times, respectively, the usual human dose. However, if overdosage occurs, discontinue therapy immediately and administer the appropriate supportive and symptomatic treatment. Refer to General Management of Acute Overdosage.

ANASTROZOLE

Rx **Arimidex** (AstraZeneca)	**Tablets:** 1 mg	Lactose. (A/Adx 1). White. Film-coated. In 30s.

Indications

➤*Breast cancer, advanced:* First-line treatment of postmenopausal women with hormone receptor positive or hormone receptor unknown locally advanced or metastatic breast cancer; treatment of advanced breast cancer in postmenopausal women with disease progression following tamoxifen therapy.

➤*Breast cancer, early:* Adjuvant treatment of postmenopausal women with hormone receptor positive early breast cancer.

➤*Unlabeled uses:* Male infertility.

Administration and Dosage

➤*Approved by the FDA:* December 27, 1995.

Patients treated with anastrozole do not require glucocorticoid or mineralocorticoid therapy. Pregnancy must be excluded before starting therapy.

1 mg once daily. In patients with advanced breast cancer, continue treatment with anastrozole until tumor progression is evident.

For adjuvant treatment of early breast cancer in postmenopausal women, the optimal duration of therapy is unknown. The median duration of therapy at the time of data analysis was 31 months; the ongoing ATAC trial is planned for 5 years of treatment.

➤*Storage/Stability:* Store at controlled room temperature, 20° to 25°C (68° to 77°F).

Actions

➤*Pharmacology:* Many breast cancers have estrogen receptors, and growth of these tumors can be stimulated by estrogens. In postmenopausal women, the principal source of circulating estrogen (primarily estradiol) is conversion of adrenally generated androstenedione to estrone by aromatase in peripheral tissues, such as adipose tissue, with further conversion of estrone to estradiol. Many breast cancers also contain aromatase; the importance of tumor-generated estrogens is uncertain.

Treatment of breast cancer has included efforts to decrease estrogen levels by ovariectomy premenopausally and by use of antiestrogens and progestational agents pre- and postmenopausally; these interventions lead to decreased tumor mass or delayed progression of tumor growth in some women.

Anastrozole is a potent and selective nonsteroidal aromatase inhibitor. It significantly lowers serum estradiol concentrations and has no detectable effect on formation of adrenal corticosteroids or aldosterone.

Clinically significant suppression of serum estradiol was seen with all doses. The recommended daily dose (1 mg) reduced estradiol by approximately 70% within 24 hours and by approximately 80% after 14 days of daily dosing. Suppression of serum estradiol was maintained for up to 6 days after cessation of daily dosing with 1 mg.

➤*Pharmacokinetics:* Inhibition of aromatase activity is primarily caused by anastrozole, the parent drug. Orally administered anastrozole is well absorbed into the systemic circulation with 83% to 85% of the dose recovered in urine or feces. Food does not affect the extent of absorption. Elimination of anastrozole is primarily via hepatic metabolism (approximately 85%) and, to a lesser extent, renal excretion (approximately 11%). Anastrozole has a mean terminal elimination half-life of approximately 50 hours in postmenopausal women. The major circulating metabolite of anastrozole, triazole, lacks pharmacologic activity. Consistent with the approximately 2-day terminal elimination half-life, plasma concentrations approach steady-state levels at about 7 days of once-daily dosing, and steady-state levels are approximately 3- to 4-fold higher than levels observed after a single dose of anastrozole. Anastrozole is 40% bound to plasma proteins.

Studies in postmenopausal women demonstrated that anastrozole is extensively metabolized, with about 10% of the dose excreted in the urine as unchanged drug within 72 hours of dosing, and the remainder (about 60% of the dose) excreted in the urine as metabolites. Metabolism of anastrozole occurs by N-dealkylation, hydroxylation, and glucuronidation. Three metabolites of anastrozole have been identified in human plasma and urine. The known metabolites are triazole, a glucuronide conjugate of hydroxyanastrozole, and a glucuronide of anastrozole itself. Several minor metabolites have not been identified.

➤*Clinical trials:*

Adjuvant treatment of breast cancer in postmenopausal women – A multicenter double-blind trial (ATAC) randomized 9366 postmenopausal women with operable breast cancer to adjuvant treatment with 1 mg anastrozole daily, tamoxifen 20 mg daily, or a combination of the 2 treatments for 5 years or until recurrence of the disease. At the time of the efficacy analysis, women had received a median of 31 months of treatment and had been followed for recurrence-free survival for a median of 33 months. The primary endpoint of the trial is recurrence-free survival, ie, time to occurrence of a distant or local recurrence, or contralateral breast primary or death from any cause.

The recommended duration of tamoxifen therapy is 5 years; continued benefit of tamoxifen after 3 years has been documented. The results of the ATAC trial in a patient population treated for a median 31 months, thus allow only a preliminary comparison of anastrozole and tamoxifen therapy. At this time, recurrence-free survival was improved in the anastrozole arm compared with the tamoxifen arm: Hazard ratio (HR) = 0.83, 95% CI 0.71 to 0.96, *P* = 0.0144. Results were essentially the same in the hormone receptor positive patients (about 84% of the patients): HR = 0.78, 95% CI 0.65 to 0.93. Recurrence-free survival in the combination treatment arm was similar to that in the tamoxifen group.

ATAC Endpoint Summary in Patients with Recurrence-Free Survival			
	Anastrozole 1 mg (N = 3125)	Tamoxifen 20 mg (N = 3116)	Anastrozole 1 mg + tamoxifen 20 mg (N = 3125)
First event (%)	10.2	12.2	12.3
Locoregional[1]	2.1	2.7	2.6
Distant	5	5.8	6.5
New contralateral primaries	0.4	1.1	0.9
Invasive	0.3	1	0.7
Ductal carcinoma in situ	0.2	< 0.1	0.2
Deaths[2]			
Death - breast cancer	0.12	0.03	0
Death - other reason	2.4	2.6	2.3

[1] Includes new primary ipsilateral breast cancer (including DCIS) and recurrences at the chest wall, axillary, and other regional lymph nodes.
[2] Includes only deaths that were first events.

First-line therapy in postmenopausal women with advanced breast cancer – Anastrozole was compared with tamoxifen in 2 double-blind, well-controlled clinical trials to assess the efficacy of each as first-line therapy for hormone receptor positive or hormone receptor unknown locally advanced or metastatic breast cancer in postmenopausal women. A total of 1021 patients were randomized to receive 1 mg anastrozole once daily or 20 mg tamoxifen once daily. Anastrozole was at least as effective as tamoxifen for objective tumor response rate in both studies and had a statistically significant advantage over tamoxifen for time to tumor progression in one of the studies.

Second-line therapy in postmenopausal women with advanced breast cancer who had disease progression following tamoxifen therapy – Anastrozole was studied in 2 well-controlled clinical trials in postmenopausal women with advanced breast cancer who had disease progression following tamoxifen therapy. Some of the patients also had received previous cytotoxic treatment. Most patients were estrogen receptor (ER)-positive. Patients were randomized to receive a single daily dose of 1 or 10 mg anastrozole or 40 mg megestrol acetate 4 times a day.

Both trials included over 375 patients. More than 33% of the patients in each treatment group had an objective response or stabilization of their disease for greater than 24 weeks. Of the 263 patients who received 1 mg anastrozole, there were 11 complete responders and 22 partial responders. In those who had an objective response, more than 80% were still responding at 6 months and more than 45% were still responding at 12 months. Both anastrozole 1 and 10 mg were similar in efficacy to megestrol acetate.

Contraindications

Hypersensitivity reaction to the drug or to any of the excipients.

Warnings

➤*ER-negative disease:* Patients with ER-negative disease and patients who did not respond to tamoxifen therapy rarely responded to anastrozole.

➤*Renal function impairment:* Anastrozole renal clearance decreased proportionally with creatinine clearance (Ccr) and was approximately 50% lower in volunteers with severe renal impairment (Ccr less than 30 mL/min/1.73 m^2) compared with controls. Because only about 10% of anastrozole is excreted unchanged in the urine, the reduction in renal clearance did not influence the total body clearance. Dosage adjustment in patients with renal insufficiency is not necessary.

➤*Hepatic function impairment:* Hepatic metabolism accounts for approximately 85% of anastrozole elimination. The apparent oral clearance (CL/F) of anastrozole was approximately 30% lower in subjects with stable hepatic cirrhosis than in control subjects with normal liver function. However, plasma anastrozole concentrations in subjects with hepatic cirrhosis were within the range of concentrations seen in healthy subjects across all clinical trials. Therefore, no dosage adjustment is needed.

➤*Carcinogenesis:* A study in rats at doses of 1 to 25 mg/kg/day (about 10 to 243 times the daily maximum recommended human dose on a mg/m^2 basis) administered by oral gavage for up to 2 years revealed an

ANASTROZOLE

increase in the incidence of hepatocellular adenoma and carcinoma and uterine stromal polyps in females and thyroid adenoma in males at the high dose. A dose-related increase was observed in the incidence of ovarian and uterine hyperplasia in females. A study in mice at oral doses of 5 to 50 mg/kg/day (about 24 to 243 times the daily maximum recommended human dose on a mg/m^2 basis) for up to 2 years produced an increase in the incidence of benign ovarian stromal, epithelial, and granulosa cell tumors at all dose levels. A dose-related increase in the incidence of ovarian hyperplasia also was observed in female mice. These ovarian changes are considered to be rodent-specific effects of aromatase inhibition and are of questionable significance to humans.

➤*Fertility impairment:* Oral administration of anastrozole to female rats (from 2 weeks before mating to pregnancy day 7) produced significant incidence of infertility and reduced numbers of viable pregnancies at 1 mg/kg/day (about 10 times the recommended human dose on a mg/m^2 basis and 9 times higher than the AUC_{0-24h} found in postmenopausal volunteers at the recommended dose). Preimplantation loss of ova or fetus was increased at doses equal to or greater than 0.02 mg/kg/day (about one-fifth the recommended human dose on a mg/m^2 basis). Recovery of fertility was observed following a 5-week nondosing period that followed 3 weeks of dosing. It is not known whether these effects observed in female rats are indicative of impaired fertility in humans.

Hypertrophy of the ovaries and the presence of follicular cysts in rats administered doses equal to or greater than 1 mg/kg/day were found in chronic studies. Hyperplastic uteri were observed in chronic studies of female dogs administered doses equal to or greater than 1 mg/kg/day. It is not known whether these effects on the reproductive organs of animals are associated with impaired fertility in humans.

➤*Pregnancy: Category D.* Anastrozole can cause fetal harm when administered to a pregnant woman. Anastrozole has been found to cross the placenta following oral administration of 0.1 mg/kg in rats and rabbits (about 1 and 1.9 times the recommended human dose on a mg/m^2 basis, respectively). Administration during organogenesis showed anastrozole to increase pregnancy loss and resorption and decrease the number of live fetuses; effects were dose-related.

There are no adequate and well-controlled studies in pregnant women. If anastrozole is used during pregnancy or if the patient becomes pregnant, apprise the patient of the potential hazard to the fetus and risk for loss of the pregnancy.

➤*Lactation:* It is not known whether anastrozole is excreted in breast milk. Exercise caution when administering to a breastfeeding woman.

➤*Children:* Safety and efficacy for use in children have not been established.

Precautions

➤*Endocrine effects:* Anastrozole does not possess direct progestogenic, androgenic, or estrogenic activity in animals but does perturb the circulating levels of progesterone, androgens, and estrogens.

➤*Lipid profile:* Mean serum total cholesterol levels increased by 0.5 mmol/L among patients receiving anastrozole. Increases in LDL cholesterol have been shown to contribute to these changes.

➤*Vaginal bleeding:* Vaginal bleeding has occurred infrequently, mainly during the first few weeks after changing from existing hormonal therapy to anastrozole. If bleeding persists, consider further evaluation.

➤*Lab test abnormalities:* During the ATAC trial, more patients receiving anastrozole were reported to have an elevated serum cholesterol compared with patients receiving tamoxifen (7% vs 3%, respectively).

Drug Interactions

➤*CYP450:* Anastrozole inhibited in vitro metabolic reactions catalyzed by cytochromes P450 1A2, 2C8/9, and 3A4, but only at relatively high concentrations. It is unlikely that coadministration of a 1 mg dose of anastrozole with other drugs will result in clinically significant inhibition of cytochrome P450-mediated metabolism of the other drugs.

➤*Tamoxifen:* Coadministration with tamoxifen reduced anastrozole concentrations by 27%.

Adverse Reactions

➤*Adjuvant therapy:* The median duration of adjuvant treatment for safety evaluation was 37.3, 36.9, and 36.5 months for patients receiving 1 mg anastrozole, 20 mg tamoxifen, and the combination of 1 mg anastrozole plus 20 mg tamoxifen, respectively.

Adverse Reactions with Anastrozole vs Tamoxifen vs Anastrozole and Tamoxifen (%)			
Adverse reaction	Anastrozole 1 mg (N = 3092)	Tamoxifen 20 mg (N = 3093)	Anastrozole 1 mg plus tamoxifen 20 mg (N = 3098)
Cardiovascular			
Vasodilation	35	40	41
Hypertension	9	8	9
Ischemic cardiovascular disease	3	2	ND[1]
Venous thromboembolic events	2	4	ND
Angina pectoris	1.7	1	ND
Deep venous thromboembolic events	1	2	ND
Ischemic cerebrovascular event	1	2	ND
MI	0.8	0.8	ND
CNS			
Mood disturbances	17	17	ND
Depression	11	11	11
Insomnia	9	8	7
Headache	9	7	7
Dizziness	6	7	6
Anxiety	5	5	5
Paresthesia	6	4	4
GI			
Nausea and vomiting	11	11	ND
Nausea	10	10	10
Constipation	7	7	7
Diarrhea	7	6	6
Dyspepsia	5	4	5
GI disorder	5	4	4
GU			
Leukorrhea	2	9	9
Urinary tract infection	6	8	7
Breast pain	7	4	6
Vulvovaginitis	6	4	4
Vaginal bleeding	5	9	ND
Vaginal discharge	3	12	ND
Endometrial cancer	0.1	0.5	ND
Metabolic/Nutritional			
Peripheral edema	8	9	9
Weight gain	8	8	9
Hypercholesterolemia	7	3	2
Musculoskeletal			
Musculoskeletal disorders[2]	30	24	ND
Arthritis	14	11	12
Arthralgia	13	8	9
Osteoporosis	7	5	6
Fracture	7	4-5	6
Bone pain	5	5	5
Arthrosis	6	4	4
Fractures of spine, hip, wrist	3	2	ND
Respiratory			
Pharyngitis	12	12	11
Cough increased	7	8	7
Dyspnea	6	6	6
Miscellaneous			
Hot flashes	35	40	ND
Asthenia	17	16	15
Pain	15	14	13
Rash	10	11	11
Lymphoedema	9	10	10
Back pain	8	8	8
Abdominal pain	7	7	7
Infection	7	7	7
Accidental injury	7	7	7
Flu syndrome	5	5	5
Chest pain	5	4	5
Sweating	4	5	5
Cataracts	4	5	ND

[1] ND = No data
[2] Refers to joint symptoms, including arthritis, arthrosis, and arthralgia.

ANASTROZOLE

►*First-line therapy:*

Adverse Reactions with Anastrozole vs Tamoxifen (%)		
Adverse reaction	Anastrozole (n = 506)	Tamoxifen (n = 511)
Cardiovascular		
Vasodilation	25	21
Hypertension	5	7
Thromboembolic disease[1]	4	6
CNS		
Headache	9	8
Dizziness	6	4
Insomnia	6	7
Depression	5	6
Hypertonia	3	5
Lethargy	1	3
GI		
GI disturbance	34	38
Nausea	19	21
Constipation	9	13
Diarrhea	8	6
Abdominal pain	8	7
Vomiting	8	7
Anorexia	5	9
Respiratory		
Cough increased	11	10
Dyspnea	10	9
Pharyngitis	10	13
Miscellaneous		
Hot flushes	26	23
Asthenia	16	16
Pain	14	14
Back pain	12	13
Peripheral edema	10	8
Bone pain	11	10
Rash	8	8
Chest pain	7	7
Flu syndrome	7	6
Pelvic pain	5	6
Tumor flare	3	4
Weight gain	2	2
Leukorrhea	2	6
Vaginal dryness	2	1
Vaginal bleeding	1	2

[1] Includes pulmonary embolism, thrombophlebitis, retinal vein thrombosis, MI, myocardial ischemia, angina pectoris, cerebrovascular accident, cerebral ischemia, and cerebral infarct.

►*Second-line therapy:* Anastrozole was generally well tolerated with less than 3.3% of the anastrozole patients and 4% of the megestrol acetate patients withdrawing because of an adverse reaction.

Adverse Reactions with Anastrozole vs Megestrol Acetate (%)		
Adverse reaction	Anastrozole 1 mg (n = 262)	Anastrozole 10 mg (n = 246)	Megestrol acetate 160 mg (n = 253)
CNS			
Headache	13	18	9
Dizziness	6	5	6
Depression	5	2	2
Paresthesia	5	6	4
GI			
GI disturbance	29	33	21
Nausea	16	20	11
Vomiting	9	11	6
Diarrhea	8	7	3
Constipation	7	7	8
Abdominal pain	7	6	7
Anorexia	7	8	4

Adverse Reactions with Anastrozole vs Megestrol Acetate (%)		
Adverse reaction	Anastrozole 1 mg (n = 262)	Anastrozole 10 mg (n = 246)	Megestrol acetate 160 mg (n = 253)
Respiratory			
Dyspnea	9	11	21
Cough increased	8	7	8
Pharyngitis	6	9	6
Miscellaneous			
Asthenia	16	13	19
Hot flushes	12-13	11-12	8-14
Pain	11	15	11
Back pain	11	11	8
Edema	7	11	14
Bone pain	6	12	8
Rash	6	6	8
Dry mouth	6	4	5
Peripheral edema	5	9	11
Pelvic pain	5	7	5
Chest pain	5	7	5
Thromboembolic disease	3	2	5
Vaginal hemorrhage	2	2	5
Vaginal dryness	2	1	1
Weight gain	2	4	12
Sweating	2	1	6
Increased appetite	0	0	5

Less frequent adverse reactions:

Cardiovascular – Hypertension, thrombophlebitis (2% to 5%).

CNS – Somnolence, confusion, insomnia, anxiety, nervousness (2% to 5%).

Dermatologic – Hair thinning, pruritus (2% to 5%).

GU – Urinary tract infection, breast pain (2% to 5%).

Hematologic – Anemia, leukopenia (2% to 5%).

Lab test abnormalities – GGT, AST, ALT, alkaline phosphatase, total cholesterol, LDL cholesterol increased (2% to 5%).

Musculoskeletal – Myalgia, arthralgia, pathological fracture (2% to 5%).

Respiratory – Sinusitis, bronchitis, rhinitis (2% to 5%).

Miscellaneous – Flu syndrome, fever, neck pain, malaise, accidental injury, infection, weight loss (2% to 5%); erythema multiforme, Stevens-Johnson syndrome (very rare).

Weight gain: Of patients treated with megestrol acetate in clinical studies, 34% experienced weight gain of 5% or more and 11% gained 10% or more. Among patients treated with 1 mg anastrozole, 13% experienced weight gain of 5% or more and 3% gained 10% or more. On average, this 5% to 10% weight gain represented between 6 and 12 lbs.

►*Postmarketing experience:*

Musculoskeletal – Joint pain/stiffness.

Overdosage

Single doses of up to 60 mg given to healthy male volunteers and up to 10 mg daily given to postmenopausal women with advanced breast cancer were well tolerated. In rats, lethality was observed after single oral doses of greater than 100 mg/kg (about 800 times the recommended human dose) and was associated with severe stomach irritation (eg, necrosis, gastritis, ulceration, hemorrhage).

There is no specific antidote to overdosage. Treatment must be symptomatic. Dialysis may be helpful because anastrozole is not highly protein bound. General supportive care, including frequent monitoring of vital signs and close observation, is indicated. Refer to General Management of Acute Overdosage.

LETROZOLE

Rx   **Femara** (Novartis)   **Tablets:** 2.5 mg   Lactose. (FV CG). Dark yellow. Film-coated. In 30s.

Indications

➤*Breast cancer, advanced:* First-line treatment of postmenopausal women with hormone receptor positive or hormone receptor unknown locally advanced or metastatic breast cancer. Letrozole also is indicated for the treatment of advanced breast cancer in postmenopausal women with disease progression following antiestrogen therapy.

Administration and Dosage

➤*Approved by the FDA:* July 30, 1997.

➤*Adult and elderly patients:* 2.5 mg once daily, without regard to meals. Continue treatment until tumor progression is evident. Patients treated with letrozole do not require glucocorticoid or mineralocorticoid replacement therapy.

➤*Renal function impairment:* No dosage adjustment is required for patients with renal impairment if Ccr is greater than or equal to 10 mL/min.

➤*Hepatic impairment:* No dosage adjustment is recommended for patients with mild to moderate hepatic impairment. Patients with severe impairment of liver function have not been studied. Because letrozole is eliminated almost exclusively by hepatic metabolism, dose patients with severe impairment of liver function with caution.

➤*Storage/Stability:* Store at 25°C (77°F); excursions permitted to 15° to 30°C (59° to 86°F).

Actions

➤*Pharmacology:* The growth of some breast cancers is stimulated or maintained by estrogens. Treatment of breast cancer thought to be hormonally responsive (eg, estrogen- or progesterone-receptor positive or receptor unknown) has included a variety of efforts to decrease estrogen levels (ovariectomy, adrenalectomy, hypophysectomy) or inhibit estrogen effects (antiestrogens and progestational agents). These interventions lead to decreased tumor mass or delayed progression of tumor growth in some women.

In postmenopausal women, estrogens mainly are derived from the action of the aromatase enzyme, which converts adrenal androgens (primarily androstenedione and testosterone) to estrone and estradiol. The suppression of estrogen biosynthesis in peripheral tissues and in the cancer tissue itself can be achieved by specifically inhibiting the aromatase enzyme.

Letrozole is a nonsteroidal competitive inhibitor of the aromatase enzyme system; it inhibits the conversion of androgens to estrogens. In adult nontumor and tumor-bearing female animals, letrozole is as effective as ovariectomy in reducing uterine weight, elevating serum luteinizing hormone (LH), and causing the regression of estrogen-dependent tumors. In contrast to ovariectomy, treatment with letrozole does not lead to an increase in serum follicle-stimulating hormone (FSH). Letrozole selectively inhibits gonadal steroidogenesis but has no significant effect on adrenal mineralocorticoid or glucocorticoid synthesis.

Letrozole inhibits the aromatase enzyme by competitively binding to the heme of the cytochrome P450 subunit of the enzyme, resulting in a reduction of estrogen biosynthesis in all tissues. Treatment of women with letrozole significantly lowers serum estrone, estradiol, and estrone sulfate and has not been shown to significantly affect adrenal corticosteroid synthesis, aldosterone synthesis, or synthesis of thyroid hormones.

➤*Pharmacokinetics:*

Absorption/Distribution – Letrozole is rapidly and completely absorbed from the GI tract; absorption is not affected by food. Letrozole's terminal elimination half-life is about 2 days and steady state plasma concentration after daily 2.5 mg dosing is reached in 2 to 6 weeks. Plasma concentrations at steady-state are 1.5 to 2 times higher than predicted from the concentrations measured after a single dose, indicating a slight nonlinearity in the pharmacokinetics of letrozole upon daily administration of 2.5 mg. These steady-state levels are maintained over extended periods; however, and continuous accumulation of letrozole does not occur. Letrozole is weakly protein bound and has a large volume of distribution (approximately 1.9 L/kg).

Metabolism/Excretion – Metabolism to a pharmacologically inactive carbinol metabolite (4, 4′-methanolbisbenzonitrile) and renal excretion of the glucuronide conjugate of this metabolite is the major pathway of letrozole clearance. About 90% of letrozole is recovered in urine; at least 75% was the glucuronide of the carbinol metabolite, about 9% was 2 unidentified metabolites, and 6% was unchanged letrozole.

In human microsomes with specific CYP isozyme activity, CYP3A4 metabolized letrozole to the carbinol metabolite while CYP2A6 formed this metabolite and its ketone analog. In human liver microsomes, letrozole strongly inhibited CYP2A6 and moderately inhibited CYP2C19.

Special populations –

Hepatic insufficiency: In a study of subjects with varying degrees of non-metastatic hepatic dysfunction, the mean AUC values of the volunteers with moderate hepatic impairment were 37% higher than in healthy subjects, but still within the range seen in subjects without impaired function.

➤*Clinical trials:*

First-line breast cancer – A recent trial was conducted comparing letrozole 2.5 mg with tamoxifen 20 mg for efficacy as first-line therapy. Median time to progression was 9.4 months for the letrozole group and 6 months in the tamoxifen group ($P = 0.0001$). An objective response (complete plus partial responses) occurred in 137 (30%) in the letrozole group and 92 (20%) in the tamoxifen group ($P = 0.0006$). No differences were seen in duration of tumor response.

The median age of this study group was 65 years, approximately 33% being 70 years of age or greater. Time to tumor progression and tumor response rates were better in patients greater than or equal to 70 years of age than in patients less than 70 years of age.

Second-line breast cancer – Letrozole initially was studied at doses of 0.1 to 5 mg daily in 181 postmenopausal estrogen/progesterone-receptor positive or unknown advanced breast cancer patients previously treated with at least antiestrogen therapy. Patients had received other hormonal therapies and also may have received cytotoxic therapy. Eight (20%) of 40 patients treated with letrozole 2.5 mg daily achieved an objective tumor response (complete or partial response).

Two large randomized controlled trials were conducted in patients with advanced breast cancer who had progressed despite antiestrogen therapy. Patients were randomized to 0.5 mg letrozole daily, 2.5 mg letrozole daily, or a comparator (megestrol acetate 160 mg daily in 1 study; aminoglutethimide 250 mg twice daily with corticosteroid supplementation in the other study). In each study, over 60% of the patients had received therapeutic antiestrogens; about 20% of these patients had an objective response.

Contraindications

Hypersensitivity to letrozole or any of its excipients.

Warnings

➤*Hepatic function impairment:* The mean AUC values of volunteers with moderate hepatic impairment receiving letrozole were 37% higher than in healthy subjects, but still within the range seen in subjects without impaired function.

➤*Carcinogenesis:* A conventional carcinogenesis study in mice at doses of 0.6 to 60 mg/kg/day (about 1 to 100 times the daily maximum recommended human dose on a mg/m² basis) administered for up to 2 years revealed a dose-related increase in the incidence of benign ovarian stromal tumors. The incidence of combined hepatocellular adenoma and carcinoma showed a significant trend in females when the high-dose group was excluded because of low survival. The carcinogenicity study in rats at oral doses of 0.1 to 10 mg/kg/day (about 0.4 to 40 times the daily maximum recommended human dose on a mg/m² basis) for up to 2 years also produced an increase in the incidence of benign ovarian stromal tumors at 10 mg/kg/day. Ovarian hyperplasia was observed in females at doses equal to or greater than 0.1 mg/kg/day.

➤*Mutagenesis:* Letrozole was not mutagenic in in vitro tests but was observed to be a potential clastogen in in vitro assays.

➤*Fertility impairment:* Repeated dosing caused sexual inactivity in females and atrophy of the reproductive tract in males and females at doses of 0.6, 0.1, and 0.03 mg/kg in mice, rats, and dogs, respectively (about 1, 0.4, and 0.4 times the daily maximum recommended human dose on a mg/m² basis, respectively).

➤*Pregnancy: Category D.* Letrozole may cause fetal harm when administered to pregnant women. Studies in rats at doses equal to or greater than 0.003 mg/kg (about 1/100 the daily maximum recommended human dose on a mg/m² basis) administered during the period of organogenesis, have shown that letrozole is embryotoxic and fetotoxic, as indicated by intrauterine mortality, increased resorption, increased postimplantation loss, decreased numbers of live fetuses and fetal anomalies including absence and shortening of renal papilla, dilation of ureter, edema, and incomplete ossification of frontal skull and metatarsals. Letrozole was teratogenic in rats. A 0.03 mg/kg dose (about 1/10 the daily maximum recommended human dose on a mg/m² basis) caused fetal domed head and cervical/centrum vertebral fusion.

Letrozole is embryotoxic at doses equal to or greater than 0.002 mg/kg and fetotoxic when administered to rabbits at 0.02 mg/kg. Fetal anomalies included incomplete ossification of the skull, sternebrae, and fore- and hindlegs.

There are no studies in pregnant women. Letrozole is indicated for postmenopausal women. If there is exposure to letrozole during pregnancy, apprise the patient of the potential hazard to the fetus and potential risk for loss of the pregnancy.

LETROZOLE

►*Lactation:* It is not known if letrozole is excreted in breast milk. Exercise caution when letrozole is administered to a nursing woman.

►*Children:* The safety and efficacy in children have not been established.

Precautions

►*Lab test abnormalities:* Moderate decreases in lymphocyte counts of uncertain clinical significance were observed in some patients receiving letrozole 2.5 mg. This depression was transient in about 50% of those affected. Two patients on letrozole developed thrombocytopenia; the relationship to the drug was unclear.

Increases in AST, ALT, and GGT greater than or equal to 5 × the upper limit of normal (ULN) and of bilirubin greater than or equal to 1.5 × the ULN most often were associated with metastatic disease in the liver. About 3% of study participants receiving letrozole had abnormalities in liver chemistries not associated with documented metastases; these abnormalities may have been related to drug therapy. In the megestrol acetate comparative study, about 8% of patients treated with megestrol acetate had abnormalities in liver chemistries that were not associated with documented liver metastases; in the aminoglutethimide study, about 10% of aminoglutethimide-treated patients had abnormalities in liver chemistries not associated with hepatic metastases.

Drug Interactions

►*Tamoxifen:* Tamoxifen may decrease letrozole plasma concentrations by 37.6%. Clinical significance is not known.

Adverse Reactions

►*First-line breast cancer:* A total of 455 patients were treated for a median time of exposure of 11 months. The incidence of adverse experiences was similar for letrozole and tamoxifen. The most frequently reported adverse experiences were bone pain, hot flushes, back pain, nausea, arthralgia, and dyspnea. Discontinuations for adverse experiences other than progression of tumor occurred in 2% of patients on letrozole and in 3% of patients on tamoxifen.

Letrozole vs Tamoxifen Adverse Reactions in First-Line Treatment (%)

Adverse reaction	Letrozole 2.5 mg (n = 455)	Tamoxifen 20 mg (n = 455)
Cardiovascular		
Edema, lower limb	5	5
Hypertension	5	4
CNS		
Headache	8	7
Insomnia	6	4
GI		
Nausea	15	16
Constipation	9	9
Diarrhea	7	4
Vomiting	7	7
Appetite decreased	4	6
Pain, abdominal	4	5
Musculoskeletal		
Pain, bone	20	18
Pain, back	17	17
Arthralgia	14	13
Pain, limb	8	7
Respiratory		
Dyspnea	14	15
Coughing	11	10
Miscellaneous		
Hot flushes	18	15
Fatigue	11	11
Chest pain	8	8
Weight decreased	6	4
Pain not otherwise specified	5	6
Breast pain	5	6
Weakness	5	3
Influenza	5	4
Alopecia/hair thinning	5	4
Postmastectomy lymphoedema	7	6

Less frequent (2% or fewer) adverse reactions:

Cardiovascular: Angina, coronary heart disease, MI, myocardial ischemia, portal vein thrombosis, pulmonary embolism, thrombophlebitis, thrombotic or hemorrhagic strokes, transient ischemic attacks, venous thrombosis.

CNS: Hemiparesis.

►*Second-line breast cancer:* Discontinuation in the megestrol acetate comparison study for adverse events other than progression of tumor occurred in 2.7% of patients on 0.5 mg letrozole, in 2.3% of patients on 2.5 mg letrozole, and in 7.9% of patients on megestrol acetate. There were fewer thromboembolic events at both letrozole doses compared with megestrol acetate (0.6% vs 4.7%). There was also less vaginal bleeding (0.3% vs 3.2%). In the aminoglutethimide comparison study, discontinuations for reasons other than tumor progression occurred in 3.1% of patients on 0.5 mg letrozole, 3.8% of patients on 2.5 mg letrozole, and 3.9% of patients on aminoglutethimide.

There are no significant differences between the high and low dose letrozole groups in either study. Most of the adverse events observed were mild to moderate. It was generally not possible to distinguish adverse reactions caused by treatment from the consequences of the patient's metastatic breast cancer, the effects of estrogen deprivation, or intercurrent illness.

Letrozole vs Megestrol Acetate vs Aminoglutethimide Adverse Reactions (5%)

Adverse reaction	Letrozole 2.5 mg (n = 359)	Letrozole 0.5 mg (n = 380)	Megestrol acetate 160 mg (n = 189)	Aminoglute-thimide 500 mg (n = 178)
CNS				
Headache	9	12	9	7
Somnolence	3	2	2	9
Dizziness	3	5	7	3
Dermatologic				
Rash[1]	5	4	3	12
Pruritus	1	2	5	3
GI				
Nausea	13	15	9	14
Vomiting	7	7	5	9
Constipation	6	7	9	7
Diarrhea	6	5	3	4
Abdominal pain	6	5	9	8
Anorexia	5	3	5	5
Dyspepsia	3	4	6	5
Musculoskeletal				
Musculoskel-etal[2]	21	22	30	14
Arthralgia	8	8	8	3
Respiratory				
Dyspnea	7	9	16	5
Coughing	6	5	7	5
Miscellaneous				
Fatigue	8	6	11	3
Chest pain	6	3	7	3
Viral infections	6	5	6	3
Hot flushes	6	5	4	3
Hypertension	5	7	5	6
Peripheral edema[3]	5	5	8	3
Asthenia	4	5	4	5
Hypercholes-terolemia	3	3	0	6
Weight increase	2	2	9	3

[1] Includes rash, erythematous rash, maculopapular rash, psoriaform rash, vesicular rash.
[2] Includes musculoskeletal pain, skeletal pain, back pain, arm pain, leg pain.
[3] Includes peripheral edema, leg edema, dependent edema, edema.

Other less frequent (fewer than 5%) adverse experiences considered consequential and reported in at least 3 patients treated with letrozole included hypercalcemia, fracture, depression, anxiety, pleural effusion, alopecia, increased sweating, and vertigo.

Overdosage

►*Symptoms:* Isolated cases of letrozole overdose have been reported. In these instances, the highest single dose ingested was 62.5 mg or 25 tablets. No serious adverse events were reported in these cases. In single dose studies the highest dose used was 30 mg, which was well tolerated. Lethality was observed in mice and rats following single oral doses that were equal to or greater than 2000 mg/kg (about 4000 to 8000 times the daily maximum recommended human dose on a mg/m^2 basis); death was associated with reduced motor activity, ataxia, and dyspnea. Lethality was observed in cats following single IV doses that were equal to or greater than 10 mg/kg (about 50 times the daily maximum recommended human dose on a mg/m^2 basis); death was preceded by depressed blood pressure and arrhythmias.

►*Treatment:* Because of the limited data available, no firm recommendations for treatment can be made. However, emesis could be induced if the patient is alert. In general, supportive care and frequent monitoring of vital signs are appropriate. Refer to General Management of Acute Overdosage.

EXEMESTANE

Rx   **Aromasin** (Pharmacia & Upjohn)   **Tablets:** 25 mg | Mannitol, methylparaben, polyvinyl alcohol. (7663). Off-white to gray. Biconvex. In 30s.

Indications

➤*Advanced breast cancer:* For the treatment of advanced breast cancer in postmenopausal women whose disease has progressed following tamoxifen therapy.

➤*Unlabeled uses:* Prevention of prostate carcinogenesis.

Administration and Dosage

➤*Approved by the FDA:* October 21, 1999.

➤*Breast cancer:* 25 mg once daily after a meal. Patients treated with exemestane do not require glucocorticoid or mineralocorticoid replacement therapy.

➤*Renal / Hepatic insufficiency:* Dosage adjustment does not appear to be necessary.

Actions

➤*Pharmacology:* Exemestane is an irreversible, steroidal aromatase inactivator, structurally related to the natural substrate androstenedione. It acts as a false substrate for the aromatase enzyme and is processed to an intermediate that binds irreversibly to the active site of the enzyme causing its inactivation, an effect also known as "suicide inhibition." Exemestane significantly lowers circulating estrogen concentrations in postmenopausal women but has no detectable effect on adrenal biosynthesis of corticosteroids or aldosterone. Exemestane has no effect on other enzymes involved in the steroidogenic pathway up to a concentration ≥ 600 times higher than that inhibiting the aromatase enzyme.

Breast cancer cell growth may be estrogen-dependent. Aromatase is the principal enzyme that converts androgens to estrogens in both pre- and postmenopausal women. While the main source of estrogen (primarily estradiol) is the ovary in premenopausal women, the principal source of circulating estrogens in postmenopausal women is from conversion of adrenal and ovarian androgens (androstenedione and testosterone) to estrogens (estrone and estradiol) by the aromatase enzyme in peripheral tissue. Estrogen deprivation through aromatase inhibition is an effective and selective treatment for some postmenopausal patients with hormone-dependent breast cancer.

➤*Pharmacokinetics:*

Absorption / Distribution – Following oral administration to healthy postmenopausal women, exemestane is rapidly absorbed.

Metabolism / Excretion – After maximum plasma concentration is reached, levels decline polyexponentially with a mean terminal half-life of ≈ 24 hours. Exemestane is extensively distributed and cleared from the systemic circulation primarily by metabolism. The pharmacokinetics of exemestane are dose proportional after single (10 to 200 mg) or repeated oral doses (0.5 to 50 mg). Following repeated daily doses of 25 mg exemestane, plasma concentrations of unchanged drug are similar to levels measured after a single dose.

Postmenopausal women with advanced breast cancer – Pharmacokinetic parameters in postmenopausal women with advanced breast cancer following single or repeated doses have been compared with those in healthy, postmenopausal women. Exemestane appears to be more rapidly absorbed in the women with breast cancer than in healthy women, with a mean T_{max} of 1.2 hours in the women with breast cancer and 2.9 hours in healthy women. After repeated dosing, the average oral clearance in women with advanced breast cancer was 45% lower than the oral clearance in healthy postmenopausal women, with corresponding higher systemic exposure. Mean AUC values following repeated doses in women with breast cancer (75.4 ng•hr/ml) were about twice those in healthy women (41.4 ng•hr/ml).

Absorption: Following oral administration of exemestane, $\geq 42\%$ was absorbed from the GI tract. Exemestane plasma levels increased by $\approx 40\%$ after a high-fat breakfast.

Distribution: Exemestane is distributed extensively into tissues. Exemestane is 90% bound to plasma proteins and the fraction bound is independent of the total concentration (albumin and α_1-acid glycoprotein). The distribution of exemestane and its metabolites into blood cells is negligible.

Metabolism: Exemestane is extensively metabolized, with levels of the unchanged drug in plasma accounting for < 10%. The initial steps in the metabolism of exemestane are oxidation of the methylene group in position 6 and reduction of the 17-keto group with subsequent formation of many secondary metabolites. Each metabolite accounts only for a limited amount of drug-related material. The metabolites are inactive or inhibit aromatase with decreased potency compared with the parent drug. One metabolite may have androgenic activity. Studies using human liver preparations indicate that cytochrome P450 3A4 (CYP 3A4) is the principal isoenzyme involved in the oxidation of exemestane.

Excretion: Following administration of exemestane to healthy postmenopausal women, the cumulative amounts excreted in urine and feces were similar ($\approx 42\%$ in urine and 42% in feces over a 1-week col-

lection period). The amount of drug excreted unchanged in urine was < 1% of the dose.

➤*Clinical trials:* 25 mg exemestane administered once daily was evaluated in a randomized, double-blind, multicenter, multinational comparative study and in 2 multicenter, single-arm studies of postmenopausal women with advanced breast cancer who had disease progression after treatment with tamoxifen for metastatic disease or as adjuvant therapy. Some patients also had received prior cytotoxic therapy, either as adjuvant treatment or for metastatic disease. The primary purpose of the 3 studies was evaluation of objective response rate (complete response and partial reponse). Time-to-tumor progression and overall survival were also assessed in the comparative trial. In the comparative study, patients were randomized to receive exemestane 25 mg once daily (n = 366) or megestrol acetate 40 mg 4 times daily (n = 403).

The objective response rates observed in the 2 treatment arms showed no difference in exemestane from megestrol acetate. Response rates for exemestane from the 2 single-arm trials were 23.4% and 28.1% There were too few deaths occurring across treatment groups to draw conclusions on overall survival differences.

Contraindications

Hypersensitivity to the drug or to any of the excipients.

Warnings

➤*Endocrine effects:* Increases in testosterone and androstenedione levels have been observed at daily doses of ≥ 200 mg. A dose-dependent decrease in sex hormone binding globulin has been observed with daily exemestane doses of ≥ 2.5 mg. Slight, nondose-dependent increases in serum luteinizing hormone and follicle-stimulating hormone levels have been observed even at low doses because of feedback at the pituitary level.

➤*Renal function impairment:* The AUC of exemestane after a single 25 mg dose was ≈ 3 times higher in subjects with moderate or severe renal insufficiency (creatinine clearance < 35 ml/min/1.73 m^2) compared with the AUC in healthy volunteers. The safety of chronic dosing in patients with moderate or severe renal impairment has not been studied. Dosage adjustment does not appear to be necessary based on experience with exemestane at repeated doses up to 200 mg daily that demonstrated a moderate increase in non-life threatening adverse events.

➤*Hepatic function impairment:* The pharmacokinetics of exemestane have been investigated in subjects with moderate or severe hepatic insufficiency (Childs-Pugh B or C). Following a single 25 mg oral dose, the AUC of exemestane was ≈ 3 times higher than that observed in healthy volunteers. The safety of chronic dosing in patients with moderate or severe hepatic impairment has not been studied. Based on experience with exemestane at repeated doses up to 200 mg daily that demonstrated a moderate increase in non-life threatening adverse events, dosage adjustment does not appear to be necessary.

➤*Mutagenesis:* Exemestane was clastogenic in human lymphocytes in vitro without metabolic activation but was not clastogenic in vivo (micronucleus assay in mouse bone marrow).

➤*Fertility impairment:* Untreated female rats showed reduced fertility when mated to males treated with 500 mg/kg/day exemestane (≈ 200 times the recommended human dose on a mg/m^2 basis) for 63 days prior to and during cohabitation. Exemestane given to female rats 14 days prior to mating and through day 15 or 20 of gestation increased the placental weights at 4 mg/kg/day (≈ 1.5 times the human dose on a mg/m^2 basis). Exemestane showed no effects on female fertility parameters (eg, ovarian function, mating behavior, conception rate) in rats given doses up to 20 mg/kg/day (≈ 8 times the human dose on a mg/m^2 basis), but mean litter size was decreased at this dose. In general toxicology studies, changes in the ovary, including hyperplasia, an increase in ovarian cysts, and a decrease in copora lutea were observed with variable frequency in mice, rats, and dogs at doses that ranged from 3 to 20 times the human dose on a mg/m^2 basis.

➤*Elderly:* Healthy postmenopausal women 43 to 68 years of age were studied in pharmacokinetic trials. Age-related alterations in exemestane pharmacokinetics were not seen over this age range. The use of exemestane in elderly patients does not require special precautions.

➤*Pregnancy: Category D.* There are no studies in pregnant women using exemestane. Exemestane is indicated for postmenopausal women. If there is exposure to exemestane during pregnancy, apprise the patient of the potential hazard to the fetus and potential risk for loss of the pregnancy.

➤*Lactation:* Exemestane is only indicated in postmenopausal women. Concentrations of exemestane and its metabolites were approximately equivalent in the milk and plasma of rats for 24 hours after a single oral dose of 1 mg/kg. It is not known whether exemestane is excreted in human breast milk.

EXEMESTANE

➤*Children:* The safety and efficacy of exemestane in pediatric patients have not been established.

Precautions

➤*Premenopausal women:* Do not administer exemestane tablets to premenopausal women.

➤*Lymphocytopenia:* Approximately 20% of patients receiving exemestane in clinical studies experienced common toxicity criteria (CTC) grade 3 or 4 lymphocytopenia. Of these patients, 89% had a pre-existing lower grade lymphopenia. Forty percent of patients either recovered or improved to a lesser severity while on treatment. Patients did not have a significant increase in viral infections, and no opportunistic infections were observed.

➤*Estrogen suppression:* Plasma estrogen (estradiol, estrone, and estrone sulfate) suppression was seen starting at a 5 mg daily dose of exemestane, with a maximum suppression of $\geq$ 85% to 95% achieved at a 25 mg dose. Exemestane 25 mg daily reduced whole body aromatization by 98% in postmenopausal women with breast cancer. After a single dose of exemestane 25 mg, the maximal suppression of circulating estrogens occurred 2 to 3 days after dosing and persisted for 4 to 5 days.

➤*Corticosteroid therapy:* Exemestane did not affect cortisol or aldosterone secretion at baseline or in response to adrenal corticotropic hormone (ACTH) at any dose up to 200 mg daily. Glucocorticoid or mineralocorticoid replacement therapy is not necessary with exemestane treatment.

➤*Lab test abnormalities:* Elevations of serum levels of AST, ALT, alkaline phosphatase, and gamma glutamyl transferase > 5 times the upper value of the normal range (ie, $\geq$ CTC grade 3) have been rarely reported but appear mostly attributable to the underlying presence of liver or bone metastases. In the comparative study, CTC grade 3 or 4 elevation of gamma glutamyl transferase without documented evidence of liver metastasis was reported in 2.7% of patients treated with exemestane and in 1.8% of patients treated with megestrol acetate.

Drug Interactions

➤*CYP 3A4:* Exemestane is extensively metabolized by CYP 3A4 and aldoketoreductases. Coadministration of ketaconazole, a potent inhibitor of CYP 3A4, has no significant effect on exemestane pharmacokinetics. Therefore, significant pharmacokinetic interactions mediated by inhibition of CYP isoenzymes appear unlikely. However, a possible decrease of exemestane plasma levels by known inducers of CYP 3A4 cannot be excluded.

➤*Drug/Food interactions:* In postmenopausal women with advanced breast cancer, exemestane plasma levels increased by $\approx$ 40% after a high-fat meal.

Adverse Reactions

A total of 1058 patients were treated with 25 mg exemestane once daily in the clinical trials program. Exemestane was generally well tolerated, and adverse events were usually mild to moderate. Only one death was considered possibly related to treatment with exemestane; an 80-year-old woman with known coronary artery disease had a MI with multiple organ failure after 9 weeks on study treatment. In the clinical trials program, 3% of the patients discontinued treatment with exemestane because of adverse events, mainly within the first 10 weeks of treatment; late discontinuation because of adverse events was uncommon (0.3%).

In the comparative study, fewer patients receiving exemestane discontinued treatment because of adverse events than those treated with megestrol acetate (2% vs 5%). The proportion of patients experiencing an excessive weight gain (> 10% of their baseline weight) was significantly higher with megestrol acetate than with exemestane (17% vs 8%).

Adverse Reactions of All Grades[1] and Causes: Exemestane vs Megestrol Acetate ($\geq$ 5%)		
Adverse reaction	Exemestane 25 mg once daily (n = 358)	Megestrol Acetate 40 mg 4 times daily (n = 400)
CNS		
Depression	13	9
Insomnia	11	9
Anxiety	10	11
Dizziness	8	6
Headache	8	7
GI		
Nausea	18	12
Vomiting	7	4
Abdominal pain	6	11
Anorexia	6	5
Constipation	5	8
Diarrhea	4	5
Increased appetite	3	6
Respiratory		
Dyspnea	10	15
Coughing	6	7
Miscellaneous		
Fatigue	22	29
Hot flashes	13	6
Pain	13	13
Edema (ie, edema, peripheral edema, leg edema)	7	6
Influenza-like symptoms	6	5
Increased sweating	6	9
Hypertension	5	6

[1] Graded according to common toxicity criteria.

Less frequent adverse events of any cause (from 2% to 5%) reported in the comparative study for patients receiving 25 mg exemestane once daily were fever, generalized weakness, paresthesia, pathological fracture, bronchitis, sinusitis, rash, itching, urinary tract infection, and lymphedema.

Additional adverse events of any cause observed in the overall clinical trials program (n = 1058) in $\geq$ 5% of patients treated with 25 mg exemestane once daily, but not in the comparative study, included pain at tumor sites (8%), asthenia (6%), and fever (5%). Adverse events of any cause reported in 2% to 5% of all patients treated with 25 mg exemestane in the overall clinical trials program, but not in the comparative study, included chest pain, hypoesthesia, confusion, dyspepsia, arthralgia, back pain, skeletal pain, infection, upper respiratory tract infection, pharyngitis, rhinitis, and alopecia.

Overdosage

Clinical trials have been conducted with exemestane given as a single dose to healthy female volunteers at doses as high as 800 mg daily for 12 weeks and to postmenopausal women with advanced breast cancer at doses as high as 600 mg. These dosages were well tolerated.

➤*Treatment:* There is no specific antidote to exemestane overdosage, and treatment must be symptomatic. General supportive care, including frequent monitoring of vital signs and close observation of the patient, is indicated. Refer to the General Management of Acute Overdosage.

ASPARAGINASE

| *Rx* | Elspar (Merck) | **Powder for Injection, lyophilized:** 10,000 IU | 80 mg mannitol. Preservative free. In 10 ml vials. |

Indications

➤*Acute lymphocytic leukemia:* Acute lymphocytic leukemia, primarily in combination with other chemotherapeutic agents, in the induction of remissions of disease in children. Do not use as the sole induction agent unless combination therapy is deemed inappropriate.

Administration and Dosage

➤*Maintenance:* Not recommended for maintenance therapy.

Because of the unpredictability of adverse reactions, use only in a hospital (see Warning Box).

➤*IV:* Give over 30 minutes through the side arm of an already running infusion of Sodium Chloride Injection or 5% Dextrose Injection. The drug has little tendency to cause phlebitis when given IV.

➤*IM:* Limit the volume at a single injection site to 2 ml. For a volume greater than 2 ml, use 2 injection sites.

➤*Induction regimens:* One of the following combination regimens is recommended for acute lymphocytic leukemia in *children*. (Day 1 is considered the first day of therapy.)

Regimen I –
Prednisone: 40 mg/m^2/day orally in 3 divided doses for 15 days, followed by tapering of the dosage as follows: 20 mg/m^2 for 2 days, 10 mg/m^2 for 2 days, 5 mg/m^2 for 2 days, 2.5 mg/m^2 for 2 days and then discontinue.
Vincristine sulfate: 2 mg/m^2 IV once weekly on days 1, 8 and 15. The maximum single dose should not exceed 2 mg.
Asparaginase: 1,000 IU/kg/day IV for 10 successive days beginning on day 22.

Regimen II –
Prednisone: 40 mg/m^2/day orally in 3 divided doses for 28 days (the total daily dose to the nearest 2.5 mg), then gradual discontinuation over 14 days.
Vincristine sulfate: 1.5 mg/m^2 IV weekly for 4 doses, on days 1, 8, 15 and 22. The maximum single dose should not exceed 2 mg.
Asparaginase: 6000 IU/m^2 IM on days 4, 7, 10, 13, 16, 19, 22, 25 and 28.

When remission is obtained with either of the above regimens, institute appropriate maintenance therapy. Do not use asparaginase as part of a maintenance regimen.

The above regimens do not preclude the need for special therapy to prevent CNS leukemia.

Asparaginase has been used in other combination regimens. Administering the drug IV concurrently with or immediately before a course of vincristine and prednisone may be associated with increased toxicity.

➤*Single agent induction therapy:* Use asparaginase as the sole induction agent only when a combined regimen is inappropriate because of toxicity or other specific patient-related factors, or in cases refractory to other therapy.

Children or adults – 200 IU/kg/day IV for 28 days. Complete remissions are of short duration, 1 to 3 months. Asparaginase has been used as the sole induction agent in other regimens.

➤*Dosage adjustments:* Carefully monitor patients undergoing induction therapy; individualize dosage. Adjustments always involve decreasing dosages of one or more agents or discontinuation. Patients who have received a course of therapy, if treated again, have an increased risk of hypersensitivity reactions. Therefore, repeat treatment only when the benefit of such therapy is weighed against the increased risk.

➤*Intradermal skin test:* Perform an intradermal skin test prior to initial administration of asparaginase and when it is given after a week or more has elapsed between doses.

Prepare the skin test solution as follows – Reconstitute a 10,000 IU vial with 5 ml of diluent. From this solution (2000 IU/ml), withdraw 0.1 ml and inject it into another vial containing 9.9 ml of diluent, yielding a skin test solution of approximately 20 IU/ml. Use 0.1 ml of this solution (about 2 IU) for the intradermal skin test. Observe the skin test site for at least 1 hour for a wheal or erythema that indicates a positive reaction. An allergic reaction even to the skin test dose may occur rarely. A negative skin test reaction does not preclude possible development of an allergic reaction.

➤*Desensitization:* Perform desensitization before giving the first treatment dose of asparaginase in positive reactors, and on retreatment of any patient. Attempt rapid desensitization of the patient by progressively increasing amounts of the drug IV. Take adequate pre-

cautions to treat an acute allergic reaction. One schedule begins with 1 IU given IV and doubles the dose every 10 minutes if no reaction has occurred, until the accumulated total amount given equals the planned doses for that day. For convenience, the following table is included to calculate the number of doses necessary to reach the patient's total dose for that day:

Asparaginase Dosing Based on Total Daily Requirements		
Injection Number[1]	Dose (IU)	Accumulated Total Dose (IU)
1	1	1
2	2	3
3	4	7
4	8	15
5	16	31
6	32	63
7	64	127
8	128	255
9	256	511
10	512	1,023
11	1,024	2,047
12	2,048	4,095
13	4,096	8,191
14	8,192	16,383
15	16,384	32,767
16	32,768	65,535
17	65,536	131,071
18	131,072	262,143

[1] For example: A patient weighing 20 kg who is to receive 200 IU/kg (total dose 4000 IU) would receive injections 1 through 12 during desensitization.

➤*Preparation of solutions:*
IV – Reconstitute the 10,000 unit vial with 5 ml Sterile Water for Injection or with Sodium Chloride Injection. Ordinary shaking during reconstitution does not inactivate the enzyme. This solution may be used for direct IV administration within 8 hours following reconstitution. For administration by infusion, dilute solutions with Sodium Chloride Injection or 5% Dextrose Injection. Infuse within 8 hours and only if clear.

Occasionally, gelatinous fiber-like particles may develop on standing. Filtration through a 5 micron filter during administration will remove the particles with no loss of potency. Some loss of potency has been observed with the use of a 0.2 micron filter.

IM – Reconstitute by adding 2 ml Sodium Chloride Injection to the 10,000 unit vial. Use the resulting solution within 8 hours and only if clear.

➤*Storage/Stability:* Store at 2° to 8°C (36° to 46°F). Because it is preservative-free, store reconstituted solution at 2° to 8°C (36° to 46°F); discard after 8 hours or sooner if cloudy.

Actions

➤*Pharmacology:* Asparaginase contains the enzyme L-asparagine amidohydrolase, type EC-2, derived from *Escherichia coli.*

In a significant number of patients with acute (particularly lymphocytic) leukemia, the malignant cells depend on exogenous asparagine for survival. Normal cells are able to synthesize asparagine and thus are affected less by the rapid depletion produced by treatment. Administration of asparaginase hydrolyzes serum asparagine to nonfunctional asparatic acid and ammonia, depriving tumor cells of a required amino acid. Tumor cell proliferation is blocked due to interruption of asparagine-dependent protein synthesis. The inhibitory activity is maximal in the postmitotic (G$_1$) phase of the cell cycle.

➤*Pharmacokinetics:*
Absorption/Distribution – Initial plasma levels of L-asparaginase following IV administration are correlated to dose. Daily administration results in a cumulative increase in plasma levels. Asparaginase serum levels following IM use are approximately one-half those achieved with IV administration. Apparent volume of distribution is approximately 70% to 80% of estimated plasma volume. There is some slow movement from vascular to extravascular, extracellular space. L-asparaginase is detected in the lymph. Cerebrospinal fluid levels usually are less than 1% of concurrent plasma levels.

Metabolism/Excretion – Plasma half-life varies from 8 to 30 hours and is not influenced by dosage. Only minimal urinary and biliary excretion occurs.

Contraindications

Anaphylactic reactions to asparaginase; pancreatitis or a history of pancreatitis.

Warnings

➤*Hematologic:* Bone marrow depression, leukopenia, thrombosis and clotting factors depressed; increase in blood ammonia during the con-

ASPARAGINASE

version of asparagine to asparatic acid by the enzyme.

➤*Bone marrow depression:* Rarely, transient bone marrow depression has been seen as evidenced by a delay in return of hemoglobin or hematocrit levels to normal in patients undergoing hematologic remission of leukemia. Marked leukopenia has been reported.

➤*Bleeding:* In addition to hypofibrinogemia, other clotting factors may be depressed. Most marked has been a decrease in factors V and VIII with a variable decrease in factors VII and IX. A decrease in circulating platelets has occurred in low incidence, which, with the increased levels of fibrin degradation products in the serum, may indicate consumption coagulopathy. Bleeding has been a problem in only a few patients; however, intracranial hemorrhage and fatal bleeding associated with low fibrinogen levels have been reported. Increased compensatory fibrinolytic activity has also occurred.

➤*Hyperglycemia:* Hyperglycemia with glucosuria and polyuria has been reported in low incidence. Serum and urine acetone are usually absent or negligible; this syndrome thus resembles hyperosmolar, nonketotic hyperglycemia. It usually responds to drug discontinuation and judicious use of IV fluid and insulin, but it may be fatal.

➤*Hepatotoxicity:* Hepatotoxicity occurs in the majority of patients. Therapy may increase preexisting liver impairment caused by prior therapy or underlying disease; asparaginase may increase the toxicity of other medications.

➤*Hypersensitivity reactions:* Reactions are frequent and may occur during the primary course of therapy. They are not completely predictable based on the intradermal skin test. Anaphylaxis and death have occurred.

Once a patient has received asparaginase, there is an increased risk of hypersensitivity reactions with retreatment. In patients found to be hypersensitive by skin testing, and in any patient previously under therapy with asparaginase, administer the drug only after successful desensitization. Even then, the possible benefit should be judged as greater than the increased risk since desensitization may also be hazardous (see Administration and Dosage).

In children with advanced leukemia, a lower incidence of anaphylaxis has occurred with IM use, although there was a higher incidence of milder hypersensitivity reactions than with IV use.

Anaphylactic reactions require the immediate use of epinephrine, oxygen and IV steroids. Refer to Management of Acute Hypersensitivity Reactions.

➤*Pregnancy:* Category C. Asparaginase has been shown to retard the weight gain of mothers and fetuses, has caused resorptions, and has resulted in dose-dependent embryotoxicity, gross abnormalities, and skeletal abnormalities in various rodent species when given in doses ranging from 0.05 to 1 times the human dose. There are no adequate and well controlled studies in pregnant women. Use during pregnancy only if the potential benefit justifies the potential risk to the fetus.

➤*Lactation:* It is not known whether this drug is excreted in breast milk. Because of potential serious adverse reactions in nursing infants, discontinue nursing or discontinue the drug, considering the importance of the drug to the mother.

➤*Children:* Asparaginase toxicity is reported to be greater in adults than in children.

Precautions

➤*Monitoring:* The fall in circulating lymphoblasts is often quite marked; normal or below normal leukocyte counts are noted frequently several days after initiating therapy and may be accompanied by a marked rise in serum uric acid. Uric acid nephropathy may develop; take appropriate preventive measures (eg, allopurinol, increased fluid intake, alkalinization of urine). Monitor peripheral blood count and bone marrow frequently.

Obtain frequent serum amylase determinations to detect early evidence of pancreatitis. If pancreatitis occurs, discontinue therapy.

Monitor blood sugar during therapy because hyperglycemia may occur (see Warnings).

➤*Infection:* Asparaginase has immunosuppressive activity in animals; consider the possibility of predisposition to infection.

Drug Interactions

Asparaginase Drug Interactions			
Precipitant drug	Object drug[*]		Description
Asparaginase	Methotrexate	↓	Asparaginase may diminish or abolish methotrexate's effect on malignant cells; this effect persists as long as plasma asparagine levels are suppressed. Do not use methotrexate with, or following asparaginase, while asparagine levels are below normal.
Vincristine and prednisone	Asparaginase	↑	IV administration of asparaginase concurrently with or immediately before a course of these drugs may be associated with increased toxicity.

[*] ↑ = Object drug increased. ↓ = Object drug decreased.

➤*Drug/Lab test interactions:* L-asparaginase may interfere with the interpretation of **thyroid function tests** by producing a rapid and marked reduction in serum concentrations of thyroxine-binding globulin within 2 days after the first dose. Serum concentrations of thyroxine-binding globulin returned to pretreatment values within 4 weeks of the last dose of L-asparaginase.

Adverse Reactions

➤*CNS:* Depression, somnolence, fatigue, coma, confusion, agitation and hallucinations (mild to severe); headache, irritability (mild); Parkinson-like syndrome with tremor and a progressive increase in muscular tone (rare). These effects usually reversed spontaneously after stopping treatment. No clear correlation exists between elevated blood ammonia levels and CNS changes.

➤*GI:* Nausea, vomiting, anorexia, abdominal cramps (usually mild). Pancreatitis, sometimes fulminant, and acute hemorrhagic pancreatitis have occurred; both may be fatal.

➤*Hepatic:* Elevations of serum glutamic-oxaloacetic transaminase (AST), serum glutamic-pyruvic transaminase (ALT), alkaline phosphatase, bilirubin (direct and indirect) and depression of serum albumin, cholesterol (total and esters) and plasma fibrinogen. Increases and decreases of total lipids; marked hypalbuminemia associated with peripheral edema. These abnormalities are usually reversible on discontinuation of therapy and some reversal may occur during the course of therapy. Fatty changes in the liver and malabsorption syndrome (see Warnings).

➤*Hypersensitivity:* Skin rash, urticaria, arthralgia, respiratory distress, and acute anaphylaxis (see Warnings).

➤*Renal:* Azotemia, usually prerenal, occurs frequently. Acute renal shut-down and fatal renal insufficiency have been reported. Proteinuria has occurred infrequently.

➤*Miscellaneous:* Chills, fever, weight loss (usually mild); fatal hyperthermia, hypoglycemia (see Warning Box).

PEGASPARGASE (PEG-L-asparaginase)

Rx	**Oncaspar** (Enzon)	**Injection:** 750 IU/ml in a phosphate buffered saline solution	Preservative free. In single-use vials.

Indications

➤*Acute lymphoblastic leukemia (ALL):* For patients with ALL who require L-asparaginase in their treatment regimen, but have developed hypersensitivity to the native forms of L-asparaginase. Pegaspargase, like L-asparaginase, is generally used in combination with other chemotherapeutic agents, such as vincristine, methotrexate, cytarabine, daunorubicin and doxorubicin. Use of pegaspargase as a single agent should only be undertaken when multi-agent chemotherapy is judged to be inappropriate for the patient.

Administration and Dosage

➤*Approved by the FDA:* February 1, 1994.

As a component of selected multiple-agent regimens, the recommended dose is 2500 IU/m² every 14 days by either the IM or IV route of administration. The preferred route of administration, however, is the IM route because of the lower incidence of hepatotoxicity, coagulopathy, and GI and renal disorders compared to the IV route.

Do not administer if there is any indication that the drug has been frozen. Although there may not be an apparent change in the appearance of the drug, pegaspargase's activity is destroyed after freezing.

➤*Dosage:* The safety and efficacy of pegaspargase have been established in patients with known previous hypersensitivity to L-asparaginase whose ages ranged from 1 to 21 years old. The recommended dose for children with a body surface area $\geq$ 0.6 m² is 2500 IU/m² administered every 14 days. The recommended dose for children with a body surface area < 0.6 m² is 82.5 IU/kg administered every 14 days.

➤*Administration:*

IM – When administering IM, limit the volume at a single injection site to 2 ml. If the volume to be administered is > 2 ml, use multiple injection sites.

IV – When administered IV, give over a period of 1 to 2 hours in 100 ml of Sodium Chloride or Dextrose Injection 5%, through an infusion that is already running.

Use as a single agent – Use of pegaspargase as the sole induction agent should be undertaken only in an unusual situation when a combined regimen, which uses other chemotherapeutic agents such as vin-

PEGASPARGASE (PEG-L-asparaginase)

cristine, methotrexate, cytarabine, daunorubicin or doxorubicin, is inappropriate because of toxicity or other specific patient-related factors, or in patients refractory to other therapy. When pegaspargase is to be used as the sole induction agent, the recommended dosage regimen is also 2500 IU/m² every 14 days.

Maintenance – When a remission is obtained, appropriate maintenance therapy may be instituted. Pegaspargase may be used as part of a maintenance regimen.

➤*Storage/Stability:* Avoid excessive agitation; do NOT shake. Keep refrigerated at 2° to 8°C (36° to 46°F). Do not use if cloudy or if precipitate is present. Do not use if stored at room temperature for > 48 hours. Do NOT freeze. Do not use product if it is known to have been frozen. Freezing destroys activity, which cannot be detected visually. Use only one dose per vial; do not re-enter the vial. Discard unused portions. Do not save unused drug for later administration.

Actions

➤*Pharmacology:* Pegaspargase is a modified version of the enzyme L-asparaginase. It is an oncolytic agent used in combination chemotherapy for the treatment of patients with acute lymphoblastic leukemia (ALL) who are hypersensitive to native forms of L-asparaginase. L-asparaginase is modified by covalently conjugating units of monomethoxypolyethylene glycol (PEG), molecular weight of 5000, to the enzyme, forming the active ingredient PEG-L-asparaginase. The L-asparaginase used in the manufacture of pegaspargase is derived from *Escherichia coli*.

Leukemic cells are unable to synthesize asparagine due to a lack of asparagine synthetase and are dependent on an exogenous source of asparagine for survival. Rapid depletion of asparagine, which results from treatment with the enzyme L-asparaginase, kills the leukemic cells. Normal cells, however, are less affected by the rapid depletion due to their ability to synthesize asparagine. This is an approach to therapy based on a specific metabolic defect in some leukemic cells which do not produce asparagine synthetase.

➤*Pharmacokinetics:* In a study in predominantly L-asparaginase-naive adult patients with leukemia and lymphoma, initial plasma levels of L-asparaginase following IV administration were determined. Plasma half-life did not appear to be influenced by dose levels, and it could not be correlated with age, sex, surface area, renal or hepatic function, diagnosis or extent of disease. Apparent volume of distribution was equal to estimated plasma volume. L-asparaginase was measurable for at least 15 days following the initial treatment with pegaspargase. The enzyme could not be detected in the urine.

In a study of newly diagnosed pediatric patients with ALL who received either a single IM injection of pegaspargase (2500 IU/m²), *E. coli* L-asparaginase (25,000 IU/m²), or *Erwinia* L-asparaginase (25,000 IU/m²), the plasma half-lives for the three forms of L-asparaginase were 5.73, 1.24 and 0.65 days, respectively.

The in vivo early leukemic cell kill after a single IM injection of pegaspargase (2500 IU/m²), native *E. coli* L-asparaginase (25,000 IU/m²) and *Erwinia* L-asparaginase (25,000 IU/m²) was studied. Bone marrow aspirates were taken before and 5 days after a single dose of one of the three different forms of L-asparaginase. The percent reduction of viable lymphoblasts at day 5 for each group was 55.7%, 57.8% and 57.9%, respectively.

In three pharmacokinetic studies, 37 relapsed ALL patients received pegaspargase at 2500 IU/m² every 2 weeks. The plasma half-life was 3.24 ± 1.83 days in nine patients who were previously hypersensitive to native L-asparaginase and 5.69 ± 3.25 days in 28 non-hypersensitive patients. The area under the curve was 9.5 ± 3.95 IU/ml/day in the previously hypersensitive patients, and 9.83 ± 5.94 IU/ml day in the non-hypersensitive patients.

➤*Clinical trials:* In four open-label studies, 42 previously hypersensitive acute leukemia patients (39 [93%] with ALL) with multiple relapses received pegaspargase at a dose of 2000 or 2500 IU/m² administered IM or IV every 14 days during induction combination chemotherapy. The reinduction response rate was 50% (36% complete remissions and 14% partial remissions). This response rate is comparable to that reported in the literature for relapsed patients treated with native L-asparaginase as part of combination chemotherapy.

Pegaspargase was also shown to have some activity as a single agent in multiply relapsed hypersensitive ALL patients, the majority of whom were pediatric. Treatment resulted in three responses (one complete remission and two partial remissions) in nine previously hypersensitive patients who would not have been able to receive any further L-asparaginase treatment.

Pegaspargase was also studied in non-hypersensitive, relapsed ALL patients who were randomized to receive two doses of pegaspargase at 2500 IU/m² every 14 days or twelve doses of *E. coli* L-asparaginase at 10,000 IU/m² 3 times a week during a 28 day induction combination chemotherapy regimen (which included vincristine and prednisone). Although the enrollment in this study was too small to be conclusive, the data showed that for 20 patients there was no significant difference between the overall response rates of 60% and 50%, respectively, or the complete remission rates of 50% and 50%, respectively.

Pegaspargase was administered during maintenance therapy regimens to 33 previously hypersensitive patients. The average number of doses received during maintenance therapy was 5.8 (range, 1 to 24) and the average duration of maintenance therapy was 126 days (range, 1 to 513).

Contraindications

Pancreatitis or a history of pancreatitis; patients who have had significant hemorrhagic events associated with prior L-asparaginase therapy; previous serious allergic reactions, such as generalized urticaria, bronchospasm, laryngeal edema, hypotension, or other unacceptable adverse reactions to pegaspargase.

Warnings

➤*Hypersensitivity reactions:* Hypersensitivity reactions to pegaspargase, including life-threatening anaphylaxis, may occur during therapy, especially in patients with known hypersensitivity to the other forms of L-asparaginase. As a routine precaution, keep patients under observation for 1 hour with resuscitation equipment and other agents necessary to treat anaphylaxis (eg, epinephrine, oxygen, IV steroids) available.

Hypersensitivity reactions to *E. coli* L-asparaginase have been reported in the literature in 3% to 73% of patients. Patients in pegaspargase clinical studies were considered to be previously hypersensitive if they experienced a systemic rash, urticaria, bronchospasm, laryngeal edema or hypotension following administration of any form of native L-asparaginase. Patients were also considered to be previously hypersensitive if they experienced local erythema, urticaria, or swelling if > 2 cm for at least 10 minutes following administration of any form of native L-asparaginase. The National Cancer Institute Common Toxicity Criteria (CTC) were used to classify the severity of the hypersensitivity reactions. These are: Grade 1 - transient rash (mild); grade 2 - mild bronchospasm (moderate); grade 3 - moderate bronchospasm or serum sickness (severe); grade 4 - hypotension or anaphylaxis (life-threatening). Additionally most transient local urticaria were considered grade 2 hypersensitivity reactions, while most sustained urticaria distant from the injection site were considered grade 3 hypersensitivity reactions. In general, the moderate to life-threatening hypersensitivity reactions were considered dose-limiting; that is, they required L-asparaginase treatment to be discontinued.

In separate studies, pegaspargase was administered IV to 48 patients and IM to 126 patients. The incidence of hypersensitivity reactions when pegaspargase was administered IM was 30% in patients who were previously hypersensitive to native L-asparaginase and 11% in non-hypersensitive patients. The incidence of hypersensitivity reactions when pegaspargase was administered IV was 60% in patients who were previously hypersensitive to native L-asparaginase and 12% in non-hypersensitive patients. Since only five previously hypersensitive patients received pegaspargase IV, no meaningful analysis of the incidence of hypersensitivity reactions was possible between either the previously hypersensitive and non-hypersensitive patients, or between the IV and IM routes of administration.

Incidence of Pegaspargase Hypersensitivity Reactions						
		CTC grade of hypersensitivity reaction				
Patient status	No.	1	2	3	4	Total
Previously hypersensitive patients	62	7	8	4	1	20 (32%)
Non-hypersensitive patients	112	5	4	1	1	11 (10%)
Total patients	174	12	12	5	2	31 (18%)

The probability of previously hypersensitive and non-hypersensitive patients completing 8 doses of therapy without developing a dose-limiting hypersensitivity reaction was 77% and 95%, respectively.

All of the 62 hypersensitive patients treated with pegaspargase in five clinical studies had previous hypersensitivity reactions to one or more of the native forms of L-asparaginase. Of the 35 patients who had previous hypersensitivity reactions to *E. coli* L-asparaginase, only 5 (14%) had dose-limiting hypersensitivity reactions. Of the 27 patients who had hypersensitivity reactions to both *E. coli* and *Erwinia* L-asparaginase, 7 (26%) had pegaspargase dose-limiting hypersensitivity reactions. The overall incidence of dose-limiting hypersensitivity reactions in 174 patients treated with pegaspargase was 9% (19% in 62 hypersensitive and 3% in 112 non-hypersensitive patients). Of the total of 9% dose-limiting hypersensitivity reactions, 1% were anaphylactic (CTC grade 4) and the other 8% were ≤ CTC grade 3.

➤*Pregnancy: Category C.* It is not known whether pegaspargase can cause fetal harm when administered to a pregnant woman or can affect reproduction capacity. Give to a pregnant woman only if clearly needed.

➤*Lactation:* It is not known whether pegaspargase is excreted in breast milk. Because of the potential for serious adverse reactions in nursing infants, decide whether to discontinue nursing or discontinue the drug, taking into account the importance of the drug to the mother.

Precautions

➤*Monitoring:* Carefully monitor and adjust the therapeutic regimen according to response and toxicity.

PEGASPARGASE (PEG-L-asparaginase)

A fall in circulating lymphoblasts is often noted after initiating therapy. This may be accompanied by a marked rise in serum uric acid. As a guide to the effects of therapy, monitor the patient's peripheral blood count and bone marrow. Obtain frequent serum amylase determinations to detect early evidence of pancreatitis. Monitor blood sugar during therapy because hyperglycemia may occur. When using pegaspargase in conjunction with hepatotoxic chemotherapy, monitor patients for liver dysfunction. Pegaspargase may affect a number of plasma proteins; therefore, monitoring of fibrinogen, PT and PTT may be indicated.

➤*Handling:* This drug may be a contact irritant, and the solution must be handled and administered with care. Gloves are recommended. Inhalation of vapors and contact with skin or mucous membranes, especially those of the eyes, must be avoided. In case of contact, wash with copious amounts of water for at least 15 minutes.

➤*Bleeding:* Patients taking pegaspargase are at higher than usual risk for bleeding problems, especially with simultaneous use of other drugs that have anticoagulant properties, such as aspirin and non-steroidal anti-inflammatories (see Drug Interactions).

➤*Infection:* Pegaspargase may have immunosuppressive activity. Therefore, it is possible that use of the drug may predispose patients to infection.

➤*Hepatic/CNS toxicity:* Severe hepatic and CNS toxicity following multi-agent chemotherapy that includes pegaspargase may occur. Caution appears warranted when treating patients with pegaspargase in combination with hepatotoxic agents, particularly when liver dysfunction is present.

Drug Interactions

Depletion of serum proteins by pegaspargase may increase the toxicity of other drugs which are protein bound. Additionally, during the period of its inhibition of protein synthesis and cell replication, pegaspargase may interfere with the action of drugs such as methotrexate, which require cell replication for their lethal effects. Pegaspargase may interfere with the enzymatic detoxification of other drugs, particularly in the liver.

Imbalances in coagulation factors have been noted with the use of pegaspargase, predisposing to bleeding or thrombosis. Use caution when administering any concurrent anticoagulant therapy, such as warfarin, heparin, dipyridamole, aspirin or nonsteroidal anti-inflammatory agents.

Adverse Reactions

Adverse reactions have occurred in adults and pediatric patients. Overall, the adult patients had a somewhat higher incidence of known L-asparaginase toxicities, except for hypersensitivity reactions, than the pediatric patients.

Excluding hypersensitivity reactions, the most frequently occurring known L-asparaginase related toxicities and adverse experiences were chemical hepatotoxicities and coagulopathies, the majority of which did not result in any significant clinical events. The incidence of significant clinical events included clinical pancreatitis (1%), hyperglycemia requiring insulin therapy (3%) and thrombosis (4%).

The following adverse reactions were reported for 174 patients in five clinical studies – Allergic reactions (which may have included rash, erythema, edema, pain, fever, chills, urticaria, dyspnea or bronchospasm), ALT increase, nausea or vomiting, fever, malaise (> 5%).

Anaphylactic reactions, dyspnea, injection site hypersensitivity, lip edema, rash, urticaria, abdominal pain, chills, pain in the extremities, hypotension, tachycardia, thrombosis, anorexia, diarrhea, jaundice, abnormal liver function test, decreased anticoagulant effect, disseminated intravascular coagulation, decreased fibrinogen, hemolytic anemia, leukopenia, pancytopenia, thrombocytopenia, increased thromboplastin, injection site pain/reaction, bilirubinemia, hyperglycemia, hyperuricemia, hypoglycemia, hypoproteinemia, peripheral edema, increased AST, arthralgia, myalgia, convulsion, headache, night sweats, paresthesia (> 1% but < 5%).

Bronchospasm, petechial rash, face edema, lesional edema, sepsis, septic shock, chest pain, endocarditis, hypertension, constipation, flatulence, GI pain, hepatomegaly, increased appetite, liver fatty deposits, coagulation disorder, increased coagulation time, decreased platelet count, purpura, increased amylase, edema, excessive thirst, hyper-ammonemia, hyponatremia, weight loss, bone pain, joint disorder, confusion, dizziness, emotional lability, somnolence, increased cough, epistaxis, upper respiratory tract infection, erythema simplex, pruritus, hematuria, increased urinary frequency, abnormal kidney function (< 1%).

➤*The following pegaspargase-related adverse reactions have been observed in patients with hematologic malignancies, primarily ALL (≈ 75%), non-Hodgkins lymphoma (≈ 13%), acute myelogenous leukemia (≈ 3%), and a variety of solid tumors (≈ 9%):*

Cardiovascular – Chest pain; subacute bacterial endocarditis; hypertension; severe hypotension; tachycardia.

CNS – Status epilepticus; temporal lobe seizures; somnolence; coma; malaise; mental status changes; dizziness; emotional lability; headache; lip numbness; finger paresthesia; mood changes; night sweats; a Parkinson-like syndrome; mild to severe confusion; disorientation; paresthesia. These side effects usually have reversed spontaneously after treatment was stopped.

Dermatologic – Itching; alopecia; fever blister; purpura; hand whiteness; fungal changes; nail whiteness and ridging; erythema simplex; jaundice; petechial rash.

GI – Anorexia; constipation; decreased appetite; diarrhea; indigestion; flatulence; gas; GI pain; mucositis; hepatomegaly; elevated gamma-glutamyltranspeptidase; increased appetite; mouth tenderness; severe colitis; nausea; vomiting.

Hematologic – Hypofibrinogenemia; prolonged prothrombin times; prolonged partial thromboplastin times; decreased antithrombin III; superficial and deep venous thrombosis; sagittal sinus thrombosis; venous catheter thrombosis; atrial thrombosis; leukopenia; agranulocytosis; pancytopenia; thrombocytopenia; disseminated intravascular coagulation; severe hemolytic anemia; anemia; clinical hemorrhage (may be fatal); easy bruisability; ecchymosis.

Hepatic – Elevations of AST, ALT and bilirubin (direct and indirect); jaundice, ascites and hypoalbuminemia, which may be associated with peripheral edema (usually are reversible on discontinuance of therapy, and some reversal may occur during the course of therapy); fatty changes in the liver; liver failure.

Hypersensitivity – These reactions may be acute or delayed, and include acute anaphylaxis, bronchospasm, dyspnea, urticaria, arthralgia, erythema, induration, edema, pain, tenderness, hives, swelling, lip edema, chills, fever and skin rashes (see Warnings).

Metabolic – Mild to severe hyperglycemia (low incidence, usually responds to discontinuation of pegaspargase and the judicious use of IV fluid and insulin); hypoglycemia; increased thirst; hyponatremia; uric acid nephropathy; hyperuricemia; hypoproteinemia; peripheral edema; hypoalbuminemia; proteinuria; weight loss; metabolic acidosis; increase in blood ammonia during the conversion of L-asparagine to aspartic acid by the enzyme.

Musculoskeletal – Diffuse and local musculoskeletal pain; arthralgia; joint stiffness; cramps.

Pancreatic: Pancreatitis, (sometimes fulminant and fatal); increased serum amylase and lipase.

Renal – Increased BUN; increased creatinine; increased urinary frequency; hematuria due to thrombopenia; severe hemorrhagic cystitis; renal dysfunction; renal failure.

Respiratory – Cough; epistaxis; severe bronchospasm; upper respiratory infection.

Miscellaneous – Localized edema; injection site reactions (including pain, swelling or redness); malaise; infection; sepsis; fatigue; septic shock.

Overdosage

Three patients received 10,000 IU/m^2 as an IV infusion. One patient experienced a slight increase in liver enzymes. A second patient developed a rash 10 minutes after the start of the infusion, which was controlled with the administration of an antihistamine and by slowing down the infusion rate. A third patient did not experience any adverse reactions.

Patient Information

Inform patients of the possibility of hypersensitivity reactions, including immediate anaphylaxis.

Pegaspargase patients are at higher than usual risk for bleeding problems. Instruct patients that the simultaneous use of pegaspargase with other drugs that may increase the risk of bleeding should be avoided (see Drug Interactions).

Pegaspargase may affect the ability of the liver to function normally in some patients. Therapy with pegaspargase may increase the toxicity of other medications (see Drug Interactions).

Pegaspargase may have immunosuppressive activity. Therefore, it is possible that use of the drug in patients may predispose the patient to infection. Patients should notify their physicians of any adverse reactions that occur.

CHROMIC PHOSPHATE P 32

| Rx | Phosphocol P 32 (Mallinckrodt) | Suspension: 15 mCi with a concentration of up to 5 mCi/ml and specific activity of up to 5 mCi/mg at time of standardization. | In 10 ml vials.[1] |

[1] With 2% benzyl alcohol, NaCl and sodium acetate.

Indications

➤*Intracavitary instillation:* Treatment of peritoneal or pleural effusions caused by metastatic disease.

➤*Interstitial injection:* Treatment of cancer.

Administration and Dosage

➤*For interstitial or intracavitary use only:* Measure dose by suitable radioactivity calibration system immediately prior to use.

The suggested dose range in the average patient (70 kg) is:

Intraperitoneal instillation – 10 to 20 mCi.

Intrapleural instillation – 6 to 12 mCi.

Interstitial use – 0.1 to 0.5 mCi/g of estimated weight of tumor.

Physical characteristics – Consult product literature for specific calibration and dosimetry information.

Actions

➤*Pharmacology:* Local irradiation by beta emission.

Chromic phosphate P 32 decays by beta emission with a physical half-life of 14.3 days. The mean energy of the beta particle is 695 keV.

Contraindications

Presence of ulcerative tumors; administration in exposed cavities or where there is evidence of loculation unless its extent is determined.

Warnings

➤*Radiopharmaceuticals:* Restrict use to physicians qualified in the safe use and handling of radionuclides produced by nuclear reactor or particle accelerator and whose experience and training have been approved by the appropriate government agency.

➤*Benzyl alcohol:* This product contains benzyl alcohol, which has been associated with fatal "gasping syndrome" in preterm infants.

➤*Pregnancy: Category C.* Use only when clearly needed and when the potential benefits outweigh the potential hazards to the fetus.

➤*Lactation:* Use only when clearly needed and when the potential benefits outweigh the potential hazards to the nursing infant.

Precautions

➤*Radioactive material:* Ensure minimum radiation exposure to the patient and occupational workers consistent with proper patient management.

➤*Intracavitary use:* Not for intravascular use.

Careful intracavitary instillation is required to avoid placing the dose of chromic phosphate P 32 into intrapleural or intraperitoneal loculations, bowel lumen or the body wall. Intestinal fibrosis or necrosis and chronic fibrosis of the body wall have resulted from unrecognized misplacement of the therapeutic agent.

➤*Large tumor masses:* Large tumor masses indicate the need for other forms of treatment; however, when other forms of treatment fail to control the effusion, chromic phosphate P 32 may be useful. In bloody effusion, treatment may be less effective.

Adverse Reactions

Transitory radiation sickness, bone marrow depression, pleuritis, peritonitis, nausea and abdominal cramping.

Radiation damage may occur if injected interstitially or into a loculation.

SODIUM IODIDE I 131

Rx	Iodotope (Bracco Diagnostics)	Capsules: Radioactivity ranging from 1 to 50 mCi per capsule at time of calibration	Blue/bluff.
		Oral solution: Radioactivity concentration of 7.05 mCi/ml at time of calibration	1 mg/ml EDTA. In vials containing ≈ 7, 14, 28, 70 or 106 mCi at time of calibration.
Rx	Sodium Iodide I 131 (Mallinckrodt)	Capsules: Radioactivity ranging from 0.75 to 100 mCi per capsule.	Various strengths.
		Oral solution: Radioactivity ranging from 3.5 to 150 mCi/vial.	0.1% sodium bisulfite and 0.2% EDTA. In vials.

Sodium Iodide I 131 is also used for treatment of hyperthyroidism. Refer to the monograph in the Endocrine/Metabolic chapter.

Indications

➤*Thyroid carcinoma:* Selected cases of thyroid carcinoma. Palliative effects may occur in patients with papillary or follicular thyroid carcinoma. Stimulation of radioiodide uptake may be achieved by giving thyrotropin. (Radioiodide will not be taken up by giant cell and spindle cell carcinoma of the thyroid or by amyloid solid carcinomas.)

➤*Hyperthyroidism:* Treatment of hyperthyroidism (see monograph in Endocrine/Metabolic chapter).

Administration and Dosage

Measure dose by a suitable radioactivity calibration system immediately prior to use.

➤*Carcinoma of the thyroid:* Individualize dosage.

Usual dose for ablation of normal thyroid tissue – 50 mCi, with subsequent therapeutic doses usually 100 to 150 mCi.

➤*Preparation of oral solution:* To prepare a stock solution use Purified Water with 0.2% sodium thiosulfate as a reducing agent. Acidic diluents may cause pH to drop below 7.5 and stimulate volatilization of iodine 131-hydriodic acid. Equipment used to prepare the stock solution must be thoroughly rinsed and free of acidic cleaning agents.

➤*Storage/Stability:* Store at room temperature (< 30°C; < 86°F).

➤*Physical characteristics:* See product literature for specific calibration and dosimetry.

Actions

➤*Pharmacology:* After rapid GI absorption, iodine 131 is primarily distributed within extracellular fluid. It is trapped and rapidly converted to protein-bound iodine by the thyroid; it is concentrated, but not protein bound, by the stomach and salivary glands. It is promptly excreted by kidneys.

About 90% of the local irradiation is caused by beta radiation and 10% is caused by gamma radiation. Iodine 131 has a physical half-life of 8.04 days.

Contraindications

Preexisting vomiting and diarrhea; women who are or may become pregnant (see Warnings).

Warnings

➤*Pregnancy: Category X.* Do not give to pregnant women (see Contraindications). Do not use in women who are or may become pregnant. Iodine 131 may cause fetal harm (eg, permanent damage to thyroid). If used during pregnancy or if patient becomes pregnant while taking this drug, inform her of the hazard to the fetus.

➤*Lactation:* Iodine 131 is excreted in breast milk; discontinue nursing during therapy. Do not resume nursing until all radiation is absent from breast milk (≈ 14 days).

➤*Children:* Safety and efficacy in children have not been established.

Precautions

➤*Radiation exposure:* Ensure minimum radiation exposure to patients and occupational workers consistent with proper patient management.

➤*Sulfite sensitivity:* Some of these products contain sulfites that may cause allergic-type reactions including anaphylactic symptoms and life-threatening or less severe asthmatic episodes in susceptible persons. The overall prevalence in the general population is unknown and probably low. It is seen more frequently in asthmatic or atopic nonasthmatic persons.

Drug Interactions

➤*Iodine, thyroid and antithyroid agents:* Uptake of iodine 131 will be affected by recent intake of stable iodine in any form, or by use of *thyroid, antithyroid* and certain other drugs. Question the patient regarding previous medication and procedures involving radiographic contrast media.

Adverse Reactions

➤*Endocrine:* Acute thyroid crises.

➤*Hematologic:* Depression of hematopoietic system with large doses; bone marrow depression; acute leukemia; anemia; blood dyscrasia; leukopenia; thrombocytopenia; death.

SODIUM IODIDE I 131

➤*Miscellaneous:* Radiation sickness (nausea, vomiting); severe sialoadenitis; increased clinical symptoms; chest pain, tachycardia, rash, hives, chromosomal abnormalities; tenderness and swelling of neck, pain on swallowing, sore throat and cough may occur around third day after treatment (usually amenable to analgesics); temporary hair thinning (may occur 2 to 3 months after treatment). Allergic reactions (infrequently).

Overdosage

➤*Symptoms:* Overdosage may result in hypothyroidism.

➤*Treatment:* Give appropriate replacement therapy.

SODIUM PHOSPHATE P 32

Rx	Sodium Phosphate P 32 (Mallinckrodt)	Injection: 0.67 mCi/ml	5mCi per vial.

Indications

➤*Leukemia:* Treatment of polycythemia vera, chronic myelocytic leukemia and chronic lymphocytic leukemia.

➤*Skeletal metastases:* Palliative treatment of selected patients with multiple areas of skeletal metastases.

Administration and Dosage

Administer IV. Do not administer as an intracavity injection. Oral administration of high-specific-activity sodium phosphate P 32 in the fasting state may equal IV administration.

Measure dose by a suitable radioactivity calibration system immediately before use.

➤*Polycythemia vera:* 1 to 8 mCi IV are given, depending upon the stage of disease and size of the patient. Individualize repeat doses.

➤*Chronic leukemia:* 6 to 15 mCi usually with concomitant hormone manipulation.

➤*Storage / Stability:* Store at room temperature, 15° to 30°C (59° to 86°F).

Actions

➤*Pharmacology:* Phosphorus is necessary to the metabolic and proliferative activity of cells. Radioactive phosphorus concentrates to a very high degree in rapidly proliferating tissue.

Sodium phosphate P 32 decays by beta emission with a physical half-life of 14.3 days. The mean energy of the sodium phosphate P 32 beta particle is 695 keV.

Contraindications

➤*Sequential therapy:* Do not use as part of sequential treatment with a chemotherapeutic agent.

➤*Polycythemia vera:* Do not administer when the leukocyte count is < 5000/mm^3 or platelet count is < 150,000/mm^3.

➤*Chronic myelocytic leukemia:* Do not administer when the leukocyte count is < 20,000/mm^3.

➤*Bone metastases:* Usually not administered when the leukocyte count is < 5000/mm^3 and the platelet count is < 100,000/mm^3.

Warnings

➤*Pregnancy: Category C.* Safey for use during pregnancy has not been established. It is not known if the drug causes fetal harm or affects reproductive ability. Use only when clearly needed and when the potential benefits outweigh the potential hazards to the fetus.

Perform examinations using radiopharmaceuticals (especially elective examinations) to women of childbearing capacity during the first 10 days following the onset of menses.

➤*Lactation:* It is not known whether sodium phosphate is excreted in breast milk. Discontinue nursing during therapy.

➤*Children:* Safety and efficacy in children have not been established.

Precautions

➤*Monitoring:* Monitor blood and bone marrow at regular intervals.

➤*Minimum exposure:* Ensure minimum radiation exposure to patients and occupational workers consistent with proper patient management.

➤*Retinoblastomas:* Sodium phosphate P 32 does not usually localize in retinoblastomas.

Overdosage

May produce serious effects on the hematopoietic system.

STRONTIUM-89 CHLORIDE

Rx	Metastron (Medi-Physics/Amersham)	Injection: 148 MBq, 4 mCi (10.9 to 22.6 mg/ml)	Preservative free. In 10 ml vials with Water for Injection.

Indications

➤*Painful skeletal metastases:* Relief of bone pain in patients with painful skeletal metastases.

Administration and Dosage

➤*Approved by the FDA:* June 19, 1993.

The recommended dose is 148 MBq, 4 mCi given by slow IV injection (1 to 2 minutes). Alternatively, a dose of 1.5 to 2.2 MBq/kg, 40 to 60 mcCi/kg may be used.

Base repeated administrations on an individual patient's response to therapy, current symptoms and hematologic status; repeat doses are generally not recommended at intervals of < 90 days.

Measure dose by suitable radioactivity calibration system immediately prior to use.

➤*Storage / Stability:* The vial is shipped in a transportation shield with an ≈ 3 mm lead wall thickness. Store the vial and its contents inside its transportation container at room temperature (15° to 25°C; 59° to 77°F).

Actions

➤*Pharmacology:* Strontium-89 is an injectable radioisotope for metastatic bone pain. Following IV injection, soluble strontium compounds behave like their calcium analogs, clearing rapidly from blood and selectively localizing in bone mineral. Uptake of strontium by bone occurs preferentially in sites of active osteogenesis; primary bone tumors and areas of metastatic involvement (blastic lesions) can accumulate significantly greater concentrations of strontium than surrounding normal bone.

Strontium-89 is retained in metastatic bone lesions much longer than in normal bone, where turnover is about 14 days. In patients with extensive skeletal metastases, well over half of the injected dose is retained in the bones.

The drug, a pure beta emitter, selectively irradiates sites of primary metastatic bone involvement with minimal effect on soft tissues distant from bone lesions.

➤*Pharmacokinetics:* Strontium-89 decays by beta emission with a physical half-life of 50.5 days. Excretion pathways are two-thirds urinary and one-third fecal in patients with bone metastases. Urinary excretion, which is higher in people without bone lesions, is greatest in the first 2 days following injection.

➤*Clinical trials:* Clinical trials have examined relief of pain in cancer patients who have received external radiation therapy for bone metastases but in whom persistent pain recurred.

Comparison of Effects of Strontium-89 vs Placebo (%)							
	Months post-treatment						
Parameter	1	2	3	4	5	6	9
Reduced pain, no increase in analgesic/ radiotherapy retreatment							
Strontium-89	71.4	78.9	60.6	59.3	36.4	63.6	—
Placebo	61.4	57.1	55.9	25	31.8	35	—
Pain free without analgesic							
Strontium-89	14.3	13.2	15.2	11.1	18.2	18.2	18.2
Placebo	6.8	8.6	5.9	0	4.5	5	0

Warnings

➤*Bone marrow toxicity:* Use of strontium-89 in patients with evidence of seriously compromised bone marrow from previous therapy or disease infiltration is not recommended unless the potential benefit of the treatment outweighs its risks. Bone marrow toxicity is to be expected following administration, particularly white blood cells (WBCs) and platelets. The extent of toxicity is variable. It is recommended that the patient's peripheral blood cell counts be monitored at least once every other week. Typically, platelets will be depressed by about 30% compared to pre-administration levels. The nadir of platelet depression in most patients is found between 12 and 16 weeks following administration of strontium-89. WBCs are usually depressed to a varying extent compared to pre-administration levels. Therefore, recovery occurs slowly, typically reaching pre-administration levels 6 months after treatment unless the patient's disease or additional therapy intervenes.

In considering repeat administration, carefully evaluate hematologic response to initial dose, current platelet level and other evidence of marrow depletion.

STRONTIUM-89 CHLORIDE

➤*Patient identification:* Verification of dose and patient identification is necessary prior to use because strontium-89 delivers a relatively high dose of radioactivity.

➤*Renal function impairment:* Strontium-89 is excreted primarily by the kidneys. In patients with renal dysfunction, weigh the possible risks of administering strontium-89 against the possible benefits.

➤*Carcinogenesis:* Strontium-89 is a potential carcinogen. Of 40 rats injected with strontium-89 in 10 consecutive monthly doses of either 250 or 350 mcCi/kg, 33 developed malignant bone tumors after a latency period of ≈ 9 months. No neoplasia was observed in control animals. Restrict treatment to patients with well documented metastatic bone disease.

➤*Pregnancy: Category D.* Strontium-89 may cause fetal harm when administered to a pregnant woman. There are no adequate and well controlled studies in pregnant women. If this drug is used during pregnancy, or if the patient becomes pregnant while receiving this drug, apprise the patient of the potential hazard to the fetus. Advise women of childbearing potential to avoid becoming pregnant.

➤*Lactation:* Because strontium acts as a calcium analog, secretion into breast milk is likely; however, it is not known whether this drug is excreted in breast milk. It is recommended that nursing be discontinued by mothers about to receive IV strontium-89.

➤*Children:* Safety and efficacy in children < 18 years of age have not been established.

Precautions

➤*Bone metastases:* Strontium-89 is not indicated for use in patients with cancer not involving bone. Confirm presence of bone metastases prior to therapy. Use with caution in patients with platelet counts < 60,000 and white cell counts < 2400.

➤*Radiopharmaceuticals:* Radiopharmaceuticals should only be used by physicians who are qualified by training and experience in the safe use and handling of radionuclides and whose experience and training have been approved by the appropriate government agency authorized to license the use of radionuclides. Like other radioactive drugs, handle with care and take safety measures to minimize radiation to clinical personnel.

➤*Onset:* In view of the delayed onset of pain relief, typically 7 to 20 days post-injection, administration to patients with very short life expectancy is not recommended.

➤*Flushing sensation:* A calcium-like flushing sensation has been observed in patients following a rapid (< 30 second injection) administration.

➤*Incontinence:* Take special precautions, such as urinary catheterization, following administration to patients who are incontinent to minimize the risk of radioactive contamination of clothing, bed linen and the patient's environment.

Adverse Reactions

One case of fatal septicemia following leukopenia was reported during clinical trials. Most severe reactions of marrow toxicity can be managed by conventional means.

A small number of patients have reported a transient increase in bone pain at 36 to 72 hours after injection. This is usually mild and self-limiting, and controllable with analgesics. One patient reported chills and fever 12 hours after injection without long-term sequelae.

Patient Information

The patient may feel a slight increase in pain for 2 or 3 days beginning 2 or 3 days after injection. The physician may suggest a temporary increase in the dose of pain medication until the pain is under control. After about 1 to 2 weeks, the pain should begin to diminish.

The patient can eat and drink normally and there is no need to avoid alcohol or caffeine unless already advised to do so. The physician may want to carry out periodic, routine blood tests.

Advise patients to tell any health practitioner who is giving them medical treatment that they have received strontium-89.

During the first week after injection, strontium-89 will be present in the blood and urine. It is therefore important to consider the following common sense precautions for 1 week: 1) Where a normal toilet is available, use in preference to a urinal. Flush the toilet twice; 2) Wipe up any spilled urine with a tissue and flush it away; 3) Always wash hands after using the toilet; 4) Immediately wash any linen or clothes that become stained with urine or blood. Wash them separately from other clothes, and rinse thoroughly; 5) If any urine collection device is used, follow instructions on its use; 6) Wash away any spilled blood if a cut occurs.

In many people who receive strontium-89, the effect lasts for several months. If pain returns, consult the physician.

SAMARIUM SM 153 LEXIDRONAM

Rx	Quadramet (Du Pont Pharma)	Injection: 1850 MBq/ml (50 mCi/ml) at calibration	Frozen, single-dose 10 ml vials. In 2 ml fill (3700 MBq) and 3 ml fill (5550 MBq).

Indications

➤*Bone lesions:* Relief of pain in patients with confirmed osteoblastic metastatic bone lesions that enhance on radionuclide bone scan.

➤*Unlabeled uses:* Ankylosing spondylitis; Paget's disease; rheumatoid arthritis.

Administration and Dosage

➤*Approved by the FDA:* March 28, 1997.

The recommended dose of samarium is 1 mCi/kg, administered IV over a period of 1 minute through a secure indwelling catheter and followed with a saline flush. Dose adjustment in patients at the extremes of weight have not been studied. Exercise caution when determining the dose in very thin or very obese patients.

Measure the dose by a suitable radioactivity calibration system, such as a radioisotope dose calibrator, immediately before administration.

Have the patient ingest (or receive by IV administration) a minimum of 500 ml (2 cups) of fluids prior to injection and void as often as possible after injection to minimize radiation exposure to the bladder.

Samarium contains calcium and may be incompatible with solutions that contain molecules that can complex with and form calcium precipitates.

Do not dilute or mix samarium with other solutions.

➤*Radiation dosimetry:* The dosimetry estimates are based on clinical biodistribution studies using methods developed for radiation dose calculations by the Medical Internal Radiation Dose (MIRD) Committee of the Society of Nuclear Medicine.

Radiation exposure is based on a urinary voiding interval of 4.8 hours. Radiation dose estimates for bone and marrow assume that radioactivity is deposited on bone surfaces, as noted in autoradiograms of biopsy bone samples in 7 patients who received samarium. Although electron emissions from Samarium–153 are abundant, with energies up to 810 keV, rapid blood clearance of samarium and low energy and abundant photon emissions generally result in low radiation doses to those parts of the body where the complex does not localize.

When blastic osseous lesions are present, significantly enhanced localization of the radiopharmaceutical will occur, with correspondingly higher doses to the lesions compared with normal bones and other organs.

Estimated Absorbed Radiation Doses of Samarium to an Average 70 kg Adult Patient		
Target organ	Rad/mCi	mGy/MBq
Bone surfaces	25	6.76
Red marrow	5.7	1.54
Urinary bladder wall	3.6	0.097
Kidneys	0.065	0.018
Whole body	0.04	0.011
Lower large intestine	0.037	0.01
Ovaries	0.032	0.0086
Muscle	0.028	0.0076
Small intestine	0.023	0.0062
Upper large intestine	0.02	0.0054
Testes	0.02	0.0054
Liver	0.019	0.0051
Spleen	0.018	0.0049
Stomach	0.015	0.0041

➤*Storage/Stability:* Thaw at room temperature before administration and use within 8 hours. Store frozen at −20° to −10°C (−4° to 14°F) in a lead shielded container.

Actions

➤*Pharmacology:* Samarium–153 lexidronam is a therapeutic agent consisting of radioactive samarium and a tetraphosphonate chelator, ethylenediaminetetramethylenephosphonic acid (EDTMP). It has an affinity for bone and concentrates in areas of bone turnover in association with hydroxyapatite. In clinical studies employing planar imaging techniques, more samarium accumulates in osteoblastic lesions than in normal bone with a lesion-to-bone ratio of ≈ 5. The mechanism of action of samarium in relieving the pain of bone metastases is not known.

Principle Radiation Emission Data of Samarium-153		
Particle	Radiation Energy (keV)[1]	Abundance
Beta	640	30%
Beta	710	50%
Beta	810	20%
Gamma	103	29%

[1] Maximum energies are listed for the beta emissions, the average beta particle is 233 keV.

SAMARIUM SM 153 LEXIDRONAM

➤*Pharmacokinetics:*

Absorption – The greater the number of metastatic lesions, the more skeletal uptake of samarium radioactivity. The relationship between skeletal uptake and the size of the metastatic lesions has not been studied. The total skeletal uptake of radioactivity is ≈ 65.5% of the injected dose. The percent of the injected dose (% ID) taken up by bone ranged from 56.3% in a patient with 5 metastatic lesions to 76.7% in a patient with 52 metastatic lesions. If the number of metastatic lesions is fixed, over the range of 0.1 to 3 mCi/kg, the % ID taken up by bone is the same regardless of the dose.

Distribution – At physiologic pH, > 90% of the complex is present as Samarium–153 $[EDTMP]^{-5}$ and < 10% as ^{153}SmH $[EDTMP]^{-4}$. The beta particle of Samarium-153 EDTMP travels an average of 3.1 mm in soft tissue and 1.7 mm in bone.

Metabolism – The complex formed by samarium and EDTMP is excreted as an intact, single species that consists of one atom of samarium and one molecule of EDTMP. Metabolic products of samarium-153 EDTMP were not detected.

Excretion –

Blood: Clearance of radioactivity from the blood demonstrated biexponential kinetics after IV injection. During the first 30 minutes, the radioactivity in the blood decreased to 15% of the injected dose with a half-life of 5.5 minutes. After 30 minutes, the radioactivity cleared from the blood more slowly with a half-life of 65.4 minutes. Less than 1% of the injected dose remained in the blood 5 hours after injection.

Urine: Samarium-153 EDTMP radioactivity was excreted in the urine after IV injection. During the first 6 hours, 34.5% was excreted. Overall, the greater the number of metastatic lesions, the less radioactivity was excreted.

Hepatic function impairment – Accumulation of activity was not detected in the liver or the intestine; this suggests that hepatobiliary excretion did not occur.

➤*Clinical trials:* Samarium was evaluated in 580 patients. Eligible patients had painful metastatic bone lesions that had failed other treatments, had ≥ 6–month expected survival and had a positive radionuclide bone scan.

The mean area under the pain curve (AUPC) decreased significantly from baseline with samarium than with placebo.

Contraindications

Hypersensitivity to EDTMP or similar phosphonate compounds.

Warnings

➤*Bone marrow suppression:* Samarium causes bone marrow suppression. Use with caution in patients with compromised bone marrow reserves. In clinical trials, white blood cell counts and platelet counts decreased to a nadir of ≈ 40% to 50% of baseline in 123 (95%) of patients within 3 to 5 weeks after samarium and tended to return to pretreatment levels by 8 weeks.

Before administering samarium, give consideration to the patient's current clinical and hematologic status and bone marrow response history to treatment with myelotoxic agents. Metastatic prostate and other cancers can be associated with disseminated intravascular coagulation (DIC); exercise caution in treating cancer patients whose platelet counts are falling or who have other clinical or laboratory findings suggesting DIC. Because of the unknown potential for additive effects on bone marrow, do not give concurrently with chemotherapy or external beam radiation therapy unless clinical benefits outweigh the risks. Use of samarium in patients with evidence of compromised bone marrow reserve from previous therapy or disease involvement is not recommended unless the potential benefits of treatment outweigh the risks. Monitor blood counts weekly for at least 8 weeks or until recovery of adequate bone marrow function.

➤*Radioactivity:* Verify the dose of radioactivity to be administered to the patient before administering samarium. Do not release patients until their radioactivity levels and exposure rates comply with federal and local regulations.

➤*Elderly:* The pharmacokinetics of samarium-153 EDTMP did not change with age.

➤*Pregnancy: Category C.* As with other radiopharmaceutical drugs, samarium can cause fetal harm when administered to a pregnant woman. Adequate and well controlled studies have not been conducted in pregnant women. Women of childbearing age should have a negative pregnancy test before administration of samarium. If this drug is used during pregnancy or if a patient becomes pregnant after taking this drug, apprise her of the potential hazard to the fetus. Advise women of childbearing potential to avoid becoming pregnant soon after receiving samarium. Advise male and female patients to use an effective method of contraception after the administration of samarium.

➤*Lactation:* It is not known whether samarium is excreted in breast milk. Because of the potential for serious adverse reactions from samarium in breastfeeding infants, make a decision to discontinue breastfeeding or discontinue the drug, taking into account the importance of the drug to the mother. If samarium is administered, it is recommended to discontinue breastfeeding.

➤*Children:* Safety and efficacy in pediatric patients < 16 years old have not been established.

Precautions

➤*Monitoring:* Because of the potential for bone marrow suppression, beginning 2 weeks after samarium administration, monitor blood counts weekly for at least 8 weeks or until recovery of adequate bone marrow function.

➤*ECG changes:* EDTMP is a chelating agent. Although the chelating effects have not been evaluated thoroughly in humans, dogs that received non-radioactive samarium EDTMP (6 times the human dose based on body weight, 3 times based on surface area) developed a variety of ECG changes (with or without the presence of hypocalcemia). Use caution and appropriate monitoring when administering samarium to patients.

➤*Skeletal effects:* Spinal cord compression frequently occurs in patients with known metastases to the cervical, thoracic or lumbar spine. In clinical studies of samarium, spinal cord compression was reported in 7% of patients who received placebo and in 8.3% of patients who received 1 mCi/kg samarium. Samarium is not indicated for treatment of spinal cord compression. Samarium administration for pain relief of metastatic bone cancer does not prevent the development of spinal cord compression. When there is a clinical suspicion of spinal cord compression, appropriate diagnostic and therapeutic measures must be taken immediately to avoid permanent disability.

➤*Incontinence:* Take special precautions with bladder catheterization in incontinent patients to minimize the risk of radioactive contamination of clothing, bed linen and the patient's environment. Urinary excretion of radioactivity occurs within ≈ 12 hours (with 35% occurring during the first 6 hours).

➤*Hypocalcemia:* Exercise caution when administering samarium to patients at risk for developing hypocalcemia.

➤*Flare reactions:* Some patients have reported a transient increase in bone pain shortly after injection (flare reaction). This is usually mild and self-limiting and occurs within 72 hours of injection. Such reactions are usually responsive to analgesics.

Drug Interactions

➤*Chemotherapy:* The potential for additive bone marrow toxicity of samarium with chemotherapy or external beam radiation has not been studied. Do not give samarium concurrently with chemotherapy or external beam radiation therapy unless the benefit outweighs the risks. Do not give samarium after either of these treatments until there has been time for adequate marrow recovery (see Warnings).

Adverse Reactions

In a subgroup of 399 patients who received samarium 1 mCi/kg, there were 23 deaths and 46 serious adverse events. The deaths occurred an average of 67 days (range, 9 to 130) after samarium. Serious events occurred an average of 46 days (range, 1 to 118) after samarium. Although most of the patient deaths and serious adverse events appear to be related to the underlying disease, the relationship of end stage disease, marrow invasion by cancer cells, previous myelotoxic treatment and samarium toxicity cannot be easily distinguished. In clinical studies, two patients with rapidly progressive prostate cancer developed thrombocytopenia and died 4 weeks after receiving samarium. One of the patients showed evidence of disseminated intravascular coagulation (DIC); the other patient experienced a fatal cerebrovascular accident, with a suspicion of DIC. The relationship of the DIC to the bone marrow suppressive effect of samarium is not known.

Samarium Adverse Reactions		
Adverse reaction	Samarium 1 mCi/kg (n = 199; %)	Placebo (n = 90; %)
Bleeding Manifestations[1]		
Ecchymosis	3	1.1
Epistaxis	2	1.1
Hematuria	5	3.3
Cardiovascular		
Arrhythmias	5	2.2
Chest pain	4	4.4
Hypertension	3	0
Hypotension	2	2.2
CNS		
Dizziness	4	1.1
Paresthesia	2	7.8
Spinal cord compression	6.5	5.5
Cerebrovascular accident/stroke	1	0
Dermatologic		
Purpura	1	0
Rash	1	2.2

SAMARIUM SM 153 LEXIDRONAM

Samarium Adverse Reactions		
Adverse reaction	Samarium 1 mCi/kg (n = 199; %)	Placebo (n = 90; %)
GI		
Abdominal pain	6	7.8
Diarrhea	6	3.3
Nausea/Vomiting	32.7	41.1
Hematologic/Lymphatic		
Coagulation disorder	1.5	0
Hemoglobin decreased	40.7	23.3
Leukopenia	59.3	6.7
Lymphadenopathy	2	0
Thrombocytopenia	69.3	8.9
Infection		
Fever/Chills	8.5	11.1
Infection, not specified	7	4.4
Oral moniliasis	2	1.1
Pneumonia	1.5	1.1
Miscellaneous		
Pain flare reaction[2]	7	5.6
Myasthenia	6.5	8.9
Pathologic fracture	2.5	2.2
Bronchitis/Cough increased	4	2.2

[1] Includes hemorrhage (GI, ocular) reported in < 1%.
[2] See Warnings.

Other adverse reactions include: Bone marrow toxicity (47%); sinus bradycardia, vasodilation (≥ 1%); alopecia, angina, congestive heart failure.

Overdosage

Overdosage with samarium has not been reported. An antidote for samarium overdosage is not known. The anticipated complications of overdosage would likely be secondary to bone marrow suppression from the radioactivity of Samrium-153 or secondary to hypocalcemia and cardiac arrhythmias related to EDTMP.

Patient Information

Advise patients who receive samarium that for several hours following administration, radioactivity will be present in excreted urine. To help protect themselves and others in their environment, precautions need to be taken for 12 hours following administration. Whenever possible, use a toilet rather than a urinal and flush the toilet several times after each use. Clean up spilled urine completely and wash hands thoroughly. If blood or urine gets onto clothing, wash the clothing separately or store for 1 to 2 weeks to allow for decay of the samarium.

Women of childbearing age should have a negative pregnancy test before administration of samarium. If this drug is used during pregnancy, or if a patient becomes pregnant after taking this drug, apprise her of the potential hazard to the fetus. Advise women of childbearing potential to avoid becoming pregnant soon after receiving samarium. Advise male and female patients to use an effective method of contraception after the administration of samarium.

CARBOPLATIN

Rx	Carboplatin (Mayne)	Injection: 10 mg/mL	In 5, 15, and 45 mL single-use vials.
Rx	Paraplatin (Bristol-Myers Squibb Oncology)		In 5 mL, 15 mL, and 45 mL single-dose vials.
Rx	Paraplatin (Bristol-Myers Squibb Oncology)	Powder for injection, lyophilized[1]: 50 mg	In single-dose vials.
		150 mg	In single-dose vials.
		450 mg	In single-dose vials.

[1] With mannitol.

WARNING

Carboplatin should be administered under the supervision of a qualified physician experienced in the use of cancer chemotherapeutic agents. Appropriate management of therapy and complications is possible only when adequate treatment facilities are readily available.

Bone marrow suppression is dose-related and may be severe, resulting in infection and/or bleeding. Anemia may be cumulative and may require transfusion support (see Warnings).

Vomiting is another frequent drug-related side effect (see Warnings).

Anaphylactic-like reactions to carboplatin have been reported and may occur within minutes of administration. Epinephrine, corticosteroids, and antihistamines have been employed to alleviate symptoms (see Warnings).

Indications

➤*Advanced ovarian carcinoma:*

Initial treatment – For the initial treatment of advanced ovarian carcinoma in established combination with other approved chemotherapeutic agents. One established combination regimen consists of carboplatin and cyclophosphamide.

Secondary treatment – For the palliative treatment of patients with ovarian carcinoma recurrent after prior chemotherapy, including patients who have been previously treated with cisplatin.

➤*Unlabeled uses:* Carboplatin, in combination with other chemotherapeutic agents, has been used for the treatment of various types of cancer such as small cell and non-small cell lung cancer, head and neck cancer, and testicular cancer. Carboplatin also has been used safely and effectively in the pediatric population.

Administration and Dosage

➤*Note:* Aluminum reacts with carboplatin (see Precautions).

➤*Carboplatin as a single agent:* Carboplatin, as a single agent, has been shown to be effective in patients with recurrent ovarian carcinoma at a dosage of 360 mg/m² IV on day 1 every 4 weeks (see *Formula dosing* for alternative dose). In general, however, do not repeat single intermittent courses of carboplatin until the neutrophil count is at least 2000/mm³ and the platelet count is at least 100,000/mm³.

➤*Combination therapy with cyclophosphamide:* In the chemotherapy of advanced ovarian cancer, an effective combination for previously untreated patients consists of: Carboplatin 300 mg/m² IV (see *Formula dosing* for alternative dose) plus cyclophosphamide 600 mg/m² IV, both on day 1 every 4 weeks for 6 cycles. Do not repeat intermittent courses of the combination until the neutrophil count is at least 2000/mm³ and the platelet count is at least 100,000/mm³.

➤*Dose adjustment:* Pretreatment platelet count and performance status are important prognostic factors for severity of myelosuppression in previously treated patients. The dose adjustments in the table below for single-agent or combination therapy are modified from controlled trials in previously treated and untreated patients with ovarian carcinoma. Blood counts were done weekly; recommendations are based on the lowest posttreatment platelet or neutrophil value.

Carboplatin Dose Adjustments		
Platelets/mm³	Neutrophils/mm³	Adjusted dose[1] from prior course
> 100,000	> 2000	125%
50,000 to 100,000	500 to 2000	No adjustment
< 50,000	< 500	75%

[1] Percentages apply to carboplatin as a single agent or to both carboplatin and cyclophosphamide in combination. In the controlled studies, dosages also were adjusted at a lower level (50% to 60%) for severe myelosuppression.

Doses greater than 125% are not recommended.

➤*Renal function impairment:* These dosing recommendations apply to the initial course of treatment. Adjust subsequent dosages according to the patient's tolerance based on degree of bone marrow suppression.

Carboplatin in Renal Insufficiency	
Baseline Ccr (mL/min)	Recommended dose on day 1
41 to 59	250 mg/m²
16 to 40	200 mg/m²
≤ 15	†

† Data too limited to permit a recommendation for treatment.

➤*Formula dosing:* Another approach for determining the initial dose of carboplatin is the use of mathematical formulas, which are based on a patient's preexisting renal function or renal function and desired platelet nadir. The use of dosing formulas, as compared with empirical dose calculation based on body surface area, allows compensation for patient variations in pretreatment renal function that might otherwise result in underdosing (in patients with above average renal function) or overdosing (in patients with impaired renal function).

A simple formula for calculating dosage, based upon a patient's glomerular filtration rate (GFR in mL/min) and carboplatin's target area under the concentration versus time curve (AUC in mg/mL•min), has been proposed by Calvert. In these studies, GFR was measured by ^{51}Cr-EDTA clearance.

Calvert formula: Total dose (mg) = (target AUC) × (GFR + 25); Note: with the Calvert formula, the total dose of carboplatin is calculated in mg, not mg/m².

The target AUC of 4 to 6 mg/mL•min using single-agent carboplatin appears to provide the most appropriate dose range in previously treated patients.

➤*Elderly:* Because renal function is often decreased in elderly patients, use formula dosing of carboplatin based on estimates of GFR in elderly patients to provide predictable plasma carboplatin AUCs and thereby minimize the risk of toxicity.

➤*Preparation of IV solutions:* Immediately before use, reconstitute the content of each vial of powder with either sterile water for injection, 5% dextrose in water, or 0.9% sodium chloride injection, according to the following schedule:

Preparation of Carboplatin Solutions		
Vial strength (mg)	Diluent volume (mL)	Concentration (mg/mL)
50	5	10
150	15	10
450	45	10

Carboplatin can be further diluted to concentrations as low as 0.5 mg/mL with 5% dextrose in water or 0.9% sodium chloride injection.

➤*Administration:* Carboplatin is usually administered by an infusion lasting at least 15 minutes. No pretreatment or posttreatment hydration or forced diuresis is required.

➤*Storage/Stability:* Store the unopened vials at controlled room temperature (15° to 30°C; 59° to 86°F). Protect from light. When prepared as directed, solutions are stable for 8 hours at room temperature (25°C; 77°F). Because no antibacterial preservative is contained in the formulations, discard solutions 8 hours after dilution.

Actions

➤*Pharmacology:* Carboplatin is a platinum coordination compound used as a cancer chemotherapeutic agent. Carboplatin, like cisplatin, produces predominantly interstrand DNA cross-links rather than DNA-protein cross-links. This effect is apparently cell-cycle nonspecific. The aquation of carboplatin, which is thought to produce the active species, occurs at a slower rate than cisplatin. Despite this difference, carboplatin and cisplatin induce equal numbers of drug-DNA cross-links, causing equivalent lesions and biological effects. Differences in potencies for carboplatin and cisplatin appear to be directly related to the difference in aquation rates.

➤*Pharmacokinetics:*

Absorption/Distribution – Carboplatin exhibits linear pharmacokinetics over the dosing range 300 to 500 mg/m². When creatinine clearance (Ccr) is approximately 60 mL/min or greater, the initial plasma half-life (alpha) is 1.1 to 2 hours, and the postdistribution plasma half-life (beta) is 2.6 to 5.9 hours. The apparent volume of distribution and mean residence time is 16 L and 3.5 hours, respectively. Carboplatin is not bound to plasma proteins. However, platinum from carboplatin becomes irreversibly bound to plasma proteins and is slowly eliminated with a minimum half-life of 5 days.

Metabolism/Excretion – Plasma levels of intact carboplatin decay in a biphasic manner after a 30-minute IV infusion of 300 to 500 mg/m². The total body clearance is 4.4 L/h. The major route of elimination is renal excretion. When Ccr is approximately 60 mL/min or greater, 65% of the dose is excreted in the urine within 12 hours and 71% within 24 hours. All of the platinum in the 24-hour urine is present as carboplatin. Only 3% to 5% of the administered platinum is excreted in the urine between 24 and 96 hours.

Special populations –

Renal function impairment: In patients with Ccr below 60 mL/min, the total body and renal clearances of carboplatin decrease as the Ccr

CARBOPLATIN

decreases. Therefore, reduce carboplatin dosages in these patients (see Administration and Dosage).

➤*Clinical trials:*

Initial treatment of ovarian cancer – Two randomized, controlled studies with carboplatin vs cisplatin, both in combination with cyclophosphamide every 28 days for 6 courses before surgical re-evaluation, demonstrated equivalent overall survival between the 2 groups.

Secondary treatment of ovarian cancer – In 2 prospective, randomized, controlled studies in patients with advanced ovarian cancer previously treated with chemotherapy, carboplatin achieved 6 clinical complete responses in 47 patients. Response duration ranged from 45 to 71 weeks or longer.

Among patients previously treated with cisplatin, those developing progressive disease while receiving cisplatin therapy may have a decreased response rate.

Contraindications

History of severe allergic reactions to cisplatin or other platinum compounds or mannitol; severe bone marrow depression (see Warnings); significant bleeding.

Warnings

➤*Bone marrow suppression:* Bone marrow suppression (leukopenia, neutropenia, and thrombocytopenia) is dose-dependent and also is the dose-limiting toxicity. Frequently monitor peripheral blood counts during carboplatin treatment and, when appropriate, until recovery is achieved. Median nadir occurs at day 21 in patients receiving single-agent carboplatin. By day 28, 90% of patients have platelet counts greater than 100,000/mm³; 74% have neutrophil counts greater than 2000/mm³; 67% have leukocyte counts greater than 4000/mm³. In general, do not repeat single intermittent courses until leukocyte, neutrophil, and platelet counts recover.

Because anemia is cumulative, transfusions may be needed during treatment with carboplatin, particularly in patients receiving prolonged therapy.

Bone marrow suppression is increased in patients who have received prior therapy, especially regimens including cisplatin. Bone marrow suppression also is increased in patients with impaired kidney function. Patients with poor performance status also have experienced a higher incidence of severe leukopenia and thrombocytopenia. Bone marrow depression may be more severe when carboplatin is combined with other bone marrow suppressing drugs or with radiotherapy. Appropriately reduce initial carboplatin dosages in these patients (see Administration and Dosage) and carefully monitor blood counts between courses. If used in combination with other bone marrow suppressing therapies, carefully manage with respect to dosage and timing to minimize additive effects.

➤*Renal toxicity:* Carboplatin has limited nephrotoxic potential, but concomitant treatment with aminoglycosides has resulted in increased renal toxicity. Exercise caution when a patient receives both drugs. Development of abnormal renal function test results is uncommon, despite the fact that carboplatin, unlike cisplatin, usually has been administered without high-volume fluid hydration or forced diuresis. Most of the reported abnormalities have been mild and approximately one half of them were reversible.

Ccr has proven to be the most sensitive measure of kidney function in patients receiving carboplatin, and it appears to be the most useful test for correlating drug clearance and bone marrow suppression. Of the patients who had a baseline value of at least 60 mL/min, 27% demonstrated a reduction below this value during therapy.

➤*Hepatic toxicity:* The incidences of abnormal liver function tests in patients with normal baseline values were reported. These abnormalities generally have been mild and reversible in approximately one half of the cases; however, the role of metastatic tumor in the liver may complicate the assessment in many patients. In a limited series of patients receiving very high doses of carboplatin and autologous bone marrow transplantation, severe abnormalities of liver function tests were reported. High dosages of carboplatin (more than 4 times the recommended dose) have resulted in severe abnormalities of liver function tests.

➤*Emesis:* Carboplatin can induce emesis that can be more severe in patients previously receiving emetogenic therapy. Carboplatin is significantly less emetogenic than cisplatin. Nausea and vomiting usually cease within 24 hours of treatment, and the incidence and intensity of emesis have been reduced by using antiemetic premedication. Although no conclusive efficacy data exist with the following schedules of carboplatin, lengthening the duration of single IV administration to 24 hours or dividing the total dose over 5 consecutive daily pulse doses has reduced emesis.

➤*Peripheral neurotoxicity:* Although peripheral neurotoxicity is infrequent, its incidence is increased in patients older than 65 years of age and in patients previously treated with cisplatin. Carboplatin therapy produces significantly fewer and less severe neurologic side effects than cisplatin therapy. Preexisting cisplatin-induced neurotoxicity does not worsen in approximately 70% of patients receiving carboplatin as secondary treatment. Although overall incidence of peripheral neurologic side effects induced by carboplatin is low, prolonged treatment, particularly in cisplatin-pretreated patients, may result in cumulative neurotoxicity.

➤*Ocular effects:* Loss of vision, which can be complete for light and colors, has been reported after the use of carboplatin with doses higher than those recommended in the package insert. Vision appears to recover totally or to a significant extent within weeks of stopping these high doses.

➤*Ototoxicity:* Clinically significant hearing loss has been reported to occur in pediatric patients when carboplatin was administered at higher than recommended doses in combination with other ototoxic agents. Concomitant treatment with aminoglycosides has resulted in increased audiologic toxicity.

➤*Hypersensitivity reactions:* Hypersensitivity to carboplatin has occurred and may occur within minutes of administration; manage with appropriate supportive therapy. There is an increased risk of allergic reactions, including anaphylaxis, in patients previously exposed to platinum therapy.

➤*Renal function impairment:* Patients with Ccr less than 60 mL/min are at increased risk of severe bone marrow suppression. In renally impaired patients who received single-agent carboplatin therapy, the incidence of severe leukopenia, neutropenia, or thrombocytopenia was approximately 25% with dosage modifications. (See Administration and Dosage). In patients with Ccr less than 60 mL/min, total body and renal clearances of carboplatin decrease as Ccr decreases. Reduce carboplatin dosages in these patients (see Administration and Dosage).

➤*Carcinogenesis:* The carcinogenic potential has not been studied, but compounds with similar mechanisms of action and mutagenicity profiles have been reported to be carcinogenic.

➤*Mutagenesis:* Carboplatin has been shown to be mutagenic both in vitro and in vivo.

➤*Elderly:* Elderly patients treated with carboplatin are more likely to develop severe thrombocytopenia than younger patients. Greater sensitivity of some older patients cannot be ruled out. Because renal function is often decreased in the elderly, consider renal function in the selection of carboplatin dosage.

➤*Pregnancy: Category D.* Carboplatin may cause fetal harm when administered to a pregnant woman. Carboplatin has been shown to be embryotoxic and teratogenic in rats. There are no adequate and well-controlled studies in pregnant women. If used during pregnancy, or if the patient becomes pregnant while receiving this drug, apprise her of the potential hazard to the fetus. Advise women of childbearing potential to avoid pregnancy.

➤*Lactation:* It is not known whether carboplatin is excreted in human milk. Because there is a possibility of toxicity in nursing infants secondary to carboplatin treatment of the mother, discontinue breastfeeding if the mother is treated with carboplatin.

➤*Children:* Safety and efficacy in pediatric patients have not been established.

Precautions

➤*Aluminum:* Aluminum can react with carboplatin, causing precipitate formation and potency loss. Do not use needles or IV administration sets containing aluminum parts that may come in contact with carboplatin for the preparation or administration of the drug.

Drug Interactions

➤*Nephrotoxic agents:* The renal effects of nephrotoxic compounds may be potentiated by carboplatin.

➤*Ototoxic agents:* Coadministration of ototoxic agents with higher than recommended carboplatin doses has resulted in clinically significant hearing loss in children (see Warnings).

Carboplatin Drug Interactions			
Precipitant drug	Object drug*		Description
Aminoglycosides	Carboplatin	↑	Coadministration has resulted in increased renal and/or audiologic toxicity. Use with caution.
Carboplatin	Aminoglycosides		
Carboplatin	Phenytoin	↓	Serum concentrations of phenytoin may be decreased, resulting in a loss of therapeutic effect. Monitor phenytoin levels and adjust dose appropriately.
Carboplatin	Warfarin	↑	The anticoagulant effect of warfarin may be increased. Monitor coagulation parameters and adjust warfarin as needed.

* ↑ = Object drug increased. ↓ = Object drug decreased.

CARBOPLATIN

Adverse Reactions

Carboplatin Adverse Reactions in Patients with Ovarian Cancer (%)		
Adverse reaction	First-line combination therapy[1] (n = 393)	Second-line single agent therapy (n = 553)
CNS		
Central neurotoxicity	26	5
Peripheral neuropathies	15	6
Ototoxicity	12	1
Other sensory side effects	5	1
GI		
Nausea and vomiting	93	92
Vomiting	83	81
Other GI side effects	46	21
Hematologic		
Thrombocytopenia		
< 100,000/mm³	66	62
< 50,000/mm³	33	35
Neutropenia		
< 2000 cells/mm³	96	67
< 1000 cells/mm³	82	21
Leukopenia		
< 4000 cells/mm³	97	85
< 2000 cells/mm³	71	26
Anemia		
< 11 g/dL	90	90
< 8 g/dL	14	21
Transfusions	35	44
Infections	16	5
Bleeding	8	5
Metabolic		
Magnesium loss	61	43
Calcium loss	16	31
Potassium loss	16	28
Sodium loss	10	47
Renal/Hepatic		
Alkaline phosphatase elevations	29	37
AST elevations	20	19
Blood urea elevations	17	22
Serum creatinine elevations	6	10
Bilirubin elevations	5	5
Miscellaneous		
Alopecia	49	2
Pain	44	23
Asthenia	41	11
Cardiovascular	19	6
Allergic	11	2
Respiratory	10	6
GU	10	2
Mucositis	8	1

[1] Combination therapy with cyclophosphamide in NCIC and SWOG studies. Combination therapy as well as treatment duration may be responsible for the differences noted with single-agent therapy.

The following incidences of adverse events are based on data from 1893 patients with various types of tumors who received carboplatin as single-agent therapy.

Hypersensitivity – Hypersensitivity (2%), including rash, urticaria, erythema, pruritus, and rarely bronchospasm and hypotension (see Warnings).

➤*Metabolic:* Abnormally decreased serum electrolyte values: Sodium (29%); magnesium (29%); calcium (22%); potassium (20%). Electrolyte supplementation was not routinely administered concomitantly with carboplatin, and these electrolyte abnormalities were rarely associated with symptoms.

➤*GI:* Vomiting (65%), severe in about ⅓ of these patients (see Warnings); nausea alone (additional 10% to 15%); pain (17%); diarrhea, constipation (6%).

➤*Hematologic:* Bone marrow suppression is the dose-limiting toxicity of carboplatin: Thrombocytopenia, platelet count less than 50,000/mm³ (25%); neutropenia, granulocyte count less than 1000/mm³ (16%); leukopenia, WBC count less than 2000/mm³ (15%) (see Warnings); infectious or hemorrhagic complications (5%); drug-related death (less than 1%); anemia (hemoglobin less than 11 g/dL) (71%) (see Warnings); transfusions (26%).

➤*Hepatic:* Alkaline phosphatase (24%); AST (15%); total bilirubin (5%). See Warnings.

➤*Miscellaneous:* Pain; asthenia; alopecia (3%); cardiovascular, respiratory, GU, and mucosal side effects (6% or less); cardiovascular events (cardiac failure, embolism, cerebrovascular accidents) (fatal in less than 1%); fever in neutropenic patients; cancer-associated hemolytic uremic syndrome (rare).

CNS – Peripheral neuropathies (4%) with mild paresthesias occurring most frequently (see Warnings); ototoxicity and other sensory abnormalities such as visual disturbances and change in taste (1%); CNS symptoms (5%) appear to be most often related to the use of antiemetics.

➤*Renal:*

Nephrotoxicity – (see Warnings): Abnormal renal function tests (blood urea nitrogen [14%]; serum creatinine [6%]).

Comparative toxicity, carboplatin vs cisplatin – In the studies when cisplatin and carboplatin were used in combination with cyclophosphamide, the pattern of toxicity exerted by the carboplatin-containing regimen was significantly different from that of the cisplatin-containing combinations. The carboplatin-containing regimens induced significantly more thrombocytopenia and, in one study, significantly more leukopenia and more need for transfusional support. In one study, the cisplatin-containing regimen produced significantly more anemia. Nonhematologic toxicities (eg, emesis, neurotoxicity, ototoxicity, renal toxicity, hypomagnesemia, alopecia) were significantly more frequent with cisplatin in both studies.

Postmarketing – Anaphylactic reactions; injection-site reactions, including redness, swelling, and pain; necrosis associated with extravasation; malaise; anorexia; hypertension.

Overdosage

There is no known antidote for carboplatin overdosage. The anticipated complications would be secondary to bone marrow suppression and/or hepatic toxicity.

CISPLATIN (CDDP)

Rx	**Cisplatin** (Various, eg, Abbott, American Pharmaceutical, Bedford Labs)	**Injection:** 1 mg/ml	In 50, 100, and 200 ml multi-dose vials.
Rx	**Platinol-AQ** (Bristol-Myers Squibb Oncology)		9 mg sodium chloride. Preservative free. In 50 and 100 ml multi-dose vials.

WARNING

Cisplatin should be administered under the supervision of a qualified physician experienced in the use of cancer chemotherapeutic agents. Appropriate management of therapy and complications is possible only when adequate diagnostic and treatment facilities are readily available.

Cumulative renal toxicity: Cumulative renal toxicity associated with cisplatin is severe (see Warnings). Other major dose-related toxicities are myelosuppression, nausea, and vomiting.

Ototoxicity: Ototoxicity, which may be more pronounced in children, and is manifested by tinnitus or loss of high frequency hearing and, occasionally, deafness, is significant.

Anaphylactic-like reactions: Anaphylactic-like reactions have occurred (see Warnings). Facial edema, bronchoconstriction, tachycardia, and hypotension may occur within minutes of cisplatin administration. Epinephrine, corticosteroids, and antihistamines have been effectively employed to alleviate symptoms (see Warnings and Adverse Reactions).

Exercise caution to prevent inadvertent cisplatin overdose. Doses > 100 mg/m²/cycle once every 3 or 4 weeks are rarely used. Care must be taken to avoid inadvertent cisplatin overdose due to confusion with carboplatin or prescribing practices that fail to differentiate daily doses from total dose per cycle.

Indications

➤*Metastatic testicular tumors:* In combination therapy in patients who have received appropriate surgical or radiotherapeutic procedures.

➤*Metastatic ovarian tumors:* In combination therapy (eg, cyclophosphamide) in patients who have received appropriate surgical or radiotherapeutic procedures. Cisplatin, as a single agent, is indicated as secondary therapy in patients refractory to standard chemotherapy who have not previously received cisplatin.

➤*Advanced bladder cancer:* As a single agent for patients with transitional cell bladder cancer no longer amenable to local treatments (eg, surgery or radiotherapy).

Administration and Dosage

For IV use only. Administer by IV infusion over 6 to 8 hours.

Note to pharmacist: Exercise caution to prevent inadvertent cisplatin overdosage. Please call prescriber if dose > 100 mg/m² per cycle. Aluminum and flip-off seal of vial have been imprinted with the following statement: Call Dr. if dose > 100 mg/m²/cycle.

➤*Metastatic testicular tumors:* The usual cisplatin dose in combination with other approved chemotherapeutic agents is 20 mg/m²/day IV for 5 days/cycle.

➤*Metastatic ovarian tumors:* In combination with cyclophosphamide:

Cisplatin – 75 to 100 mg/m² IV/cycle once every 4 weeks.

Cyclophosphamide – 600 mg/m² IV once every 4 weeks (Day 1).

In combination therapy, administer cisplatin and cyclophosphamide sequentially.

Administer cisplatin as a single agent at a dose of 100 mg/m² IV/cycle once every 4 weeks.

➤*Advanced bladder cancer:* Administer as a single agent. Give 50 to 70 mg/m² IV/cycle once every 3 or 4 weeks, depending on prior radiation therapy or chemotherapy. For heavily pretreated patients, give an initial dose of 50 mg/m²/cycle repeated every 4 weeks.

➤*Repeat courses:* Do not give a repeat course until the serum creatinine is < 1.5 mg/dl or the BUN is < 25 mg/dl or until circulating blood elements are at an acceptable level (platelets ≥ 100,000/mm³, WBC ≥ 4000/mm³). Do not give subsequent doses until an audiometric analysis indicates that auditory acuity is within normal limits.

➤*Note:* Do not use needles or IV sets containing aluminum parts for preparation or administration. Aluminum reacts with cisplatin, causing precipitation and a loss of potency.

Skin reactions associated with accidental exposure may occur. Use gloves. If solution contacts skin or mucosa, wash immediately and thoroughly with soap and water, and flush mucosa with water.

➤*Hydration:* Perform pretreatment hydration with 1 to 2 L fluid infused for 8 to 12 hours prior to dose. Then dilute the drug in 2 L of 5% Dextrose in ½ or ⅓ Normal Saline containing 37.5 g mannitol and infuse over 6 to 8 hours. If diluted solution is not to be used within 6 hours, protect from light. Do not dilute cisplatin in just 5% Dextrose Injection. Maintain adequate hydration and urinary output during the following 24 hours.

➤*Admixture compatibility:* Cisplatin and fluorouracil admixtures are stable in 0.9% Normal Saline for 1 hour.

➤*Storage/Stability:* Store at 15° to 25°C. Protect unopened container from light. Do not refrigerate. The cisplatin remaining in the amber vial following initial entry is stable for 28 days protected from light or for 7 days under fluorescent room light.

Actions

➤*Pharmacology:* Cisplatin is an inorganic heavy metal coordination complex containing a central atom of platinum surrounded by 2 chloride atoms and 2 ammonia molecules in the cis position. The antitumor effect of cisplatin has been correlated with binding to DNA, production of intrastrand crosslinks and formation of DNA adducts.

➤*Pharmacokinetics:*

Absorption/Distribution – Plasma concentrations of the parent compound, cisplatin, have a half-life of ≈ 20 to 30 minutes; the total body clearance and volume of distribution at steady-state are ≈ 15 L/hr/m² and ≈ 11 L/m², respectively. The ratios of cisplatin to total free platinum in the plasma vary considerably between patients and range from 0.5 to 1.1. Cisplatin does not undergo binding to plasma proteins; however, platinum is 90% bound to several plasma proteins including albumin, transferrin, and gamma globulin. The albumin-platinum complexes do not dissociate significantly and are slowly eliminated with a minimum half-life of ≥ 5 days.

Maximum red blood cell concentrations of platinum are reached within 90 to 150 minutes and have a terminal half-life of 36 to 47 days. Concentrations of platinum are highest in liver, prostate, and kidney, somewhat lower in bladder, muscle, testicle, pancreas, and spleen, and lowest in bowel, adrenal, heart, lung, cerebrum, and cerebellum. Platinum is present in tissues for as long as 180 days after the last administration.

Metabolism/Excretion – 90% of the drug is removed by renal mechanisms whereas < 10% is removed by biliary excretion. The parent compound, cisplatin, is excreted in the urine and accounts for 13% to 17% of the administered dose excreted within 1 hour of administration. The renal clearance of cisplatin and platinum exceed creatinine clearance, indicating active secretion by the kidney. The mean renal clearance of cisplatin is 50 to 62 ml/min/m²; platinum clearance is non-linear, variable, and dependent on dose, urine flow rate, and individual variability of active secretion and possible tubular reabsorption. Approximately 10% to 40% of the administered platinum is excreted in the urine within 24 hours with a mean of 35% to 51% excreted in the urine over 5 days.

Contraindications

Preexisting renal impairment; myelosuppression; hearing impairment; history of allergic reactions to cisplatin or other platinum-containing compounds.

Warnings

➤*Renal toxicity:* Dose-related and cumulative renal insufficiency is the major dose-limiting toxicity. Renal toxicity has been noted in 28% to 36% of patients treated with a single dose of 50 mg/m². First noted during the second week after a dose, it is manifested by elevations in BUN and creatinine, serum uric acid, or a decrease in creatinine clearance. Renal toxicity becomes more prolonged and severe with repeated courses of the drug. Renal function must return to normal before another dose can be given.

Amifostine can be used to reduce cumulative renal toxicity in patients with advanced ovarian cancer receiving repeated cisplatin administration. Refer to the individual monograph in the Antineoplastic Adjuncts section.

Impairment of renal function is associated with renal tubular damage. The administration of cisplatin using a 6- to 8-hour infusion with IV hydration and mannitol has been used to reduce nephrotoxicity. However, renal toxicity can still occur (see Precautions).

➤*Ototoxicity:* Ototoxicity has occurred in ≤ 31% of patients given a single 50 mg/m² dose. It is manifested by tinnitus or hearing loss in the high frequency range (4000 to 8000 Hz); decreased ability to hear normal conversational tones occurs occasionally. Ototoxic effects may be more severe in children. Hearing loss can be unilateral or bilateral and is more frequent and severe with repeated doses. Ototoxicity may be enhanced with prior or simultaneous cranial irradiation. It is unclear whether ototoxicity is reversible. Ototoxic effects may be related to the peak plasma concentration of cisplatin. Because ototoxicity of cisplatin is cumulative, carefully perform audiometry before starting therapy and prior to subsequent doses. Vestibular toxicity has occurred. Deafness after the initial dose of cisplatin has been reported rarely.

Ototoxicity may become more severe in patients being treated with other drugs with nephrotoxic potential.

CISPLATIN (CDDP)

➤*Hematologic:* Myelosuppression occurs in 25% to 30% of patients treated with cisplatin. The nadirs in circulating platelets and leukocytes occur between days 18 and 23 (range, 7.5 to 45); most patients recover by day 39 (range, 13 to 62). Leukopenia and thrombocytopenia are more pronounced at doses > 50 mg/m². Anemia (decrease of 2 g hemoglobin/dL) occurs at the same frequency and with the same timing as leukopenia and thrombocytopenia. Fever and infection also have been reported in patients with neutropenia.

In addition to anemia secondary to myelosuppression, a Coombs' positive hemolytic anemia has been reported. In the presence of cisplatin hemolytic anemia, a further course of treatment may be accompanied by increased hemolysis and this risk should be weighed by the treating physician.

The development of acute leukemia coincident with the use of cisplatin has rarely been reported in humans. In these reports, cisplatin was generally given in combination with other leukemogenic agents.

➤*Hepatotoxicity:* Transient elevations of liver enzymes, especially AST, as well as bilirubin, have been reported to be associated with cisplatin administration at the recommended doses.

➤*Vascular toxicities:* Vascular toxicities coincident with use of cisplatin in combination with other antineoplastic agents have occurred rarely. The events are clinically heterogeneous and may include MI, cerebrovascular accident, thrombotic microangiopathy, or cerebral arteritis. Various mechanisms have been proposed for these vascular complications. There are also reports of Raynaud's phenomenon occurring in patients treated with the combination of bleomycin and vinblastine with or without cisplatin. Hypomagnesemia developing coincident with use of cisplatin may be an added, although not essential, factor associated with this event. However, it is currently unknown if the cause of Raynaud's phenomenon in these cases is the disease, underlying vascular compromise, bleomycin, vinblastine, hypomagnesemia, or a combination of any of these factors.

➤*Hyperuricemia:* Hyperuricemia occurs at approximately the same frequency as increases in BUN and serum creatinine. It is more pronounced after doses > 50 mg/m², and peak uric acid levels generally occur 3 to 5 days after the dose. Allopurinol therapy is effective.

➤*Electrolyte disturbance:* Hypomagnesemia, hypocalcemia, hyponatremia, hypokalemia, and hypophosphatemia have occurred and are probably related to renal tubular damage. Tetany has occasionally occurred in those patients with hypocalcemia and hypomagnesemia. Generally, normal serum electrolyte levels are restored by administering supplemental electrolytes and discontinuing cisplatin.

Increased plasma iron levels and inappropriate antidiuretic hormone syndrome also have occurred.

➤*Ophthalmic effects:* Optic neuritis, papilledema, and cerebral blindness have occurred infrequently in patients receiving standard recommended cisplatin doses. Improvement or total recovery usually occurs after drug discontinuation. Steroids with or without mannitol have been used; however, efficacy has not been established.

Blurred vision and altered color perception have occurred after the use of regimens with higher doses or greater dose frequencies than those recommended. The altered color perception manifests as a loss of color discrimination, particularly in the blue-yellow axis. The only finding on funduscopic exam is irregular retinal pigmentation of the macular area.

➤*Neuropathies:* Neurotoxicity, usually characterized by peripheral neuropathy, has occurred. Severe neuropathies have occurred in patients receiving higher doses of cisplatin or greater dose frequencies than those recommended or after prolonged therapy (4 to 7 months); however, neurologic symptoms have been reported to occur after a single dose. Although symptoms and signs of cisplatin neuropathy usually develop during treatment, symptoms of neuropathy may begin 3 to 8 weeks after the last dose of cisplatin (rare). These neuropathies may be irreversible and are seen as paresthesias in a stocking-glove distribution, areflexia, and loss of proprioception and vibratory sensation. Loss of motor function also has occurred. Discontinue therapy when symptoms are first observed. Neuropathy may progress further even after stopping treatment. Preliminary evidence suggests peripheral neuropathy may be irreversible in some patients.

➤*High/Cumulative doses:* Muscle cramps, defined as localized, painful, involuntary skeletal muscle contractions of sudden onset and short duration, have occurred and were usually associated in patients receiving a relatively high cumulative dose of cisplatin and with a relatively advanced symptomatic stage of peripheral neuropathy.

➤*Hypersensitivity reactions:* Anaphylactic-like reactions have occurred. Facial edema, wheezing, tachycardia, and hypotension may occur within minutes of use in patients with prior drug exposure. Symptoms are alleviated by use of epinephrine, corticosteroids, and antihistamines. Refer to Management of Acute Hypersensitivity Reactions.

➤*Mutagenesis:* The drug is mutagenic in bacteria and produces chromosome aberrations in animal cell tissue cultures.

➤*Pregnancy: Category D.* Of 7 reported pregnancy cases, 1 infant developed profound leukopenia with neutropenia, which resolved after

10 days. The mother had developed profound neutropenia just prior to delivery. By 12 weeks of age, the child was developing normally, except for moderate bilateral hearing loss. Advise patients to avoid becoming pregnant.

➤*Lactation:* Cisplatin has been reported to be found in breast milk; patients receiving cisplatin should not breastfeed.

➤*Children:* Safety and efficacy in pediatric patients have not been established.

Precautions

➤*Monitoring:* Monitor peripheral blood counts weekly and liver function periodically. Measure serum creatinine, BUN, creatinine clearance, magnesium, sodium, calcium, and potassium levels prior to initiating therapy and prior to each subsequent course. Do not give more frequently than once every 3 to 4 weeks at the recommended dosage. Perform neurologic and auditory examinations regularly. Carefully perform audiometry before starting therapy and prior to subsequent doses.

➤*GI:* Marked nausea and vomiting occur in almost all patients and are occasionally so severe that the drug must be discontinued. Nausea and vomiting usually begin 1 to 4 hours after treatment and last up to 24 hours; nausea and anorexia may persist for up to 1 week after treatment. Metoclopramide in high doses has been used in the prophylaxis of vomiting associated with cisplatin therapy. Delayed nausea and vomiting (beginning or persisting ≥ 24 hours after chemotherapy) has occurred in patients attaining complete emetic control on the day of therapy.

Drug Interactions

Cisplatin Drug Interactions			
Precipitant drug	Object drug*		Description
Aminoglyco-sides	Cisplatin	↑	Cisplatin produces cumulative nephrotoxicity that is potentiated by aminoglycosides (see Warnings).
Loop diuretics	Cisplatin	↑	Concomitant use of loop diuretics and cisplatin may produce additive ototoxicity (see Warnings).
Cisplatin	Phenytoin	↓	Combination chemotherapy (including cisplatin) may reduce phenytoin plasma levels.

* ↑ = Object drug increased. ↓ = Object drug decreased.

Adverse Reactions

➤*CNS:* Peripheral neuropathies; seizures; dorsal column myelopathy; malaise; Lhermitte's sign; autonomic neuropathy (see Warnings).

➤*Dermatologic:* Local soft tissue toxicity has rarely been reported following extravasation of cisplatin. Severity of the local tissue toxicity appears to be related to the concentration of the cisplatin solution. Infusion of solutions with a cisplatin concentration > 0.5 mg/mL may result in tissue cellulitis, fibrosis, and necrosis.

➤*Electrolyte disturbance:* Hypomagnesemia; hypocalcemia; hyponatremia; hypokalemia; hypophosphatemia; increased plasma iron levels; antidiuretic hormone syndrome (see Warnings).

➤*GI:* Nausea, vomiting, anorexia (see Precautions); diarrhea; loss of taste.

➤*Hematologic:* Myelosuppression (25% to 30%); leukopenia; thrombocytopenia; anemia (see Warnings).

➤*Ophthalmic:* Optic neuritis, papilledema, cerebral blindness (infrequent); blurred vision; altered color perception (see Warnings).

➤*Renal:* Renal insufficiency, renal tubular damage (see Warnings).

➤*Special senses:* Tinnitus, high frequency hearing loss, vestibular toxicity (see Warnings).

➤*Miscellaneous:* Vascular toxicities (rare); hyperuricemia, ototoxicity, anaphylactic-like reactions (see Warnings); elevated AST; alopecia; asthenia.

Infrequent – Cardiac abnormalities; hiccups; rash; elevated serum amylase.

Overdosage

➤*Symptoms:* Exercise caution to prevent inadvertent overdosage with cisplatin. Acute overdosage with this drug may result in kidney failure, liver failure, deafness, ocular toxicity (including detachment of the retina), significant myelosuppression, intractable nausea and vomiting, or neuritis. In addition, death can occur following overdosage.

➤*Treatment:* No proven antidotes have been established for cisplatin overdosage. Hemodialysis, even when initiated 4 hours after the overdosage, appears to have little effect on removing platinum from the body because of cisplatin's rapid and high degree of protein binding. Management of overdosage should include general supportive measures to sustain the patient through any period of toxicity that may occur. Refer to General Management of Acute Overdosage.

OXALIPLATIN

Rx	**Eloxatin** (Sanofi-Synthelabo)	**Powder for injection, lyophilized:** 50 mg	Preservative-free. Lactose. In single-use vials.
		100 mg	Preservative-free. Lactose. In single-use vials.

WARNING

Administer oxaliplatin under the supervision of a qualified physician experienced in the use of cancer chemotherapeutic agents. Appropriate management of therapy and complications is possible only when adequate diagnostic and treatment facilities are readily available.

Anaphylactic-like reactions to oxaliplatin have been reported and may occur within minutes of oxaliplatin administration. Epinephrine, corticosteroids, and antihistamines have been employed to alleviate symptoms (see Warnings and Adverse Reactions).

Indications

➤*Metastatic carcinoma of the colon or rectum:* In combination with infusional 5-fluorouracil (5-FU)/leucovorin (LV) for the treatment of patients with metastatic carcinoma of the colon or rectum whose disease has recurred or progressed during or within 6 months of completion of first-line therapy with the combination of bolus 5-FU/LV and irinotecan.

Administration and Dosage

➤*Approved by the FDA:* August 12, 2002.

➤*Dosage:* The recommended dose schedule given every 2 weeks is as follows:

Day 1: Oxaliplatin 85 mg/m^2 IV infusion in 250 to 500 mL D5W and leucovorin 200 mg/m^2 IV infusion in D5W both given over 120 minutes at the same time in separate bags using a Y-line, followed by 5-FU 400 mg/m^2 IV bolus given over 2 to 4 minutes, followed by 5-FU 600 mg/m^2 IV infusion in 500 mL D5W (recommended) as a 22-hour continuous infusion.

Day 2: Leucovorin 200 mg/m^2 IV infusion over 120 minutes, followed by 5-FU 400 mg/m^2 IV bolus given over 2 to 4 minutes, followed by 5-FU 600 mg/m^2 IV infusion in 500 mL D5W (recommended) as a 22-hour continuous infusion.

Repeat cycle every 2 weeks.

➤*Premedication:* Premedication with antiemetics, including 5-HT$_3$ blockers with or without dexamethasone, is recommended. Prehydration is not required.

➤*Dose modification:* Prior to subsequent therapy cycles, evaluate patients for clinical toxicities and laboratory tests (see Precautions). Neuropathy was graded using a study-specific neurotoxicity scale (see Warnings). Other toxicities were graded by the National Cancer Institute Common Toxicity Criteria, Version 2.0 (NCI CTC).

Prolongation of infusion time for oxaliplatin from 2 to 6 hours decreases the C$_{max}$ by an estimated 32% and may mitigate acute toxicities. The infusion time for infusional 5-FU and leucovorin do not need to be changed.

For patients who experience persistent Grade 2 neurosensory events that do not resolve, consider a dose reduction of oxaliplatin to 65 mg/m^2. For patients with persistent Grade 3 neurosensory events, consider discontinuing therapy. The infusional 5-FU/LV regimen need not be altered.

A dose reduction of oxaliplatin to 65 mg/m^2 and infusional 5-FU by 20% (300 mg/m^2 bolus and 500 mg/m^2 22-hour infusion) is recommended for patients after recovery from Grade 3/4 GI (despite prophylactic treatment) or Grade 3/4 hematologic toxicity (neutrophils less than 1.5 × 10^9/L, platelets less than 100 × 10^9/L).

➤*Preparation for administration:* Reconstitution or final dilution must never be performed with a sodium chloride solution or other chloride-containing solutions.

The lyophilized powder is reconstituted by adding 10 mL (for the 50 mg vial) or 20 mL (for the 100 mg vial) of Water for Injection or 5% Dextrose Injection. Do not administer the reconstituted solution without further dilution. The reconstituted solution must be further diluted in an infusion solution of 250 to 500 mL of 5% Dextrose Injection.

After reconstitution in the original vial, the solution may be stored up to 24 hours under refrigeration (2° to 8°C [36° to 46°F]). After final dilution with 250 to 500 mL of 5% Dextrose Injection, the shelf life is 6 hours at room temperature (20° to 25°C [68° to 77°F]) or up to 24 hours under refrigeration (2° to 8°C [36° to 46°F]). Oxaliplatin is not light-sensitive.

➤*Incompatibilities:* Oxaliplatin is incompatible in solution with alkaline medications or media (such as basic solutions of 5-FU) and must not be mixed with these or administered simultaneously through the same infusion line. Flush the infusion line with D5W prior to administration of any concomitant medication. Do not use needles or IV administration sets containing aluminum parts that may come in contact with oxaliplatin for the preparation or mixing of the drug. Aluminum has been reported to cause degradation of platinum compounds.

➤*Handling and disposal:* As with other potentially toxic anticancer agents, exercise care in the handling and preparation of infusion solutions prepared from oxaliplatin. The use of gloves is recommended. If a solution of oxaliplatin contacts the skin, wash the skin immediately and thoroughly with soap and water. If oxaliplatin contacts the mucous membranes, flush thoroughly with water.

➤*Storage / Stability:* Store under normal lighting conditions at 25°C (77°F); excursions permitted to 15° to 30°C (59° to 86°F). After reconstitution in the original vial, the solution may be stored up to 24 hours under refrigeration (2° to 8°C [36° to 46°F]). After final dilution with 250 to 500 mL of 5% Dextrose Injection, the shelf life is 6 hours at room temperature (20° to 25°C [68° to 77°F]) or up to 24 hours under refrigeration (2° to 8°C [36° to 46°F]).

Actions

➤*Pharmacology:* Oxaliplatin undergoes nonenzymatic conversion in physiologic solutions to active derivatives via displacement of the labile oxalate ligand. Several transient reactive species are formed, including monoaquo and diaquo DACH platinum, which covalently bind with macromolecules. Both inter- and intrastrand Pt-DNA crosslinks are formed. Crosslinks are formed between the *N*7 positions of 2 adjacent guanines (GG), adjacent adenine-guanines (AG), and guanines separated by an intervening nucleotide (GNG). These crosslinks inhibit DNA replication and transcription. Cytotoxicity is cell-cycle nonspecific.

In vivo studies have shown antitumor activity of oxaliplatin against colon carcinoma. In combination with 5-FU, oxaliplatin exhibits in vitro and in vivo antiproliferative activity greater than either compound alone in several tumor models (HT29 [colon], GR [mammary], and L1210 [leukemia]).

➤*Pharmacokinetics:*

Distribution – At the end of a 2-hour infusion of oxaliplatin, approximately 15% of the administered platinum is present in the systemic circulation. The remaining 85% is rapidly distributed into tissues or eliminated in the urine. In patients, plasma protein binding of platinum is irreversible and is greater than 90%. The main binding proteins are albumin and gamma globulins. Platinum also binds irreversibly and accumulates (approximately 2-fold) in erythrocytes, where it appears to have no relevant activity. No platinum accumulation was observed in plasma ultrafiltrate following 85 mg/m^2 every 2 weeks.

Metabolism – Oxaliplatin undergoes rapid and extensive nonenzymatic biotransformation. There is no evidence of cytochrome P450-mediated metabolism in vitro.

Up to 17 platinum-containing derivatives have been observed in plasma ultrafiltrate samples from patients, including several cytotoxic species (monochloro DACH platinum, dichloro DACH platinum, and monoaquo and diaquo DACH platinum) and a number of noncytotoxic, conjugated species.

Excretion – The major route of platinum elimination is renal excretion. At 5 days after a single 2-hour infusion of oxaliplatin, urinary elimination accounted for about 54% of the platinum eliminated, with fecal excretion accounting for only about 2%. Platinum was cleared from plasma at a rate (10 to 17 L/hr) that was similar to or exceeded the average human glomerular filtration rate (GFR; 7.5 L/hr). The renal clearance of ultrafilterable platinum is significantly correlated with GFR. The reactive oxaliplatin derivatives are present as a fraction of the unbound platinum in plasma ultrafiltrate. The decline of ultrafilterable platinum levels following oxaliplatin administration is triphasic, characterized by 2 relatively short distribution phases (t½α, 0.43 hours; t½β, 16.8 hours) and a long terminal elimination phase (t½γ, 391 hours). Pharmacokinetic parameters obtained after a single 2-hour IV infusion of oxaliplatin at a dose of 85 mg/m^2 expressed as ultrafilterable platinum were C$_{max}$ of 0.814 mcg/mL and volume of distribution of 440 L.

Interpatient and intrapatient variability in ultrafilterable platinum exposure (AUC$_{0-48}$) assessed over 3 cycles was moderate to low (23% and 6%, respectively). A pharmacodynamic relationship between platinum ultrafiltrate levels and clinical safety and effectiveness has not been established.

Special populations –

Renal function impairment: The AUC$_{0-48hr}$ of platinum in the plasma ultrafiltrate increases as renal function decreases. The AUC$_{0-48hr}$ of platinum in patients with mild (Ccr 50 to 80 mL/min), moderate (Ccr 30 to less than 50 mL/min), and severe (Ccr less than 30 mL/min) renal impairment is increased by about 60%, 140%, and 190% respectively, compared with patients with normal renal function (Ccr greater than 80 mL/min).

Contraindications

History of known allergy to oxaliplatin or other platinum compounds.

Warnings

➤*Neuropathy:* Neuropathy was graded using a study-specific neurotoxicity scale, which was different than the NCI CTC. The grading scale for paresthesias/dysesthesias was the following: Grade 1, resolved and

OXALIPLATIN

did not interfere with functioning; Grade 2, interfered with function but not daily activities; Grade 3, pain or functional impairment that interfered with daily activities; Grade 4, persistent impairment that is disabling or life-threatening. Oxaliplatin is associated with the following 2 types of neuropathy:

- An acute, reversible, primarily peripheral, sensory neuropathy that is of early onset, occurring within hours or 1 to 2 days of dosing, that resolves within 14 days, and that frequently recurs with further dosing. The symptoms may be precipitated or exacerbated by exposure to cold temperature or cold objects and they usually present as transient paresthesia, dysesthesia, and hypesthesia in the hands, feet, perioral area, or throat. Jaw spasm, abnormal tongue sensation, dysarthria, eye pain, and a feeling of chest pressure also have been observed. The acute, reversible pattern of sensory neuropathy was observed in about 56% of study patients who received oxaliplatin with infusional 5-FU/LV. In any individual cycle, acute neurotoxicity was observed in approximately 30% of patients. Avoid ice (mucositis prophylaxis) during the infusion of oxaliplatin because cold temperature can exacerbate acute neurological symptoms. An acute syndrome of pharyngolaryngeal dysesthesia seen in 1% to 2% of patients is characterized by subjective sensations of dysphagia or dyspnea, without any laryngospasm or bronchospasm (no stridor or wheezing).

- A persistent (greater than 14 days), primarily peripheral, sensory neuropathy that is usually characterized by paresthesias, dysesthesias, hypesthesias, but also may include deficits in proprioception that can interfere with daily activities (eg, writing, buttoning, swallowing, and difficulty walking from impaired proprioception). These forms of neuropathy occurred in 48% of the study patients receiving oxaliplatin with infusional 5-FU/LV. Persistent neuropathy can occur without any prior acute neuropathy event. The majority of patients (80%) who developed Grade 3 persistent neuropathy progressed from prior Grade 1 or 2 events. These symptoms may improve in some patients upon discontinuation of oxaliplatin.

➤ *Pulmonary toxicity:* Oxaliplatin has been associated with pulmonary fibrosis (0.7% of study patients), which may be fatal. In cases of unexplained respiratory symptoms such as nonproductive cough, dyspnea, crackles, or radiological pulmonary infiltrates, discontinue oxaliplatin until further pulmonary investigation excludes interstitial lung disease or pulmonary fibrosis.

➤ *Hypersensitivity reactions:* As in the case for other platinum compounds, hypersensitivity and anaphylactic/anaphylactoid reactions to oxaliplatin have been reported. These allergic reactions were similar in nature and severity to those reported with other platinum-containing compounds (ie, rash; urticaria; erythema; pruritus; bronchospasm, hypotension [rare]). These reactions occur within minutes of administration; manage with appropriate supportive therapy. Drug-related deaths associated with platinum compounds from this reaction have been reported.

➤ *Renal function impairment:* The safety and effectiveness of the combination of oxaliplatin and infusional 5-FU/LV in patients with renal impairment has not been evaluated. Use the combination of oxaliplatin and infusional 5-FU/LV with caution in patients with pre-existing renal impairment because the primary route of platinum elimination is renal. Clearance of ultrafilterable platinum is decreased in patients with mild, moderate, and severe renal impairment.

➤ *Mutagenesis:* Oxaliplatin was not mutagenic to bacteria (Ames test) but was mutagenic to mammalian cells in vitro (L5178Y mouse lymphoma assay). Oxaliplatin was clastogenic in vitro (chromosome aberration in human lymphocytes) and in vivo (mouse bone marow micronucleus assay).

➤ *Fertility impairment:* Testicular damage, characterized by degeneration, hypoplasia, and atrophy, was observed in dogs administered oxaliplatin at 0.75 mg/kg/day for 5 days every 28 days for 3 cycles. A no-effect level was not identified. This daily dose is approximately one-sixth of the recommended human dose on a body surface area basis.

➤ *Elderly:* The incidence of diarrhea, dehydration, hypokalemia, and fatigue were higher in patients 65 years of age and older.

➤ *Pregnancy: Category D.* Oxaliplatin may cause fetal harm when administered to a pregnant woman. Pregnant rats were administered 1 mg/kg/day oxaliplatin (less than one-tenth the recommended human dose based on body surface area) during gestation days 1 through 5 (pre-implantation), 6 through 10, or 11 through 16 (during organogenesis). Oxaliplatin caused developmental mortality (increased early resorptions) when administered on days 6 through 10 and 11 through 16 and adversely affected fetal growth (decreased fetal weight, delayed ossification) when administered on days 6 through 10. If this drug is used during pregnancy or if the patient becomes pregnant while taking this drug, apprise the patient of the potential hazard to the fetus. Advise women of childbearing potential to avoid becoming pregnant while receiving treatment with oxaliplatin.

➤ *Lactation:* It is not known whether oxaliplatin or its derivatives are excreted in human milk. Because many drugs are excreted in human milk and because of the potential for serious adverse reactions in nursing infants from oxaliplatin, decide whether to discontinue nursing or delay the use of the drug, taking into account the importance of the drug to the mother.

➤ *Children:* The safety and efficacy of oxaliplatin in pediatric patients have not been established.

Precautions

➤ *Monitoring:* Standard monitoring of the white blood cell count with differential, hemoglobin, platelet count, and blood chemistries (including ALT, AST, bilirubin, and creatinine) is recommended before each oxaliplatin cycle (see Administration and Dosage).

➤ *GI:* The incidence of GI adverse events appears to be similar across cycles. Premedication with antiemetics, including 5-HT$_3$ blockers, is recommended. Diarrhea and mucositis may be exacerbated by the addition of oxaliplatin to infusional 5-FU/LV, and should be managed with appropriate supportive care. Because cold temperature can exacerbate acute neurological symptoms, avoid ice (mucositis prophylaxis) during the infusion of oxaliplatin.

Drug Interactions

➤ *Fluorouracil:* No pharmacokinetic interaction between 85 mg/m^2 of oxaliplatin and infusional 5-FU has been observed in patients treated every 2 weeks, but increases of 5-FU plasma concentrations by approximately 20% have been observed with doses of 130 mg/m^2 of oxaliplatin administered every 3 weeks.

➤ *Nephrotoxic agents:* Because platinum-containing species are eliminated primarily through the kidney, clearance of these products may be decreased by coadministration of potentially nephrotoxic compunds, although this has not specifically been studied.

Adverse Reactions

More than 1500 patients with advanced colorectal cancer have been treated in clinical studies with oxaliplatin either as a single agent or in combination with other medications. The most common adverse reactions were peripheral sensory neuropathies, neutropenia, nausea, emesis, and diarrhea. Four hundred and fifty patients (about 150 receiving the combination of oxaliplatin and 5-FU/LV) were studied in a randomized trial in patients with refractory and relapsed colorectal cancer. The adverse event profile in this study was similar to that seen in other studies and the adverse reactions in this trial are shown in the table below.

Thirteen percent of patients in the oxaliplatin and infusional 5-FU/LV combination arm and 18% in the infusional 5-FU/LV arm had to discontinue treatment because of adverse effects related to GI or hematologic adverse events or neuropathies. Both 5-FU and oxaliplatin are associated with GI and hematologic adverse events. When oxaliplatin is administered in combination with infusional 5-FU, the incidence of these events is increased.

The incidence of death within 30 days of treatment, regardless of causality, was 5% with the oxaliplatin and infusional 5-FU/LV combination, 8% with oxaliplatin alone, and 7% with infusional 5-FU/LV. Of the 7 deaths that occurred on the oxaliplatin and infusional 5-FU/LV combination arm within 30 days of stopping treatment, 3 may have been treatment-related, associated with GI bleeding or dehydration.

Oxaliplatin Adverse Reactions in Patients with Colorectal Cancer (%)				
	Oxaliplatin (N = 153)		Oxaliplatin + 5-FU/LV (N = 150)	
Adverse reaction	All grades (%)	Grade 3/4 (%)	All grades (%)	Grade 3/4 (%)
Any event	100	46	99	73
CNS				
Fatigue	61	9	68	7
Neuropathy	76	7	73	7
Acute	65	5	56	2
Persistent	43	3	48	6
Headache	13	< 1	17	< 1
Dizziness	7	< 1	13	< 1
Insomnia	11	< 1	9	< 1
Dermatologic				
Flushing	3	< 1	10	< 1
Rash	5	< 1	9	< 1
Alopecia	3	< 1	7	< 1
GI				
Diarrhea	46	4	67	11
Nausea	64	4	65	11
Vomiting	37	4	40	9
Stomatitis	14	0	37	3
Anorexia	20	2	29	3
Gastroesophageal reflux	1	0	5	2
Constipation	31	< 1	32	< 1
Dyspepsia	7	< 1	14	< 1
Taste perversion	5	< 1	13	< 1
Mucositis	2	< 1	7	< 1
Flatulence	3	< 1	5	< 1
GU				
Hematuria	0	< 1	6	< 1
Dysuria	1	< 1	6	< 1

OXALIPLATIN

Oxaliplatin Adverse Reactions in Patients with Colorectal Cancer (%)				
	Oxaliplatin (N = 153)		Oxaliplatin + 5-FU/LV (N = 150)	
Adverse reaction	All grades (%)	Grade 3/4 (%)	All grades (%)	Grade 3/4 (%)
Hematologic				
Anemia	64	1	81	2
Leukopenia	13	0	76	19
Neutropenia	7	0	73	44
Thrombocytopenia	30	3	64	4
Lab test abnormalities				
ALT changes	36	1	31	0
AST changes	54	4	47	0
Total bilirubin changes	13	5	13	1
Respiratory				
Dyspnea	13	7	20	4
Coughing	11	0	19	1
Rhinitis	6	< 1	15	< 1
Upper respiratory tract infection	7	< 1	10	< 1
Pharyngitis	2	< 1	9	< 1
Epistaxis	2	< 1	9	< 1
Miscellaneous				
Abdominal pain	31	7	33	4
Fever	25	1	29	1
Back pain	11	0	19	3
Edema	10	1	15	1
Pain	14	3	15	2
Injection site reaction	9	0	10	3
Thromboembolism	2	1	9	8
Hypokalemia	3	2	9	4
Dehydration	5	3	8	3
Chest pain	5	1	8	1
Febrile neutropenia	0	0	6	6
Hand-foot syndrome	1	< 1	11	< 1
Peripheral edema	5	< 1	10	< 1
Allergic reaction	3	< 1	10	< 1
Arthralgia	7	< 1	10	< 1
Abnormal lacrimation	1	< 1	7	< 1
Rigors	9	< 1	7	< 1
Hiccough	2	< 1	5	< 1

The following additional adverse events, at least possibly related to treatment and potentially important, were reported in at least 2% and less than 5% of the patients in the oxaliplatin and infusional 5-FU/LV combination arm (listed in decreasing order of frequency): Anxiety, myalgia, erythematous rash, increased sweating, conjunctivitis, weight decrease, dry mouth, rectal hemorrhage, depression, ataxia, ascites, hemorrhoids, muscle weakness, nervousness, tachycardia, abnormal micturition frequency, dry skin, pruritus, hemoptysis, purpura, vaginal hemorrhage, melena, somnolence, pneumonia, proctitis, involuntary muscle contractions, intestinal obstruction, gingivitis, tenesmus, hot flashes, enlarged abdomen, urinary incontinence.

➤*CNS:* Seventy-four percent of patients experienced neuropathy. These events can occur without any prior acute event. The majority of the patients (80%) that developed Grade 3 persistent neuropathy progressed from prior Grade 1 or 2 events. The median number of cycles administered on the oxaliplatin with infusional 5-FU/LV combination arm was 6 cycles. In clinical trials that have studied similar administration schedules of this combination regimen (median cycles ranged 10 to 12), a higher incidence (17%) of Grade 3/4 persistent neurotoxicity was observed.

➤*Dermatologic:* Extravasation may result in local pain and inflammation that may be severe and lead to complications, including necro-sis. Injection site reaction, including redness, swelling, and pain have been reported.

➤*GU:* About 10% of patients in all groups had some degree of elevation of serum creatinine. The incidence of Grade 3/4 elevations in serum creatinine in the oxaliplatin and infusional 5-FU/LV combination arm was 1%.

➤*Hematologic:* Neutropenia was frequently observed with the combination of oxaliplatin and infusional 5-FU/LV, with Grade 3 and 4 events reported in 27% and 17% of previously treated patients, respectively.

➤*Hypersensitivity:* Hypersensitivity to oxaliplatin has been observed (less than 1% Grade 3/4) in clinical studies. These allergic reactions, which can be fatal, were similar in nature and severity to those reported with other platinum-containing compounds (eg, rash; urticaria; erythema; pruritus; bronchospasm, hypotension [rare]). These reactions usually are managed with standard epinephrine, corticosteroid, and antihistamine therapy.

➤*Postmarketing:*

CNS – Loss of deep tendon reflexes; dysarthria; Lhermittes' sign; cranial nerve palsies; fasciculations.

GI – Severe diarrhea/vomiting resulting in hypokalemia, metabolic acidosis; ileus; intestinal obstruction; pancreatitis.

Hematologic – Immuno-allergic thrombocytopenia; hemolytic uremic syndrome.

Respiratory – Pulmonary fibrosis; other interstitial lung diseases.

Special senses – Decrease of visual acuity; visual field disturbance; optic neuritis; deafness.

Miscellaneous – Angioedema; anaphylactic shock.

Overdosage

There have been 4 oxaliplatin overdoses reported. One patient received two 130 mg/m^2 doses of oxaliplatin (cumulative dose of 260 mg/m^2) within a 24-hour period. The patient experienced Grade 4 thrombocytopenia (less than 25,000 cells/mm^3) without any bleeding, which resolved. Two other patients were mistakenly administered oxaliplatin instead of carboplatin. One patient received a total oxaliplatin dose of 500 mg and the other received 650 mg. The first patient experienced dyspnea, wheezing, paresthesia, profuse vomiting, and chest pain on the day of administration. She developed respiratory failure and severe bradycardia and subsequently did not respond to resuscitation efforts. The other patient also experienced dyspnea, wheezing, paresthesia, and vomiting. Her symptoms resolved with supportive care. Another patient who was mistakenly administered a 700 mg dose experienced rapid onset of dysesthesia. Inpatient supportive care was given, including hydration, electrolyte support, and platelet transfusion. Recovery occurred 15 days after the overdose. There is no known antidote for oxaliplatin overdose. In addition to thrombocytopenia, the anticipated complications of an oxaliplatin overdose include the following: Myelosuppression, nausea and vomiting, diarrhea, neurotoxicity. Monitor patients suspected of receiving an overdose, and administer supportive treatment.

Patient Information

Inform patients and patients' caregivers of the expected side effects of oxaliplatin, particularly its neurologic effects, both the acute, reversible effects and the persistent neurosensory toxicity. Inform patients that the acute neurosensory toxicity may be precipitated or exacerbated by exposure to cold or cold objects. Instruct patients to avoid cold drinks and use of ice and to cover exposed skin prior to exposure to cold temperature or cold objects.

Patients must be adequately informed of the risk of low blood cell counts and instructed to contact their physician immediately should fever, particularly if associated with persistent diarrhea, or evidence of infection develop.

Instruct patients to contact their physician if persistent vomiting, diarrhea, signs of dehydration, cough, or breathing difficulties occur, or if signs of allergic reaction appear.

MITOXANTRONE HCl

Rx **Novantrone** (Serono) | Injection: 2 mg mitoxantrone free base per ml | Preservative free. In 10, 12.5, and 15 ml multi-dose vials.[1]

[1] With 0.8% NaCl, 0.005% sodium acetate, and 0.046% acetic acid.

WARNING

Administer mitoxantrone for injection concentrate under the supervision of a physician experienced in the use of cytotoxic chemotherapy agents.

Give mitoxantrone slowly into a freely flowing IV infusion. Never give SC, IM, or intra-arterially. Severe local tissue damage may occur if there is extravasation during administration (see Adverse Reactions).

Not for intrathecal use. Severe injury with permanent sequelae can result from intrathecal administration (see Warnings).

Except for the treatment of acute nonlymphocytic leukemia, mitoxantrone therapy generally should not be given to patients with baseline neutrophil counts less than 1500 cells/mm³. In order to monitor the occurrence of bone marrow suppression, primarily neutropenia, which may be severe and result in infection, it is recommended that frequent peripheral blood cell counts be performed on all patients receiving mitoxantrone.

Myocardial toxicity, manifested in its most severe form by potentially fatal CHF, may occur either during therapy with mitoxantrone or months to years after termination of therapy. Mitoxantrone use has been associated with cardiotoxicity; this risk increases with cumulative dose. In cancer patients, the risk of symptomatic CHF was estimated to be 2.6% for patients receiving up to a cumulative dose of 140 mg/m². For this reason, monitor patients for evidence of cardiac toxicity and question them about symptoms of heart failure prior to initiation of treatment. Monitor patients with multiple sclerosis who reach a cumulative dose of 100 mg/m² for evidence of cardiac toxicity prior to each subsequent dose. Ordinarily, patients with multiple sclerosis should not receive a cumulative dose greater than 140 mg/m². Active or dormant cardiovascular disease, prior or concomitant radiotherapy to the mediastinal/pericardial area, previous therapy with other anthracyclines or anthracenediones, or concomitant use of other cardiotoxic drugs may increase the risk of cardiac toxicity. Cardiac toxicity with mitoxantrone may occur at lower cumulative doses whether or not cardiac risk factors are present (see Warnings and Administration and Dosage).

Secondary acute myelogenous leukemia (AML) has been reported in cancer patients treated with anthracyclines. Mitoxantrone is an anthracenedione, a related drug. Secondary AML has also been reported in cancer patients and multiple sclerosis patients who have been treated with mitoxantrone. The occurrence of refractory secondary leukemia is more common when anthracyclines are given in combination with DNA-damaging antineoplastic agents, when patients have been heavily pretreated with cytotoxic drugs, or when doses of anthracyclines have been escalated. The cumulative risk of developing treatment-related AML, in 1774 patients with breast cancer who received mitoxantrone concomitantly with other cytotoxic agents and radiotherapy, was estimated as 1.1% and 1.6% at 5 and 10 years, respectively (see Warnings).

Indications

➤**Multiple sclerosis (MS):** For reducing neurologic disability and/or the frequency of clinical relapses in patients with secondary (chronic) progressive, progressive relapsing, or worsening relapsing-remitting multiple sclerosis (ie, patients whose neurologic status is significantly abnormal between relapses). Mitoxantrone is not indicated in the treatment of patients with primary progressive multiple sclerosis.

The clinical patterns of multiple sclerosis in the studies were characterized as follows: Secondary progressive and progressive relapsing disease were characterized by gradual increasing disability with or without superimposed clinical relapses, and worsening relapsing-remitting disease was characterized by clinical relapses resulting in a step-wise worsening of disability.

➤**Prostate cancer:** Mitoxantrone in combination with corticosteroids is indicated as initial chemotherapy for the treatment of patients with pain related to advanced hormone-refractory prostate cancer.

➤**Acute nonlymphocytic leukemia (ANLL) in adults:** In combination with other approved drug(s) in the initial therapy of ANLL in adults. This includes myelogenous, promyelocytic, monocytic, and erythroid acute leukemias.

Administration and Dosage

➤**MS:** The recommended dosage of mitoxantrone is 12 mg/m² given as a short (approximately 5 to 15 minutes) IV infusion every 3 months.

Evaluation of left ventricular ejection fraction (LVEF) by echocardiogram or multiple gated acquisition (MUGA) scan is recommended prior to administration of the initial dose of mitoxantrone. Subsequent LVEF evaluations are recommended if signs or symptoms of CHF develop, and prior to all doses administered to patients who have received a cumulative dose of 100 mg/m² or more. Do not administer mitoxantrone

to MS patients who have received a cumulative lifetime dose of 140 mg/m² or more, or those with either LVEF of less than 50% or a clinically significant reduction in LVEF.

Monitor complete blood counts, including platelets, prior to each course of mitoxantrone and in the event that signs or symptoms of infection develop. Mitoxantrone generally should not be administered to MS patients with neutrophil counts less than 1500 cells/mm³. Monitor liver function tests prior to each course. Mitoxantrone therapy in MS patients with abnormal liver function tests is not recommended because mitoxantrone clearance is reduced by hepatic impairment and no laboratory measurement can predict drug clearance and dose adjustments.

Women with MS who are biologically capable of becoming pregnant, even if they are using birth control, should have a pregnancy test, and the results should be known before receiving each dose of mitoxantrone (see Warnings).

➤**Hormone-refractory prostate cancer:** Based on data from two Phase 3 comparative trials of mitoxantrone plus corticosteroids vs corticosteroids alone, the recommended dosage of mitoxantrone is 12 to 14 mg/m² given as a short IV infusion every 21 days.

➤**Combination initial therapy for ANLL in adults:** For induction, give 12 mg/m²/day on days 1 to 3 as an IV infusion, and give 100 mg/m² of cytarabine for 7 days as a continuous 24-hour infusion on days 1 to 7.

Most complete remissions will occur following the initial course of induction therapy. In the event of an incomplete antileukemic response, a second induction course may be given. Give mitoxantrone for 2 days and cytarabine for 5 days using the same daily dosage levels.

If severe or life-threatening nonhematologic toxicity is observed during the first induction course, withhold the second induction course until toxicity clears.

Consolidation therapy – Consolidation therapy used in 2 large randomized multicenter trials consisted of mitoxantrone 12 mg/m² given by IV infusion daily for days 1 and 2, and cytarabine 100 mg/m² for 5 days given as a continuous 24-hour infusion on days 1 to 5. The first course was given ≈ 6 weeks after the final induction course, the second was generally administered 4 weeks after the first. Severe myelosuppression occurred.

➤**Hepatic impairment:** For patients with hepatic impairment, there is at present no laboratory measurement that allows for dose adjustment recommendations.

➤**Preparation and administration:** Mitoxantrone solution must be diluted prior to use.

Dilute to at least 50 ml with either 0.9% Sodium Chloride Injection or 5% Dextrose Injection. Mitoxantrone may be further diluted into Dextrose 5% in Water, Normal Saline, or 5% Dextrose with Normal Saline, and used immediately. Do not freeze. Introduce this solution slowly into the tubing as a freely running IV infusion of 0.9% Sodium Chloride Injection or 5% Dextrose Injection over a period of not less than 3 minutes. The tubing should be attached to a butterfly needle or other suitable device and inserted preferably into a large vein. If possible, avoid veins over joints or in extremities with compromised venous or lymphatic drainage.

If extravasation occurs, stop administration immediately and restart in another vein. Carefully monitor the extravasation site for signs of necrosis or phlebitis that may require further medical attention.

If skin is accidentally exposed to mitoxantrone, rinse copiously with warm water; if the eyes are involved, use standard irrigation techniques immediately. The use of goggles, gloves, and protective gowns is recommended during preparation and administration of the drug.

➤**IV incompatibility:** Do not mix in the same infusion as heparin; a precipitate may form. Because specific compatibility data are not available, it is recommended that mitoxantrone not be mixed in the same infusion with other drugs.

➤**Storage/Stability:** Do not freeze. In the case of multidose use, after penetration of the stopper, the remaining portion of the undiluted mitoxantrone concentrate should be stored ≤ 7 days between 15° and 25°C (59° and 77°F) or 14 days under refrigeration.

Actions

➤**Pharmacology:** Mitoxantrone is a synthetic antineoplastic anthracenedione for IV use.

Mitoxantrone is a DNA-reactive agent that intercalates into deoxyribonucleic acid (DNA) through hydrogen bonding, causes crosslinks and strand breaks. Mitoxantrone also interferes with ribonucleic acid (RNA) and is a potent inhibitor of topoisomerase II, an enzyme responsible for uncoiling and repairing damaged DNA. It has a cytocidal effect on both proliferating and nonproliferating cultured human cells, suggesting lack of cell cycle phase specificity.

➤**Pharmacokinetics:**

Absorption/Distribution – Pharmacokinetics of mitoxantrone in patients following a single IV administration of mitoxantrone can be

MITOXANTRONE HCl

characterized by a 3-compartment model. The mean alpha half-life of mitoxantrone is 6 to 12 minutes, the mean beta half-life is 1.1 to 3.1 hours, and the mean gamma (terminal or elimination) half-life is 23 to 215 hours (median, approximately 75 hours). Pharmacokinetic studies have not been performed in humans receiving multiple daily dosing. Distribution to tissues is extensive: Steady-state volume of distribution exceeds $1000 \ L/m^2$. Tissue concentrations of mitoxantrone appear to exceed those in the blood during the terminal elimination phase.

In patients administered 15 to 90 mg/m^2 of mitoxantrone IV, there is a linear relationship between dose and the area under the concentration-time curve (AUC). Mitoxantrone is 78% bound to plasma proteins in the observed concentration range of 26 to 455 ng/ml. This binding is independent of concentration.

Metabolism / Excretion – Mitoxantrone is excreted in urine and feces as either unchanged drug or as inactive metabolites. In human studies, 11% and 25% of the dose were recovered in urine and feces, respectively, as either parent drug or metabolite during the 5-day period following drug administration. Of the material recovered in urine, 65% was unchanged drug. The remaining 35% was composed of monocarboxylic and dicarboxylic acid derivatives and their glucuronide conjugates. The pathways leading to the metabolism of mitoxantrone have not been elucidated.

Special populations –

Hepatic impairment: Mitoxantrone clearance is reduced by hepatic impairment. Patients with severe hepatic dysfunction (bilirubin > 3.4 mg/dl) have an AUC > 3 times greater than that of patients with normal hepatic function receiving the same dose.

➤*Clinical trials:* The benefit of consolidation therapy in ANLL patients who achieve a complete remission remains controversial. However, in the only well-controlled prospective, randomized multicenter trials with mitoxantrone in ANLL, consolidation therapy was given to all patients who achieved a complete remission. During consolidation in the US study, 2 myelosuppression-related deaths occurred in mitoxantrone patients and 1 in daunorubicin patients. However, in the foreign study, there were 8 deaths in mitoxantrone patients during consolidation that were related to the myelosuppression, and none in daunorubicin patients where less myelosuppression occurred.

Contraindications

Hypersensitivity to mitoxantrone.

Warnings

➤*Myelosuppression:* When mitoxantrone is used in high doses (more than 14 mg/m^2/day for 3 days) (eg, for treatment of leukemia), severe myelosuppression will occur. Therefore, it is recommended that mitoxantrone be administered only by physicians experienced in the chemotherapy of this disease. Laboratory and supportive services must be available for hematologic and chemistry monitoring and adjunctive therapies, including antibiotics. Blood and blood products must be available to support patients during the expected period of medullary hypoplasia and severe myelosuppression. Give particular care to assuring full hematologic recovery before undertaking consolidation therapy (if this treatment is used) and monitor patients closely during this phase. Mitoxantrone administered at any dose can cause myelosuppression.

Patients with preexisting myelosuppression as the result of prior drug therapy should not receive mitoxantrone unless it is felt that the possible benefit from such treatment warrants the risk of further medullary suppression.

➤*Cardiac:* Because of the possible danger of cardiac effects in patients previously treated with daunorubicin or doxorubicin, the benefit-to-risk ratio of mitoxantrone therapy in such patients should be determined before starting therapy. Functional cardiac changes including irreversible CHF and decreases in LVEF can occur. Cardiac toxicity may be more common in patients with prior treatment with anthracyclines, prior mediastinal radiotherapy, or with preexisting cardiovascular disease. Such patients should have regular cardiac monitoring of LVEF from the initiation of therapy. Cancer patients who received cumulative doses of 140 mg/m^2 either alone or in combination with other chemotherapeutic agents had a cumulative 2.6% probability of clinical CHF. In comparative oncology trials, the overall cumulative probability rate of moderate or severe decreases in LVEF at this dose was 13%.

MS – Functional cardiac changes may occur in patients with MS treated with mitoxantrone. In one controlled trial, 2 patients (2%) of 127 receiving mitoxantrone, 1 receiving a 5 mg/m^2 dose and the other receiving the 12 mg/m^2 dose, had LVEF values that decreased to less than 50%. An additional patient receiving 12 mg/m^2, who did not have LVEF measured, had a decrease in another echocardiographic measurement of ventricular function (fractional shortening) that led to discontinuation from the trial. There were no reports of CHF in either controlled trial.

Evaluation of LVEF (by echocardiogram or MUGA) is recommended prior to administration of the initial dose of mitoxantrone. MS patients with a baseline LVEF of less than 50% should not be treated with mitoxantrone. Subsequent LVEF evaluations are recommended if signs or symptoms of CHF develop, and prior to all doses administered to patients who have received a cumulative dose of 100 mg/m^2 or more. Mitoxantrone should not ordinarily be administered to MS patients who have received a cumulative lifetime dose of 140 mg/m^2 or more, or those with either LVEF of less than 50% or a clinically significant reduction in LVEF.

Leukemia – Acute CHF may occasionally occur in patients treated for ANLL.

Hormone-refractory prostate cancer – Functional cardiac changes such as decreases in LVEF and CHF may occur in patients with hormone-refractory prostate cancer treated with mitoxantrone.

➤*Secondary leukemia:* Secondary leukemia has been reported in cancer patients and multiple sclerosis patients treated with mitoxantrone. The largest published report involved 1774 patients with breast cancer treated with mitoxantrone in combination with methotrexate with or without mitomycin. In this study, the cumulative probability of developing secondary leukemia was estimated to be 1.1% and 1.6% at 5 and 10 years, respectively. The second largest report involved 449 patients with breast cancer treated with mitoxantrone, usually in combination with radiotherapy and/or other cytotoxic agents. In this study, the cumulative probability of developing secondary leukemia was estimated to be 2.2% at 4 years.

➤*Acute leukemia/myelodysplasia:* Topoisomerase II inhibitors, including mitoxantrone, have been associated with the development of acute leukemia and myelodysplasia.

➤*Hepatic function impairment:* Patients with MS who have hepatic impairment should ordinarily not be treated with mitoxantrone. Administer mitoxantrone with caution to other patients with hepatic impairment; a dosage adjustment may be required. In patients with severe hepatic impairment, the AUC is more than 3 times greater than the value observed in patients with normal hepatic function.

➤*Carcinogenesis:* IV treatment of rats and mice once every 21 days for 24 months with mitoxantrone resulted in an increased incidence of fibroma and external auditory canal tumors in rats at a dose of 0.03 mg/kg (0.02-fold the recommended human dose on a mg/m^2 basis), and hepatocellular adenoma in male mice at a dose of 0.1 mg/kg (0.03-fold the recommended human dose on a mg/m^2 basis). IV treatment of rats once every 21 days for 12 months with mitoxantrone resulted in an increased incidence of external auditory canal tumors in rats at a dose of 0.3 mg/kg (0.15-fold the recommended human dose on a mg/m^2 basis).

➤*Mutagenesis:* Mitoxantrone was clastogenic in the in vivo rat bone marrow assay. Mitoxantrone was also clastogenic in 2 in vitro assays; it induced DNA damage in primary rat hepatocytes and sister chromatid exchanges in Chinese hamster ovary cells. Mitoxantrone was mutagenic in bacterial and mammalian test systems (Ames/Salmonella and *E. coli* and L5178Y TK+/- mouse lymphoma).

➤*Pregnancy: Category D.* May cause fetal harm when administered to a pregnant woman. Women of childbearing potential should be advised to avoid becoming pregnant. Mitoxantrone is considered a potential human teratogen because of its mechanism of action and the developmental effects demonstrated by related agents. Treatment of pregnant rats during the organogenesis period of gestation was associated with fetal growth retardation at doses of 0.1 mg/kg/day or more (0.01 times the recommended human dose on a mg/m^2 basis). When pregnant rabbits were treated during organogenesis, an increased incidence of premature delivery was observed at doses of 0.1 mg/kg/day or more (0.01 times the recommended human dose on a mg/m^2 basis). No teratogenic effects were observed in these studies, but the maximum doses tested were well below the recommended human dose (0.02 and 0.05 times in rats and rabbits, respectively, on a mg/m^2 basis). There are no adequate and well-controlled studies in pregnant women. Women with MS who are biologically capable of becoming pregnant should have a pregnancy test prior to each dose, and the results should be known prior to administration of the drug. If this drug is used during pregnancy, or if the patient becomes pregnant while taking this drug, apprise her of the potential hazard to the fetus.

➤*Lactation:* Mitoxantrone is excreted in breast milk and significant concentrations (18 ng/ml) have been reported for 28 days after the last administration. Because of the potential for serious adverse reactions in infants, discontinue breastfeeding before starting treatment.

➤*Children:* Safety and efficacy for use in children have not been established.

Precautions

➤*Monitoring:* Frequently observe the patient and monitor hematologic and chemical laboratory parameters. Obtain a complete blood count, including platelets, prior to each course of mitoxantrone and in the event that signs and symptoms of infection develop. Liver function tests should also be performed prior to each course of therapy. Mitoxantrone in MS patients with abnormal liver function tests is not recommended because mitoxantrone clearance is reduced by hepatic impairment and no laboratory measurement can predict drug clearance and dose adjustments.

MITOXANTRONE HCl

In leukemia treatment, hyperuricemia may occur as a result of rapid lysis of tumor cells by mitoxantrone. Monitor serum uric acid levels and institute hypouricemic therapy prior to the initiation of antileukemic therapy.

Women with MS who are biologically capable of becoming pregnant, even if they are using birth control, should have a pregnancy test and the results should be known before receiving each dose of mitoxantrone (see Warnings).

▶*For IV use only:* Safety for use by routes other than IV administration has not been established.

Mitoxantrone is not indicated for SC, IM, or intra-arterial injection. There have been reports of local/regional neuropathy, some irreversible, following intra-arterial injection.

Mitoxantrone must not be given by intrathecal injection. There have been reports of neuropathy and neurotoxicity, both central and peripheral, following intrathecal injection. These reports have included seizures leading to coma and severe neurologic sequelae, and paralysis with bowel and bladder dysfunction.

▶*Systemic infections:* Treat concomitantly with or just before starting mitoxantrone.

Drug Interactions

To date, post-marketing experience has not revealed any significant drug interactions in patients who have received mitoxantrone for treatment of cancer. Information on drug interactions in patients with multiple sclerosis is limited.

Adverse Reactions

▶*Use in MS:*

Miscellaneous – Mitoxantrone was administered to 149 patients with MS in two randomized clinical trials, including 21 patients who received mitoxantrone in combination with corticosteroids.

In Study 1, the proportion of patients who discontinued treatment due to an adverse event was 9.7% (n = 6) in the 12 mg/m^2 mitoxantrone arm (leukopenia, depression, decreased LV function, bone pain and emesis, renal failure, and 1 discontinuation to prevent future complications from repeated urinary tract infections [UTIs]) compared to 3.1% (n = 2) in the placebo arm (hepatitis and MI).

Two of the 127 patients treated with mitoxantrone in Study 1 had decreased LVEF to less than 50% at some point during the 2 years of treatment. An additional patient receiving 12 mg/m^2 did not have LVEF measured, but had another echocardiographic measure of ventricular function (fractional shortening) that led to discontinuation from the study.

The proportion of patients experiencing any infection during Study 1 was 67% for the placebo group, 85% for the 5 mg/m^2 group, and 81% for the 12 mg/m^2 group. However, few of these infections required hospitalization: One placebo patient (tonsillitis), three 5 mg/m^2 patients (enteritis, UTI, viral infection), four 12 mg/m^2 patients (tonsillitis, UTI [2], endometritis).

Mitoxantrone Adverse Events Occurring in ≥ 5% of Patients (Numerically Greater Than Placebo) (Study 1; %)			
Adverse reaction	Placebo (n = 64)	5 mg/m^2 mitoxantrone (n = 65)	12 mg/m^2 mitoxantrone (n = 62)
Cardiovascular			
Arrhythmia	8	6	18
ECG abnormal	3	5	11
GI			
Nausea	20	55	76
Stomatitis	8	15	19
Diarrhea	11	25	16
Constipation	6	14	10
GU			
Menstrual disorder (% of female patients)	26	51	61
Amenorrhea (% of female patients)	3	28	43
UTI	13	29	32
Urine abnormal	6	5	11
Hematologic[1]			
Leukopenia (< 4000 cells/mm^3)	0	9	19
Granulocytopenia (< 2000 cells/mm^3)	2	6	6
Anemia	2	9	6
Metabolic/Nutritional			
Gamma-GT increased	3	3	15
AST increased[1]	8	9	8
ALT increased[1]	3	6	5
Respiratory			
Upper respiratory tract infection	52	51	53
Sinusitis	2	3	6

Mitoxantrone Adverse Events Occurring in ≥ 5% of Patients (Numerically Greater Than Placebo) (Study 1; %)			
Adverse reaction	Placebo (n = 64)	5 mg/m^2 mitoxantrone (n = 65)	12 mg/m^2 mitoxantrone (n = 62)
Miscellaneous			
Alopecia	31	38	61
Back pain	5	6	8
Headache	5	6	6

[1] Assessed using World Health Organization (WHO) toxicity criteria.

In study 2, mitoxantrone was administered once a month. Clinical adverse events most frequently reported in the mitoxantrone group included amenorrhea (53% of female patients), alopecia (33% of patients), nausea (29% of patients), and asthenia (24% of patients). The following table summarizes adverse events and laboratory abnormalities occurring in more than 5% of patients in the mitoxantrone group and numerically more frequent than in the control group.

Mitoxantrone Adverse Events Occurring More Frequently than in the Control Group (> 5%)[1]		
Event	Methylprednisolone (n = 21)	Mitoxantrone plus methylprednisolone (n = 21)
Amenorrhea (female patients)	0	53
Alopecia	0	33
Nausea	0	29
Asthenia	0	24
Pharyngitis/throat infection	5	19
Gastralgia/stomach burn/ epigastric pain	5	14
Aphthosis	0	10
Cutaneous mycosis	0	10
Rhinitis	0	10
Menorrhagia (female patients)	0	7
WBC low (< 4000 cells/mm^3)	14	100
ANC low (< 1500 cells/mm^3)	10	100
Lymphocytes low	43	95
Hemoglobin low	48	43
Platelets low (< 100,000 cells/ mm^3)	0	33
AST high	5	15
ALT high	10	15
Glucose high	5	10
Potassium low	0	10

[1] Assessed using National Cancer Institute (NCI) common toxicity criteria.

Leukopenia and neutropenia were reported in the mitoxantrone plus methylprednisolone group. Neutropenia occurred within 3 weeks after mitoxantrone administration and was always reversible. Only mild to moderate intensity infections were reported in 9 of 21 patients in the mitoxantrone plus methylprednisolone group and in 3 of 21 patients in the methylprednisolone group; none of these required hospitalization.

▶*Use in leukemia:*

Miscellaneous – The following table summarizes adverse reactions occurring in patients treated with mitoxantrone plus cytarabine in comparison with those who received daunorubicin plus cytarabine for therapy of ANLL in a large multicenter randomized prospective US trial. Adverse reactions are presented as major categories and selected of clinically significant subcategories.

Mitoxantrone Adverse Reactions				
	Induction (%)		Consolidation (%)	
Event	Mitoxantrone (n = 102)	Daunorubicin (n = 102)	Mitoxantrone (n = 55)	Daunorubicin (n = 49)
Cardiovascular	26	28	11	24
CHF	5	6	0	0
Arrhythmias	3	3	4	4
Hematologic				
Bleeding	37	41	20	6
Petechiae/ Ecchymosis	7	9	11	2
GI	88	85	58	51
Nausea/Vomiting	72	67	31	31
Diarrhea	47	47	18	8
GI hemorrhage	16	12	2	2
Abdominal pain	15	9	9	4
Mucositis/ Stomatitis	29	33	18	8
Hepatic	10	11	14	2
Jaundice	3	8	7	0

MITOXANTRONE HCl

Mitoxantrone Adverse Reactions				
	Induction (%)		Consolidation (%)	
Event	Mitoxantrone (n = 102)	Daunorubicin (n = 102)	Mitoxantrone (n = 55)	Daunorubicin (n = 49)
Infections	66	73	60	43
UTI	7	2	7	2
Pneumonia	9	7	9	0
Sepsis	34	36	31	18
Fungal infections	15	13	9	6
Pulmonary	43	43	24	14
Cough	13	9	9	2
Dyspnea	18	20	6	0
CNS	30	30	34	35
Seizures	4	4	2	8
Headache	10	9	13	8
Ophthalmic	7	6	2	4
Conjunctivitis	5	1	0	0
Miscellaneous				
Renal failure	8	6	0	2
Fever	78	71	24	18
Alopecia	37	40	22	16

Hematologic – Myelosuppression is rapid in onset and is consistent with the requirement to produce significant marrow hypoplasia in order to achieve a response in acute leukemia. The incidences of infection and bleeding seen in the US trial are consistent with those reported for other standard induction regimens.

➤*Allergic:* Hypotension, urticaria, dyspnea, and rashes have been reported occasionally. Anaphylaxis/Anaphylactoid reactions have been reported rarely.

➤*Cardiovascular:* CHF, tachycardia, ECG changes including arrhythmias, chest pain, and asymptomatic decreases in LVEF have occurred (see Warnings).

➤*Dermatologic:* Extravasation at the infusion site has been reported, which may result in erythema, swelling, pain, burning, and/or blue discoloration of the skin. Extravasation can result in tissue necrosis with resultant need for debridement and skin grafting. Phlebitis has also been reported at the site of the infusion.

➤*GI:* Nausea and vomiting occurred acutely in most patients and may have contributed to reports of dehydration, but were generally mild to moderate and could be controlled through the use of antiemetics. Stomatitis/mucositis occurred within 1 week of therapy.

➤*Hematologic:* Topoisomerase II inhibitors, including mitoxantrone, in combination with other antineoplastic agents, have been associated with the development of acute leukemia. Myelosuppression may also develop.

➤*Hormone-refractory prostate cancer:* In a randomized study in hormone-refractory prostate cancer where dose escalation was required for neutrophil counts greater than 1000/mm^3, grade 4 neutropenia (ANC less than 500/mm^3) was observed in 54% of patients treated with mitoxantrone plus low-dose prednisone. In a separate randomized trial where patients were treated with 14 mg/m^2, grade 4 neutropenia in 23% of patients treated with mitoxantrone plus hydrocortisone was observed. Neutropenic fever/infection occurred in 11% and 10% of patients receiving mitoxantrone plus corticosteroids, respectively, on the two trials. Platelets less than 50,000/mm^3 were noted in 4% and 3% of patients receiving mitoxantrone plus corticosteroids on these trials, and there was 1 patient death on mitoxantrone plus hydrocortisone due to intracranial hemorrhage after a fall.

➤*Pulmonary:* Interstitial pneumonitis has been reported in cancer patients receiving combination chemotherapy that included mitoxantrone.

Overdosage

There is no known specific antidote. Accidental overdoses have occurred. Four patients receiving 140 to 180 mg/m^2 as a single bolus injection died as a result of severe leukopenia with infection. Hematologic support and antimicrobial therapy may be required during prolonged periods of severe myelosuppression.

Although patients with severe renal failure have not been studied, mitoxantrone is extensively tissue bound and it is unlikely that the therapeutic effect or toxicity would be mitigated by peritoneal or hemodialysis.

Patient Information

Provide patients with MS with the patient package insert at the time that the decision is made to treat with mitoxantrone and prior to and in close temporal proximity to each treatment. In addition, the physician should discuss the issues addressed in the patient package insert with the patient.

Mitoxantrone may impart a blue-green color to the urine for 24 hours after administration; advise patients to expect this during therapy. Bluish discoloration of the sclera may also occur. Advise patients of the signs and symptoms of myelosuppression.

HYDROXYUREA

Rx	Mylocel (MGI Pharma)	Tablets: 1000 mg	Alcohol. (barr 979). Beige, capsule shape, biconvex, scored. Film-coated. In unit-of-use 60s.
Rx	Hydroxyurea (Various, eg, Barr, Major, Par, Roxane)	Capsules: 500 mg	In 100s and UD 100s.
Rx	Hydrea (Bristol-Myers Squibb)		Lactose. (Hydrea 830). Green and pink. In 100s.

For prescribing information on antisickling agent use, see the Hematologics chapter.

Indications

Melanoma; resistant chronic myelocytic leukemia; recurrent, metastatic, or inoperable carcinoma of the ovary.

➤*Squamous cell carcinoma:* As an adjunct to irradiation in the local control of primary squamous cell (epidermoid) carcinomas of the head and neck, excluding the lip.

➤*Unlabeled uses:*

Thrombocythemia – To reduce platelet count and prevent thrombosis in high-risk patients with essential thrombocythemia ($\approx$ 15 mg/kg/day).

HIV – Potential antiviral activity of hydroxyurea may be enhanced by didanosine.

Psoriasis – Management of refractory psoriasis (0.5 to 1.5 g daily).

Administration and Dosage

Base dosage on the patient's actual or ideal weight, whichever is less. If the patient prefers, or is unable to swallow capsules, empty the contents of the capsules into a glass of water and take immediately. Some inert material may not dissolve.

An adequate trial period to determine effectiveness is 6 weeks. When there is regression in tumor size or arrest in tumor growth, continue therapy indefinitely. Interrupt therapy if the WBC drops to < 2500/mm^3 or the platelet count to < 100,000/mm^3. In these cases, recheck counts after 3 days and resume therapy when the counts rise significantly toward normal. Because the hematopoietic rebound is prompt, it is usually necessary to omit only a few doses. If prompt rebound has not occurred during combined hydroxyurea and irradiation therapy, irradiation may also be interrupted. However, this is rare. Correct anemia with whole blood replacement; do not interrupt hydroxyurea therapy.

➤*Solid tumors:* Patients on intermittent therapy rarely require complete discontinuation of therapy because of toxicity.

Intermittent therapy – 80 mg/kg as a single dose every third day.

Continuous therapy – 20 to 30 mg/kg as a single daily dose.

➤*Concomitant irradiation therapy (carcinoma of head and neck):* 80 mg/kg as a single dose every third day. Begin hydroxyurea at least 7 days before initiation of irradiation and continue during radiotherapy and indefinitely afterwards, provided the patient is adequately observed and exhibits no unusual or severe reactions. Administer maximum irradiation dose appropriate for the therapeutic situation; adjustment of irradiation dosage is not usually necessary with concomitant hydroxyurea.

➤*Resistant chronic myelocytic leukemia:* Continuous therapy (20 to 30 mg/kg as a single daily dose) is recommended.

Actions

➤*Pharmacology:* The precise mechanism of cytotoxic action is unknown. Hydroxyurea causes an immediate inhibition of deoxyribonucleic acid (DNA) synthesis without interfering with ribonucleic acid (RNA) or protein synthesis. It interferes with the conversion of ribonucleotides to deoxyribonucleotides by blocking the ribonucleotide reductase system as a selective antimetabolite. It may also inhibit the incorporation of thymidine into DNA.

Three mechanisms have been postulated for the increased effectiveness of concomitant use of hydroxyurea with irradiation. In vitro studies suggest that hydroxyurea is lethal to normally radioresistant S-stage cells, holds other cells in the G-1 or pre-DNA synthesis stage where they are most susceptible to irradiation effects, and hinders the normal repair process of cells damaged but not killed by irradiation.

➤*Pharmacokinetics:*

Absorption/Distribution – Hydroxyurea is readily absorbed from the GI tract, reaching peak serum concentrations within $\approx$ 1 to 2 hours; by 24 hours the serum concentration is essentially zero. Hydroxyurea readily crosses the blood-brain barrier with peak CSF levels at 3 hours.

Metabolism/Excretion – About 50% of an oral dose is degraded in the liver and excreted into the urine as urea and as respiratory carbon dioxide; the remainder is excreted intact in the urine. Approximately 80% of the dose may be recovered in the urine within 12 hours.

Contraindications

Marked bone marrow depression (eg, leukopenia < 2500/mm^3 WBC or thrombocytopenia < 100,000/mm^3 platelets); severe anemia.

Warnings

➤*Erythema:* Patients who have received prior irradiation therapy may have an exacerbation of postirradiation erythema.

➤*Bone marrow suppression:* Bone marrow suppression may occur and is more common in patients with previous radiotherapy or cytotoxic antineoplastic exposure. Leukopenia is generally the first and most common manifestation; thrombocytopenia and anemia occur less often. Recovery is rapid when therapy is interrupted. Correct severe anemia with whole blood replacement before initiating hydroxyurea therapy. Do not start treatment if bone marrow function is markedly depressed.

➤*Erythrocytic abnormalities:* Self-limiting megaloblastic erythropoiesis is often seen early in hydroxyurea therapy. The morphologic changes resemble pernicious anemia but are not related to vitamin B$_{12}$ or folic acid deficiency. Hydroxyurea may delay plasma iron clearance and reduce the rate of iron utilization by erythrocytes, but it does not alter the RBC survival time.

➤*Mucositis:* Mucositis at the site is attributed to irradiation, although more severe cases may be caused by combination therapy. Treat palliatively. If severe, temporarily interrupt hydroxyurea; if extremely severe, temporarily postpone irradiation.

Control severe gastric distress by temporary interruption of hydroxyurea administration; interruption of irradiation is rarely necessary.

➤*Renal toxicity:* May temporarily impair renal tubular function accompanied by elevated serum uric acid, BUN, and creatinine levels.

➤*Renal function impairment:* Hydroxyurea is excreted by the kidneys; therefore, use with caution in patients with marked renal dysfunction.

➤*Elderly:* May be more sensitive to the effects of hydroxyurea and may require a lower dosage regimen.

➤*Pregnancy:* Category D. Drugs that affect DNA synthesis may be mutagenic. Hydroxyurea is a known teratogen in animals. Do not use in women who are or who may become pregnant, unless the potential benefits outweigh the possible hazards.

➤*Children:* Dosage regimens for children have not been established.

Precautions

➤*Monitoring:* Therapy requires close supervision. Determine the complete status of the blood, including bone marrow examination if indicated, as well as renal and liver function prior to and during treatment.

Hematology – Monitor hemoglobin, total leukocyte counts, and platelet counts at least once a week throughout therapy. If WBC decreases to < 2500/mm^3 or the platelet count to < 100,000/mm^3, interrupt therapy until values rise significantly toward normal. Treat anemia with whole blood replacement; do not interrupt therapy.

Drug Interactions

➤*Drug/Lab test interactions:* Serum uric acid, BUN, and creatinine levels may be increased by hydroxyurea.

Adverse Reactions

➤*CNS:* Headache, dizziness, disorientation, hallucinations, convulsions (rare); moderate drowsiness (large doses).

➤*Dermatologic:* Maculopapular rash; skin ulceration; facial erythema; alopecia (rare).

➤*GI:* Stomatitis; anorexia; nausea; vomiting; diarrhea; constipation.

➤*Miscellaneous:* Mucositis, renal toxicity (see Warnings); fever; chills; malaise; elevation of hepatic enzymes; abnormal BSP retention; acute pulmonary reactions (eg, diffuse pulmonary infiltrates, fever, dyspnea), dysuria (rare).

Combination therapy – Adverse reactions are similar to those using either hydroxyurea or irradiation alone, primarily bone marrow depression (anemia and leukopenia) and gastric irritation. Incidence and severity may be increased. Most patients will demonstrate concurrent leukopenia. Platelet depression (< 100,000 cells/mm^3) has occurred rarely and only in the presence of marked leukopenia.

Patient Information

Notify physician if fever, chills, sore throat, nausea, vomiting, loss of appetite, diarrhea, sores in the mouth and on the lips, unusual bleeding or bruising occur.

Medication may cause drowsiness, constipation, redness of the face, skin rash, itching, and loss of hair; notify physician if these become pronounced.

Extra fluid intake is recommended.

Contraceptive measures are recommended during therapy.

PROCARBAZINE HCl (N-Methylhydrazine; MIH)

Rx	**Matulane** (Sigma-Tau)	**Capsules:** 50 mg	Talc, mannitol, parabens. (Matulane Sigma-Tau). Ivory. In 100s.

WARNING

It is recommended that procarbazine HCl be given only by or under the supervision of a physician experienced in the use of potent antineoplastic drugs. Adequate clinical and laboratory facilities should be available to patients for proper monitoring of treatment.

Indications

➤*Hodgkin disease:* In combination with other antineoplastics for treatment of stages III and IV Hodgkin disease. Use procarbazine as part of the MOPP (nitrogen mustard, vincristine, procarbazine, prednisone) regimen.

➤*Unlabeled uses:* Procarbazine has also been shown to demonstrate activity against some non-Hodgkin lymphoma, brain tumors, small cell lung cancer, and melanoma.

Administration and Dosage

➤*Approved by the FDA:* July 22, 1969.

Base dosages on the patient's actual weight. Use estimated lean body mass (dry weight) if the patient is obese or if there has been a spurious weight gain caused by edema, ascites, or other forms of abnormal fluid retention.

The following doses are for administration of procarbazine as a single agent. When used in combination with other anticancer drugs, appropriately reduce procarbazine dosage (eg, in the MOPP regimen, the procarbazine dose is 100 mg/m^2 daily for 14 days).

➤*Adults:* To minimize nausea and vomiting, give single or divided doses of 2 to 4 mg/kg/day for the first week. Maintain daily dosage at 4 to 6 mg/kg/day until the WBC falls below 4000/mm^3, the platelets fall below 100,000/mm^3, or until maximum response is obtained. Upon evidence of hematologic toxicity, discontinue the drug until there has been satisfactory recovery, then resume treatment at 1 to 2 mg/kg/day. When maximum response is obtained, maintain the dose at 1 to 2 mg/kg/day.

➤*Children:* Close clinical monitoring is mandatory. Toxicity, evidenced by tremors, coma, and convulsions, has occurred. Individualize dosage. This dosage schedule is a guideline only: 50 mg/m^2 daily for the first week. Maintain daily dosage at 100 mg/m^2 until leukopenia or thrombocytopenia occurs or until maximum response is obtained. Upon evidence of hematologic or other toxicity, discontinue drug until there has been satisfactory response. When maximum response is attained, maintain the dose at 50 mg/m^2/day.

Actions

➤*Pharmacology:* The mode of cytotoxic action is not clear; procarbazine may inhibit protein, ribonucleic acid (RNA), and deoxyribonucleic acid (DNA) synthesis. Procarbazine may inhibit transmethylation of methyl groups of methionine into t-RNA. The absence of functional t-RNA could cause the cessation of protein synthesis and consequently DNA and RNA synthesis. In addition, procarbazine may directly damage DNA. Hydrogen peroxide, formed during the auto-oxidation of the drug, may attack protein sulfhydryl groups contained in residual protein that is tightly bound to DNA. Procarbazine does exhibit some monoamine oxidase inhibitory (MAOI) activity.

➤*Pharmacokinetics:*

Absorption/Distribution – Procarbazine is rapidly and completely absorbed from the GI tract and quickly equilibrates between plasma and cerebrospinal fluid (CSF). Following oral administration, maximum peak plasma concentrations occur within 60 minutes.

Metabolism/Excretion – Procarbazine is metabolized in the liver and kidneys to cytotoxic products. The major portion of drug is excreted in the urine as N-isopropylterephthalamic acid (approximately 70% within 24 hours following oral and IV administration). Less than 5% is excreted in urine unchanged.

After IV injection, the plasma half-life is approximately 10 minutes. Procarbazine crosses the blood-brain barrier.

Contraindications

Hypersensitivity to procarbazine; inadequate marrow reserve demonstrated by bone marrow aspiration (consider in any patient with leukopenia, thrombocytopenia, or anemia).

Warnings

➤*Hematologic effects:* If radiation or a chemotherapeutic agent known to have marrow-depressant activity has been used, an interval of 1 month or longer without such therapy is recommended before starting treatment with procarbazine. Bone marrow depression often occurs 2 to 8 weeks after the start of treatment. Toxicity common to many hydrazine derivatives includes hemolysis and the appearance of Heinz-Erlich.

Discontinue therapy if any of the following occurs: Leukopenia (WBC less than 4000/mm^3); thrombocytopenia (platelets less than 100,000/mm^3); hemorrhage or bleeding tendencies.

➤*CNS effects:* Discontinue therapy if CNS signs or symptoms such as paresthesias, neuropathies, or confusion occur.

➤*GI effects:* Discontinue therapy if stomatitis (the first small ulceration or persistent spot soreness around the oral cavity) or diarrhea with frequent bowel movements or watery stools occur.

➤*Renal/Hepatic function impairment:* Undue toxicity may occur if used in patients with known renal or hepatic function impairment. Consider hospitalization for the initial treatment course.

➤*Carcinogenesis:* Carcinogenesis in mice, rats, and monkeys has been reported including: Instances of a second nonlymphoid malignancy, including lung cancer and acute myelocytic leukemia (in patients with Hodgkin disease treated with procarbazine in combination with other chemotherapy or radiation). The risks of secondary lung cancer from treatment appear to be multiplied by tobacco use. The International Agency for Research on Cancer (IARC) considers that there is "sufficient evidence" for the human carcinogenicity of procarbazine when it is given in intensive regimens that include other antineoplastic agents but there is inadequate evidence of carcinogenicity in humans given procarbazine alone.

➤*Mutagenesis:* Procarbazine is mutagenic in a variety of bacterial and mammalian test systems.

➤*Fertility impairment:* Azoospermia and antifertility effects associated with procarbazine coadministered with other antineoplastics for treating Hodgkin disease have been reported in human clinical studies. Since these patients received multicombination therapy, it is difficult to determine to what extent procarbazine alone was involved in the male germ-cell damage. Compounds that inhibit DNA, RNA, and/or protein synthesis might be expected to have adverse effects on gametogenesis. Unscheduled DNA synthesis in the testes of rabbits and decreased fertility in male mice treated with procarbazine have been reported.

➤*Pregnancy: Category D.* Procarbazine can cause fetal harm when administered to a pregnant woman. There are no adequate and well-controlled studies in pregnant women. If this drug is used during pregnancy, inform the patient of the potential hazard to the fetus. Advise women of childbearing potential to avoid pregnancy.

Administration in the first trimester of pregnancy has been described in 5 patients; congenital malformations were observed in 4. The other pregnancy was electively terminated. When combined with other antineoplastics, procarbazine may produce gonadal dysfunction in males and females. Use only when clearly needed and when the potential benefits outweigh the potential hazards.

Procarbazine is teratogenic in the rat when given at doses approximately 4 to 13 times the maximum recommended human therapeutic dose of 6 mg/kg/day. Neurogenic tumors were noted in the offspring of rats given IV injections of 125 mg/kg procarbazine on day 22 of gestation. Compounds that inhibit DNA, RNA, and protein synthesis might be expected to have adverse effects in peri- and postnatal development.

➤*Lactation:* It is not known whether procarbazine is excreted in human milk. Because of the potential for tumorigenicity shown in animal studies, advise mothers to not nurse while receiving this drug.

➤*Children:* Close clinical monitoring is mandatory. Toxicity, evidenced by tremors, convulsions, and coma, has occurred. (See Administration and Dosage.)

Precautions

➤*Monitoring:* Obtain baseline laboratory data prior to initiation of therapy. Monitor hemoglobin, hematocrit, WBC, differential, reticulocytes, and platelets at least every 3 or 4 days. Bone marrow depression often occurs 2 to 8 weeks after the start of treatment.

Evaluate hepatic and renal function prior to initiation of therapy.

Repeat urinalysis, transaminases, alkaline phosphatase, and BUN at least weekly.

➤*Discontinue therapy:* Prompt cessation of therapy is recommended when the following occur: CNS symptoms such as paresthesias, neuropathies, or confusion; leukopenia (WBC less than 4000/mm^3); thrombocytopenia (platelets less than 100,000/mm^3); hypersensitivity reaction; stomatitis (first small ulceration or persistent spot soreness around the oral cavity); diarrhea with frequent bowel movements or watery stools; hemorrhage or bleeding tendencies.

Drug Interactions

Procarbazine Drug Interactions			
Precipitant drug	Object drug*		Description
Procarbazine	CNS depressants (ie, narcotics, hypotensive agents, phenothiazines, antihistamines, barbiturates, sedatives)	↑	Concomitant use may result in depressant effects on the CNS (ie, respiratory depression).

PROCARBAZINE HCl (N-Methylhydrazine; MIH)

Procarbazine Drug Interactions			
Precipitant drug	Object drug*		Description
Procarbazine	Ethanol	↑	Concomitant ingestion has resulted in a disulfiram-like reaction (ie, flushing of the face).
Procarbazine	Methotrexate	↑	The nephrotoxicity of methotrexate may be increased; consider an interval of ≥ 72 hours between administration of the final dose of procarbazine and the initiation of a high-dose methotrexate infusion.
Procarbazine	Sympatho-mimetics (eg, ephedrine, epinephrine)	↑	May cause an abrupt increase in blood pressure, resulting in a potentially fatal hypertensive crisis.
Procarbazine	Tricyclic antidepressants (eg, amitriptyline, imipramine)	↑	Severe toxic and fatal reactions including excitability, fluctuations in blood pressure, convulsions, and coma may occur. However, some studies report uneventful concurrent use with MAOIs.
Procarbazine	Radiation or other chemotherapy	↑	If radiation or other chemotherapy known to have marrow depressant activity has been used, wait ≥ 1 month before starting procarbazine. Interval length may also be determined by evidence of bone marrow recovery based on successive bone marrow studies.

* ↑ = Object drug increased. ↓ = Object drug decreased.

➤*Drug/Food interactions:* Ingestion of foods with high tyramine content (ie, red wine, yogurt, ripe cheese, bananas) (see the Monoamine Oxidase Inhibitors monograph) may cause an abrupt increase in blood pressure, resulting in a potentially fatal hypertensive crisis. However, none of these reactions have been currently reported.

Adverse Reactions

➤*Cardiovascular:* Hypotension; tachycardia; syncope.

➤*CNS:* Paresthesias and neuropathies; headache; dizziness; depression; apprehension; nervousness; insomnia; nightmares; hallucinations; falling; weakness; fatigue; lethargy; drowsiness; unsteadiness; ataxia; foot drop; decreased reflexes; tremors; coma; confusion; convulsions.

➤*Dermatologic:* Dermatitis; pruritus; rash; urticaria; herpes; hyperpigmentation; flushing; alopecia; diaphoresis.

➤*Endocrine:* Gynecomastia in prepubertal and early pubertal boys.

➤*GI:* Nausea, vomiting (frequent); anorexia; stomatitis; dry mouth; dysphagia; abdominal pain; hematemesis; melena; diarrhea; constipation.

➤*GU:* Hematuria; urinary frequency; nocturia.

➤*Hematologic:* Leukopenia, anemia, thrombocytopenia (frequent); pancytopenia; eosinophilia; hemolytic anemia; bleeding tendencies such as petechiae, purpura, epistaxis, hemoptysis.

➤*Hepatic:* Jaundice; hepatic dysfunction.

➤*Ophthalmic:* Retinal hemorrhage; nystagmus; photophobia; diplopia; inability to focus; papilledema.

➤*Respiratory:* Pleural effusion; pneumonitis; cough.

➤*Miscellaneous:* Pain, including myalgia and arthralgia; pyrexia; chills; intercurrent infections; edema; hoarseness; generalized allergic reactions; hearing loss; slurred speech.

Second nonlymphoid malignancies, including lung cancer, acute myelocytic leukemia, and malignant myelosclerosis and azoospermia, have been reported in patients with Hodgkin disease treated with procarbazine in combination with other chemotherapy and/or radiation. The risks of secondary lung cancer from treatment appear to be multiplied by tobacco use.

Overdosage

➤*Symptoms:* The major manifestations of overdosage with procarbazine would be anticipated to be nausea, vomiting, enteritis, diarrhea, hypotension, tremors, convulsions, and coma.

➤*Treatment:* Treatment consists of either the administration of an emetic or gastric lavage. Use general supportive measures such as IV fluids. Since the major toxicity of procarbazine is hematologic and hepatic, perform frequent complete blood counts and liver function tests throughout the recovery period and for a minimum of 2 weeks thereafter. Immediately undertake appropriate measures for correction and stabilization should abnormalities appear in any of these determinations.

Patient Information

May produce drowsiness and dizziness; patients should observe caution while driving or performing other tasks requiring alertness.

Consumption of alcoholic beverages while taking procarbazine may cause a disulfiram-like reaction.

Avoid ingestion of the following: Tyramine-containing foods (ie, red wine, yogurt, ripe cheese, bananas) (see the Monamine Oxidase Inhibitors monograph), certain cold, hay fever, or weight-reducing preparations containing sympathomimetics (see Drug Interactions). Avoid or discontinue tobacco use.

Notify physician if cough, shortness of breath, thickened bronchial secretions, fever, chills, sore throat, unusual bleeding or bruising, black tarry stools, or vomiting of blood occurs.

Medication may cause muscle or joint pain, nausea, vomiting, tiredness, weakness, constipation, headache, difficulty swallowing, loss of appetite, loss of hair, and mental depression. Notify physician if these become pronounced.

Contraceptive measures are recommended during therapy for both men and women.

TEMOZOLOMIDE

Rx	Temodar (Schering)	Capsules: 5 mg	In 5s and 20s.
		20 mg	In 5s and 20s.
		100 mg	In 5s and 20s.
		250 mg	In 5s and 20s.

Indications

➤*Anaplastic astrocytoma:* Treatment of adult patients with refractory anaplastic astrocytoma (ie, patients at first relapse who have experienced disease progression on a drug regimen containing a nitrosourea and procarbazine).

Administration and Dosage

➤*Approved by the FDA:* August 11, 1999.

Adjust the temozolomide dosage according to nadir neutrophil and platelet counts in the previous cycle and neutrophil and platelet counts at the time of initiation of the next cycle. The initial dose is 150 mg/m² orally once daily for 5 consecutive days per 28-day treatment cycle. If both the nadir and day of dosing (day 29, day 1 of next cycle) ANC are ≥ 1.5 x 10⁹/L (1500/mcl) and both the nadir and day 29 (day 1 of next cycle) platelet counts are ≥ 100 x 10⁹/L (100,000/mcl), the temozolomide dose may be increased to 200 mg/m²/day for 5 consecutive days per 28-day treatment cycle. During treatment, obtain a complete blood count on day 22 (21 days after the first dose) or within 48 hours of that day, and weekly until the ANC is > 1.5 x 10⁹/L (1500/mcl) and the platelet count exceeds 100 x 10⁹/L (100,000/mcl). Do not start the next cycle of temozolomide until the ANC and platelet count exceed these levels. If the ANC falls to < 1 x 10⁹/L (1000/mcl) or the platelet count is < 50 x 10⁹/L (50,000/mcl) during any cycle, reduce the next cycle by 50 mg/m², but not < 100 mg/m², the lowest recommended dose (see table).

Temozolomide Dosing Modifications	
Day 1	Administer 150 mg/m²/day x 5 days (starting dose) or 200 mg/m²/day x 5 days
Day 22 and Day 29 (day 1 of next cycle)	Measure ANC and platelets:
	If ANC < 1000/mcl or platelets < 50,000/mcl, postpone therapy until ANC > 1500/mcl and platelets > 100,000/mcl; reduce dose by 50 mg/m²/day for subsequent cycle.
	If ANC 1000 to 1500 /mcl or platelets 50,000 to 100,000/mcl, postpone therapy until ANC > 1500/mcl and platelets> 100,000/mcl; maintain initial dose.
	If ANC ≥ 1500/mcl and platelets ≥ 100,000/mcl, increase dose to, or maintain dose at, 200 mg/m²/day x 5 days for subsequent cycle.

Temozolomide therapy can be continued until disease progression. In the clinical trial, treatment could be continued for a maximum of 2 years, but the optimum duration of therapy is not known. For temozolomide dosage calculations based on body surface area (BSA) and for suggested capsule combinations based on daily dose, see following tables.

Daily Dose Calculations of Temozolomide by BSA[1]		
Total BSA (m²)	150 mg/m² (mg/daily)	200 mg/m² (mg daily)
0.5	75	100
0.6	90	120
0.7	105	140
0.8	120	160
0.9	135	180
1	150	200
1.1	165	220
1.2	180	240
1.3	195	260
1.4	210	280
1.5	225	300
1.6	240	320
1.7	255	340
1.8	270	360
1.9	285	380
2	300	400
2.1	315	420

Daily Dose Calculations of Temozolomide by BSA[1]		
Total BSA (m²)	150 mg/m² (mg/daily)	200 mg/m² (mg daily)
2.2	330	440
2.3	345	460
2.4	360	480
2.5	375	500

[1] Daily dose calculations by BSA for 5 consecutive days per 28-day treatment cycle for the initial chemotherapy cycle (150 mg/m²) and for subsequent chemotherapy cycles (200 mg/m²) for patients whose nadir and day of dosing (day 29, day 1 of next cycle) ANC is > 1.5 x 10⁹/L (1500/mcl) and whose nadir and day 29, day 1 of next cycle platelet count is > 100 x 10⁹/L (100,000/mcl).

Suggested Temozolomide Capsule Combinations Based on Daily Dose				
	Number of daily capsules by strength (mg)			
Total daily dose (mg)	250	100	20	5
200	0	2	0	0
205	0	2	0	1
210	0	2	0	2
215	0	2	0	3
220	0	2	1	0
225	0	2	1	1
230	0	2	1	2
235	0	2	1	3
240	0	2	2	0
245	0	2	2	1
250	1	0	0	0
255	1	0	0	1
260	1	0	0	2
265	1	0	0	3
270	1	0	1	0
275	1	0	1	1
280	1	0	1	2
285	1	0	1	3
290	1	0	2	0
295	1	0	2	1
300	0	3	0	0
305	0	3	0	1
310	0	3	0	2
315	0	3	0	3
320	0	3	1	0
325	0	3	1	1
330	1	0	4	0
335	1	0	4	1
340	0	3	2	0
345	0	3	2	1
350	1	1	0	0
355	1	1	0	1
360	1	1	0	2
365	1	1	0	3
370	1	1	1	0
375	1	1	1	1
380	1	1	1	2
385	1	1	1	3
390	1	1	2	0
395	1	1	2	1
400	0	4	0	0
405	0	4	0	1
410	0	4	0	2
415	0	4	0	3
420	0	4	1	0
425	0	4	1	1

TEMOZOLOMIDE

Suggested Temozolomide Capsule Combinations Based on Daily Dose				
	Number of daily capsules by strength (mg)			
Total daily dose (mg)	250	100	20	5
430	1	1	4	0
435	0	4	1	3
440	0	4	2	0
445	0	4	2	1
450	1	2	0	0
455	1	2	0	1
460	1	2	0	2
465	1	2	0	3
470	1	2	1	0
475	1	2	1	1
480	1	2	1	2
485	1	2	1	3
490	1	2	2	0
495	1	2	2	1
500	2	0	0	0

Absorption is affected by food; consistency of administration with respect to food is recommended. There are no dietary restrictions with temozolomide. To reduce nausea and vomiting, take temozolomide on an empty stomach. Administer at bedtime. Antiemetic therapy may be administered prior to or following temozolomide administration.

Do not open or chew temozolomide capsules. Swallow the capsules whole with a glass of water.

➤*Handling and disposal:* Temozolomide causes the rapid appearance of malignant tumors in rats. Do not open capsules. If capsules are accidentally opened or damaged, take rigorous precautions with the capsule contents to avoid inhalation or contact with the skin or mucous membranes. Consider procedures for proper handling and disposal of anticancer drugs.

Actions

➤*Pharmacology:* Temozolomide, an antineoplastic agent, is an imidazotetrazine derivative. Temozolomide is a pro-drug that undergoes rapid nonenzymatic conversion at physiologic pH to the reactive compound 3-methyl-(triazen-1-yl)imidazole-4-carboxamide (MTIC). MTIC's cytotoxicity and antiproliferative activity against tumor cells are thought to be primarily caused by methylation of specific guanine-rich areas of DNA that initiates transcription. Methylation occurs mainly at the O^6 and N^7 positions of guanine.

➤*Pharmacokinetics:*

Absorption – Temozolomide is rapidly and completely absorbed after oral administration, demonstrating a 98% oral bioavailability. Peak plasma concentrations occur in 1 hour. Food reduces the rate and extent of temozolomide absorption.

Distribution – Temozolomide has a mean apparent volume of distribution of 0.4 L/kg. It is weakly bound to human plasma proteins; the mean percent bound of drug-related total radioactivity is 15%. Penetration across the blood-brain barrier has been documented.

Metabolism – Temozolomide is spontaneously hydrolyzed at mildly alkaline pH to produce the active species, MTIC, and to the temozolomide acid metabolite. MTIC is further hydrolyzed to 5-amino-imidazole-4-carboxamide (AIC), which is known to be an intermediate in purine and nucleic acid biosynthesis and to methylhydrazine, which is believed to be the active alkylating species. Cytochrome P450 enzymes play a minor role in the metabolism of temozolomide and MTIC. Relative to the AUC of temozolomide, the exposure is 2.4% to MTIC and 23% to AIC.

Excretion – About 38% of the administered temozolomide total dose is recovered over 7 days; 37.7% in urine and 0.8% in feces. The majority of the urinary recovery includes the following: Unchanged temozolomide (5.6%), AIC (12%), temozolomide acid metabolite (2.3%), and unidentified polar metabolite(s) (17%). Overall clearance is 5.5 L/hr/m^2. Temozolomide is rapidly eliminated with a mean elimination half-life of 1.8 hours, and linear kinetics are exhibited over the therapeutic dosing range.

Special populations –

Gender: Population pharmacokinetic analysis indicates that women have an ≈ 5% lower clearance (adjusted for body surface area) for temozolomide than men. Women have higher incidences than men of Grade 4 neutropenia and thrombocytopenia in the first cycle of therapy (see Adverse Reactions).

Contraindications

Hypersensitivity reaction to any component of the product; hypersensitivity to dacarbazine (DTIC) because both drugs are metabolized to MTIC.

Warnings

➤*Myelosuppression:* Patients treated with temozolomide may experience myelosuppression. Prior to dosing, patients must have an absolute neutrophil count (ANC) ≥ 1.5 x 10^9/L and a platelet count ≥ 100 x 10^9/L. Obtain a complete blood count on day 22 (21 days after the first dose) or within 48 hours of that day, and weekly until the ANC is > 1.5 x 10^9/L and platelet count is 100 x 10^9/L. In the clinical trials, if the ANC fell to < 1 x 10^9/L or the platelet count was < 50 x 10^9/L during any cycle, the next cycle was reduced by 50 mg/m^2 but not below 100 mg/m^2. Do not administer temozolomide to patients who do not tolerate 100 mg/m^2. Elderly patients and women have been shown in clinical trials to have a higher risk of developing myelosuppression. Myelosuppression generally occurred late in the treatment cycle. The median nadirs occurred at 26 days for platelets (range, 21 to 40 days) and 28 days for neutrophils (range, 1 to 44 days). Only 14% (22/158) of patients had a neutrophil nadir and 20% (32/158) of patients had a platelet nadir that may have delayed the start of the next cycle. Neutrophil and platelet counts returned to normal, on average, within 14 days of nadir counts.

➤*Recurrent anaplastic astrocytoma:* No results are available from randomized controlled trials of recurrent anaplastic astrocytoma that demonstrate a clinical benefit resulting from treatment, such as improvement in disease-related symptoms, delayed disease progression, or improved survival.

➤*Renal function impairment:* Population pharmacokinetic analysis indicates that creatinine clearance over the range of 36 to 130 ml/min/m^2 has no effect on the clearance of temozolomide after oral administration. Exercise caution when administering temozolomide to patients with severe renal impairment. Temozolomide has not been studied in patients on dialysis.

➤*Hepatic function impairment:* In one study, the pharmacokinetics of temozolomide in patients with mild-to-moderate hepatic impairment (Child's-Pugh class I to II) were similar to those observed in patients with normal hepatic function. Exercise caution when temozolomide is administered to patients with severe hepatic impairment.

➤*Carcinogenesis:* In rats treated with 200 mg/m^2 temozolomide (equivalent to the maximum recommended daily human dose) on 5 consecutive days every 28 days for 3 cycles, mammary carcinomas were found in males and females. With 6 cycles of treatment at 25, 50, and 125 mg/m^2 (≈ ⅛ to ½ the maximum recommended daily human dose), mammary carcinomas were observed at all doses and fibrosarcomas of the heart, eye, seminal vesicles, salivary glands, abdominal cavity, uterus, and prostate; carcinoma of the seminal vesicles, schwannoma of the heart, optic nerve, and harderian gland; and adenomas of the skin, lung, pituitary, and thyroid were observed at the high dose.

➤*Mutagenesis:* Temozolomide was mutagenic in vitro in bacteria (Ames assay) and clastogenic in mammalian cells (human peripheral blood lymphocyte assays).

➤*Fertility impairment:* Multicycle toxicology studies in rats and dogs have demonstrated testicular toxicity (syncytial cells/immature sperm, testicular atrophy) at doses of 50 mg/m^2 in rats and 125 mg/m^2 in dogs (¼ and ⅝, respectively, of the maximum recommended human dose on a body surface area basis).

➤*Elderly:* Clinical studies of temozolomide did not include sufficient numbers of subjects ≥ 65 years of age to determine whether they responded differently than younger subjects. Other reported clinical experience has not identified differences in responses between the elderly and younger patients. Exercise caution when treating elderly patients. In the anaplastic astrocytoma study population, patients ≥ 70 years of age had a higher incidence of Grade 4 neutropenia and Grade 4 thrombocytopenia (2/8; 25%, and 2/10; 20%, respectively) in the first cycle of therapy than patients < 70 years of age (see Adverse Reactions).

➤*Pregnancy: Category D.* Temozolomide may cause fetal harm when administered to a pregnant woman. Five consecutive days of oral administration of 75 mg/m^2/day in rats and 150 mg/m^2/day in rabbits during organogenesis (⅜ and ¾ the maximum recommended human dose, respectively) caused numerous malformations of the external organs, soft tissues, and skeleton in both species. Doses of 150 mg/m^2/day in rats and rabbits also caused embryolethality as indicated by increased resorptions. If this drug is used during pregnancy or if the patient becomes pregnant while taking this drug, apprise her of the potential hazard to the fetus. Advise women of childbearing potential to avoid becoming pregnant during therapy with temozolomide.

➤*Lactation:* It is not known whether this drug is excreted in breast milk. Because of the potential for serious adverse reactions in nursing infants from temozolomide, patients receiving temozolomide should discontinue nursing.

➤*Children:* Safety and efficacy in pediatric patients have not been established.

Precautions

➤*Monitoring:* Obtain a complete blood count on day 22 (21 days after the first dose). Perform blood counts weekly until recovery if the ANC is < 1.5 x 10^9/L and the platelet count is < 100 x 10^9/L.

TEMOZOLOMIDE

Drug Interactions

➤*Valproic acid:* Administration of valproic acid decreases oral clearance of temozolomide by ≈ 5%. The clinical implication of this effect is not known.

➤*Drug/Food interactions:* Food reduces the rate and extent of temozolomide absorption. Mean peak plasma concentration and AUC were decreased by 32% and 9%, respectively, and T_{max} was increased 2-fold (from 1.1 to 2.25 hours) when temozolomide was administered after a modified high-fat breakfast.

Adverse Reactions

The most frequently occurring side effects were nausea, vomiting, headache, and fatigue. The adverse events were usually NCI common toxicity criteria (CTC) Grade 1 or 2 (mild-to-moderate in severity) and were self-limiting, with nausea and vomiting readily controlled with antiemetics. The incidence of severe nausea and vomiting (CTC grade 3 or 4) was 10% and 6%, respectively.

Myelosuppression – Myelosuppression (thrombocytopenia and neutropenia) was the dose-limiting adverse event. It usually occurred within the first few cycles of therapy and was not cumulative. Myelosuppression occurred late in the treatment cycle and returned to normal, on average, within 14 days of nadir counts. The median nadirs occurred at 26 days for platelets (range, 21 to 40 days) and 28 days for neutrophils (range, 1 to 44 days). Only 14% ($22/158$) of patients had a neutrophil nadir, and 20% ($32/158$) of patients had a platelet nadir, which may have delayed the start of the next cycle (see Warnings). Less than 10% of patients required hospitalization, blood transfusion, or discontinuation of therapy because of myelosuppression.

In clinical trials, there were higher rates of Grade 4 neutropenia (ANC < 500 cells/mcl) and thrombocytopenia (< 20,000 cells/mcl) in women than in men in the first cycle of therapy (12% vs 5% and 9% vs 3%, respectively).

In 932 patients, 7% (4/61) and 9.5% (6/63) of patients > 70 years of age experienced Grade 4 neutropenia or thrombocytopenia in the first cycle, respectively. For patients ≤ 70 years of age, 7% (62/871) and 5.5% (48/879) experienced Grade 4 neutropenia or thrombocytopenia in the first cycle, respectively.

Temozolomide Adverse Reactions (≥ 5%)

Adverse reaction	All events (n = 153)	Grade 3/4 (n = 79)
CNS		
Convulsions	23	5
Hemiparesis	18	6
Dizziness	12	1
Abnormal coordination	11	1
Amnesia	10	4
Insomnia	10	0
Paresthesia	9	1
Somnolence	9	3
Paresis	8	3
Ataxia	8	2
Anxiety	7	1
Dysphasia	7	1
Convulsions, local	6	0
Depression	6	0
Abnormal gait	6	1
Confusion	5	0
Dermatologic		
Rash	8	0
Pruritus	8	1
GI		
Nausea	53	10
Vomiting	42	6

Temozolomide Adverse Reactions (≥ 5%)

Adverse reaction	All events (n = 153)	Grade 3/4 (n = 79)
Constipation	33	1
Diarrhea	16	2
Abdominal pain	9	1
Anorexia	9	1
GU		
Urinary incontinence	8	2
Urinary tract infection	8	0
Micturition increased/frequency	6	0
Respiratory		
Upper respiratory tract infection	8	0
Pharyngitis	8	0
Sinusitis	6	0
Coughing	5	0
Special senses		
Diplopia	5	0
Vision abnormal[1]	5	
Miscellaneous		
Headache	41	6
Fatigue	34	4
Asthenia	13	6
Fever	13	2
Edema, peripheral	11	1
Infection, viral	11	0
Back pain	8	3
Adrenal hypercorticism	8	0
Weight increase	5	0
Myalgia	5	
Breast pain, female	6	

[1] Blurred vision, visual deficit, vision changes, vision troubles.

Temozolomide Adverse Hematologic Effects (Grade 3 to 4)

	Temozolomide[1]
Hemoglobin	4%
Neutrophils	14%
Platelets	19%
WBC	11%

[1] Change from grade 0 to 2 at baseline to grade 3 or 4 during treatment.

Overdosage

Doses of 500, 750, 1000, and 1250 mg/m² (total dose per cycle over 5 days) have been evaluated clinically in patients. Dose-limiting toxicity was hematologic and was reported at 1000 and at 1250 mg/m². Up to 1000 mg/m² has been taken as a single dose, with only the expected effects of neutropenia and thrombocytopenia resulting. In the event of an overdose, hematologic evaluation is needed. Provide supportive measures as necessary.

Patient Information

In clinical trials, the most frequently occurring adverse effects were nausea and vomiting. These were usually self-limiting or readily controlled with standard anti-emetic therapy.

There are no dietary restrictions with temozolomide. To reduce nausea and vomiting, take temozolomide on an empty stomach.

Do not open capsules. If capsules are accidentally opened or damaged, take rigorous precautions with the capsule contents to avoid inhalation or contact with the skin or mucous membranes.

Keep the medication away from children and pets.

AMIFOSTINE

Rx	**Ethyol** (MedImmune Oncology)	**Powder for Injection, lyophilized:** 500 mg (anhydrous basis)	In 10 ml single-use vials.

Indications

➤*Renal toxicity:* Reduction of cumulative renal toxicity associated with repeated administration of cisplatin in patients with advanced ovarian cancer or non-small cell lung cancer.

➤*Xerostomia:* Reduction of the incidence of moderate-to-severe xerostomia in patients undergoing postoperative radiation treatment for head and neck cancer, where the radiation port includes a substantial portion of the parotid glands.

➤*Unlabeled uses:* To prevent or reduce cisplatin-induced neurotoxicity and cyclophosphamide-induced granulocytopenia; prevent or reduce toxicity of radiation therapy to other areas; reduce toxicity of paclitaxel.

Administration and Dosage

➤*Reduction of cumulative renal toxicity with chemotherapy:* Recommended starting dose is 910 mg/m² administered once daily as a 15-minute IV infusion, starting 30 minutes prior to chemotherapy. The 15-minute infusion is better tolerated than more extended infusions.

Adequately hydrate patients prior to amifostine infusion, and keep them in a supine position during the infusion. Monitor blood pressure every 5 minutes during the infusion and thereafter as clinically indicated.

Interrupt the infusion of amifostine if the systolic blood pressure decreases significantly from the baseline value as listed in the guideline below.

Guideline for Interrupting Amifostine Infusion Due to Decrease in Systolic Blood Pressure					
	Baseline Systolic Blood Pressure (mmHg)				
	< 100	100 to 119	120 to 139	140 to 179	≥ 180
Decrease in systolic blood pressure during infusion of amifostine (mmHg)	20	25	30	40	50

If hypotension requiring interruption of therapy occurs, place patients in either the Trendelenburg or supine position and administer a Normal Saline solution using a separate IV line. If the blood pressure returns to normal within 5 minutes and the patient is asymptomatic, the infusion may be restarted so that the full dose of amifostine may be administered. If the full dose of amifostine cannot be administered, the dose of amifostine for subsequent cycles should be 740 mg/m².

It is recommended that antiemetic medication, including dexamethasone 20 mg IV and a serotonin 5HT₃ receptor antagonist, be administered prior to and in conjunction with amifostine. Additional antiemetics may be required based on the chemotherapy drugs concomitantly administered.

➤*Reduction of moderate-to-severe xerostomia from radiation of the head and neck:* 200 mg/m² administered once daily as a 3-minute IV infusion 15 to 30 minutes prior to standard fraction radiation therapy (1.8 to 2 Gy).

Adequately hydrate patients prior to amifostine infusion. Monitor blood pressure before and immediately after the infusion and as clinically indicated.

Administer antiemetic medication prior to and in conjunction with amifostine. Oral 5HT₃ receptor antagonists, alone or in combination with other antiemetics, have been used effectively in the radiotherapy setting.

➤*Reconstitution:* Reconstitute with 9.7 ml of 0.9% Sodium Chloride Injection.

➤*Admixture incompatibility:* The compatibility of amifostine with solutions other than 0.9% Sodium Chloride for Injection, or sodium chloride solutions with other additives, has not been studied and is not recommended. The use of other solutions is not recommended.

➤*Storage/Stability:* Store the lyophilized dosage form at controlled room temperature (20° to 25°C; 68° to 77°F). The reconstituted solution is chemically stable for up to 5 hours at room temperature (≈ 25°C; 77°F) or up to 24 hours under refrigeration (2° to 8°C; 36° to 46°F).

Actions

➤*Pharmacology:* Amifostine is an organic thiophosphate cytoprotective agent. This pro-drug is dephosphorylated by alkaline phosphatase in tissues to a pharmacologically active free thiol metabolite that can reduce the renal toxicity of cisplatin and for the reduction of the toxic effects of radiation on normal oral tissues. The ability to differentially protect normal tissues is attributed to the higher capillary alkaline phosphatase activity, higher pH, and better vascularity of normal tissues relative to tumor tissue. The result is a more rapid generation of the active thiol metabolite as well as a higher rate constant for uptake into cells. The higher concentration of the thiol metabolite in normal tissues is thus available to bind to, and thereby detoxify, reactive metabolites of cisplatin. The thiol metabolites also scavenge reactive oxygen species generated by exposure to cisplatin or radiation.

➤*Pharmacokinetics:* Amifostine is rapidly cleared from the plasma with a distribution half-life of less than 1 minute and an elimination half-life of approximately 8 minutes. Less than 10% of amifostine remains in the plasma 6 minutes after drug administration. Amifostine is rapidly metabolized to an active free thiol metabolite. A disulfide metabolite is produced subsequently and is less active than the free thiol. After a 10-second bolus dose of amifostine 150 mg/m², renal excretion of the parent drug and its 2 metabolites was low during the hour following drug administration, averaging 0.69%, 2.64%, and 2.22% of the administered dose for the parent, thiol, and disulfide, respectively. Measurable levels of the free thiol metabolite have been found in bone marrow cells 5 to 8 minutes after IV infusion of amifostine.

➤*Clinical trials:* A randomized, controlled trial compared 6 cycles of cyclophosphamide 1000 mg/m² and cisplatin 100 mg/m² with or without amifostine pretreatment at 910 mg/m² in 121 patients with advanced ovarian cancer. Pretreatment with amifostine significantly reduced the cumulative renal toxicity associated with cisplatin as assessed by the proportion of patients who had a 40% or greater decrease in creatinine clearance from pretreatment values, protracted elevations in serum creatinine (more than 1.5 mg/dl), or severe hypomagnesemia.

A randomized, controlled trial of standard fractionated radiation (1.8 Gy to 2 Gy/day for 5 days/week for 5 to 7 weeks) with or without amifostine, administered at 200 mg/m² as a 3-minute IV infusion 15 to 30 minutes prior to each radiation fraction, was conducted in 315 patients with head and neck cancer. Patients were required to have at least 75% of both parotid glands in the radiation field. The incidence of Grade 2 or higher acute (90 days or less from start of radiation) and late xerostomia (9 to 12 months following radiation) as assessed by RTOG Acute and Late Morbidity Scoring Criteria, was significantly reduced in patients receiving amifostine.

Contraindications

Sensitivity to aminothiol compounds.

Warnings

➤*Hypersensitivity:* Allergic manifestations including anaphylaxis and severe cutaneous reactions have been associated rarely with amifostine administration. Serious cutaneous hypersensitivity reactions have included erythema multiforme, Stevens-Johnson syndrome, toxic epidermal necrolysis, toxoderma and exfoliative dermatitis, which have been reported more frequently when amifostine is used as a radioprotectant (see Adverse Reactions). Some of these reactions have been fatal or have required hospitalization and/or discontinuation of therapy. Patients should be carefully monitored prior to, during, and after amifostine administration.

In case of severe acute allergic reactions, amifostine should be immediately and permanently discontinued. Epinephrine and other appropriate measures should be available for treatment of serious allergic events such as anaphylaxis. Amifostine should also be permanently discontinued for serious or severe cutaneous reactions or for cutaneous reactions associated with fever or other constitutional symptoms not known to be due to another etiology. Amifostine should be withheld and dermatologic consultation and biopsy considered for cutaneous reactions or mucosal lesions of unknown etiology appearing outside of the injection site or radiation port and for erythematous, edematous, or bullous lesions on the palms of the hand or soles of the feet. Reinitiation of amifostine should be at the physician's discretion based on medical judgment and appropriate dermatologic evaluation.

➤*Effectiveness of the cytotoxic regimen:* Limited data are available on the preservation of antitumor efficacy when amifostine is administered prior to cisplatin therapy in settings other than advanced ovarian cancer or non-small cell lung cancer. Although some animal data suggest interference is possible, in most tumor models, the antitumor effects of chemotherapy are not altered by amifostine. Amifostine, therefore, should not be used in patients receiving chemotherapy for malignancies in which chemotherapy can produce a significant survival benefit or cure (eg, certain malignancies of germ cell origin), except in the context of a clinical study.

➤*Effectiveness of radiotherapy:* Do not administer amifostine in patients receiving definitive radiotherapy, except during a clinical trial, due to insufficient data to exclude a tumor-protective effect in this setting. Amifostine was studied only with standard fractionated radiotherapy and when at least 75% of both parotid glands were exposed to radiation. Amifostine's effects on the incidence of xerostomia, on toxicity in the setting of combined chemotherapy and radiotherapy, and in the setting of accelerated and hyperfractionated therapy have not been systematically studied.

➤*Hypotension:* In a randomized study of patients with ovarian cancer given 910 mg/m² amifostine prior to chemotherapy, transient hypotension occurred in 62% of patients treated. Mean time of onset was 14 minutes into the infusion; mean duration was 6 minutes. In some cases, the infusion had to be prematurely terminated because of a more pronounced drop in systolic pressure. In general, blood pressure

AMIFOSTINE

returns to normal within 5 to 15 minutes. Fewer than 3% of patients discontinued amifostine because of blood pressure reductions. In the randomized study of patients with head and neck cancer given amifostine at a dose of 200 mg/m² prior to radiotherapy, hypotension was observed in 15% of patients treated.

Patients who are hypotensive or dehydrated should not receive amifostine. Patients receiving amifostine at doses recommended for chemotherapy should have antihypertensive therapy interrupted 24 hours preceding administration of amifostine. Patients receiving amifostine at doses recommended for chemotherapy who are taking antihypertensive therapy that cannot be stopped for 24 hours preceding amifostine treatment also should not receive amifostine. Adequately hydrate patients prior to amifostine infusion, and keep in a supine position during the infusion. Monitor blood pressure every 5 minutes during the infusion, and thereafter as clinically indicated. It is important that the duration of the 910 mg/m² infusion not exceed 15 minutes, as administration as a longer infusion is associated with a higher incidence of side effects. Monitor blood pressure at least before and immediately after infusions with durations < 5 minutes, and thereafter as clinically indicated. If hypotension occurs, place patient in the Trendelenburg position and give an infusion of normal saline using a separate IV line. During and after amifostine infusion, take care to monitor the blood pressure of patients whose antihypertensive medication has been interrupted since hypertension may be exacerbated by discontinuation of antihypertensive medication and other causes such as IV hydration. Guidelines for interrupting and restarting amifostine infusion if a decrease in systolic blood pressure occurs are in Administration and Dosage. Hypotension may occur during or shortly after amifostine infusion, despite adequate hydration and positioning of the patient. Hypotension has been reported to be associated with dyspnea, apnea, hypoxia, and in rare cases seizures, unconsciousness, respiratory arrest, and renal failure.

➤**Nausea and vomiting:** Administer antiemetic medication prior to and in conjunction with amifostine. When amifostine is administered with highly emetogenic chemotherapy, carefully monitor the fluid balance of the patient.

➤**Hypocalcemia:** Monitor serum calcium levels in patients at risk of hypocalcemia, such as those with nephrotic syndrome or patients receiving multiple doses. If necessary, administer calcium supplements.

➤**Elderly:** Dose selection for an elderly patient should be cautious, reflecting the greater frequency of decreased hepatic, renal, or cardiac function and of concomitant disease or other drug therapy in elderly patients.

➤**Pregnancy:** Category C. Amifostine is embryotoxic in rabbits at doses of 50 mg/kg, approximately 60% of the recommended dose in humans on a body surface area basis. There are no adequate and well-controlled studies in pregnant women. Do not use during pregnancy unless the potential benefit justifies the potential risk to the fetus.

➤**Lactation:** No information is available on the excretion of amifostine or its metabolites into breast milk. Discontinue breastfeeding if treating with amifostine.

➤**Children:** Safety and efficacy have not been established.

Precautions

➤**Monitoring:** Monitor serum calcium levels in patients at risk of hypocalcemia, such as those with nephrotic syndrome or patients receiving multiple doses of amifostine. When used prior to chemotherapy, monitor blood pressure every 5 minutes during the infusion and thereafter as clinically indicated. When used prior to radiation therapy, monitor blood pressure at least before and immediately after the infusion and thereafter as clinically indicated.

➤**Special risk:** Safety has not been established in elderly patients, or patients with preexisting cardiovascular or cerebrovascular conditions such as ischemic heart disease, arrhythmias, CHF, or history of stroke or transient ischemic attacks. Use amifostine with particular care in these and other patients in whom the common amifostine adverse effects of nausea/vomiting and hypotension may be more likely to have serious consequences.

Drug Interactions

➤**Antihypertensives:** Give special consideration to amifostine administration in patients receiving antihypertensive medications or other drugs that could cause or potentiate hypotension.

Adverse Reactions

➤**Cardiovascular:** Hypotension, usually brief systolic and diastolic, has been associated with one or more of the following adverse events: Apnea, dyspnea, hypoxia, tachycardia, bradycardia, extrasystoles, chest pain, myocardial ischemia, and convulsion. Rare cases of renal failure, MI, respiratory and cardiac arrest have been observed during or after hypotension (see Warnings).

Rare cases of arrhythmias such as atrial fibrillation/flutter and supraventricular tachycardia have been reported. These are sometimes associated with hypotension or allergic reactions.

Transient hypertension and exacerbations of pre-existing hypertension have been observed rarely after amifostine administration.

➤**GI:** Nausea and/or vomiting occur frequently after amifostine infusion and may be severe. In the ovarian cancer randomized study, the incidence of severe nausea/vomiting on day 1 of cyclophosphamide-cisplatin chemotherapy was 10% in patients who did not receive amifostine and 19% in patients who did receive amifostine. In the randomized study of patients with head and neck cancer, the incidence of severe nausea/vomiting was 8% in patients who received amifostine and 1% in patients who did not receive amifostine.

➤**Hypersensitivity:** Hypotension; fever; chills/rigors; dyspnea; cutaneous eruptions; urticaria; hypoxia; laryngeal edema; chest tightness; cardiac arrest. Other skin reactions including erythema multiforme, and in rare cases, Stevens-Johnson syndrome and toxic epidermal necrolysis, have been reported. There have been rare reports of anaphylactoid reactions.

➤**Miscellaneous:** Hypocalcemia (< 1%; see Warnings); hypotension (see Warnings); short-term, reversible loss of consciousness, seizures, syncope (rare); flushing/feeling of warmth; chills/feeling of coldness; fever; dizziness; somnolence; hiccoughs; sneezing.

Overdosage

In clinical trials, the maximum single dose of amifostine was 1300 mg/m². Children have received single doses of up to 2700 mg/m². At the higher doses, anxiety and reversible urinary retention occurred. Administration of amifostine at 2 and 4 hours after the initial dose has not led to increased nausea and vomiting or hypotension. The most likely symptom of overdosage is hypotension; manage by infusion of normal saline and other supportive measures as clinically indicated.

DEXRAZOXANE

| Rx | Zinecard (Pfizer) | Powder for Injection, lyophilized: 250 mg (10 mg/mL reconstituted) | In single-use vials with 25 mL vial sodium lactate injection. |
| | | 500 mg (10 mg/mL reconstituted) | In single-use vials with 50 mL vial sodium lactate injection. |

Indications

➤**Cardiomyopathy:** Reduction of the incidence and severity of cardiomyopathy associated with doxorubicin administration in women with metastatic breast cancer who have received a cumulative doxorubicin dose of 300 mg/m² and who would benefit from continuing therapy with doxorubicin to maintain tumor control. It is not recommended for use with the initiation of doxorubicin therapy (see Warnings).

➤**Unlabeled uses:** Cardioprotectant for other anthracyclines (epirubicin).

Administration and Dosage

➤**Approved by the FDA:** May 26, 1995.

The recommended dosage ratio of dexrazoxane:doxorubicin is 10:1 (eg, 500 mg/m² dexrazoxane:50 mg/m² doxorubicin). Dexrazoxane must be reconstituted with 0.167 Molar (M/6) sodium lactate injection to give a concentration of 10 mg dexrazoxane for each mL of sodium lactate. Administer the reconstituted solution by slow IV push or rapid drip IV infusion from a bag. After completing the infusion and prior to a total elapsed time of 30 minutes (from the beginning of the dexrazoxane infusion), give the IV injection of doxorubicin.

➤**Hepatic function impairment:** Because a doxorubicin dose reduction is recommended in the presence of hyperbilirubinemia, proportionately reduce the dexrazoxane dosage (maintaining the 10:1 ratio) in patients with hepatic impairment.

➤**Dilution:** Dilute the reconstituted dexrazoxane solution with either 0.9% sodium chloride injection or 5% dextrose injection to a concentration range of 1.3 to 5 mg/mL in IV infusion bags.

➤**Admixture incompatibility:** Do not mix dexrazoxane with other drugs.

➤**Handling and disposal:** Exercise caution in the handling and preparation of the reconstituted solution; the use of gloves is recommended. If dexrazoxane powder or solutions contact the skin or mucosa, immediately wash with soap and water.

➤**Storage/Stability:** Store at controlled room temperature, 15° to 30°C (59° to 86°F). Reconstituted and diluted solutions are stable for 6 hours at controlled room temperature or under refrigeration, 2° to 8°C (36° to 46°F). Discard unused solutions.

Actions

➤**Pharmacology:** Dexrazoxane, a derivative of EDTA, is a cardioprotective agent for use in conjunction with doxorubicin. It is a potent intracellular chelating agent. The mechanism by which dexrazoxane exerts its cardioprotective activity is not fully understood. Dexrazoxane is a cyclic derivative of EDTA that readily penetrates cell membranes. Dexrazoxane appears to be converted intracellularly to a ring-opened chelating agent

DEXRAZOXANE

that interferes with iron-mediated free radical generation thought to be responsible, in part, for anthracycline-induced cardiomyopathy.

➤*Pharmacokinetics:*

Absorption / Distribution – The mean peak plasma concentration of dexrazoxane was 36.5 mcg/mL at the end of the 15-minute infusion of a 500 mg/m^2 dose administered 15 to 30 minutes prior to the 50 mg/m^2 doxorubicin dose. Following a rapid distributive phase, dexrazoxane reaches post-distributive equilibrium within 2 to 4 hours. Dexrazoxane is not bound to plasma proteins.

Metabolism / Excretion – Metabolism studies have confirmed the presence of unchanged drug, a diacid-diamide cleavage product and 2 monoacid-monoamide ring products in the urine. Urinary excretion plays an important role in elimination; of the 500 mg/m^2 dose of dexrazoxane, 42% was excreted in the urine.

Mean Dexrazoxane Pharmacokinetic Parameters					
Doxorubicin dose (mg/m²)	Dexrazoxane dose (mg/m²)	Elimination half-life (h)	Plasma clearance (L/h/m²)	Renal clearance (L/h/m²)	Volume of distribution[1] (L/m²)
50	500	2.5	7.88	3.35	22.4
60	600	2.1	6.25	—	22

[1] At steady state.

The pharmacokinetics of dexrazoxane can be adequately described by a two-compartment open model with first-order elimination. The disposition kinetics of dexrazoxane are dose-independent, as shown by linear relationship between the area under plasma concentration-time curves and administered doses ranging from 60 to 900 mg/m^2.

Contraindications

Do not use with chemotherapy regimens that do not contain an anthracycline.

Warnings

➤*Myelosuppression:* Dexrazoxane may add to the myelosuppression caused by chemotherapeutic agents.

➤*Antitumor interference:* There is some evidence that the use of dexrazoxane concurrently with the initiation of fluorouracil, doxorubicin, and cyclophosphamide (FAC) therapy interferes with the antitumor efficacy of the regimen; this use is not recommended. In the largest of 3 breast cancer trials, patients who received dexrazoxane starting with their first cycle of FAC therapy had a lower response rate (48% vs 63%) and shorter time to progression than patients who did not receive dexrazoxane. Therefore, only use dexrazoxane in those patients who have received a cumulative doxorubicin dose of 300 mg/m^2 and are continuing with doxorubicin therapy.

➤*Anthracycline-induced cardiac toxicity:* Although clinical studies have shown that patients receiving FAC with dexrazoxane may receive a higher cumulative dose of doxorubicin before experiencing cardiac toxicity than patients receiving FAC without dexrazoxane, the use of dexrazoxane in patients who have already received a cumulative dose of doxorubicin of 300 mg/m^2 without dexrazoxane does not eliminate the potential for anthracycline-induced cardiac toxicity. Therefore, carefully monitor cardiac function.

➤*Carcinogenesis:* Secondary malignancies (primarily acute myeloid leukemia) have been reported in patients treated chronically with razoxane (razoxane is the racemic mixture of which dexrazoxane is the S(+)-enantiomer). One case of T-cell lymphoma, 1 case of B-cell lymphoma, and 6 to 8 cases of cutaneous basal cell or squamous cell carcinoma also have been reported in patients treated with razoxane.

Dexrazoxane was clastogenic to human lymphocytes in vitro and to mouse bone marrow erythrocytes in vivo (micronucleus test).

➤*Fertility impairment:* Testicular atrophy was seen with dexrazoxane administration at doses as low as 30 mg/kg/week for 6 weeks in rats (⅓ the human dose) and as low as 20 mg/kg/week for 13 weeks in dogs (approximately equal to the human dose).

➤*Elderly:* Treat elderly patients with caution because of the greater frequency of decreased hepatic, renal, or cardiac function, and concomitant disease or other drug therapy.

➤*Pregnancy:* Category C. Dexrazoxane was maternotoxic at doses of 2 mg/kg (¼₀ the human dose) and embryotoxic and teratogenic at 8 mg/kg when given daily to pregnant rats during the period of organogenesis. Teratogenic effects in the rat included imperforate anus, microphthalmia, and anophthalmia. In offspring allowed to develop to maturity, fertility was impaired in the male and female rats treated in utero during organogenesis at 8 mg/kg. In rabbits, doses of 5 mg/kg/day during organogenesis were maternotoxic, and dosages of 20 mg/kg were embryotoxic and teratogenic. Teratogenic effects in the rabbit included several skeletal malformations (eg, short tail, rib, thoracic malformations); soft tissue variations including SC, eye and cardiac hemorrhagic areas, and agenesis of the gallbladder and of the intermediate lobe of the lung. There are no adequate and well-controlled studies in pregnant women. Use during pregnancy only if the potential benefit justifies the potential risk to the fetus.

➤*Lactation:* It is not known whether dexrazoxane is excreted in breast milk. Because of the potential for serious adverse reactions in nursing infants exposed to dexrazoxane, advise mothers to discontinue nursing during dexrazoxane therapy.

➤*Children:* Safety and efficacy in children have not been established.

Precautions

➤*Monitoring:* Because dexrazoxane will always be used with cytotoxic drugs and because it may add to the myelosuppressive effects of cytotoxic drugs, frequent complete blood counts are recommended.

➤*Administration:* Do not give doxorubicin prior to dexrazoxane IV injection. Give dexrazoxane by slow IV push or rapid drip IV infusion from a bag. Give doxorubicin within 30 minutes after beginning the infusion with dexrazoxane (see Administration and Dosage).

Adverse Reactions

Dexrazoxane Adverse Reactions in Metastatic Breast Cancer Patients Receiving FAC (%)				
	FAC + Dexrazoxane		FAC + Placebo	
Adverse reaction	Courses 1 - 6 (n = 413)	Courses ≥ 7 (n = 102)	Courses 1 - 6 (n = 458)	Courses ≥ 7 (n = 99)
Dermatologic				
Alopecia	94	100	97	98
Recall skin reaction	1	1	2	0
Streaking/ Erythema	5	4	4	2
Urticaria	2	2	2	0
GI				
Anorexia	42	27	47	38
Diarrhea	21	14	24	7
Dysphagia	8	0	10	5
Esophagitis	6	3	7	4
Nausea	77	51	84	60
Stomatitis	34	26	41	28
Vomiting	59	42	72	49
Miscellaneous				
Extravasation	1	3	1	2
Fatigue/ Malaise	61	48	58	55
Fever	34	22	29	18
Hemorrhage	2	3	2	1
Infection	23	19	18	21
Neurotoxicity	17	10	13	5
Pain on injection	12	13	3	0
Phlebitis	6	3	3	5
Sepsis	17	12	14	9

The adverse experiences listed in the table are likely attributable to the FAC regimen, with the exception of pain on injection that was observed mainly with dexrazoxane.

➤*Hematologic:* Patients receiving FAC with dexrazoxane experienced more severe leukopenia, granulocytopenia, and thrombocytopenia at nadir than patients receiving FAC without dexrazoxane. However, recovery counts were similar for the 2 groups.

➤*Lab test abnormalities:* Some patients receiving FAC plus dexrazoxane or FAC plus placebo experienced marked abnormalities in hepatic or renal function tests, but the frequency and severity of abnormalities in bilirubin, alkaline phosphatase, BUN, and creatinine were similar for patients receiving FAC with or without dexrazoxane.

Overdosage

Retention of a significant dose fraction of the unchanged drug in the plasma pool, minimal tissue partitioning or binding, and availability of greater than 90% of the systemic drug levels in the unbound form suggest that dexrazoxane could be removed using conventional peritoneal or hemodialysis. Manage instances of suspected overdose with good supportive care until resolution of myelosuppression and related conditions is complete. Management of overdose should include treatment of infections, fluid regulation, and maintenance of nutritional requirements. Refer to General Management of Acute Overdosage.

Patient Information

Dexrazoxane is always used together with doxorubicin. Tell your doctor or pharmacist if any of the following occurs: fever, chills, sore throat, numbness or tingling, unusual bleeding, hair loss, nausea, vomiting, tiredness, general body discomfort, appetite loss, stomach pain, diarrhea, pain at injection site, streaking or redness of the skin, difficulty swallowing, hives.

MESNA

Rx	**Mesnex** (Bristol-Myers Squibb)	**Tablets**: 400 mg	Lactose, simethicone. (M4). White, oblong, scored. Film coated. In 10 blisters.
Rx	**Mesna** (American Pharmaceutical Partners)	**Injection**: 100 mg/mL	With 0.25 mg/mL EDTA. In 10 mL multidose vials.[1]
Rx	**Mesnex** (Bristol-Myers Squibb)		With 0.25 mg/mL EDTA. In 10 mL multidose vials.[1]

[1] With 10.4 mg benzyl alcohol as a preservative.

Indications

➤*Ifosfamide-induced hemorrhagic cystitis:* Prophylactic agent to reduce the incidence of ifosfamide-induced hemorrhagic cystitis (see Ifosfamide monograph).

➤*Unlabeled uses:* As a prophylactic agent to decrease the incidence of hemorrhagic cystitis in bone marrow transplantation patients receiving high-dose cyclophosphamide. As a uroprotective agent in a limited number of patients receiving antineoplastic regimens containing high-dose cyclophosphamide; also has been used in a limited number of patients receiving cyclophosphamide for immunologically mediated disorders (eg, systemic lupus erythematosus, polyarteritis, Wegener's granulomatosis, dermatomyositis).

Administration and Dosage

➤*Approved by the FDA:* December 30, 1988.

For the prophylaxis of ifosfamide-induced hemorrhagic cystitis, mesna may be given on a fractionated dosing schedule of 3 bolus IV injections or a single bolus injection followed by 2 mesna tablets.

➤*IV schedule:* Mesna is given as IV bolus injections in a dosage equal to 20% of the ifosfamide dosage (w/w) at the time of ifosfamide administration and 4 and 8 hours after each dose of ifosfamide. The total daily dose of mesna is 60% of the ifosfamide dose.

IV Dosing Schedule for Mesna			
	0 Hours	4 Hours	8 Hours
Ifosfamide	1.2 g/m²	-	-
Mesna injection	240 mg/m²	240 mg/m²	240 mg/m²

➤*IV and oral dosing:* Mesna injection is given as IV bolus injections in a dosage equal to 20% of the ifosfamide dosage (w/w) at the time of ifosfamide administration. Mesna tablets are given orally in a dosage equal to 40% of the ifosfamide dose 2 and 6 hours after each dose of ifosfamide. The total daily dose of mesna is 100% of the ifosfamide dose.

IV and Oral Dosing Schedule for Mesna			
	0 Hours	2 Hours	6 Hours
Ifosfamide	1.2 g/m²	-	-
Mesna injection	240 mg/m²	-	-
Mesna tablets	-	480 mg/m²	480 mg/m²

Patients who vomit within 2 hours of taking oral mesna should repeat the dose or receive IV mesna. The efficacy and safety of this ratio of IV and oral mesna has not been established as being effective for daily doses of *Ifex* higher than 2 g/m².

Repeat this dosing schedule on each day that ifosfamide is administered. When the dosage of ifosfamide is adjusted (either increased or decreased), the ratio of mesna to *Ifex* should be maintained.

➤*Preparations of IV solutions:* For IV administration, the drug can be diluted with any of the following fluids obtaining final concentrations of 20 mg mesna/mL: 5% Dextrose Injection, 5% Dextrose and 0.2% Sodium Chloride Injection, 5% Dextrose and 0.33% Sodium Chloride Injection, 5% Dextrose and 0.45% Sodium Chloride Injection, 0.92% Sodium Chloride Injection, Lactated Ringer's Injection.

➤*Admixture incompatibility/compatibility:* Mesna is not compatible with cisplatin or carboplatin. Mesna and ifosfamide are compatible in the same infusion fluid.

➤*Storage/Stability:*

Tablets – Store at controlled room temperature 20° to 25°C (68° to 77°F).

Injection – The mesna multidose vials may be stored and used for up to 8 days.

  Diluted solutions: Diluted solutions are chemically and physically stable for 24 hours at 25°C (77°F), but it is recommended that solutions of mesna be refrigerated.

Visually inspect parenteral drug products for particulate matter and discoloration prior to administration.

Actions

➤*Pharmacology:* Mesna was developed as a prophylactic agent to reduce the incidence of ifosfamide-induced hemorrhagic cystitis. In the kidney, the mesna disulfide is reduced to the free thiol compound, mesna, which reacts chemically with the urotoxic ifosfamide metabolites (acrolein and 4-hydroxy-ifosfamide), resulting in their detoxification. The first step in the detoxification process is the binding of mesna to 4-hydroxy-ifosfamide, forming a nonurotoxic 4-sulfoethylthioifosfamide. Mesna also binds to the double bonds of acrolein and other urotoxic metabolites.

➤*Pharmacokinetics:* Analogous to the physiological cysteine-cystine system, mesna is rapidly oxidized to its major metabolite, mesna disulfide (dimesna). Mesna disulfide remains in the intravascular compartment and is rapidly eliminated by the kidneys.

At doses of 2 to 4 g/m², its terminal elimination half-life is about 4 to 8 hours. As a result, repeated doses of mesna are required to maintain adequate levels of mesna in the urinary bladder during the course of elimination of the urotoxic ifosfamide metabolites.

IV-IV-IV regimen – After IV administration of 800 mg, the half-lives of mesna and dimesna in the blood are 0.36 and 1.17 hours, respectively. Approximately 32% and 33% of the administered dose is eliminated in the urine in 24 hours as mesna and dimesna, respectively. The majority of the dose recovered is eliminated within 4 hours. Mesna has a plasma clearance of 1.23 L/kg/h.

IV-oral-oral regimen – The half-life of mesna ranged from 1.2 to 8.3 hours after administration of IV plus oral doses of mesna, as recommended (see Administration and Dosage). The urinary bioavailability of oral mesna ranged from 45% to 79% of IV administered mesna. Food does not affect the urinary availability of orally administered mesna. Approximately 18% to 26% of the combined IV and oral mesna dose appears as free mesna in the urine. When compared with IV administered mesna, the IV plus oral dosing regimen increases systemic exposures (150%) and provides more sustained excretion of mesna in the urine over a 24-hour period. Approximately 5% of the mesna dose is excreted during the 12- to 24-hour interval, as compared with negligible amounts in patients given the IV regimen. The fraction of the administered dose of mesna excreted in the urine is independent of dose. Protein binding of mesna is in a moderate range (69% to 75%).

➤*Clinical trials:*

IV mesna – The hemorrhagic cystitis produced by ifosfamide is dose dependent. At a dose of 1.2 g/m² ifosfamide administered daily for 5 days, 16% to 26% of the patients who received conventional uroprophylaxis (high fluid intake, alkalinization of the urine, and administration of diuretics) developed hematuria (greater than 50 RBC/high-power field [hpf] or macrohematuria). In contrast, none of the patients who received mesna injection together with this dose of ifosfamide developed hematuria. Higher doses of ifosfamide (from 2 to 4 g/m² administered for 3 to 5 days) produced hematuria in 31% to 100% of the patients. When mesna was administered together with these doses of ifosfamide, the incidence of hematuria was less than 7%.

Oral mesna – Clinical studies comparing recommended IV and oral mesna dosing regimens demonstrated incidences of grade 3 to 4 hematuria of less than 5%. One study was an open label, randomized, 2-way crossover study comparing 3 IV doses with an initial IV dose followed by 2 oral doses of mesna in patients with cancer treated with ifosfamide at a dose of 1.2 to 2 g/m² for 3 to 5 days. Another study was a randomized, multicenter study in cancer patients receiving ifosfamide at 2 g/m² for 5 days. In both studies, development of grade 3 or 4 hematuria was the primary efficacy endpoint.

Contraindications

Hypersensitivity to mesna or other thiol compounds.

Warnings

➤*Ifosfamide toxicities:* Mesna has been developed as an agent to reduce the risk of ifosfamide-induced hemorrhagic cystitis. It will not prevent or alleviate other adverse reactions or toxicities associated with ifosfamide therapy.

➤*Hematuria:* Mesna does not prevent hemorrhagic cystitis in all patients. Up to 6% of patients treated with mesna have developed hematuria (greater than 50 RBC/hpf or WHO grade 2 and above). As a result, examine a morning specimen of urine for the presence of hematuria (microscopic evidence of red blood cells) each day prior to ifosfamide therapy. If hematuria develops when mesna is given with ifosfamide according to the recommended dosage schedule, depending on the severity of the hematuria, dosage reductions or discontinuation of ifosfamide therapy may be initiated.

Mesna must be administered with each dose of ifosfamide (see Administration and Dosage). Mesna is not effective in reducing the risk of hematuria caused by other pathological conditions such as thrombocytopenia.

➤*Hypersensitivity reactions:* Allergic reactions to mesna ranging from mild hypersensitivity to systemic anaphylactic reactions have been reported. Patients with autoimmune disorders who were treated with cyclophosphamide and mesna appeared to have a higher incidence of allergic reactions. The majority of these patients received mesna orally. Pretreatment with an antihistamine, a corticosteroid, or both may be indicated when there has been a previous allergic reaction to mesna.

MESNA

➤*Elderly:* Cautiously make dose selection for an elderly patient, reflecting the greater frequency of decreased hepatic, renal, or cardiac function, and of concomitant disease or other drug therapy. However, the ratio of ifosfamide to mesna should remain unchanged.

➤*Pregnancy: Category B.* There are no adequate and well-controlled studies in pregnant women. Because animal reproductive studies are not always predictive of human response, this drug should be used during pregnancy only if clearly needed.

➤*Lactation:* It is not known whether mesna or dimesna is excreted in breast milk. Because many drugs are excreted in human milk and because of the potential for adverse reactions in nursing infants, decide whether to discontinue nursing or to discontinue the drug, taking into account the importance of the drug to the mother.

➤*Children:* Safety and effectiveness of mesna tablets have not been established in pediatric patients. Because of the benzyl alcohol content in the mesna injection, do not use the multidose vial in neonates or infants and use with caution in older pediatric patients.

Precautions

➤*Benzyl alcohol:* Benzyl alcohol, contained in this product as a preservative, has been associated with a fatal "gasping syndrome" in premature infants.

Drug Interactions

➤*Drug/Lab test interactions:* A false positive test for urinary ketones may arise in patients treated with mesna. In this test, a red-violet color develops that, with the addition of glacial acetic acid, will return to violet.

Adverse Reactions

Mesna adverse reaction data are available from 4 phase I studies in which single IV bolus doses of 600 to 1200 mg mesna injection without concurrent chemotherapy were administered to a total of 53 subjects and single oral doses of 600 to 2400 mg of mesna tablets were administered to a total of 82 subjects.

The most frequently reported side effects (observed in 2 or more patients) for patients receiving single doses of mesna IV were the following: Headache, injection site reactions, flushing, dizziness, nausea, vomiting, somnolence, diarrhea, anorexia, fever, pharyngitis, hyperesthesia, influenza-like symptoms, coughing. Among patients who received a single 1200 mg dose as an oral solution, rigors, back pain, rash, conjunctivitis, and arthralgia also were reported. In 2 phase I multiple-dose studies where patients received mesna tablets alone or IV mesna followed by repeated doses of mesna tablets, flatulence and rhinitis were reported. In addition, constipation was reported by patients who had received repeated doses of IV mesna.

Because mesna is used in combination with ifosfamide or ifosfamide-containing chemotherapy regimens, it is difficult to distinguish the adverse reactions that may be caused by mesna from those caused by the concomitantly administered cytotoxic agents.

Adverse reactions reasonably associated with mesna administered IV and orally in 4 controlled studies in which patients received ifosfamide or ifosfamide-containing regimens are presented in the table below.

Mesna Adverse Reactions (%)		
	Mesna regimen	
Adverse reaction	IV-IV-IV (n = 119)	IV-oral-oral (n = 119)
Incidence of adverse reactions	84.9	89.1
Cardiovascular		
Chest pain	8.4	7.6
Hypotension	3.4	5
Tachycardia	0.8	5.9
CNS		
Dizziness	7.6	4.2
Headache	7.6	10.9

Mesna Adverse Reactions (%)		
	Mesna regimen	
Adverse reaction	IV-IV-IV (n = 119)	IV-oral-oral (n = 119)
Somnolence	6.7	10.1
Anxiety	5.9	3.4
Confusion	5.9	5
Insomnia	5	9.2
Dermatologic		
Alopecia	10.1	10.9
Injection site reaction	6.7	8.4
Pallor	3.4	5
Flushing	0.8	5
GI		
Nausea	54.6	53.8
Vomiting	29.4	37.8
Constipation	23.5	17.6
Anorexia	17.6	16
Abdominal pain	11.8	15.1
Diarrhea	7.6	14.3
Dyspepsia	3.4	5
Hematologic/Lymphatic		
Leukopenia	21	17.6
Thrombocytopenia	17.6	13.4
Anemia	16.8	17.6
Granulocytopenia	13.4	12.6
Hematuria[1]	6.7	5.9
Respiratory		
Dyspnea	9.2	9.2
Pneumonia	1.7	6.7
Miscellaneous		
Fatigue	20.2	20.2
Fever	20.2	15.1
Asthenia	12.6	17.6
Hypokalemia	8.4	9.2
Pain	7.6	8.4
Sweating increased	7.6	1.7
Back pain	6.7	5
Edema	6.7	7.6
Edema peripheral	6.7	6.7
Face edema	5	4.2
Coughing	4.2	8.4
Dehydration	2.5	5.9

[1] All grades.

➤*Postmarketing:* Allergic reactions, decreased platelet counts associated with allergic reactions, hypertension, hypotension, increased heart rate, increased liver enzymes, injection site reactions (including pain and erythema), limb pain, malaise, myalgia, ST-segment elevation, tachycardia, and tachypnea have been reported as part of postmarketing surveillance.

Overdosage

There is no known antidote for mesna. Oral doses of 6.1 and 4.3 g/kg were lethal to mice and rats, respectively. These doses are approximately 15 and 22 times the maximum recommended human dose on a body surface area basis. Death was preceded by diarrhea, tremor, convulsions, dyspnea, and cyanosis.

Patient Information

Advise patients taking mesna to drink at least 1 quart of liquid per day. Inform patients to report if their urine has turned pink or red, if they vomit within 2 hours of taking oral mesna, or if they miss a dose of oral mesna.

AZACITIDINE

Rx **Vidaza** (Pharmion[a])   **Powder for injection, lyophilized:** 100 mg   100 mg mannitol. In single-use vials.

[a] Pharmion Corporation, 2525 28th St., Suite 200, Boulder, CO 80301; (720) 564-9100 or (866) PHARMION; http://www.pharmion.com.

Indications

➤*Myelodysplastic syndrome (MDS):* For the treatment of patients with the following MDS subtypes: Refractory anemia or refractory anemia with ringed sideroblasts (if accompanied by neutropenia or thrombocytopenia or requiring transfusions), refractory anemia with excess blasts, refractory anemia with excess blasts in transformation, and chronic myelomonocytic leukemia.

Administration and Dosage

➤*Approved by the FDA:* May 19, 2004.

The recommended starting dose is 75 mg/m² subcutaneously, daily for 7 days, every 4 weeks. Premedicate patients for nausea and vomiting. The dose may be increased to 100 mg/m² if no beneficial effect is seen after 2 treatment cycles and if no toxicity other than nausea and vomiting has occurred. It is recommended that patients be treated for a minimum of 4 cycles; however, complete or partial response may require more than 4 treatment cycles. Treatment may be continued as long as the patient continues to benefit.

➤*Dosage adjustment:* Monitor patients for hematologic response and renal toxicities (see Precautions); delaying dosage or reduction as described below may be necessary.

For patients with baseline (start of treatment) white blood cells (WBC) greater than or equal to 3×10^9/L, absolute neutrophil counts (ANC) greater than or equal to 1.5×10^9/L, and platelets greater than or equal to 75×10^9/L, adjust the dose as follows, based on nadir counts for any given cycle.

Nadir Counts		
ANC ($\times 10^9$/L)	Platelets ($\times 10^9$/L)	% Dose in the Next Course
< 0.5	< 25	50%
0.5 to 1.5	25 to 50	67%
> 1.5	> 50	100%

For patients whose baseline counts are WBC less than 3×10^9/L, ANC less than 1.5×10^9/L, or platelets less than 75×10^9/L, base dosage adjustments on nadir counts and bone marrow biopsy cellularity at the time of the nadir as noted below, unless there is clear improvement in differentiation (percentage of mature granulocytes is higher and ANC is higher than at onset of that course) at the time of the next cycle, in which case the dose of the current treatment should be continued.

	Bone Marrow Biopsy Cellularity at Time of Nadir (%)		
	30 to 60	15 to 30	< 15
WBC or platelet nadir (% decrease in counts from baseline)	% Dose in the next course		
50 to 75	100	50	33
> 75	75	50	33

If a nadir as defined in the table above has occurred, give the next course of treatment 28 days after the start of the preceding course, providing that the WBC and platelet counts are more than 25% above the nadir and rising. If a greater than 25% increase above the nadir is not seen by day 28, reassess counts every 7 days. If a 25% increase is not seen by day 42, treat the patient with 50% of the scheduled dose.

➤*Renal function impairment/altered serum electrolytes:* If unexplained reductions in serum bicarbonate levels to less than 20 mEq/L occur, reduce the dosage by 50% on the next course. Similarly, if unexplained elevations of blood urea nitrogen (BUN) or serum creatinine occur, delay the next cycle until values return to normal or baseline and reduce the dose by 50% on the next treatment course (see Warnings).

➤*Preparation of injection:* Reconstitute azacitidine aseptically with 4 mL sterile water for injection. Inject the diluent slowly into the vial. Invert the vial 2 to 3 times and gently rotate until a uniform suspension is achieved. The suspension will be cloudy. The resulting suspension will contain 25 mg/mL azacitidine.

Immediate administration – Divide doses greater than 4 mL equally into 2 syringes.

Delayed administration – The reconstituted product may be kept in the vial or drawn into a syringe. Divide doses greater than 4 mL equally into 2 syringes.

➤*Administration:* To provide a homogenous suspension, resuspend the contents by inverting the syringe 2 to 3 times and gently rolling the syringe between the palms for 30 seconds immediately prior to administration.

Azacitidine is administered subcutaneously. Divide doses greater than 4 mL equally into 2 syringes and inject into separate sites. Rotate sites for each injection (thigh, abdomen, or upper arm). Give new injections at least one inch from an old site and never into areas where the site is tender, bruised, red, or hard.

➤*Handling and disposal:* Azacitidine is a cytotoxic drug. As with other potentially toxic compounds, exercise caution when handling and preparing azacitidine suspensions.

If reconstituted azacitidine comes into contact with the skin, immediately and thoroughly wash with soap and water. If it comes into contact with mucous membranes, flush thoroughly with water.

➤*Storage/Stability:* Store unreconstituted vials at 25°C (77°F); excursions permitted to 15° to 30°C (59° to 86°F). The reconstituted product may be held at room temperature (25°C; 77°F) for up to 1 hour but must be administered within 1 hour after reconstitution. The reconstituted product may be refrigerated immediately and may be held under refrigerated conditions (2° to 8°C; 36° to 46°F) for up to 8 hours. After removal from refrigerated conditions, the suspension may be allowed to equilibrate to room temperature for up to 30 minutes prior to administration. Properly discard unused portions of each vial. Do not save any unused portions for later administration.

Actions

➤*Pharmacology:* Azacitidine is a pyrimidine nucleoside analog of cytidine. Azacitidine is believed to exert its antineoplastic effects by causing demethylation or hypomethylation of DNA and direct cytotoxicity on abnormal hematopoietic cells in the bone marrow. The concentration of azacitidine required for maximum inhibition of DNA methylation in vitro does not cause major suppression of DNA synthesis. Hypomethylation may restore normal function to genes that are critical for differentiation and proliferation. The cytotoxic effects of azacitidine cause the death of rapidly dividing cells, including cancer cells that are no longer responsive to normal growth control mechanisms. Nonproliferating cells are relatively insensitive to azacitidine.

➤*Pharmacokinetics:*

Absorption/Distribution – The pharmacokinetics of azacitidine were studied in 6 MDS patients following a single 75 mg/m² subcutaneous dose and a single 75 mg/m² IV dose. Azacitidine is rapidly absorbed after subcutaneous administration; the peak plasma azacitidine concentration of 750 ± 403 ng/mL occurred in 0.5 hours. The bioavailability of subcutaneous azacitidine relative to IV azacitidine is approximately 89% based on area under the curve. Mean volume of distribution following IV dosing is 76 ± 26 L.

Metabolism/Excretion – An in vitro study of azacitidine incubation in human liver fractions indicated that azacitidine may be metabolized by the liver. Mean apparent subcutaneous clearance is 167 ± 49 L/h and mean half-life after subcutaneous administration is 41 ± 8 minutes. Published studies indicate that urinary excretion is the primary route of elimination of azacitidine and its metabolites. Following IV administration of radioactive azacitidine to 5 cancer patients, the cumulative urinary excretion was 85% of the radioactive dose. Fecal excretion accounted for less than 1% of administered radioactivity over 3 days. Mean excretion of radioactivity in urine following subcutaneous administration of ¹⁴C-azacitidine was 50%. The mean elimination half-lives of total radioactivity (azacitidine and its metabolites) were similar after IV and subcutaneous administrations (approximately 4 hours).

Contraindications

Known hypersensitivity to azacitidine or mannitol; patients with advanced malignant hepatic tumors (see Warnings).

Warnings

➤*Use in males:* Advise men not to father a child while receiving treatment with azacitidine.

➤*Renal function impairment:* Closely monitor patients with renal impairment for toxicity because azacitidine and its metabolites are primarily excreted by the kidneys.

➤*Hepatic function impairment:* Because azacitidine is potentially hepatotoxic in patients with severe preexisting hepatic impairment, use caution in patients with liver disease. Patients with extensive tumor burden caused by metastatic disease rarely have been reported to experience progressive hepatic coma and death during azacitidine treatment, especially in such patients with baseline albumin less than 30 g/L. Azacitidine is contraindicated in patients with advanced malignant hepatic tumors.

➤*Carcinogenesis:* Azacitidine induced tumors of the hematopoietic system in female mice at 2.2 mg/kg (6.6 mg/m²) administered intraperitoneally 3 times/week for 52 weeks. An increased incidence of tumors in the lymphoreticular system, lung, mammary glands, and skin was seen in mice treated with intraperitoneal azacitidine at 2 mg/kg (6 mg/m²) once a week for 50 weeks. A tumorigenicity study in rats dosed twice weekly at 15 or 60 mg/m² revealed an increased incidence of testicular tumors compared with controls.

➤*Mutagenesis:* Azacitidine was mutagenic in bacterial and mammalian cell systems.

➤*Fertility impairment:* Administration of azacitidine to male mice at 9.9 mg/m² daily for 3 days prior to mating with untreated female mice resulted in decreased fertility and loss of offspring during subse-

AZACITIDINE

quent embryonic and postnatal development. Treatment of male rats 3 times/week for 11 or 16 weeks at doses of 15 to 30 mg/m^2 resulted in decreased weight of the testes and epididymides, and decreased sperm counts accompanied by decreased pregnancy rates and increased loss of embryos in mated females. In a related study, male rats treated for 16 weeks at 24 mg/m^2 resulted in an increase in abnormal embryos in mated females when examined on day 2 of gestation.

➤*Elderly:* Because elderly patients are more likely to have decreased renal function, it may be useful to monitor renal function.

➤*Pregnancy: Category D.* Azacitidine may cause fetal harm when administered to a pregnant woman. Early embryotoxicity studies in mice revealed a 44% frequency of intrauterine embryonal death (increased resorption) after a single intraperitoneal injection of 6 mg/m^2 (approximately 8% of the recommended human daily dose on a mg/m^2 basis) azacitidine on gestation day 10. Developmental abnormalities in the brain have been detected in mice given azacitidine on or before gestation day 15 at doses of approximately 3 to 12 mg/m^2 (approximately 4% to 16% the recommended human daily dose on a mg/m^2 basis).

In rats, azacitidine was clearly embryotoxic when given intraperitoneally on gestation days 4 to 8 (postimplantation) at a dose of 6 mg/m^2 (approximately 8% of the recommended human daily dose on a mg/m^2 basis), although treatment in the preimplantation period (on gestation days 1 to 3) had no adverse effect on the embryos. Azacitidine caused multiple fetal abnormalities in rats after a single intraperitoneal dose of 3 to 12 mg/m^2 (approximately 8% the recommended human daily dose on a mg/m^2 basis) given on gestation days 9, 10, 11, or 12. In this study, azacitidine caused fetal death when administered at 3 to 12 mg/m^2 on gestation days 9 and 10; average live animals per litter was reduced to 9% of control at the highest dose on gestation day 9. Fetal anomalies included the following: CNS anomalies (exencephaly/encephalocele), limb anomalies (micromelia, club foot, syndactyly, oligodactyly), and others (micrognathia, gastroschisis, edema, and rib abnormalities).

There are no adequate and well-controlled studies in pregnant women using azacitidine. If this drug is used during pregnancy or if the patient becomes pregnant while taking this drug, apprise the patient of the potential hazard to the fetus. Advise women of childbearing potential to avoid becoming pregnant while receiving azacitidine treatment.

➤*Lactation:* It is not known whether azacitidine or its metabolites are excreted in human milk. Because of the potential for tumorigenicity shown for azacitidine in animal studies and the potential for serious adverse reactions, women treated with azacitidine should not nurse.

➤*Children:* Safety and efficacy have not been established.

Precautions

➤*Monitoring:* Perform complete blood counts as needed to monitor response and toxicity, but at a minimum, prior to each cycle. Obtain liver chemistries and serum creatinine prior to initiation of therapy.

➤*Hematologic toxicity:* Treatment with azacitidine is associated with neutropenia and thrombocytopenia. Perform complete blood counts as needed to monitor response and toxicity, but at a minimum, prior to each dosing cycle. After administration of the recommended dosage for the first cycle, reduce or delay dosage for subsequent cycles based on nadir counts and hematologic response (see Administration and Dosage).

➤*Renal toxicity:* Renal abnormalities ranging from elevated serum creatinine to renal failure and death have been reported rarely in patients treated with IV azacitidine in combination with other chemotherapeutic agents for non-MDS conditions. In addition, renal tubular acidosis, defined as a fall in serum bicarbonate to less than 20 mEq/L in association with an alkaline urine and hypokalemia (serum potassium less than 3 mEq/L), developed in 5 patients with chronic myelocytic leukemia treated with azacitidine and etoposide. If unexplained reductions in serum bicarbonate to less than 20 mEq/L or elevations of BUN or serum creatinine occur, reduce or hold the dosage (see Administration and Dosage).

Drug Interactions

Drug interaction studies with azacitidine have not been conducted.

Adverse Reactions

➤*Adverse reactions previously described in other sections:* Elevated serum creatinine, hepatic coma, hypokalemia, neutropenia, renal failure, renal tubular acidosis, thrombocytopenia (see Warnings and Precautions).

➤*Most common adverse reactions (subcutaneous route):* Anemia, constipation, diarrhea, ecchymosis, fatigue, injection-site erythema, leukopenia, nausea, neutropenia, pyrexia, thrombocytopenia, vomiting.

➤*Adverse reactions most frequently (more than 2%) resulting in clinical intervention (subcutaneous route):*

Discontinuation – Leukopenia (5%); thrombocytopenia (3.6%); neutropenia (2.7%).

Dose held – Leukopenia, neutropenia (4.5%); febrile neutropenia (2.7%).

Dose reduced – Leukopenia (4.5%); neutropenia (4.1%); thrombocytopenia (3.2%).

The data described below reflect exposure to azacitidine in 268 patients, including 116 exposed for 6 cycles (approximately 6 months) or more and 60 exposed for more than 12 cycles (approximately 1 year). Azacitidine was studied primarily in supportive care-controlled and uncontrolled trials (n = 150 and n = 118, respectively). Most patients received average daily doses between 50 and 100 mg/m^2.

Azacitidine Adverse Reactions (≥ 5%)[a]		
Adverse reaction	All azacitidine[b] (N = 220)	Observation[c] (N = 92)
Cardiovascular		
Cardiac murmur	10	8.7
Hypotension	6.8	2.2
Tachycardia	8.6	6.5
CNS		
Anxiety	13.2	3.3
Appetite decreased	12.7	8.7
Depression	11.8	7.6
Dizziness	18.6	5.4
Fatigue	35.9	25
Fatigue, aggravated	12.7	4.3
Headache	21.8	10.9
Hypoesthesia	5	1.1
Insomnia	10.9	4.3
Lethargy	7.7	2.2
Syncope	5.9	5.4
Dermatologic		
Dry skin	5	1.1
Erythema	16.8	4.3
Night sweats	8.6	3.3
Pallor	15.5	7.6
Pruritus	12.3	12
Rash	14.1	9.8
Skin lesion	14.5	8.7
Skin nodule	5	1.1
Sweating, increased	10.5	2.2
Urticaria	5.9	1.1
GI		
Abdominal distension	5.9	4.3
Abdominal pain	15.5	13
Abdominal pain, upper	10.5	3.3
Abdominal tenderness	11.8	1.1
Anorexia	20.5	6.5
Constipation	33.6	6.5
Diarrhea	36.4	14.1
Dyspepsia	6.8	4.3
Dysphagia	5	2.2
Gingival bleeding	9.5	4.3
Hemorrhoids	6.8	1.1
Loose stools	5.5	0
Mouth hemorrhage	5	1.1
Nausea	70.5	17.4
Oral mucosal petechiae	7.7	3.3
Stomatitis	7.7	0
Tongue ulceration	5	2.2
Vomiting	54.1	5.4
GU		
Dysuria	8.2	2.2
Urinary tract infection	7.7	5.4
Hematologic/Lymphatic		
Anemia	69.5	64.1
Anemia, aggravated	5.5	5.4
Ecchymosis	30.5	15.2
Febrile neutropenia	16.4	4.3
Hematoma	8.6	0
Leukopenia	48.2	29.3
Lymphadenopathy	9.5	3.3
Neutropenia	32.3	10.9
Petechiae	23.6	8.7
Postprocedural hemorrhage	5.9	1.1
Thrombocytopenia	65.5	45.7
Local		
Injection-site bruising	14.1	0
Injection-site erythema	35	0
Injection-site granuloma	5	0
Injection-site pain	22.7	0
Injection-site pigmentation changes	5	0
Injection-site pruritus	6.8	0

AZACITIDINE

Azacitidine Adverse Reactions (≥ 5%)[a]		
Adverse reaction	All azacitidine[b] (N = 220)	Observation[c] (N = 92)
Injection-site reaction	13.6	0
Injection-site swelling	5	0
Metabolic		
Edema, peripheral	18.6	10.9
Hypokalemia	12.7	13
Peripheral swelling	7.3	5.4
Pitting edema	14.5	9.8
Weight decreased	15.9	10.9
Musculoskeletal		
Arthralgia	22.3	3.3
Muscle cramps	5.9	3.3
Myalgia	15.9	2.2
Pain in limb	20	5.4
Respiratory		
Atelactasis	5	2.2
Breath sounds decreased	7.7	1.1
Cough	29.5	15.2
Crackles in the lung	10.5	8.7
Dyspnea	29.1	12
Dyspnea, exacerbated	5	3.3
Dyspnea, exertional	14.1	16.3
Epistaxis	16.4	9.8
Nasal congestion	5.5	1.1
Nasopharyngitis	14.5	3.3
Pharyngitis	20	7.6
Pleural effusion	6.4	6.5
Pneumonia	10.9	5.4
Postnasal drip	5.9	3.3
Productive cough	11.4	4.3
Rales	8.6	8.7
Rhinorrhea	10	2.2
Rhonchi	5.9	2.2
Sinusitis	5	3.3
Upper respiratory tract infection	12.7	4.3
Wheezing	8.6	2.2
Miscellaneous		
Back pain	18.6	7.6
Cellulitis	8.2	4.3
Chest pain	16.4	5.4
Chest wall pain	5	0
Contusion	18.6	9.8
Herpes simplex	9.1	5.4
Malaise	10.9	1.1
Pain	10.9	3.3
Postprocedural pain	5	2.2
Pyrexia	51.8	30.4
Rigors	25.5	10.9
Transfusion reaction	6.8	0
Weakness	29.1	20.7

[a] Mean azacitidine exposure = 11.4 months. Mean time in observation arm = 6.1 months.
[b] Includes events from all patients exposed to azacitidine, including patients after crossing over from observation.
[c] Includes events from observation period only; excludes any events after crossover to azacitidine.

Constipation, diarrhea, nausea, and vomiting all tended to increase in incidence with increasing doses of azacitidine. Anxiety, constipation, dizziness, epistaxis, hypokalemia, injection-site bruising, injection-site erythema, injection-site pain, insomnia, nausea, petechiae, rales, rigors, and vomiting tended to be more pronounced during the first 1 to 2 cycles of subcutaneous azacitidine treatment compared with later cycles of treatment. There did not appear to be any adverse events that increased in frequency over the course of treatment.

In clinical studies of either subcutaneous or IV azacitidine, the following serious treatment-related adverse effects occurring at a rate of less than 5% were reported.

➤*Cardiovascular:* Atrial fibrillation, cardiac failure, cardiac failure congestive, cardiorespiratory arrest, congestive cardiomyopathy, orthostatic hypotension.

➤*CNS:* Confusion, convulsions, intracranial hemorrhage.

➤*Dermatologic:* Pyoderma gangrenosum, rash pruritic, skin induration.

➤*GI:* Diverticulitis, GI hemorrhage, melena, perirectal abscess.

➤*GU:* Hematuria, loin pain, renal failure.

➤*Hematologic/Lymphatic:* Agranulocytosis, bone marrow depression, splenomegaly.

➤*Hypersensitivity:* Anaphylactic shock, hypersensitivity.

➤*Musculoskeletal:* Bone pain aggravated, muscle weakness, neck pain.

➤*Respiratory:* Hemoptysis, lung infiltration, pneumonitis, respiratory distress.

➤*Miscellaneous:* Abscess limb, bacterial infection, blastomycosis, catheter-site hemorrhage, cholecystectomy, cholecystitis, dehydration, general physical health deterioration, injection-site infection, *Klebsiella* sepsis, leukemia cutis, pharyngitis streptococcal, pneumonia *Klebsiella*, sepsis, staphylococcal bacteremia, staphylococcal infection, systemic inflammatory response syndrome, toxoplasmosis.

Overdosage

➤*Symptoms:* One case of overdose with azacitidine was reported during clinical trials. A patient experienced diarrhea, nausea, and vomiting after receiving a single IV dose of approximately 290 mg/m^2, almost 4 times the recommended starting dose. The events resolved without sequelae, and the correct dose was resumed the following day.

➤*Treatment:* In the event of overdosage, monitor the patient with appropriate blood counts and administer supportive treatment, as necessary. There is no known specific antidote for azacitidine overdosage.

Patient Information

Instruct patients to inform their physician about any underlying liver or renal disease.

Advise women of childbearing potential to avoid becoming pregnant while receiving azacitidine treatment.

Advise men not to father a child while receiving azacitidine treatment.

IRINOTECAN HCl

Rx   **Camptosar** (Pharmacia)   **Injection:** 20 mg/mL   45 mg sorbitol. In 2 and 5 mL vials.

WARNING

Administer irinotecan under the supervision of a physician who is experienced in the use of cancer chemotherapeutic agents. Appropriate management of complications is possible only when adequate diagnostic and treatment facilities are readily available.

Irinotecan can induce both early and late forms of diarrhea that appear to be mediated by different mechanisms. Both forms of diarrhea may be severe. Early diarrhea (occurring during or shortly after infusion of irinotecan) may be accompanied by chlolinergic symptoms of rhinitis, increased salivation, miosis, lacrimation, diaphoresis, flushing, and intestinal hyperperistalsis that can cause abdominal cramping. Early diarrhea and other cholinergic symptoms may be prevented or ameliorated by atropine (see Warnings). Late diarrhea (generally occurring more than 24 hours after administration of irinotecan) can be life-threatening because it may be prolonged and may lead to dehydration, electrolyte imbalance, or sepsis. Treat late diarrhea promptly with loperamide. Carefully monitor patients with diarrhea and give fluid and electrolyte replacement if they become dehydrated, or antibiotic therapy if they develop ileus, fever, or severe neutropenia (see Warnings). Interrupt administration of irinotecan and reduce subsequent doses if severe diarrhea occurs (see Administration and Dosage).

Severe myelosuppression may occur (see Warnings).

Indications

➤*Metastatic carcinoma of the colon or rectum:* First-line therapy in combination with 5-fluorouracil (5-FU) and leucovorin for patients with metastatic colon or rectal carcinomas.

It is also indicated for the treatment of metastatic carcinoma of the colon or rectum in patients whose disease has recurred or progressed following initial 5-FU-based therapy.

Administration and Dosage

➤*Approved by the FDA:* June 14, 1996.

➤*Combination agent dosage schedules:*

Irinotecan Dosage Regimens and Dose Modifications[1]

Starting dose and modified dose levels (mg/m²)		Starting dose	Dose level 1	Dose level 2
Regimen 1 6-week course with bolus 5-FU/LV (next course begins on day 43)	Irinotecan[2]	125	100	75
	LV[3]	20	20	20
	5-FU[3]	500	400	300
Regimen 2 6-week course with infusional 5-FU/LV (next course begins on day 43)	Irinotecan[4]	180	150	120
	LV[5]	200	200	200
	5-FU bolus[6]	400	320	240
	5-FU infusion[7,8]	600	480	360

[1] Dose reductions beyond dose level 2 by decrements of ≈ 20% may be warranted for patients continuing to experience toxicity. If intolerable toxicity does not develop, treatment with additional courses may be continued indefinitely as long as patients continue to experience clinical benefit.
[2] IV over 90 minutes day 1, 8, 15, 22.
[3] IV bolus day 1, 8, 15, 22.
[4] IV over 90 minutes day 1, 15, 29.
[5] IV over 2 hours day 1, 2, 15, 16, 29, 30.
[6] IV bolus day 1, 2, 15, 16, 29, 30.
[7] Infusion follows bolus administration.
[8] IV over 22 hours day 1, 2, 15, 16, 29, 30.

Do not begin a new course of therapy until the granulocyte count has recovered to greater than or equal to 1500/mm³ and the platelet count has recovered to greater than or equal to 100,000/mm³ and treatment-related diarrhea is fully resolved. Delay treatment 1 to 2 weeks to allow for recovery from treatment-related toxicities. If the patient has not recovered after a 2-week delay, consider discontinuing therapy.

Irinotecan Recommended Dose Modifications

Toxicity NCI CTC grade[1] (value)	During a course of therapy	At the start of subsequent courses of therapy[2]
No toxicity	Maintain dose level	Maintain dose level
Neutropenia		
1 (1500 to 1999/mm³)	Maintain dose level	Maintain dose level
2 (1000 to 1499/mm³)	↓ 1 dose level	Maintain dose level
3 (500 to 999/mm³)	Omit dose until resolved to ≤ grade 2, then ↓ 1 dose level	↓ 1 dose level
4 (< 500/mm³)	Omit dose until resolved to ≤ grade 2, then ↓ 2 dose levels	↓ 2 dose levels

Irinotecan Recommended Dose Modifications

Toxicity NCI CTC grade[1] (value)	During a course of therapy	At the start of subsequent courses of therapy[2]
Neutropenic fever	Omit dose until resolved, then ↓ 2 dose levels	
Other hematologic toxicities	Dose modifications for leukopenia or thrombocytopenia during a cycle of therapy and at the start of subsequent cycles of therapy are also based on NCI toxicity criteria and are the same as recommended for neutropenia above.	
Diarrhea		
1 (2 to 3 stools/day > pretreatment)	Delay dose until resolved to baseline, then give same dose	Maintain dose level
2 (4 to 6 stools/day > pretreatment)	Omit dose until resolved at baseline, then ↓ 1 dose level	Maintain dose level
3 (7 to 9 stools/day > pretreatment)	Omit dose until resolved to baseline, then ↓ 1 dose level	↓ 1 dose level
4 (≥ 10 stools/day > pretreatment)	Omit dose until resolved to baseline, then ↓ 2 dose levels	↓ 2 dose levels
Other nonhematologic toxicities[3]		
Grade 1 toxicity	Maintain dose level	Maintain dose level
Grade 2 toxicity	Omit dose until resolved to ≤ grade 1, then ↓ 1 dose level	Maintain dose level
Grade 3 toxicity	Omit dose until resolved to ≤ grade 2, then ↓ 1 dose level	↓ 1 dose level
Grade 4 toxicity	Omit dose until resolved to ≤ grade 2, then ↓ 2 dose levels	↓ 2 dose levels
	For mucositis/stomatitis, decrease only 5-FU, not irinotecan	*For mucositis/stomatitis, decrease only 5-FU, not irinotecan*

* ↓ = decrease
[1] National Cancer Institute Common Toxicity Criteria (NCI CTC).
[2] Relative to the starting dose used in the previous course.
[3] Excludes alopecia, anorexia, and asthenia.

➤*Single-agent dosage schedules:*

Irinotecan Regimens and Dose Modifications

Starting dose and modified dose levels (mg/m²)			
	Starting dose	Dose level 1	Dose level 2
Weekly regimen[1,2,3]	125	100	75
Once every 3-week regimen[3,4,5]	350	300	250

[1] Subsequent doses may be adjusted as high as 150 mg/m² or to as low as 50 mg/m² in 25 to 50 mg/m² decrements depending upon individual patient tolerance.
[2] IV over 90 minutes day 1, 8, 15, 22 then 2-week rest.
[3] If intolerable toxicity does not develop, treatment with additional courses may be continued indefinitely as long as patients continue to experience clinical benefit.
[4] Subsequent doses may be adjusted as low as 200 mg/m² in 50 mg/m² decrements depending upon individual patient tolerance.
[5] IV over 90 minutes once every 3 weeks.

Do not begin a new course of therapy until the granulocyte count has recovered to at least 1500/mm³ and the platelet count has recovered to at least 100,000/mm³ and treatment-related diarrhea is fully resolved. Delay treatment 1 to 2 weeks to allow for recovery from treatment-related toxicities. If the patient has not recovered after a 2-week delay, consider discontinuing irinotecan.

Irinotecan Recommended Dose Modifications[1]

Worst toxicity NCI grade[2] (value)	During a course of therapy Weekly	At the start of the next course of therapy (after adequate recovery) compared with the starting dose in the previous course[1] Weekly	Once every 3 weeks
No toxicity	Maintain dose level	↑ 25 mg/m² up to a maximum dose of 150 mg/m²	Maintain dose level
Neutropenia			
1 (1500 to 1999/mm³)	Maintain dose level	Maintain dose level	Maintain dose level
2 (1000 to 1499/mm³)	↓ 25 mg/m²	Maintain dose level	Maintain dose level
3 (500 to 999/mm³)	Omit dose, then ↓ 25 mg/m² when resolved to ≤ grade 2	↓ 25 mg/m²	↓ 50 mg/m²
4 (< 500/mm³)	Omit dose, then ↓ 50 mg/m² when resolved to ≤ grade 2	↓ 50 mg/m²	↓ 50 mg/m²

IRINOTECAN HCl

Irinotecan Recommended Dose Modifications[1]			
Worst toxicity NCI grade[2] (value)	During a course of therapy	At the start of the next course of therapy (after adequate recovery) compared with the starting dose in the previous course[1]	
	Weekly	Weekly	Once every 3 weeks
Neutropenic fever	Omit dose until resolved, then ↓ 50 mg/m² when resolved	↓ 50 mg/m²	↓ 50 mg/m²
Other hematologic toxicities	Dose modifications for leukopenia, thrombocytopenia, and anemia during a cycle of therapy and at the start of subsequent cycles of therapy are also based on NCI toxicity criteria and are the same as recommended for neutropenia above.		
Diarrhea			
1 (2 to 3 stools/day > pretreatment)	Maintain dose level	Maintain dose level	Maintain dose level
2 (4 to 6 stools/day > pretreatment)	↓ 25 mg/m²	Maintain dose level	Maintain dose level
3 (7 to 9 stools/day > pretreatment)	Omit dose, then ↓ 25 mg/m² when resolved to ≤ grade 2	↓ 25 mg/m²	↓ 50 mg/m²
4 (≥ 10 stools/day > pretreatment)	Omit dose, then ↓ 50 mg/m² when resolved to ≤ grade 2	↓ 50 mg/m²	↓ 50 mg/m²
Other nonhematologic toxicities[3]			
Grade 1 toxicity	Maintain dose level	Maintain dose level	Maintain dose level
Grade 2 toxicity	↓ 25 mg/m²	↓ 25 mg/m²	↓ 50 mg/m²
Grade 3 toxicity	Omit dose, then ↓ 25 mg/m² when resolved to ≤ grade 2	↓ 25 mg/m²	↓ 50 mg/m²
Grade 4 toxicity	Omit dose, then ↓ 50 mg/m² when resolved to ≤ grade 2	↓ 50 mg/m²	↓ 50 mg/m²

* ↓ = decrease ↑ = increase
[1] All dose modifications should be based on the worst preceding toxicity.
[2] National Cancer Institute Common Toxicity Criteria (NCI CTC).
[3] Excludes alopecia, anorexia, and asthenia.

Premedicating patients with antiemetic agents is recommended.

➤*Preparation:* Dilute in 5% Dextrose Injection (preferred) or 0.9% Sodium Chloride Injection to a final concentration of 0.12 to 2.8 mg/mL. As with other potentially toxic anticancer agents, exercise care in the handling and preparation of infusion solutions prepared from irinotecan injection. The use of gloves is recommended. If a solution of irinotecan contacts the skin, wash the skin immediately and thoroughly with soap and water. If irinotecan contacts the mucous membranes, flush thoroughly with water. Several published guidelines for handling and disposal of anticancer agents are available.

➤*Storage/Stability:* The solution is physically and chemically stable for up to 24 hours at room temperature (approximately 25°C) and in ambient fluorescent lighting. Solutions diluted in 5% Dextrose Injection, refrigerated (approximately 2° to 8°C; 36° to 46°F), and protected from light are physically and chemically stable for 48 hours. Refrigeration of admixtures using 0.9% Sodium Chloride Injection is not recommended because of a low and sporadic incidence of visible particulates. Freezing irinotecan and admixtures of irinotecan may result in precipitation of the drug and should be avoided. Because of possible microbial contamination during dilution, use the admixture prepared with 5% Dextrose Injection within 24 hours if refrigerated (2° to 8°C; 36° to 46°F). In the case of admixtures prepared with 5% Dextrose Injection or Sodium Chloride Injection, use the solutions within 6 hours if kept at room temperature (15° to 30°C; 59° to 86°F).

Do not add other drugs to the infusion solution. Visually inspect parenteral drug products for particulate matter and discoloration prior to administration whenever solution and container permit.

Store vials at controlled room temperature (15° to 30°C; 59° to 86°F). Protect from light. It is recommended that the vial (and backing/plastic blister remain in the carton until the time of use.

Actions

➤*Pharmacology:* Irinotecan is a derivative of camptothecin. Camptothecins interact specifically with the enzyme topoisomerase I, which relieves torsional strain in DNA by inducing reversible single-strand breaks. Irinotecan and its active metabolite SN-38 bind to the topoisomerase I-DNA complex and prevent religation of these single-strand breaks. Current research suggests that the cytotoxicity of irinotecan is due to double-strand DNA damage produced during DNA synthesis when replication enzymes interact with the ternary complex formed by

topoisomerase I, DNA, and either irinotecan or SN-38. Mammalian cells cannot efficiently repair these double-strand breaks.

In vitro cytotoxicity assays show that the potency of SN-38 relative to irinotecan varies from 2- to 2000-fold. Thus, the precise contribution of SN-38 to the activity of irinotecan is unknown.

➤*Pharmacokinetics:*

Absorption/Distribution – Over the dose range of 50 to 350 mg/m², the AUC of irinotecan increases linearly with dose; the AUC of SN-38 increases less than proportionally with dose. Maximum concentrations of the active metabolite SN-38 are generally seen within 1 hour following the end of a 90-minute infusion of irinotecan.

Irinotecan exhibits moderate plasma protein binding (30% to 68%). SN-38 is highly bound to human plasma proteins (approximately 95%). The plasma protein to which irinotecan and SN-38 predominantly binds is albumin.

Metabolism/Excretion – The metabolic conversion of irinotecan to the active metabolite SN-38 is mediated by carboxylesterase enzymes and primarily occurs in the liver. SN-38 subsequently undergoes conjugation to form a glucuronide metabolite. SN-38 glucuronide had ¹⁄₅₀ to ¹⁄₁₀₀ the activity of SN-38 in cytotoxicity assays using 2 cell lines in vitro. The disposition of irinotecan has not been fully elucidated in humans. The urinary excretion of irinotecan is 11% to 20%; SN-38, less than 1%; and SN-38 glucuronide, 3%. The cumulative biliary and urinary excretion of irinotecan and its metabolites (SN-38 and SN-38 glucuronide) over a period of 48 hours following irinotecan administration in 2 patients ranged from approximately 25% (100 mg/m²) to 50% (300 mg/m²).

Mean Irinotecan and SN-38 Pharmacokinetic Parameters in Patients with Solid Tumors								
	Irinotecan					SN-38		
Dose (mg/m²)	C_{max} (ng/mL)	AUC_{0-24}[1] (ng·h/mL)	$t_{1/2}$ (h)	V_z[2] (L/m²)	CL (L/h/m²)	C_{max} (ng/mL)	AUC_{0-24} (ng·h/mL)	$t_{1/2}$ (h)
125 (N = 64)	1660	10,200	5.8[3]	110	13.3	26.3	229	10.4[3]
340 (N = 6)	3392	20,604	11.7[4]	234	13.9	56	474	21[4]

[1] AUC_{0-24} = Area under the plasma concentration-time curve from time 0 to 24 hours after the end of the 90-minute infusion.
[2] V_z = Volume of distribution of terminal elimination phase.
[3] Plasma specimens collected for 24 hours following the end of the 90-minute infusion.
[4] Plasma specimens collected for 48 hours following the end of the 90-minute infusion. Because of the longer collection period, these values provide a more accurate reflection of the terminal elimination half-lives of irinotecan and SN-38.

Elderly – The terminal half-life of irinotecan was 6 hours in patients who were 65 years of age or older and 5.5 hours in patients younger than 65 years of age. Dose-normalized AUC_{0-24} for SN-38 in patients who were at least 65 years of age was 11% higher than in patients younger than 65 years of age. No change in the starting dose is recommended for geriatric patients receiving the weekly dosage schedule of irinotecan.

Contraindications

Hypersensitivity to irinotecan.

Warnings

➤*Toxic deaths:* Do not use in combination with the Mayo Clinic regimen of 5-FU/LV (administration for 4 to 5 consecutive days every 4 weeks) because of reports of increased toxicity, including toxic deaths. Use irinotecan as recommended.

In patients receiving either irinotecan/5-FU/LV or 5-FU/LV in the clinical trials, higher rates of hospitalization, neutropenic fever, thromboembolism, first-cycle treatment discontinuation, and early deaths were observed in patients with a baseline performance status of 2 than in patients with a baseline performance status of 0 or 1.

➤*Diarrhea:* Irinotecan injection can induce early and late forms of diarrhea that appear to be mediated by different mechanisms. Early diarrhea (occurring during or shortly after irinotecan administration) is cholinergic in nature. It is usually transient and only infrequently severe. It may be accompanied by symptoms of rhinitis, increased salivation, miosis, lacrimation, diaphoresis, flushing, and intestinal hyperperistalsis that can cause abdominal cramping. Early diarrhea may be prevented or ameliorated by atropine.

Late diarrhea (generally occurring more than 24 hours after administration of irinotecan) can be life-threatening because it may be prolonged and may lead to dehydration, electrolyte imbalance, or sepsis. Treat late diarrhea promptly with loperamide. Carefully monitor patients with diarrhea; give fluid and electrolyte replacement if they become dehydrated and antibiotic support if they develop ileus, fever, or severe neutropenia. After the first treatment, delay subsequent weekly chemotherapy treatments in patients until return of pretreatment bowel function for at least 24 hours without need for antidiarrhea medication. If grade 2, 3, or 4 late diarrhea occurs, decrease subsequent doses of irinotecan within the current cycle (see Administration and Dosage).

➤*Irradiation:* Patients who have previously received pelvic/abdominal irradiation are at an increased risk of severe myelosuppression following irinotecan administration. The concurrent administration of

IRINOTECAN HCl

irinotecan with irradiation has not been adequately studied and is not recommended.

➤*Neutropenia:* Deaths caused by sepsis following severe neutropenia have been reported in patients treated with irinotecan. Manage neutropenic complications promptly with antibiotic support. Temporarily discontinue therapy during a cycle of therapy if neutropenic fever occurs or if the absolute neutrophil count drops below 1500/mm^3. After the patient recovers to an absolute neutrophil count greater than or equal to 1500/mm^3, reduce subsequent doses of irinotecan depending upon the level of neutropenia observed. Routine administration of a colony-stimulating factor (CSF) is not necessary, but physicians may consider CSF use in patients experiencing significant neutropenia.

➤*Thromboembolism:* Thromboembolic events have been observed in patients receiving irinotecan-containing regimens; the specific cause of these events has not been determined.

➤*Orthostatic hypotension:* Dizziness sometimes may represent symptomatic evidence of orthostatic hypotension in patients with dehydration.

➤*Colitis/Ileus:* Cases of colitis complicated by ulceration, bleeding, ileus, and infection have been observed. Give patients experiencing ileus prompt antibiotic support.

➤*Hypersensitivity reactions:* Hypersensitivity reactions including severe anaphylactic or anaphylactoid reactions have been observed.

➤*Renal function impairment:* Rare cases of renal impairment and acute renal failure have been identified, usually in patients who became volume depleted from severe vomiting or diarrhea.

➤*Elderly:* Closely monitor patients older than 65 years of age because of a greater risk of late diarrhea in this population. The starting dose of irinotecan in patients 70 years of age and older for the once-every-3-week-dosage schedule should be 300 mg/m^2.

➤*Pregnancy:* Category D. Irinotecan may cause fetal harm when administered to a pregnant woman. There are no adequate and well-controlled studies in pregnant women. If the drug is used during pregnancy, or if the patient becomes pregnant while receiving the drug, apprise the patient of the potential hazard to the fetus. Advise women of childbearing potential to avoid becoming pregnant while receiving treatment with irinotecan.

➤*Lactation:* Because many drugs are excreted in breast milk and because of the potential for serious adverse reactions in nursing infants, discontinue nursing when receiving therapy with irinotecan.

➤*Children:* The safety and efficacy of irinotecan in children have not been established.

Precautions

➤*Monitoring:* Monitor the white blood cell count with differential, hemoglobin, and platelet count before each irinotecan dose.

➤*Extravasation:* Irinotecan is administered by IV infusion. Take care to avoid extravasation and monitor the infusion site for signs of inflammation. If extravasation occurs, flush the site with sterile water and apply ice.

➤*Premedication with antiemetics:* Irinotecan is emetogenic. It is recommended that patients receive premedication with antiemetic agents. In clinical studies, the majority of patients received 10 mg dexamethasone given in conjunction with another type of antiemetic agent, such as a 5-HT$_3$ blocker (eg, ondansetron, granisetron). Give antiemetic agents on the day of treatment, starting at least 30 minutes before administration of irinotecan. Consider providing patients with an antiemetic regimen (eg, prochlorperazine) for subsequent use as needed.

➤*Special risk:* In clinical trials of the weekly dosage schedule, it has been noted that patients with modestly elevated baseline serum total bilirubin levels (1 to 2 mg/dL) have had a significantly greater likelihood of experiencing first-course grade 3 or 4 neutropenia than those with bilirubin levels that were less than 1 mg/dL. Patients with abnormal glucuronidation of bilirubin, such as those with Gilbert's syndrome, may also be at greater risk of myelosuppression when receiving therapy with irinotecan. An association between baseline bilirubin elevations and an increased risk of late diarrhea has not been observed in studies of the weekly dosage schedule.

Drug Interactions

Irinotecan Drug Interactions			
Precipitant drug	Object drug*		Description
Antineoplastics	Irinotecan	↑	The adverse effects of irinotecan, such as myelosuppression and diarrhea, would be expected to be exacerbated by other antineoplastic agents having similar adverse effects.

Irinotecan Drug Interactions			
Precipitant drug	Object drug*		Description
Dexamethasone	Irinotecan	↑	Lymphocytopenia has been reported in patients receiving irinotecan, and it is possible that the administration of dexamethasone as antiemetic prophylaxis may have enhanced the likelihood of this effect. Hyperglycemia also has been reported in patients receiving irinotecan. It is probable that dexamethasone given as emetic prophylaxis contributed to hyperglycemia in some patients.
Laxatives	Irinotecan	↑	It would be expected that laxative use during therapy with irinotecan would worsen the incidence or severity of diarrhea, but this has not been studied.
Prochlorperazine	Irinotecan	↑	The incidence of akathisia in clinical trials was greater (8.5%) when prochlorperazine was administered on the same day as irinotecan than when these drugs were given on separate days (1.3%). However, the 8.5% incidence of akathisia is within the range reported for use of prochlorperazine when given as a premedication for other chemotherapeutics.
Irinotecan	Diuretics	↑	In view of the potential risk of dehydration secondary to vomiting and diarrhea induced by irinotecan, the physician may wish to withhold diuretics during dosing with irinotecan and during periods of active vomiting or diarrhea.

* ↑ = Object drug increased.

Adverse Reactions

➤*First-line combination therapy:*

Death – In Study I, 49 patients died within 30 days of study treatment: 21 received irinotecan in combination with 5-FU/LV, 15 received 5-FU/LV alone, and 13 received irinotecan alone. Deaths potentially related to treatment occurred in 2 patients who received irinotecan in combination with 5-FU/LV (2 neutropenic fever/sepsis), 3 patients who received 5-FU/LV alone (1 neutropenic fever/sepsis, 1 CNS bleeding during thrombocytopenia, 1 unknown), and 2 patients who received irinotecan alone (2 neutropenic fever).

Discontinuations because of adverse events were reported for 17 patients who received irinotecan in combination with 5-FU/LV, 14 patients who received 5-FU/LV alone, and 26 patients received irinotecan alone.

Study 1: Patients Experiencing Adverse Reactions in Combination Therapies (%)[1]					
	Irinotecan + bolus 5-FU/LV weekly × 4 every 6 wks (N = 225)		Bolus 5-FU/LV daily × 5 every 4 wks (N = 219)		Irinotecan weekly × 4 every 6 wks (N = 223)
Adverse reaction	Grade 1-4	3 & 4	1-4	3 & 4	1-4	3 & 4
Total adverse reactions	100	53.3	100	45.7	99.6	45.7
Cardiovascular						
Vasodilation	9.3	0.9	5	0	9	0
Hypotension	5.8	1.3	2.3	0.5	5.8	1.7
Thromboembolic events[2]	9.3	-	11.4	-	5.4	-
CNS						
Dizziness	23.1	1.3	16.4	0	21.1	1.8
Somnolence	12.4	1.8	4.6	1.8	9.4	1.3
Confusion	7.1	1.8	4.1	0	2.7	0
Dermatologic						
Exfoliative dermatitis	0.9	0	3.2	0.5	0	0
Rash	19.1	0	26.5	0.9	14.3	0.4
Alopecia[3]	43.1	-	26.5	-	46.1	-
GI						
Diarrhea						
Late	84.9	22.7	69.4	13.2	83	31
grade 3	-	15.1	-	5.9	-	18.4
grade 4	-	7.6	-	7.3	-	12.6
Early	45.8	4.9	31.5	1.4	43	6.7
Nausea	79.1	15.6	67.6	8.2	81.6	16.1
Abdominal pain	63.1	14.6	50.2	11.5	67.7	13
Vomiting	60.4	9.7	46.1	4.1	62.8	12.1
Anorexia	34.2	5.8	42	3.7	43.9	7.2

IRINOTECAN HCl

Study 1: Patients Experiencing Adverse Reactions in Combination Therapies (%)[1]					
	Irinotecan + bolus 5-FU/LV weekly × 4 every 6 wks (N = 225)		Bolus 5-FU/LV daily × 5 every 4 wks (N = 219)		Irinotecan weekly × 4 every 6 wks (N = 223)
Adverse reaction	Grade 1-4	3 & 4	1-4	3 & 4	1-4	3 & 4
Constipation	41.3	3.1	31.5	1.8	32.3	0.4
Mucositis	32.4	2.2	76.3	16.9	29.6	2.2
Hematologic						
Neutropenia	96.9	53.8	98.6	66.7	96.4	31.4
grade 3	-	29.8	-	23.7	-	19.3
grade 4	-	24	-	42.5	-	12.1
Leukopenia	96.9	37.8	98.6	23.3	96.4	21.5
Anemia	96.9	8.4	98.6	5.5	96.9	4.5
Neutropenic fever	-	7.1	-	14.6	-	5.8
Thrombocytopenia	96	2.6	98.6	2.7	96	1.7
Neutropenic infection	-	1.8	-	0	-	2.2
Respiratory						
Dyspnea	27.6	6.3	16	0.5	22	2.2
Cough	26.7	1.3	18.3	0	20.2	0.4
Pneumonia	6.2	2.7	1.4	1	3.6	1.3
Miscellaneous						
Increased bilirubin	87.6	7.1	92.2	8.2	83.9	7.2
Asthenia	70.2	19.5	64.4	11.9	69.1	13.9
Pain	30.7	3.1	26.9	3.6	22.9	2.2
Fever	42.2	1.7	32.4	3.6	43.5	0.4
Infection	22.2	0	16	1.4	13.9	0.4

[1] Severity of adverse events based on NCI CTC.
[2] Includes angina pectoris, arterial thrombosis, cerebral infarct, cerebrovascular accident, deep thrombophlebitis, embolus lower extremity, heart arrest, MI, myocardial ischemia, peripheral vascular disorder, pulmonary embolus, sudden death, thrombophlebitis, thrombosis, vascular disorder.
[3] Complete hair loss = grade 2.

In Study 2, 10 patients died within 30 days of last study treatment: 6 received irinotecan in combination with 5-FU/LV and 4 received 5-FU/LV alone. There was 1 potentially treatment-related death that occurred in a patient who received irinotecan in combination with 5-FU/LV (0.7%, neutropenic sepsis). Deaths from any cause within 60 days of first study treatment were reported for 3 patients who received irinotecan in combination with 5-FU/LV and 2 patients who received 5-FU/LV alone. Discontinuations because of adverse events were reported for 9 patients who received irinotecan in combination with 5-FU/LV and 1 patient who received 5-FU/LV alone.

The most clinically significant adverse events for patients receiving irinotecan-based therapy were diarrhea, nausea, vomiting, neutropenia, and alopecia. In Study I, grade 4 neutropenia, neutropenic fever (defined as grade 2 fever and grade 4 neutropenia), and mucositis were observed less often with weekly irinotecan/5-FU/LV than with monthly administration of 5-FU/LV.

Study 2: Patients Experiencing Clinically Relevant Adverse Reactions in Combination Therapies (%)[1]				
	Irinotecan + 5-FU/LV infusional days 1 and 2 every 2 wks (N = 145)		5-FU/LV infusional days 1 and 2 every 2 wks (N = 143)	
Adverse reaction	Grade 1-4	3 & 4	1-4	3 & 4
Total adverse reactions	100	72.4	100	39.2
Cardiovascular				
Hypotension	3.4	1.4	0.7	0
Thromboembolic events[2]	11.7	-	5.6	-
Dermatologic				
Hand and foot syndrome	10.3	0.7	12.6	0.7
Cutaneous signs	17.2	0.7	20.3	0
Alopecia[3]	56.6	-	16.8	-
GI				
Diarrhea				
Late	72.4	14.4	44.8	6.3
grade 3	-	10.3	-	4.2
grade 4	-	4.1	-	2.1
Cholinergic syndrome[4]	28.3	1.4	0.7	0
Nausea	66.9	2.1	55.2	3.5
Abdominal pain	17.2	2.1	16.8	0.7
Vomiting	44.8	3.5	32.2	2.8
Anorexia	35.2	2.1	18.9	0.7
Constipation	30.3	0.7	25.2	1.4
Mucositis	40	4.1	28.7	2.8

Study 2: Patients Experiencing Clinically Relevant Adverse Reactions in Combination Therapies (%)[1]				
	Irinotecan + 5-FU/LV infusional days 1 and 2 every 2 wks (N = 145)		5-FU/LV infusional days 1 and 2 every 2 wks (N = 143)	
Adverse reaction	Grade 1-4	3 & 4	1-4	3 & 4
Hematologic				
Neutropenia	82.5	46.2	47.9	13.4
grade 3	-	36.4	-	12.7
grade 4	-	9.8	-	0.7
Leukopenia	81.3	17.4	42	3.5
Anemia	97.2	2.1	90.9	2.1
Neutropenic fever	-	3.4	-	0.7
Thrombocytopenia	32.6	0	32.2	0
Neutropenic infection	-	2.1	-	0
Miscellaneous				
Asthenia	57.9	9	48.3	4.2
Dyspnea	9.7	1.4	4.9	0
Fever	22.1	0.7	25.9	0.7
Increased bilirubin	19.1	3.5	35.9	10.6
Infection	35.9	7.6	33.6	3.5
Pain	64.1	9.7	61.5	8.4

[1] Severity of adverse events based on NCI CTC.
[2] Includes angina pectoris, arterial thrombosis, cerebral infarct, cerebrovascular accident, deep thrombophlebitis, embolus lower extremity, heart arrest, MI, myocardial ischemia, peripheral vascular disorder, pulmonary embolus, sudden death, thrombophlebitis, thrombosis, vascular disorder.
[3] Complete hair loss = grade 2.
[4] Includes rhinitis, increased salivation, miosis, lacrimation, diaphoresis, flushing, abdominal cramping or diarrhea (occurring during or shortly after infusion of irinotecan).

➤*Second-line single-agent therapy:*
Weekly dosage schedule:

Adverse Reactions Occurring in > 10% of Previously Treated Irinotecan Patients with Metastatic Carcinoma of the Colon or Rectum (N = 304)[1]		
	% of patients reporting	
Adverse reaction	Grade 1-4	Grade 3 & 4
CNS		
Insomnia	19	0
Dizziness	15	0
Dermatologic		
Alopecia	60	na[2]
Sweating	16	0
Rash	13	1
GI		
Diarrhea (late)[3]	88	31
7 to 9 stools/day (grade 3)	-	16
≥ 10 stools/day (grade 4)	-	14
Nausea	86	17
Vomiting	67	12
Anorexia	55	6
Diarrhea (early)[4]	51	8
Constipation	30	2
Flatulence	12	0
Stomatitis	12	1
Dyspepsia	10	0
Hematologic		
Leukopenia	63	28
Anemia	60	7
Neutropenia	54	26
500 to < 1000/mm³ (grade 3)	-	15
< 500/mm³ (grade 4)	-	12
Metabolic/Nutritional		
Decreased body weight	30	1
Dehydration	15	4
Increased alkaline phosphatase	13	4
Increased AST	10	1
Respiratory		
Dyspnea	22	4
Increased coughing	17	0
Rhinitis	16	0
Miscellaneous		
Asthenia	76	12
Abdominal cramping/pain	57	16
Fever	45	1
Pain	24	2
Headache	17	1
Back pain	14	2
Chills	14	0
Minor infections[5]	14	0

IRINOTECAN HCl

Adverse Reactions Occurring in > 10% of Previously Treated Irinotecan Patients with Metastatic Carcinoma of the Colon or Rectum (N = 304)[1]

Adverse reaction	% of patients reporting	
	Grade 1-4	Grade 3 & 4
Vasodilation (flushing)	11	0
Edema	10	1
Abdominal enlargement	10	0

[1] Severity of adverse events of adverse events based on NCI CTC.
[2] Not applicable: Complete hair loss = NCI grade 2.
[3] Occurring > 24 hours after irinotecan administration.
[4] Occurring ≤ 24 hours after irinotecan administration.
[5] Primarily upper respiratory tract infections.

Once-every-3-week dosage schedule:

Patients Experiencing Grade 3 and 4 Adverse Reactions (%)[1]

Adverse reaction	Study 1		Study 2	
	Irinotecan N = 189	BSC[2] N = 90	Irinotecan N = 127	5-FU N = 129
Total grade 3/4 adverse reactions	79	67	69	54
Cardiovascular[3]	9	3	4	2
CNS[4]	12	13	9	4
Dermatologic				
Hand and foot syndrome	0	0	0	5
Cutaneous signs[5]	2	0	1	3
GI				
Diarrhea	22	6	22	11
Vomiting	14	8	14	5
Nausea	14	3	11	4
Abdominal pain	14	16	9	8
Constipation	10	8	8	6
Anorexia	5	7	6	4
Mucositis	2	1	2	5
Hematologic				
Leukopenia/Neutropenia	22	0	14	2
Anemia	7	6	6	3
Hemorrhage	5	3	1	3
Thrombocytopenia	1	0	4	4
Infection				
Without grade 3/4 neutropenia	8	3	1	4
With grade 3/4 neutropenia	1	0	2	0
Fever				
Without grade 3/4 neutropenia	2	1	2	0
With grade 3/4 neutropenia	2	0	4	2
Respiratory[6]	10	8	5	7
Other[7]	32	28	12	14
Miscellaneous				
Pain	19	22	17	13
Asthenia	15	19	13	12
Hepatic[8]	9	7	9	6

[1] Severity of adverse events based on NCI CTC.
[2] Best supportive care.
[3] Includes events such as dysrhythmias, ischemia, and mechanical cardiac dysfunction.
[4] Includes events such as somnolence.
[5] Includes events such as rash.
[6] Includes events such as dyspnea and cough.
[7] Includes events such as accidental injury, hepatomegaly, syncope, vertigo, and weight loss.
[8] Includes events such as ascites and jaundice.

➤*Cardiovascular:* Flushing may occur during administration. Bradycardia also may occur but has not required intervention. These effects have been attributed to the cholinergic syndrome sometimes observed during or shortly after infusion. Thromboembolic events have been observed in patients receiving irinotecan; the specific cause of these events has not been determined.

➤*Dermatologic:* Alopecia; rash.

➤*Hematologic:* Serious thrombocytopenia was uncommon. Neutropenic fever (concurrent NCI grade 4 neutropenia and fever of grade 2 or greater; 3%); NCI grade 3 or 4 anemia (7%); blood transfusions (10%). The frequency of grade 3 and 4 neutropenia was significantly higher in patients who received previous pelvic/abdominal irradiation than in those who had not received irradiation (48% vs 24%).

➤*Hepatic:* NCI grade 3 or 4 liver enzyme abnormalities (fewer than 10%). These events occurred in patients with known hepatic metastases.

➤*Respiratory:* Severe pulmonary events were infrequent; NCI grade 3 or 4 dyspnea was reported in 4% of patients. Over half of the patients with dyspnea had lung metastases; the extent to which malignant pulmonary involvement or other pre-existing lung disease may have contributed to dyspnea in these patients is unknown.

➤*Postmarketing:* The following events have been identified during postmarketing use of irinotecan in clinical practice. Cases of colitis complicated by ulceration, bleeding, ileus, or infection have been observed. There have been rare cases of renal impairment and acute renal failure, generally in patients who became infected or volume depleted from severe GI toxicities. Hypersensitivity reactions, including severe anaphylactic or anaphylactoid reactions, also have been observed (see Warnings).

Overdosage

Single doses of up to 750 mg/m^2 of irinotecan have been given. The adverse events in these patients were similar to those reported with the recommended dose and regimen. There is no known antidote for overdosage of irinotecan. Institute maximum supportive care to prevent dehydration caused by diarrhea and to treat any infectious complications.

Patient Information

Inform patients and caregivers of the expected toxic effects of irinotecan, particularly of its GI complications, such as nausea, vomiting, abdominal cramping, diarrhea, and infection. Instruct each patient to have loperamide readily available and to begin treatment for late diarrhea (generally occurring more than 24 hours after administration) at the first episode of poorly formed or loose stools or the earliest onset of bowel movements more frequent than normally expected for the patient. One dosage regimen for loperamide used in clinical trials consisted of the following (Note: This dosage regimen exceeds the usual dosage recommendations for loperamide): 4 mg at the first onset of late diarrhea and then 2 mg every 2 hours until the patient is diarrhea-free for at least 12 hours. During the night, the patient may take 4 mg loperamide every 4 hours. Premedication with loperamide is not recommended.

Avoid the use of drugs with laxative properties because of the potential for exacerbation of diarrhea. Advise patients to contact their physician to discuss any laxative use.

Instruct patients to consult their physician if any of the following occur: Diarrhea for the first time during treatment; black or bloody stools; symptoms of dehydration, such as lightheadedness, dizziness, or faintness; inability to take fluids by mouth because of nausea or vomiting; inability to get diarrhea under control within 24 hours; or fever or evidence of infection.

Patients should be alerted to the possibility of alopecia.

TOPOTECAN HCl

Rx   **Hycamtin** (GlaxoSmithKline)   **Powder for injection, lyophilized:** 4 mg (as base)   48 mg mannitol. In single-dose vials.

WARNING

Administer topotecan under the supervision of a physician experienced in the use of cancer chemotherapeutic agents. Appropriate management of complications is possible only when adequate diagnostic and treatment facilities are readily available.

Do not give topotecan therapy to patients with baseline neutrophil counts less than 1500 cells/mm^3. In order to monitor the occurrence of bone marrow suppression, primarily neutropenia that may be severe and result in infection and death, perform frequent peripheral blood cell counts on all patients receiving topotecan.

Indications

➤*Ovarian cancer:* For the treatment of patients with metastatic carcinoma of the ovary after failure of initial or subsequent chemotherapy.

➤*Small-cell lung cancer:* For the treatment of small-cell lung cancer sensitive disease after failure of first-line chemotherapy. Sensitive disease was defined as disease responding to chemotherapy but subsequently progressing at least 60 (in the Phase III study) or 90 (in the Phase II studies) days after chemotherapy.

Administration and Dosage

➤*Approved by the FDA:* May 28, 1996.

Prior to administration of the first course of topotecan, patients must have a baseline neutrophil count greater than 1500 cells/mm^3 and a platelet count greater than 100,000 cells/mm^3.

➤*Dosage:* The recommended dose of topotecan is 1.5 mg/m^2 by IV infusion over 30 minutes daily for 5 consecutive days, starting on day 1 of a 21-day course. In the absence of tumor progression, a minimum of 4 courses is recommended because tumor response may be delayed.

TOPOTECAN HCl

➤*Dosage adjustment:* In the event of severe neutropenia during any course, reduce the dose by 0.25 mg/m^2 for subsequent courses. Similarly reduce doses if the platelet count falls below 25,000 cells/mm^3. Alternatively, in the event of severe neutropenia, filgrastim (G-CSF) may be administered following the subsequent course (before resorting to dosage reduction) starting from day 6 of the course (24 hours after completion of topotecan administration).

➤*Renal function impairment:* No dosage adjustment appears to be required for treating patients with mild renal impairment (Ccr 40 to 60 mL/min). Dosage adjustment to 0.75 mg/m^2 is recommended for patients with moderate renal impairment (Ccr 20 to 39 mL/min). Insufficient data are available in patients with severe renal impairment to provide a dosage recommendation.

➤*Preparation of IV infusion:* Reconstitute each topotecan 4 mg vial with 4 mL sterile water for injection, then dilute the appropriate volume of the reconstituted solution either in 0.9% sodium chloride IV infusion or 5% dextrose IV infusion.

➤*Storage/Stability:* Protect vials from light in the original cartons between 20° and 25°C (68° and 77°F). Reconstituted vials of topotecan diluted for infusion are stable at approximately 20° to 25°C (68° to 77°F) under ambient lighting conditions for 24 hours.

Actions

➤*Pharmacology:* Topotecan HCl is a semi-synthetic derivative of camptothecin and an antitumor drug with topoisomerase I-inhibitory activity. Topoisomerase I relieves torsional strain in DNA by inducing reversible single-strand breaks. Topotecan binds to the topoisomerase I-DNA complex and prevents religation of these single-strand breaks. The cytotoxicity of topotecan is thought to be caused by double-strand DNA damage produced during DNA synthesis when replication enzymes interact with the ternary complex formed by topotecan, topoisomerase I, and DNA.

➤*Pharmacokinetics:*

Absorption/Distribution – The pharmacokinetics of topotecan have been evaluated in cancer patients following doses of 0.5 to 1.5 mg/m^2 administered as a 30 minute infusion. Topotecan exhibits multiexponential pharmacokinetics. Total exposure (AUC) is dose-proportional. The mean Vd_{ss} is between 17 and 22 L/m^2 for topotecan and 26 to 563 L/m^2 for its active lactone moiety. Topotecan is approximately 35% bound to plasma proteins.

Metabolism/Excretion – Topotecan undergoes a reversible pH-dependent hydrolysis of its lactone moiety; it is the lactone form that is pharmacologically active. In vitro studies indicate that metabolism of topotecan to an N-demethylated metabolite represents a minor metabolic pathway. Topotecan has a terminal half-life of 2 to 3 hours. Renal clearance is an important determinant of topotecan elimination with approximately 30% of the dose excreted in the urine.

Renal function impairment: In patients with mild renal impairment (Ccr 40 to 60 mL/min), topotecan plasma clearance was decreased to approximately 67%. In patients with moderate renal impairment (Ccr 20 to 39 mL/min), topotecan plasma clearance was reduced approximately 34%, with an increase in half-life. Mean half-life, estimated in 3 renally impaired patients, was approximately 5 hours. Dosage adjustment is recommended for these patients (see Administration and Dosage).

Hepatic function impairment: Plasma clearance in patients with hepatic impairment (serum bilirubin levels between 1.7 and 15 mg/dL) was decreased approximately 67%. Topotecan half-life increased slightly, from 2 to 2.5 hours, but these hepatically impaired patients tolerated the usual recommended topotecan dosage regimen.

Gender: The overall mean topotecan plasma clearance in male patients was approximately 24% higher than in female patients, largely reflecting difference in body size.

➤*Clinical trials:*

Ovarian cancer – A randomized trial compared 112 patients treated with topotecan (1.5 mg/m^2/day for 5 days starting on day 1 of a 21-day course) and 114 patients treated with paclitaxel (175 mg/m^2 over 3 hours on day 1 of a 21-day course). All patients had recurrent ovarian cancer after a platinum-containing regimen or had not responded to at least 1 prior platinum-containing regimen.

The median time to response was 7.6 weeks (range, 3.1 to 21.7) with topotecan compared with 6 weeks (range, 2.4 to 18.1) with paclitaxel. Consequently, the efficacy of topotecan may not be achieved if patients are prematurely withdrawn from treatment.

In the crossover Phase, 8 of 61 (13%) patients who received topotecan after paclitaxel had a partial response and 5 of 49 (10%) patients who received paclitaxel after topotecan had a response (2 complete responses).

Topotecan was active in ovarian cancer patients who had developed resistance to platinum-containing therapy, defined as tumor progression while on, or tumor relapse within 6 months after completion of, a platinum-containing regimen. One complete and 6 partial responses were seen in 60 patients, for a response rate of 12%. In the same study, there were no complete responders and 4 partial responders on the paclitaxel arm, for a response rate of 7%.

Small-cell lung cancer – In a phase III trial, 107 patients were treated with topotecan (1.5 mg/m^2/day for 5 days starting on day 1 of a 21-day course) and 104 patients were treated with CAV (1000 mg/m^2 cyclophosphamide, 45 mg/m^2 doxorubicin, 2 mg vincristine administered sequentially on day 1 of a 21-day course). All patients were considered sensitive to first-line chemotherapy (responders who then subsequently progressed 60 or more days after completion of first-line therapy). The time to response was similar in both arms (median 6 weeks).

The overall response rate in the topotecan group was 24% (0% complete response rate and 24% partial response rate) versus 18% (1% complete response rate and 17% partial response rate) in the CAV group. Time to response was similar in both groups with a median of 6 weeks. The median time to progression was 13.3 weeks in the topotecan group and 12.3 in the CAV group. Median survival was 25 and 24.7 weeks in the topotecan and CAV groups, respectively.

Contraindications

Hypersensitivity to topotecan or any of its ingredients; patients who are pregnant or breastfeeding; severe bone marrow depression.

Warnings

➤*Bone marrow suppression:* Bone marrow suppression (primarily neutropenia) is the dose-limiting toxicity of topotecan. Neutropenia is not cumulative over time. Administer topotecan only to patients with adequate bone marrow reserves, including baseline neutrophil counts of at least 1500 cells/mm^3 and platelet counts of at least 100,000/mm^3. WBC count decreases with increasing topotecan dose or topotecan AUC. When topotecan is administered at a dose of 1.5 mg/m^2/day for 5 days, an 80% to 90% decrease in WBC count at nadir is typically observed after the first cycle of therapy. Severe myelotoxicity has been reported when topotecan is used in combination with cisplatin.

➤*Neutropenia:* Grade 4 (less than 500 cells/mm^3) neutropenia was most common during course 1 of treatment (60%) and occurred in 39% of all courses, with a median duration of 7 days. The nadir neutrophil count occurred at a median of 12 days. Therapy-related sepsis or febrile neutropenia occurred in 23% of patients, and sepsis was fatal in 1%.

➤*Thrombocytopenia:* Grade 4 thrombocytopenia (less than 25,000/mm^3) occurred in 27% of patients and in 9% of courses, with a median duration of 5 days, platelet nadir at a median of 15 days. Platelet transfusions were given to 15% of patients and in 4% of courses.

➤*Anemia:* Severe anemia (grade 3/4, Hgb less than 8 g/dL) occurred in 37% of patients and in 14% of courses. Median nadir was at day 15. Transfusions were needed in 52% of patients and in 22% of courses.

➤*Death:* In ovarian cancer, the overall treatment-related death rate was 1%. However, in small-cell lung cancer the treatment-related death rates were 5% for topotecan and 4% for CAV (cyclophosphamide, doxorubicin, vincristine).

➤*Carcinogenesis:* Topotecan is known to be genotoxic to mammalian cells and is a probable carcinogen.

➤*Mutagenesis:* Topotecan was mutagenic to L5178Y mouse lymphoma cells and clastogenic to cultured human lymphocytes with and without metabolic activation. It also was clastogenic to mouse bone marrow.

➤*Pregnancy: Category D.* Topotecan may cause fetal harm when administered to a pregnant woman. In rabbits, a dose of 0.10 mg/kg/day (about equal to the clinical dose on a mg/m^2 basis) given on days 6 through 20 of gestation caused maternal toxicity, embryolethality, and reduced fetal body weight. In rats, a dose of 0.23 mg/kg/day (about equal to the clinical dose on a mg/m^2 basis) given for 14 days before mating through gestation day 6 caused fetal resorption, microphthalmia, preimplant loss, and mild maternal toxicity. A dose of 0.1 mg/kg/day (about half the clinical dose on a mg/m^2 basis) given to rats on days 6 through 17 of gestation caused an increase in postimplantation mortality. This dose also caused an increase in total fetal malformations. The most frequent malformations were of the eye (microphthalmia, anophthalmia, rosette formation of the retina, coloboma of the retina, ectopic orbit), brain (dilated lateral and third ventricles), skull, and vertebrae. The effects of topotecan on pregnant women have not been studied. If topotecan is used during pregnancy, or if a patient becomes pregnant while taking topotecan, warn her of the potential hazard to the fetus. Warn patients to avoid becoming pregnant.

➤*Lactation:* It is not known whether this drug is excreted in breast milk. Discontinue breastfeeding when administering topotecan.

➤*Children:* Safety and efficacy in children have not been established.

Precautions

➤*Monitoring:* Institute frequent monitoring of peripheral blood cell counts during treatment with topotecan. Do not treat patients with subsequent courses of topotecan until neutrophils recover to over 1000 cells/mm^3, platelets recover to over 100,000 cells/mm^3, and hemoglobin levels recover to 9 g/dL (with transfusion if necessary).

➤*Extravasation:* Topotecan extravasation has been associated with only mild local reactions such as erythema and bruising.

TOPOTECAN HCl

Drug Interactions

Topotecan Drug Interactions

Precipitant drug	Object drug*		Description
Cisplatin	Topotecan	↑	Myelosuppression is more severe when topotecan is given in combination with cisplatin. There are no adequate data to define a safe and effective regimen for topotecan and cisplatin in combination. Coadministration of a platinum agent on day 1 of topotecan dosing required lower doses of each agent compared with coadministration on day 5 of the topotecan dosing schedule. Greater myelosuppression also is likely to be seen when topotecan is used in combination with other cytotoxic agents, thereby necessitating a dose reduction.
Filgrastim (G-CSF)	Topotecan	↑	Coadministration can prolong the duration of neutropenia. If G-CSF is used, do not initiate until day 6 of the course of therapy, 24 hours after completion of treatment with topotecan.

* ↑ = Object drug increased.

Adverse Reactions

Data in this section are based on the combined experiences of 453 patients with metastatic ovarian carcinoma and 426 patients with small-cell lung cancer treated with topotecan.

Adverse Reactions in Patients Receiving Topotecan (%)

Hematologic adverse reactions	Incidence (n = 879)	Courses (n = 4124)
Neutropenia		
Neutrophil count < 1500 cells/mm^3	97	81
Neutrophil count < 500 cells/mm^3	78	39
Leukopenia		
Leukocyte count < 3000 cells/mm^3	97	80
Leukocyte count < 1000 cells/mm^3	32	11
Thrombocytopenia		
< 75,000 platelets/mm^3	69	42
< 25,000 platelets/mm^3	27	9
Anemia		
Hgb < 10 g/dL	89	71
Hgb < 8 g/dL	37	14
Sepsis or fever/infection with grade 4 neutropenia	23	7
Platelet transfusions	15	4
RBC transfusions	52	22

Nonhematologic Adverse Reactions in Patients Receiving Topotecan (%)

Adverse reaction	All grades		Grade 3		Grade 4	
	Patients (n = 879)	Courses (n = 4124)	Patients (n = 879)	Courses (n = 4124)	Patients (n = 879)	Courses (n = 4124)
Dermatologic						
Alopecia	49	54	NA	NA	NA	NA
Rash[1]	16	6	1	< 1	0	0
GI						
Nausea	64	42	7	2	1	< 1
Vomiting	45	22	4	1	1	< 1
Diarrhea	32	14	3	1	1	< 1
Constipation	29	15	2	1	1	< 1
Abdominal pain	22	10	2	1	2	< 1
Stomatitis	18	8	1	< 1	< 1	< 1
Anorexia	19	9	2	1	< 1	< 1
Respiratory						
Dyspnea	22	11	5	2	3	1
Coughing	15	7	1	< 1	0	0
Miscellaneous						
Headache	18	7	1	< 1	< 1	0
Fatigue	29	22	5	2	0	0
Fever	28	11	1	< 1	< 1	< 1
Pain[2]	23	11	2	1	1	< 1
Asthenia	25	13	4	1	2	< 1

[1] Includes pruritus, erythematous rash, urticaria, dermatitis, bullous eruption, and maculopapular rash.
[2] Includes body, back, and skeletal pain.

Comparative Toxicity Profiles for Ovarian Cancer Patients: Topotecan vs Paclitaxel (%)

Adverse reaction	Topotecan		Paclitaxel[1]	
	Patients (n = 112)	Courses (n = 597)	Patients (n = 114)	Courses (n = 589)
Hematologic Grade 3/4				
Grade 4 neutropenia (neutrophil count < 500 cells/mL)	80	36	21	9
Grade 3/4 anemia (Hgb < 8 g/dL)	41	16	6	2
Grade 4 thrombocytopenia (< 25,000 platelets/mL)	27	10	3	< 1
Fever/Grade 4 neutropenia	23	6	4	1
Documented sepsis	5	1	2	< 1
Death related to sepsis	2	NA	0	NA
Nonhematologic Grade 3/4				
CNS				
Arthralgia	1	< 1	3	< 1
Asthenia	5	2	3	1
Chest pain	2	< 1	1	< 1
Headache	1	< 1	2	1
Myalgia	0	0	3	2
Pain[2]	5	1	7	2
GI				
Abdominal pain	5	1	4	1
Constipation	5	1	0	0
Diarrhea	6	2	1	< 1
Intestinal obstruction	5	1	4	1
Nausea	10	3	2	< 1
Stomatitis	1	< 1	1	< 1
Vomiting	10	2	3	< 1
Miscellaneous				
Anorexia	4	1	0	0
Dyspnea	6	2	5	1
Fatigue	7	2	6	2
Malaise	2	< 1	2	< 1
Rash[3]	0	0	1	< 1
Increased hepatic enzymes[4]	1	< 1	1	< 1

[1] Premedications were not routinely used in patients randomized to topotecan, while patients receiving paclitaxel received routine pretreatment with corticosteroids, diphenhydramine, and histamine receptor type 2 blockers.
[2] Includes body, skeletal, and back pain.
[3] Includes pruritus, erythematous rash, urticaria, dermatitis, bullous eruption, and maculopapular rash.
[4] Includes increased AST and ALT.

Comparative Toxicity Profiles for Small Cell Lung Cancer Patients: Topotecan vs CAV (%)

Adverse reactions	Topotecan		CAV[1]	
	Patients (n = 107)	Courses (n = 446)	Patients (n = 104)	Courses (n = 359)
Hematologic Grade 3/4				
Grade 4 neutropenia (< 500 cells/mL)	70	38	72	51
Grade 3/4 anemia (Hgb < 8 g/dl)	42	18	20	7
Grade 3/4 thrombocytopenia (< 25,000 plts/mL)	29	10	5	1
Fever/Grade 4 neutropenia	28	9	26	13
Documented sepsis	5	1	5	1
Death related to sepsis	3	NA	1	NA
Non-Hematologic Grade 3/4				
CNS				
Asthenia	9	4	7	2
Headache	0	0	2	< 1
Pain[2]	5	2	7	4
GI				
Abdominal pain	6	1	4	2
Constipation	1	< 1	0	0
Diarrhea	1	< 1	0	0
Nausea	8	2	6	2
Stomatitis	2	< 1	1	< 1
Vomiting	3	< 1	3	1
Respiratory				
Coughing	2	1	0	0
Pneumonia	8	2	6	2

TOPOTECAN HCl

Comparative Toxicity Profiles for Small Cell Lung Cancer Patients: Topotecan vs CAV (%)				
	Topotecan		CAV[1]	
Adverse reactions	Patients (n = 107)	Courses (n = 446)	Patients (n = 104)	Courses (n = 359)
Miscellaneous				
Anorexia	3	1	4	2
Dyspnea	9	5	14	7
Fatigue	6	4	10	3
Rash[3]	1	< 1	1	< 1
Increased hepatic enzymes[4]	1	< 1	0	0

[1] Premedications were not routinely used in patients randomized to topotecan, while patients receiving CAV received routine pretreatment with corticosteroids, diphenhydramine, and histamine receptor type 2 blockers.

[2] Includes body, skeletal, and back pain.

[3] Includes pruritus, erythematous rash, urticaria, dermatitis, bullous eruption, and maculopapular rash.

[4] Includes increased AST and ALT.

➤*CNS:* Headache (18%); paresthesia (7%) was generally grade 1.

➤*Dermatologic:* Grade 2 total alopecia (31%).

➤*GI:* Nausea (64%; 8% grade 3/4); vomiting (45%; 6% grade 3/4). The prophylactic use of antiemetics was not routine in patients treated with topotecan. Diarrhea (32%; 4% grade 3/4); constipation (29%; 2% grade 3/4); abdominal pain (22%; 4% grade 3/4). Grade 3/4 abdominal pain was 6% in ovarian cancer patients and 2% in small cell lung cancer patients.

➤*Hematologic:* See Warnings.

➤*Hepatic:* Grade 1 transient elevations in hepatic enzymes (8%); greater elevations, grade 3/4 (4%); grade 3/4 elevated bilirubin (less than 2%).

➤*Respiratory:* Grade 3/4 dyspnea (4% in ovarian cancer patients, 12% in small cell lung cancer patients).

➤*Postmarketing:* Reports of adverse events in patients taking topotecan received after market introduction, which are not listed above, include the following:

Hematologic – Severe bleeding (in association with thrombocytopenia) (rare).

Dermatologic – Severe dermatitis, severe pruritus (rare).

Miscellaneous – Allergic manifestations (infrequent); anaphylactoid reactions, angioedema (rare).

Overdosage

There is no known antidote for overdosage with topotecan. The primary complication of overdosage would consist of bone marrow suppression.

One patient on a single-dose regimen of 17.5 mg/m^2 given on day 1 of a 21-day cycle had received a single dose of 35 mg/m^2. This patient experienced severe neutropenia (nadir of 320/mm^3) 14 days later but recovered without incident.

Patient Information

Topotecan may cause asthenia or fatigue. Use caution when driving or operating machinery.

ALDESLEUKIN (Interleukin-2; IL-2)

Rx	Proleukin	Powder for injection, lyophilized:	Preservative-free. In single-use vials.[1]
	(Chiron)	22 x 10^6 IU/vial (18 million IU [1.1 mg] per mL when reconstituted)	

[1] With 50 mg mannitol, 0.18 mg sodium dodecyl sulfate, and 0.17 mg monobasic and 0.89 mg dibasic sodium phosphate.

WARNING

Aldesleukin administration has been associated with capillary leak syndrome (CLS). CLS results in hypotension and reduced organ perfusion that may be severe and can result in death (see Warnings).

Restrict therapy to patients with normal cardiac and pulmonary function as defined by thallium stress testing and formal pulmonary function testing. Use extreme caution in patients with normal thallium stress tests and pulmonary function tests who have a history of prior cardiac or pulmonary disease.

Withhold aldesleukin administration in patients developing moderate to severe lethargy or somnolence; continued administration may result in coma.

CLS may be associated with cardiac arrhythmias (supraventricular and ventricular), angina, MI, respiratory insufficiency requiring intubation, GI bleeding or infarction, renal insufficiency, edema, and mental status changes.

Aldesleukin treatment is associated with impaired neutrophil function (reduced chemotaxis) and with an increased risk of disseminated infection, including sepsis and bacterial endocarditis. Adequately treat preexisting bacteria prior to initiation of therapy (see Warnings).

Indications

➤*Metastatic melanoma:* For the treatment of metastatic melanoma in adults.

➤*Metastatic renal-cell carcinoma (RCC):* For the treatment of metastatic RCC in adults.

➤*Unlabeled uses:* May be beneficial when used in combination with highly active antiretroviral therapy (HAART) in the treatment of HIV patients; in combination for treatment of cutaneous T cell lymphoma.

Administration and Dosage

➤*Approved by the FDA:* May 5, 1992.

Careful patient selection is mandatory prior to administration. Patients with more favorable ECoG performance status (ECoG PS 0) at treatment initiation respond better to aldesleukin with a higher response rate and lower toxicity. Experience in patients with ECoG PS greater than 1 is extremely limited.

The recommended aldesleukin treatment regimen is administered by a 15-minute IV infusion every 8 hours. Before initiating treatment, carefully review the prescribing information, particularly regarding patient selection, possible serious adverse events, patient monitoring, and withholding dosage.

➤*Metastatic RCC and metastatic melanoma:* Each course of treatment consists of two 5-day treatment cycles separated by a rest period: 600,000 IU/kg (0.037 mg/kg) dose administered every 8 hours by a 15-minute IV infusion for a maximum of 14 doses. Following 9 days of rest, this schedule is repeated for another 14 doses for a maximum of 28 doses per course as tolerated.

During clinical trials, doses were frequently withheld for toxicity. Metastatic RCC patients treated with this schedule received a median of 20 of the 28 doses during the first course of therapy. Metastatic melanoma patients received a median of 18 doses during the first course of therapy.

➤*Retreatment:* Evaluate patients for response approximately 4 weeks after completion of a course of therapy and again immediately prior to the scheduled start of the next treatment course. Give additional courses of treatment to patients only if there is some tumor shrinkage following the last course and retreatment is not contraindicated (see Warnings). Separate each treatment course by a rest period of at least 7 weeks from the date of hospital discharge.

➤*Dose modification:* Accomplish dose modification for toxicity by withholding or interrupting the dose rather than reducing the dose to be given. Decisions to stop, hold, or restart therapy must be made after a global assessment of the patient using the following guidelines:

Guidelines for Discontinuation of Aldesleukin Therapy

Organ system	Permanently discontinue treatment for the following toxicities:
Cardiovascular	Sustained ventricular tachycardia (≥ 5 beats)
	Cardiac rhythm disturbances not controlled or unresponsive to management
	Chest pain with ECG changes, consistent with angina or MI
	Cardiac tamponade
CNS	Coma or toxic psychosis lasting > 48 hours
	Repetitive or difficult to control seizures
GI	Bowel ischemia/perforation
	GI bleeding requiring surgery
Pulmonary	Intubation for > 72 hours
Renal	Renal failure requiring dialysis > 72 hours

Guidelines for Held Doses and Subsequent Doses of Aldesleukin

Organ system	Hold dose for:	Subsequent doses may be given if:
Cardiovascular	Atrial fibrillation, supraventricular tachycardia or bradycardia that requires treatment or is recurrent or persistent.	Patient is asymptomatic with full recovery to normal sinus rhythm.
	Systolic BP < 90 mm Hg with increasing requirements for pressors.	Systolic BP ≥ 90 mm Hg and stable or improving requirements for pressors.
	Any ECG change consistent with MI, ischemia, or myocarditis with or without chest pain; suspicion of cardiac ischemia.	Patient is asymptomatic. MI and myocarditis have been ruled out, clinical suspicion of angina is low; there is no evidence of ventricular hypokinesia.
CNS	Mental status changes, including moderate confusion or agitation.	Mental status changes completely resolved.
GI	Stool guaiac repeatedly > 3 to 4+.	Stool guaiac negative.
Hepatic	Signs of hepatic failure including encephalopathy, increasing ascites, liver pain, hypoglycemia.	All signs of hepatic failure have resolved.[1]
Pulmonary	O$_2$ saturation < 90%	O$_2$ saturation > 90%
Renal	Serum creatinine > 4.5 mg/dL or a serum creatinine of ≥ 4 mg/dL in the presence of severe volume overload, acidosis, or hyperkalemia.	Serum creatinine < 4 mg/dL, and fluid and electrolyte status is stable.
	Persistent oliguria, urine output of < 10 mL/h for 16 to 24 hours with rising serum creatinine.	Urine output > 10 mL/h with a decrease of serum creatinine > 1.5 mg/dL or normalization of serum creatinine.
Skin	Bullous dermatitis or marked worsening of preexisting skin condition (avoid topical steroid therapy).	Resolution of all signs of bullous dermatitis.
Systemic	Sepsis syndrome, patient is clinically unstable.	Sepsis syndrome has resolved, patient is clinically stable, infection is under treatment.

[1] Discontinue all further treatment for that course. If warranted, initiate a new course of treatment no sooner than 7 weeks after cessation of adverse event and hospital discharge.

➤*Reconstitution and dilutions:* Reconstitute and dilute only as recommended.

Each vial contains 22 million IU (1.3 mg) aldesleukin. Reconstitute with 1.2 mL sterile water for injection by directing diluent against the side of the vial to avoid excess foaming. Swirl; do not shake. When reconstituted as directed, each mL contains 18 million IU (1.1 mg). The resulting solution should be a clear, colorless to slightly yellow liquid.

Dilute the reconstituted aldesleukin dose in 50 mL of 5% dextrose injection and infuse over 15 minutes. In cases where the total aldesleukin dose is 1.5 mg or less (eg, a patient with a body weight of less than 40 kg), dilute the dose of aldesleukin in a smaller volume of 5% dextrose injection. Aldesleukin concentrations below 30 mcg/mL and above 70 mcg/mL have shown increased variability in drug delivery. Avoid dilution and delivery of aldesleukin outside of this concentration range. Although glass bottles and plastic (polyvinyl chloride) bags have been used in clinical trials with comparable results, it is recommended that plastic bags be used as the dilution container because experimental

ALDESLEUKIN (Interleukin-2; IL-2)

studies suggest that use of plastic containers results in more consistent drug delivery. Do not use in-line filters when administering aldesleukin.

Avoid reconstitution or dilution with bacteriostatic water for injection or 0.9% sodium chloride injection because of increased aggregation. Do not mix with other drugs.

►*Concomitant medications:* The following may be useful in the management of patients on aldesleukin therapy: Standard antipyretic therapy, including NSAIDS, started immediately prior to therapy to avoid fever; meperidine used to control the rigors associated with fever; H₂ antagonists given for prophylaxis of GI irritation and bleeding; antiemetic and antidiarrheals used as needed to treat other GI side effects. Generally, these medications are discontinued 12 hours after the last dose of aldesleukin.

►*Storage/Stability:* Before and after reconstitution and dilution, store vials in a refrigerator at 2° to 8°C (36° to 46°F). Do not freeze. Administer within 48 hours of reconstitution. Bring solution to room temperature prior to infusion. Contains no preservative. Discard unused portion. Vial is for single-use only.

Actions

►*Pharmacology:* Aldesleukin, a human recombinant interleukin-2 (IL-2) product, is a highly purified protein (lymphokine) produced by recombinant DNA technology.

Aldesleukin has been shown to possess the biological activities of human native IL-2. In vitro, the immunoregulatory properties of aldesleukin include: 1) Enhancement of lymphocyte mitogenesis and stimulation of long-term growth of human IL-2 dependent cell lines; 2) enhancement of lymphocyte cytotoxicity; 3) induction of killer cell (lymphokine-activated and natural) activity; and 4) induction of interferon-gamma production.

In vivo administration produces multiple immunological effects in a dose-dependent manner. These effects include activation of cellular immunity with profound lymphocytosis, eosinophilia, and thrombocytopenia, the production of cytokines (including tumor necrosis factor, IL-1 and gamma interferon), and inhibition of tumor growth. The exact mechanism by which aldesleukin mediates its antitumor activity is unknown.

►*Pharmacokinetics:*

Absorption/Distribution – The pharmacokinetic profile of aldesleukin is characterized by high plasma concentrations following a short IV infusion, rapid distribution into extravascular space, and elimination from the body by metabolism in the kidneys, with little or no bioactive protein excreted in the urine. Approximately 30% of the administered dose is detectable in plasma. This is consistent with animal studies demonstrating rapid (less than 1 minute) uptake of the majority of the label into the lungs, liver, kidney, and spleen. The serum distribution half-life is 13 minutes. Observed serum levels are proportional to the dose.

Metabolism/Excretion – Following the initial rapid organ distribution, the primary route of clearance of circulating aldesleukin is the kidney; it is cleared from the circulation by both glomerular filtration and peritubular extraction. This may account for the preservation of clearance in patients with rising serum creatinine values. The elimination half-life is 85 minutes following a 5 minute IV infusion. Greater than 80% of the amount of aldesleukin distributed to plasma, cleared from the circulation, and presented to the kidney is metabolized to amino acids in cells lining the proximal convoluted tubules. The mean clearance rate in cancer patients is 268 mL/min.

The solubilizing agent, sodium dodecyl sulfate, may have an effect on the kinetic properties of this product.

Contraindications

Hypersensitivity to interleukin-2 or any component of the formulation; abnormal thallium stress test or pulmonary function tests; organ allografts; retreatment in patients experiencing CLS toxicities during initial therapy (see Warnings).

Warnings

►*Autoimmunity and inflammatory reactions:* Aldesleukin has been associated with exacerbation of preexisting or initial presentation of autoimmune disease and inflammatory disorders when used concurrently with interferon-alfa. Exacerbations of Crohn disease, scleroderma, thyroiditis, hypothyroidism sometimes preceded by hyperthyroidism, inflammatory arthritis, onset of hyperglycemia and/or diabetes mellitus, oculo-bulbar myasthenia gravis, crescentic IgA glomerulonephritis, cholecystitis, cerebral vasculitis, Stevens-Johnson syndrome, and bullous pemphigoid have been reported.

►*Bacterial infections:* Aldesleukin treatment is associated with impaired neutrophil function (reduced chemotaxis) and with an increased risk of disseminated infection, including sepsis and bacterial endocarditis. Treat preexisting bacterial infections prior to initiation of therapy. Patients with indwelling central lines are at risk for infection with gram-positive microorganisms. Antibiotic prophylaxis with oxacillin, nafcillin, ciprofloxacin, or vancomycin has been associated with a reduced incidence of staphylococcal infections.

►*CLS:* Aldesleukin has been associated with CLS, which begins immediately after initiation of treatment and is marked by increased capillary permeability to protein and fluids and reduced vascular tone. In most patients, this results in a concomitant drop in mean arterial blood pressure within 2 to 12 hours after the start of treatment. With continued therapy, clinically significant hypotension (systolic blood pressure below 90 mm Hg or a 20 mm Hg drop from baseline systolic pressure) and hypoperfusion will occur. In addition, extravasation of proteins and fluids into the extravascular space will lead to the formation of edema and creation of new effusions. CLS may be associated with cardiac arrhythmias (supraventricular and ventricular), angina, MI, respiratory insufficiency requiring intubation, GI bleeding or infarction, renal insufficiency, edema, and mental status changes.

Medical management of CLS begins with careful monitoring of the patient's fluid and organ perfusion status. Frequently determine blood pressure and pulse and monitor organ function, including assessment of mental status and urine output.

Flexibility in fluid and pressor management is essential for maintaining organ perfusion and blood pressure. Consequently, use extreme caution in patients with fixed requirements for large volumes of fluid (eg, patients with hypercalcemia).

Administration of IV fluids, either colloids or crystalloids, is recommended for treatment of hypovolemia.

Clinical experience has shown that early administration of dopamine (1 to 5 mcg/kg/min) to patients manifesting CLS, before the onset of hypotension, can help maintain organ perfusion particularly to the kidney and thus preserve urine output. Carefully monitor weight and urine output. If organ perfusion and blood pressure are not sustained by dopamine therapy, the dose of dopamine may be increased to 6 to 10 mcg/kg/min, or phenylephrine HCl (1 to 5 mcg/kg/min) may be added to low-dose dopamine. Prolonged use of pressors, either in combination or as individual agents at relatively high doses, may be associated with cardiac rhythm disturbances.

Withhold treatment if patient fails to maintain organ perfusion, demonstrated by altered mental status, reduced urine output, a fall in the systolic blood pressure to below 90 mm Hg, or onset of cardiac arrhythmias. Recovery from CLS begins soon after cessation of therapy. Usually within a few hours, the blood pressure rises, organ perfusion is restored, and reabsorption of extravasated fluid and protein begins. If there has been excessive weight gain or edema formation, particularly if associated with shortness of breath from pulmonary congestion, use of diuretics once blood pressure has normalized has been shown to hasten recovery.

►*Clinical evaluation:* Because of the severe adverse events that generally accompany therapy at the recommended dosages, perform thorough clinical evaluation to identify patients with significant cardiac, pulmonary, renal, hepatic, or CNS impairment in whom aldesleukin is contraindicated.

►*CNS effects:* New neurologic signs, symptoms, and anatomic lesions following aldesleukin therapy have been reported in patients without evidence of CNS metastases. Clinical manifestations included changes in mental status, speech difficulties, cortical blindness, limb or gait ataxia, hallucinations, agitation, obtundation, and coma. Radiological findings included multiple and, less commonly, single cortical lesions on MRI and evidence of demyelination. Neurologic signs and symptoms associated with aldesleukin therapy usually improve after discontinuation of aldesleukin therapy; however, there are reports of permanent neurologic defects. One case of possible cerebral vasculitis responsive to dexamethasone has been reported. Exercise extreme caution in treating patients with known seizure disorders because aldesleukin may cause seizures.

►*CNS metastases:* Thoroughly evaluate all patients and treat CNS metastases prior to receiving therapy. Patients should be neurologically stable with a negative CT scan.

►*Retreatment:* Retreatment is contraindicated in patients who experienced the following toxicities while receiving an earlier course of therapy: Sustained ventricular tachycardia (5 beats or more); cardiac arrhythmias uncontrolled or unresponsive to management; chest pain with ECG changes, consistent with angina or myocardial infarction (MI); intubation for more than 72 hours; cardiac tamponade; renal dysfunction requiring dialysis more than 72 hours; coma or toxic psychosis lasting more than 48 hours; repetitive or difficult to control seizures; bowel ischemia/perforation; GI bleeding requiring surgery.

►*Renal/Hepatic function toxicity:* Kidney and liver function are impaired during aldesleukin treatment. Use of concomitant nephrotoxic or hepatotoxic medications may further increase toxicity to the kidney or liver. In addition, reduced kidney and liver function secondary to treatment may delay elimination of concomitant medications and increase the risk of adverse events from these drugs.

►*Hypersensitivity reactions:* Hypersensitivity reactions have been reported in patients receiving combination regimens containing sequential high-dose aldesleukin and antineoplastic agents. These reactions consisted of erythema, pruritus, and hypotension and occurred within hours of administration of chemotherapy. Refer to Management of Acute Hypersensitivity Reactions.

►*Fertility impairment:* Administering this drug to fertile persons of either sex not practicing effective contraception is not recommended.

ALDESLEUKIN (Interleukin-2; IL-2)

➤*Elderly:* Aldesleukin is excreted principally by the kidney. Because the elderly may have decreased renal function and patients with renal impairment are at an increased risk of toxicity, closely monitor patients in this age group with proper dose adjustments.

➤*Pregnancy:* Category C. Aldesleukin has been shown to have embryolethal effects in rats when given in doses at 27 to 36 times the human dose. Significant maternal toxicities were observed in pregnant rats when administered doses 2.1 to 36 times higher than the human dose during critical period of organogenesis. There are no adequate and well-controlled studies of aldesleukin in pregnant women. Use during pregnancy only if the potential benefit justifies the potential risk to the fetus.

➤*Lactation:* It is not known whether this drug is excreted in human milk. Because of the potential for serious adverse reactions in nursing infants, decide whether to discontinue nursing or to discontinue the drug, taking into the account the importance of the drug to the mother.

➤*Children:* Safety and efficacy in children younger than 18 years of age have not been established.

Precautions

➤*Monitoring:* The following clinical evaluations are recommended for all patients prior to beginning treatment and then daily during drug administration: Standard hematologic tests, including CBC, differential, and platelet counts; blood chemistries, including electrolytes and renal and hepatic function tests; chest x-rays. Serum creatinine should be 1.5 mg/dL or less prior to initiation of treatment.

All patients should have baseline pulmonary function tests with arterial blood gases. Document adequate pulmonary function (FEV_1 greater than 2 L or at least 75% of predicted for height and age) prior to initiating therapy. Screen all patients with a stress thallium study. Document normal ejection fraction and unimpaired wall motion. If a thallium stress test suggests minor wall motion abnormalities, further testing is suggested to exclude significant coronary artery disease.

Daily monitoring during therapy should include vital signs (temperature, pulse, blood pressure, respiration rate), weight, and fluid intake and output. In a patient with a decreased systolic blood pressure, especially below 90 mm Hg, conduct constant cardiac rhythm monitoring. If an abnormal complex or rhythm is seen, perform an ECG. Take vital signs hourly in these hypotensive patients.

During treatment, monitor pulmonary function on a regular basis by clinical examination, assessment of vital signs, and pulse oximetry. Further assess patients with dyspnea or clinical signs of respiratory impairment (tachypnea or rales) with arterial blood gas determination. Repeat these tests as often as clinically indicated.

Assess cardiac function daily by clinical examination and assessment of vital signs. Further assess patients with signs or symptoms of chest pain, murmurs, gallops, irregular rhythm, or palpitations with an ECG examination and cardiac enzyme evaluation. Evidence of myocardial injury, including findings compatible with MI or myocarditis, has been reported. Ventricular hypokinesia caused by myocarditis may be persistent for several months. If there is evidence of cardiac ischemia or congestive heart failure, hold aldesleukin therapy and perform a repeat thallium study.

➤*Allograft rejection:* Aldesleukin enhancement of cellular immune function may increase the risk of allograft rejection in transplant patients.

➤*Immunogenicity:* Of 77 metastatic RCC patients, 57 (74%) treated with an every-8-hour regimen developed low titers of nonneutralizing antialdesleukin antibodies. Neutralizing antibodies were not detected in this group of patients but have been detected in less than 1%. The clinical significance of anti-aldesleukin antibodies is unknown.

➤*Iodinated contrast media:* Acute, atypical adverse reactions (eg, fever, chills, nausea, vomiting, pruritus, rash, diarrhea, hypotension, edema, oliguria) have been reported in patients administered iodinated contrast media subsequent to IL-2 treatment. Symptom onset usually occurred within 1 to 4 hours following initiation of contrast media regimens administered 4 weeks to several months after IL-2 therapy.

➤*Mental status changes:* Mental status changes, including irritability, confusion, or depression, that occur while receiving aldesleukin may be indicators of bacteremia or early bacterial sepsis. Alterations in mental status caused solely by aldesleukin may progress for several days before recovery begins.

➤*Thyroid function impairment:* Hypothyroidism, sometimes preceded by hyperthyroidism, has been reported following treatment. Some patients may require thyroid replacement therapy. Changes in thyroid function may be a manifestation of autoimmunity; exercise caution when treating patients with known autoimmune disease (see Warnings).

Drug Interactions

➤*Antineoplastic agents:* Hypersensitivity reactions have been reported in patients receiving combination regimens containing sequential high-dose aldesleukin and antineoplastic agents, specifically dacarbazine, cisplatin, tamoxifen, and interferon-alfa (see Adverse Reactions).

➤*Interferon-alfa:* Exacerbations of preexisting or initial autoimmune and inflammatory disorders have been observed (see Warnings); myocardial injury including MI, myocarditis, ventricular hypokinesia, and severe rhabdomyolysis appear to be increased in patients receiving aldesleukin and interferon-alfa concurrently.

Aldesleukin Drug Interactions			
Precipitant drug	Object drug*		Description
Antihypertensives	Aldesleukin	↑	Antihypertensives may potentiate the hypotension seen with aldesleukin.
Corticosteroids	Aldesleukin	↓	Although glucocorticoids reduce the side effects of aldesleukin, coadministration may reduce the antitumor effectiveness of aldesleukin; avoid concurrent use.
Cardiotoxic agents (eg, doxorubicin)	Aldesleukin	↑	Increased toxicity in these organ systems may occur during coadministration.
Hepatotoxic agents (eg, methotrexate, asparaginase)			
Myelotoxic agents (eg, cytotoxic chemotherapy)			
Nephrotoxic agents (eg, aminoglycosides, indomethacin)			
Aldesleukin	Protease inhibitors (eg, indinavir)	↑	Protease concentrations may be elevated, increasing risk of toxicity. May need to adjust the dose of indinavir when aldesleukin is initiated or stopped.
Aldesleukin	Psychotropic agents (eg, narcotics, analgesics, sedatives, antiemetics, tranquilizers)	↔	Aldesleukin may affect CNS function. Therefore, interactions could occur following coadministration of these agents.

*↑ = Object drug increased. ↓ = Object drug decreased. ↔ = Undetermined clinical effect.

Adverse Reactions

Adverse reactions are frequent, often serious, and sometimes fatal. Should adverse events that require dose modification occur, withhold rather than reduce the dosage. In patients with both metastatic RCC and metastatic melanoma, those with ECoG PS of 1 or higher had a higher treatment-related mortality and serious adverse events. Most adverse reactions are self-limiting and usually, but not invariably, reverse or improve within 2 or 3 days of discontinuation of therapy. Examples of adverse reactions with permanent sequelae include MI, bowel perforation/infarction, and gangrene.

The rate of drug-related deaths in the 255 metastatic RCC patients who received single-agent aldesleukin was 4%; the rate of drug-related deaths in the 270 metastatic melanoma patients who received single-agent aldesleukin was 2%.

Adverse Reactions Occurring in ≥ 10% of Patients	
Adverse reaction	(n = 525)
Cardiovascular	
Arrhythmia	10
Cardiovascular disorder[1]	11
Hypotension	71
Supraventricular tachycardia	12
Tachycardia	23
Vasodilation	13
CNS	
Anxiety	12
Confusion	34
Dizziness	11
Somnolence	22
Dermatologic	
Exfoliative dermatitis	18
Pruritus	24
Rash	42
GI	
Abdomen, enlarged	10
Abdominal pain	11
Anorexia	20
Diarrhea	67
Nausea	35
Nausea and vomiting	19

ALDESLEUKIN (Interleukin-2; IL-2)

Adverse Reactions Occurring in ≥ 10% of Patients	
Adverse reaction	(n = 525)
Stomatitis	22
Vomiting	50
Hematologic/Lymphatic	
Anemia	29
Leukopenia	16
Thrombocytopenia	37
Metabolic/Nutritional	
Acidosis	12
Alkaline phosphatase increase	10
AST increase	23
Bilirubinemia	40
Creatinine increase	33
Edema	15
Hypocalcemia	11
Hypomagnesemia	12
Peripheral edema	28
Weight gain	16
Respiratory	
Cough increase	11
Dyspnea	43
Lung disorder[2]	24
Respiratory disorder[3]	11
Rhinitis	10
Miscellaneous	
Asthenia	23
Chills	52
Fever	29
Infection	13
Malaise	27
Oliguria	63
Pain	12

[1] Cardiovascular disorder: Asymptomatic ECG changes, CHF, fluctuations in blood pressure.
[2] Lung disorder: Physical findings associated with pulmonary congestion, rales, rhonchi.
[3] Respiratory disorder: ARDS, CXR infiltrates, unspecified pulmonary changes.

Life-Threatening (Grade 4) Adverse Events Occurring in > 1% of Patients	
Adverse reaction	(n = 525)
Cardiovascular	
Cardiovascular disorder[1]	1
Heart arrest	1
Hypotension	3
MI	1
Supraventricular tachycardia	1
Ventricular tachycardia	1
CNS	
Coma	2
Confusion	1
Psychosis	1
Stupor	1
GI	
Diarrhea	2
Vomiting	1
GU	
Acute kidney failure	1
Anuria	5
Oliguria	6
Hematologic	
Coagulation disorder[2]	1
Thrombocytopenia	1
Metabolic	
Acidosis	1
AST increase	1
Bilirubinemia	2
Creatinine increase	1
Respiratory	
Apnea	1
Dyspnea	1
Respiratory disorder[3]	3

Life-Threatening (Grade 4) Adverse Events Occurring in > 1% of Patients	
Adverse reaction	(n = 525)
Miscellaneous	
Fever	1
Infection	1
Sepsis	1

[1] Cardiovascular disorder: Fluctuations in blood pressure.
[2] Coagulation disorder: Intravascular coagulopathy.
[3] Respiratory disorder: ARDS, intubation, respiratory intubation.

►*Other serious events:*
Cardiovascular – Myocarditis, pericarditis, supraventricular tachycardia, transient ischemic attacks.

CNS – Cerebral edema, meningitis.

GI – Bowel necrosis, duodenal ulceration, tracheo-esophageal fistula.

Hypersensitivity – Reported in patients receiving combination regimens containing sequential high-dose aldesleukin and antineoplastic agents. These reactions consisted of erythema, pruritus, and hypotension and occurred within hours of administration of chemotherapy.

Renal – Allergic interstitial nephritis.

Special senses – Transient blindness secondary to optic neuritis.

►*Life-threatening (grade 4) events occurring in less than 1%:*
Cardiovascular – Atrial arrhythmia, AV block second-degree, bradycardia, coronary artery disorders, endocarditis, myocardial ischemia, pericardial effusion, syncope, thrombosis, ventricular extrasystoles.

CNS – Agitation, convulsion, delirium, grand mal convulsion, hyperthermia, neuropathy, paranoid reaction, shock, somnolence.

GI – Bloody diarrhea, GI disorder, GI hemorrhage, hematemesis, intestinal perforation, nausea, stomatitis, vomiting.

GU – Hyperuricemia.

Hematologic – Anemia, leukocytosis, leukopenia.

Metabolic – Hypocalcemia.

Renal – Abnormal kidney function, acute tubular necrosis, increased BUN, kidney failure.

Respiratory – Asthma, hemoptysis, hyperventilation, hypoventilation, hypoxia, lung edema, pneumothorax, respiratory acidosis.

Special senses – Mydriasis, pupillary disorder.

Miscellaneous – Abnormal liver function tests, hemorrhage, increased alkaline phosphatase, increased NPN, pancreatitis, peripheral gangrene, phlebitis.

►*Fatal events occurring in less than 1%:*
Cardiovascular – Cardiac arrest, MI, pulmonary edema, pulmonary emboli, stroke.

CNS – Malignant hyperthermia, severe depression leading to suicide.

GI – Intestinal perforation.

Respiratory – Pulmonary edema, respiratory arrest, respiratory failure.

Miscellaneous – Liver or renal failure.

►*Postmarketing:*
Cardiovascular – Cardiomyopathy, cerebral hemorrhage, fatal endocarditis, hypertension.

CNS – Cerebral lesions, encephalopathy, extrapyramidal syndrome, insomnia, neuralgia; neuritis, neuropathy (demyelination).

Dermatologic – Cellulitis, injection-site necrosis, urticaria.

GI – Cholecystitis, colitis, gastritis, intestinal obstruction.

Hepatic – Hepatitis, hepatosplenomegaly.

Musculoskeletal – Myopathy, myositis, rhabdomyolysis.

Miscellaneous – Anaphylaxis, hyperthyroidism, neutropenia, pneumonia (bacterial, fungal, viral), retroperitoneal hemorrhage.

Overdosage

►*Symptoms:* Side effects following the use of aldesleukin appear to be dose-related. Exceeding the recommended dose has been associated with a more rapid onset of expected dose-limiting toxicities.

►*Treatment:* Adverse reactions generally will reverse when the drug is stopped, particularly because its serum half-life is short. Monitor symptoms that persist after cessation of aldesleukin and treat supportively. Refer to General Management of Acute Overdosage. Life-threatening toxicities may be ameliorated by the IV administration of dexamethasone, which also may result in loss of therapeutic effect of aldesleukin.

BCG, INTRAVESICAL

Rx	**TICE BCG** (Organon)	**Powder for suspension, lyophilized:** 1 to 8 x 10^8 CFU (equivalent to $\approx$ 50 mg wet weight)	Lactose. Preservative free. In $\approx$ 50 mg vial.
Rx	**TheraCys** (Aventis Pasteur)	**Powder for suspension, lyophilized:** 10.5 $\pm$ 8.7 x 10^8 CFU (equivalent to $\approx$ 81 mg dry weight)	MSG. In 81 mg vial with 3 ml diluent vial.

BCG vaccines for tuberculosis prevention are discussed in the Biologic and Immunologics section.

WARNING

Bacillus of Calmette and Guérin (BCG) contains live, attenuated mycobacteria. Because of the potential risk for transmission, prepare, handle, and dispose of as a biohazardous material (see Precautions and Administration and Dosage).

BCG infections have been reported in health care workers, primarily from exposures resulting from accidental needle sticks or skin lacerations during the preparation of BCG for administration. Nosocomial infections have been reported in immunosuppressed patients receiving parenteral drugs that were prepared in areas in which BCG was prepared. BCG is capable of dissemination when administered by the intravesical route, and serious infections, including fatal infections, have been reported in patients receiving intravesical BCG (see Warnings, Precautions, and Adverse Reactions).

Indications

➤*Carcinoma in situ of the urinary bladder:* Treatment and prophylaxis of carcinoma in situ (CIS) of the urinary bladder and for prophylaxis of primary or recurrent stage Ta and/or T1 papillary tumors following transurethral resection (TUR) (*TheraCys, TICE BCG*); intravesical use in the treatment of CIS in the absence of an associated invasive cancer of the bladder in the following situations: 1) primary treatment of CIS with or without papillary tumors after TUR, 2) secondary treatment of CIS in patients failing to respond or relapsing after intravesical therapy with other agents, 3) primary or secondary treatment of CIS for patients with medical contraindications to radical surgery (*Pacis*).

Administration and Dosage

➤*Induction and maintenance therapy:* Allow 7 to 14 days to elapse after bladder biopsy or transurethral resection before BCG administration.

TheraCys – Do not inject SC or IV. During induction therapy, each dose is administered intravesically via catheter once a week for 6 weeks followed by maintenance therapy, consisting of 1 dose given at 3, 6, 12, 18, and 24 months after initial treatment.

TICE BCG – Do not inject SC or IV. Each dose is administered intravesically via catheter once a week for 6 weeks. This schedule may be repeated once if tumor remission is not achieved and if deemed clinically necessary. Thereafter, administer 1 dose at approximately monthly intervals for $\geq$ 6 to 12 months.

Pacis – Do not inject SC or IV. The recommended induction course is a single dose of 120 mg instilled into the bladder once weekly for 6 weeks. This schedule may be repeated if tumor remission has not been achieved and if deemed clinically necessary. The use of maintenance *Pacis* has not been studied.

➤*Administration:* Do not drink fluids for 4 hours before treatment; empty bladder prior to administration. The suspension is instilled into the bladder slowly by gravity flow, via the catheter. Do not force the flow.

During the first hour following instillation, have the patient lie for 15 minutes each in the prone and supine positions and also on each side. The patient is then allowed to be up, but needs to retain the suspension for another 60 minutes for a total of 2 hours. All patients may not be able to retain the suspension for 2 hours and should be instructed to void in less time if necessary. At the end of 2 hours, void in a seated position to avoid splashing of urine. Maintain adequate hydration.

If the bladder catheterization has been traumatic (eg, associated with bleeding), do not administer BCG and delay treatment for $\geq$ 1 to 2 weeks. Resume subsequent treatment as if no interruption in the schedule had occurred (ie, administer all doses even after a temporary halt in administration).

After use, sterilize or dispose of according to biohazardous protocol all equipment, materials, and containers used for BCG preparation and administration.

➤*Preparation of suspension:* Reconstitute and dilute immediately prior to use. If there is a delay between reconstitution and administration it must not exceed 2 hours. Treat BCG as infectious material. Prepare the suspension using sterile technique. If the preparation cannot be performed in a biocontainment hood, the pharmacist or individual responsible for mixing the agent should wear gloves, mask, and gown to avoid inadvertent exposure to broken skin or inhalation of BCG organisms. Use precautions to avoid cross-contamination of parenteral products. It should not be handled by people with an immunologic deficiency.

TheraCys – Do not remove the rubber stopper from the vial. Reconstitute only with the diluent provided to ensure proper dispersion of the organisms.

Reconstitute the lyophilized contents of 1 vial with 3 ml of diluent provided; shake gently until a fine, even suspension results. Further dilute in an additional 50 ml of the sterile, preservative free saline provided to a final volume of 53 ml.

TICE BCG – Using a small (eg, 3 ml) syringe, draw 1 ml of sterile, preservative free 0.9% sodium chloride and add to 1 vial of *TICE BCG* to resuspend. Gently swirl the vial until a homogenous suspension is obtained. Dispense the cloudy BCG suspension into the top end of a catheter-tip syringe containing 49 ml of sterile, preservative free 0.9% sodium chloride. Gently rotate the syringe. Do not filter the contents.

Pacis – Draw 1 ml of sterile diluent (preservative free 0.9% Sodium Chloride Injection) at 4° to 25°C (39° to 77°F) into a small syringe and add to 1 ampule of *Pacis* to resuspend. Leave them in contact for $\approx$ 1 minute. Then mix the suspension by withdrawing it into the syringe and expelling it gently back into the ampule 2 or 3 times. Avoid the production of foam; do not shake. Dilute the reconstituted product in an additional 49 ml of saline diluent, bringing the total volume to 50 ml. Use the suspended product immediately after preparation. Discard after 2 hours.

➤*Storage/Stability:* Keep BCG and any accompanying diluent refrigerated between 2° and 8°C (35° and 46°F). Use immediately after reconstitution and discard after 2 hours. Do not expose the freeze-dried or reconstituted BCG to sunlight, direct or indirect. Keep exposure to artificial light to a minimum. Do not use any reconstituted product that exhibits flocculation or clumping that cannot be dispersed with gentle shaking. Do not use after expiration date printed on label.

Actions

➤*Pharmacology:* BCG is a lyophilized preparation of an attenuated, live culture preparation of the Bacillus of Calmette and Guérin (BCG) strain of *Mycobacterium bovis*. BCG Live (intravesical) is used in CIS of the urinary bladder and as prophylaxis of primary or recurrent stage Ta and/or T1 papillary tumors following TUR. BCG promotes a local acute inflammatory and sub-acute granulomatous reaction with macrophage and lymphocyte infiltration in the urothelium and lamina propria of the urinary bladder. The precise mechanism of action is unknown, but the anti-tumor effect appears to be T-lymphocyte-dependent.

➤*Clinical trials:*

TheraCys vs doxorubicin HCl – A study of 285 patients compared *TheraCys* and doxorubicin in patients with CIS for complete response to treatment and survival in a randomized, multicenter clinical trial.

For patients with CIS, the complete response rate (ie, negative biopsies and urine cytology) within 6 months of the initiation of treatment was 33% with doxorubicin and 71% with *TheraCys*. The probability of being disease-free at 2 years was 23% with doxorubicin and 51% with *TheraCys*. The median disease survival was 4.9 months for doxorubicin and 30 months for *TheraCys*.

For patients with Ta/T1 papillary tumors only, the 2-year disease-free survival was 29% with doxorubicin and 50% with *TheraCys*. The median disease-free survival was 10.5 months with doxorubicin and 22.5 months with *TheraCys*.

Contraindications

Stage TaG1 papillary tumors unless they are judged to be at high risk of tumor recurrence (*TheraCys, TICE BCG*); immunosuppressed patients with congenital or acquired immune deficiencies, whether due to concurrent disease (eg, AIDS, leukemia, lymphoma, cancer therapy (eg, cytotoxic drugs, radiation), or immunosuppressive therapy (eg, corticosteroids) because of the possibility of establishing a systemic BCG infection; vaccine for the prevention of cancer; for the treatment of papillary tumors occurring alone; as an immunizing agent for the prevention of tuberculosis (*TheraCys*) (see Warnings); positive Mantoux test, unless there is evidence of an active TB infection, (*TICE BCG, Pacis*); prevention of papillary tumors after TUR or for the treatment of papillary tumors occurring alone (*Pacis*); postpone treatment until resolution of concurrent febrile illness, urinary tract infection, or gross hematuria (*Pacis*); 7 to 14 days should elapse before administering following biopsy, TUR, or traumatic catheterization (*Pacis*); active tuberculosis; papillary tumors of stages higher than T1, concurrent infections (*TICE BCG*).

Warnings

➤*Tuberculosis prevention:* Do not administer as an immunizing agent to prevent TB. These agents may cause TB sensitivity. Since this is a valuable aid in TB diagnosis, it may be useful to determine tuberculin reactivity by PPD skin testing before treatment.

➤*Management of BCG complications:* The acute, localized irritative toxicities of BCG may be accompanied by systemic manifestations

BCG, INTRAVESICAL

consistent with the "flu-like" syndrome. Systemic adverse effects of 1 to 2 days' duration (eg, malaise, fever, chills) often reflect hypersensitivity reactions that can be treated with antihistamines. However, symptoms such as fever ≥ 101.3°F (38.5°C) or acute localized inflammation such as epididymitis, prostatitis, or orchitis persisting > 2 to 3 days suggest active infection, and an evaluation for serious infectious complications considered. Refer to Management of Acute Hypersensitivity Reactions.

The irritative bladder adverse effects can usually be managed symptomatically with products such as pyridium, propantheline bromide, oxybutynin chloride, and acetaminophen. The mechanism of action of the irritative side effects has not been firmly established, but is most consistent with an immunological mechanism. There is no evidence that dose reduction or antituberculous drug therapy can prevent or lessen the irritative toxicity of BCG.

Although uncommon, serious infectious complications of intravesical BCG have been reported. The most serious infectious complication of BCG is disseminated sepsis with associated mortality. In addition, *M. bovis* infections have been reported in lung, liver, bone, bone marrow, kidney, regional lymph nodes, and prostate in patients who have received intravesical BCG. Some male GU tract infections (orchitis/epididymitis) have been resistant to multiple-drug antituberculous therapy and required orchiectomy.

Physicians using this product need to be familiar with the literature on the prevention and treatment of BCG-related complications and prepared in such emergencies to contact an infectious disease specialist with experience in treating the infectious complications of intravesical BCG.

In patients who develop persistent fever or experience an acute febrile illness consistent with severe sepsis syndrome, administer ≥ 2 antimycobacterial agents while diagnostic evaluation, including cultures, is conducted. Discontinue BCG treatment.

BCG is sensitive to the most commonly used antituberculous agents (isoniazid, rifampin, and ethambutol). BCG is also sensitive to clofazimine, cycloserine, ethionamide, para-aminosalicylic acid, rifabutin, and thiacetazone. BCG is not sensitive to pyrazinamide.

There are no data to suggest that the acute, local urinary tract toxicity common with BCG is caused by mycobacterial infection; do not use antituberculosis drugs (eg, isoniazid) to prevent or treat the local irritative toxicities of BCG.

➤*Urinary tract infection:* Do not use in the presence of a urinary tract infection because administration may result in the risk of disseminated BCG infection or in an increased severity of bladder irritation.

➤*Fever:* Do not use in the presence of a fever. If the fever is caused by an infection, withhold therapy until the patient is afebrile and off all therapy.

➤*Infection of aneurysms and prosthetic devices:* BCG infection of aneurysms and prosthetic devices (including arterial grafts, cardiac devices, and artificial joints) have been reported following intravesical administration of BCG. The risk of these ectopic BCG infections has not been determined, but is considered to be very small. The benefits of BCG therapy must be carefully weighed against the possibility of an ectopic BCG infection in patients with preexisting arterial aneurysms or prosthetic devices of any kind.

➤*Rubber latex:* The vial stopper for *TheraCys* contains natural rubber latex which may cause allergic reactions.

➤*Hypersensitivity reactions:* Systemic side effects (eg, malaise, fever, chills) of 1 to 2 days' duration may represent hypersensitivity reactions and can be treated with antihistamines.

➤*Pregnancy:* Category C. It is not known whether BCG can cause fetal harm when administered to a pregnant woman or if it affects

reproductive capacity. Give to a pregnant woman only if clearly needed. Advise women not to become pregnant while on therapy.

➤*Lactation:* It is not known whether BCG is excreted in breast milk. Because of the potential for serious adverse reactions in nursing infants, discontinue nursing or discontinue the drug, taking into account the importance of the drug to the mother.

➤*Children:* Safety and efficacy for use in children have not been established.

Precautions

➤*Monitoring:*

Allergic reactions – Assess the possibility of allergic reactions. Do not attempt administration in individuals with severe immune deficiency disease. Administer with caution to people in groups at high risk for HIV infection. Avoid in asymptomatic carriers with a positive HIV serology.

Urinary tract status – Since administration of intravesical BCG causes an inflammatory response in the bladder and has been associated with hematuria, urinary frequency, dysuria, and bacterial urinary tract infection, careful monitoring of urinary status is required. If there is an increase in the patient's existing symptoms, if symptoms persist, or if any of these symptoms develop, evaluate and manage the patient for urinary tract infection or BCG toxicity.

Infection, systemic – Closely monitor for signs and symptoms of systemic infection (see Warnings).

➤*Handling:* Contains viable attenuated mycobacteria. Handle as biohazardous. Use aseptic technique. BCG infections have been reported in health care workers, primarily from exposures resulting from accidental needle sticks or skin lacerations during the preparation of BCG for administration. Nosocomial infections have been reported in immunosuppressed patients receiving parenteral drugs that were prepared in areas in which BCG was prepared.

After usage, immediately place all equipment and materials used for instillation of the product (eg, syringes, catheters, and containers that may have come into contact with BCG) into the bladder into plastic bags labeled "Infectious Waste" and dispose of accordingly as biohazardous waste.

➤*Urine disinfection:* Disinfect urine voided for 6 hours after instillation with an equal volume of 5% sodium hypochlorite solution (undiluted household bleach) and allow to stand for 15 minutes before flushing.

➤*Transurethral resection:* Do not give intravesical BCG any sooner than 1 to 2 weeks following transurethral resection, biopsy, traumatic catherization, or gross hematuria. Fatalities caused by disseminated BCG infection and sepsis have occurred with BCG.

If the physician believes that the bladder catheterization has been traumatic (eg, associated with bleeding), or if transurethral resection, biopsy, or gross hematuria have occurred, do not administer BCG and delay treatment for ≥ 1 to 2 weeks.

Drug Interactions

➤*Bone marrow depressants/immunosuppressants/radiation:* Bone marrow depressants, immunosuppressants, or radiation may impair response to BCG.

➤*Antimicrobial therapy:* Antimicrobial therapy for other infections may interfere with the effectiveness of *TICE BCG* or *Pacis* therapy.

Adverse Reactions

Most local adverse reactions occur following the third intravesical instillation. Symptoms usually begin 4 to 6 hours after instillation and persist 24 to 72 hours.

Adverse Reactions Associated with BCG Therapy (%)						
Adverse Reaction	*Pacis*[1] (n = 292)		*TheraCys*[2] (n = 112)		*TICE BCG*[3] (n = 674)	
	Overall[4]	Grade ≥ 3	Overall	Grade ≥ 3	Overall	Grade ≥ 3
GI						
Diarrhea/GI	3	< 1	6	0	—	—
Nausea/Vomiting	—	—	16	0	3	< 1
Anorexia/Weight loss	—	—	11	0	2	< 1
GU						
Dysuria/Cystitis	60	9	52/29	4/0	60/6	11/2
Urgency/Frequency	35	7	40	2	6/40	1/7
Hematuria	34	6	39	7	26	7
Other GU symptoms	12	1	—	—	—	—
Nocturia	11	—	—	—	5	1
Urinary incontinence	7	< 1	6	0	2	0
Urinary retention	6	1	—	—	—	—
Urinary tract infection	5	1	18	1	2	1
Foreign material in urine	2	< 1	—	—	2	< 1
Irritative bladder symptoms	2	—	—	—	—	—
Urgency	—	—	18	0	—	—
Renal toxicity (NOS)	—	—	10	2	—	—

BCG, INTRAVESICAL

Adverse Reactions Associated with BCG Therapy (%)						
Adverse Reaction	*Pacis*[1] (n = 292)		*TheraCys*[2] (n = 112)		*TICE BCG*[3] (n = 674)	
	Overall[4]	Grade ≥ 3	Overall	Grade ≥ 3	Overall	Grade ≥ 3
Genital pain	—	—	10	0	—	—
Contracted bladder	—	—	5	0	—	—
Genital inflammation/abscess	—	—	—	—	2	< 1
Hematologic						
Anemia	—	—	21	0	—	—
Leukopenia	—	—	5	0	—	—
Coagulopathy	—	—	3	0	—	—
Musculoskeletal						
Arthralgia/Myalgia/Arthritis	—	—	7	1	3	< 1
Rigors	—	—	—	—	3	1
Respiratory						
Pulmonary infection	—	—	3	0	—	—
Respiratory (unclassified)	—	—	—	—	2	< 1
Miscellaneous						
Fever	13	1	38	3	20	8
Flu-like syndrome	12	1	—	—	33	9
Abdominal pain	5	1	3	0	2	1
Local pain	3	1	—	—	—	—
Not otherwise specified	2	< 1	—	—	—	—
Chills	1	—	34	3	—	—
BCG systemic infection	< 1	1	—	—	—	—
Malaise/Fatigue	—	—	40	2	7	0
Cramps/Pain	—	—	6	0	4	1
Allergy	—	—	—	—	2	< 1
Liver involvement	—	—	3	0	—	—
Systemic infection	—	—	3	0	—	—
Cardiac (unclassified)	—	—	3	0	2	1
Headache/Dizziness	—	—	2	0	2	0
Skin rash	—	—	2	0	—	—

[1] Data from a compilation of retrospective multiple studies.
[2] Data pooled from SWOG study 8216.
[3] Included 153 patients with carcinoma in situ.
[4] First course only all grades.

Overdosage

Overdosage occurs if > 1 amp/vial is given per instillation. Closely monitor for signs of systemic BCG infection. For acute local or systemic reactions suggesting active infection, consult an infectious disease specialist.

Patient Information

Advise patients to check with their physician as soon as possible if there is an increase in their existing symptoms, if their symptoms persist even after receiving a number of treatments, or if any of the following symptoms develop: Blood in urine, fever/chills, cough, skin rash, frequent urge to urinate, increased frequency of urination, increased tiredness/fatigue, joint pain, flu-like symptoms, and painful urination.

A cough that develops after administration of BCG could indicate a BCG systemic infection that is life-threatening. Notify the physician immediately.

Retain BCG in the bladder for 2 hours. Void in a seated position to avoid splashing of urine.

Disinfect urine voided for 6 hours after instillation with an equal volume of 5% sodium hypochlorite solution (undiluted household bleach); allow to disinfect for 15 minutes before flushing.

Increase fluid intake to "flush" the bladder in the hours following BCG treatment. Patients may experience burning with first void after treatment.

DENILEUKIN DIFTITOX

Rx	**Ontak** (Ligand Pharmaceuticals)	**Solution for Injection, frozen:** 150 mcg/ml	EDTA. In single-use vials.

WARNING

Denileukin diftitox should be used only by physicians experienced in the use of antineoplastic therapy and management of patients with cancer. Manage patients treated with denileukin diftitox in a facility equipped and staffed for cardiopulmonary resuscitation and where the patient can be closely monitored for an appropriate period based on his or her health status.

Indications

▶*Cutaneous T-cell lymphoma:* For the treatment of patients with persistent or recurrent cutaneous T-cell lymphoma (CTCL) whose malignant cells express the CD25 component of the IL-2 receptor. The safety and efficacy of denileukin in patients with CTCL whose malignant cells do not express the CD25 component of the IL-2 receptor have not been examined.

Administration and Dosage

▶*Approved by the FDA:* February 5, 1999.

Denileukin is for IV use only. The recommended treatment regimen (1 treatment cycle) is 9 or 18 mcg/kg/day administered IV for 5 consecutive days every 21 days. Infuse over ≥ 15 minutes. If infusional adverse reactions occur, discontinue the infusion or reduce the rate depending on the severity of the reaction. There is no clinical experience with prolonged infusion times (> 80 minutes).

The optimal duration of therapy has not been determined; however, only 2% of patients who did not demonstrate ≥ 25% decrease in tumor burden prior to the fourth course of treatment subsequently responded.

The solution in the vial may be mixed by gentle swirling; do not vigorously shake solution. After thawing, a haze may be visible. This haze should clear when the solution is at room temperature. Do not use solution unless clear, colorless, and without visible particulate matter.

▶*Preparation and administration:*
1.) Prepare and hold diluted denileukin in plastic syringes or soft plastic IV bags. Do not use a glass container because adsorption to glass may occur in the dilute state.
2.) The concentration of denileukin must be ≥ 15 mcg/ml during all steps in the preparation of the solution for IV infusion. This is best accomplished by withdrawing the calculated dose from the vial(s) and injecting it into an empty IV infusion bag. For each 1 ml of denileukin removed from the vial(s), no more than 9 ml of sterile saline without preservative should be added to the IV bag.
3.) Infuse the dose over ≥ 15 minutes.
4.) Do not administer as a bolus injection.
5.) Do not physically mix with other drugs.
6.) Do not administer through an in-line filter.
7.) Administer prepared solutions within 6 hours, using a syringe pump or IV infusion bag.
8.) Discard unused portions immediately.

▶*Storage/Stability:* Store frozen ≤ -10°C (14°F). Denileukin must be brought to room temperature, ≤ 25°C (77°F), before preparing the dose. The vials may be thawed in the refrigerator at 2° to 8°C (36° to 46°F) for ≤ 24 hours or at room temperature for 1 to 2 hours. Do not heat denileukin. Administer prepared solutions within 6 hours. Do not refreeze.

DENILEUKIN DIFTITOX

Actions

▶*Pharmacology:* Denileukin, a recombinant DNA-derived cytotoxic protein composed of the amino acid sequences for diphtheria toxin fragments A and B followed by the sequences for interleukin-2, is produced in an *Escherichia coli* expression system.

Denileukin is a fusion protein designed to direct the cytocidal action of diphtheria toxin to cells that express the IL-2 receptor. The human IL-2 receptor exists in 3 forms, low (CD25), intermediate (CD122/CD132), and high (CD25/CD122/CD132) affinity. The high-affinity form of this receptor is usually found only on activated T-lymphocytes, activated B-lymphocytes, and activated macrophages. Malignant cells expressing ≥ 1 of the subunits of the IL-2 receptor are found in certain leukemias and lymphomas including CTCL. Ex vivo studies suggest that denileukin interacts with the high-affinity IL-2 receptor on the cell surface and inhibits cellular protein synthesis, resulting in cell death within hours.

▶*Pharmacokinetics:*

Absorption/Distribution – The primary sites of distribution and accumulation of material outside the vasculature were the liver and kidneys in rats. Following the first IV dose in lymphoma patients (dose range, 3 to 31 mcg/kg/day), denileukin displayed 2-compartment behavior with a distribution half-life of ≈ 2 to 5 minutes and a terminal phase half-life of ≈ 70 to 80 minutes. Volume of distribution was similar to that of circulating blood (0.06 to 0.08 L/kg). Systemic exposure was variable but proportional to dose.

Metabolism/Excretion – Animal studies demonstrated that denileukin was metabolized by proteolytic degradation. Excreted material was < 25% of the total injected dose and consisted of low molecular weight breakdown products. Lymphoma patients demonstrated clearance rates of ≈ 1.5 to 2 ml/min/kg. No accumulation was evident between the first and fifth doses. Development of antibodies to denileukin significantly impacts clearance rates.

Immunogenicity – Prior to therapy, 39% of lymphoma patients had low titers (< 1:5) of antibody that cross-reacted with the diphtheria toxin domains of denileukin, presumably caused by prior diphtheria immunization. Development of antidenileukin antibodies was observed in 41 of 49 patients after a single course and in 33 of 34 patients after 3 cycles. Following antidenileukin antibody formation, there was a significant increase (2- to 3-fold) in clearance, which resulted in a decrease in mean systemic exposure of ≈ 75%. Changes in clearance were related to the development of antibodies.

The antibody response in all such patients was directed against the diphtheria toxin domain. A low titer of antibodies to the IL-2 portion of the denileukin molecule also developed in ≈ 50% of patients. The presence or absence of antibodies did not correlate with the risk of immediate hypersensitivity-type infusional adverse events.

▶*Clinical trials:* A randomized, double-blind study was conducted to evaluate IV infusion daily doses of 9 or 18 mcg/kg/day for 5 days every 3 weeks in 71 patients with recurrent or persistent Stage Ib to IVa CTCL. Patients received a median of 6 courses of therapy (range, 1 to 11). Overall, 30% of patients treated with denileukin experienced an objective tumor response (50% reduction in tumor burden, which was sustained for ≥ 6 weeks); 7 patients (10%) achieved a complete response and 14 patients (20%) achieved a partial response. The overall median duration of response, measured from first day of response, was 4 months with a median duration for complete response of 9 months and for partial response of 4 months. In a Phase I/II dose-escalation study, 35 patients with Stage Ia to IVb CTCL were treated with denileukin as an IV infusion at doses ranging from 3 to 31 mcg/kg/day for 5 days every 3 weeks. The overall response rate in patients with CTCL who expressed CD25 was 38%; the complete response rate was 16% and the partial response rate was 22%. There was no response in 21 patients with Hodgkin's disease.

Contraindications

Hypersensitivity to denileukin or any of its components: Diphtheria toxin, interleukin-2, or excipients.

Warnings

▶*Vascular leak syndrome:* This syndrome, characterized by ≥ 2 of the following 3 symptoms (hypotension, edema, hypoalbuminemia) was reported in 27% of patients in the clinical studies; 6% of patients were hospitalized for the management of these symptoms. The onset of symptoms in patients with vascular leak syndrome was delayed, usually occurring within the first 2 weeks of infusion and may persist or worsen after the cessation of denileukin. Take special caution in patients with preexisting cardiovascular disease.

Carefully monitor weight, edema, blood pressure, and serum albumin levels on an outpatient basis. This syndrome is usually self-limited; use treatment only if clinically indicated. The type of treatment will depend on whether edema or hypotension is the primary clinical problem. Preexisting low serum albumin levels appear to predict and may predispose patients to the syndrome (see Precautions).

▶*Hypersensitivity reactions:* Acute hypersensitivity reactions were reported in 69% of patients during or within 24 hours of infusion; approximately half of the events occurred on the first day of dosing regardless of the treatment cycle. The constellation of symptoms included ≥ 1 of the following: Hypotension (50%), back pain (30%), dyspnea (28%), vasodilation (28%), rash (25%), chest pain or tightness (24%), tachycardia (12%), dysphagia or laryngismus (5%), syncope (3%), allergic reaction (1%), or anaphylaxis (1%). These events were severe in 2% of patients. Management consists of either an interruption or a decrease in the rate of infusion (depending on the severity of the reaction); 3% of infusions were terminated prematurely and reduction in rate occurred in 4% of the infusions during the clinical trials. The administration of IV antihistamines, corticosteroids, and epinephrine may also be required; 2 subjects received epinephrine and 18 (13%) received systemic corticosteroids in the clinical studies. Have these drugs and resuscitative equipment readily available during administration. Refer to Management of Acute Hypersensitivity Reactions.

▶*Elderly:* Of the patients enrolled in the randomized 2 dosage studies, 49% were ≥ 65 years of age. These patients had response rates similar to those seen in younger patients. The following adverse events (regardless of causality) tended to be more frequent or severe in lymphoma patients who were ≥ 65 years of age: Anorexia, hypotension, anemia, confusion, rash, nausea, or vomiting.

▶*Pregnancy: Category C.* It is not known whether denileukin can cause fetal harm when administered to a pregnant woman or affect reproductive capacity. Give to a pregnant woman only if clearly needed.

▶*Lactation:* It is not known whether this drug is excreted in breast milk. Because of the potential for serious adverse reactions in nursing infants, patients receiving denileukin should discontinue nursing.

▶*Children:* Safety and efficacy in pediatric patients have not been established.

Precautions

▶*Monitoring:* Prior to administration of this product, test the patient's malignant cells for CD25 expression. A testing service for the assay of CD25 on skin biopsy samples is available. For information on this service, call (800) 964-5836.

Perform a complete blood count and a blood chemistry panel, including liver and renal function and serum albumin levels, prior to initiation of treatment and weekly during therapy.

Eighty-three percent of patients with lymphoma experienced hypoalbuminemia, which was considered moderate or severe in 17% of the affected patients. For most patients, the nadir for hypoalbuminemia occurs 1 to 2 weeks after administration. Monitor serum albumin levels prior to the initiation of each treatment course. Delay administration until serum albumin levels are ≥ 3 g/dl.

▶*Infection:* Carefully monitor patients for infections because patients with CTCL have a predisposition to cutaneous infections. Also, the binding of denileukin to activated lymphocytes and macrophages can lead to cell death and may impair immune function in patients.

Adverse Reactions

Adverse reactions were observed in 2 clinical studies of 143 patients with lymphoma, including 105 patients with CTCL, treated at doses ranging from 3 to 31 mcg/kg/day. All patients experienced ≥ 1 adverse event. Twenty-one percent of patients required hospitalization for drug-related adverse events; the most common reasons were evaluation of fever, management of vascular leak syndrome, or dehydration secondary to GI toxicity. Five percent of clinical adverse reactions were severe or life-threatening. The occurrence of adverse events tended to diminish in frequency after the first 2 courses, possibly related to antibody development.

Denileukin Adverse Reactions Occurring in Lymphoma Patients (≥ 5%; n = 143)		
Adverse reaction	All grades	Grades 3 and 4
Cardiovascular		
Hypotension	36	8
Vasodilation	22	1
Tachycardia	12	1
Thrombotic events	7	4
Hypertension	6	0
Arrhythmia	6	3
CNS		
Dizziness	22	1
Paresthesia	13	1
Nervousness	11	1
Confusion	8	6
Insomnia	9	3
Dermatologic		
Rash	34	13
Pruritus	20	3
Sweating	10	1
GI		
Nausea/vomiting	64	14
Anorexia	36	8
Diarrhea	29	3
Constipation	9	1

DENILEUKIN DIFTITOX

Denileukin Adverse Reactions Occurring in Lymphoma Patients (≥ 5%; n = 143)		
Adverse reaction	All grades	Grades 3 and 4
Dyspepsia	7	0
Dysphagia	6	1
GU		
Hematuria	10	3
Albuminuria	10	1
Pyuria	10	1
Creatinine increase	7	1
Hematologic/Lymphatic		
Anemia	18	6
Thrombocytopenia	8	2
Leukopenia	6	3
Metabolic/Nutritional		
Hypoalbuminemia	83	14
Transaminase increase	61	15
Edema	47	15
Hypocalcemia	17	3
Weight decrease	14	4
Dehydration	9	7
Hypokalemia	6	0
Musculoskeletal		
Myalgia	17	2
Arthralgia	8	1
Respiratory		
Dyspnea	29	14
Cough increase	26	2
Pharyngitis	17	0
Rhinitis	13	1
Lung disorder	8	0
Miscellaneous		
Chills/fever	81	22
Asthenia	66	22
Infection	48	24
Pain	48	13
Headache	26	3
Chest pain	24	6
Flu-like syndrome	8	0
Injection site reaction	8	1

Infectious complications – Infections of various types were reported by 48% of the study population, of which 23% were considered severe; 4% discontinued therapy because of infections. Decreased lymphocyte counts (< 900 cells/mcl) occurred in 34% of lymphoma patients. In general, lymphocyte counts dropped during the dosing period (days 1 to 5) and returned to normal by day 15. Smaller changes and more rapid recoveries were observed with subsequent courses.

Infusion-related reactions – There are 2 distinct clinical syndromes associated with denileukin infusion: An acute hypersensitivity-type symptom complex and a flu-like symptom complex. Overall, 69% of patients had infusion-related, hypersensitivity-type symptoms (see Warnings). A flu-like syndrome was experienced by 91% of patients within several hours to days after infusion. The symptom complex consists of ≥ 1 of the following: Fever or chills (81%), asthenia (66%), digestive (64%), myalgias (18%), and arthralgias (8%). In the majority of patients, these symptoms were mild-to-moderate and responded to treatment with antipyretics or anti-emetics. Antipyretics or anti-emetics were used to relieve flu-like symptoms; however, the usefulness of these agents in ameliorating toxicities or as prophylactic agents to decrease incidence of acute, flu-like toxicities has not been prospectively studied.

►*Cardiovascular:* Two patients, both of whom had known or suspected preexisting coronary artery disease, sustained acute MI while on study. Ten additional patients (7%) experienced thrombotic events. Two patients with progressive disease and multiple medical problems experienced deep-vein thrombosis. Another patient sustained a DVT and pulmonary embolus during hospitalization for management of CHF and vascular leak syndrome. One patient with a history of severe peripheral vascular disease sustained an arterial thrombosis. Six patients experienced less severe superficial thrombophlebitis. Thrombotic events were also observed in preclinical animal studies.

►*GI:* The onset of diarrhea may be delayed and the duration can be prolonged. Dehydration, usually concurrent with vomiting or anorexia, occurred in 9% of the patients. The majority of transient hepatic transaminase elevations occurred during the first course of denileukin, were self-limited, and resolved within 2 weeks.

►*Miscellaneous:*

Rash – A variety of rashes were reported, including generalized maculopapular, petechial, vesicular bullous, urticarial, or eczematous with both acute and delayed onset. Antihistamines may be effective in relieving the symptoms, but more severe rashes may require the use of topical or oral corticosteroids.

Infrequent serious adverse events – The following serious adverse events occurred at an incidence of < 5%: Pancreatitis, acute renal insufficiency, microscopic hematuria, hyperthyroidism, and hypothyroidism.

Overdosage

There is no clinical experience with accidental overdosage and no known antidote. At a dose of 31 mcg/kg/day, the dose-limiting toxicities were moderate-to-severe nausea, vomiting, fever, chills, or persistent asthenia. Doses > 31 mcg/kg/day have not been evaluated in humans. If overdose occurs, closely monitor hepatic and renal function and overall fluid balance.

LEVAMISOLE HCl

Rx	Ergamisol (Janssen)	**Tablets:** 50 mg levamisole base	(Janssen L 50). White. In blister pack 36s.

Indications

Only as adjuvant treatment in combination with fluorouracil after surgical resection in patients with Dukes' stage C colon cancer.

Administration and Dosage

Adjuvant use of levamisole and fluorouracil is limited to the following schedule:

►*Initial therapy:*

Levamisole – 50 mg orally every 8 hours for 3 days (starting 7 to 30 days post-surgery).

Fluorouracil – 450 mg/m²/day IV for 5 days concomitant with a 3 day course of levamisole (starting 21 to 34 days post-surgery).

►*Maintenance:*

Levamisole – 50 mg orally every 8 hours for 3 days every 2 weeks.

Fluorouracil – 450 mg/m²/day IV once a week beginning 28 days after the initiation of the 5 day course.

►*Treatment:* Initiate levamisole no earlier than 7 and no later than 30 days post-surgery at a dose of 50 mg every 8 hours for 3 days repeated every 14 days for 1 year. Initiate fluorouracil therapy no earlier than 21 days and no later than 35 days after surgery providing the patient is out of the hospital, ambulatory, maintaining normal oral nutrition, has well healed wounds and is fully recovered from any postoperative complications. If levamisole has been initiated from 7 to 20 days after surgery, initiate fluorouracil therapy coincident with the second course of levamisole, ie, at 21 to 34 days. If levamisole is initiated from 21 to 30 days after surgery, initiate fluorouracil simultaneously with the first course of levamisole.

Administer fluorouracil by rapid IV push at a dosage of 450 mg/m²/day for 5 consecutive days. Dosage is based on actual weight (estimated dry weight). If the patient develops any stomatitis or diarrhea (≥ 5 loose stools), discontinue this course before the full 5 doses are administered. Twenty-eight days after initiation of this course, institute weekly fluorouracil at 450 mg/m²/week and continue for a total treatment time of 1 year. If stomatitis or diarrhea develop during weekly therapy, defer the next dose of fluorouracil until these side effects have subsided. If these side effects are moderate to severe, reduce the fluorouracil dose 20% when it is resumed.

Institute dosage medications as follows: If WBC is 2500 to 3500/mm³ defer the fluorouracil dose until WBC is > 3500/mm³. If WBC is < 2500/mm³, defer the fluorouracil dose until WBC is> 3500/mm³, then resume the fluorouracil dose reduced by 20%. If WBC remains < 2500/mm³ for > 10 days despite deferring fluorouracil, discontinue administration of levamisole. Defer both drugs unless platelets are adequate (≥ 100,000/mm³).

Levamisole should not be used at doses exceeding the recommended dose or frequency. Clinical studies suggest a relationship between levamisole adverse experiences and increasing dose, and some of these (eg, agranulocytosis) may be life-threatening (see Warnings).

Before beginning this combination adjuvant treatment, the physician should become familiar with the labeling for fluorouracil.

Actions

►*Pharmacology:* Levamisole is an immunomodulator. The mechanism of action of levamisole in combination with fluorouracil is unknown. The effects of levamisole on the immune system are complex. The drug appears to restore depressed immune function rather than to stimulate response to above normal levels. Levamisole can stimulate formation of antibodies to various antigens, enhance T-cell responses by stimulating T-cell activation and proliferation, potentiate monocyte and macrophage functions including phagocytosis and chemotaxis, and increase neutrophil mobility adherence and chemotaxis. Other drugs have similar short-term effects, and the clinical relevance is unclear.

LEVAMISOLE HCl

Besides its immunomodulatory function, levamisole also inhibits alkaline phosphatase and has cholinergic activity.

➤*Pharmacokinetics:* The pharmacokinetics of levamisole have not been studied in the dosage regimen recommended with fluorouracil nor in patients with hepatic insufficiency. It appears that levamisole is rapidly absorbed from the GI tract. Mean peak plasma concentrations of 0.13 mcg/ml are attained within 1.5 to 2 hours. The plasma elimination half-life is between 3 to 4 hours. Levamisole 150 mg is extensively metabolized by the liver, and the metabolites are excreted mainly by the kidneys (70% over 3 days). The elimination half-life of metabolite excretion is 16 hours. Approximately 5% is excreted in the feces; < 5% is excreted unchanged in the urine and < 0.2% in the feces. Approximately 12% is recovered in urine as the glucuronide of p-hydroxy-levamisole.

➤*Clinical trials:* Two clinical trials having essentially the same design have demonstrated an increase in survival and a reduction in recurrence rate in patients with resected Dukes' C colon cancer treated with levamisole plus fluorouracil. After surgery patients were randomized to no further therapy, levamisole alone, or levamisole plus fluorouracil.

In one clinical trial, 262 Dukes' C colorectal cancer patients were evaluated for a minimum follow-up of 5 years. The estimated reduction in death rate was 27% for levamisole plus fluorouracil and 28% for levamisole alone. The estimated reduction in recurrence rate was 36% for levamisole plus fluorouracil and 28% for levamisole alone. In another clinical trial designed to confirm these results, 929 Dukes' C colon cancer patients were evaluated for a minimum follow-up of 2 years. The estimated reduction in death rate and recurrence rate was 33% and 41%, respectively for levamisole plus fluorouracil. The group on levamisole alone did not show advantage over the group receiving no treatment on improving recurrence or survival rates. There are presently insufficient data to evaluate the effect of the combination of levamisole plus fluorouracil in Dukes' B patients. There are also insufficient data to evaluate the effect of levamisole plus fluorouracil in patients with rectal cancer.

Contraindications

Hypersensitivity to the drug or its components.

Warnings

➤*Agranulocytosis:* Levamisole has been associated with agranulocytosis, sometimes fatal. The onset of agranulocytosis is frequently accompanied by a flu-like syndrome (eg, fever, chills); however, in a small number of patients, it is asymptomatic. A flu-like syndrome may also occur in the absence of agranulocytosis. It is essential that appropriate hematological monitoring be done routinely during therapy with levamisole and fluorouracil. Neutropenia is usually reversible following discontinuation of therapy. Instruct patients to report immediately any flu-like symptoms.

Higher than recommended doses of levamisole may be associated with an increased incidence of agranulocytosis, so do not exceed the recommended dose.

The combination of levamisole and fluorouracil has been associated with frequent neutropenia, anemia and thrombocytopenia.

➤*Fertility impairment:* In rats given 20, 60 and 180 mg/kg, copulation period was increased, duration of pregnancy was slightly increased, and fertility, pup viability and weight, lactation index and number of fetuses were decreased at 60 mg/kg.

➤*Pregnancy: Category C.* In rats, embryotoxicity was present at 160 mg/kg; in rabbits, at 180 mg/kg. There are no adequate and well controlled studies in pregnant women. Do not be administer levamisole unless the potential benefits outweigh the risks. Advise women taking the combination of levamisole and fluorouracil not to become pregnant.

➤*Lactation:* It is not known whether levamisole is excreted in breast milk; it is excreted in cows' milk. Because of the potential for serious adverse reactions in nursing infants from levamisole, decide whether to discontinue nursing or discontinue the drug, taking into account the importance of the drug to the mother.

➤*Children:* Safety and efficacy of levamisole in children have not been established.

Precautions

➤*Monitoring:* On the first day of therapy with levamisole and fluorouracil, perform a CBC with differential and platelets, electrolytes and liver function tests. Thereafter, perform a CBC with differential and platelets weekly prior to each fluorouracil treatment; perform electrolyte and liver function tests every 3 months for a total of 1 year. Institute dosage modifications (see Administration and Dosage).

Drug Interactions

➤*Alcohol:* Levamisole may produce disulfiram-like effects with concomitant alcohol.

➤*Phenytoin:* Coadministration with levamisole and fluorouracil has led to increased phenytoin plasma levels. Monitor phenytoin plasma levels and decrease the dose if necessary.

Adverse Reactions

Levamisole and Levamisole/Fluorouracil Adverse Reactions (%)		
Adverse reaction	Levamisole (n = 440)	Levamisole plus fluorouracil (n = 599)
Central and peripheral nervous system		
Dizziness	3	4
Headache	3	4
Paresthesia	2	3
Ataxia	0	2
GI		
Nausea	22	65
Diarrhea	13	52
Stomatitis	3	39
Vomiting	6	20
Anorexia	2	6
Abdominal pain	2	5
Constipation	2	3
Flatulence	< 1	2
Dyspepsia	< 1	1
Hematological		
Leukopenia		
< 2,000/mm^3	< 1	1
≥ 2,000 to <4,000/mm^3	4	19
≥ 4,000/mm^3	2	33
unscored category	0	< 1
Thrombocytopenia		
< 50,000/mm^3	0	0
≥ 50,000 to < 130,000/mm^3	1	8
≥ 130,000/mm^3	1	10
Anemia	0	6
Granulocytopenia	< 1	2
Epistaxis	0	1
Skin and appendages		
Dermatitis	8	23
Alopecia	3	22
Pruritus	1	2
Skin discoloration	0	2
Urticaria	< 1	0
Special senses		
Taste perversion	8	8
Altered sense of smell	1	1
Musculoskeletal system		
Arthralgia	5	4
Myalgia	3	2
Psychiatric		
Somnolence	3	2
Depression	1	2
Nervousness	1	2
Insomnia	1	1
Anxiety	1	1
Forgetfulness	0	1
Vision		
Abnormal tearing	0	4
Blurred vision	1	2
Conjunctivitis	< 1	2
Miscellaneous		
Fatigue	6	11
Infection	5	12
Fever	3	5
Rigors	3	5
Chest pain	< 1	1
Hyperbilirubinemia	< 1	1
Edema	1	1

LEVAMISOLE HCl

Less frequent adverse experiences included: Exfoliative dermatitis; periorbital edema; vaginal bleeding; anaphylaxis; confusion; convulsions; hallucinations; impaired concentration; renal failure; elevated serum creatinine; increased alkaline phosphatase. An encephalopathy-like syndrome has occurred.

Almost all patients receiving levamisole and fluorouracil reported adverse experiences. In a clinical trial, 66 of 463 patients (14%) discontinued the combination of levamisole plus fluorouracil because of adverse reactions; 43 (9%) developed isolated or a combination of GI toxicities (eg, nausea, vomiting, diarrhea, stomatitis, anorexia). Ten patients developed rash or pruritus. Five patients discontinued therapy because of flu-like symptoms or fever with chills; 10 patients developed CNS symptoms such as dizziness, ataxia, depression, confusion, memory loss, weakness, inability to concentrate and headache. Two patients developed reversible neutropenia and sepsis: One because of thrombocytopenia, one because of hyperbilirubinemia. One patient in the levamisole plus fluorouracil group developed agranulocytosis and sepsis, and died.

In the levamisole alone arm of the trial, 15 of 310 patients (4.8%) discontinued therapy because of adverse experiences. Six of these (2%) discontinued because of rash, six because of arthralgia/myalgia, and one each for fever and neutropenia, urinary infection and cough.

Overdosage

Fatalities have occurred in a 3-year-old child who ingested 15 mg/kg and in an adult who ingested 32 mg/kg. No further clinical information is available. In cases of overdosage, gastric lavage is recommended together with symptomatic and supportive measures. Refer to General Management of Acute Overdosage.

Patient Information

Immediately notify the physician if flu-like symptoms or malaise occurs.

TRETINOIN

Rx **Vesanoid** (Hoffmann-La Roche)   **Capsules:** 10 mg   (Vesanoid 10 Roche). Orange-yellow/reddish brown. In 100s.

WARNING

Experienced physician and institution: Patients with acute promyelocytic leukemia (APL) are at high risk in general and can have severe adverse reactions to tretinoin. Therefore, administer under the supervision of a physician who is experienced in the management of patients with acute leukemia and in a facility with laboratory and supportive services sufficient to monitor drug tolerance and to protect and maintain a patient compromised by drug toxicity, including respiratory compromise. Use of tretinoin requires that the physician concludes that the possible benefit to the patient outweighs the following adverse effects.

Retinoic acid-APL syndrome: About 25% of APL patients treated with tretinoin have experienced a syndrome called the retinoic acid-APL (RA-APL) syndrome characterized by fever, dyspnea, weight gain, radiographic pulmonary infiltrates and pleural or pericardial effusions. This syndrome has occasionally been accompanied by impaired myocardial contractility and episodic hypotension. It has been observed with or without concomitant leukocytosis. Endotracheal intubation and mechanical ventilation have been required in some cases due to progressive hypoxemia, and several patients have expired with multi-organ failure. The syndrome generally occurs during the first month of treatment, with some cases reported following the first dose.

The management of the syndrome has not been defined rigorously, but high-dose steroids given at the first suspicion of the RA-APL syndrome appear to reduce morbitity and mortality. At the first signs suggestive of the syndrome (unexplained fever, dyspnea or weight gain, abnormal chest auscultatory findings or radiographic abnormalities), immediately initiate high-dose steroids (dexamethasone 10 mg IV) every 12 hours for 3 days or until the resolution of symptoms, regardless of the leukocyte count. The majority of patients do not require termination of tretinoin therapy during treatment of the RA-APL syndrome.

Leukocytosis: During treatment, ≈ 40% of patients will develop rapidly evolving leukocytosis. Patients who present with high WBC at diagnosis (> 5 × 10⁹/L) have an increased risk of a further rapid increase in WBC counts. Rapidly evolving leukocytosis is associated with a higher risk of life-threatening complications.

If signs and symptoms of the RA-APL syndrome are present together with leukocytosis, initiate treatment with high-dose steroids immediately. Some investigators routinely add chemotherapy to tretinoin treatment in the case of patients presenting with a WBC count of > 5 × 10⁹/L or in the case of a rapid increase in WBC count for patients leukopenic start of treatment, and have reported a lower incidence of the RA-APL syndrome. Consider adding full-dose chemotherapy (including an anthracycline, if not contraindicated) to the tretinoin therapy on day 1 or 2 for patients presenting with a WBC count of > 5 × 10⁹/L or immediately, for patients presenting with a WBC count of < 5 × 10⁹/L, if the WBC count reaches ≥ 6 × 10⁹/L by day 5, or ≥ 10 × 10⁹/L by day 10 or ≥ 15 × 10⁹/L by day 28.

Teratogenic effects:

Pregnancy – Category D (see Warnings). There is a high risk that a severely deformed infant will result if tretinoin is administered during pregnancy. If, nonetheless, it is determined that tretinoin represents the best available treatment for a pregnant woman or a woman of childbearing potential, it must be assured that the patient has received full information and warnings of the risk to the fetus if she were pregnant and of the risk of possible contraception failure. She must be instructed in the need to use two reliable forms of contraception simultaneously during therapy and for 1 month following discontinuation of therapy, unless abstinence is the chosen method.

Within 1 week prior to the institution of tretinoin therapy, the patient should have blood or urine collected for a serum or urine pregnancy test with a sensitivity of at least 50 mIU/L. When possible, delay tretinoin therapy until a negative result from this test is obtained. When a delay is not possible, place the patient on two reliable forms of contraception. Repeat pregnancy testing and contraception counseling monthly throughout the period of treatment.

Indications

➤*Acute promyelocytic leukemia (APL):* Induction of remission in patients with APL, French American British (FAB) classification M3 (including the M3 variant), characterized by the presence of the t(15;17) translocation or the presence of the PML/RARα gene who are refractory to or who have relapsed from anthracycline chemotherapy, or for whom anthracycline-based chemotherapy is contraindicated. Tretinoin is for the induction of remission only. All patients should receive an accepted form of remission consolidation or maintenance therapy for APL after completion of induction therapy with tretinoin.

Administration and Dosage

➤*Approved by the FDA:* November 22, 1995.

The recommended dose is 45 mg/m²/day administered as two evenly divided doses until complete remission is documented. Discontinue therapy 30 days after achievement of complete remission or after 90 days of treatment, whichever occurs first. If after initiation of treatment the presence of the t(15:17) translocation is not confirmed by cytogenetics or by polymerase chain reaction studies and the patient has not responded to tretinoin, consider alternative therapy.

Tretinoin is for the induction of remission only. Optimal consolidation or maintenance regimens have not been determined. All patients should therefore receive a standard consolidation or maintenance chemotherapy regimen for APL after induction therapy with tretinoin unless otherwise contraindicated.

Actions

➤*Pharmacology:* Tretinoin is a retinoid that induces maturation of acute promelocytic leukemia (APL) cells in culture. Chemically, tretinoin is all-trans retinoic acid and is related to retinol (vitamin A). Tretinoin is not a cytolytic agent but instead induces cytodifferentiation and decreased proliferation of APL cells. In APL patients, tretinoin produces an initial maturation of the primitive promyelocytes derived from the leukemic clone, followed by a repopulation of the bone marrow and peripheral blood by normal, polyclonal hematopoietic cells in patients achieving complete remission (CR). The exact mechanism of action of tretinoin in APL is unknown.

➤*Pharmacokinetics:*

Absorption / Distribution – A single 45 mg/m² (≈ 80 mg) oral dose to APL patients resulted in a mean peak concentration of 347 ng/ml. Time to reach peak concentration was between 1 and 2 hours. Tretinoin is > 95% bound in plasma, predominantly to albumin.

Metabolism – Tretinoin metabolites have been identified in plasma and urine. Cytochrome P450 (CYP) enzymes have been implicated in the oxidative metabolism of tretinoin. Metabolites include 13–cis retinoic acid, 4–oxo trans retinoic acid, 4–oxo cis retinoinc acid and 4–oxo trans retinoic acid glucuronide. In APL patients, daily administration of a 45 mg/m² dose resulted in an ≈ 10–fold increase in the urinary excretion of 4–oxo trans retinoic acid glucuronide after 2 to 6 weeks of continuous dosing when compared with baseline values.

Excretion – Studies with radiolabeled drug have demonstrated that after the oral administration of 2.75 and 50 mg, > 90% of the radioactivity was recovered in the urine and feces; ≈ 63% of radioactivity was recovered in the urine within 72 hours and 31% appeared in the feces within 6 days.

Tretinoin activity is primarily due to the parent drug. In studies, orally administered drug was well absorbed into the systemic circulation, with ≈ 66% recovered in the urine. The terminal elimination half-life following initial dosing is 0.5 to 2 hours in patients with APL. There is evidence that tretinoin induces its own metabolism. Plasma concentrations decrease on average to ⅓ of their day 1 values during 1 week of continuous therapy. Mean peak concentrations decreased from 394 to 138 ng/ml, while area under the curve (AUC) values decreased from 537 to 249 ng•hr/ml during 45 mg/m² daily dosing in seven APL patients. Increasing the dose to "correct" for this change has not increased response.

➤*Clinical trials:* In 114 previously treated APL patients and in 67 previously untreated ("de novo") patients, tretinoin 45 mg/m²/day was given for up to 90 days or 30 days beyond the day that CR was reached. Complete remission occurred in 50% to 80% of relapsed patients and in 36% to 73% of de novo patients. Median survival was 5.8 to 10.8 months (relapsed) and 0.55 months (de novo).

The median time to CR was between 40 and 50 days (range, 2 to 120 days). Most patients in these studies received cytotoxic chemotherapy during the remission phase. These results compare with the 30% to 50% CR rate and ≤ 6 month median survival reported for cytotoxic chemotherapy of APL in the treatment of relapse. Ten of 15 pediatric cases achieved CR.

Contraindications

Hypersensitivity to retinoids; patients sensitive to parabens, which are used as preservatives in the gelatin capsule.

Warnings

➤*Patients without the t(15:17) translocation:* Initiation of therapy with tretinoin may be based on the morphological diagnosis of APL. Confirm the diagnosis of APL by detection of the t(15:17) genetic marker by cytogenetic studies. If these are negative, PML/RARα fusion should be sought using molecular diagnostic techniques. The response rate of other AML subtypes to tretinoin has not been demonstrated; therefore, consider alternative treatment for patients who lack the genetic marker.

TRETINOIN

➤*Retinoic acid-APL (RA-APL) syndrome:* In up to 25% of APL patients treated with tretinoin, a syndrome occurs that can be fatal (see Warning Box).

➤*Leukocytosis:* See Warning Box.

➤*Pseudotumor cerebri:* Retinoids, including tretinoin, have been associated with pseudotumor cerebri (benign intracranial hypertension), especially in children. Early signs and symptoms include papilledema, headache, nausea, vomiting, and visual disturbances. Evaluate patients with these symptoms for pseudotumor cerebri, and, if present, institute appropriate care with neurological assessment.

➤*Lipids:* Up to 60% of patients experienced hypercholesterolemia or hypertriglyceridemia, which were reversible upon completion of treatment. The clinical consequences of temporary elevation of triglycerides and cholesterol are unknown, but venous thrombosis and MI have been reported in patients who ordinarily are at low risk for such complications.

➤*Carcinogenesis:* In short-term carcinogenicity studies, tretinoin at a dose of 30 mg/kg/day ($\approx$ 2 times the human dose) increased the rate of diethylnitrosamine (DEN)-induced mouse liver adenomas and carcinomas. A 2-fold increase in the sister chromatid exchange (SCE) has been demonstrated in human diploid fibroblasts. In a 6-week toxicology study in dogs, minimal to marked testicular degeneration, with increased numbers of immature spermatozoa, were observed at 10 mg/kg/day ($\approx$ 4 times the equivalent human dose).

➤*Pregnancy:* Category D (see Warning Box). Tretinoin has teratogenic and embryotoxic effects in animals, and may be expected to cause fetal harm when administered to a pregnant woman. Tretinoin causes fetal resorptions and a decrease in live fetuses in all animals studied. Gross external, soft tissue, and skeletal alterations occurred at doses ranging from 1/20 to 4 times the human dose.

There are no adequate and well-controlled studies in pregnant women. Although experience with humans is extremely limited, increased spontaneous abortions and major human fetal abnormalities related to the use of other retinoids have been documented. Reported defects include abnormalities of the CNS, musculoskeletal system, external ear, eye, thymus and great vessels; and facial dysmorphia, cleft palate and parathyroid hormone deficiency. Some of these abnormalities were fatal. Cases of IQ scores < 85, with or without obvious CNS abnormalities, have also have been reported. All fetuses exposed during pregnancy can be affected, and there is no antepartum means of determining which fetuses are or are not affected.

Effective contraception must be used by all females during tretinoin therapy and for 1 month following discontinuation of therapy. Contraception must be used even when there is a history of infertility or menopause, unless a hysterectomy has been performed. Whenever contraception is required, it is recommended that 2 reliable forms of contraception be used simultaneously, unless abstinence is the chosen method. If pregnancy does occur during treatment, the physician and patient should discuss the desirability of continuing or terminating the pregnancy.

➤*Lactation:* It is not known whether this drug is excreted in breast milk. Because of the potential for serious adverse reactions from tretinoin in nursing infants, mothers should discontinue nursing prior to taking this drug.

➤*Children:* There are limited clinical data on the pediatric use of tretinoin. Of 15 pediatric patients (range, 1 to 16 years of age) treated with tretinoin, the incidence of complete remission was 67%. Safety and efficacy in pediatric patients < 1 year of age have not been established. Some pediatric patients experience severe headache and pseudotumor cerebri, requiring analgesic treatment and lumbar puncture for relief. Increased caution is recommended. Consider dose reduction in children experiencing serious or intolerable toxicity; however, the efficacy and safety of tretinoin at doses < 45 mg/m²/day have not been evaluated.

Precautions

➤*Monitoring:* Monitor the patient's hematologic profile, coagulation profile, liver function test results, and triglyceride and cholesterol levels frequently.

➤*Toxic side effects:* Tretinoin has potentially significant toxic side effects in APL patients. Closely observe patients undergoing therapy for signs of respiratory compromise or leukocytosis (see Warning Box). Maintain supportive care appropriate for APL patients (eg, prophylaxis for bleeding, prompt therapy for infection) during therapy.

➤*Lab test abnormalities:* Elevated liver function test results occur in 50% to 60% of patients during treatment. Carefully monitor liver function test results during treatment and give consideration to a temporary withdrawal of tretinoin if test results reach > 5 times the upper limit of normal. However, the majority of these abnormalities resolve without interruption of or after completion of treatment.

Drug Interactions

➤*Ketoconazole:* In 13 patients given ketoconazole (400 to 1200 mg) 1 hour prior to tretinoin, a 72% increase in tretinoin mean plasma AUC occurred.

As tretinoin is metabolized by the hepatic CYP system, there is a potential for alteration of pharmacokinetics in patients administered concomitant medications that are also inducers or inhibitors of this system.

➤*Drug/Food interactions:* The absorption of retinoids as a class has been shown to be enhanced when taken together with food.

Adverse Reactions

Virtually all patients experience some drug-related toxicity, especially headache, fever, weakness, and fatigue. These adverse effects are seldom permanent or irreversible nor do they usually require therapy interruption.

Typical retinoid toxicity – Most frequently reported adverse events were similar to those described in patients taking high doses of vitamin A and included headache (86%); fever (83%); skin/mucous membrane dryness, bone pain (77%); nausea/vomiting (57%); rash (54%); mucositis (26%); pruritus, increased sweating (20%); visual disturbances, ocular disorders (17%); alopecia, skin changes (14%); changed visual acuity (6%); bone inflammation, visual field defects (3%).

Ear disorders – Earache or feeling of fullness in the ears (23%); hearing loss and other unspecified auricular disorders (6%); irreversible hearing loss (< 1%).

➤*Cardiovascular:* Arrhythmias, flushing (23%); hypotension (14%); hypertension, phlebitis (11%); cardiac failure (6%); cardiac arrest, MI, enlarged heart, heart murmur, ischemia, stroke, myocarditis, pericarditis, pulmonary hypertension, secondary cardiomyopathy (3%).

➤*CNS:* Dizziness (20%); paresthesias, anxiety (17%); insomnia, depression (14%); confusion (11%); cerebral hemorrhage, intracranial hypertension, agitation (9%); hallucinations (6%); abnormal gait, agnosia, aphasia, asterixis, cerebellar edema, cerebellar disorders, convulsions, coma, CNS depression, dysarthria, encephalopathy, facial paralysis, hemiplegia, hyporeflexia, hypotaxia, no light reflex, neurologic reaction, spinal cord disorder, tremor, leg weakness, unconsciousness, dementia, forgetfulness, somnolence, slow speech (3%).

➤*GI:* GI hemorrhage (34%); abdominal pain (31%); other GI disorders (26%); diarrhea (23%); constipation (17%); dyspepsia (14%); abdominal distention (11%); hepatosplenomegaly (9%); hepatitis, ulcer, unspecified liver disorder (3%).

➤*GU:* Renal insufficiency (11%); dysuria (9%); acute renal failure, micturition frequency, renal tubular necrosis, enlarged prostate (3%).

➤*Respiratory:* The majority of these events are symptoms of the RA-APL syndrome (see Warning Box): Upper respiratory tract disorders (63%); dyspnea (60%); respiratory insufficiency (26%); pleural effusion (20%); pneumonia, rales, expiratory wheezing (14%); lower respiratory tract disorders (9%); pulmonary infiltration (6%); bronchial asthma, pulmonary/larynx edema, unspecified pulmonary disease (3%).

➤*Miscellaneous:* Erythema nodosum, basophilia, hyperhistaminemia, Sweet's syndrome, organomegaly, hypercalcemia, pancreatitis, myositis (isolated cases); malaise (66%); shivering (63%); hemorrhage (60%); infections (58%); peripheral edema (52%); pain (37%); chest discomfort (32%); edema (29%); disseminated intravascular coagulation (26%); weight increase (23%); injection site reactions, anorexia, weight decrease (17%); myalgia (14%); flank pain (9%); cellulitis (8%); face edema, fluid imbalance, pallor, lymph disorders (6%); acidosis, hypothermia, ascites (3%).

Overdosage

The maximal tolerated dose in patients with myelodysplastic syndrome or solid tumors was 195 mg/m²/day. The maximal tolerated dose in pediatric patients was lower (60 mg/m²/day). Overdosage with other retinoids has been associated with transient headache, facial flushing, cheilosis, abdominal pain, dizziness, and ataxia. These symptoms have quickly resolved without apparent residual effects.

BEXAROTENE

Rx	Targretin (Ligand Pharm.)	Capsules, soft gelatin: 75 mg	(Targretin). Off-white, oblong. In 100s.

Bexarotene is also available as a gel for cutaneous T-cell lymphoma (CTCL) lesions; refer to the monograph in the Dermatologic Agents chapter.

WARNING

Bexarotene is a member of the retinoid class of drugs that is associated with birth defects in humans. Bexarotene caused birth defects when administered orally to pregnant rats. Do not administer bexarotene to a pregnant woman.

Indications

►*Cutaneous T-cell lymphoma (CTCL):* Treatment of cutaneous manifestations of CTCL in patients who are refractory to ≥ 1 prior systemic therapy.

Administration and Dosage

►*Approved by the FDA:* December 29, 1999.

►*Initial dose:* 300 mg/m^2/day adjusted for body surface area as a single oral daily dose with a meal.

Bexarotene Initial Dose Calculation According to Body Surface Area

Initial dose level (300 mg/m^2/day)		Number of 75 mg bexarotene capsules
Body surface area (m^2)	Total daily dose (mg/day)	
0.88 to 1.12	300	4
1.13 to 1.37	375	5
1.38 to 1.62	450	6
1.63 to 1.87	525	7
1.88 to 2.12	600	8
2.13 to 2.37	675	9
2.38 to 2.62	750	10

If there is no tumor response after 8 weeks of treatment and if the initial dose of 300 mg/m^2/day is well tolerated, the dose may be escalated to 400 mg/m^2/day with careful monitoring. The 300 mg/m^2/day dose may be adjusted to 200 mg/m^2/day, then to 100 mg/m^2/day, or temporarily suspended, if necessitated by toxicity. When toxicity is controlled, doses may be carefully readjusted upward.

►*Duration of therapy:* Continue bexarotene therapy as long as the patient is deriving benefit. In CTCL clinical trials, bexarotene was administered for ≤ 97 weeks.

►*Storage/Stability:* Store at 2° to 25°C (36° to 77°F). Avoid exposing to high temperatures and humidity after the bottle is opened. Protect from light.

Actions

►*Pharmacology:* Bexarotene selectively binds and activates retinoid X receptor subtypes (RXRα, RXRβ, RXRγ). RXRs can form heterodimers with various receptor partners such as retinoic acid receptors (RARs), vitamin D receptor, thyroid receptor, and peroxisome proliferator activator receptors (PPARs). Once activated, these receptors function as transcription factors that regulate the expression of genes that control cellular differentiation and proliferation. Bexarotene inhibits the growth in vitro of some tumor cell lines of hematopoietic and squamous cell origin and induces tumor regression in vivo in some animal models. The exact mechanism of action of bexarotene in the treatment of CTCL is unknown.

►*Pharmacokinetics:*

Absorption – Bexarotene is absorbed with a T$_{max}$ of ≈ 2 hours after oral administration. Studies in patients with advanced malignancies show approximate single dose linearity within the therapeutic range and low accumulation with multiple doses. Plasma bexarotene AUC and C$_{max}$ values resulting from a 75 to 300 mg dose were 35% and 48% higher, respectively, after a fat-containing meal than after a glucose solution.

Distribution – Bexarotene is highly bound (> 99%) to plasma proteins. The plasma proteins to which bexarotene binds have not been elucidated, and the ability of bexarotene to displace drugs bound to plasma proteins and the ability of drugs to displace bexarotene binding have not been studied. The uptake of bexarotene by organs or tissues has not been evaluated.

Metabolism – Four bexarotene metabolites have been identified in plasma: 6- and 7-hydroxy-bexarotene and 6- and 7-oxo-bexarotene. In vitro studies suggest that cytochrome P450 3A4 is the major cytochrome P450 responsible for formation of the oxidative metabolites and that the oxidative metabolites may be glucuronidated. The oxidative metabolites are active in in vitro assays of retinoid receptor activation, but the relative contribution of the parent and any metabolites to the efficacy and safety of bexarotene is unknown.

Excretion – Terminal half-life of bexarotene is ≈ 7 hours. The renal elimination of bexarotene and its metabolites were examined in patients with type 2 diabetes mellitus. Neither bexarotene nor its metabolites were excreted in urine in appreciable amounts. Bexarotene is thought to be eliminated primarily through the hepatobiliary system.

Contraindications

Pregnancy; hypersensitivity to bexarotene or other product components.

Warnings

►*Lipid abnormalities:* Bexarotene induces major lipid abnormalities in most patients that must be monitored and treated during long-term therapy. About 70% of patients with CTCL who received an initial dose of ≥ 300 mg/m^2/day of bexarotene had fasting triglyceride levels > 2.5 times the upper limit of normal. About 55% had values > 800 mg/dL with a median of ≈ 1200 mg/dL. Cholesterol elevations > 300 mg/dL occurred in ≈ 60% and 75% of patients with CTCL who received an initial dose of 300 mg/m^2/day or > 300 mg/m^2/day, respectively. Decreases in high density lipoprotein (HDL) cholesterol to < 25 mg/dL were seen in ≈ 55% and 90% of patients receiving an initial dose of 300 mg/m^2/day or > 300 mg/m^2/day, respectively, of bexarotene. The effects on triglycerides, HDL cholesterol, and total cholesterol were reversible with cessation of therapy and generally mitigated by dose reduction or concomitant antihyperlipidemic therapy.

Perform fasting blood-lipid determinations before bexarotene therapy is initiated weekly until the lipid response to bexarotene is established (usually occurs within 2 to 4 weeks) and at 8-week intervals thereafter. Prior to initiating bexarotene therapy, normalize fasting triglycerides with appropriate interventions. Maintain triglyceride levels < 400 mg/dL to reduce the risk of clinical sequelae. If fasting triglycerides are elevated or become elevated during treatment, institute antihyperlipidemic therapy and, if necessary, reduce or suspend the dose of bexarotene. In the 300 mg/m^2/day initial dose group, 60% of patients were given lipid-lowering drugs. Because of a potential drug-drug interaction, gemfibrozil is not recommended for use with bexarotene (see Drug Interactions).

►*Pancreatitis:* Acute pancreatitis has been reported in 4 patients with CTCL and in 6 patients with non-CTCL cancers treated with bexarotene; the cases were associated with marked elevations of fasting serum triglycerides, the lowest being 770 mg/dL in 1 patient. One patient with advanced non-CTCL cancer died of pancreatitis. Do not treat patients with CTCL who have risk factors for pancreatitis (eg, prior pancreatitis, uncontrolled hyperlipidemia, excessive alcohol consumption, uncontrolled diabetes mellitus, biliary tract disease, medications known to increase triglyceride levels or to be associated with pancreatic toxicity).

►*Thyroid abnormalities:* Bexarotene induces biochemical evidence of clinical hypothyroidism in ≈ 50% of all patients treated, causing a reversible reduction in thyroid hormone (total thyroxine [total T4]) and thyroid-stimulating hormone (TSH) levels. The incidence of decreases in TSH and total T$_4$ were ≈ 60% and 45%, respectively, in patients with CTCL receiving an initial dose of 300 mg/m^2/day. Hypothyroidism was reported as an adverse event in 29% of patients. Consider treatment with thyroid hormone supplements in patients with laboratory evidence of hypothyroidism. Obtain baseline thyroid function tests and monitor patients during treatment.

►*Leukopenia:* A total of 18% of patients with CTCL receiving an initial dose of 300 mg/m^2/day of bexarotene had reversible leukopenia in the range of 1000 to < 3000 WBC/mm^3. Patients receiving an initial dose > 300 mg/m^2/day of bexarotene had a 43% incidence of leukopenia. Leukopenia of < 1000 WBC/mm^3 was not seen in any patient with CTCL who was treated with bexarotene. The time to onset of leukopenia was generally 4 to 8 weeks. The leukopenia observed in most patients was explained by neutropenia. In the 300 mg/m^2/day initial dose group, the incidence of NCI Grade 3 or 4 neutropenia was 12% and 4%, respectively. The leukopenia and neutropenia experienced during bexarotene therapy resolved after dose reduction or discontinuation of treatment, on average within 30 days in 93% of the patients with CTCL and 82% of patients with non-CTCL cancers. Leukopenia and neutropenia were rarely associated with severe sequelae or serious adverse events. Obtain determination of WBC with differential at baseline and periodically during treatment.

►*Cataracts:* Posterior subcapsular cataracts were observed in preclinical toxicity studies in rats and dogs administered bexarotene daily for 6 months. In 15 of 79 patients who had serial-slit lamp examinations, new cataracts or worsening of previous cataracts were found. Because of the high prevalence and rate of cataract formation in the geriatric patient population, the relationship between bexarotene and cataracts cannot be determined in the absence of an appropriate control group. Provide an appropriate ophthalmologic evaluation in patients who experience visual difficulties.

►*Hepatic function impairment:* Because < 1% of the dose is excreted in the urine unchanged and there is in vitro evidence of extensive hepatic contribution to bexarotene elimination, hepatic impairment would be expected to lead to greatly decreased clearance.

Liver function test abnormalities – For patients with CTCL receiving an initial dose of 300 mg/m^2/day of bexarotene, elevations in liver function tests (LFTs) have been observed in 5% (AST), 2% (ALT), and 0% (bilirubin). In contrast, with an initial dose > 300 mg/m^2/day of bex-

BEXAROTENE

arotene, the incidence of LFT elevations was higher at 7% (AST), 9% (ALT), and 6% (bilirubin). Two patients developed cholestasis, including 1 patient who died of liver failure. In clinical trials, elevation of LFTs resolved within 1 month in 80% of patients following a decrease in dose or discontinuation of therapy. Obtain baseline LFTs and carefully monitor LFTs after 1, 2, and 4 weeks of treatment initiation, and if stable, at least every 8 weeks therafter during treatment. Consider suspension or discontinuation of bexarotene if test results reach > 3 times the upper limit of normal values for AST, ALT, or bilirubin.

➤*Fertility impairment:* Bexarotene caused testicular degeneration when oral doses of 1.5 mg/kg/day were given to dogs for 91 days (producing ≈ ⅕ the AUC at the recommended human daily dose).

➤*Pregnancy: Category X.* Bexarotene may cause fetal harm when administered to a pregnant woman. Do not administer bexarotene to a pregnant woman or a woman who intends to become pregnant. If a woman becomes pregnant while taking bexarotene, stop therapy immediately and provide appropriate counseling.

Obtain a negative pregnancy test (eg, serum beta-human chorionic gonadotropin, beta HCG) with a sensitivity of ≥ 50 mIU/L within 1 week prior to bexarotene therapy. Repeat the pregnancy test at monthly intervals while the patient remains on bexarotene. Effective contraception must be used for 1 month prior to the initiation of therapy, during therapy, and for ≥ 1 month following discontinuation of therapy; it is recommended that 2 reliable forms of contraception be used simultaneously unless abstinence is the chosen method. Bexarotene can potentially induce metabolic enzymes and thereby theoretically reduce plasma concentrations of hormonal contraceptives (see Drug Interactions). Thus, if treatment with bexarotene is intended in a woman with childbearing potential, it is strongly recommended that one of the 2 reliable forms of contraception be nonhormonal. Initiate therapy on the second or third day of a normal menstrual period. Give no more than a 1-month supply of bexarotene to the patient so that the results of pregnancy testing can be assessed and counseling regarding avoidance of pregnancy and birth defects can be reinforced.

Male patients with sexual partners who are pregnant, possibly pregnant, or who could become pregnant must use condoms during sexual intercourse while taking bexarotene and for ≥ 1 month after the last dose of drug.

➤*Lactation:* It is not known whether bexarotene is excreted in breast milk. Because of the potential for serious adverse reactions in nursing infants from bexarotene, decide whether to discontinue nursing or to discontinue the drug, taking into account the importance of the drug to the mother.

➤*Children:* Safety and efficacy have not been established.

Precautions

➤*Monitoring:* Obtain the following lab tests prior to initiating bexarotene therapy and subsequently monitor during therapy: Lipid panel, WBC count with differential, liver function tests, and thyroid function tests (see Warnings).

➤*Vitamin A supplementation:* In clinical studies, patients were advised to limit vitamin A intake to ≤ 15,000 IU/day. Advise patients to limit vitamin A supplements to avoid potential additive toxic effects.

➤*Diabetes mellitus:* Use caution when administering bexarotene in patients using insulin, agents enhancing insulin secretion (eg, sulfonylureas), or insulin-sensitizers. Based on the mechanism of action, bexarotene could enhance the action of these agents, resulting in hypoglycemia (see Drug Interactions).

➤*Photosensitivity:* Retinoids as a class have been associated with photosensitivity. In vitro assays indicate that bexarotene is a potential photosensitizing agent. Mild phototoxicity manifested as sunburn and skin sensitivity to sunlight was observed in patients who were exposed to direct sunlight while receiving bexarotene. Advise patients to minimize exposure to sunlight and artificial ultraviolet light while receiving bexarotene.

Drug Interactions

➤*CYP450:* Bexarotene oxidative metabolites appear to be formed by cytochrome P450 3A4.

Bexarotene Drug Interactions			
Precipitant drug	Object drug*		Description
CYP450 inducers (eg, rifampin, phenytoin, phenobarbital)	Bexarotene	↓	On the basis of bexarotene metabolism, cytochrome P450 3A4 inducers may reduce plasma bexarotene concentrations.
CYP450 inhibitors (eg, ketoconazole, itraconazole, erythromycin, grapefruit juice)	Bexarotene	↑	On the basis of bexarotene metabolism, cytochrome P450 3A4 inhibitors may increase plasma bexarotene concentrations.

Bexarotene Drug Interactions			
Precipitant drug	Object drug*		Description
Gemfibrozil	Bexarotene	↑	Coadministration of bexarotene and gemfibrozil resulted in substantial increases in plasma concentrations of bexarotene. Concomitant administration of gemfibrozil with bexarotene is not recommended.
Vitamin A	Bexarotene	↑	Bexarotene is a member of the retinoids. Limit vitamin A supplements to avoid potential additive toxic effects (≤ 15,000 IU/day; see Precautions).
Bexarotene	Vitamin A		
Bexarotene	Antidiabetic agents	↑	Bexarotene may enhance antidiabetic agents, resulting in hypoglycemia (see Precautions).
Bexarotene	Tamoxifen	↓	Coadministration of bexarotene capsules and tamoxifen in women with breast cancer who were progressing on tamoxifen resulted in a modest decrease in plasma tamoxifen concentrations, possibly through an induction of cytochrome P450 3A4.
Bexarotene	Oral contraceptives	↓	Bexarotene can potentially induce metabolic enzymes and thereby theoretically reduce plasma concentrations of hormonal contraceptives. It is strongly recommended that 2 reliable forms of contraception be used concurrently, 1 of which should be nonhormonal.

* ↑ = Object drug increased. ↓ = Object drug decreased.

➤*Drug/Lab test interactions:* CA125 assay values in patients with ovarian cancer may be increased by bexarotene therapy.

➤*Drug/Food interactions:* Plasma bexarotene AUC and C_{max} values resulting from a 75 to 300 mg dose were 35% and 48% higher, respectively, after a fat-containing meal than after a glucose solution.

Adverse Reactions

Adverse events related to treatment include the following: Lipid abnormalities (eg, elevated triglycerides, elevated total and LDL cholesterol, decreased HDL cholesterol), hypothyroidism, headache, asthenia, rash, leukopenia, anemia, nausea, infection, peripheral edema, abdominal pain, and dry skin. Most adverse events occurred at a higher incidence in patients treated at starting doses of > 300 mg/m²/day.

Adverse events leading to dose reduction or study drug discontinuation in ≥ 2 patients included the following: Hyperlipemia, neutropenia/leukopenia, diarrhea, fatigue/lethargy, hypothyroidism, headache, liver function test abnormalities, rash, pancreatitis, nausea, anemia, allergic reaction, muscle spasm, pneumonia, confusion.

In 504 patients (CTCL and non-CTCL) who received bexarotene as monotherapy, drug-related serious adverse events that were fatal in 1 patient each included the following: Acute pancreatitis, subdural hematoma, liver failure.

Bexarotene Adverse Reactions (%)		
	Initial assigned dose group	
Adverse reaction	300 mg/m²/day (n = 84)	> 300 mg/m²/day (n = 53)
Dermatologic		
Rash	16.7	22.6
Dry skin	10.7	9.4
Exfoliative dermatitis	9.5	28.3
Alopecia	3.6	11.3
GI		
Nausea	15.5	7.5
Diarrhea	7.1	41.5
Vomiting	3.6	13.2
Anorexia	2.4	22.6
Hemic/Lymphatic		
Leukopenia	16.7	47.2
Anemia	6	24.5
Hypochromic anemia	3.6	13.2
Metabolic/Nutritional		
Hyperlipemia	78.6	79.2
Hypercholesteremia	32.1	62.3
Lactic dehydrogenase, increased	7.1	13.2
Miscellaneous		
Headache	29.8	41.5
Hypothyroidism	28.6	52.8
Asthenia	20.2	45.3
Infection	13.1	22.6

BEXAROTENE

Bexarotene Adverse Reactions (%)		
	Initial assigned dose group	
Adverse reaction	300 mg/m²/day (n = 84)	> 300 mg/m²/day (n = 53)
Peripheral edema	13.1	11.3
Abdominal pain	10.7	3.8
Chills	9.5	13.2
Fever	4.8	17
Insomnia	4.8	11.3
Flu syndrome	3.6	13.2
Back pain	2.4	11.3
Infection (bacterial)	1.2	13.2

Moderately-Severe and Severe Adverse Reactions with Bexarotene in ≥ 2 patients (%)				
	Initial assigned dose group			
	300 mg/m²/day (n = 84)		> 300 mg/m²/day (n = 53)	
Adverse reaction	Mod.-severe	Severe	Mod.-severe	Severe
Dermatologic				
Exfoliative dermatitis	0	1.2	5.7	1.9
Rash	1.2	2.4	1.9	0
GI				
Anorexia	0	0	5.7	0
Diarrhea	1.2	1.2	3.8	1.9
Pancreatitis	1.2	0	5.7	0
Vomiting	0	0	3.8	0
Metabolic/Nutritional				
Bilirubinemia	0	1.2	3.8	0
Hypercholesteremia	2.4	0	9.4	0
Hyperlipemia	19	7.1	32.1	9.4
AST, increased	0	0	3.8	0
ALT, increased	0	0	3.8	0
Miscellaneous				
Asthenia	1.2	0	20.8	0
Headache	3.6	0	9.4	1.9
Infection, bacterial	1.2	0	0	3.8
Peripheral edema	2.4	1.2	0	0
Hypothyroidism	1.2	1.2	3.8	0
Leukopenia	3.6	0	11.3	1.9
Pneumonia	0	0	3.8	3.8

Treatment-Emergent Abnormal Laboratory Values with Bexarotene (%)				
	Initial assigned dose			
	300 mg/m²/day (n = 83)[1]		> 300 mg/m²/day (n = 53)[1]	
Analyte	Grade 3[2]	Grade 4[2]	Grade 3	Grade 4
Triglycerides[3]	21.3	6.7	31.8	13.6
Total cholesterol[3]	18.7	6.7	15.9	29.5
Alkaline phosphatase	1.2	0	0	1.9
Hyperglycemia	1.2	0	5.7	0
Hypocalcemia	1.2	0	0	0
Hyponatremia	1.2	0	9.4	0
ALT	1.2	0	1.9	1.9
Hyperkalemia	0	0	1.9	0
Hypernatremia	0	1.2	0	0
AST	0	0	1.9	1.9
Total bilirubin	0	0	0	1.9
ANC	12	3.6	18.9	7.5

Treatment-Emergent Abnormal Laboratory Values with Bexarotene (%)				
	Initial assigned dose			
	300 mg/m²/day (n = 83)[1]		> 300 mg/m²/day (n = 53)[1]	
Analyte	Grade 3[2]	Grade 4[2]	Grade 3	Grade 4
Absolute lymphocyte count	7.2	0	15.1	0
WBC	3.6	0	11.3	0
Hemoglobin	0	0	1.9	0

[1] Number of patients with ≥ 1 analyte value postbaseline.
[2] Adapted from NCI Common Toxicity Criteria, Grade 3 and 4, Version 2. Patients are considered to have had a Grade 3 or 4 value if either of the following occurred: a) Value becomes Grade 3 or 4 during the study; b) Value is abnormal at baseline and worsens to Grade 3 or 4 on study, including all values beyond study drug discontinuation, as defined in data handling conventions.
[3] The denominator used to calculate the incidence rates for fasting Total Cholesterol and Triglycerides were n = 75 for the 300 mg/m²/day initial dose group and n = 44 for the > 300 mg/m²/day initial dose group.

In patients with CTCL receiving an initial dose of 300 mg/m²/day of bexarotene, adverse events reported at an incidence of < 10% were as follows:

➤*Cardiovascular:* Hemorrhage; hypertension; angina pectoris; chest pain; right heart failure; syncope; tachycardia.

➤*CNS:* Depression; agitation; ataxia; cerebrovascular accident; confusion; dizziness; hyperesthesia; hypesthesia; neuropathy.

➤*Dermatologic:* Skin ulcer; acne; alopecia; skin nodule; maculopapular rash; pustular rash; serous drainage; vesicular bullous rash.

➤*GI:* Constipation; dry mouth; flatulence; colitis; dyspepsia; cheilitis; gastroenteritis; gingivitis; liver failure; melena.

➤*GU:* Albuminuria; hematuria; urinary incontinence; urinary tract infection; urinary urgency; dysurea; kidney function abnormal; breast pain.

➤*Hematologic/Lymphatic:* Eosinophilia; thrombocythemia; coagulation time increased; lymphocytosis; thrombocytopenia.

➤*Metabolic:* LDH increased; creatinine increased; hypoproteinemia; hyperglycemia; weight decreased/increased; amylase increased.

➤*Musculoskeletal:* Arthralgia; myalgia; bone pain; myasthenia; arthrosis.

➤*Respiratory:* Pharyngitis; rhinitis; dyspnea; pleural effusion; bronchitis; cough increased; lung edema; hemoptysis; hypoxia.

➤*Special senses:* Dry eyes; conjunctivitis; ear pain; blepharitis; corneal lesion; keratitis; otitis externa; visual field defect.

➤*Miscellaneous:* Chills; cellulitis; sepsis; monilia.

Overdosage

Doses ≤ 1000 mg/m²/day of bexarotene have been administered in short-term studies in patients with advanced cancer without acute toxic effects. Single doses of 1500 and 720 mg/kg were tolerated without significant toxicity in rats and dogs, respectively. These doses are ≈ 30 and 50 times, respectively, the recommended human dose on a mg/m² basis.

➤*Treatment:* No clinical experience with an overdose of bexarotene has been reported. Treat any bexarotene overdose with supportive care for the signs and symptoms exhibited by the patient. Refer to General Management of Acute Overdosage.

Patient Information

Advise women of childbearing potential to avoid becoming pregnant when taking bexarotene. Effective contraception must be used for 1 month prior to the initiation of therapy, during therapy, and for ≥ 1 month following discontinuation of therapy; it is recommended that 2 reliable forms of contraception be used simultaneously unless abstinence is the chosen method.

Advise patients to limit vitamin A supplements to avoid potential additive effects.

Advise patients to minimize exposure to sunlight and artificial UV light.

RITUXIMAB

| Rx | **Rituxan** (IDEC/Genentech) | **Injection:** 10 mg/mL | Preservative free. 0.7 mg/mL polysorbate 80. In 10 and 50 mL single-use vials. |

WARNING

Fatal infusion reactions: Deaths within 24 hours of rituximab infusion have been reported. These fatal reactions followed an infusion reaction complex that included hypoxia, pulmonary infiltrates, acute respiratory distress syndrome, MI, ventricular fibrillation, or cardiogenic shock. Approximately 80% of fatal infusion reactions occurred in association with the first infusion (see Warnings and Adverse Reactions).

Patients who develop severe infusion reactions should have rituximab infusion discontinued and receive medical treatment.

Tumor lysis syndrome (TLS): Acute renal failure requiring dialysis with instances of fatal outcome has been reported in the setting of TLS following rituximab treatment (see Warnings).

Severe mucocutaneous reactions: Severe mucocutaneous reactions, some with fatal outcome, have been reported in association with rituximab treatment (see Warnings and Adverse Reactions).

Indications

➤*Non-Hodgkin's lymphoma:* Treatment of patients with relapsed or refractory low-grade or follicular, CD20-positive, B-cell non-Hodgkin's lymphoma.

Administration and Dosage

➤*Approved by the FDA:* November 26, 1997.

Do not administer as an IV push or bolus. Hypersensitivity reactions may occur (see Warnings). Consider premedication, consisting of acetaminophen and diphenhydramine, before each infusion of rituximab. Premedication may attenuate infusion-related reactions. Because transient hypotension may occur during infusion, give consideration to withholding antihypertensive medications 12 hours prior to rituximab infusion.

➤*Initial therapy:* 375 mg/m^2 given as an IV infusion once weekly for 4 or 8 doses. Rituximab may be administered in an outpatient setting.

➤*Retreatment:* Patients who subsequently develop progressive disease may be safely retreated with rituximab 375 mg/m^2 IV infusion once weekly for 4 doses. Currently, there are limited data concerning > 2 courses.

Administer the first infusion at an initial rate of 50 mg/hr. If hypersensitivity or infusion reactions do not occur, increase the infusion rate in 50 mg/hr increments every 30 minutes, to a maximum of 400 mg/hr. If hypersensitivity (non-IgE-mediated) or an infusion reaction develops, temporarily slow or interrupt the infusion (see Warning Box and Warnings). The infusion can continue at ½ the previous rate upon improvement of patient symptoms.

If the patient tolerated the first infusion well, subsequent rituximab infusions can be administered at an initial rate of 100 mg/hr, and increased by 100 mg/hr increments at 30-minute intervals, to a maximum of 400 mg/hr as tolerated. If the patient did not tolerate the first infusion well, follow guidelines under the first infusion.

➤*Compatibility/Incompatibility:* Do not mix or dilute rituximab with other drugs. No incompatibilities between rituximab and polyvinylchloride or polyethylene bags have been observed.

➤*Preparation:* Withdraw the necessary amount of rituximab and dilute to a final concentration of 1 to 4 mg/mL into an infusion bag containing either 0.9% Sodium Chloride or 5% Dextrose in Water. Gently invert the bag to mix the solution. Discard any unused portion left in the vial.

➤*Storage/Stability:* Rituximab vials are stable at 2° to 8°C (36° to 46°F). Do not use beyond expiration date stamped on carton. Protect vials from direct sunlight. Refer to Preparation for information on the stability and storage of solutions of rituximab diluted for infusion. Rituximab solutions for infusion may be stored at 2° to 8°C (36° to 46°F) for 24 hours and are stable at room temperature for an additional 24 hours. However, since rituximab solutions do not contain a preservative, store diluted solutions refrigerated at 2° to 8°C (36° to 46°F).

Actions

➤*Pharmacology:* Rituximab is a genetically engineered chimeric murine/human monoclonal antibody directed against the CD20 antigen found on the surface of normal and malignant B lymphocytes. The antibody is an IgG$_1$ kappa immunoglobulin. It binds specifically to the antigen CD20, a hydrophobic transmembrane protein located on pre-B and mature B lymphocytes. The antigen is also expressed on > 90% of B-cell non-Hodgkin's lymphomas (NHL) but is not found on hematopoietic stem cells, pro-B cells, normal plasma cells, or other normal tissues. CD20 regulates an early step(s) in the activation process for cell-cycle initiation and differentiation, and possibly functions as a calcium ion channel. CD20 is not shed from the cell surface and does not internalize upon antibody binding. Free CD20 antigen is not found in the circulation.

The Fab domain of rituximab binds to the CD20 antigen on B-lymphocytes and the Fc domain recruits immune effector functions to mediate B-cell lysis in vitro. Possible mechanisms of cell lysis include complement-dependent cytotoxicity and antibody-dependent cell mediated cytotoxicity. The antibody induces apoptosis in the DHL-4 human B-cell lymphoma line. Rituximab binding was observed on lymphoid cells in the thymus, the white pulp of the spleen, and a majority of B-lymphocytes in peripheral blood and lymph nodes. Little or no binding was observed in non-lymphoid tissues examined.

➤*Pharmacokinetics:* Administration of rituximab resulted in a rapid and sustained depletion of circulating and tissue-based B-cells. Lymph node biopsies performed 14 days after therapy showed a decrease in the percentage of B-cells in 7 of 8 patients who had received single doses of rituximab > 100 mg/m^2. Among 166 patients, circulating B-cells (measured as CD19+ cells) were depleted within the first 3 doses with sustained depletion for ≤ 6 to 9 months posttreatment in 83% of patients.

Peak and trough serum levels were inversely correlated with baseline values for the number of circulating CD20 positive B-cells and measures of disease burden. Median steady-state serum levels were higher for responders compared with nonresponders; however, no difference was found in the rate of elimination as measured by serum half-life. Serum levels were higher in patients with International Working Formulation (IWF) subtypes B, C, and D vs those with subtype A.

A wide range of half-lives may reflect the variable tumor burden among patients and the changes in CD20 positive (normal and malignant) B-cell populations upon repeated administrations.

Rituximab was detectable in the serum of patients 3 to 6 months after completion of treatment. B-cell recovery began at ≈ 6 months following completion of treatment. Median B-cell levels returned to normal by 12 months following completion of treatment.

The pharmacokinetic profile of rituximab when administered as 6 infusions of 375 mg/m^2 in combination with 6 cycles of CHOP chemotherapy was similar to that seen with rituximab alone.

There were sustained and statistically significant reductions in both IgM and IgG serum levels observed from 5 through 11 months following rituximab administration. However, only 14% were below the normal range.

➤*Clinical trials:* In 166 patients with relapsed or refractory low-grade or follicular B-cell NHL who received 375 mg/m^2 of rituximab given as an IV infusion weekly for 4 doses, the overall response rate (ORR) was 48% with a 6% complete response (CR) and a 42% partial response (PR) rate. Disease-related signs and symptoms (including B-symptoms) were present in 23% of patients at study entry and resolved in 64% of those patients. The median time to onset of response was 50 days and the median duration of response was 11.2 months (range, 1.9 to 42.1+ months).

The ORR was higher in patients with IWF B, C, and D histologic subtypes vs IWF A subtype (58% vs 12%), higher in patients whose largest lesions were < 5 cm vs > 7 cm (maximum, 21 cm) in greatest diameter (53% vs 38%), and higher in patients with chemosensitive relapse as compared with chemoresistant (defined as duration of response < 3 months) relapse (53% vs 36%). ORR in patients previously treated with autologous bone marrow transplant was 78%.

Contraindications

IgE-mediated hypersensitivity or anaphylactic reactions to murine proteins or to any component of this product (see Warnings).

Warnings

➤*Severe infusion reactions and hypersensitivity reactions:* See Warning Box, Adverse Reactions, and Hypersensitivity Reactions. Rituximab has caused severe infusion reactions. In some cases, these reactions were fatal. These severe reactions typically occurred during the first infusion with time to onset of 30 to 120 minutes. Signs and symptoms of severe infusion reactions may include hypotension, angioedema, hypoxia, or bronchospasm, and may require interruption of rituximab administration. The most severe manifestations and sequelae include pulmonary infiltrates, acute respiratory distress syndrome, MI, ventricular fibrillation, and cardiogenic shock. In the reported cases, the following factors were more frequently associated with fatal outcomes: Female gender, pulmonary infiltrates, and chronic lymphocytic leukemia or mantle cell lymphoma.

Management of severe infusion reactions – Interrupt the rituximab infusion for severe reactions and institute supportive care measures as medically indicated (eg, IV fluids, vasopressors, oxygen, bronchodilators, diphenhydramine, acetaminophen). In most cases, the infusion can be resumed at a 50% reduction in rate (eg, from 100 mg/hr to 50 mg/hr) when symptoms have completely resolved. Patients requiring close monitoring during first and all subsequent infusions include those with preexisting cardiac and pulmonary conditions, those with prior clinically significant cardiopulmonary adverse events, and those with high numbers of circulating malignant cells (≥ 25,000/m^3) with or without evidence of high tumor burden.

➤*TLS:* See Warning Box and Adverse Reactions. Rapid reduction in tumor volume followed by acute renal failure, hyperkalemia, hypocalcemia, hyperuricemia, or hyperphosphatasemia, have been reported

RITUXIMAB

within 12 to 24 hours after the first rituximab infusion. Rare instances of fatal outcome have been reported in the setting of TLS following treatment with rituximab. The risks of TLS appear to be greater in patients with high numbers of circulating malignant cells ($\geq 25,000/mm^3$) or high tumor burden. Prophylaxis for TLS should be considered for patients at high risk. Correction of electrolyte abnormalities, monitoring of renal function and fluid balance, and administration of supportive care, including dialysis, should be initiated as indicated. Following complete resolution of the complications of TLS, rituximab has been tolerated when readministered in conjunction with prophylactic therapy for TLS in a limited number of cases.

➤*Cardiac arrhythmias:* Discontinue infusions in the event of serious or life-threatening cardiac arrhythmias. Patients who develop clinically significant arrhythmias should undergo cardiac monitoring during and after subsequent infusions of rituximab. Patients with pre-existing cardiac conditions including arrhythmias and angina have had recurrences of these events during rituximab therapy; monitor these patients throughout the infusion and immediate postinfusion periods.

➤*Renal toxicity:* Rituximab administration has been associated with severe renal toxicity, including acute renal failure requiring dialysis and in some cases, has led to a fatal outcome. Renal toxicity has occurred in patients with high numbers of circulating malignant cells ($> 25,000/mm^3$) or high tumor burden who experience tumor lysis syndrome and in patients administered concomitant cisplatin therapy during clinical trials. The combination of cisplatin and rituximab is not an approved treatment regimen. If this combination is used in clinical trials, exercise extreme caution; monitor patients closely for signs of renal failure. Consider discontinuation of rituximab for those with rising serum creatinine or oliguria.

➤*Severe mucocutaneous reactions:* See Warning Box and Adverse Reactions. Mucocutaneous reactions, some with fatal outcome, have been reported in patients treated with rituximab. These reports include paraneoplastic pemphigus (an uncommon disorder that is a manifestation of the patient's underlying malignancy), Stevens-Johnson syndrome, lichenoid dermatitis, vesiculobullous dermatitis, and toxic epidermal necrolysis. The onset of the reaction in the reported cases has varied from 1 to 13 weeks following rituximab exposure. Patients experiencing a severe mucocutaneous reaction should not receive any further infusions and seek prompt medical evaluation. Skin biopsy may help to distinguish among different mucocutaneous reactions and guide subsequent treatment. The safety of readministration of rituximab to patients with any of these mucocutaneous reactions has not been determined.

➤*Hypersensitivity reactions:* Rituximab is associated with hypersensitivity reactions (non-IgE-mediated reactions), which may respond to adjustments in the infusion rate and in medical management. Hypotension, bronchospasm, and angioedema have occurred in association with rituximab infusion (see Severe Infusion Reactions). Interrupt rituximab infusion for severe hypersensitivity reactions and resume at a 50% reduction in rate (eg, from 100 to 50 mg/hr) when symptoms have completely resolved. Treatment of these symptoms with diphenhydramine and acetaminophen is recommended; additional treatment with bronchodilators or IV saline may be indicated. In most cases, patients who have experienced non-life-threatening hypersensitivity reactions have been able to complete the full course of therapy (see Administration and Dosage). Medications for the treatment of hypersensitivity reactions, (eg, epinephrine, antihistamines, corticosteroids) should be available for immediate use in the event of a reaction during administration. Refer to Management of Acute Hypersensitivity Reactions.

➤*Elderly:* Among the 331 patients enrolled in clinical studies of single agent rituximab, 24% were 65 to 75 years of age and 5% were ≥ 75 years of age. The overall response rates were higher in older (52%, age ≥ 65 years of age) vs younger (44%, age < 65 years of age) patients; however, the median duration of response, based on Kaplan-Meier estimates, was shorter in older vs younger patients: 10.1 months (range, 1.9 to 36.5+ months) vs 11.4 months (range, 2.1 to 42.1+ months), respectively. This shorter duration of response was not statistically significant. Adverse reactions, including incidence, severity, and type of adverse reaction were similar between older and younger patients.

➤*Pregnancy: Category C.* It is not known whether rituximab can cause fetal harm when administered to a pregnant woman or whether it can affect reproductive capacity. Human IgG is known to pass the placental barrier, and thus may potentially cause fetal B-cell depletion; therefore, give rituximab to a pregnant woman only if clearly needed. Individuals of child-bearing potential should use effective contraceptive methods during treatment and for ≤ 12 months following rituximab therapy.

➤*Lactation:* It is not known whether rituximab is excreted in breast milk. Because human IgG is excreted in breast milk and the potential for absorption and immunosuppression in the infant is unknown, advise women to discontinue nursing until circulating drug levels are no longer detectable.

➤*Children:* Safety and efficacy in children have not been established.

Precautions

➤*Monitoring:* Since rituximab targets all CD20-positive B lymphocytes, malignant and nonmalignant, complete blood counts (CBC), and platelet counts should be obtained at regular intervals during rituximab therapy and more frequently in patients who develop cytopenias (see Adverse Reactions). The duration of cytopenias caused by rituximab can extend well beyond the treatment period.

➤*Human antichimeric antibody (HACA) formation:* HACA was detected in 4 of 356 patients and 3 had an objective clinical response. The data reflect the percentage of patients whose test results were considered positive for antibodies to rituximab using an enzyme-linked immunosorbent assay (limit of detection = 7 ng/mL). The observed incidence of antibody positivity in an assay is highly dependent on the sensitivity and specificity of the assay and may be influenced by several factors including sample handling, concomitant medications, and underlying disease. For these reasons, comparison of the incidence of antibodies to rituximab with the incidence of antibodies to other products may be misleading.

➤*Immunization:* The safety of immunization with live viral vaccines following rituximab therapy has not been studied. The ability to generate a primary or anamnestic humoral response to vaccination is currently being studied.

Adverse Reactions

The most serious adverse reactions caused by rituximab include infusion reactions, tumor lysis syndrome, mucocutaneous reactions, hypersensitivity reactions, cardiac arrhythmias and angina, and renal failure. Refer to the Warning Box and Warnings for detailed descriptions of these reactions. Infusion reactions and lymphopenia are the most commonly occurring adverse reactions.

Because clinical trials are conducted under widely varying conditions, adverse reaction rates observed in the clinical trials of a drug cannot be directly compared to rates in the clinical trials of another drug and may not reflect the rates observed in practice. However, the adverse reaction information from clinical trials does provide a basis for identifying the adverse events that appear to be related to drug use and for approximating rates.

Additional adverse reactions have been identified during postmarketing use of rituximab. Because these reactions are reported voluntarily from a population of uncertain size, it is not always possible to reliably estimate their frequency or establish a causal relationship to rituximab exposure. Decisions to include these reactions in labeling are typically based on ≥ 1 of the following factors: 1) seriousness of the reaction, 2) frequency of reporting, or 3) strength of causal connection to rituximab.

Where specific percentages are noted, these data are based on 356 patients treated in nonrandomized, single-arm studies of rituximab administered as a single agent. Most patients received rituximab 375 mg/m^2 weekly for 4 doses. These include 39 patients with bulky disease (lesions ≥ 10 cm) and 60 patients who received > 1 course of rituximab. Thirty-seven patients received 375 mg/m^2 for 8 doses and 25 patients received doses other than 375 mg/m^2 for 4 doses and up to 500 mg/m^2 single dose in the Phase I setting. Adverse events of greater severity are referred to as Grade 3 and 4 events defined by the commonly used National Cancer Institute Common Toxicity Criteria.

Incidence of Adverse Events in Clinical Trials (Adverse Events Followed for 12 Months Following Rituximab Therapy [%; n = 356])		
Adverse reaction	All grades	Grades 3 and 4
Any adverse events	99	57
Cardiovascular	25	3
Hypotension	10	1
Hypertension	6	1
CNS	32	1
Dizziness	10	1
Anxiety	5	1
Dermatological	44	2
Night sweats	15	1
Rash	15	1
Pruritus	14	1
Urticaria	8	1
GI	37	2
Nausea	23	1
Diarrhea	10	1
Vomiting	10	1
Hemic/Lymphatic	67	48
Lymphopenia	48	40
Leukopenia	14	4
Neutropenia	14	6
Thrombocytopenia	12	2
Anemia	8	3
Metabolic/Nutritional	38	3
Angioedema	11	1
Hyperglycemia	9	1
Peripheral edema	8	0
LDH increase	7	0
Musculoskeletal	26	3
Myalgia	10	1
Arthralgia	10	1

RITUXIMAB

Incidence of Adverse Events in Clinical Trials (Adverse Events Followed for 12 Months Following Rituximab Therapy [%; n = 356])		
Adverse reaction	All grades	Grades 3 and 4
Respiratory	38	4
Increased cough	13	1
Rhinitis	12	1
Bronchospasm	8	1
Dyspnea	7	1
Sinusitis	6	0
Miscellaneous	86	10
Fever	53	1
Chills	33	3
Infection	31	4
Asthenia	26	1
Headache	19	1
Abdominal pain	14	1
Pain	12	1
Back pain	10	1
Throat irritation	9	0
Flushing	5	0

Risk factors associated with increased rates of adverse events – Administration of rituximab weekly for 8 doses resulted in higher rates of Grade 3 and 4 adverse events overall (70%) compared with administration weekly for 4 doses (57%). The incidence of Grade 3 or 4 adverse events was similar in patients retreated with rituximab compared with initial treatment (58% and 57%, respectively). The incidence of the following clinically significant adverse events was higher in patients with bulky disease (lesions ≥ 10 cm; n = 39) vs patients with lesions < 10 cm (n = 195): Abdominal pain, anemia, dyspnea, hypotension, and neutropenia.

Infusion reactions – See Warning Box and Warnings. Mild-to-moderate infusion reactions consisting of fever and chills/rigors occurred in the majority of patients during the first rituximab infusion. Other frequent infusion reactions symptoms included nausea, pruritus, angioedema, asthenia, hypotension, headache, bronchospasm, throat irritation, rhinitis, urticaria, rash, vomiting, myalgia, dizziness, and hypertension. These reactions generally occurred within 30 to 120 minutes of beginning the first infusion, and resolved with slowing or interruption of the rituximab infusion and with supportive care (diphenhydramine, acetaminophen, IV saline, and vasopressors). In an analysis of data from 356 patients with relapsed or refractory, low-grade NHL who received 4 (n = 319) or 8 (n = 37) weekly infusions of rituximab, the incidence of infusion reactions was highest during the first infusion (77%) and decreased with each subsequent infusion (30% with fourth infusion and 14% with eighth infusion).

Infectious events – Rituximab induced B-cell depletion in 70% to 80% of patients and was associated with decreased serum immunoglobulins in a minority of patients; the lymphopenia lasted a median of 14 days (range, 1 to 588 days). Infectious events occurred in 31% of patients: 19% of patients had bacterial infections, 10% had viral infections, 1% had fungal infections, and 6% were unknown infections. Incidence is not additive because a single patient may have had > 1 type of infection. Serious infectious events (Grade 3 or 4), including sepsis, occurred in 2% of patients.

Hematologic events – Grade 3 and 4 cytopenias were reported in 12% of patients treated with rituximab, these include the following: Lymphopenia (40%), neutropenia (6%), leukopenia (4%), anemia (3%), and thrombocytopenia (2%). The median duration of lymphopenia was 14 days (range, 1 to 588 days) and of neutropenia was 13 days (range, 2 to 116 days). A single occurrence of transient aplastic anemia (pure red cell aplasia) and 2 occurrences of hemolytic anemia following rituximab therapy were reported. In addition, there have been rare postmarketing reports of prolonged pancytopenia and marrow hypoplasia.

Cardiac events – See Warning Box. Grade 3 or 4 cardiac-related events include hypotension. Rare, fatal cardiac failure with symptomatic onset weeks after rituximab has also been reported. Patients who develop clinically significant cardiopulmonary events should have rituximab infusion discontinued.

Pulmonary events – See Warning Box. One hundred thirty five patients (38%) experienced pulmonary events. The most common respiratory system adverse events experienced were increased cough, rhinitis, bronchospasm, dyspnea, and sinusitis. Three pulmonary events have been reported in temporal association with rituximab infusion as a single agent: Acute bronchospasm, acute pneumonitis presenting 1 to 4 weeks post-rituximab infusion, and bronchiolitis obliterans. One case of bronchiolitis obliterans was associated with progressive pulmonary symptoms and culminated in death several months following the last rituximab infusion. The safety of resumption or continued administration of rituximab in patients with pneumonitis or bronchiolitis obliterans is unknown.

Immune/Autoimmune events – Immune/autoimmune events have been reported, including uveitis, optic neuritis in a patient with systemic vasculitis, pleuritis in a patient with a lupus-like syndrome, serum sickness with polyarticular arthritis, and vasculitis with rash.

Less commonly observed events – In clinical trials, < 5% and > 1% of the patients experienced the following events regardless of causality assessment: Agitation, anorexia, arthritis, conjunctivitis, depression, dyspepsia, edema, hyperkinesia, hypertonia, hypesthesia, hypoglycemia, injection site pain, insomnia, lacrimation disorder, malaise, nervousness, neuritis, neuropathy, paresthesia, somnolence, vertigo, weight decrease.

Overdosage

There has been no experience with overdosage. Single doses of ≤ 500 mg/m^2 have been given in controlled clinical trials.

IBRITUMOMAB TIUXETAN

Rx	**Zevalin** (Biogen Idec)	**Injection:** 3.2 mg	Preservative free. In 2 mL vials. In In-111 ibritumomab tiuxetan and Y-90 ibritumomab tiuxetan kits with 50 mM sodium acetate vial, formulation buffer vial, reaction vial, and identification labels.[1]

[1] The Indium-111 (In-111) Chloride Sterile Solution must be ordered separately from Amersham Health Inc. or Mallinckrodt, Inc. at the time the In-111 ibritumomab tiuxetan kit is ordered. The Yttrium-90 (Y-90) Chloride Sterile Solution will be shipped directly from MDS Nordion upon placement of an order for the Y-90 ibritumomab tiuxetan kit.

WARNING

Fatal infusion reactions: Deaths have occurred within 24 hours of rituximab infusion, an essential component of the ibritumomab tiuxetan therapeutic regimen. These fatalities were associated with an infusion reaction symptom complex that included hypoxia, pulmonary infiltrates, acute respiratory distress syndrome, MI, ventricular fibrillation, or cardiogenic shock. Approximately 80% of fatal infusion reactions occurred in association with the first rituximab infusion (see Warnings and Adverse Reactions). Discontinue rituximab, In-111 ibritumomab tiuxetan, and Y-90 ibritumomab tiuxetan infusions in patients who develop severe infusion reactions and give medical treatment.

Prolonged and severe cytopenias: Y-90 ibritumomab tiuxetan administration results in severe and prolonged cytopenias in most patients. Do not administer the ibritumomab tiuxetan therapeutic regimen to patients with ≥ 25% lymphoma marrow involvement or impaired bone marrow reserve (see Adverse Reactions).

Dosing: The prescribed, measured, and administered dose of Y-90 ibritumomab tiuxetan should not exceed the absolute maximum allowable dose of 32 mCi (1184 MBq).

Do not administer Y-90 ibritumomab tiuxetan to patients with altered biodistribution as determined by imaging with In-111 ibritumomab tiuxetan.

In-111 ibritumomab tiuxetan and Y-90 ibritumomab tiuxetan are radiopharmaceuticals and should be used only by physicians and other professionals qualified by training and experienced in the safe use and handling of radionuclides.

Indications

➤*Non-Hodgkin's lymphoma (NHL):* As part of the ibritumomab tiuxetan therapeutic regimen for the treatment of patients with relapsed or refractory low-grade, follicular, or transformed B-cell NHL, including patients with rituximab-refractory follicular NHL.

Administration and Dosage

➤*Approved by the FDA:* February 19, 2002.

➤*Rituximab administration:* Note that the dose of rituximab was lower when used as part of the ibritumomab tiuxetan therapeutic regimen, as compared with the dose of rituximab when used as a single agent. Do not administer rituximab as an IV push or bolus. Hypersensitivity reactions may occur (see Warnings). Consider premedication, consisting of acetaminophen and diphenhydramine, before each rituximab infusion.

➤*Dose modification:* Reduce the Y-90 ibritumomab tiuxetan dose to 0.3 mCi/kg (11.1 MBq/kg) for patients with a baseline platelet count between 100,000 and 149,000 cells/mm^3.

➤*Radionuclides:* Two separate and distinctly labeled kits are ordered for the preparation of a single dose each of In-111 ibritumomab tiuxetan and Y-90 ibritumomab tiuxetan. In-111 ibritumomab tiuxetan and Y-90 ibritumomab tiuxetan are radiopharmaceuticals and should be used only by physicians and other professionals qualified by training and experienced in the safe use and handling of radionuclides. Changing the ratio of any of the reactants in the radiolabeling process may adversely impact therapeutic results. In-111 ibritumomab tiuxetan and Y-90 ibritumomab tiuxetan should not be used in the absence of the rituximab predose.

IBRITUMOMAB TIUXETAN

➤*Ibritumomab tiuxetan therapeutic regimen administration:*

Step 1 –

First rituximab infusion: Administer rituximab at a dose of 250 mg/m^2 IV at an initial rate of 50 mg/hr. Do not mix or dilute rituximab with other drugs. If hypersensitivity or infusion-related events do not occur, escalate the infusion rate in 50 mg/hr increments every 30 minutes, to a maximum of 400 mg/hr. If hypersensitivity or an infusion-related event develops, temporarily slow or interrupt the infusion (see Warnings). The infusion can continue at 50% the previous rate upon improvement of patient symptoms.

In-111 ibritumomab tiuxetan injection: Within 4 hours following completion of the rituximab dose, 5 mCi (1.6 mg total antibody dose) of In-111 ibritumomab tiuxetan is injected IV over a period of 10 minutes.

Assess biodistribution:

First image 2 to 24 hours after In-111 ibritumomab tiuxetan;

Second image 48 to 72 hours after In-111 ibritumomab tiuxetan.

Optional: Third image 90 to 120 hours after In-111 ibritumomab tiuxetan.

If biodistribution is not acceptable, do not proceed.

Step 2 – Step 2 of the ibritumomab tiuxetan therapeutic regimen is initiated 7 to 9 days following Step 1 instructions.

Second rituximab infusion: Rituximab at a dose of 250 mg/m^2 is administered IV at an initial rate of 100 mg/hr (50 mg/hr if infusion-related events were documented during the first rituximab administration) and increased by 100 mg/hr increments at 30-minute intervals, to a maximum of 400 mg/hr, as tolerated.

Y-90 ibritumomab tiuxetan injection: Within 4 hours following completion of the rituximab dose, Y-90 ibritumomab tiuxetan at a dose of 0.4 mCi/kg (14.8 MBq/kg) actual body weight for patients with a platelet count > 150,000 cells/mm^3, and 0.3 mCi/kg (11.1 MBq/kg) actual body weight for patients with a platelet count of 100,000 to 149,000 cells/mm^3 is injected IV over a period of 10 minutes. Take precautions to avoid extravasation. Establish a free-flowing IV line prior to Y-90 ibritumomab tiuxetan injection. Close monitoring for evidence of extravasation during the injection of Y-90 ibritumomab tiuxetan is required. If any signs or symptoms of extravasation have occurred, immediately terminate the infusion and restart in another vein. The prescribed, measured, and administered dose of Y-90 ibritumomab tiuxetan must not exceed the absolute maximum allowable dose of 32 mCi (1184 MBq), regardless of the patient's body weight. Do not give Y-90 ibritumomab tiuxetan to patients with a platelet count < 100,000/mm^3 (see Warnings).

See manufacturer's product labeling for product preparation instructions.

➤*Storage/Stability:* Store at 2° to 8°C (36° to 46°F). Do not freeze.

Actions

➤*Pharmacology:* Ibritumomab tiuxetan is the immunoconjugate resulting from a stable thiourea covalent bond between the monoclonal antibody ibritumomab and the linker-chelator tiuxetan. This linker-chelator provides a high affinity, conformationally restricted chelation site for Indium-111 or Yttrium-90. The approximate molecular weight of ibritumomab tiuxetan is 148 kD.

The antibody moiety of ibritumomab tiuxetan is ibritumomab, a murine IgG$_1$ kappa monoclonal antibody directed against the CD20 antigen, which is found on the surface of normal and malignant B lymphocytes. Ibritumomab is produced in Chinese hamster ovary cells and is composed of 2 murine gamma 1 heavy chains of 445 amino acids each and 2 kappa light chains of 213 amino acids each.

Ibritumomab, like rituximab, induces apoptosis in CD20+ B-cell lines in vitro. The chelate tiuxetan, which tightly binds In-111 or Y-90, is covalently linked to the amino groups of exposed lysines and arginines contained within the antibody. The beta emission from Y-90 induces cellular damage by the formation of free radicals in the target and neighboring cells.

Ibritumomab tiuxetan binding was observed in vitro on lymphoid cells of the bone marrow, lymph node, thymus, red and white pulp of the spleen, and lymphoid follicles of the tonsil, as well as lymphoid nodules of other organs such as the large and small intestines. Binding was not observed on the nonlymphoid tissues or gonadal tissues.

➤*Pharmacokinetics:* In pharmacokinetic studies of patients receiving the ibritumomab tiuxetan therapeutic regimen, the mean effective half-life of Y-90 activity in blood was 30 hours, and the mean area under the fraction of injected activity (FIA) vs time curve in blood was 39 hours. Over 7 days, a median of 7.2% of the injected activity was excreted in urine.

In clinical studies, administration of the ibritumomab tiuxetan therapeutic regimen resulted in sustained depletion of circulating B cells. At 4 weeks, the median number of circulating B cells was 0 (range, 0 to 1084 cells/mm^3). B-cell recovery began at ≈ 12 weeks following treatment, and the median level of B cells was within the normal range (32 to 341 cells/mm^3) by 9 months after treatment. Median serum levels of IgG and IgA remained within the normal range throughout the period of B-cell depletion. Median IgM serum levels dropped below normal (median, 49 mg/dL; range, 13 to 3990 mg/dL) after treatment and recovered to normal values by 6-month posttherapy.

➤*Clinical trials:* One randomized, controlled, multicenter study compared the ibritumomab tiuxetan therapeutic regimen with treatment with rituximab. The trial was conducted in 143 patients with relapsed or refractory low-grade or follicular NHL or transformed B-cell NHL. A total of 73 patients received the ibritumomab tiuxetan therapeutic regimen and 70 patients received rituximab given as an IV infusion at 375 mg/m^2 weekly times 4 doses. The primary efficacy endpoint of the study was to determine the overall response rate (ORR) using the International Workshop Response Criteria. The ORR was significantly higher (80% vs 56%; p = 0.002) for patients treated with the ibritumomab tiuxetan therapeutic regimen. The secondary endpoints, duration of response and time to progression, were not significantly different between the 2 treatment arms.

Contraindications

Patients with known Type I hypersensitivity or anaphylactic reactions to murine proteins or to any component of this product, including rituximab, yttrium chloride, and indium chloride.

Warnings

➤*Altered biodistribution:* Do not administer Y-90 ibritumomab tiuxetan to patients with altered biodistribution of In-111 ibritumomab tiuxetan. The expected biodistribution of In-111 ibritumomab tiuxetan includes easily detectable uptake in the blood pool areas on the first day image, with less activity in the blood pool areas on the second or third day image; moderately high to high uptake in healthy liver and spleen during the first day and the second or third day image; and moderately low or very low uptake in healthy kidneys, urinary bladder, and healthy bowel on the first day image and the second or third day image. Altered biodistribution of In-111 ibritumomab tiuxetan can be characterized by diffuse uptake in normal lung more intense than the cardiac blood pool on the first day image or more intense than the liver on the second or third day image; kidneys with greater intensity than the liver on the posterior view of the second or third day image; or intense areas of uptake throughout the healthy bowel comparable to uptake by the liver on the second or third day images.

➤*Severe infusion reactions:* The ibritumomab tiuxetan therapeutic regimen may cause severe, and potentially fatal, infusion reactions. These severe reactions typically occur during the first rituximab infusion with time to onset of 30 to 120 minutes. Signs and symptoms of severe infusion reaction may include hypotension, angioedema, hypoxia, or bronchospasm, and may require interruption of rituximab, In-111 ibritumomab tiuxetan, or Y-90 ibritumomab tiuxetan administration. The most severe manifestations and sequelae may include pulmonary infiltrates, acute respiratory distress syndrome, MI, ventricular fibrillation, and cardiogenic shock.

Because the ibritumomab tiuxetan therapeutic regimen includes the use of rituximab, also see prescribing information for rituximab (*Rituxan*).

➤*Hematologic toxicity:* The most common severe adverse reactions reported with the ibritumomab tiuxetan therapeutic regimen were thrombocytopenia (61% of patients with platelet counts < 50,000 cells/mm^3) and neutropenia (57% of patients with absolute neutrophil count [ANC] < 1000 cells/mm^3) in patients with ≥ 150,000 platelets/mm^3 prior to treatment. Both incidences of severe thrombocytopenia and neutropenia increased to 78% and 74% for patients with mild thrombocytopenia at baseline (platelet count of 100,000 to 149,000 cells/mm^3). For all patients, the median time to nadir was 7 to 9 weeks and the median duration of cytopenias was 22 to 35 days. In < 5% of cases, patients experienced severe cytopenia that extended beyond the prospectively defined protocol treatment period of 12 weeks following administration of the ibritumomab tiuxetan therapeutic regimen. Some of these patients eventually recovered from cytopenia, while others experienced progressive disease, received further anticancer therapy, or died of their lymphoma without having recovered from cytopenia. The cytopenias may have influenced subsequent treatment decisions.

Hemorrhage, including fatal cerebral hemorrhage, and severe infections have occurred in a minority of patients in clinical studies. Careful monitoring for and management of cytopenias and their complications (eg, febrile neutropenia, hemorrhage) for up to 3 months after use of the ibritumomab tiuxetan therapeutic regimen are necessary. Exercise caution in treating patients with drugs that interfere with platelet function or coagulation following the ibritumomab tiuxetan therapeutic regimen and closely monitor patients receiving such agents.

Do not administer the ibritumomab tiuxetan therapeutic regimen to patients with ≥ 25% lymphoma marrow involvement or impaired bone marrow reserve (eg, prior myeloablative therapies; platelet count < 100,000 cells/mm^3; neutrophil count < 1500 cells/mm^3; hypocellular bone marrow [≤ 15% cellularity or marked reduction in bone marrow precursors]) or to patients with a history of failed stem cell collection.

➤*Viral diseases:* This product contains albumin, a derivative of human blood. Based on effective donor screening and product manufacturing processes, it carries an extremely remote risk for transmission of viral diseases. A theoretical risk for transmission of Creutzfeldt-Jakob disease (CJD) also is considered extremely remote. No cases of transmission of viral disease or CJD have ever been identified for albumin.

➤*Hypersensitivity reactions:* Anaphylactic and other hypersensitivity reactions have been reported following the IV administration of proteins to patients. Medications for the treatment of hypersensitivity

IBRITUMOMAB TIUXETAN

reactions (eg, epinephrine, antihistamines, corticosteroids) should be available for immediate use in the event of an allergic reaction during administration of ibritumomab tiuxetan. Screen patients who have received murine proteins for human antimouse antibodies (HAMA). Patients with evidence of HAMA have not been studied and may be at increased risk of allergic or serious hypersensitivity reactions during ibritumomab tiuxetan therapeutic regimen administrations.

➤*Carcinogenesis:* Radiation is a potential carcinogen and mutagen. The ibritumomab tiuxetan therapeutic regimen results in a significant radiation dose to the testes. There is a potential risk that the ibritumomab tiuxetan therapeutic regimen could cause toxic effects on the male and female gonads. Effective contraception should be used during treatment and for up to 12 months following the ibritumomab tiuxetan therapeutic regimen.

➤*Elderly:* No overall differences in safety or efficacy were observed between these subjects and younger subjects, but greater sensitivity of some older individuals cannot be ruled out.

➤*Pregnancy: Category D.* Y-90 ibritumomab tiuxetan can cause fetal harm when administered to a pregnant woman. There are no adequate and well-controlled studies in pregnant women. If this drug is used during pregnancy, or if the patient becomes pregnant while receiving this drug, apprise the patient of the potential hazard to the fetus. Advise women of childbearing age to avoid becoming pregnant.

➤*Lactation:* It is not known whether ibritumomab tiuxetan is excreted in human milk. Because human IgG is excreted in human milk and the potential for ibritumomab tiuxetan exposure in the infant is unknown, advise women to discontinue nursing and substitute formula feedings for breast feedings (see Pharmacology).

➤*Children:* The safety and efficacy of the ibritumomab tiuxetan therapeutic regimen in children have not been established.

Precautions

➤*Monitoring:* Obtain CBC and platelet counts weekly following the ibritumomab tiuxetan therapeutic regimen and until levels recover. Monitor CBC and platelet counts more frequently in patients who develop severe cytopenia, or as clinically indicated.

➤*Radionuclide precautions:* The contents of the ibritumomab tiuxetan kit are not radioactive. However, during and after radiolabeling ibritumomab tiuxetan with In-111 or Y-90, take care to minimize radiation exposure to patients and to medical personnel, consistent with institutional good radiation safety practices and patient management procedures.

➤*Immunization:* The safety of immunization with live viral vaccines following the ibritumomab tiuxetan therapeutic regimen has not been studied. Also, the ability of patients who received the ibritumomab tiuxetan therapeutic regimen to generate a primary or anamnestic humoral response to any vaccine has not been studied.

➤*Secondary malignancies:* A total of 2% of patients developed secondary malignancies following the ibritumomab tiuxetan therapeutic regimen. One patient developed a Grade 1 meningioma, 3 developed acute myelogenous leukemia, and 2 developed a myelodysplastic syndrome. The onset of a second cancer was 8 to 34 months following the ibritumomab tiuxetan therapeutic regimen and 4 to 14 years following the patients' diagnosis of NHL.

➤*Immunogenicity:* Of 211 patients who received the ibritumomab tiuxetan therapeutic regimen in clinical trials and who were followed for 90 days, there were 8 (3.8%) patients with evidence of HAMA (n = 5) or human antichimeric antibody (HACA) (n = 4) at any time during the course of the study. Two patients had low titers of HAMA prior to initiation of the ibritumomab tiuxetan therapeutic regimen; 1 remained positive without an increase in titer while the other had a negative titer posttreatment. Three patients had evidence of HACA responses prior to initiation of the ibritumomab tiuxetan; 1 had a marked increase in HACA titer while the other 2 had negative titers posttreatment. Of the 3 patients who had negative HAMA or HACA titers prior to the ibritumomab tiuxetan therapeutic regimen, 2 developed HAMA in absence of HACA titers, and 1 had HAMA and HACA positive titers posttreatment. Evidence of immunogenicity may be masked in patients who are lymphopenic. There has not been adequate evaluation of HAMA and HACA at delayed timepoints, concurrent with the recovery from lymphopenia at 6 to 12 months, to establish whether masking of the immunogenicity at early timepoints occurs. The data reflects the percentage of patients whose test results were considered positive for antibodies to ibritumomab or rituximab using kinetic enzyme immunoassays to ibritumomab or rituximab. The observed incidence of antibody positivity in an assay is highly dependent on the sensitivity and specificity of the assay and may be influenced by several factors including sample handling and concomitant medications. Comparisons of the incidence of HAMA/HACA to the ibritumomab tiuxetan therapeutic regimen with the incidence of antibodies to other products may be misleading.

Drug Interactions

No formal drug interaction studies have been performed with ibritumomab tiuxetan. Because of the frequent occurrence of severe and prolonged thrombocytopenia, weigh the potential benefits of medications that interfere with platelet function or anticoagulation against the potential increased risks of bleeding and hemorrhage. Patients receiving medications that interfere with platelet function or coagulation should have more frequent laboratory monitoring for thrombocytopenia. In addition, the transfusion practices for such patients may need to be modified given the increased risk of bleeding.

Adverse Reactions

The most serious adverse reactions caused by the ibritumomab tiuxetan therapeutic regimen include the following: Infections (predominantly bacterial in origin), allergic reactions (bronchospasm and angioedema), and hemorrhage while thrombocytopenic (resulting in deaths). In addition, patients who have received the ibritumomab tiuxetan therapeutic regimen have developed myeloid malignancies and dysplasias. Fatal infusion reactions have occurred following the infusion of rituximab.

The most common toxicities reported were the following: Neutropenia, thrombocytopenia, anemia, GI symptoms (eg, nausea, vomiting, abdominal pain, diarrhea), increased cough, dyspnea, dizziness, arthralgia, anorexia, anxiety, and ecchymosis. Hematologic toxicity was often severe and prolonged, whereas most nonhematologic toxicity was mild in severity. The following table lists adverse events that occurred in ≥ 5% of patients. The second table is a more detailed description of the incidence and duration of hematologic toxicities, according to baseline platelet count (as an indicator of bone marrow reserve).

Incidence of Adverse Reactions in ≥ 5% of Patients Receiving the Ibritumomab Tiuxetan Therapeutic Regimen (n = 349)[1]		
Adverse reaction	All grades	Grade 3/4
Any adverse event	99	89
Cardiovascular	17	3
Hypotension	6	1
CNS	27	2
Headache	12	1
Dizziness	10	< 1
Insomnia	5	0
Dermatologic	28	1
Pruritus	9	< 1
Rash	8	< 1
Flushing	6	0
GI	48	3
Nausea	31	1
Abdominal pain	16	3
Vomiting	12	0
Throat irritation	10	0
Diarrhea	9	< 1
Anorexia	8	0
Abdominal enlargement	5	0
Constipation	5	0
GU	6	< 1
Hematologic/Lymphatic	98	86
Thrombocytopenia	95	63
Neutropenia	77	60
Anemia	61	17
Ecchymosis	7	< 1
Metabolic/Nutritional	23	3
Peripheral edema	8	1
Angioedema	5	< 1
Musculoskeletal	18	1
Arthralgia	7	1
Myalgia	7	< 1
Respiratory	36	3
Dyspnea	14	2
Increased cough	10	0
Rhinitis	6	0
Bronchospasm	5	0
Special senses	7	< 1
Miscellaneous		
Asthenia	43	3
Infection	29	5
Chills	24	< 1
Fever	17	1
Pain	13	1
Back pain	8	1

[1] Adverse events were followed for a period of 12 weeks following the first rituximab infusion of the ibritumomab tiuxetan therapeutic regimen. Note: All adverse events are included, regardless of relationship.

The following adverse events (except for those noted in the above table) occurred in between 1% and 4% of patients during the treatment period: Urticaria, anxiety, dyspepsia, sweats (4%); petechia, epistaxis (3%); allergic reaction, melena (2%).

Severe or life-threatening adverse events occurred in 1% to 5% of patients (except for those noted in the above table) consisted of pancytopenia (2%); allergic reactions, GI hemorrhage, melena, tumor pain, apnea (1%). The following severe or life-threatening events occurred in < 1% of patients: Angioedema, tachycardia, urticaria, arthritis, lung

IBRITUMOMAB TIUXETAN

edema, pulmonary embolus, encephalopathy, hematemesis, subdural hematoma, vaginal hemorrhage.

➤*Hematologic:* Hematologic toxicity was the most frequently observed adverse event in clinical trials. The following table presents the incidence and duration of severe hematologic toxicity for patients with normal baseline platelet count (≥ 150,000 cells/mm³) treated with the ibritumomab tiuxetan therapeutic regimen and patients with mild thrombocytopenia (platelet count 100,000 to 149,000 cells/mm³) at baseline who were treated with a modified ibritumomab tiuxetan therapeutic regimen that included a lower specific activity Y-90 ibritumomab tiuxetan dose at 0.3 mCi/kg (11.1 MBq/kg).

Ibritumomab Tiuxetan Severe Hematologic Toxicity		
	Ibritumomab tiuxetan therapeutic regimen using 0.4 mCi/kg Y-90 dose (14.8 MBq/kg)	Modified ibritumomab tiuxetan therapeutic regimen using 0.3 mCi/kg Y-90 dose (11.1 MBq/kg)
ANC		
Median nadir (cells/mm³)	800	600
Per patient incidence ANC < 1000 cells/mm³	57%	74%
Per patient incidence ANC < 500 cells/mm³	30%	35%
Median duration (days)[1] ANC < 1000 cells/mm³	22	29
Platelets		
Median nadir (cells/mm³)	41,000	24,000
Per patient incidence Platelets < 50,000 cells/mm³	61%	78%
Per patient incidence Platelets < 10,000 cells/mm³	10%	14%
Median duration (days)[2] Platelets < 50,000 cells/mm³	24	35

[1] Median duration of neutropenia for patients with ANC < 1000 cells/mm³ (date from last laboratory value showing ANC ≥ 1000 cells/mm³ to date of first laboratory value following nadir showing ANC ≥ 1000 cells/mm³, censored at initiation of next treatment or death).

[2] Median duration of thrombocytopenia for patients with platelets < 50,000 cells/mm³ (date from last laboratory value showing platelet count ≥ 50,000 cells/mm³ to date of first laboratory value following nadir showing platelet count ≥ 50,000 cells/mm³, censored at initiation of next treatment or death).

Median time to ANC nadir was 62 days, to platelet nadir was 53 days, and to hemoglobin nadir was 68 days. Information on growth factor use and platelet transfusions is based on 211 patients for whom data were collected. Filgrastim was given to 13% of patients and erythropoietin to 8%. Platelet transfusions were given to 22% of patients and red blood cell transfusions to 20%.

➤*Miscellaneous:*

Infectious events – During the first 3 months after initiating the ibritumomab tiuxetan therapeutic regimen, 29% of patients developed infections. Three percent of patients developed serious infections comprising urinary tract infection, febrile neutropenia, sepsis, pneumonia, cellulitis, colitis, diarrhea, osteomyelitis, and upper respiratory tract infection. Life-threatening infections were reported for 2% of patients that included sepsis, empyema, pneumonia, febrile neutropenia, fever, and biliary stent-associated cholangitis. During follow-up from 3 months to 4 years after the start of treatment with ibritumomab tiuxetan, 6% of patients developed infections. Two percent of patients had serious infections comprising urinary tract infection, bacterial or viral pneumonia, febrile neutropenia, perihilar infiltrate, pericarditis, and IV drug-associated viral hepatitis. One percent of patients had life-threatening infections that included bacterial pneumonia, respiratory disease, and sepsis.

Overdosage

Doses as high as 0.52 mCi/kg (19.2 MBq/kg) of Y-90 ibritumomab tiuxetan were administered in ibritumomab tiuxetan therapeutic regimen clinical trials and severe hematological toxicities were observed. No fatalities or second organ injury resulting from overdosage administrations were documented. However, single doses up to 50 mCi (1850 MBq) of Y-90 ibritumomab tiuxetan and multiple doses of 20 mCi (740 MBq) followed by 40 mCi (1480 MBq) of Y-90 ibritumomab tiuxetan were studied in a limited number of subjects. In these trials, some patients required autologous stem cell support to manage hematological toxicity.

CETUXIMAB

Rx	**Erbitux** (Bristol-Myers Squibb)	**Injection:** 2 mg/mL	Preservative-free. In single-use 50 mL vial.[a]

[a] With 1.88 mg/mL sodium phosphate dibasic heptahydrate and 0.42 mg/mL sodium phosphate monobasic monohydrate.

WARNING

Infusion reactions: Severe infusion reactions occurred with the administration of cetuximab in approximately 3% of patients, rarely with fatal outcome (less than 1 in 1000). Approximately 90% of severe infusion reactions were associated with the first infusion of cetuximab. Severe infusion reactions are characterized by rapid onset of airway obstruction (eg, bronchospasm, stridor, hoarseness), urticaria, and hypotension (see Warnings and Adverse Reactions). Severe infusion reactions require immediate interruption of the cetuximab infusion and permanent discontinuation from further treatment (see Warnings and Administration and Dosage).

Indications

➤*Metastatic colorectal carcinoma:* Used in combination with irinotecan for the treatment of epidermal growth factor receptor (EGFR)-expressing, metastatic colorectal carcinoma in patients who are refractory to irinotecan-based chemotherapy; as a single agent for the treatment of EGFR-expressing, metastatic colorectal carcinoma in patients who are intolerant to irinotecan-based chemotherapy.

Administration and Dosage

➤*Approved by the FDA:* February 12, 2004.

Do not administer cetuximab as an IV push or bolus.

➤*Initial dose:* In combination with irinotecan or as monotherapy, 400 mg/m² as an initial loading dose (first infusion) administered as a 120-minute IV infusion (maximum infusion rate, 5 mL/min).

➤*Maintenance dose:* The recommended weekly maintenance dose (all other infusions) is 250 mg/m² infused over 60 minutes (maximum infusion rate, 5 mL/min).

➤*Premedication:* Premedication with an H_1 antagonist (eg, 50 mg diphenhydramine IV) is recommended.

➤*Dose modifications:*

Infusion reactions – If the patient experiences a mild or moderate (grade 1 or 2) infusion reaction, permanently reduce the infusion rate by 50%. Immediately and permanently discontinue cetuximab in patients who experience severe (grade 3 or 4) infusion reactions (see Warnings and Adverse Reactions).

Dermatologic toxicity and related disorders – If a patient experiences severe acneform rash, make cetuximab treatment adjustments according to the table below. In patients with mild and moderate skin toxicity, continue treatment without dose modification.

Cetuximab Dose Modification Guidelines			
Severe acneform rash occurrence	Cetuximab	Outcome	Cetuximab dose modification
1st	Delay infusion 1 to 2 weeks	Improvement	Continue at 250 mg/m²
		No improvement	Discontinue cetuximab
2nd	Delay infusion 1 to 2 weeks	Improvement	Reduce dose to 200 mg/m²
		No improvement	Discontinue cetuximab
3rd	Delay infusion 1 to 2 weeks	Improvement	Reduce dose to 150 mg/m²
		No improvement	Discontinue cetuximab
4th	Discontinue cetuximab	—	—

➤*Preparation and administration:* Administer cetuximab with the use of a low protein-binding 0.22 mcm in-line filter. The solution should be clear and colorless and may contain a small amount of easily visible, white, amorphous cetuximab particulates. Do not shake or dilute. Cetuximab can be administered via infusion pump or syringe pump.

➤*Storage/Stability:* Store vials under refrigeration at 2° to 8°C (36° to 46°F). Do not freeze. Increased particulate formation may occur at temperatures at or below 0°C. This product contains no preservatives. Preparations of cetuximab in infusion containers are chemically and physically stable for up to 12 hours at 2° to 8°C (36° to 46°F) and up to 8 hours at controlled room temperature (20° to 25°C; 68° to 77°F). Discard any remaining solution in the infusion container after 8 hours at controlled room temperature or after 12 hours at 2° to 8°C. Discard any unused portion of the vial.

Actions

➤*Pharmacology:* Cetuximab is a recombinant, human/mouse chimeric monoclonal antibody that binds specifically to the extracellular domain of the human EGFR on normal and tumor cells and competitively inhibits the binding of the epidermal growth factor (EGF) and other ligands, such as transforming growth factor-alpha. Binding of cetuximab to the EGFR blocks phosphorylation and activation of recep-

CETUXIMAB

tor-associated kinases, resulting in inhibition of cell growth, induction of apoptosis, and decreased matrix metalloproteinase and vascular endothelial growth factor reduction. The EGFR is a transmembrane glycoprotein that is a member of a subfamily of type 1 receptor tyrosine kinases. The EGFR is constitutively expressed in many normal epithelial tissues, including the skin and hair follicle. Over-expression of EGFR also is detected in many human cancers, including those of the colon and rectum.

In vitro assays and in vivo animal studies have shown that cetuximab inhibits the growth and survival of tumor cells that over-express the EGFR. No antitumor effects of cetuximab were observed in human tumor xenografts lacking EGFR expression. The addition of cetuximab to irinotecan or irinotecan plus 5-fluorouracil in animal studies resulted in an increase in antitumor effects compared with chemotherapy alone.

➤*Pharmacokinetics:*

Absorption/Distribution – The AUC increased in a greater than dose-proportional manner as the dose increased from 20 to 400 mg/m². The volume of distribution for cetuximab appeared to be independent of dose and approximated the vascular space of 2 to 3 L/m². Following a 2-hour infusion of 400 mg/m² cetuximab, the C_{max} was 184 mcg/mL. A 1-hour infusion of 250 mg/m² produced a mean C_{max} of 140 mcg/mL. Following the recommended dose regimen (400 mg/m² initial dose/ 250 mg/m² weekly dose), cetuximab concentrations reached steady-state levels by the third weekly infusion with mean peak and trough concentrations across studies ranging from 168 to 235 and 41 to 85 mcg/mL, respectively.

Metabolism/Excretion – Cetuximab clearance decreased from 0.08 to 0.02 L/h/m² as the dose increased from 20 to 200 mg/m², and at doses greater than 200 mg/m² it appeared to plateau. The mean elimination half life was 97 hours after a single 2-hour infusion of 400 mg/m² cetuximab and the mean steady-state half life was 114 hours (range, 75 to 188 hours).

Special populations –

Gender: Female patients had a 25% lower intrinsic cetuximab clearance than male patients. Dose modification based on gender is not necessary.

➤*Clinical trials:* A multicenter, randomized, controlled clinical trial was conducted in 329 patients randomized to receive either cetuximab plus irinotecan (218 patients) or cetuximab monotherapy (111 patients). In both arms of the study, cetuximab was administered as a 400 mg/m² initial dose followed by 250 mg/m² weekly until disease progression or unacceptable toxicity. All patients received a 20 mg test dose on day 1. In the cetuximab-plus-irinotecan arm, irinotecan was added to cetuximab using the same dose and schedule for irinotecan as the patient had previously failed. Acceptable irinotecan schedules were 350 mg/m² every 3 weeks, 180 mg/m² every 2 weeks, or 125 mg/m² weekly times 4 doses every 6 weeks. An Independent Radiographic Review Committee (IRC) blinded to the treatment arms assessed the progression on prior irinotecan and the response to protocol treatment for all patients.

Analyses also were conducted in 2 prespecified subpopulations: Irinotecan refractory and irinotecan and oxaliplatin failures. The irinotecan refractory population was defined as randomized patients who had received at least 2 cycles of irinotecan-based chemotherapy prior to treatment with cetuximab, and had independent confirmation of disease progression within 30 days of completion of the last cycle of irinotecan-based chemotherapy.

The irinotecan and oxaliplatin failure population was defined as irinotecan refractory patients who had previously been treated with and failed an oxaliplatin-containing regimen. The objective response rates (ORR) in these populations are presented in the following table.

Cetuximab Objective Response Rates Per Independent Review						
	Cetuximab plus irinotecan		Cetuximab monotherapy		Difference	
Populations	n	ORR (%)	n	ORR (%)	(%)	P values
All patients	218	22.9	111	10.8	12.1	0.007
Irinotecan-oxaliplatin failure	80	23.8	44	11.4	12.4	0.09
Irinotecan refractory	132	25.8	69	14.5	11.3	0.07

The median duration of response in the overall population was 5.7 months in the combination arm and 4.2 months in the monotherapy arm. Compared with patients randomized to cetuximab alone, patients randomized to cetuximab and irinotecan experienced a significantly longer median time to disease progression.

Cetuximab Time to Progression Per Independent Review				
Populations	Cetuximab plus irinotecan (median)	Cetuximab monotherapy (median)	Hazard ratio[a]	P values
All patients	4.1 mo	1.5 mo	0.54	< 0.001
Irinotecan-oxaliplatin failure	2.9 mo	1.5 mo	0.48	< 0.001
Irinotecan refractory	4 mo	1.5 mo	0.52	< 0.001

[a] Hazard ratio of cetuximab plus irinotecan: Cetuximab monotherapy.

Contraindications

No known contraindications (see Warnings).

Warnings

➤*Infusion reactions:* Severe infusion reactions occurred with the administration of cetuximab in approximately 3% of patients, rarely with fatal outcome (less than 1 in 1000). Approximately 90% of severe infusion reactions were associated with the first infusion of cetuximab despite the use of prophylactic antihistamines. These reactions were characterized by the rapid onset of airway obstruction (eg, bronchospasm, stridor, hoarseness), urticaria, and/or hypotension. Exercise caution with every cetuximab infusion, as there were patients who experienced their first severe infusion reaction during later infusions.

Severe infusion reactions require the immediate interruption of cetuximab therapy and permanent discontinuation from further treatment. Ensure that appropriate medical therapy including epinephrine, corticosteroids, IV antihistamines, bronchodilators, and oxygen are available for use in the treatment of such reactions. Carefully observe patients until the complete resolution of all signs and symptoms. In clinical trials, mild to moderate infusion reactions were managed by slowing the infusion rate of cetuximab and by continued use of antihistamine medications (eg, diphenhydramine) in subsequent doses.

➤*Pulmonary toxicity:* Interstitial lung disease (ILD) was reported in less than 0.5% of patients with advanced colorectal cancer receiving cetuximab. Interstitial pneumonitis with noncardiogenic pulmonary edema resulting in death was reported in 1 case. Two patients had pre-existing fibrotic lung disease and experienced an acute exacerbation of their disease while receiving cetuximab in combination with irinotecan. An additional case of interstitial pneumonitis was reported in a patient with head and neck cancer treated with cetuximab and cisplatin. The onset of symptoms occurred between the fourth and eleventh doses of treatment in all reported cases.

In the event of acute onset or worsening pulmonary symptoms, interrupt cetuximab therapy and promptly investigate these symptoms. If ILD is confirmed, discontinue cetuximab and appropriately treat the patient.

➤*Dermatologic toxicity:* In cynomolgus monkeys, cetuximab, when administered at doses of approximately 0.4 to 4 times the weekly human exposure, resulted in dermatologic findings including inflammation at the injection site and desquamation of the external integument. At the highest dose level, the epithelial mucosa of the nasal passage, esophagus, and tongue were similarly affected, and degenerative changes in the renal tubular epithelium occurred. Deaths caused by sepsis were observed in 50% of the animals at the highest dose level beginning after approximately 13 weeks of treatment.

In clinical studies, dermatologic toxicities, including acneform rash, skin drying and fissuring, and inflammatory and infectious sequelae (eg, blepharitis, chelitis, cellulitis, cyst) were reported. In patients with advanced colorectal cancer, acneform rash was reported in 88% of all treated patients, and was severe (grade 3 or 4) in 12% of these patients. Subsequent to the development of severe dermatologic toxicities, complications including *Staphylococcus aureus* sepsis and abscesses requiring incision and drainage were reported.

Monitor patients developing dermatologic toxicities while receiving cetuximab for the development of inflammatory or infectious sequelae, and initiate appropriate treatment of these symptoms. Institute dose modifications of any future cetuximab infusions in case of severe acneform rash (see Administration and Dosage). Consider treatment with topical and/or oral antibiotics; topical corticosteroids are not recommended.

➤*Hypersensitivity reactions:* Use with caution in patients with known hypersensitivity to cetuximab, murine proteins, or any components of this product.

➤*Fertility impairment:* A 39-week toxicity study in cynomolgus monkeys receiving 0.4 to 4 times the human dose of cetuximab revealed a tendency for impairment of menstrual cycling in treated female monkeys, including increased incidences of irregularity or absence of cycles, when compared with control animals and beginning from week 25 of treatment and continuing through the 6-week recovery period. It is not known if cetuximab can impair fertility in humans.

➤*Pregnancy: Category C.* Human IgG1 is known to cross the placental barrier; therefore, cetuximab has the potential to be transmitted from the mother to the developing fetus. It is not known whether cetuximab can cause fetal harm when administered to a pregnant woman or whether it can affect reproductive capacity. There are no adequate and well-controlled studies in pregnant women. Only give cetuximab to pregnant women, or any woman not employing adequate contraception, if the potential benefit justifies the potential risk to the fetus. Counsel all patients regarding the potential risk of cetuximab treatment to the developing fetus prior to initiation of therapy. If the patient becomes pregnant while receiving this drug, apprise her of the potential hazard to the fetus and/or the potential risk for loss of the pregnancy.

➤*Lactation:* It is not known whether cetuximab is secreted in human milk. Because human IgG1 is secreted in human milk, the potential for absorption and harm to the infant after ingestion is unknown. Based on the mean half-life of cetuximab after multiple dosing of 114 hours,

CETUXIMAB

advise women to discontinue nursing during treatment with cetuximab and for 60 days following the last dose of cetuximab.

➤*Children:* The safety and efficacy of cetuximab have not been established.

Precautions

➤*EGFR testing:* Patients enrolled in the clinical studies were required to have immunohistochemical evidence of positive EGFR expression using the *DakoCytomation EGFR pharmDx* test kit. Perform assessment for EGFR expression by laboratories with demonstrated proficiency in the specific technology being utilized. Improper assay performance, including use of suboptimally fixed tissue, failure to utilize specified reagents, deviation from specific assay instructions, and failure to include appropriate controls for assay validation can lead to unreliable results. Refer to the *DakoCytomation* test kit package insert for full instructions on assay performance.

➤*Immunogenicity:* Nonneutralizing anticetuximab antibodies were detected in 5% of evaluable patients. In patients positive for anticetuximab antibody, the median time to onset was 44 days. Although the number of seropositive patients is limited, there does not appear to be any relationship between the appearance of antibodies to cetuximab and the safety or antitumor activity of the molecule.

➤*Photosensitivity:* It is recommended that patients wear sunscreens and hats and limit sun exposure while receiving cetuximab because sunlight can exacerbate any skin reactions that may occur.

Adverse Reactions

The most serious adverse reactions associated with cetuximab were: Diarrhea (in patients receiving cetuximab plus irinotecan) (6%); dehydration (in patients receiving cetuximab plus irinotecan), fever (5%); infusion reaction, sepsis (3%); dehydration (in patients receiving cetuximab monotherapy), kidney failure (2%); dermatologic toxicity, pulmonary embolus (1%); ILD (0.5%).

Cetuximab Adverse Events (≥ 10%) in Patients with Advanced Colorectal Carcinoma				
	Cetuximab plus irinotecan (n = 354)		Cetuximab monotherapy (n = 279)	
Adverse reaction	Grades 1 to 4	Grades 3 and 4	Grades 1 to 4	Grades 3 and 4
CNS				
Depression	10	0	9	0
Headache	14	2	25	3
Insomnia	12	0	10	< 1
Dermatologic				
Acneform rash[a]	88	14	90	10
Alopecia	21	0	5	0
Conjunctivitis	14	1	7	< 1
Nail disorder	12	< 1	16	< 1
Pruritus	10	1	10	< 1
Skin disorder	15	1	5	0
GI				
Abdominal pain	45	8	25	7
Anorexia	36	4	25	3
Constipation	30	2	28	1
Diarrhea	72	22	28	2
Dyspepsia	14	0	7	0
Nausea	55	6	29	2
Stomatitis	26	2	11	< 1
Vomiting	41	7	25	3
Hematic/Lymphatic				
Anemia	16	5	10	4
Leukopenia	25	17	1	0
Metabolic/Nutritional				
Dehydration	15	6	9	2
Peripheral edema	16	1	10	< 1
Weight loss	21	0	9	1
Respiratory				
Cough increased	20	0	10	1
Dyspnea[b]	23	2	20	7

Cetuximab Adverse Events (≥ 10%) in Patients with Advanced Colorectal Carcinoma				
	Cetuximab plus irinotecan (n = 354)		Cetuximab monotherapy (n = 279)	
Adverse reaction	Grades 1 to 4	Grades 3 and 4	Grades 1 to 4	Grades 3 and 4
Miscellaneous				
Asthenia/malaise[c]	73	16	49	10
Back pain	16	3	11	3
Fever[b]	34	4	33	0
Infection	16	1	11	1
Infusion reaction[d]	19	3	25	2
Pain	23	6	19	5

[a] Acneform rash is defined as any event described as acne, dry skin, exfoliative dermatitis, maculopapular rash, pustular rash, or rash.
[b] Includes cases reported as infusion reaction.
[c] Asthenia/malaise is defined as any event described as asthenia, malaise, or somnolence.
[d] Infusion reaction is defined as any event described at any time during the clinical study as allergic reaction or anaphylactoid reaction, or any event occurring on the first day of dosing described as allergic reaction, anaphylactoid reaction, chills, chills and fever, dyspnea, or fever.

➤*Infusion reactions:* Severe, potentially fatal infusion reactions have been reported. These events include the rapid onset of airway obstruction (eg, bronchospasm, stridor, hoarseness), urticaria, and/or hypotension. In advanced colorectal cancer, severe infusion reactions were observed in 3% of patients receiving cetuximab plus irinotecan and 2% of patients receiving cetuximab monotherapy. Grade 1 and 2 infusion reactions, including chills, fever, and dyspnea usually occurring on the first day of initial dosing, were observed in 16% of patients receiving cetuximab plus irinotecan and 23% of patients receiving cetuximab monotherapy.

➤*Dermatologic toxicity and related disorders:* Nonsuppurative acneform rash described as acne, rash, maculopapular rash, pustular rash, dry skin, or exfoliative dermatitis was observed in patients receiving cetuximab plus irinotecan or cetuximab monotherapy. One or more of the dermatological adverse events were reported in 88% (14% grade 3) of patients receiving cetuximab plus irinotecan and in 90% (10% grade 3) of patients receiving cetuximab monotherapy. Acneform rash most commonly occurred on the face, upper chest, and back, but could extend to the extremities and was characterized by multiple follicular- or pustular-appearing lesions. Skin drying and fissuring were common in some instances, and were associated with inflammatory and infectious sequelae (eg, blepharitis, cellulitis, cyst). Two cases of *S. aureus* sepsis were reported. The onset of acneform rash was generally within the first 2 weeks of therapy. Although in a majority of the patients the event resolved following cessation of treatment, in nearly half of the cases the event continued beyond 28 days.

A related nail disorder, occurring in 14% of patients (0.3% grade 3), was characterized as a paronychial inflammation with associated swelling of the lateral nail folds of the toes and fingers, with the great toes and thumbs as the most commonly affected digits.

➤*Use with radiation therapy:* In a study of 21 patients with locally advanced squamous cell cancer of the head and neck, patients treated with cetuximab, cisplatin, and radiation had a 95% incidence of rash (19% grade 3). The incidence and severity of cutaneous reactions with combined modality therapy appears to be additive, particularly within the radiation port. Use appropriate caution when adding radiation to cetuximab therapy in patients with colorectal cancer.

Overdosage

Single doses of cetuximab higher than 500 mg/m^2 have not been tested. There is no experience with overdosage in human clinical trials.

Patient Information

Instruct patients to wear sunscreen and hats and to limit sun exposure while receiving cetuximab because sunlight can exacerbate any skin reactions that may occur.

Counsel all patients regarding the potential risk of cetuximab treatment to the developing fetus prior to initiation of therapy. If the patient becomes pregnant while receiving this drug, apprise her of the potential hazard to the fetus and/or the potential risk for loss of pregnancy.

BEVACIZUMAB

Rx	Avastin (Genentech)	Injection: 25 mg/mL	Preservative-free. In single-use 4 and 16 mL vials.

WARNING

GI perforation/wound healing complications: Bevacizumab administration can result in the development of GI perforation and wound dehiscence, in some instances resulting in fatality. GI perforation, sometimes associated with intra-abdominal abscess, occurred throughout treatment with bevacizumab (ie, was not correlated to duration of exposure). The incidence of GI perforation in patients receiving bolus-IFL (125 mg/m^2 irinotecan IV, 500 mg/m^2 5-fluorouracil IV, and 20 mg/m^2 leucovorin IV given once weekly for 4 weeks every 6 weeks) with bevacizumab was 2%. The typical presentation was reported as abdominal pain associated with symptoms such as constipation and vomiting. Include GI perforation in the differential diagnosis of patients receiving bevacizumab presenting with abdominal pain. Permanently discontinue bevacizumab in patients with GI perforation or wound dehiscence requiring medical intervention. The appropriate interval between termination of bevacizumab and subsequent elective surgery required to avoid the risks of impaired wound healing/wound dehiscence has not been determined (see Warnings and Administration and Dosage).

Hemorrhage: Serious and, in some cases, fatal hemoptysis has occurred in patients with nonsmall cell lung cancer treated with chemotherapy and bevacizumab. In a small study, the incidence of serious or fatal hemoptysis was 31% in patients with squamous histology and 4% in patients with adenocarcinoma receiving bevacizumab as compared with no cases in patients treated with chemotherapy alone. Do not administer bevacizumab to patients with recent hemoptysis (see Warnings and Administration and Dosage).

Indications

➤*Metastatic carcinoma:* In combination with IV 5-fluorouracil-based chemotherapy for first-line treatment of patients with metastatic carcinoma of the colon or rectum.

➤*Unlabeled uses:* Adjunctive therapy in breast cancer; renal cell carcinoma.

Administration and Dosage

➤*Approved by the FDA:* February 26, 2004.

➤*Dosage:* 5 mg/kg given once every 14 days as an IV infusion until disease progression is detected.

➤*Administration:* Do not administer as an IV push or bolus. Deliver the initial bevacizumab dose over 90 minutes as an IV infusion following chemotherapy. If the first infusion is well tolerated, the second infusion may be administered over 60 minutes. If the 60-minute infusion is well tolerated, all subsequent infusions may be administered over 30 minutes.

➤*Dose modification:*

Permanent discontinuation – Permanently discontinue bevacizumab in patients who develop GI perforation, wound dehiscence requiring medical intervention, serious bleeding, nephrotic syndrome, or hypertensive crisis.

Temporary suspension –

Proteinuria: Temporary suspension of bevacizumab is recommended in patients with evidence of moderate to severe proteinuria pending further evaluation and in patients with severe hypertension that is not controlled with medical management. The risk of continuation or temporary suspension of bevacizumab in patients with moderate to severe proteinuria is unknown.

Surgery: Suspend bevacizumab at least several weeks prior to elective surgery. Do not resume bevacizumab until the surgical incision is fully healed. Do not initiate bevacizumab for at least 28 days following major surgery. Ensure that the surgical incision is fully healed prior to initiation of bevacizumab.

➤*Preparation for administration:* Withdraw the necessary amount of bevacizumab for a dose of 5 mg/kg and dilute in a total volume of 100 mL 0.9% sodium chloride injection. Discard any unused portion because the product is preservative-free.

➤*Admixture incompatibilities:* Do not administer or mix bevacizumab infusions with dextrose solutions. No incompatibilities between bevacizumab and polyvinylchloride or polyolefin bags have been observed.

➤*Storage/Stability:* Refrigerate bevacizumab vials at 2° to 8°C (36° to 46°F). Diluted solutions for infusion may be stored at 2° to 8°C (36° to 46°F) for up to 8 hours. Protect bevacizumab vials from light. Store in the original carton until time of use. Do not freeze or shake.

Actions

➤*Pharmacology:* Bevacizumab is a recombinant, humanized, monoclonal IgG1 antibody that binds to and inhibits the biologic activity of human vascular endothelial growth factor (VEGF) in in vitro and in vivo assay systems. Bevacizumab binds VEGF and prevents the interaction of VEGF to its receptors (Flt-1 and KDR) on the surface of endothelial cells. The interaction of VEGF with its receptors leads to endothelial cell proliferation and new blood vessel formation in in vitro models of angiogenesis. Administration of bevacizumab to xenotransplant models of colon cancer in nude (athymic) mice caused reduction of microvascular growth and inhibition of metastatic disease progression.

➤*Pharmacokinetics:* The assay used to assess bevacizumab's pharmacokinetic profile did not distinguish between free bevacizumab and bevacizumab bound to VEGF ligand. Based on a population pharmacokinetic analysis of 491 patients who received 1 to 20 mg/kg bevacizumab weekly, every 2 weeks, or every 3 weeks, the estimated half life of bevacizumab was approximately 20 days (range, 11 to 50 days). The predicted time to reach steady state was 100 days. The accumulation ratio following a dose of 10 mg/kg bevacizumab every 2 weeks was 2.8.

Special populations –

Gender: After correcting for body weight, males had a higher bevacizumab clearance vs females (0.262 L/day vs 0.207 L/day). However, in a randomized study of 813 patients, there was no evidence of lesser efficacy (hazard ratio for overall survival) in males as compared with females.

Tumor burden: Patients with higher tumor burden (at or above median value of tumor surface area) had a higher bevacizumab clearance (0.249 L/day vs 0.199 L/day) than patients with tumor burdens below the median. However, in a randomized trial of 813 patients, there was no evidence of lesser efficacy (hazard ratio for overall survival) in patients with higher tumor burden as compared with patients with low tumor burden.

Contraindications

No known contraindications (see Warnings).

Warnings

➤*GI perforation/wound healing complications:* GI perforation and wound dehiscence, complicated by intra-abdominal abscesses, occurred at an increased incidence in patients receiving bevacizumab as compared with controls. Bevacizumab also has been shown to impair wound healing in preclinical animal models. In a clinical study, 0.3% of patients receiving bolus-IFL plus placebo, 2% of patients receiving bolus-IFL plus bevacizumab, and 4% of patients receiving 5-FU/LV (500 mg/m^2 5-fluorouracil and 500 mg/m^2 leucovorin weekly for 6 weeks every 8 weeks) plus bevacizumab developed GI perforation, in some instances with fatal outcome. These episodes occurred with or without intra-abdominal abscesses and at various time points during treatment. The typical presentation was reported as abdominal pain associated with symptoms such as constipation and vomiting. In addition, 0.5% of patients receiving bolus-IFL plus placebo, 1% of patients receiving bolus-IFL plus bevacizumab, and 1% of patients receiving 5-FU/LV plus bevacizumab developed a wound dehiscence during study treatment.

The appropriate interval between surgery and subsequent initiation of bevacizumab required to avoid the risks of impaired wound healing has not been determined. In a clinical study, the clinical protocol did not permit initiation of bevacizumab for at least 28 days following surgery. There was 1 patient (among 501 patients receiving bevacizumab) in whom an anastomotic dehiscence occurred when bevacizumab was initiated per protocol. In this patient, the interval between surgery and initiation of bevacizumab was greater than 2 months.

Similarly, the appropriate interval between termination of bevacizumab and subsequent elective surgery required to avoid risks of impaired wound healing has not been determined. In the same study, 39 patients who were receiving bolus-IFL plus bevacizumab underwent surgery following bevacizumab therapy and, of these patients, 15% had wound healing/bleeding complications. In the same study, 25 patients in the bolus-IFL arm underwent surgery and, of these patients, 4% had wound healing/bleeding complications. The longest interval between the last dose of study drug and dehiscence was 56 days; this occurred in a patient on the bolus-IFL plus bevacizumab arm. Ensure the interval between termination of bevacizumab and subsequent elective surgery takes into consideration the calculated half life of bevacizumab (approximately 20 days).

Discontinue bevacizumab therapy in patients with GI perforation or wound dehiscence requiring medical intervention (see Administration and Dosage).

➤*Hemorrhage:* Two distinct patterns of bleeding have occurred in patients receiving bevacizumab. The first is minor hemorrhage, most commonly grade 1 epistaxis. The second is serious, and in some cases fatal, hemorrhagic events. Serious hemorrhagic events occurred primarily in patients with nonsmall cell lung cancer. In a randomized study in patients with nonsmall cell lung cancer receiving chemotherapy with or without bevacizumab, 31% of bevacizumab-treated patients with squamous cell histology and 4% of bevacizumab-treated patients with nonsquamous histology experienced life-threatening or fatal pulmonary hemorrhage as compared with 0% of patients receiving chemotherapy alone. Of the patients experiencing events of life-threatening pulmonary hemorrhage, many had cavitation and/or necrosis of the tumor, either preexisting or developing during bevacizumab therapy. These serious hemorrhagic events occurred suddenly and presented as

BEVACIZUMAB

major or massive hemoptysis.

The risk of CNS bleeding in patients with CNS metastases receiving bevacizumab has not been evaluated because these patients were excluded from studies following development of CNS hemorrhage in a patient with a CNS metastasis in phase 1 studies.

Other serious bleeding events reported in patients receiving bevacizumab were uncommon and included GI hemorrhage, subarachnoid hemorrhage, and hemorrhagic stroke. Discontinue bevacizumab treatment in patients with serious hemorrhage (ie, requiring medical intervention) and administer aggressive medical management. Do not give bevacizumab to patients with recent hemoptysis (see Administration and Dosage).

➤Hypertension: The incidence of hypertension and severe hypertension was increased in patients receiving bevacizumab in a study (see Adverse Reactions).

Among patients with severe hypertension in the bevacizumab arms, slightly over half the patients (51%) had a diastolic reading greater than 110 associated with a systolic reading less than 200. Four months after discontinuation of therapy, persistent hypertension was present in 18 of 26 patients that received bolus-IFL plus bevacizumab and 8 of 10 patients that received bolus-IFL plus placebo. Across all clinical studies (n = 1032), development or worsening of hypertension resulted in hospitalization or discontinuation of bevacizumab in 17 patients. Four of these 17 patients developed hypertensive encephalopathy. Severe hypertension was complicated by subarachnoid hemorrhage in 1 patient.

Permanently discontinue bevacizumab in patients with hypertensive crisis. Temporary suspension is recommended in patients with severe hypertension that is not controlled with medical management (see Administration and Dosage).

➤Proteinuria: In a randomized study, the incidence and severity of proteinuria (defined as a urine dipstick reading of 1+ or greater) was increased in patients receiving bevacizumab as compared with those receiving bolus-IFL plus placebo. Urinary dipstick readings of 2+ or greater occurred in 14% of patients receiving bolus-IFL plus placebo, in 17% receiving bolus-IFL plus bevacizumab, and in 28% of patients receiving 5-FU/LV plus bevacizumab. Twenty-four-hour urine collections were obtained in patients with new onset or worsening proteinuria. None of the 118 patients receiving bolus-IFL plus placebo, 3 of 158 patients receiving bolus-IFL plus bevacizumab, and 2 of 50 patients receiving 5-FU/LV plus bevacizumab who had a 24-hour collection experienced grade 3 proteinuria (more than 3.5 g protein/24 h).

In a dose-ranging, placebo-controlled, randomized study of bevacizumab in patients with metastatic renal cell carcinoma, 24-hour urine collections were obtained in approximately half the patients enrolled. Among patients in whom 24-hour urine collections were obtained, 4 of 19 (21%) patients receiving bevacizumab at 10 mg/kg every 2 weeks, 2 of 14 (14%) receiving bevacizumab at 3 mg/kg every 2 weeks, and none of the 15 placebo patients experienced National Cancer Institute common toxicity criteria (NCI-CTC) grade 3 proteinuria (more than 3.5 g protein/24 h).

Nephrotic syndrome occurred in 5 of 1032 (0.5%) patients receiving bevacizumab in studies. One patient died and 1 required dialysis. In 3 patients, proteinuria decreased in severity several months after discontinuation of bevacizumab. No patient had normalization of urinary protein levels (by 24-hour urine) following discontinuation of bevacizumab.

Discontinue bevacizumab in patients with nephrotic syndrome (see Administration and Dosage). The safety of continued bevacizumab treatment in patients with moderate to severe proteinuria has not been evaluated. In most clinical studies, bevacizumab was interrupted for at least 2 g proteinuria/24 h and resumed when proteinuria was less than 2 g/24 h. Regularly monitor patients with moderate to severe proteinuria based on 24-hour collections until improvement and/or resolution is observed.

➤Congestive heart failure (CHF): CHF, defined as grade 2 to 4 left ventricular dysfunction, was reported in 2% of patients receiving bevacizumab in studies. CHF occurred in 14% of patients receiving bevacizumab and concurrent anthracyclines. CHF occurred in 4% of patients who received prior anthracyclines and/or left chest wall irradiation. In a controlled study, the incidence was higher in patients receiving bevacizumab plus chemotherapy as compared with patients receiving chemotherapy alone. The safety of continuation or resumption of bevacizumab in patients with cardiac dysfunction has not been studied.

➤Hypersensitivity reactions: Use bevacizumab with caution in patients with known hypersensitivity to bevacizumab or any component of this drug product.

➤Fertility impairment: Bevacizumab may impair fertility. Dose-related decreases in ovarian and uterine weights, endometrial proliferation, number of menstrual cycles, and arrested follicular development or absent corpora lutea were observed in female cynomolgus monkeys treated with 10 or 50 mg/kg bevacizumab for 13 or 26 weeks. Following a 4- or 12-week recovery period that examined only the high-dose group, trends suggestive of reversibility were noted

in the 2 females for each regimen that were assigned to recover. After the 12-week recovery period, follicular maturation arrest was no longer observed, but ovarian weights were still moderately decreased. Reduced endometrial proliferation was no longer observed at the 12-week recovery time point, but uterine weight decreases were still notable, corpora lutea were absent in 1 of 2 animals, and the number of menstrual cycles remained reduced (67%).

➤Elderly: Severe adverse events that occurred at a higher incidence (2% or more) in the elderly when compared with patients younger than 65 years of age were anemia, anorexia, asthenia, CHF, constipation, deep thrombophlebitis, dehydration, diarrhea, dyspepsia, edema, epistaxis, GI hemorrhage, hypertension, hypokalemia, hyponatremia, hypotension, increased cough, leukopenia, myocardial infarction, sepsis, and voice alteration. The effect of bevacizumab on overall survival was similar in elderly patients as compared with younger patients.

➤Pregnancy: Category C. Bevacizumab has been shown to be teratogenic in rabbits when administered in doses that are 2-fold greater than the recommended human dose on a mg/kg basis. Observed effects included decreases in maternal and fetal body weights, an increased number of fetal resorptions, and an increased incidence of specific gross and skeletal fetal alterations. Adverse fetal outcomes were observed at all doses tested.

Angiogenesis is critical to fetal development and the inhibition of angiogenesis following administration of bevacizumab is likely to result in adverse effects on pregnancy. There are no adequate and well-controlled studies in pregnant women. Use bevacizumab during pregnancy or in any woman not employing adequate contraception only if the potential benefit justifies the potential risk to the fetus. Counsel all patients regarding the potential risk of bevacizumab to the developing fetus prior to initiation of therapy. If the patient becomes pregnant while receiving bevacizumab, apprise her of the potential hazard to the fetus and/or the potential risk of loss of pregnancy. Also counsel patients who discontinue bevacizumab concerning the prolonged exposure following discontinuation of therapy (half life of approximately 20 days) and the possible effects of bevacizumab on fetal development.

➤Lactation: It is not known whether bevacizumab is secreted in human milk. Because human IgG1 is secreted into human milk, the potential for absorption and harm to the infant after ingestion is unknown. Advise women to discontinue nursing during treatment with bevacizumab and for a prolonged period following the use of bevacizumab, taking into account the half life of the product, approximately 20 days (range, 11 to 50 days).

➤Children: The safety and efficacy of bevacizumab in pediatric patients have not been studied. However, physeal dysplasia was observed in juvenile cynomolgus monkeys with open growth plates treated for 4 weeks with doses that are less than the recommended human dose based on mg/kg and exposure. The incidence and severity of physeal dysplasia were dose-related and were at least partially reversible upon cessation of treatment.

Precautions

➤Monitoring: Monitor blood pressure every 2 to 3 weeks during bevacizumab treatment. Patients who develop hypertension on bevacizumab may require blood pressure monitoring at more frequent intervals. Continue to monitor at regular intervals the blood pressure of patients with bevacizumab-induced or exacerbated hypertension who discontinue bevacizumab.

Monitor patients receiving bevacizumab for the development or worsening of proteinuria with serial urinalysis. Further assess (eg, a 24-hour urine collection) patients with a 2+ or greater urine dipstick reading (see Warnings and Administration and Dosage).

➤Infusion reactions: Infusion reactions with the first dose of bevacizumab were uncommon (less than 3%). Severe reactions during the infusion of bevacizumab occurred in 2 patients. One patient developed stridor and wheezing during their first dose. A second patient, receiving paclitaxel followed by bevacizumab, developed a grade 3 hypersensitivity reaction requiring hospitalization during their third infusion of bevacizumab. Both patients responded to medical management. Information on rechallenge is not available.

Interrupt bevacizumab infusion in all patients with severe infusion reactions and administer appropriate medical therapy. There are no data regarding the most appropriate method of identification of patients who may safely be retreated with bevacizumab after experiencing a severe infusion reaction.

➤Surgery: Do not initiate bevacizumab therapy for at least 28 days following major surgery. Ensure that the surgical incision is fully healed prior to initiation of bevacizumab. Because of the potential for impaired wound healing, suspend bevacizumab prior to elective surgery. The appropriate interval between the last dose of bevacizumab and elective surgery is unknown; however, the half life of bevacizumab is estimated to be 20 days. Ensure the interval chosen takes into consideration the half life of the drug (see Warnings).

➤Cardiovascular disease: Patients were excluded from participation in bevacizumab clinical trials, if, in the previous year, they had experienced clinically significant cardiovascular disease. Thus, the safety of bevacizumab in patients with clinically significant cardiovascular disease has not been adequately evaluated.

BEVACIZUMAB

▶*Immunogenicity:* As with all therapeutic proteins, there is a potential for immunogenicity. The incidence of antibody development in patients receiving bevacizumab has not been adequately determined because the assay sensitivity was inadequate to reliably detect lower titers. Enzyme-linked immunosorbent assays (ELISAs) were performed on sera from approximately 500 patients treated with bevacizumab, primarily in combination with chemotherapy. High-titer human antibevacizumab antibodies were not detected.

Adverse Reactions

The most serious adverse events associated with bevacizumab were CHF (see Warnings), GI perforations/wound healing complications, hemorrhage, hypertensive crises, and nephrotic syndrome. The most common severe (grade 3 to 4) adverse events among 1032 patients receiving bevacizumab in studies were asthenia, diarrhea, hypertension, leukopenia, and pain. The most common adverse events of any severity among the 742 patients receiving bevacizumab in studies were abdominal pain, anorexia, asthenia, constipation, diarrhea, dyspnea, epistaxis, exfoliative dermatitis, headache, hypertension, nausea, pain, proteinuria, stomatitis, upper respiratory tract infection, and vomiting.

Severe and life-threatening (grade 3 and 4) adverse events that occurred at a higher incidence (2% or more) in patients receiving bolus-IFL plus bevacizumab as compared with bolus-IFL plus placebo are presented in the following table.

Bevacizumab Grade 3 and 4 Adverse Events (%)

Adverse reaction	Arm 1 IFL + placebo (n = 396)	Arm 2 IFL + bevacizumab (n = 392)
Grade 3 to 4 events	74	87
Cardiovascular		
Deep vein thrombosis	5	9
Hypertension	2	12
Intra-abdominal thrombosis	1	3
Syncope	1	3
GI		
Abdominal pain	5	8
Constipation	2	4
Diarrhea	25	34
Hemic/Lymphatic		
Leukopenia	31	37
Neutropenia[a]	14	21
Miscellaneous		
Asthenia	7	10
Pain	5	8

[a] Central laboratories were collected on days 1 and 21 of each cycle. Neutrophil counts are available in 303 patients in arm 1 and 276 in arm 2.

Adverse events of any severity that occurred at a higher incidence (5% or more) in the initial phase of the study in patients receiving bevacizumab (bolus-IFL plus bevacizumab or 5-FU/LV plus bevacizumab) as compared with the bolus-IFL plus placebo arm are presented in the following table.

Bevacizumab Grade 1 to 4 Adverse Events (%)

Adverse reaction	Arm 1 IFL + placebo (n = 98)	Arm 2 IFL + bevacizumab (n = 102)	Arm 3 5-FU/LV + bevacizumab (n = 109)
Cardiovascular			
Deep vein thrombosis	3	9	6
Hypertension	14	23	34
Hypotension	7	15	7
CNS			
Abnormal gait	0	1	5
Confusion	1	1	6
Dizziness	20	26	19
Headache	19	26	26
GI			
Abdominal pain	55	61	50
Anorexia	30	43	35
Colitis	1	6	1
Constipation	29	40	29
Dry mouth	2	7	4
Dyspepsia	15	24	17
Flatulence	10	11	19
GI hemorrhage	6	24	19
Stomatitis	18	32	30
Weight loss	10	15	16
Vomiting	47	52	47
GU			
Proteinuria	24	36	36
Urinary frequency/ urgency	1	3	6

Bevacizumab Grade 1 to 4 Adverse Events (%)

Adverse reaction	Arm 1 IFL + placebo (n = 98)	Arm 2 IFL + bevacizumab (n = 102)	Arm 3 5-FU/LV + bevacizumab (n = 109)
Metabolic/Nutritional			
Bilirubinemia	0	1	6
Hypokalemia	11	12	16
Respiratory			
Dyspnea	15	26	25
Epistaxis	10	35	32
Upper respiratory tract infection	39	47	40
Voice alteration	2	9	6
Skin/Appendages			
Alopecia	26	32	6
Dry skin	7	7	20
Exfoliative dermatitis	3	3	19
Nail disorder	3	2	8
Skin discoloration	3	2	16
Skin ulcer	1	6	6
Special senses			
Excess lacrimation	2	6	18
Taste disorder	9	14	21
Miscellaneous			
Asthenia	70	74	73
Myalgia	7	8	15
Pain	55	61	62
Thrombocytopenia	0	5	5

▶*Mucocutaneous hemorrhage:* Both serious and nonserious hemorrhagic events occurred at a higher incidence in patients receiving bevacizumab (see Warnings). In the 309 patients in which grade 1 to 4 events were collected, epistaxis was common and reported in 35% of patients receiving bolus-IFL plus bevacizumab compared with 10% of patients receiving bolus-IFL plus placebo. These events were generally mild in severity (grade 1) and resolved without medical intervention. Other mild to moderate hemorrhagic events reported more frequently in patients receiving bolus-IFL plus bevacizumab when compared with those receiving bolus-IFL plus placebo included GI hemorrhage (24% vs 6%), minor gum bleeding (2% vs 0%), and vaginal hemorrhage (4% vs 2%).

▶*Thromboembolism:* In a clinical study, 18% of patients receiving bolus-IFL plus bevacizumab and 15% of patients receiving bolus-IFL plus placebo experienced a grade 3 to 4 thromboembolic event. The incidence of the following grade 3 and 4 thromboembolic events were higher in patients receiving bolus-IFL plus bevacizumab compared with patients receiving bolus-IFL plus placebo: Cerebrovascular events (4 vs 0 patients), deep venous thrombosis (34 vs 19), intra-abdominal thrombosis (13 vs 5), and myocardial infarction (6 vs 3). In contrast, the incidence of pulmonary embolism was higher in patients receiving bolus-IFL plus placebo (16 vs 20).

In the same study, 14% of patients who received bolus-IFL plus bevacizumab and 8% of patients who received bolus-IFL plus placebo had a thromboembolic event and received full-dose warfarin. Two patients in each treatment arm (4 total) developed bleeding complications. In the 2 patients treated with full-dose warfarin and bevacizumab, these events were associated with marked elevations in their international normalized ratio. Twenty-one percent of patients receiving bolus-IFL plus bevacizumab and 3% of patients receiving bolus-IFL developed an additional thromboembolic event.

▶*Other adverse events:* The following other serious adverse events are considered unusual in cancer patients receiving cytotoxic chemotherapy and occurred in at least 1 subject treated with bevacizumab in clinical studies.

GI – Anastomotic ulceration, intestinal necrosis, intestinal obstruction, mesenteric venous occlusion.

Miscellaneous – Hyponatremia, pancytopenia, polyserositis, ureteral stricture.

Overdosage

The maximum tolerated dose of bevacizumab has not been determined. The highest dose tested in humans (20 mg/kg IV) was associated with headache in 9 of 16 patients and with severe headache in 3 of 16 patients.

Patient Information

Counsel all patients regarding the potential risk of bevacizumab to the developing fetus prior to initiation of therapy. If the patient becomes pregnant while receiving bevacizumab, apprise her of the potential hazard to the fetus and/or the potential risk of loss of pregnancy. Also counsel patients who discontinue bevacizumab concerning the prolonged exposure following discontinuation of therapy (half life of approximately 20 days) and the possible effects of bevacizumab on fetal development.

TRASTUZUMAB

| Rx | **Herceptin** (Genentech) | **Powder, lyophilized:** 440 mg | Vial: Preservative free. Diluent: 20 mL vial of Bacteriostatic Water for Injection with 1.1% benzyl alcohol. |

WARNING

Cardiomyopathy: Trastuzumab administration can result in the development of ventricular dysfunction and CHF. Evaluate left ventricular function in all patients prior to and during treatment with trastuzumab. Strongly consider discontinuation of trastuzumab in patients who develop a clinically significant decrease in left ventricular function. Patients receiving trastuzumab in combination with anthracyclines and cyclophosphamide demonstrated a particularly high incidence and severity of cardiac dysfunction (see Warnings).

Hypersensitivity reactions, including anaphylaxis, infusion reactions, and pulmonary events: Trastuzumab administration can result in severe hypersensitivity reactions (including anaphylaxis), infusion reactions, and pulmonary events. Rarely, these have been fatal. In most cases, symptoms occurred during or within 24 hours of administration of trastuzumab. Interrupt trastuzumab infusion for patients experiencing dyspnea or clinically significant hypotension. Monitor patients until signs and symptoms completely resolve. Strongly consider discontinuation of trastuzumab treatment for patients who develop anaphylaxis, angioedema, or acute respiratory distress syndrome (see Warnings).

Indications

➤*Breast cancer:* For the treatment of metastatic breast cancer with tumors overexpressing the human epidermal growth factor receptor 2 (HER2) protein: 1) as a single agent in patients who have received ≥ 1 chemotherapy regimens; or 2) in combination with paclitaxel in patients who have not received chemotherapy for their metastatic disease.

Use only in patients whose tumors have HER2 protein overexpression.

Administration and Dosage

➤*Approved by the FDA:* September 25, 1998.

➤*Usual dose:* The recommended initial loading dose is 4 mg/kg infused over 90 minutes. The recommended weekly maintenance dose is 2 mg/kg and can be infused over 30 minutes if the initial loading dose was tolerated. Trastuzumab may be administered in an outpatient setting. Do not administer as an IV push or bolus.

➤*Preparation for administration:* The diluent provided has been formulated to maintain the stability and sterility of trastuzumab for up to 28 days. Other diluents have not been shown to contain effective preservatives for trastuzumab. Reconstitute each vial of trastuzumab with only 20 mL Bacteriostatic Water for Injection (BWFI), 1.1% benzyl alcohol preserved, as supplied, to yield a multidose solution containing 21 mg/mL trastuzumab. Upon reconstitution with BWFI, immediately label the vial in the area marked "Do not use after" with the date 28 days from the reconstitution date. If the patient has known hypersensitivity to benzyl alcohol, reconstitute with Sterile Water for Injection (SWFI). Use immediately and discard any unused portion. Avoid use of other reconstitution diluents.

Shaking the reconstituted trastuzumab or causing excessive foaming during the addition of diluent may result in problems with dissolution and the amount of trastuzumab that can be withdrawn from the vial.

Use appropriate aseptic technique when performing the following reconstitution steps:

1.) Using a sterile syringe, slowly inject 20 mL of the diluent into the vial containing the lyophilized cake of trastuzumab. The stream of diluent should be directed into the lyophilized cake.
2.) Swirl the vial gently to aid reconstitution. Trastuzumab may be sensitive to shear-induced stress (eg, agitation or rapid expulsion from a syringe). Do not shake.
3.) Slight foaming of the product upon reconstitution is not unusual. Allow the vial to stand undisturbed for ≈ 5 minutes. The solution should be essentially free of visible particulates, clear to slightly opalescent, and colorless to pale yellow.

Determine the dose in milligrams of trastuzumab needed, based on a loading dose of 4 mg/kg or a maintenance dose of 2 mg/kg. Calculate the volume needed from the reconstituted trastuzumab vial, withdraw this amount from the vial, and add it to an infusion bag containing 250 mL of 0.9% Sodium Chloride. Do not use Dextrose (5%) solution. Gently invert the bag to mix the solution. The reconstituted preparation results in a colorless to pale yellow transparent solution.

➤*Administration:* Treatment may be administered in an outpatient setting by infusing 4 mg/kg IV loading dose over 90 minutes. Do not administer as an IV push or bolus. Observe patients for fever and chills or other infusion-associated symptoms (see Adverse Reactions). If prior infusions are well tolerated, subsequent weekly doses of 2 mg/kg may be administered over 30 minutes.

➤*Incompatibility:* Do not mix or dilute with other drugs. Do not administer or mix with dextrose solutions.

➤*Storage/Stability:* Prior to reconstitution, vials of trastuzumab are stable at 2° to 8°C (36° to 46°F). Reconstituted trastuzumab with BWFI, as supplied, is stable for 28 days after reconstitution when stored at 2° to 8°C (36° to 46°F) and may be preserved for multiple use. Discard any remaining multi-dose reconstituted solution after 28 days. If reconstituted with unpreserved SWFI (not supplied), use immediately, and discard any unused portion. Do not freeze trastuzumab that has been reconstituted.

Trastuzumab for infusion diluted in polyvinylchloride or polyethylene bags containing 0.9% Sodium Chloride for Injection may be stored at 2° to 8°C (36° to 46°F) or at room temperature 2° to 25°C (35° to 77°F) ≤ 24 hours; however, because these solutions contain no effective preservative, refrigeration is recommended.

Actions

➤*Pharmacology:* Trastuzumab is a recombinant DNA-derived humanized monoclonal antibody that selectively binds with high affinity to the extracellular domain of the HER2. It inhibits the proliferation of human tumor cells that overexpress HER2 and mediates antibody-dependent cellular cytotoxicity (ADCC). In vitro, trastuzumab-mediated ADCC is preferentially exerted on cancer cells overexpressing HER2 compared with those that do not. The HER2 protein is overexpressed in 25% to 30% of primary breast cancers and can be detected using an immunohistochemistry-based assay of fixed tumor blocks.

➤*Pharmacokinetics:* Short duration IV infusions of 10 to 500 mg once weekly in breast cancer patients with metastatic disease demonstrated increased mean half-life and decreased clearance with increasing dose level. The half-life averaged 1.7 and 12 days at the 100 and 500 mg dose levels, respectively, and volume of distribution was 44 mL/kg. At 500 mg weekly, mean peak serum concentrations were 377 mcg/mL.

In studies using a loading dose of 4 mg/kg followed by a weekly maintenance dose of 2 mg/kg, a mean half-life of 5.8 days (range, 1 to 32 days) was observed. Between weeks 16 and 32, serum concentrations reached steady state with mean trough and peak concentrations of ≈ 79 mcg/mL and 123 mcg/mL, respectively.

Detectable concentrations of the circulating extracellular domain of the HER2 receptor (shed antigen) are found in the serum of some patients with HER2 overexpressing tumors. Baseline serum samples revealed that 64% of patients had detectable shed antigen, which ranged as high as 1880 ng/mL (median, 11 ng/mL). Patients with higher baseline shed antigen levels were more likely to have lower serum trough concentrations. However, with weekly dosing, most patients with elevated shed antigen levels achieved target serum concentrations of trastuzumab by week 6.

Mean serum trough concentrations of trastuzumab, when administered in combination with paclitaxel, were consistently elevated ≈ 1.5-fold as compared to use in combination with anthracycline plus cyclophosphamide. In primate studies, administration with paclitaxel resulted in a reduction in trastuzumab clearance.

➤*Clinical trials:* Two trials studied the safety and efficacy of trastuzumab given IV as a 4 mg/kg loading dose followed by weekly 2 mg/kg doses in patients with metastatic breast cancer whose tumors overexpressed the HER2 protein. Eligible patients had a 2+ or 3+ level of overexpression (based on a 0 to 3+ scale) by immunohistochemical assay. Both trials suggest that a 3+ level of HER2 overexpression may produce beneficial treatment effects.

A multicenter, randomized, controlled clinical trial was conducted in 469 patients not previously treated with chemotherapy for metastatic disease. Patients were randomized to receive chemotherapy alone or in combination with trastuzumab. For those who had received prior anthracycline therapy in the adjuvant setting, chemotherapy was paclitaxel (175 mg/m^2 over 3 hours every 21 days for ≥ 6 cycles); for all other patients, chemotherapy consisted of anthracycline plus cyclophosphamide (AC: doxorubicin 60 mg/m^2 or epirubicin 75 mg/m^2 plus cyclophosphamide 600 mg/m^2 every 21 days for 6 cycles).

When compared with patients receiving chemotherapy alone, patients randomized to combination therapy experienced a significantly longer time to disease progression, higher overall response rate (ORR), longer median duration of response, and higher 1-year survival rate. These were observed in patients who received trastuzumab with paclitaxel and with AC; however, the magnitude of the effects was greater in the paclitaxel subgroup.

Trastuzumab was studied as a single agent in a multicenter, open-label, single-arm clinical trial in patients who had relapsed following 1 or 2 prior chemotherapy regimens for metastatic disease. Of 222 patients enrolled, 66% had received prior adjuvant chemotherapy, 68% had received 2 prior chemotherapy regimens for metastatic disease, and 25% had received prior myeloablative treatment with hematopoietic rescue. The ORR (complete response + partial response) was 14%, with a 2% complete response rate and 12% partial response rate. Complete responses were observed only in disease limited to skin and lymph nodes.

TRASTUZUMAB

Warnings

▶*Cardiotoxicity:* Signs and symptoms of cardiac dysfunction, such as dyspnea, increased cough, paroxysmal nocturnal dyspnea, peripheral edema, S_3 gallop, or reduced ejection fraction, have been observed. CHF associated with trastuzumab therapy may be severe and has been associated with disabling cardiac failure, death, and mural thrombosis leading to stroke.

Assess baseline cardiac function including history and physical exam and ≥ 1 of the following: ECG, echocardiogram, and MUGA scan. There are no data regarding the most appropriate evaluation method for the identification of patients at risk for developing cardiotoxicity. Monitoring may not identify all patients who will develop cardiac dysfunction.

Exercise extreme caution in treating patients with preexisting cardiac dysfunction. Frequently monitor patients for deteriorating cardiac function.

The probability of cardiac dysfunction was highest in patients who received trastuzumab concurrently with anthracyclines. The data suggest that advanced age may increase the probability of cardiac dysfunction.

Preexisting cardiac disease or prior cardiotoxic therapy (eg, anthracycline or radiation therapy to the chest) may decrease the ability to tolerate trastuzumab; however, the data are not adequate to evaluate this correlation.

Strongly consider discontinuation of trastuzumab in patients who develop clinically significant CHF. In clinical trials, most patients with cardiac dysfunction responded to appropriate medical therapy, often including discontinuation of trastuzumab. The safety of continuing or resuming therapy in patients who have previously experienced cardiac toxicity has not been studied. There are insufficient data regarding discontinuation of trastuzumab therapy in patients with asymptomatic decreases in ejection fraction; closely monitor such patients for evidence of clinical deterioration.

▶*Hypersensitivity reactions, including anaphylaxis:* Severe hypersensitivity reactions have been infrequently reported in patients with trastuzumab. Signs and symptoms include anaphylaxis, urticaria, bronchospasm, angioedema, or hypotension. In some cases, the reactions have been fatal. The onset of symptoms generally occurred during an infusion, but there have also been reports of symptom onset after the completion of an infusion. Reactions were most commonly reported in association with the initial infusion.

Interrupt trastuzumab infusion in all patients with severe hypersensitivity reactions. In the event of a hypersensitivity reaction, administer appropriate medical therapy, which may include epinephrine, corticosteroids, diphenhydramine, bronchodilators, and oxygen. Evaluate and carefully monitor patients until complete resolution of signs and symptoms.

There are no data regarding the most appropriate method of identification of patients who may safely be retreated with trastuzumab after experiencing a severe hypersensitivity reaction. Trastuzumab has been readministered to some patients who fully recovered from a previous severe reaction. Prior to readministration of trastuzumab, the majority of these patients were prophylactically treated with premedications including antihistamines and/or corticosteroids. While some of these patients tolerated retreatment, others had severe reactions again despite the use of prophylactic premedications.

▶*Infusion reactions:* In the postmarketing setting, rare occurrences of severe infusion reactions leading to a fatal outcome have been associated with the use of trastuzumab.

In clinical trials, infusion reactions consisted of a symptom complex characterized by fever and chills, and on occasion included nausea, vomiting, pain (in some cases at tumor sites), headache, dizziness, dyspnea, hypotension, rash, and asthenia. These reactions were usually mild-to-moderate in severity (see Adverse Reactions).

However, in postmarketing reports, more severe adverse reactions to trastuzumab infusion were observed and included bronchospasm, hypoxia, and severe hypotension. These severe reactions were usually associated with the initial infusion of trastuzumab and generally occurred during or immediately following the infusion. However, the onset and clinical course were variable. For some patients, symptoms progressively worsened and led to further pulmonary complications (see Pulmonary Events). In other patients with acute onset of signs and symptoms, initial improvement was followed by clinical deterioration. Delayed postinfusion events with rapid clinical deterioration have also been reported. Rarely, severe infusion reactions culminated in death within hours or up to 1 week following an infusion.

Some severe reactions have been treated successfully with interruption of trastuzumab infusion and supportive therapy including oxygen, IV fluids, beta agonists, and corticosteroids.

There are no data regarding the most appropriate method of identification of patients who may safely be retreated with trastuzumab after experiencing a severe infusion reaction. Trastuzumab has been readministered to some patients who fully recovered from the previous severe reaction. Prior to readministration of trastuzumab, the majority of these patients were prophylactically treated with premedications

including antihistamines and/or corticosteroids. While some of these patients tolerated retreatment, others had severe reactions again despite the use of prophylactic premedications.

▶*Pulmonary events:* Patients with either symptomatic intrinsic pulmonary disease (eg, asthma, COPD) or patients with extensive tumor involvement of the lungs (eg, lymphangitic spread of tumor, pleural effusions, parenchymal masses), resulting in dyspnea at rest, may be at increased risk for severe pulmonary adverse events.

Severe pulmonary events leading to death have been reported rarely with the use of trastuzumab in the postmarketing setting. Signs, symptoms, and clinical findings include dyspnea, pulmonary infiltrates, pleural effusions, noncardiogenic pulmonary edema, pulmonary insufficiency and hypoxia, and acute respiratory distress syndrome. These events may or may not occur as sequelae of infusion reactions (see Infusion Reactions). Patients with symptomatic intrinsic lung disease or with extensive tumor involvement of the lungs, resulting in dyspnea at rest, may be at greater risk of severe reactions.

Other severe events reported rarely in the postmarketing setting include pneumonitis and pulmonary fibrosis.

▶*Elderly:* Trastuzumab has been administered to 133 patients who were ≥ 65 years of age. The risk of cardiac dysfunction may be increased in geriatric patients. The reported clinical experience is not adequate to determine whether older patients respond differently than younger patients.

▶*Pregnancy: Category B.* HER2 protein expression is high in many embryonic tissues including cardiac and neural tissues; in mutant mice lacking HER2, embryos died in early gestation. Placental transfer during the early (days 20 to 50 of gestation) and late (days 120 to 150 of gestation) fetal development period was observed. There are no adequate and well-controlled studies in pregnant women. Use during pregnancy only if clearly needed.

▶*Lactation:* Lactating monkeys receiving doses 25 times the weekly human maintenance dose of 2 mg/kg trastuzumab demonstrated that trastuzumab is secreted in the milk. Serum trastuzumab in infant monkeys was not associated with any adverse effects on their growth or development from birth to 3 months of age. Excretion in human breast milk is unknown. Advise women to discontinue nursing during trastuzumab therapy and for 6 months after the last dose because human IgG is excreted in breast milk, and the potential for absorption and harm to the infant is unknown.

▶*Children:* Safety and efficacy in children have not been established.

Precautions

▶*Monitoring:* Frequently monitor patients for deteriorating cardiac function. Assess baseline cardiac function including history and physical exam and ≥ 1 of the following: ECG, echocardiogram, and MUGA scan. Monitoring may not identify all patients who will develop cardiac dysfunction.

▶*Hypersensitivity:* Use trastuzumab therapy with caution in patients with known hypersensitivity to trastuzumab, Chinese Hamster ovary cell proteins, or any component of this product.

▶*Benzyl alcohol:* For patients with a known hypersensitivity to benzyl alcohol (the preservative in Bacteriostatic Water for Injection), reconstitute trastuzumab with Sterile Water for Injection, and discard following a single use.

▶*Immunogenicity:* Of the 903 patients evaluated, human anti-human antibody (HAHA) to trastuzumab was detected in 1 patient, who had no allergic manifestations.

Drug Interactions

There have been no formal drug interaction studies performed with trastuzumab in humans. Administration of paclitaxel in combination with trastuzumab resulted in a 2-fold decrease in trastuzumab clearance in a nonhuman primate study and in a 1.5-fold increase in trastuzumab serum levels in clinical studies (see Pharmacokinetics).

Adverse Reactions

Anemia and leukopenia – An increased incidence of anemia and leukopenia was observed in the treatment group receiving trastuzumab and chemotherapy, especially in the anthracycline with cyclophosphamide subgroup, compared with the treatment group receiving chemotherapy alone. The majority of these cytopenic events were mild or moderate in intensity, reversible, and none resulted in discontinuation of trastuzumab.

Hematologic toxicity is infrequent following single-agent administration with an incidence of Grade III toxicities for WBC, platelets, and hemoglobin all < 1%. No Grade IV toxicities were observed.

Diarrhea – Diarrhea was experienced by 25% of patients receiving trastuzumab. Combination treatment with chemotherapy demonstrated an increased incidence of diarrhea, primarily mild-to-moderate in severity.

Infection – An increased incidence of infections, primarily mild upper respiratory tract infections of minor clinical significance or catheter infections, was observed in patients receiving combination treatment with chemotherapy.

TRASTUZUMAB

Infusion-associated symptoms – During the first trastuzumab infusion, 40% of patients demonstrated a symptom complex most commonly consisting of chills or fever. Symptom severity was usually mild-to-moderate and was treated with acetaminophen, diphenhydramine, and meperidine (with or without reduction in the rate of trastuzumab infusion). Discontinuation was infrequent. Other signs or symptoms may include nausea, vomiting, pain (in some cases at tumor sites), rigors, headache, dizziness, dyspnea, hypotension, rash, and asthenia. The symptoms occurred infrequently with subsequent trastuzumab infusions.

Hypersensitivity reactions including anaphylaxis pulmonary events – In the postmarketing setting, severe hypersensitivity reactions (including anaphylaxis), infusion reactions, and pulmonary adverse events have been reported. These events include anaphylaxis, angioedema, bronchospasm, hypotension, hypoxia, dyspnea, pulmonary infiltrates, pleural effusions, noncardiogenic pulmonary edema, and acute respiratory distress syndrome (see Warnings).

Trastuzumab Adverse Reactions (%)					
Adverse reaction	Trastuzumab alone (n = 352)	Trastuzumab + Paclitaxel (n = 91)	Paclitaxel alone (n = 95)	Trastuzumab + AC[1] (n = 143)	AC[1] alone (n = 135)
Cardiovascular					
Any cardiac dysfunction	7[2]	11	1	28	7
Class III-IV[3]	5[2]	4	1	19	3
CHF	7	11	1	28	7
Tachycardia	5	12	4	10	5
CNS					
Headache	26	36	28	44	31
Depression	6	12	13	20	12
Dizziness	13	22	24	24	18
Insomnia	14	25	13	29	15
Neuropathy	1	13	5	4	4
Paresthesia	9	48	39	17	11
Peripheral neuritis	2	23	16	2	2
Dermatologic					
Acne	2	11	3	3	< 1
Herpes simplex	2	12	3	7	9
Rash	18	38	18	27	17
GI					
Anorexia	14	24	16	31	26
Diarrhea	25	45	29	45	26
Nausea	33	51	9	76	77
Nausea and vomiting	8	14	11	18	9
Vomiting	23	37	28	53	49
Hemic and Lymphatic					
Anemia	4	14	9	36	26
Leukopenia	3	24	17	52	34
Metabolic					
Edema	8	10	8	11	5
Peripheral edema	10	22	20	20	17
Musculoskeletal					
Arthralgia	6	37	21	8	9
Bone pain	7	24	18	7	7
Respiratory					
Cough increased	26	41	22	43	29
Dyspnea	22	27	26	42	25
Pharyngitis	12	22	14	30	18
Rhinitis	14	22	5	22	16
Sinusitis	9	21	7	13	6
Miscellaneous					
Abdominal pain	22	34	22	23	18
Accidental injury	6	13	3	9	4
Allergic reaction	3	8	2	4	2
Asthenia	42	62	57	54	55
Back pain	22	34	30	27	15
Chills	32	41	4	35	11
Fever	36	49	23	56	34
Flu syndrome	10	12	5	12	6
Infection	20	47	27	47	31
Pain	47	61	62	57	42
Urinary tract infection	5	18	14	13	7

[1] Anthracycline (doxorubicin or epirubicin) and cyclophosphamide.
[2] Trastuzumab n = 213.
[3] Classified for severity using the NY Heart Association classification system I-IV, when IV is the most severe level of cardiac failure.

Other serious adverse events – The following other serious adverse events occurred in ≥ 1 of the 958 patients treated with trastuzumab:

➤*Cardiovascular:* Vascular thrombosis; pericardial effusion; heart arrest; hypotension; syncope; hemorrhage; shock arrhythmia.

➤*CNS:* Convulsion; ataxia; confusion; manic reaction.

➤*Dermatologic:* Herpes zoster; skin ulceration.

➤*GI:* Hepatic failure; gastroenteritis; hematemesis; ileus; intestinal obstruction; colitis; esophageal ulcer; stomatitis; pancreatitis; hepatitis.

➤*GU:* Hydronephrosis; kidney failure; cervical cancer; hematuria; hemorrhagic cystitis; pyelonephritis.

➤*Hematologic:* Pancytopenia; acute leukemia; coagulation disorder; lymphangitis.

➤*Metabolic:* Hypercalcemia; hypomagnesemia; hyponatremia; hypoglycemia; growth retardation; weight loss.

➤*Musculoskeletal:* Pathological fractures; bone necrosis; myopathy.

➤*Respiratory:* Apnea; pneumothorax; asthma; hypoxia; laryngitis.

➤*Miscellaneous:* Cellulitis; anaphylactoid reaction; ascites; hydrocephalus; radiation injury; deafness; amblyopia; hypothyroidism.

Overdosage

There is no experience with overdosage in human clinical trials. Single doses > 500 mg have not been tested.

GEMTUZUMAB OZOGAMICIN

Rx **Mylotarg** (Wyeth-Ayerst)	**Powder for injection, lyophilized:** 5 mg	Preservative free. NaCl, mono/dibasic sodium phosphate. In single 20 ml vials.

WARNING

Administer under the supervision of a physician who is experienced in the use of cancer chemotherapeutic agents.

Severe myelosuppression occurs when gemtuzumab ozogamicin is used at recommended doses.

Indications

►*Acute myeloid leukemia (AML):* Treatment of patients with CD33 positive acute myeloid leukemia in first relapse who are ≥ 60 years of age and who are not considered candidates for cytotoxic chemotherapy.

Administration and Dosage

►*Approved by the FDA:* May 18, 2000.

The recommended dose of gemtuzumab ozogamicin is 9 mg/m^2, administered as a 2–hour IV infusion. Give the following prophylactic medications 1 hour before gemtuzumab ozogamicin administration; diphenhydramine 50 mg orally and acetaminophen 650 to 1000 mg orally; thereafter, 2 additional doses of acetaminophen 650 to 1000 mg orally, 1 every 4 hours as needed. Monitor vital signs during infusion and for 4 hours following infusion. The recommended treatment course with gemtuzumab ozogamicin is a total of 2 doses, 14 days apart. Full recovery from hematologic toxicities is not a requirement for administration of the second dose. Gemtuzumab ozogamicin may be administered in an outpatient setting.

►*Preparation for administration:* Protect from direct and indirect sunlight and unshielded fluorescent light during the preparation and administration of the infusion. Prepare the drug in a biologic safety hood with the fluorescent light off. Prior to reconstitution, allow drug vials to come to room temperature. Reconstitute each vial with 5 ml Sterile Water for Injection, using sterile syringes. Gently swirl each vial. The final concentration of drug in the vial is 1 mg/ml. Inspect visually for particulate matter and discoloration following reconstitution and prior to administration.

Withdraw the desired volume from each vial and inject into a 100 ml IV bag of 0.9% Sodium Chloride Injection. Place the 100 ml IV bag into a UV protectant bag. Use the resulting drug solution in the IV bag immediately.

►*Administration:* Do not administer as an IV push or bolus.

Once the reconstituted gemtuzumab ozogamicin is diluted into the IV bag containing normal saline, infuse the resulting solution over a 2–hour period. A separate IV line equipped with a low protein-binding 1.2 micron terminal filter must be used for administration of the drug. Use a UV protective bag over the IV bag during infusion. Gemtuzumab ozogamicin may be given peripherally or through a central line.

►*Storage/Stability:* Store refrigerated (2° to 8°C; 36° to 46°F). Protect from light. While in the vial, the reconstituted drug may be stored refrigerated (2° to 8°C; 36° to 46°F) and protected from light for ≤ 8 hours.

Actions

►*Pharmacology:* Gemtuzumab ozogamicin is a chemotherapy agent composed of a recombinant humanized IgG$_4$ kappa antibody conjugated with a cytotoxic antitumor antibiotic, calicheamicin, isolated from fermentation of a bacterium, *Micromonospora echinospora* sp. *calichensis*. The antibody portion of gemtuzumab ozogamicin binds specifically to the CD33 antigen. This antigen is expressed on the surface of leukemic blasts in > 80% of patients with acute myeloid leukemia (AML). CD33 is also expressed on normal and leukemic myeloid colony-forming cells, including leukemic clonogenic precursors, but it is not expressed on pluripotent hematopoietic stem cells or on nonhematopoietic cells.

Mechanism of action – Binding of the anti-CD33 antibody portion of gemtuzumab ozogamicin with the CD33 antigen results in the formation of a complex that is internalized. Upon internalization, the calicheamicin derivative is released inside the lysosomes of the myeloid cell. The released calicheamicin derivative binds to DNA in the minor groove resulting in DNA double strand breaks and cell death.

Gemtuzumab ozogamicin is cytotoxic to the CD33 positive HL-60 human leukemia cell line. It produces significant inhibition of colony formation in cultures of adult leukemic bone marrow cells. The cytotoxic effect on normal myeloid precursors leads to substantial myelosuppression, but this is reversible because pluripotent hematopoietic stem cells are spared.

►*Pharmacokinetics:* After administration of the first recommended 9 mg/m^2 dose of gemtuzumab ozogamicin, given as a 2–hour infusion, the elimination terminal half-lives of total and unconjugated calicheamicin were ≈ 45 and 100 hours, respectively. After the second 9 mg/m^2 dose, the t½ of total calicheamicin was increased to ≈ 60 hours and the area under the concentration time curve (AUC) was about twice that in the first dose period. The pharmacokinetics of unconjugated calicheamicin did not appear to change from period 1 to 2. Metabolic studies indicate hydrolytic release of the calicheamicin derivative from gemtuzumab ozogamicin. Many metabolites of this derivative were found after in vitro incubation of gemtuzumab ozogamicin in human liver microsomes and cytosol, and in HL-60 promyelocytic leukemia cells.

►*Clinical trials:* Available single-arm trial data do not provide valid comparisons with various cytotoxic regimens that have been used in relapsed acute myeloid leukemia. Response rates are in the range of rates reported with such regimens only if the CR$_p$ (complete remission including platelet transfusion independence) responses are included. Nevertheless, treatment with gemtuzumab ozogamicin can provide responses, including some of reasonable duration. The data support its use in patients for whom aggressive cytotoxic regimens would be considered unsuitable, such as many patients ≥ 60 years of age.

Contraindications

Hypersensitivity to gemtuzumab ozogamicin or any of its components: anti-CD33 antibody (hP67.6), calicheamicin derivatives, or inactive ingredients.

Warnings

The safety and efficacy of gemtuzumab ozogamicin in patients with poor performance status and organ dysfunction have not been established.

►*Myelosuppression:* Severe myelosuppression will occur in all patients given the recommended dose of this agent. Careful hematologic monitoring is required. Treat systemic infections.

►*Allergic reactions:* Gemtuzumab ozogamicin can produce a postinfusion symptom complex of fever and chills, and less commonly hypotension and dyspnea that may occur during the first 24 hours after administration. Grade 3 or 4 non-hematologic infusion-related adverse events included chills, fever, hypotension, hypertension, hyperglycemia, hypoxia, and dyspnea. Most patients received the following prophylactic medications before administration: diphenhydramine 50 mg orally and acetaminophen 650 to 1000 mg orally; thereafter, 2 additional doses of acetaminophen 650 to 1000 mg orally, 1 every 4 hours as needed. Monitor vital signs during infusion and for the 4 hours following infusion.

►*Hepatic function impairment:* Gemtuzumab ozogamicin has not been studied in patients with bilirubin > 2 mg/dl. Exercise caution when administering gemtuzumab ozogamicin in patients with hepatic impairment (see Adverse Reactions).

►*Pregnancy: Category D.* Gemtuzumab ozogamicin may cause fetal harm when administered to a pregnant woman. Daily treatment of pregnant rats with gemtuzumab ozogamicin during organogenesis caused dose-related decreases in fetal weight in association with dose-related decreases in fetal skeletal ossification beginning at 0.025 mg/kg/day. Doses of 0.06 mg/kg/day (≈ 0.04 times the recommended human single dose on a mg/m^2 basis) produced increased embryo-fetal mortality. Gross external, visceral, and skeletal alterations at the 0.06 mg/kg/day dose level included digital malformations, absence of the aortic arch, wavy ribs, anomalies of the long bones in the forelimb(s), misshapen scapula, absence of vertebral centrum, and fused sternebrae. This dose was also associated with maternal toxicity (decreased weight gain, decreased food consumption). There are no adequate and well-controlled studies in pregnant women. If gemtuzumab ozogamicin is used in pregnancy, or if the patient becomes pregnant while taking it, apprise the patient of the potential hazard to the fetus. Advise women of childbearing potential to avoid becoming pregnant while receiving treatment with gemtuzumab ozogamicin.

►*Lactation:* It is not known if gemtuzumab ozogamicin is excreted in breast milk. Because many drugs, including immunoglobulins, are excreted in breast milk, and because of the potential for serious adverse reactions in nursing infants from gemtuzumab ozogamicin, decide whether to discontinue nursing or to discontinue the drug, taking into account the importance of the drug to the mother.

►*Children:* The safety and efficacy of gemtuzumab ozogamicin in pediatric patients have not been studied.

Precautions

Do not administer as an IV push or bolus.

►*Tumor lysis syndrome:* Tumor lysis syndrome may be a consequence of leukemia treatment. Take appropriate measures (eg, hydration, allopurinol) to prevent hyperuricemia.

►*Laboratory monitoring:* Monitor electrolytes, hepatic function, complete blood counts (CBCs), and platelet counts.

Drug Interactions

There have been no formal drug interaction studies performed with gemtuzumab ozogamicin.

Adverse Reactions

Gemtuzumab ozogamicin has been administered to 142 patients with relapsed AML at 9 mg/m^2. It was generally given as 2 IV infusions separated by 14 days.

GEMTUZUMAB OZOGAMICIN

Acute Infusion-Related Adverse Reactions (%)		
Adverse reaction	Any severity	Grade 3 or 4
Chills	62	11
Fever	61	7
Nausea	38	< 1
Vomiting	32	< 1
Headache	12	< 1
Hypotension	11	4
Hypertension	6	3
Hypoxia	6	2
Dyspnea	4	1
Hyperglycemia	2	2

These symptoms generally occurred after the end of the 2–hour IV infusion and resolved after 2 to 4 hours with a supportive therapy of acetaminophen, diphenhydramine, and IV fluids. Fewer infusion-related events were observed after the second dose.

Antibody formation – Antibodies to gemtuzumab ozogamicin were not detected in a total of 142 patients in the Phase 2 clinical studies. Two patients in a Phase 1 study developed antibody titers against the calicheamicin/calicheamicin-linker portion of gemtuzumab ozogamicin after 3 doses. One patient experienced transient fever, hypotension, and dyspnea; the other patient had no clinical symptoms. No patient developed antibody responses to the hP67.6 antibody portion of gemtuzumab ozogamicin.

Myelosuppression – Severe myelosuppression is the major toxicity associated with gemtuzumab ozogamicin. During the treatment phase, 98% of patients experienced Grade 3 or 4 neutropenia. Responding patients recovered ANCs to 500/mcl by a median of 40.5 days after the first dose of gemtuzumab ozogamicin.

Anemia / Thrombocytopenia – During the treatment phase, 99% of patients experienced Grade 3 or 4 thrombocytopenia. Responding patients recovered platelet counts to 25,000/mcl by a median of 39 days after the first dose of gemtuzumab ozogamicin. Forty-seven percent of patients experienced Grade 3 or 4 anemia.

Infection – During the treatment phase, 28% of patients experienced Grade 3 or 4 infections, including opportunistic infections. The most frequent Grade 3 or 4 infection-related treatment-emergent adverse events (TEAEs) were sepsis (16%) and pneumonia (7%). Herpes simplex infection was reported in 22% of the patients.

Bleeding – During the treatment phase, 15% of patients experienced Grade 3 or 4 bleeding. The most frequent severe TEAE was epistaxis (3%). There were also reports of cerebral hemorrhage (2%), disseminated intravascular coagulation (2%), intracranial hemorrhage (2%), and hematuria (1%).

Transfusions – During the treatment phase, more transfusions were required in the NR and CR$_p$ (n = 119, total) patients compared with the CRs (n = 23).

Mucositis – A total of 35% of patients were reported to have a TEAE consistent with oral mucositis or stomatitis. During the treatment phase, 4% of patients experienced Grade 3 or 4 stomatitis/mucositis after the first dose. The mucositis events for the remaining 32% of patients were Grade 1 or 2.

Hepatotoxicity – Abnormalities of liver function were transient and generally reversible. In clinical studies, 23% of patients experienced Grade 3 or 4 hyperbilirubinemia. Nine percent of patients experienced Grade 3 or 4 abnormalities in levels of ALT, and 17% of patients experienced Grade 3 or 4 abnormalities in levels of AST. Thirteen patients had concurrent elevations of transaminases (Grade 3 to 4) and bilirubin. One patient died with liver failure in the setting of tumor lysis syndrome and multisystem organ failure 22 days after treatment. Another patient died after an episode of persistent jaundice and hepatosplenomegaly 156 days after treatment. Among 27 patients who received hematopoietic stem cell transplantations following gemtuzumab ozogamicin, 4 (3 NRs, 1 CR) died of hepatic veno-occlusive disease (VOD) 22 to 392 days following transplantation.

Dermatologic – No patients experienced alopecia. A nonspecific rash was reported in 22%.

Retreatment events – Five patients have received > 1 course of gemtuzumab ozogamicin, 4 of these patients at 9 mg/m^2. The adverse event profile for retreated patients was similar to that following their initial treatment. One of the repeat dose patients was in a Phase 1 study and received a first course of 3 doses at 1 mg/m^2 and 2 doses of a second course at 6 mg/m^2. This patient was discontinued from further dose administration as a result of an immune response to the calicheamicin/calicheamicin-linker portion of gemtuzumab ozogamicin. The 4 other retreated patients did not experience an immune response.

Dose relationship for adverse events – Dose-relationship data were generated from a small dose-escalation study. The most common clinical adverse event observed in this study was an infusion-related symptom complex of fever and chills. In general, the severity of fever, but not chills, increased as the dose level increased.

Adverse events – Adverse events (Grades 1 to 4) that occurred in ≥ 10% of the patients regardless of causality are listed in the following table:

Gemtuzumab Ozogamicin Patients with Adverse Reactions[1] (All Grades; Incidence ≥ 10%)[2]		
	Efficacy and safety studies	
Adverse reaction	All patients (n = 142)	Ages ≥ 60 (n = 80)
Cardiovascular		
Hemorrhage	10	8
Hypertension	20	20
Hypotension	20	16
Tachycardia	11	10
CNS		
Depression	9	10
Dizziness	15	11
Insomnia	15	18
Dermatologic		
Herpes simplex	22	15
Rash	22	23
Local reaction	25	25
Peripheral edema	16	21
Petechiae	20	21
GI		
Anorexia	29	31
Constipation	25	28
Diarrhea	38	38
Dyspepsia	11	11
Nausea	70	64
Stomatitis	32	25
Vomiting	63	55
GU[3]		
Hematuria	10	10
Vaginal hemorrhage	12	7
Metabolic		
Hypokalemia	31	30
Hypomagnesemia	10	4
Lactic dehydrogenase increased	13	18
Respiratory		
Cough increased	20	19
Dyspnea	32	36
Epistaxis	31	29
Pharyngitis	14	14
Pneumonia	10	10
Pulmonary physical finding[4]	11	13
Rhinitis	10	10
Miscellaneous		
Abdomen enlarged	9	11
Abdominal pain	37	29
Arthralgia	8	10
Asthenia	44	45
Back pain	15	18
Chills	73	66
Ecchymosis	13	15
Fever	85	80
Headache	35	26
Neutropenic fever	21	20
Pain	21	25
Sepsis	25	24

[1] Does not include changes in laboratory values reported as adverse events for events included in the NCI common toxicity scale.
[2] ≥ 10% limit specifies the minimum percentage threshold from ≥ 1 column for an event to be displayed in the table.
[3] Percentages for sex-specific adverse events are based on the number of patients of the relevant sex.
[4] Includes rales, rhonchi, and changes in breath sounds.

Gemtuzumab Ozogamicin Patients with Severe or NCI Grade 3 or 4 Adverse Reactions[1] (Incidence ≥ 5%)[2]		
	Efficacy and safety studies Grades 3 or 4	
Adverse reaction	All patients (n = 142)	Ages ≥ 60 (n = 80)
Cardiovascular		
Hypertension	9	11
Hypotension	8	8
Metabolic		
Hypokalemia	3	5
Lactic dehydrogenase increased	4	8
Respiratory		
Dyspnea	9	13
Pneumonia	7	6

GEMTUZUMAB OZOGAMICIN

Gemtuzumab Ozogamicin Patients with Severe or NCI Grade 3 or 4 Adverse Reactions[1] (Incidence ≥ 5%)[2]		
	Efficacy and safety studies Grades 3 or 4	
Adverse reaction	All patients (n = 142)	Ages ≥ 60 (n = 80)
Miscellaneous		
Any adverse event	91	88
Asthenia	7	10
Chills	13	15
Fever	15	14
Nausea	9	8
Neutropenic fever	7	5
Sepsis	16	16

[1] Does not include changes in laboratory values reported as adverse events for events included in the NCI common toxicity scale.

[2] ≥ 5% limit specifies the minimum percentage threshold from ≥ 1 column for an event to be displayed in the table.

Clinically important laboratory abnormalities with a Grade 3 or 4 severity are listed in the following table:

Gemtuzumab Ozogamicin Patients with Laboratory Test Results of Grade 3 or 4 Severity[1] (%)[2]		
	Efficacy and safety studies Grades 3 or 4	
Test	All patients (n = 142)	Age ≥ 60 (n = 80)
Hematologic		
Hemoglobin	47	45
WBC	96	94
Total neutrophils, absolute	98	99
Lymphocytes	93	89
Platelet count	99	99
Prothrombin time	4	4
Partial thromboplastin time	1	2

Gemtuzumab Ozogamicin Patients with Laboratory Test Results of Grade 3 or 4 Severity[1] (%)[2]		
	Efficacy and safety studies Grades 3 or 4	
Test	All patients (n = 142)	Age ≥ 60 (n = 80)
Non-hematologic		
Glucose	12	11
Creatinine	1	0
Total bilirubin	23	23
AST	17	15
ALT	9	9
Alkaline phosphatase	4	1
Calcium	12	6

[1] Severity as defined by NCI common toxicity scale version 1.

[2] Percentage is based on the number of patients receiving a particular laboratory test during the study as is indicated for each test.

There were no clinically important differences in adverse events between patients < 60 years of age and those patients ≥ 60 years of age. Laboratory parameters associated with hepatic dysfunction (eg, elevated levels of bilirubin, AST, and ALT) were more consistently observed in patients ≥ 60 years of age than those < 60 years of age.

There were no clinically important differences in adverse events between female and male patients.

Overdosage

No cases of overdose with gemtuzumab ozogamicin were reported in clinical experience. When a single dose of gemtuzumab ozogamicin was administered to animals, mortality was observed in rats at the dose of 2 mg/kg (≈ 1.3 times the recommended human dose on a mg/m² basis), and in male monkeys at the dose of 4.5 mg/kg (≈ 6 times the recommended human dose on a mg/m² basis).

➤*Treatment:* Follow general supportive measures in case of overdose. Carefully monitor blood pressure and blood counts. Gemtuzumab ozogamicin is not dialyzable.

ALEMTUZUMAB

Rx   **Campath** (Berlex)   **Solution for injection:** 30 mg/3 mL   24 mg sodium chloride, 3.5 mg dibasic sodium phosphate, 0.6 mg potassium chloride, 0.6 mg monobasic potassium phosphate, 0.056 mg EDTA. Preservative free. In amps (3s and 12s).

WARNING

Administer alemtuzumab under the supervision of a physician experienced in the use of antineoplastic therapy.

Hematologic toxicity: Serious and, in rare instances, fatal pancytopenia/marrow hypoplasia, autoimmune idiopathic thrombocytopenia, and autoimmune hemolytic anemia have occurred in patients receiving alemtuzumab therapy. Do not administer single doses of alemtuzumab > 30 mg or cumulative doses > 90 mg per week because these doses are associated with a higher incidence of pancytopenia.

Infusion reactions: Alemtuzumab can result in serious infusion reactions. Carefully monitor patients during infusions and discontinue alemtuzumab if indicated. Gradual escalation to the recommended maintenance dose is required at the initiation of therapy and after interruption of therapy for ≥ 7 days.

Infections/Opportunistic infections: Serious, sometimes fatal bacterial, viral, fungal, and protozoan infections have been reported in patients receiving alemtuzumab therapy. Prophylaxis directed against *Pneumocystis carinii* pneumonia (PCP) and herpes virus infections has been shown to decrease, but not eliminate, the occurrence of these infections.

Indications

➤*B-cell chronic lymphocytic leukemia (B-CLL):* For the treatment of B-CLL in patients who have been treated with alkylating agents and who have failed fludarabine therapy.

Administration and Dosage

➤*Approved by the FDA:* May 7, 2001.

Administer IV only. Administer over a 2-hour period. Do not administer as an IV push or bolus.

Initiate therapy at a dose of 3 mg administered as a 2-hour IV infusion daily. When the 3 mg daily dose is tolerated (eg, infusion-related toxicities are Grade 2 or less), escalate the daily dose to 10 mg and continue until tolerated. When the 10 mg dose is tolerated, the maintenance dose of 30 mg may be initiated. The maintenance dose is 30 mg/day administered 3 times/week on alternate days (ie, Monday, Wednesday, and Friday) for ≤ 12 weeks. In most patients, escalation to 30 mg can be accomplished in 3 to 7 days. Dose escalation to the recommended maintenance dose of 30 mg administered 3 times/week is required. Do not administer single doses > 30 mg or cumulative weekly doses > 90 mg because higher doses are associated with an increased incidence of pancytopenia.

➤*Concomitant medications:* Give premedication prior to the first dose, at dose escalations, and as clinically indicated. The premedication used in clinical studies was diphenhydramine 50 mg and acetaminophen 650 mg administered 30 minutes prior to alemtuzumab infusion. In cases where severe infusion-related events occur, treatment with hydrocortisone 200 mg was used in decreasing infusion-related events.

Give patients anti-infective prophylaxis to minimize the risks of serious opportunistic infections. The anti-infective regimen used in Study 1 consisted of trimethoprim/sulfamethoxazole DS twice a day 3 times/week and famciclovir or equivalent 250 mg twice a day upon initiation of alemtuzumab therapy. Continue prophylaxis for 2 months after completion of therapy or until the CD4⁺ count is ≥ 200 cells/mcL, whichever occurs later.

➤*Dose modification and reinitiation of therapy:* Discontinue alemtuzumab therapy during serious infection, serious hematologic toxicity, or other serious toxicity until the event resolves. Permanently discontinue therapy if evidence of autoimmune anemia or thrombocytopenia appears. The following table includes recommendations for dose modification for severe neutropenia or thrombocytopenia.

Dose Modification and Reinitiation of Alemtuzumab Therapy for Hematologic Toxicity	
Hematologic toxicity	Dose modification and reinitiation of therapy
For first occurrence of ANC < 250/mcL and/or platelet count ≤ 25,000/mcL	Withhold therapy. When ANC ≥ 500/mcL and platelet count ≥ 50,000/mcL, resume therapy at same dose. If delay between dosing is ≥ 7 days, initiate therapy at 3 mg and escalate to 10 mg and then to 30 mg as tolerated.
For second occurrence of ANC < 250/mcL and/or platelet count ≤ 25,000/mcL	Withhold therapy. When ANC ≥ 500/mcL and platelet count ≥ 50,000/mcL, resume therapy at 10 mg. If delay between dosing is ≥ 7 days, initiate therapy at 3 mg and escalate to 10 mg only.
For a third occurrence of ANC < 250/mcL and/or platelet count ≤ 25,000/mcL	Discontinue therapy permanently.
For a decrease in ANC and/or platelet count ≤ 50% of the baseline value in patients initiating therapy with a baseline ANC ≤ 500/mcL and/or a baseline platelet count ≤ 25,000/mcL	Withhold therapy. When ANC and platelet count return to baseline value(s), resume therapy. If the delay between dosing is ≥ 7 days, initiate therapy at 3 mg and escalate to 10 mg and then to 30 mg as tolerated.

ALEMTUZUMAB

➤*Preparation for administration:* If particulate matter is present or the solution is discolored, do not use the vial. Do not shake ampule prior to use. Withdraw the necessary amount of alemtuzumab from the ampule into a syringe. Filter with a sterile, low protein-binding, non-fiber-releasing 5 mcm filter prior to dilution.

Inject into 100 mL sterile 0.9% Sodium Chloride or 5% Dextrose in Water. Gently invert the bag to mix the solution. Discard syringe and any unused drug product.

➤*Incompatibilities:* Other drug substances should not be added or simultaneously infused through the same IV line.

➤*Storage/Stability:* Alemtuzumab contains no antimicrobial preservative. Use within 8 hours after dilution. Solutions may be stored at room temperature (15° to 30°C; 59° to 86°F) or refrigerated. Protect from light.

Prior to dilution, store at 2° to 8°C (36° to 46°F). Do not freeze. Discard if ampule has been frozen. Protect from direct sunlight.

Actions

➤*Pharmacology:* Alemtuzumab is a recombinant DNA-derived humanized monoclonal antibody (Campath-1H) that is directed against the 21-28 kD cell surface glycoprotein CD52. The Campath-1H antibody is an IgG1 kappa with human variable framework and constant regions, and complementarity-determining regions from a murine (rat) monoclonal antibody (Campath-1G). The Campath-1H antibody has an approximate molecular weight of 150 kD.

Alemtuzumab binds to CD52, a nonmodulating antigen that is present on the surface of essentially all B and T lymphocytes, a majority of monocytes, macrophages, and NK cells, and a subpopulation of granulocytes. Analysis of samples collected from multiple volunteers has not identified CD52 expression on erythrocytes or hematopoietic stem cells. The proposed mechanism of action is antibody-dependent lysis of leukemic cells following cell surface binding. Campath-1H Fab binding was observed in lymphoid tissues and the mononuclear phagocyte system. A proportion of bone marrow cells, including some CD34⁺ cells, express variable levels of CD52. Significant binding was also observed in the skin and male reproductive tract (epididymis, sperm, seminal vesicle). Mature spermatozoa stain for CD52, but neither spermatogenic cells nor immature spermatozoa show evidence of staining.

➤*Pharmacokinetics:* The pharmacokinetic profile of alemtuzumab was studied in a multicenter rising-dose trial in non-Hodgkin's lymphoma (NHL) and chronic lymphocytic leukemia (CLL). Alemtuzumab was administered once weekly for a maximum of 12 weeks. Following IV infusions over a range of doses, the maximum serum concentration (C_{max}) and the area under the curve (AUC) showed relative dose proportionality. The overall average half-life ($t_{1/2}$) over the dosing interval was ≈ 12 days. The pharmacokinetic profile of alemtuzumab administered as a 30 mg IV infusion 3 times/week was evaluated in CLL patients. Peak and trough levels of alemtuzumab rose during the first few weeks of treatment, and appeared to approach steady state by approximately week 6, although there was marked interpatient variability. The rise in serum alemtuzumab concentration corresponded with the reduction in malignant lymphocytosis.

Contraindications

Active systemic infections, underlying immunodeficiency (eg, seropositive for HIV), or known Type I hypersensitivity or anaphylactic reactions to alemtuzumab or any of its components.

Warnings

➤*Infusion-related events:* Alemtuzumab has been associated with infusion-related events including hypotension, rigors, fever, shortness of breath, bronchospasm, chills, or rash. In order to ameliorate or avoid infusion-related events, premedicate patients with an oral antihistamine and acetaminophen prior to dosing and monitor closely for infusion-related adverse events. In addition, initiate alemtuzumab at a low dose with gradual escalation to the effective dose. Careful monitoring of blood pressure and hypotensive symptoms is recommended, especially in patients with ischemic heart disease and in patients on antihypertensive medications. If therapy is interrupted for ≥ 7 days, reinstitute alemtuzumab with gradual dose escalation.

➤*Immunosuppression/Opportunistic infections:* Alemtuzumab induces profound lymphopenia. A variety of opportunistic infections have been reported in patients receiving alemtuzumab therapy. If a serious infection occurs, interrupt alemtuzumab therapy; therapy may be reinitiated following the resolution of the infection.

Anti-infective prophylaxis is recommended upon initiation of therapy and for a minimum of 2 months following the last dose of alemtuzumab or until CD4⁺ counts are ≥ 200 cells/mcL. The median time to recovery of CD4⁺ counts to ≥ 200 cells/mcL was 2 months; however, full recovery (to baseline) of CD4⁺ and CD8⁺ counts may take > 12 months.

Because of the potential for graft vs host disease (GVHD) in severely lymphopenic patients, irradiation of any blood products administered prior to recovery from lymphopenia is recommended.

➤*Hematologic toxicity:* Severe, prolonged, and in rare instances, fatal myelosuppression has occurred in patients with leukemia and lymphoma receiving alemtuzumab. Bone marrow aplasia and hypopla-

sia were observed in the clinical studies at the recommended dose. The incidence of these complications increased with doses above the recommended dose. In addition, severe and fatal autoimmune anemia and thrombocytopenia were observed in patients with CLL. Discontinue alemtuzumab for severe hematologic toxicity or in any patient with evidence of autoimmune hematologic toxicity. Following resolution of transient, nonimmune myelosuppression, alemtuzumab may be reinitiated with caution. There is no information on the safety of resumption of alemtuzumab in patients with autoimmune cytopenias or marrow aplasia.

➤*Pregnancy: Category C.* Animal reproduction studies have not been conducted with alemtuzumab. It is not known whether alemtuzumab can affect reproductive capacity or cause fetal harm when administered to a pregnant woman. However, human IgG is known to cross the placental barrier and therefore alemtuzumab may cross the placental barrier and cause fetal B and T lymphocyte depletion. Give alemtuzumab to a pregnant woman only if clearly needed.

➤*Lactation:* Excretion of alemtuzumab in breast milk has not been studied. Because many drugs including human IgG are excreted in breast milk, discontinue breastfeeding during treatment and for ≥ 3 months following the last dose of alemtuzumab.

➤*Children:* The safety and efficacy of alemtuzumab in children have not been established.

Precautions

➤*Monitoring:* Obtain complete blood counts (CBC) and platelet counts at weekly intervals during alemtuzumab therapy and more frequently if worsening anemia, neutropenia, or thrombocytopenia is observed on therapy. Assess CD4⁺ counts after treatment until recovery to ≥ 200 cells/mcL.

➤*Immunization:* Because of their immunosuppression, do not immunize patients who have recently received alemtuzumab with live viral vaccines. The safety of immunization with live viral vaccines following alemtuzumab therapy has not been studied. The ability to generate a primary or anamnestic humoral response to any vaccine following alemtuzumab therapy has not been studied.

➤*Immunogenicity:* Four (1.9%) of 211 patients evaluated for development of an immune response were found to have antibodies to alemtuzumab. The data reflect the percentage of patients whose test results were considered positive for antibody to alemtuzumab in a kinetic enzyme immunoassay, and are highly dependent on the sensitivity and specificity of the assay. The observed incidence of antibody positivity may be influenced by several additional factors, including sample handling, concomitant medications, and underlying disease. For these reasons, comparison of the incidence of antibodies to alemtuzumab with the incidence of antibodies to other products may be misleading. Patients who develop hypersensitivity to alemtuzumab may have allergic or hypersensitivity reactions to other monoclonal antibodies.

➤*Lab test abnormalities:* An immune response to alemtuzumab may interfere with subsequent diagnostic serum tests that utilize antibodies.

Adverse Reactions

Alemtuzumab Adverse Reactions in > 5% of the B-CLL Study Population During Treatment or Within 30 Days[1]		
	B-CLL studies (n = 149)	
Adverse reaction	Any grade	Grade 3 or 4
Cardiovascular		
Hypotension	32	5
Tachycardia, SVT	11	3
Hypertension	11	2
CNS		
Headache	24	1
Dysesthesias	15	—
Dizziness	12	1
Insomnia	10	—
Depression	7	1
Tremor	7	—
Somnolence	5	1
Dermatologic		
Rash, maculopapular rash, erythematous rash	40	3
Urticaria	30	5
Pruritus	24	1
Sweating increased	19	1
GI		
Nausea	54	2
Vomiting	41	4
Diarrhea	22	1
Stomatitis, ulcerative stomatitis, mucositis	14	1
Abdominal pain	11	2
Dyspepsia	10	—
Constipation	9	1

ALEMTUZUMAB

Alemtuzumab Adverse Reactions in > 5% of the B-CLL Study Population During Treatment or Within 30 Days[1]

	B-CLL studies (n = 149)	
Adverse reaction	Any grade	Grade 3 or 4
Hematologic		
Neutropenia	85	64
Anemia	80	38
Thrombocytopenia	72	50
Purpura	8	—
Epistaxis	7	1
Pancytopenia	5	3
Respiratory		
Dyspnea	26	9
Cough	25	2
Bronchitis, pneumonitis	21	13
Pneumonia	16	10
Pharyngitis	12	—
Bronchospasm	9	2
Rhinitis	7	—
Miscellaneous		
Rigors	86	16
Fever	85	19
Fatigue	34	5
Pain, skeletal pain	24	2
Anorexia	20	3
Sepsis	15	10
Asthenia	13	4
Edema, peripheral edema	13	1
Herpes simplex	11	1
Myalgias	11	—
Back pain	10	3
Chest pain	10	1
Malaise	9	1
Moniliasis	8	1
Infection (other viral or unidentified)	7	1
Temperature change sensation	5	—

[1] Data are based on 149 patients with B-CLL enrolled in studies of alemtuzumab as a single agent administered at a maintenance dosage of 30 mg IV 3 times weekly for 4 to 12 weeks.

Infusion-related adverse events resulted in discontinuation of alemtuzumab therapy in 6% of patients enrolled in Study 1 (n = 93). The most commonly reported infusion-related adverse events on this study included rigors (89%), drug-related fever (83%), nausea (47%), vomiting (33%), and hypotension (15%). Other frequently reported infusion-related events include rash (30%), fatigue (22%), urticaria (22%), dyspnea (17%), pruritus (14%), headache (13%), and diarrhea (13%). Similar types of adverse reactions were reported on the supporting studies. Acute infusion-related events were most common during the first week of therapy. Antihistamines, acetaminophen, antiemetics, meperidine, and corticosteroids as well as incremental dose escalation were used to prevent or ameliorate infusion-related events.

On Study 1, all patients were required to receive antiherpes and anti-PCP prophylaxis and were followed for infections for 6 months. Forty (43%) of 93 patients experienced 59 infections (≥ 1 infection per patient) related to alemtuzumab during treatment or within 6 months of the last dose. Of these, 37% of patients experienced 42 infections that were of Grade 3 or 4 severity; 18% were fatal. Fifty-five percent of the Grade 3 and 4 infections occurred during treatment or within 30 days of the last dose. In addition, ≥ 1 episode of febrile neutropenia (ANC ≤ 500 cells/mcL) were reported in 10% of patients.

The following types of infections were reported in Study 1: Grade 3 or 4 sepsis in 12% of patients with 1 fatality, Grade 3 or 4 pneumonia in 15% with 5 fatalities, and opportunistic infections in 17% with 4 fatalities. Candida infections were reported in 5% of patients; CMV infections in 8% (4% of Grade 3 or 4 severity); aspergillosis in 2% with fatal aspergillosis in 1%; fatal mucormycosis in 2%; fatal cryptococcal pneumonia in 1%; *Listeria monocytogenes* meningitis in 1%; disseminated herpes zoster in 1%; Grade 3 herpes simplex in 2%; and *Torulopsis* pneumonia in 1%. PCP pneumonia occurred in 1 (1%) patient who discontinued PCP prophylaxis.

In studies 2 and 3, in which antiherpes and anti-PCP prophylaxis was optional, 37 (66%) patients had 47 infections during or after receiving alemtuzumab therapy. In addition to the opportunistic infections reported above, the following types of related events were observed in these studies: interstitial pneumonitis of unknown etiology and progressive multifocal leukoencephalopathy.

Alemtuzumab therapy was permanently discontinued in 6 (6%) patients caused by pancytopenia/marrow hypoplasia. Two (2%) cases of pancytopenia/marrow hypoplasia were fatal.

Forty-four (47%) patients had ≥ 1 episode of new-onset NCI-CTC Grade 3 or 4 anemia. Sixty-two (67%) patients required RBC transfusions. In addition, erythropoietin use was reported in 19 (20%) patients. Autoimmune hemolytic anemia secondary to alemtuzumab therapy was reported in 1% of patients. Positive Coombs' test without hemolysis was reported in 2%.

Sixty-five (70%) patients had ≥ 1 episode of NCI-CTC Grade 3 or 4 neutropenia. Median duration of Grade 3 or 4 neutropenia was 28 days (range, 2 to 165 days).

Forty-eight (52%) patients had ≥ 1 episode of new-onset Grade 3 or 4 thrombocytopenia. Median duration of thrombocytopenia was 21 days (range, 2 to 165 days). Thirty-five (38%) patients required platelet transfusions for management of thrombocytopenia. Autoimmune thrombocytopenia was reported in 2% of patients with 1 fatal case of alemtuzumab-related autoimmune thrombocytopenia.

The median CD4+ at 4 weeks after initiation of alemtuzumab therapy was 2/mcL, 207/mcL at 2 months after discontinuation of alemtuzumab therapy, and 470/mcL at 6 months after discontinuation. The pattern of change in median CD8+ lymphocyte counts was similar to that of CD4+ cells. In some patients treated with alemtuzumab, CD4+ and CD8+ lymphocyte counts had not returned to baseline levels at longer than 1 year post-therapy.

►*Serious adverse events:* The following serious adverse events, defined as events that result in death, requiring or prolonging hospitalization, requiring medical intervention to prevent hospitalization, or malignancy, were reported in ≥ 1 patient treated on studies where alemtuzumab was used as a single agent (and are not reported in the previous table). These studies were conducted in patients with lymphocytic leukemia and lymphoma (n = 745) and in patients with nonmalignant diseases (n = 152) such as rheumatoid arthritis, solid organ transplant, or multiple sclerosis.

Cardiovascular – Cardiac failure; cyanosis; atrial fibrillation; cardiac arrest; ventricular arrhythmia; ventricular tachycardia; angina pectoris; coronary artery disorder; MI; pericarditis; cerebral hemorrhage; cerebrovascular disorder; deep vein thrombosis; increased capillary fragility; intracranial hemorrhage; phlebitis; subarachnoid hemorrhage; thrombophlebitis.

CNS – Abnormal gait; aphasia; coma; grand mal convulsions; paralysis; meningitis; confusion; hallucinations; nervousness; abnormal thinking; apathy.

Dermatologic – Angioedema; bullous eruption; cellulitis; purpuric rash.

GI – Duodenal ulcer; esophagitis; gingivitis; gastroenteritis; GI hemorrhage; hematemesis; hemorrhoids; intestinal obstruction; intestinal perforation; melena; paralytic ileus; peptic ulcer; pseudomembranous colitis; colitis; pancreatitis; peritonitis; hyperbilirubinemia; hepatic failure; hepatocellular damage; hypoalbuminemia; biliary pain.

GU – Abnormal renal function; acute renal failure; anuria; facial edema; hematuria; toxic nephropathy; ureteric obstruction; urinary retention; urinary tract infection.

Hematologic / Lymphatic – Coagulation disorder; disseminated intravascular coagulation; hematoma; pulmonary embolism; thrombocythemia; agranulocytosis; aplasia; decreased haptoglobin; lymphadenopathy; marrow depression; hemolysis; hemolytic anemia; splenic infarction; splenomegaly.

Metabolic / Nutritional – Acidosis; aggravated diabetes mellitus; dehydration; fluid overload; hyperglycemia; hyperkalemia; hypokalemia; hypoglycemia; hyponatremia; increased alkaline phosphatase; respiratory alkalosis.

Musculoskeletal – Arthritis or worsening arthritis; arthropathy; bone fracture; myositis; muscle atrophy; muscle weakness; osteomyelitis; polymyositis.

Respiratory – Asthma; bronchitis; chronic obstructive pulmonary disease; hemoptysis; hypoxia; pleural effusion; pleurisy; pneumothorax; pulmonary edema; pulmonary fibrosis; pulmonary infiltration; respiratory depression; respiratory insufficiency; sinusitis; stridor; throat tightness.

Miscellaneous – Allergic reactions; anaphylactoid reaction; ascites; hypovolemia; influenza-like syndrome; mouth edema; neutropenic fever; syncope; hyperthyroidism; decreased hearing; malignant lymphoma; malignant testicular neoplasm; prostatic cancer; plasma cell dyscrasia; secondary leukemia; squamous cell carcinoma; transformation to aggressive lymphoma; transformation to prolymphocytic leukemia; cervical dysplasia; abscess; bacterial infection; herpes zoster infection; *Pneumocystitis carinii* infection; otitis media; tuberculosis infection; viral infection; taste loss; endophthalmias.

Overdosage

Initial doses of alemtuzumab > 3 mg are not well tolerated. One patient who received 80 mg as an initial dose by IV infusion experienced acute bronchospasm, cough, and shortness of breath, followed by anuria and death. A review of the case suggested that tumor lysis syndrome may have played a role.

ALEMTUZUMAB

Do not administer single doses of alemtuzumab > 30 mg or as a cumulative weekly dose > 90 mg as higher doses have been associated with a higher incidence of pancytopenia.

There is no known specific antidote for alemtuzumab overdosage. Treatment consists of drug discontinuation and supportive therapy.

Patient Information

Women of childbearing potential and men of reproductive potential should use effective contraceptive methods during treatment and for a minimum of 6 months following alemtuzumab therapy.

TOSITUMOMAB AND IODINE ^{131}I-TOSITUMOMAB

Rx	**Bexxar Dosimetric Packaging**[1] (Corixa/GlaxoSmithKline)		A carton containing 2 single-use 225 mg vials and 1 single–use 35 mg vial of tositumomab. A package containing a single-use vial of ^{131}I-tositumomab.
Rx	**Tositumomab** (McKesson Biosciences)	**Injection:** 14 mg/mL	10% (w/v) maltose. Preservative-free. In 35 and 225 mg single-use vials.
Rx	**Iodine ^{131}I-Tositumomab**[2] (MDS Nordion[3])	**Injection:** 0.1 mg/mL (0.61 mCi/mL at calibration)	Preservative-free. Single-use vials.[4]
Rx	**Bexxar Therapeutic Packaging**[1] (Corixa/GlaxoSmithKline)		A carton containing 2 single-use 225 mg vials and 1 single-use 35 mg vial of tositumomab. A package containing 1 or 2 single-use vials of ^{131}I-tositumomab.
Rx	**Tositumomab** (McKesson Biosciences)	**Injection:** 14 mg/mL	10% (w/v) maltose. Preservative-free. In 35 and 225 mg single-use vials.
Rx	**Iodine ^{131}I-Tositumomab**[2] (MDS Nordion[3])	**Injection:** 1.1 mg/mL (5.6 mCi/mL at calibration)	Preservative-free. Single-use vials.[5]

[1] The components are shipped from separate sites; when ordering, ensure that the components are scheduled to arrive on the same day. The components are shipped only to individuals who are participating in the certification program.
[2] Refer to the product specification sheet for the lot specific protein concentration, activity concentration, total activity, and expiration date.
[3] MDS Nortion, 447 March Road, Ottawa, ON K2K 1X8, Canada; (613) 592-2790, (800) 267-6211.

[4] Contains 5% to 6% povidone, 1 to 2 mg/mL maltose, 0.85 to 0.95 mg/mL sodium chloride, and 0.9 to 1.3 mg/mL ascorbic acid.
[5] Contains 5% to 6% povidone, 9 to 15 mg/mL maltose, 0.85 to 0.95 mg/mL sodium chloride, and 0.9 to 1.3 mg/mL ascorbic acid.

WARNING

Hypersensitivity reactions, including anaphylaxis: Medications for the treatment of severe hypersensitivity reactions should be available for immediate use.

Prolonged and severe cytopenias: The majority of patients who received therapy experienced severe thrombocytopenia and neutropenia. Do not administer the therapeutic regimen to patients with more than 25% lymphoma marrow involvement and/or impaired bone marrow reserve.

Pregnancy: Category X. Tositumomab/^{131}I-tositumomab can cause fetal harm when administered to a pregnant woman.

Special requirements: Tositumomab/^{131}I-tositumomab contains a radioactive component and should be administered only by physicians and other health care professionals qualified by training in the safe use and handling of therapeutic radionuclides. The therapeutic regimen should be administered only by physicians who are in the process of being or have been certified by Corixa Corporation in dose calculation and administration of the therapeutic regimen.

Indications

➤*Non-Hodgkin lymphoma (NHL):* For the treatment of patients with CD20 positive, follicular NHL, with and without transformation, whose disease is refractory to rituximab and has relapsed following chemotherapy. This regimen is not indicated for the initial treatment of patients with CD20 positive NHL.

Administration and Dosage

➤*Approved by the FDA:* June 27, 2003.

The therapeutic regimen is intended as a single course of treatment. The safety of multiple courses of this drug complex, or combination of this complex with other forms of irradiation or chemotherapy have not been evaluated.

The therapeutic regimen consists of 4 components administered in 2 discrete steps: The dosimetric step, followed 7 to 14 days later by a therapeutic step. The safety of the therapeutic regimen was established only in the setting of patients receiving thyroid blocking agents and premedication to ameliorate/prevent infusion reactions. The therapeutic regimen is administered via an IV tubing set with an in-line 0.22 micron filter. The same IV tubing set and filter must be used throughout the entire dosimetric or therapeutic step. A change in filter can result in loss of drug.

➤*Dosimetric step:* Administer tositumomab 450 mg IV in 50 mL 0.9% sodium chloride over 60 minutes. Reduce the rate of infusion by 50% for mild to moderate infusional toxicity; interrupt infusion for severe infusional toxicity. After complete resolution of severe infusional toxicity, infusion may be resumed with a 50% reduction in the rate of infusion.

[131]I-tositumomab (containing 5 mCi ^{131}I and 35 mg tositumomab) IV in 30 mL 0.9% sodium chloride over 20 minutes. Reduce the rate of infusion by 50% for mild to moderate infusional toxicity; interrupt infusion for severe infusional toxicity. After complete resolution of severe infusional toxicity, infusion may be resumed with a 50% reduction in the rate of infusion.

➤*Therapeutic step:* Do not administer the therapeutic step if biodistribution is altered.

Administer tositumomab 450 mg IV in 50 mL 0.9% sodium chloride over 60 minutes. Reduce the rate of infusion by 50% for mild to moder-

ate infusional toxicity; interrupt infusion for severe infusional toxicity. After complete resolution of severe infusional toxicity, infusion may be resumed with a 50% reduction in the rate of infusion.

For ^{131}I-tositumomab, reduce the rate of infusion by 50% for mild to moderate infusional toxicity; interrupt infusion for severe infusional toxicity. After complete resolution of severe infusional toxicity, infusion may be resumed with a 50% reduction in the rate of infusion.

- In patients with 150,000 platelets/mm³ or more, the recommended dose is the activity of ^{131}I calculated to deliver 75 cGy total body irradiation and 35 mg tositumomab, administered IV over 20 minutes.
- In patients with NCI grade 1 thrombocytopenia (platelet counts = 100,000 but less than 150,000 platelets/mm³), the recommended dose is the activity of ^{131}I calculated to deliver 65 cGy total body irradiation and 35 mg tositumomab, administered IV over 20 minutes.

➤*Premedication:* The safety of the therapeutic regimen was established in studies in which all patients received the following concurrent medications.

➤*Thyroid protective agents:* Saturated solution of potassium iodide (SSKI) 4 drops orally, 3 times daily; Lugol's solution 20 drops orally, 3 times daily; or potassium iodide tablets 130 mg orally, every day. Initiate thyroid protective agents at least 24 hours prior to administration of the ^{131}I-tositumomab dosimetric dose and continue until 2 weeks after administration of the ^{131}I-tositumomab therapeutic dose.

Do not administer the dosimetric dose of ^{131}I-tositumomab to patients if they have not yet received at least 3 doses of SSKI, 3 doses of Lugol's solution, or 1 dose of 130 mg potassium iodide tablets (at least 24 hours prior to the dosimetric dose).

➤*Ameliorate/prevent infusion reactions:* Acetaminophen 650 mg orally and diphenhydramine 50 mg orally, 30 minutes prior to administration of tositumomab in the dosimetric and therapeutic steps.

➤*Preparation of therapeutic regimen and dosimetric step:* See manufacturer's product labeling for product specific preparation instructions.

➤*Storage/Stability:*

Tositumomab – Refrigerate vials of tositumomab at 2° to 8°C (36° to 46°F) prior to dilution. Protect from strong light. Do not shake. Do not freeze. Discard any unused portions left in the vial. Solutions of diluted tositumomab are stable for up to 24 hours when refrigerated at 2° to 8°C (36° to 46°F) and for up to 8 hours at room temperature. It is recommended that the diluted solution be refrigerated at 2° to 8°C (36° to 46°F) prior to administration because it does not contain preservatives. Any unused portion must be discarded. Do not freeze solutions of diluted tositumomab.

[131]I-tositumomab – Store frozen in the original lead pots. Store in a freezer at a temperature of −20°C (−4°F) or below until it is removed for thawing prior to administration.

Thawed dosimetric and therapeutic doses of ^{131}I-tositumomab are stable for up to 8 hours at 2° to 8°C (36° to 46°F) or at room temperature. Solution of ^{131}I-tositumomab diluted for infusion contains no preservatives; store refrigerated at 2° to 8°C (36° to 46°F) prior to administration, do not freeze. Any unused portion must be discarded.

Actions

➤*Pharmacology:* The tositumomab/^{131}I-tositumomab complex is an antineoplastic radioimmunotherapeutic monoclonal antibody-based regimen composed of the monoclonal antibody, tositumomab, and the radiolabeled monoclonal antibody, ^{131}I-tositumomab.

TOSITUMOMAB AND IODINE ^{131}I-TOSITUMOMAB

Tositumomab is a murine IgG$_{2a}$ lambda monoclonal antibody that binds specifically to the CD20 antigen. This antigen is a transmembrane phosphoprotein expressed on pre-B lymphocytes and at higher density on mature B lymphocytes. The antigen is also expressed on more than 90% of B-cell NHL. The recognition epitope for tositumomab is found within the extracellular domain of the CD20 antigen. CD20 does not shed from the cell surface and does not internalize following antibody binding.

Possible mechanisms of action include induction of apoptosis, complement-dependent cytotoxicity (CDC), and antibody-dependent cellular cytotoxicity (ADCC) mediated by the antibody. Additionally, cell death is associated with ionizing radiation from the radioisotope.

➤*Pharmacokinetics:* The median blood clearance following administration of 485 mg tositumomab in 110 patients with NHL was 68.2 mg/h. Patients with high tumor burden, splenomegaly, or bone marrow involvement were noted to have a faster clearance, shorter terminal half-life, and larger volume of distribution. The total body clearance, as measured by total body gamma camera counts, was dependent on the same factors noted for blood clearance.

^{131}I decays with beta and gamma emissions with a physical half-life of 8.04 days. Elimination of ^{131}I occurs by decay and excretion in the urine. Urine was collected for 49 dosimetric doses. After 5 days, the whole body clearance was 67% of the injected dose. Ninety-eight percent of the clearance was accounted for in the urine.

In clinical studies, administration of the therapeutic regimen resulted in sustained depletion of circulating CD20 positive cells. One of them was conducted in chemotherapy-naïve patients and 1 in heavily pretreated patients. At 7 weeks, the median number of circulating CD20 positive cells was 0. Lymphocyte recovery began at approximately 12 weeks following treatment. Among patients who had CD20 positive cell counts recorded at baseline and at 6 months, 14% chemotherapy naïve patients had CD20 positive cell counts below normal limits at 6 months, and 32% of heavily pretreated patients had CD20 positive cell counts below normal limits at 6 months. There was no consistent effect of the therapeutic regimen on posttreatment serum IgG, IgA, or IgM levels.

➤*Clinical trials:* The efficacy of the tositumomab/^{131}I-tositumomab regimen was evaluated in a multicenter, single-arm study in patients with low grade, transformed low grade, or follicular large-cell lymphoma whose diseases had not responded to or had progressed after rituximab therapy. All patients in the study were required to have received prior treatment with at least 4 doses of rituximab without an objective response, or to have progressed following treatment. Patients were also required to have a platelet count of at least 100,000/mm^3; an average of 25% or less of the intrabecular marrow space involved by lymphoma, and no evidence of progressive disease arising in a field irradiated with more than 3500 cGy within 1 year of completion of irradiation. Forty patients initiated treatment with the drug complex. Twenty-four patients had disease that did not respond to their last treatment with rituximab, 11 patients had disease that responded to rituximab for less than 6 months, and 5 patients had disease that responded to rituximab, with 6 months or more of a duration of response.

	Tositumomab/^{131}I-Tositumomab Patient Efficacy Outcomes			
	Objective responses to tositumomab/^{131}I-tositumomab in patients refractory to rituximab		Objective responses to tositumomab/^{131}I-tositumomab in all patients	
Response	Response rate (%) (n = 35)	Median duration of response (mo)	Response rate (%) (n = 40)	Median duration of response (mo)
Overall response	63	25	68	16
Complete response[1]	29	NR[2]	33	NR[2]

[1] Complete response rate = Pathologic and clinical complete responses
[2] NR = Not reached

Contraindications

Known hypersensitivity to murine proteins or any other component of the therapeutic regimen.

Warnings

➤*Prolonged and severe cytopenias:* The most common adverse reactions associated with the therapeutic regimen were severe or life-threatening cytopenias (NCI CTC grade 3 or 4) with 71% of the 230 patients enrolled in clinical studies experiencing grade 3 or 4 cytopenias. These consisted primarily of grade 3 or 4 thrombocytopenia (53%) and grade 3 or 4 neutropenia (63%). The time to nadir was 4 to 7 weeks, and the duration of cytopenias was approximately 30 days. Thrombocytopenia, neutropenia, and anemia persisted for more than 90 days following administration of the tositumomab-iodine drug complex in 7%, 7%, and 5% of the patients, respectively. Due to the variable onset of cytopenias, obtain complete blood counts weekly for 10 to 12 weeks. The sequelae of severe cytopenias were commonly observed in clinical studies and included infections (45%), hemorrhage (12%), a requirement for growth factors (12% G- or GM-CSF; 7% epoetin alfa) and blood product support (15% platelet transfusions; 16% red blood cell transfusions).

The safety of the therapeutic regimen has not been established in patients with more than 25% lymphoma marrow involvement, platelet count less than 100,000 cells/mm^3, or neutrophil count less than 1500 cells/mm^3.

➤*Secondary malignancies:* Myelodysplastic syndrome (MDS) and/or acute leukemia were reported in 8% of patients enrolled in the clinical studies and 2% of patients included in expanded access programs. The median time to development of MDS/leukemia was 27 months following treatment; however, the cumulative rate continues to increase. Additional malignancies were also reported in 52 of the 995 patients enrolled in clinical studies. Approximately half of these were nonmelanomatous skin cancers. The remainder, which occurred in 2 or more patients, included breast, lung, bladder, head and neck cancer, colon cancer, and melanoma, in order of decreasing incidence.

➤*Hypothyroidism:* Therapy may result in hypothyroidism. Initiate thyroid-blocking medications at least 24 hours before receiving the dosimetric dose, and continue until 14 days after the therapeutic dose. All patients must receive thyroid blocking agents; do not administer this therapeutic regimen for any patient who is unable to tolerate thyroid blocking agents. Evaluate patients for signs and symptoms of hypothyroidism and screen for biochemical evidence of hypothyroidism annually.

➤*Hypersensitivity reactions:* Hypersensitivity reactions, including anaphylaxis, were reported during and following administration of the this therapeutic regimen. Medications for the treatment of hypersensitivity reactions (eg, epinephrine, antihistamines, and corticosteroids) should be available for immediate use in the event of an allergic reaction. Screen patients who have received murine proteins for human antimouse antibodies (HAMA). Patients who are positive for HAMA may be at increased risk of anaphylaxis and serious hypersensitivity reactions during administration of the therapeutic regimen.

➤*Renal function impairment:* ^{131}I-tositumomab and ^{131}I are excreted primarily by the kidneys. Impaired renal function may decrease the rate of excretion of the radiolabeled iodine and increase patient exposure to the radioactive component of the therapeutic regimen. There are no data regarding the safety of administration of the therapeutic regimen in patients with impaired renal function.

➤*Carcinogenesis:* Radiation is a potential carcinogen. Administration of this therapeutic regimen results in delivery of a significant radiation dose to the testes. There is a potential risk that the drug complex may cause toxic effects on the male and female gonads.

➤*Elderly:* Across all studies, the overall response rate was lower in patients 65 years of age and older (41% vs 61%), and the duration of responses were shorter (10 months vs 16 months). The duration of severe hematologic toxicity was longer in those 65 years of age and older as compared to patients younger than 65 years of age. Due to limited experience, greater sensitivity of some older individuals cannot be ruled out.

➤*Pregnancy: Category X.* ^{131}I-tositumomab (a component of the therapeutic regimen) is contraindicated for use in women who are pregnant. ^{131}I may cause harm to the fetal thyroid gland when administered to pregnant women. Review of the literature has shown that transplacental passage of radioiodide may cause severe, and possibly irreversible, hypothyroidism in neonates. While there are no adequate and well-controlled studies of this drug complex in pregnant animals or humans, defer use of therapy in women of childbearing age until the possibility of pregnancy has been ruled out. If the patient becomes pregnant while being treated with the drug complex, apprise the patient of the potential hazard to the fetus. Use effective contraceptive methods during treatment and for 12 months following administration.

➤*Lactation:* Radioiodine is excreted in breast milk and may reach concentrations equal to or greater than maternal plasma concentrations. Immunoglobulins are also known to be excreted in breast milk. The absorption potential and potential for adverse effects of the monoclonal antibody component (tositumomab) in the infant are not known. Therefore, substitute formula feedings for breastfeedings before starting treatment. Advise women to discontinue nursing.

➤*Children:* The safety and efficacy of the therapeutic regimen in children have not been established.

Precautions

➤*Monitoring:* Obtain a complete blood count (CBC) with differential and platelet count prior to, and at least weekly following administration of the therapeutic regimen. Continue weekly monitoring of blood counts for a minimum of 10 weeks or, if persistent, until severe cytopenias have completely resolved. More frequent monitoring is indicated in patients with evidence of moderate or more severe cytopenias. Monitor thyroid stimulating hormone (TSH) level before treatment and annually thereafter. Measure serum creatinine levels immediately prior to administration of the therapeutic regimen.

➤*Radionuclide:* ^{131}I-tositumomab is radioactive. To minimize exposure of medical personnel and other patients, exercise caution by staying consistent with the institutional radiation safety practices and

TOSITUMOMAB AND IODINE ¹³¹I-TOSITUMOMAB

applicable federal guidelines.

➤*Immunization:* The safety of immunization with live viral vaccines following administration of the therapeutic regimen has not been studied. The ability of patients who have received this therapeutic regimen to generate a primary or anamnestic humoral response to any vaccine has not been studied.

➤*Immunogenicity:* Administration of this therapeutic regimen may result in the development of human antimurine antibodies (HAMA). The presence of HAMA may affect the accuracy of the results of in vitro and in vivo diagnostic tests and may affect the toxicity profile and efficacy of therapeutic agents that rely on murine antibody technology. Patients who are HAMA positive may be at increased risk for serious allergic reactions and other side effects if they undergo in vivo diagnostic testing or treatment with murine monoclonal antibodies.

Drug Interactions

No formal drug interaction studies have been performed. Due to the frequent occurrence of severe and prolonged thrombocytopenia, weigh the potential benefits of medications that interfere with platelet function and/or anticoagulation against the potential increased risk of bleeding and hemorrhage.

Adverse Reactions

The most serious adverse reactions observed in the clinical trials were severe and prolonged cytopenias and the sequelae of cytopenias which included infections (sepsis) and hemorrhage in thrombocytopenic patients, allergic reactions (bronchospasm and angioedema), secondary leukemia and myelodysplasia (see Warnings).

The most common adverse reactions occurring in the clinical trials included neutropenia, thrombocytopenia, and anemia that are both prolonged and severe. Less common but severe adverse reactions included pneumonia, pleural effusion, and dehydration.

Nonhematologic Adverse Reactions in 5% or more of Patients Treated with Tositumomab/¹³¹I-Tositumomab (N = 230) (%)		
Adverse reaction	All Grades (96%)	Grade 3/4 (48%)
Cardiovascular		
Hypotension	7	1
Vasodilation	5	0
CNS		
Dizziness	5	0
Headache	16	0
Somnolence	5	0
Dermatologic		
Rash	17	< 1
Pruritus	10	0
Sweating	8	< 1
GI		
Abdominal pain	15	3
Anorexia	14	0
Constipation	6	1
Diarrhea	12	0
Dyspepsia	6	< 1
Nausea	36	3
Vomiting	15	1
Metabolic		
Peripheral edema	9	0
Weight loss	6	< 1
Musculoskeletal		
Arthralgia	10	1
Myalgia	13	< 1
Respiratory		
Cough increased	21	1
Dyspnea	11	3
Pharyngitis	12	0
Pneumonia	6	0
Rhinitis	10	0
Miscellaneous		
Asthenia	46	2
Back pain	8	1
Chest pain	7	0
Chills	18	1
Fever	37	2
Hypothyroidism	7	0
Infection[1]	21	< 1
Neck pain	6	1
Pain	19	1

[1] "Infection includes" a subset of infections (eg, upper respiratory infection, pneumonia, and sepsis).

Tositumomab/¹³¹I-Tositumomab Hematologic Toxicity[a] (N = 230)	
Endpoint	Values
Platelets	
Median nadir (cells/mm³)	43,000
Per patient incidence[a] platelets < 50,000/mm³	53%
Median[b] duration of platelets < 50,000/mm³ (days)	32
Grade 3/4 without recovery to Grade 2	7%
Per patient incidence[c] platelets < 25,000/mm³	21%
ANC	
Median nadir (cells/mm³)	690
Per patient incidence[a] ANC < 1000 cells/mm³	63%
Median[b] duration of ANC < 1000 cells/mm³ (days)	31
Grade 3/4 without recovery to Grade 2	7%
Per patient incidence[c] ANC < 500 cells/mm³	25%
Hemoglobin	
Median nadir (g/dL)	10
Per patient incidence[a] < 8 g/dL	29%
Median[b] duration of hemoglobin < 8 g/dL (days)	23
Grade 3/4 without recovery to Grade 2	5%
Per patient incidence[c] hemoglobin < 6.5 g/dL	5%

[a] Grade 3/4 toxicity was assumed if patient was missing 2 or more weeks of hematology data between weeks 5 and 9.
[b] Duration of Grade 3/4 of 1000+ days (censored) was assumed for those patients with undocumented Grade 3/4 and no hematologic data on or after week 9.
[c] Grade 4 toxicity was assumed if patient had documented Grade 3 toxicity and was missing 2 or more weeks of hematology data between weeks 5 and 9.

➤*Hematologic:* Hematologic toxicity was the most frequently observed adverse event in clinical trials with the therapeutic regimen. Twenty-seven percent of the patients received 1 or more hematologic supportive care measures following the therapeutic dose. Twelve percent received G-CSF; 7% received epoetin alfa; 15% received platelet transfusions; 16% received packed red blood cell transfusions. Twelve percent of patients experienced hemorrhagic events; the majority were mild to moderate.

➤*Infections:* Forty-five percent of patients experienced 1 or more adverse events possibly related to infection. The majority were viral (eg, rhinitis, pharyngitis, flu symptoms, or herpes) or other minor infections. Eight percent of patients experienced infections that were considered serious because the patient was hospitalized to manage the infection. Documented infections included pneumonia, bacteremia, septicemia, bronchitis, and skin infections.

➤*Hypersensitivity:* Six percent experienced 1 or more of the following adverse events: Allergic reaction, face edema, injection site hypersensitivity, anaphylactoid reaction, laryngismus, and serum sickness.

➤*GI toxicity:* Thirty-eight percent of patients experienced 1 or more of the following GI adverse events: Nausea, emesis, abdominal pain, and diarrhea. These events were temporally related to the infusion of the antibody. Nausea, vomiting, and abdominal pain were often reported within days of infusion, whereas diarrhea was generally reported days to weeks after infusion.

➤*Infusional toxicity:* Symptoms, including fever, rigors or chills, sweating, hypotension, dyspnea, bronchospasm, and nausea have been reported during or within 48 hours of infusion. Twenty-nine percent of patients reported fever, rigors/chills, or sweating within 14 days following the dosimetric dose. Infusional toxicities were managed by slowing and/or temporarily interrupting the infusion. Symptomatic management was required in more severe cases.

➤*Delayed adverse reactions:*

Secondary leukemia and myelodysplastic syndrome (MDS) – There were 32 new cases of MDS/secondary leukemia reported among 3.2% of patients included in clinical studies.

Secondary malignancies – There were 52 reports of second malignancies, excluding secondary leukemias. The most common included nonmelanomatous skin cancers, breast, lung, bladder, and head and neck cancers. Some of these events included recurrence of an earlier diagnosis of cancer.

Hypothyroidism – Twelve percent of the patients included from the clinical studies had an elevated TSH level (8%) or no TSH level obtained (4%) prior to treatment. The overall incidence of hypothyroidism was 14%. New events have been observed up to 72 months post treatment.

TOSITUMOMAB AND IODINE ^{131}I-TOSITUMOMAB

Immunogenicity – Of the 220 patients who were seronegative prior to treatment, 99.5% had at least 1 posttreatment HAMA value obtained. Eleven percent seroconverted to HAMA positivity. The median time to development of HAMA was 6 months. In a study of 77 patients who were chemotherapy naïve, the incidence of conversion to HAMA seropositivity was 70%, with a median time to development of HAMA of 27 days.

Overdosage

The maximum dose of the tositumomab/^{131}I-tositumomab therapeutic regimen that was administered in clinical trials was 88 cGy. Three patients were treated with a total body dose of 85 cGy of iodine ^{131}I-tositumomab in a dose escalation study. Two of the 3 patients developed Grade 4 toxicity of 5 weeks duration with subsequent recovery. In addition, accidental overdose of the therapeutic regimen occurred in 1 patient at total body doses of 88 cGy. The patient developed Grade 3 hematologic toxicity of 18 days duration. Monitor patients who receive an accidental overdose of ^{131}I-tositumomab closely for cytopenias and radiation-related toxicity. The effectiveness of hematopoietic stem cell transplantation as a supportive care measure for marrow injury has not been studied; however, the timing of such support should take into account the pharmacokinetics of the therapeutic regimen and decay rate of the ^{131}I in order to minimize the possibility of irradiation of infused hematopoietic stem cells.

Patient Information

Inform patients that they will have a radioactive material in their body for several days upon their release from the hospital or clinic.

After discharge, provide patients with both oral and written instructions for minimizing exposure of family members, friends, and the general public.

Assess the pregnancy status of women of childbearing potential, and advise these women of the potential risks to the fetus. Instruct women who are breastfeeding to discontinue breastfeeding.

Advise patients of the potential risk of toxic effects on the male and female gonads following the therapeutic regimen, and instruct patients to use effective contraceptive methods during treatment and for 12 months following the administration of the therapeutic regimen.

Inform patients of the risks of hypothyroidism, and advise them of the importance of compliance with thyroid blocking agents and the need for life-long monitoring.

Inform patients of the risks of cytopenias and symptoms associated with cytopenia and the need for frequent monitoring.

Inform patients that certain antineoplastic agents used in the treatment of malignancy have been associated with the development of MDS, secondary leukemia, and solid tumors.

IMATIBIB MESYLATE

Rx **Gleevec** (Novartis)

Tablets: 100 mg (as base)	(NVR SA). Very dark yellow to brownish-orange, scored. Film-coated. In 100s.
400 mg (as base)	(NVR SL). Very dark yellow to brownish-orange, oval. Film-coated. In 30s.

Indications

➤*Chronic myeloid leukemia (CML):* For the treatment of newly diagnosed adult patients with Philadelphia chromosome positive CML in chronic phase; for patients with Philadelphia chromosome positive CML in blast crisis, accelerated phase, or in chronic phase after failure of interferon-alpha therapy; for children with Ph+ chronic phase CML whose disease has recurred after stem cell transplant or who are resistant to interferon-alpha therapy.

➤*Gastrointestinal stromal tumors (GIST):* For the treatment of patients with Kit (CD117)-positive, unresectable, and/or metastatic malignant GIST.

The effectiveness of imatinib in GIST is based on objective response rates. There are no controlled trials demonstrating a clinical benefit, such as improvement in disease-related symptoms or increased survival.

Administration and Dosage

➤*Approved by the FDA:* May 10, 2001.

Therapy should be initiated by a physician experienced in the treatment of patients with CML or GIST.

➤*Dosage:*

Imatinib Daily Dosing		
Indication	Adult dose (mg)	Child dose (mg/m²)
CML, chronic phase	400	260
CML, accelerated phase or blast crisis	600	N/A
GIST	400 or 600	N/A

➤*Administration:* Administer the prescribed dose orally with a meal and a large glass of water. Administer doses of 400 or 600 mg once daily, and administer doses of 800 mg as 400 mg twice daily.

In children, imatinib treatment can be given as a once daily dose or, alternatively, the daily dose may be split into 2 (once in the morning and once in the evening).

For patients unable to swallow the film-coated tablets, the tablets may be dispersed in a glass of water or apple juice. Place the required number of tablets in the appropriate volume of beverage (approximately 50 mL for a 100 mg tablet, and 200 mL for a 400 mg tablet) and stir with a spoon. Immediately administer the suspension after complete disintegration of the tablet(s).

➤*Duration:* Treatment may be continued as long as there is no evidence of progressive disease or unacceptable toxicity.

➤*Titration:* In CML, a dose increase from 400 to 600 mg in adult patients with chronic phase disease, or from 600 to 800 mg (given as 400 mg twice daily) in adult patients in accelerated phase or blast crisis may be considered in the absence of severe adverse drug reaction and severe non-leukemia-related neutropenia or thrombocytopenia in the following circumstances: Disease progression (at any time), failure to achieve a satisfactory hematologic response after at least 3 months of treatment, loss of a previously achieved hematologic or cytogenetic response, or failure to achieve a cytogenetic response after 6 to 12 months of treatment. In children with chronic phase CML, daily doses can be increased under circumstances similar to those leading to an increase in adult chronic phase disease, from 260 to 340 mg/m²/day as clinically indicated.

➤*Concomitant medications:* Increase dosage of imatinib by at least 50%, and carefully monitor clinical response in patients receiving imatinib with a potent CYP3A4 inducer, such as rifampin or phenytoin.

➤*Dose adjustment for hepatotoxicity and other nonhematologic adverse reactions:* If a severe nonhematologic adverse reaction develops (eg, severe hepatotoxicity, severe fluid retention), withhold imatinib until the event has resolved. Thereafter, treatment can be resumed as appropriate depending on the initial severity of the event.

Imatinib Dose Adjustments for Hepatotoxicity		
Toxicity	Recommendation	Dosage adjustment for next dose
Bilirubin > 3 × IULN[a]	Withhold imatinib until bilirubin levels have returned to < 1.5 × IULN	In adults, treatment with imatinib may then be continued at a reduced daily dose (300 mg if previous dose was 400 mg or 400 mg if previous dose was 600 mg). In children, daily doses can be reduced under the same circumstances from 260 to 200 mg/m²/day or from 340 to 260 mg/m²/day.
Liver transaminases > 5 × IULN	Withhold imatinib until transaminase levels have returned to < 2.5 × IULN	

[a] Institutional upper limit of normal.

➤*Dose adjustments for neutropenia and thrombocytopenia:*

Imatinib Dose Adjustments for Neutropenia and Thrombocytopenia		
Phase	ANC/Platelet value	Recommendations
Chronic phase CML (starting dose 400 mg[a]) or GIST (starting dose either 400 or 600 mg)	ANC < 1 × 10⁹/L and/or platelets < 50 × 10⁹/L	1) Stop imatinib until ANC ≥ 1.5 × 10⁹/L and platelets ≥ 75 × 10⁹/L. 2) Resume treatment with imatinib at dose of 400[a] or 600 mg. 3) If recurrence of ANC < 1 × 10⁹/L and/or platelets < 50 × 10⁹/L, repeat step 1 and resume imatinib at a reduced dose (300 mg[b] if starting dose was 400 mg[a], 400 mg if starting dose was 600 mg).
Accelerated phase CML and blast crisis (starting dose 600 mg)	ANC < 0.5 × 10⁹/L and/or platelets < 10 × 10⁹/L[c]	1) Check if cytopenia is related to leukemia (marrow aspirate or biopsy). 2) If cytopenia is unrelated to leukemia, reduce dose of imatinib to 400 mg. 3) If cytopenia persists 2 weeks, reduce further to 300 mg. 4) If cytopenia persists 4 weeks and is still unrelated to leukemia, stop imatinib until ANC ≥ 1 × 10⁹/L and platelets ≥ 20 × 10⁹/L and then resume treatment at 300 mg.

[a] Or 260 mg/m² in children.
[b] Or 200 mg/m² in children.
[c] Occurring after at least 1 month of treatment.

➤*Storage/Stability:* Store at 25°C (77°F); excursions permitted to 15° to 30°C (59° to 86°F). Protect from moisture. Dispense in a tight container.

Actions

➤*Pharmacology:* Imatinib is a protein-tyrosine kinase inhibitor that inhibits the Bcr-Abl tyrosine kinase, the constitutive abnormal tyrosine kinase created by the Philadelphia chromosome abnormality in CML. It inhibits proliferation and induces apoptosis in Bcr-Abl-positive cell lines and fresh leukemic cells from Philadelphia chromosome positive CML. In colony formation assays using ex vivo peripheral blood and bone marrow samples, imatinib shows inhibition of Bcr-Abl-positive colonies from CML patients.

In vivo, imatinib inhibits tumor growth of Bcr-Abl-transfected murine myeloid cells and Bcr-Abl-positive leukemia lines derived from CML patients in blast crisis.

Imatinib also is an inhibitor of the receptor tyrosine kinases for platelet-derived growth factor (PDGF) and stem cell factor (SCF), c-kit, and inhibits PDGF- and SCF-mediated cellular events. In vitro, imatinib inhibits proliferation and induces apoptosis in GIST cells, which express an activating c-kit mutation.

➤*Pharmacokinetics:*

Absorption/Distribution – The pharmacokinetics of imatinib have been evaluated in studies in healthy subjects and in population pharmacokinetic studies in over 900 patients. Mean imatinib AUC increased proportionally with increasing doses in the range of 25 to 1000 mg. There was no significant change in the pharmacokinetics of imatinib on repeated dosing, and accumulation is 1.5- to 2.5-fold at steady state when imatinib is dosed once daily.

Metabolism/Excretion – The main circulating active metabolite in humans is the N-demethylated piperazine derivative formed predominantly by CYP3A4. It shows in vitro potency similar to parent imatinib. The plasma AUC for this metabolite is approximately 15% of the AUC for imatinib.

Typically, clearance of imatinib in a patient 50 years of age weighing 50 kg is expected to be 8 L/h, while for a patient 50 years of age weighing 100 kg, the clearance will increase to 14 L/h. However, the interpatient variability of 40% in clearance does not warrant initial dose adjustment based on body weight and/or age, but indicates the need for close monitoring for treatment-related toxicity.

Imatinib Pharmacokinetics						
C_max	T_max	Mean absolute bioavailability	Protein binding	Metabolism pathways	Elimination t½	Routes of excretion
2.3 to 2.9 mg/mL[a]	2 to 4 h	98%	95%[b]	CYP3A4 (major); CYP1A2, 2D6, 2C9, 2C19 (minor)	≈ 18 h, ≈ 40 h[c]	68% in feces, 18% in urine[d]

[a] At steady state with 400 mg/day.
[b] Mostly to albumin and α₁-acid glycoprotein.
[c] Elimination half life for major active metabolite, the N-desmethyl derivative.
[d] Mostly as metabolites, 20% feces and 5% urine unchanged.

IMATINIB MESYLATE

➤*Clinical trials:*

Chronic phase, newly diagnosed CML – An open-label, multi-center, international phase 3 study compared efficacy of imatinib therapy vs interferon-alfa (IFN) plus cytarabine (Ara-C) combination therapy. A total of 1106 patients were randomized with 553 in each arm. The estimated rate of progression-free survival at 12 months in the intent-to-treat population was 97.2% in the imatinib arm and 80.3% in the combination therapy arm. Complete hematologic response (CHR) and cytogenetic response were secondary endpoints. A CHR was defined as white blood cells fewer than 10×10^9/L, platelets fewer than 450×10^9/L, myelocytes less than 5% in blood, no blasts and promyelocytes in blood, basophils less than 20%, and no extramedullary involvement. A complete cytogenetic response was defined as 0% Philadelphia chromosome-positive metaphases. A CHR was seen in 94.4% of the imatinib group vs 54.6% of the IFN plus Ara-C group. A complete cytogenetic response was seen in 53.7% and 2.7% of the imatinib vs the IFN plus Ara-C groups, respectively.

Contraindications

Hypersensitivity to imatinib or to any other component of the product.

Warnings

➤*GI irritation:* Imatinib is sometimes associated with GI irritation. Take with food and a large glass of water to minimize this problem.

➤*Mutagenesis:* Positive genotoxic effects were obtained for imatinib in an in vitro mammalian cell assay (Chinese hamster ovary) for clastogenicity (chromosome aberrations) in the presence of metabolic activation. Two intermediates of the manufacturing process, which also are present in the final product, are positive for mutagenesis in the Ames assay. One of these intermediates also was positive in the mouse lymphoma assay. Imatinib was not genotoxic when tested in an in vitro bacterial cell assay (Ames test), an in vitro mammalian cell assay (mouse lymphoma), and an in vivo rat micronucleus assay.

➤*Fertility impairment:* In a fertility study in male rats dosed for 70 days prior to mating, testicular and epididymal weights and percent motile sperm were decreased at 60 mg/kg, approximately three fourths the maximum clinical dose of 800 mg/day based on body surface area. This was not seen at doses of 20 mg/kg or less (one fourth the maximum human dose of 800 mg). When female rats were dosed 14 days prior to mating and through gestational day 6, there was no effect on mating or on the number of pregnant females.

➤*Elderly:* No difference was observed in the safety profile in patients older than 65 years of age as compared with younger patients, with the exception of a higher frequency of edema. The efficacy of imatinib was similar in older and younger patients.

➤*Pregnancy: Category D.* Advise women of childbearing potential to avoid becoming pregnant.

Imatinib was teratogenic in rats when administered during organogenesis at doses 100 mg/kg or more, approximately equal to the maximum clinical dose of 800 mg/day based on body surface area. Teratogenic effects included exencephaly or encephalocele and absent/reduced frontal and absent parietal bones. Female rats administered doses greater than or equal to 45 mg/kg (approximately one half the maximum human dose of 800 mg/day based on body surface area) also experienced significant postimplantation loss as evidenced by either early fetal resorption or stillbirths, nonviable pups, and early pup mortality between postpartum days 0 and 4. At doses greater than 100 mg/kg, total fetal loss was noted in all animals. These effects were not seen at doses less than or equal to 30 mg/kg (one third the maximum human dose of 800 mg).

Male and female rats were exposed in utero to a maternal imatinib dose of 45 mg/kg (approximately one half the maximum human dose of 800 mg) from day 6 of gestation and through milk during the lactation period. Body weights were reduced from birth until terminal sacrifice in these rats. Although fertility was not affected, fetal loss was seen when these male and female animals were mated.

There are no adequate and well-controlled studies in pregnant women. If imatinib is used during pregnancy, or if the patient becomes pregnant while taking imatinib, apprise the patient of the potential hazard to the fetus.

➤*Lactation:* It is not known whether imatinib or its metabolites are excreted in human milk. However, in lactating female rats administered 100 mg/kg, a dose approximately equal to the maximum clinical dose of 800 mg/day based on body surface area, imatinib and its metabolites were extensively excreted in milk at concentrations approximately 3-fold higher than in plasma. It is estimated that approximately 1.5% of a maternal dose is excreted into milk, which is equivalent to a dose to the infant of 30% of the maternal dose per unit body weight. Because many drugs are excreted in human milk and because of the potential for serious adverse reactions in nursing infants, advise women against breastfeeding while taking imatinib.

➤*Children:* The safety and efficacy of imatinib have been demonstrated only in children with Ph+ chronic phase CML with recurrence after stem cell transplantation or resistance to interferon-alpha therapy. There are no data in children younger than 3 years of age.

Precautions

➤*Dermatological toxicities:* Bullous dermatological reactions, including erythema multiforme and Stevens-Johnson syndrome, have been reported with use of imatinib. In some cases reported during post-marketing surveillance, a recurrent dermatological reaction was observed upon rechallenge. Several foreign postmarketing reports have described cases in which patients tolerated the reintroduction of imatinib therapy after resolution or improvement of the bullous reaction. In these instances, imatinib was resumed at a lower dose than that at which the reaction occurred and some patients also received concomitant treatment with corticosteroids or antihistamines.

➤*Fluid retention and edema:* Imatinib is often associated with edema and occasionally serious fluid retention (see Adverse Reactions). Weigh and monitor patients regularly for signs and symptoms of fluid retention. Carefully investigate an unexpected rapid weight gain and provide appropriate treatment. The probability of edema was increased with higher imatinib dose and age greater than 65 years of age in the CML studies. Severe superficial edema was reported in 0.9% of newly diagnosed CML patients taking imatinib and in 2% to 6% of other adult CML patients taking imatinib. In addition, other severe fluid retention (eg, pleural effusion, pericardial effusion, pulmonary edema, ascites) events were reported in 2% to 6% of other adult CML patients taking imatinib. Severe superficial edema and severe fluid retention (eg, pleural effusion, pulmonary edema, ascites) were reported in 1% to 6% of patients taking imatinib for GIST. There have been postmarketing reports, including fatalities, of cerebral edema, increased intracranial pressure, and papilledema in patients with CML treated with imatinib.

➤*Hematologic toxicity:* Treatment with imatinib is associated with anemia, neutropenia, and thrombocytopenia. Perform complete blood counts weekly for the first month, biweekly for the second month, and periodically thereafter as clinically indicated (ie, every 2 to 3 months). In CML, the occurrence of these cytopenias is dependent on the stage of disease and is more frequent in patients with accelerated phase CML or blast crisis than in patients with chronic phase CML (see Administration and Dosage).

➤*Hemorrhage:* In the newly diagnosed CML trial, 0.7% of patients had grade 3/4 hemorrhage. In the GIST clinical trial, 7 patients (5%), 4 in the 600 mg dose group and 3 in the 400 mg dose group, had a total of 8 events of common toxicity criteria (CTC) grade 3/4 GI bleeds (3 patients), intratumoral bleeds (3 patients), or both (1 patient). GI tumor sites may have been the source of GI bleeds.

➤*Hepatotoxicity:* Hepatotoxicity, occasionally severe, may occur with imatinib (see Adverse Reactions). Monitor liver function (eg, transaminases, bilirubin, alkaline phosphatase) before initiation of treatment and monthly or as clinically indicated. Manage laboratory abnormalities with interruption and/or dose reduction of imatinib therapy (see Administration and Dosage). Closely monitor patients with hepatic impairment because exposure to imatinib may be increased. As there are no clinical studies of imatinib in patients with impaired liver function, no specific advice concerning initial dosing adjustment can be given.

➤*Toxicities from long-term use:* It is important to consider potential toxicities suggested by animal studies, specifically liver and kidney toxicity and immunosuppression. Severe liver toxicity was observed in dogs treated for 2 weeks, including elevated liver enzymes, hepatocellular necrosis, bile duct necrosis, and bile duct hyperplasia. Renal toxicity was observed in monkeys treated for 2 weeks, with focal mineralization and dilation of the renal tubules and tubular nephrosis. Increased BUN and creatinine were observed in several of these animals. An increased rate of opportunistic infections was observed with chronic imatinib treatment. In a 39-week monkey study, treatment with imatinib resulted in worsening of normally suppressed malarial infections in these animals. Lymphopenia was observed in animals (as in humans).

➤*Photosensitivity:* Photosensitization (photoallergy or phototoxicity) may occur; therefore, caution patients to take protective measures (ie, sunscreens, protective clothing) against exposure to sunlight or ultraviolet light (eg, tanning beds) until tolerance is determined.

Drug Interactions

➤*Cytochrome P450:* In vitro, imatinib inhibits cytochrome P450 isoenzymes CYP3A4/5, CYP2C9, and CYP2D6. Systemic exposure to substrates of these enzymes is expected to increase when coadministered with imatinib.

IMATINIB MESYLATE

Imatinib Drug Interactions			
Precipitant drug	Object drug[*]		Description
Acetaminophen	Imatinib	↑	Increased risk of hepatoxicity may occur. There has been 1 report of fatal hepatic failure with coadministration.
Imatinib	Acetaminophen		
Inducers of CYP3A4 (eg, carbamazepine, dexamethasone, phenobarbital, phenytoin, rifampin, St. John's wort)	Imatinib	↓	Substances that induce CYP3A4 activity may increase metabolism and decrease imatinib plasma concentrations. Coadministration of multiple doses of rifampin and a single dose of imatinib increased imatinib clearance by 3.8-fold, which significantly decreased the mean C_{max} and $AUC_{(0-\infty)}$. When rifampin or other CYP3A4 inducers are indicated with imatinib, consider other therapeutic agents with less enzyme induction potential.
Inhibitors of CYP3A4 (eg, clarithromycin, erythromycin, itraconazole, ketoconazole)	Imatinib	↑	Substances that inhibit the CYP3A4 isoenzyme activity may decrease metabolism and increase imatinib concentrations. Concomitant administration with a single dose of ketoconazole resulted in an increase in the mean AUC and C_{max} of 26% and 40%, respectively, of imatinib.
Imatinib	Certain HMG-CoA reductase inhibitors (eg, simvastatin) Dihydropyridine calcium channel blockers Oral contraceptives (ie, ethinyl estradiol) Triazolobenzodiazepines	↑	Imatinib will increase plasma concentrations of other CYP3A4 metabolized drugs. Coadministration of simvastatin and imatinib resulted in an increase in the mean C_{max} and AUC of simvastatin by 2- and 3.5-fold, respectively.
Imatinib	Cyclosporine Pimozide	↑	Particular caution is recommended when administering imatinib with CYP3A4 substrates that have a narrow therapeutic window.
Imatinib	Warfarin	↑	Because warfarin is metabolized by CYP2C9 and CYP3A4, patients who require anticoagulation should receive low molecular weight or standard heparin.

[*] ↑ = Object drug increased. ↓ = Object drug decreased. ↔ = Undetermined clinical effect.

Adverse Reactions

►*CML:* The majority of imatinib-treated patients experienced adverse events at some time. Most events were of mild to moderate grade, but the drug was discontinued for drug-related adverse events in 4% of patients in chronic phase, 5% in accelerated phase, and 5% in blast crisis.

The most frequently reported drug-related adverse events were diarrhea, edema, muscle cramps, musculoskeletal pain, nausea and vomiting, and rash. Edema was most frequently periorbital or in lower limbs and was managed with diuretics, other supportive measures, or by reducing the imatinib dose (see Administration and Dosage). The frequency of severe superficial edema was 0.9% to 6%.

A variety of adverse events represent local or general fluid retention including pleural effusion, ascites, pulmonary edema, and rapid weight gain with or without superficial edema. These events appear to be dose-related, were more common in the blast crisis and accelerated phase studies (where the dose was 600 mg/day), and are more common in the elderly. These events were usually managed by interrupting imatinib treatment and with diuretics or other appropriate supportive care measures. However, a few of these events may be serious or life-threatening, and 1 patient with blast crisis died with pleural effusion, CHF, and renal failure.

Adverse events, regardless of relationship to study drug, that were reported in at least 10% of the patients treated in the imatinib studies are shown in the following tables.

Imatinib Adverse Reactions Reported in Newly Diagnosed CML Clinical Trial (≥ 10% of All Patients)[a]				
	All grades		CTC grades 3/4	
Adverse reaction	Imatinib (N = 551)	IFN + Ara-C (N = 533)	Imatinib (N = 551)	IFN + Ara-C (N = 533)
CNS				
Dizziness	13.2	23.1	0.5	3.4
Headache	28.5	41.8	0.4	3.2
Insomnia	11.4	18.4	0	2.3
GI				
Abdominal pain	23.4	22.9	2	3.6
Diarrhea	30.3	40.9	1.3	3.2
Dyspepsia	15.1	9	0	0.8
Nausea	42.5	60.8	0.4	5.1
Vomiting	14.7	26.6	0.9	3.4
Musculoskeletal				
Joint pain	26.7	38.3	2.2	6.8
Muscle cramps	35.4	9.9	1.1	0.2
Musculoskeletal pain	33.6	40.5	2.7	7.7
Myalgia	20.9	38.6	1.5	8.1
Respiratory				
Cough	12.5	21.6	0.2	0.6
Nasopharyngitis	19.2	7.7	0	0.2
Upper respiratory tract infection	12.5	7.9	0.2	0.4
Miscellaneous				
Fatigue	30.7	64.7	1.1	24
Fluid retention	54.1	10.1	0.9	0.9
Superficial edema	53.2	8.8	0.9	0.4
Other fluid retention events	3.4	1.5	0	0.6
Hemorrhage	18.9	19.9	0.7	1.3
Pharyngolaryngeal pain	14.2	11.4	0.2	0
Pyrexia	11.8	38.6	0.5	2.8
Rash	31.9	25	2	2.1
Weight increased	11.6	1.5	0.7	0.2

[a] All adverse events occurring in 10% or more of patients are listed regardless of suspected relationship to treatment.

Imatinib Adverse Reactions Reported in CML Clinical Trials (≥ 10% of All Patients in Any Trial)[a]						
	Myeloid blast crisis (n = 260)		Accelerated phase (n = 235)		Chronic phase, IFN failure (n = 532)	
Adverse reaction	All grades	Grade 3/4	All grades	Grade 3/4	All grades	Grade 3/4
CNS						
Anxiety	8	0.8	12	0	8	0.4
CNS hemorrhage	9	7	3	3	2	1
Dizziness	12	0.4	13	0	16	0.2
Headache	27	5	32	2	36	0.6
Insomnia	10	0	14	0	14	0.2
Dermatologic						
Pruritus	8	1	14	0.9	14	0.8
Skin rash	36	5	47	5	47	3
GI						
Abdominal pain	30	6	33	4	32	1
Constipation	16	2	16	0.9	9	0.4
Diarrhea	43	4	57	5	48	3
Dyspepsia	12	0	22	0	27	0
GI hemorrhage	8	4	6	5	2	0.4
Nausea	71	5	73	5	63	3
Vomiting	54	4	58	3	36	2
Musculoskeletal						
Arthralgia	25	5	34	6	40	1
Muscle cramps	28	1	47	0.4	62	2
Musculoskeletal pain	42	9	49	9	38	2
Myalgia	9	0	24	2	27	0.2
Respiratory						
Chest pain	7	2	10	0.4	11	0.8
Cough	14	0.8	27	0.9	20	0
Dyspnea	15	4	21	7	12	0.9
Nasopharyngitis	10	0	17	0	22	0.2
Pharyngitis	10	0	12	0	15	0
Pneumonia	13	7	10	7	4	1
Sinusitis	4	0.4	11	0.4	9	0.4
Upper respiratory tract infection	3	0	12	0.4	19	0

IMATINIB MESYLATE

Imatinib Adverse Reactions Reported in CML Clinical Trials (≥ 10% of All Patients in Any Trial)[a]

Adverse reaction	Myeloid blast crisis (n = 260) All grades	Myeloid blast crisis (n = 260) Grade 3/4	Accelerated phase (n = 235) All grades	Accelerated phase (n = 235) Grade 3/4	Chronic phase, IFN failure (n = 532) All grades	Chronic phase, IFN failure (n = 532) Grade 3/4
Miscellaneous						
Anorexia	14	2	17	2	7	0
Asthenia	18	5	21	5	15	0.2
Fatigue	30	4	46	4	48	1
Fluid retention	72	11	76	6	69	4
Superficial edema	66	6	74	3	67	2
Other fluid retention events[b]	22	6	15	4	7	2
Hemorrhage, any	53	19	49	11	30	2
Hypokalemia	13	4	9	2	6	0.8
Influenza	0.8	0.4	6	0	11	0.2
Liver toxicity	10	5	12	6	6	3
Night sweats	13	0.8	17	1	14	0.2
Pyrexia	41	7	41	8	21	2
Rigors	10	0	12	0.4	10	0
Weight increase	5	1	17	5	32	7

[a] All adverse events occurring in 10% or more of patients are listed regardless of suspected relationship to treatment.
[b] Other fluid retention events include anasarca, ascites, edema aggravated, fluid retention not otherwise specified, pericardial effusion, pleural effusion, and pulmonary edema.

Hematologic toxicity: Cytopenias, particularly neutropenia and thrombocytopenia, were a consistent finding in all studies, with a higher frequency at doses greater than or equal to 750 mg (phase 1 study). The occurrence of cytopenias in CML patients was also dependent on the stage of the disease, with a frequency of grade 3 or 4 neutropenia and thrombocytopenia between 2- and 3-fold higher in blast crisis and accelerated phase compared with chronic phase. In patients with newly diagnosed CML, cytopenias were less frequent than in the other CML patients. The median duration of the neutropenic and thrombocytopenic episodes varied from 2 to 3 weeks, and from 2 to 4 weeks, respectively. These events usually can be managed with either a dose reduction or an interruption of treatment with imatinib, but in rare cases require permanent discontinuation of treatment.

Hepatotoxicity: Severe elevation of transaminases or bilirubin occurred in 3% to 6% and were usually managed with dose reduction or interruption (the median duration of these episodes was approximately 1 week). Treatment was discontinued permanently because of liver laboratory abnormalities in less than 1% of patients. However, 1 patient who was taking acetaminophen regularly for fever died of acute liver failure.

Lab test abnormalities –

Imatinib Lab Abnormalities in Newly Diagnosed CML Trial (%)

CTC grades[a]	Imatinib (N = 551) Grade 3	Imatinib (N = 551) Grade 4	IFN + Ara-C (N = 533) Grade 3	IFN + Ara-C (N = 533) Grade 4
Hematology parameters				
Anemia	2.7	0.4	4.1	0.2
Neutropenia[b]	11.4	2.2	20.3	4.3
Thrombocytopenia[b]	6.9	0.2	15.8	0.6
Biochemistry parameters				
Elevated alkaline phosphatase	0.2	0	0.8	0
Elevated ALT	3.1	0.4	5.6	0
Elevated AST	2.9	0.2	3.8	0.4
Elevated bilirubin	0.2	0.5	0.2	0
Elevated creatinine	0	0	0.4	0

[a] CTC grades: Neutropenia (grade 3, at least 0.5 to 1 × 10^9/L; grade 4, less than 0.5 × 10^9/L); thrombocytopenia (grade 3, at least 10 to 50 × 10^9/L; grade 4, less than 10 × 10^9/L); anemia (grade 3, hemoglobin at least 65 to 80 g/L; grade 4, less than 65 g/L); elevated creatinine (grade 3, greater than 3 to 6 × upper limit of normal range [ULN]; grade 4, greater than 6 × ULN); elevated bilirubin (grade 3, greater than 3 to 10 × ULN; grade 4, greater than 10 × ULN); elevated alkaline phosphatase, AST, or ALT (grade 3, greater than 5 to 20 × ULN, grade 4, greater than 20 × ULN).
[b] $P < 0.001$ (difference in grade 3 plus 4 abnormalities between the 2 treatment groups).

Imatinib Lab Abnormalities in Other CML Clinical Trials (%)

CTC grade[a]	Myeloid blast crisis (n = 260) 600 mg (n = 223) 400 mg (n = 37) Grade 3	Myeloid blast crisis (n = 260) Grade 4	Accelerated phase (n = 235) 600 mg (n = 158) 400 mg (n = 77) Grade 3	Accelerated phase (n = 235) Grade 4	Chronic phase, IFN failure (n = 532) 400 mg Grade 3	Chronic phase, IFN failure (n = 532) Grade 4
Hematology parameters						
Anemia	42	11	34	7	6	1
Neutropenia	16	48	23	36	27	9
Thrombocytopenia	30	33	31	13	21	< 1
Biochemistry parameters						
Elevated alkaline phosphatase	4.6	0	5.5	0.4	0.2	0
Elevated ALT	2.3	0.4	4.3	0	2.1	0
Elevated AST	1.9	0	3	0	2.3	0
Elevated bilirubin	3.8	0	2.1	0	0.6	0
Elevated creatinine	1.5	0	1.3	0	0.2	0

[a] CTC grades: Neutropenia (grade 3, at least 0.5 to 1 × 10^9/L; grade 4, less than 0.5 × 10^9/L); thrombocytopenia (grade 3, at least 10 to 50 × 10^9/L; grade 4, less than 10 × 10^9/L); anemia (grade 3, hemoglobin at least 65 to 80 g/L; grade 4, less than 65 g/L); elevated creatinine (grade 3, greater than 3 to 6 × ULN; grade 4, greater than 6 × ULN); elevated bilirubin (grade 3, greater than 3 to 10 × ULN; grade 4, greater than 10 × ULN); elevated alkaline phosphatase, AST, or ALT (grade 3, greater than 5 to 20 × ULN, grade 4, greater than 20 × ULN).

Miscellaneous –

Elderly: With the exception of edema, where it was more frequent, there was no evidence of an increase in the incidence or severity of adverse events in older patients (65 years of age or older).

Gender: In women there was an increase in the frequency of neutropenia, as well as grade 1/2 fatigue, headache, nausea, rash, rigors, superficial edema, and vomiting.

Children: The overall safety profile of pediatric patients treated with imatinib was similar to that found in adult patients, except that musculoskeletal pain was less frequent (20.5%) and peripheral edema was not reported.

▶*GIST:* The majority of imatinib-treated patients experienced adverse events at some time. The most frequently reported adverse events were abdominal pain, diarrhea, edema, fatigue, nausea, muscle cramps, and rash. Most events were of mild to moderate severity. The drug was discontinued for adverse events in 6 patients (8%) in both dose levels studied. Superficial edema, most frequently periorbital or lower extremity edema, was managed with diuretics, other supportive measures, or by reducing the dose of imatinib (see Administration and Dosage). Severe superficial edema (CTC grade 3 or 4) was observed in 3 patients (2%), including face edema in 1 patient. Grade 3 or 4 pleural effusion or ascites was observed in 3 patients (2%).

Adverse events, regardless of relationship to study drug, that were reported in at least 10% of the patients treated with imatinib are shown in the table below. No major differences were seen in the severity of adverse events between the 400 or 600 mg treatment groups, although overall incidence of dermatitis, diarrhea, edema, headache, and muscle cramps was somewhat higher in the 600 mg treatment group.

Imatinib Adverse Reactions Reported in GIST Trial (≥ 10% of All Patients at Either Dose)[a]

Adverse reaction	All CTC grades Initial dose (mg/day) 400 mg (n = 73)	All CTC grades Initial dose (mg/day) 600 mg (n = 74)	CTC grade 3/4 Initial dose (mg/day) 400 mg (n = 73)	CTC grade 3/4 Initial dose (mg/day) 600 mg (n = 74)
CNS				
Cerebral hemorrhage	1	0	1	0
Headache	25	35	0	0
Insomnia	11	11	0	0
GI				
Abdominal pain	37	37	7	3
Diarrhea	56	60	1	4
Flatulence	16	23	0	0
GI tract hemorrhage	6	4	4	1
Nausea	53	56	3	3
Tumor hemorrhage	1	4	1	4
Vomiting	22	23	1	3
Musculoskeletal				
Muscle cramps	30	41	0	0
Musculoskeletal pain	19	11	3	0
Respiratory				
Nasopharyngitis	12	14	0	0
Upper respiratory tract infection	6	11	0	0

IMATINIB MESYLATE

Imatinib Adverse Reactions Reported in GIST Trial (≥ 10% of All Patients at Either Dose)[a]				
	All CTC grades		CTC grade 3/4	
	Initial dose (mg/day)		Initial dose (mg/day)	
Adverse reaction	400 mg (n = 73)	600 mg (n = 74)	400 mg (n = 73)	600 mg (n = 74)
Special senses				
Lacrimation increased	6	11	0	0
Taste disturbance	1	14	0	0
Miscellaneous				
Back pain	11	10	1	0
Fatigue	33	38	1	0
Fluid retention	71	76	6	3
Superficial edema	71	76	4	0
Pleural effusion or ascites	6	4	1	3
Hemorrhage, any	18	19	5	8
Pyrexia	12	5	0	0
Skin rash	26	38	3	3

[a] All adverse events occurring in 10% or more of patients are listed regardless of suspected relationship to treatment.

Imatinib Laboratory Abnormalities in GIST Trial (%)				
	400 mg (n = 73)		600 mg (n = 74)	
	CTC grade[a] 3	CTC grade 4	CTC grade 3	CTC grade 4
Hematology parameters				
Anemia	3	0	4	1
Neutropenia	3	3	5	4
Thrombocytopenia	0	0	1	0
Biochemistry parameters				
Elevated alkaline phosphatase	0	0	1	0
Elevated ALT	3	0	4	0
Elevated AST	3	0	1	1
Elevated bilirubin	1	0	1	3
Elevated creatinine	0	1	3	0
Reduced albumin	3	0	4	0

[a] CTC grades: Neutropenia (grade 3, at least 0.5 to 1×10^9/L; grade 4, less than 0.5×10^9/L); thrombocytopenia (grade 3, at least 10 to 50×10^9/L; grade 4, less than 10×10^9/L); anemia (grade 3, at least 65 to 80 g/L; grade 4, less than 65 g/L); elevated creatinine (grade 3, greater than 3 to 6 × ULN; grade 4, greater than 6 × ULN); elevated bilirubin (grade 3, greater than 3 to 10 × ULN; grade 4, greater than 10 × ULN); elevated alkaline phosphatase, AST, or ALT (grade 3, greater than 5 to 20 × ULN; grade 4, greater than 20 × ULN); albumin (grade 3, less than 20 g/L).

▶*Other adverse events:*

Cardiovascular – Cardiac failure, flushing, hypertension, hypotension, peripheral coldness, tachycardia (0.1% to 1%); pericarditis, thrombosis/embolism (less than 0.1%).

CNS – Paresthesia (1% to 10%); anxiety, depression, memory impairment, migraine, peripheral neuropathy, somnolence, syncope (0.1% to 1%); cerebral edema (including fatalities), confusion, convulsions, increased intracranial pressure (less than 0.1%).

Dermatologic – Alopecia, dry skin (1% to 10%); bullous eruption, exfoliative dermatitis, nail disorder, photosensitivity reaction, psoriasis, purpura, skin pigmentation changes (0.1% to 1%); acute generalized exanthematous pustulosis, Stevens-Johnson syndrome, vesicular rash (less than 0.1%).

GI – Abdominal distention, gastroesophageal reflux, mouth ulceration (1% to 10%); gastric ulcer, gastritis, gastroenteritis (0.1% to 1%); colitis, ileus/intestinal obstruction, pancreatitis (less than 0.1%).

GU – Breast enlargement, hematuria, menorrhagia, sexual dysfunction, urinary frequency (0.1% to 1%).

Hematologic – Pancytopenia (0.1% to 1%); aplastic anemia (less than 0.1%).

Lab test abnormalities – Blood CPK increased, blood LDH increased (0.1% to 1%).

Metabolic/Nutritional – Appetite disturbances, dehydration, gout, hypophosphatemia, weight decreased (0.1% to 1%); hyperkalemia, hyponatremia (less than 0.1%).

Musculoskeletal – Joint swelling (1% to 10%); joint and muscle stiffness, sciatica (0.1% to 1%).

Respiratory – Interstitial pneumonitis, pulmonary fibrosis (less than 0.1%).

Special senses – Conjunctivitis, vision blurred (1% to 10%); conjunctival hemorrhage, dry eye, tinnitus, vertigo (0.1% to 1%); glaucoma, macular edema, papilledema, retinal hemorrhage, vitreous hemorrhage (less than 0.1%).

Miscellaneous – Herpes simplex, herpes zoster, renal failure, sepsis (0.1% to 1%); hypersensitivity, tumor necrosis (less than 0.1%).

Overdosage

Experiences with doses greater than 800 mg are limited. An oral dose of 1200 mg/m²/day, approximately 2.5 times the human dose of 800 mg based on body surface area, was not lethal to rats following 14 days of administration. A dose of 3600 mg/m²/day, approximately 7.5 times the human dose of 800 mg, was lethal to rats after 7 to 10 administrations, because of the general deterioration of the animals with secondary degenerative histological changes in many tissues. In the event of overdosage, observe the patient and give appropriate supportive treatment.

Patient Information

Instruct patients to take this medication with a meal and a large glass of water to minimize GI upset. Do not administer with grapefruit juice.

Instruct women of childbearing potential to avoid becoming pregnant while taking this medication.

Inform patients of the common side effects including abdominal pain, diarrhea, fatigue, fluid retention, nausea, muscle cramps, and rash.

Inform patients of the potential drug interactions with acetaminophen, St. John's wort, oral contraceptives, warfarin, and anticonvulsants.

Inform patients not to breastfeed while taking this medication.

Imatinib may cause photosensitivity. Instruct patients to avoid prolonged exposure to the sun and other ultraviolet light (eg, tanning beds) and to use sunscreens and wear protective clothing until tolerance is determined.

GEFITINIB

Rx   **Iressa** (AstraZeneca)   **Tablets:** 250 mg   Lactose. (IRESSA 250). Brown. Film-coated. In 30s.

Indications

➤*Nonsmall cell lung cancer (NSCLC):* Gefitinib is indicated as monotherapy for the treatment of patients with locally advanced or metastatic non-small cell lung cancer after failure of platinum-based and docetaxel chemotherapies.

Administration and Dosage

➤*Approved by the FDA:* May 5, 2003.

➤*Dose:* The recommended daily dose of gefitinib is one 250 mg tablet with or without food. Higher doses do not give a better response and cause increased toxicity.

➤*Dosage adjustment:*

Diarrhea / Skin reactions – Patients with poorly tolerated diarrhea (sometimes associated with dehydration) or skin adverse drug reactions may be successfully managed by providing a brief (up to 14 days) therapy interruption followed by reinstatement of the 250 mg/day dose.

Pulmonary – In the event of acute onset or worsening of pulmonary symptoms (ie, dyspnea, cough, fever), interrupt gefitinib therapy, promptly investigate these symptoms, and initiate appropriate treatment. If interstitial lung disease (ILD) is confirmed, discontinue gefitinib and treat the patient appropriately.

Ocular – For patients who develop onset of new eye symptoms such as pain, medically evaluate and manage appropriately, including gefitinib therapy interruption and removal of an aberrant eyelash if present. After symptoms and eye changes have been resolved, decide on reinstatement of the 250 mg/day dose.

➤*CYP3A4 inducers:* In patients receiving a potent CYP3A4 inducer such as rifampin or phenytoin, consider a dose increase to 500 mg/day in the absence of severe adverse drug reaction, and carefully monitor clinical response and adverse events.

➤*Storage / Stability:* Store at controlled room temperature 20° to 25°C (68° to 77°F).

Actions

➤*Pharmacology:* The mechanism of the clinical antitumor action of gefitinib is not fully characterized. Gefitinib inhibits the intracellular phosphorylation of numerous tyrosine kinases associated with transmembrane cell surface receptors, including the tyrosine kinases associated with epidermal growth factor receptor (EGFR-TK). EGFR is expressed on the cell surface of many normal cells and cancer cells. No clinical studies have been performed that demonstrate a correlation between EGFR receptor expression and response to gefitinib.

➤*Pharmacokinetics:*

Absorption / Distribution – Gefitinib is slowly absorbed, with peak plasma levels occurring 3 to 7 hours after dosing and mean oral bioavailability of 60%. Gefitinib is extensively distributed throughout the body with a mean steady-state volume of distribution of 1400 L following IV administration. In vitro binding of gefitinib to human plasma proteins (serum albumin and α1-acid glycoprotein) is 90% and is independent of drug concentrations.

Metabolism / Excretion – Gefitinib undergoes extensive hepatic metabolism in humans, predominantly by CYP3A4. Three sites of biotransformation have been identified: Metabolism of the N-propoxymorpholino group; demethylation of the methoxy-substituent on the quinazoline; oxidative defluorination of the halogenated phenyl group.

Five metabolites were identified in human plasma. Only O-desmethyl gefitinib has exposure comparable to gefitinib. Although this metabolite has similar EGFR-TK activity to gefitinib in the isolated enzyme assay, it had only 1/14 of the potency of gefitinib in one of the cell-based assays.

Gefitinib is cleared primarily by the liver, with total plasma clearance and elimination half-life values of 595 mL/min and 48 hours, respectively, after IV administration. Excretion is predominantly via the feces (86%), with renal elimination of drug and metabolites accounting for less than 4% of the administered dose.

Contraindications

Severe hypersensitivity to gefitinib or any other component of the product.

Warnings

➤*Pulmonary toxicity:* Cases of ILD have been observed in patients receiving gefitinib at an overall incidence of about 1%. Approximately one third of the cases have been fatal. The reported incidence of ILD was about 2% in the Japanese post marketing experience, about 0.3% in approximately 23,000 patients treated with gefitinib in a US expanded access program, and about 1% in the studies of first-line use in NSCLC (but with similar rates in treatment and placebo groups). Reports have described the adverse event as interstitial pneumonia, pneumonitis, and alveolitis. Patients often present with the acute onset of dyspnea, sometimes associated with cough or low-grade fever, often becoming severe within a short time and requiring hospitalization. ILD has occurred in patients who have received prior radiation therapy (31% of reported cases), prior chemotherapy (57% of reported cases),

and no previous therapy (12% of reported cases). Patients with concurrent idiopathic pulmonary fibrosis whose condition worsens while receiving gefitinib have been observed to have an increased mortality compared to those without concurrent idiopathic pulmonary fibrosis.

In the event of acute onset or worsening of pulmonary symptoms (ie, dyspnea, cough, fever), interrupt gefitinib therapy and promptly investigate these symptoms. If ILD is confirmed, discontinue gefitinib and treat the patient appropriately (see Administration and Dosage).

➤*Renal function impairment:* The effect of severe renal impairment on the pharmacokinetics of gefitinib is not known. Treat patients with severe renal impairment with caution when giving gefitinib.

➤*Hepatic function impairment:* In vitro and in vivo evidence suggest that gefitinib is cleared primarily by the liver. Therefore, gefitinib exposure may be increased in patients with hepatic dysfunction. In patients with liver metastases and moderately to severely elevated biochemical liver abnormalities, however, gefitinib pharmacokinetics were similar to the pharmacokinetics of individuals without liver abnormalities. The influence of non-cancer related hepatic impairment on the pharmacokinetics of gefitinib has not been evaluated.

➤*Pregnancy: Category D.* Gefitinib may cause fetal harm when administered to a pregnant woman. A single dose study in rats showed that gefitinib crosses the placenta after an oral dose of 5 mg/kg (30 mg/mg^2, about one fifth the recommended human dose on a mg/mg^2 basis). When pregnant rats treated with 5 mg/kg from the beginning of organogenesis to the end of weaning gave birth, there was a reduction in the number of offspring born alive. This effect was more severe at 20 mg/kg and was accompanied by high neonatal mortality soon after parturition. In this study, a dose of 1 mg/kg caused no adverse effects.

In rabbits, a dose of 20 mg/kg/day (240 mg/m^2, about twice the recommended dose in humans on a mg/m^2 basis) caused reduced fetal weight.

There are no adequate and well-controlled studies in pregnant women using gefitinib. If used during pregnancy or if the patient becomes pregnant while receiving this drug, apprise the patient of the potential hazard to the fetus or potential risk for loss of the pregnancy.

➤*Lactation:* It is not known whether gefitinib is excreted in human milk. Following oral administration of carbon-14 labeled gefitinib to rats 14 days postpartum, concentrations of radioactivity in milk were higher than in blood. Levels of gefitinib and its metabolites were 11- to 19-fold higher in milk than in blood, after oral exposure of lactating rats to a dose of 5 mg/kg. Because many drugs are excreted in human milk and because of the potential for serious adverse reactions in nursing infants, advise women against breast-feeding while receiving gefitinib therapy.

➤*Children:* Safety and efficacy of gefitinib in pediatric patients have not been studied.

Precautions

➤*Hepatotoxicity:* Asymptomatic increases in liver transaminases have been observed in gefitinib treated patients; therefore, consider periodic liver function (ie, transaminases, bilirubin, and alkaline phosphatase) testing. Consider discontinuation of gefitinib if changes are severe.

Drug Interactions

➤*CYP450:* In human liver microsome studies, gefitinib had no inhibitory effect on CYP1A2, CYP2C9, and CYP3A4 activities at concentrations ranging from 2000-5000 ng/mL. At the highest concentration studied (5000 ng/mL), gefitinib inhibited CYP2C19 by 24% and CYP2D6 by 43%.

Gefitinib Drug Interactions			
Precipitant drug	Object drug*		Description
CYP3A4 inducers (eg, rifampin, phenytoin)	Gefitinib	↓	The plasma concentration of gefitinib is decreased due to an increase in its metabolism. Coadministration with rifampin caused a decrease in gefitinib AUC by 85%. Consider a dose increase of gefitinib if coadministered with a potent CYP3A4 inducer (see Administration and Dosage).
CYP3A4 inhibitors (eg, ketoconazole, itraconazole)	Gefitinib	↑	Potent CYP3A4 inhibitors decrease gefitinib metabolism and increase its plasma concentrations. Coadministration with itraconazole increased gefitinib AUC by 88%. Use with caution.
H₂ antagonist (eg, ranitidine, cimetidine) Sodium bicarbonate	Gefitinib	↓	Drugs that cause significant sustained elevations in gastric pH may reduce plasma concentrations of gefitinib and may reduce efficacy.
Gefitinib	Metoprolol	↑	Exposure to metoprolol, a substrate of CYP2D6, was increased by 30% when given with gefitinib.

GEFITINIB

Gefitinib Drug Interactions			
Precipitant drug	Object drug*		Description
Gefitinib	Warfarin	↑	INR elevations and/or bleeding events have been reported in some patients taking warfarin while on gefitinib therapy. Monitor PT or INR regularly.

* ↑ = Object drug increased. ↓ = Object drug decreased.

Adverse Reactions

Gefitinib Adverse Events (≥ 5%)		
Adverse reaction*	Gefitinib 250 mg/day (N = 102)	Gefitinib 500 mg/day (N = 114)
Diarrhea	48	67
Rash	43	54
Acne	25	33
Dry skin	13	26
Nausea	13	18
Vomiting	12	9
Pruritus	8	9
Anorexia	7	10
Asthenia	6	4
Weight loss	3	5

* A patient may have had more than 1 drug-related adverse event.

Gefitinib Adverse Events at 250 mg Dose by Worst CTC Grade (n = 102) (≥ 5%)					
Adverse reaction	All Grades	CTC Grade 1	CTC Grade 2	CTC Grade 3	CTC Grade 4
Diarrhea	48	41	6	1	0
Rash	43	39	4	0	0
Acne	25	19	6	0	0
Dry skin	13	12	1	0	0
Nausea	13	7	5	1	0
Vomiting	12	9	2	1	0
Pruritus	8	7	1	0	0
Anorexia	7	3	4	0	0
Asthenia	6	2	2	1	1

Only 2% of patients stopped therapy because of an adverse drug reaction (ADR). The onset of these ADRs occurred within the first month of therapy.

Other adverse events reported at an incidence of less than 5% in patients who received either 250 or 500 mg as monotherapy for treatment of NSCLC (along with their frequency at the 250 mg recommended dose) include the following: Peripheral edema (2%); amblyopia (2%); dyspnea (2%); conjunctivitis (1%); vesiculobullous rash (1%); mouth ulceration (1%).

►*Pulmonary:* Cases of ILD have been observed in patients receiving gefitinib at an overall incidence of about 1%. Approximately one third of the cases have been fatal. (see Warnings).

►*Miscellaneous:* In patients receiving gefitinib therapy, there were reports of eye pain and corneal erosion/ulcer, sometimes in association with aberrant eyelash growth. There were also rare reports of pancreatitis and very rare reports of corneal membrane sloughing, ocular ischemia/hemorrhage, toxic epidermal necrolysis, erythema multiforme, and allergic reactions, including angioedema and urticaria.

Data from nonclinical (in vitro and in vivo) studies indicate that gefitinib has the potential to inhibit the cardiac action potential repolarization process (eg, QT interval). The clinical relevance of these findings is unknown.

Overdosage

The acute toxicity of gefitinib up to 500 mg in clinical studies has been low. In nonclinical studies, a single dose of 12,000 mg/m^2 (about 80 times the recommended clinical dose on a mg/m^2 basis) was lethal to rats. Half this dose caused no mortality in mice.

There is no specific treatment for a gefitinib overdose and possible symptoms of overdose are not established. However, in phase 1 clinical trials, a limited number of patients were treated with daily doses of up to 1000 mg. An increase in frequency and severity of some adverse reactions was observed; mainly diarrhea and skin rash. Treat adverse reactions associated with overdose symptomatically; in particular, manage severe diarrhea appropriately.

Patient Information

Advise patients to seek medical advice promptly if they develop the folling:

1.) Severe or persistent diarrhea, nausea, anorexia, or vomiting as these have sometimes been associated with dehydration;
2.) an onset or worsening of pulmonary symptoms, (ie, shortness of breath or cough);
3.) an eye irritation; or
4.) any other new symptom.

Advise women of childbearing potential to avoid becoming pregnant.

BORTEZOMIB

Rx	Velcade (Millennium)	Powder for injection, lyophilized: 3.5 mg	35 mg mannitol. Preservative-free. Single-dose vials.

Indications

➤*Multiple myeloma:* For the treatment of multiple myeloma patients who have received at least 2 prior therapies and have demonstrated disease progression on the last therapy.

Administration and Dosage

➤*Approved by the FDA:* May 13, 2003.

The recommended dose of bortezomib is 1.3 mg/m^2/dose administered as a bolus IV injection twice weekly for 2 weeks (days 1, 4, 8, and 11) followed by a 10-day rest period (days 12 to 21).

This 3-week period is considered a treatment cycle. Separate consecutive doses by at least 72 hours.

➤*Dose modification:* Withhold bortezomib therapy at the onset of any grade 3 nonhematological or grade 4 hematological toxicities excluding neuropathy as discussed below. Once the symptoms of the toxicity have resolved, therapy may be reinitiated at a 25% reduced dose (1.3 mg/m^2/dose reduced to 1 mg/m^2/dose; 1 mg/m^2/dose reduced to 0.7 mg/m^2/dose). The following table contains the recommended dose modification for the management of patients who experience bortezomib-related neuropathic pain and/or peripheral sensory neuropathy. Treat patients with pre-existing severe neuropathy with bortezomib only after careful risk/benefit assessment.

Recommended Dose Modification for Bortezomib Related Neuropathic Pain and/or Peripheral Sensory Neuropathy	
Severity of peripheral neuropathy signs and symptoms	Modification of dose and regimen
Grade 1 (paresthesias and/or loss of reflexes) without pain or loss of function	No action.
Grade 1 with pain or grade 2 (interfering with function but not with activities of daily living)	Reduce dose to 1 mg/m^2.
Grade 2 with pain or grade 3 (interfering with activities of daily living)	Withhold bortezomib therapy until toxicity resolves. When toxicity resolves reinitiate with a reduced dose of bortezomib at 0.7 mg/m^2 and change treatment schedule to once weekly.
Grade 4 (permanent sensory loss that interferes with function)	Discontinue bortezomib.

➤*Reconstitution:* Prior to use, the contents of each vial must be reconstituted with 3.5 mL of normal (0.9%) saline, sodium chloride injection.

Use caution during handling and preparation. Use of gloves and other protective clothing to prevent skin contact is recommended.

➤*Storage/Stability:* Unopened vials of bortezomib are stable until the date indicated on the package when stored in the original package, protected from light, and at controlled room temperature 25°C (77°F); excursions permitted to 15° to 30°C (59° to 86°F).

When reconstituted, bortezomib may be stored at 25°C (77°F); excursions permitted to 15° to 30°C (59° to 86°F). Administer reconstituted bortezomib within 8 hours of preparation. The reconstituted material may be stored in the original vial and/or the syringe prior to administration. The product may be stored for up to 3 hours in a syringe; however, total storage time for the reconstituted material must not exceed 8 hours when exposed to normal indoor lighting.

Actions

➤*Pharmacology:* Bortezomib, a modified dipeptidyl boronic acid, is a reversible inhibitor of the chymotrypsin-like activity of the 26S proteasome in mammalian cells. The 26S proteasome is a large protein complex that degrades ubiquitinated proteins. The ubiquitin-proteasome pathway plays an essential role in regulating the intracellular concentration of specific proteins, thereby maintaining homeostasis within cells. Inhibition of the 26S proteasome prevents this targeted proteolysis, which can affect multiple signaling cascades within the cell. This disruption of normal homeostatic mechanisms can lead to cell death. Experiments have demonstrated that bortezomib is cytotoxic to a variety of cancer cell types in vitro. Bortezomib causes a delay in tumor growth in vivo in nonclinical tumor models, including multiple myeloma.

➤*Pharmacokinetics:*

Absorption/Distribution – Following IV administration of 1.3 mg/m^2 dose, the median estimated maximum plasma concentration of bortezomib was 509 ng/mL (range, 109 to 1300 ng/mL) in 8 patients with multiple myeloma and creatinine clearance values ranging from 31 to 169 mL/min. The binding of bortezomib to human plasma proteins averaged 83% over the concentration range of 100 to 1000 ng/mL.

Metabolism/Excretion – In vitro studies with human liver microsomes and human cDNA-expressed cytochrome P450 isozymes indicate that bortezomib is primarily oxidatively metabolized via cytochrome P450 enzymes 3A4, 2D6, 2C19, 2C9, and 1A2. The major metabolic

pathway is deboronation to form 2 deboronated metabolites that subsequently undergo hydroxylation to several metabolites. Deboronated-bortezomib metabolites are inactive as 26S proteasome inhibitors. Pooled plasma data from 8 patients at 10 and 30 minutes after dosing indicate that the plasma levels of metabolites are low compared with the parent drug. In patients with advanced malignancies, the mean elimination half-life of bortezomib after the first dose ranged from 9 to 15 hours at doses ranging from 1.45 to 2 mg/m^2.

Contraindications

Hypersensitivity to bortezomib, boron, or mannitol.

Warnings

➤*Peripheral neuropathy:* Bortezomib treatment causes a peripheral neuropathy that is predominantly sensory, although cases of mixed sensorimotor neuropathy also have been reported. Patients with pre-existing symptoms (ie, numbness, pain, or a burning feeling in the feet or hands) and/or signs of peripheral neuropathy may experience worsening during treatment with bortezomib. Monitor patients for symptoms of neuropathy, such as a burning sensation, hyperesthesia, hypesthesia, paresthesia, discomfort, or neuropathic pain. Patients experiencing new or worsening peripheral neuropathy may require change in the dose and schedule of bortezomib (see Administration and Dosage). Limited follow-up data regarding the outcome of peripheral neuropathy are available. Of the patients who experienced treatment-emergent neuropathy, more than 70% had previously been treated with neurotoxic agents and more than 80% of these patients had signs or symptoms of peripheral neuropathy at baseline.

Caution patients about the use of concomitant medications that may be associated with peripheral neuropathy (eg, amiodarone, antivirals, isoniazid, nitrofurantoin, statins) or with a decrease in blood pressure.

➤*Hypotension:* Bortezomib treatment can cause orthostatic/postural hypotension in about 12% of patients. These events are observed throughout therapy. Use caution when treating patients with a history of syncope, patients receiving medication known to be associated with hypotension, and patients who are dehydrated. Management of orthostatic/postural hypotension may include adjustment of antihypertensive medications, hydration, or administration of mineralocorticoids.

➤*Thrombocytopenia:* Thrombocytopenia, which occurred in about 40% of patients throughout therapy, was maximal at day 11 and usually recovered by the next cycle. Frequently monitor complete blood counts including platelet counts throughout treatment. Onset is most common in cycles 1 and 2 but can continue throughout therapy. There have been reports of GI and intracerebral hemorrhage in association with bortezomib-induced thrombocytopenia. Bortezomib treatment may be temporarily discontinued if patients experience grade 4 thrombocytopenia. Bortezomib may be reinitiated at a reduced dose after resolution of thrombocytopenia (see Administration and Dosage).

➤*Renal function impairment:* No clinical information is available on the use of bortezomib in patients with Ccr values less than 13 mL/min and patients on hemodialysis. Closely monitor these patients for toxicities when treated with bortezomib.

➤*Hepatic function impairment:* Bortezomib is metabolized by liver enzymes and bortezomib's clearance may decrease in patients with hepatic impairment. Closely monitor these patients for toxicities when treated with bortezomib.

➤*Mutagenesis:* Bortezomib showed clastogenic activity (structural chromosomal aberrations) in the in vitro chromosomal aberration assay using Chinese hamster ovary cells.

➤*Fertility impairment:* In the 6-month rat toxicity study, degenerative effects in the ovary were observed at doses of 0.3 mg/m^2 or more (one-fourth of the recommended clinical dose), and degenerative changes in the testes occurred at 1.2 mg/m^2. Bortezomib could have a potential effect on either male or female fertility.

➤*Elderly:* Of patients 65 years of age or older, 19% experienced responses vs 32% in patients under 65 years of age. Across the 256 patients analyzed for safety, the incidence of grade 3 or 4 events reported was 74%, 80%, and 85% for patients 50 years of age or younger, 51 to 65 years of age, and older than 65 years of age, respectively.

➤*Pregnancy:* Category D. Women of childbearing potential should avoid becoming pregnant while being treated with bortezomib.

Pregnant rabbits given bortezomib during organogenesis at a dose of 0.05 mg/kg (0.6 mg/m^2) experienced significant postimplantation loss and decreased number of live fetuses. Live fetuses from these litters also showed significant decreases in fetal weight. The dose is approximately 0.5 times the clinical dose of 1.3 mg/m^2 based on body surface area.

No placental transfer studies have been conducted with bortezomib. There are no adequate and well-controlled studies in pregnant women. If bortezomib is used during pregnancy, or if the patient becomes pregnant while receiving this drug, apprise the patient of the potential hazard to the fetus.

BORTEZOMIB

▶*Lactation:* It is not known whether bortezomib is excreted in human milk. Because many drugs are excreted in human milk and because of the potential for serious adverse reactions in nursing infants from bortezomib, advise women against breastfeeding while being treated with bortezomib.

▶*Children:* The safety and efficacy of bortezomib in children have not been established.

Precautions

▶*Monitoring:* Frequently monitor complete blood counts, including platelet counts, throughout treatment.

▶*GI effects:* Bortezomib treatment can cause nausea, diarrhea, constipation, and vomiting, sometimes requiring use of antiemetics and antidiarrheals. Administer fluid and electrolyte replacement to prevent dehydration.

Drug Interactions

Bortezomib Drug Interactions			
Precipitant drug	Object drug*		Description
CYP450 inducers or inhibitors	Bortezomib	↑↓	Bortezomib is a substrate for cytochrome P450 3A4, 2D6, 2C19, 2C9, and 1A2. Closely monitor patients for toxicities or reduced efficacy when bortezomib is coadministered with drugs that are inducers/inhibitors of cytochrome P450 3A4.
Bortezomib	CYP450 2C19 substrates	↑	Bortezomib may inhibit 2C19 isoenzyme activity and increase exposure to drugs that are substrates for this isoenzyme.
Bortezomib	Oral hypoglycemic agents	↑↓	Coadministration has resulted in hypo- and hyperglycemia. Closely monitor blood glucose levels and adjust dose of antidiabetic medication if necessary.

* ↑ = Object drug increased. ↓ = Object drug decreased.

Adverse Reactions

Two studies evaluated 228 patients with multiple myeloma receiving bortezomib 1.3 mg/m^2/dose twice weekly for 2 weeks followed by a 10-day rest period (21-day treatment cycle length) for a maximum of 8 treatment cycles.

The most commonly reported adverse events were asthenic conditions (eg, fatigue, malaise, weakness) (65%), nausea (64%), diarrhea (51%), appetite decreased (including anorexia) (43%), constipation (43%), thrombocytopenia (43%), peripheral neuropathy (including peripheral sensory neuropathy and peripheral neuropathy aggravated) (37%), pyrexia (36%), vomiting (36%), and anemia (32%). Fourteen percent of patients experienced at least 1 episode of grade 4 toxicity, with the most common toxicity being thrombocytopenia (3%) and neutropenia (3%). See table below.

A total of 113 (50%) of the 228 patients experienced serious adverse events during the studies. The most commonly reported serious adverse events included pyrexia (7%), pneumonia (7%), diarrhea (6%), vomiting (5%), dehydration (5%), and nausea (4%).

Adverse events thought to be drug-related and leading to discontinuation occurred in 18% of patients. The reasons for discontinuation included peripheral neuropathy (5%), thrombocytopenia (4%), diarrhea (2%), and fatigue (2%).

Two deaths were reported and considered to be possibly related to the drug: 1 case of cardiopulmonary arrest and 1 case of respiratory failure.

Most Commonly Reported Adverse Events with Bortezomib (≥ 10% Overall)			
	All patients (N = 228)		
Adverse reaction	All events	Grade 3 events	Grade 4 events
CNS			
Anxiety	14	0	0
Dizziness (excluding vertigo)	21	1	0
Headache	28	4	0
Insomnia	27	1	0
Peripheral neuropathy[1]	37	14	0
Dermatologic			
Pruritus	11	0	0
Rash	21	< 1	0
GI			
Abdominal pain	13	2	0
Appetite decreased[2]	43	3	0
Constipation[2]	43	2	0
Diarrhea[2]	51	7	< 1
Dyspepsia	13	0	0
Nausea[2]	64	6	0
Vomiting[2]	36	7	< 1

Most Commonly Reported Adverse Events with Bortezomib (≥ 10% Overall)			
	All patients (N = 228)		
Adverse reaction	All events	Grade 3 events	Grade 4 events
Hematologic			
Anemia	32	9	0
Neutropenia[3]	24	13	3
Thrombocytopenia[4]	43	27	3
Musculoskeletal			
Arthralgia	26	5	0
Bone pain	14	2	0
Muscle cramps	14	< 1	0
Myalgia	14	2	0
Respiratory			
Cough	17	< 1	0
Dyspnea	22	3	< 1
Pneumonia	10	5	0
Upper respiratory tract infection	18	0	0
Special senses			
Dysgeusia	13	< 1	0
Vision blurred	11	< 1	0
Miscellaneous			
Asthenic conditions[5]	65	18	< 1
Back pain	14	4	0
Dehydration	18	7	0
Edema	25	1	0
Herpes zoster	11	< 1	0
Hypotension[6]	12	4	0
Pain in limb	26	7	0
Paresthesia and dysesthesia	23	3	0
Pyrexia (> 38°C, 100°F)	36	4	0
Rigors	12	< 1	0

[1] New onset or worsening of existing neuropathy was noted throughout the cycles of treatment. Six percent of patients discontinued bortezomib because of neuropathy. More than 80% of all study patients had signs or symptoms of peripheral neuropathy at baseline evaluation. The incidence of grade 3 neuropathy was 5% (2 of 41 patients) in patients without baseline neuropathy. Symptoms may improve or return to baseline in some patients upon discontinuation of bortezomib. The complete time-course of this toxicity has not been fully characterized.

[2] The majority of patients experienced GI adverse events during the studies, including nausea, diarrhea, constipation, and vomiting. Grade 3 or 4 GI events occurred in 21% of patients and were considered serious in 13% of patients.

[3] The incidence of febrile neutropenia was less than 1%.

[4] Thrombocytopenia was characterized by a dose-related decrease in platelet count during the bortezomib dosing period (days 1 to 11) with a return to baseline in platelet count during the rest period (days 12 to 21) in each treatment cycle. Four percent of patients discontinued bortezomib treatment due to thrombocytopenia of any grade.

[5] Asthenia was predominantly reported as grade 1 or 2. The first onset of fatigue was most often reported during the first and second cycles of therapy. Two percent of patients discontinued treatment because of fatigue.

[6] Most events were grade 1 or 2 in severity. Patients developing orthostatic hypotension did not have evidence of orthostatic hypotension at study entry; half had pre-existing hypertension and one third had evidence of peripheral neuropathy. Doses of antihypertensive medications may need to be adjusted in patients receiving bortezomib. Four percent of patients experienced hypotension, including orthostatic hypotension, and had a concurrent syncopal event.

▶*Serious adverse events:* In approximately 580 patients, the following serious adverse events (not described above) were reported, considered at least possibly related to study medication, and in at least 1 patient treated with bortezomib administered as monotherapy or in combination with other chemotherapeutics. These studies were conducted in patients with hematological malignancies and in solid tumors.

Cardiovascular – Atrial fibrillation aggravated, atrial flutter, cardiac amyloidosis, cardiac arrest, cardiac failure congestive, cerebrovascular accident, deep venous thrombosis, myocardial ischemia, MI, pericardial effusion, peripheral embolism, pulmonary edema, pulmonary embolism, ventricular tachycardia.

CNS – Ataxia, coma, dizziness, dysarthria, dysautonomia, cranial palsy, grand mal convulsion, hemorrhagic stroke, motor dysfunction, spinal cord compression, transient ischemic attack.

GI – Ascites, dysphagia, fecal impaction, gastritis hemorrhagic, GI hemorrhage, hematemesis, ileus paralytic, large intestinal obstruction, paralytic intestinal obstruction, small intestinal obstruction, large intestinal perforation, stomatitis, melena, pancreatitis acute.

Hepatic – Hyperbilirubinemia, portal vein thrombosis.

Hypersensitivity – Anaphylactic reaction, drug hypersensitivity, immune complex mediated hypersensitivity.

Metabolic/Nutritional – Hypocalcemia, hyperuricemia, hypokalemia, hyponatremia, tumor lysis syndrome.

Psychiatric – Agitation, confusion, psychotic disorder, suicidal ideation.

Renal/GU – Calculus renal, bilateral hydronephrosis, bladder spasm, hematuria, urinary incontinence, urinary retention, acute and chronic

BORTEZOMIB

renal failure, glomerular nephritis proliferative.

Respiratory – Acute respiratory distress syndrome, atelectasis, chronic obstructive airway disease exacerbated, dyspnea, dyspnea exertional, epistaxis, hemoptysis, hypoxia, lung infiltration, pleural effusion, pneumonitis, respiratory distress, respiratory failure.

Miscellaneous – Bacteremia, disseminated intravascular coagulation, skeletal fracture, subdural hematoma.

Overdosage

Cardiovascular safety pharmacology studies in monkeys show that lethal IV doses are associated with decreases in blood pressure, increases in heart rate, increases in contractility, and ultimately terminal hypotension. In monkeys, doses of 3 mg/m^2 and greater (approximately twice the recommended clinical dose) resulted in progressive hypotension starting at 1 hour and progressing to death by 12 to 14 hours following drug administration.

No cases of overdosage with bortezomib were reported during clinical trials. Single doses of up to 2 mg/m^2/week have been administered in adults. In the event of overdosage, monitor the patient's vital signs and give appropriate supportive care to maintain blood pressure and body temperature.

There is no known antidote for bortezomib overdosage.

Patient Information

Because bortezomib may be associated with fatigue, dizziness, syncope, orthostatic/postural hypotension, diplopia, or blurred vision, patients should be cautious when operating machinery, including automobiles.

Advise patients to use effective contraceptive measures to prevent pregnancy and to avoid breastfeeding during treatment with bortezomib.

Because patients receiving bortezomib therapy may experience vomiting and/or diarrhea, advise patients of appropriate measures to avoid dehydration. Instruct patients to seek medical advice if they experience symptoms of dizziness, lightheadedness, or fainting spells.

Caution patients about the use of concomitant medications that may be associated with peripheral neuropathy (eg, amiodarone, antivirals, isoniazid, nitrofurantoin, statins), or with a decrease in blood pressure.

Instruct patients to contact their physician if they experience new or worsening symptoms of peripheral neuropathy.

PORFIMER SODIUM

Rx	**Photofrin** (Axican Scandipharm)	**Cake or powder for injection (freeze-dried):** 75 mg	Preservative-free. In vials.

Indications

➤*Esophageal cancer:* For palliation of patients with completely obstructing esophageal cancer, or of patients with partially obstructing esophageal cancer who cannot be satisfactorily treated with Nd:YAG laser therapy.

➤*Endobronchial non-small cell lung cancer (NSCLC):* For treatment of microinvasive endobronchial NSCLC in patients for whom surgery and radiotherapy are not indicated; reduction of obstruction and palliation of symptoms in patients with completely or partially obstructing endobronchial NSCLC.

➤*Barrett esophagus (BE):* For ablation of high-grade dysplasia (HGD) in BE patients who do not undergo esophagectomy.

➤*Unlabeled uses:* For treatment of AIDS-related cutaneous Kaposi sarcoma, primary or recurrent basal cell carcinoma, and squamous cell carcinoma.

Administration and Dosage

➤*Approved by the FDA:* December 27, 1995.

Photodynamic therapy (PDT) with porfimer is a 2-stage process requiring administration of drug and light by trained practitioners. The first stage is the IV injection of porfimer, followed 40 to 50 hours later by illumination with laser lights constituting the second stage of therapy. A second laser light application may be given 96 to 120 hours after injection, preceded by gentle debridement of residual tumor (see Laser light administration). In clinical studies, debridement via endoscopy was required 2 days after the initial light application.

➤*Porfimer administration:* Administer 2 mg/kg porfimer as a single slow IV injection over 3 to 5 minutes.

Esophageal and endobronchial cancer – For treatment of esophageal and endobronchial cancer, patients may receive a second course of PDT a minimum of 30 days after the initial therapy; up to 3 courses of PDT (each separated by a minimum of 30 days) can be given. Before each course of treatment, evaluate esophageal cancer patients for the presence of a tracheoesophageal/bronchoesophageal fistula (see Contraindications).

In patients with endobronchial lesions who have recently undergone radiotherapy, allow sufficient time (approximately 4 weeks) between therapies to ensure that acute inflammation produced by radiotherapy has subsided prior to PDT (see Precautions, Use with radiotherapy). Evaluate all patients for the possibility that the tumor may be eroding into a major blood vessel.

Barrett esophagus – For the ablation of HGD BE, patients may receive an additional course of PDT at a minimum of 90 days after the initial therapy; up to 3 courses of PDT (each injection separated by a minimum of 90 days) can be given to a previously treated segment that still shows high-grade dysplasia, low-grade dysplasia, or Barrett metaplasia, or to a new segment if the initial Barrett segment was more than 7 cm in length. Both residual and additional segments may be treated in the same light session(s) provided that the total length of the segments treated with the balloon/diffuser combination is not greater than 7 cm. In the case of a previously treated esophageal segment, if it has not sufficiently healed and/or histological assessment of biopsies is not clear, the subsequent course of PDT may be delayed for an additional 1 to 2 months.

➤*Preparation of solution:* Reconstitute each vial of porfimer with 31.8 mL of either 5% dextrose injection or 0.9% sodium chloride injection, resulting in a final concentration of 2.5 mg/mL and a pH in the range of 7 to 8. Shake well until dissolved. Do not mix porfimer with other drugs in the same solution. Porfimer has been formulated with an overage to deliver the 75 mg labeled quantity. Protect the reconstituted product from bright light and use immediately. Reconstituted porfimer is an opaque solution in which detection of particulate matter by visual inspection is extremely difficult.

➤*Extravasation:* Take precautions to prevent extravasation at the injection site. If extravasation occurs, take care to protect the area from light. There is no known benefit from injecting the extravasation site with another substance.

➤*Laser light administration:*

Esophageal and endobronchial cancer – Initiate 630 nm wavelength laser light delivery to the patient 40 to 50 hours following injection with porfimer. A second laser light treatment may be given as early as 96 hours or as late as 120 hours after the initial injection with porfimer. Do not give additional injections of porfimer for such retreatment with laser light. Before providing a second laser light treatment, debride the residual tumor. Vigorous debridement may cause tumor bleeding.

The laser system must be approved for a stable power output delivery at a wavelength of 630 ± 3 nm. Light is delivered to the tumor by cylindrical *OPTIGUIDE* fiber optic diffusers passed through the operating channel of an endoscope/bronchoscope. Before use, carefully read instructions for the fiber optic and selected laser system. Porfimer photoactivation is controlled by the total light dose delivered.

OPTIGUIDE cylindrical diffusers are available in several lengths. The choice of diffuser tip length depends on the length of the tumor. Size diffuser length to avoid exposure of nonmalignant tissue to light and to prevent overlapping of previously treated malignant tissue.

Esophageal cancer – Deliver a light dose of 300 J/cm of diffuser length. The total power output at the fiber tip is set to deliver the appropriate light dose using exposure times of 12 minutes and 30 seconds.

Endobronchial cancer – The light dose should be 200 J/cm of diffuser length. The total power output at the fiber tip is set to deliver the appropriate light dose using exposure times of 8 minutes and 20 seconds. For noncircumferential endobronchial tumors that are soft enough to penetrate, interstitial fiber placement is preferred to intraluminal activation because this method results in less exposure of the healthy bronchial mucosa to light. It is important to perform a debridement 2 to 3 days after each light administration to minimize the potential for obstruction caused by necrotic debris. Refer to the *OPTIGUIDE* instructions for complete instructions concerning the fiber optic diffuser.

Barrett esophagus – Deliver light approximately 40 to 50 hours after porfimer administration by an *OPTIGUIDE* fiber optic diffuser passed through the central channel of a centering balloon. The choice of fiber optic/balloon diffuser combination will depend on the length of Barrett mucosa to be treated.

Fiber Optic Diffuser/Balloon Combination*		
Treated Barrett mucosa length (cm)	Fiber optic diffuser size (cm)	Balloon window size (cm)
6 to 7	9	7
4 to 5	7	5
1 to 3	5	3

* Whenever possible, the BE segment selected for treatment should include normal tissue margins of a few millimeters at the proximal and distal ends.

Light doses: Photoactivation is controlled by the total light dose delivered. The objective is to expose and treat all areas of HGD and the entire length of BE. The light dose administered will be 130 J/cm of diffuser length using a centering balloon. Based on the pivotal clinical study, acceptable light intensity for the balloon/diffuser combinations ranges from 200 to 270 mW/cm of diffuser.

Light dose calculation: To calculate the light dose, the following specific light dosimetry equation applies for all fiber optic diffusers:

$$\text{Light dose (J/cm)} = \frac{\text{Power Output from Diffuser (w)} \times \text{Treatment time (s)}}{\text{Diffuser Length (cm)}}$$

Fiber Optic Power Outputs and Treatment Times Required to Deliver 130 J/cm of Diffuser Length Using the Centering Balloon					
Balloon window length (cm)	Diffuser length (cm)	Light intensity (mW/cm)	Required power output from diffuser* (mW)	Treatment time (secs)	Treatment time (min:sec)
3	5	270	1350	480	8:00
5	7	270	1900	480	8:00
7	9	270	2440	480	8:00
		200	1800	650	10:50

* As measured by immersing the diffuser into the cuvet in the power meter and slowly increasing the laser power. Note: No more than 1.5 times the required diffuser power output should be needed from the laser. If more than this is required, check the system.

Use short fiber diffusers (up to 2.5 cm) to pretreat nodules with 50 J/cm diffuser length prior to regular balloon treatment in the first laser light session or for the treatment of "skip" areas (ie, an area that does not show sufficient mucosal response) after the first light session. For this treatment, the fiber optic diffuser is used without a centering balloon, and a light intensity of 400 mW/cm should be used. For nodule pretreatment and treatment of skipped areas, take care to minimize exposure to normal tissue as it also is sensitized.

Short Fiber Optic Diffuser to be Used Without a Centering Balloon to Deliver 50 J/cm of Diffuser Length at a Light Intensity of 400 mW/cm			
Diffuser length (cm)	Required power output from diffuser* (mW)	Treatment time (sec)	Treatment time (min:sec)
1.0	400	125	2:05
1.5	600	125	2:05
2.0	800	125	2:05
2.5	1000	125	2:05

* As measured by immersing the diffuser into the cuvet in the power meter and slowly increasing the laser power. Note: No more than 1.5 times the required diffuser power output should be needed from the laser. If more than this is required, check the system.

A maximum of 7 cm of esophageal mucosa is treated at the first light session using an appropriate size of centering balloon and fiber optic diffuser. Whenever possible, the segment selected for the first light application should contain all the areas of HGD. Also, whenever pos-

PORFIMER SODIUM

sible, the BE segment selected for the first light application should include normal tissue margin of a few millimeters at the proximal and distal ends.

Nodules are to be pretreated at a light dose of 50 J/cm of diffuser length with a short (2.5 cm) fiber optic diffuser placed directly against the nodule followed by standard balloon application as described above.

Repeat light application: A second laser light application may be given to a previously treated segment that shows a skip area using a short (2.5 cm) fiber optic diffuser at the light dose of 50 J/cm of the diffuser length. Patients with BE greater than 7 cm should have the remaining untreated length of Barrett epithelium treated with a second PDT course at least 90 days later.

HGD in BE of 7 cm			
Procedure	Study day	Light delivery devices	Treatment intent
Porfimer injection	Day 1	NA	Uptake of photosensitizer
Laser light application	Day 3[*]	3, 5, or 7 cm balloon (130 J/cm)	Photoactivation
Laser light application (optional)	Day 5	Short (2.5 cm) fiber optic diffuser (50 J/cm)	Treatment of skip areas only

[*] Discrete nodules will receive an initial light application of 50 J/cm (using a short diffuser) before the balloon light application.

➤*Handling spills and disposal:* Wipe up porfimer spills with a damp cloth. Avoid skin and eye contact because of potential photosensitivity reactions upon exposure to light; use rubber gloves and eye protection. Dispose of all contaminated materials in a polyethylene bag in a manner consistent with local regulations.

➤*Accidental exposure:* Because of its potential to induce photosensitivity, porfimer might be an eye and skin irritant in the presence of bright light. Avoid contact with the eyes and skin during preparation and administration. Any overexposed person must be protected from bright light.

➤*Storage/Stability:* Store at controlled room temperature of 20° to 25°C (68° to 77°F). Protect reconstituted porfimer from bright light, and use immediately. Do not mix porfimer with other drugs in the same solution.

Actions

➤*Pharmacology:* Porfimer is a photosensitizing agent used in the PDT of tumors and of HGD in BE. The cytotoxic and antitumor actions of porfimer are light- and oxygen-dependent. PDT with porfimer is a 2-stage process. The first stage is the IV injection of porfimer. Clearance from a variety of tissues occurs over 40 to 72 hours, but tumors, skin, and organs of the reticuloendothelial system (including liver and spleen) retain porfimer for a longer period. Illumination with 630 nm wavelength laser light constitutes the second stage of therapy. Tumor selectivity in treatment occurs through a combination of selective retention of porfimer sodium and selective delivery of light. Cellular damage caused by porfimer PDT is a consequence of the propagation of radical reactions. Radical initiation may occur after porfimer absorbs light to form a porphyrin-excited state. Spin transfer from porfimer to molecular oxygen may then generate singlet oxygen. Subsequent radical reactions can form superoxide and hydroxyl radicals. Tumor death also occurs through ischemic necrosis secondary to vascular occlusion that appears to be partly mediated by thromboxane A_2 release. The laser treatment induces a photochemical, not a thermal, effect.

➤*Pharmacokinetics:* Following a 2 mg/kg dose to 4 male cancer patients, the average peak plasma concentration was approximately 15 mcg/mL, elimination half-life was approximately 250 hours, steady-state volume of distribution was approximately 0.49 L/kg, and total plasma clearance was approximately 0.051 mL/min/kg. The mean plasma concentration at 48 hours was approximately 2.6 mcg/mL.

Porfimer was approximately 90% protein bound in human serum in vitro. The binding was independent of concentration over the range of 20 to 100 mcg/mL.

➤*Clinical trials:*

Esophageal cancer – PDT with porfimer was utilized in a study of 17 patients with completely obstructing esophageal carcinoma. After a single course of therapy, 94% of patients obtained an objective tumor response and 76% experienced some palliation of their dysphagia. Eleven (65%) received clinically important benefit from PDT. Clinically important benefit was defined hierarchically as a complete tumor response (3 patients), achievement of normal swallowing (2 patients went from grade 5 dysphagia to grade 1), or achievement of a marked improvement of 2 or more grades of dysphagia with minimal adverse reactions (6 patients). The median duration of benefit in these patients was 69 or more days. The median survival for these 11 patients was 115 days.

Endobronchial cancer – The safety and efficacy of porfimer PDT was evaluated in the treatment of microinvasive endobronchial tumors in 62 inoperable patients in 3 noncomparative studies. The complete tumor response rate, biopsy-proven at least 3 months after treatment, was 50%, median time to tumor recurrence was more than 2.7 years,

median survival was 2.9 years, and disease-specific survival was 4.1 years.

BE – A randomized, controlled study was conducted to assess the efficacy of PDT with porfimer for injection plus omeprazole (porfimer PDT + OM) in producing complete ablation of HGD in patients with BE compared with control patients receiving omeprazole alone (OM only). A total of 208 patients who had biopsy-proven HGD in BE were enrolled in the study. Patients randomized to the porfimer PDT + OM treatment received up to 3 courses of treatment separated by at least 90 days. Each course consisted of IV administration of 2 mg/kg of porfimer followed 40 to 50 hours later by a 630 nm laser light dose of 130 J/cm delivered using a centering balloon. A second laser light dose of 50 J/cm could be administered without a centering balloon 96 to 120 hours after the injection of porfimer for treatment of skip areas. Because centering balloons are up to 7 cm in length, patients with more extensive HGD were treated with 2 or 3 courses. Both the porfimer PDT treatment group and the control group received 20 mg of omeprazole twice daily to decrease reflux esophagitis.

The quality of response in the porfimer PDT + OM group was significantly better than that measured in the OM-only group. Seventy-two (52%) patients in the porfimer PDT + OM group achieved a CR1 response as compared with only 5 (7%) patients in the OM-only group. Eighty-one (59%) patients in the porfimer PDT + OM group achieved a CR2 or better response as compared with 10 (14%) patients in the OM-only group. The probability of maintaining a complete response (CR3 or better) by the end of the follow-up period was 53% in the porfimer PDT + OM group and only 13% in the OM-only group.

The time to patients' progression to cancer was significantly longer in the porfimer PDT + OM group than in the OM-only group.

Contraindications

➤*Porfimer:* Porphyria or in patients with known allergies to porphyrins.

➤*PDT:* Existing tracheoesophageal or bronchoesophageal fistula; tumors eroding into a major blood vessel.

Warnings

➤*Fistula:* PDT is not recommended if the esophageal tumor is eroding into the trachea or bronchial tree and the likelihood of tracheoesophageal or bronchoesophageal fistula resulting from treatment is sufficiently high.

If the endobronchial tumor invades deeply into the bronchial wall, the possibility exists for fistula formation upon resolution of tumor.

➤*Esophageal varices:* Treat patients with esophageal varices with extreme caution. Do not administer light directly to the variceal area because of a high risk of bleeding.

➤*Treatment-induced inflammation:* Use PDT with extreme caution for endobronchial tumors in locations where treatment-induced inflammation could obstruct the main airway (eg, long or circumferential tumors of the trachea, tumors of the carina that involve both mainstem bronchi circumferentially, or circumferential tumors in the mainstem bronchus in patients with prior pneumonectomy).

➤*Photosensitivity:* All patients who receive porfimer will be photosensitive and must observe precautions to avoid exposure of skin and eyes to direct sunlight or bright indoor light (eg, examination lamps, including dental lamps, operating room lamps, unshaded light bulbs at close proximity) for at least 30 days. The photosensitivity is caused by residual drug that will be present in all parts of the skin. Exposure of the skin to ambient indoor light is beneficial because the remaining drug will be gradually and safely inactivated through a photobleaching reaction. Therefore, advise patients not to stay in a darkened room during this period and encourage them to expose their skin to ambient indoor light.

The level of photosensitivity will vary for different areas of the body, depending on the extent of previous exposure to light. Before exposing any area of skin to direct sunlight or bright indoor light, the patient should test it for residual photosensitivity. Instruct the patient to expose a small area of skin to sunlight for 10 minutes. If no photosensitivity reaction (erythema, edema, blistering) occurs within 24 hours, the patient can gradually resume normal outdoor activities, initially continuing to exercise caution and gradually allowing increased exposure. If some photosensitivity reaction occurs with the limited skin test, have the patient continue precautions for another 2 weeks before retesting. The tissue around the eyes may be more sensitive, and therefore, it is not recommended that the face be used for testing. If patients travel to a different geographical area with greater sunshine, they should retest their level of photosensitivity.

UV (ultraviolet) sunscreens are of no value in protecting against photosensitivity reactions, because photoactivation is caused by visible light.

➤*Mutagenesis:* Porfimer caused less than 2-fold, but significant, increases in sister chromatid exchange in CHO cells irradiated with visible light and a 3-fold increase in Chinese hamster lung fibroblasts irradiated with near UV light. Porfimer PDT caused an increase in thymidine kinase mutants and DNA-protein cross-links in mouse L5178Y cells, and caused a light-dose dependent increase in DNA-strand

PORFIMER SODIUM

breaks in malignant human cervical carcinoma cells but not in normal cells.

➤*Elderly:* Approximately 70% of patients treated with PDT using porfimer in clinical trials were older than 60 years of age. There was no apparent difference in effectiveness or safety in these patients compared with younger people. Dose modification based on age is not required.

➤*Pregnancy: Category C.* There are no adequate and well-controlled studies in pregnant women. Use during pregnancy only if the potential benefit justifies the potential risk to the fetus. Women of childbearing potential should practice an effective method of contraception during therapy.

In rats, porfimer 8 mg/kg/day (0.64 times the clinical dose) for 10 days caused maternal and fetal toxicity resulting in increased resorptions, decreased litter size, delayed ossification, and reduced fetal weight. When given to rabbits during organogenesis at 4 mg/kg/day (0.65 times the clinical dose) for 13 days, maternal toxicity occurred, resulting in increased resorptions, decreased litter size, and reduced fetal body weight. Porfimer given to rats during late pregnancy through lactation at 4 mg/kg/day (0.32 times the clinical dose) for at least 42 days caused a reversible decrease in growth of offspring.

➤*Lactation:* It is not known whether this drug is excreted in breast milk. Because of the potential for serious adverse reactions in nursing infants, women receiving porfimer must not breastfeed.

➤*Children:* Safety and efficacy in children have not been established.

Precautions

➤*Monitoring:* The risk of overlooking cancer in BE patients and the need for rigorous monitoring, despite the endoscopic appearance of complete squamous cell re-epithelialization, is very important. It is recommended that endoscopic biopsy surveillance be conducted every 3 months until 4 consecutive negative evaluations for HGD have been recorded; further follow-up may be scheduled every 6 to 12 months. Assess patients for the possibility that a tumor may be eroding into a pulmonary blood vessel.

➤*Ocular sensitivity:* Ocular discomfort, commonly described as sensitivity to sun, bright lights, or car headlights, has been reported in patients who received porfimer. For 30 days when outdoors, patients should wear dark sunglasses that have an average white light transmittance of less than 4%.

➤*Chest pain:* As a result of PDT treatment, patients may complain of substernal chest pain because of inflammatory responses within the area of treatment. Such pain may be of sufficient intensity to warrant the short-term use of opiate analgesics.

➤*Esophageal strictures:* Esophageal strictures as a result of PDT of HGD in BE are common adverse events. An esophageal stricture was defined as a fixed lumen narrowing with solid-food dysphagia and requiring dilation. Esophageal strictures were reported in 38% of patients enrolled in the 3 clinical studies. Overall, esophageal strictures occurred within 6 months following PDT and were manageable through dilations. Multiple dilations of esophageal strictures may be required. Take special care during dilation to avoid perforation of the esophagus. A high proportion of patients who developed an esophageal stricture received a nodule pretreatment prior to developing the event (49%) and/or had a mucosal segment treated twice. Therefore, nodule pretreatment and retreating the same mucosal segment more than once may influence the risk of developing an esophageal stricture.

➤*Use with radiotherapy:* If PDT is to be used before or after radiotherapy, allot sufficient time between the 2 therapies to ensure that the inflammatory response produced by the first treatment has subsided before commencing the second treatment. The inflammatory response from PDT will depend on tumor size and extent of surrounding healthy tissue that receives light. Allow 2 to 4 weeks after PDT before commencing radiotherapy. Similarly, if PDT is to be given after radiotherapy, the acute inflammatory reaction from radiotherapy usually subsides within 4 weeks after completing radiotherapy, after which PDT may be given.

➤*Respiratory distress:* Closely monitor patients with endobronchial lesions between the laser light therapy and the mandatory debridement bronchoscopy for any evidence of respiratory distress. Inflammation, mucositis, and necrotic debris may cause obstruction of the airway. If respiratory distress occurs, carry out immediate bronchoscopy to remove secretions and debris to open the airway.

➤*Long-term dosing:* Long-term dosing caused discoloration of testes and ovaries, hypertrophy of the testes, and decreased body weight in the parent rats.

➤*Extravasation:* Take precautions to prevent extravasation at the injection site. If extravasation occurs, take care to protect the area from light. There is no known benefit from injecting the extravasation site with another substance.

➤*Special risk:* PDT is not suitable for emergency treatment of patients with severe acute respiratory distress caused by an obstructing endobronchial lesion because 40 to 50 hours are required between injection with porfimer and laser light treatment. PDT also is not suit-

able for patients with esophageal or gastric varices, or patients with esophageal ulcers greater than 1 cm in diameter.

Drug Interactions

➤*Photosensitizing agents:* It is possible that concomitant use of other photosensitizing agents (eg, tetracyclines, sulfonamides, phenothiazines, sulfonylureas, hypoglycemic agents, thiazide diuretics, griseofulvin, fluoroquinolones) could increase the risk of photosensitivity reaction.

➤*Miscellaneous:* Compounds that quench active oxygen species or scavenge radicals (eg, dimethyl sulfoxide, β-carotene, ethanol, formate, mannitol) would be expected to decrease PDT activity. Preclinical data also suggest that tissue ischemia, allopurinol, calcium channel blockers, and some prostaglandin synthesis inhibitors could interfere with porfimer PDT. Drugs that decrease clotting, vasoconstriction, or platelet aggregation (eg, thromboxane A_2 inhibitors) could decrease the efficacy of PDT. Glucocorticoid hormones given before or concomitantly with PDT may decrease the efficacy of the treatment.

Adverse Reactions

Systemically induced effects associated with PDT with porfimer consist of photosensitivity and mild constipation. All patients who receive porfimer will be photosensitive and must observe precautions to avoid sunlight and bright indoor light (see Warnings). Photosensitivity reactions (mostly mild to moderate erythema) occurred in approximately 20% of cancer patients and in 68% of HGD in BE treated with porfimer. These reactions also included: swelling, itching, burning sensation, feeling hot, or blisters. In a single study of 24 healthy subjects, some evidence of photosensitivity reactions occurred in all subjects. Other less common skin manifestations also were reported in areas where photosensitivity reactions had occurred, such as increased hair growth, skin discolorations, skin nodules, increased wrinkles, and increased skin fragility. These manifestations may be attributable to a pseudoporphyria state (temporary drug-induced cutaneous porphyria). Most toxicities associated with this therapy are local effects seen in the region of illumination and occasionally in surrounding tissues. The local adverse reactions are characteristic of an inflammatory response induced by the photodynamic effect.

➤*Esophageal cancer:*

Porfimer-PDT Adverse Reactions in Obstructing Esophageal Cancer Patients (≥ 5%)	
Adverse reaction	% of Patients (n = 88)
Cardiovascular	
Chest pain	22
Atrial fibrillation	10
Cardiac failure	7
Hypotension	7
Tachycardia	6
Hypertension	6
Chest pain (substernal)	5
CNS	
Insomnia	14
Anorexia	8
Confusion	8
Anxiety	7
Asthenia	6
GI	
Constipation	24
Nausea	24
Abdominal pain	20
Vomiting	17
Dysphagia	10
Esophageal edema/ tumor bleeding	8
Hematemesis	8
Dyspepsia	6
Esophageal stricture	6
Diarrhea	5
Eructation	5
Esophagitis	5
Melena	5
Metabolic/Nutritional	
Weight decrease	9
Dehydration	7
Respiratory	
Pleural effusion	32
Dyspnea	20
Pneumonia	18
Pharyngitis	11
Respiratory insufficiency	10
Cough	7
Tracheoesophageal fistula	6

PORFIMER SODIUM

Porfimer-PDT Adverse Reactions in Obstructing Esophageal Cancer Patients (≥ 5%)

Adverse reaction	% of Patients (n = 88)
Miscellaneous	
Anemia	32
Fever	31
Pain	22
Photosensitivity	19
Back pain	11
Moniliasis	9
UTI	7
Edema, peripheral	7
Edema, generalized	5
Surgical complication	5

Location of the tumor was a prognostic factor for the following 3 adverse events: Upper third of the esophagus (esophageal edema), middle third (atrial fibrillation), and lower third, the most vascular region (anemia). Also, patients with large tumors (larger than 10 cm) were more likely to experience anemia. Two of 17 patients with complete esophageal obstruction from tumor experienced esophageal perforations that were possibly treatment-associated; these perforations occurred during subsequent endoscopies.

Serious and other notable adverse events observed in less than 5% of PDT-treated patients with obstructing esophageal cancer include the following:

Cardiovascular – Angina pectoris; bradycardia; MI; sick sinus syndrome; supraventricular tachycardia.

GI – Esophageal perforation; gastric ulcer; ileus; jaundice; peritonitis.

Respiratory – Bronchitis; bronchospasm; laryngotracheal edema; pneumonitis; pulmonary hemorrhage; pulmonary edema; respiratory failure; stridor.

Miscellaneous – Sepsis has occurred occasionally. The temporal relationship of some GI, cardiovascular, and respiratory events to the administration of light was suggestive of mediastinal inflammation in some patients. Vision-related events of abnormal vision, diplopia, eye pain, and photophobia have been reported. PDT with porfimer may result in anemia because of tumor bleeding.

►*Endobronchial cancer:*

Porfimer-PDT Adverse Reactions with Superficial Endobronchial Tumor Patients (≥ 5%)

Adverse reaction	PDT with Porfimer (n = 90)
Patients with ≥ 1 adverse reaction	49
Photosensitivity reaction	22
Exudate	22
Obstruction	21
Edema	18
Stricture	11
Ulceration	9
Cough	9
Dyspnea	7

In patients with superficial endobronchial tumors, 44 of 90 patients (49%) experienced an adverse event, two-thirds of which were related to the respiratory system. The most common reaction to therapy was a mucositis reaction in one-fifth of the patients that manifested as edema, exudate, and obstruction. The obstruction (mucus plug) is easily removed with suction or forceps. Mucositis can be minimized by avoiding exposure of healthy tissue to excessive light. Three patients experienced life-threatening dyspnea: 1 was given a double dose of light, 1 was treated concurrently in both mainstem bronchi, and 1 had prior pneumonectomy and was treated in the sole remaining airway. Stent placement was required in 3% of the patients because of endobronchial stricture. Fatal hemoptysis occurred within 30 days of treatment in 1 patient with superficial tumors (1%).

Obstructing endobronchial cancer – Patients who have received radiation therapy have a higher incidence of fatal massive hemoptysis after treatment with PDT and after other forms of local treatment. In controlled studies comparing PDT with Nd:YAG laser for palliation of obstructing endobronchial cancer, the incidence of fatal massive hemoptysis in patients previously treated with radiotherapy was 21% (6/29) in patients treated with PDT and 10% (3/29) in patients treated with Nd:YAG. In patients with no prior radiotherapy, the overall incidence of fatal massive hemoptysis was less than 1%.

Other serious or notable adverse events were observed in less than 5% of PDT-treated patients with endobronchial cancer; their relationship to therapy is uncertain. In the respiratory system, pulmonary thrombosis, pulmonary embolism, and lung abscess have occurred. Cardiac failure, sepsis, and possible cerebrovascular accident also have been reported in one patient each.

►*Barrett esophagus:*

Adverse Events Reported in ≥ 5% of BE Patients with HGD Treated with Porfimer PDT

Adverse reaction	Treatment groups			
	HGD porfimer PDT + OM N = 219	HGD OM only N = 69	Other[1] porfimer PDT N = 99	Total porfimer PDT N = 318
Cardiovascular				
Chest discomfort	6	1	21	11
Hypertension	5	1	0	3
CNS				
Headache	8	9	2	6
Fatigue	6	3	0	4
Insomnia	5	4	1	4
Depression	5	4	0	3
Anxiety	5	1	0	3
Dermatologic				
Photosensitivity reaction	46	0	16	37
Rash	6	4	7	7
Pruritus	6	1	1	4
Sunburn	4	0	6	4
GI				
Esophageal stricture[2]	39	0	37	38
Vomiting	33	6	35	34
Nausea	28	7	64	39
Esophageal narrowing[3]	27	6	16	24
Dysphagia	23	1	27	24
Constipation	21	7	9	17
Abdominal pain (upper, lower, NOS)	15	6	8	12
Diarrhea	10	10	6	9
Hiccup	8	0	1	6
Esophageal pain	7	0	9	8
Dyspepsia	5	4	6	6
Odynophagia	6	0	4	5
Eructation	5	0	4	5
Metabolic/Nutritional				
Dehydration	11	3	8	10
Decreased weight	8	3	3	6
Anorexia	3	3	8	4
Musculoskeletal				
Back pain	7	6	1	5
Arthralgia	5	9	1	3
Respiratory				
Pleural effusion	11	0	15	13
Dyspnea	7	4	4	6
Sinusitis	5	4	2	4
Bronchitis	5	4	2	4
Miscellaneous				
Chest pain	32	12	40	35
Pyrexia	21	4	13	19
Pain	8	3	7	8
Post-procedural pain	7	1	14	9
Increased body temperature	4	0	8	5

[1] Includes patients with Barrett metaplasia, indefinite dysplasia, LGD, and adenocarcinoma at baseline.
[2] In the controlled clinical trial, an esophageal stricture was defined as a fixed lumen narrowing with solid-food dysphagia that required dilations; in the uncontrolled clinical trials, an esophageal stricture was defined as any dilated esophageal narrowing.
[3] An esophageal narrowing was defined as an undilated esophageal stenosis.

In the porfimer PDT + OM group, severe treatment-associated adverse events included chest pain of noncardiac origin, dysphagia, nausea, vomiting, regurgitation, and heartburn. The severity of these symptoms decreased within 4 to 6 weeks following treatment.

Photosensitivity reactions – The majority of photosensitivity reactions occurred within 90 days following porfimer injection and were of mild (69%) or moderate (24%) intensity. Almost all (98%) of the photo-

PORFIMER SODIUM

sensitivity reactions were considered to be associated with treatment. Fourteen (10%) patients reported severe reactions, all of which resolved. The typical reaction was described as skin disorder, sunburn, or rash, and mostly affected the face, hands, and neck. Associated symptoms and signs were swelling, pruritus, erythema, blisters, itching, burning sensation, and feeling of heat.

Esophageal stenosis/strictures – The majority of esophageal stenosis and strictures reported in the porfimer PDT + OM group were of mild (55%) or moderate (37%) intensity, while approximately 8% were of severe intensity. The majority of esophageal strictures were reported during course 2 of treatment. All esophageal strictures were considered to be associated with treatment. Most esophageal strictures were manageable through dilations (see Precautions).

Overdosage

Effects of overdosage on the duration of photosensitivity are unknown. Two 2 mg/kg doses given 2 days apart (10 patients) and three 2 mg/kg doses given within 2 weeks (1 patient) were tolerated without notable adverse reactions. Do not give laser treatment if an overdose of porfimer is administered. In the event of an overdose, instruct patients to protect their eyes and skin from direct sunlight or bright indoor lights for 30 days. At this time, have patients test for residual photosensitivity. Porfimer is not dialyzable.

➤*Overdose of laser light following porfimer injection:* Increased symptoms and damage to healthy tissue might be expected following an overdose of light. Light doses of 2 to 3 times the recommended dose have been administered to a few patients with superficial endobron-chial tumors. One patient experienced life-threatening dyspnea and the others had no notable complications.

Patient Information

Advise patients that this medicine will be prepared and administered by a health care provider in a medical setting.

Advise patients to contact a doctor if they experience severe chest pain, difficulty breathing, or abnormal blood loss.

Inform patients this drug will cause sensitivity to the sun, bright lights, or car headlights. For 30 days, they should avoid exposure of skin and eyes to direct sunlight from skylights or undraped windows or bright indoor light.

Instruct patients to test skin for sensitivity before exposing skin to bright indoor light or direct sunlight. To test the skin, expose a small skin area to sunlight for 10 minutes. If no sensitivity reactions (eg, rash, swelling, blistering) occur within 24 hours, gradually resume normal outdoor activities.

If patients must go out during daylight hours, instruct them to cover the skin as much as possible (long-sleeved shirts, slacks, gloves, socks) and wear dark sunglasses even on cloudy days or when in a car.

Contraceptive measures (birth control) are recommended during treatment to avoid birth defects. Instruct patients to inform their doctor if they are pregnant, become pregnant, are planning to become pregnant, or if they are breastfeeding.

Inform patients that lab tests may be required to monitor treatment and to keep appointments.

MITOTANE (o,p'-DDD)

Rx	Lysodren (Bristol-Myers Squibb Oncology)	**Tablets:** 500 mg	Scored. In 100s.

WARNING

Temporarily discontinue mitotane immediately following shock or severe trauma because the prime action of mitotane is adrenal suppression. Administer exogenous steroids in such circumstances because the depressed adrenal may not start to function immediately.

Indications

➤*Adrenal cortical carcinoma:* For the treatment of inoperable adrenal cortical carcinoma (functional and nonfunctional).

➤*Unlabeled uses:* For the treatment of Cushing syndrome secondary to pituitary disorders.

Administration and Dosage

Start at 2 to 6 g/day in divided doses, 3 or 4 times daily. Increase dose incrementally to 9 to 10 g/day. If severe side effects appear, reduce the dose until the maximum tolerated dose is achieved. If the patient can tolerate higher doses and if improved clinical response appears possible, increase the dose until adverse reactions interfere. Maximum tolerated dose varies from 2 to 16 g/day (usually 9 to 10 g). The highest doses used in studies were 18 to 19 g/day.

Continue treatment as long as clinical benefits are observed (ie, maintenance of clinical status or slowing of growth of metastatic lesions). If no clinical benefits are observed after 3 months at the maximum tolerated dose, consider the case a clinical failure. However, 10% of the patients who showed a measurable response required more than 3 months at the maximum tolerated dose. Early diagnosis and prompt institution of treatment improve the probability of a positive clinical response. Clinical effectiveness can be shown by reductions in tumor mass, pain, weakness, or anorexia and steroid symptoms.

➤*Intermittent therapy:* A number of patients have been treated intermittently, restarting treatment when severe symptoms reappeared. Patients often do not respond after the third or fourth such course. Continuous treatment with the maximum possible dosage may be the best approach.

➤*Storage/Stability:* Store at room temperature (15° to 30°C; 59° to 86°F).

Actions

➤*Pharmacology:* Mitotane is an adrenal cytotoxic agent, although it can cause adrenal inhibition without cellular destruction. The primary action is upon the adrenal cortex. The production of adrenal steroids is reduced. The biochemical mechanism of action is unknown. Data suggest the drug modifies the peripheral metabolism of steroids and directly suppresses the adrenal cortex.

Use of mitotane alters the extra-adrenal metabolism of cortisol, leading to a reduction in measurable 17-hydroxycorticosteroids, even though plasma levels of corticosteroids do not fall. The drug causes increased formation of 6-β-hydroxycortisol.

➤*Pharmacokinetics:*

Absorption/Distribution – Approximately 40% of oral mitotane is absorbed; it can be found in most body tissues but is primarily stored in fat. Blood levels become undetectable after 6 to 9 weeks.

Metabolism/Excretion – Approximately 10% of the dose is recovered in the urine as a water-soluble metabolite. A variable amount of metabolite (1% to 17%) is excreted in the bile and the balance is stored in the tissues. Following discontinuation of mitotane, the plasma terminal half-life ranged from 18 to 159 days. No unchanged mitotane has been found in urine or bile.

Contraindications

Hypersensitivity to mitotane.

Warnings

➤*Shock or severe trauma:* Temporarily discontinue mitotane immediately following shock or severe trauma because adrenal suppression is its prime action. Use exogenous steroids in such circumstances because the depressed adrenal may not start to secrete steroids immediately.

➤*Tumor tissue:* Surgically remove all possible tumor tissue from large metastatic masses before administration to minimize the possibility of infarction and hemorrhage in the tumor caused by a rapid, cytotoxic effect of the drug.

➤*Long-term therapy:* Continuous administration of high doses may lead to brain damage and impairment of function. Conduct behavioral and neurological assessments at regular intervals when continuous treatment exceeds 2 years.

➤*Hepatic function impairment:* Administer with care to patients with liver disease other than metastatic lesions of the adrenal cortex. Interference with mitotane metabolism may occur, causing drug accumulation.

➤*Carcinogenesis:* The carcinogenic and mutagenic potential is unknown. However, the mechanism of action suggests the drug probably has less carcinogenic potential than other cytotoxic chemotherapeutic drugs.

➤*Pregnancy: Category C.* Safety for use during pregnancy has not been established. Use only when clearly needed and when the potential benefits outweigh the potential hazards to the fetus.

➤*Lactation:* It is not known whether mitotane is excreted in breast milk. Because of the potential for adverse reactions in nursing infants, decide whether to discontinue nursing or discontinue the drug.

➤*Children:* Safety and effectiveness have not been established.

Precautions

➤*Adrenal insufficiency:* A substantial percentage of patients show signs of adrenal insufficiency. Watch for this condition, and institute steroid therapy if necessary. The metabolism of exogenous steroids is modified with mitotane; somewhat higher doses than replacement therapy may be required.

Drug Interactions

Use mitotane with caution in patients receiving drugs susceptible to the influence of hepatic enzyme induction.

MITOTANE (o,p'-DDD)

Mitotane Drug Interactions			
Precipitant drug	Object drug*		Description
Mitotane	Corticosteroids	↓	Corticosteroid metabolism may be altered by mitotane; higher dosages may be required.
Mitotane	Warfarin	↓	The metabolism of warfarin may be accelerated by the mechanism of hepatic microsomal enzyme induction, leading to an increase in dosage requirements of warfarin. Monitor patients for a change in anticoagulant dosage requirements when administering mitotane to patients on coumarin-type anticoagulants.
Spironolactone	Mitotane	↓	Adrenolytic effects of mitotane may be blocked by spironolactone; observe for diminished clinical signs of mitotane; consider discontinuation of spironolactone.

*↓ = Object drug decreased.

➤*Drug/Lab test interactions:* Protein-bound iodine (PBI) levels and urinary 17-hydroxycorticosteroids may be decreased by mitotane.

Adverse Reactions

➤*Cardiovascular:* Hypertension, orthostatic hypotension, and flushing (infrequent).

➤*CNS:* Primarily depression as manifested by lethargy and somnolence (25%), and dizziness or vertigo (15%).

➤*Dermatologic:* Skin toxicity (approximately 15%). Primarily transient skin rashes. In some instances, this side effect subsided while patients were maintained on the drug.

➤*GI:* Anorexia, nausea or vomiting, and diarrhea (80%).

➤*GU:* Hematuria, hemorrhagic cystitis, and albuminuria (infrequent).

➤*Ophthalmic:* Visual blurring, diplopia, lens opacity, and toxic retinopathy (infrequent).

➤*Miscellaneous:* Generalized aching, hyperpyrexia, and lowered PBI (infrequent).

Patient Information

Instruct patient to notify a physician if nausea, vomiting, loss of appetite, diarrhea, mental depression, skin rash, or darkening of the skin occurs.

Medication may cause aching muscles, fever, flushing, or muscle twitching; advise patient to notify a physician if these become pronounced.

May produce drowsiness, dizziness, and tiredness; advise patient to observe caution when driving or performing other tasks requiring alertness.

Contraceptive measures are recommended during therapy.

ARSENIC TRIOXIDE

Rx	**Trisenox** (Cell Therapeutics, Inc.)	Injection: 1 mg/1 ml	Preservative-free. In 10s.

WARNING

Experienced physician and institution: Administer arsenic trioxide injection under the supervision of a physician who is experienced in the management of patients with acute leukemia.

APL differentiation syndrome: Some patients with acute promyelocytic leukemia (APL) treated with arsenic trioxide have experienced symptoms similar to a syndrome called retinoic-acid-acute promyelocytic leukemia (RA-APL) or APL differentiation syndrome, characterized by fever, dyspnea, weight gain, pulmonary infiltrates, and pleural or pericardial effusions, with or without leukocytosis. This syndrome can be fatal. The management of the syndrome has not been fully studied, but high-dose steroids have been used at the first suspicion of the APL differentiation syndrome and appear to mitigate signs and symptoms. At the first signs that could suggest the syndrome (eg, unexplained fever, dyspnea, weight gain, abnormal chest auscultatory findings, radiographic abnormalities), immediately initiate high-dose steroids (10 mg dexamethasone IV twice daily), irrespective of the leukocyte count and continued for ≥ 3 days until signs and symptoms have abated. The majority of patients do not require termination of arsenic trioxide therapy during treatment of the APL differentiation syndrome.

ECG abnormalities: Arsenic trioxide can cause QT interval prolongation and complete atrioventricular block. QT prolongation can lead to a torsade de pointes-type ventricular arrhythmia, which can be fatal. The risk of torsade de pointes is related to the extent of QT prolongation, concomitant administration of QT prolonging drugs, a history of torsade de pointes, preexisting QT interval prolongation, CHF, administration of potassium-wasting diuretics, or other conditions that result in hypokalemia or hypomagnesemia. One patient (also receiving amphotericin B) had torsade de pointes during induction therapy for relapsed APL with arsenic trioxide.

ECG and electrolyte monitoring recommendations: Prior to initiating therapy with arsenic trioxide, perform a 12-lead ECG and assess serum electrolytes (eg, potassium, calcium, magnesium) and creatinine; correct preexisting electrolyte abnormalities and, if possible, discontinue drugs that are known to prolong the QT interval. For QTc > 500 msec, complete corrective measures and reassess the QTc with serial ECGs prior to considering using arsenic trioxide. During therapy with arsenic trioxide, keep potassium concentrations > 4 mEq/dl and magnesium concentrations > 1.8 mg/dl. Reassess patients who reach an absolute QT interval value > 500 msec and take immediate action to correct concomitant risk factors, if any, while considering the risk/benefit of continuing vs suspending arsenic trioxide therapy. If syncope or rapid or irregular heartbeat develops, hospitalize the patient for monitoring, assess serum electrolytes, temporarily discontinue arsenic trioxide therapy until the QTc interval regresses to < 460 msec, electrolyte abnormalities are corrected, and the syncope and irregular heartbeat cease. There are no data on the effect of arsenic trioxide on the QTc interval during the infusion.

Indications

➤*Acute promyelocytic leukemia:* Arsenic trioxide is indicated for the induction of remission and consolidation in patients with APL who are refractory to, or have relapsed from, retinoid and anthracycline chemotherapy, and whose APL is characterized by the presence of the t(15;17) translocation or PML/RAR-alpha gene expression.

The response rate of other acute myelogenous leukemia subtypes to arsenic trioxide has not been examined.

Administration and Dosage

➤*Approved by the FDA:* September 25, 2000.

For IV use only.

Dilute arsenic trioxide with 100 to 250 ml 5% Dextrose Injection or 0.9% Sodium Chloride Injection immediately after withdrawal from the ampule. The ampule is for single use and does not contain any preservatives. Discard unused portions of each ampule properly. Do not save any unused portions for later administration. Do not mix arsenic trioxide with other medications.

Administer arsenic trioxide IV over 1 to 2 hours. The infusion duration may be extended up to 4 hours if acute vasomotor reactions are observed. A central venous catheter is not required.

Arsenic trioxide is recommended to be given according to the following schedule:

➤*Induction treatment schedule:* Administer arsenic trioxide IV at a dose of 0.15 mg/kg/day until bone marrow remission. Total induction dose should not exceed 60 doses.

➤*Consolidation treatment schedule:* Begin consolidation treatment 3 to 6 weeks after completion of induction therapy. Administer arsenic trioxide IV at a dose of 0.15 mg/kg/day for 25 doses over a period of up to 5 weeks.

➤*Storage/Stability:* Store at 25°C (77°F); excursions permitted to 15° to 30°C (59° to 86°F). Do not freeze.

Do not use beyond expiration date printed on the label.

After dilution, arsenic trioxide is chemically and physically stable when stored for 24 hours at room temperature and 48 hours when refrigerated.

Actions

➤*Pharmacology:* The mechanism of action of arsenic trioxide is not completely understood. Arsenic trioxide causes morphological changes and DNA fragmentation characteristic of apoptosis in NB4 human promyelocytic leukemia cells in vitro. Arsenic trioxide also causes damage or degradation of the fusion protein PML/RAR alpha.

The pharmacokinetics of trivalent arsenic, the active species of arsenic trioxide, has not been characterized.

➤*Pharmacokinetics:*

Metabolism – The metabolism of arsenic trioxide involves reduction of pentavalent arsenic to trivalent arsenic by arsenate reductase and methylation of trivalent arsenic to monomethylarsonic acid and monomethylarsonic acid to dimethylarsinic acid by methyltransferases. The main site of methylation reactions appears to be the liver. Arsenic is stored mainly in the liver, kidney, heart, lung, hair, and nails.

ARSENIC TRIOXIDE

Excretion – Disposition of arsenic following IV administration has not been studied. Trivalent arsenic is mostly methylated in humans and excreted in urine.

Contraindications

Hypersensitivity to arsenic.

Warnings

Administer arsenic trioxide under the supervision of a physician who is experienced in the management of patients with acute leukemia.

➤*APL differentiation syndrome:* Nine of 40 patients with APL treated with arsenic trioxide at a dose of 0.15 mg/kg experienced the APL differentiation syndrome.

➤*Hyperleukocytosis:* Treatment with arsenic trioxide has been associated with the development of hyperleukocytosis ($\geq 10 \times 10^3$/mcl) in 20 of 40 patients. A relationship did not exist between baseline WBC counts and development of hyperleukocytosis nor baseline WBC counts and peak WBC counts. Hyperleukocytosis was not treated with additional chemotherapy. WBC counts during consolidation were not as high as during induction treatment.

➤*QT prolongation:* Expect QT/QTc prolongation during treatment with arsenic trioxide; torsade de pointes as well as complete heart block have been reported. Over 460 ECG tracings from 40 patients with refractory or relapsed APL treated with arsenic trioxide were evaluated for QTc prolongation. Sixteen of 40 patients (40%) had ≥ 1 ECG tracing with a QTc interval > 500 msec. Prolongation of the QTc was observed between 1 and 5 weeks after arsenic trioxide infusion, and then returned towards baseline by the end of 8 weeks after arsenic trioxide infusion. In these ECG evaluations, women did not experience more pronounced QT prolongation than men, and there was no correlation with age.

➤*Complete AV block:* Complete AV block has been reported with arsenic trioxide in the published literature, including a case of a patient with APL.

➤*Renal/Hepatic function impairment:* The safety and efficacy of arsenic trioxide in patients with renal or hepatic impairment have not been studied. Particular caution is needed in patients with renal failure receiving arsenic trioxide, as renal excretion is the main route of elimination of arsenic.

➤*Mutagenesis:* Trivalent arsenic produced an increase in the incidence of chromosome aberrations and micronuclei in bone marrow cells of mice.

➤*Fertility impairment:* The effect of arsenic on fertility has not been adequately studied.

➤*Pregnancy: Category D.* Arsenic trioxide may cause fetal harm when administered to a pregnant woman. Studies in pregnant mice, rats, hamsters, and primates have shown that inorganic arsenicals cross the placental barrier when given orally or by injection. The reproductive toxicity of arsenic trioxide has been studied in a limited manner. An increase in resorptions, neural-tube defects, anophthalmia, and microphthalmia were observed in rats administered 10 mg/kg of arsenic trioxide on gestation day 9 ($\approx$ 10 times the recommended human daily dose on a mg/m^2 basis). Similar findings occurred in mice administered a 10 mg/kg dose of a related trivalent arsenic, sodium arsenite, ($\approx$ 5 times the projected human dose on a mg/m^2 basis) on gestation days 6, 7, 8, or 9. IV injection of 2 mg/kg sodium arsenite (approximately equivalent to the projected human daily dose on a mg/m^2 basis) on gestation day 7 (the lowest dose tested) resulted in neural-tube defects in hamsters.

There are no studies in pregnant women using arsenic trioxide. If this drug is used during pregnancy, or if the patient becomes pregnant while taking this drug, apprise the patient of the potential harm to the fetus. One patient who became pregnant while receiving arsenic trioxide had a miscarriage. Advise women of childbearing potential to avoid becoming pregnant.

➤*Lactation:* Arsenic is excreted in human breast milk. Because of the potential for serious adverse reactions in nursing infants from arsenic trioxide, decide whether to discontinue nursing or to discontinue the drug, taking into account the importance of the drug to the mother.

➤*Children:* There are limited clinical data on the pediatric use of arsenic trioxide. Of 5 patients < 18 years of age (age range, 5 to 16 years) treated with arsenic trioxide at the recommended dose of 0.15 mg/kg/day, 3 achieved a complete response.

Safety and efficacy of arsenic trioxide in pediatric patients < 5 years of age have not been studied.

Precautions

➤*Monitoring:* Monitor the patient's electrolyte, hematologic, and coagulation profile at least twice weekly, and more frequently for clinically unstable patients during the induction phase, and at least weekly during the consolidation phase. Obtain ECGs weekly, and more frequently for clinically unstable patients, during induction and consolidation.

Drug Interactions

No formal assessments of pharmacokinetic drug-drug interactions between arsenic trioxide and other agents have been conducted. The methyltransferases responsible for metabolizing arsenic trioxide are not members of the cytochrome P450 family of isoenzymes.

Caution is advised when arsenic trioxide is coadministered with other medications that can prolong the QT interval (eg, certain antiarrhythmics, thioridazine) or lead to electrolyte abnormalities (eg, diuretics, amphotericin B).

Adverse Reactions

Forty patients in the Phase 2 study received the recommended dose of 0.15 mg/kg, of which 29 completed both induction and consolidation treatment cycles. An additional 12 patients with relapsed or refractory APL received doses generally similar to the recommended dose. Most patients experienced some drug-related toxicity, most commonly leukocytosis, GI (eg, nausea, vomiting, diarrhea, abdominal pain), fatigue, edema, hyperglycemia, dyspnea, cough, rash or itching, headaches, and dizziness. These adverse effects have not been observed to be permanent or irreversible, nor do they usually require interruption of therapy.

Serious adverse events (SAEs), grade 3 or 4 according to version 2 of the NCI Common Toxicity Criteria, were common. Those SAEs attributed to arsenic trioxide in the Phase 2 study of 40 patients with refractory or relapsed APL included APL differentiation syndrome (n = 3); hyperleukocytosis (n = 3); QTc interval $\geq$ 500 msec (n = 16, 1 with torsade de pointes); atrial dysrhythmias (n = 2); and hyperglycemia (n = 2).

The following table describes the adverse events that were observed in patients treated for APL with arsenic trioxide at the recommended dose at a rate of $\geq$ 5%. Similar adverse event profiles were seen in the other patient populations who received arsenic trioxide.

Arsenic Trioxide Adverse Events at a Dose of 0.15 mg/kg/day ($\geq$ 5%; n = 40)		
Adverse reaction	All adverse events, any grade % (n)	Grade 3 and 4 events % (n)
Cardiovascular		
Tachycardia	55 (22)	—
ECG QT corrected interval prolonged> 500 msec	38 (16)	—
Hypotension	25 (10)	5 (2)
Hypertension	10 (4)	—
Palpitations	10 (4)	—
ECG abnormal other than QT interval prolongation	7 (3)	—
CNS		
Headache	60 (24)	3 (1)
Insomnia	43 (17)	3 (1)
Paresthesia	33 (13)	5 (2)
Anxiety	30 (12)	—
Depression	20 (8)	—
Dizziness (excluding vertigo)	23 (9)	—
Tremor	13 (5)	—
Convulsion	8 (3)	5 (2)
Somnolence	8 (3)	—
Agitation	5 (2)	—
Coma	5 (2)	5 (2)
Confusion	5 (2)	—
Dermatologic		
Dermatitis	43 (17)	—
Pruritus	33 (13)	2 (1)
Injection site pain	20 (8)	—
Ecchymosis	20 (8)	—
Dry skin	15 (6)	—
Erythema, nonspecific	13 (5)	—
Increased sweating	13 (5)	—
Injection site erythema	13 (5)	—
Injection site edema	10 (4)	—
Flushing	10 (4)	—
Pallor	10 (4)	—
Facial edema	8 (3)	—
Night sweats	8 (3)	—
Petechiae	8 (3)	—
Hyperpigmentation	8 (3)	—
Skin lesions, nonspecific	8 (3)	—
Urticaria	8 (3)	—
Local exfoliation	5 (2)	—
Eyelid edema	5 (2)	—

ARSENIC TRIOXIDE

Arsenic Trioxide Adverse Events at a Dose of 0.15 mg/kg/day (≥ 5%; n = 40)		
Adverse reaction	All adverse events, any grade % (n)	Grade 3 and 4 events % (n)
GI		
Nausea	75 (30)	—
Vomiting	58 (23)	—
Abdominal pain (lower and upper)	58 (23)	10 (4)
Diarrhea	53 (21)	—
Sore throat	40 (14)	—
Constipation	28 (11)	3 (1)
Anorexia	23 (9)	—
Appetite, decreased	15 (6)	—
Loose stools	10 (4)	—
Dyspepsia	10 (4)	—
Oral blistering	8 (3)	—
Fecal incontinence	8 (3)	—
GI hemorrhage	8 (3)	—
Dry mouth	8 (3)	—
Abdominal tenderness	8 (3)	—
Diarrhea hemorrhagic	8 (3)	—
Abdominal distension	8 (3)	—
Oral candidiasis	5 (2)	—
GU		
Vaginal hemorrhage	13 (5)	—
Intermenstrual bleeding	8 (3)	—
Renal failure	8 (3)	3 (1)
Renal impairment	8 (3)	—
Oliguria	5 (2)	—
Incontinence	5 (2)	—
Hematologic/Lymphatic		
Leukocytosis	50 (20)	3 (1)
Anemia	20 (8)	5 (2)
Thrombocytopenia	19 (7)	12 (5)
Febrile neutropenia	13 (5)	8 (3)
Neutropenia	10 (4)	10 (4)
Disseminated intravascular coagulation	8 (3)	8 (3)
Lymphadenopathy	8 (3)	—
Metabolic/Nutritional		
Hypokalemia	50 (20)	13 (5)
Hypomagnesemia	45 (18)	13 (5)
Hyperglycemia	45 (18)	13 (5)
ALT, increased	20 (8)	5 (2)
Hyperkalemia	18 (7)	5 (2)
AST, increased	13 (5)	3 (1)
Hypocalcemia	10 (4)	—
Hypoglycemia	8 (3)	—
Acidosis	5 (2)	—
Musculoskeletal		
Arthralgia	33 (13)	8 (3)
Myalgia	25 (10)	5 (2)
Bone pain	23 (9)	10 (4)
Back pain	18 (7)	3 (1)
Neck pain	13 (5)	—
Limb pain	13 (5)	5 (2)

Arsenic Trioxide Adverse Events at a Dose of 0.15 mg/kg/day (≥ 5%; n = 40)		
Adverse reaction	All adverse events, any grade % (n)	Grade 3 and 4 events % (n)
Ophthalmic		
Eye irritation	10 (4)	—
Blurred vision	10 (4)	—
Dry eye	8 (3)	—
Painful red eye	5 (2)	—
Respiratory		
Cough	65 (26)	—
Dyspnea	53 (21)	10 (4)
Epistaxis	25 (10)	—
Hypoxia	23 (9)	10 (4)
Pleural effusion	20 (8)	3 (1)
Sinusitis	20 (8)	—
Postnasal drip	13 (5)	—
Wheezing	13 (5)	—
Upper respiratory tract infection	13 (5)	3 (1)
Decreased breath sounds	10 (4)	—
Crepitations	10 (4)	—
Rales	10 (4)	—
Hemoptysis	8 (3)	—
Tachypnea	8 (3)	—
Rhonchi	8 (3)	—
Special senses		
Earache	8 (3)	—
Tinnitus	5 (2)	—
Miscellaneous		
Fatigue	63 (25)	5 (2)
Fever	63 (25)	5 (2)
Edema, nonspecific	40 (16)	—
Rigors	38 (15)	—
Chest pain	25 (10)	5 (2)
Pain, nonspecific	15 (6)	3 (1)
Weight gain	13 (5)	—
Herpes simplex	13 (5)	—
Weakness	10 (4)	5 (2)
Hemorrhage	8 (3)	—
Weight loss	8 (3)	—
Bacterial infection, nonspecific	8 (3)	3 (1)
Herpes zoster	8 (3)	—
Nasopharyngitis	5 (2)	—
Drug hypersensitivity	5 (2)	3 (1)
Sepsis	5 (2)	5 (2)

➤*Chronic effects:* Potential adverse effects of chronic arsenic trioxide therapy may include dermatologic changes, polyneuropathy, and cardiac toxicities. More studies are needed to assess chronic therapeutic toxicities of arsenic trioxide.

Overdosage

➤*Symptoms:* If symptoms suggestive of serious acute arsenic toxicity (eg, convulsions, muscle weakness, confusion) appear, immediately discontinue arsenic trioxide therapy and consider chelation therapy.

➤*Treatment:* A conventional protocol for acute arsenic intoxication includes dimercaprol administered at a dose of 3 mg/kg IM every 4 hours until immediate life-threatening toxicity has subsided. Thereafter, 250 mg penicillamine orally, up to a maximum frequency of 4 times/day (≤ 1 g/day), may be given.

TALC POWDER, STERILE

Rx	**Sclerosol** (Bryan)	**Aerosol:** 4 g talc	CFC-12. In single-use aluminum canister with 2 delivery tubes of 15 and 25 cm.
	Sterile Talc Powder (Bryan)	**Powder:** 5 g talc	In 100 mL glass bottle.

Indications

➤*Malignant pleural effusion:* To prevent recurrence of malignant pleural effusions in symptomatic patients.

➤*Unlabeled uses:* Benign pleural effusions; pneumothorax.

Administration and Dosage

➤*Approved by the FDA:* December 24, 1997.

Administer after adequate drainage of the effusion. Success of the pleurodesis is related to the completeness of the drainage of the pleural fluid as well as full reexpansion of the lung, both of which will promote symphysis of the pleural surfaces.

➤*Aerosol:* 4 to 8 g dose administered during thoracoscopy or open thoracotomy delivered intrapleurally from the spray canister (1 to 2 cans), which delivers talc at a rate of 0.4 g/second.

Administration – Shake canister well before usage. Remove protective cap and securely attach actuator button with its delivery tube (either 15 or 25 cm) to the valve stem of canister.

Insert delivery tube through pleural trocar, taking care not to place the distal end of the delivery tube adjacent to the lung parenchyma or directly against the chest wall. While firmly holding the delivery tube and pleural trocar together in one hand, gently apply pressure to the actuator button on the canister. Talc aerosol is not delivered by metered dose but depends on the extent and duration of manual compression of the actuator button on the canister. Point the distal end of the delivery tube in several different directions while administering short bursts in order to distribute the talc powder equally and extensively on all visceral and parietal pleural surfaces. For optimal distribution, always maintain the talc aerosol canister in the upright position. After application, discard the canister and delivery tube. The duration of chest tube drainage following talc sclerosis is dictated by the clinical situation.

➤*Powder:* 5 g dissolved in 50 to 100 mL sodium chloride injection, administered intrapleurally via chest tube. The optimal dose for effective pleurodesis is unknown; 5 g was the dose most frequently reported in the published literature.

Preparation – Using a 16-gauge needle attached to a 60 mL *LuerLok* syringe, measure and slowly draw up 50 mL of sodium chloride injection. Vent the talc bottle using a needle. Slowly inject the 50 mL sodium chloride injection into the bottle. For doses greater than 5 g, repeat this procedure with a second bottle. Swirl the bottle to disperse the talc powder and continue swirling to avoid settling of the talc in the slurry. Divide the content of each bottle into two 60 mL irrigation syringes by withdrawing 25 mL of the slurry into each syringe with continuous swirling. Add a sufficient quantity of sodium chloride injection to each syringe, up to a total volume of 50 mL in each syringe. Draw air into each syringe to the 60 mL mark to serve as a headspace for mixing prior to administration.

Each syringe contains 2.5 g sterile talc in 50 mL sodium chloride injection. Once the slurry has been made, use within 12 hours or discard and prepare a fresh slurry. Label the syringes appropriately, noting the expiration date and time with the statements "For pleurodesis only – Not for IV administration" and "Shake well before use."

Prior to administration, completely and continuously agitate the syringes to evenly redisperse the talc and avoid settlement. Immediately prior to administration, vent the 10 mL air headspace from each syringe. Attach the adapter and place a syringe tip on the adapter. Maintain continuous agitation of the syringes. Shake well before instillation.

Administration – Administer the talc slurry through the chest tube by gently applying pressure to the syringe plunger and empty the contents of the syringe into the chest cavity. After the talc slurry has been administered through the chest tube into the pleural cavity, the chest tube may be flushed with 10 to 25 mL sodium chloride solution to ensure the complete talc dose is delivered.

Following introduction of the talc slurry, the chest drainage tube is clamped and the patient is asked to move, at 20- to 30-minute intervals, from supine to alternating decubitus positions so that over a period of approximately 2 hours the talc is distributed within the chest cavity. Recent evidence suggests this step may not be necessary. At the end of this period, the chest drainage tube is unclamped, and the excess saline is removed by the routine continual external suction on the tube.

➤*Storage/Stability:*

Aerosol – Contents under pressure. Do not puncture or incinerate container. Store between 15° to 30°C (59° to 86°F). Protect against sunlight and do not expose to a temperature above 49°C (120°F) or the canister may rupture. Avoid freezing. Shake well before using.

Powder – Store at room temperature (18° to 25°C). Protect against sunlight.

Actions

➤*Pharmacology:* Sterile talc powder is a sclerosing agent for intrapleural administration. The therapeutic action of talc instilled into the pleural cavity is believed to result from induction of an inflammatory reaction. This reaction promotes adherence of the visceral to the parietal pleura, obliterating the pleural space and preventing reaccumulation of pleural fluid. The extent of talc systemically absorbed after intrapleural administration has not been adequately studied. Systemic exposure could be affected by the integrity of the visceral pleura and, therefore, could be increased if talc is administered immediately following lung resection or biopsy.

➤*Clinical trials:* The following prospective, randomized studies were designed to evaluate the risk of recurrence of malignant pleural effusions in patients with a variety of solid tumors.

Clinical Trials Evaluating Talc Powder for the Treatment of Malignant Pleural Effusions			
Treatment	Tumor	Response rate (*P* value[1])	Minimum of duration of response
Talc slurry 10 g/250 mL normal saline vs chest tube drainage	Variety	64% vs 41% *P* = 0.29	3 months
Talc slurry 5 g/50 mL normal saline vs bleomycin 1 mg/kg/50 mL normal saline	Variety	79% vs 75% *P* = 1	NA
Talc slurry 5 g/150 mL normal saline[2] vs bleomycin 1 unit/kg/150 mL normal saline[2]	Variety	64% vs 56% *P* = 0.77	NA
Talc slurry 5 g/50 mL normal saline plus lidocaine 2% 10 mL vs talc insufflation 5 g powder	Variety	90% vs 96% *P* = 0.61	NA
Talc poudrage vs tetracycline solution	Breast	61% vs 43% *P* = 0.345	12 months
Talc poudrage vs mustine solution	Breast	78% vs 39% *P* = 0.016	6 months

[1] Two-sided *P* value based on Fisher's exact test.
[2] Plus lidocaine 1%, 10 mL.

Warnings

➤*Pregnancy: Category B.* There are no adequate and well-controlled studies in pregnant women. Do not use during pregnancy unless clearly needed.

➤*Children:* Safety and efficacy in pediatric patients have not been established.

Precautions

➤*Future procedures:* Consider the possibility of future diagnostic and therapeutic procedures involving the hemithorax to be treated prior to administering talc. Sclerosis of the pleural space may preclude subsequent diagnostic procedures of the pleura on the treated side. Talc sclerosis may complicate or preclude future ipsilateral lung resective surgery, including pneumonectomy for transplantation purposes.

➤*Potentially curable malignancies:* Talc has no known antineoplastic activity. Do not use for potentially curable malignancies where systemic therapy would be more appropriate (eg, a malignant effusion secondary to a potentially curable lymphoma).

➤*Pulmonary complications:* Acute pneumonitis or acute respiratory distress syndrome (ARDS) have been rarely reported in association with intrapleural talc administration. It is unclear whether these were causally related to talc. Talc was not applied thoracoscopically or by insufflation in any of the reported cases. Three of 4 case reports of ARDS have occurred after treatment with 10 g talc administered via intrapleural chest tube instillation. One patient died 1 month post-treatment, and 2 patients recovered without further sequelae.

IV administration of talc is a well-recognized cause of pulmonary hypertension and pulmonary lung parenchymal disease, but these complications have not been reported after intrapleural administration. Pulmonary diseases (eg, silicosis or asbestosis-like diseases, chronic bronchitis, bronchogenic carcinoma, and pleural plaques) have been reported in association with inhaled talc.

➤*Aerosol:* The contents of the talc aerosol canister are under pressure. Do not puncture the canister and do not use or store near heat or open flame.

Drug Interactions

The efficacy of a second sclerosing agent after prior talc pleurodesis may be diminished by the absorptive properties of talc.

TALC POWDER, STERILE

Adverse Reactions

Talc administration has been described in more than 2000 patients. Patients with malignant pleural effusions were treated with talc via poudrage or slurry. In general, with respect to reported adverse experiences, it is difficult to distinguish the effects of talc from the effects of the procedures associated with its administration. The most reported common adverse experiences were fever and pain. Almost all of the cases of fever and over half of the cases of pain were in patients who received diagnostic biopsies at the time of talc administration.

►*Cardiovascular:* Asystolic arrest, hypotension, hypovolemia, myocardial infarction, tachycardia (rare).

►*Respiratory:* ARDS, bronchopleural fistula, dyspnea, hemoptysis, hypoxemia, pneumonia, pulmonary emboli, unilateral pulmonary edema (rare).

►*Miscellaneous:* Infection at the site of thoracostomy or thoracoscopy, localized bleeding, subcutaneous emphysema; empyema (rare).

Overdosage

►*Symptoms:* Overdosages have not been reported. Potential exists for pulmonary complications.

►*Treatment:* Excessive talc may be partially removed with saline lavage.

The following is a list of available diagnostic aids for professional office use or for use by patients at home (when noted). Those tests requiring special equipment and used primarily by commercial laboratories are not included. For complete information on specific uses, directions and characteristics of these products, consult the manufacturers' package literature.

ACETONE (Ketone) TESTS
To detect the presence of ketones.

Acetest (Bayer Corp)	**Reagent tablets** for urine, whole blood, serum or plasma tests	In 100s.
Chemstrip K (Boehringer Mannheim)	**Reagent strips** for urine tests	In 25s.
Ketostix (Bayer Corp)[1]	**Reagent strips** for urine tests	In 50s, 100s and UD 20s.

[1] For use by patient at home.

ALBUMIN TESTS
To detect the presence of protein.

Albustix (Bayer Corp)	**Reagent strips** for urine tests	In 100s.
Chemstrip Micral (Boehringer Mannheim)	**Reagent strips** for urine tests	In 30s.

BACTERIURIA TESTS
To detect nitrate, nitrite, uropathogens, total bacterial or gram-negative bacterial counts.

Microstix-3 (Bayer Corp)	**Reagent strips** for urine tests	In test kits containing 25 reagent strips, 25 incubation pouches and 25 ID labels.
Uricult (LifeSign LLC)	**Culture paddles** for urine tests	In 10s.
Isocult for Bacteriuria (Remel)	**Culture paddles** for urine tests	In 12s.
UTI Urinary Tract Infection Urine Test Strips (Consumers Choice Systems)	**Test strips** for urine tests	In 6 strips and 6 cups.

BILIRUBIN TESTS
To detect the presence of bilirubin.

Ictotest (Bayer Corp)	**Reagent tablets** for urine tests	In 100s.

BLOOD UREA NITROGEN TESTS
To estimate amounts of urea nitrogen.

Azostix (Bayer Corp)	**Reagent strips** for whole blood tests	In 25s.

CANDIDA TESTS
To detect *Candida albicans*.

Isocult for *Candida* (Remel)	**Culture paddles** for vaginal specimen tests	In 4s.
CandidaSure (LifeSign LLC)	**Reagent slides** for vaginal specimen tests	In kits containing 20 slides.

CHLAMYDIA TRACHOMATIS TESTS
To detect and identify *Chlamydia trachomatis*.

Chlamydiazyme (Abbott)	**Reagent kit** for enzyme immunoassay	In kits containing 100 and 500 tests.
MicroTrak *Chlamydia Trachomatis* (Syva)	**Slide tests** for urogenital, rectal, conjunctival or nasopharyngeal specimens	In kits containing 60 tests.
Amplicor (Roche Diagnostics Systems)	**Reagent kit** for endocervical, male urethral and male urine specimens	In kits containing 10, 96 and 100 tests.
Sure Cell Chlamydia (Kodak)	**Reagent kit** for endocervical, urethral, male urine or ocular specimens	In kits containing 10, 25 and 100 tests.
Clearview Chlamydia (Wampole)	**Color-label immunoassay** for endocervical specimens	In 20s.

CHOLESTEROL TESTS
To estimate cholesterol levels. For use by patient at home.

Advanced Care Cholesterol Test (Johnson & Johnson)	**Cassette** for blood test	In kits containing test cassette, result chart, lancet, gauze pad, adhesive bandage, instruction booklet and question and answer booklet.

COLOR ALLERGY SCREENING TESTS
For determination of immunoglobulin E.

CAST (Biomerica)	**Reagent sticks** for serum tests	In kits containing reagent sticks for 25 tests.

CRYPTOCOCCAL ANTIGEN TESTS
For the qualitative or quantitative determination of *Cryptococcus neoformans* antigen.

Crypto-LA (Wampole)	**Slide tests** for CSF and serum	In 70s.

DRUGS OF ABUSE TESTS
For detecting drugs of abuse (marijuana, cocaine, amphetamine, methamphetamine, phencyclidine, codeine, morphine, and heroin).

otc	**Dr. Brown's Home Drug Testing System** (Personal Health and Hygiene)	**Collection kit:** 1 urine specimen collection kit	In 1s.

GASTROINTESTINAL TESTS

For determination of GI disorders.

Entero-Test (HDC Corp)	**String capsules** for collection of duodenal fluid	In packages containing 25 capsules, pH sticks and color charts.
Entero-Test Pediatric Capsules (HDC Corp)	**String capsules** for collection of duodenal fluid	In packages containing 25 capsules, pH sticks and color charts.
Gastro-Test (HDC Corp)	**String capsules** for collection of stomach acid	In packages containing 25 capsules, pH sticks and color charts.
Pyloriset (LifeSign LLC)	**Reagent kit** for serum test	In kits containing 20 latex reagents, positive and negative controls, dilution buffers, mixing sticks and test cards.

H. PYLORI TESTS

For use in the detection of gastric urease as an aid in the diagnosis of *H. pylori* infection in the human stomach. The test utilizes a liquid scintillation counter for the measurement of $^{14}CO_2$ in breath samples.

PYtest (Tri-Med Specialties, Inc.)	**Capsules** 14c urea	Clear, gelatin. In UD packages of 1s, 10s, and 100s. In *PYtest Kit* containing a capsule and breath collection equipment.

GLUCOSE, BLOOD TESTS

To determine blood glucose levels. For use by patient at home.

Chemstrip bG (Boehringer Mannheim)	**Reagent strips** for blood tests	In 25s, 50s and 100s.
Diascan (Home Diagnostics)		In 50s for use with *Diascan Color Chart* (provided) or *Diascan Blood Glucose Meter*.
Glucostix (Bayer Corp)		In 50s, 100s and UD 25s for use with bottle label color blocks, *Glucometer* II, *Glucometer* II *With Memory, Glucometer M* or *Glucometer QA Blood Glucose Meters*.
Glucofilm (Bayer Corp)		In 25s, 50s and 100s for use with *Glucometer 3, Glucometer QA* or *Glucometer M+ Blood Glucose Meters*.
Glucometer Encore (Bayer Corp)		In 50s for use with *Glucometer Encore Blood Glucose Meter* or *Glucometer M+ Blood Glucose Meters*.
Glucometer Elite (Bayer Corp)		In 25s and 50s with code strips for use with *Glucometer Elite Blood Glucose Meter*.
Accu-Chek Advantage (Boehringer Mannheim)		In 50s to be used with *Accu-Chek Advantage Blood Glucose Monitoring System*.
One Touch (LifeScan)		In 25s, 50s and 100s for use with *One Touch Basic Blood Glucose Monitoring System* or *One Touch* II *Blood Glucose Monitoring System*.
First Choice (Polymer Technology)		In 25s, 50s and 100s for use with *Glucometer* II, *Glucometer* II *With Memory, Glucometer 3, Diascan, One Touch, One Touch* II or *One Touch Basic Meters*.

GLUCOSE, URINE TESTS

To measure glucose in urine. For use by patient at home.

Clinitest (Bayer Corp)	**Reagent tablets** for urine tests	In 36s and 100s with color charts and sets containing 36 tablets, 1 test tube, 1 dropper and color chart.
Chemstrip bG (Boehringer Mannheim)	**Reagent strips** for urine tests	In 100s.
Chemstrip uG (Boehringer Mannheim)		In 100s.
Clinistix (Bayer Corp)		In 50s.
Diastix (Bayer Corp)		In 50s and 100s.

GONORRHEA TESTS

Used as a presumptive test for *Neisseria gonorrhoeae*.

Biocult-GC (Orion Diagnostica)	**Culture paddles** for endocervical, oropharyngeal, anterior urethra or anal cultures	In kits containing vials, CO_2-generating tablets, swabs, reagent and specimen ID labels.
Gonozyme Diagnostic (Abbott)	**Reagent kit** for urogenital swab specimens	In test kits containing reagent, reaction trays, assay tubes with identifying racks and cover seals for 100 tests.
LCx Assay (Abbott)	**Reagent kit** in endocervical, male urethral and urine swab specimens.	In kits containing swabs, vials and reagent for 100 tests.
Isocult for *Neisseria gonorrhoeae* (Remel)	**Culture paddles** for endocervical, rectal and urethral cultures	In test kits containing culture tubes, CO_2-generating tablets, reagent and information sheet for 12 tests.
MicroTrak *Neisseria gonorrhoeae* Culture Confirmation Test (Syva)	**Reagent kit** for endocervical, urethral, rectal, conjunctival and pharyngeal cultures	In test kits containing reagent, reconstitution diluent and mounting fluid for 85 tests.

HEMATOCRIT/HEMOGLOBIN TESTS

To determine hematocrit/hemoglobin measurement.

Stat-Crit (Wampole)	**Electrode device** for blood samples	In 120s for use with *STAT-CRIT* instrument kit.

HEMOGLOBIN, GLYCATED (HbA$_{1c}$) TESTS

In diabetes (Type 1 or 2) for the quantitative measurement of glycated hemoglobin levels.

A1cNow (Metrika)	**Kit** for blood samples	In 1-pack test kit with monitor, lancets, and dilution kit and in 10-pack professional use kits.

HUMAN IMMUNODEFICIENCY VIRUS (HIV) TESTS
For the detection of HIV.

HIV-1 LA Recombigen HIV-1 Latex Agglutination Test (Cambridge Biotech)	**Reagent kit** for blood, serum, plasma or capillary sample tests	In kits containing vial, diluent, card and transfer loop for 100 tests.
HIVAB HIV-1 EIA (Abbott)	**Reagent kit** for serum or plasma tests	In kits containing reagents for 100 tests.
HIVAG-1 (Abbott)	**Reagent kit** for serum or plasma tests	In kits containing reagents for 100 tests.
Amplicor HIV-1 Monitor (Roche)	**Reagent kit** for plasma HIV-1 tests	In kits containing reagents for 24 tests.
Confide (Direct Access Diagnostics)	**Reagent kit** for HIV blood tests	In kit containing materials to draw blood sample, a test card and a protective mailer for 1 test.
HIVAB HIV-1/HIV-2 (rDNA) EIA (Abbott)	**In vitro enzyme immunoassay** for qualitative detection of antibodies to human immunodeficiency viruses type 1 or type 2 in human serum or plasma.	In 100, 1000 and 5000 test kits.
OraSure (Epitope)[1]	**Reagent kit** for oral fluid tests	In kit containing collection pad, vial and reagent for 1 test.
OraSure HIV-1 (Epitope)	**Collection kit** for oral specimen collection	In kit containing cotton fiber on stick with collection vial.

[1] For use by patient at home.

MONONUCLEOSIS TESTS
For qualitative and quantitative identification of heterophilic antibodies for the diagnosis of infectious mononucleosis.

Mono-Diff (Wampole)	**Reagent kit** for serum or plasma tests	In kits containing reagent, absorbent I and II, positive control serum, calibrated capillary tubes and bulbs, disposable stirrers and disposable card slides for 20 tests.
Mono-Latex (Wampole)	**Reagent kit** for serum or plasma tests	In kits containing reagent latex, positive control, negative control, capillary tubes and bulbs, black glass slide and disposable stirrers for 20 and 50 tests.
Mono-Plus (Wampole)	**Reagent kit** for serum or plasma tests	In kits containing *micro-plus* test devices and *mono-plus* developer solution for 30 tests.
Monospot (Meridian Diagnostics)	**Slide test** for serum or plasma	In kits containing reagents I and II, indicator cells, positive and negative control serum, glass slide, microcapillary pipettes, rubber bulbs, plastic pipettes and wooden applicators for 20 tests.
Monosticon Dri-Dot (Organon Teknika)	**Slide test** for serum, plasma or whole blood tests	In kits containing test slides, positive and negative I.M. serum controls, dropper bottle and *dispenstirs* for 25 and 100 tests.
Mono-Test (Wampole)	**Slide test** for serum or plasma	In kits containing reagent, positive and negative control serums, calibrated capillary tubes and bulbs, glass slides, disposable stirrers and card slides for 40 and 100 tests.
Quantaffirm (Organon Teknika)	**Reagent kit** for serum tests	In test kits containing vials and reagent for 4 tests.

OCCULT BLOOD SCREENING TESTS
To detect occult blood.

ColoCare (Helena Labs)[1]	**Kit** for fecal specimens	In kits containing 3 tests.
ColoScreen (Helena Labs)	**Slide tests** for fecal specimens	In kits containing slides, monitors, tape, developer, specimen applicators and mailing envelopes for 100 tests.
EZ Detect (Biomerica)[1]	**Kit** for fecal specimens	In kits containing 5 test tissues, control and control card for 48 tests.
Hemoccult II Dispensapak (SmithKline Diagnostics)[1]	**Slide tests** for fecal specimens	In kits containing slides, applicators and developer for 100 tests.
Hemoccult II Dispensapak Plus (SmithKline Diagnostics)[1]	**Slide tests** for fecal specimens	In kits containing slides, sample collection tissues, applicators and mailing pouch for 40 tests.
Hemoccult II (SmithKline Diagnostics)	**Slide tests** for fecal specimens	In kits containing developer and applicators for 102 and 1020 tests.
Hemoccult Slides (SmithKline Diagnostics)	**Slide tests** for fecal specimens	In kits containing developer and applicators for 100 and 1000 tests.
Hemoccult Tape (SmithKline Diagnostics)	**Tape** for fecal specimens	In kits containing tape dispenser and developer for 100 tests.
Hemoccult SENSA (SmithKline Diagnostics)	**Slide tests** for fecal specimens	In 100s and 1000s with developer and applicators.
Hemoccult II SENSA (SmithKline Diagnostics)	**Slide tests** for fecal specimens	In kits containing slides, tissues, applicators and mailing pouches for 40 tests.
HemeSelect Reagent (SmithKline Diagnostics)	**Reagent kit** for fecal specimens	In kits containing vials, diluent, Hb positive control, microtiter plate and droppers for 40 tests. *For use with HemeSelect Sample Collection Kit.*
HemeSelect Collection (SmithKline Diagnostics)[1]	**Collection kit** for fecal specimens	In kits containing sample collection card, applicator, self-sealing sample bag and instructions. *For use with the HemeSelect Reagent Kit.*
Hema-Chek (Bayer Corp)[1]	**Slide tests** for fecal specimens	In kits containing slide pak, developer, control and applicator sticks for 100 and 300 tests.
Hematest (Bayer Corp)	**Reagent tablets** for fecal specimens	In packages containing reagent tablets and filter paper for 100 tests.
Hemastix (Bayer Corp)	**Reagent strips** for urine specimens	In 50s.
Gastroccult (SmithKline Diagnostics)	**Slide tests** for gastric specimens	In kits containing slides, developer and applicators for 40 tests.

[1] For use by patient at home.

OVULATION TESTS

To measure luteinizing hormone for prediction of ovulation.

Answer Ovulation (Carter Wallace)[1]	**Kit** for urine tests	In kits containing vial, droppers, clear tube, urine collection containers, test well, stand and clear tube holder for 5 tests.
Clearplan Easy (Whitehall)[1]	**Kit** for urine tests	In kits containing sticks for 5 tests.
OvuQUICK Self-Test (Quidel)[1]	**Kit** for urine tests	In kits containing urine cup, droppers, reconstitution buffer, enzyme conjugate, test pad labels, test pad, foil pouch, substrate and stop solution for 6 tests.
OvuKIT Self-Test (Quidel)[1]	**Kit** for urine tests	In kits containing test stick, vials, urine cups and test stick holder for 6 and 9 tests.
Color Ovulation Test (Biomerica)[1]	**Kit** for urine tests	In 9 day test kits.
First Response Ovulation Predictor (Carter Wallace)[1]	**Kit** for urine tests	In kits containing vial, droppers, clear tube, urine collection containers, test well, stand and clear tube holder for 5 tests.
Conceive Ovulation Predictor (Quidel)	**Cassettes** for urine tests	In kits containing cassettes, foil pouches, plastic cups and droppers for 5 tests.
QTest Ovulation (Quidel)	**Kit** for urine tests	In kits containing teststrips, teststrip holders, urine collection cups, glass vials, reagents, solutions and droppers for 5 tests.
OvuGen (BioGenex)	**Kit** for urine tests	In kits of 6 and 10.

[1] For use by patient at home.

PREGNANCY TESTS

To detect the presence of human chorionic gonadotropin.

Advance (Ortho)[1]	**Stick** for urine test	In 1s.
Answer One-Step Pregnancy Test (Carter Wallace)[1]	**Stick** for urine test	In 1s.
Answer Plus (Carter Wallace)[1]	**Kit** for urine test	In kits containing urine collection cup, filter dropper, vial, test well, test tray and tube for 1 test.
Answer Quick & Simple (Carter Wallace)[1]	**Kit** for urine test	In kits containing dropper, tube and color key for 2 tests.
Conceive Pregnancy (Quidel)[1]	**Kit** for urine test	In kits containing tape cassette, dropper, plastic cup for 1 and 2 tests.
Clearblue Easy (Whitehall)[1]	**Stick** for urine test	In 1s.
e.p.t. Quick Stick (Parke-Davis)[1]	**Stick** for urine test	In 1s.
Fact Plus (Ortho)[1]	**Kit** for urine test	In kits containing test disk, urine collection cup and urine dropper.
First Response (Carter Wallace)[1]	**Stick** for urine test	In 1s.
Fortel Midstream (Biomerica)	**Stick** for urine test	In 1s.
Fortel Plus (Biomerica)[1]	**Kit** for urine test	In kits containing urine collection cup, test device, dropper and absorbent packet.
One Step Midstream (Biocare International)[1]	**Stick** for urine test	In 1s.
Midstream Pregnancy Test Kit (Goldline)	**Kit** for urine test	In 1s.
Pregnosis (Roche)[1]	**Slide tests** for urine	In kits containing reagents, droppers, pipettes, applicator stick and slide for 50 and 200 tests.
Nimbus Quick Strip (Biomerica)[1]	**Test strips** for urine	In 25s.
RapidVue (Quidel)[1]	**Kit** for urine test	In kits containing cup, dropper and test cassette.
QTest (Quidel)[1]	**Stick** for urine test	In kits containing vial, test stick, reagent, developer and solution for 1 test.
UCG Slide (Wampole)	**Slide tests** for urine	In kits containing latex reagent, antibody reagent, slide stirrers and plastic cup for 30, 100, 300 and 1000 tests.
Abbott TestPack hCG-Urine Plus (Abbott)	**Kit** for urine test	In kits containing reaction dish and transfer pipette. In 20s.
Nimbus (Biomerica)	**Kit** for urine test	In kits containing tube, conjugate and pipettes for 25, 50 and 100 tests.
Nimbus Plus (Biomerica)	**Kit** for urine test	In kits containing test devices and droppers for 25 tests.
Unistep hCG (Orion Diagnostica)	**Kit** for urine test	In kits containing hCG reaction packs and droppers for 25 and 50 tests.
QuickVue (Quidel)	**Cassettes** for urine test	In kits containing test cassettes and pipettes 25 and 75 tests.
SureCell Pregnancy (Kodak)	**Kit** for urine test	In kits containing reagents for 10, 25 and 100 tests.
SureCell hCG-Urine Test (Kodak)	**Kit** for urine test	In 10s, 25s and 100s.
UCG Beta-Slide Monoclonal II (Wampole)	**Slide tests** for urine	In kits containing slide test and reagent for 50, 100 and 300 tests.

[1] For use by patient at home.

RHEUMATOID FACTOR TEST

To detect rheumatoid factor in blood.

Rheumatex (Wampole)	**Slide tests** for blood	In kits containing reagents and slides for 100 and 200 tests.
Rheumaton (Wampole)	**Slide tests** for serum or synovial fluid	In kits containing reagent, positive and negative control, tubes, bulbs and slides for 20, 50 and 150 tests.

SICKLE CELL TEST

To detect hemoglobin S.

Sickledex (Ortho)	**Kit** for blood tests	In kits containing reagents and solution for 12 and 100 tests.

STAPHYLOCOCCUS TEST

To determine the presence of *Staphylococcus aureus*.

Isocult for *Staphylococcus aureus* (Remel)	**Culture paddles** for exudate	In kits containing reagents for 12 tests.

STREPTOCOCCI TESTS

To detect beta-hemolytic group A streptococci, group B streptococci, streptococcal pharyngitis, antibodies to DNase-B, *Streptococcus pneumoniae* and streptococcal extracellular antigens.

Sure Cell Streptococci (Kodak)	**Kit** for the detection of group A streptococcal antigen from throat swabs and blood	In kits containing test cells, extraction blocks, reagents, dye solutions, filter and swabs for 25 and 100 tests.
Culturette 10 Minute Group A Strep ID (Becton Dickinson)	**Slide test** for the detection of group A streptococcal antigen from throat swabs	In kits containing reagents and test slides for 55 and 200 tests.
Isocult for *Streptococcal pharyngitis* (Remel)	**Culture paddles** for the detection of streptococcal pharyngitis from throat swabs	In kits culture paddles and reagents for 12 tests.
Respiracult-Strep (LifeSign LLC)	**Culture paddles** for the detection of group A beta-hemolytic streptococci from throat and nasopharyngeal sources	In kits containing reagents and culture paddles for 25 and 50 tests.
Streptonase-B (Wampole)	**Kit** for the detection of antibodies to DNase-B in serum	In kits containing reagents and tubes for 10 tests.
Test Pack (Abbott)	**Kit** for the detection of group A streptococci from throat specimens	In kits containing reagents, extraction tubes and swabs for 40 and 80 tests.
Bactigen B Streptococcus-CS (Wampole)	**Slide tests** for the detection of group B streptococcus antigen from vaginal and cervical swabs	In kits containing reagents, slides, droppers and stirrers for 48 tests.
Streptozyme (Wampole)	**Slide tests** for the detection of streptococcal extracellular antigens in blood, plasma and serum	In kits containing reagents, tubes, positive and negative control serum, bulbs and slides for 15, 50 and 150 tests.
Detect-A-Strep (Antibodies Inc.)	**Slide tests** for the detection of streptococcal antigen from throat swabs	In kits containing reagents and test plates for 6 tests.

TOXOPLASMOSIS TEST

To detect the presence of *Toxoplasma gondii* in blood.

TPM Test (Wampole)	**Kit** for blood test	In kits including reagents for 120 tests.

VIRUS TESTS

To detect human T-Lymphotropic type 1, HSV-1, HSV-2, herpes, rotavirus, rubella and C-reactive protein.

Human T-Lymphotropic Virus Type I EIA (Abbott)	**Reagent kit** for serum or plasma tests	In kits containing reagents, vials and reaction trays for 100 tests.
MicroTrak HSV 1/HSV 2 Culture Identification/Typing Test (Syva)	**Culture test** for tissue	1 test per kit.
MicroTrak HSV1/HSV2 Direct Specimen Identification/Typing Test (Syva)	**Slide test** for external lesions	In kits containing reagent for 60 tests.
Sure Cell Herpes (Kodak)	**Reagent kit** for genital, rectal, oral or dermal swabs	In 10s and 25s.
Rubazyme for Rubella (Abbott)	**Reagent kit** for serum test	In kits containing reagents and diluent for 1 and 5 tests.
Virogen Herpes (Wampole)	**Slide test** for the detection of herpes simplex virus antigens directly from lesions or cell culture	In kits containing reagents, stirrers, slides and slide covers for 100 tests.
Virogen Rotatest for Rotavirus (Wampole)	**Slide test** for fecal specimens	In kits containing reagents, extraction buffer and slides for 50 tests.
Immunex C-Reactive Protein (Wampole)	**Kit** for blood tests	In kits containing reagents and slides for 100 tests.
Impact Rubella (Wampole)	**Slide test** for serum	In kits containing reagents and slides for 100, 500 and 5000 tests.

COMBINATION TESTS

To detect a multiplicity of conditions, including *Haemophilus influenzae* type b, *Neisseria meningitidis* serogroups A/B/C/Y/W135, *Streptococcus pneumoniae*, *Salmonella*, *Shigella*, *N. gonorrhoeae*, *T. vaginalis* and Candida.

Bactigen Meningitis Panel (Wampole)	**Slide test** for cerebrospinal fluid, serum, urine and blood	In 54s.
Bactigen *Salmonella-Shigella* (Wampole)	**Slide test** for cultures	In kits containing reagents, dispenser cannulae, droppers, slides and stirrers for 96 tests.
Isocult for *N. gonorrhoeae* and *Candida* (Remel)	**Culture test** for endocervical rectal, urethral, pharyngeal and vaginal specimens	In 12s.
Isocult for *T. vaginalis* and *Candida* (Remel)	**Culture test** for vaginal and urethral cultures	In kits containing culture tubes and reagents for 12 tests.

SODIUM AND pH URINE TEST

Used for the quantitative detection of Na and pH in urine and for the qualitative detection of bladder tumor associated antigen in urine.

BTA stat Test (Polymedco, Inc.)	**Kit** for bladder cancer test	In kits containing 30 foil packages with a BTA stat device, disposable dropper, and disposable desiccant pouch.

MULTIPLE URINE TEST PRODUCTS
To make simultaneous determinations of two or more urine tests.

Product & Distributor	Glucose	Protein	pH	Blood	Ketones	Bilirubin	Urobilinogen	Nitrite	Leukocytes	How Supplied
Chemstrip 2 GP (Boehringer Mannheim)	X	X								In 100s.
Uristix (Bayer Corp)	X	X								In 100s.
Combistix (Bayer Corp)	X	X	X							In 100s.
Hema-Combistix (Bayer Corp)	X	X	X	X						In 100s.
Uristix 4 (Bayer Corp)	X	X						X	X	In 100s.
Chemstrip 4 the OB (Boehringer Mannheim)	X	X			X				X	In 100s.
Chemstrip uGK (Boehringer Mannheim)	X				X					In 50s.
Keto-Diastix (Bayer Corp)	X				X					In 50s and 100s.
Chemstrip 6 (Boehringer Mannheim)	X	X	X	X	X				X	In 100s.
Labstix (Bayer Corp)	X	X	X	X	X					In 100s.
Bili-Labstix (Bayer Corp)	X	X	X	X	X	X				In 100s.
Chemstrip 7 (Boehringer Mannheim)	X	X	X	X	X	X			X	In 100s.
Multistix (Bayer Corp)	X	X	X	X	X	X	X			In 100s.
Multistix SG[1] (Bayer Corp)	X	X	X	X	X	X	X			In 100s.
Multistix 7 (Bayer Corp)	X	X	X	X	X			X	X	In 100s.
Multistix 8 SG[1] (Bayer Corp)	X	X	X	X	X			X	X	In 100s.
Chemstrip 8 (Boehringer Mannheim)	X	X	X	X	X	X	X		X	In 100s.
N-Multistix (Bayer Corp)	X	X	X	X	X	X	X	X		In 100s.
N-Multistix SG[1] (Bayer Corp)	X	X	X	X	X	X	X	X		In 100s.
Multistix 9 SG[1] (Bayer Corp)	X	X	X	X	X	X		X	X	In 100s.
Multistix 10 SG[1] (Bayer Corp)	X	X	X	X	X	X	X	X	X	In 100s.
Chemstrip 10 With SG[1] (Boehringer Mannheim)	X	X	X	X	X	X	X	X	X	In 100s.
Chemstrip 9 (Boehringer Mannheim)	X	X	X	X	X	X	X	X	X	In 100s.
Multistix 9 (Bayer Corp)	X	X	X	X	X	X	X	X	X	In 100s.
Chemstrip 2 LN (Boehringer Mannheim)								X	X	In 100s.
Multistix 2 (Bayer Corp)								X	X	In 100s.
Biotel Kidney (Biotel)		X		X						In 12s.

[1] Also tests specific gravity.

The following is a list of available diagnostic aids for professional office use or for use by patients at home (when noted). Those tests requiring special equipment and used primarily by commercial laboratories are not included. For complete information on specific uses, directions and characteristics of these products, consult the manufacturers' package literature.

AMINOHIPPURATE SODIUM (PAH)

For the estimation of renal plasma flow and to measure the functional capacity of the renal tubular secretory mechanism.

Rx	**Aminohippurate Sodium** (Merck)	**Injection:** 20% aqueous solution	In 10 ml vials.

HYSTEROSCOPY FLUID

For use with the hysteroscope as an aid in distending the uterine cavity and in irrigating and visualizing its surfaces.

Rx	**Hyskon** (Pharmacia & Upjohn)	**Solution:** 32% w/v dextran 70 in 10% w/v dextrose	In 100 and 250 ml.

INDIGOTINDISULFONATE SODIUM INJECTION

For localizing ureteral orifices during cystoscopy and ureteral catheterization.

Rx	**Indigo Carmine** (American Regent)	**Solution ampules for injection:** 0.8% aqueous solution	In 5 ml amps.

INDOCYANINE GREEN

For determining cardiac output, hepatic function and liver blood flow and for ophthalmic angiography.

Rx	**Cardio-Green** (Becton Dickinson)	**Powder**	In 25 and 50 mg vials with solvent.

INULIN

For measurement of glomerular filtration rate (GFR).

Rx	**Inulin Injection** (Iso-Tex Diagnostics)	**Injection:** 100 mg per ml	In 50 ml vials.[1]

[1] With 0.9% Sodium Chloride in Water for Injection.

MANNITOL

For measurement of glomerular filtration rate (GFR). For therapeutic indications, refer to monographs in the Cardiovasculars and Anti-Infectives chapters.

Rx	**Mannitol IV** (Various, eg, Kendall McGaw)	**Injection:** 10%	In 1000 ml.
Rx	**Mannitol IV** (Various, eg, Abbott, Kendall McGaw)	**Injection:** 15%	In 150 and 500 ml.
Rx	**Mannitol IV** (Various, eg, Abbott, Kendall McGaw)	**Injection:** 20%	In 250 and 500 ml.
Rx	**Mannitol IV** (Various, eg, American Regent, Astra, IMS, Pasadena, Schein, Steris)	**Injection:** 25%	In 50 ml vials and syringes.

SODIUM IODIDE I^{123}

Rx	**Sodium Iodide I-123** (Mallinckrodt Medical)	**Capsules:** 3.7 MBq	Sucrose. Red/white. In 1s, 3s, and 5s.
		7.4 MBq	Sucrose. Green/white. In 1s, 3s, and 5s.

Indications

As a diagnostic procedure in evaluating thyroid function or morphology.

Administration and Dosage

The recommended oral dose for the average patient (70 kg) is 3.7 to 14.8 MBq (100 to 400 mcCi). The lower part of the dosage range is recommended for uptake studies alone, and the higher part, 14.8 MBq, for thyroid imaging. The determination of I^{123} concentration in the thyroid gland may be initiated at 6 hours after administering the dose; measure according to standardized procedures.

Measure the patient dose by a suitable radioactivity calibration system immediately prior to administration. Can be given up to 30 hours after calibration time and date. Thereafter, discard according to standard safety procedures. Wear waterproof gloves at all times when handling capsules or container.

➤*Storage/Stability:* The contents of the vial are radioactive and adequate shielding and handling precautions must be maintained. Dispense and preserve capsules in tightly closed containers that are adequately shielded. Control the storage and disposal of Sodium Iodide I^{123} capsules in a manner that is in compliance with the appropriate regulations of the government agency authorized to license the use of this radionuclide. Store at room temperature (15° to 30°C; 59° to 86°F).

Actions

➤*Pharmacology:* Sodium Iodide I^{123} (Na^{123} I) is readily absorbed from the upper GI tract. The iodide is distributed primarily within the extracellular fluid of the body. It is trapped and organically bound by the thyroid and concentrated by the stomach, choroid plexus, and salivary glands. It is excreted by the kidneys.

The fraction of the administered dose that is accumulated in the thyroid gland may be a measure of thyroid function in the absence of unusually high or low iodine intake or administration of certain drugs that influence iodine accumulation by the thyroid gland. Accordingly, question the patient carefully regarding previous medications or procedures involving radiographic media. Healthy subjects can accumulate ≈ 10% to 50% of the administered iodine dose in the thyroid gland; however, normal and abnormal ranges are established by individual physician's criteria.

Warnings

➤*Pregnancy:* Category C. It is not known whether Sodium Iodide I^{123} can cause fetal harm when administered to a pregnant woman or can affect reproductive capacity. Give to a pregnant woman only if clearly needed. Do not study females of childbearing age unless the benefits anticipated from the test outweigh the possible risk of exposure to the amount of ionizing radiation associated with the test. Ideally, perform examinations using radiopharmaceuticals, especially those elective in nature, during the first few (≈ 10) days following onset of menses.

➤*Lactation:* Because I^{123} is excreted in breast milk, substitute formula feeding for breastfeeding if the agent must be administered to the mother during lactation.

➤*Children:* Safety and efficacy are not established. Do not study children unless benefits anticipated from the test outweigh possible risk of exposure to the amount of ionizing radiation associated with the test.

Precautions

➤*Radioactivity:* Capsule contents are radioactive. Shield preparation adequately at all times.

➤*Administration:* Do not use after expiration time and date stated on the label. Administer prescribed Sodium Iodide I^{123} dose as soon as practical from time of receipt of product (ie, as close to calibration time as possible), in order to minimize the fraction of radiation exposure due to the relative increase of radionuclidic contaminants with time.

➤*Handle with care:* Use appropriate safety measures to minimize radiation exposure to clinical personnel. Take care to minimize radiation exposure to the patient consistent with proper patient management.

Radiopharmaceuticals should be used only by physicians who are qualified by training and experience in the safe use and handling of radionuclides, and whose experience and training have been approved by the appropriate government agency authorized to license the use of radionuclides.

Adverse Reactions

Although rare, reactions include the following, in decreasing order of frequency: Nausea; vomiting; chest pain; tachycardia; itching skin; rash; hives.

THYROTROPIN ALFA

Rx	**Thyrogen** (Genzyme)	**Powder for injection, lyophilized:** 1.1 mg thyrotropin alfa (≥ 4 IU)/vial	Kit of two 1.1 mg single-use vials of thyrotropin alfa and two 10 mL vials of diluent.[1]

[1] 36 mg mannitol, 5.1 mg sodium phosphate, 2.4 mg NaCl.

Indications

➤*Adjunctive diagnostic tool for serum thyroglobulin (Tg) testing:* For use as an adjunctive diagnostic tool for serum Tg testing with or without radioiodine imaging in the follow-up of patients with well-differentiated thyroid cancer.

Other potential clinical uses – May be used in patients with an undetectable Tg on thyroid hormone suppressive therapy to exclude the diagnosis of residual or recurrent thyroid cancer.

May be used in patients requiring serum Tg testing and radioiodine imaging who are unwilling to undergo thyroid hormone withdrawal testing and whose treating physician believes that use of a less sensitive test is justified.

May be used in patients who are either unable to mount an adequate endogenous thyroid stimulating hormone (TSH) response to thyroid hormone withdrawal or in whom withdrawal is medically contraindicated.

It is not recommended to stimulate radioiodine uptake for the purposes of ablative radiotherapy of thyroid cancer.

Administration and Dosage

➤*Approved by the FDA:* November 30, 1998.

Administer thyrotropin alfa IM only. Do not administer IV.

After reconstitution with 1.2 mL Sterile Water for Injection, administer a 1 mL solution (0.9 mg thyrotropin alfa) by IM injection to the buttock. Reconstitute the powder immediately prior to use with 1.2 mL of the diluent provided.

➤*Usual dose:* 0.9 mg IM may be administered every 24 hours for 2 doses or every 72 hours for 3 doses.

➤*Adjunctive thyroid testing:* For radioiodine imaging, administer radioiodine 24 hours following the final thyrotropin alfa injection. Perform scanning 48 hours after radioiodine administration (72 hours after the final injection of thyrotropin alfa).

For serum Tg testing, obtain the serum sample 72 hours after the final injection of thyrotropin alfa.

➤*Storage/Stability:* Store at 2° to 8°C (36° to 46°F). If necessary, the reconstituted solution can be stored for up to 24 hours between 2° to 8°C (36° to 46°F), while avoiding microbial contamination.

After reconstitution with the accompanying Sterile Water for Injection visually inspect each vial for particulate matter or discoloration before use. Do not use any vial exhibiting particulate matter or discoloration.

Do not use after the expiration date on the vial. Protect from light.

Actions

➤*Pharmacology:* Thyrotropin alfa (recombinant human thyroid stimulating hormone) is a heterodimeric glycoprotein produced by recombinant DNA technology. It has comparable biochemical properties to the human pituitary TSH. Binding of thyrotropin alfa to TSH receptors on normal thyroid epithelial cells or on well-differentiated thyroid cancer tissue stimulates iodine uptake and organification, and synthesis and secretion of thyroglobulin (Tg), triiodothyronine (T$_3$), and thyroxine (T$_4$).

➤*Pharmacokinetics:* The pharmacokinetics of thyrotropin alfa were studied in 16 patients with well-differentiated thyroid cancer given a single 0.9 mg IM dose. Mean peak concentrations of ≈ 116 mU/L were reached between 3 and 24 hours after injection (median of 10 hours). The mean apparent elimination half-life was ≈ 25 hours. The organ(s) of TSH clearance in humans have not been identified, but studies of pituitary-derived TSH suggest the involvement of the liver and kidneys.

Warnings

➤*Pregnancy:* Category C. It is not known whether thyrotropin alfa can cause fetal harm when administered to a pregnant woman or can affect reproductive capacity. Give thyrotropin alfa to a pregnant woman only if clearly needed.

➤*Lactation:* It is not known whether the drug is excreted in human milk. Because many drugs are excreted in milk, exercise caution when administering thyrotropin alfa to a nursing woman.

➤*Children:* Safety and efficacy in pediatric patients < 16 years of age have not been established.

THYROTROPIN ALFA

Precautions

►*Diagnosis:* Even when thyrotropin alfa-stimulated Tg testing is performed in combination with radioiodine imaging, there remains a meaningful risk of missing a diagnosis of thyroid cancer or of underestimating the extent of disease. Therefore, thyroid hormone withdrawal Tg testing with radioiodine imaging remains the standard diagnostic modality to assess the presence, location, and extent of thyroid cancer.

A newly detectable Tg level or a Tg level rising over time after thyrotropin alfa, or a high index of suspicion of metastatic disease, even in the setting of a negative or low-stage thyrotropin alfa radioiodine scan, should prompt further evaluation such as thyroid hormone withdrawal to definitively establish the location and extent of thyroid cancer. On the other hand, none of the 31 patients studied with undetectable thyrotropin alfa Tg levels (< 2.5 ng/mL) had metastatic disease. Therefore, an undetectable thyrotropin alfa Tg level suggests the absence of clinically significant disease.

►*Thyroglobulin antibodies:* Tg antibodies may confound the Tg assay and render Tg levels uninterpretable. Therefore, in such cases, even with a negative or low-stage thyrotropin alfa radioiodine scan, give consideration to evaluating patients further with, for example, a confirmatory thyroid hormone withdrawal scan to determine the location and extent of thyroid cancer.

►*Previous treatment with bovine TSH:* Exercise caution when thyrotropin alfa is administered to patients who have been previously treated with bovine TSH and, in particular, to those patients who have experienced hypersensitivity reactions to bovine TSH.

►*Special risk:* Thyrotropin alfa is known to cause a transient but significant rise in serum thyroid hormone concentration. Therefore, exercise caution in patients with a known history of heart disease and with significant residual thyroid tissue.

Adverse Reactions

Thyrotropin Alfa Adverse Events (≥ 1%)	
Adverse reaction	n = 381
CNS	
Headache	7.3
Dizziness	1.6
Paresthesia	1.6
GI	
Nausea	10.5
Vomiting	2.1
Nausea and vomiting	1.3

Thyrotropin Alfa Adverse Events (≥ 1%)	
Adverse reaction	n = 381
Miscellaneous	
Asthenia	3.4
Chills	1
Fever	1
Flu syndrome	1

Post-marketing –

Hypersensitivity: There have been several reports of hypersensitivity reactions consisting of urticaria, rash, pruritus, and flushing. However, in clinical trials no patients have developed antibodies to thyrotropin alfa, either after single or repeated (27 patients) use of the product.

Four patients out of 55 (7.3%) with CNS metastases who were followed in a special treatment protocol experienced acute hemiplegia, hemiparesis, or pain 1 to 3 days after thyrotropin alfa administration. The symptoms were attributed to local edema or focal hemorrhage at the site of the cerebral or spinal cord metastases. In addition, 1 case each of acute visual loss and of dysphagia secondary to laryngeal edema, requiring tracheotomy, have been reported 24 hours after thyrotropin alfa administration in patients with metastases to the optic nerve and paratracheal areas, respectively. Pretreatment with corticosteroids may be considered under such circumstances.

A 77-year-old nonthyroidectomized patient with a history of heart disease and spinal metastases who received 4 thyrotropin alfa injections over 6 days in a special treatment protocol experienced a fatal MI 24 hours after he received the last thyrotropin alfa injection. The event was likely related to thyrotropin alfa-induced hyperthyroidism.

Overdosage

There has been no reported experience of overdose in humans. However, in clinical trials, 3 patients experienced symptoms after receiving thyrotropin alfa doses higher than those recommended. Two patients had nausea after a 2.7 mg IM dose, and in 1 of these patients, the event was accompanied by weakness, dizziness, and headache. Another patient experienced nausea, vomiting, and hot flashes after a 3.6 mg IM dose.

In addition, 1 patient experienced symptoms after receiving thyrotropin alfa IV. This patient received 0.3 mg thyrotropin alfa as a single IV bolus and 15 minutes later experienced severe nausea, vomiting, diaphoresis, hypotension (BP decreased from 115/66 mmHg to 81/44 mmHg), and tachycardia (pulse increased from 75 to 117 bpm).

GONADORELIN HCl

| *Rx* | **Factrel** (Wyeth-Ayerst) | **Powder for injection, lyophilized:** 100 mcg (as HCl)/vial.[1] | With 2 mL sterile diluent.[2] |
| | | 500 mcg (as HCl)/vial.[1] | |

[1] With 100 mg lactose. [2] With 2% benzyl alcohol.

Indications

Evaluating functional capacity and response of the gonadotropes of the anterior pituitary; the luteinizing hormone (LH) response is useful in testing suspected gonadotropin deficiency; evaluating residual gonadotropic function of pituitary following removal of pituitary tumor by surgery or irradiation.

Administration and Dosage

➤*Adults:* 100 mcg SC or IV. In females, perform the test in the early follicular phase (days 1 to 7) of the menstrual cycle.

For specific test methodology and interpretation of test results, refer to manufacturer's full prescribing product information.

➤*Preparation of solution:* Reconstitute 100 mcg vial with 1 mL and the 500 mcg vial with 2 mL of accompanying diluent. Prepare immediately before use.

➤*Storage/Stability:* After reconstitution, store at room temperature (≈ 25°C; ≈ 77°F); use within 1 day. Discard unused solution and diluent.

Actions

➤*Pharmacology:* Gonadorelin is a synthetic luteinizing hormone-releasing hormone (LH-RH), also referred to as gonadotropin-releasing hormone (GnRH). It is structurally identical to natural LH-RH.

Gonadorelin has gonadotropin-releasing effects on the anterior pituitary. Normal baseline LH levels are 5 to 25 mIU/mL in postpubertal males and postpubertal and premenopausal females, but levels vary with assay method.

In menopausal and postmenopausal females, the baseline LH levels are elevated; maximum LH increases are exaggerated when compared with premenopausal levels.

Patients with clinically diagnosed or suspected pituitary or hypothalamic dysfunction often had subnormal or no LH responses following administration.

Contraindications

Hypersensitivity to gonadorelin or any of the components of the product.

Warnings

➤*Hypersensitivity and allergic reactions:* Hypersensitivity and allergic reactions have rarely occurred following multiple-dose administration (see Adverse Reactions). Refer to Management of Acute Hypersensitivity Reactions.

➤*Pregnancy: Category B.* No adequate and well-controlled studies have been conducted in pregnant women. Repetitive, high doses of gonadorelin may cause luteolysis and inhibition of spermatogenesis. Safety for use during pregnancy has not been established; use only when clearly needed.

Precautions

➤*Antibody formation:* Antibody formation has rarely occurred after chronic administration of large doses.

Drug Interactions

➤*Androgen, estrogen, glucocorticoid, and progestin:* Androgen-, estrogen-, glucocorticoid-, and progestin-containing preparations directly affect pituitary secretion of the gonadotropins. Do not conduct tests during administration of these agents.

➤*Digoxin and oral contraceptives:* May suppress gonadotropin levels.

➤*Levodopa and spironolactone:* May transiently elevate gonadotropin levels.

➤*Phenothiazines and dopamine antagonists:* Increase prolactin which may blunt the response to gonadorelin.

Adverse Reactions

➤*Systemic:* Headache; nausea; lightheadedness; abdominal discomfort; flushing (rare).

➤*Local:* Swelling, with occasional pain, and pruritus at the SC injection site may occur. Local and generalized skin rash have been noted after chronic SC administration.

Rare instances of hypersensitivity reaction (bronchospasm, tachycardia, flushing, urticaria, induration at injection site) and anaphylactic reactions have occurred following multiple-dose administration.

Overdosage

Gonadorelin has been administered parenterally in doses up to 3 mg twice daily for 28 days without any signs or symptoms of overdosage. Treat symptomatically as needed. Refer to General Management of Acute Overdosage.

TOLBUTAMIDE SODIUM

| *Rx* | **Orinase Diagnostic** (Pharmacia) | **Powder for Injection:** 1 g (as sodium)/vial | In vials. |

Indications

As an aid in the diagnosis of pancreatic islet cell adenoma. Accurate differential diagnosis of spontaneous hypoglycemia is essential to avoid subtotal pancreatic resection in patients in whom surgery is not indicated.

Administration and Dosage

For IV use only.

➤*Fajans test:*
1.) Eat a high carbohydrate diet of 150 to 300 g/day for at least 3 days prior to test.
2.) On the morning of the test, after an overnight fast, obtain a fasting blood specimen.
3.) Inject 20 mL tolbutamide solution IV at a constant rate over 2 to 3 minutes.
4.) Withdraw blood specimens at the following intervals (in minutes) after the midpoint of the injection: 20, 30, 45, 60, 90, 120, 150, and 180. The determination of serum insulin levels before, and at 10, 20, and 30 minutes after the IV administration, provides a specific and safer test for insulinoma, and permits the performance of the test in the presence of moderate fasting hypoglycemia, because interpretation is not based on the decline of the blood glucose.
5.) Blood glucose determinations are made by the true glucose procedures.
6.) Terminate the procedure with readily assimilable carbohydrates or breakfast.

➤*Interpretation of results:*

Healthy subjects – A decrease in blood sugar (38% to 79% of the fasting level) may be expected. At 90 to 120 minutes, 78% to 100% of the initial level may be seen. Similar responses occur in patients with functional hyperinsulinism.

Insulinoma patients – Minimum blood sugar levels of 17% to 50% of fasting values are seen. In 90 to 180 minutes, levels range from 40% to 64%. Patients with liver disease may show the same type of blood glucose response as patients with insulinomas; use appropriate laboratory and clinical tests to distinguish between these conditions.

Inject 1 g IV at a constant rate over 2 to 3 minutes.

For specific test methodology (Fajans test) and interpretation of test results, refer to the manufacturer's full prescribing product information.

➤*Storage/Stability:* Use within 1 hour after reconstitution, but only if solution is complete and clear.

Actions

➤*Pharmacokinetics:* Patients with functioning insulinomas exhibit hypoglycemic responses to IV tolbutamide, which are distinctive from responses of normal individuals.

Administration of 1 g to healthy subjects results in a rapid fall in blood sugar levels for 30 to 45 minutes, followed by a secondary rise into the normal range in the ensuing 90 to 180 minutes. The initial hypoglycemia results from the rapid release of insulin from the pancreatic beta cells, while the secondary rise is due to activation of counter-regulatory factors. Serum insulin levels rise from a fasting mean value of 19 microU/mL to a peak mean value of ≈ 40 microU/mL (range, 27 to 89), 20 minutes after injection.

In contrast, patients with insulinomas exhibit tolbutamide-induced blood sugar decreases of greater magnitude associated with an excessive, prompt rise in serum insulin (118 to 1055 microU/mL). The magnitude of blood sugar fall in these patients is of greater significance than the persistence of hypoglycemia for 3 hours after administration. Persistent tolbutamide-induced hypoglycemia, rather than degree of blood sugar decrease, is important in the diagnosis of pancreatic islet cell adenomas.

Contraindications

Children (see Warnings); previous allergy to tolbutamide or related sulfonylureas.

Warnings

➤*False-positive:* Responses occurred in a few patients with liver disease, alcohol hypoglycemia, idiopathic hypoglycemia of infancy, severe undernutrition, azotemia, sarcoma, and other extrapancreatic insulin-producing tumors.

TOLBUTAMIDE SODIUM

➤*Hypoglycemia:* May develop, particularly in patients with fasting hypoglycemic blood sugar levels. If it occurs, terminate the test immediately; inject 12.5 to 25 g glucose IV in a 25% to 50% solution.

➤*Anaphylaxis:* Epinephrine and other resuscitative drugs should be available. Refer to Management of Acute Hypersensitivity Reactions.

➤*Renal/Hepatic function impairment:* Use cautiously because severe and prolonged hypoglycemia following oral tolbutamide has occurred.

➤*Pregnancy:* Category C.

Teratogenic effects – Tolbutamide sodium was teratogenic in rats given doses 25 to 100 times the human dose (increased mortality in offspring and ocular and bony abnormalities). There are no adequate and well controlled studies in pregnant women. Tolbutamide is not recommended for the treatment of pregnant diabetic patients. Consider the possible hazards of the use in women of childbearing potential who might become pregnant while using the drug.

Nonteratogenic effects – Prolonged severe hypoglycemia (4 to 10 days) occurred in neonates born to mothers who were receiving a sulfonylurea drug at the time of delivery. This has occurred more frequently with the use of agents with prolonged half-lives. Use of the drug in pregnant patients is not recommended.

➤*Lactation:* Tolbutamide is excreted in small amounts in the breast milk of nursing mothers. Because of the potential for serious adverse reactions in nursing infants, discontinue nursing or discontinue the drug.

➤*Children:* Not recommended in children because of the lack of data to establish ideal dosage and the inability to interpret results.

Precautions

➤*Test dose-induced hypoglycemic symptoms:* Are usually not severe; however, certain nondiabetics may develop moderate to severe symptoms. To avoid this occurrence, terminate the diagnostic test by administering carbohydrates immediately after obtaining the 30 minute blood sample, especially in the testing of persons with atherosclerosis.

Use only a true glucose procedure (Somogyi-Nelson, Modified Folin-Wu, AutoAnalyzer, or glucose oxidase) to eliminate highly variable amounts of nonglucose-reducing substances as a major source of error.

Drug Interactions

➤*Salicylates, sulfonamides, oxyphenbutazone, phenylbutazone, probenecid, and MAOIs:* May interfere with results of a tolbutamide tolerance test.

Since the tolbutamide diagnostic test involves a single injection, drug interactions that may occur with chronic tolbutamide use may not occur in this situation. However, for further information refer to the Sulfonylureas monograph.

➤*Drug/Lab test interactions:* On rare occasions, urine containing the tolbutamide metabolite may give a false-positive reaction for **albumin** by the usual test (acidification after boiling). Circumvent this problem by using bromphenol reagent strips.

Adverse Reactions

Rare – Mild shoulder pain or slight burning sensation along the course of the vein during the IV injection may occur. It lasts no more than 2 to 3 minutes, is attributed to venospasm and may be obviated by administering the solution over 2 to 3 min.

Thrombophlebitis with thrombosis – Thrombophlebitis with thrombosis of the injected vein occurs in 0.8% to 2.4% of patients. These are usually painless, detectable only by careful palpation and may not appear for 1 or 2 weeks after injection. No sequelae have been noted. The vein gradually shrinks or recanalizes.

Overdosage

The dose which may cause hypoglycemia is variable; usual therapeutic doses have caused symptomatic hypoglycemia.

➤*Symptoms:* Overdose of sulfonylureas, including tolbutamide, will produce symptoms of hypoglycemia. Seizures may occur with marked hypoglycemia.

Mild – Sweating; trembling; weakness; fatigue; nervousness; hunger; nausea.

Severe – Lethargy; confusion; stupor; loss of consciousness; coma.

➤*Treatment:* Treat mild symptoms of hypoglycemia without loss of consciousness with oral glucose and adjustment in drug dosage and meal patterns. Continue monitoring until the patient is out of danger. Severe hypoglycemic reactions with coma, seizure or other neurological impairment are rare, but require immediate hospitalization; give a rapid IV injection of 50% dextrose solution. Repeat as needed. Follow by a continuous infusion of 10% dextrose solution to maintain the blood glucose level above 100 mg/dl. Closely monitor patients in hospital for a minimum of 24 to 48 hours, since hypoglycemia may recur after apparent clinical recovery.

Overdosage with sulfonylurea drugs has not responded to peritoneal dialysis or hemodialysis. Experience, however, is quite limited.

METHACHOLINE CHLORIDE

Rx	Provocholine (Methapharm)	Solution for inhalation (after reconstitution of powder): 100 mg per 5 ml	In 5 ml vials.

WARNING

Methacholine is a bronchoconstrictor for diagnostic purposes only. Perform inhalation challenge under the supervision of a physician trained in and thoroughly familiar with all aspects of the technique, all contraindications, warnings and precautions of methacholine challenge and the management of respiratory distress. Have emergency equipment and medication immediately available to treat acute respiratory distress.

Administer only by inhalation; severe bronchoconstriction and reduction in respiratory function can result. Patients with severe hyperreactivity of the airways can experience bronchoconstriction at a dosage as low as 0.025 mg/ml (0.125 cumulative units). If severe bronchoconstriction occurs, reverse immediately by administration of a rapid-acting inhaled bronchodilator (β-agonist). Do not perform methacholine challenge in any patient with clinically apparent asthma, wheezing or very low baseline pulmonary function tests (ie, FEV_1 < 1 to 1.5 L or < 70% of the predicted values). Consult standard nomograms for predicted values.

Indications

➤*Bronchial airway hyperreactivity diagnosis:* For the diagnosis of bronchial airway hyperreactivity in subjects who do not have clinically apparent asthma.

Administration and Dosage

Administer by inhalation only.

Before inhalation challenge is begun, perform baseline pulmonary function tests. The subject to be challenged must have an FEV_1 of at least 70% of the predicted value.

The target level for a positive challenge is a 20% reduction in the FEV_1 compared with the baseline value after inhalation of the control sodium chloride solution. Calculate and record the target value before challenge is started.

➤*Procedure:* Perform the challenge by giving a subject ascending serial concentrations of methacholine. At each concentration, five breaths are administered by a nebulizer that permits intermittent delivery time of 0.6 seconds by either a Y-tube or a breath-actuated timing device (dosimeter).

At each of five inhalations of a serial concentration, the subject begins at functional residual capacity (FRC) and slowly and completely inhales the dose delivered. Within 5 minutes, FEV_1 values are determined. The procedure ends either when there is a ≥ 20% reduction in the FEV_1 compared with the baseline sodium chloride solution value (ie, a positive response) or if 188.88 total cumulative units have been given (see table below) and FEV_1 has been reduced by ≤ 14% (ie, a negative response). If there is a reduction of 15% to 19% in FEV_1 vs baseline, either repeat the challenge at that concentration or give a higher concentration as long as dosage administered does not result in total cumulative units > 188.88.

The following is a suggested schedule for administration of methacholine challenge. Calculate cumulative units by multiplying number of breaths by concentration given. Total cumulative units is the sum of cumulative units for each concentration given.

Suggested Methacholine Administration Schedule				
Vial	Serial concentration	Number of breaths	Cumulative units per concentration	Total cumulative units
E	0.025 mg/ml	5	0.125	0.125
D	0.25 mg/ml	5	1.25	1.375
C	2.5 mg/ml	5	12.5	13.88
B	10 mg/ml	5	50	63.88
A	25 mg/ml	5	125	188.88

An inhaled β-agonist may be administered after methacholine challenge to expedite the return of the FEV_1 to baseline and to relieve the discomfort of the subject. Most patients revert to normal pulmonary function within 5 minutes following bronchodilators or within 30 to 45 minutes without any bronchodilator.

➤*Dilutions:* (Do not inhale powder. Do not handle this material if you have asthma or hay fever.) Make all dilutions with 0.9% sodium chloride injection containing 0.4% phenol (pH 7). Use a bacterial-retentive filter (porosity 0.22 μ) when transferring solution from vial to nebulizer. After adding the sodium chloride solution, shake each vial to obtain a clear solution.

METHACHOLINE CHLORIDE

Vial A – Add 4 ml of 0.9% sodium chloride injection containing 0.4% phenol (pH 7) to the 5 ml vial containing 100 mg (25 mg/ml).

Vial B – Remove 3 ml from vial A, transfer to another vial and add 4.5 ml of the 0.9% sodium chloride solution (10 mg/ml). An alternative method of preparing vial B is to remove 1 ml from vial A and add 1.5 ml 0.9% sodium chloride solution.

Vial C – Remove 1 ml from vial A, transfer to another vial and add 9 ml of the 0.9% sodium chloride solution (2.5 mg/ml). This step depletes contents of vial A if the first dilution method under vial B directions is used.

Vial D – Remove 1 ml from vial C, transfer to another vial and add 9 ml of the 0.9% sodium chloride solution (0.25 mg/ml).

Vial E – Remove 1 ml from vial D, transfer to another vial and add 9 ml of the 0.9% sodium chloride solution (0.025 mg/ml).

➤*Storage / Stability:* Store dilutions A through D in refrigerator 2° to 8°C (36° to 46°F) for up to 2 weeks, then discard the vials. Freezing does not affect the stability of dilutions A through D. Vial E must be prepared on the day of the challenge. Store the unreconstituted powder at 15° to 30°C (59° to 86°F).

Actions

➤*Pharmacology:* Methacholine is a parasympathomimetic (cholinergic) bronchoconstrictor, the β-methyl homolog of acetylcholine, and differs from the latter primarily in its greater duration and selectivity of action. Bronchial smooth muscle contains significant parasympathetic innervation. Bronchoconstriction occurs when the vagus nerve is stimulated releasing acetylcholine from the nerve endings. Muscle constriction is essentially confined to the local site of release because acetylcholine is rapidly inactivated by acetylcholinesterase. Compared with acetylcholine, methacholine is more slowly hydrolyzed by acetylcholinesterase and is almost totally resistant to inactivation by nonspecific cholinesterase or pseudocholinesterase. Asthmatics are markedly more sensitive to inhaled methacholine-induced bronchoconstriction than are healthy subjects. This difference is the pharmacologic basis for the methacholine inhalation challenge.

Contraindications

Hypersensitivity to methacholine or other parasympathomimetics; repeated administration other than challenge with increasing doses; patients receiving any β-adrenergic blocking agent because, in such patients, responses to methacholine can be exaggerated or prolonged, and may not respond as readily to treatment.

Warnings

➤*Pregnancy: Category C.* It is not known whether this drug can cause fetal harm when administered to a pregnant patient or can affect reproductive capacity. Give to a pregnant woman only if clearly needed. In females of childbearing potential, perform inhalation challenge either within 10 days following the onset of menses or within 2 weeks of a negative pregnancy test.

➤*Lactation:* It is not known whether inhaled methacholine is excreted in breast milk. Do not administer to nursing women.

➤*Children:* Safety and efficacy for use in children < 5 years of age have not been established.

Precautions

➤*Special risk patients:* Do not administer to patients with epilepsy, cardiovascular disease accompanied by bradycardia, vagotonia, peptic ulcer disease, thyroid disease, urinary tract obstruction or other conditions that could be adversely affected by a cholinergic agent unless the benefit to the individual outweighs the potential risk.

Adverse Reactions

Inhalation – Headache, throat irritation, lightheadedness, itching (one case each).

Oral / Injection – Nausea; vomiting; substernal pain or pressure; hypotension; fainting; transient complete heart block.

Overdosage

➤*Symptoms:* When administered orally or by injection, overdosage with methacholine can result in a syncopal reaction with cardiac arrest and loss of consciousness.

➤*Treatment:* Treat serious toxic reactions with 0.5 to 1 mg atropine sulfate, IM or IV.

Patient Information

Instruct patients about symptoms that may occur as a result of the test, and explain how to manage such symptoms.

Female patients should inform physician of pregnancy, the date of last onset of menses or the date and result of last pregnancy test.

SECRETIN

Rx	**SecreFlo** (Repligen)	**Powder for injection, lyophilized:** 16 mcg of purified secretin	In vials[1].

[1] With 20 mg mannitol, 15 mg L-cysteine.

Indications

➤*Pancreatic secretion stimulation:* For the stimulation of pancreatic secretions, including bicarbonate, to aid in the diagnosis of pancreatic exocrine dysfunction.

For the stimulation of pancreatic secretions to facilitate the identification of the ampulla of Vater and accessory papilla during endoscopic retrograde cholangiopancreatography (ERCP).

➤*Gastrin secretions:* For the stimulation of gastrin secretion to aid in the diagnosis of gastrinoma.

Administration and Dosage

➤*Approved by the FDA:* April 4, 2002.

➤*Preparation for administration:* Dissolve the contents of the secretin vial in 8 mL of sodium chloride injection to yield a concentration of 2 mcg/mL. Shake vigorously to ensure dissolution. Use immediately after reconstitution. Discard any unused portion after reconstitution.

➤*Dosage:*

To stimulate pancreatic secretions, including bicarbonate, to aid in the diagnosis of exocrine pancreas dysfunction – 0.2 mcg/kg by IV injection over 1 minute.

Stimulation of gastrin secretion to aid in the diagnosis of gastrinoma – 0.4 mcg/kg by IV injection over 1 minute.

Facilitation of the identification of the ampulla of Vater and accessory papilla during ERCP to aid in cannulation of the pancreatic ducts – 0.2 mcg/kg by IV injection over 1 minute.

➤*Administration:*

To stimulate pancreatic secretions, including bicarbonate, to aid in the diagnosis of exocrine pancreas dysfunction – A radiopaque, double-lumen tube is passed through the mouth following a 12- to 15-hour fast. Under fluoroscopic control, the opening of the proximal lumen of the tube is placed in the gastric antrum and the opening of the distal lumen just beyond the papilla of Vater. The positioning of the tube must be confirmed and the tube secured prior to secretin testing. Intermittent negative pressure of 25 to 40 mm Hg is applied to both lumens and maintained throughout the test. When duodenal contents have a pH greater than or equal to 6, a baseline sample of duodenal fluids is collected for a 10-minute period. A test dose of 0.2 mcg (0.1 mL) secretin is injected IV to test for possible allergies. After 1 minute, if there are no untoward reactions, secretin at a dose of 0.2 mcg/kg is injected IV over 1 minute. Duodenal fluid is collected for 60 minutes thereafter. The aspirate is divided into 4 collection periods of 15 minutes each. The duodenal lumen of the tube is cleared with an injection of air after collection of each sample. Wide variation in volume of the aspirate is indicative of incomplete aspiration. Each sample of duodenal fluid is to be chilled and subsequently analyzed for volume and bicarbonate concentration. Exocrine pancreas dysfunction typically associated with chronic pancreatitis is indicated if the peak bicarbonate concentration for any sample is less than 80 mEq/L.

Stimulation of gastrin to aid in the diagnosis of gastrinoma – The patient should have fasted for at least 12 hours prior to beginning the test. Before injecting secretin, 2 blood samples are drawn for determination of fasting serum gastrin levels (baseline values). Subsequently, a test dose of secretin 0.2 mcg (0.1 mL) is injected IV to test for possible allergies. If there are no untoward reactions, 0.4 mcg/kg of secretin is administered IV over 1 minute; postinjection blood samples are collected after 1, 2, 5, 10, and 30 minutes for determination of serum gastrin concentrations. Gastrinoma is strongly suspected in patients who show an increase in serum gastrin concentration of more than 110 pg/mL over basal levels on any of the postinjection samples.

Facilitation of the identification of the ampulla of Vater and accessory papilla during ERCP – When difficulty is encountered by the endoscopist in identifying the ampulla of Vater or in indentifying the accessory papilla in patients with pancreas divisum, administration of secretin at a dose of 0.2 mcg/kg IV over 1 minute results in visible excretion of pancreatic fluid from the orifices of these papillae, enabling their identification and facilitating cannulation.

➤*Storage/Stability:* Store the unreconstituted product at –20°C (freezer).

Actions

➤*Pharmacology:* The primary action of secretin is to increase the volume and bicarbonate content of secreted pancreatic juices. In the validated cat bioassay, which was used to define and quantitate the biological activity of secretin and as the release test for the biologically-derived porcine secretin (bPS) product, secretin demonstrates a potency of approximately 5000 clinical units (CU)/mg of peptide as opposed to 3000 CU/mg for bPS. As a pure peptide drug product, secretin dosing is expressed by weight in micrograms. The relationship of micrograms of secretin to biological activity is 0.2 mcg = 1 CU.

➤*Pharmacokinetics:* After IV bolus administration of 0.4 mcg/kg, secretin concentration rapidly declines to baseline secretin levels within 60 to 90 minutes. The elimination half-life of secretin is 27 minutes. The clearance of secretin is approximately 487 mL/min, and the volume of distribution is approximately 2 L.

➤*Clinical trials:* Two small studies examined the relationship of peak bicarbonate concentration observed in 3 groups of patients: Normal healthy subjects; patients with chronic pancreatitis; patients with a past medical history of chronic pancreatitis and abnormal secretin-stimulation test results but with sufficient recovery of exocrine pancreas function to have currently normal test results. Secretin was compared with bPS. All 12 normal subjects had peak bicarbonate concentrations greater than 80 mEq/L, while all patients with chronic pancreatitis had peak bicarbonate concentrations less than 80 mEq/L.

A volume response of less than 2 mL/kg/h, bicarbonate concentration of less than 80 mEq/L, and bicarbonate output of less than 0.2 mEq/kg/h are consistent with impaired pancreatic function.

In 3 crossover studies evaluating 21 different patients with a documented history of chronic pancreatitis, secretin was compared with bPS. All of the patients treated with either drug had peak concentrations of less than 80 mEq/L.

In 2 crossover studies, 8 patients with tissue-confirmed gastrinoma received secretin. Results of serum gastrin concentrations were compared with those for bPS. Serum gastrin concentrations exceeded 110 pg/mL from basal levels in all patients for both drugs tested.

Contraindications

Do not give secretin to patients suffering from acute pancreatitis until the episode has subsided.

Warnings

➤*Hypersensitivity reactions:* Because of a potential allergic reaction to secretin, give patients an IV test dose of 0.2 mcg (0.1 mL). If no allergic reaction is noted after 1 minute, the recommended dose for the specific indication (see Administration and Dosage) may be injected slowly over 1 minute. A test dose is especially important in patients with a history of atopic allergy and/or asthma. Have appropriate measures for the treatment of acute hypersensitivity reactions immediately available. No allergic reactions were observed after the test dose or full dose of secretin in more than 981 patients.

➤*Elderly:* Greater sensitivity of some older individuals cannot be ruled out.

➤*Pregnancy: Category C.* Give secretin to a pregnant woman only if clearly needed.

➤*Lactation:* It is not known whether secretin is excreted in human milk. Because many drugs are excreted in human milk, exercise caution when secretin is administered to a nursing woman.

➤*Children:* Safety and efficacy in pediatric patients have not been established.

Precautions

➤*Special risk:* Patients who have undergone vagotomy, who are receiving anticholinergic agents at the time of secretin stimulation testing, or who have inflammatory bowel disease may be hyporesponsive to secretin stimulation. This response does not indicate pancreatic disease. A greater than normal volume response to secretin stimulation, which may mask coexisting pancreatic disease, is occasionally encountered in patients with alcoholic or other liver disease.

Drug Interactions

The concomitant use of anticholinergic agents may make patients hyporesponsive (ie, may produce a false-positive result).

Adverse Reactions

Occasional, mild adverse events have been noted in association with the use of secretin in clinical studies of more than 981 patients and 24 volunteer subjects.

Secretin Adverse Reactions (%)	
Adverse reaction	n = 981
Cardiovascular	
Decreased blood pressure	6
Bradycardia (mild)	2
Thready pulse	1
CNS	
Lightheadedness	3
Headache	2
Numbness/tingling in extremities	2
Fatigue	1

SECRETIN

Secretin Adverse Reactions (%)	
Adverse reaction	n = 981
Possible seizure	1
Dermatologic	
Diaphoresis	6
Flushing	6
Pallor	1
Rash, abdominal	1
Urticaria 2° contrast material (prior to secretin administration)	1
GI	
Nausea	8
Abdominal discomfort	7
Burning in stomach	3
Abdominal cramps	2
Diarrhea	1
Hunger pangs	1
Vomiting	1

Secretin Adverse Reactions (%)	
Adverse reaction	n = 981
Miscellaneous	
Bleeding, sphincter-ectomy	6
Bleeding, upper GI 2° to endoscopic abrasion	2
Endoscopic perforation of pancreatic duct	2
Transient respiratory distress	2
Bloating	1
Fever	1
Hot sensation	1
Leukocytoplastic vasculitis	1
Transient low O_2 saturation	1

Overdosage

A single IV dose of 20 mcg/kg of secretin was not lethal to mice or rabbits.

SIMETHICONE COATED CELLULOSE SUSPENSION

Rx **SonoRx** (Bracco Diagnostics)   **Oral suspension:** 7.5 mg/mL simethicone-coated cellulose   Fructose. Orange flavor. In 400 mL single-dose glass bottles.

Indications

➤*Diagnostic ultrasound imaging agent:* An orally administered gas shadowing reduction agent used to enhance the delineation of upper abdominal anatomy in conjunction with ultrasound imaging. Simethicone coated cellulose suspension (SCCS) is not indicated as a therapeutic antiflatuence or GI motility agent.

Administration and Dosage

➤*Approved by the FDA:* October 29, 1998.

The recommended dose of SCCS is 400 mL administered orally over 15 minutes. Take after fasting for at least 4 hours.

➤*Imaging:* Begin abdominal ultrasound imaging within 10 minutes after completing the ingestion of SCCS.

➤*Drug preparation:* Prior to administration, invert the container of SCCS and shake vigorously to resuspend any material that has settled. Let the suspension stand unopened for 2 minutes before administration to the patient to allow excess air to escape.

➤*Storage/Stability:* Store at controlled room temperature 20° to 25°C (68° to 77°F). Do not freeze.

Actions

➤*Pharmacology:* SCCS is an aqueous suspension diagnostic ultrasound imaging agent that consists of 22-micron cellulose fibers coated with 0.25% simethicone and is intended for oral administration. SCCS, when resuspended, acts locally within the GI tract to adsorb and disperse gas within the bowel lumen.

➤*Pharmacokinetics:*

Metabolism – Metabolic studies of simethicone coated cellulose were not conducted. Cellulose is not metabolized by humans.

Excretion – The cellulose component of SCCS is eliminated in the feces. The kinetics of SCCS were evaluated in a vehicle control study of 10 healthy volunteers; 7 received SCCS, 3 received the control. Silicon measurements in the blood and urine were monitored as the surrogate marker for simethicone. Silicon was measured over 5 days before dosing, and at 15 and 30 minutes, and 1, 2, 3, 6, 10, 15, 24, and 48 hours after dosing. In these subjects, the concentrations of silicon detected in the blood (6.04 to 7.47 mcg/mL) in 2 of the SCCS treated subjects before SCCS were similar to those detected in the blood after SCCS (5.61 to 11.42 mcg/mL).

The other 5 SCCS-treated subjects did not have silicon detected in the blood before SCCS, and 2 of the 5 had levels of silicon detected after SCCS; however, these levels were similar to those subjects who had silicon detected in the blood before and after SCCS. Urine levels of silicon in all subjects were similar before and after SCCS. The silicon levels in the blood and urine before and after the control were similar to those before and after SCCS.

Special populations – The pharmacokinetics and rate of fecal elimination was studied in 15 patients with impaired bowel motility or impaired bowel mucosa. Of these patients, 12 received SCCS and 3 received the vehicle. In these patients, the detection of silicon, as a surrogate marker for simethicone, in the blood and urine was similar to that of the healthy volunteers reported in the preceding pharmacokinetics section.

As in the healthy volunteers, the cellulose component of SCCS was eliminated in feces. Based on the fraction of ingested fiber that was eliminated in feces following the administration of SCCS, the rate of fecal elimination of cellulose appears to be lower in the patients with impaired bowel motility or impaired bowel mucosa than in the healthy volunteers.

Contraindications

As with other large-volume oral contrast agents, SCCS is contraindicated in patients with known or suspected intestinal perforation and obstruction (see Warnings); allergy to its active or inactive ingredients.

Warnings

➤*Aspiration:* The ingestion of SCCS may cause vomiting that could be associated with aspiration. Of the 385 patients or healthy volunteers who received SCCS, nausea was reported in 3.4% and vomiting in 2.1%. Patients who have a tracheoesophageal fistula may aspirate. Take precautions to avoid aspiration.

➤*Peritoneal tissues:* The effects of SCCS on human peritoneal tissues have not been studied. In rats, throughout a 3-month study observation period, after the intraperitoneal injection of SCCS at the lowest test dose of 5 mL/kg, capsular granulomatous inflammation of the spleen, liver, and kidneys, accumulation of cellulose in the red pulp of the spleen and glomeruli of the kidneys were observed. The effects of SCCS on human peritoneal tissues are not known.

➤*Pregnancy: Category B.* Adequate and well-controlled clinical studies have not been conducted in pregnant women. Use in pregnancy only if essential.

➤*Lactation:* Studies have not been conducted to determine whether SCCS is excreted in breast milk. Exercise caution when administering to a nursing woman.

➤*Children:* Safety and efficacy in children have not been established. Dose adjustments for the capacity of the upper GI tract have not been studied.

Precautions

➤*GI effects:* SCCS is associated with nausea, vomiting, and abdominal pain. In patients who have these symptoms before the ingestion of SCCS, the symptoms could increase in severity. This could confound the ability to distinguish adverse effects of SCCS from the signs and symptoms of obstruction or perforation and from any preexisting conditions.

Patients who have a current or recent history of hiatal hernia, esophageal reflux, nausea, vomiting, or abdominal pain may not be able to tolerate SCCS. Studies have not been conducted in these patients.

➤*Fluid shifts/intake:* Give SCCS with caution to patients who cannot tolerate large fluid shifts and who are on specific fluid intake requirements.

Adverse Reactions

Of the 448 subjects evaluated, 18% who received SCCS and 12% who received a control agent reported at least 1 adverse event. Of the subjects who received SCCS, at least 1 adverse event was reported in 19% of patients and 8% of healthy volunteers. Deaths or serious adverse events were not reported during the study observation period.

Gastrointestinal Function Tests

SIMETHICONE COATED CELLULOSE SUSPENSION

The most frequently reported adverse events were associated with the digestive system. Diarrhea was reported in 5.5%, nausea in 3.4%, and vomiting in 2.1% of subjects who received SCCS. Orange-colored stools may occur.

Simethicone Coated Cellulose Suspension Adverse Reactions (> 0.5%)		
Adverse reaction	SCCS control (n = 385)	Control agent (n = 138)
GI		
Diarrhea	5.5	2.9
Nausea	3.4	0.7
Vomiting	2.1	0
Eructation	1	0.7
Dyspepsia	0.5	1.4
Flatulence	0.5	0
Respiratory		
Pharyngitis	0.5	0
Rhinitis	0.5	0
Miscellaneous		
Abdominal pain	2.1	0.7
Headache	1.8	0.7
Back pain	1	0.7
Chest pain	0.8	0.7
Rash	0.5	0
Ear pain	0.5	0
Chills	0.5	0

The following additional adverse events were reported in less than 0.5% of people who received SCCS:

➤*Cardiovascular:* Bradycardia; hematoma; hypertension; pallor; palpitations; tachycardia.

➤*CNS:* Hypertonia; somnolence.

➤*GI:* Dysphagia; dry mouth; melena.

➤*Hematologic / Lymphatic:* Ecchymosis; lymphadenopathy.

➤*Respiratory:* Epistaxis; pneumothorax; sinusitis.

➤*Miscellaneous:* Asthenia; fever; malaise; neck pain; pelvic pain; pain; hypoglycemia; dysuria.

Patient Information

Instruct patients who are candidates to receive SCCS to inform the physician if they are pregnant or breastfeeding.

Inform patients of the following:

SCCS is prescribed for delineation of abdominal anatomy during ultrasound imaging.

• SCCS can cause nausea, vomiting, diarrhea, abdominal pain, or other GI discomfort.

• For most patients, complete elimination of SCCS occurs within 24 to 48 hours following administration.

• Feces may appear orange-colored until SCCS is completely eliminated.

Ask patients if they are able to drink approximately 400 mL (14 oz or 1 pt) over a 15-minute period. Ask patients if they have a hiatal hernia or problems with regurgitation when they lie on their backs after eating.

SINCALIDE

Rx	**Kinevac** (Bracco Diagnostics)	**Powder for injection, lyophilized:** 5 mcg/vial for reconstitution (1 mcg/mL when reconstituted)	In vials.

Indications

➤*Gallbladder contraction stimulation:* To stimulate gallbladder contraction, as may be assessed by contrast agent cholecystography or ultrasonography, or to obtain by duodenal aspiration a sample of concentrated bile for analysis of cholesterol, bile salts, phospholipids, and crystals.

➤*Pancreatic secretion stimulation:* To stimulate pancreatic secretion (especially in conjunction with secretin) prior to obtaining a duodenal aspirate for analysis of enzyme activity, composition, and cytology.

➤*Barium meal transit time acceleration:* To accelerate the transit of a barium meal through the small bowel, thereby decreasing the time and extent of radiation associated with fluoroscopy and X-ray examination of the intestinal tract.

Administration and Dosage

➤*Contraction of the gallbladder:* A dose of 0.02 mcg/kg (1.4 mcg/70 kg) is injected IV over 30 to 60 seconds; if satisfactory gallbladder contraction does not occur in 15 minutes, a second dose (0.04 mcg/kg) may be given. To reduce the intestinal side effects, an IV infusion may be prepared at a dose of 0.12 mcg/kg in 100 mL of Sodium Chloride Injection and given at a rate of 2 mL/min; alternatively, an IM dose of 0.1 mcg/kg may be given. When sincalide is used in cholecystography, roentgenograms are usually taken at 5-minute intervals after the injection. For visualization of the cystic duct, it may be necessary to take roentgenograms at 1-minute intervals during the first 5 minutes after the injection.

➤*Barium meal transit time acceleration:* To accelerate the transit time of a barium meal through the small bowel, administer sincalide after the barium meal is beyond the proximal jejunum. (Sincalide, like cholecystoidnin, may cause pyloric contraction.) The recommended dose is 0.04 mcg/kg sincalide (2.8 mcg/70 kg) injected IV over a 30- to 60-second interval; if satisfactory transit of the barium meal has not occurred in 30 minutes, a second dose of 0.04 mcg/kg sincalide may be administered. For reduction of side effects, a 30-minute IV infusion of sincalide (0.12 mcg/kg [8.4 mcg/70 kg] diluted to approximately 100 mL with Sodium Chloride Injection) may be administered.

➤*Pancreatic secretion stimulation:* Secretin dose of 0.25 units/kg is infused IV over 60 minutes. Thirty minutes after initiating secretin, give a separate IV infusion of sincalide at a total dose of 0.02 mcg/kg over 30 minutes. For example, the total dose for a 70 kg patient is 1.4 mcg sincalide; therefore, dilute 1.4 mL reconstituted sincalide solution to 30 mL with Sodium Chloride Injection and administer at a rate of 1 mL/min.

➤*Preparation of solution:* To reconstitute, add 5 mL Sterile Water for Injection to the vial; make any additional dilution with 0.9% Sodium Chloride for Injection. The solution may be kept at room temperature. Use within 24 hours after reconstitution; discard any unused portion.

➤*Storage / Stability:* Store at room temperature 15° to 30° C (59° to 86° F) prior to reconstitution.

Actions

➤*Pharmacology:* Sincalide IV substantially reduces gallbladder size by causing it to contract. The evacuation of bile that results is similar to the physiological response to endogenous cholecystokinin. Bolus IV administration causes a prompt contraction of the gallbladder that becomes maximal in 5 to 15 minutes, as compared with the stimulus of a fatty meal, which causes a progressive contraction that becomes maximal after approximately 40 minutes. Generally, a 40% reduction in radiographic area of the gallbladder is satisfactory, although some patients will show area reduction of 60% to 70%.

Like cholecystokinin, sincalide stimulates pancreatic secretion; concurrent administration with secretin increases the volume of pancreatic secretion and the output of bicarbonate and protein (enzymes) by the gland. This combined effect of secretin and sincalide permits the assessment of specific pancreatic function through measurement and analysis of the duodenal aspirate. The parameters determined are the following: Volume of the secretion; bicarbonate concentration; amylase content (which parallels the content of trypsin and total protein).

Cholecystokinin and sincalide stimulate intestinal motility and may cause pyloric contraction, which retards gastric emptying.

Contraindications

Hypersensitivity to sincalide; intestinal obstruction.

Warnings

➤*Pregnancy: Category B.* Reproduction studies in rats in which sincalide was administered SC at doses up to 12.5 times the maximum recommended human dose revealed no evidence of harm to the fetus due to sincalide. However, there are no adequate and well-controlled studies in pregnant women. Because animal reproduction studies are not always predictive of human response, use this drug during pregnancy only if clearly needed.

Do not administer sincalide to pregnant women near term because of its effect on smooth muscle; the possibility of prematurely inducing labor exists.

➤*Lactation:* It is not known whether this drug is excreted in human milk. Because many drugs are excreted in human milk, exercise caution when sincalide is administered to a nursing woman.

➤*Children:* The safety for use in children has not been established.

Precautions

Stimulation of gallbladder contraction in patients with small gallbladder stones may lead to the evacuation of the stones, resulting in their lodging in the cystic duct or in the common bile duct. The risk is minimal because sincalide, when given as directed, does not ordinarily cause complete contraction of the gallbladder.

Adverse Reactions

Reactions to sincailde are generally mild and of short duration. The most frequent adverse reactions were abdominal discomfort or pain, and nausea; rapid IV injection of 0.04 mcg/kg sincalide expectably

SINCALIDE

causes transient abdominal cramping. These phenomena are usually manifestations of the physiologic action of the drug, including delayed gastric emptying and increased intestinal motility. These reactions occurred in approximately 20% of patients; they are not to be construed as necessarily indicating an abnormality of the biliary tract unless there is other clinical or radiologic evidence of disease.

The incidence of other adverse reactions, including vomiting, flushing, sweating, rash, hypotension, hypertension, shortness of breath, urge to defecate, headache, diarrhea, sneezing, and numbness was less than 1%; dizziness was reported in approximately 2% of patients. These manifestations are usually lessened by slower injection rate.

Overdosage

➤*Symptoms:* GI symptoms (abdominal cramps, nausea, vomiting, and diarrhea) should be expected. Hypotension with dizziness or fainting might also occur. Starting with single bolus IV injection comparable with the human dose of 0.4 mg/kg, sincalide caused hypotension and bradycardia in dogs. Higher doses injected once or repeatedly in dogs caused syncope and ECG changes in addition. These effects were attributed to sincalide-induced vagal stimulation in that all were prevented by pretreatment with atropine or bilateral vagotomy.

➤*Treatment:* Treat overdosage symptoms symptomatically over a short duration.

BENZYLPENICILLOYL-POLYLYSINE

Rx	**Pre-Pen** (Hollister-Stier)	**Solution:** 0.25 ml per amp.	In single-dose amps.

Indications

An adjunct in assessing the risk of administering penicillin (benzylpenicillin or penicillin G) in adults with a history of clinical penicillin hypersensitivity. A negative skin test is associated with an incidence of allergic reactions of < 5% after the administration of penicillin; the incidence may be > 20% in the presence of a positive skin test.

Administration and Dosage

►*Scratch testing:* Perform skin testing on the inner volar aspect of the forearm. *Always* apply the skin test material first by the scratch technique. After preparing the skin surface, use a sterile 20 gauge needle to make a 3 to 5 mm scratch on the epidermis. Very little pressure is required to break the epidermal continuity. If bleeding occurs, prepare a second site and scratch more lightly with the needle, sufficient to produce a nonbleeding scratched surface. Apply a small drop of solution to the scratch and rub gently with an applicator, toothpick or the side of the needle.

Interpretation of test results – Observe for the appearance of a wheal, erythema and itching at the test site during the next 15 minutes, then wipe off the solution over the scratch. A positive reaction consists of development of a pale wheal, usually with pseudopods, surrounding the scratch site within 10 minutes. It varies in diameter from 5 to 15 mm (or more). This wheal may be surrounded by erythema and accompanied by itching. The most sensitive individuals develop itching instantly, and the wheal and erythema promptly appear. As soon as a positive response is clearly evident, wipe off the solution over the scratch. If the scratch test is either negative or equivocally positive (< 5 mm wheal, little or no erythema, no itching), perform an intradermal test.

►*Intradermal test:* Using a tuberculin syringe with a ⅜" to ⅝", 26 to 30 gauge, short bevel needle, withdraw the contents of the ampule. Prepare a sterile skin test area on the upper, outer arm, sufficiently below the deltoid muscle to permit proximal application of a tourniquet, if necessary. Inject an amount of benzylpenicilloyl-polylysine sufficient to raise the smallest possible perceptible bleb. This volume will be 0.01 to 0.02 ml. Using a separate syringe and needle, inject a like amount of saline as a control at least 1½ inches from the test site.

Interpretation of test results – Most skin reactions develop within 5 to 15 minutes.

Negative (−): No increase in size of original bleb or no greater reaction than the control site.

Ambiguous (±): Wheal only slightly larger than initial injection bleb, with or without accompanying erythematous flare and larger than the control site.

Positive (+): Itching and marked increase in size of original bleb. Wheal may exceed 20 mm in diameter and exhibit pseudopods.

The control site should be completely reactionless. If it exhibits a wheal greater than 2 to 3 mm, repeat the test. If the same reaction is observed, consult a physician experienced with allergy skin testing.

►*Storage / Stability:* Stable only when kept under refrigeration; discard test materials subjected to ambient temperatures for over a day.

Actions

►*Pharmacology:* Benzylpenicilloyl-polylysine is a skin test antigen that reacts specifically with benzylpenicilloyl skin sensitizing antibodies (reagins: IgE class) to produce an immediate wheal and flare reaction at a skin test site. Individuals exhibiting a positive response possess reagins against the benzylpenicilloyl group.

Individuals who have previously received therapeutic penicillin may have positive skin test reactions to benzylpenicilloyl-polylysine and to other non-benzylpenicilloyl haptenes of minor determinants. The major metabolite of penicillin is the penicilloyl group; this "major determinant" is thought to be responsible for accelerated reactions, but not anaphylaxis. Other breakdown products or "minor determinants" are felt to be responsible for anaphylaxis and immediate systemic reactions. Virtually everyone who receives penicillin develops specific anti-

bodies, but skin tests to penicillin and penicillin-derived reagents become positive in less than 10% of patients who have tolerated penicillin in the past; allergic responses are infrequent (< 1%).

Many individuals reacting positively will not develop a systemic allergic reaction on subsequent exposure to therapeutic penicillin; this skin test facilitates assessing the local allergic skin reactivity to benzylpenicilloyl.

Contraindications

Systemic or marked local reaction to previous administration. Do not test patients known to be extremely hypersensitive to penicillin.

Warnings

►*Systemic allergic reactions:* Systemic allergic reactions rarely follow a skin test. Avoid by making the first application by scratch test. Use the intradermal route only if the scratch test is entirely negative. Do not perform skin testing with penicillin or other penicillin derived reagents simultaneously.

►*Pregnancy:* Safety for use during pregnancy has not been established. Use only when clearly needed and when potential benefits outweigh potential hazards.

Precautions

Allergic reactions are predominantly dermatologic. Data are insufficient to document that a decreased incidence of anaphylactic reactions following penicillin administration will occur in patients with a negative skin test. Similarly, data are insufficient to determine the value of this skin test as a means of assessing the risk of administering therapeutic penicillin (when penicillin is the drug of choice) in adult patients with no history of clinical penicillin hypersensitivity or in pediatric patients.

No reagent, test or combination of tests will completely assure a reaction to penicillin therapy will not occur.

Data are insufficient to assess the potential danger of sensitization to penicillin from repeated skin testing.

There are no data to assess the clinical value of benzylpenicilloyl-polylysine skin test where exposure to penicillin is suspected as a cause of a drug reaction and in patients who are undergoing routine allergy evaluation.

There are no data relating the clinical value of skin tests to the risk of administering semisynthetic penicillins (phenoxymethyl penicillin, ampicillin, carbenicillin, dicloxacillin, methicillin, nafcillin, oxacillin) and cephalosporin-derived antibiotics.

Consider the following clinical outcomes when the decision to administer or not to administer penicillin is based in part on the skin test: (1) An allergic reaction to penicillin may occur in a patient with a negative skin test. (2) A patient may have an anaphylactic reaction to penicillin in the presence of a negative skin test and a negative history of clinical penicillin hypersensitivity. (3) If penicillin is the absolute drug of choice in a life-threatening situation, successful desensitization with therapeutic penicillin may be possible, despite a positive skin test or a positive history of clinical penicillin hypersensitivity.

Adverse Reactions

►*Hypersensitivity:* Have epinephrine 1:1000 immediately available. Refer to Management of Acute Hypersensitivity Reactions.

►*Local:* Occasional intense inflammatory response at the skin test site.

►*Systemic:* Generalized erythema, pruritus, urticaria, angioneurotic edema, dyspnea or hypotension. The usual methods of treating a skin test antigen-induced reaction (application of a venous occlusion tourniquet proximal to the skin test site and administration of epinephrine or antihistamine) are recommended and will usually control the reaction. Systemic allergic reactions following skin test procedures usually are of short duration and controllable, but observe the patient for several hours.

DIPYRIDAMOLE

Rx	**Dipyridamole** (Various, eg, American Pharm., Bedford, ESI Lederle)	**Injection:** 5 mg/ml[1]	In 2 and 10 ml vials.

[1] With 50 mg polyethylene glycol 600 and 2 mg tartaric acid.

Dipyridamole oral is used as an antiplatelet agent. Refer to the individual monograph in the Hematologic Agents chapter.

Indications

As an alternative to exercise in thallium myocardial perfusion imaging for the evaluation of coronary artery disease in patients who cannot exercise adequately.

Administration and Dosage

Adjust dose according to weight of patient. Recommended dose is 0.142 mg/kg/min (0.57 mg/kg total) infused over 4 min. Although maximum tolerated dose is not determined, clinical experience suggests a total dose > 60 mg is not needed for any patient. Prior to IV use, dilute

in at least a 1:2 ratio with 0.5N NaCl Injection, 1N NaCl Injection, or 5% Dextrose Injection for a total volume of ≈ 20 to 50 ml. Infusion of undiluted dipyridamole may cause local irritation. Inject thallium-201 within 5 minutes after the 4 minute dipyridamole infusion.

►*Storage / Stability:* Avoid freezing. Protect from direct light.

Actions

►*Pharmacology:* Dipyridamole for IV injection is a coronary vasodilator used for the evaluation of coronary artery disease. The mechanism of vasodilation has not been fully elucidated, but may result from inhibition of adenosine uptake, an important mediator of coronary vasodilation. How dipyridamole-induced vasodilation leads to abnormalities in thallium distribution ventriculation function is also uncertain, but presumably represents a "steal" phenomenon in which

DIPYRIDAMOLE

relatively intact vessels dilate, and sustain enhanced flow, leaving reduced pressure and flow across areas of hemodynamically important coronary vascular constriction.

In a study of 10 patients with angiographically normal or minimally stenosed coronary vessels, IV dipyridamole 0.56 mg/kg infused over 4 minutes resulted in an average fivefold increase in coronary blood flow velocity compared to resting coronary flow velocity. The mean time to peak flow velocity was 6.5 minutes from the start of the 4 minute infusion. Cardiovascular responses, when given to patients in the supine position, include a mild but significant increase in heart rate of ≈ 20% and mild, but significant decreases in both systolic and diastolic blood pressure of ≈ 2% to 8%, with vital signs returning to baseline values in ≈ 30 minutes.

➤*Pharmacokinetics:* Plasma dipyridamole concentrations decline in a triexponential fashion following IV infusion with half-lives averaging 3 to 12 minutes, 33 to 62 minutes and 11.6 to 15 hours. The mean dipyridamole serum concentration is 4.6 ± 1.3 mcg/ml 2 minutes after a 4 minute 0.568 mg/kg infusion. The average plasma protein binding of dipyridamole is ≈ 99%, primarily to α_1-glycoprotein. Dipyridamole is metabolized in the liver to the glucuronic acid conjugate and excreted with the bile. Average total body clearance is 2.3 to 3.5 ml/min/kg, with apparent volume of distribution at steady state of 1 to 2.5 L/kg and a central apparent volume of 3 to 5 L.

➤*Clinical trials:* In a study of about 1100 patients who underwent coronary arteriography and IV dipyridamole-assisted thallium imaging, the sensitivity of the dipyridamole test (true positive dipyridamole divided by the total number of patients with positive angiography) was about 85%. The specificity (true negative divided by the number of patients with negative angiograms) was about 50%. In a subset of patients who had exercise thallium imaging as well as dipyridamole thallium imaging, sensitivity and specificity of the two tests were almost identical.

Contraindications

Hypersensitivity to dipyridamole.

Warnings

➤*Cardiotoxicity and bronchospasm:* Serious adverse reactions have included fatal and non-fatal myocardial infarction, ventricular fibrillation, symptomatic ventricular tachycardia, transient cerebral ischemia and bronchospasm.

In a study of 3911 patients given IV dipyridamole as an adjunct to thallium myocardial perfusion imaging, two types of serious adverse events occurred: Four cases of myocardial infarction (0.1%; two fatal, two non-fatal); and six cases of severe bronchospasm (0.2%). Although the incidence was small (0.3%; 10 of 3911), the potential clinical information to be gained through use of IV dipyridamole thallium imaging must be weighed against the patient risk. Patients with a history of unstable angina may be at a greater risk for severe myocardial ischemia, and patients with a history of asthma may be at a greater risk for bronchospasm.

When thallium myocardial perfusion imaging is performed with IV dipyridamole, parenteral aminophylline should be readily available for relieving adverse events such as bronchospasm or chest pain. Monitor vital signs during, and for 10 to 15 minutes following, the IV infusion of dipyridamole, and obtain an ECG tracing using at least one chest lead. Should severe chest pain or bronchospasm occur, administer parenteral aminophylline by slow IV injection (50 to 100 mg over 30 to 60 seconds) in doses ranging from 50 to 250 mg. In the case of severe hypotension, place the patient in a supine position with the head tilted down, if necessary, before administration of aminophylline. If 250 mg does not relieve chest pain symptoms within a few minutes, SL nitroglycerin may be administered. If chest pain continues despite use of aminophylline and nitroglycerin, consider the possibility of myocardial infarction. If the clinical condition of a patient with an adverse event permits a 1 minute delay in the use of aminophylline, thallium-201 may be injected and allowed to circulate for 1 minute before the injection of aminophylline. This will allow initial thallium perfusion imaging to be performed before reversal of the pharmacologic effects of dipyridamole on the coronary circulation.

➤*Fertility impairment:* A significant reduction in number of corpora lutea with consequent reduced implantations and live fetuses occurred in rats after 1250 mg/day.

➤*Pregnancy: Category B.* There are no adequate and well controlled studies in pregnant women. Use during pregnancy only if clearly needed.

➤*Lactation:* Dipyridamole is excreted in breast milk.

➤*Children:* Safety and efficacy in children have not been established.

Drug Interactions

Theophylline may abolish the coronary vasodilation induced by IV dipyridamole. This could lead to a false negative thallium imaging result.

Adverse Reactions

Adverse reaction information is derived from a study of 3911 patients, from spontaneous reports and from the published literature.

IV Dipyridamole Adverse Reactions (>1%)	
Adverse Reaction	Incidence (%)
Chest pain/angina pectoris	19.7
Headache	12.2
Dizziness	11.8
ECG abnormalities/ST-T changes	7.5
ECG abnormalities/extrasystoles	5.2
Hypotension	4.6
Nausea	4.6
Flushing	3.4
ECG abnormalities/tachycardia	3.2
Dyspnea	2.6
Pain unspecified	2.6
Blood pressure lability	1.6
Hypertension	1.5
Paresthesia	1.3
Fatigue	1.2

➤*Other adverse reactions (≤ 1%):*

Cardiovascular – ECG abnormalities unspecified (0.8%); arrhythmia unspecified (0.6%); palpitation (0.3%); ventricular tachycardia (see Warnings), bradycardia (0.2%); myocardial infarction (see Warnings), AV block, syncope, orthostatic hypotension, atrial fibrillation, supraventricular tachycardia (0.1%); ventricular arrhythmia unspecified (see Warnings), heart block unspecified, cardiomyopathy, edema (0.03%).

CNS – Hypothesia (0.5%); hypertonia (0.3%); nervousness/anxiety (0.2%); tremor (0.1%); abnormal coordination, somnolence, dysphonia, migraine, vertigo (0.03%).

GI – Dyspepsia (1%); dry mouth (0.8%); abdominal pain (0.7%); flatulence (0.6%); vomiting (0.4%); eructation (0.1%); dysphagia, tenesmus, increased appetite (0.03%).

Respiratory – Pharyngitis (0.3%); bronchospasm (0.2%, see Warnings); hyperventilation, rhinitis (0.1%); coughing, pleural pain (0.03%).

Miscellaneous – Myalgia (0.9%); back pain (0.6%); injection site reaction unspecified, diaphoresis (0.4%); asthenia, malaise, arthralgia (0.3%); injection site pain, rigor, earache, tinnitus, vision abnormalities unspecified, dysgeusia (0.1%); thirst, depersonalization, eye pain, renal pain, perineal pain, breast pain, intermittent claudication, leg cramping (0.03%).

Overdosage

It is unlikely that overdosage will occur because of the nature of use (ie, single IV administration in controlled settings).

SERMORELIN ACETATE

Rx	**Geref** (Serono Labs)	**Powder for Injection, lyophilized**: 50 mcg (as the acetate)[1]	In amps with 2 ml of 0.9% Sodium Chloride Injection as a diluent in vials.

[1] With 5 mg mannitol, 0.66 mg monobasic sodium phosphate and 0.04 mg dibasic sodium phosphate; may contain up to 1% albumin (Human).

Indications

As a single IV injection for evaluating the ability of the somatotroph of the pituitary gland to secrete growth hormone.

Administration and Dosage

➤*Approved by the FDA:* 1991.

Individualize dosage for each patient according to weight. Administer in a single IV dose of 1 mcg/kg in the morning following an overnight fast.

➤*Children (or subjects < 50 kg):*
1.) Reconstitute the contents of one 50 mcg amp with a minimum of 0.5 ml of the accompanying sterile diluent.
2.) Draw venous blood samples for GH determinations 15 minutes before and immediately prior to administration.
3.) Administer a bolus of 1 mcg/kg IV followed by a 3 ml normal saline flush.
4.) Draw venous blood samples for GH determinations at 15, 30, 45 and 60 minutes after administration.

➤*Adults (or subjects > 50 kg):*
1.) Determine the number of amps needed, based on a dose of 1 mcg/kg.
2.) Reconstitute the contents of each amp with a minimum of 0.5 ml of the accompanying sterile diluent.
3.) Follow steps 2 through 4 in the Children's section.

➤*Storage/Stability:* The lyophilized product must be stored under refrigeration (2° to 8°C; 36° to 46°F). Use immediately after reconstitution. Discard unused material.

SERMORELIN ACETATE

Actions

►*Pharmacology:* Sermorelin is for diagnostic use only. It increases plasma growth hormone (GH) concentrations by direct stimulation of the pituitary gland to release GH. Sermorelin is an acetate salt of a synthetic, 29-amino acid polypeptide that is the amino-terminal segment of the naturally occurring human growth hormone-releasing hormone (GHRH or GRH) consisting of 44 amino acid residues. Sermorelin appears to be equivalent to GRH (1-44) in its ability to stimulate growth hormone secretion in humans. It has also been called GRH (1-29) and GHRH (1-29).

Because baseline GH levels are generally very low (< 4 ng/ml), provocative tests may be useful in determining the functional GH-secreting capability of the pituitary somatotroph. Adults and children with normal responses to standard provocative tests of GH secretion were used to define the range of normal plasma GH-level responses to sermorelin. It was found that the absolute peak GH level following sermorelin infusion and the time elapsed from infusion to that peak are appropriate measures to evaluate the response to GH infusion. Doses used in children and adults in these studies ranged from 0.3 to 6.06 mcg/kg with a majority of patients receiving 1 mcg/kg. Based on these studies and published reports, 1 mcg/kg was chosen as the recommended dose for diagnostic purposes.

►*Clinical trials:* A total of 71 sermorelin injection tests were performed on 47 boys and 24 girls who showed normal responses to standard, indirect provocative tests such as clonidine, L-dopa and arginine. The GH peak plasma response to sermorelin was 28 ± 15 ng/ml and the time to this peak was 30 ± 27 minutes.

Of all children who had GH responses of > 7 ng/ml to standard provocative tests, 96% also had responses to sermorelin of > 7 ng/ml. In 77 patients who failed to respond to standard provocative tests, mean GH peak responses to sermorelin were significantly lower compared to the mean GH peak response of normal control children. However, 53% of the children who failed to respond to standard tests had a GH response to sermorelin of > 7 ng/ml suggesting that clinical GH deficiency is frequently not due to somatotroph failure.

Preliminary studies have demonstrated an age-related decline in GH responsiveness to GRH in persons > 40 years old, but the normal range of GH response to sermorelin in older adults has not been established.

Contraindications

Hypersensitivity to sermorelin or any of the excipients.

Warnings

►*Antibody formation:* Has occurred in humans after chronic SC administration of large doses of sermorelin. Approximately one in four patients given repeated doses of one or more of the three forms of GRH (1-29, 1-40 and 1-44) has developed antibodies to GRH. The clinical significance of these antibodies is unknown. One patient who developed antibodies to GRH (1-44) also experienced an allergic reaction described as severe redness, swelling and urticaria at the injection sites. No long-lasting effects from this reaction were reported. No symptomatic allergic reactions to GRH (1-29) have been reported.

►*GH deficiency:* A normal plasma GH response to sermorelin demonstrates that the somatotroph is intact. However, a normal response does not exclude GH deficiency because this deficiency is frequently the result of hypothalamic dysfunction in the presence of an intact somatotroph. The sermorelin stimulation test is most easily interpreted when there is a subnormal response to conventional provocative testing and a normal response to sermorelin. Such findings suggest that hypothalamic dysfunction is the cause for the growth hormone deficiency. When both conventional and sermorelin testing result in subnormal GH responses, the site of dysfunction cannot be determined with certainty because some patients with GH deficiency due to hypothalamic dysfunction require repeated sermorelin administration before demonstrating a normal response.

►*Acromegaly:* The sermorelin test has not been found useful in the diagnosis of acromegaly.

►*Hypersensitivity reactions:* Although hypersensitivity reactions have been observed with other polypeptide hormones, to date no such reactions have been reported following the administration of a single dose of sermorelin.

►*Pregnancy: Category C.* Sermorelin produces minor variations in fetuses of rats and rabbits when given in SC doses of 50, 150 and 500 mcg/kg. In the rat teratology study, external malformations (thin tail) were observed in the higher dose groups, and there was an increase in minor skeletal variants at the high dose. Some visceral malformations (hydroureter) were observed in all treatment groups, with the incidence greatest in the high-dose group. In rabbits, minor skeletal anomalies were significantly greater in the treated animals than in the controls. There are no adequate and well controlled studies in pregnant women. Use sermorelin during pregnancy only if the potential benefit justifies the potential risk to the fetus.

►*Lactation:* It is not known whether this drug is excreted in breast milk. Exercise caution when administering to a nursing woman.

Precautions

►*Subnormal GH response:* Obesity, hyperglycemia and elevated plasma fatty acids generally are associated with subnormal GH responses to sermorelin.

Drug Interactions

The sermorelin test should not be conducted in the presence of drugs that directly affect the pituitary secretion of somatotropin. These include preparations that contain or release somatostatin, insulin, glucocorticoids, or cyclooxygenase inhibitors such as aspirin or indomethacin. Somatotropin levels may be transiently elevated by clonidine, levodopa and insulin-induced hypoglycemia. Response to sermorelin may be blunted in patients who are receiving muscarinic antagonists (atropine) or who are hypothyroid or being treated with antithyroid medications such as propylthiouracil. Discontinue exogenous growth hormone therapy at least 1 week before administering the test.

Adverse Reactions

The following adverse reactions, in decreasing order of frequency, have occurred following sermorelin administration: Transient warmth or flushing of the face; injection site pain; redness or swelling at injection site; nausea; headache; vomiting; strange taste in the mouth; paleness; tightness in the chest. Antibody formation has been reported (see Warnings).

Overdosage

Changes of heart rate and blood pressure have occurred with the various GRH peptides in IV doses exceeding 10 mcg/kg. Cardiovascular collapse is a conceivable, but as of yet, unreported, complication of overdosage with GRH (1-29).

ADENOSINE

| *Rx* | **Adenoscan** (Fujisawa) | **Injection:** 3 mg/ml | Preservative-free. In 30 ml single-dose vials. |

For information on the use of adenosine as an antiarrhythmic agent, refer to the monograph in the Cardiovascular Agents chapter.

Indications

►*Diagnostic aid:* Adjunct to thallium-201 myocardial perfusion scintigraphy in patients unable to exercise adequately.

Administration and Dosage

For IV infusion only. Safety and efficacy of the intracoronary route have not been established.

Adenosine should be given as a continuous peripheral intravenous infusion.

The recommended IV dose for adults is 140 mcg/kg/min infused for 6 minutes (total dose of 0.84 mg/kg).

Inject the required dose of thallium-201 at the midpoint of the adenosine infusion (ie, after the first 3 minutes of adenosine). Thallium-201 is physically compatible with adenosine and may be injected into the adenosine infusion set.

The injection should be as close to the venous access as possible to prevent an inadvertent increase in the dose of adenosine (the contents of the IV tubing) being administered.

The following adenosine infusion nomogram may be used to determine the appropriate infusion rate corrected for total body weight:

Adenosine Infusion Rate Based on Weight		
Patient weight		Infusion rate ml/min
kg	lbs	
45	99	2.1
50	110	2.3
55	121	2.6
60	132	2.8
65	143	3
70	154	3.3
75	165	3.5
80	176	3.8
85	187	4
90	198	4.2

This nomogram was derived from the following general formula:

$$\frac{0.14 \text{ (mg/kg/min)} \times \text{total body weight (kg)}}{\text{Adenosine concentration (3 mg/ml)}} = \text{infusion rate (ml/min)}$$

►*Storage/Stability:* Store at controlled room temperature 15° to 30°C (59° to 86°F). Do not refrigerate as crystallization may occur. If crystallization has occurred, dissolve crystals by warming to room temperature. The solution must be clear at the time of use.

ADENOSINE

Actions

▶*Pharmacology:* Adenosine is an endogenous nucleoside occurring in all cells of the body. Adenosine is a potent vasodilator in most vascular beds, except in renal afferent arterioles and hepatic veins where it produces vasoconstriction. Adenosine is thought to exert its effects through activation of purine receptors (cell-surface A_1- and A_2-adenosine receptors). Although the exact mechanism by which adenosine receptor activation relaxes vascular smooth muscle is not known, there is evidence to support both inhibition of the slow inward calcium current reducing calcium uptake and activation of adenylate cyclase through A_2-receptors in smooth muscle cells. Adenosine may also lessen vascular tone by modulating sympathetic neurotransmission.

Myocardial uptake of thallium-201 is directly proportional to coronary blood flow. Since adenosine significantly increases blood flow in normal coronary arteries with little or no increase in stenotic arteries, adenosine causes relatively less thallium-201 uptake in vascular territories supplied by stenotic coronary arteries (ie, a greater difference is seen after adenosine between areas served by normal vessels and areas served by stenotic vessels than is seen prior to adenosine).

Hemodynamics – Adenosine produces a direct negative chronotropic, dromotropic and inotropic effect on the heart, presumably due to A_1-receptor agonism, and produces peripheral vasodilation, presumably due to A_2-receptor agonism. The net effect of adenosine in humans is typically a mild to moderate reduction in systolic, diastolic and mean arterial blood pressure associated with a reflex increase in heart rate. Rarely, significant hypotension and tachycardia have been observed.

▶*Pharmacokinetics:* Adenosine IV is rapidly cleared from the circulation via cellular uptake, primarily by erythrocytes and vascular endothelial cells. Intracellular adenosine is rapidly metabolized either via polyphorylation to adenosine monophosphate by adenosine kinase or via deamination to inosine by adenosine deaminase in the cytosol. These intracellular metabolites are not vasoactive. Inosine formed by deamination of adenosine can leave the cell intact or can be degraded to hypoxanthine, xanthine and ultimately uric acid. Adenosine monophosphate formed by phosphorylation of adenosine is incorporated into the high-energy phosphate pool. As adenosine requires no hepatic or renal function for its activation or inactivation, hepatic and renal failure would not be expected to alter its effectiveness or tolerability.

Contraindications

Second- or third-degree AV block (except in patients with a functioning artificial pacemaker); sinus node disease, such as sick sinus syndrome or symptomatic bradycardia (except in patients with a functioning artificial pacemaker); suspected bronchoconstrictive or bronchospastic lung disease (eg, asthma); hypersensitivity to adenosine.

Warnings

▶*Cardiac effects:* Fatal cardiac arrest, sustained ventricular tachycardia (requiring resuscitation) and nonfatal myocardial infarction have been reported coincident with adenosine infusion. Patients with unstable angina may be at greater risk.

Sinoatrial and atrioventricular nodal block – Adenosine exerts a direct depressant effect on the SA and AV nodes and has the potential to cause AV block, or sinus bradycardia. Approximately 6.3% of patients develop AV block with adenosine, including first-degree (2.9%), second-degree (2.6%) and third-degree (0.8%) heart block. All episodes of AV block have been asymptomatic and transient, and did not require intervention. Use with caution in patients with preexisting first-degree AV block or bundle branch block and avoid in patients with high-grade AV block or sinus node dysfunction (except in patients with a functional artificial pacemaker). Discontinue in any patient who develops persistent or symptomatic high-grade AV block. Sinus pause has been rarely observed with adenosine infusions.

Hypotension – Adenosine is a potent peripheral vasodilator and can cause significant hypotension. Patients with an intact baroreceptor reflex mechanism are able to maintain blood pressure and tissue perfusion in response to adenosine by increasing heart rate and cardiac output. However, use with caution in patients with autonomic dysfunction, stenotic valvular heart disease, pericarditis or pericardial effusions, stenotic carotid artery disease with cerebrovascular insufficiency, or uncorrected hypovolemia, due to the risk of hypotensive complications in these patients. Discontinue in any patient who develops persistent or symptomatic hypotension.

Hypertension – Increases in systolic and diastolic pressure have been observed (as great as 140 mm Hg systolic in one case) concomitant with adenosine infusion; most increases resolved spontaneously within several minutes, but in some cases, hypertension lasted for several hours.

▶*Bronchoconstriction:* Adenosine is a respiratory stimulant and, with IV administration, increases minute ventilation (Ve) and reduces arterial PCO_2 causing respiratory alkalosis. Approximately 28% of patients experience breathlessness (dyspnea) or an urge to breathe deeply. These complaints are transient and rarely require intervention. Adenosine given by inhalation may cause bronchoconstriction in asthmatic patients, presumably due to mast cell degranulation and histamine release. These effects have not been observed in healthy subjects.

Adenosine has been given to a limited number of patients with asthma and mild to moderate exacerbation of their symptoms has occurred. Respiratory compromise has occurred during adenosine infusion in patients with obstructive pulmonary disease. Use with caution in patients with obstructive lung disease not associated with bronchoconstriction (eg, emphysema, bronchitis) and avoid in patients with bronchoconstriction or bronchospasm (eg, asthma). Discontinue in any patient who develops severe respiratory difficulties.

Adenosine produces a variety of chromosomal alterations. In rats and mice, adenosine caused decreased spermatogenesis and increased numbers of abnormal sperm, a reflection of the ability of adenosine to produce chromosomal damage.

▶*Pregnancy:* Category C. It is not known whether adenosine can cause fetal harm when administered to pregnant women; use during pregnancy only if clearly needed.

▶*Children:* Safety and efficacy in patients < 18 years of age have not been established.

Drug Interactions

Whenever possible, drugs that might inhibit or augment the effects of adenosine should be withheld for at least five half-lives, prior to the use of adenosine.

Adenosine Drug Interactions			
Precipitant drug	Object drug*		Description
Cardioactive agents	Adenosine	↑	Because of the potential for additive or synergistic depressant effects on the SA and AV nodes, use with caution in the presence of these agents.
Methylxanthines (eg, caffeine and theophylline)	Adenosine	↓	The vasoactive effect of adenosine is inhibited by adenosine receptor antagonists, such as methylxanthines.

* ↑ = Object drug increased. ↓ = Object drug decreased.

Adverse Reactions

Despite the short half-life of adenosine, 10.6% of the side effects listed occurred several hours after the infusion terminated. Also, 8.4% of the side effects that began coincident with the infusion persisted for up to 24 hours after the infusion was complete. In many cases, it is not possible to know whether these late adverse events are the result of adenosine infusion.

Adenosine Adverse Reactions (≥ 1%) (n = 1421)	
Adverse reaction	%
Flushing	44
Chest discomfort	40
Dyspnea or urge to breathe deeply	28
Headache	18
Throat, neck or jaw discomfort	15
GI discomfort	13
Lightheadedness/dizziness	12
Upper extremity discomfort	4
ST segment depression	3
First-degree AV block	3
Second-degree AV block	3
Paresthesia	2
Hypotension	2
Nervousness	2
Arrhythmias	1

The following adverse events occurred in < 1% of patients: Back discomfort; lower extremity discomfort; weakness.

▶*Cardiovascular:* Nonfatal myocardial infarction; life-threatening ventricular arrhythmia; third-degree AV block; bradycardia; palpitation; sinus exit block; sinus pause; sweating; T-wave changes, hypertension (systolic blood pressure > 200 mm Hg).

▶*CNS:* Drowsiness; emotional instability; tremors.

▶*GU:* Vaginal pressure; urgency.

▶*Pulmonary:* Cough.

▶*Special senses:* Blurred vision; dry mouth; ear discomfort; metallic taste; nasal congestion; scotomata; tongue discomfort.

Overdosage

The half-life of adenosine is < 10 seconds and side effects (when they occur) usually resolve quickly when the infusion is discontinued, although delayed or persistent effects have been observed. Methylxanthines, such as caffeine and theophylline, are competitive adenosine receptor antagonists and theophylline has been used to effectively terminate persistent side effects. In controlled clinical trials, theophylline (50 to 125 mg slow IV injection) was needed to abort adenosine side effects in < 2% of patients.

ARGININE HCl

Rx   **R-Gene 10** (Pharmacia & Upjohn)   **Injection:** 10% arginine HCl (950 mOsmol/L)   With 47.5 mEq chloride ion per 100 ml. In 300 ml.

Indications

➤*Diagnostic aid:* An IV stimulant to the pituitary for the release of human growth hormone (HGH) in patients where the measurement of pituitary reserve for HGH can be of diagnostic usefulness. It can be used as a diagnostic aid in such conditions as panhypopituitarism, pituitary dwarfism, chromophobe adenoma, postsurgical craniopharyngioma, hypophysectomy, pituitary trauma, acromegaly, gigantism and problems of growth and stature.

Administration and Dosage

Administer IV.

➤*Dose:*

Adults – 300 ml.

Children – 5 ml/kg.

➤*Test procedure:* For successful administration of the test for measurement of pituitary reserve of human growth hormone, clinical conditions and procedures should be as follows:

1.) Schedule the test in the morning following a normal night's sleep and an overnight fast which should continue throughout the test period. Place patient at bed rest, and for at least 30 minutes before the infusion begins, take care to minimize apprehension and distress. This is particularly important in children.
2.) Infuse through an indwelling needle or soft catheter placed in an antecubital vein or other suitable vein. Take blood samples by venipuncture from the contralateral arm. A desirable schedule for drawing blood samples is at –30, 0, 30, 60, 90, 120 and 150 minutes. Promptly centrifuge blood samples and store the plasma at -20°C (-4°F) until assayed by one of the published radioimmunoassay procedures.
3.) Infuse arginine beginning at zero time at a uniform rate which will permit the recommended dose to be administered in 30 minutes.

➤*Interpretation of results:* Infusion IV often induces a pronounced rise in the plasma level of human growth hormone in subjects with intact pituitary function. This rise is usually diminished or absent in patients with impairment of this function.

Expected Plasma Levels of HGH with Arginine		
Patient	Control range (ng/ml)	Range of peak response to arginine (ng/ml)
Normal	0-6	10-30
Pituitary deficient	0-4	0-10

The above ranges are based on the mean values of plasma HGH levels calculated from the data of several clinical investigators and reflect their experiences with various methods of radioimmunoassay. Upon gaining experience with this diagnostic test, each clinician will establish his own ranges for control and peak levels of HGH.

Diagnostic test results showing a deficiency of pituitary reserve for HGH should be confirmed by a second test with arginine, or confirmed with the insulin hypoglycemia test. A waiting period of 1 day is advised between tests.

➤*Storage/Stability:* Invert and inspect each bottle before use to be sure that its contents are clear. Discard any flask in which its contents are not clear or which lacks a vacuum.

Actions

➤*Pharmacology:* Infusion IV often induces a pronounced rise in the plasma level of HGH in subjects with intact pituitary function. This rise is usually diminished or absent in patients with impairment of this function.

Contraindications

Persons having highly allergic tendencies.

Warnings

Arginine is a diagnostic aid and not intended for therapeutic use.

➤*Route of administration:* Always administer by IV injection due to the drug's hypertonicity.

➤*Deficiency of pituitary reserve for HGH:* If the insulin hypoglycemia test has indicated a deficiency of pituitary reserve for HGH, a test with arginine is advisable to confirm the negative response. This can be done after a waiting period of 1 day. As patients may not respond during the first test, the unresponsive patient should be tested again to confirm the negative result. A second test can be performed after a waiting period of 1 day. Some patients who respond to arginine do not respond to insulin and vice versa. The rate of false positive responses is approximately 32%, and the rate of false negatives is approximately 27%.

➤*Hypersensitivity reactions:* Have a suitable antihistaminic drug available in case of an allergic reaction. Refer to Management of Acute Hypersensitivity Reactions.

➤*Pregnancy: Category B.* Do not use this drug during pregnancy.

➤*Lactation:* It is not known whether IV administration of arginine could result in significant quantities of arginine in breast milk. Systemically administered amino acids are secreted into breast milk in quantities not likely to have a deleterious effect on the infant. Nevertheless, exercise caution when arginine is administered to nursing women.

Precautions

Arginine is a hypertonic (950 mOsmol/L) and acidic (average pH of 5.6) solution that can irritate tissues. Use care to ensure administration of arginine through a patent catheter within a patent vein.

➤*Excessive infusion rates:* May result in local irritation and flushing, nausea or vomiting. Inadequate dosing or prolongation of the infusion period may diminish the stimulus to the pituitary and nullify the test.

➤*Nitrogen:* Arginine has a high content of metabolizable nitrogen; consider the temporary effect of a high load of nitrogen upon the kidneys when administered.

➤*Chloride:* The chloride ion content is 47.5 mEq/100 ml of solution; consider the effect of infusing this amount of chloride into patients with electrolyte imbalance before the test is undertaken.

➤*Growth hormone levels:* Basal and post-stimulation levels of growth hormone are elevated in patients who are pregnant or who are taking oral contraceptives.

Adverse Reactions

Approximately 3% of patients reported nonspecific side effects consisting of nausea, vomiting, headache, flushing, numbness and local venous irritation.

One patient had an allergic reaction manifested as a confluent macular rash with reddening and swelling of the hands and face. The rash subsided rapidly after the infusion was terminated and 50 mg diphenhydramine was administered. One patient had an apparent decrease in platelet count from 150,000 to 60,000. One patient with a history of acrocyanosis had an exacerbation of this condition following infusion.

Overdosage

An overdosage may cause a transient metabolic acidosis with hyperventilation. The acidosis will be compensated and the base deficit will return to normal following completion of the infusion. If the condition persists, determine the deficit and correct by a calculated dose of an alkalizing agent.

CORTICORELIN OVINE TRIFLUTATE

Rx   **Acthrel** (Ferring)   **Cake, lyophilized:** 100 mcg corticorelin ovine (as trifluoroacetate)[1]   In 5 ml single-dose vials with diluent.

[1] With 0.88 mg ascorbic acid, 10 mg lactose and 26 mg cysteine hydrochloride monohydrate.

Indications

➤*Cushing's syndrome, differential diagnosis:* Differentiating pituitary and ectopic production of ACTH in patients with ACTH-dependent Cushing's syndrome.

Administration and Dosage

➤*Approved by the FDA:* May 23, 1996 (1PV classification).

➤*Test methodology:* To evaluate the status of the pituitary-adrenal axis in the differentiation of a pituitary source from an ectopic source of excessive ACTH secretion, a corticorelin test procedure requires a minimum of five blood samples.

Procedure –

1.) Draw venous blood samples 15 minutes before and immediately prior to corticorelin administration. The ACTH baseline is obtained by averaging the values of the two samples.
2.) Administer corticorelin as an IV infusion over a 30- to 60-second interval at a dose of 1 mcg/kg. Higher dosages are not recommended (see Precautions).
3.) Draw blood samples at 15, 30, and 60 minutes after administration.

Cortisol determinations may be performed on the same blood samples for the same time points as outlined above.

➤*Dosage:* A single IV dose of corticorelin at 1 mcg/kg is recommended for the testing of pituitary corticotrophin function. A dose of 1 mcg/kg is

CORTICORELIN OVINE TRIFLUTATE

the lowest dose that produces maximal cortisol responses and significant (though apparently sub-maximal) ACTH responses. Doses > 1 mcg/kg are not recommended. Some adverse effects can be reduced by administering the drug as an infusion over 30 seconds instead of as a bolus injection.

If a repeat evaluation using the corticorelin stimulation test with corticorelin is needed, it is recommended that the repeat test be carried out at the same time of day as the original test because there are differences in basal levels and peak response levels following morning or evening administration (see Pharmacokinetics).

►*Interpretation of test results:* The interpretations of the ACTH and cortisol responses following corticorelin administration requires a knowledge of the clinical status of the individual patient, understanding of hypothalamic-pituitary-adrenal physiology, and familiarity with the normal hormonal ranges and the standards used by the laboratory that performs the ACTH and cortisol assays.

Cushing's disease – A hyper response to corticorelin is seen in the majority of patients, despite high basal cortisol levels. This response pattern indicates an impairment of the negative feedback of cortisol on the pituitary. Patients with pituitary-dependent Cushing's disease tested with corticorelin do not show the negative correlation between basal and stimulated levels of ACTH and cortisol that is found in healthy subjects. A positive correlation between basal ACTH levels and maximum ACTH increments after corticorelin administration has been found in Cushing's disease patients.

Ectopic ACTH secretion – Patients with Cushing's syndrome caused by ectopic ACTH secretion are found to have very high basal levels of ACTH and cortisol, which were not further stimulated by corticorelin. However, there have been rare instances of patients with ectopic sources of ACTH that have responded to the corticorelin test.

►*Reconstitution:* Reconstitute corticorelin with 2 ml of 0.9% Sodium Chloride Injection by injecting 2 ml of the saline diluent into the lyophilized drug product cake. Avoid bubble formation. DO NOT SHAKE the vial. Instead, roll the vial to dissolve the drug product. The resulting sterile solution contains 50 mcg corticorelin ovine triflutate/ml.

►*Storage/Stability:* Corticorelin is stable in the lyophilized form when stored refrigerated at 2° to 8°C (36° to 45°F) and protected from light. The reconstituted solution is stable up to 8 hours under refrigerated conditions. Discard unused reconstituted solution.

Actions

►*Pharmacology:* Corticorelin ovine triflutate causes a rapid and sustained release of plasma ACTH levels with a similar cortisol response. In addition, it causes a concomitant and prolonged release of the related proopiomelanocortin peptides β- and γ- lipotropins and β-endorphin. When corticorelin is administered to patients with pituitary-related hypercortisolism, plasma ACTH and cortisol levels increase indicating impairment of the negative feedback of cortisol on the pituitary. This method of stimulation testing is used to differentiate between etiologies of ACTH-dependent hypercortisolism.

Approximately 83% of patients with hypercortisolism (Cushing's syndrome) have ACTH-dependent hypersecretion of cortisol. Hypercortisolism in these patients is: 1) caused by pituitary hypersecretion of ACTH (Cushing's disease) from an adenoma or nonadenomatous hyperplasia; or 2) occurs secondary to ectopic secretion of ACTH. Cushing's syndrome caused by the autonomous cortisol secretion by an adrenal tumor is referred to as ACTH-independent and is less common.

After confirmation of Cushing's syndrome and ruling out autonomous adrenal hyperfunction, the corticorelin test is used as an aid in establishing the source of excessive ACTH secretion in ACTH-dependent hypercortisolism. Cushing's disease (ACTH of pituitary origin) is confirmed by an increase in plasma ACTH and cortisol levels following corticorelin injection, whereas patients with ectopic ACTH secretion will exhibit little or no response.

►*Pharmacokinetics:*

Absorption/Distribution – Plasma ACTH levels in healthy subjects increased 2 minutes after IV doses of ≥ 0.3 mcg/kg and reached peak levels after 10 to 15 minutes. Plasma cortisol levels increased within 10 minutes and peaked at 30 to 60 minutes. As the dose was increased, the rises in plasma ACTH and cortisol were more sustained and exhibited a biphasic response with a second lower peak at 2 to 3 hours. Graded IV doses (0.01, 0.03, 0.1, 0.3, 1, 3, 10, 30 mcg/kg) produced a linear increase in plasma immunoreactive corticorelin (IR-corticorelin ovine triflutate). The duration of mean plasma ACTH increase after 0.3, 3, and 30 mcg/kg was 4, 7 and 8 hours, respectively, with a similar but more prolonged effect on plasma cortisol. The mean volume of distribution for IR-corticorelin ovine triflutate is 6.2 L.

Basal levels and peak responses in individual patients differ following morning or evening administration. Combined data from 9 trials conducted in the morning and 4 conducted in the evening are presented in

the table below showing the basal and peak levels of ACTH and cortisol following the administration of 1 mcg/kg or 100 mcg.

Basal and Peak Levels of ACTH and Cortisol in Healthy Subjects after 1 mcg/kg or 100 mcg of Corticorelin					
Time of day	No. of subjects	ACTH concentration mean (range) pg/ml		Cortisol concentration mean (range) mcg/dl	
		Basal	Peak	Basal	Peak
a.m.	143	28 (16-65)	68 (39-114)	11 (8-13)	21 (17-25)
p.m.	70	9 (8-13)	30 (25-42)	4 (2-6)	16 (15-18)

Continuous infusion does not abolish the circadian rhythm of plasma ACTH and cortisol, but does appear to desensitize the corticotropin. However, intermittent doses (25 mcg every 4 hours for 72 hours) elicit the expected ACTH and cortisol responses.

Metabolism/Excretion – The plasma clearance of IR-corticorelin ovine triflutate exhibits a biexponential decay with α- and β-half lives of 11.5 and 73 minutes and a clearance of $\approx$ 95 L/m^2/day. Corticorelin does not appear to be bound by a specific plasma protein.

►*Clinical trials:* In one study of 29 healthy volunteers, plasma ACTH and cortisol levels over a corticorelin dose range of 0.001 to 30 mcg/kg showed a more direct dose-dependent relationship for ACTH than for cortisol. The threshold dose was determined to be 0.03 mcg/kg with a half-maximal dose of 0.3 to 1 mcg/kg and a maximally effective dose of 3 to 10 mcg/kg.

Warnings

►*Pregnancy: Category C.* It is not known whether corticorelin ovine triflutate can cause fetal harm when administered to a pregnant woman or can affect reproductive capacity. Give to a pregnant woman only if clearly needed.

►*Lactation:* It is not known whether corticorelin is secreted in breast milk. Exercise caution when corticorelin is administered to a nursing woman.

►*Children:* Only a few tests have been performed on children. Dosage was 1 mcg/kg. Patient studies have involved only children with multiple hypothalamic or pituitary hormone deficiencies or tumors. No differences in response to the corticorelin test have been reported in the children studied.

Precautions

►*Dose-dependent effects:* The severity of adverse effects to a corticorelin injection appears to be dose-dependent. Dosages > 1 mcg/kg are not recommended. While few adverse effects have been observed at the 1 mcg/kg or 100 mcg dose, higher doses have been associated with transient tachycardia, decreased blood pressure, loss of consciousness and asystole. These symptoms can be substantially reduced by administering the drug as a 30–second IV infusion instead of a bolus injection.

►*Flushing/Cardiovascular effects:* Flushing of the face, neck and upper chest beginning almost immediately and lasting 3 to 5 minutes has occurred. Recipients have also reported an urge to take a deep breath, which occurs with a timing similar to that of flushing. Higher doses (≥ 3 mcg/kg) are associated with more prolonged flushing, tachycardia, hypotension, dyspnea and "chest compression" or tightness. The cardiovascular effects occurred 2 to 3 minutes after injection and lasted for 30 to 60 minutes. The flushing was more prolonged, lasting up to 4 hours in some subjects. All signs and symptoms could be reduced by administering the drug as a 30–second infusion instead of by bolus injection.

Drug Interactions

►*Dexamethasone:* The plasma ACTH response to corticorelin is inhibited or blunted in healthy subjects pretreated with dexamethasone.

►*Heparin:* The use of a heparin solution to maintain IV cannula patency during the corticorelin test is not recommended. A possible interaction between corticorelin and heparin may have been responsible for a major hypotensive reaction that occurred after corticorelin administration.

Adverse Reactions

Flushing of the face, neck and upper chest (16%); urge to take a deep breath (6%); prolonged flushing; tachycardia; hypotension; dyspnea; "chest compression" or tightness; significant increases in heart rate and decreases in blood pressure (see Precautions).

Overdosage

Symptoms of overdose include severe facial flushing, cardiovascular changes and dyspnea. In the event of toxic overdoses, treat adverse effects symptomatically.

METYRAPONE

| *Rx* | **Metopirone** (Novartis) | **Capsules:** 250 mg | (CIBA LN) Soft gelatin. White to yellowish white. Oblong. In 18s. |

Indications

➤*Diagnostic aid:* A diagnostic drug for testing hypothalamic-pituitary adrenocorticotropic hormone (ACTH) function.

Administration and Dosage

➤*Approved by the FDA:* January 25, 1962.

➤*Single-dose short test:* This test, usually given on an outpatient basis, determines plasma 11–desoxycortisol and ACTH levels after a single dose of metyrapone. Give adults and children 30 mg/kg (maximum 3 g metyrapone) at midnight with yogurt or milk. The blood sample for the assay is taken early the following morning (7:30 am to 8 am). Freeze the plasma as soon as possible. Then give the patient a prophylactic dose of 50 mg cortisone acetate.

Interpretation – Normal values will depend on the method used to determine ACTH and 11–desoxycortisol levels. An intact ACTH reserve is generally indicated by an increase in plasma ACTH to at least 44 pmol/L (200 ng/L) or by an increase in 11–desoxycortisol to > 0.2 mcmol/L (70 mcg/L). Hospitalize patients with suspected adrenocortical insufficiency overnight as a precautionary measure.

➤*Multiple-dose test:*
• Day 1: Control period – Collect 24-hour urine for measurement of 17-hydroxycorticosteroids (17-OHCS) or 17-ketogenic steroids (17-KGS).
• Day 2: ACTH test to determine the ability of adrenals to respond – Standard ACTH test such as infusion of 50 units ACTH over 8 hours and measurement of 24-hour urinary steroids. If results indicate adequate response, the metyrapone test may proceed.
• Day 3 to 4: Rest period.
• Day 5: Administration of metyrapone (recommended with milk or snack). Adults: 750 mg orally, every 4 hours for 6 doses. A single dose is approximately equivalent to 15 mg/kg. Children: 15 mg/kg orally every 4 hours for 6 doses. A minimal single dose of 250 mg is recommended.
• Day 6: After administration of metyrapone – Determination of 24-hour urinary steroids for effect.

Interpretation –
ACTH Test: The normal 24-hour urinary excretion of 17–OHCS ranges from 3 to 12 mg. Following continuous IV infusion of 50 units ACTH over a period of 8 hours, 17-OHCS excretion increases to 15 to 45 mg per 24 hours.

➤*Metyrapone response:*
Normal response – In patients with a normally functioning pituitary, administration of metyrapone is followed by a 2- to 4-fold increase of 17–OHCS excretion or doubling of 17-KGS excretion.

Subnormal response – Subnormal response in patient without adrenal insufficiency is indicative of some degree of impairment of pituitary function, either panhypopituitarism or partial hypopituitarism (limited pituitary reserve).

Panhypopituitarism: Panhypopituitarism is readily diagnosed by the classical clinical and chemical evidence of hypogonadism, hypothyroidism, and hypoadrenocorticism. These patients usually have subnormal basal urinary steroid levels. Depending upon the duration of the disease and degree of adrenal atrophy, they may fail to respond to exogenous ACTH in the normal manner. Administration of metyrapone is not essential in the diagnosis, but if given, it will not induce an appreciable increase in urinary steroids.

Partial hypopituitarism: Partial hypopituitarism or limited pituitary reserve is the more difficult diagnosis as these patients do not present the classical signs and symptoms of hypopituitarism. Measurements of target organ functions often are normal under basal conditions. The response to exogenous ACTH is usually normal, producing the expected rise of urinary steroids (17-OHCS or 17-KGS).

However, the response to metyrapone is subnormal; that is, no significant increase in 17-OHCS or 17-KGS excretion occurs.

This failure to respond to metyrapone may be interpreted as evidence of impaired pituitary-adrenal reserve. In view of the normal response to exogenous ACTH, the failure to respond to metyrapone is inferred to be related to a defect in the CNS-pituitary mechanism which normally regulates ACTH secretions. Presumably, the ACTH-secreting mechanism of these individuals are already working at their maximal rates to meet everyday conditions and possess limited "reserve" capacities to secrete additional ACTH either in response to stress or to decreased cortisol levels occurring as a result of metyrapone administration.

Subnormal response in patients with Cushing's syndrome is suggestive of either autonomous adrenal tumors that suppress the ACTH-releasing capacity of the pituitary or nonendocrine ACTH-secreting tumors.

➤*Excessive response:* An excessive excretion of 17-OHCS or 17-KGS after administration of metyrapone is suggestive of Cushing's syndrome associated with adrenal hyperplasia. These patients have an elevated excretion of urinary corticosteroids under basal conditions and will often, but not invariably, show a "supernormal" response to ACTH and also to metyrapone, excreting more than 35 mg per 24 hours of either 17-OHCS or 17-KGS.

Actions

➤*Pharmacology:* Metyrapone is an inhibitor of endogenous adrenal corticosteroid synthesis. The pharmacological effect of metyrapone is to reduce cortisol and corticosterone production by inhibiting the 11–β-hydroxylation reaction in the adrenal cortex. Removal of the strong inhibitory feedback mechanism exerted by cortisol results in an increase in ACTH production by the pituitary. With continued blockade of the enzymatic steps leading to production of cortisol and corticosterone, there is a marked increase in adrenocortical secretion of their immediate precursors, 11-desoxycortisol and desoxycorticosterone, which are weak suppressors of ACTH release, and a corresponding elevation of these steroids in the plasma and of their metabolites in the urine. These metabolites are readily determined by measuring urinary 17-OHCS or 17-KGS. Because of these actions, metyrapone is used as a diagnostic test, with urinary 17-OHCS measured as an index of pituitary ACTH responsiveness. Metyrapone may also suppress biosynthesis of aldosterone, resulting in a mild natriuresis.

The response to metyrapone does not occur immediately. Following oral administration, peak steroid excretion occurs during the subsequent 24–hour period.

➤*Pharmacokinetics:*

Absorption – Metyrapone is absorbed rapidly and well when administered orally as prescribed. Peak plasma concentrations are usually reached 1 hour after administration. After administration of 750 mg, mean peak plasma concentrations are 3.7 mcg/ml, falling to 0.5 mcg/ml 4 hours after administration. Following a single 2000 mg dose, mean peak plasma concentrations of metyrapone in plasma are 7.3 mcg/ml.

Metabolism – The major biotransformation is a reduction of the ketone to metyrapol, an active alcohol metabolite. Eight hours after a single oral dose, the ratio of metyrapone to metyrapol in the plasma is 1:1.5. Metyrapone and metyrapol are both conjugated with glucuronide.

Excretion – Metyrapone is rapidly eliminated from the plasma. The mean terminal elimination half-life is 1.9 hours. Metyrapol takes about twice as long as metyrapone to be eliminated from the plasma. After administration of 4.5 g metyrapone (750 mg every 4 hours), an average of 5.3% of the dose was excreted in the urine in the form of metyrapone (9.2% free and 90.8% as glucuronide) and 38.5% in the form of metyrapol (8.1% free and 91.9% as glucuronide) within 72 hours after the first dose was given.

Contraindications

Adrenal cortical insufficiency; hypersensitivity to metyrapone or any of its excipients.

Warnings

➤*Acute adrenal insufficiency:* Metyrapone may induce acute adrenal insufficiency in patients with reduced adrenal secretory capacity.

➤*Pregnancy: Category C.* A subnormal response to metyrapone may occur in pregnant women. The metyrapone test was administered to 20 pregnant women in their second and third trimester of pregnancy and evidence was found that the fetal pituitary responded to the enzymatic block. It is not known if metyrapone can affect reproduction capacity. Give to a pregnant women only if clearly needed.

➤*Lactation:* It is not known whether this drug is excreted in breast milk. Exercise caution when administering to a nursing woman.

➤*Children:* See Administration and Dosage.

Precautions

➤*Response of adrenals:* Ability of adrenals to respond to exogenous ACTH should be demonstrated before metyrapone is employed as a test.

➤*Hypo-/Hyperthyroidism:* In the presence of hypo- or hyperthyroidism, response to the metyrapone test may be subnormal.

➤*Hazardous tasks:* Since metyrapone may cause dizziness and sedation, patients should exercise caution when driving or operating machinery.

METYRAPONE

Drug Interactions

Metyrapone Drug Interactions			
Precipitant drug	Object drug[*]		Description
Corticosteroids	Metyrapone	↓	Drugs affecting pituitary or adrenocortical function, including all corticosteroid therapy, must be discontinued prior to and during testing with metyrapone.
Phenytoin	Metyrapone	↓	The metabolism of metyrapone is accelerated by phenytoin; therefore, results of the test may be inaccurate in patients taking phenytoin within 2 weeks before.
Estrogens	Metyrapone	↓	A subnormal response may occur in patients on estrogen therapy.
Metyrapone	Acetaminophen	↑	Metyrapone inhibits the glucuronidation of acetaminophen and could possibly potentiate acetaminophen toxicity.

[*] ↑ = Object drug increased. ↓ = Object drug decreased.

Adverse Reactions

➤*CNS:* Headache; dizziness; sedation.

➤*Dermatologic:* Allergic rash.

➤*GI:* Nausea; vomiting; abdominal discomfort or pain.

➤*Hematologic:* Rarely, decreased white blood cell count or bone marrow depression.

Overdosage

➤*Symptoms:* One case has been recorded in which a 6-year-old girl died after 2 doses of 2 g metyrapone.

Oral LD_{50} in animals (mg/kg): Rats, 521; maximum tolerated IV dose in 1 dog, 300.

The clinical picture of poisoning with metyrapone is characterized by GI symptoms and by signs of acute adrenocortical insufficiency.

Cardiovascular – Cardiac arrhythmias; hypotension; dehydration.

CNS – Anxiety; confusion; weakness; impairment of consciousness.

GI – Nausea; vomiting; epigastric pain; diarrhea.

Lab test abnormalities – Hyponatremia; hypochloremia; hyperkalemia.

In patients under treatment with insulin or oral antidiabetics, the signs and symptoms of acute poisoning with metyrapone may be aggravated or modified.

➤*Treatment:* There is no specific antidote. Besides general measures to eliminate the drug and reduce its absorption, immediately administer a large dose of hydrocortisone together with saline and glucose infusions. For a few days, monitor blood pressure and fluid and electrolyte balance.

ARBUTAMINE

GenESA (Gensia Automedics)	**Injection**: 0.05 mg/ml	Sodium metabisulfite. In a 20 ml prefilled syringe.

Indications

➤*Coronary artery disease, diagnosis:* In patients with suspected coronary artery disease (CAD) who cannot exercise adequately, stress induction with arbutamine is indicated as an aid in diagnosing the presence or absence of CAD.

Administration and Dosage

➤*Approved by the FDA:* September 12, 1997.

Before using the *GenESA System*, it is essential to read and understand the *GenESA System Directions For Use.*

Arbutamine 0.05 mg/ml must be administered from the prefilled syringe and must not be diluted or transferred to another syringe. Arbutamine is intended for direct IV infusion only with the *GenESA* device.

Select the desired rate of heart rate (HR) rise (HR slope: Low, 4 bpm/min; medium, 8 bpm/min; high, 12 bpm/min). Alternatively select any value from 4 to 12 bpm/min and the maximum HR to be achieved [HR target - estimated by the device as $(220 - age) \times 85\%$, or adjusted manually by the operator for each patient test]. Base the choice of HR slope on the desired duration of the test and the rate of HR rise judged to be most appropriate. The use of the medium slope is supported for a majority of patients.

Upon starting the test, the *GenESA* device administers a small dose of arbutamine (0.1 mcg/kg/min for 1 minute) and measures the patient's HR response. The device then calculates the difference between the desired and actual HR response, and maintains or modifies the infusion rate. The maximum infusion rate delivered by the *GenESA* device is 0.8 mcg/kg/min and the maximum total dose is 10 mcg/kg. The *GenESA* device includes a "HOLD HR" feature that, when activated, allows HR to be maintained at approximately the current level for up to 5 minutes.

Terminate the infusion of arbutamine when a diagnostic endpoint (eg, ST segment deviation on ECG) has been reached, if clinically significant symptoms or arrhythmias occur, or if clinically appropriate for any other reason. The *GenESA* device will stop drug delivery when the maximum HR limit has been reached or after a total of 10 mcg/kg arbutamine has been delivered. Following completion of the infusion, monitor the patient using the *GenESA* device or other means, until HR and blood pressure have returned to acceptable levels.

Heart rate saturation is an endpoint of the *GenESA System* test. If such a flattening or plateau of the HR response is detected when the HR is ≤ 40 bpm above the baseline level, restart of the arbutamine infusion is allowed. If the HR is > 40 bpm above baseline and an HR saturation occurs, restart of the arbutamine infusion is prevented by the *GenESA* device because it is unlikely that any further clinically significant increase in HR will occur and potential risk exists for serious cardiac arrhythmias (see Warnings).

Actions

➤*Pharmacology:* Arbutamine is a synthetic catecholamine with chronotropic and inotropic properties. By increasing cardiac work through its positive chronotropic and inotropic actions, arbutamine acts as a cardiac stress agent to mimic exercise and provoke myocardial ischemia in patients with compromised coronary arteries. It also probably limits regional subendocardial perfusion, and hence tissue oxygenation, by its increase in HR. The delivery system adjusts the rate of arbutamine delivery to achieve a selected increase in HR.

Arbutamine is a sympathomimetic that exhibits mixed β_{1+2} adrenoceptor agonist and mild α_1–adrenoceptors activity. Arbutamine displays 10–fold greater affinity for β-receptors and 5-fold lower binding at the α-receptor level compared with dobutamine. The β-agonist activity of arbutamine provides cardiac stress by increasing HR, cardiac contractility and systolic blood pressure (SBP).

Some α-receptor activity is retained in vivo, such that the degree of hypotension observed for given chronotropic activity is less with arbutamine than with isoproterenol, a specific β-agonist.

➤*Pharmacokinetics:*

Absorption/Distribution – Because of sensitivity limitations of the arbutamine assay, the pharmacokinetics have been characterized only for the first 20 to 30 minutes after the termination of IV infusions of ≤ 0.3 mcg/kg/min. The onset of effect on HR after start of arbutamine infusion is rapid (≈ 1 minute), the half-life is ≈ 8 minutes, plasma clearance is ≈ 4 L/hr/kg and volume of distribution is 0.74 L/kg. Plasma protein binding is ≈ 58%.

Metabolism/Excretion – Arbutamine is mainly (> 75%) eliminated by metabolism, principally to methoxyarbutamine, which is excreted in free or conjugated form in urine. Ketoarbutamine has been tentatively identified as another metabolite. Total plasma declined with a half-life of 1.8 hours, probably caused by metabolites with longer half-lives than arbutamine. The rapid onset of effect and rapid decline in HR following termination of infusion (time for a 50% decrease is 13 to 16 minutes) suggest that the pharmacological activity resides primarily with the parent compound. Following IV infusion, 84% of the total dose is excreted in the urine within 48 hours, with 9% excreted in feces.

Contraindications

Idiopathic hypertrophic subaortic stenosis; history of recurrent sustained ventricular tachycardia; CHF (NYHA Class III or IV); previous manifestation of hypersensitivity to arbutamine. The *GenESA System* must not be used in the presence of an implanted cardiac pacemaker or automated cardioverter/defibrillator.

Warnings

➤*Administration:* Arbutamine must not be administered without the use of the *GenESA* device. The *GenESA System* delivers arbutamine through a closed-loop, computer-controlled drug-delivery system to elicit acute cardiovascular responses.

ARBUTAMINE

➤*Cardiac events:* Arbutamine administration was associated with serious cardiac adverse events, including 3 episodes of ventricular fibrillation, 1 episode of sustained ventricular tachycardia, 3 episodes of atrial fibrillation, 1 myocardial infarction and 2 cases of severe angina. The incidence of serious adverse events is thus low (< 5%). Nevertheless, the potential information to be gained through the use of arbutamine must be weighed against the potential risks to each patient.

Arbutamine is not recommended in patients with unstable angina, mechanical left ventricular outflow obstruction such as severe valvular aortic stenosis, uncontrolled systemic hypertension, a cardiac transplant, a history of cerebrovascular accident or peripheral vascular disorder resulting in cerebral or aortic aneurysm.

➤*Arrhythmias:* Arbutamine may precipitate or exacerbate supraventricular and ventricular arrhythmias and its administration is not recommended in patients with a history of sustained arrhythmias of this nature, or in patients taking certain antiarrhythmic agents, particularly Class 1 agents (eg, quinidine, lidocaine).

Most arrhythmias were self-limiting and all resolved without sequelae. If any arrhythmias are of clinical concern, discontinue drug infusion immediately and administer appropriate therapy (eg, IV β-blockers; see Overdosage), if necessary. The *GenESA* device is not designed to detect arrhythmias; therefore appropriate monitoring equipment must be used during the test. The *GenESA* device administers arbutamine based on HR response and it is possible that, in the presence of an arrhythmia, the *GenESA* device may register an inaccurate HR. Monitor ECG carefully and take appropriate action in the event of inaccurate HR detection.

➤*Hemodynamic effects:* Arbutamine may cause rapid increase or paradoxical decreases in HR and SBP. Discontinuation of arbutamine infusion results in reversal of these effects. The infusion may be restarted if considered clinically appropriate. In patients with known or suspected CAD, mean maximum increase in HR was 52 bpm and the mean maximum increase in SBP was 36 mmHg. After termination of arbutamine infusion, HR decreased, with 50% of the HR increase gone within 16 minutes.

In 19 patients (12 with and 7 without a stenosis ≥ 50% in 1 or more major coronary arteries) the cardiac hemodynamic effects of arbutamine were assessed using invasive techniques. Cardiac contractility, cardiac output and total systemic vascular resistance (SVR) were determined at low stress (a mean HR increase from baseline of 25 bpm) and at peak stress (a mean HR increase from baseline of 40 bpm). At low stress, cardiac contractility and output had increased by 66% and 45%, respectively, from baseline, and they rose to 80% and 63% above baseline at peak stress. Total SVR decreased from baseline by 41% at low stress and by 48% at peak stress. By 15 minutes after the end of the infusion, cardiac contractility and SVR were within ≈ 15% of baseline, and cardiac output was 29% above baseline.

Left ventricular ejection fraction (LVEF), assessed by echocardiography, was evaluated in a study of 156 patients with known or suspected CAD tested using arbutamine infusion and exercise. With an increase in HR from baseline of ≈ 20 bpm, the relative increase in LVEF was 22%. At the end of the arbutamine infusion, when the mean increase in HR from baseline was 59 bpm, the relative increase in LVEF was 23%. By comparison, the relative increase in LVEF at the end of the exercise was 14%.

➤*Beta blockers:* The effects of arbutamine on HR and SBP are attenuated by concurrent use of beta blockers. Depending on the beta blocker, evidence of this attenuation is still present 23 hours after the last dose. In patients in whom beta blockers had been withdrawn for a minimum of 48 hours prior to receiving arbutamine, the HR and the SBP responses to arbutamine were similar to those seen in patients who had not received beta blockers for at least 2 weeks prior to arbutamine.

➤*Special risk patients:* Arbutamine is not recommended in patients with narrow-angle glaucoma or uncontrolled hyperthyroidism.

➤*Hypersensitivity reactions:* Reactions suggestive of hypersensitivity have been reported occasionally with the administration of other catecholamines (eg, dobutamine).

➤*Renal/Hepatic function impairment:* The acute use of arbutamine for diagnostic testing makes it unlikely that alterations in renal or hepatic function will influence the safety and diagnostic efficacy of the test.

➤*Pregnancy: Category B.* There are no adequate and well-controlled studies in pregnant women. Use during pregnancy only if clearly needed.

Precautions

➤*Monitoring:* Monitor ECG and blood pressure continuously. The *GenESA* device provides such monitoring capabilities but a diagnostic-quality ECG machine must also be used to monitor the ECG.

➤*Potassium levels:* Arbutamine can produce a transient reduction in serum potassium concentration, rarely to hypokalemic levels. Overall, changes in serum potassium in patients with clinically significant arrhythmias were not clearly different from those seen in other patients.

➤*ECG changes:* Arbutamine infusion is associated with a transient increase in corrected QT interval, as measured from the surface ECG. This effect did not appear to be associated with an increased incidence of arrhythmias.

➤*Sulfite sensitivity:* Arbutamine contains sodium metabisulfite, a sulfite that may cause allergic-type reactions, including anaphylactic symptoms and life-threatening or less severe asthmatic episodes, in certain susceptible individuals. The overall prevalence of sulfite sensitivity in the general population is unknown and probably low; it is seen more frequently in asthmatic than nonasthmatic individuals.

Drug Interactions

Beta blockers may attenuate the response to arbutamine and should be withdrawn at least 48 hours before conducting a test (see Warnings).

Avoid concomitant administration with **digoxin**, **atropine** (or other anticholinergic drugs) or **tricyclic antidepressants**. Because arbutamine dosing is based on the HR response of the patient, the use of atropine to enhance the chronotropic response to arbutamine is not recommended.

Adverse Reactions

Serious events include ventricular and atrial fibrillation and severe cardiac ischemia (see Warnings).

Most Frequent Adverse Reactions with Arbutamine (%)	
Adverse reaction	Incidence (n = 2082)
Tremor	15
Angina pectoris	12
Cardiac arrhythmias	12
Ventricular	6
Supraventricular	4
Headache	9
Hypotension	6
Chest pain	4
Dizziness	4
Dyspnea	4
Palpitation	4
Flushing	3
Hot flushes	3
Nausea	3
Paresthesia	2
Anxiety	1.9
Pain (non-specific)	1.8
Increased sweating	1.5
Fatigue	1.3
Taste perversion	1.3
Dry mouth	1.1
Hypoesthesia	1
Vasodilation	1

Incidence of Arrhythmias with Arbutamine (%)	
Arrhythmia	Incidence (n = 2082)
Total patients experiencing arrhythmias[1]	12
Ventricular	6.2
Ventricular fibrillation	0.1
Ventricular tachycardia	1.8
Other ventricular[2]	5.1
Supraventricular	3.8
Supraventricular tachycardia	1.9
Atrial fibrillation	1
Other supraventricular[3]	1.2
Junctional	0.8
Bradycardia	1.1
Sinus tachycardia	0.9
Heart block[4]	0.1
Sinus arrhythmia	0.05

[1] Patients may have experienced > 1 arrhythmia.
[2] Includes premature ventricular contractions (PVCs), couplets, triplets (rate ≤ 100 bpm), multifocal PVCs, ventricular bigeminy/trigeminy and idioventricular rhythm.
[3] Includes premature atrial contractions and atrial arrhythmias (coronary sinus rhythm).
[4] Includes sinoatrial block and right bundle branch block.

Other adverse events include the following:

➤*Cardiovascular:* ST segment depression (0.6%); hypertension (0.4%); myocardial ischemia (0.1%; see Warnings).

➤*Psychiatric:* Nervousness (0.7%); agitation (0.2%).

➤*Respiratory:* Coughing (0.2%); bronchospasm (0.1%).

➤*Miscellaneous:* Asthenia (0.4%); twitching (0.3%); rash, malaise, rigors (0.2%); back pain/abdominal pain (0.1%); abnormal lacrimation; injection site reaction.

ARBUTAMINE

Overdosage

Because arbutamine delivery is controlled by the *GenESA* device to give a defined increase in HR, overdosage is unlikely to occur. The maximum total dose permitted by the *GenESA* device is 10 mcg/kg. If overdosage occurs, it should be short-lived, as arbutamine is metabolized rapidly, and most effects would be extensions of arbutamine's pharmacologic effects.

➤*Symptoms:* The symptoms of toxicity due to excessive dosing are those of catecholamine excess: Tremor, headache, flushing, hypotension, dizziness, paresthesia, nausea, hot flushes, angina, increased sweating and anxiety. The positive chronotropic and inotropic effects of arbutamine on the myocardium may cause tachyarrhythmias, hypertension, myocardial infarction and ventricular fibrillation. If arbutamine is ingested, unpredictable absorption may occur from the mouth and GI tract.

➤*Treatment:* Initial actions include discontinuing administration, establishing an airway and ensuring adequate oxygenation and ventilation. Severe signs or symptoms (angina, tachyarrhythmias, ST segment abnormalities, hypotension) may be successfully treated with an IV β-blocker. Other treatment, such as sublingual nitrates, should be used if considered clinically appropriate. Given the rapid elimination of arbutamine, forced diuresis, peritoneal dialysis, hemodialysis or charcoal hemoperfusion are unlikely to be required for arbutamine overdosage.

CAPROMAB PENDETIDE

Rx	**ProstaScint** (Cytogen)	**Kit:** Each contains 0.5 mg capromab pendetide/ml of sodium phosphate buffered saline and 1 vial of 82 mg sodium acetate in 2 ml Sterile Water for Injection	Preservative free. Includes 1 sterile 0.22 mcm *Millex GV filter*, prescribing information, and 2 identification labels.

Indications

➤*Prostate cancer:* As a diagnostic imaging agent in newly-diagnosed patients with biopsy-proven prostate cancer, thought to be clinically-localized after standard diagnostic evaluation (eg, chest x-ray, bone scan, CT scan, or MRI), who are at high risk for pelvic lymph node metastases. It is not indicated in patients who are not at high risk.

➤*Post-prostatectomy patients:* As a diagnostic imaging agent in post-prostatectomy patients with a rising PSA and a negative or equivocal standard metastatic evaluation in whom there is a high clinical suspicion of occult metastatic disease. The imagine performance following radiation therapy has not been studied.

Consider the information provided by capromab in conjunction with other diagnostic information. Confirm scans that are positive for metastatic disease histologically in patients who are otherwise candidates for surgery or radiation therapy unless medically contraindicated. Do not use scans that are negative for metastatic disease in lieu of histological confirmation.

It is not indicated as a screening tool for carcinoma of the prostate nor for readministration for assessment of response to treatment.

Administration and Dosage

The patient dose of the radiolabel must be measured in a dose calibrator prior to administration.

The recommended dose of capromab pendetide is 0.5 mg radiolabeled with 5 mCi of Indium In 111 chloride. Each dose is IV administered over 5 minutes. Do not mix with any other medication during its administration. Indium In 111 capromab may be readministered following infiltration or a technically inadequate scan; however, it is not indicated for readministration for assessment of response to treatment.

Each kit is a unit dose package. After radiolabeling with Indium In 111, administer the entire Indium In 111 capromab dose to the patient. Reducing the dose of Indium In 111, unlabeled capromab, or Indium In 111 capromab may adversely impact imaging results and is, therefore, not recommended. Inspect parenteral drug products visually for particulate matter and discoloration prior to administration whenever solution and container permit.

For further dosing information, see kit instructions.

SATUMOMAB PENDETIDE

Rx	**OncoScint CR/OV** (Cytogen)	**Kit:** Each contains 1 mg satumomab pendetide/2 ml sodium phosphate buffered saline and 136 mg sodium acetate trihydrate/2 ml of Sterile Water for Injection.	Preservative free. Includes 0.22 mcm *Millex GV* filter, prescribing information, and 2 identification labels.

Indications

➤*Extrahepatic malignant disease:* As a diagnostic imaging agent for determining the extent and location of extrahepatic malignant disease in patients with known colorectal or ovarian cancer. Clinical studies suggest that this imaging agent should be used after completion of standard diagnostic tests when additional information regarding disease extent could aid in patient management. The diagnostic images acquired with satumomab should be interpreted in conjunction with a review of information obtained from other appropriate tests.

➤*Human antimouse antibody (HAMA)-negative patients:* For readministration to HAMA-negative patients who are at risk of recurrence. Ordering physicians should be aware that HAMA-positive patients have alterations in the biodistribution of the radioimmunoconjugate and in the quality of imaging. Therefore, it is vital that before any repeat use of satumomab, determine HAMA levels in pre-infusion sera. Evaluate the results with respect to the patient's clinical situation and follow the guidelines.

➤*Dose repetition:* Do not repeat satumomab to people whose HAMA levels is > 400 ng/ml because of the possibility of infusional reactions, and uniformly altered biodistribution and poor quality images. In general, if HAMA values are < 50 ng/ml, most subjects will image normally.

Altered biodistribution may occur in 3% to 4% (3/80 samples) of cases for unknown reasons unrelated to HAMA level. If HAMA values are between 50 and 400 ng/ml, there is a higher incidence of subjects who will show altered biodistribution (7/13 samples) and uninformative imaging; in this range the frequency of HAMA interference with imaging has yet to be determined.

Satumomab is not indicated as a screening test for ovarian or colorectal cancer.

Administration and Dosage

The dose of satumomab is 1 mg radiolabeled with 5 mCi of Indium In 111 chloride. Each dose is administered intravenously over 5 minutes and should not be mixed with any other medication during its administration. Measure the patient dose of the radiolabel in a dose calibrator prior to administration.

Each kit is a unit dose package. Administer the entire satumomab dose to the patients after radiolabeling with Indium In 111. Reducing the dose of either component may adversely impact imaging results and is, therefore, not recommended.

For further dosing information, see kit instructions.

CANDIDA ALBICANS SKIN TEST ANTIGEN

| *Rx* | **Candin** (Allermed) | **Injection:** Prepared from the culture filtrate and cells of two strains of *Candida albicans*. | In 1 ml multidose vial. |

Indications

▶*Reduced cellular hypersensitivity:* For use as a recall antigen for detecting delayed-type hypersensitivity (DTH) by intracutaneous (intradermal) testing. The product may be useful in evaluating the cellular immune response in patients suspected of having reduced cellular hypersensitivity. Because some persons with normal cellular immunity are not hypersensitive to *Candida albicans*, a response rate < 100% to the antigen is to be expected in healthy individuals. Therefore, the concurrent use of other licensed DTH skin test antigens is recommended.

▶*HIV:* Antigens of *C. albicans* are useful in the assessment of diminished cellular immunity in persons infected with HIV. Responses to DTH antigens have prognostic value in patients with cancer. Because HIV infection can modify the DTH response to tuberculin, it is advisable to skin test HIV-infected patients at high risk of tuberculosis with antigens in addition to tuberculin, to assess their competency to react to tuberculin. (See Warnings.)

Administration and Dosage

▶*Approved by the FDA:* November 27, 1995.

▶*Test method:* C. albicans skin test antigen is administered intradermally, on the volar surface of the forearm or on the outer aspect of the upper arm. The test dose is 0.1 ml. Cleanse the skin with 70% alcohol before applying the skin test. (See Precautions.)

▶*Interpretation:* A positive DTH reaction consists of induration ≥ 5 mm. The time required for the induration response to reach maximum intensity varies with the individual. The reaction usually begins within 24 hours and peaks between 24 and 48 hours. Read the skin test after 48 hours by visually inspecting the test site and palpating the indurated area. Measure across two diameters. Report the mean of the longest and midpoint diameters of the indurated area as the DTH response. For example, a reaction that is 10 mm (longest diameter) by 8 mm (midpoint orthogonal diameter) has a sum of 18 mm and a mean of 9 mm. The DTH response is therefore 9 mm.

▶*Storage / Stability:* Store between 2° to 8°C (35° to 46°F). Do not freeze.

Actions

▶*Pharmacology:* The potency of *C. albicans* is measured by dose-response skin tests in healthy adults. The procedure involves concurrent (side-by-side) testing of production lots with an internal reference (IR), using sensitive adults who have been previously screened and qualified to serve as test subjects. The induration response at 48 hours elicited by 0.1 ml of a production lot is measured and compared to the response elicited by 0.1 ml of the IR. The test is satisfactory if the potency of the production lot does not differ more than ± 20% from the potency of the IR, when analyzed by the paired t-test.

Cellular or DTH can be assessed by intracutaneous testing with bacterial, viral and fungal antigens to which most healthy persons are sensitized. A positive skin test denotes prior antigenic exposure, T-cell competency and an intact inflammatory response. The reaction usually peaks 48 hours after antigen is introduced into the skin and is manifest as induration at the test site.

Recall antigens may be useful in evaluating DTH by eliciting positive induration reactions 48 to 72 hours after intracutaneous administration. Except for mumps skin test antigen, most commonly used recall antigens were developed for other purposes, and the size of the reaction elicited may not be directly related to cellular immunity because of variability in antigen source and dose and skin test administration and measurement techniques. Useful antigens are those which elicit a reaction size > 5 mm in > 50% of healthy individuals. The combination of results from skin testing with more than one antigen should result in detection of DTH in at least 95% of healthy subjects.

The inflammatory response associated with the DTH reaction is characterized by an infiltration of lymphocytes and macrophages at the site of antigen deposition. Specific cell types that appear to play a major role in the DTH response include CD4+ and CD8+ T-lymphocytes which leave the recirculating lymphocyte pool in response to exogenous antigen. Both CD4+ and CD8+ lymphocytes have been recovered from DTH reactions elicited by *Candida* antigen.

▶*Clinical trials:* The incidence of DTH reactions to unstandardized *Candida* antigens has been reported to vary from 52% to 89%, depending on the strength of the antigen and the mm induration required for a positive test.

In one group of 18 healthy adults, 78% of the individuals reacted to *C. albicans* with an induration response of ≥ 5 mm at 48 hours. In a second study of 35 subjects, 60% had induration reactions > 5 mm at 48 hours. In this study, 65% of males tested positive compared to 53% of females; the mean induration in responding males was 12.8 mm and in responding females was 13 mm. When subjects in these studies were tested with two reagents, *C. albicans* and mumps skin test antigen, 92% were positive to at least one antigen, a higher response rate than to either antigen used alone.

In another study, the skin test responses of adults with HIV infection were compared to those of healthy control subjects. The responses in HIV-infected patients who did not meet the definition of AIDS were less than in uninfected subjects, but the differences were not statistically significant. A significant difference was found between AIDS patients and uninfected controls in both mean induration and proportion with ≥ 5 mm response.

In a related study involving 20 male patients diagnosed with AIDS, one subject responded to *C. albicans*. In this study, 65% of the male control subjects had DTH reactions > 5 mm to *C. albicans*. The mean induration response at 48 hours for control subjects was 8.33 mm, compared to 1.78 mm for the AIDS subjects.

In a published study of DTH anergy, 479 subjects (334 males and 145 females) infected with HIV and being screened for tuberculosis were skin tested with several additional antigens, including *C. albicans*. Only 12% reacted to tuberculin (≥ 5 mm), 57% reacted to *C. albicans* (≥ 3 mm) and 60% reacted to either tuberculin or *C. albicans* or both. In this study, a 3 mm induration response to *C. albicans* was considered positive. In conclusion, HIV-infected subjects, testing with other DTH antigens, increases the accuracy of interpretation of negative tuberculin reactions.

In another study of 18 patients with lung cancer, *C. albicans* elicited a positive induration response in 28%. In a second series of 20 patients with metastatic cancer, no reactions ≥ 5 mm were observed.

Contraindications

History of a previous unacceptable adverse reaction to this antigen or to a similar product (eg, extreme hypersensitivity or allergy).

Warnings

▶*Type I allergy:* The product should not be used to diagnose or treat Type I allergy to *C. albicans*.

▶*Immunodeficiency:* Immunodeficiency states, such as advanced HIV infection or cancer, can modify the DTH response to tuberculin. It may be advisable to skin test patients at high risk of tuberculosis with antigens in addition to tuberculin to confirm the patient's state of cellular immunity.

▶*Local reactions:* Usually subside within hours or days after administration of the skin test. In some patients, skin discoloration may persist for several weeks. Local reactions may be treated with a cold compress and topical steroids. Severe loval reactions may require additional measures as appropriate.

In persons with a bleeding tendency, bruising and non-specific induration may occur due to the trauma of the skin test.

▶*Systemic reactions to C. albicans:* Systemic reactions to *C. albicans* have not been observed. However, all foreign antigens have the remote possibility of causing type I anaphylaxis and even death when injected intradermally. Systemic reactions usually occur within 30 minutes after the injection of antigen.

▶*Hypersensitivity reactions:* As has been observed with other, unstandardized antigens used for DTH skin testing, it is possible that some patients may have exquisite immediate hypersensitivity to *C. albicans*. These reactions are characterized by the presence of an edematous hive surrounded by a zone of erythema. They occur ≈ 15 to 20 minutes after the intradermal injection of the antigen. The size of the immediate reaction varies depending on the sensitivity of the individual. Immediate hypersensitivity reactions have been reported in 17% to 22% of patients, with erythema of 10 to 24 mm in diameter, and in another 5% to 13% of patients, with erythema of 5 to 9 mm. When using this product, have available the facilities and medications necessary to treat all potential local and systemic side effects. Refer to Management of Acute Hypersensitivity Reactions.

▶*Elderly:* C. albicans has not been adequately studied in elderly patients. However, the DTH response to *C. albicans* may be diminished in elderly patients, since the aging process is known to alter cell-mediated immunity.

▶*Pregnancy: Category C.* It is not known whether *C. albicans* can cause fetal harm when administered to a pregnant woman or can affect reproduction capacity. Give to pregnant women only if clearly needed. Problems in pregnancy are unlikely.

▶*Lactation:* It is not known whether *C. albicans* is excreted in breast milk. Problems in breastfeeding are unlikely.

▶*Children:* The safety and efficacy in children has not been established.

Precautions

▶*Route of administration:* Inject the antigen intradermally as superficially as possible causing a distinct, sharply defined bleb at the skin test site. An unreliable reaction may result if the product is injected subcutaneously. It must not be given IV. Do not inject into a blood vessel.

CANDIDA ALBICANS SKIN TEST ANTIGEN

Drug Interactions

➤*Corticosteroids:* Pharmacologic doses of corticosteroids may variably suppress the DTH skin test response after 2 weeks of therapy. The mechanism of suppression is believed to involve a decrease in monocytes and lymphocytes, particularly T-cells. The skin test response usually returns to the pretreatment level within several weeks after steroid therapy is discontinued.

Adverse Reactions

➤*Systemic:* Sneezing; coughing; itching; shortness of breath; abdominal cramps; vomiting; diarrhea; tachycardia; hypotension; respiratory failure. Progression of the delayed reaction to vesiculation, necrosis and ulceration is possible (see Warnings).

➤*Local:* Redness; swelling; bruising; pruritus; excoriation; discoloration of the skin; rash; vesiculation; bullae dermal exfoliation; cellulitis (severe). (See Warnings.)

COCCIDIOIDIN

Rx	**BioCox** (Iatric)	**Injection:** 1:100 w/v	0.01% thimerosal. Mycelial derivative. In 1 ml 10-test multidose vial.
	Spherulin (ALK)		0.01% thimerosal. Spherule derivative. In 1 ml 10-test multidose vial.
Rx	**BioCox** (Iatric)	**Injection:** 1:10 w/v	0.01% thimerosal. Mycelial derivative. In 10-test multidose vial.
	Spherulin (ALK)		0.01% thimerosal. Spherule derivative. In 10-test multidose vial.

Indications

For detection of delayed hypersensitivity to *Coccidioides immitis.* Serves as an aid in the diagnosis of coccidioidomycosis. The skin test is a valuable diagnostic tool to differentiate coccidioidomycosis from the common cold, influenza and other mycotic or bacterial infections (eg, blastomycosis, histoplasmosis, tuberculosis, sarcoidosis).

➤*Unlabeled uses:* In endemic areas (eg, the southwestern US), coccidioidin may be a useful addition to anergy skin-test panels to assess competence of recipients' cell-mediated immunity, but use of mycelial coccidioidin may obscure the results of other fungal assays.

Administration and Dosage

➤*Test method:* Inject 0.1 ml of a 1:100 dilution intradermally on the flexor surface of the forearm. Use a weaker 1:1000 or 1:10,000 dilution if erythema nodosum is evident.

Perform the 1:10 dilution skin test only on persons nonreactive to the 1:100 dilution.

➤*Interpretation:* Consider the following points in interpretation: (1) A positive reaction may cause a transitory rise in titer of complement fixation antibody to histoplasma antigens, but not to coccidioidin; (2) coccidioidin may elicit skin test cross-reactions in individuals infected with *Histoplasma, Blastomyces* and possibly other fungi; (3) coccidioidin may boost level of skin sensitivity to coccidioidin in already sensitive individuals; (4) the skin test may be negative in severe forms of disease (anergy) or when prolonged periods of time have passed since infection.

Positive reaction – Induration of ≥ 5 mm. Erythema without induration is considered negative. Read tests both at 24 and 48 hours because some reactions may fade after 36 hours. A positive test reaction indicates present or past infection with *Coccidioides immitis.*

Negative reaction – A negative test (< 5 mm induration) means the individual has not been sensitized to coccidioidin or has lost sensitivity.

➤*Storage/Stability:* Store at 2° to 8°C (36° to 46°F). Discard if frozen. Product can tolerate 14 days at room temperature. Refrigerate dilutions after compounding and discard within 24 hours.

Actions

➤*Pharmacology:* Positive skin tests result from activation of sensitized T-lymphocytes, a delayed-hypersensitivity reaction involving cellular immunity. Coccidioidin deposited in the skin reacts with sensitized lymphocytes, causing the release of mediators that induce the inflammatory, edematous reaction recognized as a positive reaction. The reaction depends on the person having been previously sensitized to coccidioidin.

Spherule-derived coccidioidin may detect significantly more infected persons than mycelium-derived coccidioidin. Nonetheless, 50% false-negative rates have occurred in patients with disseminated disease. Coccidioidin tests are highly specific, implying that few healthy test recipients will test falsely positive. Mycelium- and spherule-derived products are probably equally specific.

Contraindications

Hypersensitivity to thimerosal; patients with erythema nodosum.

Warnings

➤*Immunodeficiency:* Persons receiving immunosuppressive therapy or with other immunodeficiencies (especially those involving cell-mediated immunity) may have a diminished skin-test response to this and other diagnostic antigens.

➤*Hypersensitivity reactions:* Because of the possibility of an immediate systemic allergic reaction, observe the patient for 15 minutes after the injection. Have epinephrine available in case an acute hypersensitivity reaction occurs. See also Management of Acute Hypersensitivity Reactions.

➤*Pregnancy: Category C.* Use only if clearly needed. It is unlikely that coccidioidin crosses the placenta.

➤*Lactation:* It is not likely that coccidioidin is excreted in breast milk.

➤*Children:* Safety and efficacy of mycelial coccidioidin have not been specifically established in children, but spherule-derived coccidioidin is safe and effective in children, including those < 5 years of age.

Drug Interactions

Coccidioidin Drug Interactions

Precipitant drug	Object drug[a]		Description
Immunosuppressants	Coccidioidin	↑	Reactivity to any delayed-hypersensitivity test may be suppressed in persons receiving corticosteroids or other immunosuppressive drugs, or in persons who were recently immunized with live virus vaccines (eg, measles, mumps, rubella, poliovirus). If delayed-hypersensitivity skin testing is indicated, perform it either preceding or simultaneous with immunization or 4 to 6 weeks after immunization.
Cimetidine	Coccidioidin	↑	Several weeks of cimetidine therapy may augment or enhance delayed-hypersensitivity responses to skin test antigens, although this effect was not consistently observed. The effect may be mediated through cimetidine binding to suppressor T-lymphocytes.

[a] ↑ = Object drug increased.

➤*Drug/Lab test interactions:* A positive reaction to *BioCox* may cause a rise in titers of complement-fixing antibodies against *Emmonsiella capsulata (Histoplasma capsulatum)* and coccidioidin. Unlike *BioCox, Spherulin* does not induce humoral antibodies nor does it affect complement-fixation titers for either histoplasmosis or coccidioidomycosis. Either coccidioidin may boost existing hypersensitivity in recipients, manifested after a subsequent test.

Adverse Reactions

➤*Local:* An occasional patient may develop an immediate local wheal reaction. Occasionally, large local reactions may lead to vesiculation, local tissue necrosis and scar formation.

➤*Systemic:* Patients with great sensitivity may rarely develop a systemic reaction consisting of fever or erythema nodosum. There are no reports that skin testing can cause a recrudescence of the disease.

HISTAMINE PHOSPHATE

Rx	Histatrol (Center Laboratories)	Scratch/Prick: 1 mg/ml histamine base as the phosphate (2.75 mg/ml histamine phosphate)	Glycerin 50% w/v, 0.4% phenol. In 5 ml vials.
		Multi-Test: 1 mg/ml histamine base as the phosphate	Glycerin 50% w/v. In 5 ml vials.
		Intradermal: 0.1 mg/ml histamine base as the phosphate (0.275 mg/ml histamine phosphate)	Glycerin free. 0.4% phenol. In 5 ml vials.

Indications

➤*Allergenic skin testing:* For use as a positive control in evaluation of allergenic skin testing.

Administration and Dosage

➤*Interpretation:* The patient's response is based on the size of erythema (degree of redness) and size of wheal (smooth, slightly elevated area) which appear after 15 to 20 minutes.

Prick, puncture, and scratch testing – Use histamine base 1 mg/ml (histamine phosphate 2.75 mg/ml) to give a positive reaction. In a large population, the NHANES II survey reports a mean (average of length and width) wheal of 4.4 mm and a mean erythema of 18.4 mm. Interpret all positive reactions against an appropriate negative control.

Intradermal skin testing – Use histamine base 0.1 mg/ml (histamine phosphate 0.275 mg/ml) or 0.01 mg/ml to give a positive reaction. In 2 successive years of testing, the Committee on Standardization of the American College of Allergy reported positive reactions at histamine base doses ≥ 0.01 mg/ml. Mean sum of diameter (sum of length and width) of wheals were ≈ 14 mm and sum of erythema was ≈ 52 mm following 0.01 ml intradermal doses of 0.01 mg/ml histamine base. When 0.01 ml of 0.1 mg/ml histamine base was injected, the sum of crossed diameters of wheal ranged from 15 to 20 mm and the sum of crossed diameters of erythema ranged from 60 to 80 mm. The available 0.1 mg/ml concentration must be diluted to achieve this dose. Interpret all positive reactions against an appropriate negative control.

➤*Storage/Stability:* Refrigerate and protect vials from light.

Actions

➤*Pharmacology:* Histamine acts as a potent vasodilator when released from mast cells during an allergic reaction. It is largely responsible for the immediate skin test reaction of a sensitive patient when challenged with an offending allergen.

Contraindications

Do not inject histamine into individuals with hypotension, severe hypertension, or severe cardiac, pulmonary, or renal disease.

Warnings

➤*Intracutaneous testing:* Use caution in intracutaneous testing to avoid injection into a venule or capillary.

➤*Bronchial disease:* Small doses by any route of administration may precipitate asthma in patients with bronchial disease.

➤*Hypersensitivity reactions:* Epinephrine injection (1:1000) and injectable antihistamines should be available for immediate use in the event the patient exhibits a severe response. A tourniquet can be applied above the test site to slow absorption if a severe response occurs.

➤*Pregnancy: Category C.* There are no adequate and well-controlled studies in pregnant women. However, based on histamine's known ability to contract uterine muscle, avoid exposure or repeated doses. Use histamine phosphate during pregnancy only if the potential benefit justifies the potential risk to the fetus or mother.

➤*Children:* Histamine solutions for percutaneous testing have been given safely in infants and young children. Therefore, anticipate small skin test reactions in children < 6 years of age. Safety and efficacy for intracutaneous testing in children < 6 years of age have not been established.

Drug Interactions

➤*Antiallergic drugs:* In the period of 24 hours prior to testing, the patient should not have taken any antiallergic drugs. The pharmacologic action of such agents interferes with the skin test response.

Adverse Reactions

Following the injection of large doses of histamine, systemic reactions may include flushing, dizziness, headache, bronchial constriction, urticaria, asthma, marked hypertension or hypotension, abdominal cramps, vomiting, metallic taste, and local or generalized allergic manifestations.

Overdosage

➤*Symptoms:* A large SC dose of histamine phosphate may cause severe occipital headache, blurred vision, anginal pain, a rapid drop in blood pressure, and cyanosis of the face.

➤*Treatment:* Give epinephrine injection SC or IM in case of emergency due to severe reactions (see Warnings). An antihistamine preparation may be given IM to ameliorate systemic reaction to overdose.

HISTOPLASMIN

Rx	Histoplasmin, Diluted (Parke-Davis)	Injection: 1:100 w/v (P-D) or v/v (ALK). Standardized sterile filtrate from cultures of *Histoplasma capsulatum*	0.5% phenol, polysorbate 80. Mycelial derivative. In 1 ml, 10 test multidose vials.
Rx	Histolyn-CYL (ALK Labs)		0.4% phenol, polysorbate 80, human serum albumin. Controlled yeast lysate. In 1.3 ml multidose vials.

Indications

An aid in diagnosing histoplasmosis, in detecting delayed hypersensitivity to *Histoplasma capsulatum* and in differentiating possible histoplasmosis from coccidioidomycosis, sarcoidosis and other mycotic or bacterial infections, and in interpreting x-rays showing pulmonary infiltration and calcification. It may also be useful in epidemiological studies of persons with exposure to histoplasmosis and other infectious diseases.

➤*Unlabeled uses:* In endemic areas (eg, the Ohio and Mississippi River valleys), histoplasmin may be a useful addition to anergy skin test panels to assess competence of recipients' cell-mediated immunity, but use of mycelial histoplasmin may obscure the results of other fungal assays.

Administration and Dosage

Inject intradermally only.

The two forms of histoplasmin are generically inequivalent. Mycelial histoplasmin is more likely to boost complement-fixing antibody titers than yeast-lysate histoplasmin.

➤*Test method:* Inject 0.1 ml intradermally into the flexor surface of the forearm. Use a tuberculin syringe and a 26-gauge, 3/8 inch or 27-gauge, 1/2 inch needle. If correctly injected, a small bleb will rise over the needle point. Read reactions 48 to 72 hours after injection. The usual delayed skin test reaction appears in 24 hours and reaches a maximum in 48 to 72 hours.

➤*Interpretation:* Describe and measure the reaction in terms of millimeters of induration and degree of reaction (from slight induration to vesiculation and necrosis). A reaction of ≥ 5 mm induration is positive. In case of doubt and if clinically indicated, repeat the test only after obtaining serum for antibody titer.

Positive reaction – May indicate a past infection or a mild, subacute or chronic infection with *H. capsulatum* or immunologically related organisms, such as *Blastomyces* or *Coccidioides* species. It may also denote improvement in cases of serious illness of symptomatic histoplasmosis that previously may have been histoplasmin-negative.

Differential diagnosis – Histoplasmin is of little value in diagnosing acute fulminating infections because a negative reaction usually occurs. In mild infections, repeatedly negative reactions may suggest the exclusion of *Histoplasma* as the causative agent. Employ the tuberculin test in conjunction with histoplasmin to exclude the possibility of tuberculosis. The histoplasmin skin test sometimes causes elevation of serum antibody titers to histoplasmin.

To distinguish lesions associated with histoplasmin sensitivity from other causes, consider: (1) Skin sensitivity to histoplasmin but not tuberculin; (2) lesions must persist for 2 months (to exclude transient pneumonic lesions); and (3) laboratory and clinical examinations to exclude tuberculosis, Boeck's sarcoid, sarcoidosis, Hodgkin's disease, etc. These criteria may help interpret roentgenographic findings.

➤*Storage/Stability:* Store at 2° to 8°C (36° to 46°F).

Actions

➤*Pharmacology:* Positive skin tests result from activation of sensitized T-lymphocytes, a delayed-hypersensitivity reaction involving cellular immunity. Histoplasmin antigens deposited in the skin react with sensitized lymphocytes, causing the release of mediators that induce the inflammatory, edematous reaction recognized as a positive reaction. The reaction depends on the person having been previously sensitized to histoplasmin.

The sensitivity of mycelial histoplasmin is not described, but some infected test recipients will test falsely negative. Yeast-lysate histoplasmin tests are 83% sensitive, implying that 17% of infected test recipients will test falsely negative. Most patients with acute or chronic

HISTOPLASMIN

pulmonary histoplasmosis react positively to the test. However in critically ill people or those with disseminated disease, the frequency of positive reactions falls to about 50%. In epidemic histoplasmosis, the rate of positive reactions may approach 100%.

The specificity of mycelial histoplasmin is not described, but some uninfected test recipients will test falsely positive. Mycelial histoplasmin may cross-react and yield false-positive responses to *Blastomyces, Coccidioides* and related fungi. Yeast-lysate histoplasmin tests are highly specific, implying that few uninfected test recipients will test falsely positive.

Warnings

➤*Immunodeficiency:* Persons receiving immunosuppressive therapy or with other immunodeficiencies (especially those involving cell-mediated immunity) may have a diminished skin-test response to this and other diagnostic antigens.

➤*Hypersensitivity reactions:* Have epinephrine immediately available in case an anaphylactoid or acute hypersensitivity reaction occurs. See also Management of Acute Hypersensitivity Reactions.

Do not administer histoplasmin to known histoplasmin-positive reactors because of the severity of reactions (eg, vesiculation, ulceration, necrosis) that may occur at the test site in very highly hypersensitive individuals.

➤*Pregnancy: Category C.* Use only if clearly needed. It is unlikely that histoplasmin crosses the placenta.

➤*Lactation:* It is unlikely that histoplasmin is excreted in breast milk.

➤*Children:* Safety and efficacy of mycelial histoplasmin have not been established, but yeast-lysate histoplasmin has been routinely administered to children with no special safety problems noted.

Precautions

➤*Monitoring:* If serological studies are indicated, draw the blood sample prior to administering the skin test or within 48 to 96 hours following the skin-test injection. After this time period, a rise in titer associated with a positive skin test may occur.

➤*Local reactions:* Greater than recommended doses (eg, > 0.1 ml) may produce severe erythema and induration followed by necrosis and ulceration that may last for several weeks.

Drug Interactions

Histoplasmin Drug Interactions

Precipitant drug	Object drug[a]		Description
Cimetidine	Histoplasmin	↑	Several weeks of cimetidine therapy may augment or enhance delayed-hypersensitivity responses to skin test antigens, although this effect was not consistently observed. The effect may be mediated through cimetidine binding to suppressor T-lymphocytes.
Immunosuppressants Vaccines, virus	Histoplasmin	↓	Reactivity to any delayed-hypersensitivity test may be suppressed in persons receiving corticosteroids or other immunosuppressive drugs, or in persons who were recently immunized with live virus vaccines (eg, measles, mumps, rubella, poliovirus). If delayed-hypersensitivity skin testing is indicated, perform it either preceding or simultaneously with immunization or 4 to 6 weeks after immunization.

[a] ↑ = Object drug increased.   ↓ = Object drug decreased.

Adverse Reactions

➤*Local:* In highly sensitive individuals, vesiculation, ulceration or necrosis may occur at the test site and may result in scarring. Cold packs or topical steroids may provide symptomatic relief of the associated pain, pruritus and discomfort.

➤*Hypersensitivity:* Urticaria, angioedema, shortness of breath and excessive perspiration (see Warnings).

MUMPS SKIN TEST ANTIGEN (MSTA)

Rx	**MSTA** (Pasteur-Mérieux Connaught)	**Injection:** 40 complement-fixing units/ml	0.012 M glycine, < 1:8000 formaldehyde solution, and 1:10,000 thimerosal. In 1 ml vials (10 tests).

Indications

➤*Delayed hypersensitivity testing:* For detection of delayed hypersensitivity to mumps antigens and assessment of cell-mediated immunity. Because most of the population (except the very young) have had contact or infection with mumps virus, they usually demonstrate a delayed cutaneous hypersensitivity to mumps skin test antigen if an adequate cellular immune system exists; 67% to 90% of healthy adults demonstrate a delayed hypersensitivity reaction.

Administration and Dosage

Must be given intradermally. If it is injected SC, no reaction or an unreliable reaction may occur.

➤*Test method:* Shake vial well before withdrawing each dose. Inject 0.1 ml intradermally on the inner surface of the forearm after suitable preparation of the skin. Examine the reaction in 48 to 72 hours.

➤*Interpretation:* Positive reaction consists of a mean diameter of induration ≥ 5 mm (ie, the average of the longest width and the longest length). A positive test implies previous antigenic exposure and, indirectly, T-lymphocyte competence and an intact inflammatory response, and confirms the integrity of the cellular immune response.

➤*Negative reaction:* If the test has been given correctly, it probably indicates either anergy or nonsensitivity.

➤*Pseudopositive reactions:* May develop in persons sensitive to egg protein.

➤*Storage/Stability:* Store between 2° and 8°C (36° to 46°F). Discard if frozen. Product can tolerate ≤ 4 days at ≤ 37°C (100°F). Do not freeze.

Actions

➤*Pharmacology:* Positive skin tests result from activation of sensitized T-lymphocytes, a delayed-hypersensitivity reaction involving cellular immunity. MSTA deposited in the skin reacts with sensitized lymphocytes, causing the release of mediators that induce the inflammatory, edematous reaction recognized as a positive reaction. The reaction depends on the person having been previously sensitized to mumps.

When used to assess delayed hypersensitivity reactivity in a group of 90 cancer patients, MSTA was essentially 100% sensitive (as confirmed by reaction to at least 1 other delayed hypersensitivity test antigen), implying that no immunocompetent test recipients would test falsely negative.

Contraindications

Generally, do not administer this product to anyone with a history of hypersensitivity, especially anaphylactic reactions, to eggs, egg products, or thimerosal.

Warnings

➤*Immunodeficiency:* Persons receiving immunosuppressive therapy or with other immunodeficiencies (especially those involving cell-mediated immunity) may have a diminished skin-test response to this and other diagnostic antigens. Tuberculosis, bacterial or viral infection, malnutrition, malignancy, and immunosuppression may suppress skin-test responsiveness.

➤*Hypersensitivity reactions:* Mumps skin test antigen is propagated in eggs and also contains thimerosal as a preservative. Do not administer to anyone with a history of hypersensitivity (allergy) to eggs, egg products, or thimerosal. Epinephrine injection (1:1000) must be immediately available to combat unexpected anaphylactic or other allergic reactions. See also Management of Acute Hypersensitivity Reactions.

➤*Elderly:* Skin-test responsiveness may be delayed or reduced in magnitude in older people.

➤*Pregnancy: Category C.* It is unlikely that MSTA crosses the placenta. It is not known whether MSTA can cause fetal harm when administered to a pregnant woman or can affect reproductive capacity. Give to a pregnant woman only if clearly needed.

➤*Lactation:* It is unlikely that MSTA is excreted into breast milk. It is not known whether this drug is excreted in human milk. Exercise caution when MSTA is administered to a nursing women.

➤*Children:* Safety and efficacy in children have not been established.

Precautions

➤*Mumps:* MSTA was initially used to determine susceptibility to mumps. It is no longer considered effective for identifying immunity to mumps virus infection. Safety and efficacy have not been established in young adults who have been immunized with live mumps vaccine.

MUMPS SKIN TEST ANTIGEN (MSTA)

Drug Interactions

Mumps Skin-Test Antigen Drug Interactions

Precipitant drug	Object drug[a]		Description
Cimetidine	MSTA	↑	Several weeks of cimetidine therapy may augment or enhance delayed hypersensitivity responses to skin-test antigens, although this effect was not consistently observed. The effect may be mediated through cimetidine binding to suppressor T-lymphocytes.
Immunosuppressants	MSTA	↓	Reactivity to any delayed hypersensitivity test may be suppressed in people receiving corticosteroids or other immunosuppressive drugs, or in people who were recently immunized with live virus vaccines (eg, measles, mumps, rubella, poliovirus). If delayed hypersensitivity skin testing is indicated, perform it either preceding or simultaneously with immunization, or 4 to 6 weeks after immunization.
Vaccines, viral	MSTA		

[a] ↑ = Object drug increased.   ↓ = Object drug decreased.

Adverse Reactions

Local reactions may include tenderness, pruritus, vesiculation, and rash. Sloughing, necrosis, abscess formation, or regional lymphadenopathy may be associated with unusually large delayed hypersensitivity reactions. Adverse reactions may include nausea, anorexia, headache, unsteadiness, drowsiness, sweating, sensation of warmth, and lymphadenopathy.

Indications

►*Diagnostic:* For the evaluation of general immune competence or to determine sensitivity to a particular antigen. See individual agents for specific indications.

Actions

►*Pharmacology:* Delayed hypersensitivity skin testing with multiple antigens is a tool used to determine patients' sensitivity to various antigens or to determine general cellular immune competence. Immunocompetent patients who have previously been exposed to or have a history of sensitivity to antigens represented in the skin test antigen panel will normally exhibit a cutaneous delayed hypersensitivity immune response (Type IV) resulting in inflammation with erythema and itching at the site of application. Negative responses imply either immunologic incompetence (anergy) or no previous exposure.

Following primary contact, the antigen binds to epidermal Langerhans cells and is processed and presented to helper T-lymphocytes (T-cells). Circulating T-cells react with the antigens and induce a specific immune response which includes mitosis (blastogenesis) and the release of many soluble mediators (lymphokines) including interleukin-2. Interleukin-2 stimulates the production of other lymphocytes, chemotactic factors that recruit macrophages, basophils, eosinophils, and migration inhibitory factor. The resulting inflammation produces a papular, vesicular, or bullous response with erythema and itching at the site of application. A positive response normally appears within 9 to 96 hours; however, the intensity of the inflammation usually reaches its peak 24 to 72 hours after antigen application and resolves within a few days to a couple of weeks.

Reactivity to skin test antigens derived from microorganisms may decrease or disappear temporarily as a result of febrile illness, bacterial or viral infections, or live virus vaccination. Malnutrition, malignancy, and immunosuppression induced by drug therapy or other immunodeficiences may suppress responsiveness to delayed-type hypersensitivity skin test antigens.

Contraindications

Application on acneiform, infected, or inflamed skin; use of any antigen in patients with a history of systemic reaction to that antigen.

Warnings

►*Hypersensitivity reactions:* Carefully evaluate any patient with a known history of severe systemic or local reaction to any of the antigen components or inactive substances. Although severe systemic reactions are rare, do not use any antigen in patients with a history of systemic reactions to that antigen. Patients extremely sensitive to specific antigens may exhibit extreme reactions that may be bullous or ulcerative with pronounced erythema, infiltration, and coalescing vesicles. Have epinephrine available in case of severe reactions. Refer to General Management of Acute Hypersensitivity Reactions.

►*Carcinogenesis:* Some products contain antigens derived from substances which are known or suspected carcinogens including nickel refinery dust, nickel sulfite, and formaldehyde (known carcinogens); and nickel sulfate, potassium dichromate, cobalt dichloride, epoxy resin, and thiuram mix (suspected carcinogens). The potential effects of using very low concentrations of these substances for single or multiple applications are currently unknown.

►*Pregnancy: Category C.* It is not known whether skin test antigens can cause fetal harm when administered to a pregnant woman or can affect reproductive capacity. Pregnancy may result in a decreased level of sensitivity to the test antigens. Use in a pregnant woman only if clearly needed.

►*Lactation:* It is not known, but is unlikely that skin test antigens appear in breast milk. Use caution when administering to a nursing woman.

►*Children:* The safety and efficacy of skin test antigens in children have not been established.

Precautions

►*Immunodeficiency:* People receiving immunosuppressive therapy may have a diminished skin test response (see Drug Interactions). Certain medical conditions (eg, malnutrition, malignancy, diabetes mellitus, uremia, acquired immune deficiency disorders) can also contribute to immunodeficiency and may suppress skin test responsiveness.

Febrile illness, tuberculosis, bacterial or viral infection, or live virus vaccination may decrease or hinder responsiveness to skin test antigens derived from microorganisms.

Drug Interactions

Medications or procedures which may induce an immunodeficient state and decrease reactivity include corticosteroids, chemotherapeutic agents, antilymphocyte globulin, and irradiation.

Adverse Reactions

Adverse reactions are normally mild and usually occur only at the site of test application. Vesiculation, ulceration, or necrosis at the test site may occur in highly sensitive subjects. Systemic reactions may occur in patients highly sensitive to allergenic components. Development of a severe test reaction may be treated with a topical corticosteroid or, in rare cases, with a systemic corticosteroid; have epinephrine available for serious systemic reactions.

Adverse events reported in patients being tested with multiple skin test antigens (patch testing) for the diagnosis of contact dermatitis included erythema, hyperpigmentation, pruritus, scarring, and urticaria.

Patient Information

Inform patients of the types of test site reactions that may be expected. Itching and burning may be severe in extremely sensitive patients.

ALLERGEN PATCH TESTING

| Rx | T.R.U.E. Test (GlaxoWellcome) | Allergen-containing patches. In multipack cartons (5s). |

For additional information, refer to the Skin Test Antigens, Multiple Introduction.

Indications

►*Contact dermatitis:* Primarily as an aid in the diagnosis of allergic contact dermatitis in patients whose histories suggest sensitivity to ≥ 1 of the substances included on the test panels. May also be used adjunctively to evaluate other eczemas (atopic, seborrheic, venous, palmar, and plantar hyperkeratotic eczema, vesiculosis, or neurodermatitis) and other dermatologic diseases that do not heal, such as leg ulcers and psoriasis, to determine whether there may be a contact hypersensitivity component.

Administration and Dosage

The test is best applied on the upper part of the back. Apply to healthy skin that is free of acne, scars, dermatitis, or any other condition that may interfere with interpretation of test results. Discontinue use of topical steroids on the test site or oral steroids (equivalent to ≥ 15 mg prednisolone) for ≥ 2 weeks prior to testing. Topical steroids on nontest areas may be appropriate. Instruct patients to avoid extreme physical activity or mechanical action that may result in reduced adhesion or loss of patch test material. Avoid getting the area around the patch wet. Minimize exposure to the sun in order to prevent a sun-induced skin reaction that may interfere with interpretation of test results. Older patients may exhibit an increased frequency of cutaneous allergies.

►*Application:* Apply patches taken directly from the refrigerator or allow them to come to room temperature (15 to 20 minutes) prior to application. Remove protective plastic covering from test panel 1.1. Position the allergen patch test on the upper left side of the patient's back (≈ 5 cm from the midline) so that #1 allergen is in the upper left corner. Avoid applying on the margin of the scapula; smooth outward toward the edges. With a medical marking pen, indicate on the skin the location of the 2 notches on the panel.

Repeat the process with test panel 2.1 on the upper right side of the patient's back so that #13 allergen is in the upper left corner. Have the patient wear the patch test for a minimum of 48 hours.

►*Interpretation:* A positive test reaction should meet the criteria for an allergic reaction (papular or vesicular erythema and infiltration).

The reaction should be read at 72 to 96 hours, when allergic reactions are fully developed and mild irritant reactions have faded. If reading at 48 hours is considered, another reading at 72 to 96 hours is recommended. Advise patients to report reactions occurring after 7 days to detect potential sensitizations. Note that p-phenylenediamine may turn the patch test area black on some patients. This is because the allergen is a dye and does not represent an allergic reaction. Discoloration may remain for approximately ≤ 2 weeks.

Neomycin sulfate and p-phenylenediamine sometimes cause reactions that may not appear until 4 or 5 days (or later) after the application. Instruct patients to report this. An additional office visit will verify a late reaction.

False negatives – False-negative results may be caused by insufficient patch contact with the skin, sensitization to a substance not present in the test panel, or premature evaluation of the test.

False positives – A false-positive result may occur when an irritant reaction (patchy follicular or homogeneous erythema without infiltration) cannot be differentiated from an allergic reaction. If an irritant reaction cannot be distinguished, a retest may be considered in a few weeks or months.

A test reaction that appears 7 days or later with no preceding reaction may be a sign of contact sensitization.

Dermatitis flare up may occur in some patients. Excited skin syndrome (angry back) consists of a hyperreactive state of the skin in which false-positive patch test reactions concur with dermatitis at a distant body site or with adjacent strong positive skin test reactions. On rare occa-

ALLERGEN PATCH TESTING

sions, it may be necessary to remove the test strip from the patient because of severe itching or burning sensations.

Evaluate test results carefully in patients with multiple, positive, concomitant patch test results. To determine false positives, retesting at a later date may be considered.

➤*Storage / Stability:* Store between 2° and 8°C (36° and 46°F).

Actions

➤*Pharmacology:* The patch test system contains 23 of the most common allergens suspected of causing allergic contact dermatitis and a negative control. They represent ≈ 80% of the most common allergens. Nickel sulfate normally induces the greatest number of positive patch test responses when screening prospective patients.

The allergens are homogenized in ≥ 1 of the following materials to produce the allergen films that coat the patches: Hydroxypropyl cellulose, methylcellulose, polyvidone, and β-cyclodextrin. Butylhydroxyanisole (BHA) and butylhydroxytoluene (BHT) have been added to the colophony patch. No other excipients are used. Panel 1.1 chemical allergen components include the following: Nickel sulfate; wool alcohols (lanolin); neomycin sulfate; potassium dichromate; caine mix (benzocaine, tetracaine HCl, dibucaine HCl); fragrance mix (geraniol, cinnamaldehyde, hydroxycit-ronellal, cinnamyl alcohol, eugenol, isoeugenol, α-amylcinnamaldehyde, and oak moss); colophony (from the resin of pine trees); paraben mix (5 ester derivatives of parahydroxybenzoic acid); negative control (uncoated polyester patch); balsam of Peru; ethylenediamine dihydrochloride; cobalt dichloride. The chemical allergens of panel 2.2 include the following: P-tert-butylphenol formaldehyde resin; epoxy resin; carba mix (diphenylguanidine, zincdibutyldithiocarbamate, zincdiethyldithiocarbamate); black rubber mix (paraphenylenediamine derivatives); Cl+ Me-isothiazolinone; quaternium-15; mercaptobenzothiazole; p-phenylenediamine (a blue-black aniline dye); formaldehyde; mercapto mix (3 benzothiazole sulfenamide derivatives); thimerosal (a preservative that contains mercury); thiuram mix (tetramethylthiuram monosulfide, tetramethylthiuram disulfide, disulfiram, dipentamethylenethiuram disulfide).

The frequency of positive responses to the various allergens can change depending on the specific patient population as well as occupational and environmental influences.

Contraindications

Extensive ongoing contact dermatitis.

TUBERCULIN PURIFIED PROTEIN DERIVATIVE (Mantoux; PPD; Tuberculin skin test [TST])

Rx	**Aplisol** (Monarch)	Injection: 5 TU[a]/0.1 mL	In 1 mL (10 tests) and 5 mL (50 tests) vials.[b]
Rx	**Tubersol** (Aventis Pasteur)		In 1 mL (10 tests) and 5 mL (50 tests) vials.[c]

[a] TU = tuberculin units.
[b] With potassium and sodium phosphates, 0.35% phenol, and polysorbate 80.
[c] In isotonic phosphate buffer saline with 0.28% phenol and polysorbate 80.

Indications

➤*Tuberculosis (TB):* Skin test to aid in the diagnosis of TB infection with or without a history of BCG vaccination.

The 5 tuberculin units (TU) dose of tuberculin PPD intradermally (Mantoux) is recommended as the standard tuberculin test, and tuberculin PPD is recommended by the American Lung Association as an aid in the detection of infection with *Mycobacterium tuberculosis*.

Administration and Dosage

The purified protein fraction is isolated from culture filtrates of a human strain of *M. tuberculosis*.

Take special care to ensure the product is given intradermally and on the volar (flexor) aspect of the forearm. Do not administer IV, IM, or SC.

Tuberculin reactivity may indicate prior infection or disease with *M. tuberculosis* and does not necessarily indicate the presence of active TB disease. Evaluate individuals showing tuberculin reactions considered positive by current guidelines by other diagnostic means, such as x-ray examination of the chest and microbiological examination of the sputum.

➤*Test method:* The recommended test dose is 0.1 mL injected intradermally into the volar (flexor) surface of the forearm with a 1 mL syringe calibrated in tenths and fitted with a short, ¼ to ½ inch, 26- or 27-gauge needle.

Insert the point of the needle into the epidermal (most superficial) layers of the skin with the needle bevel pointing upward. If performed properly, a definite pale bleb will rise at the needle point, about 10 mm in diameter. The bleb will disperse within minutes. If the injection was performed improperly, (ie, no bleb formed), then repeat the test immediately at least 5 cm (2 in) from the first site.

➤*Interpretation:* Read 48 to 72 hours after administration. Measure the diameter of the induration transversely to the long axis of the forearm and record in millimeters. Disregard any erythema. Interpret the reaction as follows:

Positive – An induration of at least 5 mm is classified as positive for people who have human immunodeficiency virus (HIV) infection or risk factors of HIV infection but unknown HIV status; those who have had recent close contact with people who have active TB; or people who have fibrotic chest radiographs consistent with healed TB.

An induration of at least 10 mm is classified as positive for all people who do not meet any of the criteria above but have other risk factors for TB (high-risk groups and high prevalence groups, as defined by the CDC).

An induration of greater than or equal to 15 is considered positive in people who do not meet any of the above criteria.

Recent conversion –
  Less than 35 years of age: An increase of at least 10 mm within a 2-year period.
  Greater than or equal to 35 years of age: An increase of at least 15 mm within a 2-year period.

Inconclusive – Induration of 5 to 9 mm. Retest using a different injection site. In the case of known contacts, interpret an induration measuring 5 mm or even smaller as positive. Rule out cross-reaction from other mycobacterial infection.

➤*Retesting:* Any individual who does not show a positive reaction to an initial injection of 5 TU or a second test with 5 TU may be considered as tuberculin negative.

➤*Storage/Stability:* Store at 2° to 8°C (35° to 46°F). Do not freeze. Discard product if exposed to freezing. Tuberculin solutions can be adversely affected by exposure to light. Store this product in the dark except when doses are actually being withdrawn from the vial.

Discard vials in use for more than 30 days because of possible oxidation and degradation that may affect potency.

Actions

➤*Pharmacology:* The reaction to intradermally injected tuberculin is a delayed (cellular) hypersensitivity reaction. The reaction, which characteristically shows a delayed course, reaching its peak more than 48 to 72 hours after administration, consists of induration caused by cellular infiltration of lymphocytes. Clinically, a delayed hypersensitivity reaction to tuberculin is a manifestation of previous infection with *M. tuberculosis* or a variety of non-TB bacteria. Sensitization may be induced by natural mycobacterial infection or by vaccination with BCG vaccine.

The sensitization following infection with mycobacteria occurs primarily in the regional lymph nodes. Small lymphocytes (T lymphocytes) proliferate in response to the antigenic stimulus to give rise to specifically sensitized lymphocytes. After about 6 weeks, these lymphocytes enter the blood stream and circulate for years. Subsequent restimulation of these sensitized lymphocytes with the same or a similar antigen,

such as the intradermal injection of tuberculin, evokes a local reaction caused by infiltration of these cells.

Characteristically, delayed hypersensitivity reactions to tuberculin begin at 5 to 6 hours, are maximal at 48 to 72 hours, and subside over a period of days. Immediate hypersensitivity (allergic) reactions to tuberculin or to constituents of the diluent also may occur, but these allergic reactions have no diagnostic importance.

In geriatric patients or in patients receiving a tuberculin skin test for the first time, the reaction may develop more slowly and may not be maximal until after 72 hours. Because their immune systems are immature, many neonates and infants less than 6 weeks of age who are infected with *M. tuberculosis* do not react at all to tuberculin tests.

Contraindications

Hypersensitivity to tuberculin PPD or any component of the formulation; tuberculin-positive reactors (see Warnings).

Warnings

➤*Tuberculin positive reactors:* Do not administer to known tuberculin-positive reactors because of the severity of reactions (eg, vesiculation, ulceration, necrosis) that may occur at the test site.

➤*HIV infection:* Because tuberculin skin test results are less reliable as CD4 counts decline in HIV-infected individuals, complete screening as early as possible after HIV infection occurs. Periodically screen those HIV-infected patients at high risk for continuing exposure to TB-patients for TB infection. If they have TB symptoms or if they are exposed to a patient who has pulmonary TB, promptly evaluate HIV-infected people for TB. Because active disease can develop rapidly in HIV-infected people, give the highest priority for contact investigation to people potentially coinfected with HIV and TB.

➤*SC injection:* Avoid injecting SC. If this occurs, a general febrile reaction or acute inflammation around old tuberculous lesions may occur in sensitive individuals and no local reaction will develop; the test cannot be interpreted.

➤*Immunodeficiency:* Skin test responsiveness may be suppressed during or for as much as 6 weeks following viral infection, live viral vaccination, miliary or pulmonary TB infection, bacterial infection, severe febrile illness, malnutrition, sarcoidosis, malignancy, or immunosuppression (eg, corticosteroids or other immunosuppressive pharmacotherapy). In most patients who are very sick with TB, a previously negative tuberculin test becomes positive after a few weeks of chemotherapy. When of diagnostic importance, accept a negative test as proof that hypersensitivity is absent only after normal reactivity to common antigens has been demonstrated, such as with an anergy test panel.

➤*Hypersensitivity reactions:* Have epinephrine immediately available. See also Management of Acute Hypersensitivity Reactions.

➤*Pregnancy: Category C* (Tuberculin). Animal reproduction studies have not been conducted. However, the Advisory Council for Elimination of Tuberculosis states that tuberculin skin testing is considered valid and safe throughout pregnancy. No teratogenic effects of testing during pregnancy have been documented.

The risk of unrecognized TB and the close postpartum contact between a mother with active disease and an infant leaves the infant in grave danger of TB and complications such as tuberculous meningitis. Therefore, the prescribing physician should consider if the potential benefits outweigh the possible risks for performing the tuberculin test on a pregnant woman or a woman of childbearing age, particularly in certain high-risk populations.

➤*Children:* There is no age contraindication of tuberculin skin testing of infants. Because their immune systems are immature, many infants under 6 weeks of age who are infected with *M. tuberculosis* do not react to the tuberculin test. Older infants and children develop tuberculin sensitivity 6 weeks or more after initial infection. Very young children are at increased risk for active TB once infected; therefore, during contact investigations, give priority with regard to skin testing and evaluation for preventive therapy to infants and young children who have been exposed to people with active TB. Give these children preventive therapy if their reactions to a tuberculin skin test measure 5 mm or more. A cutoff of 10 mm is appropriate for children where TB case rates are high. A cutoff of 15 mm is used for children with minimal risk exposure to TB.

Precautions

➤*Active TB:* Administer the tuberculin skin test with caution, or not at all, in people with documented active TB or documented treatment in the past because of the severity of reactions (eg, vesiculation, ulceration, necrosis) that may occur at the test site.

➤*Altered reactivity:* Reactivity to the test may be depressed or suppressed for as long as 5 to 6 weeks in individuals who have received

TUBERCULIN PURIFIED PROTEIN DERIVATIVE
(Mantoux; PPD; Tuberculin skin test [TST])

recent immunization with certain live virus vaccines (ie, measles, mumps, rubella, oral polio, yellow fever, varicella), who have had viral infections (eg, rubeola, influenza, mumps), or who are receiving corticosteroids or immunosuppressive agents.

►*Booster effect:* Infection of an individual with tubercle bacilli or other mycobacteria results in a delayed hypersensitivity response to tuberculin that is demonstrated by the skin test. The delayed hypersensitivity response may gradually wane over a period of years. If a person receives a tuberculin test at this time (after several years), the response may be a reaction that is not significant. The stimulus of the test may boost or increase the size of the reaction to a second test, sometimes causing an apparent conversion or development of sensitivity.

Tuberculin reactivity may indicate prior infection or disease with *M. tuberculosis* and does not necessarily indicate the presence of active tuberculous disease. Individuals showing a tuberculin reaction should be further evaluated with other diagnostic procedures.

►*False negative reaction:* Not all infected people will have a delayed hypersensitivity reaction to a tuberculin test. A large number of factors have been reported to cause a decreased ability to respond to the tuberculin test in the presence of tuberculous infection, including the following: Viral infections (ie, measles, mumps, chickenpox, HIV), live virus vaccinations (ie, measles, mumps, rubella, oral polio, yellow fever), overwhelming TB, other bacterial infections, drugs (eg, corticosteroids, many other immunosuppressive agents), and malignancy.

Anything that impairs or attenuates cell mediated immunity potentially can cause a false negative tuberculin reaction (ie, viral infections [particularly HIV] live virus vaccines, severe protein malnutrition, lymphoma, leukemia, sarcoidosis, use of glucocorticosteroids, other immunosuppressant drugs).

►*Previous BCG vaccination:* Consider the possibility that the skin test sensitivity also may be due to a previous contact with atypical mycobacteria or previous BCG vaccination.

BCG vaccination may produce a PPD reaction that cannot be distinguished reliably from a reaction caused by infection with *M. tuberculosis*. For a person who was vaccinated with BCG, the probability that a PPD reaction results from infection with *M. tuberculosis* increases (1) as the size of the reaction increases, (2) when the person is a contact of a person with TB, (3) when the person's country of origin has a high prevalence of TB, and (4) as the length of time between vaccination and

PPD testing increases. For example, a PPD test reaction of greater than or equal to 10 mm probably can be attributed to *M. tuberculosis* infection in an adult who was vaccinated with BCG as a child and who is from a country with high prevalence of TB.

Drug Interactions

Reactivity to the test may be depressed or suppressed for up to 6 weeks in individuals who are receiving corticosteroids or immunosuppressive agents.

Reactivity to PPD may be depressed temporarily by certain live virus vaccines (ie, measles, mumps, rubella, oral polio, yellow fever, varicella). Therefore, if a tuberculin test is to be performed, administer it either before or simultaneously, at separate sites, with these vaccines in combined form or as separate antigens, or postpone testing for 4 to 6 weeks.

Adverse Reactions

►*Local:*

Very rare – Vesiculation, ulceration, or necrosis may appear at the test site in highly sensitive people. Cold packs or topical steroid preparations may be employed for symptomatic relief of the associated pain, pruritus, and discomfort.

Strongly positive reactions may result in scarring at the test site.

Uncommon – Immediate erythematous or other reactions may occur at the injection site.

►*Systemic:*

Systemic – Rare systemic allergic reactions have been reported that were manifested by immediate skin rash or generalized rash within 24 hours. Two of the reported cases had concurrent symptoms of upper respiratory stridor. These reactions were treated with epinephrine and steroids and resolved.

Patient Information

Instruct patients to report to their health care provider adverse events such as vesiculation, ulceration, or necrosis, which may appear at the test site in highly sensitive patients.

Inform the patient that pain, pruritus, and discomfort at the site may occur.

Inform the patient of the need to return for the reading of the test.

Inform the patient of the need to maintain a personal immunization record.

Indications

Consult individual monographs for specific indications.

Actions

►*Pharmacology:* Radiopaque agents are usually grouped according to osmolality (high or low), structure (monomeric or dimeric ring structure), and ion tendency (nonionic or ionic).

High-osmolality contrast media (HOCM) have an osmolality in solution between 1200 and 2400 mOsm/kg H_2O and are ionic monomers.

Low-osmolality contrast media (LOCM) are classified as ionic dimers (ie, ioxaglate), nonionic monomers, or nonionic dimers. Because of lower toxicities, nonionic monomers are becoming the more preferred contrast media. Ioversol and iohexal are 2 of the newer nonionic monomers and are more hydrophilic, thus possibly producing less toxicity. The nonionic dimers are still mostly in the developmental stages, but they are of limited clinical use because of their viscosity approaching that of plasma. The osmolality of LOCM is ≈ 290 to 860 mOsm/kg H_2O. LOCM agents are generally more costly than HOCM agents, but are less toxic.

The most important characteristic of contrast media is the iodine content. The relatively high atomic weight of iodine contributes sufficient radiodensity for radiographic contrast with surrounding tissues. Barium, one of the noniodine-containing contrast media, is an insoluble material that, because of its density, provides a positive contrast during x-ray examination.

Paramagnetic agents – Paramagnetic agents enhance the use of magnetic resonance imaging (MRI). When administered in living organisms, these agents influence the longitudinal or spin-lattice time (T_1) and the transverse or spin-spin relaxation time (T_2). By lowering the T_1 and T_2 values in tissues that retain them, the signal intensity and the image contrast are enhanced upon exposure to a strong magnetic field.

Nonionic vs ionic agents – Iohexol, iopamidol, ioversol, and iodixanol are nonionic iodine contrast media. The other iodinated contrast media currently available are ionic. The nonionic compounds are more hydrophilic than ionic agents, resulting in decreased protein-binding and tissue-binding propensities. The nonionic media have a lower osmolality than the ionic contrast media (1 to 3 times the osmolality of human serum vs 5 to 8) and are associated with a lower incidence of adverse effects. The nonionic media are also associated with a lower incidence of anaphylactoid reactions.

Pharmacokinetic Parameters of IV Radiopaque Agents			
Radiopaque agent	Osmolality (mOsm/kg H_2O)	Viscosity (cps)	
Ionic agents			
Diatrizoate meglumine 30%	633	1.94[a]	1.42[b]
Diatrizoate meglumine 60%	1415	6.17[a]	4.12[b]
Diatrizoate meglumine 66% and diatrizoate sodium 10% (Hypaque-76)	2016	-	9.0[b]
Diatrizoate meglumine 66% and diatrizoate sodium 10% (MD-76 R)	1551	16.4[a]	10.5[b]
Diatrizoate meglumine 66% and diatrizoate sodium 10% (RenoCal-76)	1870	15.0[a]	9.1[b]
Diatrizoate sodium 50%	1515	3.25[a]	2.34[b]
Iothalamate meglumine 30%	600	2.0[a]	1.5[b]
Iothalamate meglumine 43%	1000	3.0[a]	2.0[b]
Iothalamate meglumine 60%	1400	6.0[a]	4.0[b]
Ioxaglate meglumine 39.3% and ioxaglate sodium 19.6%	600	15.7[a]	7.5[b]
Nonionic agents			
Gadodiamide	789	2.0[c]	1.4[b]
Gadoteridol	630	2.0[c]	1.3[b]
Gadoversetamide	1110	3.1[c]	2.0[b]
Iodixanol 270	290	12.7[c]	6.3[b]
Iodixanol 320	290	26.6[c]	11.8[b]
Iohexol 140	322	2.3[c]	1.5[b]
Iohexol 180	408	3.1[c]	2.0[b]
Iohexol 240	520	5.8[c]	3.4[b]
Iohexol 300	672	11.8[c]	6.3[b]
Iohexol 350	844	20.4[c]	10.4[b]
Iopamidol 41%	413	3.3[c]	2.0[b]
Iopamidol 51%	524	5.1[c]	3.0[b]
Iopamidol 61%	616	8.8[b]	4.7[b]
Iopamidol 76%	796	20.9[c]	9.4[b]
Iopromide 150	328	2.3[c]	1.5[b]
Iopromide 240	483	4.9[c]	2.8[b]
Iopromide 300	607	9.2[c]	4.9[b]
Iopromide 370	774	22.0[c]	10.0[b]
Ioversol 34%	355	2.7[a]	1.9[b]
Ioversol 51%	502	4.6[a]	3.0[b]
Ioversol 64%	651	8.2[a]	5.5[b]

Pharmacokinetic Parameters of IV Radiopaque Agents			
Radiopaque agent	Osmolality (mOsm/kg H_2O)	Viscosity (cps)	
Ioversol 68%	702	9.9[a]	5.8[b]
Ioversol 74%	792	14.3[a]	9.0[b]
Paramagnetic agents			
Ferumoxides	340	-	-
Gadopentetate dimeglumine	1960	4.9[c]	2.9[b]
Mangofodipir trisodium	298	-	0.8[b]

[a] Viscosity at 25°C.
[b] Viscosity at 37°C.
[c] Viscosity at 20°C.

Contraindications

Consult package inserts for individual contraindications.

►*Barium sulfate:* Barium sulfate products are contraindicated in patients with known or suspected obstruction of the colon, known or suspected GI tract perforation, suspected tracheoesophageal fistula, obstructing lesions of the small intestine, pyloric stenosis, inflammation or neoplastic lesions of the rectum, recent rectal biopsy, or known hypersensitivity to barium sulfate formulations.

Do not use barium sulfate suspensions for infants with swallowing disorders or for newborns with complete duodenal or jejunal obstruction or when distal small bowel or colon obstruction is suspected. Barium sulfate suspension is not recommended for very small preterm infants and young children when there is a possibility of leakage from the GI tract, such as necrotizing enterocolitis, unexplained pneumoperitoneum, gasless abdomen, other bowel perforation, esophageal perforation, or postoperative anastomosea.

Known hypersensitivity or allergy to latex is a contraindication for the use of enema tips with latex retention cuffs. The use of retention cuff enema tip is not necessary or desirable in patients with normal sphincter tone. The presence of adequate sphincter tone can be judged by preliminary rectal digital examination.

Warnings

►*Inadvertent intrathecal administration:* Serious adverse reactions have been reported because of the inadvertent intrathecal administration of iodinated contrast media that are not indicated for intrathecal use. These serious adverse reactions include death, convulsions, cerebral hemorrhage, coma, paralysis, arachnoiditis, acute renal failure, cardiac arrest, seizures, rhabdomyolysis, hyperthermia, and brain edema. Special attention must be given to ensure that the drug product is not administered intrathecally.

►*Blood coagulation inhibition:* Nonionic iodinated contrast media inhibit blood coagulation in vitro less than ionic contrast media. Clotting has been reported when blood remains in contact with syringes containing nonionic contrast media.

►*Thromboembolic events:* Serious, rarely fatal, thromboembolic events causing MI and stroke have been reported during angiographic procedures with ionic and nonionic contrast media. Therefore, meticulous IV administration technique is necessary, particularly during angiographic procedures, to minimize thromboembolic events. Numerous factors, including length of procedure, catheter and syringe material, underlying disease state, and concomitant medications may contribute to the development of thromboembolic events. For these reasons, meticulous angiographic techniques are recommended, including close attention to guidewire and catheter manipulation, use of manifold systems and 3-way stopcocks, frequent catheter flushing with heparinized saline solutions and minimizing the length of the procedures. The use of plastic syringes in place of glass syringes has been reported to decrease but not eliminate the likelihood of in vitro clotting.

►*Cardiac shunts (perflutren):* Exercise extreme caution when considering administering activated perflutren in patients who have cardiac shunts.

►*Pulmonary vascular diseases (perflutren):* Administer with caution in patients with chronic pulmonary vascular disease such as severe emphysema, pulmonary vasculitis, or other causes of reduced pulmonary vascular cross-sectional area.

►*Neurologic sequelae:* Serious neurologic sequelae, including permanent paralysis, can occur following cerebral arteriography, selective spinal arteriography, and arteriography of vessels supplying the spinal cord. A cause-effect relationship to the contrast medium has not been established because the patients' preexisting condition and procedural technique are causative factors in themselves. Do not inject contrast media arterially following the administration of vasopressors because they strongly potentiate neurologic effects.

►*Special risk patients:* Exercise caution in patients with severely impaired renal function, combined renal and hepatic disease, severe thyrotoxicosis, myelomatosis, or anuria, particularly when large doses are administered.

►*Nephrotoxicity:* Toxicity ranges from transient tubular enzymuria to irreversible oliguric renal failure. Incidence is estimated at ≤ 1% in healthy patients, to 30% to 70% in patients with major risk factors such as preexisting renal insufficiency, diabetes, and conditions associated with decreased renal blood flow. Preventive measures include avoiding use of radiographic contrast media in high-risk patients, and using the smallest effective dose; also ensure adequate hydration before procedure and discontinue other nephrotoxic agents. Some experts recommend the use of LOCM.

➤*Pheochromocytoma:* Perform administration of radiopaque materials to patients known or suspected of having pheochromocytoma with extreme caution. If, in the opinion of the physician, the possible benefits of such procedures outweigh the considered risks, the procedures may be performed; however, keep the amount of radiopaque medium injected to an absolute minimum. Assess the blood pressure throughout the procedure, and have measures for treatment of a hypertensive crisis available.

➤*Sickle cell disease/Hyperthyroidism:* Contrast media may promote sickling in individuals who are homozygous for sickle cell disease when administered intravascularly. Reports of thyroid storm following the IV use of iodinated radiopaque agents in patients with hyperthyroidism or with an autonomously functioning thyroid nodule, suggest that this additional risk be evaluated in such patients before use of any contrast medium.

➤*Hyperthyroidism:* Cases of hyperthyroidism have been reported with the use of oral contrast media. Some of these patients reportedly had multinodular goiters, which may have been responsible for the increased hormone synthesis in response to excess iodine. Exercise caution when administering enteral GI radiopaque agents to hyperthyroid and euthyroid goiterous patients.

➤*Hypersensitivity reactions:* The risk of a reaction to a nonionic LOCM is estimated to be ≥ 5 times lower than with conventional agents. Risk factors for an immediate reaction include the following: Previous immediate reaction, environmental allergies (ie, food or hay fever), asthma, CHF, use of beta-blockers, current or previous use of interleukin-2, and high anxiety state. Most guidelines suggest the use

of LOCM in those who have a history of previous reactions, asthma, allergies, or who have a history of cardiac dysfunction. Pretreatment regimens may include prednisone, diphenhydramine, with or without ephedrine.

Reports of delayed reactions have ranged from 2.1% to 31% and were mostly mild and required no specific treatment. The most common symptoms included headache, itching, rash, and urticaria, with most developing within 6 hours after administration. Those patients who have been treated with interleukin-2 may have a higher tendency to delayed reactions. Refer to Management of Acute Hypersensitivity Reactions.

Patient Information

➤*Oral and rectal iodinated agents:* Take all medication with water after a fat-free dinner the evening before the test. Thereafter, take only water until the test is completed.

Inform physician of pregnancy or allergy to iodine, any foods, or x-ray materials.

These agents may cause mild and transient abdominal cramping, nausea, vomiting, diarrhea, skin rashes, itching, heartburn, dizziness, or headache.

Consult physician if thyroid tests are planned; iodine may interfere.

➤*Parenteral iodinated agents:* Prior to these procedures, notify physician if any of the following conditions exist: Pregnancy; diabetes; multiple myeloma; pheochromocytoma; homozygous sickle cell disease; thyroid disease; allergy to any drugs or food; reactions to previous injections of dyes used for x-ray procedures. Also notify physician if taking any other medications, including *otc* drugs or natural products.

These agents are to be given only by personnel experienced in their use, and only in facilities with proper equipment to deal with possible untoward effects.

Oral Cholecystographic Agents

IOPANOIC ACID (66.68% iodine)

Rx	Telepaque (Nycomed)	**Tablets:** 500 mg iopanoic acid, 333.4 mg iodine	Off-white, scored. In 6s.

For complete prescribing information, refer to product package labeling.

Indications
Oral cholecystography; cholangiography.

GI Contrast Agents (Iodinated)

DIATRIZOATE SODIUM (59.87% iodine)

Rx	**Hypaque Sodium** (Nycomed)	**Powder:** 600 mg iodine/g	In 10 g bottles and 250 g cans with measuring spoon.[a]

[a] With polysorbate 80.

For complete prescribing information, refer to product package labeling.

Indications
For radiographic examination of the GI tract following oral or rectal administration.

DIATRIZOATE MEGLUMINE 66% and DIATRIZOATE SODIUM 10% (36.7% iodine)

Rx	Gastrografin (Bracco Diagnostics)	**Solution:** 660 mg diatrizoate meglumine, 100 mg diatrizoate sodium, and 367 mg iodine/mL	Lemon flavor. In 120 mL bottles.[a]
Rx	MD-Gastroview (Mallinckrodt)		Vanilla-lemon flavor. In 120 and 240 mL bottles.[b]

[a] With EDTA, polysorbate 80, saccharin, simethicone. [b] With EDTA, saccharin.

For complete prescribing information, refer to product package labeling.

Indications
Radiographic examination of segments of the GI tract and for computed tomography.

GI Contrast Agents (Miscellaneous)

BARIUM SULFATE

Rx	Baro-cat (Mallinckrodt)	**Suspension:** 1.5%	Pineapple-banana flavor. In 300, 900, and 1900 mL bottles.[a]
Rx	Prepcat (Mallinckrodt)		Strawberry flavor. In 450 mL bottles.[a]
Rx	Bear·E·Yum CT (Mallinckrodt)		In 200 and 1900 mL bottles.[a]
Rx	Cheetah (Mallinckrodt)	**Suspension:** 2.2%	In 250, 450, 900, and 1900 mL bottles.[b]
Rx	Medescan (Mallinckrodt)	**Suspension:** 2.3%	In 250, 450, and 1900 mL bottles.[c]
Rx	Enecat CT (Mallinckrodt)	**Concentrated suspension:** 5%	In 110 mL with 480 mL bottle for dilution with flexible tubing, clamp, and enema tip.[a]
Rx	Tomocat (Mallinckrodt)		Strawberry flavor. In 145 mL with 480 mL bottle for dilution, 225 mL with 1000 mL bottle for dilution, and enema kit in 110 mL with 480 mL bottle for dilution with flexible tubing, clamp, and enema tip.[a]
Rx	EntroEase (Mallinckrodt)	**Suspension:** 13%	In 600 mL.[d]
Rx	Entrobar (Mallinckrodt)	**Suspension:** 50%	In 500 mL with or without kit.[d]
Rx	Liquid Barosperse (Mallinckrodt)	**Suspension:** 60%	Vanilla flavor. In 355 and 1900 mL bottles.[d]
Rx	Bear·E·Yum GI (Mallinckrodt)		In 200 mL.[d]
Rx	HD 85 (Mallinckrodt)	**Suspension:** 85%	Raspberry flavor. In 150 and 450 mL kits and 1900 mL bottles.[e]
Rx	Imager ac (Mallinckrodt)	**Suspension:** 100%	In 650 mL bottles with enema tip-tubing assemblies with kit and 1900 mL bottles.[f]
Rx	Flo-Coat (Mallinckrodt)		In 1850 mL bottles.[d]
Rx	Medebar Plus (Mallinckrodt)		In 1900 mL bottles and 650 mL bottles with enema tip-tubing assemblies.[d]

GI Contrast Agents (Miscellaneous)

BARIUM SULFATE

Rx	Epi-C (Mallinckrodt)	Suspension: 150%	Spearmint flavor. In 450 mL bottles.[d]
Rx	Liqui-Coat HD (Mallinckrodt)	Suspension: 210%	Vanilla-raspberry flavor. In UD 150 mL bottles.[b]
Rx	Barium Sulfate, USP (Various, eg, Humco)	Powder for suspension	In 1 lb.
Rx	EntroEase Dry (Mallinckrodt)	Powder for suspension: 92%	In 90 g.
Rx	Barosperse (Mallinckrodt)	Powder for suspension: 95%	Vanilla flavor. In UD 225 and 900 g bottles, and 340 and 454 g enema kits, and 25 lb bulk.[d]
Rx	Tonopaque (Mallinckrodt)		Cherry flavor. In UD 180 and 1200 g bottles and 25 lb container.[a]
Rx	Barobag (Mallinckrodt)	Powder for suspension: 97%	In 340 and 454 g kits.[d]
Rx	Baricon (Mallinckrodt)	Powder for suspension: 98%	Lemon-vanilla flavor. In UD 340 g.[g]
Rx	Enhancer (Mallinckrodt)		Lemon-vanilla flavor. In UD 312 g.[g]
Rx	HD 200 Plus (Mallinckrodt)		Strawberry flavor. In UD 312 g.[g]
Rx	Intropaste (Mallinckrodt)	Paste: 70%	In 454 g tubes.[h]
Rx	Anatrast (Mallinckrodt)	Paste: 100%	In 500 g tubes and enema tip assemblies.[i]

[a] With simethicone, sorbitol.
[b] With simethicone, sorbitol, saccharin, sodium benzoate.
[c] With sorbitol, saccharin, sodium benzoate.
[d] With simethicone.
[e] With simethicone, saccharin.

[f] With simethicone, sorbitol, sodium benzoate.
[g] With simethicone, sorbitol, sucrose.
[h] With simethicone, sorbitol, saccharin, parabens.
[i] With simethicone, sorbitol, parabens.

For complete prescribing information, refer to product package labeling.

Indications

For computed tomography of the GI tract; double-contrast colon and stomach examinations.

➤ *Medebar Plus:* X-ray diagnosis of the GI tract; may administer without dilution for double-contrast colon, single-contrast esophagus, small bowel, and enteroclysis examinations; may use aqueous dilutions for single-contrast stomach and single-contrast colon examinations.

➤ *Anatrast:* Defecography.

➤ *Intropaste, EntroEase:* X-ray examination of the esophagus.

➤ *Entrobar:* Small bowel contrast x-ray examinations.

➤ *Liquid Barosperse:* X-ray diagnosis of the GI tract; may administer suspension without dilution for esophageal swallow or filled stomach examinations; may administer aqueous dilutions rectally for routine filled colon studies or given orally for filled stomach or enteroclysis procedures.

➤ *Bear•E•Yum GI:* X-ray diagnosis of the GI tract; may administer without dilution for filled stomach examinations; may administer aqueous dilutions rectally for routine filled colon studies or given orally for filled stomach or enteroclysis procedures.

➤ *HD 85:* X-ray diagnosis of the GI tract; may administer suspension without dilution for double-contrast colon examinations; may administer aqueous dilutions rectally for routine filled colon studies or given orally for esophageal swallow, filled stomach, or enteroclysis procedures.

FERUMOXSIL

Rx	GastroMARK (Mallinckrodt)	Suspension: 175 mcg iron/mL	In 300 mL bottles.[a]

[a] With sorbitol, saccharin, parabens.

For complete prescribing information, refer to product package labeling.

Indications

In adult patients for oral use with MRI to enhance the delineation of the bowel to distinguish it from organs and tissues that are adjacent to the upper regions of the GI tract.

RADIOPAQUE POLYVINYL CHLORIDE

Rx	Sitzmarks (Konsyl)	Capsules: Contains 24 radiopaque rings (1 mm × 4.5 mm)	In 10s.

For complete prescribing information, refer to product package labeling.

Indications

For adult patients with severe constipation who have otherwise negative GI evaluations.

SODIUM BICARBONATE AND TARTARIC ACID

Rx	Baros (Mallinckrodt)	Granules: 460 mg sodium bicarbonate and 420 mg tartaric acid/g	Simethicone. In 3 g plastic ampules.

For complete prescribing information, refer to product package labeling.

Indications

For use in double-contrast examinations of the stomach.

Parenteral Agents

DIATRIZOATE MEGLUMINE 30% (14.1% iodine)

Rx	Reno-Dip (Bracco Diagnostics)	Injection: 300 mg diatrizoate meglumine and 141 mg iodine/mL	In 300 mL bottles[a] with or without infusion set.

[a] With EDTA.

For complete prescribing information, refer to product package labeling.

Indications

Computed tomography; drip infusion pyelography and venography.

DIATRIZOATE MEGLUMINE 60% (28.2% iodine)

Rx	Hypaque Meglumine 60% (Nycomed)	Injection: 600 mg diatrizoate meglumine and 282 mg iodine/mL	In 50 and 100 mL vials, 150 mL fill in 200 mL bottles, and 200 mL fill in 200 mL bottles.[a]
Rx	Reno-60 (Bracco Diagnostics)		In 10 and 50 mL vials, 100 mL bottles, and 150 mL bottles with and without infusion sets.[a]

[a] With EDTA.

For complete prescribing information, refer to product package labeling.

Indications

Excretory urography, cerebral angiography, peripheral arteriography, venography, operative, T-tube, or percutaneous transhepatic cholangiography, splenoportography, arthrography, discography, and computed tomography.

Parenteral Agents

DIATRIZOATE MEGLUMINE 52% and DIATRIZOATE SODIUM 8% (29.3% iodine)

Rx	**Renografin-60** (Bracco Diagnostics)	**Injection:** 520 mg diatrizoate meglumine, 80 mg diatrizoate sodium, and 292.5 mg iodine/mL	In 10 and 50 mL vials and 100 mL bottles.[a]

[a] With EDTA.

For complete prescribing information, refer to product package labeling.

Indications

Urography; angiography; arteriography; venography; cholangiography; splenoportography; arthrography; discography; computed tomography.

DIATRIZOATE MEGLUMINE 66% and DIATRIZOATE SODIUM 10% (37% iodine)

Rx	**Hypaque-76** (Nycomed)	**Injection:** 660 mg diatrizoate meglumine, 100 mg diatrizoate sodium, and 370 mg iodine/mL	In 50 mL vials, 200 mL bottles, and 100 and 150 mL in 200 mL dilution bottles.[a]
Rx	**MD-76 R** (Mallinckrodt)		In 50 mL vials, 100, 150, and 200 mL bottles, and 125 mL power injector syringes.[a]
Rx	**RenoCal-76** (Bracco Diagnostics)		In 50 mL vials, 100, 150, and 200 mL bottles.[a]

[a] With EDTA.

For complete prescribing information, refer to product package labeling.

Indications

Urography, aortography, angiocardiography, ventriculography, angiography, arteriography, computed tomography; nephrotomography (*RenoCal-76* only); venography (*Hypaque-76* only).

DIATRIZOATE SODIUM 50% (30% iodine)

Rx	**Hypaque Sodium 50%** (Nycomed)	**Injection:** 500 mg diatrizoate sodium and 300 mg iodine/mL	In 50 mL vials.[a]

[a] With EDTA.

For complete prescribing information, refer to product package labeling.

Indications

Excretory urography; angiography; aortography; venography; cholangiography; hysterosalpingography; splenoportography; computed tomography.

IOTHALAMATE MEGLUMINE 30% (14.1% iodine)

Rx	**Conray 30** (Mallinckrodt)	**Injection:** 300 mg iothalamate meglumine and 141 mg iodine/mL	In 50 mL vials and 150 and 300 mL bottles.[a]

[a] With EDTA.

For complete prescribing information, refer to product package labeling.

Indications

Urography; computed tomography; angiography.

IOTHALAMATE MEGLUMINE 43% (20.2% iodine)

Rx	**Conray 43** (Mallinckrodt)	**Injection:** 430 mg iothalamate meglumine and 202 mg iodine/mL	In 50 and 100 mL vials, 150, 200, and 250 mL bottles, and 50 mL prefilled syringes.[a]

[a] With EDTA.

For complete prescribing information, refer to product package labeling.

Indications

Venography; urography; computed tomography; angiography.

IOTHALAMATE MEGLUMINE 60% (28.2% iodine)

Rx	**Conray** (Mallinckrodt)	**Injection:** 600 mg iothalamate meglumine and 282 mg iodine/mL	In 30, 50, and 100 mL vials, 100, 150, and 200 mL bottles, and 50 and 125 mL prefilled power injector syringes.[a]

[a] With EDTA.

For complete prescribing information, refer to product package labeling.

Indications

Urography; angiography; arteriography; venography; arthrography; cholangiography; cholangiopancreatography; computed tomography; angiotomography.

IOXAGLATE MEGLUMINE 39.3% and IOXAGLATE SODIUM 19.6% (32% iodine)

Rx	**Hexabrix** (Mallinckrodt)	**Injection:** 393 mg ioxaglate meglumine, 196 mg ioxaglate sodium, and 320 mg iodine/mL	In 20, 30, and 50 mL vials, 150 mL bottles, 75 mL fill in 150 mL bottles, 100 mL fill in 150 mL bottles, 200 mL fill in 250 mL bottles, and 125 mL power injector syringes, 50 mL fill in 125 mL power injector syringes, and 100 mL fill in 125 mL powder injector syringes.[a]

[a] With EDTA.

For complete prescribing information, refer to product package labeling.

Indications

Pediatric angiocardiography; arteriography; ventriculography; aortography; angiography; venography; phlebography; urography; computed tomography; arthrography; hysterosalpingography.

IODIPAMIDE MEGLUMINE 52% (25.7% iodine)

Rx	**Cholografin Meglumine** (Bracco Diagnostics)	**Injection:** 520 mg iodipamide meglumine and 257 mg iodine/mL	In 20 mL vials.[a]

[a] With EDTA.

For complete prescribing information, refer to product package labeling.

Indications

Cholangiography; cholecystography.

GADODIAMIDE

Rx	**Omniscan** (Nycomed)	**Injection:** 287 mg/mL	Preservative-free. In 10, 20, and 50 mL vials, 5 mL fill in 10 mL vials, 15 mL fill in 20 mL vials, 10 mL fill in 20 mL prefilled syringes, 15 mL fill in 20 mL prefilled syringes, and 20 mL prefilled syringes.

For complete prescribing information, refer to product package labeling.

Indications

➤*CNS:* For IV use in MRI to visualize lesions with abnormal vascularity (or those thought to cause abnormalities in the blood-brain barrier) in the brain (intracranial lesions), spine, and associated tissues.

➤*Body (intrathoracic [noncardiac], intra-abdominal, pelvic, and retroperitoneal regions):* For IV administration to facilitate the visualization of lesions with abnormal vascularity within the thoracic (noncardiac), abdominal, and pelvic cavities, and the retroperitoneal space.

GADOTERIDOL

Rx	**ProHance** (Bracco Diagnostics)	**Injection:** 279.3 mg/mL	Preservative-free. In 5 mL fill in 15 mL vials, 10, 15, and 20 mL fill in 30 mL vials, and 10 and 17 mL fill in 20 mL prefilled syringes.

For complete prescribing information, refer to product package labeling.

Indications

➤*CNS:* For use in MRI in adults and children > 2 years of age to visualize lesions with abnormal vascularity in the brain (intracranial lesions), spine, and associated tissues.

➤*Extracranial/Extraspinal tissues:* For use in MRI in adults to visualize lesions in the head and neck.

GADOVERSETAMIDE

Rx	**OptiMARK** (Mallinckrodt)	**Injection:** 330.9 mg gadoversetamide	Preservative-free. In 50 mL bottles.

For complete prescribing information, refer to product package labeling.

Indications

➤*CNS:* For use with MRI in patients with abnormal blood-brain barrier or abnormal vascularity of the brain, spine, and associated tissues.

➤*Hepatic:* For use with MRI to provide contrast enhancement and facilitate visualization of lesions with abnormal vascularity in the liver of patients who are highly suspect for liver structural abnormalities on computed tomography.

IODIXANOL

Rx	**Visipaque 270** (Nycomed)	**Injection:** 550 mg iodixanol and 270 mg iodine/mL	In 50 mL vials, 50, 100, and 200 mL bottles, 150 mL fill in 200 mL bottles, and 100, 150, and 200 mL flexible containers.[a]
Rx	**Visipaque 320** (Nycomed)	**Injection:** 652 mg iodixanol and 320 mg iodine/mL	In 50 mL vials, 50, 100, and 200 mL bottles, 150 mL fill in 200 mL bottles, and 100, 150, and 200 mL flexible containers.[a]

[a] With EDTA.

For complete prescribing information, refer to product package labeling.

Indications

➤*Intra-arterial:* Intra-arterial digital subtraction angiography (*Visipaque 270* only); angiocardiography (left ventriculography and selective coronary arteriography), peripheral arteriography, visceral arteriography, cerebral arteriography (*Visipaque 320* only).

➤*IV:* CECT imaging of the head and body, excretory urography; peripheral venography (*Visipaque 270* only).

IOHEXOL

Rx	**Omnipaque 140** (Nycomed)	**Injection:** 302 mg iohexol equivalent to 140 mg iodine/mL	In 50 mL vials and bottles.[a]
Rx	**Omnipaque 240** (Nycomed)	**Injection:** 518 mg iohexol equivalent to 240 mg iodine/mL	In 10, 20, and 50 mL vials, 50 mL bottles, 100, 150, and 200 mL flexible containers, 50 mL prefilled syringes, 100 mL fill in 100 mL bottles, 150 mL fill in 200 mL bottles, and 200 mL fill in 200 mL bottles.[a]
Rx	**Omnipaque 300** (Nycomed)	**Injection:** 647 mg iohexol equivalent to 300 mg iodine/mL	In 10, 30, and 50 mL vials, 50 mL bottles, 100 and 150 mL flexible containers, 50 mL prefilled syringes, 75 mL fill in 100 mL bottles, 100 mL fill in 100 mL bottles, 125 mL fill in 200 mL bottles, 150 mL fill in 200 mL bottles, 125 mL fill in 150 mL flexible containers.[a]
Rx	**Omnipaque 350** (Nycomed)	**Injection:** 755 mg iohexol equivalent to 350 mg iodine/mL	In 50 mL vials, 50 mL bottles, 100, 150, and 200 mL flexible containers, 50 mL prefilled syringes, 75 mL fill in 100 mL bottles, 100 mL fill in 100 mL bottles, 125 mL fill in 200 mL bottles, 150 mL fill in 200 mL bottles, 200 mL fill in 200 mL bottles, 250 mL fill in 300 mL bottles, 125 mL fill in 150 mL flexible containers.[a]

[a] With EDTA.

For complete prescribing information, refer to product package labeling.

Indications

➤*Intrathecal:*

Adults –
 Omnipaque 180, Omnipaque 240, Omnipaque 300: Myelography (lumbar, thoracic, cervical, total columnar), and computerized tomography (myelography, cisternography, ventriculography).

Children –
 Omnipaque 180: Myelography (lumbar, thoracic, cervical, total columnar), computerized tomography (myelography, cisternography).

➤*Intravascular:*

Adults –
 Omnipaque 350: Angiocardiography (ventriculography, selective coronary arteriography); aortography; computed tomographic head and body imaging; IV digital subtraction angiography of the head, neck, abdominal, renal, and peripheral vessels; peripheral arteriography; excretory urography.
 Omnipaque 300: Aortography, computed tomographic head and body imaging, cerebral arteriography, peripheral venography (phlebography), excretory urography.
 Omnipaque 240: Computed tomographic head imaging, peripheral venography (phlebography).
 Omnipaque 140: Intra-arterial digital subtraction angiography of the head, neck, abdominal, renal, and peripheral vessels.

Children –
 Omnipaque 350: Angiocardiography (ventriculography, pulmonary arteriography, venography); studies of the collateral arteries and aortography.
 Omnipaque 300: Angiocardiography (ventriculography), excretory urography, and computed tomographic head imaging.
 Omnipaque 240: Computed tomographic head imaging.

IOPAMIDOL 41% (20% iodine)

Rx	**Isovue-200** (Bracco Diagnostics)	**Injection:** 408 mg iopamidol and 200 mg iodine/mL	In 50 mL vials, 100 mL bottles, and 200 mL bottles with infusion set.[a]
	Isovue-M 200 (Bracco Diagnostics)		In 10 and 20 mL vials.[a] *For intrathecal use.*

[a] With EDTA.

For complete prescribing information, refer to product package labeling.

Indications

➤*Isovue-200:* Angiography; arteriography; ventriculography; angiocardiography; aortography; venography; computed tomography; urography.

➤*Isovue-M 200:*

Adults – Myelography; computed tomography; cisternography; ventriculography.

Children > 2 years of age – Thoraco-lumbar myelography.

Parenteral Agents

IOPAMIDOL 51% (25% iodine)

Rx	**Isovue-250** (Bracco Diagnostics)	**Injection:** 510 mg iopamidol and 250 mg iodine/mL	In 50 mL vials, 100, 150, and 200 mL bottles, 150 mL power injector syringes.[a]

[a] With EDTA.

For complete prescribing information, refer to product package labeling.

Indications

Angiography; arteriography; ventriculography; angiocardiography; aortography; venography; urography; computed tomography.

IOPAMIDOL 61% (30% iodine)

Rx	**Isovue-300** (Bracco Diagnostics)	**Injection:** 612 mg iopamidol and 300 mg iodine/mL	In 30 and 50 mL vials, 75 and 100 mL bottles, 150 mL bottles with or without administration sets, 100 and 150 mL power injector syringes.[a]
Rx	**Isovue-M 300** (Bracco Diagnostics)		In 15 mL vials.[a] *For intrathecal use.*

[a] With EDTA.

For complete prescribing information, refer to product package labeling.

Indications

Angiography, arteriography, ventriculography, angiocardiography, aortography, venography, urography, computed tomography; myelography, cisternography (*Isovue-M 300* only).

IOPAMIDOL 76% (37% iodine)

Rx	**Isovue-370** (Bracco Diagnostics)	**Injection:** 755 mg iopamidol and 370 mg iodine/mL	In 20, 30, and 50 mL vials, 50, 75, 100, 125, 150, 175, and 200 mL bottles, 75 and 100 mL power injector syringes.[a]

[a] With EDTA.

For complete prescribing information, refer to product package labeling.

Indications

Angiography; arteriography; ventriculography; angiocardiography; aortography; venography; urography; computed tomography.

IOPROMIDE

Rx	**Ultravist 150** (Berlex)	**Injection:** 311.70 mg iopromide and 150 mg iodine/mL	In 50 mL vials.[a]
Rx	**Ultravist 240** (Berlex)	**Injection:** 498.72 mg iopromide and 240 mg iodine/mL	In 50 and 100 mL vials and 200 mL fill in 250 mL vials.[a]
Rx	**Ultravist 300** (Berlex)	**Injection:** 623.4 mg iopromide and 300 mg iodine/mL	In 50, 100, and 150 mL vials.[a]
Rx	**Ultravist 370** (Berlex)	**Injection:** 768.86 mg iopromide and 370 mg iodine/mL	In 50, 100, and 150 mL vials, and 200 mL fill in 250 mL vials.[a]

[a] With EDTA.

For complete prescribing information, refer to product package labeling.

Indications

➤*Ultravist 150:* Intra-arterial digital subtraction angiography.

➤*Ultravist 240:* Peripheral venography.

➤*Ultravist 300:* Cerebral arteriography; peripheral arteriography; contrast enhanced computed tomographic (CECT) imaging of the head and body; excretory urography.

➤*Ultravist 370:* Coronary arteriography; left ventriculography; visceral angiography; aortography.

IOVERSOL 34% (16% iodine)

Rx	**Optiray 160** (Mallinckrodt)	**Injection:** 339 mg ioversol and 160 mg iodine/mL	In 50 and 100 mL bottles.[a]

[a] With EDTA.

For complete prescribing information, refer to product package labeling.

Indications

Angiography.

IOVERSOL 51% (24% iodine)

Rx	**Optiray 240** (Mallinckrodt)	**Injection:** 509 mg ioversol and 240 mg iodine/mL	In 50, 100, and 150 mL bottles, 200 mL fill in 250 mL bottles, 50 mL hand-held syringes, and 125 mL power injector syringes.[a]

[a] With EDTA.

For complete prescribing information, refer to product package labeling.

Indications

Angiography; venography; computed tomography; urography.

IOVERSOL 64% (30% iodine)

Rx	**Optiray 300** (Mallinckrodt)	**Injection:** 636 mg ioversol and 300 mg iodine/mL	In 50, 100, and 150 mL bottles, 200 mL fill in 250 mL bottles, 50 mL hand-held syringes, and 100 mL fill in 125 mL power injector syringes.[a]

[a] With EDTA.

For complete prescribing information, refer to product package labeling.

Indications

Angiography; arteriography; venography; urography; computed tomography.

IOVERSOL 68% (32% iodine)

Rx	**Optiray 320** (Mallinckrodt)	**Injection:** 678 mg ioversol and 320 mg iodine/mL	In 20 and 30 mL vials, 50, 100, and 150 mL bottles, 75 mL fill in 100 mL bottles, 200 mL fill in 250 mL bottles, 30 and 50 mL hand-held syringes, 50 mL fill in 125 mL power injector syringes, 75 mL fill in 125 mL power injector syringes, 100 mL fill in 125 mL power injector syringes, and 125 mL power injector syringes.[a]

[a] With EDTA.

For complete prescribing information, refer to product package labeling.

Indications

➤*Adults:* Angiography; arteriography; venography; aortography; ventriculography; computed tomography; urography.

➤*Children:* Angiocardiography; computed tomography; urography.

IOVERSOL 74% (35% iodine)

Rx	**Optiray 350** (Mallinckrodt)	**Injection:** 741 mg ioversol and 350 mg iodine/mL	In 50, 100, and 150 mL bottles, 75 mL fill in 100 mL bottles, 200 mL fill in 250 mL bottles, 30 and 50 mL hand-held syringes, 50 mL fill in 125 mL power injector syringes, 75 mL fill in 125 mL power injector syringes, 100 mL fill in 125 mL power injector syringes, and 125 mL power injector syringes.[a]

[a] With EDTA.

For complete prescribing information, refer to product package labeling.

Indications

Arteriography, ventriculography, computed tomography, urography, angiography, venography; angiocardiography (in children).

FERUMOXIDES

Rx	**Feridex I.V.** (Berlex)	**Injectable solution:** 11.2 mg iron/mL (56 mg of iron/vial)	In 5 mL single-dose vials with administration filter.

For complete prescribing information, refer to product package labeling.

Indications

As an adjunct to MRI (in adult patients) to enhance the T2-weighted images used in the detection and evaluation of lesions of the liver that are associated with an alteration in the reticuloendothelial system.

GADOPENTETATE DIMEGLUMINE

Rx	**Magnevist** (Berlex)	**Injection:** 469.01 mg/mL	Preservative-free. In 5, 10, 15, and 20 mL single-dose vials, 10, 15, and 20 mL pre-filled disposable syringes, and 100 mL pharmacy bulk packages.

For complete prescribing information, refer to product package labeling.

Indications

➤*CNS:* With MRI in adults and children ≥ 2 years of age to visualize lesions with abnormal vascularity in the brain (intracranial lesions), spine, and associated tissues.

➤*Extracranial/Extraspinal tissues:* For use with MRI in adults and children ≥ 2 years of age to facilitate visualization of lesions with abnormal vascularity in the head and neck.

➤*Body:* For use with MRI in adults and children ≥ 2 years of age to facilitate visualization of lesions with abnormal vascularity in the body (excluding the heart).

MANGAFODIPIR TRISODIUM

Rx	**Teslascan** (Nycomed)	**Injection:** 37.9 mg (50 mcmol)/mL	Preservative-free. In 10 mL vials.

For complete prescribing information, refer to product package labeling.

Indications

As an adjunct to MRI in patients to enhance the T_1-weighted images used in the detection, localization, characterization, and evaluation of lesions of the liver.

HUMAN ALBUMIN MICROSPHERES

Rx	**Optison** (Mallinckrodt)	**Injectable suspension:** Each mL contains 5 to 8 × 10^8 human albumin microspheres, 10 mg albumin human, 0.22 ± 0.11 mg/mL octafluoropropane in 0.9% aqueous sodium chloride	In 3 mL fill in single-use 3 mL vials.

For complete prescribing information, refer to product package labeling.

Indications

For use in patients with suboptimal echocardiograms to opacify the left ventricle and to improve the delineation of the left ventricular endocardial borders.

PERFLUTREN

Rx	**Definity** (Bristol-Myers Squibb)	**Injection:** 6.52 mg/mL octafluoropropane in lipid-coated microspheres	Preservative-free. In single-use 2 mL vials.[a]

[a] Requires activation with a *Vialmix* (not included).

For complete prescribing information, refer to product package labeling.

Indications

To opacify the left ventricular chamber and to improve the delineation of the left ventricular endocardial border in patients with suboptimal echocardiography.

ISOSULFAN BLUE

Rx	**Lymphazurin 1%** (United States Surgical Corp.)	**Injection:** 10 mg/mL	Preservative-free. In 5 mL vials.

For complete prescribing information, refer to product package labeling.

Indications

Delineates the lymphatic vessels. It is an adjunct to lymphography for visualization of the lymphatic system draining the region of injection.

PENTETREOTIDE

Rx	**OctreoScan** (Mallinckrodt)	**Kit:** 10 mcg pentetreotide and Indium In111 Chloride Sterile Solution	In 10 mL vials.

For complete prescribing information, refer to product package labeling.

Indications

For the scintigraphic localization of primary and metastatic neuroendocrine tumors bearing somatostatin receptors.

Miscellaneous Agents

DIATRIZOATE MEGLUMINE 18% (8.5% iodine)

Rx	**Cystografin Dilute** (Bracco Diagnostics)	**Injection:** 180 mg diatrizoate meglumine and 85 mg iodine/mL	In 300 mL bottles with or without administration sets.[a]

[a] With EDTA.

For complete prescribing information, refer to product package labeling.

Indications

Retrograde cystourethrography.

DIATRIZOATE MEGLUMINE 30% (14.1% iodine)

Rx	**Cystografin** (Bracco Diagnostics)	**Injection:** 300 mg diatrizoate meglumine and 141 mg iodine/mL	In 100 mL fill in 200 mL and 300 mL fill in 400 mL.[a]
Rx	**Hypaque-Cysto** (Nycomed)		Preservative-free. In 100 mL in a pediatric 300 mL dilution bottle and 250 mL in a 500 mL dilution bottle.[a]
Rx	**Reno-30** (Bracco Diagnostics)		In 50 mL multiple-dose vials.[b]

[a] With EDTA.   [b] With EDTA and parabens.

For complete prescribing information, refer to product package labeling.

Indications

Retrograde cystourethrography (*Cystografin* and *Hypaque-Cysto*); retrograde or ascending pyelography (*Reno-30*).

IOTHALAMATE MEGLUMINE 17.2% (8.1% iodine)

Rx	**Cysto-Conray** II (Mallinckrodt)	**Injection:** 172 mg iothalamate meglumine equivalent to 81 mg iodine/mL	In 250 and 500 mL bottles.[a]

[a] With EDTA.

For complete prescribing information, refer to product package labeling.

Indications

Retrograde cystography; cystourethrography.

IOTHALAMATE MEGLUMINE 43% (20.2% iodine)

Rx	**Cysto-Conray** (Mallinckrodt)	**Injection:** 430 mg iothalamate meglumine equivalent to 202 mg iodine/mL	In 50 and 100 mL vials and 250 mL bottles.[a]

[a] With EDTA.

For complete prescribing information, refer to product package labeling.

Indications

Retrograde cystography; cystourethrography; retrograde pyelography.

DIATRIZOATE MEGLUMINE 52.7% and IODIPAMIDE MEGLUMINE 26.8% (38% iodine)

Rx	**Sinografin** (Bracco Diagnostics)	**Injection:** 527 mg diatrizoate meglumine, 268 mg iodipamide meglumine, and 380 mg iodine/mL	In 10 mL vials.[a]

[a] With EDTA.

For complete prescribing information, refer to product package labeling.

Indications

Hysterosalpingography.

ETHIODIZED OIL (37% iodine)

Rx	**Ethiodol** (Savage)	**Injection:** 475 mg iodine/mL	In 10 mL amps.[a]

[a] With 1% poppyseed oil.

For complete prescribing information, refer to product package labeling.

Indications

Hysterosalpingography; lymphography.

POTASSIUM PERCHLORATE

Rx	**Perchloracap** (Mallinckrodt)	**Capsules:** 200 mg	(NDC 19-N025). Gray. In 100s.

For complete prescribing information, refer to product package labeling.

Indications

To minimize the accumulation of pertechnetate Tc 99m in the choroid plexus and in the salivary and thyroid glands of patients receiving sodium pertechnetate Tc 99m for brain and blood pool imaging and placenta localization.

▶*Unlabeled uses:* Treatment of hyperthyroidism.

The Orphan Drug Act defines an orphan drug as a drug or biological product for the diagnosis, treatment, or prevention of a rare disease or condition. A rare disease is one that affects less than 200,000 people in the United States or one that affects greater than 200,000 people but for which there is no reasonable expectation that the cost of developing the drug and making it available will be recovered from sales of that drug in the United States.

The FDA Office of Orphan Products Development (OOPD) provides an information package that includes an overview of the FDA's orphan drug program, a brief description of the orphan products grant program, and a current list of designated orphan products. OOPD's information package also contains a directory sheet listing sources of information about the treatment of rare diseases, patient organiza-

tions, and availability of orphan drugs. Requests for the Rare Disease Information Directory or the entire orphan drugs information package may be made by contacting OOPD:

Office of Orphan Products Development (HF-35)
Food and Drug Administration
5600 Fishers Lane
Rockville, MD 20857
(301) 827-3666 or (800) 300-7469; fax: (301) 443-4915
Internet: http://www.fda.gov/orphan/

Those agents that have been approved for marketing or whose specific indication has been approved for marketing are denoted with the footnote a.

Orphan Drugs		
Drug (*Trade name*)	Proposed use	Sponsor
(+/-)-7-[3-(4-acetyl-3-methoxy-2-propylphenoxy)propoxy]-3,4-dihydro-8-propyl-2H-1-benzopyran-2-2 carboxylic acid	To prevent serious adverse events associated with vascular leak syndrome caused by interleukin-2 therapy	BioMedicines
(1S)-1-(9-deazahypoxanthin-9-yl)-1,4-dideoxy-1,4-imino-D-ribitol-hydrochloride	T-cell non-Hodgkin lymphoma	BioCryst Pharm
(4S)-4-ethyl-4-hydroxy-3, 14-dioxo-3,4,12,14-tetrahydro-1-H-pyrano[3?,4?:6,7]-indolizino-[1,2-b]-quinoline-11-carbaldehyde O-(tert-butyl)-(E)-oxime (*Gimatecan*)	Malignant glioma	Sigma-Tau Res
[5,10,15,20-tetrakis(1,3-diethylimidazolium-2-yl)porphyrinato] manganese(III)pentachloride	Amyotrophic lateral sclerosis	Aeolus Pharm
1,1'-[1,4-phenylenebis(methylene)]-bis-1,4,8,11-tetraazacyclotetradecan	With filgrastim to improve the yield of progentor cells in the apheresis product for subsequent stem cell transplantation following myelosuppressive or myeloablative chemotherapy	AnorMED
1,5-(Butylimino)-1,5 dideoxy,D-glucitol	Fabry disease	Oxford GlycoSciences
1-(11-dodecylamino-10-hydroxyundecyl)-3-7-dimethylxanthine hydrogen methanesulfonate	Hormone refractory prostate carcinoma	Cell Therapeutics
111Indium pentetreotide (*SomatoTher*)	Somatostatin receptor-positive neuroendocrine tumors	Louisiana State Univ Medical Center Foundation
166Ho-DOTMP	Multiple myeloma	NeoRx
2'-3'-dideoxyadenosine	AIDS	National Cancer Inst
2',3',5'-tri-o-acetyluridine	Mitochondrial disease	Repligen
2'-deoxycytidine	Host-protective agent in acute myelogenous leukemia	Steven Grant, MD
2-0-Butyryl-1-0-octyl-myo-inositol 3,4,5,6-tetrakisphosphate	Cystic fibrosis	Inologic
2-0-desulfated heparin (*Aeropin*)	Cystic fibrosis	Kennedy and Hoidal, MDs
2-(3-diethylaminopropyl)-8,8-dipropyl-2-azaspiro[4,5]decan dimaleate (*Atiprimod*)	Multiple myeloma and associated bone resorption	Callisto Pharm
24,25 dihydroxycholecalciferol	Uremic osteodystrophy	Lemmon
2-chloroethyl-3-sarcosinamide-1-nitrosourea (*Sarmustine*)	Malignant glioma	Pangene
		Lawrence Panasci, MD
2-methoxyestradiol (*Panzem*)	Multiple myeloma	EntreMed
3-(3,5-dimethyl-1H-2ylmethylene)-1,3-dihydro-indol-2-one	Kaposi sarcoma; von Hippel-Lindau disease	Sugen
3,4-diaminopyridine	Lambert-Eaton myasthenic syndrome	Jacobus Pharm
3-(4'aminoisoindoline-1'-one)-1-piperidine-2,6-dione (CC-5013) (*Revimid*)	Multiple myeloma; myelodysplastic syndromes	Celgene
3,5,3'-triiodothyroacetate	Well-differentiated papillary, follicular, or combined papillary/follicular carcinomas of the thyroid gland	Elliot Danforth Jr., MD
3'-azido-2',3'dideoxyuridine (*AZDU*)	AIDS	Berlex Labs
4,5-dibromorhodamine 123 (*Theralux Irradiation Device*)	Chronic myelogenous leukemia	Celmed BioSciences
4-aminosalicylic acid	Mild to moderate ulcerative colitis in patients intolerant to sulfasalazine	Warren Beeken, MD
(*Pamisyl*)		Parke-Davis
(*Rezipas*)		Squibb
40SD02	Chronic iron overload resulting from conventional transfusional treatment of beta-thalassemia major and sickle cell anemia	Biomedical Frontiers
5,5',5''-[Phosphinothioylidyne-tris(imino-2,1-ethanediyl)]tris[5-methylchelidoninium]trihydroide hexahydrochloride	Pancreatic cancer	Now Pharm AG
5,6-dihydro-5-azacytidine	Malignant mesothelioma	ILEX Oncology
506U78	Chronic lymphocytic leukemia	GlaxoSmithKline

Orphan Drugs		
Drug (*Trade name*)	Proposed use	Sponsor
5a8, monoclonal antibody to CD4	Postexposure prophylaxis for occupational exposure to human immunodeficiency virus (HIV)	Biogen
5-aza-2'-deoxycytidine	Acute leukemia	SuperGen
6-hydroxymethylacylfulvene	Histologically confirmed advanced or metastatic pancreatic cancer	MGI Pharma
8-cyclopentyl 1,3-dipropylxanthine	Cystic fibrosis	SciClone Pharm
8-methoxsalen (*Uvadex*)	In conjunction with the UVAR photopheresis system to treat diffuse systemic sclerosis; to prevent acute rejection of cardiac allografts	Therakos
9-cis retinoic acid (*Panretin*)	To prevent retinal detachment caused by proliferative vitreoretinopathy	Allergan
	Acute promyelocytic leukemia	Ligand Pharm
9-nitro-20-(S)-camptothecin (*Camvirex*)	Pancreatic cancer	SuperGen
	Pediatric HIV infection/AIDS	NovoMed Pharm
90Y-hPAMA4 (*PAN-Cide*)	Pancreatic cancer	Immunomedics
a-(3-aminophthalimido) glutaramide (*Actimid*[a])	Multiple myeloma	Celgene
Abetimus	Lupus nephritis	La Jolla Pharm
ACA125	Epithelial ovarian cancer	CellControl Biomedical Labs
Acetylcysteine (*Acetadote*)[a]	IV treatment for moderate to severe acetaminophen overdose	Ligand
(*Mucomyst/Mucomyst 10 IV*)		Bristol-Myers Squibb
Acid sphingomyelinase	Niemann-Pick disease type B	Genzyme
Aconiazide	Tuberculosis	Lincoln Diagnostics
Adeno-associated viral-based vector cystic fibrosis gene therapy	Cystic fibrosis	Targeted Genetics
Adeno-associated viral vector containing the gene for human coagulation Factor IX (*Coagulin-B*)	Intrahepatic and IM treatment of moderate to severe hemophilia	Avigen
Adenosine	With BCNU (carmustine) in the treatment of brain tumors	Medco Res
Adenovirus-based vector Factor VIII complementary DNA to somatic cells (*MiniAdFVIII*)	Hemophilia A	GenStar Therapeutics
Adenovirus-mediated herpes simplex virus-thymidine kinase gene	With gancyclovir in the treatment of malignant glioma	Ark Therapeutics Ltd
Aerosolized pooled immune globulin	Respiratory syncytial virus lower respiratory tract disease	Pediatric Pharm
α-Galactosidase A (*Plant-Produced Human α-Galactosidase*)	Fabry disease	Large Scale Biology
AI-RSA	Autoimmune uveitis	AutoImmune
Albendazole (*Albenza*)	Hydatid disease (cystic echinococcosis caused by *Echinococcus granulosus* larvae or alveolar echinococcosis caused by *E. multilocularis* larvae);[a] neurocysticercosis caused by *Taenia solium* as: 1) Chemotherapy of parenchymal, subarachnoidal, and racemose (cysts in spinal fluid) neurocysticercosis in symptomatic cases and 2) prophylaxis of epilepsy and other sequelae in asymptomatic neurocysticercosis[a]	SmithKline Beecham
Albuterol	To prevent paralysis caused by spinal cord injury	MotoGen
Aldesleukin (*Proleukin*)	Metastatic renal cell carcinoma[a]; metastatic melanoma[a]; primary immunodeficiency disease associated with T-cell defects; acute myelogenous leukemia; non-Hodgkin lymphoma	Chiron
Alemtuzumab (*Campath*)	Chronic lymphocytic leukemia[a]	Millennium and ILEX Partners, LP
Alendronate (*Fosamax*)	Osteogenesis imperfecta in pediatric patients 4 years of age and older	Merck
Alendronate disodium (*Fosamax*)	Bone manifestations of Gaucher disease	Richard J. Wenstrup, MD
Alglucerase injection (*Ceredase*)	Replacement therapy in Gaucher disease type I,[a] II, and III	Genzyme
Alitretinoin (*Panretin*)	Topical treatment of cutaneous lesions in AIDS-related Kaposi sarcoma[a]	Ligand Pharm
Allantoin (*Alwextin*)	Skin blistering and erosions associated with inherited epidermolysis bullosa	Alwyn Co.
Allogeneic human retinal pigment epithelial cells on gelatin microcarriers (*Spheramine*)	Hoehn and Yahr stage 3 and 4 Parkinson disease	Titan Pharm
Allogeneic peripheral blood mononuclear cells (sensitized against patient alloantigens by mixed lymphocyte culture) (*CYTOIMPLANT*)	Pancreatic cancer	Applied Immunotherapeutics LLC
Allogenic thymic tissue for transplantation, cultured, partially T-cell depleted	Therapy for primary immune deficiency resulting from athymia associated with complete DiGeorge syndrome	Duke University Medical Center
Allopurinol riboside	Chagas disease; cutaneous and visceral leishmaniasis	Burroughs Wellcome
Allopurinol sodium (*Aloprim for Injection*)	Ex-vivo preservation of cadaveric kidneys for transplantation	Burroughs Wellcome
	Management of patients with leukemia, lymphoma, and solid tumor malignancies who are receiving cancer therapy that causes elevations of serum and urinary uric acid levels and who cannot tolerate oral therapy[a]	Catalytica Pharm

Orphan Drugs		
Drug (*Trade name*)	Proposed use	Sponsor
Alpha-1-antitrypsin (recombinant DNA origin)	Supplementation therapy for alpha-1-antitrypsin deficiency in the ZZ phenotype population	Chiron
Alpha₁-proteinase inhibitor (human) (*Prolastin*)	To slow the progression of emphysema in alpha₁-antitrypsin deficient patients	Aventis Behring LLC
	Replacement therapy in the alpha₁-proteinase inhibitor congenital deficiency state[a]	Bayer
Alpha-galactosidase A (*CC-Galactosidase*)	Alpha-galactosidase A deficiency (Fabry disease)	Orphan Medical
(*Fabrase*)	Fabry disease	Robert J. Desnick, MD
(*Replagal*)	Long-term enzyme replacement therapy for treatment of Fabry disease	Transkaryotic Therapies
Alpha-melanocyte stimulating hormone	To prevent and treat intrinsic acute renal failure caused by ischemia	National Institute of Diabetes, and Digestive and Kidney Diseases
Alprostadil	For severe peripheral arterial occlusive disease (critical limb ischemia) when other procedures, grafts, or angioplasty are not indicated	Schwarz Pharma
Alteplase (*Activase*)	Intraventricular hemorrhage associated with intracerebral hemorrhage	Daniel F. Hanley, MD
Altretamine (*Hexalen*)	Advanced ovarian adenocarcinoma[a]	Medimmune Oncology
AMG 531	Immune thrombocytopenic purpura	Amgen
Amifostine (*Ethyol*)	To reduce the incidence of moderate to severe xerostomia in postoperative radiation treatment for head and neck cancer[a]; to reduce the incidence and severity of toxicities associated with cisplatin administration; myelodysplastic syndromes; chemoprotective agent for the following: Cisplatin in metastatic melanoma, cisplatin in advanced ovarian carcinoma,[a] cyclophosphamide in advanced ovarian carcinoma	MedImmune Oncology
Amiloride HCl solution for inhalation	Cystic fibrosis	GlaxoWellcome R&D
Aminocaproic acid (*Caprogel*)	Topical treatment of traumatic hyphema of the eye	Eastern Virginia Medical School
Aminosalicylate sodium	Crohn disease	Syncom Pharm
Aminosalicylic acid (*Paser Granules*)	Tuberculosis infections[a]	Jacobus Pharm
Aminosidine (*Gabbromicina*)	Tuberculosis; *Mycobacterium avium* complex	Thomas P. Kanyok, PharmD
(*Paromomycin*)	Visceral leishmaniasis (kala-azar)	
Amiodarone (*Amio-Aqueous*)	Incessant ventricular tachycardia	Academic Pharm
Amiodarone HCl (*Cordarone*)	Acute treatment and prophylaxis of life-threatening ventricular tachycardia or ventricular fibrillation[a]	Wyeth-Ayerst Labs
Ammonium tetrathiomolybdate	Wilson disease	George J. Brewer, MD
Amphotericin B lipid complex (*Abelcet*)	Invasive protothecosis, sporotrichosis, coccidioidomycosis, zygomycosis, and candidiasis; invasive fungal infections[a]	Liposome
Amsacrine (*Amsidyl*)	Acute adult leukemia	Warner-Lambert
Anagrelide (*Agrylin*)	Polycythemia vera; essential thrombocythemia[a]; thrombocytosis in chronic myelogenous leukemia	Roberts Pharm
Ananain, comosain (*Vianain*)	Enzymatic debridement of severe burns	Genzyme
Anaritide acetate (*Auriculin*)	Acute renal failure; improvement of early renal allograft function following renal transplantation	Scios
Ancestim (*Stemgen*)	With filgrastim to decrease the number of phereses required to collect peripheral blood progenitor cells capable of providing rapid multilineage hematopoietic reconstitution following myelosuppressive or myeloablative therapy	Amgen
Ancrod (*Viprinex*)	To establish and maintain anticoagulation in heparin-intolerant patients undergoing cardiopulmonary bypass	Knoll Pharm
Angiotensin 1-7 (*MARstem*)	Neutropenia associated with autologous bone marrow transplantation; myelodysplastic syndrome	Maret Pharm
Anti pan T lymphocyte monoclonal antibody (*Anti-t Lymphocyte Immunotoxin Xmmly-h65-rta*)	In-vivo treatment of bone marrow recipients to prevent graft rejection and graft vs host disease; ex-vivo treatment to eliminate mature T-cells from potential bone marrow grafts	Xoma
Antiangiogenic components extracted from marine cartilage (*Neovastat [AE-941]*)	Renal cell carcinoma	AEterna Labs
Anti-CD23 IgG1, kappa monoclonal antibody	Chronic lymphocytic leukemia	IDEC Pharm
Anti-CD45 monoclonal antibodies	To prevent acute graft rejection of human organ transplants	Baxter Healthcare
Anti-CEA Sheep-human chimeric monoclonal antibody labeled w/iodine-131 (KAb201)	Pancreatic cancer	KS Biomedix Ltd
Anti-cytomegalovirus monoclonal antibodies	To prevent/treat human cytomegalovirus infection in bone marrow and organ transplantation and in AIDS	Biomedical Res Inst
Antiepilepsirine	Drug-resistant generalized tonic-clonic epilepsy in children and adults	Children's Hospital, Columbus, OH
Antihemophilic factor (human) (*Alphanate*)	von Willebrand disease	Alpha Therapeutic

Orphan Drugs		
Drug (*Trade name*)	Proposed use	Sponsor
Antihemophilic factor (recombinant) (*Kogenate*)	Prophylaxis/Treatment of bleeding in hemophilia A[a] or for prophylaxis when surgery is required in these patients[a]	Bayer
(*ReFacto*)	To control/prevent hemorrhagic episodes; for surgical prophylaxis in patients with hemophilia A (congenital factor VIII deficiency or classic hemophilia)	Genetics Institute
Antihemophilic factor/von Willebrand factor complex (human), dried, pasteurized (*Humate-P*)	To treat/prevent bleeding in hemophilia A (classical hemophilia) in adult patients; treat spontaneous and trauma-induced bleeding episodes in severe von Willebrand disease, and in mild to moderate von Willebrand disease where use of desmopressin is known or suspected to be inadequate in adult and pediatric patients[a]	Aventis Behring LLC
Anti-interferon-gamma Fab from goats	Immunologic corneal allograft rejection	Advanced Biotherapy
Antimelanoma antibody XMMME-001-DTPA 111 Indium (*Antimelanoma Antibody XMMME-001-DTPA 111 Indium*)	Diagnostic use in imaging systemic and nodal melanoma metastasis	Xoma
Antimelanoma antibody XMMME-001-RTA (*Antimelanoma Antibody XMMME-001-RTA*)	Stage III melanoma not amenable to surgical resection	Xoma
Antipyrine test	For use as an index of hepatic drug metabolizing capacity	Upsher-Smith Labs
Antisense 20-mer phosphorothioate oligonucleotide [complementary to the coding region of R2 component of the human ribonucleotide reductase mRNA] (*GTI-2040*)	Renal cell carcinoma	Lorus Therapeutics
Anti-tap-72 immunotoxin (*Xomazyme-791*)	Metastatic colorectal adenocarcinoma	Xoma
Antithrombin III (human) (*Antithrombin III human*)	To prevent/arrest episodes of thrombosis in congenital AT-III deficiency and/or to prevent the occurrence of thrombosis in AT-III deficiency who have undergone trauma or who are about to undergo surgery or parturition	American National Red Cross
(*ATnativ*)	Hereditary antithrombin III deficiency in connection with surgical or obstetrical procedures or thromboembolism[a]	Pharmacia & Upjohn AB
(*Thrombate III*)	Replacement therapy in congenital deficiency of AT-III to prevent and treat thrombosis and pulmonary emboli[a]	Bayer
Antithrombin III (human) concentrate IV (*Kybernin P*)	Prophylaxis/Treatment of thromboembolic episodes in genetic AT-III deficiency	Aventis Behring LLC
Anti-thymocyte globulin (Rabbit) (*Thymoglobulin*)	Myelodysplastic syndrome (MDS)	SangStat Medical
Anti-thymocyte serum (*Nashville Rabbit Anti-thymocyte Serum*)	Allograft rejection, including solid organ (kidney, liver, heart, lung, pancreas) and bone marrow transplantation	Applied Medical Res
Antivenin crotaline (pit-viper) equine immune F(ab)2 (*Antivipmyn*)	Envenomation by Crotaline snakes	Rare Disease Therapeutics
Antivenin crotalidae polyvalent immune Fab (ovine) (*CroFab*)	Envenomations inflicted by North American crotalid snakes[a]	Protherics
Antivenom (crotalidae) purified (avian)	Envenomation by poisonous snakes belonging to the *Crotalidae* family	Ophidian Pharm
AP1903	Acute graft vs host disease in patients undergoing bone marrow transplantation	Ariad Gene Therapeutics
APL 400-020 V-Beta DNA vaccine	Cutaneous T-cell lymphoma	Wyeth-Lederle Vaccines & Pediatrics
Apomorphine	Treatment of the on-off fluctuations associated with late-stage Parkinson disease	Pentech Pharm
	Rescue treatment for early morning motor dysfunction in late-stage Parkinson disease	Scherer DDS
Apomorphine HCl (*Apokyn*)	Treatment of the on-off fluctuations associated with late-stage Parkinson disease	Mylan
Aprotinin (*Trasylol*)	Prophylaxis to reduce perioperative blood loss and the homologous blood transfusion requirement in patients undergoing cardiopulmonary bypass surgery in the course of repeat coronary artery bypass graft (CABG) surgery, and in selected cases of primary CABG surgery when the risk of bleeding is especially high (impaired hemostasis), or where transfusion is unavailable or unacceptable[a]	Bayer
Arcitumomab (*99m Tc-labeled CEA-Scan*)	Diagnosis and localization of primary, residual, recurrent, and metastatic medullary thyroid carcinoma	Immunomedics
Arginine butyrate	Beta-hemoglobinopathies and beta-thalassemia	Susan P. Perrine, MD
	Sickle cell disease and beta-thalassemia	Vertex Pharm
Arsenic trioxide (*Trisenox*)	Acute promyelocytic leukemia[a]; chronic myeloid leukemia; multiple myeloma; myelodysplastic syndrome; acute myelocytic leukemia subtypes M0, M1, M2, M4, M5, M6, and M7; chronic lymphocytic leukemia; liver cancer	Cell Therapeutics
Artesunate	Malaria	World Health Organization
As-101	AIDS	NPDC-AS101
AT1001	Fabry disease	Amicus Therapeutics
Atomoxetine HCl (*Strattera*)	Tourette syndrome	Eli Lilly
Atovaquone (*Mepron*)	AIDS-associated *Pneumocystis carinii* pneumonia (PCP)[a]; to prevent PCP in high-risk, HIV-infected patients (defined by $\geq$ 1 episode of PCP and/or a peripheral CD4+ lymphocyte count $\leq$ 200/mm^3)[a]; treatment and suppression of *Toxoplasma gondii* encephalitis; primary prophylaxis of HIV-infected people at high risk for developing *T. gondii* encephalitis	GlaxoWellcome GlaxoWellcome R & D

Orphan Drugs

Drug (*Trade name*)	Proposed use	Sponsor
Augmerosen (*Genasense*)	Multiple myeloma; acute myelocytic leukemia; chronic lymphocytic leukemia	Genta
Autologous antigen presenting cells pulsed with autologous tumor Ig idiotype (*Mylovenge*)	Multiple myeloma	Dendreon
Autologous dendritic cells pulsed with autologous glioblastoma multi-forme acid-eluted tumor antigens (*DCVax-Brain*)	Glioblastoma multiforme	Northwest Biotherapeutics
Autologous DNP-conjugated tumor vaccine (*M-Vax*)	Adjuvant therapy in melanoma patients with surgically resectable lymph node metastasis (stage III and limited stage IV disease)	Avax Technologies
Autologous tumor-derived gp96 heat shock protein-peptide complex (*Oncophage*)	Renal cell carcinoma; metastatic melanoma	Antigenics
Autolymphocyte therapy	Renal cell carcinoma	Cytogen
Azacitadine	Myelodysplastic syndromes	Pharmion
Azathioprine (*Imuran*)	Oral manifestations of graft vs host disease	Oral Solutions
Aztreonam	Inhalation therapy for control of gram-negative bacteria in the respiratory tract with cystic fibrosis	Corus Pharma
B lymphocyte stimulator (*BLyS*)	Common variable immunodeficiency	Human Genome Sciences
Bacitracin (*Altracin*)	Antibiotic-associated pseudomembranous enterocolitis caused by toxins A and B elaborated by *Clostridium difficile*	AL Labs
Baclofen (*Lioresal Intrathecal*)	Intractable spasticity caused by multiple sclerosis or spinal cord injury	Infusaid
	Intractable spasticity caused by spinal cord injury, multiple sclerosis, and other spinal diseases (eg, spinal ischemia, spinal tumor, transverse myelitis, cervical spondylosis, degenerative myelopathy)[a]; spasticity associated with cerebral palsy	Medtronic
	Dystonia	Medronic Neurological
Basiliximab (*Simulect*)	Prophylaxis of solid organ rejection[a]	Novartis
Beclomethasone 17,21-dipropionate	To prevent GI graft vs host disease	Enteron Pharm
Beclomethasone dipropionate	Oral administration for intestinal graft vs host disease	George B. McDonald, MD
Benzoate and phenylacetate (*Ucephan*)	Adjunctive therapy to prevent/treat hyperammonemia in patients with urea cycle enzymopathy caused by carbamylphosphate synthetase, ornithine, transcarbamylase, or argininosuccinate synthetase deficiency[a]	Immunex
Benzoate/Phenylacetate (*Ammonul*)	Acute hyperammonemia and associated encephalopathy in patients with deficiencies in enzymes of the urea cycle	Medicis Pharm
Benzophenone-3, octylmethyoxycin-namate, avobenzone, titanium diox-ide, zinc oxide (*Total Block VL SPF 75*)	To prevent visible light-induced skin photosensitivity as a result of porfimer sodium photody-namic therapy	Fallien Cosmeceuticals Ltd
Benzydamine HCl (*Tantum*)	Prophylactic treatment of oral mucositis resulting from radiation therapy for head and neck cancer	Angelini Pharm
Benzylpenicillin, benzylpenicilloic, benzylpenilloic acid (*Pre-Pen/MDM*)	To assess risk of penicillin administration when it is the preferred drug of choice in adult patients who have previously received penicillin and in adults who have a history of clinical penicillin sensitivity	Hollister-Stier Labs LLC
Beractant (*Survanta Intratracheal Suspension*)	To prevent/treat neonatal respiratory distress syndrome (RDS)[a]; for full-term newborns with res-piratory failure caused by meconium aspiration syndrome, persistent pulmonary hypertension of the newborn, or pneumonia and sepsis	Ross
Beraprost	Pulmonary arterial hypertension associated with any New York Heart Association classification (class I, II, III, or IV)	United Therapeutics
Beta alethine (*Betathine*)	Multiple myeloma; metastatic melanoma	Dovetail Tech
Betaine (*Cystadane*)	Homocystinuria[a]	Orphan Medical
Bethandidine sulfate	To prevent recurrence of primary ventricular fibrillation; treat primary ventricular fibrillation	Medco Res
Bexarotene (*Targretin*)	Cutaneous manifestations of cutaneous T-cell lymphoma in patients who are refractory to ≥ 1 prior systemic therapy[a]	Ligand Pharm
Bifidobacterium longum infantis 35624	Pediatric Crohn disease	Alimentary Health Ltd
Bindarit	Lupus nephritis	Angelini Pharm
Bioartificial liver system utilizing xenogenic hepatocytes in a hollow fiber bioreactor cartridge (BAL)	In acute liver failure presenting with encephalopathy deteriorating beyond Parson grade 2	Excorp Medical
Bis(4-fluorophenyl)phenylacetamide	Sickle cell disease	ICAgen
Bleomycin (*Blenoxane*)	Pancreatic cancer	Genetronics
Bleomycin sulfate (*Blenoxane*)	Malignant pleural effusion[a]	Bristol-Myers Squibb Pharm Res Inst
BMY-45622	Ovarian cancer	Bristol-Myers Squibb
Bortezomib (*Velcade*)	Multiple myeloma[a]	Millennium Pharm
Bosentan (*Tracleer*)	Pulmonary arterial hypertension[a]	Actelion Life Sciences

Orphan Drugs

Drug (*Trade name*)	Proposed use	Sponsor
Botulinum toxin type A	Synkinetic closure of the eyelid associated with VII cranial nerve aberrant regeneration	Botulinim Toxin Res
(*Botox*)	Blepharospasm and strabismus associated with dystonia in adults ≥ 12 years of age[a]; cervical dystonia[a]; dynamic muscle contracture in pediatric cerebral palsy	Allergan
(*Dysport*)	Spasmodic torticollis (cervical dystonia); dynamic muscle contractures in pediatric cerebral palsy; essential blepharospasm	Ipsen Limited
Botulinum toxin type B (*NeuroBloc*)	Cervical dystonia[a]	Elan Pharm
Botulinum toxin type F	Spasmodic torticollis (cervical dystonia); essential blepharospasm	Ipsen Limited
Botulism immune globulin (*BabyBIG*)	Infant botulism[a]	CA Dept Health Services
Bovine colostrum	AIDS-related diarrhea	Donald Hastings, DVM
Bovine immunoglobulin concentrate, *Cryptosporidium parvum* (*Sporidin-G*)	Treatment and symptomatic relief of *Cryptosporidium parvum* infection of the GI tract in immunocompromised patients	GalaGen
Bovine whey protein concentrate (*Immuno-C*)	Cryptosporidiosis caused by *Cryptosporidium parvum* in the GI tract of patients who are immunodeficient/immunocompromised or immunocompetent	Biomune Systems
Branched chain amino acids	Amyotrophic lateral sclerosis	Mount Sinai Medical Center
Brimonidine (*Alphagan*)	Anterior ischemic optic neuropathy	Allergan
Bromhexine (*Bisolvon*)	Mild to moderate keratoconjunctivitis sicca in Sjogren syndrome	Boehringer Ingelheim
Broxuridine (*Broxine/Neomark*)	Radiation sensitizer in the treatment of primary brain tumors	NeoPharm
Bryostatin-1	With paclitaxel in the treatment of esophageal cancer	GPC Biotech
Buffered intrathecal electrolyte/dextrose injection (*Elliotts B Solution*)	Diluent in intrathecal administration of methotrexate and cytarabine for prevention or treatment of meningeal leukemia or lymphocytic lymphoma[a]	Orphan Medical
Buprenorphine HCl (*Subutex*)	Opiate addictions in opiate users[a]	Reckitt Benckiser Pharm
Buprenorphine in combination with naloxone (*Suboxone*)	Opiate addiction in opiate users[a]	Reckitt Benckiser Pharm
Busulfan (*Busulfex*)	Preparative therapy in the treatment of malignancies with bone marrow transplantation[a]	Orphan Medical
(*Partaject*)	Preparative therapy for pediatric patients undergoing bone marrow transplantation	SuperGen
(*Spartaject*)	Preparative therapy for malignancies treated with bone marrow transplantation	Sparta Pharm
	Primary brain malignancies	SuperGen
(*Spartaject-Busulfan*)	Intrathecal therapy for neoplastic meningitis	SuperGen
Butyrylcholinesterase	Reduction and clearance of toxic blood levels of cocaine encountered during a drug overdose; postsurgical apnea	Shire Labs
BW 12C	Sickle cell disease	Burroughs Wellcome
C1 esterase inhibitor (human)	To prevent and treat angioedema caused by C1-esterase inhibitor deficiency	Alpha Therapeutic
C1-esterase inhibitor, human, pasteurized (*Berinert P*)	To prevent and/or treat acute attacks of hereditary angioedema	Aventis Behring LLC
C1-inhibitor (*C1-Inhibitor [human] Vapor Heated, Immuno*)	To treat acute attacks of angioedema; to prevent acute attacks of angioedema, including short-term prophylaxis for patients requiring dental or other surgical procedures	Baxter Healthcare
Caffeine (*Cafcit*)	Apnea of prematurity[a]	OPR Development, LP
Calcitonin-human for injection (*Cibacalcin*)	Symptomatic Paget disease (osteitis deformans)[a]	Novartis
Calcitonin-salmon nasal spray (*Miacalcin Nasal Spray*)	Symptomatic Paget disease (osteitis deformans)	Sandoz Pharm
Calcium acetate (*Phos-Lo*)	Hyperphosphatemia in end-stage renal disease	Pharmedic
	Hyperphosphatemia in end-stage renal failure[a]	Braintree Labs
Calcium carbonate (*R & D Calcium Carbonate/600*)	Hyperphosphatemia in end-stage renal disease	R & D Labs
Calcium gluconate (*Calgonate*)	A wash for hydrofluoric acid spills on human skin	Calgonate
Calcium gluconate gel (*H-F Gel*)	Emergency topical treatment of hydrogen fluoride (hydrofluoric acid) burns	LTR Pharm
Calcium gluconate gel 2.5%	Emergency topical treatment of hydrogen fluoride (hydrofluoric acid) burns	Paddock Labs
Calfactant (*Infasurf*)	Acute respiratory distress syndrome	ONY
Capsaicin	Painful HIV-associated neuropathy; erythromelalgia	NeurogesX
Carbamic acid,[[4-[[3-[[4-[1-(4-hydroxyphenyl)-1-methyl-ethyl]phenoxy]methyl]phenyl]methoxy]phenyl]iminomethyl]-,ethyl ester	Management of cystic fibrosis	Boeringer Ingelheim
Carbamylglutamic acid	N-acetylglutamate synthetase deficiency	Orphan Europe
Carbovir	AIDS and symptomatic HIV infection with CD4 count < 200/mm³	GlaxoWellcome
Carboxypeptidase G2	To treat patients at risk of methotrexate toxicity	Protherics

Orphan Drugs		
Drug (*Trade name*)	Proposed use	Sponsor
Carmustine	Intracranial malignancies	Direct Therapeutics
Cascara sagrada fluid extract	For oral drug overdosage to speed lower bowel evacuation	Intramed
CD4 human truncated 369 AA poly-peptide (*Soluble T4*)	AIDS	SmithKline Beecham
CD5-T lymphocyte immunotoxin (*Xomazyme-H65*)	Graft vs host disease and/or rejection in bone marrow transplant recipients	Xoma
CDP571	Crohn disease	Celltech Chiroscience Ltd
Cells produced using the Aastrom-Replicelle System and SC-I Therapy Kit	For patients receiving high-dose chemotherapy who are unable to generate an acceptable dose of peripheral blood stem cells and have a sufficient bone marrow aspirate without morphological evidence of tumor	Aastrom Biosciences
Centruroides immune F(ab)2 (*Alacramyn*)	Scorpion envenomations requiring medical attention	Silanes Labs SA de CV
Ceramide trihexosidase/alpha-galactosidase A (*Fabrazyme*)	Fabry disease[a]	Genzyme
Cetiedil citrate injection	Sickle cell disease crisis	Baker Cummins Pharm
Cetuximab	Squamous cell cancer of the head and neck in patients who express epidermal growth factor receptor	ImClone Systems
Chenodeoxycholic acid (*Chenofalk*)	Cerebrotendinous xanthomatosis	Dr. Falk Pharma GmbH
Chenodiol (*Chenix*)	Radiolucent stones in well-opacifying gallbladders where elective surgery would be undertaken except for presence of increased surgical risk caused by systemic disease or age[a]	Solvay
Chimeric (human-murine) G250 IgG monoclonal antibody	Renal cell carcinoma	Wilex Biotechnology GmbH
Chimeric, humanized monoclonal antibody to *Staphylococcus*	Prophylaxis of *Staphylococcus epidermidis* sepsis in low birth weight ($\leq$ 1500 g) infants	Biosynexus
Chimeric M-T412 (human-murine) IgG monoclonal anti-CD4	Multiple sclerosis	Centocor
Chlorhexidine gluconate mouth rinse (*Peridex*)	Amelioration of oral mucositis associated with cytoreductive therapy used in conditioning patients for bone marrow transplantation therapy	Procter & Gamble
Cholic acid (3 alpha, 7 alpha, 12 alpha trihydroxy 5-beta cholanolic acid) (*Falkochol*)	Inborn errors of cholesterol and bile acid synthesis and metabolism	Dr. Falk Pharma GmbH
Choline chloride (*Intrachol*)	Choline deficiency (specifically the choline deficiency, hepatic steatosis, and cholestasis associated with long-term parenteral nutrition)	Orphan Medical
Chondrocyte-alginate gel suspension	To correct vesicoureteral reflux in the pediatric population	Curis
Chondroitinase	Patients undergoing vitrectomy	Bausch & Lomb
Ciliary neurotrophic factor	Amyotrophic lateral sclerosis	Regeneron Pharm
Ciliary neurotrophic factor, recombinant human	Motor neuron disease (including amyotrophic lateral sclerosis, progressive muscular atrophy, progressive bulbar palsy, and primary lateral sclerosis); spinal muscular atrophies	Syntex-Synergen Neuroscience
Cinacalcet	Hypercalcemia in patients with parathyroid carcinoma	Amgen
Cisplatin/Epinephrine (*IntraDose*)	Metastatic malignant melanoma; squamous cell carcinoma of the head and neck	Matrix Pharm
Citric acid, glucono-delta-lactone, and magnesium carbonate (*Renacidin Irrigation*)	Renal and bladder calculi of the apatite or struvite variety[a]	United-Guardian
Civamide (*Zucapsaicin*)	Postherpetic neuralgia of the trigeminal nerve	Winston Labs
Cladribine (*Leustatin Injection*)	Hairy-cell leukemia[a]; chronic lymphocytic leukemia; non-Hodgkin lymphoma; acute myeloid leukemia	RW Johnson Pharm Res Inst
(*Mylinax*)	Chronic progressive multiple sclerosis	
Clindamycin (*Cleocin*)	To treat and prevent *Pneumocystis carinii* pneumonia associated with AIDS	Pharmacia & Upjohn Pfizer
Clofarabine (*Clofarex*)	Acute lymphoblastic and myelogenous leukemia	Ilex Products
Clofazimine (*Lamprene*)	Lepromatous leprosy, including dapsone-resistant lepromatous leprosy and lepromatous leprosy complicated by erythema nodosum leprosum[a]	Novartis
Clonazepam (*Klonopin*)	Hyperekplexia (startle disease)	Hoffmann-La Roche
Clonidine (*Duraclon*)	For continuous epidural administration as adjunctive therapy with intraspinal opiates for pain in cancer patients tolerant or unresponsive to intraspinal opiates[a]	Roxane Labs
Clostridial collagenase	Advanced (involutional or residual stage) Dupuytren disease	L. Hurst, MD and M. Badalamente, PhD
Clotrimazole	Sickle cell disease	Carlo Brugnara, MD
Coagulation factor VIIa (recombinant) (*NovoSeven*)	Bleeding episodes in hemophilia A or B patients with inhibitors to Factor VIII or Factor IX[a]	Novo Nordisk
Coagulation factor IX (*Mononine*)	Replacement treatment and prophylaxis of hemorrhagic complications of hemophilia B[a]	Armour Pharm
Coagulation factor IX (human) (*AlphaNine*)	Replacement therapy in hemophilia B for prevention and control of bleeding episodes and during surgery to correct defective hemostasis[a]	Alpha Therapeutic
Coagulation factor IX (recombinant) (*BeneFix*)	Hemophilia B[a]	Genetics Inst

Orphan Drugs		
Drug (*Trade name*)	Proposed use	Sponsor
Coenzyme Q10	Huntington disease	Vitaline
Colchicine	Arrest the progression of neurologic disability caused by chronic progressive multiple sclerosis	Pharmacontrol
Colfosceril palmitate, cetyl alcohol, tyloxapol (*Exosurf*)	Adult respiratory distress syndrome	GlaxoSmithKline
(*Exosurf Neonatal for Intratracheal Suspension*)	To prevent hyaline membrane disease (respiratory distress syndrome) in infants born at ≤ 32 weeks gestation[a]; to treat established hyaline membrane disease at all gestational ages[a]	GlaxoWellcome
Collagenase (lyophilized) for injection (*Plaquase*)	Peyronie disease	Advance Biofactures
Combretastatin A4 phosphate	Anaplastic thyroid cancer, medullary thyroid cancer, and stage VI papillary or follicular thyroid cancer	OXiGENE
Conjugate of human transferrin and a mutant diphtheria toxin (CRM 107) (*TransMID*)	Malignant tumors of the CNS	INTELLIgene Expressions
Conjugated bile acids (*COBARTin*)	Steatorrhea in short bowel syndrome	Jarrow Formulas
Corticorelin ovine triflutate (*Acthrel*)	To differentiate between pituitary and ectopic production of adrenocorticotropic hormone (ACTH) in ACTH-dependent Cushing syndrome[a]	Ferring Labs
Corticotropin-releasing factor, human (*Xerecept*)	Peritumoral brain edema	Neurobiological Technologies
Coumarin (*Onkolox*)	Renal cell carcinoma	Drossapharm Ltd
Creatine (*Creapure*)	Amyotrophic lateral sclerosis	Avicena Group
Cromolyn sodium (*Gastrocrom*)	Mastocytosis[a]	Fisons
Cromolyn sodium 4% ophthalmic solution (*Opticrom 4% Ophthalmic Solution*)	Vernal keratoconjunctivitis[a]	Fisons
***Cryptosporidium* hyperimmune bovine colostrum IgG concentrate**	Diarrhea in AIDS patients caused by infection with *Cryptosporidium parvum*	ImmuCell
CT-2584 mesylate	Adult soft tissue sarcoma; malignant mesothelioma	Cell Therapeutics
CY-1503 (*Cylexin*)	Postischemic pulmonary reperfusion edema following surgical treatment for chronic thrombo-embolic pulmonary hypertension; for neonates and infants undergoing cardiopulmonary bypass during surgical repair of congenital heart lesions	Cytel
CY-1899	Chronic active hepatitis B infection in HLA-A2 positive patients	Cytel
Cyclosporin	Prophylaxis of acute rejection in patients requiring allogenic lung transplant	Chiron
Cyclosporine	Refractory acute rejection in patients requiring allogenic lung transplants	Chiron
Cyclosporine 2% ophthalmic ointment	Treatment of patients at high risk of graft rejection following penetrating keratoplasty; corneal melting syndromes of known or presumed immunologic etiopathogenesis, including Mooren ulcer	Allergan
Cyclosporine in combination with omega-3 polyunsaturated fatty acids	To prevent solid organ graft rejection	RTP Pharma
Cyclosporine ophthalmic (*Optimmune*)	Severe keratoconjunctivitis sicca associated with Sjogren syndrome	University of Georgia
Cyproterone acetate (*Androcur*)	Severe hirsutism	Berlex Labs
Cysteamine (*Cystagon*)	Nephropathic cystinosis	Jess G. Thoene, MD
	Nephropathic cystinosis[a]	Mylan
Cysteamine HCl	Corneal cystine crystal accumulation in cystinosis patients	Sigma-Tau Pharm
Cystic fibrosis gene therapy	Cystic fibrosis	Genzyme
Cystic fibrosis Tr gene therapy (recombinant adenovirus) (*AdGVCFTR.10*)	Cystic fibrosis	GenVec
Cystic fibrosis transmembrane con-ductance regulator	Cystic fibrosis transmembrane conductance regulator protein replacement therapy in cystic fibrosis	Genzyme
Cystic fibrosis transmembrane con-ductance regulator gene	Cystic fibrosis	Genetic Therapy
Cytarabine liposomal (*DepoCyt*)	Neoplastic meningitis[a]	DepoTech
Cytomegalovirus immune globulin IV (human) (*CytoGam*)	With ganciclovir sodium for the treatment of cytomegalovirus pneumonia in bone marrow transplant patients	Bayer
	Prevention or attenuation of primary cytomegalovirus disease in immunosuppressed recipients of organ transplants[a]	MA Public Health Bio Labs
Daclizumab (*Zenapax*)	To prevent acute renal allograft rejection[a]	Hoffmann-LaRoche
Dantrolene sodium (*Dantrium*)	Neuroleptic malignant syndrome	Norwich Eaton Pharm
Dapsone	Prophylaxis of toxoplasmosis in severely immunocompromised patients with CD4 counts < 100	Jacobus Pharm
Dapsone, USP (*Dapsone*)	Prophylaxis of *Pneumocystis carinii* pneumonia (PCP); with trimethoprim for treatment of PCP	Jacobus Pharm
Daunorubicin citrate liposome injection (*DaunoXome*)	Advanced HIV-associated Kaposi sarcoma[a]	NeXstar
Debrase (*Debridase*)	Debridement of acute, deep dermal burns in hospitalized patients	MediWound Ltd

Orphan Drugs		
Drug (*Trade name*)	Proposed use	Sponsor
Decitabine	Myelodysplastic syndromes; chronic myelogenous leukemia; sickle cell anemia	SuperGen
Deferasirox	Chronic iron overload in patients with transfusion-dependent anemias	Novartis
Deferiprone (*Ferriprox*)	Iron overload in patients with hematologic disorders requiring chronic transfusion therapy	Apotex Res
Defibrotide	Thrombotic thrombocytopenic purpura	Crinos
	Hepatic veno-occlusive disease	Gentium SpA
Dehydroepiandrosterone (DHEA) (*Fidelin*)	Systemic lupus erythematosus (SLE) and reduction of steroid use in steroid-dependent SLE patients	Genelabs Tech
	Replacement therapy in patients with adrenal insufficiency	Paladin Labs
Dehydroepiandrosterone sulfate sodium	To treat serious burns requiring hospitalization; to accelerate re-epithelialization of donor sites in those hospitalized burn patients who must undergo autologous skin grafting	Pharmadigm
Denileukin diftitox (*Ontak*)	Persistent or recurrent cutaneous T-cell lymphoma whose malignant cells express the CD25 component of the IL-2 receptor[a]	Ligand Pharm
Deoxyribose, phosphorothioate	Advanced malignant melanoma (stages II, III, and IV)	Genta
Desmopressin acetate	Mild hemophilia A and von Willebrand disease[a]	Aventis Behring LLC
Dexamethasone	Used in posterior segment drug delivery system in idiopathic intermediate uveitis	Oculex Pharm
Dexrazoxane (*Zinecard*)	T prevent cardiomyopathy associated with doxorubicin administration[a]	Pharmacia & Upjohn
Dextran 1	Cystic fibrosis	BCY LifeSciences
Dextran 70 (*Dehydrex*)	Recurrent corneal erosion unresponsive to conventional therapy	Holles Labs
Dextran and deferoxamine (*Bio-Rescue*)	Acute iron poisoning	Biomedical Frontiers
Dextran sulfate (inhaled, aerosolized) (*Uendex*)	As an adjunct to the treatment of cystic fibrosis	Kennedy and Hoidal, MDs
Dextran sulfate sodium	AIDS	Ueno Fine Chemicals
DHA-paclitaxel (*Taxoprexin*)	Pancreatic cancer; metastatic malignant melanoma; adenocarcinoma of the stomach or lower esophagus	Protarga
Dianeal peritoneal dialysis solution with 1.1% amino acids (*Nutrineal [Peritoneal Dialysis Solution with 1.1% Amino Acid]*)	Nutritional supplement for malnourishment in patients undergoing continuous ambulatory peritoneal dialysis	Baxter Healthcare
Diazepam viscous solution for rectal administration	For the management of selected, refractory patients with epilepsy on stable regimens of antiepileptic drugs who require intermittent use of diazepam to control bouts of increased seizure activity[a]	Xcel
Diaziquone	Primary brain malignancies (grade III and IV astrocytomas)	Warner-Lambert
Dideoxyinosine	AIDS	Bristol-Myers Squibb
Diethyldithiocarbamate (*Imuthiol*)	AIDS	Connaught Labs
Diferuloylmethane	Cystic fibrosis	Seer Pharm
Digitoxin	Soft tissue sarcomas; ovarian cancer	PrimeCyte
Digoxin immune FAB (ovine) (*Digibind*)	To treat potentially life-threatening digitalis intoxication in patients refractory to management by conventional therapy[a]	GlaxoWellcome
(*Digidote*)	Life-threatening acute cardiac glycoside intoxication manifested by conduction disorders, ectopic ventricular activity, and, in some cases, hyperkalemia	Boehringer Mannheim
Dihydrotestosterone (*Androgel-DHT*)	Weight loss in AIDS with HIV-associated wasting	Unimed
Dimethyl sulfoxide	Topical treatment for the prevention of soft tissue injury following extravasation of cytotoxic drugs; palmar-plantar-erythrodysesthesia syndrome	Cancer Technologies
	Increased intracranial pressure in patients with severe, closed-head injury (traumatic brain coma) for whom no other effective treatment is available	Pharma 21
	Cutaneous manifestations of scleroderma	Research Industries
Dipalmitoylphosphatidylcholine/ Phosphatidylglycerol (*ALEC*)	To prevent/treat neonatal respiratory distress syndrome	Forum Products
Diphenylcyclopenone	Chronic severe forms of alopecia areata (alopecia totalis/alopecia universalis)	Lloyd E. King, Jr.
Disaccharide tripeptide glycerol dipalmitoyl (*Immther*)	Pulmonary and hepatic metastases in colorectal adenocarcinoma	ImmunoTherapeutics
Disodium clodronate	Hypercalcemia of malignancy	Discovery Experimental & Development
Disodium clodronate tetrahydrate (*Bonefos*)	Increased bone resorption caused by malignancy	Anthra Pharm
Disodium silibinin dihemisuccinate (*Legalon*)	Hepatic intoxication by *Amanita phalloides* (mushroom poisoning)	Pharmaquest
DMP 777	Therapeutic management of lung disease attributable to cystic fibrosis	DuPont
DNA-lipid complex (DMRIE/DOPE)/ plasmid vector (VCL-1102, Vical) expressing human interleukin-2 (*Leuvectin*)	Renal cell carcinoma	Vical
DNP-modified autologous tumor vaccine (*O-Vax*)	Adjuvant therapy for the treatment of ovarian cancer	AVAX Technologies
Docosahexanoic acid-paclitaxel (*Taxoprexin*)	Hormone-refractory prostate cancer	Protarga

Orphan Drugs		
Drug (*Trade name*)	Proposed use	Sponsor
Dornase alfa (*Pulmozyme*)	Reduces mucous viscosity and enables the clearance of airway secretions in cystic fibrosis[a]	Genentech
Doxorubicin liposome (*Doxil*)	Ovarian cancer[a]	Alza
D-peptide of the sequence AKRHH-GYKRKFH-NH2 (*PulmaDex*)	Cystic fibrosis	Demegen
Dronabinol (*Marinol*)	Stimulation of appetite and prevention of weight loss in patients with a confirmed diagnosis of AIDS[a]	Unimed
Duramycin	Cystic fibrosis	MoliChem Medicines
Dynamine	Lambert-Eaton myasthenic syndrome; hereditary motor and sensory neuropathy type I (Charcot-Marie-Tooth disease)	Mayo Foundation
Eculizumab	Idiopathic membranous glomerular nephropathy; paroxysmal nocturnal hemoglobinuria	Alexion Pharm
Eflornithine HCl (*Ornidyl*)	*Trypanosoma brucei* gambiense infection (sleeping sickness)[a]	Hoechst Marion Roussel
	Pneumocystis carinii pneumonia in AIDS	Marion Merrell Dow
Elcatonin	Intrathecal treatment of intractable pain	Innapharma
Enadoline HCl	Severe head injury	Warner-Lambert
Encapsulated porcine islet preparation (*BetaRx*)	For patients with type I diabetes already on immunosuppression	VivoRx
Enisoprost	In organ transplantation to diminish the nephrotoxicity induced by cyclosporine; with cyclosporine in organ transplantation to reduce acute transplant rejection	G.D. Searle
Epidermal growth factor (human)	Acceleration of corneal epithelial regeneration and healing of stromal tissue in nonhealing corneal defects	Chiron Vision
	To promote cutaneous wound healing in extreme burn treatment protocols	Ethicon
Epirubicin (*Ellence*)	Breast cancer[a]	Pharmacia & Upjohn
Epoetin alfa	Myelodysplastic syndrome	Johnson & Johnson Pharm R & D
(*Epogen*)	Anemia associated with end-stage renal disease[a] or HIV infection or treatment[a]	Amgen
(*Procrit*)	Anemia associated with end-stage renal disease; anemia of prematurity in preterm infants; HIV-associated anemia related to HIV infection or treatment	RW Johnson Pharm Res Inst
Epoetin beta (*Marogen*)	Anemia associated with end-stage renal disease	Chugai-USA
Epoprostenol (*Cycloprostin*)	Replacement of heparin in patients requiring hemodialysis and who are at increased risk of hemorrhage	Upjohn
(*Flolan*)	Primary pulmonary hypertension[a]; secondary pulmonary hypertension caused by intrinsic precapillary pulmonary vascular disease[a]; replacement of heparin in patients requiring hemodialysis and who are at increased risk of hemorrhage	GlaxoSmithKline
Epratuzumab (*LymphoCIDE*)	Non-Hodgkin lymphoma	Amgen
Erlotinib HCl (*Tarceva*)	Malignant gliomas	Genentech
Erwinia L-asparaginase	Alternative to *Escherichia coli* asparaginase in those situations where repeat courses of asparaginase therapy for acute lymphoblastic leukemia are required or when allergic reactions force the discontinuance of the *E. coli* preparation	Lyphomed
(*Erwinase*)	Acute lymphocytic leukemia	Porton International
Erythropoietin (recombinant human)	Anemia associated with end-stage renal disease	McDonnell Douglas
		Organon Teknika
Etanercept (*Enbrel*)	Reduction in signs and symptoms of moderately to severely active polyarticular-course juvenile rheumatoid arthritis where there has been inadequate response to ≥ 1 disease-modifying antirheumatic drug[a]; Wegener granulomatosis	Immunex
Ethanolamine oleate (*Ethamolin*)	To prevent rebleeding of esophageal varices that have recently bled[a]	Block Drug
Ethinyl estradiol, USP	Turner syndrome	Bio-Technology General
Ethiofos	A chemoprotective agent for cisplatin and cyclophosphamide in ovarian cancer	US Bioscience
Ethyl eicosapentaenoate	Huntington disease	Laxdale Ltd
Etidronate disodium (*Didronel*)	Hypercalcemia of malignancy inadequately managed by dietary modification and/or oral hydration[a]	MGI Pharma
(*Didronel IV Infusion*)	To prevent/treat degenerative metabolic bone disease in patients who require long-term (≥ 6 months) total parenteral nutrition	
Etiocholanedione	Aplastic anemia; Prader-Willi syndrome	SuperGen
Exemestane (*Aromasin*)	Advanced breast cancer in postmenopausal women whose disease has progressed following tamoxifen therapy[a]	Pharmacia & Upjohn
Exisulind	Suppression and control of colonic adenomatous polyps in the inherited disease adenomatous polyposis coli	Cell Pathways
Factor XIII [A2] homodimer, recombinant DNA orgin	Congenital FXIII deficiency; prophylaxis of bleeding associated with congenital FXIII deficiency	ZymoGenetics
Factor XIII concentrate (human) pasteurized (*Fibrogammin P*)	Congenital Factor XIII deficiency	Aventis Behring LLC
Factor XIII, recombinant	Congenital Factor XIII deficiency	Zymogenetics
Fampridine (*Neurelan*)	For the relief of symptoms of multiple sclerosis; chronic, incomplete spinal cord injury	Acorda Therapeutics

Orphan Drugs		
Drug (*Trade name*)	Proposed use	Sponsor
Felbamate (*Felbatol*)	Lennox-Gastaut syndrome[a]	Wallace Labs
Ferric hexacyanoferrate (II) "Prussian Blue"	Known or suspected internal contamination with radioactive or nonradioactive cesium or thallium	Degussa AG
FIAU	Adjunctive treatment of chronic active hepatitis B	Oclassen Pharm
Fibrinogen (human)	Control of bleeding and prophylactic treatment of patients deficient in fibrinogen	Alpha Therapeutics
Fibronectin (human plasma-derived)	For nonhealing corneal ulcers or epithelial defects unresponsive to conventional therapy and the underlying cause has been eliminated	Melville Biologics
Fibronectin (plasma-derived)	For nonhealing corneal ulcers or epithelial defects unresponsive to conventional therapy and for which any infectious cause of the defect has been eliminated	Chiron Vision
Filgrastim (*Neupogen*)	Severe chronic neutropenia (absolute neutrophil count < 500/mm³)[a]; neutropenia associated with bone marrow transplants[a]; AIDS patients with cytomegalovirus retinitis being treated with ganciclovir; mobilization of peripheral blood progenitor cells for collection in patients who will receive myeloablative or myelosuppressive chemotherapy[a]; to reduce duration of neutropenia, fever, antibiotic use, and hospitalization following induction and consolidation treatment for acute myeloid leukemia[a]; myelodysplastic syndrome	Amgen
Flucinolone	Uveitis involving the posterior segment of the eye	Bausch & Lomb
Fludarabine phosphate (*Fludara*)	Treatment and management of non-Hodgkin lymphoma; chronic lymphocytic leukemia (CLL) including refractory CLL[a]	Berlex Labs
Flumecinol (*Zixoryn*)	Hyperbilirubinemia in newborn infants unresponsive to phototherapy	Farmacon
Flunarizine (*Sibelium*)	Alternating hemiplegia	Janssen Res
Fluorouracil	With interferon alpha-2a, recombinant, for advanced colorectal and esophageal carcinomas	Hoffmann-La Roche
	Glioblastoma multiforme	Ethypharm SA
(*Adrucil*)	With leucovorin for metastatic adenocarcinoma of the colon and rectum	Lederle Labs
Fluoxetine (*Prozac*)	Autism	Eric Hollander, MD
Follitropin alfa, recombinant (*Gonal-F*)	Induction of spermatogenesis in men with primary and secondary hypogonadotropic hypogonadism in whom the cause of infertility is not caused by primary testicular failure[a]	Serono Labs
Fomepizole (*Antizol*)	Methanol or ethylene glycol poisoning[a]	Orphan Medical
Fosphenytoin (*Cerebyx*)	Acute treatment of patients with status epilepticus of the grand mal type[a]	Warner-Lambert
Fructose-1,6-diphosphate (*Cordox*)	For painful vaso-occlusive episodes associated with sickle cell disease	Questcor Pharm
G17DT immunogen	Adenocarcinoma of the pancreas; gastric cancer	Aphton
Gabapentin (*Neurontin*)	Amyotrophic lateral sclerosis	Warner-Lambert
Gallium nitrate injection (*Ganite*)	Hypercalcemia of malignancy[a]	Solopak Pharm
Gamma hydroxybutyrate	Narcolepsy and auxiliary symptoms of cataplexy, sleep paralysis, hypnagogic hallucinations, and automatic behavior	Biocraft Labs
Gamma hydroxybutyric acid	Narcolepsy and auxiliary symptoms of cataplexy, sleep paralysis, hypnagogic hallucinations, and automatic behavior	Sigma Chemical
Gammalinolenic acid	Juvenile rheumatoid arthritis	Robert B. Zurier, MD
Ganaxolone	Infantile spasms	Purdue Pharma LP
Ganciclovir intravitreal implant (*Vitrasert Implant*)	Cytomegalovirus retinitis[a]	Bausch & Lomb Surgical, Chiron Vision Products
Ganciclovir sodium (*Cytovene*)	Cytomegalovirus retinitis in immunocompromised patients with AIDS[a]	Syntex (USA)
Gancyclovir	Severe human cytomegalovirus infections in specific immunosuppressed patient populations	Burroughs Wellcome
Gangliosides as sodium salts (*Cronassial*)	Retinitis pigmentosa	Fidia Pharm
Gavilimomab	Acute graft vs host disease	Abgenix
Gemtuzumab ozogamicin (*Mylotarg*)	CD33-positive acute myeloid leukemia[a]	Wyeth-Ayerst Labs
Gene plasmid hVEGF165 driven by human cytomegalovirus, and [2,3-bis(oleoyl)propyl]trimethyl ammonium and dioleoyl phosphatidyl ethanolamine (*Trinam*)	To prevent complications caused by neointimal hyperplasia disease in certain vascular anastomoses	Ark Therapeutics
Gentamicin impregnated PMMA beads on surgical wire (*Septopal*)	Chronic osteomyelitis of posttraumatic, postoperative, or hematogenous origin	Lipha Pharm
Gentamicin liposome injection (*Maitec*)	Disseminated *Mycobacterium avium*-intracellulare infection	Liposome
Glatiramer acetate (*Copaxone*)	Multiple sclerosis[a]	Teva
Glatiramer acetate for injection (*Copaxone*)	Primary-progressive multiple sclerosis	Teva
Glutamine	With human growth hormone in the treatment of short bowel syndrome (nutrient malabsorption from the GI tract resulting from an inadequate absorptive surface)	Nutritional Restart Pharm
Glyceol	To decrease intracranial hypertension and/or alleviate cerebral edema in patients who may benefit from osmotherapy	Chugai Pharm

Orphan Drugs		
Drug (*Trade name*)	Proposed use	Sponsor
Glyceryl trioleate and glyceryl trierucate	Adrenoleukodystrophy	Hugo W. Moser, MD
Gonadorelin acetate (*Lutrepulse*)	Ovulation induction in women with hypothalamic amenorrhea caused by a deficiency or absence in quantity or pulse pattern of endogenous GnRH secretion[a]	Ferring Labs
Gossypol	Cancer of the adrenal cortex	Marcus M. Reidenberg, MD
Gp100 adenoviral gene therapy	Metastatic melanoma	Genzyme
Granulocyte macrophage-colony stimulating factor (*Leucomax*)	Neutropenia caused by hairy cell leukemia; neutropenia associated with bone marrow transplants; severe thermal injuries in patients with > 40% full or partial thickness burns; myelodysplastic syndrome; chronic lymphocytic leukemia to increase granulocyte count	Schering
Group B streptococcus immune globulin	Disseminated group B streptococcal infection in neonates	North American Biologicals
Growth hormone releasing factor	Long-term treatment of children who have growth failure caused by a lack of adequate endogenous growth hormone secretion	Valeant Pharm
Guanethidine monosulfate (*Ismelin*)	Moderate to severe sympathetic reflex dystrophy and causalgia	Novartis
Guanfacine (*Tenex*)	Fragile X syndrome	Watson Labs
Gusperimus (*Spanidin*)	Acute renal graft rejection episodes	Bristol-Myers Squibb Pharm Res Inst
h5G1.1-mAb	Dermatomyositis	Alexion Pharm
Halofantrine (*Halfan*)	Mild to moderate acute malaria caused by susceptible strains of *Plasmodium falciparum* and *P. vivax*[a]	SmithKline Beecham
Halofuginone (*Stenorol*)	Systemic sclerosis	Collgard Biopharmaceuticals Ltd
Heme arginate (*Normosang*)	Symptomatic stage of acute porphyria; myelodysplastic syndromes	Berlex Labs
Hemin (*Panhematin*)	Amelioration of recurrent attacks of acute intermittent porphyria (AIP) temporarily related to the menstrual cycle in susceptible women and similar symptoms that occur in other patients with AIP, porphyria variegata, and hereditary coproporphyria[a]	Abbott Labs
Hemin and zinc mesoporphyrin (*Hemex*)	Acute porphyric syndromes	Herbert L. Bonkovsky, MD
Heparin, oral unfractionated	Sickle cell disease	TRF Technologies
Hepatitis B immune globulin IV (human) (*Nabi-HB*)	Prophylaxis against hepatitis B virus reinfection in liver transplant patients	NABI
Hepatitis C virus immune globulin (human)	Prophylaxis of hepatitis C infection in liver transplant recipients	NABI
HepeX-B	To prevent hepatitis B virus reinfection in liver transplant patients	XTL Biopharmaceuticals
Herpes simplex virus gene	Primary and metastatic brain tumors	Genetic Therapy
Herpes simplex virus, genetically engineered (G207)	Malignant glioma	MediGene
Histamine (*Maxamine*)	Adjunctive to cytokine therapy in treatment of acute myeloid leukemia and malignant melanoma	Maxim Pharm
Histrelin	Treatment of acute intermittent porphyria, hereditary coproporphyria, and variegate porphyria	Karl E. Anderson, MD
Histrelin acetate (*Supprelin Injection*)	Central precocious puberty[a]	Roberts Pharm
HIV neutralizing antibodies (*Immupath*)	AIDS	Hemacare
HLA-B7/Beta2M DNA Lipid (DMRIE/ DOPE) Complex (*Allovectin-7*)	Invasive and metastatic melanoma (stages II, III, IV)	Vical Incorporated
Homoharringtonine	Chronic myelogenous leukemia	American BioScience
HPA-23	AIDS	Rhone-Poulenc Rorer
Hsp E7	Recurrent respiratory papillomatosis	StressGen Biotechnologies
Hu1D10, humanized, monoclonal antibody (*Remitogen*)	1D10+ B cell non-Hodgkin lymphoma	Protein Design Labs
Human acid precursor alpha-glucosidase, recombinant	Glycogen storage disease type II	Pharming/Genzyme LLC
Human anti-transforming growth factor beta 1 monoclonal antibody	Systemic sclerosis	Genzyme
Human anti-tumor necrosis factor alpha monoclonal antibody	Uveitis of the posterior segment of noninfectious etiology, and uveitis of the anterior segment of noninfectious etiology and refractory to conventional therapy	Centocor
Human gammaglobulin	Juvenile rheumatoid arthritis; GI disturbances (eg, constipation, diarrhea, abdominal pain) associated with regression-onset autism in pediatric patients; idiopathic inflammatory myopathies	Protein Therapeutics
Human IgM monoclonal antibody (C-58) to cytomegalovirus (*Centovir*)	Cytomegalovirus infections in allogenic bone marrow transplant patients; prophylaxis of cytomegalovirus infections in bone marrow transplant patients	Centocor
Human immunodeficiency virus immune globulin (*Hivig*)	AIDS; HIV-infected pregnant women and pediatric patients; infants of HIV-infected mothers	NABI
Human T-lymphotropic virus type III Gp 160 antigens (*Vaxsyn HIV-1*)	AIDS	MicroGeneSys

Orphan Drugs		
Drug (*Trade name*)	Proposed use	Sponsor
Humanized anti-CD2 monoclonal antibody	Graft vs host disease	MedImmune
Humanized anti-human CD2 MAb (*MEDI-507*)	Induction of donor-specific immunologic unresponsiveness resulting in prophylaxis of organ rejection without the need for chronic immunosuppressive therapy in allogeneic renal transplants	Biotransplant
Humanized anti-tac (*Zenapax*)	To prevent acute graft vs host disease following bone marrow transplantation	Hoffmann-La Roche
Humanized MAb (IDEC-131) to CD40L	Systemic lupus erythematosus	Idec Pharm
Humanized monoclonal antibody against Shiga-like toxin II	To prevent the development of or to decrease the incidence and severity of hemolytic uremic syndrome and associated sequelae of Shiga-like toxin-producing *Escherichia coli*	Teijin America
Hyaluronic acid	Emphysema caused by alpha-1 antitrypsin deficiency	Exhale Therapeutics
Hydroxocobalamin (*Cyanokit*)	Acute cyanide poisoning	Orphan Medical
		EMD Pharm
Hydroxycobalamin/Sodium thiosulfate	Severe acute cyanide poisoning	Alan H. Hall, MD
Hydroxyurea (*Droxia*)	Sickle cell anemia as shown by the presence of hemoglobin S[a]	Bristol-Myers Squibb Pharm Res Inst
Hypericin	Glioblastoma multiforme; cutaneous T-cell lymphoma	Nexell Therapeutics
I(131)-TM-601 (chlorotoxin)	Malignant glioma	TransMolecular
Ibritumomab tiuxetan (*Zevalin*)	B-cell non-Hodgkin lymphoma[a]	IDEC Pharm
Ibuprofen IV solution (*Salprofen*)	To prevent/treat patent ductus arteriosus	Farmacon-IL LLC
Icatbant	Angioedema	Jerini AG
Icodextrin 7.5% with electrolytes peritoneal dialysis solution (*Extraneal [with 7.5% Icodextrin] Peritoneal Dialysis Solution*)	End-stage renal disease requiring peritoneal dialysis treatment[a]	Baxter Healthcare
Idarubicin (*Idamycin*)	Myelodysplastic syndromes; chronic myelogenous leukemia	Pharmacia & Upjohn
Idarubicin HCl for injection (*Idamycin*)	Acute lymphoblastic leukemia in pediatric patients	Pharmacia & Upjohn
	Acute myelogenous leukemia (acute nonlymphocytic leukemia)[a]	Adria Labs
IDN 6556	Patients undergoing solid organ transplantation	Idun Pharm
Idoxuridine	Nonparenchymatous sarcomas	NeoPharm
Iduronate-2-sulfatase	Long-term enzyme replacement therapy for mucopolysaccharidosis II (Hunter syndrome)	Transkaryotic Therapies
Ifosfamide (*Ifex*)	Testicular cancer[a]; bone sarcomas; soft tissue sarcomas	Bristol-Myers Squibb Pharm Res Inst
IL-4 pseudomonas toxin fusion protein (IL-4(38-37)-PE38KDEL)	Astrocytic glioma	Neurocrine Biosciences
IL-13-PE38QQR	Malignant glioma	NeoPharm
Iloprost solution for infusion	Heparin-associated thrombocytopenia; Raynaud phenomenon secondary to systemic sclerosis	Berlex Labs
Imatinib mesylate (*Gleevec*)	Chronic myelogenous leukemia[a]; GI stromal tumors[a]	Novartis
Imciromab pentetate (*Myoscint*)	To detect early necrosis as an indication of rejection of orthotopic cardiac transplants	Centocor
Imexon	Multiple myeloma; metastatic malignant melanoma; pancreatic adenocarcinoma	AmpliMed
Imiglucerase (*Cerezyme*)	Replacement therapy in patients with types I, II, and III Gaucher disease[a]	Genzyme
Immune globulin IV (human) (*Gamimune N*)	Infection prophylaxis in pediatric patients with HIV[a]	Bayer
(*Immuno, Iveegam*)	Acute myocarditis; polymyositis/dermatomyositis; juvenile rheumatoid arthritis	Immuno Clin Res
Imported fire ant venom, allergenic extract	Skin testing for victims of fire ant stings to confirm fire ant sensitivity and, if positive, as immunotherapy for prevention of IgE-mediated anaphylactic reactions	ALK Labs
Indium In-111 altumomab pentetate (*Hybri-ceaker*)	To detect suspected and previously unidentified tumor foci of recurrent colorectal carcinoma	Hybritech
Indium In 111 murine monoclonal antibody FAB to myosin (*Myoscint*)	To aid in diagnosis of myocarditis	Centocor
Infliximab (*Remicade*)	Moderately to severely active Crohn disease for the reduction of the signs and symptoms in patients who have an inadequate response to conventional therapy; fistulizing Crohn disease for the reduction in the number of draining enterocutaneous fistula(s)[a]; chronic sarcoidosis; giant cell arteritis; juvenile rheumatoid arthritis; Crohn disease and ulcerative colitis in pediatric (0 to 16 years of age) patients	Centocor
INGN 201 (*Advexin*)	Head and neck cancer	Introgen Therapeutics
INH-A00021 (*Veronate*)	To reduce (prevent) nosocomial bacteremia caused by staphylococci in very low birth weight infants	Inhibitex
Inolimomab (*Leukotac*)	Graft vs host disease	Opi
Inosine pranobex (*Isoprinosine*)	Subacute sclerosing panencephalitis	Newport Pharm
Interferon alfa-1b	Multiple myeloma	Ernest C. Borden
Interferon alfa-2a (recombinant) (*Roferon-A*)	AIDS-related Kaposi sarcoma[a]; renal-cell carcinoma; with fluorouracil for esophageal carcinoma or advanced colorectal cancer; with teceleukin for metastatic renal cell carcinoma or metastatic malignant melanoma; chronic myelogenous leukemia[a]	Hoffmann-La Roche

Orphan Drugs		
Drug (*Trade name*)	Proposed use	Sponsor
Interferon alfa-2b (recombinant) (*Intron A*)	AIDS-related Kaposi sarcoma[a]; metastatic renal cell carcinoma; chronic myelogenous leukemia; laryngeal (respiratory) papillomatosis; acute hepatitis B; primary malignant brain tumors; invasive carcinoma of the cervix; carcinoma in situ of the urinary bladder; chronic delta hepatitis; ovarian carcinoma	Schering
Interferon alfa-n1 (*Wellferon*)	AIDS-related Kaposi sarcoma	Burroughs Wellcome
	Human papillomavirus in severe resistant/recurrent respiratory (laryngeal) papillomatosis	Glaxo Wellcome
Interferon beta-1a (recombinant human) (*Avonex*)	Acute non-A, non-B hepatitis; primary brain tumors; juvenile rheumatoid arthritis; multiple sclerosis[a]; pulmonary fibrosis	Biogen
(*Betaseron*)	Multiple sclerosis[a]	Berlex Labs and Chiron
	AIDS	Berlex Labs
(*r-HuIFN-beta*)	Systemic treatment of cutaneous T-cell lymphoma and cutaneous malignant melanoma; intralesional and/or systemic treatment of AIDS-related Kaposi sarcoma	Biogen
(*R-IFN-beta*)	Systemic treatment of metastatic renal cell carcinoma	Biogen
(*Rebif*)	Symptomatic patients with AIDS (including CD4 T-cell counts < 200 cells/mm^3); secondary progressive multiple sclerosis	Serono Labs
Interferon gamma-1b (*Actimmune*)	Renal cell carcinoma	Genentech
	Chronic granulomatous disease[a]; delaying time to disease progression in patients with severe, malignant osteopetrosis[a]; idiopathic pulmonary fibrosis	InterMune
Interleukin-1 alpha, human recombinant	Hematopoietic potentiation in aplastic anemia; promotion of early engraftment in bone marrow transplantation	Immunex
Interleukin-1 receptor antagonist (human recombinant) (*Antril*)	Juvenile rheumatoid arthritis; to prevent/treat graft vs host disease in transplant recipients	Amgen
Interleukin-2 (*Teceleukin*)	Alone or with interferon alfa-2a for metastatic renal-cell carcinoma; alone or with interferon alfa-2a for metastatic malignant melanoma	Hoffmann-La Roche
Interleukin-3 human (recombinant)	Promotion of erythropoiesis in Diamond-Blackfan anemia (congenital pure red cell aplasia)	Immunex
	Sequential administration with sargramostim to accelerate neutrophil and platelet recovery in patients undergoing autologous bone marrow transplantation for Hodgkin disease or non-Hodgkin lymphoma	Sandoz Pharm
Intraoral fluoride releasing system (IFRS)	To prevent dental caries caused by radiation-induced xerostomia in head and neck cancer	Digestive Care
Iobenguane sulfate I 131	Diagnostic adjunct in patients with pheochromocytoma[a]	University of Michigan
Iodine I 123 murine monoclonal antibody to alpha-fetoprotein	Detection of hepatocellular carcinoma and hepatoblastoma and alpha-fetoprotein-producing germ-cell tumors	Immunomedics
Iodine I 123 murine monoclonal antibody to hCG	Detection of hCG-producing tumors (eg, germ-cell, trophoblastic-cell tumors)	Immunomedics
Iodine I 131 6B-iodomethyl-19-norcholesterol	Adrenal cortical imaging	David E. Kuhl, MD
Iodine I 131 bis(indium-diethylenetri-aminepentaacetic acid)tyrosyllysine/hMN-14x m734 F(ab')2 bispecific monoclonal antibody (*Pentacea*)	Small-cell lung cancer	IBC Pharm
Iodine I 131 Lym-1 monoclonal antibody	B-cell lymphoma	Lederle Labs
Iodine I 131 murine monoclonal antibody IgG2a to B cell (*Immurait, LI-2-I-131*)	B-cell leukemia and B-cell lymphoma	Immunomedics
Iodine I 131 murine monoclonal antibody to alpha-fetoprotein	Hepatocellular carcinoma and hepatoblastoma; alpha-fetoprotein-producing germ-cell tumors	Immunomedics
Iodine I 131 murine monoclonal antibody to hCG	hCG-producing tumors (eg, germ-cell, trophoblastic-cell tumors)	Immunomedics
Iodine I 131 radiolabeled chimeric MAb tumor necrosis treatment (TNT-1B) (*131IchTNT-1*)	Glioblastoma multiforme and anaplastic astrocytoma	Peregrine Pharm
Irofulven	Renal cell carcinoma; ovarian cancer	MGI Pharma
Iron(III)-hexacyanoferrate(II) (*Radiogardase*)	Known or suspected internal contamination with radioactive or nonradioactive cesium or thallium[a]	Heyl Chemisch-Pharmzeutische
Isobutyramide	Sickle cell disease and beta-thalassemia	Alpha Therapeutics
(*Isobutyramide Oral Solution*)	Beta-hemoglobinopathies and beta-thalassemia syndromes	Susan P. Perrine, MD
Japanese encephalitis vaccine (live, attenuated)	To prevent Japanese encephalitis	Boran Pharm
Ketoconazole (*Nizoral*)	With cyclosporine A to diminish the nephrotoxicity induced by cyclosporine in organ transplantation	Pharmedic
L-2-oxothiazolidine-4-carboxylic acid (*Procysteine*)	Adult respiratory distress syndrome; amyotrophic lateral sclerosis	Transcend Therapeutics
L-5-hydroxytryptophan	Tetrahydrobiopterin deficiency	Watson Labs
L-baclofen	Trigeminal neuralgia	Gerhard Fromm, MD
(*Neuralgon*)	Trigeminal neuralgia; intractable spasticity from spinal cord injury or multiple sclerosis; intractable spasticity in children with cerebral palsy	Pharmascience
L-cycloserine	Gaucher disease	Meir Lev, MD
L-cysteine	To prevent and lessen photosensitivity in erythropoietic protoporphyria	Orphan Pharm USA
L-glutamine	Sickle cell disease	Orphan Drugs International LLC

Orphan Drugs		
Drug (*Trade name*)	Proposed use	Sponsor
L-glutamyl-L-tryptophan	AIDS-related Kaposi sarcoma	Cytran
L-leucovorin (*Isovorin*)	With high-dose methotrexate in the treatment of osteosarcoma; in combination chemotherapy with the approved agent 5-fluorouracil in the palliative treatment of metastatic adenocarcinoma of the colon and rectum	Lederle Labs
L-threonine	Spasticity associated with familial spastic paraparesis	Interneuron Pharm
(*Threostat*)	Amyotrophic lateral sclerosis	Tyson & Assoc
Lactic acid (*Aphthaid*)	Severe aphthous stomatitis in severely, terminally immunocompromised patients	Frontier Pharm
Lactic acid bacteria (*Lactobacilli, Bifidobacteria,* and *Streptococcus* sp.)	Chronic active pouchitis; to prevent disease relapse in patients with chronic pouchitis	VSL Pharm
Lactobin (*Lactobin*)	AIDS-associated diarrhea unresponsive to initial antidiarrheal therapy	Roxane Labs
Lactoferrin alpha	To prevent and treat graft vs host disease	Agennix
Lamotrigine (*Lamictal*)	Lennox-Gastaut syndrome[a]	GlaxoWellcome R & D
Lanreotide, Somatostatin (*Ipstyl*)	Acromegaly	IPSEN
Laronidase (*Aldurazyme*)	Patients with mucopolysaccharidosis-I[a]	BioMarin Pharm
Latrodectus immune F(ab)2 (*Aracmyn*)	Black widow spider envenomations	Rare Disease Therapeutics
Leflunomide	To prevent acute and chronic rejection in patients with solid organ transplants	James W. Williams, MD
Lepirudin (*Refludan*)	Heparin-associated thrombocytopenia type II[a]	Hoechst Marion Roussel
Leucovorin (*Leucovorin calcium*)	With 5-fluorouracil for metastatic colorectal cancer[a]; rescue use after high-dose methotrexate therapy in the treatment of osteosarcoma[a]	Immunex
Leucovorin calcium (*Wellcovorin*)	With 5-fluorouracil for the treatment of metastatic colorectal cancer	GlaxoWellcome R & D
Leupeptin	As an adjunct to microsurgical peripheral nerve repair	Neuromuscular Adjuncts
Leuprolide acetate (*Lupron Injection*)	Central precocious puberty[a]	Tap Pharm
Levocabastine HCl ophthalmic suspension 0.05%	Vernal keratoconjunctivitis	Iolab Pharm
Levocarnitine (*Carnitor*)	Genetic carnitine deficiency[a]; primary and secondary carnitine deficiency of genetic origin[a]; to prevent/treat secondary carnitine deficiency in valproic acid toxicity; pediatric cardiomyopathy; to treat zidovudine-induced mitochondrial myopathy; manifestations of carnitine deficiency in patients with end-stage renal disease who require dialysis[a]	Sigma-Tau Pharm
Levodopa and carbidopa (*Duodopa*)	Late-stage Parkinson disease	Nouvel Pharma
Levomethadyl acetate HCl (*ORLAAM*)	Heroin addiction suitable for maintenance on opiate agonists[a]	Biodevelopment
Lidocaine patch 5% (*Lidoderm Patch*)	To relieve allodynia (painful hypersensitivity) and chronic pain in postherpetic neuralgia[a]	Teikoku Pharma USA
Lintuzumab (*Zamyl*)	Acute myelogenous leukemia	Protein Design Labs
Liothyronine sodium injection (*Triostat*)	Myxedema coma/precoma[a]	SmithKline Beecham
Lipase, amylase, and protease (*TheraCLEC-Total*)	Pancreatic insufficiency	Altus Biologics
Lipid/DNA human cystic fibrosis gene	Cystic fibrosis	Genzyme
Liposomal amphotericin B (*AmBisome*)	Cryptococcal meningitis[a]; visceral leishmaniasis[a]; histoplasmosis	Fujisawa USA
Liposomal-cis-bis-neodecanoato-trans-R,R-1,2-diaminocyclohexane-Pt (II)	Malignant mesothelioma	Antigenics
Liposomal cyclosporin A (*Cyclospire*)	For aerosolized administration to prevent/treat lung allograft rejection and pulmonary rejection events associated with bone marrow transplantation	Vernon Knight, MD
Liposomal N-Acetylglucosminyl-N-Acetylmuramyl-L-Ala-D-isoGln-L-Ala-glycerolidpalmitoyl (*ImmTher*)	Osteosarcoma; Ewing sarcoma	Endorex
Liposomal nystatin (*Nyotran*)	Invasive fungal infections	Antigenics
Liposomal p-ethoxy growth receptor bound protein-2 antisense product	Chronic myelogenous leukemia	Interpath Pharm
Liposomal prostaglandin E1 injection	Acute respiratory distress syndrome	Liposome
Liposome encapsulated recombinant interleukin-2	Brain and CNS tumors; kidney and renal pelvis cancers	Biomira USA
Lisofylline	To treat patients undergoing induction therapy for acute myeloid leukemia	Cell Therapeutics
Lodoxamide tromethamine (*Alomide Ophthalmic Solution*)	Vernal keratoconjunctivitis[a]	Alcon Labs
Loxoribine	Common variable immunodeficiency	RW Johnson Pharm
Lucinactant (*Surfaxin*)	Meconium aspiration syndrome in newborn infants; respiratory distress syndrome in premature infants; acute adult respiratory distress syndrome	Discovery Labs
Lysine acetylsalicylate injectable	Pain and fever secondary to sickle cell disease crisis	GD Searle

Orphan Drugs

Drug (Trade name)	Proposed use	Sponsor
Mafenide acetate solution (*Sulfamylon solution*)	Adjunctive topical antimicrobial agent to control bacterial infection when used under moist dressings over meshed autografts on excised burn wounds[a]	Mylan
Mafosfamide	Neoplastic meningitis	Baxter Oncology GmbH
Marijuana	HIV-associated wasting syndrome	Multidisciplinary Assoc for Psychedelic Studies
MART-1 adenoviral gene therapy for malignant melanoma	Metastatic melanoma	Genzyme
Matrix metalloproteinase inhibitor (*Galardin*)	Corneal ulcers	Glycomed
MaxAdFVIII	Hemophilia A	GenStar Therapeutics
Mazindol (*Sanorex*)	Duchenne muscular dystrophy	Platon J. Collipp, MD
Mecamylamine (*Inversine*)	Tourette syndrome	Targacept
Mecasermin	Growth hormone insufficiency syndrome	Genentech
(*Myotrophin*)	Amyotrophic lateral sclerosis	Cephalon
Medroxyprogesterone acetate (*Hematrol*)	Immune thrombocytopenic purpura	InKine Pharm
Mefloquine HCl (*Lariam*)	Acute malaria caused by *Plasmodium falciparum* and *P. vivax*[a]; prophylaxis of *P. falciparum* malaria resistant to other available drugs[a]	Hoffman-La Roche
(*Mephaquin*)	To prevent/treat chloroquine-resistant *Falciparum* malaria	Mepha AG
Megestrol acetate (*Megace*)	Anorexia, cachexia, or significant weight loss (≥ 10% of baseline body weight) with confirmed diagnosis of AIDS[a]	Bristol-Myers Squibb Pharm Res Inst
Melanoma cell vaccine	Invasive melanoma	CancerVax
Melanoma vaccine (*Melacine*)	Stage III-IV melanoma	Ribi ImmunoChem Res
Melatonin	Circadian rhythm sleep disorders in blind people with no light perception	Robert Sack, MD
Meloxicam (*Mobic*)	Juvenile rheumatoid arthritis	Boehringer Ingelheim
Melphalan (*Alkeran for Injection*)	Hyperthermic regional limb perfusion to treat metastatic melanoma of the extremity; multiple myeloma for whom oral therapy is inappropriate[a]	GlaxoWellcome
Meropenem (*Merrem IV*)	Manage acute pulmonary exacerbations in cystic fibrosis patients caused by respiratory tract infections with susceptible organisms	Zeneca
Mesna	Inhibition of the urotoxic effects induced by oxazaphosphorine compounds (eg, cyclophosphamide)	Asta Medica
(*Mesnex*)	As a prophylactic to reduce the incidence of ifosfamide-induced hemorrhagic cystitis[a]	Degussa
Methionine/L-methionine	AIDS myelopathy	Alessandro Di Rocco, MD
Methotrexate (*Rheumatrex*)	Juvenile rheumatoid arthritis	Wyeth-Ayerst Labs
Methotrexate sodium (*Methotrexate*)	Osteogenic sarcoma[a]	Lederle Labs
Methotrexate with laurocapram (*Methotrexate/Azone*)	Topical treatment of *Mycosis fungoides*	Durham Pharm
Methoxsalen (*Uvadex*)	Used in conjunction with the UVAR photopheresis system to treat graft vs host disease	Therakos
Methylbicyclone	Cystic fibrosis	Sucampo Pharm
Methylnaltrexone	Chronic opioid-induced constipation unresponsive to conventional therapy	University of Chicago
Metreleptin	Metabolic disorders secondary to lipodystrophy; leptin deficiency secondary to generalized lipodystrophy and partial familial lipodystrophy	Amgen
Metronidazole (*Metrogel*)	Perioral dermatitis	Galderma Labs
Metronidazole (topical) (*Flagyl*)	Grade III and IV anaerobically infected, decubitus ulcers	Searle
(*Metrogel*)	Acne rosacea[a]	Galderma Labs
Microbubble contrast agent (*Filmix Neurosonographic Contrast Agent*)	Intraoperative aid in the identification and localization of intracranial tumors	Cav-Con
Midodrine HCl (*Amatine*)	Symptomatic orthostatic hypotension[a]	Schier Ridgewood FKA
Miglustat (*Zavesca*)	Gaucher disease[a]	Actelion Pharm
Minocycline HCl (*Minocin Intravenous*)	Chronic malignant pleural effusion	Lederle Labs
Mitoguazone (*apep*)	Diffuse non-Hodgkin lymphoma, including AIDS-related diffuse non-Hodgkin lymphoma	ILEX Oncology
Mitolactol	Adjuvant therapy in the treatment of primary brain tumors; recurrent invasive or metastatic squamous carcinoma of the cervix	Biopharmaceutics
Mitomycin-C	Refractory glaucoma as an adjunct to ab externo glaucoma surgery	IOP
Mitoxantrone (*Novantrone*)	Progressive-relapsing multiple sclerosis[a]; secondary-progressive multiple sclerosis[a]	Immunex
	Hormone-refractory prostate cancer[a]	Serono Labs
Mitoxantrone HCl (*Novantrone*)	Acute myelogenous leukemia (acute nonlymphocytic leukemia)[a]	Lederle Labs

Orphan Drugs		
Drug (*Trade name*)	Proposed use	Sponsor
MN14 monoclonal antibody to carcinoembryonic antigen (*Cea-Cide*)	Small-cell lung cancer; pancreatic cancer	Immunomedics
Modafinil (*Provigil*)	Excessive daytime sleepiness in narcolepsy[a]	Cephalon
Molgramostim (*Leucomax*)	Aplastic anemia; AIDS patients with neutropenia caused by the disease, AZT, or ganciclovir	Schering
Monarsen	Myasthenia gravis	Medica Venture Partners
Monoclonal Ab(murine) anti-idiotype melanoma-associated antigen (*Melimmune*)	Invasive cutaneous melanoma	IDEC Pharm
Monoclonal antibodies (murine or human) to B-cell lymphoma	B-cell lymphoma	IDEC Pharm
Monoclonal antibody 17-1a (*Panorex*)	Pancreatic cancer	Centocor
Monoclonal antibody-B43.13 (*Ovarex MAb-B43.13*)	Epithelial ovarian cancer	AltaRex US
Monoclonal antibody for immunization against lupus nephritis	Lupus nephritis	VivoRx Autoimmune
Monoclonal antibody to cytomegalovirus (human)	Treatment of cytomegalovirus retinitis in AIDS; prophylaxis of cytomegalovirus disease in solid organ transplantation	Protein Design Labs
Monoclonal antibody to hepatitis B virus (human)	Prophylaxis of hepatitis B reinfection in liver transplantation secondary to end-stage chronic hepatitis B infection	Protein Design Labs
Monoclonal antiendotoxin antibody XMMEn-0e5	Gram-negative sepsis that has progressed to shock	Pfizer
Monoctanoin (*Moctanin*)	Dissolution of cholesterol gallstones retained in the common bile duct[a]	Ethitek Pharm
Monolaurin (*Glylorin*)	Congenital primary ichthyosis	GlaxoWellcome
Morphine sulfate concentrate (preservative free) (*Infumorph*)	In microinfusion devices for intraspinal administration for intractable chronic pain[a]	Elkins-Sinn
Motexafin gadolinium (*Xcytrin*)	With whole brain radiation for the treatment of brain metastases arising from solid tumors	Pharmacyclics
MTC-DOX for injection	Hepatocellular carcinoma	FeRx
Mucoid exopolysaccharide *Pseudomonas* hyperimmune globulin (*MEP IGIV*)	To prevent and treat pulmonary infections caused by *Pseudomonas aeruginosa* in cystic fibrosis	North American Biologicals
Multi-vitamin infusion (neonatal formula)	To establish and maintain total parenteral nutrition in very low birth weight infants	Astra Pharm
Muramyltripeptide, phosphatidyl-ethanolamine encased in multi-lamellar liposomes	Children and adolescent osteosarcoma	Immuno-Designed Molecules
Murine MAb (Lym-1) and Iodine 131-I radiolabeled murine MAb (Lym-1) to human B-cell lymphoma (*Oncolym*)	B-cell non-Hodgkin lymphoma	Peregrine Pharm
Murine MAb to polymorphic epithelial mucin, human milk fat globule 1 (*Theragyn*)	Adjunctive treatment for ovarian cancer	Antisoma plc
Mx-dnG1 or Rexin-G retroviral vector (*Rexin-G*)	Pancreatic cancer	Epeius Biotechnologies
Mycobacterium avium sensitin RS-10	In the diagnosis of invasive *Mycobacterium avium* disease in immunocompetent individuals	Statens Seruminstitut
Mycobacterium with immunomodulator, heat killed (*CADI Mw*)	Adjunctive to multi-drug therapy in the management of multibacillary leprosy	CPL, Inc.
Myelin	Multiple sclerosis	Autoimmune
Myristoylated recombinant SCR1-3 of human complement reseptor type I (*APT070*)	To prevent delayed graft function in solid organ transplant	Adprotech
N-[4-bromo-2-(1H-1,2,3,4-tetrazol-5-yl)phenyl]-N'-[3,5-bis(trifluoro-methyl)phenyl]urea	Sickle cell disease	NeuroSearch A/S
N-acetylcysteinate lysine (*Nacystelyn Dry Powder Inhaler*)	Management of cystic fibrosis	Galephar Pharm Res
N-acetylcysteine	Acute liver failure	William M. Lee, MD, FACP
N-acetylprocainamide	To prevent life-threatening ventricular arrhythmias in documented procainamide-induced lupus	NAPA of the Bahamas
(*Napa*)	Lower the defibrillation energy requirement sufficiently to allow automatic implantable cardioverter defibrillator therapy in patients who could otherwise not use the device	Medco Res
N-acetylgalactosamine-4-sulfatase, recombinant human	Mucopolysaccharidosis type VI (Maroteaux-Lamy syndrome)	BioMarin Pharm
N-acetyl-sarcosyl-glycyl-L-valyl-D-alloisoleucyl-L-threonyl-L-norvaly-L-isoleucyl-L-arginyl-L-prolylethyl-aminde acetate	Soft tissue sarcoma	Abbott
Nafarelin acetate (*Synarel Nasal Solution*)	Central precocious puberty[a]	Syntex (USA)

Drug (Trade name)	Proposed use	Sponsor
Naltrexone HCl (*Trexan*)	Blockade of the pharmacological effects of exogenous opioids as an adjunct to maintain opioid-free state in detoxified, formerly opioid-dependent individuals[a]	DuPont Pharm
Natural human lymphoblastoid interferon-alpha	Polycythemia vera	Amarillo Biosciences
	Papillomavirus warts in the oral cavity of HIV-positive patients; Behcet disease	Atrix Labs
NDROGE	Postanoxic intention myoclonus	Watson Labs
Nebacumab (*Centoxin*)	Gram-negative bacteremia that has progressed to endotoxin shock	Centocor
Neurotrophin-1	Motor neuron disease/amyotrophic lateral sclerosis	Arthur Dale Ericsson, MD
NG-29 (*Somatrel*)	Diagnostic measure of the capacity of the pituitary gland to release growth hormone	Ferring Labs
Nifedipine	Interstitial cystitis	Jonathan Fleischmann, MD
Niprisan (*Hemoxin*)	Sickle cell disease	Xechem
Nitazoxanide (*Alinia*)	Intestinal giardiasis[a]; cryptosporidiosis[a]	Romark Labs
(*Cryptaz*)	Intestinal amebiasis	
Nitisinone (*Orfadin*)	Tyrosinemia type 1[a]; alkaptonuria	Swedish Orphan AB
Nitric oxide (*INOmax*)	Persistent pulmonary hypertension in the newborn[a]; acute adult respiratory distress syndrome	INO Therapeutics
Nitroprusside	To prevent and treat cerebral vasospasm following subarachnoid hemorrhage	Jeffrey Evan Thomas, MD
Nolatrexed (*THYMITAQ*)	Hepatocellular carcinoma	Zarix
Novel acting thrombolytic (NAT)	Peripheral arterial occlusion	Amgen
NZ-1002	Enzyme replacement therapy in patients with all subtypes of mucopolysaccharidosis I	Novazyme Pharm
Octavalent *Pseudomonas aeruginosa* O-polysaccharide-toxin A conjugate (*Aerugen*)	To prevent *Pseudomonas aeruginosa* infections in cystic fibrosis	Orphan Europe
Octreotide (*Sandostatin LAR*)	Acromegaly[a]; severe diarrhea and flushing associated with malignant carcinoid tumors[a]; diarrhea associated with vasoactive intestinal peptide tumors (VIPoma)[a]	Novartis
Ofloxacin (*Ocuflox Ophthalmic Solution*)	Bacterial corneal ulcers[a]	Allergan
Oglufanide disodium	Ovarian cancer	Cytran
OM 401 (*Drepanol*)	Prophylactic treatment of sickle cell disease	Omex International
Omega-3 (n-3) polyunsaturated fatty acid (with all double bonds in the cis configuration)	To prevent organ graft rejection	Research Triangle Pharm
Omega-3 (n-3) polyunsaturated fatty acids (*Omacor*)	IgA nephropathy	Pronova Biocare, AS
Oncorad Ov103	Ovarian cancer	Cytogen
Oprelvekin (*Neumega*)	To prevent severe chemotherapy-induced thrombocytopenia[a]	Genetics Institute
Orgotein for injection	Familial amyotrophic lateral sclerosis associated with a mutation of the gene (on chromosome 21q) for copper, zinc superoxide dismutase	Oxis International
Oxaliplatin	Ovarian cancer	Debio Pharm SA
Oxandrolone	Constitutional delay of growth and puberty	Bio-Technology General
(*Hepandrin*)	For moderate/severe acute alcoholic hepatitis in the presence of moderate protein calorie malnutrition	
(*Oxandrin*)	Duchenne and Becker muscular dystrophy; adjunctive therapy for AIDS patients with HIV-wasting syndrome; short stature associated with Turner syndrome	
Oxybate (*Xyrem*)	Narcolepsy[a]	Orphan Medical
Oxymorphone (*Numorphan H.P.*)	To relieve severe intractable pain in narcotic-tolerant patients	DuPont Merck
Oxypurinol	Hyperuricemia in patients intolerant to allopurinol	Cardiome Pharma
P1, P4-Di(uridine 5′-tetraphosphate), tetrasodium salt	Cystic fibrosis	Inspire Pharm
p1-(uridine 5′-)-p4-(2′-deoxycytidine 5′-) tetraphosphate, tetrasodium salt	Cystic fibrosis	Inspire Pharm
PA mAb (*Abthrax*)	Treat anthrax	Human Genome Sciences
Paclitaxel (*Paxene*)	AIDS-related Kaposi sarcoma	Baker Norton Pharm
(*Taxol*)[a]		Bristol-Myers Squibb Pharm Res Inst
Papain, trypsin, and chymotrypsin (*Wobe-Mugos*)	Multiple myeloma	Marlyn Nutraceuticals
Papaverine topical gel	Sexual dysfunction in spinal cord injury	Pharmedic
Parvovirus B19 (recombinant VP1 and VP2; *Spodoptera frugiperda* cells) vaccine (*MEDI-491*)	To prevent transient aplastic crisis in patients with sickle cell anemia	MedImmune

Orphan Drugs		
Drug (*Trade name*)	Proposed use	Sponsor
Patul-end	Patulous eustachian tube	Ear Foundation
Pegademase bovine (*Adagen*)	Enzyme replacement for adenosine deaminase deficiency in patients with severe combined immunodeficiency[a]	Enzon
Pegaspargase (*Oncaspar*)	Acute lymphocytic leukemia[a]	Enzon
PEG-glucocerebrosidase (*Lysodase*)	Chronic enzyme replacement therapy in Gaucher disease patients deficient in glucocerebrosidase	National Institute of Mental Health, NIH
Peginterferon alfa-2a (*PEGASYS*)	Renal cell carcinoma; chronic myelogenous leukemia	Hoffmann-La Roche
PEG-interleukin-2	Primary immunodeficiencies associated with T-cell defects	Chiron
Pegvisomant (*Somavert*)	Acromegaly[a]	Sensus
Pegylated arginine deiminase (*Hepacid*)	Hepatocellular carcinoma	Phoenix Pharmacologics
(*Melanocid*)	Invasive malignant melanoma	
Pegylated recombinant human mega-karyocyte growth and development factor (*MEGAGEN*)	To reduce the period of thrombocytopenia in patients undergoing hematopoietic stem cell transplantation	Amgen
Peldesine	Cutaneous T-cell lymphoma	BioCryst Pharm
Pemetrexed disodium (*Alimta*)	Malignant pleural mesothelioma	Eli Lilly
Pentamidine isethionate	*Pneumocystis carinii* pneumonia	Aventis Behring
(*Nebupent*)	*Pneumocystis carinii* pneumonia prevention in high-risk patients[a]	Fujisawa USA
(*Pentam 300*)	*Pneumocystis carinii* pneumonia[a]	Fujisawa USA
Pentamidine isethionate (inhalation) (*Pneumopent*)	To prevent *Pneumocystis carinii* pneumonia in high-risk patients	Fisons
Pentastarch (*Pentaspan*)	Adjunctive in leukapheresis to improve the harvesting and increase the yield of leukocytes by centrifugal means[a]	DuPont Pharm
Pentosan polysulphate sodium (*Elmiron*)	Interstitial cystitis[a]	Alza
Pentostatin (*Nipent*)	Chronic lymphocytic leukemia; cutaneous T-cell lymphoma; peripheral T-cell lymphomas	SuperGen
Pentostatin for injection (*Nipent*)	Hairy-cell leukemia[a]	SuperGen
Perflubron (*LiquiVent*)	Acute adult respiratory distress syndrome	Alliance Pharm
Perfosfamide (*Pergamid*)	Ex-vivo treatment of autologous bone marrow and subsequent reinfusion in acute myelogenous leukemia, also referred to as acute nonlymphocytic leukemia	Scios Nova
Pergolide (*Permax*)	Tourette syndrome	Floyd R. Sallee, MD, PhD
Phenylacetate	Adjunctive to surgery, radiation therapy, and chemotherapy for the treatment of patients with primary or recurrent malignant glioma	Elan Drug Delivery
Phenylalanine ammonia-lyase (*Phenylase*)	Hyperphenylalaninemia	Ibex Technologies
Phenylbutyrate	Acute promyelocytic leukemia	Elan Drug Delivery
Phenylephrine	Ileal pouch anal anastomosis related fecal incontinence	SLA Pharma
Phosphocysteamine	Cystinosis	Medea Res Labs
Pilocarpine HCl (*Salagen*)	Xerostomia induced by radiation therapy for head and neck cancer[a]; xerostomia and keratoconjunctivitis sicca in Sjogren syndrome[a]	MGI Pharma
Piracetam (*Nootropil*)	Myoclonus	UCB Pharma
Pirfenidone	Idiopathic pulmonary fibrosis	InterMune
Piritrexim isethionate	Infections caused by *Pneumocystis carinii*, *Toxoplasma gondii*, and *Mycobacterium avium-intracellulare*	Burroughs Wellcome
Polifeprosan 20 with carmustine (*Gliadel*)	Malignant glioma[a]	Guilford Pharm
Poloxamer 188 (*Flocor*)	Vasospasm in subarachnoid hemorrhage patients following surgical repair of a ruptured cerebral aneurysm; sickle cell crisis; severe burns requiring hospitalization	CytRx
Poloxamer 331 (*Protox*)	Initial therapy for toxoplasmosis in AIDS patients	CytRx
Poly I: poly C12U (*Ampligen*)	AIDS; renal cell carcinoma; chronic fatigue syndrome; invasive metastatic melanoma (stage IIB, III, IV)	Hemispherx Biopharma
Poly-ICLC	Primary brain tumors	Oncovir
Polyethylene glycol (PEG)-uricase	To control the clinical consequences of hyperuricemia in patients with severe gout in whom conventional therapy is contraindicated or has been ineffective	Bio-Technology General
Polyethylene glycol-modified uricase (*Zurase*)	Tumor lysis syndrome in cancer patients undergoing chemotherapy; prophylaxis of hyperuricemia in cancer patients prone to develop tumor lysis syndrome during chemotherapy	Phoenix Pharmacologics
Polyinosinic-polycytidilic acid (*Poly-ICLC*)	Adjuvant to smallpox vaccination; flavivirus infections including those caused by West Nile, Japanese encephalitis, dengue, St. Louis encephalitis, yellow fever, Murray valley, and Banzai viruses	Oncovir
Polyinosinic-polycytidilic acid (*Poly-ICLC*) (*Hiltonol*)	Orthopox virus infections	Oncovir
Polymeric oxygen	Sickle cell anemia	Capmed USA

Orphan Drugs		
Drug (*Trade name*)	Proposed use	Sponsor
Porcine fetal neural dopaminergic cells and/or precursors aseptically prepared and coated with anti-MHC-1 Ab for intracerebral implantation (*NeuroCell-PD*)	Hoehn and Yahr stage 4 and 5 Parkinson disease	Diacrin/Genzyme LLC
Porcine fetal neural dopaminergic cells and/or precursors aseptically prepared for intracerebral implantation (*NeuroCell-PD*)	Hoehn and Yahr stage 4 and 5 Parkinson disease	Diacrin/Genzyme LLC
Porcine fetal neural gabaergic cells and/or precursors aseptically prepared and coated with anti-MHC-1 Ab for intracerebral implantation (*NeuroCell-HD*)	Huntington disease	Diacrin/Genzyme LLC
Porcine fetal neural gabaergic cells and/or precursors aseptically prepared for intracerebral implantation for Huntington disease (*NeuroCell-HD*)	Huntington disease	Diacrin/Genzyme LLC
Porcine Sertoli cells aseptically prepared for intracerebral co-implantation with fetal neural tissue (*N-Graft*)	Hoehn and Yahr stage 4 and 5 Parkinson disease	Titan Pharm
Porfimer (*Photofrin*)	Ablation of high-grade dysplasia in Barrett esophagus in patients who are not considered to be candidates for esophagectomy[a]	Axcan Scandipharm
Porfimer sodium (*Photofrin*)	Photodynamic therapy of patients with primary or recurrent obstructing (partially or completely) esophageal carcinoma[a]; photodynamic therapy of patients with transitional cell carcinoma in situ of the urinary bladder	QLT Phototherapeutics
Porfiromycin (*Promycin*)	Head, neck, and cervical cancer	Boehringer Ingelheim
Potassium citrate (*Urocit-K*)	To prevent uric acid nephrolithiasis[a]; to prevent calcium renal stones in patients with hypocitraturia[a]; to avoid the complication of calcium stone formation in uric lithiasis[a]	University of Texas Health Sciences Center at Dallas
Potassium citrate and citric acid	Dissolution and control of uric acid and cysteine calculi in the urinary tract	Willen Drug
Pr-122 (redox-phenytoin)	Emergency rescue treatment of status epilepticus, grand mal type	Pharmos
PR-225 (redox-acyclovir)	Herpes simplex encephalitis in AIDS	Pharmos
PR-239 (redox penicillin G)	AIDS-associated neurosyphilis	Pharmos
Pr-320 (molecusol-carbamazepine)	Emergency rescue treatment of status epilepticus, grand mal type	Pharmos
Pramiracetam sulfate	Management of cognitive dysfunction and enhancement of antidepressant activity with electroconvulsive therapy	Cambridge Neuroscience
Praziquantel	Neurocysticercosis	EM Pharm
Prednimustine (*Sterecyt*)	Malignant non-Hodgkin lymphomas	Pharmacia
Primaquine phosphate	With clindamycin HCl in AIDS-associated *Pneumocystis carinii* pneumonia	Sanofi Winthrop
Progesterone	Establish and maintain pregnancy in women undergoing in vitro fertilization or embryo transfer procedures	Watson Labs
Propamidine isethionate 0.1% ophthalmic solution (*Brolene*)	Acanthamoeba keratitis	Bausch & Lomb
Prostaglandin E1 enol ester (AS-013)	Fontaine stage IV chronic, critical limb ischemia	Mitsubishi Pharma
Prostaglandin E1 in lipid emulsion (*Lipo-PGE1*)	Ischemic ulceration of the lower limbs caused by peripheral arterial disease	Alpha Therapeutic
Protaxel	Ovarian cancer	Biophysica
Protein C concentrate (*Protein C Concentrate [human] Vapor Heated, Immuno*)	Replacement therapy in patients with congenital or acquired protein C deficiency to prevent/treat warfarin-induced skin necrosis during oral anticoagulation; to prevent and treat purpura fulminans in meningococcemia	Immuno Clin Res
	Replacement therapy in congenital protein C deficiency to prevent and treat thrombosis, pulmonary emboli, and purpura fulminans	Baxter Healthcare
Protirelin	To prevent infant respiratory distress syndrome associated with prematurity	UCB Pharma
Protirelin injection	Amyotrophic lateral sclerosis	Abbott Labs
Pulmonary surfactant replacement	To prevent and treat infant respiratory distress syndrome	Scios Nova
Pulmonary surfactant replacement, porcine (*Curosurf*)	To prevent and treat respiratory distress syndrome in premature infants	Dey Labs
Purified extract of *Pseudomonas aeruginosa* (*ImmuDyn*)	Immune thrombocytopenic purpura where it is required to increase platelet counts	DynaGen
Purified type II collagen (*Colloral*)	Juvenile rheumatoid arthritis	AutoImmune
pVGI.1(VEGF2)	Thromboangiitis obliterans	Vascular Genetics
Pyruvate	Interstitial lung disease	Cellular Sciences
Quinacrine HCl	To prevent recurrence of pneumothorax in high-risk patients	Lyphomed
R-etodolac	Chronic lymphocytic leukemia	Salmedix
(R)-N-[2-(6-chloro-5-methoxy-1H-indol-3-yl)propyl]acetamide	Circadian rhythm sleep disorders in blind people with no light perception; neuroleptic-induced tardive dyskinesia in patients with schizophrenia	Phase 2 Discovery

Orphan Drugs		
Drug (*Trade name*)	Proposed use	Sponsor
Rasburicase (*Elitek*)	Malignancy-associated or chemotherapy-induced hyperuricemia[a]	Sanofi-Synthelabo
Recombinant adeno-associated virus alpha 1-antitrypsin vector (*rAAV-AAT*)	Alpha1-antitrypsin deficiency	Applied Genetic Technologies
Recombinant bactericidal/ permeability-increasing protein (*Neuprex*)	Severe meningococcal disease	Xoma
Recombinant glycine2-human glucagon-like peptide-2	Short bowel syndrome	NPS Allelix
Recombinant human acid alpha-glucosidase	Glycogen storage disease type II	Genzyme
Recombinant human alpha-1 anti-trypsin (rAAT)	Cystic fibrosis	Arriva Pharm
		PPL Therapeutics (Scotland) Ltd
	To delay progression of chronic obstructive pulmonary disease resulting from AAT deficiency-mediated emphysema and bronchiectasis	Baxter Healthcare
Recombinant human alpha-fetoprotein (rhAFP)	Myasthenia gravis	Merrimack Pharm
Recombinant human antithrombin III	Antithrombin III-dependent heparin resistance requiring anticoagulation	AT III LLC
Recombinant human C1-esterase inhibitor	Prophylactic treatment of angioedema caused by hereditary or acquired C1-esterase inhibitor deficiency; treatment of acute attacks of angioedema caused by hereditary or acquired C1-esterase inhibitor deficiency	Pharming NV
Recombinant human CD4 immuno-globulin G	AIDS resulting from HIV-1 infection	Genentech
Recombinant human Clara Cell 10kDa protein	To prevent neonatal bronchopulmonary dysplasia in premature neonates with respiratory distress syndrome	Claragen
Recombinant human endostatin protein	Neuroendocrine tumors; metastatic melanoma	EntreMed
Recombinant human fibroblast growth factor-20	Radiation-induced oral mucositis	CuraGen
Recombinant human gelsolin	Respiratory symptoms of cystic fibrosis; acute and chronic respiratory symptoms of bronchiectasis	Biogen
Recombinant human highly phosphorylated acid alpha-glucosidase	For enzyme replacement therapy in patients with all subtypes of glycogen storage disease type II (GSDII, Pompe disease)	Novazyme Pharm
Recombinant human insulin-like growth factor-I	Postpoliomyelitis syndrome	Cephalon
(*IGF-1*)	Growth hormone receptor deficiency; antibody-mediated growth hormone resistance with isolated growth hormone deficiency la	Pharmacia & Upjohn
(*PV802*)	Short-bowel syndrome as a result of resection of the small bowel or congenital dysfunction of the intestines	GroPep Pty Ltd
Recombinant human insulin-like growth factor-I/insulin-like growth factor binding protein-3	Major burns that require hospitalization	Celtrix Pharm
(*SomatoKine*)	Growth hormone insensitivity syndrome	
Recombinant human interleukin-12	Renal cell carcinoma	Genetics Institute
Recombinant human keratinocyte growth factor	To reduce the incidence and severity of radiation-induced xerostomia	Amgen
Recombinant human luteinizing hormone (*LHadi*)	With recombinant human follicle stimulating hormone for women with chronic anovulation caused by hypogonadotropic hypogonadism	Serono Labs
Recombinant human monoclonal antibody to hsp90 (*Mycograb*)	Invasive candidiasis	NeuTec Pharma plc
Recombinant human nerve growth factor	HIV-associated sensory neuropathy	Genentech
Recombinant human neutrophil inhibitor (hNE)	Cystic fibrosis	Dyax
Recombinant human porphobilinogen deaminase (*Porphozyme*)	Acute intermittent porphyria attacks	HemeBiotech A/S
Recombinant human porphobilinogen deaminase, erythropoetic form	To prevent acute intermittent porphyria attacks	HemeBiotech A/S
Recombinant human relaxin	Progressive systemic sclerosis	Connetics
Recombinant human thrombopoietin	To accelerate platelet recovery in patients undergoing hematopoietic stem-cell transplantation	Genentech
Recombinant humanized MAb 5c8	To prevent and treat Factor VIII/Factor IX inhibitors in hemophilia A or B; to prevent rejection of solid organ transplants; to prevent rejection of pancreatic islet cell transplants; immune thrombocytopenic purpura; systemic lupus erythematosus	Biogen
Recombinant inhibitor of human plasma kallikrein	Angioedema	Dyax
Recombinant methionyl brain-derived neurotrophic factor	Amyotrophic lateral sclerosis	Amgen
Recombinant methionyl human stem cell factor	Primary bone marrow failure	Amgen
Recombinant retroviral vector - glucocerebrosidase	Enzyme replacement therapy for types I, II, or III Gaucher disease	Genetic Therapy

Orphan Drugs		
Drug (*Trade name*)	Proposed use	Sponsor
Recombinant secretory leucocyte protease inhibitor	Congenital alpha-1 antitrypsin deficiency; cystic fibrosis	Amgen
Recombinant soluble human CD4 (rCD4)	AIDS	Genentech
(*Receptin*)		Biogen
Recombinant T-cell receptor ligand	Patients with multiple sclerosis who are HLA-DR2 positive and autoreactive to myelin oligodendrocyte glycoprotein residues 35-55	Virogenomics
Recombinant urate oxidase	Prophylaxis of chemotherapy-induced hyperuricemia	Sanofi-Synthelabo
Recombinant vaccinia (human papillomavirus) (*TA-HPV*)	Cervical cancer	Xenova Res Ltd
Reduced L-glutathione (*Cachexon*)	AIDS-associated cachexia	Telluride Pharm
Remacemide (*Ecovia*)	Huntington disease	AstraZeneca LP
Repertaxin	To prevent delayed graft function in solid organ transplant	Dompe s.p.a.
Repository corticotropin or adreno-corticotropic hormone (*H.P. Acthar Gel*)	Infantile spasms	Questcor
Resiniferatoxin	Intractable pain at end-stage disease	Andrew J. Mannes, MD
Respiratory syncytial virus (RSV) immune globulin (human) (*Hypermune RSV*)	To treat respiratory syncytial virus lower respiratory tract infections in hospitalized infants and young children	MedImmune
(*Respigam*)	Prophylaxis of respiratory syncytial virus (RSV) lower respiratory tract infections in infants and young children at high risk of RSV disease[a]	MedImmune and MA Public Health Biologics
Retroviral gamma-c cDNA containing vector	X-linked severe combined immune deficiency disease	AVAX Tech
Retroviral vector, R-GC and GC gene 1750	Gaucher disease	Genzyme
Reviparin sodium (*Clivarine*)	Deep vein thrombosis that may lead to pulmonary embolism in pediatric patients; long-term treatment of acute deep vein thrombosis with or without pulmonary embolism in pregnant patients	Knoll AG
RGG0853, E1A lipid complex	Ovarian cancer	Targeted Genetics
rhIGF-I/rhIGFBP-3 (*SomatoKine*)	Extreme insulin-resistance syndromes (type A, Rabson-Mendenhall syndrome, Leprechaunism, type B syndrome)	Insmed
Rho (D) immune globulin IV (human) (*WinRho SD*)	Immune thrombocytopenic purpura[a]	Rh Pharm
rhuMAb VEGF (bevacizumab) (*Avastin*)	Renal cell carcinoma	Genentech
Ribavirin (*Rebetol*)	Chronic hepatitis C in pediatric patients[a]	Schering
(*Virazole*)	Hemorrhagic fever with renal syndrome	Valeant
Ricin (blocked) conjugated murine MCA (anti-B4)	B-cell leukemia and B-cell lymphoma; ex vivo purging of leukemic cells from the bone marrow of non-T-cell acute lymphocytic leukemia patients who are in complete remission	ImmunoGen
Ricin (blocked) conjugated murine MCA (anti-my9)	Myeloid leukemia, including acute myelogenous leukemia, and blast crisis of chronic myeloid leukemia; ex vivo treatment of autologous bone marrow and subsequent reinfusion in acute myelogenous leukemia	ImmunoGen
Ricin (blocked) conjugated murine MCA (n901)	Small-cell lung cancer	ImmunoGen
Ricin (blocked) conjugated murine monoclonal antibody (CD6)	Cutaneous T-cell lymphomas, acute T-cell leukemia-lymphoma, and related mature T-cell malignancies	ImmunoGen
Rifabutin	To treat disseminated *Mycobacterium avium* complex disease	Pfizer
(*Mycobutin*)	To prevent disseminated *Mycobacterium avium* complex disease in advanced HIV infection[a]	Adria Labs
Rifalazil	Pulmonary tuberculosis	PathoGenesis
Rifampin (*Rifadin IV*)	Antituberculosis treatment when oral doseform is not feasible[a]	Hoechst Marion Roussel
Rifampin, isoniazid, pyrazinamide (*Rifater*)	Short-course treatment of tuberculosis[a]	Hoechst Marion Roussel
Rifapentine (*Priftin*)	Pulmonary tuberculosis[a]; *Mycobacterium avium* complex (MAC) in patients with AIDS; prophylaxis of MAC in patients with AIDS and a CD4+ count ≤ 75/mm³	Hoechst Marion Roussel
Rifaximin (*Normix*)	Hepatic encephalopathy	Salix Pharm
RII Retinamide	Myelodysplastic syndromes	Sparta Pharm
Riluzole (*Rilutek*)	Amyotrophic lateral sclerosis[a]; Huntington disease	Rhone-Poulenc Rorer
Rituximab (*Rituxan*)	Non-Hodgkin B-cell lymphoma[a]; chronic lymphocytic leukemia	IDEC Pharm
	Immune thrombocytopenic purpura	Genentech
Roquinimex (*Linomide*)	To prolong time to relapse in leukemia patients who have undergone autologous bone marrow transplantation	Pharmacia & Upjohn
rSP-C lung surfactant (*Venticute*)	Adult respiratory distress syndrome	Byk Gulden Pharm
Rubitecan	HIV- and AIDS-infected pediatric patients	SuperGen
S(-)-3-[3-amino-phthalimido]-glutaramide	Multiple myeloma	EntreMed

Orphan Drugs		
Drug (*Trade name*)	Proposed use	Sponsor
Sacrosidase (*Sucraid*)	Congenital sucrase-isomaltase deficiency[a]	Orphan Medical
S-adenosylmethionine	AIDS-myelopathy	Alessandro Di Rocco, MD
Sargramostim (*Leukine*)	Neutropenia associated with bone marrow transplant, graft failure, and delay of engraftment and for promotion of early engraftment[a]; to reduce neutropenia and leukopenia and decrease the incidence of death caused by infection in patients with acute myelogenous leukemia[a]	Immunex
Satumomab pendetide (*OncoScint CR/OV*)	Detect ovarian carcinoma[a]	Cytogen
SB-408075	Pancreatic cancer	SmithKline Beecham
SC-1 monoclonal antibody	CD55 (sc-1) positive gastric tumors	H3 Pharma
SCH 58500	Primary ovarian cancer	Schering
Secalciferol (*Osteo-D*)	Familial hypophosphatemic rickets	Teva Pharm USA
Secretory leukocyte protease inhibitor	Bronchopulmonary dysplasia	Synergen
Selegiline HCl (*Eldepryl*)	Adjuvant to levodopa and carbidopa in idiopathic Parkinson disease (paralysis agitans), postencephalitic Parkinsonism, and symptomatic Parkinsonism[a]	Somerset Pharm
Sermorelin acetate (*Geref*)	Idiopathic or organic growth hormone deficiency in children with growth failure[a]; adjunctive to gonadotropin in ovulation induction in anovulatory or oligo-ovulatory infertility after failure of clomiphene citrate or gonadotropin alone; AIDS-associated catabolism/weight loss	Serono Labs
***Serratia marcescens* extract (polyribosomes)** (*Imuvert*)	Primary brain malignancies	Cell Technology
SGN-30 (anti-CD30 mAb)	Hodgkin disease	Seattle Genetics
Short chain fatty acid enema (*Colomed*)	Chronic radiation proctitis	Richard I. Breuer, MD
Short chain fatty acid solution (*Colomed*)	Active phase of ulcerative colitis with involvement restricted to the left side of the colon	Richard I. Breuer, MD
Silver sulfadiazine and cerium nitrate (*Flammacerium*)	To prevent mortality in severely burned patients	Synthes (USA)
Siplizumab	T-cell lymphomas	Medimmune Oncology
SK&F 110679	Long-term treatment of children who have growth failure caused by a lack of adequate endogenous growth hormone secretion	SmithKline Beecham
Sodium 1,3-propanedisulfonate	Secondary amyloidosis	Neurochem
Sodium dichloroacetate	Congenital lactic acidosis	Peter W. Stacpoole, PhD, MD
		Questcor Pharm
	Lactic acidosis in severe malaria; homozygous familial hypercholesterolemia	Peter W. Stacpoole, PhD, MD
	Antidote in managing systemic monochloroacetic acid poisoning	EBD Group
(*Ceresine*)	Severe head injury	Questcor Pharm
Sodium monomercaptoundecahydro-closo-dodecaborate	In conjunction with a thermal or epithermal neutron beam in boron nuclear capture therapy of glioblastoma multiforme	Theragenics
(*Borocell*)	In boron neutron capture therapy in glioblastoma multiforme	Neutron Technology & Neutron R & D Partner
Sodium phenylbutyrate	Adjunctive to surgery, radiation therapy, and chemotherapy for primary or recurrent malignant glioma	Elan Drug Delivery
(*Buphenyl*)	The following urea cycle disorders: Carbamylphosphate synthetase deficiency; ornithine transcarbamylase deficiency[a]; arginiosuccinic acid synthetase deficiency; sickling disorders including S-S, S-C, and S-thalassemia hemoglobinopathy	Medicis Pharm
Sodium pyruvate	Cystic fibrosis	Cellular Sciences
Sodium tetradecyl sulfate (*Sotradecol*)	Bleeding esophageal varices	Elkins-Sinn
Sodium thiosulfate	To prevent platinum-induced ototoxicity in pediatric patients	Adherex Technologies
Soluble complement receptor type 1	To prevent postcardiopulmonary bypass syndrome in children undergoing cardiopulmonary bypass	Avant Immunotherapeutics
Soluble recombinant human complement receptor type 1	To prevent and reduce adult respiratory distress syndrome	T Cell Sciences
Somatostatin	Bleeding esophageal varices	UCB Pharm
(*Zecnil*)	Adjunctive to nonoperative management of secreting cutaneous fistulas of the stomach, duodenum, small intestine (jejunum and ileum), or pancreas	Ferring Labs
Somatrem for injection (*Protropin*)	Long-term treatment of children with growth failure caused by lack of adequate endogenous growth hormone secretion[a]; short stature associated with Turner syndrome	Genentech
Somatropin (*Biotropin*)	Cachexia associated with AIDS	Bio-Technology General
(*Genotropin*)	Adults with growth hormone deficiency[a]	Pharmacia & Upjohn
(*Humatrope*)	Short stature associated with Turner syndrome[a]	Eli Lilly
(*Norditropin*)	Adjunctive in ovulation induction in women with infertility caused by hypogonadotropic hypogonadism or bilateral tubal occlusion or unexplained infertility who are undergoing in vivo or in vitro fertilization procedures; short stature associated with Turner syndrome	Novo Nordisk Pharm
(*Nutropin*)	Long-term treatment of children with growth failure caused by lack of adequate endogenous growth hormone secretion[a]	Genentech

Drug (*Trade name*)	Proposed use	Sponsor
Somatropin for injection (*Nutropin*)	Growth retardation associated with chronic renal failure[a]; short stature associated with Turner syndrome[a]; replacement therapy for growth hormone deficiency in adults after epiphyseal closure[a]	Genentech
(*Humatrope*)	Long-term treatment of children who have growth failure caused by inadequate secretion of normal endogenous growth hormone[a]	Eli Lilly
(*Serostim*)	AIDS-associated catabolism/weight loss[a]	Serono Labs
Somatropin (rDNA) (*Genotropin*)	Growth failure in children who were born small for gestational age[a]; short stature in patients with Prader-Willi syndrome[a]	Pharmacia & Upjohn
(*Nutropin Depot*)	Long-term treatment of children who have growth failure caused by a lack of adequate endogenous growth hormone secretion	Genentech
(*Saizen*)	Enhancement of nitrogen retention in hospitalized patients suffering from severe burns; idiopathic or organic growth hormone deficiency in children with growth failure	Serono Labs
(*Serostim*)	Alone or with glutamine in short bowel syndrome	Serono Labs
Somatropin (rDNA) for injection (*Serostim*)	Children with AIDS-associated failure-to-thrive, including AIDS-associated wasting	Serono Labs
Somatropin (rDNA origin) injection (*Norditropin*)	Growth failure in children caused by inadequate growth hormone secretion	Novo Nordisk
Sorivudine (*BRAVAVIR*)	Herpes zoster (shingles) in immunocompromised patients	Bristol-Myers Squibb
Sotalol HCl (*Betapace*)	To prevent and treat[a] life-threatening ventricular tachyarrhythmias	Berlex Labs
Spiramycin (*Rovamycine*)	Symptomatic relief and parasitic cure of chronic cryptosporidiosis in immunodeficiency	Rhone-Poulenc Rorer
Squalamine lactate	Ovarian cancer refractory or resistant to standard chemotherapy	Genaera
SS1(dsFv)-PE38	Malignant mesothelioma; epithelial ovarian cancer	NeoPharm
***Staphylococcus aureus* immune globulin (human)** (*Altastaph*)	Prophylaxis against *Staphylococcus aureus* infections in low birth weight neonates	NABI
ST1-RTA immunotoxin (SR 44163)	To prevent acute graft vs host disease in allogenic bone marrow transplantation; treat B-chronic lymphocytic leukemia	Sanofi Winthrop
SU101	Malignant glioma; ovarian cancer	Sugen
Suberoylanilide hydroxamic acid	Multiple myeloma	Aton Pharma
Succimer (*Chemet*)	To prevent cystine kidney stones in patients with homozygous cystinuria who are prone to stone development; mercury intoxication	Sanofi Winthrop
(*Chemet capsules*)	Lead poisoning in children[a]	Bock Pharmacal
Sucralfate	Oral mucositis and stomatitis following radiation therapy for head and neck cancer	Fuisz Tech
Sucralfate suspension	Oral complications of chemotherapy in bone marrow transplants; oral ulcerations and dysphagia in epidermolysis bullosa	Darby Pharm
Sulfadiazine	With pyrimethamine for *Toxoplasma gondii* encephalitis in patients with and without AIDS[a]	Eon Labs
Sulfapyridine	Dermatitis herpetiformis	Jacobus Pharm
Superoxide dismutase (human)	To protect donor organ tissue from damage or injury mediated by oxygen-derived free radicals that are generated during the necessary periods of ischemia (hypoxia, anoxia) and especially reperfusion associated with the operative procedure	Pharmacia-Chiron Partnership
Superoxide dismutase (recombinant human) (*Oxsodrol*)	To prevent reperfusion injury to donor organ tissue	Bio-Technology General
Suramin (*Metaret*)	Hormone-refractory prostate cancer	Warner-Lambert
Surface active extract of saline lavage of bovine lungs (*Infasurf*)	To prevent and treat respiratory failure caused by pulmonary surfactant deficiency in preterm infants	ONY
Surfactant (human) (amniotic fluid derived) (*Human Surf*)	To prevent and treat neonatal respiratory distress syndrome	T. Allen Merritt, MD
Synsorb Pk	Verocytotoxogenic *Escherichia coli* infections	Synsorb Biotech
Synthetic human parathyroid hormone 1-34	Hypoparathyroidism	Orphan Pharm US
Synthetic human secretin	To evaluate exocrine pancreas function; obtaining desquamated pancreatic cells for cytopathologic examination in pancreatic carcinoma; diagnosing gastrinoma associated with Zollinger-Ellison syndrome; with diagnostic procedures for pancreatic disorders to increase pancreatic fluid secretion	ChiRhoClin
Synthetic porcine secretin	To evaluate exocrine pancreas function[a]; obtaining desquamated pancreatic cells for cytopathologic examination in pancreatic carcinoma; diagnosing gastrinoma associated with Zollinger-Ellison syndrome[a]; with diagnostic procedures for pancreatic disorders to increase pancreatic fluid secretion[a]	ChiRhoClin
T4 endonuclease V, liposome encapsulated	To prevent cutaneous neoplasms and other skin abnormalities in xeroderma pigmentosum	AGI Dermatics
Tacrolimus (*Prograf*)	Prophylaxis of graft vs host disease	Fujisawa USA
TAK-603	Crohn disease	Tap Holdings
Talc, sterile (*Steritalc*)	Malignant pleural effusion; pneumothorax	Novatech SA
Talc powder, sterile (*Sclerosol Intrapleural Aerosol*)	Malignant pleural effusion[a]	Bryan

Orphan Drugs		
Drug (*Trade name*)	Proposed use	Sponsor
T-cell depleted stem cell enriched cellular product from peripheral blood stem cells	Chronic granulomatous disease	Nexell Therapeutics
Technetium Tc99m anti-melanoma murine monoclonal antibody (*Oncotrac Melanoma Imaging Kit*)	To detect, by imaging, metastases of malignant melanoma	NeoRx
Technetium Tc99m murine monoclonal antibody (IgG2a) to B cell (*LymphoScan*)	Diagnostic imaging in evaluating the extent of disease in patients with histologically confirmed diagnosis of non-Hodgkin B-cell lymphoma, acute B-cell lymphoblastic leukemia (in children and adults), and chronic B-cell lymphocytic leukemia	Immunomedics
Technetium Tc99m murine monoclonal antibody to hCG (*Immuraid, hCG-Tc-99m*)	To detect human chorionic gonadotropin-producing tumors such as germ-cell and trophoblastic cell tumors	Immunomedics
Technetium Tc99m murine monoclonal antibody to human AFP (*AFP-Scan*)	To detect alpha-fetoprotein producing germ-cell tumors; detect hepatocellular carcinoma and hepatoblastoma	Immunomedics
(*Immuraid*)	To detect hepatocellular carcinoma and hepatoblastoma	
Technetium Tc99m pterotetramide	Identification of ovarian carcinomas	Endocyte
Technetium Tc99m rh-Annexin V (*Apomate*)	Diagnosis or assessment of rejection status in heart, heart-lung, single lung, or bilateral lung transplants	Theseus Imaging
Temoporfin (*Foscan*)	Palliative treatment of recurrent, refractory, or second primary squamous cell carcinomas of the head and neck considered to be incurable with surgery or radiotherapy	Scotia Pharm
Temozolomide (*Temodal*)	Advanced metastatic melanoma	Schering-Plough Res Inst
(*Temodar*)	Recurrent malignant glioma[a]	
Teniposide (*Vumon for Injection*)	Refractory childhood acute lymphocytic leukemia[a]	Bristol-Myers Squibb Pharm Res Inst
Teriparatide (*Parathar*)	Diagnostic agent for patients with clinical and laboratory evidence of hypocalcemia caused by hypoparathyroidism or pseudohypoparathyroidism	Rhone-Poulenc Rorer
	Idiopathic osteoporosis	Henri Beaufour Institute USA
Terlipressin (*Glypressin*)	Bleeding esophageal varices	Ferring Labs
Testosterone (*Androgel*)	Weight loss in AIDS patients with HIV-associated wasting	Unimed
(*TheraDerm Testosterone Transdermal System*)	Physiologic testosterone replacement in androgen-deficient, HIV-positive patients with an associated weight loss	Watson Labs
Testosterone propionate ointment 2%	Vulvar dystrophies	Star Pharm
Testosterone sublingual	Constitutional delay of growth and puberty in boys	Bio-Technology General
Tetrabenazine	Moderate/Severe tardive dyskinesia; Huntington disease	Prestwick Pharm
Tetrahydrobiopterin	Hyperphenylalaninemia	Biomarin Pharm
Tetraiodothyroacetic acid	Suppression of thyroid stimulating hormone in patients with well-differentiated cancer of the thyroid gland	Elliot Danforth Jr., MD
Tezacitabine	Adenocarcinoma of the esophagus and stomach	Chiron
TGF(beta)2-specific phosphorothioate antisense oligodeoxynucleotide (*Oncomun*)	Malignant glioma	Antisense Pharma GmbH
Thalidomide	To treat and prevent recurrent aphthous ulcers in severely, terminally immunocompromised patients; to treat/prevent graft vs host disease	Andrulis Res
	Clinical manifestations of mycobacterial infection caused by *Mycobacterium tuberculosis* and nontuberculous mycobacteria; primary brain malignancies; severe recurrent aphthous stomatitis in severely, terminally immunocompromised patients; Kaposi sarcoma	Celgene
	To treat and prevent graft vs host disease in bone marrow transplantation; to treat and maintain reactional lepromatous leprosy	Pediatric Pharm
(*Synovir*)	HIV-associated wasting syndrome	Celgene
(*Thalomid*)	Erythema nodosum leprosum[a]; multiple myeloma; Crohn disease	Celgene
Thymalfasin (*Zadaxin*)	Chronic active hepatitis B; DiGeorge anomaly with immune defects; hepatocellular carcinoma	SciClone Pharm
Thymoxamine HCl	To reverse phenylephrine-induced mydriasis in patients who have narrow anterior angles and are at risk of developing an acute attack of angle-closure glaucoma following mydriasis	Iolab Pharm
Thyrotropin alfa (*Thyrogen*)	Well-differentiated papillary, follicular, or combined papillary/follicular carcinomas of the thyroid; adjunct in the diagnosis of thyroid cancer[a]	Genzyme
Tiapride	Tourette syndrome	Sanofi-Synthelabo
Tiazofurin (2-Beta-D-ribofuranosyl-4-thiazolecarboxamide)	Chronic myelogenous leukemia	Ribapharm
Tin ethyl etiopurpurin	To prevent access graft disease in hemodialysis patients	Miravant Medical Technologies
Tinidazole	Giardiasis; amebiasis	Presutti Labs
Tiopronin (*Thiola*)	To prevent cystine nephrolithiasis in patients with homozygous cystinuria[a]	Charles Y. C. Pak, MD
Tirapazamine	Head and neck cancer	Sanofi-Synthelabo
Tiratricol (*Triacana*)	With levothyroxine to suppress thyroid stimulating hormone in patients with well-differentiated thyroid cancer who are intolerant to adequate doses of levothyroxine alone	Laphal Labs
Tizanidine HCl (*Zanaflex*)	Spasticity associated with multiple sclerosis and spinal cord injury	Athena Neurosciences

Orphan Drugs		
Drug (*Trade name*)	Proposed use	Sponsor
Tobramycin (*Tobi*)	Bronchiectasis patients infected with *Pseudomonas aeruginosa*	Chiron
Tobramycin for inhalation (*TOBI*)	Bronchopulmonary infections of *P. aeruginosa* in cystic fibrosis patients[a]	Pathogenesis
Tocophersolan oral solution (vitamin E-tpgs)	Vitamin E deficiency resulting from malabsorption caused by prolonged cholestatic hepatobiliary disease	Sterling Winthrop
Topiramate (*Topamax*)	Lennox-Gastaut syndrome[a]	RW Johnson Pharm Res Inst
Toralizumab	Immune thrombocytopenic purpura	IDEC Pharm
Toremifene (*Fareston*)	Hormonal therapy of metastatic breast carcinoma[a]; desmoid tumors	Orion
Tositumomab and iodine I 131 tositumomab (*Bexxar*)	Non-Hodgkin B-cell lymphoma[a]	Corixa
Tranexamic acid (*Cyklokapron*)	Patients with congenital coagulopathies who are undergoing surgical procedures (eg, dental extractions)[a]; undergoing prostatectomy where there is hemorrhage or risk of hemorrhage as a result of increased fibrinolysis or fibrinogenolysis; hereditary angioneurotic edema	Pharmacia
Tranilast (*Rizaben*)	Malignant glioma	Angiogen Pharm
Transforming growth factor-beta 2	Full-thickness macular holes	Celtrix Pharm
Transgenic human alpha 1 antitrypsin	Emphysema secondary to alpha 1 antitrypsin deficiency	PPL Therapeutics (Scotland) Ltd
Trastuzumab (*Herceptin*)	Pancreatic cancer that overexpresses p185HER2	Genentech
Treosulfan (*Ovastat*)	Ovarian cancer	Medac GmbH
Treprostinil (*Remodulin*)	Treatment of pulmonary arterial hypertension[a]	United Therapeutics
Tretinoin	Squamous metaplasia of the ocular surface epithelia (conjunctiva and/or cornea) with mucous deficiency and keratinization	Hannan Ophthalmic Marketing Service
(*ATRA-IV*)	Acute and chronic leukemia; T-cell non-Hodgkin lymphoma	Antigenics
(*Vesanoid*)	Acute promyelocytic leukemia[a]	Hoffmann-La Roche
Tri-antennary glycotripeptide derivative of 5-fluorodeoxyuridine monophosphate	Hepatocellular carcinoma	Cell Works
Trientine HCl (*Syprine*)	Wilson disease intolerant or inadequately responsive to penicillamine[a]	Merck Sharp & Dohme Res
Trimetrexate glucuronate (*Neutrexin*)	Metastatic carcinoma of head and neck (buccal cavity, pharynx, larynx); metastatic colorectal adenocarcinoma; pancreatic adenocarcinoma; *Pneumocystis carinii* pneumonia in AIDS patients[a]; advanced non-small-cell carcinoma of the lung; metastatic osteogenic sarcoma	Medimmune Oncology
Triptorelin pamoate (*Decapeptyl Injection*)	In palliative treatment of advanced ovarian carcinoma of epithelial origin	Debio R.A.
Trisaccharides A and B (*Biosynject*)	Moderate to very severe clinical forms of transfusion reactions arising from ABO incompatible transfusions of blood, blood products, and blood derivatives; moderate to severe clinical forms of hemolytic disease in newborns arising from placental transfer of antibodies against blood groups A and B; ABO-incompatible solid organ transplantation including kidney, heart, liver, and pancreas; to prevent ABO hemolytic reactions arising from ABO-incompatible bone marrow transplantation	Chembiomed Ltd
Trisodium citrate concentration (*Hemocitrate*)	Used in leukapheresis procedures	Hemotec Medical
Tumor necrosis factor-binding protein I	Symptomatic AIDS patients including all patients with CD4 T-cell counts < 200 cells/mm^3	Serono Labs
Tumor necrosis factor-binding protein II	Symptomatic AIDS patients including all patients with CD4 T-cell counts < 200 cells/mm^3	Serono Labs
Tyloxapol (*Supervent*)	Cystic fibrosis	Kennedy and Hoidal, MDs
Ubiquinone (*Ubi-Q-Gel*)	Mitochondrial cytopathies	Gel-Tec, Division of Tishcon
Unconjugated chimeric (human-murine) G250 IgG monoclonal antibody	Renal cell carcinoma	Wilex Biotechnology GmbH
Uridine 5′-triphosphate	Cystic fibrosis; facilitate removal of lung secretions in primary ciliary dyskinesia	Inspire Pharm
Urofollitropin (*Fertinex*)	For the initiation and reinitiation of spermatogenesis in adult males with reproductive failure caused by hypothalamic or pituitary dysfunction, hypogonadotropic hypogonadism	Serono Labs
(*Metrodin*)	Ovulation induction in patients with polycystic ovarian disease who have an elevated luteinizing hormone/follicle-stimulating hormone ratio and who have failed to respond to adequate clomiphene citrate therapy[a]	
Urogastrone	To accelerate corneal epithelial regeneration and healing of stromal incisions from corneal transplant surgery	Chiron Vision
Ursodiol (*Actigall*)	Management of clinical signs and symptoms associated with primary biliary cirrhosis	Novartis
(*URSO*)	Primary biliary cirrhosis[a]	Axcan Pharma
Valine, isoleucine, and leucine (*VIL*)	Hyperphenylalaninemia	Leas Res Products
Valrubicin (*Valstar*)	Carcinoma in situ of the urinary bladder[a]	Anthra Pharm
Vapreotide (*Octastatin*)	GI and pancreatic fistulas; to prevent early postoperative complications following pancreatic resection; esophageal variceal hemorrhage patients with portal hypertension	Debiopharm S.A.

Drug (*Trade name*)	Proposed use	Sponsor
Vapreotide pamoate (*Sanvar*)	Acromegaly	H3 Pharma
Vasoactive intestinal peptide	Acute respiratory distress syndrome	Sami I. Said, MD
Vasoactive intestinal polypeptide	Acute esophageal food impaction	Research Triangle Pharm
Vigabatrin (*Sabril*)	Infantile spasms	Aventis
Viloxazine HCl (*Catatrol*)	Narcolepsy; cataplexy	Stuart Pharm
Virulizin (*Virulizin*)	Pancreatic cancer	Lorus Therapeutics
Xenogeneic hepatocytes (*HepatAssist Liver Assist System*)	Severe liver failure	Circe Biomedical
XL119	Bile duct tumors	Exelixis
Yttrium-90 radiolabeled humanized monoclonal anti-carcinoembryonic antigen IgG antibody (*Cea-Cide*)	Ovarian carcinoma	Immunomedics
Zalcitabine	AIDS	National Cancer Inst, DCT
(*Hivid*)	AIDS[a]	Hoffman-La Roche
Zidovudine (*Retrovir*)	AIDS[a]; AIDS-related complex[a]	GlaxoWellcome
Zinc acetate (*Galzin*)	Wilson disease[a]	Lemmon
Zoledronate (*Zometa, Zabel*)	Tumor-induced hypercalcemia[a]	Novartis

[a] Approved for marketing.

ABETIMUS SODIUM (*Riquent* by La Jolla Pharmaceutical) – An immunomodulator

➤*Actions:*

Pharmacology – Abetimus is awaiting approval for the treatment of patients with systemic lupus erythematosus (SLE) at risk of renal disease. Autoantibodies against double-stranded DNA (anti-dsDNA) have been implicated in the pathogenesis of renal disease in patients with SLE. Increased levels of circulating anti-dsDNA often precede renal flares.

Abetimus is an immunomodulant designed to lower anti-dsDNA. Abetimus is a synthetic oligonucleotide conjugate with a molecular weight of approximately 54 kDaltons. It is composed of 4 double-stranded 20-mer oligonucleotides. Each oligonucleotide is attached through an aliphatic linker to a center, branched platform of triethylene glycol.

Abetimus reduces circulating anti-dsDNA by at least 2 mechanisms. It acutely depletes circulating anti-dsDNA by forming small, soluble complexes with the anti-dsDNA. It also acts by inducing highly selective B lymphocyte tolerance. This is done by cross linking anti-dsDNA receptors on B cells resulting in B cell anergy. The high-affinity autoantibodies produce the greatest response, but the affinity to abetimus declines with repeated administration.

Following IV administration in patients with SLE anti-dsDNA titers rapidly decline and remain below baseline for up to 4 weeks.

Pharmacokinetics – The plasma half-life of abetimus is approximately 1 hour.

Clinical trials – Abetimus was assessed in a phase 3, randomized, placebo-controlled study enrolling patients with SLE and an anti-dsDNA of 15 units/mL or greater. At baseline, at least 1 immunosuppressive agent was being used by 48% of patients in the abetimus group and 42% of patients in the placebo group; 83% of patients in both groups were on prednisone. Patients were randomized to receive 100 mg abetimus or placebo weekly for up to 22 months. Compared with placebo, abetimus was associated with a significant reduction in anti-dsDNA from baseline ($P = 0.0001$). Reductions in anti-dsDNA were correlated with increases in C3 ($P < 0.0001$). The intent-to-treat population consisted of patients with high-affinity anti-dsDNA (145 patients in the abetimus group and 153 patients in the placebo group). The incidence of renal flares did not differ in this analysis (12% on abetimus vs 16% on placebo), nor did the incidence of major SLE flares (24% on abetimus vs 31% on placebo). Use of high-dose corticosteroids and/or cyclophosphamide also was similar in the 2 groups (23% on abetimus and 24% on placebo). The median time to renal flare was 123 months in the abetimus group compared with 89 months in the placebo group. Subgroup analysis was performed with 43 of the patients with impaired renal function (serum creatinine of 1.5 mg/dL or greater at baseline; 20 patients in the abetimus group and 23 in the placebo group). Eight patients with impaired renal function experienced a renal flare (2 of 20 [10%] on abetimus and 6 of 23 [26%] on placebo). Among patients experiencing a sustained reduction in anti-dsDNA during this study, the incidence of renal flare was reduced. Renal flares occurred in 41 patients in this study, with 5 (12%) occurring in patients with sustained antibody reductions and 38 (88%) occurring in patients without sustained reductions. Abetimus appears most likely to reduce renal flares in SLE patients with a history of renal disease and impaired renal function and in those patients achieving sustained reductions in anti-dsDNA.

➤*Adverse Reactions:* Adverse events observed in abetimus clinical trials have been consistent with SLE. Adverse events occurred with similar frequency and were of similar type and severity in abetimus- and placebo-treated groups.

➤*Summary:* Abetimus is a unique therapy that may reduce the incidence of renal flares in patients with SLE. The greatest reduction in renal flares was observed in patients with a history of renal disease and impaired renal function and in patients achieving sustained reductions in anti-dsDNA titers. Additional data will be necessary to determine the optimal population to be treated with abetimus. An NDA was filed with the FDA in December 2004.

ACAMPROSATE (*Campral* by Forest Laboratories) – A psychotropic drug for the treatment of alcohol (ethanol) dependence

➤*Actions:*

Pharmacology – The mechanism by which acamprosate reduces alcohol intake and relapses is unclear. Acamprosate inhibits neuronal hyperexcitability by antagonizing excitatory amino acids. It has been proposed that acamprosate may act as a partial co-agonist of N-methyl-D-aspartate (NMDA) receptors, enhancing their activation at low levels of activation by endogenous activators, but inhibiting activation when levels of endogenous activators are high, such as alcohol withdrawal.

Pharmacokinetics – Acamprosate is rapidly, but incompletely, absorbed after oral administration. The mean absolute oral bioavailability was 11% after multiple-dose administration. The time to maximum plasma concentration with 666 mg tid or 1000 mg bid occurred at 3.5 to 9.5 hours after administration. Acamprosate is not bound to plasma proteins and has a moderate volume of distribution of 20 L. It is not metabolized; rather it is eliminated as unchanged drug in the urine and possibly by biliary excretion. The elimination half-life of acamprosate was ≈ 33 hours after multiple oral doses. Steady-state is reached after 5 to 7 days. Pharmacokinetic differences were not seen between male and female patients or in those with mild to moderate hepatic insufficiency or chronic alcoholism compared with healthy volunteers. The elimination of acamprosate is decreased in patients with renal insufficiency.

Clinical trials – Acamprosate has been compared with placebo in several double-blind studies. Outcomes of these trials included rate of study completion, rate of abstinence for the interval preceding each study visit, rate of total abstinence, time to relapse of drinking, and cumulative abstinence duration. Short-term efficacy (ie, < 6 months) has been studied in 4 trials. Acamprosate was shown to be superior in efficacy compared with placebo in 3 of 4 studies. The authors of the fourth study suggest several reasons for lack of efficacy, including the patient population and possible subtherapeutic dosages. Six-month efficacy has been studied in 6 trials. Five trials demonstrated superior efficacy for acamprosate vs placebo. A sixth trial did not demonstrate a treatment effect for acamprosate; however, treatment was instituted after a long interval post-detoxification. Long-term efficacy (ie, > 6 months) was demonstrated in 5 trials, but craving was not reduced in these clinical trials relative to placebo.

Acamprosate was compared with naltrexone in a randomized, single-blind, 12-month trial conducted in male patients between 18 and 65 years of age. After completing detoxification, 157 patients received naltrexone 50 mg/day (n = 77) or acamprosate 1665 to 1998 mg/day in 3 divided doses (n = 80). If difficult-to-control relapses occurred during the study period, patients were treated with disulfiram until relapse was fully over (2 to 3 weeks). The mean number of days to first alcohol consumption was 44 for naltrexone patients and 39 for acamprosate patients (P = 0.34). The mean number of days to first relapse (≥ 5 drinks/day) was longer for naltrexone (63 days) than acamprosate (42 days) (P = 0.02). Naltrexone patients also consumed fewer drinks at a time (4 vs 9, P = 0.01), had more days of abstinence (243 vs 180, P = 0.03), and had lower craving scores than acamprosate patients (11.3 vs 15.3, P = 0.01). In addition, the number of naltrexone patients treated with disulfiram (17 patients, 22%) was fewer than acamprosate patients (42 patients, 52%) (P = 0.0002).

➤*Drug Interactions:* Food decreases the absorption of acamprosate compared with a fasting state. Pharmacokinetic interactions were not observed when acamprosate was administered with alcohol, diazepam, imipramine, or disulfiram.

➤*Adverse Reactions:* In double-blind trials, diarrhea was the only side effect that consistently occurred more frequently than placebo (10%). This adverse effect appeared to be dose-dependent in 1 study; however, this was not supported by data from a second dose-response study.

➤*Summary:* Acamprosate is marketed in 23 European countries, but is currently in phase III trials in the US. Acamprosate is more effective than placebo for prolonging abstinence and reducing the rate of relapse. Naltrexone was shown to be superior in efficacy to acamprosate in one head-to-head trial in patients with moderate dependence. Acamprosate should be started as soon as possible after withdrawal from alcohol consumption. The recommended dose is 1.3 g/day in patients < 60 kg and 2 g/day in patients ≥ 60 kg, given in divided doses. Treatment with two 500 mg tablets twice daily is bioequivalent to two 333 mg tablets 3 times/day. It should not be administered to patients with renal insufficiency. Adverse events were similar to placebo in clinical trials and drug interactions are absent with several medications often used concomitantly for alcohol dependence.

ACETORPHAN (by Laboratoire Bioproject, Paris, France) – An enkephalinase inhibitor

➤*Actions:*

Pharmacology – Acetorphan is a lipophilic inhibitor of enkephalinase, a peptidase present in the GI tract and the CNS. By inhibiting enkephalinase, endogenous enkephalin concentrations increase, giving acetorphan varied therapeutic indications.

Acetorphan is used for symptomatic treatment of acute diarrhea in adults. Treatment should not last more than 7 days. Acetorphan administration does not obviate the need for hydration when relevant.

Pharmacokinetics – Available pharmacokinetic data in humans are limited to the dosing information included below.

Clinical trials – A double-blind, crossover design evaluated the ability of acetorphan to prevent diarrhea in patients receiving castor oil. Acetorphan was administered 45 minutes after the castor oil. Castor oil was selected to induce an experimental secretory diarrhea. Six subjects were studied. Prophylactic acetorphan significantly reduced the mean number of stools during the following 24 hours by 50% and the stool weight by 37%. No side effects other than nausea and discomfort, which were noted in all subjects, were reported.

One hundred ninety-nine patients randomly received acetorphan or placebo after being diagnosed with infectious diarrhea. Patients took 2 capsules (100 mg each) upon enrollment in the study and 1 capsule after each unformed stool for a maximum of 10 days. No other therapies were initiated during the trial with the exception of acetaminophen as needed. Patients receiving acetorphan experienced a significantly shorter duration of diarrhea. Of the patients still experiencing diarrhea on day 10, 7% received acetorphan, and 24% received placebo. Side effects were similar between the 2 groups.

One study compared the efficacy of acetorphan (100 mg 3 times/day) and loperamide (eg, *Imodium A-D*; 1.33 mg 3 times/day) in the treatment of infectious diarrhea. Therapy continued until resolution of diarrhea or for a maximum of 7 days. Thirty-seven patients received acetorphan, and 32 patients received loperamide. The mean duration of diarrhea did not differ between the 2 groups. However, abdominal distension and constipation were significantly more common in the loperamide group.

Another study compared the efficacy of acetorphan and clonidine (eg, *Catapres*) in suppressing opiate withdrawal symptoms. Nineteen heroin or synthetic opiate addicts were treated with 50 mg IV acetorphan twice daily or 0.075 mg clonidine 5 times/day; they displayed opioid withdrawal syndrome within 24 hours after a hospital admission. Changes in the overall Opiate Withdrawal Scale did not differ between the 2 groups; however, diarrhea and lacrimation were more improved in the acetorphan group. No side effects were noted in the acetorphan group; 1 clonidine patient experienced severe hypotension.

Published studies evaluating analgesic activity are only in the animal model. The potential for a new analgesic mechanism of action makes acetorphan a promising agent. Acetorphan has been shown to have minimal abuse potential and withdrawal is not precipitated upon abrupt discontinuation of the drug in animals.

Finally, a possible role in the treatment of gastroesophageal reflux disease (GERD) has been suggested based on the results of a study evaluating the drug's effects on the lower esophageal sphincter.

➤*Adverse Reactions:* No side effects significantly different from placebo have been identified in the clinical trials.

➤*Summary:* Acetorphan is not commercially available in the US, but it is available in France as 100 mg capsules. However, recent research suggests it will provide a novel antidiarrheal agent with minimal side effects. Several potential additional indications are currently being investigated, such as the treatment of opioid withdrawal, GERD, and analgesia.

AIDS DRUGS IN DEVELOPMENT

AIDS Drugs in Development			
Drug	Drug type	FDA status	Treatment sponsor
Adipose redistribution syndrome			
Serostim[2] (somatropin [rDNA origin])	growth hormone	Phase II/III	Serono
AIDS			
ACT (activated cellular therapy)	other	Phase II	Neoprobe
BMS-234475	nd[1]	Phase I	Bristol-Myers Squibb
Cytolin	nontoxid AIDS monoclonal antibody	Phase I/II	CytoDyn Inc.
MDX-240	virus-specific bispecific antibody	Phase I/II	Medarex Inc.
SPD 754	nd[1]	Phase I	Shire Pharmaceutical
SPD 756	nd[1]	Phase I	Shire Pharmaceutical
Tipranavir	protease inhibitor	Phase II	Boehringer-Ingelheim Pharmaceuticals
Aphthous ulcers			
Thalomid (thalidomide)[2]	nd[1]	Phase III	Celgene
Cachexia			
Testosterone[2]	anabolic steroid	Phase II	TheraTech
CMV infection			
Benzimidavir (1263W94)	CMV-DNA inhibitor	Phase II	GlaxoSmithKline
T902611 (T611)	nd[1]	Phase I	Tularik
CMV retinitis			
GW275175	CMV-DNA maturation inhibitor	Phase I	GlaxoSmithKline
Dementia			
Memantine[2]	NMDA receptor antagonist/neuroprotective agent	Phase II	Neurobiological Technologies
Diarrhea			
DiffGAM	nd[1]	Phase II	Immucell
Letrazurile	nd[1]	Phase II	Janssen Pharmaceutica
Synsorb CD (due to *Clostridium difficile*)	GI	Phase II	Synsorb Biotech
Fungal infections			
FK463[1]	nd[1]	Phase III	Fujisawa
Oramed[1]	nd[1]	Phase II	Biosyn
Posaconazole[1] (oral triazole)	nd[1]	Phase III	Schering-Plough
Hepatitis B co-infection			
Entecavir (BMS 200475)	nd[1]	Phase II	Bristol-Myers Squibb
Herpes co-infection			
Forvade (cidofovir gel)	antiviral	Phase I/II completed	Gilead Sciences
ME-609 cream	nd[1]	Phase II completed	Medivir
HIV infection			
AIDS vaccine	vaccine	Phase I	United Biomedical
Alferon N (interferon alfa-n3)[2] injection	nd[1]	Phase III	Interferon Sciences
ALVAC-E120TMG (vCP1521)	nd[1]	Phase II	Aventis Pasteur
ALVAC-MN120TMG (vCP205)	nd[1]	Phase I/II	Aventis Pasteur
Amdoxovir	nucleoside analog	Phase II	Gilead
Ampligen	nucleic acid	Phase II	HemispheRx Biopharma
Ancer 20 injection	nd[1]	Phase I	Zeria USA
Anticort[2] (procaine HCl)	nd[1]	Phase II completed	Samaritan
Aztec (zidovudine) controlled-release	antiviral	Phase III completed	Verex Pharmaceuticals
BAY 50-4798	nd[1]	Phase I	Bayer
Beta-L-Fd4C	nd[1]	Phase II	Achillion Pharmaceuticals
BMS-234475	second generation protease inhibitor	Phase II	Bristol-Myers Squibb
BMS 561390	NNRTI[3]	Phase II	Bristol-Myers Squibb
Calanolide A	NNRTI[3]	Phase I/II	Sarawak MediChem
CCR5	receptor antagonist	Phase I	Schering-Plough
Crixivan in *NanoCrystal* formulation (indinavir)	protease inhibitor	Phase II	NanoSystems LLC/Merck and Co. Inc.
CS-92	NRTI[4]	Phase I/II	Triangle Pharmaceuticals
Cytolin	nd[1]	Phase I/II	Amerimmune Pharmaceuticals
Epivir/lamivudine (once-daily dosing)	nd[1]	application submitted	GlaxoSmithKline
Epivir and *Ziagen* combination tablet	nd[1]	Phase III	GlaxoSmithKline
GEM 92	nd[1]	Phase I	Hybridon
HGP-30 and sargramostim[2]	nd[1]	Phase I	Cel-Sci Corp./Immunex Corp.
HGTV43	gene therapy	Phase I	Enzo Biochem
HIV Therapeutic	nd[1]	Phase I	United Biomedical

~ Bibliography Available on Request ~

AIDS Drugs in Development

Drug	Drug type	FDA status	Treatment sponsor
HIV-IT	nd[1]	Phase II	Chiron Viagene
IL-2	nd[1]	Phase I/II	Bayer
ISIS 5320	nd[1]	Phase I	Isis Pharmaceuticals, Inc.
L-708,906	integrase inhibitor	nd[1]	nd[1]
MIV-150	NNRTI[3]	Phase I	Chiron
MIV-310[2]	nd[1]	Phase II	Medivir
Multikine	immunotherapeutic agent	Phase I	Cel-Sci Corp.
PA-457	budding inhibitor	preclinical	Panacos Pharmaceuticals
Pro 542	recombinant fusion inhibitor	Phase II	Progenics/Genzyme Transgenics
Pro 2000 gel	antiviral agent/microbicide	Phase II	Interneuron
Proleukin[2] (aldesleukin) interleukin-2 (IL-2)	interleukin	Phase III	Chiron
Rev 123	nd[1]	Phase I/II	Novartis
S-1360 (GW810781)	integrase inhibitor	Phase II	GlaxoSmithKline
Savvy	vaginal gel microbicide and spermicide	Phase I/II	Biosyn
T-1249	fusion inhibitor	Phase I/II	Trimeris
TAT antagonist	antiviral	Phase I/II	Hoffman-LaRoche
Timunox (thymopentin)	immunomodulator	Phase III	Immunobiology Research Institute
Tipranavir	nonpeptidic protease inhibitor	Phase III	Boehringer-Ingelheim Pharmaceuticals
TM 114	protease inhibitor	Phase II	Tibotec
TMC125	NNRTI[3]	Phase II	Tibotec
TNX-355	anti-CD4 monoclonal antibody	Phase I	Tanox
Tucaresol (immunopotentiator)	immunomodulator/immunopotentiator	Phase II	GlaxoWellcome
Tumor necrosis factor (TNF)	antiviral	Phase I	Immunex
UK-427,857	entry inhibitor	Phase I	nd[1]
Ushercell	nd[1]	Phase I	Polydex
VX-175 (GW433908)	protease inhibitor	Phase III	Vertex Pharmaceuticals
VX-385	nd[1]	Phase I	Vertex Pharmaceuticals
WF10 OXO[2]	nd[1]	Phase III	Chemie
Zerit (stavudine) extended-release	nd[1]	application submitted	Bristol-Myers Squibb

HIV infection and AIDS

Drug	Drug type	FDA status	Treatment sponsor
Abavca/Perthon	plant derivative	Phase I/II	Advanced Plant Pharmaceuticals
Ampligen	nd[1]	Phase II/III	HemispheRx Biopharma
Capravirine	NNRTI[3]	Phase II	Agouron Pharmaceuticals
Emtriva and *Viread*	nd[1]	Research stage	Gilead
GS 4338	nd[1]	Research stage	Gilead
GS 7340	nd[1]	Phase I	Gilead
HE 2000	cellular energy regulators	Phase II	Hollis-Eden Pharmaceuticals
T-1249	peptide fusion inhibitor	Phase I/II	Trimeris
Tipranavir	protease inhibitor	Phase III	Boehringer-Ingelheim Pharmaceuticals
Zadaxin	nd[1]	Phase II	SciClone

HIV wasting

Drug	Drug type	FDA status	Treatment sponsor
Androderm[2]	testosterone replacement	Phase III	SmithKline Beecham
Androgel DHT (dihydrotestosterone gel)	steroid	Phase II	Unimed
Thalomid[2] (thalidomide)	TNF-alpha selective inhibitor	Phase III	Celgene

HPV co-infection

Drug	Drug type	FDA status	Treatment sponsor
Low-dose oral interferon alpha	nd[1]	Phase I	Atrix Laboratories
Multikine (leukocyte interleukin injection)	interleukin	Phase I	Cel-Sci Corp.
Veldona Lozenge (interferon alpha)	natural human interferon alpha	Phase III	Amarillo Biosciences

Kaposi sarcoma

Drug	Drug type	FDA status	Treatment sponsor
A-007	nd[1]	Phase I	Dekk-Tec
Panretin (alitretinoin) oral	retinoic acid	Phase II	Ligand Pharmaceuticals
BMS 275291	nd[1]	Phase I/II	National Cancer Institute
Cidofovir[2]	antiviral	Phase II completed	Gilead Sciences
Interleukin-12	interleukin	Phase II	National Cancer Institute
Metastat (4-dedimethysancycline)	matrix metallo proteinase inhibitor	Phase II	CollaGenex Pharmaceuticals
Panretin and interferon	nd[1]	Phase I/II	Ligand Pharmaceuticals
Paxene (paclitaxel), *Taxol*[2]	nd[1]	Phase III/Phase II/III	IVAX/National Cancer Institute
SU5416	angiogenesis inhibitor	Phase II completed	SUGEN

~ Bibliography Available on Request ~

AIDS Drugs in Development			
Drug	Drug type	FDA status	Treatment sponsor
Thalidomide[2]	cytokine-selective inhibitor	Phase II completed	National Cancer Institute
Virulizin	macrophage activator	Phase III	Imutec Pharma
Lymphomas			
Bryostatin	nd[1]	Phase I	National Cancer Institute
Proleukin[2] (aldesleukin, interleukin-2 [IL-2])	nd[1]	Phase II	National Cancer Institute
Rituxan (rituximab)	nd[1]	Phase II	National Cancer Institute/IDEC Pharmaceuticals
Virulizin	macrophage activator	Phase III	Imutec Pharma
Mycobacterial infection			
MiKasome (amikasin)	nd[1]	Phase II	NeXstar Pharmaceuticals
Mycobacterial avium complex			
Rifalazil (PA-1648)	rifampin derivative	Phase II	PathoGenesis
Non-Hodgkin lymphoma			
ATRA-IV (tretinoin)	liposomal all-transretinoic acid	Phase II	Aronex Pharmaceuticals
G3139	antisense compound	Phase I/II	Genta
LymphoCide	nd[1]	Phase III	Immunomedics
Proleukin[2] (aldesleukin, interleukin-2 [IL-2])	nd[1]	Phase II	National Cancer Institute
Rituxan (rituximab)	nd[1]	Phase II	National Cancer Institute/IDEC Pharmaceuticals
Pain			
DPI3290	nd[1]	Phase II	Ardent
Morphelan ROER (morphine sulfate rapid-onset extended-release)	nd[1]	application submitted	Elan Pharmaceuticals/Ligand Pharmaceuticals
Ziconotide	nd[1]	application submitted	Elan Pharmaceuticals
PCP infection			
Dapsone[2]	nd[1]	Phase III	Jacobus
Dapsone/pyrimethamine/folinic acid[2]	nd[1]	Phase III	Jacobus
Dapsone/trimethoprim[2]	nd[1]	Phase III	Jacobus
DB 289	nd[1]	Phase I	Immtech
Pediatric HIV			
Combivir[2] (zidovudine/lamivudine)	nucleoside analog reverse transcriptase inhibitor combination	nd[1]	GlaxoSmithKline
Crixivan[2] (indinavir)	protease inhibitor	nd[1]	Merck
Fortovase[2] (saquinavir)	protease inhibitor	nd[1]	Roche
HIV-1 immunogen	nd[1]	Phase I completed	Agouron Pharmaceuticals
Hivid[2] (zalcitabine, ddC)	NRTI[4]	nd[1]	Roche
Invirase[2] (saquinavir)	protease inhibitor	nd[1]	Roche
MKC-442	nd[1]	Phase II	Triangle Pharmaceuticals
Rescriptor[2] (delavirdine)	NNRTI[3]	Phase II	Pfizer
Viread (tenofovir disoproxil fumarate)	nucleoside analog reverse transcriptase inhibitor	Phase I	Gilead Sciences
Progressive multifocal leukoencephalopathy (PML)			
Topotecan (hycamtin)[1,2]	semi-synthetic derivative of camptothecin, toposiomerase I-inhibitor	Phase II completed	GlaxoSmithKline
Vaccines			
AIDS vaccine	multi-envelope HIV vaccine component	Phase I	St. Jude Children's Research Hospital
Aidsvax	vaccine	Phase III	VaxGen
ALVAC (vCP1452)	vaccine	Phase II	Aventis Pasteur
ALVAC (vCP1521)	vaccine	Phase II	Aventis Pasteur
Genevax-HIV/APL-400-003 (end/rev) facilitated DNA-based vaccine	vaccine	Phase I	Wyeth
Genevax-HIV/APL-400-047 (gag/pol) facilitated DNA-based vaccine	vaccine	Phase I	Wyeth
HIV vaccine	vaccine	Phase I	GlaxoSmithKline
HIV-1 peptide vaccine	vaccine	Phase I	National Cancer Institute
Remune	vaccine	Phase III	Immune Response
TBC-3B	vaccine, recombinant	Phase I	Therion Biologics

[1] nd = no data.
[2] Approved for other indications; refer to individual monographs.

[3] NNRTI = Non-nucleoside reverse transcriptase inhibitor.
[4] NRTI = Nucleoside reverse transcriptase inhibitor.

►*Summary:* Acquired Immunodeficiency Syndrome (AIDS) is an immunodeficiency state caused by an infection with the human immunodeficiency virus, HIV. There are several drugs being studied for HIV, AIDS, and AIDS-related illnesses. Listed above are some antiviral, cytokine, immunomodulating drugs, and vaccines currently undergoing clinical trials.

ALICAFORSEN (by ISIS) – An antisense inhibitor of ICAM-1

➤*Actions:*

Pharmacology – Alicaforsen is a 20-base antisense phosphorothioate oligodeoxynucleotide that selectively inhibits cytokine-induced intercellular adhesion molecule 1 (ICAM-1) expression in various human cells in vitro and in vivo. This drug is designed to hybridize to a sequence in the 3′ untranslated region of human ICAM-1 mRNA. The heterodimer formed by alicaforsen and mRNA serves as a substrate for mRNase H, an enzyme family that cleaves RNA in DNA-RNA heterodimers. In vitro, alicaforsen specifically reduces ICAM-1 mRNA thereby reducing ICAM-1 protein expression. A parenteral form of this drug is currently undergoing Phase 3 trials for treatment of Crohn disease. Phase 2 trials are being performed on an enema formulation for the treatment of ulcerative colitis and a topical preparation for psoriasis.

Pharmacokinetics – The metabolism and pharmacokinetics of alicaforsen have not been well defined, but it appears to follow a one-compartment model. Distribution into tissue is the primary route of clearance. Half-life, AUC, volume of distribution, C_{max}, and plasma clearance appear to be dose-dependent, indicating a saturable component to alicaforsen's distribution. Gender may also have an effect on kinetic profile of alicaforsen. In 1 study, men had plasma clearance rates up to 37% higher than women, resulting in a shorter half-life of 0.94 hours for 70 kg men vs 1.14 hours for 70 kg women. C_{max} and AUC values were higher in women than in men. Another study noted that men had a 20% higher plasma clearance of alicaforsen than women, resulting in lower AUC values in men versus women (55.5 µg.h/mL vs. 64.6 µg.h/mL). Volume of distribution might also be gender-dependent, which may be explained by differences in body fat composition since alicaforsen is poorly distributed into adipose tissue. Metabolism of alicaforsen was not altered by sex or exogenous estrogen therapy in 1 study.

Clinical trials –

Crohn disease: Alicaforsen was compared with placebo in a randomized, controlled trial of 299 patients 14 to 80 years of age with steroid-dependent Crohn disease. Enrolled patients had moderately active disease (Crohn disease activity index [CDAI] 200 to 350) for at least 3 months prior to trial participation despite 10 to 40 mg of prednisone or equivalent with at least 1 unsuccessful steroid taper attempt within the previous 2 years and at study onset. Stable doses of aminosalicylates were allowed during the study, but immunosuppressants were excluded in the prior 4 weeks. Patients were stratified based on their current steroid dose (prednisone equivalent of 10 to 19 or 20 to 40 mg/day) and then randomized to receive placebo (n = 101) or 1 of 2 alicaforsen regimens, administered as 2 mg/kg IV infusions 3 times weekly for 2 (n = 99) or 4 weeks (n = 99). The maximum dose permitted was 200 mg. Baseline steroid doses were maintained in the high-dose stratum until day eight, at which time they were placed on prednisone 20 mg/day. The doses were then tapered by 2.5 mg/day/week as tolerated. Patients in the low-dose stratum were maintained on their baseline steroid doses and then placed on a taper regimen identical to the high-dose stratum to sustain dosage by study week with the high dose stratum. These patients were then placed on a taper regimen identical to the high dose group. At week 14, 64% of placebo patients and 78% of alicaforsen patients had successfully discontinued steroid therapy. The primary endpoint of steroid-free disease remission (CDAI less than 150, steroid dose = 0) was achieved by similar proportions of patients in each of the 3 treatment groups: 19.2% of the 2-week group, 21.2% of the 4-week group, and 18.8% of the placebo group. Patients with higher baseline steroid doses had a higher rate of steroid-free disease remission. Secondary endpoints, including decreased steroid doses and quality of life, were achieved by a similar number of patients in all 3 groups as well. Although not statistically significant, patients with higher alicaforsen AUC values had increased response rates, suggesting that alicaforsen may be effective if given at high enough doses.

In a double-blind, placebo-controlled trial, 20 patients 18 to 80 years of age with moderate Crohn disease (CDAI of 200 to 350) received 13 doses of alicaforsen or placebo over a 26-day period and were followed for an additional 5 months. At the conclusion of the treatment period, 7 of 15 alicaforsen patients (2 of 3 receiving 0.5 mg/kg, 1 of 3 receiving 1 mg/kg, and 4 of 9 receiving 2 mg/kg) were in remission vs 1 placebo patient. Five of the 7 alicaforsen-treated remitters were still in remission 6 months after therapy. Three of these patients were successfully weaned off of steroids and 1 was maintained at 10 mg/day. Mean corticosteroid doses decreased in alicaforsen patients throughout the study period, while placebo patients experienced increased steroid doses after the treatment period. Mean CDAI scores were not significantly different between the 3 groups throughout the study.

➤*Adverse Reactions:* Infusion-related reactions including fever/chills, nausea, vomiting, headaches, myalgia/arthralgia, increased diarrhea, and facial flushing were reported. Hypersensitivity reactions have occurred in a small number of study patients. Transient, clinically silent post-infusion aPTT prolongation has been noted in several trials.

➤*Summary:* Studies conducted to date, both in vitro and in vivo, suggest that alicaforsen is a novel agent with anti-inflammatory potential. Based on clinical trials, alicaforsen can reduce steroid requirements in patients with moderate Crohn disease and might induce disease remission in some patients. Alicaforsen appears to be well tolerated with a low incidence of side effects. Phase 3 trials were discontinued in 1999 due to lack of efficacy to support an NDA filing. ISIS reinstated Phase 3 studies in November 2001 and are ongoing at this time in the US, Europe, and Canada.

ALVIMOPAN (by Adolor/GlaxoSmithKline) – An opioid receptor antagonist

➤*Actions:*

Pharmacology – Alvimopan is a peripherally selective, mu opioid receptor antagonist used to reduce or prevent adverse GI side effects of opioid analgesics without reversing analgesia. The activation of peripheral receptors within the GI tract is particularly important because the magnitude of bowel dysfunction correlates more closely with opioid concentrations in the enteric nervous system than with concentrations in the CNS. When administered, opioids may delay gastric emptying, increase tone of GI smooth muscle, induce spasm and provoke colic, inhibit propulsive contractions, and decrease GI transit. These effects typically lead to constipation, bloating, nausea, vomiting, and abdominal distention.

Unlike other opioid antagonists, alvimopan is restricted in activity to the GI tract, therefore not antagonizing the desired central effects of analgesia. Other antagonists my reverse adverse effects of opioids on GI function, but these antagonists are centrally active, therefore antagonizing analgesia and precipitating symptoms of opioid withdrawal in morphine-dependent subjects.

Pharmacokinetics – Administered orally, alvimopan has very limited systemic absorption and a long duration of action. Because of its large size, alvimopan does not cross the blood-brain barrier and does not possess inherent prokinetic effects. No other data is available.

Clinical trials – Clinical trials have been performed to assess the effects of alvimopan on morphine-induced delay in GI transit, examine effects on morphine analgesia, and evaluate the length of recovery time of GI function after surgery.

In a double-blind, placebo-controlled, crossover trial, 14 patients were randomized to receive placebo plus IV saline, placebo plus 0.05 mg/kg IV morphine sulfate, or alvimopan plus 0.05 mg/kg IV morphine sulfate. Each participant received all 3 treatments in order to evaluate effects on GI transit time. IV morphine prolonged GI transit time from 69 to 103 minutes (P = 0.005). Oral administration of 2 mg alvimopan prevented the morphine-induced increase in GI transit (P = 0.004) and produced average transit times of 76 minutes.

A randomized, double-blind study enrolling 45 patients was performed to assess the effect of alvimopan on morphine analgesia. Patients were assigned to receive 4 mg oral alvimopan and 0.15 mg/kg IV morphine, oral placebo and 0.15 mg/kg IV morphine, or oral placebo and IV saline. Measurement included categorical pain scores, visual analog scale (VAS) pain score, pain relief scores, and pupil diameter. Results showed VAS scores to be significantly reduced by morphine with or without alvimopan, whereas IV saline solution did not affect VAS scores. Categorical pain and relief scores also showed significant analgesia with morphine that was unaffected by alvimopan. Morphine constricted pupil size whereas alvimopan did not affect pupil size. However, IV saline solution did not result in pupil constriction.

The effects of alvimopan on postoperative GI function and length of hospitalization were studied in patients undergoing major abdominal surgery. Seventy-nine patients were randomly given 1 mg alvimopan, 6 mg alvimopan, or identical placebo capsules. All patients received opioids for postoperative pain. Patients given the 6 mg alvimopan had significantly faster recovery of GI function than those given placebo. The median time to the first passage of flatus decreased from 70 to 49 hours (P = 0.03), the median time to first bowel movement decreased from 111 to 70 hours (P = 0.01), and discharge time decreased from 91 to 68 hours (P = 0.03). The 1 mg alvimopan group did not see such prominent improvements, indicating that dosing is a key factor in treatment.

➤*Summary:* Alvimopan is a novel medication shown to decrease GI side effects of opioid medications. Because activity is peripherally selective and does not cross the blood-brain barrier, these side effects can be reduced without compromising the effects of analgesia. This unique medication could play a significant role in treating adverse GI side effects from opioid medications, speeding recovery of bowel function after surgery, and shortening the duration of hospitalization. Optimal dosing and common side effects have not been established at this time. Alvimopan is currently in phase 3 clinical trials and an NDA is expected to be filed in 2003. Adolor and GlaxoSmithKline will jointly develop and market alvimopan.

AMSACRINE (*Amsidyl* by Parke-Davis) – A dye derivative for the treatment of acute leukemia and lymphoma

➤*Actions:*

Pharmacology – Amsacrine is an acridine dye derivative for the treatment of acute leukemia and lymphoma. It inhibits DNA synthesis by a mechanism similar to the anthracyclines, via intercalation with base pairs in the DNA molecule. The precise mechanism of action is not well understood; however, it is thought that amsacrine may also interact with cellular membranes and interfere with the enzyme topoisomerase II.

Pharmacokinetics – Amsacrine has demonstrated biphasic elimination characteristics. Its distribution half-life is 0.15 to 1.4 hours. The terminal half-life is 4.7 to 9 hours. Elimination is via hepatic metabolism and biliary excretion. More than 80% of an administered dose is excreted via the biliary route into the feces. Approximately 2% to 10% of the dose is excreted in the urine unchanged. Changes in hepatic function significantly reduce clearance and increase the elimination half-life. In patients with severe hepatic dysfunction, the elimination half-life is 17.2 hours. The major metabolite, which appears inactive, is an amsacrine-glutathione 5' conjugate.

The volume of distribution is 1.7 to 2.6 L/kg. Amsacrine is highly plasma protein bound (96.4% to 97.7%), however, 2 hours after administration 50% plasma protein binding has also been reported. High levels of amsacrine have been found distributed in the gallbladder, kidney and lower levels in the lung, testes, muscle, fat, spleen, bladder, pancreas, colon, prostate, brain and cerebrospinal fluid.

Clinical trials –

Acute myelogenous leukemia (AML): Amsacrine and cytarabine were compared in 48 patients with AML in relapse. Patients were treated with either amsacrine 75 mg/m^2 daily for 7 days or high-dose cytarabine 3 g/m^2 every 12 hours for 6 days. Response rates in both groups were similar, with 3 of 23 amsacrine-treated patients and 3 of 25 cytarabine-treated patients achieving complete remission. All patients achieved remissions after only 1 course of therapy. Failures appeared to be primarily due to the inability to reduce the leukemic population (absolute drug resistance) or regrowth of leukemia (relative drug resistance), with over half the patients demonstrating drug resistance. Overall response rates with both agents were low. In another study,

therapy with amsacrine administered as a continuous infusion at a dose of 90 mg/m^2/day for 5 days produced no complete responses in 21 patients with refractory or relapsed AML. Other studies have reported response rates of 15% to 29% for reinduction of complete remission.

Acute promyelocytic leukemia (APL): An amsacrine, cytarabine and thioguanine regimen was compared with a daunorubicin, cytarabine, thioguanine regimen in a small number of patients with APL. Complete remission was achieved in 7 of 7 patients receiving the amsacrine regimen and 5 of 9 patients receiving the daunorubicin regimen, suggesting amsacrine may effectively replace daunorubicin in some APL chemotherapy regimens.

Acute lymphoblastic leukemia (ALL): In patients with refractory or relapsed ALL, amsacrine alone was demonstrated to be as effective as a combination regimen with cytarabine and thioguanine. Complete remissions were achieved in 3 of 11 amsacrine-treated patients and 3 of 13 cytarabine-treated patients. Amsacrine plus high-dose cytarabine was also evaluated in ALL. As in other types of leukemia, this combination produced good remission rates but does not appear to impact long-term survival.

➤*Adverse Reactions:* Common adverse effects include myelosuppression, stomatitis/mucositis, nausea and vomiting, alopecia, phlebitis, diarrhea, hypersensitivity reactions, hepatoxicity, hyperbilirubinemia, hypoalbuminemia, mild hepatic dysfunction, elevations in alkaline phosphatase and transaminase levels, serious cardiac arrhythmias (ventricular tachycardia, supraventricular tachyarrhythmias), QT interval prolongation, hypokalemia, transient hypomagnesemia, acute myocardial necrosis, presented as an acute myocardial infarction, congestive heart failure, sudden death and seizures.

The most common adverse effects of the combination cytarabine and amsacrine regimens have included nausea and vomiting, ocular discomfort, mucositis, hepatic dysfunction, cutaneous erythremia and cerebellar dysfunction.

➤*Summary:* Amsacrine appears to be an active agent in the treatment of refractory/relapsed acute leukemia when administered alone or in combination with other chemotherapeutic agents, especially cytarabine. Amsacrine therapy has been demonstrated to improve the rate of complete remissions, but duration of survival has not been shown to improve. The role of amsacrine may be most effective in combination with other agents to induce remissions prior to bone marrow transplantation. An NDA has been filed with the FDA.

ANCESTIM (*Stemgen* by Amgen) – A hematopoietic growth factor

➤*Actions:*

Pharmacology – Ancestim is a recombinant human stem cell factor (SCF), also called *c-kit* ligand, Steel factor, and mast-cell growth factor. It exists as a soluble circulating glycoprotein and a membrane-bound molecule expressed on stromal cells in the bone marrow microenvironment. In combination with other cytokines, SCF induces proliferation and increases receptiveness to lineage commitment of primitive and mature hematopoietic progenitors. Administration of recombinant human SCF is associated with the mobilization of peripheral blood progenitor cells (PBPC). Ancestim alone is not sufficient to increase PBPC harvest to achieve hematapoietic recovery. When administered in combination with filgrastim (*Neupogen*), it synergistically increases the number of PBPCs in the peripheral blood. It also acts synergistically with other hematopoietic growth factors, including sargramostim (*Leukine*), erythropoietin (epoetin alfa; *Epogen, Procrit*), interleukin-3, interleukin-6, and interleukin-7.

Clinical trials –

Non-Hodgkin's lymphoma: In 38 patients with non-Hodgkin's lymphoma who were eligible for autologous transplantation, patients were treated with filgrastim alone or in combination with ancestim to mobilize PBPCs for 7 days, with apheresis performed on days 5 through 7. Three to 10 days after apheresis, patients began a 4-day regimen of high-dose chemotherapy and then received PBPC reinfusion and filgrastim until engraftment. Overall, the total mononuclear cell count, CD34+ cell content, granulocyte-macrophage colony-forming cells (GM-CFC) and burst-forming units-erythroid (BFU-E) per kg in the apheresis were similar in the 2 treatment groups.

Breast cancer: Breast cancer patients (n=215) having at least 1 prior cycle of cytotoxic chemotherapy at least 3 weeks before enrollment received either filgrastim alone (10 mcg/kg/day for 7 days) or in combination with ancestim 5 to 30 mcg/kg/day for 7, 10, or 13 days. Patients were then treated with high-dose chemotherapy followed by infusions of PBPCs on days 0 to 2 and filgrastim until absolute neutrophil count recovery. The median number of CD34+ cells collected was greater for patients treated with the combination. There were more CD34+ cells harvested in the groups receiving ancestim 20 and 25 mcg/kg/day 7-day treatment courses than with filgrastim alone.

The effects of ancestim plus filgrastim on PBPC harvest were compared with the effects of filgrastim alone in 62 patients with early-stage

breast cancer. Concurrent therapy resulted in increased levels of PBPCs, which allowed for greater levels of PBPCs to be obtained by apheresis than with filgrastim alone. Pretreatment for several days with ancestim prior to initiation of filgrastim enhanced cell mobilization and allowed for collection of more cells than with concurrent ancestim plus filgrastim. Hematologic recovery following high-dose chemotherapy was rapid in each treatment group.

Multiple myeloma: In a study of patients with multiple myeloma, treatment with ancestim plus filgrastim was more effective than filgrastim alone for mobilizing PBPC. The combination therapy required fewer apheresis collections to achieve the target number of CD34+ cells.

Ovarian carcinoma: The effects of ancestim in PBPC mobilization and collection were evaluated in 48 patients with ovarian carcinoma. Forty-eight hours after chemotherapy, patients received filgrastim alone or with ancestim (5, 10, 15, or 20 mcg/kg/day). The combination of filgrastim plus ancestim 20 mcg/kg/day produced a 5.8-fold increase in long-term culture-initiating cells compared to the use of filgrastim alone. A 3-fold increase in CD34+ cells and up to a 64-fold increase in CD34+/33- cells were observed with the combination compared with the use of filgrastim alone.

➤*Adverse Reactions:* Injection site reactions including erythema, pruritus, swelling, and hyperpigmentation (> 80%); mild-to-moderate allergic reactions, including rash, respiratory symptoms (cough, hoarseness, laryngospasm), and itching (15%); urticaria; dermatographia; angioedema; hypotension. The major toxicity has been an anaphylactic-type reaction, which occurred in 33 of 564 patients studied; the reaction was severe, but not life-threatening, in 76% of those patients.

➤*Summary:* The administration of ancestim with filgrastim can increase mobilization and collection of PBPCs. Greater benefit may be achieved with the combination in patients who have received extensive chemotherapy. Ancestim should not be routinely used in all patients who will be undergoing PBPC collection. Additional studies are necessary to determine which patients may benefit from the effects of ancestim. Ancestim may offer an economic advantage if it allows for faster hematologic recovery, fewer days of growth factor administration, and fewer apheresis collections. The optimal dose has not been established. However, 1 large clinical trial demonstrated the optimal dose to be ancestim SC 20 mcg/kg/day plus filgrastim 10 mcg/kg/day, with daily apheresis beginning on day 5. Ancestim was recommended for approval by the FDA's Biological Response Modifiers Advisory Committee in July 1998.

ARTESUNATE (sponsored by the World Health Organization) – An antimalarial agent

➤*Actions:*

Pharmacology – Artesunate rectal capsules are undergoing FDA review for use in the emergency treatment of acute malaria in patients who cannot take medication by mouth and for whom parenteral treatment is not available. They are not to be used in settings where it is possible to provide immediate therapy with oral or parenteral antimalarials. Artesunate is a water-soluble derivative of artemisinin. Artemisinin is a sesquiterpene lactone endoperoxide isolated from the Chinese medicinal herb qinghao, *Artemisia annua* L. (sweet wormwood). Artesunate acts by increasing the oxidant stress on the plasmodia within the erythrocyte. Artesunate exerts this effect by increasing production of activated oxygen species (oxygen radicals) within the erythrocyte. Artesunate is highly active against *Plasmodium falciparum*, including multidrug-resistant strains; however, sensitivity has declined in regions where mefloquine resistance is prevalent. Artesunate also is highly active against *Plasmodium vivax*.

Pharmacokinetics – Artesunate is metabolized rapidly to an active metabolite dihydroartemisinin (DHA) by blood esterases and hepatic metabolism. The artesunate half-life is 2 to 3 minutes. From 25% to 72% of the total artesunate dose is converted to DHA. DHA is primarily excreted in the urine. The AUC of artesunate following oral administration is much lower than that achieved following rectal artesunate administration; however, the AUC of DHA is similar. Artesunate is 59% plasma protein bound; DHA is 43% plasma protein bound.

Clinical trials – Three pivotal studies were submitted to the FDA in which a single dose of rectal artesunate was administered during the first 24 hours of therapy and compared with a standard antimalarial regimen for 24 hours. These studies were performed in health care settings in Thailand, Malawi, and South Africa, and patients received full adjunctive therapy with fluid, transfusions, antipyretics, and anticonvulsants as needed. Two studies enrolled pediatric patients and 1 enrolled adults. Patients were treated with rectal artesunate 10 mg/kg as a single dose for the first 24 hours, or a regimen with a comparator agent (oral artesunate or parenteral quinine). In the study conducted in Thailand, patients received rectal or oral artesunate followed by oral artesunate plus mefloquine. In the studies conducted in Malawi and South Africa, patients received rectal artesunate or parenteral quinine, followed by oral sulfadoxine-pyrimethamine or parenteral quinine if unable to receive oral therapy. Parasitemia was the primary endpoint in these studies. At 24 hours, clinical success rates were similar in the patients receiving artesunate to those receiving the comparator agents. Parasitological success (parasite count less than or equal to 10% of

baseline) was similar in the study comparing rectal and oral artesunate (73% and 71.4%), and much greater with artesunate in the studies comparing rectal artesunate with parenteral quinine (88% vs 13.6%, $P < 0.0001$, and 84.6% vs 25%, $P = 0.0034$). At 28 days, recrudescence or reinfection occurred in none of the evaluable patients in the study conducted in Thailand, 45.3% of artesunate-treated patients and 22.7% of quinine-treated patients in the study conducted in Malawi, and 8% of artesunate-treated patients and 25% of quinine-treated patients in the study conducted in South Africa. An FDA advisory committee recommended that additional studies large enough to detect a mortality benefit be conducted. An ongoing, double-blind, placebo-controlled field study currently is evaluating rectal artesunate administered according to the proposed indication in patients as young as 6 months of age. As of March 2002, a total of 3366 patients had been enrolled.

➤*Drug Interactions:* Artesunate alters the pharmacokinetics of mefloquine. When oral artesunate has been administered with oral mefloquine, the mefloquine peak concentration has been reduced, the clearance has been increased, and the volume of distribution has been expanded. In another study, administration of oral mefloquine on the third day of a 3-day oral artesunate regimen resulted in a 72% increase in mefloquine bioavailability compared with administration on day 1. Administration of mefloquine at the conclusion of artesunate administration may minimize the potential for interactions and also reduces the risk of vomiting associated with mefloquine.

➤*Adverse Reactions:* Adverse events occurring during rectal artesunate therapy have included abdominal pain, vomiting, diarrhea, and pruritus. The incidence and nature of adverse events observed in artesunate studies have been difficult to distinguish from the signs and symptoms of severe falciparum malaria.

➤*Summary:* Rectal artesunate offers an opportunity to initiate antimalarial therapy earlier in order to reduce malaria mortality. For the emergency treatment of malaria, the recommended dose is a single 10 mg/kg dose within the first 24 hours, followed by appropriate antimalarial therapy. Therapy with artesunate rectal capsules alone is not indicated for the therapy of malaria; supplemental oral or parenteral therapy must supplement the initial artesunate regimen. The results of ongoing studies should provide additional information on its effects on mortality in these at-risk populations. The available studies suggest artesunate therapy is useful in quickly lowering parasite counts. Rectal artesunate should be made widely available in those regions with endemic malaria and limited health care resources. The WHO submitted for approval of rectal artesunate suppositories under orphan drug status and with expedited review. In July 2002, an FDA advisory committee unanimously recommended accelerated approval.

CARPROFEN (*Rimadyl* by Roche) – A nonsteroidal anti-inflammatory drug

➤*Actions:*

Pharmacology – Carprofen [(D,L)-6-chloro-alpha-methylcarbazole-2-acetic acid] is a member of the arylpropionic acid class of nonsteroidal anti-inflammatory drugs (NSAIDs), which includes ibuprofen (eg, *Motrin*), naproxen (eg, *Naprosyn*), and others. The drug also possesses analgesic and antipyretic activity.

Although the site and exact mechanism of action of the NSAIDs has not been fully elucidated, most investigators agree that these drugs owe their analgesic and anti-inflammatory activity, as well as their gastric irritant properties, to their ability to inhibit prostaglandin synthetase. Carprofen is considered to be a less potent inhibitor of prostaglandin biosynthesis than naproxen or ibuprofen and is only 1% to 4% as potent as indomethacin (eg, *Indocin*).

Considerable evidence suggests that the anti-inflammatory activity of carprofen is due primarily to the D-isomer; the L-isomer is only about one-seventh as potent.

Pharmacokinetics –

Absorption/Distribution: Carprofen is rapidly and extensively absorbed after oral administration. Peak concentrations of approximately 6 to 12 mcg/mL are achieved in 1 to 3 hours; absolute bioavailability is approximately 90%. Ingestion of food results in a slight reduction in the rate of absorption as well as the peak plasma concentration. However, the total amount of the drug absorbed is not reduced. Peak plasma concentrations may be higher in the elderly. Carprofen is highly protein bound (> 98%). In patients with osteoarthritis (OA) or rheumatoid arthritis (RA), the drug enters the synovial fluid rapidly, where it may achieve concentrations in excess of plasma concentrations.

Metabolism: Approximately 65% to 70% of an administered dose is metabolized by direct conjugation to an ester glucuronide. The elimination half-life ($t\frac{1}{2}$) is between 13 to 25 hours. Despite the extensive hepatic metabolism, no difference has been observed in pharmacokinetics between cirrhotics and healthy volunteers. Thus, dosage adjustments are unnecessary in patients with renal or hepatic insufficiency.

Excretion: Most of an orally administered dose of carprofen (65% to

70%) is eliminated in the urine as the glucuronide metabolite; only 3% to 12% of a dose is excreted unchanged. The remainder of the drug is excreted in the feces after undergoing extensive enterohepatic recycling.

Clinical trials – Carprofen is effective in a variety of clinical settings including treatment of rheumatoid arthritis, osteoarthritis, ankylosing spondylitis, extra-articular inflammatory processes (eg, tendonitis, bursitis), acute pain syndromes (eg, dental and post-traumatic pain) and acute gouty arthritis. Dosages have ranged from 150 to 600 mg/day in 2 or 3 divided doses. The few available comparative studies have usually shown carprofen to be equal to, or superior to, aspirin up to 3600 mg/day. Comparisons with indomethacin 75 to 150 mg/day have usually shown the lower doses (up to 300 mg/day) of carprofen to be slightly less effective but better tolerated than indomethacin. Larger doses of carprofen (400 to 600 mg/day) have been used in the treatment of OA; however, the use of larger doses may not produce any additional response over lower doses.

➤*Adverse Reactions:*

Dermatologic – Cutaneous reactions such as eczema, skin rash, urticaria, and photosensitivity have occurred in 6% to 10% of patients.

GI – GI effects have occurred in approximately 15% of patients. Pain, nausea, heartburn, and dyspepsia are most common, while diarrhea is uncommon (approximately 1%). More serious GI side effects such as peptic ulceration are rare. Carprofen has been used along with antacids in patients with active peptic ulcer disease and has been well tolerated.

Hepatic enzyme elevation – Hepatic enzyme elevation occurred in 1.4% of patients in European trials and in as many as 14% of patients in large American trials. These enzyme elevations are usually asymptomatic.

Renal or urinary – Renal or urinary adverse reactions including urinary frequency, dysuria, burning, hematuria, nephritis, proteinuria, and acute renal failure occurred in 3.4% of 1521 patients in premarketing clinical trials.

➤*Summary:* Carprofen appears to be an effective NSAID that offers convenient twice daily dosing. Despite a low incidence of serious GI side effects, the drug does not appear superior to currently available agents.

Carprofen was approved by the FDA December 31, 1987. However, Roche has made a decision not to market carprofen at this time.

CELIPROLOL HCl (*Selecor* by Aventis) – A cardioselective beta-adrenergic blocking agent

➤*Actions:*

Pharmacology – Celiprolol is a third-generation, cardioselective, hydrophilic beta-adrenoreceptor blocking agent. It possesses weak vasodilating and bronchodilating effects attributed to partial, selective β_2-adrenoreceptor agonist activity and, possibly, direct papaverine-like smooth muscle relaxation. There is evidence for intrinsic sympathomimetic activity (ISA) at the β_2-receptor. The drug is devoid of membrane stabilizing activity (MSA, or quinidine-like effect). Weak alpha$_2$-antagonist properties also are present but are not considered clinically significant at therapeutic doses.

At therapeutic doses, celiprolol reduces heart rate and blood pressure. While the drug dose not generally produce any ECG changes, it can increase the AV nodal functional refractory period. Celiprolol does not appear to alter pulmonary function, nor inhibit bronchodilation induced by agents such as aminophylline (eg, *Phyllocontin*), albuterol (eg, *Proventil*), and ipratropium (*Atrovent*). Triglycerides, LDL cholesterol, and total cholesterol are decreased in some patients while HDL is increased; it appears that total lipid levels are not increased. A reduction in fibrinogen levels has occurred, which may be of some benefit in hypertensive patients with hypercoagulability.

Pharmacokinetics – Following oral administration, absorption is nonlinear and dose-dependent. Bioavailability ranges from 30% to 70% following a single 100 mg dose and averages 74% after a 400 mg dose. Single-dose bioavailability is reduced by chlorthalidone (eg, *Hygroton*), hydrochlorothiazide (eg, *Esidrix*), and theophylline (eg, *Theo-Dur*). Food also has reduced bioavailability in some studies, but data are conflicting. Peak plasma concentrations and pharmacodynamic activity are seen 2 to 4 hours after oral administration; pharmacodynamic activity persists for 24 hours. Protein binding is ≈ 25% and the drug follows a hydrophilic pattern of distribution.

Celiprolol is largely unmetabolized and is excreted unchanged in urine and feces. It does not undergo first-pass hepatic metabolism and there are no significant active metabolites. Approximately 15% (range, 3% to 22%) of an oral dose and 50% of an IV dose is recovered in the urine within 3 days, the rest being excreted in the feces. Steady-state concentrations are achieved after 2 to 3 days. The predominant mode of excretion of active drug is renal; renal dysfunction may cause a reduction in systemic clearance and the need for dose reduction. Bioavailability is decreased and the extent of renal elimination increased in patients with cirrhosis. The pharmacokinetics are not significantly different in the elderly. The elimination half-life averages 4 to 5 hours. Placental transfer averages 3% at steady state compared with 18% for propranolol (eg, *Inderal*) and 6% for atenolol (*Tenormin*).

Clinical trials – Celiprolol is a safe and effective drug for treatment of hypertension and angina. In doses of 200 to 500 mg once daily in the morning, celiprolol reduces blood pressure to comparable levels seen with other β-blockers, calcium blockers, and ACE inhibitors. In comparative trials in patients with mild to moderate hypertension, a 200 to 600 mg dose was similar in efficacy to 80 to 160 mg/day propranolol or 100 mg/day atenolol. In patients with angina, celiprolol 300 to 600 mg/day was as effective as propranolol 80 to 160 mg/day or atenolol 50 to 100 mg/day in improving exercise performance, reducing the number of angina attacks and nitroglycerin requirements, and increasing the time to, or reducing the degree of, ST segment depression. The addition of a diuretic to doses of 200 to 400 mg/day may be more effective at controlling blood pressure than the use of celiprolol monotherapy in doses of 300 to 600 mg/day.

➤*Adverse Reactions:* In a study of > 2300 patients, side effects were mild. GI symptoms (eg, nausea, abdominal discomfort, diarrhea), the most frequently reported complaints, were responsible for drug discontinuation in 13 patients. Cardiovascular symptoms included development of a modest degree of CHF, AV nodal block, and bradycardia. Other side effects included: Headache (6%); fatigue (4%); dizziness (3%); insomnia (1%); Raynaud's phenomenon; orthostatic hypotension; bronchial obstruction; tremor; rash; muscle cramps; impotence.

➤*Summary:* Celiprolol appears to be well tolerated and effective for the treatment of hypertension and angina. Its combination of cardioselectivity, β_2-agonist activity, hydrophilicity and long duration of action make it unique among currently available drugs in this class. Whether these properties will be useful in the myriad of other applications for which β-blockers have been used (eg, post-MI prophylaxis, migraine, selected arrhythmias) will require additional experience. Celiprolol is currently available in Europe.

CILAZAPRIL (*Inhibace* by Roche/Glaxo) – A non-sulfhydryl-containing ACE inhibitor

➤*Actions:*

Pharmacology – Cilazapril is a potent, structurally new, non-sulfhydryl-containing orally active angiotensin-converting enzyme (ACE) inhibitor prodrug under investigation for use in patients with hypertension and CHF. Following oral administration, cilazapril is de-esterified in the liver and other tissues to the active diacid form, cilazaprilat. Cilazaprilat is ≈ 10 times more potent than captopril (*Capoten*) and 5 times more potent than enalaprilat, the active form of enalapril (*Vasotec*).

ACE inhibitors block the enzymatic conversion of angiotensin I to the potent vasoconstrictor angiotensin II. While this inhibition also results in reduced metabolism of bradykinin, alterations in the prostaglandin system and reductions in plasma aldosterone and antidiuretic hormone, these responses do not appear to be responsible for the primary therapeutic effects of these agents. Blockade of angiotensin II production reduces supine and standing blood pressure in hypertensive patients. In patients with CHF, the vasodilatory response reduces afterload, leading to an increase in cardiac output. These beneficial responses may be facilitated by the responses mentioned above.

After administration of cilazapril, ACE activity, angiotensin II and plasma aldosterone concentrations, total peripheral resistance, blood pressure (systolic, diastolic, and mean), and the response to exogenous angiotensin I are all reduced, while heart rate, baroreceptor reflex sensitivity, cardiovascular reflexes, and glomerular filtration rate are usually unchanged.

Pharmacokinetics – Cilazapril is rapidly absorbed after oral administration, with peak levels of the parent compound achieved at ≈ 1 hour. Conversion to cilazaprilat, the active form, is rapid and extensive, with peak levels attained at ≈ 1.8 hours with 57% absolute bioavailability of the active compound. In contrast to some other ACE inhibitors, the bioavailability is not significantly reduced by food. After single doses of 0.5, 1, 2.5, and 5 mg, peak plasma levels of cilazaprilat were 5.4, 12.4, 37.7, and 94.2 ng/mL, respectively, indicating that greater than proportional increases in the active compound are achieved over this dose range. The elimination of cilazaprilat is biphasic, with an initial half-life of 1 to 2 hours controlled by the rate of conversion to this active form, followed by a prolonged terminal elimination half-life of 30 to 50 hours. The volume of distribution is ≈ 20 L.

Clearance of cilazaprilat is almost exclusively renal. Patients with severe renal or hepatic impairment may require smaller or less frequent doses. One study suggests that hypertensive patients undergoing hemodialysis can be controlled on 0.5 mg cilazapril postdialysis. Presence of CHF or advanced age has not been shown to significantly alter pharmacokinetic parameters.

Clinical trials – Clinical trials in > 4500 hypertensive patients have evaluated the efficacy of cilazapril. Single daily doses of 2.5 to 5 mg are as effective as single daily doses of the following: 25 to 50 mg hydrochlorothiazide (HCTZ; eg, *Esidrix*); 50 to 100 mg atenolol (*Tenormin*); 80 to 160 mg sustained-release propranolol (eg, *Inderal LA*); and 10 to 20 mg enalapril. In patients with mild to moderate hypertension, a 5 mg cilazapril dose produces a maximal effect, which can be enhanced by the addition of 12.5 to 25 mg HCTZ. In patients with severe hypertension, including patients with left ventricular hypertrophy, the mean effective dose was 10 mg in combination with 12.5 to 25 mg HCTZ/day.

➤*Drug Interactions:* Indomethacin (eg, *Indocin*) considerably attenuates the antihypertensive activity of cilazapril. This attenuation was most pronounced when cilazapril was added to indomethacin, while the addition of indomethacin to a stable cilazapril regimen resulted in a degree of attenuation of effect, which was considered to be clinically insignificant. Thus, the significance of this interaction appears to be dependent on the order of drug administration.

➤*Adverse Reactions:* Cilazapril appears to be well tolerated. In controlled trials of cilazapril monotherapy in > 3500 patients, the most frequently reported side effects were: Headache (4.5%); dizziness (3.3%); fatigue (1.7%); cough (1.6%); chest pain (0.8%); rash, somnolence (0.6%). In patients ≥ 65 years of age, cough, dizziness, palpitations and somnolence occurred slightly more frequently than in younger patients. The addition of HCTZ in an additional 1000 patients resulted in a slightly higher incidence of dizziness, cough and somnolence, while the incidence of other side effects was comparable to cilazapril monotherapy.

➤*Summary:* Cilazapril is a long-acting, potent ACE inhibitor. It appears to be well tolerated, while offering the advantage of once-daily dosing; this property may make it a useful addition to a class of drugs whose safety and efficacy continue to be confirmed in a variety of disease states. An NDA for cilazapril was filed in September 1989 for hypertension. Roche and Glaxo will comarket cilazapril as *Inhibace*. On August 13, 1992, the FDA classified cilazapril as "approvable".

CILOMILAST

CILOMILAST (*Ariflo* by GlaxoSmithKline) – A Phosphodiesterase Type-IV Inhibitor

➤*Actions:*

Pharmacology – Cilomilast is under review for use in the maintenance of lung function in patients with COPD who are poorly responsive to albuterol. It also has been studied in the treatment of asthma. Cilomilast is an orally active phosphodiesterase (PDE) IV-specific inhibitor. It is more potent, but produces less emetogenic effects compared with previously developed oral PDE-IV inhibitors. (Theophylline is a non-selective PDE inhibitor.) PDE-IV is an enzyme that metabolizes cyclic 3',5'-adenosine monophosphate in inflammatory and immune cells, and in airway smooth muscle cells. Based on its mechanism, it was believed that cilomilast could produce bronchodilation and reduce inflammation in patients with airway disease. In vitro cilomilast produced suppression of eosinophils, neutrophils, basophils, and T-cells. Anti-inflammatory effects have been observed in vivo, as administration of cilomilast 15 mg twice daily for 12 weeks in patients with COPD was associated with reductions in CD8+ ($P = 0.001$) and CD68+ ($P < 0.05$) airway tissue inflammatory cells. Acute bronchodilatory effects were not observed, however, following single-dose administration of cilomilast 15 mg in patients with COPD.

Pharmacokinetics – Following oral administration on an empty stomach, the peak cilomilast levels are reached within 1 to 2 hours. Administration with food results in a delay in the time to peak of 2 to 4 hours and a reduction in the peak concentration by approximately 40%; however, overall extent of absorption (reflected by the AUC) is not altered by administration with food. Oral bioavailability is approximately 100%. Cilomilast is 99.5% plasma protein bound, primarily to albumin. The terminal elimination half-life of cilomilast is 6 to 8 hours. Cilomilast undergoes extensive hepatic metabolism via oxidation, acyl glucuronidation, and decyclopentylation, with subsequent glucuronidation or sulfation. The primary enzyme responsible for cilomilast metabolism is CYP2C8. Metabolites do not appear to contribute to the activity of cilomilast. Approximately 1% of the dose is excreted in the urine as unchanged cilomilast. Cilomilast is contraindicated in patients with severe hepatic impairment and should be used with caution in patients with mild or moderate hepatic impairment. Cilomilast plasma concentrations were unchanged in patients with renal impairment; however, reductions in protein binding and intrinsic clearance resulted in an increase in the AUC of unbound cilomilast and an increase in the elimination half-life.

Clinical trials – Cilomilast 15 mg twice daily was evaluated in 4 large, double-blind, placebo-controlled, 24-week studies enrolling patients with COPD. Enrolled patients were poorly responsive to inhaled albuterol, defined as an improvement in FEV_1 of 15% or less or 200 mL or less after albuterol administration. Patients using ipratropium at study enrollment could continue its use, and all patients received as-needed inhaled albuterol. Additional COPD medications were permitted for less than 14 days to treat COPD exacerbations. The primary outcomes were change from baseline in trough FEV_1 and in St. George's Respiratory Questionnaire score averaged over 24 weeks (a reduction in score reflects improvement in health status; a 4-point change is considered a clinically relevant change). Secondary outcomes included COPD exacerbations, forced vital capacity (FVC), exercise tolerance, postexercise breathlessness, and summary symptom score. In a combined analysis of 3 of the studies enrolling 2058 patients, the incidence of exacerbation-free survival was greater in the cilomilast-treated patients than the placebo-treated patients. During the 24-week studies, 58% of placebo-treated patients and 65.1% of cilomilast-treated patients experienced no exacerbations of any kind ($P = 0.006$), and 68.2% of placebo-treated patients and 75.7% of cilomilast-treated patients experienced no level 2 or 3 exacerbations (requiring physician treatment or hospitalization, $P = 0.001$). The pooled analysis of the 4 clinical trials (n = 2883) places the exacerbation-free rate (level 2 or 3 exacerbation, requiring physician treatment or hospitalization) at 72.3% with placebo and 75.7% with cilomilast therapy; relative risk of 0.88 (95% CI 0.75, 1.03; $P = 0.1008$).

➤*Drug Interactions:* Increased GI adverse effects were observed when erythromycin was administered concurrently with cilomilast. No pharmacokinetic interaction was observed. If erythromycin must be added to the cilomilast regimen, it should be done with caution and the patient monitored for GI adverse effects.

➤*Adverse Reactions:* The most frequently observed adverse reactions include nausea (16%), diarrhea (14%), abdominal pain (12%), vomiting (6%), dyspepsia (7%), and headache (8%). GI tolerance was improved when cilomilast was administered with food.

➤*Summary:* Cilomilast has some activity in COPD; however, further studies are necessary to better characterize its activity. The recommended dose is 15 mg twice daily, and it should be taken with food to improve GI tolerance. An NDA for cilomilast 15 mg tablets was filed in December 2002. In September 2003 the FDA's Pulmonary-Allergy Drugs Advisory Committee recommended that further long-term efficacy studies are necessary to recommend approval.

CISAPRIDE

CISAPRIDE (*Propulsid* by Janssen) – Available through investigational limited access program

➤*Indications:* Cisapride was voluntarily withdrawn from the US market in July 2000 because of the risk of serious cardiac arrhythmias and death. This drug is available to licensed physicians in the US through an investigational limited access program within the following treatment protocols:
- *Adults*: Gastroesophageal reflux disease (GERD), gastroparesis, pseudo-obstruction, or severe chronic constipation refractory to standard therapy.
- *Pediatrics*: Refractory GERD or acute, life-threatening symptoms secondary to GERD, severe chronic constipation, and pseudo-obstruction unresponsive to appropriate therapy.
- *Neonates*: Enteral feeding intolerance.

To be enrolled in the investigational limited access program, patients must have failed all standard therapeutic modalities and have undergone an appropriate diagnostic evaluation, including radiologic examinations or endoscopy. In addition, physicians must perform a baseline screening assessment, including physical examination, laboratory tests, and ECG to screen for contraindicated risk factors. A physician evaluation (under the care of or by consultation with a gastroenterologist) and follow-up testing must be repeated at regular intervals according to the protocol.

➤*Contraindications:* Serious cardiac arrhythmias including ventricular tachycardia, ventricular fibrillation, torsades de pointes, and QT prolongation have been reported in patients taking cisapride with other drugs that inhibit cytochrome P450 3A4 or that prolong the QT interval. Some of these events have been fatal. Concomitant oral or IV administration of these drugs with cisapride is contraindicated. Cisapride is also contraindicated in patients with disorders that may predispose them to arrhythmias; patients in whom an increase in GI motility could be harmful (eg, in the presence of GI hemorrhage, mechanical obstruction, or perforation); and known hypersensitivity or intolerance to the drug.

➤*Drug Interactions:* Numerous drug classes and agents increase the risk of developing serious cardiac arrhythmias. Cisapride is contraindicated in patients taking certain macrolide antibiotics (eg, clarithromycin, erythromycin, troleandomycin), certain antifungals (eg, fluconazole, itraconazole, ketoconazole), protease inhibitors (eg, indinavir, ritonavir), phenothiazines (eg, proclorperazine, promethazine), class IA and class III antiarrhythmics (eg, quinidine, procainamide, sotalol), tricyclic antidepressants (eg, amitriptyline), certain antidepressants (eg, nefazodone, maprotiline), certain antipsychotic medications (eg, sertindole), bepridil, sparfloxacin, and grapefruit juice. Certain anticholinergic agents (eg, belladonna alkaloids, dicyclomine), oral anticoagulants, H_2-receptor antagonists, and diuretics (eg, furosemide, thiazides) also interact with cisapride. The preceding lists are not comprehensive.

➤*Adverse Reactions:* Serious cardiac arrhythmias including ventricular tachycardia, ventricular fibrillation, torsades de pointes, and QT prolongation have been reported in ongoing postmarketing surveillance. From July 1993 through May 1999, 341 such cases have been reported, including 80 fatalities. In ≈ 85% of these cases, the events occurred when cisapride was used in patients with known risk factors. In clinical trials, the following adverse experiences were reported in > 1% of patients treated with cisapride and at least as often on cisapride as on placebo: Headache, diarrhea, abdominal pain, nausea, constipation, flatulence, dyspepsia, rhinitis, sinusitis, coughing, viral infection, upper respiratory tract infection, pain, fever, urinary tract infection, micturition frequency, insomnia, anxiety, nervousness, rash, pruritus, arthralgia, abnormal vision, and vaginitis.

➤*Summary:* Cisapride is no longer commercially distributed in the US. Cisapride is available in the US only through an investigational limited access program.

Complete information on enrolling patients or receiving additonal information regarding the cisapride investigational limited access program sponsored by Janssen Pharmaceutica may be obtained by calling toll-free (877)795-4247.

~ Bibliography Available on Request ~

CLOBAZAM (*Frisium* by Aventis) and NITRAZEPAM (Mogadon by Roche) – Two investigational benzodiazepines

►*Actions:*

Pharmacology – Clobazam and nitrazepam are investigational benzodiazepine derivatives. The profile of these agents parallels those of approved benzodiazepines; subtle differences account for individual product distinction.

Clobazam: Clobazam is structurally and pharmacologically related to approved benzodiazepines. Antianxiety and anticonvulsant properties are similar to diazepam; the usual adult dose is 20 to 30 mg/day. Initially, clobazam is effective against all varieties of epilepsy; however, efficacy decreases within a few days to a few weeks in approximately one-third of patients. Success also has been demonstrated in cyclic exacerbations of epilepsy associated with menstruation. Clobazam is a weak hypnotic agent.

Nitrazepam: Nitrazepam has been widely used for many years in Europe and Canada as a sedative/hypnotic in doses of 2.5 to 10 mg, and in the management of myoclonic seizures of childhood epilepsy. Its structure and clinical effects are also analogous to other benzodiazepines.

Pharmacokinetics –

Clobazam: The pharmacokinetics are independent of dose and concentration. Oral clobazam is 87% absorbed. Concomitant administration with alcohol increases clobazam's bioavailability by 50%. Food may slow the rate but does not alter total absorption. Absorption is not influenced by age or sex. Clobazam is 85% bound to human serum protein; peak serum concentrations occur 1 to 4 hours after ingestion. It is metabolized via dealkylation and hydroxylation to a pharmacologically active metabolite, N-desmethylclobazam, and several inactive metabolites. The mean half-life of the unchanged drug is 18 hours, and up to

77 hours for metabolites. Clobazam is 81% to 97% excreted in the urine; accumulation is expected in impaired renal function.

Nitrazepam: Nitrazepam is 80% bioavailable following oral administration. Absorption is rapid: 0.5 to 5 hours to peak concentration; concomitant administration with food decreases peak levels by 30%. Nitrazepam is lipophilic and is widely distributed in the body; 10% to 15% is found in the cerebrospinal fluid; 85% to 90% is plasma protein bound. It crosses the placenta and is found in breast milk (50% and about 50% to 100% of maternal plasma concentration, respectively). Metabolism is extensive and excretion is urinary, primarily as inactive metabolites; only 1 is excreted as the unchanged drug. The elimination half-life is approximately 30 hours.

►*Adverse Reactions:*

Clobazam – The most frequent (10% to 44%) side effects include: Drowsiness, hangover effects, dizziness, weakness, and lightheadedness. Less frequent (5% to 10%) adverse reactions include: Weight gain, orthostatic hypotension, syncope, headache, dry mouth, and incoordination.

Nitrazepam – The frequency of adverse reactions increases with age and dosage and parallels those of other benzodiazepines. The most common include: Fatigue, dizziness, lightheadedness, drowsiness, lethargy, mental confusion, staggering, ataxia, and falling. Nightmares, insomnia, agitation, rash, pruritus, headache, and GI disturbances also have been reported. The hangover effect is also common and may be a function of nitrazepam's long half-life.

►*Summary:* Nitrazepam and clobazam appear to be safe and effective agents with antianxiety, anticonvulsant, and hypnotic properties. These agents have long elimination half-lives; this enhances the potential for drug accumulation and increases the potential for residual side effects. These agents are unlikely to replace established benzodiazepine derivatives; however, they may provide viable therapeutic alternatives.

DOMPERIDONE (*Motilium* by Janssen Pharmaceutica) – An antiemetic

►*Actions:*

Pharmacology – Acute nausea and vomiting induced by cytotoxic chemotherapy are frequent and serious toxicities distressful to cancer patients. Symptoms can be so pronounced and refractory that they interfere with therapeutic measures and patient nutrition. Available antiemetics block the chemoreceptor trigger zone (CTZ) (neuroleptics), sedate the vomiting centers (antihistamines), block afferent impulses at the vomiting center (anticholinergics), act peripherally and in the CNS (metoclopramide), or by less defined central mechanisms (cannabinoids). These agents are effective in most patients; however, side effects (eg, drowsiness, dry mouth, hypotension, extrapyramidal effects) are limitations. Domperidone, an investigational antiemetic, appears to act with minimum adverse effects.

Domperidone is chemically unrelated to the butyrophenones, phenothiazines, or metoclopramide; however, it shares pharmacological properties with these agents. In the medulla it produces a direct blocking effect of dopamine receptors in the CTZ. Like metoclopramide and haloperidol, domperidone is a peripheral dopamine antagonist; however, it contrasts in that it does not cross the blood-brain barrier and produce CNS effects. It selectively blocks peripheral dopamine receptors in the GI wall, thus enhancing normal synchronized GI peristalsis and motility in the proximal portion of the GI tract; it also may counteract anticholinergic-induced relaxation of the lower esophageal sphincter (LES).

Pharmacokinetics – Peak plasma levels are achieved within 30 minutes following IM or oral administration and between 1 to 4 hours after rectal administration. Approximately 40% of a dose is rapidly distributed into peripheral compartments. It is metabolized in the liver and eliminated in the urine, primarily as conjugates. Less than 1% appears in the urine as unchanged drug. Excretion is almost complete within 4 days. The duration of activity is between 2 and 4 hours following IV administration.

Clinical trials – The effectiveness of domperidone in the treatment of nausea and vomiting associated with cytotoxic chemotherapy has been evaluated. Several double-blind studies were conducted in patients with Hodgkin's disease. Domperidone 16 mg IV was preferred and superior to placebo; it was effective and well tolerated, and decreased the duration of nausea and vomiting by greater than ⅓ when injected

1 hour before the start of cytostatic treatment. Domperidone, 1 to 40 mg IV daily, was administered with chemotherapy infusion in 172 patients. Vomiting induced by agents considered to be moderate emetics (eg, cyclophosphamide, 5-fluorouracil, vinblastine) was reduced; however, patients with emesis induced by doxorubicin or mechlorethamine did not respond as well. The higher dosages of domperidone did not achieve a proportionally augmented response rate. In another study, 4 mg domperidone IV produced excellent or good response in 72% of patients receiving varied chemotherapy; poor responses occurred in patients receiving dacarbazine. When 12 mg domperidone IV was compared with 10 mg metoclopramide IV, both drugs produced a good or excellent response in 70% of patients; however, metoclopramide had a higher incidence of side effects. Domperidone 1 mg/kg IV or metoclopramide 0.5 mg/kg IV was used to prevent chemotherapy-induced nausea and vomiting in children. In the random crossover trial, domperidone decreased nausea and vomiting to a significantly greater extent than metoclopramide.

Domperidone has been compared favorably to cimetidine in 20 gastric ulcer patients; it also may have value in treating symptoms of gastroesophageal reflux and postoperative- or bromocriptine-induced nausea and vomiting.

►*Adverse Reactions:* Domperidone does not appear to produce significant side effects or toxicities. Doses of 40 mg IV or 100 mg orally have not been reported to produce CNS or cardiovascular side effects, only facial flushing, headache, slight somnolence, and dry mouth. Unlike metoclopramide, domperidone does not cross the blood-brain barrier; therefore, the incidence of extrapyramidal or psychotropic effects should be low. Yet there have been isolated reports of idiosyncratic extrapyramidal reactions. Domperidone does not stimulate aldosterone secretion.

►*Summary:* Domperidone selectively blocks peripheral dopamine receptors in the GI wall and in the CTZ. Its major advantage appears to be the lack of significant side effects; it may be an effective alternative to available antiemetics, including metoclopramide. Domperidone, like other antiemetics, produces variable effects on cytotoxic chemotherapy-induced nausea and vomiting, depending on the agent administered. There is limited or no data available comparing domperidone to more standard antiemetic agents other than metoclopramide. Domperidone was developed in Belgium by Janssen Pharmaceutica; it is available in Europe.

DULOXETINE (*Cymbalta* by Eli Lilly) – An antidepressant

➤Actions:

Pharmacology – Duloxetine has been submitted to the FDA for approval for use in the treatment of major depressive disorder. Duloxetine is a dual uptake inhibitor; it blocks the reuptake of serotonin and norepinephrine. Duloxetine and venlafaxine produce dose-dependent inhibited binding of the serotonin and norepinephrine transporter radioligands. In vitro, duloxetine has a higher affinity than venlafaxine for the various serotonin and norepinephrine transporters. The norepinephrine/serotonin selectivity ratio for duloxetine for human transporters is 9.4; this ratio is 30 for venlafaxine.

Pharmacokinetics – Duloxetine's pharmacokinetic parameters are best characterized by a 1-compartment open model with dose-dependent linear changes in plasma concentrations. Peak plasma concentrations occur within 6 hours of oral administration. Administration with food or at bedtime delays the peak plasma concentrations by 4 hours. However, food has no effect on the peak plasma concentration, while bedtime administration resulted in a 28.7% reduction in peak plasma concentrations and a 17.8% reduction in the area-under-the-curve (AUC). Duloxetine is highly protein bound (greater than 95%). The mean oral clearance of duloxetine is 114 L/h, its apparent volume of distribution is 1943 L, and the half-life is 12.5 to 14 hours (9.2 to 19.1 hours); however, there is a high variability because of the drug's extensive biotransformation. Steady-state plasma concentrations are achieved within 3 days.

Clinical trials – A multicenter, double-blind, placebo-controlled study was conducted with 173 patients to evaluate the efficacy of duloxetine in the treatment of major depressive disorder. Patients were randomly assigned to treatment with duloxetine, fluoxetine, and placebo. The initial dose of the duloxetine was 20 mg twice daily. This dose was forced titrated at weekly intervals to 120 mg daily over 3 weeks. The dose of the fluoxetine was 20 mg once daily combined with a placebo dose. The HAM-D17 after 8 weeks of therapy in those patients with a baseline HAM-D17 score of less than 19 was reduced by 6.16 with duloxetine, by 5 with fluoxetine, and by 5.15 with placebo. While patients with a baseline HAM-D17 score of greater than or equal to 19 experienced a 9.3 score reduction with duloxetine, 7.77 reduction with fluoxetine, and 6.72 reduction with placebo. The response rate, calculated using the last observation carried forward (LOCF), was 49% with duloxetine (P = 0.167 vs placebo), 45% with fluoxetine (P = 0.393 vs placebo), and 36% with placebo after 8 weeks of therapy. The estimated probability of remission was 56% (P = 0.02 vs placebo) with duloxetine, 30% with fluoxetine, and 32% with placebo. While the remission rate, using LOCF analysis, was 43% (P = 0.072 vs placebo), 30% (P = 0.815 vs placebo), and 27%, respectively. Duloxetine was better than fluoxetine (P = 0.041) in improving anxiety based on the results of the HAM-D17 anxiety subscale. In the primary endpoint and other secondary endpoints, duloxetine was not better than fluoxetine, but there was a trend toward better numerical improvements in the score with the duloxetine therapy.

Duloxetine is useful in the treatment of major depressive disorder and may be able to decrease comorbid chronic pain in some patients. Animal studies indicate that duloxetine might be useful in the treatment of urinary incontinence by increasing bladder capacity and increasing periurethral striated muscle electromyogram activity.

➤Drug Interactions: Duloxetine appears to inhibit the CYP2D6 isozyme but does not affect drugs metabolized by the CYP1A2 isozyme. The bioavailability of duloxetine can be significantly decreased with activated charcoal. Concurrent use in patients taking monoamine oxidase inhibitors (MAOIs) is contraindicated.

➤Adverse Reactions: Adverse effects have included insomnia, headache, somnolence, dry mouth, tremor, asthenia, nausea, constipation, diarrhea, anorexia, dizziness, sweating, flu, rhinitis, and agitation. A few patients reported abnormal ejaculation, rash, and migraine. Like other antidepressants, duloxetine alters sleep architecture. It causes an increase in rapid eye movement (REM) sleep latency and decreases REM time after 7 days of therapy. Like venlafaxine, duloxetine can increase heart rate and blood pressure. Duloxetine therapy may cause a decrease in weight.

➤Summary: Duloxetine is effective in the treatment of major depressive disorder. Its antidepressant effects are a result of the inhibition of serotonin and norepinephrine reuptake, which is a mechanism of action similar to venlafaxine. The dose of duloxetine used in the clinical trials was 20 to 120 mg daily, administered once or twice daily. The most recently published double-blind studies used 60 mg once daily and 60 mg twice daily. Concurrent use in patients taking MAOIs is contraindicated. Lilly filed a New Drug Application for duloxetine with the FDA in December 2001. The FDA issued approvable letters in 2002 and 2003.

EXENATIDE (by Amylin Pharmaceuticals/Eli Lilly) – An Incretin Mimetic Agent

➤Actions:

Pharmacology – Exenatide (synthetic exendin-4), a 39-amino acid, is a glucagon-like peptide-1 (GLP-1) agonist derived from the venom of the Gila monster lizard. It is currently being evaluated as a subcutaneous injectable treatment to improve glucose control in type 2 diabetic patients who are not using insulin and are not achieving target levels with diet and oral medications. Normally, human GLP-1 functions as an incretin hormone to promote insulin secretion in response to food intake. Similar to this peptide, exenatide binds and activates the GLP-l receptor to promote GLP-l-like glucoregulation and to mimic the antidiabetic effects of GLP-1. In general, the actions of exenatide include glucose-dependent enhancement of insulin secretion, glucose-dependent suppression of inappropriately high glucagon secretion, glycosylated hemoglobin level reduction, gastric emptying delay, food intake reduction, weight gain suppression, and insulin sensitizing effect. Exenatide thus decreases the risk of hyperglycemic episodes by increasing the precision of glucose/insulin secretion coupling as well as maintaining normal glucose-sensing control mechanisms. Furthermore, exenatide appears to promote beta cell proliferation and neogenesis from precursor cells in in vitro and in vivo models.

Pharmacokinetics – Exenatide is metabolized by dipeptidyl peptidase IV. In comparison with native GLP-1, it is less resistant to NH_2-terminal degradation by this enzyme because of the presence of a glycine amino acid at position 2. In one study, peak concentration of exenatide was reached 2 to 3 hours after administration (0.08 mcg/kg subcutaneously) and was still detectable at 6 hours postdose. The half-life and C_{max} for subjects without detectable anti-exenatide antibodies was 202 ± 182 min and 163 ± 86 pg/mL, respectively, on day 1 and 226 ± 170 min and 159 ± 81 pg/mL, respectively, on day 28 (n = 63; mean $\pm$ SD). The half-life and C_{max} for subjects with detectable anti-exenatide antibodies was 125 ± 42 min and 172 ± 57 pg/mL, respectively, on day 1 and 373 ± 250 min and 357 ± 215 pg/mL, respectively, on day 28.

Clinical trials – One hundred and nine inadequately controlled type 2 diabetic patients who were unable to achieve HbA_{1c} less than 7% despite receiving sulfonylureas and/or metformin, were examined in a phase 2, 4-arm, placebo-controlled, randomized, multicenter, triple-blind study with exenatide. In this trial, subcutaneous exenatide was administered 2 or 3 times/day at a dose of 0.08 mcg/kg. Results from this study demonstrated a dose-dependent decrease in plasma glucose levels, improved insulin production, and decreased glucagon secretion. In addition, significantly lowered postprandial hypoglycemia was seen throughout the treatment. At day 28, 90% of exenatide-treated patients showed a reduction of at least 0.5% in their HbA_{1c} levels as compared with 33% of the placebo-treated patients. Postprandial plasma glucagon concentrations and rate of gastric emptying were reduced in a dose-dependent manner. Moreover, studies also showed that postprandial plasma glucose concentrations were substantially lowered following a *Sustacal* meal challenge while subcutaneous doses below 0.1 mcg/kg were well tolerated. Results from the first of the 3 phase 3 trials, reported in August 2003, confirmed that in a 7-month study of 336 randomized patients, exenatide produced significant, dose-dependent reductions in the primary glucose control endpoint and significant reduction in body weight. No difference was observed in rates of mild to moderate hypoglycemia between placebo and exenatide. The average HbA_{1c} entry was 8.2%. However, at the end of the study, 46% of the subjects receiving the highest exenatide dose (10 mcg twice daily) reduced their average HbA_{1c} level to the recommended target range of less than or equal to 7% (average of 7.3%).

➤Adverse Reactions: The most commonly reported side effect was a dose-dependent transient nausea. It tended to occur mostly upon initiation of therapy and usually subsided over the first week. One study showed a 34% reduction in nausea when target dose was achieved through gradual dose titration. Other side effects included a small and acute transient rise in serum cortisol concentration on the first day of treatment and mild, transient hypoglycemia when used in combination with sulfonylureas.

➤Summary: Exenatide is the first member of a new class of therapeutic medications known as incretin mimetic agents. It is a potent peptide that exerts several antidiabetic actions and is being investigated for the treatment of type 2 diabetic patients who are not able to achieve target glucose levels with either diet and/or oral medication. Exenatide is currently in phase 3 clinical studies. An NDA is expected to be filed in 2004.

~ Bibliography Available on Request ~

EXISULIND (*Aptosyn* by Cell Pathways) – A Selective Apoptotic Antineoplastic Drug

➤*Actions:*

Pharmacology – Exisulind (sulindac sulphone) was being evaluated by the FDA for the treatment of familial adenomatous polyposis (FAP); the FDA notified Cell Pathways on September 22, 2000, that the drug was non-approvable. Exisulind also is being evaluated for use in a number of other conditions, including Gardner's syndrome; sporadic colonic adenomatous polyps; Barrett's esophagus; prostate, breast, and lung cancer; and other solid tumors.

Pharmacokinetics – Exisulind reaches peak serum concentration within 2 to 2.5 hours after oral administration. The absorption half-life is 0.7 hours. Its elimination half-life ranges from 4.88 to 6.81 hours. The total body clearance of exisulind is 8.2 to 10.1 L/hr and its apparent volume of distribution is 58.8 to 69.3 L.

Clinical trials –

FAP: A phase I study was conducted in patients with FAP. All of the patients had undergone a subtotal colectomy ≥ 3 years prior to the study. In addition, each patient had to have ≥ 5 rectal polyps at the time of study enrollment. No NSAIDs were allowed for ≥ 2 weeks prior to the study and throughout the course of the study. Patients were treated with 200, 300, or 400 mg oral exisulind twice daily for ≥ 4 months. Dose escalation was allowed after a minimum of 2 weeks if toxicities did not occur. If toxicity occurred, it was possible to lower the dose of exisulind. Effectiveness and safety analysis included a sigmoidoscopic evaluation. The number of polyps in each rectal segment was counted and biopsies were obtained from normal-appearing mucosa in each segment. Twenty patients were enrolled in the study, but only 18 were evaluable. The number of polyps at baseline and after 1 month of therapy was similar in all treatment groups. No increase in polyp count occurred with the 300 and 400 mg twice daily dosing regimen after 4 to 6 months. However, the number of polyps increased in those patients treated with 200 mg twice daily after 4 to 6 months (> 50%).

A placebo-controlled study (n = 34) of patients with FAP was designed to show a difference in polyp formation rates in patients who historically formed between 10 and 40 new polyps per year. Patients were treated with 600 mg/day exisulind. The exisulind therapy resulted in a 53% reduction in the number of polyps formed compared with placebo after 1 year. Patients were then enrolled in an open-label extension study. At 6-month intervals, the number of rectal polyps was determined and removed. After 6 months of therapy, the original placebo-treated patients had a median reduction in polyps of 50%. Those previously treated with exisulind had an additional 50% reduction in polyp formation, which represented a 75% reduction over the 18-month observation period.

Other uses: Exisulind has shown promising results in mammary carcinogenesis and hepatocellular carcinoma in rat models or in vitro cell lines. Further studies will be necessary to determine if exisulind will be valuable in the treatment of mammary cancer.

A small phase I study (n = 18) was conducted to assess the safety and pharmacokinetics of exisulind in patients with FAP plus colonic adenomas. Three cohorts of 6 patients were treated with either 200, 300, or 400 mg exisulind twice daily for 6 months. Three of the patients in the 400 mg twice daily group had to have the medication discontinued or the dose reduced because of grade 2 or 3 hepatic toxicity and a fourth patient develped grade 1 hepatotoxicity. The number of polyps increased in the patients treated with 200 mg twice daily. The number of polyps in the 300 mg and 400/200 mg (patients started on 400 mg then reduced to 200 mg) groups remained stable with a regression in some polyps.

➤*Adverse Reactions:* The most common GI adverse reactions included nausea, vomiting, diarrhea, changes in the frequency or consistency of bowel movements, abdominal pain, and dyspepsia, and were found to be dose related. A dose-limiting hepatic toxicity occurred with the 400 mg twice daily regimen.

➤*Summary:* The adult dose is 150 mg 4 times/day. Less frequent administration does not produce the same benefits on polyp formation. The ability to decrease the number and size of polyps and cause regression in the colorectal adenomas with exisulind is encouraging, but it is still too early to determine if exisulind can replace, delay the need for, or limit the anatomical extent of proctocolectomy and prevent carcinoma development. Until these data are available for review, exisulind (if approved) could only be considered an adjunct to surgical management of the disease.

FENOTEROL HBr (*Berotec* by Boehringer Ingelheim) – A β_2 agonist

➤*Actions:*

Pharmacology – Fenoterol HBr is a β_2-adrenergic agonist undergoing investigation in the US as a bronchodilating agent. It has been available outside the US since the early 1970s as a metered dose inhaler (MDI), a solution for nebulization, a powder for inhalation, and an oral dosage form.

Stimulation of β_2-adrenoreceptors activates adenyl cyclase, which converts adenosine triphosphate into cAMP. Increased levels of cAMP inhibit mediator release and produce bronchodilation. Although controversial, an increase in mucociliary transport also may occur. In addition, β_2 stimulation causes vasodilation of peripheral blood vessels. This effect can result in a baroreceptor-mediated reflex-positive chronotropic response (increase in heart rate) and stimulation of skeletal muscle, leading to tremor. Fenoterol has greater β_2 selectivity than metaproterenol, but it is approximately equal in selectivity to albuterol and terbutaline. Bronchoselectivity is enhanced by administering fenoterol by inhalation; this allows for use of a lower dose to achieve a therapeutic effect and reduce dose-related side effects.

Usual therapeutic doses (200 to 400 mcg) of inhaled fenoterol do not significantly affect the cardiovascular system; however, marked cardiovascular effects have been observed after oral, SC, IM, or IV administration. Fenoterol prevents immediate antigen-induced bronchospasm but does not prevent delayed allergic reactions. A transient reduction in serum potassium levels (representing the uptake of potassium into the intracellular space) and an increase in serum glucose levels have been observed, but the clinical significance remains unclear.

Pharmacokinetics – Approximately 60% of an oral dose is absorbed, with peak plasma levels reached in 2 hours. After inhalation, fenoterol appears to undergo a 2-stage absorption process; the first stage is independent of dose, while the second is similar to that seen after oral administration. This is consistent with the observation that, when a drug is administered by inhalation, as much as 90% of the dose is swallowed. Fenoterol undergoes extensive first-pass metabolism. The half-life of total radioactive-labeled drug is 7 hours; however, this does not represent a true half-life for the parent compound. Although maximum effect of inhaled fenoterol is not achieved for 1 to 2 hours, 60% of the maximal response is seen within the first few minutes. The duration of action is ≈ 4 to 6 hours. However, because the lower therapeutic dose produces near maximal bronchodilatation, increasing the dose to near maximal effective concentrations will increase the duration of action without affecting the intensity of the peak response. After oral administration, < 2% of the dose is eliminated unchanged in the urine; the balance is excreted as acid conjugates in the urine and feces (40%).

Clinical trials – Clinical trials have established the efficacy of fenoterol for maintenance therapy in patients with moderate to severe asthma, therapy of chronic obstructive pulmonary disease (COPD), protection against exercise-induced asthma, and treatment of acute asthma attacks. It is difficult to evaluate many of the studies because they are single-dose studies, or because they do not compare equipotent doses when evaluated against albuterol and terbutaline. However, at equipotent doses (1 puff fenoterol [200 mcg/puff] = 2 puffs albuterol [100 mcg/puff] = 2 puffs terbutaline [250 mcg/puff]), there appears to be no clinically significant difference in duration of action, bronchoselectivity, or therapeutic efficacy among the 3 agents. The dose of fenoterol used to treat an acute asthma attack is 200 mcg (1 puff) repeated once in 5 minutes for children, and 1 to 3 puffs for adults. Maintenance therapy is 1 to 2 puffs 2 to 4 times/day for adults; give 1 puff twice daily to children. Increasing an inhaled dose of fenoterol to > 600 mcg (3 puffs) does not appear to increase the therapeutic response but may increase the incidence of side effects. In one study, an 800 mcg dose increased the heart rate 10% with a slow return to baseline over 2 hours. Although inhaled bronchodilators have many advantages, as many as 10% of the patients may not receive maximal therapeutic benefit due to improper MDI use.

➤*Adverse Reactions:* After inhalation of therapeutic doses of fenoterol, side effects are rare. After oral therapy, skeletal muscle tremor, tachycardia, palpitations and nervousness occur occasionally. Fenoterol is not recommended for use in patients with hyperthyroidism. Use with caution in patients with cardiovascular disease, diabetes mellitus, and hepatic or renal dysfunction.

➤*Summary:* Fenoterol by inhalation appears to be a safe and effective treatment for prophylaxis of exercise-induced bronchospasm, acute attacks of mild to moderate asthma, and maintenance therapy for chronic asthma or COPD. However, no apparent advantage of fenoterol over equipotent doses of the currently available β_2-selective agonists, albuterol or terbutaline, has yet been demonstrated. Further information on this product can be received from Boehringer Ingelheim Canada.

FENRETINIDE (by McNeil Pharmaceuticals) – A synthetic retinoid

➤*Actions:*

Pharmacology – Fenretinide (N-4-hydroxyphenylretinamide) is a synthetic retinoid currently under evaluation for use in prevention of breast, bladder, oral, and skin cancer. It does not act like other retinoids, because its activity does not correlate with cellular retinoic acid-binding proteins. However, it is believed that fenretinide is metabolized to an agent that competes for cellular retinoic acid-binding protein binding sites.

Pharmacokinetics – Peak levels are achieved in 3 to 9 hours following oral administration. Bioavailability is significantly increased by administration after a meal (189%), particularly after a high-fat meal (200% to 300%). The elimination half-life is 17.4 to 27 hours. Fenretinide was present in very low amounts (at the limits of detectability) 50 days after discontinuation of treatment for 1 year with 200 mg/day. Levels were undetectable 6 days after the last dose following 1 month of treatment at that dose. After 5 years of continuous treatment, fenretinide concentrations were at the limits of detectability at 6 and 12 months after discontinuation, while levels of the metabolite were 5 times higher. Retinol concentrations returned to baseline after 1 month.

Clinical trials – The effects of fenretinide were evaluated in 149 women who received fenretinide for at least 4 years in a breast cancer chemoprevention trial. Evaluation was done by mammographies performed at baseline and then once a year. The results of mammographies after 4 years of fenretinide therapy reported no substantial changes in breast parenchymal patterns, except in 1 patient who demonstrated improvement (P2 to P1 Wolfe's classification). Preliminary studies are evaluating the effects of combination tamoxifen (eg, *Nolvadex*) and fenretinide in patients with previously untreated metastatic breast cancer.

One trial involved patients with previously untreated homogenous or nonhomogenous oral leukoplakias that had a benign postoperative histology following laser resection. Patients were randomized to receive fenretinide 200 mg/day for a maximum of 52 weeks (with a 3-day drug holiday at the end of each month) or no treatment. Of 153 patients in this study (74 treated with fenretinide and 79 in the control group), 19 patients had recurrences (9 in the control group and 10 in the fenretinide group), and 15 had new localizations (12 in the control group and 3 in the fenretinide group). The overall risk of recurrence and new localization was 6% in the fenretinide group and 30% in the control group.

Another report described the treatment of oral lichen planus (2 patients) and leukoplakias (6 patients) with topical fenretinide. Eight patients applied fenretinide twice daily by opening a 100 mg capsule and applying its contents to the affected sites after brushing teeth. Responses were apparent in all patients within 15 days. After 1 month of therapy, 2 patients had complete response and the other 6 had a > 75% response. No side effects were observed.

Results of a small study evaluating fenretinide effects on the outcomes of previously-resected superficial bladder cancer have been reported. Twelve patients were treated with fenretinide 200 mg/day and were compared with 17 non-randomized, untreated controls. The proportion of patients with DNA aneuploid stemlines in bladder washed cells decreased from 7 of 12 (58%) to 5 of 11 (45%) in the fenretinide group, but increased from 7 of 17 (41%) to 10 of 17 (59%) in the control group. Positive or suspicious cytologic examinations were present in 3 of 12 fenretinide-treated patients prior to therapy, but all reverted to normal. Positive or suspicious cytologic examinations increased from 4 of 17 to 6 of 17 during the study in the control group. These data suggest fenretinide may affect DNA content and abnormal cytology in patients with previously-resected superficial bladder cancer. Additional studies are necessary to further evaluate the effects of fenretinide in bladder cancer, including patients with previous bladder papillomas or transitional cell carcinoma.

It also has been suggested that fenretinide be evaluated as chemoprevention in patients with cervical dysplasia or previous basal cell or squamous cell actinic keratoses.

➤*Summary:* Insufficient information on the effects of fenretinide in cancer chemoprevention are available at this time. Fenretinide does appear to be better tolerated than currently-available retinoids under evaluation for cancer chemoprevention. Fenretinide is currently in phase III trials by McNeil.

FLUPIRTINE MALEATE

FLUPIRTINE MALEATE – A nonnarcotic analgesic

➤*Actions:*

Pharmacology – Flupirtine maleate, a triaminopyridine derivative, is a nonnarcotic analgesic structurally unrelated to other analgesic agents. Although its exact mechanism of action is not known, flupirtine lacks affinity for any type of opiate receptor and therefore, has a mechanism that differs from the opiates. Flupirtine also appears to lack some of the side effects of the opiates including constipation, respiratory depression, withdrawal phenomena, development of tolerance, and abuse potential. It is suggested that flupirtine is a medium to strong analgesic; its duration of action is comparable with codeine, and it is up to 3 times as potent as codeine and propoxyphene (eg, *Darvon*), up to twice as potent as meperidine (eg, *Demerol*), and approximately 10 times as potent as acetaminophen (eg, *Tylenol*).

Pharmacokinetics – The pharmacokinetics of flupirtine have not been well defined. The drug appears to have linear kinetics. A dosage of 100 mg 3 times/day achieves average steady-state blood levels equivalent to the peak for a single 200 mg dose. In one study of 55 patients, the analgesic effect occurred within 45 minutes to 2 hours; the duration of action was 4 to 6 hours. The half-life of flupirtine appears to be 7 to 10 hours.

In 13 elderly patients receiving 100 mg flupirtine 3 times/day for 12 days, the mean elimination half-life was higher than in healthy young subjects (mean, 18.6 hours on day 12 vs 6.5 hours). This was associated with an increased maximum serum concentration and reduced clearance in the elderly subjects.

In 12 patients with renal impairment, the half-life of flupirtine was higher compared with healthy subjects (mean, 9.8 hours vs 6.5 hours) following a single oral 100 mg dose.

Flupirtine peak levels and area under the curve may be higher in patients with primary biliary cirrhosis. In a study of ten patients, flupirtine did not induce hepatic microsomal enzymes.

Clinical trials – Flupirtine is effective in the treatment of pain resulting from various procedures or conditions including episiotomy, cancer, and postoperative and dental pain. Dosages used have ranged from 100 to 600 mg/day; the most common dosages were 100 mg once daily or 100 mg 3 times/day. Capsules were used in most studies although the suppository form also was used. Analgesic efficacy of flupirtine was judged to be as effective as other analgesics used in the studies including acetaminophen, codeine, pentazocine (*Talwin NX*), oxycodone plus acetaminophen (eg, *Percocet*), naproxen (eg, *Naprosyn*), and diclofenac (*Voltaren*). Flupirtine appears to have no tolerance or addiction potential. In one study, the average number of capsules taken per month remained constant for 12 months, as did the analgesic effect.

Flupirtine significantly reduced seizure frequency in 8 of 9 patients with minimal side effects; however, because other derivatives of the drug may have greater activity, no further studies in the treatment of epilepsy are planned at this time.

➤*Adverse Reactions:* Flupirtine does not appear to share the common side effects of the opiates such as respiratory depression and constipation. The drug is generally well tolerated. In a study of 55 patients, the most common adverse effects were dizziness (11%), drowsiness (9% to 10%), pruritus (9%), and dry mouth (5%). Other side effects that occurred included: Pain in forehead; sensation of excessive fullness in stomach; muscular tremor; nausea; other GI disturbances (eg, vomiting, abdominal discomfort).

➤*Summary:* Flupirtine is a nonnarcotic analgesic that compares favorably in efficacy with other available analgesics. However, at this time, it offers no clear advantage over the nonsteroidal anti-inflammatory agents except perhaps in the GI and CNS side effect profile. It does offer an advantage over the opiates in side effect profile, abuse potential, withdrawal phenomena, and development of tolerance. The average dose appears to be 100 mg 1 to 3 times/day. It has been used in capsule and suppository formulations.

An NDA was filed for flupirtine by Carter-Wallace in April 1986. At one time, a 1989 approval was anticipated; however, there has been no recent projected approval date and Carter-Wallace is no longer interested in pursuing this product.

~ Bibliography Available on Request ~

INSULIN DETEMIR (by Novo Nordisk) – A long-acting insulin

➤*Actions:*

Pharmacology – Insulin detemir has been submitted to the FDA for approval as a treatment for patients with Type 1 diabetes mellitus or Type 2 diabetes mellitus who require basal (long-acting) insulin to control their hyperglycemia. Insulin detemir (Lys^{B29}-tetradecanoyl, des-(B30) human insulin; NN304) is a neutral, soluble insulin preparation in which the B29 lysine residue has been covalently bound to a 14-carbon fatty acid. The fatty acid extension facilitates the compounds ability to reservedly bind to albumin in the plasma, thereby prolonging the activity of insulin detemir by delaying its appearance in the interstitial fluid and delaying its action at insulin sensitive tissues.

The time-action profile of insulin detemir 0.15, 0.3, and 0.6 units/kg administered SC have been compared with that of NPH insulin 0.3 units/kg administered SC in 11 healthy volunteers. Peak insulin detemir concentrations were reached after 4 to 6 hours. A pronounced peak in metabolic effect was not observed with insulin detemir, in contrast with NPH insulin. Insulin detemir also demonstrated a slower onset of action. In a similar study, insulin detemir 0.3 and 0.6 units/kg also have been compared with NPH insulin 0.3 and 0.6 units/kg and placebo in 10 healthy volunteers. NPH insulin was more active at these doses than the equal doses of insulin detemir. As in the other study, insulin detemir was associated with a flatter activity profile. A similar crossover study has also been conducted comparing single doses of insulin detemir (0.1, 0.2, 0.4, 0.8, and 1.6 units/kg) and NPH insulin (0.3 units/kg) administered SC in 12 patients with Type 1 diabetes. While NPH insulin demonstrated peak activity around 6 to 8 hours, a flatter glucose infusion rate profile was observed for insulin detemir. The duration of action for the 0.4 unit/kg insulin detemir dose was 20 hours. In another study enrolling 6 patients with Type 1 diabetes, the peak action of insulin detemir was observed at 600 to 660 minutes after SC injection.

Pharmacokinetics – Insulin detemir is rapidly absorbed following SC administration, but slowly transported to the peripheral tissue. Insulin detemir is more than 98% bound to albumin in the plasma and more than 96% bound in the interstitial fluid. Only the free insulin detemir is available to cross the endothelial barrier. Peak plasma concentrations occur within 3 to 6 hours then decline to baseline within 24 hours. Maximal metabolic effect occurs within 6 to 11 hours after injection. The half-life of insulin detemir is 4 to 6 hours.

Clinical trials – Insulin detemir and NPH insulin were compared with a 6-month open-label study enrolling 747 patients with Type 1 diabetes. Patients were randomized 2:1 to therapy with insulin detemir or NPH insulin as basal insulin in conjunction with regular human insulin as bolus insulin. At baseline the mean age was 40.5 years, mean duration of diabetes was 16.9 years, mean body mass index was 25.2 kg/m², and mean HbA_{1C} was 8.35%. After 6 months glycemic control was similar (mean difference in HbA_{1C} [insulin detemir - NPH] was − 0.12% [95% CI − 0.25, 0.02]). Fasting plasma glucose levels were lower in patients treated with insulin detemir (− 1.16 mmol/L, P = 0.001). The overall risk of hypoglycemia was similar in the 2 groups, although nocturnal hypoglycemia risk was 26% lower in patients receiving insulin detemir (P = 0.003). Patients lost a mean 0.2 kg in the insulin detemir group, but gained a mean of 0.4 kg in the NPH group after 6 months of therapy (baseline adjusted mean difference 0.5 kg, P = 0.003).

➤*Adverse Reactions:* Hypoglycemia is the most common adverse effect associated with insulin detemir therapy. SC injections of insulin detemir were well-tolerated.

➤*Summary:* Insulin detemir is a long-acting insulin formulation that will provide an alternative to NPH insulin and insulin glargine. Compared with NPH insulin, insulin detemir has a flat activity profile and does not produce peak insulin concentrations like that observed with NPH insulin. Comparisons with insulin glargine are not available. However, it appears that insulin detemir produces a similar type of flat activity profile as insulin glargine. Administer insulin detemir once or twice daily as a SC injection; however, insulin detemir is intended for once-daily SC administration at bedtime in most patients. The optimal dose and conversion factor for conversion from other long-acting insulin formulations have not been established. A New Drug Application was filed in December 2002 and an approvable letter was issued by the FDA in October 2003.

LACIDIPINE (*Lacipil* by GlaxoSmithKline) – A dihydropyridine calcium antagonist

➤*Actions:*

Pharmacology – Lacidipine, a 1,4 dihydropyridine calcium channel blocker, is a selective vasodilator that exerts little effect on myocardial contractility. The dose required to impair cardiac function is approximately 50 times greater than that needed for significant blood pressure reduction. Electrocardiographic studies indicate that it has no effect on SA node function or AV node conduction. Lacidipine effectively reduces blood pressure and decreases systemic vascular resistance by dilating peripheral and coronary arteries. This may lead to reflex tachycardia during the early stages of therapy. In addition to its cardiovascular effects, lacidipine has been shown in animal studies to have mild diuretic and natriuretic effects. In vitro studies also have demonstrated antioxidant activity and a possible tissue protective effect. As with other calcium channel blockers, there is some evidence to suggest activity toward inhibiting atherosclerosis. Lacidipine has been shown via a rat model to decrease infarct size following cerebral artery occlusion. The drug does not appear to affect carbohydrate or lipid metabolism.

Pharmacokinetics – Lacidipine is rapidly absorbed after oral administration and undergoes extensive first-pass metabolism. Virtually no parent drug is excreted in the urine or feces. Of the 2 primary metabolites, neither possesses pharmacologic activity. Due to the first-pass effect, the absolute bioavailability of lacidipine is < 20. Its high lipophilicity results in a prolonged pharmacologic effect, thus facilitating a single daily dose regimen. The elimination half-life ranges from 2 to 10 hours after a single dose, but increases to 12 to 15 hours at steady state. Plasma protein binding exceeds 90%. Volume of distribution after a single dose is ≈ 1 to 2 L/kg.

Metabolism of lacidipine is decreased in elderly patients and in those with liver impairment. The elimination of the drug appears to be unaffected by renal function.

Clinical trials – Dose titration studies involving over 400 patients with mild to moderate hypertension demonstrate a minimum response rate of 77%, as defined by the achievement of a diastolic blood pressure (DBP) ≤ 90 mmHg or a reduction in DBP of ≥ 15 mmHg. Doses of lacidipine ranged from 2 to 8 mg, administered once daily. One study treated 96 hypertensive patients with lacidipine, starting at a dose of 4 mg for 1 month. If DBP was not controlled after 1 month, the dose was increased to 8 mg. If DBP was not controlled after the second month, a beta blocker was added to the regimen. At 2 months, mean values for DBP and systolic blood pressure (SBP) dropped significantly. After 5 months, 87% of the patients were controlled: 63% on 4 mg, 21% on 8 mg, and 3% with combination therapy.

Studies have compared lacidipine 2 to 6 mg/day to hydrochlorothiazide (eg, *Esidrix*) 25 to 50 mg/day, atenolol (eg, *Tenormin*) 50 to 100 mg/day, sustained-release nifedipine (eg, *Procardia XL*) 20 to 40 mg twice daily and enalapril (*Vasotec*) 10 to 20 mg/day. In all cases, the differences in mean decrease for both SBP and DBP were not significantly different. In studies comparing lacidipine 4 mg/day to other long-acting dihydropyridine calcium antagonists, lacidipine showed greater antihypertensive effect than amlodipine (*Norvasc*) 10 mg/day and similar efficacy to that of isradipine 5 mg/day; further study is needed to clarify this issue.

➤*Adverse Reactions:* Adverse effects for lacidipine correspond to those expected for the dihydropyridine calcium antagonists, mostly due to the vasodilatory properties of these drugs: Headache (15%); flushing (10%); edema (8%); dizziness (6%); palpitations (5%); fatigue (4%); gastric irritation (3%). Generally, the side effects are mild and diminish over time. In most cases, they appear to be dose-related. Less common effects include paresthesia, impotence, and changes in liver function tests. The tolerability of lacidipine compares favorably to nifedipine; further study is needed to compare lacidipine with newer long-acting drugs in the class (eg, amlodipine).

➤*Summary:* Lacidipine appears to be a safe, effective agent for first-line treatment of mild to moderate hypertension. The recommended starting dose is 2 to 4 mg, titrated as needed up to 8 mg/day. Elderly patients and those with liver impairment should be started at 2 mg/day. Future clinical trials may elucidate additional beneficial effects of lacidipine and perhaps define new therapeutic roles for the drug.

Lacidipine is marketed as an antihypertensive drug in Europe by GlaxoSmithKline and other companies. It can be found under a variety of trade names, including *Lacipil*, *Viapres*, *Lacirex*, and *Motens*.

~ *Bibliography Available on Request* ~

LEVOSIMENDAN (*Simdax* by Orion Pharma) – A Calcium Sensitizer

➤*Actions:*

Pharmacology – Levosimendan is a calcium sensitizer developed for the treatment of decompensated heart failure. It sensitizes troponin C to calcium and is dependent on calcium concentration. It increases the effects of calcium on cardiac myofilaments during systole when calcium concentration is increased. Normal diastolic relaxation occurs because of decreasing calcium concentration and sensitization. Levosimendan also opens ATP-sensitive potassium channels on vascular smooth muscle, causing coronary and systemic vasodilation. These dual mechanisms result in an increase in cardiac output without an increase in myocardial oxygen demand.

Pharmacokinetics – Levosimendan is well absorbed with a bioavailability of 85%; however, an oral formulation is not available. Approximately 97% of levosimendan is protein bound, mostly to albumin. The elimination half-life of levosimendan is 1 hour. Elimination is mainly by conjugation and excretion takes place in the urine and feces. A linear relationship is seen between the dose administered and the plasma concentration of levosimendan.

An active metabolite, OR-1896, is formed by acetylation and accounts for approximately 5% of the total plasma concentration of levosimendan. Peak concentration of OR-1896 is achieved 1 to 2 days after cessation of a 24-hour infusion of levosimendan. OR-1896 has a half-life of approximately 80 hours, and its pharmacologic effects may last for approximately 1 week. The duration of effect of levosimendan may be increased in rapid acetylators because of an increase in the formation of OR-1896. Levosimendan is not metabolized by cytochrome-P isoenzymes.

Renal dysfunction has little effect on levosimendan concentration but does prolong the half-life of OR-1896. The elimination half-life of levosimendan is slightly prolonged by liver cirrhosis; however, the effects on the production or metabolism of OR-1896 are unknown.

Clinical trials – A randomized, double-blind, dose-ranging study comparing levosimendan with placebo enrolled 504 patients with decompensated heart failure complicating acute myocardial infarction. The patients were randomized to receive either placebo or 1 of 4 dose regimens of levosimendan: 6 mcg/kg loading dose plus 0.1 mcg/kg/min continuous infusion; 12 mcg/kg loading dose plus 0.2 mcg/kg/min continuous infusion; 24 mcg/kg loading dose plus 0.2 mcg/kg/min continuous infusion; 24 mcg/kg loading dose plus 0.4 mcg/kg/min continuous infusion. The combined risk of death and worsening heart failure was lower for the 6-hour infusion compared with placebo (2% vs 5.9%, respectively; $P = 0.033$) and for 24 hours after the start of the infusion (4% vs 8.8%, respectively; $P = 0.044$). Sinus tachycardia was most common in the highest levosimendan dose group (5%). Myocardial rupture occurred more frequently with placebo than with levosimendan (3.9% vs 0.25%, respectively; $P = 0.027$).

A randomized, double-blind, double-dummy, parallel-group clinical trial comparing levosimendan with dobutamine enrolled 203 patients with low-output heart failure that required treatment with an IV inotropic agent. Patients were treated with either a loading dose of 24 mcg/kg levosimendan over 10 minutes followed by a continuous infusion of 0.1 mcg/kg/min levosimendan, or a continuous infusion of 5 mcg/kg/min dobutamine without a loading dose. At 24 hours, hemodynamic performance had improved in 28% of the levosimendan patients vs 15% of the dobutamine patients ($P = 0.022$). In the levosimendan group, 8% of the patients died within 31 days compared with 17% of the dobutamine group ($P = 0.049$). The most common adverse events seen with levosimendan use were headache or migraine (14%) and hypotension (9%). Rate and rhythm disorders and angina pectoris, chest pain, or myocardial ischemia occurred more frequently in the dobutamine group.

➤*Adverse Reactions:* The most common adverse reactions reported in clinical trials were headache, hypotension, and dizziness related to vasodilatory effects of levosimendan. Levosimendan was associated with tachycardia and ventricular extrasystoles in studies vs placebo. When compared with dobutamine, levosimendan was associated with increased incidence of headache and hypotension.

➤*Summary:* Studies conducted to date suggest that levosimendan is a unique positive inotropic agent for use in decompensated heart failure. Based on clinical data, levosimendan is more efficacious than dobutamine and appears to be associated with fewer adverse events. Levosimendan has been approved in several European countries. It is currently in phase 3 trials in the United States.

LOFEXIDINE HCl (by Britannia Pharmaceuticals Limited) – An α_2 adrenergic agonist for the treatment of opioid withdrawal symptoms

➤*Actions:*

Pharmacology – Lofexidine is a centrally acting α_2 adrenergic agonist. It is structurally related to clonidine, which has been used in the treatment of opiate withdrawal syndrome. Adrenergic agonists effectively suppress withdrawal symptoms, which may originate from adrenergic hyperactivity in the locus caeruleus.

Pharmacokinetics – Lofexidine exhibits a biphasic decline in plasma concentration. First phase half-life ranges from 1.3 to 3.7 hours; second phase half-life ranges from 9 to 18.3 hours.

Clinical trials – One randomized, double-blind study examined clinical response to methadone or lofexidine in treating 86 polydrug-abusing opiate addicts experiencing withdrawal. In this study, 42 patients received 0.6 mg lofexidine initially, increasing by 0.4 mg/day for 3 days. After the titration, patients were maintained on 2 mg/day for 3 days, followed by downward titration of 0.4 mg/day for 3 days. Investigators concluded that lofexidine and methadone are clinically equivalent with regard to overall treatment retention, although patients receiving lofexidine experienced more withdrawal symptoms than those receiving methadone.

Another randomized, double-blind study compared lofexidine with clonidine in treating 80 heroin addicts undergoing opiate withdrawal. Forty patients received four 0.2 mg lofexidine capsules during the first day of treatment. The investigator adjusted subsequent dosing based on evaluation of withdrawal symptoms and blood pressure. The maximum daily dose was 1.6 mg lofexidine. The results indicated that lofexidine and clonidine are equally effective in managing opiate withdrawal syndrome, and that fewer patients receiving lofexidine therapy experienced significant hypotension than patients in the clonidine group. Lofexidine therapy was withheld on 10.1% of patient-days due to hypotension, compared with 20.9% of patient-days during clonidine therapy.

This product is available in the United Kingdom. The recommended initial dose is 0.2 mg twice daily and may be increased by 0.2 to 0.4 mg/day to 2.4 mg maximum daily dose. Recommended duration of therapy is 7 to 10 days.

➤*Drug Interactions:* CNS depression associated with alcohol, barbiturates, and other sedatives may be enhanced with lofexidine administration. Lofexidine efficacy may be reduced with coadministration of tricyclic antidepressants.

➤*Adverse Reactions:* In clinical trials, the most common side effects associated with lofexidine therapy included dry mouth, dizziness, bradycardia, sedation, hypotension, lethargy, and headache. The risk of hypotension increases with increasing doses. Rebound hypertension may occur with sudden withdrawal. Avoid use of this agent in patients with cerebrovascular disease, ischemic heart disease, bradycardia, renal impairment, or history of depression.

➤*Summary:* The relief of acute opiate withdrawal syndrome is only one goal in a complex strategy for successful opiate addiction treatment. Effective therapy also must address social and psychological issues.

Adrenergic agonists have been studied for opiate withdrawal treatment for > 20 years and provide a nonnarcotic alternative for this use. Among agents in this class, lofexidine appears to be safer for withdrawal syndrome. Several small trials have been published that examine the use of lofexidine for suppression of opiate withdrawal symptoms; however, additional larger studies are needed. Lofexidine currently is being evaluated in phase III trials for this indication.

MILNACIPRAN (*Ixel* by Cypress Bioscience) – A Serotonin Norepinephrine Reuptake Inhibitor

➤*Actions:*

Pharmacology – Milnacipran is a cyclopropane derivative currently being considered for use in fibromyalgia and depression. It inhibits norepinephrine and serotonin reuptake at presynaptic sites. The drug does not interact with postsynaptic receptors, including adrenergic and muscarinic receptors, leading to significantly improved patient tolerance.

Pharmacokinetics – Milnacipran is rapidly and extensively absorbed from the GI tract with an absolute bioavailability of greater than 85%. Maximum plasma concentrations were observed in nearly 2 hours after administration, with indistinguishable profiles between IV or orally administered drug. The drug is excreted via active tubular secretion and the elimination half-life is 8 hours. Milnacipran has a low affinity for plasma proteins, binding only 13%. The main product of metabolism is the glucuronic acid conjugate and is present in plasma concentrations similar to the parent drug. Other metabolites are considered clinically insignificant. Cytochrome P450 enzymes are not implicated in the metabolism of milnacipran. The drug is not influenced by either age or liver insufficiency. Since the drug and its main metabolite are excreted via active tubular secretion, adjust the dose of milnacipran in patients with renal impairment.

Clinical trials – Milnacipran has been shown to be an effective antidepressant in controlled trials. The efficacy of milnacipran has been compared with both standard tricyclic antidepressants (imipramine, amitriptyline, clomipramine) and selective serotonin reuptake inhibitors (SSRIs) (fluoxetine, fluvoxamine). Studies comparing tricyclics and milnacipran have shown comparable efficacy. However, in a 26-week, double-blind, randomized, parallel study of 107 patients comparing clomipramine with milnacipran, milnacipran was shown to be inferior with respect to the rate of responders. The mean change in the Hamilton Depression Rating Scale (HAMD) score between the baseline and the last rating ranged from 23.7 to 12 in the milnacipran-treated patients and from 23.1 to 8 in the clomipramine-treated patients. In a 6-week, randomized, double-blind comparison of milnacipran with imipramine in 109 patients, milnacipran and imipramine were shown to be of equivalent efficacy. The reduction in HAMD scores was not significantly different. The mean change in score for the milnacipran group was 17.3 and 15.7 for the imipramine group. The overall reporting of adverse events was lower with milnacipran, while there were significantly more withdrawals from the imipramine group because of adverse events.

In a 6-week, randomized, parallel-group study comparing milnacipran with fluvoxamine in 113 patients, milnacipran was shown to be of superior efficacy with a decreased incidence of adverse events. The overall HAMD scores decreased by a mean of 62.1% for the milnacipran group and by 49.3% in the fluvoxamine group ($P = 0.05$).

A 12-week, phase 2 study of milnacipran for the treatment of fibromyalgia pain was completed in 125 patients. Patients who received milnacipran experienced statistical improvement in pain scores compared with those who received placebo. Other symptoms that showed statistical improvement were fatigue, mood, physical function, and patient global scores.

➤*Adverse Reactions:* Milnacipran has been shown to have a superior adverse event profile over tricyclic antidepressants and are generally better tolerated than the SSRIs. The most common adverse reactions experienced are abdominal pain, anxiety, constipation, dose-related nausea, dry mouth, dysuria, somnolence, tremor, and vertigo.

➤*Summary:* Milnacipran is a serotonin norepinephrine reuptake inhibitor that has been shown to be safe and effective for the treatment of depression. While being comparable in efficacy to the tricyclic antidepressants and superior in efficacy to the SSRIs, milnacipran is much less likely to cause adverse events. Milnacipran is currently undergoing phase 3 trials for use in the treatment of fibromyalgia syndrome, while being studied in preclinical trials for use in the treatment of irritable bowel syndrome.

NITRENDIPINE (*Baypress* by Bayer) – A Type II calcium channel blocking agent

➤*Actions:*

Pharmacology – Nitrendipine is a 1,4-dihydropyridine derivative calcium entry blocker, structurally similar to nifedipine. It is further classified as a type II calcium antagonist because, at usual doses and concentrations, it is devoid of electrophysiologic effects but is a potent peripheral vasodilator. Relaxation of peripheral vascular smooth muscle occurs as a result of inhibition of calcium influx across cellular membranes.

Nitrendipine causes a decrease in systolic and diastolic blood pressure, primarily due to arteriolar dilation. Significant peripheral venodilation is unlikely, because postural hypotension is usually not seen. Reflex increases in heart rate, AV nodal conduction, and myocardial contractility occur frequently at therapeutic doses and may precipitate myocardial ischemia in patients with coronary artery disease. Plasma renin activity and catecholamine concentrations increase during therapy with nitrendipine; however, the fact that it reduces the pressor response to norepinephrine but affects no change in responses to angiotensin II may explain its greater effectiveness in the treatment of low-renin hypertension. Nitrendipine does not alter glomerular filtration rate (GFR), renal blood flow, or plasma aldosterone levels. A short-term, modest diuretic and natriuretic effect has been observed on initiation of therapy.

The dose/response relationship for this effect appears to be flat; a 10 mg dose produces maximum diuresis. It is unlikely that this has any therapeutic implications during long-term therapy. Preliminary data suggest that nitrendipine has no effect on blood glucose, total cholesterol, triglyceride, or uric acid levels.

Pharmacokinetics – Available pharmacokinetic data are based on experience with small numbers of patients using assays of varying sensitivity; data vary.

Nitrendipine appears to be well absorbed after oral administration. Peak serum concentrations are seen at 1 to 2 hours; peak effect is seen at approximately 4 hours. The distribution half-life ($t\frac{1}{2}$-α) is approximately 1 hour. Beta elimination half-life ($t\frac{1}{2}$-β) averages 8 to 11 hours. Nitrendipine is metabolized by the liver to an inactive pyridine analog and to several more polar metabolites that are excreted in the urine. Dosage adjustments appear to be necessary in patients with hepatic dysfunction, but specific guidelines are not established. A single-dose study in 16 patients with various degrees of renal dysfunction found no alterations in any kinetic parameters; dosage adjustments appear unnecessary in renal patients.

Clinical trials – Nitrendipine is effective in the treatment of mild to moderate hypertension (diastolic blood pressure 90 to 114 mmHg). Initial data suggest that the drug is particularly useful in low-renin hypertension, which accounts for 20% to 30% of the hypertensive population. Doses of 10 to 80 mg/day have been used, administered as a single dose or in 2 to 3 divided doses per day. Although a single daily dose will decrease blood pressure for 24 hours, most patients require twice-daily dosing for optimal blood pressure control. Due to reflex increases in heart rate and contractility, concomitant β-blocker therapy may be required in some patients. It has not been determined whether nitrendipine, like verapamil and nifedipine, tends to be more effective in older patients.

➤*Adverse Reactions:* Nitrendipine has a side effect profile similar to nifedipine. The side effect reported most frequently is headache. Fatigue, peripheral edema, flushing, palpitations, dizziness, polyuria, and mild elevations in liver function (in 2 patients) also have occurred.

➤*Summary:* Nitrendipine is a potent vasodilator that effectively reduces blood pressure when given 1 to 3 times/day. The drug appears most useful in low-renin hypertensives. Biochemical abnormalities common to other currently used antihypertensives (eg, hypokalemia, hyperglycemia, increased uric acid and lipids) are not seen with this class of drugs and may represent an advantage over β-blockers and diuretics. Although most patients will require twice-daily dosing, the only other available dihydropyridine (nifedipine) usually requires dosing 3 to 4 times/day.

A New Drug Application (NDA) is pending with the FDA for an antihypertensive indication. Nitrendipine will be comarketed by Miles and Roche; however, there are no plans to market nitrendipine at this time.

OMAPATRILAT (by Bristol-Myers Squibb) – A vasopeptidase inhibitor (VPI)

➤*Actions:*

Pharmacology – Omapatrilat is a vasopeptidase inhibitor (VPI) that simultaneously inhibits neural endopeptidase and angiotensin-converting enzyme. Oral administration of omapatrilat showed potent and long-lasting antihypertensive effects in low-, normal-, and high-renin animal models.

Omapatrilat has been shown to be a potent antihypertensive agent and to increase cardiac output, decrease left ventricular end-diastolic and peak systolic pressures, and decrease peripheral vascular resistance in patients with heart failure. The efficacy of omapatrilat suggests a utility in a broad range of patient types. The ability of vasopeptidase inhibition to lower arterial pressure, regardless of renin activation or sodium status, suggests a synergistic interplay between potentiation of the natriuretic peptide system (NPS) and inhibition of the renin-angiotensin-aldosterone system (RAAS).

Pharmacokinetics – Omapatrilat has an oral bioavailability of ≈ 30%, with a protein binding of 80%. It may be given with or without food, and it has a very large volume of distribution (1800 L), suggesting tissue penetration. The time to maximum concentration of an oral dose is ≈ 2 hours. Omapatrilat's effective half-life is 14 to 19 hours.

This drug is metabolized in the liver, forms disulphide bonds with endogenous thiols, and is extensively metabolized via amide hydrolysis, glucuronidation, S-oxidation, and S-methylation. There are no active metabolites of omapatrilat found in plasma. Approximately 80% of an IV dose and 64% of an oral dose were recovered in urine, with < 1% excreted as unchanged drug. Renal function does not appear to influence the disposition or excretion of omapatrilat and hemodialysis does not contribute to its clearance.

Biotransformation data based on in vivo and in vitro studies suggest that cytochrome P450 is not involved in the metabolism of omapatrilat. Several studies have shown that omapatrilat does not inhibit P450 isoenzymes CYP-1A2, CYP-3A4, CYP-2C19, CYP-2D6, and CYP-2C9. Omapatrilat has no known interaction with other medications.

Clinical trials – In a parallel, dose-finding, placebo-controlled trial, 174 patients with mild to moderate hypertension were divided into groups of ≈ 25 each and given daily doses of 1, 5, 12.5, 30, or 75 mg omapatrilat or placebo. The main efficacy end-point was the change from baseline in the average 24-hour ambulatory diastolic blood pressure on the last day of the double-blind treatment period. Omapatrilat produced dose-dependent decreases in the average 24-hour ambulatory blood pressure. Omapatrilat produced greater reductions in systolic blood pressure than diastolic pressure. Seven days after discontinuation of treatment, trough seated blood pressure was still decreased compared with baseline in all active drug groups. This may mean that rebound hypertension is unlikely with discontinuation or interruption of therapy. In patients ≥ 65 years of age, as well as in African-Americans, omapatrilat significantly reduced systolic and diastolic blood pressure. No changes in heart rate were associated with the antihypertensive effects of omapatrilat.

Another randomized, double-blind, multicenter trial of 369 patients with NYHA class II-IV heart failure evaluated the efficacy of omapatrilat 2.5, 5, 10, 20, or 40 mg/day for 12 weeks. Omapatrilat was administered once daily for 12 weeks; the first 190 patients received doses of 2.5, 5, or 10 mg, and the last 179 patients received doses of 2.5, 20, or 40 mg. Ejection fraction improved in a dose-dependent fashion and heart rate decreased with omapatrilat. Cardiac index remained unchanged while arterial pressure also decreased in a dose-related manner. The combined incidence of cointervention for heart failure, hospitalization, or death was 34% with 2.5 mg omapatrilat and 19% with 40 mg omapatrilat.

➤*Adverse Reactions:* Side effects were investigated in 1 clinical trial comparing omapatrilat with lisinopril in 573 patients with class II-IV CHF. More adverse events related to the GI tract (nausea, vomiting, constipation, and diarrhea), as well as neurological symptoms (eg, dizziness, vision disturbances, and hypotension) were noted with omapatrilat as compared with lisinopril.

In data submitted for the New Drug Application for omapatrilat, 44 instances of angioedema occurred among > 6000 patients, and 4 cases were severe enough to require intubation.

➤*Summary:* Omapatrilat represents a new class of pharmacologic agents that alter the balance of circulating and local humoral factors in favor of vasodilation. Omapatrilat offers the promise to be an important new advancement in the treatment of hypertension and heart failure. However, because of the instances of angioedema, additional studies are necessary to further define its place in therapy for efficacy and adverse effects. The FDA issued an approvable letter in 2002.

PHENFORMIN – Available under IND exemption

➤*Indications:* May be used only in patients with adult-onset, nonketotic diabetics who meet all of the following criteria: In addition to elevated blood glucose, have symptoms such as polydipsia; symptoms are not controlled with diet and sulfonylureas or patient cannot take sulfonylureas because of nontolerance or allergy; symptoms are controlled by phenformin; there are no underlying risk factors that contraindicate the use; (a) his/her occupation is such that the risk of hypoglycemia from insulin would threaten his/her job or be a hazard to him/her or others, or (b) patient cannot take insulin because of disability and has no practical way to receive assistance.

Phenformin also is available under a separate IND for a dermatological condition called atrophie blanche or livedo vasculitis.

➤*Contraindications:* Although there is no absolute way to predict the population at risk for lactic acidosis, the following are recognized contraindications: Insulin-dependent diabetes; hypersensitivity to phenformin; renal disease with even mild degrees of impaired renal function; liver disease; history of lactic acidosis; alcohol abuse; any acute medical situation such as cardiovascular collapse (shock), CHF, MI, surgery or septicemia; disease states that may be associated with hypoxemia; complications of diabetes such as metabolic acidosis, coma, infection or gangrene; acute GI disturbances (vomiting or diarrhea), which are likely to result in dehydration and prerenal azotemia.

➤*Adverse Reactions:* Lactic acidosis in patients taking phenformin has been estimated to occur in 0.25 to 4 cases per 1000 phenformin treatment years. Lactic acidosis is characterized by elevated lactate levels, increased lactate-to-pyruvate ratio and decreased blood pH. In many of the reported cases, azotemia ranging from mild to severe was present.

Nausea, vomiting, hyperventilation, malaise, or abdominal pain may herald the onset of lactic acidosis. Instruct the patient to discontinue phenformin and notify the physician immediately if any of these symptoms occur.

Warn patients against using alcohol while receiving phenformin, because ethanol and phenformin potentiate the tendency of each to cause elevated blood lactate levels.

➤*Summary:* The biguanide hypoglycemic agent, phenformin, was removed from the US market on October 23, 1977, as a result of concern over the unacceptably high risk of lactic acidosis associated with its use. Phenformin is now available only through an Investigational New Drug (IND) Application, which must be filed with the US Food and Drug Administration. Use of phenformin is restricted to specific clearly defined situations and requires registration and reporting to the FDA. Complete information on use of phenformin, physician sponsor applications, patient consent forms, and request forms for ordering phenformin tablets or capsules are available from:

Center for Drug Evaluation and Research
Division of Metabolism and Endocrine
Drug Products (HFD-510)
Room 14-B-19
5600 Fishers Lane
Rockville, Maryland 20857
301-443-3510

Although phenformin has been removed from the market because of the potential for adverse effects, a select group of patients may require use of this agent. Careful patient selection is necessary to assure a reasonable risk-benefit ratio. Supplies of phenformin are available to practicing physicians from the FDA under an IND exemption.

~ Bibliography Available on Request ~

PINACIDIL (*Pindac* by Lilly) – An antihypertensive agent

►*Actions:*

Pharmacology – Pinacidil is a vasodilator under investigation for use as an antihypertensive agent. Pinacidil acts at the level of the precapillary, arteriolar (resistance) vessels, causing direct relaxation of vascular smooth muscle. Its vasodilator effect is not altered by blockade of β-adrenergic, cholinergic, or histaminic receptors, or by the presence of prostaglandin inhibitors such as indomethacin.

When compared with other vasodilators with similar sites of action (eg, minoxidil [*Loniten*], guancydine, diazoxide [*Hyperstat*]), pinacidil, at comparable levels of blood pressure reduction, produces quantitatively identical increases in heart rate, reflex sympathetic mediated cardiac contractility, and cardiac output. However, when compared with hydralazine (another precapillary arteriolar vasodilator), pinacidil, at doses that produce equivalent reductions in total peripheral resistance, is a more potent blood pressure lowering agent. Because blood pressure is a function of the cardiac output multiplied by the total peripheral resistance, this difference may be explained by the fact that hydralazine appears to have a direct (as well as the indirect) cardiostimulatory effect that offsets some of the blood pressure reduction caused by vasodilation. As would be expected from their differing effects on cardiac output, pinacidil produces less of an increase in myocardial oxygen consumption than hydralazine.

Although an active metabolite has been identified, it does not appear to contribute significantly to the overall antihypertensive activity.

There is a linear correlation between pinacidil drug levels and the fall in mean blood pressure and total peripheral resistance; minimal therapeutic levels are 50 ng/mL.

Pharmacokinetics –

Absorption/Distribution: Available data are complicated by the fact that at least 2 different oral formulations have been used in clinical trials. However, in general, bioavailability approaches 100% after oral administration, with both peak serum levels and effect occurring at 1 hour. Coadministration of food does not alter bioavailability but slightly delays absorption. Approximately 60% of a dose is protein bound.

Metabolism/Excretion: Pinacidil is metabolized by the liver to a number of metabolites, the most significant being the active metabolite, pinacidil N-oxide. Within the first 24 hours, 55% to 60% of an administered dose appears in the urine as pinacidil or the N-oxide, 20% to 30% is excreted in the urine as other metabolites and 3% is recovered in the feces. The elimination half-life (t½) varies between 1.5 to 3 hours. Average clearance values are 42 ± 5 L/hr.

Although exact dosage guidelines have not been established, patients with liver disease should have therapy initiated slowly, at low doses, and with careful blood pressure monitoring. Eight patients with chronic, stable cirrhosis showed a 50% reduction in clearance, prolongation of the half-life and a decrease in the percentage of parent compound converted to the N-oxide metabolite.

Clinical trials – Only a limited number of clinical studies, each involving only a few patients, have been published. This may reflect that pinacidil is not considered to be a first- or second-line drug in the stepped-care approach.

Pinacidil use has generally been confined to patients with moderate to severe hypertension. It is safe and effective, especially when added to a regimen of a diuretic and β-blocker in patients who failed the initial combination regimen. Pinacidil has been particularly effective in selected patients with renal impairment (dialysis and non-dialysis patients) with drug-resistant, non-volume dependent hypertension.

Although most studies have used doses of 10 to 100 mg twice daily, some clinicians feel that the drug may require 3 times/day dosing. The most effective dose range appears to be 12.5 or 25 mg twice daily.

►*Adverse Reactions:* Pinacidil appears to be well tolerated. Only a few reports of mild side effects (eg, dizziness, headache, facial flushing) have been noted.

Edema has occurred in 23.5% to 45.2% of patients on doses of pinacidil alone of 25 to 50 mg. Concomitant diuretics may be required in most patients.

Two patients developed positive anti-nuclear antibody (ANA) titers while receiving pinacidil. Neither had clinical manifestations of a lupus-like syndrome, and a direct cause and effect relationship could not be linked to pinacidil; further studies are necessary to investigate the potential for pinacidil to cause a drug-induced lupus syndrome.

►*Summary:* Pinacidil appears to be a promising alternative agent for the treatment of moderate to severe hypertension. However, further studies are needed to clarify the drug's optimal dosing schedule, long-term side effects, and optimal drug combinations.

The FDA's Cardio-Renal Drugs Advisory Committee recommended approval of pinacidil on May 28, 1987, with the stipulation that it be used concomitantly with diuretics. The drug was approved by the FDA in December 1989; however, Lilly has no plans to market pinacidil at this time.

PIRENZEPINE HCl (*Gastrozepine* by Boehringer Ingelheim) – An antiulcer agent

►*Actions:*

Pharmacology – Pirenzepine is a tricyclic benzodiazepine antiulcer agent comparable to standard antiulcer agents such as cimetidine and ranitidine. However, its uniqueness and mechanism of action hinge on *selective* antimuscarinic activity for gastric acid secretory cells.

Pirenzepine selectively suppresses basal and stimulated acid and pepsin secretion with lesser effects on other muscarinic sites (eg, salivary secretion) compared with atropine and other classic anticholinergic agents. Controlled trials show that 50 mg, 2 to 3 times/day, inhibits acid secretion at least up to 4.5 hours after dosing. Higher doses inhibit esophageal and colonic motility and decrease lower esophageal sphincter pressure. Pirenzepine also may have cytoprotective effects; however, this is of questionable significance because it has little or no effect on gastric mucus and endogenous gastric prostaglandin production.

Pharmacokinetics – Pirenzepine is a hydrophilic molecule that has systemic bioavailability after oral dosing of 20% to 30%. Approximately 10% of the drug is protein bound. Little drug is found in the brain; brain to serum concentration is 1 to 10.

At least 80% is renally excreted unchanged. Most metabolites are of a desmethyl variety. The parent molecule has a half-life of about 10 hours.

These data indicate the potential for few CNS effects and the need to adjust dosage in patients with impaired renal function.

Clinical trials – Numerous short-term (1 to 6 weeks) studies have been conducted comparing pirenzepine with placebo and other antiulcer drugs in ulcer patients. In small doses (50 to 75 mg/day), duodenal ulcer healing percentages with pirenzepine are not superior to placebo. Doses of 100 to 150 mg/day produce healing in 70% to 90% of patients. Statistically significant symptomatic improvement (decreased antacid use and pain) occurs with both dosage levels.

Short-term double-blind studies comparing duodenal ulcer healing rates of pirenzepine (100 to 150 mg/day) and cimetidine (1 g/day) produced similar results (60% to 79% for pirenzepine and 53% to 85% for cimetidine). A single study comparing pirenzepine (100 mg/day) to cimetidine (1 g/day) and ranitidine (300 mg/day) found similar rates of ulcer healing. However, pirenzepine showed a slower effect on symptom disappearance.

Fewer studies have been conducted in patients with gastric ulcer. Double-blind studies comparing pirenzepine with placebo show a need to use adequate doses (100 to 150 mg/day). Pirenzepine and cimetidine have produced similar healing rates (50% vs 48%) in patients with gastric ulcer, but more studies are indicated.

Trials were performed comparing maintenance doses of pirenzepine (30 to 50 mg/day) to placebo and cimetidine (400 mg/day) in duodenal ulcer patients for 12 months. Results indicate statistically significant reductions in ulcer recurrences for active treatment groups vs placebo (24% recurrence in active treatment group vs 80 in placebo-treated patients). No difference was demonstrated in recurrence rates between pirenzepine and cimetidine patients.

Combined use of pirenzepine with ranitidine or cimetidine shows more effective inhibition of gastric acid secretion than with use of a single agent. Such combinations may be useful in peptic ulcer conditions resistant to single drug therapy and in the Zollinger-Ellison syndrome.

►*Adverse Reactions:* Pirenzepine is well tolerated with few reported adverse effects. Dry mouth is the most common effect, but nausea, vomiting, diarrhea, constipation, increased appetite, anorexia, tiredness, and difficulty of accommodation have all occurred. Daily doses of less than 150 mg seem to significantly reduce the incidence of at least some of these problems.

►*Summary:* In clinical studies, pirenzepine is equally effective as cimetidine in the treatment of peptic ulcer disease. Its low incidence of side effects and selective inhibition of muscarinic gastric acid secretion will make it a valuable addition to existing agents used to treat ulcers. Pirenzepine is currently available in some European countries; expected date of availability in the US is unknown. A New Drug Application is pending.

PRAMLINTIDE ACETATE (*Symlin* by Amylin Pharmaceuticals) – An amylin analog

➤*Actions:*

Pharmacology – Pramlintide is a stable, nonaggregating, synthetic analog of endogenous amylin. Amylin is a 37-amino acid peptide secreted from pancreatic beta cells with insulin in response to nutrient intake. Pramlintide differs from amylin by only 3 amino acids. In animal models, pramlintide delays gastric emptying associated with vagal stimulation, secondary to centrally mediated activity. In healthy subjects, gastric emptying half-time was increased from 112 minutes with placebo to 169 minutes with 30 mcg pramlintide and 177 minutes with 60 mcg pramlintide. At 120 minutes after meal ingestion, 47% of the meal was retained with placebo, compared with 72% retained with 30 mcg pramlintide. Small bowel and colonic transport are not affected.

Pharmacokinetics – Following IV doses of 30, 100, and 300 mcg as 2-minute boluses or 2-hour infusions, peak pramlintide concentrations and pramlintide AUC increased with increasing dose. Peak concentrations were higher following the bolus dose, but AUC, half-life, and clearance values were comparable. The distribution phase half-life is ≈ 3 to 12 minutes. The terminal elimination half-life is 20 to 47 minutes. Steady-state volume of distribution is 56 L. Clearance is ≈ 1 L/min.

Clinical trials –

Type I diabetes mellitus: Pramlintide was evaluated in a 1-year, double-blind, placebo-controlled study enrolling 479 patients with type I diabetes mellitus. In addition to their usual insulin therapy, patients were treated with SC pramlintide 60 mcg 3 times/day, pramlintide 60 mcg 4 times/day, or placebo. Mean baseline HbA_{1C} was 8.9%. The average change in HbA_{1C} from baseline compared with placebo was -0.4% in the pramlintide 3 times/day group and -0.3% in the pramlintide 4 times/day group ($P \leq 0.001$). The mean total daily insulin dose was reduced in the pramlintide group but increased in the placebo group ($P = 0.0002$). In 60 pramlintide-treated patients who maintained a stable total daily insulin dose over the course of the study, the change in HbA_{1C} from baseline compared with placebo was -0.7% for both pramlintide groups and was consistent over time ($P \leq 0.02$). Patients in the pramlintide groups lost weight, with mean reductions of 1.4 kg in the 3 times/day group and 1.7 kg in the 4 times/day group, compared with placebo ($P = 0.005$). Among ≈ 40% of patients at study entry with a body mass index > 27, the weight loss was even greater: -3.2 kg in the 3 times/day group and -2 kg in the 4 times/day group, compared with placebo ($P < 0.003$).

Type II diabetes mellitus: In a 1-year, double-blind, placebo-controlled study enrolling 498 patients, pramlintide also was demonstrated to improve glycemic control and increase weight loss. Patients were treated with insulin plus SC pramlintide 90 mcg twice daily, pramlintide 120 mcg twice daily, or placebo. Mean baseline HbA_{1C} was 9.1%. In the 120 mcg group, the average change in HbA_{1C} was -0.4% at 26 weeks and -0.6% at 52 weeks, compared with placebo ($P < 0.003$). In the 90 mcg group, the average change in HbA_{1C} was -0.3% at 26 and 52 weeks, compared with placebo ($P < 0.15$). The average change in HbA_{1C} from weeks 4 to 52 compared with placebo was -0.4% in the 120 mcg group ($P < 0.001$) and -0.3% in the 90 mcg group ($P = 0.033$). At 52 weeks, mean weight was decreased by 1.2 kg in the 120 mcg pramlintide group and decreased by 0.5 kg in the 90 mcg group, compared with a 0.7 kg weight gain in the placebo group.

➤*Drug Interactions:* No drug interactions have been reported, but use pramlintide with caution with other medications that can decrease or increase blood glucose levels.

➤*Adverse Reactions:* Adverse effects have included nausea, vomiting, dyspepsia, and anorexia. With continued administration, nausea and anorexia were reported to occur less frequently. Hypoglycemia has occurred with similar frequency in pramlintide- and placebo-treated patients.

➤*Summary:* Pramlintide has been administered as an SC injection in the anterior abdominal wall 15 minutes prior to meals 4 times/day. Less frequent dosing may be possible in some patients. Pramlintide may be useful in the treatment of some patients who require insulin therapy. Pramlintide is not a substitute for insulin, but is complementary to the action of the insulin. It appears to delay gastric emptying, resulting in reduced serum fructosamine and 24-hour plasma glucose concentrations. It also may improve glucose levels in patients with type II diabetes mellitus poorly controlled (HbA_{1C} levels > 8%) by diet or oral hypoglycemic medications. The new drug application for pramlintide was submitted to the FDA in December 2000. The FDA issued an approvable letter in 2003.

RAMOPLANIN

RAMOPLANIN (by Vicuron/Genome Therapeutics) – A glycolipodepsipeptide antibiotic

➤*Actions:*

Pharmacology – Ramoplanin is an oral, nonabsorbable glycolipodepsipeptide currently undergoing investigation in the United States for use as an antibiotic to prevent bloodstream infections caused by vancomycin-resistant enterococci (VRE) in patients who have GI colonization with VRE. Ramoplanin has a broad spectrum of activity and is bactericidal against many gram-positive aerobic and anaerobic bacteria, including vancomycin-resistant *Enterococcus faecium*, *Enterococcus faecalis*, and *Clostridium difficile*. It inhibits bacterial cell wall biosynthesis by interfering with peptidoglycan production. The N-acetylglucosaminyltransferase-catalyzed conversion of lipid intermediate I to lipid intermediate II, a step that occurs before the transglycosylation and transpeptidation reactions, is inhibited by ramoplanin. Ramoplanin's mechanism of action is distinct from that of glycopeptides – it does not complex with the D-Ala-D-Ala sequence of cell wall precursors.

Pharmacokinetics – Ramoplanin is not absorbed through the oral route and, therefore, is not absorbed into the bloodstream. Instead, ramoplanin remains in the GI tract where it exerts its bacteriocidal effects on VRE.

Clinical trials – The in vitro activity of ramoplanin was compared with that of teicoplanin, vancomycin (eg, *Vancocin*), linezolid (eg, *Zyvox*), and 5 other agents against 300 gram-positive and 54 gram-negative strains of intestinal anaerobes. Overall, ramoplanin had excellent activity against *C. difficile* and most gram-positive enteric anaerobes, including vancomycin-resistant strains but is largely inactive against gram-negative anaerobes.

In another trial, the in vitro activity of ramoplanin was compared with linezolid (*Zyvox*)-resistant and quinupristin/dalfopristin (*Synercid*)-resistant VRE. The MIC and killing curves of 7 linezolid-resistant and 2 quinupristin/dalfopristin-resistant VRE were evaluated against linezolid and quinupristin/dalfopristin susceptible VRE. Ramoplanin showed consistent in vitro activity (MIC of 0.125 to 0.25 mcg/mL) against VRE, including linezolid and quinupristin/dalfopristin-resistant isolates while time-kill curves demonstrated the bactericidal activity of ramoplanin against all 3 VRE in the study.

In vivo trials with ramoplanin that have been published to date are limited. In one randomized, double-blind, placebo-controlled study involving 68 patients, the safety and efficacy of oral ramoplanin was compared with placebo for the suppression of VRE in patients with asymptomatic GI colonization. Patients received either 100 mg ramoplanin, 400 mg ramoplanin, or placebo orally, twice daily for 7 days. The outcomes were accessed by comparing the proportion of people per group from whom VRE was not recovered in each active-drug treatment group with that in the placebo-treated group on days 7, 14, and 21 after treatment. By day 7, 90% of the patients treated with 400 mg ramoplanin had no detectable levels of VRE while all placebo-treated patients remained colonized. However, by day 21 (2 weeks after the end of therapy) only 29% of the patients treated with 400 mg ramoplanin remained free of detectable levels of VRE compared with 25% of placebo-treated patients.

A phase 2 study is underway to evaluate the safety and efficacy of ramoplanin for the treatment of *C. difficile*-associated diarrhea (CDAD). One in vivo study to date has evaluated the efficacy of ramoplanin against vancomycin (eg, *Vancocin*) and metronidazole (eg, *Flagyl*) for the prevention and treatment of CDAD in the hamster model. Hamsters were treated with a single SC injection of 100 mg/kg clindamycin (eg, *Cleocin*) and then received either 50 mg/kg ramoplanin or 50 mg/kg vancomycin once daily for 5 days. Another group of hamsters were treated with both clindamycin 100 mg/kg and *C. difficile* and then received either 25, 50, or 100 mg/kg ramoplanin, 25, 50, or 100 mg/kg vancomycin, or 100, 200, or 400 mg/kg metronidazole once daily for 5 days. Overall, treatment with ramoplanin showed higher survival rates than hamsters treated with vancomycin. Furthermore, high dose ramoplanin was superior to vancomycin at all doses in the clindamycin and *C. difficile*-induced colitis hamster model. Metronidazole showed no dose response and was the least effective agent.

➤*Adverse Reactions:* In the multiple dose study, ramoplanin was well tolerated and the occurrence of adverse events was similar across all treatment groups. Three patients developed diarrhea, 2 developed abdominal pain, 1 developed dyspepsia, 1 developed flatulence, and 1 developed nausea. Four deaths occurred during the 21-day study and an additional 8 patients died after completion of the study, but the investigators concluded the deaths to be directly related to the patients' underlying medical conditions and not to VRE infection nor to ramoplanin.

➤*Summary:* Ramoplanin has been given fast-track status from the FDA and appears to be a promising glycolipodepsipeptide antibiotic with a novel mechanism of action. Ramoplanin appears to be effective and well tolerated for the prevention of VRE bloodstream infections and is active against many gram-positive aerobic and anaerobic bacteria, including *C. difficile*. An NDA is not expected to be filed before spring/summer 2005.

~ Bibliography Available on Request ~

REBOXETINE MESYLATE (*Vestra* by Pharmacia) – An antidepressant

►*Actions:*

Pharmacology – Reboxetine is a selective norepinephrine reuptake inhibitor. It is chemically unrelated to the tricyclic or tetracyclic antidepressants, the monoamine oxidase inhibitors (MAOIs), or the selective serotonin reuptake inhibitors (SSRIs). It is an equimolar mixture of 2 enantiomers, but the (R,R)-enantiomer does not have any apparent pharmacologic effects. It has weak affinity for serotonin and dopamine and little affinity for muscarinic, histaminergic, or adrenergic receptors.

Pharmacokinetics – Peak plasma levels of reboxetine occur within 2 hours of oral administration. Administration of reboxetine with a high-fat meal results in a 2- to 3-hour delay in peak plasma concentrations, a small decrease in peak plasma concentrations (16.8%), and no change in the extent of absorption. The elimination half-life of reboxetine is 12 to 16 hours. The drug is extensively metabolized by the liver and excreted in the urine. Reboxetine is primarily metabolized by CYP 3A4 and not metabolized by cytochrome P450 2D6. It does not inhibit or induce the CYP 1A2, 2C9, 2C19, 2D6, 2E1, and 3A4 isoenzymes at therapeutic concentrations. Higher concentrations may inhibit CYP 3A4 and 2D6, but these concentrations are above those required for a therapeutic effect. The fraction excreted unchanged in the urine is 0.09. The pharmacokinetic values of reboxetine are similar in young, middle-aged, and elderly patients. However, patients ≥ 75 years of age may have an increased AUC and decreased plasma clearance. Decreased hepatic function can decrease the metabolic clearance of reboxetine, but it does not increase the systemic exposure to the drug. Patients with alcoholic liver disease have decreased clearance, increased half-life, and increased systemic exposure to the drug; therefore, a reduction in dose is warranted in patients with hepatic insufficiency. The clearance of reboxetine decreases with renal dysfunction, and the AUC is increased. Therefore, a dosage reduction may be necessary in patients with severe renal dysfunction.

►*Drug Interactions:* Reboxetine has no effects on cytochrome P450 enzymes 1A2, 2C, 2D6, or 3A4 in therapeutic concentrations. Other antidepressants with no effects on these enzymes are bupropion (*Wellbutrin*), mirtazapine (*Remeron*), and venlafaxine (*Effexor*). Citalopram (*Celexa*), fluoxetine (*Prozac*), fluvoxamine (*Luvox*), nefazodone (*Serzone*), paroxetine (*Paxil*), and sertraline (*Zoloft*) inhibit at least 1 of these isoenzymes to some extent. Reboxetine is metabolized by the CYP 3A4 isoenzyme, so inhibitors (eg, ketoconazole [*Nizoral*], erythromycin [*E-mycin*]) and inducers (eg, rifampin [*Rifadin*], phenytoin [*Dilantin*]) of this isoenzyme may affect the metabolism of reboxetine. An interaction between reboxetine and MAOIs may occur because it has been reported with other antidepressants. To avoid this potential interaction, do not use reboxetine in combination with an MAOI within 7 days of initiating or 14 days of discontinuing therapy with an MAOI.

►*Adverse Reactions:* Adverse effects reported with reboxetine therapy have included dry mouth, dizziness, headache, nausea, constipation, insomnia, somnolence, tremor, diaphoresis, urinary hesitancy or retention, agitation, anxiety, nervousness, tachycardia, and reduced blood pressure. Reboxetine has minimal effect on psychomotor and cognitive function compared with tricyclic antidepressants. Reboxetine plus ethanol does not adversely affect the cognitive function or psychomotor performance of the patient.

►*Summary:* Like all newer antidepressant medications, reboxetine is better tolerated than the older tricyclic antidepressants. Reboxetine will offer clinicians an alternative agent for those patients who fail to respond to an SSRI or who are unable to tolerate a tricyclic antidepressant. Reboxetine also may be more effective in improving social functioning for some patients. The usual starting dosage of reboxetine was 4 mg twice daily. If necessary, the dose can be increased after 3 weeks. The dosages of reboxetine used in the clinical trials ranged from 4 to 12 mg/day. The drug is generally given in equally divided doses twice daily. The dosage used in elderly patients was 4 to 6 mg/day. The maximum recommended dosage in the US will be 10 mg/day. The starting dosage in patients with hepatic or renal dysfunction should be 2 mg twice daily; the maximum recommended dosage in these patients will be 6 mg/day. The safety and efficacy of reboxetine in children have not been established. Reboxetine is an effective antidepressant with efficacy and tolerability comparable with the other antidepressants.

REMOXIPRIDE (*Roxiam* by Astra/Merck) – An antipsychotic agent

►*Actions:*

Pharmacology – Remoxipride, a substituted benzamide, is an atypical antipsychotic agent. It is a weak, but selective, dopamine-2 (D_2) receptor antagonist. D_2 receptors are thought to act in an inhibitory manner on adenylate cyclase, while dopamine-1 (D_1) receptors are associated with adenylate cyclase stimulation. The presynaptic dopamine "autoreceptors", which regulate the synthesis and release of dopamine, appear to be of the D_2 subtype. Many investigators have suggested that it is blockade of the D_2 receptor that mediates the clinical effects of most antipsychotic agents.

Remoxipride has a marked affinity for sigma receptors, which mediate opioid effects; clinical significance is unknown. There is a wide range between the dose that blocks apomorphine-induced hyperactivity and the dose that produces catalepsy, suggesting a favorable separation between the dose associated with antipsychotic effects and that producing extrapyramidal symptoms. The administration of remoxipride causes a significant, transient increase in prolactin release; however, prolonged administration (> 15 days) results in a reduction in this response.

Pharmacokinetics – Remoxipride is almost completely absorbed after oral administration with a bioavailability of 96% for both standard and controlled release (CR) formulations. There is no first-pass metabolism. Plasma levels peak within 1 to 2 hours after administration of standard formulations and within 2 to 6 hours after CR formulations and are linearly related to dose. Volume of distribution averages 0.5 to 0.7 L/kg. Protein binding averages 80%. CSF levels average 6% to 17% of total plasma levels. Breast milk concentrations are ≈ 30% of those in plasma.

Approximately 70% of an administered dose is metabolized in the liver to 6 inactive oxidized metabolites. Plasma concentrations of unchanged remoxipride are higher in slow debrisoquine metabolizers. Between 10% and 40% of an oral dose is excreted unchanged in the urine. Plasma elimination half-life averages 4 to 7 hours.

Remoxipride is a weak base (pKa 8.9). Urinary elimination is reduced and plasma half-life is prolonged in alkaline urine (pH 7.2). Conversely, acidification of urine (pH 5.2) results in increased urinary elimination and a reduction in half-life. Mean plasma concentrations are increased and the half-life is prolonged in the elderly, in patients with creatinine clearances < 25 mL/min, and in severe liver disease. Most investigators recommend initiating therapy with 50% the usual dose in the elderly.

Clinical trials – Remoxipride is an effective treatment for chronic schizophrenia and acute exacerbations of chronic schizophrenia. Improvement was documented in positive (eg, thought disturbances, hostility/suspiciousness, hallucinations, delusions) and negative (eg, emotional withdrawal, motor retardation) symptoms. In doses of 150 to 600 mg/day, remoxipride had similar antipsychotic efficacy to haloperidol (eg, *Haldol*) 5 to 45 mg/day and thioridazine (eg, *Mellaril*) 150 to 750 mg/day.

In most clinical trials, therapy was initiated with 300 mg/day. Patients responded to total daily doses of 300 to 450 mg/day (maximum dose, 600 mg/day) during initiation of therapy, and were tapered to usual maintenance doses of 150 to 300 mg/day. Dosage adjustments were made no more frequently than every 3 days and were based on patient response.

Remoxipride also may be effective in the treatment of acute mania.

►*Adverse Reactions:* Remoxipride, like other atypical antipsychotic agents (eg, clozapine [*Clozaril*]), causes less frequent extrapyramidal symptoms (EPS) than the classic antipsychotic agents (eg, haloperidol). Long-term, comparative trials reported an EPS incidence of 2% to 15% and 7% to 27% in the remoxipride- and haloperidol-treated groups, respectively. Pooled data from 9 comparative trials with haloperidol also showed a lower incidence of insomnia, tiredness/drowsiness, difficulty in concentration, and dry mouth in the remoxipride-treated group. Although isolated reports of cardiovascular effects such as postural hypotension are documented, they are not considered to be clinically significant.

►*Summary:* Available data suggests that remoxipride is a safe and effective treatment for schizophrenia. Its favorable side effect profile makes it an important therapeutic option for patients unable to tolerate traditional antipsychotic agents. Additional comparative and long-term studies are necessary to clarify its overall role in the treatment of schizophrenia and evaluate its potential to cause tardive dyskinesia.

An NDA for remoxipride was filed in December 1988. However, because of recent reports of aplastic anemia, including 1 death, in European patients, Astra/Merck notified investigators to discontinue use of the drug. The company has recommended restricting the use of the drug to patients who have failed other antipsychotics. The drug, which will be marketed as *Roxiam* by Astra/Merck, is currently available in the UK, Denmark, and Luxembourg. The NDA was withdrawn in December 1993.

~ Bibliography Available on Request ~

RITANSERIN (by Janssen) – A specific central serotonin S₂-antagonist

►Actions:

Pharmacology – Ritanserin is a specific, long-acting central serotonin S_2-antagonist that does not affect norepinephrine, acetylcholine, or central dopamine antagonism, but does antagonize peripheral histamine. Ritanserin improves sleep quality, decreases fatigue, increases energy levels, improves depressed mood and anxiety and appears to lack abuse potential. Ritanserin 10 mg twice daily also improves neuroleptic-induced akathisia in patients resistant to traditional therapy (eg, anticholinergics, benzodiazepines, beta-blockers). These actions of ritanserin have caused researchers to investigate its effects in the treatment of anxiety, schizophrenia, alcoholism, drug abuse, depressive disorders, and Parkinsonism.

Pharmacokinetics – The oral bioavailability is about 75%. Following oral administration, very little drug is recovered unchanged in the urine after a 5 mg IV dose suggesting that it is extensively metabolized by the liver. In a study involving 9 healthy volunteers, peak plasma concentrations occurred within 2.39 hours after oral administration. Steady-state plasma concentrations are achieved within 1 week after initiating dosing and the half-life is ≈ 40 hours. Ritanserin is usually administered with or after a meal to decrease the incidence of transient side effects (eg, dizziness, tiredness, lightheadedness) that have been reported in 10% of patients.

Clinical trials – A trial involving 33 patients was conducted to determine the effectiveness of ritanserin in decreasing the negative symptoms in type II schizophrenia over a 6-week period. Patients initially received 10 mg ritanserin. Doses were increased by 10 mg increments to 30 mg as tolerated. The average total dose at the end of the study was 26 mg. Ritanserin significantly improved several negative symptoms such as facial expressions, global affective flattening, and relationships with friends and peers and also caused significant reductions in scores for emotional withdrawal and depressive mood compared with placebo. Three patients in the ritanserin group dropped out of the study because of lack of efficacy and one due to side effects (eg, unrest).

In another study, 9 patients with acute schizophrenia received 10 mg ritanserin twice daily for 4 weeks. Five of the nine patients experienced a 50% decrease in comprehensive psychological rating scale scores, and scores for negative symptoms also decreased significantly from base

line. No extrapyramidal side effects or akathisia that could be attributed to ritanserin were reported.

Several studies have examined the ability of ritanserin to affect the motor symptoms of Parkinson's disease. Initial studies demonstrated that ritanserin significantly reduced tremor. In contrast, 2 recent studies determined that ritanserin (range, 5 to 30 mg/day) had a positive effect on dyskinesias but not tremor.

Ritanserin's effect on dysthymia has been studied compared with placebo, amitriptyline (eg, *Elavil*), and imipramine (eg, *Tofranil*). Ritanserin was superior to placebo and equal to amitriptyline and imipramine for up to 8 weeks (n > 300).

Several studies have determined that ritanserin is effective in relieving anxiety, decreasing fatigue, and increasing energy in patients with generalized anxiety disorders compared with placebo, and 10 mg ritanserin appears to have equal efficacy to lorazepam (eg, *Ativan*). The antianxiety effects occurred after 2 to 4 weeks of treatment.

Ritanserin decreases craving for alcohol and cocaine. One study involving 39 patients concluded that 5 mg ritanserin decreased desire and craving for alcohol but did not change the amount of alcohol intake during 14 days of the study. Another small study (n = 5) suggested that patients receiving 10 mg ritanserin for 28 days not only had no desire to drink but also demonstrated improvement in mood. Several large scale double-blind studies that will include> 900 patients with various types of alcohol dependence are currently underway.

Slow wave sleep (SWS) patterns were significantly improved in several studies when ritanserin was given to patients with alcoholism and depressive disorders; one study found that ritanserin did not affect SWS in 12 depressed patients.

►Adverse Reactions:
Ritanserin appears to be well tolerated. Observed side effects in clinical trials were minimal, with 10% of patients reporting transient dizziness, tiredness, and lightheadedness.

►Summary:
Although ritanserin shows promise in the treatment of a variety of psychiatric illnesses including anxiety, schizophrenia, alcoholism, drug abuse, depressive disorders, and Parkinsonism, it is still undergoing clinical trials and has not been approved by the FDA. The dosing range used in the studies was from 5 to 30 mg/day in adults. Side effects are minimal and mild and there seems to be a lack of clinically significant changes in vital signs, laboratory values, ECGs, or mood evaluations. Research in the US has been discontinued.

ROXATIDINE ACETATE (*Roxin* by Hoechst-Roussel) – An agent for peptic ulcers

►Actions:

Pharmacology – Roxatidine acetate is a potent, selective, histamine H_2RA (H_2 receptor antagonist) that is structurally unrelated to cimetidine (eg, *Tagamet*) or ranitidine (eg, *Zantac*). Its potency is 3 to 6 times that of cimetidine and twice that of ranitidine. Basal gastric acid secretion is inhibited by > 90% 3 hours after a single 50 mg dose and by 86% 4 to 6 hours after a 75 mg dose. Unlike cimetidine, ranitidine, or famotidine (eg, *Pepcid*), roxatidine has a mucosal protective effect in animal models. It has no direct effect on serum gastrin levels (unlike cimetidine or ranitidine) and no antiandrogenic effect.

Pharmacokinetics – Roxatidine acetate is well absorbed with a bioavailability of > 95%. After administration, it is rapidly converted to roxatidine, its active metabolite, by esterases in the small intestine, plasma, and liver. The peak concentration occurs 3 hours after oral administration, with food and antacids having little or no clinical effect on its pharmacokinetics. Its volume of distribution is 3.2 L/kg after a single dose and 1.7 L/kg at steady state. Plasma protein binding is 6% to 7%. Elimination is primarily renal with 96% eliminated as roxatidine. The clearance is 21 to 29 L/hr and the half-life is 4 to 8 hours. Other than roxatidine, 9 other inactive metabolites have been identified. Because it is renally eliminated, the dose of roxatidine must be adjusted in patients with severe renal dysfunction.

The pharmacokinetic parameters of a single dose of 150 mg roxatidine were evaluated in 31 patients with varying degrees of renal dysfunction (control group, mild chronic renal failure [CRF], moderate CRF, severe CRF, or uremia). The half-life increased 12 hours in patients with uremia (Ccr < 7 mL/min), with the T_{max} doubling (2.08 hours vs 4.05 hours, respectively). In patients with renal failure, there can be an increase in half-life by 140% to 200% with peak plasma concentrations increasing by 50% to 70%. Data on the effects of hemodialysis are conflicting, ranging from no effect to a marked reduction in plasma concentration.

Clinical trials –

Duodenal ulcers (DU): 75 mg roxatidine twice daily is effective for the treatment of DU. Six-week healing rates were between 73% to 90%, with 8-week rates being between 87% to 95%.

The efficacy of roxatidine was evaluated in 356 patients with active DU in a multicenter, double-blind trial. Patients were randomized to

receive roxatidine (150 mg at bedtime, n = 170) or placebo (n = 170) for 4 weeks; antacids were administered as needed for pain relief. Four-week ulcer healing rates were 68% for patients receiving roxatidine compared with 30% for placebo; roxatidine was also better at decreasing abdominal pain.

Roxatidine also is effective as maintenance therapy for the prevention of DU. In one trial, 105 patients with healed duodenal ulcers received 75 mg roxatidine at bedtime for 6 months as preventive therapy. Ulcer relapse rates were 18% after 3 months and 35% after 6 months. Relapse rates were higher in smokers. In another trial evaluating 372 patients with healed duodenal ulcers, cumulative ulcer relapse rates at 12 months were 35% for patients receiving roxatidine (75 mg at bedtime) vs 66% for placebo. Most patients who relapsed did so within 6 months. When patients relapsed, they were asymptomatic in 26% of patients receiving roxatidine vs 16% of patients receiving placebo. The study showed that roxatidine 75 mg at bedtime is effective as preventive therapy for DU.

Gastric ulcers (GU): In small, noncomparative trials in patients with gastric ulcers, 75 mg roxatidine twice daily had ulcer healing rates ranging from 77% to 96% at 8 weeks. In a double-blind, multicenter trial, patients with GU were randomized to receive 75 mg roxatidine twice daily (n = 172) or 150 mg at bedtime (n = 171). Both dosing regimens were found to produce symptomatic pain relief and to have comparable ulcer healing rates (84% and 86% at 8 weeks, respectively).

►Adverse Reactions:
The most common adverse effects are hypersensitivity reactions (rash), GI (diarrhea, constipation, nausea), or involve the CNS (headache, dizziness, fatigue).

►Summary:
Roxatidine acetate is a potent, selective H_2 receptor antagonist that is effective for treatment of and maintenance therapy for duodenal and gastric ulcers. It is generally well tolerated with the primary side effects involving the GI, cutaneous, or central nervous systems.

For the treatment of peptic ulcer disease, roxatidine should be dosed 75 mg twice daily or 150 mg at bedtime for 8 weeks. For prevention of DU or GU recurrence, the dose is 75 mg at bedtime. Decrease dose in patients with renal dysfunction; treatment doses of 75 mg once daily for a Ccr between 20 and 40 mL/min and 75 mg every other day for a CCr of < 20 ml/min have been suggested.

Hoechst-Roussel has filed an NDA for *Roxin*.

SERTINDOLE (*Serdolect* by Lundbeck A/S [Denmark]) – An antipsychotic agent

➤*Actions:*

Pharmacology – Sertindole is a new "atypical" antipsychotic agent with unique pharmacologic properties compared with traditional agents. The mechanism of action of sertindole is via its strong antagonism of dopamine D_2, serotonin 5-HT$_2$, and norepinephrine alpha$_1$ receptors. Sertindole appears to have low extrapyramidal symptoms (EPS) potential, does not cause anticholinergic side effects, does not inhibit cognitive functioning and has potent anxiolytic activity.

Pharmacokinetics –

Immunocompromised patients: Sertindole is slowly absorbed from the GI tract with a peak plasma concentration achieved after 8 to 10 hours. Following a single oral dose, the elimination half-life is approximately 60 hours, but there is great patient variability with 10% of subjects demonstrating half-lives > 100 hours after administration of a single dose. Due to sertindole's long half-life, steady-state concentrations are not reached until after 3 to 4 weeks. The long half-life of sertindole should allow for once-daily dosing. Sertindole is characterized by non-linear kinetics. Increasing the dose by 20% can increase plasma concentrations by approximately 40%. Sertindole is significantly bound to plasma proteins (> 99%), with only a small amount of the drug being renally excreted; therefore, sertindole will presumably not be eliminated by dialysis. In vitro studies have shown that sertindole is predominately metabolized by the hepatic cytochrome P450 3A4 isoform system and eliminated via the GI tract. Sertindole has 2 metabolites, norsertindole and Lu 28-092, but the activity of these metabolites has not been established.

Clinical trials – In 7 phase I trials, over 100 healthy patients received sertindole 0.5 to 32 mg as a single dose or in escalating dosing for up to 14 days. These studies demonstrated that, overall, sertindole was safe and well tolerated.

Three phase II studies examined the efficacy of sertindole in doses of 4 to 24 mg/day. The first was a pilot, double-blind, randomized, placebo-controlled, multi-center study designed to compare the efficacy of sertindole (n = 27) and placebo (n = 11) in patients diagnosed with schizophrenia or schizoaffective disorder. The study concluded that sertindole was effective in most patients at a dose of 16 or 20 mg/day and this therapy was associated with minimal adverse effects.

The second and third phase II studies were randomized, double-blind, multi-centered, and placebo-controlled with identical study designs except that each study had 4 different treatment groups: 8, 12, or 20 mg/day of sertindole or placebo in the second trial, and the third study had 4 or 12 mg/day sertindole, placebo, or 8 mg haloperidol (eg, *Haldol*) twice daily. All patients taking sertindole were titrated upwards starting with 4 mg/day and increasing by 4 mg every third day until the desired dose was reached. The titration phase lasted 12 days and the maintenance phase period was 28 days. Patients enrolled in both studies had to have a previous response to antipsychotic drugs. There were 205 patients enrolled in the second trial and 109 in the third; 153 patients completed at least 13% of the total 40 days of the second trial and were included in the final analysis (107 completed the entire study). Only the 20 mg sertindole group significantly improved in all efficacy parameters compared with placebo. Sertindole 20 mg was equally efficacious to haloperidol but caused fewer side effects.

In a long term, open-label study, sertindole 4 to 24 mg/day was administered to 170 patients for up to 2 years to determine its safety and efficacy. The mean exposure to sertindole was 121 days (range, 2 to 532 days) and the most common dose administered was 20 mg/day (33%).

➤*Adverse Reactions:* Adverse effects observed during phase I trials included lethargy, drowsiness, nasal congestion, sexual dysfunction, GI complaints, dizziness, lightheadedness, mild tremor, orthostatic hypotension, syncope, dystonia, postural hypotension, and cogwheel rigidity. No patients experienced EPS. The most common adverse effects experienced during phase II trials that occurred more often with sertindole 20 mg/day than with placebo included: Headache, nasal congestion (26%); dry ejaculation (17%); constipation, dizziness, somnolence (11%). Dry ejaculation was the only side effect that was found to be significantly greater than placebo (P < 0.05). Adverse effects experienced during the long-term study were similar, but incidence rates were higher.

➤*Summary:* Sertindole should provide an effective and safe alternative treatment when therapy with traditional antipsychotics have failed due to lack of efficacy or intolerable side effects. Additional trials are necessary to establish long-term safety, especially the incidence of tardive dyskinesia, and efficacy of sertindole. The drug, which will be available from Lundbeck A/S (Denmark), became "approvable" in 1998.

SOLIFENACIN SUCCINATE (*Vesicare* by Yamanouchi Pharma America) – An anticholinergic agent

➤*Actions:*

Pharmacology – Solifenacin has been submitted for FDA approval for the treatment of overactive bladder with symptoms of urinary incontinence, urgency, and frequency. Solifenacin is an anticholinergic agent, which is a muscarinic receptor antagonist. It has greater affinity for the M3 receptor than the M1 or M2 receptors. In mice and rat models, solifenacin has greater selectivity for bladder muscle cells and colon muscle cells than salivary gland cells. Activity at submandibular gland cells was lower with solifenacin than with tolterodine, oxybutynin, or atropine. In animal models of irritable bowel syndrome, solifenacin reduced stress-induced diarrhea and morphine-induced constipation.

Pharmacokinetics – Following oral administration, peak solifenacin concentrations were reached within 3 to 6 hours. The bioavailability of oral solifenacin was 88%. Ingestion of solifenacin with a high-fat meal had no impact on solifenacin pharmacokinetics. The solifenacin terminal half-life was 40 to 55 hours. Steady-state concentrations were reached after approximately 10 days of consecutive dosing. Solifenacin is metabolized via CYP3A4. Three percent to 10% of the dose was excreted unchanged in the urine. In elderly subjects the mean time to peak was increased to 5 to 9 hours and the mean half-life was 48 to 82 hours.

Clinical trials – A study compared 2 doses of solifenacin with placebo and tolterodine in 1077 patients with symptoms of overactive bladder. Following a 2-week, single-blind, placebo run-in period, patients were randomized to therapy with placebo (267 patients), tolterodine 2 mg twice daily (263 patients), or solifenacin 5 mg (279 patients), or 10 mg (268 patients) once daily for 12 weeks. The primary study endpoint was the mean change from baseline in mean number of micturitions per 24 hours. Micturition frequency was reduced by 1.2 micturitions per 24 hours (10%) in the placebo group, 2.2 micturitions per 24 hours (18%, P < 0.001) in the solifenacin 5 mg group, 2.6 micturitions per 24 hours (21%, P < 0.001) in the solifenacin 10 mg group, and 1.9 micturitions per 24 hours (15%, P < 0.05) in the tolterodine group. Urgency episodes per 24 hours were reduced by 1.4 episodes (26%) in the placebo group,

2.8 episodes (49%, P < 0.001) in the solifenacin 5 mg group, 3.1 episodes (53%, P < 0.001) in the solifenacin 10 mg group, and 2 episodes (37%) in the tolterodine group. Episodes of urge incontinence per 24 hours were reduced by 0.6 episodes (29%) in the placebo group, 1.4 episodes (59%, P < 0.01) in the solifenacin 5 mg group, 1.3 episodes (62%, P < 0.01) in the solifenacin 10 mg group, and 0.9 episodes (47%) in the tolterodine group. Dry mouth occurred in 4.9% of placebo-treated patients, 14.3% of patients treated with 5 mg solifenacin, 21.3% of patients treated with 10 mg solifenacin, and 19.4% of patients treated with tolterodine. Overall, solifenacin was well tolerated and highly effective relative to placebo and tolterodine.

➤*Drug Interactions:* Administration of ketoconazole concomitantly with a single 10 mg solifenacin dose resulted in a 40% increase in the solifenacin peak concentration, a 55% increase in the solifenacin half-life, and a 100% increase in the solifenacin AUC. Despite the increase in solifenacin levels, the incidence of adverse reactions was not increased. Further studies are necessary to assess the impact of CYP3A4 inhibitors on solifenacin levels and side effects following repeated solifenacin doses.

➤*Adverse Reactions:* Adverse events associated with solifenacin have included dry mouth, constipation, blurred vision, headache, and somnolence. In a dose-finding study, dry mouth occurred in 8% of placebo-treated patients, 9% of patients treated with solifenacin 2.5 mg, 12% treated with solifenacin 5 mg, 33% treated with solifenacin 10 mg, and 48% treated with solifenacin 20 mg.

➤*Summary:* Solifenacin will offer an alternative to oxybutynin for the treatment of overactive bladder with urinary incontinence, urgency, or frequency. It appears to be associated with a lower incidence of dry mouth and other anticholinergic side effects than oxybutynin prompt-release tablets. It will compete with tolterodine, trospium, and sustained-release and transdermal oxybutynin formulations, which are also associated with fewer anticholinergic side effects. The optimal dosage for solifenacin has not been established. In clinical trials it appears effective and generally well tolerated at doses of 5 to 10 mg once daily. A New Drug Application for solifenacin was filed in December 2002.

TEICOPLANIN (*Targocid* by Aventis) – A glycopeptide antibiotic

➤*Actions:*

Pharmacology – Teicoplanin (teichomycin A2) is a glycopeptide antibiotic complex structurally related to vancomycin (eg, *Vancocin*). It has a similar spectrum of activity but a longer half-life, which allows less frequent dosing. It may be administered by IM and IV injection and brief (30 minute) infusion. Teicoplanin is a mixture of 6 closely related glycopeptide components designated as teicoplanin-A2 (1 through 5) and teicoplanin-A3. The components of the A2 complex account for 90% to 95% of teicoplanin. The drug interferes with cell wall synthesis in susceptible organisms by inhibiting peptidoglycan polymerization.

Like vancomycin, teicoplanin is active only against gram-positive organisms. It is bactericidal against most susceptible strains, with the possible exception of some coagulase-negative staphylococci (which may show reduced susceptibility), where it may be bacteriostatic. It has equivalent or superior activity (based on MIC data) to vancomycin against staphylococci, including both methicillin-sensitive and -resistant *S. aureus*, *S. epidermidis*, streptococci (including viridans group, and groups B, C, F, and G), enterococci, and many anaerobic gram-positive bacteria, including *Clostridium difficile*, *C. perfringens*, *Listeria monocytogenes*, and *Corynebacterium jeikeium*. Vancomycin-resistant enterococci may be resistant to teicoplanin.

Teicoplanin is usually synergistic with aminoglycosides and imipenem, and additive with rifampin (eg, *Rifadin*). A postantibiotic effect of 2.4 to 4.1 hours has been reported with both methicillin-sensitive and -resistant strains of *S. aureus*.

Pharmacokinetics – Like vancomycin, teicoplanin is minimally absorbed after oral administration; this route is acceptable only for the treatment of pseudomembranous colitis. Following IM administration of 3 mg/kg, peak levels of 5 to 7 mcg/mL are achieved at 2 to 4 hours; bioavailability is 90%. Peak serum levels after IV administration are dependent on the dose and the method of administration. Following administration of 3 mg/kg, peak levels after a 30-second injection or a 30-minute infusion average 53 and 20 mcg/mL, respectively. Trough (24 hour) levels are not influenced. The drug is widely distributed in most tissues and fluids (with the exception of the CSF), although the rate and extent varies. Volume of distribution (Vd) at steady state averages 0.6 to 0.8 L/kg. Protein binding is 90%.

The drug does not appear to undergo metabolism and is excreted in the urine almost entirely by glomerular filtration. The terminal elimination half-life averages 45 to 70 hours. In patients with renal dysfunction and the elderly, the elimination half-life is increased but the Vd is unchanged. Current dosing recommendations for renal impairment state that usual doses be given for the first 3 days. Thereafter, either the dose is reduced or the interval prolonged, based on the degree of renal insufficiency according to the following scheme: Creatinine clearance (Ccr) 40 to 60 mL/min, half the dose or twice the interval; Ccr < 40 mL/min, one-third the dose or triple the interval.

Clinical trials – Reported response rates by type of infection are: Skin and soft tissue (90%); septicemia, bone and joint (89%); endocarditis (83%); respiratory tract (77%). Other applications in which the drug has demonstrated efficacy include: Endocarditis prophylaxis in dental surgery; Hickman catheter and other indwelling device-related infections; neurosurgical shunt ventriculitis; chronic ambulatory peritoneal dialysis (CAPD)-related peritonitis (added to dialysate); surgical prophylaxis; presumed gram-positive infections in immunocompromised patients. The usual loading and maintenance doses of 6 mg/kg followed by 3 mg/kg/24 hours may need to be increased in children and in the treatment of *S. aureus* endocarditis and septicemia. A reduction in efficacy has been noted in diabetics, immunocompromised patients, and when foreign bodies are present.

➤*Adverse Reactions:* The overall incidence of side effects is 10.3%. Most commonly reported effects include: Non-specific complaints (fatigue, headache, diarrhea) (5.1%); injection-site intolerance (pain, redness, phlebitis) (3%); hypersensitivity skin reactions (pruritus, urticaria, maculopapular rash) (2.4%); hematologic abnormalities (eosinophilia, reversible neutropenia, increased platelet count) (2.2%); transient elevation of LFTs (1.7%); nephrotoxicity (0.35% to 0.6%); high-frequency hearing loss, which may be irreversible (0.28%); bronchospasm (0.2%); anaphylactoid reactions (0.07%). Teicoplanin does not appear to cause the dose or infusion rate-related histamine release associated with the "red man syndrome," as does vancomycin. Concomitant use of an aminoglycoside appears to increase the incidence of nephrotoxicity.

➤*Summary:* Teicoplanin appears to be a safe and effective alternative to vancomycin. Potential advantages appear to be the availability of IM administration, reduced infusion times, and volume requirements, lack of infusion-related reactions and once daily dosing. The NDA for teicoplanin was filed in March 1991. The FDA has given the drug a "1A" priority review rating. Teicoplanin is currently available in 13 countries.

TEZOSENTAN

TEZOSENTAN (*Veletri* by Genentech) – A dual endothelin receptor antagonist

➤*Actions:*

Pharmacology – Tezosentan is a dual endothelin receptor antagonist that displays high affinity to endothelin-A and endothelin-B receptors. Endothelin is a potent vasoconstrictor and is responsible for increasing resistance in blood vessels. Because of its ability to block endothelin receptors and produce vasodilation, tezosentan is being studied for possible use in patients with acute heart failure, pulmonary edema, and hepatorenal syndrome.

Pharmacokinetics – Tezosentan is available in a parenteral dosage form only. Initial studies show that tezosentan most likely follows a standard 2-compartment model. One study demonstrates the half-lives of the 2 disposition phases to be approximately 6 minutes and 3.2 hours.

Tezosentan is metabolized in the liver and excreted almost exclusively in the bile. Less than 5% of the total dose is cleared renally. It has 1 metabolite that is formed by hydroxylation of the isopropyl side chain, and it is thought to be 10 times less potent than the parent compound. Therefore, it is currently considered to be clinically insignificant.

Clinical trials – Tezosentan is currently undergoing phase 3 clinical trials. Several studies have been performed and several others are currently ongoing. The randomized IV tezosentan (RITZ) trials have been completed with mixed outcomes. The initial trial RITZ-2 showed that tezosentan had a positive effect on cardiac index and pulmonary capillary wedge pressure (PCWP) in patients with acute heart failure. This double-blind study randomized 184 patients with NYHA III/IV heart failure to standard therapy plus placebo, 50 mg/h tezosentan, or 100 mg/h tezosentan. Cardiac index increased by approximately 0.4 L/min/m^2 in both tezosentan groups, which was significant compared with placebo ($P < 0.0001$). The patients' PCWP decreased by approximately 3.9 mm Hg in both tezosentan groups and was significant compared with placebo ($P < 0.0001$). However, later studies in the RITZ series showed that tezosentan produced no significant added benefit in improving clinical symptoms or mortality compared with the current standard of therapy in patients with acute heart failure. In addition, more patients in the tezosentan groups suffered from adverse effects in these trials. In the RITZ-1 trial, 669 patients with acute decompensated heart failure were randomized in a double-blind, placebo-controlled study. Three hundred thirty-eight patients were assigned to the standard treatment group plus placebo while 331 where assigned to the standard treatment plus 50 mg/h tezosentan group. Tezosentan did not produce significant improvement in dyspnea at 24 hours. In addition, tezosentan was unable to show significant improvement in time to death or worsening heart failure during the first 24 hours. The RITZ-4 trial evaluated the use of tezosentan in patients with acute heart failure associated with acute coronary syndrome. This double-blind, placebo-controlled study randomized 193 patients to receive standard therapy plus placebo or 25 mg/h tezosentan for 1 hour followed by 50 mg/h for 23 hours up to 48 hours. Improvement in the primary endpoint, which was a composite of death, worsening heart failure, recurrent ischemia, or recurrent or new MI within the first 72 hours of drug treatment was not significant ($P = 0.52$). Finally, the RITZ-5 trial evaluated the use of tezosentan in pulmonary edema. The primary endpoint was a change in SO$_2$ from baseline over the first hour. In this double-blind, placebo-controlled study, 84 patients were randomized to receive standard therapy plus placebo or 50 mg/h tezosentan for 30 minutes followed by a maintenance dose of 50 to 100 mg/h for a total of 24 hours. The conclusions for the primary endpoint did not show significant improvement in SO$_2$.

Researchers have hypothesized that an inappropriately high dose may be responsible for the significant adverse effects of tezosentan. The lack of improving clinical symptoms and mortality may be the result of patients responding well to conventional therapy, making it difficult to determine any additional effects of new therapy. Currently, tezosentan is undergoing morbidity and mortality trials in patients with acute heart failure (Veritas 1 and Veritas 2). The trials are expected to be concluded in the spring of 2005.

➤*Drug Interactions:* One study has shown that concomitant administration of tezosentan and cyclosporin may lead to increased exposure to tezosentan. The mechanism for this effect has not been completely elucidated but is thought to be related to the inhibition of transport proteins in the liver.

➤*Adverse Reactions:* In general, clinical studies investigating the use of tezosentan have shown that a nitrate-like headache was the most common adverse effect of tezosentan. Hypotension, dizziness, nausea, vomiting, and decreased renal function also were observed.

➤*Summary:* Tezosentan is a dual endothelin antagonist that has shown promising efficacy in increasing cardiac index and reducing pulmonary capillary wedge pressure. It has not shown significant improvement in clinical symptoms or mortality at the doses that have been selected in past phase 3 clinical trials. New morbidity and mortality studies are currently underway to evaluate its efficacy in the treatment of acute heart failure.

TIBOLONE

TIBOLONE (*Xyvion* by Organon) – A synthetic steroid

➤*Actions:*

Pharmacology – Tibolone is a synthetic steroid with weak estrogenic, progestogenic, and androgenic activity, structurally related to nor-ethynodrel. It inhibits osteoclastic activity and increases trabecular and cortical bone mass in postmenopausal women. Compared with placebo, tibolone reduced serum alkaline phosphatase, osteocalcin, serum albumin, calcium, and phosphate concentrations, and suppressed the urinary calcium:creatinine and hydroxypyroline:creatinine ratios. In the endometrium, tibolone is transformed by 3β-hydroxysteroid dehydrogenase isomerase into the D-4 metabolite. This metabolite does not have estrogenic activity but does have intrinsic progestogenic activity, therefore not stimulating the endometrium. Tibolone therapy does not require an additional progestogen to protect the endometrium.

Pharmacokinetics – Tibolone given orally is rapidly absorbed, appearing in the plasma within 30 minutes and peaking in 4 hours. Metabolism is mainly in the liver and excretion occurs in the urine and feces. The elimination half-life is ≈ 45 hours.

Clinical trials – Tibolone was an effective synthetic steroid for the treatment of menopausal symptoms and the prevention of osteoporosis in controlled clinical trials. Its efficacy seems to be equivalent to combined hormone replacement therapy (HRT), with similar reductions in vasomotor symptoms and increased spinal bone mineral density. Tibolone also was reported to be effective in reducing vasomotor symptoms and bone loss when used as add-back therapy in patients undergoing therapy for endometriosis or uterine leiomyomata with gonadotropin-releasing hormone analog. Studies were also performed concerning tibolone and its effects on lipids. Tibolone reduced HDL-cholesterol and triglycerides to a greater extent than combined HRT, while producing an overall reduction in total cholesterol comparable with that of transdermal estradiol. Tibolone also has been studied to assess its effects on sexuality. Tibolone was associated with an increase in the frequency of sexual interest, frequency of orgasm, general sexual satisfaction, sexual responsiveness, and a reduction in the frequency of dyspareunia. The most commonly studied dosage has been 2.5 mg once daily, continuously.

➤*Adverse Reactions:* The most common side effects include edema, nausea, breast tenderness, vaginal spotting or bleeding, bloating, leg pain, headache, and weight gain. Although weight gain is reported as a side effect, tibolone has been demonstrated to prevent total body fat and lean muscle mass changes associated with menopause without weight changes in a small study. Bleeding occurs in 10% to 15% of women during the first month of treatment and ≈ 4% after 6 months of treatment. The rate of amenorrhea in one 6-year study was 90% after the first 6 months of therapy with tibolone and 91% in the control group. Breakthrough bleeding is more likely to occur in patients who are younger, recently menopausal, and with detectable estradiol levels. Weight gain, increased blood pressure, or impairment of glycemic control were not observed in a group of postmenopausal women with type 2 diabetes treated with tibolone 2.5 mg/day for 2 months. Similarly, a lack of effect on glucose tolerance was observed in another study enrolling healthy women.

➤*Summary:* Tibolone will offer an alternative for the treatment of menopausal symptoms and prevention of osteoporosis. Tibolone increases bone mineral density to an extent comparable with that achieved with estrogen replacement therapy. It has been associated with a high degree of amenorrhea, comparable with that achieved with combined continuous estrogen/progestogen regimens. Added weak androgenic activity may provide added benefits in some patients, although more data are necessary to evaluate this effect. The lipid profile, particularly the considerable drop in HDL-cholesterol, may limit its use, although therapy also has been associated with a significant drop in triglycerides, which may be beneficial in others. Tibolone is commercially available in Europe under the trade name *Livial*.

TIRILAZAD

TIRILAZAD (*Freedox* by Upjohn) – A 21-aminosteroid antioxidant

➤*Actions:*

Pharmacology – Tirilazad mesylate is a 21-aminosteroid (also referred to as lazaroids) with distinct antioxidant properties. It does not manifest glucocorticoid activity. Tirilazad acts as a cytoprotective agent that oxidizes peroxyl radicals and stabilizes cell membranes. It also helps to preserve the membrane content of vitamin E (alphatocopherol), another important antioxidant. As a result of its ability to prevent lipid peroxidation in cell membranes, tirilazad promotes tissue survival in the vicinity of a CNS injury.

Because of the high content of polyunsaturated lipids in neuronal membranes, the CNS is particularly susceptible to the destructive effects of oxygen radicals. Tissue injury occurring during CNS trauma or a stroke increases oxygen radical production, which in turn leads to damaging lipid peroxidation reactions. Such oxygen radical-mediated processes appear to be involved in posttraumatic brain edema, spinal axonal degeneration and microvascular damage. The progressive secondary tissue destruction, which follows the precipitating event, may be amenable to therapy with antioxidants.

Pharmacokinetics – Tirilazad is administered in a citrate solution as an IV infusion over not > 30 minutes. It is a lipophilic substance that distributes extensively to tissue, with a volume of distribution of ≈ 1.7 L/kg. The drug appears to follow a multicompartment elimination pattern. Following a single dose, the half-life is ≈ 3.75 hours. However, upon multiple dosing, a terminal elimination half-life of 35 hours has been observed. Elimination occurs via hepatic metabolism. The clearance of tirilazad is roughly equal to hepatic plasma flow.

Clinical trials – In numerous neurological studies of animal models, tirilazad has shown distinct promise as a useful therapeutic agent for brain and spinal injury, aneurysmal subarachnoid hemorrhage (SAH), and stroke. Phase III clinical trials are currently being conducted in each of these areas.

The second National Acute Spinal Cord Injury Study (NASCIS 2) demonstrated that patients treated with high-dose methylprednisolone (eg, *Solu-Medrol*; 8 to 9 g/day) within 8 hours of injury, experienced significantly greater neurological improvement than those treated with placebo. The efficacy of methylprednisolone in slowing the progression of CNS damage is believed to be due to its antioxidant properties rather than its glucocorticoid activity. For this reason, in NASCIS 3 (an ongoing follow-up study), 1 of the 3 treatment arms involves 2 g methylprednisolone bolus, followed by 2.5 mg/kg tirilazad infusion every 6 hours for a total of 48 hours.

To date, most of the clinical efficacy trials conducted with tirilazad have studied its use in SAH. Upjohn has submitted 3 double-blind, randomized, placebo controlled study results to the FDA in support of an NDA for tirilazad in the treatment of SAH. However, an FDA committee determined that these studies did not confirm efficacy; 1 study showed an improvement in males, but this was not replicated in another study, and there were no differences in females.

Tirilazad and newer, more potent antioxidants also may be studied in other neurologic conditions in which peroxidative mechanisms have been implicated. These include Alzheimer's disease, Parkinson's disease, and multiple sclerosis.

➤*Adverse Reactions:* Tirilazad has been safe in elderly patients (≈ 66 years of age) with acute ischemic stroke at doses < 6 mg/kg/day for 3 days. In healthy volunteers, tirilazad had no effect on cerebral blood flow or oxygen metabolism. Studies have failed to show any significant glucocorticoid effect to be caused by the drug. Up to 50% of subjects in 1 study exhibited a moderate, transient increase in serum alanine transaminase. The most noted side effect has been mild to moderate pain at the injection site, occurring in 60% to 80% of patients.

Studies involving tirilazad and both nimodipine (*Nimotop*) and cimetidine (eg, *Tagamet*) have failed to identify a clinically significant drug interaction with either of those drugs.

➤*Summary:* Tirilazad is a potent antioxidant, similar in structure to other steroids, but without glucocorticoid activity. Because of its ability to prevent oxygen radical-mediated lipid peroxidation, it may prove to be useful in preventing progressive neuronal degeneration and associated complications following brain and spinal injury, SAH, and stroke.

Upjohn submitted a new drug application in June 1994 for tirilazad with the indication of SAH. Due to the lack of serious side effects that have been documented thus far, and the considerable potential benefit that this drug possesses as a therapeutic agent in areas greatly in need of new treatment modalities, approval is anticipated. However, on September 26, 1994, the FDA's Peripheral and Central Nervous System Drugs Advisory Committee decided that the studies for tirilazad did not confirm efficacy and that further studies would be necessary. A Treatment IND program was discussed as a possibility.

TROSPECTOMYCIN (*Spexil* by Upjohn) – An aminocyclitol antibiotic

➤Actions:

Pharmacology – Trospectomycin is a water soluble analog of spectinomycin (*Trobicin*) that is 8 to 10 times more potent and has a broader spectrum of activity. It has good gram-positive and gram-negative aerobic and anaerobic activity, including in vitro activity against *Staphylococci*, *Streptococci*, *Peptostreptococci*, *Peptococci*, *Haemophilus*, *Gardnerella*, *Neisseria*, *Bacteroides*, *Chlamydia*, *Mycoplasma*, and *Ureaplasma*. It has moderate activity against Enterobacteriaceae and no activity against *Pseudomonas*.

Trospectomycin acts by binding to the 30S component of the ribosome unit thereby inhibiting protein synthesis. It has a greater affinity for the 30S ribosome unit than spectinomycin and therefore has higher activity. Cross-resistance to spectinomycin has been observed in vitro.

Pharmacokinetics – Patients (n = 128) were randomized to receive trospectomycin (75 to 1000 mg) by IM injection or by 20 minute IV infusion. The IM product was 100% bioavailable. The mean peak plasma concentration and AUC were linear relative to dose, and the half-life was 2.1 hours. Serum concentrations were < 2 mcg/mL 12 hours postdose, suggesting 2 to 3 times/day dosing as the MIC for most organisms is between 2 to 4 mcg/mL. In another trial, trospectomycin was administered by IV infusion. While almost no drug was found in the feces, 48% to 62% was recovered in the urine during the first 48 hours, suggesting that the drug is slowly released from tissues. The half-life of 2.18 hours did not change with increasing dose.

Clinical trials – The in vitro activity of trospectomycin was compared with that of amikacin (eg, *Amikin*), cephalothin (eg, *Keflin*), and vancomycin (eg, *Vancocin*) against 342 gram-positive organisms. Vancomycin was the most active agent overall, and trospectomycin was better than amikacin, especially for *Staphylococci* and *Streptococci*.

The activity of trospectomycin, clindamycin (eg, *Cleocin*), metronidazole (eg, *Flagyl*), imipenem (*Primaxin*), cefoxitin (*Mefoxin*), and piperacillin (*Pipracil*) was evaluated against 72 strains of *Bacteroides*. Trospectomycin had very good activity and was comparable with imipenem and metronidazole. Its activity was greater than that of piperacillin and cefoxitin. In another trial, trospectomycin was comparable with clindamycin and cefoxitin against *Bacteroides fragilis*, and there was no cross-resistance between the 3 drugs. Of the organisms tested, 90% to 100% were resistant to ampicillin (eg, *Polycillin*) and cefaclor (eg, *Ceclor*), and > 50% were resistant to doxycycline (eg, *Vibramycin*). None of the organisms tested were resistant to trospectomycin.

The effect of trospectomycin and several other antibiotics was evaluated against *Mycoplasma pneumoniae*, *M. hominis*, and *Ureaplasma urealyticum*. Trospectomycin and spectinomycin were equivalent to tetracycline (eg, *Achromycin*) against *M. pneumoniae* but less active against *M. hominis*. It was concluded that trospectomycin is active against *Mycoplasma*-induced respiratory or genital infections.

To date, published in vivo trials with trospectomycin are limited. The efficacy of a single 1 g IM dose was evaluated in 10 men with uncomplicated *C. trachomatis* urethritis. All were culture-positive at follow-up on days 4 to 8. On follow-up on days 21 to 28, 6 of the 8 men were still culture-positive. It was concluded that a single IM dose for the treatment of uncomplicated *C. trachomatis* urethritis is not effective.

➤Adverse Reactions: In one study, mild, transient and local reactions were seen in 20% of subjects receiving trospectomycin vs 22% with placebo; none of the reactions were thought to be drug-related. Overall, mild and transient side effects were seen in 32% of 64 subjects receiving trospectomycin; 12 had dizziness or lightheadedness and 17 who received > 600 mg had perioral/facial numbness. Results from a similar trial using IM injection were comparable.

In a multiple-dose trial involving 10 healthy males, trospectomycin caused significantly more pain at the injection site. There was also a significant increase in perioral paresthesias with increasing doses (especially at the 500 and 750 mg doses). Perioral paresthesias were mild and transient, were seen shortly after dosing and lasted about 1 to 2 hours. Tolerance did not develop over the 7 days of the study. Clinically significant orthostatic hypotension occurred after the first dose in patients receiving 500 or 750 mg but was not seen with subsequent dosing.

➤Summary: Trospectomycin is an injectable aminocyclitol aminoglycoside that is structurally related to spectinomycin. It has good gram-positive and gram-negative aerobic and anaerobic activity and may prove to be useful for the treatment of upper respiratory tract infections, bacterial vaginitis, pelvic inflammatory disease, and gonorrhea. Overall, it appears to be well tolerated and the major side effects are pain at the injection site and perioral paresthesias.

VALSPODAR

VALSPODAR (*Amdray* by Novartis) – A P-glycoprotein (P-gp) inhibitor

➤Actions:

Pharmacology – Valspodar (SDZ PSC 833), a cyclosporine analog, is employed in reversing classic multidrug resistance (MDR) to natural product-derived cytotoxic agents. MDR results from overexpression of the multidrug resistance gene (MDR-1) leading to overproduction of P-gp. P-gp is believed to function as a transmembrane efflux pump that prevents the intracellular accumulation of certain cytotoxic agents, such as anthracyclines, epidophyllotoxins, vinca alkaloids, and taxanes. Valspodar acts as a P-gp inhibitor, thus preventing drug resistance. In addition, valspodar is believed to influence clearance of some chemotherapeutic agents.

Pharmacokinetics – Valspodar is metabolized by cytochrome P450 3A. It can be administered by IV infusion or orally. The following 3 oral formulations have been tested: An oral solution, microemulsion oral solution, and microemulsion capsule. The microemulsion formulas have a greater bioavailability when compared with the conventional oral solution (≈ 54% and ≈ 52% for the microemulsion oral solution and capsule, respectively, as compared with ≈ 29% for the conventional oral solution). The microemulsion formulas also display a higher C_{max} and a lower t_{max} compared with the conventional oral solution.

Clinical trials – In a phase II study, researchers evaluating 2 regimens involving valspodar, mitoxantrone (*Novantrone*), and etoposide (eg, *VePesid*) for treatment of refractory and relapsed acute myelogenous leukemia (AML) concluded that their results of 32% of patients achieving complete remission appeared "encouraging." However, no comparison was made to a control or reference study. Additional studies are necessary.

➤Drug Interactions:

Digoxin (eg, Lanoxin) – Valspodar, given in a single oral dose to healthy subjects with steady-state levels of digoxin, increased digoxin AUC (in all of the subjects) and C_{max} (in 11 of the 12 subjects), while decreasing digoxin renal clearance (in 11 of the 12 subjects). Coadministration of digoxin and valspodar orally for 5 days in healthy subjects increased digoxin AUC (in all of the subjects) and C_{max} (in 11 of the 12 subjects), and decreased renal and nonrenal clearance of digoxin.

Paclitaxel (Taxol) – Valspodar slightly increases peak plasma levels and AUC of paclitaxel and significantly prolongs the paclitaxel elimination phase.

Etoposide – Valspodar decreased the clearance of etoposide by 57% when administered concomitantly.

➤Adverse Reactions: Valspodar lacks immunosuppressive and nephrotoxic qualities. Transient hyperbilirubinemia appears to be the most frequent adverse effect of valspodar among several studies. Reversible cerebellar ataxia also has been observed.

➤Summary: Valspodar is a P-gp inhibitor currently in phase III clinical studies for treatment of AML, decreasing chemotherapy resistance in relapsing multiple myeloma, and reducing drug resistance or inhibiting drug resistance development in ovarian cancer. Additional studies to demonstrate efficacy are warranted.

~ Bibliography Available on Request ~

VESNARINONE (*Arkin-Z* by Otsuka) – An inotropic agent for CHF

►*Actions:*

Pharmacology – Vesnarinone, a quinolinone derivative, is an oral inotropic agent with little to no effect on heart rate or myocardial oxygen consumption. The mechanism of action is largely unknown. It may be related to a slight inhibition of PDE III, which causes an increase in cyclic AMP and finally an increase in the inward calcium current. There is also a reduction in the potassium current.

In addition, vesnarinone inhibits the production and release of cytokines such as TNF-alpha, IL-1, IL-2, and IFN-gamma. This inhibition may relate directly to its efficacy as an inotropic agent. Increased concentrations of TNF-alpha are seen in patients with chronic heart failure. These increased concentrations depress myocardial contractility, alter muscle membrane potential, decrease blood pressure, and precipitate pulmonary edema. Therefore, reducing the concentration of TNF-alpha is beneficial in patients with heart failure.

Interestingly, vesnarinone also inhibits the replication of HIV-1 in peripheral blood lymphocytes and in chronically infected macrophages, suggesting that it may be useful in treating patients with HIV-1 disease.

Pharmacokinetics – The pharmacokinetic parameters of vesnarinone were evaluated in 21 healthy male volunteers in a 2-phase, nonblinded trial. In phase I, subjects received vesnarinone in a sequentially ascending single dose ranging from 7.5 to 240 mg. In phase II, 3 subjects received vesnarinone 30 mg/day for 15 days. The elimination half-life was 44.7 ± 1.2 hour and the clearance 0.284 ± 0.018 L/hr. The drug was fairly extensively metabolized, with only 11% to 27% (mean, 17.7%) being excreted unchanged in the urine. The authors concluded that elimination of vesnarinone is dose-dependent and that plasma concentrations are proportional to the dose administered.

Clinical trials – In 2 small, uncontrolled trials, vesnarinone was administered to a total of 20 patients with CHF; significant hemodynamic and functional improvement was seen. In a small, placebo controlled study, 8 patients with chronic, stable, moderate CHF received vesnarinone 60 mg/day or placebo for 4 to 8 weeks. Patients were then crossed over to the alternate treatment group. Symptomatic improvement was noted in 4 patients while receiving vesnarinone. In addition, vesnarinone caused an increase in contractility of the left ventricle. Mild to moderate dyspnea and fatigue on exertion was seen in all patients while receiving placebo. In 2 placebo-controlled, double-blind trials, a total of 159 patients with CHF were randomized to receive vesnarinone 60 mg/day or placebo for 12 weeks. In both trials, there was an improvement in the quality of life and a reduction in the severity or progression of heart failure in patients receiving vesnarinone.

The long-term use of vesnarinone was evaluated in a double-blind trial involving 477 patients with CHF. Patients were randomized to receive vesnarinone 60 mg/day or placebo for 6 months. Patients receiving vesnarinone experienced an improvement in their quality of life and a reduction in morbidity and mortality when compared with patients receiving placebo. In the initial design of this trial, patients also could be randomized to receive vesnarinone 120 mg/day. However, this treatment group was stopped after the first 253 patients had been enrolled because of a significant increase in mortality. These results suggest that vesnarinone may have a narrow therapeutic window.

►*Adverse Reactions:* The primary side effect noted with vesnarinone use is reversible neutropenia seen in 2.5% of patients. Other reported side effects include: Reversible agranulocytosis; palpitations; dyspnea; gastric discomfort; nausea; headache; skin rash.

►*Summary:* Vesnarinone is a new positive inotropic agent that appears to be effective in the management of CHF. Because of its unique mechanism of action involving inhibition of cytokines, vesnarinone may prove to be a useful alternative in the long-term management of this patient population. It appears to be well tolerated with the exception of the relatively high incidence of reversible neutropenia. Because of this potentially serious toxicity, the clinical utility of vesnarinone remains to be determined.

Although vesnarinone is currently available in Japan, all research ended in the US on July 31, 1996.

VIGABATRIN (*Sabril* by Aventis) – An anticonvulsant agent

►*Actions:*

Pharmacology – Vigabatrin is a second generation antiepileptic that appears to exert its mechanism of action via increasing brain GABA levels by inhibition of GABA metabolism. These effects on GABA appear to be dose-related. Vigabatrin has an S(+)-enantiomer that inhibits GABA-T, whereas the R(-)-enantiomer has almost no effect. Vigabatrin's mechanism of action also may be attributed to its ability to decrease excitation-related amino acids, aspartate, glutamate, and glutamine concentrations in the brain, but these same changes do not occur in the CSF.

Pharmacokinetics – Although the exact bioavailability of vigabatrin is not known, following oral administration about 80% of the dose is recovered in the urine. In healthy volunteers, its absorption was rapid and peak plasma concentrations occurred within the first 2 hours. When vigabatrin was administered with food, its approximate bioavailability was $92\% \pm 11\%$. Vigabatrin has a volume of distribution of about 0.8 L/kg, is not bound to plasma proteins, and distributes into the CSF. The drug does not appear to be metabolized by the liver, or influence hepatic metabolism. The elimination half-life observed in 24 volunteers was ≈ 7 hours and does not appear to be significantly affected by single or multiple dosing, and appears to be similar in adults and children. Dosing adjustments may be necessary in patients with renal impairment (Ccr less than 60 mL/min) and in the elderly.

Clinical trials – When traditional antiepileptic therapies including add on treatments are used, up to 25% of patients still experience seizures. The studies examining the efficacy of vigabatrin as an antiepileptic medication were primarily add-on trials in patients with resistant epilepsy. Reductions in seizure frequency have been observed in patients with partial and complex partial seizures, but reductions have been observed less frequently with primary generalized seizures, and no reductions (and even worsening) of absence and myoclonic seizures. In a meta-analysis of 9 European trials, of the patients with complex partial seizures, 72% showed a > 25% decrease in seizure frequency over a 7- to 12-week period. When combining all clinical trials (including European studies) examining the efficacy of vigabatrin in treatment of resistant partial complex epilepsy, between 33% and 61% of patients experienced a > 50% reduction in seizure frequency at doses between 1 and 4 g/day.

The use of vigabatrin in doses ranging from 50 to 150 mg/kg/day also has been studied as add-on therapy in children with partial, generalized, Lennox-Gaustaut syndrome and West syndrome. Results appear similar to those in adults; children with partial seizures appeared to respond better with rates between 38% and 49% of patients experiencing between a 50% to 100% reduction in seizure frequency. Vigabatrin also has been examined in the use of intractable infantile spasms and was found to be effective in reducing spasms > 50% in 30 patients (71%), with complete relief of spasms in 16 patients (38%). Caution should be used in the interpretation of these results since great variability can occur with the incidence of infantile seizures over time.

►*Drug Interactions:* One of the major advantages of vigabatrin is the fact that it does not appear to be metabolized by the liver, nor influence hepatic metabolism. Therefore, the typical drug interactions observed with traditional anticonvulsants are not seen with vigabatrin. However, vigabatrin was shown to decrease phenytoin (eg, *Dilantin*) levels by 20% to 30% in clinical trials. No mechanism of action could account for the decreased levels; therefore, phenytoin levels should be monitored if vigabatrin is added. Vigabatrin does not appear to interact with phenobarbital, primidone, carbamazepine (eg, *Tegretol*), or valproate (eg, *Depakene*) to any clinically significant degree.

►*Adverse Reactions:* Vigabatrin appears to be well tolerated with minimal side effects and when they do occur, they are mild. In a trial of 254 patients who received vigabatrin from 12 months to > 2 years, up to 75% of patients reported no side effects. Data from pooled studies indicate that the most common side effects are: Somnolence; fatigue; irritability; dizziness; headache; depression; confusion; poor concentration; abdominal pain; anorexia (some trials have reported weight gain). In the studies involving children, the main side effects observed were agitation and insomnia, with a similar number of patients reporting a lack of side effects (79%).

►*Summary:* Vigabatrin appears to be effective in the treatment of complex partial seizures, less effective for primary generalized seizures, and not effective (and may even worsen) absence and myoclonic seizures. The dosing range is from 1 to 4 g/day in adults, with 2 to 3 g appearing to be the most optimal, and a dose of 50 to 150 mg/kg/day in children. Side effects are minimal and mild and there seems to be a lack of clinically significant drug interactions, except that observed with phenytoin.

Vigabatrin is already available in Europe and Canada and has been deemed approvable in the US.

~ Bibliography Available on Request ~

VILOXAZINE (*Catatrol* by AstraZeneca) – A bicyclic antidepressant

➤*Actions:*

Pharmacology – Viloxazine is a bicyclic antidepressant agent. It has noradrenergic reuptake blocking properties and acts, in part, as an amphetamine-like central stimulant. Overall sympathomimetic, sedative and anticholinergic activity is less than that seen with the tricyclic antidepressants (eg, imipramine [eg, *Tofranil*]). Conflicting data has been reported on the effects of viloxazine on the seizure threshold, with some reports indicating that seizure risk is greater, while others claiming it is less than that seen with traditional tricyclics. Rapid eye movement (REM) sleep and overall sleep time is markedly reduced with viloxazine. It does not appear to potentiate the effects of alcohol.

Pharmacokinetics – Viloxazine is rapidly and almost completely (85%) absorbed after oral administration in the small intestine. Peak blood levels occur 1 to 4 hours after ingestion; however, no correlation has been established between blood levels and clinical response. Volume of distribution averages 0.78 L/kg. The elimiriation half-life ranges from 2 to 5 hours. The drug is extensively metabolized by hydroxylation and oxidation to inactive metabolites in the liver. Only 12% to 15% of the parent compound is eliminated unchanged by the kidneys. In patients > 60 years of age, there appears to be a reduction in viloxazine clearance, possibly due to decreased hepatic metabolism. Specific dosage guidelines in the elderly and patients with hepatic dysfunction have not been established.

Clinical trials – Viloxazine was an effective antidepressant in controlled clinical trials of hospitalized and outpatient populations with depression. Its efficacy appears to be equivalent to imipramine, with a 60% response rate. Published trials have not examined whether efficacy rates vary with specific types of depression. Viloxazine also has been studied in small groups of patients with narcolepsy and cataplexy (a form of narcolepsy characterized by periods of momentary paralysis); this appears to be a potential target population. Fewer sleep attacks were reported during treatment.

➤*Drug Interactions:* Viloxazine decreases the elimination rate of theophylline (eg, *Theo-Dur*), carbamazepine (eg, *Tegretol*), and phenytoin (eg, *Dilantin*), possibly by competing for the same microsomal enzymes. When viloxazine was added to a stable regimen of these drugs, theophylline toxicity was reported (no levels available), carbamazepine levels increased by 55%, and those of its active metabolite by 16%, and phenytoin levels increased by an average of 36%.

➤*Adverse Reactions:* Nausea is the most commonly reported side effect, with an average incidence of 19%, but some studies have reported an incidence as high as 50%. Nausea progressing to vomiting was reported in 4.7% of patients. These effects may be minimized by initiating therapy with low doses accompanied by slow, upward dose titration. Headache is also commonly reported. Less frequently reported side effects include: Insomnia; taste disturbances; hypomania; mania; dizziness; tachycardia; ataxia; tremor; confusion; restlessness; dry mouth; constipation; drowsiness; difficult micturition; seizures. The anticholinergic-related side effects appear to occur less frequently than with the tricyclic agents.

➤*Summary:* Viloxazine is a safe and effective antidepressant with a somewhat different side effect profile than the tricyclic antidepressants, although it is most likely to be used in patients with narcolepsy or cataplexy. Available data has not established whether viloxazine has any advantages over currently available agents. Additional studies in specific populations of patients are needed to establish its place in therapy. Viloxazine currently has orphan drug status for the treatment of cataplexy and narcolepsy.

VINDESINE SULFATE (*Eldisine* by Lilly) – An antineoplastic

➤*Actions:*

Pharmacology – Vindesine sulfate (Lilly 99094, NSC-245467, DAVA, desacetyl vinblastine amide sulfate) is a synthetic vinca alkaloid derived from vinblastine sulfate, but more closely resembling the activity of vincristine.

A large number of studies support its utility in a diverse group of cancer types. Major and dose-limiting toxicities include myelosuppression and neurotoxicity.

The mechanism of vindesine's anticancer action is probably like that of the other vinca alkaloids; it is cell-cycle specific and blocks mitosis with metaphase arrest. Vinca alkaloids bind specifically to cellular microtubules of the mitotic apparatus and disrupt their function. This leads to inability of the dividing cell to correctly segregate chromosomes and ultimately, to cell death.

Pharmacokinetics – Vindesine sulfate appears to have similar pharmacokinetics to vincristine and vinblastine. The triphasic clearance profile of IV vindesine is summarized below:

IV Vindesine Clearance

Phase	Half-life (minutes)	Volume of distribution (liters)
Alpha (α)	3 ± 1	5 ± 2
Beta (β)	99 ± 45	58 ± 51
Gamma (γ)	1213 ± 493	598 ± 294

Elimination in the urine in the first 24 hours accounts for 13.2% of the total dose administered. The remainder is sequestered in the body or eliminated in the bile.

Clinical trials – Overall, vindesine demonstrates good activity in difficult-to-treat and refractory cancer types. Responses to vindesine in patients who have received vincristine or vinblastine therapy suggest a lack of cross-resistance between these agents. Doses have ranged from 3 to 4.5 mg/m^2 as an IV bolus every 1 to 2 weeks *or* 1 to 2 mg/m^2/day for 2 to 10 days every 2 to 3 weeks. The results of clinical studies are summarized below:

Vindesine Clinical Studies

Cancer type	Number of patients treated	Response rate Range (%)	Response rate Average (%)	Complete number of patients
Colorectal	33	6	6	1
Esophageal	76	17 to 55	43	0
Leukemias	26	15 to 61	38	4
Lung	234	17 to 43	30	10
Lymphoma	61	34 to 50	41	4
Metastatic breast	120	0 to 28	18	0
Total	550	0 to 61	29	19

➤*Adverse Reactions:* Major dose-limiting toxicities include myelosuppression and neuropathy. The primary hematologic toxicity is leukopenia, which is reversible with dosage reduction or discontinuation. Anemia and thrombocytopenia occur but are rarely severe. Neurotoxicity appears to be a function of cumulative dose. Patients with hepatic dysfunction and those over 60 years of age may be at greater risk. Neurotoxic manifestations include peripheral paresthesia, decreased tendon reflexes, muscle weakness and myalgia, headache, parotid and jaw pain, constipation, and paralytic ileus.

Other side effects include: Nausea; vomiting; stomatitis; hoarseness; transient hepatic dysfunction; inappropriate antidiuretic hormone secretion; fever; skin rash; alopecia; local cellulitis. Vindesine sulfate is a potent vesicant; avoid extravasation into the SC tissues.

➤*Summary:* Vindesine sulfate is a vinca alkaloid that demonstrates promise for a wide variety of cancer types; however, its full extent of activity remains to be determined. Its major toxicities are similar to those of its family, myelotoxicity and neurotoxicity.

~ Bibliography Available on Request ~

XIMELAGATRAN (*Exanta* by AstraZeneca Pharmaceuticals LP) – An Anticoagulant

➤*Actions:*

Pharmacology – Ximelagatran is an oral, direct, thrombin inhibitor being evaluated as an anticoagulant for prevention of stroke, as a consequence of atrial fibrillation, for primary and secondary prevention and treatment of a venous thromboembolic event (VTE) and for secondary prevention of post-MI. Ximelagatran, a small-molecule prodrug, is converted to its active form melagatran in vivo. Melagatran's anticoagulant effects are reversible and include inhibition of platelet activation and aggregation and reduction of fibrinolysis. Inhibition of circulating and clot-bound thrombin occurs via binding to the active site. Furthermore, this inhibition has been shown to decrease the amount of thrombin generation, most likely because of a reduction of thrombin-mediated positive feedback of the coagulation system.

Pharmacokinetics – Ximelagatran is rapidly absorbed and converted to melagatran postadministration. The bioavailability of melagatran is approximately 20%, peak levels are achieved within 2 hours, and its half-life ranges between 3 and 4 hours. The majority of melagatran is excreted unchanged via the kidney within 12 hours of administration.

Clinical trials – Several randomized, multicenter trials (Melagatran for thrombin inhibition in orthopedic surgery [METHRO], Expanded prophylaxis evaluation surgery study [EXPRESS], *Exanta* used to lessen thrombosis [EXULT]) to determine the efficacy and safety of ximelagatran for VTE prophylaxis in patients undergoing orthopedic hip or knee surgeries have been performed. Ximelagatran was compared with standard regimens of either warfarin or enoxaparin in these studies. A randomized, double-blind, multicenter, dose-finding study enrolling 443 patients evaluated ximelagatran for the prevention of VTE post-knee surgery. In this study, no significant difference was observed in the incidence of VTE between ximelagatran and enoxaparin. However, in a second randomized, double-blind, multicenter trial enrolling 1,557 patients designed to evaluate ximelagatran in the prevention of VTE post-hip surgery, ximelagatran exhibited a small but significantly higher incidence of VTE compared with enoxaparin (3.3%, 95% CI). Comparison for VTE prevention post-knee surgery in 3 different randomized, double-blind, multicenter trials enrolling a total of 4,337 patients showed ximelagatran to have comparable efficacy to warfarin at doses of 24 mg twice daily and higher efficacy at doses of 36 mg twice daily (EXULT A: 20.3% with ximelagatran vs 27.6% with warfarin, P = 0.003; EXULT B: 22.5% vs 31%, P < 0.001).

Thrombin inhibitor in venous thromboembolism (THRIVE) is a randomized, double-blind, multicenter trial enrolling 1,233 patients that evaluated the efficacy and safety of ximelagatran as compared with placebo in the extended secondary prevention of venous thromboembolism after 6 months of warfarin therapy. Over an 18-month follow-up, ximelagatran significantly reduced the recurrence rate of VTE (2.8% risk with ximelagatran vs 12.6% risk with placebo, P < 0.001) with continued reduction of risk over time.

The safety and efficacy of ximelagatran in prevention of stroke in patients with nonvalvular atrial fibrillation has been evaluated in randomized trials (stroke prevention using the oral direct thrombin inhibitor ximelagatran in patients with nonvalvular atrial fibrillation [SPORTIF]). A total of 7,329 participants randomized in SPORTIF III and IV trials had a diagnosis of atrial fibrillation plus at least 1 risk factor for stroke. Trial results have shown ximelagatran to have comparable efficacy to warfarin in prevention of stroke and systemic embolic events among high-risk patients.

A randomized, placebo-controlled, multicenter dose-finding study (Efficacy and safety of the oral direct thrombin inhibitor ximelagatran in patients with recent myocardial damage [ESTEEM]) to compare the effectiveness of ximelagatran with placebo for prevention of severe ischemia, nonfatal MI, and death in patients with history of a recent MI was performed. A total of 1,900 patients were randomized to receive 1 of 4 doses of oral ximelagatran twice daily or placebo for 6 months. All patients also received up to 160 mg of acetylsalicylic acid (ASA) once daily. Ximelagatran in combination with ASA was more effective than ASA alone when the composite endpoint of death, non-fatal MI, and severe recurrent ischemia were evaluated (12.7% vs 16.3%, respectively; P = 0.036). Additionally, incidence of major bleeding with ximelagatran was higher when compared with placebo (1.8% vs 0.9%, respectively).

➤*Adverse Reactions:* Ximelagatran has been associated with few adverse events in clinical trials. The incidence of bleeding is similar to that observed with warfarin or enoxaparin. Asymptomatic elevations of ALT have occurred at rates higher than those associated with warfarin; however, the elevated levels have spontaneously decreased with continued treatment or post-discontinuation of the drug.

➤*Summary:* Ximelagatran is an oral, direct, thrombin inhibitor that has proven effective in prevention of stroke as a consequence of atrial fibrillation in primary and secondary prevention and treatment of a VTE and in secondary prevention of post-MI. Its convenient route of oral administration and predictable pharmacokinetic and pharmacodynamic profile provide an advantage in its use over that of currently available anticoagulants; however, these benefits will most likely be weighed against its twice-daily dosing, higher cost, and incidence of hepatic effects. AstraZeneca Pharmaceuticals LP filed an NDA for ximelagatran in December 2003. Phase 3 trials are in progress. Ximelagatran is currently approved in France.

ZICONOTIDE (by Elan Pharmaceuticals) – A unique non-narcotic analgesic

➤*Actions:*

Pharmacology – Ziconotide (SNX-111) is a non-opioid analgesic being evaluated for the treatment of chronic intractable pain. It is an omega-conotoxin that is synthetically derived from a substance isolated from cone-snail venom, and appears to be 100 to 1000 times more potent than morphine. Ziconotide is a voltage-sensitive, N-type neuronal calcium channel blocker that reversibly blocks critical openings in nerve cells, thus interrupting pain transmission from the spinal cord to the brain. Because it is selective for pain-associated channels through which calcium travels, it does not interfere with channels that transmit normal sensations. Therefore, the pain is relieved without numbness. Initial animal models showed that it acts synergistically with morphine without producing tolerance or cross-tolerance to morphine analgesia.

Pharmacokinetics – Pharmacokinetic data on ziconotide have not been published. Current administration is intrathecal (including through an implantable pump), but Elan is developing epidural administration.

Clinical trials – There are no published clinical trials on the use of ziconotide for the treatment of chronic pain. In a phase II, randomized, double-blind study, researchers evaluated ziconotide for the treatment of acute postoperative pain. Results showed the high-dose (7 mcg/hr) ziconotide group required significantly fewer additional analgesics than the low-dose (0.7 mcg/hr) group and the placebo group, but also produced more significant adverse effects. The low-dose ziconotide group required fewer additional morphine equivalents compared with the placebo group, but this was not statistically significant. Also, chronic administration of ziconotide for 7 days did not produce tolerance to the antinociceptive effects when compared with morphine controls.

Ziconotide also has been evaluated as a possible treatment for severe spasticity after spinal cord injury. Two case reports showed a significant decrease in spasticity, but only one of the patients had successful pain relief. The other patient developed side effects that prohibited an increase in the dosage, and, therefore, was unable to obtain pain relief.

The FDA's acceptance of Elan's NDA for ziconotide was based on the initial results from an unpublished phase III clinical trial in > 700 patients with intractable pain, in which ziconotide produced significant pain relief in 57% of patients.

➤*Adverse Reactions:* The most commonly reported adverse effects were dizziness, blurred vision, sedation, nausea, and lateral-gaze nystagmus. These effects were dose-dependent and usually resolved with sympathetic treatment or dosage reduction. Other less common adverse reactions included dysmetria, confusion, hallucinations, agitation, disorientation, hypotension, rash, and liver enzyme elevations. These effects may take days to weeks to completely resolve after the discontinuation of ziconotide. Although ziconotide may be absent from CSF after discontinuation, it appears to remain active in the tissues for extended periods of time. To lessen the likelihood of these effects, one author proposed extending the time between dosage elevations and starting with very low doses. Patients did not show signs of tolerance or addiction to ziconotide even after several months of treatment.

➤*Summary:* Ziconotide selectively blocks the N-type neuronal calcium channels, therefore inhibiting nerve impulse from the spine to the brain. Initial clinical trials show ziconotide to be a safe and effective treatment option for chronic intractable pain. Adverse effects appear to be minor and manageable with dose reduction and symptomatic care. Ziconotide's advantages over traditional opiates are that it does not appear to be addictive or produce tolerance to its analgesic effects. The main disadvantage is the route of administration: Ziconotide is currently administered by the intrathecal route with the option of an implantable pump. Elan is currently developing epidural administration. More clinical trials are needed to further evaluate the safety and effectiveness of ziconotide. Elan received an FDA approvable letter on June 28, 2000.

FDA NEW DRUG CLASSIFICATION

The FDA developed an alpha-numeric drug classification to aid in the prioritization of a new drug review. The use of numbers identify the drug's chemical classification; letters identify the assessment of thera-peutic potential or review priority. This system was revised in 1992. When the classification for a new drug is known, it is listed in paren-theses following the approval date for the drug at the beginning of the Administration and Dosage section of the monograph.

FDA Classification System for Newly Approved Drugs	
Chemical Ranking	
1 =	New chemical entity not previously marketed in US
2 =	New salt form of a drug currently on US market
3 =	New dosage formulation of a drug currently on US market
4 =	New combination of drugs already available in US
5 =	New manufacturer (ie, generic drug)
6 =	New indication for drug already approved
7 =	Marketed drug without an approved NDA (drugs marketed prior to 1938)
Therapeutic Potential/Review Priority	
A =	Represents significant therapeutic gain over drugs currently available *(replaced by "P" ranking in 1992)*
AA =	Represents important therapeutic gain for drugs indicated for AIDS
B =	Represents modest therapeutic advances in drug therapy *(replaced by "P" ranking in 1992)*
C =	Represents little or no therapeutic gain in drug class *(replaced by "S" ranking in 1992)*
E =	Drug used to treat life-threatening or severely debilitated patients
P =	Priority; represents a therapeutic gain or provides improved treatment over marketed drugs OR has mod-est advantages compared to marketed agents (this category was initiated in first quarter of 1992)
S =	Standard; has similar therapeutic properties when compared to marketed drugs (this category was initi-ated in the first quarter of 1992)

CONTROLLED SUBSTANCES

CONTROLLED SUBSTANCES

The Controlled Substances Act of 1970 regulates the manufacturing, distribution and dispensing of drugs that have abuse potential. The Drug Enforcement Administration (DEA) within the US Department of Justice is the chief federal agency responsible for enforcing the act.

➤*DEA Schedules:* Drugs under jurisdiction of the Controlled Sub-stances Act are divided into five schedules based on their potential for abuse and physical and psychological dependence. All controlled sub-stances listed in *Drug Facts and Comparisons®* are identified by sched-ule as follows:

Schedule I *(c-ı):* High abuse potential and no accepted medical use (eg, heroin, marijuana, LSD).

Schedule II *(c-ıı):* High abuse potential with severe dependence liability (eg, narcotics, amphetamines, dronabinol, some barbiturates).

Schedule III *(c-ııı):* Less abuse potential than schedule II drugs and moderate dependence liability (eg, nonbarbiturate sedatives, nonam-phetamine stimulants, limited amounts of certain narcotics).

Schedule IV *(c-ıv):* Less abuse potential than schedule III drugs and limited dependence liability (eg, some sedatives, antianxiety agents, nonnarcotic analgesics).

Schedule V *(c-v):* Limited abuse potential. Primarily small amounts of narcotics (codeine) used as antitussives or antidiarrheals. Under fed-eral law, limited quantities of certain *c-v* drugs may be purchased with-out a prescription directly from a pharmacist if allowed under state statutes. The purchaser must be at least 18 years of age and must fur-nish suitable identification. All such transactions must be recorded by the dispensing pharmacist.

➤*Registration:* Prescribing physicians and dispensing pharmacies must be registered with the DEA, PO Box 28083, Central Station, Washington, DC 20005.

➤*Inventory:* Separate records must be kept of purchases and dispens-ing of controlled substances. An inventory of controlled substances must be made every 2 years.

➤*Prescriptions:* Prescriptions for controlled substances must be writ-ten in ink and include: Date; name and address of the patient; name, address and DEA number of the physician. Oral prescriptions must be promptly committed to writing. Controlled substance prescriptions may not be dispensed or refilled more than 6 months after the date issued or be refilled more than five times. A written prescription signed by the physician is required for schedule II drugs. In case of emergency, oral prescriptions for schedule II substances may be filled; however, the physician must provide a signed prescription within 72 hours. Schedule II prescriptions cannot be refilled. A triplicate order form is necessary for the transfer of controlled substances in schedule II. Forms are avail-able for the individual prescriber at no charge from the DEA.

➤*State Laws:* In many cases state laws are more restrictive than fed-eral laws and therefore impose additional requirements (eg, triplicate prescription forms).

The rational use of any medication requires a risk versus benefit assessment. Among the myriad of risk factors which complicate this assessment, pregnancy is one of the most perplexing.

The FDA has established five categories to indicate the potential of a systemically absorbed drug for causing birth defects. The key differentiation among the categories rests upon the degree (reliability) of documentation and the risk vs benefit ratio. Pregnancy Category X is particularly notable in that if any data exists that may implicate a drug as a teratogen and the risk vs benefit ratio does not support use of the drug, the drug is contraindicated during pregnancy. These categories are summarized below:

FDA Pregnancy Categories	
Pregnancy Category	**Definition**
A	Controlled studies show no risk. Adequate, well-controlled studies in pregnant women have failed to demonstrate risk to the fetus.
B	No evidence of risk in humans. Either animal findings show risk, but human findings do not; or if no adequate human studies have been done, animal findings are negative.
C	Risk cannot be ruled out. Human studies are lacking, and animal studies are either positive for fetal risk or lacking. However, potential benefits may justify the potential risks.
D	Positive evidence of risk. Investigational or post-marketing data show risk to the fetus. Nevertheless, potential benefits may outweigh the potential risks. If needed in a life-threatening situation or a serious disease, the drug may be acceptable if safer drugs cannot be used or are ineffective.
X	Contraindicated in pregnancy. Studies in animals or human, or investigational or post-marketing reports have shown fetal risk which clearly outweighs any possible benefit to the patient.

Regardless of the designated Pregnancy Category or presumed safety, no drug should be administered during pregnancy unless it is clearly needed and potential benefits outweigh potential hazards to the fetus.

ANTIHYPERTENSIVES

►*Definition of hypertension:* Hypertension is defined as a systolic blood pressure (SBP) of greater than 140 mm Hg, diastolic blood pressure (DBP) of greater than 90 mm Hg, or the use of an antihypertensive medication. The classification of prehypertension recognizes the relationship between blood pressure (BP) and the risk of cardiovascular disease (CVD) events and calls for increased education of health care professionals and the public in order to reduce BP levels. Patients with SBP of 120 to 139 or a DBP of 80 to 89 should be considered prehypertensive and are at an increased risk for developing hypertension. These patients require health promoting lifestyle modifications to prevent CVD. In individuals 40 to 70 years of age, each elevation of 20 mm Hg in SBP or every 10 mm Hg in DBP doubles the risk of CVD across the entire BP range from 115/75 to 185/115 mm Hg. As a result, identifying and treating high BP decreases cardiovascular mortality and morbidity in these patients and protects against hypertension related complications of stroke, coronary events, heart failure, renal disease progression, progression to more severe hypertension, and all-cause mortality. In order to identify high-risk individuals, the following table presents the classification of adult BP.

Classification of BP for Adults ≥ 18 Years of Age[1]			
Category	Systolic (mm Hg)		Diastolic (mm Hg)
Normal	< 120	and	< 80
Prehypertension[2]	120 to 139	or	80 to 89
Hypertension,[3] Stage 1	140 to 159	or	90 to 99
Hypertension,[3] Stage 2	≥ 160	or	≥ 100

[1] Not taking antihypertensive drugs and not acutely ill. When systolic and diastolic BPs fall into 2 different categories, select the higher category to classify the individual's BP status.
[2] Require health promoting lifestyle modifications to prevent CVD.
[3] Based on the average of ≥ 2 readings taken at each of ≥ 2 visits after an initial screening; also requires health promoting lifestyle modifications.

►*BP measurement:* Measure BP in a standardized fashion using equipment that meets certification criteria.
- Seat patients in a chair with their backs supported and their arms bared and supported at heart level. Tell patients to refrain from smoking or ingesting caffeine during the 30 minutes preceding the measurement.
- Under special circumstances, measuring BP in the supine and standing positions may be indicated.
- Begin measurement after 5 minutes or more of rest.
- Use the appropriate cuff size to ensure accurate measurement. Make sure the bladder within the cuff encircles at least 80% of the arm. Many adults will require a large adult cuff.
- Take measurements preferably with a mercury sphygmomanometer; otherwise, a recently calibrated aneroid manometer or a validated electronic device can be used.
- Record SBP and DBP. The first appearance of sound (phase 1) is used to define SBP. The disappearance of sound (phase 5) is used to define DBP.
- Take the average of 2 or more readings separated by 2 minutes. If the first 2 readings differ by more than 5 mm Hg, obtain an average additional reading.

►*Risk stratification:*

Major Cardiovascular Disease (CVD) Risk Factors
General
Hypertension
Cigarette smoking
Obesity (body mass index ≥ 30 kg/m²)
Physical inactivity
Dyslipidemia
Diabetes mellitus
Microalbuminuria or estimated GFR < 60 mL/min
Age (> 55 years for men, > 65 years for women)
Family history of premature cardiovascular disease (women 65 years of age or men < 55 years of age)
Target organ damage
Heart disease
Left ventricular hypertrophy
Angina/prior MI
Heart failure
Prior coronary revascularization
Brain
Stroke or transient ischemic attack
Chronic kidney disease
Peripheral arterial disease
Retinopathy

Assess for Identifiable Causes of Hypertension
Sleep apnea
Drug induced/related
Chronic kidney disease
Primary aldosteronism
Renovascular disease
Cushing syndrome or steroid therapy
Pheochromocytoma
Coarctation of aorta
Thyroid/parathyroid disease

►*Pharmacotherapy:* The use of pharmacologic agents to reduce BP has demonstrated decreases in cardiovascular morbidity and mortality protection against stroke, coronary events, heart failure, renal disease progression, progression to more severe hypertension, and all-cause mortality.

Goals of therapy: The ultimate goal is to reduce cardiovascular complications and renal morbidity and mortality. In patients 50 years of age or older, the primary focus should be on achieving the SBP goal, then the DBP goal will automatically fall into place. SBP and DBP treatment to targets of less than 140/90 mm Hg is associated with a decrease in CVD complications. In hypertensive diabetes or renal disease patients, the BP goal is less than 130/80 mm Hg.

Prevention and management: Reduction of morbidity and mortality may be attained by achieving and maintaining SBP 140 mm Hg or less and DBP 90 mm Hg or less if tolerated and controlling other modifiable risk factors for cardiovascular disease. This may be accomplished by lifestyle modification alone or with pharmacologic therapy.

Lifestyle modifications: Prescribe lifestyle modifications for all patients with prehypertension and hypertension.
- Lifestyle modifications offer the potential for preventing hypertension, lowering BP, and reducing other cardiovascular risk factors at little cost and with minimal risk. Strongly encourage patients to adopt these lifestyle modifications, particularly if they have additional risk factors for premature cardiovascular disease, such as dyslipidemia or diabetes mellitus. Even when lifestyle modifications alone are not adequate in controlling hypertension, they may reduce the number and dosage of antihypertensive medications needed to manage the condition.

Lifestyle Modifications for Hypertension Management[1,2]		
Modification	Recommendation	Approximate SBP reduction
Weight loss	Maintain normal body weight index	5 to 20 mm Hg per 10 kg of weight loss
Institute DASH eating plan	Start a diet rich in vegetables, fruit, and low fat dietary products with a decreased content of saturated and total fat	8 to 14 mm Hg
Dietary sodium restriction	Reduce dietary sodium intake to 2.4 g sodium or 6 g sodium chloride	2 to 8 mm Hg
Limit alcohol consumption	Limit alcohol intake to less than 30 mL ethanol (eg, 720 mL beer, 300 mL wine, or 90 mL 80 proof whiskey) per day or 15 mL ethanol in women and lighter weight individuals	2 to 4 mm Hg
Physical activity	Regular aerobic activity at least 30 minutes/day on most days of the week.	4 to 9 mm Hg

[1] For overall cardiovascular risk, discontinue tobacco use.
[2] Effects of these modifications are time and dose dependent and may be enhanced for some individuals.

Considerations for individualizing drug therapy: The table below describes compelling indications that require certain antihypertensive drug classes for high-risk conditions. The drug selections for each compelling indication are based on favorable clinical data.

Compelling Indications for Individual Drug Classes	
Compelling indication[1]	Recommended drug therapy[2]
Heart failure	Thiazide, BB, ACEI, ARB, ALDO ant
Post-MI	BB, ACEI, ALDO ant
High CVD risk	Thiazide, BB, ACEI, CCB
Diabetes	Thiazide, BB, ACEI, ARB, CCB
Chronic kidney disease	ACEI, ARB
Recurrent stroke prevention	Thiazide, ACEI

[1] Compelling indications for antihypertensive drugs are based on benefits from clinical study outcomes; the compelling indication is managed in parallel with the BP.
[2] BB = beta blocker; ACEI = angiotensin converting enzyme inhibitor; ARB = angiotensin receptor blocker; CCB = calcium channel blocker; ALDO ant = aldosterone antagonist.

ANTIHYPERTENSIVES

Initial drug therapy: When a decision has been made to begin antihypertensive therapy and there are no compelling indications for another type of drug, choose a thiazide-type diuretic, either alone or in combination with 1 of the other classes (eg, ACEI, ARB, BB, CCB). Numerous randomized controlled trials have shown a reduction in morbidity and mortality with these agents. The majority of patients who are hypertensive will require treatment with 2 or more antihypertensive medications in order to achieve their BP goals of less than 140/90 mm Hg or less than 130/80 mm Hg for patients with diabetes or chronic kidney disease. When BP is more than 20/10 mm Hg above goal BP, consider initiating therapy with 2 drugs, 1 of which is usually a thiazide-type diuretic, either as separate drugs or in fixed-dose combinations. Use caution and observe those patients at risk for orthostatic hypotension, such as diabetic patients and the elderly.

Follow-up recommendations: Once antihypertensive therapy is initiated, follow-ups at monthly intervals are necessary until BP goal is reached. Patients with stage 2 hypertension or with complicating comorbid conditions will require more frequent visits. Once BP is controlled and at goal, follow-up visits should take place at 3- to 6-month intervals. Comorbidities, such as heart failure and diabetes will also dictate the frequency of office visits and laboratory tests. Monitor serum potassium and creatinine levels at least once or twice per year. Consider low-dose aspirin therapy only once BP is controlled.

►*Special patient populations:*

Race: Most black people are at greater risk for the development of high BP, type 2 diabetes, coronary heart disease, left ventricular hypertension, stroke, and end-stage renal disease. As monotherapy, BBs, ARBs, and ACEIs may produce less BP lowering effects than thiazide diuretics and CCBs. Consider the following antihypertensive combinations: BB/diuretic, ACEI/diuretic, ACEI/CCB, or ARB/diuretic. For patients with uncomplicated hypertension, the target BP is less than 140/90 mm Hg, and for patients with high risk for cardiovascular events in association with type 2 diabetes or renal insufficiency, the target BP goal is less than 130/80 mm Hg. When prescribing ACEIs for black patients, it is important to note that there appears to be an increased risk for ACEI-associated angioedema and/or cough.

Resistant hypertension: Failure to reach BP goal in patients who followed proper treatment is known as resistant hypertension. Consider a consultation with a BP specialist if target BP cannot be achieved. See table for causes of resistant hypertension.

Causes of Resistant Hypertension
Improper BP measurement
Volume overload and pseudotolerance
Excess sodium intake
Volume retention from kidney disease
Inadequate diuretic therapy
Drug-induced or other causes
Nonadherence
Inadequate doses
Inappropriate combinations
Nonsteroidal anti-inflammatory drugs; cyclooxygenase 2 inhibitors
Cocaine, amphetamines, other illicit drugs
Sympathomimetics (decongestants, anoretics)
Oral contraceptives
Adrenal steroids
Cyclosporine and tacrolimus
Erythropoietin
Licorice (including some chewing tobacco)
Selected over the counter dietary supplements and medicines (eg, ephedra, ma haung, bitter orange)
Associated conditions
Obesity
Excess alcohol intake
Identifiable causes of hypertension

Hypertensive emergencies: Patients with marked BP elevations that also have acute target-organ damage (eg, encephalopathy, MI, unstable angina, pulmonary edema, eclampsia, stroke, head trauma, life-threatening arterial bleed, aortic dissection) require parenteral drug therapy and hospitalization. Patients with BP elevation without target-organ damage do not require hospitalization, but should receive immediate oral antihypertensive therapy while being carefully evaluated and monitored for precipitating causes or hypertension-induced heart or kidney disease.

Considerations for Individualizing Antihypertensive Drug Therapy[1]	
Indication	Drug therapy
May have favorable effects on comorbid conditions[2]	
Angina	Beta blockers, CCB
Atrial tachycardia and fibrillation	Beta blockers, CCB (non-DHP)
Cyclosporine-induced hypertension (caution with the dose of cyclosporine)	CCB
Diabetes mellitus (types 1 and 2) with proteinuria	ACE 1 (preferred), CCB
Diabetes mellitus (type 2)	Low-dose diuretics
Dyslipidemia	Alpha blockers
Essential tremor	Beta blockers (non-CS)
Heart failure	Carvedilol, losartan potassium
Hyperthyroidism	Beta blockers
Migraine	Beta blockers (non-CS), CCB (non-DHP)
MI	Diltiazem HCl, verapamil HCl
Osteoporosis	Thiazides
Preoperative hypertension	Beta blockers
Prostatism (BPH)	Alpha blockers
Renal insufficiency (caution in renovascular hypertension and creatinine ≥ 265.2 mmol/L [3 mg/dL])	ACEI
May have unfavorable effects on comorbid conditions[2,3]	
Bronchospastic disease	Beta blockers[4]
Depression	Beta blockers, central alpha agonists, reserpine[4]
Diabetes mellitus (types 1 and 2)	Beta blockers, high-dose diuretics
Dyslipidemia	Beta blockers (non-ISA), diuretics (high-dose)
Gout	Diuretics
2° or 3° heart block	Beta blockers,[4] CCB (non-DHP)[4]
Heart failure	Beta blockers (except carvedilol), CCB (except amlodipine besylate, felodipine)
Liver disease	Labetalol HCl, methyldopa[4]
Peripheral vascular disease	Beta blockers
Pregnancy	ACEI,[4] angiotensin II receptor blockers[4]
Renal insufficiency	Potassium-sparing agents
Renovascular disease	ACEI, angiotensin II receptor blockers

[1] ACEI= angiotensin-converting enzyme inhibitors; BPH = benign prostatic hyperplasia; CCB = calcium channel blocker; DHP = dihydropyridine; ISA = intrinsic sympathomimetic activity; MI = myocardial infarction; non-CS = noncardioselective.
[2] Conditions and drugs are listed in alphabetical order.
[3] These drugs may be used with special monitoring unless contraindicated.
[4] Contraindicated.

ALGORITHM FOR TREATMENT OF HYPERTENSION*

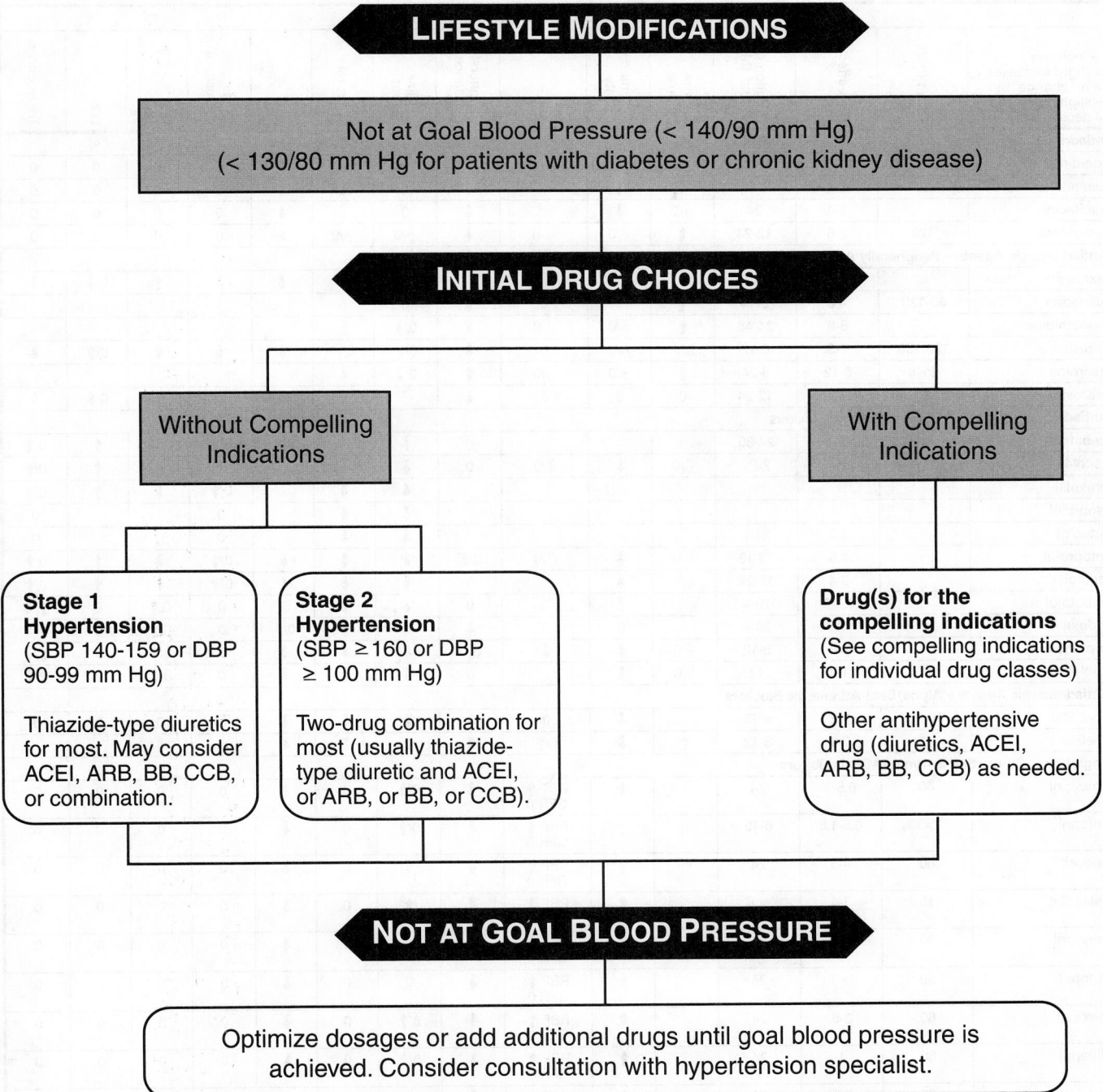

LIFESTYLE MODIFICATIONS

Not at Goal Blood Pressure (< 140/90 mm Hg)
(< 130/80 mm Hg for patients with diabetes or chronic kidney disease)

INITIAL DRUG CHOICES

Without Compelling Indications

With Compelling Indications

Stage 1 Hypertension
(SBP 140-159 or DBP 90-99 mm Hg)

Thiazide-type diuretics for most. May consider ACEI, ARB, BB, CCB, or combination.

Stage 2 Hypertension
(SBP ≥ 160 or DBP ≥ 100 mm Hg)

Two-drug combination for most (usually thiazide-type diuretic and ACEI, or ARB, or BB, or CCB).

Drug(s) for the compelling indications
(See compelling indications for individual drug classes)

Other antihypertensive drug (diuretics, ACEI, ARB, BB, CCB) as needed.

NOT AT GOAL BLOOD PRESSURE

Optimize dosages or add additional drugs until goal blood pressure is achieved. Consider consultation with hypertension specialist.

DBP, diastolic blood pressure; SBP, systolic blood pressure.
Drug abbreviations: ACEI, angiotensin converting enzyme inhibitor; ARB, angiotensin receptor blocker; BB, beta blocker; CCB, calcium channel blocker.

* *The Seventh Report of the Joint National Committee on Prevention, Detection, Evaluation, and Treatment of High Blood Pressure.* National Institutes of Health. May 2003.

ANTIHYPERTENSIVES

Agents used in hypertension therapy are listed in the following tables:

Pharmacological Effects of Antihypertensive Agents

Legend: ↑ = increase · ⇧ = slight increases · 0 = no change · ⇩ = slight decrease · ↓ = decrease

Agent	Onset (min)	Peak effect[1] (h)	Duration of action[2] (h)	Plasma volume	Plasma renin activity	RBF GFR[3]	Peripheral resistance	Cardiac output	Heart rate	LVH	Total cholesterol	HDL	LDL	Triglycerides
Antiadrenergic Agents – Centrally Acting														
Clonidine	30-60	2-5	12-24	↑	⇩	⇩/0	↓	⇩/0	↓	↓	0	0	0	0
Guanabenz	60	2-4	6-12	0	↓	0	↓	0	↓	↓	0	0	0	0
Guanfacine		1-4	24	⇩/0	↓		↓	0	⇩	↓	0	0	0	0
Methyldopa	120	2-6	12-24	↑	⇩/0	⇩/0	↓	⇩/0	⇩/0	↓	0	0	0	0
Antiadrenergic Agents – Peripherally Acting														
Doxazosin		2-3								↓	↓	↑	0/↓	↓
Guanadrel	30-120	4-6	9-14	↑		0	↓	0	↓					
Guanethidine		6-8	24-48	↑	⇩/0	⇩/0	↓	0/↓	↓					
Prazosin	120-130	1-3	6-12	0/⇧	⇩/0	0	↓	0/⇧	0/⇧	↓	↓	↑	0/↑	↓
Reserpine	days	6-12	6-24	↑	⇩/0	⇩/0	↑	0/↓	↓					
Terazosin	15	1-2	12-24	0	0	0	↓	⇧	⇧	↓	↓	↑	0/↓	↓
Antiadrenergic Agents – Beta-Adrenergic Blockers														
Acebutolol		3-8	24-30		⇩			↓	↓	0/↓	0/↑	↓	↑	0/↑
Atenolol		2-4	24 +		⇩/0	↓/0	0	↓	↓	↓	0/↑	↓	↑	0/↑
Betaxolol								↓	↓		0/↑	↓	↑	0/↑
Bisoprolol								↓	↓		0			0
Carteolol		1-3	24 +					↓	↓		0			0
Metoprolol		1.5	13-19	⇩/0	↓	⇩/0	0/↓	↓	↓	↓	0/↑	↓	↑	0/↑
Nadolol		3-4	17-24	⇩/0	↓	0	0	↓	↓	↓	0/↑	↓	↑	0/↑
Penbutolol		1.5-3	20 +	↓	⇩	0		↓	↓	0	0/↑	0	0	↑/↓
Pindolol		1	24 +	0	0	0	↓	⇩	⇩	0/↓	0	0/↑	0	↑/↓
Propranolol		2-4	8-12	⇩/0	↓	⇩/0	↓	↓	↓	0	0/↑	0	0	↑/↓
Timolol		1-3	12	⇩/0	↓		0	↓	↓	↓	0/↑	0	0	↑/↓
Antiadrenergic Agents – Alpha/Beta-Adrenergic Blockers														
Carvedilol	30-60	1-2	> 15	↓	0	↓	↓	↓	↓	0	0	0	0	0
Labetalol		2-4	8-12	↑	↓	0/↑	↓	0	↓	↓				
Angiotensin-Converting Enzyme (ACE) Inhibitors														
Benazepril	60	0.5-1	24		↑	RBF ↑, GFR 0	↓	0/↑	0	↓	0	0	0	0
Captopril	15-30	0.5-1.5	6-12	⇧	↑	RBF ↑, GFR 0	↓	0/↑	0	↓	0	0	0	0
Enalapril	60	4-6	24	0/⇧	↑	RBF ↑, GFR 0	↓	↑	0	↓	0	0	0	0
Enalaprilat	15	3-4	≈ 6		↑	RBF ↑, GFR 0	↓	↑	0	↓	0	0	0	0
Fosinopril	60	≈ 3	24		↑	RBF ↑, GFR 0	↓	0/↑	0	↓	0	0	0	0
Lisinopril	60	≈ 7	24		↑	RBF ↑, GFR 0	↓	0	0	↓	0	0	0	0
Moexipril	60	3-6	24		↑	RBF ↑, GFR 0	↓	0/↑	0	↓	0	0	0	0
Quinapril	60	1	24		↑	RBF ↑, GFR 0	↓	0/↑	0	↓	0	0	0	0
Perindopril	60	3-7	24		↑	GFR 0	↓	0/↑	0	↓	0	0	0	0
Ramipril	60-120	1	24		↑	RBF ↑, GFR 0	↓	0/↑	0	↓	0	0	0	0
Trandolapril	120-240	6-8	24		↑	RBF ↑, GFR 0	↓	0/↑	0	↓	0	0	0	0
Angiotensin II Receptor Antagonists														
Candesartan	120-180	6-8	> 24	↓	↑	RBF ⇧, GFR 0	↓	↑	0	↓	0	0	0	0
Eprosartan	60-120	1-3	24	↓	↑	RBF ⇧, GFR 0	↓	↑	0	↓	0	0	0	0
Irbesartan	90-120	3-6	24	↓	↑	RBF ⇧[4], GFR 0	↓	↑	0	↓	0	0	0	0
Losartan	120-180	6	24	↓	↑	RBF ⇧[4], GFR 0	↓	↑	0	↓	0	0	0	0
Telmisartan	180	3-9	24	↓	↑	RBF ⇧[4], GFR 0	↓	↑	0	↓	0	0	0	0
Valsartan	120	6	24	↓	↑	RBF ⇧[4], GFR 0	↓	↑	0	↓	0	0	0	0
Olmesartan		1-2	24	↓	↑	RBF ⇧[4], GFR 0	↓	↑	0	↓	0	0	0	0

ANTIHYPERTENSIVES

Pharmacological Effects of Antihypertensive Agents

Legend:
- ↑ = increase
- ⇑ = slight increases
- 0 = no change
- ⇓ = slight decrease
- ↓ = decrease

	Onset (min)	Peak effect[1] (h)	Duration of action[2] (h)	Plasma volume	Plasma renin activity	RBF GFR[3]	Peripheral resistance	Cardiac output	Heart rate	LVH	Total cholesterol	HDL	LDL	Triglycerides
Calcium Channel Blocking Agents														
Amlodipine	gradual	6-12	> 24	0	0	↑	↓↓↓	0	0	↓	0	0	0	0
Diltiazem SR	30-60	6-11			0		↓	0-↑	↓-0	↓	0	0	0	0
Felodipine	120-300	2.5-5			0		↓↓↓	↑	↑	↓	0	0	0	0
Isradipine	120	1.5					↓↓↓	↑	↑/↓	↓	0	0	0	0
Nicardipine	20	0.5-2			⇑/↑	↑	↓	↑	↑	↓	0	0/⇑	0	0
Nifedipine SR	20	6				RBF↑ GFR↑	↓↓↓	↑↑	↑	↓	0	0	0	0
Nisoldipine		1.5[5]			0		↓	⇑	⇑	↓	0	0	0	0
Verapamil	30	1-2.2			0/⇑	RBF↑ GFR⇑	↓	↑/↓	↑/↓	↓	0	0/⇑	0	0
Diuretics														
Amiloride	120	6-10	24	↓	↑	0	↓	↓	0					
Loop diuretics	within 60	1-2	4-8	↓	↑	↑	↓	↓	0	0/↓	↑	0	↑	↑
Spironolactone	24-48 hr	48-72	48-72	↓	↑	0	↓	0	0					
Thiazides and derivatives	60-120	4-12	6-72	↓	↑	↓	↓	↓	0	0/↓	↑	0	↑	↑
Triamterene	2-4 hr	6-8	12-16											
Vasodilators														
Hydralazine	45	0.5-2	6-8	↑	↑	↑	↓	↑	↑	↑				
Minoxidil	30	2-3	24-72	↑	↑	0	↓	↑	↑	↑				
Agents For Pheochromocytoma														
Phentolamine	immed.		5-10 min	⇑	↑	↑	↓	0/↑	↑					
Phenoxy-benzamine	gradual	2-3	24 +	⇑	↑	↑	↓	↑	↓					
Metyrosine		6 +	2-3 days				↓		↓					
Agents For Hypertensive Emergencies/Urgencies														
Captopril[6]				⇑	↑	RBF↑ GFR 0	↓	0/↑	0					
Clonidine	< 5			↑	⇓	⇓/0	↓	⇓/0	↓	↓				
Diazoxide	1-2	5 min	< 12	↑	↑	↑	↓	↑	↑					
Enalaprilat[6]					↑	RBF↑ GFR 0	↓	↑	0					
Esmolol	1-2	5	10-20	0	0		↓	↓	⇓			NA		
Fenoldopam	5		30-60		↑	RBF⇑ GFR 0	⇓		⇑					
Hydralazine	10-20		3-6											
Labetalol	5-10		3-6	↑	↓	0/↑	↓	0	↓					
Nicardipine (IV)	1-5		3-6		⇑/↑	⇑	↓	↑	↑					
Nitroglycerin (IV)[6]	immed.		transient	0	0		↓	↑	↑					
Nitroprusside	0.5-1		3-5 min	↑	↑	0	↓	⇓	⇑					
Phentolamine[6]	1-2		3-10 min											
Miscellaneous Agents														
Tolazoline[6]							↓							
Eplerenone		1.5	> 24	↓	↑		↓		0		⇓	⇑		↑

[1] Peak clinical effect following a single oral dose, except where indicated.
[2] Duration of action is frequently dose-dependent.
[3] Renal blood flow and glomerular filtration rate.
[4] Experimental and small clinical studies indicate that angiotensin II receptor antagonists have effects on renal function similar to ACEIs.
[5] Immediate release; 6 to 12 hours for extended release.
[6] Unlabeled use.

H. PYLORI AGENTS

Helicobacter pylori is found in ≈ 100% of chronic active antral gastritis cases, 90% to 95% of duodenal ulcer patients, and 50% to 80% of gastric ulcer patients. The treatment of documented *H. pylori* infection in patients with confirmed peptic ulcer on first presentation or recurrence has been recommended by the National Institutes of Health in a 1994 Consensus Conference. Once *H. pylori* eradication has been achieved, reinfection rates are < 0.5% per year, and ulcer recurrence rates are dramatically reduced.

Numerous clinical trials have been done to determine the optimal regimen for *H. pylori* eradication, with cure rates ranging from ≈ 70% to 90%. There remains no gold standard of therapy to date. Base selection of the most appropriate therapy on consideration of treatment efficacy, cost, safety, drug-interaction potential, antibiotic resistance, tolerability, and convenience of administration. The FDA has approved 5 combination regimens for the treatment of *H. pylori* infection in patients with active duodenal ulcer. Studies have found that regimens consisting of a proton pump inhibitor (ie, lansoprazole or omeprazole) in conjunction with 2 antibiotics administered for 14 days are associated with cure rates that exceed 90%; this is in contrast to cure rates of 70% to 80% found with other regimens (eg, dual therapy, bismuth-based triple therapies).

Several studies have concluded that cure of *H. pylori* significantly reduces the risk of recurrent ulcer disease, obviating the need for continued maintenance therapy in patients with a history of uncomplicated disease. Make the decision to continue maintenance antisecretory therapy in patients with a history of complicated ulcer disease following successful *H. pylori* treatment on an individual basis.

The following is a brief description of the individual agents used in *H. pylori* eradication regimens and their role in eradication. Consult the individual drug monographs for complete prescribing information.

➤*Amoxicillin:* Amoxicillin works by inhibiting the synthesis of bacterial cell walls. It demonstrates topical activity and is stable in an acid environment but is most active at a neutral pH. *H. pylori* is very sensitive to amoxicillin in vitro and in vivo. Bacterial resistance to amoxicillin has not been reported. More common adverse effects include diarrhea, along with other GI effects, and hypersensitivity or allergic reactions. Take without regard to meals.

➤*Tetracycline:* This agent works by inhibiting bacterial protein synthesis. It acts topically and is active at a low pH. *H. pylori* is very sensitive to tetracycline. Bacterial resistance to tetracycline has not been reported. Adverse effects include diarrhea, along with other GI effects, esophageal ulcers, and photosensitivity reactions. Take on an empty stomach with plenty of water. Do not give simultaneously with dairy products (eg, milk, cheese), antacids, laxatives, or iron-containing products. If these agents are used, take them at least 2 hours before or after tetracycline.

➤*Metronidazole:* The exact mechanism of this agent is not well understood. It demonstrates selective toxicity to anaerobic or microaerophilic microorganisms and for anoxic or hypoxic cells. The drug diffuses into the cells and leads to the development of compounds that bind to DNA and inhibit synthesis, causing cell death. The activity of metronidazole is relatively independent of pH. Primary metronidazole resistance has been observed in 20% to 73% of *H. pylori* strains isolated and has been shown to significantly decrease *H. pylori* cure rates following treatment with a metronidazole-containing regimen. Adverse effects of metronidazole include metallic taste, nausea, peripheral neuropathy, and a disulfiram-type reaction manifested by flushing, nausea, tachycardia, vomiting, and other GI symptoms when used with alcohol. Metronidazole can be taken with food to minimize GI upset.

➤*Clarithromycin:* Clarithromycin is a macrolide antibiotic that inhibits bacterial protein synthesis. It is more acid-stable than erythromycin, better absorbed, and more effective against *H. pylori*. Resistance can develop when clarithromycin is used alone. It is generally < 8%. Adverse effects include abnormal taste, diarrhea, and nausea. Clarithromycin may be taken without regard to meals.

➤*Bismuth:* Bismuth compounds are topical compounds that disrupt the integrity of bacterial cell walls. The mechanism and role of bismuth in *H. pylori* eradication is multifactorial. Bismuth compounds are thought to lyse *H. pylori* near the gastric surface; prevent the adhesion of *H. pylori* to the gastric epithelium; inhibit its urease, phospholipase, and proteolytic activity; and decrease resistance development when used with antimicrobial agents such as metronidazole. Adverse effects of bismuth compounds may include a temporary and harmless darkening of the tongue and stool, diarrhea, and the potential for CNS toxici-

ties when used in high doses. Take bismuth compounds without regard to meals.

➤*Antisecretory agents (H₂ antagonists, proton pump inhibitors):* Provide rapid symptom relief and accelerated ulcer healing when used with antimicrobial agents for *H. pylori* eradication. Proton pump inhibitors may have a direct effect on inhibiting the growth of *H. pylori* and also appear to have a synergistic effect when combined with antimicrobial agents.

➤*Eradication of H. pylori:*

Single antimicrobial agents: Monotherapy is not recommended because of the potential for the development of antimicrobial resistance.

Dual therapy:

• *Proton pump inhibitors plus amoxicillin* – Significant variation exists among numerous studies that have been conducted to date with eradication rates ranging from 30% to 80%. Therefore, dual therapy with these 2 agents is not recommended.

• *Proton pump inhibitors plus clarithromycin* – A number of studies have looked at the use of these agents in combination for *H. pylori* eradication, and the overall eradication appears to be ≈ 71%. Currently, the American College of Gastroenterology recommends adding a second antimicrobial agent to this regimen to enhance successful eradication.

Double antimicrobial therapy plus an antisecretory drug:

Regimens Used in the Eradication of *H. pylori*		
Regimen	Dosing	Duration
Metronidazole + Clarithromycin + Omeprazole OR Lansoprazole	500 mg twice daily with meals 500 mg twice daily with meals 20 mg twice daily with meals 30 mg twice daily with meals	2 weeks
Amoxicillin + Clarithromycin + Omeprazole OR Lansoprazole	1 g twice daily with meals 500 mg twice daily with meals 20 mg twice daily before meals 30 mg twice daily with meals	2 weeks
Metronidazole + Omeprazole + Amoxicillin	500 mg twice daily with meals 20 mg twice daily before meals 1 g twice daily with meals	2 weeks

Triple-therapy regimens: These regimens have proved to be very effective in eradicating *H. pylori*. The primary disadvantage of these regimens is compliance because of the variety and number of medications used. Likewise, adverse effects are more common in patients taking these regimens compared with alternatives.

Regimens Used in the Eradication of *H. Pylori*		
Regimen	Dosing	Duration
Bismuth subsalicylate +	525 mg 4 times/day with meals and at bedtime	2 weeks
Metronidazole +	250 mg 4 times/day with meals and at bedtime	1 week
Tetracycline +	500 mg 4 times/day	2 weeks
H₂-receptor antagonist	As directed[1]	2 weeks + additional 2 weeks
Bismuth subsalicylate +	525 mg 4 times/day with meals and at bedtime	2 weeks
Metronidazole +	500 mg 3 times/day with meals and at bedtime	2 weeks
Tetracycline +	500 mg 4 times/day	2 weeks
Omeprazole OR	20 mg/day before meals	2 weeks
Lansoprazole	30 mg/day	2 weeks
Ranitidine bismuth citrate +	400 mg 2 times/day with meals and at bedtime	2 weeks
Clarithromycin +	500 mg 2 times/day	2 weeks
Amoxicillin OR	1 g 2 times/day with meals and at bedtime	2 weeks
Metronidazole OR	500 mg 2 times/day with meals and at bedtime	2 weeks
Tetracycline	500 mg 2 times/day	2 weeks

[1] See individual monographs for dosing instructions.

Quadruple therapy regimens (2 antibiotics, bismuth, antisecretory agent): Like triple therapy regimens, these have proven to be effective in *H. pylori* eradication. The primary disadvantage of these regimens is compliance. In addition, because of the variety and number of medications used, adverse effects are more common in patients taking these regimens compared with alternatives.

H. PYLORI AGENTS

FDA-Approved Therapies for *H. pylori* Infection	
Regimen	Dosing
Lansoprazole +	30 mg 2 times daily for 10 to 14 days[1]
Clarithromycin +	500 mg 2 times daily for 10 to 14 days[1]
Amoxicillin	1 g 2 times daily for 10 to 14 days[1]
Omeprazole +	20 mg 2 times daily for 10 days
Clarithromycin +	500 mg 2 times daily for 10 days
Amoxicillin	1 g 2 times daily for 10 days
Omeprazole +	40 mg once daily for 2 weeks
Clarithromycin	500 mg 3 times daily for 2 weeks
Omeprazole	Follow by 20 mg once daily for additional 2 weeks
Ranitidine bismuth citrate +	400 mg 2 daily for 2 weeks
Clarithromycin	500 mg 3 times daily for 2 weeks
Ranitidine bismuth citrate	Follow by 400 mg 2 times daily for additional 2 weeks
Bismuth subsalicylate +	525 mg 4 times daily for 2 weeks
Metronidazole +	250 mg 4 times daily for 2 weeks
Tetracycline +	500 mg 4 times daily for 2 weeks
Histamine-2 (H$_2$)-receptor antagonist	Dose as directed[2] for 2 weeks + additional 2 weeks
Lansoprazole +	30 mg 3 times daily for 2 weeks
Amoxicillin	1 g 3 times daily for 2 weeks

[1] Therapy associated with ≥ 90% *H. pylori* eradication rate.
[2] See individual monographs for dosing instructions.

►*Practice Guidelines from the American College of Gastroenterology:* In the 1996 Consensus Statement on Medical Treatment of Peptic Ulcer Disease, the American College of Gastroenterology does not recommend single-antibiotic combinations of either clarithromycin or amoxicillin with proton pump inhibitors because efficacy is < 70% (cure), and a high-dose, 2–week treatment period is required. The Consensus Statement recommends a two-antibiotic combination of clarithromycin, metronidazole or amoxicillin in regimens that do not employ a bismuth compound. In addition, the American College of Gastroenterology suggests adding either tetracycline or amoxicillin to the recently approved ranitidine-bismuth citrate-clarithromycin combination to enhance successful *H. pylori* eradication. Combining a proton pump inhibitor, either omeprazole or lansoprazole, with two antibiotics is thought to enhance effectiveness and allow for a shorter duration of treatment.

There are a number of factors that limit the effectiveness of regimens designed to eradicate *H. pylori*. The first, antibiotic resistance, is seen with metronidazole and clarithromycin but has not been reported with bismuth, amoxicillin or tetracycline. Because prior antibiotic exposure predicts drug resistance in individuals, take this factor into consideration when selecting a regimen. Although data are limited, studies have demonstrated that eradication of *H. pylori* is possible with metronidazole-containing regimens despite the presence of resistant organisms, but eradication rates are significantly lower. Alternatively, the American College of Gastroenterology suggests possible drug regimens to employ in cases of metronidazole resistance. These include bismuth, clarithromycin, and tetracycline or omeprazole, amoxicillin, and clarithromycin. On the other hand, clarithromycin resistance is more bothersome because resistant organisms do not respond favorably to clarithromycin-containing regimens.

Second, mild adverse effects (eg, diarrhea, metallic taste, black stools) do occur in ≈ 30% to 50% of patients. Therefore, shorter treatment periods in this group of patients may be better tolerated.

Finally, patient compliance is often a problem because of cumbersome regimens and adverse effects.

►*Maintenance therapy with antisecretory agents:* Several studies have concluded that cure of *H. pylori* significantly reduces the risk of recurrent ulcer disease, obviating the need for continued maintenance therapy in patients with a history of uncomplicated disease. The decision to continue maintenance antisecretory therapy in patients with a history of complicated ulcer disease following successful *H. pylori* treatment should be made on an individual basis. Factors to be considered that may favor the continuation of antisecretory therapy include: The presence of comorbid illness or the use of medications (eg, NSAIDs, anticoagulant therapy) that may increase risk of recurrence or complications, and severity of the previous ulcer-related complications.

►*Confirming successful eradication:* Confirming successful eradication is important in patients with a history of complicated or refractory ulcers but is controversial in those with uncomplicated ulcers who remain asymptomatic after therapy.

►*Refractory ulcers in patients receiving antibiotic therapy for H. pylori eradication:* Refractory ulcers in patients receiving antibiotic therapy for *H. pylori* eradication is often due to failure to successfully eradicate *H. pylori* infection. Resistance patterns, as well as noncompliance, and concurrent NSAID use may play a role in refractory cases.

RABIES PROPHYLAXIS PRODUCTS

Although rabies rarely affects humans in the US, every year ≈ 16,000 to 39,000 people receive postexposure prophylaxis. Appropriate management depends on the interpretation of the risk of infection and the efficacy and risk of prophylactic treatment. There are 2 types of immunizing products: Vaccines and globulins. Use both types of products concurrently for rabies postexposure prophylaxis.

➤*Vaccines:* Vaccines induce an active immune response that requires about 7 to 10 days to develop, and usually persists for ≥ 2 years.

➤*Human Diploid Cell Rabies Vaccine (HDCV):* An inactivated virus vaccine prepared from fixed rabies virus grown in human diploid cell culture.

➤*Rabies Vaccine, Adsorbed (RVA):* A cell culture-derived vaccine prepared from the Kissling strain of rabies virus adapted to a diploid cell line of the fetal rhesus lung.

➤*Purified Chick Embryo Cell Vaccine (PCEC):* An inactivated virus, it is prepared from the fixed rabies virus strain Flury LEP grown in primary cultures of chicken fibroblasts.

Four formulations of 3 inactivated rabies vaccines are currently licensed for preexposure and postexposure prophylaxis in the US. When used as indicated, all 3 types of rabies vaccines are considered equally safe and efficacious. The potency of 1 dose is ≥ 2.5 IU per 1 ml of rabies virus antigen, which is the World Health Organization recommended standard. A full 1 ml dose can be used for both preexposure and postexposure prophylaxis. However, only the Imovax Rabies I.D. vaccine (HDCV) has been evaluated and approved by the FDA for the intradermal dose and route for preexposure vaccination. Therefore, do not use RVA and PCEC intradermally. Usually, an immunization series is initiated and completed with 1 vaccine product. No clinical studies have been conducted that document a change in efficacy or the frequency of adverse reactions when the series is completed with a second vaccine product.

➤*Globulins:* Globulins provide rapid passive immune protection that persists for a short time (half-life of about 21 days).

Rabies Immune Globulin, Human (RIG): Antirabies gamma globulin, concentrated from plasma of hyperimmunized human donors.

➤*Rationale of treatment:* Individually evaluate each possible rabies exposure. Consult local or state public health officials if questions arise about the need for prophylaxis. Consider the following factors before specific treatment is initiated:

Species of biting animal: Carnivorous animals (especially skunks, foxes, coyotes, raccoons, dogs and cats) and bats are more likely to be infective than other animals. Unless the animal is tested and shown not rabid, initiate postexposure prophylaxis upon bite or non-bite exposure to these animals. If treatment has been initiated and subsequent testing shows the exposing animal is not rabid, treatment can be discontinued.

Since the likelihood that a domestic dog or cat is infected with rabies varies from region to region, the need for postexposure prophylaxis also varies. Bites of rabbits, hares, squirrels, chipmunks, rats, mice, hamsters, guinea pigs, gerbils and other rodents are rarely found to be infected with rabies and have not been known to cause human rabies in the US. In these cases, consult state or local health departments before a decision is made to initiate postexposure antirabies prophylaxis.

Circumstances of biting incident: An unprovoked attack is more likely to mean that the animal is rabid. Bites inflicted during attempts to feed or handle an apparently healthy animal should generally be regarded as provoked.

Type of exposure: Rabies is transmitted by introducing the virus into open cuts or wounds in skin via mucous membranes. The likelihood of rabies infection varies with the nature and extent of the exposure.
• *Bite* – Any penetration of the skin by teeth.
• *Nonbite* – Scratches, abrasions, open wounds or mucous membranes contaminated with saliva or other potentially infectious material, such as brain tissue from a rabid animal. There have been two instances of airborne rabies acquired in laboratories and two probable airborne rabies cases acquired in one bat-infested cave.

Casual contact with a rabid animal, such as petting it (without a bite or nonbite exposure), is not an indication for prophylaxis.

The only documented cases of rabies due to human-to-human transmission occurred in 8 patients who received corneal transplants from persons who died of rabies undiagnosed at the time of death.

➤*Preexposure prophylaxis:* Preexposure immunization does not eliminate the need for prompt postexposure prophylaxis following an exposure; it only reduces the postexposure regimen.

Consider preexposure immunization for persons in high-risk groups: Veterinarians, animal handlers, certain laboratory workers and persons, especially children, spending time (eg, ≥ 1 month) in foreign countries where rabies is a constant threat. Also consider others whose vocational or avocational pursuits bring them into contact with potentially rabid dogs, cats, foxes, skunks or bats. Pre-exposure immunization of immunosuppressed persons is not recommended.

Preexposure prophylaxis is given for several reasons. First, it may provide protection to persons with inapparent exposure to rabies. Secondly, it may protect persons whose postexposure therapy might be expected to be delayed. Finally, although it does not eliminate the need for additional therapy after a rabies exposure, it simplifies therapy by eliminating the need for globulin and decreasing the number of doses of vaccine needed. This is of particular importance for persons at high risk of being exposed in countries where the available rabies immunizing products may carry a higher risk of adverse reactions.

Preexposure immunization: Preexposure immunization consists of 3 doses of HDCV, RVA, or PCEC 1 ml/dose, IM (ie, deltoid area), one each on days 0, 7 and 21 or 28. The intradermal dose is 0.1 ml in the deltoid area of either arm on days 0, 7 and 21 or 28. Administration of routine booster doses of vaccine depends on exposure risk category as noted below.

Criteria for Preexposure Immunization

Risk category	Nature of risk	Typical populations	Preexposure regimen
Continuous	Virus present continuously, often in high concentrations. Aerosol, bite or nonbite exposure possible. Specific exposures may go unrecognized.	Rabies research lab workers,[1] rabies biologics production workers.	Primary preexposure immunization course. Serology every 6 months. Booster immunization when antibody titer falls below acceptable level.[2]
Frequent	Exposure usually episodic, with source recognized or unrecognized. Aerosol, bite or nonbite exposure.	Rabies diagnostic lab workers,[1] spelunkers, veterinarians and staff and animal control and wildlife workers in rabies epizootic areas.	Primary preexposure immunization course. Serology every 2 years. Booster immunization when antibody titer falls below acceptable level.
Infrequent (greater than population-at-large)	Exposure nearly always episodic with source recognized. Bite or nonbite exposure.	Veterinarians and animal control wildlife workers in areas of low rabies endemicity. Travelers to foreign rabies epizootic areas. Veterinary students.	Primary preexposure immunization course. No routine booster immunization or serology.
Rare (population-at-large)	Exposure always episodic, or bite with source recognized.	US population-at-large, including individuals in rabies epi-zootic areas.	No preexposure immunization.

[1] Judgment of relative risk and extra monitoring of immunization status of laboratory workers is the responsibility of the laboratory supervisor (see US Department of Health and Human Services' *Biosafety in Microbiological and Biomedical Laboratories,*1984).

[2] Preexposure booster immunization consists of one dose of HDCV, PCEC, or RVA 1 ml/dose, IM or 0.1 ml ID day 0 only. Acceptable antibody level is 1:5 titer (complete inhibition in RFFIT at 1:5 dilution). Boost if titer falls below 1:5.

➤*Postexposure prophylaxis:*

Local wound treatment: Immediate and thorough washing of all bite wounds and scratches with soap and water is perhaps the most effective means of preventing rabies. Give tetanus and a virucidal agent such as povidone-iodine solution irrigation prophylaxis and control bacterial infection as indicated.

Immunization: Postexposure antirabies immunization should always include both passive immunization (preferably RIG) and vaccine, with one exception: Persons previously immunized with HDCV in recommended preexposure or postexposure regimens or with other types of vaccines and who have a documented adequate rabies antibody titer should receive only vaccine. The globulin/vaccine combination is recommended for both bite and nonbite exposures, regardless of the interval between exposure and treatment.

Treatment: Use the following recommendations as a guide in conjunction with knowledge of the circumstances of the situation. Consult public health officials with questions about the need for rabies prophylaxis.

RABIES PROPHYLAXIS PRODUCTS

	Treatment Recommendations for Postexposure Rabies	
Animal species	Condition of animal at time of attack	Treatment of exposed person[1]
Domestic: Dogs, cats and ferrets	Healthy & available for 10 days of observation	None, unless animal develops rabies[2]
	Rabid/suspected rabid	RIG and vaccine[3]
	Unknown (escaped)	Consult public health officials. If treatment is indicated, give RIG and vaccine[3]
Wild: Skunk, bat, fox, coyote, raccoon, bobcat and other carnivores	Regard as rabid unless proven negative by laboratory test[3]	Consider immediate vaccination[3]
Other: Livestock, rodents, rabbits and hares, large rodents and other mammals	Consider individually: Bites of squirrels, hamsters, guinea pigs, gerbils, chipmunks, rats, mice, other rodents, rabbits and hares almost never call for antirabies prophylaxis. Consult public health officials.	

[1] If treatment is indicated, administer both RIG and vaccine as soon as possible, regardless of the interval from exposure.
[2] Begin treatment with RIG and vaccine at first sign of rabies in biting domestic animals during the usual holding period of 10 days. Kill and test the symptomatic animal immediately.
[3] Kill and test animal as soon as possible. Holding for observation is not recommended. Discontinue vaccine if fluorescent antibody tests of animal are negative.

Treatment Schedule for Postexposure Rabies Prophylaxis	
Vaccination status	Treatment[1]
Not previously vaccinated	*Local wound cleansing:* All postexposure treatment should begin with immediate, thorough cleansing of each wound with soap and water. If available, a virucidal agent such as povidone-iodine solution should be used to irrigate the wounds.
	Rabies immune globulin: Give 20 IU/kg. If anatomically feasible, infiltrate the full dose around the wound(s) and inject the balance IM at an anatomical site distant from vaccine administration. Do not give RIG through the same syringe or into the same anatomical site as rabies vaccine. Because RIG may partially suppress active induction of antirabies antibody, give no more than the recommended dose.
	Rabies vaccine: Give 1 ml IM in the deltoid area[2] on days 0, 3, 7, 14 and 28.
Previously vaccinated[3]	*Local wound cleansing:* All postexposure treatments begin with immediate, thorough cleansing of each wound with soap and water. If available, a virucidal agent such as povidone-iodine solution should be used to irrigate the wounds.
	Do not administer RIG.
	Rabies vaccine: Give 1 ml IM in the deltoid area on days 0 and 3.

[1] These regimens apply to all age groups, including children.
[2] The deltoid area is the only acceptable site of vaccination for adults and older children. For younger children, the outer aspect of the thigh may be used. Vaccine should never be administered in the gluteal area.
[3] Any person with a history of pre- or postexposure vaccination with HDCV, PCEC or RVA; or with both a history of vaccination with any other type of rabies vaccine and a documented history of antibody response to that vaccination.

Recommendations for Postexposure Immunization
2 doses of HDVC, 1 ml/dose, IM, one each on days 0 and 3.
RIG, 20 IU/kg. If anatomically feasible, infiltrate the full dose in the area around and into the wounds. Administer remaining volume IM at a distant site. Five doses of HDCV, RVA or PCEC, 1 ml/dose, IM, one each on days 0, 3, 7, 14 and 28.

➤*Passive immunization:* Administer RIG once at the beginning of antirabies therapy. If not given when vaccination was begun, RIG can be given through the seventh day after the first dose of vaccine. After that, RIG is not indicated, since an antibody response is presumed to have occurred. The recommended RIG dose is 20 IU/kg ($\approx$ 9 IU/lb). If anatomically feasible, infiltrate the full dose in the area around and into the wound. Because RIG may partially suppress active production of antibody, do not exceed the recommended dose.

➤*Active immunization:* Administer the vaccine in conjunction with RIG on day 0. Give five 1 ml doses of the vaccine IM in the deltoid area. For children the anterolateral aspect of the thigh is also acceptable. Do not use gluteal area. Administer the first dose as soon as possible after the exposure; give an additional dose on each of days 3, 7, 14 and 28 after the first dose (day 0). WHO recommends a sixth dose at 90 days after the first dose. In unusual instances (eg, an immunosuppressed patient), serologic testing is indicated.

➤*Previously immunized persons:* When an immunized person who was vaccinated by the recommended regimen with HDCV, PCEC or RVA or who had previously demonstrated rabies antibody is exposed to rabies, that person should receive two doses of HDCV, PCEC or RVA 1 ml/dose, IM, one immediately and one 3 days later. If the person's immune status is not known, postexposure antirabies treatment may be necessary. If antibody can be demonstrated in a serum sample collected before vaccine is given, treatment can be discontinued after at least two doses of the vaccine.

Rapid intervention is essential to minimize morbidity and mortality in an acute toxic ingestion. Institute measures to prevent absorption and hasten elimination as appropriate; however, symptomatic and supportive care takes precedence over other therapy. It is assumed that basic life support measures, (eg, cardiopulmonary resuscitation [CPR]) have been instituted. Specific antidotes are discussed in the overdosage section of individual or group monographs. The discussion below outlines procedures used in the management of acute overdosage of orally ingested systemic drugs. **Consultation with a regional poison control center is highly recommended.**

ADVANCED LIFE SUPPORT MEASURES

➤*Adequate Airway:* Adequate Airway must be established and maintained, generally via oropharyngeal or endotracheal airways, cricothyrotomy or tracheostomy.

➤*Ventilation:* Ventilation may then be performed via mouth-to-mouth insufflation, hand-operated bag (ambu bag) or by mechanical ventilator.

➤*Circulation:* Circulation must be maintained.

• *Hypotension:* If hypotension/hypoperfusion occurs, place the patient in shock position (head lowered, feet elevated); specific therapy may include:

Establish IV access and initiate IV fluids (eg, 0.9% or 0.45% Saline, Lactated Ringer's, Dextrose). A maintenance flow rate is generally 100 to 200 ml/hour; individualize as necessary.

Plasma, plasma protein fractions, whole blood or plasma expanders may be required.

Severe hypotension may require judicious use of cardiovascular active agents. The most commonly recommended agents are dopamine, dobutamine and norepinephrine.

• *Arrhythmia* treatment is dictated by the offending drug.

• *Hypertension,* sometimes severe, may occur. (See Nitroprusside and Diazoxide, Parenteral in the Agents for Hypertensive Emergencies section.)

➤*Seizures:* Simple isolated seizures may require only observation and supportive care. Repetitive seizures or status epilepticus require therapy. Give IV diazepam or lorazepam followed by fosphenytoin and/or phenobarbital. General anesthesia with or without neuromuscular blockade may be necessary for seizures refractory to standard therapy.

REDUCTION OF DRUG ABSORPTION

➤*Gastric decontamination:* is generally recommended as soon as possible; however, this is generally not very effective unless employed within the first 1 to 2 hours after ingestion. Gastric lavage and the administration of activated charcoal are the two most commonly employed methods for gastric decontamination.

• *Gastric lavage* may be used within 1 to 2 hours of ingestion of an acute overdose. Airway protection via endotracheal intubation is appropriate for the patient without a gag reflex or comatose patients. Position the patient on left side, face down and use a large bore tube. Instill warm water or saline 300 to 360 ml for adults. Avoid water for infants and children; use warm saline or 5% to 6% polyethylene glycol solution. Repeat instillations until lavage solution returns clear. Add charcoal before removing the tube.

• Activated charcoal Absorption, using activated charcoal alone or following gastric lavage, is appropriate for many significant toxic ingestions. It adsorbs a wide variety of toxins and is most effective when given within 1 to 2 hours of ingestion. The adult dose is 50 to 100 g of activated charcoal mixed in 240 ml of water; the pediatric dose is 1 g/kg, or 25 to 50 g in 120 ml of water.

➤*Cathartics:* Cathartics are generally not used alone in the treatment of acute overdose. More often they are administered with activated charcoal to increase the elimination of the charcoal-poison complex. The administration of a saline cathartic (eg, magnesium citrate) or an osmotic cathartic (eg, sorbitol) with activated charcoal has the most rapid effect.

➤*Whole bowel irrigation (WBI):* Whole bowel irrigation utilizes rapid administration of large volumes of lavage solutions, such as PEG. The dose is 4 to 6 L over 1 to 2 hours for adults and 0.5 L/hr for children. It may be useful to remove certain sustained-release dosage forms, cocaine-containing condoms or balloons, or toxins for which activated charcoal is ineffective (eg, iron, lithium).

ELIMINATION OF ABSORBED DRUG

➤*Interruption of enterohepatic circulation:* Interruption of enterohepatic circulation by "gastric dialysis" uses scheduled doses of activated charcoal for 1 to 2 days. Gastric dialysis not only interrupts the enterohepatic cycle of some drugs, but also creates an osmotic gradient, drawing drug from the plasma back into the gastrointestinal lumen where it is bound by the charcoal and excreted in the feces.

➤*Diuresis:* Diuresis may be effective as identified in the individual drug monographs.

• *Alkaline diuresis* promotes elimination of weak acids (eg, barbiturates, salicylates) and is accomplished by the administration of IV sodium bicarbonate.

➤*Dialysis:* Dialysis is indicated in a minority of severe overdose cases. Drug factors that alter dialysis effectiveness include volume of distribution, drug compartmentalization, protein binding and lipid/water solubility.

• *Hemodialysis* may be used as a supportive measure when the patient is having complications (eg, severe metabolic acidosis, electrolyte imbalances, renal failure).

• *Peritoneal dialysis* is generally less effective than hemodialysis.

• *Charcoal hemoperfusion* may be useful when a drug can be adsorbed by charcoal (eg, theophylline, barbiturates).

Poison Control Center: _____

Type I hypersensitivity reactions (immediate hypersensitivity or anaphylaxis) are immunologic responses to a foreign antigen to which a patient has been previously sensitized. Anaphylactoid reactions are not immunologically mediated; however, symptoms and treatment are similar.

SIGNS AND SYMPTOMS

Acute hypersensitivity reactions typically begin within 1 to 30 minutes of exposure to the offending antigen. Tingling sensations and a generalized flush may proceed to a fullness in the throat, chest tightness or a "feeling of impending doom." Generalized urticaria and sweating are common. *Severe* reactions include life-threatening involvement of the airway and cardiovascular system.

TREATMENT

Appropriate and immediate treatment is imperative. The following general measures are commonly employed:

➤*Epinephrine:* 1:1000, 0.2 to 0.5 mg (0.2 to 0.5 ml) SC is the primary treatment. In children, administer 0.01 mg/kg or 0.1 mg. Doses may be repeated every 5 to 15 minutes if needed. A succession of small doses is more effective and less dangerous than a single large dose. Additionally, 0.1 mg may be introduced into an injection site where the offending drug was administered. If appropriate, the use of a tourniquet above the site of injection of the causative agent may slow its absorption and distribution. However, remove or loosen the tourniquet every 10 to 15 minutes to maintain circulation.

Epinephrine IV (generally indicated in the presence of hypotension) is often recommended in a 1:10,000 dilution, 0.3 to 0.5 mg over 5 minutes; repeat every 15 minutes, if necessary. In children, inject 0.1 to 0.2 mg or 0.01 mg/kg/dose over 5 minutes; repeat every 30 minutes.

A conservative IV epinephrine protocol includes 0.1 mg of a 1:100,000 dilution (0.1 mg of a 1:1000 dilution mixed in 10 ml normal saline) given over 5 to 10 minutes. If an IV infusion is necessary, administer at a rate of 1 to 4 mcg/min. In children, infuse 0.1 to 1.5 (maximum) mcg/kg/min.

Dilute epinephrine 1:10,000 may be administered through an endotracheal tube, if no other parenteral access is available, directly into the bronchial tree. It is rapidly absorbed there from the capillary bed of the lung.

➤*Airway:* Ensure a patent airway via endotracheal intubation or cricothyrotomy (ie, inferior laryngotomy, used prior to tracheotomy) and administer oxygen. Severe respiratory difficulty may respond to IV aminophylline or to other bronchodilators.

➤*Hypotension:* The patient should be recumbent with feet elevated. Depending upon the severity, consider the following measures:
• Establish a patent IV catheter in a suitable vein.
• Administer IV fluids (eg, Normal Saline, Lactated Ringer's).
• Administer plasma expanders.
• Administer cardioactive agents (see group and individual monographs). Commonly recommended agents include dopamine, dobutamine, norepinephrine and phenylephrine.

➤*Adjunctive therapy:* does not alter acute reactions, but may modify an ongoing or slow-onset process and shorten the course of the reaction.
• *Antihistamines: Diphenhydramine* – 50 to 100 mg IM or IV, continued orally at 5 mg/kg/day or 50 mg every 6 hours for 1 to 2 days. For children, give 5 mg/kg/day, maximum 300 mg/day.
Chlorpheniramine: (adults, 10 to 20 mg; children, 5 to 10 mg) IM or slowly IV.
Hydroxyzine: 10 to 25 mg orally or 25 to 50 mg IM 3 to 4 times daily.
• *Corticosteroids*, eg, hydrocortisone IV 100 to 1000 mg or equivalent, followed by 7 mg/kg/day IV or oral for 1 to 2 days. The role of corticosteroids is controversial.
• *H$_2$ antagonists: Cimetidine – Children,* 25 to 30 mg/kg/day IV in six divided doses; *adults,* 300 mg every 6 hours. *Ranitidine* – 50 mg IV over 3 to 5 minutes. May be of value in addition to H$_1$ antihistamines, although this opinion is not universally shared.

INTERNATIONAL SYSTEM OF UNITS

INTERNATIONAL SYSTEM OF UNITS

The *Système international d'unités* (International System of Units) or *SI* is a modernized version of the metric system. The primary goal of the conversion to SI units is to revise the present confused measurement system and to improve test-result communications.

The SI has 7 basic units from which other units are derived:

Base Units of SI		
Physical quantity	Base unit	SI symbol
length	meter	m
mass	kilogram	kg
time	second	s
amount of substance	mole	mol
thermodynamic temperature	kelvin	K
electric current	ampere	A
luminous intensity	candela	cd

Combinations of these base units can express any property, although, for simplicity, special names are given to some of these derived units.

Representative Derived Units		
Derived unit	Name and symbol	Derivation from base units
area	square meter	m^2
volume	cubic meter	m^3
force	newton (N)	$kg \cdot m \cdot s^{-2}$
pressure	pascal (Pa)	$kg \cdot m^{-1} \cdot s^{-2}$ (N/m^2)
work, energy	joule (J)	$kg \cdot m^2 \cdot s^{-2}$ (N·m)
mass density	kilogram per cubic meter	kg/m^3
frequency	hertz (Hz)	1 cycle/s^{-1}
temperature degree	Celsius (°C)	°C = °K − 273.15
concentration		
mass	kilogram/liter	kg/L
substance	mole/liter	mol/L
molality	mole/kilogram	mol/kg
density	kilogram/liter	kg/L

Prefixes to the base unit are used in this system to form decimal multiples and submultiples. The preferred multiples and submultiples listed below change the quantity by increments of 10^3 or 10^{-3}. The exceptions to these recommended factors are within the middle rectangle.

Prefixes and Symbols for Decimal Multiples and Submultiples		
Factor	Prefix	Symbol
10^{18}	exa	E
10^{15}	peta	P
10^{12}	tera	T
10^{9}	giga	G
10^{6}	mega	M
10^{3}	kilo	k
10^{2}	hecto	h
10^{1}	deka	da
10^{-1}	deci	d
10^{-2}	centi	c
10^{-3}	milli	m
10^{-6}	micro	μ
10^{-9}	nano	n
10^{-12}	pico	p
10^{-15}	femto	f
10^{-18}	atto	a

To convert drug concentrations to or from SI units:

Conversion factor (CF) = $\dfrac{1000}{\text{mol wt}}$

Conversion *to* SI units: $\mu g/ml$ x CF = $\mu mol/L$

Conversion *from* SI units: $\mu mol/L \div CF = \mu g/ml$

In the following tables, normal reference values for commonly requested laboratory tests are listed in traditional units and in SI units. The tables are a guideline only. Values are method dependent and "normal values" may vary between laboratories.

	Blood, Plasma or Serum	
	Reference Value	
Determination	Conventional Units	SI Units
Ammonia (NH_3) – diffusion	20-120 mcg/dl	12-70 mcmol/L
Ammonia Nitrogen	15–45 µg/dl	11–32 µmol/L
Amylase	35-118 IU/L	0.58-1.97 mckat/L
Anion Gap ($Na^+-[Cl^-+HCO_3^-]$) (P)	7–16 mEq/L	7–16 mmol/L
Antinuclear antibodies	negative at 1:10 dilution of serum	negative at 1:10 dilution of serum
Antithrombin III (AT III)	80-120 U/dl	800-1200 U/L
Bicarbonate: Arterial Venous	21–28 mEq/L 22–29 mEq/L	21–28 mmol/L 22–29 mmol/L
Bilirubin: Conjugated (direct) Total	≤ 0.2 mg/dl 0.1-1 mg/dl	≤ 4 mcmol/L 2-18 mcmol/L
Calcitonin	< 100 pg/ml	< 100 ng/L
Calcium: Total Ionized	8.6-10.3 mg/dl 4.4-5.1 mg/dl	2.2-2.74 mmol/L 1-1.3 mmol/L
Carbon dioxide content (plasma)	21-32 mmol/L	21-32 mmol/L
Carcinoembryonic antigen	< 3 ng/ml	< 3 mcg/L
Chloride	95-110 mEq/L	95-110 mmol/L
Coagulation screen: Bleeding time Prothrombin time Partial thromboplastin time (activated) Protein C Protein S	3-9.5 min 10-13 sec 22-37 sec 0.7-1.4 µ/ml 0.7-1.4 µ/ml	180-570 sec 10-13 sec 22-37 sec 700-1400 U/ml 700-1400 U/ml
Copper, total	70-160 mcg/dl	11-25 mcmol/L
Corticotropin (ACTH adrenocorticotropic hormone) – 0800 hr	< 60 pg/ml	< 13.2 pmol/L
Cortisol: 0800 hr 1800 hr 2000 hr	5-30 mcg/dl 2-15 mcg/dl ≤ 50% of 0800 hr	138-810 nmol/L 50-410 nmol/L ≤ 50% of 0800 hr
Creatine kinase: Female Male	20-170 IU/L 30-220 IU/L	0.33-2.83 mckat/L 0.5-3.67 mckat/L
Creatine kinase isoenzymes, MB fraction	0-12 IU/L	0-0.2 mckat/L
Creatinine	0.5-1.7 mg/dl	44-150 mcmol/L
Fibrinogen (coagulation factor I)	150-360 mg/dl	1.5-3.6 g/L
Follicle-stimulating hormone (FSH): Female Midcycle Male	2-13 mIU/ml 5-22 mIU/ml 1-8 mIU/ml	2-13 IU/L 5-22 IU/L 1-8 IU/L
Glucose, fasting	65-115 mg/dl	3.6-6.3 mmol/L

Glucose Tolerance Test (Oral)	mg/dL		mmol/L	
	Normal	Diabetic	Normal	Diabetic
Fasting	70-105	> 140	3.9-5.8	> 7.8
60 min	120-170	≥ 200	6.7-9.4	≥11.1
90 min	100-140	≥ 200	5.6-7.8	≥ 11.1
120 min	70-120	≥ 140	3.9-6.7	≥ 7.8

(γ) - Glutamyltransferase (GGT): Male Female	9-50 units/L 8-40 units/L	9-50 units/L 8-40 units/L
Haptoglobin	44-303 mg/dl	0.44-3.03 g/L

Hematologic tests:
Fibrinogen
Hematocrit (Hct), female
   male
Hemoglobin A_{1C}
Hemoglobin (Hb), female
   male
Leukocyte count (WBC)
Erythrocyte count (RBC), female
   male
Mean corpuscular volume (MCV)
Mean corpuscular hemoglobin (MCH)
Mean corpuscular hemoglobin concentrate (MCHC)
Erythrocyte sedimentation rate (sedrate, ESR)
	200-400 mg/dl
	36%-44.6%
	40.7%-50.3%
	5.3%-7.5% of total Hgb
	12.1-15.3 g/dl
	13.8-17.5 g/dl
	3800-9800/mcl
	3.5-5 × 10^6/mcl
	4.3-5.9 × 10^6/mcl
	80-97.6 mcm^3
	27-33 pg/cell
	33-36 g/dl
	≤ 30 mm/hr
		2-4 g/L
		0.36-0.446 fraction of 1
		0.4-0.503 fraction of 1
		0.053-0.075
		121-153 g/L
		138-175 g/L
		3.8-9.8 x 10^9/L
		3.5-5 x 10^{12}/L
		4.3-5.9 x 10^{12}/L
		80-97.6 fl
		1.66-2.09 fmol/cell
		20.3-22 mmol/L
		≤ 30 mm/hr

Erythrocyte enzymes: Glucose-6-phosphate dehydroge nase (G-6-PD) Ferritin Folic acid: normal Platelet count Reticulocytes Vitamin B_{12}	250-5000 units/10^6 cells 10-383 ng/ml > 3.1-12.4 ng/ml 150-450 × 10^3/mcl 0.5%-1.5% of erythrocytes 223-1132 pg/ml	250-5000 mcunits/cell 23-862 pmol/L 7-28.1 nmol/L 150-450 × 10^9/L 0.005-0.015 165-835 pmol/L
Iron: Female Male	30-160 mcg/dl 45-160 mcg/dl	5.4-31.3 mcmol/L 8.1-31.3 mcmol/L
Iron binding capacity	220-420 mcg/dl	39.4-75.2 mcmol/L
Isocitrate Dehydrogenase	1.2-7 units/L	1.2-7 units/L

Blood, Plasma or Serum		
Determination	**Reference Value**	
	Conventional Units	**SI Units**
Isoenzymes		
Fraction 1	14%-26% of total	0.14-0.26 fraction of total
Fraction 2	29%-39% of total	0.29-0.39 fraction of total
Fraction 3	20%-26% of total	0.20-0.26 fraction of total
Fraction 4	8%-16% of total	0.08-0.16 fraction of total
Fraction 5	6%-16% of total	0.06-0.16 fraction of total
Lactate dehydrogenase	100-250 IU/L	1.67-4.17 mckat/L
Lactic acid (lactate)	6-19 mg/dl	0.7-2.1 mmol/L
Lead	≤ 50 mcg/dl	≤ 2.41 mcmol/L
Lipase	10-150 units/L	10-150 units/L
Lipids:		
Total Cholesterol		
Desirable	< 200 mg/dl	< 5.2 mmol/L
Borderline-high	200-239 mg/dl	< 5.2-6.2 mmol/L
High	> 239 mg/dl	> 6.2 mmol/L
LDL		
Desirable	< 130 mg/dl	< 3.36 mmol/L
Borderline-high	130-159 mg/dl	3.36-4.11 mmol/L
High	> 159 mg/dl	> 4.11 mmol/L
HDL (low)	< 35 mg/dl	< 0.91 mmol/L
Triglycerides		
Desirable	< 200 mg/dl	< 2.26 mmol/L
Borderline-high	200-400 mg/dl	2.26-4.52 mmol/L
High	400-1000 mg/dl	4.52-11.3 mmol/L
Very high	> 1000 mg/dl	> 11.3 mmol/L
Magnesium	1.3-2.2 mEq/L	0.65-1.1 mmol/L
Osmolality	280-300 mOsm/kg	280-300 mmol/kg
Oxygen saturation (arterial)	94%-100%	0.94-1 fraction of 1
PCO_2, arterial	35-45 mm Hg	4.7-6 kPa
pH, arterial	7.35-7.45	7.35-7.45
PO_2, arterial: Breathing room air[1]	80-105 mm Hg	10.6-14 kPa
On 100% O_2	> 500 mm Hg	
Phosphatase (acid), total at 37°C	0.13-0.63 IU/L	2.2-10.5 IU/L or 2.2-10.5 mckat/L
Phosphatase alkaline[2]	20-130 IU/L	20-130 IU/L or 0.33-2.17 mckat/L
Phosphorus, inorganic,[3] (phosphate)	2.5-5 mg/dl	0.8-1.6 mmol/L
Potassium	3.5-5 mEq/L	3.5-5 mmol/L
Progesterone		
Female	0.1-1.5 ng/ml	0.32-4.8 nmol/L
Follicular phase	0.1-1.5 ng/ml	0.32-4.8 nmol/L
Luteal phase	2.5-28 ng/ml	8-89 nmol/L
Male	< 0.5 ng/ml	< 1.6 nmol/L
Prolactin	1.4-24.2 ng/ml	1.4-24.2 mcg/L
Prostate specific antigen	0-4 ng/ml	0-4 ng/ml
Protein: Total	6-8 g/dl	60-80 g/L
Albumin	3.6-5 g/dl	36-50 g/L
Globulin	2.3-3.5 g/dl	23-35 g/L
Rheumatoid factor	< 60 IU/ml	< 60 kIU/L
Sodium	135-147 mEq/L	135-147 mmol/L
Testosterone: Female	6-86 ng/dl	0.21-3 nmol/L
Male	270-1070 ng/dl	9.3-37 nmol/L
Thyroid Hormone Function Tests:		
Thyroid-stimulating hormone (TSH)	0.35-6.2 mcU/ml	0.35-6.2 mU/L
Thyroxine-binding globulin capacity	10-26 mcg/dl	100-260 mcg/dl
Total triiodothyronine (T_3)	75-220 ng/dl	1.2-3.4 nmol/L
Total thyroxine by RIA (T_4)	4-11 mcg/dl	51-142 nmol/L
T_3 resin uptake	25%-38%	0.25-0.38 fraction of 1
Transaminase, AST (aspartate aminotransferase, SGOT)	11-47 IU/L	0.18-0.78 mckat/L
Transaminase, ALT (alanine aminotrans ferase, SGPT)	7-53 IU/L	0.12-0.88 mckat/L
Transferrin	220-400 mg/dL	2.20-4.00 g/L
Urea nitrogen (BUN)	8-25 mg/dl	2.9-8.9 mmol/L
Uric acid	3-8 mg/dl	179-476 mcmol/L
Vitamin A (retinol)	15-60 mcg/dl	0.52-2.09 mcmol/L
Zinc	50-150 mcg/dl	7.7-23 mcmol/L

[1] Age dependent   [2] Infants and adolescents up to 104 U/L   [3] Infants in the first year up to 6 mg/dl

Urine		
Determination	**Reference Value**	
	Conventional Units	**SI Units**
Calcium[1]	50-250 mcg/day	1.25-6.25 mmol/day
Catecholamines: Epinephrine	< 20 mcg/day	< 109 nmol/day

	Urine	
	Reference Value	
Determination	Conventional Units	SI Units
Norepinephrine	< 100 mcg/day	< 590 nmol/day
Catecholamines, 24-hr	< 110 µg	< 650 nmol
Copper[1]	15-60 mcg/day	0.24-0.95 mcmol/day
Creatinine: Child	8-22 mg/kg	71-195 µmol/kg
Adolescent	8-30 mg/kg	71-265 µmol/kg
Female	0.6-1.5 g/day	5.3-13.3 mmol/day
Male	0.8-1.8 g/day	7.1-15.9 mmol/day
pH	4.5-8	4.5-8
Phosphate[1]	0.9-1.3 g/day	29-42 mmol/day
Potassium[1]	25-100 mEq/day	25-100 mmol/day
Protein		
Total	1-14 mg/dL	10-140 mg/L
At rest	50-80 mg/day	50-80 mg/day
Protein, quantitative	< 150 mg/day	< 0.15 g/day
Sodium[1]	100-250 mEq/day	100-250 mmol/day
Specific Gravity, random	1.002-1.030	1.002-1.030
Uric Acid, 24-hr	250-750 mg	1.48-4.43 mmol

[1] Diet dependent

	Drug Levels†		
		Reference Value	
Drug Determination		Conventional Units	SI Units
Aminoglycosides	Amikacin		
	(trough)	1-8 mcg/ml	1.7-13.7 mcmol/L
	(peak)	20-30 mcg/ml	34-51 mcmol/L
	Gentamicin		
	(trough)	0.5-2 mcg/ml	1-4.2 mcmol/L
	(peak)	6-10 mcg/ml	12.5-20.9 mcmol/L
	Kanamycin		
	(trough)	5-10 mcg/ml	nd
	(peak)	20-25 mcg/ml	nd
	Netilmicin		
	(trough)	0.5-2 mcg/ml	nd
	(peak)	6-10 mcg/ml	nd
	Streptomycin		
	(trough)	< 5 mcg/ml	nd
	(peak)	5-20 mcg/ml	nd
	Tobramycin		
	(trough)	0.5-2 mcg/ml	1.1-4.3 mcmol/L
	(peak)	5-20 mcg/ml	12.8-21.8 mcmol/L
Antiarrhythmics	Amiodarone	0.5-2.5 mcg/ml	1.5-4 mcmol/L
	Bretylium	0.5-1.5 mcg/ml	nd
	Digitoxin	9-25 mcg/L	11.8-32.8 nmol/L
	Digoxin	0.8-2 ng/ml	0.9-2.5 nmol/L
	Disopyramide	2-8 mcg/ml	6-18 mcmol/L
	Flecainide	0.2-1 mcg/ml	nd
	Lidocaine	1.5-6 mcg/ml	4.5-21.5 mcmol/L
	Mexiletine	0.5-2 mcg/ml	nd
	Procainamide	4-8 mcg/ml	17-34 mcmol/ml
	Propranolol	50-200 ng/ml	190-770 nmol/L
	Quinidine	2-6 mcg/ml	4.6-9.2 mcmol/L
	Tocainide	4-10 mcg/ml	nd
	Verapamil	0.08-0.3 mcg/ml	nd
Anti-convulsants	Carbamazepine	4-12 mcg/ml	17-51 mcmol/L
	Phenobarbital	10-40 mcg/ml	43-172 mcmol/L
	Phenytoin	10-20 mcg/ml	40-80 mcmol/L
	Primidone	4-12 mcg/ml	18-55 mcmol/L
	Valproic acid	40-100 mcg/ml	280-700 mcmol/L
Antidepressants	Amitriptyline	110-250 ng/ml[3]	500-900 nmol/L
	Amoxapine	200-500 ng/ml	nd
	Bupropion	25-100 ng/ml	nd
	Clomipramine	80-100 ng/ml	nd
	Desipramine	115-300 ng/ml	nd
	Doxepin	110-250 ng/ml[3]	nd
	Imipramine	225-350 ng/ml[3]	nd
	Maprotiline	200-300 ng/ml	nd
	Nortriptyline	50-150 ng/ml	nd
	Protriptyline	70-250 ng/ml	nd
	Trazodone	800-1600 ng/ml	nd

	Drug Levels†		
		Reference Value	
Drug Determination		Conventional Units	SI Units
Antipsychotics	Chlorpromazine	50-300 ng/ml	150-950 nmol/L
	Fluphenazine	0.13-2.8 ng/ml	nd
	Haloperidol	5-20 ng/ml	nd
	Perphenazine	0.8-1.2 ng/ml	nd
	Thiothixene	2-57 ng/ml	nd
Miscellaneous	Amantadine	300 ng/ml	nd
	Amrinone	3.7 mcg/ml	nd
	Chlorampheni-col	10-20 mcg/ml	31-62 mcmol/L
	Cyclosporine[1]	250-800 ng/ml (whole blood, RIA)	nd
		50-300 ng/ml (plasma, RIA)	nd
	Ethanol[2]	0 mg/dl	0 mmol/L
	Hydralazine	100 ng/ml	nd
	Lithium	0.6-1.2 mEq/L	0.6-1.2 mmol/L
	Salicylate	100-300 mg/L	724-2172 mcmol/L
	Sulfonamide	5-15 mg/dl	nd
	Terbutaline	0.5-4.1 ng/ml	nd
	Theophylline	10-20 mcg/ml	55-110 mcmol/L
	Vancomycin		
	(trough)	5-15 ng/ml	nd
	(peak)	20-40 mcg/ml	nd

† The values given are generally accepted as desirable for treatment without toxicity for most patients. However, exceptions are not uncommon.
[1] 24 hour trough values [2] Toxic: 50-100 mg/dl (10.9-21.7 mmol/L) [3] Parent drug plus N-desmethyl metabolite
nd – No data available

The following is adopted from the Seventh Report of the Joint National Committee on Prevention, Detection, Evaluation, and Treatment of High Blood Pressure, National Institutes of Health.

Classification of Blood Pressure*			
	Reference Value		
Category	Systolic (mm Hg)		Diastolic (mm Hg)
Normal	< 120	and	< 80
Prehypertension	120-139	or	80-89
Stage 1 Hypertension	140-159	or	90--99
Stage 2 Hypertension	≥ 160	or	≥ 100

* For adults age 18 and older who are not taking antihypertensive drugs and not acutely ill. When systolic and diastolic blood pressures fall into different categories, the higher category should be selected to classify the individual's blood pressure status.

The classification is based on the average of two or more readings properly measured taken at each of two or more visits after an initial reading.

Source: The Seventh Report of the Joint National Committee on Prvention, Detection, Evaluation, and Treatment of High Blood Pressure. JAMA 2003;289:2560-2571.

To calculate milliequivalent weight: $mEq = \dfrac{\text{gram molecular weight/valence}}{1000}$

$mEq = \dfrac{mg}{eq\ wt}$ equivalent weight or eq wt $= \dfrac{\text{gram molecular weight}}{\text{valence}}$

Commonly used mEq weights			
Chloride	35.5 mg = 1 mEq	Magnesium	12 mg = 1 mEq
Sodium	23 mg = 1 mEq	Potassium	39 mg = 1 mEq
Calcium	20 mg = 1 mEq		

To convert temperature °C ↔ °F: $\dfrac{°C}{°F - 32} = \dfrac{5}{9}$ or $°C = \dfrac{5}{9}(°F - 32)$

$$°F = 32 + \dfrac{9}{5}\ °C$$

To calculate creatinine clearance (Ccr) from serum creatinine:

Male: $Ccr = \dfrac{\text{weight (kg)} \times (140 - \text{age})}{72 \times \text{serum creatinine (mg/dL)}}$ Female: Ccr = 0.85 × calculation for males

To calculate ideal body weight (kg):

Male = 50 kg + 2.3 kg (each inch > 5 ft)   Female = 45.5 kg + 2.3 kg (each inch > 5 ft)

To calculate body surface area (BSA) in adults and children:

1) *Dubois method:*

SA (cm^2) = wt (kg)$^{0.425}$ × ht (cm)$^{0.725}$ × 71.84

SA (m^2) = K × $\sqrt[3]{wt^2\ (kg)}$ (common K value 0.1 for toddlers, 0.103 for neonates)

2) *Simplified method:*

$$BSA\ (m^2) = \sqrt{\dfrac{\text{ht (cm)} \times \text{wt (kg)}}{3600}}$$

To approximate surface area (m^2) of children from weight (kg):

Weight range (kg)	≈ Surface area (m^2)
1 to 5	(0.05 × kg) + 0.05
6 to 10	(0.04 × kg) + 0.10
11 to 20	(0.03 × kg) + 0.20
21 to 40	(0.02 × kg) + 0.40

Suggested Weights for Adults	
Height*	Weight in pounds†
4'10"	91-119
4'11"	94-124
5'0"	97-128
5'1"	101-132
5'2"	104-137
5'3"	107-141
5'4"	111-146
5'5"	114-150
5'6"	118-155
5'7"	121-160
5'8"	125-164
5'9"	129-169
5'10"	132-174
5'11"	136-179
6'0"	140-184
6'1"	144-189
6'2"	148-195
6'3"	152-200
6'4"	156-205
6'5"	160-211
6'6"	164-216

* Without shoes.   † Without clothes.

The higher weights in the ranges generally apply to people with more muscle and bone. Source: Nutrition and Your Health: Dietary Guidelines for Americans, 4th ed, 1995. US Department of Agriculture, US Department of Health and Human Services. At press time, these new guidelines had not been officially released. It is possible some changes to this chart will occur.

►*Standard Medical Abbreviations used in medical orders:*

Abbreviation	Meaning	Abbreviation	Meaning	Abbreviation	Meaning
≈	approximately equals	ADME	absorption, distribution, metabolism and elimination	ARC	AIDS-related complex
Δ	delta			ARDS	adult respiratory distress syndrome
ε	epsilon; molar absorption coefficient	admov	apply (*admove*)	ARF	acute renal failure
Ω	omega; ohm	ADP	adenosine diphosphate	Arg	arginine
5-HIAA	5-hydroxyindoleacetic acid	ADR	adverse drug reaction	ARV	AIDS-related virus
5-HT	5-hydroxytryptamine (serotonin)	ADRRS	Adverse Drug Reaction Reporting System	as	left ear (*aurio sinister*)
6-MP	6-mercaptopurine	ad sat	to saturation (*ad saturatum, ad saturandum*)	ASHD	arteriosclerotic heart disease
17-OHCS	17-hydroxycorticosteroids	adst feb	when fever is present (*adstante febre*)	ASHP	American Society of Hospital Pharmacists
α	alpha			Asn	asparagine
A	ampere(s)	ad us.	ext for external use (*ad usum externum*)	Asp	aspartic acid
Å	angstrom(s)	adv	against (*adversum*)	AST	aspartate aminotransferase, serum (previously SGOT)
aa	of each (ana)	aer	aerosol		
āā	of each (ana)	Ag	antigen; silver (*argentum*)	atm	standard atmosphere
AA	Alcoholics Anonymous; amino acid	agit. Ante us.	shake before using (*agita ante usum*)	ATN	acute tubular necrosis
AACP	American Association of Clinical Pharmacy; American Association of Colleges of Pharmacy	agit. Bene	shake well (*agita bene*)	ATP	adenosine triphosphate
		AHA	American Hospital Association	ATPase	adenosine triphosphatase
				ATPD	ambient temperature and pressure, saturated
AARP	American Association of Retired Persons	AID	artificial insemination donor	at wt	atomic weight
Ab	antibody	AIDS	acquired immunodeficiency syndrome	au	each ear (*aures utrae*)
ABGs	arterial blood gases			AU	gold (*aurum*)
abs feb	when fever is absent (*absente febre*)	AJHP	*American Journal of Hospital Pharmacy*	AUC	area under the plasma concentration-time curve
ABVD	Adriamycin (doxorubicin), bleomycin, vinblastine, (and) dacarbazine	al	left ear (*aurio laeva*)	AV	atrioventricular
		ala	alanine	A-V	arteriovenous; atrioventricular (block, bundle, conduction, dissociation, extrasystole)
		ALL	acute lymphocytic leukemia		
ac	before meals or food (*ante cibum*)	ALT	alanine aminotransferase, serum (previously SGPT)	AW	atomic weight
ACCP	American College of Clinical Pharmacy	alt hor	every other hour (*alternis horis*)	AWP	average wholesale price
ACD	acid-citrate-dextrose			ax.	axis
ACE	angiotensin-converting enzyme	A.M.	before noon; morning (*ante meridiem*)	β	beta
ACEI	angiotensin-converting enzyme inhibitor	AMA	American Medical Association	BAC	blood-alcohol concentration
ACh	acetylcholine			BADL	basic activities of daily life
ACIP	Advisory Committee on Immunization Practices	AML	acute myelogenous leukemia	BBB	blood brain barrier
		AMP	adenosine monophosphate	BDZ	benzodiazepine
ACLS	advanced cardiac life support	ANA	antinuclear antibody(ies)	bib	drink (*bibe*)
ACPE	American Council on Pharmaceutical Education	ANC	acid neutralizing capacity	bid	twice daily; two times a day (*bis in die*)
		ANDA	abbreviated new drug application	bm	bowel movement
ACS	American Chemical Society	ANOVA	analysis of variance	BMR	basal metabolic rate
ACT	activated clotting time	ANUG	acute necrotizing ulcerative gingivitis	bp	boiling point
ACTH	adrenocorticotropic hormone			BP	blood pressure
		APA	antipernicious anemia (factor)	BPH	benign prostatic hypertrophy
ad to;	to; up to (*ad*)	APAP	acetaminophen	bpm	beats per minute
a.d.	right ear (*aurio dextra*)	APC	antigen presenting cell(s)	BSA	body surface area
ADE	adverse drug experience	APhA	American Pharmaceutical Association	BT	bleeding time
ADH	antidiuretic hormone			BUN	blood urea nitrogen
adhib	to be administered (*adhibendus*)	aPTT	activated partial thromboplastin time	C	centigrade
ad lib	as desired, at pleasure (*ad libitum*)	aq	water (*aqua*)	C.	*clostridium*
				c	gallon (*cong*)
				c̄	with (*cum*)
ADLs	activities of daily living	aq. dest	distilled water (*aqua destillata*)	°C	degrees Celsius

Abbreviation	Meaning	Abbreviation	Meaning	Abbreviation	Meaning
Ca	calcium	COG	center of gravity	det	give (*detur*)
CA	cancer; carcinoma; cardiac arrest; chronologic age; croup-associated	comp	compound (*compositus*)	DHHS	Department of Health and Human Services
		COMT	catecholamine-o-methyl transferase	DIC	disseminated intravascular coagulation
CAD	coronary artery disease	cont rem	let the medicine be continued (*continuetur remedium*)	dieb alt	every other day (*diebus alternis*)
Cal	Calorie (kilocalorie)				
cAMP	cyclic adenosine monophosphate	COPD	chronic obstructive pulmonary disease	dil	dilute (*dilue*)
caps	capsule (*capsula*)	CPAP	continuous positive airway pressure	dim	one-half (*dimidius*)
CAS	Chemical Abstracts Service			dir prop	with proper direction (*directione propria*)
CAT	computerized axial tomography	CPK	creatine phosphokinase	div in par aeq	divide into equal parts (*divide in partes aequales*)
		CPR	cardiopulmonary resuscitation		
cath	catheterize	CQI	continuous quality improvement	DIS	drug information source
CBA	cost-benefit analysis			disp	dispense (*dispensa*)
CBC	complete blood count	Cr	creatinine; chromium	div	divide
CC	chief complaint	CrCl	creatinine clearance	DJD	degenerative joint disease
cc	cubic centimeter	CRD	chronic respiratory disease	DKA	diabetic ketoacidosis
CCBs	calcium channel blockers			dl	deciliter (100 ml)
CCU	coronary care unit; critical care unit	CRF	chronic renal failure	DMD	Doctor of Dental Medicine
		CRH	corticotropin-releasing hormone	DMSO	dimethyl sulfoxide
CD4	T-helper lymphocytes and macrophages			DNA	deoxyribonucleic acid
		crm	cream	DNR	do not resuscitate
CDC	Centers for Disease Control and Prevention	CRNA	Certified Registered Nurse Anesthetist	DNS	Director of Nursing Service; Doctor of Nursing Services
CEA	cost effectiveness analysis	C&S	culture and sensitivity		
CF	cystic fibrosis	CSA	Controlled Substances Act; cyclosporin A	DO	Doctor of Osteopathy
CFC	chlorofluorocarbon			DOA	dead on arrival
CFU	colony-forming units	CSF	cerebrospinal fluid; colony-stimulating factors	DP	Doctor of Podiatry
CHD	coronary heart disease			DPH	Doctor of Public Health; Doctor of Public Hygiene
CHF	congestive heart failure	CSP	cellulose sodium phosphate		
Ci	curie			DPI	dry powder inhaler
CK	creatinine kinase	ct	clotting time	DPM	Doctor of Physical Medicine; Doctor of Podiatric Medicine
Cl	chlorine	CT	computerized tomography		
Cl_{cr}	creatinine clearance	CTZ	chemoreceptor trigger zone		
cm	centimeter; cream			DPS	disintegrations per second
Cm	curium	cu	cubic	DRG	diagnosis-related groups
cm^2	square centimeter(s)	Cu	copper (*cuprum*)	DRI	Dietary Reference Intakes
cm^3	cubic centimeter	CV	cardiovascular	drp	drop(s)
CMA	Certified Medical Assistant	CVA	cerebrovascular accident	DrPh	Doctor of Public Health; Doctor of Public Hygiene
		CVP	central venous pressure		
CMC	carpometacarpal	CXR	chest x-ray	DRR	Drug Regimen Review
CMI	cell-mediated immunity	cyl	cylinder; cylindrical (lens)	DT	delirium tremens
CML	chronic myelocytic leukemia	cys	cysteine	dtd	give of such a dose (*dentur tales doses*)
		d	day (*dies*)		
C_{max}	maximum effective plasma concentration	D5W	Dextrose 5% in Water Solution	DTP	diphtheria, tetanus toxoids & pertussis vaccine
C_{min}	minimum effective plasma concentration	D10W	Dextrose 10% in Water Solution	DTRs	deep tendon reflexes
				DUB	dysfunctional uterine bleeding
CMT	Certified Medical Transcriptionist	D&C	dilation and curettage; designation applied to dyes permitted for use in drugs and cosmetics		
CMV	cytomegalovirus I			DUE	Drug Usage Evaluations
CMVIG	cytomegalovirus immune globulin			DUR	Drug Utilization Review
		D&E	dilation and evacuation	dur dol	while pain lasts (*durante dolore*)
CN	cranial nerve	DC	Doctor of Chiropractic		
CNM	Certified Nurse Midwife	DDS	Doctor of Dental Surgery	DVA	Department of Veterans Affairs
CNS	central nervous system	DEA	Drug Enforcement Administration		
CO	cardiac output			DVM	Doctor of Veterinary Medicine
CO_2	carbon dioxide	deglut	swallow (*degluttiatur*)		
CoA	coenzyme A	DERM	dermatologic	DVT	deep venous thrombosis
				E.	*Enterococcus; Escherichia*
				EBV	Epstein-Barr virus

Abbreviation	Meaning	Abbreviation	Meaning	Abbreviation	Meaning
EC	enteric coated	FD&C	designation applied to dyes permitted for use in foods, drugs and cosmetics; Food, Drug and Cosmetic Act	h	hour (*hora*)
ECG	electrocardiogram			H_2	histamine 2
ECT	electroconvulsive therapy			H_2O	water
ed.	editor			HA	hyaluronic acid
ED	emergency department; effective dose	Fe	iron (*ferrum*)	Hb	hemoglobin
ED_{50}	median-effective dose	FEF	forced expiratory flow	HbF	fetal hemoglobin
EDTA	ethylenediamine tetraacetic acid	FET	forced expiratory time	HBIG	hepatitis B immune specific globulin
		FEV_1	forced expiratory volume in 1 second	HCFA	Health Care Financing Administration
EEG	electroencephalogram				
EENT	eye, ear, nose, and throat	fl oz	fluid ounce(s)	HCG	human chorionic gonadotropin
EF	ejection fraction	Fru	fructose		
eg	for example (*exempli gratia*)	FSH	follicle-stimulating hormone	HCl	hydrochloric acid
				HCN	hydrogen cyanide
EIA	enzyme immunoassay	ft	make; let be made (*fac, fiat, fiant*)	Hct	hematocrit
EKG	electrocardiogram			hd	bedtime (*hora decubitus*)
el	elixir	ft	foot (feet)	HDL	high-density lipoprotein
ELISA	enzyme-linked immunosorbent assay	ft^2	square foot (feet)	HEMA	hematologic
		FTC	Federal Trade Commission	HEME	hematologic
elix	elixir			hep	hepatic
EMIT	enzyme-multiplied immunoassay test	FTI	free-thyroxine index	HEPA	high efficiency particulate air
		FUO	fever of unknown origin		
emp	as directed	FVC	forced vital capacity	Hg	mercury (*hydragyrum*)
ENL	erythema nodosum leprosum	γ	gamma	Hgb	hemoglobin
		g	gram (*gramma*)	HGH	human pituitary growth hormone
ENT	ear, nose, throat	G-6-P	glucose-6-phosphate		
EPA	Environmental Protection Agency	G-6-PD	glucose-6-phosphate dehydrogenase	*Hib.*	*Haemophilus influenzae*
EPAP	expiratory positive airway pressure	GABA	gamma-aminobutyric acid	*His.*	*Haemophilus influenzae* type b
		Gal	galactose		
EPO	erythropoietin	gal	gallon	HIV	human immunodeficiency virus
EPS	extrapyramidal syndrome (or symptoms)	G-CSF	granulocyte colony-stimulating factor	HLA	human leukocyte antigen
ER	emergency room; estrogen receptor; extended release; endoplasmic reticulum	GERD	gastroesophageal reflux disease	HMG-CoA	3-hydroxy-3-methylglutaryl coenzyme A
		GFR	glomerular filtration rate	HMO	health maintenance organization
ESR	erythrocyte sedimentation rate; electron spin resonance	GGTP	gamma glutamyl transpeptidase	hor decub	at bedtime (*hora decubitus*)
		GH	growth hormone		
et	and	GHRF	growth hormone-releasing factor	hor som	at bedtime (*hora somni*)
ET	via endotracheal tube			HPA	hypothalamic-pituitary-adrenocortical (axis)
et al.	for 3 or more co-authors or co-workers (*et alii*)	GHRH	growth hormone-releasing hormone	HPLC	high performance liquid chromatography
ex aq	in water	GI	gastrointestinal		
ext rel	extended release	GLC	gas-liquid chromatography	HPLC/MS	high performance liquid chromatography/mass spectrometry
F	fluorine				
f	make; let be made (*fac, fiat, fiant*)	gln	glutamine	HPMC	hydroxypropylmethylcellulose
		glu	glutamic acid; glutamyl		
°F	degrees Fahrenheit	gly	glycine	HPV	human papillomavirus
Fab	fragment of immunoglobulin G involved in antigen binding	Gm	gram (*gramma*)	HR	heart rate
		gr	grain (*granum*)	hr	hour
		grad	gradually (*gradatim*)	hs	at bedtime (*hora somni*)
FAO	Food and Agriculture Organization	gran	granule(s)	HSA	human serum albumin
FAS	fetal alcohol syndrome	GRAS	generally regarded as safe*	HSV-1	herpes simplex virus type 1
FBS	fasting blood sugar	gtt	a drop (*gutta*)	HSV-2	herpes simplex virus type 2
FDA	Food and Drug Administration	GU	genitourinary		
		guttat	drop by drop (*guttatim*)	Hz	hertz
		Gyn	gynecology	I	iodine
		H.	*Haemophilus; Helicobacter*	IADL	instrumental activities of daily living

Abbreviation	Meaning	Abbreviation	Meaning	Abbreviation	Meaning
I/O	intake/output	JCAHO	Joint Commission on Accreditation of Health-care Organizations	MADD	Mothers Against Drunk Drivers
IBW	ideal body weight			man pr	early morning; first thing in the morning (*mane primo*)
IC	intracoronary	K	potassium (*kalium*); kelvin		
ICD	International Classification of Diseases of the World Health Organization	kcal	kilocalorie(s)	MAO	monoamine oxidase
		keV	kiloelectronvolt(s)	MAOI	monoamine oxidase inhibitor
ICF	intracellular fluid	kg	kilogram	MAP	mean arterial pressure
ICP	intracranial pressure	kJ	kilojoule(s)	max	maximum
ICU	intensive care unit	*Kleb.*	*Klebsiella*	MBC	minimum bactericidal concentration
ID	intradermal; infective dose	KVO	keep vein open	MBD	minimal brain dysfunction
IDDM	insulin-dependent diabetes mellitus (type 1 diabetes)	L	liter	mcg	microgram
		L.	*Legionella*; *Listeria*	MCH	mean corpuscular hemoglobin
IDU	idoxuridine	lb	pound		
IFN	interferon	LBW	low body weight	MCHC	mean corpuscular hemoglobin concentration
Ig	immunoglobulin	LD	lethal dose	mCi	millicurie
IL	interleukin	LD-50	a dose lethal to 50% of the specified animals or microorganisms	MCT	medium-chain triglyceride
Ile	isoleucine			MCV	mean corpuscular volume
IM	intramuscular	LDH	lactate dehydrogenase	MD	Doctor of Medicine (*Medicinae Doctor*)
in	inch(es)	LDL	low-density lipoprotein		
in²	square inch(es)	LE	lupus erythematosus	MDI	metered dose inhaler
IND	Investigational New Drug	Leu	leucine	m dict	as directed (*more dicto*)
in d	daily (*in dies*)	LFT	liver function test	MDR	minimum daily requirements
INDA	Investigational New Drug Application	LH	luteinizing hormone		
		liq	liquid (*liquor*)	MEC	minimum effective concentration
Inh	inhaled	LM	Licentiate in Midwifery		
INH	isoniazid	LOC	level of consciousness	MEDLARS	Medical Literature Analysis and Retrieval System
Inhal	inhalation	Lot	lotion		
Inj	injection	LPN	Licensed Practical Nurse	MEDLINE	National Library of Medicine medical database
INR	International Normalizing Ratio	Lr	lawrencium		
		LSD	lysergic acid diethylamide	mEq	milliequivalent
int cib	between meals (*inter cibos*)	LTCF	long-term care facility	Met	methionine
		LTM	long-term memory	MeV	megaelectronvolt(s)
IOP	intraocular pressure	LUQ	left upper quadrant (of abdomen)	Mg	magnesium
IP	intraperitoneal(ly)			mg	milligram
IPA	International Pharmaceutical Abstracts	LVEDP	left ventricular end-diastolic pressure	MHC	major histocompatibility complex
IPPB	intermittent positive pressure breathing	LVET	left ventricular ejection time	MI	myocardial infarction
IPV	poliovirus vaccine inactivated	LVF	left ventricular function	MIA	metabolite bacterial inhibition assay
		LVN	Licensed Visiting Nurse; Licensed Vocational Nurse	MIC	minimum inhibitory concentration
IQ	intelligence quotient				
ISA	intrinsic sympathomimetic activity	LVP	large-volume parenterals	MID	minimal infecting dose
		Lw	former symbol for lawrencium (see Lr)	min	minute
ISF	interstitial fluid			min.	minimum
ISI	Institute for Scientific Information	Lys	lysine	MIP	maximum inspiratory pressure
		μm	micrometer		
ISO	International Organization for Standardization	μg	microgram	mixt	a mixture (*mixtura*)
		m	meter	MJ	mejajoule(s)
IT	intrathecal(ly)	M	mix (*misce*)	ml	milliliter
IU	international unit(s)	M	molar (strength of a solution)	mm	millimeter
IUD	intrauterine device			mm²	square millimeter(s)
IV	intravenous	*M.*	*Moraxella*; *Mycobacterium*; *Mycoplasma*	mm³	cubic millimeter(s)
IVF	intravascular fluid			mmHg	millimeters of mercury
IVP	intravenous piggyback	m²	square meter (of body surface area)	mmol	millimole
J	joule(s)			MMR	measles, mumps and rubella virus vaccine, live
JCAH	Joint Commission on Accreditation of Hospitals	m³	cubic meter(s)		
		MA	mental age		
		MAC	maximum allowable cost		

Abbreviation	Meaning	Abbreviation	Meaning	Abbreviation	Meaning
MMWR	*Morbidity and Mortality Weekly Report*	NMS	neuroleptic malignant syndrome	part aeq	equal parts/amounts (*partes aequales*)
Mn	manganese	NMT	not more than (on prescriptions)	part vic	in divided doses (*partitis vicibus*)
Mo	molybdenum	no	number (*numerus*)	PAS	para-aminosalicylic acid
mo	month	noc	in the night (*nocturnal*)	PAW	pulmonary arterial wedge
mol	mole(s)	noc maneq	at night and the morning (*nocte maneque*)	PAWP	pulmonary artery wedge pressure
mor dict	in the manner stated (*more dicto*)	non rep	do not repeat; no refills (*non repetatur*)	Pb	lead (*plumbum*)
mor sol	as usual; as customary (*more solito*)	NPN	nonprotein nitrogen	PBP	penicillin-binding protein
mOsm	milliosmole	NPO	nothing by mouth	pc	after meals (*post cibum; post cibos*)
MPH	Master of Public Health	NS	normal saline (as in solution)	PCA	patient-controlled analgesia
MRI	magnetic resonance imaging	NSAIA	nonsteroidal anti-inflammatory agent	pCO_2	plasma partial pressure of carbon dioxide
mRNA	messenger RNA	NSAID	nonsteroidal anti-inflammatory drug	PCP	phencyclidine
MS	mass spectrometry; mitral stenosis; multiple sclerosis	NTD	neutral tube defect	PCR	polymerase chain reaction
MW	molecular weight	O	a pint (*octarius*)	PDGF	platelet-derived growth factor
N	normal (strength of a solution)	OB/GYN	obstetrics and gynecology	PDLL	poorly differentiated lymphocytic lymphoma
N.	*Neisseria*	OBRA	Omnibus Budget Reconciliation Act of 1990	PE	pulmonary embolism
Na	sodium (*natrium*)	OBS	organic brain syndrome	PEEP	positive end expiratory pressure
NABP	National Association of Boards of Pharmacy	OC	oral contraceptive	PEG	polyethylene glycol
NABPLEX	National Association of Boards of Pharmacy Licensing Exam	Oct	a pint (*octarius*)	PERLA	pupils equal, react to light and accommodation
NAD	nicotinamide-adenine dinucleotide phosphate	od	right eye (*oculus dexter*)	PET	positron emission tomography
NADH	reduced form of nicotine adenine dinucleotide	OD	Doctor of Optometry; overdose	pg	picogram(s)
NADP	nicotinamide-adenine dinucleotide phosphate	Oint	ointment	PG	prostaglandin
NADPH	nicotinamide-adenine dinucleotide phosphate (reduced form)	ol	left eye (*oculus laevus*)	PGA	prostaglandin A
		omn hor	at every hour (*omni hora*)	PGB	prostaglandin B
NAPA	*N*-acetyl procainamide	Ophth	ophthalmic	PGE	prostaglandin E
NARD	National Association of Retail Druggists - Now NCPA; National Assoc. of Community Pharmacists	os	left eye (*oculus sinister*)	PGF	prostaglandin F
		OSHA	Occupational Safety and Health Administration	pH	the negative logarithm of the hydrogen ion concentration
nb	note well (*nota bene*)	OT	occupational therapy	PharmD	Doctor of Pharmacy (*Pharmaciae Doctor*)
nCi	nanocurie(s)	otc	over-the-counter (nonprescription)	PhD	Doctor of Philosophy (*Philosophiae Doctor*)
NCPA	National Assoc. of Community Pharmacists	OPV	oral poliovirus vaccine, live	Phe	phenylalanine
ND	Doctor of Naturopathic Medicine	ou	each eye (*oculo uterque*)	PhG	German Pharmacopeia (*Pharmacopoeia Germanica*)
NDA	new drug application	o/w	oil-in-water (emulsion)		
NF	National Formulary	oz	ounce	PHS	Public Health Service
ng	nanogram	P	phosphorus	pKa	the negative logarithm of the dissociation constant
NG	nasogastric	*P*	probability		
NK	natural killer (cells); killer T cells	P&T	pharmacy and therapeutics (committee)	PKU	phenylketonuria
		Pa	pascal(s)	PMA	Pharmaceutical Manufacturers Association
NIDDM	non-insulin dependent diabetes mellitus (type 2 diabetes)	PA	Physician Assistant; Physician's Assistant	PMN	polymorphonuclear leukocyte
		PABA	para-aminobenzoic acid	PMR	patient medication record
NIH	National Institutes of Health	PAC	premature atrial contraction	PMS	premenstrual syndrome
NLM	National Library of Medicine	$PaCO_2$	arterial plasma partial pressure of carbon dioxide	PND	paroxysmal nocturnal dyspnea
nm	nanometer(s)	PAD	premature atrial depolarization	po	by mouth; orally (*per os*)
		PAF	platelet-activating factor		
		PaO_2	partial alveolar oxygen	pO_2	oxygen pressure (tension)

Abbreviation	Meaning	Abbreviation	Meaning	Abbreviation	Meaning
POR	problem-oriented medical record	qs ad	a sufficient quantity to make	Ser	serine
POS	point of service	qt	quart	sf	sugar free
post cib	after meals (*post cibos*)	qv	as much as you wish (*quam volueris*)	SGGT	serum gamma-glutamyl transferase
PPD	purified protein derivative of tuberculin	R&D	research and development	SGOT	(see AST)
PPI	patient package insert	RA	rheumatoid arthritis	SGPT	(see ALT)
ppm	parts per million	RAI	radioactive iodine	*Sh.*	*Shigella*
PPO	preferred provider organization	RAS	renin-angiotension system; reticular-activating system	SIADH	syndrome of inappropriate secretion of antidiuretic hormone
pr	per rectum	RAST	radioallergosorbent test	SIDS	sudden infant death syndrome
Pr.	*Proteus*	RBC	red blood (cell) count	Sig	label; let it be printed (*signa*)
prn	as needed; when required (*pro re nata*)	RDA	Recommended Dietary (Daily) Allowance	SI units	International System of Units
Pro	proline	RDS	respiratory distress syndrome	SK	streptokinase
pro rat. Aet.	According to patient's age (*pro ratione aetatis*)	RDW	red-cell distribution width	SL	sublingual(ly)
Ps.	*Pseudomonas*	RE	reticuloendothelial	SLE	systemic lupus erythematosus
PSA	prostate-specific antigen	rem	radio equivalent man	SMA	sequential multiple analysis
PSP	phenolsulfonphthalein	REM	rapid eye movement	Sn	tin (*stannum*)
PSVT	paroxysmal supraventricular tachycardia	rep	let it be repeated (*repetatur*)	SNF	skilled nursing facility
pt	pint	RES	reticuloendothelial system	sol	solution (*solutio*)
PT	prothrombin time; pharmacy and therapeutics; physical therapy	RF	releasing factor	soln	solution
		Rh	Rhesus (RH blood group)	solv	dissolve
PTH	parathyroid hormone	RIA	radioimmunoassay	sp	species
PTT	partial thromboplastin time	RN	Registered Nurse	SPECT	single photon emission computerized tomography
PUD	peptic ulcer disease	RNA	ribonucleic acid		
pulv	a powder (*pulvis*)	ROM	range of motion	sp gr	specific gravity
PUVA	oral administration of psoralen and subsequent exposure to ultraviolet light of A wavelengths (UVA)	RPh	registered pharmacist	SPF	sun protection factor
		rpm	revolutions per minute	sq	square
		rps	revolutions per second	SR	sedimentation rate; sustained-release
		RR	respiratory rate		
PVC	premature ventricular contraction; polyvinyl chloride	RT$_3$U	total serum thyroxine concentration	ss	one-half (*semis*)
		RUL	right upper lobe (of lung)	s̅s̅	one-half (*semis*)
PVD	peripheral vascular disease; premature ventricular depolarizations	RUQ	right upper quadrant (of abdomen)	SSRI	selective serotonin reuptake inhibitors
		Rx	prescription only; take; a recipe (*recipe*)	*Staph.*	*Staphylococcus*
pwdr	powder	*S.*	*Salmonella; Serratia*	stat	immediately; at once (*statim*)
q	every	s	second	STM	short-term memory
Q	volume of blood flow	s	without (*sine*)	STP	standard temperature and pressure
QA	quality assurance	s̅	without (*sine*)		
qad	every other day (*quoque alternis die*)	S&S	signs and symptoms	*Str.*	*Streptococcus*
QC	quality control	S-A	sinoatrial	STD	sexually transmitted disease
qd	every day (*quaque die*)	sa	according to art (*secundum artem*)	supp	suppository (*suppositorium*)
qh	every hour (*quaque hora*)	sat	saturated (*sataratus*)	suppl	supplement(s)
q hr	every hour	Sb	antimony (*stibium*)	susp	suspension
qid	four times daily (*quarter in die*)	SBE	self breast examination; subacute bacterial endocarditis	SV	stroke volume
ql	as much as desired (*quantum libet*)			syr	syrup (*syrupus*)
qod	every other day	SC	subcutaneous(ly)	t$_{1/2}$	half-life
q 2 hr	every 2 hours	S$_{cr}$	serum creatinine	T$_3$	triiodothyronine
qs	a sufficient quantity (*quantum sufficiat*)	SD	standard deviation; streptodornase	T$_4$	thyroxine
				tab	tablet (*tabella*)
		Se	selenium	tal	such
qs	as much as is enough (*quantum satis*)	sec	second	tal dos	such doses

Abbreviation	Meaning	Abbreviation	Meaning	Abbreviation	Meaning
TB	tuberculosis	tr	tincture	V_c	volume of distribution of the central compartment
TBC	thyroxine-binding globulin	trit	triturate (*tritura*)	V_d	volume of distribution (one compartment)
TBP	thyroxine-binding proteins	tRNA	transfer RNA		
TBPA	thyroxine-binding pre-albumin	Trp	tryptophan	$V_{d\beta}$	volume of distribution of the β phase
		TSA	tumor-specific antigens		
TBW	total body weight	TSH	thyroid-stimulating hormone	V_{dss}	steady-state apparent volume of distribution
TCA	tricyclic antidepressant				
TD_{50}	median toxic dose	tsp	teaspoonful	VHDL	very high density lipoprotein
TEEC	transesophageal echocardiography	TSS	toxic shock syndrome		
		TSTA	tumor-specific transplantation antigen	VLDL	very low density lipoprotein
TEN	toxic epidermal necrolysis				
TENS	transcutaneous electrical nerve stimulation	TT	thrombin time	VMA	vanillylmandelic acid
		TV	tidal volume	vol	volume
TG	total triglycerides	Tyr	tyrosine	VS	vital signs
THC	tetrahydrocannabinol	U	unit	v/v	volume in volume
Thr	threonine	ud	as directed	v/w	volume in weight
TIA	transient ischemic attack	UD	unit-dose package	wa	while awake
tid	three times daily (*ter in die*)	UK	United Kingdom	WBC	white blood (cell) count
		ung	ointment (*unguentum*)	WBCT	whole blood clotting time
tbsp	tablespoonful	URI	upper respiratory infection	WDLL	well-differentiated lymphocytic lymphoma
tinct	tincture				
TLC	total lung capacity; thin layer chromatography	USAN	United States Adopted Name(s)	WFI	water for injection
		USP	*United States Pharmacopeia*	WHO	World Health Organization
T_{max}	time to maximum concentration				
TMJ	temporomandibular joint	USPHS	United States Public Health Service	wk	week
TNF	tumor necrosis factor			WNL	within normal limits
TNM	tumor, node, metastasis (tumor staging)	ut dict	as directed (*ut dictum*)	w/o	water in oil
		UTI	urinary tract infection	wt	weight
top	topical(ly)	UVA	ultraviolet A wave	w/v	weight in volume
TOPV	trivalent oral polio vaccine	V	volt	w/w	weight in weight
tPA	tissue plasminogen activator	VA	Veterans Administration	yo	years old
		vag	vaginal(ly)	yr	year
TPN	total parenteral nutrition	Val	valine	ZE	Zollinger-Ellison
TPR	temperature, pulse, respirations	var	variety	Zn	zinc
TQM	total quality management	VC	vital capacity		

MANUFACTURER/DISTRIBUTOR ABBREVIATIONS

This listing includes only those manufacturers whose names are abbreviated in *Drug Facts and Comparisons®*. It is not a complete list of all manufacturers whose products are listed in this book.

B-D	Becton, Dickinson & Co.	B-D	Becton, Dickinson & Co.	B-D	Becton, Dickinson & Co.
B-I	Boehringer Ingelheim	McNeil-CPC	McNeil Consumer Products Company	Schwarz Pharma K-U	Schwarz Pharma Inc.
B-Mannheim	Boehringer Mannheim				
B-M Squibb	Bristol-Myers Squibb	Mead-J	Mead Johnson Nutritional	SK-Beecham, SKB	SmithKline Beecham
Hickam	Dow B. Hickam				
Inter. Ethical	International Ethical Labs	Merck	Merck & Co.	URL	United Research Labs
		P-D	Parke-Davis	Warner-C	Warner Chilcott
IMS	International Medication Systems	PBH	PBH Wesley Jessen	Warner-L	Warner-Lambert
		P & G	Procter & Gamble	W-A	Wyeth-Ayerst
J & J	Johnson & Johnson	RPR	Rhone-Poulenc Rorer		

00089, 55298, 55326
3M Personal Healthcare Prods.
3M Center
Building 275-5W-05
St. Paul, MN 55144-1000
651-733-1110
800-364-3577
www.mmm.com

00089
3M Pharmaceuticals
3M Center
Building 275-5W-05
St. Paul, MN 55144-1000
651-773-1110
800-364-3577
www.mmm.com

63801
7 Oaks Pharmaceutical Corp.
161 Harry Stanley Dr.
Easley, SC 29640
864-850-1700
877-723-6725
www.7oakspharma.com

A & D Medical
1555 McCandless Drive
Milpitas, CA 95035
408-263-5333
888-726-9966
www.andmedical.com

AAI Pharma (Headquarters)
2320 Scientific Park Drive
Wilmington, NC 28405
910-254-7350
800-575-4224
www.aaipharma.com

12463
Abana Pharmaceuticals, Inc.
See Jones Pharma Incorporated

Abbott Diagnostics
10 Abbott Park Rd.
Abbott Park, IL 60064-6154
800-323-9100

Abbott Hospital Products
100 Abbott Park Rd.
Abbott Park, IL 60064-6154
847-937-6100
800-615-0187

00074
Abbott Laboratories
Pharmaceutical Division
100 Abbott Park Rd.
Abbott Park, IL 60064-6154
800-633-9110
www.abbott.com

Aber Pharmaceuticals, Inc.
10511 Old Ridge Road
Ashland, VA 23005

Able Laboratories, Inc.
6 Hollywood Ct.
South Plainfield, NJ 07080
908-754-2253
www.able.com

Academic Pharmaceuticals, Inc.
21 N. Skokie Valley Highway
Lake Bluff, IL 60044
847-735-1170

Access Pharmaceuticals
2600 Stemmons Freeway
Dallas, TX 75207-2107
214-905-5100
www.accesspharma.com

Acme United Corp.
1931 Black Rock Turnpike
Fairfield, CT 06825
203-332-7330
800-835-2263
www.acmeunited.com

Actelion Pharmaceuticals US, Inc.
601 Gateway Blvd.
Suite 100
South San Francisco, CA 94080
650-624-6900
www.actelion.com

53014
Adams Laboratories, Inc.
14801 Sovereign Road
Fort Worth, TX 76155-2645
817-354-3858
800-770-5270
www.adamslabs.com

Adria Laboratories
See Pharmacia Corp.

Advance
2201-F 5th Avenue
Ronkonkoma, NY 11779
631-981-4600

00062
Advance Biofactures Corp.
Biospecifics Technologies
35 Wilbur Street
Lynbrook, NY 11563
516-593-7000
www.biospecifics.com

10888
Advanced Nutritional Technology
6988 Sierra Ct.
Dublin, CA 94568
925-803-1168
800-624-6543
www.antlab.com

Advanced Polymer Systems
See AP Pharma

Advanced Vision Research
7 Alfred St.
Suite 330
Woburn, MA 01801
781-932-8327
800-579-8327
www.theratears.com

Aero Pharmaceuticals
3848 FAU Blvd., Suite 100
Boca Raton, FL 33431
800-223-6837

63010
Agouron Pharmaceuticals
See Pfizer

A.H. Robins Consumer Products
See Whitehall-Robins Healthcare

00031
A.H. Robins, Inc.
See Whitehall-Robins Healthcare

Aid-Pack USA
See NutraMax Products, Inc.

17478
Akorn, Inc.
2500 Millbrook Dr.
Buffalo Grove, IL 60089
847-279-6100
800-535-7155
www.akorn.com

41383
AKPharma, Inc.
6840 Old Egg Harbor Rd.
Pleasantville, NJ 08232
609-645-0767
800-994-4711
www.akpharma.com

A.L. Labs
See Alpharma USPD, Inc.

Alberto Culver
2525 Armitage Avenue
Melrose Park, IL 60160
708-450-3000
www.alberto.com

00065, 00998
Alcon Laboratories, Inc.
6201 S. Freeway
Ft. Worth, TX 76134-2009
817-568-7128
800-862-5266
www.alconlabs.com

Aligen
2415 Jerusalem Avenue
N. Bellmore, NY 11710

Aligon Pharmaceuticals
1860 County Road 95
Helena, AL 35080
205-663-0521

Alimenterics Inc
301 American Road
Morris Plains, NJ 07950

ALK Abello
1700 Royston Lane
Round Rock, TX 78664
888-255-3744

38697
ALK Laboratories, Inc.
27 Village Lane
Wallingford, CT 06492
203-949-2727
800-325-7354

Allegiance Healthcare Corp.
1430 Waukegan Road
McGaw Park, IL 60085
847-689-8410
800-964-5227
www.allegiance.net

00173
Allen & Hanburys
See GlaxoSmithKline, Inc.

Allendale Pharmaceuticals, Inc.
73 Franklin Turnpike
Allendale, NJ 07401
888-343-4499
www.allendalepharm.com

Allercreme
See Carme, Inc.

Allerderm Laboratories, Inc.
P.O. Box 2070
Petaluma, CA 94953-2070
707-664-8777
800-926-4568
www.allerderm.com

00023, 11980
Allergan, Inc.
2525 DuPont Dr.
Irvine, CA 92623-9534
714-246-4500
800-433-8871
www.allergan.com

Allergy Laboratories, Inc.
P.O. Box 348
Oklahoma City, OK 73101-0348
405-235-1451
800-654-3971
www.allergylabs.com

Allermed
7203 Convoy Court
San Diego, CA 92111
858-292-1060
800-221-2748
www.allermed.com

Alliance Pharmaceutical Corp.
6175 Lusk Blvd.
San Diego, CA 92121
858-410-5200
www.allp.com

Allied Pharmacy
801 Stadium Dr.
Suite 111
Arlington, TX 76111
817-226-5050

54569
Allscripts, Inc.
2401 Commerce Dr.
Libertyville, IL 60048-4464
847-680-3515
800-654-0889
www.allscripts.com

Almay, Inc.
1501 Williamsboro St.
Oxford, NC 27565
919-603-2953
800-992-5629
www.almay.com

Alpha 1 Biomedicals, Inc.
See Arriva Pharmaceuticals

49669
Alpha Therapeutic Corp.
5555 Valley Blvd.
Los Angeles, CA 90032
323-225-2221
800-421-0008
www.alphather.com

Alpharma Purepac Pharmaceuticals
200 Elmora Avenue
Elizabeth, NJ 07207
800-432-8534
www.alpharma.com
www.purepac.com

Alpharma USPD, Inc.
7205 Windsor Blvd.
Baltimore, MD 21244
410-298-1000
800-638-9096
www.alpharmaUSPD.com

51641
Alra Laboratories, Inc.
3850 Clearview Ct.
Gurnee, IL 60031
847-244-4238
800-248-2572

Altana Inc.
See Fougera Company

AltaRex Corp.
1601 Tupelo Rd., Suite 350
Waltham, MA 02451
781-672-0138
888-801-6665
www.altarex.com

00731
Alto Pharmaceuticals, Inc.
15810 Gulf Blvd.
Redington Beach, FL 33708
800-330-2891

Alva-Amco Pharmacal Cos, Inc.
7711 Merrimac Avenue
Nile, IL 60714
800-792-2582
www.alva-amco.com

17314
Alza Corp.
1900 Charleston Rd.
Mountain View, CA 94039
650-564-5000
www.alza.com

Amarin Pharmaceuticals
2 Belvedere Place, Suite 350
Mill Valley, CA 94941
908-580-5535
866-426-2746
www.amarinpharma.com

AMBI Pharmaceuticals, Inc.
See Nutrition 21

10038
Ambix Laboratories
210 Orchard St.
E. Rutherford, NJ 07073
201-939-2200
www.ambixlabs.com

89709, 90605
Amcon Laboratories
40 N. Rock Hill Rd.
St. Louis, MO 63119
314-961-5758
800-255-6161
www.amconlabs.com

Amend Drug and Chemical Corporation
See Ruger Chemical

Americal Pharmaceutical, Inc.
See Akorn, Inc.

51201
American Dermal Corp.
See Aventis Pharmaceuticals

American Generics, Inc.
34 West Fulton Street
Gloversville, NY 12078
518-725-1800

American Health Packaging
2550 John Glenn Avenue A
Columbus, OH 43217
614-492-8177
800-707-4621
www.amerisourcebergen.com

American Home Products
See Wyeth Pharmaceuticals

American Lecithin Company
115 Hurley Rd., Unit 2B
Oxford, CT 06478
203-262-7100
800-364-4416
www.americanlecithin.com

11649
American Medical Industries
330 E. Third St., Suite 2
Dell Rapids, SD 57022
605-428-5501

American Pharmaceutical Co.
1340 N. Jefferson St.
Anaheim, CA 92807
714-579-7545

63323
American Pharmaceutical Partners, Inc.
10866 Wilshire Blvd.
Suite 1270
Los Angeles, CA 90024
310-826-8505
800-551-7176
www.appdrugs.com

52769
American Red Cross
1616 N. Ft. Myers Dr.
17th Floor
Arlington, VA 22209
800-446-8883
www.redcross.org/plasma

American Red Cross (National Headquarters)
431 18th Street, NW
Washington, DC 20006
202-303-4498
www.redcross.org

00517
American Regent Labs., Inc.
See Luitpold Pharmaceuticals, Inc.

Ameriderm Laboratories, Inc.
13 Kentucky Avenue
Paterson, NJ 07503
800-455-7211
www.ameriderm.aol.com

Amerilab Technologies
3101 Louisiana Avenue North
New Hope, MN 55427
763-525-1262
www.amerilabtech.com

AmerisourceBergen
1300 Morris Dr.
Chesterbrook, PA 19087
800-829-3132
www.amerisourcebergen.com

Amerx Health Care Corp.
1150 Cleveland St.
Suite 410
Clearwater, FL 33755
727-443-0530
800-448-9599
www.amerigel.com

55513
Amgen Inc.
1 Amgen Center Dr.
Thousand Oaks, CA 91320
805-447-1000
800-282-6436
www.amgen.com

52152
Amide Pharmaceuticals, Inc.
101 E. Main St.
Little Falls, NJ 07424
973-890-1440
www.amide.com

Amkas Laboratories Inc.
4217 Commercial Way
Glenview, IL 60025
847-296-5075

Amphastar Pharmaceuticals, Inc.
11570 6th St.
Rancho Cucamonga, CA 91730
800-423-4136
www.amphastar.com

53926
AMSCO Scientific
See Steris Laboratories

Anabolic Inc.
17802 Gillette Avenue
Irvine, CA 92614
949-863-0340
800-445-6849
www.anaboliclabs.com

Anaquest
See Baxter

Andrew Jergens Company
2535 Spring Grove Ave.
Cincinnati, OH 45214
513-421-1400
800-222-3553
800-742-8798
www.jergens.com

Andrulis Pharmaceutical Corp.
P.O. Box 2135
Bethesda, MD 20817
301-419-2400

Andrx Laboratories, Inc.
6311 Ridgewood Rd. SW401
Box 15
Jackson, MS 39211
601-898-0751
888-898-0751
www.andrx.com

62037
Andrx Pharmaceuticals, Inc.
4001 S.W. 47th Ave.
Ft. Lauderdale, FL 33314
954-581-7500
800-621-7143
www.andrx.com

Angelini Pharmaceuticals, Inc.
50 Tice Blvd.
Woodcliff Lake, NJ 07677
201-489-4100
www.angelinipharmaceuticals.com

Ansell Healthcare, Inc.
200 Schulz Dr.
Red Bank, NJ 07701
732-345-5400
www.ansell.com

Antares Pharma
707 Eagleview Boulevard
Suite 414
Exton, PA 19341
610-458-6200

Anthra Pharmaceuticals, Inc.
103 Carnegie Center
Suite 102
Princeton, NJ 08540
609-514-1060
www.anthra.com

Antibodies, Inc.
P.O. Box 1560
Davis, CA 95617
530-758-4400
800-824-8540
www.antibodiesinc.com

Antigenics Inc.
630 5th Ave.
Suite 2100
New York, NY 10111
212-332-4774
www.aronex-pharm.com

AP Pharma
123 Saginaw Drive
Redwood City, CA 94063
650-366-2626
www.appharma.com

48028
Aplicare Inc.
50 E. Industrial Rd.
Branford, CT 06405
800-760-3236

Apollon Inc.
1 Great Valley Parkway
Malvern, PA 19355

60505
Apotex Corp.
2400 N. Commerce Pkwy.
Suite 400
Weston, FL 33326
847-821-8005
800-706-5575
www.apotexcorp.com

Apotex USA
616 Heathrow Dr.
Lincolnshire, IL 60069
847-821-8005
800-706-5575
www.apotexcorp.com

Apothecary Products, Inc.
11750 12th Ave. S.
Burnsville, MN 55337
952-890-1940
800-328-2742
www.apothecaryproducts.com

00003, 00015
Apothecon, Inc.
(Bristol-Myers Squibb)
P.O. Box 4500
Princeton, NJ 08540
609-897-2000
800-321-1335
www.bms.com

48723
Apothecus, Inc.
220 Townsend Sq.
Oyster Bay, NY 11771
516-624-8200
800-227-2393
www.info@apothecus.com

Applied Analytical Industries
2320 Scientific Park Drive
Wilmington, NC 28405
910-254-7000
800-575-4224
www.aai.de/

Applied Biotech, Inc.
10237 Flanders Ct.
San Diego, CA 92121
858-587-6771
www.abiapogent.com

Applied Genetics Inc. Dermatics
205 Buffalo Ave.
Freeport, NY 11520
516-868-9026
www.agiderm.com

Applied Medical Research
308 15th Ave. N.
Nashville, TN 37203
615-327-0670

Approved Drug
See Health for Life Brands, Inc.

00275
Arco Pharmaceuticals, Inc.
See Nature's Bounty, Inc.

00070
Arcola Laboratories
500 Arcola Rd.
P.O. Box 1200
Collegeville, PA 19426
800-207-8049

Armour Pharmaceutical
See Aventis Behring

Aronex Pharmaceuticals, Inc.
See Antigenics Inc.
www.aronex.com

Arrow International Corp.
   Headquarters
2400 Bernville Rd.
Reading, PA 19605
610-378-0131
800-523-8446
www.arrowintl.com

Asafi Pharmaceutical
P.O. Box 801764
Santa Clarita, CA 91380-1764
661-294-9509
www.asafi.com
www.home.aid.com

59439
Ascent Pediatrics, Inc.
8125 North Haden Road
Scottsdale, AZ 85258
602-808-8800
www.ascentpediatrics.com

AstraZeneca LP
1800 Concord Pike
Wilmington, DE 19850
800-456-3669
800-237-8898
www.AstraZeneca-us.com

59075
Athena Neurosciences, Inc.
See Elan Pharmaceuticals

Athlon Pharmaceuticals, Inc.
301 Snow Drive
Birmingham, AL 35209
205-986-7111

59702
Atley Pharmaceuticals, Inc.
10511 Old Ridge Rd.
Ashland, VA 23005
804-227-2250
www.atley.com

AutoImmune, Inc.
1199 Madia St.
Pasadena, CA 91103
626-792-1235
www.autoimmuneinc.com

Auxilium Pharmaceuticals, Inc.
160 W. Germantown Pike
Suite D5
Norristown, PA 19401
610-278-6316

00053
Aventis Behring L.L.C.
1020 First Ave.
P.O. Box 61501
King of Prussia, PA 19406
610-878-4000
800-504-5434
www.aventisbehring.com

44184
Aventis Pasteur
Discovery Drive
Swiftwater, PA 18370
570-839-7187
800-822-2463
www.us.aventispasteur.com

Aventis Pharmaceuticals
300 Somerset Corporate Blvd.
Bridgewater, NJ 08807
800-633-1610
800-207-8049
www.aventis.com

Axcan Scandipharm
22 Inverness Center Pkwy.
Suite 310
Birmingham, AL 35242
205-991-8085
800-950-8085
www.axcanscandipharm.com

B. Braun Medical Inc.
901 Marcon Blvd.
Allentown, PA 18109
610-266-0500
800-227-2862
www.bbraunusa.com

Bajamar Chemical Co., Inc.
9609 Dielman Rock Island
St. Louis, MO 63132
314-997-3414
888-242-3414
www.vesselvite.com

58174
Baker Cummins
Dermatologicals
See Baker Norton Pharmaceuticals

00575, 11414
Baker Norton Pharmaceuticals
4400 Biscayne Blvd.
Miami, FL 33137
800-327-4114
www.ivax.com

Ballard Medical Products
12050 S. Lone Peak Pkwy.
Draper, UT 84020
801-572-6800
800-528-5591
www.kchealthcare.com

Ballay Pharmaceuticals, Inc.
200 Stillwater
P.O. Box 1356
Wimberley, TX 78676
512-847-6458

Banner Pharmacaps
4125 Premiere Dr.
High Point, NC 27265
336-812-8700
800-447-1140
www.banpharm.com

Bard
See C.R. Bard

Barr/Duramed
See Barr Laboratories

00555
Barr Laboratories, Inc.
2 Quaker Rd.
Pomona, NY 10970
845-362-1100
800-222-0190
www.barrlabs.com

10116
Bartor Pharmacal Co.
70 High St.
Rye, NY 10580
914-967-4219

58887
Basel Pharmaceuticals
See Novartis Pharmaceuticals

BASF Corporation
3000 Continental Drive North
Mount Olive, NJ 07828
973-426-2600
800-526-1072
www.basf.com/usa

10119
Bausch & Lomb Personal
Products Division
1400 N. Goodman St.
P.O. Box 450
Rochester, NY 14692-0450
585-338-6000
800-553-5340
www.bausch.com

24208, 57782
Bausch & Lomb
Pharmaceuticals
8500 Hidden River Pkwy.
Tampa, FL 33637
813-975-7770
800-323-0000
www.bausch.com

Bausch & Lomb Surgical
180 Via Verde
San Dimas, CA 91773
800-338-2020
www.bausch.com

Baxa Corporation
14445 Grasslands Dr.
Inglewood, CO 80112
303-690-4204
800-567-2292
www.baxa.com

00944
Baxter Healthcare Corporation
1 Baxter Parkway
Deerfield, IL 60015
800-422-9837
www.baxter.com

Baxter Healthcare Corporation
Anesthesia Critical Care
   Pharmaceuticals
95 Spring Street
New Providence, NJ 07974
800-667-0959
www.baxter.com

Baxter Healthcare Corporation
Baxter Bioscience
1627 Lake Cook Road
Deerfield, IL 60015
800-423-2090
www.baxter.com

Baxter Healthcare Corporation
Clintec Nutrition
1 Baxter Pkwy.
Deerfield, IL 60015
800-422-2751
www.nutriforum.com

Baxter Healthcare Corporation
Medication Delivery
Route 120 and Wilson Road
Round Lake, IL 60073
800-229-0001
www.baxter.com

Baxter Hyland Immuno
See Baxter Healthcare Corporation,
   Baxter Bioscience

Baxter Pharm. Prods., Inc.
   (Baxter PPI)
See Baxter Healthcare, Anesthesia
   Critical Care Pharmaceuticals

00118
Bayer Allergy Products
See Hollister-Stier

Bayer Biological
See Bayer Corp.

12843, 16500
Bayer Consumer Care Division
36 Columbia Rd.
P.O. Box 1910
Morristown, NJ 07962
800-331-4536
www.bayercare.com

00026, 00161, 00192
Bayer Corp.
400 Morgan Lane
West Haven, CT 06516
203-937-2000
800-288-8371
www.bayer.com

00193
Bayer Diagnostics
430 S. Beiger St.
Mishawaka, IN 46544
219-256-3390
800-248-2637
www.bayerdiag.com
www.glucometer.com

31280
BD (Becton Dickinson & Co.)
1 Becton Dr.
Franklin Lakes, NJ 07417
201-847-6800
888-237-2762
www.bd.com

00011
BD Biosciences
2350 Qume Drive
San Jose, CA 95131
800-223-8226
www.bdbiosciences.com

BD Diagnostic Systems &
   Medical Supplies
7 Loveton Circle
Sparks, MD 21152
410-316-4000
www.bd.com

BDI Marketing
9700 N. Michigan Road
Carmel, IN 46220
317-228-0000
800-428-1717
www.bdi-marketing.com

BDI Pharmaceuticals, Inc.
See BDI Marketing

00486
Beach Pharm.
5220 S. Manhattan Ave.
Tampa, FL 33611
800-322-8210

Beckman Coulter, Inc.
See Coulter Corp.

Becton Dickinson & Co.
See BD

Becton Dickinson Microbiology
   Systems
7 Loveton Circle
Sparks, MD 21152
410-316-4000
800-638-8663
www.bd.com

55390
Bedford Laboratories
300 Northfield Rd.
Bedford, OH 44146
440-232-3320
800-562-4797
www.bedfordlabs.com

10356
Beiersdorf, Inc.
360 Martin Luther King Dr.
South Norwalk, CT 06856-5529
203-853-8008
800-233-2340
www.beiersdorf.com

Bergen Brunswig Drug Co.
4000 Metropolitan Dr.
Orange, CA 92868
714-385-4000
800-841-4662
www.amerisourcebergen.net

50419
Berlex Laboratories, Inc.
6 West Belt
Wayne, NJ 07470
973-694-4100
888-237-5394
www.berlex.com

58337
Berna Products Corp.
4216 Ponce De Leon Blvd.
Coral Gables, FL 33146
305-443-2900
800-533-5899
www.bernaproducts.com

Bertek Pharmaceuticals, Inc.
P.O. Box 5047
Sugarland, TX 77478
281-240-1000
800-231-3052
www.bertek.com

Best Generics
See Goldline Consumer, Inc.

Beta Dermaceuticals
P.O. Box 691106
San Antonio, TX 78269-1106
210-349-9326
800-434-2382
www.beta-derm.com

00283
Beutlich Pharmaceuticals
1541 Shields Dr.
Waukegan, IL 60085
847-473-1100
800-238-8542
www.beutlich.com

00225
B. F. Ascher and Co.
15501 West 109th St.
Lenexa, KS 66219
913-888-1880
800-324-1880

Bi-Coastal Pharmaceutical Corp.
130 Maple Avenue
Red Bank, NJ 07701
732-530-6606
www.bicoastalpharm.com

Biocare International, Inc.
2643 Grand Ave.
Bellmore, NY 11710

Biocore Medical Technologies
11800 Tech Road
Suite 240
Silver Spring, MD 20904
301-625-6818
888-689-5655
www.biocore.com

00332
Biocraft Laboratories, Inc.
See Teva Pharmaceuticals USA

BioCryst Pharmaceuticals, Inc.
2190 Parkway Lake Dr.
Birmingham, AL 35244
205-444-4600
www.biocryst.com

Biofilm, Inc.
3121 Scott St.
Vista, CA 92083-8323
760-727-9030
800-848-5900
www.biofilm.com

Biogen
See Biogen Idec

Biogen Idec
14 Cambridge Center
Cambridge, MA 02142
617-679-2000
800-262-4363
www.biogen.com

BioGenex Laboratories
4600 Norris Canyon Rd.
Suite 400
San Ramon, CA 94583
925-275-0550
800-421-4149
www.biogenex.com

Bioglan Pharmaceuticals
7 Great Valley Parkway
Suite 301
Malvern, PA 19355
610-232-2000
888-246-4526
www.bioglan.com

Bioline Labs, Inc.
See Ivax Corporation

Biomedical Frontiers, Inc.
1095 10th Avenue, S.E.
Minneapolis, MN 55414
612-378-0228

Biomerica, Inc.
1533 Monrovia Ave.
Newport Beach, CA 92663
949-645-2111
800-854-3002
www.biomerica.com

Biomerieux
100 Randolpe St.
Durham, NC 27712
916-620-2000
800-432-9682

Biomira USA, Inc.
1002 East Park Blvd.
Newport Beach, CA 92663
609-655-5300
www.biomira.com

Biomolecular Sciences, Inc.
13428 Maxella Avenue 285
Marina del Ray, CA 90292
310-301-9439
800-260-3587
www.genomicwhey.com

Bionexus, Ltd.
30 Brown Road
Ithaca, NY 14850
607-266-9492
800-835-0869
www.bionexs.com

Bioniche Pharma Group
231 Dundas Street East
P.O. Box 1570
Belleville, Ontario
Canada K8N5J2
613-966-8058
www.bioniche.com

Biopharmaceutics, Inc.
See Feminique Corp.

Biopharm Labs
10 H Runway Road
Levittown, PA 19057
215-949-3711
www.biopharm.de/

Biopure Corp.
11 Hurley
Cambridge, MA 02141
617-234-6500
www.biopure.com

53191
Biospecifics Technologies Corp.
35 Wilbur Street
Lynbrook, NY 11563
516-593-7000
www.biospecifics.com

BioStar, Inc.
See ThermoElectron
www.biostar.ca/

BIO-TECH Pharmacal, Inc.
P.O. Box 1992
Fayetteville, AR 72702
479-443-9148
800-345-1199
www.bio-tech-pharm.com

Bio-Technology General Corp.
1 Tower Center
East Brunswick, NJ 08816
800-284-2480
www.btgc.com

Biotrol International
650 S. Taylor Avenue
Suite 20
Louisville, CO 80027
303-673-0341
800-822-8550
www.biotrol.com

BioVail Pharmaceuticals, Inc.
170 Southport Dr.
Morrisville, NC 27560
919-674-2600
877-357-4276
www.biovail.com

BIRA Corp.
2525 Quicksilver
McDonald, PA 15057
724-796-1820

50289
Birchwood Laboratories, Inc.
7900 Fuller Rd.
Eden Prairie, MN 53344
952-937-7900
800-328-6156
www.birchlabs.com

12136
Bird Products Corp.
1100 Bird Center Dr.
Palm Springs, CA 92262
760-778-7200
800-328-4139
www.viasyscriticalcare.com

00165
Blaine Pharmaceuticals
1515 Production Dr.
Burlington, KY 41005
859-283-9437
800-633-9353
www.blainepharma.com

00154
Blair Laboratories
See Purdue Frederick Co.

50486
Blairex Labs, Inc.
1600 Brian Drive
Columbus, IN 47201
812-378-1864
800-252-4739
www.blairex.com

Blansett Pharmacal Co., Inc.
P.O. Box 638
14 Parkstone Circle
N. Little Rock, AR 72115
501-758-8635
www.blansett.com

10157
Blistex Inc.
1800 Swift Dr.
Oak Brook, IL 60523
630-571-2870
888-784-2472
www.blistex.com

10158
Block Drug Co., Inc.
See GlaxoSmithKline Consumer
Healthcare, L.P.
www.blockdrug.com

10160
Bluco Inc.
28350 Schoolcraft
Livonia, MI 48150
734-513-4500
800-832-4464
www.blucoinc.com

Boca Pharmacal, Inc.
6601 Lyons Rd.
Coconut Creek, FL 33073
800-354-8460
www.bocamedicalproducts.com

00563
Bock Pharmacal Co.
See Sanofi-Synthelabo, Inc.

00597
Boehringer Ingelheim Pharmaceuticals, Inc.
900 Ridgebury Rd.
Ridgefield, CT 06877-0368
203-798-9988
800-542-6257
www.boehringer-ingelheim.com

53169
Boehringer Mannheim
See Roche Laboratories

Boericke & Tafel
2381 Circadian Way
Santa Rose, CA 95407
707-571-8202
800-876-9505

Bone Care Center
1600 Aspen Commons
Middleton, WI 53562
608-662-7800
888-389-3300
www.bonecare.com

Bone Care International
1600 Aspen Commons
Middleton, WI 53562
888-389-4242
www.bonecare.com

Bonnie Bell
18519 Detroit Avenue
P.O. Box 770349
Lakewood, OH 44107
216-221-0800
800-321-1006
www.bonniebell.com

Boots Pharmaceuticals, Inc.
See Abbott Laboratories
www.boots.co.uk/frontpage.html

Botanical Laboratories
1441 W. Smith Rd.
Ferndale, WA 98248
360-384-5656
888-977-8008
www.botlab.com

00003
Bracco Diagnostics, Inc.
P.O. Box 5250
Princeton, NJ 08543
609-514-2200
800-631-5244
www.bracco.com

Bradley Pharmaceutical
383 Rt. 46 West
Fairfield, NJ 07004
800-929-9300
www.bradpharm.com

52268
Braintree Laboratories, Inc.
P.O. Box 850929
Braintree, MA 02185-0929
781-843-2202
800-874-6756
www.braintreelabs.com

45617
Breath Asure, Inc.
See Health Assure, Inc.
www.breathasure.com

51991
Breckenridge Pharmaceutical, Inc.
1141 S. Rogers Circle
Suite 3
Boca Raton, FL 33487
561-367-8512
800-466-2700
www.breckenridgepharma.com

72363
Brimms Inc.
See Shield Manufacturing

Brioschi
19-01 Pollitt Drive
Fairlawn, NJ 07410
201-796-4226
www.brioschi-usa.com

Bristol-Myers Oncology/Virology
P.O. Box 4500
Princeton, NJ 08540
800-426-7644
www.bmsoncology.com

19810
Bristol-Myers Products
P.O. Box 4000
Princeton, NJ 08543-4000
800-468-7746
www.bms.com

00003, 00015, 00087
Bristol-Myers Squibb Company
P.O. Box 4500
Princeton, NJ 08540
609-897-2000
800-321-1335
www.bms.com
www.bmsoncology.com

63256
Bryan Corporation
4 Plympton St.
Woburn, MA 01801
781-935-0004
800-343-7711
www.bryancorp.com

BSN, Jobst
5825 Carnegie Blvd.
Charlotte, NC 28209
800-221-7573
www.jobst.com

BTG Pharmaceutical Corporation
One Tower Center Blvd. 14th Floor
East Brunswick, NJ 08816
732-418-9300
800-284-2480
www.btgc.com

Burroughs Wellcome Co.
See GlaxoSmithKline

00398
C & M Pharmacal, Inc.
1721 Maple Lane Ave.
Hazel Park, MI 48030
248-548-7846
800-423-5173
www.genesispharm.com

Cag Nutrition
See ConAgra Functional Foods, Inc.

Calmoseptine, Inc.
16602 Burke Lane
Huntington Beach, CA 92647
800-800-3405
www.calmoseptineointment.com

Calwood Nutritionals, Inc.
500 McCormick Drive
Suite J
Glen Burnie, MD 21061
410-590-4890
800-479-9942
www.calwoodnutritionals.com

00147
Camall Co., Inc.
P.O. Box 989
Traverse City, MI 49685
800-521-6720

Cambrex Bioscience
5901 East Lombard Street
Baltimore, MD 21224
410-563-9200
877-676-5888
www.marathonbio.com

Cambridge NeuroScience
See Baxter Health Care

43656
Cambridge Nutraceuticals
See Baxter Nutrition

Can-Am Care Corp.
3780 Manfell Rd., Suite T50
Alpharetta, GA 30022
800-461-7448

64543
Capellon Pharmaceuticals, Ltd.
7509 Flagstone Street
Ft. Worth, TX 76118
817-595-5820
www.capellon.com

57664
Caraco Pharmaceutical Laboratories Ltd.
1150 Elijah McCoy Dr.
Detroit, MI 48202
313-871-8400
800-818-4555
www.caraco.com

Cardinal Health, Inc.
7000 Cardinal Place
Dublin, OH 43017
614-617-5000
800-234-8701
www.cardinal-health.com

Care Technologies, Inc.
10 Corbin Dr.
Darien, CT 06820
800-783-1919
www.lice.com

Carma Labs, Inc.
5801 W. Airways Ave.
Franklin, WI 53132
414-421-7707
www.carma-labs.com

Carme, Inc.
920 Airpark Road
Napa, CA 94558
707-226-3900
www.senetekplc@aol.com

Carnation
See Nestle Instant Nutrition

00086
Carnrick Laboratories
See Elan Pharmaceuticals

46287
Carolina Medical Products
8026 US 264 Alternate
Farmville, NC 27828
252-753-7111
800-227-6637
www.carolinamedical.com

Carrington Laboratories, Inc.
2001 Walnut Hill Lane
Irving, TX 75038
972-518-1300
800-527-5216
www.carringtonlabs.com

Carter Products
See Church & Dwight Co.

00164
Carter-Wallace, Inc.
See Med Pointe

00132
C.B. Fleet Co., Inc.
4615 Murray Place
P.O. Box 11349
Lynchburg, VA 24502
434-522-8429
800-999-9711
www.cbfleet.com

CCA Industries, Inc.
200 Murray Hill Pkwy.
East Rutherford, NJ 07073
800-524-2720
www.ccaindustries.com

Cebert Pharmaceuticals, Inc.
1200 Corporate Drive
Suite 370
Birmingham, AL 35242
205-981-0201
www.cebert.com

Celestial Seasonings, Inc.
4600 Sleepytime Dr.
Boulder, CO 80301
303-530-5300
800-525-0347
www.celestialseasonings.com

Celgene Corp.
7 Powder Horn Dr.
Warren, NJ 07059
732-271-1001
800-890-4619
www.celgene.com

Cell Pathways
See OSI Pharmaceuticals
www.cellpathways.com

Cell Therapeutics
501 Elliott Ave. West
Suite 400
Seattle, WA 98119
206-272-4000
800-215-2355
www.ctiseattle.com

Cellcor, Inc.
200 Wells Avenue
Newton, MA 02159

Cellegy Pharmaceuticals, Inc.
349 Oyster Pointe Blvd.
Suite 200
South San Francisco, CA 94080
650-616-2200
www.cellegy.com

Celltech Pharmaceutical Co.
755 Jefferson Rd.
Rochester, NY 14623
585-475-9000
800-234-5535
www.celltechgroup.com

Celtrix Pharmaceuticals, Inc.
2033 Gateway Pl., Suite 600
San Jose, CA 95110
408-988-2500

00053
Centeon
See Aventis Behring

Center Laboratories
See ALK Abello

00268
Center Pharmaceuticals, Inc.
See ALK Abello

Centers for Disease Control and Prevention
1600 Clifton Rd. N.E.
Atlanta, GA 30333
404-639-3670
www.cdc.gov

Centocor, Inc.
200 Great Valley Pkwy.
Malvern, PA 19355
610-651-6000
800-457-6399
www.centocor.com

00131
Central Pharmaceuticals, Inc.
See Schwarz Pharma

00436
Century Pharmaceuticals, Inc.
10377 Hague Rd.
Indianapolis, IN 46256-3399
317-849-4210

Cephalon, Inc.
145 Brandywine Pkwy.
West Chester, PA 19380
610-344-0200
800-782-3656
www.cephalon.com

Cera Products
8265-I Patuxent Range Road
Jessup, MD 20794
301-490-4941
888-ceralyte
www.ceralyte.com

00173
Cerenex Pharmaceuticals
See GlaxoSmithKline

Cervical Cap Ltd.
430 Monterey Ave.
Suite 1B
Los Gatos, CA 95030
408-395-2100
www.cervicalcap.com

10223
Cetylite Industries, Inc.
9051 River Rd.
Pennsauken, NJ 08110
865-665-6111
800-257-7740
www.cetylite.com

Chantal Pharmaceutical
12121 Wilshire Blvd.
Suite 1120
Los Angeles, CA 90025

54429
Chase Laboratories
See Banner Pharmacaps

49447
Chattem Consumer Products
1715 W. 38th St.
Chattanooga, TN 37409
423-821-4571
800-366-6833
www.chattem.com

ChemTrak, Inc.
929 East Arques Avenue
Sunnyvale, CA 94086

Chesapeake Biological Labs., Inc.
1111 S. Paca St.
Baltimore, MD 21230
410-843-5000
800-441-4225
www.cblinc.com

00521
Chesebrough-Ponds USA, Inc.
See Unilever Home and Personal Care USA

Cheshire Pharmaceutical Systems
6225 Shiloh Rd.
Alpharetta, GA 30005

Chester Labs
1900 Section Road
Suite A
Cincinnati, OH 45237

Chew-Rite Co.
265 S. Pioneer Blvd.
Springboro, OH 45066
937-746-5509

Chiesi Pharmaceuticals, Inc.
150 Danbury Rd.
Ridgefield, CT 06877
203-438-3390

Children's Hospital of Columbus
700 Children's Dr.
Columbus, OH 43205
614-722-2000
www.columbuschildrens.com

Chilton Labs., Inc.
299B Fairfield Ave.
Fairfield , NJ 07004
973-575-1992

53905
Chiron Therapeutics
4560 Horton St.
Emeryville, CA 94608
510-655-8730
800-244-7668
www.chiron.com

Chiron Vision
See Bausch & Lomb Surgical

Chronimed Inc.
10900 Red Circle Dr.
Minnetonka, MN 55343
952-979-3600
www.chronimed.com

Church & Dwight Co.
469 N. Harrison Street
Princeton, NJ 08543
800-833-9532
www.churchdwight.com

00083
Ciba-Geigy Pharmaceuticals
See Novartis Pharmaceuticals

00346
Ciba Vision Corporation
11460 Johns Creek Pkwy.
Duluth, GA 30097
770-476-3937
800-845-6585
www.cibavision.com

Cima Labs
10000 Valley View Road
Eden Prairie, MN 55344
952-947-8700
www.cimalabs.com

00677, 00725, 71114
Circa Pharmaceuticals, Inc.
See Watson Laboratories, Inc.

94503
Cirrus Healthcare Products, L.L.C.
60 Main St.
Cold Spring Harbor, NY 11724
631-692-7600
800-327-6151
www.cirrushealthcare.com

CIS-US, Inc.
10 DeAngelo Dr.
Bedford, MA 01730
781-275-7120
800-221-7554
www.cisusinc.com

Citra Anticoagulants
55 Messina Drive
Braintree, MA 02184
781-848-2174
800-299-3411

Claragen, Inc.
12300 Washington Avenue
Suite 200
Rockville, MD 20852
301-231-7022
www.claragen.com

45802
Clay-Park Labs, Inc.
1700 Bathgate Ave.
Bronx, NY 10457
718-901-2800
800-933-5550
www.claypark.com

Clear Technologies
See Care Technologies Inc.

55553
Clint Pharmaceuticals
629 Shute Lane
Old Hickory, TN 37138
615-882-0042
800-677-5022

Clintec Nutrition
See Baxter Healthcare Corporation

Closure Medical Corp
5250 Greensdairy Road
Raleigh, NC 27616
919-876-7800
www.closuremed.com

57145
CNS, Inc.
7615 Smethand Ln.
Eden Prairie, MN 55344
952-229-1500
www.cns.com

Coats Aloe
2146 Merrit Drive
Garland, TX 75041
972-278-9651
800-486-ALOE
www.coatsaloe.com

Colgate Oral Pharmaceuticals
1 Colgate Way
Canton, MA 02021
781-821-2880
800-821-2880
www.colgateprofessional.com

Colgate-Palmolive Co.
300 Park Ave.
New York, NY 10022
212-310-2000
800-221-4607
www.colgate.com

Collagen Corp.
See INAMED Corp.

27280
CollaGenex Pharmaceuticals, Inc.
41 University Dr.
Suite 200
Newtown, PA 18940
215-579-7388
888-339-5678
www.cgpi@collagenex.com

Coloplast
1955 West Oak Circle
Marietta, GA 30062
800-533-0464
www.us.coloplast.com

Colorado Biolabs
404 N Street
P.O. Box 125
Cozad, NE 69130
888-442-0067
www.coloradobiolabs.com

00837, 21406
Columbia Laboratories, Inc.
354 Eisenhower Parkway
Plaza 1, 2nd Floor
Livingston, NJ 07039
973-994-3999
www.columbialabs.com

11509
Combe, Inc.
1101 Westchester Ave.
White Plains, NY 10604
914-694-5454
800-431-2610
www.combe.com

CompliMed Medical Research Group
1441 West Smith Rd.
Ferndale, WA 98248
360-384-5656
888-977-8008
www.complimed.com

ConAgra Functional Foods, Inc.
1218 E. Hartman Ave.
Omaha, NE 68110
402-455-0634
888-828-4242
www.culturelle.com

Conair Interplak Division
1 Cummings Point Rd.
Stamford, CT 06902
800-726-6247
www.conair.com

Con-Cise Contact Lens Co.
14450 Doolittle Dr.
San Leandro, CA 94577
510-483-9400
800-772-3911
www.con-cise.com

20254
Concord Laboratories
140 New Dutch Lane
Fairfield, NJ 07004
973-227-6757

11793, 49281, 50361
Connaught Labs
See Aventis Pasteur

00007
Connetics Corporation
3290 W. Bayshore Rd.
Palo Alto, CA 94303
650-843-2800
800-280-2879
www.connetics.com

43786
Consep Inc.
See Woodstream Corp.

00223
Consolidated Midland Corp.
20 Main St.
Brewster, NY 10509
845-279-6108

18149
Consumers Choice Systems, Inc.
2370 130th Ave. NE
Suite 101
Bellevue, WA 98005
425-883-6310

34044
Continental Consumer Products
770 Forest
Suite B
Birmingham, MI 48009
800-542-5903

33130
Continental Quest Research
220 W. Carmel Dr.
Carmel, IN 46032
317-843-2501
800-451-5773
www.continentalquest.com

Contract Pharmacal Corp.
135 Adams Ave.
Hauppauge, NY 11788
631-231-4610
www.cpchealth.com

00003
ConvaTec
P.O. Box 5254
Princeton, NJ 08543
908-904-2200
800-422-8811
www.convatec.com

Cooke Pharma, Inc.
See Unither Pharma

59426
CooperVision
200 Willow Brook Office Park
Fairport, NY 14450
585-385-6810
800-538-7850
www.coopervisionhydron.com

38245
Copley Pharmaceutical
See Teva Pharmaceuticals USA

COR Therapeutics, Inc.
See Millennium Pharmaceuticals

Cord Labs
See Geneva Pharmaceuticals

Corixa
1124 Columbia St.
Suite 200
Seattle, WA 98104
206-754-5711
www.corixa.com

Coulter Corp.
(Beckman Coulter, Inc.)
11800 S.W. 147 Ave.
P.O. Box 169015
Miami, FL 33196
305-380-3800
800-327-6531
www.coulter.com

C.R. Bard
730 Central Avenue
Murray Hill, NJ 07974
908-277-8000
www.crbard.com

08011
C.R. Bard, Inc.
Urological Division
8195 Industrial Blvd.
Covington, GA 30014
800-526-4455
www.crbard.com

Creomulsion
See Summit Industries, Inc.

C.S. Dent & Co Division
See Grandpa Brands Company

CTEX Pharmaceuticals Inc.
See Andrx Labs

Cumberland Swan, Inc.
One Swan Drive
Smyrna, TN 37167
615-459-8900
www.cumberlandswan.com

55326
Curatek Pharmaceuticals
See 3M Pharmaceuticals

Cutis Pharma, Inc.
100 Cummings Ctr.
Suite 421C
Beverly, MA 01915
978-867-1010
www.cutispharma.com

Cutter Biologicals
See Bayer Corp.

Cyanotech Corp.
73-4460 Queen Kaahamanu Hwy.
Suite 102
Kailua-Kona, HI 96740
808-326-1353
800-395-1353
www.cyanotech.com

Cyclin Pharmaceuticals Inc.
1289 Demingy Way
Madison, WI 53725
800-558-7046
800-982-1186
www.womenshealth.com

Cygnus, Inc.
400 Penobscot Dr.
Redwood City, CA 94063
650-369-4300
www.cygn.com

54799
Cynacon/OCuSOFT
5311 Ave. North
Rosenburg, TX 77471
800-233-5469
www.ocusoft.com

Cypress Pharmaceutical, Inc.
135 Industrial Blvd.
Madison, MS 39110
601-856-4393
800-856-4393
www.cypressrx.com

Cypros Pharmaceutical Corp.
See Questcor Pharmaceuticals, Inc.

Cytogen Corporation
650 College Rd. East
3rd Floor
Princeton, NJ 08540
609-750-8200
800-833-3533
www.cytogen.com

23731
Cytosol Laboratories
55 Messina Dr.
Braintree, MA 02184
781-848-9386
800-288-3858
www.cytosol.com

Cytosol Ophthalmics
P.O. Box 1408
1325 William White Pl.
Lenoir, NC 28645
828-758-2343
800-234-5166
www.cytosol.com

CytRx Corp.
11726 San Vicente Blvd.
Suite 650
Los Angeles, CA 90049
310-826-5648
www.cytrx.com

Daiichi Pharm. Corp.
11 Philips Pkwy.
Montvale, NJ 07645-1810
201-573-7000
877-324-4244
www.daiichius.com

Danbury Pharmacal
(Watson Laboratories)
1033 Stoneleigh Ave.
Carmel, NY 10512
914-767-2000
800-553-4044
www.watson.com

Danco Labs., LLC
P.O. Box 4816
New York, NY 10185
212-424-1950
877-432-7596
www.earlyoptionpill.com

D & K Healthcare Resources
8235 Forsyth Blvd.
St. Louis, MO 63105
314-727-3485
www.dkwd.com

00689
Daniels Pharmaceuticals, Inc.
See Jones Pharma Incorporated

58869
Dartmouth Pharmaceuticals
(Elan Pharmaceuticals)
38 Church Ave.
Wareham, MA 02571
508-295-2200
800-414-3566
www.ilovemynails.com

00938
Davis and Geck Care Products
See Kendall Health Care Products

Davol, Inc.
100 Sockanossett Crossroad
Cranston, RI 02920
401-463-7000
www.davol.com

52041
Dayton Laboratories
7760 NW 56th St.
Miami, FL 33166
305-594-0988
800-446-0255

Debio Pharmaceuticals S.A.
17, Rue des Terreaux
Case Postale 211 CH-1000
Lausanne 9
Switzerland 0041 21 321 0111
www.debio.com

Degussa Corp.
379 Enterpace Pkwy.
Parsippany, NJ 07054-0677
973-541-8000
877-273-2668
www.degussa.com

Deliz Pharmaceutical
Corporation
P.O. Box 29765
San Juan, PR 00929
787-272-2211

10310
Del Pharmaceuticals
565 Broad Hollow Rd.
Farmingdale, NY 11735
516-844-2020
800-645-9888
www.dellabs.com

00316
Del Ray Laboratories
349 Lasecox Road
Johnson City, TN 37604
800-334-4286

48532
Delmont Laboratories, Inc.
P.O. Box 269
Swarthmore, PA 19081
610-543-3365
800-562-5541
www.delmont.com

Delta Pharmaceuticals
2 Davis Dr.
P.O. Box 12278
Research Triangle Park, NC 29063

Den-Mat Corporation
2727 Skyway Dr.
Santa Maria, CA 93455
805-922-8491
800-433-6628
www.den-mat.com

00295
Denison Labs., Inc.
P.O. Box 1305
Pawtucket, RI 02862
401-723-5500

49336
Dental Herb Co.
1000 Holland Dr., Suite 7
Boca Raton, FL 33487
561-241-4262
800-747-4372
www.dentalherbcompany.com

DepoTech Corp.
(SkyePharma)
10450 Science Center
San Diego, CA 92121-1119
858-625-2424
www.skyepharma.com

Derma Science
214 Carnegie Center
Suite 100
Princeton, NJ 08540
609-514-4744
800-825-4325
www.dermasciences.com

Dermalogix Partners
P.O. Box 1510
Scarborough, ME 04070
207-883-4103
www.dermalogix.com

Dermarite
3 East 26th Street
Paterson, NJ 07513
973-569-9000
800-337-6296
www.dermarite.com

00066
Dermik Laboratories, Inc.
(Arcola)
1050 Westlake Dr.
Berwin, PA 193126
484-595-2700
800-666-6030
www.dermik.com

DeRoyal Industries, Inc.
200 DeBusk Lane
Powell, TN 37849
423-938-7828
800-337-6925
www.deroyal.com

DexGen Pharmaceuticals, Inc.
P.O. Box 675
Manasquan, NJ 08736
732-223-8811
877-339-4361
www.dexgen.com

49502
Dey Laboratories, Inc.
2751 Napa Valley Corporate Dr.
Napa, CA 94558
707-224-3200
800-755-5560
www.deyinc.com

DHS, Inc.
11525 N. Fulton Ind. Blvd.
Alpharetta, GA 30004
770-751-1787
800-392-7771

Diacrin Corp
Bldg. 96, 13th St.
Charlestown, MA 02129
617-242-9100
www.diacrin.com

Dial Corporation
15501 N. Dial Blvd.
Scottsdale, AZ 85260
480-754-3425
www.dialcorp.com

DiaPharma Group, Inc.
8948 Beckett Rd.
West Chester, OH 45069-2939
513-860-9324
800-526-5224
www.diapharma.com

Diatide, Inc.
See Berlex Laboratories

Dickinson Brands, Inc.
31 East High Street
East Hampton, CT 06424
860-267-2279
888-860-2279
www.witchhazel.com

Digestive Care Inc.
1120 Win Dr.
Bethlehem, PA 18017
610-882-5950

Discovery Laboratories, Inc.
350 S Main St.
Suite 307
Doylestown, PA 18901
215-340-4699
www.discoverylabs.com

Discus Dental Inc.
8550 Higuera St.
Culver City, CA 90232
310-845-8200
800-273-2847
www.discusdental.com

00777
Dista Products Co.
See Eli Lilly and Co.

Dixon-Shane
256 Geiger Rd.
Philadelphia, PA 19115
215-673-3415
800-262-7770
www.dixonshane.com

DJ Pharma, Inc.
See BioVail

10337
Doak Dermatologics
See Bradley Pharmaceuticals

Dolisos America, Inc.
3014 Rigel Ave.
Las Vegas, NM 89102
800-365-4767
www.dolisos.com

25358
Donell DerMedex
See Donell Inc.

Donell Inc.
501 Fifth Avenue
Suite 1214
New York, NY 10017
212-682-0666
877-853-9605
www.cxproducts.com

Dover Pharmaceutical, Inc.
P.O. Box 809
Islington, MA 02090
800-777-6847

00514
Dow Hickam, Inc.
See Bertek Pharmaceuticals, Inc.

Dow Pharmaceutical Sciences
1330A Redwood Way
Petaluma, CA 94954
707-793-2600
www.dowpharm.com

Dreir Pharmaceuticals, Inc.
9602 N. 122nd Place
Scottsdale, AZ 85259
480-607-3584
800-541-4044
www.dreirpharmaceuticals.com

Dr. Reddy's Laboratories, Inc.
One Park Way
Upper Saddle River, NJ 07458
201-760-2880
www.drreddys.com

Drug Abuse Sciences
25954 Eden Landing Rd.
Hayward, CA 94545
510-529-3200
www.drugabusesciences.com

DSC Laboratories
1979 Latimer Dr.
Muskegon, MI 49442
800-492-5988
www.dsclab.com

00094
DuPont Pharmaceuticals Co.
See Bristol-Myers Squibb

51479
Dura/Elan Pharmaceuticals
See Elan Pharmaceuticals

51285
Duramed Pharmaceuticals
See Barr Laboratories

Durex Consumer Products
3585 Engineering Dr.
Suite 200
Norcross, GA 30092
770-582-2222
888-566-3468
www.durex.com

Durham Pharmacal Corp.
See Steifel Consumer Healthcare

DUSA Pharmaceuticals, Inc.
25 Upton
Wilmington, MA 01887
978-657-7500
www.dusapharma.com

DynaGen Inc.
See Able Laboratories, Inc.

Eagle Vision, Inc.
8500 Wolf Lake Dr.
Suite 110
P.O. Box 34877
Memphis, TN 38184
901-380-7000
800-222-7584
www.eaglevis.com

Eastman Kodak Co.
343 State St.
Rochester, NY 14650
585-724-4000
800-242-2424
www.kodak.com

Eaton Medical Corp.
1401 Heistan Place
Memphis, TN 38104
901-274-0000
800-253-4740
www.easyeyes.com

19458
Eckerd Drug Corp.
P.O. Box 4689
Clearwater, FL 33758
800-325-3737
www.eckerd.com

Ecological Formulas, Inc.
1061-B Shary Circle, Suite B
Concord, CA 94518
800-888-4585

38130
Econo Med Pharmaceuticals
4305 Sartin Rd.
Burlington, NC 27217-7522
336-226-1091
800-327-6007

55053
Econolab
See Breckenridge Pharmaceuticals

00095, 59010
ECR Pharmaceuticals
3969 Deep Rock Rd.
P.O. Box 71600
Richmond, VA 23233
804-527-1950
800-527-1955
www.ecrpharmaceuticals.com

Edwards Lifescience
6864 S. 300 West
Midvale, UT 84047
800-453-8432
800-562-0200

00485
Edwards Pharmaceuticals, Inc.
111 Mulberry St.
Ripley, MS 38663
800-543-9560

55806
Effcon Laboratories
1800 Sandy Plains Pkwy.
Suite 102
P.O. Box 7499
Marietta, GA 30065-1499
770-428-7011
800-722-2428
www.effcon.com

00168
E. Fougera Co.
60 Baylis Rd.
Melville, NY 11747
800-432-6673
www.fougera.com

Eisai Inc.
500 Frank W. Burr Blvd.
Teaneck, NJ 07666
201-692-1100
888-793-4724
www.eisai.com

Elan Pharmaceuticals
7475 Lusk Blvd.
San Diego, CA 92121
858-457-2553
800-859-8586
www.elan.com

00002, 59075
Eli Lilly and Co.
Lilly Corp. Center
Indianapolis, IN 46285
317-276-2000
800-545-5979
www.lilly.com

00641
Elkins-Sinn, Inc.
See Wyeth-Ayerst

EM Industries, Inc.
See EMD Chemicals, Inc.

00802
Emerson Laboratories
See Humco Holding Group, Inc.

Enamelon, Inc.
7 Cedar Brook Dr.
Cranbury, NJ 08512

60951
Endo Laboratories, Inc.
100 Painters Dr.
Chadds Ford, PA 19317
610-558-9800
800-462-3636
www.endo.com

Endurance Products Co.
9914 SW Tigard St.
P.O. Box 230489
Tigard, OR 97281
800-483-2532
www.endur.com

62333
EnviroDerm Pharmaceuticals, Inc.
46 Christa McAuliffe Blvd.
Plymouth, MA 02360
508-747-9601
800-991-DERM
www.enviroderm.com

57665
Enzon, Inc.
685 Route 202/206
Bridgewater, NJ 08854
908-541-8600
www.enzon.com

00185, 00536
Eon Labs Manufacturing, Inc.
227-15 N. Conduit Ave.
Laurelton, NY 11413
718-276-8600
800-526-0225
www.eonlabs.com

Epitope Inc.
See OraSure Technologies

E.R. Squibb & Sons, Inc.
See Bristol-Myers Squibb Co.

00005, 59911
ESI Lederle Generics
See Wyeth Pharmaceuticals

ESP Pharma
2035 Lincoln Hwy.
Suite 2150
Edison, NJ 08817
866-437-7742
www.esppharma.com

58177
Ethex Corp.
10888 Metro Ct.
St. Louis, MO 63043-2413
314-567-3307
800-321-1705
www.ethex.com

Ethicon, Inc.
(Johnson & Johnson)
US Route 22 West
Somerville, NJ 08876-0151
908-218-0707
800-255-2500
www.ethiconinc.com

Eurand America, Inc.
845 Center Dr.
Vandalia, OH 45377
937-898-9669
www.eurand.com

Eurand International S.P.A.
20060 Pessano con Bornagio
Milan, Italy
39-02-954281
www.eurand.com

Evans Vaccines Ltd.
Florey House
The Oxford Science Park
Oxford, UK OX 44GA
44 8547 451 500
www.evansvaccines.com

Evenflo Company, Inc.
1801 Commerce Drive
Piqua, OH 45356
800-223-5921
www.evenflo.com

00642
Everett Laboratories, Inc.
29 Spring St.
West Orange, NJ 07052
973-324-0200
www.everettlabs.com

Excellium Pharmaceutical
3-G Oak Road
Fairfield, NJ 07004
973-276-9600

Excelsior Medical Corporation
P.O. Box 299
Long Branch, NJ 07740
800-487-4276

Eye Care & Cure Corporation
1140 N. Rosemont Boulevard
Tucson, AZ 85712
520-321-1262
800-486-6169
www.eyecareandcure.com

E-Z-EM
717 Main St.
Westbury, NY 11590
516-333-8230
800-544-4624
www.ezem.com

Falcon Ophthalmics, Inc.
6201 S. Freeway
Fort Worth, TX 76134
817-551-8710
800-343-2133
www.alconlabs.com

Farmacon, Inc.
90 Grove St.
Suite 109
Ridgefield, CT 06877-4118
203-431-9989

60976
Faro Pharmaceuticals, Inc.
Houston, TX 77043
877-994-3276
800-480-1985

99766
Faulding USA
See Mayne Pharma (USA) Inc.

The F.C. Sturtevant Company
P.O. Box 607
Bronxville, NY 10708
914-337-5131
888-871-5661
www.columbiapowder.com

11423
Female Health Co.
515 N. State St.
Chicago, IL 60610
312-595-9123
800-884-1601

Feminique Corp.
990 Station Rd.
Bellport, NY 11713
631-286-5800

00496
Ferndale Laboratories, Inc.
780 W. Eight Mile Rd.
Ferndale, MI 48220-1218
248-548-0900
888-548-0900
www.ferndalelabs.com

Ferraris Medical Ltd.
4 Harforde Court
John Tate Road
Hertford, UK SG13 7NW
+44 (0) 1992 526300
www.ferrarismedical.com

Ferring Pharmaceuticals Inc.
400 Rella Blvd.
Suffern, NY 10901
888-793-6367
888-337-7464
www.ferringusa.com

FH Faulding & Co. Ltd.
See Mayne Group Limited

31795
Fibertone
See Naturally Vitamins Co.

**Fidia Pharmaceutical
Corporation**
2000 K St. N.W. #700
Washington, DC 20006
202-371-9898
www.fidiapharma.com

00421
Fielding Pharmaceutical Co.
11551 Adie Road
Maryland Heights, MO 63043
314-567-5462
800-776-3435
www.fieldingcompany.com

**First Horizon Pharmaceutical
Corp.**
6195 Shiloh Rd.
Alpharetta, GA 30005
770-442-9707
800-849-9707
www.firsthorizonpharm.com

First Quality Products
80 Cuttermill Road
Suite 500
Great Neck, NY 11021
516-929-3030
www.firstquality.com

First Scientific Inc.
Lake Forest Plaza
2222 Francisco Dr., 510-174
El Dorado Hills, CA 95762
916-491-5088
800-767-2208
www.freshcleanse.com

51687
Fischer Pharmaceuticals, Inc.
7040 W. Palmetto Park Rd. #4
Suite 606
Boca Raton, FL 33433-3407
561-338-3338
800-782-0222
www.dr-fischer.com

Fiske Industries
527 Route 303
Orangeburg, NY 10962
845-398-3340
800-248-8033
www.cosmeticsolutions.com

00585
Fison Corp.
See Celltech Pharmaceutical Co.

54323
Flanders, Inc.
P.O. Box 80428
Charleston, SC 29416
www.flandersbuttocksointment.com
843-571-3363

00256
Fleming & Co.
1733 Gilsinn Lane
Fenton, MO 63026-2918
636-343-5206
www.flemingcompany.com

Flents Products Company
5401 S. Graham Road
St. Charles, MI 48655
989-865-8221
800-262-8221
www.flents.com

Flex-Power
1563 Solano Avenue
Berkeley, CA 94706
866-FLEXPOWER
866-353-9769

00288
Fluoritab Corp.
P.O. Box 507
Temperance, MI 48182-0507
734-847-3985

FNC Medical Corporation
5600 Everglades
Units B & C
Ventura, CA 93003
805-644-7578
800-440-2888
www.fncmedical.com

Forest Laboratories, Inc.
909 Third Ave.
New York, NY 10022
212-421-7850
800-947-5227
www.frx.com
www.forestpharm.com

Forest Laboratories Ireland Ltd
See Forest Pharmaceutical, Inc.

00258, 00456, 00535
Forest Pharmaceutical, Inc.
13600 Shoreline
St. Louis, MO 63045
314-493-7000
800-678-1605
www.forestpharm.com

Forte Pharma
See Eon Labs Manufacturing, Inc.

Fournier Research
9 Law Dr.
P.O. Box 340
Fairfield, NY 07004
973-683-0024

Free Radical Sciences, Inc.
245 First St.
Cambridge, MA 02142
617-374-1200

10432
Freeda Vitamins, Inc.
36 E. 41st St.
New York, NY 10017-6203
212-685-4980
800-777-3737
www.freedavitamins.com

**Fresenius Medical Care North
America**
95 Hayden Avenue
Lexington, MA 02420
781-402-9000
www.fmc-ag.com

Fuisz Technologies, Ltd.
14555 Avion at Lakeside
Suite 250
Chantilly, VA 22151
703-803-3260

00469, 57317
Fujisawa Healthcare, Inc.
3 Parkway N.
Deerfield, IL 60015-2548
847-317-8800
800-888-7704
www.fujisawa.com

00713
G & W Laboratories
111 Coolidge St.
South Plainfield, NJ 07080-3895
908-753-2000
800-922-1038
www.gwlabs.com

Galagen Nutrition Medical, Inc.
See Hormel Healthlabs

00299
Galderma Laboratories, Inc.
14501 N. Freeway
Ft. Worth, TX 76177
817-961-5000
800-582-8225
www.galdermausa.com

Galen Pharma
Seagoe Industrial Estate
Craigavon, UK BT63 5UA
028 3833 4974
www.galen.co.uk

Gallipot, Inc.
2020 Silver Bell Rd.
St. Paul, MN 55122
651-681-9517
800-423-6967
www.gallipot.com

00254
Gambro, Inc.
10810 W. Collins Ave.
Lakewood, CO 80215-4498
303-232-6800
800-525-2623
www.gambro.com

57844
Gate Pharmaceuticals
1090 Horsham Rd.
North Wales, PA 19454-1090
215-591-3046
800-292-4283
www.gatepharma.com

00386
Gebauer Co.
9410 St. Catherine Ave.
Cleveland, OH 44104-5226
216-271-5252
800-321-9348
www.gebauerco.com

00028
Geigy Pharmaceuticals
See Novartis Pharmaceuticals

Geist Pharmaceutical, L.L.C.
20 N. Meridian St.
Suite 9500
Indianapolis, IN 46204
317-833-0700
888-644-3478
www.geistrx.com

Gel-Kam
P.O. Box 80009
Dallas, TX 75380
214-233-2800

Gel-Tech
See Matrix Initiatives, Inc.
www.zicam.com

Gen-King
See Kinray

52761
GenDerm Corp.
See Medicis Pharmaceutical Corp.

50242
Genentech, Inc.
1 DNA Way
S. San Francisco, CA 94080-4990
650-225-1000
800-551-2231
www.gene.com

52584
General Injectables & Vaccines
U.S. Hwy. 52 S.
P.O. Box 9
Bastian, VA 24314-0009
276-688-4121
800-521-7468
www.giv.com

00918
General Medical Corp.
See McKesson Medical-Surgical

General Nutrition Inc.
300 6th Ave.
Pittsburgh, PA 15222
412-288-4600
888-462-2548
www.gnc.com

98318
Genesis Nutrition
1816 Wall St.
Florence, SC 29501
843-665-6928
800-451-7933
www.genesisnutrition.com

Genesis Pharmaceuticals
9 Campus Drive, Suite 7
Parsippany, NJ 07054
800-459-8663
www.genesispharm.com

Genetic Therapy, Inc.
938 Clopper Rd.
Gaithersburg, MD 20878
301-590-2626

Genetics Institute
35 Cambridge Park Dr.
Cambridge, MA 02140
617-503-7332
888-446-3344
www.genetics.com

**Geneva Pharmaceutical
Technology Corporation**
2400 Route 130N
Dayton, NJ 08810
732-274-2400
www.genevarx.com

00781
Geneva Pharmaceuticals
See Sandoz

GenpharmInternational, Inc.
See Medarex, Inc.

00703
**Gensia Sicor Pharmaceuticals,
Inc.**
19 Hughes
Irvine, CA 92618
949-445-0218
800-729-9991
www.gensiasicor.com

GenVec, Inc.
65 W. Watkins Mill Rd.
Gaithersburg, MD 20878
240-632-0740
www.genvec.com

58468
Genzyme Corp.
One Kendall Square
Building 1400
Cambridge, MA 02139
617-252-7500
800-326-7002
www.genzyme.com

Geodesic MediTech, Inc.
2921 Sandy Pointe No. 3
Del Mar, CA 92014
858-792-1100
888-357-9399

Gerber Products Company
445 State St.
Fremont, MI 49413-0001
800-443-7237
www.gerber.com

Geriatric Pharmaceutical Corp.
See Roberts Pharmaceutical Corp.

Geri-Care Products
250 Moonachie Avenue
Moonachie, NJ 07074-1897
201-440-0409
800-654-8322
geri-careproducts.com

Geritrex Corporation
144 Kingsbridge Road East
Mount Vernin, NY 10550
914-668-4003
800-736-3437
www.geritrex@aol.com

Gilead Sciences
333 Lakeside Dr.
Foster City, CA 94404
650-574-3000
800-445-3235
www.gilead.com

59366
Glades Pharmaceuticals
6340 Sugarloaf Parkway, Suite 400
Duluth, GA 30097
866-436-0318
888-445-2337
www.glades.com

GlaxoSmithKline
1 Franklin Plaza
Philadelphia, PA 19102
215-751-4000
888-825-5249
www.gsk.com

**GlaxoSmithKline Consumer
Healthcare, L.P.**
100 Beecham Dr.
Pittsburgh, PA 15205
800-245-1040
www.gsk.com

GlaxoSmithKline Pharm.
5 Moore Dr.
P.O. Box 13398
Research Triangle Park, NC 27709
919-248-2100
888-825-5249
www.gsk.com

00081, 00173
GlaxoWellcome, Inc.
See GlaxoSmithKline

00516
Glenwood, Inc.
111 Cedar Land
P.O. Box 5419
Englewood, NJ 07631
201-569-0050
800-542-0772
www.glenwood-llc.com

00115
Global Pharmaceuticals, Inc.
3735 Castor & Kensington Aves.
Philadelphia, PA 19124
215-289-2220
www.globalphar.com

Global Source
5371 Hiatus Rd.
Sunrise, FL 33351
954-747-8977
www.globalvitamin.com

GM Pharmaceutical
P.O. Box 150312
Arlington, TX 76015
817-461-8230

GML Industries, LLC
51 Monarch Dr.
P.O. Box 1973
Denison, TX 75020
903-463-7321
877-828-4633
www.gml-industries.com

60429
Golden State Medical Supply
1799 Eastman Avenue
Ventura, CA 93003
805-477-9866
www.gsms.us

Goldline Consumer
See Ivax Corporation

00182
Goldline Laboratories, Inc.
See Ivax Pharmaceuticals

74684
Goody's Manufacturing Corp.
See GlaxoSmithKline Consumer
Healthcare, L.P.

10481
Gordon Laboratories
6801 Ludlow St.
Upper Darby, PA 19082-2408
610-734-2011
800-356-7870
www.gordonlabs.com

12165
**Graham Field Health Products
Inc.**
2935 NE Parkway
Atlanta, GA 30360
800-347-5678
www.grahamfield.com

Grandpa Brands Company
1820 Airport Exchange Blvd.
Erlanger, KY 41018
859-647-0777
800-684-1468
www.grandpabrands.com

00152
Gray Pharmaceutical Co.
See Purdue Frederick Co.

Great American Nutrition
2002 S. 5070 West
Salt Lake City, UT 84104
800-223-5326
www.weider.com

51301
Great Southern Laboratories
10863 Rockley Rd.
Houston, TX 77099
281-530-3077

Green Turtle Bay Vitamin Co.
56 High St.
P.O. Box 642
Summit, NJ 07901
908-277-2240
800-887-8535
www.energywave.com

59762
Greenstone Limited
See Pfizer, Inc.

22840
Greer Laboratories, Inc.
P.O. Box 800
Lenoir, NC 28645-0800
828-754-5327
800-378-3906
www.greerlabs.com

Grifols USA, Inc.
2410 Lillyvale Avenue
Los Angeles, CA 90032
888-GRIFOLS (888-474-3657
800-421-0008

Guardian Drug Company
P.O. Box 915
Dayton, NJ 08810
609-860-2600
www.guardiandrug.com

Guardian Laboratories
230 Marcus Blvd.
P.O. Box 18050
Hauppage, NY 11788
631-273-0900
800-645-5566
www.u-g.com

Guilford Pharmaceuticals, Inc.
6611 Tributary St.
Baltimore, MD 21224
410-631-6300
800-453-3746
www.guilfordpharm.com

Gum-Tech Industries, Inc.
See Matrix Initiatives, Inc.

Gynetics
3371 Route One
Suite 200
Lawrenceville, NJ 08648
609-919-1931
800-311-7378
www.gynetics.com

Halocarbon Products Corporation
887 Kinderkamack Rd.
P.O. Box 661
River Edge, NJ 07661
201-262-8899
www.halocarbon.com

00879
Halsey Drug Co.
(Watson)
695 N. Perryville Rd.
Rockford, IL 61107
815-399-2060
800-336-2750
www.halseydrug.com

Hannan Ophthalmic Marketing Services, Inc.
34 Sherrill Rd.
Nashville, MA 02050
781-834-8111

52512
Harmony Laboratories
1109 S. Main
P.O. Box 39
Landis, NC 28088
704-857-0707
800-245-6284

Hart Health & Safety
P.O. Box 94044
Seattle, WA 98124
800-234-4278
www.harthealth.com

Harvard Drug Corp.
31778 Enterprise Drive
Livonia, MI 48150
800-875-0123
www.harvarddrugs.com

Harvest Pharmaceuticals, Inc.
1881 Grove Avenue
P.O. Box 3587
Radford, VA 24141
800-455-5525

52637
Hauser Pharmaceutical Inc.
4401 E. U.S. Hwy. 30
Valparaiso, IN 46383
800-441-2309
www.hauserpharmaceutical.com

63717
Hawthorn Pharmaceuticals Inc.
See Cypress Pharmaceutical, Inc.

HDC Corporation
628 Gibraltar Ct.
Milpitas, CA 95035
408-942-7340
800-227-8162
www.hdccorp.com

Health & Medical Techniques
See Graham Field Health Products Inc.

Health Assure, Inc.
26635 West Agoura Road
Suite 205
Calabasas, CA 91302
818-706-6100
www.healthassure.com

50383
Health Care Products
369 Bayview Ave.
Amityville, NY 11701
631-789-8455
800-899-3116
www.diabeticproducts.com

Health Enterprises
90 George Leven Drive
N. Attleboro, MA 02760
508-695-0727
www.healthenterprises.com

00598
Health for Life Brands, Inc.
1643 E. Genessee St.
Syracuse, NY 13210
315-478-6303
800-448-5255

Health-Mark Diagnostics
3341 S.W. 15th St.
Pompano Beach, FL 33069
954-984-8881

Health Products Corp.
1060 Nepper Han
Yonkers, NY 10703
914-423-2900

Healthcare Direct Services
15424 N. Nebraska Ave.
Lutz, FL 33549
813-948-3005
800-729-8446
www.hcdsales.com

51662
Healthfirst Corp.
22316 70th Ave. W., Unit A
Mountlake Terrace, WA 98043-2184
425-771-5733
800-331-1984
www.healthfirstcorp.com

00064
Healthpoint Medical
3909 Hulen St.
Ft. Worth, TX 76107
817-900-4105
800-441-8227
www.healthpoint.com

Heel Inc.
11025 LH Lafontaine
Anjou, QC H1J 2Z4
514-353-4335
888-879-4335

Helena Laboratories
1530 Lindbergh Dr.
Beaumont, TX 77707
409-842-3714
800-231-5663
www.helena.com

Hemacare Corp.
21101 Oxnard St.
Woodland Hills, CA 91367
817-310-0717
www.hemacare.com

Hemagen Diagnostics, Inc.
9033 Red Branch Rd.
Columbia, MD 21045
443-367-5500
800-495-2180
www.hemagen.com

HemispheRx Biopharma, Inc.
1 Penn Center
1617 John F. Kennedy Blvd.
Suite 660
Philadelphia, PA 19103
215-988-0080
www.hemispherx.net

Hemotec Medical Products, Inc.
P.O. Box 19255
Johnston, RI 02919
401-934-2571

Henry Schein, Inc.
135 Duryea Rd.
Melville, NY 11747
631-843-5500
www.henryschein.com

Herald Pharmacal Inc.
See Allergan, Inc.

Herbert Laboratories
See Allergan, Inc.

Heritage Consumer Products, LLC.
141 South Ave.
Suite 2
Fanwood, NJ 07023
800-344-7239

50383
Hi-Tech Pharmacal Co. Inc.
369 Bayview Ave.
Amityville, NY 11701
631-789-8228
www.hitechpharm.com

28105
Hill Dermaceuticals, Inc.
2650 S. Mellonville Ave.
Sanford, FL 32773
800-344-5707
www.hillderm.com

Hillestad Pharmaceuticals
178 U.S. Highway 51 N
P.O. Box 1700
Woodruff, WI 54568-1700
800-535-7742
www.hillestadlabs.com

17808
Himmel Pharmaceuticals, Inc.
P.O. Box 5479
Lake Worth, FL 33466
561-585-0070
800-535-3823

Hisamitsu America
3528 Torrance Boulevard
Suite 112
Torrance, CA 90503
www.salponas-usa.com

00839
H.L. Moore Drug Exchange, Inc.
See Moore Medical Corp.

00039, 00068, 00088
Hoechst-Marion Roussel
See Aventis Pharmaceuticals

Hoffman-LaRoche
See Roche Laboratories

58573
Hogil Pharmaceutical Corp.
2 Manhattansville Rd.
Purchase, NY 10577
914-696-7600
www.hogil.com

47992
Holles Laboratories, Inc.
30 Forest Notch
Cohasset, MA 02025-1198
781-383-0005
800-356-4015

Hollister-Stier
3525 N. Regal
Spokane, WA 99207
800-992-1120
www.hollister-stier.com

Home Access Health Corporation
2401 W. Hassell Rd.
Suite 1510
Hoffman Estates, IL 60195-5200
847-781-2500
www.homeaccess.com

Home Diagnostics
51 James Way
Eatontown, NJ 07724

Hope Pharmaceuticals
8260 E. Gelding Dr.
Suite 104
Scottsdale, AZ 85260
480-607-1970
800-755-9595
www.hopepharm.com

59630
Horizon Pharmaceutical Corp.
See First Horizon Pharmaceutical Corp.

Hormel Healthlabs
1 Hormel Place
Austin, MN 55912
800-866-7757
www.hormelhealthlabs.com

Hospak Unit Dose Products
5910 Creekside Lane
Rockford, IL 61114
815-877-6480
866-846-7725
www.hospak@rockford.com

58407
Houba
(Halsey Drug Co.)
16235 State Rd. 17
Culver, IN 46511
574-842-3305

Huckaby Pharmacal, Inc.
11802 Brinley Ave.
Suite 201
Louisville, KY 40243
502-243-4000
888-206-5525
www.huckabypharmacal.com

Humanicare International
9 Elkins Road
East Brunswick, NJ 08816
732-613-9000
800-631-5270
www.humanicare.com

00395
Humco Holding Group, Inc.
7400 Alumax
Texarkana, TX 75501
903-831-7808
800-662-3435
www.humco.com

Humphreys (Dickinson Brands)
63 Meadow Road
Rutherford, NJ 07070
201-933-7744

Hybritech
(Beckman Coulter)
7330 Carroll Rd.
San Diego, CA 92121
858-578-9800
www.beckmancoulter.com

Hyland Immuno
See Baxter Healthcare Corporation, Baxter Bioscience

Hyland Laboratories, Inc.
See Standard Homeopathic Co.

Hyland Therapeutics
See Baxter Hyland Immuno

Hynson, Westcott & Dunning
See Becton Dickinson Microbiology
  Systems

Hyperion Medical, Inc.
1130 Celebration Boulevard
Celebration, FL 34747
407-566-1520
800-743-8111
www.hyperionmedical.com

Hypoguard USA, Inc.
7301 Ohms Lane
Suite 200
Edina, MN 55439
952-646-3200
www.hypoguard.com

00314
Hyrex Pharmaceuticals
3494 Democrat Rd.
Memphis, TN 38118
901-794-9050
800-238-5282

Iatric Corp.
2330 S. Industrial Park Ave.
Tempe, AZ 85282
602-966-7248
800-528-4401

ICI Pharmaceuticals
See AstraZeneca L.P.

ICN Canada Ltd.
Montreal, Quebec
Canada

ICN Pharmaceuticals
3300 Hyland Avenue
Costa Mesa, CA 92626
714-545-0100
800-548-5100
www.icnpharm.com

IDEC Pharmaceuticals
See Biogen Idec

Ilex Oncology Inc.
4545 Horizon Hill Blvd.
San Antonio, TX 78229
210-949-8200
www.ilexonc.com

Immucell Corp.
56 Evergreen Dr.
Portland, ME 04103
207-878-2770
800-466-8235
www.immucell.com

00205, 58406
Immunex Corp.
See Amgen, Inc.

54129
Immuno U.S., Inc.
(Baxter Healthcare Corp.)
1200 Parkdale Rd.
Rochester, MI 48307-1744
248-652-4760
www.baxter.com

Immunobiology Research Inst.
Route 22 East
P.O. Box 999
Annandale, NJ 08801-0999
908-730-1700

ImmunoGen
128 Sidney St.
Cambridge, MA 02139
617-995-2500
www.immunogen.com

Immunomedics Inc.
300 American Rd.
Morris Plains, NJ 07950
973-605-8200
www.immunomedics.com

Immunotec Research Ltd.
292 Adrien Patenaude
Vandreuil-Dorion, QC J7V 5V5
514-424-9992

Impax Laboratories, Inc.
30831 Huntwood Ave.
Hayward, CA 94544
510-476-2000
www.impaxlabs.com

00548
I.M.S., Ltd.
See Celltech Pharmaceutical Co.

IMX Pharmaceuticals, Inc.
2295 Corporate Blvd.
Boca Raton, FL 33431
561-998-5660

INAMED Corporation
5540 Ekwill Drive
Santa Barbara, CA 93111
805-683-6761
800-722-2007
www.inamed.com

Inbrand
1169 Canton Road
Marietta, GA 30066
770-422-3036

Indevus Pharmaceuticals, Inc.
99 Hayden Ave.
Suite 200
Lexington, MA 02421
781-861-8444
www.indevus.com

InKine Pharmaceutical
  Company, Inc.
1787 Sentry Pkwy.
West Bldg. 18, Suite 440
Blue Bell, PA 19422
215-283-6850
www.inkine.com

Inner Health Group
6203 Woodlake Ctr.
San Antonio, TX 78244
210-661-9257
800-381-4697
www.michaelshealth.com

Innovite, Inc.
See Endurance Products Company

InnoZen, Inc.
6429 Independence Avenue
Woodland Hills, CA 91367
818-593-4880
800-599-8892

INO Therapeutics, Inc.
6th State Route 173
Clinton, NJ 08809
908-238-6600
877-566-94466
www.inotherapeutics.com

Insource
P.O. Box 39
Bland, VA 24315
276-688-0211
800-366-3829
www.insourceonline.com

Inspire Pharmaceuticals, Inc.
4222 Emperor Blvd.
Suite 470
Durham, NC 27703
919-941-9777
www.inspirepharm.com

Integrated Therapeutics
9755 S.W. Commerce Circle
Suite B2
Wilsonville, OR 97080
800-869-9705
www.integrativeinc.com

Integrity Pharmaceutical
  Corporaton
9084 Technology Drive
Suite 600
Fishers, IN 46038
317-558-2820
800-823-6878
www.integritypharma.com

Interchem Corp.
120 Route 17 N., Suite 115
P.O. Box 1579
Paramus, NJ 07653
201-261-7333
800-261-7332
www.interchem.com

Intercure, Inc.
400 Kelby Street, Parker Plaza
12th Floor
Fort Lee, NJ 07024
201-720-7750
www.intercure.com

Interferon Sciences
783 Jersey Ave.
New Brunswick, NJ 08901
732-249-3250
888-728-4372
www.interferonsciences.com

Intermax Pharmaceuticals, Inc.
228 Sherwood Ave.
Farmingdale, NY 11735
631-777-3318

InterMune Pharmaceuticals,
  Inc.
3280 Bayside Blvd.
Bayshore, CA 94005
415-466-2200
www.intermune.com

11584
International Ethical Labs
Reparto Metropolitano
Avenue Americo Miranda #1021
Rio Piedras, PR 00921
787-765-3510

International Laboratory
  Technology Corp.
3389 Sheridan St.
Suite 149
Hollywood, FL 33021

International Labs
2350 31st Street South
St. Petersburg, FL 33712
727-327-4094
www.internationallabs.com

International Medications
  Systems, Ltd.
1886 Santa Anita Ave.
South El Monte, CA 91733
800-423-4136
www.ims-limited.com

Interneuron Pharmaceuticals,
  Inc.
See Indevus Pharmaceuticals, Inc.

Interpharm Ltd.
99b Cobbold Road
Unit 1
Willesden, London, UK NW 10 9SL
020 8830 0803
www.interpharm.co.uk

00814
Interstate Drug Exchange
See Henry Schein, Inc.

Intramed Corp
4333 Orange St., #3610
Riverside, CA 92501
909-328-9999
www.intramed.com

52189
Invamed, Inc.
See Geneva Pharmaceuticals

Inveresk Research, Inc.
11000 Weston Pkwy.
Suite 100
Cary, NC 27513
919-460-9005
800-988-9845
www.inveresk.com

Inverness Medical Innovations
51 Sawyer Rd.
Suite 200
Waltham, MA 02453
781-647-3900
800-899-7353
www.invernessmedical.com

00258
Inwood Laboratories
See Forest Laboratories

Iolab Pharmaceuticals
See Ciba Vision Corp.

61646
Iomed
See IoPharm

IOP, Inc.
3151 Airway Ave.
Suite I-1
Costa Mesa, CA 92626
714-549-1185
800-535-3545
www.iopinc.com

IoPharm
7552 Pebble Dr.
Ft. Worth, TX 76118
817-595-5820

54921
IPR Pharmaceuticals, Inc.
P.O. Box 1967
Carolina, PR 00984
787-750-5353
800-477-6385

Isis Pharmaceuticals
2292 Faraday Ave.
Carlsbad, CA 92008
760-931-9200
www.isispharm.com

50914
Iso-Tex Diagnostics, Inc.
1511 County Rd. 129
P.O. Box 909
Friendswood, TX 77546
281-482-1231
800-447-4839
www.isotexdiagnostics.com

Ivax Corporation
4400 Biscayne Blvd.
Miami, FL 33137
305-575-6000
www.ivaxpharmaceuticals.com

Ivax Pharmaceuticals, Inc.
4400 Biscayne Blvd.
Miami, FL 33137
305-575-6000
800-327-4114
www.ivaxpharmaceuticals.com

Ivy Corporation
P.O. Box 596
W. Caldwell, NJ 07006
800-443-8856

16837
**J & J Merck Consumer Pharm.
Co.**
7050 Camp Hill Rd.
Ft. Washington, PA 19034
215-273-7000
800-523-3484
www.jnj-merck.com

49938
Jacobus Pharmaceutical Co.
37 Cleveland Lane
P.O. Box 5920
Princeton, NJ 08540
609-921-7447

Jamol Labs
13 Ackerman Avenue
Emerson, NJ 07630
201-262-6363

50458
Janssen Pharmaceutica
1125 Trenton-Harbourton Rd.
Titusville, NJ 08560-0200
609-730-2000
800-526-7736
www.janssen.com

J.B. Williams Company, Inc.
65 Harristown Rd.
Glen Rock, NJ 07452-3317
201-251-8100
800-254-8656

Jergens
See The Andrew Jergens Company

**Jerome Stevens
Pharmaceuticals, Inc.**
60 Da Vinci Drive
Bohemia, NY 11234
516-567-1113

00304
J.J. Balan, Inc.
5725 Foster Ave.
Brooklyn, NY 11234
800-552-2526
www.jjbalan.com

JMI-Canton Pharmaceuticals
See Jones Pharma Incorporated

00137
Johnson & Johnson
One Johnson & Johnson Plz.
New Brunswick, NJ 08933
732-524-0400
www.jnj.com

**Johnson & Johnson Consumers'
Products Company**
199 Grandview Rd.
Skillman, NJ 08558-9418
732-524-0400
800-526-3967
www.jnj.com

56091
Johnson & Johnson Medical
2500 E. Arbrook Blvd.
Arlington, TX 76014
800-423-5850
www.jnjmedical.com

00252, 52604, 00689
Jones Pharma Incorporated
See King Pharmaceuticals, Inc.

88395
J. R. Carlson Laboratories
15 College Dr.
Arlington Heights, IL 60004-1985
847-255-1600
888-234-5656
www.carlsonlabs.com

10106
J.T. Baker, Inc.
See Mallinckrodt-Baker, Inc.

KabiVitrum, Inc.
See Pharmacia Corp.

Kanetta Pharmacal
90 Park Ave.
New York, NY 10016
212-907-2690
800-372-6634

00588
Keene Pharmaceuticals, Inc.
303 South Mockingbird
P.O. Box 7
Keene, TX 76059-0007
817-645-8083
800-541-0530

28851
Kendall Health Care Products
15 Hampshire St.
Mansfield, MA 02048
508-261-8000
800-962-9888
www.kendallhq.com

Kendall-McGaw Labs, Inc.
See B. Braun Medical Inc.

00482
Kenwood Laboratories
See Bradley Pharmaceuticals

(The) Key Company
1313 West Essex
St. Louis, MO 63122
314-965-6699
800-325-9592
www.thekeycompany.com

00085
Key Pharmaceuticals
See Schering-Plough Corp.

Kiel Laboratories, Inc.
2225 Centennial
Gainesville, GA 30504
770-534-0079
www.kielpharm.com

Kimberly-Clark
351 Phelps Drive
Irving, TX 75038
972-281-1200
www.kimberly-clark.com

60793
King Pharmaceuticals, Inc.
501 Fifth St.
Bristol, TN 37620
423-989-8000
800-776-3637
www.kingpharm.com

55299
Kingswood Laboratories, Inc.
10375 Hague Rd.
Indianapolis, IN 46256
317-849-9513
800-968-7772

Kinray
152-35 10th Ave.
Whitestone, NY 11357
718-767-1234
800-854-6729

58223
Kirkman Laboratories, Inc.
6400 SW Rosewood
Lake Oswego, OR 97035
503-694-1600
800-245-8282
www.kirkmanlabs.com

31600
Kiwi Brands, Inc.
(Sara Lee Household & Body Care)
447 Old Swede Rd.
Douglassville, PA 19518
610-385-3041

KLI Corp.
1119 Third Ave. S.W.
Carmel, IN 46032
317-846-7452
800-308-7452
www.entertainers-secret.com

00044, 00048, 00524
Knoll Pharmaceuticals
See Abbott Laboratories

Kodak Dental
343 State St.
Rochester, NY 14650
716-724-5631
800-933-8031
www.kodak.com

(Eastman) Kodak Co.
343 State St.
Rochester, NY 14650
585-724-4000
www.kodak.com

Konec, Inc.
3840 East 44th Street
Suite 609
Tucson, AZ 85713
520-571-9119
www.konec-inc.com

00224
Konsyl Pharmaceuticals
4200 S. Hulen
Suite 513
Ft. Worth, TX 76109
817-763-8011
800-356-6795
www.konsyl.com

Kos Pharmaceutics, Inc.
1001 Brickell Bay Dr.
25th Floor
Miami, FL 33131
305-577-3464
www.kospharm.com

55505
Kramer Laboratories, Inc.
8778 S.W. 8th St.
Miami, FL 33174-9990
302-223-1287
800-824-4894
www.kramerlabs.com

Kremers Urban
P.O. Box 427
Mequon, WI 53092
414-238-5205
800-625-5710

K-Tech USA, Inc.
80 S. W. 8th Street
Miami, FL 33130
305-373-8248

K.V. Pharmaceutical Co.
2503 S. Hanley Rd.
St. Louis, MO 63144
314-645-6600
www.kvpharmaceutical.com

La Haye Laboratories, Inc.
See U.S. Neutraceuticals, LLC

Lacrimedics, Inc.
P.O. Box 1209
Eastsound, WA 98245
360-376-7095
800-367-8327
www.lacrimedics.com

41383
Lactaid, Inc.
7050 Camp Hill Rd.
Ft. Washington, PA 19034
215-273-7000
800-522-8243
www.lactaid.com

59081
Lafayette Pharmaceuticals, Inc.
See Mallinckrodt-Baker, Inc.

Lake Consumer Products
730 Corporate Woods Pkwy.
Vernon Hills, IL 60061
847-793-0230
800-537-8658
www.lakeconsumer.com

L.A.M. Pharmaceutical Corp.
755 Center Street
Unit 5
Lewiston, NY 14092
716-754-2002
877-526-7717
www.lampharm.com

Lane Labs
25 Commerce Drive
Allendale, NJ 07401
201-236-9090
800-526-3005
www.lanelabs.com

00527
Lannett Co., Inc.
9000 State Rd.
Philadelphia, PA 19136
215-333-9000
800-325-9994
www.lannett.com

Lansinoh Laboratories
333 Fairfax Street
Suite 400
Alexandria, VA 22314
703-299-1100
www.lansinoh.com

Lantiseptic
See Summit Industries, Inc.

00277
Laser, Inc.
2200 W. 97th Place
P.O. Box 905
Crown Point, IN 46307
219-663-1165
800-325-0925

10651
Lavoptik Co., Inc.
661 Western Ave.
St. Paul, MN 55103
612-489-0760

Layton Bioscience, Inc.
709 E. Evelyn Ave.
Sunnyvale, CA 94086
408-616-1000
www.laytonbio.com

LecTec Corporation
10701 Red Circle Dr.
Minnetonka, MN 55343
952-933-2291
800-777-2291
www.lectec.com

Lederle Consumer Health
See Wyeth Consumer Health

Lederle Labs
401 N. Middleton Rd.
Pearl River, NY 10965
914-732-5000
800-395-9938

**Lederle Pharmaceutical
   Division**
See Wyeth-Ayerst Labs

Lederle-Praxis Biologicals
See Legere Pharmaceuticals, Inc.

23558
Lee Pharmaceuticals
1434 Santa Anita Ave.
South Elmonte, CA 91733
800-950-5337
www.leepharmaceuticals.com

Leeming
See Pfizer US Pharmaceutical
   Group

25332
Legere Pharmaceuticals, Inc.
7326 E. Evans Rd.
Scottsdale, AZ 85260
602-991-4033
800-528-3144

19200
Lehn & Fink
See Reckitt & Colman

Leiner Health Products
901 East 233rd St.
Carson, CA 90745
310-835-8400
www.leiner.com

Leiras Pharmaceuticals, Inc.
2345 Waukegan Rd.
Suite N-135
Bannockburn, IL 60015

Lek Pharmaceuticals, Inc.
115 North 3rd Street
Suite 301
Wilmington, NC 28401
910-362-0021
866-542-4360
www.lek.si

00093, 00332
Lemmon Co.
See Teva Pharmaceuticals USA

Liberty Medical Supply
10045 South Federal Highway
Port St. Lucie, FL 34952
www.libertymedical.com

Liberty Pharmaceutical
8881 Liberty Lane
Port St. Lucie, FL 34952
www.libertymedical.com

Life Cycle Ventures, Inc.
220 Lake Dr.
Newark, DE 19702
609-493-3000

Lifescan, Inc.
1000 Gibraltar
Milpitas, CA 95035-6312
408-263-9789
800-524-7226
www.lifescan.com

LifeSign LLC
71 Veronica Ave.
P.O. Box 218
Somerset, NJ 08875-0218
908-246-3366
800-526-2125
www.lifesignmed.com

LifeStyle
712 Ginesi Dr.
Morganville, NJ 07751
800-622-7376
732-972-9205

Ligand Pharmaceuticals, Inc.
10275 Science Center Dr.
San Diego, CA 92121
858-550-7500
800-964-5836
www.ligand.com

00002, 59075
Lilly and Co.
See Eli Lilly and Co.

Lilly France S.A.
F-67640
Fegersheim, France

Lincoln Diagnostics
P.O. Box 1128
Decatur, IL 62525
217-877-2531
800-537-1336
www.lincolndiagnostics.com

Line One Laboratories
Pasadena, CA 91107
626-577-3428
www.lineonelabsusa.com

Lipha Pharmaceuticals, Inc.
9 West 57th St.
Suite 3825
New York, NY 10019

60799
Liposome Co.
See Elan Pharmaceuticals

Liverite Products Inc.
15405 Redhill Avenue
Suite C
Tustin, CA 92780
888-425-5483
www.liverite.com

Llorens Pharmaceutical
P.O. Box 720008
Miami, FL 33172
866-595-5598
www.llorenspharm.com

LNK International, Inc.
60 Arkay Dr.
Hauppauge, NY 11788
516-435-3500

Lobana Laboratories
(Ulmer Pharmacal)
1614 Industry Ave.
P.O. Box 408
Park Rapids, MN 56470
612-559-0601
800-848-5637
www.lobanaproducts.com

Lobob Laboratories
1440 Atteberry Lane
San Jose, CA 95131
408-432-0580
800-835-6262
www.loboblabs.com

Loch Pharmaceuticals
See Bedford Laboratories

Logimedix
1675 N. Commerce Parkway
Weston, FL 33326
800-821-0047
www.logimedix.com

Loma Lux Laboratories
P.O. Box 702418
Tulsa, OK 74170-2418
918-664-9882
800-316-9636
www.lomalux.com

L'Oreal Suncare Research
575 Fifth Avenue
26th Floor
New York, NY 10017
212-984-4109
800-322-2036
www.lorealparisusa.com

00273
Lorvic Corp.
See Young Dental Mfg.

59417
Lotus Biochemical Corporation
See New River Pharma

LSI America Corporation
4732 Twin Valley Dr.
Austin, TX 78731-3537
512-451-3738
800-720-5936
www.ondrox.com

Luitpold Pharmaceuticals, Inc.
1 Luitpold Dr.
Shirley, NY 11967
631-924-4000
800-645-1706
www.luitpold.com

Lunsco
Route 2, Box 62
Pulaski, VA 24301
540-980-4358

Luyties Pharmacal Co.
P.O. Box 8080
Richford, VT 05476
800-325-8080
www.1800homeopathy.com

00374
Lyne Laboratories
10 Burke Dr.
Brockton, MA 02301
508-583-8700
800-525-0450
www.lyne.com

MAGNA Pharmaceuticals, Inc.
11802 Brinley Avenue
Suite 201
Louisville, KY 40243
502-254-5552
888-206-5525
www.magnaweb.com

**Magno-Humphries Laboratories,
   Inc.**
8800 S.W. Commercial St.
Tigard, OR 97223
503-254-5464
www.magno-humphries.com

Majestic Drug
4996 Main Street
Route 42
South Fallsburg, NY 12779
845-436-0011
800-238-0220
www.majesticdrug.com

00904
Major Pharmaceuticals, Inc.
31778 Enterprise Dr.
Livonia, MI 48150
734-525-8700
800-688-9696

10106
Mallinckrodt Baker, Inc.
222 Red School Lane
Phillipsburg, NJ 08865
908-859-2151
800-582-2537
www.jtbaker.com

00406
Mallinckrodt Chemical
2nd St.
St. Louis, MO 63042
314-539-1216
800-325-8888
www.mallinckrodt.com

00019
Mallinckrodt, Inc.
675 McDonnell Blvd.
Hazelwood, MO 63042
314-654-2000
800-554-5343
www.mallinckrodt.com

Manloe Labs, Inc.
(New Horizons Distributing)
6320 S. Sandhill Rd.
Suite 10
Las Vegas, NV 89120
702-449-7154
800-777-4876

10706
Manne
P.O. Box 825
Johns Island, SC 29457
800-517-0228

Marathon Biopharmaceuticals
See Cambrex Bioscience

Marin Pharmaceuticals
1730 N.W. 79th Avenue
Miami, FL 33126
305-593-5333

Marion Merrell Dow
9300 Ward Parkway
P.O. Box 8480
Kansas City, MO 64114
816-966-4000

Marlex Pharmaceuticals, Inc.
50 McCullough Dr.
Southgate Center
New Castle, DE 19720
302-328-3355
www.marlexpharm.com

Marlin Industries
P.O. Box 560
Grover City, CA 93483-0560
805-473-2743
800-423-5926

12939
Marlop Pharmaceuticals, Inc.
230 Marshall St.
Elizabeth, NJ 07206
908-355-8854

10712
Marlyn Nutraceuticals, Inc.
4404 E. Ellwood
Phoenix, AZ 85040
480-991-0200
888-766-4406
www.naturally.com

00682
Marnel Pharmaceuticals, Inc.
206 Luke St.
Lafayette, LA 70506
337-232-1396

00209
Marsam Pharmaceuticals, Inc.
See Watson Pharmaceuticals, Inc.

52555
Martec Pharmaceutical, Inc.
1800 N. Topping Avenue
Box 33510
Kansas City, MO 64120-3510
816-241-4144
800-822-6782
www.martec-kc.com

12758
Mason Pharmaceuticals, Inc.
4425 Jamboree/Suite 250
Newport Beach, CA 92660
949-851-6860
800-366-2454

11845
Mason Vitamins, Inc.
5105 N.W. 159th St.
Miami Lakes, FL 33014-6370
305-624-5557
800-327-6005
www.masonvitamins.com

14362
Mass. Public Health Bio. Lab.
305 South St.
Jamaica Plains, MA 02130-3597
617-983-6400

Matrix Initiatives, Inc.
2375 Camelback
Suite 500
Phoenix, AZ 85016
602-387-5353
800-808-4866
www.zicam.com

Matrix Laboratories, Inc.
See Chiron

Mayer Laboratories
646 Kennedy Street
Building C
Oakland, CA 94606
510-437-8989
www.mayerlabs.com

Mayne Group Ltd.
Level 21/390 St. Kilda Rd.
Melbourne, Australia 3004
+6139868-0700
www.maynegroup.com

Mayne Pharma (USA) Inc.
650 From Road
Mack-Cali Centre II, Second Floor
Paramus, NJ 07652
201-225-5500
www.maynepharma.com/us

Mayo Foundation
200 1st St. S.W.
Rochester, MN 55905
507-284-2511
www.mayo.edu

00259
Mayrand, Inc.
See Merz Pharmaceuticals

00264
McGaw, Inc.
See B. Braun Medical Inc.

49072
McGuff Pharmaceuticals, Inc.
2921 W. MacArthur Blvd., Suite 141
Santa Ana, CA 92704
877-444-1133
www.mcguff.com

McKesson Drug Co.
1 Post St.
San Francisco, CA 94104
415-983-8300
www.mckesson.com

McKesson Medical-Surgical
8741 Landmark Rd.
Richmond, VA 23228
804-264-7500
www.mckgenmed.com

00045
McNeil Consumer & Specialty Pharmaceuticals
7050 Camp Hill Rd.
Mail Stop 278
Ft. Washington, PA 19034-2292
215-273-7000
800-962-5357
www.tylenol.com

McNeil Pharmaceutical
See Ortho-McNeil

MCR American Pharmaceuticals
16206 Flight Path Dr.
Brooksville, FL 34604
352-754-8587
www.mcramerican.com

MD Pharmaceutical
3130 S. Harbor Blvd. #320
Santa Ana, CA 92704
714-755-4400

58607
ME Pharmaceuticals, Inc.
2800 Southweast Parkway
Richmond, IN 47374
765-962-4410
800-637-4276
www.mepharm.com

Mead Johnson Laboratories
See Bristol-Myers Squibb

00087
Mead Johnson Nutritionals
2400 W. Lloyd Expressway
Evansville, IN 47721-7189
812-429-5000
www.meadjohnson.com

Mead Johnson Oncology
See Bristol-Myers Oncology/Virolgy

45565
Med-Derm Pharmaceuticals
P.O. Box 1452
Johnson City, TN 37605
423-926-4413
800-334-4286
www.delrayderm.com

53978
Med-Pro, Inc.
210 E. 4th St.
Lexington, NE 68850
308-324-4571
800-447-6060
www.med-pro-inc.com

Medac GmbH c/o Princeton Regulatory Assoc.
116 Village Blvd., Suite 200
Princeton, NJ 08540
609-951-9596

Medarex, Inc.
707 State Rd.
Princeton, NJ 08540
609-430-2880
www.medarex.com

Medchem Products
160 New Boston St.
Woburn, MA 01801
781-932-5000

11940
Medco Lab, Inc.
P.O. Box 864
Sioux City, IA 51102-5333
712-255-8770
www.medcolabs.com

Medcon Biolab Technologies, Inc.
50 Brigham Hill Road
Grafton, MA 01519
508-839-4203
800-443-6332
www.ilexpaste.com

Medco Research, Inc.
See King Pharmaceuticals Inc.

00585
Medeva Pharmaceuticals
See Celltech Pharmaceutical Co.

Medi Aid Corp.
See Baxa Corporation

Medi-Plex Pharm., Inc.
See ECR Pharmaceuticals

Medical Action Industries
800 Prime Place
Hauppauge, NY 11788
631-231-4600
800-645-7042

Medical Nutrition
10 West Forest Avenue
Englewood, NJ 07531
201-569-1188

00576
Medical Products Panamericana
647 W. Flagler St.
Miami, FL 33130
305-545-6524

(The) Medicines Company
1 Cambridge Center
Cambridge, MA 02142
617-225-9099
800-264-4662
www.angiomax.com

Medicis Dermatologics, Inc.
See Medicis Pharmaceutical Corp.

99207
Medicis Pharmaceutical Corp.
8125 N. Hayden Dr.
Scottsdale, AZ 85258
602-808-8800
800-550-5115
www.medicis.com

Medicore Inc.
2337 W. 76th St.
Hialeah, FL 33016
305-558-4000

60574
MedImmune, Inc.
35 W. Watkins Mill Rd.
Gaithersburg, MD 20878
877-633-4411
www.medimmune.com

Mediniche
167 Lamp & Lantern Village/PMB 300
Chesterfield, MO 63017
314-542-9539
www.mediniche.com

Medisca Inc.
661 Route 3, Unit C
Plattsburgh, NY 12901
518-561-0109
800-932-1039
www.medisca.com

MediSense, Inc.
See Abbott

Medix Pharmaceuticals Americas, Inc. (MPA)
12505 Starkey Rd.
Suite M
Largo, FL 33773
888-242-3463
800-672-7811
www.biafine.com

Med Pointe Healthcare, Inc.
265 Davidson Ave., Suite 300
Somerset, NJ 08873-4120
732-564-2200
www.medpointeinc.com

00348, 75137
Medtech Laboratories, Inc.
3510 N. Lake Creek
Jackson, WY 83001-1108
307-739-8208
800-443-4908
www.medtechinc.com

58281
Medtronic Inc.
710 Medtronic Pkwy.
Minneapolis, MN 55432
763-514-4000
800-328-0810
www.medtronic.com

MedVantx, Inc.
9171 Towne Center Drive/Suite 100
San Diego, CA 92122-6231
858-625-2990
www.medvantx.com

Meijer
2929 Walker Avenue N.W.
Grand Rapids, NJ 49544
616-453-6711
www.meijer.com

Melville Biologics
(Precision Pharma Services)
155 Duryea Rd.
Melville, NY 11747
631-752-7320

Menicon America
1840 Gateway Dr.
2nd Floor
San Mateo, CA 94404
650-378-1424
800-MENICON
www.menicon.com

22200
Mennen Co.
See Colgate-Palmolive Co.

Menper Distributors, Inc.
6500 N.W. 35th Ave.
Miami, FL 33147
305-551-7204

10742
Mentholatum Co., Inc.
707 Sterling Dr.
Orchard Park, NY 14127
716-677-2500
800-688-7660
www.mentholatum.com

Mentor Urology
5425 Hollister Avenue
Santa Barbara, CA 93111
805-681-6000
800-525-0245
www.mentorcorp.com

00006
Merck & Co.
1 Merck Dr.
White House Station, NJ 08889
908-423-1000
800-672-6372
www.merck.com

Merck Human Health (a division of Merck & Co)
770 Sumneytown Pike
West Point, PA 19486-0004
215-652-5000

Meretek Diagnostics, Inc.
2655 Crescent Dr./Suite C
Lafayette, CO 80026
720-479-6400
800-MERETEK
www.meretek.com

00394
Mericon Industries, Inc.
8819 N. Pioneer Rd.
Peoria, IL 61615
309-693-2150
800-242-6464

Meridian Chemical & Equipment
1316 Commerce Dr.
Decatur, AL 35601
256-350-1297
800-687-7850
www.letcoin.com

Meridian Medical Technologies
10240 Old Columbian Rd.
Columbia, MD 21046
410-309-6830
800-638-8093
www.meridianmeds.com

Merieux Institute, Inc.
See Aventis

30727
Merit Pharmaceuticals
2611 San Fernando Rd.
Los Angeles, CA 90065
213-227-4831
800-334-0514
www.meritpharms.com

Merkle GmBh Omnibusverkehr
Ulmer Weg 28/ 89558 Bohmenkirch
Germany
07332/922133

Merrell-Dow
See Aventis

Merz Pharmaceuticals
4215 Tudor Lane
Greensboro, NC 27410
336-856-2003
800-421-9657
www.merzusa.com

Methapharm, Inc. (Corporate Office)
131 Clarence St.
Brantford, Ontario, Canada N3T2V6
800-287-7686
www.methapharm.com

Methapharm, Inc. (Head Office)
2825 University Dr.
Suite 240
Coral Springs, FL 33065
519-751-3602
800-287-7686
www.methapharm.com

Metrika, Inc.
510 Oakmead Pkwy.
Sunnyvale, CA 94085
408-524-2255
877-212-4968
www.A1cNow.com

Met-Rx USA
6111 Broken Sound Parkway, N.W.
Boca Raton, FL 33487
800-556-3879
www.metrx.com

MGI Pharma, Inc.
5775 W. Old Shakopee Rd./Suite 110
Bloomington, MN 55437-3174
952-346-4700
800-562-0679
www.mgipharma.com

Michigan Department of Health
320 S. Walnut
Lansing, MI 48913
517-373-3740

MicroGeneSys, Inc.
1000 Research Pkwy.
Meriden, CT 06450-7159
203-686-0800
800-488-7099

Micron Technology, Inc.
8000 S. Federal Way
Boise, ID 83707
208-368-4000

00682, 46672
Mikart, Inc.
1750 Chattahoochee Ave.
Atlanta, GA 30318
404-354-4510
www.mikart.com

Miles, Inc.
See Bayer Corp.

00396, 34567
Milex Products, Inc.
4311 N. Normandy
Chicago, IL 60634
773-736-5500
800-621-1278
www.milexproducts.com

Millennium Pharmaceuticals, Inc.
75 Sidney St.
Cambridge, MA 02139
617-679-7000
www.millennium.com

17204
Miller Pharmacal Group, Inc.
350 Randy Rd., Suite #2
Carol Stream, IL 60188
630-871-9557
800-323-2935
www.millerpharmacal.com

Minrad Inc.
3950 Schelden Circle
Bethlehem, PA 18017
716-855-1068

00276
Misemer Pharmaceuticals, Inc.
See Edwards Pharmaceuticals, Inc.

00178
Mission Pharmacal Company
P.O. Box 786099
San Antonio, TX 78278-6099
210-696-8400
800-531-3333
www.missionpharmacal.com

Miza Pharmaceuticals
4950 Younge St.
Suite 2001
P.O. Box 118
Toronto, Ontario
Canada M2N 6K1
416-927-0600

Miza Pharmaceuticals USA
40 Main St.
P.O. Box 210
Fairton, NJ 08320-0210
856-451-9350

Molnlycke Healthcare
826 Newtown-Yardley Road
Newtown, PA 18940
267-685-2000
800-882-4582
www.molnlyckehc.com

Monaghan Medical Corporation
5 Latour Ave.
Suite 1600
P.O. Box 2805
Plattsburgh, NY 12901
518-561-7330
800-833-9653
www.monaghanmed.com

53169
Monarch Pharmaceuticals
501 5th St.
Bristol, TN 37620
423-989-8000
800-776-3637
www.monarchpharm.com

Monticello Drug Co.
1604 Stockton Co.
Jacksonville, FL 32204
904-384-3666
800-735-0666
www.monticellocompanies.com

Moore Medical Corp.
389 John Downey Dr.
P.O. Box 2740
New Britain, CT 06050-1500
800-234-1464
www.mooremedical.com

Morepen Laboratories Limited
4th Floor
Antriksh Bhawan 22
Kasturba Gandhi Marg
New Delhi, India 110001
+91-11-23324443
www.morepen.com

00426, 00832, 60432
Morton Grove Pharmaceuticals, Inc.
6451 W. Main St.
Morton Grove, IL 60053
847-967-5600
800-346-6854
www.mgp-online.com

Morton International
100 Independence Mall West
Philadelphia, PA 19106
215-592-3000
www.rohmhaas.com

Morton Salt
123 N. Wacker Dr.
Chicago, IL 60606
312-807-2000
www.mortonsalt.com

MotherSOY International, Inc.
424 S. Kentucky Ave.
Evansville, IN 47714
812-424-5432
888-769-0769
www.mothersoy.com

Mount Sinai Medical Ctr.
1 Gustave L. Levy Place
New York, NY 10029-6574
212-241-6500

Mova Pharmaceutical
5 Cedar Book Dr.
Cranberry, NJ 08512
609-409-8320
www.movapharm.com

Movo Pharmaceuticals
P.O. Box 8639
Caguas, PR 00726
787-746-8500
800-468-5201

MPM Medical Inc.
2301 Crown Ct.
Irving, TX 75038
972-893-4090
800-232-5512
www.mpmmedicalinc.com

MSD
See Merck & Co.

MTI Biotech
2625 North Loop Drive/Suite 2150
Ames, IA 50010
877-465-8836
www.mtibiotech.com

54964
Murdock, Madaus, Schwabe
See Nature's Way

00451
Muro Pharmaceutical, Inc.
890 East St.
Tewksbury, MA 01876-9987
978-851-5981
800-225-0974
www.muropharm.com

00150
Murray Drug Corp.
1103 Northwood Dr.
Murray, KY 42071
270-753-6654

53489
Mutual Pharmaceutical Co., Inc.
(United Research Laboratories)
1100 Orthodox St.
Philadelphia, PA 19124
215-288-6500
800-523-3684
www.urlmutual.com

00378
Mylan Pharmaceuticals, Inc.
781 Chestnut Ridge Rd.
Morgantown, WV 26505
304-599-2595
800-826-9526
www.mylan.com

05973
Nabi
5800 Park of Commerce Blvd. NW
Boca Raton, FL 33487
561-989-5800
800-635-1766
www.nabi.com

05745
Nastech Pharmaceutical Co., Inc.
3450 Montevilla Pkwy.
Bothell, WA 98021
425-908-3600

National Medical Products, Inc.
57 Parker St.
Irvine, CA 92618
949-768-1147
www.jtip.com

National Vitamin Co., Inc.
2075 West Scranton Ave.
Porterville, CA 93257-8358
559-781-8871
800-538-5828
www.nationalvitamin.com

53983
NaTREN, Inc.
3105 Willow Lane
Westlake Village, CA 91361
805-371-4737
800-992-3323
www.natren.com

Natrol, Inc.
21411 Prairie St.
Chatsworth, CA 91311
800-326-1520
www.natrol.com

Naturally Vitamins Co.
4404 E. Elwood St.
Phoenix, AZ 85040
480-991-0200
800-899-4499
www.naturallyvitamins.com

Nature Smart
1500 East 128th Ave.
Thornton, CO 80241

Nature's Best
550 N. Kingsbury St.
Unit 514
Chicago, IL 60610
800-584-8544
www.naturesbestenzyme.com

25077
Nature's Bounty, Inc.
90 Orville Dr.
Bohemia, NY 11716
631-244-2055
800-645-5412
www.naturesbounty.com

Nature's Sunshine Products, Inc.
75 East 1700 South
Provo, UT 84606
801-342-4305
800-223-8225
www.naturessunshine.com

Nature's Way
1375 North Mountain Springs Pkwy.
Springvale, UT 84663
801-489-1500
800-926-8883
www.naturesway.com

74312
NBTY, Inc.
See Nature's Bounty, Inc.

Neil Labs
55 Lake Drive
East Windsor, NJ 08520
609-448-5500
www.neillabs.com

Nelson Neutraceuticals
(formerly NCI Medical Foods)
5801 Ayala Avenue
Irwindale, CA 91706
626-815-3393
800-869-1515

NeoRx Corp.
300 Elliot Ave. West, Suite 500
Seattle, WA 98119
206-281-7001
www.neorx.com

Nephro-Tech, Inc.
P.O. Box 16106
Shawnee, KS 66203
785-883-4108
800-879-4755
www.nephrotech.com

00487
Nephron Pharmaceuticals Corp.
4121 SW 34th St.
Orlando, FL 32811-5459
407-246-1389
800-443-4313
www.nephronpharm.com

Nestle Clinical Nutrition
3 Parkway N.
Suite 500
Deerfield, IL 60015
847-317-2800
800-388-0300
www.nestleclinicalnutrition.com

Nestle Infant Nutrition
P.O. Box AW
Wilkes-Barre, PA 18703
800-628-2229
www.verybestbaby.com

Neurex Pharmaceuticals
See Elan Pharmaceuticals

NeuroGenesis
120 Park Ave.
League City, TX 77573
800-345-8912
www.neurogenesis.com

10812, 70501
Neutrogena Corporation
5760 W. 96th St.
Los Angeles, CA 90045-5595
310-642-1150
800-582-4048
www.neutrogena.com

Neutron Technology Corp.
See Micron Technology, Inc.

New Halsey Drug Co., Inc.
See Halsey Drug Co.

New Mark Laboratories
P.O. Box 6321
Edison, NJ 08818
732-417-1870
800-338-8079

New River Pharma
100 5th St.
Suite 410
Bristol, TN 37620
423-989-9192
800-455-5525

New World Trading Corp.
P.O. Box 952
DeBary, FL 32713
407-556-0608

56146
NeXstar Pharmaceuticals, Inc.
2860 Wilderness Place
Boulder, CO 80301
303-444-5893
800-403-3945

NF Formulas
9755 S.W. Commerce Circle/Suite B2
Wilsonville, OR 97070
503-682-9755
800-931-1709
www.integrativeinc.com

59016
Niche Pharmaceuticals, Inc.
209 N. Oak St.
P.O. Box 449
Roanoke, TX 76262
817-491-2770
800-677-0355
www.niche-inc.com

Nion Corp.
15501 E. First St.
Irwindale, CA 91706

Nnodum Corporation
886 Clinton Springs Ave.
Cincinnati, OH 45229
513-861-2329
888-301-9457
www.zikspain.com

Nolco Pharmaceuticals
Villas Del Senorial
San Juan, PR 00926

51801
Nomax, Inc.
40 N. Rock Hill Rd.
St. Louis, MO 63119
314-961-2500
www.nomax.com

Noramco Inc.
1440 Olympic Dr.
Athens, GA 30601
706-353-4400
www.noramco.com

Norcliff Thayer
See SmithKline Beecham Consumer Healthcare

10118
Norstar Consumer Products Co., Inc.
5517 Ninety-fifth Ave.
Kenosha, WI 53144
262-652-8505
888-282-5164
www.norstarcpc.com

North American Biologicals, Inc.
See Nabi

North American Vaccine, Inc.
See Baxter

Northern Research Laboratories, Inc.
4225 White Bear Pkwy.
Suite 600
St. Paul, MN 55110
651-653-3380
888-884-4675
www.northernresearch.com

Novartis Consumer Health
200 Kimball Dr.
Parsippany, NJ 07054-0622
973-503-8000
888-452-0051
www.novartis.com

Novartis Nutrition
1600 Utica Ave. S.
Suite 600
Minneapolis, MN 55416
800-999-9978
www.novartis.com

Novartis Ophthalmics, Inc.
11695 Johns Creek Parkway
Duluth, GA 30097-1556
866-393-6336
www.novartisophthalmics.com

Novartis Pharma AG
CH 4402
Basale, Switzerland
41613241111

00028, 00067, 00083, 58887
Novartis Pharmaceuticals Corp.
59 Route 10
East Hanover, NJ 04936
973-781-8300
888-669-6682
www.us-novartis.com

Novavax, Inc.
8320 Guilford Road, Suite C
Columbia, MD 21046
301-854-3900
www.novavax.com

Noven Pharmaceuticals
11960 SW 144th St.
Miami, FL 33186
305-253-5099
888-253-5099
www.noven.com

00169
Novo Nordisk
100 College Rd. West
Princeton, NJ 08540
609-987-5800
www.novonordisk-us.com

00362
Novocol
See Septodont, Inc.

55953
Novopharm USA, Inc.
165 E. Commerce Dr., Suite 100
Schaumburg, IL 60173
847-882-4200
800-426-0769

55499
Numark Laboratories, Inc.
164 Northfield Avenue
Edison, NJ 08818
732-417-1870
800-338-8079
www.numarklabs.com

Nutra Cea
1261 Hawk's Flight Court
El Dorado Hills, CA 95762
877-723-1700
www.nutracea.com

Nutraceutical Solutions
6704 Ranger Avenue
Corpus Christi, TX 78415
800-856-7040
www.eliquidsolutions.com

NutraMax Laboratories, Inc.
2208 Lakeside Blvd.
Edgewood, MD 21040
410-776-4000
800-925-5187
www.nutramaxlabs.com

NutraMax Products
51 Blackburn Dr.
Gloucester, MA 01930
978-282-1800
www.nutramax.com

Nutri Vention
6203 Woodlake Center
San Antonio, TX 78244
210-661-8589
800-390-7940

NutriSoy International, Inc.
See MotherSOY International, Inc.

Nutrition 21
4 Manhattanville Road
Purchase, NY 10577
914-701-4500
www.nutrition21.com

Nutrition Medical, Inc.
See Hormel Healthlabs

Nutro Laboratories
650 Hadley Rd.
South Plainfield, NJ 07080
908-754-9300

00407
Nycomed Amersham
101 Carnegie Center
Princeton, NJ 08540-6231
609-514-6000
800-654-0118
www.nycomed-amersham.com

10797
Oakhurst Co.
3000 Hempstead Turnpike
Levittown, NY 11756
516-731-5380
800-831-1135

55515
Oclassen Pharmaceuticals, Inc.
See Watson Pharm

O'Connor, Inc.
See Columbia Laboratories, Inc.

51944
Ocumed, Inc.
119 Harrison Ave.
Roseland, NJ 07068
973-226-2330

Odyssey Pharmaceuticals, Inc.
72 DeForest Ave.
East Hanover, NJ 07936
877-427-9068
www.odysseypharm.com

OHM Laboratories, Inc.
1385 Ohm Labs
New Brunswick, NJ 08902
732-418-2235
800-527-6481

10019
Ohmeda Pharmaceuticals
See Baxter Healthcare

Omnii Oral Pharmaceuticals
1500 N. Florida Mango Rd.
Suite 1
West Palm Beach, FL 33409
561-689-1140
800-445-3386

ONY, Inc.
1576 Sweet Home Rd.
Amherst, NY 14228
716-636-9096
877-274-4669

Optics Laboratory, Inc.
9480 Telstar Ave. #3
El Monte, CA 91731
626-350-1926
800-968-6788

Optikem International
2172 S. Jason St.
Denver, CO 80223
303-936-1137
800-525-1752

50520
Optimox Corp.
P.O. Box 3378
Torrance, CA 90510
310-618-9370
800-223-1601
www.optimox.com

52238
Optopics Laboratories Corp.
See Miza Pharmaceuticals USA

00041
Oral-B Laboratories
600 Clipper Dr.
Belmont, CA 94002
650-598-5000
800-446-7252
www.oral-b.com

OraPharma, Inc.
732 Louis Dr.
Warminster, PA 18974
215-956-2200

Orasure Technologies
220 East First Street
Bethlehem, PA 18015
610-882-1820
www.orasure.com

Organogenesis Inc.
150 Dan Rd.
Canton, MA 02021
781-575-0775
617-575-0440

00052
Organon, Inc.
375 Mt. Pleasant Ave.
West Orange, NJ 07052
973-325-4500
800-631-1253
www.organon-usa.com

Organon Teknika Corp.
See Biomerieux

Orion Corp.
Koivumankkaantie
6 Ovi 73 02200
Espoo, Finland
358-9-429-2745

Orion Diagnostica
(Lifesign)
71 Veronica Ave.
P.O. Box 218
Somerset, NJ 08875-0218
800-526-2125

Orphan Medical, Inc.
13911 Ridgedale Dr.
Suite 250
Minnetonka, MN 55305
888-867-7426

Orphan Pharmaceuticals USA
See Rare Disease Therapeutics

59676
Ortho Biotech, Inc.
430 Route 22 East
P.O. Box 6914
Bridgewater, NJ 08807-0914
800-325-7504
www.orthobiotech.com

Ortho-Clinical Diagnostics
100 Indigo Creek Dr.
Rochester, NY 14626
800-828-6316
www.orthoclinical.com

00062
Ortho-McNeil Pharmaceutical
1000 Route 202
P.O. Box 300
Raritan, NJ 08869
908-218-6000
800-631-5273
www.ortho-mcneil.com

**Ortho Neutrogena –
Dermatological**
199 Grandview Rd.
Skillman, NJ 08558
800-426-7762

OSI Pharmaceuticals
58 South Service Road
Suite 110
Melville, NY 11747
631-962-2000
www.osip.com

Otis Clapp & Sons Inc.
115 Shawmut Rd.
Canton, MA 02021
800-777-6847
781-821-5400

59148
**Otsuka America
Pharmaceutical, Inc.**
2440 Research Blvd.
Suite 250
Rockville, MD 20850
301-417-0900
800-562-3974
www.otsuka.com

Ovation Pharm
One Overlook Pt., Suite 110
Lincolnshire, IL 60069
888-514-5204
847-282-1001

Owen/Galderma
See Galderma Laboratories, Inc.

Owen Mumford Inc.
1755 A West Oak Commons Ct.
Marietta, GA 30062
770-977-2226
800-421-6936
www.owenmumford.com

**Oxford Pharmaceutical
Services, Inc.**
1 US Highway 46 West
Totowa, NJ 07512
973-256-0600
877-284-9120
www.oxfordpharm.com

Oxis International
6040 N. Cutter Circle
Suite 317
Portland, OR 97217
503-283-3911
800-547-3686
www.oxis.com

Oxypure Inc.
3550 Morris St. N.
St. Petersburg, FL 33713
888-216-8930

00574
P&S Laboratories, Inc.
210 W. 131st St.
Los Angeles, CA 90061
800-624-9659

Paddock Laboratories
3490 Quebec Ave. N.
Minneapolis, MN 55427
763-546-4676
800-328-5113
www.paddocklabs.com

53159
Palisades Pharmaceuticals, Inc.
See Glenwood, Inc.

Pamlab, LLC
P.O. Box 8950
Mandeville, LA 70470-8950
985-893-4097

Pan American Laboratories
P.O. Box 8950
Mandeville, LA 70470-8950
985-893-4097
www.panamericanlabs.com

49884
Par Pharmaceutical, Inc.
300 Tice Blvd., 3rd Floor
Woodcliff Lake, NJ 07677
201-802-4200
800-828-9393
www.parpharm.com

Parenta Pharmaceuticals, Inc.
One Southern Ct.
West Columbia, SC 89169
803-791-1171

00071
Parke-Davis
A Pfizer Company
235 East 42nd Street
New York, NY 10017
800-438-1985

Parkedale Pharmaceuticals
501 5th St.
Bristol, TN 37620
800-776-3637
800-336-7783

Parker Lab, Inc.
286 Eldridge Rd.
Fairfield, NJ 07004
973-276-9500

50930
Parnell Pharmaceuticals, Inc.
1525 Francisco Blvd., Suite 15
San Rafael, CA 94901
415-256-1800
800-457-4276
www.parnellpharm.com

10865
Parthenon Co., Inc.
3311 W. 2400 S.
Salt Lake City, UT 84119
801-972-5184
800-453-8898

00418
Pasadena Research Labs
See Taylor Pharmaceuticals

Pascal Co., Inc.
2929 N.E. Northrup Way
P.O. Box 1478
Bellevue, WA 98009-1478
425-827-4694

11793, 49281, 50361
**Pasteur-Mérieux-Connaught
Labs**
See Aventis

PathoGenesis Corp.
See Chiron Therapeutics

PD-RX Pharmaceuticals, Inc.
727 N. Ann Arbor Ave.
Oklahoma City, OK 73127
405-942-3040
800-299-7379
www.pdrx.com

Peachtree Pharm
See UCB

PediaMed Pharmaceuticals, Inc.
782 Springdale Dr.
Suite 120
Exton, PA 19341
484-875-9375

Pediatric Pharmaceuticals
120 Wood Ave. S., Suite 300
Iselin, NJ 08830
732-603-7708
www.pediatricpharm.com

00884
Pedinol Pharmacal, Inc.
30 Banfi Plaza N.
Farmingdale, NY 11735
631-293-9500
800-733-4665
www.pedinol.com

10974
Pegasus Laboratories, Inc.
8809 Ely Rd.
Pensacola, FL 32514
850-478-2770

Penederm, Inc.
See Bertek

Penetech Pharm
3315 Algonquin Rd., Suite 310
Rolling Meadows, IL 60008
847-255-0303

Pennex Pharmaceutical, Inc.
See Morton Grove
    Pharmaceuticals, Inc.

Pentech Pharmaceuticals, Inc
417 Harvester Ct.
Wheeling, IL 60090
847-459-9122

Permeable Technologies, Inc.
See LifeStyle

Perrigo Company
515 Eastern Ave.
Allegan, MI 49010
269-673-8451
800-719-9260
www.perrigo.com

00096
Person and Covey, Inc.
616 Allen Ave.
Glendale, CA 91201
818-240-1030
800-423-2341
www.personandcovey.com

Personal Care
225 Summit Ave.
Montvale, NJ 07645-1574
201-573-5633
800-816-5742

Personal Products Company
199 Grandview Rd.
Skillman, NJ 08558
908-218-8625
800-582-6097
www.jnj.com

00927
Pfeiffer Co.
71 Southwest
Atlanta, GA 30315
404-614-0255
800-342-6450

Pfipharmecs
See Pfizer US Pharmaceutical
    Group

Pfizer Consumer Health
235 E. 42nd St.
New York, NY 10017
212-573-5656
800-332-1240
www.pfizer.com

00069, 00663, 74300
Pfizer US Pharmaceutical Group
235 E. 42nd St.
New York, NY 10017
800-438-1985
www.pfizer.com

Pharma 21
503-494-8474

Pharma Medica
966 Pantera Drive, Unit 31
Mississauga, Ontario, Canada
    L4W2S1
877-742-7621

Pharma Pac
513 Sandydale Dr.
Nipomo, CA 93444
805-929-1333
800-841-5554
www.pharmapac.com

Pharma-Tek, Inc.
See X-Gen Pharmaceuticals

Pharmaderm
4126 Steve Reynolds Blvd.
Norcross, GA 30093
866-377-6457
678-287-1500

00121
Pharmaceutical Associates, Inc.
201 Delaware St.
Greenville, SC 29605
864-277-7282
800-845-8210

Pharmaceutical Basics, Inc.
See Rosemont Pharmaceutical Corp.

51655
**Pharmaceutical Corp of America
    (PCA)**
6210 Technology Center Dr.
Indianapolis, IN 46278
317-616-4498

21659
Pharmaceutical Labs, Inc.
6704 Ranger Ave.
Corpus Christi, TX 78415
361-854-0755
800-856-7040

45334
Pharmaceutical Specialties, Inc.
P.O. Box 6298
Rochester, MN 55903
507-288-8500
800-325-8232
www.psico.com

00013, 00016
Pharmacia Corp.
A Division of Pfizer
235 East 42nd Street
New York, NY 10017
800-323-4204
www.pnu.com

**Pharmacia & Upjohn Consumer
    Healthcare**
7000 Portage Rd.
Kalamazoo, MI 49001
269-833-9599
800-717-2824

Pharmadigm, Inc.
2401 Foothill Dr.
Salt Lake City, UT 84109
801-464-6100
www.pharmadigm.com

Pharmafair
See Bausch & Lomb
    Pharmaceuticals

55422
Pharmakon Laboratories, Inc.
6050 Jet Port Industrial Blvd.
Tampa, FL 33634
813-886-3216
800-888-4045
www.pharmakonlabs.com

Pharmanex
75 West Center
Provo, UT 84601
801-345-9800
800-487-1000
www.pharmanex.com

Pharmascience Lab
6111 Royal Mount Ave.
Montreal, Quebec H4 P2 T4
514-340-9735
800-340-9735
www.pharmscience.com

00813
Pharmavite
P.O. Box 9606
Mission Hills, CA 91346-9606
800-276-2878
www.naturemade.com

Pharmedix
25590 Seaboard Lane
Hayward, CA 94545
800-486-1811

Pharmelle
890 N. Lafayette St.
Florissant, MO 63031
314-830-4150

Pharmics, Inc.
2702 S. 3600 West, Suite H
Salt Lake City, UT 84119
801-966-4138
800-456-4138
www.pharmics.com

Pharmion Corporation
4865 Riverbend Rd.
Boulder, CO 80301
720-564-9100

PharmPak, Inc.
1221 Andersen Dr. Ste. B
San Rafael, CA 94901
415-455-9981
800-541-6315

Phillips Gulf Corporation
See Healthcare Direct Services

Phoenix Laboratories
140 Lauman Ln.
Hicksville, NY 11801
516-822-1230

Physicians Total Care
5415 S. 125th East Ave.
Suite 205
Tulsa, OK 74146
918-254-2273
800-759-3650
www.physicianstotalcare.com

PhytoPharmica, Inc.
825 Challenger Dr.
Green Bay, WI 54311
920-469-1313
www.phytopharmica.com

Playtex Co.
75 Commerce Dr.
Allendale, NJ 07401-1600
201-785-8000
800-816-5742
www.playtex.com

Pliva
72 Eagle Rock Ave.
P.O. Box 371
East Hanover, NJ 07936
973-386-5566
800-922-0547

Plough, Inc.
See Schering-Plough HealthCare
    Products

Poly Pharmaceuticals, Inc.
P.O. Box 93
Quitman, MS 39355
800-882-1041

00998
PolyMedica Corporation
11 State Street
Woburn, MA 01801
781-933-2020
www.polymedica.com

47144
Polymer Technology Corp.
100 Research Dr.
Wilmington, MA 01887
978-658-6111

Portal Pharmaceutical
67 East Mendez Vigo
Myaguez, PR 00680
787-832-6645

Porton Product Limited
See Speywood Pharmaceuticals, Inc.

Powderject Vaccines
585 Science Dr.
Madison, WI 53711
608-231-3150

**Praecis Pharmaceuticals
    Incorporated**
830 Winter Street
Waltham, MA 02451-1420
877-PRAECIS
877-772-3247

Prasco Laboratories
7155 E. Kemper Rd.
Cincinnati, OH 45249
513-469-1414

59012
Pratt Pharmaceuticals
See Pfizer

Premier
See Advanced Polymer Systems

Press Chem & Pharm Lab
P.O. Box 09103
Columbus, OH 43209
614-863-2802

Prestige Brands
26811 S. Bay Dr., Suite 300
Bonita Springs, FL 34134
239-948-8545

00684
Primedics Laboratories
14131 S. Avalon
Los Angeles, CA 90061
323-770-3005

Princeton Pharm. Products
See Bristol-Myers Squibb Co.

Priority Healthcare
250 Technology Park, Suite 124
Lake Mary, FL 32748
407-804-6700
866-474-8326

37000
Procter & Gamble Co.
8500 Governors Hill Dr.
Cincinnati, OH 45249
800-448-4878
www.pg.com

00149
Procter & Gamble Pharm.
11450 Grooms Rd.
Cincinnati, OH 45242
513-335-3321
800-448-4878
www.pg.com

ProCyte Corporation
P.O. Box 808
Redmond, WA 98073-0808
425-869-1239
800-848-3668
www.procyte.com

ProEthic Laboratories, LLC
5531 Perimeter Pkwy. Ct.
Mongomery, AL 36115
334-288-1288
866-776-3844

Prometheus Laboratories, Inc.
5739 Pacific Center Blvd.
San Diego, CA 92121
858-824-0895
888-423-5227

ProMetic Pharma USA, Inc.
5436 W. 78th St.
Indianapolis, IN 46368
317-334-5600

Propharma
7760 N.W. 56 St.
Miami, FL 33166
305-592-9216
800-446-0255

Propst Pharmaceuticals
130 Vintage Dr.
Huntsville, AL 35811
256-704-6394

Protein Design Labs, Inc.
34801 Campus Dr.
Fremont, CA 94555
510-574-1400
www.pdl.com

Protein Sciences Corp.
1000 Research Pkwy.
Meriden, CT 06450-7159
203-686-0800
800-488-7099
www.proteinsciences.com

Protherics Inc.
5214 Maryland Way
Suite 405
Brentwood, TN 37027
615-327-1027
www.protherics.com

PRX Pharm
1 Ram Ridge Road
Spring Valley, NY 10977
845-425-7100
800-423-1032

Psychemedics Corp.
1280 Massachusetts Ave.
Cambridge, MA 02138
617-868-7455
800-628-8073
www.psychemedics.com

PTS Labs
4342 West 12th St.
Houston, TX 77055
713-680-2291

Purdue Frederick Co.
One Stamford Forum
201 Tressor Blvd.
Stamford, CT 06091-3431
203-588-8000
800-877-5666
www.purduepharma.com

00228
Purepac Pharmaceutical Co.
See Faulding

Purilens, Inc.
See The LifeStyle Company, Inc.

Puritan's Pride
1233 Montauk Hwy.
P.O. Box 9001
Oakdale, NY 11769-9001
800-645-9584
www.puritanspride.com

Q-Pharma, Inc.
120 W. Dayton
Suite C-7
Edmonds, WA 98020
425-778-5404

QLT, Inc.
887 Great Northern Way
Vancouver, BC V5T 4T5
Canada
604-707-7000
800-663-5486
www.qlt-pdt.com

00603
Qualitest Pharmaceuticals
1236 Jordan Rd.
Huntsville, AL 35811
256-859-4011

Qualitest Prod.
130 Vintage Dr.
Huntsville, AL 35811
256-859-4011
800-444-4011

Quality Care Pharm, Inc.
3000 W. Warner Ave.
Santa Ana, CA 92704
714-754-5800

Quality Care Products, LLC
7560 Lewis Ave.
Temperance, MI 48182
734-847-3847

Questcor Pharmaceuticals, Inc.
3260 Whipple Rd.
Union City, CA 94587
510-400-0700
www.questcor.com

Quidel Corp.
10165 McKellar Ct.
San Diego, CA 92121
858-552-1100
800-874-1517
www.quidel.com

Quigley Corp.
470 Park Avenue S.
New York, NY 10016
212-725-4500
www.quigleyco.com

Quintessa Corporation
P.O. Box 808
Lancaster, CA 93584
661-940-5600

54391
R & D Laboratories, Inc.
3925 E. Watkins
Phoenix, AZ 85034
800-927-1034
www.mdlabs.com

R & R Registrations
P.O. Box 262069
San Diego, CA 92196
858-586-0751

R.A. McNeil Company
1210 East Dallas Rd.
Chattanooga, TN 37405
423-265-8240
800-755-3038

Ranbaxy Pharmaceuticals Inc.
600 College Rd. E.
Princeton, NJ 08540
609-720-9200
888-726-2299
www.ranbaxy.com

30103
Randob Laboratories, Ltd.
6 Walnut St.
P.O. Box 440
Cornwall, NY 12518
548-534-2197

Rare Disease Therapeutics
1101 Kermit Dr., Suite 608
Nashville, TN 37217
615-399-0700

Reckitt & Colman
See Reckitt Benckiser Pharm

10952
Reckitt Benckiser Pharm
10710 Midlothien Turnpike
Richmond, VA 23235
804-379-1090
800-444-7599

Recsei Laboratories
330 S. Kellogg
Building M
Goleta, CA 93117-3875
805-964-2912

48028
Redi-Products Labs, Inc.
See Aplicare, Inc.

00021
Reed & Carnrick
See Schwarz Pharma

10956
Reese Pharmaceutical Co., Inc.
10617 Frank Ave.
Cleveland, OH 44106-0157
216-231-6441
800-321-7178

Regeneron Pharmaceuticals
777 Old Saw Mill River Rd.
Tarrytown, NY 10591
914-347-7400
www.regeneron.com

Regent Laboratories
700 W. Hillsboro Blvd.
#2-206
Deerfield Beach, FL 33441
800-872-1525

Reid Rowell
See Solvay Pharmaceuticals

Reliant Pharmaceuticals
110 Allen Rd.
Liberty Corner, NJ 07938
908-580-1200
www.reliantrx.com

Remel, Inc.
12076 Santa Fe Dr.
Lenexa, KS 66215
913-888-0939
800-255-6730
www.remelinc.com

Repligen
41 Seyon Street, Building #1
Waltham, MA 02494
781-250-0111
781-250-0115

10961
Requa, Inc.
540 Barnum Building 2
Bridgeport, CT 06608
800-321-1085
www.requa.com

Research Industries Corp.
See Edwards Lifesciences

Research Triangle Institute
P.O. Box 133
Riverdale, NJ 07457
973-839-2518
www.rti.org

60575
Respa Pharmaceuticals, Inc.
P.O. Box 88222
Carol Stream, IL 60188
630-462-9986

Resperonics
1501 Ardmore Blvd.
Pittsburgh, PA 15211
412-731-2100

Rexall Group
6111 Broken Sound Pkwy. NW
Boca Raton, FL 33457
800-255-7399

00122
Rexall Sundown, Inc.
6111 Broken Sound Pkwy. NW
Boca Raton, FL 33487
561-241-9400
800-327-0908
www.rexallsundown.com

Rgene Therapeutics, Inc.
2170 Buckthorne Pl.
Suite 170
Houston, TX 77380
713-367-5443

RH Pharmaceuticals, Inc.
(Cangene Corp.)
104 Chancellor Matheson Rd.
Manitoba, Canada R3T 5Y3
204-989-6850

Rhone-Poulenc Rorer Consumer, Inc.
See Aventis Pharmaceuticals

00075, 00083
Rhone-Poulenc Rorer Pharmaceuticals, Inc.
See Aventis Pharmaceuticals

Ribi
See Corixa Corporation

Richardson-Vicks, Inc.
See Procter & Gamble Co.

12071
Richie Pharmacal, Inc.
119 State Ave.
P.O. Box 460
Glasgow, KY 42141
502-651-6159
800-627-0250
www.richiepharmacal.com

Richmond Pharm
3510 Mayland Court
Richmond, VA 23233
804-270-4498

Ricola USA, Inc.
51 Gibraltar Dr.
Morris Plains, NJ 07950
973-984-6811
www.ricolausa.com

54807
R.I.D., Inc.
609 N. Mednik Ave.
Los Angeles, CA 90022-1320
323-268-0635

R.I.J. Pharmaceutical Corp.
40 Commercial Ave.
Middletown, NY 10941
845-692-5799

Rising Pharm
411 Sette Drive, #N3
Paramus, NJ 07652
201-262-4200

Rite Aid Corp.
30 Hunter Ln.
Capitol Hill, PA 17011
717-761-2633
www.riteaid.com

54092
Roberts Pharmaceutical Corp.
(Shire U.S.)
7900 Tannersgate Dr.
Florence, KY 41042
800-828-2088

Roche Diagnostic Systems, Inc.
1080 U.S. Hwy. 202
Somerville, NJ 08876-3771
908-253-7200
800-428-5074
www.rocheusa.com

00004, 00033, 00140, 18393, 42987
Roche Laboratories
340 Kingsland St.
Nutley, NJ 07110-1199
973-235-5000
800-526-6367
www.rocheusa.com

Rodlen Laboratories
100 Fairway Drive, Suite 134
Vernon Hills, IL 60061
847-362-8200

00049
Roerig
See Pfizer

Romark Laboratories
6200 Courtney Campbell Causeway
Suite 880
Tampa, FL 33607
813-282-8544
www.romarklabs.com

00832
Rosemont Pharmaceutical Corp.
301 S. Cherokee St.
Denver, CO 80223
800-445-8091

00074
Ross Products Division, Abbott Labs
625 Cleveland
Columbus, OH 43215
800-986-8510
www.rosslabs.com

00054
Roxane Laboratories, Inc.
1809 Wilson Road
Columbus, OH 43216
800-848-0120
www.roxane.com

51875
Royce Laboratories, Inc.
(Watson Laboratories)
3530 NW 165th St.
Miami, FL 33014
305-624-1500
800-677-6923

RP
645 Martinsville Road, Suite 200
Basking Ridge, NJ 07920
908-580-1500

R.P. Scherer-North America
See Cardinal Health

00536
Rugby Labs, Inc.
2170 Satellite Blvd.
Suite 300
Duluth, GA 30097
678-584-5678

Russ Pharmaceuticals
See UCB Pharmaceuticals, Inc.

RX Elite
1404 N. Mait St., Suite 200
Meridian, ID 83642
208-288-5550

46500
Rydelle Laboratories
(S.C. Johnson)
1525 Howe St.
Racine, WI 53403-5011
414-631-2000
800-558-5252

Rystan, Inc.
47 Center Ave.
P.O. Box 214
Little Falls, NJ 07424-0214
973-256-3737

65649
Salix Pharmaceuticals, Inc.
3600 W. Bayshore Rd.
Palo Alto, CA 94303
650-849-5900

00043
Sandoz Consumer
506 Carnegie Center Dr., Suite 400
Princeton, NJ 08540
609-627-8500
800-525-8747
www.us.sandoz.com

00212
Sandoz Nutrition Corp.
506 Carnegie Center Dr., Suite 400
Princeton, NJ 08540
609-627-8500
800-525-8747
www.us.sandoz.com

00078
Sandoz Pharmaceuticals
506 Carnegie Center Dr., Suite 400
Princeton, NJ 08540
609-627-8500
800-525-8747
www.us.sandoz.com

SangStat Medical Corp.
6300 Dumbarton Circle
Fremont, CA 94555
510-789-4300
www.sangstat.com

Sankyo Pharma
2 Hilton Ct.
Parsippany, NJ 07054-1296
973-359-2600
www.sankyopharma.com

00024
Sanofi-Synthelabo, Inc.
90 Park Ave.
New York, NY 10016
212-551-4000
800-223-1062
www.sanofi-synthelabous.com

Santen, Inc.
555 Gateway Rd.
Napa, CA 94558
707-254-1750
800-611-2011

00281
Savage Laboratories
60 Baylis Rd.
Melville, NY 11747-2006
631-454-9071
800-231-0206
www.savagelabs.com

Savient Pharmaceuticals, Inc.
70 Wood Avenue
South Iselin, NJ 08830
723-632-8800

S C Johnson
1525 Howe Street
Racine, WI 53403-5011
800-494-4855

Scandinavian Natural Health & Beauty Products
13 N. 7th St.
Perkasie, PA 18944
215-453-2505
800-288-2844
www.scandinaviannaturals.com

11012
Schaffer Laboratories
3128 Pacific Coast Hwy #98
Torrance, CA 90505
800-231-ORAL
www.schafferlabs.com

00364, 00591
Schein Pharmaceutical, Inc.
See Watson

00274, 00032
Scherer Laboratories, Inc.
2301 Ohio Dr.
Suite 234
Plano, TX 75093
800-310-5357

00085, 11017, 41100, 54092
Schering-Plough Corp.
2000 Galloping Hill Rd.
Kenilworth, NJ 07033-0530
908-298-4000
www.sch-plough.com

00085, 11017, 41000, 41100
Schering-Plough HealthCare Products
110 Allen Rd.
Liberty Corner, NJ 07938
908-604-1746
800-842-4090
www.schering-plough.com

00234
Schmid Products Co.
See Durex Consumer Products

Scholl, Inc.
See Schering-Plough HealthCare Products

00021, 00091, 00131, 62175
Schwarz Pharma
P.O. Box 2038
Milwaukee, WI 53201
800-558-5114
www.schwarzusa.com

Schwarzkopf & Dep Inc.
2101 E. Via Arado
Rancho Dominguez, CA 90220
310-604-0777
800-326-2855

SciClone Pharmaceuticals, Inc.
901 Mariner's Island Blvd.
Suite 205
San Mateo, CA 94404
650-358-3456
www.sciclone.com

Scios Nova
820 W. Maude Ave.
Sunnyvale, CA 94085
408-616-8200
www.sciosinc.com

00372
Scot-Tussin Pharmacal, Inc.
50 Clemence St.
P.O. Box 8217
Cranston, RI 02920-0217
401-942-8555
800-638-7268
www.scot-tussin.com

SDA Laboratories
280 Railroad Ave.
Greenwich, CT 06830
203-861-0005

SDR Pharmaceuticals, Inc.
Andover, NJ 07821
973-786-7996

00014, 00025
Searle
See Pharmacia Corp.

00551
Seatrace Pharmaceuticals
P.O. Box 7200
Gadsden, AL 35906
256-442-5023

Sepracor
84 Waterford Drive
Marlboro, MA 01752
508-481-6700
800-245-5961
www.sepracor.com

Septodont, Inc.
245 C Quinley Blvd.
New Castle, DE 19720
302-328-1102
800-872-8305
www.septodontinc.com

61471
Sequus Pharmaceuticals, Inc.
960 Hamilton Ct.
Menlo Park, CA 94025
650-323-9011
800-323-9051

50694
Seres Laboratories
3331B Industrial Dr.
Santa Rosa, CA 95403
707-526-4526
www.sereslabs.com

44087
Serono Laboratories, Inc.
One Technology Place
Rockland, MA 02370
800-283-8088
www.seronousa.com

Seyer Pharmatec, Inc.
413 St. George St.
San Juan, PR 00936
787-728-7044
787-728-7055

Shaklee Corp.
4747 Willow Rd.
Pleasanton, CA 94588
925-924-2000
www.shaklee.com

Sheffield Laboratories
170 Broad St.
New London, CT 06320
860-442-4451
800-222-1087

08884
Sherwood Davis & Geck
See Kendall Health Care Products

08884
Sherwood Medical
See Kendall Health Care Products

Shield Manufacturing, Inc.
425 Fillmore Ave.
Tonawanda, NY 14150
800-828-7669
www.shieldsports.com

Shinogi Qualicaps, Inc.
6505 Frunz Warner Parkway
Whitsett, NC 27377-9215
336-449-3900

58521
Shire US, Inc.
One Riverfront Place
Newport, KY 41071
859-669-8000
www.shiregroup.com

SHS North America
9900 Belward Campus Dr.
Suite 100, P.O. Box 117
Rockville, MD 20850
301-795-2300
800-636-2283
www.SHSNA.com

50111
Sidmak Laboratories, Inc.
See Pliva

54482
Sigma-Tau Pharmaceuticals
800 S. Frederick Ave.
Suite 300
Gaithersburg, MD 20877-4150
301-948-1041
800-447-0169
www.sigmatau.com

54838
Silarx Pharmaceuticals, Inc.
19 West St.
Spring Valley, NY 10977
845-352-4020
888-9SILARX

Similisan
108 N. Ridge St.
P.O. Box 7429
Breckenridge, CO 80424
970-547-5060
800-240-9780

Sirius Laboratories, Inc.
100 Fairway Dr.
Suite 130
Vernon Hills, IL 60061
847-968-2424

SkinMedica, Inc.
5909 Sea Lion Place, Ste. H
Carlsbad, CA 92008
760-448-3600
866-867-0110
www.skinmedica.com

SkyePharma Inc.
10 East 63rd Street
New York, NY 10021
212-753-5780
www.skyepharma.com

Slim Fast Foods Co.
777 S. Flagler Dr.
West Tower
Suite 1400
P.O. Box 3625
West Palm Beach, FL 33401
561-833-9920

Smith & Nephew Ortho
1450 Brooks Rd.
Memphis, TN 38116
800-821-5700
www.smithnephew.com

Smith & Nephew United
See Smith & Nephew Ortho

08026
Smith & Nephew Wound Management
P.O. Box 81
101 Hessle Rd.
Hull
HU32BN UK
www.smithnephew.com

00766
SmithKline Beecham Consumer Healthcare
1500 Littleton Rd.
Parsippany, NJ 07084
973-889-2100
www.sb.com

00978
SmithKline Diagnostics
4300 N. Harbor Blvd.
Fullerton, CA 92834
800-877-6242

Snuva, Inc.
715 South Boulevard
Oak Park, IL 60302
708-725-3783
800-250-4258
www.snuva.com

33984
Solgar Co., Inc.
500 Willow Tree Rd.
Leonia, NJ 07605
201-944-2311
800-645-2246
www.solgar.com

00032
Solvay Pharmaceuticals
901 Sawyer Rd.
Marietta, GA 30062-2224
770-578-9000
800-241-1643
www.solvaypharmaceuticals.com

39506
Somerset Pharmaceuticals
2202 N.W. Shore Blvd.
Suite 450
Tampa, FL 33602
813-288-0040
800-892-8889
www.somersetpharm.com

Southwest Technologies
1746 Levee Road
North Kansas City, MO 64116
816-221-2442
800-247-9951
www.swtechinc.com

Southwood Pharmaceuticals
60 Empire Drive
Lake Forest, CA 92630
800-442-4443
www.southwoodpharm.com

Sovereign Pharmaceuticals
7590 Sand St.
Ft. Worth, TX 76118
817-284-0429

Sparta Pharmaceuticals
111 Rock Rd.
Horsham, PA 19044-2310
215-442-1700

Spear Dermatology Products
1247 Sussex Turnpike, Suite 120
Randolph, NJ 07869
973-895-6447
866-507-7327

Specialty Medical Supplies
10191 W. Sample Rd., Ste. 104
Coral Spring, FL 33065
954-752-5603

38137
Spectrum Chemical Mfg. Corp.
14422 S. San Pedro St.
Gardena, CA 90248-9985
310-516-8000
800-772-8786
www.spectrumchemical.com

Spenco Medical Corporation
P.O. Box 2501
Waco, TX 76702
520-325-1554
800-877-3626
www.spenco.com

55688
Speywood Pharmaceuticals, Inc.
30401 Agoura Rd.
Suite 102
Agoura Hills, CA 91301
818-879-2200

S.S.S. Company
71 University Avenue S.W.
P.O. Box 4447
Atlanta, GA 30315
404-521-0857
800-237-3843

St. Jude Medical, Inc.
1 Lillehei Plaza
St. Paul, MN 55117-1761
612-483-2000

Stada Pharmaceuticals, Inc.
5 Cedar Brook Dr.
Cranbury, NJ 08512
609-409-5999
800-542-6682
www.stadausa.com

Stanback Co.
(GlaxoSmithKline)
200 North 16th St.
Philadelphia, PA 19101
704-633-9231
800-338-5428
www.gsk.com

53385
Standard Drug Co.
1279 N. 7th St.
Riverton, IL 62561
217-629-9884

Standard Homeopathic Co.
210 W. 131st St.
P.O. Box 61067
Los Angeles, CA 90061
310-768-0700
800-624-9659

00076
Star Pharmaceuticals, Inc.
1990 N.W. 44th St.
Pompano Beach, FL 33064-8712
954-971-9704
800-845-7827
www.starpharm.com

51318
Stellar Pharmacal Corp.
See Star Pharmaceuticals, Inc.

Stephan Company
1850 W. McNab Rd.
Ft. Lauderdale, FL 33309
954-971-0600
800-327-4963

00402
Steris Laboratories, Inc.
See Watson Laboratories

Sterling Health
15070 Beltwood Pkwy.
Dallas, TX 75001-3715
972-991-9293

Sterling Winthrop
See Sanofi-Synthelabo

Stewart-Jackson Pharmacal
4587 Demaskis Rd.
Memphis, TN 38118
800-367-1395

Stiefel Consumer Healthcare
Route 145
Oak Hill, NY 12460
518-239-4195
888-438-7426

00145
Stiefel Laboratories, Inc.
6340 Sugarloaf Parkway, Suite 400
Duluth, GA 30097
800-633-7647
888-784-3335
www.stiefel.com

57706
Storz
See Bausch & Lomb Surgical

58980
Stratus Pharmaceuticals, Inc.
14377 S.W. 142nd St.
P.O. Box 4632
Miami, FL 33186-6727
305-254-6793
800-442-7882
www.stratuspharmaceuticals.com

Stuart Pharmaceuticals
See AstraZeneca L.P.

Sugen Inc.
(Informagen, Inc.)
375 Little Bay Rd.
Newington, NH 03801
www.informagen.com

Summa Rx Laboratories
2940 FM 3028
Mineral Wells, TX 76067
940-325-0771
800-537-7319

11086
Summers Laboratories, Inc.
103 G.P. Clement Dr.
Collegeville, PA 19426-2044
610-454-1471
800-533-7546
www.sumlab.com

Summit Industries, Inc.
2901 W. Lawrence Ave.
Chicago, IL 60625
773-588-2444
800-729-9729
www.summitindustries.net

57267
Summit Pharmaceuticals
See Novartis Pharmaceuticals Corp.

Sunrise Medical HHG, Inc.
240 Motor Parkway
Hauppauge, NY 11788
613-435-1515
800-782-0282

SuperGen, Inc.
4140 Dublin Blvd.
Suite 200
Dublin, CA 94568
925-560-0100
800-353-1075
www.supergen.com

Superior Pharmaceutical Co.
1385 Kemper Meadow Dr.
Cincinnati, OH 45240
800-826-5035
www.superiorpharm.com

11704
Survival Technical, Inc.
See Meridian Medical Technologies

Swiss-American Products, Inc.
4641 Nall Rd.
Dallas, TX 75244
972-385-2900
800-633-8872

Swiss Bioceutical
2533 N. Carson St., Ste. 3573
Carson City, NV 89706
775-841-7020

Syncom Pharmaceuticals, Inc.
66 Hanover Rd.
Florham Park, NJ 07932
973-822-9222
800-400-0056

Synergen, Inc.
See Amgen Inc.

00033, 18393, 42987
Syntex Laboratories
See Roche Laboratories

Synthon Pharmaceuticals, Ltd.
6330 Quadrangle Drive
Suite 305
Chapel Hill, NC 27517
800-576-4459

Syva Co.
1717 Deerfield Rd.
Deerfield, IL 60015
847-267-5300
800-227-9948

**Takeda Chemical Industries,
Ltd.**
1-1 Doshomachi 4-Chome Chuo-Ku
Osaka, Japan

**Takeda Pharmaceuticals
America, Inc.**
475 Half Day Rd., Suite 500
Lincolnshire, IL 60069
847-383-3000

Tambrands, Inc.
777 Westchester Avenue
White Plains, NY
914-696-6000

Tanning Research Labs, Inc.
1190 U.S. 1 N.
Ormond Beach, FL 32174
386-677-9559
800-874-4844
www.htropic.com

Tanox Inc.
10301 Stella Link
Houston, TX 77025-5497
713-664-2288
www.tanox.com

00300
TAP Pharmaceuticals
2355 Waukegan Rd.
Deerfield, IL 60015
800-621-1020

Targeted Genetics Corp.
1100 Olive Way, Ste. 100
Seattle, WA 98101
206-623-7612
www.targen.com

51672
Taro Pharmaceuticals USA, Inc.
5 Skyline Dr.
Hawthorne, NY 10532-9998
914-345-9001
800-544-1449
www.taropharma.com

Taylor Pharmacal
(Akorn)
2500 Millbrook Dr.
Buffalo Grove, IL 60089
847-279-6100
800-932-5676

00418
Taylor Pharmaceuticals
(Akorn)
2500 Millbrook Dr.
Buffalo Grove, IL 60089
847-279-6100
800-223-9851

TEAMM Pharmaceuticals, Inc.
3000 Aerial Center Parkway
Suite 110
Morrisville, NC 27560
919-481-9020
866-481-9020
www.teammpharma.com

83926
Tec Laboratories, Inc.
615 Water Ave. S.E.
P.O. Box 1958
Albany, OR 97321-0512
541-926-4577
800-482-4464
www.teclabsinc.com

Teikoku Seiyaku Co. Ltd.
567 Sanbonmatsu Ochi Cho
Kagawa Ohkawa Gun, Japan
7692695

Telluride Pharm. Corp.
300 Valley Road
Hillsborough, NJ 08844-4656
908-369-1800
908-369-1331
www.tellpharm.com

Tel-Test, Inc.
P.O. Box 1421
Friendswood, TX 77546
281-482-2762
800-631-0600
www.tel-test.com

Terumo Medical Corporation
2101 Cottontail Lane
Somerset, NJ 08873
732-302-4900
800-283-7866
www.terumomedical.com

TestPak, Inc.
125 Algonquin Parkway
Whippany, NJ 07981
973-887-4440
973-887-9098

Teva Marion Partners
10236 Marion Park Dr.
P.O. Box 9627
Kansas City, MO 64134
816-966-5000
800-362-7466

00093, 00332
Teva Pharmaceuticals USA
1090 Horsham Rd.
P.O. Box 1090
North Wales, PA 19454-1090
215-591-3000
800-545-8800
www.tevausa.com

Textilease Medique Products Co.
900 Lively Blvd.
Wood Dale, IL 60191
630-694-4100
800-634-7680
www.textileasemedique.com

49158
Thames Pharmacal, Inc.
2100 Fifth Ave.
Ronkonkoma, NY 11779-6933
516-737-1155
800-225-1003

Ther-Rx Corporation
13622 Lakefront Dr.
Earth City, MO 63045
314-209-1517
877-567-7676

Therakos, Inc.
437 Creameway
Exton, PA 19341
610-280-1000

Therapeutic Antibodies, Inc.
(Protherics)
5214 Maryland Way
Suite 405
Brentwood, TN 37027
615-327-1027

Therasense
1370 S. Loop Rd.
Alameda, CA 94502
510-749-5400
www.therasense.com

11290
Thompson Medical Co., Inc.
See Chattem Consumer Products

T/I Pharmaceuticals, Inc.
See Fischer Pharmaceuticals, Inc.

49483
Time-Cap Labs, Inc.
7 Michael Avenue
Farmingdale, NY 11735
631-753-9090

Tishcon Corp.
30 New York Ave.
Westbury, NY 11590
516-333-3050
800-848-8442
www.tishcon.com

Tom's of Maine, Inc.
P.O. Box 710
Kennebunk, ME 04043
207-985-2944
800-775-2388
www.tomsofmaine.com

Topco Assoc. Inc.
7711 Gross Point Rd.
Skokie, IL 60077
847-676-3030

Topix Pharmaceuticals
5200 New Horizons Blvd.
North Amityville, NY 11701-1144
800-445-2595

Transdermal Technologies, Inc.
1368 North Killian Drive
Lake Park, FL 33403
561-848-2345

Trask Industries, Inc.
163 Farrell Street
Somerset, NJ 08873
800-579-3131

Tri-Med Laboratories
68 Veronica Ave.
Somerset, NJ 08873
732-249-6363

Tri Tec Laboratories
1000 Robins Rd.
Lynchburg, VA 24504-3558
804-845-7073

Triage Pharmaceuticals
See Health for Life Brands, Inc.

Trigen Laboratories, Inc.
207 Kiley Drive
Salisbury, MD 21802
410-860-8500

Trimen, Inc.
P.O. Box 309
New Oxford, PA 17350
717-624-4770
800-233-7120

Trinity Technologies
572 Washington Street
Wellesley, MA 02482-6418
781-235-2223

79511
Triton Consumer Products, Inc.
561 W. Golf Rd.
Arlington Heights, IL 60005-3904
847-228-7650
800-942-2009
www.mg217.com

Truxton
136 Harding Avenue
P.O. Box 1081
Bellmawr, NJ 08099
856-933-2333

Tweezerman
55 Sea Cliff Ave.
Glen Cove, NY 11542-3695
516-676-7772
800-645-3340

Twinlab Corp.
150 Motor Pkwy.
Hauppauge, NY 11788
631-467-3140
800-645-5626
www.twinlab.com

Tyler, Inc.
(Integrated Therapies Inc.)
2204 North Birdsdale
Gresham, OR 97030
503-661-5401
800-869-9705

53335
Tyson Nutraceuticals
12832 S. Chadron Ave.
Hawthorne, CA 90250-5525
310-675-1080
800-799-3233
www.tysonnutraceuticals.com

UAD Laboratories, Inc.
See Forest Pharmaceutical, Inc.

UCB Pharmaceuticals, Inc.
1950 Lake Park Dr.
Smyrna, GA 30080
770-803-2177
800-477-7877
www.ucb.be

51079
UDL Laboratories, Inc.
1718 Northrock Ct.
Rockford, IL 61103
815-282-1201
800-435-5272
www.udllabs.com

00127
Ulmer Pharmacal Co.
1614 Industry Ave.
P.O. Box 408
Park Rapids, MN 56470
218-732-2656
800-848-5637

Ultimed
287 East Sixth St.
St. Paul, MN 55101
651-291-7909

Unico Holdings, Inc.
1830 2nd Ave. N.
Lake Worth, FL 33461
800-367-4477

Unigen Pharmaceuticals, Inc.
1221 Tech Court
Westminster, MD 21157
410-751-2108

Unilever Home and Personal Care USA
33 Benedict Place
Greenwich, CT 06836
203-661-2000
800-243-5320
www.unileverusa.com

41785
Unimed Pharmaceuticals
4 Parkway North
Deerfield, IL 60015
847-282-5400
800-742-7366
www.unimed.com

Unipath Diagnostics Co.
47 Hulfish St.
Suite 400
Princeton, NJ 08542
609-430-2727
800-321-3279
www.unipath.com

00327
United Guardian Laboratories
P.O. Box 18050
Hauppauge, PA 19124
631-273-0900
800-645-5566

00677
United Research Laboratories (URL)
See Mutual Pharmaceutical Company

Unither Pharma
(United Therapeutics Corp.)
1110 Spring St.
Silver Spring, MD 20910
301-608-9292
888-808-6838
www.unitherpharma.com

Univax Biologics
See Nabi

00009
Upjohn Co.
See Pharmacia Corp.

00245
Upsher-Smith Labs, Inc.
14905 23rd Ave. N.
Minneapolis, MN 55447-4709
612-473-4412
800-328-3344
www.upsher-smith.com

URL
See Mutual Pharmaceutical Company

Urocare Products, Inc.
2735 Melbourne Avenue
Pomona, CA 91767-1931
909-621-6013
800-423-4441
www.urocare.com

UroCor, Inc.
405 Research Parkway
Oklahoma City, OK 73104
405-290-4000
800-634-9330
www.dianon.com

Urologix
14405 21st Ave. N.
Minneapolis, MN 55447
763-475-1400
800-475-1403
www.urologix.com

Urometrics, Inc.
2022 Ferry Street
Suite 3125
Anoka, MN 55303
763-323-1968
877-774-1442
www.urometrics.com

58178
US Bioscience
100 Front St.
Suite 400
West Conshohocken, PA 19428
215-832-4553
800-447-3969
www.usbio.com

US DenTek Corp.
307 Excellence Way
Maryville, TN 37801
865-983-1300
800-433-6835

US Dermatologics
133 Franklin Corner Rd.
Lawrenceville, NJ 08648
609-219-1166
877-873-3762
www.usderm.com

U.S. Neutraceuticals, LLC
2751 Nutra Lane
Eustis, FL 32726
352-357-2004
877-729-7256
www.usnutra.com

52747
US Pharmaceutical Corp.
2401-C Mellon Ct.
Decatur, GA 30035
770-987-4745

US Surgical Corp.
150 Glover Ave.
Norwalk, CT 06856
203-845-1000
800-722-8772
www.ussurg.com

USA Nutritionals
513 Commack Rd.
Deerpark, NY 11729
631-643-0600
800-722-7570
www.USANutritionals.com

ValMed, Inc.
221 Spring Street
Shewsbury, MA 01545
508-393-1599

Value in Pharmaceuticals
3000 Alt Blvd.
Grand Island, NY 14072
716-773-4600
800-724-3784
www.vippharm.com

Van Den Bergh Foods Company
(Unilever Home and Personal Care USA)
75 Merritt Blvd.
Trumbull, CT 06611
203-381-3500

Vangard Labs, Inc.
P.O. Box 1268
Glasgow, KY 42142-1268
800-825-4123

Ventlab Corporation
2934 Highway 601 North
Mocksville, NC 27028
336-492-2636
www.ventlab.com

VersaPharm Inc.
1775 W. Oak Pkwy.
Suite 800
Marietta, GA 30062-2260
770-499-8100
800-548-0700
www.versapharm.com

Vertex Pharmaceuticals, Inc.
130 Waverly St.
Cambridge, MA 02139-4211
617-576-3111
www.vpharm.com

Verum Pharmaceuticals
1000 Park Forty Plaza
Suite 300
Research Triangle Park, NC 27713
866-358-3786

Vetco Inc.
105 Baylis Rd.
Melville, NY 11747
631-755-1155
800-754-8853

53258
VHA Inc.
220 E. Las Colinas Blvd.
Irving, TX 75039
972-830-0000
800-842-7587

23900
Vicks Health Care Products
See Procter & Gamble Co.

25866
Vicks Pharmacy Products
See Procter & Gamble Co.

Viratek
See AstraZeneca L.P.

Virco Pharmaceuticals Inc.
P.O. Box 11117
Blacksburg, VA 24062
540-552-1968
888-968-4726

54891
Vision Pharmaceuticals, Inc.
P.O. Box 400
Mitchell, SD 57301-0400
605-996-3356
800-325-6789
www.visionpharm.com

VistaPharm
224 Cahaba Valley Dr.
Suite B-3
Birmingham, AL 35242
205-981-1387
www.vistapharm.com

Vita-Rx Corp
P.O. Box 8229
Columbus, GA 31908
706-568-1881

Vital Care Group
8935 NW 27 St.
Miami, FL 33172
305-620-4007

54022
Vitaline Corp.
(Integrated Therapeutics, Inc.)
9725 Southwest Commerce Cir.
Suite A9
Wilsonville, OR 97070
541-482-9231
800-648-4755
www.vitaline.com

Vitality Inc.
8935 NW 27 St.
Miami, FL 33172
305-620-4007

Vital Signs Inc.
20 Campus Road
Totowa, NJ 07512
800-932-0760

Vitamin Research Product, Inc.
3579 Hwy. 50 E.
Carson City, NV 89701
775-884-1300
800-877-2447
www.vrp.com

Vitamin Science Inc.
914 Westwood Blvd.
Los Angeles, CA 90024
310-443-9952
800-480-VITE

Vivus Inc.
1172 Castro Street
Mountainview, CA 94043
650-934-5200
888-345-6873
www.vivus.com

59310
Wakefield Pharmaceuticals, Inc.
310 Maxwell Rd.
Suite 100
Alpharetta, GA 30004
404-664-1661

Wal-Med, Inc.
11302 164th Street East
Puyallup, WA 98374
877-542-3688

00037
Wallace Laboratories
(Carter Wallace)
Half Acre Rd.
Cranbury, NJ 08512-0181
609-655-6000
800-526-3840
www.wallacelabs.com

Wallace Pharmaceuticals
265 Davidson Avenue
Suite 300
Somerset, NJ 08873-4120
732-564-2200
www.wallacepharmaceuticals.com

00017
Wampole Laboratories
Half Acre Rd.
P.O. Box 1001
Cranbury, NJ 08512
609-655-6000
800-257-9525
www.wampolelabs.com

00047, 00430
Warner Chilcott Laboratories
100 Enterprise Dr.
Suite 280
Rockaway, NJ 07866
800-521-8813
800-424-5202
www.wclabs.com

11370, 12546, 12547, 00071, 00501
Warner Lambert
182 Tabor Rd.
Morris Plains, NJ 07950
973-385-2000
800-524-2624
www.pfizer.com

Warner Lambert Consumer
Healthcare
(Pfizer Pharmaceuticals)
182 Tabor Rd.
Morris Plains, NJ 07950
973-385-2000
800-524-2624
www.pfizer.com

59930
Warrick Pharmaceutical, Corp.
(Schering Plough Corp.)
12125 Moya Blvd.
Reno, NV 89506
800-547-3869

Watson Laboratories
1033 Stoneleigh Avenue
Carmel, NY 10512
914-767-2000
800-553-4044
www.watsonpharm.com

00047, 52544, 51875, 55515
Watson Pharmaceuticals
311 Bonnie Circle Dr.
Corona, CA 92880
909-493-5300
800-272-5525
www.watsonpharm.com

W. E. Bassett
100 Trap Falls Road
Shelton, CT 06484-4647
203-929-8483

59196
WE Pharmaceuticals, Inc.
P.O. Box 1142
Ramona, CA 92065
619-788-9155
800-262-9555
www.weez.com

Weider Nutrition International,
Inc.
2002 S. 5070 W.
Salt Lake City, UT 84104
801-975-5000
800-453-9542
www.weider.com

Weleda
175 North Rt. 9W
P.O. Box 249
Congers, NY 10920
845-268-8572

Wellspring Pharmaceutical
1430 Route 34
Neptune, NJ 07753
732-938-5885

Wendt Laboratories
P.O. Box 1142
Belle Plaine, MN 56011
800-328-5890

00917
Wesley Pharmacal, Inc.
114 Railroad Dr.
Ivyland, PA 18974
215-953-1680

59591
West Point Pharma
See Endo Laboratories, Inc.

Western Research Laboratories
21602 N. 21st Ave.
Phoenix, AZ 85027
623-879-8537
877-797-7997

00003, 00072
West-Ward Pharmaceutical
Corp.
465 Industrial Way W.
Eatontown, NJ 07724
732-542-1191
800-631-2174

Westwood Squibb
Pharmaceuticals
(Bristol-Myers Squibb)
100 Forest Ave.
Buffalo, NY 14213
716-887-7667
800-333-0950
www.westwoodsquibb.com

W. F. Young
302 Benton Drive
East Longmeadow, MA 06484-4674
413-526-9999

11444
W.F. Young, Inc.
111 Lyman St.
P.O. Box 14
Springfield, MA 01102
413-737-0201
800-628-9653
www.absorbine.com

50474
Whitby Pharmaceuticals, Inc.
See UCB Pharmaceuticals, Inc.

00031, 00573
Whitehall-Robins Healthcare
See Wyeth Consumers Health

White Labs, Inc.
7564 Trade Street
San Diego, CA 92121
858-693-3441
www.whitelabs.com

Willen Pharmaceuticals
See Baker Norton
    Pharmaceuticals

William Labs
P.O. Box 101
Oradell, NJ 07649
973-772-4004

Wintec
4280 Technology Drive
Fremont, CA 94538
510-360-6300
www.wintecind.com

Winthrop Consumer
See Bayer Consumer Care Division

Winthrop Pharmaceuticals
See Sanofi-Synthelabo

12120
Wisconsin Pharmacal Co.
(WPC Brands)
1 Repel Rd.
Jackson, WI 53037
262-677-4121
800-558-6614
www.wispharm.com

Wm. Wrigley Jr. Co.
410 N. Michigan Ave.
Chicago, IL 60611
312-644-2121
866-787-7277

Women First Healthcare Inc.
12220 El Camino Real
Suite 400
San Diego, CA 92130
858-509-1171
www.womenfirst.com

Women's Capital Corp.
1990 M St. NW
Suite 250
Washington, DC 20036
800-330-1271
www.go2planb.com

Woodside Biomedical Inc.
1915 Aston Ave., Suite 102
Carlsbad, CA 92008
760-804-6900
888-297-9728
www.woodsidebiomedical.com

Woodward Laboratories, Inc.
11132 Winners Circle
Suite 100
Los Alamitos, CA 90720
562-598-0800
www.woodwardlabs.com

Wraser Pharmaceuticals
P.O. Box 3262
Ridgeland, MS 39158
601-605-0664
www.wraser.com

Wyeth-Ayerst Laboratories
P.O. Box 8299
Philadelphia, PA 19101
610-688-4400
800-995-4603
www.wyeth.com

Wyeth Consumer Health
5 Giralda Farms
Madison, NJ 07940
973-660-5500
800-322-3129

00008, 00031
Wyeth Pharmaceuticals
555 East Lancaster Ave.
St. David's, PA 19087
610-902-1200
800-995-4603
www.wyeth.com

X-Gen Pharmaceuticals
P.O. Box 1920
Huntington, NY 11743
516-757-5522
866-390-4411
www.pharma-tek.com

50962
Xactdose, Inc.
See Alpharma USPD, Inc.

Xanodyne Pharmacal, Inc.
7300 Turfway Road
Suite 300
Florence, KY 41042
877-926-6396

Xcel Pharmaceuticals
6363 Greenwich Drive
Suite 100
San Diego, CA 92122
858-202-2700
877-361-2719
www.xcelpharmaceuticals.com

Xoma
2910 Seventh St.
Berkeley, CA 94710
510-644-1170
800-544-9662
www.xoma.com

00116
Xttrium Laboratories, Inc.
415 W. Pershing Rd.
Chicago, IL 60609
773-268-5800
800-587-3721
www.xttrium.com

York Pharmaceuticals, Inc.
1201 Douglas Avenue
Kansas City, KS 66103
913-321-1070

64855
Young Again Products
3608-B Oleander Dr. #310
Wilmington, NC 28403
910-392-6775

60077, 00273
Young Dental Mfg.
13705 Shoreline Ct. E.
Earth City, MO 63045
314-344-0010
800-325-1881
www.youngdental.com

Zee Medical, Inc.
22 Corporate Park
Irvine, CA 92606

00310, 00163, 00187
Zeneca Pharmaceuticals
See AstraZeneca L.P.

00172, 00182
**Zenith Goldline
  Pharmaceuticals**
See Ivax Pharmaceutical

Zenith Laboratories
140 LeGrand Ave.
Northvale, NJ 07647-2403

51284
Zila Pharmaceuticals, Inc.
5227 N. 7th St.
Phoenix, AZ 85014
602-266-6700
800-922-7887
www.zila.com

ZLB Bioplasma
801 North Brand Blvd.
Suite 1150
Glendale, CA 91203
866-244-2952
www.zlbusa.com

Zoetica Pharmaceutical Group
214 Carnegie Center
Suite 106
Princeton, NJ 08540

Zonagen, Inc.
2408 Timberloch Pl., B-4
The Woodlands, TX 77380
281-367-5892
www.zonagen.com

Zyber Pharmaceuticals, Inc.
P.O. Box 40
Gonzales, LA 70707
225-647-3002
800-793-2145

ZymeTx, Inc.
800 Research Parkway
Suite 100
Oklahoma City, OK 73104
405-271-1314
888-817-1314
ww.zymetx.com

Zymogenetics, Inc.
1201 Eastlake Ave. E.
Seattle, WA 98102
206-442-6600

This **Index** lists all generic names (in bold face), brand names, and group names included in Drug Facts and Comparisons®. Additionally, many synonyms, pharmacological actions, and therapeutic uses for the agents listed are included.

Entries with a prefix preceding the number are found in the ancillary chapters. A prefix of KU indicates the Keeping Up section, a prefix of A indicates placement in the Appendix section.

INDEX

INDEX

INDEX

INDEX

INDEX

This index contains a comprehensive listing of drug trade names unique to Canada. The generic equivalent follows the Canadian trade name in bold. Accessing a *Drug Facts and Comparisons®* (*DFC*) monograph using a Canadian trade name will be a two step process. Use the Canadian Drug List to determine the generic, then use the Index to find the page number of the *DFC* drug monograph.

Apo-Ticlopidine (Apotex), see **Ticlopidine HCl**

Apo-Timol (Apotex), see **Timolol Maleate**

Apo-Timop (Apotex), see **Timolol Maleate**

Apo-Tobramycin (Apotex), see **Tobramycin**

Apo-Tolbutamide (Apotex), see **Tolbutamide**

Apo-Trazodone (Apotex), see **Trazodone HCl**

Apo-Trazodone D (Apotex), see **Trazodone HCl**

Apo-Triazide (Apotex), see **Hydrochlorothiazide/ Triamterene, Diuretic Combinations**

Apo-Triazo (Apotex), see **Triazolam**

Apo-Trifluoperazine (Apotex), see **Trifluoperazine HCl**

Apo-Trihex (Apotex), see **Trihexyphenidyl HCl**

Apo-Trimethoprim (Apotex), see **Triomethoprim**

Apo-Trimip (Apotex), see **Trimipramine Maleate**

Apo-Valproic (Apotex), see **Valproic Acid**

Apo-Verap (Apotex), see **Verapamil HCl**

Apo-Warfarin (Apotex), see **Warfarin Sodium**

Aquatain (Whitehall-Robins), see **Emollients**

Aralen (Sanofi-Synthalbo), see **Chloroquine Phosphate**

Aristospan (Stiefel/Glades), see **Triamcinolone Hexacetonide**

Asaphen (Pharmascience), see **Aspirin**

Asaphen E.C. (Pharmascience), see **Aspirin**

Atacand Plus (AstraZeneca), see **Candesartan Cilexetil/Hydrochloro- thiazide**

Atasol (Carter-Horner), see **Acetaminophen**

Atasol-8 (Carter-Horner), see **Acetaminophen/Caffeine Citrate/Codeine Phosphate, Narcotic Analgesic Combinations**

Atasol-15 (Carter-Horner), see **Acetaminophen/Caffeine Citrate/Codeine Phosphate, Narcotic Analgesic Combinations**

Atasol-30 (Carter-Horner), see **Acetaminophen/Caffeine Citrate/Codeine Phosphate, Narcotic Analgesic Combinations**

Auralgan (Whitehall-Robins), see **Antipyrine/Benzocaine, Otic Preparations**

Avaxim (Aventis Pasteur), see **Hepatitis A Vaccine, Inactivated**

AvaximPediatric (Aventis Pasteur), see **Hepatitis A Vaccine, Inactivated**

Baciguent (Johnson &

Johnson), see **Bacitracin**

Balminil Codeine + Decongestant + Expectorant (Rougier), see **Codeine Phosphate/Guaifenesin/ Pseudoephedrine HCl Antitussive and Expectorant Combinations, Upper Respiratory Combinations**

Balminil Cough and Flu (Rougier), see **Dextromethorphan HBr/Acetaminophen/ Guaifenesin/Pseudo- ephedrine HCl Antitussive and Expectorant Combinations, Upper Respiratory Combinations**

Balminil DM (Rougier), see **Dextromethorphan HBr**

Balminil DM Children (Rougier), see **Dextromethorphan HBr**

Balminil DM + Decongestant (Rougier), see **Dextromethorphan HBr/Pseudoephedrine HCl**

Balminil DM + Decongestant + Expectorant (Rougier), see **Dextromethorphan HBr/Guaifenesin/ Pseudoephedrine HCl**

Balminil DM + Expectorant (Rougier), see **Dextromethorphan HBr/Guaifenesin, Cough Preparations**

Balminil Expectorant (Rougier), see **Guaifenesin**

Balminil Nasal Decongestant (Rougier), see **Xylometazoline HCl**

Barriere-HC (Shire), see **Hydrocortisone**

Bellergal Spacetabs (Novartis Pharmaceuticals), see **Belladonna/Ergotamine/ Phenobarbital, Gastrointestinal Anticholinergic Combinations**

Bengay Arthritis Extra Strength (Pfizer Consumer Healthcare), see **Rubs and Liniments**

Bengay Ice Extra Strength (Pfizer Consumer Healthcare), see **Rubs and Liniments**

Bengay Muscle Pain Regular Strength (Original) (Pfizer Consumer Healthcare), see **Rubs and Liniments**

Bengay Muscle Pain Ultra Strength (Pfizer Consumer Healthcare), see **Rubs and Liniments**

Benoxyl 5% (Steifel), see **Benzoyl Peroxide**

Benoxyl 10% (Steifel), see **Benzoyl Peroxide**

Benoxyl 20% (Steifel), see **Benzoyl Peroxide**

Bentylol (Aventis Pharma), see **Dicyclomine HCl**

Benuryl (ICN), see **Probenecid**

Benylin 2 Cold and Flu with Codeine (Non-prescription) (Pfizer Consumer Healthcare), see **Codeine Phosphate/ Guaifenesin/Pseudo- ephedrine HCl**

Benylin DM (Pfizer Consumer Healthcare), see **Dextromethorphan HBr**

Benylin DM 12 Hour Nightime (Pfizer Consumer Healthcare), see **Dextromethorphan HBr**

Benylin DM For Children (Pfizer Consumer Healthcare), see **Dextromethorphan HBr**

Benylin DM For Children 12 Hour Bedtime (Pfizer Consumer Healthcare), see **Dextromethorphan HBr**

Benylin DM-D (Adult) (Pfizer Consumer Healthcare), see **Dextromethorphan HBr/Pseudoephedrine HCl, Respiratory Combinations**

Benylin DM-D-E (Pfizer Consumer Healthcare), see **Dextromethorphan HBr/Guaifenesin/ Pseudoephedrine HCl, Respiratory Combinations**

Benylin DM-D-E Extra Strength (Pfizer Consumer Healthcare), see **Dextromethorphan HBr/Guaifenesin/Pseudo- ephedrine HCl Antitussive and Expectorant Combinations, Upper Respiratory Combinations**

Benylin DM-D For Children (Pfizer Consumer Healthcare), see **Dextromethorphan HBr/Pseudoephedrine HCl, Respiratory Combinations**

Benylin DM-E (Pfizer Consumer Healthcare), see **Dextromethorphan HBr/Guaifenesin, Respiratory Combinations**

Benylin DM-E Extra Strength (Pfizer Consumer Healthcare), see **Dextromethorphan HBr/Guaifenesin Antitussives with Expectorants, Upper Respiratory Combinations**

Benylin E Extra Strength (Pfizer Consumer Healthcare), see **Guaifenesin**

Benztropine Omega (Omega), see **Benztropine Mesylate**

Betacaine (Canderm Pharma), see **Lidocaine HCl**

Betaderm (Taro), see **Betamethasone Valerate**

Betaject (Sabex), see **Betamethasone Sodium Phosphate/Betamethasone Acetate**

Betaloc (AstraZeneca), see **Metoprolol Tartrate**

Betaloc Durules (AstraZeneca), see **Metoprolol Tartrate**

Betaxin (Abbott), see **Thiamine HCl**

Betnesol Preparations (Shire), see **Betamethasone Sodium Phosphate**

Biaxin BID (Abbott), see, **Clarithromycin**

Biobase (Odan), see **Ethyl Alcohol, Miscellaneous Antiseptics**

Biobase-G (Odan), see **Ethyl Alcohol/Glycolic Acid, Miscellaneous Antiseptics**

Biolon (Ophtapharma), see **Sodium Hyaluronate**

Biquin Durules (AstraZeneca), see **Quinidine Sulfate**

Bonamine (Pfizer Consumer Healthcare), see **Meclizine HCl**

Brevicon 0.5/35 (Pfizer), see **Ethinyl Estradiol/Norethindrone Contraceptive Hormones**

Brevicon 1/35 (Pfizer), see **Ethinyl Estradiol/Norethindrone Contraceptive Hormones**

Bricanyl Turbuhaler (AstraZeneca), see **Terbutaline Sulfate**

Bufferin Extra-Strength (Bristol-Myers Squibb), see **Aspirin**

Bugs Bunny and Friends (Bayer Consumer), see **Multivitamins with Minerals**

Burinex (LEO), see **Bumetanide**

Buscopan (Boehringer Ingelheim), see **Hyoscine HBr**

Caelyx (Schering), see **Doxorubicin HCl**

Calcite 500 (Riva), see **Calcium Carbonate**

Calcite D-500 (Riva), see **Calcium Carbonate/ Vitamin D**

Calcium 500 (Trianon), see **Calcium Carbonate**

Calcium 500 mg with Vitamin D (Novopharm), see **Calcium and Vitamin D, Nutritional Combination Products**

Calcium D 500 (Trianon), see **Calcium/Vitamin D Combinations**

Calcium Oyster Shell (Novopharm), see **Calcium Carbonate, Minerals**

Calmylin Original With Codeine (Rougier), see **Ammonium Chloride/ Codeine Phosphate/ Diphenhydramine HCl, Cough Preparations**

Calmylin With Codeine (Rougier), see **Codeine Phosphate/Guaifenesin/ Pseudoephedrine HCl, Cough Preparations**

Caltine (Ferring), see **Calcitonin (Salmon)**

Candistatin (Westwood-Squibb), see **Nystatin**

Canesten Topical (Bayer Consumer), see **Clotrimazole**

Canesten Vaginal (Bayer Consumer), see **Clotrimazole**

Dimetapp Extra Strength DM Cough & Cold Liquid (Whitehall-Robins), see **Brompheniramine Maleate/Phenylephrine HCl/Dextromethorphan HBr**

Dimetapp Nighttime Cold Extra Strength (Whitehall-Robins), see **Chlorpheniramine Maleate/Phenylephrine HCl/Acetaminophen Decongestant, Antihistamine, and Analgesic Combinations, Upper Respiratory Combinations**

Dimetapp Oral Infant Cold Drops (Whitehall-Robins), see **Brompheniramine Maleate/Phenylephrine HCl, Respiratory Combinations**

Diodoquin (Glenwood), see **Iodoquinol**

Diofluor Injection (Dioptic), see **Fluorescein Sodium**

Diofluor Strips (Dioptic), see **Fluorescein Sodium**

Diovol (Carter-Horner), see **Aluminum Hydroxide/Magnesium Hydroxide, Antacid Combinations**

Diovol Ex (Carter-Horner), see **Aluminum Hydroxide/Magnesium Hydroxide, Antacid Combinations**

Diovol Plus (Carter-Horner), see **Aluminum Hydroxide/Magnesium Hydroxide/Simethicone, Antacid Combinations**

Diovol Plus AF (Carter-Horner), see **Calcium Carbonate/Magnesium Hydroxide/Simethicone, Antacid Combinations**

Diprolene Glycol (Schering), see **Betamethasone Dipropionate**

Dixarit (Boehringer Ingelheim), see **Clonidine HCl**

Doak Oil (TCD), see **Isopropyl Palmitate/Mineral Oil/Tar Distillate, Tar-Containing Products, Bath Preparations**

Doak Oil Forte (TCD), see **Isopropyl Palmitate/Mineral Oil/Tar Distillate Tar-Containing Products, Bath Preparations**

Doxycin (Riva), see **Doxycycline Hyclate**

Dristan (Whitehall-Robins), see **Acetaminophen/Chlorpheniramine Maleate/Phenylephrine HCl, Respiratory Combinations**

Dristan Extra Strength (Whitehall-Robins), see **Acetaminophen/Chlorpheniramine Maleate/Phenylephrine HCl, Respiratory Combinations**

Dristan Long Lasting, Nasal Mist/Spray (Whitehall-Robins), see **Oxymetazoline HCl Nasal Decongestants**

Dristan N.D. (Whitehall-Robins), see **Acetaminophen/Pseudoephedrine HCl, Respiratory Combinations**

Dristan N.D. Extra Strength (Whitehall-Robins), see **Acetaminophen/Pseudoephedrine HCl, Respiratory Combinations**

Duofilm Gel for Kids (Stiefel), see **Salicylic Acid**

Duoforte 27 (Stiefel), see **Salicylic Acid**

Duonalc (ICN), see **Isopropyl Alcohol, Miscellaneous Topical Antiseptics**

Duonalc-E Mild (ICN), see **Ethyl Alcohol, Miscellaneous Topical Antiseptics**

Duonalc-E Solution (ICN), see **Ethyl Alcohol/Isopropyl Alcohol, Miscellaneous Topical Antiseptics**

Duragesic (Janssen-Ortho), see **Fentanyl Transdermal System**

Duralith (Janssen-Ortho), see **Lithium Carbonate**

Ecostatin (Westwood-Squibb), see **Econazole Nitrate**

EES 600 (Abbott), see **Erythromycin Ethylsuccinate**

Elocom (Schering), see **Mometasone Furoate**

Eltor 120 (Aventis Pharma), see **Pseudoephedrine HCl**

Eltroxin (GlaxoSmithKline), see **Levothyroxine Sodium**

EMLA Patch (AstraZeneca), see **Lidocaine and Prilocaine, Local Anesthetics, Topical Combinations**

Emo-Cort (TCD), see **Hydrocortisone**

Endantadine (Linson Pharma), see **Amantadine HCl**

Endodan (Linson Pharma), see **Aspirin/Oxycodone HCl, Analgesic Combinations**

Enfalac Fer-In-Sol (Mead Johnson Nutritionals), see **Ferrous Sulfate**

Enfalac Lactofree (Mead Johnson Nutritionals), see **Infant Foods, Specialized**

Enfalac Nutramigen (Mead Johnson Nutritionals), see **Infant Foods**

Enfalac Poly-Vi-Sol (Mead Johnson Nutritionals), see **Multivitamins Drops and Liquids**

Enfalac Pregestimil (Mead Johnson Nutritionals), see **Infant Foods**

Enfalac Prosobee Soy (Mead Johnson Nutritionals), see **Infant Foods**

Enfalac Tri-Vi-Sol (Mead Johnson Nutritionals), see **Multivitamins Drops and Liquids**

Enfalac Tri-Vi-Sol with Fluoride (Mead Johnson Nutritionals), see **Multivitamins with Fluoride**

Entocort Capsules (AstraZeneca), see **Budesonide**

Entocort Enema (AstraZeneca), see **Budesonide**

Epaxal (Berna Products), see **Hepatitis A Vaccine, Inactivated**

Epiject I.V. (Abbott), see **Valproic Acid**

Epi-Lyt AHA Medicated Lotion (Stiefel), see **Glycerin/Lactic Acid Emollients**

Epival (Abbott), see **Divalproex Sodium**

Epival ER (Abbott), see **Divalproex Sodium**

Eprex (Janssen-Ortho), see **Epoetin Alfa**

Erybid (Abbott), see **Erythromycin**

Estradot (Novartis Pharmaceuticals), see **Estradiol**

Estrogel (Schering), see **Estradiol Hemihydrate**

Etibi (ICN), see **Ethambutol HCl**

Euflex (Schering), see **Flutamide**

Euglucon (Pharmascience), see **Glyburide**

Eumovate (GlaxoSmithKline Consumer Healthcare), see **Clobetasone 17-Butyrate**

Evra (Janssen-Ortho), see **Ethinyl Estradiol/Norelgestromin**

Eyestil (Ophtapharma), see **Sodium Hyaluronate**

Ezetrol (Merck Frosst), see **Ezetimibe**

Ferodan (Odan), see **Ferrous Sulfate**

Fiorinal-C1/4 (Paladin), see **Aspirin/Butalbital/Caffeine/Codeine Phosphate, Analgesic Combinations**

Fiorinal-C1/2 (Paladin), see **Aspirin/Butalbital/Caffeine/Codeine Phosphate, Analgesic Combinations**

Flamazine (Smith & Nephew), see **Silver Sulfadiazine**

Florazole ER (Ferring), **Metronidazole**

Florinef (Shire), see **Fludrocortisone Acetate**

Floven HFA (GlaxoSmithKline), see **Fluticasone Propionate**

Fluoderm (Taro), see **Fluocinolone Acetonide**

Fluor-A-Day (Pharmascience), see **Sodium Fluoride**

Fluotic (Aventis Pharma), see **Sodium Fluoride**

Fluphenazine Omega (Omega), see **Fluphenazine Decanoate**

Fluviral S/F (Shire Bioligics), see **Influenza Virus Vaccine, Inactivated**

Follow-Up (Nestle), see **Infant Foods**

Fortovase Roche (Roche), see **Saquinavir**

Froben (Abbott), see **Flurbiprofen**

Froben SR (Abbott), see **Flurbiprofen**

Furosemide Special (Sabex), see **Furosemide**

FXT (Oryx), see **Fluoxetine HCl**

Gastrolyte (Aventis Pharma), see **Dextrose With Electrolytes**

Gaviscon Heartburn Relief Formula Liquid (GlaxoSmithKline Consumer Healthcare), see **Aluminum Hydroxide/Sodium Alginate, Antacid Combinations**

Gelusil Extra Strength (Pfizer Consumer Healthcare), see **Aluminum Hydroxide/Magnesium Hydroxide, Antacid Combinations**

Gen-Acebutolol (Genpharm), see **Acebutolol HCl**

Gen-Acebutolol Type S (Genpharm), see **Acebutolol HCl**

Gen-Acyclovir (Genpharm), see **Acyclovir**

Gen-Alprazolam (Genpharm), see **Alprazolam**

Gen-Amantadine (Antiparkinsonian) (Genpharm), see **Amantadine HCl**

Gen-Amantadine (Antiviral) (Genpharm), see **Amantadine HCl**

Gen-Amiodarone (Genpharm), see **Amiodarone HCl**

Gen-Amoxicillin (Genpharm), see **Amoxicillin Trihydrate**

Gen-Atenolol (Genpharm), see **Atenolol**

Gen-Azathioprine (Genpharm), see **Azathioprine**

Gen-Baclofen (Genpharm), see **Baclofen**

Gen-Beclo AQ (Genpharm), see **Beclomethasone Dipropionate**

Gen-Budesonide AQ. (Genpharm), see **Budesonide**

Gen-Buspirone (Genpharm), see **Buspirone HCl**

Gen-Captopril (Genpharm), see **Captopril**

Gen-Carbamazepine CR (Genpharm), see **Carbamazepine**

Gen-Cimetidine (Genpharm), see **Cimetidine**

Gen-Clobetasol Cream/Ointment (Genpharm), see **Clobetasol 17-Propionate**

Lithane (Pfizer),
see **Lithium Carbonate**

Loestrin 1.5/30 (Galen Chemicals), see **Ethinyl Estradiol/Norethindrone Acetate, Monophasic Oral Contraceptives, Sex Hormones**

Lomine (Riva),
see **Dicyclomine HCl**

Losec (AstraZeneca),
see **Omeprazole Magnesium**

Lotriderm (Schering), see **Betamethasone Dipropionate/Clotrimazole Corticosteroid/Antifungal Combinations**

Lovenox HP (Aventis Pharma),
see **Enoxaparin Sodium**

Loxapac (Sabex), see **Loxapine**

Lozide (Servier), see **Indapamide Hemihydrate**

Lupron Depot 3.75 mg/11.25 mg (Tap Pharmaceuticals), see **Leuprolide Acetate**

Lupron/Lupron Depot 3.75 mg/7.5 mg (Tap Pharmaceuticals), see **Leuprolide Acetate**

Lupron/Lupron Depot 7.5 mg/22.5 mg/30 mg (Tap Pharmaceuticals), see **Leuprolide Acetate**

Lyderm (TaroPharma), see **Fluocinonide**

Lyteprep (E-Z-EM Canada), see **Polyethylene Glycol/Electrolyte, Bowel Evacuants**

Maltlevol-M (Carter-Horner), see **Multiple Vitamins And Minerals**

Maltlevol-12 (Carter-Horner), see **Multiple Vitamins**

Marvelon (Organon), see **Desogestrel/Ethinyl Estradiol, Oral Contraceptives**

Materna (Whitehall-Robins), see **Multivitamins with Minerals**

Maxalt RPD (Merck Frosst), see **Rizatriptan Benzoate**

MD-76 (tyco Healthcare), see **Diatrizoate Meglumine/Diatrizoate Sodium**

Megace OS (Bristol), see **Megestrol Acetate**

Mesasal (GlaxoSmithKline Consumer Healthcare), see **5-Aminosalicylic Acid**

M-Eslon (Aventis Pharma), see **Morphine Sulfate**

Mestinon-SR (ICN), see **Pyridostigmine Bromide**

Metadol (Pharmascience), see **Methadone HCl**

Meted (Medicis), see **Salicylic Acid/Sulfur, Antiseborrheic Combinations**

Methoxacet (Rougier), see **Acetaminophen/Methocarbamol, Analgesic Combinations**

Methoxisal (Rougier), see **Aspirin/Methocarbamol, Analgesic Combinations**

Metoclopramide Omega (Omega), see **Metoclopramide**

Miacalcin NS (Novartis Pharmaceuticals), see **Calcitonin-Salmon**

Micardis Plus (Boehringer Ingelheim), see **Hydrochlorothiazide/Telmisartan Antihypertensive Combinations**

Micozole (Taro), see **Miconazole Nitrate**

Micronor (Janssen-Ortho), see **Norethindrone**

Midol Extra Strength (Bayer Consumer), see **Acetaminophen/Caffeine/Pyrilamine Maleate, Analgesic Combinations**

Midol PMS Extra Strength (Bayer Consumer), see **Acetaminophen/Pamabrom/Pyrilamine Maleate, Analgesic Combinations**

Midol Regular (Bayer Consumer), see **Aspirin/Caffeine, Analgesic Combinations**

Minestrin 1/20 (Galen Chemicals), see **Ethinyl Estradiol/Norethindrone Acetate, Oral Contraceptives**

Minirin (Ferring), see **Desmopression Acetate**

Min-Ovral 21 (Wyeth Canada), see **Ethinyl Estradiol/Levonorgestrel, Oral Contraceptives**

Min-Ovral 28 (Wyeth Canada), see **Ethinyl Estradiol/Levonorgestrel, Oral Contraceptives**

Mobicox (Boehringer Ingelheim), see **Meloxicam**

Modecate (Squibb), see **Fluphenazine Decanoate**

Modecate Concentrate (Squibb), see **Fluphenazine Decanoate**

Moduret (Merck Frosst), see **Amiloride HCl/Hydrochlorothiazide, Diuretic Combinations**

Moisturel (Westwood-Squibb), see **Dimethicone/Petrolatum Emollients, Miscellaneous**

Monistat 1 Combination Pack (McNeil Consumer Healthcare), see **Miconazole Nitrate**

Monistat 1 Vaginal Ovule (McNeil Consumer Healthcare), see **Miconazole Nitrate**

Monistat 3 Vaginal Ovules (McNeil Consumer Healthcare), see **Miconazole Nitrate**

Monistat Derm Cream (McNeil Consumer Healthcare), see **Miconazole Nitrate**

Monitan (Wyeth Canada), see **Acebutolol HCl**

Monocor (Biovail Pharmaceuticals), see **Bisoprolol Fumarate**

Morphine HP (Sabex), see **Morphine Sulfate**

Morphine LP Epidural (Sabex), see **Morphine Sulfate**

M.O.S.-Sulfate (ICN), see **Morphine Sulfate**

Motrin IB Extra Strength (McNeil Consumer Healthcare), see **Ibuprofen**

Motrin IB Super Strength (McNeil Consumer Healthcare), see **Ibuprofen**

Multi-12 (Sabex), see **Multivitamins, Parenteral**

Multi-12/K1 (Sabex), see **Multivitamins, Parenteral**

Mutacol (Berna Products), see **Cholera Vaccine Live Oral**

Mylanta Double Strength Plain (Pfizer Consumer Healthcare), see **Aluminum Hydroxide/Magnesium Hydroxide, Antacid Combinations**

Mylanta Extra Strength (Pfizer Consumer Healthcare), see **Aluminum Hydroxide/Magnesium Hydroxide/Simethicone, Antacid Combinations**

Mylanta Regular Strength (Pfizer Consumer Healthcare), see **Aluminum Hydroxide/Magnesium Hydroxide/Simethicone, Antacid Combinations**

Myocet (Elan), see **Doxorubicin HCl**

Nalcrom (Aventis Pharma), see **Cromolyn Sodium**

Neosporin Eye and Ear Solution (GlaxoSmithKline), see **Neomycin and Polymyxin B Sulfates and Gramicidin Ophthalmic Solution**

Neosporin Irrigating Solution (GlaxoSmithKline), see **Neomycin Sulfate/Polymyxin B Sulfate, Topical Anti-infective Combinations**

Neosporin Ointment (GlaxoSmithKline), see **Neomycin and Polymyxin B Sulfates and Bacitracin Zinc Ophthalmic Ointment**

NeoStrata Canada Astringent Acne Treatment (Canderm Pharma), see **Salicylic Acid**

Neostrata Canada Blemish Spot Gel (Canderm Pharma), see **Salicylic Acid**

Neostrata Canada HQ (Canderm Pharma), see **Hydroquinone**

Neostrata Canada HQ Plus Gel (Canderm Pharma), see **Hydroquinone**

NeoVisc (Stellar), see **Sodium Hyaluronate**

Nesacaine-CE (AstraZeneca), see **Chloroprocaine HCl**

Nicorette Gum Plus (Pfizer Consumer Healthcare), see **Nicotine**

NidaGel (3M Pharmaceuticals), see **Metronidazole**

Nipride (Mayne Pharma), see **Sodium Nitroprusside**

Nitrazadon (ICN), see **Nitrazepam**

Nitrolingual Pumpspray (Aventis Pharma), see **Nitroglycerin**

Nix Creme Rinse (Insight Pharma), see **Permethrin**

Nix Dermal Cream (GlaxoSmithKline Consumer Healthcare), see **Permethrin**

Nolvadex-D (AstraZeneca), see **Tamoxifen Citrate**

Norvir Sec (Abbott), see **Ritonavir**

Novahistex DH (Aventis Pharma), see **Hydrocodone Bitartrate/Phenylephrine HCl, Cough Preparations**

Novamilor (Novopharm), see **Amiloride HCl/Hydrochlorothiazide, Diuretic Combinations**

Novamoxin (Novopharm), see **Amoxicillin Trihydrate**

Novasen (Novopharm), see **Aspirin**

Novo-5 ASA (Novopharm), see **5-Aminosalicylic Acid**

Novo-Acebutolol (Novopharm), see **Acebutolol HCl**

Novo-Alendronate (Novopharm), see **Alendronate Sodium**

Novo-Alprazol (Novopharm), see **Alprazolam**

Novo-Amiodarone (Novopharm), see **Amiodarone HCl**

Novo-Ampicillin (Novopharm), see **Ampicillin**

Novo-Atenol (Novopharm), see **Atenolol**

Novo-Buspirone (Novopharm), see **Buspirone HCl**

Novo-Captoril (Novopharm), see **Captopril**

Novo-Carbamaz (Novopharm), see **Carbamazepine**

Novo-Cefaclor (Novopharm), see **Cefaclor**

Novo-Cefadroxil (Novopharm), see **Cefadroxil**

Novo-Cholamine (Novopharm), see **Cholestyramine Resin**

Novo-Cholamine Light (Novopharm), see **Cholestyramine Resin**

Novo-Cimetine (Novopharm), see **Cimetidine**

Novo-Clindamycin (Novopharm), see **Clindamycin**

Novo-Clobazam (Novopharm), see **Clobazam**

Novo-Clobetasol (Novopharm), see **Clobetasol 17-Propionate**

Novo-Clonazepam (Novopharm), see **Clonazepam**

Novo-Clonidine (Novopharm), see **Clonidine HCl**

Novo-Clopate (Novopharm), see **Clorazepate Dipotassium**

Novo-Cloxin (Novopharm), see **Cloxacillin Sodium**

Novo-Cycloprine (Novopharm), see **Cyclobenzaprine HCl**

Novo-Difenac (Novopharm), see **Diclofenac Sodium**

Novo-Difenac-K (Novopharm), see **Diclofenac Potassium**

Novo-Difenac SR (Novopharm), see **Diclofenac Sodium**

Novo-Diflunisal (Novopharm), see **Diflunisal**

Novo-Diltazem (Novopharm), see **Diltiazem HCl**

Novo-Diltiazem CD (Novopharm), see **Diltiazem HCl**

Novo-Diltazem SR (Novopharm), see **Diltiazem HCl**

Novo-Dimenate (Novopharm), see **Dimenhydrinate**

Novo-Divalproex (Novopharm), see **Divalproex Sodium Valproic Acid and Derivatives**

Novo-Docusate Calcium (Novopharm), see **Docusate Calcium**

Novo-Docusate Sodium (Novopharm), see **Docusate Sodium**

Novo-Doxazosin (Novopharm), see **Doxazosin Mesylate**

Novo-Doxepin (Novopharm), see **Doxepin HCl**

Novo-Doxylin (Novopharm), see **Doxycycline Hyclate**

Novo-Famotidine (Novopharm), see **Famotidine**

Novo-Ferrogluc (Novopharm), see **Ferrous Gluconate**

Novo-Fluconazole (Novopharm), see **Fluconazole**

Novo-Fluoxetine (Novopharm), see **Fluoxetine HCl**

Novo-Flurprofen (Novopharm), see **Flurbiprofen**

Novo-Flutamide (Novopharm), see **Flutamide**

Novo-Fluvoxamine (Novopharm), see **Fluvoxamine Maleate**

Novo-Furantoin (Novopharm), see **Nitrofurantoin**

Novo-Gabapentin (Novopharm), see **Gabapentin**

Novo-Gemfibrozil (Novopharm), see **Gemfibrozil**

Novo-Glyburide (Novopharm), see **Glyburide**

Novo-Hydroxyzin (Novopharm), see **Hydroxyzine HCl**

Novo-Hylazin (Novopharm), see **Hydralazine HCl**

Novo-Indapamide (Novopharm), see **Indapamide**

Novo-Ipramide (Novopharm), see **Ipratropium Bromide**

Novo-Keto (Novopharm), see **Ketoprofen**

Novo-Ketoconazole (Novopharm), see **Ketoconazole**

Novo-Ketorolac (Novopharm), see **Ketorolac Tromethamine**

Novo-Ketotifen (Novopharm), see **Ketotifen Fumarate**

Novo-Levobunolol (Novopharm), see **Levobunolol HCl**

Novo-Levocarbidopa (Novopharm), see **Carbidopa/Levodopa**

Novo-Lexin (Novopharm), see **Cephalexin**

Novolinge 10/90 (Novo Nordisk), see **Insulin Injection (Human)/Insulin Isophane (Human)**

Novolinge 20/80 (Novo Nordisk), see **Insulin Injection (Human)/Insulin Isophane (Human)**

Novolinge 30/70 (Novo Nordisk), see **Insulin Injection (Human)/Insulin Isophane (Human)**

Novolinge 40/60 (Novo Nordisk), see **Insulin Injection (Human)/Insulin Isophane (Human)**

Novolinge 50/50 (Novo Nordisk), see **Insulin Injection (Human)/Insulin Isophane (Human)**

Novolinge NPH (Novo Nordisk), see **Insulin Isophane (Human)**

Novolinge Toronto (Novo Nordisk), see **Insulin Injection (Human)**

Novo-Loperamide (Novopharm), see **Loperamide HCl**

Novo-Lorazem (Novopharm), see **Lorazepam**

Novo-Lovastatin (Novopharm), see **Lovastatin**

Novo-Maprotiline (Novopharm), see **Maprotiline HCl**

Novo-Medrone (Novopharm), see **Medroxyprogesterone Acetate**

Novo-Metformin (Novopharm), see **Metformin HCl**

Novo-Methacin (Novopharm), see **Indomethacin**

Novo-Metoprol (Novopharm), see **Metoprolol Tartrate**

Novo-Mexiletine (Novopharm), see **Mexiletine HCl**

Novo-Minocycline (Novopharm), see **Minocycline HCl**

Novo-Misoprostol (Novopharm), see **Misoprostol**

Novo-Nadolol (Novopharm), see **Nadolol**

Novo-Naprox (Novopharm), see **Naproxen**

Novo-Naprox-EC (Novopharm), see **Naproxen**

Novo-Naprox Sodium (Novopharm), see **Naproxen Sodium**

Novo-Naprox Sodium DS (Novopharm), see **Naproxen Sodium**

Novo-Naprox SR (Novopharm), see **Naproxen Sodium**

Novo-Nifedin (Novopharm), see **Nifedipine**

Novo-Nizatidine (Novopharm), see **Nizatidine**

Novo-Norfloxacin (Novopharm), see **Norfloxacin**

Novo-Nortriptyline (Novopharm), see **Nortriptyline HCl**

Novo-Oxybutynin (Novopharm), see **Oxybutynin Chloride**

Novo-Pen-VK (Novopharm), see **Penicillin V Potassium**

Novo-Peridol (Novopharm), see **Haloperidol**

Novo-Pheniram (Novopharm), see **Chlorpheniramine Maleate**

Novo-Pindol (Novopharm), see **Pindolol**

Novo-Pirocam (Novopharm), see **Piroxicam**

Novo-Pravastatin (Novopharm), see **Pravastatin Sodium**

Novo-Prazin (Novopharm), see **Prazosin HCl**

Novo-Profen (Novopharm), see **Ibuprofen**

Novo-Ranidine (Novopharm), see **Ranitidine HCl**

NovoRapid (Novo Nordisk), see **Insulin Aspart**

Novo-Selegiline (Novopharm), see **Selegiline HCl**

Novo-Sertraline (Novopharm), see **Sertraline HCl**

Novo-Sotalol (Novopharm), see **Sotalol HCl**

Novo-Spiroton (Novopharm), see **Spironolactone**

Novo-Spirozine (Novopharm), see **Hydrochlorothiazide/ Spironolactone, Diuretic Combinations**

Novo-Sucralate (Novopharm), see **Sucralfate**

Novo-Sundac (Novopharm), see **Sulindac**

Novo-Tamoxifen (Novopharm), see **Tamoxifen Citrate**

Novo-Temazepam (Novopharm), see **Temazepam**

Novo-Terazosin (Novopharm), see **Terazosin HCl**

Novo-Terbinafine (Novopharm), see **Terbinafine HCl**

Novo-Theophyl SR (Novopharm), see **Theophylline**

Novo-Ticlopidine (Novopharm), see **Ticlopidine HCl**

Novo-Timol (Novopharm), see **Timolol Maleate**

Novo-Trazodone (Novopharm), see **Trazodone HCl**

Novo-Triamzide (Novopharm), see **Hydrochlorothiazide/ Triamterene, Diuretic Combinations**

Novo-Trimel (Novopharm), see **Sulfamethoxazole/ Trimethoprim**

Novo-Trimel DS (Novopharm), see **Sulfamethoxazole/ Trimethoprim**

Novo-Valproic (Novopharm), see **Valproic Acid**

Novo-Veramil SR (Novopharm), see **Verapamil HCl**

Nozinan (Aventis Pharma), see **Methotrimeprazine Maleate**

Nu-Acebutolol (Nu-Pharm), see **Acebutolol HCl**

Nu-Acyclovir (Nu-Pharm), see **Acyclovir**

Nu-Alpraz (Nu-Pharm), see **Alprazolam**

Nu-Amilzide (Nu-Pharm), see **Amiloride HCl/ Hydrochlorothiazide Diuretic Combinations**

Nu-Amoxi (Nu-Pharm), see **Amoxicillin Trihydrate**

Nu-Ampi (Nu-Pharm), see **Ampicillin Trihydrate**

Nu-Atenol (Nu-Pharm), see **Atenolol**

Nu-Baclo (Nu-Pharm), see **Baclofen**

Nubain (Bristol-Myers Squibb), see **Nalbuphine HCl**

Nu-Beclomethasone (Nu-Pharm), see **Beclomethasone Dipropionate**

Nu-Buspirone (Nu-Pharm), see **Buspirone HCl**

Nu-Capto (Nu-Pharm), see **Captopril**

Nu-Carbamazepine (Nu-Pharm), see **Carbamazepine**

Nu-Cefaclor (Nu-Pharm), see **Cefaclor**

Nu-Cephalex (Nu-Pharm), see **Cephalexin**

Nu-Cimet (Nu-Pharm), see **Cimetidine**

Nu-Clonazepam (Nu-Pharm), see **Clonazepam**

Nu-Clonidine (Nu-Pharm), see **Clonidine HCl**

Nu-Cloxi (Nu-Pharm), see **Cloxacillin Sodium**

Nu-Cotrimox (Nu-Pharm), see **Sulfamethoxazole/ Trimethoprim**

Nu-Cromolyn (Nu-Pharm), see **Cromolyn Sodium**

Nu-Cyclobenzaprine (Nu-Pharm), see **Cyclobenzaprine HCl**

Nu-Desipramine (Nu-Pharm), see **Desipramine HCl**

Nu-Diclo (Nu-Pharm), see **Diclofenac Sodium**

Nu-Diclo-SR (Nu-Pharm), see **Diclofenac Sodium**

Nu-Diflunisal (Nu-Pharm), see **Diflunisal**

Nu-Diltiaz (Nu-Pharm), see **Diltiazem HCl**

Nu-Diltiaz-CD (Nu-Pharm), see **Diltiazem HCl**

Nu-Divalproex (Nu-Pharm), see **Divalproex Sodium, Valproic Acid and Derivatives**

Nu-Doxycycline (Nu-Pharm), see **Doxycycline Hyclate**

Nu-Erythromycin-S (Nu-Pharm), see **Erythromycin Stearate**

Nu-Famotidine (Nu-Pharm), see **Famotidine**

Nu-Fenofibrate (Nu-Pharm), see **Fenofibrate**

Nu-Fluoxetine (Nu-Pharm), see **Fluoxetine HCl**

ratio-Doxycycline (ratiopharm), see **Doxycycline**

ratio-Ectosone (ratiopharm), see **Betamethasone Valerate**

ratio-Emtec-30 (ratiopharm), see **Acetaminophen/Codeine Narcotic Analgesic Combinations**

ratio-Famotidine (ratiopharm), see **Famotidine**

ratio-Flunisolide (ratiopharm), see **Flunisolide**

ratio-Fluoxetine (ratiopharm), see **Fluoxetine HCl**

ratio-Flurbiprofen (ratiopharm), see **Flurbiprofen**

ratio-Fluvoxamine (ratiopharm), see **Fluvoxamine**

ratio-Gentamicin (ratiopharm), see **Gentamicin**

ratio-Glyburide (ratiopharm), see **Glyburide**

ratio-Indomethacin (ratiopharm), see **Indomethacin**

ratio-Ipratropium (ratiopharm), see **Ipratropium Bromide**

ratio-Ipratropium UDV (ratiopharm), see **Ipratropium Bromide**

ratio-Ketorolac (ratiopharm), see **Ketorolac Tromethamine**

ratio-Lactulose (ratiopharm), see **Lactulose**

ratio-Lamotrigine (ratiopharm), see **Lamotrigine**

ratio-Lenoltec No. 4 (ratiopharm), see **Acetaminophen/Codeine Phosphate Narcotic Analgesic Combinations**

ratio-Levobunolol (ratiopharm), see **Levobunolol HCl**

ratio-Lovastatin (ratiopharm), see **Lovastatin**

ratio-Metformin (ratiopharm), see **Metformin HCl**

ratio-Methotrexate (ratiopharm), see **Methotrexate**

ratio-Methylphenidate (ratiopharm), see **Methylphenidate HCl**

ratio-Minocycline (ratiopharm), see **Minocycline**

ratio-Morphine SR (ratiopharm), see **Morphine Sulfate**

ratio-MPA (ratiopharm), see **Medroxyprogesterone Acetate**

ratio-Nadolol (ratiopharm), see **Nadolol**

ratio-Naproxen (ratiopharm), see **Naproxen**

ratio-Nortriptyline (ratiopharm), see **Nortriptyline HCl**

ratio-Nystatin (ratiopharm), see **Nystatin**

ratio-Oxycocet (ratiopharm), see **Acetaminophen/Oxycodone Narcotic Analgesic Combinations**

ratio-Ocycodan (ratiopharm), see **Aspirin/Oxycodone Narcotic Analgesic Combinations**

ratio-Pentoxifylline (ratiopharm), see **Pentoxifylline**

ratio-Pravastatin (ratiopharm), see **Pravastatin Sodium**

ratio-Prednisolone (ratiopharm), see **Prednisolone Acetate Ophthalmic**

ratio-Ranitidine (ratiopharm), see **Ranitidine HCl**

ratio-Salbutamol (ratiopharm), see **Albuterol**

ratio-Salbutamol HFA (ratiopharm), see **Albuterol**

ratio-Sertraline (ratiopharm), see **Sertraline HCl**

ratio-Simvastatin (ratiopharm), see **Simvastatin**

ratio-Sotalol (ratiopharm), see **Sotalol HCl**

ratio-Sulfasalazine (ratiopharm), see **Sulfasalazine**

ratio-Tecnal (ratiopharm), see **Aspirin/Butalbital/Caffeine Nonnarcotic Analgesic Combinations**

ratio-Temazepam (ratiopharm), see **Temazepam**

ratio-Terazosin (ratiopharm), see **Terazosin HCl**

ratio-Timolol (ratiopharm), see **Timolol Maleate**

ratio-Topilene (ratiopharm), see **Betamethasone Dipropionate**

ratio-Topisone (ratiopharm), see **Betamethasone Dipropionate**

ratio-Trazodone (ratiopharm), see **Trazodone HCl**

ratio-Trazodone Dividose (ratiopharm), see **Trazodone HCl**

ratio-Tryptophan (ratiopharm), see **L-Tryptophan**

ratio-Valproic (ratiopharm), see **Valproic Acid**

Reactine (Pfizer Consumer Healthcare), see **Cetirizine HCl**

Reactine Allergy & Sinus (Pfizer Consumer Healthcare), see **Cetirizine HCl/Pseudoephedrine HCl**

Rejuva-A (Stiefel), see **Tretinoin**

Renedil (Aventis Pharma), see **Felodipine**

Retisol-A (Stiefel), see **Tretinoin**

Revitalose-C-1000 (Rivex Pharma), see **Vitamin C**

Rhinocort Turbuhaler (AstraZeneca), see **Budesonide**

Rhodacine (Rhoxalpharma), see **Indomethacin**

Rho-Nitro Pumpspray (Rhodiapharm), see **Nitroglycerin**

Rhodis (Rhodiapharm), see **Ketoprofen**

Rhodis EC (Rhodiapharm), see **Ketoprofen**

Rhodis SR (Rhodiapharm), see **Ketoprofen**

Rhotral (Rhodiapharm), see **Acebutolol HCl**

Rhotrimine (Rhodiapharm), see **Trimipramine Maleate**

Rhovail (Rhodiapharm), see **Ketoprofen**

Rhoxal-amiodarone (Rhoxalpharma), see **Amiodarone HCl**

Rhoxal-atenolol (Rhoxalpharma), see **Atenolol**

Rhoxal-bisoprolol (Rhoxalpharma), see **Bisoprolol Fumarate**

Rhoxal-clonazepam (Rhoxalpharma), see **Clonazepam**

Rhoxal-cyclosporine (Rhoxalpharma), see **Cyclosporine**

Rhoxal-diltiazem CD (Rhoxalpharma), see **Diltiazem HCl**

Rhoxal-estradiol derm (Rhoxalpharma), see **Estradiol Transdermal System**

Rhoxal-fluoxetine (Rhoxalpharma), see **Fluoxetine HCl**

Rhoxal-fluvoxamine (Rhoxalpharma), see **Fluvoxamine Maleate**

Rhoxal-glyburide (Rhoxalpharma), see **Glyburide**

Rhoxal-loperamide (Rhoxalpharma), see **Loperamide HCl**

Rhoxal-lovastatin (Rhoxalpharma), see **Lovastatin**

Rhoxal-metformin (Rhoxalpharma), see **Metformin HCl**

Rhoxal-metformin FC (Rhoxalpharma), see **Metformin HCl**

Rhoxal-metoprolol (Type L) (Rhoxalpharma), see **Metoprolol Tartrate**

Rhoxal-minocycline (Rhoxalpharma), see **Minocycline HCl**

Rhoxal-nabumetone (Rhoxalpharma), see **Nabumetone**

Rhoxal-orphenadrine (Rhoxalpharma), see **Orphenadrine Citrate**

Rhoxal-pravastatin (Rhoxalpharma), see **Pravastatin Sodium**

Rhoxal-ranitidine (Rhoxalpharma), see **Ranitidine HCl**

Rhoxal-salbutamol (Rhoxalpharma), see **Albuterol Sulfate**

Rhoxal-simvastatin (Rhoxalpharma), see **Simvastatin**

Rhoxal-sotalol (Rhoxalpharma), see **Sotalol HCl**

Rhoxal-ticlopidine (Rhoxalpharma), see **Ticlopidine HCl**

Rhoxal-timolol (Rhoxalpharma), see **Timolol Maleate**

Rhoxal-valproic (Rhoxalpharma), see **Valproic Acid**

Rhoxal-valproic EC (Rhoxalpharma), see **Valproic Acid**

Riva-Loperamide (Riva), see **Loperamide HCl**

Rivanase AQ (Riva), see **Beclomethasone Dipropionate**

Rivasol (Riva), see **Zinc Sulfate Monohydrate**

Rivotril (Roche), see **Clonazepam**

Robaxacet (Whitehall-Robins), see **Acetaminophen/ Methocarbamol, Analgesic Combinations**

Robaxacet Extra Strength (Whitehall-Robins), see **Acetaminophen/ Methocarbamol, Analgesic Combinations**

Robaxisal Extra Strength (Whitehall-Robins), see **Aspirin/Methocarbamol, Skeletal Muscle Relaxant Combinations**

Robitussin Children's (Whitehall-Robins), see **Dextromethorphan HBr**

Robitussin Children's Cough and Cold (Whitehall-Robins), see **Dextromethorphan HBr/Pseudoephedrine HCl**

Robitussin Cough, Cold & Flu Liqui-Gels (Whitehall-Robins), see **Acetaminophen/ Dextromethorphan HBr/ Guaifenesin/ Pseudoephedrine HCl, Cough Preparations**

Robitussin Extra Strength (Whitehall-Robins), see **Guaifenesin**

Robitussin Extra Strength Cough & Cold (Whitehall-Robins), see **Dextromethorphan HBr/Guaifenesin/Pseudo-ephedrine HCl Antitussive and Expectorant Combinations, Upper Respiratory Combinations**

Robitussin Extra Strength DM (Whitehall-Robins), see **Dextromethorphan HBr/Guaifenesin Antitussives with Expectorants, Upper Respiratory Combinations**

Robitussin With Codeine (Whitehall-Robins), see **Codeine Phosphate/ Guaifenesin/Pheniramine Maleate, Cough Preparations**

Rofact (ICN), see **Rifampin**

Rogitine (Paladin), see **Phentolamine**

Royvac (Waymar), see **Bisacodyl/Magnesium Citrate, Miscellaneous Bowel Evacuants**

Rythmodan (Aventis Pharma), see **Disopyramide**

Rythmodan-LA (Aventis Pharma), see **Disopyramide Phosphate**

SAB-Prednase (Sabex), see **Prednisolone Sodium Phosphate**

Salazopyrin (Pfizer), see **Sulfasalazine**

Salazopyrin En-Tabs (Pfizer), see **Sulfasalazine**

Salofalk (Axcan Pharma), see **5-Aminosalicylic Acid**

Sandimmune I.V. (Novartis Pharmaceuticals), see **Cyclosporine**

Sans-Acne (Galderma), see **Erythromycin/Ethyl Alcohol, Topical Antibiotics**

Sarna HC (Steifel), see **Hydrocortisone**

Sarna-P (Steifel), see **Pramoxine HCl**

Seaford Liquid Multivite (Seaford), see **Multivitamins with Minerals**

Sebcur (Dermtek), see **Salicylic Acid**

Sebcur/T (Dermtek), see **Coal Tar/Salicylic Acid, Antiseborrheic Combinations**

Sebulex (Westwood-Squibb), see **Salicylic Acid/Sulfur, Antiseborrheic Combinations**

Secaris (Pharmascience), see **Polyethylene Glycol/Propylene Glycol**

Selax (Odan), see **Docusate Sodium**

Select 1/35 (Dispensapharm), see **Ethinyl Estradiol/Norethindrone, Oral Contraceptives**

Senna Laxative Pills Extra Strength Peristaltic Stimulant (Tanta), see **Sennosides**

Senna Laxative Pills Regular Strength Peristaltic Stimulant (Tanta), see **Sennosides**

Senna-S Tablets Peristaltic Stimulant-Surfactant (Tanta), see **Docusate Sodium/Sennosides**

Senna Tablets Peristaltic Stimulant (Tanta), see **Sennosides**

Sensorcaine with Epinephrine (AstraZeneca), see **Bupivacaine HCl with Epinephrine 1:200,000 Injectable Local Anesthetics**

Sevorane AF (Abbott), see **Sevoflurane**

Similac Advance LF (Abbott), see **Lactose-Free Infant Formulas**

Simply Sleep (McNeil Consumer Healthcare), see **Diphenhydramine HCl**

Sinutab Nightime (Pfizer Consumer Healthcare), see **Acetaminophen/Diphenhydramine/Pseudoephedrine HCl, Respiratory Combinations**

Sinutab Sinus and Allergy (Pfizer Consumer Healthcare), see **Acetaminophen/Chlorpheniramine Maleate/Pseudoephedrine HCl, Respiratory Combinations**

Sinutab Sinus Non Drowsy (Pfizer Consumer Healthcare), see **Acetaminophen/Pseudoephedrine HCl Decongestant and Analgesic Combinations, Upper Respiratory Combinations**

Sinutab With Codeine (Pfizer Consumer Healthcare), see **Acetaminophen/Chlorpheniramine Maleate/Codeine/Pseudoephedrine HCl, Cough Preparations**

SMA, Preemie (Nestle), see **Infant Foods**

Soflax (Pharmascience), see **Docusate Sodium**

Solugel 4 (Steifel), see **Benzoyl Peroxide**

Solugel 8 (Steifel), see **Benzoyl Peroxide**

Soluver (Dermtek), see **Salicylic Acid**

Soluver Plus (Dermtek), see **Salicylic Acid**

Sotacor (Bristol), see **Sotalol HCl**

Starnoc (Servier), see **Zaleplon**

Stemetil (Aventis Pharma), see **Prochlorperazine Mesylate**

Stieprox (Steifel), see **Ciclopirox**

Stieva-A (Steifel), see **Tretinoin**

Stilamin (Serono), see **Somatostatin**

Stresstabs Plus (Whitehall-Robins), see **Vitamins With Minerals**

Sudafed Cold & Cough Extra Strength (Pfizer Consumer Healthcare), see **Acetaminophen/Dextromethorphan HBr/Pseudoephedrine HCl Pediatric Antitussive Combinations, Upper Respiratory Combinations**

Sudafed Cold & Flu (Pfizer Consumer Healthcare), see **Acetaminophen/Dextromethorphan HBr/Guaifenesin/Pseudoephedrine HCl, Cough Preparations**

Sudafed Decongestant Children's Chewable (Pfizer Consumer Healthcare), see **Pseudoephedrine HCl**

Sudafed Decongestant 12 Hour (Pfizer Consumer Healthcare), see **Pseudoephedrine HCl**

Sudafed Decongestant Extra Strength (Pfizer Consumer Healthcare), see **Pseudoephedrine HCl**

Sudafed Head Cold And Sinus Extra Strength (Pfizer Consumer Healthcare), see **Acetaminophen/Pseudoephedrine HCl, Respiratory Combinations**

Sudafed Sinus Advance (Pfizer Consumer Healthcare), see **Ibuprofen/Pseudoephedrine HCl Decongestant and Analgesic Combinations, Upper Respiratory Combinations**

Sulcrate (Aventis Pharma), see **Sucralfate**

Sulcrate Suspension Plus (Aventis Pharma), see **Sucralfate**

Supeudol (Sabex), see **Oxycodone HCl**

Synphasic (Pfizer), see **Ethinyl Estradiol/Norethindrone, Oral Contraceptives**

Tamofen (Aventis Pharma), see **Tamoxifen Citrate**

Targel (Odan), see **Coal Tar**

Taro-Carbamazepine (Taro), see **Carbamazepine**

Taro-Sone (Taro), see **Betamethasone Dipropionate**

Taro-Warfarin (Taro), see **Warfarin Sodium**

Tazocin (Wyeth Canada), see **Piperacillin Sodium with Tazobactam Sodium**

Td Adsorbed (Aventis Pasteur), see **Diphtheria and Tetanus Toxoids, Adsorbed, Adult, Agents for Active Immunization**

Teardrops (Novartis Ophthalmics), see **Artificial Tears**

Tears Encore (Dioptic), see **Polysorbate 80, Artificial Tears**

Tebrazid (ICN), see **Pyrazinamide**

Tersa-Tar (TCD), see **Tar Distillate, Antiseborrheics**

Tiamol (TaroPharma), see **Fluocinonide**

Tolectin (Janssen-Ortho), see **Tolmetin Sodium**

Topsyn (Medicis), see **Fluocinonide**

Toradol IM (Roche), see **Ketorolac Tromethamine**

Transderm-V (Novartis Pharmaceuticals), see **Scopolamine**

Trans-Plantar (Westwood-Squibb), see **Salicylic Acid**

Travasol with Electrolytes (Baxter), see **Amino Acids/Dextrose/Electrolytes Crystalline Amino Acid Infusions with Electrolytes in Dextrose, Intravenous Nutritional Therapy**

Travasol without Electrolytes (Baxter), see **Amino Acids/Dextrose Crystalline Amino Acid Infusions with Dextrose, Intravenous Nutritional Therapy**

Triaderm (Taro), see **Triamcinolone Acetonide**

Trianal (Trianon), see **Aspirin/Butalbital/Caffeine, Analgesic Combinations**

Trianal C1/4 (Trianon), see **Aspirin/Butalbital/Caffeine/Codeine Phosphate, Analgesic Combinations**

Trianal C1/2 (Trianon), see **Aspirin/Butalbital/Caffeine/Codeine Phosphate, Analgesic Combinations**

Triatec-8 (Trianon), see **Acetaminophen/Caffeine Citrate/Codeine Phosphate, Analgesic Combinations**

Triatec-8 Strong (Trianon), see **Acetaminophen/Caffeine Citrate/Codeine Phosphate, Analgesic Combinations**

Triatec-30 (Trianon), see **Acetaminophen/Codeine Phosphate, Analgesic Combinations**

Tri-Cyclen (Janssen-Ortho), see **Ethinyl Estradiol/Norgestimate, Oral Contraceptives**

Trikacide (Pharmascience), see **Metronidazole**

Triphasil 21 (Wyeth Canada), see **Ethinyl Estradiol/Levonorgestrel Triphasic Oral Contraceptives**

Triphasil 28 (Wyeth Canada), see **Ethinyl Estradiol/Levonorgestrel Triphasic Oral Contraceptives**

Triquilar 21 (Berlex Canada), see **Ethinyl Estradiol/Levonorgestrel, Oral Contraceptives**

Triquilar 28 (Berlex Canada), see **Ethinyl Estradiol/Levonorgestrel, Oral Contraceptives**

Trisan (Dermtek), see **Triclosan**

Trombovar (E-Z-EM Canada), see **Sodium Tetradecyl Sulfate**

Tryptan (ICN), see **L-Tryptophan**

Tylenol Aches And Strains (McNeil Consumer Healthcare), see **Acetaminophen/Chlorzoxazone, Skeletal Muscle Relaxant Combinations**

Tylenol Allergy Sinus (Multi-Symptom Relief) (McNeil Consumer Healthcare), see **Acetaminophen/Chlorpheniramine Maleate/Pseudoephedrine HCl, Respiratory Combinations**

Tylenol Allergy Sinus (Nighttime Relief) (McNeil Consumer Healthcare), see **Acetaminophen/Pseudo-ephedrine HCl/ Diphenhydramine HCl Decongestant, Antihistamine, and Analgesic Combinations, Upper Respiratory Combinations**

Tylenol Cold & Flu (Nighttime Relief) (McNeil Consumer Healthcare), see **Dextromethorphan HBr/ Pseudoephedrine HCl/ Acetaminophen/Chlor-pheniramine Maleate Antitussive Combinations, Upper Respiratory Combinations**

Tylenol Cold Caplets Extra Strength (Daytime) (McNeil Consumer Healthcare), see **Acetaminophen/ Dextromethorphan HBr/ Pseudoephedrine HCl, Cough Preparations**

Tylenol Cold Caplets Extra Strength (Nighttime) (McNeil Consumer Healthcare), see **Acetaminophen/ Chlorpheniramine Maleate/ Dextromethorphan HBr/ Pseudoephedrine HCl, Cough Preparations**

Tylenol Cold Caplets Regular Strength (Chest Congestion) (McNeil Consumer Healthcare), see **Dextromethorphan HBr/Acetaminophen/ Guaifenesin/Pseudoephedrine HCl Antitussive and Expectorant Combinations, Upper Respiratory Combinations**

Tylenol Cold Caplets Regular Strength (Daytime) (McNeil Consumer Healthcare), see **Acetaminophen/Dextro-methorphan HBr/Pseudo-ephedrine HCl, Cough Preparations**

Tylenol Cold Caplets Regular Strength (Nighttime) (McNeil Consumer Healthcare), see **Acetaminophen/Chlorphen-iramine Maleate/Dextro-methorphan HBr/Pseudo-ephedrine HCl, Cough Preparations**

Tylenol Cold Suspension Children's (McNeil Consumer Healthcare), see **Acetaminophen/Chlorphen-iramine Maleate/ Pseudoephdedrine HCl Decongestant, Antihistamine and Analgesic, Upper Respiratory Combinations**

Tylenol Cold Suspension Children's DM (McNeil Consumer Healthcare), see **Acetaminophen/Chlorphen-iramine Maleate/Dextro-methorphan HBr/Pseudo-ephedrine HCl, Antitussive Combinations, Cough Preparations**

Tylenol Cold Suspension Infant's (McNeil Consumer Healthcare), see **Acetaminophen/Chlorphen-iramine Maleate/Pseudo-ephedrine HCl Decongestant, Antihistamine and Analgesic, Upper Respiratory Combinations**

Tylenol Cold Tablets Children's Chewable (McNeil Consumer Healthcare), see **Acetaminophen/Chlorphen-iramine Maleate/Pseudo-ephedrine HCl Decongestant, Antihistamine and Analgesic, Upper Respiratory Combinations**

Tylenol Cold Tablets Children's DM Chewable (McNeil Consumer Healthcare), see **Acetaminophen/Chlorphen-iramine Maleate/ Dextromethorphan HBr/Pseudoephedrine HCl, Antitussive Combinations, Cough Preparations**

Tylenol Cold Tablets Junior Strength DM (McNeil Consumer Healthcare), see **Acetaminophen/ Chlorpheniramine Maleate/ Dextromethorphan HBr/ Pseudoephedrine HCl, Cough Preparations**

Tylenol Cough (McNeil Consumer Healthcare), see **Acetaminophen/ Dextromethorphan HBr, Antitussive Combinations**

Tylenol Decongestant (McNeil Consumer Healthcare), see **Acetaminophen/ Pseudoephedrine HCl, Respiratory Combinations**

Tylenol Elixir with Codeine (Janssen-Ortho/McNeil Consumer Healthcare), see **Acetaminophen/Codeine, Analgesic Combinations**

Tylenol Flu (Daytime Relief) (McNeil Consumer Healthcare), see **Dextromethorphan HBr/ Acetaminophen/Pseudo-ephedrine HCl Antitussive Combinations, Upper Respiratory Combinations**

Tylenol Flu (Nighttime Relief) (McNeil Consumer Healthcare), see **Acetaminophen/ Pseudoephedrine HCl/Diphenhydramine HCl Decongestant, Antihistamine, and Analgesic Combinations, Upper Respiratory Combinations**

Tylenol Menstrual (McNeil Consumer Healthcare), see **Acetaminophen/Pamabrom/ Pyrilamine Maleate, Nonnarcotic Analgesic Combinations**

Tylenol No. 1 (Janssen-Ortho/McNeil Consumer Healthcare), see **Acetaminophen/Caffeine/ Codeine Phosphate, Narcotic Analgesic Combinations**

Tylenol No. 1 Forte (Janssen-Ortho/McNeil Consumer Healthcare), see **Acetaminophen/Caffeine/ Codeine Phosphate, Narcotic Analgesic Combinations**

Tylenol Sinus Children's (McNeil Consumer Healthcare), see **Acetaminophen/Pseudo-ephedrine HCl Pediatric Decongestant and Analgesic Combinations, Upper Respiratory Combinations**

Tylenol Sinus Extra Strength (Daytime Relief) (McNeil Consumer Healthcare), see **Acetaminophen/Pseudo-ephedrine HCl Decongestant and Analgesic Combinations, Upper Respiratory Combinations**

Tylenol Sinus Extra Strength (Nighttime Relief) (McNeil Consumer Healthcare), see **Acetaminophen/Pseudo-ephedrine HCl/Doxylamine Succinate Decongestant, Antihistamine, and Analgesic Combinations, Upper Respiratory Combinations**

Tylenol Sinus Regular Strength (McNeil Consumer Healthcare), see **Acetaminophen/ Pseudoephedrine HCl, Respiratory Combinations**

Ultramop Capsules (Canderm Pharma), see **Methoxsalen**

Ultramop Lotion (Canderm Pharma), see **Methoxsalen**

Ultraquin (Canderm Pharma), see **Hydroquinone**

Unidet (Pfizer), see **Tolterodine Tartrate**

Unisom Extra Strength (Pfizer Consumer Healthcare), see **Diphenhydramine HCl**

Unisom Extra Strength Sleepgels (Pfizer Consumer Healthcare), see **Diphenhydramine HCl**

Unitron PEG (Schering), see **Peginterferon alfa-2b**

Uremol 10 (TCD), see **Urea, Topical**

Uremol 20 (TCD), see **Urea, Topical**

Uremol HC (TCD), see **Hydrocortisone Acetate**

UriSec (Odan), see **Urea, Topical**

Uromitexan (Baxter), see **Mesna**

Valisone Scalp Lotion (Schering), see **Betamethasone Valerate**

Valium Roche Oral (Roche), see **Diazepam**

Valtaxin (Paladin), see **Valrubicin**

Vamin N (Baxter), see **Amino Acid/Electrolyte IV Nutritionals**

Vaponefrin (Aventis Pharma), see **Epinephrine HCl**

Varilrix (GlaxoSmithKline), see **Varicella Virus Vaccine**

Varivax III (Merck Frosst), see **Varicella Virus Vaccine**

Vasocon (Novartis Ophthalmics), see **Naphazoline HCl**

Vaxigrip (Aventis Pasteur), see **Influenza Virus Vaccine**

Ventodisk (GlaxoSmithKline), see **Albuterol**

Ventolin Diskus (GlaxoSmithKline), see **Albuterol**

Ventolin Oral Liquid (GlaxoSmithKline), see **Albuterol**

Versel (TCD), see **Selenium Sulfide**

Visine Original Eye Drops (Pfizer Consumer Healthcare), see **Tetrahydrozoline HCl**

Visine Workplace Eye Drops (Pfizer Consumer Healthcare), see **Oxymetazoline HCl**

Viskazide (Novartis Pharmaceuticals), see **Hydrochlorothiazide/ Pindolol, Antihypertensive Combinations**

Vitalux Time Release (Novartis Ophthalmics), see **Multivitamins with Minerals**

Vita 3B (Riva), see **Vitamin B**

Vita 3B + C (Riva), see **Multiple Vitamins**

Vivotif (Berna Products), see **Typhoid Vaccine (Live Oral Attenuated Ty21a)**

Vivotif L (Berna Products), see **Typhoid Vaccine (Live Oral Attenuated Ty21a)**

Voltaren Ophtha (Novartis Ophthalmics), see **Diclofenac Sodium**

Voltaren Rapide (Novartis Pharmaceuticals), see **Diclofenac Potassium**

Wake-up Tablets (Adrem), see **Caffeine**

Wartec (Paladin), see **Podofilox**

Winpred (ICN), see **Prednisone**

Xanax TS (Pfizer), see **Alprazolam**

Xatral (Sanofi-Synthelabo), see **Alfuzosin HCl**

X-Tar (Dormer), see **Coal Tar/Menthol/Salicylic Acid, Antiseborrheic Combinations**

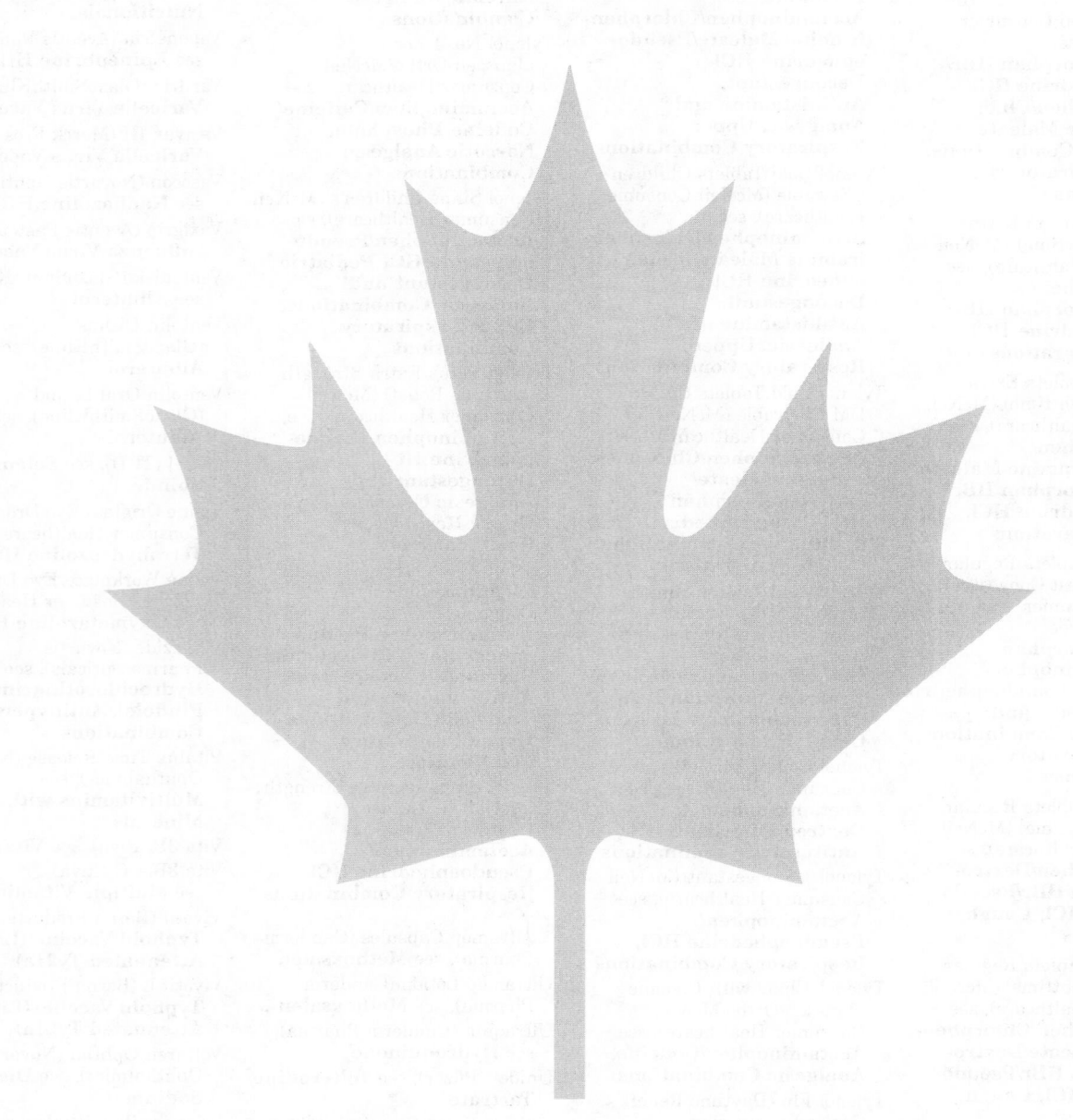